EXPERT

2019

ICD-10-CM Expert for Physicians

The complete official code set

Codes valid from October 1, 2018
through September 30, 2019

Power up your coding
optum360coding.com

OPTUM360°®

Publisher's Notice

The *ICD-10-CM Expert for Physicians: The Complete Official Code Set* is designed to be an accurate and authoritative source regarding coding and every reasonable effort has been made to ensure accuracy and completeness of the content. However, Optum360 makes no guarantee, warranty, or representation that this publication is accurate, complete or without errors. It is understood that Optum360 is not rendering any legal or other professional services or advice in this publication and that Optum360 bears no liability for any results or consequences that may arise from the use of this book.

Acknowledgments

Marianne Randall, CPC, *Product Manager*
Karen Schmidt, BSN, *Technical Director*
Anita Schmidt, BS, RHIT, AHIMA-approved ICD-10-CM/PCS Trainer, *Clinical Technical Editor*
Leanne Patterson, CPC, *Clinical Technical Editor*
Anne Kenney, BA, MBA, CCA, CCS, *Clinical Technical Editor*
Karen Krawzik, RHIT, CCS, AHIMA-approved ICD-10-CM/PCS Trainer, *Clinical Technical Editor*
Peggy Willard, CCS, AHIMA-approved ICD-10-CM/PCS Trainer, *Clinical Technical Editor*
Dr. Vikas Kumar, BHMS, CPC, CPC-H, *Clinical Technical Editor*
Stacy Perry, *Manager, Desktop Publishing*
Lisa Singley, *Project Manager*
Tracy Betzler, *Senior Desktop Publishing Specialist*
Hope M. Dunn, *Senior Desktop Publishing Specialist*
Katie Russell, *Desktop Publishing Specialist*
Kate Holden, *Editor*

Our Commitment to Accuracy

Optum360 is committed to producing accurate and reliable materials.

To report corrections, please visit www.optum360coding.com/accuracy or email accuracy@optum.com. You can also reach customer service by calling 1.800.464.3649, option 1.

Anita Schmidt, BS, RHIT, AHIMA-approved ICD-10-CM/PCS Trainer

Ms. Schmidt has expertise in Level I Adult and Pediatric Trauma hospital coding, specializing in ICD-9-CM, ICD-10-CM/PCS, DRG, and CPT coding. Her experience includes analysis of medical record documentation, assignment of ICD-10-CM and PCS codes, DRG validation, as well as CPT code assignments for same-day surgery cases. She has conducted coding training and auditing, including DRG validation, conducted electronic health record training, and worked with clinical documentation specialists to identify documentation needs and potential areas for physician education. Most recently she has been developing content for resource and educational products related to ICD-10-CM and ICD-10-PCS. Ms. Schmidt is an AHIMA-approved ICD-10-CM/PCS trainer, and is an active member of the American Health Information Management Association (AHIMA) and the Minnesota Health Information Management Association (MHIMA).

Leanne Patterson, CPC

Ms. Patterson has more than 10 years of experience in the health care profession. She has an extensive background in professional component coding, with expertise in E/M coding and auditing, and HIPAA compliance. Her experience includes general surgery coding, serving as director of compliance, conducting chart-to-claim audits and physician education. She has been responsible for coding and denial management in large multispecialty physician practices, and most recently served as a practice manager where she supervised implementation of a new EHR system. Ms. Patterson is credentialed by the American Academy of Professional Coders (AAPC) as a Certified Professional Coder (CPC).

2019 ICD-10-CM Official Guidelines for Coding and Reporting

Optum360 is pleased to provide you with this 2019 ICD-10-CM codebook that INCLUDES the 2019 Official Guidelines for Coding and Reporting.

Contents

Preface

ICD-10-CM Official Preface

This FY 2019 update of the International Statistical Classification of Diseases and Related Health Problems, 10th revision, Clinical Modification (ICD-10-CM) is being published by the United States government in recognition of its responsibility to promulgate this classification throughout the United States for morbidity coding. The International Statistical Classification of Diseases and Related Health Problems, 10th Revision (ICD-10), published by the World Health Organization (WHO), is the foundation of ICD-10-CM. ICD-10 continues to be the classification used in cause-of-death coding in the United States. The ICD-10-CM is comparable with the ICD-10. The WHO Collaborating Center for the Family of International Classifications in North America, housed at the Centers for Disease Control and Prevention's National Center for Health Statistics (NCHS), has responsibility for the implementation of ICD and other WHO-FIC classifications and serves as a liaison with the WHO, fulfilling international obligations for comparable classifications and the national health data needs of the United States. The historical background of ICD and ICD-10 can be found in the Introduction to the International Classification of Diseases and Related Health Problems (ICD-10), 2010, World Health Organization, Geneva, Switzerland.

ICD-10-CM is the United States' clinical modification of the World Health Organization's ICD-10. The term "clinical" is used to emphasize the modification's intent: to serve as a useful tool in the area of classification of morbidity data for indexing of health records, medical care review, and ambulatory and other health care programs, as well as for basic health statistics. To describe the clinical picture of the patient the codes must be more precise than those needed only for statistical groupings and trend analysis.

Characteristics of ICD-10-CM

ICD-10-CM far exceeds its predecessors in the number of concepts and codes provided. The disease classification has been expanded to include health-related conditions and to provide greater specificity at the sixth and seventh character level. The sixth and seventh characters are not optional and are intended for use in recording the information documented in the clinical record.

ICD-10-CM extensions, interpretations, modifications, addenda, or errata other than those approved by the Centers for Disease Control and Prevention are not to be considered official and should not be utilized. Continuous maintenance of the ICD-10- CM is the responsibility of the aforementioned agencies. However, because the ICD-10- CM represents the best in contemporary thinking of clinicians, nosologists, epidemiologists, and statisticians from both public and private sectors, when future modifications are considered, advice will be sought from all stakeholders.

All official authorized addenda since the last complete update (October 1, 2017) have been included in this revision. For more detailed information please see the complete official authorized addenda to ICD-10-CM, including the "ICD-10-CM Official Guidelines for Coding and Reporting," and a description of the ICD-10-CM updating and maintenance process.

Official Updates

The National Center for Health Statistics (NCHS), a section of the Centers for Disease Control and Prevention (CDC), is the agency charged with maintaining and updating ICD-10-CM. The 2019 official addendum was posted to the Centers for Medicare and Medicaid Services (CMS) website on June 11, 2018, identifying the changes to the ICD-10-CM code set for fiscal 2019. A summary of changes is provided below:

48 Codes Changed from Valid to Invalid

Note: Validity changes are the result of new codes being added to the classification, changing a previously valid code to an invalid code, creating a new subcategory.

C43.11	C43.12	C4A.11	C4A.12	C44.102
C44.109	C44.112	C44.119	C44.122	C44.129
C44.192	C44.199	D03.11	D03.12	D04.11
D04.12	D22.11	D22.12	D23.11	D23.12
E72.8	E78.4	F53	G51.3	G71.0
H57.8	I63.8	K35.2	K35.3	K35.89
K61.3	K83.0	M79.1	N35.8	N35.9
O86.0	P02.7	P04.1	P04.8	P74.2
P74.3	P74.4	Q51.2	Q93.5	R82.99
R93.8	Z04.8	Z13.4		

3 Codes Deleted from the Classification

T81.4XXA	Infection following a procedure, initial encounter
T81.4XXD	Infection following a procedure, subsequent encounter
T81.4XXS	Infection following a procedure, sequela

279 New Codes Added

C43.111	Malignant melanoma of right upper eyelid, including canthus
C43.112	Malignant melanoma of right lower eyelid, including canthus
C43.121	Malignant melanoma of left upper eyelid, including canthus
C43.122	Malignant melanoma of left lower eyelid, including canthus
C4A.111	Merkel cell carcinoma of right upper eyelid, including canthus
C4A.112	Merkel cell carcinoma of right lower eyelid, including canthus
C4A.121	Merkel cell carcinoma of left upper eyelid, including canthus
C4A.122	Merkel cell carcinoma of left lower eyelid, including canthus
C44.1021	Unspecified malignant neoplasm of skin of right upper eyelid, including canthus
C44.1022	Unspecified malignant neoplasm of skin of right lower eyelid, including canthus
C44.1091	Unspecified malignant neoplasm of skin of left upper eyelid, including canthus
C44.1092	Unspecified malignant neoplasm of skin of left lower eyelid, including canthus
C44.1121	Basal cell carcinoma of skin of right upper eyelid, including canthus
C44.1122	Basal cell carcinoma of skin of right lower eyelid, including canthus
C44.1191	Basal cell carcinoma of skin of left upper eyelid, including canthus
C44.1192	Basal cell carcinoma of skin of left lower eyelid, including canthus
C44.1221	Squamous cell carcinoma of skin of right upper eyelid, including canthus
C44.1222	Squamous cell carcinoma of skin of right lower eyelid, including canthus
C44.1291	Squamous cell carcinoma of skin of left upper eyelid, including canthus
C44.1292	Squamous cell carcinoma of skin of left lower eyelid, including canthus
C44.131	Sebaceous cell carcinoma of skin of unspecified eyelid, including canthus
C44.1321	Sebaceous cell carcinoma of skin of right upper eyelid, including canthus
C44.1322	Sebaceous cell carcinoma of skin of right lower eyelid, including canthus
C44.1391	Sebaceous cell carcinoma of skin of left upper eyelid, including canthus
C44.1392	Sebaceous cell carcinoma of skin of left lower eyelid, including canthus
C44.1921	Other specified malignant neoplasm of skin of right upper eyelid, including canthus
C44.1922	Other specified malignant neoplasm of skin of right lower eyelid, including canthus
C44.1991	Other specified malignant neoplasm of skin of left upper eyelid, including canthus
C44.1992	Other specified malignant neoplasm of skin of left lower eyelid, including canthus
D03.111	Melanoma in situ of right upper eyelid, including canthus
D03.112	Melanoma in situ of right lower eyelid, including canthus
D03.121	Melanoma in situ of left upper eyelid, including canthus
D03.122	Melanoma in situ of left lower eyelid, including canthus
D04.111	Carcinoma in situ of skin of right upper eyelid, including canthus
D04.112	Carcinoma in situ of skin of right lower eyelid, including canthus
D04.121	Carcinoma in situ of skin of left upper eyelid, including canthus
D04.122	Carcinoma in situ of skin of left lower eyelid, including canthus
D22.111	Melanocytic nevi of right upper eyelid, including canthus
D22.112	Melanocytic nevi of right lower eyelid, including canthus
D22.121	Melanocytic nevi of left upper eyelid, including canthus
D22.122	Melanocytic nevi of left lower eyelid, including canthus
D23.111	Other benign neoplasm of skin of right upper eyelid, including canthus
D23.112	Other benign neoplasm of skin of right lower eyelid, including canthus
D23.121	Other benign neoplasm of skin of left upper eyelid, including canthus
D23.122	Other benign neoplasm of skin of left lower eyelid, including canthus
E72.81	Disorders of gamma aminobutyric acid metabolism
E72.89	Other specified disorders of amino-acid metabolism

279 New Codes Added (continued)

Code	Description
E75.26	Sulfatase deficiency
E78.41	Elevated Lipoprotein(a)
E78.49	Other hyperlipidemia
E88.02	Plasminogen deficiency
F12.23	Cannabis dependence with withdrawal
F12.93	Cannabis use, unspecified with withdrawal
F53.0	Postpartum depression
F53.1	Puerperal psychosis
F68.A	Factitious disorder imposed on another
G51.31	Clonic hemifacial spasm, right
G51.32	Clonic hemifacial spasm, left
G51.33	Clonic hemifacial spasm, bilateral
G51.39	Clonic hemifacial spasm, unspecified
G71.00	Muscular dystrophy, unspecified
G71.01	Duchenne or Becker muscular dystrophy
G71.02	Facioscapulohumeral muscular dystrophy
G71.09	Other specified muscular dystrophies
H01.00A	Unspecified blepharitis right eye, upper and lower eyelids
H01.00B	Unspecified blepharitis left eye, upper and lower eyelids
H01.01A	Ulcerative blepharitis right eye, upper and lower eyelids
H01.01B	Ulcerative blepharitis left eye, upper and lower eyelids
H01.02A	Squamous blepharitis right eye, upper and lower eyelids
H01.02B	Squamous blepharitis left eye, upper and lower eyelids
H02.151	Paralytic ectropion of right upper eyelid
H02.152	Paralytic ectropion of right lower eyelid
H02.153	Paralytic ectropion of right eye, unspecified eyelid
H02.154	Paralytic ectropion of left upper eyelid
H02.155	Paralytic ectropion of left lower eyelid
H02.156	Paralytic ectropion of left eye, unspecified eyelid
H02.159	Paralytic ectropion of unspecified eye, unspecified eyelid
H02.20A	Unspecified lagophthalmos right eye, upper and lower eyelids
H02.20B	Unspecified lagophthalmos left eye, upper and lower eyelids
H02.20C	Unspecified lagophthalmos, bilateral, upper and lower eyelids
H02.21A	Cicatricial lagophthalmos right eye, upper and lower eyelids
H02.21B	Cicatricial lagophthalmos left eye, upper and lower eyelids
H02.21C	Cicatricial lagophthalmos, bilateral, upper and lower eyelids
H02.22A	Mechanical lagophthalmos right eye, upper and lower eyelids
H02.22B	Mechanical lagophthalmos left eye, upper and lower eyelids
H02.22C	Mechanical lagophthalmos, bilateral, upper and lower eyelids
H02.23A	Paralytic lagophthalmos right eye, upper and lower eyelids
H02.23B	Paralytic lagophthalmos left eye, upper and lower eyelids
H02.23C	Paralytic lagophthalmos, bilateral, upper and lower eyelids
H02.881	Meibomian gland dysfunction right upper eyelid
H02.882	Meibomian gland dysfunction right lower eyelid
H02.883	Meibomian gland dysfunction of right eye, unspecified eyelid
H02.884	Meibomian gland dysfunction left upper eyelid
H02.885	Meibomian gland dysfunction left lower eyelid
H02.886	Meibomian gland dysfunction of left eye, unspecified eyelid
H02.889	Meibomian gland dysfunction of unspecified eye, unspecified eyelid
H02.88A	Meibomian gland dysfunction right eye, upper and lower eyelids
H02.88B	Meibomian gland dysfunction left eye, upper and lower eyelids
H10.821	Rosacea conjunctivitis, right eye
H10.822	Rosacea conjunctivitis, left eye
H10.823	Rosacea conjunctivitis, bilateral
H10.829	Rosacea conjunctivitis, unspecified eye
H57.811	Brow ptosis, right
H57.812	Brow ptosis, left
H57.813	Brow ptosis, bilateral
H57.819	Brow ptosis, unspecified
H57.89	Other specified disorders of eye and adnexa
I63.81	Other cerebral infarction due to occlusion or stenosis of small artery
I63.89	Other cerebral infarction
I67.850	Cerebral autosomal dominant arteriopathy with subcortical infarcts and leukoencephalopathy
I67.858	Other hereditary cerebrovascular disease
K35.20	Acute appendicitis with generalized peritonitis, without abscess
K35.21	Acute appendicitis with generalized peritonitis, with abscess
K35.30	Acute appendicitis with localized peritonitis, without perforation or gangrene
K35.31	Acute appendicitis with localized peritonitis and gangrene, without perforation
K35.32	Acute appendicitis with perforation and localized peritonitis, without abscess
K35.33	Acute appendicitis with perforation and localized peritonitis, with abscess
K35.890	Other acute appendicitis without perforation or gangrene
K35.891	Other acute appendicitis without perforation, with gangrene
K61.31	Horseshoe abscess
K61.39	Other ischiorectal abscess
K61.5	Supralevator abscess
K82.A1	Gangrene of gallbladder in cholecystitis
K82.A2	Perforation of gallbladder in cholecystitis
K83.01	Primary sclerosing cholangitis
K83.09	Other cholangitis
M79.10	Myalgia, unspecified site
M79.11	Myalgia of mastication muscle
M79.12	Myalgia of auxiliary muscles, head and neck
M79.18	Myalgia, other site
N35.016	Post-traumatic urethral stricture, male, overlapping sites
N35.116	Postinfective urethral stricture, not elsewhere classified, male, overlapping sites

279 New Codes Added (continued)

N35.811	Other urethral stricture, male, meatal
N35.812	Other urethral bulbous stricture, male
N35.813	Other membranous urethral stricture, male
N35.814	Other anterior urethral stricture, male, anterior
N35.816	Other urethral stricture, male, overlapping sites
N35.819	Other urethral stricture, male, unspecified site
N35.82	Other urethral stricture, female
N35.911	Unspecified urethral stricture, male, meatal
N35.912	Unspecified bulbous urethral stricture, male
N35.913	Unspecified membranous urethral stricture, male
N35.914	Unspecified anterior urethral stricture, male
N35.916	Unspecified urethral stricture, male, overlapping sites
N35.919	Unspecified urethral stricture, male, unspecified site
N35.92	Unspecified urethral stricture, female
N99.116	Postprocedural urethral stricture, male, overlapping sites
O30.131	Triplet pregnancy, trichorionic/triamniotic, first trimester
O30.132	Triplet pregnancy, trichorionic/triamniotic, second trimester
O30.133	Triplet pregnancy, trichorionic/triamniotic, third trimester
O30.139	Triplet pregnancy, trichorionic/triamniotic, unspecified trimester
O30.231	Quadruplet pregnancy, quadrachorionic/quadra-amniotic, first trimester
O30.232	Quadruplet pregnancy, quadrachorionic/quadra-amniotic, second trimester
O30.233	Quadruplet pregnancy, quadrachorionic/quadra-amniotic, third trimester
O30.239	Quadruplet pregnancy, quadrachorionic/quadra-amniotic, unspecified trimester
O30.831	Other specified multiple gestation, number of chorions and amnions are both equal to the number of fetuses, first trimester
O30.832	Other specified multiple gestation, number of chorions and amnions are both equal to the number of fetuses, second trimester
O30.833	Other specified multiple gestation, number of chorions and amnions are both equal to the number of fetuses, third trimester
O30.839	Other specified multiple gestation, number of chorions and amnions are both equal to the number of fetuses, unspecified trimester
O86.00	Infection of obstetric surgical wound, unspecified
O86.01	Infection of obstetric surgical wound, superficial incisional site
O86.02	Infection of obstetric surgical wound, deep incisional site
O86.03	Infection of obstetric surgical wound, organ and space site
O86.04	Sepsis following an obstetrical procedure
O86.09	Infection of obstetric surgical wound, other surgical site
P02.70	Newborn affected by fetal inflammatory response syndrome
P02.78	Newborn affected by other conditions from chorioamnionitis
P04.11	Newborn affected by maternal antineoplastic chemotherapy
P04.12	Newborn affected by maternal cytotoxic drugs
P04.13	Newborn affected by maternal use of anticonvulsants
P04.14	Newborn affected by maternal use of opiates
P04.15	Newborn affected by maternal use of antidepressants
P04.16	Newborn affected by maternal use of amphetamines
P04.17	Newborn affected by maternal use of sedative-hypnotics
P04.1A	Newborn affected by maternal use of anxiolytics
P04.18	Newborn affected by other maternal medication
P04.19	Newborn affected by maternal use of unspecified medication
P04.40	Newborn affected by maternal use of unspecified drugs of addiction
P04.42	Newborn affected by maternal use of hallucinogens
P04.81	Newborn affected by maternal use of cannabis
P04.89	Newborn affected by other maternal noxious substances
P35.4	Congenital Zika virus disease
P74.21	Hypernatremia of newborn
P74.22	Hyponatremia of newborn
P74.31	Hyperkalemia of newborn
P74.32	Hypokalemia of newborn
P74.41	Alkalosis of newborn
P74.421	Hyperchloremia of newborn
P74.422	Hypochloremia of newborn
P74.49	Other transitory electrolyte disturbance of newborn
Q51.20	Other doubling of uterus, unspecified
Q51.21	Other complete doubling of uterus
Q51.22	Other partial doubling of uterus
Q51.28	Other doubling of uterus, other specified
Q93.51	Angelman syndrome
Q93.59	Other deletions of part of a chromosome
Q93.82	Williams syndrome
R82.991	Hypocitraturia
R82.992	Hyperoxaluria
R82.993	Hyperuricosuria
R82.994	Hypercalciuria
R82.998	Other abnormal findings in urine
R93.811	Abnormal radiologic findings on diagnostic imaging of right testicle
R93.812	Abnormal radiologic findings on diagnostic imaging of left testicle
R93.813	Abnormal radiologic findings on diagnostic imaging of testicles, bilateral
R93.819	Abnormal radiologic findings on diagnostic imaging of unspecified testicle
R93.89	Abnormal findings on diagnostic imaging of other specified body structures
T43.641A	Poisoning by ecstasy, accidental (unintentional), initial encounter
T43.641D	Poisoning by ecstasy, accidental (unintentional), subsequent encounter
T43.641S	Poisoning by ecstasy, accidental (unintentional), sequela
T43.642A	Poisoning by ecstasy, intentional self-harm, initial encounter
T43.642D	Poisoning by ecstasy, intentional self-harm, subsequent encounter
T43.642S	Poisoning by ecstasy, intentional self-harm, sequela

279 New Codes Added (continued)

T43.643A	Poisoning by ecstasy, assault, initial encounter
T43.643D	Poisoning by ecstasy, assault, subsequent encounter
T43.643S	Poisoning by ecstasy, assault, sequela
T43.644A	Poisoning by ecstasy, undetermined, initial encounter
T43.644D	Poisoning by ecstasy, undetermined, subsequent encounter
T43.644S	Poisoning by ecstasy, undetermined, sequela
T74.51XA	Adult forced sexual exploitation, confirmed, initial encounter
T74.51XD	Adult forced sexual exploitation, confirmed, subsequent encounter
T74.51XS	Adult forced sexual exploitation, confirmed, sequela
T74.52XA	Child sexual exploitation, confirmed, initial encounter
T74.52XD	Child sexual exploitation, confirmed, subsequent encounter
T74.52XS	Child sexual exploitation, confirmed, sequela
T74.61XA	Adult forced labor exploitation, confirmed, initial encounter
T74.61XD	Adult forced labor exploitation, confirmed, subsequent encounter
T74.61XS	Adult forced labor exploitation, confirmed, sequela
T74.62XA	Child forced labor exploitation, confirmed, initial encounter
T74.62XD	Child forced labor exploitation, confirmed, subsequent encounter
T74.62XS	Child forced labor exploitation, confirmed, sequela
T76.51XA	Adult forced sexual exploitation, suspected, initial encounter
T76.51XD	Adult forced sexual exploitation, suspected, subsequent encounter
T76.51XS	Adult forced sexual exploitation, suspected, sequela
T76.52XA	Child sexual exploitation, suspected, initial encounter
T76.52XD	Child sexual exploitation, suspected, subsequent encounter
T76.52XS	Child sexual exploitation, suspected, sequela
T76.61XA	Adult forced labor exploitation, suspected, initial encounter
T76.61XD	Adult forced labor exploitation, suspected, subsequent encounter
T76.61XS	Adult forced labor exploitation, suspected, sequela
T76.62XA	Child forced labor exploitation, suspected, initial encounter
T76.62XD	Child forced labor exploitation, suspected, subsequent encounter
T76.62XS	Child forced labor exploitation, suspected, sequela
T81.40XA	Infection following a procedure, unspecified, initial encounter
T81.40XD	Infection following a procedure, unspecified, subsequent encounter
T81.40XS	Infection following a procedure, unspecified, sequela
T81.41XA	Infection following a procedure, superficial incisional surgical site, initial encounter
T81.41XD	Infection following a procedure, superficial incisional surgical site, subsequent encounter
T81.41XS	Infection following a procedure, superficial incisional surgical site, sequela
T81.42XA	Infection following a procedure, deep incisional surgical site, initial encounter
T81.42XD	Infection following a procedure, deep incisional surgical site, subsequent encounter
T81.42XS	Infection following a procedure, deep incisional surgical site, sequela
T81.43XA	Infection following a procedure, organ and space surgical site, initial encounter
T81.43XD	Infection following a procedure, organ and space surgical site, subsequent encounter
T81.43XS	Infection following a procedure, organ and space surgical site, sequela
T81.44XA	Sepsis following a procedure, initial encounter
T81.44XD	Sepsis following a procedure, subsequent encounter
T81.44XS	Sepsis following a procedure, sequela
T81.49XA	Infection following a procedure, other surgical site, initial encounter
T81.49XD	Infection following a procedure, other surgical site, subsequent encounter
T81.49XS	Infection following a procedure, other surgical site, sequela
Y07.6	Multiple perpetrators of maltreatment and neglect
Z04.81	Encounter for examination and observation of victim following forced sexual exploitation
Z04.82	Encounter for examination and observation of victim following forced labor exploitation
Z04.89	Encounter for examination and observation for other specified reasons
Z13.30	Encounter for screening examination for mental health and behavioral disorders, unspecified
Z13.31	Encounter for screening for depression
Z13.32	Encounter for screening for maternal depression
Z13.39	Encounter for screening examination for other mental health and behavioral disorders
Z13.40	Encounter for screening for unspecified developmental delays
Z13.41	Encounter for autism screening
Z13.42	Encounter for screening for global developmental delays (milestones)
Z13.49	Encounter for screening for other developmental delays
Z20.821	Contact with and (suspected) exposure to Zika virus
Z28.83	Immunization not carried out due to unavailability of vaccine
Z62.813	Personal history of forced labor or sexual exploitation in childhood
Z83.430	Family history of elevated lipoprotein(a)
Z83.438	Family history of other disorder of lipoprotein metabolism and other lipidemia
Z91.42	Personal history of forced labor or sexual exploitation

143 Code Descriptions Revised

Note: Each code is listed with its revised description only. Please refer to the full FY 2019 official addenda code files at https://www.cdc.gov/nchs/icd/icd10cm.htm for the specific changes made to the codes listed.

E67.1	Hypercarotenemia
E72.53	Primary hyperoxaluria
F68.10	Factitious disorder imposed on self, unspecified
F68.11	Factitious disorder imposed on self, with predominantly psychological signs and symptoms

143 Code Descriptions Revised (continued)

F68.12	Factitious disorder imposed on self, with predominantly physical signs and symptoms
F68.13	Factitious disorder imposed on self, with combined psychological and physical signs and symptoms
H04.201	Unspecified epiphora, right side
H04.202	Unspecified epiphora, left side
H04.203	Unspecified epiphora, bilateral
H04.209	Unspecified epiphora, unspecified side
H04.221	Epiphora due to insufficient drainage, right side
H04.222	Epiphora due to insufficient drainage, left side
H04.223	Epiphora due to insufficient drainage, bilateral
H04.229	Epiphora due to insufficient drainage, unspecified side
I63.219	Cerebral infarction due to unspecified occlusion or stenosis of unspecified vertebral artery
I63.239	Cerebral infarction due to unspecified occlusion or stenosis of unspecified carotid artery
I63.333	Cerebral infarction due to thrombosis of bilateral posterior cerebral arteries
I63.343	Cerebral infarction due to thrombosis of bilateral cerebellar arteries
J84.848	Other interstitial lung diseases of childhood
K43.5	Parastomal hernia without obstruction or gangrene
L98.495	Non-pressure chronic ulcer of skin of other sites with muscle involvement without evidence of necrosis
L98.496	Non-pressure chronic ulcer of skin of other sites with bone involvement without evidence of necrosis
L98.498	Non-pressure chronic ulcer of skin of other sites with other specified severity
M26.621	Arthralgia of right temporomandibular joint
M50.01	Cervical disc disorder with myelopathy, high cervical region
M50.11	Cervical disc disorder with radiculopathy, high cervical region
M50.21	Other cervical disc displacement, high cervical region
M50.31	Other cervical disc degeneration, high cervical region
M50.81	Other cervical disc disorders, high cervical region
M50.91	Cervical disc disorder, unspecified, high cervical region
M86.621	Other chronic osteomyelitis, right humerus
M86.622	Other chronic osteomyelitis, left humerus
M86.629	Other chronic osteomyelitis, unspecified humerus
N63.0	Unspecified lump in unspecified breast
O00.212	Left ovarian pregnancy with intrauterine pregnancy
Q66.89	Other specified congenital deformities of feet
R40.2330	Coma scale, best motor response, abnormal flexion, unspecified time
R40.2331	Coma scale, best motor response, abnormal flexion, in the field [EMT or ambulance]
R40.2332	Coma scale, best motor response, abnormal flexion, at arrival to emergency department
R40.2333	Coma scale, best motor response, abnormal flexion, at hospital admission
R40.2334	Coma scale, best motor response, abnormal flexion, 24 hours or more after hospital admission
S62.626A	Displaced fracture of middle phalanx of right little finger, initial encounter for closed fracture
S62.626B	Displaced fracture of middle phalanx of right little finger, initial encounter for open fracture
S62.626D	Displaced fracture of middle phalanx of right little finger, subsequent encounter for fracture with routine healing
S62.626G	Displaced fracture of middle phalanx of right little finger, subsequent encounter for fracture with delayed healing
S62.626K	Displaced fracture of middle phalanx of right little finger, subsequent encounter for fracture with nonunion
S62.626P	Displaced fracture of middle phalanx of right little finger, subsequent encounter for fracture with malunion
S62.626S	Displaced fracture of middle phalanx of right little finger, sequela
S62.627A	Displaced fracture of middle phalanx of left little finger, initial encounter for closed fracture
S62.627B	Displaced fracture of middle phalanx of left little finger, initial encounter for open fracture
S62.627D	Displaced fracture of middle phalanx of left little finger, subsequent encounter for fracture with routine healing
S62.627G	Displaced fracture of middle phalanx of left little finger, subsequent encounter for fracture with delayed healing
S62.627K	Displaced fracture of middle phalanx of left little finger, subsequent encounter for fracture with nonunion
S62.627P	Displaced fracture of middle phalanx of left little finger, subsequent encounter for fracture with malunion
S62.627S	Displaced fracture of middle phalanx of left little finger, sequela
S62.628A	Displaced fracture of middle phalanx of other finger, initial encounter for closed fracture
S62.628B	Displaced fracture of middle phalanx of other finger, initial encounter for open fracture
S62.628D	Displaced fracture of middle phalanx of other finger, subsequent encounter for fracture with routine healing
S62.628G	Displaced fracture of middle phalanx of other finger, subsequent encounter for fracture with delayed healing
S62.628K	Displaced fracture of middle phalanx of other finger, subsequent encounter for fracture with nonunion
S62.628P	Displaced fracture of middle phalanx of other finger, subsequent encounter for fracture with malunion
S62.628S	Displaced fracture of middle phalanx of other finger, sequela
S62.629A	Displaced fracture of middle phalanx of unspecified finger, initial encounter for closed fracture
S62.629B	Displaced fracture of middle phalanx of unspecified finger, initial encounter for open fracture
S62.629D	Displaced fracture of middle phalanx of unspecified finger, subsequent encounter for fracture with routine healing
S62.629G	Displaced fracture of middle phalanx of unspecified finger, subsequent encounter for fracture with delayed healing
S62.629K	Displaced fracture of middle phalanx of unspecified finger, subsequent encounter for fracture with nonunion
S62.629P	Displaced fracture of middle phalanx of unspecified finger, subsequent encounter for fracture with malunion
S62.629S	Displaced fracture of middle phalanx of unspecified finger, sequela
S62.654A	Nondisplaced fracture of middle phalanx of right ring finger, initial encounter for closed fracture
S62.654B	Nondisplaced fracture of middle phalanx of right ring finger, initial encounter for open fracture

143 Code Descriptions Revised (continued)

S62.654D   Nondisplaced fracture of middle phalanx of right ring finger, subsequent encounter for fracture with routine healing

S62.654G   Nondisplaced fracture of middle phalanx of right ring finger, subsequent encounter for fracture with delayed healing

S62.654K   Nondisplaced fracture of middle phalanx of right ring finger, subsequent encounter for fracture with nonunion

S62.654P   Nondisplaced fracture of middle phalanx of right ring finger, subsequent encounter for fracture with malunion

S62.654S   Nondisplaced fracture of middle phalanx of right ring finger, sequela

S62.655A   Nondisplaced fracture of middle phalanx of left ring finger, initial encounter for closed fracture

S62.655B   Nondisplaced fracture of middle phalanx of left ring finger, initial encounter for open fracture

S62.655D   Nondisplaced fracture of middle phalanx of left ring finger, subsequent encounter for fracture with routine healing

S62.655G   Nondisplaced fracture of middle phalanx of left ring finger, subsequent encounter for fracture with delayed healing

S62.655K   Nondisplaced fracture of middle phalanx of left ring finger, subsequent encounter for fracture with nonunion

S62.655P   Nondisplaced fracture of middle phalanx of left ring finger, subsequent encounter for fracture with malunion

S62.655S   Nondisplaced fracture of middle phalanx of left ring finger, sequela

S62.656A   Nondisplaced fracture of middle phalanx of right little finger, initial encounter for closed fracture

S62.656B   Nondisplaced fracture of middle phalanx of right little finger, initial encounter for open fracture

S62.656D   Nondisplaced fracture of middle phalanx of right little finger, subsequent encounter for fracture with routine healing

S62.656G   Nondisplaced fracture of middle phalanx of right little finger, subsequent encounter for fracture with delayed healing

S62.656K   Nondisplaced fracture of middle phalanx of right little finger, subsequent encounter for fracture with nonunion

S62.656P   Nondisplaced fracture of middle phalanx of right little finger, subsequent encounter for fracture with malunion

S62.656S   Nondisplaced fracture of middle phalanx of right little finger, sequela

S62.657A   Nondisplaced fracture of middle phalanx of left little finger, initial encounter for closed fracture

S62.657B   Nondisplaced fracture of middle phalanx of left little finger, initial encounter for open fracture

S62.657D   Nondisplaced fracture of middle phalanx of left little finger, subsequent encounter for fracture with routine healing

S62.657G   Nondisplaced fracture of middle phalanx of left little finger, subsequent encounter for fracture with delayed healing

S62.657K   Nondisplaced fracture of middle phalanx of left little finger, subsequent encounter for fracture with nonunion

S62.657P   Nondisplaced fracture of middle phalanx of left little finger, subsequent encounter for fracture with malunion

S62.657S   Nondisplaced fracture of middle phalanx of left little finger, sequela

S62.658A   Nondisplaced fracture of middle phalanx of other finger, initial encounter for closed fracture

S62.658B   Nondisplaced fracture of middle phalanx of other finger, initial encounter for open fracture

S62.658D   Nondisplaced fracture of middle phalanx of other finger, subsequent encounter for fracture with routine healing

S62.658G   Nondisplaced fracture of middle phalanx of other finger, subsequent encounter for fracture with delayed healing

S62.658K   Nondisplaced fracture of middle phalanx of other finger, subsequent encounter for fracture with nonunion

S62.658P   Nondisplaced fracture of middle phalanx of other finger, subsequent encounter for fracture with malunion

S62.658S   Nondisplaced fracture of middle phalanx of other finger, sequela

S62.659A   Nondisplaced fracture of middle phalanx of unspecified finger, initial encounter for closed fracture

S62.659B   Nondisplaced fracture of middle phalanx of unspecified finger, initial encounter for open fracture

S62.659D   Nondisplaced fracture of middle phalanx of unspecified finger, subsequent encounter for fracture with routine healing

S62.659G   Nondisplaced fracture of middle phalanx of unspecified finger, subsequent encounter for fracture with delayed healing

S62.659K   Nondisplaced fracture of middle phalanx of unspecified finger, subsequent encounter for fracture with nonunion

S62.659P   Nondisplaced fracture of middle phalanx of unspecified finger, subsequent encounter for fracture with malunion

S62.659S   Nondisplaced fracture of middle phalanx of unspecified finger, sequela

S99.101A   Unspecified physeal fracture of right metatarsal, initial encounter for closed fracture

S99.101B   Unspecified physeal fracture of right metatarsal, initial encounter for open fracture

S99.101D   Unspecified physeal fracture of right metatarsal, subsequent encounter for fracture with routine healing

S99.101G   Unspecified physeal fracture of right metatarsal, subsequent encounter for fracture with delayed healing

S99.101K   Unspecified physeal fracture of right metatarsal, subsequent encounter for fracture with nonunion

S99.101P   Unspecified physeal fracture of right metatarsal, subsequent encounter for fracture with malunion

S99.101S   Unspecified physeal fracture of right metatarsal, sequela

S99.132A   Salter-Harris Type III physeal fracture of left metatarsal, initial encounter for closed fracture

S99.132B   Salter-Harris Type III physeal fracture of left metatarsal, initial encounter for open fracture

S99.132D   Salter-Harris Type III physeal fracture of left metatarsal, subsequent encounter for fracture with routine healing

S99.132G   Salter-Harris Type III physeal fracture of left metatarsal, subsequent encounter for fracture with delayed healing

S99.132K   Salter-Harris Type III physeal fracture of left metatarsal, subsequent encounter for fracture with nonunion

S99.132P   Salter-Harris Type III physeal fracture of left metatarsal, subsequent encounter for fracture with malunion

S99.132S   Salter-Harris Type III physeal fracture of left metatarsal, sequela

T81.11XA   Postprocedural cardiogenic shock, initial encounter

T81.11XD   Postprocedural cardiogenic shock, subsequent encounter

T81.11XS   Postprocedural cardiogenic shock, sequela

143 Code Descriptions Revised (continued)

V00.821A	Fall from baby stroller, initial encounter
V00.821D	Fall from baby stroller, subsequent encounter
V00.821S	Fall from baby stroller, sequela
V00.822A	Baby stroller colliding with stationary object, initial encounter
V00.822D	Baby stroller colliding with stationary object, subsequent encounter
V00.822S	Baby stroller colliding with stationary object, sequela
V00.828A	Other accident with baby stroller, initial encounter
V00.828D	Other accident with baby stroller, subsequent encounter
V00.828S	Other accident with baby stroller, sequela
Y92.000	Kitchen of unspecified non-institutional (private) residence as the place of occurrence of the external cause
Y93.23	Activity, snow (alpine) (downhill) skiing, snowboarding, sledding, tobogganing and snow tubing
Z40.03	Encounter for prophylactic removal of fallopian tube(s)
Z68.43	Body mass index (BMI) 50-59.9, adult
Z77.123	Contact with and (suspected) exposure to radon and other naturally occurring radiation
Z77.29	Contact with and (suspected) exposure to other hazardous substances

Proprietary Updates

The following proprietary features have also been added:

- 300+ new definitions that describe, in lay terms, a specific condition or disease process
- 90+ new coding tips that provide coding advice beyond the code classification
- Updated *AHA Coding Clinic* references through second quarter 2018
- Conversion table of ICD-10-CM codes
- Updated pharmacology list
- New QPP icon identifying CMS Quality Payment Program (QPP) claims-based codes applicable to the Merit-based Incentive Payment System (MIPS)
- New appendix outlining Medicare's QPP and the MIPS track

Conversion Table of ICD-10-CM Codes

Code Assignment Beginning 10/1/2018	Previous Code(s) Assignment
C43.111	C43.11
C43.112	C43.11
C43.121	C43.12
C43.122	C43.12
C4A.111	C4A.11
C4A.112	C4A.11
C4A.121	C4A.12
C4A.122	C4A.12
C44.1021	C44.102
C44.1022	C44.102
C44.1091	C44.109
C44.1092	C44.109
C44.1121	C44.112
C44.1122	C44.112
C44.1191	C44.119
C44.1192	C44.119
C44.1221	C44.122
C44.1222	C44.122
C44.1291	C44.129
C44.1292	C44.129
C44.131	C44.19
C44.1321	C44.19
C44.1322	C44.19
C44.1391	C44.19
C44.1392	C44.19
C44.1921	C44.192
C44.1922	C44.192
C44.1991	C44.199
C44.1992	C44.199
D03.111	D03.11
D03.112	D03.11
D03.121	D03.12
D03.122	D03.12
D04.111	D04.11
D04.112	D04.11
D04.121	D04.12
D04.122	D04.12
D22.111	D22.11
D22.112	D22.11
D22.121	D22.12
D22.122	D22.12
D23.111	D23.11
D23.112	D23.11
D23.121	D23.12

Code Assignment Beginning 10/1/2018	Previous Code(s) Assignment
D23.122	D23.12
E72.81	E72.8
E72.89	E72.8
E75.26	E75.29
E78.41	E78.4
E78.49	E78.4
E88.02	E88.09
F12.23	F12.288
F12.93	F12.988
F53.0	F53
F53.1	F53
F68.A	F68.10
G51.31	G51.3
G51.32	G51.3
G51.33	G51.3
G51.39	G51.3
G71.00	G71.0
G71.01	G71.0
G71.02	G71.0
G71.09	G71.0
H01.00A	H01.001 and H01.002
H01.00B	H01.004 and H01.005
H01.01A	H01.011 and H01.012
H01.01B	H01.014 and H01.015
H01.02A	H01.021 and H01.022
H01.02B	H01.024 and H01.025
H02.151	H02.101–H02.106; H02.109
H02.152	H02.101–H02.106; H02.109
H02.153	H02.101–H02.106; H02.109
H02.154	H02.101–H02.106; H02.109
H02.155	H02.101–H02.106; H02.109
H02.156	H02.101–H02.106; H02.109
H02.159	H02.101–H02.106; H02.109
H02.20A	H02.201 and H02.202
H02.20B	H02.204 and H02.205
H02.20C	H02.201, H02.202, H02.204 and H02.205
H02.21A	H02.211 and H02.212
H02.21B	H02.214 and H02.215
H02.21C	H02.211, H02.212, H02.214 and H02.215
H02.22A	H02.221 and H02.222
H02.22B	H02.224 and H02.225
H02.22C	H02.221, H02.222, H02.224 and H02.225
H02.23A	H02.231 and H02.232
H02.23B	H02.234 and H02.235

Code Assignment Beginning 10/1/2018	Previous Code(s) Assignment	Code Assignment Beginning 10/1/2018	Previous Code(s) Assignment
H02.23C	H02.231, H02.232, H02.234 and H02.235	N35.812	N35.8
H02.881	H02.89	N35.813	N35.8
H02.882	H02.89	N35.814	N35.8
H02.883	H02.89	N35.816	N35.8
H02.884	H02.89	N35.819	N35.8
H02.885	H02.89	N35.82	N35.8
H02.886	H02.89	N35.911	N35.9
H02.889	H02.89	N35.912	N35.9
H02.88A	H02.89	N35.913	N35.9
H02.88B	H02.89	N35.914	N35.9
H10.821	H10.89	N35.916	N35.9
H10.822	H10.89	N35.919	N35.9
H10.823	H10.89	N35.92	N35.9
H10.829	H10.89	N99.116	N99.114
H57.811	H57.8	O30.131	O30.101
H57.812	H57.8	O30.132	O30.101
H57.813	H57.8	O30.133	O30.101
H57.819	H57.8	O30.139	O30.101
H57.89	H57.8	O30.231	O30.201
I63.81	I63.8	O30.232	O30.201
I63.89	I63.8	O30.233	O30.201
I67.850	I67.89	O30.239	O30.201
I67.858	I67.89	O30.831	O30.801
K35.20	K35.2	O30.832	O30.801
K35.21	K35.2	O30.833	O30.801
K35.30	K35.3	O30.839	O30.801
K35.31	K35.3	O86.00	O86.0
K35.32	K35.3	O86.01	O86.0
K35.33	K35.3	O86.02	O86.0
K35.890	K35.89	O86.03	O86.0
K35.891	K35.89	O86.04	O86.0
K61.31	K61.3	O86.09	O86.0
K61.39	K61.3	P02.70	P02.7
K61.5	K61.3	P02.78	P02.7
K82.A1	K81.0	P04.11	P04.1
K82.A2	K82.2 and K81.9	P04.12	P04.1
K83.01	K83.0	P04.13	P04.1
K83.09	K83.0	P04.14	P04.1
M79.10	M79.1	P04.15	P04.1
M79.11	M79.1	P04.16	P04.1
M79.12	M79.1	P04.17	P04.1
M79.18	M79.1	P04.1A	P04.1
N35.016	N35.014	P04.18	P04.1
N35.116	N35.114	P04.19	P04.1
N35.811	N35.8	P04.40	P04.49
		P04.42	P04.49

Code Assignment Beginning 10/1/2018	Previous Code(s) Assignment	Code Assignment Beginning 10/1/2018	Previous Code(s) Assignment
PØ4.81	PØ4.8	T74.61XA	T74.11XA
PØ4.89	PØ4.8	T74.61XD	T74.11XD
P35.4	P35.8 and A92.5	T74.61XS	T74.11XS
P74.21	P74.2	T74.62XA	T74.12XA
P74.22	P74.2	T74.62XD	T74.12XD
P74.31	P74.3	T74.62XS	T74.12XS
P74.32	P74.3	T76.51XA	T76.21XA
P74.41	P74.4	T76.51XD	T76.21XD
P74.421	P74.4	T76.51XS	T76.21XS
P74.422	P74.4	T76.52XA	T76.22XA
P74.49	P74.4	T76.52XD	T76.22XD
Q51.2Ø	Q51.2	T76.52XS	T76.22XS
Q51.21	Q51.2	T76.61XA	T76.11XA
Q51.22	Q51.2	T76.61XD	T76.11XD
Q51.28	Q51.2	T76.61XS	T76.11XS
Q93.51	Q93.5	T76.62XA	T76.12XA
Q93.59	Q93.5	T76.62XD	T76.12XD
Q93.82	Q93.89	T76.62XS	T76.12XS
R82.991	R82.99	T81.40XA	T81.4XXA
R82.992	R82.99	T81.40XD	T81.4XXD
R82.993	R82.99	T81.40XS	T81.4XXS
R82.994	R82.99	T81.41XA	T81.4XXA
R82.998	R82.99	T81.41XD	T81.4XXD
R93.811	R93.8	T81.41XS	T81.4XXS
R93.812	R93.8	T81.42XA	T81.4XXA
R93.813	R93.8	T81.42XD	T81.4XXD
R93.819	R93.8	T81.42XS	T81.4XXS
R93.89	R93.8	T81.43XA	T81.4XXA
T43.641A	T43.621A	T81.43XD	T81.4XXD
T43.641D	T43.621D	T81.43XS	T81.4XXS
T43.641S	T43.621S	T81.44XA	T81.4XXA
T43.642A	T43.622A	T81.44XD	T81.4XXD
T43.642D	T43.622D	T81.44XS	T81.4XXS
T43.642S	T43.622S	T81.49XA	T81.4XXA
T43.643A	T43.623A	T81.49XD	T81.4XXD
T43.643D	T43.623D	T81.49XS	T81.4XXS
T43.643S	T43.623S	Y07.6	YØ7.59
T43.644A	T43.624A	ZØ4.81	ZØ4.8
T43.644D	T43.624D	ZØ4.82	ZØ4.8
T43.644S	T43.624S	ZØ4.89	ZØ4.8
T74.51XA	T74.21XA	Z13.3Ø	Z13.8
T74.51XD	T74.21XD	Z13.31	Z13.8
T74.51XS	T74.21XS	Z13.32	Z13.8
T74.52XA	T74.22XA	Z13.39	Z13.8
T74.52XD	T74.22XD	Z13.4Ø	Z13.4
T74.52XS	T74.22XS	Z13.41	Z13.4

Code Assignment Beginning 10/1/2018	Previous Code(s) Assignment
Z13.42	Z13.4
Z13.49	Z13.4
Z20.821	Z20.828
Z28.83	Z28.89
Z62.813	Z62.810
Z83.430	Z83.49
Z83.438	Z83.49
Z91.42	Z91.410

Introduction

History of ICD-10-CM

The ICD-10-CM classification system was developed by the National Center for Health Statistics (NCHS) as a clinical modification to the ICD-10 system developed by the World Health Organization (WHO), primarily as a unique system for use in the United States for morbidity and mortality reporting. Although ICD-10 replaced ICD-9 for use in coding and classifying mortality data from death certificates beginning January 1, 1999, ICD-10-CM implementation was postponed many years until legislation to replace ICD-9-CM, volumes 1 and 2, with ICD-10-CM was approved.

ICD-10 is the copyrighted product of the World Health Organization (WHO), which has authorized the development of a clinical modification (CM) of ICD-10 for use in the United States. However, all modifications to the ICD-10 must conform to WHO conventions for ICD. The development of ICD-10-CM included comprehensive evaluation by a Technical Advisory Panel and extensive consultation with physician groups, clinical coders, and other industry experts.

The ICD-10-CM draft and crosswalk between ICD-9-CM and ICD-10-CM were made available on the Centers for Medicare and Medicaid Services (CMS) website for public comment. The initial public comment period extended from December 1997 through February 1998. A field test for ICD-10-CM was conducted in the summer of 2003 jointly by the American Hospital Association (AHA) and the American Health Information Management Association (AHIMA). Public comments and suggestions were reviewed and additional modifications to ICD-10-CM were made. Revisions were made to ICD-10-CM based on the established update process for ICD-10-CM (the ICD-10-CM Coordination and Maintenance Committee) and the World Health Organization's ICD-10 (the Update and Revision Committee).

These revisions to ICD-10-CM have included:

- Information relevant to ambulatory and managed care encounters
- Expanded injury codes
- Creation of combination diagnosis/symptom codes to reduce the number of codes needed to fully describe a condition
- The addition of 6th and 7th character classifications
- Incorporation of common 4th and 5th character classifications
- Classifications specific to laterality
- Classification refinement for increased data granularity

This new structure allows for further expansion than was possible with the ICD-9-CM classification system.

The Department of Health and Human Services (HHS) published the final rule regarding the adoption of both ICD-10-CM and ICD-10-PCS in the January 16, 2009, *Federal Register* (45 CFR part 162 [CMS—0013—F]). The initial compliance date for implementation of ICD-10-CM and ICD-10-PCS as a replacement for ICD-9-CM was set at October 1, 2013. On April 17, 2012, the Department of Health and Human Services (HHS) released a notice to postpone the date by which certain health care entities have to comply with International Classification of Diseases, 10th Revision diagnosis and procedure codes (ICD-10). The compliance date for implementation of ICD-10-CM and ICD-10-PCS as a replacement for ICD-9-CM was changed to October 1, 2014. On April 1, 2014, Congress enacted the Protecting Access to Medicare Act of 2014, which contained a provision to delay the implementation of ICD-10-CM/PCS by at least one year, prohibiting the Department of Health and Human Services (HHS) from adopting the ICD-10-CM/PCS code sets as the mandatory standard until October 1, 2015. Eventually, the ICD-10-CM/PCS code sets were implemented in their entirety on October 1, 2015, and volumes 1 and 2 of ICD-9-CM were retired.

ICD-10-CM: The Complete Official Code Set

ICD-10-CM for Physicians: The Complete Official Code Set 2019 edition includes many of the enhancements described below in direct response to requests from our subscribers.

As you review the content, you will find the following:

- Optum360 Exclusive feature — Check Placeholder Alert symbol, indicating the need for one or more "filler" X character assignments in the 5th and/or 6th character position, in order to appropriately assign a required character in the 7th character position

- Optum360 Exclusive feature — Key word differentiation by the use of a green font that highlights the differentiating terms in similar code descriptions in a given category

- Optum360 Exclusive color coding, symbols, and footnotes that alert coders to coding and reimbursement issues, including the majority of the Medicare code edits

- Optum360 Exclusive feature — Exclusive *following* references and Check Additional Character symbol in the indexes. The *following* references (designed and used exclusively by Optum360) help coders locate those alphanumeric codes that are out of sequence in the tabular section.

- Optum360 Exclusive feature — Exclusive shaded guides in the index that help users easily follow the indent levels for the subterms under a main term

- Illustrations throughout the tabular list and at the back of the book that feature anatomy and terminology included in the ICD-10-CM classification system

- Optum360 Exclusive feature — Detailed Muscle/Tendon tables that correspond to codes in chapters 13 and 19

- The complete ICD-10-CM Official Guidelines for Coding and Reporting, published by the U.S. Department of Health and Human Services and approved by the cooperating parties (American Health Information Management Association, National Center for Health Statistics, Centers for Medicare and Medicaid Services, American Hospital Association)

- Optum360 Exclusive feature — Official chapter-specific guidelines with coding examples at the beginning of each chapter

- All the official ICD-10-CM codes, indexes, notes, footnotes, and symbols

- Check 4th, 5th, 6th, and 7th character symbols that identify codes that require the addition of a 4th, 5th, 6th, or 7th character for code specificity and validity

- Color coding and symbol legend at the bottom of each page

Please review "How to Use *ICD-10-CM Expert for Physicians*" in this section to learn about the features that will help you assign and report correct codes, ensuring appropriate reimbursement.

This International Classification of Diseases, 10th Revision, Clinical Modification (ICD-10-CM) is being published by the United States Government in recognition of its responsibility to promulgate this classification throughout the United States for morbidity coding. This code book represents an adaptation of ICD-10 that was created specifically for use in the United States. Revisions to ICD-10-CM will be made based on the established update process for ICD-10-CM (the ICD-10-CM Coordination and Maintenance Committee) and the World Health Organization's ICD-10 (the Update and Revision Committee).

Use of Official Sources

The *ICD-10-CM Expert for Physicians* contains the official U.S. Department of Health and Human Services, Tenth Revision, Clinical Modification, ICD-10-CM codes, effective for the current year.

Much of the color coding and many of the symbols that identify coding and reimbursement issues are derived from official federal government sources, including the Integrated Outpatient Code Editor (IOCE), version 19.2.

For the most current IOCE documents please refer to the following: https://www.cms.gov/Medicare/Coding/OutpatientCodeEdit/OCEQtrReleaseSpecs.html.

Steps to Correct Coding

1. Before beginning to use this code book, review section I.A., "Conventions for the ICD-10-CM," and section I.B., "General Coding Guidelines," of the ICD-10-CM Official Guidelines for Coding and Reporting.

2. Look up the main term in the alphabetic index and scan the subterm entries as appropriate. Review continued lines and additional subterms that may appear in the next column or on the next page.

3. Note all parenthetical terms (nonessential modifiers) that help in code selection but do not affect code assignment. Shaded vertical guidelines in the index are provided to help determine the indentation level for each subterm in relation to the main terms.

4. Pay close attention to the following instructions in the index:
   - "See," "see also," and "see category" cross-references
   - "With"/"without" notes
   - "Omit code" notes
   - "Due to" subterms
   - Other instructions found in note boxes, such as "code by site"
   - *Following* references and Check Additional Character symbol in the indexes. The *following* references (designed and used exclusively by Optum360) help coders locate those alphanumeric codes that are out of sequence in the tabular section.

5. Do not code from the alphabetic index without verifying the accuracy of the code in the tabular list. Locate the code in the alphanumerically arranged tabular list.

6. To determine the appropriateness of the code selection and proper coding, read all instructional material:
   - "Includes" and both types of "Excludes" notes
   - "Use additional code" and "code first underlying disease" instructions
   - "Code also"
   - 4th, 5th, and 6th character requirements and 7th character extension requirements
   - Age and sex symbols

7. Consult the official ICD-10-CM guidelines, which govern the use of specific codes. These guidelines provide both general and chapter-specific coding guidance.

8. Confirm and assign the correct code.

Organization
This book is organized in the following manner:

Introduction
The introductory material in this book includes the ICD-10-CM Official Preface, the history of ICD-10-CM as well as an overview of the classification system.

Official ICD-10-CM Conventions and Guidelines
Included in this section are the *2019 Official Guidelines for Coding and Reporting.* This section also provides an explanation of the conventions and guidelines regulating the appropriate assignment and reporting of ICD-10-CM codes. This coding guidance is presented by the National Center for Health Statistics (NCHS), a governmental agency of the Centers for Disease Control and Prevention (CDC), within the United States Department of Health and Human Services (DHHS).

Alphabetic Index to Diseases
The Alphabetic Index to Diseases is arranged in alphabetic order by disease — by specific illness, injury, eponym, abbreviation, or other descriptive diagnostic term. The Index also lists diagnostic terms for other reasons for encounters with health care professionals.

Neoplasm Table
The Neoplasm Table provides the proper code based upon histology of the neoplasm and site.

Table of Drugs and Chemicals
The Table of Drugs and Chemicals lists the drug and the specific codes that identify the drug and the intent. No additional external cause of injury and poisoning code is assigned in ICD-10-CM.

Index to External Causes
The Alphabetic Index to External Causes of Injuries is arranged in alphabetic order by main term indicating the event.

Tabular List of Diseases
ICD-10-CM codes and descriptors are arranged numerically within the tabular list of diseases within 21 separate chapters according to body system or nature of injury and disease. Classifications that were previously considered supplemental to ICD-9-CM (e.g., V codes and E codes) are incorporated into the tabular listing of ICD-10-CM as individual chapters. Chapters 20, "External Causes of Morbidity," and 21, "Factors Influencing Health Status and Contact with Health Services," include chapter-specific guidelines.

Appendixes

The additional resources described below have been included as appendixes for the *ICD-10-CM Expert for Physicians*. These resources further instruct the professional coder on the appropriate application of the ICD-10-CM code set.

Appendix A: 10 Steps to Correct Coding

This step-by-step tutorial walks the coder through the process of locating the correct code in the alphabetic index and verifying it in the tabular section while following applicable conventions and guidelines. Detailed examples are provided and explained along with advice for proper sequencing.

Appendix B: Valid 3-character ICD-10-CM Codes

The user may consult this table to confirm that no further specificity, such as the use of 4th, 5th, 6th, or 7th characters or placeholders (X), is necessary. All ICD-10-CM codes that are valid at the three-character level are listed.

Appendix C: Pharmacology List 2019

This reference is a comprehensive but not all-inclusive list of pharmacological agents used to treat acute and/or chronic conditions. Drugs are listed in alphabetical order by their brand and/or generic names along with their drug action and indications for which they may commonly be prescribed. Some drugs have also been mapped to their appropriate Z code for long-term drug use.

Appendix D: Z Codes for Long-Term Drug Use with Associated Drugs

This resource correlates Z codes that are used to identify current long-term drug use with a list of drugs that are typically categorized to that class of drug.

Note: These tables are not all-inclusive but list some of the more commonly used drugs.

Appendix E: Z Codes Only as Principal/First-Listed Diagnosis

Chapter 21, "Factors Influencing Health Status and Contact with Health Services," provides codes to deal with encounters for circumstances other than a disease or injury. Many of these codes may be reported *only* as the principal/first-listed diagnosis. This resource lists all of these codes in one table for quick and easy reference to ensure accurate reporting.

Appendix F: Centers for Medicare & Medicaid Services Hierarchical Condition Categories (CMS-HCC)

This resource provides the framework behind the Centers for Medicare and Medicaid Services' (CMS) Medicare Advantage (MA) program, a risk-adjustment model developed as a means of compensating health care plans with large numbers of Medicare Part C beneficiaries. It includes a brief synopsis of the evolution of the program from its inception; insight into the various elements needed to predict risk, including the principles used to develop the hierarchical condition categories (HCCs), which make up one of the fundamental components of the risk-adjustment model. This appendix also outlines the audit process used to ensure the accuracy of payments made to MA plans.

Appendix G: Centers for Medicare & Medicaid Services Quality Payment Program

This resource provides an overview of the Medicare Access and CHIP Reauthorization Act (MACRA), which replaced Medicare's sustainable growth rate (SGR) methodology with the Quality Payment Program (QPP). It summarizes the Merit-based Incentive Payment System (MIPS) track used by those who opt to participate in traditional Medicare and not an advanced alternative payment model (APM). This includes eligibility requirements and an overview of the four performance categories that combine to make up the MIPS.

Illustrations

This section includes illustrations of normal anatomy with ICD-10-CM specific terminology.

Overview of ICD-10-CM Official Conventions

This is an overview of the ICD-10-CM official conventions, which are general rules for using the classification system, independent of the guidelines. The official conventions and instructions of the classification, which take precedence over the guidelines, are incorporated within the alphabetic index and tabular list as instructional notes and are applicable regardless of the health care setting. For the full version of the official conventions, see the ICD-10-CM Official Guidelines for Coding and Reporting, section I.A., which is included in this book.

Format

ICD-10-CM is divided into two main parts: the index, an alphabetical list of terms and their corresponding code, and the tabular list, a sequential, alphanumeric list of codes divided into chapters based on body system or condition. The index contains the Index to Diseases and Injuries (main index) and the Index to External Causes of Injury. Also included in the main index is the Neoplasm Table and a Table of Drugs and Chemicals.

The tabular list contains categories, subcategories, and valid codes. ICD-10-CM is an alphanumeric classification system. The 1st character of a three-character category is a letter. The 2nd and 3rd characters may be numbers or alpha characters. A three-character category without further subclassification is equivalent to a valid three-character code. Subcategories are either four or five characters. Subcategory characters include either letters or numbers. Codes may be three, four, five, six, or seven characters in length, in which each level of subdivision after a category is a subcategory. The final level of subdivision is a valid code. The final character in a code may be either a letter or a number.

The ICD-10-CM uses the letter "X" as a placeholder. A placeholder "X" is used as a 5th character placeholder at certain six-character codes to allow for future expansion, without disturbing the 6th character structure. For instance, an initial encounter for accidental poisoning by penicillin is coded to T36.0X1A. The "X" in the 5th character position is a placeholder, or filler character.

Similarly, certain categories have applicable 7th character extensions. In these cases, the 7th character extension is required for all codes within the category, or as otherwise instructed in the tabular list notations. 7th character extensions must always be the last character in the data field. If a code is not a full six characters in length, a dummy placeholder "X" must be used to fill in the empty characters when a 7th character extension is required.

Punctuation

[]   In the tabular list, brackets are used to enclose synonyms, alternative wording, or explanatory phrases. In the index, brackets are used to identify manifestation codes.

( )   Parentheses are used in both the index and tabular list to enclose nonessential modifiers; supplementary words that may be present or absent in the statement of a disease or procedure without affecting the code number to which it is assigned.

:   Colons are used in the tabular list after an incomplete term that needs one or more of the modifiers following the colon to make it assignable to a given category.

Abbreviations

NEC
The abbreviation NEC, "Not elsewhere classifiable" represents "other specified" in the ICD-10-CM. An index entry that states NEC directs the coder to an "other specified" code in the tabular list. Codes titled "Other" or "Other specified" in the tabular list (usually a code with a 4th or 6th character 8 and 5th character 9) are for use when the information in the medical record provides detail for which a specific code does not exist.

NOS
The abbreviation NOS, "Not otherwise specified," in the tabular list may be interpreted as "unspecified." Codes in the tabular list with "Unspecified" in the title (usually a code with a 4th or 6th character 9 and 5th character Ø) are for use when the information in the medical record is insufficient to assign a more specific code.

Typeface

Boldface
Boldface type is used for main term entries in the alphabetic index, and all codes and descriptions in the tabular list.

General Notes

The following conventions and notes appear only in the tabular list of diseases:

Includes Notes
The word INCLUDES appears immediately under certain categories to further define, clarify, or give examples of the content of a code category.

Inclusion Terms
Lists of inclusion terms are included under certain codes. These terms indicate some of the conditions for which that code number may be used. Inclusion terms may be synonyms with the code title, or, in the case of "other specified" codes, the terms may also provide a list of various conditions included within a classification code. The inclusion terms are not exhaustive. The index may provide additional terms that may also be assigned to a given code.

Excludes Notes
ICD-10-CM has two types of excludes notes. Each note has a different definition for use. However, they are similar in that they both indicate that codes excluded from each other are independent of each other.

Excludes 1
An EXCLUDES1 note is a "pure" excludes. It means "NOT CODED HERE!" An Excludes 1 note indicates mutually exclusive codes: two conditions that cannot be reported together. For example, a congenital form of a disease may not be reported with the acquired form of the same condition. The code excluded should never be reported with the applicable codes listed above the excludes notation.

An exception to the Excludes 1 definition is when the two conditions are unrelated to each other. If it is not clear whether the two conditions involving an Excludes 1 note are related or not, query the provider. For example, code F45.8 Other somatoform disorders, has an Excludes 1 note for "sleep related teeth grinding (G47.63)" because "teeth grinding" is an inclusion term under F45.8. Only one of these two codes should be assigned for teeth grinding. However psychogenic dysmenorrhea is also an inclusion term under F45.8, and a patient could have both this condition and sleep-related teeth grinding. In this case, the two conditions are clearly unrelated to each other, so it would be appropriate to report F45.8 and G47.63 together.

Excludes 2
An EXCLUDES 2 note means "NOT INCLUDED HERE." An Excludes 2 note indicates that although the excluded condition is not part of the condition it is excluded from, a patient may have both conditions at the same time. Therefore, when an Excludes 2 note appears under a code, it may be acceptable to use both the code and the excluded code together if supported by the medical documentation.

Note
NOTE The term "NOTE" appears as an icon and precedes the instructional information. These notes function as alerts to highlight coding instructions within the text.

Default Codes
In the index, the default code is the code listed next to the main term. The default code represents the condition most commonly associated with the main term. This code may be assigned when documentation does not facilitate reporting a more specific code. Alternatively, it may provide an unspecified code for the condition.

Syndromes
Follow the alphabetic index guidance when coding syndromes. In the absence of index guidance, assign codes for the documented manifestations of the syndrome.

And
When the term "and" is used in a narrative statement or code title it may be interpreted as "and/or."

With
The word "with" or "in" should be interpreted to mean "associated with" or "due to" when it appears in a code title, the Alphabetic Index (either under a main term or subterm), or an instructional note in the Tabular List. The classification presumes a causal relationship between the two conditions linked by these terms in the Alphabetic Index or Tabular List. These conditions should be coded as related even in the absence of provider documentation explicitly linking them, unless the documentation clearly states the conditions are unrelated or when another guideline exists that specifically requires a documented linkage between two conditions (e.g., sepsis guideline for "acute organ dysfunction that is not clearly associated with the sepsis"). For conditions not specifically linked by these relational terms in the classification or when a guideline requires that a linkage between two conditions be explicitly documented, provider documentation must link the conditions in order to code them as related.

The word "with" in the Alphabetic Index is sequenced immediately following the main term, not in alphabetical order.

See and See Also
When the instruction "See" follows a main term in the alphabetic index, it indicates that another term must be referenced in order to locate the correct code. The instructional note "See also" simply provides alternative terms that may be useful in determining the correct code but is not necessary to follow if the main term supplies the appropriate code.

Instructional Notes Used in the Tabular List
In the tabular section, the following instructional notes appear in red type for emphasis:

Code First/Use additional code:
These instructional notes provide sequencing instruction. They may appear independently of each other or to designate certain etiology/manifestation paired codes. These instructions signal the coder that an additional code should be reported to provide a more complete picture of that diagnosis.

In etiology/manifestation coding, ICD-10-CM requires the underlying condition to be sequenced first, followed by the manifestation. In these situations, codes with "In diseases classified elsewhere" in the code description are never permitted as a first-listed or principal diagnosis code and must be sequenced following the underlying condition code.

Code Also:
A "code also" note alerts the coder that more than one code may be required to fully describe the condition. The sequencing depends on the circumstances of the encounter. Factors that may determine sequencing include severity and reason for the encounter.

Code Assignment and Clinical Criteria
Diagnosis code assignment must be based on the provider's diagnostic statement that the condition exists and is not based on clinical criteria the provider used to establish the diagnosis. Conflicting documentation must be queried.

Additional Annotations

Code-Level Notations

The tabular section of ICD-10-CM has various colors, symbol, and other tabular annotations that may help in code selection, provide clinical or coding information, or alert the coder to reimbursement issues affected by the diagnosis code assignment. Some codes may have more than one annotation. For quick reference to the meanings of the colors and symbols, look at the color/symbol legend at the bottom of each page in the tabular list.

Italics

Italicized type is used for all exclusion notes and to identify manifestation codes, those codes that should not be reported as first-listed (principal) diagnoses.

Color Coding/Symbols

New Code
This ● icon identifies the codes that are new to the classification system for the current year. The new code icon is to the left of the code.

Revised Code Title
This ▲ icon to the left of a code alerts the user to a change in that code's title. This change may be as simple as adding or removing punctuation, which may or may not change the intent of the code, to adding or removing specific terms from a code description that completely alter the circumstances in which the code would be used.

Revised Text
The revised text ►◄ "bow ties" alert the user to changes in parenthetical notes for the current year. Revised text may include the following:

- A change in a current parenthetical description
- A change in the code(s) associated with a current parenthetical note
- A change in how a current parenthetical note is classified (e.g., an Excludes 1 note that changed to an Excludes 2 note)
- Addition of a new parenthetical note(s) to a code

Deleted Text
~~Strikethrough~~ on code description(s) and/or code note(s) indicates a deletion from the classification for the current year.

Additional Characters Required
√4ᵗʰ This symbol indicates that the code requires a 4th character.

√5ᵗʰ This symbol indicates that the code requires a 5th character.

√6ᵗʰ This symbol indicates that the code requires a 6th character.

√7ᵗʰ This symbol indicates that the code requires a 7th character.

> √5ᵗʰ **H60.3** Other infective otitis externa
> > √6ᵗʰ **H60.31** Diffuse otitis externa
> > > **H60.311** Diffuse otitis externa, right ear
> > > **H60.312** Diffuse otitis externa, left ear
> > > **H60.313** Diffuse otitis externa, bilateral
> > > **H60.319** Diffuse otitis externa, unspecified ear ▽

√x7ᵗʰ This symbol indicates that the code requires a 7th character following the placeholder "X". Codes with fewer than six characters that require a 7th character must contain placeholder "X" to fill in the empty character(s).

> √x7ᵗʰ **T16.1** Foreign body in right ear

Key Word

Green font is used throughout the Tabular List of Diseases to differentiate the key words that appear in similar code descriptions in a given category or subcategory.

For example, refer to the list of codes below from category H55:

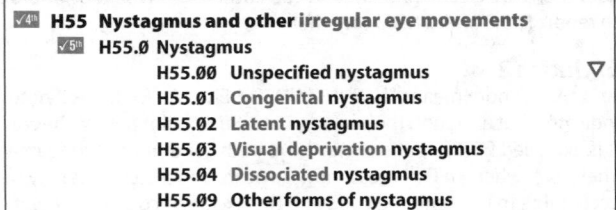

> √4ᵗʰ **H55 Nystagmus and other irregular eye movements**
> > √5ᵗʰ **H55.0 Nystagmus**
> > > **H55.00** Unspecified nystagmus ▽
> > > **H55.01** Congenital nystagmus
> > > **H55.02** Latent nystagmus
> > > **H55.03** Visual deprivation nystagmus
> > > **H55.04** Dissociated nystagmus
> > > **H55.09** Other forms of nystagmus

The portion of the code description that appears in **green font** in the tabular list helps the coder quickly identify the key terms and the correct code. This convention is especially useful when the codes describe laterality, such as the following codes from subcategory H40.22:

> √6ᵗʰ **H40.22 Chronic angle-closure glaucoma**
> Chronic primary angle-closure glaucoma
> > √7ᵗʰ **H40.221** Chronic angle-closure glaucoma, right eye
> > √7ᵗʰ **H40.222** Chronic angle-closure glaucoma, left eye
> > √7ᵗʰ **H40.223** Chronic angle-closure glaucoma, bilateral
> > √7ᵗʰ **H40.229** Chronic angle-closure glaucoma, unspecified eye ▽

The key word convention is used only in those categories in which there are multiple codes with very similar descriptions with only a few words that differentiate them.

Medicare Code Edits

Medicare Administrative Contractors and many payers use Medicare code edits to check the coding accuracy on claims. The coding edit information in this manual reflects those edits used for outpatient institutional providers, which also include hospitals that are subject to the outpatient prospective payment system (OPPS). These edits have been updated to reflect changes in the Integrated Outpatient Code Editor (IOCE), version 19.2.

Age and Sex Edit
The age and sex edits below are used to detect inconsistencies between the patient's age and/or sex and the patient's diagnosis. The following edit symbols appear in the tabular list to the right of the code description.

Ⓝ **Newborn Age: 0**

These diagnoses are intended for newborns and neonates and the patient's age must be 0 years.

> **N47.0** Adherent prepuce, newborn Ⓝ♂

Ⓟ **Pediatric Age: 0-17**

These diagnoses are intended for children and the patient's age must be between 0 and 17 years.

> **L21.1** Seborrheic infantile dermatitis Ⓟ

Ⓜ **Maternity Age: 12-55**

These diagnoses are intended for childbearing patients between the age of 12 and 55 years.

> **O02.9** Abnormal product of conception, unspecified Ⓜ♀▽

A Adult Age: 15-124

These diagnoses are intended for patients between the age of 15 and 124 years.

R54	Age-related physical debility	A
	Frailty	
	Old age	
	Senescence	
	Senile asthenia	
	Senile debility	
	EXCLUDES 1 age-related cognitive decline (R41.81)	
	sarcopenia (M62.84)	
	senile psychosis (F03)	
	senility NOS (R41.81)	

♂ Male diagnosis only

Q98.0	Klinefelter syndrome karyotype 47, XXY	♂

♀ Female diagnosis only

N35.12	Postinfective urethral stricture, not elsewhere classified, female	♀

Manifestation Code

These codes appear in italic type, with a **blue color bar** over the title. A manifestation code cannot be reported as a first-listed or principal diagnosis. By definition, a manifestation code represents a demonstration of some aspect of an underlying disease, which is separately classifiable. In the alphabetic index, these codes are listed as the secondary code in brackets. The underlying disease code is listed first.

G32.89	*Other specified degenerative disorders of nervous system in diseases classified elsewhere*
	Degenerative encephalopathy in diseases classified elsewhere

Medicare Advantage Risk Adjustment Edits

Medicare Advantage plans provided as part of the Medicare Part C program use a risk-adjustment model to plan for future healthcare costs of Medicare Part C participants. The risk-adjustment model measures disease burden by assigning certain ICD-10-CM diagnosis codes to hierarchical condition categories (HCC). The HCC information in this manual has been updated to reflect the CMS-HCC model category for v22 of the CMS-HCC risk-adjustment software.

HCC CMS-HCC Condition

This symbol indicates that the condition is considered a CMS-HCC diagnosis. All HCC conditions that are appropriately documented are used in the risk-adjustment model for Medicare Advantage to provide a means of comparing quality of care across Medicare Part C participants as well as predict future healthcare costs.

The HCC icon appears to the right of the code description.

Y62.2	Failure of sterile precautions during kidney dialysis and other perfusion	HCC

Medicare Quality Payment Program Edits

In an effort to repeal the Medicare sustainable growth rate (SGR), focus on quality of patient outcomes, and control Medicare spending, Congress passed the Medicare Access and CHIP Reauthorization Act (MACRA) in 2015. MACRA repealed the Medicare SGR methodology used for updating the Medicare physician fee schedule (MPFS) and replaced it with the Quality Payment Program (QPP). Under the QPP, providers who demonstrate success at controlling costs while providing high-quality care to their patients are eligible to earn increased payments and avoid negative payment adjustments. The QPP information in this manual reflects 2018 claims-based diagnosis codes published by CMS for reporting quality measures.

Q QPP Condition

This symbol indicates that the condition is recognized as a quality measure for claims-based reporting under the Merit-based Incentive Payment System (MIPS).

G44.52	New daily persistent headache (NDPH)	Q

Other Code-Level Notations
▽ Unspecified Code

Use these codes when neither the diagnostic statement nor the documentation provides enough information to assign a more specific diagnosis code. These codes may be stated as "Unspecified" or "Not otherwise specified (NOS)."

Note: Do not assign these codes when a more specific diagnosis has been determined.

D04.9	Carcinoma in situ of skin, unspecified	▽

PDx PDx Symbol

This symbol identifies a Z code that generally is for use as a first-listed (or principal) diagnosis only but may be used as an additional diagnosis if the patient has more than one encounter on the same day or there is more than one reason for the encounter.

The instructions for Z code use contained in the ICD-10-CM official coding guidelines identify those Z codes that can be used only as a PDx. All other Z codes may either be SDx or PDx, depending upon circumstances of the encounter, by meeting the definition of first-listed or principal diagnosis, and by following any specific Z code guidelines in section I.C.21 a-c. The responsibility of those assigning the Z codes as PDx is to make sure the circumstances of the encounter meet the definition of first-listed or principal diagnosis, follow all coding instructions, and follow the Z code specific guidelines. Optum360 does not include any SDx edit since there is no official source for it and the Z code use is determined by circumstances of the encounter.

Note: Please note that the symbols indicating the Z code "principal or first-listed only" designation and the Z codes that may be principal or first-listed diagnoses included in the official coding guidelines [section I.C.21.c.16] are consistent with reporting guidelines for health care encounters *excluding acute care inpatient admissions*. These Z code edits are often in conflict with the inpatient prospective payment system (IPPS) edits. For example, code Z34.90 Encounter for supervision of normal pregnancy, unspecified, unspecified trimester, may be an appropriate primary reason for an outpatient encounter. However, supervision for a normal pregnancy is not an acceptable principal diagnosis or reason for an inpatient admission and will have an unacceptable principal diagnosis edit under the inpatient prospective payment system (IPPS).

Z51.12	Encounter for antineoplastic immunotherapy	PDx

AHA This symbol precedes official citations from AHA's *Coding Clinic for ICD-10-CM/PCS*. Similar to the parenthetical notes, AHA references are placed in a hierarchical pattern at the chapter, code block, category, subcategory, or valid code level. This means that the information found in the reference applies to one or more codes depending on where the citation is placed.

The citations appear in purple type and are listed with the most current citation first. *Coding Clinic* citations included in this edition have been updated through second quarter 2018.

> **I15.1 Hypertension secondary to other renal disorders**
> AHA: 2016, 3Q, 22

DEF This symbol precedes a definition of a condition or disease.

The definition appears in purple type under the code.

> ✓5ᵗʰ **M51.4 Schmorl's nodes**
> **DEF:** Irregular bone defect in the margin of the vertebral body that causes herniation into the end plate of the vertebral body.

TIP This symbol precedes coding advice that is not readily available within the ICD-10-CM classification. It may relate official coding guidelines, indexing nuances, or advice from *AHA's Coding Clinic for ICD-10-CM/PCS*.

The tip appears in brown type under the code.

> **P15.8 Other specified birth injuries**
> **TIP:** Use for any injury of newborn from scalpel.

Footnotes

Certain codes in the tabular section have a numerical superscript located to the upper left of the code. This numerical superscript corresponds to a specific footnote description.

For example:

> [1] ✓7ᵗʰ **M48.51 Collapsed vertebra, not elsewhere classified, occipito-atlanto-axial region** ᴴᶜᶜ

The footnote description for numerical superscript 1 is "HCC with 7th character indicating initial encounter." This means that a collapsed occipito-atlanto-axial vertebra would be considered an HCC only when the 7th character represents an initial encounter, such as 7th character A, B, or C, depending on the category. In previous editions the footnote description was provided at the bottom of the same page on which a numerical superscript was found. For convenience, beginning with the 2019 edition, the footnote descriptions are no longer provided on the tabular page but have been placed on the front cover.

The following list also provides the footnote descriptions of all numerical superscripts found in the Tabular List of Diseases:

1 These codes are considered an HCC when reported with a 7th character indicating an initial encounter (7th character A, B, or C).

2 These codes are considered an HCC when reported with a 7th character indicating an initial encounter (7th character A or B) OR sequela.

3 These codes are considered an HCC when reported with a 7th character indicating sequela.

Chapter-Level Notations

Chapter-Specific Guidelines with Coding Examples

Each chapter begins with the Official Guidelines for Coding and Reporting specific to that chapter, where provided. Coding examples specific to outpatient care settings have been provided to illustrate the coding and/or sequencing guidance in these guidelines.

Muscle and Tendon Table

ICD-10-CM categorizes certain muscles and tendons in the upper and lower extremities by their action (e.g., extension or flexion) as well as their anatomical location. The Muscle/Tendon table is provided at the beginning of chapter 13 and chapter 19 to help users when code selection depends on the action of the muscle and/or tendon.

Note: This table is not all-inclusive, and proper code assignment should be based on the provider's documentation.

Index Notations

▽ Subterms under main terms may continue to next column or page. This warning statement is a reminder to always check for additional subterms and information that may continue onto the next page or column before making a final selection.

Following References

The Index includes following references to assist in locating "out-of-sequence" codes in the tabular list. "Out-of-sequence" codes contain an alphabetic character (letter) in the 3rd or 4th character position. These codes are placed according to the classification rules — the placement of the codes according to condition — not according to alphabetic or numeric sequencing rules.

Examples:

> **Carcinoma** (malignant) (*see also* Neoplasm, by site, malignant)
> neuroendocrine (*see also* Tumor, neuroendocrine)
> high grade, any site C7A.1 (*following* C75)
> poorly differentiated, any site C7A.1 (*following* C75)

In the tabular rubric, C7A is included after rubric C75 and before C76.

> **Gout, chronic** (*see also* Gout, gouty) M1A.9 ✓ (*following* M08)
> drug-induced M1A.20 ✓ (*following* M08)
> ankle M1A.27- ✓ (*following* M08)
> elbow M1A.22- ✓ (*following* M08)

In the tabular rubric, M1A is included after rubric M08 and before M10.

2019 ICD-10-CM Official Guidelines for Coding and Reporting

Narrative changes appear in **bold** text

Items underlined have been moved within the guidelines since the FY 2018 version

Italics are used to indicate revisions to heading changes

The Centers for Medicare and Medicaid Services (CMS) and the National Center for Health Statistics (NCHS), two departments within the U.S. Federal Government's Department of Health and Human Services (DHHS) provide the following guidelines for coding and reporting using the International Classification of Diseases, 10th Revision, Clinical Modification (ICD-10-CM). These guidelines should be used as a companion document to the official version of the ICD-10-CM as published on the NCHS website. The ICD-10-CM is a morbidity classification published by the United States for classifying diagnoses and reason for visits in all health care settings. The ICD-10-CM is based on the ICD-10, the statistical classification of disease published by the World Health Organization (WHO).

These guidelines have been approved by the four organizations that make up the Cooperating Parties for the ICD-10-CM: the American Hospital Association (AHA), the American Health Information Management Association (AHIMA), CMS, and NCHS.

These guidelines are a set of rules that have been developed to accompany and complement the official conventions and instructions provided within the ICD-10-CM itself. The instructions and conventions of the classification take precedence over guidelines. These guidelines are based on the coding and sequencing instructions in the Tabular List and Alphabetic Index of ICD-10-CM, but provide additional instruction. Adherence to these guidelines when assigning ICD-10-CM diagnosis codes is required under the Health Insurance Portability and Accountability Act (HIPAA). The diagnosis codes (Tabular List and Alphabetic Index) have been adopted under HIPAA for all healthcare settings. A joint effort between the healthcare provider and the coder is essential to achieve complete and accurate documentation, code assignment, and reporting of diagnoses and procedures. These guidelines have been developed to assist both the healthcare provider and the coder in identifying those diagnoses that are to be reported. The importance of consistent, complete documentation in the medical record cannot be overemphasized. Without such documentation accurate coding cannot be achieved. The entire record should be reviewed to determine the specific reason for the encounter and the conditions treated.

The term encounter is used for all settings, including hospital admissions. In the context of these guidelines, the term provider is used throughout the guidelines to mean physician or any qualified health care practitioner who is legally accountable for establishing the patient's diagnosis. Only this set of guidelines, approved by the Cooperating Parties, is official.

The guidelines are organized into sections. Section I includes the structure and conventions of the classification and general guidelines that apply to the entire classification, and chapter-specific guidelines that correspond to the chapters as they are arranged in the classification. Section II includes guidelines for selection of principal diagnosis for non-outpatient settings. Section III includes guidelines for reporting additional diagnoses in non-outpatient settings. Section IV is for outpatient coding and reporting. It is necessary to review all sections of the guidelines to fully understand all of the rules and instructions needed to code properly.

Section I. Conventions, general coding guidelines and chapter specific guidelines

The conventions, general guidelines and chapter-specific guidelines are applicable to all health care settings unless otherwise indicated. The conventions and instructions of the classification take precedence over guidelines.

A. Conventions for the ICD-10-CM

The conventions for the ICD-10-CM are the general rules for use of the classification independent of the guidelines. These conventions are incorporated within the Alphabetic Index and Tabular List of the ICD-10-CM as instructional notes.

1. The Alphabetic Index and Tabular List

The ICD-10-CM is divided into the Alphabetic Index, an alphabetical list of terms and their corresponding code, and the Tabular List, a structured list of codes divided into chapters based on body system or condition. The Alphabetic Index consists of the following parts: the Index of Diseases and Injury, the Index of External Causes of Injury, the Table of Neoplasms and the Table of Drugs and Chemicals.

See Section I.C2. General guidelines

See Section I.C.19. Adverse effects, poisoning, underdosing and toxic effects

2. Format and Structure:

The ICD-10-CM Tabular List contains categories, subcategories and codes. Characters for categories, subcategories and codes may be either a letter or a number. All categories are 3 characters. A three-character category that has no further subdivision is equivalent to a code. Subcategories are either 4 or 5 characters. Codes may be 3, 4, 5, 6 or 7 characters. That is, each level of subdivision after a category is a subcategory. The final level of subdivision is a code. Codes that have applicable 7th characters are still referred to as codes, not subcategories. A code that has an applicable 7th character is considered invalid without the 7th character.

The ICD-10-CM uses an indented format for ease in reference.

3. Use of codes for reporting purposes

For reporting purposes only codes are permissible, not categories or subcategories, and any applicable 7th character is required.

4. Placeholder character

The ICD-10-CM utilizes a placeholder character "X". The "X" is used as a placeholder at certain codes to allow for future expansion. An example of this is at the poisoning, adverse effect and underdosing codes, categories T36-T50.

Where a placeholder exists, the X must be used in order for the code to be considered a valid code.

5. 7th Characters

Certain ICD-10-CM categories have applicable 7th characters. The applicable 7th character is required for all codes within the category, or as the notes in the Tabular List instruct. The 7th character must always be the 7th character in the data field. If a code that requires a 7th character is not 6 characters, a placeholder X must be used to fill in the empty characters.

6. Abbreviations

a. Alphabetic Index abbreviations

NEC "Not elsewhere classifiable"

This abbreviation in the Alphabetic Index represents "other specified." When a specific code is not available for a condition, the Alphabetic Index directs the coder to the "other specified" code in the Tabular List.

NOS "Not otherwise specified"

This abbreviation is the equivalent of unspecified.

b. Tabular List abbreviations

NEC "Not elsewhere classifiable"

This abbreviation in the Tabular List represents "other specified". When a specific code is not available for a condition, the Tabular List includes an NEC entry under a code to identify the code as the "other specified" code.

NOS "Not otherwise specified"

This abbreviation is the equivalent of unspecified.

7. Punctuation

[ ] Brackets are used in the Tabular List to enclose synonyms, alternative wording or explanatory phrases. Brackets are used in the Alphabetic Index to identify manifestation codes.

( ) Parentheses are used in both the Alphabetic Index and Tabular List to enclose supplementary words that may be present or absent in the statement of a disease or procedure without affecting the code number to which it is assigned. The terms within the parentheses are referred to as nonessential modifiers. The nonessential modifiers in the Alphabetic Index to Diseases apply to subterms following a main term except when a nonessential modifier and a subentry are mutually exclusive, the subentry takes precedence. For example, in the ICD-10-CM Alphabetic Index under the main term Enteritis, "acute" is a nonessential modifier and "chronic" is a subentry. In this case, the nonessential modifier "acute" does not apply to the subentry "chronic".

: Colons are used in the Tabular List after an incomplete term which needs one or more of the modifiers following the colon to make it assignable to a given category.

8. Use of "and"

See Section I.A.14. Use of the term "And"

9. Other and Unspecified codes

a. "Other" codes

Codes titled "other" or "other specified" are for use when the information in the medical record provides detail for which a specific code does not exist. Alphabetic Index entries with NEC in the line designate "other" codes in the Tabular List. These Alphabetic Index entries represent specific disease entities for which no specific code exists so the term is included within an "other" code.

b. "Unspecified" codes

Codes titled "unspecified" are for use when the information in the medical record is insufficient to assign a more specific code. For those categories for which an unspecified code is not provided, the "other specified" code may represent both other and unspecified.

See Section I.B.18 Use of Signs/Symptom/Unspecified Codes

10. Includes Notes

This note appears immediately under a three character code title to further define, or give examples of, the content of the category.

11. Inclusion terms

List of terms is included under some codes. These terms are the conditions for which that code is to be used. The terms may be synonyms of the code title, or, in the case of "other specified" codes, the terms are a list of the various conditions assigned to that code. The inclusion terms are not necessarily exhaustive. Additional terms found only in the Alphabetic Index may also be assigned to a code.

12. Excludes Notes

The ICD-10-CM has two types of excludes notes. Each type of note has a different definition for use but they are all similar in that they indicate that codes excluded from each other are independent of each other.

a. Excludes1

A type 1 Excludes note is a pure excludes note. It means "NOT CODED HERE!" An Excludes1 note indicates that the code excluded should never be used at the same time as the code above the Excludes1 note. An Excludes1 is used when two conditions cannot occur together, such as a congenital form versus an acquired form of the same condition.

An exception to the Excludes1 definition is the circumstance when the two conditions are unrelated to each other. If it is not clear whether the two conditions involving an Excludes1 note are related or not, query the provider. For example, code F45.8, Other somatoform disorders, has an Excludes1 note for "sleep related teeth grinding (G47.63)," because "teeth grinding" is an inclusion term under F45.8. Only one of these two codes should be assigned for teeth grinding. However psychogenic dysmenorrhea is also an inclusion term under F45.8, and a patient could have both this condition and sleep related teeth grinding. In this case, the two conditions are clearly unrelated to each other, and so it would be appropriate to report F45.8 and G47.63 together.

b. Excludes2

A type 2 Excludes note represents "Not included here." An excludes2 note indicates that the condition excluded is not part of the condition represented by the code, but a patient may have both conditions at the same time. When an Excludes2 note appears under a code, it is acceptable to use both the code and the excluded code together, when appropriate.

13. Etiology/manifestation convention ("code first", "use additional code" and "in diseases classified elsewhere" notes)

Certain conditions have both an underlying etiology and multiple body system manifestations due to the underlying etiology. For such conditions, the ICD-10-CM has a coding convention that requires the underlying condition be sequenced first, if applicable, followed by the manifestation. Wherever such a combination exists, there is a "use additional code" note at the etiology code, and a "code first" note at the manifestation code. These instructional notes indicate the proper sequencing order of the codes, etiology followed by manifestation.

In most cases the manifestation codes will have in the code title, "in diseases classified elsewhere." Codes with this title are a component of the etiology/ manifestation convention. The code title indicates that it is a manifestation code. "In diseases classified elsewhere" codes are never permitted to be used as first-listed or principal diagnosis codes. They must be used in conjunction with an underlying condition code and they must be listed following the underlying condition. See category F02, Dementia in other diseases classified elsewhere, for an example of this convention.

There are manifestation codes that do not have "in diseases classified elsewhere" in the title. For such codes, there is a "use additional code" note at the etiology code and a "code first" note at the manifestation code, and the rules for sequencing apply.

In addition to the notes in the Tabular List, these conditions also have a specific Alphabetic Index entry structure. In the Alphabetic Index both conditions are listed together with the etiology code first followed by the manifestation codes in brackets. The code in brackets is always to be sequenced second.

An example of the etiology/manifestation convention is dementia in Parkinson's disease. In the Alphabetic Index, code G20 is listed first, followed by code F02.80 or F02.81 in brackets. Code G20 represents the underlying etiology, Parkinson's disease, and must be sequenced first, whereas code F02.80 and F02.81 represent the manifestation of dementia in diseases classified elsewhere, with or without behavioral disturbance.

"Code first" and "Use additional code" notes are also used as sequencing rules in the classification for certain codes that are not part of an etiology/ manifestation combination.

See Section I.B.7. Multiple coding for a single condition.

14. "And"

The word "and" should be interpreted to mean either "and" or "or" when it appears in a title.

For example, cases of "tuberculosis of bones", "tuberculosis of joints" and "tuberculosis of bones and joints" are classified to subcategory A18.0, Tuberculosis of bones and joints.

15. "With"

The word "with" or "in" should be interpreted to mean "associated with" or "due to" when it appears in a code title, the Alphabetic Index **(either under a main term or subterm),** or an instructional note in the Tabular List. The classification presumes a causal relationship between the two conditions linked by these terms in the Alphabetic Index or Tabular List. These conditions should be coded as related even in the absence of provider documentation explicitly linking them, unless the documentation clearly states the conditions are unrelated or when another guideline exists that specifically requires a documented linkage between two conditions (e.g., sepsis guideline for "acute organ dysfunction that is not clearly associated with the sepsis").

For conditions not specifically linked by these relational terms in the classification or when a guideline requires that a linkage between two conditions be explicitly documented, provider documentation must link the conditions in order to code them as related.

The word "with" in the Alphabetic Index is sequenced immediately following the main term, not in alphabetical order.

16. "See" and "See Also"

The "see" instruction following a main term in the Alphabetic Index indicates that another term should be referenced. It is necessary to go to the main term referenced with the "see" note to locate the correct code.

A "see also" instruction following a main term in the Alphabetic Index instructs that there is another main term that may also be referenced that may provide additional Alphabetic Index entries that may be useful. It is not necessary to follow the "see also" note when the original main term provides the necessary code.

17. "Code also" note

A "code also" note instructs that two codes may be required to fully describe a condition, but this note does not provide sequencing direction. The sequencing depends on the circumstances of the encounter.

18. Default codes

A code listed next to a main term in the ICD-10-CM Alphabetic Index is referred to as a default code. The default code represents that condition that is most commonly associated with the main term, or is the unspecified code for the condition. If a condition is documented in a medical record (for example, appendicitis) without any additional information, such as acute or chronic, the default code should be assigned.

19. Code assignment and Clinical Criteria

The assignment of a diagnosis code is based on the provider's diagnostic statement that the condition exists. The provider's statement that the patient has a particular condition is sufficient. Code assignment is not based on clinical criteria used by the provider to establish the diagnosis.

B. General Coding Guidelines

1. Locating a code in the ICD-10-CM

To select a code in the classification that corresponds to a diagnosis or reason for visit documented in a medical record, first locate the term in the Alphabetic Index, and then verify the code in the Tabular List. Read and be guided by instructional notations that appear in both the Alphabetic Index and the Tabular List.

It is essential to use both the Alphabetic Index and Tabular List when locating and assigning a code. The Alphabetic Index does not always provide the full code. Selection of the full code, including laterality and any applicable 7th character can only be done in the Tabular List. A dash (-) at the end of an Alphabetic Index entry indicates that additional characters are required. Even if a dash is not included at the Alphabetic Index entry, it is necessary to refer to the Tabular List to verify that no 7th character is required.

2. Level of Detail in Coding

Diagnosis codes are to be used and reported at their highest number of characters available.

ICD-10-CM diagnosis codes are composed of codes with 3, 4, 5, 6 or 7 characters. Codes with three characters are included in ICD-10-CM as the heading of a category of codes that may be further subdivided by the use of fourth and/or fifth characters and/or sixth characters, which provide greater detail.

A three-character code is to be used only if it is not further subdivided. A code is invalid if it has not been coded to the full number of characters required for that code, including the 7th character, if applicable.

3. Code or codes from A00.0 through T88.9, Z00-Z99.8

The appropriate code or codes from A00.0 through T88.9, Z00-Z99.8 must be used to identify diagnoses, symptoms, conditions, problems, complaints or other reason(s) for the encounter/visit.

4. Signs and symptoms

Codes that describe symptoms and signs, as opposed to diagnoses, are acceptable for reporting purposes when a related definitive diagnosis has not been established (confirmed) by the provider. Chapter 18 of ICD-10-CM, Symptoms, Signs, and Abnormal Clinical and Laboratory Findings, Not Elsewhere Classified (codes R00.0 - R99) contains many, but not all, codes for symptoms.

See Section I.B.18 Use of Signs/Symptom/Unspecified Codes

5. Conditions that are an integral part of a disease process

Signs and symptoms that are associated routinely with a disease process should not be assigned as additional codes, unless otherwise instructed by the classification.

6. Conditions that are not an integral part of a disease process

Additional signs and symptoms that may not be associated routinely with a disease process should be coded when present.

7. Multiple coding for a single condition

In addition to the etiology/manifestation convention that requires two codes to fully describe a single condition that affects multiple body systems, there are other single conditions that also require more than one code. "Use additional code" notes are found in the Tabular List at codes that are not part of an etiology/manifestation pair where a secondary code is useful to fully describe a condition. The sequencing rule is the same as the etiology/manifestation pair, "use additional code" indicates that a secondary code should be added, if known.

For example, for bacterial infections that are not included in chapter 1, a secondary code from category B95, Streptococcus, Staphylococcus, and Enterococcus, as the cause of diseases classified elsewhere, or B96, Other bacterial agents as the cause of diseases classified elsewhere, may be required to identify the bacterial organism causing the infection. A "use additional code" note will normally be found at the infectious disease code, indicating a need for the organism code to be added as a secondary code.

"Code first" notes are also under certain codes that are not specifically manifestation codes but may be due to an underlying cause. When there is a "code first" note and an underlying condition is present, the underlying condition should be sequenced first, if known.

"Code, if applicable, any causal condition first" notes indicate that this code may be assigned as a principal diagnosis when the causal condition is unknown or not applicable. If a causal condition is known, then the code for that condition should be sequenced as the principal or first-listed diagnosis.

Multiple codes may be needed for sequela, complication codes and obstetric codes to more fully describe a condition. See the specific guidelines for these conditions for further instruction.

8. Acute and Chronic Conditions

If the same condition is described as both acute (subacute) and chronic, and separate subentries exist in the Alphabetic Index at the same indentation level, code both and sequence the acute (subacute) code first.

9. Combination Code

A combination code is a single code used to classify:

> Two diagnoses, or
>
> A diagnosis with an associated secondary process (manifestation)
>
> A diagnosis with an associated complication

Combination codes are identified by referring to subterm entries in the Alphabetic Index and by reading the inclusion and exclusion notes in the Tabular List.

Assign only the combination code when that code fully identifies the diagnostic conditions involved or when the Alphabetic Index so directs. Multiple coding should not be used when the classification provides a combination code that clearly identifies all of the elements documented in the diagnosis. When the combination code lacks necessary specificity in describing the manifestation or complication, an additional code should be used as a secondary code.

10. Sequela (Late Effects)

A sequela is the residual effect (condition produced) after the acute phase of an illness or injury has terminated. There is no time limit on when a sequela code can be used. The residual may be apparent early, such as in cerebral infarction, or it may occur months or years later, such as that due to a previous injury. Examples of sequela include: scar formation resulting from a burn, deviated septum due to a nasal fracture, and infertility due to tubal occlusion from old tuberculosis. Coding of sequela generally requires two codes sequenced in the following order: the condition or nature of the sequela is sequenced first. The sequela code is sequenced second.

An exception to the above guidelines are those instances where the code for the sequela is followed by a manifestation code identified in the Tabular List and title, or the sequela code has been expanded (at the fourth, fifth or sixth character levels) to include the manifestation(s). The code for the acute phase of an illness or injury that led to the sequela is never used with a code for the late effect.

See Section I.C.9. Sequelae of cerebrovascular disease

See Section I.C.15. Sequelae of complication of pregnancy, childbirth and the puerperium

See Section I.C.19. Application of 7th characters for Chapter 19

11. Impending or Threatened Condition

Code any condition described at the time of discharge as "impending" or "threatened" as follows:

> If it did occur, code as confirmed diagnosis.

If it did not occur, reference the Alphabetic Index to determine if the condition has a subentry term for "impending" or "threatened" and also reference main term entries for "Impending" and for "Threatened."

If the subterms are listed, assign the given code.

If the subterms are not listed, code the existing underlying condition(s) and not the condition described as impending or threatened.

12. Reporting Same Diagnosis Code More than Once

Each unique ICD-10-CM diagnosis code may be reported only once for an encounter. This applies to bilateral conditions when there are no distinct codes identifying laterality or two different conditions classified to the same ICD-10-CM diagnosis code.

13. Laterality

Some ICD-10-CM codes indicate laterality, specifying whether the condition occurs on the left, right or is bilateral. If no bilateral code is provided and the condition is bilateral, assign separate codes for both the left and right side. If the side is not identified in the medical record, assign the code for the unspecified side.

When a patient has a bilateral condition and each side is treated during separate encounters, assign the "bilateral" code (as the condition still exists on both sides), including for the encounter to treat the first side. For the second encounter for treatment after one side has previously been treated and the condition no longer exists on that side, assign the appropriate unilateral code for the side where the condition still exists (e.g., cataract surgery performed on each eye in separate encounters). The bilateral code would not be assigned for the subsequent encounter, as the patient no longer has the condition in the previously-treated site. If the treatment on the first side did not completely resolve the condition, then the bilateral code would still be appropriate.

14. Documentation *by Clinicians Other than the Patient's Provider*

Code assignment is based on the documentation by patient's provider (i.e., physician or other qualified healthcare practitioner legally accountable for establishing the patient's diagnosis). There are a few exceptions, such as codes for the Body Mass Index (BMI), depth of non-pressure chronic ulcers, pressure ulcer stage, coma scale, and NIH stroke scale (NIHSS) codes, code assignment may be based on medical record documentation from clinicians who are not the patient's provider (i.e., physician or other qualified healthcare practitioner legally accountable for establishing the patient's diagnosis), since this information is typically documented by other clinicians involved in the care of the patient (e.g., a dietitian often documents the BMI, a nurse often documents the pressure ulcer stages, and an emergency medical technician often documents the coma scale). However, the associated diagnosis (such as overweight, obesity, acute stroke, or pressure ulcer) must be documented by the patient's provider. If there is conflicting medical record documentation, either from the same clinician or different clinicians, the patient's attending provider should be queried for clarification.

For social determinants of health, such as information found in categories Z55-Z65, Persons with potential health hazards related to socioeconomic and psychosocial circumstances, code assignment may be based on medical record documentation from clinicians involved in the care of the patient who are not the patient's provider since this information represents social information, rather than medical diagnoses.

The BMI, coma scale, NIHSS codes **and categories Z55-Z65** should only be reported as secondary diagnoses.

15. Syndromes

Follow the Alphabetic Index guidance when coding syndromes. In the absence of Alphabetic Index guidance, assign codes for the documented manifestations of the syndrome. Additional codes for manifestations that are not an integral part of the disease process may also be assigned when the condition does not have a unique code.

16. Documentation of Complications of Care

Code assignment is based on the provider's documentation of the relationship between the condition and the care or procedure, unless otherwise instructed by the classification. The guideline extends to any complications of care, regardless of the chapter the code is located in. It is important to note that not all conditions that occur during or following medical care or surgery are classified as complications. There must be a cause-and-effect relationship between the care provided and the condition, and an indication in the documentation that it is a complication. Query the provider for clarification, if the complication is not clearly documented.

17. **Borderline Diagnosis**

If the provider documents a "borderline" diagnosis at the time of discharge, the diagnosis is coded as confirmed, unless the classification provides a specific entry (e.g., borderline diabetes). If a borderline condition has a specific index entry in ICD-10-CM, it should be coded as such. Since borderline conditions are not uncertain diagnoses, no distinction is made between the care setting (inpatient versus outpatient). Whenever the documentation is unclear regarding a borderline condition, coders are encouraged to query for clarification.

18. **Use of Sign/Symptom/Unspecified Codes**

Sign/symptom and "unspecified" codes have acceptable, even necessary, uses. While specific diagnosis codes should be reported when they are supported by the available medical record documentation and clinical knowledge of the patient's health condition, there are instances when signs/symptoms or unspecified codes are the best choices for accurately reflecting the healthcare encounter. Each healthcare encounter should be coded to the level of certainty known for that encounter.

If a definitive diagnosis has not been established by the end of the encounter, it is appropriate to report codes for sign(s) and/or symptom(s) in lieu of a definitive diagnosis. When sufficient clinical information isn't known or available about a particular health condition to assign a more specific code, it is acceptable to report the appropriate "unspecified" code (e.g., a diagnosis of pneumonia has been determined, but not the specific type). Unspecified codes should be reported when they are the codes that most accurately reflect what is known about the patient's condition at the time of that particular encounter. It would be inappropriate to select a specific code that is not supported by the medical record documentation or conduct medically unnecessary diagnostic testing in order to determine a more specific code.

19. **Coding for Healthcare Encounters in Hurricane Aftermath**

a. **Use of External Cause of Morbidity Codes**

An external cause of morbidity code should be assigned to identify the cause of the injury(ies) incurred as a result of the hurricane. The use of external cause of morbidity codes is supplemental to the application of ICD-10-CM codes. External cause of morbidity codes are never to be recorded as a principal diagnosis (first-listed in non-inpatient settings). The appropriate injury code should be sequenced before any external cause codes. The external cause of morbidity codes capture how the injury or health condition happened (cause), the intent (unintentional or accidental; or intentional, such as suicide or assault), the place where the event occurred, the activity of the patient at the time of the event, and the person's status (e.g., civilian, military). They should not be assigned for encounters to treat hurricane victims' medical conditions when no injury, adverse effect or poisoning is involved. External cause of morbidity codes should be assigned for each encounter for care and treatment of the injury. External cause of morbidity codes may be assigned in all health care settings. For the purpose of capturing complete and accurate ICD-10-CM data in the aftermath of the hurricane, a healthcare setting should be considered as any location where medical care is provided by licensed healthcare professionals.

b. **Sequencing of External Causes of Morbidity Codes**

Codes for cataclysmic events, such as a hurricane, take priority over all other external cause codes except child and adult abuse and terrorism and should be sequenced before other external cause of injury codes. Assign as many external cause of morbidity codes as necessary to fully explain each cause. For example, if an injury occurs as a result of a building collapse during the hurricane, external cause codes for both the hurricane and the building collapse should be assigned, with the external causes code for hurricane being sequenced as the first external cause code. For injuries incurred as a direct result of the hurricane, assign the appropriate code(s) for the injuries, followed by the code X37.0-, Hurricane (with the appropriate 7th character), and any other applicable external cause of injury codes. Code X37.0- also should be assigned when an injury is incurred as a result of flooding caused by a levee breaking related to the hurricane. Code X38.-, Flood (with the appropriate 7th character), should be assigned when an injury is from flooding resulting directly from the storm. Code X36.0.-, Collapse of dam or man-made structure, should not be assigned when the cause of the collapse is due to the hurricane. Use of code X36.0- is limited to collapses of man-made structures due to earth surface movements, not due to storm surges directly from a hurricane.

c. **Other External Causes of Morbidity Code Issues**

For injuries that are not a direct result of the hurricane, such as an evacuee that has incurred an injury as a result of a motor vehicle accident, assign the appropriate external cause of morbidity code(s) to describe the cause of the injury, but do not assign code X37.0-, Hurricane. If it is not clear whether the injury was a direct result of the hurricane, assume the injury is due to the hurricane and assign code X37.0-, Hurricane, as well as any other applicable external cause of morbidity codes. In addition to code X37.0-, Hurricane, other possible applicable external cause of morbidity codes include:

W54.0-, Bitten by dog

X30-, Exposure to excessive natural heat

X31-, Exposure to excessive natural cold

X38-, Flood

d. **Use of Z codes**

Z codes (other reasons for healthcare encounters) may be assigned as appropriate to further explain the reasons for presenting for healthcare services, including transfers between healthcare facilities. The ICD-10-CM Official Guidelines for Coding and Reporting identify which codes maybe assigned as principal or first-listed diagnosis only, secondary diagnosis only, or principal/first-listed or secondary (depending on the circumstances). Possible applicable Z codes include:

Z59.0, Homelessness

Z59.1, Inadequate housing

Z59.5, Extreme poverty

Z75.1, Person awaiting admission to adequate facility elsewhere

Z75.3, Unavailability and inaccessibility of health-care facilities

Z75.4, Unavailability and inaccessibility of other helping agencies

Z76.2, Encounter for health supervision and care of other healthy infant and child

Z99.12, Encounter for respirator [ventilator] dependence during power failure

The external cause of morbidity codes and the Z codes listed above are not an all-inclusive list. Other codes may be applicable to the encounter based upon the documentation. Assign as many codes as necessary to fully explain each healthcare encounter. Since patient history information may be very limited, use any available documentation to assign the appropriate external cause of morbidity and Z codes.

C. Chapter-Specific Coding Guidelines

In addition to general coding guidelines, there are guidelines for specific diagnoses and/or conditions in the classification. Unless otherwise indicated, these guidelines apply to all health care settings. Please refer to Section II for guidelines on the selection of principal diagnosis.

1. **Chapter 1: Certain Infectious and Parasitic Diseases (A00-B99)**

a. **Human Immunodeficiency Virus (HIV) Infections**

1) **Code only confirmed cases**

Code only confirmed cases of HIV infection/illness. This is an exception to the hospital inpatient guideline Section II, H.

In this context, "confirmation" does not require documentation of positive serology or culture for HIV; the provider's diagnostic statement that the patient is HIV positive, or has an HIV-related illness is sufficient.

2) **Selection and sequencing of HIV codes**

(a) **Patient admitted for HIV-related condition**

If a patient is admitted for an HIV-related condition, the principal diagnosis should be B20, Human immunodeficiency virus [HIV] disease followed by additional diagnosis codes for all reported HIV-related conditions.

(b) **Patient with HIV disease admitted for unrelated condition**

If a patient with HIV disease is admitted for an unrelated condition (such as a traumatic injury), the code for the unrelated condition (e.g., the nature of injury code) should be the principal diagnosis. Other diagnoses would be B20 followed by additional diagnosis codes for all reported HIV-related conditions.

(c) Whether the patient is newly diagnosed
Whether the patient is newly diagnosed or has had previous admissions/encounters for HIV conditions is irrelevant to the sequencing decision.

(d) Asymptomatic human immunodeficiency virus
Z21, Asymptomatic human immunodeficiency virus [HIV] infection status, is to be applied when the patient without any documentation of symptoms is listed as being "HIV positive," "known HIV," "HIV test positive," or similar terminology. Do not use this code if the term "AIDS" is used or if the patient is treated for any HIV-related illness or is described as having any condition(s) resulting from his/her HIV positive status; use B20 in these cases.

(e) Patients with inconclusive HIV serology
Patients with inconclusive HIV serology, but no definitive diagnosis or manifestations of the illness, may be assigned code R75, Inconclusive laboratory evidence of human immunodeficiency virus [HIV].

(f) Previously diagnosed HIV-related illness
Patients with any known prior diagnosis of an HIV-related illness should be coded to B20. Once a patient has developed an HIV-related illness, the patient should always be assigned code B20 on every subsequent admission/encounter. Patients previously diagnosed with any HIV illness (B20) should never be assigned to R75 or Z21, Asymptomatic human immunodeficiency virus [HIV] infection status.

(g) HIV Infection in Pregnancy, Childbirth and the Puerperium
During pregnancy, childbirth or the puerperium, a patient admitted (or presenting for a health care encounter) because of an HIV-related illness should receive a principal diagnosis code of O98.7-, Human immunodeficiency [HIV] disease complicating pregnancy, childbirth and the puerperium, followed by B20 and the code(s) for the HIV-related illness(es). Codes from Chapter 15 always take sequencing priority.

Patients with asymptomatic HIV infection status admitted (or presenting for a health care encounter) during pregnancy, childbirth, or the puerperium should receive codes of O98.7- and Z21.

(h) Encounters for testing for HIV
If a patient is being seen to determine his/her HIV status, use code Z11.4, Encounter for screening for human immunodeficiency virus [HIV]. Use additional codes for any associated high risk behavior.

If a patient with signs or symptoms is being seen for HIV testing, code the signs and symptoms. An additional counseling code Z71.7, Human immunodeficiency virus [HIV] counseling, may be used if counseling is provided during the encounter for the test.

When a patient returns to be informed of his/her HIV test results and the test result is negative, use code Z71.7, Human immunodeficiency virus [HIV] counseling.

If the results are positive, see previous guidelines and assign codes as appropriate.

b. Infectious agents as the cause of diseases classified to other chapters
Certain infections are classified in chapters other than Chapter 1 and no organism is identified as part of the infection code. In these instances, it is necessary to use an additional code from Chapter 1 to identify the organism. A code from category B95, Streptococcus, Staphylococcus, and Enterococcus as the cause of diseases classified to other chapters, B96, Other bacterial agents as the cause of diseases classified to other chapters, or B97, Viral agents as the cause of diseases classified to other chapters, is to be used as an additional code to identify the organism. An instructional note will be found at the infection code advising that an additional organism code is required.

c. Infections resistant to antibiotics
Many bacterial infections are resistant to current antibiotics. It is necessary to identify all infections documented as antibiotic resistant. Assign a code from category Z16, Resistance to antimicrobial drugs, following the infection code only if the infection code does not identify drug resistance.

d. Sepsis, Severe Sepsis, and Septic Shock
1) Coding of Sepsis and Severe Sepsis
(a) Sepsis
For a diagnosis of sepsis, assign the appropriate code for the underlying systemic infection. If the type of infection or causal organism is not further specified, assign code A41.9, Sepsis, unspecified organism.

A code from subcategory R65.2, Severe sepsis, should not be assigned unless severe sepsis or an associated acute organ dysfunction is documented.

(i) Negative or inconclusive blood cultures and sepsis
Negative or inconclusive blood cultures do not preclude a diagnosis of sepsis in patients with clinical evidence of the condition; however, the provider should be queried.

(ii) Urosepsis
The term urosepsis is a nonspecific term. It is not to be considered synonymous with sepsis. It has no default code in the Alphabetic Index. Should a provider use this term, he/she must be queried for clarification.

(iii) Sepsis with organ dysfunction
If a patient has sepsis and associated acute organ dysfunction or multiple organ dysfunction (MOD), follow the instructions for coding severe sepsis.

(iv) Acute organ dysfunction that is not clearly associated with the sepsis
If a patient has sepsis and an acute organ dysfunction, but the medical record documentation indicates that the acute organ dysfunction is related to a medical condition other than the sepsis, do not assign a code from subcategory R65.2, Severe sepsis. An acute organ dysfunction must be associated with the sepsis in order to assign the severe sepsis code. If the documentation is not clear as to whether an acute organ dysfunction is related to the sepsis or another medical condition, query the provider.

(b) Severe sepsis
The coding of severe sepsis requires a minimum of 2 codes: first a code for the underlying systemic infection, followed by a code from subcategory R65.2, Severe sepsis. If the causal organism is not documented, assign code A41.9, Sepsis, unspecified organism, for the infection. Additional code(s) for the associated acute organ dysfunction are also required.

Due to the complex nature of severe sepsis, some cases may require querying the provider prior to assignment of the codes.

2) Septic shock
(a) Septic shock generally refers to circulatory failure associated with severe sepsis, and therefore, it represents a type of acute organ dysfunction.
For cases of septic shock, the code for the systemic infection should be sequenced first, followed by code R65.21, Severe sepsis with septic shock or code T81.12, Postprocedural septic shock. Any additional codes for the other acute organ dysfunctions should also be assigned. As noted in the sequencing instructions in the Tabular List, the code for septic shock cannot be assigned as a principal diagnosis.

3) Sequencing of severe sepsis
If severe sepsis is present on admission, and meets the definition of principal diagnosis, the underlying systemic infection should be assigned as principal diagnosis followed by the appropriate code from subcategory R65.2 as required by the sequencing rules in the Tabular List. A code from subcategory R65.2 can never be assigned as a principal diagnosis.

When severe sepsis develops during an encounter (it was not present on admission), the underlying systemic infection and the appropriate code from subcategory R65.2 should be assigned as secondary diagnoses.

Severe sepsis may be present on admission, but the diagnosis may not be confirmed until sometime after admission. If the documentation is not clear whether severe sepsis was present on admission, the provider should be queried.

4) Sepsis and severe sepsis with a localized infection
If the reason for admission is both sepsis or severe sepsis and a localized infection, such as pneumonia or cellulitis, a code(s) for the underlying systemic infection should be assigned first and the

code for the localized infection should be assigned as a secondary diagnosis. If the patient has severe sepsis, a code from subcategory R65.2 should also be assigned as a secondary diagnosis. If the patient is admitted with a localized infection, such as pneumonia, and sepsis/severe sepsis doesn't develop until after admission, the localized infection should be assigned first, followed by the appropriate sepsis/severe sepsis codes.

5) **Sepsis due to a postprocedural infection**

(a) **Documentation of causal relationship**
As with all postprocedural complications, code assignment is based on the provider's documentation of the relationship between the infection and the procedure.

(b) **Sepsis due to a postprocedural infection**
For i**nfections following a procedure, a code from** T81.**40, to T81.43** Infection following a procedure, or **a code from** O86.**00 to O86.03,** Infection of obstetric surgical wound, **that identifies the site of the infection** should be coded first, **if known. Assign an additional code for sepsis following a procedure (T81.44) or sepsis following an obstetrical procedure (O86.04). Use an additional code to identify the infectious agent.** If the patient has severe sepsis, the appropriate code from subcategory R65.2 should also be assigned with the additional code(s) for any acute organ dysfunction.

For infections following infusion, transfusion, therapeutic injection, or immunization, a code from subcategory T80.2, Infections following infusion, transfusion, and therapeutic injection, or code T88.0-, Infection following immunization, should be coded first, followed by the code for the specific infection. If the patient has severe sepsis, the appropriate code from subcategory R65.2 should also be assigned, with the additional codes(s) for any acute organ dysfunction.

(c) **Postprocedural infection and postprocedural septic shock**
If a postprocedural infection has resulted in postprocedural septic shock, **assign the codes indicated above for sepsis due to a postprocedural infection, followed by code T81.12-, Postprocedural septic shock. Do not assign code R65.21, Severe sepsis with septic shock. Additional code(s) should be assigned for any acute organ dysfunction.**

6) **Sepsis and severe sepsis associated with a noninfectious process (condition)**
In some cases a noninfectious process (condition), such as trauma, may lead to an infection which can result in sepsis or severe sepsis. If sepsis or severe sepsis is documented as associated with a noninfectious condition, such as a burn or serious injury, and this condition meets the definition for principal diagnosis, the code for the noninfectious condition should be sequenced first, followed by the code for the resulting infection. If severe sepsis is present, a code from subcategory R65.2 should also be assigned with any associated organ dysfunction(s) codes. It is not necessary to assign a code from subcategory R65.1, Systemic inflammatory response syndrome (SIRS) of non-infectious origin, for these cases.

If the infection meets the definition of principal diagnosis, it should be sequenced before the non-infectious condition. When both the associated non-infectious condition and the infection meet the definition of principal diagnosis, either may be assigned as principal diagnosis.

Only one code from category R65, Symptoms and signs specifically associated with systemic inflammation and infection, should be assigned. Therefore, when a non-infectious condition leads to an infection resulting in severe sepsis, assign the appropriate code from subcategory R65.2, Severe sepsis. Do not additionally assign a code from subcategory R65.1, Systemic inflammatory response syndrome (SIRS) of non-infectious origin.

See Section I.C.18. SIRS due to non-infectious process

7) **Sepsis and septic shock complicating abortion, pregnancy, childbirth, and the puerperium**
See Section I.C.15. Sepsis and septic shock complicating abortion, pregnancy, childbirth and the puerperium

8) **Newborn sepsis**
See Section I.C.16. f. Bacterial sepsis of Newborn

e. **Methicillin Resistant Staphylococcus aureus (MRSA) Conditions**
1) **Selection and sequencing of MRSA codes**
(a) **Combination codes for MRSA infection**
When a patient is diagnosed with an infection that is due to methicillin resistant *Staphylococcus aureus* (MRSA), and that infection has a combination code that includes the causal organism (e.g., sepsis, pneumonia) assign the appropriate combination code for the condition (e.g., code A41.02, Sepsis due to Methicillin resistant Staphylococcus aureus or code J15.212, Pneumonia due to Methicillin resistant Staphylococcus aureus). Do not assign code B95.62, Methicillin resistant Staphylococcus aureus infection as the cause of diseases classified elsewhere, as an additional code, because the combination code includes the type of infection and the MRSA organism. Do not assign a code from subcategory Z16.11, Resistance to penicillins, as an additional diagnosis.
See Section C.1. for instructions on coding and sequencing of sepsis and severe sepsis.

(b) **Other codes for MRSA infection**
When there is documentation of a current infection (e.g., wound infection, stitch abscess, urinary tract infection) due to MRSA, and that infection does not have a combination code that includes the causal organism, assign the appropriate code to identify the condition along with code B95.62, Methicillin resistant Staphylococcus aureus infection as the cause of diseases classified elsewhere for the MRSA infection. Do not assign a code from subcategory Z16.11, Resistance to penicillins.

(c) **Methicillin susceptible Staphylococcus aureus (MSSA) and MRSA colonization**
The condition or state of being colonized or carrying MSSA or MRSA is called colonization or carriage, while an individual person is described as being colonized or being a carrier. Colonization means that MSSA or MSRA is present on or in the body without necessarily causing illness. A positive MRSA colonization test might be documented by the provider as "MRSA screen positive" or "MRSA nasal swab positive".
Assign code Z22.322, Carrier or suspected carrier of Methicillin resistant Staphylococcus aureus, for patients documented as having MRSA colonization. Assign code Z22.321, Carrier or suspected carrier of Methicillin susceptible Staphylococcus aureus, for patient documented as having MSSA colonization. Colonization is not necessarily indicative of a disease process or as the cause of a specific condition the patient may have unless documented as such by the provider.

(d) **MRSA colonization and infection**
If a patient is documented as having both MRSA colonization and infection during a hospital admission, code Z22.322, Carrier or suspected carrier of Methicillin resistant Staphylococcus aureus, and a code for the MRSA infection may both be assigned.

f. **Zika virus infections**
1) **Code only confirmed cases**
Code only a confirmed diagnosis of Zika virus (A92.5, Zika virus disease) as documented by the provider. This is an exception to the hospital inpatient guideline Section II, H. In this context, "confirmation" does not require documentation of the type of test performed; the physician's diagnostic statement that the condition is confirmed is sufficient. This code should be assigned regardless of the stated mode of transmission.

If the provider documents "suspected", "possible" or "probable" Zika, do not assign code A92.5. Assign a code(s) explaining the reason for encounter (such as fever, rash, or joint pain) or Z20.**821**, Contact with and (suspected) exposure to **Zika virus**.

2. **Chapter 2: Neoplasms (C00-D49)**
General guidelines
Chapter 2 of the ICD-10-CM contains the codes for most benign and all malignant neoplasms. Certain benign neoplasms, such as prostatic adenomas, may be found in the specific body system chapters. To properly code a neoplasm it is necessary to determine from the record if the neoplasm is benign, in-situ, malignant, or of uncertain histologic behavior. If malignant, any secondary (metastatic) sites should also be determined.

Primary malignant neoplasms overlapping site boundaries

A primary malignant neoplasm that overlaps two or more contiguous (next to each other) sites should be classified to the subcategory/code .8 ('overlapping lesion'), unless the combination is specifically indexed elsewhere. For multiple neoplasms of the same site that are not contiguous such as tumors in different quadrants of the same breast, codes for each site should be assigned.

Malignant neoplasm of ectopic tissue

Malignant neoplasms of ectopic tissue are to be coded to the site of origin mentioned, e.g., ectopic pancreatic malignant neoplasms involving the stomach are coded to malignant neoplasm of pancreas, unspecified (C25.9).

The neoplasm table in the Alphabetic Index should be referenced first. However, if the histological term is documented, that term should be referenced first, rather than going immediately to the Neoplasm Table, in order to determine which column in the Neoplasm Table is appropriate. For example, if the documentation indicates "adenoma," refer to the term in the Alphabetic Index to review the entries under this term and the instructional note to "see also neoplasm, by site, benign." The table provides the proper code based on the type of neoplasm and the site. It is important to select the proper column in the table that corresponds to the type of neoplasm. The Tabular List should then be referenced to verify that the correct code has been selected from the table and that a more specific site code does not exist.

See Section I.C.21. Factors influencing health status and contact with health services, Status, for information regarding Z15.0, codes for genetic susceptibility to cancer.

a. **Treatment directed at the malignancy**

If the treatment is directed at the malignancy, designate the malignancy as the principal diagnosis.

The only exception to this guideline is if a patient admission/encounter is solely for the administration of chemotherapy, immunotherapy or external beam radiation therapy, assign the appropriate Z51.-- code as the first-listed or principal diagnosis, and the diagnosis or problem for which the service is being performed as a secondary diagnosis.

b. **Treatment of secondary site**

When a patient is admitted because of a primary neoplasm with metastasis and treatment is directed toward the secondary site only, the secondary neoplasm is designated as the principal diagnosis even though the primary malignancy is still present.

c. **Coding and sequencing of complications**

Coding and sequencing of complications associated with the malignancies or with the therapy thereof are subject to the following guidelines:

1) **Anemia associated with malignancy**

When admission/encounter is for management of an anemia associated with the malignancy, and the treatment is only for anemia, the appropriate code for the malignancy is sequenced as the principal or first-listed diagnosis followed by the appropriate code for the anemia (such as code D63.0, Anemia in neoplastic disease**).**

2) **Anemia associated with chemotherapy, immunotherapy and radiation therapy**

When the admission/encounter is for management of an anemia associated with an adverse effect of the administration of chemotherapy or immunotherapy and the only treatment is for the anemia, the anemia code is sequenced first followed by the appropriate codes for the neoplasm and the adverse effect (T45.1X5-, Adverse effect of antineoplastic and immunosuppressive drugs).

When the admission/encounter is for management of an anemia associated with an adverse effect of radiotherapy, the anemia code should be sequenced first, followed by the appropriate neoplasm code and code Y84.2, Radiological procedure and radiotherapy as the cause of abnormal reaction of the patient, or of later complication, without mention of misadventure at the time of the procedure.

3) **Management of dehydration due to the malignancy**

When the admission/encounter is for management of dehydration due to the malignancy and only the dehydration is being treated (intravenous rehydration), the dehydration is sequenced first, followed by the code(s) for the malignancy.

4) **Treatment of a complication resulting from a surgical procedure**

When the admission/encounter is for treatment of a complication resulting from a surgical procedure, designate the complication as the principal or first-listed diagnosis if treatment is directed at resolving the complication.

d. **Primary malignancy previously excised**

When a primary malignancy has been previously excised or eradicated from its site and there is no further treatment directed to that site and there is no evidence of any existing primary malignancy **at that site**, a code from category Z85, Personal history of malignant neoplasm, should be used to indicate the former site of the malignancy. Any mention of extension, invasion, or metastasis to another site is coded as a secondary malignant neoplasm to that site. The secondary site may be the principal or first-listed with the Z85 code used as a secondary code.

e. **Admissions/Encounters involving chemotherapy, immunotherapy and radiation therapy**

1) **Episode of care involves surgical removal of neoplasm**

When an episode of care involves the surgical removal of a neoplasm, primary or secondary site, followed by adjunct chemotherapy or radiation treatment during the same episode of care, the code for the neoplasm should be assigned as principal or first-listed diagnosis**.**

2) **Patient admission/encounter solely for administration of chemotherapy, immunotherapy and radiation therapy**

If a patient admission/encounter is solely for the administration of chemotherapy, immunotherapy or external beam radiation therapy assign code Z51.0, Encounter for antineoplastic radiation therapy, or Z51.11, Encounter for antineoplastic chemotherapy, or Z51.12, Encounter for antineoplastic immunotherapy as the first-listed or principal diagnosis. If a patient receives more than one of these therapies during the same admission more than one of these codes may be assigned, in any sequence.

The malignancy for which the therapy is being administered should be assigned as a secondary diagnosis.

If a patient admission/encounter is for the insertion or implantation of radioactive elements (e.g., brachytherapy) the appropriate code for the malignancy is sequenced as the principal or first-listed diagnosis. Code Z51.0 should not be assigned.

3) **Patient admitted for radiation therapy, chemotherapy or immunotherapy and develops complications**

When a patient is admitted for the purpose of external beam radiotherapy, immunotherapy or chemotherapy and develops complications such as uncontrolled nausea and vomiting or dehydration, the principal or first-listed diagnosis is Z51.0, Encounter for antineoplastic radiation therapy, or Z51.11, Encounter for antineoplastic chemotherapy, or Z51.12, Encounter for antineoplastic immunotherapy followed by any codes for the complications.

When a patient is admitted for the purpose of insertion or implantation of radioactive elements (e.g., brachytherapy)and develops complications such as uncontrolled nausea and vomiting or dehydration, the principal or first-listed diagnosis is the appropriate code for the malignancy followed by any codes for the complications.

f. **Admission/encounter to determine extent of malignancy**

When the reason for admission/encounter is to determine the extent of the malignancy, or for a procedure such as paracentesis or thoracentesis, the primary malignancy or appropriate metastatic site is designated as the principal or first-listed diagnosis, even though chemotherapy or radiotherapy is administered.

g. **Symptoms, signs, and abnormal findings listed in Chapter 18 associated with neoplasms**

Symptoms, signs, and ill-defined conditions listed in Chapter 18 characteristic of, or associated with, an existing primary or secondary site malignancy cannot be used to replace the malignancy as principal or first-listed diagnosis, regardless of the number of admissions or encounters for treatment and care of the neoplasm.

See section I.C.21. Factors influencing health status and contact with health services, Encounter for prophylactic organ removal.

h. **Admission/encounter for pain control/management**

See Section I.C.6. for information on coding admission/encounter for pain control/management.

i. **Malignancy in two or more noncontiguous sites**
A patient may have more than one malignant tumor in the same organ. These tumors may represent different primaries or metastatic disease, depending on the site. Should the documentation be unclear, the provider should be queried as to the status of each tumor so that the correct codes can be assigned.

j. **Disseminated malignant neoplasm, unspecified**
Code C80.0, Disseminated malignant neoplasm, unspecified, is for use only in those cases where the patient has advanced metastatic disease and no known primary or secondary sites are specified. It should not be used in place of assigning codes for the primary site and all known secondary sites.

k. **Malignant neoplasm without specification of site**
Code C80.1, Malignant (primary) neoplasm, unspecified, equates to Cancer, unspecified. This code should only be used when no determination can be made as to the primary site of a malignancy. This code should rarely be used in the inpatient setting.

l. **Sequencing of neoplasm codes**
1) **Encounter for treatment of primary malignancy**
If the reason for the encounter is for treatment of a primary malignancy, assign the malignancy as the principal/first-listed diagnosis. The primary site is to be sequenced first, followed by any metastatic sites.

2) **Encounter for treatment of secondary malignancy**
When an encounter is for a primary malignancy with metastasis and treatment is directed toward the metastatic (secondary) site(s) only, the metastatic site(s) is designated as the principal/first-listed diagnosis. The primary malignancy is coded as an additional code.

3) **Malignant neoplasm in a pregnant patient**
When a pregnant woman has a malignant neoplasm, a code from subcategory O9A.1-, Malignant neoplasm complicating pregnancy, childbirth, and the puerperium, should be sequenced first, followed by the appropriate code from Chapter 2 to indicate the type of neoplasm.

4) **Encounter for complication associated with a neoplasm**
When an encounter is for management of a complication associated with a neoplasm, such as dehydration, and the treatment is only for the complication, the complication is coded first, followed by the appropriate code(s) for the neoplasm.

The exception to this guideline is anemia. When the admission/encounter is for management of an anemia associated with the malignancy, and the treatment is only for anemia, the appropriate code for the malignancy is sequenced as the principal or first-listed diagnosis followed by code D63.0, Anemia in neoplastic disease.

5) **Complication from surgical procedure for treatment of a neoplasm**
When an encounter is for treatment of a complication resulting from a surgical procedure performed for the treatment of the neoplasm, designate the complication as the principal/first-listed diagnosis. See guideline regarding the coding of a current malignancy versus personal history to determine if the code for the neoplasm should also be assigned.

6) **Pathologic fracture due to a neoplasm**
When an encounter is for a pathological fracture due to a neoplasm, and the focus of treatment is the fracture, a code from subcategory M84.5, Pathological fracture in neoplastic disease, should be sequenced first, followed by the code for the neoplasm.

If the focus of treatment is the neoplasm with an associated pathological fracture, the neoplasm code should be sequenced first, followed by a code from M84.5 for the pathological fracture.

m. **Current malignancy versus personal history of malignancy**
When a primary malignancy has been excised but further treatment, such as an additional surgery for the malignancy, radiation therapy or chemotherapy is directed to that site, the primary malignancy code should be used until treatment is completed.

When a primary malignancy has been previously excised or eradicated from its site, there is no further treatment (of the malignancy) directed to that site, and there is no evidence of any existing primary malignancy **at that site**, a code from category Z85, Personal history of malignant neoplasm, should be used to indicate the former site of the malignancy.

Subcategories Z85.0 – Z85.7 should only be assigned for the former site of a primary malignancy, not the site of a secondary malignancy. Codes from subcategory Z85.8-, may be assigned for the former site(s) of either a primary or secondary malignancy included in this subcategory.
See Section I.C.21. Factors influencing health status and contact with health services, History (of)

n. **Leukemia, Multiple Myeloma, and Malignant Plasma Cell Neoplasms in remission versus personal history**
The categories for leukemia, and category C90, Multiple myeloma and malignant plasma cell neoplasms, have codes indicating whether or not the leukemia has achieved remission. There are also codes Z85.6, Personal history of leukemia, and Z85.79, Personal history of other malignant neoplasms of lymphoid, hematopoietic and related tissues. If the documentation is unclear as to whether the leukemia has achieved remission, the provider should be queried.
See Section I.C.21. Factors influencing health status and contact with health services, History (of)

o. **Aftercare following surgery for neoplasm**
See Section I.C.21. Factors influencing health status and contact with health services, Aftercare

p. **Follow-up care for completed treatment of a malignancy**
See Section I.C.21. Factors influencing health status and contact with health services, Follow-up

q. **Prophylactic organ removal for prevention of malignancy**
See Section I.C. 21, Factors influencing health status and contact with health services, Prophylactic organ removal

r. **Malignant neoplasm associated with transplanted organ**
A malignant neoplasm of a transplanted organ should be coded as a transplant complication. Assign first the appropriate code from category T86.-, Complications of transplanted organs and tissue, followed by code C80.2, Malignant neoplasm associated with transplanted organ. Use an additional code for the specific malignancy.

3. **Chapter 3: Disease of the blood and blood-forming organs and certain disorders involving the immune mechanism (D50-D89)**
Reserved for future guideline expansion

4. **Chapter 4: Endocrine, Nutritional, and Metabolic Diseases (E00-E89)**
a. **Diabetes mellitus**
The diabetes mellitus codes are combination codes that include the type of diabetes mellitus, the body system affected, and the complications affecting that body system. As many codes within a particular category as are necessary to describe all of the complications of the disease may be used. They should be sequenced based on the reason for a particular encounter. Assign as many codes from categories E08 – E13 as needed to identify all of the associated conditions that the patient has.

1) **Type of diabetes**
The age of a patient is not the sole determining factor, though most type 1 diabetics develop the condition before reaching puberty. For this reason type 1 diabetes mellitus is also referred to as juvenile diabetes.

2) **Type of diabetes mellitus not documented**
If the type of diabetes mellitus is not documented in the medical record the default is E11.-, Type 2 diabetes mellitus.

3) **Diabetes mellitus and the use of insulin and oral hypoglycemics**
If the documentation in a medical record does not indicate the type of diabetes but does indicate that the patient uses insulin, code E11.-, Type 2 diabetes mellitus, should be assigned. An additional code should be assigned from category Z79 to identify the long-term (current) use of insulin or oral hypoglycemic drugs. If the patient is treated with both oral medications and insulin, only the code for long-term (current) use of insulin should be assigned. Code Z79.4 should not be assigned if insulin is given temporarily to bring a type 2 patient's blood sugar under control during an encounter.

4) **Diabetes mellitus in pregnancy and gestational diabetes**
See Section I.C.15. Diabetes mellitus in pregnancy.
See Section I.C.15. Gestational (pregnancy induced) diabetes

5) **Complications due to insulin pump malfunction**

(a) **Underdose of insulin due to insulin pump failure**
An underdose of insulin due to an insulin pump failure should be assigned to a code from subcategory T85.6, Mechanical complication of other specified internal and external prosthetic devices, implants and grafts, that specifies the type of pump malfunction, as the principal or first-listed code, followed by code T38.3X6-, Underdosing of insulin and oral hypoglycemic [antidiabetic] drugs. Additional codes for the type of diabetes mellitus and any associated complications due to the underdosing should also be assigned.

(b) **Overdose of insulin due to insulin pump failure**
The principal or first-listed code for an encounter due to an insulin pump malfunction resulting in an overdose of insulin, should also be T85.6-, Mechanical complication of other specified internal and external prosthetic devices, implants and grafts, followed by code T38.3X1-, Poisoning by insulin and oral hypoglycemic [antidiabetic] drugs, accidental (unintentional).

6) **Secondary diabetes mellitus**
Codes under categories E08, Diabetes mellitus due to underlying condition, E09, Drug or chemical induced diabetes mellitus, and E13, Other specified diabetes mellitus, identify complications/manifestations associated with secondary diabetes mellitus. Secondary diabetes is always caused by another condition or event (e.g., cystic fibrosis, malignant neoplasm of pancreas, pancreatectomy, adverse effect of drug, or poisoning).

(a) **Secondary diabetes mellitus and the use of insulin or oral hypoglycemic drugs**
For patients with secondary diabetes mellitus who routinely use insulin or oral hypoglycemic drugs, an additional code from category Z79 should be assigned to identify the long-term (current) use of insulin or oral hypoglycemic drugs. If the patient is treated with both oral medications and insulin, only the code for long-term (current) use of insulin should be assigned. Code Z79.4 should not be assigned if insulin is given temporarily to bring a secondary diabetic patient's blood sugar under control during an encounter.

(b) **Assigning and sequencing secondary diabetes codes and its causes**
The sequencing of the secondary diabetes codes in relationship to codes for the cause of the diabetes is based on the Tabular List instructions for categories E08, E09 and E13.

(i) **Secondary diabetes mellitus due to pancreatectomy**
For postpancreatectomy diabetes mellitus (lack of insulin due to the surgical removal of all or part of the pancreas), assign code E89.1, Postprocedural hypoinsulinemia. Assign a code from category E13 and a code from subcategory Z90.41, Acquired absence of pancreas, as additional codes.

(ii) **Secondary diabetes due to drugs**
Secondary diabetes may be caused by an adverse effect of correctly administered medications, poisoning or sequela of poisoning.
See section I.C.19.e for coding of adverse effects and poisoning, and section I.C.20 for external cause code reporting.

5. **Chapter 5: Mental, Behavioral and Neurodevelopmental disorders (F01–F99)**

a. **Pain disorders related to psychological factors**
Assign code F45.41, for pain that is exclusively related to psychological disorders. As indicated by the Excludes 1 note under category G89, a code from category G89 should not be assigned with code F45.41.

Code F45.42, Pain disorders with related psychological factors, should be used with a code from category G89, Pain, not elsewhere classified, if there is documentation of a psychological component for a patient with acute or chronic pain.
See Section I.C.6. Pain

b. **Mental and behavioral disorders due to psychoactive substance use**

1) **In Remission**
Selection of codes for "in remission" for categories F10-F19, Mental and behavioral disorders due to psychoactive substance use (categories F10-F19 with -.11, -.21) requires the provider's clinical judgment. The appropriate codes for "in remission" are assigned only on the basis of provider documentation (as defined in the Official Guidelines for Coding and Reporting), unless otherwise instructed by the classification.

Mild substance use disorders in early or sustained remission are classified to the appropriate codes for substance abuse in remission, and moderate or severe substance use disorders in early or sustained remission are classified to the appropriate codes for substance dependence in remission.

2) **Psychoactive Substance Use, Abuse and Dependence**
When the provider documentation refers to use, abuse and dependence of the same substance (e.g. alcohol, opioid, cannabis, etc.), only one code should be assigned to identify the pattern of use based on the following hierarchy:

- If both use and abuse are documented, assign only the code for abuse
- If both abuse and dependence are documented, assign only the code for dependence
- If use, abuse and dependence are all documented, assign only the code for dependence
- If both use and dependence are documented, assign only the code for dependence.

3) **Psychoactive Substance Use, *Unspecified***
As with all other **unspecified** diagnoses, the codes for **unspecified** psychoactive substance use (F10.9-, F11.9-, F12.9-, F13.9-, F14.9-, F15.9-, F16.9-, **F18.9-, F19.9-**) should only be assigned based on provider documentation and when they meet the definition of a reportable diagnosis (see Section III, Reporting Additional Diagnoses). These codes are to be used only when the psychoactive substance use is associated with a physical, mental or behavioral disorder, and such a relationship is documented by the provider.

c. **Factitious Disorder**
Factitious disorder imposed on self or Munchausen's syndrome is a disorder in which a person falsely reports or causes his or her own physical or psychological signs or symptoms. For patients with documented factitious disorder on self or Munchausen's syndrome, assign the appropriate code from subcategory F68.1-, Factitious disorder imposed on self.
Munchausen's syndrome by proxy (MSBP) is a disorder in which a caregiver (perpetrator) falsely reports or causes an illness or injury in another person (victim) under his or her care, such as a child, an elderly adult, or a person who has a disability. The condition is also referred to as "factitious disorder imposed on another" or "factitious disorder by proxy." The perpetrator, not the victim, receives this diagnosis. Assign code F68.A, Factitious disorder imposed on another, to the perpetrator's record. For the victim of a patient suffering from MSBP, assign the appropriate code from categories T74, Adult and child abuse, neglect and other maltreatment, confirmed, or T76, Adult and child abuse, neglect and other maltreatment, suspected.
See Section I.C.19.f. Adult and child abuse, neglect and other maltreatment

6. **Chapter 6: Diseases of the Nervous System (G00-G99)**

a. **Dominant/nondominant side**
Codes from category G81, Hemiplegia and hemiparesis, and subcategories G83.1, Monoplegia of lower limb, G83.2, Monoplegia of upper limb, and G83.3, Monoplegia, unspecified, identify whether the dominant or nondominant side is affected. Should the affected side be documented, but not specified as dominant or nondominant, and the classification system does not indicate a default, code selection is as follows:

- For ambidextrous patients, the default should be dominant.
- If the left side is affected, the default is non-dominant.
- If the right side is affected, the default is dominant.

b. **Pain - Category G89**

1) **General coding information**
Codes in category G89, Pain, not elsewhere classified, may be used in conjunction with codes from other categories and

chapters to provide more detail about acute or chronic pain and neoplasm-related pain, unless otherwise indicated below.

If the pain is not specified as acute or chronic, post-thoracotomy, postprocedural, or neoplasm-related, do not assign codes from category G89.

A code from category G89 should not be assigned if the underlying (definitive) diagnosis is known, unless the reason for the encounter is pain control/ management and not management of the underlying condition.

When an admission or encounter is for a procedure aimed at treating the underlying condition (e.g., spinal fusion, kyphoplasty), a code for the underlying condition (e.g., vertebral fracture, spinal stenosis) should be assigned as the principal diagnosis. No code from category G89 should be assigned.

(a) **Category G89 Codes as Principal or First-Listed Diagnosis**

Category G89 codes are acceptable as principal diagnosis or the first-listed code:

- When pain control or pain management is the reason for the admission/encounter (e.g., a patient with displaced intervertebral disc, nerve impingement and severe back pain presents for injection of steroid into the spinal canal). The underlying cause of the pain should be reported as an additional diagnosis, if known.

- When a patient is admitted for the insertion of a neurostimulator for pain control, assign the appropriate pain code as the principal or first-listed diagnosis. When an admission or encounter is for a procedure aimed at treating the underlying condition and a neurostimulator is inserted for pain control during the same admission/encounter, a code for the underlying condition should be assigned as the principal diagnosis and the appropriate pain code should be assigned as a secondary diagnosis.

(b) **Use of Category G89 Codes in Conjunction with Site Specific Pain Codes**

(i) **Assigning Category G89 and Site-Specific Pain Codes**

Codes from category G89 may be used in conjunction with codes that identify the site of pain (including codes from chapter 18) if the category G89 code provides additional information. For example, if the code describes the site of the pain, but does not fully describe whether the pain is acute or chronic, then both codes should be assigned.

(ii) **Sequencing of Category G89 Codes with Site-Specific Pain Codes**

The sequencing of category G89 codes with site-specific pain codes (including chapter 18 codes), is dependent on the circumstances of the encounter/admission as follows:

- If the encounter is for pain control or pain management, assign the code from category G89 followed by the code identifying the specific site of pain (e.g., encounter for pain management for acute neck pain from trauma is assigned code G89.11, Acute pain due to trauma, followed by code M54.2, Cervicalgia, to identify the site of pain).

- If the encounter is for any other reason except pain control or pain management, and a related definitive diagnosis has not been established (confirmed) by the provider, assign the code for the specific site of pain first, followed by the appropriate code from category G89.

2) **Pain due to devices, implants and grafts**

See Section I.C.19. Pain due to medical devices

3) **Postoperative Pain**

The provider's documentation should be used to guide the coding of postoperative pain, as well as *Section III. Reporting Additional Diagnoses and Section IV. Diagnostic Coding and Reporting in the Outpatient Setting.*

The default for post-thoracotomy and other postoperative pain not specified as acute or chronic is the code for the acute form.

Routine or expected postoperative pain immediately after surgery should not be coded.

(a) **Postoperative pain not associated with specific postoperative complication**

Postoperative pain not associated with a specific postoperative complication is assigned to the appropriate postoperative pain code in category G89.

(b) **Postoperative pain associated with specific postoperative complication**

Postoperative pain associated with a specific postoperative complication (such as painful wire sutures) is assigned to the appropriate code(s) found in Chapter 19, Injury, poisoning, and certain other consequences of external causes. If appropriate, use additional code(s) from category G89 to identify acute or chronic pain (G89.18 or G89.28).

4) **Chronic pain**

Chronic pain is classified to subcategory G89.2. There is no time frame defining when pain becomes chronic pain. The provider's documentation should be used to guide use of these codes.

5) **Neoplasm Related Pain**

Code G89.3 is assigned to pain documented as being related, associated or due to cancer, primary or secondary malignancy, or tumor. This code is assigned regardless of whether the pain is acute or chronic.

This code may be assigned as the principal or first-listed code when the stated reason for the admission/encounter is documented as pain control/pain management. The underlying neoplasm should be reported as an additional diagnosis.

When the reason for the admission/encounter is management of the neoplasm and the pain associated with the neoplasm is also documented, code G89.3 may be assigned as an additional diagnosis. It is not necessary to assign an additional code for the site of the pain.

See Section I.C.2 for instructions on the sequencing of neoplasms for all other stated reasons for the admission/encounter (except for pain control/pain management).

6) **Chronic pain syndrome**

Central pain syndrome (G89.0) and chronic pain syndrome (G89.4) are different than the term "chronic pain," and therefore codes should only be used when the provider has specifically documented this condition.

See Section I.C.5. Pain disorders related to psychological factors

7. **Chapter 7: Diseases of the Eye and Adnexa (H00-H59)**

a. **Glaucoma**

1) **Assigning Glaucoma Codes**

Assign as many codes from category H40, Glaucoma, as needed to identify the type of glaucoma, the affected eye, and the glaucoma stage.

2) **Bilateral glaucoma with same type and stage**

When a patient has bilateral glaucoma and both eyes are documented as being the same type and stage, and there is a code for bilateral glaucoma, report only the code for the type of glaucoma, bilateral, with the seventh character for the stage.

When a patient has bilateral glaucoma and both eyes are documented as being the same type and stage, and the classification does not provide a code for bilateral glaucoma (i.e. subcategories H40.10 and H40.20) report only one code for the type of glaucoma with the appropriate seventh character for the stage.

3) **Bilateral glaucoma stage with different types or stages**

When a patient has bilateral glaucoma and each eye is documented as having a different type or stage, and the classification distinguishes laterality, assign the appropriate code for each eye rather than the code for bilateral glaucoma.

When a patient has bilateral glaucoma and each eye is documented as having a different type, and the classification does not distinguish laterality (i.e. subcategories H40.10 and H40.20), assign one code for each type of glaucoma with the appropriate seventh character for the stage.

When a patient has bilateral glaucoma and each eye is documented as having the same type, but different stage, and the classification does not distinguish laterality (i.e. subcategories H40.10 and H40.20), assign a code for the type of glaucoma for each eye with the seventh character for the specific glaucoma stage documented for each eye.

4) Patient admitted with glaucoma and stage evolves during the admission

If a patient is admitted with glaucoma and the stage progresses during the admission, assign the code for highest stage documented.

5) Indeterminate stage glaucoma

Assignment of the seventh character "4" for "indeterminate stage" should be based on the clinical documentation. The seventh character "4" is used for glaucomas whose stage cannot be clinically determined. This seventh character should not be confused with the seventh character "Ø", unspecified, which should be assigned when there is no documentation regarding the stage of the glaucoma.

b. Blindness

If "blindness" or "low vision" of both eyes is documented but the visual impairment category is not documented, assign code H54.3, Unqualified visual loss, both eyes. If "blindness" or "low vision" in one eye is documented but the visual impairment category is not documented, assign a code from H54.6-, Unqualified visual loss, one eye. If "blindness" or "visual loss" is documented without any information about whether one or both eyes are affected, assign code H54.7, Unspecified visual loss.

8. Chapter 8: Diseases of the Ear and Mastoid Process (H60-H95)

Reserved for future guideline expansion

9. Chapter 9: Diseases of the Circulatory System (IØØ-I99)

a. Hypertension

The classification presumes a causal relationship between hypertension and heart involvement and between hypertension and kidney involvement, as the two conditions are linked by the term "with" in the Alphabetic Index. These conditions should be coded as related even in the absence of provider documentation explicitly linking them, unless the documentation clearly states the conditions are unrelated.

For hypertension and conditions not specifically linked by relational terms such as "with," "associated with" or "due to" in the classification, provider documentation must link the conditions in order to code them as related.

1) Hypertension with Heart Disease

Hypertension with heart conditions classified to I50.- or **I51.4-I51.7, I51.89, I51.9**, are assigned to a code from category I11, Hypertensive heart disease. Use additional code(s) from category I5Ø, Heart failure, to identify the type(s) of heart failure in those patients with heart failure.

The same heart conditions (I50.-, **I51.4-I51.7, I51.89, I51.9**) with hypertension are coded separately if the provider has **documented they are unrelated to the hypertension**. Sequence according to the circumstances of the admission/encounter.

2) Hypertensive Chronic Kidney Disease

Assign codes from category I12, Hypertensive chronic kidney disease, when both hypertension and a condition classifiable to category N18, Chronic kidney disease (CKD), are present. CKD should not be coded as hypertensive if the **provider indicates the CKD is not related to the hypertension**.

The appropriate code from category N18 should be used as a secondary code with a code from category I12 to identify the stage of chronic kidney disease.

See Section I.C.14. Chronic kidney disease.

If a patient has hypertensive chronic kidney disease and acute renal failure, an additional code for the acute renal failure is required.

3) Hypertensive Heart and Chronic Kidney Disease

Assign codes from combination category I13, Hypertensive heart and chronic kidney disease, when there is hypertension with both heart and kidney involvement. If heart failure is present, assign an additional code from category I5Ø to identify the type of heart failure.

The appropriate code from category N18, Chronic kidney disease, should be used as a secondary code with a code from category I13 to identify the stage of chronic kidney disease.

See Section I.C.14. Chronic kidney disease.

The codes in category I13, Hypertensive heart and chronic kidney disease, are combination codes that include hypertension, heart disease and chronic kidney disease. The Includes note at I13 specifies that the conditions included at I11 and I12 are included together in I13. If a patient has hypertension, heart disease and chronic kidney disease, then a code from I13 should be used, not individual codes for hypertension, heart disease and chronic kidney disease, or codes from I11 or I12.

For patients with both acute renal failure and chronic kidney disease, an additional code for acute renal failure is required.

4) Hypertensive Cerebrovascular Disease

For hypertensive cerebrovascular disease, first assign the appropriate code from categories I60-I69, followed by the appropriate hypertension code.

5) Hypertensive Retinopathy

Subcategory H35.Ø, Background retinopathy and retinal vascular changes, should be used with a code from category I1Ø- I15, Hypertensive disease to include the systemic hypertension. The sequencing is based on the reason for the encounter.

6) Hypertension, Secondary

Secondary hypertension is due to an underlying condition. Two codes are required: one to identify the underlying etiology and one from category I15 to identify the hypertension. Sequencing of codes is determined by the reason for admission/encounter.

7) Hypertension, Transient

Assign code RØ3.Ø, Elevated blood pressure reading without diagnosis of hypertension, unless patient has an established diagnosis of hypertension. Assign code O13.-, Gestational [pregnancy-induced] hypertension without significant proteinuria, or O14.-, Pre-eclampsia, for transient hypertension of pregnancy.

8) Hypertension, Controlled

This diagnostic statement usually refers to an existing state of hypertension under control by therapy. Assign the appropriate code from categories I1Ø-I15, Hypertensive diseases.

9) Hypertension, Uncontrolled

Uncontrolled hypertension may refer to untreated hypertension or hypertension not responding to current therapeutic regimen. In either case, assign the appropriate code from categories I1Ø-I15, Hypertensive diseases.

10) Hypertensive Crisis

Assign a code from category I16, Hypertensive crisis, for documented hypertensive urgency, hypertensive emergency or unspecified hypertensive crisis. Code also any identified hypertensive disease (I10-I15). The sequencing is based on the reason for the encounter.

11) Pulmonary Hypertension

Pulmonary hypertension is classified to category I27, Other pulmonary heart diseases. For secondary pulmonary hypertension (I27.1, I27.2-), code also any associated conditions or adverse effects of drugs or toxins. The sequencing is based on the reason for the encounter, **except for adverse effects of drugs (See Section I.C.19.e.).**

b. Atherosclerotic Coronary Artery Disease and Angina

ICD-10-CM has combination codes for atherosclerotic heart disease with angina pectoris. The subcategories for these codes are I25.11, Atherosclerotic heart disease of native coronary artery with angina pectoris and I25.7, Atherosclerosis of coronary artery bypass graft(s) and coronary artery of transplanted heart with angina pectoris.

When using one of these combination codes it is not necessary to use an additional code for angina pectoris. A causal relationship can be assumed in a patient with both atherosclerosis and angina pectoris, unless the documentation indicates the angina is due to something other than the atherosclerosis.

If a patient with coronary artery disease is admitted due to an acute myocardial infarction (AMI), the AMI should be sequenced before the coronary artery disease.

See Section I.C.9. Acute myocardial infarction (AMI)

c. Intraoperative and Postprocedural Cerebrovascular Accident

Medical record documentation should clearly specify the cause-and-effect relationship between the medical intervention and the cerebrovascular accident in order to assign a code for intraoperative or postprocedural cerebrovascular accident.

Proper code assignment depends on whether it was an infarction or hemorrhage and whether it occurred intraoperatively or postoperatively. If it was a cerebral hemorrhage, code assignment depends on the type of procedure performed.

d. Sequelae of Cerebrovascular Disease

1) Category I69, Sequelae of Cerebrovascular disease

Category I69 is used to indicate conditions classifiable to categories I60-I67 as the causes of sequela (neurologic deficits), themselves classified elsewhere. These "late effects" include neurologic deficits that persist after initial onset of conditions classifiable to categories I60-I67. The neurologic deficits caused by cerebrovascular disease may be present from the onset or may arise at any time after the onset of the condition classifiable to categories I60-I67.

Codes from category I69, Sequelae of cerebrovascular disease, that specify hemiplegia, hemiparesis and monoplegia identify whether the dominant or nondominant side is affected. Should the affected side be documented, but not specified as dominant or nondominant, and the classification system does not indicate a default, code selection is as follows:

- For ambidextrous patients, the default should be dominant.
- If the left side is affected, the default is non-dominant.
- If the right side is affected, the default is dominant.

2) Codes from category I69 with codes from I60-I67

Codes from category I69 may be assigned on a health care record with codes from I60-I67, if the patient has a current cerebrovascular disease and deficits from an old cerebrovascular disease.

3) Codes from category I69 and Personal history of transient ischemic attack (TIA) and cerebral infarction (Z86.73)

Codes from category I69 should not be assigned if the patient does not have neurologic deficits.

See Section I.C.21. 4. History (of) for use of personal history codes

e. Acute myocardial infarction (AMI)

1) Type 1 ST elevation myocardial infarction (STEMI) and non-ST elevation myocardial infarction (NSTEMI)

The ICD-10-CMcodes for type 1 acute myocardial infarction (AMI) identify the site, such as anterolateral wall or true posterior wall. Subcategories I21.0-I21.2 and code I21.3 are used for type 1 ST elevation myocardial infarction (STEMI). Code I21.4, Non-ST elevation (NSTEMI) myocardial infarction, is used for type 1 non ST elevation myocardial infarction (NSTEMI) and nontransmural MIs.

If a type 1 NSTEMI evolves to STEMI, assign the STEMI code. If a type 1 STEMI converts to NSTEMI due to thrombolytic therapy, it is still coded as STEMI.

For encounters occurring while the myocardial infarction is equal to, or less than, four weeks old, including transfers to another acute setting or a postacute setting, and the myocardial infarction meets the definition for "other diagnoses" (see Section III, Reporting Additional Diagnoses), codes from category I21 may continue to be reported. For encounters after the 4 week time frame and the patient is still receiving care related to the myocardial infarction, the appropriate aftercare code should be assigned, rather than a code from category I21. For old or healed myocardial infarctions not requiring further care, code I25.2, Old myocardial infarction, may be assigned.

2) Acute myocardial infarction, unspecified

Code I21.9, Acute myocardial infarction, unspecified, is the default for unspecified acute myocardial infarction or unspecified type. If only type 1 STEMI or transmural MI without the site is documented, assign code I21.3, ST elevation (STEMI) myocardial infarction of unspecified site.

3) AMI documented as nontransmural or subendocardial but site provided

If an AMI is documented as nontransmural or subendocardial, but the site is provided, it is still coded as a subendocardial AMI.

See Section I.C.21.3 for information on coding status post administration of tPA in a different facility within the last 24 hours.

4) Subsequent acute myocardial infarction

A code from category I22, Subsequent ST elevation (STEMI) and non-ST elevation (NSTEMI) myocardial infarction, is to be used when a patient who has suffered a type 1 or unspecified AMI has a new AMI within the 4 week time frame of the initial AMI. A code

from category I22 must be used in conjunction with a code from category I21. The sequencing of the I22 and I21 codes depends on the circumstances of the encounter.

Do not assign code I22 for subsequent myocardial infarctions other than type 1 or unspecified. For subsequent type 2 AMI assign only code I21.A1. For subsequent type 4 or type 5 AMI, assign only code I21.A9.

If a subsequent myocardial infarction of one type occurs within 4 weeks of a myocardial infarction of a different type, assign the appropriate codes from category I21 to identify each type. Do not assign a code from I22. Codes from category I22 should only be assigned if both the initial and subsequent myocardial infarctions are type 1 or unspecified.

5) Other Types of Myocardial Infarction

The ICD-10-CM provides codes for different types of myocardial infarction. Type 1 myocardial infarctions are assigned to codes I21.0-I21.4 **and I21.9**.

Type 2 myocardial infarction (myocardial infarction due to demand ischemia or secondary to ischemic balance), is assigned to code I21.A1, Myocardial infarction type 2 with a code for the underlying cause. Do not assign code I24.8, Other forms of acute ischemic heart disease, for the demand ischemia. Sequencing of type 2 AMI or the underlying cause is dependent on the circumstances of admission. When a type 2 AMI code is described as NSTEMI or STEMI, only assign code I21.A1. Codes I21.01-I21.4 should only be assigned for type 1 AMIs.

Acute myocardial infarctions type 3, 4a, 4b, 4c and 5 are assigned to code I21.A9, Other myocardial infarction type.

The "Code also" and "Code first" notes should be followed related to complications, and for coding of postprocedural myocardial infarctions during or following cardiac surgery.

10. Chapter 10: Diseases of the Respiratory System (J00-J99)

a. Chronic Obstructive Pulmonary Disease [COPD] and Asthma

1) Acute exacerbation of chronic obstructive bronchitis and asthma

The codes in categories J44 and J45 distinguish between uncomplicated cases and those in acute exacerbation. An acute exacerbation is a worsening or a decompensation of a chronic condition. An acute exacerbation is not equivalent to an infection superimposed on a chronic condition, though an exacerbation may be triggered by an infection.

b. Acute Respiratory Failure

1) Acute respiratory failure as principal diagnosis

A code from subcategory J96.0, Acute respiratory failure, or subcategory J96.2, Acute and chronic respiratory failure, may be assigned as a principal diagnosis when it is the condition established after study to be chiefly responsible for occasioning the admission to the hospital, and the selection is supported by the Alphabetic Index and Tabular List. However, chapter-specific coding guidelines (such as obstetrics, poisoning, HIV, newborn) that provide sequencing direction take precedence.

2) Acute respiratory failure as secondary diagnosis

Respiratory failure may be listed as a secondary diagnosis if it occurs after admission, or if it is present on admission, but does not meet the definition of principal diagnosis.

3) Sequencing of acute respiratory failure and another acute condition

When a patient is admitted with respiratory failure and another acute condition, (e.g., myocardial infarction, cerebrovascular accident, aspiration pneumonia), the principal diagnosis will not be the same in every situation. This applies whether the other acute condition is a respiratory or nonrespiratory condition. Selection of the principal diagnosis will be dependent on the circumstances of admission. If both the respiratory failure and the other acute condition are equally responsible for occasioning the admission to the hospital, and there are no chapter-specific sequencing rules, the guideline regarding two or more diagnoses that equally meet the definition for principal diagnosis *(Section II, C.)* may be applied in these situations.

If the documentation is not clear as to whether acute respiratory failure and another condition are equally responsible for occasioning the admission, query the provider for clarification.

c. Influenza due to certain identified influenza viruses

Code only confirmed cases of influenza due to certain identified influenza viruses (category J09), and due to other identified influenza virus (category J10). This is an exception to the hospital inpatient guideline Section II, H. (Uncertain Diagnosis).

In this context, "confirmation" does not require documentation of positive laboratory testing specific for avian or other novel influenza A or other identified influenza virus. However, coding should be based on the provider's diagnostic statement that the patient has avian influenza, or other novel influenza A, for category J09, or has another particular identified strain of influenza, such as H1N1 or H3N2, but not identified as novel or variant, for category J10.

If the provider records "suspected" or "possible" or "probable" avian influenza, or novel influenza, or other identified influenza, then the appropriate influenza code from category J11, Influenza due to unidentified influenza virus, should be assigned. A code from category J09, Influenza due to certain identified influenza viruses, should not be assigned nor should a code from category J10, Influenza due to other identified influenza virus.

d. Ventilator associated Pneumonia
1) Documentation of Ventilator associated Pneumonia
As with all procedural or postprocedural complications, code assignment is based on the provider's documentation of the relationship between the condition and the procedure.

Code J95.851, Ventilator associated pneumonia, should be assigned only when the provider has documented ventilator associated pneumonia (VAP). An additional code to identify the organism (e.g., Pseudomonas aeruginosa, code B96.5) should also be assigned. Do not assign an additional code from categories J12-J18 to identify the type of pneumonia.

Code J95.851 should not be assigned for cases where the patient has pneumonia and is on a mechanical ventilator and the provider has not specifically stated that the pneumonia is ventilator-associated pneumonia. If the documentation is unclear as to whether the patient has a pneumonia that is a complication attributable to the mechanical ventilator, query the provider.

2) Ventilator associated Pneumonia Develops after Admission
A patient may be admitted with one type of pneumonia (e.g., code J13, Pneumonia due to Streptococcus pneumonia) and subsequently develop VAP. In this instance, the principal diagnosis would be the appropriate code from categories J12-J18 for the pneumonia diagnosed at the time of admission. Code J95.851, Ventilator associated pneumonia, would be assigned as an additional diagnosis when the provider has also documented the presence of ventilator associated pneumonia.

11. Chapter 11: Diseases of the Digestive System (K00-K95)
Reserved for future guideline expansion

12. Chapter 12: Diseases of the Skin and Subcutaneous Tissue (L00-L99)
a. Pressure ulcer stage codes
1) Pressure ulcer stages
Codes from category L89, Pressure ulcer, identify the site of the pressure ulcer as well as the stage of the ulcer.

The ICD-10-CM classifies pressure ulcer stages based on severity, which is designated by stages 1-4, unspecified stage and unstageable.

Assign as many codes from category L89 as needed to identify all the pressure ulcers the patient has, if applicable.

See Section I.B.14 for pressure ulcer stage documentation by clinicians other than patient's provider

2) Unstageable pressure ulcers
Assignment of the code for unstageable pressure ulcer (L89.--0) should be based on the clinical documentation. These codes are used for pressure ulcers whose stage cannot be clinically determined (e.g., the ulcer is covered by eschar or has been treated with a skin or muscle graft) and pressure ulcers that are documented as deep tissue injury but not documented as due to trauma. This code should not be confused with the codes for unspecified stage (L89.--9). When there is no documentation regarding the stage of the pressure ulcer, assign the appropriate code for unspecified stage (L89.--9).

3) Documented pressure ulcer stage
Assignment of the pressure ulcer stage code should be guided by clinical documentation of the stage or documentation of the terms found in the Alphabetic Index. For clinical terms describing the stage that are not found in the Alphabetic Index, and there is no documentation of the stage, the provider should be queried.

4) Patients admitted with pressure ulcers documented as healed
No code is assigned if the documentation states that the pressure ulcer is completely healed.

5) Patients admitted with pressure ulcers documented as healing
Pressure ulcers described as healing should be assigned the appropriate pressure ulcer stage code based on the documentation in the medical record. If the documentation does not provide information about the stage of the healing pressure ulcer, assign the appropriate code for unspecified stage.

If the documentation is unclear as to whether the patient has a current (new) pressure ulcer or if the patient is being treated for a healing pressure ulcer, query the provider.

For ulcers that were present on admission but healed at the time of discharge, assign the code for the site and stage of the pressure ulcer at the time of admission.

6) Patient admitted with pressure ulcer evolving into another stage during the admission
If a patient is admitted to an inpatient hospital with a pressure ulcer at one stage and it progresses to a higher stage, two separate codes should be assigned: one code for the site and stage of the ulcer on admission and a second code for the same ulcer site and the highest stage reported during the stay.

b. Non-Pressure Chronic Ulcers
1) Patients admitted with non-pressure ulcers documented as healed
No code is assigned if the documentation states that the non-pressure ulcer is completely healed.

2) Patients admitted with non-pressure ulcers documented as healing
Non-pressure ulcers described as healing should be assigned the appropriate non-pressure ulcer code based on the documentation in the medical record. If the documentation does not provide information about the severity of the healing non-pressure ulcer, assign the appropriate code for unspecified severity.

If the documentation is unclear as to whether the patient has a current (new) non-pressure ulcer or if the patient is being treated for a healing non-pressure ulcer, query the provider.

For ulcers that were present on admission but healed at the time of discharge, assign the code for the site and severity of the non-pressure ulcer at the time of admission.

3) Patient admitted with non-pressure ulcer that progresses to another severity level during the admission
If a patient is admitted to an inpatient hospital with a non-pressure ulcer at one severity level and it progresses to a higher severity level, two separate codes should be assigned: one code for the site and severity level of the ulcer on admission and a second code for the same ulcer site and the highest severity level reported during the stay.

See Section I.B.14 for pressure ulcer stage documentation by clinicians other than patient's provider

13. Chapter 13: Diseases of the Musculoskeletal System and Connective Tissue (M00-M99)
a. Site and laterality
Most of the codes within Chapter 13 have site and laterality designations. The site represents the bone, joint or the muscle involved. For some conditions where more than one bone, joint or muscle is usually involved, such as osteoarthritis, there is a "multiple sites" code available. For categories where no multiple site code is provided and more than one bone, joint or muscle is involved, multiple codes should be used to indicate the different sites involved.
1) Bone versus joint
For certain conditions, the bone may be affected at the upper or lower end, (e.g., avascular necrosis of bone, M87, Osteoporosis, M80, M81). Though the portion of the bone affected may be at the joint, the site designation will be the bone, not the joint.

b. Acute traumatic versus chronic or recurrent musculoskeletal conditions
Many musculoskeletal conditions are a result of previous injury or trauma to a site, or are recurrent conditions. Bone, joint or muscle conditions that are the result of a healed injury are usually found in chapter 13. Recurrent bone, joint or muscle conditions are also usually

found in chapter 13. Any current, acute injury should be coded to the appropriate injury code from chapter 19. Chronic or recurrent conditions should generally be coded with a code from chapter 13. If it is difficult to determine from the documentation in the record which code is best to describe a condition, query the provider.

c. Coding of Pathologic Fractures

7th character A is for use as long as the patient is receiving active treatment for the fracture. While the patient may be seen by a new or different provider over the course of treatment for a pathological fracture, assignment of the 7th character is based on whether the patient is undergoing active treatment and not whether the provider is seeing the patient for the first time.

7th character D is to be used for encounters after the patient has completed active treatment for the fracture and is receiving routine care for the fracture during the healing or recovery phase. The other 7th characters, listed under each subcategory in the Tabular List, are to be used for subsequent encounters for treatment of problems associated with the healing, such as malunions, nonunions, and sequelae.

Care for complications of surgical treatment for fracture repairs during the healing or recovery phase should be coded with the appropriate complication codes.

See Section I.C.19. Coding of traumatic fractures.

d. Osteoporosis

Osteoporosis is a systemic condition, meaning that all bones of the musculoskeletal system are affected. Therefore, site is not a component of the codes under category M81, Osteoporosis without current pathological fracture. The site codes under category M80, Osteoporosis with current pathological fracture, identify the site of the fracture, not the osteoporosis.

1) Osteoporosis without pathological fracture

Category M81, Osteoporosis without current pathological fracture, is for use for patients with osteoporosis who do not currently have a pathologic fracture due to the osteoporosis, even if they have had a fracture in the past. For patients with a history of osteoporosis fractures, status code Z87.310, Personal history of (healed) osteoporosis fracture, should follow the code from M81.

2) Osteoporosis with current pathological fracture

Category M80, Osteoporosis with current pathological fracture, is for patients who have a current pathologic fracture at the time of an encounter. The codes under M80 identify the site of the fracture. A code from category M80, not a traumatic fracture code, should be used for any patient with known osteoporosis who suffers a fracture, even if the patient had a minor fall or trauma, if that fall or trauma would not usually break a normal, healthy bone.

14. Chapter 14: Diseases of Genitourinary System (N00-N99)

a. Chronic kidney disease

1) Stages of chronic kidney disease (CKD)

The ICD-10-CM classifies CKD based on severity. The severity of CKD is designated by stages 1-5. Stage 2, code N18.2, equates to mild CKD; stage 3, code N18.3, equates to moderate CKD; and stage 4, code N18.4, equates to severe CKD. Code N18.6, End stage renal disease (ESRD), is assigned when the provider has documented end-stage-renal disease (ESRD).

If both a stage of CKD and ESRD are documented, assign code N18.6 only.

2) Chronic kidney disease and kidney transplant status

Patients who have undergone kidney transplant may still have some form of chronic kidney disease (CKD) because the kidney transplant may not fully restore kidney function. Therefore, the presence of CKD alone does not constitute a transplant complication. Assign the appropriate N18 code for the patient's stage of CKD and code Z94.0, Kidney transplant status. If a transplant complication such as failure or rejection or other transplant complication is documented, see section I.C.19.g for information on coding complications of a kidney transplant. If the documentation is unclear as to whether the patient has a complication of the transplant, query the provider.

3) Chronic kidney disease with other conditions

Patients with CKD may also suffer from other serious conditions, most commonly diabetes mellitus and hypertension. The sequencing of the CKD code in relationship to codes for other

contributing conditions is based on the conventions in the Tabular List.

See I.C.9. Hypertensive chronic kidney disease.

See I.C.19. Chronic kidney disease and kidney transplant complications.

15. Chapter 15: Pregnancy, Childbirth, and the Puerperium (O00-O9A)

a. General Rules for Obstetric Cases

1) Codes from chapter 15 and sequencing priority

Obstetric cases require codes from chapter 15, codes in the range O00-O9A, Pregnancy, Childbirth, and the Puerperium. Chapter 15 codes have sequencing priority over codes from other chapters. Additional codes from other chapters may be used in conjunction with chapter 15 codes to further specify conditions. Should the provider document that the pregnancy is incidental to the encounter, then code Z33.1, Pregnant state, incidental, should be used in place of any chapter 15 codes. It is the provider's responsibility to state that the condition being treated is not affecting the pregnancy.

2) Chapter 15 codes used only on the maternal record

Chapter 15 codes are to be used only on the maternal record, never on the record of the newborn.

3) Final character for trimester

The majority of codes in Chapter 15 have a final character indicating the trimester of pregnancy. The timeframes for the trimesters are indicated at the beginning of the chapter. If trimester is not a component of a code, it is because the condition always occurs in a specific trimester, or the concept of trimester of pregnancy is not applicable. Certain codes have characters for only certain trimesters because the condition does not occur in all trimesters, but it may occur in more than just one.

Assignment of the final character for trimester should be based on the provider's documentation of the trimester (or number of weeks) for the current admission/encounter. This applies to the assignment of trimester for pre-existing conditions as well as those that develop during or are due to the pregnancy. The provider's documentation of the number of weeks may be used to assign the appropriate code identifying the trimester.

Whenever delivery occurs during the current admission, and there is an "in childbirth" option for the obstetric complication being coded, the "in childbirth" code should be assigned.

4) Selection of trimester for inpatient admissions that encompass more than one trimester

In instances when a patient is admitted to a hospital for complications of pregnancy during one trimester and remains in the hospital into a subsequent trimester, the trimester character for the antepartum complication code should be assigned on the basis of the trimester when the complication developed, not the trimester of the discharge. If the condition developed prior to the current admission/encounter or represents a pre-existing condition, the trimester character for the trimester at the time of the admission/encounter should be assigned.

5) Unspecified trimester

Each category that includes codes for trimester has a code for "unspecified trimester." The "unspecified trimester" code should rarely be used, such as when the documentation in the record is insufficient to determine the trimester and it is not possible to obtain clarification.

6) 7th character for Fetus Identification

Where applicable, a 7th character is to be assigned for certain categories (O31, O32, O33.3 - O33.6, O35, O36, O40, O41, O60.1, O60.2, O64, and O69) to identify the fetus for which the complication code applies.

Assign 7th character "0":

- For single gestations
- When the documentation in the record is insufficient to determine the fetus affected and it is not possible to obtain clarification.
- When it is not possible to clinically determine which fetus is affected.

b. Selection of OB Principal or First-listed Diagnosis

1) Routine outpatient prenatal visits

For routine outpatient prenatal visits when no complications are present, a code from category Z34, Encounter for supervision of normal pregnancy, should be used as the first-listed diagnosis.

These codes should not be used in conjunction with chapter 15 codes.

2) Supervision of High-Risk Pregnancy

Codes from category O09, Supervision of high-risk pregnancy, are intended for use only during the prenatal period. For complications during the labor or delivery episode as a result of a high-risk pregnancy, assign the applicable complication codes from Chapter 15. If there are no complications during the labor or delivery episode, assign code O80, Encounter for full-term uncomplicated delivery.

For routine prenatal outpatient visits for patients with high-risk pregnancies, a code from category O09, Supervision of high-risk pregnancy, should be used as the first-listed diagnosis. Secondary chapter 15 codes may be used in conjunction with these codes if appropriate.

3) Episodes when no delivery occurs

In episodes when no delivery occurs, the principal diagnosis should correspond to the principal complication of the pregnancy which necessitated the encounter. Should more than one complication exist, all of which are treated or monitored, any of the complications codes may be sequenced first.

4) When a delivery occurs

When an obstetric patient is admitted and delivers during that admission, the condition that prompted the admission should be sequenced as the principal diagnosis. If multiple conditions prompted the admission, sequence the one most related to the delivery as the principal diagnosis. A code for any complication of the delivery should be assigned as an additional diagnosis. In cases of cesarean delivery, if the patient was admitted with a condition that resulted in the performance of a cesarean procedure, that condition should be selected as the principal diagnosis. If the reason for the admission was unrelated to the condition resulting in the cesarean delivery, the condition related to the reason for the admission should be selected as the principal diagnosis.

5) Outcome of delivery

A code from category Z37, Outcome of delivery, should be included on every maternal record when a delivery has occurred. These codes are not to be used on subsequent records or on the newborn record.

c. Pre-existing conditions versus conditions due to the pregnancy

Certain categories in Chapter 15 distinguish between conditions of the mother that existed prior to pregnancy (pre-existing) and those that are a direct result of pregnancy. When assigning codes from Chapter 15, it is important to assess if a condition was pre-existing prior to pregnancy or developed during or due to the pregnancy in order to assign the correct code.

Categories that do not distinguish between pre-existing and pregnancy-related conditions may be used for either. It is acceptable to use codes specifically for the puerperium with codes complicating pregnancy and childbirth if a condition arises postpartum during the delivery encounter.

d. Pre-existing hypertension in pregnancy

Category O10, Pre-existing hypertension complicating pregnancy, childbirth and the puerperium, includes codes for hypertensive heart and hypertensive chronic kidney disease. When assigning one of the O10 codes that includes hypertensive heart disease or hypertensive chronic kidney disease, it is necessary to add a secondary code from the appropriate hypertension category to specify the type of heart failure or chronic kidney disease.

See Section I.C.9. Hypertension.

e. Fetal Conditions Affecting the Management of the Mother

1) Codes from categories O35 and O36

Codes from categories O35, Maternal care for known or suspected fetal abnormality and damage, and O36, Maternal care for other fetal problems, are assigned only when the fetal condition is actually responsible for modifying the management of the mother, i.e., by requiring diagnostic studies, additional observation, special care, or termination of pregnancy. The fact that the fetal condition exists does not justify assigning a code from this series to the mother's record.

2) In utero surgery

In cases when surgery is performed on the fetus, a diagnosis code from category O35, Maternal care for known or suspected fetal abnormality and damage, should be assigned identifying the fetal condition. Assign the appropriate procedure code for the procedure performed.

No code from Chapter 16, the perinatal codes, should be used on the mother's record to identify fetal conditions. Surgery performed in utero on a fetus is still to be coded as an obstetric encounter.

f. HIV Infection in Pregnancy, Childbirth and the Puerperium

During pregnancy, childbirth or the puerperium, a patient admitted because of an HIV-related illness should receive a principal diagnosis from subcategory O98.7-, Human immunodeficiency [HIV] disease complicating pregnancy, childbirth and the puerperium, followed by the code(s) for the HIV-related illness(es).

Patients with asymptomatic HIV infection status admitted during pregnancy, childbirth, or the puerperium should receive codes of O98.7- and Z21, Asymptomatic human immunodeficiency virus [HIV] infection status.

g. Diabetes mellitus in pregnancy

Diabetes mellitus is a significant complicating factor in pregnancy. Pregnant women who are diabetic should be assigned a code from category O24, Diabetes mellitus in pregnancy, childbirth, and the puerperium, first, followed by the appropriate diabetes code(s) (E08-E13) from Chapter 4.

h. Long term use of insulin and oral hypoglycemics

See section I.C.4.a.3 for information on the long term use of insulin and oral hypoglycemic.

i. Gestational (pregnancy induced) diabetes

Gestational (pregnancy induced) diabetes can occur during the second and third trimester of pregnancy in women who were not diabetic prior to pregnancy. Gestational diabetes can cause complications in the pregnancy similar to those of pre-existing diabetes mellitus. It also puts the woman at greater risk of developing diabetes after the pregnancy. Codes for gestational diabetes are in subcategory O24.4, Gestational diabetes mellitus. No other code from category O24, Diabetes mellitus in pregnancy, childbirth, and the puerperium, should be used with a code from O24.4.

The codes under subcategory O24.4 include diet controlled, insulin controlled, and controlled by oral hypoglycemic drugs. If a patient with gestational diabetes is treated with both diet and insulin, only the code for insulin-controlled is required. If a patient with gestational diabetes is treated with both diet and oral hypoglycemic medications, only the code for "controlled by oral hypoglycemic drugs" is required. Code Z79.4, Long-term (current) use of insulin or code Z79.84, Long-term (current) use of oral hypoglycemic drugs, should not be assigned with codes from subcategory O24.4.

An abnormal glucose tolerance in pregnancy is assigned a code from subcategory O99.81, Abnormal glucose complicating pregnancy, childbirth, and the puerperium.

j. Sepsis and septic shock complicating abortion, pregnancy, childbirth and the puerperium

When assigning a chapter 15 code for sepsis complicating abortion, pregnancy, childbirth, and the puerperium, a code for the specific type of infection should be assigned as an additional diagnosis. If severe sepsis is present, a code from subcategory R65.2, Severe sepsis, and code(s) for associated organ dysfunction(s) should also be assigned as additional diagnoses.

k. Puerperal sepsis

Code O85, Puerperal sepsis, should be assigned with a secondary code to identify the causal organism (e.g., for a bacterial infection, assign a code from category B95-B96, Bacterial infections in conditions classified elsewhere). A code from category A40, Streptococcal sepsis, or A41, Other sepsis, should not be used for puerperal sepsis. If applicable, use additional codes to identify severe sepsis (R65.2-) and any associated acute organ dysfunction.

l. Alcohol, tobacco and drug use during pregnancy, childbirth and the puerperium

1) Alcohol use during pregnancy, childbirth and the puerperium

Codes under subcategory O99.31, Alcohol use complicating pregnancy, childbirth, and the puerperium, should be assigned for any pregnancy case when a mother uses alcohol during the pregnancy or postpartum. A secondary code from category F10, Alcohol related disorders, should also be assigned to identify manifestations of the alcohol use.

    2) **Tobacco use during pregnancy, childbirth and the puerperium**

    Codes under subcategory O99.33, Smoking (tobacco) complicating pregnancy, childbirth, and the puerperium, should be assigned for any pregnancy case when a mother uses any type of tobacco product during the pregnancy or postpartum. A secondary code from category F17, Nicotine dependence, should also be assigned to identify the type of nicotine dependence.

    3) **Drug use during pregnancy, childbirth and the puerperium**

    Codes under subcategory O99.32, Drug use complicating pregnancy, childbirth, and the puerperium, should be assigned for any pregnancy case when a mother uses drugs during the pregnancy or postpartum. This can involve illegal drugs, or inappropriate use or abuse of prescription drugs. Secondary code(s) from categories F11-F16 and F18-F19 should also be assigned to identify manifestations of the drug use.

m. **Poisoning, toxic effects, adverse effects and underdosing in a pregnant patient**

A code from subcategory O9A.2, Injury, poisoning and certain other consequences of external causes complicating pregnancy, childbirth, and the puerperium, should be sequenced first, followed by the appropriate injury, poisoning, toxic effect, adverse effect or underdosing code, and then the additional code(s) that specifies the condition caused by the poisoning, toxic effect, adverse effect or underdosing.

See Section I.C.19. Adverse effects, poisoning, underdosing and toxic effects.

n. **Normal Delivery, Code O80**

    1) **Encounter for full term uncomplicated delivery**

    Code O80 should be assigned when a woman is admitted for a full-term normal delivery and delivers a single, healthy infant without any complications antepartum, during the delivery, or postpartum during the delivery episode. Code O80 is always a principal diagnosis. It is not to be used if any other code from chapter 15 is needed to describe a current complication of the antenatal, delivery, or perinatal period. Additional codes from other chapters may be used with code O80 if they are not related to or are in any way complicating the pregnancy.

    2) **Uncomplicated delivery with resolved antepartum complication**

    Code O80 may be used if the patient had a complication at some point during the pregnancy, but the complication is not present at the time of the admission for delivery.

    3) **Outcome of delivery for O80**

    Z37.0, Single live birth, is the only outcome of delivery code appropriate for use with O80.

o. **The Peripartum and Postpartum Periods**

    1) **Peripartum and Postpartum periods**

    The postpartum period begins immediately after delivery and continues for six weeks following delivery. The peripartum period is defined as the last month of pregnancy to five months postpartum.

    2) **Peripartum and postpartum complication**

    A postpartum complication is any complication occurring within the six-week period.

    3) **Pregnancy-related complications after 6 week period**

    Chapter 15 codes may also be used to describe pregnancy-related complications after the peripartum or postpartum period if the provider documents that a condition is pregnancy related.

    4) **Admission for routine postpartum care following delivery outside hospital**

    When the mother delivers outside the hospital prior to admission and is admitted for routine postpartum care and no complications are noted, code Z39.0, Encounter for care and examination of mother immediately after delivery, should be assigned as the principal diagnosis.

    5) **Pregnancy associated cardiomyopathy**

    Pregnancy associated cardiomyopathy, code O90.3, is unique in that it may be diagnosed in the third trimester of pregnancy but may continue to progress months after delivery. For this reason, it is referred to as peripartum cardiomyopathy. Code O90.3 is only for use when the cardiomyopathy develops as a result of pregnancy in a woman who did not have pre-existing heart disease.

p. **Code O94, Sequelae of complication of pregnancy, childbirth, and the puerperium**

    1) **Code O94**

    Code O94, Sequelae of complication of pregnancy, childbirth, and the puerperium, is for use in those cases when an initial complication of a pregnancy develops a sequelae requiring care or treatment at a future date.

    2) **After the initial postpartum period**

    This code may be used at any time after the initial postpartum period.

    3) **Sequencing of Code O94**

    This code, like all sequela codes, is to be sequenced following the code describing the sequelae of the complication.

q. **Termination of Pregnancy and Spontaneous abortions**

    1) **Abortion with Liveborn Fetus**

    When an attempted termination of pregnancy results in a liveborn fetus, assign code Z33.2, Encounter for elective termination of pregnancy and a code from category Z37, Outcome of Delivery.

    2) **Retained Products of Conception following an abortion**

    Subsequent encounters for retained products of conception following a spontaneous abortion or elective termination of pregnancy, without complications are assigned O03.4, Incomplete spontaneous abortion without complication, or code O07.4, Failed attempted termination of pregnancy without complication. This advice is appropriate even when the patient was discharged previously with a discharge diagnosis of complete abortion. If the patient has a specific complication associated with the spontaneous abortion or elective termination of pregnancy in addition to retained products of conception, assign the appropriate complication in category O03 or O07 instead of code O03.4 or O07.4

    3) **Complications leading to abortion**

    Codes from Chapter 15 may be used as additional codes to identify any documented complications of the pregnancy in conjunction with codes in categories in O04, O07 and O08.

r. **Abuse in a pregnant patient**

For suspected or confirmed cases of abuse of a pregnant patient, a code(s) from subcategories O9A.3, Physical abuse complicating pregnancy, childbirth, and the puerperium, O9A.4, Sexual abuse complicating pregnancy, childbirth, and the puerperium, and O9A.5, Psychological abuse complicating pregnancy, childbirth, and the puerperium, should be sequenced first, followed by the appropriate codes (if applicable) to identify any associated current injury due to physical abuse, sexual abuse, and the perpetrator of abuse.

See Section I.C.19. Adult and child abuse, neglect and other maltreatment.

16. **Chapter 16: Certain Conditions Originating in the Perinatal Period (P00-P96)**

For coding and reporting purposes the perinatal period is defined as before birth through the 28th day following birth. The following guidelines are provided for reporting purposes.

a. **General Perinatal Rules**

    1) **Use of Chapter 16 Codes**

    Codes in this chapter are <u>never</u> for use on the maternal record. Codes from Chapter 15, the obstetric chapter, are never permitted on the newborn record. Chapter 16 codes may be used throughout the life of the patient if the condition is still present.

    2) **Principal Diagnosis for Birth Record**

    When coding the birth episode in a newborn record, assign a code from category Z38, Liveborn infants according to place of birth and type of delivery, as the principal diagnosis. A code from category Z38 is assigned only once, to a newborn at the time of birth. If a newborn is transferred to another institution, a code from category Z38 should not be used at the receiving hospital.

    A code from category Z38 is used only on the newborn record, not on the mother's record.

    3) **Use of Codes from other Chapters with Codes from Chapter 16**

    Codes from other chapters may be used with codes from chapter 16 if the codes from the other chapters provide more specific detail. Codes for signs and symptoms may be assigned when a definitive diagnosis has not been established. If the reason for the encounter is a perinatal condition, the code from chapter 16 should be sequenced first.

4) Use of Chapter 16 Codes after the Perinatal Period

Should a condition originate in the perinatal period, and continue throughout the life of the patient, the perinatal code should continue to be used regardless of the patient's age.

5) Birth process or community acquired conditions

If a newborn has a condition that may be either due to the birth process or community acquired and the documentation does not indicate which it is, the default is due to the birth process and the code from Chapter 16 should be used. If the condition is community-acquired, a code from Chapter 16 should not be assigned.

6) Code all clinically significant conditions

All clinically significant conditions noted on routine newborn examination should be coded. A condition is clinically significant if it requires:

- clinical evaluation; or
- therapeutic treatment; or
- diagnostic procedures; or
- extended length of hospital stay; or
- increased nursing care and/or monitoring; or
- has implications for future health care needs

Note: The perinatal guidelines listed above are the same as the general coding guidelines for "additional diagnoses", except for the final point regarding implications for future health care needs. Codes should be assigned for conditions that have been specified by the provider as having implications for future health care needs.

b. Observation and Evaluation of Newborns for Suspected Conditions not Found

1) Use of Z05 codes

Assign a code from category Z05, Observation and evaluation of newborns and infants for suspected conditions ruled out, to identify those instances when a healthy newborn is evaluated for a suspected condition that is determined after study not to be present. Do not use a code from category Z05 when the patient has identified signs or symptoms of a suspected problem; in such cases code the sign or symptom.

2) Z05 on Other than the Birth Record

A code from category Z05 may also be assigned as a principal or first-listed code for readmissions or encounters when the code from category Z38 code no longer applies. Codes from category Z05 are for use only for healthy newborns and infants for which no condition after study is found to be present.

3) Z05 on a birth record

A code from category Z05 is to be used as a secondary code after the code from category Z38, Liveborn infants according to place of birth and type of delivery.

c. Coding Additional Perinatal Diagnoses

1) Assigning codes for conditions that require treatment

Assign codes for conditions that require treatment or further investigation, prolong the length of stay, or require resource utilization.

2) Codes for conditions specified as having implications for future health care needs

Assign codes for conditions that have been specified by the provider as having implications for future health care needs.

Note: This guideline should not be used for adult patients.

d. Prematurity and Fetal Growth Retardation

Providers utilize different criteria in determining prematurity. A code for prematurity should not be assigned unless it is documented. Assignment of codes in categories P05, Disorders of newborn related to slow fetal growth and fetal malnutrition, and P07, Disorders of newborn related to short gestation and low birth weight, not elsewhere classified, should be based on the recorded birth weight and estimated gestational age.

When both birth weight and gestational age are available, two codes from category P07 should be assigned, with the code for birth weight sequenced before the code for gestational age.

e. Low birth weight and immaturity status

Codes from category P07, Disorders of newborn related to short gestation and low birth weight, not elsewhere classified, are for use for a child or adult who was premature or had a low birth weight as a newborn and this is affecting the patient's current health status.

See Section I.C.21. Factors influencing health status and contact with health services, Status.

f. Bacterial Sepsis of Newborn

Category P36, Bacterial sepsis of newborn, includes congenital sepsis. If a perinate is documented as having sepsis without documentation of congenital or community acquired, the default is congenital and a code from category P36 should be assigned. If the P36 code includes the causal organism, an additional code from category B95, Streptococcus, Staphylococcus, and Enterococcus as the cause of diseases classified elsewhere, or B96, Other bacterial agents as the cause of diseases classified elsewhere, should not be assigned. If the P36 code does not include the causal organism, assign an additional code from category B96. If applicable, use additional codes to identify severe sepsis (R65.2-) and any associated acute organ dysfunction.

g. Stillbirth

Code P95, Stillbirth, is only for use in institutions that maintain separate records for stillbirths. No other code should be used with P95. Code P95 should not be used on the mother's record.

17. Chapter 17: Congenital malformations, deformations, and chromosomal abnormalities (Q00-Q99)

Assign an appropriate code(s) from categories Q00-Q99, Congenital malformations, deformations, and chromosomal abnormalities when a malformation/deformation or chromosomal abnormality is documented. A malformation/deformation/or chromosomal abnormality may be the principal/first-listed diagnosis on a record or a secondary diagnosis.

When a malformation/deformation or chromosomal abnormality does not have a unique code assignment, assign additional code(s) for any manifestations that may be present.

When the code assignment specifically identifies the malformation/deformation or chromosomal abnormality, manifestations that are an inherent component of the anomaly should not be coded separately. Additional codes should be assigned for manifestations that are not an inherent component.

Codes from Chapter 17 may be used throughout the life of the patient. If a congenital malformation or deformity has been corrected, a personal history code should be used to identify the history of the malformation or deformity. Although present at birth, malformation/deformation/or chromosomal abnormality may not be identified until later in life. Whenever the condition is diagnosed by the physician, it is appropriate to assign a code from codes Q00-Q99. For the birth admission, the appropriate code from category Z38, Liveborn infants, according to place of birth and type of delivery, should be sequenced as the principal diagnosis, followed by any congenital anomaly codes, Q00- Q99.

18. Chapter 18: Symptoms, signs, and abnormal clinical and laboratory findings, not elsewhere classified (R00-R99)

Chapter 18 includes symptoms, signs, abnormal results of clinical or other investigative procedures, and ill-defined conditions regarding which no diagnosis classifiable elsewhere is recorded. Signs and symptoms that point to a specific diagnosis have been assigned to a category in other chapters of the classification.

a. Use of symptom codes

Codes that describe symptoms and signs are acceptable for reporting purposes when a related definitive diagnosis has not been established (confirmed) by the provider.

b. Use of a symptom code with a definitive diagnosis code

Codes for signs and symptoms may be reported in addition to a related definitive diagnosis when the sign or symptom is not routinely associated with that diagnosis, such as the various signs and symptoms associated with complex syndromes. The definitive diagnosis code should be sequenced before the symptom code.

Signs or symptoms that are associated routinely with a disease process should not be assigned as additional codes, unless otherwise instructed by the classification.

c. Combination codes that include symptoms

ICD-10-CM contains a number of combination codes that identify both the definitive diagnosis and common symptoms of that diagnosis.

When using one of these combination codes, an additional code should not be assigned for the symptom.

d. Repeated falls

Code R29.6, Repeated falls, is for use for encounters when a patient has recently fallen and the reason for the fall is being investigated.

Code Z91.81, History of falling, is for use when a patient has fallen in the past and is at risk for future falls. When appropriate, both codes R29.6 and Z91.81 may be assigned together.

e. **Coma scale**

The coma scale codes (R40.2-) can be used in conjunction with traumatic brain injury codes, acute cerebrovascular disease or sequelae of cerebrovascular disease codes. These codes are primarily for use by trauma registries, but they may be used in any setting where this information is collected. The coma scale may also be used to assess the status of the central nervous system for other non-trauma conditions, such as monitoring patients in the intensive care unit regardless of medical condition. The coma scale codes should be sequenced after the diagnosis code(s).

These codes, one from each subcategory, are needed to complete the scale. The 7th character indicates when the scale was recorded. The 7th character should match for all three codes.

At a minimum, report the initial score documented on presentation at your facility. This may be a score from the emergency medicine technician (EMT) or in the emergency department. If desired, a facility may choose to capture multiple coma scale scores.

Assign code R40.24, Glasgow coma scale, total score, when only the total score is documented in the medical record and not the individual score(s).

Do not report codes for individual or total Glasgow coma scale scores for a patient with a medically induced coma or a sedated patient.

See Section I.B.14 for coma scale documentation by clinicians other than patient's provider

f. **Functional quadriplegia**

GUIDELINE HAS BEEN DELETED EFFECTIVE OCTOBER 1, 2017

g. **SIRS due to Non-Infectious Process**

The systemic inflammatory response syndrome (SIRS) can develop as a result of certain non-infectious disease processes, such as trauma, malignant neoplasm, or pancreatitis. When SIRS is documented with a noninfectious condition, and no subsequent infection is documented, the code for the underlying condition, such as an injury, should be assigned, followed by code R65.10, Systemic inflammatory response syndrome (SIRS) of non-infectious origin without acute organ dysfunction, or code R65.11, Systemic inflammatory response syndrome (SIRS) of non-infectious origin with acute organ dysfunction. If an associated acute organ dysfunction is documented, the appropriate code(s) for the specific type of organ dysfunction(s) should be assigned in addition to code R65.11. If acute organ dysfunction is documented, but it cannot be determined if the acute organ dysfunction is associated with SIRS or due to another condition (e.g., directly due to the trauma), the provider should be queried.

h. **Death NOS**

Code R99, Ill-defined and unknown cause of mortality, is only for use in the very limited circumstance when a patient who has already died is brought into an emergency department or other healthcare facility and is pronounced dead upon arrival. It does not represent the discharge disposition of death.

i. **NIHSS Stroke Scale**

The NIH stroke scale (NIHSS) codes (R29.7- -) can be used in conjunction with acute stroke codes (I63) to identify the patient's neurological status and the severity of the stroke. The stroke scale codes should be sequenced after the acute stroke diagnosis code(s).

At a minimum, report the initial score documented. If desired, a facility may choose to capture multiple stroke scale scores.

See Section I.B.14 for NIHSS stroke scale documentation by clinicians other than patient's provider

19. **Chapter 19: Injury, poisoning, and certain other consequences of external causes (S00-T88)**

a. **Application of 7th Characters in Chapter 19**

Most categories in chapter 19 have a 7th character requirement for each applicable code. Most categories in this chapter have three 7th character values (with the exception of fractures): A, initial encounter, D, subsequent encounter and S, sequela. Categories for traumatic fractures have additional 7th character values. While the patient may be seen by a new or different provider over the course of treatment for an injury, assignment of the 7th character is based on whether the patient is undergoing active treatment and not whether the provider is seeing the patient for the first time.

For complication codes, active treatment refers to treatment for the condition described by the code, even though it may be related to an earlier precipitating problem. For example, code T84.50XA, Infection and inflammatory reaction due to unspecified internal joint prosthesis, initial encounter, is used when active treatment is provided for the infection, even though the condition relates to the prosthetic device, implant or graft that was placed at a previous encounter.

7th character "A", initial encounter is used for each encounter where the patient is receiving active treatment for the condition.

7th character "D" subsequent encounter is used for encounters after the patient has completed active treatment of the condition and is receiving routine care for the condition during the healing or recovery phase.

The aftercare Z codes should not be used for aftercare for conditions such as injuries or poisonings, where 7th characters are provided to identify subsequent care. For example, for aftercare of an injury, assign the acute injury code with the 7th character "D" (subsequent encounter).

7th character "S", sequela, is for use for complications or conditions that arise as a direct result of a condition, such as scar formation after a burn. The scars are sequelae of the burn. When using 7th character "S", it is necessary to use both the injury code that precipitated the sequela and the code for the sequela itself. The "S" is added only to the injury code, not the sequela code. The 7th character "S" identifies the injury responsible for the sequela. The specific type of sequela (e.g. scar) is sequenced first, followed by the injury code.

See Section I.B.10 Sequelae, (Late Effects)

b. **Coding of Injuries**

When coding injuries, assign separate codes for each injury unless a combination code is provided, in which case the combination code is assigned. Codes from category T07, Unspecified multiple injuries should not be assigned in the inpatient setting unless information for a more specific code is not available. Traumatic injury codes (S00-T14.9) are not to be used for normal, healing surgical wounds or to identify complications of surgical wounds.

The code for the most serious injury, as determined by the provider and the focus of treatment, is sequenced first.

1) **Superficial injuries**

Superficial injuries such as abrasions or contusions are not coded when associated with more severe injuries of the same site.

2) **Primary injury with damage to nerves/blood vessels**

When a primary injury results in minor damage to peripheral nerves or blood vessels, the primary injury is sequenced first with additional code(s) for injuries to nerves and spinal cord (such as category S04), and/or injury to blood vessels (such as category S15). When the primary injury is to the blood vessels or nerves, that injury should be sequenced first.

c. **Coding of Traumatic Fractures**

The principles of multiple coding of injuries should be followed in coding fractures. Fractures of specified sites are coded individually by site in accordance with both the provisions within categories S02, S12, S22, S32, S42, S49, S52, S59, S62, S72, S79, S82, S89, S92 and the level of detail furnished by medical record content.

A fracture not indicated as open or closed should be coded to closed. A fracture not indicated whether displaced or not displaced should be coded to displaced.

More specific guidelines are as follows:

1) **Initial vs. Subsequent Encounter for Fractures**

Traumatic fractures are coded using the appropriate 7th character for initial encounter (A, B, C) for each encounter where the patient is receiving active treatment for the fracture. The appropriate 7th character for initial encounter should also be assigned for a patient who delayed seeking treatment for the fracture or nonunion.

Fractures are coded using the appropriate 7th character for subsequent care for encounters after the patient has completed active treatment of the fracture and is receiving routine care for the fracture during the healing or recovery phase.

Care for complications of surgical treatment for fracture repairs during the healing or recovery phase should be coded with the appropriate complication codes.

Care of complications of fractures, such as malunion and nonunion, should be reported with the appropriate 7th character for subsequent care with nonunion (K, M, N,) or subsequent care with malunion (P, Q, R).

Malunion/nonunion: The appropriate 7th character for initial encounter should also be assigned for a patient who delayed seeking treatment for the fracture or nonunion.

The open fracture designations in the assignment of the 7th character for fractures of the forearm, femur and lower leg, including ankle are based on the Gustilo open fracture classification. When the Gustilo classification type is not specified for an open fracture, the 7th character for open fracture type I or II should be assigned (B, E, H, M, Q).

A code from category M80, not a traumatic fracture code, should be used for any patient with known osteoporosis who suffers a fracture, even if the patient had a minor fall or trauma, if that fall or trauma would not usually break a normal, healthy bone.

See Section I.C.13. Osteoporosis.

The aftercare Z codes should not be used for aftercare for traumatic fractures. For aftercare of a traumatic fracture, assign the acute fracture code with the appropriate 7th character.

2) Multiple fractures sequencing

Multiple fractures are sequenced in accordance with the severity of the fracture.

d. Coding of Burns and Corrosions

The ICD-10-CM makes a distinction between burns and corrosions. The burn codes are for thermal burns, except sunburns, that come from a heat source, such as a fire or hot appliance. The burn codes are also for burns resulting from electricity and radiation. Corrosions are burns due to chemicals. The guidelines are the same for burns and corrosions.

Current burns (T20-T25) are classified by depth, extent and by agent (X code). Burns are classified by depth as first degree (erythema), second degree (blistering), and third degree (full-thickness involvement). Burns of the eye and internal organs (T26-T28) are classified by site, but not by degree.

1) Sequencing of burn and related condition codes

Sequence first the code that reflects the highest degree of burn when more than one burn is present.

a. When the reason for the admission or encounter is for treatment of external multiple burns, sequence first the code that reflects the burn of the highest degree.

b. When a patient has both internal and external burns, the circumstances of admission govern the selection of the principal diagnosis or first-listed diagnosis.

c. When a patient is admitted for burn injuries and other related conditions such as smoke inhalation and/or respiratory failure, the circumstances of admission govern the selection of the principal or first-listed diagnosis.

2) Burns of the same *anatomic* site

Classify burns of the same **anatomic** site **and on the same side** but of different degrees to the subcategory identifying the highest degree recorded in the diagnosis **(e.g., for second and third degree burns of right thigh, assign only code T24.311-).**

3) Non-healing burns

Non-healing burns are coded as acute burns.

Necrosis of burned skin should be coded as a non-healed burn.

4) Infected Burn

For any documented infected burn site, use an additional code for the infection.

5) Assign separate codes for each burn site

When coding burns, assign separate codes for each burn site. Category T30, Burn and corrosion, body region unspecified is extremely vague and should rarely be used.

Codes for burns of "multiple sites" should only be assigned when the medical record documentation does not specify the individual sites.

6) Burns and Corrosions Classified According to Extent of Body Surface Involved

Assign codes from category T31, Burns classified according to extent of body surface involved, or T32, Corrosions classified according to extent of body surface involved, when the site of the burn is not specified or when there is a need for additional data. It is advisable to use category T31 as additional coding when needed to provide data for evaluating burn mortality, such as that needed by burn units. It is also advisable to use category T31 as an additional code for reporting purposes when there is

mention of a third-degree burn involving 20 percent or more of the body surface.

Categories T31 and T32 are based on the classic "rule of nines" in estimating body surface involved: head and neck are assigned nine percent, each arm nine percent, each leg 18 percent, the anterior trunk 18 percent, posterior trunk 18 percent, and genitalia one percent. Providers may change these percentage assignments where necessary to accommodate infants and children who have proportionately larger heads than adults, and patients who have large buttocks, thighs, or abdomen that involve burns.

7) Encounters for treatment of sequela of burns

Encounters for the treatment of the late effects of burns or corrosions (i.e., scars or joint contractures) should be coded with a burn or corrosion code with the 7th character "S" for sequela.

8) Sequelae with a late effect code and current burn

When appropriate, both a code for a current burn or corrosion with 7th character "A" or "D" and a burn or corrosion code with 7th character "S" may be assigned on the same record (when both a current burn and sequelae of an old burn exist). Burns and corrosions do not heal at the same rate and a current healing wound may still exist with sequela of a healed burn or corrosion.

See Section I.B.10 Sequela (Late Effects)

9) Use of an external cause code with burns and corrosions

An external cause code should be used with burns and corrosions to identify the source and intent of the burn, as well as the place where it occurred.

e. Adverse Effects, Poisoning, Underdosing and Toxic Effects

Codes in categories T36-T65 are combination codes that include the substance that was taken as well as the intent. No additional external cause code is required for poisonings, toxic effects, adverse effects and underdosing codes.

1) Do not code directly from the Table of Drugs

Do not code directly funderdosinrom the Table of Drugs and Chemicals. Always refer back to the Tabular List.

2) Use as many codes as necessary to describe

Use as many codes as necessary to describe completely all drugs, medicinal or biological substances.

3) If the same code would describe the causative agent

If the same code would describe the causative agent for more than one adverse reaction, poisoning, toxic effect or underdosing, assign the code only once.

4) If two or more drugs, medicinal or biological substances

If two or more drugs, medicinal or biological substances are reported, code each individually unless a combination code is listed in the Table of Drugs and Chemicals.

5) The occurrence of drug toxicity is classified in ICD-10-CM as follows:

(a) Adverse Effect

When coding an adverse effect of a drug that has been correctly prescribed and properly administered, assign the appropriate code for the nature of the adverse effect followed by the appropriate code for the adverse effect of the drug (T36-T50). The code for the drug should have a 5th or 6th character "5" (for example T36.0X5-) Examples of the nature of an adverse effect are tachycardia, delirium, gastrointestinal hemorrhaging, vomiting, hypokalemia, hepatitis, renal failure, or respiratory failure.

(b) Poisoning

When coding a poisoning or reaction to the improper use of a medication (e.g., overdose, wrong substance given or taken in error, wrong route of administration), first assign the appropriate code from categories T36-T50. The poisoning codes have an associated intent as their 5th or 6th character (accidental, intentional self-harm, assault and undetermined. If the intent of the poisoning is unknown or unspecified, code the intent as accidental intent. The undetermined intent is only for use if the documentation in the record specifies that the intent cannot be determined. Use additional code(s) for all manifestations of poisonings.

If there is also a diagnosis of abuse or dependence of the substance, the abuse or dependence is assigned as an additional code.

Examples of poisoning include:

(i) Error was made in drug prescription
Errors made in drug prescription or in the administration of the drug by provider, nurse, patient, or other person.

(ii) Overdose of a drug intentionally taken
If an overdose of a drug was intentionally taken or administered and resulted in drug toxicity, it would be coded as a poisoning.

(iii) Nonprescribed drug taken with correctly prescribed and properly administered drug
If a nonprescribed drug or medicinal agent was taken in combination with a correctly prescribed and properly administered drug, any drug toxicity or other reaction resulting from the interaction of the two drugs would be classified as a poisoning.

(iv) Interaction of drug(s) and alcohol
When a reaction results from the interaction of a drug(s) and alcohol, this would be classified as poisoning.

See Section I.C.4. if poisoning is the result of insulin pump malfunctions.

(c) Underdosing
Underdosing refers to taking less of a medication than is prescribed by a provider or a manufacturer's instruction. **Discontinuing the use of a prescribed medication on the patient's own initiative (not directed by the patient's provider) is also classified as an underdosing.** For underdosing, assign the code from categories T36-T50 (fifth or sixth character "6").

Codes for underdosing should never be assigned as principal or first-listed codes. If a patient has a relapse or exacerbation of the medical condition for which the drug is prescribed because of the reduction in dose, then the medical condition itself should be coded.

Noncompliance (Z91.12-, Z91.13- **and Z91.14-**) or complication of care (Y63.6-Y63.9) codes are to be used with an underdosing code to indicate intent, if known.

(d) Toxic Effects
When a harmful substance is ingested or comes in contact with a person, this is classified as a toxic effect. The toxic effect codes are in categories T51-T65.

Toxic effect codes have an associated intent: accidental, intentional self-harm, assault and undetermined.

f. Adult and child abuse, neglect and other maltreatment
Sequence first the appropriate code from categories T74, Adult and child abuse, neglect and other maltreatment, confirmed) or T76, Adult and child abuse, neglect and other maltreatment, suspected) for abuse, neglect and other maltreatment, followed by any accompanying mental health or injury code(s).

If the documentation in the medical record states abuse or neglect it is coded as confirmed (T74.-). It is coded as suspected if it is documented as suspected (T76.-).

For cases of confirmed abuse or neglect an external cause code from the assault section (X92-Y09) should be added to identify the cause of any physical injuries. A perpetrator code (Y07) should be added when the perpetrator of the abuse is known. For suspected cases of abuse or neglect, do not report external cause or perpetrator code.

If a suspected case of abuse, neglect or mistreatment is ruled out during an encounter code Z04.71, Encounter for examination and observation following alleged physical adult abuse, ruled out, or code Z04.72, Encounter for examination and observation following alleged child physical abuse, ruled out, should be used, not a code from T76.

If a suspected case of alleged rape or sexual abuse is ruled out during an encounter code Z04.41, Encounter for examination and observation following alleged adult rape or code Z04.42, Encounter for examination and observation following alleged child rape, should be used, not a code from T76.

If a suspected case of forced sexual exploitation or forced labor exploitation is ruled out during an encounter, code Z04.81, Encounter for examination and observation of victim following forced sexual exploitation, or code Z04.82, Encounter for examination and observation of victim following forced labor exploitation, should be used, not a code from T76.
See Section I.C.15. Abuse in a pregnant patient.

g. Complications of care
1) General guidelines for complications of care
(a) Documentation of complications of care
See Section I.B.16. for information on documentation of complications of care.

2) Pain due to medical devices
Pain associated with devices, implants or grafts left in a surgical site (for example painful hip prosthesis) is assigned to the appropriate code(s) found in Chapter 19, Injury, poisoning, and certain other consequences of external causes. Specific codes for pain due to medical devices are found in the T code section of the ICD-10-CM. Use additional code(s) from category G89 to identify acute or chronic pain due to presence of the device, implant or graft (G89.18 or G89.28).

3) Transplant complications
(a) Transplant complications other than kidney
Codes under category T86, Complications of transplanted organs and tissues, are for use for both complications and rejection of transplanted organs. A transplant complication code is only assigned if the complication affects the function of the transplanted organ. Two codes are required to fully describe a transplant complication: the appropriate code from category T86 and a secondary code that identifies the complication.

Pre-existing conditions or conditions that develop after the transplant are not coded as complications unless they affect the function of the transplanted organs.

See I.C.21. for transplant organ removal status
See I.C.2. for malignant neoplasm associated with transplanted organ.

(b) Kidney transplant complications
Patients who have undergone kidney transplant may still have some form of chronic kidney disease (CKD) because the kidney transplant may not fully restore kidney function. Code T86.1- should be assigned for documented complications of a kidney transplant, such as transplant failure or rejection or other transplant complication. Code T86.1- should not be assigned for post kidney transplant patients who have chronic kidney (CKD) unless a transplant complication such as transplant failure or rejection is documented. If the documentation is unclear as to whether the patient has a complication of the transplant, query the provider.

Conditions that affect the function of the transplanted kidney, other than CKD, should be assigned a code from subcategory T86.1, Complications of transplanted organ, Kidney, and a secondary code that identifies the complication.

For patients with CKD following a kidney transplant, but who do not have a complication such as failure or rejection, *see section I.C.14. Chronic kidney disease and kidney transplant status.*

4) Complication codes that include the external cause
As with certain other T codes, some of the complications of care codes have the external cause included in the code. The code includes the nature of the complication as well as the type of procedure that caused the complication. No external cause code indicating the type of procedure is necessary for these codes.

5) Complications of care codes within the body system chapters
Intraoperative and postprocedural complication codes are found within the body system chapters with codes specific to the organs and structures of that body system. These codes should be sequenced first, followed by a code(s) for the specific complication, if applicable.

20. Chapter 20: External Causes of Morbidity (V00-Y99)
The external causes of morbidity codes should never be sequenced as the first-listed or principal diagnosis.

External cause codes are intended to provide data for injury research and evaluation of injury prevention strategies. These codes capture how the injury or health condition happened (cause), the intent (unintentional or accidental; or intentional, such as suicide or assault), the place where the event occurred the activity of the patient at the time of the event, and the person's status (e.g., civilian, military).

There is no national requirement for mandatory ICD-10-CM external cause code reporting. Unless a provider is subject to a state-based external cause code reporting mandate or these codes are required by a particular payer, reporting of ICD-10-CM codes in Chapter 20, External Causes of Morbidity, is not required. In the absence of a mandatory reporting requirement, providers are encouraged to voluntarily report external cause codes, as they provide valuable data for injury research and evaluation of injury prevention strategies.

a. General External Cause Coding Guidelines

1) Used with any code in the range of A00.0-T88.9 Z00-Z99

An external cause code may be used with any code in the range of A00.0-T88.9, Z00-Z99, classification that represents a health condition due to an external cause. Though they are most applicable to injuries, they are also valid for use with such things as infections or diseases due to an external source, and other health conditions, such as a heart attack that occurs during strenuous physical activity.

2) External cause code used for length of treatment

Assign the external cause code, with the appropriate 7th character (initial encounter, subsequent encounter or sequela) for each encounter for which the injury or condition is being treated.

Most categories in chapter 20 have a 7th character requirement for each applicable code. Most categories in this chapter have three 7th character values: A, initial encounter, D, subsequent encounter and S, sequela. While the patient may be seen by a new or different provider over the course of treatment for an injury or condition, assignment of the 7th character for external cause should match the 7th character of the code assigned for the associated injury or condition for the encounter.

3) Use the full range of external cause codes

Use the full range of external cause codes to completely describe the cause, the intent, the place of occurrence, and if applicable, the activity of the patient at the time of the event, and the patient's status, for all injuries, and other health conditions due to an external cause.

4) Assign as many external cause codes as necessary

Assign as many external cause codes as necessary to fully explain each cause. If only one external code can be recorded, assign the code most related to the principal diagnosis.

5) The selection of the appropriate external cause code

The selection of the appropriate external cause code is guided by the Alphabetic Index of External Causes and by Inclusion and Exclusion notes in the Tabular List.

6) External cause code can never be a principal diagnosis

An external cause code can never be a principal (first-listed) diagnosis.

7) Combination external cause codes

Certain of the external cause codes are combination codes that identify sequential events that result in an injury, such as a fall which results in striking against an object. The injury may be due to either event or both. The combination external cause code used should correspond to the sequence of events regardless of which caused the most serious injury.

8) No external cause code needed in certain circumstances

No external cause code from Chapter 20 is needed if the external cause and intent are included in a code from another chapter (e.g. T36.0X1- Poisoning by penicillins, accidental (unintentional)).

b. Place of Occurrence Guideline

Codes from category Y92, Place of occurrence of the external cause, are secondary codes for use after other external cause codes to identify the location of the patient at the time of injury or other condition.

Generally, a place of occurrence code is assigned only once, at the initial encounter for treatment. However, in the rare instance that a new injury occurs during hospitalization, an additional place of occurrence code may be assigned. No 7th characters are used for Y92.

Do not use place of occurrence code Y92.9 if the place is not stated or is not applicable.

c. Activity Code

Assign a code from category Y93, Activity code, to describe the activity of the patient at the time the injury or other health condition occurred.

An activity code is used only once, at the initial encounter for treatment. Only one code from Y93 should be recorded on a medical record.

The activity codes are not applicable to poisonings, adverse effects, misadventures or sequela.

Do not assign Y93.9, Unspecified activity, if the activity is not stated.

A code from category Y93 is appropriate for use with external cause and intent codes if identifying the activity provides additional information about the event.

d. Place of Occurrence, Activity, and Status Codes Used with other External Cause Code

When applicable, place of occurrence, activity, and external cause status codes are sequenced after the main external cause code(s). Regardless of the number of external cause codes assigned, generally there should be only one place of occurrence code, one activity code, and one external cause status code assigned to an encounter. However, in the rare instance that a new injury occurs during hospitalization, an additional place of occurrence code may be assigned.

e. If the Reporting Format Limits the Number of External Cause Codes

If the reporting format limits the number of external cause codes that can be used in reporting clinical data, report the code for the cause/intent most related to the principal diagnosis. If the format permits capture of additional external cause codes, the cause/intent, including medical misadventures, of the additional events should be reported rather than the codes for place, activity, or external status.

f. Multiple External Cause Coding Guidelines

More than one external cause code is required to fully describe the external cause of an illness or injury. The assignment of external cause codes should be sequenced in the following priority:

If two or more events cause separate injuries, an external cause code should be assigned for each cause. The first-listed external cause code will be selected in the following order:

External codes for child and adult abuse take priority over all other external cause codes.

See Section I.C.19., Child and Adult abuse guidelines.

External cause codes for terrorism events take priority over all other external cause codes except child and adult abuse.

External cause codes for cataclysmic events take priority over all other external cause codes except child and adult abuse and terrorism.

External cause codes for transport accidents take priority over all other external cause codes except cataclysmic events, child and adult abuse and terrorism.

Activity and external cause status codes are assigned following all causal (intent) external cause codes.

The first-listed external cause code should correspond to the cause of the most serious diagnosis due to an assault, accident, or self-harm, following the order of hierarchy listed above.

g. Child and Adult Abuse Guideline

Adult and child abuse, neglect and maltreatment are classified as assault. Any of the assault codes may be used to indicate the external cause of any injury resulting from the confirmed abuse.

For confirmed cases of abuse, neglect and maltreatment, when the perpetrator is known, a code from Y07, Perpetrator of maltreatment and neglect, should accompany any other assault codes.

See Section I.C.19. Adult and child abuse, neglect and other maltreatment

h. Unknown or Undetermined Intent Guideline

If the intent (accident, self-harm, assault) of the cause of an injury or other condition is unknown or unspecified, code the intent as accidental intent. All transport accident categories assume accidental intent.

1) Use of undetermined intent

External cause codes for events of undetermined intent are only for use if the documentation in the record specifies that the intent cannot be determined.

i. Sequelae (Late Effects) of External Cause Guidelines

1) Sequelae external cause codes

Sequela are reported using the external cause code with the 7th character "S" for sequela. These codes should be used with any report of a late effect or sequela resulting from a previous injury.

See Section I.B.10 Sequela (Late Effects)

2) **Sequela external cause code with a related current injury**
A sequela external cause code should never be used with a related current nature of injury code.

3) **Use of sequela external cause codes for subsequent visits**
Use a late effect external cause code for subsequent visits when a late effect of the initial injury is being treated. Do not use a late effect external cause code for subsequent visits for follow-up care (e.g., to assess healing, to receive rehabilitative therapy) of the injury when no late effect of the injury has been documented.

j. **Terrorism Guidelines**
1) **Cause of injury identified by the Federal Government (FBI) as terrorism**
When the cause of an injury is identified by the Federal Government (FBI) as terrorism, the first-listed external cause code should be a code from category Y38, Terrorism. The definition of terrorism employed by the FBI is found at the inclusion note at the beginning of category Y38. Use additional code for place of occurrence (Y92.-). More than one Y38 code may be assigned if the injury is the result of more than one mechanism of terrorism.

2) **Cause of an injury is suspected to be the result of terrorism**
When the cause of an injury is suspected to be the result of terrorism a code from category Y38 should not be assigned. Suspected cases should be classified as assault.

3) **Code Y38.9, Terrorism, secondary effects**
Assign code Y38.9, Terrorism, secondary effects, for conditions occurring subsequent to the terrorist event. This code should not be assigned for conditions that are due to the initial terrorist act.

It is acceptable to assign code Y38.9 with another code from Y38 if there is an injury due to the initial terrorist event and an injury that is a subsequent result of the terrorist event.

k. **External cause status**
A code from category Y99, External cause status, should be assigned whenever any other external cause code is assigned for an encounter, including an Activity code, except for the events noted below. Assign a code from category Y99, External cause status, to indicate the work status of the person at the time the event occurred. The status code indicates whether the event occurred during military activity, whether a non-military person was at work, whether an individual including a student or volunteer was involved in a non-work activity at the time of the causal event.

A code from Y99, External cause status, should be assigned, when applicable, with other external cause codes, such as transport accidents and falls. The external cause status codes are not applicable to poisonings, adverse effects, misadventures or late effects.

Do not assign a code from category Y99 if no other external cause codes (cause, activity) are applicable for the encounter.

An external cause status code is used only once, at the initial encounter for treatment. Only one code from Y99 should be recorded on a medical record.

Do not assign code Y99.9, Unspecified external cause status, if the status is not stated.

21. **Chapter 21: Factors influencing health status and contact with health services (Z00-Z99)**
Note: The chapter specific guidelines provide additional information about the use of Z codes for specified encounters.

a. **Use of Z codes in any healthcare setting**
Z codes are for use in any healthcare setting. Z codes may be used as either a first-listed (principal diagnosis code in the inpatient setting) or secondary code, depending on the circumstances of the encounter. Certain Z codes may only be used as first-listed or principal diagnosis.

b. **Z Codes indicate a reason for an encounter**
Z codes are not procedure codes. A corresponding procedure code must accompany a Z code to describe any procedure performed.

c. **Categories of Z Codes**
1) **Contact/Exposure**
Category Z20 indicates contact with, and suspected exposure to, communicable diseases. These codes are for patients who do not show any sign or symptom of a disease but are suspected to have been exposed to it by close personal contact with an infected individual or are in an area where a disease is epidemic.

Category Z77, Other contact with and (suspected) exposures hazardous to health, indicates contact with and suspected exposures hazardous to health.

Contact/exposure codes may be used as a first-listed code to explain an encounter for testing, or, more commonly, as a secondary code to identify a potential risk.

2) **Inoculations and vaccinations**
Code Z23 is for encounters for inoculations and vaccinations. It indicates that a patient is being seen to receive a prophylactic inoculation against a disease. Procedure codes are required to identify the actual administration of the injection and the type(s) of immunizations given. Code Z23 may be used as a secondary code if the inoculation is given as a routine part of preventive health care, such as a well-baby visit.

3) **Status**
Status codes indicate that a patient is either a carrier of a disease or has the sequelae or residual of a past disease or condition. This includes such things as the presence of prosthetic or mechanical devices resulting from past treatment. A status code is informative, because the status may affect the course of treatment and its outcome. A status code is distinct from a history code. The history code indicates that the patient no longer has the condition.

A status code should not be used with a diagnosis code from one of the body system chapters, if the diagnosis code includes the information provided by the status code. For example, code Z94.1, Heart transplant status, should not be used with a code from subcategory T86.2, Complications of heart transplant. The status code does not provide additional information. The complication code indicates that the patient is a heart transplant patient.

For encounters for weaning from a mechanical ventilator, assign a code from subcategory J96.1, Chronic respiratory failure, followed by code Z99.11, Dependence on respirator [ventilator] status.

The status Z codes/categories are:

Z14   Genetic carrier

Genetic carrier status indicates that a person carries a gene, associated with a particular disease, which may be passed to offspring who may develop that disease. The person does not have the disease and is not at risk of developing the disease.

Z15   Genetic susceptibility to disease

Genetic susceptibility indicates that a person has a gene that increases the risk of that person developing the disease.

Codes from category Z15 should not be used as principal or first-listed codes. If the patient has the condition to which he/she is susceptible, and that condition is the reason for the encounter, the code for the current condition should be sequenced first. If the patient is being seen for follow-up after completed treatment for this condition, and the condition no longer exists, a follow-up code should be sequenced first, followed by the appropriate personal history and genetic susceptibility codes. If the purpose of the encounter is genetic counseling associated with procreative management, code Z31.5, Encounter for genetic counseling, should be assigned as the first-listed code, followed by a code from category Z15. Additional codes should be assigned for any applicable family or personal history.

Z16   Resistance to antimicrobial drugs

This code indicates that a patient has a condition that is resistant to antimicrobial drug treatment. Sequence the infection code first.

Z17   Estrogen receptor status

Z18   Retained foreign body fragments

Z19   Hormone sensitivity malignancy status

Z21   Asymptomatic HIV infection status

This code indicates that a patient has tested positive for HIV but has manifested no signs or symptoms of the disease.

Z22   Carrier of infectious disease

Carrier status indicates that a person harbors the specific organisms of a disease without manifest symptoms and is capable of transmitting the infection.

Z28.3   Underimmunization status

Z33.1   Pregnant state, incidental

This code is a secondary code only for use when the pregnancy is in no way complicating the reason for visit. Otherwise, a code from the obstetric chapter is required.

Z66   Do not resuscitate

This code may be used when it is documented by the provider that a patient is on do not resuscitate status at any time during the stay.

Z67   Blood type

Z68   Body mass index (BMI)

BMI codes should only be assigned when the associated diagnosis (such as overweight or obesity) meets the definition of a reportable diagnosis (see Section III, Reporting Additional Diagnoses). **Do not assign BMI codes during pregnancy.** *See Section I.B.14 for BMI documentation by clinicians other than the patient's provider.*

Z74.01   Bed confinement status

Z76.82   Awaiting organ transplant status

Z78   Other specified health status

Code Z78.1, Physical restraint status, may be used when it is documented by the provider that a patient has been put in restraints during the current encounter. Please note that this code should not be reported when it is documented by the provider that a patient is temporarily restrained during a procedure.

Z79   Long-term (current) drug therapy

Codes from this category indicate a patient's continuous use of a prescribed drug (including such things as aspirin therapy) for the long-term treatment of a condition or for prophylactic use. It is not for use for patients who have addictions to drugs. This subcategory is not for use of medications for detoxification or maintenance programs to prevent withdrawal symptoms in patients with drug dependence (e.g., methadone maintenance for opiate dependence). Assign the appropriate code for the drug dependence instead.

Assign a code from Z79 if the patient is receiving a medication for an extended period as a prophylactic measure (such as for the prevention of deep vein thrombosis) or as treatment of a chronic condition (such as arthritis) or a disease requiring a lengthy course of treatment (such as cancer). Do not assign a code from category Z79 for medication being administered for a brief period of time to treat an acute illness or injury (such as a course of antibiotics to treat acute bronchitis).

Z88   Allergy status to drugs, medicaments and biological substances

Except: Z88.9, Allergy status to unspecified drugs, medicaments and biological substances status

Z89   Acquired absence of limb

Z90   Acquired absence of organs, not elsewhere classified

Z91.0-   Allergy status, other than to drugs and biological substances

Z92.82   Status post administration of tPA (rtPA) in a different facility within the last 24 hours prior to admission to a current facility

Assign code Z92.82, Status post administration of tPA (rtPA) in a different facility within the last 24 hours prior to admission to current facility, as a secondary diagnosis when a patient is received by transfer into a facility and documentation indicates they were administered tissue plasminogen activator (tPA) within the last 24 hours prior to admission to the current facility.

This guideline applies even if the patient is still receiving the tPA at the time they are received into the current facility.

The appropriate code for the condition for which the tPA was administered (such as cerebrovascular disease or myocardial infarction) should be assigned first.

Code Z92.82 is only applicable to the receiving facility record and not to the transferring facility record.

Z93   Artificial opening status

Z94   Transplanted organ and tissue status

Z95   Presence of cardiac and vascular implants and grafts

Z96   Presence of other functional implants

Z97   Presence of other devices

Z98   Other postprocedural states

Assign code Z98.85, Transplanted organ removal status, to indicate that a transplanted organ has been previously removed. This code should not be assigned for the encounter in which the transplanted organ is removed. The complication necessitating removal of the transplant organ should be assigned for that encounter.

See section I.C19. for information on the coding of organ transplant complications.

Z99   Dependence on enabling machines and devices, not elsewhere classified

Note: Categories Z89-Z90 and Z93-Z99 are for use only if there are no complications or malfunctions of the organ or tissue replaced, the amputation site or the equipment on which the patient is dependent.

4)   **History (of)**

There are two types of history Z codes, personal and family. Personal history codes explain a patient's past medical condition that no longer exists and is not receiving any treatment, but that has the potential for recurrence, and therefore may require continued monitoring.

Family history codes are for use when a patient has a family member(s) who has had a particular disease that causes the patient to be at higher risk of also contracting the disease.

Personal history codes may be used in conjunction with follow-up codes and family history codes may be used in conjunction with screening codes to explain the need for a test or procedure. History codes are also acceptable on any medical record regardless of the reason for visit. A history of an illness, even if no longer present, is important information that may alter the type of treatment ordered.

The history Z code categories are:

Z80   Family history of primary malignant neoplasm

Z81   Family history of mental and behavioral disorders

Z82   Family history of certain disabilities and chronic diseases (leading to disablement)

Z83   Family history of other specific disorders

Z84   Family history of other conditions

Z85   Personal history of malignant neoplasm

Z86   Personal history of certain other diseases

Z87   Personal history of other diseases and conditions

Z91.4-   Personal history of psychological trauma, not elsewhere classified

Z91.5   Personal history of self-harm

Z91.81 History of falling

Z91.82 Personal history of military deployment

Z92   Personal history of medical treatment

Except: Z92.0, Personal history of contraception

Except: Z92.82, Status post administration of tPA (rtPA) in a different facility within the last 24 hours prior to admission to a current facility

5)   **Screening**

Screening is the testing for disease or disease precursors in seemingly well individuals so that early detection and treatment can be provided for those who test positive for the disease (e.g., screening mammogram).

The testing of a person to rule out or confirm a suspected diagnosis because the patient has some sign or symptom is a diagnostic examination, not a screening. In these cases, the sign or symptom is used to explain the reason for the test.

A screening code may be a first-listed code if the reason for the visit is specifically the screening exam. It may also be used as an additional code if the screening is done during an office visit for other health problems. A screening code is not necessary if the screening is inherent to a routine examination, such as a pap smear done during a routine pelvic examination.

Should a condition be discovered during the screening then the code for the condition may be assigned as an additional diagnosis.

The Z code indicates that a screening exam is planned. A procedure code is required to confirm that the screening was performed.

The screening Z codes/categories:

Z11   Encounter for screening for infectious and parasitic diseases

Z12   Encounter for screening for malignant neoplasms

Z13   Encounter for screening for other diseases and disorders
    Except: Z13.9, Encounter for screening, unspecified

Z36   Encounter for antenatal screening for mother

6) Observation

There are three observation Z code categories. They are for use in very limited circumstances when a person is being observed for a suspected condition that is ruled out. The observation codes are not for use if an injury or illness or any signs or symptoms related to the suspected condition are present. In such cases the diagnosis/symptom code is used with the corresponding external cause code.

The observation codes are to be used as principal diagnosis only. The only exception to this is when the principal diagnosis is required to be a code from category Z38, Liveborn infants according to place of birth and type of delivery. Then a code from category Z05, Encounter for observation and evaluation of newborn for suspected diseases and conditions ruled out, is sequenced after the Z38 code. Additional codes may be used in addition to the observation code, but only if they are unrelated to the suspected condition being observed.

Codes from subcategory Z03.7, Encounter for suspected maternal and fetal conditions ruled out, may either be used as a first-listed or as an additional code assignment depending on the case. They are for use in very limited circumstances on a maternal record when an encounter is for a suspected maternal or fetal condition that is ruled out during that encounter (for example, a maternal or fetal condition may be suspected due to an abnormal test result). These codes should not be used when the condition is confirmed. In those cases, the confirmed condition should be coded. In addition, these codes are not for use if an illness or any signs or symptoms related to the suspected condition or problem are present. In such cases the diagnosis/symptom code is used.

Additional codes may be used in addition to the code from subcategory Z03.7, but only if they are unrelated to the suspected condition being evaluated.

Codes from subcategory Z03.7 may not be used for encounters for antenatal screening of mother. *See Section I.C.21. Screening.*

For encounters for suspected fetal condition that are inconclusive following testing and evaluation, assign the appropriate code from category O35, O36, O40 or O41.

The observation Z code categories:

Z03   Encounter for medical observation for suspected diseases and conditions ruled out

Z04   Encounter for examination and observation for other reasons
    Except: Z04.9, Encounter for examination and observation for unspecified reason

Z05   Encounter for observation and evaluation of newborn for suspected diseases and conditions ruled out

7) Aftercare

Aftercare visit codes cover situations when the initial treatment of a disease has been performed and the patient requires continued care during the healing or recovery phase, or for the long-term consequences of the disease. The aftercare Z code should not be used if treatment is directed at a current, acute disease. The diagnosis code is to be used in these cases. Exceptions to this rule are codes Z51.0, Encounter for antineoplastic radiation therapy,

and codes from subcategory Z51.1, Encounter for antineoplastic chemotherapy and immunotherapy. These codes are to be first-listed, followed by the diagnosis code when a patient's encounter is solely to receive radiation therapy, chemotherapy, or immunotherapy for the treatment of a neoplasm. If the reason for the encounter is more than one type of antineoplastic therapy, code Z51.0 and a code from subcategory Z51.1 may be assigned together, in which case one of these codes would be reported as a secondary diagnosis.

The aftercare Z codes should also not be used for aftercare for injuries. For aftercare of an injury, assign the acute injury code with the appropriate 7th character (for subsequent encounter).

The aftercare codes are generally first-listed to explain the specific reason for the encounter. An aftercare code may be used as an additional code when some type of aftercare is provided in addition to the reason for admission and no diagnosis code is applicable. An example of this would be the closure of a colostomy during an encounter for treatment of another condition.

Aftercare codes should be used in conjunction with other aftercare codes or diagnosis codes to provide better detail on the specifics of an aftercare encounter visit, unless otherwise directed by the classification. Should a patient receive multiple types of antineoplastic therapy during the same encounter, code Z51.0, Encounter for antineoplastic radiation therapy, and codes from subcategory Z51.1, Encounter for antineoplastic chemotherapy and immunotherapy, may be used together on a record. The sequencing of multiple aftercare codes depends on the circumstances of the encounter.

Certain aftercare Z code categories need a secondary diagnosis code to describe the resolving condition or sequelae. For others, the condition is included in the code title.

Additional Z code aftercare category terms include fitting and adjustment, and attention to artificial openings.

Status Z codes may be used with aftercare Z codes to indicate the nature of the aftercare. For example code Z95.1, Presence of aortocoronary bypass graft, may be used with code Z48.812, Encounter for surgical aftercare following surgery on the circulatory system, to indicate the surgery for which the aftercare is being performed. A status code should not be used when the aftercare code indicates the type of status, such as using Z43.0, Encounter for attention to tracheostomy, with Z93.0, Tracheostomy status.

The aftercare Z category/codes:

Z42   Encounter for plastic and reconstructive surgery following medical procedure or healed injury

Z43   Encounter for attention to artificial openings

Z44   Encounter for fitting and adjustment of external prosthetic device

Z45   Encounter for adjustment and management of implanted device

Z46   Encounter for fitting and adjustment of other devices

Z47   Orthopedic aftercare

Z48   Encounter for other postprocedural aftercare

Z49   Encounter for care involving renal dialysis

Z51   Encounter for other aftercare and medical care

8) Follow-up

The follow-up codes are used to explain continuing surveillance following completed treatment of a disease, condition, or injury. They imply that the condition has been fully treated and no longer exists. They should not be confused with aftercare codes, or injury codes with a 7th character for subsequent encounter, that explain ongoing care of a healing condition or its sequelae. Follow-up codes may be used in conjunction with history codes to provide the full picture of the healed condition and its treatment. The follow-up code is sequenced first, followed by the history code.

A follow-up code may be used to explain multiple visits. Should a condition be found to have recurred on the follow-up visit, then the diagnosis code for the condition should be assigned in place of the follow-up code.

The follow-up Z code categories:

Z08   Encounter for follow-up examination after completed treatment for malignant neoplasm

Z09   Encounter for follow-up examination after completed treatment for conditions other than malignant neoplasm

Z39   Encounter for maternal postpartum care and examination

9) Donor

Codes in category Z52, Donors of organs and tissues, are used for living individuals who are donating blood or other body tissue. These codes are only for individuals donating for others, not for self-donations. They are not used to identify cadaveric donations.

10) Counseling

Counseling Z codes are used when a patient or family member receives assistance in the aftermath of an illness or injury, or when support is required in coping with family or social problems.

The counseling Z codes/categories:

Z30.0-   Encounter for general counseling and advice on contraception

Z31.5   Encounter for procreative genetic counseling

Z31.6-   Encounter for general counseling and advice on procreation

Z32.2   Encounter for childbirth instruction

Z32.3   Encounter for childcare instruction

Z69   Encounter for mental health services for victim and perpetrator of abuse

Z70   Counseling related to sexual attitude, behavior and orientation

Z71   Persons encountering health services for other counseling and medical advice, not elsewhere classified

Z76.81 Expectant mother prebirth pediatrician visit

11) Encounters for Obstetrical and Reproductive Services

See Section I.C.15. Pregnancy, Childbirth, and the Puerperium, for further instruction on the use of these codes.

Z codes for pregnancy are for use in those circumstances when none of the problems or complications included in the codes from the Obstetrics chapter exist (a routine prenatal visit or postpartum care). Codes in category Z34, Encounter for supervision of normal pregnancy, are always first-listed and are not to be used with any other code from the OB chapter.

Codes in category Z3A, Weeks of gestation, may be assigned to provide additional information about the pregnancy. Category Z3A codes should not be assigned for pregnancies with abortive outcomes (categories O00-O08), elective termination of pregnancy (code Z33.2), nor for postpartum conditions, as category Z3A is not applicable to these conditions. The date of the admission should be used to determine weeks of gestation for inpatient admissions that encompass more than one gestational week.

The outcome of delivery, category Z37, should be included on all maternal delivery records. It is always a secondary code. Codes in category Z37 should not be used on the newborn record.

Z codes for family planning (contraceptive) or procreative management and counseling should be included on an obstetric record either during the pregnancy or the postpartum stage, if applicable.

Z codes/categories for obstetrical and reproductive services:

Z30   Encounter for contraceptive management

Z31   Encounter for procreative management

Z32.2   Encounter for childbirth instruction

Z32.3   Encounter for childcare instruction

Z33   Pregnant state

Z34   Encounter for supervision of normal pregnancy

Z36   Encounter for antenatal screening of mother

Z3A   Weeks of gestation

Z37   Outcome of delivery

Z39   Encounter for maternal postpartum care and examination

Z76.81 Expectant mother prebirth pediatrician visit

12) Newborns and Infants

See Section I.C.16. Newborn (Perinatal) Guidelines, for further instruction on the use of these codes.

Newborn Z codes/categories:

Z76.1   Encounter for health supervision and care of foundling

Z00.1-   Encounter for routine child health examination

Z38   Liveborn infants according to place of birth and type of delivery

13) Routine and administrative examinations

The Z codes allow for the description of encounters for routine examinations, such as, a general check-up, or, examinations for administrative purposes, such as, a pre-employment physical. The codes are not to be used if the examination is for diagnosis of a suspected condition or for treatment purposes. In such cases the diagnosis code is used. During a routine exam, should a diagnosis or condition be discovered, it should be coded as an additional code. Pre-existing and chronic conditions and history codes may also be included as additional codes as long as the examination is for administrative purposes and not focused on any particular condition.

Some of the codes for routine health examinations distinguish between "with" and "without" abnormal findings. Code assignment depends on the information that is known at the time the encounter is being coded. For example, if no abnormal findings were found during the examination, but the encounter is being coded before test results are back, it is acceptable to assign the code for "without abnormal findings." When assigning a code for "with abnormal findings," additional code(s) should be assigned to identify the specific abnormal finding(s).

Pre-operative examination and pre-procedural laboratory examination Z codes are for use only in those situations when a patient is being cleared for a procedure or surgery and no treatment is given.

The Z codes/categories for routine and administrative examinations:

Z00   Encounter for general examination without complaint, suspected or reported diagnosis

Z01   Encounter for other special examination without complaint, suspected or reported diagnosis

Z02   Encounter for administrative examination

     Except: Z02.9, Encounter for administrative examinations, unspecified

Z32.0-   Encounter for pregnancy test

14) Miscellaneous Z codes

The miscellaneous Z codes capture a number of other health care encounters that do not fall into one of the other categories. Certain of these codes identify the reason for the encounter; others are for use as additional codes that provide useful information on circumstances that may affect a patient's care and treatment.

Prophylactic Organ Removal

For encounters specifically for prophylactic removal of an organ (such as prophylactic removal of breasts due to a genetic susceptibility to cancer or a family history of cancer), the principal or first-listed code should be a code from category Z40, Encounter for prophylactic surgery, followed by the appropriate codes to identify the associated risk factor (such as genetic susceptibility or family history).

If the patient has a malignancy of one site and is having prophylactic removal at another site to prevent either a new primary malignancy or metastatic disease, a code for the malignancy should also be assigned in addition to a code from subcategory Z40.0, Encounter for prophylactic surgery for risk factors related to malignant neoplasms. A Z40.0 code should not be assigned if the patient is having organ removal for treatment of a malignancy, such as the removal of the testes for the treatment of prostate cancer.

Miscellaneous Z codes/categories:

Z28   Immunization not carried out

     Except: Z28.3, Underimmunization status

Z29   Encounter for other prophylactic measures

Z40   Encounter for prophylactic surgery

Z41   Encounter for procedures for purposes other than remedying health state

   Except: Z41.9, Encounter for procedure for purposes other than remedying health state, unspecified

Z53   Persons encountering health services for specific procedures and treatment, not carried out

Z55   Problems related to education and literacy

Z56   Problems related to employment and unemployment

Z57   Occupational exposure to risk factors

Z58   Problems related to physical environment

Z59   Problems related to housing and economic circumstances

Z60   Problems related to social environment

Z62   Problems related to upbringing

Z63   Other problems related to primary support group, including family circumstances

Z64   Problems related to certain psychosocial circumstances

Z65   Problems related to other psychosocial circumstances

Z72   Problems related to lifestyle

   Note: These codes should be assigned only when the documentation specifies that the patient has an associated problem

Z73   Problems related to life management difficulty

Z74   Problems related to care provider dependency

   Except: Z74.01, Bed confinement status

Z75   Problems related to medical facilities and other health care

Z76.0 Encounter for issue of repeat prescription

Z76.3 Healthy person accompanying sick person

Z76.4 Other boarder to healthcare facility

Z76.5 Malingerer [conscious simulation]

Z91.1- Patient's noncompliance with medical treatment and regimen

Z91.83 Wandering in diseases classified elsewhere

Z91.84- Oral health risk factors

Z91.89 Other specified personal risk factors, not elsewhere classified

See Section I.B.14 for Z55-Z65 Persons with potential health hazards related to socioeconomic and psychosocial circumstances, documentation by clinicians other than the patient's provider.

15) **Nonspecific Z codes**

   Certain Z codes are so non-specific, or potentially redundant with other codes in the classification, that there can be little justification for their use in the inpatient setting. Their use in the outpatient setting should be limited to those instances when there is no further documentation to permit more precise coding. Otherwise, any sign or symptom or any other reason for visit that is captured in another code should be used.

   Nonspecific Z codes/categories:

   Z02.9 Encounter for administrative examinations, unspecified

   Z04.9 Encounter for examination and observation for unspecified reason

   Z13.9 Encounter for screening, unspecified

   Z41.9 Encounter for procedure for purposes other than remedying health state, unspecified

   Z52.9 Donor of unspecified organ or tissue

   Z86.59 Personal history of other mental and behavioral disorders

   Z88.9 Allergy status to unspecified drugs, medicaments and biological substances status

   Z92.0 Personal history of contraception

16) **Z Codes That May Only be Principal/First-Listed Diagnosis**

   The following Z codes/categories may only be reported as the principal/first-listed diagnosis, except when there are multiple encounters on the same day and the medical records for the encounters are combined:

   Z00   Encounter for general examination without complaint, suspected or reported diagnosis

      Except: Z00.6

Z01   Encounter for other special examination without complaint, suspected or reported diagnosis

Z02   Encounter for administrative examination

Z03   Encounter for medical observation for suspected diseases and conditions ruled out

Z04   Encounter for examination and observation for other reasons

Z33.2 Encounter for elective termination of pregnancy

Z31.81 Encounter for male factor infertility in female patient

Z31.83 Encounter for assisted reproductive fertility procedure cycle

Z31.84 Encounter for fertility preservation procedure

Z34   Encounter for supervision of normal pregnancy

Z39   Encounter for maternal postpartum care and examination

Z38   Liveborn infants according to place of birth and type of delivery

Z40   Encounter for prophylactic surgery

Z42   Encounter for plastic and reconstructive surgery following medical procedure or healed injury

Z51.0 Encounter for antineoplastic radiation therapy

Z51.1- Encounter for antineoplastic chemotherapy and immunotherapy

Z52   Donors of organs and tissues

   Except: Z52.9, Donor of unspecified organ or tissue

Z76.1 Encounter for health supervision and care of foundling

Z76.2 Encounter for health supervision and care of other healthy infant and child

Z99.12 Encounter for respirator [ventilator] dependence during power failure

Section II. Selection of Principal Diagnosis

The circumstances of inpatient admission always govern the selection of principal diagnosis. The principal diagnosis is defined in the Uniform Hospital Discharge Data Set (UHDDS) as "that condition established after study to be chiefly responsible for occasioning the admission of the patient to the hospital for care."

The UHDDS definitions are used by hospitals to report inpatient data elements in a standardized manner. These data elements and their definitions can be found in the July 31, 1985, Federal Register (Vol. 50, No, 147), pp. 31038-40.

Since that time the application of the UHDDS definitions has been expanded to include all non-outpatient settings (acute care, short term, long term care and psychiatric hospitals; home health agencies; rehab facilities; nursing homes, etc). The UHDDS definitions also apply to hospice services (all levels of care).

In determining principal diagnosis, coding conventions in the ICD-10-CM, the Tabular List and Alphabetic Index take precedence over these official coding guidelines.

(See Section I.A., Conventions for the ICD-10-CM)

The importance of consistent, complete documentation in the medical record cannot be overemphasized. Without such documentation the application of all coding guidelines is a difficult, if not impossible, task.

A. **Codes for symptoms, signs, and ill-defined conditions**

   Codes for symptoms, signs, and ill-defined conditions from Chapter 18 are not to be used as principal diagnosis when a related definitive diagnosis has been established.

B. **Two or more interrelated conditions, each potentially meeting the definition for principal diagnosis.**

   When there are two or more interrelated conditions (such as diseases in the same ICD-10-CM chapter or manifestations characteristically associated with a certain disease) potentially meeting the definition of principal diagnosis, either condition may be sequenced first, unless the circumstances of the admission, the therapy provided, the Tabular List, or the Alphabetic Index indicate otherwise.

C. **Two or more diagnoses that equally meet the definition for principal diagnosis**

   In the unusual instance when two or more diagnoses equally meet the criteria for principal diagnosis as determined by the circumstances of admission, diagnostic workup and/or therapy provided, and the

Alphabetic Index, Tabular List, or another coding guidelines does not provide sequencing direction, any one of the diagnoses may be sequenced first.

D. Two or more comparative or contrasting conditions

In those rare instances when two or more contrasting or comparative diagnoses are documented as "either/or" (or similar terminology), they are coded as if the diagnoses were confirmed and the diagnoses are sequenced according to the circumstances of the admission. If no further determination can be made as to which diagnosis should be principal, either diagnosis may be sequenced first.

E. A symptom(s) followed by contrasting/comparative diagnoses

GUIDELINE HAS BEEN DELETED EFFECTIVE OCTOBER 1, 2014

F. Original treatment plan not carried out

Sequence as the principal diagnosis the condition, which after study occasioned the admission to the hospital, even though treatment may not have been carried out due to unforeseen circumstances.

G. Complications of surgery and other medical care

When the admission is for treatment of a complication resulting from surgery or other medical care, the complication code is sequenced as the principal diagnosis. If the complication is classified to the T80-T88 series and the code lacks the necessary specificity in describing the complication, an additional code for the specific complication should be assigned.

H. Uncertain Diagnosis

If the diagnosis documented at the time of discharge is qualified as "probable", "suspected", "likely", "questionable", "possible", or "still to be ruled out", or other similar terms indicating uncertainty, code the condition as if it existed or was established. The bases for these guidelines are the diagnostic workup, arrangements for further workup or observation, and initial therapeutic approach that correspond most closely with the established diagnosis.

Note: This guideline is applicable only to inpatient admissions to short-term, acute, long-term care and psychiatric hospitals.

I. Admission from Observation Unit

1. Admission Following Medical Observation

When a patient is admitted to an observation unit for a medical condition, which either worsens or does not improve, and is subsequently admitted as an inpatient of the same hospital for this same medical condition, the principal diagnosis would be the medical condition which led to the hospital admission.

2. Admission Following Post-Operative Observation

When a patient is admitted to an observation unit to monitor a condition (or complication) that develops following outpatient surgery, and then is subsequently admitted as an inpatient of the same hospital, hospitals should apply the Uniform Hospital Discharge Data Set (UHDDS) definition of principal diagnosis as "that condition established after study to be chiefly responsible for occasioning the admission of the patient to the hospital for care."

J. Admission from Outpatient Surgery

When a patient receives surgery in the hospital's outpatient surgery department and is subsequently admitted for continuing inpatient care at the same hospital, the following guidelines should be followed in selecting the principal diagnosis for the inpatient admission:

- If the reason for the inpatient admission is a complication, assign the complication as the principal diagnosis.
- If no complication, or other condition, is documented as the reason for the inpatient admission, assign the reason for the outpatient surgery as the principal diagnosis.
- If the reason for the inpatient admission is another condition unrelated to the surgery, assign the unrelated condition as the principal diagnosis.

K. Admissions/Encounters for Rehabilitation

When the purpose for the admission/encounter is rehabilitation, sequence first the code for the condition for which the service is being performed. For example, for an admission/encounter for rehabilitation for right-sided dominant hemiplegia following a cerebrovascular infarction, report code I69.351, Hemiplegia and hemiparesis following cerebral infarction affecting right dominant side, as the first-listed or principal diagnosis.

If the condition for which the rehabilitation service is being provided is no longer present, report the appropriate aftercare code as the first-listed or principal diagnosis, unless the rehabilitation service is being provided following an injury. For rehabilitation services following active treatment of an injury, assign the injury code with the appropriate seventh character for subsequent encounter as the first-listed or principal diagnosis. For example, if a patient with severe degenerative osteoarthritis of the hip,

underwent hip replacement and the current encounter/admission is for rehabilitation, report code Z47.1, Aftercare following joint replacement surgery, as the first-listed or principal diagnosis. If the patient requires rehabilitation post hip replacement for right intertrochanteric femur fracture, report code S72.141D, Displaced intertrochanteric fracture of right femur, subsequent encounter for closed fracture with routine healing, as the first-listed or principal diagnosis.

See Section I.C.21.c.7, Factors influencing health states and contact with health services, Aftercare.

See Section I.C.19.a for additional information about the use of 7th characters for injury codes.

Section III. Reporting Additional Diagnoses

GENERAL RULES FOR OTHER (ADDITIONAL) DIAGNOSES

For reporting purposes the definition for "other diagnoses" is interpreted as additional conditions that affect patient care in terms of requiring:

clinical evaluation; or
therapeutic treatment; or
diagnostic procedures; or
extended length of hospital stay; or
increased nursing care and/or monitoring.

The UHDDS item #11-b defines Other Diagnoses as "all conditions that coexist at the time of admission, that develop subsequently, or that affect the treatment received and/or the length of stay. Diagnoses that relate to an earlier episode which have no bearing on the current hospital stay are to be excluded." UHDDS definitions apply to inpatients in acute care, short-term, long term care and psychiatric hospital setting. The UHDDS definitions are used by acute care short-term hospitals to report inpatient data elements in a standardized manner. These data elements and their definitions can be found in the July 31, 1985, Federal Register (Vol. 50, No, 147), pp. 31038-40.

Since that time the application of the UHDDS definitions has been expanded to include all non-outpatient settings (acute care, short term, long term care and psychiatric hospitals; home health agencies; rehab facilities; nursing homes, etc). The UHDDS definitions also apply to hospice services (all levels of care).

The following guidelines are to be applied in designating "other diagnoses" when neither the Alphabetic Index nor the Tabular List in ICD-10-CM provide direction. The listing of the diagnoses in the patient record is the responsibility of the attending provider.

A. Previous conditions

If the provider has included a diagnosis in the final diagnostic statement, such as the discharge summary or the face sheet, it should ordinarily be coded. Some providers include in the diagnostic statement resolved conditions or diagnoses and status-post procedures from previous admission that have no bearing on the current stay. Such conditions are not to be reported and are coded only if required by hospital policy.

However, history codes (categories Z80-Z87) may be used as secondary codes if the historical condition or family history has an impact on current care or influences treatment.

B. Abnormal findings

Abnormal findings (laboratory, x-ray, pathologic, and other diagnostic results) are not coded and reported unless the provider indicates their clinical significance. If the findings are outside the normal range and the attending provider has ordered other tests to evaluate the condition or prescribed treatment, it is appropriate to ask the provider whether the abnormal finding should be added.

Please note: This differs from the coding practices in the outpatient setting for coding encounters for diagnostic tests that have been interpreted by a provider.

C. Uncertain Diagnosis

If the diagnosis documented at the time of discharge is qualified as "probable", "suspected", "likely", "questionable", "possible", or "still to be ruled out" or other similar terms indicating uncertainty, code the condition as if it existed or was established. The bases for these guidelines are the diagnostic workup, arrangements for further workup or observation, and initial therapeutic approach that correspond most closely with the established diagnosis.

Note: This guideline is applicable only to inpatient admissions to short-term, acute, long-term care and psychiatric hospitals.

Section IV.Diagnostic Coding and Reporting Guidelines for Outpatient Services

These coding guidelines for outpatient diagnoses have been approved for use by hospitals/ providers in coding and reporting hospital-based outpatient services and provider-based office visits. Guidelines in Section I, Conventions, general coding guidelines and chapter-specific guidelines, should also be applied for outpatient services and office visits.

Information about the use of certain abbreviations, punctuation, symbols, and other conventions used in the ICD-10-CM Tabular List (code numbers and titles), can be found in Section IA of these guidelines, under "Conventions Used in the Tabular List." Section I.B. contains general guidelines that apply to the entire classification. Section I.C. contains chapter-specific guidelines that correspond to the chapters as they are arranged in the classification. Information about the correct sequence to use in finding a code is also described in Section I.

The terms encounter and visit are often used interchangeably in describing outpatient service contacts and, therefore, appear together in these guidelines without distinguishing one from the other.

Though the conventions and general guidelines apply to all settings, coding guidelines for outpatient and provider reporting of diagnoses will vary in a number of instances from those for inpatient diagnoses, recognizing that:

The Uniform Hospital Discharge Data Set (UHDDS) definition of principal diagnosis does not apply to hospital-based outpatient services and provider-based office visits.

Coding guidelines for inconclusive diagnoses (probable, suspected, rule out, etc.) were developed for inpatient reporting and do not apply to outpatients.

A. Selection of first-listed condition

In the outpatient setting, the term first-listed diagnosis is used in lieu of principal diagnosis.

In determining the first-listed diagnosis the coding conventions of ICD-10-CM, as well as the general and disease specific guidelines take precedence over the outpatient guidelines.

Diagnoses often are not established at the time of the initial encounter/visit. It may take two or more visits before the diagnosis is confirmed.

The most critical rule involves beginning the search for the correct code assignment through the Alphabetic Index. Never begin searching initially in the Tabular List as this will lead to coding errors.

1. Outpatient Surgery

When a patient presents for outpatient surgery (same day surgery), code the reason for the surgery as the first-listed diagnosis (reason for the encounter), even if the surgery is not performed due to a contraindication.

2. Observation Stay

When a patient is admitted for observation for a medical condition, assign a code for the medical condition as the first-listed diagnosis.

When a patient presents for outpatient surgery and develops complications requiring admission to observation, code the reason for the surgery as the first reported diagnosis (reason for the encounter), followed by codes for the complications as secondary diagnoses.

B. Codes from A00.0 through T88.9, Z00-Z99

The appropriate code(s) from A00.0 through T88.9, Z00-Z99 must be used to identify diagnoses, symptoms, conditions, problems, complaints, or other reason(s) for the encounter/visit.

C. Accurate reporting of ICD-10-CM diagnosis codes

For accurate reporting of ICD-10-CM diagnosis codes, the documentation should describe the patient's condition, using terminology which includes specific diagnoses as well as symptoms, problems, or reasons for the encounter. There are ICD-10-CM codes to describe all of these.

D. Codes that describe symptoms and signs

Codes that describe symptoms and signs, as opposed to diagnoses, are acceptable for reporting purposes when a diagnosis has not been established (confirmed) by the provider. Chapter 18 of ICD-10-CM, Symptoms, Signs, and Abnormal Clinical and Laboratory Findings Not Elsewhere Classified (codes R00-R99) contain many, but not all codes for symptoms.

E. Encounters for circumstances other than a disease or injury

ICD-10-CM provides codes to deal with encounters for circumstances other than a disease or injury. The Factors Influencing Health Status and Contact with Health Services codes (Z00-Z99) are provided to deal with occasions when circumstances other than a disease or injury are recorded as diagnosis or problems.

See Section I.C.21. Factors influencing health status and contact with health services.

F. Level of Detail in Coding

1. ICD-10-CM codes with 3, 4, 5, 6 or 7 characters

ICD-10-CM is composed of codes with 3, 4, 5, 6 or 7 characters. Codes with three characters are included in ICD-10-CM as the heading of a category of codes that may be further subdivided by the use of fourth, fifth, sixth or seventh characters to provide greater specificity.

2. Use of full number of characters required for a code

A three-character code is to be used only if it is not further subdivided. A code is invalid if it has not been coded to the full number of characters required for that code, including the 7th character, if applicable.

G. ICD-10-CM code for the diagnosis, condition, problem, or other reason for encounter/visit

List first the ICD-10-CM code for the diagnosis, condition, problem, or other reason for encounter/visit shown in the medical record to be chiefly responsible for the services provided. List additional codes that describe any coexisting conditions. In some cases the first-listed diagnosis may be a symptom when a diagnosis has not been established (confirmed) by the physician.

H. Uncertain diagnosis

Do not code diagnoses documented as "probable", "suspected," "questionable," "rule out," or "working diagnosis" or other similar terms indicating uncertainty. Rather, code the condition(s) to the highest degree of certainty for that encounter/visit, such as symptoms, signs, abnormal test results, or other reason for the visit.

Please note: This differs from the coding practices used by short-term, acute care, long-term care and psychiatric hospitals.

I. Chronic diseases

Chronic diseases treated on an ongoing basis may be coded and reported as many times as the patient receives treatment and care for the condition(s)

J. Code all documented conditions that coexist

Code all documented conditions that coexist at the time of the encounter/visit, and require or affect patient care treatment or management. Do not code conditions that were previously treated and no longer exist. However, history codes (categories Z80-Z87) may be used as secondary codes if the historical condition or family history has an impact on current care or influences treatment.

K. Patients receiving diagnostic services only

For patients receiving diagnostic services only during an encounter/visit, sequence first the diagnosis, condition, problem, or other reason for encounter/visit shown in the medical record to be chiefly responsible for the outpatient services provided during the encounter/visit. Codes for other diagnoses (e.g., chronic conditions) may be sequenced as additional diagnoses.

For encounters for routine laboratory/radiology testing in the absence of any signs, symptoms, or associated diagnosis, assign Z01.89, Encounter for other specified special examinations. If routine testing is performed during the same encounter as a test to evaluate a sign, symptom, or diagnosis, it is appropriate to assign both the Z code and the code describing the reason for the non-routine test.

For outpatient encounters for diagnostic tests that have been interpreted by a physician, and the final report is available at the time of coding, code any confirmed or definitive diagnosis(es) documented in the interpretation. Do not code related signs and symptoms as additional diagnoses.

Please note: This differs from the coding practice in the hospital inpatient setting regarding abnormal findings on test results.

L. Patients receiving therapeutic services only

For patients receiving therapeutic services only during an encounter/visit, sequence first the diagnosis, condition, problem, or other reason for encounter/visit shown in the medical record to be chiefly responsible for the outpatient services provided during the encounter/visit. Codes for other diagnoses (e.g., chronic conditions) may be sequenced as additional diagnoses.

The only exception to this rule is that when the primary reason for the admission/encounter is chemotherapy or radiation therapy, the appropriate Z code for the service is listed first, and the diagnosis or problem for which the service is being performed listed second.

M. Patients receiving preoperative evaluations only

For patients receiving preoperative evaluations only, sequence first a code from subcategory Z01.81, Encounter for pre-procedural examinations, to describe the pre-op consultations. Assign a code for the condition to describe the reason for the surgery as an additional diagnosis. Code also any findings related to the pre-op evaluation.

N. Ambulatory surgery

For ambulatory surgery, code the diagnosis for which the surgery was performed. If the postoperative diagnosis is known to be different from the preoperative diagnosis at the time the diagnosis is confirmed, select the postoperative diagnosis for coding, since it is the most definitive.

O. Routine outpatient prenatal visits

See Section I.C.15. Routine outpatient prenatal visits.

P. Encounters for general medical examinations with abnormal findings

The subcategories for encounters for general medical examinations, Z00.0- and encounter for routine child health examination, Z00.12-, provide codes for with and without abnormal findings. Should a general medical examination result in an abnormal finding, the code for general medical examination with abnormal finding should be assigned as the first-listed diagnosis. An examination with abnormal findings refers to a condition/diagnosis that is newly identified or a change in severity of a chronic condition (such as uncontrolled hypertension, or an acute exacerbation of chronic obstructive pulmonary disease) during a routine physical examination. A secondary code for the abnormal finding should also be coded.

Q. Encounters for routine health screenings

See Section I.C.21. Factors influencing health status and contact with health services, Screening

Appendix I. Present on Admission Reporting Guidelines

Introduction

These guidelines are to be used as a supplement to the *ICD-10-CM Official Guidelines for Coding and Reporting* to facilitate the assignment of the Present on Admission (POA) indicator for each diagnosis and external cause of injury code reported on claim forms (UB-04 and 837 Institutional).

These guidelines are not intended to replace any guidelines in the main body of the *ICD-10-CM Official Guidelines for Coding and Reporting*. The POA guidelines are not intended to provide guidance on when a condition should be coded, but rather, how to apply the POA indicator to the final set of diagnosis codes that have been assigned in accordance with Sections I, II, and III of the official coding guidelines. Subsequent to the assignment of the ICD-10-CM codes, the POA indicator should then be assigned to those conditions that have been coded.

As stated in the Introduction to the *ICD-10-CM Official Guidelines for Coding and Reporting,* a joint effort between the healthcare provider and the coder is essential to achieve complete and accurate documentation, code assignment, and reporting of diagnoses and procedures. The importance of consistent, complete documentation in the medical record cannot be overemphasized. Medical record documentation from any provider involved in the care and treatment of the patient may be used to support the determination of whether a condition was present on admission or not. In the context of the official coding guidelines, the term "provider" means a physician or any qualified healthcare practitioner who is legally accountable for establishing the patient's diagnosis.

These guidelines are not a substitute for the provider's clinical judgment as to the determination of whether a condition was/was not present on admission. The provider should be queried regarding issues related to the linking of signs/symptoms, timing of test results, and the timing of findings.

Please see the CDC website for the detailed list of ICD-10-CM codes that do not require the use of a POA indicator (https://www.cdc.gov/nchs/icd/icd10cm.htm). The codes and categories on this exempt list are for circumstances regarding the healthcare encounter or factors influencing health status that do not represent a current disease or injury or that describe conditions that are always present on admission.

General Reporting Requirements

All claims involving inpatient admissions to general acute care hospitals or other facilities that are subject to a law or regulation mandating collection of present on admission information.

Present on admission is defined as present at the time the order for inpatient admission occurs -- conditions that develop during an outpatient encounter, including emergency department, observation, or outpatient surgery, are considered as present on admission.

POA indicator is assigned to principal and secondary diagnoses (as defined in Section II of the Official Guidelines for Coding and Reporting) and the external cause of injury codes.

Issues related to inconsistent, missing, conflicting or unclear documentation must still be resolved by the provider.

If a condition would not be coded and reported based on UHDDS definitions and current official coding guidelines, then the POA indicator would not be reported.

Reporting Options

    Y - Yes

    N - No

    U - Unknown

    W – Clinically undetermined

    Unreported/Not used – (Exempt from POA reporting)

Reporting Definitions

    Y = present at the time of inpatient admission

    N = not present at the time of inpatient admission

    U = documentation is insufficient to determine if condition is present on admission

    W = provider is unable to clinically determine whether condition was present on admission or not

Timeframe for POA Identification and Documentation

There is no required timeframe as to when a provider (per the definition of "provider" used in these guidelines) must identify or document a condition to be present on admission. In some clinical situations, it may not be possible for a provider to make a definitive diagnosis (or a condition may not be recognized or reported by the patient) for a period of time after admission. In some cases it may be several days before the provider arrives at a definitive diagnosis. This does not mean that the condition was not present on admission. Determination of whether the condition was present on admission or not will be based on the applicable POA guideline as identified in this document, or on the provider's best clinical judgment.

If at the time of code assignment the documentation is unclear as to whether a condition was present on admission or not, it is appropriate to query the provider for clarification.

Assigning the POA Indicator

Condition is on the "Exempt from Reporting" list

    Leave the "present on admission" field blank if the condition is on the list of ICD-10-CM codes for which this field is not applicable. This is the only circumstance in which the field may be left blank.

POA Explicitly Documented

    Assign Y for any condition the provider explicitly documents as being present on admission.

    Assign N for any condition the provider explicitly documents as not present at the time of admission.

Conditions diagnosed prior to inpatient admission

    Assign "Y" for conditions that were diagnosed prior to admission (example: hypertension, diabetes mellitus, asthma)

Conditions diagnosed during the admission but clearly present before admission

    Assign "Y" for conditions diagnosed during the admission that were clearly present but not diagnosed until after admission occurred.

    Diagnoses subsequently confirmed after admission are considered present on admission if at the time of admission they are documented as suspected, possible, rule out, differential diagnosis, or constitute an underlying cause of a symptom that is present at the time of admission.

Condition develops during outpatient encounter prior to inpatient admission

    Assign Y for any condition that develops during an outpatient encounter prior to a written order for inpatient admission.

Documentation does not indicate whether condition was present on admission

    Assign "U" when the medical record documentation is unclear as to whether the condition was present on admission. "U" should not be routinely assigned and used only in very limited circumstances. Coders are encouraged to query the providers when the documentation is unclear.

Documentation states that it cannot be determined whether the condition was or was not present on admission

    Assign "W" when the medical record documentation indicates that it cannot be clinically determined whether or not the condition was present on admission.

Chronic condition with acute exacerbation during the admission

If a single code identifies both the chronic condition and the acute exacerbation, see POA guidelines pertaining to codes that contain multiple clinical concepts.

If a single code only identifies the chronic condition and not the acute exacerbation (e.g., acute exacerbation of chronic leukemia), assign "Y."

Conditions documented as possible, probable, suspected, or rule out at the time of discharge

If the final diagnosis contains a possible, probable, suspected, or rule out diagnosis, and this diagnosis was based on signs, symptoms or clinical findings suspected at the time of inpatient admission, assign "Y."

If the final diagnosis contains a possible, probable, suspected, or rule out diagnosis, and this diagnosis was based on signs, symptoms or clinical findings that were not present on admission, assign "N".

Conditions documented as impending or threatened at the time of discharge

If the final diagnosis contains an impending or threatened diagnosis, and this diagnosis is based on symptoms or clinical findings that were present on admission, assign "Y".

If the final diagnosis contains an impending or threatened diagnosis, and this diagnosis is based on symptoms or clinical findings that were not present on admission, assign "N".

Acute and Chronic Conditions

Assign "Y" for acute conditions that are present at time of admission and N for acute conditions that are not present at time of admission.

Assign "Y" for chronic conditions, even though the condition may not be diagnosed until after admission.

If a single code identifies both an acute and chronic condition, see the POA guidelines for codes that contain multiple clinical concepts.

Codes That Contain Multiple Clinical Concepts

Assign "N" if at least one of the clinical concepts included in the code was not present on admission (e.g., COPD with acute exacerbation and the exacerbation was not present on admission; gastric ulcer that does not start bleeding until after admission; asthma patient develops status asthmaticus after admission).

Assign "Y" if all of the clinical concepts included in the code were present on admission (e.g., duodenal ulcer that perforates prior to admission).

For infection codes that include the causal organism, assign "Y" if the infection (or signs of the infection) were present on admission, even though the culture results may not be known until after admission (e.g., patient is admitted with pneumonia and the provider documents Pseudomonas as the causal organism a few days later).

Same Diagnosis Code for Two or More Conditions

When the same ICD-10-CM diagnosis code applies to two or more conditions during the same encounter (e.g. two separate conditions classified to the same ICD-10-CM diagnosis code):

Assign "Y" if all conditions represented by the single ICD-10-CM code were present on admission (e.g. bilateral unspecified age-related cataracts).

Assign "N" if any of the conditions represented by the single ICD-10-CM code was not present on admission (e.g. traumatic secondary and recurrent hemorrhage and seroma is assigned to a single code T79.2, but only one of the conditions was present on admission).

Obstetrical conditions

Whether or not the patient delivers during the current hospitalization does not affect assignment of the POA indicator. The determining factor for POA assignment is whether the pregnancy complication or obstetrical condition described by the code was present at the time of admission or not.

If the pregnancy complication or obstetrical condition was present on admission (e.g., patient admitted in preterm labor), assign "Y".

If the pregnancy complication or obstetrical condition was not present on admission (e.g., 2nd degree laceration during delivery, postpartum hemorrhage that occurred during current hospitalization, fetal distress develops after admission), assign "N".

If the obstetrical code includes more than one diagnosis and any of the diagnoses identified by the code were not present on admission assign "N". (e.g., Category O11, Pre-existing hypertension with pre-eclampsia)

Perinatal conditions

Newborns are not considered to be admitted until after birth. Therefore, any condition present at birth or that developed in utero is considered present at admission and should be assigned "Y". This includes conditions that occur during delivery (e.g., injury during delivery, meconium aspiration, exposure to streptococcus B in the vaginal canal).

Congenital conditions and anomalies

Assign "Y" for congenital conditions and anomalies except for categories Q00-Q99, Congenital anomalies, which are on the exempt list. Congenital conditions are always considered present on admission.

External cause of injury codes

Assign "Y" for any external cause code representing an external cause of morbidity that occurred prior to inpatient admission (e.g., patient fell out of bed at home, patient fell out of bed in emergency room prior to admission)

Assign "N" for any external cause code representing an external cause of morbidity that occurred during inpatient hospitalization (e.g., patient fell out of hospital bed during hospital stay, patient experienced an adverse reaction to a medication administered after inpatient admission).

A

Aarskog's syndrome Q87.1
Abandonment — *see* Maltreatment
Abasia (-astasia) (hysterical) F44.4
Abderhalden-Kaufmann-Lignac syndrome (cystinosis) E72.04
Abdomen, abdominal (*see also* condition)
  muscle deficiency syndrome Q79.4
  angina K55.1
  acute R10.0
Abdominalgia — *see* Pain, abdominal
Abduction contracture, hip or other joint — *see* Contraction, joint
Aberrant (congenital) (*see also* Malposition, congenital)
  hepatic duct Q44.5
  endocrine gland NEC Q89.2
  breast Q83.8
  artery (peripheral) Q27.8
    basilar NEC Q28.1
    cerebral Q28.3
    coronary Q24.5
    digestive system Q27.8
    eye Q15.8
    lower limb Q27.8
    precerebral Q28.1
    pulmonary Q25.79
    renal Q27.2
    retina Q14.1
    specified site NEC Q27.8
    subclavian Q27.8
    upper limb Q27.8
    vertebral Q28.1
  adrenal gland Q89.1
  pancreas Q45.3
  parathyroid gland Q89.2
  pituitary gland Q89.2
  sebaceous glands, mucous membrane, mouth, congenital Q38.6
  spleen Q89.09
  subclavian artery Q27.8
  thymus (gland) Q89.2
  thyroid gland Q89.2
  vein (peripheral) NEC Q27.8
    cerebral Q28.3
    digestive system Q27.8
    lower limb Q27.8
    precerebral Q28.1
    specified site NEC Q27.8
    upper limb Q27.8
Aberration
  distantial — *see* Disturbance, visual
  mental F99
Abetalipoproteinemia E78.6
Abiotrophy R68.89
Ablatio, ablation
  retinae — *see* Detachment, retina
Ablepharia, ablepharon Q10.3
Abnormal, abnormality, abnormalities (*see also* Anomaly)
  acid-base balance (mixed) E87.4
  albumin R77.0
  alphafetoprotein R77.2
  alveolar ridge K08.9
  anatomical relationship Q89.9
  apertures, congenital, diaphragm Q79.1
  auditory perception H93.29- ☑
    diplacusis — *see* Diplacusis
    hyperacusis — *see* Hyperacusis
    recruitment — *see* Recruitment, auditory
    threshold shift — *see* Shift, auditory threshold
  autosomes Q99.9
    fragile site Q95.5
  basal metabolic rate R94.8
  biosynthesis, testicular androgen E29.1
  bleeding time R79.1
  blood level (of)
    cobalt R79.0
    copper R79.0
    iron R79.0
    lithium R78.89
    magnesium R79.0

Abnormal, abnormality, abnormalities — *continued*
  blood level — *continued*
    mineral NEC R79.0
    zinc R79.0
  blood pressure
    elevated R03.0
    low reading (nonspecific) R03.1
  blood sugar R73.09
  blood-gas level R79.81
  bowel sounds R19.15
    absent R19.11
    hyperactive R19.12
  brain scan R94.02
  breathing R06.9
  caloric test R94.138
  cerebrospinal fluid R83.9
    cytology R83.6
    drug level R83.2
    enzyme level R83.0
    hormones R83.1
    immunology R83.4
    microbiology R83.5
    nonmedicinal level R83.3
    specified type NEC R83.8
  chemistry, blood R79.9
    C-reactive protein R79.82
    drugs — *see* Findings, abnormal, in blood
    gas level R79.81
    minerals R79.0
    pancytopenia D61.818
    PTT R79.1
    specified NEC R79.89
    toxins — *see* Findings, abnormal, in blood
  chest sounds (friction) (rales) R09.89
  chromosome, chromosomal Q99.9
    with more than three X chromosomes, female Q97.1
    analysis result R89.8
      bronchial washings R84.8
      cerebrospinal fluid R83.8
      cervix uteri NEC R87.89
      nasal secretions R84.8
      nipple discharge R89.8
      peritoneal fluid R85.89
      pleural fluid R84.8
      prostatic secretions R86.8
      saliva R85.89
      seminal fluid R86.8
      sputum R84.8
      synovial fluid R89.8
      throat scrapings R84.8
      vagina R87.89
      vulva R87.89
      wound secretions R89.8
    dicentric replacement Q93.2
    ring replacement Q93.2
    sex Q99.8
      female phenotype Q97.9
        specified NEC Q97.8
      male phenotype Q98.9
        specified NEC Q98.8
      structural male Q98.6
    specified NEC Q99.8
  clinical findings NEC R68.89
  coagulation D68.9
    newborn, transient P61.6
    profile R79.1
    time R79.1
  communication — *see* Fistula
  conjunctiva, vascular H11.41- ☑
  coronary artery Q24.5
  cortisol-binding globulin E27.8
  course, eustachian tube Q17.8
  creatinine clearance R94.4
  cytology
    anus R85.619
      atypical squamous cells cannot exclude high grade squamous intraepithelial lesion (ASC-H) R85.611
      atypical squamous cells of undetermined significance (ASC-US) R85.610
      cytologic evidence of malignancy R85.614

Abnormal, abnormality, abnormalities — *continued*
  cytology — *continued*
    anus — *continued*
      high grade squamous intraepithelial lesion (HGSIL) R85.613
      human papillomavirus (HPV) DNA test
        high risk positive R85.81
        low risk postive R85.82
      inadequate smear R85.615
      low grade squamous intraepithelial lesion (LGSIL) R85.612
      satisfactory anal smear but lacking transformation zone R85.616
      specified NEC R85.618
      unsatisfactory smear R85.615
      female genital organs — *see* Abnormal, Papanicolaou (smear)
  dark adaptation curve H53.61
  dentofacial NEC — *see* Anomaly, dentofacial
  development, developmental Q89.9
    central nervous system Q07.9
  diagnostic imaging
    abdomen, abdominal region NEC R93.5
    biliary tract R93.2
    bladder R93.41
    breast R92.8
    central nervous system NEC R90.89
    cerebrovascular NEC R90.89
    coronary circulation R93.1
    digestive tract NEC R93.3
    gastrointestinal (tract) R93.3
    genitourinary organs R93.89
    head R93.0
    heart R93.1
    intrathoracic organ NEC R93.89
    kidney R93.42- ☑
    limbs R93.6
    liver R93.2
    lung (field) R91.8
    musculoskeletal system NEC R93.7
    renal pelvis R93.41
    retroperitoneum R93.5
    site specified NEC R93.89
    skin and subcutaneous tissue R93.89
    skull R93.0
    testis R93.81- ☑
    ureter R93.41
    urinary organs specified NEC R93.49
  direction, teeth, fully erupted M26.30
  ear ossicles, acquired NEC H74.39- ☑
    ankylosis — *see* Ankylosis, ear ossicles
    discontinuity — *see* Discontinuity, ossicles, ear
    partial loss — *see* Loss, ossicles, ear (partial)
  Ebstein Q22.5
  echocardiogram R93.1
  echoencephalogram R90.81
  echogram — *see* Abnormal, diagnostic imaging
  electrocardiogram [ECG] [EKG] R94.31
  electroencephalogram [EEG] R94.01
  electrolyte — *see* Imbalance, electrolyte
  electromyogram [EMG] R94.131
  electro-oculogram [EOG] R94.110
  electrophysiological intracardiac studies R94.39
  electroretinogram [ERG] R94.111
  erythrocytes
    congenital, with perinatal jaundice D58.9
  feces (color) (contents) (mucus) R19.5
  finding — *see* Findings, abnormal, without diagnosis
  fluid
    amniotic — *see* Abnormal, specimen, specified
    cerebrospinal — *see* Abnormal, cerebrospinal fluid
    peritoneal — *see* Abnormal, specimen, digestive organs
    pleural — *see* Abnormal, specimen, respiratory organs
    synovial — *see* Abnormal, specimen, specified
    thorax (bronchial washings) (pleural fluid) — *see* Abnormal, specimen, respiratory organs
    vaginal — *see* Abnormal, specimen, female genital organs
  form
    teeth K00.2

▼ Subterms under main terms may continue to next column or page   ☑ Additional Character Required — Refer to the Tabular List for Character Selection   1

Aarskog's syndrome — Abnormal, abnormality, abnormalities

Abnormal, abnormality, abnormalities —
    continued
    form — *continued*
      uterus — *see* Anomaly, uterus
    function studies
      auditory R94.120
      bladder R94.8
      brain R94.09
      cardiovascular R94.30
      ear R94.128
      endocrine NEC R94.7
      eye NEC R94.118
      kidney R94.4
      liver R94.5
      nervous system
        central NEC R94.09
        peripheral NEC R94.138
      pancreas R94.8
      placenta R94.8
      pulmonary R94.2
      special senses NEC R94.128
      spleen R94.8
      thyroid R94.6
      vestibular R94.121
    gait — *see* Gait
      hysterical F44.4
    gastrin secretion E16.4
    globulin R77.1
      cortisol-binding E27.8
      thyroid-binding E07.89
    glomerular, minor (*see also* N00-N07 with fourth character .0) N05.0
    glucagon secretion E16.3
    glucose tolerance (test) (non-fasting) R73.09
    gravitational (G) forces or states (effect of) T75.81 ☑
    hair (color) (shaft) L67.9
      specified NEC L67.8
    hard tissue formation in pulp (dental) K04.3
    head movement R25.0
    heart
      rate R00.9
        specified NEC R00.8
      shadow R93.1
      sounds NEC R01.2
    hemoglobin (disease) (*see also* Disease, hemoglobin) D58.2
      trait — *see* Trait, hemoglobin, abnormal
    histology NEC R89.7
    immunological findings R89.4
      in serum R76.9
        specified NEC R76.8
    increase in appetite R63.2
    involuntary movement — *see* Abnormal, movement, involuntary
    jaw closure M26.51
    karyotype R89.8
    kidney function test R94.4
    knee jerk R29.2
    leukocyte (cell) (differential) NEC D72.9
    liver function test R94.5
    loss of
      height R29.890
      weight R63.4
    mammogram NEC R92.8
      calcification (calculus) R92.1
      microcalcification R92.0
    Mantoux test R76.11
    movement (disorder) (*see also* Disorder, movement)
      head R25.0
      involuntary R25.9
        fasciculation R25.3
        of head R25.0
        spasm R25.2
        specified type NEC R25.8
        tremor R25.1
    myoglobin (Aberdeen) (Annapolis) R89.7
    neonatal screening P09
    oculomotor study R94.113
    palmar creases Q82.8
    Papanicolaou (smear)
      anus R85.619
        atypical squamous cells cannot exclude high grade squamous intraepithelial lesion (ASC-H) R85.611
        atypical squamous cells of undetermined significance (ASC-US) R85.610
        cytologic evidence of malignancy R85.614

Abnormal, abnormality, abnormalities —
    continued
    Papanicolaou — *continued*
      anus — *continued*
        high grade squamous intraepithelial lesion (HGSIL) R85.613
        human papillomavirus (HPV) DNA test
          high risk positive R85.81
          low risk postive R85.82
        inadequate smear R85.615
        low grade squamous intraepithelial lesion (LGSIL) R85.612
        satisfactory anal smear but lacking transformation zone R85.616
        specified NEC R85.618
        unsatisfactory smear R85.615
      bronchial washings R84.6
      cerebrospinal fluid R83.6
      cervix R87.619
        atypical squamous cells cannot exclude high grade squamous intraepithelial lesion (ASC-H) R87.611
        atypical squamous cells of undetermined significance (ASC-US) R87.610
        cytologic evidence of malignancy R87.614
        high grade squamous intraepithelial lesion (HGSIL) R87.613
        inadequate smear R87.615
        low grade squamous intraepithelial lesion (LGSIL) R87.612
        non-atypical endometrial cells R87.618
        satisfactory cervical smear but lacking transformation zone R87.616
        specified NEC R87.618
        thin preparaton R87.619
        unsatisfactory smear R87.615
      nasal secretions R84.6
      nipple discharge R89.6
      peritoneal fluid R85.69
      pleural fluid R84.6
      prostatic secretions R86.6
      saliva R85.69
      seminal fluid R86.6
      sites NEC R89.6
      sputum R84.6
      synovial fluid R89.6
      throat scrapings R84.6
      vagina R87.629
        atypical squamous cells cannot exclude high grade squamous intraepithelial lesion (ASC-H) R87.621
        atypical squamous cells of undetermined significance (ASC-US) R87.620
        cytologic evidence of malignancy R87.624
        high grade squamous intraepithelial lesion (HGSIL) R87.623
        inadequate smear R87.625
        low grade squamous intraepithelial lesion (LGSIL) R87.622
        specified NEC R87.628
        thin preparation R87.629
        unsatisfactory smear R87.625
      vulva R87.69
      wound secretions R89.6
    partial thromboplastin time (PTT) R79.1
    pelvis (bony) — *see* Deformity, pelvis
    percussion, chest (tympany) R09.89
    periods (grossly) — *see* Menstruation
    phonocardiogram R94.39
    plantar reflex R29.2
    plasma
      protein R77.9
        specified NEC R77.8
      viscosity R70.1
    pleural (folds) Q34.0
    posture R29.3
    product of conception O02.9
      specified type NEC O02.89
    prothrombin time (PT) R79.1
    pulmonary
      artery, congenital Q25.79
      function, newborn P28.89
      test results R94.2
    pulsations in neck R00.2
    pupillary H21.56- ☑
      function (reaction) (reflex) — *see* Anomaly, pupil, function
    radiological examination — *see* Abnormal, diagnostic imaging

Abnormal, abnormality, abnormalities —
    continued
    red blood cell(s) (morphology) (volume) R71.8
    reflex — *see* Reflex
    renal function test R94.4
    response to nerve stimulation R94.130
    retinal correspondence H53.31
    retinal function study R94.111
    rhythm, heart (*see also* Arrhythmia)
    saliva — *see* Abnormal, specimen, digestive organs
    scan
      kidney R94.4
      liver R93.2
      thyroid R94.6
    secretion
      gastrin E16.4
      glucagon E16.3
    semen, seminal fluid — *see* Abnormal, specimen, male genital organs
    serum level (of)
      acid phosphatase R74.8
      alkaline phosphatase R74.8
      amylase R74.8
      enzymes R74.9
        specified NEC R74.8
      lipase R74.8
      triacylglycerol lipase R74.8
    shape
      gravid uterus — *see* Anomaly, uterus
    sinus venosus Q21.1
    size, tooth, teeth K00.2
    spacing, tooth, teeth, fully erupted M26.30
    specimen
      digestive organs (peritoneal fluid) (saliva) R85.9
        cytology R85.69
        drug level R85.2
        enzyme level R85.0
        histology R85.7
        hormones R85.1
        immunology R85.4
        microbiology R85.5
        nonmedicinal level R85.3
        specified type NEC R85.89
      female genital organs (secretions) (smears) R87.9
        cytology R87.69
          cervix R87.619
            human papillomavirus (HPV) DNA test
              high risk positive R87.810
              low risk positive R87.820
            inadequate (unsatisfactory) smear R87.615
            non-atypical endometrial cells R87.618
            specified NEC R87.618
          vagina R87.629
            human papillomavirus (HPV) DNA test
              high risk positive R87.811
              low risk positive R87.821
            inadequate (unsatisfactory) smear R87.625
          vulva R87.69
        drug level R87.2
        enzyme level R87.0
        histological R87.7
        hormones R87.1
        immunology R87.4
        microbiology R87.5
        nonmedicinal level R87.3
        specified type NEC R87.89
      male genital organs (prostatic secretions) (semen) R86.9
        cytology R86.6
        drug level R86.2
        enzyme level R86.0
        histological R86.7
        hormones R86.1
        immunology R86.4
        microbiology R86.5
        nonmedicinal level R86.3
        specified type NEC R86.8
      nipple discharge — *see* Abnormal, specimen, specified
      respiratory organs (bronchial washings) (nasal secretions) (pleural fluid) (sputum) R84.9
        cytology R84.6
        drug level R84.2
        enzyme level R84.0
        histology R84.7
        hormones R84.1
        immunology R84.4

Abnormal, abnormality, abnormalities — *continued*
  specimen — *continued*
    respiratory organs — *continued*
      microbiology R84.5
      nonmedicinal level R84.3
      specified type NEC R84.8
    specified organ, system and tissue NOS R89.9
      cytology R89.6
      drug level R89.2
      enzyme level R89.0
      histology R89.7
      hormones R89.1
      immunology R89.4
      microbiology R89.5
      nonmedicinal level R89.3
      specified type NEC R89.8
    synovial fluid — *see* Abnormal, specimen, specified
    thorax (bronchial washings) (pleural fluids) — *see* Abnormal, specimen, respiratory organs
    vagina (secretion) (smear) R87.629
    vulva (secretion) (smear) R87.69
    wound secretion — *see* Abnormal, specimen, specified
    spermatozoa — *see* Abnormal, specimen, male genital organs
  sputum (amount) (color) (odor) R09.3
  stool (color) (contents) (mucus) R19.5
    bloody K92.1
    guaiac positive R19.5
  synchondrosis Q78.8
  thermography (*see also* Abnormal, diagnostic imaging) R93.89
  thyroid-binding globulin E07.89
  tooth, teeth (form) (size) K00.2
  toxicology (findings) R78.9
  transport protein E88.09
  tumor marker NEC R97.8
  ultrasound results — *see* Abnormal, diagnostic imaging
  umbilical cord complicating delivery O69.9 ☑
  urination NEC R39.198
  urine (constituents) R82.90
    bile R82.2
    cytological examination R82.8
    drugs R82.5
    fat R82.0
    glucose R81
    heavy metals R82.6
    hemoglobin R82.3
    histological examination R82.8
    ketones R82.4
    microbiological examination (culture) R82.79
    myoglobin R82.1
    positive culture R82.79
    protein — *see* Proteinuria
    specified substance NEC R82.998
      chromoabnormality NEC R82.91
    substances nonmedical R82.6
  uterine hemorrhage — *see* Hemorrhage, uterus
  vectorcardiogram R94.39
  visually evoked potential (VEP) R94.112
  white blood cells D72.9
    specified NEC D72.89
  X-ray examination — *see* Abnormal, diagnostic imaging
Abnormity (any organ or part) — *see* Anomaly
Abocclusion M26.29
  hemolytic disease (newborn) P55.1
  incompatibility reaction ABO — *see* Complication(s), transfusion, incompatibility reaction, ABO
Abolition, language R48.8
Aborter, habitual or recurrent — *see* Loss (of), pregnancy, recurrent
Abortion (complete) (spontaneous) O03.9
  with
    retained products of conception — *see* Abortion, incomplete
  attempted (elective) (failed) O07.4
    complicated by O07.30
      afibrinogenemia O07.1
      cardiac arrest O07.36
      chemical damage of pelvic organ(s) O07.34
      circulatory collapse O07.31
      cystitis O07.38
      defibrination syndrome O07.1
      electrolyte imbalance O07.33
      embolism (air) (amniotic fluid) (blood clot) (fat) (pulmonary) (septic) (soap) O07.2
      endometritis O07.0

Abortion — *continued*
  attempted — *continued*
    complicated by — *continued*
      genital tract and pelvic infection O07.0
      hemolysis O07.1
      hemorrhage (delayed) (excessive) O07.1
      infection
        genital tract or pelvic O07.0
        urinary tract tract O07.38
      intravascular coagulation O07.1
      laceration of pelvic organ(s) O07.34
      metabolic disorder O07.33
      oliguria O07.32
      oophoritis O07.0
      parametritis O07.0
      pelvic peritonitis O07.0
      perforation of pelvic organ(s) O07.34
      renal failure or shutdown O07.32
      salpingitis or salpingo-oophoritis O07.0
      sepsis O07.37
      shock O07.31
      specified condition NEC O07.39
      tubular necrosis (renal) O07.32
      uremia O07.32
      urinary tract infection O07.38
      venous complication NEC O07.35
        embolism (air) (amniotic fluid) (blood clot) (fat) (pulmonary) (septic) (soap) O07.2
  complicated (by) (following) O03.80
    afibrinogenemia O03.6
    cardiac arrest O03.86
    chemical damage of pelvic organ(s) O03.84
    circulatory collapse O03.81
    cystitis O03.88
    defibrination syndrome O03.6
    electrolyte imbalance O03.83
    embolism (air) (amniotic fluid) (blood clot) (fat) (pulmonary) (septic) (soap) O03.7
    endometritis O03.5
    genital tract and pelvic infection O03.5
    hemolysis O03.6
    hemorrhage (delayed) (excessive) O03.6
    infection
      genital tract or pelvic O03.5
      urinary tract O03.88
    intravascular coagulation O03.6
    laceration of pelvic organ(s) O03.84
    metabolic disorder O03.83
    oliguria O03.82
    oophoritis O03.5
    parametritis O03.5
    pelvic peritonitis O03.5
    perforation of pelvic organ(s) O03.84
    renal failure or shutdown O03.82
    salpingitis or salpingo-oophoritis O03.5
    sepsis O03.87
    shock O03.81
    specified condition NEC O03.89
    tubular necrosis (renal) O03.82
    uremia O03.82
    urinary tract infection O03.88
    venous complication NEC O03.85
      embolism (air) (amniotic fluid) (blood clot) (fat) (pulmonary) (septic) (soap) O03.7
  failed — *see* Abortion, attempted
  habitual or recurrent N96
    with current abortion — *see* categories O03-O04
    without current pregnancy N96
    care in current pregnancy O26.2- ☑
  incomplete (spontaneous) O03.4
    complicated (by) (following) O03.30
      afibrinogenemia O03.1
      cardiac arrest O03.36
      chemical damage of pelvic organ(s) O03.34
      circulatory collapse O03.31
      cystitis O03.38
      defibrination syndrome O03.1
      electrolyte imbalance O03.33
      embolism (air) (amniotic fluid) (blood clot) (fat) (pulmonary) (septic) (soap) O03.2
      endometritis O03.0
      genital tract and pelvic infection O03.0
      hemolysis O03.1
      hemorrhage (delayed) (excessive) O03.1
      infection
        genital tract or pelvic O03.0
        urinary tract O03.38
      intravascular coagulation O03.1
      laceration of pelvic organ(s) O03.34

Abortion — *continued*
  incomplete — *continued*
    complicated — *continued*
      metabolic disorder O03.33
      oliguria O03.32
      oophoritis O03.0
      parametritis O03.0
      pelvic peritonitis O03.0
      perforation of pelvic organ(s) O03.34
      renal failure or shutdown O03.32
      salpingitis or salpingo-oophoritis O03.0
      sepsis O03.37
      shock O03.31
      specified condition NEC O03.39
      tubular necrosis (renal) O03.32
      uremia O03.32
      urinary infection O03.38
      venous complication NEC O03.35
        embolism (air) (amniotic fluid) (blood clot) (fat) (pulmonary) (septic) (soap) O03.2
  induced (encounter for) Z33.2
    complicated by O04.80
      afibrinogenemia O04.6
      cardiac arrest O04.86
      chemical damage of pelvic organ(s) O04.84
      circulatory collapse O04.81
      cystitis O04.88
      defibrination syndrome O04.6
      electrolyte imbalance O04.83
      embolism (air) (amniotic fluid) (blood clot) (fat) (pulmonary) (septic) (soap) O04.7
      endometritis O04.5
      genital tract and pelvic infection O04.5
      hemolysis O04.6
      hemorrhage (delayed) (excessive) O04.6
      infection
        genital tract or pelvic O04.5
        urinary tract O04.88
      intravascular coagulation O04.6
      laceration of pelvic organ(s) O04.84
      metabolic disorder O04.83
      oliguria O04.82
      oophoritis O04.5
      parametritis O04.5
      pelvic peritonitis O04.5
      perforation of pelvic organ(s) O04.84
      renal failure or shutdown O04.82
      salpingitis or salpingo-oophoritis O04.5
      sepsis O04.87
      shock O04.81
      specified condition NEC O04.89
      tubular necrosis (renal) O04.82
      uremia O04.82
      urinary tract infection O04.88
      venous complication NEC O04.85
        embolism (air) (amniotic fluid) (blood clot) (fat) (pulmonary) (septic) (soap) O04.7
  missed O02.1
  spontaneous — *see* Abortion (complete) (spontaneous)
    threatened O20.0
  threatened (spontaneous) O20.0
  tubal O00.10- ☑
    with intrauterine pregnancy O00.11- ☑
Abortus fever A23.1
Aboulomania F60.7
Abrami's disease D59.8
Abramov-Fiedler myocarditis (acute isolated myocarditis) I40.1
Abrasion T14.8 ☑
  abdomen, abdominal (wall) S30.811 ☑
  alveolar process S00.512 ☑
  ankle S90.51- ☑
  antecubital space — *see* Abrasion, elbow
  anus S30.817 ☑
  arm (upper) S40.81- ☑
  auditory canal — *see* Abrasion, ear
  auricle — *see* Abrasion, ear
  axilla — *see* Abrasion, arm
  back, lower S30.810 ☑
  breast S20.11- ☑
  brow S00.81 ☑
  buttock S30.810 ☑
  calf — *see* Abrasion, leg
  canthus — *see* Abrasion, eyelid
  cheek S00.81 ☑
    internal S00.512 ☑
  chest wall — *see* Abrasion, thorax
  chin S00.81 ☑

Abrasion — *continued*
clitoris S30.814 ☑
cornea S05.0- ☑
costal region — *see* Abrasion, thorax
dental K03.1
digit(s)
  foot — *see* Abrasion, toe
  hand — *see* Abrasion, finger
ear S00.41- ☑
elbow S50.31- ☑
epididymis S30.813 ☑
epigastric region S30.811 ☑
epiglottis S10.11 ☑
esophagus (thoracic) S27.818 ☑
  cervical S10.11 ☑
eyebrow — *see* Abrasion, eyelid
eyelid S00.21- ☑
face S00.81 ☑
finger(s) S60.41- ☑
  index S60.41- ☑
  little S60.41- ☑
  middle S60.41- ☑
  ring S60.41- ☑
flank S30.811 ☑
foot (except toe(s) alone) S90.81- ☑
  toe — *see* Abrasion, toe
forearm S50.81- ☑
  elbow only — *see* Abrasion, elbow
forehead S00.81 ☑
genital organs, external
  female S30.816 ☑
  male S30.815 ☑
groin S30.811 ☑
gum S00.512 ☑
hand S60.51- ☑
head S00.91 ☑
  ear — *see* Abrasion, ear
  eyelid — *see* Abrasion, eyelid
  lip S00.511 ☑
  nose S00.31 ☑
  oral cavity S00.512 ☑
  scalp S00.01 ☑
  specified site NEC S00.81 ☑
heel — *see* Abrasion, foot
hip S70.21- ☑
inguinal region S30.811 ☑
interscapular region S20.419 ☑
jaw S00.81 ☑
knee S80.21- ☑
labium (majus) (minus) S30.814 ☑
larynx S10.11 ☑
leg (lower) S80.81- ☑
  knee — *see* Abrasion, knee
  upper — *see* Abrasion, thigh
lip S00.511 ☑
lower back S30.810 ☑
lumbar region S30.810 ☑
malar region S00.81 ☑
mammary — *see* Abrasion, breast
mastoid region S00.81 ☑
mouth S00.512 ☑
nail
  finger — *see* Abrasion, finger
  toe — *see* Abrasion, toe
nape S10.81 ☑
nasal S00.31 ☑
neck S10.91 ☑
  specified site NEC S10.81 ☑
  throat S10.11 ☑
nose S00.31 ☑
occipital region S00.01 ☑
oral cavity S00.512 ☑
orbital region — *see* Abrasion, eyelid
palate S00.512 ☑
palm — *see* Abrasion, hand
parietal region S00.01 ☑
pelvis S30.810 ☑
penis S30.812 ☑
perineum
  female S30.814 ☑
  male S30.810 ☑
periocular area — *see* Abrasion, eyelid
phalanges
  finger — *see* Abrasion, finger
  toe — *see* Abrasion, toe
pharynx S10.11 ☑

Abrasion — *continued*
pinna — *see* Abrasion, ear
popliteal space — *see* Abrasion, knee
prepuce S30.812 ☑
pubic region S30.810 ☑
pudendum
  female S30.816 ☑
  male S30.815 ☑
sacral region S30.810 ☑
scalp S00.01 ☑
scapular region — *see* Abrasion, shoulder
scrotum S30.813 ☑
shin — *see* Abrasion, leg
shoulder S40.21- ☑
skin NEC T14.8 ☑
sternal region S20.319 ☑
submaxillary region S00.81 ☑
submental region S00.81 ☑
subungual
  finger(s) — *see* Abrasion, finger
  toe(s) — *see* Abrasion, toe
supraclavicular fossa S10.81 ☑
supraorbital S00.81 ☑
temple S00.81 ☑
temporal region S00.81 ☑
testis S30.813 ☑
thigh S70.31- ☑
thorax, thoracic (wall) S20.91 ☑
  back S20.41- ☑
  front S20.31- ☑
throat S10.11 ☑
thumb S60.31- ☑
toe(s) (lesser) S90.416 ☑
  great S90.41- ☑
tongue S00.512 ☑
tooth, teeth (dentifrice) (habitual) (hard tissues) (occupational) (ritual) (traditional) K03.1
trachea S10.11 ☑
tunica vaginalis S30.813 ☑
tympanum, tympanic membrane — *see* Abrasion, ear
uvula S00.512 ☑
vagina S30.814 ☑
vocal cords S10.11 ☑
vulva S30.814 ☑
wrist S60.81- ☑
Abrism — *see* Poisoning, food, noxious, plant
Abruptio placentae O45.9- ☑
with
  afibrinogenemia O45.01- ☑
  coagulation defect O45.00- ☑
    specified NEC O45.09- ☑
  disseminated intravascular coagulation O45.02- ☑
  hypofibrinogenemia O45.01- ☑
  specified NEC O45.8- ☑
Abruption, placenta — *see* Abruptio placentae
Abscess (connective tissue) (embolic) (fistulous) (infective) (metastatic) (multiple) (pernicious) (pyogenic) (septic) L02.91
with
  diverticular disease (intestine) K57.80
    with bleeding K57.81
    large intestine K57.20
      with
        bleeding K57.21
        small intestine K57.40
          with bleeding K57.41
      small intestine K57.00
        with
          bleeding K57.01
          large intestine K57.40
            with bleeding K57.41
  lymphangitis — *code by* site under Abscess
abdomen, abdominal
  cavity K65.1
  wall L02.211
abdominopelvic K65.1
accessory sinus — *see* Sinusitis
adrenal (capsule) (gland) E27.8
alveolar K04.7
  with sinus K04.6
amebic A06.4
  brain (and liver or lung abscess) A06.6
  genitourinary tract A06.82
  liver (without mention of brain or lung abscess) A06.4
  lung (and liver) (without mention of brain abscess) A06.5

Abscess — *continued*
amebic — *continued*
  specified site NEC A06.89
  spleen A06.89
anerobic A48.0
ankle — *see* Abscess, lower limb
anorectal K61.2
antecubital space — *see* Abscess, upper limb
antrum (chronic) (Highmore) — *see* Sinusitis, maxillary
anus K61.0
apical (tooth) K04.7
  with sinus (alveolar) K04.6
appendix K35.33
areola (acute) (chronic) (nonpuerperal) N61.1
  puerperal, postpartum or gestational — *see* Infection, nipple
arm (any part) — *see* Abscess, upper limb
artery (wall) I77.89
atheromatous I77.2
auricle, ear — *see* Abscess, ear, external
axilla (region) L02.41- ☑
  lymph gland or node L04.2
back (any part, except buttock) L02.212
Bartholin's gland N75.1
  with
    abortion — *see* Abortion, by type complicated by, sepsis
    ectopic or molar pregnancy O08.0
    following ectopic or molar pregnancy O08.0
Bezold's — *see* Mastoiditis, acute
bilharziasis B65.1
bladder (wall) — *see* Cystitis, specified type NEC
bone (subperiosteal) (*see also* Osteomyelitis, specified type NEC)
  accessory sinus (chronic) — *see* Sinusitis
  chronic or old — *see* Osteomyelitis, chronic
  jaw (lower) (upper) M27.2
  mastoid — *see* Mastoiditis, acute, subperiosteal
  petrous — *see* Petrositis
  spinal (tuberculous) A18.01
    nontuberculous — *see* Osteomyelitis, vertebra
bowel K63.0
brain (any part) (cystic) (otogenic) G06.0
  amebic (with abscess of any other site) A06.6
  gonococcal A54.82
  pheomycotic (chromomycotic) B43.1
  tuberculous A17.81
breast (acute) (chronic) (nonpuerperal) N61.1
  newborn P39.0
  puerperal, postpartum, gestational — *see* Mastitis, obstetric, purulent
broad ligament N73.2
  acute N73.0
  chronic N73.1
Brodie's (localized) (chronic) M86.8X- ☑
bronchi J98.09
buccal cavity K12.2
bulbourethral gland N34.0
bursa M71.00
  ankle M71.07- ☑
  elbow M71.02- ☑
  foot M71.07- ☑
  hand M71.04- ☑
  hip M71.05- ☑
  knee M71.06- ☑
  multiple sites M71.09
  pharyngeal J39.1
  shoulder M71.01- ☑
  specified site NEC M71.08
  wrist M71.03- ☑
buttock L02.31
canthus — *see* Blepharoconjunctivitis
cartilage — *see* Disorder, cartilage, specified type NEC
cecum K35.33
cerebellum, cerebellar G06.0
  sequelae G09
cerebral (embolic) G06.0
  sequelae G09
cervical (meaning neck) L02.11
  lymph gland or node L04.0
cervix (stump) (uteri) — *see* Cervicitis
cheek (external) L02.01
  inner K12.2
chest J86.9
  with fistula J86.0
  wall L02.213
chin L02.01
choroid — *see* Inflammation, chorioretinal

4

☑ **Additional Character Required** — Refer to the Tabular List for Character Selection   ▽ **Subterms under main terms may continue to next column or page**

Abscess — *continued*
  circumtonsillar J36
  cold (lung) (tuberculous) (*see also* Tuberculosis, abscess, lung)
    articular — *see* Tuberculosis, joint
  colon (wall) K63.0
  colostomy K94.02
  conjunctiva — *see* Conjunctivitis, acute
  cornea H16.31- ☑
  corpus
    cavernosum N48.21
    luteum — *see* Oophoritis
  Cowper's gland N34.0
  cranium G06.0
  cul-de-sac (Douglas') (posterior) — *see* Peritonitis, pelvic, female
  cutaneous — *see* Abscess, by site
  dental K04.7
    with sinus (alveolar) K04.6
  dentoalveolar K04.7
    with sinus K04.6
  diaphragm, diaphragmatic K65.1
  Douglas' cul-de-sac or pouch — *see* Peritonitis, pelvic, female
  Dubois A50.59
  ear (middle) (*see also* Otitis, media, suppurative)
    acute — *see* Otitis, media, suppurative, acute
    external H60.0- ☑
  entamebic — *see* Abscess, amebic
  enterostomy K94.12
  epididymis N45.4
  epidural G06.2
    brain G06.0
    spinal cord G06.1
  epiglottis J38.7
  epiploon, epiploic K65.1
  erysipelatous — *see* Erysipelas
  esophagus K20.8
  ethmoid (bone) (chronic) (sinus) J32.2
  external auditory canal — *see* Abscess, ear, external
  extradural G06.2
    brain G06.0
      sequelae G09
    spinal cord G06.1
  extraperitoneal K68.19
  eye — *see* Endophthalmitis, purulent
  eyelid H00.03- ☑
  face (any part, except ear, eye and nose) L02.01
  fallopian tube — *see* Salpingitis
  fascia M72.8
  fauces J39.1
  fecal K63.0
  femoral (region) — *see* Abscess, lower limb
  filaria, filarial — *see* Infestation, filarial
  finger (any) (*see also* Abscess, hand)
    nail — *see* Cellulitis, finger
  foot L02.61- ☑
  forehead L02.01
  frontal sinus (chronic) J32.1
  gallbladder K81.0
  genital organ or tract
    female (external) N76.4
    male N49.9
      multiple sites N49.8
      specified NEC N49.8
  gestational mammary O91.11- ☑
  gestational subareolar O91.11- ☑
  gingival — *see* Peridontitis, localized
  gland, glandular (lymph) (acute) — *see* Lymphadenitis, acute
  gluteal (region) L02.31
  gonorrheal — *see* Gonococcus
  groin L02.214
  gum — *see* Peridontitis, localized
  hand L02.51- ☑
  head NEC L02.811
    face (any part, except ear, eye and nose) L02.01
  heart — *see* Carditis
  heel — *see* Abscess, foot
  helminthic — *see* Infestation, helminth
  hepatic (cholangitic) (hematogenic) (lymphogenic) (pyelphlebitic) K75.0
    amebic A06.4
  hip (region) — *see* Abscess, lower limb
  horseshoe K61.31
  ileocecal K35.33
  ileostomy (bud) K94.12
  iliac (region) L02.214

Abscess — *continued*
  iliac — *continued*
    fossa K35.33
  infraclavicular (fossa) — *see* Abscess, upper limb
  inguinal (region) L02.214
    lymph gland or node L04.1
  intersphincteric K61.4
  intestine, intestinal NEC K63.0
    rectal K61.1
  intra-abdominal (*see also* Abscess, peritoneum) K65.1
    following procedure T81.43 ☑
      obstetrical O86.03
    postprocedural T81.49 ☑
      retroperitoneal K68.11
  intracranial G06.0
  intramammary — *see* Abscess, breast
  intramuscular, following procedure T81.42 ☑
    obstetrical O86.02
  intraorbital — *see* Abscess, orbit
  intraperitoneal K65.1
  intrasphincteric (anus) K61.4
  intraspinal G06.1
  intratonsillar J36
  ischiorectal (fossa) (specified NEC) K61.39
  jaw (bone) (lower) (upper) M27.2
  joint — *see* Arthritis, pyogenic or pyemic
    spine (tuberculous) A18.01
      nontuberculous — *see* Spondylopathy, infective
  kidney N15.1
    with calculus N20.0
      with hydronephrosis N13.6
    puerperal (postpartum) O86.21
  knee (*see also* Abscess, lower limb)
    joint M00.9
  labium (majus) (minus) N76.4
  lacrimal
    caruncle — *see* Inflammation, lacrimal, passages, acute
    gland — *see* Dacryoadenitis
    passages (duct) (sac) — *see* Inflammation, lacrimal, passages, acute
  lacunar N34.0
  larynx J38.7
  lateral (alveolar) K04.7
    with sinus K04.6
  leg (any part) — *see* Abscess, lower limb
  lens H27.8
  lingual K14.0
    tonsil J36
  lip K13.0
  Littre's gland N34.0
  liver (cholangitic) (hematogenic) (lymphogenic) (pyle-phlebitic) (pyogenic) K75.0
    amebic (due to Entamoeba histolytica) (dysenteric) (tropical) A06.4
    with
      brain abscess (and liver or lung abscess) A06.6
      lung abscess A06.5
  loin (region) L02.211
  lower limb L02.41- ☑
  lumbar (tuberculous) A18.01
    nontuberculous L02.212
  lung (miliary) (putrid) J85.2
    with pneumonia J85.1
      due to specified organism (see Pneumonia, in (due to))
    amebic (with liver abscess) A06.5
      with
        brain abscess A06.6
        pneumonia A06.5
  lymph, lymphatic, gland or node (acute) (*see also* Lymphadenitis, acute)
    mesentery I88.0
  malar M27.2
  mammary gland — *see* Abscess, breast
  marginal, anus K61.0
  mastoid — *see* Mastoiditis, acute
  maxilla, maxillary M27.2
    molar (tooth) K04.7
      with sinus K04.6
    premolar K04.7
    sinus (chronic) J32.0
  mediastinum J85.3
  meibomian gland — *see* Hordeolum
  meninges G06.2
  mesentery, mesenteric K65.1
  mesosalpinx — *see* Salpingitis
  mons pubis L02.215

Abscess — *continued*
  mouth (floor) K12.2
  muscle — *see* Myositis, infective
  myocardium I40.0
  nabothian (follicle) — *see* Cervicitis
  nasal J32.9
  nasopharyngeal J39.1
  navel L02.216
    newborn P38.9
      with mild hemorrhage P38.1
      without hemorrhage P38.9
  neck (region) L02.11
    lymph gland or node L04.0
  nephritic — *see* Abscess, kidney
  nipple N61.1
    associated with
      lactation — *see* Pregnancy, complicated by
      pregnancy — *see* Pregnancy, complicated by
  nose (external) (fossa) (septum) J34.0
    sinus (chronic) — *see* Sinusitis
  omentum K65.1
  operative wound T81.49 ☑
  orbit, orbital — *see* Cellulitis, orbit
  otogenic G06.0
  ovary, ovarian (corpus luteum) — *see* Oophoritis
  oviduct — *see* Oophoritis
  palate (soft) K12.2
    hard M27.2
  palmar (space) — *see* Abscess, hand
  pancreas (duct) — *see* Pancreatitis, acute
  parafrenal N48.21
  parametric, parametrium N73.2
    acute N73.0
    chronic N73.1
  paranephric N15.1
  parapancreatic — *see* Pancreatitis, acute
  parapharyngeal J39.0
  pararectal K61.1
  parasinus — *see* Sinusitis
  parauterine (*see also* Disease, pelvis, inflammatory) N73.2
  paravaginal — *see* Vaginitis
  parietal region (scalp) L02.811
  parodontal — *see* Peridontitis, aggressive, localized
  parotid (duct) (gland) K11.3
    region K12.2
  pectoral (region) L02.213
  pelvis, pelvic
    female — *see* Disease, pelvis, inflammatory
    male, peritoneal K65.1
  penis N48.21
    gonococcal (accessory gland) (periurethral) A54.1
  perianal K61.0
  periapical K04.7
    with sinus (alveolar) K04.6
  periappendicular K35.33
  pericardial I30.1
  pericecal K35.33
  pericemental — *see* Peridontitis, aggressive, localized
  pericholecystic — *see* Cholecystitis, acute
  pericoronal — *see* Peridontitis, aggressive, localized
  peridental — *see* Peridontitis, aggressive, localized
  perimetric (*see also* Disease, pelvis, inflammatory) N73.2
  perinephric, perinephritic — *see* Abscess, kidney
  perineum, perineal (superficial) L02.215
    urethra N34.0
  periodontal (parietal) — *see* Peridontitis, aggressive, localized
    apical K04.7
  periosteum, periosteal (*see also* Osteomyelitis, specified type NEC)
    with osteomyelitis (*see also* Osteomyelitis, specified type NEC)
      acute — *see* Osteomyelitis, acute
      chronic — *see* Osteomyelitis, chronic
  peripharyngeal J39.0
  peripleuritic J86.9
    with fistula J86.0
  periprostatic N41.2
  perirectal K61.1
  perirenal (tissue) — *see* Abscess, kidney
  perisinuous (nose) — *see* Sinusitis
  peritoneum, peritoneal (perforated) (ruptured) K65.1
    with appendicitis (*see also* Appendicitis) K35.33
    pelvic
      female — *see* Peritonitis, pelvic, female
      male K65.1
    postoperative T81.49 ☑

☑ Subterms under main terms may continue to next column or page   ☑ Additional Character Required — Refer to the Tabular List for Character Selection   5

Index

Abscess — Abscess

Abscess — *continued*
peritoneum, peritoneal — *continued*
   puerperal, postpartum, childbirth O85
   tuberculous A18.31
peritonsillar J36
perityphlic K35.33
periureteral N28.89
periurethral N34.0
   gonococcal (accessory gland) (periurethral) A54.1
periuterine (*see also* Disease, pelvis, inflammatory) N73.2
perivesical — *see* Cystitis, specified type NEC
petrous bone — *see* Petrositis
phagedenic NOS L02.91
   chancroid A57
pharynx, pharyngeal (lateral) J39.1
pilonidal L05.01
pituitary (gland) E23.6
pleura J86.9
   with fistula J86.0
popliteal — *see* Abscess, lower limb
postcecal K35.33
postlaryngeal J38.7
postnasal J34.0
postoperative (any site) (*see also* Infection, postoperative wound) T81.49 ☑
   retroperitoneal K68.11
postpharyngeal J39.0
posttonsillar J36
post-typhoid A01.09
pouch of Douglas — *see* Peritonitis, pelvic, female
premammary — *see* Abscess, breast
prepatellar — *see* Abscess, lower limb
prostate N41.2
   gonococcal (acute) (chronic) A54.22
psoas muscle K68.12
puerperal — *code by* site under Puerperal, abscess
pulmonary — *see* Abscess, lung
pulp, pulpal (dental) K04.01
   irreversible K04.02
   reversible K04.01
rectovaginal septum K63.0
rectovesical — *see* Cystitis, specified type NEC
rectum K61.1
renal — *see* Abscess, kidney
retina — *see* Inflammation, chorioretinal
retrobulbar — *see* Abscess, orbit
retrocecal K65.1
retrolaryngeal J38.7
retromammary — *see* Abscess, breast
retroperitoneal NEC K68.19
   postprocedural K68.11
retropharyngeal J39.0
retrouterine — *see* Peritonitis, pelvic, female
retrovesical — *see* Cystitis, specified type NEC
root, tooth K04.7
   with sinus (alveolar) K04.6
round ligament (*see also* Disease, pelvis, inflammatory) N73.2
rupture (spontaneous) NOS L02.91
sacrum (tuberculous) A18.01
   nontuberculous M46.28
salivary (duct) (gland) K11.3
scalp (any part) L02.811
scapular — *see* Osteomyelitis, specified type NEC
sclera — *see* Scleritis
scrofulous (tuberculous) A18.2
scrotum N49.2
seminal vesicle N49.0
septal, dental K04.7
   with sinus (alveolar) K04.6
serous — *see* Periostitis
shoulder (region) — *see* Abscess, upper limb
sigmoid K63.0
sinus (accessory) (chronic) (nasal) (*see also* Sinusitis)
   intracranial venous (any) G06.0
Skene's duct or gland N34.0
skin — *see* Abscess, by site
specified site NEC L02.818
spermatic cord N49.1
sphenoidal (sinus) (chronic) J32.3
spinal cord (any part) (staphylococcal) G06.1
   tuberculous A17.81
spine (column) (tuberculous) A18.01
   epidural G06.1
   nontuberculous — *see* Osteomyelitis, vertebra
spleen D73.3
   amebic A06.89

Abscess — *continued*
stitch T81.41
   following an obstetrical procedure O86.01
subarachnoid G06.2
   brain G06.0
   spinal cord G06.1
subareolar — *see* Abscess, breast
subcecal K35.33
subcutaneous (*see also* Abscess, by site)
   following procedure T81.41 ☑
     obstetrical O86.01
   pheomycotic (chromomycotic) B43.2
subdiaphragmatic K65.1
subdural G06.2
   brain G06.0
     sequelae G09
   spinal cord G06.1
sub-fascial, following an obstetrical procedure O86.02
subgaleal L02.811
subhepatic K65.1
sublingual K12.2
   gland K11.3
submammary — *see* Abscess, breast
submandibular (region) (space) (triangle) K12.2
   gland K11.3
submaxillary (region) L02.01
   gland K11.3
submental L02.01
   gland K11.3
subperiosteal — *see* Osteomyelitis, specified type NEC
subphrenic K65.1
   following an obstetrical procedure O86.03
   postoperative T81.43 ☑
suburethral N34.0
sudoriparous L75.8
supraclavicular (fossa) — *see* Abscess, upper limb
supralevator K61.5
suprapelvic, acute N73.0
suprarenal (capsule) (gland) E27.8
sweat gland L74.8
tear duct — *see* Inflammation, lacrimal, passages, acute
temple L02.01
temporal region L02.01
temporosphenoidal G06.0
tendon (sheath) M65.00
   ankle M65.07- ☑
   foot M65.07- ☑
   forearm M65.03- ☑
   hand M65.04- ☑
   lower leg M65.06- ☑
   pelvic region M65.05- ☑
   shoulder region M65.01- ☑
   specified site NEC M65.08
   thigh M65.05- ☑
   upper arm M65.02- ☑
testis N45.4
thigh — *see* Abscess, lower limb
thorax J86.9
   with fistula J86.0
throat J39.1
thumb (*see also* Abscess, hand)
   nail — *see* Cellulitis, finger
thymus (gland) E32.1
thyroid (gland) E06.0
toe (any) (*see also* Abscess, foot)
   nail — *see* Cellulitis, toe
tongue (staphylococcal) K14.0
tonsil(s) (lingual) J36
tonsillopharyngeal J36
tooth, teeth (root) K04.7
   with sinus (alveolar) K04.6
   supporting structures NEC — *see* Periodontitis, aggressive, localized
trachea J39.8
trunk L02.219
   abdominal wall L02.211
   back L02.212
   chest wall L02.213
   groin L02.214
   perineum L02.215
   umbilicus L02.216
tubal — *see* Salpingitis
tuberculous — *see* Tuberculosis, abscess
tubo-ovarian — *see* Salpingo-oophoritis
tunica vaginalis N49.1
umbilicus L02.216
upper
   limb L02.41- ☑

Abscess — *continued*
upper — *continued*
   respiratory J39.8
urethral (gland) N34.0
urinary N34.0
uterus, uterine (wall) (*see also* Endometritis)
   ligament (*see also* Disease, pelvis, inflammatory) N73.2
   neck — *see* Cervicitis
uvula K12.2
vagina (wall) — *see* Vaginitis
vaginorectal — *see* Vaginitis
vas deferens N49.1
vermiform appendix K35.33
vertebra (column) (tuberculous) A18.01
   nontuberculous — *see* Osteomyelitis, vertebra
vesical — *see* Cystitis, specified type NEC
vesico-uterine pouch — *see* Peritonitis, pelvic, female
vitreous (humor) — *see* Endophthalmitis, purulent
vocal cord J38.3
von Bezold's — *see* Mastoiditis, acute
vulva N76.4
vulvovaginal gland N75.1
web space — *see* Abscess, hand
wound T81.49 ☑
wrist — *see* Abscess, upper limb
Absence (of) (organ or part) (complete or partial)
adrenal (gland) (congenital) Q89.1
   acquired E89.6
albumin in blood E88.09
alimentary tract (congenital) Q45.8
   upper Q40.8
alveolar process (acquired) — *see* Anomaly, alveolar
ankle (acquired) Z89.44- ☑
anus (congenital) Q42.3
   with fistula Q42.2
aorta (congenital) Q25.41
appendix, congenital Q42.8
arm (acquired) Z89.20- ☑
   above elbow Z89.22- ☑
     congenital (with hand present) — *see* Agenesis, arm, with hand present
     and hand — *see* Agenesis, forearm, and hand
   below elbow Z89.21- ☑
     congenital (with hand present) — *see* Agenesis, arm, with hand present
     and hand — *see* Agenesis, forearm, and hand
   congenital — *see* Defect, reduction, upper limb
   shoulder (following explanation of shoulder joint prosthesis) (joint) (with or without presence of antibiotic-impregnated cement spacer) Z89.23- ☑
     congenital (with hand present) — *see* Agenesis, arm, with hand present
artery (congenital) (peripheral) Q27.8
   brain Q28.3
   coronary Q24.5
   pulmonary Q25.79
   specified NEC Q27.8
   umbilical Q27.0
atrial septum (congenital) Q21.1
auditory canal (congenital) (external) Q16.1
auricle (ear), congenital Q16.0
bile, biliary duct, congenital Q44.5
bladder (acquired) Z90.6
   congenital Q64.5
bowel sounds R19.11
brain Q00.0
   part of Q04.3
breast(s) (and nipple(s)) (acquired) Z90.1- ☑
   congenital Q83.8
broad ligament Q50.6
bronchus (congenital) Q32.4
canaliculus lacrimalis, congenital Q10.4
cerebellum (vermis) Q04.3
cervix (acquired) (with uterus) Z90.710
   with remaining uterus Z90.712
   congenital Q51.5
chin, congenital Q18.8
cilia (congenital) Q10.3
   acquired — *see* Madarosis
clitoris (congenital) Q52.6
coccyx, congenital Q76.49
cold sense R20.8
congenital
   lumen — *see* Atresia
   organ or site NEC — *see* Agenesis
   septum — *see* Imperfect, closure

Absence — *continued*
  corpus callosum Q04.0
  cricoid cartilage, congenital Q31.8
  diaphragm (with hernia), congenital Q79.1
  digestive organ(s) or tract, congenital Q45.8
    acquired NEC Z90.49
    upper Q40.8
  ductus arteriosus Q28.8
  duodenum (acquired) Z90.49
    congenital Q41.0
  ear, congenital Q16.9
    acquired H93.8- ☑
    auricle Q16.0
    external Q16.0
    inner Q16.5
    lobe, lobule Q17.8
    middle, except ossicles Q16.4
      ossicles Q16.3
    ossicles Q16.3
  ejaculatory duct (congenital) Q55.4
  endocrine gland (congenital) NEC Q89.2
    acquired E89.89
  epididymis (congenital) Q55.4
    acquired Z90.79
  epiglottis, congenital Q31.8
  esophagus (congenital) Q39.8
    acquired (partial) Z90.49
  eustachian tube (congenital) Q16.2
  extremity (acquired) Z89.9
    congenital Q73.0
    knee (following explantation of knee joint prosthe-
        sis) (joint) (with or without presence of antibi-
        otic-impregnated cement spacer) Z89.52- ☑
    lower (above knee) Z89.619
      below knee Z89.51- ☑
    upper — *see* Absence, arm
  eye (acquired) Z90.01
    congenital Q11.1
    muscle (congenital) Q10.3
  eyeball (acquired) Z90.01
  eyelid (fold) (congenital) Q10.3
    acquired Z90.01
  face, specified part NEC Q18.8
  fallopian tube(s) (acquired) Z90.79
    congenital Q50.6
  family member (causing problem in home) NEC (*see
      also* Disruption, family) Z63.32
  femur, congenital — *see* Defect, reduction, lower limb,
      longitudinal, femur
  fibrinogen (congenital) D68.2
    acquired D65
  finger(s) (acquired) Z89.02- ☑
    congenital — *see* Agenesis, hand
  foot (acquired) Z89.43- ☑
    congenital — *see* Agenesis, foot
  forearm (acquired) — *see* Absence, arm, below elbow
  gallbladder (acquired) Z90.49
    congenital Q44.0
  gamma globulin in blood D80.1
    hereditary D80.0
  genital organs
    acquired (female) (male) Z90.79
    female, congenital Q52.8
      external Q52.71
      internal NEC Q52.8
    male, congenital Q55.8
  genitourinary organs, congenital NEC
    female Q52.8
    male Q55.8
  globe (acquired) Z90.01
    congenital Q11.1
  glottis, congenital Q31.8
  hand and wrist (acquired) Z89.11- ☑
    congenital — *see* Agenesis, hand
  head, part (acquired) NEC Z90.09
  heat sense R20.8
  hip (following explantation of hip joint prosthesis)
      (joint) (with or without presence of antibiotic-
      impregnated cement spacer) Z89.62- ☑
  hymen (congenital) Q52.4
  ileum (acquired) Z90.49
    congenital Q41.2
  immunoglobulin, isolated NEC D80.3
    IgA D80.2
    IgG D80.3
    IgM D80.4
  incus (acquired) — *see* Loss, ossicles, ear
    congenital Q16.3

Absence — *continued*
  inner ear, congenital Q16.5
  intestine (acquired) (small) Z90.49
    congenital Q41.9
      specified NEC Q41.8
    large Z90.49
      congenital Q42.9
        specified NEC Q42.8
  iris, congenital Q13.1
  jejunum (acquired) Z90.49
    congenital Q41.1
  joint
    acquired
      hip (following explantation of hip joint prosthe-
          sis) (with or without presence of antibiotic-
          impregnated cement spacer) Z89.62- ☑
      knee (following explantation of knee joint pros-
          thesis) (with or without presence of antibi-
          otic-impregnated cement spacer)
          Z89.52- ☑
      shoulder (following explantation of shoulder
          joint prosthesis) (with or without presence
          of antibiotic-impregnated cement spacer)
          Z89.23- ☑
    congenital NEC Q74.8
  kidney(s) (acquired) Z90.5
    congenital Q60.2
      bilateral Q60.1
      unilateral Q60.0
  knee (following explantation of knee joint prosthesis)
      (joint) (with or without presence of antibiotic-
      impregnated cement spacer) Z89.52- ☑
  labyrinth, membranous Q16.5
  larynx (congenital) Q31.8
    acquired Z90.02
  leg (acquired) (above knee) Z89.61- ☑
    below knee (acquired) Z89.51- ☑
    congenital — *see* Defect, reduction, lower limb
  lens (acquired) (*see also* Aphakia)
    congenital Q12.3
    post cataract extraction Z98.4- ☑
  limb (acquired) — *see* Absence, extremity
  lip Q38.6
  liver (congenital) Q44.7
  lung (fissure) (lobe) (bilateral) (unilateral) (congenital)
      Q33.3
    acquired (any part) Z90.2
  menstruation — *see* Amenorrhea
  muscle (congenital) (pectoral) Q79.8
    ocular Q10.3
  neck, part Q18.8
  neutrophil — *see* Agranulocytosis
  nipple(s) (with breast(s)) (acquired) Z90.1- ☑
    congenital Q83.2
  nose (congenital) Q30.1
    acquired Z90.09
  organ
    of Corti, congenital Q16.5
    or site, congenital NEC Q89.8
      acquired NEC Z90.89
  osseous meatus (ear) Q16.4
  ovary (acquired)
    bilateral Z90.722
    congenital
      bilateral Q50.02
      unilateral Q50.01
    unilateral Z90.721
  oviduct (acquired)
    bilateral Z90.722
    congenital Q50.6
    unilateral Z90.721
  pancreas (congenital) Q45.0
    acquired Z90.410
      complete Z90.410
      partial Z90.411
      total Z90.410
  parathyroid gland (acquired) E89.2
    congenital Q89.2
  patella, congenital Q74.1
  penis (congenital) Q55.5
    acquired Z90.79
  pericardium (congenital) Q24.8
  pituitary gland (congenital) Q89.2
    acquired E89.3
  prostate (acquired) Z90.79
    congenital Q55.4
  pulmonary valve Q22.0
  punctum lacrimale (congenital) Q10.4

Absence — *continued*
  radius, congenital — *see* Defect, reduction, upper limb,
      longitudinal, radius
  rectum (congenital) Q42.1
    with fistula Q42.0
    acquired Z90.49
  respiratory organ NOS Q34.9
  rib (acquired) Z90.89
    congenital Q76.6
  sacrum, congenital Q76.49
  salivary gland(s), congenital Q38.4
  scrotum, congenital Q55.29
  seminal vesicles (congenital) Q55.4
    acquired Z90.79
  septum
    atrial (congenital) Q21.1
    between aorta and pulmonary artery Q21.4
    ventricular (congenital) Q20.4
  sex chromosome
    female phenotype Q97.8
    male phenotype Q98.8
  skull bone (congenital) Q75.8
    with
      anencephaly Q00.0
      encephalocele — *see* Encephalocele
      hydrocephalus Q03.9
        with spina bifida — *see* Spina bifida, by site,
            with hydrocephalus
      microcephaly Q02
  spermatic cord, congenital Q55.4
  spine, congenital Q76.49
  spleen (congenital) Q89.01
    acquired Z90.81
  sternum, congenital Q76.7
  stomach (acquired) (partial) Z90.3
    congenital Q40.2
  superior vena cava, congenital Q26.8
  teeth, tooth (congenital) K00.0
    acquired (complete) K08.109
      class I K08.101
      class II K08.102
      class III K08.103
      class IV K08.104
      due to
        caries K08.139
          class I K08.131
          class II K08.132
          class III K08.133
          class IV K08.134
        periodontal disease K08.129
          class I K08.121
          class II K08.122
          class III K08.123
          class IV K08.124
        specified NEC K08.199
          class I K08.191
          class II K08.192
          class III K08.193
          class IV K08.194
        trauma K08.119
          class I K08.111
          class II K08.112
          class III K08.113
          class IV K08.114
      partial K08.409
        class I K08.401
        class II K08.402
        class III K08.403
        class IV K08.404
        due to
          caries K08.439
            class I K08.431
            class II K08.432
            class III K08.433
            class IV K08.434
          periodontal disease K08.429
            class I K08.421
            class II K08.422
            class III K08.423
            class IV K08.424
          specified NEC K08.499
            class I K08.491
            class II K08.492
            class III K08.493
            class IV K08.494
          trauma K08.419
            class I K08.411
            class II K08.412
            class III K08.413

Absence — *continued*
  teeth, tooth — *continued*
    acquired — *continued*
      partial — *continued*
        due to — *continued*
          trauma — *continued*
            class IV K08.414
  tendon (congenital) Q79.8
  testis (congenital) Q55.0
    acquired Z90.79
  thumb (acquired) Z89.01- ☑
    congenital — *see* Agenesis, hand
  thymus gland Q89.2
  thyroid (gland) (acquired) E89.0
    cartilage, congenital Q31.8
    congenital E03.1
  toe(s) (acquired) Z89.42- ☑
    with foot — *see* Absence, foot and ankle
    congenital — *see* Agenesis, foot
    great Z89.41- ☑
  tongue, congenital Q38.3
  trachea (cartilage), congenital Q32.1
  transverse aortic arch, congenital Q25.49
  tricuspid valve Q22.4
  umbilical artery, congenital Q27.0
  upper arm and forearm with hand present, congenital
    — *see* Agenesis, arm, with hand present
  ureter (congenital) Q62.4
    acquired Z90.6
  urethra, congenital Q64.5
  uterus (acquired) Z90.710
    with cervix Z90.710
    with remaining cervical stump Z90.711
    congenital Q51.0
  uvula, congenital Q38.5
  vagina, congenital Q52.0
  vas deferens (congenital) Q55.4
    acquired Z90.79
  vein (peripheral) congenital NEC Q27.8
    cerebral Q28.3
    digestive system Q27.8
    great Q26.8
    lower limb Q27.8
    portal Q26.5
    precerebral Q28.1
    specified site NEC Q27.8
    upper limb Q27.8
  vena cava (inferior) (superior), congenital Q26.8
  ventricular septum Q20.4
  vertebra, congenital Q76.49
  vulva, congenital Q52.71
  wrist (acquired) Z89.12- ☑
Absorbent system disease I87.8
Absorption
  carbohydrate, disturbance K90.49
  chemical — *see* Table of Drugs and Chemicals
    through placenta (newborn) P04.9
      environmental substance P04.6
      nutritional substance P04.5
      obstetric anesthetic or analgesic drug P04.0
  drug NEC — *see* Table of Drugs and Chemicals
    addictive
      through placenta (newborn) (*see also* Newborn,
        affected by, maternal, use of) P04.40
        cocaine P04.41
        hallucinogens P04.42
        specified drug NEC P04.49
    medicinal
      through placenta (newborn) P04.19
    through placenta (newborn) P04.19
      obstetric anesthetic or analgesic drug P04.0
  fat, disturbance K90.49
    pancreatic K90.3
  noxious substance — *see* Table of Drugs and Chemicals
  protein, disturbance K90.49
  starch, disturbance K90.49
  toxic substance — *see* Table of Drugs and Chemicals
  uremic — *see* Uremia
Abstinence symptoms, syndrome
  alcohol F10.239
    with delirium F10.231
  cocaine F14.23
  neonatal P96.1
  nicotine — *see* Dependence, drug, nicotine, with,
    withdrawal
  opioid F11.93
    with dependence F11.23
  psychoactive NEC F19.939

Abstinence symptoms, syndrome — *continued*
  psychoactive — *continued*
    with
      delirium F19.931
      dependence F19.239
        with
          delirium F19.231
          perceptual disturbance F19.232
        uncomplicated F19.230
      perceptual disturbance F19.932
    uncomplicated F19.930
  sedative F13.939
    with
      delirium F13.931
      dependence F13.239
        with
          delirium F13.231
          perceptual disturbance F13.232
        uncomplicated F13.230
      perceptual disturbance F13.932
    uncomplicated F13.930
  stimulant NEC F15.93
    with dependence F15.23
Abulia R68.89
Abulomania F60.7
Abuse
  adult — *see* Maltreatment, adult
    as reason for
      couple seeking advice (including offender) Z63.0
  alcohol (non-dependent) F10.10
    with
      anxiety disorder F10.180
      intoxication F10.129
        with delirium F10.121
        uncomplicated F10.120
      mood disorder F10.14
      other specified disorder F10.188
      psychosis F10.159
        delusions F10.150
        hallucinations F10.151
      sexual dysfunction F10.181
      sleep disorder F10.182
      unspecified disorder F10.19
    counseling and surveillance Z71.41
    in remission (early) (sustained) F10.11
  amphetamine (or related substance) — *see* Abuse,
    drug, stimulant NEC
  analgesics (non-prescribed) (over the counter) F55.8
  antacids F55.0
  antidepressants — *see* Abuse, drug, psychoactive NEC
  anxiolytic — *see* Abuse, drug, sedative
  barbiturates — *see* Abuse, drug, sedative
  caffeine — *see* Abuse, drug, stimulant NEC
  cannabis, cannabinoids — *see* Abuse, drug, cannabis
  child — *see* Maltreatment, child
  cocaine — *see* Abuse, drug, cocaine
  drug NEC (non-dependent) F19.10
    with sleep disorder F19.182
    amphetamine type — *see* Abuse, drug, stimulant
      NEC
    analgesics (non-prescribed) (over the counter) F55.8
    antacids F55.0
    antidepressants — *see* Abuse, drug, psychoactive
      NEC
    anxiolytics — *see* Abuse, drug, sedative
    barbiturates — *see* Abuse, drug, sedative
    caffeine — *see* Abuse, drug, stimulant NEC
    cannabis F12.10
      with
        anxiety disorder F12.180
        intoxication F12.129
          with
            delirium F12.121
            perceptual disturbance F12.122
          uncomplicated F12.120
        other specified disorder F12.188
        psychosis F12.159
          delusions F12.150
          hallucinations F12.151
        unspecified disorder F12.19
      in remission (early) (sustained) F12.11
    cocaine F14.10
      with
        anxiety disorder F14.180
        intoxication F14.129
          with
            delirium F14.121
            perceptual disturbance F14.122

Abuse — *continued*
  drug — *continued*
    cocaine — *continued*
      with — *continued*
        intoxication — *continued*
          uncomplicated F14.120
        mood disorder F14.14
        other specified disorder F14.188
        psychosis F14.159
          delusions F14.150
          hallucinations F14.151
        sexual dysfunction F14.181
        sleep disorder F14.182
        unspecified disorder F14.19
      in remission (early) (sustained) F14.11
    counseling and surveillance Z71.51
    hallucinogen F16.10
      with
        anxiety disorder F16.180
        flashbacks F16.183
        intoxication F16.129
          with
            delirium F16.121
            perceptual disturbance F16.122
          uncomplicated F16.120
        mood disorder F16.14
        other specified disorder F16.188
        perception disorder, persisting F16.183
        psychosis F16.159
          delusions F16.150
          hallucinations F16.151
        unspecified disorder F16.19
      in remission (early) (sustained) F16.11
    hashish — *see* Abuse, drug, cannabis
    herbal or folk remedies F55.1
    hormones F55.3
    hypnotics — *see* Abuse, drug, sedative
    in remission (early) (sustained) F19.11
    inhalant F18.10
      with
        anxiety disorder F18.180
        dementia, persisting F18.17
        intoxication F18.129
          with delirium F18.121
          uncomplicated F18.120
        mood disorder F18.14
        other specified disorder F18.188
        psychosis F18.159
          delusions F18.150
          hallucinations F18.151
        unspecified disorder F18.19
      in remission (early) (sustained) F18.11
    laxatives F55.2
    LSD — *see* Abuse, drug, hallucinogen
    marihuana — *see* Abuse, drug, cannabis
    morphine type (opioids) — *see* Abuse, drug, opioid
    opioid F11.10
      with
        intoxication F11.129
          with
            delirium F11.121
            perceptual disturbance F11.122
          uncomplicated F11.120
        mood disorder F11.14
        other specified disorder F11.188
        psychosis F11.159
          delusions F11.150
          hallucinations F11.151
        sexual dysfunction F11.181
        sleep disorder F11.182
        unspecified disorder F11.19
      in remission (early) (sustained) F11.11
    PCP (phencyclidine) (or related substance) — *see*
      Abuse, drug, hallucinogen
    psychoactive NEC F19.10
      with
        amnestic disorder F19.16
        anxiety disorder F19.180
        dementia F19.17
        intoxication F19.129
          with
            delirium F19.121
            perceptual disturbance F19.122
          uncomplicated F19.120
        mood disorder F19.14
        other specified disorder F19.188
        psychosis F19.159
          delusions F19.150
          hallucinations F19.151

Abuse — continued
  drug — continued
    psychoactive — continued
      with — continued
        sexual dysfunction F19.181
        sleep disorder F19.182
        unspecified disorder F19.19
    sedative, hypnotic or anxiolytic F13.10
      with
        anxiety disorder F13.180
        intoxication F13.129
          with delirium F13.121
          uncomplicated F13.120
        mood disorder F13.14
        other specified disorder F13.188
        psychosis F13.159
          delusions F13.150
          hallucinations F13.151
        sexual dysfunction F13.181
        sleep disorder F13.182
        unspecified disorder F13.19
      in remission (early) (sustained) F13.11
    solvent — see Abuse, drug, inhalant
    steroids F55.3
    stimulant NEC F15.10
      with
        anxiety disorder F15.180
        intoxication F15.129
          with
            delirium F15.121
            perceptual disturbance F15.122
          uncomplicated F15.120
        mood disorder F15.14
        other specified disorder F15.188
        psychosis F15.159
          delusions F15.150
          hallucinations F15.151
        sexual dysfunction F15.181
        sleep disorder F15.182
        unspecified disorder F15.19
      in remission (early) (sustained) F15.11
    tranquilizers — see Abuse, drug, sedative
    vitamins F55.4
  hallucinogens — see Abuse, drug, hallucinogen
  hashish — see Abuse, drug, cannabis
  herbal or folk remedies F55.1
  hormones F55.3
  hypnotic — see Abuse, drug, sedative
  inhalant — see Abuse, drug, inhalant
  laxatives F55.2
  LSD — see Abuse, drug, hallucinogen
  marihuana — see Abuse, drug, cannabis
  morphine type (opioids) — see Abuse, drug, opioid
  non-psychoactive substance NEC F55.8
    antacids F55.0
    folk remedies F55.1
    herbal remedies F55.1
    hormones F55.3
    laxatives F55.2
    steroids F55.3
    vitamins F55.4
  opioids — see Abuse, drug, opioid
  PCP (phencyclidine) (or related substance) — see
    Abuse, drug, hallucinogen
  physical (adult) (child) — see Maltreatment
  psychoactive substance — see Abuse, drug, psychoac-
    tive NEC
  psychological (adult) (child) — see Maltreatment
  sedative — see Abuse, drug, sedative
  sexual — see Maltreatment
  solvent — see Abuse, drug, inhalant
  steroids F55.3
  vitamins F55.4
Acalculia R48.8
  developmental F81.2
Acanthamebiasis (with) B60.10
  conjunctiva B60.12
  keratoconjunctivitis B60.13
  meningoencephalitis B60.11
  other specified B60.19
Acanthocephaliasis B83.8
Acanthocheilonemiasis B74.4
Acanthocytosis E78.6
Acantholysis L11.9
Acanthosis (acquired) (nigricans) L83
  benign Q82.8
  congenital Q82.8
  seborrheic L82.1

Acanthosis — continued
  seborrheic — continued
    inflamed L82.0
  tongue K14.3
Acapnia E87.3
Acarbia E87.2
Acardia, acardius Q89.8
Acardiacus amorphus Q89.8
Acardiotrophia I51.4
Acariasis B88.0
  scabies B86
Acarodermatitis (urticarioides) B88.0
Acarophobia F40.218
Acatalasemia, acatalasia E80.3
Acathisia (drug induced) G25.71
Accelerated atrioventricular conduction I45.6
Accentuation of personality traits (type A) Z73.1
Accessory (congenital)
  adrenal gland Q89.1
  anus Q43.4
  appendix Q43.4
  atrioventricular conduction I45.6
  auditory ossicles Q16.3
  auricle (ear) Q17.0
  biliary duct or passage Q44.5
  bladder Q64.79
  blood vessels NEC Q27.9
    coronary Q24.5
  bone NEC Q79.8
  breast tissue, axilla Q83.1
  carpal bones Q74.0
  cecum Q43.4
  chromosome(s) NEC (nonsex) Q92.9
    with complex rearrangements NEC Q92.5
      seen only at prometaphase Q92.8
    13 — see Trisomy, 13
    18 — see Trisomy, 18
    21 — see Trisomy, 21
    partial Q92.9
    sex
      female phenotype Q97.8
  coronary artery Q24.5
  cusp(s), heart valve NEC Q24.8
    pulmonary Q22.3
  cystic duct Q44.5
  digit(s) Q69.9
  ear (auricle) (lobe) Q17.0
  endocrine gland NEC Q89.2
  eye muscle Q10.3
  eyelid Q10.3
  fallopian tube (fimbria) (ostium) Q50.6
  finger(s) Q69.0
  foreskin N47.8
  frontonasal process Q75.8
  gallbladder Q44.1
  genital organ(s)
    female Q52.8
      external Q52.79
      internal NEC Q52.8
    male Q55.8
  genitourinary organs NEC Q89.8
    female Q52.8
    male Q55.8
  hallux Q69.2
  heart Q24.8
    valve NEC Q24.8
      pulmonary Q22.3
  hepatic ducts Q44.5
  hymen Q52.4
  intestine (large) (small) Q43.4
  kidney Q63.0
  lacrimal canal Q10.6
  leaflet, heart valve NEC Q24.8
  ligament, broad Q50.6
  liver Q44.7
    duct Q44.5
  lobule (ear) Q17.0
  lung (lobe) Q33.1
  muscle Q79.8
  navicular of carpus Q74.0
  nervous system, part NEC Q07.8
  nipple Q83.3
  nose Q30.8
  organ or site not listed — see Anomaly, by site
  ovary Q50.31
  oviduct Q50.6
  pancreas Q45.3

Accessory — continued
  parathyroid gland Q89.2
  parotid gland (and duct) Q38.4
  pituitary gland Q89.2
  preauricular appendage Q17.0
  prepuce N47.8
  renal arteries (multiple) Q27.2
  rib Q76.6
    cervical Q76.5
  roots (teeth) K00.2
  salivary gland Q38.4
  sesamoid bones Q74.8
    foot Q74.2
    hand Q74.0
  skin tags Q82.8
  spleen Q89.09
  sternum Q76.7
  submaxillary gland Q38.4
  tarsal bones Q74.2
  teeth, tooth K00.1
  tendon Q79.8
  thumb Q69.1
  thymus gland Q89.2
  thyroid gland Q89.2
  toes Q69.2
  tongue Q38.3
  tooth, teeth K00.1
  tragus Q17.0
  ureter Q62.5
  urethra Q64.79
  urinary organ or tract NEC Q64.8
  uterus Q51.28
  vagina Q52.10
  valve, heart NEC Q24.8
    pulmonary Q22.3
  vertebra Q76.49
  vocal cords Q31.8
  vulva Q52.79
Accident
  birth — see Birth, injury
  cardiac — see Infarct, myocardium
  cerebral I63.9
  cerebrovascular (embolic) (ischemic) (thrombotic) I63.9
    aborted I63.9
    hemorrhagic — see Hemorrhage, intracranial, intrac-
      erebral
    old (without sequelae) Z86.73
      with sequelae (of) — see Sequelae, infarction,
        cerebral
  coronary — see Infarct, myocardium
  craniovascular I63.9
  vascular, brain I63.9
Accidental — see condition
Accommodation (disorder) (see also condition)
  hysterical paralysis of F44.89
  insufficiency of H52.4
  paresis — see Paresis, of accommodation
  spasm — see Spasm, of accommodation
Accouchement — see Delivery
Accreta placenta O43.21- ☑
Accretio cordis (nonrheumatic) I31.0
Accretions, tooth, teeth K03.6
Acculturation difficulty Z60.3
Accumulation secretion, prostate N42.89
Acephalia, acephalism, acephalus, acephaly Q00.0
Acephalobrachia monster Q89.8
Acephalochirus monster Q89.8
Acephalogaster Q89.8
Acephalostomus monster Q89.8
Acephalothorax Q89.8
Acerophobia F40.298
Acetonemia R79.89
  in Type 1 diabetes E10.10
    with coma E10.11
Acetonuria R82.4
Achalasia (cardia) (esophagus) K22.0
  congenital Q39.5
  pylorus Q40.0
  sphincteral NEC K59.8
Ache(s) — see Pain
Acheilia Q38.6
Achillobursitis — see Tendinitis, Achilles
Achillodynia — see Tendinitis, Achilles
Achlorhydria, achlorhydric (neurogenic) K31.83
  anemia D50.8
  diarrhea K31.83
  psychogenic F45.8
  secondary to vagotomy K91.1

Achluophobia F40.228
Acholia K82.8
Acholuric jaundice (familial) (splenomegalic) (see also Spherocytosis)
  acquired D59.8
Achondrogenesis Q77.0
Achondroplasia (osteosclerosis congenita) Q77.4
Achroma, cutis L80
Achromat (ism), achromatopsia (acquired) (congenital) H53.51
Achromia, congenital — see Albinism
Achromia parasitica B36.0
Achylia gastrica K31.89
  psychogenic F45.8
Acid
  burn — see Corrosion
  deficiency
    amide nicotinic E52
    ascorbic E54
    folic E53.8
    nicotinic E52
    pantothenic E53.8
  intoxication E87.2
  peptic disease K30
  phosphatase deficiency E83.39
  stomach K30
    psychogenic F45.8
Acidemia E87.2
  argininosuccinic E72.22
  isovaleric E71.110
  metabolic (newborn) P19.9
    first noted before onset of labor P19.0
    first noted during labor P19.1
    noted at birth P19.2
  methylmalonic E71.120
  pipecolic E72.3
  propionic E71.121
Acidity, gastric (high) K30
  psychogenic F45.8
Acidocytopenia — see Agranulocytosis
Acidocytosis D72.1
Acidopenia — see Agranulocytosis
Acidosis (lactic) (respiratory) E87.2
  in Type 1 diabetes E10.10
    with coma E10.11
  kidney, tubular N25.89
  lactic E87.2
  metabolic NEC E87.2
    with respiratory acidosis E87.4
    hyperchloremic, of newborn P74.421
    late, of newborn P74.0
  mixed metabolic and respiratory, newborn P84
  newborn P84
  renal (hyperchloremic) (tubular) N25.89
  respiratory E87.2
    complicated by
      metabolic
        acidosis E87.4
        alkalosis E87.4
Aciduria
  4-hydroxybutyric E72.81
  argininosuccinic E72.22
  gamma-hydroxybutyric E72.81
  glutaric (type I) E72.3
    type II E71.313
    type III E71.5- ☑
  orotic (congenital) (hereditary) (pyrimidine deficiency) E79.8
    anemia D53.0
Acladiosis (skin) B36.0
Aclasis, diaphyseal Q78.6
Acleistocardia Q21.1
Aclusion — see Anomaly, dentofacial, malocclusion
Acne L70.9
  artificialis L70.8
  atrophica L70.2
  cachecticorum (Hebra) L70.8
  conglobata L70.1
  cystic L70.0
  decalvans L66.2
  excoriée (des jeunes filles) L70.5
  frontalis L70.2
  indurata L70.0
  infantile L70.4
  keloid L73.0
  lupoid L70.2
  necrotic, necrotica (miliaris) L70.2
  neonatal L70.4

Acne — continued
  nodular L70.0
  occupational L70.8
  picker's L70.5
  pustular L70.0
  rodens L70.2
  rosacea L71.9
  specified NEC L70.8
  tropica L70.3
  varioliformis L70.2
  vulgaris L70.0
Acnitis (primary) A18.4
Acosta's disease T70.29 ☑
Acoustic — see condition
Acousticophobia F40.298
Acquired (see also condition)
  immunodeficiency syndrome (AIDS) B20
Acrania Q00.0
Acroangiodermatitis I78.9
Acroasphyxia, chronic I73.89
Acrobystitis N47.7
Acrocephalopolysyndactyly Q87.0
Acrocephalosyndactyly Q87.0
Acrocephaly Q75.0
Acrochondrohyperplasia — see Syndrome, Marfan's
Acrocyanosis I73.8 ☑
  newborn P28.2
    meaning transient blue hands and feet — omit code
Acrodermatitis L30.8
  atrophicans (chronica) L90.4
  continua (Hallopeau) L40.2
  enteropathica (hereditary) E83.2
  Hallopeau's L40.2
  infantile papular L44.4
  perstans L40.2
  pustulosa continua L40.2
  recalcitrant pustular L40.2
Acrodynia — see Poisoning, mercury
Acromegaly, acromegalia E22.0
Acromelalgia I73.81
Acromicria, acromikria Q79.8
Acronyx L60.0
Acropachy, thyroid — see Thyrotoxicosis
Acroparesthesia (simple) (vasomotor) I73.89
Acropathy, thyroid — see Thyrotoxicosis
Acrophobia F40.241
Acroposthitis N47.7
Acroscleriasis, acroscleroderma, acrosclerosis — see Sclerosis, systemic
Acrosphacelus I96
Acrospiroma, eccrine — see Neoplasm, skin, benign
Acrostealgia — see Osteochondropathy
Acrotrophodynia — see Immersion
ACTH ectopic syndrome E24.3
Actinic — see condition
Actinobacillosis, actinobacillus A28.8
  mallei A24.0
  muris A25.1
Actinomyces israelii (infection) — see Actinomycosis
Actinomycetoma (foot) B47.1
Actinomycosis, actinomycotic A42.9
  with pneumonia A42.0
  abdominal A42.1
  cervicofacial A42.2
  cutaneous A42.89
  gastrointestinal A42.1
  pulmonary A42.0
  sepsis A42.7
  specified site NEC A42.89
Actinoneuritis G62.82
Action, heart
  disorder I49.9
  irregular I49.9
    psychogenic F45.8
Activated protein C resistance D68.51
Activation
  mast cell (disorder) (syndrome) D89.40
    idiopathic D89.42
    monoclonal D89.41
    secondary D89.43
    specified type NEC D89.49
Active — see condition
Acute (see also condition)
  abdomen R10.0
  gallbladder — see Cholecystitis, acute
Acyanotic heart disease (congenital) Q24.9
Acystia Q64.5

Adair-Dighton syndrome (brittle bones and blue sclera, deafness) Q78.0
Adamantinoblastoma — see Ameloblastoma
Adamantinoma (see also Cyst, calcifying odontogenic)
  long bones C40.90
    lower limb C40.2- ☑
    upper limb C40.0- ☑
  malignant C41.1
    jaw (bone) (lower) C41.1
      upper C41.0
  tibial C40.2- ☑
Adamantoblastoma — see Ameloblastoma
Adams-Stokes (-Morgagni) disease or syndrome I45.9
Adaption reaction — see Disorder, adjustment
Addiction (see also Dependence) F19.20
  alcohol, alcoholic (ethyl) (methyl) (wood) (without remission) F10.20
    with remission F10.21
  drug — see Dependence, drug
  ethyl alcohol (without remission) F10.20
    with remission F10.21
  heroin — see Dependence, drug, opioid
  methyl alcohol (without remission) F10.20
    with remission F10.21
  methylated spirit (without remission) F10.20
    with remission F10.21
  morphine (-like substances) — see Dependence, drug, opioid
  nicotine — see Dependence, drug, nicotine
  opium and opioids — see Dependence, drug, opioid
  tobacco — see Dependence, drug, nicotine
Addison-Biermer anemia (pernicious) D51.0
Addisonian crisis E27.2
Addison's
  anemia (pernicious) D51.0
  disease (bronze) or syndrome E27.1
    tuberculous A18.7
  keloid L94.0
Addison-Schilder complex E71.528
Additional (see also Accessory)
  chromosome(s) Q99.8
    21 — see Trisomy, 21
    sex — see Abnormal, chromosome, sex
Adduction contracture, hip or other joint — see Contraction, joint
Adenitis (see also Lymphadenitis)
  acute, unspecified site L04.9
  axillary I88.9
    acute L04.2
    chronic or subacute I88.1
  Bartholin's gland N75.8
  bulbourethral gland — see Urethritis
  cervical I88.9
    acute L04.0
    chronic or subacute I88.1
  chancroid (Hemophilus ducreyi) A57
  chronic, unspecified site I88.1
  Cowper's gland — see Urethritis
  due to Pasteurella multocida (P. septica) A28.0
  epidemic, acute B27.09
  gangrenous L04.9
  gonorrheal NEC A54.89
  groin I88.9
    acute L04.1
    chronic or subacute I88.1
  infectious (acute) (epidemic) B27.09
  inguinal I88.9
    acute L04.1
    chronic or subacute I88.1
  lymph gland or node, except mesenteric I88.9
    acute — see Lymphadenitis, acute
    chronic or subacute I88.1
  mesenteric (acute) (chronic) (nonspecific) (subacute) I88.0
  parotid gland (suppurative) — see Sialoadenitis
  salivary gland (any) (suppurative) — see Sialoadenitis
  scrofulous (tuberculous) A18.2
  Skene's duct or gland — see Urethritis
  strumous, tuberculous A18.2
  subacute, unspecified site I88.1
  sublingual gland (suppurative) — see Sialoadenitis
  submandibular gland (suppurative) — see Sialoadenitis
  submaxillary gland (suppurative) — see Sialoadenitis
  tuberculous — see Tuberculosis, lymph gland
  urethral gland — see Urethritis
  Wharton's duct (suppurative) — see Sialoadenitis
Adenoacanthoma — see Neoplasm, malignant, by site

☑ **Additional Character Required** — Refer to the Tabular List for Character Selection   ▽ **Subterms under main terms may continue to next column or page**

Adenoameloblastoma — see Cyst, calcifying odontogenic

Adenocarcinoid (tumor) — see Neoplasm, malignant, by site

Adenocarcinoma (see also Neoplasm, malignant, by site)
  acidophil
    specified site — see Neoplasm, malignant, by site
    unspecified site C75.1
  adrenal cortical C74.0- ☑
  alveolar — see Neoplasm, lung, malignant
  apocrine
    breast — see Neoplasm, breast, malignant
    in situ
      breast D05.8- ☑
      specified site NEC — see Neoplasm, skin, in situ
      unspecified site D04.9
    specified site NEC — see Neoplasm, skin, malignant
    unspecified site C44.99
  basal cell
    specified site — see Neoplasm, skin, malignant
    unspecified site C08.9
  basophil
    specified site — see Neoplasm, malignant, by site
    unspecified site C75.1
  bile duct type C22.1
    liver C22.1
    specified site NEC — see Neoplasm, malignant, by site
    unspecified site C22.1
  bronchiolar — see Neoplasm, lung, malignant
  bronchioloalveolar — see Neoplasm, lung, malignant
  ceruminous C44.29- ☑
  cervix, in situ (see also Carcinoma, cervix uteri, in situ) D06.9
  chromophobe
    specified site — see Neoplasm, malignant, by site
    unspecified site C75.1
  diffuse type
    specified site — see Neoplasm, malignant, by site
    unspecified site C16.9
  duct
    infiltrating
      with Paget's disease — see Neoplasm, breast, malignant
      specified site — see Neoplasm, malignant, by site
      unspecified site (female) C50.91- ☑
        male C50.92- ☑
    specified site — see Neoplasm, malignant, by site
    unspecified site
      female C56.9
      male C61
  eosinophil
    specified site — see Neoplasm, malignant, by site
    unspecified site C75.1
  follicular
    with papillary C73
    moderately differentiated C73
    specified site — see Neoplasm, malignant, by site
    trabecular C73
    unspecified site C73
    well differentiated C73
  Hurthle cell C73
  in
    adenomatous
      polyposis coli C18.9
  infiltrating duct
    with Paget's disease — see Neoplasm, breast, malignant
    specified site — see Neoplasm, by site, malignant
    unspecified site (female) C50.91- ☑
      male C50.92- ☑
  inflammatory
    specified site — see Neoplasm, by site, malignant
    unspecified site (female) C50.91- ☑
      male C50.92- ☑
  intestinal type
    specified site — see Neoplasm, malignant, by site
    unspecified site C16.9
  intracystic papillary
  intraductal
    breast D05.1- ☑
    noninfiltrating
      breast D05.1- ☑

Adenocarcinoma — continued
  intraductal — continued
    noninfiltrating — continued
      papillary
        with invasion
          specified site — see Neoplasm, malignant, by site, malignant
          unspecified site (female) C50.91- ☑
            male C50.92- ☑
        breast D05.1- ☑
        specified site NEC — see Neoplasm, in situ, by site
        unspecified site D05.1- ☑
      specified site NEC — see Neoplasm, in situ, by site
      unspecified site D05.1- ☑
    papillary
      with invasion
        specified site — see Neoplasm, malignant, by site
        unspecified site (female) C50.91- ☑
          male C50.92- ☑
      breast D05.1- ☑
      specified site — see Neoplasm, in situ, by site
      unspecified site D05.1- ☑
    specified site NEC — see Neoplasm, in situ, by site
    unspecified site D05.1- ☑
  islet cell
    with exocrine, mixed
      specified site — see Neoplasm, malignant, by site
      unspecified site C25.9
    pancreas C25.4
    specified site NEC — see Neoplasm, malignant, by site
    unspecified site C25.4
  lobular
    in situ
      breast D05.0- ☑
      specified site NEC — see Neoplasm, in situ, by site
      unspecified site D05.0- ☑
    specified site — see Neoplasm, malignant, by site
    unspecified site (female) C50.91- ☑
      male C50.92- ☑
  mucoid (see also Neoplasm, malignant, by site)
    cell
      specified site — see Neoplasm, malignant, by site
      unspecified site C75.1
  nonencapsulated sclerosing C73
  papillary
    with follicular C73
    follicular variant C73
    intraductal (noninfiltrating)
      with invasion
        specified site — see Neoplasm, malignant, by site
        unspecified site (female) C50.91- ☑
          male C50.92- ☑
      breast D05.1- ☑
      specified site NEC — see Neoplasm, in situ, by site
      unspecified site D05.1- ☑
    serous
      specified site — see Neoplasm, malignant, by site
      unspecified site C56.9
  papillocystic
    specified site — see Neoplasm, malignant, by site
    unspecified site C56.9
  pseudomucinous
    specified site — see Neoplasm, malignant, by site
    unspecified site C56.9
  renal cell C64- ☑
  sebaceous — see Neoplasm, skin, malignant
  serous (see also Neoplasm, malignant, by site)
    papillary
      specified site — see Neoplasm, malignant, by site
      unspecified site C56.9
  sweat gland — see Neoplasm, skin, malignant
  water-clear cell C75.0

Adenocarcinoma-in-situ (see also Neoplasm, in situ, by site)
  breast D05.9- ☑

Adenofibroma
  clear cell — see Neoplasm, benign, by site
  endometrioid D27.9
    borderline malignancy D39.10
    malignant C56- ☑
  mucinous
    specified site — see Neoplasm, benign, by site
    unspecified site D27.9
  papillary
    specified site — see Neoplasm, benign, by site
    unspecified site D27.9
  prostate — see Enlargement, enlarged, prostate
  serous
    specified site — see Neoplasm, benign, by site
    unspecified site D27.9
  specified site — see Neoplasm, benign, by site
  unspecified site D27.9

Adenofibrosis
  breast — see Fibroadenosis, breast
  endometrioid N80.0

Adenoiditis (chronic) J35.02
  with tonsillitis J35.03
  acute J03.90
    recurrent J03.91
    specified organism NEC J03.80
      recurrent J03.81
    staphylococcal J03.80
      recurrent J03.81
    streptococcal J03.00
      recurrent J03.01

Adenoids — see condition

Adenolipoma — see Neoplasm, benign, by site

Adenolipomatosis, Launois-Bensaude E88.89

Adenolymphoma
  specified site — see Neoplasm, benign, by site
  unspecified site D11.9

Adenoma (see also Neoplasm, benign, by site)
  acidophil
    specified site — see Neoplasm, benign, by site
    unspecified site D35.2
  acidophil-basophil, mixed
    specified site — see Neoplasm, benign, by site
    unspecified site D35.2
  adrenal (cortical) D35.00
    clear cell D35.00
    compact cell D35.00
    glomerulosa cell D35.00
    heavily pigmented variant D35.00
    mixed cell D35.00
  alpha-cell
    pancreas D13.7
    specified site NEC — see Neoplasm, benign, by site
    unspecified site D13.7
  alveolar D14.30
  apocrine
    breast D24- ☑
    specified site NEC — see Neoplasm, skin, benign, by site
    unspecified site D23.9
  basal cell D11.9
  basophil
    specified site — see Neoplasm, benign, by site
    unspecified site D35.2
  basophil-acidophil, mixed
    specified site — see Neoplasm, benign, by site
    unspecified site D35.2
  beta-cell
    pancreas D13.7
    specified site NEC — see Neoplasm, benign, by site
    unspecified site D13.7
  bile duct D13.4
    common D13.5
    extrahepatic D13.5
    intrahepatic D13.4
    specified site NEC — see Neoplasm, benign, by site
    unspecified site D13.4
  black D35.00
  bronchial D38.1
    cylindroid type — see Neoplasm, lung, malignant
  ceruminous D23.2- ☑
  chief cell D35.1
  chromophobe
    specified site — see Neoplasm, benign, by site
    unspecified site D35.2
  colloid
    specified site — see Neoplasm, benign, by site
    unspecified site D34

Adenoma — continued
- duct
- eccrine, papillary — see Neoplasm, skin, benign
- endocrine, multiple
  - single specified site — see Neoplasm, uncertain behavior, by site
  - two or more specified sites D44- ☑
  - unspecified site D44.9
- endometrioid (see also Neoplasm, benign)
  - borderline malignancy — see Neoplasm, uncertain behavior, by site
- eosinophil
  - specified site — see Neoplasm, benign, by site
  - unspecified site D35.2
- fetal
  - specified site — see Neoplasm, benign, by site
  - unspecified site D34
- follicular
  - specified site — see Neoplasm, benign, by site
  - unspecified site D34
- hepatocellular D13.4
- Hurthle cell D34
- islet cell
  - pancreas D13.7
  - specified site NEC — see Neoplasm, benign, by site
  - unspecified site D13.7
- liver cell D13.4
- macrofollicular
  - specified site — see Neoplasm, benign, by site
  - unspecified site D34
- malignant, malignum — see Neoplasm, malignant, by site
- microcystic
  - pancreas D13.6
  - specified site NEC — see Neoplasm, benign, by site
  - unspecified site D13.6
- microfollicular
  - specified site — see Neoplasm, benign, by site
  - unspecified site D34
- mucoid cell
  - specified site — see Neoplasm, benign, by site
  - unspecified site D35.2
- multiple endocrine
  - single specified site — see Neoplasm, uncertain behavior, by site
  - two or more specified sites D44- ☑
  - unspecified site D44.9
- nipple D24- ☑
- papillary (see also Neoplasm, benign, by site)
  - eccrine — see Neoplasm, skin, benign, by site
- Pick's tubular
  - specified site — see Neoplasm, benign, by site
  - unspecified site
    - female D27.9
    - male D29.20
- pleomorphic
  - carcinoma in — see Neoplasm, salivary gland, malignant
  - specified site — see Neoplasm, malignant, by site
  - unspecified site C08.9
- polypoid (see also Neoplasm, benign)
  - adenocarcinoma in — see Neoplasm, malignant, by site
  - adenocarcinoma in situ — see Neoplasm, in situ, by site
- prostate — see Neoplasm, benign, prostate
- rete cell D29.20
- sebaceous — see Neoplasm, skin, benign
- Sertoli cell
  - specified site — see Neoplasm, benign, by site
  - unspecified site
    - female D27.9
    - male D29.20
- skin appendage — see Neoplasm, skin, benign
- sudoriferous gland — see Neoplasm, skin, benign
- sweat gland — see Neoplasm, skin, benign
- testicular
  - specified site — see Neoplasm, benign, by site
  - unspecified site
    - female D27.9
    - male D29.20
- tubular (see also Neoplasm, benign, by site)
  - adenocarcinoma in — see Neoplasm, malignant, by site
  - adenocarcinoma in situ — see Neoplasm, in situ, by site

Adenoma — continued
- tubular (see also Neoplasm, benign, by site) — continued
  - Pick's
    - specified site — see Neoplasm, benign, by site
    - unspecified site
      - female D27.9
      - male D29.20
- tubulovillous (see also Neoplasm, benign, by site)
  - adenocarcinoma in — see Neoplasm, malignant, by site
  - adenocarcinoma in situ — see Neoplasm, in situ, by site
- villous — see Neoplasm, uncertain behavior, by site
  - adenocarcinoma in — see Neoplasm, malignant, by site
  - adenocarcinoma in situ — see Neoplasm, in situ, by site
- water-clear cell D35.1

Adenomatosis
- endocrine (multiple) E31.20
  - single specified site — see Neoplasm, uncertain behavior, by site
- erosive of nipple D24- ☑
- pluriendocrine — see Adenomatosis, endocrine
- pulmonary D38.1
  - malignant — see Neoplasm, lung, malignant
- specified site — see Neoplasm, benign, by site
- unspecified site D12.6

Adenomatous
- goiter (nontoxic) E04.9
  - with hyperthyroidism — see Hyperthyroidism, with, goiter, nodular
  - toxic — see Hyperthyroidism, with, goiter, nodular

Adenomyoma (see also Neoplasm, benign, by site)
- prostate — see Enlarged, prostate

Adenomyometritis N80.0

Adenomyosis N80.0

Adenopathy (lymph gland) R59.9
- generalized R59.1
- inguinal R59.0
- localized R59.0
- mediastinal R59.0
- mesentery R59.0
- syphilitic (secondary) A51.49
- tracheobronchial R59.0
  - tuberculous A15.4
    - primary (progressive) A15.7
- tuberculous (see also Tuberculosis, lymph gland)
  - tracheobronchial A15.4
    - primary (progressive) A15.7

Adenosalpingitis — see Salpingitis

Adenosarcoma — see Neoplasm, malignant, by site

Adenosclerosis I88.8

Adenosis (sclerosing) breast — see Fibroadenosis, breast

Adenovirus, as cause of disease classified elsewhere B97.0

Adentia (complete) (partial) — see Absence, teeth

Adherent (see also Adhesions)
- labia (minora) N90.89
- pericardium (nonrheumatic) I31.0
  - rheumatic I09.2
- placenta (with hemorrhage) O72.0
  - without hemorrhage O73.0
- prepuce, newborn N47.0
- scar (skin) L90.5
- tendon in scar L90.5

Adhesions, adhesive (postinfective) K66.0
- with intestinal obstruction K56.50
  - complete K56.52
  - incomplete K56.51
  - partial K56.51
- abdominal (wall) — see Adhesions, peritoneum
- appendix K38.8
- bile duct (common) (hepatic) K83.8
- bladder (sphincter) N32.89
- bowel — see Adhesions, peritoneum
- cardiac I31.0
  - rheumatic I09.2
- cecum — see Adhesions, peritoneum
- cervicovaginal N88.1
  - congenital Q52.8
  - postpartal O90.89
    - old N88.1
- cervix N88.1
- ciliary body NEC — see Adhesions, iris
- clitoris N90.89
- colon — see Adhesions, peritoneum

Adhesions, adhesive — continued
- common duct K83.8
- congenital (see also Anomaly, by site)
  - fingers — see Syndactylism, complex, fingers
  - omental, anomalous Q43.3
  - peritoneal Q43.3
  - tongue (to gum or roof of mouth) Q38.3
- conjunctiva (acquired) H11.21- ☑
  - congenital Q15.8
- cystic duct K82.8
- diaphragm — see Adhesions, peritoneum
- due to foreign body — see Foreign body
- duodenum — see Adhesions, peritoneum
- ear
  - middle H74.1- ☑
- epididymis N50.89
- epidural — see Adhesions, meninges
- epiglottis J38.7
- eyelid H02.59
- female pelvis N73.6
- gallbladder K82.8
- globe H44.89
- heart I31.0
  - rheumatic I09.2
- ileocecal (coil) — see Adhesions, peritoneum
- ileum — see Adhesions, peritoneum
- intestine (see also Adhesions, peritoneum)
  - with obstruction K56.50
    - complete K56.52
    - incomplete K56.51
    - partial K56.51
- intra-abdominal — see Adhesions, peritoneum
- iris H21.50- ☑
  - anterior H21.51- ☑
  - goniosynechiae H21.52- ☑
  - posterior H21.54- ☑
  - to corneal graft T85.898 ☑
- joint — see Ankylosis
  - knee M23.8X
  - temporomandibular M26.61- ☑
- labium (majus) (minus), congenital Q52.5
- liver — see Adhesions, peritoneum
- lung J98.4
- mediastinum J98.59
- meninges (cerebral) (spinal) G96.12
  - congenital Q07.8
  - tuberculous (cerebral) (spinal) A17.0
- mesenteric — see Adhesions, peritoneum
- nasal (septum) (to turbinates) J34.89
- ocular muscle — see Strabismus, mechanical
- omentum — see Adhesions, peritoneum
- ovary N73.6
  - congenital (to cecum, kidney or omentum) Q50.39
- paraovarian N73.6
- pelvic (peritoneal)
  - female N73.6
    - postprocedural N99.4
  - male — see Adhesions, peritoneum
  - postpartal (old) N73.6
  - tuberculous A18.17
- penis to scrotum (congenital) Q55.8
- periappendiceal (see also Adhesions, peritoneum)
- pericardium (nonrheumatic) I31.0
  - focal I31.8
  - rheumatic I09.2
  - tuberculous A18.84
- pericholecystic K82.8
- perigastric — see Adhesions, peritoneum
- periovarian N73.6
- periprostatic N42.89
- perirectal — see Adhesions, peritoneum
- perirenal N28.89
- peritoneum, peritoneal (postinfective)
  - with obstruction (intestinal) K56.50
    - complete K56.52
    - incomplete K56.51
    - partial K56.51
  - congenital Q43.3
  - pelvic, female N73.6
    - postprocedural N99.4
  - postpartal, pelvic N73.6
  - postprocedural K66.0
  - to uterus N73.6
- peritubal N73.6
- periureteral N28.89
- periuterine N73.6
- perivesical N32.89
- perivesicular (seminal vesicle) N50.89

☑ Additional Character Required — Refer to the Tabular List for Character Selection   ⏷ Subterms under main terms may continue to next column or page

Adhesions, adhesive — *continued*
　pleura, pleuritic J94.8
　　tuberculous NEC A15.6
　pleuropericardial J94.8
　postoperative (gastrointestinal tract) K66.0
　　with obstruction (*see also* Obstruction, intestine, postoperative) K91.30
　　due to foreign body accidentally left in wound — *see* Foreign body, accidentally left during a procedure
　　pelvic peritoneal N99.4
　　urethra — *see* Stricture, urethra, postprocedural
　　vagina N99.2
　postpartal, old (vulva or perineum) N90.89
　preputial, prepuce N47.5
　pulmonary J98.4
　pylorus — *see* Adhesions, peritoneum
　sciatic nerve — *see* Lesion, nerve, sciatic
　seminal vesicle N50.89
　shoulder (joint) — *see* Capsulitis, adhesive
　sigmoid flexure — *see* Adhesions, peritoneum
　spermatic cord (acquired) N50.89
　　congenital Q55.4
　spinal canal G96.12
　stomach — *see* Adhesions, peritoneum
　subscapular — *see* Capsulitis, adhesive
　temporomandibular M26.61- ☑
　tendinitis (*see also* Tenosynovitis, specified type NEC)
　　shoulder — *see* Capsulitis, adhesive
　testis N44.8
　tongue, congenital (to gum or roof of mouth) Q38.3
　　acquired K14.8
　trachea J39.8
　tubo-ovarian N73.6
　tunica vaginalis N44.8
　uterus N73.6
　　internal N85.6
　　to abdominal wall N73.6
　vagina (chronic) N89.5
　　postoperative N99.2
　vitreomacular H43.82- ☑
　vitreous H43.89
　vulva N90.89
Adiaspiromycosis B48.8
Adie (-Holmes) **pupil or syndrome** — *see* Anomaly, pupil, function, tonic pupil
Adiponecrosis neonatorum P83.88
Adiposis (*see also* Obesity)
　cerebralis E23.6
　dolorosa E88.2
Adiposity (*see also* Obesity)
　heart — *see* Degeneration, myocardial
　localized E65
Adiposogenital dystrophy E23.6
Adjustment
　disorder — *see* Disorder, adjustment
　implanted device — *see* Encounter (for), adjustment (of)
　prosthesis, external — *see* Fitting
　reaction — *see* Disorder, adjustment
Administration of tPA (rtPA) in a different facility within the last 24 hours prior to admission to current facility Z92.82
Admission (for) (*see also* Encounter (for))
　adjustment (of)
　　artificial
　　　arm Z44.00- ☑
　　　　complete Z44.01- ☑
　　　　partial Z44.02- ☑
　　　eye Z44.2 ☑
　　　leg Z44.10- ☑
　　　　complete Z44.11- ☑
　　　　partial Z44.12- ☑
　　brain neuropacemaker Z46.2
　　　implanted Z45.42
　　breast
　　　implant Z45.81 ☑
　　　prosthesis (external) Z44.3 ☑
　　colostomy belt Z46.89
　　contact lenses Z46.0
　　cystostomy device Z46.6
　　dental prosthesis Z46.3
　　device NEC
　　　abdominal Z46.89
　　　implanted Z45.89
　　　　cardiac Z45.09

Admission — *continued*
　adjustment — *continued*
　　device — *continued*
　　　implanted — *continued*
　　　　cardiac — *continued*
　　　　　defibrillator (with synchronous cardiace pacemaker) Z45.02
　　　　　pacemaker (cardiac resynchronization therapy (CRT-P)) Z45.018
　　　　　　pulse generator Z45.010
　　　　　resynchronization therapy defibrillator (CRT-D) Z45.02
　　　　hearing device Z45.328
　　　　　bone conduction Z45.320
　　　　　cochlear Z45.321
　　　　infusion pump Z45.1
　　　　nervous system Z45.49
　　　　　CSF drainage Z45.41
　　　　　hearing device — *see* Admission, adjustment, device, implanted, hearing device
　　　　　neuropacemaker Z45.42
　　　　　visual substitution Z45.31
　　　　specified NEC Z45.89
　　　　vascular access Z45.2
　　　　visual substitution Z45.31
　　　nervous system Z46.2
　　　　implanted — *see* Admission, adjustment, device, implanted, nervous system
　　　orthodontic Z46.4
　　　prosthetic Z44.9
　　　　arm — *see* Admission, adjustment, artificial, arm
　　　　breast Z44.3 ☑
　　　　dental Z46.3
　　　　eye Z44.2 ☑
　　　　leg — *see* Admission, adjustment, artificial, leg
　　　　specified type NEC Z44.8
　　　substitution
　　　　auditory Z46.2
　　　　　implanted — *see* Admission, adjustment, device, implanted, hearing device
　　　　nervous system Z46.2
　　　　　implanted — *see* Admission, adjustment, device, implanted, nervous system
　　　　visual Z46.2
　　　　　implanted Z45.31
　　　urinary Z46.6
　　hearing aid Z46.1
　　　implanted — *see* Admission, adjustment, device, implanted, hearing device
　　ileostomy device Z46.89
　　intestinal appliance or device NEC Z46.89
　　neuropacemaker (brain) (peripheral nerve) (spinal cord) Z46.2
　　　implanted Z45.42
　　orthodontic device Z46.4
　　orthopedic (brace) (cast) (device) (shoes) Z46.89
　　pacemaker (cardiac resynchronization therapy (CRT-P))
　　　cardiac Z45.018
　　　　pulse generator Z45.010
　　　nervous system Z46.2
　　　　implanted Z45.42
　　portacath (port-a-cath) Z45.2
　　prosthesis Z44.9
　　　arm — *see* Admission, adjustment, artificial, arm
　　　breast Z44.3 ☑
　　　dental Z46.3
　　　eye Z44.2 ☑
　　　leg — *see* Admission, adjustment, artificial, leg
　　　specified NEC Z44.8
　　spectacles Z46.0
　aftercare (*see also* Aftercare) Z51.89
　　postpartum
　　　immediately after delivery Z39.0
　　　routine follow-up Z39.2
　　radiation therapy (antineoplastic) Z51.0
　attention to artificial opening (of) Z43.9
　　artificial vagina Z43.7
　　colostomy Z43.3
　　cystostomy Z43.5
　　enterostomy Z43.4
　　gastrostomy Z43.1
　　ileostomy Z43.2
　　jejunostomy Z43.4
　　nephrostomy Z43.6

Admission — *continued*
　attention to artificial opening — *continued*
　　specified site NEC Z43.8
　　　intestinal tract Z43.4
　　　urinary tract Z43.6
　　tracheostomy Z43.0
　　ureterostomy Z43.6
　　urethrostomy Z43.6
　breast augmentation or reduction Z41.1
　breast reconstruction following mastectomy Z42.1
　change of
　　dressing (nonsurgical) Z48.00
　　neuropacemaker device (brain) (peripheral nerve) (spinal cord) Z46.2
　　　implanted Z45.42
　　surgical dressing Z48.01
　circumcision, ritual or routine (in absence of diagnosis) Z41.2
　clinical research investigation (control) (normal comparison) (participant) Z00.6
　contraceptive management Z30.9
　cosmetic surgery NEC Z41.1
　counseling (*see also* Counseling)
　　dietary Z71.3
　　gestational carrier Z31.7
　　HIV Z71.7
　　human immunodeficiency virus Z71.7
　　nonattending third party Z71.0
　　procreative management NEC Z31.69
　delivery, full-term, uncomplicated O80
　　cesarean, without indication O82
　desensitization to allergens Z51.6
　dietary surveillance and counseling Z71.3
　ear piercing Z41.3
　examination at health care facility (adult) (*see also* Examination) Z00.00
　　with abnormal findings Z00.01
　　clinical research investigation (control) (normal comparison) (participant) Z00.6
　　dental Z01.20
　　　with abnormal findings Z01.21
　　donor (potential) Z00.5
　　ear Z01.10
　　　with abnormal findings NEC Z01.118
　　eye Z01.00
　　　with abnormal findings Z01.01
　　general, specified reason NEC Z00.8
　　hearing Z01.10
　　　with abnormal findings NEC Z01.118
　　　infant or child (over 28 days old) Z00.129
　　　　with abnormal findings Z00.121
　　postpartum checkup Z39.2
　　psychiatric (general) Z00.8
　　requested by authority Z04.6
　　vision Z01.00
　　　with abnormal findings Z01.01
　　　infant or child (over 28 days old) Z00.129
　　　　with abnormal findings Z00.121
　fitting (of)
　　artificial
　　　arm — *see* Admission, adjustment, artificial, arm
　　　eye Z44.2 ☑
　　　leg — *see* Admission, adjustment, artificial, leg
　　brain neuropacemaker Z46.2
　　　implanted Z45.42
　　breast prosthesis (external) Z44.3 ☑
　　colostomy belt Z46.89
　　contact lenses Z46.0
　　cystostomy device Z46.6
　　dental prosthesis Z46.3
　　dentures Z46.3
　　device NEC
　　　abdominal Z46.89
　　　nervous system Z46.2
　　　　implanted — *see* Admission, adjustment, device, implanted, nervous system
　　　orthodontic Z46.4
　　　prosthetic Z44.9
　　　　breast Z44.3 ☑
　　　　dental Z46.3
　　　　eye Z44.2 ☑
　　　substitution
　　　　auditory Z46.2
　　　　　implanted — *see* Admission, adjustment, device, implanted, hearing device
　　　　nervous system Z46.2
　　　　　implanted — *see* Admission, adjustment, device, implanted, nervous system

Admission — *continued*
  fitting — *continued*
    device — *continued*
      substitution — *continued*
        visual Z46.2
          implanted Z45.31
      hearing aid Z46.1
      ileostomy device Z46.89
      intestinal appliance or device NEC Z46.89
      neuropacemaker (brain) (peripheral nerve) (spinal cord) Z46.2
        implanted Z45.42
      orthodontic device Z46.4
      orthopedic device (brace) (cast) (shoes) Z46.89
      prosthesis Z44.9
        arm — *see* Admission, adjustment, artificial, arm
        breast Z44.3 ☑
        dental Z46.3
        eye Z44.2 ☑
        leg — *see* Admission, adjustment, artificial, leg
        specified type NEC Z44.8
      spectacles Z46.0
  follow-up examination Z09
  intrauterine device management Z30.431
    initial prescription Z30.014
  mental health evaluation Z00.8
    requested by authority Z04.6
  observation — *see* Observation
  Papanicolaou smear, cervix Z12.4
    for suspected malignant neoplasm Z12.4
  plastic and reconstructive surgery following medical procedure or healed injury NEC Z42.8
  plastic surgery, cosmetic NEC Z41.1
  postpartum observation
    immediately after delivery Z39.0
    routine follow-up Z39.2
  poststerilization (for restoration) Z31.0
    aftercare Z31.42
  procreative management Z31.9
  prophylactic (measure) — (*see also* Encounter, prophylactic measures)
    organ removal Z40.00
      breast Z40.01
      fallopian tube(s) Z40.03
        with ovary(s) Z40.02
      ovary(s) Z40.02
      specified organ NEC Z40.09
      testes Z40.09
    vaccination Z23
  psychiatric examination (general) Z00.8
    requested by authority Z04.6
  radiation therapy (antineoplastic) Z51.0
  reconstructive surgery following medical procedure or healed injury NEC Z42.8
  removal of
    cystostomy catheter Z43.5
    drains Z48.03
    dressing (nonsurgical) Z48.00
    implantable subdermal contraceptive Z30.46
    intrauterine contraceptive device Z30.432
    neuropacemaker (brain) (peripheral nerve) (spinal cord) Z46.2
      implanted Z45.42
    staples Z48.02
    surgical dressing Z48.01
    sutures Z48.02
    ureteral stent Z46.6
  respirator [ventilator] use during power failure Z99.12
  restoration of organ continuity (poststerilization) Z31.0
    aftercare Z31.42
  sensitivity test (*see also* Test, skin)
    allergy NEC Z01.82
    Mantoux Z11.1
  tuboplasty following previous sterilization Z31.0
    aftercare Z31.42
  vasoplasty following previous sterilization Z31.0
    aftercare Z31.42
  vision examination Z01.00
    with abnormal findings Z01.01
    infant or child (over 28 days old) Z00.129
      with abnormal findings Z00.121
  waiting period for admission to other facility Z75.1
Adnexitis (suppurative) — *see* Salpingo-oophoritis
Adolescent X-linked adrenoleukodystrophy E71.521
Adrenal (gland) — *see* condition
Adrenalism, tuberculous A18.7
Adrenalitis, adrenitis E27.8
  autoimmune E27.1

Adrenalitis, adrenitis — *continued*
  meningococcal, hemorrhagic A39.1
Adrenarche, premature E27.0
Adrenocortical syndrome — *see* Cushing's, syndrome
Adrenogenital syndrome E25.9
  acquired E25.8
  congenital E25.0
  salt loss E25.0
Adrenogenitalism, congenital E25.0
Adrenoleukodystrophy E71.529
  neonatal E71.511
  X-linked E71.529
    Addison only phenotype E71.528
    Addison-Schilder E71.528
    adolescent E71.521
    adrenomyeloneuropathy E71.522
    childhood cerebral E71.520
    other specified E71.528
Adrenomyeloneuropathy E71.522
Adventitious bursa — *see* Bursopathy, specified type NEC
Adverse effect — *see* Table of Drugs and Chemicals, categories T36-T50, with 6th character 5
Advice — *see* Counseling
Adynamia (episodica) (hereditary) (periodic) G72.3
Aeration lung imperfect, newborn — *see* Atelectasis
Aerobullosis T70.3 ☑
Aerocele — *see* Embolism, air
Aerodermectasia
  subcutaneous (traumatic) T79.7 ☑
Aerodontalgia T70.29 ☑
Aeroembolism T70.3 ☑
Aerogenes capsulatus infection A48.0
Aero-otitis media T70.0 ☑
Aerophagy, aerophagia (psychogenic) F45.8
Aerophobia F40.228
Aerosinusitis T70.1 ☑
Aerotitis T70.0 ☑
Affection — *see* Disease
Afibrinogenemia (*see also* Defect, coagulation) D68.8
  acquired D65
  congenital D68.2
  following ectopic or molar pregnancy O08.1
  in abortion — *see* Abortion, by type, complicated by, afibrinogenemia
  puerperal O72.3
African
  sleeping sickness B56.9
  tick fever A68.1
  trypanosomiasis B56.9
    gambian B56.0
    rhodesian B56.1
Aftercare (*see also* Care) Z51.89
  following surgery (for) (on)
    amputation Z47.81
    attention to
      drains Z48.03
      dressings (nonsurgical) Z48.00
        surgical Z48.01
      sutures Z48.02
    circulatory system Z48.812
    delayed (planned) wound closure Z48.1
    digestive system Z48.815
    explantation of joint prosthesis (staged procedure)
      hip Z47.32
      knee Z47.33
      shoulder Z47.31
    genitourinary system Z48.816
    joint replacement Z47.1
    neoplasm Z48.3
    nervous system Z48.811
    oral cavity Z48.814
    organ transplant
      bone marrow Z48.290
      heart Z48.21
      heart-lung Z48.280
      kidney Z48.22
      liver Z48.23
      lung Z48.24
      multiple organs NEC Z48.288
      specified NEC Z48.298
    orthopedic NEC Z47.89
    planned wound closure Z48.1
    removal of internal fixation device Z47.2
    respiratory system Z48.813
    scoliosis Z47.82
    sense organs Z48.810
    skin and subcutaneous tissue Z48.817

Aftercare — *continued*
  following surgery — *continued*
    specified body system
      circulatory Z48.812
      digestive Z48.815
      genitourinary Z48.816
      nervous Z48.811
      oral cavity Z48.814
      respiratory Z48.813
      sense organs Z48.810
      skin and subcutaneous tissue Z48.817
      teeth Z48.814
      specified NEC Z48.89
      spinal Z47.89
      teeth Z48.814
    fracture — *code to* fracture with seventh character D
    involving
      removal of
        drains Z48.03
        dressings (nonsurgical) Z48.00
        staples Z48.02
        surgical dressings Z48.01
        sutures Z48.02
    neuropacemaker (brain) (peripheral nerve) (spinal cord) Z46.2
      implanted Z45.42
    orthopedic NEC Z47.89
    postprocedural — *see* Aftercare, following surgery
After-cataract — *see* Cataract, secondary
Agalactia (primary) O92.3
  elective, secondary or therapeutic O92.5
Agammaglobulinemia (acquired) (secondary) (nonfamilial) D80.1
  with
    immunoglobulin-bearing B-lymphocytes D80.1
    lymphopenia D81.9
  autosomal recessive (Swiss type) D80.0
  Bruton's X-linked D80.0
  common variable (CVAgamma) D80.1
  congenital sex-linked D80.0
  hereditary D80.0
  lymphopenic D81.9
  Swiss type (autosomal recessive) D80.0
  X-linked (with growth hormone deficiency) (Bruton) D80.0
Aganglionosis (bowel) (colon) Q43.1
Age (old) — *see* Senility
Agenesis
  adrenal (gland) Q89.1
  alimentary tract (complete) (partial) NEC Q45.8
    upper Q40.8
  anus, anal (canal) Q42.3
    with fistula Q42.2
  aorta Q25.41
  appendix Q42.8
  arm (complete) Q71.0- ☑
    with hand present Q71.1- ☑
  artery (peripheral) Q27.9
    brain Q28.3
    coronary Q24.5
    pulmonary Q25.79
    specified NEC Q27.8
    umbilical Q27.0
  auditory (canal) (external) Q16.1
  auricle (ear) Q16.0
  bile duct or passage Q44.5
  bladder Q64.5
  bone Q79.9
  brain Q00.0
    part of Q04.3
  breast (with nipple present) Q83.8
    with absent nipple Q83.0
  bronchus Q32.4
  canaliculus lacrimalis Q10.4
  carpus — *see* Agenesis, hand
  cartilage Q79.9
  cecum Q42.8
  cerebellum Q04.3
  cervix Q51.5
  chin Q18.8
  cilia Q10.3
  circulatory system, part NOS Q28.9
  clavicle Q74.0
  clitoris Q52.6
  coccyx Q76.49
  colon Q42.9
    specified NEC Q42.8
  corpus callosum Q04.0

Agenesis — *continued*
cricoid cartilage Q31.8
diaphragm (with hernia) Q79.1
digestive organ(s) or tract (complete) (partial) NEC Q45.8
upper Q40.8
ductus arteriosus Q28.8
duodenum Q41.0
ear Q16.9
auricle Q16.0
lobe Q17.8
ejaculatory duct Q55.4
endocrine (gland) NEC Q89.2
epiglottis Q31.8
esophagus Q39.8
eustachian tube Q16.2
eye Q11.1
adnexa Q15.8
eyelid (fold) Q10.3
face
bones NEC Q75.8
specified part NEC Q18.8
fallopian tube Q50.6
femur — *see* Defect, reduction, lower limb, longitudinal, femur
fibula — *see* Defect, reduction, lower limb, longitudinal, fibula
finger (complete) (partial) — *see* Agenesis, hand
foot (and toes) (complete) (partial) Q72.3- ☑
forearm (with hand present) — *see* Agenesis, arm, with hand present
and hand Q71.2- ☑
gallbladder Q44.0
gastric Q40.2
genitalia, genital (organ(s))
female Q52.8
external Q52.71
internal NEC Q52.8
male Q55.8
glottis Q31.8
hair Q84.0
hand (and fingers) (complete) (partial) Q71.3- ☑
heart Q24.8
valve NEC Q24.8
pulmonary Q22.0
hepatic Q44.7
humerus — *see* Defect, reduction, upper limb
hymen Q52.4
ileum Q41.2
incus Q16.3
intestine (small) Q41.9
large Q42.9
specified NEC Q42.8
iris (dilator fibers) Q13.1
jaw M26.09
jejunum Q41.1
kidney(s) (partial) Q60.2
bilateral Q60.1
unilateral Q60.0
labium (majus) (minus) Q52.71
labyrinth, membranous Q16.5
lacrimal apparatus Q10.4
larynx Q31.8
leg (complete) Q72.0- ☑
with foot present Q72.1- ☑
lower leg (with foot present) — *see* Agenesis, leg, with foot present
and foot Q72.2- ☑
lens Q12.3
limb (complete) Q73.0
lower — *see* Agenesis, leg
upper — *see* Agenesis, arm
lip Q38.0
liver Q44.7
lung (fissure) (lobe) (bilateral) (unilateral) Q33.3
mandible, maxilla M26.09
metacarpus — *see* Agenesis, hand
metatarsus — *see* Agenesis, foot
muscle Q79.8
eyelid Q10.3
ocular Q15.8
musculoskeletal system NEC Q79.8
nail(s) Q84.3
neck, part Q18.8
nerve Q07.8
nervous system, part NEC Q07.8
nipple Q83.2
nose Q30.1

Agenesis — *continued*
nuclear Q07.8
organ
of Corti Q16.5
or site not listed — *see* Anomaly, by site
osseous meatus (ear) Q16.1
ovary
bilateral Q50.02
unilateral Q50.01
oviduct Q50.6
pancreas Q45.0
parathyroid (gland) Q89.2
parotid gland(s) Q38.4
patella Q74.1
pelvic girdle (complete) (partial) Q74.2
penis Q55.5
pericardium Q24.8
pituitary (gland) Q89.2
prostate Q55.4
punctum lacrimale Q10.4
radioulnar — *see* Defect, reduction, upper limb
radius — *see* Defect, reduction, upper limb, longitudinal, radius
rectum Q42.1
with fistula Q42.0
renal Q60.2
bilateral Q60.1
unilateral Q60.0
respiratory organ NEC Q34.8
rib Q76.6
roof of orbit Q75.8
round ligament Q52.8
sacrum Q76.49
salivary gland Q38.4
scapula Q74.0
scrotum Q55.29
seminal vesicles Q55.4
septum
atrial Q21.1
between aorta and pulmonary artery Q21.4
ventricular Q20.4
shoulder girdle (complete) (partial) Q74.0
skull (bone) Q75.8
with
anencephaly Q00.0
encephalocele — *see* Encephalocele
hydrocephalus Q03.9
with spina bifida — *see* Spina bifida, by site, with hydrocephalus
microcephaly Q02
spermatic cord Q55.4
spinal cord Q06.0
spine Q76.49
spleen Q89.01
sternum Q76.7
stomach Q40.2
submaxillary gland(s) (congenital) Q38.4
tarsus — *see* Agenesis, foot
tendon Q79.8
testicle Q55.0
thymus (gland) Q89.2
thyroid (gland) E03.1
cartilage Q31.8
tibia — *see* Defect, reduction, lower limb, longitudinal, tibia
tibiofibular — *see* Defect, reduction, lower limb, specified type NEC
toe (and foot) (complete) (partial) — *see* Agenesis, foot
tongue Q38.3
trachea (cartilage) Q32.1
ulna — *see* Defect, reduction, upper limb, longitudinal, ulna
upper limb — *see* Agenesis, arm
ureter Q62.4
urethra Q64.5
urinary tract NEC Q64.8
uterus Q51.0
uvula Q38.5
vagina Q52.0
vas deferens Q55.4
vein(s) (peripheral) Q27.9
brain Q28.3
great NEC Q26.8
portal Q26.5
vena cava (inferior) (superior) Q26.8
vermis of cerebellum Q04.3
vertebra Q76.49
vulva Q52.71

Ageusia R43.2
Agitated — *see* condition
Agitation R45.1
Aglossia (congenital) Q38.3
Aglossia-adactylia syndrome Q87.0
Aglycogenosis E74.00
Agnosia (body image) (other senses) (tactile) R48.1
developmental F88
verbal R48.1
auditory R48.1
developmental F80.2
developmental F80.2
visual (object) R48.3
Agoraphobia F40.00
with panic disorder F40.01
without panic disorder F40.02
Agrammatism R48.8
Agranulocytopenia — *see* Agranulocytosis
Agranulocytosis (chronic) (cyclical) (genetic) (infantile) (periodic) (pernicious) (*see also* Neutropenia) D70.9
congenital D70.0
cytoreductive cancer chemotherapy sequela D70.1
drug-induced D70.2
due to cytoreductive cancer chemotherapy D70.1
due to infection D70.3
secondary D70.4
drug-induced D70.2
due to cytoreductive cancer chemotherapy D70.1
Agraphia (absolute) R48.8
with alexia R48.0
developmental F81.81
Ague (dumb) — *see* Malaria
Agyria Q04.3
Ahumada-del Castillo syndrome E23.0
Aichomophobia F40.298
AIDS (related complex) B20
Ailment heart — *see* Disease, heart
Ailurophobia F40.218
AIN — *see* Neoplasia, intraepithelial, anal
Ainhum (disease) L94.6
AIPHI (acute idiopathic pulmonary hemorrhage in infants (over 28 days old)) R04.81
Air
anterior mediastinum J98.2
compressed, disease T70.3 ☑
conditioner lung or pneumonitis J67.7
embolism (artery) (cerebral) (any site) T79.0 ☑
with ectopic or molar pregnancy O08.2
due to implanted device NEC — *see* Complications, by site and type, specified NEC
following
abortion — *see* Abortion by type, complicated by, embolism
ectopic or molar pregnancy O08.2
infusion, therapeutic injection or transfusion T80.0 ☑
in pregnancy, childbirth or puerperium — *see* Embolism, obstetric
traumatic T79.0 ☑
hunger, psychogenic F45.8
rarefied, effects of — *see* Effect, adverse, high altitude
sickness T75.3 ☑
Airplane sickness T75.3 ☑
Akathisia (drug-induced) (treatment-induced) G25.71
neuroleptic induced (acute) G25.71
tardive G25.71
Akinesia R29.898
Akinetic mutism R41.89
Akureyri's disease G93.3
Alactasia, congenital E73.0
Alagille's syndrome Q44.7
Alastrim B03
Albers-Schönberg syndrome Q78.2
Albert's syndrome — *see* Tendinitis, Achilles
Albinism, albino E70.30
with hematologic abnormality E70.339
Chédiak-Higashi syndrome E70.330
Hermansky-Pudlak syndrome E70.331
other specified E70.338
I E70.320
II E70.321
ocular E70.319
autosomal recessive E70.311
other specified E70.318
X-linked E70.310
oculocutaneous E70.329
other specified E70.328

Albinism, albino — *continued*
 oculocutaneous — *continued*
  tyrosinase (ty) negative E70.320
  tyrosinase (ty) positive E70.321
 other specified E70.39
Albinismus E70.30
Albright (-McCune)(-Sternberg) syndrome Q78.1
Albuminous — *see* condition
Albuminuria, albuminuric (acute) (chronic) (subacute)
 (*see also* Proteinuria) R80.9
 complicating pregnancy — *see* Proteinuria, gestational
  with
    gestational hypertension — *see* Pre-eclampsia
    pre-existing hypertension — *see* Hypertension,
     complicating pregnancy, pre-existing,
     with, pre-eclampsia
 gestational — *see* Proteinuria, gestational
  with
    gestational hypertension — *see* Pre-eclampsia
    pre-existing hypertension — *see* Hypertension,
     complicating pregnancy, pre-existing,
     with, pre-eclampsia
 orthostatic R80.2
 postural R80.2
 pre-eclamptic — *see* Pre-eclampsia
 scarlatinal A38.8
Albuminurophobia F40.298
Alcaptonuria E70.29
Alcohol, alcoholic, alcohol-induced
 addiction (without remission) F10.20
  with remission F10.21
 amnestic disorder, persisting F10.96
  with dependence F10.26
 anxiety disorder F10.980
 bipolar and related disorder F10.94
 brain syndrome, chronic F10.97
  with dependence F10.27
 cardiopathy I42.6
 counseling and surveillance Z71.41
  family member Z71.42
 delirium (acute) (tremens) (withdrawal) F10.231
  with intoxication F10.921
   in
     abuse F10.121
     dependence F10.221
 dementia F10.97
  with dependence F10.27
 depressive disorder F10.94
 deterioration F10.97
  with dependence F10.27
 hallucinosis (acute) F10.951
  in
    abuse F10.151
    dependence F10.251
 insanity F10.959
 intoxication (acute) (without dependence) F10.129
  with
    delirium F10.121
    dependence F10.229
     with delirium F10.221
     uncomplicated F10.220
    uncomplicated F10.120
 jealousy F10.988
 Korsakoff's, Korsakov's, Korsakow's F10.26
 liver K70.9
  acute — *see* Disease, liver, alcoholic, hepatitis
 major neurocognitive disorder, amnestic-confabulatory
  type F10.96
 major neurocognitive disorder, nonamnestic-confabu-
  latory type F10.97
 mania (acute) (chronic) F10.959
 mild neurocognitive disorder F10.988
 paranoia, paranoid (type) psychosis F10.950
 pellagra E52
 poisoning, accidental (acute) NEC — *see* Table of Drugs
  and Chemicals, alcohol, poisoning
 psychosis — *see* Psychosis, alcoholic
 psychotic disorder F10.959
 sexual dysfunction F10.981
 sleep disorder F10.982
 withdrawal (without convulsions) F10.239
  with delirium F10.231
Alcoholism (chronic) (without remission) F10.20
 with
   psychosis — *see* Psychosis, alcoholic
   remission F10.21
 Korsakov's F10.96
  with dependence F10.26

Alder (-Reilly) **anomaly or syndrome** (leukocyte granulation) D72.0
Aldosteronism E26.9
 familial (type I) E26.02
 glucocorticoid-remediable E26.02
 primary (due to (bilateral) adrenal hyperplasia) E26.09
 primary NEC E26.09
 secondary E26.1
 specified NEC E26.89
Aldosteronoma D44.10
Aldrich (-Wiskott) **syndrome** (eczema-thrombocytopenia) D82.0
Alektorophobia F40.218
Aleppo boil B55.1
Aleukemic — *see* condition
Aleukia
 congenital D70.0
 hemorrhagica D61.9
  congenital D61.09
 splenica D73.1
Alexia R48.0
 developmental F81.0
 secondary to organic lesion R48.0
Algoneurodystrophy M89.00
 ankle M89.07- ☑
 foot M89.07- ☑
 forearm M89.03- ☑
 hand M89.04- ☑
 lower leg M89.06- ☑
 multiple sites M89.0- ☑
 shoulder M89.01- ☑
 specified site NEC M89.08
 thigh M89.05- ☑
 upper arm M89.02- ☑
Algophobia F40.298
Alienation, mental — *see* Psychosis
Alkalemia E87.3
Alkalosis E87.3
 metabolic E87.3
  with respiratory acidosis E87.4
  of newborn P74.41
 respiratory E87.3
Alkaptonuria E70.29
Allen-Masters syndrome N83.8
Allergy, allergic (reaction) (to) T78.40 ☑
 air-borne substance NEC (rhinitis) J30.89
 alveolitis (extrinsic) J67.9
  due to
    Aspergillus clavatus J67.4
    Cryptostroma corticale J67.6
    organisms (fungal, thermophilic actinomycete)
     growing in ventilation (air conditioning)
     systems J67.7
  specified type NEC J67.8
 anaphylactic reaction or shock T78.2 ☑
 angioneurotic edema T78.3 ☑
 animal (dander) (epidermal) (hair) (rhinitis) J30.81
 bee sting (anaphylactic shock) — *see* Toxicity, venom,
  arthropod, bee
 biological — *see* Allergy, drug
 colitis (*see also* Colitis, allergic) K52.29
 dander (animal) (rhinitis) J30.81
 dandruff (rhinitis) J30.81
 dental restorative material (existing) K08.55
 dermatitis — *see* Dermatitis, contact, allergic
 diathesis — *see* History, allergy
 drug, medicament & biological (any) (external) (internal) T78.40 ☑
  correct substance properly administered — *see* Table of Drugs and Chemicals, by drug, adverse
   effect
  wrong substance given or taken NEC (by accident)
   — *see* Table of Drugs and Chemicals, by drug,
   poisoning
  due to pollen J30.1
 dust (house) (stock) (rhinitis) J30.89
  with asthma — *see* Asthma, allergic extrinsic
 eczema — *see* Dermatitis, contact, allergic
 epidermal (animal) (rhinitis) J30.81
 feathers (rhinitis) J30.89
 food (any) (ingested) NEC T78.1 ☑
  anaphylactic shock — *see* Shock, anaphylactic, due
   to food
  dermatitis — *see* Dermatitis, due to, food
  dietary counseling and surveillance Z71.3
  in contact with skin L23.6
  rhinitis J30.5

Allergy, allergic — *continued*
 food — *continued*
  status (without reaction) Z91.018
   eggs Z91.012
   milk products Z91.011
   peanuts Z91.010
   seafood Z91.013
   specified NEC Z91.018
 gastrointestinal — *see also* specific type of allergic reaction
  meaning colitis (*see also* Colitis, allergic) K52.29
  meaning gastroenteritis (*see also* Gastroenteritis,
   allergic) K52.29
  meaning other adverse food reaction not elsewhere
   classified T78.1 ☑
 grain J30.1
 grass (hay fever) (pollen) J30.1
  asthma — *see* Asthma, allergic extrinsic
 hair (animal) (rhinitis) J30.81
 history (of) — *see* History, allergy
 horse serum — *see* Allergy, serum
 inhalant (rhinitis) J30.89
  pollen J30.1
 kapok (rhinitis) J30.89
 medicine — *see* Allergy, drug
 milk protein (*see also* Allergy, food) Z91.011
  anaphylactic reaction T78.07 ☑
  dermatitis L27.2
  enterocolitis syndrome K52.21
  enteropathy K52.22
  gastroenteritis K52.29
  gastroesophageal reflux (*see also* Reaction, adverse,
   food) K21.9
   with esophagitis K21.0
  proctocolitis K52.82
 nasal, seasonal due to pollen J30.1
 pneumonia J82
 pollen (any) (hay fever) J30.1
  asthma — *see* Asthma, allergic extrinsic
 primrose J30.1
 primula J30.1
 proctocolitis K52.82
 purpura D69.0
 ragweed (hay fever) (pollen) J30.1
  asthma — *see* Asthma, allergic extrinsic
 rose (pollen) J30.1
 seasonal NEC J30.2
 Senecio jacobae (pollen) J30.1
 serum (*see also* Reaction, serum) T80.69 ☑
  anaphylactic shock T80.59 ☑
 shock (anaphylactic) T78.2 ☑
  due to
    administration of blood and blood products
     T80.51 ☑
    adverse effect of correct medicinal substance
     properly administered T88.6 ☑
    immunization T80.52 ☑
    serum NEC T80.59 ☑
    vaccination T80.52 ☑
 specific NEC T78.49 ☑
 tree (any) (hay fever) (pollen) J30.1
  asthma — *see* Asthma, allergic extrinsic
 upper respiratory J30.9
 urticaria L50.0
 vaccine — *see* Allergy, serum
 wheat — *see* Allergy, food
Allescheriasis B48.2
Alligator skin disease Q80.9
Allocheiria, allochiria R20.8
Almeida's disease — *see* Paracoccidioidomycosis
Alopecia (hereditaria) (seborrheica) L65.9
 androgenic L64.9
  drug-induced L64.0
  specified NEC L64.8
 areata L63.9
  ophiasis L63.2
  specified NEC L63.8
  totalis L63.0
  universalis L63.1
 cicatricial L66.9
  specified NEC L66.8
 circumscripta L63.9
 congenital, congenitalis Q84.0
 due to cytotoxic drugs NEC L65.8
 mucinosa L65.2
 postinfective NEC L65.8
 postpartum L65.0
 premature L64.8

☑ **Additional Character Required** — **Refer to the Tabular List for Character Selection**   ᴺᴱᶜ **Subterms under main terms may continue to next column or page**

Alopecia — *continued*
  specific (syphilitic) A51.32
  specified NEC L65.8
  syphilitic (secondary) A51.32
  totalis (capitis) L63.0
  universalis (entire body) L63.1
  X-ray L58.1
Alpers' disease G31.81
Alpine sickness T70.29
Alport syndrome Q87.81
ALTE (apparent life threatening event) **in newborn and infant** R68.13
Alteration (of), **Altered**
  awareness
    transient R40.4
    unintended under general anesthesia, during procedure T88.53 ☑
  mental status R41.82
  pattern of family relationships affecting child Z62.898
  sensation
    following
      cerebrovascular disease I69.998
        cerebral infarction I69.398
        intracerebral hemorrhage I69.198
        nontraumatic intracranial hemorrhage NEC I69.298
        specified disease NEC I69.898
        subarachnoid hemorrhage I69.098
Alternating — *see* condition
Altitude, high (effects) — *see* Effect, adverse, high altitude
Aluminosis (of lung) J63.0
Alveolitis
  allergic (extrinsic) — *see* Pneumonitis, hypersensitivity
  due to
    Aspergillus clavatus J67.4
    Cryptostroma corticale J67.6
  fibrosing (cryptogenic) (idiopathic) J84.112
  jaw M27.3
  sicca dolorosa M27.3
Alveolus, alveolar — *see* condition
Alymphocytosis D72.810
  thymic (with immunodeficiency) D82.1
Alymphoplasia, thymic D82.1
Alzheimer's disease or sclerosis — *see* Disease, Alzheimer's
Amastia (with nipple present) Q83.8
  with absent nipple Q83.0
Amathophobia F40.228
Amaurosis (acquired) (congenital) (*see also* Blindness)
  fugax G45.3
  hysterical F44.6
  Leber's congenital H35.50
  uremic — *see* Uremia
Amaurotic idiocy (infantile) (juvenile) (late) E75.4
Amaxophobia F40.248
Ambiguous genitalia Q56.4
Amblyopia (congenital) (ex anopsia) (partial) (suppression) H53.00- ☑
  anisometropic — *see* Amblyopia, refractive
  deprivation H53.01- ☑
  hysterical F44.6
  nocturnal (*see also* Blindness, night)
    vitamin A deficiency E50.5
  refractive H53.02- ☑
  strabismic H53.03- ☑
  suspect H53.04- ☑
  tobacco H53.8
  toxic NEC H53.8
  uremic — *see* Uremia
Ameba, amebic (histolytica) (*see also* Amebiasis)
  abscess (liver) A06.4
Amebiasis A06.9
  with abscess — *see* Abscess, amebic
  acute A06.0
  chronic (intestine) A06.1
    with abscess — *see* Abscess, amebic
  cutaneous A06.7
  cutis A06.7
  cystitis A06.81
  genitourinary tract NEC A06.82
  hepatic — *see* Abscess, liver, amebic
  intestine A06.0
  nondysenteric colitis A06.2
  skin A06.7
  specified site NEC A06.89
Ameboma (of intestine) A06.3

Amelia Q73.0
  lower limb — *see* Agenesis, leg
  upper limb — *see* Agenesis, arm
Ameloblastoma (*see also* Cyst, calcifying odontogenic)
  long bones C40.9- ☑
    lower limb C40.2- ☑
    upper limb C40.0- ☑
  malignant C41.1
    jaw (bone) (lower) C41.1
      upper C41.0
  tibial C40.2- ☑
Amelogenesis imperfecta K00.5
  nonhereditaria (segmentalis) K00.4
Amenorrhea N91.2
  hyperhormonal E28.8
  primary N91.0
  secondary N91.1
Amentia — *see* Disability, intellectual
  Meynert's (nonalcoholic) F04
American
  leishmaniasis B55.2
  mountain tick fever A93.2
Ametropia — *see* Disorder, refraction
AMH (asymptomatic microscopic hematuria) R31.21
Amianthosis J61
Amimia R48.8
Amino-acid disorder E72.9
  anemia D53.0
Aminoacidopathy E72.9
Aminoaciduria E72.9
Amnesia R41.3
  anterograde R41.1
  auditory R48.8
  dissociative F44.0
    with dissociative fugue F44.1
  hysterical F44.0
  postictal in epilepsy — *see* Epilepsy
  psychogenic F44.0
  retrograde R41.2
  transient global G45.4
Amnes(t)ic syndrome (post-traumatic) F04
  induced by
    alcohol F10.96
      with dependence F10.26
    psychoactive NEC F19.96
      with
        abuse F19.16
        dependence F19.26
    sedative F13.96
      with dependence F13.26
Amnion, amniotic — *see* condition
Amnionitis — *see* Pregnancy, complicated by
Amok F68.8
Amoral traits F60.89
Amphetamine (or other stimulant) **-induced**
  anxiety disorder F15.980
  bipolar and related disorder F15.94
  delirium F15.921
  depressive disorder F15.94
  obsessive-compulsive and related disorder F15.988
  psychotic disorder F15.959
  sexual dysfunction F15.981
  sleep disorder F15.982
  stimulant withdrawal F15.23
Ampulla
  lower esophagus K22.8
  phrenic K22.8
Amputation (*see also* Absence, by site, acquired)
  neuroma (postoperative) (traumatic) — *see* Complications, amputation stump, neuroma
  stump (surgical)
    abnormal, painful, or with complication (late) — *see* Complications, amputation stump
    healed or old NOS Z89.9
  traumatic (complete) (partial)
    arm (upper) (complete) S48.91- ☑
      at
        elbow S58.01- ☑
          partial S58.02- ☑
        shoulder joint (complete) S48.01- ☑
          partial S48.02- ☑
      between
        elbow and wrist (complete) S58.11- ☑
          partial S58.12- ☑
        shoulder and elbow (complete) S48.11- ☑
          partial S48.12- ☑
      partial S48.92- ☑

Amputation — *continued*
  traumatic — *continued*
    breast (complete) S28.21- ☑
      partial S28.22- ☑
    clitoris (complete) S38.211 ☑
      partial S38.212 ☑
    ear (complete) S08.11- ☑
      partial S08.12- ☑
    finger (complete) (metacarpophalangeal) S68.11- ☑
      index S68.11- ☑
      little S68.11- ☑
      middle S68.11- ☑
      partial S68.12- ☑
        index S68.12- ☑
        little S68.12- ☑
        middle S68.12- ☑
        ring S68.12- ☑
      ring S68.11- ☑
      thumb — *see* Amputation, traumatic, thumb
      transphalangeal (complete) S68.61- ☑
        index S68.61- ☑
        little S68.61- ☑
        middle S68.61- ☑
        partial S68.62- ☑
          index S68.62- ☑
          little S68.62- ☑
          middle S68.62- ☑
          ring S68.62- ☑
        ring S68.61- ☑
    foot (complete) S98.91- ☑
      at ankle level S98.01- ☑
        partial S98.02- ☑
      midfoot S98.31- ☑
        partial S98.32- ☑
      partial S98.92- ☑
    forearm (complete) S58.91- ☑
      at elbow level (complete) S58.01- ☑
        partial S58.02- ☑
      between elbow and wrist (complete) S58.11- ☑
        partial S58.12- ☑
      partial S58.92- ☑
    genital organ(s) (external)
      female (complete) S38.211 ☑
        partial S38.212 ☑
      male
        penis (complete) S38.221 ☑
          partial S38.222 ☑
        scrotum (complete) S38.231 ☑
          partial S38.232 ☑
        testes (complete) S38.231 ☑
          partial S38.232 ☑
    hand (complete) (wrist level) S68.41- ☑
      finger(s) alone — *see* Amputation, traumatic, finger
      partial S68.42- ☑
      thumb alone — *see* Amputation, traumatic, thumb
      transmetacarpal (complete) S68.71- ☑
        partial S68.72- ☑
    head
      ear — *see* Amputation, traumatic, ear
      nose (partial) S08.812 ☑
        complete S08.811 ☑
      part S08.89 ☑
        scalp S08.0 ☑
    hip (and thigh) (complete) S78.91- ☑
      at hip joint (complete) S78.01- ☑
        partial S78.02- ☑
      between hip and knee (complete) S78.11- ☑
        partial S78.12- ☑
      partial S78.92- ☑
    labium (majus) (minus) (complete) S38.21- ☑
      partial S38.21- ☑
    leg (lower) S88.91- ☑
      at knee level S88.01- ☑
        partial S88.02- ☑
      between knee and ankle S88.11- ☑
        partial S88.12- ☑
      partial S88.92- ☑
    nose (partial) S08.812 ☑
      complete S08.811 ☑
    penis (complete) S38.221 ☑
      partial S38.222 ☑
    scrotum (complete) S38.231 ☑
      partial S38.232 ☑
    shoulder — *see* Amputation, traumatic, arm

Amputation — continued
  traumatic — continued
    shoulder — *see* Amputation, traumatic, arm — *continued*
      at shoulder joint — *see* Amputation, traumatic, arm, at shoulder joint
    testes (complete) S38.231 ☑
      partial S38.232 ☑
    thigh — *see* Amputation, traumatic, hip
    thorax, part of S28.1 ☑
      breast — *see* Amputation, traumatic, breast
    thumb (complete) (metacarpophalangeal) S68.01- ☑
      partial S68.02- ☑
      transphalangeal (complete) S68.51- ☑
        partial S68.52- ☑
    toe (lesser) S98.13- ☑
      great S98.11- ☑
        partial S98.12- ☑
      more than one S98.21- ☑
        partial S98.22- ☑
      partial S98.14- ☑
    vulva (complete) S38.211 ☑
      partial S38.212 ☑
Amputee (bilateral) (old) Z89.9
Amsterdam dwarfism Q87.1
Amusia R48.8
  developmental F80.89
Amyelencephalus, amyelencephaly Q00.0
Amyelia Q06.0
Amygdalitis — *see* Tonsillitis
Amygdalolith J35.8
Amyloid heart (disease) E85.4 [I43]
Amyloidosis (generalized) (primary) E85.9
  with lung involvement E85.4 [J99]
  familial E85.2
  genetic E85.2
  heart E85.4 [I43]
  hemodialysis-associated E85.3
  light chain (AL) E85.81
  liver E85.4 [K77]
  localized E85.4
  neuropathic heredofamilial E85.1
  non-neuropathic heredofamilial E85.0
  organ limited E85.4
  Portuguese E85.1
  pulmonary E85.4 [J99]
  secondary systemic E85.3
  senile systemic (SSA) E85.82
  skin (lichen) (macular) E85.4 [L99]
  specified NEC E85.89
  subglottic E85.4 [J99]
  wild-type transthyretin-related (ATTR) E85.82
Amylopectinosis (brancher enzyme deficiency) E74.03
Amylophagia — *see* Pica
Amyoplasia congenita Q79.8
Amyotonia M62.89
  congenita G70.2
Amyotrophia, amyotrophy, amyotrophic G71.8
  congenita Q79.8
  diabetic — *see* Diabetes, amyotrophy
  lateral sclerosis G12.21
  neuralgic G54.5
  spinal progressive G12.25
Anacidity, gastric K31.83
  psychogenic F45.8
Anaerosis of newborn P28.89
Analbuminemia E88.09
Analgesia — *see* Anesthesia
Analphalipoproteinemia E78.6
Anaphylactic
  purpura D69.0
  shock or reaction — *see* Shock, anaphylactic
Anaphylactoid shock or reaction — *see* Shock, anaphylactic
Anaphylactoid syndrome of pregnancy O88.01- ☑
Anaphylaxis — *see* Shock, anaphylactic
Anaplasia cervix (see also Dysplasia, cervix) N87.9
Anaplasmosis, human A77.49
Anarthria R47.1
Anasarca R60.1
  cardiac — *see* Failure, heart, congestive
  lung J18.2
  newborn P83.2
  nutritional E43
  pulmonary J18.2
  renal N04.9

Anastomosis
  aneurysmal — *see* Aneurysm
  arteriovenous ruptured brain I60.8
  intestinal K63.89
    complicated NEC K91.89
      involving urinary tract N99.89
  retinal and choroidal vessels (congenital) Q14.8
Anatomical narrow angle H40.03- ☑
Ancylostoma, ancylostomiasis (braziliense) (caninum) (ceylanicum) (duodenale) B76.0
  Necator americanus B76.1
Andersen's disease (glycogen storage) E74.09
Anderson-Fabry disease E75.21
Andes disease T70.29 ☑
Andrews' disease (bacterid) L08.89
Androblastoma
  benign
    specified site — *see* Neoplasm, benign, by site
    unspecified site
      female D27.9
      male D29.20
  malignant
    specified site — *see* Neoplasm, malignant, by site
    unspecified site
      female C56.9
      male C62.90
  specified site — *see* Neoplasm, uncertain behavior, by site
  tubular
    with lipid storage
      specified site — *see* Neoplasm, benign, by site
      unspecified site
        female D27.9
        male D29.20
    specified site — *see* Neoplasm, benign, by site
    unspecified site
      female D27.9
      male D29.20
  unspecified site
    female D39.10
    male D40.10
Androgen insensitivity syndrome (see also Syndrome, androgen insensitivity) E34.50
Androgen resistance syndrome (see also Syndrome, androgen insensitivity) E34.50
Android pelvis Q74.2
  with disproportion (fetopelvic) O33.3 ☑
    causing obstructed labor O65.3
Androphobia F40.290
Anectasis, pulmonary (newborn) — *see* Atelectasis
Anemia (essential) (general) (hemoglobin deficiency) (infantile) (primary) (profound) D64.9
  with (due to) (in)
    disorder of
      anaerobic glycolysis D55.2
      pentose phosphate pathway D55.1
    koilonychia D50.9
  achlorhydric D50.8
  achrestic D53.1
  Addison (-Biermer) (pernicious) D51.0
  agranulocytic — *see* Agranulocytosis
  amino-acid-deficiency D53.0
  aplastic D61.9
    congenital D61.09
    drug-induced D61.1
    due to
      drugs D61.1
      external agents NEC D61.2
      infection D61.2
      radiation D61.2
    idiopathic D61.3
    red cell (pure) D60.9
      chronic D60.0
      congenital D61.01
      specified type NEC D60.8
      transient D60.1
    specified type NEC D61.89
    toxic D61.2
  aregenerative
    congenital D61.09
  asiderotic D50.9
  atypical (primary) D64.9
  Baghdad spring D55.0
  Balantidium coli A07.0
  Biermer's (pernicious) D51.0
  blood loss (chronic) D50.0
    acute D62
  bothriocephalus B70.0 [D63.8]

Anemia — continued
  brickmaker's B76.9 [D63.8]
  cerebral I67.89
  childhood D58.9
  chlorotic D50.8
  chronic
    blood loss D50.0
    hemolytic D58.9
      idiopathic D59.9
    simple D53.9
  chronica congenita aregenerativa D61.09
  combined system disease NEC D51.0 [G32.0]
    due to dietary vitamin B12 deficiency D51.3 [G32.0]
  complicating pregnancy, childbirth or puerperium — *see* Pregnancy, complicated by (management affected by), anemia
  congenital P61.4
    aplastic D61.09
    due to isoimmunization NOS P55.9
    dyserythropoietic, dyshematopoietic D64.4
    following fetal blood loss P61.3
    Heinz body D58.2
    hereditary hemolytic NOS D58.9
    pernicious D51.0
    spherocytic D58.0
  Cooley's (erythroblastic) D56.1
  cytogenic D51.0
  deficiency D53.9
    2, 3 diphosphoglycurate mutase D55.2
    2, 3 PG D55.2
    6 phosphogluconate dehydrogenase D55.1
    6-PGD D55.1
    amino-acid D53.0
    combined B12 and folate D53.1
    enzyme D55.9
      drug-induced (hemolytic) D59.2
      glucose-6-phosphate dehydrogenase (G6PD) D55.0
      glycolytic D55.2
      nucleotide metabolism D55.3
      related to hexose monophosphate (HMP) shunt pathway NEC D55.1
      specified type NEC D55.8
    erythrocytic glutathione D55.1
    folate D52.9
      dietary D52.0
      drug-induced D52.1
    folic acid D52.9
      dietary D52.0
      drug-induced D52.1
    G SH D55.1
    G6PD D55.0
    GGS-R D55.1
    glucose-6-phosphate dehydrogenase D55.0
    glutathione reductase D55.1
    glyceraldehyde phosphate dehydrogenase D55.2
    hexokinase D55.2
    iron D50.9
      secondary to blood loss (chronic) D50.0
    nutritional D53.9
      with
        poor iron absorption D50.8
        specified deficiency NEC D53.8
    phosphofructo-aldolase D55.2
    phosphoglycerate kinase D55.2
    PK D55.2
    protein D53.0
    pyruvate kinase D55.2
    transcobalamin II D51.2
    triose-phosphate isomerase D55.2
    vitamin B12 NOS D51.9
      dietary D51.3
      due to
        intrinsic factor deficiency D51.0
        selective vitamin B12 malabsorption with proteinuria D51.1
      pernicious D51.0
      specified type NEC D51.8
  Diamond-Blackfan (congenital hypoplastic) D61.01
  dibothriocephalus B70.0 [D63.8]
  dimorphic D53.1
  diphasic D53.1
  Diphyllobothrium (Dibothriocephalus) B70.0 [D63.8]
  due to (in) (with)
    antineoplastic chemotherapy D64.81
    blood loss (chronic) D50.0
      acute D62
    chemotherapy, antineoplastic D64.81
    chronic disease classified elsewhere NEC D63.8

Anemia — *continued*
  due to — *continued*
    chronic kidney disease D63.1
    deficiency
      amino-acid D53.0
      copper D53.8
      folate (folic acid) D52.9
        dietary D52.0
        drug-induced D52.1
      molybdenum D53.8
      protein D53.0
      zinc D53.8
    dietary vitamin B12 deficiency D51.3
    disorder of
      glutathione metabolism D55.1
      nucleotide metabolism D55.3
    drug — *see* Anemia, by type (*see also* Table of Drugs and Chemicals)
    end stage renal disease D63.1
    enzyme disorder D55.9
    fetal blood loss P61.3
    fish tapeworm (D.latum) infestation B70.0 [D63.8]
    hemorrhage (chronic) D50.0
      acute D62
    impaired absorption D50.9
    loss of blood (chronic) D50.0
      acute D62
    myxedema E03.9 [D63.8]
    Necator americanus B76.1 [D63.8]
    prematurity P61.2
    selective vitamin B12 malabsorption with proteinuria D51.1
    transcobalamin II deficiency D51.2
  Dyke-Young type (secondary) (symptomatic) D59.1
  dyserythropoietic (congenital) D64.4
  dyshematopoietic (congenital) D64.4
  Egyptian B76.9 [D63.8]
  elliptocytosis — *see* Elliptocytosis
  enzyme-deficiency, drug-induced D59.2
  epidemic (*see also* Ancylostomiasis) B76.9 [D63.8]
  erythroblastic
    familial D56.1
    newborn (*see also* Disease, hemolytic) P55.9
    of childhood D56.1
  erythrocytic glutathione deficiency D55.1
  erythropoietin-resistant anemia (EPO resistant anemia) D63.1
  Faber's (achlorhydric anemia) D50.9
  factitious (self-induced blood letting) D50.0
  familial erythroblastic D56.1
  Fanconi's (congenital pancytopenia) D61.09
  favism D55.0
  fish tapeworm (D. latum) infestation B70.0 [D63.8]
  folate (folic acid) deficiency D52.9
  glucose-6-phosphate dehydrogenase (G6PD) deficiency D55.0
  glutathione-reductase deficiency D55.1
  goat's milk D52.0
  granulocytic — *see* Agranulocytosis
  Heinz body, congenital D58.2
  hemolytic D58.9
    acquired D59.9
      with hemoglobinuria NEC D59.6
      autoimmune NEC D59.1
      infectious D59.4
      specified type NEC D59.8
      toxic D59.4
    acute D59.9
      due to enzyme deficiency specified type NEC D55.8
      Lederer's D59.1
    autoimmune D59.1
      drug-induced D59.0
    chronic D58.9
      idiopathic D59.9
    cold type (secondary) (symptomatic) D59.1
    congenital (spherocytic) — *see* Spherocytosis
    due to
      cardiac conditions D59.4
      drugs (nonautoimmune) D59.2
        autoimmune D59.0
      enzyme disorder D55.9
        drug-induced D59.2
      presence of shunt or other internal prosthetic device D59.4
    familial D58.9
    hereditary D58.9
      due to enzyme disorder D55.9
        specified type NEC D55.8

Anemia — *continued*
  hemolytic — *continued*
    hereditary — *continued*
      specified type NEC D58.8
    idiopathic (chronic) D59.9
    mechanical D59.4
    microangiopathic D59.4
    nonautoimmune D59.4
      drug-induced D59.2
    nonspherocytic
      congenital or hereditary NEC D55.8
        glucose-6-phosphate dehydrogenase deficiency D55.0
        pyruvate kinase deficiency D55.2
        type
          I D55.1
          II D55.2
      type
        I D55.1
        II D55.2
    secondary D59.4
      autoimmune D59.1
    specified (hereditary) type NEC D58.8
    Stransky-Regala type (*see also* Hemoglobinopathy) D58.8
    symptomatic D59.4
      autoimmune D59.1
    toxic D59.4
    warm type (secondary) (symptomatic) D59.1
  hemorrhagic (chronic) D50.0
    acute D62
  Herrick's D57.1
  hexokinase deficiency D55.2
  hookworm B76.9 [D63.8]
  hypochromic (idiopathic) (microcytic) (normoblastic) D50.9
    due to blood loss (chronic) D50.0
      acute D62
    familial sex-linked D64.0
    pyridoxine-responsive D64.3
    sideroblastic, sex-linked D64.0
  hypoplasia, red blood cells D61.9
    congenital or familial D61.01
  hypoplastic (idiopathic) D61.9
    congenital or familial (of childhood) D61.01
  hypoproliferative (refractory) D61.9
  idiopathic D64.9
    aplastic D61.3
    hemolytic, chronic D59.9
  in (due to) (with)
    chronic kidney disease D63.1
    end stage renal disease D63.1
    failure, kidney (renal) D63.1
    neoplastic disease (*see also* Neoplasm) D63.0
  intertropical (*see also* Ancylostomiasis) D63.8
  iron deficiency D50.9
    secondary to blood loss (chronic) D50.0
      acute D62
    specified type NEC D50.8
  Joseph-Diamond-Blackfan (congenital hypoplastic) D61.01
  Lederer's (hemolytic) D59.1
  leukoerythroblastic D61.82
  macrocytic D53.9
    nutritional D52.0
    tropical D52.8
  malarial (*see also* Malaria) B54 [D63.8]
  malignant (progressive) D51.0
  malnutrition D53.9
  marsh (*see also* Malaria) B54 [D63.8]
  Mediterranean (with other hemoglobinopathy) D56.9
  megaloblastic D53.1
    combined B12 and folate deficiency D53.1
    hereditary D51.1
    nutritional D52.0
    orotic aciduria D53.0
    refractory D53.1
    specified type NEC D53.1
  megalocytic D53.1
  microcytic (hypochromic) D50.9
    due to blood loss (chronic) D50.0
      acute D62
    familial D56.8
  microdrepanocytosis D57.40
  microelliptopoikilocytic (Rietti-Greppi- Micheli) D56.9
  miner's B76.9 [D63.8]
  myelodysplastic D46.9
  myelofibrosis D75.81
  myelogenous D64.89

Anemia — *continued*
  myelopathic D64.89
  myelophthisic D61.82
  myeloproliferative D47.Z9 (*following* D47.4)
  newborn P61.4
    due to
      ABO (antibodies, isoimmunization, maternal/fetal incompatibility) P55.1
      Rh (antibodies, isoimmunization, maternal/fetal incompatibility) P55.0
    following fetal blood loss P61.3
    posthemorrhagic (fetal) P61.3
  nonspherocytic hemolytic — *see* Anemia, hemolytic, nonspherocytic
  normocytic (infectional) D64.9
    due to blood loss (chronic) D50.0
      acute D62
    myelophthisic D61.82
  nutritional (deficiency) D53.9
    with
      poor iron absorption D50.8
      specified deficiency NEC D53.8
    megaloblastic D52.0
  of prematurity P61.2
  orotaciduric (congenital) (hereditary) D53.0
  osteosclerotic D64.89
  ovalocytosis (hereditary) — *see* Elliptocytosis
  paludal (*see also* Malaria) B54 [D63.8]
  pernicious (congenital) (malignant) (progressive) D51.0
  pleochromic D64.89
    of sprue D52.8
  posthemorrhagic (chronic) D50.0
    acute D62
    newborn P61.3
  postoperative (postprocedural)
    due to (acute) blood loss D62
      chronic blood loss D50.0
    specified NEC D64.9
  postpartum O90.81
  pressure D64.89
  progressive D64.9
    malignant D51.0
    pernicious D51.0
  protein-deficiency D53.0
  pseudoleukemica infantum D64.89
  pure red cell D60.9
    congenital D61.01
  pyridoxine-responsive D64.3
  pyruvate kinase deficiency D55.2
  refractory D46.4
    with
      excess of blasts D46.20
        1 (RAEB 1) D46.21
        2 (RAEB 2) D46.22
        in transformation (RAEB T) — *see* Leukemia, acute myeloblastic
      hemochromatosis D46.1
      sideroblasts (ring) (RARS) D46.1
    megaloblastic D53.1
    sideroblastic D46.1
    sideropenic D50.9
    without ring sideroblasts, so stated D46.0
    without sideroblasts without excess of blasts D46.0
  Rietti-Greppi-Micheli D56.9
  scorbutic D53.2
  secondary to
    blood loss (chronic) D50.0
      acute D62
    hemorrhage (chronic) D50.0
      acute D62
  semiplastic D61.89
  sickle-cell — *see* Disease, sickle-cell
  sideroblastic D64.3
    hereditary D64.0
    hypochromic, sex-linked D64.0
    pyridoxine-responsive NEC D64.3
    refractory D46.1
    secondary (due to)
      disease D64.1
      drugs and toxins D64.2
    specified type NEC D64.3
  sideropenic (refractory) D50.9
    due to blood loss (chronic) D50.0
      acute D62
  simple chronic D53.9
  specified type NEC D64.89
  spherocytic (hereditary) — *see* Spherocytosis
  splenic D64.89
  splenomegalic D64.89

Anemia — *continued*
  stomatocytosis D58.8
  syphilitic (acquired) (late) A52.79 [D63.8]
  target cell D64.89
  thalassemia D56.9
  thrombocytopenic — *see* Thrombocytopenia
  toxic D61.2
  tropical B76.9 [D63.8]
    macrocytic D52.8
  tuberculous A18.89 [D63.8]
  vegan D51.3
  vitamin
    B12 deficiency (dietary) pernicious D51.0
    B6-responsive D64.3
  von Jaksch's D64.89
  Witts' (achlorhydric anemia) D50.8
Anemophobia F40.228
Anencephalus, anencephaly Q00.0
Anergasia — *see* Psychosis, organic
Anesthesia, anesthetic R20.0
  complication or reaction NEC (*see also* Complications, anesthesia) T88.59 ☑
    due to
      correct substance properly administered — *see* Table of Drugs and Chemicals, by drug, adverse effect
      overdose or wrong substance given — *see* Table of Drugs and Chemicals, by drug, poisoning
    unintended awareness under general anesthesia during procedure T88.53 ☑
      personal history of Z92.84
  cornea H18.81- ☑
  dissociative F44.6
  functional (hysterical) F44.6
  hyperesthetic, thalamic G89.0
  hysterical F44.6
  local skin lesion R20.0
  sexual (psychogenic) F52.1
  shock (due to) T88.2 ☑
  skin R20.0
  testicular N50.9
Anetoderma (maculosum) (of) L90.8
  Jadassohn-Pellizzari L90.2
  Schweniger-Buzzi L90.1
Aneurin deficiency E51.9
Aneurysm (anastomotic) (artery) (cirsoid) (diffuse) (false) (fusiform) (multiple) (saccular) I72.9
  abdominal (aorta) I71.4
    ruptured I71.3
    syphilitic A52.01
  aorta, aortic (nonsyphilitic) I71.9
    abdominal I71.4
      ruptured I71.3
    arch I71.2
      ruptured I71.1
    arteriosclerotic I71.9
      ruptured I71.8
    ascending I71.2
      ruptured I71.1
    congenital Q25.43
    descending I71.9
      abdominal I71.4
        ruptured I71.3
      ruptured I71.8
      thoracic I71.2
        ruptured I71.1
    root Q25.43
    ruptured I71.8
    sinus, congenital Q25.43
    syphilitic A52.01
    thoracic I71.2
      ruptured I71.1
    thoracoabdominal I71.6
      ruptured I71.5
    thorax, thoracic (arch) I71.2
      ruptured I71.1
    transverse I71.2
      ruptured I71.1
    valve (heart) (*see also* Endocarditis, aortic) I35.8
  arteriosclerotic I72.9
    cerebral I67.1
      ruptured — *see* Hemorrhage, intracranial, subarachnoid
  arteriovenous (congenital) (*see also* Malformation, arteriovenous)
    acquired I77.0
      brain I67.1

Aneurysm — *continued*
  arteriovenous (*see also* Malformation, arteriovenous) — *continued*
    acquired — *continued*
      coronary I25.41
      pulmonary I28.0
    brain Q28.2
      ruptured I60.8
    peripheral — *see* Malformation, arteriovenous, peripheral
    precerebral vessels Q28.0
    specified site NEC (*see also* Malformation, arteriovenous)
      acquired I77.0
  basal — *see* Aneurysm, brain
  basilar (trunk) I72.5
  berry (congenital) (nonruptured) I67.1
    ruptured I60.7
  brain I67.1
    arteriosclerotic I67.1
      ruptured — *see* Hemorrhage, intracranial, subarachnoid
    arteriovenous (congenital) (nonruptured) Q28.2
      acquired I67.1
        ruptured I60.8
      ruptured I60.8
    berry (congenital) (nonruptured) I67.1
      ruptured (*see also* Hemorrhage, intracranial, subarachnoid) I60.7
    congenital Q28.3
      ruptured I60.7
    meninges I67.1
      ruptured I60.8
    miliary (congenital) (nonruptured) I67.1
      ruptured (*see also* Hemorrhage, intracranial, subarachnoid) I60.7
    mycotic I33.0
    ruptured — *see* Hemorrhage, intracranial, subarachnoid
    syphilitic (hemorrhage) A52.05
  cardiac (false) (*see also* Aneurysm, heart) I25.3
  carotid artery (common) (external) I72.0
    internal (intracranial) I67.1
      extracranial portion I72.0
    ruptured into brain I60.0- ☑
    syphilitic A52.09
      intracranial A52.05
  cavernous sinus I67.1
    arteriovenous (congenital) (nonruptured) Q28.3
      ruptured I60.8
  celiac I72.8
  central nervous system, syphilitic A52.05
  cerebral — *see* Aneurysm, brain
  chest — *see* Aneurysm, thorax
  circle of Willis I67.1
    congenital Q28.3
      ruptured I60.6
    ruptured I60.6
  common iliac artery I72.3
  congenital (peripheral) Q27.8
    aorta (root) (sinus) Q25.43
    brain Q28.3
      ruptured I60.7
    coronary Q24.5
    digestive system Q27.8
    lower limb Q27.8
    pulmonary Q25.79
    retina Q14.1
    specified site NEC Q27.8
    upper limb Q27.8
  conjunctiva — *see* Abnormality, conjunctiva, vascular
  conus arteriosus — *see* Aneurysm, heart
  coronary (arteriosclerotic) (artery) I25.41
    arteriovenous, congenital Q24.5
    congenital Q24.5
    ruptured — *see* Infarct, myocardium
    syphilitic A52.06
    vein I25.89
  cylindroid (aorta) I71.9
    ruptured I71.8
    syphilitic A52.01
  ductus arteriosus Q25.0
  endocardial, infective (any valve) I33.0
  femoral (artery) (ruptured) I72.4
  gastroduodenal I72.8
  gastroepiploic I72.8
  heart (wall) (chronic or with a stated duration of over 4 weeks) I25.3

Aneurysm — *continued*
  heart — *continued*
    valve — *see* Endocarditis
  hepatic I72.8
  iliac (common) (artery) (ruptured) I72.3
  infective I72.9
    endocardial (any valve) I33.0
  innominate (nonsyphilitic) I72.8
    syphilitic A52.09
  interauricular septum — *see* Aneurysm, heart
  interventricular septum — *see* Aneurysm, heart
  intrathoracic (nonsyphilitic) I71.2
    ruptured I71.1
    syphilitic A52.01
  lower limb I72.4
  lung (pulmonary artery) I28.1
  mediastinal (nonsyphilitic) I72.8
    syphilitic A52.09
  miliary (congenital) I67.1
    ruptured — *see* Hemorrhage, intracerebral, subarachnoid, intracranial
  mitral (heart) (valve) I34.8
  mural — *see* Aneurysm, heart
  mycotic I72.9
    endocardial (any valve) I33.0
    ruptured, brain — *see* Hemorrhage, intracerebral, subarachnoid
  myocardium — *see* Aneurysm, heart
  neck I72.0
  pancreaticoduodenal I72.8
  patent ductus arteriosus Q25.0
  peripheral NEC I72.8
    congenital Q27.8
      digestive system Q27.8
      lower limb Q27.8
      specified site NEC Q27.8
      upper limb Q27.8
  popliteal (artery) (ruptured) I72.4
  precerebral
    congenital (nonruptured) Q28.1
    specified site, NEC I72.5
  pulmonary I28.1
    arteriovenous Q25.72
      acquired I28.0
    syphilitic A52.09
    valve (heart) — *see* Endocarditis, pulmonary
  racemose (peripheral) I72.9
    congenital — *see* Aneurysm, congenital
  radial I72.1
  Rasmussen NEC A15.0
  renal (artery) I72.2
  retina (*see also* Disorder, retina, microaneurysms)
    congenital Q14.1
    diabetic — *see* Diabetes, microaneurysms, retinal
  sinus of Valsalva Q25.49
  specified NEC I72.8
  spinal (cord) I72.8
    syphilitic (hemorrhage) A52.09
  splenic I72.8
  subclavian (artery) (ruptured) I72.8
    syphilitic A52.09
  superior mesenteric I72.8
  syphilitic (aorta) A52.01
    central nervous system A52.05
    congenital (late) A50.54 [I79.0]
    spine, spinal A52.09
  thoracoabdominal (aorta) I71.6
    ruptured I71.5
    syphilitic A52.01
  thorax, thoracic (aorta) (arch) (nonsyphilitic) I71.2
    ruptured I71.1
    syphilitic A52.01
  traumatic (complication) (early), specified site — *see* Injury, blood vessel
  tricuspid (heart) (valve) I07.8
  ulnar I72.1
  upper limb (ruptured) I72.1
  valve, valvular — *see* Endocarditis
  venous (*see also* Varix) I86.8
    congenital Q27.8
      digestive system Q27.8
      lower limb Q27.8
      specified site NEC Q27.8
      upper limb Q27.8
  ventricle — *see* Aneurysm, heart
  vertebral artery I72.6
  visceral NEC I72.8
Angelman syndrome Q93.51

20

☑ **Additional Character Required** — Refer to the Tabular List for Character Selection
▽ **Subterms under main terms may continue to next column or page**

Anger R45.4
Angiectasis, angiectopia I99.8
Angiitis I77.6
  allergic granulomatous M3Ø.1
  hypersensitivity M31.Ø
  necrotizing M31.9
    specified NEC M31.8
  nervous system, granulomatous I67.7
Angina (attack) (cardiac) (chest) (heart) (pectoris) (syndrome) (vasomotor) I2Ø.9
  with
    atherosclerotic heart disease — see Arteriosclerosis, coronary (artery),
    documented spasm I2Ø.1
  abdominal K55.1
  accelerated — see Angina, unstable
  agranulocytic — see Agranulocytosis
  angiospastic — see Angina, with documented spasm
  aphthous BØ8.5
  crescendo — see Angina, unstable
  croupous JØ5.Ø
  cruris I73.9
  de novo effort — see Angina, unstable
  diphtheritic, membranous A36.Ø
  equivalent I2Ø.8
  exudative, chronic J37.Ø
  following acute myocardial infarction I23.7
  gangrenous diphtheritic A36.Ø
  intestinal K55.1
  Ludovici K12.2
  Ludwig's K12.2
  malignant diphtheritic A36.Ø
  membranous JØ5.Ø
    diphtheritic A36.Ø
    Vincent's A69.1
  mesenteric K55.1
  monocytic — see Mononucleosis, infectious
  of effort — see Angina, specified NEC
  phlegmonous J36
    diphtheritic A36.Ø
  post-infarctional I23.7
  pre-infarctional — see Angina, unstable
  Prinzmetal — see Angina, with documented spasm
  progressive — see Angina, unstable
  pseudomembranous A69.1
  pultaceous, diphtheritic A36.Ø
  spasm-induced — see Angina, with documented spasm
  specified NEC I2Ø.8
  stable I2Ø.8
  stenocardia — see Angina, specified NEC
  stridulous, diphtheritic A36.2
  tonsil J36
  trachealis JØ5.Ø
  unstable I2Ø.Ø
  variant — see Angina, with documented spasm
  Vincent's A69.1
  worsening effort — see Angina, unstable
Angioblastoma — see Neoplasm, connective tissue, uncertain behavior
Angiocholecystitis — see Cholecystitis, acute
Angiocholitis (see also Cholecystitis, acute) K83.Ø9
Angiodysgenesis spinalis G95.19
Angiodysplasia (cecum) (colon) K55.2Ø
  with bleeding K55.21
  duodenum (and stomach) K31.819
    with bleeding K31.811
  stomach (and duodenum) K31.819
    with bleeding K31.811
Angioedema (allergic) (any site) (with urticaria) T78.3 ☑
  hereditary D84.1
Angioendothelioma — see Neoplasm, uncertain behavior, by site
  benign D18.ØØ
    intra-abdominal D18.Ø3
    intracranial D18.Ø2
    skin D18.Ø1
    specified site NEC D18.Ø9
  bone — see Neoplasm, bone, malignant
  Ewing's — see Neoplasm, bone, malignant
Angioendotheliomatosis C85.8- ☑
Angiofibroma (see also Neoplasm, benign, by site)
  juvenile
    specified site — see Neoplasm, benign, by site
    unspecified site D1Ø.6
Angiohemophilia (A) (B) D68.Ø
Angioid streaks (choroid) (macula) (retina) H35.33
Angiokeratoma — see Neoplasm, skin, benign
  corporis diffusum E75.21

Angioleiomyoma — see Neoplasm, connective tissue, benign
Angiolipoma (see also Lipoma)
  infiltrating — see Lipoma
Angioma (see also Hemangioma, by site)
  capillary I78.1
  hemorrhagicum hereditaria I78.Ø
  intra-abdominal D18.Ø3
  intracranial D18.Ø2
  malignant — see Neoplasm, connective tissue, malignant
  plexiform D18.ØØ
    intra-abdominal D18.Ø3
    intracranial D18.Ø2
    skin D18.Ø1
    specified site NEC D18.Ø9
  senile I78.1
  serpiginosum L81.7
  skin D18.Ø1
  specified site NEC D18.Ø9
  spider I78.1
  stellate I78.1
  venous Q28.3
Angiomatosis Q82.8
  bacillary A79.89
  encephalotrigeminal Q85.8
  hemorrhagic familial I78.Ø
  hereditary familial I78.Ø
  liver K76.4
Angiomyolipoma — see Lipoma
Angiomyoliposarcoma — see Neoplasm, connective tissue, malignant
Angiomyoma — see Neoplasm, connective tissue, benign
Angiomyosarcoma — see Neoplasm, connective tissue, malignant
Angiomyxoma — see Neoplasm, connective tissue, uncertain behavior
Angioneurosis F45.8
Angioneurotic edema (allergic) (any site) (with urticaria) T78.3 ☑
  hereditary D84.1
Angiopathia, angiopathy I99.9
  cerebral I67.9
    amyloid E85.4 [I68.Ø]
  diabetic (peripheral) — see Diabetes, angiopathy
  peripheral I73.9
    diabetic — see Diabetes, angiopathy
    specified type NEC I73.89
  retinae syphilitica A52.Ø5
  retinalis (juvenilis)
    diabetic — see Diabetes, retinopathy
    proliferative — see Retinopathy, proliferative
Angiosarcoma (see also Neoplasm, connective tissue, malignant)
  liver C22.3
Angiosclerosis — see Arteriosclerosis
Angiospasm (peripheral) (traumatic) (vessel) I73.9
  brachial plexus G54.Ø
  cerebral G45.9
  cervical plexus G54.2
  nerve
    arm — see Mononeuropathy, upper limb
      axillary G54.Ø
      median — see Lesion, nerve, median
      ulnar — see Lesion, nerve, ulnar
    axillary G54.Ø
    leg — see Mononeuropathy, lower limb
    median — see Lesion, nerve, median
    plantar — see Lesion, nerve, plantar
    ulnar — see Lesion, nerve, ulnar
Angiospastic disease or edema I73.9
Angiostrongyliasis
  due to
    Parastrongylus
      cantonensis B83.2
      costaricensis B81.3
    intestinal B81.3
Anguillulosis — see Strongyloidiasis
Angulation
  cecum — see Obstruction, intestine
  coccyx (acquired) (see also subcategory) M43.8 ☑
    congenital NEC Q76.49
  femur (acquired) (see also Deformity, limb, specified type NEC, thigh)
    congenital Q74.2
  intestine (large) (small) — see Obstruction, intestine
  sacrum (acquired) (see also subcategory) M43.8 ☑
    congenital NEC Q76.49

Angulation — continued
  sigmoid (flexure) — see Obstruction, intestine
  spine — see Dorsopathy, deforming, specified NEC
  tibia (acquired) (see also Deformity, limb, specified type NEC, lower leg)
    congenital Q74.2
  ureter N13.5
    with infection N13.6
  wrist (acquired) (see also Deformity, limb, specified type NEC, forearm)
    congenital Q74.Ø
Angulus infectiosus (lips) K13.Ø
Anhedonia R45.84
  sexual F52.Ø
Anhidrosis L74.4
Anhydration E86.Ø
Anhydremia E86.Ø
Anidrosis L74.4
Aniridia (congenital) Q13.1
Anisakiasis (infection) (infestation) B81.Ø
Anisakis larvae infestation B81.Ø
Aniseikonia H52.32
Anisocoria (pupil) H57.Ø2
  congenital Q13.2
Anisocytosis R71.8
Anisometropia (congenital) H52.31
Ankle — see condition
Ankyloblepharon (eyelid) (acquired) (see also Blepharophimosis)
  filiforme (adnatum) (congenital) Q1Ø.3
  total Q1Ø.3
Ankyloglossia Q38.1
Ankylosis (fibrous) (osseous) (joint) M24.6Ø
  ankle M24.67- ☑
  arthrodesis status Z98.1
  cricoarytenoid (cartilage) (joint) (larynx) J38.7
  dental KØ3.5
  ear ossicles H74.31- ☑
  elbow M24.62- ☑
  foot M24.67- ☑
  hand M24.64- ☑
  hip M24.65- ☑
  incostapedial joint (infectional) — see Ankylosis, ear ossicles
  jaw (temporomandibular) M26.61- ☑
  knee M24.66- ☑
  lumbosacral (joint) M43.27
  postoperative (status) Z98.1
  produced by surgical fusion, status Z98.1
  sacro-iliac (joint) M43.28
  shoulder M24.61- ☑
  spine (joint) (see also Fusion, spine)
    spondylitic — see Spondylitis, ankylosing
  surgical Z98.1
  temporomandibular M26.61- ☑
  tooth, teeth (hard tissues) KØ3.5
  wrist M24.63- ☑
Ankylostoma — see Ancylostoma
Ankylostomiasis — see Ancylostomiasis
Ankylurethria — see Stricture, urethra
Annular (see also condition)
  detachment, cervix N88.8
  organ or site, congenital NEC — see Distortion
  pancreas (congenital) Q45.1
Anodontia (complete) (partial) (vera) KØØ.Ø
  acquired KØ8.1Ø ☑
Anomaly, anomalous (congenital) (unspecified type) Q89.9
  abdominal wall NEC Q79.59
  acoustic nerve QØ7.8
  adrenal (gland) Q89.1
  Alder (-Reilly) (leukocyte granulation) D72.Ø
  alimentary tract Q45.9
    upper Q4Ø.9
  alveolar M26.7Ø
    hyperplasia M26.79
      mandibular M26.72
      maxillary M26.71
    hypoplasia M26.79
      mandibular M26.74
      maxillary M26.73
    ridge (process) M26.79
    specified NEC M26.79
  ankle (joint) Q74.2
  anus Q43.9
  aorta (arch) NEC Q25.4Ø
    coarctation (preductal) (postductal) Q25.1

Anomaly, anomalous — *continued*
- aortic cusp or valve Q23.9
- appendix Q43.8
- apple peel syndrome Q41.1
- aqueduct of Sylvius Q03.0
  - with spina bifida — *see* Spina bifida, with hydrocephalus
- arm Q74.0
- arteriovenous NEC
  - coronary Q24.5
  - gastrointestinal Q27.33
    - acquired — *see* Angiodysplasia
- artery (peripheral) Q27.9
  - basilar NEC Q28.1
  - cerebral Q28.3
  - coronary Q24.5
  - digestive system Q27.8
  - eye Q15.8
  - great Q25.9
    - specified NEC Q25.8
  - lower limb Q27.8
  - peripheral Q27.9
    - specified NEC Q27.8
  - pulmonary NEC Q25.79
  - renal Q27.2
  - retina Q14.1
  - specified site NEC Q27.8
  - subclavian Q27.8
    - origin Q25.48
  - umbilical Q27.0
  - upper limb Q27.8
  - vertebral NEC Q28.1
- aryteno-epiglottic folds Q31.8
- atrial
  - bands or folds Q20.8
  - septa Q21.1
- atrioventricular
  - excitation I45.6
  - septum Q21.0
- auditory canal Q17.8
- auricle
  - ear Q17.8
    - causing impairment of hearing Q16.9
  - heart Q20.8
- Axenfeld's Q15.0
- back Q89.9
- band
  - atrial Q20.8
  - heart Q24.8
  - ventricular Q24.8
- Bartholin's duct Q38.4
- biliary duct or passage Q44.5
- bladder Q64.70
  - absence Q64.5
  - diverticulum Q64.6
  - exstrophy Q64.10
    - cloacal Q64.12
    - extroversion Q64.19
    - specified type NEC Q64.19
    - supravesical fissure Q64.11
  - neck obstruction Q64.31
  - specified type NEC Q64.79
- bone Q79.9
  - arm Q74.0
  - face Q75.9
  - leg Q74.2
  - pelvic girdle Q74.2
  - shoulder girdle Q74.0
  - skull Q75.9
    - with
      - anencephaly Q00.0
      - encephalocele — *see* Encephalocele
      - hydrocephalus Q03.9
        - with spina bifida — *see* Spina bifida, by site, with hydrocephalus
      - microcephaly Q02
- brain (multiple) Q04.9
  - vessel Q28.3
- breast Q83.9
- broad ligament Q50.6
- bronchus Q32.4
- bulbus cordis Q21.9
- bursa Q79.9
- canal of Nuck Q52.4
- canthus Q10.3
- capillary Q27.9
- cardiac Q24.9
  - chambers Q20.9
    - specified NEC Q20.8

Anomaly, anomalous — *continued*
- cardiac — *continued*
  - septal closure Q21.9
    - specified NEC Q21.8
  - valve NEC Q24.8
    - pulmonary Q22.3
- cardiovascular system Q28.8
- carpus Q74.0
- caruncle, lacrimal Q10.6
- cascade stomach Q40.2
- cauda equina Q06.3
- cecum Q43.9
- cerebral Q04.9
  - vessels Q28.3
- cervix Q51.9
- Chédiak-Higashi (-Steinbrinck) (congenital gigantism of peroxidase granules) E70.330
- cheek Q18.9
- chest wall Q67.8
  - bones Q76.9
- chin Q18.9
- chordae tendineae Q24.8
- choroid Q14.3
  - plexus Q07.8
- chromosomes, chromosomal Q99.9
  - D (1) — *see* condition, chromosome 13
  - E (3) — *see* condition, chromosome 18
  - G — *see* condition, chromosome 21
  - sex
    - female phenotype Q97.8
    - gonadal dysgenesis (pure) Q99.1
    - Klinefelter's Q98.4
    - male phenotype Q98.9
    - Turner's Q96.9
  - specified NEC Q99.8
- cilia Q10.3
- circulatory system Q28.9
- clavicle Q74.0
- clitoris Q52.6
- coccyx Q76.49
- colon Q43.9
- common duct Q44.5
- communication
  - coronary artery Q24.5
  - left ventricle with right atrium Q21.0
- concha (ear) Q17.3
- connection
  - portal vein Q26.5
  - pulmonary venous Q26.4
    - partial Q26.3
    - total Q26.2
  - renal artery with kidney Q27.2
- cornea (shape) Q13.4
- coronary artery or vein Q24.5
- cranium — *see* Anomaly, skull
- cricoid cartilage Q31.8
- cystic duct Q44.5
- dental
  - alveolar — *see* Anomaly, alveolar
  - arch relationship M26.20
    - specified NEC M26.29
- dentofacial M26.9
  - alveolar — *see* Anomaly, alveolar
  - dental arch relationship M26.20
    - specified NEC M26.29
  - functional M26.50
    - specified NEC M26.59
  - jaw size M26.00
    - macrogenia M26.05
    - mandibular
      - hyperplasia M26.03
      - hypoplasia M26.04
    - maxillary
      - hyperplasia M26.01
      - hypoplasia M26.02
    - microgenia M26.06
    - specified type NEC M26.09
  - jaw-cranial base relationship M26.10
    - asymmetry M26.12
      - maxillary M26.11
    - specified type NEC M26.19
  - malocclusion M26.4
    - dental arch relationship NEC M26.29
    - jaw size — *see* Anomaly, dentofacial, jaw size
    - jaw-cranial base relationship — *see* Anomaly, dentofacial, jaw-cranial base relationship
  - specified type NEC M26.89
  - temporomandibular joint M26.60- ☑

Anomaly, anomalous — *continued*
- dentofacial — *continued*
  - temporomandibular joint — *continued*
    - adhesions M26.61- ☑
    - ankylosis M26.61- ☑
    - arthralgia M26.62- ☑
    - articular disc M26.63- ☑
    - specified type NEC M26.69
  - tooth position, fully erupted M26.30
    - specified NEC M26.39
- dermatoglyphic Q82.8
- diaphragm (apertures) NEC Q79.1
- digestive organ(s) or tract Q45.9
  - lower Q43.9
  - upper Q40.9
- distance, interarch (excessive) (inadequate) M26.25
- distribution, coronary artery Q24.5
- ductus
  - arteriosus Q25.0
  - botalli Q25.0
- duodenum Q43.9
- dura (brain) Q04.9
  - spinal cord Q06.9
- ear (external) Q17.9
  - causing impairment of hearing Q16.9
  - inner Q16.5
  - middle (causing impairment of hearing) Q16.4
  - ossicles Q16.3
- Ebstein's (heart) (tricuspid valve) Q22.5
- ectodermal Q82.9
- Eisenmenger's (ventricular septal defect) Q21.8
- ejaculatory duct Q55.4
- elbow Q74.0
- endocrine gland NEC Q89.2
- epididymis Q55.4
- epiglottis Q31.8
- esophagus Q39.9
- eustachian tube Q17.8
- eye Q15.9
  - anterior segment Q13.9
    - specified NEC Q13.89
  - posterior segment Q14.9
    - specified NEC Q14.8
  - ptosis (eyelid) Q10.0
  - specified NEC Q15.8
- eyebrow Q18.8
- eyelid Q10.3
  - ptosis Q10.0
- face Q18.9
  - bone(s) Q75.9
- fallopian tube Q50.6
- fascia Q79.9
- femur NEC Q74.2
- fibula NEC Q74.2
- finger Q74.0
- fixation, intestine Q43.3
- flexion (joint) NOS Q74.9
  - hip or thigh Q65.89
- foot NEC Q74.2
  - varus (congenital) Q66.3
- foramen
  - Botalli Q21.1
  - ovale Q21.1
- forearm Q74.0
- forehead Q75.8
- form, teeth K00.2
- fovea centralis Q14.1
- frontal bone — *see* Anomaly, skull
- gallbladder (position) (shape) (size) Q44.1
- Gartner's duct Q52.4
- gastrointestinal tract Q45.9
- genitalia, genital organ(s) or system
  - female Q52.9
    - external Q52.70
    - internal NOS Q52.9
  - male Q55.9
    - hydrocele P83.5
    - specified NEC Q55.8
- genitourinary NEC
  - female Q52.9
  - male Q55.9
- Gerbode Q21.0
- glottis Q31.8
- granulation or granulocyte, genetic (constitutional) (leukocyte) D72.0
- gum Q38.6
- gyri Q07.9
- hair Q84.2
- hand Q74.0

Anomaly, anomalous — *continued*
- hard tissue formation in pulp K04.3
- head — *see* Anomaly, skull
- heart Q24.9
  - auricle Q20.8
  - bands or folds Q24.8
  - fibroelastosis cordis I42.4
  - obstructive NEC Q22.6
  - patent ductus arteriosus (Botalli) Q25.0
  - septum Q21.9
    - auricular Q21.1
    - interatrial Q21.1
    - interventricular Q21.0
      - with pulmonary stenosis or atresia, dextraposition of aorta and hypertrophy of right ventricle Q21.3
    - specified NEC Q21.8
    - ventricular Q21.0
      - with pulmonary stenosis or atresia, dextraposition of aorta and hypertrophy of right ventricle Q21.3
  - tetralogy of Fallot Q21.3
  - valve NEC Q24.8
    - aortic
      - bicuspid valve Q23.1
      - insufficiency Q23.1
      - stenosis Q23.0
        - subaortic Q24.4
    - mitral
      - insufficiency Q23.3
      - stenosis Q23.2
    - pulmonary Q22.3
      - atresia Q22.0
      - insufficiency Q22.2
      - stenosis Q22.1
        - infundibular Q24.3
        - subvalvular Q24.3
    - tricuspid
      - atresia Q22.4
      - stenosis Q22.4
  - ventricle Q20.8
- heel NEC Q74.2
- Hegglin's D72.0
- hemianencephaly Q00.0
- hemicephaly Q00.0
- hemicrania Q00.0
- hepatic duct Q44.5
- hip NEC Q74.2
- hourglass stomach Q40.2
- humerus Q74.0
- hydatid of Morgagni
  - female Q50.5
  - male (epididymal) Q55.4
    - testicular Q55.29
- hymen Q52.4
- hypersegmentation of neutrophils, hereditary D72.0
- hypophyseal Q89.2
- ileocecal (coil) (valve) Q43.9
- ileum Q43.9
- ilium NEC Q74.2
- integument Q84.9
  - specified NEC Q84.8
- interarch distance (excessive) (inadequate) M26.25
- intervertebral cartilage or disc Q76.49
- intestine (large) (small) Q43.9
  - with anomalous adhesions, fixation or malrotation Q43.3
- iris Q13.2
- ischium NEC Q74.2
- jaw — *see* Anomaly, dentofacial
  - alveolar — *see* Anomaly, alveolar
- jaw-cranial base relationship — *see* Anomaly, dentofacial, jaw-cranial base relationship
- jejunum Q43.8
- joint Q74.9
  - specified NEC Q74.8
- Jordan's D72.0
- kidney(s) (calyx) (pelvis) Q63.9
  - artery Q27.2
  - specified NEC Q63.8
- Klippel-Feil (brevicollis) Q76.1
- knee Q74.1
- labium (majus) (minus) Q52.70
- labyrinth, membranous Q16.5
- lacrimal apparatus or duct Q10.6
- larynx, laryngeal (muscle) Q31.9
  - web (bed) Q31.0
- lens Q12.9
- leukocytes, genetic D72.0

Anomaly, anomalous — *continued*
- leukocytes, genetic — *continued*
  - granulation (constitutional) D72.0
- lid (fold) Q10.3
- ligament Q79.9
  - broad Q50.6
  - round Q52.8
- limb Q74.9
  - lower NEC Q74.2
    - reduction deformity — *see* Defect, reduction, lower limb
  - upper Q74.0
- lip Q38.0
- liver Q44.7
  - duct Q44.5
- lower limb NEC Q74.2
- lumbosacral (joint) (region) Q76.49
  - kyphosis — *see* Kyphosis, congenital
  - lordosis — *see* Lordosis, congenital
- lung (fissure) (lobe) Q33.9
- mandible — *see* Anomaly, dentofacial
- maxilla — *see* Anomaly, dentofacial
- May (-Hegglin) D72.0
- meatus urinarius NEC Q64.79
- meningeal bands or folds Q07.9
  - constriction of Q07.8
  - spinal Q06.9
- meninges Q07.9
  - cerebral Q04.8
  - spinal Q06.9
- meningocele Q05.9
- mesentery Q45.9
- metacarpus Q74.0
- metatarsus NEC Q74.2
- middle ear Q16.4
  - ossicles Q16.3
- mitral (leaflets) (valve) Q23.9
  - insufficiency Q23.3
  - specified NEC Q23.8
  - stenosis Q23.2
- mouth Q38.6
- Müllerian (*see also* Anomaly, by site)
  - uterus NEC Q51.818
- multiple NEC Q89.7
- muscle Q79.9
  - eyelid Q10.3
- musculoskeletal system, except limbs Q79.9
- myocardium Q24.8
- nail Q84.6
- narrowness, eyelid Q10.3
- nasal sinus (wall) Q30.8
- neck (any part) Q18.9
- nerve Q07.9
  - acoustic Q07.8
  - optic Q07.8
- nervous system (central) Q07.9
- nipple Q83.9
- nose, nasal (bones) (cartilage) (septum) (sinus) Q30.9
  - specified NEC Q30.8
- ocular muscle Q15.8
- omphalomesenteric duct Q43.0
- opening, pulmonary veins Q26.4
- optic
  - disc Q14.2
  - nerve Q07.8
- opticociliary vessels Q13.2
- orbit (eye) Q10.7
- organ Q89.9
  - of Corti Q16.5
- origin
  - artery
    - innominate Q25.8
    - pulmonary Q25.79
    - renal Q27.2
    - subclavian Q25.48
- osseous meatus (ear) Q16.1
- ovary Q50.39
- oviduct Q50.6
- palate (hard) (soft) NEC Q38.5
- pancreas or pancreatic duct Q45.3
- papillary muscles Q24.8
- parathyroid gland Q89.2
- paraurethral ducts Q64.79
- parotid (gland) Q38.4
- patella Q74.1
- Pelger-Huët (hereditary hyposegmentation) D72.0
- pelvic girdle NEC Q74.2
- pelvis (bony) NEC Q74.2
  - rachitic E64.3

Anomaly, anomalous — *continued*
- penis (glans) Q55.69
- pericardium Q24.8
- peripheral vascular system Q27.9
- Peter's Q13.4
- pharynx Q38.8
- pigmentation L81.9
  - congenital Q82.8
- pituitary (gland) Q89.2
- pleural (folds) Q34.0
- portal vein Q26.5
  - connection Q26.5
- position, tooth, teeth, fully erupted M26.30
  - specified NEC M26.39
- precerebral vessel Q28.1
- prepuce Q55.69
- prostate Q55.4
- pulmonary Q33.9
  - artery NEC Q25.79
  - valve Q22.3
    - atresia Q22.0
    - insufficiency Q22.2
    - specified type NEC Q22.3
    - stenosis Q22.1
      - infundibular Q24.3
      - subvalvular Q24.3
  - venous connection Q26.4
    - partial Q26.3
    - total Q26.2
- pupil Q13.2
  - function H57.00
    - anisocoria H57.02
    - Argyll Robertson pupil H57.01
    - miosis H57.03
    - mydriasis H57.04
    - specified type NEC H57.09
    - tonic pupil H57.05- ☑
- pylorus Q40.3
- radius Q74.0
- rectum Q43.9
- reduction (extremity) (limb)
  - femur (longitudinal) — *see* Defect, reduction, lower limb, longitudinal, femur
  - fibula (longitudinal) — *see* Defect, reduction, lower limb, longitudinal, fibula
  - lower limb — *see* Defect, reduction, lower limb
  - radius (longitudinal) — *see* Defect, reduction, upper limb, longitudinal, radius
  - tibia (longitudinal) — *see* Defect, reduction, lower limb, longitudinal, tibia
  - ulna (longitudinal) — *see* Defect, reduction, upper limb, longitudinal, ulna
  - upper limb — *see* Defect, reduction, upper limb
- refraction — *see* Disorder, refraction
- renal Q63.9
  - artery Q27.2
  - pelvis Q63.9
    - specified NEC Q63.8
- respiratory system Q34.9
  - specified NEC Q34.8
- retina Q14.1
- rib Q76.6
  - cervical Q76.5
- Rieger's Q13.81
- rotation — *see* Malrotation
  - hip or thigh Q65.89
- round ligament Q52.8
- sacroiliac (joint) NEC Q74.2
- sacrum NEC Q76.49
  - kyphosis — *see* Kyphosis, congenital
  - lordosis — *see* Lordosis, congenital
- saddle nose, syphilitic A50.57
- salivary duct or gland Q38.4
- scapula Q74.0
- scrotum — *see* Malformation, testis and scrotum
- sebaceous gland Q82.9
- seminal vesicles Q55.4
- sense organs NEC Q07.8
- sex chromosomes NEC (*see also* Anomaly, chromosomes)
  - female phenotype Q97.8
  - male phenotype Q98.9
- shoulder (girdle) (joint) Q74.0
- sigmoid (flexure) Q43.9
- simian crease Q82.8
- sinus of Valsalva Q25.49
- skeleton generalized Q78.9
- skin (appendage) Q82.9

Anomaly, anomalous — *continued*
  skull Q75.9
    with
      anencephaly Q00.0
      encephalocele — *see* Encephalocele
      hydrocephalus Q03.9
        with spina bifida — *see* Spina bifida, by site,
          with hydrocephalus
      microcephaly Q02
  specified organ or site NEC Q89.8
  spermatic cord Q55.4
  spine, spinal NEC Q76.49
    column NEC Q76.49
      kyphosis — *see* Kyphosis, congenital
      lordosis — *see* Lordosis, congenital
    cord Q06.9
    nerve root Q07.8
  spleen Q89.09
    agenesis Q89.01
  stenonian duct Q38.4
  sternum NEC Q76.7
  stomach Q40.3
  submaxillary gland Q38.4
  tarsus NEC Q74.2
  tendon Q79.9
  testis — *see* Malformation, testis and scrotum
  thigh NEC Q74.2
  thorax (wall) Q67.8
    bony Q76.9
  throat Q38.8
  thumb Q74.0
  thymus gland Q89.2
  thyroid (gland) Q89.2
    cartilage Q31.8
  tibia NEC Q74.2
    saber A50.56
  toe Q74.2
  tongue Q38.3
  tooth, teeth K00.9
    eruption K00.6
    position, fully erupted M26.30
    spacing, fully erupted M26.30
  trachea (cartilage) Q32.1
  tragus Q17.9
  tricuspid (leaflet) (valve) Q22.9
    atresia or stenosis Q22.4
    Ebstein's Q22.5
  Uhl's (hypoplasia of myocardium, right ventricle) Q24.8
  ulna Q74.0
  umbilical artery Q27.0
  urachus Q64.4
  ureter Q62.8
    obstructive NEC Q62.39
      cecoureterocele Q62.32
      orthotopic ureterocele Q62.31
  urethra Q64.70
    absence Q64.5
    double Q64.74
    fistula to rectum Q64.73
    obstructive Q64.39
      stricture Q64.32
    prolapse Q64.71
    specified type NEC Q64.79
  urinary tract Q64.9
  uterus Q51.9
    with only one functioning horn Q51.4
  uvula Q38.5
  vagina Q52.4
  valleculae Q31.8
  valve (heart) NEC Q24.8
    coronary sinus Q24.5
    inferior vena cava Q24.8
    pulmonary Q22.3
    sinus coronario Q24.5
    venae cavae inferioris Q24.8
  vas deferens Q55.4
  vascular Q27.9
    brain Q28.3
    ring Q25.45
  vein(s) (peripheral) Q27.9
    brain Q28.3
    cerebral Q28.3
    coronary Q24.5
    developmental Q28.3

Anomaly, anomalous — *continued*
  vein(s) — *continued*
    great Q26.9
      specified NEC Q26.8
  vena cava (inferior) (superior) Q26.9
  venous — *see* Anomaly, vein(s)
  venous return Q26.8
  ventricular
    bands or folds Q24.8
    septa Q21.0
  vertebra Q76.49
    kyphosis — *see* Kyphosis, congenital
    lordosis — *see* Lordosis, congenital
  vesicourethral orifice Q64.79
  vessel(s) Q27.9
    optic papilla Q14.2
    precerebral Q28.1
  vitelline duct Q43.0
  vitreous body or humor Q14.0
  vulva Q52.70
  wrist (joint) Q74.0
Anomia R48.8
Anonychia (congenital) Q84.3
  acquired L60.8
Anophthalmos, anophthalmus (congenital) (globe)
  Q11.1
  acquired Z90.01
Anopia, anopsia H53.46- ☑
  quadrant H53.46- ☑
Anorchia, anorchism, anorchidism Q55.0
Anorexia R63.0
  hysterical F44.89
  nervosa F50.00
    atypical F50.9
    binge-eating type F50.2
      with purging F50.02
    restricting type F50.01
Anorgasmy, psychogenic (female) F52.31
  male F52.32
Anosmia R43.0
  hysterical F44.6
  postinfectional J39.8
Anosognosia R41.89
Anosteoplasia Q78.9
Anovulatory cycle N97.0
Anoxemia R09.02
  newborn P84
Anoxia (pathological) R09.02
  altitude T70.29 ☑
  cerebral G93.1
    complicating
      anesthesia (general) (local) or other sedation
        T88.59 ☑
        in labor and delivery O74.3
        in pregnancy O29.21- ☑
        postpartum, puerperal O89.2
      delivery (cesarean) (instrumental) O75.4
    during a procedure G97.81
    newborn P84
    resulting from a procedure G97.82
  due to
    drowning T75.1 ☑
    high altitude T70.29 ☑
  heart — *see* Insufficiency, coronary
  intrauterine P84
  myocardial — *see* Insufficiency, coronary
  newborn P84
  spinal cord G95.11
  systemic (by suffocation) (low content in atmosphere)
    — *see* Asphyxia, traumatic
Anteflexion — *see* Anteversion
Antenatal
  care (normal pregnancy) Z34.90
  screening (encounter for) of mother (*see also* En-
    counter, antenatal screening) Z36.9
Antepartum — *see* condition
Anterior — *see* condition
Antero-occlusion M26.220
Anteversion
  cervix — *see* Anteversion, uterus
  femur (neck), congenital Q65.89
  uterus, uterine (cervix) (postinfectional) (postpartal,
    old) N85.4
    congenital Q51.818
    in pregnancy or childbirth — *see* Pregnancy, com-
      plicated by
Anthophobia F40.228
Anthracosilicosis J60

Anthracosis (lung) (occupational) J60
  lingua K14.3
Anthrax A22.9
  with pneumonia A22.1
  cerebral A22.8
  colitis A22.2
  cutaneous A22.0
  gastrointestinal A22.2
  inhalation A22.1
  intestinal A22.2
  meningitis A22.8
  pulmonary A22.1
  respiratory A22.1
  sepsis A22.7
  specified manifestation NEC A22.8
Anthropoid pelvis Q74.2
  with disproportion (fetopelvic) O33.0
Anthropophobia F40.10
  generalized F40.11
Antibodies, maternal (blood group) — *see* Isoimmunization, affecting management of pregnancy
  anti-D — *see* Isoimmunization, affecting management
    of pregnancy, Rh
  newborn P55.0
Antibody
  anticardiolipin R76.0
    with
      hemorrhagic disorder D68.312
      hypercoagulable state D68.61
  antiphosphatidylglycerol R76.0
    with
      hemorrhagic disorder D68.312
      hypercoagulable state D68.61
  antiphosphatidylinositol R76.0
    with
      hemorrhagic disorder D68.312
      hypercoagulable state D68.61
  antiphosphatidylserine R76.0
    with
      hemorrhagic disorder D68.312
      hypercoagulable state D68.61
  antiphospholipid R76.0
    with
      hemorrhagic disorder D68.312
      hypercoagulable state D68.61
Anticardiolipin syndrome D68.61
Anticoagulant, circulating (intrinsic) (*see also* Disorder,
  hemorrhagic) D68.318
  drug-induced (extrinsic) (*see also* Disorder, hemorrhag-
    ic) D68.32
  iatrogenic D68.32
Antidiuretic hormone syndrome E22.2
Antimonial cholera — *see* Poisoning, antimony
Antiphospholipid
  antibody
    with hemorrhagic disorder D68.312
  syndrome D68.61
Antisocial personality F60.2
Antithrombinemia — *see* Circulating anticoagulants
Antithromboplastinemia D68.318
Antithromboplastinogenemia D68.318
Antitoxin complication or reaction — *see* Complications, vaccination
Antlophobia F40.228
Antritis J32.0
  maxilla J32.0
    acute J01.00
      recurrent J01.01
  stomach K29.60
    with bleeding K29.61
Antrum, antral — *see* condition
Anuria R34
  calculous (impacted) (recurrent) (*see also* Calculus,
    urinary) N20.9
  following
    abortion — *see* Abortion by type complicated by,
      renal failure
    ectopic or molar pregnancy O08.4
  newborn P96.0
  postprocedural N99.0
  postrenal N13.8
  traumatic (following crushing) T79.5 ☑
Anus, anal — *see* condition
Anusitis K62.89
Anxiety F41.9
  depression F41.8
  episodic paroxysmal F41.0
  generalized F41.1

☑ Additional Character Required — Refer to the Tabular List for Character Selection   ▽ Subterms under main terms may continue to next column or page

Anxiety — *continued*
  hysteria F41.8
  neurosis F41.1
  panic type F41.0
  reaction F41.1
  separation, abnormal (of childhood) F93.0
  specified NEC F41.8
  state F41.1
Aorta, aortic — *see* condition
Aortectasia — *see* Ectasia, aorta
  with aneurysm — *see* Aneurysm, aorta
Aortitis (nonsyphilitic) (calcific) I77.6
  arteriosclerotic I70.0
  Doehle-Heller A52.02
  luetic A52.02
  rheumatic — *see* Endocarditis, acute, rheumatic
  specific (syphilitic) A52.02
  syphilitic A52.02
    congenital A50.54 [I79.1]
Apathetic thyroid storm — *see* Thyrotoxicosis
Apathy R45.3
Apeirophobia F40.228
Apepsia K30
  psychogenic F45.8
Aperistalsis, esophagus K22.0
Apertognathia M26.29
Apert's syndrome Q87.0
Aphagia R13.0
  psychogenic F50.9
Aphakia (acquired) (postoperative) H27.0- ☑
  congenital Q12.3
Aphasia (amnestic) (global) (nominal) (semantic) (syntactic) R47.01
  acquired, with epilepsy (Landau-Kleffner syndrome)
    — *see* Epilepsy, specified NEC
  auditory (developmental) F80.2
  developmental (receptive type) F80.2
    expressive type F80.1
    Wernicke's F80.2
  following
    cerebrovascular disease I69.920
      cerebral infarction I69.320
      intracerebral hemorrhage I69.120
      nontraumatic intracranial hemorrhage NEC
        I69.220
      specified disease NEC I69.820
      subarachnoid hemorrhage I69.020
    primary progressive G31.01 [F02.80]
      with behavioral disturbance G31.01 [F02.81]
    progressive isolated G31.01 [F02.80]
      with behavioral disturbance G31.01 [F02.81]
  sensory F80.2
  syphilis, tertiary A52.19
  Wernicke's (developmental) F80.2
Aphonia (organic) R49.1
  hysterical F44.4
  psychogenic F44.4
Aphthae, aphthous (*see also* condition)
  Bednar's K12.0
  cachectic K14.0
  epizootic B08.8
  fever B08.8
  oral (recurrent) K12.0
  stomatitis (major) (minor) K12.0
  thrush B37.0
  ulcer (oral) (recurrent) K12.0
    genital organ(s) NEC
      female N76.6
      male N50.89
    larynx J38.7
Apical — *see* condition
Apiphobia F40.218
Aplasia (*see also* Agenesis)
  abdominal muscle syndrome Q79.4
  alveolar process (acquired) — *see* Anomaly, alveolar
    congenital Q38.6
  aorta (congenital) Q25.41
  axialis extracorticalis (congenita) E75.29
  bone marrow (myeloid) D61.9
    congenital D61.01
  brain Q00.0
    part of Q04.3
  bronchus Q32.4
  cementum K00.4
  cerebellum Q04.3
  cervix (congenital) Q51.5
  congenital pure red cell D61.01
  corpus callosum Q04.0

Aplasia — *continued*
  cutis congenita Q84.8
  erythrocyte congenital D61.01
  extracortical axial E75.29
  eye Q11.1
  fovea centralis (congenital) Q14.1
  gallbladder, congenital Q44.0
  iris Q13.1
  labyrinth, membranous Q16.5
  limb (congenital) Q73.8
    lower — *see* Defect, reduction, lower limb
    upper — *see* Agenesis, arm
  lung, congenital (bilateral) (unilateral) Q33.3
  pancreas Q45.0
  parathyroid-thymic D82.1
  Pelizaeus-Merzbacher E75.29
  penis Q55.5
  prostate Q55.4
  red cell (with thymoma) D60.9
    acquired D60.9
      due to drugs D60.9
    adult D60.9
    chronic D60.0
    congenital D61.01
    constitutional D61.01
    due to drugs D60.9
    hereditary D61.01
    of infants D61.01
    primary D61.01
    pure D61.01
      due to drugs D60.9
    specified type NEC D60.8
    transient D60.1
  round ligament Q52.8
  skin Q84.8
  spermatic cord Q55.4
  spleen Q89.01
  testicle Q55.0
  thymic, with immunodeficiency D82.1
  thyroid (congenital) (with myxedema) E03.1
  uterus Q51.0
  ventral horn cell Q06.1
Apnea, apneic (of) (spells) R06.81
  newborn NEC P28.4
    obstructive P28.4
    sleep (central) (obstructive) (primary) P28.3
  prematurity P28.4
  sleep G47.30
    central (primary) G47.31
      idiopathic G47.31
      in conditions classified elsewhere G47.37
    obstructive (adult) (pediatric) G47.33
      hypopnea G47.33
    primary central G47.31
    specified NEC G47.39
Apneumatosis, newborn P28.0
Apocrine metaplasia (breast) — *see* Dysplasia, mammary, specified type NEC
Apophysitis (bone) (*see also* Osteochondropathy)
  calcaneus M92.8
  juvenile M92.9
Apoplectiform convulsions (cerebral ischemia) I67.82
Apoplexia, apoplexy, apoplectic
  adrenal A39.1
  heart (auricle) (ventricle) — *see* Infarct, myocardium
  heat T67.0 ☑
  hemorrhagic (stroke) — *see* Hemorrhage, intracranial
  meninges, hemorrhagic — *see* Hemorrhage, intracranial, subarachnoid
  uremic N18.9 [I68.8]
Appearance
  bizarre R46.1
  specified NEC R46.89
  very low level of personal hygiene R46.0
Appendage
  epididymal (organ of Morgagni) Q55.4
  intestine (epiploic) Q43.8
  preauricular Q17.0
  testicular (organ of Morgagni) Q55.29
Appendicitis (pneumococcal) (retrocecal) K37
  with
    gangrene K35.891
    perforation NOS K35.32
    peritoneal abscess K35.33
    peritonitis NEC K35.33
      generalized (with perforation or rupture) K35.20
        with abscess K35.21
      localized K35.30

Appendicitis — *continued*
  with — *continued*
    peritonitis — *continued*
      localized — *continued*
        with
          gangrene K35.31
          perforation K35.32
            and abscess K35.33
        rupture (with localized peritonitis) K35.32
  acute (catarrhal) (fulminating) (gangrenous) (obstructive) (retrocecal) (suppurative) K35.80
    with
      gangrene K35.891
      peritoneal abscess K35.33
      peritonitis NEC K35.33
        generalized (with perforation or rupture) K35.20
          with abscess K35.21
        localized K35.30
          with
            gangrene K35.31
            perforation K35.32
              and abscess K35.33
    specified NEC K35.890
      with gangrene K35.891
  amebic A06.89
  chronic (recurrent) K36
  exacerbation — *see* Appendicitis, acute
  gangrenous — *see* Appendicitis, acute
  healed (obliterative) K36
  interval K36
  neurogenic K36
  obstructive K36
  recurrent K36
  relapsing K36
  ruptured NOS (with localized peritonitis) K35.32
  subacute (adhesive) K36
  subsiding K36
  suppurative — *see* Appendicitis, acute
  tuberculous A18.32
Appendicopathia oxyurica B80
Appendix, appendicular (*see also* condition)
  epididymis Q55.4
  Morgagni
    female Q50.5
    male (epididymal) Q55.4
      testicular Q55.29
  testis Q55.29
Appetite
  depraved — *see* Pica
  excessive R63.2
  lack or loss (*see also* Anorexia) R63.0
    nonorganic origin F50.89
    psychogenic F50.89
  perverted (hysterical) — *see* Pica
Apple peel syndrome Q41.1
Apprehension state F41.1
Apprehensiveness, abnormal F41.9
Approximal wear K03.0
Apraxia (classic) (ideational) (ideokinetic) (ideomotor) (motor) (verbal) R48.2
  following
    cerebrovascular disease I69.990
      cerebral infarction I69.390
      intracerebral hemorrhage I69.190
      nontraumatic intracranial hemorrhage NEC
        I69.290
      specified disease NEC I69.890
      subarachnoid hemorrhage I69.090
    oculomotor, congenital H51.8
Aptyalism K11.7
Apudoma — *see* Neoplasm, uncertain behavior, by site
Aqueous misdirection H40.83- ☑
Arabicum elephantiasis — *see* Infestation, filarial
Arachnitis — *see* Meningitis
Arachnodactyly — *see* Syndrome, Marfan's
Arachnoiditis (acute) (adhesive) (basal) (brain) (cerebrospinal) — *see* Meningitis
Arachnophobia F40.210
Arboencephalitis, Australian A83.4
Arborization block (heart) I45.5
ARC (AIDS-related complex) B20
Arch
  aortic Q25.49
  bovine Q25.49
Arches — *see* condition
Arcuate uterus Q51.810
Arcuatus uterus Q51.810

Arcus (cornea) senilis — *see* Degeneration, cornea, senile
Arc-welder's lung J63.4
Areflexia R29.2
Areola — *see* condition
Argentaffinoma (*see also* Neoplasm, uncertain behavior, by site)
   malignant — *see* Neoplasm, malignant, by site
   syndrome E34.0
Argininemia E72.21
Arginosuccinic aciduria E72.22
Argyll Robertson phenomenon, pupil or syndrome (syphilitic) A52.19
   atypical H57.09
   nonsyphilitic H57.09
Argyria, argyriasis
   conjunctival H11.13- ☑
   from drug or medicament — *see* Table of Drugs and Chemicals, by substance
Argyrosis, conjunctival H11.13- ☑
Arhinencephaly Q04.1
Ariboflavinosis E53.0
Arm — *see* condition
Arnold-Chiari disease, obstruction or syndrome (type II) Q07.00
   with
      hydrocephalus Q07.02
         with spina bifida Q07.03
      spina bifida Q07.01
         with hydrocephalus Q07.03
   type III — *see* Encephalocele
   type IV Q04.8
Aromatic amino-acid metabolism disorder E70.9
   specified NEC E70.8
Arousals, confusional G47.51
Arrest, arrested
   cardiac I46.9
      complicating
         abortion — *see* Abortion, by type, complicated by, cardiac arrest
         anesthesia (general) (local) or other sedation — *see* Table of Drugs and Chemicals, by drug
            in labor and delivery O74.2
            in pregnancy O29.11- ☑
               postpartum, puerperal O89.1
         delivery (cesarean) (instrumental) O75.4
      due to
         cardiac condition I46.2
         specified condition NEC I46.8
      intraoperative I97.71- ☑
      newborn P29.81
      personal history, successfully resuscitated Z86.74
      postprocedural I97.12- ☑
         obstetric procedure O75.4
   cardiorespiratory — *see* Arrest, cardiac
   circulatory — *see* Arrest, cardiac
   deep transverse O64.0 ☑
   development or growth
      bone — *see* Disorder, bone, development or growth
      child R62.50
      tracheal rings Q32.1
   epiphyseal
      complete
         femur M89.15- ☑
         humerus M89.12- ☑
         tibia M89.16- ☑
         ulna M89.13- ☑
         forearm M89.13- ☑
            specified NEC M89.13- ☑
            ulna — *see* Arrest, epiphyseal, by type, ulna
         lower leg M89.16- ☑
            specified NEC M89.168
            tibia — *see* Arrest, epiphyseal, by type, tibia
      partial
         femur M89.15- ☑
         humerus M89.12- ☑
         tibia M89.16- ☑
         ulna M89.13- ☑
      specified NEC M89.18
   granulopoiesis — *see* Agranulocytosis
   growth plate — *see* Arrest, epiphyseal
   heart — *see* Arrest, cardiac
   legal, anxiety concerning Z65.3
   physeal — *see* Arrest, epiphyseal
   respiratory R09.2
      newborn P28.81
   sinus I45.5
   spermatogenesis (complete) — *see* Azoospermia

Arrest, arrested — *continued*
   spermatogenesis — *see* Azoospermia — *continued*
      incomplete — *see* Oligospermia
   transverse (deep) O64.0 ☑
Arrhenoblastoma
   benign
      specified site — *see* Neoplasm, benign, by site
      unspecified site
         female D27.9
         male D29.20
   malignant
      specified site — *see* Neoplasm, malignant, by site
      unspecified site
         female C56.9
         male C62.90
   specified site — *see* Neoplasm, uncertain behavior, by site
   unspecified site
      female D39.10
      male D40.10
Arrhythmia (auricle) (cardiac) (juvenile) (nodal) (reflex) (sinus) (supraventricular) (transitory) (ventricle) I49.9
   block I45.9
   extrasystolic I49.49
   newborn
      bradycardia P29.12
      occurring before birth P03.819
         before onset of labor P03.810
         during labor P03.811
      tachycardia P29.11
   psychogenic F45.8
   specified NEC I49.8
   vagal R55
   ventricular re-entry I47.0
Arrillaga-Ayerza syndrome (pulmonary sclerosis with pulmonary hypertension) I27.0
Arsenical pigmentation L81.8
   from drug or medicament — *see* Table of Drugs and Chemicals
Arsenism — *see* Poisoning, arsenic
Arterial — *see* condition
Arteriofibrosis — *see* Arteriosclerosis
Arteriolar sclerosis — *see* Arteriosclerosis
Arteriolith — *see* Arteriosclerosis
Arteriolitis I77.6
   necrotizing, kidney I77.5
   renal — *see* Hypertension, kidney
Arteriolosclerosis — *see* Arteriosclerosis
Arterionephrosclerosis — *see* Hypertension, kidney
Arteriopathy I77.9
   cerebral autosomal dominant, with subcortical infarcts and leukoencephalopathy (CADASIL) I67.850
Arteriosclerosis, arteriosclerotic (diffuse) (obliterans) (of) (senile) (with calcification) I70.90
   aorta I70.0
   arteries of extremities — *see* Arteriosclerosis, extremities
   brain I67.2
   bypass graft
      coronary — *see* Arteriosclerosis, coronary, bypass graft
      extremities — *see* Arteriosclerosis, extremities, bypass graft
   cardiac — *see* Disease, heart, ischemic, atherosclerotic
   cardiopathy — *see* Disease, heart, ischemic, atherosclerotic
   cardiorenal — *see* Hypertension, cardiorenal
   cardiovascular — *see* Disease, heart, ischemic, atherosclerotic
   carotid (*see also* Occlusion, artery, carotid) I65.2- ☑
   central nervous system I67.2
   cerebral I67.2
   cerebrovascular I67.2
   coronary (artery)
      due to
         calcified coronary lesion (severely) I25.84
         lipid rich plaque I25.83
      bypass graft I25.810
         with
            angina pectoris I25.709
               with documented spasm I25.701
               specified type NEC I25.708
               unstable I25.700
            ischemic chest pain I25.709
         autologous artery I25.810
            with
               angina pectoris I25.729
                  with documented spasm I25.721

Arteriosclerosis, arteriosclerotic — *continued*
   coronary — *continued*
      bypass graft — *continued*
         autologous artery — *continued*
            with — *continued*
               angina pectoris — *continued*
                  specified type I25.728
                  unstable I25.720
               ischemic chest pain I25.729
         autologous vein I25.810
            with
               angina pectoris I25.719
                  with documented spasm I25.711
                  specified type I25.718
                  unstable I25.710
               ischemic chest pain I25.719
         nonautologous biological I25.810
            with
               angina pectoris I25.739
                  with documented spasm I25.731
                  specified type I25.738
                  unstable I25.730
               ischemic chest pain I25.739
         specified type NEC I25.810
            with
               angina pectoris I25.799
                  with documented spasm I25.791
                  specified type I25.798
                  unstable I25.790
               ischemic chest pain I25.799
      native vessel
         with
            angina pectoris I25.119
               with documented spasm I25.111
               specified type NEC I25.118
               unstable I25.110
            ischemic chest pain I25.119
      transplanted heart I25.811
         bypass graft I25.812
            with
               angina pectoris I25.769
                  with documented spasm I25.761
                  specified type I25.768
                  unstable I25.760
               ischemic chest pain I25.769
         native coronary artery I25.811
            with
               angina pectoris I25.759
                  with documented spasm I25.751
                  specified type I25.758
                  unstable I25.750
               ischemic chest pain I25.759
   extremities (native arteries) I70.209
      bypass graft I70.309
         autologous vein graft I70.409
            leg I70.409
               with
                  gangrene (and intermittent claudication, rest pain and ulcer) I70.469
                  intermittent claudication I70.419
                  rest pain (and intermittent claudication) I70.429
            bilateral I70.403
               with
                  gangrene (and intermittent claudication, rest pain and ulcer) I70.463
                  intermittent claudication I70.463
                  rest pain (and intermittent claudication) I70.423
                  specified type NEC I70.493
            left I70.402
               with
                  gangrene (and intermittent claudication, rest pain and ulcer) I70.462
                  intermittent claudication I70.412
                  rest pain (and intermittent claudication) I70.422
                  ulceration (and intermittent claudication and rest pain) I70.449
                     ankle I70.443
                     calf I70.442
                     foot site NEC I70.445
                     heel I70.444
                     lower leg NEC I70.448
                     midfoot I70.444
                     thigh I70.441
                specified type NEC I70.492

☑ Additional Character Required — Refer to the Tabular List for Character Selection   ▽ Subterms under main terms may continue to next column or page

Arteriosclerosis, arteriosclerotic — *continued*
  extremities — *continued*
    bypass graft — *continued*
      autologous vein graft — *continued*
        leg — *continued*
          right I70.401
            with
              gangrene (and intermittent claudication, rest pain and ulcer) I70.461
              intermittent claudication I70.411
              rest pain (and intermittent claudication) I70.421
              ulceration (and intermittent claudication and rest pain) I70.439
                ankle I70.433
                calf I70.432
                foot site NEC I70.435
                heel I70.434
                lower leg NEC I70.438
                midfoot I70.434
                thigh I70.431
            specified type NEC I70.491
          specified type NEC I70.499
        specified NEC I70.408
          with
            gangrene (and intermittent claudication, rest pain and ulcer) I70.468
            intermittent claudication I70.418
            rest pain (and intermittent claudication) I70.428
            ulceration (and intermittent claudication and rest pain) I70.45
          specified type NEC I70.498
    leg I70.309
      with
        gangrene (and intermittent claudication, rest pain and ulcer) I70.369
        intermittent claudication I70.319
        rest pain (and intermittent claudication) I70.329
      bilateral I70.303
        with
          gangrene (and intermittent claudication, rest pain and ulcer) I70.363
          intermittent claudication I70.313
          rest pain (and intermittent claudication) I70.323
        specified type NEC I70.393
      left I70.302
        with
          gangrene (and intermittent claudication, rest pain and ulcer) I70.362
          intermittent claudication I70.312
          rest pain (and intermittent claudication) I70.322
          ulceration (and intermittent claudication and rest pain) I70.349
            ankle I70.343
            calf I70.342
            foot site NEC I70.345
            heel I70.344
            lower leg NEC I70.348
            midfoot I70.344
            thigh I70.341
        specified type NEC I70.392
      right I70.301
        with
          gangrene (and intermittent claudication, rest pain and ulcer) I70.361
          intermittent claudication I70.311
          rest pain (and intermittent claudication) I70.321
          ulceration (and intermittent claudication and rest pain) I70.339
            ankle I70.333
            calf I70.332
            foot site NEC I70.335
            heel I70.334
            lower leg NEC I70.338
            midfoot I70.334
            thigh I70.331
        specified type NEC I70.391
      specified type NEC I70.399
    nonautologous biological graft I70.509
      leg I70.509
        with
          gangrene (and intermittent claudication, rest pain and ulcer) I70.569

Arteriosclerosis, arteriosclerotic — *continued*
  extremities — *continued*
    bypass graft — *continued*
      nonautologous biological graft — *continued*
        leg — *continued*
          with — *continued*
            intermittent claudication I70.519
            rest pain (and intermittent claudication) I70.529
          bilateral I70.503
            with
              gangrene (and intermittent claudication, rest pain and ulcer) I70.563
              intermittent claudication I70.513
              rest pain (and intermittent claudication) I70.523
            specified type NEC I70.593
          left I70.502
            with
              gangrene (and intermittent claudication, rest pain and ulcer) I70.562
              intermittent claudication I70.512
              rest pain (and intermittent claudication) I70.522
              ulceration (and intermittent claudication and rest pain) I70.549
                ankle I70.543
                calf I70.542
                foot site NEC I70.545
                heel I70.544
                lower leg NEC I70.548
                midfoot I70.544
                thigh I70.541
            specified type NEC I70.592
          right I70.501
            with
              gangrene (and intermittent claudication, rest pain and ulcer) I70.561
              intermittent claudication I70.511
              rest pain (and intermittent claudication) I70.521
              ulceration (and intermittent claudication and rest pain) I70.539
                ankle I70.533
                calf I70.532
                foot site NEC I70.535
                heel I70.534
                lower leg NEC I70.538
                midfoot I70.534
                thigh I70.531
            specified type NEC I70.591
          specified type NEC I70.599
        specified NEC I70.508
          with
            gangrene (and intermittent claudication, rest pain and ulcer) I70.568
            intermittent claudication I70.518
            rest pain (and intermittent claudication) I70.528
            ulceration (and intermittent claudication and rest pain) I70.55
          specified type NEC I70.598
      nonbiological graft I70.609
        leg I70.609
          with
            gangrene (and intermittent claudication, rest pain and ulcer) I70.669
            intermittent claudication I70.619
            rest pain (and intermittent claudication) I70.629
          bilateral I70.603
            with
              gangrene (and intermittent claudication, rest pain and ulcer) I70.663
              intermittent claudication I70.613
              rest pain (and intermittent claudication) I70.623
            specified type NEC I70.693
          left I70.602
            with
              gangrene (and intermittent claudication, rest pain and ulcer) I70.662
              intermittent claudication I70.612

Arteriosclerosis, arteriosclerotic — *continued*
  extremities — *continued*
    bypass graft — *continued*
      nonbiological graft — *continued*
        leg — *continued*
          left — *continued*
            with — *continued*
              rest pain (and intermittent claudication) I70.622
              ulceration (and intermittent claudication and rest pain) I70.649
                ankle I70.643
                calf I70.642
                foot site NEC I70.645
                heel I70.644
                lower leg NEC I70.648
                midfoot I70.644
                thigh I70.641
            specified type NEC I70.692
          right I70.601
            with
              gangrene (and intermittent claudication, rest pain and ulcer) I70.661
              intermittent claudication I70.611
              rest pain (and intermittent claudication) I70.621
              ulceration (and intermittent claudication and rest pain) I70.639
                ankle I70.633
                calf I70.632
                foot site NEC I70.635
                heel I70.634
                lower leg NEC I70.638
                midfoot I70.634
                thigh I70.631
            specified type NEC I70.691
          specified type NEC I70.699
        specified NEC I70.608
          with
            gangrene (and intermittent claudication, rest pain and ulcer) I70.668
            intermittent claudication I70.618
            rest pain (and intermittent claudication) I70.628
            ulceration (and intermittent claudication and rest pain) I70.65
          specified type NEC I70.698
    specified graft NEC I70.709
      leg I70.709
        with
          gangrene (and intermittent claudication, rest pain and ulcer) I70.769
          intermittent claudication I70.719
          rest pain (and intermittent claudication) I70.729
        bilateral I70.703
          with
            gangrene (and intermittent claudication, rest pain and ulcer) I70.763
            intermittent claudication I70.713
            rest pain (and intermittent claudication) I70.723
          specified type NEC I70.793
        left I70.702
          with
            gangrene (and intermittent claudication, rest pain and ulcer) I70.762
            intermittent claudication I70.712
            rest pain (and intermittent claudication) I70.722
            ulceration (and intermittent claudication and rest pain) I70.749
              ankle I70.743
              calf I70.742
              foot site NEC I70.745
              heel I70.744
              lower leg NEC I70.748
              midfoot I70.744
              thigh I70.741
          specified type NEC I70.792
        right I70.701
          with
            gangrene (and intermittent claudication, rest pain and ulcer) I70.761
            artermittent claudication I70.711

Arteriosclerosis, arteriosclerotic — *continued*
  extremities — *continued*
    bypass graft — *continued*
      specified graft — *continued*
        leg — *continued*
          right — *continued*
            with — *continued*
              rest pain (and intermittent claudication) I70.721
              ulceration (and intermittent claudication and rest pain) I70.739
                ankle I70.733
                calf I70.732
                foot site NEC I70.735
                heel I70.734
                lower leg NEC I70.738
                midfoot I70.734
                thigh I70.731
            specified type NEC I70.791
        specified type NEC I70.799
    specified NEC I70.708
      with
        gangrene (and intermittent claudication, rest pain and ulcer) I70.768
        intermittent claudication I70.718
        rest pain (and intermittent claudication) I70.728
        ulceration (and intermittent claudication and rest pain) I70.75
      specified type NEC I70.798
    specified NEC I70.308
      with
        gangrene (and intermittent claudication, rest pain and ulcer) I70.368
        intermittent claudication I70.318
        rest pain (and intermittent claudication) I70.328
        ulceration (and intermittent claudication and rest pain) I70.35
      specifiec type NEC I70.398
    leg I70.209
      with
        gangrene (and intermittent claudication, rest pain and ulcer) I70.269
        intermittent claudication I70.219
        rest pain (and intermittent claudication) I70.229
      bilateral I70.203
        with
          gangrene (and intermittent claudication, rest pain and ulcer) I70.263
          intermittent claudication I70.213
          rest pain (and intermittent claudication) I70.223
        specified type NEC I70.293
      left I70.202
        with
          gangrene (and intermittent claudication, rest pain and ulcer) I70.262
          intermittent claudication I70.212
          rest pain (and intermittent claudication) I70.222
          ulceration (and intermittent claudication and rest pain) I70.249
            ankle I70.243
            calf I70.242
            foot site NEC I70.245
            heel I70.244
            lower leg NEC I70.248
            midfoot I70.244
            thigh I70.241
        specified type NEC I70.292
      right I70.201
        with
          gangrene (and intermittent claudication, rest pain and ulcer) I70.261
          intermittent claudication I70.211
          rest pain (and intermittent claudication) I70.221
          ulceration (and intermittent claudication and rest pain) I70.239
            ankle I70.233
            calf I70.232
            foot site NEC I70.235
            heel I70.234
            lower leg NEC I70.238
            midfoot I70.234
            thigh I70.231
        specified type NEC I70.291

Arteriosclerosis, arteriosclerotic — *continued*
  extremities — *continued*
    leg — *continued*
      specified type NEC I70.299
    specified site NEC I70.208
      with
        gangrene (and intermittent claudication, rest pain and ulcer) I70.268
        intermittent claudication I70.218
        rest pain (and intermittent claudication) I70.228
        ulceration (and intermittent claudication and rest pain) I70.25
      specified type NEC I70.298
  generalized I70.91
  heart (disease) — *see* Arteriosclerosis, coronary (artery),
  kidney — *see* Hypertension, kidney
  medial — *see* Arteriosclerosis, extremities
  mesenteric (artery) K55.1
  Mönckeberg's — *see* Arteriosclerosis, extremities
  myocarditis I51.4
  peripheral (of extremities) — *see* Arteriosclerosis, extremities
  pulmonary (idiopathic) I27.0
  renal (arterioles) (*see also* Hypertension, kidney)
    artery I70.1
  retina (vascular) I70.8 [H35.0-] ☑
  specified artery NEC I70.8
  spinal (cord) G95.19
  vertebral (artery) I67.2
Arteriospasm I73.9
Arteriovenous — *see* condition
Arteritis I77.6
  allergic M31.0
  aorta (nonsyphilitic) I77.6
    syphilitic A52.02
  aortic arch M31.4
  brachiocephalic M31.4
  brain I67.7
    syphilitic A52.04
  cerebral I67.7
    in systemic lupus erythematosus M32.19
    listerial A32.89
    syphilitic A52.04
    tuberculous A18.89
  coronary (artery) I25.89
    rheumatic I01.8
      chronic I09.89
    syphilitic A52.06
  cranial (left) (right), giant cell M31.6
  deformans — *see* Arteriosclerosis
  giant cell NEC M31.6
    with polymyalgia rheumatica M31.5
  necrosing or necrotizing M31.9
    specified NEC M31.8
  nodosa M30.0
  obliterans — *see* Arteriosclerosis
  pulmonary I28.8
  rheumatic — *see* Fever, rheumatic
  senile — *see* Arteriosclerosis
  suppurative I77.2
  syphilitic (general) A52.09
    brain A52.04
    coronary A52.06
    spinal A52.09
  temporal, giant cell M31.6
  young female aortic arch syndrome M31.4
Artery, arterial (*see also* condition)
  abscess I77.89
  single umbilical Q27.0
Arthralgia (allergic) (*see also* Pain, joint)
  in caisson disease T70.3 ☑
  temporomandibular M26.62- ☑
Arthritis, arthritic (acute) (chronic) (nonpyogenic) (subacute) M19.90
  allergic — *see* Arthritis, specified form NEC
  ankylosing (crippling) (spine) (*see also* Spondylitis, ankylosing)
    sites other than spine — *see* Arthritis, specified form NEC
  atrophic — *see* Osteoarthritis
    spine — *see* Spondylitis, ankylosing
  back — *see* Spondylopathy, inflammatory
  blennorrhagic (gonococcal) A54.42
  Charcot's — *see* Arthropathy, neuropathic
    diabetic — *see* Diabetes, arthropathy, neuropathic
    syringomyelic G95.0
  chylous (filarial) (*see also* category M01) B74.9

Arthritis, arthritic — *continued*
  climacteric (any site) NEC — *see* Arthritis, specified form NEC
  crystal (-induced) — *see* Arthritis, in, crystals
  deformans — *see* Osteoarthritis
  degenerative — *see* Osteoarthritis
  due to or associated with
    acromegaly E22.0
    brucellosis — *see* Brucellosis
    caisson disease T70.3 ☑
    diabetes — *see* Diabetes, arthropathy
    dracontiasis (*see also* category M01) B72
    enteritis NEC
      regional — *see* Enteritis, regional
    erysipelas (*see also* category M01) A46
    erythema
      epidemic A25.1
      nodosum L52
    filariasis NOS B74.9
    glanders A24.0
    helminthiasis (*see also* category M01) B83.9
    hemophilia D66 [M36.2]
    Henoch- (Schönlein) purpura D69.0 [M36.4]
    human parvovirus (*see also* category M01) B97.6
    infectious disease NEC M01 ☑
    leprosy (*see also* category M01) (*see also* Leprosy) A30.9
    Lyme disease A69.23
    mycobacteria (*see also* category M01) A31.8
    parasitic disease NEC (*see also* category M01) B89
    paratyphoid fever (*see also* category M01) (*see also* Fever, paratyphoid) A01.4
    rat bite fever (*see also* category M01) A25.1
    regional enteritis — *see* Enteritis, regional
    respiratory disorder NOS J98.9
    serum sickness (*see also* Reaction, serum) T80.69 ☑
    syringomyelia G95.0
    typhoid fever A01.04
  epidemic erythema A25.1
  febrile — *see* Fever, rheumatic
  gonococcal A54.42
  gouty (acute) — *see* Gout
  in (due to)
    acromegaly (*see also* subcategory M14.8-) E22.0
    amyloidosis (*see also* subcategory M14.8-) E85.4
    bacterial disease (*see also* subcategory M01) A49.9
    Behçet's syndrome M35.2
    caisson disease (*see also* subcategory M14.8-) T70.3 ☑
    coliform bacilli (Escherichia coli) — *see* Arthritis, in, pyogenic organism NEC
    crystals M11.9
      dicalcium phosphate — *see* Arthritis, in, crystals, specified type NEC
      hydroxyapatite M11.0- ☑
      pyrophosphate — *see* Arthritis, in, crystals, specified type NEC
      specified type NEC M11.80
        ankle M11.87- ☑
        elbow M11.82- ☑
        foot joint M11.87- ☑
        hand joint M11.84- ☑
        hip M11.85- ☑
        knee M11.86- ☑
        multiple sites M11.8- ☑
        shoulder M11.81- ☑
        vertebrae M11.88
        wrist M11.83- ☑
    dermatoarthritis, lipoid E78.81
    dracontiasis (dracunculiasis) (*see also* category M01) B72
    endocrine disorder NEC (*see also* subcategory M14.8-) E34.9
    enteritis, infectious NEC (*see also* category M01) A09
      specified organism NEC (*see also* category M01) A08.8
    erythema
      multiforme (*see also* subcategory M14.8-) L51.9
      nodosum (*see also* subcategory M14.8-) L52
    gout — *see* Gout
    helminthiasis NEC (*see also* category M01) B83.9
    hemochromatosis (*see also* subcategory M14.8-) E83.118
    hemoglobinopathy NEC D58.2 [M36.3]
    hemophilia NEC D66 [M36.2]
    Hemophilus influenzae M00.8- ☑ [B96.3]
    Henoch (-Schönlein) purpura D69.0 [M36.4]

Arthritis, arthritic — *continued*
  in — *continued*
    hyperparathyroidism NEC (*see also* subcategory M14.8-) E21.3
    hypersensitivity reaction NEC T78.49 ☑ [M36.4]
    hypogammaglobulinemia (*see also* subcategory M14.8-) D80.1
    hypothyroidism NEC (*see also* subcategory M14.8-) E03.9
    infection — *see* Arthritis, pyogenic or pyemic
      spine — *see* Spondylopathy, infective
    infectious disease NEC M01 ☑
    leprosy (*see also* category M01) A30.9
    leukemia NEC C95.9- [M36.1]
    lipoid dermatoarthritis E78.81
    Lyme disease A69.23
    Mediterranean fever, familial (*see also* subcategory M14.8-) M04.1
    Meningococcus A39.83
    metabolic disorder NEC (*see also* subcategory M14.8-) E88.9
    multiple myelomatosis C90.0- ☑ [M36.1]
    mumps B26.85
    mycosis NEC (*see also* category M01) B49
    myelomatosis (multiple) C90.0- ☑ [M36.1]
    neurological disorder NEC G98.0
    ochronosis (*see also* subcategory M14.8-) E70.29
    O'nyong-nyong (*see also* category M01) A92.1
    parasitic disease NEC (*see also* category M01) B89
    paratyphoid fever (*see also* category M01) A01.4
    Pseudomonas — *see* Arthritis, pyogenic, bacterial NEC
    psoriasis L40.50
    pyogenic organism NEC — *see* Arthritis, pyogenic, bacterial NEC
    Reiter's disease — *see* Reiter's disease
    respiratory disorder NEC (*see also* subcategory M14.8-) J98.9
    reticulosis, malignant (*see also* subcategory M14.8-) C86.0
    rubella B06.82
    Salmonella (arizonae) (cholerae-suis) (enteritidis) (typhimurium) A02.23
    sarcoidosis D86.86
    specified bacteria NEC — *see* Arthritis, pyogenic, bacterial NEC
    sporotrichosis B42.82
    syringomyelia G95.0
    thalassemia NEC D56.9 [M36.3]
    tuberculosis — *see* Tuberculosis, arthritis
    typhoid fever A01.04
    urethritis, Reiter's — *see* Reiter's disease
    viral disease NEC (*see also* category M01) B34.9
  infectious or infective (*see also* Arthritis, pyogenic or pyemic)
    spine — *see* Spondylopathy, infective
  juvenile M08.90
    with systemic onset — *see* Still's disease
    ankle M08.97- ☑
    elbow M08.92- ☑
    foot joint M08.97- ☑
    hand joint M08.94- ☑
    hip M08.95- ☑
    knee M08.96- ☑
    multiple site M08.99
    pauciarticular M08.40
      ankle M08.47- ☑
      elbow M08.42- ☑
      foot joint M08.47- ☑
      hand joint M08.44- ☑
      hip M08.45- ☑
      knee M08.46- ☑
      shoulder M08.41- ☑
      vertebrae M08.48
      wrist M08.43- ☑
    psoriatic L40.54
    rheumatoid — *see* Arthritis, rheumatoid, juvenile
    shoulder M08.91- ☑
    specified type NEC M08.80
      ankle M08.87- ☑
      elbow M08.82- ☑
      foot joint M08.87- ☑
      hand joint M08.84- ☑
      hip M08.85- ☑
      knee M08.86- ☑
      multiple site M08.89
      shoulder M08.81- ☑

Arthritis, arthritic — *continued*
  juvenile — *continued*
    specified type — *continued*
      specified joint NEC M08.88
      vertebrae M08.88
      wrist M08.83- ☑
    wrist M08.93- ☑
  meaning osteoarthritis — *see* Osteoarthritis
  meningococcal A39.83
  menopausal (any site) NEC — *see* Arthritis, specified form NEC
  mutilans (psoriatic) L40.52
  mycotic NEC (*see also* category M01) B49
  neuropathic (Charcot) — *see* Arthropathy, neuropathic
    diabetic — *see* Diabetes, arthropathy, neuropathic
    nonsyphilitic NEC G98.0
    syringomyelic G95.0
  ochronotic (*see also* subcategory M14.8-) E70.29
  palindromic (any site) — *see* Rheumatism, palindromic
  pneumococcal M00.10
    ankle M00.17- ☑
    elbow M00.12- ☑
    foot joint — *see* Arthritis, pneumococcal, ankle
    hand joint M00.14- ☑
    hip M00.15- ☑
    knee M00.16- ☑
    multiple site M00.19
    shoulder M00.11- ☑
    vertebra M00.18
    wrist M00.13- ☑
  postdysenteric — *see* Arthropathy, postdysenteric
  postmeningococcal A39.84
  postrheumatic, chronic — *see* Arthropathy, postrheumatic, chronic
  primary progressive (*see also* Arthritis, specified form NEC)
    spine — *see* Spondylitis, ankylosing
  psoriatic L40.50
  purulent (any site except spine) — *see* Arthritis, pyogenic or pyemic
    spine — *see* Spondylopathy, infective
  pyogenic or pyemic (any site except spine) M00.9
    bacterial NEC M00.80
      ankle M00.87- ☑
      elbow M00.82- ☑
      foot joint — *see* Arthritis, pyogenic, bacterial NEC, ankle
      hand joint M00.84- ☑
      hip M00.85- ☑
      knee M00.86- ☑
      multiple site M00.89
      shoulder M00.81- ☑
      vertebra M00.88
      wrist M00.83- ☑
    pneumococcal — *see* Arthritis, pneumococcal
    spine — *see* Spondylopathy, infective
    staphylococcal — *see* Arthritis, staphylococcal
    streptococcal — *see* Arthritis, streptococcal NEC
      pneumococcal — *see* Arthritis, pneumococcal
  reactive — *see* Reiter's disease
  rheumatic (*see also* Arthritis, rheumatoid)
    acute or subacute — *see* Fever, rheumatic
  rheumatoid M06.9
    with
      carditis — *see* Rheumatoid, carditis
      endocarditis — *see* Rheumatoid, carditis
      heart involvement NEC — *see* Rheumatoid, carditis
      lung involvement — *see* Rheumatoid, lung
      myocarditis — *see* Rheumatoid, carditis
      myopathy — *see* Rheumatoid, myopathy
      pericarditis — *see* Rheumatoid, carditis
      polyneuropathy — *see* Rheumatoid, polyneuropathy
      rheumatoid factor — *see* Arthritis, rheumatoid, seropositive
      splenoadenomegaly and leukopenia — *see* Felty's syndrome
      vasculitis — *see* Rheumatoid, vasculitis
      visceral involvement NEC — *see* Rheumatoid, arthritis, with involvement of organs NEC
    juvenile (with or without rheumatoid factor) M08.00
      ankle M08.07- ☑
      elbow M08.02- ☑
      foot joint M08.07- ☑
      hand joint M08.04- ☑
      hip M08.05- ☑

Arthritis, arthritic — *continued*
  rheumatoid — *continued*
    juvenile — *continued*
      knee M08.06- ☑
      multiple sites M08.09
      shoulder M08.01- ☑
      vertebra M08.08
      wrist M08.03- ☑
    seronegative M06.00
      ankle M06.07- ☑
      elbow M06.02- ☑
      foot joint M06.07- ☑
      hand joint M06.04- ☑
      hip M06.05- ☑
      knee M06.06- ☑
      multiple site M06.09
      shoulder M06.01- ☑
      vertebra M06.08
      wrist M06.03- ☑
    seropositive M05.9
      specified NEC M05.80
        ankle M05.87- ☑
        elbow M05.82- ☑
        foot joint M05.87- ☑
        hand joint M05.84- ☑
        hip M05.85- ☑
        knee M05.86- ☑
        multiple sites M05.89
        shoulder M05.81- ☑
        vertebra — *see* Spondylitis, ankylosing
        wrist M05.83- ☑
      without organ involvement M05.70
        ankle M05.77- ☑
        elbow M05.72- ☑
        foot joint M05.77- ☑
        hand joint M05.74- ☑
        hip M05.75- ☑
        knee M05.76- ☑
        multiple sites M05.79
        shoulder M05.71- ☑
        vertebra — *see* Spondylitis, ankylosing
        wrist M05.73- ☑
    specified type NEC M06.80
      ankle M06.87- ☑
      elbow M06.82- ☑
      foot joint M06.87- ☑
      hand joint M06.84- ☑
      hip M06.85- ☑
      knee M06.86- ☑
      multiple site M06.89
      shoulder M06.81- ☑
      vertebra M06.88
      wrist M06.83- ☑
    spine — *see* Spondylitis, ankylosing
  rubella B06.82
  scorbutic (*see also* subcategory M14.8-) E54
  senile or senescent — *see* Osteoarthritis
  septic (any site except spine) — *see* Arthritis, pyogenic or pyemic
    spine — *see* Spondylopathy, infective
  serum (nontherapeutic) (therapeutic) — *see* Arthropathy, postimmunization
  specified form NEC M13.80
    ankle M13.87- ☑
    elbow M13.82- ☑
    foot joint M13.87- ☑
    hand joint M13.84- ☑
    hip M13.85- ☑
    knee M13.86- ☑
    multiple site M13.89
    shoulder M13.81- ☑
    specified joint NEC M13.88
    wrist M13.83- ☑
  spine (*see also* Spondylopathy, inflammatory)
    infectious or infective NEC — *see* Spondylopathy, infective
    Marie-Strümpell — *see* Spondylitis, ankylosing
    pyogenic — *see* Spondylopathy, infective
    rheumatoid — *see* Spondylitis, ankylosing
    traumatic (old) — *see* Spondylopathy, traumatic
    tuberculous A18.01
  staphylococcal M00.00
    ankle M00.07- ☑
    elbow M00.02- ☑
    foot joint — *see* Arthritis, staphylococcal, ankle
    hand joint M00.04- ☑

☜ **Subterms under main terms may continue to next column or page**   ☑ **Additional Character Required — Refer to the Tabular List for Character Selection**   **29**

Arthritis, arthritic — Arthritis, arthritic

Arthritis, arthritic — *continued*
  staphylococcal — *continued*
    hip M00.05- ☑
    knee M00.06- ☑
    multiple site M00.09
    shoulder M00.01- ☑
    vertebra M00.08
    wrist M00.03- ☑
  streptococcal NEC M00.20
    ankle M00.27- ☑
    elbow M00.22- ☑
    foot joint — *see* Arthritis, streptococcal, ankle
    hand joint M00.24- ☑
    hip M00.25- ☑
    knee M00.26- ☑
    multiple site M00.29
    shoulder M00.21- ☑
    vertebra M00.28
    wrist M00.23- ☑
  suppurative — *see* Arthritis, pyogenic or pyemic
  syphilitic (late) A52.16
    congenital A50.55 [M12.80]
  syphilitica deformans (Charcot) A52.16
  temporomandibular M26.69
  toxic of menopause (any site) — *see* Arthritis, specified form NEC
  transient — *see* Arthropathy, specified form NEC
  traumatic (chronic) — *see* Arthropathy, traumatic
  tuberculous A18.02
    spine A18.01
  uratic — *see* Gout
  urethritica (Reiter's) — *see* Reiter's disease
  vertebral — *see* Spondylopathy, inflammatory
  villous (any site) — *see* Arthropathy, specified form NEC
Arthrocele — *see* Effusion, joint
Arthrodesis status Z98.1
Arthrodynia (*see also* Pain, joint)
Arthrodysplasia Q74.9
Arthrofibrosis, joint — *see* Ankylosis
Arthrogryposis (congenital) Q68.8
  multiplex congenita Q74.3
Arthrokatadysis M24.7
Arthropathy (*see also* Arthritis) M12.9
  Charcot's — *see* Arthropathy, neuropathic
    diabetic — *see* Diabetes, arthropathy, neuropathic
    syringomyelic G95.0
  cricoarytenoid J38.7
  crystal (-induced) — *see* Arthritis, in, crystals
  diabetic NEC — *see* Diabetes, arthropathy
  distal interphalangeal, psoriatic L40.51
  enteropathic M07.60
    ankle M07.67- ☑
    elbow M07.62- ☑
    foot joint M07.67- ☑
    hand joint M07.64- ☑
    hip M07.65- ☑
    knee M07.66- ☑
    multiple site M07.69
    shoulder M07.61- ☑
    vertebra M07.68
    wrist M07.63- ☑
  following intestinal bypass M02.00
    ankle M02.07- ☑
    elbow M02.02- ☑
    foot joint M02.07- ☑
    hand joint M02.04- ☑
    hip M02.05- ☑
    knee M02.06- ☑
    multiple site M02.09
    shoulder M02.01- ☑
    vertebra M02.08
    wrist M02.03- ☑
  gouty (*see also* Gout)
    in (due to)
      Lesch-Nyhan syndrome E79.1 [M14.8-] ☑
      sickle-cell disorders D57- ☑ [M14.8-] ☑
  hemophilic NEC D66 [M36.2]
    in (due to)
      hyperparathyroidism NEC E21.3 [M14.8-] ☑
      metabolic disease NOS E88.9 [M14.8-] ☑
  in (due to)
    acromegaly E22.0 [M14.8-] ☑
    amyloidosis E85.4 [M14.8-] ☑
    blood disorder NOS D75.9 [M36.3]
    diabetes — *see* Diabetes, arthropathy
    endocrine disease NOS E34.9 [M14.8-] ☑

Arthropathy — *continued*
  in — *continued*
    erythema
      multiforme L51.9 [M14.8-] ☑
      nodosum L52 [M14.8-] ☑
    hemochromatosis E83.118 [M14.8-] ☑
    hemoglobinopathy NEC D58.2 [M36.3]
    hemophilia NEC D66 [M36.2]
    Henoch-Schönlein purpura D69.0 [M36.4]·
    hyperthyroidism E05.90 [M14.8-] ☑
    hypothyroidism E03.9 [M14.8-] ☑
    infective endocarditis I33.0 [M12.80]
    leukemia NEC C95.9- ☑ [M36.1]
    malignant histiocytosis C96.A [M36.1]
    metabolic disease NOS E88.9 [M14.8-] ☑
    multiple myeloma C90.0- ☑ [M36.1]
    neoplastic disease NOS (*see also* Neoplasm) D49.9 [M36.1]
    nutritional deficiency (*see also* subcategory M14.8-) E63.9
    psoriasis NOS L40.50
    sarcoidosis D86.86
    syphilis (late) A52.77
      congenital A50.55 [M12.80]
    thyrotoxicosis (*see also* subcategory M14.8-) E05.90
    ulcerative colitis K51.90 [M07.60]
    viral hepatitis (postinfectious) NEC B19.9 [M12.80]
    Whipple's disease (*see also* subcategory M14.8-) K90.81
  Jaccoud — *see* Arthropathy, postrheumatic, chronic
  juvenile — *see* Arthritis, juvenile
    psoriatic L40.54
  mutilans (psoriatic) L40.52
  neuropathic (Charcot) M14.60
    ankle M14.67- ☑
    diabetic — *see* Diabetes, arthropathy, neuropathic
    elbow M14.62- ☑
    foot joint M14.67- ☑
    hand joint M14.64- ☑
    hip M14.65- ☑
    knee M14.66- ☑
    multiple site M14.69
    nonsyphilitic NEC G98.0
    shoulder M14.61- ☑
    syringomyelic G95.0
    vertebra M14.68
    wrist M14.63- ☑
  osteopulmonary — *see* Osteoarthropathy, hypertrophic, specified NEC
  postdysenteric M02.10
    ankle M02.17- ☑
    elbow M02.12- ☑
    foot joint M02.17- ☑
    hand joint M02.14- ☑
    hip M02.15- ☑
    knee M02.16- ☑
    multiple site M02.19
    shoulder M02.11- ☑
    vertebra M02.18
    wrist M02.13- ☑
  postimmunization M02.20
    ankle M02.27- ☑
    elbow M02.22- ☑
    foot joint M02.27- ☑
    hand joint M02.24- ☑
    hip M02.25- ☑
    knee M02.26- ☑
    multiple site M02.29
    shoulder M02.21- ☑
    vertebra M02.28
    wrist M02.23- ☑
  postinfectious NEC B99 ☑ [M12.80]
    in (due to)
      enteritis due to Yersinia enterocolitica A04.6 [M12.80]
      syphilis A52.77
      viral hepatitis NEC B19.9 [M12.80]
  postrheumatic, chronic (Jaccoud) M12.00
    ankle M12.07- ☑
    elbow M12.02- ☑
    foot joint M12.07- ☑
    hand joint M12.04- ☑
    hip M12.05- ☑
    knee M12.06- ☑
    multiple site M12.09
    shoulder M12.01- ☑
    specified joint NEC M12.08

Arthropathy — *continued*
  postrheumatic, chronic — *continued*
    vertebrae M12.08
    wrist M12.03- ☑
  psoriatic NEC L40.59
    interphalangeal, distal L40.51
  reactive M02.9
    in (due to)
      infective endocarditis I33.0 [M02.9]
    specified type NEC M02.80
      ankle M02.87- ☑
      elbow M02.82- ☑
      foot joint M02.87- ☑
      hand joint M02.84- ☑
      hip M02.85- ☑
      knee M02.86- ☑
      multiple site M02.89
      shoulder M02.81- ☑
      vertebra M02.88
      wrist M02.83- ☑
  specified form NEC M12.80
    ankle M12.87- ☑
    elbow M12.82- ☑
    foot joint M12.87- ☑
    hand joint M12.84- ☑
    hip M12.85- ☑
    knee M12.86- ☑
    multiple site M12.89
    shoulder M12.81- ☑
    specified joint NEC M12.88
    vertebrae M12.88
    wrist M12.83- ☑
  syringomyelic G95.0
  tabes dorsalis A52.16
  tabetic A52.16
  transient — *see* Arthropathy, specified form NEC
  traumatic M12.50
    ankle M12.57- ☑
    elbow M12.52- ☑
    foot joint M12.57- ☑
    hand joint M12.54- ☑
    hip M12.55- ☑
    knee M12.56- ☑
    multiple site M12.59
    shoulder M12.51- ☑
    specified joint NEC M12.58
    vertebrae M12.58
    wrist M12.53- ☑
Arthropyosis — *see* Arthritis, pyogenic or pyemic
Arthrosis (deformans) (degenerative) (localized) (*see also* Osteoarthritis) M19.90
  spine — *see* Spondylosis
Arthus' phenomenon or reaction T78.41 ☑
  due to
    drug — *see* Table of Drugs and Chemicals, by drug
Articular — *see* condition
Articulation, reverse (teeth) M26.24
Artificial
  insemination complication — *see* Complications, artificial, fertilization
  opening status (functioning) (without complication) Z93.9
    anus (colostomy) Z93.3
    colostomy Z93.3
    cystostomy Z93.50
      appendico-vesicostomy Z93.52
      cutaneous Z93.51
      specified NEC Z93.59
    enterostomy Z93.4
    gastrostomy Z93.1
    ileostomy Z93.2
    intestinal tract NEC Z93.4
    jejunostomy Z93.4
    nephrostomy Z93.6
    specified site NEC Z93.8
    tracheostomy Z93.0
    ureterostomy Z93.6
    urethrostomy Z93.6
    urinary tract NEC Z93.6
    vagina Z93.8
  vagina status Z93.8
Arytenoid — *see* condition
Asbestosis (occupational) J61
Ascariasis B77.9
  with
    complications NEC B77.89
    intestinal complications B77.0

Ascariasis — *continued*
  with — *continued*
    pneumonia, pneumonitis B77.81
Ascaridosis, ascariasis — *see* Ascariasis
Ascaris (infection) (infestation) (lumbricoides) — *see* Ascariasis
Ascending — *see* condition
ASC-H (atypical squamous cells cannot exclude high grade squamous intraepithelial lesion on cytologic smear)
  anus R85.611
  cervix R87.611
  vagina R87.621
Aschoff's bodies — *see* Myocarditis, rheumatic
Ascites (abdominal) R18.8
  cardiac (*see also* Failure, heart, right) I50.810
  chylous (nonfilarial) I89.8
    filarial — *see* Infestation, filarial
  due to
    cirrhosis, alcoholic K70.31
    hepatitis
      alcoholic K70.11
      chronic active K71.51
    S. japonicum B65.2
  heart (*see also* Failure, heart, right) I50.810
  malignant R18.0
  pseudochylous R18.8
  syphilitic A52.74
  tuberculous A18.31
ASC-US (atypical squamous cells of undetermined significance on cytologic smear)
  anus R85.610
  cervix R87.610
  vagina R87.620
Aseptic — *see* condition
Asherman's syndrome N85.6
Asialia K11.7
Asiatic cholera — *see* Cholera
Asimultagnosia (simultanagnosia) R48.3
Askin's tumor — *see* Neoplasm, connective tissue, malignant
Asocial personality F60.2
Asomatognosia R41.4
Aspartylglucosaminuria E77.1
Asperger's disease or syndrome F84.5
Aspergilloma — *see* Aspergillosis
Aspergillosis (with pneumonia) B44.9
  bronchopulmonary, allergic B44.81
  disseminated B44.7
  generalized B44.7
  pulmonary NEC B44.1
    allergic B44.81
    invasive B44.0
  specified NEC B44.89
  tonsillar B44.2
Aspergillus (flavus) (fumigatus) (infection) (terreus) — *see* Aspergillosis
Aspermatogenesis — *see* Azoospermia
Aspermia (testis) — *see* Azoospermia
Asphyxia, asphyxiation (by) R09.01
  antenatal P84
  birth P84
  bunny bag — *see* Asphyxia, due to, mechanical threat to breathing, trapped in bed clothes
  crushing S28.0 ☑
  drowning T75.1 ☑
  gas, fumes, or vapor — *see* Table of Drugs and Chemicals
  inhalation — *see* Inhalation
  intrauterine P84
  local I73.00
    with gangrene I73.01
  mucus (*see also* Foreign body, respiratory tract, causing asphyxia)
  newborn P84
  pathological R09.01
  postnatal P84
    mechanical — *see* Asphyxia, due to, mechanical threat to breathing
  prenatal P84
  reticularis R23.1
  strangulation — *see* Asphyxia, due to, mechanical threat to breathing
  submersion T75.1 ☑
  traumatic T71.9 ☑
    due to
      crushed chest S28.0 ☑

Asphyxia, asphyxiation — *continued*
  traumatic — *continued*
    due to — *continued*
      foreign body (in) — *see* Foreign body, respiratory tract, causing asphyxia
      low oxygen content of ambient air T71.20 ☑
        due to
          being trapped in
            low oxygen environment T71.29 ☑
            in car trunk T71.221 ☑
              circumstances undetermined T71.224 ☑
              done with intent to harm by another person T71.223 ☑
                self T71.222 ☑
            in refrigerator T71.231 ☑
              circumstances undetermined T71.234 ☑
              done with intent to harm by another person T71.233 ☑
                self T71.232 ☑
      cave-in T71.21 ☑
      mechanical threat to breathing (accidental) T71.191 ☑
        circumstances undetermined T71.194 ☑
        done with intent to harm by
          another person T71.193 ☑
          self T71.192 ☑
        hanging T71.161 ☑
          circumstances undetermined T71.164 ☑
          done with intent to harm by
            another person T71.163 ☑
            self T71.162 ☑
      plastic bag T71.121 ☑
        circumstances undetermined T71.124 ☑
        done with intent to harm by
          another person T71.123 ☑
          self T71.122 ☑
      smothering
        in furniture T71.151 ☑
          circumstances undetermined T71.154 ☑
          done with intent to harm by
            another person T71.153 ☑
            self T71.152 ☑
        under
          another person's body T71.141 ☑
            circumstances undetermined T71.144 ☑
            done with intent to harm T71.143 ☑
          pillow T71.111 ☑
            circumstances undetermined T71.114 ☑
            done with intent to harm by
              another person T71.113 ☑
              self T71.112 ☑
      trapped in bed clothes T71.131 ☑
        circumstances undetermined T71.134 ☑
        done with intent to harm by
          another person T71.133 ☑
          self T71.132 ☑
  vomiting, vomitus — *see* Foreign body, respiratory tract, causing asphyxia
Aspiration
  amniotic (clear) fluid (newborn) P24.10
    with
      pneumonia (pneumonitis) P24.11
      respiratory symptoms P24.11
  blood
    newborn (without respiratory symptoms) P24.20
      with
        pneumonia (pneumonitis) P24.21
        respiratory symptoms P24.21
      specified age NEC — *see* Foreign body, respiratory tract
  bronchitis J69.0
  food or foreign body (with asphyxiation) — *see* Asphyxia, food
  liquor (amnii) (newborn) P24.10
    with
      pneumonia (pneumonitis) P24.11
      respiratory symptoms P24.11
  meconium (newborn) (without respiratory symptoms) P24.00
    with
      pneumonitis (pneumonitis) P24.01
      respiratory symptoms P24.01

Aspiration — *continued*
  milk (newborn) (without respiratory symptoms) P24.30
    with
      pneumonia (pneumonitis) P24.31
      respiratory symptoms P24.31
    specified age NEC — *see* Foreign body, respiratory tract
  mucus (*see also* Foreign body, by site, causing asphyxia)
    newborn P24.10
      with
        pneumonia (pneumonitis) P24.11
        respiratory symptoms P24.11
  neonatal P24.9
    specific NEC (without respiratory symptoms) P24.80
      with
        pneumonia (pneumonitis) P24.81
        respiratory symptoms P24.81
  newborn P24.9
    specific NEC (without respiratory symptoms) P24.80
      with
        pneumonia (pneumonitis) P24.81
        respiratory symptoms P24.81
  pneumonia J69.0
  pneumonitis J69.0
  syndrome of newborn — *see* Aspiration, by substance, with pneumonia
  vernix caseosa (newborn) P24.80
    with
      pneumonia (pneumonitis) P24.81
      respiratory symptoms P24.81
  vomitus (*see also* Foreign body, respiratory tract)
    newborn (without respiratory symptoms) P24.30
      with
        pneumonia (pneumonitis) P24.31
        respiratory symptoms P24.31
Asplenia (congenital) Q89.01
  postsurgical Z90.81
Assam fever B55.0
Assault, sexual — *see* Maltreatment
Assmann's focus NEC A15.0
Astasia (-abasia) (hysterical) F44.4
Asteatosis cutis L85.3
Astereognosia, astereognosis R48.1
Asterixis R27.8
  in liver disease K71.3
Asteroid hyalitis — *see* Deposit, crystalline
Asthenia, asthenic R53.1
  cardiac (*see also* Failure, heart) I50.9
    psychogenic F45.8
  cardiovascular (*see also* Failure, heart) I50.9
    psychogenic F45.8
  heart (*see also* Failure, heart) I50.9
    psychogenic F45.8
  hysterical F44.4
  myocardial (*see also* Failure, heart) I50.9
    psychogenic F45.8
  nervous F48.8
  neurocirculatory F45.8
  neurotic F48.8
  psychogenic F48.8
  psychoneurotic F48.8
  psychophysiologic F48.8
  reaction (psychophysiologic) F48.8
  senile R54
Asthenopia (*see also* Discomfort, visual)
  hysterical F44.6
  psychogenic F44.6
Asthenospermia — *see* Abnormal, specimen, male genital organs
Asthma, asthmatic (bronchial) (catarrh) (spasmodic) J45.909
  with
    chronic obstructive bronchitis J44.9
      with
        acute lower respiratory infection J44.0
        exacerbation (acute) J44.1
    chronic obstructive pulmonary disease J44.9
      with
        acute lower respiratory infection J44.0
        exacerbation (acute) J44.1
    exacerbation (acute) J45.901
    hay fever — *see* Asthma, allergic extrinsic
    rhinitis, allergic — *see* Asthma, allergic extrinsic
    status asthmaticus J45.902
  allergic extrinsic J45.909
    with
      exacerbation (acute) J45.901
      status asthmaticus J45.902

▽ Subterms under main terms may continue to next column or page   ☑ Additional Character Required — Refer to the Tabular List for Character Selection   **31**

Ascariasis — Asthma, asthmatic

Asthma, asthmatic — *continued*
- atopic — *see* Asthma, allergic extrinsic
- cardiac — *see* Failure, ventricular, left
- cardiobronchial I50.1
- childhood J45.909
  - with
    - exacerbation (acute) J45.901
    - status asthmaticus J45.902
- chronic obstructive J44.9
  - with
    - acute lower respiratory infection J44.0
    - exacerbation (acute) J44.1
- collier's J60
- cough variant J45.991
- detergent J69.8
- due to
  - detergent J69.8
  - inhalation of fumes J68.3
- eosinophilic J82
- extrinsic, allergic — *see* Asthma, allergic extrinsic
- grinder's J62.8
- hay — *see* Asthma, allergic extrinsic
- heart I50.1
- idiosyncratic — *see* Asthma, nonallergic
- intermittent (mild) J45.20
  - with
    - exacerbation (acute) J45.21
    - status asthmaticus J45.22
- intrinsic, nonallergic — *see* Asthma, nonallergic
- Kopp's E32.8
- late-onset J45.909
  - with
    - exacerbation (acute) J45.901
    - status asthmaticus J45.902
- mild intermittent J45.20
  - with
    - exacerbation (acute) J45.21
    - status asthmaticus J45.22
- mild persistent J45.30
  - with
    - exacerbation (acute) J45.31
    - status asthmaticus J45.32
- Millar's (laryngismus stridulus) J38.5
- miner's J60
- mixed J45.909
  - with
    - exacerbation (acute) J45.901
    - status asthmaticus J45.902
- moderate persistent J45.40
  - with
    - exacerbation (acute) J45.41
    - status asthmaticus J45.42
- nervous — *see* Asthma, nonallergic
- nonallergic (intrinsic) J45.909
  - with
    - exacerbation (acute) J45.901
    - status asthmaticus J45.902
- persistent
  - mild J45.30
    - with
      - exacerbation (acute) J45.31
      - status asthmaticus J45.32
  - moderate J45.40
    - with
      - exacerbation (acute) J45.41
      - status asthmaticus J45.42
  - severe J45.50
    - with
      - exacerbation (acute) J45.51
      - status asthmaticus J45.52
- platinum J45.998
- pneumoconiotic NEC J64
- potter's J62.8
- predominantly allergic J45.909
- psychogenic F54
- pulmonary eosinophilic J82
- red cedar J67.8
- Rostan's I50.1
- sandblaster's J62.8
- sequoiosis J67.8
- severe persistent J45.50
  - with
    - exacerbation (acute) J45.51
    - status asthmaticus J45.52
- specified NEC J45.998
- stonemason's J62.8
- thymic E32.8
- tuberculous — *see* Tuberculosis, pulmonary

Asthma, asthmatic — *continued*
- Wichmann's (laryngismus stridulus) J38.5
- wood J67.8

Astigmatism (compound) (congenital) H52.20- ☑
- irregular H52.21- ☑
- regular H52.22- ☑

Astraphobia F40.220

Astroblastoma
- specified site — *see* Neoplasm, malignant, by site
- unspecified site C71.9

Astrocytoma (cystic)
- anaplastic
  - specified site — *see* Neoplasm, malignant, by site
  - unspecified site C71.9
- fibrillary
  - specified site — *see* Neoplasm, malignant, by site
  - unspecified site C71.9
- fibrous
  - specified site — *see* Neoplasm, malignant, by site
  - unspecified site C71.9
- gemistocytic
  - specified site — *see* Neoplasm, malignant, by site
  - unspecified site C71.9
- juvenile
  - specified site — *see* Neoplasm, malignant, by site
  - unspecified site C71.9
- pilocytic
  - specified site — *see* Neoplasm, malignant, by site
  - unspecified site C71.9
- piloid
  - specified site — *see* Neoplasm, malignant, by site
  - unspecified site C71.9
- protoplasmic
  - specified site — *see* Neoplasm, malignant, by site
  - unspecified site C71.9
- specified site NEC — *see* Neoplasm, malignant, by site
- subependymal D43.2
  - giant cell
    - specified site — *see* Neoplasm, uncertain behavior, by site
    - unspecified site D43.2
  - specified site — *see* Neoplasm, uncertain behavior, by site
  - unspecified site D43.2
- unspecified site C71.9

Astroglioma
- specified site — *see* Neoplasm, malignant, by site
- unspecified site C71.9

Asymbolia R48.8

Asymmetry (*see also* Distortion)
- between native and reconstructed breast N65.1
- face Q67.0
- jaw (lower) — *see* Anomaly, dentofacial, jaw-cranial base relationship, asymmetry

Asynergia, asynergy R27.8
- ventricular I51.89

Asystole (heart) — *see* Arrest, cardiac

At risk
- for
  - dental caries Z91.849
    - high Z91.843
    - low Z91.841
    - moderate Z91.842
  - falling Z91.81

Ataxia, ataxy, ataxic R27.0
- acute R27.8
- brain (hereditary) G11.9
- cerebellar (hereditary) G11.9
  - with defective DNA repair G11.3
  - alcoholic G31.2
  - early-onset G11.1
  - in
    - alcoholism G31.2
    - myxedema E03.9 [G13.2]
    - neoplastic disease (*see also* Neoplasm) D49.9 [G32.81]
    - specified disease NEC G32.81
  - late-onset (Marie's) G11.2
- cerebral (hereditary) G11.9
- congenital nonprogressive G11.0
- family, familial — *see* Ataxia, hereditary
- following
  - cerebrovascular disease I69.993
    - cerebral infarction I69.393
    - intracerebral hemorrhage I69.193
    - nontraumatic intracranial hemorrhage NEC I69.293
    - specified disease NEC I69.893

Ataxia, ataxy, ataxic — *continued*
- following — *continued*
  - cerebrovascular disease — *continued*
    - subarachnoid hemorrhage I69.093
  - Friedreich's (heredofamilial) (cerebellar) (spinal) G11.1
- gait R26.0
  - hysterical F44.4
- general R27.8
- gluten M35.9 [G32.81]
  - with celiac disease K90.0 [G32.81]
- hereditary G11.9
  - with neuropathy G60.2
  - cerebellar — *see* Ataxia, cerebellar
  - spastic G11.4
  - specified NEC G11.8
  - spinal (Friedreich's) G11.1
- heredofamilial — *see* Ataxia, hereditary
- Hunt's G11.1
- hysterical F44.4
- locomotor (progressive) (syphilitic) (partial) (spastic) A52.11
  - diabetic — *see* Diabetes, ataxia
- Marie's (cerebellar) (heredofamilial) (late-onset) G11.2
- nonorganic origin F44.4
- nonprogressive, congenital G11.0
- psychogenic F44.4
- Roussy-Lévy G60.0
- Sanger-Brown's (hereditary) G11.2
- spastic hereditary G11.4
- spinal
  - hereditary (Friedreich's) G11.1
  - progressive (syphilitic) A52.11
- spinocerebellar, X-linked recessive G11.1
- telangiectasia (Louis-Bar) G11.3

Ataxia-telangiectasia (Louis-Bar) G11.3

Atelectasis (massive) (partial) (pressure) (pulmonary) J98.11
- newborn P28.10
  - due to resorption P28.11
  - partial P28.19
  - primary P28.0
  - secondary P28.19
- primary (newborn) P28.0
- tuberculous — *see* Tuberculosis, pulmonary

Atelocardia Q24.9

Atelomyelia Q06.1

Atheroembolism
- of
  - extremities
    - lower I75.02- ☑
    - upper I75.01- ☑
  - kidney I75.81
  - specified NEC I75.89

Atheroma, atheromatous (*see also* Arteriosclerosis) I70.90
- aorta, aortic I70.0
  - valve (*see also* Endocarditis, aortic) I35.8
- aorto-iliac I70.0
- artery — *see* Arteriosclerosis
- basilar (artery) I67.2
- carotid (artery) (common) (internal) I67.2
- cerebral (arteries) I67.2
- coronary (artery) I25.10
  - with angina pectoris — *see* Arteriosclerosis, coronary (artery),
  - degeneration — *see* Arteriosclerosis
- heart, cardiac — *see* Disease, heart, ischemic, atherosclerotic
- mitral (valve) I34.8
- myocardium, myocardial — *see* Disease, heart, ischemic, atherosclerotic
- pulmonary valve (heart) (*see also* Endocarditis, pulmonary) I37.8
- tricuspid (heart) (valve) I36.8
- valve, valvular — *see* Endocarditis
- vertebral (artery) I67.2

Atheromatosis — *see* Arteriosclerosis

Atherosclerosis (*see also* Arteriosclerosis)
- coronary
  - artery I25.10
    - with angina pectoris — *see* Arteriosclerosis, coronary (artery),
    - due to
      - calcified coronary lesion (severely) I25.84
      - lipid rich plaque I25.83
- transplanted heart I25.811
  - bypass graft I25.812

Atherosclerosis — *continued*
  transplanted heart — *continued*
    bypass graft — *continued*
      with angina pectoris — *see* Arteriosclerosis,
        coronary (artery),
      native coronary artery I25.811
        with angina pectoris — *see* Arteriosclerosis,
          coronary (artery),
Athetosis (acquired) R25.8
  bilateral (congenital) G80.3
  congenital (bilateral) (double) G80.3
  double (congenital) G80.3
  unilateral R25.8
Athlete's
  foot B35.3
  heart I51.7
Athrepsia E41
Athyrea (acquired) (*see also* Hypothyroidism)
  congenital E03.1
Atonia, atony, atonic
  bladder (sphincter) (neurogenic) N31.2
  capillary I78.8
  cecum K59.8
    psychogenic F45.8
  colon — *see* Atony, intestine
  congenital P94.2
  esophagus K22.8
  intestine K59.8
    psychogenic F45.8
  stomach K31.89
    neurotic or psychogenic F45.8
  uterus (during labor) O62.2
    with hemorrhage (postpartum) O72.1
    postpartum (with hemorrhage) O72.1
      without hemorrhage O75.89
Atopy — *see* History, allergy
Atransferrinemia, congenital E88.09
Atresia, atretic
  alimentary organ or tract NEC Q45.8
    upper Q40.8
  ani, anus, anal (canal) Q42.3
    with fistula Q42.2
  aorta (ring) Q25.29
  aortic (orifice) (valve) Q23.0
    arch Q25.21
    congenital with hypoplasia of ascending aorta and
      defective development of left ventricle (with
      mitral stenosis) Q23.4
    in hypoplastic left heart syndrome Q23.4
  aqueduct of Sylvius Q03.0
    with spina bifida — *see* Spina bifida, with hydro-
      cephalus
  artery NEC Q27.8
    cerebral Q28.3
    coronary Q24.5
    digestive system Q27.8
    eye Q15.8
    lower limb Q27.8
    pulmonary Q25.5
    specified site NEC Q27.8
    umbilical Q27.0
    upper limb Q27.8
  auditory canal (external) Q16.1
  bile duct (common) (congenital) (hepatic) Q44.2
    acquired — *see* Obstruction, bile duct
  bladder (neck) Q64.39
    obstruction Q64.31
  bronchus Q32.4
  cecum Q42.8
  cervix (acquired) N88.2
    congenital Q51.828
    in pregnancy or childbirth — *see* Anomaly, cervix,
      in pregnancy or childbirth
      causing obstructed labor O65.5
  choana Q30.0
  colon Q42.9
    specified NEC Q42.8
  common duct Q44.2
  cricoid cartilage Q31.8
  cystic duct Q44.2
    acquired K82.8
      with obstruction K82.0
  digestive organs NEC Q45.8
  duodenum Q41.0
  ear canal Q16.1
  ejaculatory duct Q55.4
  epiglottis Q31.8
  esophagus Q39.0

Atresia, atretic — *continued*
  esophagus — *continued*
    with tracheoesophageal fistula Q39.1
  eustachian tube Q17.8
  fallopian tube (congenital) Q50.6
    acquired N97.1
  follicular cyst N83.0- ☑
  foramen of
    Luschka Q03.1
      with spina bifida — *see* Spina bifida, with hydro-
        cephalus
    Magendie Q03.1
      with spina bifida — *see* Spina bifida, with hydro-
        cephalus
  gallbladder Q44.1
  genital organ
    external
      female Q52.79
      male Q55.8
    internal
      female Q52.8
      male Q55.8
  glottis Q31.8
  gullet Q39.0
    with tracheoesophageal fistula Q39.1
  heart valve NEC Q24.8
    pulmonary Q22.0
    tricuspid Q22.4
  hymen Q52.3
    acquired (postinfective) N89.6
  ileum Q41.2
  intestine (small) Q41.9
    large Q42.9
      specified NEC Q42.8
  iris, filtration angle Q15.0
  jejunum Q41.1
  lacrimal apparatus Q10.4
  larynx Q31.8
  meatus urinarius Q64.33
  mitral valve Q23.2
    in hypoplastic left heart syndrome Q23.4
  nares (anterior) (posterior) Q30.0
  nasopharynx Q34.8
  nose, nostril Q30.0
    acquired J34.89
  organ or site NEC Q89.8
  osseous meatus (ear) Q16.1
  oviduct (congenital) Q50.6
    acquired N97.1
  parotid duct Q38.4
    acquired K11.8
  pulmonary (artery) Q25.5
    valve Q22.0
  pulmonic Q22.0
  pupil Q13.2
  rectum Q42.1
    with fistula Q42.0
  salivary duct Q38.4
    acquired K11.8
  sublingual duct Q38.4
    acquired K11.8
  submandibular duct Q38.4
    acquired K11.8
  submaxillary duct Q38.4
    acquired K11.8
  thyroid cartilage Q31.8
  trachea Q32.1
  tricuspid valve Q22.4
  ureter Q62.10
    pelvic junction Q62.11
    vesical orifice Q62.12
  ureteropelvic junction Q62.11
  ureterovesical orifice Q62.12
  urethra (valvular) Q64.39
    stricture Q64.32
  urinary tract NEC Q64.8
  uterus Q51.818
    acquired N85.8
  vagina (congenital) Q52.4
    acquired (postinfectional) (senile) N89.5
  vas deferens Q55.3
  vascular NEC Q27.8
    cerebral Q28.3
    digestive system Q27.8
    lower limb Q27.8
    specified site NEC Q27.8
    upper limb Q27.8
  vein NEC Q27.8
    digestive system Q27.8

Atresia, atretic — *continued*
  vein — *continued*
    great Q26.8
    lower limb Q27.8
    portal Q26.5
    pulmonary Q26.4
      partial Q26.3
      total Q26.2
    specified site NEC Q27.8
    upper limb Q27.8
  vena cava (inferior) (superior) Q26.8
  vesicourethral orifice Q64.31
  vulva Q52.79
    acquired N90.5
Atrichia, atrichosis — *see* Alopecia
Atrophia (*see also* Atrophy)
  cutis senilis L90.8
    due to radiation L57.8
  gyrata of choroid and retina H31.23
  senilis R54
    dermatological L90.8
      due to radiation (nonionizing) (solar) L57.8
  unguium L60.3
    congenita Q84.6
Atrophie blanche (en plaque) (de Milian) L95.0
Atrophoderma, atrophodermia (of) L90.9
  diffusum (idiopathic) L90.4
  maculatum L90.8
    et striatum L90.8
      due to syphilis A52.79
    syphilitic A51.39
  neuriticum L90.8
  Pasini and Pierini L90.3
  pigmentosum Q82.1
  reticulatum symmetricum faciei L66.4
  senile L90.8
    due to radiation (nonionizing) (solar) L57.8
  vermiculata (cheeks) L66.4
Atrophy, atrophic (of)
  adrenal (capsule) (gland) E27.49
    primary (autoimmune) E27.1
  alveolar process or ridge (edentulous) K08.20
  anal sphincter (disuse) N81.84
  appendix K38.8
  arteriosclerotic — *see* Arteriosclerosis
  bile duct (common) (hepatic) K83.8
  bladder N32.89
    neurogenic N31.8
  blanche (en plaque) (of Milian) L95.0
  bone (senile) NEC (*see also* Disorder, bone, specified
    type NEC)
    due to
      tabes dorsalis (neurogenic) A52.11
  brain (cortex) (progressive) G31.9
    frontotemporal circumscribed G31.01 [F02.80]
      with behavioral disturbance G31.01 [F02.81]
    senile NEC G31.1
  breast N64.2
    obstetric — *see* Disorder, breast, specified type NEC
  buccal cavity K13.79
  cardiac — *see* Degeneration, myocardial
  cartilage (infectional) (joint) — *see* Disorder, cartilage,
    specified NEC
  cerebellar — *see* Atrophy, brain
  cerebral — *see* Atrophy, brain
  cervix (mucosa) (senile) (uteri) N88.8
    menopausal N95.8
  Charcot-Marie-Tooth G60.0
  choroid (central) (macular) (myopic) (retina) H31.10- ☑
    diffuse secondary H31.12- ☑
    gyrate H31.23
    senile H31.11- ☑
  ciliary body — *see* Atrophy, iris
  conjunctiva (senile) H11.89
  corpus cavernosum N48.89
  cortical — *see* Atrophy, brain
  cystic duct K82.8
  Déjérine-Thomas G23.8
  disuse NEC — *see* Atrophy, muscle
  Duchenne-Aran G12.21
  ear H93.8- ☑
  edentulous alveolar ridge K08.20
  endometrium (senile) N85.8
    cervix N88.8
  enteric K63.89
  epididymis N50.89
  eyeball — *see* Disorder, globe, degenerated condition,
    atrophy

Atrophy, atrophic — *continued*
- eyelid (senile) — *see* Disorder, eyelid, degenerative
- facial (skin) L90.9
- fallopian tube (senile) N83.32- ☑
  - with ovary N83.33- ☑
- fascioscapulohumeral (Landouzy- Déjérine) G71.02
- fatty, thymus (gland) E32.8
- gallbladder K82.8
- gastric K29.40
  - with bleeding K29.41
- gastrointestinal K63.89
- glandular I89.8
- globe H44.52- ☑
- gum — *see* Recession, gingival
- hair L67.8
- heart (brown) — *see* Degeneration, myocardial
- hemifacial Q67.4
  - Romberg G51.8
- infantile E41
  - paralysis, acute — *see* Poliomyelitis, paralytic
- intestine K63.89
- iris (essential) (progressive) H21.26- ☑
  - specified NEC H21.29
- kidney (senile) (terminal) (*see also* Sclerosis, renal) N26.1
  - congenital or infantile Q60.5
    - bilateral Q60.4
    - unilateral Q60.3
  - hydronephrotic — *see* Hydronephrosis
- lacrimal gland (primary) H04.14- ☑
  - secondary H04.15- ☑
- Landouzy-Déjérine G71.02
- laryngitis, infective J37.0
- larynx J38.7
- Leber's optic (hereditary) H47.22
- lip K13.0
- liver (yellow) K72.90
  - with coma K72.91
  - acute, subacute K72.00
    - with coma K72.01
  - chronic K72.10
    - with coma K72.11
- lung (senile) J98.4
- macular (dermatological) L90.8
  - syphilitic, skin A51.39
    - striated A52.79
- mandible (edentulous) K08.20
  - minimal K08.21
  - moderate K08.22
  - severe K08.23
- maxilla K08.20
  - minimal K08.24
  - moderate K08.25
  - severe K08.26
- muscle, muscular (diffuse) (general) (idiopathic) (primary) M62.50
  - ankle M62.57- ☑
  - Duchenne-Aran G12.21
  - foot M62.57- ☑
  - forearm M62.53- ☑
  - hand M62.54- ☑
  - infantile spinal G12.0
  - lower leg M62.56- ☑
  - multiple sites M62.59
  - myelopathic — *see* Atrophy, muscle, spinal
  - myotonic G71.11
  - neuritic G58.9
  - neuropathic (peroneal) (progressive) G60.0
  - pelvic (disuse) N81.84
  - peroneal G60.0
  - progressive (bulbar) G12.21
    - adult G12.1
    - infantile (spinal) G12.0
    - spinal G12.25
      - adult G12.1
      - infantile G12.0
  - pseudohypertrophic G71.02
  - shoulder region M62.51- ☑
  - specified site NEC M62.58
  - spinal G12.9
    - adult form G12.1
    - Aran-Duchenne G12.21
    - childhood form, type II G12.1
    - distal G12.1
    - hereditary NEC G12.1
    - infantile, type I (Werdnig-Hoffmann) G12.0
    - juvenile form, type III (Kugelberg- Welander) G12.1

Atrophy, atrophic — *continued*
- muscle, muscular — *continued*
  - spinal — *continued*
    - progressive G12.25
    - scapuloperoneal form G12.1
    - specified NEC G12.8
  - syphilitic A52.78
  - thigh M62.55- ☑
  - upper arm M62.52- ☑
- myocardium — *see* Degeneration, myocardial
- myometrium (senile) N85.8
  - cervix N88.8
- myopathic NEC — *see* Atrophy, muscle
- myotonia G71.11
- nail L60.3
- nasopharynx J31.1
- nerve (*see also* Disorder, nerve)
  - abducens — *see* Strabismus, paralytic, sixth nerve
  - accessory G52.8
  - acoustic or auditory H93.3 ☑
  - cranial G52.9
    - eighth (auditory) H93.3 ☑
    - eleventh (accessory) G52.8
    - fifth (trigeminal) G50.8
    - first (olfactory) G52.0
    - fourth (trochlear) — *see* Strabismus, paralytic, fourth nerve
    - second (optic) H47.20
    - sixth (abducens) — *see* Strabismus, paralytic, sixth nerve
    - tenth (pneumogastric) (vagus) G52.2
    - third (oculomotor) — *see* Strabismus, paralytic, third nerve
    - twelfth (hypoglossal) G52.3
  - hypoglossal G52.3
  - oculomotor — *see* Strabismus, paralytic, third nerve
  - olfactory G52.0
  - optic (papillomacular bundle)
    - syphilitic (late) A52.15
      - congenital A50.44
  - pneumogastric G52.2
  - trigeminal G50.8
  - trochlear — *see* Strabismus, paralytic, fourth nerve
  - vagus (pneumogastric) G52.2
- neurogenic, bone, tabetic A52.11
- nutritional E41
- old age R54
- olivopontocerebellar G23.8
- optic (nerve) H47.20
  - glaucomatous H47.23- ☑
  - hereditary H47.22
  - primary H47.21- ☑
  - specified type NEC H47.29- ☑
  - syphilitic (late) A52.15
    - congenital A50.44
- orbit H05.31- ☑
- ovary (senile) N83.31- ☑
  - with fallopian tube N83.33- ☑
- oviduct (senile) — *see* Atrophy, fallopian tube
- palsy, diffuse (progressive) G12.22
- pancreas (duct) (senile) K86.89
- parotid gland K11.0
- pelvic muscle N81.84
- penis N48.89
- pharynx J39.2
- pluriglandular E31.8
  - autoimmune E31.0
- polyarthritis M15.9
- prostate N42.89
- pseudohypertrophic (muscle) G71.02
- renal (*see also* Sclerosis, renal) N26.1
- retina, retinal (postinfectional) H35.89
- rhinitis J31.0
- salivary gland K11.0
- scar L90.5
- sclerosis, lobar (of brain) G31.09 [F02.80]
  - with behavioral disturbance G31.09 [F02.81]
- scrotum N50.89
- seminal vesicle N50.89
- senile R54
  - due to radiation (nonionizing) (solar) L57.8
- skin (patches) (spots) L90.9
  - degenerative (senile) L90.8
  - due to radiation (nonionizing) (solar) L57.8
  - senile L90.8
- spermatic cord N50.89
- spinal (acute) (cord) G95.89
  - muscular — *see* Atrophy, muscle, spinal

Atrophy, atrophic — *continued*
- spinal — *continued*
  - paralysis G12.20
    - acute — *see* Poliomyelitis, paralytic
    - meaning progressive muscular atrophy G12.21
- spine (column) — *see* Spondylopathy, specified NEC
- spleen (senile) D73.0
- stomach K29.40
  - with bleeding K29.41
- striate (skin) L90.6
  - syphilitic A52.79
- subcutaneous L90.9
- sublingual gland K11.0
- submandibular gland K11.0
- submaxillary gland K11.0
- Sudeck's — *see* Algoneurodystrophy
- suprarenal (capsule) (gland) E27.49
  - primary E27.1
- systemic affecting central nervous system
  - in
    - myxedema E03.9 [G13.2]
    - neoplastic disease (*see also* Neoplasm) D49.9 [G13.1]
    - specified disease NEC G13.8
- tarso-orbital fascia, congenital Q10.3
- testis N50.0
- thenar, partial — *see* Syndrome, carpal tunnel
- thymus (fatty) E32.8
- thyroid (gland) (acquired) E03.4
  - with cretinism E03.1
  - congenital (with myxedema) E03.1
- tongue (senile) K14.8
  - papillae K14.4
- trachea J39.8
- tunica vaginalis N50.89
- turbinate J34.89
- tympanic membrane (nonflaccid) H73.82- ☑
  - flaccid H73.81- ☑
- upper respiratory tract J39.8
- uterus, uterine (senile) N85.8
  - cervix N88.8
  - due to radiation (intended effect) N85.8
    - adverse effect or misadventure N99.89
- vagina (senile) N95.2
- vas deferens N50.89
- vascular I99.8
- vertebra (senile) — *see* Spondylopathy, specified NEC
- vulva (senile) N90.5
- Werdnig-Hoffmann G12.0
- yellow — *see* Failure, hepatic

Attack, attacks
- with alteration of consciousness (with automatisms) — *see* Epilepsy, localization-related, symptomatic, with complex partial seizures
- Adams-Stokes I45.9
- akinetic — *see* Epilepsy, generalized, specified NEC
- angina — *see* Angina
- atonic — *see* Epilepsy, generalized, specified NEC
- benign shuddering G25.83
- cataleptic — *see* Catalepsy
- coronary — *see* Infarct, myocardium
- cyanotic, newborn P28.2
- drop NEC R55
- epileptic — *see* Epilepsy
- heart — *see* infarct, myocardium
- hysterical F44.9
- jacksonian — *see* Epilepsy, localization-related, symptomatic, with simple partial seizures
- myocardium, myocardial — *see* Infarct, myocardium
- myoclonic — *see* Epilepsy, generalized, specified NEC
- panic F41.0
- psychomotor — *see* Epilepsy, localization-related, symptomatic, with complex partial seizures
- salaam — *see* Epilepsy, spasms
- schizophreniform, brief F23
- shuddering, benign G25.83
- Stokes-Adams I45.9
- syncope R55
- transient ischemic (TIA) G45.9
  - specified NEC G45.8
- unconsciousness R55
  - hysterical F44.89
- vasomotor R55
- vasovagal (paroxysmal) (idiopathic) R55
- without alteration of consciousness — *see* Epilepsy, localization-related, symptomatic, with simple partial seizures

Attention (to)
  artificial
    opening (of) Z43.9
      digestive tract NEC Z43.4
        colon Z43.3
        ilium Z43.2
        stomach Z43.1
      specified NEC Z43.8
      trachea Z43.0
      urinary tract NEC Z43.6
        cystostomy Z43.5
        nephrostomy Z43.6
        ureterostomy Z43.6
        urethrostomy Z43.6
      vagina Z43.7
    colostomy Z43.3
    cystostomy Z43.5
    deficit disorder or syndrome F98.8
      with hyperactivity — see Disorder, attention-deficit
        hyperactivity
    gastrostomy Z43.1
    ileostomy Z43.2
    jejunostomy Z43.4
    nephrostomy Z43.6
    surgical dressings Z48.01
    sutures Z48.02
    tracheostomy Z43.0
    ureterostomy Z43.6
    urethrostomy Z43.6
Attrition
  gum — see Recession, gingival
  tooth, teeth (excessive) (hard tissues) K03.0
Atypical, atypism (see also condition)
  cells (on cytologcial smear) (endocervical) (endometrial)
    (glandular)
      cervix R87.619
      vagina R87.629
  cervical N87.9
  endometrium N85.9
    hyperplasia N85.00
  parenting situation Z62.9
Auditory — see condition
Aujeszky's disease B33.8
Aurantiasis, cutis E67.1
Auricle, auricular (see also condition)
  cervical Q18.2
Auriculotemporal syndrome G50.8
Austin Flint murmur (aortic insufficiency) I35.1
Australian
  Q fever A78
  X disease A83.4
Autism, autistic (childhood) (infantile) F84.0
  atypical F84.9
  spectrum disorder F84.0
Autodigestion R68.89
Autoerythrocyte sensitization (syndrome) D69.2
Autographism L50.3
Autoimmune
  disease (systemic) M35.9
  inhibitors to clotting factors D68.311
  lymphoproliferative syndrome [ALPS] D89.82
  thyroiditis E06.3
Autointoxication R68.89
Automatism G93.89
  with temporal sclerosis G93.81
  epileptic — see Epilepsy, localization-related, symp-
    tomatic, with complex partial seizures
  paroxysmal, idiopathic — see Epilepsy, localization-
    related, symptomatic, with complex partial
    seizures
Autonomic, autonomous
  bladder (neurogenic) N31.2
  hysteria seizure F44.5
Autosensitivity, erythrocyte D69.2
Autosensitization, cutaneous L30.2
Autosome — see condition by chromosome involved
Autotopagnosia R48.1
Autotoxemia R68.89
Autumn — see condition
Avellis' syndrome G46.8
Aversion
  oral R63.3
    newborn P92.- ☑
    nonorganic origin F98.2 ☑
  sexual F52.1
Aviator's
  disease or sickness — see Effect, adverse, high altitude
  ear T70.0 ☑

Avitaminosis (multiple) (see also Deficiency, vitamin)
  E56.9
  B E53.9
    with
      beriberi E51.11
      pellagra E52
  B2 E53.0
  B6 E53.1
  B12 E53.8
  D E55.9
    with rickets E55.0
  G E53.0
  K E56.1
  nicotinic acid E52
AVNRT (atrioventricular nodal re-entrant tachycardia)
  I47.1
AVRT (atrioventricular nodal re-entrant tachycardia) I47.1
Avulsion (traumatic)
  blood vessel — see Injury, blood vessel
  bone — see Fracture, by site
  cartilage (see also Dislocation, by site)
    symphyseal (inner), complicating delivery O71.6
  external site other than limb — see Wound, open, by
    site
  eye S05.7- ☑
  head (intracranial)
    external site NEC S08.89 ☑
    scalp S08.0 ☑
  internal organ or site — see Injury, by site
  joint (see also Dislocation, by site)
    capsule — see Sprain, by site
  kidney S37.06- ☑
  ligament — see Sprain, by site
  limb (see also Amputation, traumatic, by site)
    skin and subcutaneous tissue — see Wound, open,
      by site
  muscle — see Injury, muscle
  nerve (root) — see Injury, nerve
  scalp S08.0 ☑
  skin and subcutaneous tissue — see Wound, open, by
    site
  spleen S36.032 ☑
  symphyseal cartilage (inner), complicating delivery
    O71.6
  tendon — see Injury, muscle
  tooth S03.2 ☑
Awareness of heart beat R00.2
Axenfeld's
  anomaly or syndrome Q15.0
  degeneration (calcareous) Q13.4
Axilla, axillary (see also condition)
  breast Q83.1
Axonotmesis — see Injury, nerve
Ayerza's disease or syndrome (pulmonary artery scle-
    rosis with pulmonary hypertension) I27.0
Azoospermia (organic) N46.01
  due to
    drug therapy N46.021
    efferent duct obstruction N46.023
    infection N46.022
    radiation N46.024
    specified cause NEC N46.029
    systemic disease N46.025
Azotemia R79.89
  meaning uremia N19
Azygos
  continuation inferior vena cava Q26.8
  lobe (lung) Q33.1

B

Baastrup's disease — see Kissing spine
Babesiosis B60.0
Babington's disease (familial hemorrhagic telangiecta-
    sia) I78.0
Babinski's syndrome A52.79
Baby
  crying constantly R68.11
  floppy (syndrome) P94.2
Bacillary — see condition
Bacilluria R82.71
Bacillus (see also Infection, bacillus)
  abortus infection A23.1
  anthracis infection A22.9
  coli infection (see also Escherichia coli) B96.20
  Flexner's A03.1

Bacillus — continued
  mallei infection A24.0
  Shiga's A03.0
  suipestifer infection — see Infection, salmonella
Back — see condition
Backache (postural) M54.9
  sacroiliac M53.3
  specified NEC M54.89
Backflow — see Reflux
Backward reading (dyslexia) F81.0
Bacteremia R78.81
  with sepsis — see Sepsis
Bactericholia — see Cholecystitis, acute
Bacterid, bacteride (pustular) L40.3
Bacterium, bacteria, bacterial
  agent NEC, as cause of disease classified elsewhere
    B96.89
  in blood — see Bacteremia
  in urine — see Bacteriuria
Bacteriuria, bacteruria R82.71
  asymptomatic R82.71
Bacteroides
  fragilis, as cause of disease classified elsewhere B96.6
Bad
  heart — see Disease, heart
  trip
    due to drug abuse — see Abuse, drug, hallucinogen
    due to drug dependence — see Dependence, drug,
      hallucinogen
Baelz's disease (cheilitis glandularis apostematosa) K13.0
Baerensprung's disease (eczema marginatum) B35.6
Bagasse disease or pneumonitis J67.1
Bagassosis J67.1
Baker's cyst — see Cyst, Baker's
Bakwin-Krida syndrome (metaphyseal dysplasia) Q78.5
Balancing side interference M26.56
Balanitis (circinata) (erosiva) (gangrenosa) (phagedenic)
    (vulgaris) N48.1
  amebic A06.82
  candidal B37.42
  due to Haemophilus ducreyi A57
  gonococcal (acute) (chronic) A54.23
  xerotica obliterans N48.0
Balanoposthitis N47.6
  gonococcal (acute) (chronic) A54.23
  ulcerative (specific) A63.8
Balanorrhagia — see Balanitis
Balantidiasis, balantidiosis A07.0
Bald tongue K14.4
Baldness (see also Alopecia)
  male-pattern — see Alopecia, androgenic
Balkan grippe A78
Balloon disease — see Effect, adverse, high altitude
Balo's disease (concentric sclerosis) G37.5
Bamberger-Marie disease — see Osteoarthropathy,
    hypertrophic, specified type NEC
Bancroft's filariasis B74.0
Band(s)
  adhesive — see Adhesions, peritoneum
  anomalous or congenital (see also Anomaly, by site)
    heart (atrial) (ventricular) Q24.8
    intestine Q43.3
    omentum Q43.3
  cervix N88.1
  constricting, congenital Q79.8
  gallbladder (congenital) Q44.1
  intestinal (adhesive) — see Adhesions, peritoneum
  obstructive
    intestine K56.50
      complete K56.52
      incomplete K56.51
      partial K56.51
    peritoneum K56.50
      complete K56.52
      incomplete K56.51
      partial K56.51
  periappendiceal, congenital Q43.3
  peritoneal (adhesive) — see Adhesions, peritoneum
  uterus N73.6
    internal N85.6
  vagina N89.5
Bandemia D72.825
Bandl's ring (contraction), complicating delivery O62.4
Bangkok hemorrhagic fever A91
Bang's disease (brucella abortus) A23.1
Bankruptcy, anxiety concerning Z59.8
Bannister's disease T78.3 ☑

Bannister's disease — *continued*
  hereditary D84.1
Banti's disease or syndrome (with cirrhosis) (with portal hypertension) K76.6
Bar, median, prostate — *see* Enlargement, enlarged, prostate
Barcoo disease or rot — *see* Ulcer, skin
Barlow's disease E54
Barodontalgia T70.29 ☑
Baron Münchausen syndrome — *see* Disorder, factitious
Barosinusitis T70.1 ☑
Barotitis T70.0 ☑
Barotrauma T70.29 ☑
  odontalgia T70.29 ☑
  otitic T70.0 ☑
  sinus T70.1 ☑
Barraquer (-Simons) **disease or syndrome** (progressive lipodystrophy) E88.1
Barré-Guillain disease or syndrome G61.0
Barrel chest M95.4
Barré-Liéou syndrome (posterior cervical sympathetic) M53.0
Barrett's
  disease — *see* Barrett's, esophagus
  esophagus K22.70
    with dysplasia K22.719
      high grade K22.711
      low grade K22.710
    without dysplasia K22.70
  syndrome — *see* Barrett's, esophagus
  ulcer K22.10
    with bleeding K22.11
    without bleeding K22.10
Bársony (-Polgár) (-Teschendorf) **syndrome** (corkscrew esophagus) K22.4
Barth syndrome E78.71
Bartholinitis (suppurating) N75.8
  gonococcal (acute) (chronic) (with abscess) A54.1
Bartonellosis A44.9
  cutaneous A44.1
  mucocutaneous A44.1
  specified NEC A44.8
  systemic A44.0
Barton's fracture S52.56- ☑
Bartter's syndrome E26.81
Basal — *see* condition
Basan's (hidrotic) ectodermal dysplasia Q82.4
Baseball finger — *see* Dislocation, finger
Basedow's disease (exophthalmic goiter) — *see* Hyperthyroidism, with, goiter
Basic — *see* condition
Basilar — *see* condition
Bason's (hidrotic) ectodermal dysplasia Q82.4
Basopenia — *see* Agranulocytosis
Basophilia D72.824
Basophilism (cortico-adrenal) (Cushing's) (pituitary) E24.0
Bassen-Kornzweig disease or syndrome E78.6
Bat ear Q17.5
Bateman's
  disease B08.1
  purpura (senile) D69.2
Bathing cramp T75.1 ☑
Bathophobia F40.248
Batten (-Mayou) **disease** E75.4
  retina E75.4 [H36]
Batten-Steinert syndrome G71.11
Battered — *see* Maltreatment
Battey Mycobacterium infection A31.0
Battle exhaustion F43.0
Battledore placenta O43.19- ☑
Baumgarten-Cruveilhier cirrhosis, disease or syndrome K74.69
Bauxite fibrosis (of lung) J63.1
Bayle's disease (general paresis) A52.17
Bazin's disease (primary) (tuberculous) A18.4
Beach ear — *see* Swimmer's, ear
Beaded hair (congenital) Q84.1
Béal conjunctivitis or syndrome B30.2
Beard's disease (neurasthenia) F48.8
Beat(s)
  atrial, premature I49.1
  ectopic I49.49
  elbow — *see* Bursitis, elbow
  escaped, heart I49.49
  hand — *see* Bursitis, hand
  knee — *see* Bursitis, knee

Beat(s) — *continued*
  premature I49.40
    atrial I49.1
    auricular I49.1
    supraventricular I49.1
Beau's
  disease or syndrome — *see* Degeneration, myocardial
  lines (transverse furrows on fingernails) L60.4
Bechterev's syndrome — *see* Spondylitis, ankylosing
Becker's
  cardiomyopathy I42.8
  disease
    idiopathic mural endomyocardial disease I42.3
    myotonia congenita, recessive form G71.12
  dystrophy G71.01
  pigmented hairy nevus D22.5
Beck's syndrome (anterior spinal artery occlusion) I65.8
Beckwith-Wiedemann syndrome Q87.3
Bed confinement status Z74.01
Bed sore — *see* Ulcer, pressure, by site
Bedbug bite(s) — *see* Bite(s), by site, superficial, insect
Bedclothes, asphyxiation or suffocation by — *see* Asphyxia, traumatic, due to, mechanical, trapped
Bednar's
  aphthae K12.0
  tumor — *see* Neoplasm, malignant, by site
Bedridden Z74.01
Bedsore — *see* Ulcer, pressure, by site
Bedwetting — *see* Enuresis
Bee sting (with allergic or anaphylactic shock) — *see* Toxicity, venom, arthropod, bee
Beer drinker's heart (disease) I42.6
Begbie's disease (exophthalmic goiter) — *see* Hyperthyroidism, with, goiter
Behavior
  antisocial
    adult Z72.811
    child or adolescent Z72.810
  disorder, disturbance — *see* Disorder, conduct
  disruptive — *see* Disorder, conduct
  drug seeking Z76.5
  inexplicable R46.2
  marked evasiveness R46.5
  obsessive-compulsive R46.81
  overactivity R46.3
  poor responsiveness R46.4
  self-damaging (life-style) Z72.89
  sleep-incompatible Z72.821
  slowness R46.4
  specified NEC R46.89
  strange (and inexplicable) R46.2
  suspiciousness R46.5
  type A pattern Z73.1
  undue concern or preoccupation with stressful events R46.6
  verbosity and circumstantial detail obscuring reason for contact R46.7
Behçet's disease or syndrome M35.2
Behr's disease — *see* Degeneration, macula
Beigel's disease or morbus (white piedra) B36.2
Bejel A65
Bekhterev's syndrome — *see* Spondylitis, ankylosing
Belching — *see* Eructation
Bell's
  mania F30.8
  palsy, paralysis G51.0
    infant or newborn P11.3
  spasm G51.3- ☑
Bence Jones albuminuria or proteinuria NEC R80.3
Bends T70.3 ☑
Benedikt's paralysis or syndrome G46.3
Benign (*see also* condition)
  prostatic hyperplasia — *see* Hyperplasia, prostate
Bennett's fracture (displaced) S62.21- ☑
Benson's disease — *see* Deposit, crystalline
Bent
  back (hysterical) F44.4
  nose M95.0
    congenital Q67.4
Bereavement (uncomplicated) Z63.4
Bergeron's disease (hysterical chorea) F44.4
Berger's disease — *see* Nephropathy, IgA
Beriberi (dry) E51.11
  heart (disease) E51.12
  polyneuropathy E51.11
  wet E51.12
    involving circulatory system E51.11

Berlin's disease or edema (traumatic) S05.8X- ☑
Berlock (berloque) **dermatitis** L56.2
Bernard-Horner syndrome G90.2
Bernard-Soulier disease or thrombopathia D69.1
Bernhardt (-Roth) **disease** — *see* Mononeuropathy, lower limb, meralgia paresthetica
Bernheim's syndrome — *see* Failure, heart, right
Bertielliasis B71.8
Berylliosis (lung) J63.2
Besnier-Boeck (-Schaumann) **disease** — *see* Sarcoidosis
Besnier's
  lupus pernio D86.3
  prurigo L20.0
Bestiality F65.89
Best's disease H35.50
Betalipoproteinemia, broad or floating E78.2
Beta-mercaptolactate-cysteine disulfiduria E72.09
Betting and gambling Z72.6
  pathological (compulsive) F63.0
Bezoar T18.9 ☑
  intestine T18.3 ☑
  stomach T18.2 ☑
Bezold's abscess — *see* Mastoiditis, acute
Bianchi's syndrome R48.8
Bicornate or bicornis uterus Q51.3
  in pregnancy or childbirth O34.00
    causing obstructed labor O65.5
Bicuspid aortic valve Q23.1
Biedl-Bardet syndrome Q87.89
Bielschowsky (-Jansky) disease E75.4
Biermer's (pernicious) anemia or disease D51.0
Biett's disease L93.0
Bifid (congenital)
  apex, heart Q24.8
  clitoris Q52.6
  kidney Q63.8
  nose Q30.2
  patella Q74.1
  scrotum Q55.29
  toe NEC Q74.2
  tongue Q38.3
  ureter Q62.8
  uterus Q51.3
  uvula Q35.7
Biforis uterus (suprasimplex) Q51.3
Bifurcation (congenital)
  gallbladder Q44.1
  kidney pelvis Q63.8
  renal pelvis Q63.8
  rib Q76.6
  tongue, congenital Q38.3
  trachea Q32.1
  ureter Q62.8
  urethra Q64.74
  vertebra Q76.49
Big spleen syndrome D73.1
Bigeminal pulse R00.8
Bilateral — *see* condition
Bile
  duct — *see* condition
  pigments in urine R82.2
Bilharziasis (*see also* Schistosomiasis)
  chyluria B65.0
  cutaneous B65.3
  galacturia B65.0
  hematochyluria B65.0
  intestinal B65.1
  lipemia B65.9
  lipuria B65.0
  oriental B65.2
  piarhemia B65.9
  pulmonary NOS B65.9 [J99]
    pneumonia B65.9 [J17]
  tropical hematuria B65.0
  vesical B65.0
Biliary — *see* condition
Bilirubin metabolism disorder E80.7
  specified NEC E80.6
Bilirubinemia, familial nonhemolytic E80.4
Bilirubinuria R82.2
Biliuria R82.2
Bilocular stomach K31.2
Binswanger's disease I67.3
Biparta, bipartite
  carpal scaphoid Q74.0
  patella Q74.1
  vagina Q52.10

☑ **Additional Character Required** — Refer to the Tabular List for Character Selection   ▽ Subterms under main terms may continue to next column or page

Bird
  face Q75.8
  fancier's disease or lung J67.2
Birth
  complications in mother — *see* Delivery, complicated
  compression during NOS P15.9
  defect — *see* Anomaly
  immature (less than 37 completed weeks) — *see* Preterm, newborn
    extremely (less than 28 completed weeks) — *see* Immaturity, extreme
  inattention, at or after — *see* Maltreatment, child, neglect
  injury NOS P15.9
    basal ganglia P11.1
    brachial plexus NEC P14.3
    brain (compression) (pressure) P11.2
    central nervous system NOS P11.9
    cerebellum P11.1
    cerebral hemorrhage P10.1
    external genitalia P15.5
    eye P15.3
    face P15.4
    fracture
      bone P13.9
        specified NEC P13.8
      clavicle P13.4
      femur P13.2
      humerus P13.3
      long bone, except femur P13.3
      radius and ulna P13.3
      skull P13.0
      spine P11.5
      tibia and fibula P13.3
    intracranial P11.2
      laceration or hemorrhage P10.9
        specified NEC P10.8
    intraventricular hemorrhage P10.2
    laceration
      brain P10.1
      by scalpel P15.8
      peripheral nerve P14.9
    liver P15.0
    meninges
      brain P11.1
      spinal cord P11.5
    nerve
      brachial plexus P14.3
      cranial NEC (except facial) P11.4
      facial P11.3
      peripheral P14.9
      phrenic (paralysis) P14.2
    paralysis
      facial nerve P11.3
      spinal P11.5
    penis P15.5
    rupture
      spinal cord P11.5
    scalp P12.9
    scalpel wound P15.8
    scrotum P15.5
    skull NEC P13.1
      fracture P13.0
    specified type NEC P15.8
    spinal cord P11.5
    spine P11.5
    spleen P15.1
    sternomastoid (hematoma) P15.2
    subarachnoid hemorrhage P10.3
    subcutaneous fat necrosis P15.6
    subdural hemorrhage P10.0
    tentorial tear P10.4
    testes P15.5
    vulva P15.5
  lack of care, at or after — *see* Maltreatment, child, neglect
  neglect, at or after — *see* Maltreatment, child, neglect
  palsy or paralysis, newborn, NOS (birth injury) P14.9
  premature (infant) — *see* Preterm, newborn
  shock, newborn P96.89
  trauma — *see* Birth, injury
  weight
    low (2499 grams or less) — *see* Low, birthweight
      extremely (999 grams or less) — *see* Low, birthweight, extreme
    4000 grams to 4499 grams P08.1
    4500 grams or more P08.0
Birthmark Q82.5

Birt-Hogg-Dube syndrome Q87.89
Bisalbuminemia E88.09
Biskra's button B55.1
Bite(s) (animal) (human)
  abdomen, abdominal
    wall S31.159 ☑
      with penetration into peritoneal cavity S31.659 ☑
      epigastric region S31.152 ☑
        with penetration into peritoneal cavity S31.652 ☑
      left
        lower quadrant S31.154 ☑
          with penetration into peritoneal cavity S31.654 ☑
        upper quadrant S31.151 ☑
          with penetration into peritoneal cavity S31.651 ☑
      periumbilic region S31.155 ☑
        with penetration into peritoneal cavity S31.655 ☑
      right
        lower quadrant S31.153 ☑
          with penetration into peritoneal cavity S31.653 ☑
        upper quadrant S31.150 ☑
          with penetration into peritoneal cavity S31.650 ☑
      superficial NEC S30.871 ☑
        insect S30.861 ☑
    alveolar (process) — *see* Bite, oral cavity
    amphibian (venomous) — *see* Venom, bite, amphibian
    animal (*see also* Bite, by site)
      venomous — *see* Venom
    ankle S91.05- ☑
      superficial NEC S90.57- ☑
        insect S90.56- ☑
    antecubital space — *see* Bite, elbow
    anus S31.835 ☑
      superficial NEC S30.877 ☑
        insect S30.867 ☑
    arm (upper) S41.15- ☑
      lower — *see* Bite, forearm
      superficial NEC S40.87- ☑
        insect S40.86- ☑
    arthropod NEC — *see* Venom, bite, arthropod
    auditory canal (external) (meatus) — *see* Bite, ear
    auricle, ear — *see* Bite, ear
    axilla — *see* Bite, arm
    back (*see also* Bite, thorax, back)
      lower S31.050 ☑
        with penetration into retroperitoneal space S31.051 ☑
      superficial NEC S30.870 ☑
        insect S30.860 ☑
    bedbug — *see* Bite(s), by site, superficial, insect
    breast S21.05- ☑
      superficial NEC S20.17- ☑
        insect S20.16- ☑
    brow — *see* Bite, head, specified site NEC
    buttock S31.805 ☑
      left S31.825 ☑
      right S31.815 ☑
      superficial NEC S30.870 ☑
        insect S30.860 ☑
    calf — *see* Bite, leg
    canaliculus lacrimalis — *see* Bite, eyelid
    canthus, eye — *see* Bite, eyelid
    centipede — *see* Toxicity, venom, arthropod, centipede
    cheek (external) S01.45- ☑
      internal — *see* Bite, oral cavity
      superficial NEC S00.87 ☑
        insect S00.86 ☑
    chest wall — *see* Bite, thorax
    chigger B88.0
    chin — *see* Bite, head, specified site NEC
    clitoris — *see* Bite, vulva
    costal region — *see* Bite, thorax
    digit(s)
      hand — *see* Bite, finger
      toe — *see* Bite, toe
    ear (canal) (external) S01.35- ☑
      superficial NEC S00.47- ☑
        insect S00.46- ☑
    elbow S51.05- ☑
      superficial NEC S50.37- ☑

Bite(s) — *continued*
  elbow — *continued*
    superficial — *continued*
      insect S50.36- ☑
  epididymis — *see* Bite, testis
  epigastric region — *see* Bite, abdomen
  epiglottis — *see* Bite, neck, specified site NEC
  esophagus, cervical S11.25 ☑
    superficial NEC S10.17 ☑
      insect S10.16 ☑
  eyebrow — *see* Bite, eyelid
  eyelid S01.15- ☑
    superficial NEC S00.27- ☑
      insect S00.26- ☑
  face NEC — *see* Bite, head, specified site NEC
  finger(s) S61.259 ☑
    with
      damage to nail S61.359 ☑
    index S61.258 ☑
      with
        damage to nail S61.358 ☑
      left S61.251 ☑
        with
          damage to nail S61.351 ☑
      right S61.250 ☑
        with
          damage to nail S61.350 ☑
      superficial NEC S60.478 ☑
        insect S60.46- ☑
    little S61.25- ☑
      with
        damage to nail S61.35- ☑
      superficial NEC S60.47- ☑
        insect S60.46- ☑
    middle S61.25- ☑
      with
        damage to nail S61.35- ☑
      superficial NEC S60.47- ☑
        insect S60.46- ☑
    ring S61.25- ☑
      with
        damage to nail S61.35- ☑
      superficial NEC S60.47- ☑
        insect S60.46- ☑
    superficial NEC S60.479 ☑
      insect S60.469 ☑
    thumb — *see* Bite, thumb
  flank — *see* Bite, abdomen, wall
  flea — *see* Bite, by site, superficial, insect
  foot (except toe(s) alone) S91.35- ☑
    superficial NEC S90.87- ☑
      insect S90.86- ☑
    toe — *see* Bite, toe
  forearm S51.85- ☑
    elbow only — *see* Bite, elbow
    superficial NEC S50.87- ☑
      insect S50.86- ☑
  forehead — *see* Bite, head, specified site NEC
  genital organs, external
    female S31.552 ☑
      superficial NEC S30.876 ☑
        insect S30.866 ☑
      vagina and vulva — *see* Bite, vulva
    male S31.551 ☑
      penis — *see* Bite, penis
      scrotum — *see* Bite, scrotum
      superficial NEC S30.875 ☑
        insect S30.865 ☑
      testes — *see* Bite, testis
  groin — *see* Bite, abdomen, wall
  gum — *see* Bite, oral cavity
  hand S61.45- ☑
    finger — *see* Bite, finger
    superficial NEC S60.57- ☑
      insect S60.56- ☑
    thumb — *see* Bite, thumb
  head S01.95 ☑
    cheek — *see* Bite, cheek
    ear — *see* Bite, ear
    eyelid — *see* Bite, eyelid
    lip — *see* Bite, lip
    nose — *see* Bite, nose
    oral cavity — *see* Bite, oral cavity
    scalp — *see* Bite, scalp
    specified site NEC S01.85 ☑
      superficial NEC S00.87 ☑

◢ Subterms under main terms may continue to next column or page   ☑ Additional Character Required — Refer to the Tabular List for Character Selection   37

Bird — Bite

Bite(s) — *continued*
  head — *continued*
    specified site — *continued*
      superficial — *continued*
        insect S00.86 ☑
      superficial NEC S00.97 ☑
        insect S00.96 ☑
    temporomandibular area — *see* Bite, cheek
  heel — *see* Bite, foot
  hip S71.05- ☑
    superficial NEC S70.27- ☑
      insect S70.26- ☑
  hymen S31.45 ☑
  hypochondrium — *see* Bite, abdomen, wall
  hypogastric region — *see* Bite, abdomen, wall
  inguinal region — *see* Bite, abdomen, wall
  insect — *see* Bite, by site, superficial, insect
  instep — *see* Bite, foot
  interscapular region — *see* Bite, thorax, back
  jaw — *see* Bite, head, specified site NEC
  knee S81.05- ☑
    superficial NEC S80.27- ☑
      insect S80.26- ☑
  labium (majus) (minus) — *see* Bite, vulva
  lacrimal duct — *see* Bite, eyelid
  larynx S11.015 ☑
    superficial NEC S10.17 ☑
      insect S10.16 ☑
  leg (lower) S81.85- ☑
    ankle — *see* Bite, ankle
    foot — *see* Bite, foot
    knee — *see* Bite, knee
    superficial NEC S80.87- ☑
      insect S80.86- ☑
    toe — *see* Bite, toe
    upper — *see* Bite, thigh
  lip S01.551 ☑
    superficial NEC S00.571 ☑
      insect S00.561 ☑
  lizard (venomous) — *see* Venom, bite, reptile
  loin — *see* Bite, abdomen, wall
  lower back — *see* Bite, back, lower
  lumbar region — *see* Bite, back, lower
  malar region — *see* Bite, head, specified site NEC
  mammary — *see* Bite, breast
  marine animals (venomous) — *see* Toxicity, venom, marine animal
  mastoid region — *see* Bite, head, specified site NEC
  mouth — *see* Bite, oral cavity
  nail
    finger — *see* Bite, finger
    toe — *see* Bite, toe
  nape — *see* Bite, neck, specified site NEC
  nasal (septum) (sinus) — *see* Bite, nose
  nasopharynx — *see* Bite, head, specified site NEC
  neck S11.95 ☑
    involving
      cervical esophagus — *see* Bite, esophagus, cervical
      larynx — *see* Bite, larynx
      pharynx — *see* Bite, pharynx
      thyroid gland S11.15 ☑
      trachea — *see* Bite, trachea
    specified site NEC S11.85 ☑
      superficial NEC S10.87 ☑
        insect S10.86 ☑
    superficial NEC S10.97 ☑
      insect S10.96 ☑
    throat S11.85 ☑
      superficial NEC S10.17 ☑
        insect S10.16 ☑
  nose (septum) (sinus) S01.25 ☑
    superficial NEC S00.37 ☑
      insect S00.36 ☑
  occipital region — *see* Bite, scalp
  oral cavity S01.552 ☑
    superficial NEC S00.572 ☑
      insect S00.562 ☑
  orbital region — *see* Bite, eyelid
  palate — *see* Bite, oral cavity
  palm — *see* Bite, hand
  parietal region — *see* Bite, scalp
  pelvis S31.050 ☑
    with penetration into retroperitoneal space S31.051 ☑
    superficial NEC S30.870 ☑

Bite(s) — *continued*
  pelvis — *continued*
    superficial — *continued*
      insect S30.860 ☑
  penis S31.25 ☑
    superficial NEC S30.872 ☑
      insect S30.862 ☑
  perineum
    female — *see* Bite, vulva
    male — *see* Bite, pelvis
  periocular area (with or without lacrimal passages) — *see* Bite, eyelid
  phalanges
    finger — *see* Bite, finger
    toe — *see* Bite, toe
  pharynx S11.25 ☑
    superficial NEC S10.17 ☑
      insect S10.16 ☑
  pinna — *see* Bite, ear
  poisonous — *see* Venom
  popliteal space — *see* Bite, knee
  prepuce — *see* Bite, penis
  pubic region — *see* Bite, abdomen, wall
  rectovaginal septum — *see* Bite, vulva
  red bug B88.0
  reptile NEC (*see also* Venom, bite, reptile)
    nonvenomous — *see* Bite, by site
    snake — *see* Venom, bite, snake
  sacral region — *see* Bite, back, lower
  sacroiliac region — *see* Bite, back, lower
  salivary gland — *see* Bite, oral cavity
  scalp S01.05 ☑
    superficial NEC S00.07 ☑
      insect S00.06 ☑
  scapular region — *see* Bite, shoulder
  scrotum S31.35 ☑
    superficial NEC S30.873 ☑
      insect S30.863 ☑
  sea-snake (venomous) — *see* Toxicity, venom, snake, sea snake
  shin — *see* Bite, leg
  shoulder S41.05- ☑
    superficial NEC S40.27- ☑
      insect S40.26- ☑
  snake (*see also* Venom, bite, snake)
    nonvenomous — *see* Bite, by site
  spermatic cord — *see* Bite, testis
  spider (venomous) — *see* Toxicity, venom, spider
    nonvenomous — *see* Bite, by site, superficial, insect
  sternal region — *see* Bite, thorax, front
  submaxillary region — *see* Bite, head, specified site NEC
  submental region — *see* Bite, head, specified site NEC
  subungual
    finger(s) — *see* Bite, finger
    toe — *see* Bite, toe
  superficial — *see* Bite, by site, superficial
  supraclavicular fossa S11.85 ☑
  supraorbital — *see* Bite, head, specified site NEC
  temple, temporal region — *see* Bite, head, specified site NEC
  temporomandibular area — *see* Bite, cheek
  testis S31.35 ☑
    superficial NEC S30.873 ☑
      insect S30.863 ☑
  thigh S71.15- ☑
    superficial NEC S70.37- ☑
      insect S70.36- ☑
  thorax, thoracic (wall) S21.95 ☑
    back S21.25- ☑
      with penetration into thoracic cavity S21.45- ☑
    breast — *see* Bite, breast
    front S21.15- ☑
      with penetration into thoracic cavity S21.35- ☑
    superficial NEC S20.97 ☑
      back S20.47- ☑
      front S20.37- ☑
      insect S20.96 ☑
        back S20.46- ☑
        front S20.36- ☑
  throat — *see* Bite, neck, throat
  thumb S61.05- ☑
    with
      damage to nail S61.15- ☑
    superficial NEC S60.37- ☑
      insect S60.36- ☑

Bite(s) — *continued*
  thyroid S11.15 ☑
    superficial NEC S10.87 ☑
      insect S10.86 ☑
  toe(s) S91.15- ☑
    with
      damage to nail S91.25- ☑
    great S91.15- ☑
      with
        damage to nail S91.25- ☑
    lesser S91.15- ☑
      with
        damage to nail S91.25- ☑
    superficial NEC S90.47- ☑
      great S90.47- ☑
      insect S90.46- ☑
        great S90.46- ☑
  tongue S01.552 ☑
  trachea S11.025 ☑
    superficial NEC S10.17 ☑
      insect S10.16 ☑
  tunica vaginalis — *see* Bite, testis
  tympanum, tympanic membrane — *see* Bite, ear
  umbilical region S31.155 ☑
  uvula — *see* Bite, oral cavity
  vagina — *see* Bite, vulva
  venomous — *see* Venom
  vocal cords S11.035 ☑
    superficial NEC S10.17 ☑
      insect S10.16 ☑
  vulva S31.45 ☑
    superficial NEC S30.874 ☑
      insect S30.864 ☑
  wrist S61.55- ☑
    superficial NEC S60.87- ☑
      insect S60.86- ☑
Biting, cheek or lip K13.1
Biventricular failure (heart) I50.82
Björck (-Thorson) **syndrome** (malignant carcinoid) E34.0
Black
  death A20.9
  eye S00.1- ☑
  hairy tongue K14.3
  heel (foot) S90.3- ☑
  lung (disease) J60
  palm (hand) S60.22- ☑
Blackfan-Diamond anemia or syndrome (congenital hypoplastic anemia) D61.01
Blackhead L70.0
Blackout R55
Bladder — *see* condition
Blast (air) (hydraulic) (immersion) (underwater)
  blindness S05.8X- ☑
  injury
    abdomen or thorax — *see* Injury, by site
    ear (acoustic nerve trauma) — *see* Injury, nerve, acoustic, specified type NEC
    syndrome NEC T70.8 ☑
Blastoma — *see* Neoplasm, malignant, by site
  pulmonary — *see* Neoplasm, lung, malignant
Blastomycosis, blastomycotic B40.9
  Brazilian — *see* Paracoccidioidomycosis
  cutaneous B40.3
  disseminated B40.7
  European — *see* Cryptococcosis
  generalized B40.7
  keloidal B48.0
  North American B40.9
  primary pulmonary B40.0
  pulmonary B40.2
    acute B40.0
    chronic B40.1
  skin B40.3
  South American — *see* Paracoccidioidomycosis
  specified NEC B40.89
Bleb(s) R23.8
  emphysematous (lung) (solitary) J43.9
  endophthalmitis H59.43
  filtering (vitreous), after glaucoma surgery Z98.83
  inflamed (infected), postprocedural H59.40
    stage 1 H59.41
    stage 2 H59.42
    stage 3 H59.43
  lung (ruptured) J43.9
    congenital — *see* Atelectasis
    newborn P25.8
  subpleural (emphysematous) J43.9

38   ☑ **Additional Character Required** — **Refer to the Tabular List for Character Selection**   ▽ **Subterms under main terms may continue to next column or page**

Bite — Bleb

Blebitis, postprocedural H59.40
  stage 1 H59.41
  stage 2 H59.42
  stage 3 H59.43
Bleeder (familial) (hereditary) — see Hemophilia
Bleeding (see also Hemorrhage)
  anal K62.5
  anovulatory N97.0
  atonic, following delivery O72.1
  capillary I78.8
    puerperal O72.2
  contact (postcoital) N93.0
  due to uterine subinvolution N85.3
  ear — see Otorrhagia
  excessive, associated with menopausal onset N92.4
  familial — see Defect, coagulation
  following intercourse N93.0
  gastrointestinal K92.2
  hemorrhoids — see Hemorrhoids
  intermenstrual (regular) N92.3
    irregular N92.1
  intraoperative — see Complication, intraoperative, hemorrhage
  irregular N92.6
  menopausal N92.4
  newborn, intraventricular — see Newborn, affected by, hemorrhage, intraventricular
  nipple N64.59
  nose R04.0
  ovulation N92.3
  postclimacteric N95.0
  postcoital N93.0
  postmenopausal N95.0
  postoperative — see Complication, postprocedural, hemorrhage
  preclimacteric N92.4
  pre-pubertal vaginal N93.1
  puberty (excessive, with onset of menstrual periods) N92.2
  rectum, rectal K62.5
    newborn P54.2
  tendencies — see Defect, coagulation
  throat R04.1
  tooth socket (post-extraction) K91.840
  umbilical stump P51.9
  uterus, uterine NEC N93.9
    climacteric N92.4
    dysfunctional or functional N93.8
    menopausal N92.4
    preclimacteric or premenopausal N92.4
    unrelated to menstrual cycle N93.9
  vagina, vaginal (abnormal) N93.9
    dysfunctional or functional N93.8
    newborn P54.6
    pre-pubertal N93.1
  vicarious N94.89
Blennorrhagia, blennorrhagic — see Gonorrhea
Blennorrhea (acute) (chronic) (see also Gonorrhea)
  inclusion (neonatal) (newborn) P39.1
  lower genitourinary tract (gonococcal) A54.00
  neonatorum (gonococcal ophthalmia) A54.31
Blepharelosis — see Entropion
Blepharitis (angularis) (ciliaris) (eyelid) (marginal) (nonulcerative) H01.009
  herpes zoster B02.39
  left H01.006
    lower H01.005
    upper H01.004
    upper and lower H01.00B
  right H01.003
    lower H01.002
    upper H01.001
    upper and lower H01.00A
  squamous H01.029
    left H01.026
      lower H01.025
      upper H01.024
      upper and lower H01.02B
    right H01.023
      lower H01.022
      upper H01.021
      upper and lower H01.02A
  ulcerative H01.019
    left H01.016
      lower H01.015
      upper H01.014
      upper and lower H01.01B
    right H01.013

Blepharitis — continued
  ulcerative — continued
    right — continued
      lower H01.012
      upper H01.011
      upper and lower H01.01A
Blepharochalasis H02.30
  congenital Q10.0
  left H02.36
    lower H02.35
    upper H02.34
  right H02.33
    lower H02.32
    upper H02.31
Blepharoclonus H02.59
Blepharoconjunctivitis H10.50- ☑
  angular H10.52- ☑
  contact H10.53- ☑
  ligneous H10.51- ☑
Blepharophimosis (eyelid) H02.529
  congenital Q10.3
  left H02.526
    lower H02.525
    upper H02.524
  right H02.523
    lower H02.522
    upper H02.521
Blepharoptosis H02.40- ☑
  congenital Q10.0
  mechanical H02.41- ☑
  myogenic H02.42- ☑
  neurogenic H02.43- ☑
  paralytic H02.43- ☑
Blepharopyorrhea, gonococcal A54.39
Blepharospasm G24.5
  drug induced G24.01
Blighted ovum O02.0
Blind (see also Blindness)
  bronchus (congenital) Q32.4
  loop syndrome K90.2
    congenital Q43.8
  sac, fallopian tube (congenital) Q50.6
  spot, enlarged — see Defect, visual field, localized, scotoma, blind spot area
  tract or tube, congenital NEC — see Atresia, by site
Blindness (acquired) (congenital) (both eyes) H54.0X- ☑
  blast S05.8X- ☑
  color — see Deficiency, color vision
  concussion S05.8X- ☑
  cortical H47.619
    left brain H47.612
    right brain H47.611
  day H53.11
  due to injury (current episode) S05.9- ☑
    sequelae — code to injury with seventh character S
  eclipse (total) — see Retinopathy, solar
  emotional (hysterical) F44.6
  face H53.16
  hysterical F44.6
  legal (both eyes) (USA definition) H54.8
  mind R48.8
  night H53.60
    abnormal dark adaptation curve H53.61
    acquired H53.62
    congenital H53.63
    specified type NEC H53.69
    vitamin A deficiency E50.5
  one eye (other eye normal) H54.40
    left (normal vision on right) H54.42- ☑
      low vision on right H54.12- ☑
    low vision, other eye H54.10
    right (normal vision on left) H54.41- ☑
      low vision on left H54.11- ☑
  psychic R48.8
  river B73.01
  snow — see Photokeratitis
  sun, solar — see Retinopathy, solar
  transient — see Disturbance, vision, subjective, loss, transient
  traumatic (current episode) S05.9- ☑
  word (developmental) F81.0
    acquired R48.0
    secondary to organic lesion R48.0
Blister (nonthermal)
  abdominal wall S30.821 ☑
  alveolar process S00.522 ☑

Blister — continued
  ankle S90.52- ☑
  antecubital space — see Blister, elbow
  anus S30.827 ☑
  arm (upper) S40.82- ☑
  auditory canal — see Blister, ear
  auricle — see Blister, ear
  axilla — see Blister, arm
  back, lower S30.820 ☑
  beetle dermatitis L24.89
  breast S20.12- ☑
  brow S00.82 ☑
  calf — see Blister, leg
  canthus — see Blister, eyelid
  cheek S00.82 ☑
    internal S00.522 ☑
  chest wall — see Blister, thorax
  chin S00.82 ☑
  costal region — see Blister, thorax
  digit(s)
    foot — see Blister, toe
    hand — see Blister, finger
  due to burn — see Burn, by site, second degree
  ear S00.42- ☑
  elbow S50.32- ☑
  epiglottis S10.12 ☑
  esophagus, cervical S10.12 ☑
  eyebrow — see Blister, eyelid
  eyelid S00.22- ☑
  face S00.82 ☑
  fever B00.1
  finger(s) S60.429 ☑
    index S60.42- ☑
    little S60.42- ☑
    middle S60.42- ☑
    ring S60.42- ☑
  foot (except toe(s) alone) S90.82- ☑
    toe — see Blister, toe
  forearm S50.82- ☑
    elbow only — see Blister, elbow
  forehead S00.82 ☑
  fracture — omit code
  genital organ
    female S30.826 ☑
    male S30.825 ☑
  gum S00.522 ☑
  hand S60.52- ☑
  head S00.92 ☑
    ear — see Blister, ear
    eyelid — see Blister, eyelid
    lip S00.521 ☑
    nose S00.32 ☑
    oral cavity S00.522 ☑
    scalp S00.02 ☑
    specified site NEC S00.82 ☑
  heel — see Blister, foot
  hip S70.22- ☑
  interscapular region S20.429 ☑
  jaw S00.82 ☑
  knee S80.22- ☑
  larynx S10.12 ☑
  leg (lower) S80.82- ☑
    knee — see Blister, knee
    upper — see Blister, thigh
  lip S00.521 ☑
  malar region S00.82 ☑
  mammary — see Blister, breast
  mastoid region S00.82 ☑
  mouth S00.522 ☑
  multiple, skin, nontraumatic R23.8
  nail
    finger — see Blister, finger
    toe — see Blister, toe
  nasal S00.32 ☑
  neck S10.92 ☑
    specified site NEC S10.82 ☑
    throat S10.12 ☑
  nose S00.32 ☑
  occipital region S00.02 ☑
  oral cavity S00.522 ☑
  orbital region — see Blister, eyelid
  palate S00.522 ☑
  palm — see Blister, hand
  parietal region S00.02 ☑
  pelvis S30.820 ☑
  penis S30.822 ☑

Blister — *continued*
  periocular area — *see* Blister, eyelid
  phalanges
    finger — *see* Blister, finger
    toe — *see* Blister, toe
  pharynx S10.12 ☑
  pinna — *see* Blister, ear
  popliteal space — *see* Blister, knee
  scalp S00.02 ☑
  scapular region — *see* Blister, shoulder
  scrotum S30.823 ☑
  shin — *see* Blister, leg
  shoulder S40.22-
  sternal region S20.329 ☑
  submaxillary region S00.82 ☑
  submental region S00.82 ☑
  subungual
    finger(s) — *see* Blister, finger
    toe(s) — *see* Blister, toe
  supraclavicular fossa S10.82 ☑
  supraorbital S00.82 ☑
  temple S00.82 ☑
  temporal region S00.82 ☑
  testis S30.823 ☑
  thermal — *see* Burn, second degree, by site
  thigh S70.32-
  thorax, thoracic (wall) S20.92 ☑
    back S20.42-
    front S20.32-
  throat S10.12 ☑
  thumb S60.32-
  toe(s) S90.42- ☑
    great S90.42-
  tongue S00.522 ☑
  trachea S10.12 ☑
  tympanum, tympanic membrane — *see* Blister, ear
  upper arm — *see* Blister, arm (upper)
  uvula S00.522 ☑
  vagina S30.824 ☑
  vocal cords S10.12 ☑
  vulva S30.824 ☑
  wrist S60.82- ☑
Bloating R14.0
Bloch-Sulzberger disease or syndrome Q82.3
Block, blocked
  alveolocapillary J84.10
  arborization (heart) I45.5
  arrhythmic I45.9
  atrioventricular (incomplete) (partial) I44.30
    with atrioventricular dissociation I44.2
    complete I44.2
      congenital Q24.6
    congenital Q24.6
    first degree I44.0
    second degree (types I and II) I44.1
    specified NEC I44.39
    third degree I44.2
    types I and II I44.1
  auriculoventricular — *see* Block, atrioventricular
  bifascicular (cardiac) I45.2
  bundle-branch (complete) (false) (incomplete) I45.4
    bilateral I45.2
    left I44.7
      with right bundle branch block I45.2
      hemiblock I44.60
        anterior I44.4
        posterior I44.5
      incomplete I44.7
        with right bundle branch block I45.2
    right I45.10
      with
        left bundle branch block I45.2
        left fascicular block I45.2
      specified NEC I45.19
      Wilson's type I45.19
  cardiac I45.9
  conduction I45.9
    complete I44.2
  fascicular (left) I44.60
    anterior I44.4
    posterior I44.5
    right I45.0
    specified NEC I44.69
  foramen Magendie (acquired) G91.1
    congenital Q03.1
      with spina bifida — *see* Spina bifida, by site, with hydrocephalus

Block, blocked — *continued*
  heart I45.9
    bundle branch I45.4
      bilateral I45.2
    complete (atrioventricular) I44.2
    congenital Q24.6
    first degree (atrioventricular) I44.0
    second degree (atrioventricular) I44.1
    specified type NEC I45.5
    third degree (atrioventricular) I44.2
  hepatic vein I82.0
  intraventricular (nonspecific) I45.4
    bundle branch
      bilateral I45.2
  kidney N28.9
    postcystoscopic or postprocedural N99.0
  Mobitz (types I and II) I44.1
  myocardial — *see* Block, heart
  nodal I45.5
  organ or site, congenital NEC — *see* Atresia, by site
  portal (vein) I81
  second degree (types I and II) I44.1
  sinoatrial I45.5
  sinoauricular I45.5
  third degree I44.2
  trifascicular I45.3
  tubal N97.1
  vein NOS I82.90
  Wenckebach (types I and II) I44.1
Blockage — *see* Obstruction
Blocq's disease F44.4
Blood
  constituents, abnormal R78.9
  disease D75.9
  donor — *see* Donor, blood
  dyscrasia D75.9
    with
      abortion — *see* Abortion, by type, complicated by, hemorrhage
      ectopic pregnancy O08.1
      molar pregnancy O08.1
    following ectopic or molar pregnancy O08.1
    newborn P61.9
    puerperal, postpartum O72.3
  flukes NEC — *see* Schistosomiasis
  in
    feces K92.1
      occult R19.5
    urine — *see* Hematuria
  mole O02.0
  occult in feces R19.5
  pressure
    decreased, due to shock following injury T79.4 ☑
    examination only Z01.30
    fluctuating I99.8
    high — *see* Hypertension
      borderline R03.0
      incidental reading, without diagnosis of hypertension R03.0
    low (*see also* Hypotension)
      incidental reading, without diagnosis of hypotension R03.1
  spitting — *see* Hemoptysis
  staining cornea — *see* Pigmentation, cornea, stromal
  transfusion
    reaction or complication — *see* Complications, transfusion
  type
    A (Rh positive) Z67.10
      Rh negative Z67.11
    AB (Rh positive) Z67.30
      Rh negative Z67.31
    B (Rh positive) Z67.20
      Rh negative Z67.21
    O (Rh positive) Z67.40
      Rh negative Z67.41
    Rh (positive) Z67.90
      negative Z67.91
  vessel rupture — *see* Hemorrhage
  vomiting — *see* Hematemesis
Blood-forming organs, disease D75.9
Bloodgood's disease — *see* Mastopathy, cystic
Bloom (-Machacek)(-Torre) **syndrome** Q82.8
Blount's disease or osteochondrosis — *see* Osteochondrosis, juvenile, tibia
Blue
  baby Q24.9
  diaper syndrome E72.09

Blue — *continued*
  dome cyst (breast) — *see* Cyst, breast
  dot cataract Q12.0
  nevus D22.9
  sclera Q13.5
    with fragility of bone and deafness Q78.0
  toe syndrome I75.02- ☑
Blueness — *see* Cyanosis
Blues, postpartal O90.6
  baby O90.6
Blurring, visual H53.8
Blushing (abnormal) (excessive) R23.2
BMI — *see* Body, mass index
Boarder, hospital NEC Z76.4
  accompanying sick person Z76.3
  healthy infant or child Z76.2
  foundling Z76.1
Bockhart's impetigo L01.02
Bodechtel-Guttman disease (subacute sclerosing panencephalitis) A81.1
Boder-Sedgwick syndrome (ataxia-telangiectasia) G11.3
Body, bodies
  Aschoff's — *see* Myocarditis, rheumatic
  asteroid, vitreous — *see* Deposit, crystalline
  cytoid (retina) — *see* Occlusion, artery, retina
  drusen (degenerative) (macula) (retinal) (*see also* Degeneration, macula, drusen)
    optic disc — *see* Drusen, optic disc
  foreign — *see* Foreign body
  loose
    joint, except knee — *see* Loose, body, joint
      knee M23.4- ☑
    sheath, tendon — *see* Disorder, tendon, specified type NEC
  mass index (BMI)
    adult
      19.9 or less Z68.1
      20.0-20.9 Z68.20
      21.0-21.9 Z68.21
      22.0-22.9 Z68.22
      23.0-23.9 Z68.23
      24.0-24.9 Z68.24
      25.0-25.9 Z68.25
      26.0-26.9 Z68.26
      27.0-27.9 Z68.27
      28.0-28.9 Z68.28
      29.0-29.9 Z68.29
      30.0-30.9 Z68.30
      31.0-31.9 Z68.31
      32.0-32.9 Z68.32
      33.0-33.9 Z68.33
      34.0-34.9 Z68.34
      35.0-35.9 Z68.35
      36.0-36.9 Z68.36
      37.0-37.9 Z68.37
      38.0-38.9 Z68.38
      39.0-39.9 Z68.39
      40.0-44.9 Z68.41
      45.0-49.9 Z68.42
      50.0-59.9 Z68.43
      60.0-69.9 Z68.44
      70 and over Z68.45
    pediatric
      5th percentile to less than 85th percentile for age Z68.52
      85th percentile to less than 95th percentile for age Z68.53
      greater than or equal to ninety-fifth percentile for age Z68.54
      less than fifth percentile for age Z68.51
  Mooser's A75.2
  rice (*see also* Loose, body, joint)
    knee M23.4- ☑
  rocking F98.4
Boeck's
  disease or sarcoid — *see* Sarcoidosis
  lupoid (miliary) D86.3
Boerhaave's syndrome (spontaneous esophageal rupture) K22.3
Boggy
  cervix N88.8
  uterus N85.8
Boil (*see also* Furuncle, by site)
  Aleppo B55.1
  Baghdad B55.1
  Delhi B55.1
  lacrimal
    gland — *see* Dacryoadenitis

☑ **Additional Character Required** — Refer to the Tabular List for Character Selection   ▽ **Subterms under main terms may continue to next column or page**

Boil — *continued*
  lacrimal — *continued*
    passages (duct) (sac) — *see* Inflammation, lacrimal, passages, acute
    Natal B55.1
    orbit, orbital — *see* Abscess, orbit
    tropical B55.1
Bold hives — *see* Urticaria
Bombé, iris — *see* Membrane, pupillary
Bone — *see* condition
Bonnevie-Ullrich syndrome (*see also* Turner's syndrome) Q87.1
Bonnier's syndrome H81.8 ☑
Bonvale dam fever T73.3 ☑
Bony block of joint — *see* Ankylosis
BOOP (bronchiolitis obliterans organized pneumonia) J84.89
Borderline
  diabetes mellitus R73.03
  hypertension R03.0
  osteopenia M85.8- ☑
  pelvis, with obstruction during labor O65.1
  personality F60.3
Borna disease A83.9
Bornholm disease B33.0
Boston exanthem A88.0
Botalli, ductus (patent) (persistent) Q25.0
Bothriocephalus latus infestation B70.0
Botulism (foodborne intoxication) A05.1
  infant A48.51
  non-foodborne A48.52
  wound A48.52
Bouba — *see* Yaws
Bouchard's nodes (with arthropathy) M15.2
Bouffée délirante F23
Bouillaud's disease or syndrome (rheumatic heart disease) I01.9
Bourneville's disease Q85.1
Boutonniere deformity (finger) — *see* Deformity, finger, boutonniere
Bouveret (-Hoffmann) **syndrome** (paroxysmal tachycardia) I47.9
Bovine heart — *see* Hypertrophy, cardiac
Bowel — *see* condition
Bowen's
  dermatosis (precancerous) — *see* Neoplasm, skin, in situ
  disease — *see* Neoplasm, skin, in situ
  epithelioma — *see* Neoplasm, skin, in situ
  type
    epidermoid carcinoma-in-situ — *see* Neoplasm, skin, in situ
    intraepidermal squamous cell carcinoma — *see* Neoplasm, skin, in situ
Bowing
  femur (*see also* Deformity, limb, specified type NEC, thigh)
    congenital Q68.3
  fibula (*see also* Deformity, limb, specified type NEC, lower leg)
    congenital Q68.4
  forearm — *see* Deformity, limb, specified type NEC, forearm
  leg(s), long bones, congenital Q68.5
  radius — *see* Deformity, limb, specified type NEC, forearm
  tibia (*see also* Deformity, limb, specified type NEC, lower leg)
    congenital Q68.4
Bowleg(s) (acquired) M21.16- ☑
  congenital Q68.5
  rachitic E64.3
Boyd's dysentery A03.2
Brachial — *see* condition
Brachycardia R00.1
Brachycephaly Q75.0
Bradley's disease A08.19
Bradyarrhythmia, cardiac I49.8
Bradycardia (sinoatrial) (sinus) (vagal) R00.1
  neonatal P29.12
  reflex G90.09
  tachycardia syndrome I49.5
Bradykinesia R25.8
Bradypnea R06.89
Bradytachycardia I49.5
Brailsford's disease or osteochondrosis — *see* Osteochondrosis, juvenile, radius

Brain (*see also* condition)
  death G93.82
  syndrome — *see* Syndrome, brain
Branched-chain amino-acid disorder E71.2
Branchial — *see* condition
  cartilage, congenital Q18.2
Branchiogenic remnant (in neck) Q18.0
Brandt's syndrome (acrodermatitis enteropathica) E83.2
Bravais-jacksonian epilepsy — *see* Epilepsy, localization-related, symptomatic, with simple partial seizures
Braxton Hicks contractions — *see* False, labor
Brazilian leishmaniasis B55.2
BRBPR K62.5
Break, retina (without detachment) H33.30- ☑
  with retinal detachment — *see* Detachment, retina
  horseshoe tear H33.31- ☑
  multiple H33.33- ☑
  round hole H33.32- ☑
Breakdown
  device, graft or implant (*see also* Complications, by site and type, mechanical) T85.618 ☑
    arterial graft NEC — *see* Complication, cardiovascular device, mechanical, vascular
    breast (implant) T85.41 ☑
    catheter NEC T85.618 ☑
      cystostomy T83.010 ☑
      dialysis (renal) T82.41 ☑
        intraperitoneal T85.611 ☑
      Hopkins T83.018 ☑
      ileostomy T83.018 ☑
      infusion NEC T82.514 ☑
        cranial T85.610- ☑
        epidural T85.610 ☑
        intrathecal T85.610 ☑
        spinal T85.610 ☑
        subarachnoid T85.610 ☑
        subdural T85.610 ☑
      nephrostomy T83.012 ☑
      urethral indwelling T83.011 ☑
      urinary NEC T83.018 ☑
      urostomy T83.018 ☑
    electronic (electrode) (pulse generator) (stimulator)
      bone T84.310 ☑
      cardiac T82.119 ☑
        electrode T82.110 ☑
        pulse generator T82.111 ☑
        specified type NEC T82.118 ☑
      nervous system — *see* Complication, prosthetic device, mechanical, electronic nervous system stimulator
      urinary — *see* Complication, genitourinary, device, urinary, mechanical
    fixation, internal (orthopedic) NEC — *see* Complication, fixation device, mechanical
    gastrointestinal — *see* Complications, prosthetic device, mechanical, gastrointestinal device
    genital NEC T83.418 ☑
      intrauterine contraceptive device T83.31 ☑
      penile prosthesis (cylinder) (implanted) (pump) (resevoir) T83.410 ☑
      testicular prosthesis T83.411 ☑
    heart NEC — *see* Complication, cardiovascular device, mechanical
    intrathecal infusion pump T85.615 ☑
    joint prosthesis — *see* Complications..., joint prosthesis, internal, mechanical, by site
    nervous system, specified device NEC T85.615 ☑
    ocular NEC — *see* Complications, prosthetic device, mechanical, ocular device
    orthopedic NEC — *see* Complication, orthopedic, device, mechanical
    specified NEC T85.618 ☑
    subcutaneous device pocket
      nervous system prosthetic device, implant, or graft T85.890 ☑
      other internal prosthetic device, implant, or graft T85.898 ☑
    sutures, permanent T85.612 ☑
      used in bone repair — *see* Complications, fixation device, internal (orthopedic), mechanical
    urinary NEC T83.118 ☑
      graft T83.21 ☑
      sphincter, implanted T83.111 ☑
      stent (ileal conduit) (nephroureteral) T83.113 ☑

Breakdown — *continued*
  device, graft or implant (*see also* Complications, by site and type, mechanical) — *continued*
    urinary — *continued*
      stent — *continued*
        ureteral indwelling T83.112 ☑
      vascular NEC — *see* Complication, cardiovascular device, mechanical
      ventricular intracranial shunt T85.01 ☑
  nervous F48.8
  perineum O90.1
  respirator J95.850
    specified NEC J95.859
  ventilator J95.850
    specified NEC J95.859
Breast (*see also* condition)
  buds E30.1
    in newborn P96.89
  dense R92.2
  nodule (*see also* Lump, breast) N63.0
Breath
  foul R19.6
  holder, child R06.89
  holding spell R06.89
  shortness R06.02
Breathing
  labored — *see* Hyperventilation
  mouth R06.5
    causing malocclusion M26.5 ☑
  periodic R06.3
    high altitude G47.32
Breathlessness R06.81
Breda's disease — *see* Yaws
Breech presentation (mother) O32.1 ☑
  causing obstructed labor O64.1 ☑
  footling O32.8 ☑
    causing obstructed labor O64.8 ☑
  incomplete O32.8 ☑
    causing obstructed labor O64.8 ☑
Breisky's disease N90.4
Brennemann's syndrome I88.0
Brenner
  tumor (benign) D27.9
    borderline malignancy D39.1- ☑
    malignant C56 ☑
    proliferating D39.1- ☑
Bretonneau's disease or angina A36.0
Breus' mole O02.0
Brevicollis Q76.49
Brickmakers' anemia B76.9 [D63.8]
Bridge, myocardial Q24.5
Bright red blood per rectum (BRBPR) K62.5
Bright's disease (*see also* Nephritis)
  arteriosclerotic — *see* Hypertension, kidney
Brill (-Zinsser) **disease** (recrudescent typhus) A75.1
  flea-borne A75.2
  louse-borne A75.1
Brill-Symmers' disease C82.90
Brion-Kayser disease — *see* Fever, parathyroid
Briquet's disorder or syndrome F45.0
Brissaud's
  infantilism or dwarfism E23.0
  motor-verbal tic F95.2
Brittle
  bones disease Q78.0
  nails L60.3
    congenital Q84.6
Broad (*see also* condition)
  beta disease E78.2
  ligament laceration syndrome N83.8
Broad- or floating-betalipoproteinemia E78.2
Brock's syndrome (atelectasis due to enlarged lymph nodes) J98.19
Brocq-Duhring disease (dermatitis herpetiformis) L13.0
Brodie's abscess or disease M86.8X- ☑
Broken
  arches (*see also* Deformity, limb, flat foot)
  arm (meaning upper limb) — *see* Fracture, arm
  back — *see* Fracture, vertebra
  bone — *see* Fracture
  implant or internal device — *see* Complications, by site and type, mechanical
  leg (meaning lower limb) — *see* Fracture, leg
  nose S02.2 ☑
  tooth, teeth — *see* Fracture, tooth
Bromhidrosis, bromidrosis L75.0
Bromidism, bromism G92

Bromidism, bromism — *continued*
due to
    correct substance properly administered — *see* Table of Drugs and Chemicals, by drug, adverse effect
    overdose or wrong substance given or taken — *see* Table of Drugs and Chemicals, by drug, poisoning
chronic (dependence) F13.20
Bromidrosiphobia F40.298
Bronchi, bronchial — *see* condition
Bronchiectasis (cylindrical) (diffuse) (fusiform) (localized) (saccular) J47.9
with
    acute
        bronchitis J47.0
        lower respiratory infection J47.0
    exacerbation (acute) J47.1
congenital Q33.4
tuberculous NEC — *see* Tuberculosis, pulmonary
Bronchiolectasis — *see* Bronchiectasis
Bronchiolitis (acute) (infective) (subacute) J21.9
with
    bronchospasm or obstruction J21.9
    influenza, flu or grippe — *see* Influenza, with, respiratory manifestations NEC
chemical (chronic) J68.4
    acute J68.0
chronic (fibrosing) (obliterative) J44.9
due to
    external agent — *see* Bronchitis, acute, due to
    human metapneumovirus J21.1
    respiratory syncytial virus J21.0
    specified organism NEC J21.8
fibrosa obliterans J44.9
influenzal — *see* Influenza, with, respiratory manifestations NEC
obliterans J42
    with organizing pneumonia (BOOP) J84.89
obliterative (chronic) (subacute) J44.9
    due to fumes or vapors J68.4
    due to chemicals, gases, fumes or vapors (inhalation) J68.4
respiratory, interstitial lung disease J84.115
Bronchitis (diffuse) (fibrinous) (hypostatic) (infective) (membranous) J40
with
    influenza, flu or grippe — *see* Influenza, with, respiratory manifestations NEC
    obstruction (airway) (lung) J44.9
    tracheitis (15 years of age and above) J40
        acute or subacute J20.9
        chronic J42
        under 15 years of age J20.9
acute or subacute (with bronchospasm or obstruction) J20.9
    with
        bronchiectasis J47.0
        chronic obstructive pulmonary disease J44.0
    chemical (due to gases, fumes or vapors) J68.0
    due to
        fumes or vapors J68.0
        Haemophilus influenzae J20.1
        Mycoplasma pneumoniae J20.0
        radiation J70.0
        specified organism NEC J20.8
        Streptococcus J20.2
        virus
            coxsackie J20.3
            echovirus J20.7
            parainfluenzae J20.4
            respiratory syncytial J20.5
            rhinovirus J20.6
    viral NEC J20.8
allergic (acute) J45.909
    with
        exacerbation (acute) J45.901
        status asthmaticus J45.902
arachidic T17.528 ☑
aspiration (due to fumes or vapors) J68.0
asthmatic J45.9 ☑
    chronic J44.9
        with
            acute lower respiratory infection J44.0
            exacerbation (acute) J44.1
capillary — *see* Pneumonia, broncho
caseous (tuberculous) A15.5
Castellani's A69.8

Bronchitis — *continued*
catarrhal (15 years of age and above) J40
    acute — *see* Bronchitis, acute
    chronic J41.0
    under 15 years of age J20.9
chemical (acute) (subacute) J68.0
    chronic J68.4
    due to fumes or vapors J68.0
        chronic J68.4
chronic J42
    with
        airways obstruction J44.9
        tracheitis (chronic) J42
    asthmatic (obstructive) J44.9
    catarrhal J41.0
    chemical (due to fumes or vapors) J68.4
    due to
        chemicals, gases, fumes or vapors (inhalation) J68.4
        radiation J70.1
        tobacco smoking J41.0
    emphysematous J44.9
    mucopurulent J41.1
    non-obstructive J41.0
    obliterans J44.9
    obstructive J44.9
    purulent J41.1
    simple J41.0
croupous — *see* Bronchitis, acute
due to gases, fumes or vapors (chemical) J68.0
emphysematous (obstructive) J44.9
exudative — *see* Bronchitis, acute
fetid J41.1
grippal — *see* Influenza, with, respiratory manifestations NEC
in those under 15 years age — *see* Bronchitis, acute
    chronic — *see* Bronchitis, chronic
influenzal — *see* Influenza, with, respiratory manifestations NEC
mixed simple and mucopurulent J41.8
moulder's J62.8
mucopurulent (chronic) (recurrent) J41.1
    acute or subacute J20.9
    simple (mixed) J41.8
obliterans (chronic) J44.9
obstructive (chronic) (diffuse) J44.9
pituitous J41.1
pneumococcal, acute or subacute J20.2
pseudomembranous, acute or subacute — *see* Bronchitis, acute
purulent (chronic) (recurrent) J41.1
    acute or subacute — *see* Bronchitis, acute
putrid J41.1
senile (chronic) J42
simple and mucopurulent (mixed) J41.8
smokers' J41.0
spirochetal NEC A69.8
subacute — *see* Bronchitis, acute
suppurative (chronic) J41.1
    acute or subacute — *see* Bronchitis, acute
tuberculous A15.5
under 15 years of age — *see* Bronchitis, acute
    chronic — *see* Bronchitis, chronic
viral NEC, acute or subacute (*see also* Bronchitis, acute) J20.8
Bronchoalveolitis J18.0
Bronchoaspergillosis B44.1
Bronchocele meaning goiter E04.0
Broncholithiasis J98.09
    tuberculous NEC A15.5
Bronchomalacia J98.09
    congenital Q32.2
Bronchomycosis NOS B49 [J99]
    candidal B37.1
Bronchopleuropneumonia — *see* Pneumonia, broncho
Bronchopneumonia — *see* Pneumonia, broncho
Bronchopneumonitis — *see* Pneumonia, broncho
Bronchopulmonary — *see* condition
Bronchopulmonitis — *see* Pneumonia, broncho
Bronchorrhagia (see Hemoptysis)
Bronchorrhea J98.09
    acute J20.9
    chronic (infective) (purulent) J42
Bronchospasm (acute) J98.01
    with
        bronchiolitis, acute J21.9
        bronchitis, acute (conditions in J20) — *see* Bronchitis, acute

Bronchospasm — *continued*
    due to external agent — *see* condition, respiratory, acute, due to
    exercise induced J45.990
Bronchospirochetosis A69.8
    Castellani A69.8
Bronchostenosis J98.09
Bronchus — *see* condition
Brontophobia F40.220
Bronze baby syndrome P83.88
Brooke's tumor — *see* Neoplasm, skin, benign
Brown enamel of teeth (hereditary) K00.5
Brown's sheath syndrome H50.61- ☑
Brown-Séquard disease, paralysis or syndrome G83.81
Bruce sepsis A23.0
Brucellosis (infection) A23.9
    abortus A23.1
    canis A23.3
    dermatitis A23.9
    melitensis A23.0
    mixed A23.8
    sepsis A23.9
        melitensis A23.0
        specified NEC A23.8
    suis A23.2
Bruck-de Lange disease Q87.1
Bruck's disease — *see* Deformity, limb
BRUE (brief resolved unexplained event) R68.13
Brugsch's syndrome Q82.8
Bruise (skin surface intact) (*see also* Contusion)
    with
        open wound — *see* Wound, open
    internal organ — *see* Injury, by site
    newborn P54.5
    scalp, due to birth injury, newborn P12.3
    umbilical cord O69.5 ☑
Bruit (arterial) R09.89
    cardiac R01.1
Brush burn — *see* Abrasion, by site
Bruton's X-linked agammaglobulinemia D80.0
Bruxism
    psychogenic F45.8
    sleep related G47.63
Bubbly lung syndrome P27.0
Bubo I88.8
    blennorrhagic (gonococcal) A54.89
    chancroidal A57
    climatic A55
    due to Haemophilus ducreyi A57
    gonococcal A54.89
    indolent (nonspecific) I88.8
    inguinal (nonspecific) I88.8
        chancroidal A57
        climatic A55
        due to H. ducreyi A57
        infective I88.8
    scrofulous (tuberculous) A18.2
    soft chancre A57
    suppurating — *see* Lymphadenitis, acute
    syphilitic (primary) A51.0
        congenital A50.07
    tropical A55
    virulent (chancroidal) A57
Bubonic plague A20.0
Bubonocele — *see* Hernia, inguinal
Buccal — *see* condition
Buchanan's disease or osteochondrosis M91.0
Buchem's syndrome (hyperostosis corticalis) M85.2
Bucket-handle fracture or tear (semilunar cartilage) — *see* Tear, meniscus
Budd-Chiari syndrome (hepatic vein thrombosis) I82.0
Budgerigar fancier's disease or lung J67.2
Buds
    breast E30.1
        in newborn P96.89
Buerger's disease (thromboangiitis obliterans) I73.1
Bulbar — *see* condition
Bulbus cordis (left ventricle) (persistent) Q21.8
Bulimia (nervosa) F50.2
    atypical F50.9
    normal weight F50.9
Bulky
    stools R19.5
    uterus N85.2
Bulla (e) R23.8
    lung (emphysematous) (solitary) J43.9

Burn — *continued*
  finger — *continued*
    multiple sites — *continued*
      with thumb — *continued*
        first degree T23.149 ☑
        left T23.042 ☑
          first degree T23.142 ☑
          second degree T23.242 ☑
          third degree T23.342 ☑
        right T23.041 ☑
          first degree T23.141 ☑
          second degree T23.241 ☑
          third degree T23.341 ☑
        second degree T23.249 ☑
        third degree T23.349 ☑
      first degree T23.139 ☑
      left T23.032 ☑
        first degree T23.132 ☑
        second degree T23.232 ☑
        third degree T23.332 ☑
      right T23.031 ☑
        first degree T23.131 ☑
        second degree T23.231 ☑
        third degree T23.331 ☑
      second degree T23.239 ☑
      third degree T23.339 ☑
    right T23.021 ☑
      first degree T23.121 ☑
      second degree T23.221 ☑
      third degree T23.321 ☑
    second degree T23.229 ☑
    third degree T23.329 ☑
  flank — *see* Burn, abdominal wall
  foot T25.029 ☑
    first degree T25.129 ☑
    left T25.022 ☑
      first degree T25.122 ☑
      second degree T25.222 ☑
      third degree T25.322 ☑
    multiple with ankle — *see* Burn, lower, limb, multiple, ankle and foot
    right T25.021 ☑
      first degree T25.121 ☑
      second degree T25.221 ☑
      third degree T25.321 ☑
    second degree T25.229 ☑
    third degree T25.329 ☑
  forearm T22.019 ☑
    first degree T22.119 ☑
    left T22.012 ☑
      first degree T22.112 ☑
      second degree T22.212 ☑
      third degree T22.312 ☑
    right T22.011 ☑
      first degree T22.111 ☑
      second degree T22.211 ☑
      third degree T22.311 ☑
    second degree T22.219 ☑
    third degree T22.319 ☑
  forehead T20.06 ☑
    first degree T20.16 ☑
    second degree T20.26 ☑
    third degree T20.36 ☑
  fourth degree — *code as* Burn, third degree, by site
  friction — *see* Burn, by site
  from swallowing caustic or corrosive substance NEC — *see* Corrosion, by site
  full thickness skin loss — *code as* Burn, third degree, by site
  gastrointestinal tract NEC T28.2 ☑
    from swallowing caustic or corrosive substance T28.7 ☑
  genital organs
    external
      female T21.07 ☑
        first degree T21.17 ☑
        second degree T21.27 ☑
        third degree T21.37 ☑
      male T21.06 ☑
        first degree T21.16 ☑
        second degree T21.26 ☑
        third degree T21.36 ☑
    internal T28.3 ☑
      from caustic or corrosive substance T28.8 ☑
  groin — *see* Burn, abdominal wall
  hand(s) T23.009 ☑

Burn — *continued*
  hand(s) — *continued*
    back — *see* Burn, dorsum of hand
    finger — *see* Burn, finger
    first degree T23.109 ☑
    left T23.002 ☑
      first degree T23.102 ☑
      second degree T23.202 ☑
      third degree T23.302 ☑
    multiple sites with wrist T23.099 ☑
      first degree T23.199 ☑
      left T23.092 ☑
        first degree T23.192 ☑
        second degree T23.292 ☑
        third degree T23.392 ☑
      right T23.091 ☑
        first degree T23.191 ☑
        second degree T23.291 ☑
        third degree T23.391 ☑
      second degree T23.299 ☑
      third degree T23.399 ☑
    palm — *see* Burn, palm
    right T23.001 ☑
      first degree T23.101 ☑
      second degree T23.201 ☑
      third degree T23.301 ☑
    second degree T23.209 ☑
    third degree T23.309 ☑
    thumb — *see* Burn, thumb
  head (and face) (and neck) T20.00 ☑
    cheek — *see* Burn, cheek
    chin — *see* Burn, chin
    ear — *see* Burn, ear
    eye(s) only — *see* Burn, eye
    first degree T20.10 ☑
    forehead — *see* Burn, forehead
    lip — *see* Burn, lip
    multiple sites T20.09 ☑
      first degree T20.19 ☑
      second degree T20.29 ☑
      third degree T20.39 ☑
    neck — *see* Burn, neck
    nose — *see* Burn, nose
    scalp — *see* Burn, scalp
    second degree T20.20 ☑
    third degree T20.30 ☑
  hip(s) — *see* Burn, thigh
  inhalation — *see* Burn, respiratory tract
    caustic or corrosive substance (fumes) — *see* Corrosion, respiratory tract
  internal organ(s) T28.40 ☑
    alimentary tract T28.2 ☑
      esophagus T28.1 ☑
    eardrum T28.41 ☑
    esophagus T28.1 ☑
    from caustic or corrosive substance (swallowing) NEC — *see* Corrosion, by site
    genitourinary T28.3 ☑
    mouth T28.0 ☑
    pharynx T28.0 ☑
    respiratory tract — *see* Burn, respiratory tract
    specified organ NEC T28.49 ☑
  interscapular region — *see* Burn, back, upper
  intestine (large) (small) T28.2 ☑
  knee T24.029 ☑
    first degree T24.129 ☑
    left T24.022 ☑
      first degree T24.122 ☑
      second degree T24.222 ☑
      third degree T24.322 ☑
    right T24.021 ☑
      first degree T24.121 ☑
      second degree T24.221 ☑
      third degree T24.321 ☑
    second degree T24.229 ☑
    third degree T24.329 ☑
  labium (majus) (minus) — *see* Burn, genital organs, external, female
  lacrimal apparatus, duct, gland or sac — *see* Burn, eye, specified site NEC
  larynx T27.0 ☑
    with lung T27.1 ☑
  leg(s) (lower) (upper) — *see* Burn, lower, limb
  lightning — *see* Burn, by site

Burn — *continued*
  limb(s)
    lower (except ankle or foot alone) — *see* Burn, lower, limb
    upper — *see* Burn, upper limb
  lip(s) T20.02 ☑
    first degree T20.12 ☑
    second degree T20.22 ☑
    third degree T20.32 ☑
  lower
    back — *see* Burn, back
    limb T24.009 ☑
      ankle — *see* Burn, ankle
      calf — *see* Burn, calf
      first degree T24.109 ☑
      foot — *see* Burn, foot
      hip — *see* Burn, thigh
      knee — *see* Burn, knee
      left T24.002 ☑
        first degree T24.102 ☑
        second degree T24.202 ☑
        third degree T24.302 ☑
      multiple sites, except ankle and foot T24.099 ☑
        ankle and foot T25.099 ☑
          first degree T25.199 ☑
          left T25.092 ☑
            first degree T25.192 ☑
            second degree T25.292 ☑
            third degree T25.392 ☑
          right T25.091 ☑
            first degree T25.191 ☑
            second degree T25.291 ☑
            third degree T25.391 ☑
          second degree T25.299 ☑
          third degree T25.399 ☑
        first degree T24.199 ☑
        left T24.092 ☑
          first degree T24.192 ☑
          second degree T24.292 ☑
          third degree T24.392 ☑
        right T24.091 ☑
          first degree T24.191 ☑
          second degree T24.291 ☑
          third degree T24.391 ☑
        second degree T24.299 ☑
        third degree T24.399 ☑
      right T24.001 ☑
        first degree T24.101 ☑
        second degree T24.201 ☑
        third degree T24.301 ☑
      second degree T24.209 ☑
      thigh — *see* Burn, thigh
      third degree T24.309 ☑
      toe — *see* Burn, toe
  lung (with larynx and trachea) T27.1 ☑
  mouth T28.0 ☑
  neck T20.07 ☑
    first degree T20.17 ☑
    second degree T20.27 ☑
    third degree T20.37 ☑
  nose (septum) T20.04 ☑
    first degree T20.14 ☑
    second degree T20.24 ☑
    third degree T20.34 ☑
  ocular adnexa — *see* Burn, eye
  orbit region — *see* Burn, eyelid
  palm T23.059 ☑
    first degree T23.159 ☑
    left T23.052 ☑
      first degree T23.152 ☑
      second degree T23.252 ☑
      third degree T23.352 ☑
    right T23.051 ☑
      first degree T23.151 ☑
      second degree T23.251 ☑
      third degree T23.351 ☑
    second degree T23.259 ☑
    third degree T23.359 ☑
  partial thickness — *code as* Burn, unspecified degree, by site
  pelvis — *see* Burn, trunk
  penis — *see* Burn, genital organs, external, male
  perineum
    female — *see* Burn, genital organs, external, female
    male — *see* Burn, genital organs, external, male
  periocular area — *see* Burn, eyelid

Burns' disease or osteochondrosis — see Osteochondrosis, juvenile, ulna
Bursa — see condition
Bursitis M71.9
  Achilles — see Tendinitis, Achilles
  adhesive — see Bursitis, specified NEC
  ankle — see Enthesopathy, lower limb, ankle, specified type NEC
  calcaneal — see Enthesopathy, foot, specified type NEC
  collateral ligament, tibial — see Bursitis, tibial collateral
  due to use, overuse, pressure (see also Disorder, soft tissue, due to use, specified type NEC)
    specified NEC — see Disorder, soft tissue, due to use, specified NEC
  Duplay's M75.0 ✓
  elbow NEC M70.3- ✓
    olecranon M70.2- ✓
  finger — see Disorder, soft tissue, due to use, specified type NEC, hand
  foot — see Enthesopathy, foot, specified type NEC
  gonococcal A54.49
  gouty — see Gout
  hand M70.1- ✓
  hip NEC M70.7- ✓
    trochanteric M70.6- ✓
  infective NEC M71.10
    abscess — see Abscess, bursa
    ankle M71.17- ✓
    elbow M71.12- ✓
    foot M71.17- ✓
    hand M71.14- ✓
    hip M71.15- ✓
    knee M71.16- ✓
    multiple sites M71.19
    shoulder M71.11- ✓
    specified site NEC M71.18
    wrist M71.13- ✓
  ischial — see Bursitis, hip
  knee NEC M70.5- ✓
    prepatellar M70.4- ✓
  occupational NEC (see also Disorder, soft tissue, due to, use)
  olecranon — see Bursitis, elbow, olecranon
  pharyngeal J39.1
  popliteal — see Bursitis, knee
  prepatellar M70.4- ✓
  radiohumeral M77.8
  rheumatoid M06.20
    ankle M06.27- ✓
    elbow M06.22- ✓
    foot joint M06.27- ✓
    hand joint M06.24- ✓
    hip M06.25- ✓
    knee M06.26- ✓
    multiple site M06.29
    shoulder M06.21- ✓
    vertebra M06.28
    wrist M06.23- ✓
  scapulohumeral — see Bursitis, shoulder
  semimembranous muscle (knee) — see Bursitis, knee
  shoulder M75.5- ✓
    adhesive — see Capsulitis, adhesive
  specified NEC M71.50
    ankle M71.57- ✓
    due to use, overuse or pressure — see Disorder, soft tissue, due to, use
    elbow M71.52- ✓
    foot M71.57- ✓
    hand M71.54- ✓
    hip M71.55- ✓
    knee M71.56- ✓
    shoulder — see Bursitis, shoulder
    specified site NEC M71.58
    tibial collateral M76.4- ✓
    wrist M71.53- ✓
  subacromial — see Bursitis, shoulder
  subcoracoid — see Bursitis, shoulder
  subdeltoid — see Bursitis, shoulder
  syphilitic A52.78
  Thornwaldt, Tornwaldt J39.2
  tibial collateral M76.4- ✓
  toe — see Enthesopathy, foot, specified type NEC
  trochanteric (area) — see Bursitis, hip, trochanteric
  wrist — see Bursitis, hand
Bursopathy M71.9
  specified type NEC M71.80

Bursopathy — continued
  specified type — continued
    ankle M71.87- ✓
    elbow M71.82- ✓
    foot M71.87- ✓
    hand M71.84- ✓
    hip M71.85- ✓
    knee M71.86- ✓
    multiple sites M71.89
    shoulder M71.81- ✓
    specified site NEC M71.88
    wrist M71.83- ✓
Burst stitches or sutures (complication of surgery) T81.31 ✓
  external operation wound T81.31 ✓
  internal operation wound T81.32 ✓
Buruli ulcer A31.1
Bury's disease L95.1
Buschke's
  disease B45.3
  scleredema — see Sclerosis, systemic
Busse-Buschke disease B45.3
Buttock — see condition
Button
  Biskra B55.1
  Delhi B55.1
  oriental B55.1
Buttonhole deformity (finger) — see Deformity, finger, boutonniere
Bwamba fever A92.8
Byssinosis J66.0
Bywaters' syndrome T79.5 ✓

C

Cachexia R64
  cancerous R64
  cardiac — see Disease, heart
  dehydration E86.0
  due to malnutrition R64
  exophthalmic — see Hyperthyroidism
  heart — see Disease, heart
  hypophyseal E23.0
  hypopituitary E23.0
  lead — see Poisoning, lead
  malignant R64
  marsh — see Malaria
  nervous F48.8
  old age R54
  paludal — see Malaria
  pituitary E23.0
  renal N28.9
  saturnine — see Poisoning, lead
  senile R54
  Simmonds' E23.0
  splenica D73.0
  strumipriva E03.4
  tuberculous NEC — see Tuberculosis
CADASIL (cerebral autosomal dominant arteriopathy with subcortical infarcts and leukoencephalopathy) I67.850
Café, au lait spots L81.3
Caffeine-induced
  anxiety disorder F15.980
  sleep disorder F15.982
Caffey's syndrome Q78.8
Caisson disease T70.3 ✓
Cake kidney Q63.1
Caked breast (puerperal, postpartum) O92.79
Calabar swelling B74.3
Calcaneal spur — see Spur, bone, calcaneal
Calcaneo-apophysitis M92.8
Calcareous — see condition
Calcicosis J62.8
Calciferol (vitamin D) deficiency E55.9
  with rickets E55.0
Calcification
  adrenal (capsule) (gland) E27.49
    tuberculous E35 [B90.8]
  aorta I70.0
  artery (annular) — see Arteriosclerosis
  auricle (ear) — see Disorder, pinna, specified type NEC
  basal ganglia G23.8
  bladder N32.89
    due to Schistosoma hematobium B65.0
  brain (cortex) — see Calcification, cerebral
  bronchus J98.09

Calcification — continued
  bursa M71.40
    ankle M71.47- ✓
    elbow M71.42- ✓
    foot M71.47- ✓
    hand M71.44- ✓
    hip M71.45- ✓
    knee M71.46- ✓
    multiple sites M71.49
    shoulder M75.3- ✓
    specified site NEC M71.48
    wrist M71.43- ✓
  cardiac — see Degeneration, myocardial
  cerebral (cortex) G93.89
    artery I67.2
  cervix (uteri) N88.8
  choroid plexus G93.89
  conjunctiva — see Concretion, conjunctiva
  corpora cavernosa (penis) N48.89
  cortex (brain) — see Calcification, cerebral
  dental pulp (nodular) K04.2
  dentinal papilla K00.4
  fallopian tube N83.8
  falx cerebri G96.19
  gallbladder K82.8
  general E83.59
  heart (see also Degeneration, myocardial)
    valve — see Endocarditis
  idiopathic infantile arterial (IIAC) Q28.8
  intervertebral cartilage or disc (postinfective) — see Disorder, disc, specified NEC
  intracranial — see Calcification, cerebral
  joint — see Disorder, joint, specified type NEC
  kidney N28.89
    tuberculous N29 [B90.1]
  larynx (senile) J38.7
  lens — see Cataract, specified NEC
  lung (active) (postinfectional) J98.4
    tuberculous B90.9
  lymph gland or node (postinfectional) I89.8
    tuberculous (see also Tuberculosis, lymph gland) B90.8
  mammographic R92.1
  massive (paraplegic) — see Myositis, ossificans, in, quadriplegia
  medial — see Arteriosclerosis, extremities
  meninges (cerebral) (spinal) G96.19
  metastatic E83.59
  Mönckeberg's — see Arteriosclerosis, extremities
  muscle M61.9
    due to burns — see Myositis, ossificans, in, burns
    paralytic — see Myositis, ossificans, in, quadriplegia
    specified type NEC M61.40
      ankle M61.47- ✓
      foot M61.47- ✓
      forearm M61.43- ✓
      hand M61.44- ✓
      lower leg M61.46- ✓
      multiple sites M61.49
      pelvic region M61.45- ✓
      shoulder region M61.41- ✓
      specified site NEC M61.48
      thigh M61.45- ✓
      upper arm M61.42- ✓
  myocardium, myocardial — see Degeneration, myocardial
  ovary N83.8
  pancreas K86.89
  penis N48.89
  periarticular — see Disorder, joint, specified type NEC
  pericardium (see also Pericarditis) I31.1
  pineal gland E34.8
  pleura J94.8
    postinfectional J94.8
    tuberculous NEC B90.9
  pulpal (dental) (nodular) K04.2
  sclera H15.89
  spleen D73.89
  subcutaneous L94.2
  suprarenal (capsule) (gland) E27.49
  tendon (sheath) (see also Tenosynovitis, specified type NEC)
    with bursitis, synovitis or tenosynovitis — see Tendinitis, calcific
  trachea J39.8
  ureter N28.89
  uterus N85.8

Calcification — continued
  vitreous — see Deposit, crystalline
Calcified — see Calcification
Calcinosis (interstitial) (tumoral) (universalis) E83.59
  with Raynaud's phenomenon, esophageal dysfunction, sclerodactyly, telangiectasia (CREST syndrome) M34.1
  circumscripta (skin) L94.2
  cutis L94.2
Calciphylaxis (see also Calcification, by site) E83.59
Calcium
  deposits — see Calcification, by site
  metabolism disorder E83.50
  salts or soaps in vitreous — see Deposit, crystalline
Calciuria R82.994
Calculi — see Calculus
Calculosis, intrahepatic — see Calculus, bile duct
Calculus, calculi, calculous
  ampulla of Vater — see Calculus, bile duct
  anuria (impacted) (recurrent) (see also Calculus, urinary) N20.9
  appendix K38.1
  bile duct (common) (hepatic) K80.50
    with
      calculus of gallbladder — see Calculus, gallbladder and bile duct
      cholangitis K80.30
        with
          cholecystitis — see Calculus, bile duct, with cholecystitis
          obstruction K80.31
        acute K80.32
          with
            chronic cholangitis K80.36
              with obstruction K80.37
            obstruction K80.33
        chronic K80.34
          with
            acute cholangitis K80.36
              with obstruction K80.37
            obstruction K80.35
      cholecystitis (with cholangitis) K80.40
        with obstruction K80.41
        acute K80.42
          with
            chronic cholecystitis K80.46
              with obstruction K80.47
            obstruction K80.43
        chronic K80.44
          with
            acute cholecystitis K80.46
              with obstruction K80.47
            obstruction K80.45
  biliary (see also Calculus, gallbladder)
    specified NEC K80.80
      with obstruction K80.81
  bilirubin, multiple — see Calculus, gallbladder
  bladder (encysted) (impacted) (urinary) (diverticulum) N21.0
  bronchus J98.09
  calyx (kidney) (renal) — see Calculus, kidney
  cholesterol (pure) (solitary) — see Calculus, gallbladder
  common duct (bile) — see Calculus, bile duct
  conjunctiva — see Concretion, conjunctiva
  cystic N21.0
    duct — see Calculus, gallbladder
  dental (subgingival) (supragingival) K03.6
  diverticulum
    bladder N21.0
    kidney N20.0
  epididymis N50.89
  gallbladder K80.20
    with
      bile duct calculus — see Calculus, gallbladder and bile duct
      cholecystitis K80.10
        with obstruction K80.11
        acute K80.00
          with
            chronic cholecystitis K80.12
              with obstruction K80.13
            obstruction K80.01
        chronic K80.10
          with
            acute cholecystitis K80.12
              with obstruction K80.13
            obstruction K80.11
      specified NEC K80.18

Calculus, calculi, calculous — continued
  gallbladder — continued
    with — continued
      cholecystitis — continued
        specified — continued
          with obstruction K80.19
        obstruction K80.21
  gallbladder and bile duct K80.70
    with
      cholecystitis K80.60
        with obstruction K80.61
        acute K80.62
          with
            chronic cholecystitis K80.66
              with obstruction K80.67
              obstruction K80.63
        chronic K80.64
          with
            acute cholecystitis K80.66
              with obstruction K80.67
            obstruction K80.65
      obstruction K80.71
  hepatic (duct) — see Calculus, bile duct
  ileal conduit N21.8
  intestinal (impaction) (obstruction) K56.49
  kidney (impacted) (multiple) (pelvis) (recurrent) (staghorn) N20.0
    with calculus, ureter N20.2
    congenital Q63.8
  lacrimal passages — see Dacryolith
  liver (impacted) — see Calculus, bile duct
  lung J98.4
  mammographic R92.1
  nephritic (impacted) (recurrent) — see Calculus, kidney
  nose J34.89
  pancreas (duct) K86.89
  parotid duct or gland K11.5
  pelvis, encysted — see Calculus, kidney
  prostate N42.0
  pulmonary J98.4
  pyelitis (impacted) (recurrent) N20.0
    with hydronephrosis N13.2
  pyelonephritis (impacted) (recurrent) N20 ☑
    with hydronephrosis N13.2
  renal (impacted) (recurrent) — see Calculus, kidney
  salivary (duct) (gland) K11.5
  seminal vesicle N50.89
  staghorn — see Calculus, kidney
  Stensen's duct K11.5
  stomach K31.89
  sublingual duct or gland K11.5
    congenital Q38.4
  submandibular duct, gland or region K11.5
  submaxillary duct, gland or region K11.5
  suburethral N21.8
  tonsil J35.8
  tooth, teeth (subgingival) (supragingival) K03.6
  tunica vaginalis N50.89
  ureter (impacted) (recurrent) N20.1
    with calculus, kidney N20.2
      with hydronephrosis N13.2
        with infection N13.6
  urethra (impacted) N21.1
  urinary (duct) (impacted) (passage) (tract) N20.9
    with hydronephrosis N13.2
      with infection N13.6
    in (due to)
    lower N21.9
      specified NEC N21.8
  vagina N89.8
  vesical (impacted) N21.0
  Wharton's duct K11.5
  xanthine E79.8 [N22]
Calicectasis N28.89
Caliectasis N28.89
California
  disease B38.9
  encephalitis A83.5
Caligo cornea — see Opacity, cornea, central
Callositas, callosity (infected) L84
Callus (infected) L84
  bone — see Osteophyte
    excessive, following fracture — code as Sequelae of fracture
CALME (childhood asymmetric labium majus enlargement) N90.61
Calorie deficiency or malnutrition (see also Malnutrition) E46

Calvé-Perthes disease — see Legg-Calvé-Perthes disease
Calvé's disease — see Osteochondrosis, juvenile, spine
Calvities — see Alopecia, androgenic
Cameroon fever — see Malaria
Camptocormia (hysterical) F44.4
Camurati-Engelmann syndrome Q78.3
Canal (see also condition)
  atrioventricular common Q21.2
Canaliculitis (lacrimal) (acute) (subacute) H04.33- ☑
  Actinomyces A42.89
  chronic H04.42- ☑
Canavan's disease E75.29
Canceled procedure (surgical) Z53.9
  because of
    contraindication Z53.09
      smoking Z53.01
    left against medical advice (AMA) Z53.21
    patient's decision Z53.20
      for reasons of belief or group pressure Z53.1
      specified reason NEC Z53.29
    specified reason NEC Z53.8
Cancer (see also Neoplasm, by site, malignant)
  bile duct type liver C22.1
  blood — see Leukemia
  breast (see also Neoplasm, breast, malignant) C50.91- ☑
  hepatocellular C22.0
  lung (see also Neoplasm, lung, malignant) C34.90
  ovarian (see also Neoplasm ovary, malignant) C56.9
  unspecified site (primary) C80.1
Cancer (o)phobia F45.29
Cancerous — see Neoplasm, malignant, by site
Cancrum oris A69.0
Candidiasis, candidal B37.9
  balanitis B37.42
  bronchitis B37.1
  cheilitis B37.83
  congenital P37.5
  cystitis B37.41
  disseminated B37.7
  endocarditis B37.6
  enteritis B37.82
  esophagitis B37.81
  intertrigo B37.2
  lung B37.1
  meningitis B37.5
  mouth B37.0
  nails B37.2
  neonatal P37.5
  onychia B37.2
  oral B37.0
  osteomyelitis B37.89
  otitis externa B37.84
  paronychia B37.2
  perionyxis B37.2
  pneumonia B37.1
  proctitis B37.82
  pulmonary B37.1
  pyelonephritis B37.49
  sepsis B37.7
  skin B37.2
  specified site NEC B37.89
  stomatitis B37.0
  systemic B37.7
  urethritis B37.41
  urogenital site NEC B37.49
  vagina B37.3
  vulva B37.3
  vulvovaginitis B37.3
Candidid L30.2
Candidosis — see Candidiasis
Candiru infection or infestation B88.8
Canities (premature) L67.1
  congenital Q84.2
Canker (mouth) (sore) K12.0
  rash A38.9
Cannabinosis J66.2
Cannabis induced
  anxiety disorder F12.980
  psychotic disorder F12.959
  sleep disorder F12.988
Canton fever A75.9
Cantrell's syndrome Q87.89
Capillariasis (intestinal) B81.1
  hepatic B83.8
Capillary — see condition
Caplan's syndrome — see Rheumatoid, lung

Capsule

Capsule — *see* condition
Capsulitis (joint) (*see also* Enthesopathy)
  adhesive (shoulder) M75.0- ☑
  hepatic K65.8
  labyrinthine — *see* Otosclerosis, specified NEC
  thyroid E06.9
Caput
  crepitus Q75.8
  medusae I86.8
  succedaneum P12.81
Car sickness T75.3 ☑
Carapata (disease) A68.0
Carate — *see* Pinta
Carbon lung J60
Carbuncle L02.93
  abdominal wall L02.231
  anus K61.0
  auditory canal, external — *see* Abscess, ear, external
  auricle ear — *see* Abscess, ear, external
  axilla L02.43- ☑
  back (any part) L02.232
  breast N61.1
  buttock L02.33
  cheek (external) L02.03
  chest wall L02.233
  chin L02.03
  corpus cavernosum N48.21
  ear (any part) (external) (middle) — *see* Abscess, ear, external
  external auditory canal — *see* Abscess, ear, external
  eyelid — *see* Abscess, eyelid
  face NEC L02.03
  femoral (region) — *see* Carbuncle, lower limb
  finger — *see* Carbuncle, hand
  flank L02.231
  foot L02.63- ☑
  forehead L02.03
  genital — *see* Abscess, genital
  gluteal (region) L02.33
  groin L02.234
  hand L02.53- ☑
  head NEC L02.831
  heel — *see* Carbuncle, foot
  hip — *see* Carbuncle, lower limb
  kidney — *see* Abscess, kidney
  knee — *see* Carbuncle, lower limb
  labium (majus) (minus) N76.4
  lacrimal
    gland — *see* Dacryoadenitis
    passages (duct) (sac) — *see* Inflammation, lacrimal, passages, acute
  leg — *see* Carbuncle, lower limb
  lower limb L02.43- ☑
  malignant A22.0
  navel L02.236
  neck L02.13
  nose (external) (septum) J34.0
  orbit, orbital — *see* Abscess, orbit
  palmar (space) — *see* Carbuncle, hand
  partes posteriores L02.33
  pectoral region L02.233
  penis N48.21
  perineum L02.235
  pinna — *see* Abscess, ear, external
  popliteal — *see* Carbuncle, lower limb
  scalp L02.831
  seminal vesicle N49.0
  shoulder — *see* Carbuncle, upper limb
  specified site NEC L02.838
  temple (region) L02.03
  thumb — *see* Carbuncle, hand
  toe — *see* Carbuncle, foot
  trunk L02.239
    abdominal wall L02.231
    back L02.232
    chest wall L02.233
    groin L02.234
    perineum L02.235
    umbilicus L02.236
  umbilicus L02.236
  upper limb L02.43- ☑
  urethra N34.0
  vulva N76.4
Carbunculus — *see* Carbuncle
Carcinoid (tumor) — *see* Tumor, carcinoid
Carcinoidosis E34.0

Carcinoma (malignant) (*see also* Neoplasm, by site, malignant)
  acidophil
    specified site — *see* Neoplasm, malignant, by site
    unspecified site C75.1
  acidophil-basophil, mixed
    specified site — *see* Neoplasm, malignant, by site
    unspecified site C75.1
  adnexal (skin) — *see* Neoplasm, skin, malignant
  adrenal cortical C74.0- ☑
  alveolar — *see* Neoplasm, lung, malignant
    cell — *see* Neoplasm, lung, malignant
  ameloblastic C41.1
    upper jaw (bone) C41.0
  apocrine
    breast — *see* Neoplasm, breast, malignant
    specified site NEC — *see* Neoplasm, skin, malignant
    unspecified site C44.99
  basal cell (pigmented) (*see also* Neoplasm, skin, malignant) C44.91
    fibro-epithelial — *see* Neoplasm, skin, malignant
    morphea — *see* Neoplasm, skin, malignant
    multicentric — *see* Neoplasm, skin, malignant
  basaloid
  basal-squamous cell, mixed — *see* Neoplasm, skin, malignant
  basophil
    specified site — *see* Neoplasm, malignant, by site
    unspecified site C75.1
  basophil-acidophil, mixed
    specified site — *see* Neoplasm, malignant, by site
    unspecified site C75.1
  basosquamous — *see* Neoplasm, skin, malignant
  bile duct
    with hepatocellular, mixed C22.0
    liver C22.1
    specified site NEC — *see* Neoplasm, malignant, by site
    unspecified site C22.1
  branchial or branchiogenic C10.4
  bronchial or bronchogenic — *see* Neoplasm, lung, malignant
  bronchiolar — *see* Neoplasm, lung, malignant
  bronchioloalveolar — *see* Neoplasm, lung, malignant
  C cell
    specified site — *see* Neoplasm, malignant, by site
    unspecified site C73
  ceruminous C44.29- ☑
  cervix uteri
    in situ D06.9
      endocervix D06.0
      exocervix D06.1
      specified site NEC D06.7
  chorionic
    specified site — *see* Neoplasm, malignant, by site
    unspecified site
      female C58
      male C62.90
  chromophobe
    specified site — *see* Neoplasm, malignant, by site
    unspecified site C75.1
  cloacogenic
    specified site — *see* Neoplasm, malignant, by site
    unspecified site C21.2
  diffuse type
    specified site — *see* Neoplasm, malignant, by site
    unspecified site C16.9
  duct (cell)
    with Paget's disease — *see* Neoplasm, breast, malignant
    infiltrating
      with lobular carcinoma (in situ)
        specified site — *see* Neoplasm, malignant, by site
        unspecified site (female) C50.91- ☑
          male C50.92- ☑
      specified site — *see* Neoplasm, malignant, by site
        unspecified site (female) C50.91- ☑
          male C50.92- ☑
  ductal
    with lobular
      specified site — *see* Neoplasm, malignant, by site
      unspecified site (female) C50.91- ☑
        male C50.92- ☑

Carcinoma — *continued*
  ductular, infiltrating
    specified site — *see* Neoplasm, malignant, by site
    unspecified site (female) C50.91- ☑
      male C50.92- ☑
  embryonal
    liver C22.7
  endometrioid
    specified site — *see* Neoplasm, malignant, by site
    unspecified site
      female C56.9
      male C61
  eosinophil
    specified site — *see* Neoplasm, malignant, by site
    unspecified site C75.1
  epidermoid (*see also* Neoplasm, skin, malignant)
    in situ, Bowen's type — *see* Neoplasm, skin, in situ
  fibroepithelial, basal cell — *see* Neoplasm, skin, malignant
  follicular
    with papillary (mixed) C73
    moderately differentiated C73
    pure follicle C73
    specified site — *see* Neoplasm, malignant, by site
    trabecular C73
    unspecified site C73
    well differentiated C73
  generalized, with unspecified primary site C80.0
  glycogen-rich — *see* Neoplasm, breast, malignant
  granulosa cell C56- ☑
  hepatic cell C22.0
  hepatocellular C22.0
    with bile duct, mixed C22.0
    fibrolamellar C22.0
  hepatocholangiolitic C22.0
  Hurthle cell C73
  in
    adenomatous
      polyposis coli C18.9
    pleomorphic adenoma — *see* Neoplasm, salivary glands, malignant
    situ — *see* Carcinoma-in-situ
  infiltrating
    duct
      with lobular
        specified site — *see* Neoplasm, malignant, by site
        unspecified site (female) C50.91- ☑
          male C50.92- ☑
      with Paget's disease — *see* Neoplasm, breast, malignant
      specified site — *see* Neoplasm, malignant
      unspecified site (female) C50.91- ☑
        male C50.92- ☑
    ductular
      specified site — *see* Neoplasm, malignant
      unspecified site (female) C50.91- ☑
        male C50.92- ☑
    lobular
      specified site — *see* Neoplasm, malignant
      unspecified site (female) C50.91- ☑
        male C50.92- ☑
  inflammatory
    specified site — *see* Neoplasm, malignant
    unspecified site (female) C50.91- ☑
      male C50.92- ☑
  intestinal type
    specified site — *see* Neoplasm, malignant, by site
    unspecified site C16.9
  intracystic
    noninfiltrating — *see* Neoplasm, in situ, by site
  intraductal (noninfiltrating)
    with Paget's disease — *see* Neoplasm, breast, malignant
    breast D05.1- ☑
    papillary
      with invasion
        specified site — *see* Neoplasm, malignant, by site
        unspecified site (female) C50.91- ☑
          male C50.92- ☑
      breast D05.1- ☑
      specified site NEC — *see* Neoplasm, in situ, by site
      unspecified site (female) D05.1- ☑
    specified site NEC — *see* Neoplasm, in situ, by site
    unspecified site (female) D05.1- ☑

☑ **Additional Character Required — Refer to the Tabular List for Character Selection**   ☝ **Subterms under main terms may continue to next column or page**

Carcinoma — *continued*
- intraepidermal — *see* Neoplasm, in situ
  - squamous cell, Bowen's type — *see* Neoplasm, skin, in situ
- intraepithelial — *see* Neoplasm, in situ, by site
  - squamous cell — *see* Neoplasm, in situ, by site
- intraosseous C41.1
  - upper jaw (bone) C41.0
- islet cell
  - with exocrine, mixed
    - specified site — *see* Neoplasm, malignant, by site
    - unspecified site C25.9
  - pancreas C25.4
  - specified site NEC — *see* Neoplasm, malignant, by site
  - unspecified site C25.4
- juvenile, breast — *see* Neoplasm, breast, malignant
- large cell
  - small cell
    - specified site — *see* Neoplasm, malignant, by site
    - unspecified site C34.90
- Leydig cell (testis)
  - specified site — *see* Neoplasm, malignant, by site
  - unspecified site
    - female C56.9
    - male C62.90
- lipid-rich (female) C50.91- ☑
  - male C50.92- ☑
- liver cell C22.0
- liver NEC C22.7
- lobular (infiltrating)
  - with intraductal
    - specified site — *see* Neoplasm, malignant, by site
    - unspecified site (female) C50.91- ☑
      - male C50.92- ☑
  - noninfiltrating
    - breast D05.0- ☑
    - specified site NEC — *see* Neoplasm, in situ, by site
    - unspecified site D05.0- ☑
  - specified site — *see* Neoplasm, malignant, by site
  - unspecified site (female) C50.91- ☑
    - male C50.92- ☑
- medullary
  - with
    - amyloid stroma
      - specified site — *see* Neoplasm, malignant, by site
      - unspecified site C73
    - lymphoid stroma
      - specified site — *see* Neoplasm, malignant, by site
      - unspecified site (female) C50.91- ☑
        - male C50.92- ☑
- Merkel cell C4A.9 (*following* C43)
  - anal margin C4A.51 (*following* C43)
  - anal skin C4A.51 (*following* C43)
  - canthus C4A.1- ☑ (*following* C43)
  - ear and external auricular canal C4A.2- ☑ (*following* C43)
  - external auricular canal C4A.2- ☑ (*following* C43)
  - eyelid, including canthus C4A.1- ☑ (*following* C43)
  - face C4A.30 (*following* C43)
    - specified NEC C4A.39 (*following* C43)
  - hip C4A.7- ☑ (*following* C43)
  - lip C4A.0 (*following* C43)
  - lower limb, including hip C4A.7- ☑ (*following* C43)
  - neck C4A.4 (*following* C43)
  - nodal presentation C7B.1 (*following* C75)
  - nose C4A.31 (*following* C43)
  - overlapping sites C4A.8 (*following* C43)
  - perianal skin C4A.51 (*following* C43)
  - scalp C4A.4 (*following* C43)
  - secondary C7B.1 (*following* C75)
  - shoulder C4A.6- ☑ (*following* C43)
  - skin of breast C4A.52 (*following* C43)
  - trunk NEC C4A.59 (*following* C43)
  - upper limb, including shoulder C4A.6- ☑ (*following* C43)
  - visceral metastatic C7B.1 (*following* C75)
- metastatic — *see* Neoplasm, secondary, by site
- metatypical — *see* Neoplasm, skin, malignant
- morphea, basal cell — *see* Neoplasm, skin, malignant

Carcinoma — *continued*
- mucoid
  - cell
    - specified site — *see* Neoplasm, malignant, by site
    - unspecified site C75.1
- neuroendocrine (*see also* Tumor, neuroendocrine)
  - high grade, any site C7A.1 (*following* C75)
  - poorly differentiated, any site C7A.1 (*following* C75)
- nonencapsulated sclerosing C73
- noninfiltrating
  - intracystic — *see* Neoplasm, in situ, by site
  - intraductal
    - breast D05.1- ☑
    - papillary
      - breast D05.1- ☑
      - specified site NEC — *see* Neoplasm, in situ, by site
      - unspecified site D05.1- ☑
    - specified site — *see* Neoplasm, in situ, by site
    - unspecified site D05.1- ☑
  - lobular
    - breast D05.0- ☑
    - specified site NEC — *see* Neoplasm, in situ, by site
    - unspecified site (female) D05.0- ☑
- oat cell
  - specified site — *see* Neoplasm, malignant, by site
  - unspecified site C34.90
- odontogenic C41.1
  - upper jaw (bone) C41.0
- papillary
  - with follicular (mixed) C73
  - follicular variant C73
  - intraductal (noninfiltrating)
    - with invasion
      - specified site — *see* Neoplasm, malignant, by site
      - unspecified site (female) C50.91- ☑
        - male C50.92- ☑
    - breast D05.1- ☑
    - specified site NEC — *see* Neoplasm, in situ, by site
    - unspecified site D05.1- ☑
  - serous
    - specified site — *see* Neoplasm, malignant, by site
    - surface
      - specified site — *see* Neoplasm, malignant, by site
      - unspecified site C56.9
    - unspecified site C56.9
- papillocystic
  - specified site — *see* Neoplasm, malignant, by site
  - unspecified site C56.9
- parafollicular cell
  - specified site — *see* Neoplasm, malignant, by site
  - unspecified site C73
- pilomatrix — *see* Neoplasm, skin, malignant
- pseudomucinous
  - specified site — *see* Neoplasm, malignant, by site
  - unspecified site C56.9
- renal cell C64- ☑
- Schmincke — *see* Neoplasm, nasopharynx, malignant
- Schneiderian
  - specified site — *see* Neoplasm, malignant, by site
  - unspecified site C30.0
- sebaceous — *see* Neoplasm, skin, malignant
- secondary (*see also* Neoplasm, secondary, by site)
  - Merkel cell C7B.1 (*following* C75)
- secretory, breast — *see* Neoplasm, breast, malignant
- serous
  - papillary
    - specified site — *see* Neoplasm, malignant, by site
    - unspecified site C56.9
  - surface, papillary
    - specified site — *see* Neoplasm, malignant, by site
    - unspecified site C56.9
- Sertoli cell
  - specified site — *see* Neoplasm, malignant, by site
  - unspecified site C62.90
    - female C56.9
    - male C62.90
- skin appendage — *see* Neoplasm, skin, malignant

Carcinoma — *continued*
- small cell
  - fusiform cell
    - specified site — *see* Neoplasm, malignant, by site
    - unspecified site C34.90
  - intermediate cell
    - specified site — *see* Neoplasm, malignant, by site
    - unspecified site C34.90
  - large cell
    - specified site — *see* Neoplasm, malignant, by site
    - unspecified site C34.90
- solid
  - with amyloid stroma
    - specified site — *see* Neoplasm, malignant, by site
    - unspecified site C73
  - microinvasive
    - specified site — *see* Neoplasm, malignant, by site
    - unspecified site C53.9
- sweat gland — *see* Neoplasm, skin, malignant
- theca cell C56.- ☑
- thymic C37
- unspecified site (primary) C80.1
- water-clear cell C75.0

Carcinoma-in-situ (*see also* Neoplasm, in situ, by site)
- breast NOS D05.9- ☑
  - specified type NEC D05.8- ☑
- epidermoid (*see also* Neoplasm, in situ, by site)
  - with questionable stromal invasion
    - cervix D06.9
    - specified site NEC — *see* Neoplasm, in situ, by site
    - unspecified site D06.9
  - Bowen's type — *see* Neoplasm, skin, in situ
- intraductal
  - breast D05.1- ☑
  - specified site NEC — *see* Neoplasm, in situ, by site
  - unspecified site D05.1- ☑
- lobular
  - with
    - infiltrating duct
      - breast (female) C50.91- ☑
        - male C50.92- ☑
      - specified site NEC — *see* Neoplasm, malignant
      - unspecified site (female) C50.91- ☑
        - male C50.92- ☑
    - intraductal
      - breast D05.8- ☑
      - specified site NEC — *see* Neoplasm, in situ, by site
      - unspecified site (female) D05.8- ☑
  - breast D05.0- ☑
  - specified site NEC — *see* Neoplasm, in situ, by site
  - unspecified site D05.0- ☑
- squamous cell (*see also* Neoplasm, in situ, by site)
  - with questionable stromal invasion
    - cervix D06.9
    - specified site NEC — *see* Neoplasm, in situ, by site
    - unspecified site D06.9

Carcinomaphobia F45.29
Carcinomatosis C80.0
- peritonei C78.6
- unspecified site (primary) (secondary) C80.0
Carcinosarcoma — *see* Neoplasm, malignant, by site
- embryonal — *see* Neoplasm, malignant, by site
Cardia, cardial — *see* condition
Cardiac (*see also* condition)
- death, sudden — *see* Arrest, cardiac
- pacemaker
  - in situ Z95.0
  - management or adjustment Z45.018
- tamponade I31.4
Cardialgia — *see* Pain, precordial
Cardiectasis — *see* Hypertrophy, cardiac
Cardiochalasia K21.9
Cardiomalacia I51.5
Cardiomegalia glycogenica diffusa E74.02 [I43]
Cardiomegaly (*see also* Hypertrophy, cardiac)
- congenital Q24.8
- glycogen E74.02 [I43]
- idiopathic I51.7
Cardiomyoliposis I51.5

⛉ **Subterms under main terms may continue to next column or page**   ☑ **Additional Character Required** — Refer to the Tabular List for Character Selection   **49**

Index

Carcinoma — Cardiomyoliposis

Cardiomyopathy (familial) (idiopathic) I42.9
  alcoholic I42.6
  amyloid E85.4 [I43]
    transthyretin-related (ATTR) familial E85.4
  arteriosclerotic — see Disease, heart, ischemic,
    atherosclerotic
  beriberi E51.12
  cobalt-beer I42.6
  congenital I42.4
  congestive I42.0
  constrictive NOS I42.5
  dilated I42.0
  due to
    alcohol I42.6
    beriberi E51.12
    cardiac glycogenosis E74.02 [I43]
    drugs I42.7
    external agents NEC I42.7
    Friedreich's ataxia G11.1
    myotonia atrophica G71.11 [I43]
    progressive muscular dystrophy G71.09 [I43]
  glycogen storage E74.02 [I43]
  hypertensive — see Hypertension, heart
  hypertrophic (nonobstructive) I42.2
    obstructive I42.1
      congenital Q24.8
  in
    Chagas' disease (chronic) B57.2
      acute B57.0
    sarcoidosis D86.85
  ischemic I25.5
  metabolic E88.9 [I43]
    thyrotoxic E05.90 [I43]
      with thyroid storm E05.91 [I43]
  newborn I42.8
    congenital I42.4
  nutritional E63.9 [I43]
    beriberi E51.12
  obscure of Africa I42.8
  peripartum O90.3
  postpartum O90.3
  restrictive NEC I42.5
  rheumatic I09.0
  secondary I42.9
  stress induced I51.81
  takotsubo I51.81
  thyrotoxic E05.90 [I43]
    with thyroid storm E05.91 [I43]
  toxic NEC I42.7
  transthyretin-related (ATTR) familial amyloid E85.4
  tuberculous A18.84
  viral B33.24
Cardionephritis — see Hypertension, cardiorenal
Cardionephropathy — see Hypertension, cardiorenal
Cardionephrosis — see Hypertension, cardiorenal
Cardiopathia nigra I27.0
Cardiopathy (see also Disease, heart) I51.9
  idiopathic I42.9
  mucopolysaccharidosis E76.3 [I52]
Cardiopericarditis — see Pericarditis
Cardiophobia F45.29
Cardiorenal — see condition
Cardiorrhexis — see Infarct, myocardium
Cardiosclerosis — see Disease, heart, ischemic,
  atherosclerotic
Cardiosis — see Disease, heart
Cardiospasm (esophagus) (reflex) (stomach) K22.0
  congenital Q39.5
    with megaesophagus Q39.5
Cardiostenosis — see Disease, heart
Cardiosymphysis I31.0
Cardiovascular — see condition
Carditis (acute) (bacterial) (chronic) (subacute) I51.89
  meningococcal A39.50
  rheumatic — see Disease, heart, rheumatic
  rheumatoid — see Rheumatoid, carditis
  viral B33.20
Care (of) (for) (following)
  child (routine) Z76.2
  family member (handicapped) (sick)
    creating problem for family Z63.6
    provided away from home for holiday relief Z75.5
    unavailable, due to
      absence (person rendering care) (sufferer) Z74.2
      inability (any reason) of person rendering care
        Z74.2
  foundling Z76.1
  holiday relief Z75.5

Care — continued
  improper — see Maltreatment
  lack of (at or after birth) (infant) — see Maltreatment,
    child, neglect
  lactating mother Z39.1
  palliative Z51.5
  postpartum
    immediately after delivery Z39.0
    routine follow-up Z39.2
  respite Z75.5
  unavailable, due to
    absence of person rendering care Z74.2
    inability (any reason) of person rendering care Z74.2
  well-baby Z76.2
Caries
  bone NEC A18.03
  dental (dentino enamel junction) (early childhood) (of
    dentine) (pre-eruptive) (recurrent) (to the pulp)
    K02.9
    arrested (coronal) (root) K02.3
    chewing surface
      limited to enamel K02.51
      penetrating into dentin K02.52
      penetrating into pulp K02.53
    coronal surface
      chewing surface
        limited to enamel K02.51
        penetrating into dentin K02.52
        penetrating into pulp K02.53
      pit and fissure surface
        limited to enamel K02.51
        penetrating into dentin K02.52
        penetrating into pulp K02.53
      smooth surface
        limited to enamel K02.61
        penetrating into dentin K02.62
        penetrating into pulp K02.63
    pit and fissure surface
      limited to enamel K02.51
      penetrating into dentin K02.52
      penetrating into pulp K02.53
    primary, cervical origin K02.52
    root K02.7
    smooth surface
      limited to enamel K02.61
      penetrating into dentin K02.62
      penetrating into pulp K02.63
  external meatus — see Disorder, ear, external, specified
    type NEC
  hip (tuberculous) A18.02
  initial (tooth)
    chewing surface K02.51
    pit and fissure surface K02.51
    smooth surface K02.61
  knee (tuberculous) A18.02
  labyrinth H83.8 ☑
  limb NEC (tuberculous) A18.03
  mastoid process (chronic) — see Mastoiditis, chronic
    tuberculous A18.03
  middle ear H74.8 ☑
  nose (tuberculous) A18.03
  orbit (tuberculous) A18.03
  ossicles, ear — see Abnormal, ear ossicles
  petrous bone — see Petrositis
  root (dental) (tooth) K02.7
  sacrum (tuberculous) A18.01
  spine, spinal (column) (tuberculous) A18.01
  syphilitic A52.77
    congenital (early) A50.02 [M90.80]
  tooth, teeth — see Caries, dental
  tuberculous A18.03
  vertebra (column) (tuberculous) A18.01
Carious teeth — see Caries, dental
Carneous mole O02.0
Carnitine insufficiency E71.40
Carotenemia (dietary) E67.1
Carotenosis (cutis) (skin) E67.1
Carotid body or sinus syndrome G90.01
Carotidynia G90.01
Carpal tunnel syndrome — see Syndrome, carpal tunnel
Carpenter's syndrome Q87.0
Carpopedal spasm — see Tetany
Carr-Barr-Plunkett syndrome Q97.1
Carrier (suspected) of
  amebiasis Z22.1
  bacterial disease NEC Z22.39
    diphtheria Z22.2
    intestinal infectious NEC Z22.1

Carrier of — continued
  bacterial disease — continued
    intestinal infectious — continued
      typhoid Z22.0
    meningococcal Z22.31
    sexually transmitted Z22.4
    specified NEC Z22.39
    staphylococcal (Methicillin susceptible) Z22.321
      Methicillin resistant Z22.322
    streptococcal Z22.338
      group B Z22.330
        complicating pregnancy or delivery
          O99.82- ☑
    typhoid Z22.0
  cholera Z22.1
  diphtheria Z22.2
  gastrointestinal pathogens NEC Z22.1
  genetic Z14.8
    cystic fibrosis Z14.1
    hemophilia A (asymptomatic) Z14.01
      symptomatic Z14.02
  gestational, pregnant Z33.1
  gonorrhea Z22.4
  HAA (hepatitis Australian-antigen) B18.8
  HB (c)(s)-AG B18.1
  hepatitis (viral) B18.9
    Australia-antigen (HAA) B18.8
    B surface antigen (HBsAg) B18.1
      with acute delta- (super)infection B17.0
    C B18.2
    specified NEC B18.8
  human T-cell lymphotropic virus type-1 (HTLV-1) infec-
    tion Z22.6
  infectious organism Z22.9
    specified NEC Z22.8
  meningococci Z22.31
  Salmonella typhosa Z22.0
  serum hepatitis — see Carrier, hepatitis
  staphylococci (Methicillin susceptible) Z22.321
    Methicillin resistant Z22.322
  streptococci Z22.338
    group B Z22.330
      complicating pregnancy or delivery O99.82- ☑
  syphilis Z22.4
  typhoid Z22.0
  venereal disease NEC Z22.4
Carrion's disease A44.0
Carter's relapsing fever (Asiatic) A68.1
Cartilage — see condition
Caruncle (inflamed)
  conjunctiva (acute) — see Conjunctivitis, acute
  labium (majus) (minus) N90.89
  lacrimal — see Inflammation, lacrimal, passages
  myrtiform N89.8
  urethral (benign) N36.2
Cascade stomach K31.2
Caseation lymphatic gland (tuberculous) A18.2
Cassidy (-Scholte) syndrome (malignant carcinoid) E34.0
Castellani's disease A69.8
Castration, traumatic, male S38.231 ☑
Casts in urine R82.998
Cat
  cry syndrome Q93.4
  ear Q17.3
  eye syndrome Q92.8
Catabolism, senile R54
Catalepsy (hysterical) F44.2
  schizophrenic F20.2
Cataplexy (idiopathic) — see Narcolepsy
Cataract (cortical) (immature) (incipient) H26.9
  with
    neovascularization — see Cataract, complicated
  age-related — see Cataract, senile
  anterior
    and posterior axial embryonal Q12.0
    pyramidal Q12.0
  associated with
    galactosemia E74.21 [H28]
    myotonic disorders G71.19 [H28]
  blue Q12.0
  central Q12.0
  cerulean Q12.0
  complicated H26.20
    with
      neovascularization H26.21- ☑
      ocular disorder H26.22- ☑
      glaucomatous flecks H26.23- ☑
  congenital Q12.0

Cataract — *continued*
  coraliform Q12.0
  coronary Q12.0
  crystalline Q12.0
  diabetic — *see* Diabetes, cataract
  drug-induced H26.3- ☑
  due to
    ocular disorder — *see* Cataract, complicated
    radiation H26.8
  electric H26.8
  extraction status Z98.4- ☑
  glass-blower's H26.8
  heat ray H26.8
  heterochromic — *see* Cataract, complicated
  hypermature — *see* Cataract, senile, morgagnian type
  in (due to)
    chronic iridocyclitis — *see* Cataract, complicated
    diabetes — *see* Diabetes, cataract
    endocrine disease E34.9 [H28]
    eye disease — *see* Cataract, complicated
    hypoparathyroidism E20.9 [H28]
    malnutrition-dehydration E46 [H28]
    metabolic disease E88.9 [H28]
    myotonic disorders G71.19 [H28]
    nutritional disease E63.9 [H28]
  infantile — *see* Cataract, presenile
  irradiational — *see* Cataract, specified NEC
  juvenile — *see* Cataract, presenile
  malnutrition-dehydration E46 [H28]
  morgagnian — *see* Cataract, senile, morgagnian type
  myotonic G71.19 [H28]
  myxedema E03.9 [H28]
  nuclear
    embryonal Q12.0
    sclerosis — *see* Cataract, senile, nuclear
  presenile H26.00- ☑
    combined forms H26.06- ☑
    cortical H26.01- ☑
    lamellar — *see* Cataract, presenile, cortical
    nuclear H26.03- ☑
    specified NEC H26.09
    subcapsular polar (anterior) H26.04- ☑
      posterior H26.05- ☑
    zonular — *see* Cataract, presenile, cortical
  secondary H26.40
    Soemmering's ring H26.41- ☑
    specified NEC H26.49- ☑
    to eye disease — *see* Cataract, complicated
  senile H25.9
    brunescens — *see* Cataract, senile, nuclear
    combined forms H25.81- ☑
    coronary — *see* Cataract, senile, incipient
    cortical H25.01- ☑
    hypermature — *see* Cataract, senile, morgagnian type
    incipient (mature) (total) H25.09- ☑
      cortical — *see* Cataract, senile, cortical
      subcapsular — *see* Cataract, senile, subcapsular
    morgagnian type (hypermature) H25.2- ☑
    nuclear (sclerosis) H25.1- ☑
    polar subcapsular (anterior) (posterior) — *see* Cataract, senile, incipient
    punctate — *see* Cataract, senile, incipient
    specified NEC H25.89
    subcapsular polar (anterior) H25.03- ☑
      posterior H25.04- ☑
  snowflake — *see* Diabetes, cataract
  specified NEC H26.8
  toxic — *see* Cataract, drug-induced
  traumatic H26.10- ☑
    localized H26.11- ☑
    partially resolved H26.12- ☑
    total H26.13- ☑
  zonular (perinuclear) Q12.0
Cataracta (*see also* Cataract)
  brunescens — *see* Cataract, senile, nuclear
  centralis pulverulenta Q12.0
  cerulea Q12.0
  complicata — *see* Cataract, complicated
  congenita Q12.0
  coralliformis Q12.0
  coronaria Q12.0
  diabetic — *see* Diabetes, cataract
  membranacea
    accreta — *see* Cataract, secondary
    congenita Q12.0
  nigra — *see* Cataract, senile, nuclear

Cataracta — *continued*
  sunflower — *see* Cataract, complicated
Catarrh, catarrhal (acute) (febrile) (infectious) (inflammation) (*see also* condition) J00
  bronchial — *see* Bronchitis
  chest — *see* Bronchitis
  chronic J31.0
  due to congenital syphilis A50.03
  enteric — *see* Enteritis
  eustachian H68.009
  fauces — *see* Pharyngitis
  gastrointestinal — *see* Enteritis
  gingivitis K05.00
    nonplaque induced K05.01
    plaque induced K05.00
  hay — *see* Fever, hay
  intestinal — *see* Enteritis
  larynx, chronic J37.0
  liver B15.9
    with hepatic coma B15.0
  lung — *see* Bronchitis
  middle ear, chronic — *see* Otitis, media, nonsuppurative, chronic, serous
  mouth K12.1
  nasal (chronic) — *see* Rhinitis
  nasobronchial J31.1
  nasopharyngeal (chronic) J31.1
    acute J00
  pulmonary — *see* Bronchitis
  spring (eye) (vernal) — *see* Conjunctivitis, acute, atopic
  summer (hay) — *see* Fever, hay
  throat J31.2
  tubotympanal (*see also* Otitis, media, nonsuppurative)
    chronic — *see* Otitis, media, nonsuppurative, chronic, serous
Catatonia (schizophrenic) F20.2
Catatonic
  disorder due to known physiologic condition F06.1
  schizophrenia F20.2
  stupor R40.1
Cat-scratch (*see also* Abrasion)
  disease or fever A28.1
Cauda equina — *see* condition
Cauliflower ear M95.1- ☑
Causalgia (upper limb) G56.4- ☑
  lower limb G57.7- ☑
Cause
  external, general effects T75.89 ☑
Caustic burn — *see* Corrosion, by site
Cave-in, injury
  crushing (severe) — *see* Crush
  suffocation — *see* Asphyxia, traumatic, due to low oxygen, due to cave-in
Cavernitis (penis) N48.29
Cavernositis N48.29
Cavernous — *see* condition
Cavitation of lung (*see also* Tuberculosis, pulmonary)
  nontuberculous J98.4
Cavities, dental — *see* Caries, dental
Cavity
  lung — *see* Cavitation of lung
  optic papilla Q14.2
  pulmonary — *see* Cavitation of lung
Cavovarus foot, congenital Q66.1
Cavus foot (congenital) Q66.7
  acquired — *see* Deformity, limb, foot, specified NEC
Cazenave's disease L10.2
Cecitis K52.9
  with perforation, peritonitis, or rupture K65.8
Cecum — *see* condition
Celiac
  artery compression syndrome I77.4
  disease (with steatorrhea) K90.0
  infantilism K90.0
Cell(s), **cellular** (*see also* condition)
  in urine R82.998
Cellulitis (diffuse) (phlegmonous) (septic) (suppurative) L03.90
  abdominal wall L03.311
  anaerobic A48.0
  ankle — *see* Cellulitis, lower limb
  anus K61.0
  arm — *see* Cellulitis, upper limb
  auricle (ear) — *see* Cellulitis, ear
  axilla L03.11- ☑
  back (any part) L03.312

Cellulitis — *continued*
  breast (acute) (nonpuerperal) (subacute) N61.0
    nipple N61.0
  broad ligament
    acute N73.0
  buttock L03.317
  cervical (meaning neck) L03.221
  cervix (uteri) — *see* Cervicitis
  cheek (external) L03.211
    internal K12.2
  chest wall L03.313
  chronic L03.90
  clostridial A48.0
  corpus cavernosum N48.22
  digit
    finger — *see* Cellulitis, finger
    toe — *see* Cellulitis, toe
  Douglas' cul-de-sac or pouch
    acute N73.0
  drainage site (following operation) T81.49 ☑
  ear (external) H60.1- ☑
  eosinophilic (granulomatous) L98.3
  erysipelatous — *see* Erysipelas
  external auditory canal — *see* Cellulitis, ear
  eyelid — *see* Abscess, eyelid
  face NEC L03.211
  finger (intrathecal) (periosteal) (subcutaneous) (subcuticular) L03.01- ☑
  foot — *see* Cellulitis, lower limb
  gangrenous — *see* Gangrene
  genital organ NEC
    female (external) N76.4
    male N49.9
      multiple sites N49.8
      specified NEC N49.8
  gluteal (region) L03.317
  gonococcal A54.89
  groin L03.314
  hand — *see* Cellulitis, upper limb
  head NEC L03.811
    face (any part, except ear, eye and nose) L03.211
  heel — *see* Cellulitis, lower limb
  hip — *see* Cellulitis, lower limb
  jaw (region) L03.211
  knee — *see* Cellulitis, lower limb
  labium (majus) (minus) — *see* Vulvitis
  lacrimal passages — *see* Inflammation, lacrimal, passages
  larynx J38.7
  leg — *see* Cellulitis, lower limb
  lip K13.0
  lower limb L03.11- ☑
    toe — *see* Cellulitis, toe
  mouth (floor) K12.2
  multiple sites, so stated L03.90
  nasopharynx J39.1
  navel L03.316
    newborn P38.9
      with mild hemorrhage P38.1
      without hemorrhage P38.9
  neck (region) L03.221
  nipple (acute) (nonpuerperal) (subacute) N61.0
  nose (septum) (external) J34.0
  orbit, orbital H05.01- ☑
  palate (soft) K12.2
  pectoral (region) L03.313
  pelvis, pelvic (chronic)
    female (*see also* Disease, pelvis, inflammatory) N73.2
      acute N73.0
    following ectopic or molar pregnancy O08.0
    male K65.0
  penis N48.22
  perineal, perineum L03.315
  periorbital L03.213
  perirectal K61.1
  peritonsillar J36
  periurethral N34.0
  periuterine (*see also* Disease, pelvis, inflammatory) N73.2
    acute N73.0
  pharynx J39.1
  preseptal L03.213
  rectum K61.1
  retroperitoneal K68.9
  round ligament
    acute N73.0
  scalp (any part) L03.811
  scrotum N49.2

Cellulitis — *continued*
seminal vesicle N49.0
shoulder — *see* Cellulitis, upper limb
specified site NEC L03.818
submandibular (region) (space) (triangle) K12.2
gland K11.3
submaxillary (region) K12.2
gland K11.3
thigh — *see* Cellulitis, lower limb
thumb (intrathecal) (periosteal) (subcutaneous) (subcuticular) — *see* Cellulitis, finger
toe (intrathecal) (periosteal) (subcutaneous) (subcuticular) L03.03- ☑
tonsil J36
trunk L03.319
abdominal wall L03.311
back (any part) L03.312
buttock L03.317
chest wall L03.313
groin L03.314
perineal, perineum L03.315
umbilicus L03.316
tuberculous (primary) A18.4
umbilicus L03.316
upper limb L03.11- ☑
axilla — *see* Cellulitis, axilla
finger — *see* Cellulitis, finger
thumb — *see* Cellulitis, finger
vaccinal T88.0 ☑
vocal cord J38.3
vulva — *see* Vulvitis
wrist — *see* Cellulitis, upper limb
Cementoblastoma, benign — *see* Cyst, calcifying odontogenic
Cementoma — *see* Cyst, calcifying odontogenic
Cementoperiostitis — *see* Periodontitis
Cementosis K03.4
Central auditory processing disorder H93.25
Central pain syndrome G89.0
Cephalematocele, cephal (o)hematocele
newborn P52.8
birth injury P10.8
traumatic — *see* Hematoma, brain
Cephalematoma, cephalhematoma (calcified)
newborn (birth injury) P12.0
traumatic — *see* Hematoma, brain
Cephalgia, cephalalgia (*see also* Headache)
histamine G44.009
intractable G44.001
not intractable G44.009
trigeminal autonomic (TAC) NEC G44.099
intractable G44.091
not intractable G44.099
Cephalic — *see* condition
Cephalitis — *see* Encephalitis
Cephalocele — *see* Encephalocele
Cephalomenia N94.89
Cephalopelvic — *see* condition
Cerclage (with cervical incompetence) in pregnancy — *see* Incompetence, cervix, in pregnancy
Cerebellitis — *see* Encephalitis
Cerebellum, cerebellar — *see* condition
Cerebral — *see* condition
Cerebritis — *see* Encephalitis
Cerebro-hepato-renal syndrome Q87.89
Cerebromalacia — *see* Softening, brain
sequelae of cerebrovascular disease I69.398
Cerebroside lipidosis E75.22
Cerebrospasticity (congenital) G80.1
Cerebrospinal — *see* condition
Cerebrum — *see* condition
Ceroid-lipofuscinosis, neuronal E75.4
Cerumen (accumulation) (impacted) H61.2- ☑
Cervical (*see also* condition)
auricle Q18.2
dysplasia in pregnancy — *see* Abnormal, cervix, in pregnancy or childbirth
erosion in pregnancy — *see* Abnormal, cervix, in pregnancy or childbirth
fibrosis in pregnancy — *see* Abnormal, cervix, in pregnancy or childbirth
fusion syndrome Q76.1
rib Q76.5
shortening (complicating pregnancy) O26.87- ☑
Cervicalgia M54.2
Cervicitis (acute) (chronic) (nonvenereal) (senile (atrophic)) (subacute) (with ulceration) N72

Cervicitis — *continued*
with
abortion — *see* Abortion, by type complicated by genital tract and pelvic infection
ectopic pregnancy O08.0
molar pregnancy O08.0
chlamydial A56.09
gonococcal A54.03
herpesviral A60.03
puerperal (postpartum) O86.11
syphilitic A52.76
trichomonal A59.09
tuberculous A18.16
Cervicocolpitis (emphysematosa) (*see also* Cervicitis) N72
Cervix — *see* condition
Cesarean delivery, previous, affecting management of pregnancy O34.219
classical (vertical) scar O34.212
low transverse scar O34.211
Céstan (-Chenais) paralysis or syndrome G46.3
Céstan-Raymond syndrome I65.8
Cestode infestation B71.9
specified type NEC B71.8
Cestodiasis B71.9
Chabert's disease A22.9
Chacaleh E53.8
Chafing L30.4
Chagas' (-Mazza) disease (chronic) B57.2
with
cardiovascular involvement NEC B57.2
digestive system involvement B57.30
megacolon B57.32
megaesophagus B57.31
other specified B57.39
megacolon B57.32
megaesophagus B57.31
myocarditis B57.2
nervous system involvement B57.40
meningitis B57.41
meningoencephalitis B57.42
other specified B57.49
specified organ involvement NEC B57.5
acute (with) B57.1
cardiovascular NEC B57.0
myocarditis B57.0
Chagres fever B50.9
Chairridden Z74.09
Chalasia (cardiac sphincter) K21.9
Chalazion H00.19
left H00.16
lower H00.15
upper H00.14
right H00.13
lower H00.12
upper H00.11
Chalcosis (*see also* Disorder, globe, degenerative, chalcosis)
cornea — *see* Deposit, cornea
crystalline lens — *see* Cataract, complicated
retina H35.89
Chalicosis (pulmonum) J62.8
Chancre (any genital site) (hard) (hunterian) (mixed) (primary) (seronegative) (seropositive) (syphilitic) A51.0
congenital A50.07
conjunctiva NEC A51.2
Ducrey's A57
extragenital A51.2
eyelid A51.2
lip A51.2
nipple A51.2
Nisbet's A57
of
carate A67.0
pinta A67.0
yaws A66.0
palate, soft A51.2
phagedenic A57
simple A57
soft A57
bubo A57
palate A51.2
urethra A51.0
yaws A66.0
Chancroid (anus) (genital) (penis) (perineum) (rectum) (urethra) (vulva) A57

Chandler's disease (osteochondritis dissecans, hip) — *see* Osteochondritis, dissecans, hip
Change(s) (in) (of) (*see also* Removal)
arteriosclerotic — *see* Arteriosclerosis
bone (*see also* Disorder, bone)
diabetic — *see* Diabetes, bone change
bowel habit R19.4
cardiorenal (vascular) — *see* Hypertension, cardiorenal
cardiovascular — *see* Disease, cardiovascular
circulatory I99.9
cognitive (mild) (organic) R41.89
color, tooth, teeth
during formation K00.8
posteruptive K03.7
contraceptive device Z30.433
corneal membrane H18.30
Bowman's membrane fold or rupture H18.31- ☑
Descemet's membrane
fold H18.32- ☑
rupture H18.33- ☑
coronary — *see* Disease, heart, ischemic
degenerative, spine or vertebra — *see* Spondylosis
dental pulp, regressive K04.2
dressing (nonsurgical) Z48.00
surgical Z48.01
heart — *see* Disease, heart
hip joint — *see* Derangement, joint, hip
hyperplastic larynx J38.7
hypertrophic
nasal sinus J34.89
turbinate, nasal J34.3
upper respiratory tract J39.8
indwelling catheter Z46.6
inflammatory (*see also* Inflammation)
sacroiliac M46.1
job, anxiety concerning Z56.1
joint — *see* Derangement, joint
life — *see* Menopause
mental status R41.82
minimal (glomerular) (*see also* N00-N07 with fourth character .0) N05.0
myocardium, myocardial — *see* Degeneration, myocardial
of life — *see* Menopause
pacemaker Z45.018
pulse generator Z45.010
personality (enduring) F68.8
due to (secondary to)
general medical condition F07.0
secondary (nonspecific) F60.89
regressive, dental pulp K04.2
renal — *see* Disease, renal
retina H35.9
myopic (*see also* Myopia, degenerative) H44.2- ☑
sacroiliac joint M53.3
senile (*see also* condition) R54
sensory R20.8
skin R23.9
acute, due to ultraviolet radiation L56.9
specified NEC L56.8
chronic, due to nonionizing radiation L57.9
specified NEC L57.8
cyanosis R23.0
flushing R23.2
pallor R23.1
petechiae R23.3
specified change NEC R23.8
swelling — *see* Mass, localized
texture R23.4
trophic
arm — *see* Mononeuropathy, upper limb
leg — *see* Mononeuropathy, lower limb
vascular I99.9
vasomotor I73.9
voice R49.9
psychogenic F44.4
specified NEC R49.8
Changing sleep-work schedule, affecting sleep G47.26
Changuinola fever A93.1
Chapping skin T69.8 ☑
Charcot-Marie-Tooth disease, paralysis or syndrome G60.0
Charcot's
arthropathy — *see* Arthropathy, neuropathic
cirrhosis K74.3
disease (tabetic arthropathy) A52.16
joint (disease) (tabetic) A52.16

Index

Charcot's — *continued*
  joint — *continued*
    diabetic — *see* Diabetes, with, arthropathy
    syringomyelic G95.0
  syndrome (intermittent claudication) I73.9
CHARGE association Q89.8
Charley-horse (quadriceps) M62.831
  traumatic (quadriceps) S76.11- ☑
Charlouis' disease — *see* Yaws
Cheadle's disease E54
Checking (of)
  cardiac pacemaker (battery) (electrode(s)) Z45.018
    pulse generator Z45.010
  implantable subdermal contraceptive Z30.46
  intrauterine contraceptive device Z30.431
  wound Z48.0- ☑
    due to injury — code to Injury, by site, using appropriate seventh character for subsequent encounter
Check-up — *see* Examination
Chédiak-Higashi (-Steinbrinck) **syndrome** (congenital gigantism of peroxidase granules) E70.330
Cheek — *see* condition
Cheese itch B88.0
Cheese-washer's lung J67.8
Cheese-worker's lung J67.8
Cheilitis (acute) (angular) (catarrhal) (chronic) (exfoliative) (gangrenous) (glandular) (infectional) (suppurative) (ulcerative) (vesicular) K13.0
  actinic (due to sun) L56.8
    other than from sun L59.8
  candidal B37.83
Cheilodynia K13.0
Cheiloschisis — *see* Cleft, lip
Cheilosis (angular) K13.0
  with pellagra E52
  due to
    vitamin B2 (riboflavin) deficiency E53.0
Cheiromegaly M79.89
Cheiropompholyx L30.1
Cheloid — *see* Keloid
Chemical burn — *see* Corrosion, by site
Chemodectoma — *see* Paraganglioma, nonchromaffin
Chemosis, conjunctiva — *see* Edema, conjunctiva
Chemotherapy (session) (for)
  cancer Z51.11
  neoplasm Z51.11
Cherubism M27.8
Chest — *see* condition
Cheyne-Stokes breathing (respiration) R06.3
Chiari's
  disease or syndrome (hepatic vein thrombosis) I82.0
  malformation
    type I G93.5
    type II — *see* Spina bifida
  net Q24.8
Chicago disease B40.9
Chickenpox — *see* Varicella
Chiclero ulcer or sore B55.1
Chigger (infestation) B88.0
Chignon (disease) B36.8
  newborn (from vacuum extraction) (birth injury) P12.1
Chilaiditi's syndrome (subphrenic displacement, colon) Q43.3
Chilblain(s) (lupus) T69.1 ☑
Child
  custody dispute Z65.3
Childbirth — *see* Delivery
Childhood
  cerebral X-linked adrenoleukodystrophy E71.520
  period of rapid growth Z00.2
Chill(s) R68.83
  with fever R50.9
  congestive in malarial regions B54
  without fever R68.83
Chilomastigiasis A07.8
Chimera 46,XX/46,XY Q99.0
Chin — *see* condition
Chinese dysentery A03.9
Chionophobia F40.228
Chitral fever A93.1
Chlamydia, chlamydial A74.9
  cervicitis A56.09
  conjunctivitis A74.0
  cystitis A56.01
  endometritis A56.11
  epididymitis A56.19

Chlamydia, chlamydial — *continued*
  female
    pelvic inflammatory disease A56.11
    pelviperitonitis A56.11
  orchitis A56.19
  peritonitis A74.81
  pharyngitis A56.4
  proctitis A56.3
  psittaci (infection) A70
  salpingitis A56.11
  sexually-transmitted infection NEC A56.8
  specified NEC A74.89
  urethritis A56.01
  vulvovaginitis A56.02
Chlamydiosis — *see* Chlamydia
Chloasma (skin) (idiopathic) (symptomatic) L81.1
  eyelid H02.719
    hyperthyroid E05.90 [H02.719]
      with thyroid storm E05.91 [H02.719]
    left H02.716
      lower H02.715
      upper H02.714
    right H02.713
      lower H02.712
      upper H02.711
Chloroma C92.3- ☑
Chlorosis D50.9
  Egyptian B76.9 [D63.8]
  miner's B76.9 [D63.8]
Chlorotic anemia D50.8
Chocolate cyst (ovary) N80.1
Choked
  disc or disk — *see* Papilledema
  on food, phlegm, or vomitus NOS — *see* Foreign body, by site
  while vomiting NOS — *see* Foreign body, by site
Chokes (resulting from bends) T70.3 ☑
Choking sensation R09.89
Cholangiectasis K83.8
Cholangiocarcinoma
  with hepatocellular carcinoma, combined C22.0
  liver C22.1
  specified site NEC — *see* Neoplasm, malignant, by site
  unspecified site C22.1
Cholangiohepatitis K83.8
  due to fluke infestation B66.1
Cholangiohepatoma C22.0
Cholangiolitis (acute) (chronic) (extrahepatic) (gangrenous) (intrahepatic) K83.09
  paratyphoidal — *see* Fever, paratyphoid
  typhoidal A01.09
Cholangioma D13.4
  malignant — *see* Cholangiocarcinoma
Cholangitis (ascending) (recurrent) (secondary) (stenosing) (suppurative) K83.09
  with calculus, bile duct — *see* Calculus, bile duct, with cholangitis
  chronic nonsuppurative destructive K74.3
  primary K83.09
    sclerosing K83.01
  sclerosing K83.09
Cholecystectasia K82.8
Cholecystitis K81.9
  with
    calculus, stones in
      bile duct (common) (hepatic) — *see* Calculus, bile duct, with cholecystitis
      cystic duct — *see* Calculus, gallbladder, with cholecystitis
      gallbladder — *see* Calculus, gallbladder, with cholecystitis
    choledocholithiasis — *see* Calculus, bile duct, with cholecystitis
    cholelithiasis — *see* Calculus, gallbladder, with cholecystitis
    gangrene of gallbladder K82.A1
    perforation of gallbladder K82.A2
  acute (emphysematous) (gangrenous) (suppurative) K81.0
    with
      calculus, stones in
        cystic duct — *see* Calculus, gallbladder, with cholecystitis, acute
        gallbladder — *see* Calculus, gallbladder, with cholecystitis, acute
      choledocholithiasis — *see* Calculus, bile duct, with cholecystitis, acute

Cholecystitis — *continued*
  acute — *continued*
    with — *continued*
      cholelithiasis — *see* Calculus, gallbladder, with cholecystitis, acute
      chronic cholecystitis K81.2
        with gallbladder calculus K80.12
          with obstruction K80.13
    chronic K81.1
      with acute cholecystitis K81.2
        with gallbladder calculus K80.12
          with obstruction K80.13
  emphysematous (acute) — *see* Cholecystitis, acute
  gangrenous — *see* Cholecystitis, acute
  paratyphoidal, current A01.4
  suppurative — *see* Cholecystitis, acute
  typhoidal A01.09
Cholecystolithiasis — *see* Calculus, gallbladder
Choledochitis (suppurative) K83.09
Choledocholith — *see* Calculus, bile duct
Choledocholithiasis (common duct) (hepatic duct) — *see* Calculus, bile duct
  cystic — *see* Calculus, gallbladder
  typhoidal A01.09
Cholelithiasis (cystic duct) (gallbladder) (impacted) (multiple) — *see* Calculus, gallbladder
  bile duct (common) (hepatic) — *see* Calculus, bile duct
  hepatic duct — *see* Calculus, bile duct
  specified NEC K80.80
    with obstruction K80.81
Cholemia (*see also* Jaundice)
  familial (simple) (congenital) E80.4
  Gilbert's E80.4
Choleperitoneum, choleperitonitis K65.3
Cholera (Asiatic) (epidemic) (malignant) A00.9
  antimonial — *see* Poisoning, antimony
  classical A00.0
  due to Vibrio cholerae 01 A00.9
    biovar cholerae A00.0
    biovar eltor A00.1
    el tor A00.1
  el tor A00.1
Cholerine — *see* Cholera
Cholestasis NEC K83.1
  with hepatocyte injury K71.0
  due to total parenteral nutrition (TPN) K76.89
  pure K71.0
Cholesteatoma (ear) (middle) (with reaction) H71.9- ☑
  attic H71.0- ☑
  external ear (canal) H60.4- ☑
  mastoid H71.2- ☑
  postmastoidectomy cavity (recurrent) — *see* Complications, postmastoidectomy, recurrent cholesteatoma
  recurrent (postmastoidectomy) — *see* Complications, postmastoidectomy, recurrent cholesteatoma
  tympanum H71.1- ☑
Cholesteatosis, diffuse H71.3- ☑
Cholesteremia E78.00
Cholesterin in vitreous — *see* Deposit, crystalline
Cholesterol
  deposit
    retina H35.89
    vitreous — *see* Deposit, crystalline
  elevated (high) E78.00
    with elevated (high) triglycerides E78.2
    screening for Z13.220
  imbibition of gallbladder K82.4
Cholesterolemia (essential) (pure) E78.00
  familial E78.01
  hereditary E78.01
Cholesterolosis, cholesterosis (gallbladder) K82.4
  cerebrotendinous E75.5
Cholocolic fistula K82.3
Choluria R82.2
Chondritis M94.8X9
  aurical H61.03- ☑
  costal (Tietze's) M94.0
  external ear H61.03- ☑
  patella, posttraumatic — *see* Chondromalacia, patella
  pinna H61.03- ☑
  purulent M94.8X- ☑
  tuberculous NEC A18.02
    intervertebral A18.01
Chondroblastoma (*see also* Neoplasm, bone, benign)
  malignant — *see* Neoplasm, bone, malignant
Chondrocalcinosis M11.20

Charcot's — Chondrocalcinosis

Chondrocalcinosis — *continued*
- ankle M11.27- ☑
- elbow M11.22- ☑
- familial M11.10
  - ankle M11.17- ☑
  - elbow M11.12- ☑
  - foot joint M11.17- ☑
  - hand joint M11.14- ☑
  - hip M11.15- ☑
  - knee M11.16- ☑
  - multiple site M11.19
  - shoulder M11.11- ☑
  - vertebrae M11.18
  - wrist M11.13- ☑
- foot joint M11.27- ☑
- hand joint M11.24- ☑
- hip M11.25- ☑
- knee M11.26- ☑
- multiple site M11.29
- shoulder M11.21- ☑
- specified type NEC M11.20
  - ankle M11.27- ☑
  - elbow M11.22- ☑
  - foot joint M11.27- ☑
  - hand joint M11.24- ☑
  - hip M11.25- ☑
  - knee M11.26- ☑
  - multiple site M11.29
  - shoulder M11.21- ☑
  - vertebrae M11.28
  - wrist M11.23- ☑
- vertebrae M11.28
- wrist M11.23- ☑

Chondrodermatitis nodularis helicis or anthelicis — *see* Perichondritis, ear

Chondrodysplasia Q78.9
- with hemangioma Q78.4
- calcificans congenita Q77.3
- fetalis Q77.4
- metaphyseal (Jansen's) (McKusick's) (Schmid's) Q78.8
- punctata Q77.3

Chondrodystrophy, chondrodystrophia (familial) (fetalis) (hypoplastic) Q78.9
- calcificans congenita Q77.3
- myotonic (congenital) G71.13
- punctata Q77.3

Chondroectodermal dysplasia Q77.6

Chondrogenesis imperfecta Q77.4

Chondrolysis M94.35- ☑

Chondroma (*see also* Neoplasm, cartilage, benign)
- juxtacortical — *see* Neoplasm, bone, benign
- periosteal — *see* Neoplasm, bone, benign

Chondromalacia (systemic) M94.20
- acromioclavicular joint M94.21- ☑
- ankle M94.27- ☑
- elbow M94.22- ☑
- foot joint M94.27- ☑
- glenohumeral joint M94.21- ☑
- hand joint M94.24- ☑
- hip M94.25- ☑
- knee M94.26- ☑
  - patella M22.4- ☑
- multiple sites M94.29
- patella M22.4- ☑
- rib M94.28
- sacroiliac joint M94.259
- shoulder M94.21- ☑
- sternoclavicular joint M94.21- ☑
- vertebral joint M94.28
- wrist M94.23- ☑

Chondromatosis (*see also* Neoplasm, cartilage, uncertain behavior)
- internal Q78.4

Chondromyxosarcoma — *see* Neoplasm, cartilage, malignant

Chondro-osteodysplasia (Morquio-Brailsford type) E76.219

Chondro-osteodystrophy E76.29

Chondro-osteoma — *see* Neoplasm, bone, benign

Chondropathia tuberosa M94.0

Chondrosarcoma — *see* Neoplasm, cartilage, malignant
- juxtacortical — *see* Neoplasm, bone, malignant
- mesenchymal — *see* Neoplasm, connective tissue, malignant
- myxoid — *see* Neoplasm, cartilage, malignant

Chordee (nonvenereal) N48.89
- congenital Q54.4

Chordee — *continued*
- gonococcal A54.09

Chorditis (fibrinous) (nodosa) (tuberosa) J38.2

Chordoma — *see* Neoplasm, vertebral (column), malignant

Chorea (chronic) (gravis) (posthemiplegic) (senile) (spasmodic) G25.5
- with
  - heart involvement I02.0
    - active or acute (conditions in I01-) I02.0
    - rheumatic I02.9
      - with valvular disorder I02.0
    - rheumatic heart disease (chronic) (inactive)(quiescent) — *code to* rheumatic heart condition involved
- drug-induced G25.4
- habit F95.8
- hereditary G10
- Huntington's G10
- hysterical F44.4
- minor I02.9
  - with heart involvement I02.0
- progressive G25.5
  - hereditary G10
- rheumatic (chronic) I02.9
  - with heart involvement I02.0
- Sydenham's I02.9
  - with heart involvement — *see* Chorea, with rheumatic heart disease
- nonrheumatic G25.5

Choreoathetosis (paroxysmal) G25.5

Chorioadenoma (destruens) D39.2

Chorioamnionitis O41.12- ☑

Chorioangioma D26.7

Choriocarcinoma — *see* Neoplasm, malignant, by site
- combined with
  - embryonal carcinoma — *see* Neoplasm, malignant, by site
  - other germ cell elements — *see* Neoplasm, malignant, by site
  - teratoma — *see* Neoplasm, malignant, by site
- specified site — *see* Neoplasm, malignant, by site
- unspecified site
  - female C58
  - male C62.90

Chorioencephalitis (acute) (lymphocytic) (serous) A87.2

Chorioepithelioma — *see* Choriocarcinoma

Choriomeningitis (acute) (lymphocytic) (serous) A87.2

Chorionepithelioma — *see* Choriocarcinoma

Chorioretinitis (*see also* Inflammation, chorioretinal)
- disseminated (*see also* Inflammation, chorioretinal, disseminated)
  - in neurosyphilis A52.19
- Egyptian B76.9 [D63.8]
- focal (*see also* Inflammation, chorioretinal, focal)
- histoplasmic B39.9 [H32]
- in (due to)
  - histoplasmosis B39.9 [H32]
  - syphilis (secondary) A51.43
    - late A52.71
  - toxoplasmosis (acquired) B58.01
    - congenital (active) P37.1 [H32]
  - tuberculosis A18.53
- juxtapapillary, juxtapapillaris — *see* Inflammation, chorioretinal, focal, juxtapapillary
- leprous A30.9 [H32]
- miner's B76.9 [D63.8]
- progressive myopia (degeneration) (*see also* Myopia, degenerative) H44.2- ☑
- syphilitic (secondary) A51.43
  - congenital (early) A50.01 [H32]
    - late A50.32
  - late A52.71
- tuberculous A18.53

Chorioretinopathy, central serous H35.71- ☑

Choroid — *see* condition

Choroideremia H31.21

Choroiditis — *see* Chorioretinitis

Choroidopathy — *see* Disorder, choroid

Choroidoretinitis — *see* Chorioretinitis

Choroidoretinopathy, central serous — *see* Chorioretinopathy, central serous

Christian-Weber disease M35.6

Christmas disease D67

Chromaffinoma (*see also* Neoplasm, benign, by site)
- malignant — *see* Neoplasm, malignant, by site

Chromatopsia — *see* Deficiency, color vision

Chromhidrosis, chromidrosis L75.1

Chromoblastomycosis — *see* Chromomycosis

Chromoconversion R82.91

Chromomycosis B43.9
- brain abscess B43.1
- cerebral B43.1
- cutaneous B43.0
- skin B43.0
- specified NEC B43.8
- subcutaneous abscess or cyst B43.2

Chromophytosis B36.0

Chromosome — *see* Anomaly, by chromosome involved
- D (1) — *see* Anomaly, chromosome 13
- E (3) — *see* Anomaly, chromosome 18
- G — *see* Anomaly, chromosome 21

Chromotrichomycosis B36.8

Chronic — *see* condition
- fracture — *see* Fracture, pathological

Churg-Strauss syndrome M30.1

Chyle cyst, mesentery I89.8

Chylocele (nonfilarial) I89.8
- filarial (*see also* Infestation, filarial) B74.9 [N51]
- tunica vaginalis N50.89
  - filarial (*see also* Infestation, filarial) B74.9 [N51]

Chylomicronemia (fasting) (with hyperprebetalipoproteinemia) E78.3

Chylopericardium I31.3
- acute I30.9

Chylothorax (nonfilarial) I89.8
- filarial (*see also* Infestation, filarial) B74.9 [J91.8]

Chylous — *see* condition

Chyluria (nonfilarial) R82.0
- due to
  - bilharziasis B65.0
  - Brugia (malayi) B74.1
    - timori B74.2
  - schistosomiasis (bilharziasis) B65.0
  - Wuchereria (bancrofti) B74.0
- filarial — *see* Infestation, filarial

Cicatricial (deformity) — *see* Cicatrix

Cicatrix (adherent) (contracted) (painful) (vicious) (*see also* Scar) L90.5
- adenoid (and tonsil) J35.8
- alveolar process M26.79
- anus K62.89
- auricle — *see* Disorder, pinna, specified type NEC
- bile duct (common) (hepatic) K83.8
- bladder N32.89
- bone — *see* Disorder, bone, specified type NEC
- brain G93.89
- cervix (postoperative) (postpartal) N88.1
- common duct K83.8
- cornea H17.9
  - tuberculous A18.59
- duodenum (bulb), obstructive K31.5
- esophagus K22.2
- eyelid — *see* Disorder, eyelid function
- hypopharynx J39.2
- lacrimal passages — *see* Obstruction, lacrimal
- larynx J38.7
- lung J98.4
- middle ear H74.8 ☑
- mouth K13.79
- muscle M62.89
  - with contracture — *see* Contraction, muscle NEC
- nasopharynx J39.2
- palate (soft) K13.79
- penis N48.89
- pharynx J39.2
- prostate N42.89
- rectum K62.89
- retina — *see* Scar, chorioretinal
- semilunar cartilage — *see* Derangement, meniscus
- seminal vesicle N50.89
- skin L90.5
  - infected L08.89
  - postinfective L90.5
  - tuberculous B90.8
- specified site NEC L90.5
- throat J39.2
- tongue K14.8
- tonsil (and adenoid) J35.8
- trachea J39.8
- tuberculous NEC B90.9
- urethra N36.8
- uterus N85.8
- vagina N89.8
  - postoperative N99.2
- vocal cord J38.3

Cicatrix — *continued*
   wrist, constricting (annular) L90.5
CIDP (chronic inflammatory demyelinating polyneuropathy) G61.81
CIN — *see* Neoplasia, intraepithelial, cervix
CINCA (chronic infantile neurological, cutaneous and articular syndrome) M04.2
Cinchonism — *see* Deafness, ototoxic
   correct substance properly administered — *see* Table of Drugs and Chemicals, by drug, adverse effect
   overdose or wrong substance given or taken — *see* Table of Drugs and Chemicals, by drug, poisoning
Circle of Willis — *see* condition
Circular — *see* condition
Circulating anticoagulants (*see also* Disorder, hemorrhagic) D68.318
   due to drugs (*see also* Disorder, hemorrhagic) D68.32
   following childbirth O72.3
Circulation
   collateral, any site I99.8
   defective (lower extremity) I99.9
     congenital Q28.9
   embryonic Q28.9
   failure (peripheral) R57.9
     newborn P29.89
   fetal, persistent P29.38
   heart, incomplete Q28.9
Circulatory system — *see* condition
Circulus senilis (cornea) — *see* Degeneration, cornea, senile
Circumcision (in absence of medical indication) (ritual) (routine) Z41.2
Circumscribed — *see* condition
Circumvallate placenta O43.11- ☑
Cirrhosis, cirrhotic (hepatic) (liver) K74.60
   alcoholic K70.30
     with ascites K70.31
   atrophic — *see* Cirrhosis, liver
   Baumgarten-Cruveilhier K74.69
   biliary (cholangiolitic) (cholangitic) (hypertrophic) (obstructive) (pericholangiolitic) K74.5
     due to
       Clonorchiasis B66.1
       flukes B66.3
     primary K74.3
     secondary K74.4
   cardiac (of liver) K76.1
   Charcot's K74.3
   cholangiolitic, cholangitic, cholostatic (primary) K74.3
   congestive K76.1
   Cruveilhier-Baumgarten K74.69
   cryptogenic (liver) K74.69
   due to
     hepatolenticular degeneration E83.01
     Wilson's disease E83.01
     xanthomatosis E78.2
   fatty K76.0
     alcoholic K70.0
   Hanot's (hypertrophic) K74.3
   hepatic — *see* Cirrhosis, liver
   hypertrophic K74.3
   Indian childhood K74.69
   kidney — *see* Sclerosis, renal
   Laennec's K70.30
     with ascites K70.31
     alcoholic K70.30
       with ascites K70.31
     nonalcoholic K74.69
   liver K74.60
     alcoholic K70.30
       with ascites K70.31
       fatty K70.0
     congenital P78.81
     syphilitic A52.74
   lung (chronic) J84.10
   macronodular K74.69
     alcoholic K70.30
       with ascites K70.31
   micronodular K74.69
     alcoholic K70.30
       with ascites K70.31
   mixed type K74.69
   monolobular K74.3
   nephritis — *see* Sclerosis, renal
   nutritional K74.69
     alcoholic K70.30
       with ascites K70.31
   obstructive — *see* Cirrhosis, biliary

Cirrhosis, cirrhotic — *continued*
   ovarian N83.8
   pancreas (duct) K86.89
   pigmentary E83.110
   portal K74.69
     alcoholic K70.30
       with ascites K70.31
   postnecrotic K74.69
     alcoholic K70.30
       with ascites K70.31
   pulmonary J84.10
   renal — *see* Sclerosis, renal
   spleen D73.2
   stasis K76.1
   Todd's K74.3
   unilobar K74.3
   xanthomatous (biliary) K74.5
     due to xanthomatosis (familial) (metabolic) (primary) E78.2
Cistern, subarachnoid R93.0
Citrullinemia E72.23
Citrullinuria E72.23
Civatte's disease or poikiloderma L57.3
Clam digger's itch B65.3
Clammy skin R23.1
Clap — *see* Gonorrhea
Clarke-Hadfield syndrome (pancreatic infantilism) K86.89
Clark's paralysis G80.9
Clastothrix L67.8
Claude Bernard-Horner syndrome G90.2
   traumatic — *see* Injury, nerve, cervical sympathetic
Claude's disease or syndrome G46.3
Claudicatio venosa intermittens I87.8
Claudication (intermittent) I73.9
   cerebral (artery) G45.9
   spinal cord (arteriosclerotic) G95.19
     syphilitic A52.09
   venous (axillary) I87.8
Claustrophobia F40.240
Clavus (infected) L84
Clawfoot (congenital) Q66.89
   acquired — *see* Deformity, limb, clawfoot
Clawhand (acquired) (*see also* Deformity, limb, clawhand)
   congenital Q68.1
Clawtoe (congenital) Q66.89
   acquired — *see* Deformity, toe, specified NEC
Clay eating — *see* Pica
Cleansing of artificial opening — *see* Attention to, artificial, opening
Cleft (congenital) — *see also* Imperfect, closure
   alveolar process M26.79
   branchial (persistent) Q18.2
     cyst Q18.0
       fistula Q18.0
       sinus Q18.0
   cricoid cartilage, posterior Q31.8
   cyst Q18.0
     fistula Q18.0
     sinus Q18.0
   foot Q72.7 ☑
   hand Q71.6 ☑
   lip (unilateral) Q36.9
     with cleft palate Q37.9
       hard Q37.1
         with soft Q37.5
       soft Q37.3
         with hard Q37.5
       bilateral Q36.0
         with cleft palate Q37.8
           hard Q37.0
             with soft Q37.4
           soft Q37.2
             with hard Q37.4
     median Q36.1
   nose Q30.2
   palate Q35.9
     with cleft lip (unilateral) Q37.9
       bilateral Q37.8
     hard Q35.1
       with
         cleft lip (unilateral) Q37.1
           bilateral Q37.0
         soft Q35.5
           with cleft lip (unilateral) Q37.5
             bilateral Q37.4
     medial Q35.5
     soft Q35.3

Cleft — *continued*
   palate — *continued*
     soft — *continued*
       with
         cleft lip (unilateral) Q37.3
           bilateral Q37.2
         hard Q35.5
           with cleft lip (unilateral) Q37.5
             bilateral Q37.4
   penis Q55.69
   scrotum Q55.29
   thyroid cartilage Q31.8
   uvula Q35.7
Cleidocranial dysostosis Q74.0
Cleptomania F63.2
Clicking hip (newborn) R29.4
Climacteric (female) (*see also* Menopause)
   arthritis (any site) NEC — *see* Arthritis, specified form NEC
   depression (single episode) F32.89
     recurrent episode F33.8
   male (symptoms) (syndrome) NEC N50.89
   melancholia (single episode) F32.89
     recurrent episode F33.8
   paranoid state F22
   polyarthritis NEC — *see* Arthritis, specified form NEC
   symptoms (female) N95.1
Clinical research investigation (clinical trial) (control subject) (normal comparison) (participant) Z00.6
Clitoris — *see* condition
Cloaca (persistent) Q43.7
Clonorchiasis, clonorchis infection (liver) B66.1
Clonus R25.8
Closed bite M26.29
Clostridium (C.) **perfringens, as cause of disease classified elsewhere** B96.7
Closure
   congenital, nose Q30.0
   cranial sutures, premature Q75.0
   defective or imperfect NEC — *see* Imperfect, closure
   fistula, delayed — *see* Fistula
   foramen ovale, imperfect Q21.1
   hymen N89.6
   interauricular septum, defective Q21.1
   interventricular septum, defective Q21.0
   lacrimal duct (*see also* Stenosis, lacrimal, duct)
     congenital Q10.5
   nose (congenital) Q30.0
     acquired M95.0
   of artificial opening — *see* Attention to, artificial, opening
   vagina N89.5
   valve — *see* Endocarditis
   vulva N90.5
Clot (blood) (*see also* Embolism)
   artery (obstruction) (occlusion) — *see* Embolism
   bladder N32.89
   brain (intradural or extradural) — *see* Occlusion, artery, cerebral
   circulation I74.9
   heart (*see also* Infarct, myocardium)
     not resulting in infarction I51.3
   vein — *see* Thrombosis
Clouded state R40.1
   epileptic — *see* Epilepsy, specified NEC
   paroxysmal — *see* Epilepsy, specified NEC
Cloudy antrum, antra J32.0
Clouston's (hidrotic) **ectodermal dysplasia** Q82.4
Clubbed nail pachydermoperiostosis M89.40 [L62]
Clubbing of finger(s) (nails) R68.3
Clubfinger R68.3
   congenital Q68.1
Clubfoot (congenital) Q66.89
   acquired — *see* Deformity, limb, clubfoot
   equinovarus Q66.0
   paralytic — *see* Deformity, limb, clubfoot
Clubhand (congenital) (radial) Q71.4- ☑
   acquired — *see* Deformity, limb, clubhand
Clubnail R68.3
   congenital Q84.6
Clump, kidney Q63.1
Clumsiness, clumsy child syndrome F82
Cluttering F80.81
Clutton's joints A50.51 [M12.80]
Coagulation, intravascular (diffuse) (disseminated) (*see also* Defibrination syndrome)

Coagulation, intravascular — *continued*
  complicating abortion — *see* Abortion, by type, complicated by, intravascular coagulation
  following ectopic or molar pregnancy O08.1
Coagulopathy (*see also* Defect, coagulation)
  consumption D65
  intravascular D65
    newborn P60
Coalition
  calcaneo-scaphoid Q66.89
  tarsal Q66.89
Coalminer's
  elbow — *see* Bursitis, elbow, olecranon
  lung or pneumoconiosis J60
Coalworker's lung or pneumoconiosis J60
Coarctation
  aorta (preductal) (postductal) Q25.1
  pulmonary artery Q25.71
Coated tongue K14.3
Coats' disease (exudative retinopathy) — *see* Retinopathy, exudative
Cocaine-induced
  anxiety disorder F14.980
  bipolar and related disorder F14.94
  depressive disorder F14.94
  obsessive-compulsive and related disorder F14.988
  psychotic disorder F14.959
  sexual dysfunction F14.981
  sleep disorder F14.982
Cocainism — *see* Disorder, cocaine use
Coccidioidomycosis B38.9
  cutaneous B38.3
  disseminated B38.7
  generalized B38.7
  meninges B38.4
  prostate B38.81
  pulmonary B38.2
    acute B38.0
    chronic B38.1
  skin B38.3
  specified NEC B38.89
Coccidioidosis — *see* Coccidioidomycosis
Coccidiosis (intestinal) A07.3
Coccydynia, coccygodynia M53.3
Coccyx — *see* condition
Cochin-China diarrhea K90.1
Cockayne's syndrome Q87.1
Cocked up toe — *see* Deformity, toe, specified NEC
Cock's peculiar tumor L72.3
Codman's tumor — *see* Neoplasm, bone, benign
Coenurosis B71.8
Coffee-worker's lung J67.8
Cogan's syndrome H16.32- ☑
  oculomotor apraxia H51.8
Coitus, painful (female) N94.10
  male N53.12
  psychogenic F52.6
Cold J00
  with influenza, flu, or grippe — *see* Influenza, with, respiratory manifestations NEC
  agglutinin disease or hemoglobinuria (chronic) D59.1
  bronchial — *see* Bronchitis
  chest — *see* Bronchitis
  common (head) J00
  effects of T69.9 ☑
    specified effect NEC T69.8 ☑
  excessive, effects of T69.9 ☑
    specified effect NEC T69.8 ☑
  exhaustion from T69.8 ☑
  exposure to T69.9 ☑
    specified effect NEC T69.8 ☑
  head J00
  injury syndrome (newborn) P80.0
  on lung — *see* Bronchitis
  rose J30.1
  sensitivity, auto-immune D59.1
  symptoms J00
  virus J00
Coldsore B00.1
Colibacillosis A49.8
  as the cause of other disease (*see also* Escherichia coli) B96.20
  generalized A41.50
Colic (bilious) (infantile) (intestinal) (recurrent) (spasmodic) R10.83
  abdomen R10.83
    psychogenic F45.8

Colic — *continued*
  appendix, appendicular K38.8
  bile duct — *see* Calculus, bile duct
  biliary — *see* Calculus, bile duct
  common duct — *see* Calculus, bile duct
  cystic duct — *see* Calculus, gallbladder
  Devonshire NEC — *see* Poisoning, lead
  gallbladder — *see* Calculus, gallbladder
  gallstone — *see* Calculus, gallbladder
    gallbladder or cystic duct — *see* Calculus, gallbladder
  hepatic (duct) — *see* Calculus, bile duct
  hysterical F45.8
  kidney N23
  lead NEC — *see* Poisoning, lead
  mucous K58.9
    with diarrhea K58.0
    psychogenic F54
  nephritic N23
  painter's NEC — *see* Poisoning, lead
  pancreas K86.89
  psychogenic F45.8
  renal N23
  saturnine NEC — *see* Poisoning, lead
  ureter N23
  urethral N36.8
    due to calculus N21.1
  uterus NEC N94.89
    menstrual — *see* Dysmenorrhea
  worm NOS B83.9
Colicystitis — *see* Cystitis
Colitis (acute) (catarrhal) (chronic) (noninfective) (hemorrhagic) (*see also* Enteritis) K52.9
  allergic K52.29
    with
      food protein-induced enterocolitis syndrome K52.21
      proctocolitis K52.82
  amebic (acute) (*see also* Amebiasis) A06.0
    nondysenteric A06.2
  anthrax A22.2
  bacillary — *see* Infection, Shigella
  balantidial A07.0
  Clostridium difficile
    not specified as recurrent A04.72
    recurrent A04.71
  coccidial A07.3
  collagenous K52.831
  cystica superficialis K52.89
  dietary counseling and surveillance (for) Z71.3
  dietetic (*see also* Colitis, allergic) K52.29
  drug-induced K52.1
  due to radiation K52.0
  eosinophilic K52.82
  food hypersensitivity (*see also* Colitis, allergic) K52.29
  giardial A07.1
  granulomatous — *see* Enteritis, regional, large intestine
  indeterminate, so stated K52.3
  infectious — *see* Enteritis, infectious
  ischemic K55.9
    acute (subacute) (*see also* Ischemia, intestine, acute) K55.039
    chronic K55.1
    due to mesenteric artery insufficiency K55.1
    fulminant (acute) (*see also* Ischemia, intestine, acute) K55.039
  left sided K51.50
    with
      abscess K51.514
      complication K51.519
        specified NEC K51.518
      fistula K51.513
      obstruction K51.512
      rectal bleeding K51.511
  lymphocytic K52.832
  membranous
    psychogenic F54
  microscopic K52.839
    specified NEC K52.838
  mucous — *see* Syndrome, irritable, bowel
    psychogenic F54
  noninfective K52.9
    specified NEC K52.89
  polyposa — *see* Polyp, colon, inflammatory
  protozoal A07.9
  pseudomembranous
    not specified as recurrent A04.72
    recurrent A04.71

Colitis — *continued*
  pseudomucinous — *see* Syndrome, irritable, bowel
  regional — *see* Enteritis, regional, large intestine
    infectious A09
  segmental — *see* Enteritis, regional, large intestine
  septic — *see* Enteritis, infectious
  spastic K58.9
    with diarrhea K58.0
    psychogenic F54
  staphylococcal A04.8
    foodborne A05.0
  subacute ischemic (*see also* Ischemia, intestine, acute) K55.039
  thromboulcerative (*see also* Ischemia, intestine, acute) K55.039
  toxic NEC K52.1
    due to Clostridium difficile
      not specified as recurrent A04.72
      recurrent A04.71
  transmural — *see* Enteritis, regional, large intestine
  trichomonal A07.8
  tuberculous (ulcerative) A18.32
  ulcerative (chronic) K51.90
    with
      complication K51.919
        abscess K51.914
        fistula K51.913
        obstruction K51.912
        rectal bleeding K51.911
        specified complication NEC K51.918
    enterocolitis — *see* Enterocolitis, ulcerative
    ileocolitis — *see* Ileocolitis, ulcerative
    mucosal proctocolitis — *see* Proctocolitis, mucosal
    proctitis — *see* Proctitis, ulcerative
    pseudopolyposis — *see* Polyp, colon, inflammatory
    psychogenic F54
    rectosigmoiditis — *see* Rectosigmoiditis, ulcerative
    specified type NEC K51.80
      with
        complication K51.819
          abscess K51.814
          fistula K51.813
          obstruction K51.812
          rectal bleeding K51.811
          specified complication NEC K51.818
Collagenosis, collagen disease (nonvascular) (vascular) M35.9
  cardiovascular I42.8
  reactive perforating L87.1
  specified NEC M35.8
Collapse R55
  adrenal E27.2
  cardiorespiratory R57.0
  cardiovascular R57.0
    newborn P29.89
  circulatory (peripheral) R57.9
    during or after labor and delivery O75.1
    following ectopic or molar pregnancy O08.3
    newborn P29.89
  during or
    after labor and delivery O75.1
    resulting from a procedure, not elsewhere classified T81.10 ☑
  external ear canal — *see* Stenosis, external ear canal
  general R55
  heart — *see* Disease, heart
  heat T67.1 ☑
  hysterical F44.89
  labyrinth, membranous (congenital) Q16.5
  lung (massive) (*see also* Atelectasis) J98.19
    pressure due to anesthesia (general) (local) or other sedation T88.2 ☑
      during labor and delivery O74.1
      in pregnancy O29.02- ☑
      postpartum, puerperal O89.09
  myocardial — *see* Disease, heart
  nervous F48.8
  neurocirculatory F45.8
  nose M95.0
  postoperative T81.10 ☑
  pulmonary (*see also* Atelectasis) J98.19
    newborn — *see* Atelectasis
  trachea J39.8
  tracheobronchial J98.09
  valvular — *see* Endocarditis
  vascular (peripheral) R57.9
    during or after labor and delivery O75.1
    following ectopic or molar pregnancy O08.3

Collapse — *continued*
  vascular — *continued*
    newborn P29.89
  vertebra M48.50- ☑
    cervical region M48.52- ☑
    cervicothoracic region M48.53- ☑
    in (due to)
      metastasis — *see* Collapse, vertebra, in, specified
        disease NEC
      osteoporosis (*see also* Osteoporosis) M80.88 ☑
        cervical region M80.88 ☑
        cervicothoracic region M80.88 ☑
        lumbar region M80.88 ☑
        lumbosacral region M80.88 ☑
        multiple sites M80.88 ☑
        occipito-atlanto-axial region M80.88 ☑
        sacrococcygeal region M80.88 ☑
        thoracic region M80.88 ☑
        thoracolumbar region M80.88 ☑
      specified disease NEC M48.50- ☑
        cervical region M48.52- ☑
        cervicothoracic region M48.53- ☑
        lumbar region M48.56- ☑
        lumbosacral region M48.57- ☑
        occipito-atlanto-axial region M48.51- ☑
        sacrococcygeal region M48.58- ☑
        thoracic region M48.54- ☑
        thoracolumbar region M48.55- ☑
    lumbar region M48.56- ☑
    lumbosacral region M48.57- ☑
    occipito-atlanto-axial region M48.51- ☑
    sacrococcygeal region M48.58- ☑
    thoracic region M48.54- ☑
    thoracolumbar region M48.55- ☑
Collateral (*see also* condition)
  circulation (venous) I87.8
  dilation, veins I87.8
Colles' fracture S52.53- ☑
Collet (-Sicard) syndrome G52.7
Collier's asthma or lung J60
Collodion baby Q80.2
Colloid nodule (of thyroid) (cystic) E04.1
Coloboma (iris) Q13.0
  eyelid Q10.3
  fundus Q14.8
  lens Q12.2
  optic disc (congenital) Q14.2
    acquired H47.31- ☑
Coloenteritis — *see* Enteritis
Colon — *see* condition
Colonization
  MRSA (Methicillin resistant Staphylococcus aureus)
    Z22.322
  MSSA (Methicillin susceptible Staphylococcus aureus)
    Z22.321
  status — *see* Carrier (suspected) of
Coloptosis K63.4
Color blindness — *see* Deficiency, color vision
Colostomy
  attention to Z43.3
  fitting or adjustment Z46.89
  malfunctioning K94.03
  status Z93.3
Colpitis (acute) — *see* Vaginitis
Colpocele N81.5
Colpocystitis — *see* Vaginitis
Colpospasm N94.2
Column, spinal, vertebral — *see* condition
Coma R40.20
  with
    motor response (none) R40.231 ☑
      abnormal extensor posturing to pain or noxious
        stimuli (< 2 years of age) R40.232 ☑
      abnormal flexure posturing to pain or noxious
        stimuli (0-5 years of age) R40.233 ☑
      extensor posturing to pain or noxious stimuli (2-
        5 years of age) R40.232 ☑
      flexion/decorticate posturing (< 2 years of age)
        R40.233 ☑
      localizes pain (2-5 years of age) R40.235 ☑
      normal or spontaneous movement (< 2 years of
        age) R40.236 ☑
      obeys commands (2-5 years of age) R40.236 ☑
      score of
        1 R40.231 ☑
        2 R40.232 ☑

Coma — *continued*
  with — *continued*
    motor response — *continued*
      score of — *continued*
        3 R40.233 ☑
        4 R40.234 ☑
        5 R40.235 ☑
        6 R40.236 ☑
      withdraws from pain or noxious stimuli (0-5 years
        of age) R40.234 ☑
      withdraws to touch (< 2 years of age) R40.235 ☑
    opening of eyes (never) R40.211 ☑
      in response to
        pain R40.212 ☑
        sound R40.213 ☑
      score of
        1 R40.211 ☑
        2 R40.212 ☑
        3 R40.213 ☑
        4 R40.214 ☑
      spontaneous R40.214 ☑
    verbal response (none) R40.221 ☑
      confused conversation R40.224 ☑
      cooing or babbling or crying appropriately (<2
        years of age) R40.225 ☑
      inappropriate crying or screaming (< 2 years of
        age) R40.223 ☑
      inappropriate words (2-5 years of age)
        R40.224 ☑
      incomprehensible sounds (2-5 years of age)
        R40.222 ☑
      incomprehensible words R40.222 ☑
      irritable cries (< 2 years of age) R40.224 ☑
      moans/grunts to pain; restless (< 2 years old)
        R40.222 ☑
      oriented R40.225 ☑
      score of
        1 R40.221 ☑
        2 R40.222 ☑
        3 R40.223 ☑
        4 R40.224 ☑
        5 R40.225 ☑
      screaming (2-5 years of age) R40.223 ☑
      uses appropriate words (2-5 years of age)
        R40.225 ☑
  eclamptic — *see* Eclampsia
  epileptic — *see* Epilepsy
  Glasgow, scale score — *see* Glasgow coma scale
  hepatic — *see* Failure, hepatic, by type, with coma
  hyperglycemic (diabetic) — *see* Diabetes, by type, with
    hyperosmolarity, with coma
  hyperosmolar (diabetic) — *see* Diabetes, by type, with
    hyperosmolarity, with coma
  hypoglycemic (diabetic) — *see* Diabetes, by type, with
    hypoglycemia, with coma
    nondiabetic E15
  in diabetes — *see* Diabetes, coma
  insulin-induced — *see* Coma, hypoglycemic
  ketoacidotic (diabetic) — *see* Diabetes, by type, with
    ketoacidosis, with coma
  myxedematous E03.5
  newborn P91.5
  persistent vegetative state R40.3
  specified NEC, without documented Glasgow coma
    scale score, or with partial Glasgow coma scale
    score reported R40.244 ☑
Comatose — *see* Coma
Combat fatigue F43.0
Combined — *see* condition
Comedo, comedones (giant) L70.0
Comedocarcinoma (*see also* Neoplasm, breast, malignant)
  noninfiltrating
    breast D05.8- ☑
    specified site — *see* Neoplasm, in situ, by site
    unspecified site D05.8- ☑
Comedomastitis — *see* Ectasia, mammary duct
Comminuted fracture — *code as* Fracture, closed
Common
  arterial trunk Q20.0
  atrioventricular canal Q21.2
  atrium Q21.1
  cold (head) J00
  truncus (arteriosus) Q20.0
  variable immunodeficiency — *see* Immunodeficiency,
    common variable
  ventricle Q20.4

Commotio, commotion (current)
  brain — *see* Injury, intracranial, concussion
  cerebri — *see* Injury, intracranial, concussion
  retinae S05.8X- ☑
  spinal cord — *see* Injury, spinal cord, by region
  spinalis — *see* Injury, spinal cord, by region
Communication
  between
    base of aorta and pulmonary artery Q21.4
    left ventricle and right atrium Q20.5
    pericardial sac and pleural sac Q34.8
    pulmonary artery and pulmonary vein, congenital
      Q25.72
  congenital between uterus and digestive or urinary
    tract Q51.7
Compartment syndrome (deep) (posterior) (traumatic)
  T79.A0 ☑ (*following* T79.7)
  abdomen T79.A3 ☑ (*following* T79.7)
  lower extremity (hip, buttock, thigh, leg, foot, toes)
    T79.A2 ☑ (*following* T79.7)
  nontraumatic
    abdomen M79.A3 (*following* M79.7)
    lower extremity (hip, buttock, thigh, leg, foot, toes)
      M79.A2- ☑ (*following* M79.7)
    specified site NEC M79.A9 (*following* M79.7)
    upper extremity (shoulder, arm, forearm, wrist,
      hand, fingers) M79.A1- ☑ (*following* M79.7)
  specified site NEC T79.A9 ☑ (*following* T79.7)
  upper extremity (shoulder, arm, forearm, wrist, hand,
    fingers) T79.A1- ☑ (*following* T79.7)
Compensation
  failure — *see* Disease, heart
  neurosis, psychoneurosis — *see* Disorder, factitious
Complaint (*see also* Disease)
  bowel, functional K59.9
    psychogenic F45.8
  intestine, functional K59.9
    psychogenic F45.8
  kidney — *see* Disease, renal
  miners' J60
Complete — *see* condition
Complex
  Addison-Schilder E71.528
  cardiorenal — *see* Hypertension, cardiorenal
  Costen's M26.69
  disseminated mycobacterium avium- intracellulare
    (DMAC) A31.2
  Eisenmenger's (ventricular septal defect) I27.83
  hypersexual F52.8
  jumped process, spine — *see* Dislocation, vertebra
  primary, tuberculous A15.7
  Schilder-Addison E71.528
  subluxation (vertebral) M99.19
    abdomen M99.19
    acromioclavicular M99.17
    cervical region M99.11
    cervicothoracic M99.11
    costochondral M99.18
    costovertebral M99.18
    head region M99.10
    hip M99.15
    lower extremity M99.16
    lumbar region M99.13
    lumbosacral M99.13
    occipitocervical M99.10
    pelvic region M99.15
    pubic M99.15
    rib cage M99.18
    sacral region M99.14
    sacrococcygeal M99.14
    sacroiliac M99.14
    specified NEC M99.19
    sternochondral M99.18
    sternoclavicular M99.17
    thoracic region M99.12
    thoracolumbar M99.12
    upper extremity M99.17
  Taussig-Bing (transposition, aorta and overriding pul-
    monary artery) Q20.1
Complication(s) (from) (of)
  accidental puncture or laceration during a procedure
    (of) — *see* Complications, intraoperative (in-
    traprocedural), puncture or laceration
  amputation stump (surgical) (late) NEC T87.9
    dehiscence T87.81
    infection or inflammation T87.40
      lower limb T87.4- ☑
      upper limb T87.4- ☑

Complication(s) — *continued*
- amputation stump — *continued*
  - necrosis T87.50
    - lower limb T87.5- ☑
    - upper limb T87.5- ☑
  - neuroma T87.30
    - lower limb T87.3- ☑
    - upper limb T87.3- ☑
  - specified type NEC T87.89
- anastomosis (and bypass) (see also Complications, prosthetic device or implant)
  - intestinal (internal) NEC K91.89
    - involving urinary tract N99.89
  - urinary tract (involving intestinal tract) N99.89
  - vascular — *see* Complications, cardiovascular device or implant
- anesthesia, anesthetic (see also Anesthesia, complication) T88.59 ☑
  - brain, postpartum, puerperal O89.2
  - cardiac
    - in
      - labor and delivery O74.2
      - pregnancy O29.19-
    - postpartum, puerperal O89.1
  - central nervous system
    - in
      - labor and delivery O74.3
      - pregnancy O29.29-
    - postpartum, puerperal O89.2
  - difficult or failed intubation T88.4 ☑
    - in pregnancy O29.6-
  - failed sedation (conscious) (moderate) during procedure T88.52 ☑
  - general, unintended awareness during procedure T88.53 ☑
  - hyperthermia, malignant T88.3 ☑
  - hypothermia T88.51 ☑
  - intubation failure T88.4 ☑
  - malignant hyperthermia T88.3 ☑
  - pulmonary
    - in
      - labor and delivery O74.1
      - pregnancy NEC O29.09- ☑
    - postpartum, puerperal O89.09
  - shock T88.2 ☑
  - spinal and epidural
    - in
      - labor and delivery NEC O74.6
        - headache O74.5
      - pregnancy NEC O29.5X- ☑
    - postpartum, puerperal NEC O89.5
      - headache O89.4
  - unintended awareness under general anesthesia during procedure T88.53 ☑
- anti-reflux device — *see* Complications, esophageal anti-reflux device
- aortic (bifurcation) graft — *see* Complications, graft, vascular
- aortocoronary (bypass) graft — *see* Complications, coronary artery (bypass) graft
- aortofemoral (bypass) graft — *see* Complications, extremity artery (bypass) graft
- arteriovenous
  - fistula, surgically created T82.9 ☑
    - embolism T82.818 ☑
    - fibrosis T82.828 ☑
    - hemorrhage T82.838 ☑
    - infection or inflammation T82.7 ☑
    - mechanical
      - breakdown T82.510 ☑
      - displacement T82.520 ☑
      - leakage T82.530 ☑
      - malposition T82.520 ☑
      - obstruction T82.590 ☑
      - perforation T82.590 ☑
      - protrusion T82.590 ☑
    - pain T82.848 ☑
    - specified type NEC T82.898 ☑
    - stenosis T82.858 ☑
    - thrombosis T82.868 ☑
  - shunt, surgically created T82.9 ☑
    - embolism T82.818 ☑
    - fibrosis T82.828 ☑
    - hemorrhage T82.838 ☑
    - infection or inflammation T82.7 ☑
    - mechanical
      - breakdown T82.511 ☑

Complication(s) — *continued*
- arteriovenous — *continued*
  - shunt, surgically created — *continued*
    - mechanical — *continued*
      - displacement T82.521 ☑
      - leakage T82.531 ☑
      - malposition T82.521 ☑
      - obstruction T82.591 ☑
      - perforation T82.591 ☑
      - protrusion T82.591 ☑
    - pain T82.848 ☑
    - specified type NEC T82.898 ☑
    - stenosis T82.858 ☑
    - thrombosis T82.868 ☑
- arthroplasty — *see* Complications, joint prosthesis
- artificial
  - fertilization or insemination N98.9
    - attempted introduction (of)
      - embryo in embryo transfer N98.3
      - ovum following in vitro fertilization N98.2
    - hyperstimulation of ovaries N98.1
    - infection N98.0
    - specified NEC N98.8
  - heart T82.9 ☑
    - embolism T82.817 ☑
    - fibrosis T82.827 ☑
    - hemorrhage T82.837 ☑
    - infection or inflammation T82.7 ☑
    - mechanical
      - breakdown T82.512 ☑
      - displacement T82.522 ☑
      - leakage T82.532 ☑
      - malposition T82.522 ☑
      - obstruction T82.592 ☑
      - perforation T82.592 ☑
      - protrusion T82.592 ☑
    - pain T82.847 ☑
    - specified type NEC T82.897 ☑
    - stenosis T82.857 ☑
    - thrombosis T82.867 ☑
  - opening
    - cecostomy — *see* Complications, colostomy
    - colostomy — *see* Complications, colostomy
    - cystostomy — *see* Complications, cystostomy
    - enterostomy — *see* Complications, enterostomy
    - gastrostomy — *see* Complications, gastrostomy
    - ileostomy — *see* Complications, enterostomy
    - jejunostomy — *see* Complications, enterostomy
    - nephrostomy — *see* Complications, stoma, urinary tract
    - tracheostomy — *see* Complications, tracheostomy
    - ureterostomy — *see* Complications, stoma, urinary tract
    - urethrostomy — *see* Complications, stoma, urinary tract
- balloon implant or device
  - gastrointestinal T85.9 ☑
    - embolism T85.818 ☑
    - fibrosis T85.828 ☑
    - hemorrhage T85.838 ☑
    - infection and inflammation T85.79 ☑
    - pain T85.848 ☑
    - specified type NEC T85.898 ☑
    - stenosis T85.858 ☑
    - thrombosis T85.868 ☑
  - vascular (counterpulsation) T82.9 ☑
    - embolism T82.818 ☑
    - fibrosis T82.828 ☑
    - hemorrhage T82.838 ☑
    - infection or inflammation T82.7 ☑
    - mechanical
      - breakdown T82.513 ☑
      - displacement T82.523 ☑
      - leakage T82.533 ☑
      - malposition T82.523 ☑
      - obstruction T82.593 ☑
      - perforation T82.593 ☑
      - protrusion T82.593 ☑
    - pain T82.848 ☑
    - specified type NEC T82.898 ☑
    - stenosis T82.858 ☑
    - thrombosis T82.868 ☑
- bariatric procedure
  - gastric band procedure K95.09
    - infection K95.01

Complication(s) — *continued*
- bariatric procedure — *continued*
  - specified procedure NEC K95.89
    - infection K95.81
- bile duct implant (prosthetic) T85.9 ☑
  - embolism T85.818 ☑
  - fibrosis T85.828 ☑
  - hemorrhage T85.838 ☑
  - infection and inflammation T85.79 ☑
  - mechanical
    - breakdown T85.510 ☑
    - displacement T85.520 ☑
    - malfunction T85.510 ☑
    - malposition T85.520 ☑
    - obstruction T85.590 ☑
    - perforation T85.590 ☑
    - protrusion T85.590 ☑
    - specified NEC T85.590 ☑
  - pain T85.848 ☑
  - specified type NEC T85.898 ☑
  - stenosis T85.858 ☑
  - thrombosis T85.868 ☑
- bladder device (auxiliary) — *see* Complications, genitourinary, device or implant, urinary system
- bleeding (postoperative) — *see* Complication, postoperative, hemorrhage
  - intraoperative — *see* Complication, intraoperative, hemorrhage
- blood vessel graft — *see* Complications, graft, vascular
- bone
  - device NEC T84.9 ☑
    - embolism T84.81 ☑
    - fibrosis T84.82 ☑
    - hemorrhage T84.83 ☑
    - infection or inflammation T84.7 ☑
    - mechanical
      - breakdown T84.318 ☑
      - displacement T84.328 ☑
      - malposition T84.328 ☑
      - obstruction T84.398 ☑
      - perforation T84.398 ☑
      - protrusion T84.398 ☑
    - pain T84.84 ☑
    - specified type NEC T84.89 ☑
    - stenosis T84.85 ☑
    - thrombosis T84.86 ☑
  - graft — *see* Complications, graft, bone
  - growth stimulator (electrode) — *see* Complications, electronic stimulator device, bone
  - marrow transplant — *see* Complications, transplant, bone, marrow
- brain neurostimulator (electrode) — *see* Complications, electronic stimulator device, brain
- breast implant (prosthetic) T85.9 ☑
  - capsular contracture T85.44 ☑
  - embolism T85.818 ☑
  - fibrosis T85.828 ☑
  - hemorrhage T85.838 ☑
  - infection and inflammation T85.79 ☑
  - mechanical
    - breakdown T85.41 ☑
    - displacement T85.42 ☑
    - leakage T85.43 ☑
    - malposition T85.42 ☑
    - obstruction T85.49 ☑
    - perforation T85.49 ☑
    - protrusion T85.49 ☑
    - specified NEC T85.49 ☑
  - pain T85.848 ☑
  - specified type NEC T85.898 ☑
  - stenosis T85.858 ☑
  - thrombosis T85.868 ☑
- bypass (see also Complications, prosthetic device or implant)
  - aortocoronary — *see* Complications, coronary artery (bypass) graft
  - arterial (see also Complications, graft, vascular)
    - extremity — *see* Complications, extremity artery (bypass) graft
- cardiac (see also Disease, heart)
  - device, implant or graft T82.9 ☑
    - embolism T82.817 ☑
    - fibrosis T82.827 ☑
    - hemorrhage T82.837 ☑
    - infection or inflammation T82.7 ☑
      - valve prosthesis T82.6

☑ **Additional Character Required** — Refer to the Tabular List for Character Selection ▽ Subterms under main terms may continue to next column or page

Complication(s) — *continued*
  cardiac (*see also* Disease, heart) — *continued*
    device, implant or graft — *continued*
      mechanical
        breakdown T82.519 ☑
          specified device NEC T82.518 ☑
        displacement T82.529 ☑
          specified device NEC T82.528 ☑
        leakage T82.539 ☑
          specified device NEC T82.538 ☑
        malposition T82.529 ☑
          specified device NEC T82.528 ☑
        obstruction T82.599 ☑
          specified device NEC T82.598 ☑
        perforation T82.599 ☑
          specified device NEC T82.598 ☑
        protrusion T82.599 ☑
          specified device NEC T82.598 ☑
      pain T82.847 ☑
      specified type NEC T82.897 ☑
      stenosis T82.857 ☑
      thrombosis T82.867 ☑
  cardiovascular device, graft or implant T82.9 ☑
    aortic graft — *see* Complications, graft, vascular
    arteriovenous
      fistula, artificial — *see* Complication, arteriovenous, fistula, surgically created
      shunt — *see* Complication, arteriovenous, shunt, surgically created
    artificial heart — *see* Complication, artificial, heart
    balloon (counterpulsation) device — *see* Complication, balloon implant, vascular
    carotid artery graft — *see* Complications, graft, vascular
    coronary bypass graft — *see* Complication, coronary artery (bypass) graft
    dialysis catheter (vascular) — *see* Complication, catheter, dialysis
    electronic T82.9 ☑
      electrode T82.9 ☑
        embolism T82.817 ☑
        fibrosis T82.827 ☑
        hemorrhage T82.837 ☑
        infection T82.7 ☑
        mechanical
          breakdown T82.110 ☑
          displacement T82.120 ☑
          leakage T82.190 ☑
          obstruction T82.190 ☑
          perforation T82.190 ☑
          protrusion T82.190 ☑
          specified type NEC T82.190 ☑
        pain T82.847 ☑
        specified NEC T82.897 ☑
        stenosis T82.857 ☑
        thrombosis T82.867 ☑
      embolism T82.817 ☑
      fibrosis T82.827 ☑
      hemorrhage T82.837 ☑
      infection T82.7 ☑
      mechanical
        breakdown T82.119 ☑
        displacement T82.129 ☑
        leakage T82.199 ☑
        obstruction T82.199 ☑
        perforation T82.199 ☑
        protrusion T82.199 ☑
        specified type NEC T82.199 ☑
      pain T82.847 ☑
      pulse generator T82.9 ☑
        embolism T82.817 ☑
        fibrosis T82.827 ☑
        hemorrhage T82.837 ☑
        infection T82.7 ☑
        mechanical
          breakdown T82.111 ☑
          displacement T82.121 ☑
          leakage T82.191 ☑
          obstruction T82.191 ☑
          perforation T82.191 ☑
          protrusion T82.191 ☑
          specified type NEC T82.191 ☑
        pain T82.847 ☑
        specified NEC T82.897 ☑
        stenosis T82.857 ☑
        thrombosis T82.867 ☑

Complication(s) — *continued*
  cardiovascular device, graft or implant — *continued*
    electronic — *continued*
      specified condition NEC T82.897 ☑
      specified device NEC T82.9 ☑
        embolism T82.817 ☑
        fibrosis T82.827 ☑
        hemorrhage T82.837 ☑
        infection T82.7 ☑
        mechanical
          breakdown T82.118 ☑
          displacement T82.128 ☑
          leakage T82.198 ☑
          obstruction T82.198 ☑
          perforation T82.198 ☑
          protrusion T82.198 ☑
          specified type NEC T82.198 ☑
        pain T82.847 ☑
        specified NEC T82.897 ☑
        stenosis T82.857 ☑
        thrombosis T82.867 ☑
      stenosis T82.857 ☑
      thrombosis T82.867 ☑
    extremity artery graft — *see* Complication, extremity artery (bypass) graft
    femoral artery graft — *see* Complication, extremity artery (bypass) graft
    heart
      transplant — *see* Complication, transplant, heart
      valve — *see* Complication, prosthetic device, heart valve
        graft — *see* Complication, heart, valve, graft
    heart-lung transplant — *see* Complication, transplant, heart, with lung
    infection or inflammation T82.7 ☑
    umbrella device — *see* Complication, umbrella device, vascular
    vascular graft (or anastomosis) — *see* Complication, graft, vascular
  carotid artery (bypass) graft — *see* Complications, graft, vascular
  catheter (device) NEC (*see also* Complications, prosthetic device or implant)
    cranial infusion
      infection and inflammation T85.735 ☑
      mechanical
        breakdown T85.610 ☑
        displacement T85.620 ☑
        leakage T85.630 ☑
        malfunction T85.690 ☑
        malposition T85.620 ☑
        obstruction T85.690 ☑
        perforation T85.690 ☑
        protrusion T85.690 ☑
        specified NEC T85.690 ☑
    cystostomy T83.9 ☑
      embolism T83.81 ☑
      fibrosis T83.82 ☑
      hemorrhage T83.83 ☑
      infection and inflammation T83.510 ☑
      mechanical
        breakdown T83.010 ☑
        displacement T83.020 ☑
        leakage T83.030 ☑
        malposition T83.020 ☑
        obstruction T83.090 ☑
        perforation T83.090 ☑
        protrusion T83.090 ☑
        specified NEC T83.090 ☑
      pain T83.84 ☑
      specified type NEC T83.89 ☑
      stenosis T83.85 ☑
      thrombosis T83.86 ☑
    dialysis (vascular) T82.9 ☑
      embolism T82.818 ☑
      fibrosis T82.828 ☑
      hemorrhage T82.838 ☑
      infection and inflammation T82.7 ☑
      intraperitoneal — *see* Complications, catheter, intraperitoneal
      mechanical
        breakdown T82.41 ☑
        displacement T82.42 ☑
        leakage T82.43 ☑
        malposition T82.42 ☑
        obstruction T82.49 ☑

Complication(s) — *continued*
  catheter (*see also* Complications, prosthetic device or implant) — *continued*
    dialysis — *continued*
      mechanical — *continued*
        perforation T82.49 ☑
        protrusion T82.49 ☑
      pain T82.848 ☑
      specified type NEC T82.898 ☑
      stenosis T82.858 ☑
      thrombosis T82.868 ☑
    epidural infusion T85.9 ☑
      embolism T85.810 ☑
      fibrosis T85.820 ☑
      hemorrhage T85.830 ☑
      infection and inflammation T85.735 ☑
      mechanical
        breakdown T85.610 ☑
        displacement T85.620 ☑
        leakage T85.630 ☑
        malfunction T85.610 ☑
        malposition T85.620 ☑
        obstruction T85.690 ☑
        perforation T85.690 ☑
        protrusion T85.690 ☑
        specified NEC T85.690 ☑
      pain T85.840 ☑
      specified type NEC T85.890 ☑
      stenosis T85.850 ☑
      thrombosis T85.860 ☑
    intraperitoneal dialysis T85.9 ☑
      embolism T85.818 ☑
      fibrosis T85.828 ☑
      hemorrhage T85.838 ☑
      infection and inflammation T85.71 ☑
      mechanical
        breakdown T85.611 ☑
        displacement T85.621 ☑
        leakage T85.631 ☑
        malfunction T85.611 ☑
        malposition T85.621 ☑
        obstruction T85.691 ☑
        perforation T85.691 ☑
        protrusion T85.691 ☑
        specified NEC T85.691 ☑
      pain T85.848 ☑
      specified type NEC T85.898 ☑
      stenosis T85.858 ☑
      thrombosis T85.868 ☑
    intrathecal infusion
      infection and inflammation T85.735 ☑
      mechanical
        breakdown T85.610 ☑
        displacement T85.620 ☑
        leakage T85.630 ☑
        malfunction T85.690 ☑
        malposition T85.620 ☑
        obstruction T85.690 ☑
        perforation T85.690 ☑
        protrusion T85.690 ☑
        specified NEC T85.690 ☑
    intravenous infusion T82.9 ☑
      embolism T82.818 ☑
      fibrosis T82.828 ☑
      hemorrhage T82.838 ☑
      infection or inflammation T82.7 ☑
      mechanical
        breakdown T82.514 ☑
        displacement T82.524 ☑
        leakage T82.534 ☑
        malposition T82.524 ☑
        obstruction T82.594 ☑
        perforation T82.594 ☑
        protrusion T82.594 ☑
      pain T82.848 ☑
      specified type NEC T82.898 ☑
      stenosis T82.858 ☑
      thrombosis T82.868 ☑
    spinal infusion
      infection and inflammation T85.735 ☑
      mechanical
        breakdown T85.610 ☑
        displacement T85.620 ☑
        leakage T85.630 ☑
        malfunction T85.690 ☑
        malposition T85.620 ☑

Complication(s) — *continued*
  catheter (*see also* Complications, prosthetic device or implant) — *continued*
    spinal infusion — *continued*
      mechanical — *continued*
        obstruction T85.690 ☑
        perforation T85.690 ☑
        protrusion T85.690 ☑
        specified NEC T85.690 ☑
      subarachnoid infusion
        infection and inflammation T85.735 ☑
        mechanical
          breakdown T85.610 ☑
          displacement T85.620 ☑
          leakage T85.630 ☑
          malfunction T85.690 ☑
          malposition T85.620 ☑
          obstruction T85.690 ☑
          perforation T85.690 ☑
          protrusion T85.690 ☑
          specified NEC T85.690 ☑
      subdural infusion T85.9 ☑
        embolism T85.810 ☑
        fibrosis T85.820 ☑
        hemorrhage T85.830 ☑
        infection and inflammation T85.735 ☑
        mechanical
          breakdown T85.610 ☑
          displacement T85.620 ☑
          leakage T85.630 ☑
          malfunction T85.610 ☑
          malposition T85.620 ☑
          obstruction T85.690 ☑
          perforation T85.690 ☑
          protrusion T85.690 ☑
          specified NEC T85.690 ☑
        pain T85.840 ☑
        specified type NEC T85.890 ☑
        stenosis T85.850 ☑
        thrombosis T85.860 ☑
    urethral T83.9 ☑
      displacement T83.028 ☑
      embolism T83.81 ☑
      fibrosis T83.82 ☑
      hemorrhage T83.83 ☑
      indwelling
        breakdown T83.011 ☑
        displacement T83.021 ☑
        infection and inflammation T83.511 ☑
        leakage T83.031 ☑
        specified complication NEC T83.091 ☑
      infection and inflammation T83.511 ☑
      leakage T83.038 ☑
      malposition T83.028 ☑
      mechanical
        breakdown T83.011 ☑
      obstruction (mechanical) T83.091 ☑
      pain T83.84 ☑
      perforation T83.091 ☑
      protrusion T83.091 ☑
      specified type NEC T83.091 ☑
      stenosis T83.85 ☑
      thrombosis T83.86 ☑
    urinary NEC
      breakdown T83.018 ☑
      displacement T83.028 ☑
      infection and inflammation T83.518 ☑
      leakage T83.038 ☑
      specified complication NEC T83.098 ☑
  cecostomy (stoma) — *see* Complications, colostomy
  cesarean delivery wound NEC O90.89
    disruption O90.0
    hematoma O90.2
    infection (following delivery) O86.00
  chemotherapy (antineoplastic) NEC T88.7 ☑
  chin implant (prosthetic) — *see* Complication, prosthetic device or implant, specified NEC
  circulatory system I99.8
    intraoperative I97.88
    postprocedural I97.89
      following cardiac surgery (*see also* Infarct, myocardium, associated with revascularization procedure) I97.19- ☑
        postcardiotomy syndrome I97.0
      hypertension I97.3
      lymphedema after mastectomy I97.2

Complication(s) — *continued*
  circulatory system — *continued*
    postprocedural — *continued*
      postcardiotomy syndrome I97.0
      specified NEC I97.89
  colostomy (stoma) K94.00
    hemorrhage K94.01
    infection K94.02
    malfunction K94.03
    mechanical K94.03
    specified complication NEC K94.09
  contraceptive device, intrauterine — *see* Complications, intrauterine, contraceptive device
  cord (umbilical) — *see* Complications, umbilical cord
  corneal graft — *see* Complications, graft, cornea
  coronary artery (bypass) graft T82.9 ☑
    atherosclerosis — *see* Arteriosclerosis, coronary (artery),
    embolism T82.818 ☑
    fibrosis T82.828 ☑
    hemorrhage T82.838 ☑
    infection and inflammation T82.7 ☑
    mechanical
      breakdown T82.211 ☑
      displacement T82.212 ☑
      leakage T82.213 ☑
      malposition T82.212 ☑
      obstruction T82.218 ☑
      perforation T82.218 ☑
      protrusion T82.218 ☑
      specified NEC T82.218 ☑
    pain T82.848 ☑
    specified type NEC T82.898 ☑
    stenosis T82.858 ☑
    thrombosis T82.868 ☑
  counterpulsation device (balloon), intra- aortic — *see* Complications, balloon implant, vascular
  cystostomy (stoma) N99.518
    catheter — *see* Complications, catheter, cystostomy
    hemorrhage N99.510
    infection N99.511
    malfunction N99.512
    specified type NEC N99.518
  delivery (*see also* Complications, obstetric) O75.9
    procedure (instrumental) (manual) (surgical) O75.4
    specified NEC O75.89
  dialysis (peritoneal) (renal) (*see also* Complications, infusion)
    catheter (vascular) — *see* Complication, catheter, dialysis
    peritoneal, intraperitoneal — *see* Complications, catheter, intraperitoneal
  dorsal column (spinal) neurostimulator — *see* Complications, electronic stimulator device, spinal cord
  drug NEC T88.7 ☑
  ear procedure (*see also* Disorder, ear)
    intraoperative H95.88
      hematoma — *see* Complications, intraoperative, hemorrhage (hematoma) (of), ear
      hemorrhage — *see* Complications, intraoperative, hemorrhage (hematoma) (of), ear
      laceration — *see* Complications, intraoperative, puncture or laceration..., ear
      specified NEC H95.88
    postoperative H95.89
      external ear canal stenosis H95.81- ☑
      hematoma — *see* Complications, postprocedural, hematoma (of), ear
      hemorrhage — *see* Complications, postprocedural, hemorrhage (of), ear
      postmastoidectomy — *see* Complications, postmastoidectomy
      seroma — *see* Complications, postprocedural, seroma (of), mastoid process
      specified NEC H95.89
  ectopic pregnancy O08.9
    damage to pelvic organs O08.6
    embolism O08.2
    genital infection O08.0
    hemorrhage (delayed) (excessive) O08.1
    metabolic disorder O08.5
    renal failure O08.4
    shock O08.3
    specified type NEC O08.0
    venous complication NEC O08.7

Complication(s) — *continued*
  electronic stimulator device
    bladder (urinary) — *see* Complications, electronic stimulator device, urinary
    bone T84.9 ☑
      breakdown T84.310 ☑
      displacement T84.320 ☑
      embolism T84.81 ☑
      fibrosis T84.82 ☑
      hemorrhage T84.83 ☑
      infection or inflammation T84.7 ☑
      malfunction T84.310 ☑
      malposition T84.320 ☑
      mechanical NEC T84.390 ☑
      obstruction T84.390 ☑
      pain T84.84 ☑
      perforation T84.390 ☑
      protrusion T84.390 ☑
      specified type NEC T84.89 ☑
      stenosis T84.85 ☑
      thrombosis T84.86 ☑
    brain T85.9 ☑
      embolism T85.810 ☑
      fibrosis T85.820 ☑
      hemorrhage T85.830 ☑
      infection and inflammation T85.731 ☑
      mechanical
        breakdown T85.110 ☑
        displacement T85.120 ☑
        leakage T85.190 ☑
        malposition T85.120 ☑
        obstruction T85.190 ☑
        perforation T85.190 ☑
        protrusion T85.190 ☑
        specified NEC T85.190 ☑
      pain T85.840 ☑
      specified type NEC T85.890 ☑
      stenosis T85.850 ☑
      thrombosis T85.860 ☑
    cardiac (defibrillator) (pacemaker) — *see* Complications, cardiovascular device or implant, electronic
    generator (brain) (gastric) (peripheral) (sacral) (spinal)
      breakdown T85.113 ☑
      displacement T85.123 ☑
      leakage T85.193 ☑
      malposition T85.123 ☑
      obstruction T85.193 ☑
      perforation T85.193 ☑
      protrusion T85.193 ☑
      specified type NEC T85.193 ☑
    muscle T84.9 ☑
      breakdown T84.418 ☑
      displacement T84.428 ☑
      embolism T84.81 ☑
      fibrosis T84.82 ☑
      hemorrhage T84.83 ☑
      infection or inflammation T84.7 ☑
      mechanical NEC T84.498 ☑
      pain T84.84 ☑
      specified type NEC T84.89 ☑
      stenosis T84.85 ☑
      thrombosis T84.86 ☑
    nervous system T85.9 ☑
      brain — *see* Complications, electronic stimulator device, brain
      cranial nerve — *see* Complications, electronic stimulator device, peripheral nerve
      embolism T85.810 ☑
      fibrosis T85.820 ☑
      gastric nerve — *see* Complications, electronic stimulator device, peripheral nerve
      hemorrhage T85.830 ☑
      infection and inflammation T85.738 ☑
      mechanical
        breakdown T85.118 ☑
        displacement T85.128 ☑
        leakage T85.199 ☑
        malposition T85.128 ☑
        obstruction T85.199 ☑
        perforation T85.199 ☑
        protrusion T85.199 ☑
        specified NEC T85.199 ☑
      pain T85.840 ☑

  ☑ **Additional Character Required** — **Refer to the Tabular List for Character Selection**   ▽ **Subterms under main terms may continue to next column or page**

Complication(s) — *continued*
- electronic stimulator device — *continued*
  - nervous system — *continued*
    - peripheral nerve — *see* Complications, electronic stimulator device, peripheral nerve
    - sacral nerve — *see* Complications, electronic stimulator device, peripheral nerve
    - specified type NEC T85.890 ☑
    - spinal cord — *see* Complications, electronic stimulator device, spinal cord
    - stenosis T85.850 ☑
    - thrombosis T85.860 ☑
    - vagal nerve — *see* Complications, electronic stimulator device, peripheral nerve
  - peripheral nerve T85.9 ☑
    - embolism T85.810 ☑
    - fibrosis T85.820 ☑
    - hemorrhage T85.830 ☑
    - infection and inflammation T85.732 ☑
    - mechanical
      - breakdown T85.111 ☑
      - displacement T85.121 ☑
      - leakage T85.191 ☑
      - malposition T85.121 ☑
      - obstruction T85.191 ☑
      - perforation T85.191 ☑
      - protrusion T85.191 ☑
      - specified NEC T85.191 ☑
    - pain T85.840 ☑
    - specified type NEC T85.890 ☑
    - stenosis T85.850 ☑
    - thrombosis T85.860 ☑
  - spinal cord T85.9 ☑
    - embolism T85.810 ☑
    - fibrosis T85.820 ☑
    - hemorrhage T85.830 ☑
    - infection and inflammation T85.733 ☑
    - mechanical
      - breakdown T85.112 ☑
      - displacement T85.122 ☑
      - leakage T85.192 ☑
      - malposition T85.122 ☑
      - obstruction T85.192 ☑
      - perforation T85.192 ☑
      - protrusion T85.192 ☑
      - specified NEC T85.192 ☑
    - pain T85.840 ☑
    - specified type NEC T85.890 ☑
    - stenosis T85.850 ☑
    - thrombosis T85.860 ☑
  - urinary T83.9 ☑
    - embolism T83.81 ☑
    - fibrosis T83.82 ☑
    - hemorrhage T83.83 ☑
    - infection and inflammation T83.598 ☑
    - mechanical
      - breakdown T83.110 ☑
      - displacement T83.120 ☑
      - malposition T83.120 ☑
      - perforation T83.190 ☑
      - protrusion T83.190 ☑
      - specified NEC T83.190 ☑
    - pain T83.84 ☑
    - specified type NEC T83.89 ☑
    - stenosis T83.85 ☑
    - thrombosis T83.86 ☑
- electroshock therapy T88.9 ☑
- specified NEC T88.8 ☑
- endocrine E34.9
  - postprocedural
    - adrenal hypofunction E89.6
    - hypoinsulinemia E89.1
    - hypoparathyroidism E89.2
    - hypopituitarism E89.3
    - hypothyroidism E89.0
    - ovarian failure E89.40
      - asymptomatic E89.40
      - symptomatic E89.41
    - specified NEC E89.89
    - testicular hypofunction E89.5
- endodontic treatment NEC M27.59
- enterostomy (stoma) K94.10
  - hemorrhage K94.11
  - infection K94.12
  - malfunction K94.13
  - mechanical K94.13

Complication(s) — *continued*
- enterostomy — *continued*
  - specified complication NEC K94.19
- episiotomy, disruption O90.1
- esophageal anti-reflux device T85.9 ☑
  - embolism T85.818 ☑
  - fibrosis T85.828 ☑
  - hemorrhage T85.838 ☑
  - infection and inflammation T85.79 ☑
  - mechanical
    - breakdown T85.511 ☑
    - displacement T85.521 ☑
    - malfunction T85.511 ☑
    - malposition T85.521 ☑
    - obstruction T85.591 ☑
    - perforation T85.591 ☑
    - protrusion T85.591 ☑
    - specified NEC T85.591 ☑
  - pain T85.848 ☑
  - specified type NEC T85.898 ☑
  - stenosis T85.858 ☑
  - thrombosis T85.868 ☑
- esophagostomy K94.30
  - hemorrhage K94.31
  - infection K94.32
  - malfunction K94.33
  - mechanical K94.33
  - specified complication NEC K94.39
- extracorporeal circulation T80.90 ☑
- extremity artery (bypass) graft T82.9 ☑
  - arteriosclerosis — *see* Arteriosclerosis, extremities, bypass graft
  - embolism T82.818 ☑
  - fibrosis T82.828 ☑
  - hemorrhage T82.838 ☑
  - infection and inflammation T82.7 ☑
  - mechanical
    - breakdown T82.318 ☑
      - femoral artery T82.312 ☑
    - displacement T82.328 ☑
      - femoral artery T82.322 ☑
    - leakage T82.338 ☑
      - femoral artery T82.332 ☑
    - malposition T82.328 ☑
      - femoral artery T82.322 ☑
    - obstruction T82.398 ☑
      - femoral artery T82.392 ☑
    - perforation T82.398 ☑
      - femoral artery T82.392 ☑
    - protrusion T82.398 ☑
      - femoral artery T82.392 ☑
  - pain T82.848 ☑
  - specified type NEC T82.898 ☑
  - stenosis T82.858 ☑
  - thrombosis T82.868 ☑
- eye H57.9
  - corneal graft — *see* Complications, graft, cornea
  - implant (prosthetic) T85.9 ☑
    - embolism T85.818 ☑
    - fibrosis T85.828 ☑
    - hemorrhage T85.838 ☑
    - infection and inflammation T85.79 ☑
    - mechanical
      - breakdown T85.318 ☑
      - displacement T85.328 ☑
      - leakage T85.398 ☑
      - malposition T85.328 ☑
      - obstruction T85.398 ☑
      - perforation T85.398 ☑
      - protrusion T85.398 ☑
      - specified NEC T85.398 ☑
    - pain T85.848 ☑
    - specified type NEC T85.898 ☑
    - stenosis T85.858 ☑
    - thrombosis T85.868 ☑
  - intraocular lens — *see* Complications, intraocular lens
  - orbital prosthesis — *see* Complications, orbital prosthesis
- female genital N94.9
  - device, implant or graft NEC — *see* Complications, genitourinary, device or implant, genital tract
- femoral artery (bypass) graft — *see* Complication, extremity artery (bypass) graft
- fixation device, internal (orthopedic) T84.9 ☑
  - infection and inflammation T84.60 ☑

Complication(s) — *continued*
- fixation device, internal — *continued*
  - infection and inflammation — *continued*
    - arm T84.61- ☑
      - humerus T84.61- ☑
      - radius T84.61- ☑
      - ulna T84.61- ☑
    - leg T84.629 ☑
      - femur T84.62- ☑
      - fibula T84.62- ☑
      - tibia T84.62- ☑
    - specified site NEC T84.89 ☑
    - spine T84.63 ☑
  - mechanical
    - breakdown
      - limb T84.119 ☑
        - carpal T84.210 ☑
        - femur T84.11- ☑
        - fibula T84.11- ☑
        - humerus T84.11- ☑
        - metacarpal T84.210 ☑
        - metatarsal T84.213 ☑
        - phalanx
          - foot T84.213 ☑
          - hand T84.210 ☑
        - radius T84.11- ☑
        - tarsal T84.213 ☑
        - tibia T84.11- ☑
        - ulna T84.11- ☑
      - specified bone NEC T84.218 ☑
      - spine T84.216 ☑
    - displacement
      - limb T84.129 ☑
        - carpal T84.220 ☑
        - femur T84.12- ☑
        - fibula T84.12- ☑
        - humerus T84.12- ☑
        - metacarpal T84.220 ☑
        - metatarsal T84.223 ☑
        - phalanx
          - foot T84.223 ☑
          - hand T84.220 ☑
        - radius T84.12- ☑
        - tarsal T84.223 ☑
        - tibia T84.12- ☑
        - ulna T84.12- ☑
      - specified bone NEC T84.228 ☑
      - spine T84.226 ☑
    - malposition — *see* Complications, fixation device, internal, mechanical, displacement
    - obstruction — *see* Complications, fixation device, internal, mechanical, specified type NEC
    - perforation — *see* Complications, fixation device, internal, mechanical, specified type NEC
    - protrusion — *see* Complications, fixation device, internal, mechanical, specified type NEC
    - specified type NEC
      - limb T84.199 ☑
        - carpal T84.290 ☑
        - femur T84.19- ☑
        - fibula T84.19- ☑
        - humerus T84.19- ☑
        - metacarpal T84.290 ☑
        - metatarsal T84.293 ☑
        - phalanx
          - foot T84.293 ☑
          - hand T84.290 ☑
        - radius T84.19- ☑
        - tarsal T84.293 ☑
        - tibia T84.19- ☑
        - ulna T84.19- ☑
      - specified bone NEC T84.298 ☑
      - vertebra T84.296 ☑
  - specified type NEC T84.89 ☑
  - embolism T84.81 ☑
  - fibrosis T84.82 ☑
  - hemorrhage T84.83 ☑
  - pain T84.84 ☑
  - specified complication NEC T84.89 ☑
  - stenosis T84.85 ☑
  - thrombosis T84.86 ☑
- following
  - acute myocardial infarction NEC I23.8
    - aneurysm (false) (of cardiac wall) (of heart wall) (ruptured) I23.3
    - angina I23.7

Complication(s) — *continued*
  following — *continued*
    acute myocardial infarction — *continued*
      atrial
        septal defect I23.1
        thrombosis I23.6
      cardiac wall rupture I23.3
      chordae tendinae rupture I23.4
      defect
        septal
          atrial (heart) I23.1
          ventricular (heart) I23.2
      hemopericardium I23.0
      papillary muscle rupture I23.5
      rupture
        cardiac wall I23.3
          with hemopericardium I23.0
        chordae tendineae I23.4
        papillary muscle I23.5
      specified NEC I23.8
      thrombosis
        atrium I23.6
        auricular appendage I23.6
        ventricle (heart) I23.6
      ventricular
        septal defect I23.2
        thrombosis I23.6
    ectopic or molar pregnancy O08.9
      cardiac arrest O08.81
      sepsis O08.82
      specified type NEC O08.89
      urinary tract infection O08.83
    termination of pregnancy — *see* Abortion
  gastrointestinal K92.9
    bile duct prosthesis — *see* Complications, bile duct implant
    esophageal anti-reflux device — *see* Complications, esophageal anti-reflux device
    postoperative
      colostomy — *see* Complications, colostomy
      dumping syndrome K91.1
      enterostomy — *see* Complications, enterostomy
      gastrostomy — *see* Complications, gastrostomy
      malabsorption NEC K91.2
      obstruction (*see also* Obstruction, intestine, postoperative) K91.30
      postcholecystectomy syndrome K91.5
      specified NEC K91.89
      vomiting after GI surgery K91.0
    prosthetic device or implant
      bile duct prosthesis — *see* Complications, bile duct implant
      esophageal anti-reflux device — *see* Complications, esophageal anti-reflux device
      specified type NEC
        embolism T85.818 ☑
        fibrosis T85.828 ☑
        hemorrhage T85.838 ☑
        mechanical
          breakdown T85.518 ☑
          displacement T85.528 ☑
          malfunction T85.518 ☑
          malposition T85.528 ☑
          obstruction T85.598 ☑
          perforation T85.598 ☑
          protrusion T85.598 ☑
          specified NEC T85.598 ☑
        pain T85.848 ☑
        specified complication NEC T85.898 ☑
        stenosis T85.858 ☑
        thrombosis T85.868 ☑
  gastrostomy (stoma) K94.20
    hemorrhage K94.21
    infection K94.22
    malfunction K94.23
    mechanical K94.23
    specified complication NEC K94.29
  genitourinary
    device or implant T83.9 ☑
      genital tract T83.9 ☑
        infection or inflammation T83.69 ☑
        intrauterine contraceptive device — *see* Complications, intrauterine, contraceptive device
        mechanical — *see* Complications, by device, mechanical
        mesh — *see* Complications, mesh

Complication(s) — *continued*
  genitourinary — *continued*
    device or implant — *continued*
      genital tract — *continued*
        penile prosthesis — *see* Complications, prosthetic device, penile
        specified type NEC T83.89 ☑
          embolism T83.81 ☑
          fibrosis T83.82 ☑
          hemorrhage T83.83 ☑
          pain T83.84 ☑
          specified complication NEC T83.89 ☑
          stenosis T83.85 ☑
          thrombosis T83.86 ☑
        vaginal mesh — *see* Complications, mesh
      urinary system T83.9 ☑
        cystostomy catheter — *see* Complication, catheter, cystostomy
        electronic stimulator — *see* Complications, electronic stimulator device, urinary
        indwelling urethral catheter — *see* Complications, catheter, urethral, indwelling
        infection or inflammation T83.598 ☑
          indwelling urethral catheter T83.511 ☑
        kidney transplant — *see* Complication, transplant, kidney
        organ graft — *see* Complication, graft, urinary organ
        specified type NEC T83.89 ☑
          embolism T83.81 ☑
          fibrosis T83.82 ☑
          hemorrhage T83.83 ☑
          mechanical T83.198 ☑
            breakdown T83.118 ☑
            displacement T83.128 ☑
            malfunction T83.118 ☑
            malposition T83.128 ☑
            obstruction T83.198 ☑
            perforation T83.198 ☑
            protrusion T83.198 ☑
            specified NEC T83.198 ☑
          sphincter implant — *see* Complications, implant, urinary sphincter
          sphincter, implanted T83.191 ☑
          stent (ileal conduit) (nephroureteral) T83.193 ☑
          pain T83.84 ☑
          specified complication NEC T83.89 ☑
          stenosis T83.85 ☑
          thrombosis T83.86 ☑
          ureteral indwelling T83.192 ☑
    postprocedural
      pelvic peritoneal adhesions N99.4
      renal failure N99.0
      specified NEC N99.89
      stoma — *see* Complications, stoma, urinary tract
      urethral stricture — *see* Stricture, urethra, postprocedural
      vaginal
        adhesions N99.2
        vault prolapse N99.3
  graft (bypass) (patch) (*see also* Complications, prosthetic device or implant)
    aorta — *see* Complications, graft, vascular
    arterial — *see* Complication, graft, vascular
    bone T86.839
      failure T86.831
      infection T86.832
      mechanical T84.318 ☑
        breakdown T84.318 ☑
        displacement T84.328 ☑
        protrusion T84.398 ☑
        specified type NEC T84.398 ☑
      rejection T86.830
      specified type NEC T86.838
    carotid artery — *see* Complications, graft, vascular
    cornea T86.849
      failure T86.841
      infection T86.842
      mechanical T85.398 ☑
        breakdown T85.318 ☑
        displacement T85.328 ☑
        protrusion T85.398 ☑
        specified type NEC T85.398 ☑
      rejection T86.840
      retroprosthetic membrane T85.398 ☑
      specified type NEC T86.848

Complication(s) — *continued*
  graft (*see also* Complications, prosthetic device or implant) — *continued*
    femoral artery (bypass) — *see* Complication, extremity artery (bypass) graft
    genital organ or tract — *see* Complications, genitourinary, device or implant, genital tract
    muscle T84.9 ☑
      breakdown T84.410 ☑
      displacement T84.420 ☑
      embolism T84.81 ☑
      fibrosis T84.82 ☑
      hemorrhage T84.83 ☑
      infection and inflammation T84.7 ☑
      mechanical NEC T84.490 ☑
      pain T84.84 ☑
      specified type NEC T84.89 ☑
      stenosis T84.85 ☑
      thrombosis T84.86 ☑
    nerve — *see* Complication, prosthetic device or implant, specified NEC
    skin — *see* Complications, prosthetic device or implant, skin graft
    tendon T84.9 ☑
      breakdown T84.410 ☑
      displacement T84.420 ☑
      embolism T84.81 ☑
      fibrosis T84.82 ☑
      hemorrhage T84.83 ☑
      infection and inflammation T84.7 ☑
      mechanical NEC T84.490 ☑
      pain T84.84 ☑
      specified type NEC T84.89 ☑
      stenosis T84.85 ☑
      thrombosis T84.86 ☑
    urinary organ T83.9 ☑
      embolism T83.81 ☑
      fibrosis T83.82 ☑
      hemorrhage T83.83 ☑
      infection and inflammation T83.598 ☑
        indwelling urethral catheter T83.511 ☑
      mechanical
        breakdown T83.21 ☑
        displacement T83.22 ☑
        erosion T83.24 ☑
        exposure T83.25 ☑
        leakage T83.23 ☑
        malposition T83.22 ☑
        obstruction T83.29 ☑
        perforation T83.29 ☑
        protrusion T83.29 ☑
        specified NEC T83.29 ☑
      pain T83.84 ☑
      specified type NEC T83.89 ☑
      stenosis T83.85 ☑
      thrombosis T83.86 ☑
    vascular T82.9 ☑
      embolism T82.818 ☑
      femoral artery — *see* Complication, extremity artery (bypass) graft
      fibrosis T82.828 ☑
      hemorrhage T82.838 ☑
      mechanical
        breakdown T82.319 ☑
          aorta (bifurcation) T82.310 ☑
          carotid artery T82.311 ☑
          specified vessel NEC T82.318 ☑
        displacement T82.329 ☑
          aorta (bifurcation) T82.320 ☑
          carotid artery T82.321 ☑
          specified vessel NEC T82.328 ☑
        leakage T82.339 ☑
          aorta (bifurcation) T82.330 ☑
          carotid artery T82.331 ☑
          specified vessel NEC T82.338 ☑
        malposition T82.329 ☑
          aorta (bifurcation) T82.320 ☑
          carotid artery T82.321 ☑
          specified vessel NEC T82.328 ☑
        obstruction T82.399 ☑
          aorta (bifurcation) T82.390 ☑
          carotid artery T82.391 ☑
          specified vessel NEC T82.398 ☑
        perforation T82.399 ☑
          aorta (bifurcation) T82.390 ☑
          carotid artery T82.391 ☑

☑ **Additional Character Required** — **Refer to the Tabular List for Character Selection**   ▽ Subterms under main terms may continue to next column or page

Complication(s) — *continued*
  graft (*see also* Complications, prosthetic device or implant) — *continued*
    vascular — *continued*
      mechanical — *continued*
        perforation — *continued*
          specified vessel NEC T82.398 ☑
        protrusion T82.399 ☑
          aorta (bifurcation) T82.390 ☑
          carotid artery T82.391 ☑
          specified vessel NEC T82.398 ☑
      pain T82.848 ☑
      specified complication NEC T82.898 ☑
      stenosis T82.858 ☑
      thrombosis T82.868 ☑
  heart I51.9
    assist device
      infection and inflammation T82.7 ☑
    following acute myocardial infarction — *see* Complications, following, acute myocardial infarction
    postoperative — *see* Complications, circulatory system
    transplant — *see* Complication, transplant, heart and lung(s) — *see* Complications, transplant, heart, with lung
    valve
      graft (biological) T82.9 ☑
        embolism T82.817 ☑
        fibrosis T82.827 ☑
        hemorrhage T82.837 ☑
        infection and inflammation T82.7 ☑
        mechanical T82.228 ☑
          breakdown T82.221 ☑
          displacement T82.222 ☑
          leakage T82.223 ☑
          malposition T82.222 ☑
          obstruction T82.228 ☑
          perforation T82.228 ☑
          protrusion T82.228 ☑
        pain T82.847 ☑
        specified type NEC T82.897 ☑
        stenosis T82.857 ☑
        thrombosis T82.867 ☑
      prosthesis T82.9 ☑
        embolism T82.817 ☑
        fibrosis T82.827 ☑
        hemorrhage T82.837 ☑
        infection or inflammation T82.6 ☑
        mechanical T82.09 ☑
          breakdown T82.01 ☑
          displacement T82.02 ☑
          leakage T82.03 ☑
          malposition T82.02 ☑
          obstruction T82.09 ☑
          perforation T82.09 ☑
          protrusion T82.09 ☑
        pain T82.847 ☑
        specified type NEC T82.897 ☑
          mechanical T82.09 ☑
        stenosis T82.857 ☑
        thrombosis T82.867 ☑
  hematoma
    intraoperative — *see* Complication, intraoperative, hemorrhage
    postprocedural — *see* Complication, postprocedural, hematoma
  hemodialysis — *see* Complications, dialysis
  hemorrhage
    intraoperative — *see* Complication, intraoperative, hemorrhage
    postprocedural — *see* Complication, postprocedural, hemorrhage
  ileostomy (stoma) — *see* Complications, enterostomy
  immunization (procedure) — *see* Complications, vaccination
  implant (*see also* Complications, by site and type)
    urinary sphincter T83.9 ☑
      embolism T83.81 ☑
      fibrosis T83.82 ☑
      hemorrhage T83.83 ☑
      infection and inflammation T83.591 ☑
      mechanical
        breakdown T83.111 ☑
        displacement T83.121 ☑
        leakage T83.191 ☑

Complication(s) — *continued*
  implant (*see also* Complications, by site and type) — *continued*
    urinary sphincter — *continued*
      mechanical — *continued*
        malposition T83.121 ☑
        obstruction T83.191 ☑
        perforation T83.191 ☑
        protrusion T83.191 ☑
        specified NEC T83.191 ☑
      pain T83.84 ☑
      specified type NEC T83.89 ☑
      stenosis T83.85 ☑
      thrombosis T83.86 ☑
  infusion (procedure) T80.90 ☑
    air embolism T80.0 ☑
    blood — *see* Complications, transfusion
    catheter — *see* Complications, catheter
    infection T80.29 ☑
    pump — *see* Complications, cardiovascular, device or implant
    sepsis T80.29 ☑
    serum reaction (*see also* Reaction, serum) T80.69 ☑
      anaphylactic shock (*see also* Shock, anaphylactic) T80.59 ☑
    specified type NEC T80.89 ☑
  inhalation therapy NEC T81.81 ☑
  injection (procedure) T80.90 ☑
    drug reaction — *see* Reaction, drug
    infection T80.29 ☑
    sepsis T80.29 ☑
    serum (prophylactic) (therapeutic) — *see* Complications, vaccination
    specified type NEC T80.89 ☑
    vaccine (any) — *see* Complications, vaccination
  inoculation (any) — *see* Complications, vaccination
  insulin pump
    infection and inflammation T85.72 ☑
    mechanical
      breakdown T85.614 ☑
      displacement T85.624 ☑
      leakage T85.633 ☑
      malposition T85.624 ☑
      obstruction T85.694 ☑
      perforation T85.694 ☑
      protrusion T85.694 ☑
      specified NEC T85.694 ☑
  intestinal pouch NEC K91.858
  intraocular lens (prosthetic) T85.9 ☑
    embolism T85.818 ☑
    fibrosis T85.828 ☑
    hemorrhage T85.838 ☑
    infection and inflammation T85.79 ☑
    mechanical
      breakdown T85.21 ☑
      displacement T85.22 ☑
      malposition T85.22 ☑
      obstruction T85.29 ☑
      perforation T85.29 ☑
      protrusion T85.29 ☑
      specified NEC T85.29 ☑
    pain T85.848 ☑
    specified type NEC T85.898 ☑
    stenosis T85.858 ☑
    thrombosis T85.868 ☑
  intraoperative (intraprocedural)
    cardiac arrest (*see also* Infarct, myocardium, associated with revascularization procedure)
      during cardiac surgery I97.710
      during other surgery I97.711
    cardiac functional disturbance NEC (*see also* Infarct, myocardium, associated with revascularization procedure)
      during cardiac surgery I97.790
      during other surgery I97.791
    hemorrhage (hematoma) (of)
      circulatory system organ or structure
        during cardiac bypass I97.411
        during cardiac catheterization I97.410
        during other circulatory system procedure I97.418
        during other procedure I97.42
      digestive system organ
        during procedure on digestive system K91.61
        during procedure on other organ K91.62

Complication(s) — *continued*
  intraoperative — *continued*
    hemorrhage — *continued*
      ear
        during procedure on ear and mastoid process H95.21
        during procedure on other organ H95.22
      endocrine system organ or structure
        during procedure on endocrine system organ or structure E36.01
        during procedure on other organ E36.02
      eye and adnexa
        during ophthalmic procedure H59.11- ☑
        during other procedure H59.12- ☑
      genitourinary organ or structure
        during procedure on genitourinary organ or structure N99.61
        during procedure on other organ N99.62
      mastoid process
        during procedure on ear and mastoid process H95.21
        during procedure on other organ H95.22
      musculoskeletal structure
        during musculoskeletal surgery M96.810
        during non-orthopedic surgery M96.811
        during orthopedic surgery M96.810
      nervous system
        during a nervous system procedure G97.31
        during other procedure G97.32
      respiratory system
        during other procedure J95.62
        during procedure on respiratory system organ or structure J95.61
      skin and subcutaneous tissue
        during a dermatologic procedure L76.01
        during a procedure on other organ L76.02
      spleen
        during a procedure on other organ D78.02
        during a procedure on the spleen D78.01
    puncture or laceration (accidental) (unintentional) (of)
      brain
        during a nervous system procedure G97.48
        during other procedure G97.49
      circulatory system organ or structure
        during circulatory system procedure I97.51
        during other procedure I97.52
      digestive system
        during procedure on digestive system K91.71
        during procedure on other organ K91.72
      ear
        during procedure on ear and mastoid process H95.31
        during procedure on other organ H95.32
      endocrine system organ or structure
        during procedure on endocrine system organ or structure E36.11
        during procedure on other organ E36.12
      eye and adnexa
        during ophthalmic procedure H59.21- ☑
        during other procedure H59.22- ☑
      genitourinary organ or structure
        during procedure on genitourinary organ or structure N99.71
        during procedure on other organ N99.72
      mastoid process
        during procedure on ear and mastoid process H95.31
        during procedure on other organ H95.32
      musculoskeletal structure
        during musculoskeletal surgery M96.820
        during non-orthopedic surgery M96.821
        during orthopedic surgery M96.820
      nervous system
        during a nervous system procedure G97.48
        during other procedure G97.49
      respiratory system
        during other procedure J95.72
        during procedure on respiratory system organ or structure J95.71
      skin and subcutaneous tissue
        during a dermatologic procedure L76.11
        during a procedure on other organ L76.12
      spleen
        during a procedure on other organ D78.12
        during a procedure on the spleen D78.11
    specified NEC
      circulatory system I97.88
      digestive system K91.81

Complication(s) — *continued*
  intraoperative — *continued*
    specified — *continued*
      ear H95.88
      endocrine system E36.8
      eye and adnexa H59.88
      genitourinary system N99.81
      mastoid process H95.88
      musculoskeletal structure M96.89
      nervous system G97.81
      respiratory system J95.88
      skin and subcutaneous tissue L76.81
      spleen D78.81
  intraperitoneal catheter (dialysis) (infusion) — *see* Complications, catheter, intraperitoneal
  intrathecal infusion pump
    infection and inflammation T85.738 ☑
    mechanical
      breakdown T85.615 ☑
      displacement T85.625 ☑
      leakage T85.635 ☑
      malfunction T85.695 ☑
      malposition T85.625 ☑
      obstruction T85.695 ☑
      perforation T85.695 ☑
      protrusion T85.695 ☑
      specified NEC T85.695 ☑
  intrauterine
    contraceptive device
      embolism T83.81 ☑
      fibrosis T83.82 ☑
      hemorrhage T83.83 ☑
      infection and inflammation T83.69 ☑
      mechanical
        breakdown T83.31 ☑
        displacement T83.32 ☑
        malposition T83.32 ☑
        obstruction T83.39 ☑
        perforation T83.39 ☑
        protrusion T83.39 ☑
        specified NEC T83.39 ☑
      pain T83.84 ☑
      specified type NEC T83.89 ☑
      stenosis T83.85 ☑
      thrombosis T83.86 ☑
    procedure (fetal), to newborn P96.5
  jejunostomy (stoma) — *see* Complications, enterostomy
  joint prosthesis, internal T84.9 ☑
    breakage (fracture) T84.01- ☑
    dislocation T84.02- ☑
    fracture T84.01- ☑
    infection or inflammation T84.50 ☑
      hip T84.5- ☑
      knee T84.5- ☑
      specified joint NEC T84.59 ☑
    instability T84.02- ☑
    malposition — *see* Complications, joint prosthesis, mechanical, displacement
    mechanical
      breakage, broken T84.01- ☑
      dislocation T84.02- ☑
      fracture T84.01- ☑
      instability T84.02- ☑
      leakage — *see* Complications, joint prosthesis, mechanical, specified NEC
      loosening T84.039 ☑
        hip T84.03- ☑
        knee T84.03- ☑
        specified joint NEC T84.038 ☑
      obstruction — *see* Complications, joint prosthesis, mechanical, specified NEC
      perforation — *see* Complications, joint prosthesis, mechanical, specified NEC
      osteolysis T84.059 ☑
        hip T84.05- ☑
        knee T84.05- ☑
        other specified joint T84.058 ☑
      protrusion — *see* Complications, joint prosthesis, mechanical, specified NEC
      specified complication NEC T84.099 ☑
        hip T84.09- ☑
        knee T84.09- ☑
        other specified joint T84.098 ☑
      subluxation T84.02- ☑
      wear of articular bearing surface T84.069 ☑

Complication(s) — *continued*
  joint prosthesis, internal — *continued*
    mechanical — *continued*
      wear of articular bearing surface — *continued*
        hip T84.06- ☑
        knee T84.06- ☑
        other specified joint T84.068 ☑
      specified joint NEC T84.89 ☑
        embolism T84.81 ☑
        fibrosis T84.82 ☑
        hemorrhage T84.83 ☑
        pain T84.84 ☑
        specified complication NEC T84.89 ☑
        stenosis T84.85 ☑
        thrombosis T84.86 ☑
      subluxation T84.02- ☑
  kidney transplant — *see* Complications, transplant, kidney
  labor O75.9
    specified NEC O75.89
  liver transplant (immune or nonimmune) — *see* Complications, transplant, liver
  lumbar puncture G97.1
    cerebrospinal fluid leak G97.0
    headache or reaction G97.1
  lung transplant — *see* Complications, transplant, lung
    and heart — *see* Complications, transplant, lung, with heart
  male genital N50.9
    device, implant or graft — *see* Complications, genitourinary, device or implant, genital tract
    postprocedural or postoperative — *see* Complications, genitourinary, postprocedural
      specified NEC N99.89
  mastoid (process) procedure
    intraoperative H95.88
      hematoma — *see* Complications, intraoperative, hemorrhage (hematoma) (of), mastoid process
      hemorrhage — *see* Complications, intraoperative, hemorrhage (hematoma) (of), mastoid process
      laceration — *see* Complications, intraoperative, puncture or laceration, mastoid process
      specified NEC H95.88
    postmastoidectomy — *see* Complications, postmastoidectomy
    postoperative H95.89
      external ear canal stenosis H95.81 ☑
      hematoma — *see* Complications, postprocedural, hematoma (of), mastoid process
      hemorrhage — *see* Complications, postprocedural, hemorrhage (of), mastoid process
      postmastoidectomy — *see* Complications, postmastoidectomy
      seroma — *see* Complications, postprocedural, seroma (of), mastoid process
      specified NEC H95.89
  mastoidectomy cavity — *see* Complications, postmastoidectomy
  mechanical — *see* Complications, by site and type, mechanical
  medical procedures (*see also* Complication(s), intraoperative) T88.9 ☑
  metabolic E88.9
    postoperative E89.89
      specified NEC E89.89
  molar pregnancy NOS O08.9
    damage to pelvic organs O08.6
    embolism O08.2
    genital infection O08.0
    hemorrhage (delayed) (excessive) O08.1
    metabolic disorder O08.5
    renal failure O08.4
    shock O08.3
    specified type NEC O08.0
    venous complication NEC O08.7
  musculoskeletal system (*see also* Complication, intraoperative (intraprocedural), by site)
    device, implant or graft NEC — *see* Complications, orthopedic, device or implant
    internal fixation (nail) (plate) (rod) — *see* Complications, fixation device, internal
    joint prosthesis — *see* Complications, joint prosthesis
    post radiation M96.89
      kyphosis M96.2

Complication(s) — *continued*
  musculoskeletal system (*see also* Complication, intraoperative, by site) — *continued*
    post radiation — *continued*
      scoliosis M96.5
      specified complication NEC M96.89
    postoperative (postprocedural) M96.89
      with osteoporosis — *see* Osteoporosis
      fracture following insertion of device — *see* Fracture, following insertion of orthopedic implant, joint prosthesis or bone plate
      joint instability after prosthesis removal M96.89
      lordosis M96.4
      postlaminectomy syndrome NEC M96.1
        kyphosis M96.3
      pseudarthrosis M96.0
      specified complication NEC M96.89
  nephrostomy (stoma) — *see* Complications, stoma, urinary tract, external NEC
  nervous system G98.8
    central G96.9
    device, implant or graft (*see also* Complication, prosthetic device or implant, specified NEC)
      electronic stimulator (electrode(s)) — *see* Complications, electronic stimulator device
      specified NEC
        infection and inflammation T85.738 ☑
        mechanical T85.695 ☑
          breakdown T85.615 ☑
          displacement T85.625 ☑
          leakage T85.635 ☑
          malfunction T85.695 ☑
          malposition T85.625 ☑
          obstruction T85.695 ☑
          perforation T85.695 ☑
          protrusion T85.695 ☑
          specified NEC T85.695 ☑
      ventricular shunt — *see* Complications, ventricular shunt
    electronic stimulator (electrode(s)) — *see* Complications, electronic stimulator device
    postprocedural G97.82
      intracranial hypotension G97.2
      specified NEC G97.82
      spinal fluid leak G97.0
  newborn, due to intrauterine (fetal) procedure P96.5
  nonabsorbable (permanent) sutures — *see* Complication, sutures, permanent
  obstetric O75.9
    procedure (instrumental) (manual) (surgical) specified NEC O75.4
    specified NEC O75.89
    surgical wound NEC O90.89
      hematoma O90.2
      infection O86.00
  ocular lens implant — *see* Complications, intraocular lens
  ophthalmologic
    postprocedural bleb — *see* Blebitis
  orbital prosthesis T85.9 ☑
    embolism T85.818 ☑
    fibrosis T85.828 ☑
    hemorrhage T85.838 ☑
    infection and inflammation T85.79 ☑
    mechanical
      breakdown T85.31- ☑
      displacement T85.32- ☑
      malposition T85.32- ☑
      obstruction T85.39- ☑
      perforation T85.39- ☑
      protrusion T85.39- ☑
      specified NEC T85.39- ☑
    pain T85.848 ☑
    specified type NEC T85.898 ☑
    stenosis T85.858 ☑
    thrombosis T85.868 ☑
  organ or tissue transplant (partial) (total) — *see* Complications, transplant
  orthopedic (*see also* Disorder, soft tissue)
    device or implant T84.9 ☑
      bone
        device or implant — *see* Complication, bone, device NEC
        graft — *see* Complication, graft, bone
      breakdown T84.418 ☑
      displacement T84.428 ☑

Complication(s) — *continued*
orthopedic (*see also* Disorder, soft tissue) — *continued*
   device or implant — *continued*
     electronic bone stimulator — *see* Complications, electronic stimulator device, bone
     embolism T84.81 ☑
     fibrosis T84.82 ☑
     fixation device — *see* Complication, fixation device, internal
     hemorrhage T84.83 ☑
     infection or inflammation T84.7 ☑
     joint prosthesis — *see* Complication, joint prosthesis, internal
     malfunction T84.418 ☑
     malposition T84.428 ☑
     mechanical NEC T84.498 ☑
     muscle graft — *see* Complications, graft, muscle
     obstruction T84.498 ☑
     pain T84.84 ☑
     perforation T84.498 ☑
     protrusion T84.498 ☑
     specified complication NEC T84.89 ☑
     stenosis T84.85 ☑
     tendon graft — *see* Complications, graft, tendon
     thrombosis T84.86 ☑
   fracture (following insertion of device) — *see* Fracture, following insertion of orthopedic implant, joint prosthesis or bone plate
   postprocedural M96.89
     fracture — *see* Fracture, following insertion of orthopedic implant, joint prosthesis or bone plate
     postlaminectomy syndrome NEC M96.1
       kyphosis M96.3
       lordosis M96.4
     postradiation
       kyphosis M96.2
       scoliosis M96.5
     pseudarthrosis post-fusion M96.0
     specified type NEC M96.89
pacemaker (cardiac) — *see* Complications, cardiovascular device or implant, electronic
pancreas transplant — *see* Complications, transplant, pancreas
penile prosthesis (implant) — *see* Complications, prosthetic device, penile
perfusion NEC T80.90 ☑
perineal repair (obstetrical) NEC O90.89
   disruption O90.1
   hematoma O90.2
   infection (following delivery) O86.09
phototherapy T88.9 ☑
   specified NEC T88.8 ☑
postmastoidectomy NEC H95.19- ☑
   cyst, mucosal H95.13- ☑
   granulation H95.12- ☑
   inflammation, chronic H95.11- ☑
   recurrent cholesteatoma H95.0- ☑
postoperative — *see* Complications, postprocedural
   circulatory — *see* Complications, circulatory system
   ear — *see* Complications, ear
   endocrine — *see* Complications, endocrine
   eye — *see* Complications, eye
   lumbar puncture G97.1
     cerebrospinal fluid leak G97.0
   nervous system (central) (peripheral) — *see* Complications, nervous system
   respiratory system — *see* Complications, respiratory system
postprocedural (*see also* Complications, surgical procedure)
   cardiac arrest (*see also* Infarct, myocardium, associated with revascularization procedure)
     following cardiac surgery I97.120
     following other surgery I97.121
   cardiac functional disturbance NEC (*see also* Infarct, myocardium, associated with revascularization procedure)
     following cardiac surgery I97.190
     following other surgery I97.191
   cardiac insufficiency
     following cardiac surgery I97.110
     following other surgery I97.111
   chorioretinal scars following retinal surgery H59.81- ☑

Complication(s) — *continued*
postprocedural (*see also* Complications, surgical procedure) — *continued*
   following cataract surgery
     cataract (lens) fragments H59.02- ☑
     cystoid macular edema H59.03- ☑
     specified NEC H59.09- ☑
     vitreous (touch) syndrome H59.01- ☑
   heart failure
     following cardiac surgery I97.130
     following other surgery I97.131
   hematoma (of)
     circulatory system organ or structure
       following cardiac bypass I97.631
       following cardiac catheterization I97.630
       following other circulatory system procedure I97.638
       following other procedure I97.621
     digestive system
       following procedure on digestive system K91.870
       following procedure on other organ K91.871
     ear
       following other procedure H95.52
       following procedure on ear and mastoid process H95.51
     endocrine system
       following endocrine system procedure E89.820
       following other procedure E89.821
     eye and adnexa
       following ophthalmic procedure H59.33- ☑
       following other procedure H59.34- ☑
     genitourinary organ or structure
       following procedure on genitourinary organ or structure N99.840
       following procedure on other organ N99.841
     mastoid process
       following other procedure H95.52
       following procedure on ear and mastoid process H95.51
     musculoskeletal structure
       following musculoskeletal surgery M96.840
       following non-orthopedic surgery M96.841
       following orthopedic surgery M96.840
     nervous system
       following nervous system procedure G97.61
       following other procedure G97.62
     respiratory system
       following other procedure J95.861
       following procedure on respiratory system organ or structure J95.860
     skin and subcutaneous tissue
       following dermatologic procedure L76.31
       following procedure on other organ L76.32
     spleen
       following procedure on other organ D78.32
       following procedure on the spleen D78.31
   hemorrhage (of)
     circulatory system organ or structure
       following cardiac bypass I97.611
       following cardiac catheterization I97.610
       following other circulatory system procedure I97.618
       following other procedure I97.620
     digestive system
       following procedure on digestive system K91.840
       following procedure on other organ K91.841
     ear
       following other procedure H95.42
       following procedure on ear and mastoid process H95.41
     endocrine system
       following endocrine system procedure E89.810
       following other procedure E89.811
     eye and adnexa
       following ophthalmic procedure H59.31- ☑
       following other procedure H59.32- ☑
     genitourinary organ or structure
       following procedure on genitourinary organ or structure N99.820
       following procedure on other organ N99.821
     mastoid process
       following other procedure H95.42
       following procedure on ear and mastoid process H95.41

Complication(s) — *continued*
postprocedural (*see also* Complications, surgical procedure) — *continued*
   hemorrhage — *continued*
     musculoskeletal structure
       following musculoskeletal surgery M96.830
       following non-orthopedic surgery M96.831
       following orthopedic surgery M96.830
     nervous system
       following nervous system procedure G97.51
       following other procedure G97.52
     respiratory system
       following a respiratory system procedure J95.830
       following other procedure J95.831
     skin and subcutaneous tissue
       following a procedure on other organ L76.22
       following dermatologic procedure L76.21
     spleen
       following procedure on other organ D78.22
       following procedure on the spleen D78.21
   seroma (of)
     circulatory system organ or structure
       following cardiac bypass I97.641
       following cardiac catheterization I97.640
       following other circulatory system procedure I97.648
       following other procedure I97.622
     digestive system
       following procedure on digestive system K91.872
       following procedure on other organ K91.873
     ear
       following other procedure H95.54
       following procedure on ear and mastoid process H95.53
     endocrine system
       following endocrine system procedure E89.822
       following other procedure E89.823
     eye and adnexa
       following ophthalmic procedure H59.35- ☑
       following other procedure H59.36- ☑
     genitourinary organ or structure
       following procedure on genitourinary organ or structure N99.842
       following procedure on other organ N99.843
     mastoid process
       following other procedure H95.54
       following procedure on ear and mastoid process H95.53
     musculoskeletal structure
       following musculoskeletal surgery M96.842
       following non-orthopedic surgery M96.843
       following orthopedic surgery M96.842
     nervous system
       following nervous system procedure G97.63
       following other procedure G97.64
     respiratory system
       following other procedure J95.863
       following procedure on respiratory system organ or structure J95.862
     skin and subcutaneous tissue
       following dermatologic procedure L76.33
       following procedure on other organ L76.34
     spleen
       following procedure on other organ D78.34
       following procedure on the spleen D78.33
   specified NEC
     circulatory system I97.89
     digestive K91.89
     ear H95.89
     endocrine E89.89
     eye and adnexa H59.89
     genitourinary N99.89
     mastoid process H95.89
     metabolic E89.89
     musculoskeletal structure M96.89
     nervous system G97.82
     respiratory system J95.89
     skin and subcutaneous tissue L76.82
     spleen D78.89
pregnancy NEC — *see* Pregnancy, complicated by
prosthetic device or implant T85.9 ☑
   bile duct — *see* Complications, bile duct implant
   breast — *see* Complications, breast implant

▽ Subterms under main terms may continue to next column or page   ☑ Additional Character Required — Refer to the Tabular List for Character Selection   65

Complication — Complication

Complication(s) — *continued*
  prosthetic device or implant — *continued*
    bulking agent
      ureteral
        erosion T83.714 ☑
        exposure T83.724 ☑
      urethral
        erosion T83.713 ☑
        exposure T83.723 ☑
    cardiac and vascular NEC — *see* Complications, cardiovascular device or implant
    corneal transplant — *see* Complications, graft, cornea
    electronic nervous system stimulator — *see* Complications, electronic stimulator device
    epidural infusion catheter — *see* Complications, catheter, epidural
    esophageal anti-reflux device — *see* Complications, esophageal anti-reflux device
    genital organ or tract — *see* Complications, genitourinary, device or implant, genital tract
      specified NEC T83.79- ☑
    heart valve — *see* Complications, heart, valve, prosthesis
    infection or inflammation T85.79 ☑
      intestine transplant T86.892
      liver transplant T86.43
      lung transplant T86.812
      pancreas transplant T86.892
      skin graft T86.822
    intraocular lens — *see* Complications, intraocular lens
    intraperitoneal (dialysis) catheter — *see* Complications, catheter, intraperitoneal
    joint — *see* Complications, joint prosthesis, internal
    mechanical NEC T85.698 ☑
      dialysis catheter (vascular) (*see also* Complication, catheter, dialysis, mechanical)
        peritoneal — *see* Complication, catheter, intraperitoneal, mechanical
      gastrointestinal device T85.598 ☑
      ocular device T85.398 ☑
      subdural (infusion) catheter T85.690 ☑
      suture, permanent T85.692 ☑
        that for bone repair — *see* Complications, fixation device, internal (orthopedic), mechanical
      ventricular shunt
        breakdown T85.01 ☑
        displacement T85.02 ☑
        leakage T85.03 ☑
        malposition T85.02 ☑
        obstruction T85.09 ☑
        perforation T85.09 ☑
        protrusion T85.09 ☑
        specified NEC T85.09 ☑
    mesh
      erosion (to surrounding organ or tissue) T83.718 ☑
        urethral (into pelvic floor muscles) T83.712 ☑
        vaginal (into pelvic floor muscles) T83.711 ☑
      exposure (into surrounding organ or tissue) T83.728 ☑
        urethral (through urethral wall) T83.722 ☑
        vaginal (into vagina) (through vaginal wall) T83.721 ☑
    orbital — *see* Complications, orbital prosthesis
    penile T83.9 ☑
      embolism T83.81 ☑
      fibrosis T83.82 ☑
      hemorrhage T83.83 ☑
      infection and inflammation T83.61 ☑
      mechanical
        breakdown T83.410 ☑
        displacement T83.420 ☑
        leakage T83.490 ☑
        malposition T83.420 ☑
        obstruction T83.490 ☑
        perforation T83.490 ☑
        protrusion T83.490 ☑
        specified NEC T83.490 ☑
      pain T83.84 ☑
      specified type NEC T83.89 ☑
      stenosis T83.85 ☑
      thrombosis T83.86 ☑

Complication(s) — *continued*
  prosthetic device or implant — *continued*
    prosthetic materials NEC
      erosion (to surrounding organ or tissue) T83.718 ☑
      exposure (into surrounding organ or tissue) T83.728 ☑
    skin graft T86.829
      artificial skin or decellularized allodermis
        embolism T85.818 ☑
        fibrosis T85.828 ☑
        hemorrhage T85.838 ☑
        infection and inflammation T85.79 ☑
        mechanical
          breakdown T85.613 ☑
          displacement T85.623 ☑
          malfunction T85.613 ☑
          malposition T85.623 ☑
          obstruction T85.693 ☑
          perforation T85.693 ☑
          protrusion T85.693 ☑
          specified NEC T85.693 ☑
        pain T85.848 ☑
        specified type NEC T85.898 ☑
        stenosis T85.858 ☑
        thrombosis T85.868 ☑
      failure T86.821
      infection T86.822
      rejection T86.820
      specified NEC T86.828
    sling
      urethral (female) (male)
        erosion T83.712 ☑
        exposure T83.722 ☑
    specified NEC T85.9 ☑
      embolism T85.818 ☑
      fibrosis T85.828 ☑
      hemorrhage T85.838 ☑
      infection and inflammation T85.79 ☑
      mechanical
        breakdown T85.618 ☑
        displacement T85.628 ☑
        leakage T85.638 ☑
        malfunction T85.618 ☑
        malposition T85.628 ☑
        obstruction T85.698 ☑
        perforation T85.698 ☑
        protrusion T85.698 ☑
        specified NEC T85.698 ☑
      pain T85.848 ☑
      specified type NEC T85.898 ☑
      stenosis T85.858 ☑
      thrombosis T85.868 ☑
    subdural infusion catheter — *see* Complications, catheter, subdural
    sutures — *see* Complications, sutures
    urinary organ or tract NEC — *see* Complications, genitourinary, device or implant, urinary system
    vascular — *see* Complications, cardiovascular device or implant
    ventricular shunt — *see* Complications, ventricular shunt (device)
  puerperium — *see* Puerperal
  puncture, spinal G97.1
    cerebrospinal fluid leak G97.0
    headache or reaction G97.1
  pyelogram N99.89
  radiation
    kyphosis M96.2
    scoliosis M96.5
  reattached
    extremity (infection) (rejection)
      lower T87.1X- ☑
      upper T87.0X- ☑
    specified body part NEC T87.2
  reconstructed breast
    asymmetry between native and reconstructed breast N65.1
    deformity N65.0
    disproportion between native and reconstructed breast N65.1
    excess tissue N65.0
    misshapen N65.0
  reimplant NEC (*see also* Complications, prosthetic device or implant)

Complication(s) — *continued*
  reimplant (*see also* Complications, prosthetic device or implant) — *continued*
    limb (infection) (rejection) — *see* Complications, reattached, extremity
    organ (partial) (total) — *see* Complications, transplant
    prosthetic device NEC — *see* Complications, prosthetic device
  renal N28.9
    allograft — *see* Complications, transplant, kidney
    dialysis — *see* Complications, dialysis
  respirator
    mechanical J95.850
      specified NEC J95.859
  respiratory system J98.9
    device, implant or graft — *see* Complication, prosthetic device or implant, specified NEC
    lung transplant — *see* Complications, prosthetic device or implant, lung transplant
    postoperative J95.89
      air leak J95.812
      Mendelson's syndrome (chemical pneumonitis) J95.4
      pneumothorax J95.811
      pulmonary insufficiency (acute) (after nonthoracic surgery) J95.2
        chronic J95.3
        following thoracic surgery J95.1
      respiratory failure (acute) J95.821
        acute and chronic J95.822
      specified NEC J95.89
      subglottic stenosis J95.5
      tracheostomy complication — *see* Complications, tracheostomy
    therapy T81.89 ☑
  sedation during labor and delivery O74.9
    cardiac O74.2
    central nervous system O74.3
    pulmonary NEC O74.1
  shunt (*see also* Complications, prosthetic device or implant)
    arteriovenous — *see* Complications, arteriovenous, shunt
    ventricular (communicating) — *see* Complications, ventricular shunt
  skin
    graft T86.829
      failure T86.821
      infection T86.822
      rejection T86.820
      specified type NEC T86.828
  spinal
    anesthesia — *see* Complications, anesthesia, spinal
    catheter (epidural) (subdural) — *see* Complications, catheter
    puncture or tap G97.1
      cerebrospinal fluid leak G97.0
      headache or reaction G97.1
  stent
    bile duct — *see* Complications, bile duct prosthesis
    ureteral indwelling
      breakdown T83.112 ☑
      displacement T83.122 ☑
      leakage T83.192 ☑
      malposition T83.122 ☑
      obstruction T83.192 ☑
      perforation T83.192 ☑
      protrusion T83.192 ☑
      specified NEC T83.192 ☑
    urinary NEC (ileal conduit) (nephroureteral) T83.193 ☑
      embolism T83.81 ☑
      fibrosis T83.82 ☑
      hemorrhage T83.83 ☑
      infection and inflammation T83.593 ☑
      mechanical
        breakdown T83.113 ☑
        displacement T83.123 ☑
        leakage T83.193 ☑
        malposition T83.123 ☑
        obstruction T83.193 ☑
        perforation T83.193 ☑
        protrusion T83.193 ☑
        specified NEC T83.193 ☑
      pain T83.84 ☑
      specified type NEC T83.89 ☑

☑ **Additional Character Required** — Refer to the Tabular List for Character Selection   ⁜ **Subterms under main terms may continue to next column or page**

Complication(s) — *continued*
  stent — *continued*
    urinary — *continued*
      stenosis T83.85 ☑
      thrombosis T83.86 ☑
    vascular
      end stent stenosis — *see* Restenosis, stent
      in stent stenosis — *see* Restenosis, stent
  stoma
    digestive tract
      colostomy — *see* Complications, colostomy
      enterostomy — *see* Complications, enterostomy
      esophagostomy — *see* Complications, esophagostomy
      gastrostomy — *see* Complications, gastrostomy
    urinary tract N99.528
      continent N99.538
        hemorrhage N99.530
        herniation N99.533
        infection N99.531
        malfunction N99.532
        specified type NEC N99.538
        stenosis N99.534
      cystostomy — *see* Complications, cystostomy
      external NOS N99.528
      hemorrhage N99.520
      herniation N99.523
      incontinent N99.528
        hemorrhage N99.520
        herniation N99.523
        infection N99.521
        malfunction N99.522
        specified type NEC N99.528
        stenosis N99.524
      infection N99.521
      malfunction N99.522
      specified type NEC N99.528
      stenosis N99.524
  stomach banding — *see* Complication(s), bariatric procedure
  stomach stapling — *see* Complication(s), bariatric procedure
  surgical material, nonabsorbable — *see* Complication, suture, permanent
  surgical procedure (on) T81.9 ☑
    amputation stump (late) — *see* Complications, amputation stump
    cardiac — *see* Complications, circulatory system
    cholesteatoma, recurrent — *see* Complications, postmastoidectomy, recurrent cholesteatoma
    circulatory (early) — *see* Complications, circulatory system
    digestive system — *see* Complications, gastrointestinal
    dumping syndrome (postgastrectomy) K91.1
    ear — *see* Complications, ear
    elephantiasis or lymphedema I97.89
      postmastectomy I97.2
    emphysema (surgical) T81.82 ☑
    endocrine — *see* Complications, endocrine
    eye — *see* Complications, eye
    fistula (persistent postoperative) T81.83 ☑
    foreign body inadvertently left in wound (sponge) (suture) (swab) — *see* Foreign body, accidentally left during a procedure
    gastrointestinal — *see* Complications, gastrointestinal
    genitourinary NEC N99.89
    hematoma
      intraoperative — *see* Complication, intraoperative, hemorrhage
      postprocedural — *see* Complication, postprocedural, hematoma
    hemorrhage
      intraoperative — *see* Complication, intraoperative, hemorrhage
      postprocedural — *see* Complication, postprocedural, hemorrhage
    hepatic failure K91.82
    hyperglycemia (postpancreatectomy) E89.1
    hypoinsulinemia (postpancreatectomy) E89.1
    hypoparathyroidism (postparathyroidectomy) E89.2
    hypopituitarism (posthypophysectomy) E89.3
    hypothyroidism (post-thyroidectomy) E89.0
    intestinal obstruction (*see also* Obstruction, intestine, postoperative) K91.30
    intracranial hypotension following ventricular shunting (ventriculostomy) G97.2

Complication(s) — *continued*
  surgical procedure — *continued*
    lymphedema I97.89
      postmastectomy I97.2
    malabsorption (postsurgical) NEC K91.2
      osteoporosis — *see* Osteoporosis, postsurgical malabsorption
    mastoidectomy cavity NEC — *see* Complications, postmastoidectomy
    metabolic E89.89
      specified NEC E89.89
    musculoskeletal — *see* Complications, musculoskeletal system
    nervous system (central) (peripheral) — *see* Complications, nervous system
    ovarian failure E89.40
      asymptomatic E89.40
      symptomatic E89.41
    peripheral vascular — *see* Complications, surgical procedure, vascular
    postcardiotomy syndrome I97.0
    postcholecystectomy syndrome K91.5
    postcommissurotomy syndrome I97.0
    postgastrectomy dumping syndrome K91.1
    postlaminectomy syndrome NEC M96.1
      kyphosis M96.3
    postmastectomy lymphedema syndrome I97.2
    postmastoidectomy cholesteatoma — *see* Complications, postmastoidectomy, recurrent cholesteatoma
    postvagotomy syndrome K91.1
    postvalvulotomy syndrome I97.0
    pulmonary insufficiency (acute) J95.2
      chronic J95.3
      following thoracic surgery J95.1
    reattached body part — *see* Complications, reattached
    respiratory — *see* Complications, respiratory system
    shock (hypovolemic) T81.19 ☑
    spleen (postoperative) D78.89
      intraoperative D78.81
    stitch abscess T81.41 ☑
    subglottic stenosis (postsurgical) J95.5
    testicular hypofunction E89.5
    transplant — *see* Complications, organ or tissue transplant
    urinary NEC N99.89
    vaginal vault prolapse (posthysterectomy) N99.3
    vascular (peripheral)
      artery T81.719 ☑
        mesenteric T81.710 ☑
        renal T81.711 ☑
        specified NEC T81.718 ☑
      vein T81.72 ☑
    wound infection T81.49 ☑
  suture, permanent (wire) NEC T85.9 ☑
    with repair of bone — *see* Complications, fixation device, internal
    embolism T85.818 ☑
    fibrosis T85.828 ☑
    hemorrhage T85.838 ☑
    infection and inflammation T85.79 ☑
    mechanical
      breakdown T85.612 ☑
      displacement T85.622 ☑
      malfunction T85.612 ☑
      malposition T85.622 ☑
      obstruction T85.692 ☑
      perforation T85.692 ☑
      protrusion T85.692 ☑
      specified NEC T85.692 ☑
    pain T85.848 ☑
    specified type NEC T85.898 ☑
    stenosis T85.858 ☑
    thrombosis T85.868 ☑
  tracheostomy J95.00
    granuloma J95.09
    hemorrhage J95.01
    infection J95.02
    malfunction J95.03
    mechanical J95.03
    obstruction J95.03
    specified type NEC J95.09
    tracheo-esophageal fistula J95.04
  transfusion (blood) (lymphocytes) (plasma) T80.92 ☑
    air emblism T80.0 ☑
    circulatory overload E87.71

Complication(s) — *continued*
  transfusion — *continued*
    febrile nonhemolytic transfusion reaction R50.84
    hemochromatosis E83.111
    hemolysis T80.89 ☑
    hemolytic reaction (antigen unspecified) T80.919 ☑
    incompatibility reaction (antigen unspecified) T80.919 ☑
      ABO T80.30 ☑
        delayed serologic (DSTR) T80.39 ☑
        hemolytic transfusion reaction (HTR) (unspecified time after transfusion) T80.319 ☑
          acute (AHTR) (less than 24 hours after transfusion) T80.310 ☑
          delayed (DHTR) (24 hours or more after transfusion) T80.311 ☑
        specified NEC T80.39 ☑
      acute (antigen unspecified) T80.910 ☑
      delayed (antigen unspecified) T80.911 ☑
      delayed serologic (DSTR) T80.89 ☑
      non-ABO (minor antigens (Duffy) (K) (Kell) (Kidd) (Lewis) (M) (N) (P) (S)) T80.A0 ☑ (*following* T80.4)
        delayed serologic (DSTR) T80.A9 ☑ (*following* T80.4)
        hemolytic transfusion reaction (HTR) (unspecified time after transfusion) T80.A19 ☑ (*following* T80.4)
          acute (AHTR) (less than 24 hours after transfusion) T80.A10 ☑ (*following* T80.4)
          delayed (DHTR) (24 hours or more after transfusion) T80.A11 ☑ (*following* T80.4)
        specified NEC T80.A9 ☑ (*following* T80.4)
      Rh (antigens (C) (c) (D) (E) (e)) (factor) T80.40 ☑
        delayed serologic (DSTR) T80.49 ☑
        hemolytic transfusion reaction (HTR) (unspecified time after transfusion) T80.419 ☑
          acute (AHTR) (less than 24 hours after transfusion) T80.410 ☑
          delayed (DHTR) (24 hours or more after transfusion) T80.411 ☑
        specified NEC T80.49 ☑
    infection T80.29 ☑
      acute T80.22- ☑
    reaction NEC T80.89 ☑
    sepsis T80.29 ☑
    shock T80.89 ☑
  transplant T86.90
    bone T86.839
      failure T86.831
      infection T86.832
      rejection T86.830
      specified type NEC T86.838
    bone marrow T86.00
      failure T86.02
      infection T86.03
      rejection T86.01
      specified type NEC T86.09
    cornea T86.849
      failure T86.841
      infection T86.842
      rejection T86.840
      specified type NEC T86.848
    failure T86.92
    heart T86.20
      with lung T86.30
      cardiac allograft vasculopathy T86.290
        failure T86.32
        infection T86.33
        rejection T86.31
        specified type NEC T86.39
      failure T86.22
      infection T86.23
      rejection T86.21
      specified type NEC T86.298
    infection T86.93
    intestine T86.859
      failure T86.851
      infection T86.852
      rejection T86.850
      specified type NEC T86.858
    kidney T86.10
      failure T86.12
      infection T86.13
      rejection T86.11
      specified type NEC T86.19

Complication(s) — *continued*
  transplant — *continued*
    liver T86.40
      failure T86.42
      infection T86.43
      rejection T86.41
      specified type NEC T86.49
    lung T86.819
      with heart T86.30
        failure T86.32
        infection T86.33
        rejection T86.31
        specified type NEC T86.39
      failure T86.811
      infection T86.812
      rejection T86.810
      specified type NEC T86.818
    malignant neoplasm C80.2
    pancreas T86.899
      failure T86.891
      infection T86.892
      rejection T86.890
      specified type NEC T86.898
    peripheral blood stem cells T86.5
    post-transplant lymphoproliferative disorder (PTLD) D47.Z1 (*following* D47.4)
    rejection T86.91
    skin T86.829
      failure T86.821
      infection T86.822
      rejection T86.820
      specified type NEC T86.828
    specified
      tissue T86.899
        failure T86.891
        infection T86.892
        rejection T86.890
        specified type NEC T86.898
      type NEC T86.99
    stem cell (from peripheral blood) (from umbilical cord) T86.5
    umbilical cord stem cells T86.5
  trauma (early) T79.9 ☑
    specified NEC T79.8 ☑
  ultrasound therapy NEC T88.9 ☑
  umbilical cord NEC
    complicating delivery O69.9 ☑
    specified NEC O69.89 ☑
  umbrella device, vascular T82.9 ☑
    embolism T82.818 ☑
    fibrosis T82.828 ☑
    hemorrhage T82.838 ☑
    infection or inflammation T82.7 ☑
    mechanical
      breakdown T82.515 ☑
      displacement T82.525 ☑
      leakage T82.535 ☑
      malposition T82.525 ☑
      obstruction T82.595 ☑
      perforation T82.595 ☑
      protrusion T82.595 ☑
    pain T82.848 ☑
    specified type NEC T82.898 ☑
    stenosis T82.858 ☑
    thrombosis T82.868 ☑
  urethral catheter — *see* Complications, catheter, urethral, indwelling
  vaccination T88.1 ☑
    anaphylaxis NEC T80.52 ☑
    arthropathy — *see* Arthropathy, postimmunization
    cellulitis T88.0 ☑
    encephalitis or encephalomyelitis G04.02
    infection (general) (local) NEC T88.0 ☑
    meningitis G03.8
    myelitis G04.02
    protein sickness T80.62 ☑
    rash T88.1 ☑
    reaction (allergic) T88.1 ☑
      serum T80.62 ☑
    sepsis T88.0 ☑
    serum intoxication, sickness, rash, or other serum reaction NEC T80.62 ☑
      anaphylactic shock T80.52 ☑
    shock (allergic) (anaphylactic) T80.52 ☑
    vaccinia (generalized) (localized) T88.1 ☑
  vas deferens device or implant — *see* Complications, genitourinary, device or implant, genital tract

Complication(s) — *continued*
  vascular I99.9
    device or implant T82.9 ☑
      embolism T82.818 ☑
      fibrosis T82.828 ☑
      hemorrhage T82.838 ☑
      infection or inflammation T82.7 ☑
      mechanical
        breakdown T82.519 ☑
          specified device NEC T82.518 ☑
        displacement T82.529 ☑
          specified device NEC T82.528 ☑
        leakage T82.539 ☑
          specified device NEC T82.538 ☑
        malposition T82.529 ☑
          specified device NEC T82.528 ☑
        obstruction T82.599 ☑
          specified device NEC T82.598 ☑
        perforation T82.599 ☑
          specified device NEC T82.598 ☑
        protrusion T82.599 ☑
          specified device NEC T82.598 ☑
      pain T82.848 ☑
      specified type NEC T82.898 ☑
      stenosis T82.858 ☑
      thrombosis T82.868 ☑
    dialysis catheter — *see* Complication, catheter, dialysis
    following infusion, therapeutic injection or transfusion T80.1 ☑
    graft T82.9 ☑
      embolism T82.818 ☑
      fibrosis T82.828 ☑
      hemorrhage T82.838 ☑
      mechanical
        breakdown T82.319 ☑
          aorta (bifurcation) T82.310 ☑
          carotid artery T82.311 ☑
          specified vessel NEC T82.318 ☑
        displacement T82.329 ☑
          aorta (bifurcation) T82.320 ☑
          carotid artery T82.321 ☑
          specified vessel NEC T82.328 ☑
        leakage T82.339 ☑
          aorta (bifurcation) T82.330 ☑
          carotid artery T82.331 ☑
          specified vessel NEC T82.338 ☑
        malposition T82.329 ☑
          aorta (bifurcation) T82.320 ☑
          carotid artery T82.321 ☑
          specified vessel NEC T82.328 ☑
        obstruction T82.399 ☑
          aorta (bifurcation) T82.390 ☑
          carotid artery T82.391 ☑
          specified vessel NEC T82.398 ☑
        perforation T82.399 ☑
          aorta (bifurcation) T82.390 ☑
          carotid artery T82.391 ☑
          specified vessel NEC T82.398 ☑
        protrusion T82.399 ☑
          aorta (bifurcation) T82.390 ☑
          carotid artery T82.391 ☑
          specified vessel NEC T82.398 ☑
      pain T82.848 ☑
      specified complication NEC T82.898 ☑
      stenosis T82.858 ☑
      thrombosis T82.868 ☑
    postoperative — *see* Complications, postoperative, circulatory
    vena cava device (filter) (sieve) (umbrella) — *see* Complications, umbrella device, vascular
  ventilation therapy NEC T81.81 ☑
  ventilator
    mechanical J95.850
      specified NEC J95.859
  ventricular (communicating) shunt (device) T85.9 ☑
    embolism T85.810 ☑
    fibrosis T85.820 ☑
    hemorrhage T85.830 ☑
    infection and inflammation T85.730 ☑
    mechanical
      breakdown T85.01 ☑
      displacement T85.02 ☑
      leakage T85.03 ☑
      malposition T85.02 ☑
      obstruction T85.09 ☑

Complication(s) — *continued*
  ventricular shunt — *continued*
    mechanical — *continued*
      perforation T85.09 ☑
      protrusion T85.09 ☑
      specified NEC T85.09 ☑
    pain T85.840 ☑
    specified type NEC T85.890 ☑
    stenosis T85.850 ☑
    thrombosis T85.860 ☑
  wire suture, permanent (implanted) — *see* Complications, suture, permanent
Compressed air disease T70.3 ☑
Compression
  with injury — *code by* Nature of injury
  artery I77.1
    celiac, syndrome I77.4
  brachial plexus G54.0
  brain (stem) G93.5
    due to
      contusion (diffuse) — *see* Injury, intracranial, diffuse
        focal — *see* Injury, intracranial, focal
      injury NEC — *see* Injury, intracranial, diffuse
      traumatic — *see* Injury, intracranial, diffuse
  bronchus J98.09
  cauda equina G83.4
  celiac (artery) (axis) I77.4
  cerebral — *see* Compression, brain
  cervical plexus G54.2
  cord
    spinal — *see* Compression, spinal
    umbilical — *see* Compression, umbilical cord
  cranial nerve G52.9
    eighth H93.3 ☑
    eleventh G52.8
    fifth G50.8
    first G52.0
    fourth — *see* Strabismus, paralytic, fourth nerve
    ninth G52.1
    second — *see* Disorder, nerve, optic
    seventh G51.8
    sixth — *see* Strabismus, paralytic, sixth nerve
    tenth G52.2
    third — *see* Strabismus, paralytic, third nerve
    twelfth G52.3
  diver's squeeze T70.3 ☑
  during birth (newborn) P15.9
  esophagus K22.2
  eustachian tube — *see* Obstruction, eustachian tube, cartilaginous
  facies Q67.1
  fracture
    nontraumatic NOS — *see* Collapse, vertebra
    pathological — *see* Fracture, pathological
    traumatic — *see* Fracture, traumatic
  heart — *see* Disease, heart
  intestine — *see* Obstruction, intestine
  laryngeal nerve, recurrent G52.2
    with paralysis of vocal cords and larynx J38.00
      bilateral J38.02
      unilateral J38.01
  lumbosacral plexus G54.1
  lung J98.4
  lymphatic vessel I89.0
  medulla — *see* Compression, brain
  nerve (*see also* Disorder, nerve) G58.9
    arm NEC — *see* Mononeuropathy, upper limb
    axillary G54.0
    cranial — *see* Compression, cranial nerve
    leg NEC — *see* Mononeuropathy, lower limb
    median (in carpal tunnel) — *see* Syndrome, carpal tunnel
    optic — *see* Disorder, nerve, optic
    plantar — *see* Lesion, nerve, plantar
    posterior tibial (in tarsal tunnel) — *see* Syndrome, tarsal tunnel
    root or plexus NOS (in) G54.9
      intervertebral disc disorder NEC — *see* Disorder, disc, with, radiculopathy
        with myelopathy — *see* Disorder, disc, with, myelopathy
      neoplastic disease (*see also* Neoplasm) D49.9 [G55]
      spondylosis — *see* Spondylosis, with radiculopathy
    sciatic (acute) — *see* Lesion, nerve, sciatic

Index

Complication — Compression

Compression — *continued*
- nerve (*see also* Disorder, nerve) — *continued*
  - sympathetic G90.8
  - traumatic — *see* Injury, nerve
  - ulnar — *see* Lesion, nerve, ulnar
  - upper extremity NEC — *see* Mononeuropathy, upper limb
  - spinal (cord) G95.20
    - by displacement of intervertebral disc NEC (*see also* Disorder, disc, with, myelopathy)
    - nerve root NOS G54.9
      - due to displacement of intervertebral disc NEC — *see* Disorder, disc, with, radiculopathy
      - with myelopathy — *see* Disorder, disc, with, myelopathy
    - specified NEC G95.29
    - spondylogenic (cervical) (lumbar, lumbosacral) (thoracic) — *see* Spondylosis, with myelopathy NEC
      - anterior — *see* Syndrome, anterior, spinal artery, compression
    - traumatic — *see* Injury, spinal cord, by region
  - subcostal nerve (syndrome) — *see* Mononeuropathy, upper limb, specified NEC
  - sympathetic nerve NEC G90.8
  - syndrome T79.5 ☑
  - trachea J39.8
  - ulnar nerve (by scar tissue) — *see* Lesion, nerve, ulnar
  - umbilical cord
    - complicating delivery O69.2 ☑
      - cord around neck O69.1 ☑
      - prolapse O69.0 ☑
      - specified NEC O69.2 ☑
  - ureter N13.5
  - vein I87.1
  - vena cava (inferior) (superior) I87.1

Compulsion, compulsive
- gambling F63.0
- neurosis F42.8
- personality F60.5
- states F42.8
- swearing F42.8
  - in Gilles de la Tourette's syndrome F95.2
- tics and spasms F95.9

Concato's disease (pericardial polyserositis) A19.9
- nontubercular I31.1
- pleural — *see* Pleurisy, with effusion

Concavity chest wall M95.4

Concealed penis Q55.64

Concern (normal) **about sick person in family** Z63.6

Concrescence (teeth) K00.2

Concretio cordis I31.1
- rheumatic I09.2

Concretion (*see also* Calculus)
- appendicular K38.1
- canaliculus — *see* Dacryolith
- clitoris N90.89
- conjunctiva H11.12- ☑
- eyelid — *see* Disorder, eyelid, specified type NEC
- lacrimal passages — *see* Dacryolith
- prepuce (male) N47.8
- salivary gland (any) K11.5
- seminal vesicle N50.89
- tonsil J35.8

Concussion (brain) (cerebral) (current) S06.0X9 ☑
- with
  - loss of consciousness of 30 minutes or less S06.0X1 ☑
  - loss of consciousness of unspecified duration S06.0X9 ☑
  - blast (air) (hydraulic) (immersion) (underwater)
    - abdomen or thorax — *see* Injury, blast, by site
    - ear with acoustic nerve injury — *see* Injury, nerve, acoustic, specified type NEC
- cauda equina S34.3 ☑
- conus medullaris S34.02 ☑
- ocular S05.8X- ☑
- spinal (cord)
  - cervical S14.0 ☑
  - lumbar S34.01 ☑
  - sacral S34.02 ☑
  - thoracic S24.0 ☑
- syndrome F07.81
- without loss of consciousness S06.0X0 ☑

Condition — *see* Disease

Conditions arising in the perinatal period — *see* Newborn, affected by

Conduct disorder — *see* Disorder, conduct

Condyloma A63.0
- acuminatum A63.0
- gonorrheal A54.09
- latum A51.31
- syphilitic A51.31
  - congenital A50.07
- venereal, syphilitic A51.31

Conflagration (*see also* Burn)
- asphyxia (by inhalation of gases, fumes or vapors) (*see also* Table of Drugs and Chemicals) T59.9- ☑

Conflict (with) (*see also* Discord)
- family Z73.9
- marital Z63.0
  - involving divorce or estrangement Z63.5
- parent-child Z62.820
  - parent-adopted child Z62.821
  - parent-biological child Z62.820
  - parent-foster child Z62.822
- social role NEC Z73.5

Confluent — *see* condition

Confusion, confused R41.0
- epileptic F05
- mental state (psychogenic) F44.89
- psychogenic F44.89
- reactive (from emotional stress, psychological trauma) F44.89

Confusional arousals G47.51

Congelation T69.9 ☑

Congenital (*see also* condition)
- aortic septum Q25.49
- intrinsic factor deficiency D51.0
- malformation — *see* Anomaly

Congestion, congestive
- bladder N32.89
- bowel K63.89
- brain G93.89
- breast N64.59
- bronchial J98.09
- catarrhal J31.0
- chest R09.89
- chill, malarial — *see* Malaria
- circulatory NEC I99.8
- duodenum K31.89
- eye — *see* Hyperemia, conjunctiva
- facial, due to birth injury P15.4
- general R68.89
- glottis J37.0
- heart — *see* Failure, heart, congestive
- hepatic K76.1
- hypostatic (lung) — *see* Edema, lung
- intestine K63.89
- kidney N28.89
- labyrinth H83.8 ☑
- larynx J37.0
- liver K76.1
- lung R09.89
  - active or acute — *see* Pneumonia
- malaria, malarial — *see* Malaria
- nasal R09.81
- nose R09.81
- orbit, orbital (*see also* Exophthalmos)
  - inflammatory (chronic) — *see* Inflammation, orbit
- ovary N83.8
- pancreas K86.89
- pelvic, female N94.89
- pleural J94.8
- prostate (active) N42.1
- pulmonary — *see* Congestion, lung
- renal N28.89
- retina H35.81
- seminal vesicle N50.1
- spinal cord G95.19
- spleen (chronic) D73.2
- stomach K31.89
- trachea — *see* Tracheitis
- urethra N36.8
- uterus N85.8
  - with subinvolution N85.3
- venous (passive) I87.8
- viscera R68.89

Congestive — *see* Congestion

Conical
- cervix (hypertrophic elongation) N88.4
- cornea — *see* Keratoconus
- teeth K00.2

Conjoined twins Q89.4

Conjugal maladjustment Z63.0

Conjugal maladjustment — *continued*
- involving divorce or estrangement Z63.5

Conjunctiva — *see* condition

Conjunctivitis (staphylococcal) (streptococcal) NOS H10.9
- Acanthamoeba B60.12
- acute H10.3- ☑
  - atopic H10.1- ☑
  - chemical (*see also* Corrosion, cornea) H10.21- ☑
  - mucopurulent H10.02- ☑
    - follicular H10.01- ☑
  - pseudomembranous H10.22- ☑
  - serous except viral H10.23- ☑
    - viral — *see* Conjunctivitis, viral
  - toxic H10.21- ☑
- adenoviral (acute) (follicular) B30.1
- allergic (acute) — *see* Conjunctivitis, acute, atopic
  - chronic H10.45
    - vernal H10.44
- anaphylactic — *see* Conjunctivitis, acute, atopic
- Apollo B30.3
- atopic (acute) — *see* Conjunctivitis, acute, atopic
- Béal's B30.2
- blennorrhagic (gonococcal) (neonatorum) A54.31
- chemical (acute) (*see also* Corrosion, cornea) H10.21- ☑
- chlamydial A74.0
  - due to trachoma A71.1
  - neonatal P39.1
- chronic (nodosa) (petrificans) (phlyctenular) H10.40- ☑
  - allergic H10.45
    - vernal H10.44
  - follicular H10.43- ☑
  - giant papillary H10.41- ☑
  - simple H10.42- ☑
  - vernal H10.44
- coxsackievirus 24 B30.3
- diphtheritic A36.86
- due to
  - dust — *see* Conjunctivitis, acute, atopic
  - filariasis B74.9
  - mucocutaneous leishmaniasis B55.2
- enterovirus type 70 (hemorrhagic) B30.3
- epidemic (viral) B30.9
  - hemorrhagic B30.3
- gonococcal (neonatorum) A54.31
- granular (trachomatous) A71.1
  - sequelae (late effect) B94.0
- hemorrhagic (acute) (epidemic) B30.3
- herpes zoster B02.31
- in (due to)
  - Acanthamoeba B60.12
  - adenovirus (acute) (follicular) B30.1
  - Chlamydia A74.0
  - coxsackievirus 24 B30.3
  - diphtheria A36.86
  - enterovirus type 70 (hemorrhagic) B30.3
  - filariasis B74.9
  - gonococci A54.31
  - herpes (simplex) virus B00.53
    - zoster B02.31
  - infectious disease NEC B99 ☑
  - meningococci A39.89
  - mucocutaneous leishmaniasis B55.2
  - rosacea H10.82- ☑
  - syphilis (late) A52.71
  - zoster B02.31
- inclusion A74.0
- infantile P39.1
  - gonococcal A54.31
- Koch-Weeks' — *see* Conjunctivitis, acute, mucopurulent
- light — *see* Conjunctivitis, acute, atopic
- ligneous — *see* Blepharoconjunctivitis, ligneous
- meningococcal A39.89
- mucopurulent — *see* Conjunctivitis, acute, mucopurulent
- neonatal P39.1
  - gonococcal A54.31
- Newcastle B30.8
- of Béal B30.2
- parasitic
  - filariasis B74.9
  - mucocutaneous leishmaniasis B55.2
- Parinaud's H10.89
- petrificans H10.89
- rosacea H10.82- ☑
- specified NEC H10.89
- swimming-pool B30.1
- trachomatous A71.1
  - acute A71.0

Conjunctivitis — *continued*
  trachomatous — *continued*
    sequelae (late effect) B94.0
  traumatic NEC H10.89
  tuberculous A18.59
  tularemic A21.1
  tularensis A21.1
  viral B30.9
    due to
      adenovirus B30.1
      enterovirus B30.3
    specified NEC B30.8
Conjunctivochalasis H11.82- ☑
Connective tissue — *see* condition
Conn's syndrome E26.01
Conradi (-Hunermann) **disease** Q77.3
Consanguinity Z84.3
  counseling Z71.89
Conscious simulation (of illness) Z76.5
Consecutive — *see* condition
Consolidation lung (base) — *see* Pneumonia, lobar
Constipation (atonic) (neurogenic) (simple) (spastic)
    K59.00
  chronic K59.09
    idiopathic K59.04
  drug-induced K59.03
  functional K59.04
  outlet dysfunction K59.02
  psychogenic F45.8
  slow transit K59.01
  specified NEC K59.09
Constitutional (*see also* condition)
  substandard F60.7
Constitutionally substandard F60.7
Constriction (*see also* Stricture)
  auditory canal — *see* Stenosis, external ear canal
  bronchial J98.09
  duodenum K31.5
  esophagus K22.2
  external
    abdomen, abdominal (wall) S30.841 ☑
    alveolar process S00.542 ☑
    ankle S90.54- ☑
    antecubital space — *see* Constriction, external, forearm
    arm (upper) S40.84- ☑
    auricle — *see* Constriction, external, ear
    axilla — *see* Constriction, external, arm
    back, lower S30.840 ☑
    breast S20.14- ☑
    brow S00.84 ☑
    buttock S30.840 ☑
    calf — *see* Constriction, external, leg
    canthus — *see* Constriction, external, eyelid
    cheek S00.84 ☑
      internal S00.542 ☑
    chest wall — *see* Constriction, external, thorax
    chin S00.84 ☑
    clitoris S30.844 ☑
    costal region — *see* Constriction, external, thorax
    digit(s)
      foot — *see* Constriction, external, toe
      hand — *see* Constriction, external, finger
    ear S00.44- ☑
    elbow S50.34- ☑
    epididymis S30.843 ☑
    epigastric region S30.841 ☑
    esophagus, cervical S10.14 ☑
    eyebrow — *see* Constriction, external, eyelid
    eyelid S00.24- ☑
    face S00.84 ☑
    finger(s) S60.44- ☑
      index S60.44- ☑
      little S60.44- ☑
      middle S60.44- ☑
      ring S60.44- ☑
    flank S30.841 ☑
    foot (except toe(s) alone) S90.84- ☑
      toe — *see* Constriction, external, toe
    forearm S50.84- ☑
      elbow only — *see* Constriction, external, elbow
    forehead S00.84 ☑
    genital organs, external
      female S30.846 ☑
      male S30.845 ☑
    groin S30.841 ☑
    gum S00.542 ☑

Constriction — *continued*
  external — *continued*
    hand S60.54- ☑
    head S00.94 ☑
      ear — *see* Constriction, external, ear
      eyelid — *see* Constriction, external, eyelid
      lip S00.541 ☑
      nose S00.34 ☑
      oral cavity S00.542 ☑
      scalp S00.04 ☑
      specified site NEC S00.84 ☑
    heel — *see* Constriction, external, foot
    hip S70.24- ☑
    inguinal region S30.841 ☑
    interscapular region S20.449 ☑
    jaw S00.84 ☑
    knee S80.24- ☑
    labium (majus) (minus) S30.844 ☑
    larynx S10.14 ☑
    leg (lower) S80.84- ☑
      knee — *see* Constriction, external, knee
      upper — *see* Constriction, external, thigh
    lip S00.541 ☑
    lower back S30.840 ☑
    lumbar region S30.840 ☑
    malar region S00.84 ☑
    mammary — *see* Constriction, external, breast
    mastoid region S00.84 ☑
    mouth S00.542 ☑
    nail
      finger — *see* Constriction, external, finger
      toe — *see* Constriction, external, toe
    nasal S00.34 ☑
    neck S10.94 ☑
      specified site NEC S10.84 ☑
      throat S10.14 ☑
    nose S00.34 ☑
    occipital region S00.04 ☑
    oral cavity S00.542 ☑
    orbital region — *see* Constriction, external, eyelid
    palate S00.542 ☑
    palm — *see* Constriction, external, hand
    parietal region S00.04 ☑
    pelvis S30.840 ☑
    penis S30.842 ☑
    perineum
      female S30.844 ☑
      male S30.840 ☑
    periocular area — *see* Constriction, external, eyelid
    phalanges
      finger — *see* Constriction, external, finger
      toe — *see* Constriction, external, toe
    pharynx S10.14 ☑
    pinna — *see* Constriction, external, ear
    popliteal space — *see* Constriction, external, knee
    prepuce S30.842 ☑
    pubic region S30.840 ☑
    pudendum
      female S30.846 ☑
      male S30.845 ☑
    sacral region S30.840 ☑
    scalp S00.04 ☑
    scapular region — *see* Constriction, external, shoulder
    scrotum S30.843 ☑
    shin — *see* Constriction, external, leg
    shoulder S40.24- ☑
    sternal region S20.349 ☑
    submaxillary region S00.84 ☑
    submental region S00.84 ☑
    subungual
      finger(s) — *see* Constriction, external, finger
      toe(s) — *see* Constriction, external, toe
    supraclavicular fossa S10.84 ☑
    supraorbital S00.84 ☑
    temple S00.84 ☑
    temporal region S00.84 ☑
    testis S30.843 ☑
    thigh S70.34- ☑
    thorax, thoracic (wall) S20.94 ☑
      back S20.44- ☑
      front S20.34- ☑
    throat S10.14 ☑
    thumb S60.34- ☑
    toe(s) (lesser) S90.44- ☑
      great S90.44- ☑

Constriction — *continued*
  external — *continued*
    tongue S00.542 ☑
    trachea S10.14 ☑
    tunica vaginalis S30.843 ☑
    uvula S00.542 ☑
    vagina S30.844 ☑
    vulva S30.844 ☑
    wrist S60.84- ☑
  gallbladder — *see* Obstruction, gallbladder
  intestine — *see* Obstruction, intestine
  larynx J38.6
    congenital Q31.8
      specified NEC Q31.8
      subglottic Q31.1
  organ or site, congenital NEC — *see* Atresia, by site
  prepuce (acquired) (congenital) N47.1
  pylorus (adult hypertrophic) K31.1
    congenital or infantile Q40.0
    newborn Q40.0
  ring dystocia (uterus) O62.4
  spastic (*see also* Spasm)
    ureter N13.5
  ureter N13.5
    with infection N13.6
  urethra — *see* Stricture, urethra
  visual field (peripheral) (functional) — *see* Defect, visual field
Constrictive — *see* condition
Consultation
  medical — *see* Counseling, medical
  religious Z71.81
  specified reason NEC Z71.89
  spiritual Z71.81
  without complaint or sickness Z71.9
    feared complaint unfounded Z71.1
    specified reason NEC Z71.89
Consumption — *see* Tuberculosis
Contact (with) (*see also* Exposure (to))
  acariasis Z20.7
  AIDS virus Z20.6
  air pollution Z77.110
  algae and algae toxins Z77.121
  algae bloom Z77.121
  anthrax Z20.810
  aromatic amines Z77.020
  aromatic (hazardous) compounds NEC Z77.028
  aromatic dyes NOS Z77.028
  arsenic Z77.010
  asbestos Z77.090
  bacterial disease NEC Z20.818
  benzene Z77.021
  blue-green algae bloom Z77.121
  body fluids (potentially hazardous) Z77.21
  brown tide Z77.121
  chemicals (chiefly nonmedicinal) (hazardous) NEC Z77.098
  cholera Z20.09
  chromium compounds Z77.018
  communicable disease Z20.9
    bacterial NEC Z20.818
    specified NEC Z20.89
    viral NEC Z20.828
    Zika virus Z20.821
  cyanobacteria bloom Z77.121
  dyes Z77.098
  Escherichia coli (E. coli) Z20.01
  fiberglass — *see* Table of Drugs and Chemicals, fiber-glass
  German measles Z20.4
  gonorrhea Z20.2
  hazardous metals NEC Z77.018
  hazardous substances NEC Z77.29
  hazards in the physical environment NEC Z77.128
  hazards to health NEC Z77.9
  HIV Z20.6
  HTLV-III/LAV Z20.6
  human immunodeficiency virus (HIV) Z20.6
  infection Z20.9
    specified NEC Z20.89
  infestation (parasitic) NEC Z20.7
  intestinal infectious disease NEC Z20.09
    Escherichia coli (E. coli) Z20.01
  lead Z77.011
  meningococcus Z20.811
  mold (toxic) Z77.120
  nickel dust Z77.018
  noise Z77.122

Conjunctivitis — Contact

70   ☑ **Additional Character Required** — Refer to the Tabular List for Character Selection   ▽ **Subterms under main terms may continue to next column or page**

▼ Subterms under main terms may continue to next column or page   ☑ Additional Character Required — Refer to the Tabular List for Character Selection   71

Contact — Contusion

Contusion — *continued*
- brow S00.83 ☑
- buttock S30.0 ☑
- canthus, eye S00.1- ☑
- cauda equina S34.3 ☑
- cerebellar, traumatic S06.37- ☑
- cerebral S06.33- ☑
    - left side S06.32- ☑
    - right side S06.31- ☑
- cheek S00.83 ☑
    - internal S00.532 ☑
- chest (wall) — *see* Contusion, thorax
- chin S00.83 ☑
- clitoris S30.23 ☑
- colon — *see* Injury, intestine, large, contusion
- common bile duct S36.13 ☑
- conjunctiva S05.1- ☑
    - with foreign body (in conjunctival sac) — *see* Foreign body, conjunctival sac
- conus medullaris (spine) S34.139 ☑
- cornea — *see* Contusion, eyeball
    - with foreign body — *see* Foreign body, cornea
- corpus cavernosum S30.21 ☑
- cortex (brain) (cerebral) — *see* Injury, intracranial, diffuse
    - focal — *see* Injury, intracranial, focal
- costal region — *see* Contusion, thorax
- cystic duct S36.13 ☑
- diaphragm S27.802 ☑
- duodenum S36.420 ☑
- ear S00.43- ☑
- elbow S50.0- ☑
    - with forearm — *see* Contusion, forearm
- epididymis S30.22 ☑
- epigastric region S30.1 ☑
- epiglottis S10.0 ☑
- esophagus (thoracic) S27.812 ☑
    - cervical S10.0 ☑
- eyeball S05.1- ☑
- eyebrow S00.1- ☑
- eyelid (and periocular area) S00.1- ☑
- face NEC S00.83 ☑
- fallopian tube S37.529 ☑
    - bilateral S37.522 ☑
    - unilateral S37.521 ☑
- femoral triangle S30.1 ☑
- finger(s) S60.00 ☑
    - with damage to nail (matrix) S60.10 ☑
    - index S60.02- ☑
        - with damage to nail S60.12- ☑
    - little S60.05- ☑
        - with damage to nail S60.15- ☑
    - middle S60.03- ☑
        - with damage to nail S60.13- ☑
    - ring S60.04- ☑
        - with damage to nail S60.14- ☑
    - thumb — *see* Contusion, thumb
- flank S30.1 ☑
- foot (except toe(s) alone) S90.3- ☑
    - toe — *see* Contusion, toe
- forearm S50.1- ☑
    - elbow only — *see* Contusion, elbow
- forehead S00.83 ☑
- gallbladder S36.122 ☑
- genital organs, external
    - female S30.202 ☑
    - male S30.201 ☑
- globe (eye) — *see* Contusion, eyeball
- groin S30.1 ☑
- gum S00.532 ☑
- hand S60.22- ☑
    - finger(s) — *see* Contusion, finger
    - wrist — *see* Contusion, wrist
- head S00.93 ☑
    - ear — *see* Contusion, ear
    - eyelid — *see* Contusion, eyelid
    - lip S00.531 ☑
    - nose S00.33 ☑
    - oral cavity S00.532 ☑
    - scalp S00.03 ☑
    - specified part NEC S00.83 ☑
- heart (*see also* Injury, heart) S26.91 ☑
- heel — *see* Contusion, foot
- hepatic duct S36.13 ☑
- hip S70.0- ☑
- ileum S36.428 ☑

Contusion — *continued*
- iliac region S30.1 ☑
- inguinal region S30.1 ☑
- interscapular region S20.229 ☑
- intra-abdominal organ S36.92 ☑
    - colon — *see* Injury, intestine, large, contusion
    - liver S36.112 ☑
    - pancreas — *see* Contusion, pancreas
    - rectum S36.62 ☑
    - small intestine — *see* Injury, intestine, small, contusion
    - specified organ NEC S36.892 ☑
    - spleen — *see* Contusion, spleen
    - stomach S36.32 ☑
- iris (eye) — *see* Contusion, eyeball
- jaw S00.83 ☑
- jejunum S36.428 ☑
- kidney S37.01- ☑
    - major (greater than 2 cm) S37.02- ☑
    - minor (less than 2 cm) S37.01- ☑
- knee S80.0- ☑
- labium (majus) (minus) S30.23 ☑
- lacrimal apparatus, gland or sac S05.8X- ☑
- larynx S10.0 ☑
- leg (lower) S80.1- ☑
    - knee — *see* Contusion, knee
- lens — *see* Contusion, eyeball
- lip S00.531 ☑
- liver S36.112 ☑
- lower back S30.0 ☑
- lumbar region S30.0 ☑
- lung S27.329 ☑
    - bilateral S27.322 ☑
    - unilateral S27.321 ☑
- malar region S00.83 ☑
- mastoid region S00.83 ☑
- membrane, brain — *see* Injury, intracranial, diffuse
    - focal — *see* Injury, intracranial, focal
- mesentery S36.892 ☑
- mesosalpinx S37.892 ☑
- mouth S00.532 ☑
- muscle — *see* Contusion, by site
- nail
    - finger — *see* Contusion, finger, with damage to nail
    - toe — *see* Contusion, toe, with damage to nail
- nasal S00.33 ☑
- neck S10.93 ☑
    - specified site NEC S10.83 ☑
    - throat S10.0 ☑
- nerve — *see* Injury, nerve
- newborn P54.5
- nose S00.33 ☑
- occipital
    - lobe (brain) — *see* Injury, intracranial, diffuse
        - focal — *see* Injury, intracranial, focal
    - region (scalp) S00.03 ☑
- orbit (region) (tissues) S05.1- ☑
- ovary S37.429 ☑
    - bilateral S37.422 ☑
    - unilateral S37.421 ☑
- palate S00.532 ☑
- pancreas S36.229 ☑
    - body S36.221 ☑
    - head S36.220 ☑
    - tail S36.222 ☑
- parietal
    - lobe (brain) — *see* Injury, intracranial, diffuse
        - focal — *see* Injury, intracranial, focal
    - region (scalp) S00.03 ☑
- pelvic organ S37.92 ☑
    - adrenal gland S37.812 ☑
    - bladder S37.22 ☑
    - fallopian tube — *see* Contusion, fallopian tube
    - kidney — *see* Contusion, kidney
    - ovary — *see* Contusion, ovary
    - prostate S37.822 ☑
    - specified organ NEC S37.892 ☑
    - ureter S37.12 ☑
    - urethra S37.32 ☑
    - uterus S37.62 ☑
- pelvis S30.0 ☑
- penis S30.21 ☑
- perineum
    - female S30.23 ☑
    - male S30.0 ☑
- periocular area S00.1- ☑

Contusion — *continued*
- peritoneum S36.81 ☑
- periurethral tissue — *see* Contusion, urethra
- pharynx S10.0 ☑
- pinna — *see* Contusion, ear
- popliteal space — *see* Contusion, knee
- prepuce S30.21 ☑
- prostate S37.822 ☑
- pubic region S30.1 ☑
- pudendum
    - female S30.202 ☑
    - male S30.201 ☑
- quadriceps femoris — *see* Contusion, thigh
- rectum S36.62 ☑
- retroperitoneum S36.892 ☑
- round ligament S37.892 ☑
- sacral region S30.0 ☑
- scalp S00.03 ☑
    - due to birth injury P12.3
- scapular region — *see* Contusion, shoulder
- sclera — *see* Contusion, eyeball
- scrotum S30.22 ☑
- seminal vesicle S37.892 ☑
- shoulder S40.01- ☑
- skin NEC T14.8 ☑
- small intestine — *see* Injury, intestine, small, contusion
- spermatic cord S30.22 ☑
- spinal cord — *see* Injury, spinal cord, by region
    - cauda equina S34.3 ☑
    - conus medullaris S34.139 ☑
- spleen S36.029 ☑
    - major S36.021 ☑
    - minor S36.020 ☑
- sternal region S20.219 ☑
- stomach S36.32 ☑
- subconjunctival S05.1- ☑
- subcutaneous NEC T14.8 ☑
- submaxillary region S00.83 ☑
- submental region S00.83 ☑
- subperiosteal NEC T14.8 ☑
- subungual
    - finger — *see* Contusion, finger, with damage to nail
    - toe — *see* Contusion, toe, with damage to nail
- supraclavicular fossa S10.83 ☑
- supraorbital S00.83 ☑
- suprarenal gland S37.812 ☑
- temple (region) S00.83 ☑
- temporal
    - lobe (brain) — *see* Injury, intracranial, diffuse
        - focal — *see* Injury, intracranial, focal
    - region S00.83 ☑
- testis S30.22 ☑
- thigh S70.1- ☑
- thorax (wall) S20.20 ☑
    - back S20.22- ☑
    - front S20.21- ☑
- throat S10.0 ☑
- thumb S60.01- ☑
    - with damage to nail S60.11- ☑
- toe(s) (lesser) S90.12- ☑
    - with damage to nail S90.22- ☑
    - great S90.11- ☑
        - with damage to nail S90.21- ☑
- tongue S00.532 ☑
- trachea (cervical) S10.0 ☑
    - thoracic S27.52 ☑
- tunica vaginalis S30.22 ☑
- tympanum, tympanic membrane — *see* Contusion, ear
- ureter S37.12 ☑
- urethra S37.32 ☑
- urinary organ NEC S37.892 ☑
- uterus S37.62 ☑
- uvula S00.532 ☑
- vagina S30.23 ☑
- vas deferens S37.892 ☑
- vesical S37.22 ☑
- vocal cord(s) S10.0 ☑
- vulva S30.23 ☑
- wrist S60.21- ☑

Conus (congenital) (any type) Q14.8
- cornea — *see* Keratoconus
- medullaris syndrome G95.81

Conversion hysteria, neurosis or reaction F44.9

Converter, tuberculosis (test reaction) R76.11

Conviction (legal), **anxiety concerning** Z65.0

Conviction (legal), **anxiety concerning** — *continued*
  with imprisonment Z65.1
Convulsions (idiopathic) (*see also* Seizure(s)) R56.9
  apoplectiform (cerebral ischemia) I67.82
  dissociative F44.5
  epileptic — *see* Epilepsy
  epileptiform, epileptoid — *see* Seizure, epileptiform
  ether (anesthetic) — *see* Table of Drugs and Chemicals,
      by drug
  febrile R56.00
    with status epilepticus G40.901
    complex R56.01
      with status epilepticus G40.901
    simple R56.00
  hysterical F44.5
  infantile P90
    epilepsy — *see* Epilepsy
  jacksonian — *see* Epilepsy, localization-related, symp-
      tomatic, with simple partial seizures
  myoclonic G25.3
  newborn P90
  obstetrical (nephritic) (uremic) — *see* Eclampsia
  paretic A52.17
  post traumatic R56.1
  psychomotor — *see* Epilepsy, localization-related,
      symptomatic, with complex partial seizures
  recurrent R56.9
  reflex R25.8
  scarlatinal A38.8
  tetanus, tetanic — *see* Tetanus
  thymic E32.8
Convulsive (*see also* Convulsions)
Cooley's anemia D56.1
Coolie itch B76.9
Cooper's
  disease — *see* Mastopathy, cystic
  hernia — *see* Hernia, abdomen, specified site NEC
Copra itch B88.0
Coprophagy F50.89
Coprophobia F40.298
Coproporphyria, hereditary E80.29
Cor
  biloculare Q20.8
  bovis, bovinum — *see* Hypertrophy, cardiac
  pulmonale (chronic) I27.81
    acute I26.09
  triatriatum, triatrium Q24.2
  triloculare Q20.8
    biatrium Q20.4
    biventriculare Q21.1
Corbus' disease (gangrenous balanitis) N48.1
Cord (*see also* condition)
  around neck
    complicating delivery O69.81 ☑
      with compression O69.1 ☑
  bladder G95.89
    tabetic A52.19
Cordis ectopia Q24.8
Corditis (spermatic) N49.1
Corectopia Q13.2
Cori's disease (glycogen storage) E74.03
Corkhandler's disease or lung J67.3
Corkscrew esophagus K22.4
Corkworker's disease or lung J67.3
Corn (infected) L84
Cornea (*see also* condition)
  donor Z52.5
  plana Q13.4
Cornelia de Lange syndrome Q87.1
Cornu cutaneum L85.8
Cornual gestation or pregnancy O00.80
  with intrauterine pregnancy O00.81
Coronary (artery) — *see* condition
Coronavirus, as cause of disease classified elsewhere
    B97.29
  SARS-associated B97.21
Corpora (*see also* condition)
  amylacea, prostate N42.89
  cavernosa — *see* condition
Corpulence — *see* Obesity
Corpus — *see* condition
Corrected transposition Q20.5
Corrosion (injury) (acid) (caustic) (chemical) (lime) (exter-
    nal) (internal) T30.4
  abdomen, abdominal (muscle) (wall) T21.42 ☑
    first degree T21.52 ☑
    second degree T21.62 ☑

Corrosion — *continued*
  abdomen, abdominal — *continued*
    third degree T21.72 ☑
  above elbow T22.439 ☑
    first degree T22.539 ☑
    left T22.432 ☑
      first degree T22.532 ☑
      second degree T22.632 ☑
      third degree T22.732 ☑
    right T22.431 ☑
      first degree T22.531 ☑
      second degree T22.631 ☑
      third degree T22.731 ☑
    second degree T22.639 ☑
    third degree T22.739 ☑
  alimentary tract NEC T28.7 ☑
  ankle T25.419 ☑
    first degree T25.519 ☑
    left T25.412 ☑
      first degree T25.512 ☑
      second degree T25.612 ☑
      third degree T25.712 ☑
    multiple with foot — *see* Corrosion, lower, limb,
        multiple, ankle and foot
    right T25.411 ☑
      first degree T25.511 ☑
      second degree T25.611 ☑
      third degree T25.711 ☑
    second degree T25.619 ☑
    third degree T25.719 ☑
  anus — *see* Corrosion, buttock
  arm(s) (meaning upper limb(s)) — *see* Corrosion, upper
      limb
  axilla T22.449 ☑
    first degree T22.549 ☑
    left T22.442 ☑
      first degree T22.542 ☑
      second degree T22.642 ☑
      third degree T22.742 ☑
    right T22.441 ☑
      first degree T22.541 ☑
      second degree T22.641 ☑
      third degree T22.741 ☑
    second degree T22.649 ☑
    third degree T22.749 ☑
  back (lower) T21.44 ☑
    first degree T21.54 ☑
    second degree T21.64 ☑
    third degree T21.74 ☑
    upper T21.43 ☑
      first degree T21.53 ☑
      second degree T21.63 ☑
      third degree T21.73 ☑
  blisters — *code as* Corrosion, second degree, by site
  breast(s) — *see* Corrosion, chest wall
  buttock(s) T21.45 ☑
    first degree T21.55 ☑
    second degree T21.65 ☑
    third degree T21.75 ☑
  calf T24.439 ☑
    first degree T24.539 ☑
    left T24.432 ☑
      first degree T24.532 ☑
      second degree T24.632 ☑
      third degree T24.732 ☑
    right T24.431 ☑
      first degree T24.531 ☑
      second degree T24.631 ☑
      third degree T24.731 ☑
    second degree T24.639 ☑
    third degree T24.739 ☑
  canthus (eye) — *see* Corrosion, eyelid
  cervix T28.8 ☑
  cheek T20.46 ☑
    first degree T20.56 ☑
    second degree T20.66 ☑
    third degree T20.76 ☑
  chest wall T21.41 ☑
    first degree T21.51 ☑
    second degree T21.61 ☑
    third degree T21.71 ☑
  chin T20.43 ☑
    first degree T20.53 ☑
    second degree T20.63 ☑
    third degree T20.73 ☑
  colon T28.7 ☑

Corrosion — *continued*
  conjunctiva (and cornea) — *see* Corrosion, cornea
  cornea (and conjunctiva) T26.6- ☑
  deep necrosis of underlying tissue — *code as* Corrosion,
      third degree, by site
  dorsum of hand T23.469 ☑
    first degree T23.569 ☑
    left T23.462 ☑
      first degree T23.562 ☑
      second degree T23.662 ☑
      third degree T23.762 ☑
    right T23.461 ☑
      first degree T23.561 ☑
      second degree T23.661 ☑
      third degree T23.761 ☑
    second degree T23.669 ☑
    third degree T23.769 ☑
  ear (auricle) (external) (canal) T20.41 ☑
    drum T28.91 ☑
    first degree T20.51 ☑
    second degree T20.61 ☑
    third degree T20.71 ☑
  elbow T22.429 ☑
    first degree T22.529 ☑
    left T22.422 ☑
      first degree T22.522 ☑
      second degree T22.622 ☑
      third degree T22.722 ☑
    right T22.421 ☑
      first degree T22.521 ☑
      second degree T22.621 ☑
      third degree T22.721 ☑
    second degree T22.629 ☑
    third degree T22.729 ☑
  entire body — *see* Corrosion, multiple body regions
  epidermal loss — *code as* Corrosion, second degree,
      by site
  epiglottis T27.4 ☑
  erythema, erythematous — *code as* Corrosion, first
      degree, by site
  esophagus T28.6 ☑
  extent (percentage of body surface)
    less than 10 percent T32.0
    10-19 percent (0-9 percent third degree) T32.10
      with 10-19 percent third degree T32.11
    20-29 percent (0-9 percent third degree) T32.20
      with
          10-19 percent third degree T32.21
          20-29 percent third degree T32.22
    30-39 percent (0-9 percent third degree) T32.30
      with
          10-19 percent third degree T32.31
          20-29 percent third degree T32.32
          30-39 percent third degree T32.33
    40-49 percent (0-9 percent third degree) T32.40
      with
          10-19 percent third degree T32.41
          20-29 percent third degree T32.42
          30-39 percent third degree T32.43
          40-49 percent third degree T32.44
    50-59 percent (0-9 percent third degree) T32.50
      with
          10-19 percent third degree T32.51
          20-29 percent third degree T32.52
          30-39 percent third degree T32.53
          40-49 percent third degree T32.54
          50-59 percent third degree T32.55
    60-69 percent (0-9 percent third degree) T32.60
      with
          10-19 percent third degree T32.61
          20-29 percent third degree T32.62
          30-39 percent third degree T32.63
          40-49 percent third degree T32.64
          50-59 percent third degree T32.65
          60-69 percent third degree T32.66
    70-79 percent (0-9 percent third degree) T32.70
      with
          10-19 percent third degree T32.71
          20-29 percent third degree T32.72
          30-39 percent third degree T32.73
          40-49 percent third degree T32.74
          50-59 percent third degree T32.75
          60-69 percent third degree T32.76
          70-79 percent third degree T32.77
    80-89 percent (0-9 percent third degree) T32.80
      with
          10-19 percent third degree T32.81

Corrosion — *continued*
 extent — *continued*
  80-89 percent — *continued*
   with — *continued*
    20-29 percent third degree T32.82
    30-39 percent third degree T32.83
    40-49 percent third degree T32.84
    50-59 percent third degree T32.85
    60-69 percent third degree T32.86
    70-79 percent third degree T32.87
    80-89 percent third degree T32.88
  90 percent or more (0-9 percent third degree) T32.90
   with
    10-19 percent third degree T32.91
    20-29 percent third degree T32.92
    30-39 percent third degree T32.93
    40-49 percent third degree T32.94
    50-59 percent third degree T32.95
    60-69 percent third degree T32.96
    70-79 percent third degree T32.97
    80-89 percent third degree T32.98
    90-99 percent third degree T32.99
 extremity — *see* Corrosion, limb
 eye(s) and adnexa T26.9-
  with resulting rupture and destruction of eyeball T26.7-
  conjunctival sac — *see* Corrosion, cornea
  cornea — *see* Corrosion, cornea
  lid — *see* Corrosion, eyelid
  periocular area — *see* Corrosion eyelid
  specified site NEC T26.8-
 eyeball — *see* Corrosion, eye
 eyelid(s) T26.5-
 face — *see* Corrosion, head
 finger T23.429
  first degree T23.529
  left T23.422
   first degree T23.522
   second degree T23.622
   third degree T23.722
  multiple sites (without thumb) T23.439
   with thumb T23.449
    first degree T23.549
    left T23.442
     first degree T23.542
     second degree T23.642
     third degree T23.742
    right T23.441
     first degree T23.541
     second degree T23.641
     third degree T23.741
    second degree T23.649
    third degree T23.749
   first degree T23.539
   left T23.432
    first degree T23.532
    second degree T23.632
    third degree T23.732
   right T23.431
    first degree T23.531
    second degree T23.631
    third degree T23.731
   second degree T23.639
   third degree T23.739
  right T23.421
   first degree T23.521
   second degree T23.621
   third degree T23.721
  second degree T23.629
  third degree T23.729
 flank — *see* Corrosion, abdomen
 foot T25.429
  first degree T25.529
  left T25.422
   first degree T25.522
   second degree T25.622
   third degree T25.722
  multiple with ankle — *see* Corrosion, lower, limb, multiple, ankle and foot
  right T25.421
   first degree T25.521
   second degree T25.621
   third degree T25.721
  second degree T25.629
  third degree T25.729
 forearm T22.419

Corrosion — *continued*
 forearm — *continued*
  first degree T22.519
  left T22.412
   first degree T22.512
   second degree T22.612
   third degree T22.712
  right T22.411
   first degree T22.511
   second degree T22.611
   third degree T22.711
  second degree T22.619
  third degree T22.719
 forehead T20.46
  first degree T20.56
  second degree T20.66
  third degree T20.76
 fourth degree — *code as* Corrosion, third degree, by site
 full thickness skin loss — *code as* Corrosion, third degree, by site
 gastrointestinal tract NEC T28.7
 genital organs
  external
   female T21.47
    first degree T21.57
    second degree T21.67
    third degree T21.77
   male T21.46
    first degree T21.56
    second degree T21.66
    third degree T21.76
  internal T28.8
 groin — *see* Corrosion, abdominal wall
 hand(s) T23.409
  back — *see* Corrosion, dorsum of hand
  finger — *see* Corrosion, finger
  first degree T23.509
  left T23.402
   first degree T23.502
   second degree T23.602
   third degree T23.702
  multiple sites with wrist T23.499
   first degree T23.599
   left T23.492
    first degree T23.592
    second degree T23.692
    third degree T23.792
   right T23.491
    first degree T23.591
    second degree T23.691
    third degree T23.791
   second degree T23.699
   third degree T23.799
  palm — *see* Corrosion, palm
  right T23.401
   first degree T23.501
   second degree T23.601
   third degree T23.701
  second degree T23.609
  third degree T23.709
  thumb — *see* Corrosion, thumb
 head (and face) (and neck) T20.40
  cheek — *see* Corrosion, cheek
  chin — *see* Corrosion, chin
  ear — *see* Corrosion, ear
  eye(s) only — *see* Corrosion, eye
  first degree T20.50
  forehead — *see* Corrosion, forehead
  lip — *see* Corrosion, lip
  multiple sites T20.49
   first degree T20.59
   second degree T20.69
   third degree T20.79
  neck — *see* Corrosion, neck
  nose — *see* Corrosion, nose
  scalp — *see* Corrosion, scalp
  second degree T20.60
  third degree T20.70
 hip(s) — *see* Corrosion, lower, limb
 inhalation — *see* Corrosion, respiratory tract
 internal organ(s) (*see also* Corrosion, by site) T28.90
  alimentary tract T28.7
   esophagus T28.6
  esophagus T28.6
  genitourinary T28.8

Corrosion — *continued*
 internal organ(s) (*see also* Corrosion, by site) — *continued*
  mouth T28.5
  pharynx T28.5
  specified organ NEC T28.99
 interscapular region — *see* Corrosion, back, upper
 intestine (large) (small) T28.7
 knee T24.429
  first degree T24.529
  left T24.422
   first degree T24.522
   second degree T24.622
   third degree T24.722
  right T24.421
   first degree T24.521
   second degree T24.621
   third degree T24.721
  second degree T24.629
  third degree T24.729
 labium (majus) (minus) — *see* Corrosion, genital organs, external, female
 lacrimal apparatus, duct, gland or sac — *see* Corrosion, eye, specified site NEC
 larynx T27.4
  with lung T27.5
 leg(s) (meaning lower limb(s)) — *see* Corrosion, lower limb
 limb(s)
  lower — *see* Corrosion, lower, limb
  upper — *see* Corrosion, upper limb
 lip(s) T20.42
  first degree T20.52
  second degree T20.62
  third degree T20.72
 lower
  back — *see* Corrosion, back
  limb T24.409
   ankle — *see* Corrosion, ankle
   calf — *see* Corrosion, calf
   first degree T24.509
   foot — *see* Corrosion, foot
   knee — *see* Corrosion, knee
   left T24.402
    first degree T24.502
    second degree T24.602
    third degree T24.702
   multiple sites, except ankle and foot T24.499
    ankle and foot T25.499
     first degree T25.599
     left T25.492
      first degree T25.592
      second degree T25.692
      third degree T25.792
     right T25.491
      first degree T25.591
      second degree T25.691
      third degree T25.791
     second degree T25.699
     third degree T25.799
    first degree T24.599
    left T24.492
     first degree T24.592
     second degree T24.692
     third degree T24.792
    right T24.491
     first degree T24.591
     second degree T24.691
     third degree T24.791
    second degree T24.699
    third degree T24.799
   right T24.401
    first degree T24.501
    second degree T24.601
    third degree T24.701
   second degree T24.609
   thigh — *see* Corrosion, thigh
   third degree T24.709
 lung (with larynx and trachea) T27.5
 mouth T28.5
 neck T20.47
  first degree T20.57
  second degree T20.67
  third degree T20.77
 nose (septum) T20.44
  first degree T20.54

☑ **Additional Character Required** — Refer to the Tabular List for Character Selection   Subterms under main terms may continue to next column or page

⚐ Subterms under main terms may continue to next column or page   ☑ Additional Character Required — Refer to the Tabular List for Character Selection   75

Corrosion — Corrosion

Corrosion — *continued*
- upper limb — *continued*
  - third degree T22.70 ☑
  - wrist — *see* Corrosion, hand
- uterus T28.8 ☑
- vagina T28.8 ☑
- vulva — *see* Corrosion, genital organs, external, female
- wrist T23.479 ☑
  - first degree T23.579 ☑
  - left T23.472 ☑
    - first degree T23.572 ☑
    - second degree T23.672 ☑
    - third degree T23.772 ☑
  - multiple sites with hand T23.499 ☑
    - first degree T23.599 ☑
    - left T23.492 ☑
      - first degree T23.592 ☑
      - second degree T23.692 ☑
      - third degree T23.792 ☑
    - right T23.491 ☑
      - first degree T23.591 ☑
      - second degree T23.691 ☑
      - third degree T23.791 ☑
    - second degree T23.699 ☑
    - third degree T23.799 ☑
  - right T23.471 ☑
    - first degree T23.571 ☑
    - second degree T23.671 ☑
    - third degree T23.771 ☑
  - second degree T23.679 ☑
  - third degree T23.779 ☑

Corrosive burn — *see* Corrosion
Corsican fever — *see* Malaria
Cortical — *see* condition
Cortico-adrenal — *see* condition
Coryza (acute) J00
- with grippe or influenza — *see* Influenza, with, respiratory manifestations NEC
- syphilitic
  - congenital (chronic) A50.05

Costen's syndrome or complex M26.69
Costiveness — *see* Constipation
Costochondritis M94.0
Cot death R99
Cotard's syndrome F22
Cotia virus B08.8
Cotton wool spots (retinal) H35.81
Cotungo's disease — *see* Sciatica
Cough (affected) (chronic) (epidemic) (nervous) R05
- with hemorrhage — *see* Hemoptysis
- bronchial R05
  - with grippe or influenza — *see* Influenza, with, respiratory manifestations NEC
- functional F45.8
- hysterical F45.8
- laryngeal, spasmodic R05
- psychogenic F45.8
- smokers' J41.0
- tea taster's B49

Counseling (for) Z71.9
- abuse NEC
  - perpetrator Z69.82
  - victim Z69.81
- alcohol abuser Z71.41
  - family Z71.42
- child abuse
  - nonparental
    - perpetrator Z69.021
    - victim Z69.020
  - parental
    - perpetrator Z69.011
    - victim Z69.010
- consanguinity Z71.89
- contraceptive Z30.09
- dietary Z71.3
- drug abuser Z71.51
  - family member Z71.52
- exercise Z71.82
- family Z71.89
- fertility preservation (prior to cancer therapy) (prior to removal of gonads) Z31.62
- for non-attending third party Z71.0
  - related to sexual behavior or orientation Z70.2
- genetic
  - nonprocreative Z71.83
  - procreative NEC Z31.5
- gestational carrier Z31.7

Counseling — *continued*
- health (advice) (education) (instruction) — *see* Counseling, medical
- human immunodeficiency virus (HIV) Z71.7
- impotence Z70.1
- insulin pump use Z46.81
- medical (for) Z71.9
  - boarding school resident Z59.3
  - consanguinity Z71.89
  - feared complaint and no disease found Z71.1
  - human immunodeficiency virus (HIV) Z71.7
  - institutional resident Z59.3
  - on behalf of another Z71.0
    - related to sexual behavior or orientation Z70.2
  - person living alone Z60.2
  - specified reason NEC Z71.89
- natural family planning
  - procreative Z31.61
  - to avoid pregnancy Z30.02
- perpetrator (of)
  - abuse NEC Z69.82
  - child abuse
    - non-parental Z69.021
    - parental Z69.011
  - rape NEC Z69.82
  - spousal abuse Z69.12
- procreative NEC Z31.69
  - fertility preservation (prior to cancer therapy) (prior to removal of gonads) Z31.62
  - using natural family planning Z31.61
- promiscuity Z70.1
- rape victim Z69.81
- religious Z71.81
- sex, sexual (related to) Z70.9
  - attitude(s) Z70.0
  - behavior or orientation Z70.1
  - combined concerns Z70.3
  - non-responsiveness Z70.1
  - on behalf of third party Z70.2
  - specified reason NEC Z70.8
- specified reason NEC Z71.89
- spiritual Z71.81
- spousal abuse (perpetrator) Z69.12
  - victim Z69.11
- substance abuse Z71.89
  - alcohol Z71.41
  - drug Z71.51
  - tobacco Z71.6
- tobacco use Z71.6
- use (of)
  - insulin pump Z46.81
- victim (of)
  - abuse Z69.81
  - child abuse
    - by parent Z69.010
    - non-parental Z69.020
    - rape NEC Z69.81

Coupled rhythm R00.8
Couvelaire syndrome or uterus (complicating delivery) O45.8X- ☑
Cowperitis — *see* Urethritis
Cowper's gland — *see* condition
Cowpox B08.010
- due to vaccination T88.1 ☑
Coxa
- magna M91.4- ☑
- plana M91.2- ☑
- valga (acquired) (*see also* Deformity, limb, specified type NEC, thigh)
  - congenital Q65.81
  - sequelae (late effect) of rickets E64.3
- vara (acquired) (*see also* Deformity, limb, specified type NEC, thigh)
  - congenital Q65.82
  - sequelae (late effect) of rickets E64.3
Coxalgia, coxalgic (nontuberculous) (*see also* Pain, joint, hip)
- tuberculous A18.02
Coxitis — *see* Monoarthritis, hip
Coxsackie (virus) (infection) B34.1
- as cause of disease classified elsewhere B97.11
- carditis B33.20
- central nervous system NEC A88.8
- endocarditis B33.21
- enteritis A08.39
- meningitis (aseptic) A87.0
- myocarditis B33.22
- pericarditis B33.23

Coxsackie — *continued*
- pharyngitis B08.5
- pleurodynia B33.0
- specific disease NEC B33.8
Crabs, meaning pubic lice B85.3
Crack baby P04.41
Cracked nipple N64.0
- associated with
  - lactation O92.13
  - pregnancy O92.11- ☑
  - puerperium O92.12
Cracked tooth K03.81
Cradle cap L21.0
Craft neurosis F48.8
Cramp(s) R25.2
- abdominal — *see* Pain, abdominal
- bathing T75.1 ☑
- colic R10.83
  - psychogenic F45.8
- due to immersion T75.1 ☑
- fireman T67.2 ☑
- heat T67.2 ☑
- immersion T75.1 ☑
- intestinal — *see* Pain, abdominal
  - psychogenic F45.8
- leg, sleep related G47.62
- limb (lower) (upper) NEC R25.2
  - sleep related G47.62
- linotypist's F48.8
  - organic G25.89
- muscle (limb) (general) R25.2
  - due to immersion T75.1 ☑
  - psychogenic F45.8
- occupational (hand) F48.8
  - organic G25.89
- salt-depletion E87.1
- sleep related, leg G47.62
- stoker's T67.2 ☑
- swimmer's T75.1 ☑
- telegrapher's F48.8
  - organic G25.89
- typist's F48.8
  - organic G25.89
- uterus N94.89
  - menstrual — *see* Dysmenorrhea
- writer's F48.8
  - organic G25.89
Cranial — *see* condition
Craniocleidodysostosis Q74.0
Craniofenestria (skull) Q75.8
Craniolacunia (skull) Q75.8
Craniopagus Q89.4
Craniopathy, metabolic M85.2
Craniopharyngeal — *see* condition
Craniopharyngioma D44.4
Craniorachischisis (totalis) Q00.1
Cranioschisis Q75.8
Craniostenosis Q75.0
Craniosynostosis Q75.0
Craniotabes (cause unknown) M83.8
- neonatal P96.3
- rachitic E64.3
- syphilitic A50.56
Cranium — *see* condition
Craw-craw — *see* Onchocerciasis
Creaking joint — *see* Derangement, joint, specified type NEC
Creeping
- eruption B76.9
- palsy or paralysis G12.22
Crenated tongue K14.8
Creotoxism A05.9
Crepitus
- caput Q75.8
- joint — *see* Derangement, joint, specified type NEC
Crescent or conus choroid, congenital Q14.3
CREST syndrome M34.1
Cretin, cretinism (congenital) (endemic) (nongoitrous) (sporadic) E00.9
- pelvis
  - with disproportion (fetopelvic) O33.0
    - causing obstructed labor O65.0
- type
  - hypothyroid E00.1
  - mixed E00.2
  - myxedematous E00.1
  - neurological E00.0

☑ **Additional Character Required — Refer to the Tabular List for Character Selection**   ▽ **Subterms under main terms may continue to next column or page**

Creutzfeldt-Jakob disease or syndrome (with dementia) A81.00
  familial A81.09
  iatrogenic A81.09
  specified NEC A81.09
  sporadic A81.09
  variant (vCJD) A81.01
Crib death R99
Cribriform hymen Q52.3
Cri-du-chat syndrome Q93.4
Crigler-Najjar disease or syndrome E80.5
Crime, victim of Z65.4
Crimean hemorrhagic fever A98.0
Criminalism F60.2
Crisis
  abdomen R10.0
  acute reaction F43.0
  addisonian E27.2
  adrenal (cortical) E27.2
  celiac K90.0
  Dietl's N13.8
  emotional (see also Disorder, adjustment)
    acute reaction to stress F43.0
    specific to childhood and adolescence F93.8
  glaucomatocyclitic — see Glaucoma, secondary, inflammation
  heart — see Failure, heart
  nitritoid I95.2
    correct substance properly administered — see Table of Drugs and Chemicals, by drug, adverse effect
    overdose or wrong substance given or taken — see Table of Drugs and Chemicals, by drug, poisoning
  oculogyric H51.8
    psychogenic F45.8
  Pel's (tabetic) A52.11
  psychosexual identity F64.2
  renal N28.0
  sickle-cell D57.00
    with
      acute chest syndrome D57.01
      splenic sequestration D57.02
    state (acute reaction) F43.0
  tabetic A52.11
  thyroid — see Thyrotoxicosis with thyroid storm
  thyrotoxic — see Thyrotoxicosis with thyroid storm
Crocq's disease (acrocyanosis) I73.89
Crohn's disease — see Enteritis, regional
Crooked septum, nasal J34.2
Cross syndrome E70.328
Crossbite (anterior) (posterior) M26.24
Cross-eye — see Strabismus, convergent concomitant
Croup, croupous (catarrhal) (infectious) (inflammatory) (nondiphtheritic) J05.0
  bronchial J20.9
  diphtheritic A36.2
  false J38.5
  spasmodic J38.5
    diphtheritic A36.2
  stridulous J38.5
    diphtheritic A36.2
Crouzon's disease Q75.1
Crowding, tooth, teeth, fully erupted M26.31
CRST syndrome M34.1
Cruchet's disease A85.8
Cruelty in children (see also Disorder, conduct)
Crural ulcer — see Ulcer, lower limb
Crush, crushed, crushing T14.8 ☑
  abdomen S38.1 ☑
  ankle S97.0- ☑
  arm (upper) (and shoulder) S47.- ☑
    axilla — see Crush, arm
  back, lower S38.1 ☑
  buttock S38.1 ☑
  cheek S07.0 ☑
  chest S28.0 ☑
  cranium S07.1 ☑
  ear S07.0 ☑
  elbow S57.0- ☑
  extremity
    lower
      ankle — see Crush, ankle
      below knee — see Crush, leg
      foot — see Crush, foot
      hip — see Crush, hip
      knee — see Crush, knee

Crush, crushed, crushing — continued
  extremity — continued
    lower — continued
      thigh — see Crush, thigh
      toe — see Crush, toe
    upper
      below elbow S67.9- ☑
      elbow — see Crush, elbow
      finger — see Crush, finger
      forearm — see Crush, forearm
      hand — see Crush, hand
      thumb — see Crush, thumb
      upper arm — see Crush, arm
      wrist — see Crush, wrist
  face S07.0 ☑
  finger(s) S67.1- ☑
    with hand (and wrist) — see Crush, hand, specified site NEC
    index S67.19- ☑
    little S67.19- ☑
    middle S67.19- ☑
    ring S67.19- ☑
    thumb — see Crush, thumb
  foot S97.8- ☑
    toe — see Crush, toe
  forearm S57.8- ☑
  genitalia, external
    female S38.002 ☑
      vagina S38.03 ☑
      vulva S38.03 ☑
    male S38.001 ☑
      penis S38.01 ☑
      scrotum S38.02 ☑
      testis S38.02 ☑
  hand (except fingers alone) S67.2- ☑
    with wrist S67.4- ☑
  head S07.9 ☑
    specified NEC S07.8 ☑
  heel — see Crush, foot
  hip S77.0- ☑
    with thigh S77.2- ☑
  internal organ (abdomen, chest, or pelvis) NEC T14.8 ☑
  knee S87.0- ☑
  labium (majus) (minus) S38.03 ☑
  larynx S17.0 ☑
  leg (lower) S87.8- ☑
    knee — see Crush, knee
  lip S07.0 ☑
  lower
    back S38.1 ☑
    leg — see Crush, leg
  neck S17.9 ☑
  nerve — see Injury, nerve
  nose S07.0 ☑
  pelvis S38.1 ☑
  penis S38.01 ☑
  scalp S07.8 ☑
  scapular region — see Crush, arm
  scrotum S38.02 ☑
  severe, unspecified site T14.8 ☑
  shoulder (and upper arm) — see Crush, arm
  skull S07.1 ☑
  syndrome (complication of trauma) T79.5 ☑
  testis S38.02 ☑
  thigh S77.1- ☑
    with hip S77.2- ☑
  throat S17.8 ☑
  thumb S67.0- ☑
    with hand (and wrist) — see Crush, hand, specified site NEC
  toe(s) S97.10- ☑
    great S97.11- ☑
    lesser S97.12- ☑
  trachea S17.0 ☑
  vagina S38.03 ☑
  vulva S38.03 ☑
  wrist S67.3- ☑
    with hand S67.4- ☑
Crusta lactea L21.0
Crusts R23.4
Crutch paralysis — see Injury, brachial plexus
Cruveilhier-Baumgarten cirrhosis, disease or syndrome K74.69
Cruveilhier's atrophy or disease G12.8
Crying (constant) (continuous) (excessive)
  child, adolescent, or adult R45.83

Crying — continued
  infant (baby) (newborn) R68.11
Cryofibrinogenemia D89.2
Cryoglobulinemia (essential) (idiopathic) (mixed) (primary) (purpura) (secondary) (vasculitis) D89.1
  with lung involvement D89.1 [J99]
Cryptitis (anal) (rectal) K62.89
Cryptococcosis, cryptococcus (infection) (neoformans) B45.9
  bone B45.3
  cerebral B45.1
  cutaneous B45.2
  disseminated B45.7
  generalized B45.7
  meningitis B45.1
  meningocerebralis B45.1
  osseous B45.3
  pulmonary B45.0
  skin B45.2
  specified NEC B45.8
Cryptopapillitis (anus) K62.89
Cryptophthalmos Q11.2
  syndrome Q87.0
Cryptorchid, cryptorchism, cryptorchidism Q53.9
  bilateral Q53.20
    abdominal Q53.211
    perineal Q53.22
  unilateral Q53.10
    abdominal Q53.111
    perineal Q53.12
Cryptosporidiosis A07.2
  hepatobiliary B88.8
  respiratory B88.8
Cryptostromosis J67.6
Crystalluria R82.998
Cubitus
  congenital Q68.8
  valgus (acquired) M21.0- ☑
    congenital Q68.8
    sequelae (late effect) of rickets E64.3
  varus (acquired) M21.1- ☑
    congenital Q68.8
    sequelae (late effect) of rickets E64.3
Cultural deprivation or shock Z60.3
Curling esophagus K22.4
Curling's ulcer — see Ulcer, peptic, acute
Curschmann (-Batten) (-Steinert) **disease or syndrome** G71.11
Curse, Ondine's — see Apnea, sleep
Curvature
  organ or site, congenital NEC — see Distortion
  penis (lateral) Q55.61
  Pott's (spinal) A18.01
  radius, idiopathic, progressive (congenital) Q74.0
  spine (acquired) (angular) (idiopathic) (incorrect) (postural) — see Dorsopathy, deforming
    congenital Q67.5
    due to or associated with
      Charcot-Marie-Tooth disease (see also subcategory M49.8) G60.0
      osteitis
        deformans M88.88
        fibrosa cystica (see also subcategory M49.8) E21.0
      tuberculosis (Pott's curvature) A18.01
    sequelae (late effect) of rickets E64.3
    tuberculous A18.01
Cushingoid due to steroid therapy E24.2
  correct substance properly administered — see Table of Drugs and Chemicals, by drug, adverse effect
  overdose or wrong substance given or taken — see Table of Drugs and Chemicals, by drug, poisoning
Cushing's
  syndrome or disease E24.9
    drug-induced E24.2
    iatrogenic E24.2
    pituitary-dependent E24.0
    specified NEC E24.8
  ulcer — see Ulcer, peptic, acute
Cusp, Carabelli — omit code
Cut (external) (see also Laceration)
  muscle — see Injury, muscle
Cutaneous (see also condition)
  hemorrhage R23.3
  larva migrans B76.9
Cutis (see also condition)
  hyperelastica Q82.8
    acquired L57.4

Cutis — *continued*
laxa (hyperelastica) — *see* Dermatolysis
marmorata R23.8
osteosis L94.2
pendula — *see* Dermatolysis
rhomboidalis nuchae L57.2
verticis gyrata Q82.8
acquired L91.8
Cyanosis R23.0
due to
patent foramen botalli Q21.1
persistent foramen ovale Q21.1
enterogenous D74.8
paroxysmal digital — *see* Raynaud's disease
with gangrene I73.01
retina, retinal H35.89
Cyanotic heart disease I24.9
congenital Q24.9
Cycle
anovulatory N97.0
menstrual, irregular N92.6
Cyclencephaly Q04.9
Cyclical vomiting (*see also* Vomiting, cyclical) G43.A0
(*following* G43.7)
psychogenic F50.89
Cyclitis (*see also* Iridocyclitis) H20.9
chronic — *see* Iridocyclitis, chronic
Fuchs' heterochromic H20.81- ☑
granulomatous — *see* Iridocyclitis, chronic
lens-induced — *see* Iridocyclitis, lens-induced
posterior H30.2- ☑
Cycloid personality F34.0
Cyclophoria H50.54
Cyclopia, cyclops Q87.0
Cyclopism Q87.0
Cyclosporiasis A07.4
Cyclothymia F34.0
Cyclothymic personality F34.0
Cyclotropia H50.41- ☑
Cylindroma (*see also* Neoplasm, malignant, by site)
eccrine dermal — *see* Neoplasm, skin, benign
skin — *see* Neoplasm, skin, benign
Cylindruria R82.998
Cynanche
diphtheritic A36.2
tonsillaris J36
Cynophobia F40.218
Cynorexia R63.2
Cyphosis — *see* Kyphosis
Cyprus fever — *see* Brucellosis
Cyst (colloid) (mucous) (simple) (retention)
adenoid (infected) J35.8
adrenal gland E27.8
congenital Q89.1
air, lung J98.4
allantoic Q64.4
alveolar process (jaw bone) M27.40
amnion, amniotic O41.8X- ☑
aneurysmal M27.49
anterior
chamber (eye) — *see* Cyst, iris
nasopalatine K09.1
antrum J34.1
anus K62.89
apical (tooth) (periodontal) K04.8
appendix K38.8
arachnoid, brain (acquired) G93.0
congenital Q04.6
arytenoid J38.7
Baker's M71.2- ☑
ruptured M66.0
tuberculous A18.02
Bartholin's gland N75.0
bile duct (common) (hepatic) K83.5
bladder (multiple) (trigone) N32.89
blue dome (breast) — *see* Cyst, breast
bone (local) NEC M85.60
aneurysmal M85.50
ankle M85.57- ☑
foot M85.57- ☑
forearm M85.53- ☑
hand M85.54- ☑
jaw M27.49
lower leg M85.56- ☑
multiple site M85.59
neck M85.58
rib M85.58

Cyst — *continued*
bone — *continued*
aneurysmal — *continued*
shoulder M85.51- ☑
skull M85.58
specified site NEC M85.58
thigh M85.55- ☑
toe M85.57- ☑
upper arm M85.52- ☑
vertebra M85.58
solitary M85.40
ankle M85.47- ☑
fibula M85.46- ☑
foot M85.47- ☑
hand M85.44- ☑
humerus M85.42- ☑
jaw M27.49
neck M85.48
pelvis M85.45- ☑
radius M85.43- ☑
rib M85.48
shoulder M85.41- ☑
skull M85.48
specified site NEC M85.48
tibia M85.46- ☑
toe M85.47- ☑
ulna M85.43- ☑
vertebra M85.48
specified type NEC M85.60
ankle M85.67- ☑
foot M85.67- ☑
forearm M85.63- ☑
hand M85.64- ☑
jaw M27.40
developmental (nonodontogenic) K09.1
odontogenic K09.0
latent M27.0
lower leg M85.66- ☑
multiple site M85.69
neck M85.68
rib M85.68
shoulder M85.61- ☑
skull M85.68
specified site NEC M85.68
thigh M85.65- ☑
toe M85.67- ☑
upper arm M85.62- ☑
vertebra M85.68
brain (acquired) G93.0
congenital Q04.6
hydatid B67.99 [G94]
third ventricle (colloid), congenital Q04.6
branchial (cleft) Q18.0
branchiogenic Q18.0
breast (benign) (blue dome) (pedunculated) (solitary) N60.0- ☑
involution — *see* Dysplasia, mammary, specified type NEC
sebaceous — *see* Dysplasia, mammary, specified type NEC
broad ligament (benign) N83.8
bronchogenic (mediastinal) (sequestration) J98.4
congenital Q33.0
buccal K09.8
bulbourethral gland N36.8
bursa, bursal NEC M71.30
with rupture — *see* Rupture, synovium
ankle M71.37- ☑
elbow M71.32- ☑
foot M71.37- ☑
hand M71.34- ☑
hip M71.35- ☑
multiple sites M71.39
pharyngeal J39.2
popliteal space — *see* Cyst, Baker's
shoulder M71.31- ☑
specified site NEC M71.38
wrist M71.33- ☑
calcifying odontogenic D16.5
upper jaw (bone) (maxilla) D16.4
canal of Nuck (female) N94.89
congenital Q52.4
canthus — *see* Cyst, conjunctiva
carcinomatous — *see* Neoplasm, malignant, by site
cauda equina G95.89
cavum septi pellucidi — *see* Cyst, brain
celomic (pericardium) Q24.8

Cyst — *continued*
cerebellopontine (angle) — *see* Cyst, brain
cerebellum — *see* Cyst, brain
cerebral — *see* Cyst, brain
cervical lateral Q18.0
cervix NEC N88.8
embryonic Q51.6
nabothian N88.8
chiasmal optic NEC — *see* Disorder, optic, chiasm
chocolate (ovary) N80.1
choledochus, congenital Q44.4
chorion O41.8X- ☑
choroid plexus G93.0
ciliary body — *see* Cyst, iris
clitoris N90.7
colon K63.89
common (bile) duct K83.5
congenital NEC Q89.8
adrenal gland Q89.1
epiglottis Q31.8
esophagus Q39.8
fallopian tube Q50.4
kidney Q61.00
more than one (multiple) Q61.02
specified as polycystic Q61.3
adult type Q61.2
infantile type NEC Q61.19
collecting duct dilation Q61.11
solitary Q61.01
larynx Q31.8
liver Q44.6
lung Q33.0
mediastinum Q34.1
ovary Q50.1
oviduct Q50.4
periurethral (tissue) Q64.79
prepuce Q55.69
salivary gland (any) Q38.4
sublingual Q38.6
submaxillary gland Q38.6
thymus (gland) Q89.2
tongue Q38.3
ureterovesical orifice Q62.8
vulva Q52.79
conjunctiva H11.44- ☑
cornea H18.89- ☑
corpora quadrigemina G93.0
corpus
albicans N83.29- ☑
luteum (hemorrhagic) (ruptured) N83.1- ☑
Cowper's gland (benign) (infected) N36.8
cranial meninges G93.0
craniobuccal pouch E23.6
craniopharyngeal pouch E23.6
cystic duct K82.8
Cysticercus — *see* Cysticercosis
Dandy-Walker Q03.1
with spina bifida — *see* Spina bifida
dental (root) K04.8
developmental K09.0
eruption K09.0
primordial K09.0
dentigerous (mandible) (maxilla) K09.0
dermoid — *see* Neoplasm, benign, by site
with malignant transformation C56.- ☑
implantation
external area or site (skin) NEC L72.0
iris — *see* Cyst, iris, implantation
vagina N89.8
vulva N90.7
mouth K09.8
oral soft tissue K09.8
sacrococcygeal — *see* Cyst, pilonidal
developmental K09.1
odontogenic K09.0
oral region (nonodontogenic) K09.1
ovary, ovarian Q50.1
dura (cerebral) G93.0
spinal G96.19
ear (external) Q18.1
echinococcal — *see* Echinococcus
embryonic
cervix uteri Q51.6
fallopian tube Q50.4
vagina Q52.4
endometrium, endometrial (uterus) N85.8
ectopic — *see* Endometriosis
enterogenous Q43.8

☑ **Additional Character Required — Refer to the Tabular List for Character Selection**   🔺 **Subterms under main terms may continue to next column or page**

Cyst — continued
- epidermal, epidermoid (inclusion) (see also Cyst, skin) L72.0
  - mouth K09.8
  - oral soft tissue K09.8
- epididymis N50.3
- epiglottis J38.7
- epiphysis cerebri E34.8
- epithelial (inclusion) L72.0
- epoophoron Q50.5
- eruption K09.0
- esophagus K22.8
- ethmoid sinus J34.1
- external female genital organs NEC N90.7
- eyelid (sebaceous) H02.829
  - infected — see Hordeolum
  - left H02.826
    - lower H02.825
    - upper H02.824
  - right H02.823
    - lower H02.822
    - upper H02.821
- eye NEC H57.89
  - congenital Q15.8
- fallopian tube N83.8
  - congenital Q50.4
- fimbrial (twisted) Q50.4
- fissural (oral region) K09.1
- follicle (graafian) (hemorrhagic) N83.0- ☑
  - nabothian N88.8
- follicular (atretic) (hemorrhagic) (ovarian) N83.0- ☑
  - dentigerous K09.0
  - odontogenic K09.0
  - skin L72.9
    - specified NEC L72.8
- frontal sinus J34.1
- gallbladder K82.8
- ganglion — see Ganglion
- Gartner's duct Q52.4
- gingiva K09.0
- gland of Moll — see Cyst, eyelid
- globulomaxillary K09.1
- graafian follicle (hemorrhagic) N83.0- ☑
- granulosal lutein (hemorrhagic) N83.1- ☑
- hemangiomatous D18.00
  - intra-abdominal D18.03
  - intracranial D18.02
  - skin D18.01
  - specified site NEC D18.09
- hemorrhagic M27.49
- hydatid (see also Echinococcus) B67.90
  - brain B67.99 [G94]
  - liver (see also Cyst, liver, hydatid) B67.8
  - lung NEC B67.99 [J99]
  - Morgagni
    - female Q50.5
    - male (epididymal) Q55.4
      - testicular Q55.29
  - specified site NEC B67.99
- hymen N89.8
  - embryonic Q52.4
- hypopharynx J39.2
- hypophysis, hypophyseal (duct) (recurrent) E23.6
  - cerebri E23.6
- implantation (dermoid)
  - external area or site (skin) NEC L72.0
  - iris — see Cyst, iris, implantation
  - vagina N89.8
  - vulva N90.7
- incisive canal K09.1
- inclusion (epidermal) (epithelial) (epidermoid) (squamous) L72.0
  - not of skin — code under Cyst, by site
- intestine (large) (small) K63.89
- intracranial — see Cyst, brain
- intraligamentous (see also Disorder, ligament)
  - knee — see Derangement, knee
- intrasellar E23.6
- iris H21.309
  - exudative H21.31- ☑
  - idiopathic H21.30- ☑
  - implantation H21.32- ☑
  - parasitic H21.33- ☑
  - pars plana (primary) H21.34- ☑
    - exudative H21.35- ☑
- jaw (bone) M27.40
  - aneurysmal M27.49
  - developmental (odontogenic) K09.0

Cyst — continued
- jaw — continued
  - fissural K09.1
  - hemorrhagic M27.49
  - traumatic M27.49
- joint NEC — see Disorder, joint, specified type NEC
- kidney (acquired) N28.1
  - calyceal — see Hydronephrosis
  - congenital Q61.00
    - more than one (multiple) Q61.02
      - specified as polycystic Q61.3
        - adult type (autosomal dominant) Q61.2
        - infantile type (autosomal recessive) NEC Q61.19
          - collecting duct dilation Q61.11
  - pyelogenic — see Hydronephrosis
  - simple N28.1
  - solitary (single) Q61.01
    - acquired N28.1
- labium (majus) (minus) N90.7
  - sebaceous N90.7
- lacrimal (see also Disorder, lacrimal system, specified NEC)
  - gland H04.13- ☑
  - passages or sac — see Disorder, lacrimal system, specified NEC
- larynx J38.7
- lateral periodontal K09.0
- lens H27.8
  - congenital Q12.8
- lip (gland) K13.0
- liver (idiopathic) (simple) K76.89
  - congenital Q44.6
  - hydatid B67.8
    - granulosus B67.0
    - multilocularis B67.5
- lung J98.4
  - congenital Q33.0
  - giant bullous J43.9
- lutein N83.1- ☑
- lymphangiomatous D18.1
- lymphoepithelial, oral soft tissue K09.8
- macula — see Degeneration, macula, hole
- malignant — see Neoplasm, malignant, by site
- mammary gland — see Cyst, breast
- mandible M27.40
  - dentigerous K09.0
  - radicular K04.8
- maxilla M27.40
  - dentigerous K09.0
  - radicular K04.8
- medial, face and neck Q18.8
- median
  - anterior maxillary K09.1
  - palatal K09.1
- mediastinum, congenital Q34.1
- meibomian (gland) — see Chalazion
  - infected — see Hordeolum
- membrane, brain G93.0
- meninges (cerebral) G93.0
  - spinal G96.19
- meniscus, knee — see Derangement, knee, meniscus, cystic
- mesentery, mesenteric K66.8
  - chyle I89.8
- mesonephric duct
  - female Q50.5
  - male Q55.4
- milk N64.89
- Morgagni (hydatid)
  - female Q50.5
  - male (epididymal) Q55.4
    - testicular Q55.29
- mouth K09.8
- Müllerian duct Q50.4
  - appendix testis Q55.29
  - cervix Q51.6
  - fallopian tube Q50.4
  - female Q50.4
  - male Q55.29
  - prostatic utricle Q55.4
  - vagina (embryonal) Q52.4
- multilocular (ovary) D39.10
  - benign — see Neoplasm, benign, by site
- myometrium N85.8
- nabothian (follicle) (ruptured) N88.8
- nasoalveolar K09.1
- nasolabial K09.1

Cyst — continued
- nasopalatine (anterior) (duct) K09.1
- nasopharynx J39.2
- neoplastic — see Neoplasm, uncertain behavior, by site
  - benign — see Neoplasm, benign, by site
- nervous system NEC G96.8
- neuroenteric (congenital) Q06.8
- nipple — see Cyst, breast
- nose (turbinates) J34.1
  - sinus J34.1
- odontogenic, developmental K09.0
- omentum (lesser) K66.8
  - congenital Q45.8
- ora serrata — see Cyst, retina, ora serrata
- oral
  - region K09.9
    - developmental (nonodontogenic) K09.1
    - specified NEC K09.8
  - soft tissue K09.9
    - specified NEC K09.8
- orbit H05.81- ☑
- ovary, ovarian (twisted) N83.20- ☑
  - adherent N83.20- ☑
  - chocolate N80.1
  - corpus
    - albicans N83.29- ☑
    - luteum (hemorrhagic) N83.1- ☑
  - dermoid D27.9
  - developmental Q50.1
  - due to failure of involution NEC N83.20- ☑
  - endometrial N80.1
  - follicular (graafian) (hemorrhagic) N83.0- ☑
  - hemorrhagic N83.20- ☑
  - in pregnancy or childbirth O34.8- ☑
    - with obstructed labor O65.5
  - multilocular D39.10
  - pseudomucinous D27.9
  - retention N83.29- ☑
  - serous N83.20- ☑
  - specified NEC N83.29- ☑
  - theca lutein (hemorrhagic) N83.1- ☑
  - tuberculous A18.18
- oviduct N83.8
- palate (median) (fissural) K09.1
- palatine papilla (jaw) K09.1
- pancreas, pancreatic (hemorrhagic) (true) K86.2
  - congenital Q45.2
  - false K86.3
- paralabral
  - hip M24.85- ☑
  - shoulder S43.43- ☑
- paramesonephric duct Q50.4
  - female Q50.4
  - male Q55.29
- paranephric N28.1
- paraphysis, cerebri, congenital Q04.6
- parasitic B89
- parathyroid (gland) E21.4
- paratubal N83.8
- paraurethral duct N36.8
- paroophoron Q50.5
- parotid gland K11.6
- parovarian Q50.5
- pelvis, female N94.89
  - in pregnancy or childbirth O34.8- ☑
    - causing obstructed labor O65.5
- penis (sebaceous) N48.89
- periapical K04.8
- pericardial (congenital) Q24.8
  - acquired (secondary) I31.8
- pericoronal K09.0
- periodontal K04.8
  - lateral K09.0
- peripelvic (lymphatic) N28.1
- peritoneum K66.8
  - chylous I89.8
- periventricular, acquired, newborn P91.1
- pharynx (wall) J39.2
- pilar L72.11
- pilonidal (infected) (rectum) L05.91
  - with abscess L05.01
  - malignant C44.59- ☑
- pituitary (duct) (gland) E23.6
- placenta O43.19- ☑
- pleura J94.8
- popliteal — see Cyst, Baker's
- porencephalic Q04.6

▽ Subterms under main terms may continue to next column or page   ☑ Additional Character Required — Refer to the Tabular List for Character Selection   79

Cyst — Cyst

Cyst — *continued*
  porencephalic — *continued*
    acquired G93.Ø
  postanal (infected) — *see* Cyst, pilonidal
  postmastoidectomy cavity (mucosal) — *see* Complications, postmastoidectomy, cyst
  preauricular Q18.1
  prepuce N47.4
    congenital Q55.69
  primordial (jaw) KØ9.Ø
  prostate N42.83
  pseudomucinous (ovary) D27.9
  pupillary, miotic H21.27- ☑
  radicular (residual) KØ4.8
  radiculodental KØ4.8
  ranular K11.8
  Rathke's pouch E23.6
  rectum (epithelium) (mucous) K62.89
  renal — *see* Cyst, kidney
  residual (radicular) KØ4.8
  retention (ovary) N83.29- ☑
    salivary gland K11.6
  retina H33.19- ☑
    ora serrata H33.11- ☑
    parasitic H33.12- ☑
  retroperitoneal K68.9
  sacrococcygeal (dermoid) — *see* Cyst, pilonidal
  salivary gland or duct (mucous extravasation or retention) K11.6
  Sampson's N8Ø.1
  sclera H15.89
  scrotum L72.9
    sebaceous L72.3
  sebaceous (duct) (gland) L72.3
    breast — *see* Dysplasia, mammary, specified type NEC
    eyelid — *see* Cyst, eyelid
    genital organ NEC
      female N94.89
      male N5Ø.89
    scrotum L72.3
  semilunar cartilage (knee) (multiple) — *see* Derangement, knee, meniscus, cystic
  seminal vesicle N5Ø.89
  serous (ovary) N83.2Ø- ☑
  sinus (accessory) (nasal) J34.1
  Skene's gland N36.8
  skin L72.9
    breast — *see* Dysplasia, mammary, specified type NEC
    epidermal, epidermoid L72.Ø
    epithelial L72.Ø
    eyelid — *see* Cyst, eyelid
    genital organ NEC
      female N9Ø.7
      male N5Ø.89
    inclusion L72.Ø
    scrotum L72.9
    sebaceous L72.3
    sweat gland or duct L74.8
  solitary
    bone — *see* Cyst, bone, solitary
    jaw M27.4Ø
    kidney N28.1
  spermatic cord N5Ø.89
  sphenoid sinus J34.1
  spinal meninges G96.19
  spleen NEC D73.4
    congenital Q89.Ø9
    hydatid (*see also* Echinococcus) B67.99 [D77]
  Stafne's M27.Ø
  subarachnoid intrasellar R93.Ø
  subcutaneous, pheomycotic (chromomycotic) B43.2
  subdural (cerebral) G93.Ø
    spinal cord G96.19
  sublingual gland K11.6
  submandibular gland K11.6
  submaxillary gland K11.6
  suburethral N36.8
  suprarenal gland E27.8
  suprasellar — *see* Cyst, brain
  sweat gland or duct L74.8
  synovial (*see also* Cyst, bursa)
    ruptured — *see* Rupture, synovium
  tarsal — *see* Chalazion
  tendon (sheath) — *see* Disorder, tendon, specified type NEC
  testis N44.2

Cyst — *continued*
  testis — *continued*
    tunica albuginea N44.1
  theca lutein (ovary) N83.1- ☑
  Thornwaldt's J39.2
  thymus (gland) E32.8
  thyroglossal duct (infected) (persistent) Q89.2
  thyroid (gland) EØ4.1
  thyrolingual duct (infected) (persistent) Q89.2
  tongue K14.8
  tonsil J35.8
  tooth — *see* Cyst, dental
  Tornwaldt's J39.2
  trichilemmal (proliferating) L72.12
  trichodermal L72.12
  tubal (fallopian) N83.8
    inflammatory — *see* Salpingitis, chronic
  tubo-ovarian N83.8
    inflammatory N7Ø.13
  tunica
    albuginea testis N44.1
    vaginalis N5Ø.89
  turbinate (nose) J34.1
  Tyson's gland N48.89
  urachus, congenital Q64.4
  ureter N28.89
  ureterovesical orifice N28.89
  urethra, urethral (gland) N36.8
  uterine ligament N83.8
  uterus (body) (corpus) (recurrent) N85.8
    embryonic Q51.818
      cervix Q51.6
  vagina, vaginal (implantation) (inclusion) (squamous cell) (wall) N89.8
    embryonic Q52.4
  vallecula, vallecular (epiglottis) J38.7
  vesical (orifice) N32.89
  vitreous body H43.89
  vulva (implantation) (inclusion) N9Ø.7
    congenital Q52.79
    sebaceous gland N9Ø.7
  vulvovaginal gland N9Ø.7
  wolffian
    female Q5Ø.5
    male Q55.4
Cystadenocarcinoma — *see* Neoplasm, malignant, by site
  bile duct C22.1
  endometrioid — *see* Neoplasm, malignant, by site
    specified site — *see* Neoplasm, malignant, by site
    unspecified site
      female C56.9
      male C61
  mucinous
    papillary
      specified site — *see* Neoplasm, malignant, by site
      unspecified site C56.9
    specified site — *see* Neoplasm, malignant, by site
    unspecified site C56.9
  papillary
    mucinous
      specified site — *see* Neoplasm, malignant, by site
      unspecified site C56.9
    pseudomucinous
      specified site — *see* Neoplasm, malignant, by site
      unspecified site C56.9
    serous
      specified site — *see* Neoplasm, malignant, by site
      unspecified site C56.9
    specified site — *see* Neoplasm, malignant, by site
    unspecified site C56.9
  pseudomucinous
    papillary
      specified site — *see* Neoplasm, malignant, by site
      unspecified site C56.9
    specified site — *see* Neoplasm, malignant, by site
    unspecified site C56.9
  serous
    papillary
      specified site — *see* Neoplasm, malignant, by site
      unspecified site C56.9
    specified site — *see* Neoplasm, malignant, by site

Cystadenocarcinoma — *continued*
  serous — *continued*
    unspecified site C56.9
Cystadenofibroma
  clear cell — *see* Neoplasm, benign, by site
  endometrioid D27.9
    borderline malignancy D39.1- ☑
    malignant C56.- ☑
  mucinous
    specified site — *see* Neoplasm, benign, by site
    unspecified site D27.9
  serous
    specified site — *see* Neoplasm, benign, by site
    unspecified site D27.9
  specified site — *see* Neoplasm, benign, by site
  unspecified site D27.9
Cystadenoma (*see also* Neoplasm, benign, by site)
  bile duct D13.4
  endometrioid — *see* Neoplasm, benign, by site
    borderline malignancy — *see* Neoplasm, uncertain behavior, by site
  malignant — *see* Neoplasm, malignant, by site
  mucinous
    borderline malignancy
      ovary C56.- ☑
      specified site NEC — *see* Neoplasm, uncertain behavior, by site
      unspecified site C56.9
    papillary
      borderline malignancy
        ovary C56.- ☑
        specified site NEC — *see* Neoplasm, uncertain behavior, by site
        unspecified site C56.9
      specified site — *see* Neoplasm, benign, by site
      unspecified site D27.9
    specified site — *see* Neoplasm, benign, by site
    unspecified site D27.9
  papillary
    borderline malignancy
      ovary C56.- ☑
      specified site NEC — *see* Neoplasm, uncertain behavior, by site
      unspecified site C56.9
    lymphomatosum
      specified site — *see* Neoplasm, benign, by site
      unspecified site D11.9
    mucinous
      borderline malignancy
        ovary C56.- ☑
        specified site NEC — *see* Neoplasm, uncertain behavior, by site
        unspecified site C56.9
      specified site — *see* Neoplasm, benign, by site
      unspecified site D27.9
    pseudomucinous
      borderline malignancy
        ovary C56.- ☑
        specified site NEC — *see* Neoplasm, uncertain behavior, by site
        unspecified site C56.9
      specified site — *see* Neoplasm, benign, by site
      unspecified site D27.9
    serous
      borderline malignancy
        ovary C56.- ☑
        specified site NEC — *see* Neoplasm, uncertain behavior, by site
        unspecified site C56.9
      specified site — *see* Neoplasm, benign, by site
      unspecified site D27.9
    specified site — *see* Neoplasm, benign, by site
    unspecified site D27.9
  pseudomucinous
    borderline malignancy
      ovary C56.- ☑
      specified site NEC — *see* Neoplasm, uncertain behavior, by site
      unspecified site C56.9
    papillary
      borderline malignancy
        ovary C56.- ☑
        specified site NEC — *see* Neoplasm, uncertain behavior, by site
        unspecified site C56.9
      specified site — *see* Neoplasm, benign, by site
      unspecified site D27.9
    specified site — *see* Neoplasm, benign, by site

Cystadenoma — *continued*
  pseudomucinous — *continued*
    unspecified site D27.9
  serous
    borderline malignancy
      ovary C56.- ☑
      specified site NEC — *see* Neoplasm, uncertain
          behavior, by site
      unspecified site C56.9
    papillary
      borderline malignancy
        ovary C56.- ☑
        specified site NEC — *see* Neoplasm, uncertain
            behavior, by site
        unspecified site C56.9
      specified site — *see* Neoplasm, benign, by site
      unspecified site D27.9
    specified site — *see* Neoplasm, benign, by site
    unspecified site D27.9
Cystathionine synthase deficiency E72.11
Cystathioninemia E72.19
Cystathioninuria E72.19
Cystic (*see also* condition)
  breast (chronic) — *see* Mastopathy, cystic
  corpora lutea (hemorrhagic) N83.1- ☑
  duct — *see* condition
  eyeball (congenital) Q11.0
  fibrosis — *see* Fibrosis, cystic
  kidney (congenital) Q61.9
    adult type Q61.2
    infantile type NEC Q61.19
      collecting duct dilatation Q61.11
    medullary Q61.5
  liver, congenital Q44.6
  lung disease J98.4
    congenital Q33.0
  mastitis, chronic — *see* Mastopathy, cystic
  medullary, kidney Q61.5
  meniscus — *see* Derangement, knee, meniscus, cystic
  ovary N83.20- ☑
Cysticercosis, cysticerciasis B69.9
  with
    epileptiform fits B69.0
    myositis B69.81
  brain B69.0
  central nervous system B69.0
  cerebral B69.0
  ocular B69.1
  specified NEC B69.89
Cysticercus cellulose infestation — *see* Cysticercosis
Cystinosis (malignant) E72.04
Cystinuria E72.01
Cystitis (exudative) (hemorrhagic) (septic) (suppurative)
    N30.90
  with
    fibrosis — *see* Cystitis, chronic, interstitial

Cystitis — *continued*
  with — *continued*
    hematuria N30.91
    leukoplakia — *see* Cystitis, chronic, interstitial
    malakoplakia — *see* Cystitis, chronic, interstitial
    metaplasia — *see* Cystitis, chronic, interstitial
    prostatitis N41.3
  acute N30.00
    with hematuria N30.01
    of trigone N30.30
      with hematuria N30.31
  allergic — *see* Cystitis, specified type NEC
  amebic A06.81
  bilharzial B65.9 [N33]
  blennorrhagic (gonococcal) A54.01
  bullous — *see* Cystitis, specified type NEC
  calculous N21.0
  chlamydial A56.01
  chronic N30.20
    with hematuria N30.21
    interstitial N30.10
      with hematuria N30.11
    of trigone N30.30
      with hematuria N30.31
    specified NEC N30.20
      with hematuria N30.21
  cystic (a) — *see* Cystitis, specified type NEC
  diphtheritic A36.85
  echinococcal
    granulosus B67.39
    multilocularis B67.69
  emphysematous — *see* Cystitis, specified type NEC
  encysted — *see* Cystitis, specified type NEC
  eosinophilic — *see* Cystitis, specified type NEC
  follicular — *see* Cystitis, of trigone
  gangrenous — *see* Cystitis, specified type NEC
  glandularis — *see* Cystitis, specified type NEC
  gonococcal A54.01
  incrusted — *see* Cystitis, specified type NEC
  interstitial (chronic) — *see* Cystitis, chronic, interstitial
  irradiation N30.40
    with hematuria N30.41
  irritation — *see* Cystitis, specified type NEC
  malignant — *see* Cystitis, specified type NEC
  of trigone N30.30
    with hematuria N30.31
  panmural — *see* Cystitis, chronic, interstitial
  polyposa — *see* Cystitis, specified type NEC
  prostatic N41.3
  puerperal (postpartum) O86.22
  radiation — *see* Cystitis, irradiation
  specified type NEC N30.80
    with hematuria N30.81
  subacute — *see* Cystitis, chronic
  submucous — *see* Cystitis, chronic, interstitial
  syphilitic (late) A52.76

Cystitis — *continued*
  trichomonal A59.03
  tuberculous A18.12
  ulcerative — *see* Cystitis, chronic, interstitial
Cystocele (-urethrocele)
  female N81.10
    with prolapse of uterus — *see* Prolapse, uterus
    lateral N81.12
    midline N81.11
    paravaginal N81.12
  in pregnancy or childbirth O34.8- ☑
    causing obstructed labor O65.5
  male N32.89
Cystolithiasis N21.0
Cystoma (*see also* Neoplasm, benign, by site)
  endometrial, ovary N80.1
  mucinous
    specified site — *see* Neoplasm, benign, by site
    unspecified site D27.9
  serous
    specified site — *see* Neoplasm, benign, by site
    unspecified site D27.9
  simple (ovary) N83.29- ☑
Cystoplegia N31.2
Cystoptosis N32.89
Cystopyelitis — *see* Pyelonephritis
Cystorrhagia N32.89
Cystosarcoma phyllodes D48.6- ☑
  benign D24- ☑
  malignant — *see* Neoplasm, breast, malignant
Cystostomy
  attention to Z43.5
  complication — *see* Complications, cystostomy
  status Z93.50
    appendico-vesicostomy Z93.52
    cutaneous Z93.51
    specified NEC Z93.59
Cystourethritis — *see* Urethritis
Cystourethrocele (*see also* Cystocele)
  female N81.10
    with uterine prolapse — *see* Prolapse, uterus
    lateral N81.12
    midline N81.11
    paravaginal N81.12
  male N32.89
Cytomegalic inclusion disease
  congenital P35.1
Cytomegalovirus infection B25.9
Cytomycosis (reticuloendothelial) B39.4
Cytopenia D75.9
  refractory
    with multilineage dysplasia D46.A (*following* D46.2)
      and ring sideroblasts (RCMD RS) D46.B (*following*
          D46.2)
Czerny's disease (periodic hydrarthrosis of the knee) —
    see Effusion, joint, knee

D

Da Costa's syndrome F45.8
Daae (-Finsen) **disease** (epidemic pleurodynia) B33.Ø
Dabney's grip B33.Ø
Dacryoadenitis, dacryadenitis HØ4.ØØ- ☑
  acute HØ4.Ø1- ☑
  chronic HØ4.Ø2- ☑
Dacryocystitis HØ4.3Ø- ☑
  acute HØ4.32- ☑
  chronic HØ4.41- ☑
  neonatal P39.1
  phlegmonous HØ4.31- ☑
  syphilitic A52.71
    congenital (early) A5Ø.Ø1
  trachomatous, active A71.1
    sequelae (late effect) B94.Ø
Dacryocystoblenorrhea — *see* Inflammation, lacrimal, passages, chronic
Dacryocystocele — *see* Disorder, lacrimal system, changes
Dacryolith, dacryolithiasis HØ4.51- ☑
Dacryoma — *see* Disorder, lacrimal system, changes
Dacryopericystitis — *see* Dacryocystitis
Dacryops HØ4.11- ☑
Dacryostenosis (*see also* Stenosis, lacrimal)
  congenital Q1Ø.5
Dactylitis
  bone — *see* Osteomyelitis
  sickle-cell D57.ØØ
    Hb C D57.219
    Hb SS D57.ØØ
    specified NEC D57.819
  skin LØ8.9
  syphilitic A52.77
  tuberculous A18.Ø3
Dactylolysis spontanea (ainhum) L94.6
Dactylosymphysis Q7Ø.9
  fingers — *see* Syndactylism, complex, fingers
  toes — *see* Syndactylism, complex, toes
Damage
  arteriosclerotic — *see* Arteriosclerosis
  brain (nontraumatic) G93.9
    anoxic, hypoxic G93.1
      resulting from a procedure G97.82
    child NEC G8Ø.9
    due to birth injury P11.2
  cardiorenal (vascular) — *see* Hypertension, cardiorenal
  cerebral NEC — *see* Damage, brain
  coccyx, complicating delivery O71.6
  coronary — *see* Disease, heart, ischemic
  eye, birth injury P15.3
  liver (nontraumatic) K76.9
    alcoholic K7Ø.9
    due to drugs — *see* Disease, liver, toxic
    toxic — *see* Disease, liver, toxic
  medication T88.7 ☑
  pelvic
    joint or ligament, during delivery O71.6
    organ NEC
      during delivery O71.5
      following ectopic or molar pregnancy OØ8.6
  renal — *see* Disease, renal
  subendocardium, subendocardial — *see* Degeneration, myocardial
  vascular I99.9
Dana-Putnam syndrome (subacute combined sclerosis with pernicious anemia) — *see* Degeneration, combined
Danbolt (-Cross) **syndrome** (acrodermatitis enteropathica) E83.2
Dandruff L21.Ø
Dandy-Walker syndrome QØ3.1
  with spina bifida — *see* Spina bifida
Danlos' syndrome Q79.6
Darier (-White) **disease** (congenital) Q82.8
  meaning erythema annulare centrifugum L53.1
Darier-Roussy sarcoid D86.3
Darling's disease or histoplasmosis B39.4
Darwin's tubercle Q17.8
Dawson's (inclusion body) **encephalitis** A81.1

De Beurmann (-Gougerot) **disease** B42.1
De la Tourette's syndrome F95.2
De Lange's syndrome Q87.1
De Morgan's spots (senile angiomas) I78.1
De Quervain's
  disease (tendon sheath) M65.4
  syndrome E34.51
  thyroiditis (subacute granulomatous thyroiditis) EØ6.1
De Toni-Fanconi (-Debré) **syndrome** E72.Ø9
  with cystinosis E72.Ø4
Dead
  fetus, retained (mother) O36.4 ☑
    early pregnancy OØ2.1
  labyrinth H83.2 ☑
  ovum, retained OØ2.Ø
Deaf nonspeaking NEC H91.3
Deafmutism (acquired) (congenital) NEC H91.3
  hysterical F44.6
  syphilitic, congenital (*see also* subcategory) H94.8 A5Ø.Ø9
Deafness (acquired) (complete) (hereditary) (partial) H91.9- ☑
  with blue sclera and fragility of bone Q78.Ø
  auditory fatigue — *see* Deafness, specified type NEC
  aviation T7Ø.Ø ☑
    nerve injury — *see* Injury, nerve, acoustic, specified type NEC
  boilermaker's H83.3 ☑
  central — *see* Deafness, sensorineural
  conductive H9Ø.2
    and sensorineural
      mixed H9Ø.8
        bilateral H9Ø.6
    bilateral H9Ø.Ø
    unilateral H9Ø.1- ☑
      with restricted hearing on the contralateral side H9Ø.A- ☑
  congenital H9Ø.5
    with blue sclera and fragility of bone Q78.Ø
  due to toxic agents — *see* Deafness, ototoxic
  emotional (hysterical) F44.6
  functional (hysterical) F44.6
  high frequency H91.9- ☑
  hysterical F44.6
  low frequency H91.9- ☑
  mental R48.8
  mixed conductive and sensorineural H9Ø.8
    bilateral H9Ø.6
    unilateral H9Ø.7- ☑
  nerve — *see* Deafness, sensorineural
  neural — *see* Deafness, sensorineural
  noise-induced (*see also* subcategory) H83.3 ☑
    nerve injury — *see* Injury, nerve, acoustic, specified type NEC
  nonspeaking H91.3
  ototoxic H91.Ø ☑
  perceptive — *see* Deafness, sensorineural
  psychogenic (hysterical) F44.6
  sensorineural H9Ø.5
    and conductive
      bilateral H9Ø.6
      mixed H9Ø.8
        bilateral H9Ø.6
    bilateral H9Ø.3
    unilateral H9Ø.4- ☑
      with restricted hearing on the contralateral side H9Ø.A- ☑
  sensory — *see* Deafness, sensorineural
  specified type NEC H91.8 ☑
  sudden (idiopathic) H91.2- ☑
  syphilitic A52.15
  transient ischemic H93.Ø1- ☑
  traumatic — *see* Injury, nerve, acoustic, specified type NEC
  word (developmental) H93.25
Death (cause unknown) (of) (unexplained) (unspecified cause) R99
  brain G93.82
  cardiac (sudden) (with successful resuscitation) — *code to* underlying disease
    family history of Z82.41
    personal history of Z86.74

Death — *continued*
  family member (assumed) Z63.4
Debility (chronic) (general) (nervous) R53.81
  congenital or neonatal NOS P96.9
  nervous R53.81
  old age R54
  senile R54
Débove's disease (splenomegaly) R16.1
Decalcification
  bone — *see* Osteoporosis
  teeth KØ3.89
Decapsulation, kidney N28.89
Decay
  dental — *see* Caries, dental
  senile R54
  tooth, teeth — *see* Caries, dental
Deciduitis (acute)
  following ectopic or molar pregnancy OØ8.Ø
Decline (general) — *see* Debility
  cognitive, age-associated R41.81
Decompensation
  cardiac (acute) (chronic) — *see* Disease, heart
  cardiovascular — *see* Disease, cardiovascular
  heart — *see* Disease, heart
  hepatic — *see* Failure, hepatic
  myocardial (acute) (chronic) — *see* Disease, heart
  respiratory J98.8
Decompression sickness T7Ø.3 ☑
Decrease (d)
  absolute neutrophile count — *see* Neutropenia
  blood
    platelets — *see* Thrombocytopenia
    pressure RØ3.1
      due to shock following
        injury T79.4 ☑
        operation T81.19 ☑
  estrogen E28.39
    postablative E89.4Ø
      asymptomatic E89.4Ø
      symptomatic E89.41
  fragility of erythrocytes D58.8
  function
    lipase (pancreatic) K9Ø.3
    ovary in hypopituitarism E23.Ø
    parenchyma of pancreas K86.89
    pituitary (gland) (anterior) (lobe) E23.Ø
      posterior (lobe) E23.Ø
  functional activity R68.89
  glucose R73.Ø9
  hematocrit R71.Ø
  hemoglobin R71.Ø
  leukocytes D72.819
    specified NEC D72.818
  libido R68.82
  lymphocytes D72.81Ø
  platelets D69.6
  respiration, due to shock following injury T79.4 ☑
  sexual desire R68.82
  tear secretion NEC — *see* Syndrome, dry eye
  tolerance
    fat K9Ø.49
    glucose R73.Ø9
    pancreatic K9Ø.3
    salt and water E87.8
  vision NEC H54.7
  white blood cell count D72.819
    specified NEC D72.818
Decubitus (ulcer) — *see* Ulcer, pressure, by site
  cervix N86
Deepening acetabulum — *see* Derangement, joint, specified type NEC, hip
Defect, defective Q89.9
  3-beta-hydroxysteroid dehydrogenase E25.Ø
  11-hydroxylase E25.Ø
  21-hydroxylase E25.Ø
  abdominal wall, congenital Q79.59
  antibody immunodeficiency D8Ø.9
  aorticopulmonary septum Q21.4
  atrial septal (ostium secundum type) Q21.1
    following acute myocardial infarction (current complication) I23.1
    ostium primum type Q21.2

Defect, defective — *continued*
  atrioventricular
    canal Q21.2
    septum Q21.2
  auricular septal Q21.1
  bilirubin excretion NEC E80.6
  biosynthesis, androgen (testicular) E29.1
  bulbar septum Q21.0
  catalase E80.3
  cell membrane receptor complex (CR3) D71
  circulation I99.9
    congenital Q28.9
    newborn Q28.9
  coagulation (factor) (*see also* Deficiency, factor) D68.9
    with
      ectopic pregnancy O08.1
      molar pregnancy O08.1
    acquired D68.4
    antepartum with hemorrhage — *see* Hemorrhage, antepartum, with coagulation defect
    due to
      liver disease D68.4
      vitamin K deficiency D68.4
    hereditary NEC D68.2
    intrapartum O67.0
    newborn, transient P61.6
    postpartum O99.13
      with hemorrhage O72.3
    specified type NEC D68.8
  complement system D84.1
  conduction (heart) I45.9
    bone — *see* Deafness, conductive
  congenital, organ or site not listed — *see* Anomaly, by site
  coronary sinus Q21.1
  cushion, endocardial Q21.2
  degradation, glycoprotein E77.1
  dental bridge, crown, fillings — *see* Defect, dental restoration
  dental restoration K08.50
    specified NEC K08.59
  dentin (hereditary) K00.5
  Descemet's membrane, congenital Q13.89
  developmental (*see also* Anomaly)
    cauda equina Q06.3
  diaphragm
    with elevation, eventration or hernia — *see* Hernia, diaphragm
    congenital Q79.1
      with hernia Q79.0
      gross (with hernia) Q79.0
  ectodermal, congenital Q82.9
  Eisenmenger's Q21.8
  enzyme
    catalase E80.3
    peroxidase E80.3
  esophagus, congenital Q39.9
  extensor retinaculum M62.89
  fibrin polymerization D68.2
  filling
    bladder R93.41
    kidney R93.42- ☑
    renal pelvis R93.41
    stomach R93.3
    ureter R93.41
    urinary organs, specified NEC R93.49
  GABA (gamma aminobutyric acid) metabolic E72.81
  Gerbode Q21.0
  glycoprotein degradation E77.1
  Hageman (factor) D68.2
  hearing — *see* Deafness
  high grade F70
  interatrial septal Q21.1
  interauricular septal Q21.1
  interventricular septal Q21.0
    with dextroposition of aorta, pulmonary stenosis and hypertrophy of right ventricle Q21.3
    in tetralogy of Fallot Q21.3
  learning (specific) — *see* Disorder, learning
  lymphocyte function antigen-1 (LFA-1) D84.0
  lysosomal enzyme, post-translational modification E77.0
  major osseous M89.70
    ankle M89.77- ☑
    carpus M89.74- ☑
    clavicle M89.71- ☑
    femur M89.75- ☑
    fibula M89.76- ☑

Defect, defective — *continued*
  major osseous — *continued*
    fingers M89.74- ☑
    foot M89.77- ☑
    forearm M89.73- ☑
    hand M89.74- ☑
    humerus M89.72- ☑
    lower leg M89.76- ☑
    metacarpus M89.74- ☑
    metatarsus M89.77- ☑
    multiple sites M89.79
    pelvic region M89.75- ☑
    pelvis M89.75- ☑
    radius M89.73- ☑
    scapula M89.71- ☑
    shoulder region M89.71- ☑
    specified NEC M89.78
    tarsus M89.77- ☑
    thigh M89.75- ☑
    tibia M89.76- ☑
    toes M89.77- ☑
    ulna M89.73- ☑
  mental — *see* Disability, intellectual
  modification, lysosomal enzymes, post-translational E77.0
  obstructive, congenital
    renal pelvis Q62.39
    ureter Q62.39
      atresia — *see* Atresia, ureter
      cecoureterocele Q62.32
      megaureter Q62.2
      orthotopic ureterocele Q62.31
  osseous, major M89.70
    ankle M89.77- ☑
    carpus M89.74- ☑
    clavicle M89.71- ☑
    femur M89.75- ☑
    fibula M89.76- ☑
    fingers M89.74- ☑
    foot M89.77- ☑
    forearm M89.73- ☑
    hand M89.74- ☑
    humerus M89.72- ☑
    lower leg M89.76- ☑
    metacarpus M89.74- ☑
    metatarsus M89.77- ☑
    multiple sites M89.9
    pelvic region M89.75- ☑
    pelvis M89.75- ☑
    radius M89.73- ☑
    scapula M89.71- ☑
    shoulder region M89.71- ☑
    specified NEC M89.78
    tarsus M89.77- ☑
    thigh M89.75- ☑
    tibia M89.76- ☑
    toes M89.77- ☑
    ulna M89.73- ☑
  osteochondral NEC (*see also* Deformity) M95.8
  ostium
    primum Q21.2
    secundum Q21.1
  peroxidase E80.3
  placental blood supply — *see* Insufficiency, placental
  platelets, qualitative D69.1
    constitutional D68.0
  postural NEC, spine — *see* Dorsopathy, deforming
  reduction
    limb Q73.8
      lower Q72.9- ☑
        absence — *see* Agenesis, leg
          foot — *see* Agenesis, foot
        longitudinal
          femur Q72.4- ☑
          fibula Q72.6- ☑
          tibia Q72.5- ☑
        specified type NEC Q72.89- ☑
        split foot Q72.7- ☑
      specified type NEC Q73.8
      upper Q71.9- ☑
        absence — *see* Agenesis, arm
          forearm — *see* Agenesis, forearm
          hand — *see* Agenesis, hand
        lobster-claw hand Q71.6- ☑
        longitudinal
          radius Q71.4- ☑

Defect, defective — *continued*
  reduction — *continued*
    limb — *continued*
      upper — *continued*
        longitudinal — *continued*
          ulna Q71.5- ☑
        specified type NEC Q71.89- ☑
  renal pelvis Q63.8
    obstructive Q62.39
  respiratory system, congenital Q34.9
  restoration, dental K08.50
    specified NEC K08.59
  retinal nerve bundle fibers H35.89
  septal (heart) NOS Q21.9
    acquired (atrial) (auricular) (ventricular) (old) I51.0
    atrial Q21.1
      concurrent with acute myocardial infarction — *see* Infarct, myocardium
      following acute myocardial infarction (current complication) I23.1
    ventricular (*see also* Defect, ventricular septal) Q21.0
  sinus venosus Q21.1
  speech R47.9
    developmental F80.9
    specified NEC R47.89
  Taussig-Bing (aortic transposition and overriding pulmonary artery) Q20.1
  teeth, wedge K03.1
  vascular (local) I99.9
    congenital Q27.9
  ventricular septal Q21.0
    concurrent with acute myocardial infarction — *see* Infarct, myocardium
    following acute myocardial infarction (current complication) I23.2
    in tetralogy of Fallot Q21.3
  vision NEC H54.7
  visual field H53.40
    bilateral
      heteronymous H53.47
      homonymous H53.46- ☑
    generalized contraction H53.48- ☑
    localized
      arcuate H53.43- ☑
      scotoma (central area) H53.41- ☑
        blind spot area H53.42- ☑
      sector H53.43- ☑
      specified type NEC H53.45- ☑
  voice R49.9
    specified NEC R49.8
  wedge, tooth, teeth (abrasion) K03.1
Deferentitis N49.1
  gonorrheal (acute) (chronic) A54.23
Defibrination (syndrome) D65
  antepartum — *see* Hemorrhage, antepartum, with coagulation defect, disseminated intravascular coagulation
  following ectopic or molar pregnancy O08.1
  intrapartum O67.0
  newborn P60
  postpartum O72.3
Deficiency, deficient
  3-beta hydroxysteroid dehydrogenase E25.0
  5-alpha reductase (with male pseudohermaphroditism) E29.1
  11-hydroxylase E25.0
  21-hydroxylase E25.0
  abdominal muscle syndrome Q79.4
  AC globulin (congenital) (hereditary) D68.2
    acquired D68.4
  accelerator globulin (Ac G) (blood) D68.2
  acid phosphatase E83.39
  activating factor (blood) D68.2
  adenosine deaminase (ADA) D81.3
  aldolase (hereditary) E74.19
  alpha-1-antitrypsin E88.01
  amino-acids E72.9
  anemia — *see* Anemia
  aneurin E51.9
  antibody with
    hyperimmunoglobulinemia D80.6
    near-normal immunoglobins D80.6
  antidiuretic hormone E23.2
  anti-hemophilic
    factor (A) D66
      B D67
      C D68.1
    globulin (AHG) NEC D66

Deficiency, deficient — *continued*
  antithrombin (antithrombin III) D68.59
  ascorbic acid E54
  attention (disorder) (syndrome) F98.8
    with hyperactivity — *see* Disorder, attention-deficit
        hyperactivity
  autoprothrombin
    C D68.2
    I D68.2
    II D67
  beta-glucuronidase E76.29
  biotin E53.8
  biotin-dependent carboxylase D81.819
  biotinidase D81.810
  brancher enzyme (amylopectinosis) E74.03
  C1 esterase inhibitor (C1-INH) D84.1
  calciferol E55.9
    with
        adult osteomalacia M83.8
        rickets — *see* Rickets
  calcium (dietary) E58
  calorie, severe E43
    with marasmus E41
        and kwashiorkor E42
  cardiac — *see* Insufficiency, myocardial
  carnitine E71.40
    due to
        hemodialysis E71.43
        inborn errors of metabolism E71.42
        Valproic acid therapy E71.43
    iatrogenic E71.43
    muscle palmityltransferase E71.314
    primary E71.41
    secondary E71.448
  carotene E50.9
  central nervous system G96.8
  ceruloplasmin (Wilson) E83.01
  choline E53.8
  Christmas factor D67
  chromium E61.4
  clotting (blood) (*see also* Deficiency, coagulation factor)
      D68.9
  clotting factor NEC (hereditary) (*see also* Deficiency,
      factor) D68.2
  coagulation NOS D68.9
    with
        ectopic pregnancy O08.1
        molar pregnancy O08.1
    acquired (any) D68.4
    antepartum hemorrhage — *see* Hemorrhage, an-
        tepartum, with coagulation defect
    clotting factor NEC (*see also* Deficiency, factor) D68.2
    due to
        hyperprothrombinemia D68.4
        liver disease D68.4
        vitamin K deficiency D68.4
    newborn, transient P61.6
    postpartum O72.3
    specified NEC D68.8
  cognitive F09
  color vision H53.50
    achromatopsia H53.51
    acquired H53.52
    deuteranomaly H53.53
    protanomaly H53.54
    specified type NEC H53.59
    tritanomaly H53.55
  combined glucocorticoid and mineralocorticoid E27.49
  contact factor D68.2
  copper (nutritional) E61.0
  corticoadrenal E27.40
    primary E27.1
  craniofacial axis Q75.0
  cyanocobalamin E53.8
  debrancher enzyme (limit dextrinosis) E74.03
  dehydrogenase
    long chain/very long chain acyl CoA E71.310
    medium chain acyl CoA E71.311
    short chain acyl CoA E71.312
  diet E63.9
  dihydropyrimidine dehydrogenase (DPD) E88.89
  disaccharidase E73.9
  edema — *see* Malnutrition, severe
  endocrine E34.9
  energy-supply — *see* Malnutrition
  enzymes, circulating NEC E88.09
  ergosterol E55.9

Deficiency, deficient — *continued*
  ergosterol — *continued*
    with
        adult osteomalacia M83.8
        rickets — *see* Rickets
  essential fatty acid (EFA) E63.0
  factor (*see also* Deficiency, coagulation)
    Hageman D68.2
    I (congenital) (hereditary) D68.2
    II (congenital) (hereditary) D68.2
    IX (congenital) (functional) (hereditary) (with func-
        tional defect) D67
    multiple (congenital) D68.8
        acquired D68.4
    V (congenital) (hereditary) D68.2
    VII (congenital) (hereditary) D68.2
    VIII (congenital) (functional) (hereditary) (with
        functional defect) D66
        with vascular defect D68.0
    X (congenital) (hereditary) D68.2
    XI (congenital) (hereditary) D68.1
    XII (congenital) (hereditary) D68.2
    XIII (congenital) (hereditary) D68.2
  femoral, proximal focal (congenital) — *see* Defect, re-
      duction, lower limb, longitudinal, femur
  fibrinase D68.2
  fibrinogen (congenital) (hereditary) D68.2
    acquired D65
  fibrin-stabilizing factor (congenital) (hereditary) D68.2
    acquired D68.4
  folate E53.8
  folic acid E53.8
  foreskin N47.3
  fructokinase E74.11
  fructose 1,6-diphosphatase E74.19
  fructose-1-phosphate aldolase E74.19
  GABA (gamma aminobutyric acid) transaminase E72.81
  GABA-T (gamma aminobutyric acid transaminase)
      E72.81
  galactokinase E74.29
  galactose-1-phosphate uridyl transferase E74.29
  gammaglobulin in blood D80.1
    hereditary D80.0
  glass factor D68.2
  glucocorticoid E27.49
    mineralocorticoid E27.49
  glucose-6-phosphatase E74.01
  glucose-6-phosphate dehydrogenase anemia D55.0
  glucuronyl transferase E80.5
  glycogen synthetase E74.09
  gonadotropin (isolated) E23.0
  growth hormone (idiopathic) (isolated) E23.0
  Hageman factor D68.2
  hemoglobin D64.9
  hepatophosphorylase E74.09
  homogentisate 1,2-dioxygenase E70.29
  hormone
    anterior pituitary (partial) NEC E23.0
        growth E23.0
    growth (isolated) E23.0
    pituitary E23.0
    testicular E29.1
  hypoxanthine- (guanine)-phosphoribosyltransferase
      (HG- PRT) (total H-PRT) E79.1
  immunity D84.9
    cell-mediated D84.8
        with thrombocytopenia and eczema D82.0
    combined D81.9
    humoral D80.9
    IgA (secretory) D80.2
    IgG D80.3
    IgM D80.4
  immuno — *see* Immunodeficiency
  immunoglobulin, selective
    A (IgA) D80.2
    G (IgG) (subclasses) D80.3
    M (IgM) D80.4
  inositol (B complex) E53.8
  intrinsic
    factor (congenital) D51.0
    sphincter N36.42
        with urethral hypermobility N36.43
  iodine E61.8
    congenital syndrome — *see* Syndrome, iodine-defi-
        ciency, congenital
  iron E61.1
    anemia D50.9
  kalium E87.6
  kappa-light chain D80.8

Deficiency, deficient — *continued*
  labile factor (congenital) (hereditary) D68.2
    acquired D68.4
  lacrimal fluid (acquired) (*see also* Syndrome, dry eye)
    congenital Q10.6
  lactase
    congenital E73.0
    secondary E73.1
  Laki-Lorand factor D68.2
  lecithin cholesterol acyltransferase E78.6
  lipocaic K86.89
  lipoprotein (familial) (high density) E78.6
  liver phosphorylase E74.09
  lysosomal alpha-1, 4 glucosidase E74.02
  magnesium E61.2
  major histocompatibility complex
    class I D81.6
    class II D81.7
  manganese E61.3
  menadione (vitamin K) E56.1
    newborn P53
  mental (familial) (hereditary) — *see* Disability, intellec-
      tual
  methylenetetrahydrofolate reductase (MTHFR) E72.12
  mevalonate kinase M04.1
  mineralocorticoid E27.49
    with glucocorticoid E27.49
  mineral NEC E61.8
  molybdenum (nutritional) E61.5
  moral F60.2
  multiple nutrient elements E61.7
  multiple sulfatase (MSD) E75.26
  muscle
    carnitine (palmityltransferase) E71.314
    phosphofructokinase E74.09
  myoadenylate deaminase E79.2
  myocardial — *see* Insufficiency, myocardial
  myophosphorylase E74.04
  NADH diaphorase or reductase (congenital) D74.0
  NADH-methemoglobin reductase (congenital) D74.0
  natrium E87.1
  niacin (amide) (-tryptophan) E52
  nicotinamide E52
  nicotinic acid E52
  number of teeth — *see* Anodontia
  nutrient element E61.9
    multiple E61.7
    specified NEC E61.8
  nutrition, nutritional E63.9
    sequelae — *see* Sequelae, nutritional deficiency
    specified NEC E63.8
  of interleukin 1 receptor antagonist [DIRA] M04.8
  ornithine transcarbamylase E72.4
  ovarian E28.39
  oxygen — *see* Anoxia
  pantothenic acid E53.8
  parathyroid (gland) E20.9
  perineum (female) N81.89
  phenylalanine hydroxylase E70.1
  phosphoenolpyruvate carboxykinase E74.4
  phosphofructokinase E74.19
  phosphomannomutase E74.8
  phosphomannose isomerase E74.8
  phosphomannosyl mutase E74.8
  phosphorylase kinase, liver E74.09
  pituitary hormone (isolated) E23.0
  plasma thromboplastin
    antecedent (PTA) D68.1
    component (PTC) D67
  plasminogen (type 1) (type 2) E88.02
  platelet NEC D69.1
    constitutional D68.0
  polyglandular E31.8
    autoimmune E31.0
  potassium (K) E87.6
  prepuce N47.3
  proaccelerin (congenital) (hereditary) D68.2
    acquired D68.4
  proconvertin factor (congenital) (hereditary) D68.2
    acquired D68.4
  protein (*see also* Malnutrition) E46
    anemia D53.0
    C D68.59
    S D68.59
  prothrombin (congenital) (hereditary) D68.2
    acquired D68.4
  Prower factor D68.2
  pseudocholinesterase E88.09

Deficiency, deficient — *continued*
PTA (plasma thromboplastin antecedent) D68.1
PTC (plasma thromboplastin component) D67
purine nucleoside phosphorylase (PNP) D81.5
pyracin (alpha) (beta) E53.1
pyridoxal E53.1
pyridoxamine E53.1
pyridoxine (derivatives) E53.1
pyruvate
    carboxylase E74.4
    dehydrogenase E74.4
riboflavin (vitamin B2) E53.Ø
salt E87.1
secretion
    ovary E28.39
    salivary gland (any) K11.7
    urine R34
selenium (dietary) E59
serum antitrypsin, familial E88.Ø1
short stature homeobox gene (SHOX)
    with
        dyschondrosteosis Q78.8
        short stature (idiopathic) E34.3
        Turner's syndrome Q96.9
sodium (Na) E87.1
SPCA (factor VII) D68.2
sphincter, intrinsic N36.42
    with urethral hypermobility N36.43
stable factor (congenital) (hereditary) D68.2
    acquired D68.4
Stuart-Prower (factor X) D68.2
succinic semialdehyde dehydrogenase E72.81
sucrase E74.39
sulfatase E75.26
sulfite oxidase E72.19
thiamin, thiaminic (chloride) E51.9
    beriberi (dry) E51.11
        wet E51.12
thrombokinase D68.2
    newborn P53
thyroid (gland) — *see* Hypothyroidism
tocopherol E56.Ø
tooth bud KØØ.Ø
transcobalamine II (anemia) D51.2
vanadium E61.6
vascular I99.9
vasopressin E23.2
vertical ridge KØ6.8
viosterol — *see* Deficiency, calciferol
vitamin (multiple) NOS E56.9
    A E5Ø.9
        with
            Bitot's spot (corneal) E5Ø.1
            follicular keratosis E5Ø.8
            keratomalacia E5Ø.4
            manifestations NEC E5Ø.8
            night blindness E5Ø.5
            scar of cornea, xerophthalmic E5Ø.6
            xeroderma E5Ø.8
            xerophthalmia E5Ø.7
            xerosis
                conjunctival E5Ø.Ø
                    and Bitot's spot E5Ø.1
                cornea E5Ø.2
                    and ulceration E5Ø.3
        sequelae E64.1
    B (complex) NOS E53.9
        with
            beriberi (dry) E51.11
                wet E51.12
            pellagra E52
    B1 NOS E51.9
        beriberi (dry) E51.11
            with circulatory system manifestations E51.11
                wet E51.12
    B12 E53.8
    B2 (riboflavin) E53.Ø
    B6 E53.1
    C E54
        sequelae E64.2
    D E55.9
        with
            adult osteomalacia M83.8
            rickets — *see* Rickets
            25-hydroxylase E83.32
    E E56.Ø
    folic acid E53.8
    G E53.Ø
    group B E53.9

Deficiency, deficient — *continued*
vitamin — *continued*
    group B — *continued*
        specified NEC E53.8
        H (biotin) E53.8
        K E56.1
            of newborn P53
        nicotinic E52
        P E56.8
        PP (pellagra-preventing) E52
        specified NEC E56.8
        thiamin E51.9
            beriberi — *see* Beriberi
zinc, dietary E6Ø
Deficit (*see also* Deficiency)
    attention and concentration R41.84Ø
        disorder — *see* Attention, deficit
        following
            cerebral infarction I69.31Ø
            cerebrovascular disease I69.91Ø
                specified disease NEC I69.81Ø
            nontraumatic
                intracerebral hemorrhage I69.11Ø
                specified intracranial hemorrhage NEC I69.21Ø
                subarachnoid hemorrhage I69.Ø1Ø
    cognitive
        communication R41.841
        emotional
            following
                cerebral infarction I69.315
                cerebrovascular disease I69.915
                    specified disease NEC I69.815
                nontraumatic
                    intracerebral hemorrhage I69.115
                    specified intracranial hemorrhage NEC I69.215
                    subarachnoid hemorrhage I69.Ø15
        following
            cerebral infarction I69.319
            cerebrovascular disease I69.919
                specified disease NEC I69.819
            nontraumatic
                intracerebral hemorrhage I69.119
                specified intracranial hemorrhage NEC I69.219
                subarachnoid hemorrhage I69.Ø19
        social
            following
                cerebral infarction I69.315
                cerebrovascular disease I69.915
                    specified disease NEC I69.815
                nontraumatic
                    intracerebral hemorrhage I69.115
                    specified intracranial hemorrhage NEC I69.215
                    subarachnoid hemorrhage I69.Ø15
    cognitive NEC R41.89
        following
            cerebral infarction I69.318
            cerebrovascular disease I69.918
                specified disease NEC I69.818
            nontraumatic
                intracerebral hemorrhage I69.118
                specified intracranial hemorrhage NEC I69.218
                subarachnoid hemorrhage I69.Ø18
    concentration R41.84Ø
    executive function R41.844
        following
            cerebral infarction I69.314
            cerebrovascular disease I69.914
                specified disease NEC I69.814
            nontraumatic
                intracerebral hemorrhage I69.114
                specified intracranial hemorrhage NEC I69.214
                subarachnoid hemorrhage I69.Ø14
    frontal lobe R41.844
        following
            cerebral infarction I69.314
            cerebrovascular disease I69.914
                specified disease NEC I69.814
            nontraumatic
                intracerebral hemorrhage I69.114
                specified intracranial hemorrhage NEC I69.214
                subarachnoid hemorrhage I69.Ø14
    memory
        following
            cerebral infarction I69.311
            cerebrovascular disease I69.911
                specified disease NEC I69.811

Deficit — *continued*
    memory — *continued*
        following — *continued*
            nontraumatic
                intracerebral hemorrhage I69.111
                specified intracranial hemorrhage NEC I69.211
                subarachnoid hemorrhage I69.Ø11
    neurologic NEC R29.818
        ischemic
            reversible (RIND) I63.9
                prolonged (PRIND) I63.9
    oxygen RØ9.Ø2
    prolonged reversible ischemic neurologic (PRIND) I63.9
    psychomotor R41.843
        following
            cerebral infarction I69.313
            cerebrovascular disease I69.913
                specified disease NEC I69.813
            nontraumatic
                intracerebral hemorrhage I69.113
                specified intracranial hemorrhage NEC I69.213
                subarachnoid hemorrhage I69.Ø13
    visuospatial R41.842
        following
            cerebral infarction I69.312
            cerebrovascular disease I69.912
                specified disease NEC I69.812
            nontraumatic
                intracerebral hemorrhage I69.112
                specified intracranial hemorrhage NEC I69.212
                subarachnoid hemorrhage I69.Ø12
Deflection
    radius — *see* Deformity, limb, specified type NEC, forearm
    septum (acquired) (nasal) (nose) J34.2
    spine — *see* Curvature, spine
    turbinate (nose) J34.2
Defluvium
    capillorum — *see* Alopecia
    ciliorum — *see* Madarosis
    unguium L6Ø.8
Deformity Q89.9
    abdomen, congenital Q89.9
    abdominal wall
        acquired M95.8
        congenital Q79.59
    acquired (unspecified site) M95.9
    adrenal gland Q89.1
    alimentary tract, congenital Q45.9
        upper Q4Ø.9
    ankle (joint) (acquired) (*see also* Deformity, limb, lower leg)
        abduction — *see* Contraction, joint, ankle
        congenital Q68.8
        contraction — *see* Contraction, joint, ankle
        specified type NEC — *see* Deformity, limb, foot, specified NEC
    anus (acquired) K62.89
        congenital Q43.9
    aorta (arch) (congenital) Q25.4Ø
        acquired I77.89
    aortic
        arch, acquired I77.89
        cusp or valve (congenital) Q23.8
            acquired (*see also* Endocarditis, aortic) I35.8
    arm (acquired) (upper) (*see also* Deformity, limb, upper arm)
        congenital Q68.8
        forearm — *see* Deformity, limb, forearm
    artery (congenital) (peripheral) NOS Q27.9
        acquired I77.89
        coronary (acquired) I25.9
            congenital Q24.5
        umbilical Q27.Ø
    atrial septal Q21.1
    auditory canal (external) (congenital) (*see also* Malformation, ear, external)
        acquired — *see* Disorder, ear, external, specified type NEC
    auricle
        ear (congenital) (*see also* Malformation, ear, external)
            acquired — *see* Disorder, pinna, deformity
    back — *see* Dorsopathy, deforming
    bile duct (common) (congenital) (hepatic) Q44.5
        acquired K83.8
    biliary duct or passage (congenital) Q44.5
        acquired K83.8

▽ Subterms under main terms may continue to next column or page   ☑ **Additional Character Required** — Refer to the Tabular List for Character Selection   **85**

Deficiency, deficient — Deformity

Deformity — continued

bladder (neck) (trigone) (sphincter) (acquired) N32.89
  congenital Q64.79
bone (acquired) NOS M95.9
  congenital Q79.9
  turbinate M95.0
brain (congenital) Q04.9
  acquired G93.89
  reduction Q04.3
breast (acquired) N64.89
  congenital Q83.9
  reconstructed N65.0
bronchus (congenital) Q32.4
  acquired NEC J98.09
bursa, congenital Q79.9
canaliculi (lacrimalis) (acquired) (see also Disorder, lacrimal system, changes)
  congenital Q10.6
canthus, acquired — see Disorder, eyelid, specified type NEC
capillary (acquired) I78.8
cardiovascular system, congenital Q28.9
caruncle, lacrimal (acquired) (see also Disorder, lacrimal system, changes)
  congenital Q10.6
cascade, stomach K31.2
cecum (congenital) Q43.9
  acquired K63.89
cerebral, acquired G93.89
  congenital Q04.9
cervix (uterus) (acquired) NEC N88.8
  congenital Q51.9
cheek (acquired) M95.2
  congenital Q18.9
chest (acquired) (wall) M95.4
  congenital Q67.8
  sequelae (late effect) of rickets E64.3
chin (acquired) M95.2
  congenital Q18.9
choroid (congenital) Q14.3
  acquired H31.8
  plexus Q07.8
    acquired G96.19
cicatricial — see Cicatrix
cilia, acquired — see Disorder, eyelid, specified type NEC
clavicle (acquired) M95.8
  congenital Q68.8
clitoris (congenital) Q52.6
  acquired N90.89
clubfoot — see Clubfoot
coccyx (acquired) — see subcategory M43.8 ☑
colon (congenital) Q43.9
  acquired K63.89
concha (ear), congenital (see also Malformation, ear, external)
  acquired — see Disorder, pinna, deformity
cornea (acquired) H18.70
  congenital Q13.4
  descemetocele — see Descemetocele
  ectasia — see Ectasia, cornea
  specified NEC H18.79- ☑
  staphyloma — see Staphyloma, cornea
coronary artery (acquired) I25.9
  congenital Q24.5
cranium (acquired) — see Deformity, skull
cricoid cartilage (congenital) Q31.8
  acquired J38.7
cystic duct (congenital) Q44.5
  acquired K82.8
Dandy-Walker Q03.1
  with spina bifida — see Spina bifida
diaphragm (congenital) Q79.1
  acquired J98.6
digestive organ NOS Q45.9
ductus arteriosus Q25.0
duodenal bulb K31.89
duodenum (congenital) Q43.9
  acquired K31.89
dura — see Deformity, meninges
ear (acquired) (see also Disorder, pinna, deformity)
  congenital (external) Q17.9
    internal Q16.5
    middle Q16.4
      ossicles Q16.3
    ossicles Q16.3
ectodermal (congenital) NEC Q84.9
ejaculatory duct (congenital) Q55.4

Deformity — continued

ejaculatory duct — continued
  acquired N50.89
elbow (joint) (acquired) (see also Deformity, limb, upper arm)
  congenital Q68.8
  contraction — see Contraction, joint, elbow
endocrine gland NEC Q89.2
epididymis (congenital) Q55.4
  acquired N50.89
epiglottis (congenital) Q31.8
  acquired J38.7
esophagus (congenital) Q39.9
  acquired K22.8
eustachian tube (congenital) NEC Q17.8
eye, congenital Q15.9
eyebrow (congenital) Q18.8
eyelid (acquired) (see also Disorder, eyelid, specified type NEC)
  congenital Q10.3
face (acquired) M95.2
  congenital Q18.9
fallopian tube, acquired N83.8
femur (acquired) — see Deformity, limb, specified type NEC, thigh
fetal
  with fetopelvic disproportion O33.7 ☑
  causing obstructed labor O66.3
finger (acquired) M20.00- ☑
  boutonniere M20.02- ☑
  congenital Q68.1
  flexion contracture — see Contraction, joint, hand
  mallet finger M20.01- ☑
  specified NEC M20.09- ☑
  swan-neck M20.03- ☑
flexion (joint) (acquired) (see also Deformity, limb, flexion) M21.20
  congenital NOS Q74.9
    hip Q65.89
foot (acquired) (see also Deformity, limb, lower leg)
  cavovarus (congenital) Q66.1
  congenital NOS Q66.9
    specified type NEC Q66.89
  specified type NEC — see Deformity, limb, foot, specified NEC
  valgus (congenital) Q66.6
    acquired — see Deformity, valgus, ankle
  varus (congenital) NEC Q66.3
    acquired — see Deformity, varus, ankle
forearm (acquired) (see also Deformity, limb, forearm)
  congenital Q68.8
forehead (acquired) M95.2
  congenital Q75.8
frontal bone (acquired) M95.2
  congenital Q75.8
gallbladder (congenital) Q44.1
  acquired K82.8
gastrointestinal tract (congenital) NOS Q45.9
  acquired K63.89
genitalia, genital organ(s) or system NEC
  female (congenital) Q52.9
    acquired N94.89
    external Q52.70
  male (congenital) Q55.9
    acquired N50.89
globe (eye) (congenital) Q15.8
  acquired H44.89
gum, acquired NEC K06.8
hand (acquired) — see Deformity, limb, hand
  congenital Q68.1
head (acquired) M95.2
  congenital Q75.8
heart (congenital) Q24.9
  septum Q21.9
    auricular Q21.1
    ventricular Q21.0
  valve (congenital) NEC Q24.8
    acquired — see Endocarditis
heel (acquired) — see Deformity, foot
hepatic duct (congenital) Q44.5
  acquired K83.8
hip (joint) (acquired) (see also Deformity, limb, thigh)
  congenital Q65.9
  due to (previous) juvenile osteochondrosis — see Coxa, plana
  flexion — see Contraction, joint, hip
hourglass — see Contraction, hourglass
humerus (acquired) M21.82- ☑

Deformity — continued

humerus — continued
  congenital Q74.0
hypophyseal (congenital) Q89.2
ileocecal (coil) (valve) (acquired) K63.89
  congenital Q43.9
ileum (congenital) Q43.9
  acquired K63.89
ilium (acquired) M95.5
  congenital Q74.2
integument (congenital) Q84.9
intervertebral cartilage or disc (acquired) — see Disorder, disc, specified NEC
intestine (large) (small) (congenital) NOS Q43.9
  acquired K63.89
intrinsic minus or plus (hand) — see Deformity, limb, specified type NEC, forearm
iris (acquired) H21.89
  congenital Q13.2
ischium (acquired) M95.5
  congenital Q74.2
jaw (acquired) (congenital) M26.9
joint (acquired) NEC M21.90
  congenital Q68.8
  elbow M21.92- ☑
  hand M21.94- ☑
  hip M21.95- ☑
  knee M21.96- ☑
  shoulder M21.92- ☑
  wrist M21.93- ☑
kidney(s) (calyx) (pelvis) (congenital) Q63.9
  acquired N28.89
  artery (congenital) Q27.2
    acquired I77.89
Klippel-Feil (brevicollis) Q76.1
knee (acquired) NEC (see also Deformity, limb, lower leg)
  congenital Q68.2
labium (majus) (minus) (congenital) Q52.79
  acquired N90.89
lacrimal passages or duct (congenital) NEC Q10.6
  acquired — see Disorder, lacrimal system, changes
larynx (muscle) (congenital) Q31.8
  acquired J38.7
  web (glottic) Q31.0
leg (upper) (acquired) NEC (see also Deformity, limb, thigh)
  congenital Q68.8
  lower leg — see Deformity, limb, lower leg
lens (acquired) H27.8
  congenital Q12.9
lid (fold) (acquired) (see also Disorder, eyelid, specified type NEC)
  congenital Q10.3
ligament (acquired) — see Disorder, ligament
  congenital Q79.9
limb (acquired) M21.90
  clawfoot M21.53- ☑
  clawhand M21.51- ☑
  clubfoot M21.54- ☑
  clubhand M21.52- ☑
  congenital, except reduction deformity Q74.9
  flat foot M21.4- ☑
  flexion M21.20
    ankle M21.27- ☑
    elbow M21.22- ☑
    finger M21.24- ☑
    hip M21.25- ☑
    knee M21.26- ☑
    shoulder M21.21- ☑
    toe M21.27- ☑
    wrist M21.23- ☑
  foot
    claw — see Deformity, limb, clawfoot
    club — see Deformity, limb, clubfoot
    drop M21.37- ☑
    flat — see Deformity, limb, flat foot
    specified NEC M21.6X- ☑
  forearm M21.93- ☑
  hand M21.94- ☑
  lower leg M21.96- ☑
  specified type NEC M21.80
    forearm M21.83- ☑
    lower leg M21.86- ☑
    thigh M21.85- ☑
    upper arm M21.82- ☑
  thigh M21.95- ☑

Deformity — *continued*
  limb — *continued*
    unequal length M21.70
      short site is
        femur M21.75- ☑
        fibula M21.76- ☑
        humerus M21.72- ☑
        radius M21.73- ☑
        tibia M21.76- ☑
        ulna M21.73- ☑
      upper arm M21.92- ☑
    valgus — *see* Deformity, valgus
    varus — *see* Deformity, varus
    wrist drop M21.33- ☑
  lip (acquired) NEC K13.0
    congenital Q38.0
  liver (congenital) Q44.7
    acquired K76.89
  lumbosacral (congenital) (joint) (region) Q76.49
    acquired — *see* subcategory M43.8 ☑
    kyphosis — *see* Kyphosis, congenital
    lordosis — *see* Lordosis, congenital
  lung (congenital) Q33.9
    acquired J98.4
  lymphatic system, congenital Q89.9
  Madelung's (radius) Q74.0
  mandible (acquired) (congenital) M26.9
  maxilla (acquired) (congenital) M26.9
  meninges or membrane (congenital) Q07.9
    cerebral Q04.8
      acquired G96.19
    spinal cord (congenital) G96.19
      acquired G96.19
  metacarpus (acquired) — *see* Deformity, limb, forearm
    congenital Q74.0
  metatarsus (acquired) — *see* Deformity, foot
    congenital Q66.9
  middle ear (congenital) Q16.4
    ossicles Q16.3
  mitral (leaflets) (valve) I05.8
    parachute Q23.2
    stenosis, congenital Q23.2
  mouth (acquired) K13.79
    congenital Q38.6
  multiple, congenital NEC Q89.7
  muscle (acquired) M62.89
    congenital Q79.9
      sternocleidomastoid Q68.0
  musculoskeletal system (acquired) M95.9
    congenital Q79.9
    specified NEC M95.8
  nail (acquired) L60.8
    congenital Q84.6
  nasal — *see* Deformity, nose
  neck (acquired) M95.3
    congenital Q18.9
      sternocleidomastoid Q68.0
  nervous system (congenital) Q07.9
  nipple (congenital) Q83.9
    acquired N64.89
  nose (acquired) (cartilage) M95.0
    bone (turbinate) M95.0
    congenital Q30.9
      bent or squashed Q67.4
    saddle M95.0
      syphilitic A50.57
    septum (acquired) J34.2
      congenital Q30.8
    sinus (wall) (congenital) Q30.8
      acquired M95.0
    syphilitic (congenital) A50.57
      late A52.73
  ocular muscle (congenital) Q10.3
    acquired — *see* Strabismus, mechanical
  opticociliary vessels (congenital) Q13.2
  orbit (eye) (acquired) H05.30
    atrophy — *see* Atrophy, orbit
    congenital Q10.7
    due to
      bone disease NEC H05.32- ☑
      trauma or surgery H05.33- ☑
    enlargement — *see* Enlargement, orbit
    exostosis — *see* Exostosis, orbit
  organ of Corti (congenital) Q16.5
  ovary (congenital) Q50.39
    acquired N83.8
  oviduct, acquired N83.8
  palate (congenital) Q38.5

Deformity — *continued*
  palate — *continued*
    acquired M27.8
    cleft (congenital) — *see* Cleft, palate
  pancreas (congenital) Q45.3
    acquired K86.89
  parathyroid (gland) Q89.2
  parotid (gland) (congenital) Q38.4
    acquired K11.8
  patella (acquired) — *see* Disorder, patella, specified
    NEC
  pelvis, pelvic (acquired) (bony) M95.5
    with disproportion (fetopelvic) O33.0
      causing obstructed labor O65.0
    congenital Q74.2
    rachitic sequelae (late effect) E64.3
  penis (glans) (congenital) Q55.69
    acquired N48.89
  pericardium (congenital) Q24.8
    acquired — *see* Pericarditis
  pharynx (congenital) Q38.8
    acquired J39.2
  pinna, acquired (*see also* Disorder, pinna, deformity)
    congenital Q17.9
  pituitary (congenital) Q89.2
  posture — *see* Dorsopathy, deforming
  prepuce (congenital) Q55.69
    acquired N47.8
  prostate (congenital) Q55.4
    acquired N42.89
  pupil (congenital) Q13.2
    acquired — *see* Abnormality, pupillary
  pylorus (congenital) Q40.3
    acquired K31.89
  rachitic (acquired), old or healed E64.3
  radius (acquired) (*see also* Deformity, limb, forearm)
    congenital Q68.8
  rectum (congenital) Q43.9
    acquired K62.89
  reduction (extremity) (limb), congenital (*see also* con-
      dition and site) Q73.8
    brain Q04.3
    lower — *see* Defect, reduction, lower limb
    upper — *see* Defect, reduction, upper limb
  renal — *see* Deformity, kidney
  respiratory system (congenital) Q34.9
  rib (acquired) M95.4
    congenital Q76.6
    cervical Q76.5
  rotation (joint) (acquired) — *see* Deformity, limb,
      specified site NEC
    congenital Q74.9
    hip — *see* Deformity, limb, specified type NEC, thigh
      congenital Q65.89
  sacroiliac joint (congenital) — *see* subcategory Q74.2
    acquired — *see* subcategory M43.8 ☑
  sacrum (acquired) — *see* subcategory M43.8 ☑
  saddle
    back — *see* Lordosis
    nose M95.0
      syphilitic A50.57
  salivary gland or duct (congenital) Q38.4
    acquired K11.8
  scapula (acquired) M95.8
    congenital Q68.8
  scrotum (congenital) (*see also* Malformation, testis and
      scrotum)
    acquired N50.89
  seminal vesicles (congenital) Q55.4
    acquired N50.89
  septum, nasal (acquired) J34.2
  shoulder (joint) (acquired) — *see* Deformity, limb, up-
      per arm
    congenital Q74.0
    contraction — *see* Contraction, joint, shoulder
  sigmoid (flexure) (congenital) Q43.9
    acquired K63.89
  skin (congenital) Q82.9
  skull (acquired) M95.2
    congenital Q75.8
      with
        anencephaly Q00.0
        encephalocele — *see* Encephalocele
        hydrocephalus Q03.9
          with spina bifida — *see* Spina bifida, by
            site, with hydrocephalus
        microcephaly Q02

Deformity — *continued*
  soft parts, organs or tissues (of pelvis)
    in pregnancy or childbirth NEC O34.8- ☑
      causing obstructed labor O65.5
  spermatic cord (congenital) Q55.4
    acquired N50.89
      torsion — *see* Torsion, spermatic cord
  spinal — *see* Dorsopathy, deforming
    column (acquired) — *see* Dorsopathy, deforming
    congenital Q67.5
    cord (congenital) Q06.9
      acquired G95.89
    nerve root (congenital) Q07.9
  spine (acquired) (*see also* Dorsopathy, deforming)
    congenital Q67.5
    rachitic E64.3
    specified NEC — *see* Dorsopathy, deforming, speci-
      fied NEC
  spleen
    acquired D73.89
    congenital Q89.09
  Sprengel's (congenital) Q74.0
  sternocleidomastoid (muscle), congenital Q68.0
  sternum (acquired) M95.4
    congenital NEC Q76.7
  stomach (congenital) Q40.3
    acquired K31.89
  submandibular gland (congenital) Q38.4
  submaxillary gland (congenital) Q38.4
    acquired K11.8
  talipes — *see* Talipes
  testis (congenital) (*see also* Malformation, testis and
      scrotum)
    acquired N44.8
      torsion — *see* Torsion, testis
  thigh (acquired) (*see also* Deformity, limb, thigh)
    congenital NEC Q68.8
  thorax (acquired) (wall) M95.4
    congenital Q67.8
    sequelae of rickets E64.3
  thumb (acquired) (*see also* Deformity, finger)
    congenital NEC Q68.1
  thymus (tissue) (congenital) Q89.2
  thyroid (gland) (congenital) Q89.2
    cartilage Q31.8
    acquired J38.7
  tibia (acquired) (*see also* Deformity, limb, specified type
      NEC, lower leg)
    congenital NEC Q68.8
    saber (syphilitic) A50.56
  toe (acquired) M20.6- ☑
    congenital Q66.9
    hallux rigidus M20.2- ☑
    hallux valgus M20.1- ☑
    hallux varus M20.3- ☑
    hammer toe M20.4- ☑
    specified NEC M20.5X- ☑
  tongue (congenital) Q38.3
    acquired K14.8
  tooth, teeth K00.2
  trachea (rings) (congenital) Q32.1
    acquired J39.8
  transverse aortic arch (congenital) Q25.49
  tricuspid (leaflets) (valve) I07.8
    atresia or stenosis Q22.4
    Ebstein's Q22.5
  trunk (acquired) M95.8
    congenital Q89.9
  ulna (acquired) (*see also* Deformity, limb, forearm)
    congenital NEC Q68.8
  urachus, congenital Q64.4
  ureter (opening) (congenital) Q62.8
    acquired N28.89
  urethra (congenital) Q64.79
    acquired N36.8
  urinary tract (congenital) Q64.9
    urachus Q64.4
  uterus (congenital) Q51.9
    acquired N85.8
  uvula (congenital) Q38.5
  vagina (acquired) N89.8
    congenital Q52.4
  valgus NEC M21.00
    ankle M21.07- ☑
    elbow M21.02- ☑
    hip M21.05- ☑
    knee M21.06- ☑
  valve, valvular (congenital) (heart) Q24.8

Deformity — *continued*
valve, valvular — *continued*
acquired — *see* Endocarditis
varus NEC M21.10
ankle M21.17- ☑
elbow M21.12- ☑
hip M21.15 ☑
knee M21.16- ☑
tibia — *see* Osteochondrosis, juvenile, tibia
vas deferens (congenital) Q55.4
acquired N50.89
vein (congenital) Q27.9
great Q26.9
vertebra — *see* Dorsopathy, deforming
vertical talus (congenital) Q66.80
left foot Q66.82
right foot Q66.81
vesicourethral orifice (acquired) N32.89
congenital NEC Q64.79
vessels of optic papilla (congenital) Q14.2
visual field (contraction) — *see* Defect, visual field
vitreous body, acquired H43.89
vulva (congenital) Q52.79
acquired N90.89
wrist (joint) (acquired) (*see also* Deformity, limb, forearm)
congenital Q68.8
contraction — *see* Contraction, joint, wrist

Degeneration, degenerative
adrenal (capsule) (fatty) (gland) (hyaline) (infectional)
E27.8
amyloid (*see also* Amyloidosis) E85.9
anterior cornua, spinal cord G12.29
anterior labral S43.49- ☑
aorta, aortic I70.0
fatty I77.89
aortic valve (heart) — *see* Endocarditis, aortic
arteriovascular — *see* Arteriosclerosis
artery, arterial (atheromatous) (calcareous) (*see also*
Arteriosclerosis)
cerebral, amyloid E85.4 [I68.0]
medial — *see* Arteriosclerosis, extremities
articular cartilage NEC — *see* Derangement, joint, articular cartilage, by site
atheromatous — *see* Arteriosclerosis
basal nuclei or ganglia G23.9
specified NEC G23.8
bone NEC — *see* Disorder, bone, specified type NEC
brachial plexus G54.0
brain (cortical) (progressive) G31.9
alcoholic G31.2
arteriosclerotic I67.2
childhood G31.9
specified NEC G31.89
cystic G31.89
congenital Q04.6
in
alcoholism G31.2
beriberi E51.2
cerebrovascular disease I67.9
congenital hydrocephalus Q03.9
with spina bifida (*see also* Spina bifida)
Fabry-Anderson disease E75.21
Gaucher's disease E75.22
Hunter's syndrome E76.1
lipidosis
cerebral E75.4
generalized E75.6
mucopolysaccharidosis — *see* Mucopolysaccharidosis
myxedema E03.9 [G32.89]
neoplastic disease (*see also* Neoplasm)
D49.6 [G32.89]
Niemann-Pick disease E75.249 [G32.89]
sphingolipidosis E75.3 [G32.89]
vitamin B12 deficiency E53.8 [G32.89]
senile NEC G31.1
breast N64.89
Bruch's membrane — *see* Degeneration, choroid
capillaries (fatty) I78.8
amyloid E85.89 [I79.8]
cardiac (*see also* Degeneration, myocardial)
valve, valvular — *see* Endocarditis
cardiorenal — *see* Hypertension, cardiorenal
cardiovascular (*see also* Disease, cardiovascular)
renal — *see* Hypertension, cardiorenal
cerebellar NOS G31.9
alcoholic G31.2

Degeneration, degenerative — *continued*
cerebellar — *continued*
primary (hereditary) (sporadic) G11.9
cerebral — *see* Degeneration, brain
cerebrovascular I67.9
due to hypertension I67.4
cervical plexus G54.2
cervix N88.8
due to radiation (intended effect) N88.8
adverse effect or misadventure N99.89
chamber angle H21.21- ☑
changes, spine or vertebra — *see* Spondylosis
chorioretinal (*see also* Degeneration, choroid)
hereditary H31.20
choroid (colloid) (drusen) H31.10- ☑
atrophy — *see* Atrophy, choroidal
hereditary — *see* Dystrophy, choroidal, hereditary
ciliary body H21.22- ☑
cochlear — *see* subcategory H83.8 ☑
combined (spinal cord) (subacute) E53.8 [G32.0]
with anemia (pernicious) D51.0 [G32.0]
due to dietary vitamin B12 deficiency
D51.3 [G32.0]
in (due to)
vitamin B12 deficiency E53.8 [G32.0]
anemia D51.9 [G32.0]
conjunctiva H11.10
concretions — *see* Concretion, conjunctiva
deposits — *see* Deposit, conjunctiva
pigmentations — *see* Pigmentation, conjunctiva
pinguecula — *see* Pinguecula
xerosis — *see* Xerosis, conjunctiva
cornea H18.40
calcerous H18.43
band keratopathy H18.42- ☑
familial, hereditary — *see* Dystrophy, cornea
hyaline (of old scars) H18.49
keratomalacia — *see* Keratomalacia
nodular H18.45- ☑
peripheral H18.46- ☑
senile H18.41- ☑
specified type NEC H18.49
cortical (cerebellar) (parenchymatous) G31.89
alcoholic G31.2
diffuse, due to arteriopathy I67.2
corticobasal G31.85
cutis L98.8
amyloid E85.4 [L99]
dental pulp K04.2
disc disease — *see* Degeneration, intervertebral disc
NEC
dorsolateral (spinal cord) — *see* Degeneration, combined
extrapyramidal G25.9
eye, macular (*see also* Degeneration, macula)
congenital or hereditary — *see* Dystrophy, retina
facet joints — *see* Spondylosis
fatty
liver NEC K76.0
alcoholic K70.0
grey matter (brain) (Alpers') G31.81
heart (*see also* Degeneration, myocardial)
amyloid E85.4 [I43]
atheromatous — *see* Disease, heart, ischemic,
atherosclerotic
ischemic — *see* Disease, heart, ischemic
hepatolenticular (Wilson's) E83.01
hepatorenal K76.7
hyaline (diffuse) (generalized)
localized — *see* Degeneration, by site
infrapatellar fat pad M79.4
intervertebral disc NOS
with
myelopathy — *see* Disorder, disc, with,
myelopathy
radiculitis or radiculopathy — *see* Disorder, disc,
with, radiculopathy
cervical, cervicothoracic — *see* Disorder, disc, cervical, degeneration
with
myelopathy — *see* Disorder, disc, cervical,
with myelopathy
neuritis, radiculitis or radiculopathy — *see*
Disorder, disc, cervical, with neuritis
lumbar region M51.36
with
myelopathy M51.06

Degeneration, degenerative — *continued*
intervertebral disc — *continued*
lumbar region — *continued*
with — *continued*
neuritis, radiculitis, radiculopathy or sciatica
M51.16
lumbosacral region M51.37
with
neuritis, radiculitis, radiculopathy or sciatica
M51.17
sacrococcygeal region M53.3
thoracic region M51.34
with
myelopathy M51.04
neuritis, radiculitis, radiculopathy M51.14
thoracolumbar region M51.35
with
myelopathy M51.05
neuritis, radiculitis, radiculopathy M51.15
intestine, amyloid E85.4
iris (pigmentary) H21.23- ☑
ischemic — *see* Ischemia
joint disease — *see* Osteoarthritis
kidney N28.89
amyloid E85.4 [N29]
cystic, congenital Q61.9
fatty N28.89
polycystic Q61.3
adult type (autosomal dominant) Q61.2
infantile type (autosomal recessive) NEC Q61.1
collecting duct dilatation Q61.11
Kuhnt-Junius (*see also* Degeneration, macula)
H35.32- ☑
lens — *see* Cataract
lenticular (familial) (progressive) (Wilson's) (with cirrhosis of liver) E83.01
liver (diffuse) NEC K76.89
amyloid E85.4 [K77]
cystic K76.89
congenital Q44.6
fatty NEC K76.0
alcoholic K70.0
hypertrophic K76.89
parenchymatous, acute or subacute K72.00
with coma K72.01
pigmentary K76.89
toxic (acute) K71.9
lung J98.4
lymph gland I89.8
hyaline I89.8
macula, macular (acquired) (age-related) (senile)
H35.30
angioid streaks H35.33
atrophic age-related H35.31- ☑
congenital or hereditary — *see* Dystrophy, retina
cystoid H35.35- ☑
drusen H35.36- ☑
dry age-related H35.31- ☑
exudative H35.32- ☑
hole H35.34- ☑
nonexudative H35.31- ☑
puckering H35.37- ☑
toxic H35.38- ☑
wet age-related H35.32- ☑
membranous labyrinth, congenital (causing impairment of hearing) Q16.5
meniscus — *see* Derangement, meniscus
mitral — *see* Insufficiency, mitral
Mönckeberg's — *see* Arteriosclerosis, extremities
motor centers, senile G31.1
multi-system G90.3
mural — *see* Degeneration, myocardial
muscle (fatty) (fibrous) (hyaline) (progressive) M62.
heart — *see* Degeneration, myocardial
myelin, central nervous system G37.9
myocardial, myocardium (fatty) (hyaline) (senile) I5
with rheumatic fever (conditions in I00) I09.0
active, acute or subacute I01.2
with chorea I02.0
inactive or quiescent (with chorea) I09.0
hypertensive — *see* Hypertension, heart
rheumatic — *see* Degeneration, myocardial, wit
rheumatic fever
syphilitic A52.06
nasal sinus (mucosa) J32.9
frontal J32.1
maxillary J32.0
nerve — *see* Disorder, nerve

☑ **Additional Character Required** — **Refer to the Tabular List for Character Selection**   ☞ **Subterms under main terms may continue to next column or pa**

Degeneration, degenerative — *continued*
　nervous system G31.9
　　alcoholic G31.2
　　amyloid E85.4 [G99.8]
　　autonomic G90.9
　　fatty G31.89
　　specified NEC G31.89
　nipple N64.89
　olivopontocerebellar (hereditary) (familial) G23.8
　osseous labyrinth — *see* subcategory H83.8 ☑
　ovary N83.8
　　cystic N83.20- ☑
　　microcystic N83.20- ☑
　pallidal pigmentary (progressive) G23.0
　pancreas K86.89
　　tuberculous A18.83
　penis N48.89
　pigmentary (diffuse) (general)
　　localized — *see* Degeneration, by site
　　pallidal (progressive) G23.0
　pineal gland E34.8
　pituitary (gland) E23.6
　popliteal fat pad M79.4
　posterolateral (spinal cord) — *see* Degeneration, combined
　pulmonary valve (heart) I37.8
　pulp (tooth) K04.2
　pupillary margin H21.24- ☑
　renal — *see* Degeneration, kidney
　retina H35.9
　　hereditary (cerebroretinal) (congenital) (juvenile) (macula) (peripheral) (pigmentary) — *see* Dystrophy, retina
　　Kuhnt-Junius (*see also* Degeneration, macula) H35.32- ☑
　　macula (cystic) (exudative) (hole) (nonexudative) (pseudohole) (senile) (toxic) — *see* Degeneration, macula
　　peripheral H35.40
　　　lattice H35.41- ☑
　　　microcystoid H35.42- ☑
　　　paving stone H35.43- ☑
　　　secondary
　　　　pigmentary H35.45- ☑
　　　　vitreoretinal H35.46- ☑
　　　senile reticular H35.44- ☑
　　pigmentary (primary) (*see also* Dystrophy, retina)
　　　secondary — *see* Degeneration, retina, peripheral, secondary
　　posterior pole — *see* Degeneration, macula
　saccule, congenital (causing impairment of hearing) Q16.5
　senile R54
　　brain G31.1
　　cardiac, heart or myocardium — *see* Degeneration, myocardial
　　motor centers G31.1
　　vascular — *see* Arteriosclerosis
　sinus (cystic) (*see also* Sinusitis)
　　polypoid J33.1
　skin L98.8
　　amyloid E85.4 [L99]
　　colloid L98.8
　spinal (cord) G31.89
　　amyloid E85.4 [G32.89]
　　combined (subacute) — *see* Degeneration, combined
　　dorsolateral — *see* Degeneration, combined
　　familial NEC G31.89
　　fatty G31.89
　　funicular — *see* Degeneration, combined
　　posterolateral — *see* Degeneration, combined
　　subacute combined — *see* Degeneration, combined
　　tuberculous A17.81
　spleen D73.0
　　amyloid E85.4 [D77]
　stomach K31.89
　striatonigral G23.2
　suprarenal (capsule) (gland) E27.8
　synovial membrane (pulpy) — *see* Disorder, synovium, specified type NEC
　tapetoretinal — *see* Dystrophy, retina
　thymus (gland) E32.8
　　fatty E32.8
　thyroid (gland) E07.89
　tricuspid (heart) (valve) I07.9
　tuberculous NEC — *see* Tuberculosis
　turbinate J34.89

Degeneration, degenerative — *continued*
　uterus (cystic) N85.8
　vascular (senile) — *see* Arteriosclerosis
　　hypertensive — *see* Hypertension
　vitreoretinal, secondary — *see* Degeneration, retina, peripheral, secondary, vitreoretinal
　vitreous (body) H43.81- ☑
　Wallerian — *see* Disorder, nerve
　Wilson's hepatolenticular E83.01
Deglutition
　paralysis R13.0
　　hysterical F44.4
　pneumonia J69.0
Degos' disease I77.89
Dehiscence (of)
　amputation stump T87.81
　cesarean wound O90.0
　closure of
　　cornea T81.31 ☑
　　craniotomy T81.32 ☑
　　fascia (muscular) (superficial) T81.32 ☑
　　internal organ or tissue T81.32 ☑
　　laceration (external) (internal) T81.33 ☑
　　ligament T81.32 ☑
　　mucosa T81.31 ☑
　　muscle or muscle flap T81.32 ☑
　　ribs or rib cage T81.32 ☑
　　skin and subcutaneous tissue (full-thickness) (superficial) T81.31 ☑
　　skull T81.32 ☑
　　sternum (sternotomy) T81.32 ☑
　　tendon T81.32 ☑
　　traumatic laceration (external) (internal) T81.33 ☑
　episiotomy O90.1
　operation wound NEC T81.31 ☑
　　external operation wound (superficial) T81.31 ☑
　　internal operation wound (deep) T81.32 ☑
　perineal wound (postpartum) O90.1
　traumatic injury wound repair T81.33 ☑
　wound T81.30 ☑
　　traumatic repair T81.33 ☑
Dehydration E86.0
　newborn P74.1
Déjérine-Roussy syndrome G89.0
Déjérine-Sottas disease or neuropathy (hypertrophic) G60.0
Déjérine-Thomas atrophy G23.8
Delay, delayed
　any plane in pelvis
　　complicating delivery O66.9
　birth or delivery NOS O63.9
　closure, ductus arteriosus (Botalli) P29.38
　coagulation — *see* Defect, coagulation
　conduction (cardiac) (ventricular) I45.9
　delivery, second twin, triplet, etc O63.2
　development R62.50
　　global F88
　　intellectual (specific) F81.9
　　language F80.9
　　　due to hearing loss F80.4
　　learning F81.9
　　pervasive F84.9
　　physiological R62.50
　　　specified stage NEC R62.0
　　reading F81.0
　　sexual E30.0
　　speech F80.9
　　　due to hearing loss F80.4
　　spelling F81.81
　ejaculation F52.32
　gastric emptying K30
　menarche E30.0
　menstruation (cause unknown) N91.0
　milestone R62.0
　passage of meconium (newborn) P76.0
　primary respiration P28.9
　puberty (constitutional) E30.0
　separation of umbilical cord P96.82
　sexual maturation, female E30.0
　sleep phase syndrome G47.21
　union, fracture — *see* Fracture, by site
　vaccination Z28.9
Deletion(s)
　autosome Q93.9
　　identified by fluorescence in situ hybridization (FISH) Q93.89
　　identified by in situ hybridization (ISH) Q93.89

Deletion(s) — *continued*
　chromosome
　　with complex rearrangements NEC Q93.7
　　part of NEC Q93.59
　　seen only at prometaphase Q93.89
　　short arm
　　　22q11.2 Q93.81
　　　4 Q93.3
　　　5p Q93.4
　　specified NEC Q93.89
　　long arm chromosome 18 or 21 Q93.89
　　with complex rearrangements NEC Q93.7
　microdeletions NEC Q93.88
Delhi boil or button B55.1
Delinquency (juvenile) (neurotic) F91.8
　group Z72.810
Delinquent immunization status Z28.3
Delirium, delirious (acute or subacute) (not alcohol- or drug-induced) (with dementia) R41.0
　alcoholic (acute) (tremens) (withdrawal) F10.921
　　with intoxication F10.921
　　　in
　　　　abuse F10.121
　　　　dependence F10.221
　due to (secondary to)
　　alcohol
　　　intoxication F10.921
　　　　in
　　　　　abuse F10.121
　　　　　dependence F10.221
　　　withdrawal F10.231
　　amphetamine intoxication F15.921
　　　in
　　　　abuse F15.121
　　　　dependence F15.221
　　anxiolytic
　　　intoxication F13.921
　　　　in
　　　　　abuse F13.121
　　　　　dependence F13.221
　　　withdrawal F13.231
　　cannabis intoxication (acute) F12.921
　　　in
　　　　abuse F12.121
　　　　dependence F12.221
　　cocaine intoxication (acute) F14.921
　　　in
　　　　abuse F14.121
　　　　dependence F14.221
　　general medical condition F05
　　hallucinogen intoxication F16.921
　　　in
　　　　abuse F16.121
　　　　dependence F16.221
　　hypnotic
　　　intoxication F13.921
　　　　in
　　　　　abuse F13.121
　　　　　dependence F13.221
　　　withdrawal F13.231
　　inhalant intoxication (acute) F18.921
　　　in
　　　　abuse F18.121
　　　　dependence F18.221
　　multiple etiologies F05
　　opioid intoxication (acute) F11.921
　　　in
　　　　abuse F11.121
　　　　dependence F11.221
　　other (or unknown) substance F19.921
　　phencyclidine intoxication (acute) F16.921
　　　in
　　　　abuse F16.121
　　　　dependence F16.221
　　psychoactive substance NEC intoxication (acute) F19.921
　　　in
　　　　abuse F19.121
　　　　dependence F19.221
　　sedative
　　　intoxication F13.921
　　　　in
　　　　　abuse F13.121
　　　　　dependence F13.221
　　　withdrawal F13.231
　　unknown etiology F05
　exhaustion F43.0
　hysterical F44.89
　postprocedural (postoperative) F05

Delirium, delirious — *continued*
  puerperal F05
  thyroid — *see* Thyrotoxicosis with thyroid storm
  traumatic — *see* Injury, intracranial
  tremens (alcohol-induced) F10.231
    sedative-induced F13.231
Delivery (childbirth) (labor)
  arrested active phase O62.1
  cesarean (for)
    abnormal
      pelvis (bony) (deformity) (major) NEC with dispro-
          portion (fetopelvic) O33.0
        with obstructed labor O65.0
      presentation or position O32.9 ☑
    abruptio placentae (*see also* Abruptio placentae)
        O45.9- ☑
    acromion presentation O32.2 ☑
    atony, uterus O62.2
    breech presentation O32.1 ☑
      incomplete O32.8 ☑
    brow presentation O32.3 ☑
    cephalopelvic disproportion O33.9
    cerclage O34.3- ☑
    chin presentation O32.3 ☑
    cicatrix of cervix O34.4- ☑
    contracted pelvis (general)
      inlet O33.2
      outlet O33.3 ☑
    cord presentation or prolapse O69.0 ☑
    cystocele O34.8- ☑
    deformity (acquired) (congenital)
      pelvic organs or tissues NEC O34.8- ☑
      pelvis (bony) NEC O33.0
    disproportion NOS O33.9
    eclampsia — *see* Eclampsia
    face presentation O32.3 ☑
    failed
      forceps O66.5
      induction of labor O61.9
        instrumental O61.1
        mechanical O61.1
        medical O61.0
        specified NEC O61.8
        surgical O61.1
      trial of labor NOS O66.40
        following previous cesarean delivery O66.41
      vacuum extraction O66.5
      ventouse O66.5
    fetal-maternal hemorrhage O43.01- ☑
    hemorrhage (intrapartum) O67.9
      with coagulation defect O67.0
      specified cause NEC O67.8
    high head at term O32.4 ☑
    hydrocephalic fetus O33.6
    incarceration of uterus O34.51- ☑
    incoordinate uterine action O62.4
    increased size, fetus O33.5 ☑
    inertia, uterus O62.2
      primary O62.0
      secondary O62.1
    lateroversion, uterus O34.59- ☑
    mal lie O32.9 ☑
    malposition
      fetus O32.9 ☑
      pelvic organs or tissues NEC O34.8- ☑
      uterus NEC O34.59- ☑
    malpresentation NOS O32.9 ☑
    oblique presentation O32.2 ☑
    occurring after 37 completed weeks of gestation
        but before 39 completed weeks gestation due
        to (spontaneous) onset of labor O75.82
    oversize fetus O33.5 ☑
    pelvic tumor NEC O34.8- ☑
    placenta previa O44.0- ☑
      complete O44.0- ☑
        with hemorrhage O44.1- ☑
    placental insufficiency O36.51- ☑
    planned, occurring after 37 completed weeks of
        gestation but before 39 completed weeks
        gestation due to (spontaneous) onset of labor
        O75.82
    polyp, cervix O34.4- ☑
      causing obstructed labor O65.5
    poor dilatation, cervix O62.0
    pre-eclampsia O14.94
      mild O14.04
      moderate O14.04

Delivery — *continued*
  cesarean — *continued*
    pre-eclampsia — *continued*
      severe O14.14
        with hemolysis, elevated liver enzymes and
            low platelet count (HELLP) O14.24
    previous
      cesarean delivery O34.219
        classical (vertical) scar O34.212
        low transverse scar O34.211
      surgery (to)
        cervix O34.4- ☑
        gynecological NEC O34.8- ☑
        rectum O34.7- ☑
        uterus O34.29
        vagina O34.6- ☑
    prolapse
      arm or hand O32.2 ☑
      uterus O34.52- ☑
    prolonged labor NOS O63.9
    rectocele O34.8- ☑
    retroversion
      uterus O34.53- ☑
    rigid
      cervix O34.4- ☑
      pelvic floor O34.8- ☑
      perineum O34.7- ☑
      vagina O34.6- ☑
      vulva O34.7- ☑
    sacculation, pregnant uterus O34.59- ☑
    scar(s)
      cervix O34.4- ☑
      cesarean delivery O34.219
        classical (vertical) O34.212
        low transverse O34.211
      transmural uterine O34.29
      uterus O34.29
    Shirodkar suture in situ O34.3- ☑
    shoulder presentation O32.2 ☑
    stenosis or stricture, cervix O34.4- ☑
    streptococcus group B (GBS) carrier state O99.824
    transmural uterine scar O34.29
    transverse presentation or lie O32.2 ☑
    tumor, pelvic organs or tissues NEC O34.8- ☑
      cervix O34.4- ☑
    umbilical cord presentation or prolapse O69.0 ☑
    without indication O82
  completely normal case O80
  complicated O75.9
    by
      abnormal, abnormality (of)
        forces of labor O62.9
          specified type NEC O62.8
        glucose O99.814
        uterine contractions NOS O62.9
      abruptio placentae (*see also* Abruptio placentae)
          O45.9- ☑
      abuse
        physical O9A.32 (*following* O99)
        psychological O9A.52 (*following* O99)
        sexual O9A.42 (*following* O99)
      adherent placenta O72.0
        without hemorrhage O73.0
      alcohol use O99.314
      anemia (pre-existing) O99.02
      anesthetic death O74.8
      annular detachment of cervix O71.3
      atony, uterus O62.2
      attempted vacuum extraction and forceps O66.5
      Bandl's ring O62.4
      bariatric surgery status O99.844
      biliary tract disorder O26.62
      bleeding — *see* Delivery, complicated by, hem-
          orrhage
      blood disorder NEC O99.12
      cervical dystocia (hypotonic) O62.2
        primary O62.0
        secondary O62.1
      circulatory system disorder O99.42
      compression of cord (umbilical) NEC O69.2 ☑
      condition NEC O99.89
      contraction, contracted ring O62.4
      cord (umbilical)
        around neck
          with compression O69.1 ☑
          without compression O69.81 ☑
        bruising O69.5 ☑
        complication O69.9 ☑

Delivery — *continued*
  complicated — *continued*
    by — *continued*
      cord — *continued*
        complication — *continued*
          specified NEC O69.89 ☑
          compression NEC O69.2 ☑
          entanglement O69.2 ☑
            without compression O69.82 ☑
          hematoma O69.5 ☑
          presentation O69.0 ☑
          prolapse O69.0 ☑
          short O69.3 ☑
          thrombosis (vessels) O69.5 ☑
          vascular lesion O69.5 ☑
      Couvelaire uterus O45.8X- ☑
      damage to (injury to) NEC
        perineum O71.82
        periurethral tissue O71.82
        vulva O71.82
      delay following rupture of membranes (sponta-
          neous) — *see* Pregnancy, complicated by,
          premature rupture of membranes
      depressed fetal heart tones O76
      diabetes O24.92
        gestational O24.429
          diet controlled O24.420
          insulin controlled O24.424
          oral drug controlled (antidiabetic) (hypo-
              glycemic) O24.425
        pre-existing O24.32
          specified NEC O24.82
          type 1 O24.02
          type 2 O24.12
      diastasis recti (abdominis) O71.89
      dilatation
        bladder O66.8
        cervix incomplete, poor or slow O62.0
      disease NEC O99.89
      disruptio uteri — *see* Delivery, complicated by,
          rupture, uterus
      drug use O99.324
      dysfunction, uterus NOS O62.9
        hypertonic O62.4
        hypotonic O62.2
          primary O62.0
          secondary O62.1
        incoordinate O62.4
      eclampsia O15.1
      embolism (pulmonary) — *see* Embolism, obste-
          ric
      endocrine, nutritional or metabolic disease NEC
          O99.284
      failed
        attempted vaginal birth after previous cesar-
            an delivery O66.41
        induction of labor O61.9
          instrumental O61.1
          mechanical O61.1
          medical O61.0
          specified NEC O61.8
          surgical O61.1
        trial of labor O66.40
      female genital mutilation O65.5
      fetal
        abnormal acid-base balance O68
        acidemia O68
        acidosis O68
        alkalosis O68
        death, early O02.1
        deformity O66.3
        heart rate or rhythm (abnormal) (non-reassu-
            ing) O76
        hypoxia O77.8
        stress O77.9
          due to drug administration O77.1
          electrocardiographic evidence of O77.8
          specified NEC O77.8
          ultrasound evidence of O77.8
      fever during labor O75.2
      gastric banding status O99.844
      gastric bypass status O99.844
      gastrointestinal disease NEC O99.62
      gestational
        diabetes O24.429
          diet controlled O24.420
          insulin (and diet) controlled O24.424

☑ **Additional Character Required** — Refer to the Tabular List for Character Selection   ▼ Subterms under main terms may continue to next column or pag

Delivery — continued
- complicated — continued
  - by — continued
    - prolapse — continued
      - uterus O34.52- ☑
    - prolonged labor O63.9
      - first stage O63.0
      - second stage O63.1
    - protozoal disease (maternal) O98.62
    - respiratory disease NEC O99.52
    - retained membranes or portions of placenta O72.2
      - without hemorrhage O73.1
    - retarded birth O63.9
    - retention of secundines (with hemorrhage) O72.0
      - without hemorrhage O73.0
      - partial O72.2
        - without hemorrhage O73.1
    - rupture
      - bladder (urinary) O71.5
      - cervix O71.3
      - pelvic organ NEC O71.5
      - urethra O71.5
      - uterus (during or after labor) O71.1
        - before labor O71.0- ☑
    - separation, pubic bone (symphysis pubis) O71.6
    - shock O75.1
    - shoulder presentation O64.4 ☑
    - skin disorder NEC O99.72
    - spasm, cervix O62.4
    - stenosis or stricture, cervix O65.5
    - streptococcus group B (GBS) carrier state O99.824
    - subluxation of symphysis (pubis) O26.72
    - syphilis (maternal) O98.12
    - tear — see Delivery, complicated by, laceration
    - tetanic uterus O62.4
    - trauma (obstetrical) (see also Delivery, complicated, by, damage to) O71.9
      - non-obstetric O9A.22 (following O99)
      - periurethral O71.82
      - specified NEC O71.89
    - tuberculosis (maternal) O98.02
    - tumor, pelvic organs or tissues NEC O65.5
    - umbilical cord around neck
      - with compression O69.1 ☑
      - without compression O69.81 ☑
    - uterine inertia O62.2
      - during latent phase of labor O62.0
      - primary O62.0
      - secondary O62.1
    - vasa previa O69.4 ☑
    - velamentous insertion of cord O43.12- ☑
  - specified complication NEC O75.89
- delayed NOS O63.9
  - following rupture of membranes
    - artificial O75.5
  - second twin, triplet, etc. O63.2
- forceps, low following failed vacuum extraction O66.5
- missed (at or near term) O36.4 ☑
- normal O80
- obstructed — see Delivery, complicated by, obstructed labor
- precipitate O62.3
- preterm (see also Pregnancy, complicated by, preterm labor) O60.10 ☑
- spontaneous O80
- term pregnancy NOS O80
- uncomplicated O80
- vaginal, following previous cesarean delivery O34.219
  - classical (vertical) scar O34.212
  - low transverse scar O34.211

Delusions (paranoid) — see Disorder, delusional
Dementia (degenerative (primary)) (old age) (persisting) F03.90
- with
  - aggressive behavior F03.91
  - behavioral disturbance F03.91
  - combative behavior F03.91
  - Lewy bodies G31.83 [F02.80]
    - with behavioral disturbance G31.83 [F02.81]
  - Parkinsonism G31.83 [F02.80]
    - with behavioral disturbance G31.83 [F02.81]
  - Parkinson's disease G20 [F02.80]
    - with behavioral disturbance G20 [F02.81]
  - violent behavior F03.91
- alcoholic F10.97
  - with dependence F10.27
- Alzheimer's type — see Disease, Alzheimer's

Dementia — continued
- arteriosclerotic — see Dementia, vascular
- atypical, Alzheimer's type — see Disease, Alzheimer's, specified NEC
- congenital — see Disability, intellectual
- frontal (lobe) G31.09 [F02.80]
  - with behavioral disturbance G31.09 [F02.81]
- frontotemporal G31.09 [F02.80]
  - with behavioral disturbance G31.09 [F02.81]
  - specified NEC G31.09 [F02.80]
    - with behavioral disturbance G31.09 [F02.81]
- Huntington's disease or chorea G10
  - with dementia G10 [F02.80]
- in (due to)
  - with behavioral disturbance G31.83 [F02.81]
  - alcohol F10.97
    - with dependence F10.27
  - Alzheimer's disease — see Disease, Alzheimer's
  - arteriosclerotic brain disease — see Dementia, vascular
  - cerebral lipidoses E75.- ☑ [F02.80]
    - with behavioral disturbance E75.- ☑ [F02.81]
  - Creutzfeldt-Jakob disease (see also Creutzfeldt-Jakob disease or syndrome (with dementia)) A81.00
  - epilepsy G40.- ☑ [F02.80]
    - with behavioral disturbance G40.- ☑ [F02.81]
  - hepatolenticular degeneration E83.01 [F02.80]
    - with behavioral disturbance E83.01 [F02.81]
  - human immunodeficiency virus (HIV) disease B20 [F02.80]
    - with behavioral disturbance B20 [F02.81]
  - Huntington's disease or chorea G10 [F02.80]
    - with behavioral disturbance G10 [F02.81]
  - hypercalcemia E83.52 [F02.80]
    - with behavioral disturbance E83.52 [F02.81]
  - hypothyroidism, acquired E03.9 [F02.80]
    - with behavioral disturbance E03.9 [F02.81]
    - due to iodine deficiency E01.8 [F02.80]
      - with behavioral disturbance E01.8 [F02.81]
  - inhalants F18.97
    - with dependence F18.27
  - multiple
    - etiologies F03 ☑
    - sclerosis G35 [F02.80]
      - with behavioral disturbance G35 [F02.81]
  - neurosyphilis A52.17 [F02.80]
    - with behavioral disturbance A52.17 [F02.81]
    - juvenile A50.49 [F02.80]
      - with behavioral disturbance A50.49 [F02.81]
  - niacin deficiency E52 [F02.80]
    - with behavioral disturbance E52 [F02.81]
  - paralysis agitans G20 [F02.80]
    - with behavioral disturbance G20 [F02.81]
  - Parkinson's disease G20 [F02.80]
    - with behavioral disturbance G20 [F02.81]
  - pellagra E52 [F02.80]
    - with behavioral disturbance E52 [F02.81]
  - Pick's G31.01 [F02.80]
    - with behavioral disturbance G31.01 [F02.81]
  - polyarteritis nodosa M30.0 [F02.80]
    - with behavioral disturbance M30.0 [F02.81]
  - psychoactive drug F19.97
    - with dependence F19.27
    - inhalants F18.97
      - with dependence F18.27
    - sedatives, hypnotics or anxiolytics F13.97
      - with dependence F13.27
  - sedatives, hypnotics or anxiolytics F13.97
    - with dependence F13.27
  - systemic lupus erythematosus M32.- ☑ [F02.80]
    - with behavioral disturbance M32.- ☑ [F02.81]
  - trypanosomiasis
    - African B56.9 [F02.80]
      - with behavioral disturbance B56.9 [F02.81]
  - unknown etiology F03 ☑
  - vitamin B12 deficiency E53.8 [F02.80]
    - with behavioral disturbance E53.8 [F02.81]
  - volatile solvents F18.97
    - with dependence F18.27
- infantile, infantilis F84.3
- Lewy body G31.83 [F02.80]
  - with behavioral disturbance G31.83 [F02.81]
- multi-infarct — see Dementia, vascular
- paralytica, paralytic (syphilitic) A52.17 [F02.80]
  - with behavioral disturbance A52.17 [F02.81]
  - juvenilis A50.45
- paretic A52.17
- praecox — see Schizophrenia

Dementia — continued
- presenile F03 ☑
  - Alzheimer's type — see Disease, Alzheimer's, early onset
- primary degenerative F03 ☑
- progressive, syphilitic A52.17
- senile F03 ☑
  - with acute confusional state F05
  - Alzheimer's type — see Disease, Alzheimer's, late onset
  - depressed or paranoid type F03 ☑
- vascular (acute onset) (mixed) (multi-infarct) (subcortical) F01.50
  - with behavioral disturbance F01.51
Demineralization, bone — see Osteoporosis
Demodex folliculorum (infestation) B88.0
Demophobia F40.248
Demoralization R45.3
Demyelination, demyelinization
- central nervous system G37.9
  - specified NEC G37.8
- corpus callosum (central) G37.1
- disseminated, acute G36.9
  - specified NEC G36.8
- global G35
- in optic neuritis G36.0
Dengue (classical) (fever) A90
- hemorrhagic A91
- sandfly A93.1
Dennie-Marfan syphilitic syndrome A50.45
Dens evaginatus, in dente or invaginatus K00.2
Dense breasts R92.2
Density
- increased, bone (disseminated) (generalized) (spotted) — see Disorder, bone, density and structure, specified type NEC
- lung (nodular) J98.4
Dental (see also condition)
- examination Z01.20
  - with abnormal findings Z01.21
- restoration
  - aesthetically inadequate or displeasing K08.56
  - defective K08.50
    - specified NEC K08.59
  - failure of marginal integrity K08.51
  - failure of periodontal anatomical integrity K08.54
Dentia praecox K00.6
Denticles (pulp) K04.2
Dentigerous cyst K09.0
Dentin
- irregular (in pulp) K04.3
- opalescent K00.5
- secondary (in pulp) K04.3
- sensitive K03.89
Dentinogenesis imperfecta K00.5
Dentinoma — see Cyst, calcifying odontogenic
Dentition (syndrome) K00.7
- delayed K00.6
- difficult K00.7
- precocious K00.6
- premature K00.6
- retarded K00.6
Dependence (on) (syndrome) F19.20
- with remission F19.21
- alcohol (ethyl) (methyl) (without remission) F10.20
  - with
    - amnestic disorder, persisting F10.26
    - anxiety disorder F10.280
    - dementia, persisting F10.27
    - intoxication F10.229
      - with delirium F10.221
      - uncomplicated F10.220
    - mood disorder F10.24
    - psychotic disorder F10.259
      - with
        - delusions F10.250
        - hallucinations F10.251
    - remission F10.21
    - sexual dysfunction F10.281
    - sleep disorder F10.282
    - specified disorder NEC F10.288
    - withdrawal F10.239
      - with
        - delirium F10.231
        - perceptual disturbance F10.232
      - uncomplicated F10.230
  - counseling and surveillance Z71.41
- amobarbital — see Dependence, drug, sedative

☑ **Additional Character Required** — Refer to the Tabular List for Character Selection   ⬚ Subterms under main terms may continue to next column or page

Dependence — continued
amphetamine(s) (type) — see Dependence, drug, stimulant NEC
amytal (sodium) — see Dependence, drug, sedative
analgesic NEC F55.8
anesthetic (agent) (gas) (general) (local) NEC — see Dependence, drug, psychoactive NEC
anxiolytic NEC — see Dependence, drug, sedative
barbital(s) — see Dependence, drug, sedative
barbiturate(s) (compounds) (drugs classifiable to T42) — see Dependence, drug, sedative
benzedrine — see Dependence, drug, stimulant NEC
bhang — see Dependence, drug, cannabis
bromide(s) NEC — see Dependence, drug, sedative
caffeine — see Dependence, drug, stimulant NEC
cannabis (sativa) (indica) (resin) (derivatives) (type) — see Dependence, drug, cannabis
chloral (betaine) (hydrate) — see Dependence, drug, sedative
chlordiazepoxide — see Dependence, drug, sedative
coca (leaf) (derivatives) — see Dependence, drug, cocaine
cocaine — see Dependence, drug, cocaine
codeine — see Dependence, drug, opioid
combinations of drugs F19.20
dagga — see Dependence, drug, cannabis
demerol — see Dependence, drug, opioid
dexamphetamine — see Dependence, drug, stimulant NEC
dexedrine — see Dependence, drug, stimulant NEC
dextromethorphan — see Dependence, drug, opioid
dextromoramide — see Dependence, drug, opioid
dextro-nor-pseudo-ephedrine — see Dependence, drug, stimulant NEC
dextrorphan — see Dependence, drug, opioid
diazepam — see Dependence, drug, sedative
dilaudid — see Dependence, drug, opioid
D-lysergic acid diethylamide — see Dependence, drug, hallucinogen
drug NEC F19.20
  with sleep disorder F19.282
  cannabis F12.20
    with
      anxiety disorder F12.280
      intoxication F12.229
        with
          delirium F12.221
          perceptual disturbance F12.222
        uncomplicated F12.220
      other specified disorder F12.288
      psychosis F12.259
        delusions F12.250
        hallucinations F12.251
      unspecified disorder F12.29
      withdrawal F12.23
    in remission F12.21
  cocaine F14.20
    with
      anxiety disorder F14.280
      intoxication F14.229
        with
          delirium F14.221
          perceptual disturbance F14.222
        uncomplicated F14.220
      mood disorder F14.24
      other specified disorder F14.288
      psychosis F14.259
        delusions F14.250
        hallucinations F14.251
      sexual dysfunction F14.281
      sleep disorder F14.282
      unspecified disorder F14.29
      withdrawal F14.23
    in remission F14.21
    withdrawal symptoms in newborn P96.1
  counseling and surveillance Z71.51
  hallucinogen F16.20
    with
      anxiety disorder F16.280
      flashbacks F16.283
      intoxication F16.229
        with delirium F16.221
        uncomplicated F16.220
      mood disorder F16.24
      other specified disorder F16.288
      perception disorder, persisting F16.283
      psychosis F16.259
        delusions F16.250

Dependence — continued
drug — continued
  hallucinogen — continued
    with — continued
      psychosis — continued
        hallucinations F16.251
      unspecified disorder F16.29
    in remission F16.21
  in remission F19.21
  inhalant F18.20
    with
      anxiety disorder F18.280
      dementia, persisting F18.27
      intoxication F18.229
        with delirium F18.221
        uncomplicated F18.220
      mood disorder F18.24
      other specified disorder F18.288
      psychosis F18.259
        delusions F18.250
        hallucinations F18.251
      unspecified disorder F18.29
    in remission F18.21
  nicotine F17.200
    with disorder F17.209
      in remission F17.201
      specified disorder NEC F17.208
      withdrawal F17.203
    chewing tobacco F17.220
      with disorder F17.229
        in remission F17.221
        specified disorder NEC F17.228
        withdrawal F17.223
    cigarettes F17.210
      with disorder F17.219
        in remission F17.211
        specified disorder NEC F17.218
        withdrawal F17.213
    specified product NEC F17.290
      with disorder F17.299
        remission F17.291
        specified disorder NEC F17.298
        withdrawal F17.293
  opioid F11.20
    with
      intoxication F11.229
        with
          delirium F11.221
          perceptual disturbance F11.222
        uncomplicated F11.220
      mood disorder F11.24
      other specified disorder F11.288
      psychosis F11.259
        delusions F11.250
        hallucinations F11.251
      sexual dysfunction F11.281
      sleep disorder F11.282
      unspecified disorder F11.29
      withdrawal F11.23
    in remission F11.21
  psychoactive NEC F19.20
    with
      amnestic disorder F19.26
      anxiety disorder F19.280
      dementia F19.27
      intoxication F19.229
        with
          delirium F19.221
          perceptual disturbance F19.222
        uncomplicated F19.220
      mood disorder F19.24
      other specified disorder F19.288
      psychosis F19.259
        delusions F19.250
        hallucinations F19.251
      sexual dysfunction F19.281
      sleep disorder F19.282
      unspecified disorder F19.29
      withdrawal F19.239
        with
          delirium F19.231
          perceptual disturbance F19.232
        uncomplicated F19.230
  sedative, hypnotic or anxiolytic F13.20
    with
      amnestic disorder F13.26
      anxiety disorder F13.280
      dementia, persisting F13.27
      intoxication F13.229

Dependence — continued
drug — continued
  sedative, hypnotic or anxiolytic — continued
    with — continued
      intoxication — continued
        with delirium F13.221
        uncomplicated F13.220
      mood disorder F13.24
      other specified disorder F13.288
      psychosis F13.259
        delusions F13.250
        hallucinations F13.251
      sexual dysfunction F13.281
      sleep disorder F13.282
      unspecified disorder F13.29
      withdrawal F13.239
        with
          delirium F13.231
          perceptual disturbance F13.232
        uncomplicated F13.230
    in remission F13.21
  stimulant NEC F15.20
    with
      anxiety disorder F15.280
      intoxication F15.229
        with
          delirium F15.221
          perceptual disturbance F15.222
        uncomplicated F15.220
      mood disorder F15.24
      other specified disorder F15.288
      psychosis F15.259
        delusions F15.250
        hallucinations F15.251
      sexual dysfunction F15.281
      sleep disorder F15.282
      unspecified disorder F15.29
      withdrawal F15.23
    in remission F15.21
ethyl
  alcohol (without remission) F10.20
    with remission F10.21
  bromide — see Dependence, drug, sedative
  carbamate F19.20
  chloride F19.20
  morphine — see Dependence, drug, opioid
ganja — see Dependence, drug, cannabis
glue (airplane) (sniffing) — see Dependence, drug, inhalant
glutethimide — see Dependence, drug, sedative
hallucinogenics — see Dependence, drug, hallucinogen
hashish — see Dependence, drug, cannabis
hemp — see Dependence, drug, cannabis
heroin (salt) (any) — see Dependence, drug, opioid
hypnotic NEC — see Dependence, drug, sedative
Indian hemp — see Dependence, drug, cannabis
inhalants — see Dependence, drug, inhalant
khat — see Dependence, drug, stimulant NEC
laudanum — see Dependence, drug, opioid
LSD (-25) (derivatives) — see Dependence, drug, hallucinogen
luminal — see Dependence, drug, sedative
lysergic acid — see Dependence, drug, hallucinogen
maconha — see Dependence, drug, cannabis
marihuana — see Dependence, drug, cannabis
meprobamate — see Dependence, drug, sedative
mescaline — see Dependence, drug, hallucinogen
methadone — see Dependence, drug, opioid
methamphetamine(s) — see Dependence, drug, stimulant NEC
methaqualone — see Dependence, drug, sedative
methyl
  alcohol (without remission) F10.20
    with remission F10.21
  bromide — see Dependence, drug, sedative
  morphine — see Dependence, drug, opioid
  phenidate — see Dependence, drug, stimulant NEC
  sulfonal — see Dependence, drug, sedative
morphine (sulfate) (sulfite) (type) — see Dependence, drug, opioid
narcotic (drug) NEC — see Dependence, drug, opioid
nembutal — see Dependence, drug, sedative
neraval — see Dependence, drug, sedative
neravan — see Dependence, drug, sedative
neurobarb — see Dependence, drug, sedative
nicotine — see Dependence, drug, nicotine
nitrous oxide F19.20

Index

Dependence — Derangement

Dependence — continued
- nonbarbiturate sedatives and tranquilizers with similar effect — see Dependence, drug, sedative
- on
  - artificial heart (fully implantable) (mechanical) Z95.812
  - aspirator Z99.0
  - care provider (because of) Z74.9
    - impaired mobility Z74.09
    - need for
      - assistance with personal care Z74.1
      - continuous supervision Z74.3
      - no other household member able to render care Z74.2
    - specified reason NEC Z74.8
  - machine Z99.89
    - enabling NEC Z99.89
    - specified type NEC Z99.89
  - renal dialysis (hemodialysis) (peritoneal) Z99.2
  - respirator Z99.11
  - ventilator Z99.11
  - wheelchair Z99.3
- opiate — see Dependence, drug, opioid
- opioids — see Dependence, drug, opioid
- opium (alkaloids) (derivatives) (tincture) — see Dependence, drug, opioid
- oxygen (long-term) (supplemental) Z99.81
- paraldehyde — see Dependence, drug, sedative
- paregoric — see Dependence, drug, opioid
- PCP (phencyclidine) (or related substance) — see Dependence, drug, hallucinogen
- pentobarbital — see Dependence, drug, sedative
- pentobarbitone (sodium) — see Dependence, drug, sedative
- pentothal — see Dependence, drug, sedative
- peyote — see Dependence, drug, hallucinogen
- phencyclidine (PCP) (or related substance) — see Dependence, drug, hallucinogen
- phenmetrazine — see Dependence, drug, stimulant NEC
- phenobarbital — see Dependence, drug, sedative
- polysubstance F19.20
- psilocibin, psilocin, psilocyn, psilocyline — see Dependence, drug, hallucinogen
- psychostimulant NEC — see Dependence, drug, stimulant NEC
- secobarbital — see Dependence, drug, sedative
- seconal — see Dependence, drug, sedative
- sedative NEC — see Dependence, drug, sedative
- specified drug NEC — see Dependence, drug
- stimulant NEC — see Dependence, drug, stimulant NEC
- substance NEC — see Dependence, drug
- supplemental oxygen Z99.81
- tobacco — see Dependence, drug, nicotine
  - counseling and surveillance Z71.6
- tranquilizer NEC — see Dependence, drug, sedative
- vitamin B6 E53.1
- volatile solvents — see Dependence, drug, inhalant

Dependency
- care-provider Z74.9
- passive F60.7
- reactions (persistent) F60.7

Depersonalization (in neurotic state) (neurotic) (syndrome) F48.1

Depletion
- extracellular fluid E86.9
- plasma E86.1
- potassium E87.6
  - nephropathy N25.89
- salt or sodium E87.1
  - causing heat exhaustion or prostration T67.4 ☑
  - nephropathy N28.9
- volume NOS E86.9

Deployment (current) (military) status Z56.82
- in theater or in support of military war, peacekeeping and humanitarian operations Z56.82
- personal history of Z91.82
  - military war, peacekeeping and humanitarian deployment (current or past conflict) Z91.82
  - returned from Z91.82

Depolarization, premature I49.40
- atrial I49.1
- junctional I49.2
- specified NEC I49.49
- ventricular I49.3

Deposit
- bone in Boeck's sarcoid D86.89
- calcareous, calcium — see Calcification

Deposit — continued
- cholesterol
  - retina H35.89
  - vitreous (body) (humor) — see Deposit, crystalline
- conjunctiva H11.11- ☑
- cornea H18.00- ☑
  - argentous H18.02- ☑
  - due to metabolic disorder H18.03- ☑
  - Kayser-Fleischer ring H18.04- ☑
  - pigmentation — see Pigmentation, cornea
- crystalline, vitreous (body) (humor) H43.2- ☑
- hemosiderin in old scars of cornea — see Pigmentation, cornea, stromal
- metallic in lens — see Cataract, specified NEC
- skin R23.8
- tooth, teeth (betel) (black) (green) (materia alba) (orange) (tobacco) K03.6
- urate, kidney — see Calculus, kidney

Depraved appetite — see Pica

Depressed
- HDL cholesterol E78.6

Depression (acute) (mental) F32.9
- agitated (single episode) F32.2
- anaclitic — see Disorder, adjustment
- anxiety F41.8
  - persistent F34.1
- arches (see also Deformity, limb, flat foot)
- atypical (single episode) F32.89
  - recurrent episode F33.8
- basal metabolic rate R94.8
- bone marrow D75.89
- central nervous system R09.2
- cerebral R29.818
  - newborn P91.4
- cerebrovascular I67.9
- chest wall M95.4
- climacteric (single episode) F32.89
  - recurrent episode F33.8
- endogenous (without psychotic symptoms) F33.2
  - with psychotic symptoms F33.3
- functional activity R68.89
- hysterical F44.89
- involutional (single episode) F32.89
  - recurrent episode F33.8
- major F32.9
  - with psychotic symptoms F32.3
  - recurrent — see Disorder, depressive, recurrent
- manic-depressive — see Disorder, depressive, recurrent
- masked (single episode) F32.89
- medullary G93.89
- menopausal (single episode) F32.89
  - recurrent episode F33.8
- metatarsus — see Depression, arches
- monopolar F33.9
- nervous F34.1
- neurotic F34.1
- nose M95.0
- postnatal (NOS) F53.0
- postpartum (NOS) F53.0
- post-psychotic of schizophrenia F32.89
- post-schizophrenic F32.89
- psychogenic (reactive) (single episode) F32.9
- psychoneurotic F34.1
- psychotic (single episode) F32.3
  - recurrent F33.3
- reactive (psychogenic) (single episode) F32.9
  - psychotic (single episode) F32.3
- recurrent — see Disorder, depressive, recurrent
- respiratory center G93.89
- seasonal — see Disorder, depressive, recurrent
- senile F03 ☑
- severe, single episode F32.2
- situational F43.21
- skull Q67.4
- specified NEC (single episode) F32.89
- sternum M95.4
- visual field — see Defect, visual field
- vital (recurrent) (without psychotic symptoms) F33.2
  - with psychotic symptoms F33.3
  - single episode F32.2

Deprivation
- cultural Z60.3
- effects NOS T73.9 ☑
  - specified NEC T73.8 ☑
- emotional NEC Z65.8
  - affecting infant or child — see Maltreatment, child, psychological
- food T73.0 ☑

Deprivation — continued
- protein — see Malnutrition
- sleep Z72.820
- social Z60.4
  - affecting infant or child — see Maltreatment, child, psychological
- specified NEC T73.8 ☑
- vitamins — see Deficiency, vitamin
- water T73.1 ☑

Derangement
- ankle (internal) — see Derangement, joint, ankle
- cartilage (articular) NEC — see Derangement, joint, articular cartilage, by site
  - recurrent — see Dislocation, recurrent
- cruciate ligament, anterior, current injury — see Sprain, knee, cruciate, anterior
- elbow (internal) — see Derangement, joint, elbow
- hip (joint) (internal) (old) — see Derangement, joint, hip
- joint (internal) M24.9
  - ankylosis — see Ankylosis
  - articular cartilage M24.10
    - ankle M24.17- ☑
    - elbow M24.12- ☑
    - foot M24.17- ☑
    - hand M24.14- ☑
    - hip M24.15- ☑
    - knee NEC M23.9- ☑
    - loose body — see Loose, body
    - shoulder M24.11- ☑
    - wrist M24.13- ☑
  - contracture — see Contraction, joint
  - current injury (see also Dislocation)
    - knee, meniscus or cartilage — see Tear, meniscus
  - dislocation
    - pathological — see Dislocation, pathological
    - recurrent — see Dislocation, recurrent
  - knee — see Derangement, knee
  - ligament — see Disorder, ligament
  - loose body — see Loose, body
  - recurrent — see Dislocation, recurrent
  - specified type NEC M24.80
    - ankle M24.87- ☑
    - elbow M24.82- ☑
    - foot joint M24.87- ☑
    - hand joint M24.84- ☑
    - hip M24.85- ☑
    - shoulder M24.81- ☑
    - wrist M24.83- ☑
  - temporomandibular M26.69
- knee (recurrent) M23.9- ☑
  - ligament disruption, spontaneous M23.60- ☑
    - anterior cruciate M23.61- ☑
    - capsular M23.67- ☑
    - instability, chronic M23.5- ☑
    - lateral collateral M23.64- ☑
    - medial collateral M23.63- ☑
    - posterior cruciate M23.62- ☑
  - loose body M23.4- ☑
  - meniscus M23.30- ☑
    - cystic M23.00- ☑
      - lateral M23.002
        - anterior horn M23.04- ☑
        - posterior horn M23.05- ☑
        - specified NEC M23.06- ☑
      - medial M23.005
        - anterior horn M23.01- ☑
        - posterior horn M23.02- ☑
        - specified NEC M23.03- ☑
    - degenerate — see Derangement, knee, meniscus, specified NEC
    - detached — see Derangement, knee, meniscus, specified NEC
    - due to old tear or injury M23.20- ☑
      - lateral M23.20- ☑
        - anterior horn M23.24- ☑
        - posterior horn M23.25- ☑
        - specified NEC M23.26- ☑
      - medial M23.20- ☑
        - anterior horn M23.21- ☑
        - posterior horn M23.22- ☑
        - specified NEC M23.23- ☑
    - retained — see Derangement, knee, meniscus, specified NEC
    - specified NEC M23.30- ☑
      - lateral M23.30- ☑

Derangement — *continued*
  knee — *continued*
    meniscus — *continued*
      specified — *continued*
        lateral — *continued*
          anterior horn M23.34- ☑
          posterior horn M23.35- ☑
          specified NEC M23.36- ☑
        medial M23.30- ☑
          anterior horn M23.31- ☑
          posterior horn M23.32- ☑
          specified NEC M23.33- ☑
      old M23.8X- ☑
      specified NEC — *see* subcategory M23.8 ☑
   low back NEC — *see* Dorsopathy, specified NEC
   meniscus — *see* Derangement, knee, meniscus
   mental — *see* Psychosis
   patella, specified NEC — *see* Disorder, patella, derangement NEC
   semilunar cartilage (knee) — *see* Derangement, knee, meniscus, specified NEC
   shoulder (internal) — *see* Derangement, joint, shoulder
Dercum's disease E88.2
Derealization (neurotic) F48.1
Dermal — *see* condition
Dermaphytid — *see* Dermatophytosis
Dermatitis (eczematous) L30.9
  ab igne L59.0
  acarine B88.0
  actinic (due to sun) L57.8
   other than from sun L59.8
  allergic — *see* Dermatitis, contact, allergic
  ambustionis, due to burn or scald — *see* Burn
  amebic A06.7
  ammonia L22
  arsenical (ingested) L27.8
  artefacta L98.1
   psychogenic F54
  atopic L20.9
   psychogenic F54
   specified NEC L20.89
  autoimmune progesterone L30.8
  berlock, berloque L56.2
  blastomycotic B40.3
  blister beetle L24.89
  bullous, bullosa L13.9
   mucosynechial, atrophic L12.1
   seasonal L30.8
   specified NEC L13.8
  calorica L59.0
   due to burn or scald — *see* Burn
  caterpillar L24.89
  cercarial B65.3
  combustionis L59.0
   due to burn or scald — *see* Burn
  congelationis T69.1 ☑
  contact (occupational) L25.9
   allergic L23.9
    due to
     adhesives L23.1
     cement L23.5
     chemical products NEC L23.5
     chromium L23.0
     cosmetics L23.2
     dander (cat) (dog) L23.81
     drugs in contact with skin L23.3
     dyes L23.4
     food in contact with skin L23.6
     hair (cat) (dog) L23.81
     insecticide L23.5
     metals L23.0
     nickel L23.0
     plants, non-food L23.7
     plastic L23.5
     rubber L23.5
     specified agent NEC L23.89
    due to
     cement L25.3
     chemical products NEC L25.3
     cosmetics L25.0
     dander (cat) (dog) L23.81
     drugs in contact with skin L25.1
     dyes L25.2
     food in contact with skin L25.4
     hair (cat) (dog) L23.81
     plants, non-food L25.5
     specified agent NEC L25.8
    irritant L24.9

Dermatitis — *continued*
  contact — *continued*
   irritant — *continued*
    due to
     cement L24.5
     chemical products NEC L24.5
     cosmetics L24.3
     detergents L24.0
     drugs in contact with skin L24.4
     food in contact with skin L24.6
     oils and greases L24.1
     plants, non-food L24.7
     solvents L24.2
     specified agent NEC L24.89
  contusiformis L52
  diabetic — *see* E08-E13 with .620
  diaper L22
  diphtheritica A36.3
  dry skin L85.3
  due to
   acetone (contact) (irritant) L24.2
   acids (contact) (irritant) L24.5
   adhesive(s) (allergic) (contact) (plaster) L23.1
    irritant L24.5
   alcohol (irritant) (skin contact) (substances in category T51) L24.2
    taken internally L27.8
   alkalis (contact) (irritant) L24.5
   arsenic (ingested) L27.8
   carbon disulfide (contact) (irritant) L24.2
   caustics (contact) (irritant) L24.5
   cement L25.3
   cereal (ingested) L27.2
   chemical(s) NEC L25.3
    taken internally L27.8
   chlorocompounds L24.2
   chromium (contact) (irritant) L24.81
   coffee (ingested) L27.2
   cold weather L30.8
   cosmetics (contact) L25.0
    allergic L23.2
    irritant L24.3
   cyclohexanes L24.2
   dander (cat) (dog) L23.81
   Demodex species B88.0
   Dermanyssus gallinae B88.0
   detergents (contact) (irritant) L24.0
   dichromate L24.81
   drugs and medicaments (generalized) (internal use) L27.0
    external — *see* Dermatitis, due to, drugs, in contact with skin
    in contact with skin L25.1
     allergic L23.3
     irritant L24.4
    localized skin eruption L27.1
    specified substance — *see* Table of Drugs and Chemicals
   dyes (contact) L25.2
    allergic L23.4
    irritant L24.89
   epidermophytosis — *see* Dermatophytosis
   esters L24.2
   external irritant NEC L24.9
   fish (ingested) L27.2
   flour (ingested) L27.2
   food (ingested) L27.2
    in contact with skin L25.4
   fruit (ingested) L27.2
   furs (allergic) (contact) L23.81
   glues — *see* Dermatitis, due to, adhesives
   glycols L24.2
   greases NEC (contact) (irritant) L24.1
   hair (cat) (dog) L23.81
   hot
    objects and materials — *see* Burn
    weather or places L59.0
   hydrocarbons L24.2
   infrared rays L59.8
   ingestion, ingested substance L27.9
    chemical NEC L27.8
    drugs and medicaments — *see* Dermatitis, due to, drugs
    food L27.2
    specified NEC L27.8
   insecticide in contact with skin L24.5
   internal agent L27.9

Dermatitis — *continued*
  due to — *continued*
   internal agent — *continued*
    drugs and medicaments (generalized) — *see* Dermatitis, due to, drugs
    food L27.2
   irradiation — *see* Dermatitis, due to, radioactive substance
   ketones L24.2
   lacquer tree (allergic) (contact) L23.7
   light (sun) NEC L57.8
    acute L56.8
    other L59.8
   Liponyssoides sanguineus B88.0
   low temperature L30.8
   meat (ingested) L27.2
   metals, metal salts (contact) (irritant) L24.81
   milk (ingested) L27.2
   nickel (contact) (irritant) L24.81
   nylon (contact) (irritant) L24.5
   oils NEC (contact) (irritant) L24.1
   paint solvent (contact) (irritant) L24.2
   petroleum products (contact) (irritant) (substances in T52.0) L24.2
   plants NEC (contact) L25.5
    allergic L23.7
    irritant L24.7
   plasters (adhesive) (any) (allergic) (contact) L23.1
    irritant L24.5
   plastic (contact) L25.3
   preservatives (contact) — *see* Dermatitis, due to, chemical, in contact with skin
   primrose (allergic) (contact) L23.7
   primula (allergic) (contact) L23.7
   radiation L59.8
    nonionizing (chronic exposure) L57.8
    sun NEC L57.8
     acute L56.8
   radioactive substance L58.9
    acute L58.0
    chronic L58.1
   radium L58.9
    acute L58.0
    chronic L58.1
   ragweed (allergic) (contact) L23.7
   Rhus (allergic) (contact) (diversiloba) (radicans) (toxicodendron) (venenata) (verniciflua) L23.7
   rubber (contact) L24.5
   Senecio jacobaea (allergic) (contact) L23.7
   solvents (contact) (irritant) (substances in category T52) L24.2
   specified agent NEC (contact) L25.8
    allergic L23.89
    irritant L24.89
   sunshine NEC L57.8
    acute L56.8
   tetrachlorethylene (contact) (irritant) L24.2
   toluene (contact) (irritant) L24.2
   turpentine (contact) L24.2
   ultraviolet rays (sun NEC) (chronic exposure) L57.8
    acute L56.8
   vaccine or vaccination L27.0
    specified substance — *see* Table of Drugs and Chemicals
   varicose veins — *see* Varix, leg, with, inflammation
   X-rays L58.9
    acute L58.0
    chronic L58.1
  dyshydrotic L30.1
  dysmenorrheica N94.6
  escharotica — *see* Burn
  exfoliative, exfoliativa (generalized) L26
   neonatorum L00
  eyelid (*see also* Dermatosis, eyelid)
   allergic H01.119
    left H01.116
     lower H01.115
     upper H01.114
    right H01.113
     lower H01.112
     upper H01.111
   contact — *see* Dermatitis, eyelid, allergic
   due to
    Demodex species B88.0
    herpes (zoster) B02.39
     simplex B00.59
   eczematous H01.139
    left H01.136

Index

Dermatitis — Detachment

Dermatitis — *continued*
 eyelid (*see also* Dermatosis, eyelid) — *continued*
  eczematous — *continued*
   left — *continued*
    lower H01.135
    upper H01.134
   right H01.133
    lower H01.132
    upper H01.131
 facta, factitia, factitial L98.1
  psychogenic F54
 flexural NEC L20.82
 friction L30.4
 fungus B36.9
  specified type NEC B36.8
 gangrenosa, gangrenous infantum L08.0
 harvest mite B88.0
 heat L59.0
 herpesviral, vesicular (ear) (lip) B00.1
 herpetiformis (bullous) (erythematous) (pustular)
   (vesicular) L13.0
  juvenile L12.2
  senile L12.0
 hiemalis L30.8
 hypostatic, hypostatica — *see* Varix, leg, with, inflammation
 infectious eczematoid L30.3
 infective L30.3
 irritant — *see* Dermatitis, contact, irritant
 Jacquet's (diaper dermatitis) L22
 Leptus B88.0
 lichenified NEC L28.0
 medicamentosa (generalized) (internal use) — *see*
   Dermatitis, due to drugs
 mite B88.0
 multiformis L13.0
  juvenile L12.2
 napkin L22
 neurotica L13.0
 nummular L30.0
 papillaris capillitii L73.0
 pellagrous E52
 perioral L71.0
 photocontact L56.2
 polymorpha dolorosa L13.0
 pruriginosa L13.0
 pruritic NEC L30.8
 psychogenic F54
 purulent L08.0
 pustular
  contagious B08.02
  subcorneal L13.1
 pyococcal L08.0
 pyogenica L08.0
 repens L40.2
 Ritter's (exfoliativa) L00
 Schamberg's L81.7
 schistosome B65.3
 seasonal bullous L30.8
 seborrheic L21.9
  infantile L21.1
  specified NEC L21.8
 sensitization NOS L23.9
 septic L08.0
 solare L57.8
 specified NEC L30.8
 stasis I87.2
  with
   varicose ulcer — *see* Varix, leg, with ulcer, with
     inflammation
   varicose veins — *see* Varix, leg, with, inflamma-
     tion
  due to postthrombotic syndrome — *see* Syndrome,
    postthrombotic
 suppurative L08.0
 traumatic NEC L30.4
 trophoneurotica L13.0
 ultraviolet (sun) (chronic exposure) L57.8
  acute L56.8
 varicose — *see* Varix, leg, with, inflammation
 vegetans L10.1
 verrucosa B43.0
 vesicular, herpesviral B00.1
Dermatoarthritis, lipoid E78.81
Dermatochalasis, eyelid H02.839
 left H02.836
  lower H02.835
  upper H02.834

Dermatochalasis, eyelid — *continued*
 right H02.833
  lower H02.832
  upper H02.831
Dermatofibroma (lenticulare) — *see* Neoplasm, skin,
   benign
 protuberans — *see* Neoplasm, skin, uncertain behavior
Dermatofibrosarcoma (pigmented) (protuberans) —
   see Neoplasm, skin, malignant
Dermatographia L50.3
Dermatolysis (exfoliativa) (congenital) Q82.8
 acquired L57.4
 eyelids — *see* Blepharochalasis
 palpebrarum — *see* Blepharochalasis
 senile L57.4
Dermatomegaly NEC Q82.8
Dermatomucosomyositis M33.10
 with
  myopathy M33.12
  respiratory involvement M33.11
  specified organ involvement NEC M33.19
Dermatomycosis B36.9
 furfuracea B36.0
 specified type NEC B36.8
Dermatomyositis (acute) (chronic) (*see also* Dermatopolymyositis)
 adult (*see also* Dermatomyositis, specified NEC) M33.10
 in (due to) neoplastic disease (*see also* Neoplasm)
   D49.9 [M36.0]
 juvenile M33.00
  with
   myopathy M33.02
   respiratory involvement M33.01
   specified organ involvement NEC M33.09
  without myopathy M33.03
 specified NEC M33.10
  with
   myopathy M33.12
   respiratory involvement M33.11
   specified organ involvement NEC M33.19
  without myopathy M33.13
Dermatoneuritis of children — *see* Poisoning, mercury
Dermatophilosis A48.8
Dermatophytid L30.2
Dermatophyte — *see* Dermatophytosis
Dermatophytosis (epidermophyton) (infection) (Microsporum) (tinea) (Trichophyton) B35.9
 beard B35.0
 body B35.4
 capitis B35.0
 corporis B35.4
 deep-seated B35.8
 disseminated B35.8
 foot B35.3
 granulomatous B35.8
 groin B35.6
 hand B35.2
 nail B35.1
 perianal (area) B35.6
 scalp B35.0
 specified NEC B35.8
Dermatopolymyositis M33.90
 with
  myopathy M33.92
  respiratory involvement M33.91
  specified organ involvement NEC M33.99
 in neoplastic disease (*see also* Neoplasm) D49.9 [M36.0]
 juvenile M33.00
  with
   myopathy M33.02
   respiratory involvement M33.01
   specified organ involvement NEC M33.09
 specified NEC M33.10
  myopathy M33.12
  respiratory involvement M33.11
  specified organ involvement NEC M33.19
 without myopathy M33.93
Dermatopolyneuritis — *see* Poisoning, mercury
Dermatorrhexis Q79.6
 acquired L57.4
Dermatosclerosis (*see also* Scleroderma)
 localized L94.0
Dermatosis L98.9
 Andrews' L08.89
 Bowen's — *see* Neoplasm, skin, in situ
 bullous L13.9
  specified NEC L13.8
 exfoliativa L26

Dermatosis — *continued*
 eyelid (noninfectious)
  dermatitis — *see* Dermatitis, eyelid
  discoid lupus erythematosus — *see* Lupus, erythe-
    matosus, eyelid
  xeroderma — *see* Xeroderma, acquired, eyelid
 factitial L98.1
 febrile neutrophilic L98.2
 gonococcal A54.89
 herpetiformis L13.3
  juvenile L12.2
 linear IgA L13.8
 menstrual NEC L98.8
 neutrophilic, febrile L98.2
 occupational — *see* Dermatitis, contact
 papulosa nigra L82.1
 pigmentary L81.9
  progressive L81.7
  Schamberg's L81.7
 psychogenic F54
 purpuric, pigmented L81.7
 pustular, subcorneal L13.1
 transient acantholytic L11.1
Dermographia, dermographism L50.3
Dermoid (cyst) (*see also* Neoplasm, benign, by site)
 with malignant transformation C56- ☑
 due to radiation (nonionizing) L57.8
Dermopathy
 infiltrative with thyrotoxicosis — *see* Thyrotoxicosis
 nephrogenic fibrosing L90.8
Dermophytosis — *see* Dermatophytosis
Descemetocele H18.73- ☑
Descemet's membrane — *see* condition
Descending — *see* condition
Descensus uteri — *see* Prolapse, uterus
Desert
 rheumatism B38.0
 sore — *see* Ulcer, skin
Desertion (newborn) — *see* Maltreatment
Desmoid (extra-abdominal) (tumor) — *see* Neoplasm,
   connective tissue, uncertain behavior
 abdominal D48.1
Despondency F32.9
Desquamation, skin R23.4
Destruction, destructive (*see also* Damage)
 articular facet (*see also* Derangement, joint, specifie?
    type NEC)
  knee M23.8X- ☑
  vertebra — *see* Spondylosis
 bone (*see also* Disorder, bone, specified type NEC)
  syphilitic A52.77
 joint (*see also* Derangement, joint, specified type NE?
  sacroiliac M53.3
 rectal sphincter K62.89
 septum (nasal) J34.89
 tuberculous NEC — *see* Tuberculosis
 tympanum, tympanic membrane (nontraumatic) —
    see Disorder, tympanic membrane, specified NE?
 vertebral disc — *see* Degeneration, intervertebral di?
Destructiveness (*see also* Disorder, conduct)
 adjustment reaction — *see* Disorder, adjustment
Desultory labor O62.2
Detachment
 cartilage — *see* Sprain
 cervix, annular N88.8
  complicating delivery O71.3
 choroid (old) (postinfectional) (simple) (spontaneou?
    H31.40- ☑
  hemorrhagic H31.41- ☑
  serous H31.42- ☑
 ligament — *see* Sprain
 meniscus (knee) (*see also* Derangement, knee, men?
    cus, specified NEC)
  current injury — *see* Tear, meniscus
  due to old tear or injury — *see* Derangement, kne?
    meniscus, due to old tear
 retina (without retinal break) (serous) H33.2- ☑
  with retinal:
   break H33.00- ☑
    giant H33.03- ☑
    multiple H33.02- ☑
    single H33.01- ☑
   dialysis H33.04- ☑
  pigment epithelium — *see* Degeneration, retina?
    separation of layers, pigment epithelium d?
    tachment

☑ **Additional Character Required** — **Refer to the Tabular List for Character Selection**   ▽ Subterms under main terms may continue to next column or pa?

Detachment — *continued*
  retina — *continued*
    rhegmatogenous — *see* Detachment, retina, with
      retinal, break
    specified NEC H33.8
    total H33.05- ☑
    traction H33.4- ☑
    vitreous (body) H43.81 ☑
Detergent asthma J69.8
Deterioration
  epileptic F06.8
  general physical R53.81
  heart, cardiac — *see* Degeneration, myocardial
  mental — *see* Psychosis
  myocardial, myocardium — *see* Degeneration, myocardial
    dial
  senile (simple) R54
Deuteranomaly (anomalous trichromat) H53.53
Deuteranopia (complete) (incomplete) H53.53
Development
  abnormal, bone Q79.9
  arrested R62.50
    bone — *see* Arrest, development or growth, bone
    child R62.50
    due to malnutrition E45
  defective, congenital (*see also* Anomaly, by site)
    cauda equina Q06.3
    left ventricle Q24.8
      in hypoplastic left heart syndrome Q23.4
    valve Q24.8
      pulmonary Q22.3
  delayed (*see also* Delay, development) R62.50
    arithmetical skills F81.2
    language (skills) (expressive) F80.1
    learning skill F81.9
    mixed skills F88
    motor coordination F82
    reading F81.0
    specified learning skill NEC F81.89
    speech F80.9
    spelling F81.81
    written expression F81.81
  imperfect, congenital (*see also* Anomaly, by site)
    heart Q24.9
    lungs Q33.6
  incomplete
    bronchial tree Q32.4
    organ or site not listed — *see* Hypoplasia, by site
    respiratory system Q34.9
  sexual, precocious NEC E30.1
  tardy, mental (*see also* Disability, intellectual) F79
Developmental — *see* condition
  testing, infant or child — *see* Examination, child
Devergie's disease (pityriasis rubra pilaris) L44.0
Deviation (in)
  conjugate palsy (eye) (spastic) H51.0
  esophagus (acquired) K22.8
  eye, skew H51.8
  midline (jaw) (teeth) (dental arch) M26.29
    specified site NEC — *see* Malposition
  nasal septum J34.2
    congenital Q67.4
  opening and closing of the mandible M26.53
  organ or site, congenital NEC — *see* Malposition, congenital
  septum (nasal) (acquired) J34.2
    congenital Q67.4
  sexual F65.9
    bestiality F65.89
    erotomania F52.8
    exhibitionism F65.2
    fetishism, fetishistic F65.0
      transvestism F65.1
    frotteurism F65.81
    masochism F65.51
    multiple F65.89
    necrophilia F65.89
    nymphomania F52.8
    pederosis F65.4
    pedophilia F65.4
    sadism, sadomasochism F65.52
    satyriasis F52.8
    specified type NEC F65.89
    transvestism F64.1
    voyeurism F65.3
  teeth, midline M26.29
  trachea J39.8
  ureter, congenital Q62.61

Device
  cerebral ventricle (communicating) in situ Z98.2
  contraceptive — *see* Contraceptive, device
  drainage, cerebrospinal fluid, in situ Z98.2
Devic's disease G36.0
Devil's
  grip B33.0
  pinches (purpura simplex) D69.2
Devitalized tooth K04.99
Devonshire colic — *see* Poisoning, lead
Dextraposition, aorta Q20.3
  in tetralogy of Fallot Q21.3
Dextrinosis, limit (debrancher enzyme deficiency) E74.03
Dextrocardia (true) Q24.0
  with
    complete transposition of viscera Q89.3
    situs inversus Q89.3
Dextrotransposition, aorta Q20.3
d-glycericacidemia E72.59
Dhat syndrome F48.8
Dhobi itch B35.6
Di George's syndrome D82.1
Di Guglielmo's disease C94.0- ☑
Diabetes, diabetic (mellitus) (sugar) E11.9
  with
    amyotrophy E11.44
    arthropathy NEC E11.618
    autonomic (poly)neuropathy E11.43
    cataract E11.36
    Charcot's joints E11.610
    chronic kidney disease E11.22
    circulatory complication NEC E11.59
    complication E11.8
      specified NEC E11.69
    dermatitis E11.620
    foot ulcer E11.621
    gangrene E11.52
    gastroparalysis E11.43
    gastroparesis E11.43
    glomerulonephrosis, intracapillary E11.21
    glomerulosclerosis, intercapillary E11.21
    hyperglycemia E11.65
    hyperosmolarity E11.00
      with coma E11.01
    hypoglycemia E11.649
      with coma E11.641
    ketoacidosis E11.10
      with coma E11.11
    kidney complications NEC E11.29
    Kimmelsteil-Wilson disease E11.21
    loss of protective sensation (LOPS) — *see* Diabetes, by type, with neuropathy
    mononeuropathy E11.41
    myasthenia E11.44
    necrobiosis lipoidica E11.620
    nephropathy E11.21
    neuralgia E11.42
    neurologic complication NEC E11.49
    neuropathic arthropathy E11.610
    neuropathy E11.40
    ophthalmic complication NEC E11.39
    oral complication NEC E11.638
    osteomyelitis E11.69
    periodontal disease E11.630
    peripheral angiopathy E11.51
      with gangrene E11.52
    polyneuropathy E11.42
    renal complication NEC E11.29
    renal tubular degeneration E11.29
    retinopathy E11.319
      with macular edema E11.311
        resolved following treatment E11.37 ☑
      nonproliferative E11.329 ☑
        with macular edema E11.321 ☑
        mild E11.329 ☑
          with macular edema E11.321 ☑ ⁎
        moderate E11.339 ☑
          with macular edema E11.331 ☑
        severe E11.349 ☑
          with macular edema E11.341 ☑
      proliferative E11.359 ☑
        with
          combined traction retinal detachment and rhegmatogenous retinal detachment E11.354 ☑
          macular edema E11.351 ☑
          stable proliferative diabetic retinopathy E11.355 ☑

Diabetes, diabetic — *continued*
  with — *continued*
    retinopathy — *continued*
      proliferative — *continued*
        with — *continued*
          traction retinal detachment involving the macula E11.352 ☑
          traction retinal detachment not involving the macula E11.353 ☑
        resolved following treatment E09.37 ☑
    skin complication NEC E11.628
    skin ulcer NEC E11.622
  brittle — *see* Diabetes, type 1
  bronzed E83.110
  complicating pregnancy — *see* Pregnancy, complicated by, diabetes
  dietary counseling and surveillance Z71.3
  due to
    autoimmune process — *see* Diabetes, type 1
    immune mediated pancreatic islet beta-cell destruction — *see* Diabetes, type 1
  due to drug or chemical E09.9
    with
      amyotrophy E09.44
      arthropathy NEC E09.618
      autonomic (poly)neuropathy E09.43
      cataract E09.36
      Charcot's joints E09.610
      chronic kidney disease E09.22
      circulatory complication NEC E09.59
      complication E09.8
        specified NEC E09.69
      dermatitis E09.620
      foot ulcer E09.621
      gangrene E09.52
      gastroparalysis E09.43
      gastroparesis E09.43
      glomerulonephrosis, intracapillary E09.21
      glomerulosclerosis, intercapillary E09.21
      hyperglycemia E09.65
      hyperosmolarity E09.00
        with coma E09.01
      hypoglycemia E09.649
        with coma E09.641
      ketoacidosis E09.10
        with coma E09.11
      kidney complications NEC E09.29
      Kimmelstiel-Wilson disease E09.21
      mononeuropathy E09.41
      myasthenia E09.44
      necrobiosis lipoidica E09.620
      nephropathy E09.21
      neuralgia E09.42
      neurologic complication NEC E09.49
      neuropathic arthropathy E09.610
      neuropathy E09.40
      ophthalmic complication NEC E09.39
      oral complication NEC E09.638
      periodontal disease E09.630
      peripheral angiopathy E09.51
        with gangrene E09.52
      polyneuropathy E09.42
      renal complication NEC E09.29
      renal tubular degeneration E09.29
      retinopathy E09.319
        with macular edema E09.311
        resolved following treatment E09.37 ☑
        nonproliferative E09.329 ☑
          with macular edema E09.321 ☑
          mild E09.329 ☑
            with macular edema E09.321 ☑
          moderate E09.339 ☑
            with macular edema E09.331 ☑
          severe E09.349 ☑
            with macular edema E09.341 ☑
        proliferative E09.359 ☑
          with
            combined traction retinal detachment and rhegmatogenous retinal detachment E09.354 ☑
            macular edema E09.351 ☑
            stable proliferative diabetic retinopathy E09.355 ☑
            traction retinal detachment involving the macula E09.352 ☑
            traction retinal detachment not involving the macula E09.353 ☑
    skin complication NEC E09.628

Diabetes, diabetic — *continued*
  due to drug or chemical — *continued*
    with — *continued*
      skin ulcer NEC E09.622
  due to underlying condition E08.9
    with
      amyotrophy E08.44
      arthropathy NEC E08.618
      autonomic (poly)neuropathy E08.43
      cataract E08.36
      Charcot's joints E08.610
      chronic kidney disease E08.22
      circulatory complication NEC E08.59
      complication E08.8
        specified NEC E08.69
      dermatitis E08.620
      foot ulcer E08.621
      gangrene E08.52
      gastroparalysis E08.43
      gastroparesis E08.43
      glomerulonephrosis, intracapillary E08.21
      glomerulosclerosis, intercapillary E08.21
      hyperglycemia E08.65
      hyperosmolarity E08.00
        with coma E08.01
      hypoglycemia E08.649
        with coma E08.641
      ketoacidosis E08.10
        with coma E08.11
      kidney complications NEC E08.29
      Kimmelsteil-WIlson disease E08.21
      mononeuropathy E08.41
      myasthenia E08.44
      necrobiosis lipoidica E08.620
      nephropathy E08.21
      neuralgia E08.42
      neurologic complication NEC E08.49
      neuropathic arthropathy E08.610
      neuropathy E08.40
      ophthalmic complication NEC E08.39
      oral complication NEC E08.638
      periodontal disease E08.630
      peripheral angiopathy E08.51
        with gangrene E08.52
      polyneuropathy E08.42
      renal complication NEC E08.29
      renal tubular degeneration E08.29
      retinopathy E08.319
        with macular edema E08.311
        resolved following treatment E08.37 ☑
        nonproliferative E08.329 ☑
          with macular edema E08.321 ☑
          mild E08.329 ☑
            with macular edema E08.321 ☑
          moderate E08.339 ☑
            with macular edema E08.331 ☑
          severe E08.349 ☑
            with macular edema E08.341 ☑
        proliferative E08.359 ☑
          with
            combined traction retinal detachment and rhegmatogenous retinal detachment E08.354 ☑
            macular edema E08.351 ☑
            stable proliferative diabetic retinopathy E08.355 ☑
            traction retinal detachment involving the macula E08.352 ☑
            traction retinal detachment not involving the macula E08.353 ☑
      skin complication NEC E08.628
      skin ulcer NEC E08.622
  gestational (in pregnancy) O24.419
    affecting newborn P70.0
    diet controlled O24.410
    in childbirth O24.429
      diet controlled O24.420
      insulin (and diet) controlled O24.424
      oral drug controlled (antidiabetic) (hypoglycemic) O24.425
    insulin (and diet) controlled O24.414
    oral drug controlled (antidiabetic) (hypoglycemic) O24.415
    puerperal O24.439
      diet controlled O24.430
      insulin (and diet) controlled O24.434
      oral drug controlled (antidiabetic) (hypoglycemic) O24.435

Diabetes, diabetic — *continued*
  hepatogenous E13.9
  idiopathic — *see* Diabetes, type 1
  inadequately controlled — *code to* Diabetes, by type, with hyperglycemia
  insipidus E23.2
    nephrogenic N25.1
    pituitary E23.2
    vasopressin resistant N25.1
  insulin dependent — *code to* type of diabetes
  juvenile-onset — *see* Diabetes, type 1
  ketosis-prone — *see* Diabetes, type 1
  latent R73.03
  neonatal (transient) P70.2
  non-insulin dependent — *code to* type of diabetes
  out of control — *code to* Diabetes, by type, with hyperglycemia
  phosphate E83.39
  poorly controlled — *code to* Diabetes, by type, with hyperglycemia
  postpancreatectomy — *see* Diabetes, specified type NEC
  postprocedural — *see* Diabetes, specified type NEC
  secondary diabetes mellitus NEC — *see* Diabetes, specified type NEC
  specified type NEC E13.9
    with
      amyotrophy E13.44
      arthropathy NEC E13.618
      autonomic (poly)neuropathy E13.43
      cataract E13.36
      Charcot's joints E13.610
      chronic kidney disease E13.22
      circulatory complication NEC E13.59
      complication E13.8
        specified NEC E13.69
      dermatitis E13.620
      foot ulcer E13.621
      gangrene E13.52
      gastroparalysis E13.43
      gastroparesis E13.43
      glomerulonephrosis, intracapillary E13.21
      glomerulosclerosis, intercapillary E13.21
      hyperglycemia E13.65
      hyperosmolarity E13.00
        with coma E13.01
      hypoglycemia E13.649
        with coma E13.641
      ketoacidosis E13.10
        with coma E13.11
      kidney complications NEC E13.29
      Kimmelsteil-Wilson disease E13.21
      mononeuropathy E13.41
      myasthenia E13.44
      necrobiosis lipoidica E13.620
      nephropathy E13.21
      neuralgia E13.42
      neurologic complication NEC E13.49
      neuropathic arthropathy E13.610
      neuropathy E13.40
      ophthalmic complication NEC E13.39
      oral complication NEC E13.638
      periodontal disease E13.630
      peripheral angiopathy E13.51
        with gangrene E13.52
      polyneuropathy E13.42
      renal complication NEC E13.29
      renal tubular degeneration E13.29
      retinopathy E13.319
        with macular edema E13.311
        resolved following treatment E13.37 ☑
        nonproliferative E13.329 ☑
          with macular edema E13.321 ☑
          mild E13.329 ☑
            with macular edema E13.321 ☑
          moderate E13.339 ☑
            with macular edema E13.331 ☑
          severe E13.349 ☑
            with macular edema E13.341 ☑
        proliferative E13.359 ☑
          with
            combined traction retinal detachment and rhegmatogenous retinal detachment E13.354 ☑
            macular edema E13.351 ☑
            stable proliferative diabetic retinopathy E13.355 ☑

Diabetes, diabetic — *continued*
  specified type — *continued*
    with — *continued*
      retinopathy — *continued*
        proliferative — *continued*
          with — *continued*
            traction retinal detachment involving the macula E13.352 ☑
            traction retinal detachment not involving the macula E13.353 ☑
      skin complication NEC E13.628
      skin ulcer NEC E13.622
  steroid-induced — *see* Diabetes, due to, drug or chemical
  type 1 E10.9
    with
      amyotrophy E10.44
      arthropathy NEC E10.618
      autonomic (poly)neuropathy E10.43
      cataract E10.36
      Charcot's joints E10.610
      chronic kidney disease E10.22
      circulatory complication NEC E10.59
      complication E10.8
        specified NEC E10.69
      dermatitis E10.620
      foot ulcer E10.621
      gangrene E10.52
      gastroparalysis E10.43
      gastroparesis E10.43
      glomerulonephrosis, intracapillary E10.21
      glomerulosclerosis, intercapillary E10.21
      hyperglycemia E10.65
      hypoglycemia E10.649
        with coma E10.641
      ketoacidosis E10.10
        with coma E10.11
      kidney complications NEC E10.29
      Kimmelsteil-Wilson disease E10.21
      mononeuropathy E10.41
      myasthenia E10.44
      necrobiosis lipoidica E10.620
      nephropathy E10.21
      neuralgia E10.42
      neurologic complication NEC E10.49
      neuropathic arthropathy E10.610
      neuropathy E10.40
      ophthalmic complication NEC E10.39
      oral complication NEC E10.638
      osteomyelitis E10.69
      periodontal disease E10.630
      peripheral angiopathy E10.51
        with gangrene E10.52
      polyneuropathy E10.42
      renal complication NEC E10.29
      renal tubular degeneration E10.29
      retinopathy E10.319
        with macular edema E10.311
        resolved following treatment E10.37 ☑
        nonproliferative E10.329 ☑
          with macular edema E10.321 ☑
          mild E10.329 ☑
            with macular edema E10.321 ☑
          moderate E10.339 ☑
            with macular edema E10.331 ☑
          severe E10.349 ☑
            with macular edema E10.341 ☑
        proliferative E10.359 ☑
          with
            combined traction retinal detachment and rhegmatogenous retinal detachment E10.354 ☑
            macular edema E10.351 ☑
            stable proliferative diabetic retinopathy E10.355 ☑
            traction retinal detachment involving the macula E10.352 ☑
            traction retinal detachment not involving the macula E10.353 ☑
      skin complication NEC E10.628
      skin ulcer NEC E10.622
  type 2 E11.9
    with
      amyotrophy E11.44
      arthropathy NEC E11.618
      autonomic (poly)neuropathy E11.43
      cataract E11.36
      Charcot's joints E11.610

Diabetes, diabetic — *continued*
  type 2 — *continued*
    with — *continued*
      chronic kidney disease E11.22
      circulatory complication NEC E11.59
      complication E11.8
        specified NEC E11.69
      dermatitis E11.620
      foot ulcer E11.621
      gangrene E11.52
      gastroparalysis E11.43
      gastroparesis E11.43
      glomerulonephrosis, intracapillary E11.21
      glomerulosclerosis, intercapillary E11.21
      hyperglycemia E11.65
      hyperosmolarity E11.00
        with coma E11.01
      hypoglycemia E11.649
        with coma E11.641
      ketoacidosis E11.10
        with coma E11.11
      kidney complications NEC E11.29
      Kimmelstiel-Wilson disease E11.21
      mononeuropathy E11.41
      myasthenia E11.44
      necrobiosis lipoidica E11.620
      nephropathy E11.21
      neuralgia E11.42
      neurologic complication NEC E11.49
      neuropathic arthropathy E11.610
      neuropathy E11.40
      ophthalmic complication NEC E11.39
      oral complication NEC E11.638
      osteomyelitis E11.69
      periodontal disease E11.630
      peripheral angiopathy E11.51
        with gangrene E11.52
      polyneuropathy E11.42
      renal complication NEC E11.29
      renal tubular degeneration E11.29
      retinopathy E11.319
        with macular edema E11.311
        resolved following treatment E11.37 ☑
        nonproliferative E11.329 ☑
          with macular edema E11.321 ☑
          mild E11.329 ☑
            with macular edema E11.321 ☑
          moderate E11.339 ☑
            with macular edema E11.331 ☑
          severe E11.349 ☑
            with macular edema E11.341 ☑
        proliferative E11.359 ☑
          with
            combined traction retinal detachment
              and rhegmatogenous retinal
              detachment E11.354 ☑
            macular edema E11.351 ☑
            stable proliferative diabetic retinopa-
              thy E11.355 ☑
            traction retinal detachment involving
              the macula E11.352 ☑
            traction retinal detachment not involv-
              ing the macula E11.353 ☑
      skin complication NEC E11.628
      skin ulcer NEC E11.622
  uncontrolled
    meaning
      hyperglycemia — *see* Diabetes, by type, with,
        hyperglycemia
      hypoglycemia — *see* Diabetes, by type, with,
        hypoglycemia
Diacyclothrombopathia D69.1
Diagnosis deferred R69
Dialysis (intermittent) (treatment)
  noncompliance (with) Z91.15
  renal (hemodialysis) (peritoneal), status Z99.2
  retina, retinal — *see* Detachment, retina, with retinal,
    dialysis
Diamond-Blackfan anemia (congenital hypoplastic)
  D61.01
Diamond-Gardener syndrome (autoerythrocyte sensi-
  tization) D69.2
Diaper rash L22
Diaphoresis (excessive) R61
Diaphragm — *see* condition
Diaphragmalgia R07.1
Diaphragmatitis, diaphragmitis J98.6
Diaphysial aclasis Q78.6

Diaphysitis — *see* Osteomyelitis, specified type NEC
Diarrhea, diarrheal (disease) (infantile) (inflammatory)
  R19.7
  achlorhydric K31.83
  allergic K52.29
    due to
      colitis — *see* Colitis, allergic
      enteritis — *see* Enteritis, allergic
  amebic (*see also* Amebiasis) A06.0
    with abscess — *see* Abscess, amebic
    acute A06.0
    chronic A06.1
    nondysenteric A06.2
  bacillary — *see* Dysentery, bacillary
  balantidial A07.0
  cachectic NEC K52.89
  Chilomastix A07.8
  choleriformis A00.1
  chronic (noninfectious) K52.9
  coccidial A07.3
  Cochin-China K90.1
    strongyloidiasis B78.0
  Dientamoeba A07.8
  dietetic (*see also* Diarrhea, allergic) K52.29
  drug-induced K52.1
  due to
    bacteria A04.9
      specified NEC A04.8
    Campylobacter A04.5
    Capillaria philippinensis B81.1
    Clostridium difficile
      not specified as recurrent A04.72
      recurrent A04.71
    Clostridium perfringens (C) (F) A04.8
    Cryptosporidium A07.2
    drugs K52.1
    Escherichia coli A04.4
      enteroaggregative A04.4
      enterohemorrhagic A04.3
      enteroinvasive A04.2
      enteropathogenic A04.0
      enterotoxigenic A04.1
      specified NEC A04.4
    food hypersensitivity (*see also* Diarrhea, allergic)
      K52.29
    Necator americanus B76.1
    S. japonicum B65.2
    specified organism NEC A08.8
      bacterial A04.8
      viral A08.39
    Staphylococcus A04.8
    Trichuris trichiuria B79
    virus — *see* Enteritis, viral
    Yersinia enterocolitica A04.6
  dysenteric A09
  endemic A09
  epidemic A09
  flagellate A07.9
  Flexner's (ulcerative) A03.1
  functional K59.1
    following gastrointestinal surgery K91.89
    psychogenic F45.8
  Giardia lamblia A07.1
  giardial A07.1
  hill K90.1
  infectious A09
  malarial — *see* Malaria
  mite B88.0
  mycotic NEC B49
  neonatal (noninfectious) P78.3
  nervous F45.8
  neurogenic K59.1
  noninfectious K52.9
  postgastrectomy K91.1
  postvagotomy K91.1
  protozoal A07.9
    specified NEC A07.8
  psychogenic F45.8
  specified
    bacterium NEC A04.8
    virus NEC A08.39
  strongyloidiasis B78.0
  toxic K52.1
  trichomonal A07.8
  tropical K90.1
  tuberculous A18.32
  viral — *see* Enteritis, viral

Diastasis
  cranial bones M84.88
    congenital NEC Q75.8
  joint (traumatic) — *see* Dislocation
  muscle M62.00
    ankle M62.07- ☑
    congenital Q79.8
    foot M62.07- ☑
    forearm M62.03- ☑
    hand M62.04- ☑
    lower leg M62.06- ☑
    pelvic region M62.05- ☑
    shoulder region M62.01- ☑
    specified site NEC M62.08
    thigh M62.05- ☑
    upper arm M62.02- ☑
  recti (abdomen)
    complicating delivery O71.89
    congenital Q79.59
Diastema, tooth, teeth, fully erupted M26.32
Diastematomyelia Q06.2
Diataxia, cerebral G80.4
Diathesis
  allergic — *see* History, allergy
  bleeding (familial) D69.9
  cystine (familial) E72.00
  gouty — *see* Gout
  hemorrhagic (familial) D69.9
    newborn NEC P53
  spasmophilic R29.0
Diaz's disease or osteochondrosis (juvenile) (talus) —
  see Osteochondrosis, juvenile, tarsus
Dibothriocephalus, dibothriocephaliasis (latus) (infection) (infestation) B70.0
  larval B70.1
Dicephalus, dicephaly Q89.4
Dichotomy, teeth K00.2
Dichromat, dichromatopsia (congenital) — *see* Deficiency, color vision
Dichuchwa A65
Dicroceliasis B66.2
Didelphia, didelphys — *see* Double uterus
Didymytis N45.1
  with orchitis N45.3
Dietary
  inadequacy or deficiency E63.9
  surveillance and counseling Z71.3
Dietl's crisis N13.8
Dieulafoy lesion (hemorrhagic)
  duodenum K31.82
  esophagus K22.8
  intestine (colon) K63.81
  stomach K31.82
Difficult, difficulty (in)
  acculturation Z60.3
  feeding R63.3
    newborn P92.9
      breast P92.5
      specified NEC P92.8
    nonorganic (infant or child) F98.29
  intubation, in anesthesia T88.4 ☑
  mechanical, gastroduodenal stoma K91.89
    causing obstruction (*see also* Obstruction, intestine,
      postoperative) K91.30
  micturition
    need to immediately re-void R39.191
    position dependent R39.192
    specified NEC R39.198
  reading (developmental) F81.0
    secondary to emotional disorders F93.9
  spelling (specific) F81.81
    with reading disorder F81.89
    due to inadequate teaching Z55.8
  swallowing — *see* Dysphagia
  walking R26.2
  work
    conditions NEC Z56.5
    schedule Z56.3
Diffuse — *see* condition
Digestive — *see* condition
Dihydropyrimidine dehydrogenase disease (DPD)
  E88.89
Diktyoma — *see* Neoplasm, malignant, by site
Dilaceration, tooth K00.4
Dilatation
  anus K59.8
    venule — *see* Hemorrhoids

Dilatation — continued
aorta (focal) (general) — *see* Ectasia, aorta
  with aneuysm — *see* Aneurysm, aorta
  congenital Q25.44
artery — *see* Aneurysm
bladder (sphincter) N32.89
  congenital Q64.79
blood vessel I99.8
bronchial J47.9
  with
    exacerbation (acute) J47.1
    lower respiratory infection J47.0
calyx (due to obstruction) — *see* Hydronephrosis
capillaries I78.8
cardiac (acute) (chronic) (*see also* Hypertrophy, cardiac)
  congenital Q24.8
    valve NEC Q24.8
      pulmonary Q22.3
    valve — *see* Endocarditis
cavum septi pellucidi Q06.8
cervix (uteri) (*see also* Incompetency, cervix)
  incomplete, poor, slow complicating delivery O62.0
colon K59.39
  congenital Q43.1
  psychogenic F45.8
  toxic K59.31
common duct (acquired) K83.8
  congenital Q44.5
cystic duct (acquired) K82.8
  congenital Q44.5
duct, mammary — *see* Ectasia, mammary duct
duodenum K59.8
esophagus K22.8
  congenital Q39.5
  due to achalasia K22.0
eustachian tube, congenital Q17.8
gallbladder K82.8
gastric — *see* Dilatation, stomach
heart (acute) (chronic) (*see also* Hypertrophy, cardiac)
  congenital Q24.8
  valve — *see* Endocarditis
ileum K59.8
  psychogenic F45.8
jejunum K59.8
  psychogenic F45.8
kidney (calyx) (collecting structures) (cystic) (parenchyma) (pelvis) (idiopathic) N28.89
lacrimal passages or duct — *see* Disorder, lacrimal system, changes
lymphatic vessel I89.0
mammary duct — *see* Ectasia, mammary duct
Meckel's diverticulum (congenital) Q43.0
  malignant — *see* Table of Neoplasms, small intestine, malignant
myocardium (acute) (chronic) — *see* Hypertrophy, cardiac
organ or site, congenital NEC — *see* Distortion
pancreatic duct K86.89
pericardium — *see* Pericarditis
pharynx J39.2
prostate N42.89
pulmonary
  artery (idiopathic) I28.8
  valve, congenital Q22.3
pupil H57.04
rectum K59.39
saccule, congenital Q16.5
salivary gland (duct) K11.8
sphincter ani K62.89
stomach K31.89
  acute K31.0
  psychogenic F45.8
submaxillary duct K11.8
trachea, congenital Q32.1
ureter (idiopathic) N28.82
  congenital Q62.2
  due to obstruction N13.4
urethra (acquired) N36.8
vasomotor I73.9
vein I86.8
ventricular, ventricle (acute) (chronic) (*see also* Hypertrophy, cardiac)
  cerebral, congenital Q04.8
venule NEC I86.8
vesical orifice N32.89
Dilated, dilation — *see* Dilatation
Diminished, diminution
hearing (acuity) — *see* Deafness

Diminished, diminution — *continued*
sense or sensation (cold) (heat) (tactile) (vibratory) R20.8
vision NEC H54.7
vital capacity R94.2
Diminuta taenia B71.0
Dimitri-Sturge-Weber disease Q85.8
Dimple
congenital sacral Q82.6
parasacral Q82.6
pilonidal or postanal — *see* Cyst, pilonidal
Dioctophyme renalis (infection) (infestation) B83.8
Dipetalonemiasis B74.4
Diphallus Q55.69
Diphtheria, diphtheritic (gangrenous) (hemorrhagic) A36.9
carrier (suspected) Z22.2
cutaneous A36.3
faucial A36.0
infection of wound A36.3
laryngeal A36.2
myocarditis A36.81
nasal, anterior A36.89
nasopharyngeal A36.1
neurological complication A36.89
pharyngeal A36.0
specified site NEC A36.89
tonsillar A36.0
Diphyllobothriasis (intestine) B70.0
larval B70.1
Diplacusis H93.22- ☑
Diplegia (upper limbs) G83.0
congenital (cerebral) G80.8
facial G51.0
lower limbs G82.20
spastic G80.1
Diplococcus, diplococcal — *see* condition
Diplopia H53.2
Dipsomania F10.20
with
  psychosis — *see* Psychosis, alcoholic
  remission F10.21
Dipylidiasis B71.1
DIRA (deficiency of interleukin 1 receptor antagonist) M04.8
Direction, teeth, abnormal, fully erupted M26.30
Dirofilariasis B74.8
Dirt-eating child F98.3
Disability, disabilities
heart — *see* Disease, heart
intellectual F79
with
  autistic features F84.9
mild (I.Q. 50-69) F70
moderate (I.Q. 35-49) F71
profound (I.Q. under 20) F73
severe (I.Q. 20-34) F72
specified level NEC F78
knowledge acquisition F81.9
learning F81.9
limiting activities Z73.6
spelling, specific F81.81
Disappearance of family member Z63.4
Disarticulation — *see* Amputation
meaning traumatic amputation — *see* Amputation, traumatic
Discharge (from)
abnormal finding in — *see* Abnormal, specimen
breast (female) (male) N64.52
diencephalic autonomic idiopathic — *see* Epilepsy, specified NEC
ear (*see also* Otorrhea)
  blood — *see* Otorrhagia
excessive urine R35.8
nipple N64.52
penile R36.9
postnasal R09.82
prison, anxiety concerning Z65.2
urethral R36.9
  without blood R36.0
  hematospermia R36.1
vaginal N89.8
Discitis, diskitis M46.40
cervical region M46.42
cervicothoracic region M46.43
lumbar region M46.46
lumbosacral region M46.47
multiple sites M46.49

Discitis, diskitis — *continued*
occipito-atlanto-axial region M46.41
pyogenic — *see* Infection, intervertebral disc, pyogenic
sacrococcygeal region M46.48
thoracic region M46.44
thoracolumbar region M46.45
Discoid
meniscus (congenital) Q68.6
semilunar cartilage (congenital) — *see* Derangement, knee, meniscus, specified NEC
Discoloration
nails L60.8
teeth (posteruptive) K03.7
  during formation K00.8
Discomfort
chest R07.89
visual H53.14- ☑
Discontinuity, ossicles, ear H74.2- ☑
Discord (with)
boss Z56.4
classmates Z55.4
counselor Z64.4
employer Z56.4
family Z63.8
fellow employees Z56.4
in-laws Z63.1
landlord Z59.2
lodgers Z59.2
neighbors Z59.2
probation officer Z64.4
social worker Z64.4
teachers Z55.4
workmates Z56.4
Discordant connection
atrioventricular (congenital) Q20.5
ventriculoarterial Q20.3
Discrepancy
centric occlusion maximum intercuspation M26.55
leg length (acquired) — *see* Deformity, limb, unequal length
  congenital — *see* Defect, reduction, lower limb
uterine size date O26.84- ☑
Discrimination
ethnic Z60.5
political Z60.5
racial Z60.5
religious Z60.5
sex Z60.5
Disease, diseased (*see also* Syndrome)
absorbent system I87.8
acid-peptic K30
Acosta's T70.29 ☑
Adams-Stokes (-Morgagni) (syncope with heart block) I45.9
Addison's anemia (pernicious) D51.0
adenoids (and tonsils) J35.9
adrenal (capsule) (cortex) (gland) (medullary) E27.9
  hyperfunction E27.0
  specified NEC E27.8
ainhum L94.6
airway
  obstructive, chronic J44.9
    due to
      cotton dust J66.0
      specific organic dusts NEC J66.8
  reactive — *see* Asthma
akamushi (scrub typhus) A75.3
Albers-Schönberg (marble bones) Q78.2
Albert's — *see* Tendinitis, Achilles
alimentary canal K63.9
alligator-skin Q80.9
  acquired L85.0
alpha heavy chain C88.3
alpine T70.29 ☑
altitude T70.20 ☑
alveolar ridge
  edentulous K06.9
    specified NEC K06.8
alveoli, teeth K08.9
Alzheimer's G30.9 [F02.80]
  with behavioral disturbance G30.9 [F02.81]
  early onset G30.0 [F02.80]
    with behavioral disturbance G30.0 [F02.81]
  late onset G30.1 [F02.80]
    with behavioral disturbance G30.1 [F02.81]
  specified NEC G30.8 [F02.80]
    with behavioral disturbance G30.8 [F02.81]
amyloid — *see* Amyloidosis

☑ **Additional Character Required** — Refer to the Tabular List for Character Selection   ▽ Subterms under main terms may continue to next column or page

Disease, diseased — *continued*
- Andersen's (glycogenosis IV) E74.09
- Andes T70.29 ☑
- Andrews' (bacterid) L08.89
- angiospastic I73.9
  - cerebral G45.9
  - vein I87.8
- anterior
  - chamber H21.9
  - horn cell G12.29
- antiglomerular basement membrane (anti- GBM) antibody M31.0
  - tubulo-interstitial nephritis N12
- antral — *see* Sinusitis, maxillary
- anus K62.9
  - specified NEC K62.89
- aorta (nonsyphilitic) I77.9
  - syphilitic NEC A52.02
- aortic (heart) (valve) I35.9
  - rheumatic I06.9
- Apollo B30.3
- aponeuroses — *see* Enthesopathy
- appendix K38.9
  - specified NEC K38.8
- aqueous (chamber) H21.9
- Arnold-Chiari — *see* Arnold-Chiari disease
- arterial I77.9
  - occlusive — *see* Occlusion, by site
    - due to stricture or stenosis I77.1
- arteriocardiorenal — *see* Hypertension, cardiorenal
- arteriolar (generalized) (obliterative) I77.9
- arteriorenal — *see* Hypertension, kidney
- arteriosclerotic (*see also* Arteriosclerosis)
  - cardiovascular — *see* Disease, heart, ischemic, atherosclerotic
  - coronary (artery) — *see* Disease, heart, ischemic, atherosclerotic
  - heart — *see* Disease, heart, ischemic, atherosclerotic
- artery I77.9
  - cerebral I67.9
  - coronary I25.10
    - with angina pectoris — *see* Arteriosclerosis, coronary (artery)
- arthropod-borne NOS (viral) A94
  - specified type NEC A93.8
- atticoantral, chronic H66.20
  - left H66.22
    - with right H66.23
  - right H66.21
    - with left H66.23
- auditory canal — *see* Disorder, ear, external
- auricle, ear NEC — *see* Disorder, pinna
- Australian X A83.4
- autoimmune (systemic) NOS M35.9
  - hemolytic (cold type) (warm type) D59.1
    - drug-induced D59.0
  - thyroid E06.3
- autoinflammatory M04.9
  - NOD2-associated M04.8
  - specified type NEC M04.8
- aviator's — *see* Effect, adverse, high altitude
- Ayerza's (pulmonary artery sclerosis with pulmonary hypertension) I27.0
- Babington's (familial hemorrhagic telangiectasia) I78.0
- bacterial A49.9
  - specified NEC A48.8
  - zoonotic A28.9
    - specified type NEC A28.8
- Baelz's (cheilitis glandularis apostematosa) K13.0
- bagasse J67.1
- balloon — *see* Effect, adverse, high altitude
- Bang's (brucella abortus) A23.1
- Bannister's T78.3 ☑
- barometer makers' — *see* Poisoning, mercury
- Barraquer (-Simons') (progressive lipodystrophy) E88.1
- Barrett's — *see* Barrett's, esophagus
- Bartholin's gland N75.9
- basal ganglia G25.9
  - degenerative G23.9
    - specified NEC G23.8
  - specified NEC G25.89
- Basedow's (exophthalmic goiter) — *see* Hyperthyroidism, with, goiter (diffuse)
- Bateman's B08.1
- Batten-Steinert G71.11
- Battey A31.0
- Beard's (neurasthenia) F48.8

Disease, diseased — *continued*
- Becker
  - idiopathic mural endomyocardial I42.3
  - myotonia congenita G71.12
- Begbie's (exophthalmic goiter) — *see* Hyperthyroidism, with, goiter (diffuse)
- behavioral, organic F07.9
- Beigel's (white piedra) B36.2
- Benson's — *see* Deposit, crystalline
- Bernard-Soulier (thrombopathy) D69.1
- Bernhardt (-Roth) — *see* Mononeuropathy, lower limb, meralgia paresthetica
- Biermer's (pernicious anemia) D51.0
- bile duct (common) (hepatic) K83.9
  - with calculus, stones — *see* Calculus, bile duct
  - specified NEC K83.8
- biliary (tract) K83.9
  - specified NEC K83.8
- Billroth's — *see* Spina bifida
- bird fancier's J67.2
- black lung J60
- bladder N32.9
  - in (due to)
    - schistosomiasis (bilharziasis) B65.0 [N33]
  - specified NEC N32.89
- bleeder's D66
- blood D75.9
  - forming organs D75.9
  - vessel I99.9
- Bloodgood's — *see* Mastopathy, cystic
- Bodechtel-Guttmann (subacute sclerosing panencephalitis) A81.1
- bone (*see also* Disorder, bone)
  - aluminum M83.4
  - fibrocystic NEC
    - jaw M27.49
- bone-marrow D75.9
- Borna A83.9
- Bornholm (epidemic pleurodynia) B33.0
- Bouchard's (myopathic dilatation of the stomach) K31.0
- Bouillaud's (rheumatic heart disease) I01.9
- Bourneville (-Brissaud) (tuberous sclerosis) Q85.1
- Bouveret (-Hoffmann) (paroxysmal tachycardia) I47.9
- bowel K63.9
  - functional K59.9
    - psychogenic F45.8
- brain G93.9
  - arterial, artery I67.9
  - arteriosclerotic I67.2
  - congenital Q04.9
  - degenerative — *see* Degeneration, brain
  - inflammatory — *see* Encephalitis
  - organic G93.9
    - arteriosclerotic I67.2
  - parasitic NEC B71.9 [G94]
  - senile NEC G31.1
  - specified NEC G93.89
- breast (*see also* Disorder, breast) N64.9
  - cystic (chronic) — *see* Mastopathy, cystic
  - fibrocystic — *see* Mastopathy, cystic
  - Paget's
    - female, unspecified side C50.91- ☑
    - male, unspecified side C50.92- ☑
  - specified NEC N64.89
- Breda's — *see* Yaws
- Bretonneau's (diphtheritic malignant angina) A36.0
- Bright's — *see* Nephritis
  - arteriosclerotic — *see* Hypertension, kidney
- Brill's (recrudescent typhus) A75.1
- Brill-Zinsser (recrudescent typhus) A75.1
- Brion-Kayser — *see* Fever, paratyphoid
- broad
  - beta E78.2
  - ligament (noninflammatory) N83.9
    - inflammatory — *see* Disease, pelvis, inflammatory
    - specified NEC N83.8
- Brocq-Duhring (dermatitis herpetiformis) L13.0
- Brocq's
  - meaning
    - dermatitis herpetiformis L13.0
    - prurigo L28.2
- bronchopulmonary J98.4
- bronchus NEC J98.09
- bronze Addison's E27.1
  - tuberculous A18.7
- budgerigar fancier's J67.2
- Buerger's (thromboangiitis obliterans) I73.1

Disease, diseased — *continued*
- bullous L13.9
  - chronic of childhood L12.2
  - specified NEC L13.8
- Bürger-Grütz (essential familial hyperlipemia) E78.3
- bursa — *see* Bursopathy
- caisson T70.3 ☑
- California — *see* Coccidioidomycosis
- capillaries I78.9
  - specified NEC I78.8
- Carapata A68.0
- cardiac — *see* Disease, heart
- cardiopulmonary, chronic I27.9
- cardiorenal (hepatic) (hypertensive) (vascular) — *see* Hypertension, cardiorenal
- cardiovascular (atherosclerotic) I25.10
  - with angina pectoris — *see* Arteriosclerosis, coronary (artery),
  - congenital Q28.9
  - hypertensive — *see* Hypertension, heart
  - newborn P29.9
    - specified NEC P29.89
  - renal (hypertensive) — *see* Hypertension, cardiorenal
  - syphilitic (asymptomatic) A52.00
- cartilage — *see* Disorder, cartilage
- Castellani's A69.8
- Castleman (unicentric) (multicentric) D47.Z2
  - HHV-8-associated (*see also* Herpesvirus, human, 8) D47.Z2
- cat-scratch A28.1
- Cavare's (familial periodic paralysis) G72.3
- cecum K63.9
- celiac (adult) (infantile) (with steatorrhea) K90.0
- cellular tissue L98.9
- central core G71.2
- cerebellar, cerebellum — *see* Disease, brain
- cerebral (*see also* Disease, brain)
  - degenerative — *see* Degeneration, brain
- cerebrospinal G96.9
- cerebrovascular I67.9
  - acute I67.89
    - embolic I63.4- ☑
    - thrombotic I63.3- ☑
  - arteriosclerotic I67.2
  - hereditary NEC I67.858
  - specified NEC I67.89
- cervix (uteri) (noninflammatory) N88.9
  - inflammatory — *see* Cervicitis
  - specified NEC N88.8
- Chabert's A22.9
- Chandler's (osteochondritis dissecans, hip) — *see* Osteochondritis, dissecans, hip
- Charlouis — *see* Yaws
- Chédiak-Steinbrinck (-Higashi) (congenital gigantism of peroxidase granules) E70.330
- chest J98.9
- Chiari's (hepatic vein thrombosis) I82.0
- Chicago B40.9
- Chignon B36.8
- chigo, chigoe B88.1
- childhood granulomatous D71
- Chinese liver fluke B66.1
- chlamydial A74.9
  - specified NEC A74.89
- cholecystic K82.9
- choroid H31.9
  - specified NEC H31.8
- Christmas D67
- chronic bullous of childhood L12.2
- chylomicron retention E78.3
- ciliary body H21.9
  - specified NEC H21.89
- circulatory (system) NEC I99.8
  - newborn P29.9
  - syphilitic A52.00
    - congenital A50.54
- coagulation factor deficiency (congenital) — *see* Defect, coagulation
- coccidioidal — *see* Coccidioidomycosis
- cold
  - agglutinin or hemoglobinuria D59.1
    - paroxysmal D59.6
  - hemagglutinin (chronic) D59.1
- collagen NOS (nonvascular) (vascular) M35.9
  - specified NEC M35.8
- colon K63.9
  - functional K59.9

Disease, diseased — continued
colon — continued
  functional — continued
    congenital Q43.2
  ischemic (see also Ischemia, intestine, acute) K55.039
colonic inflammatory bowel, unclassified (IBDU) K52.3
combined system — see Degeneration, combined
compressed air T70.3 ☑
Concato's (pericardial polyserositis) A19.9
  nontubercular I31.1
  pleural — see Pleurisy, with effusion
conjunctiva H11.9
  chlamydial A74.0
  specified NEC H11.89
  viral B30.9
    specified NEC B30.8
connective tissue, systemic (diffuse) M35.9
  in (due to)
    hypogammaglobulinemia D80.1 [M36.8]
    ochronosis E70.29 [M36.8]
  specified NEC M35.8
Conor and Bruch's (boutonneuse fever) A77.1
Cooper's — see Mastopathy, cystic
Cori's (glycogenosis III) E74.03
corkhandler's or corkworker's J67.3
cornea H18.9
  specified NEC H18.89- ☑
coronary (artery) — see Disease, heart, ischemic, atherosclerotic
  congenital Q24.5
  ostial, syphilitic (aortic) (mitral) (pulmonary) A52.03
corpus cavernosum N48.9
  specified NEC N48.89
Cotugno's — see Sciatica
coxsackie (virus) NEC B34.1
cranial nerve NOS G52.9
Creutzfeldt-Jakob — see Creutzfeldt-Jakob disease or syndrome
Crocq's (acrocyanosis) I73.89
Crohn's — see Enteritis, regional
Curschmann G71.11
cystic
  breast (chronic) — see Mastopathy, cystic
  kidney, congenital Q61.9
  liver, congenital Q44.6
  lung J98.4
    congenital Q33.0
cytomegalic inclusion (generalized) B25.9
  with pneumonia B25.0
  congenital P35.1
cytomegaloviral B25.9
  specified NEC B25.8
Czerny's (periodic hydrarthrosis of the knee) — see Effusion, joint, knee
Daae (-Finsen) (epidemic pleurodynia) B33.0
Darling's — see Histoplasmosis capsulati
de Quervain's (tendon sheath) M65.4
  thyroid (subacute granulomatous thyroiditis) E06.1
Débove's (splenomegaly) R16.1
deer fly — see Tularemia
Degos' I77.89
demyelinating, demyelinizating (nervous system) G37.9
  multiple sclerosis G35
  specified NEC G37.8
dense deposit (see also N00-N07 with fourth character .6) N05.6
deposition, hydroxyapatite — see Disease, hydroxyapatite deposition
Devergie's (pityriasis rubra pilaris) L44.0
Devic's G36.0
diaphorase deficiency D74.0
diaphragm J98.6
diarrheal, infectious NEC A09
digestive system K92.9
  specified NEC K92.89
disc, degenerative — see Degeneration, intervertebral disc
discogenic (see also Displacement, intervertebral disc NEC)
  with myelopathy — see Disorder, disc, with, myelopathy
diverticular — see Diverticula
Dubois (thymus) A50.59 [E35]
Duchenne-Griesinger G71.01
Duchenne's
  muscular dystrophy G71.01
  pseudohypertrophy, muscles G71.01
ductless glands E34.9

Disease, diseased — continued
Duhring's (dermatitis herpetiformis) L13.0
duodenum K31.9
  specified NEC K31.89
Dupré's (meningism) R29.1
Dupuytren's (muscle contracture) M72.0
Durand-Nicholas-Favre (climatic bubo) A55
Duroziez's (congenital mitral stenosis) Q23.2
ear — see Disorder, ear
Eberth's — see Fever, typhoid
Ebola (virus) A98.4
Ebstein's heart Q22.5
Echinococcus — see Echinococcus
echovirus NEC B34.1
Eddowes' (brittle bones and blue sclera) Q78.0
edentulous (alveolar) ridge K06.9
  specified NEC K06.8
Edsall's T67.2 ☑
Eichstedt's (pityriasis versicolor) B36.0
Eisenmenger's (irreversible) I27.83
Ellis-van Creveld (chondroectodermal dysplasia) Q77.6
end stage renal (ESRD) N18.6
  due to hypertension I12.0
endocrine glands or system NEC E34.9
endomyocardial (eosinophilic) I42.3
English (rickets) E55.0
enteroviral, enterovirus NEC B34.1
  central nervous system NEC A88.8
epidemic B99.9
  specified NEC B99.8
epididymis N50.9
Erb (-Landouzy) G71.02
Erdheim-Chester (ECD) E88.89
esophagus K22.9
  functional K22.4
    psychogenic F45.8
  specified NEC K22.8
Eulenburg's (congenital paramyotonia) G71.19
eustachian tube — see Disorder, eustachian tube
external
  auditory canal — see Disorder, ear, external
  ear — see Disorder, ear, external
extrapyramidal G25.9
  specified NEC G25.89
eye H57.9
  anterior chamber H21.9
  inflammatory NEC H57.89
  muscle (external) — see Strabismus
  specified NEC H57.89
  syphilitic — see Oculopathy, syphilitic
eyeball H44.9
  specified NEC H44.89
eyelid — see Disorder, eyelid
  specified NEC — see Disorder, eyelid, specified type NEC
eyeworm of Africa B74.3
facial nerve (seventh) G51.9
  newborn (birth injury) P11.3
Fahr (of brain) G23.8
Fahr Volhard (of kidney) I12.- ☑
fallopian tube (noninflammatory) N83.9
  inflammatory — see Salpingo-oophoritis
  specified NEC N83.8
familial periodic paralysis G72.3
Fanconi's (congenital pancytopenia) D61.09
fascia NEC (see also Disorder, muscle)
  inflammatory — see Myositis
  specified NEC M62.89
Fauchard's (periodontitis) — see Periodontitis
Favre-Durand-Nicolas (climatic bubo) A55
Fede's K14.0
Feer's — see Poisoning, mercury
female pelvic inflammatory (see also Disease, pelvis, inflammatory) N73.9
  syphilitic (secondary) A51.42
  tuberculous A18.17
Fernels' (aortic aneurysm) I71.9
fibrocaseous of lung — see Tuberculosis, pulmonary
fibrocystic — see Fibrocystic disease
Fiedler's (leptospiral jaundice) A27.0
fifth B08.3
file-cutter's — see Poisoning, lead
fish-skin Q80.9
  acquired L85.0
Flajani (-Basedow) (exophthalmic goiter) — see Hyperthyroidism, with, goiter (diffuse)
flax-dresser's J66.1
fluke — see Infestation, fluke

Disease, diseased — continued
foot and mouth B08.8
foot process N04.9
Forbes' (glycogenosis III) E74.03
Fordyce-Fox (apocrine miliaria) L75.2
Fordyce's (ectopic sebaceous glands) (mouth) Q38.6
Forestier's (rhizomelic pseudopolyarthritis) M35.3
  meaning ankylosing hyperostosis — see Hyperostosis, ankylosing
Fothergill's
  neuralgia — see Neuralgia, trigeminal
  scarlatina anginosa A38.9
Fournier (gangrene) N49.3
  female N76.89
fourth B08.8
Fox (-Fordyce) (apocrine miliaria) L75.2
Francis' — see Tularemia
Franklin C88.2
Frei's (climatic bubo) A55
Friedreich's
  combined systemic or ataxia G11.1
  myoclonia G25.3
frontal sinus — see Sinusitis, frontal
fungus NEC B49
Gaisböck's (polycythemia hypertonica) D75.1
gallbladder K82.9
  calculus — see Calculus, gallbladder
  cholecystitis — see Cholecystitis
  cholesterolosis K82.4
  fistula — see Fistula, gallbladder
  hydrops K82.1
  obstruction — see Obstruction, gallbladder
  perforation K82.2
  specified NEC K82.8
gamma heavy chain C88.2
Gamna's (siderotic splenomegaly) D73.2
Gamstorp's (adynamia episodica hereditaria) G72.3
Gandy-Nanta (siderotic splenomegaly) D73.2
ganister J62.8
gastric — see Disease, stomach
gastroesophageal reflux (GERD) K21.9
  with esophagitis K21.0
gastrointestinal (tract) K92.9
  amyloid E85.4
  functional K59.9
    psychogenic F45.8
  specified NEC K92.89
Gee (-Herter) (-Heubner) (-Thaysen) (nontropical sprue) K90.0
genital organs
  female N94.9
  male N50.9
Gerhardt's (erythromelalgia) I73.81
Gibert's (pityriasis rosea) L42
Gierke's (glycogenosis I) E74.01
Gilles de la Tourette's (motor-verbal tic) F95.2
gingiva K06.9
  plaque induced K05.00
  specified NEC K06.8
gland (lymph) I89.9
Glanzmann's (hereditary hemorrhagic thrombasthenia) D69.1
glass-blower's (cataract) — see Cataract, specified NEC
  salivary gland hypertrophy K11.1
Glisson's — see Rickets
globe H44.9
  specified NEC H44.89
glomerular (see also Glomerulonephritis)
  with edema — see Nephrosis
  acute — see Nephritis, acute
  chronic — see Nephritis, chronic
  minimal change N05.0
  rapidly progressive N01.9
glycogen storage E74.00
  Andersen's E74.09
  Cori's E74.03
  Forbes' E74.03
  generalized E74.00
  glucose-6-phosphatase deficiency E74.01
  heart E74.02 [I43]
  hepatorenal E74.09
  Hers' E74.09
  liver and kidney E74.09
  McArdle's E74.04
  muscle phosphofructokinase E74.09
  myocardium E74.02 [I43]
  Pompe's E74.02
  Tauri's E74.09

☑ **Additional Character Required** — Refer to the Tabular List for Character Selection
▽ Subterms under main terms may continue to next column or page

Disease, diseased — *continued*
  glycogen storage — *continued*
    type Ø E74.Ø9
    type I E74.Ø1
    type II E74.Ø2
    type III E74.Ø3
    type IV E74.Ø9
    type V E74.Ø4
    type VI-XI E74.Ø9
    Von Gierke's E74.Ø1
  Goldstein's (familial hemorrhagic telangiectasia) I78.Ø
  gonococcal NOS A54.9
  graft-versus-host (GVH) D89.813
    acute D89.81Ø
    acute on chronic D89.812
    chronic D89.811
  grainhandler's J67.8
  granulomatous (childhood) (chronic) D71
  Graves' (exophthalmic goiter) — *see* Hyperthyroidism, with, goiter (diffuse)
  Griesinger's — *see* Ancylostomiasis
  Grisel's M43.6
  Gruby's (tinea tonsurans) B35.Ø
  Guillain-Barré G61.Ø
  Guinon's (motor-verbal tic) F95.2
  gum KØ6.9
  gynecological N94.9
  H (Hartnup's) E72.Ø2
  Haff — *see* Poisoning, mercury
  Hageman (congenital factor XII deficiency) D68.2
  hair (color) (shaft) L67.9
    follicles L73.9
      specified NEC L73.8
  Hamman's (spontaneous mediastinal emphysema) J98.2
  hand, foot and mouth BØ8.4
  Hansen's — *see* Leprosy
  Hantavirus, with pulmonary manifestations B33.4
    with renal manifestations A98.5
  Harada's H3Ø.81- ☑
  Hartnup (pellagra-cerebellar ataxia-renal aminoaciduria) E72.Ø2
  Hart's (pellagra-cerebellar ataxia-renal aminoaciduria) E72.Ø2
  Hashimoto's (struma lymphomatosa) EØ6.3
  Hb — *see* Disease, hemoglobin
  heart (organic) I51.9
    with
      pulmonary edema (acute) (*see also* Failure, ventricular, left) I5Ø.1
      rheumatic fever (conditions in IØØ)
        active IØ1.9
          with chorea IØ2.Ø
          specified NEC IØ1.8
        inactive or quiescent (with chorea) IØ9.9
          specified NEC IØ9.89
    amyloid E85.4 [I43]
    aortic (valve) I35.9
    arteriosclerotic or sclerotic (senile) — *see* Disease, heart, ischemic, atherosclerotic
    artery, arterial — *see* Disease, heart, ischemic, atherosclerotic
    beer drinkers' I42.6
    beriberi (wet) E51.12
    black I27.Ø
    congenital Q24.9
      cyanotic Q24.9
      specified NEC Q24.8
    coronary — *see* Disease, heart, ischemic
    cryptogenic I51.9
    fibroid — *see* Myocarditis
    functional I51.89
      psychogenic F45.8
    glycogen storage E74.Ø2 [I43]
    gonococcal A54.83
    hypertensive — *see* Hypertension, heart
    hyperthyroid (*see also* Hyperthyroidism) EØ5.9Ø [I43]
      with thyroid storm EØ5.91 [I43]
    ischemic (chronic or with a stated duration of over 4 weeks) I25.9
      atherosclerotic (of) I25.1Ø
        with angina pectoris — *see* Arteriosclerosis, coronary (artery)
        coronary artery bypass graft — *see* Arteriosclerosis, coronary (artery), cardiomyopathy I25.5

Disease, diseased — *continued*
  heart — *continued*
    ischemic — *continued*
      diagnosed on ECG or other special investigation, but currently presenting no symptoms I25.6
      silent I25.6
      specified form NEC I25.89
    kyphoscoliotic I27.1
    meningococcal A39.5Ø
      endocarditis A39.51
      myocarditis A39.52
      pericarditis A39.53
    mitral IØ5.9
      specified NEC IØ5.8
    muscular — *see* Degeneration, myocardial
    psychogenic (functional) F45.8
    pulmonary (chronic) I27.9
      in schistosomiasis B65.9 [I52]
      specified NEC I27.89
    rheumatic (chronic) (inactive) (old) (quiescent) (with chorea) IØ9.9
      active or acute IØ1.9
        with chorea (acute) (rheumatic) (Sydenham's) IØ2.Ø
      specified NEC IØ9.89
    senile — *see* Myocarditis
    syphilitic A52.Ø6
      aortic A52.Ø3
        aneurysm A52.Ø1
      congenital A5Ø.54 [I52]
    thyrotoxic (*see also* Thyrotoxicosis) EØ5.9Ø [I43]
      with thyroid storm EØ5.91 [I43]
    valve, valvular (obstructive) (regurgitant) (*see also* Endocarditis)
      congenital NEC Q24.8
        pulmonary Q22.3
    vascular — *see* Disease, cardiovascular
  heavy chain NEC C88.2
    alpha C88.3
    gamma C88.2
    mu C88.2
  Hebra's
    pityriasis
      maculata et circinata L42
      rubra pilaris L44.Ø
    prurigo L28.2
  hematopoietic organs D75.9
  hemoglobin or Hb
    abnormal (mixed) NEC D58.2
      with thalassemia D56.9
    AS genotype D57.3
    Bart's D56.Ø
    C (Hb-C) D58.2
      with other abnormal hemoglobin NEC D58.2
      elliptocytosis D58.1
      Hb-S D57.2- ☑
      sickle-cell D57.2- ☑
      thalassemia D56.8
    Constant Spring D58.2
    D (Hb-D) D58.2
    E (Hb-E) D58.2
    E-beta thalassemia D56.5
    elliptocytosis D58.1
    H (Hb-H) (thalassemia) D56.Ø
      with other abnormal hemoglobin NEC D56.9
      Constant Spring D56.Ø
    I thalassemia D56.9
    M D74.Ø
    S or SS D57.1
    SC D57.2- ☑
    SD D57.8- ☑
    SE D57.8- ☑
    spherocytosis D58.Ø
    unstable, hemolytic D58.2
  hemolytic (newborn) P55.9
    autoimmune (cold type) (warm type) D59.1
    drug-induced D59.Ø
    due to or with
      incompatibility
        ABO (blood group) P55.1
        blood (group) (Duffy) (K) (Kell) (Kidd) (Lewis) (M) (S) NEC P55.8
        Rh (blood group) (factor) P55.Ø
      Rh negative mother P55.Ø
    specified type NEC P55.8
    unstable hemoglobin D58.2
  hemorrhagic D69.9

Disease, diseased — *continued*
  hemorrhagic — *continued*
    newborn P53
  Henoch (-Schönlein) (purpura nervosa) D69.Ø
  hepatic — *see* Disease, liver
  hepatolenticular E83.Ø1
  heredodegenerative NEC
    spinal cord G95.89
  herpesviral, disseminated BØØ.7
  Hers' (glycogenosis VI) E74.Ø9
  Herter (-Gee) (-Heubner) (nontropical sprue) K9Ø.Ø
  Heubner-Herter (nontropical sprue) K9Ø.Ø
  high fetal gene or hemoglobin thalassemia D56.9
  Hildenbrand's — *see* Typhus
  hip (joint) M25.9
    congenital Q65.89
    suppurative MØØ.9
    tuberculous A18.Ø2
  His (-Werner) (trench fever) A79.Ø
  Hodgson's I71.2
    ruptured I71.1
  Holla — *see* Spherocytosis
  hookworm B76.9
    specified NEC B76.8
  host-versus-graft D89.813
    acute D89.81Ø
    acute on chronic D89.812
    chronic D89.811
  human immunodeficiency virus (HIV) B2Ø
  Huntington's G1Ø
    with dementia G1Ø [FØ2.8Ø]
  Hutchinson's (cheiropompholyx) — *see* Hutchinson's disease
  hyaline (diffuse) (generalized)
    membrane (lung) (newborn) P22.Ø
    adult J8Ø
  hydatid — *see* Echinococcus
  hydroxyapatite deposition M11.ØØ
    ankle M11.Ø7- ☑
    elbow M11.Ø2- ☑
    foot joint M11.Ø7- ☑
    hand joint M11.Ø4- ☑
    hip M11.Ø5- ☑
    knee M11.Ø6- ☑
    multiple site M11.Ø9
    shoulder M11.Ø1- ☑
    vertebra M11.Ø8
    wrist M11.Ø3- ☑
  hyperkinetic — *see* Hyperkinesia
  hypertensive — *see* Hypertension
  hypophysis E23.7
  Iceland G93.3
  I-cell E77.Ø
  immune D89.9
  immunoproliferative (malignant) C88.9
    small intestinal C88.3
    specified NEC C88.8
  inclusion B25.9
    salivary gland B25.9
  infectious, infective B99.9
    congenital P37.9
      specified NEC P37.8
      viral P35.9
        specified type NEC P35.8
    specified NEC B99.8
  inflammatory
    penis N48.29
      abscess N48.21
      cellulitis N48.22
    prepuce N47.7
      balanoposthitis N47.6
    tubo-ovarian — *see* Salpingo-oophoritis
  intervertebral disc (*see also* Disorder, disc)
    with myelopathy — *see* Disorder, disc, with, myelopathy
    cervical, cervicothoracic — *see* Disorder, disc, cervical
    with
      myelopathy — *see* Disorder, disc, cervical, with myelopathy
      neuritis, radiculitis or radiculopathy — *see* Disorder, disc, cervical, with neuritis
      specified NEC — *see* Disorder, disc, cervical, specified type NEC
    lumbar (with)
      myelopathy M51.Ø6
      neuritis, radiculitis, radiculopathy or sciatica M51.16

Disease, diseased — *continued*
  intervertebral disc (*see also* Disorder, disc) — *continued*
    lumbar — *continued*
      specified NEC M51.86
    lumbosacral (with)
      neuritis, radiculitis, radiculopathy or sciatica M51.17
      specified NEC M51.87
    specified NEC — *see* Disorder, disc, specified NEC
    thoracic (with)
      myelopathy M51.04
      neuritis, radiculitis or radiculopathy M51.14
      specified NEC M51.84
    thoracolumbar (with)
      myelopathy M51.05
      neuritis, radiculitis or radiculopathy M51.15
      specified NEC M51.85
  intestine K63.9
    functional K59.9
      psychogenic F45.8
      specified NEC K59.8
    organic K63.9
    protozoal A07.9
    specified NEC K63.89
  iris H21.9
    specified NEC H21.89
  iron metabolism or storage E83.10
  island (scrub typhus) A75.3
  itai-itai — *see* Poisoning, cadmium
  Jakob-Creutzfeldt — *see* Creutzfeldt-Jakob disease or syndrome
  jaw M27.9
    fibrocystic M27.49
    specified NEC M27.8
  jigger B88.1
  joint (*see also* Disorder, joint)
    Charcot's — *see* Arthropathy, neuropathic (Charcot)
    degenerative — *see* Osteoarthritis
      multiple M15.9
      spine — *see* Spondylosis
    hypertrophic — *see* Osteoarthritis
    sacroiliac M53.3
    specified NEC — *see* Disorder, joint, specified type NEC
    spine NEC — *see* Dorsopathy
    suppurative — *see* Arthritis, pyogenic or pyemic
  Jourdain's (acute gingivitis) K05.00
    nonplaque induced K05.01
    plaque induced K05.00
  Kaschin-Beck (endemic polyarthritis) M12.10
    ankle M12.17- ☑
    elbow M12.12- ☑
    foot joint M12.17- ☑
    hand joint M12.14- ☑
    hip M12.15- ☑
    knee M12.16- ☑
    multiple site M12.19
    shoulder M12.11- ☑
    vertebra M12.18
    wrist M12.13- ☑
  Katayama B65.2
  Kedani (scrub typhus) A75.3
  Keshan E59
  kidney (functional) (pelvis) N28.9
    chronic N18.9
      hypertensive — *see* Hypertension, kidney
      stage 1 N18.1
      stage 2 (mild) N18.2
      stage 3 (moderate) N18.3
      stage 4 (severe) N18.4
      stage 5 N18.5
    complicating pregnancy — *see* Pregnancy, complicated by, renal disease
    cystic (congenital) Q61.9
    fibrocystic (congenital) Q61.8
    hypertensive — *see* Hypertension, kidney
    in (due to)
      schistosomiasis (bilharziasis) B65.9 [N29]
    multicystic Q61.4
    polycystic Q61.3
      adult type Q61.2
      childhood type NEC Q61.19
        collecting duct dilatation Q61.11
  Kimmelstiel (-Wilson) (intercapillary polycystic (congenital) glomerulosclerosis) — *see* E08-E13 with .21
  Kinnier Wilson's (hepatolenticular degeneration) E83.01
  kissing — *see* Mononucleosis, infectious

Disease, diseased — *continued*
  Klebs' (*see also* Glomerulonephritis) N05- ☑
  Klippel-Feil (brevicollis) Q76.1
  Köhler-Pellegrini-Stieda (calcification, knee joint) — *see* Bursitis, tibial collateral
  Kok Q89.8
  König's (osteochondritis dissecans) — *see* Osteochondritis, dissecans
  Korsakoff's (nonalcoholic) F04
    alcoholic F10.96
      with dependence F10.26
  Kostmann's (infantile genetic agranulocytosis) D70.0
  kuru A81.81
  Kyasanur Forest A98.2
  labyrinth, ear — *see* Disorder, ear, inner
  lacrimal system — *see* Disorder, lacrimal system
  Lafora's — *see* Epilepsy, generalized, idiopathic
  Lancereaux-Mathieu (leptospiral jaundice) A27.0
  Landry's G61.0
  Larrey-Weil (leptospiral jaundice) A27.0
  larynx J38.7
  legionnaires' A48.1
    nonpneumonic A48.2
  Lenegre's I44.2
  lens H27.9
    specified NEC H27.8
  Lev's (acquired complete heart block) I44.2
  Lewy body (dementia) G31.83 [F02.80]
    with behavioral disturbance G31.83 [F02.81]
  Lichtheim's (subacute combined sclerosis with pernicious anemia) D51.0
  Lightwood's (renal tubular acidosis) N25.89
  Lignac's (cystinosis) E72.04
  lip K13.0
  lipid-storage E75.6
    specified NEC E75.5
  Lipschütz's N76.6
  liver (chronic) (organic) K76.9
    alcoholic (chronic) K70.9
      acute — *see* Disease, liver, alcoholic, hepatitis
      cirrhosis K70.30
        with ascites K70.31
      failure K70.40
        with coma K70.41
      fatty liver K70.0
      fibrosis K70.2
      hepatitis K70.10
        with ascites K70.11
      sclerosis K70.2
    cystic, congenital Q44.6
    drug-induced (idiosyncratic) (toxic) (predictable) (unpredictable) — *see* Disease, liver, toxic
    end stage K72.90
      due to hepatitis — *see* Hepatitis
    fatty, nonalcoholic (NAFLD) K76.0
      alcoholic K70.0
    fibrocystic (congenital) Q44.6
    fluke
      Chinese B66.1
      oriental B66.1
      sheep B66.3
    gestational alloimmune (GALD) P78.84
    glycogen storage E74.09 [K77]
    in (due to)
      schistosomiasis (bilharziasis) B65.9 [K77]
    inflammatory K75.9
      alcoholic K70.1 ☑
      specified NEC K75.89
    polycystic (congenital) Q44.6
    toxic K71.9
      with
        cholestasis K71.0
        cirrhosis (liver) K71.7
        fibrosis (liver) K71.7
        focal nodular hyperplasia K71.8
        hepatic granuloma K71.8
        hepatic necrosis K71.10
          with coma K71.11
        hepatitis NEC K71.6
          acute K71.2
          chronic
            active K71.50
              with ascites K71.51
            lobular K71.4
            persistent K71.3
          lupoid K71.50
            with ascites K71.51
        peliosis hepatis K71.8

Disease, diseased — *continued*
  liver — *continued*
    toxic — *continued*
      with — *continued*
        veno-occlusive disease (VOD) of liver K71.8
      veno-occlusive K76.5
  Lobo's (keloid blastomycosis) B48.0
  Lobstein's (brittle bones and blue sclera) Q78.0
  Ludwig's (submaxillary cellulitis) K12.2
  lumbosacral region M53.87
  lung J98.4
    black J60
    congenital Q33.9
    cystic J98.4
      congenital Q33.0
    fibroid (chronic) — *see* Fibrosis, lung
    fluke B66.4
      oriental B66.4
    in
      amyloidosis E85.4 [J99]
      sarcoidosis D86.0
      Sjögren's syndrome M35.02
      systemic
        lupus erythematosus M32.13
        sclerosis M34.81
    interstitial J84.9
      of childhood, specified NEC J84.848
      respiratory bronchiolitis J84.115
      specified NEC J84.89
    obstructive (chronic) J44.9
      with
        acute
          bronchitis J44.0
          exacerbation NEC J44.1
          lower respiratory infection J44.0
        alveolitis, allergic J67.9
        asthma J44.9
        bronchiectasis J47.9
          with
            exacerbation (acute) J47.1
            lower respiratory infection J47.0
        bronchitis J44.9
          with
            exacerbation (acute) J44.1
            lower respiratory infection J44.0
        emphysema J43.9
        hypersensitivity pneumonitis J67.9
      decompensated J44.1
        with
          exacerbation (acute) J44.1
    polycystic J98.4
      congenital Q33.0
    rheumatoid (diffuse) (interstitial) — *see* Rheumatoid, lung
  Lutembacher's (atrial septal defect with mitral stenosis) Q21.1
  Lyme A69.20
  lymphatic (gland) (system) (channel) (vessel) I89.9
  lymphoproliferative D47.9
    specified NEC D47.Z9 (*following* D47.4)
    T-gamma D47.Z9 (*following* D47.4)
    X-linked D82.3
  Magitot's M27.2
  malarial — *see* Malaria
  malignant (*see also* Neoplasm, malignant, by site)
  Manson's B65.1
  maple bark J67.6
  maple-syrup-urine E71.0
  Marburg (virus) A98.3
  Marion's (bladder neck obstruction) N32.0
  Marsh's (exophthalmic goiter) — *see* Hyperthyroidism with, goiter (diffuse)
  mastoid (process) — *see* Disorder, ear, middle
  Mathieu's (leptospiral jaundice) A27.0
  Maxcy's A75.2
  McArdle (-Schmid-Pearson) (glycogenosis V) E74.04
  mediastinum J98.59
  medullary center (idiopathic) (respiratory) G93.89
  Meige's (chronic hereditary edema) Q82.0
  meningococcal — *see* Infection, meningococcal
  mental F99
    organic F09
  mesenchymal M35.9
  mesenteric embolic (*see also* Ischemia, intestine, acute) K55.039
  metabolic, metabolism E88.9
    bilirubin E80.7
  metal-polisher's J62.8

104

☑ **Additional Character Required** — **Refer to the Tabular List for Character Selection**   ▽ **Subterms under main terms may continue to next column or page**

Disease, diseased — *continued*
- metastatic (*see also* Neoplasm, secondary, by site) C79.9
- microvascular - code to condition
- microvillus
  - atrophy Q43.8
  - inclusion (MVD) Q43.8
- middle ear — *see* Disorder, ear, middle
- Mikulicz' (dryness of mouth, absent or decreased lacrimation) K11.8
- Milroy's (chronic hereditary edema) Q82.0
- Minamata — *see* Poisoning, mercury
- minicore G71.2
- Minor's G95.19
- Minot's (hemorrhagic disease, newborn) P53
- Minot-von Willebrand-Jürgens (angiohemophilia) D68.0
- Mitchell's (erythromelalgia) I73.81
- mitral (valve) I05.9
  - nonrheumatic I34.9
- mixed connective tissue M35.1
- moldy hay J67.0
- Monge's T70.29 ☑
- Morgagni-Adams-Stokes (syncope with heart block) I45.9
- Morgagni's (syndrome) (hyperostosis frontalis interna) M85.2
- Morton's (with metatarsalgia) — *see* Lesion, nerve, plantar
- Morvan's G60.8
- motor neuron (bulbar) (mixed type) (spinal) G12.20
  - amyotrophic lateral sclerosis G12.21
  - familial G12.24
  - progressive bulbar palsy G12.22
  - specified NEC G12.29
- moyamoya I67.5
- mu heavy chain disease C88.2
- multicore G71.2
- muscle (*see also* Disorder, muscle)
  - inflammatory — *see* Myositis
  - ocular (external) — *see* Strabismus
- musculoskeletal system, soft tissue — *see also* Disorder, soft tissue
  - specified NEC — *see* Disorder, soft tissue, specified type NEC
- mushroom workers' J67.5
- mycotic B49
- myelodysplastic, not classified C94.6
- myeloproliferative, not classified C94.6
  - chronic D47.1
- myocardium, myocardial (*see also* Degeneration, myocardial) I51.5
  - primary (idiopathic) I42.9
- myoneural G70.9
- Naegeli's D69.1
- nails L60.9
  - specified NEC L60.8
- Nairobi (sheep virus) A93.8
- nasal J34.9
- nemaline body G71.2
- nerve — *see* Disorder, nerve
- nervous system G98.8
  - autonomic G90.9
  - central G96.9
    - specified NEC G96.8
  - congenital Q07.9
  - parasympathetic G90.9
  - specified NEC G98.8
  - sympathetic G90.9
  - vegetative G90.9
- neuromuscular system G70.9
- Newcastle B30.8
- Nicolas (-Durand)-Favre (climatic bubo) A55
- nipple N64.9
  - Paget's C50.01- ☑
    - female C50.01- ☑
    - male C50.02- ☑
- Nishimoto (-Takeuchi) I67.5
- nonarthropod-borne NOS (viral) B34.9
  - enterovirus NEC B34.1
- nonautoimmune hemolytic D59.4
  - drug-induced D59.2
- Nonne-Milroy-Meige (chronic hereditary edema) Q82.0
- nose J34.9
- nucleus pulposus — *see* Disorder, disc
- nutritional E63.9
- oast-house-urine E72.19
  - ocular
    - herpesviral B00.50
    - zoster B02.30

Disease, diseased — *continued*
- obliterative vascular I77.1
- Ohara's — *see* Tularemia
- Opitz's (congestive splenomegaly) D73.2
- Oppenheim-Urbach (necrobiosis lipoidica diabeticorum) — *see* E08-E13 with .620
- optic nerve NEC — *see* Disorder, nerve, optic
- orbit — *see* Disorder, orbit
- Oriental liver fluke B66.1
- Oriental lung fluke B66.4
- Ormond's N13.5
- Oropouche virus A93.0
- Osler-Rendu (familial hemorrhagic telangiectasia) I78.0
- osteofibrocystic E21.0
- Otto's M24.7
- outer ear — *see* Disorder, ear, external
- ovary (noninflammatory) N83.9
  - cystic N83.20- ☑
  - inflammatory — *see* Salpingo-oophoritis
  - polycystic E28.2
  - specified NEC N83.8
- Owren's (congenital) — *see* Defect, coagulation
- pancreas K86.9
  - cystic K86.2
  - fibrocystic E84.9
  - specified NEC K86.89
- panvalvular I08.9
  - specified NEC I08.8
- parametrium (noninflammatory) N83.9
- parasitic B89
  - cerebral NEC B71.9 [G94]
  - intestinal NOS B82.9
  - mouth B37.0
  - skin NOS B88.9
  - specified type — *see* Infestation
  - tongue B37.0
- parathyroid (gland) E21.5
  - specified NEC E21.4
- Parkinson's G20
- parodontal K05.6
- Parrot's (syphilitic osteochondritis) A50.02
- Parry's (exophthalmic goiter) — *see* Hyperthyroidism, with, goiter (diffuse)
- Parson's (exophthalmic goiter) — *see* Hyperthyroidism, with, goiter (diffuse)
- Paxton's (white piedra) B36.2
- pearl-worker's — *see* Osteomyelitis, specified type NEC
- Pellegrini-Stieda (calcification, knee joint) — *see* Bursitis, tibial collateral
- pelvis, pelvic N94.9
  - female NOS N94.9
    - specified NEC N94.89
  - gonococcal (acute) (chronic) A54.24
  - inflammatory (female) N73.9
    - acute N73.0
    - chlamydial A56.11
    - chronic N73.1
    - specified NEC N73.8
    - syphilitic (secondary) A51.42
      - late A52.76
    - tuberculous A18.17
  - organ, female N94.9
  - peritoneum, female NEC N94.89
- penis N48.9
  - inflammatory N48.29
    - abscess N48.21
    - cellulitis N48.22
  - specified NEC N48.89
- periapical tissues NOS K04.90
- periodontal K05.6
  - specified NEC K05.5
- periosteum — *see* Disorder, bone, specified type NEC
- peripheral
  - arterial I73.9
  - autonomic nervous system G90.9
  - nerves — *see* Polyneuropathy
  - vascular NOS I73.9
- peritoneum K66.9
  - pelvic, female NEC N94.89
  - specified NEC K66.8
- persistent mucosal (middle ear) H66.20
  - left H66.22
    - with right H66.23
  - right H66.21
    - with left H66.23
- Petit's — *see* Hernia, abdomen, specified site NEC
- pharynx J39.2
  - specified NEC J39.2

Disease, diseased — *continued*
- Phocas' — *see* Mastopathy, cystic
- photochromogenic (acid-fast bacilli) (pulmonary) A31.0
  - nonpulmonary A31.9
- Pick's G31.01 [F02.80]
  - with behavioral disturbance G31.01 [F02.81]
  - brain G31.01 [F02.80]
    - with behavioral disturbance G31.01 [F02.81]
  - of pericardium (pericardial pseudocirrhosis of liver) I31.1
- pigeon fancier's J67.2
- pineal gland E34.8
- pink — *see* Poisoning, mercury
- Pinkus' (lichen nitidus) L44.1
- pinworm B80
- Piry virus A93.8
- pituitary (gland) E23.7
- pituitary-snuff-taker's J67.8
- pleura (cavity) J94.9
  - specified NEC J94.8
- pneumatic drill (hammer) T75.21 ☑
- Pollitzer's (hidradenitis suppurativa) L73.2
- polycystic
  - kidney or renal Q61.3
    - adult type Q61.2
    - childhood type NEC Q61.19
      - collecting duct dilatation Q61.11
  - liver or hepatic Q44.6
  - lung or pulmonary J98.4
    - congenital Q33.0
  - ovary, ovaries E28.2
  - spleen Q89.09
- polyethylene T84.05- ☑
- Pompe's (glycogenosis II) E74.02
- Posadas-Wernicke B38.9
- Potain's (pulmonary edema) — *see* Edema, lung
- prepuce N47.8
  - inflammatory N47.7
    - balanoposthitis N47.6
- Pringle's (tuberous sclerosis) Q85.1
- prion, central nervous system A81.9
  - specified NEC A81.89
- prostate N42.9
  - specified NEC N42.89
- protozoal B64
  - acanthamebiasis — *see* Acanthamebiasis
  - African trypanosomiasis — *see* African trypanosomiasis
  - babesiosis B60.0
  - Chagas disease — *see* Chagas disease
  - intestine, intestinal A07.9
  - leishmaniasis — *see* Leishmaniasis
  - malaria — *see* Malaria
  - naegleriasis B60.2
  - pneumocystosis B59
  - specified organism NEC B60.8
  - toxoplasmosis — *see* Toxoplasmosis
- pseudo-Hurler's E77.0
- psychiatric F99
- psychotic — *see* Psychosis
- Puente's (simple glandular cheilitis) K13.0
- puerperal (*see also* Puerperal) O90.89
- pulmonary (*see also* Disease, lung)
  - artery I28.9
  - chronic obstructive J44.9
    - with
      - acute bronchitis J44.0
      - exacerbation (acute) J44.1
      - lower respiratory infection (acute) J44.0
    - decompensated J44.1
      - with
        - exacerbation (acute) J44.1
  - heart I27.9
    - specified NEC I27.89
  - hypertensive (vascular) (*see also* Hypertension, pulmonary) I27.20
    - NEC I27.2 ☑
    - primary (idiopathic) I27.0
  - valve I37.9
    - rheumatic I09.89
- pulp (dental) NOS K04.90
- pulseless M31.4
- Putnam's (subacute combined sclerosis with pernicious anemia) D51.0
- Pyle (-Cohn) (metaphyseal dysplasia) Q78.5
- ragpicker's or ragsorter's A22.1
- Raynaud's — *see* Raynaud's disease
- reactive airway — *see* Asthma

Disease, diseased — *continued*
Reclus' (cystic) — *see* Mastopathy, cystic
rectum K62.9
  specified NEC K62.89
Refsum's (heredopathia atactica polyneuritiformis)
  G60.1
renal (functional) (pelvis) (*see also* Disease, kidney)
  N28.9
  with
    edema — *see* Nephrosis
    glomerular lesion — *see* Glomerulonephritis
      with edema — *see* Nephrosis
    interstitial nephritis N12
  acute N28.9
  chronic (*see also* Disease, kidney, chronic) N18.9
  cystic, congenital Q61.9
  diabetic — *see* E08-E13 with .22
  end-stage (failure) N18.6
    due to hypertension I12.0
  fibrocystic (congenital) Q61.8
  hypertensive — *see* Hypertension, kidney
  lupus M32.14
  phosphate-losing (tubular) N25.0
  polycystic (congenital) Q61.3
    adult type Q61.2
    childhood type NEC Q61.19
      collecting duct dilatation Q61.11
  rapidly progressive N01.9
  subacute N01.9
Rendu-Osler-Weber (familial hemorrhagic telangiectasia) I78.0
renovascular (arteriosclerotic) — *see* Hypertension,
  kidney
respiratory (tract) J98.9
  acute or subacute NOS J06.9
    due to
      chemicals, gases, fumes or vapors (inhalation)
        J68.3
      external agent J70.9
        specified NEC J70.8
      radiation J70.0
      smoke inhalation J70.5
    noninfectious J39.8
  chronic NOS J98.9
    due to
      chemicals, gases, fumes or vapors J68.4
      external agent J70.9
        specified NEC J70.8
      radiation J70.1
    newborn P27.9
      specified NEC P27.8
  due to
    chemicals, gases, fumes or vapors J68.9
      acute or subacute NEC J68.3
      chronic J68.4
    external agent J70.9
      specified NEC J70.8
  newborn P28.9
    specified type NEC P28.89
  upper J39.9
    acute or subacute J06.9
    noninfectious NEC J39.8
    specified NEC J39.8
    streptococcal J06.9
retina, retinal H35.9
  Batten's or Batten-Mayou E75.4 [H36]
  specified NEC H35.89
rheumatoid — *see* Arthritis, rheumatoid
rickettsial NOS A79.9
  specified type NEC A79.89
Riga (-Fede) (cachectic aphthae) K14.0
Riggs' (compound periodontitis) — *see* Periodontitis
Ritter's L00
Rivalta's (cervicofacial actinomycosis) A42.2
Robles' (onchocerciasis) B73.01
Roger's (congenital interventricular septal defect) Q21.0
Rosenthal's (factor XI deficiency) D68.1
Ross River B33.1
Rossbach's (hyperchlorhydria) K30
Rotes Quérol — *see* Hyperostosis, ankylosing
Roth (-Bernhardt) — *see* Mononeuropathy, lower limb,
  meralgia paresthetica
Runeberg's (progressive pernicious anemia) D51.0
sacroiliac NEC M53.3
salivary gland or duct K11.9
  inclusion B25.9
  specified NEC K11.8
  virus B25.9

Disease, diseased — *continued*
sandworm B76.9
Schimmelbusch's — *see* Mastopathy, cystic
Schmorl's — *see* Schmorl's disease or nodes
Schönlein (-Henoch) (purpura rheumatica) D69.0
Schottmüller's — *see* Fever, paratyphoid
Schultz's (agranulocytosis) — *see* Agranulocytosis
Schwalbe-Ziehen-Oppenheim G24.1
Schwartz-Jampel G71.13
sclera H15.9
  specified NEC H15.89
scrofulous (tuberculous) A18.2
scrotum N50.9
sebaceous glands L73.9
semilunar cartilage, cystic (*see also* Derangement, knee,
  meniscus, cystic)
seminal vesicle N50.9
serum NEC (*see also* Reaction, serum) T80.69 ☑
sexually transmitted A64
  anogenital
    herpesviral infection — *see* Herpes, anogenital
    warts A63.0
  chancroid A57
  chlamydial infection — *see* Chlamydia
  gonorrhea — *see* Gonorrhea
  granuloma inguinale A58
  specified organism NEC A63.8
  syphilis — *see* Syphilis
  trichomoniasis — *see* Trichomoniasis
Sézary C84.1- ☑
shimamushi (scrub typhus) A75.3
shipyard B30.0
sickle-cell D57.1
  with crisis (vasoocclusive pain) D57.00
    with
      acute chest syndrome D57.01
      splenic sequestration D57.02
  elliptocytosis D57.8- ☑
  Hb-C D57.20
    with crisis (vasoocclusive pain) D57.219
      with
        acute chest syndrome D57.211
        splenic sequestration D57.212
    without crisis D57.20
  Hb-SD D57.80
    with crisis D57.819
      with
        acute chest syndrome D57.811
        splenic sequestration D57.812
  Hb-SE D57.80
    with crisis D57.819
      with
        acute chest syndrome D57.811
        splenic sequestration D57.812
  specified NEC D57.80
    with crisis D57.819
      with
        acute chest syndrome D57.811
        splenic sequestration D57.812
  spherocytosis D57.80
    with crisis D57.819
      with
        acute chest syndrome D57.811
        splenic sequestration D57.812
  thalassemia D57.40
    with crisis (vasoocclusive pain) D57.419
      with
        acute chest syndrome D57.411
        splenic sequestration D57.412
    without crisis D57.40
silo-filler's J68.8
  bronchitis J68.0
  pneumonitis J68.0
  pulmonary edema J68.1
simian B B00.4
Simons' (progressive lipodystrophy) E88.1
sin nombre virus B33.4
sinus — *see* Sinusitis
Sirkari's B55.0
sixth B08.20
  due to human herpesvirus 6 B08.21
  due to human herpesvirus 7 B08.22
skin L98.9
  due to metabolic disorder NEC E88.9 [L99]
  specified NEC L98.8
slim (HIV) B20
small vessel I73.9

Disease, diseased — *continued*
Sneddon-Wilkinson (subcorneal pustular dermatosis)
  L13.1
South African creeping B88.0
spinal (cord) G95.9
  congenital Q06.9
  specified NEC G95.89
spine (*see also* Spondylopathy)
  joint — *see* Dorsopathy
  tuberculous A18.01
spinocerebellar (hereditary) G11.9
  specified NEC G11.8
spleen D73.9
  amyloid E85.4 [D77]
  organic D73.9
  polycystic Q89.09
  postinfectional D73.89
sponge-diver's — *see* Toxicity, venom, marine animal,
  sea anemone
Startle Q89.8
Steinert's G71.11
Sticker's (erythema infectiosum) B08.3
Stieda's (calcification, knee joint) — *see* Bursitis, tibial
  collateral
Stokes' (exophthalmic goiter) — *see* Hyperthyroidism,
  with, goiter (diffuse)
Stokes-Adams (syncope with heart block) I45.9
stomach K31.9
  functional, psychogenic F45.8
  specified NEC K31.89
stonemason's J62.8
storage
  glycogen — *see* Disease, glycogen storage
  mucopolysaccharide — *see* Mucopolysaccharidosis
striatopallidal system NEC G25.89
Stuart-Prower (congenital factor X deficiency) D68.2
Stuart's (congenital factor X deficiency) D68.2
subcutaneous tissue — *see* Disease, skin
supporting structures of teeth K08.9
  specified NEC K08.89
suprarenal (capsule) (gland) E27.9
  hyperfunction E27.0
  specified NEC E27.8
sweat glands L74.9
  specified NEC L74.8
Sweeley-Klionsky E75.21
Swift (-Feer) — *see* Poisoning, mercury
swimming-pool granuloma A31.1
Sylvest's (epidemic pleurodynia) B33.0
sympathetic nervous system G90.9
synovium — *see* Disorder, synovium
syphilitic — *see* Syphilis
systemic tissue mast cell C96.20
tanapox (virus) B08.71
Tangier E78.6
Tarral-Besnier (pityriasis rubra pilaris) L44.0
Tauri's E74.09
tear duct — *see* Disorder, lacrimal system
tendon, tendinous (*see also* Disorder, tendon)
  nodular — *see* Trigger finger
terminal vessel I73.9
testis N50.9
thalassemia Hb-S — *see* Disease, sickle-cell, thalassemia
Thaysen-Gee (nontropical sprue) K90.0
Thomsen G71.12
throat J39.2
  septic J02.0
thromboembolic — *see* Embolism
thymus (gland) E32.9
  specified NEC E32.8
thyroid (gland) E07.9
  heart (*see also* Hyperthyroidism) E05.90 [I43]
    with thyroid storm E05.91 [I43]
  specified NEC E07.89
Tietze's M94.0
tongue K14.9
  specified NEC K14.8
tonsils, tonsillar (and adenoids) J35.9
tooth, teeth K08.9
  hard tissues K03.9
    specified NEC K03.89
  pulp NEC K04.99
  specified NEC K08.89
Tourette's F95.2
trachea NEC J39.8
tricuspid I07.9
  nonrheumatic I36.9
triglyceride-storage E75.5

Disease, diseased — *continued*
- trophoblastic — *see* Mole, hydatidiform
- tsutsugamushi A75.3
- tube (fallopian) (noninflammatory) N83.9
  - inflammatory — *see* Salpingitis
  - specified NEC N83.8
- tuberculous NEC — *see* Tuberculosis
- tubo-ovarian (noninflammatory) N83.9
  - inflammatory — *see* Salpingo-oophoritis
  - specified NEC N83.8
- tubotympanic, chronic — *see* Otitis, media, suppurative, chronic, tubotympanic
- tubulo-interstitial N15.9
  - specified NEC N15.8
- tympanum — *see* Disorder, tympanic membrane
- Uhl's Q24.8
- Underwood's (sclerema neonatorum) P83.0
- Unverricht (-Lundborg) — *see* Epilepsy, generalized, idiopathic
- Urbach-Oppenheim (necrobiosis lipoidica diabeticorum) — *see* E08-E13 with .620
- ureter N28.9
  - in (due to)
    - schistosomiasis (bilharziasis) B65.0 [N29]
- urethra N36.9
  - specified NEC N36.8
- urinary (tract) N39.9
  - bladder N32.9
    - specified NEC N32.89
  - specified NEC N39.8
- uterus (noninflammatory) N85.9
  - infective — *see* Endometritis
  - inflammatory — *see* Endometritis
  - specified NEC N85.8
- uveal tract (anterior) H21.9
  - posterior H31.9
- vagabond's B85.1
- vagina, vaginal (noninflammatory) N89.9
  - inflammatory NEC N76.89
  - specified NEC N89.8
- valve, valvular I38
  - multiple I08.9
    - specified NEC I08.8
- van Creveld-von Gierke (glycogenosis I) E74.01
- vas deferens N50.9
- vascular I99.9
  - arteriosclerotic — *see* Arteriosclerosis
  - ciliary body NEC — *see* Disorder, iris, vascular
  - hypertensive — *see* Hypertension
  - iris NEC — *see* Disorder, iris, vascular
  - obliterative I77.1
    - peripheral I73.9
  - occlusive I99.8
  - peripheral (occlusive) I73.9
    - in diabetes mellitus — *see* E08-E13 with .51
- vasomotor I73.9
- vasospastic I73.9
- vein I87.9
- venereal (*see also* Disease, sexually transmitted) A64
  - chlamydial NEC A56.8
    - anus A56.3
    - genitourinary NOS A56.2
    - pharynx A56.4
    - rectum A56.3
  - fifth A55
  - sixth A55
  - specified nature or type NEC A63.8
- vertebra, vertebral (*see also* Spondylopathy)
  - disc — *see* Disorder, disc
- vibration — *see* Vibration, adverse effects
- viral, virus (*see also* Disease, by type of virus) B34.9
  - arbovirus NOS A94
  - arthropod-borne NOS A94
  - congenital P35.9
    - specified NEC P35.8
  - Hanta (with renal manifestations) (Dobrava) (Puumala) (Seoul) A98.5
    - with pulmonary manifestations (Andes) (Bayou) (Bermejo) (Black Creek Canal) (Choclo) (Juquitiba) (Laguna negra) (Lechiguanas) (New York) (Oran) (Sin nombre) B33.4
  - Hantaan (Korean hemorrhagic fever) A98.5
  - human immunodeficiency (HIV) B20
  - Kunjin A83.4
  - nonarthropod-borne NOS B34.9
  - Powassan A84.8
  - Rocio (encephalitis) A83.6

Disease, diseased — *continued*
- viral, virus (*see also* Disease, by type of virus) — *continued*
  - Sin nombre (Hantavirus) (cardio)-pulmonary syndrome) B33.4
  - Tahyna B33.8
  - vesicular stomatitis A93.8
  - vitreous H43.9
    - specified NEC H43.89
  - vocal cord J38.3
- Volkmann's, acquired T79.6 ☑
- von Eulenburg's (congenital paramyotonia) G71.19
- von Gierke's (glycogenosis I) E74.01
- von Graefe's — *see* Strabismus, paralytic, ophthalmoplegia, progressive
- von Willebrand (-Jürgens) (angiohemophilia) D68.0
- Vrolik's (osteogenesis imperfecta) Q78.0
- vulva (noninflammatory) N90.9
  - inflammatory NEC N76.89
  - specified NEC N90.89
- Wallgren's (obstruction of splenic vein with collateral circulation) I87.8
- Wassilieff's (leptospiral jaundice) A27.0
- wasting NEC R64
  - due to malnutrition E41
- Waterhouse-Friderichsen A39.1
- Wegner's (syphilitic osteochondritis) A50.02
- Weil's (leptospiral jaundice of lung) A27.0
- Weir Mitchell's (erythromelalgia) I73.81
- Werdnig-Hoffmann G12.0
- Wermer's E31.21
- Werner-His (trench fever) A79.0
- Werner-Schultz (neutropenic splenomegaly) D73.81
- Wernicke-Posadas B38.9
- whipworm B79
- white blood cells D72.9
  - specified NEC D72.89
- white matter R90.82
- white-spot, meaning lichen sclerosus et atrophicus L90.0
  - penis N48.0
  - vulva N90.4
- Wilkie's K55.1
- Wilkinson-Sneddon (subcorneal pustular dermatosis) L13.1
- Willis' — *see* Diabetes
- Wilson's (hepatolenticular degeneration) E83.01
- woolsorter's A22.1
- yaba monkey tumor B08.72
- yaba pox (virus) B08.72
- Zika virus A92.5
  - congenital P35.4
- zoonotic, bacterial A28.9
  - specified type NEC A28.8

Disfigurement (due to scar) L90.5
Disgerminoma — *see* Dysgerminoma
DISH (diffuse idiopathic skeletal hyperostosis) — *see* Hyperostosis, ankylosing
Disinsertion, retina — *see* Detachment, retina
Dislocatable hip, congenital Q65.6
Dislocation (articular)
- with fracture — *see* Fracture
- acromioclavicular (joint) S43.10- ☑
  - with displacement
    - 100%-200% S43.12- ☑
    - more than 200% S43.13- ☑
  - inferior S43.14- ☑
  - posterior S43.15- ☑
- ankle S93.0- ☑
- astragalus — *see* Dislocation, ankle
- atlantoaxial S13.121 ☑
- atlantooccipital S13.111 ☑
- atloidooccipital S13.111 ☑
- breast bone S23.29 ☑
- capsule, joint — *code by* site under Dislocation
- carpal (bone) — *see* Dislocation, wrist
- carpometacarpal (joint) NEC S63.05- ☑
  - thumb S63.04- ☑
- cartilage (joint) — *code by* site under Dislocation
- cervical spine (vertebra) — *see* Dislocation, vertebra, cervical
- chronic — *see* Dislocation, recurrent
- clavicle — *see* Dislocation, acromioclavicular joint
- coccyx S33.2 ☑
- congenital NEC Q68.8
- coracoid — *see* Dislocation, shoulder
- costal cartilage S23.29 ☑
- costochondral S23.29 ☑

Dislocation — *continued*
- cricoarytenoid articulation S13.29 ☑
- cricothyroid articulation S13.29 ☑
- dorsal vertebra — *see* Dislocation, vertebra, thoracic
- ear ossicle — *see* Discontinuity, ossicles, ear
- elbow S53.10- ☑
  - congenital Q68.8
  - pathological — *see* Dislocation, pathological NEC, elbow
  - radial head alone — *see* Dislocation, radial head
  - recurrent — *see* Dislocation, recurrent, elbow
  - traumatic S53.10- ☑
    - anterior S53.11- ☑
    - lateral S53.14- ☑
    - medial S53.13- ☑
    - posterior S53.12- ☑
    - specified type NEC S53.19- ☑
- eye, nontraumatic — *see* Luxation, globe
- eyeball, nontraumatic — *see* Luxation, globe
- femur
  - distal end — *see* Dislocation, knee
  - proximal end — *see* Dislocation, hip
- fibula
  - distal end — *see* Dislocation, ankle
  - proximal end — *see* Dislocation, knee
- finger S63.25- ☑
  - index S63.25- ☑
  - interphalangeal S63.27- ☑
    - distal S63.29- ☑
      - index S63.29- ☑
      - little S63.29- ☑
      - middle S63.29- ☑
      - ring S63.29- ☑
    - index S63.27- ☑
    - little S63.27- ☑
    - middle S63.27- ☑
    - proximal S63.28- ☑
      - index S63.28- ☑
      - little S63.28- ☑
      - middle S63.28- ☑
      - ring S63.28- ☑
    - ring S63.27- ☑
  - little S63.25- ☑
  - metacarpophalangeal S63.26- ☑
    - index S63.26- ☑
    - little S63.26- ☑
    - middle S63.26- ☑
    - ring S63.26- ☑
  - middle S63.25- ☑
  - recurrent — *see* Dislocation, recurrent, finger
  - ring S63.25- ☑
  - thumb — *see* Dislocation, thumb
- foot S93.30- ☑
  - recurrent — *see* Dislocation, recurrent, foot
  - specified site NEC S93.33- ☑
  - tarsal joint S93.31- ☑
  - tarsometatarsal joint S93.32- ☑
  - toe — *see* Dislocation, toe
- fracture — *see* Fracture
- glenohumeral (joint) — *see* Dislocation, shoulder
- glenoid — *see* Dislocation, shoulder
- habitual — *see* Dislocation, recurrent
- hip S73.00- ☑
  - anterior S73.03- ☑
    - obturator S73.02- ☑
  - central S73.04- ☑
  - congenital (total) Q65.2
    - bilateral Q65.1
    - partial Q65.5
      - bilateral Q65.4
      - unilateral Q65.3- ☑
    - unilateral Q65.0- ☑
  - developmental M24.85- ☑
  - pathological — *see* Dislocation, pathological NEC, hip
  - posterior S73.01- ☑
  - recurrent — *see* Dislocation, recurrent, hip
- humerus, proximal end — *see* Dislocation, shoulder
- incomplete — *see* Subluxation, by site
- incus — *see* Discontinuity, ossicles, ear
- infracoracoid — *see* Dislocation, shoulder
- innominate (pubic junction) (sacral junction) S33.39 ☑
  - acetabulum — *see* Dislocation, hip
- interphalangeal (joint(s))
  - finger S63.279 ☑
    - distal S63.29- ☑

Dislocation — Dislocation

Dislocation — *continued*
  interphalangeal(s) — *continued*
    finger — *continued*
      distal — *continued*
        index S63.29- ☑
        little S63.29- ☑
        middle S63.29- ☑
        ring S63.29- ☑
      index S63.27- ☑
      little S63.27- ☑
      middle S63.27- ☑
      proximal S63.28- ☑
        index S63.28- ☑
        little S63.28- ☑
        middle S63.28- ☑
        ring S63.28- ☑
      ring S63.27- ☑
    foot or toe — *see* Dislocation, toe
    thumb S63.12- ☑
  jaw (cartilage) (meniscus) S03.0- ☑
  joint prosthesis — *see* Complications, joint prosthesis, mechanical, displacement, by site
  knee S83.106 ☑
    cap — *see* Dislocation, patella
    congenital Q68.2
    old M23.8X- ☑
    patella — *see* Dislocation, patella
    pathological — *see* Dislocation, pathological NEC, knee
    proximal tibia
      anteriorly S83.11- ☑
      laterally S83.14- ☑
      medially S83.13- ☑
      posteriorly S83.12- ☑
    recurrent (*see also* Derangement, knee, specified NEC)
    specified type NEC S83.19- ☑
  lacrimal gland H04.16- ☑
  lens (complete) H27.10
    anterior H27.12- ☑
    congenital Q12.1
    ocular implant — *see* Complications, intraocular lens
    partial H27.11- ☑
    posterior H27.13- ☑
    traumatic S05.8X- ☑
  ligament — *code by* site under Dislocation
  lumbar (vertebra) — *see* Dislocation, vertebra, lumbar
  lumbosacral (vertebra) (*see also* Dislocation, vertebra, lumbar)
    congenital Q76.49
  mandible S03.0- ☑
  meniscus (knee) — *see* Tear, meniscus
    other sites - code by site under Dislocation
  metacarpal (bone)
    distal end — *see* Dislocation, finger
    proximal end S63.06- ☑
  metacarpophalangeal (joint)
    finger S63.26- ☑
      index S63.26- ☑
      little S63.26- ☑
      middle S63.26- ☑
      ring S63.26- ☑
    thumb S63.11- ☑
  metatarsal (bone) — *see* Dislocation, foot
  metatarsophalangeal (joint(s)) — *see* Dislocation, toe
  midcarpal (joint) S63.03- ☑
  midtarsal (joint) — *see* Dislocation, foot
  neck S13.20 ☑
    specified site NEC S13.29 ☑
    vertebra — *see* Dislocation, vertebra, cervical
  nose (septal cartilage) S03.1 ☑
  occipitoatloid S13.111 ☑
  old — *see* Derangement, joint, specified type NEC
  ossicles, ear — *see* Discontinuity, ossicles, ear
  partial — *see* Subluxation, by site
  patella S83.006 ☑
    congenital Q74.1
    lateral S83.01- ☑
    recurrent (nontraumatic) M22.0- ☑
      incomplete M22.1- ☑
    specified type NEC S83.09- ☑
  pathological NEC M24.30
    ankle M24.37- ☑
    elbow M24.32- ☑
    foot joint M24.37- ☑

Dislocation — *continued*
  pathological — *continued*
    hand joint M24.34- ☑
    hip M24.35- ☑
    knee M24.36- ☑
    lumbosacral joint — *see* subcategory M53.2 ☑
    pelvic region — *see* Dislocation, pathological, hip
    sacroiliac — *see* subcategory M53.2 ☑
    shoulder M24.31- ☑
    wrist M24.33- ☑
  pelvis NEC S33.30 ☑
    specified NEC S33.39 ☑
  phalanx
    finger or hand — *see* Dislocation, finger
    foot or toe — *see* Dislocation, toe
  prosthesis, internal — *see* Complications, prosthetic device, by site, mechanical
  radial head S53.006 ☑
    anterior S53.01- ☑
    posterior S53.02- ☑
    specified type NEC S53.09- ☑
  radiocarpal (joint) S63.02- ☑
  radiohumeral (joint) — *see* Dislocation, radial head
  radioulnar (joint)
    distal S63.01- ☑
    proximal — *see* Dislocation, elbow
  radius
    distal end — *see* Dislocation, wrist
    proximal end — *see* Dislocation, radial head
  recurrent M24.40
    ankle M24.47- ☑
    elbow M24.42- ☑
    finger M24.44- ☑
    foot joint M24.47- ☑
    hand joint M24.44- ☑
    hip M24.45- ☑
    knee M24.46- ☑
      patella — *see* Dislocation, patella, recurrent
    patella — *see* Dislocation, patella, recurrent
    sacroiliac — *see* subcategory M53.2 ☑
    shoulder M24.41- ☑
    toe M24.47- ☑
    vertebra (*see also* subcategory) M43.5 ☑
      atlantoaxial M43.4
        with myelopathy M43.3
    wrist M24.43- ☑
  rib (cartilage) S23.29 ☑
  sacrococcygeal S33.2 ☑
  sacroiliac (joint) (ligament) S33.2 ☑
    congenital Q74.2
    recurrent — *see* subcategory M53.2 ☑
  sacrum S33.2 ☑
  scaphoid (bone) (hand) (wrist) — *see* Dislocation, wrist
    foot — *see* Dislocation, foot
  scapula — *see* Dislocation, shoulder, girdle, scapula
  semilunar cartilage, knee — *see* Tear, meniscus
  septal cartilage (nose) S03.1 ☑
  septum (nasal) (old) J34.2
  sesamoid bone — *code by* site under Dislocation
  shoulder (blade) (ligament) (joint) (traumatic) S43.006 ☑
    acromioclavicular — *see* Dislocation, acromioclavicular
    chronic — *see* Dislocation, recurrent, shoulder
    congenital Q68.8
    girdle S43.30- ☑
      scapula S43.31- ☑
      specified site NEC S43.39- ☑
    humerus S43.00- ☑
      anterior S43.01- ☑
      inferior S43.03- ☑
      posterior S43.02- ☑
    pathological — *see* Dislocation, pathological NEC, shoulder
    recurrent — *see* Dislocation, recurrent, shoulder
    specified type NEC S43.08- ☑
  spine
    cervical — *see* Dislocation, vertebra, cervical
    congenital Q76.49
    due to birth trauma P11.5
    lumbar — *see* Dislocation, vertebra, lumbar
    thoracic — *see* Dislocation, vertebra, thoracic
  spontaneous — *see* Dislocation, pathological
  sternoclavicular (joint) S43.206 ☑
    anterior S43.21- ☑
    posterior S43.22- ☑

Dislocation — *continued*
  sternum S23.29 ☑
  subglenoid — *see* Dislocation, shoulder
  symphysis pubis S33.4 ☑
  talus — *see* Dislocation, ankle
  tarsal (bone(s)) (joint(s)) — *see* Dislocation, foot
  tarsometatarsal (joint(s)) — *see* Dislocation, foot
  temporomandibular (joint) S03.0- ☑
  thigh, proximal end — *see* Dislocation, hip
  thorax S23.20 ☑
    specified site NEC S23.29 ☑
    vertebra — *see* Dislocation, vertebra
  thumb S63.10- ☑
    interphalangeal joint — *see* Dislocation, interphalangeal (joint), thumb
    metacarpophalangeal joint — *see* Dislocation, metacarpophalangeal (joint), thumb
  thyroid cartilage S13.29 ☑
  tibia
    distal end — *see* Dislocation, ankle
    proximal end — *see* Dislocation, knee
  tibiofibular (joint)
    distal — *see* Dislocation, ankle
    superior — *see* Dislocation, knee
  toe(s) S93.106 ☑
    great S93.10- ☑
      interphalangeal joint S93.11- ☑
      metatarsophalangeal joint S93.12- ☑
    interphalangeal joint S93.119 ☑
    lesser S93.106 ☑
      interphalangeal joint S93.11- ☑
      metatarsophalangeal joint S93.12- ☑
    metatarsophalangeal joint S93.12- ☑
  tooth S03.2 ☑
  trachea S23.29 ☑
  ulna
    distal end S63.07- ☑
    proximal end — *see* Dislocation, elbow
  ulnohumeral (joint) — *see* Dislocation, elbow
  vertebra (articular process) (body) (traumatic)
    cervical S13.101 ☑
      atlantoaxial joint S13.121 ☑
      atlantooccipital joint S13.111 ☑
      atloidooccipital joint S13.111 ☑
      joint between
        C0 and C1 S13.111 ☑
        C1 and C2 S13.121 ☑
        C2 and C3 S13.131 ☑
        C3 and C4 S13.141 ☑
        C4 and C5 S13.151 ☑
        C5 and C6 S13.161 ☑
        C6 and C7 S13.171 ☑
        C7 and T1 S13.181 ☑
      occipitoatloid joint S13.111 ☑
    congenital Q76.49
    lumbar S33.101 ☑
      joint between
        L1 and L2 S33.111 ☑
        L2 and L3 S33.121 ☑
        L3 and L4 S33.131 ☑
        L4 and L5 S33.141 ☑
    nontraumatic — *see* Displacement, intervertebral disc
    partial — *see* Subluxation, by site
    recurrent NEC — *see* subcategory M43.5 ☑
    thoracic S23.101 ☑
      joint between
        T1 and T2 S23.111 ☑
        T2 and T3 S23.121 ☑
        T3 and T4 S23.123 ☑
        T4 and T5 S23.131 ☑
        T5 and T6 S23.133 ☑
        T6 and T7 S23.141 ☑
        T7 and T8 S23.143 ☑
        T8 and T9 S23.151 ☑
        T9 and T10 S23.153 ☑
        T10 and T11 S23.161 ☑
        T11 and T12 S23.163 ☑
        T12 and L1 S23.171 ☑
  wrist (carpal bone) S63.006 ☑
    carpometacarpal joint — *see* Dislocation, carpometacarpal (joint)
    distal radioulnar joint — *see* Dislocation, radioulnar (joint), distal
    metacarpal bone, proximal — *see* Dislocation, metacarpal (bone), proximal end

☑ **Additional Character Required — Refer to the Tabular List for Character Selection**   ▽ **Subterms under main terms may continue to next column or page**

Dislocation — continued
- wrist — continued
  - midcarpal — see Dislocation, midcarpal (joint)
  - radiocarpal joint — see Dislocation, radiocarpal (joint)
  - recurrent — see Dislocation, recurrent, wrist
  - specified site NEC S63.09- ☑
  - ulna — see Dislocation, ulna, distal end
- xiphoid cartilage S23.29 ☑

Disorder (of) (see also Disease)
- acantholytic L11.9
  - specified NEC L11.8
- acute
  - psychotic — see Psychosis, acute
  - stress F43.0
- adjustment (grief) F43.20
  - with
    - anxiety F43.22
      - with depressed mood F43.23
    - conduct disturbance F43.24
      - with emotional disturbance F43.25
    - depressed mood F43.21
      - with anxiety F43.23
    - other specified symptom F43.29
- adrenal (capsule) (gland) (medullary) E27.9
  - specified NEC E27.8
- adrenogenital E25.9
  - drug-induced E25.8
  - iatrogenic E25.8
  - idiopathic E25.8
- adult personality (and behavior) F69
  - specified NEC F68.8
- affective (mood) — see Disorder, mood
- aggressive, unsocialized F91.1
- alcohol use
  - mild F10.10
    - with
      - alcohol intoxication F10.129
        - delirium F10.121
      - alcohol-induced
        - anxiety disorder F10.180
        - bipolar and related disorder F10.14
        - depressive disorder F10.14
        - psychotic disorder F10.159
        - sexual dysfunction F10.181
        - sleep disorder F10.182
    - in remission (early) (sustained) F10.11
  - moderate or severe F10.20
    - with
      - alcohol intoxication F10.229
        - delirium F10.221
      - alcohol-induced
        - anxiety disorder F10.280
        - bipolar and related disorder F10.24
        - depressive disorder F10.24
        - major neurocognitive disorder, amnestic-confabulatory type F10.26
        - major neurocognitive disorder, non-amnestic-confabulatory type F10.27
        - mild neurocognitive disorder F10.288
        - psychotic disorder F10.259
        - sexual dysfunction F10.281
        - sleep disorder F10.282
      - in remission (early) (sustained) F10.21
- alcohol-related F10.99
  - with
    - amnestic disorder, persisting F10.96
    - anxiety disorder F10.980
    - dementia, persisting F10.97
    - intoxication F10.929
      - with delirium F10.921
      - uncomplicated F10.920
    - mood disorder F10.94
    - other specified F10.988
    - psychotic disorder F10.959
      - with
        - delusions F10.950
        - hallucinations F10.951
    - sexual dysfunction F10.981
    - sleep disorder F10.982
- allergic — see Allergy
- alveolar NEC J84.09
- amino-acid
  - cystathioninuria E72.19
  - cystinosis E72.04
  - cystinuria E72.01
  - glycinuria E72.09

Disorder — continued
- amino-acid — continued
  - homocystinuria E72.11
  - metabolism — see Disturbance, metabolism, amino-acid
  - specified NEC E72.89
  - neonatal, transitory P74.8
  - renal transport NEC E72.09
  - transport NEC E72.09
- amnesic, amnestic
  - alcohol-induced F10.96
    - with dependence F10.26
  - due to (secondary to) general medical condition F04
  - psychoactive NEC-induced F19.96
    - with
      - abuse F19.16
      - dependence F19.26
  - sedative, hypnotic or anxiolytic-induced F13.96
    - with dependence F13.26
- amphetamine (or other stimulant) use
  - mild
    - with
      - amphetamine, cocaine, or other stimulant intoxication
        - with perceptual disturbances F15.122
        - without perceptual disturbances F15.129
      - amphetamine (or other stimulant) -induced
        - anxiety disorder F15.180
        - bipolar and related disorder F15.14
        - depressive disorder F15.14
        - obsessive-compulsive and related disorder F15.188
        - psychotic disorder F15.159
        - sexual dysfunction F15.181
      - intoxication delirium F15.121
  - moderate or severe
    - with
      - amphetamine, cocaine, or other stimulant intoxication
        - with perceptual disturbances F15.222
        - without perceptual disturbances F15.229
      - amphetamine (or other stimulant) -induced
        - anxiety disorder F15.280
        - bipolar and related disorder F15.24
        - depressive disorder F15.24
        - obsessive-compulsive and related disorder F15.288
        - psychotic disorder F15.259
        - sexual dysfunction F15.281
      - intoxication delirium F15.221
- amphetamine-type substance use
  - mild F15.10
    - in remission (early) (sustained) F15.11
  - moderate F15.20
    - in remission (early) (sustained) F15.21
  - severe F15.20
    - in remission (early) (sustained) F15.21
- anaerobic glycolysis with anemia D55.2
- anxiety F41.9
  - due to (secondary to)
    - alcohol F10.980
      - in
        - abuse F10.180
        - dependence F10.280
    - amphetamine F15.980
      - in
        - abuse F15.180
        - dependence F15.280
    - anxiolytic F13.980
      - in
        - abuse F13.180
        - dependence F13.280
    - caffeine F15.980
      - in
        - abuse F15.180
        - dependence F15.280
    - cannabis F12.980
      - in
        - abuse F12.180
        - dependence F12.280
    - cocaine F14.980
      - in
        - abuse F14.180
        - dependence F14.180
    - general medical condition F06.4
    - hallucinogen F16.980
      - in
        - abuse F16.180
        - dependence F16.280

Disorder — continued
- anxiety — continued
  - due to — continued
    - hypnotic F13.980
      - in
        - abuse F13.180
        - dependence F13.280
    - inhalant F18.980
      - in
        - abuse F18.180
        - dependence F18.280
    - phencyclidine F16.980
      - in
        - abuse F16.180
        - dependence F16.280
    - psychoactive substance NEC F19.980
      - in
        - abuse F19.180
        - dependence F19.280
    - sedative F13.980
      - in
        - abuse F13.180
        - dependence F13.280
    - volatile solvents F18.980
      - in
        - abuse F18.180
        - dependence F18.280
  - generalized F41.1
  - illness F45.21
  - mixed
    - with depression (mild) F41.8
    - specified NEC F41.3
  - organic F06.4
  - phobic F40.9
    - of childhood F40.8
  - specified NEC F41.8
- aortic valve — see Endocarditis, aortic
- aromatic amino-acid metabolism E70.9
  - specified NEC E70.8
- arteriole NEC I77.89
- artery NEC I77.89
- articulation — see Disorder, joint
- attachment (childhood)
  - disinhibited F94.2
  - reactive F94.1
- attention-deficit hyperactivity (adolescent) (adult) (child) F90.9
  - combined
    - presentation F90.2
    - type F90.2
  - hyperactive
    - impulsive presentation F90.1
    - type F90.1
  - inattentive
    - presentation F90.0
    - type F90.0
  - specified type NEC F90.8
- attention-deficit without hyperactivity (adolescent) (adult) (child) F98.8
- auditory processing (central) H93.25
- autism spectrum F84.0
- autistic F84.0
- autoimmune D89.89
- autonomic nervous system G90.9
  - specified NEC G90.8
- avoidant
  - child or adolescent F40.10
  - restrictive food intake F50.82
- balance
  - acid-base E87.8
    - mixed E87.4
  - electrolyte E87.8
  - fluid NEC E87.8
- behavioral (disruptive) — see Disorder, conduct
- beta-amino-acid metabolism E72.89
- bile acid and cholesterol metabolism E78.70
  - Barth syndrome E78.71
  - other specified E78.79
  - Smith-Lemli-Opitz syndrome E78.72
- bilirubin excretion E80.6
- binge eating F50.81
- binocular
  - movement H51.9
    - convergence
      - excess H51.12
      - insufficiency H51.11
    - internuclear ophthalmoplegia — see Ophthalmoplegia, internuclear
    - palsy of conjugate gaze H51.0

Disorder — continued
  binocular — continued
    movement — continued
      specified type NEC H51.8
    vision NEC — see Disorder, vision, binocular
  bipolar (I) (type I) F31.9
    and related due to a known physiological condition
      with
        manic features F06.33
        manic- or hypomanic-like episodes F06.33
        mixed features F06.34
    current (or most recent) episode
      depressed F31.9
        with psychotic features F31.5
        without psychotic features F31.30
          mild F31.31
          moderate F31.32
          severe (without psychotic features) F31.4
            with psychotic features F31.5
      hypomanic F31.0
      manic F31.9
        with psychotic features F31.2
        without psychotic features F31.10
          mild F31.11
          moderate F31.12
          severe (without psychotic features)
            F31.13
            with psychotic features F31.2
      mixed F31.60
        mild F31.61
        moderate F31.62
        severe (without psychotic features) F31.63
          with psychotic features F31.64
        severe depression (without psychotic features)
          F31.4
          with psychotic features F31.5
    in remission (currently) F31.70
      in full remission
        most recent episode
          depressed F31.76
          hypomanic F31.72
          manic F31.74
          mixed F31.78
      in partial remission
        most recent episode
          depressed F31.75
          hypomanic F31.71
          manic F31.73
          mixed F31.77
    organic F06.30
    single manic episode F30.9
      mild F30.11
      moderate F30.12
      severe (without psychotic symptoms) F30.13
        with psychotic symptoms F30.2
    specified NEC F31.89
  bipolar II (type 2) F31.81
  bladder N32.9
    functional NEC N31.9
    in schistosomiasis B65.0 [N33]
    specified NEC N32.89
  bleeding D68.9
  blood D75.9
    in congenital early syphilis A50.09 [D77]
  body dysmorphic F45.22
  bone M89.9
    continuity M84.9
      specified type NEC M84.80
        ankle M84.87- ☑
        fibula M84.86- ☑
        foot M84.87- ☑
        hand M84.84- ☑
        humerus M84.82- ☑
        neck M84.88
        pelvis M84.859
        radius M84.83- ☑
        rib M84.88
        shoulder M84.81- ☑
        skull M84.88
        thigh M84.85- ☑
        tibia M84.86- ☑
        ulna M84.83- ☑
        vertebra M84.88
    density and structure M85.9
      cyst (see also Cyst, bone, specified type NEC)
        aneurysmal — see Cyst, bone, aneurysmal
        solitary — see Cyst, bone, solitary

Disorder — continued
  bone — continued
    density and structure — continued
      diffuse idiopathic skeletal hyperostosis — see
        Hyperostosis, ankylosing
      fibrous dysplasia (monostotic) — see Dysplasia,
        fibrous, bone
      fluorosis — see Fluorosis, skeletal
      hyperostosis of skull M85.2
      osteitis condensans — see Osteitis, condensans
      specified type NEC M85.8- ☑
        ankle M85.87- ☑
        foot M85.87- ☑
        forearm M85.83- ☑
        hand M85.84- ☑
        lower leg M85.86- ☑
        multiple sites M85.89
        neck M85.88
        rib M85.88
        shoulder M85.81- ☑
        skull M85.88
        thigh M85.85- ☑
        upper arm M85.82- ☑
        vertebra M85.88
    development and growth NEC M89.20
      carpus M89.24- ☑
      clavicle M89.21- ☑
      femur M89.25- ☑
      fibula M89.26- ☑
      finger M89.24- ☑
      humerus M89.22- ☑
      ilium M89.259
      ischium M89.259
      metacarpus M89.24- ☑
      metatarsus M89.27- ☑
      multiple sites M89.29
      neck M89.28
      radius M89.23- ☑
      rib M89.28
      scapula M89.21- ☑
      skull M89.28
      tarsus M89.27- ☑
      tibia M89.26- ☑
      toe M89.27- ☑
      ulna M89.23- ☑
      vertebra M89.28
    specified type NEC M89.8X- ☑
  brachial plexus G54.0
  branched-chain amino-acid metabolism E71.2
    specified NEC E71.19
  breast N64.9
    agalactia — see Agalactia
    associated with
      lactation O92.70
        specified NEC O92.79
      pregnancy O92.20
        specified NEC O92.29
      puerperium O92.20
        specified NEC O92.29
    cracked nipple — see Cracked nipple
    galactorrhea — see Galactorrhea
    hypogalactia O92.4
    lactation disorder NEC O92.79
    mastitis — see Mastitis
    nipple infection — see Infection, nipple
    retracted nipple — see Retraction, nipple
    specified type NEC N64.89
  Briquet's F45.0
  bullous, in diseases classified elsewhere L14
  caffeine use
    mild
      with
        caffeine-induced
          anxiety disorder F15.180
          sleep disorder F15.182
    moderate or severe
      with
        caffeine-induced
          anxiety disorder F15.280
          sleep disorder F15.282
  cannabis use
    mild F12.10
      with
        cannabis intoxication delirium F12.121
          with perceptual disturbances F12.122
          without perceptual disturbances F12.129

Disorder — continued
  cannabis use — continued
    mild — continued
      with — continued
        cannabis-induced
          anxiety disorder F12.180
          psychotic disorder F12.159
          sleep disorder F12.188
      in remission (early) (sustained) F12.11
    moderate or severe F12.20
      with
        cannabis intoxication
          with perceptual disturbances F12.222
          without perceptual disturbances F12.229
        cannabis-induced
          anxiety disorder F12.280
          psychotic disorder F12.259
          sleep disorder F12.288
        delirium F12.221
      in remission (early) (sustained) F12.21
  carbohydrate
    absorption, intestinal NEC E74.39
    metabolism (congenital) E74.9
      specified NEC E74.8
  cardiac, functional I51.89
  carnitine metabolism E71.40
  cartilage M94.9
    articular NEC — see Derangement, joint, articular
      cartilage
    chondrocalcinosis — see Chondrocalcinosis
    specified type NEC M94.8X- ☑
      articular — see Derangement, joint, articular
        cartilage
      multiple sites M94.8X0
  catatonia (due to known physiological condition) (with
    another mental disorder) F06.1
  catatonic
    due to (secondary to) known physiological condition
      F06.1
    organic F06.1
  central auditory processing H93.25
  cervical
    region NEC M53.82
    root (nerve) NEC G54.2
  character NOS F60.9
  childhood disintegrative NEC F84.3
  cholesterol and bile acid metabolism E78.70
    Barth syndrome E78.71
    other specified E78.79
    Smith-Lemli-Opitz syndrome E78.72
  choroid H31.9
    atrophy — see Atrophy, choroid
    degeneration — see Degeneration, choroid
    detachment — see Detachment, choroid
    dystrophy — see Dystrophy, choroid
    hemorrhage — see Hemorrhage, choroid
    rupture — see Rupture, choroid
    scar — see Scar, chorioretinal
    solar retinopathy — see Retinopathy, solar
    specified type NEC H31.8
  ciliary body — see Disorder, iris
    degeneration — see Degeneration, ciliary body
  coagulation (factor) (see also Defect, coagulation) D68.9
    newborn, transient P61.6
  cocaine use
    mild F14.10
      with
        amphetamine, cocaine, or other stimulant
          intoxication
          with perceptual disturbances F14.122
          without perceptual disturbances F14.129
        cocaine intoxication delirium F14.121
        cocaine-induced
          anxiety disorder F14.180
          bipolar and related disorder F14.14
          depressive disorder F14.14
          obsessive-compulsive and related disor-
            der F14.188
          psychotic disorder F14.159
          sexual dysfunction F14.181
          sleep disorder F14.182
      in remission (early) (sustained) F14.11
    moderate or severe F14.20
      with
        amphetamine, cocaine, or other stimulant
          intoxication
          with perceptual disturbances F14.222
          without perceptual disturbances F14.229

110
☑ Additional Character Required — Refer to the Tabular List for Character Selection
▽ Subterms under main terms may continue to next column or page

Disorder — continued
  cocaine use — continued
    moderate or severe — continued
      with — continued
        cocaine intoxication delirium F14.221
        cocaine-induced
          anxiety disorder F14.280
          bipolar and related disorder F14.24
          depressive disorder F14.24
          obsessive-compulsive and related disor-
            der F14.288
          psychotic disorder F14.259
          sexual dysfunction F14.281
          sleep disorder F14.282
      in remission (early) (sustained) F14.21
  coccyx NEC M53.3
  cognitive F09
    due to (secondary to) general medical condition F09
    persisting R41.89
      due to
        alcohol F10.97
          with dependence F10.27
        anxiolytics F13.97
          with dependence F13.27
        hypnotics F13.97
          with dependence F13.27
        sedatives F13.97
          with dependence F13.27
        specified substance NEC F19.97
          with
            abuse F19.17
            dependence F19.27
  communication F80.9
    social pragmatic F80.82
  conduct (childhood) F91.9
    adjustment reaction — see Disorder, adjustment
    adolescent onset type F91.2
    childhood onset type F91.1
    compulsive F63.9
    confined to family context F91.0
    depressive F91.8
    group type F91.2
    hyperkinetic — see Disorder, attention-deficit hy-
      peractivity
    oppositional defiance F91.3
    socialized F91.2
    solitary aggressive type F91.1
    specified NEC F91.8
    unsocialized (aggressive) F91.1
  conduction, heart I45.9
  congenital glycosylation (CDG) E74.8
  conjunctiva H11.9
    infection — see Conjunctivitis
  connective tissue, localized L94.9
    specified NEC L94.8
  conversion (functional neurological symptom disorder)
    with
      abnormal movement F44.4
      anesthesia or sensory loss F44.6
      attacks or seizures F44.5
      mixed symptoms F44.7
      special sensory symptoms F44.6
      speech symptoms F44.4
      swallowing symptoms F44.4
      weakness or paralysis F44.4
  convulsive (secondary) — see Convulsions
  cornea H18.9
    deformity — see Deformity, cornea
    degeneration — see Degeneration, cornea
    deposits — see Deposit, cornea
    due to contact lens H18.82- ☑
      specified as edema — see Edema, cornea
    edema — see Edema, cornea
    keratitis — see Keratitis
    keratoconjunctivitis — see Keratoconjunctivitis
    membrane change — see Change, corneal mem-
      brane
    neovascularization — see Neovascularization,
      cornea
    scar — see Opacity, cornea
    specified type NEC H18.89- ☑
    ulcer — see Ulcer, cornea
  corpus cavernosum N48.9
  cranial nerve — see Disorder, nerve, cranial
  cyclothymic F34.0
  defiant oppositional F91.3
  delusional (persistent) (systematized) F22
    induced F24

Disorder — continued
  depersonalization F48.1
  depressive F32.9
    due to known physiological condition
      with
        depressive features F06.31
        major depressive-like episode F06.32
        mixed features F06.34
    major F32.9
      with psychotic symptoms F32.3
      in remission (full) F32.5
        partial F32.4
      recurrent F33.9
        with psychotic features F33.3
      single episode F32.9
        mild F32.0
        moderate F32.1
        severe (without psychotic symptoms) F32.2
          with psychotic symptoms F32.3
    organic F06.31
    persistent F34.1
    recurrent F33.9
      current episode
        mild F33.0
        moderate F33.1
        severe (without psychotic symptoms) F33.2
          with psychotic symptoms F33.3
      in remission F33.40
        full F33.42
        partial F33.41
      specified NEC F33.8
    single episode — see Episode, depressive
    specified NEC F32.89
  developmental F89
    arithmetical skills F81.2
    coordination (motor) F82
    expressive writing F81.81
    language F80.9
      expressive F80.1
      mixed receptive and expressive F80.2
      receptive type F80.2
      specified NEC F80.89
    learning F81.9
      arithmetical F81.2
      reading F81.0
    mixed F88
    motor coordination or function F82
    pervasive F84.9
      specified NEC F84.8
    phonological F80.0
    reading F81.0
    scholastic skills (see also Disorder, learning)
      mixed F81.89
    specified NEC F88
    speech F80.9
      articulation F80.0
      specified NEC F80.89
    written expression F81.81
  diaphragm J98.6
  digestive (system) K92.9
    newborn P78.9
      specified NEC P78.89
    postprocedural — see Complication, gastrointestinal
    psychogenic F45.8
  disc (intervertebral) M51.9
    with
      myelopathy
        cervical region M50.00
        cervicothoracic region M50.03
        high cervical region M50.01
        lumbar region M51.06
        mid-cervical region M50.020
        sacrococcygeal region M53.3
        thoracic region M51.04
        thoracolumbar region M51.05
      radiculopathy
        cervical region M50.10
        cervicothoracic region M50.13
        high cervical region M50.11
        lumbar region M51.16
        lumbosacral region M51.17
        mid-cervical region M50.120
        sacrococcygeal region M53.3
        thoracic region M51.14
        thoracolumbar region M51.15
    cervical M50.90
      with
        myelopathy M50.00
          C2-C3 M50.01

Disorder — continued
  disc — continued
    cervical — continued
      with — continued
        myelopathy — continued
          C3-C4 M50.01
          C4-C5 M50.021
          C5-C6 M50.022
          C6-C7 M50.023
          C7-T1 M50.03
          cervicothoracic region M50.03
          high cervical region M50.01
          mid-cervical region M50.020
        neuritis, radiculitis or radiculopathy M50.10
          C2-C3 M50.11
          C3-C4 M50.11
          C4-C5 M50.121
          C5-C6 M50.122
          C6-C7 M50.123
          C7-T1 M50.13
          cervicothoracic region M50.13
          high cervical region M50.11
          mid-cervical region M50.120
      C2-C3 M50.91
      C3-C4 M50.91
      C4-C5 M50.921
      C5-C6 M50.922
      C6-C7 M50.923
      C7-T1 M50.93
      cervicothoracic region M50.93
      degeneration M50.30
        C2-C3 M50.31
        C3-C4 M50.31
        C4-C5 M50.321
        C5-C6 M50.322
        C6-C7 M50.323
        C7-T1 M50.33
        cervicothoracic region M50.33
        high cervical region M50.31
        mid-cervical region M50.320
      displacement M50.20
        C2-C3 M50.21
        C3-C4 M50.21
        C4-C5 M50.221
        C5-C6 M50.222
        C6-C7 M50.223
        C7-T1 M50.23
        cervicothoracic region M50.23
        high cervical region M50.21
        mid-cervical region M50.220
      high cervical region M50.91
      mid-cervical region M50.920
      specified type NEC M50.80
        C2-C3 M50.81
        C3-C4 M50.81
        C4-C5 M50.821
        C5-C6 M50.822
        C6-C7 M50.823
        C7-T1 M50.83
        cervicothoracic region M50.83
        high cervical region M50.81
        mid-cervical region M50.820
    specified NEC
      lumbar region M51.86
      lumbosacral region M51.87
      sacrococcygeal region M53.3
      thoracic region M51.84
      thoracolumbar region M51.85
  disinhibited attachment (childhood) F94.2
  disintegrative, childhood NEC F84.3
  disruptive F91.9
    mood dysregulation F34.81
    specified NEC F91.8
  disruptive behavior — see Disorder, conduct
  dissocial personality F60.2
  dissociative F44.9
    affecting
      motor function F44.4
        and sensation F44.7
      sensation F44.6
        and motor function F44.7
    brief reactive F43.0
    due to (secondary to) general medical condition
      F06.8
    mixed F44.7
    organic F06.8
    other specified NEC F44.89
  double heterozygous sickling — see Disease, sickle-cell
  dream anxiety F51.5

Disorder — *continued*

drug induced hemorrhagic D68.32
drug related F19.99
  abuse — *see* Abuse, drug
  dependence — *see* Dependence, drug
dysmorphic body F45.22
dysthymic F34.1
ear H93.9- ☑
  bleeding — *see* Otorrhagia
  deafness — *see* Deafness
  degenerative H93.09-
  discharge — *see* Otorrhea
  external H61.9- ☑
    auditory canal stenosis — *see* Stenosis, external ear canal
    exostosis — *see* Exostosis, external ear canal
    impacted cerumen — *see* Impaction, cerumen
    otitis — *see* Otitis, externa
    perichondritis — *see* Perichondritis, ear
    pinna — *see* Disorder, pinna
    specified type NEC H61.89- ☑
  inner H83.9- ☑
    vestibular dysfunction — *see* Disorder, vestibular function
  middle H74.9- ☑
    adhesive H74.1- ☑
    ossicle — *see* Abnormal, ear ossicles
    polyp — *see* Polyp, ear (middle)
    specified NEC, in diseases classified elsewhere H75.8- ☑
  postprocedural — *see* Complications, ear, procedure
  specified NEC, in diseases classified elsewhere H94.8- ☑
eating (adult) (psychogenic) F50.9
  anorexia — *see* Anorexia
  binge F50.81
  bulimia F50.2
  child F98.29
    pica F98.3
    rumination disorder F98.21
  pica F50.89
    childhood F98.3
electrolyte (balance) NEC E87.8
  with
    abortion — *see* Abortion by type complicated by specified condition NEC
    ectopic pregnancy O08.5
    molar pregnancy O08.5
  acidosis (metabolic) (respiratory) E87.2
  alkalosis (metabolic) (respiratory) E87.3
elimination, transepidermal L87.9
  specified NEC L87.8
emotional (persistent) F34.9
  of childhood F93.9
    specified NEC F93.8
endocrine E34.9
  postprocedural E89.89
    specified NEC E89.89
erectile (male) (organic) (*see also* Dysfunction, sexual, male, erectile) N52.9
  nonorganic F52.21
erythematous — *see* Erythema
esophagus K22.9
  functional K22.4
  psychogenic F45.8
eustachian tube H69.9- ☑
  infection — *see* Salpingitis, eustachian
  obstruction — *see* Obstruction, eustachian tube
  patulous — *see* Patulous, eustachian tube
  specified NEC H69.8- ☑
exhibitionistic F65.2
extrapyramidal G25.9
  in deseases classified elsewhere — *see* category G26
  specified type NEC G25.89
eye H57.9
  postprocedural — *see* Complication, postprocedural, eye
eyelid H02.9
  cyst — *see* Cyst, eyelid
  degenerative H02.70
    chloasma — *see* Chloasma, eyelid
    madarosis — *see* Madarosis
    specified type NEC H02.79
    vitiligo — *see* Vitiligo, eyelid
    xanthelasma — *see* Xanthelasma
  dermatochalasis — *see* Dermatochalasis

Disorder — *continued*

eyelid — *continued*
  edema — *see* Edema, eyelid
  elephantiasis — *see* Elephantiasis, eyelid
  foreign body, retained — *see* Foreign body, retained, eyelid
  function H02.59
    abnormal innervation syndrome — *see* Syndrome, abnormal innervation
    blepharochalasis — *see* Blepharochalasis
    blepharoclonus — *see* Blepharoclonus
    blepharophimosis — *see* Blepharophimosis
    blepharoptosis — *see* Blepharoptosis
    lagophthalmos — *see* Lagophthalmos
    lid retraction — *see* Retraction, lid
  hypertrichosis — *see* Hypertrichosis, eyelid
  specified type NEC H02.89
  vascular H02.879
    left H02.876
      lower H02.875
      upper H02.874
    right H02.873
      lower H02.872
      upper H02.871
factitious
  by proxy F68.A
  imposed on another F68.A
  imposed on self F68.10
    with predominantly
      psychological symptoms F68.11
        with physical symptoms F68.13
      physical symptoms F68.12
        with psychological symptoms F68.13
factor, coagulation — *see* Defect, coagulation
fatty acid
  metabolism E71.30
    specified NEC E71.39
  oxidation
    LCAD E71.310
    MCAD E71.311
    SCAD E71.312
    specified deficiency NEC E71.318
feeding (infant or child) (*see also* Disorder, eating) R63.3
  or eating disorder F50.9
  specified NEC F50.9
feigned (with obvious motivation) Z76.5
  without obvious motivation — *see* Disorder, factitious
female
  hypoactive sexual desire F52.0
  orgasmic F52.31
  sexual interest/arousal F52.22
fetishistic F65.0
fibroblastic M72.9
  specified NEC M72.8
fluency
  adult onset F98.5
  childhood onset F80.81
  following
    cerebral infarction I69.323
    cerebrovascular disease I69.923
      specified disease NEC I69.823
    intracerebral hemorrhage I69.123
    nontraumatic intracranial hemorrhage NEC I69.223
    subarachnoid hemorrhage I69.023
  in conditions classified elsewhere R47.82
fluid balance E87.8
follicular (skin) L73.9
  specified NEC L73.8
frotteuristic F65.81
fructose metabolism E74.10
  essential fructosuria E74.11
  fructokinase deficiency E74.11
  fructose-1, 6-diphosphatase deficiency E74.19
  hereditary fructose intolerance E74.12
  other specified E74.19
functional polymorphonuclear neutrophils D71
gallbladder, biliary tract and pancreas in diseases classified elsewhere K87
gambling F63.0
gamma aminobutyric acid (GABA) metabolism E72.81
gamma-glutamyl cycle E72.89
gastric (functional) K31.9
  motility K30
  psychogenic F45.8
  secretion K30
gastrointestinal (functional) NOS K92.9

Disorder — *continued*

gastrointestinal — *continued*
  newborn P78.9
  psychogenic F45.8
gender-identity or -role F64.9
  childhood F64.2
  effect on relationship F66
  of adolescence or adulthood F64.0
    nontranssexual F64.8
  specified NEC F64.8
  uncertainty F66
genito-pelvic pain penetration F52.6
genitourinary system
  female N94.9
  male N50.9
  psychogenic F45.8
globe H44.9
  degenerated condition H44.50
    absolute glaucoma H44.51- ☑
    atrophy H44.52- ☑
    leucocoria H44.53- ☑
  degenerative H44.30
    chalcosis H44.31- ☑
    myopia (*see also* Myopia, degenerative) H44.2- ☑
    siderosis H44.32- ☑
    specified type NEC H44.39- ☑
  endophthalmitis — *see* Endophthalmitis
  foreign body, retained — *see* Foreign body, intraocular, old, retained
  hemophthalmos — *see* Hemophthalmos
  hypotony H44.40
    due to
      ocular fistula H44.42- ☑
      specified disorder NEC H44.43- ☑
    flat anterior chamber H44.41- ☑
    primary H44.44- ☑
  luxation — *see* Luxation, globe
  specified type NEC H44.89
glomerular (in) N05.9
  amyloidosis E85.4 [N08]
  cryoglobulinemia D89.1 [N08]
  disseminated intravascular coagulation D65 [N08]
  Fabry's disease E75.21 [N08]
  familial lecithin cholesterol acyltransferase deficiency E78.6 [N08]
  Goodpasture's syndrome M31.0
  hemolytic-uremic syndrome D59.3
  Henoch (-Schönlein) purpura D69.0 [N08]
  malariae malaria B52.0
  microscopic polyangiitis M31.7 [N08]
  multiple myeloma C90.0- ☑ [N08]
  mumps B26.83
  schistosomiasis B65.9 [N08]
  sepsis NEC A41.- ☑ [N08]
    streptococcal A40.- ☑ [N08]
  sickle-cell disorders D57.- ☑ [N08]
  strongyloidiasis B78.9 [N08]
  subacute bacterial endocarditis I33.0 [N08]
  syphilis A52.75
  systemic lupus erythematosus M32.14
  thrombotic thrombocytopenic purpura M31.1 [N08]
  Waldenström macroglobulinemia C88.0 [N08]
  Wegener's granulomatosis M31.31
gluconeogenesis E74.4
glucosaminoglycan metabolism — *see* Disorder, metabolism, glucosaminoglycan
glycine metabolism E72.50
  d-glycericacidemia E72.59
  hyperhydroxyprolinemia E72.59
  hyperoxaluria R82.992
    primary E72.53
  hyperprolinemia E72.59
  non-ketotic hyperglycinemia E72.51
  oxalosis E72.53
  oxaluria E72.53
  sarcosinemia E72.59
  trimethylaminuria E72.52
glycoprotein metabolism E77.9
  specified NEC E77.8
habit (and impulse) F63.9
  involving sexual behavior NEC F65.9
  specified NEC F63.89
hallucinogen use
  mild F16.10
    with
      hallucinogen intoxication delirium F16.121

Disorder — *continued*
  hallucinogen use — *continued*
    mild — *continued*
      with — *continued*
        hallucinogen-induced
          anxiety disorder F16.180
          bipolar and related disorder F16.14
          depressive disorder F16.14
          psychotic disorder F16.159
        other hallucinogen intoxication F16.129
        in remission (early) (sustained) F16.11
    moderate or severe F16.20
      with
        hallucinogen intoxication delirium F16.221
        hallucinogen-induced
          anxiety disorder F16.280
          bipolar and related disorder F16.24
          depressive disorder F16.24
          psychotic disorder F16.259
        other hallucinogen intoxication F16.229
        in remission (early) (sustained) F16.21
  heart action I49.9
  hematological D75.9
    newborn (transient) P61.9
      specified NEC P61.8
  hematopoietic organs D75.9
  hemorrhagic NEC D69.9
    drug-induced D68.32
    due to
      extrinsic circulating anticoagulants D68.32
      increase in
        anti-IIa D68.32
        anti-Xa D68.32
      intrinsic
        circulating anticoagulants D68.318
        increase in
          anti-IXa D68.318
          antithrombin D68.318
          anti-VIIIa D68.318
          anti-XIa D68.318
    following childbirth O72.3
  hemostasis — *see* Defect, coagulation
  histidine metabolism E70.40
    histidinemia E70.41
    other specified E70.49
  hoarding F42.3
  hyperkinetic — *see* Disorder, attention-deficit hyperactivity
  hyperleucine-isoleucinemia E71.19
  hypervalinemia E71.19
  hypoactive sexual desire F52.0
  hypochondriacal F45.20
    body dysmorphic F45.22
    neurosis F45.21
    other specified F45.29
  identity
    dissociative F44.81
    illness anxiety F45.21
    of childhood F93.8
  immune mechanism (immunity) D89.9
    specified type NEC D89.89
  impaired renal tubular function N25.9
    specified NEC N25.89
  impulse (control) F63.9
  inflammatory
    pelvic, in diseases classified elsewhere — *see* category N74
    penis N48.29
      abscess N48.21
      cellulitis N48.22
  inhalant use
    mild F18.10
      with
        inhalant intoxication F18.129
        inhalant intoxication delirium F18.121
        inhalant-induced
          anxiety disorder F18.180
          depressive disorder F18.14
          major neurocognitive disorder F18.17
          mild neurocognitive disorder F18.188
          psychotic disorder F18.159
        in remission (early) (sustained) F18.11
    moderate or severe F18.20
      with
        inhalant intoxication F18.229
        inhalant intoxication delirium F18.221
        inhalant-induced
          anxiety disorder F18.280
          depressive disorder F18.24

Disorder — *continued*
  inhalant use — *continued*
    moderate or severe — *continued*
      with — *continued*
        inhalant-induced — *continued*
          major neurocognitive disorder F18.27
          mild neurocognitive disorder F18.288
          psychotic disorder F18.259
        in remission (early) (sustained) F18.21
  integument, newborn P83.9
    specified NEC P83.88
  intermittent explosive F63.81
  internal secretion pancreas — *see* Increased, secretion, pancreas, endocrine
  intestine, intestinal
    carbohydrate absorption NEC E74.39
      postoperative K91.2
    functional NEC K59.9
      postoperative K91.89
    psychogenic F45.8
    vascular K55.9
      chronic K55.1
      specified NEC K55.8
  intraoperative (intraprocedural) — *see* Complications, intraoperative
  involuntary emotional expression (IEED) F07.89
  iris H21.9
    adhesions — *see* Adhesions, iris
    atrophy — *see* Atrophy, iris
    chamber angle recession — *see* Recession, chamber angle
    cyst — *see* Cyst, iris
    degeneration — *see* Degeneration, iris
    in diseases classified elsewhere H22
    iridodialysis — *see* Iridodialysis
    iridoschisis — *see* Iridoschisis
    miotic pupillary cyst — *see* Cyst, pupillary
    pupillary
      abnormality — *see* Abnormality, pupillary
      membrane — *see* Membrane, pupillary
    specified type NEC H21.89
    vascular NEC H21.1X- ☑
  iron metabolism E83.10
    specified NEC E83.19
  isovaleric acidemia E71.110
  jaw, developmental M27.0
    temporomandibular (*see also* Anomaly, dentofacial, temporomandibular joint) M26.60- ☑
  joint M25.9
    derangement — *see* Derangement, joint
    effusion — *see* Effusion, joint
    fistula — *see* Fistula, joint
    hemarthrosis — *see* Hemarthrosis
    instability — *see* Instability, joint
    osteophyte — *see* Osteophyte
    pain — *see* Pain, joint
    psychogenic F45.8
    specified type NEC M25.80
      ankle M25.87- ☑
      elbow M25.82- ☑
      foot joint M25.87- ☑
      hand joint M25.84- ☑
      hip M25.85- ☑
      knee M25.86- ☑
      shoulder M25.81- ☑
      wrist M25.83- ☑
    stiffness — *see* Stiffness, joint
  ketone metabolism E71.32
  kidney N28.9
    functional (tubular) N25.9
    in
      schistosomiasis B65.9 [N29]
    tubular function N25.9
      specified NEC N25.89
  lacrimal system H04.9
    changes H04.69
      fistula — *see* Fistula, lacrimal
    gland H04.19
      atrophy — *see* Atrophy, lacrimal gland
      cyst — *see* Cyst, lacrimal, gland
      dacryops — *see* Dacryops
      dislocation — *see* Dislocation, lacrimal gland
      dry eye syndrome — *see* Syndrome, dry eye
      infection — *see* Dacryoadenitis
    granuloma — *see* Granuloma, lacrimal
    inflammation — *see* Inflammation, lacrimal
    obstruction — *see* Obstruction, lacrimal

Disorder — *continued*
  lacrimal system — *continued*
    specified NEC H04.89
  lactation NEC O92.79
  language (developmental) F80.9
    expressive F80.1
    mixed receptive and expressive F80.2
    receptive F80.2
  late luteal phase dysphoric N94.89
  learning (specific) F81.9
    acalculia R48.8
    alexia R48.0
    mathematics F81.2
    reading F81.0
    specified
      with impairment in
        mathematics F81.2
        reading F81.0
        written expression F81.81
      specified NEC F81.89
      spelling F81.81
      written expression F81.81
  lens H27.9
    aphakia — *see* Aphakia
    cataract — *see* Cataract
    dislocation — *see* Dislocation, lens
    specified type NEC H27.8
  ligament M24.20
    ankle M24.27- ☑
    attachment, spine — *see* Enthesopathy, spinal
    elbow M24.22- ☑
    foot joint M24.27- ☑
    hand joint M24.24- ☑
    hip M24.25- ☑
    knee — *see* Derangement, knee, specified NEC
    shoulder M24.21- ☑
    vertebra M24.28
    wrist M24.23- ☑
  ligamentous attachments (*see also* Enthesopathy)
    spine — *see* Enthesopathy, spinal
  lipid
    metabolism, congenital E78.9
    storage E75.6
      specified NEC E75.5
  lipoprotein
    deficiency (familial) E78.6
    metabolism E78.9
      specified NEC E78.89
  liver K76.9
    malarial B54 [K77]
  low back (*see also* Dorsopathy, specified NEC)
  lumbosacral
    plexus G54.1
    root (nerve) NEC G54.4
  lung, interstitial, drug-induced J70.4
    acute J70.2
    chronic J70.3
  lymphoproliferative, post-transplant (PTLD) D47.Z1
    (*following* D47.4)
  lysine and hydroxylysine metabolism E72.3
  major neurocognitive — *see* Dementia, in (due to)
  male
    erectile (organic) (*see also* Dysfunction, sexual, male, erectile) N52.9
      nonorganic F52.21
    hypoactive sexual desire F52.0
    orgasmic F52.32
  manic F30.9
    organic F06.33
  mast cell activation — *see* Activation, mast cell
  mastoid (*see also* Disorder, ear, middle)
    postprocedural — *see* Complications, ear, procedure
  meniscus — *see* Derangement, knee, meniscus
  menopausal N95.9
    specified NEC N95.8
  menstrual N92.6
    psychogenic F45.8
    specified NEC N92.5
  mental (or behavioral) (nonpsychotic) F99
    due to (secondary to)
      amphetamine
        due to drug abuse — *see* Abuse, drug, stimulant
        due to drug dependence — *see* Dependence, drug, stimulant
      brain disease, damage and dysfunction F09
      caffeine use

Disorder — *continued*
  mental — *continued*
    due to — *continued*
      caffeine use — *continued*
        due to drug abuse — *see* Abuse, drug, stimulant
        due to drug dependence — *see* Dependence, drug, stimulant
      cannabis use
        due to drug abuse — *see* Abuse, drug, cannabis
        due to drug dependence — *see* Dependence, drug, cannabis
      general medical condition F09
      sedative or hypnotic use
        due to drug abuse — *see* Abuse, drug, sedative
        due to drug dependence — *see* Dependence, drug, sedative
      tobacco (nicotine) use — *see* Dependence, drug, nicotine
    following organic brain damage F07.9
      frontal lobe syndrome F07.0
      personality change F07.0
      postconcussional syndrome F07.81
      specified NEC F07.89
    infancy, childhood or adolescence F98.9
    neurotic — *see* Neurosis
    organic or symptomatic F09
    presenile, psychotic F03 ☑
    problem NEC
    psychoneurotic — *see* Neurosis
    psychotic — *see* Psychosis
    puerperal F53.0
    senile, psychotic NEC F03 ☑
  metabolic, amino acid, transitory, newborn P74.8
  metabolism NOS E88.9
    amino-acid E72.9
      aromatic E70.9
        albinism — *see* Albinism
        histidine E70.40
          histidinemia E70.41
          other specified E70.49
        hyperphenylalaninemia E70.1
          classical phenylketonuria E70.0
        other specified E70.8
        tryptophan E70.5
        tyrosine E70.20
          hypertyrosinemia E70.21
          other specified E70.29
      branched chain E71.2
        3-methylglutaconic aciduria E71.111
        hyperleucine-isoleucinemia E71.19
        hypervalinemia E71.19
        isovaleric acidemia E71.110
        maple syrup urine disease E71.0
        methylmalonic acidemia E71.120
        organic aciduria NEC E71.118
        other specified E71.19
        proprionate NEC E71.128
        proprionic acidemia E71.121
      glycine E72.50
        d-glycericacidemia E72.59
        hyperhydroxyprolinemia E72.59
        hyperoxaluria R82.992
          primary E72.53
        hyperprolinemia E72.59
        non-ketotic hyperglycinemia E72.51
        other specified E72.59
        sarcosinemia E72.59
        trimethylaminuria E72.52
      hydroxylysine E72.3
      lysine E72.3
      ornithine E72.4
      other specified E72.89
        beta-amino acid E72.89
        gamma-glutamyl cycle E72.89
      straight-chain E72.89
      sulfur-bearing E72.10
        homocystinuria E72.11
        methylenetetrahydrofolate reductase deficiency E72.12
        other specified E72.19
    bile acid and cholesterol metabolism E78.70
    bilirubin E80.7
      specified NEC E80.6
    calcium E83.50
      hypercalcemia E83.52

  metabolism — *continued*
    calcium — *continued*
      hypocalcemia E83.51
      other specified E83.59
    carbohydrate E74.9
      specified NEC E74.8
    cholesterol and bile acid metabolism E78.70
    congenital E88.9
    copper E83.00
      specified type NEC E83.09
      Wilson's disease E83.01
    cystinuria E72.01
    fructose E74.10
    galactose E74.20
    glucosaminoglycan E76.9
      mucopolysaccharidosis — *see* Mucopolysaccharidosis
      specified NEC E76.8
    glutamine E72.89
    glycine E72.50
    glycogen storage (hepatorenal) E74.09
    glycoprotein E77.9
      specified NEC E77.8
    glycosaminoglycan E76.9
      specified NEC E76.8
    in labor and delivery O75.89
    iron E83.10
    isoleucine E71.19
    leucine E71.19
    lipoid E78.9
    lipoprotein E78.9
      specified NEC E78.89
    magnesium E83.40
      hypermagnesemia E83.41
      hypomagnesemia E83.42
      other specified E83.49
    mineral E83.9
      specified NEC E83.89
    mitochondrial E88.40
      MELAS syndrome E88.41
      MERRF syndrome (myoclonic epilepsy associated with ragged-red fibers) E88.42
      other specified E88.49
    ornithine E72.4
    phosphatases E83.30
    phosphorus E83.30
      acid phosphatase deficiency E83.39
      hypophosphatasia E83.39
      hypophosphatemia E83.39
        familial E83.31
      other specified E83.39
      pseudovitamin D deficiency E83.32
    plasma protein NEC E88.09
    porphyrin — *see* Porphyria
    postprocedural E89.89
      specified NEC E89.89
    purine E79.9
      specified NEC E79.8
    pyrimidine E79.9
      specified NEC E79.8
    pyruvate E74.4
    serine E72.89
    sodium E87.8
    specified NEC E88.89
    threonine E72.89
    valine E71.19
    zinc E83.2
  methylmalonic acidemia E71.120
  micturition NEC (*see also* Difficulty, micturition) R39.198
    feeling of incomplete emptying R39.14
    hesitancy R39.11
    poor stream R39.12
    psychogenic F45.8
    split stream R39.13
    straining R39.16
    urgency R39.15
  mild neurocognitive G31.84
  mitochondrial metabolism E88.40
  mitral (valve) — *see* Endocarditis, mitral
  mixed
    anxiety and depressive F41.8
    of scholastic skills (developmental) F81.89
    receptive expressive language F80.2
  mood F39
    bipolar — *see* Disorder, bipolar
    depressive — *see* Disorder, depressive
    due to (secondary to)
      alcohol F10.94

  mood — *continued*
    due to — *continued*
      amphetamine F15.94
        in
          abuse F15.14
          dependence F15.24
      anxiolytic F13.94
        in
          abuse F13.14
          dependence F13.24
      cocaine F14.94
        in
          abuse F14.14
          dependence F14.24
      general medical condition F06.30
      hallucinogen F16.94
        in
          abuse F16.14
          dependence F16.24
      hypnotic F13.94
        in
          abuse F13.14
          dependence F13.24
      inhalant F18.94
        in
          abuse F18.14
          dependence F18.24
      opioid F11.94
        in
          abuse F11.14
          dependence F11.24
      phencyclidine (PCP) F16.94
        in
          abuse F16.14
          dependence F16.24
      physiological condition F06.30
        with
          depressive features F06.31
          major depressive-like episode F06.32
          manic features F06.33
          mixed features F06.34
      psychoactive substance NEC F19.94
        in
          abuse F19.14
          dependence F19.24
      sedative F13.94
        in
          abuse F13.14
          dependence F13.24
      volatile solvents F18.94
        in
          abuse F18.14
          dependence F18.24
    manic episode F30.9
      with psychotic symptoms F30.2
      in remission (full) F30.4
        partial F30.3
      specified type NEC F30.8
      without psychotic symptoms F30.10
        mild F30.11
        moderate F30.12
        severe F30.13
    organic F06.30
      right hemisphere F07.89
    persistent F34.9
      cyclothymia F34.0
      dysthymia F34.1
      specified type NEC F34.89
    recurrent F39
    right hemisphere organic F07.89
  movement G25.9
    drug-induced G25.70
      akathisia G25.71
      specified NEC G25.79
    hysterical F44.4
    in diseases classified elsewhere — *see* category G26
    periodic limb G47.61
      sleep related G47.61
    sleep related NEC G47.69
    specified NEC G25.89
    stereotyped F98.4
    treatment-induced G25.9
  multiple personality F44.81
  muscle M62.9
    attachment, spine — *see* Enthesopathy, spinal
    in trichinellosis — *see* Trichinellosis, with muscle disorder
    psychogenic F45.8

Disorder — *continued*
  muscle — *continued*
    specified type NEC M62.89
    tone, newborn P94.9
      specified NEC P94.8
  muscular
    attachments (*see also* Enthesopathy)
      spine — *see* Enthesopathy, spinal
    urethra N36.44
  musculoskeletal system, soft tissue — *see* Disorder, soft tissue
    postprocedural M96.89
    psychogenic F45.8
  myoneural G70.9
    due to lead G70.1
    specified NEC G70.89
    toxic G70.1
  myotonic NEC G71.19
  nail, in diseases classified elsewhere L62
  neck region NEC — *see* Dorsopathy, specified NEC
  neonatal onset multisystemic inflammatory (NOMID) M04.2
  nerve G58.9
    abducent NEC — *see* Strabismus, paralytic, sixth nerve
    accessory G52.8
    acoustic — *see* subcategory H93.3 ☑
    auditory — *see* subcategory H93.3 ☑
    auriculotemporal G50.8
    axillary G54.0
    cerebral — *see* Disorder, nerve, cranial
    cranial G52.9
      eighth — *see* subcategory H93.3 ☑
      eleventh G52.8
      fifth G50.9
      first G52.0
      fourth NEC — *see* Strabismus, paralytic, fourth nerve
      multiple G52.7
      ninth G52.1
      second NEC — *see* Disorder, nerve, optic
      seventh NEC G51.8
      sixth NEC — *see* Strabismus, paralytic, sixth nerve
      specified NEC G52.8
      tenth G52.2
      third NEC — *see* Strabismus, paralytic, third nerve
      twelfth G52.3
    entrapment — *see* Neuropathy, entrapment
    facial G51.9
      specified NEC G51.8
    femoral — *see* Lesion, nerve, femoral
    glossopharyngeal NEC G52.1
    hypoglossal G52.3
    intercostal G58.0
    lateral
      cutaneous of thigh — *see* Mononeuropathy, lower limb, meralgia paresthetica
      popliteal — *see* Lesion, nerve, popliteal
    lower limb — *see* Mononeuropathy, lower limb
    medial popliteal — *see* Lesion, nerve, popliteal, medial
    median NEC — *see* Lesion, nerve, median
    multiple G58.7
    oculomotor NEC — *see* Strabismus, paralytic, third nerve
    olfactory G52.0
    optic NEC H47.09- ☑
      hemorrhage into sheath — *see* Hemorrhage, optic nerve
      ischemic H47.01- ☑
    peroneal — *see* Lesion, nerve, popliteal
    phrenic G58.8
    plantar — *see* Lesion, nerve, plantar
    pneumogastric G52.2
    posterior tibial — *see* Syndrome, tarsal tunnel
    radial — *see* Lesion, nerve, radial
    recurrent laryngeal G52.2
    root G54.9
      cervical G54.2
      lumbosacral G54.1
      specified NEC G54.8
      thoracic G54.3
    sciatic NEC — *see* Lesion, nerve, sciatic
    specified NEC G58.8
      lower limb — *see* Mononeuropathy, lower limb, specified NEC
      upper limb — *see* Mononeuropathy, upper limb, specified NEC

Disorder — *continued*
  nerve — *continued*
    sympathetic G90.9
    tibial — *see* Lesion, nerve, popliteal, medial
    trigeminal G50.9
      specified NEC G50.8
    trochlear NEC — *see* Strabismus, paralytic, fourth nerve
    ulnar — *see* Lesion, nerve, ulnar
    upper limb — *see* Mononeuropathy, upper limb
    vagus G52.2
  nervous system G98.8
    autonomic (peripheral) G90.9
      specified NEC G90.8
    central G96.9
      specified NEC G96.8
    parasympathetic G90.9
    specified NEC G98.8
    sympathetic G90.9
    vegetative G90.9
  neurocognitive R41.9
    major
      with
        aggressive behavior F01.51
        combative behavior F01.51
        violent behavior F01.51
      due to vascular disease, with behavioral disturbance F01.51
      in (due to) (other diseases classified elsewhere) (*see also* Dementia, in (due to)) F02.80
        with
          aggressive behavior F02.81
          combative behavior F02.81
          violent behavior F02.81
        without behavioral disturbance F01.50
    mild G31.84
  neurodevelopmental F89
    specified NEC F88
  neurohypophysis NEC E23.3
  neurological NEC R29.818
  neuromuscular G70.9
    hereditary NEC G71.9
    specified NEC G70.89
    toxic G70.1
  neurotic F48.9
    specified NEC F48.8
  neutrophil, polymorphonuclear D71
  nicotine use — *see* Dependence, drug, nicotine
  nightmare F51.5
  non-rapid eye movement sleep arousal
    sleep terror type F51.4
    sleepwalking type F51.3
  nose J34.9
    specified NEC J34.89
  obsessive-compulsive F42.9
    and related disorder due to a known physiological condition F06.8
  odontogenesis NOS K00.9
  opioid use
    with
      opioid-induced psychotic disorder F11.959
        with
          delusions F11.950
          hallucinations F11.951
      due to drug abuse — *see* Abuse, drug, opioid
      due to drug dependence — *see* Dependence, drug, opioid
    mild F11.10
      with
        opioid-induced
          anxiety disorder F11.188
          depressive disorder F11.14
          sexual dysfunction F11.181
        opioid intoxication
          with perceptual disturbances F11.122
          delirium F11.121
          without perceptual disturbances F11.129
      in remission (early) (sustained) F11.11
    moderate or severe F11.20
      with
        opioid-induced
          anxiety disorder F11.288
          anxiety disorder F11.988
          depressive disorder F11.24
          depressive disorder F11.94
          sexual dysfunction F11.281
          sexual dysfunction F11.981

Disorder — *continued*
  opioid use — *continued*
    moderate or severe — *continued*
      with — *continued*
        opioid intoxication
          with perceptual disturbances F11.222
          delirium F11.221
          without perceptual disturbances F11.229
      in remission (early) (sustained) F11.21
  oppositional defiant F91.3
  optic
    chiasm H47.49
      due to
        inflammatory disorder H47.41
        neoplasm H47.42
        vascular disorder H47.43
    disc H47.39- ☑
      coloboma — *see* Coloboma, optic disc
      drusen — *see* Drusen, optic disc
      pseudopapilledema — *see* Pseudopapilledema
    radiations — *see* Disorder, visual, pathway
    tracts — *see* Disorder, visual, pathway
  orbit H05.9
    cyst — *see* Cyst, orbit
    deformity — *see* Deformity, orbit
    edema — *see* Edema, orbit
    enophthalmos — *see* Enophthalmos
    exophthalmos — *see* Exophthalmos
    hemorrhage — *see* Hemorrhage, orbit
    inflammation — *see* Inflammation, orbit
    myopathy — *see* Myopathy, extraocular muscles
    retained foreign body — *see* Foreign body, orbit, old
    specified type NEC H05.89
  organic
    anxiety F06.4
    catatonic F06.1
    delusional F06.2
    dissociative F06.8
    emotionally labile (asthenic) F06.8
    mood (affective) F06.30
    schizophrenia-like F06.2
  orgasmic (female) F52.31
    male F52.32
  ornithine metabolism E72.4
  overanxious F41.1
    of childhood F93.8
  pain
    with related psychological factors F45.42
    exclusively related to psychological factors F45.41
    genito-pelvic penetration disorder F52.6
  pancreatic internal secretion E16.9
    specified NEC E16.8
  panic F41.0
    with agoraphobia F40.01
  papulosquamous L44.9
    in diseases classified elsewhere L45
    specified NEC L44.8
  paranoid F22
    induced F24
    shared F24
  paraphilic F65.9
    specified NEC F65.89
  parathyroid (gland) E21.5
    specified NEC E21.4
  parietoalveolar NEC J84.09
  paroxysmal, mixed R56.9
  patella M22.9- ☑
    chondromalacia — *see* Chondromalacia, patella
    derangement NEC M22.3X- ☑
    recurrent
      dislocation — *see* Dislocation, patella, recurrent
      subluxation — *see* Dislocation, patella, recurrent, incomplete
    specified NEC M22.8X- ☑
  patellofemoral M22.2X- ☑
  pedophilic F65.4
  pentose phosphate pathway with anemia D55.1
  perception, due to hallucinogens F16.983
    in
      abuse F16.183
      dependence F16.283
  peripheral nervous system NEC G64
  peroxisomal E71.50
    biogenesis
      neonatal adrenoleukodystrophy E71.511
      specified disorder NEC E71.518
      Zellweger syndrome E71.510

Disorder — *continued*
    peroxisomal — *continued*
        rhizomelic chondrodysplasia punctata E71.540
        specified form NEC E71.548
            group 1 E71.518
            group 2 E71.53
            group 3 E71.542
        X-linked adrenoleukodystrophy E71.529
            adolescent E71.521
            adrenomyeloneuropathy E71.522
            childhood E71.520
            specified form NEC E71.528
        Zellweger-like syndrome E71.541
    persistent
        (somatoform) pain F45.41
        affective (mood) F34.9
    personality (*see also* Personality) F60.9
        affective F34.0
        aggressive F60.3
        amoral F60.2
        anankastic F60.5
        antisocial F60.2
        anxious F60.6
        asocial F60.2
        asthenic F60.7
        avoidant F60.6
        borderline F60.3
        change (secondary) due to general medical condition F07.0
        compulsive F60.5
        cyclothymic F34.0
        dependent (passive) F60.7
        depressive F34.1
        dissocial F60.2
        emotional instability F60.3
        expansive paranoid F60.0
        explosive F60.3
        following organic brain damage F07.9
        histrionic F60.4
        hyperthymic F34.0
        hypothymic F34.1
        hysterical F60.4
        immature F60.89
        inadequate F60.7
        labile F60.3
        mixed (nonspecific) F60.89
        moral deficiency F60.2
        narcissistic F60.81
        negativistic F60.89
        obsessional F60.5
        obsessive (-compulsive) F60.5
        organic F07.9
        overconscientious F60.5
        paranoid F60.0
        passive (-dependent) F60.7
        passive-aggressive F60.89
        pathological NEC F60.9
        pseudosocial F60.2
        psychopathic F60.2
        schizoid F60.1
        schizotypal F21
        self-defeating F60.7
        specified NEC F60.89
        type A F60.5
        unstable (emotional) F60.3
    pervasive, developmental F84.9
    phencyclidine use
        mild F16.10
            with
                phencyclidine intoxication F16.129
                phencyclidine intoxication delirium F16.121
                phencyclidine-induced
                    anxiety disorder F16.180
                    bipolar and related disorder F16.14
                    depressive disorder F16.14
                    psychotic disorder F16.159
            in remission (early) (sustained) F16.11
        moderate or severe F16.20
            with
                phencyclidine intoxication F16.229
                phencyclidine intoxication delirium F16.221
                phencyclidine-induced
                    anxiety disorder F16.280
                    bipolar and related disorder F16.14
                    depressive disorder F16.24
                    psychotic disorder F16.259
            in remission (early) (sustained) F16.21
    phobic anxiety, childhood F40.8
    phosphate-losing tubular N25.0

Disorder — *continued*
    pigmentation L81.9
        choroid, congenital Q14.3
        diminished melanin formation L81.6
        iron L81.8
        specified NEC L81.8
    pinna (noninfective) H61.10- ☑
        deformity, acquired H61.11- ☑
        hematoma H61.12- ☑
        perichondritis — *see* Perichondritis, ear
        specified type NEC H61.19- ☑
    pituitary gland E23.7
        iatrogenic (postprocedural) E89.3
        specified NEC E23.6
    platelets D69.1
    plexus G54.9
        specified NEC G54.8
    polymorphonuclear neutrophils D71
    porphyrin metabolism — *see* Porphyria
    postconcussional F07.81
    posthallucinogen perception F16.983
        in
            abuse F16.183
            dependence F16.283
    postmenopausal N95.9
        specified NEC N95.8
    postprocedural (postoperative) — *see* Complications, postprocedural
    post-transplant lymphoproliferative D47.Z1 (*following* D47.4)
    post-traumatic stress (PTSD) F43.10
        acute F43.11
        chronic F43.12
    premenstrual dysphoric (PMDD) F32.81
    prepuce N47.8
    propionic acidemia E71.121
    prostate N42.9
        specified NEC N42.89
    psychogenic NOS (*see also* condition) F45.9
        anxiety F41.8
        appetite F50.9
        asthenic F48.8
        cardiovascular (system) F45.8
        compulsive F42.8
        cutaneous F54
        depressive F32.9
        digestive (system) F45.8
        dysmenorrheic F45.8
        dyspneic F45.8
        endocrine (system) F54
        eye NEC F45.8
        feeding — *see* Disorder, eating
        functional NEC F45.8
        gastric F45.8
        gastrointestinal (system) F45.8
        genitourinary (system) F45.8
        heart (function) (rhythm) F45.8
        hyperventilatory F45.8
        hypochondriacal — *see* Disorder, hypochondriacal
        intestinal F45.8
        joint F45.8
        learning F81.9
        limb F45.8
        lymphatic (system) F45.8
        menstrual F45.8
        micturition F45.8
        monoplegic NEC F44.4
        motor F44.4
        muscle F45.8
        musculoskeletal F45.8
        neurocirculatory F45.8
        obsessive F42.8
        occupational F48.8
        organ or part of body NEC F45.8
        paralytic NEC F44.4
        phobic F40.9
        physical NEC F45.8
        rectal F45.8
        respiratory (system) F45.8
        rheumatic F45.8
        sexual (function) F52.9
        skin (allergic) (eczematous) F54
        sleep F51.9
        specified part of body NEC F45.8
        stomach F45.8
    psychological F99
        associated with
            disease classified elsewhere F54

Disorder — *continued*
    psychological — *continued*
        associated with — *continued*
            sexual
                development F66
                relationship F66
            uncertainty about gender identity F64.9
    psychomotor NEC F44.4
        hysterical F44.4
    psychoneurotic (*see also* Neurosis)
        mixed NEC F48.8
    psychophysiologic — *see* Disorder, somatoform
    psychosexual F65.9
        development F66
        identity of childhood F64.2
    psychosomatic NOS — *see* Disorder, somatoform
        multiple F45.0
        undifferentiated F45.1
    psychotic — *see* Psychosis
        transient (acute) F23
    puberty E30.9
        specified NEC E30.8
    pulmonary (valve) — *see* Endocarditis, pulmonary
    purine metabolism E79.9
    pyrimidine metabolism E79.9
    pyruvate metabolism E74.4
    reactive attachment (childhood) F94.1
    reading R48.0
        developmental (specific) F81.0
    receptive language F80.2
    receptor, hormonal, peripheral (*see also* Syndrome, androgen insensitivity) E34.50
    recurrent brief depressive F33.8
    reflex R29.2
    refraction H52.7
        aniseikonia H52.32
        anisometropia H52.31
        astigmatism — *see* Astigmatism
        hypermetropia — *see* Hypermetropia
        myopia — *see* Myopia
        presbyopia H52.4
        specified NEC H52.6
    relationship F68.8
        due to sexual orientation F66
    REM sleep behavior G47.52
    renal function, impaired (tubular) N25.9
    resonance R49.9
        specified NEC R49.8
    respiratory function, impaired (*see also* Failure, respiration)
        postprocedural — *see* Complication, postoperative, respiratory system
        psychogenic F45.8
    retina H35.9
        angioid streaks H35.33
        changes in vascular appearance H35.01- ☑
        degeneration — *see* Degeneration, retina
        dystrophy (hereditary) — *see* Dystrophy, retina
        edema H35.81
        hemorrhage — *see* Hemorrhage, retina
        ischemia H35.82
        macular degeneration — *see* Degeneration, macula
        microaneurysms H35.04- ☑
        microvascular abnormality NEC H35.09
        neovascularization — *see* Neovascularization, retina
        retinopathy — *see* Retinopathy
        separation of layers H35.70
            central serous chorioretinopathy H35.71- ☑
            pigment epithelium detachment (serous) H35.72- ☑
                hemorrhagic H35.73- ☑
        specified type NEC H35.89
        telangiectasis — *see* Telangiectasis, retina
        vasculitis — *see* Vasculitis, retina
    retroperitoneal K68.9
    right hemisphere organic affective F07.89
    rumination (infant or child) F98.21
    sacrum, sacrococcygeal NEC M53.3
    schizoaffective F25.9
        bipolar type F25.0
        depressive type F25.1
        manic type F25.0
        mixed type F25.0
        specified NEC F25.8
    schizoid of childhood F84.5
    schizophrenia spectrum and other psychotic disorder F29
        specified NEC F28

☑ **Additional Character Required** — Refer to the Tabular List for Character Selection   ▼ Subterms under main terms may continue to next column or page

Disorder — *continued*
  schizophreniform F20.81
    brief F23
  schizotypal (personality) F21
  secretion, thyrocalcitonin E07.0
  sedative, hypnotic, or anxiolytic use
    mild F13.10
      with
        sedative, hypnotic, or anxiolytic intoxication F13.129
        sedative, hypnotic, or anxiolytic intoxication delirium F13.121
        sedative, hypnotic, or anxiolytic-induced
          anxiety disorder F13.180
          bipolar and related disorder F13.14
          depressive disorder F13.14
          psychotic disorder F13.159
          sexual dysfunction F13.181
      in remission (early) (sustained) F13.11
    moderate or severe F13.20
      with
        sedative, hypnotic, or anxiolytic intoxication F13.229
        sedative, hypnotic, or anxiolytic intoxication delirium F13.221
        sedative, hypnotic, or anxiolytic-induced
          anxiety disorder F13.280
          bipolar and related disorder F13.24
          depressive disorder F13.24
          major neurocognitive disorder F13.27
          mild neurocognitive disorder F13.288
          psychotic disorder F13.259
          sexual dysfunction F13.281
      in remission (early) (sustained) F13.21
  seizure (*see also* Epilepsy) G40.909
    intractable G40.919
      with status epilepticus G40.911
  semantic pragmatic F80.89
    with autism F84.0
  sense of smell R43.1
    psychogenic F45.8
  separation anxiety, of childhood F93.0
  sexual
    aversion F52.1
    function, psychogenic F52.9
    interest/arousal, female F52.22
    masochism F65.51
    maturation F66
    nonorganic F52.9
    preference (*see also* Deviation, sexual) F65.9
      fetishistic transvestism F65.1
    relationship F66
    sadism F65.52
  shyness, of childhood and adolescence F40.10
  sibling rivalry F93.8
  sickle-cell (sickling) (homozygous) — *see* Disease, sickle-cell
    heterozygous D57.3
    specified type NEC D57.8- ☑
    trait D57.3
  sinus (nasal) J34.9
    specified NEC J34.89
  skin L98.9
    atrophic L90.9
      specified NEC L90.8
    granulomatous L92.9
      specified NEC L92.8
    hypertrophic L91.9
      specified NEC L91.8
    infiltrative NEC L98.6
    newborn P83.9
      specified NEC P83.88
    picking F42.4
    psychogenic (allergic) (eczematous) F54
  sleep G47.9
    breathing-related — *see* Apnea, sleep
    circadian rhythm G47.20
      advance sleep phase type G47.22
      delayed sleep phase type G47.21
      due to
        alcohol
          abuse F10.182
          dependence F10.282
          use F10.982
        amphetamines
          abuse F15.182
          dependence F15.282
          use F15.982

Disorder — *continued*
  sleep — *continued*
    circadian rhythm — *continued*
      due to — *continued*
        caffeine
          abuse F15.182
          dependence F15.282
          use F15.982
        cocaine
          abuse F14.182
          dependence F14.282
          use F14.982
        drug NEC
          abuse F19.182
          dependence F19.282
          use F19.982
        opioid
          abuse F11.182
          dependence F11.282
          use F11.982
        psychoactive substance NEC
          abuse F19.182
          dependence F19.282
          use F19.982
        sedative, hypnotic, or anxiolytic
          abuse F13.182
          dependence F13.282
          use F13.982
        stimulant NEC
          abuse F15.182
          dependence F15.282
          use F15.982
      free running type G47.24
      in conditions classified elsewhere G47.27
      irregular sleep wake type G47.23
      jet lag type G47.25
      non-24-hour sleep-wake type G47.24
      shift work type G47.26
      specified NEC G47.29
    due to
      alcohol
        abuse F10.182
        dependence F10.282
        use F10.982
      amphetamine
        abuse F15.182
        dependence F15.282
        use F15.982
      anxiolytic
        abuse F13.182
        dependence F13.282
        use F13.982
      caffeine
        abuse F15.182
        dependence F15.282
        use F15.982
      cocaine
        abuse F14.182
        dependence F14.282
        use F14.982
      drug NEC
        abuse F19.182
        dependence F19.282
        use F19.982
      hypnotic
        abuse F13.182
        dependence F13.282
        use F13.982
      opioid
        abuse F11.182
        dependence F11.282
        use F11.982
      psychoactive substance NEC
        abuse F19.182
        dependence F19.282
        use F19.982
      sedative
        abuse F13.182
        dependence F13.282
        use F13.982
      stimulant NEC
        abuse F15.182
        dependence F15.282
        use F15.982
    emotional F51.9
    excessive somnolence — *see* Hypersomnia
    hypersomnia type — *see* Hypersomnia
    initiating or maintaining — *see* Insomnia
    nightmares F51.5

Disorder — *continued*
  sleep — *continued*
    nonorganic F51.9
      specified NEC F51.8
    parasomnia type G47.50
      specified NEC G47.8
    terrors F51.4
    walking F51.3
    sleep-wake pattern or schedule (*see also* Disorder, sleep, circadian rhythm) G47.9
    specified NEC G47.8
  social
    anxiety (of childhood) F40.10
      generalized F40.11
    functioning in childhood F94.9
      specified NEC F94.8
    pragmatic F80.82
  soft tissue M79.9
    ankle M79.9
    due to use, overuse and pressure M70.90
      ankle M70.97- ☑
      bursitis — *see* Bursitis
      foot M70.97- ☑
      forearm M70.93- ☑
      hand M70.94- ☑
      lower leg M70.96- ☑
      multiple sites M70.99
      pelvic region M70.95- ☑
      shoulder region M70.91- ☑
      specified site NEC M70.98
      specified type NEC M70.80
        ankle M70.87- ☑
        foot M70.87- ☑
        forearm M70.83- ☑
        hand M70.84- ☑
        lower leg M70.86- ☑
        multiple sites M70.89
        pelvic region M70.85- ☑
        shoulder region M70.81- ☑
        specified site NEC M70.88
        thigh M70.85- ☑
        upper arm M70.82- ☑
      thigh M70.95- ☑
      upper arm M70.92- ☑
    foot M79.9
    forearm M79.9
    hand M79.9
    lower leg M79.9
    multiple sites M79.9
    occupational — *see* Disorder, soft tissue, due to use, overuse and pressure
    pelvic region M79.9
    shoulder region M79.9
    specified type NEC M79.89
    thigh M79.9
    upper arm M79.9
  somatic symptom F45.1
  somatization F45.0
  somatoform F45.9
    pain (persistent) F45.41
    somatization (multiple) (long-lasting) F45.0
    specified NEC F45.8
    undifferentiated F45.1
  somnolence, excessive — *see* Hypersomnia
  specific
    arithmetical F81.2
    developmental, of motor F82
    reading F81.0
    speech and language F80.9
    spelling F81.81
    written expression F81.81
  speech R47.9
    articulation (functional) (specific) F80.0
    developmental F80.9
    specified NEC R47.89
  speech-sound F80.0
  spelling (specific) F81.81
  spine (*see also* Dorsopathy)
    ligamentous or muscular attachments, peripheral — *see* Enthesopathy, spinal
    specified NEC — *see* Dorsopathy, specified NEC
  stereotyped, habit or movement F98.4
  stimulant use (other) (unspecified)
    mild F15.10
      in remission (early) (sustained) F15.11
    moderate or severe F15.20
      in remission (early) (sustained) F15.21
  stomach (functional) — *see* Disorder, gastric

Disorder — *continued*
  stress F43.9
    acute F43.0
    post-traumatic F43.10
      acute F43.11
      chronic F43.12
  substance use (other) (unknown)
    mild F19.10
      with substance-induced
        anxiety disorder F19.180
        bipolar and related disorder F19.14
        depressive disorder F19.14
        major neurocognitive disorder F19.17
        mild neurocognitive disorder F19.188
        obsessive-compulsive and related disorder F19.188
        sexual dysfunction F19.181
        substance intoxication F19.129
        substance intoxication delirium F19.121
    moderate or severe F19.20
      with substance-induced
        anxiety disorder F19.280
        bipolar and related disorder F19.24
        depressive disorder F19.24
        major neurocognitive disorder F19.27
        mild neurocognitive disorder F19.288
        obsessive-compulsive and related disorder F19.288
        sexual dysfunction F19.281
      in remission (early) (sustained) F19.21
      substance intoxication F19.229
      substance intoxication delirium F19.221
  sulfur-bearing amino-acid metabolism E72.10
  sweat gland (eccrine) L74.9
    apocrine L75.9
      specified NEC L75.8
    specified NEC L74.8
  synovium M67.90
    acromioclavicular M67.91- ☑
    ankle M67.97- ☑
    elbow M67.92- ☑
    foot M67.97- ☑
    forearm M67.93- ☑
    hand M67.94- ☑
    hip M67.95- ☑
    knee M67.96- ☑
    multiple sites M67.99
    rupture — *see* Rupture, synovium
    shoulder M67.91- ☑
    specified type NEC M67.80
      acromioclavicular M67.81- ☑
      ankle M67.87- ☑
      elbow M67.82- ☑
      foot M67.87- ☑
      hand M67.84- ☑
      hip M67.85- ☑
      knee M67.86- ☑
      multiple sites M67.89
      wrist M67.83- ☑
    synovitis — *see* Synovitis
    upper arm M67.92- ☑
    wrist M67.93- ☑
  temperature regulation, newborn P81.9
    specified NEC P81.8
  temporomandibular joint M26.60- ☑
  tendon M67.90
    acromioclavicular M67.91- ☑
    ankle M67.97- ☑
    contracture — *see* Contracture, tendon
    elbow M67.92- ☑
    foot M67.97- ☑
    forearm M67.93- ☑
    hand M67.94- ☑
    hip M67.95- ☑
    knee M67.96- ☑
    multiple sites M67.99
    rupture — *see* Rupture, tendon
    shoulder M67.91- ☑
    specified type NEC M67.80
      acromioclavicular M67.81- ☑
      ankle M67.87- ☑
      elbow M67.82- ☑
      foot M67.87- ☑
      hand M67.84- ☑
      hip M67.85- ☑
      knee M67.86- ☑
      multiple sites M67.89

Disorder — *continued*
  tendon — *continued*
    specified type — *continued*
      trunk M67.88
      wrist M67.83- ☑
    synovitis — *see* Synovitis
    tendinitis — *see* Tendinitis
    tenosynovitis — *see* Tenosynovitis
    trunk M67.98
    upper arm M67.92- ☑
    wrist M67.93- ☑
  thoracic root (nerve) NEC G54.3
  thyrocalcitonin hypersecretion E07.0
  thyroid (gland) E07.9
    function NEC, neonatal, transitory P72.2
    iodine-deficiency related E01.8
    specified NEC E07.89
  tic — *see* Tic
  tobacco use
    chewing tobacco (mild) (moderate) (severe)
      in remission (early) (sustained) F17.221
    cigarettes (mild) (moderate) (severe)
      in remission (early) (sustained) F17.211
    mild Z72.0
      in remission (early) (sustained) F17.201
    moderate F17.200
      in remission (early) (sustained) F17.201
    severe F17.200
      in remission (early) (sustained) F17.201
    specified product NEC (mild) (moderate) (severe)
      in remission (early) (sustained) F17.291
  tooth K08.9
    development K00.9
      specified NEC K00.8
    eruption K00.6
  Tourette's F95.2
  trance and possession F44.89
  transvestic F65.1
  trauma and stressor-related F43.9
    other specified F43.8
  tricuspid (valve) — *see* Endocarditis, tricuspid
  tryptophan metabolism E70.5
  tubular, phosphate-losing N25.0
  tubulo-interstitial (in)
    brucellosis A23.9 [N16]
    cystinosis E72.04
    diphtheria A36.84
    glycogen storage disease E74.00 [N16]
    leukemia NEC C95.9- ☑ [N16]
    lymphoma NEC C85.9- ☑ [N16]
    mixed cryoglobulinemia D89.1 [N16]
    multiple myeloma C90.0- ☑ [N16]
    Salmonella infection A02.25
    sarcoidosis D86.84
    sepsis A41.9 [N16]
      streptococcal A40.9 [N16]
    systemic lupus erythematosus M32.15
    toxoplasmosis B58.83
    transplant rejection T86.91 [N16]
    Wilson's disease E83.01 [N16]
  tubulo-renal function, impaired N25.9
    specified NEC N25.89
  tympanic membrane H73.9- ☑
    atrophy — *see* Atrophy, tympanic membrane
    infection — *see* Myringitis
    perforation — *see* Perforation, tympanum
    specified NEC H73.89- ☑
  unsocialized aggressive F91.1
  urea cycle metabolism E72.20
    argininemia E72.21
    arginosuccinic aciduria E72.22
    citrullinemia E72.23
    ornithine transcarbamylase deficiency E72.4
    other specified E72.29
  ureter (in) N28.9
    schistosomiasis B65.0 [N29]
    tuberculosis A18.11
  urethra N36.9
    specified NEC N36.8
  urinary system N39.9
    specified NEC N39.8
  valve, heart
    aortic — *see* Endocarditis, aortic
    mitral — *see* Endocarditis, mitral
    pulmonary — *see* Endocarditis, pulmonary
    rheumatic
      aortic — *see* Endocarditis, aortic, rheumatic
      mitral — *see* Endocarditis, mitral

Disorder — *continued*
  valve, heart — *continued*
    rheumatic — *continued*
      pulmonary — *see* Endocarditis, pulmonary, rheumatic
      tricuspid — *see* Endocarditis, tricuspid
    tricuspid — *see* Endocarditis, tricuspid
  vestibular function H81.9- ☑
    specified NEC — *see* subcategory H81.8 ☑
    in diseases classified elsewhere H82.- ☑
  vertigo — *see* Vertigo
  vision, binocular H53.30
    abnormal retinal correspondence H53.31
    diplopia H53.2
    fusion with defective stereopsis H53.32
    simultaneous perception H53.33
    suppression H53.34
  visual
    cortex
      blindness H47.619
        left brain H47.612
        right brain H47.611
      due to
        inflammatory disorder H47.629
          left brain H47.622
          right brain H47.621
        neoplasm H47.639
          left brain H47.632
          right brain H47.631
        vascular disorder H47.649
          left brain H47.642
          right brain H47.641
    pathway H47.9
      due to
        inflammatory disorder H47.51- ☑
        neoplasm H47.52- ☑
        vascular disorder H47.53- ☑
      optic chiasm — *see* Disorder, optic, chiasm
  vitreous body H43.9
    crystalline deposits — *see* Deposit, crystalline
    degeneration — *see* Degeneration, vitreous
    hemorrhage — *see* Hemorrhage, vitreous
    opacities — *see* Opacity, vitreous
    prolapse — *see* Prolapse, vitreous
    specified type NEC H43.89
  voice R49.9
    specified type NEC R49.8
  volatile solvent use
    due to drug abuse — *see* Abuse, drug, inhalant
    due to drug dependence — *see* Dependence, drug, inhalant
  voyeuristic F65.3
  white blood cells D72.9
    specified NEC D72.89
  withdrawing, child or adolescent F40.10
Disorientation R41.0
Displacement, displaced
  acquired traumatic of bone, cartilage, joint, tendon NEC — *see* Dislocation
  adrenal gland (congenital) Q89.1
  appendix, retrocecal (congenital) Q43.8
  auricle (congenital) Q17.4
  bladder (acquired) N32.89
    congenital Q64.19
  brachial plexus (congenital) Q07.8
  brain stem, caudal (congenital) Q04.8
  canaliculus (lacrimalis), congenital Q10.6
  cardia through esophageal hiatus (congenital) Q40.1
  cerebellum, caudal (congenital) Q04.8
  cervix — *see* Malposition, uterus
  colon (congenital) Q43.3
  device, implant or graft (*see also* Complications, by site and type, mechanical) T85.628 ☑
    arterial graft NEC — *see* Complication, cardiovascular device, mechanical, vascular
    breast (implant) T85.42 ☑
    catheter NEC T85.628 ☑
      dialysis (renal) T82.42 ☑
        intraperitoneal T85.621 ☑
      infusion NEC T82.524 ☑
        spinal (epidural) (subdural) T85.620 ☑
      urinary
        cystostomy T83.020 ☑
        Hopkins T83.028 ☑
        ileostomy T83.028 ☑
        indwelling T83.021 ☑
        nephrostomy T83.022 ☑

☑ **Additional Character Required** — Refer to the Tabular List for Character Selection   ▽ **Subterms under main terms may continue to next column or page**

Displacement, displaced — *continued*
  device, implant or graft (*see also* Complications, by site and type, mechanical) — *continued*
    catheter — *continued*
      urinary — *continued*
        specified NEC T83.028 ☑
        urostomy T83.028 ☑
    electronic (electrode) (pulse generator) (stimulator) — *see* Complication, electronic stimulator
    fixation, internal (orthopedic) NEC — *see* Complication, fixation device, mechanical
    gastrointestinal — *see* Complications, prosthetic device, mechanical, gastrointestinal device
    genital NEC T83.428 ☑
      intrauterine contraceptive device (string) T83.32 ☑
      penile prosthesis (cylinder) (implanted) (pump) (reservoir) T83.420 ☑
      testicular prosthesis T83.421 ☑
    heart NEC — *see* Complication, cardiovascular device, mechanical
    joint prosthesis — *see* Complications, joint prosthesis, mechanical
    ocular — *see* Complications, prosthetic device, mechanical, ocular device
    orthopedic NEC — *see* Complication, orthopedic, device or graft, mechanical
    specified NEC T85.628 ☑
    urinary NEC T83.128 ☑
      graft T83.22 ☑
      sphincter, implanted T83.121 ☑
      stent (ileal conduit) (nephroureteral) T83.123 ☑
      ureteral indwelling T83.122 ☑
    vascular NEC — *see* Complication, cardiovascular device, mechanical
    ventricular intracranial shunt T85.02 ☑
  electronic stimulator
    bone T84.320 ☑
    cardiac — *see* Complications, cardiac device, electronic
    nervous system — *see* Complication, prosthetic device, mechanical, electronic nervous system stimulator
    urinary — *see* Complications, electronic stimulator, urinary
  esophageal mucosa into cardia of stomach, congenital Q39.8
  esophagus (acquired) K22.8
    congenital Q39.8
  eyeball (acquired) (lateral) (old) — *see* Displacement, globe
    congenital Q15.8
    current — *see* Avulsion, eye
  fallopian tube (acquired) N83.4- ☑
    congenital Q50.6
    opening (congenital) Q50.6
  gallbladder (congenital) Q44.1
  gastric mucosa (congenital) Q40.2
  globe (acquired) (old) (lateral) H05.21- ☑
    current — *see* Avulsion, eye
  heart (congenital) Q24.8
    acquired I51.89
  hymen (upward) (congenital) Q52.4
  intervertebral disc NEC
    with myelopathy — *see* Disorder, disc, with, myelopathy
    cervical, cervicothoracic (with) M50.20
      myelopathy — *see* Disorder, disc, cervical, with myelopathy
      neuritis, radiculitis or radiculopathy — *see* Disorder, disc, cervical, with neuritis
    due to trauma — *see* Dislocation, vertebra
    lumbar region M51.26
      with
        myelopathy M51.06
        neuritis, radiculitis, radiculopathy or sciatica M51.16
    lumbosacral region M51.27
      with
        neuritis, radiculitis, radiculopathy or sciatica M51.17
    sacrococcygeal region M53.3
    thoracic region M51.24
      with
        myelopathy M51.04
        neuritis, radiculitis, radiculopathy M51.14
    thoracolumbar region M51.25

Displacement, displaced — *continued*
  intervertebral disc — *continued*
    thoracolumbar region — *continued*
      with
        myelopathy M51.05
        neuritis, radiculitis, radiculopathy M51.15
  intrauterine device (string) T83.32 ☑
  kidney (acquired) N28.83
    congenital Q63.2
  lachrymal, lacrimal apparatus or duct (congenital) Q10.6
  lens, congenital Q12.1
  macula (congenital) Q14.1
  Meckel's diverticulum Q43.0
    malignant — *see* Table of Neoplasms, small intestine, malignant
  nail (congenital) Q84.6
    acquired L60.8
  opening of Wharton's duct in mouth Q38.4
  organ or site, congenital NEC — *see* Malposition, congenital
  ovary (acquired) N83.4- ☑
    congenital Q50.39
    free in peritoneal cavity (congenital) Q50.39
    into hernial sac N83.4- ☑
  oviduct (acquired) N83.4- ☑
    congenital Q50.6
  parathyroid (gland) E21.4
  parotid gland (congenital) Q38.4
  punctum lacrimale (congenital) Q10.6
  sacro-iliac (joint) (congenital) Q74.2
    current injury S33.2 ☑
    old — *see* subcategory M53.2 ☑
  salivary gland (any) (congenital) Q38.4
  spleen (congenital) Q89.09
  stomach, congenital Q40.2
  sublingual duct Q38.4
  tongue (downward) (congenital) Q38.3
  tooth, teeth, fully erupted M26.30
    horizontal M26.33
    vertical M26.34
  trachea (congenital) Q32.1
  ureter or ureteric opening or orifice (congenital) Q62.62
  uterine opening of oviducts or fallopian tubes Q50.6
  uterus, uterine — *see* Malposition, uterus
  ventricular septum Q21.0
    with rudimentary ventricle Q20.4

Disproportion
  between native and reconstructed breast N65.1
  fiber-type G71.2
Disruptio uteri — *see* Rupture, uterus
Disruption (of)
  ciliary body NEC H21.89
  closure of
    cornea T81.31 ☑
    craniotomy T81.32 ☑
    fascia (muscular) (superficial) T81.32 ☑
    internal organ or tissue T81.32 ☑
    laceration (external) (internal) T81.33 ☑
    ligament T81.32 ☑
    mucosa T81.31 ☑
    muscle or muscle flap T81.32 ☑
    ribs or rib cage T81.32 ☑
    skin and subcutaneous tissue (full-thickness) (superficial) T81.31 ☑
    skull T81.32 ☑
    sternum (sternotomy) T81.32 ☑
    tendon T81.32 ☑
    traumatic laceration (external) (internal) T81.33 ☑
  family Z63.8
    due to
      absence of family member due to military deployment Z63.31
      absence of family member NEC Z63.32
      alcoholism and drug addiction in family Z63.72
      bereavement Z63.4
      death (assumed) or disappearance of family member Z63.4
      divorce or separation Z63.5
      drug addiction in family Z63.72
      return of family member from military deployment (current or past conflict) Z63.71
      stressful life events NEC Z63.79
  iris NEC H21.89
  ligament(s) (*see also* Sprain)
    knee
      current injury — *see* Dislocation, knee
      old (chronic) — *see* Derangement, knee, instability

Disruption — *continued*
  ligament(s) (*see also* Sprain) — *continued*
    knee — *continued*
      spontaneous NEC — *see* Derangement, knee, disruption ligament
    ossicular chain — *see* Discontinuity, ossicles, ear
  pelvic ring (stable) S32.810 ☑
    unstable S32.811 ☑
  traumatic injury wound repair T81.33 ☑
  wound T81.30 ☑
    episiotomy O90.1
    operation T81.31 ☑
      cesarean O90.0
      external operation wound (superficial) T81.31 ☑
      internal operation wound (deep) T81.32 ☑
    perineal (obstetric) O90.1
    traumatic injury repair T81.33 ☑
Dissatisfaction with
  employment Z56.9
  school environment Z55.4
Dissecting — *see* condition
Dissection
  aorta I71.00
    abdominal I71.02
    thoracic I71.01
    thoracoabdominal I71.03
  artery I77.70
    basilar (trunk) I77.75
    carotid I77.71
    cerebral (nonruptured) I67.0
      ruptured — *see* Hemorrhage, intracranial, subarachnoid
    coronary I25.42
    extremity
      lower I77.77
      upper I77.76
    iliac I77.72
    precerebral
      congenital (nonruptured) Q28.1
      specified site NEC I77.75
    renal I77.73
    specified NEC I77.79
    vertebral I77.74
  precerebral artery, congenital (nonruptured) Q28.1
    Heartland A93.8
  traumatic — *see* Wound, open, by site
  vascular I99.8
  wound — *see* Wound, open
Disseminated — *see* condition
Dissociation
  auriculoventricular or atrioventricular (AV) (any degree) (isorhythmic) I45.89
    with heart block I44.2
  interference I45.89
Dissociative reaction, state F44.9
Dissolution, vertebra — *see* Osteoporosis
Distension, distention
  abdomen R14.0
  bladder N32.89
  cecum K63.89
  colon K63.89
  gallbladder K82.8
  intestine K63.89
  kidney N28.89
  liver K76.89
  seminal vesicle N50.89
  stomach K31.89
    acute K31.0
    psychogenic F45.8
  ureter — *see* Dilatation, ureter
  uterus N85.8
Distoma hepaticum infestation B66.3
Distomiasis B66.9
  bile passages B66.3
  hemic B65.9
  hepatic B66.3
    due to Clonorchis sinensis B66.1
  intestinal B66.5
  liver B66.3
    due to Clonorchis sinensis B66.1
  lung B66.4
  pulmonary B66.4
Distomolar (fourth molar) K00.1
Disto-occlusion (Division I) (Division II) M26.212
Distortion(s) (congenital)
  adrenal (gland) Q89.1
  arm NEC Q68.8
  bile duct or passage Q44.5

Distortion(s) — *continued*
bladder Q64.79
brain Q04.9
cervix (uteri) Q51.9
chest (wall) Q67.8
bones Q76.8
clavicle Q74.0
clitoris Q52.6
coccyx Q76.49
common duct Q44.5
coronary Q24.5
cystic duct Q44.5
ear (auricle) (external) Q17.3
inner Q16.5
middle Q16.4
ossicles Q16.3
endocrine NEC Q89.2
eustachian tube Q17.8
eye (adnexa) Q15.8
face bone(s) NEC Q75.8
fallopian tube Q50.6
femur NEC Q68.8
fibula NEC Q68.8
finger(s) Q68.1
foot Q66.9
genitalia, genital organ(s)
female Q52.8
external Q52.79
internal NEC Q52.8
gyri Q04.8
hand bone(s) Q68.1
heart (auricle) (ventricle) Q24.8
valve (cusp) Q24.8
hepatic duct Q44.5
humerus NEC Q68.8
hymen Q52.4
intrafamilial communications Z63.8
jaw NEC M26.89
labium (majus) (minus) Q52.79
leg NEC Q68.8
lens Q12.8
liver Q44.7
lumbar spine Q76.49
with disproportion O33.8
causing obstructed labor O65.0
lumbosacral (joint) (region) Q76.49
kyphosis — *see* Kyphosis, congenital
lordosis — *see* Lordosis, congenital
nerve Q07.8
nose Q30.8
organ
of Corti Q16.5
or site not listed — *see* Anomaly, by site
ossicles, ear Q16.3
oviduct Q50.6
pancreas Q45.3
parathyroid (gland) Q89.2
pituitary (gland) Q89.2
radius NEC Q68.8
sacroiliac joint Q74.2
sacrum Q76.49
scapula Q74.0
shoulder girdle Q74.0
skull bone(s) NEC Q75.8
with
anencephalus Q00.0
encephalocele — *see* Encephalocele
hydrocephalus Q03.9
with spina bifida — *see* Spina bifida, with hydrocephalus
microcephaly Q02
spinal cord Q06.8
spine Q76.49
kyphosis — *see* Kyphosis, congenital
lordosis — *see* Lordosis, congenital
spleen Q89.09
sternum NEC Q76.7
thorax (wall) Q67.8
bony Q76.8
thymus (gland) Q89.2
thyroid (gland) Q89.2
tibia NEC Q68.8
toe(s) Q66.9
tongue Q38.3
trachea (cartilage) Q32.1
ulna NEC Q68.8
ureter Q62.8
urethra Q64.79

Distortion(s) — *continued*
urethra — *continued*
causing obstruction Q64.39
uterus Q51.9
vagina Q52.4
vertebra Q76.49
kyphosis — *see* Kyphosis, congenital
lordosis — *see* Lordosis, congenital
visual (*see also* Disturbance, vision)
shape and size H53.15
vulva Q52.79
wrist (bones) (joint) Q68.8
Distress
abdomen — *see* Pain, abdominal
acute respiratory R06.03
syndrome (adult) (child) J80
epigastric R10.13
fetal P84
complicating pregnancy — *see* Stress, fetal
gastrointestinal (functional) K30
psychogenic F45.8
intestinal (functional) NOS K59.9
psychogenic F45.8
maternal, during labor and delivery O75.0
relationship, with spouse or intimate partner Z63.0
respiratory (adult) (child) R06.03
newborn P22.9
specified NEC P22.8
orthopnea R06.01
psychogenic F45.8
shortness of breath R06.02
specified type NEC R06.09
Distribution vessel, atypical Q27.9
coronary artery Q24.5
precerebral Q28.1
Districhiasis L68.8
Disturbance(s) (*see also* Disease)
absorption K90.9
calcium E58
carbohydrate K90.49
fat K90.49
pancreatic K90.3
protein K90.49
starch K90.49
vitamin — *see* Deficiency, vitamin
acid-base equilibrium E87.8
mixed E87.4
activity and attention (with hyperkinesis) — *see* Disorder, attention-deficit hyperactivity
amino acid transport E72.00
assimilation, food K90.9
auditory nerve, except deafness — *see* subcategory H93.3 ☑
behavior — *see* Disorder, conduct
blood clotting (mechanism) (*see also* Defect, coagulation) D68.9
cerebral
nerve — *see* Disorder, nerve, cranial
status, newborn P91.9
specified NEC P91.88
circulatory I99.9
conduct (*see also* Disorder, conduct) F91.9
adjustment reaction — *see* Disorder, adjustment
compulsive F63.9
disruptive F91.9
hyperkinetic — *see* Disorder, attention-deficit hyperactivity
socialized F91.2
specified NEC F91.8
unsocialized F91.1
coordination R27.8
cranial nerve — *see* Disorder, nerve, cranial
deep sensibility — *see* Disturbance, sensation
digestive K30
psychogenic F45.8
electrolyte (*see also* Imbalance, electrolyte)
newborn, transitory P74.49
hyperammonemia P74.6
hyperchloremia P74.421
hyperchloremic metabolic acidosis P74.421
hypochloremia P74.422
potassium balance
hyperkalemia P74.31
hypokalemia P74.32
sodium balance
hypernatremia P74.21
hyponatremia P74.22
specified type NEC P74.49

Disturbance(s) — *continued*
emotions specific to childhood and adolescence F93.9
with
anxiety and fearfulness NEC F93.8
elective mutism F94.0
oppositional disorder F91.3
sensitivity (withdrawal) F40.10
shyness F40.10
social withdrawal F40.10
involving relationship problems F93.8
mixed F93.8
specified NEC F93.8
endocrine (gland) E34.9
neonatal, transitory P72.9
specified NEC P72.8
equilibrium R42
fructose metabolism E74.10
gait — *see* Gait
hysterical F44.4
psychogenic F44.4
gastrointestinal (functional) K30
psychogenic F45.8
habit, child F98.9
hearing, except deafness and tinnitus — *see* Abnormal, auditory perception
heart, functional (conditions in I44-I50)
due to presence of (cardiac) prosthesis I97.19- ☑
postoperative I97.89
cardiac surgery (*see also* Infarct, myocardium, associated with revascularization procedure) I97.19- ☑
hormones E34.9
innervation uterus (parasympathetic) (sympathetic) N85.8
keratinization NEC
gingiva K05.10
nonplaque induced K05.11
plaque induced K05.10
lip K13.0
oral (mucosa) (soft tissue) K13.29
tongue K13.29
learning (specific) — *see* Disorder, learning
memory — *see* Amnesia
mild, following organic brain damage F06.8
mental F99
associated with diseases classified elsewhere F54
metabolism E88.9
with
abortion — *see* Abortion, by type with other specified complication
ectopic pregnancy O08.5
molar pregnancy O08.5
amino-acid E72.9
aromatic E70.9
branched-chain E71.2
straight-chain E72.89
sulfur-bearing E72.10
ammonia E72.20
arginine E72.21
argininosuccinic acid E72.22
carbohydrate E74.9
cholesterol E78.9
citrulline E72.23
cystathionine E72.19
general E88.9
glutamine E72.89
histidine E70.40
homocystine E72.19
hydroxylysine E72.3
in labor or delivery O75.89
iron E83.10
lipoid E78.9
lysine E72.3
methionine E72.19
neonatal, transitory P74.9
calcium and magnesium P71.9
specified type NEC P71.8
carbohydrate metabolism P70.9
specified type NEC P70.8
specified NEC P74.8
ornithine E72.4
phosphate E83.39
sodium NEC E87.8
threonine E72.89
tryptophan E70.5
tyrosine E70.20
urea cycle E72.20
motor R29.2

☑ **Additional Character Required — Refer to the Tabular List for Character Selection**   ▽ **Subterms under main terms may continue to next column or page**

Disturbance(s) — *continued*
　nervous, functional R45.0
　neuromuscular mechanism (eye), due to syphilis A52.15
　nutritional E63.9
　　nail L60.3
　ocular motion H51.9
　　psychogenic F45.8
　oculogyric H51.8
　　psychogenic F45.8
　oculomotor H51.9
　　psychogenic F45.8
　olfactory nerve R43.1
　optic nerve NEC — *see* Disorder, nerve, optic
　oral epithelium, including tongue NEC K13.29
　perceptual due to
　　alcohol withdrawal F10.232
　　amphetamine intoxication F15.922
　　　in
　　　　abuse F15.122
　　　　dependence F15.222
　　anxiolytic withdrawal F13.232
　　cannabis intoxication (acute) F12.922
　　　in
　　　　abuse F12.122
　　　　dependence F12.222
　　cocaine intoxication (acute) F14.922
　　　in
　　　　abuse F14.122
　　　　dependence F14.222
　　hypnotic withdrawal F13.232
　　opioid intoxication (acute) F11.922
　　　in
　　　　abuse F11.122
　　　　dependence F11.222
　　phencyclidine intoxication (acute) F16.122
　　sedative withdrawal F13.232
　personality (pattern) (trait) (*see also* Disorder, personality) F60.9
　　following organic brain damage F07.9
　polyglandular E31.9
　　specified NEC E31.8
　potassium balance, newborn
　　hyperkalemia P74.31
　　hypokalemia P74.32
　psychogenic F45.9
　psychomotor F44.4
　psychophysical visual H53.16
　pupillary — *see* Anomaly, pupil, function
　reflex R29.2
　rhythm, heart I49.9
　salivary secretion K11.7
　sensation (cold) (heat) (localization) (tactile discrimination) (texture) (vibratory) NEC R20.9
　　hysterical F44.6
　　skin R20.9
　　　anesthesia R20.0
　　　hyperesthesia R20.3
　　　hypoesthesia R20.1
　　　paresthesia R20.2
　　　specified type NEC R20.8
　　smell R43.9
　　　and taste (mixed) R43.8
　　　anosmia R43.0
　　　parosmia R43.1
　　　specified NEC R43.8
　　taste R43.9
　　　and smell (mixed) R43.8
　　　parageusia R43.2
　　　specified NEC R43.8
　sensory — *see* Disturbance, sensation
　situational (transient) (*see also* Disorder, adjustment)
　　acute F43.0
　sleep G47.9
　　nonorganic origin F51.9
　smell — *see* Disturbance, sensation, smell
　sociopathic F60.2
　sodium balance, newborn
　　hypernatremia P74.21
　　hyponatremia P74.22
　speech R47.9
　　developmental F80.9
　　specified NEC R47.89
　stomach (functional) K31.9
　sympathetic (nerve) G90.9
　taste — *see* Disturbance, sensation, taste
　temperature
　　regulation, newborn P81.9
　　　specified NEC P81.8
　　sense R20.8

Disturbance(s) — *continued*
　temperature — *continued*
　　sense — *continued*
　　　hysterical F44.6
　tooth
　　eruption K00.6
　　formation K00.4
　　structure, hereditary NEC K00.5
　touch — *see* Disturbance, sensation
　vascular I99.9
　　arteriosclerotic — *see* Arteriosclerosis
　vasomotor I73.9
　vasospastic I73.9
　vision, visual H53.9
　　following
　　　cerebral infarction I69.398
　　　cerebrovascular disease I69.998
　　　　specified NEC I69.898
　　　intracerebral hemorrhage I69.198
　　　nontraumatic intracranial hemorrhage NEC I69.298
　　　specified disease NEC I69.898
　　　subarachnoid hemorrhage I69.098
　　psychophysical H53.16
　　specified NEC H53.8
　　subjective H53.10
　　　day blindness H53.11
　　　discomfort H53.14- ☑
　　　distortions of shape and size H53.15
　　　loss
　　　　sudden H53.13- ☑
　　　　transient H53.12- ☑
　　　specified type NEC H53.19
　voice R49.9
　　psychogenic F44.4
　　specified NEC R49.8
Diuresis R35.8
Diver's palsy, paralysis or squeeze T70.3 ☑
Diverticulitis (acute) K57.92
　bladder — *see* Cystitis
　ileum — *see* Diverticulitis, intestine, small
　intestine K57.92
　　with
　　　abscess, perforation or peritonitis K57.80
　　　　with bleeding K57.81
　　　bleeding K57.93
　　congenital Q43.8
　　large K57.32
　　　with
　　　　abscess, perforation or peritonitis K57.20
　　　　　with bleeding K57.21
　　　　bleeding K57.33
　　　　small intestine K57.52
　　　　　with
　　　　　　abscess, perforation or peritonitis K57.40
　　　　　　　with bleeding K57.41
　　　　　　bleeding K57.53
　　small K57.12
　　　with
　　　　abscess, perforation or peritonitis K57.00
　　　　　with bleeding K57.01
　　　　bleeding K57.13
　　　　large intestine K57.52
　　　　　with
　　　　　　abscess, perforation or peritonitis K57.40
　　　　　　　with bleeding K57.41
　　　　　　bleeding K57.53
Diverticulosis K57.90
　with bleeding K57.91
　large intestine K57.30
　　with
　　　bleeding K57.31
　　　small intestine K57.50
　　　　with bleeding K57.51
　small intestine K57.10
　　with
　　　bleeding K57.11
　　　large intestine K57.50
　　　　with bleeding K57.51
Diverticulum, diverticula (multiple) K57.90
　appendix (noninflammatory) K38.2
　bladder (sphincter) N32.3
　　congenital Q64.6
　bronchus (congenital) Q32.4
　　acquired J98.09
　calyx, calyceal (kidney) N28.89

Diverticulum, diverticula — *continued*
　cardia (stomach) K31.4
　cecum — *see* Diverticulosis, intestine, large
　　congenital Q43.8
　colon — *see* Diverticulosis, intestine, large
　　congenital Q43.8
　duodenum — *see* Diverticulosis, intestine, small
　　congenital Q43.8
　epiphrenic (esophagus) K22.5
　esophagus (congenital) Q39.6
　　acquired (epiphrenic) (pulsion) (traction) K22.5
　eustachian tube — *see* Disorder, eustachian tube, specified NEC
　fallopian tube N83.8
　gastric K31.4
　heart (congenital) Q24.8
　ileum — *see* Diverticulosis, intestine, small
　jejunum — *see* Diverticulosis, intestine, small
　kidney (pelvis) (calyces) N28.89
　　with calculus — *see* Calculus, kidney
　Meckel's (displaced) (hypertrophic) Q43.0
　　malignant — *see* Table of Neoplasms, small intestine, malignant
　midthoracic K22.5
　organ or site, congenital NEC — *see* Distortion
　pericardium (congenital) (cyst) Q24.8
　　acquired I31.8
　pharyngoesophageal (congenital) Q39.6
　　acquired K22.5
　pharynx (congenital) Q38.7
　rectosigmoid — *see* Diverticulosis, intestine, large
　　congenital Q43.8
　rectum — *see* Diverticulosis, intestine, large
　Rokitansky's K22.5
　seminal vesicle N50.89
　sigmoid — *see* Diverticulosis, intestine, large
　　congenital Q43.8
　stomach (acquired) K31.4
　　congenital Q40.2
　trachea (acquired) J39.8
　ureter (acquired) N28.89
　　congenital Q62.8
　ureterovesical orifice N28.89
　urethra (acquired) N36.1
　　congenital Q64.79
　ventricle, left (congenital) Q24.8
　vesical N32.3
　　congenital Q64.6
　Zenker's (esophagus) K22.5
Division
　cervix uteri (acquired) N88.8
　glans penis Q55.69
　labia minora (congenital) Q52.79
　ligament (partial or complete) (current) (*see also* Sprain)
　　with open wound — *see* Wound, open
　muscle (partial or complete) (current) (*see also* Injury, muscle)
　　with open wound — *see* Wound, open
　nerve (traumatic) — *see* Injury, nerve
　spinal cord — *see* Injury, spinal cord, by region
　vein I87.8
Divorce, causing family disruption Z63.5
Dix-Hallpike neurolabyrinthitis — *see* Neuronitis, vestibular
Dizziness R42
　hysterical F44.89
　psychogenic F45.8
DMAC (disseminated mycobacterium avium- intracellulare complex) A31.2
DNR (do not resuscitate) Z66
Doan-Wiseman syndrome (primary splenic neutropenia) — *see* Agranulocytosis
Doehle-Heller aortitis A52.02
Dog bite — *see* Bite
Dohle body panmyelopathic syndrome D72.0
Dolichocephaly Q67.2
Dolichocolon Q43.8
Dolichostenomelia — *see* Syndrome, Marfan's
Donohue's syndrome E34.8
Donor (organ or tissue) Z52.9
　blood (whole) Z52.000
　　autologous Z52.010
　　specified component (lymphocytes) (platelets) NEC Z52.008
　　　autologous Z52.018
　　　specified donor NEC Z52.098
　　specified donor NEC Z52.090
　stem cells Z52.001

Donor — *continued*
  blood — *continued*
    stem cells — *continued*
      autologous Z52.011
      specified donor NEC Z52.091
  bone Z52.20
    autologous Z52.21
    marrow Z52.3
    specified type NEC Z52.29
  cornea Z52.5
  egg (Oocyte) Z52.819
    age 35 and over Z52.812
      anonymous recipient Z52.812
      designated recipient Z52.813
    under age 35 Z52.810
      anonymous recipient Z52.810
      designated recipient Z52.811
  kidney Z52.4
  liver Z52.6
  lung Z52.89
  lymphocyte — *see* Donor, blood, specified components NEC
  Oocyte — *see* Donor, egg
  platelets Z52.008
  potential, examination of Z00.5
  semen Z52.89
  skin Z52.10
    autologous Z52.11
    specified type NEC Z52.19
  specified organ or tissue NEC Z52.89
  sperm Z52.89
Donovanosis A58
Dorsalgia M54.9
  psychogenic F45.41
  specified NEC M54.89
Dorsopathy M53.9
  deforming M43.9
    specified NEC — *see* subcategory M43.8 ☑
  specified NEC M53.80
    cervical region M53.82
    cervicothoracic region M53.83
    lumbar region M53.86
    lumbosacral region M53.87
    occipito-atlanto-axial region M53.81
    sacrococcygeal region M53.88
    thoracic region M53.84
    thoracolumbar region M53.85
Double
  albumin E88.09
  aortic arch Q25.45
  auditory canal Q17.8
  auricle (heart) Q20.8
  bladder Q64.79
  cervix Q51.820
    with doubling of uterus (and vagina) Q51.10
      with obstruction Q51.11
  inlet ventricle Q20.4
  kidney with double pelvis (renal) Q63.0
  meatus urinarius Q64.75
  monster Q89.4
  outlet
    left ventricle Q20.2
    right ventricle Q20.1
  pelvis (renal) with double ureter Q62.5
  tongue Q38.3
  ureter (one or both sides) Q62.5
    with double pelvis (renal) Q62.5
  urethra Q64.74
  urinary meatus Q64.75
  uterus Q51.20
    with
      doubling of cervix (and vagina) Q51.10
        with obstruction Q51.11
    complete Q51.21
    in pregnancy or childbirth O34.59- ☑
      causing obstructed labor O65.5
    partial Q51.22
    specified NEC Q51.28
  vagina Q52.10
    with doubling of uterus (and cervix) Q51.10
      with obstruction Q51.11
  vision H53.2
  vulva Q52.79
Douglas' pouch, cul-de-sac — *see* condition
Down syndrome Q90.9
  meiotic nondisjunction Q90.0
  mitotic nondisjunction Q90.1
  mosaicism Q90.1

Down syndrome — *continued*
  translocation Q90.2
DPD (dihydropyrimidine dehydrogenase deficiency) E88.89
Dracontiasis B72
Dracunculiasis, dracunculosis B72
Dream state, hysterical F44.89
Drepanocytic anemia — *see* Disease, sickle-cell
Dresbach's syndrome (elliptocytosis) D58.1
Dreschlera (hawaiiensis) (infection) B43.8
Dressler's syndrome I24.1
Drift, ulnar — *see* Deformity, limb, specified type NEC, forearm
Drinking (alcohol)
  excessive, to excess NEC (without dependence) F10.10
    habitual (continual) (without remission) F10.20
      with remission F10.21
Drip, postnasal (chronic) R09.82
  due to
    allergic rhinitis — *see* Rhinitis, allergic
    common cold J00
    gastroesophageal reflux — *see* Reflux, gastroesophageal
    nasopharyngitis — *see* Nasopharyngitis
    other known condition — *code to* condition
    sinusitis — *see* Sinusitis
Droop
  facial R29.810
    cerebrovascular disease I69.992
      cerebral infarction I69.392
      intracerebral hemorrhage I69.192
      nontraumatic intracranial hemorrhage NEC I69.292
      specified disease NEC I69.892
      subarachnoid hemorrhage I69.092
Drop (in)
  attack NEC R55
  finger — *see* Deformity, finger
  foot — *see* Deformity, limb, foot, drop
  hematocrit (precipitous) R71.0
  hemoglobin R71.0
  toe — *see* Deformity, toe, specified NEC
  wrist — *see* Deformity, limb, wrist drop
Dropped heart beats I45.9
Dropsy, dropsical (*see also* Hydrops)
  abdomen R18.8
  brain — *see* Hydrocephalus
  cardiac, heart — *see* Failure, heart, congestive
  gangrenous — *see* Gangrene
  heart — *see* Failure, heart, congestive
  kidney — *see* Nephrosis
  lung — *see* Edema, lung
  newborn due to isoimmunization P56.0
  pericardium — *see* Pericarditis
Drowned, drowning (near) T75.1 ☑
Drowsiness R40.0
Drug
  abuse counseling and surveillance Z71.51
  addiction — *see* Dependence
  dependence — *see* Dependence
  habit — *see* Dependence
  harmful use — *see* Abuse, drug
  induced fever R50.2
  overdose — *see* Table of Drugs and Chemicals, by drug, poisoning
  poisoning — *see* Table of Drugs and Chemicals, by drug, poisoning
  resistant organism infection (*see also* Resistant, organism, to, drug) Z16.30
  therapy
    long term (current) (prophylactic) — *see* Therapy, drug long-term (current) (prophylactic)
    short term — *omit code*
  wrong substance given or taken in error — *see* Table of Drugs and Chemicals, by drug, poisoning
Drunkenness (without dependence) F10.129
  acute in alcoholism F10.229
  chronic (without remission) F10.20
    with remission F10.21
  pathological (without dependence) F10.129
    with dependence F10.229
  sleep F51.9
Drusen
  macula (degenerative) (retina) — *see* Degeneration, macula, drusen
  optic disc H47.32- ☑
Dry, dryness (*see also* condition)

Dry, dryness — *continued*
  larynx J38.7
  mouth R68.2
    due to dehydration E86.0
  nose J34.89
  socket (teeth) M27.3
  throat J39.2
DSAP L56.5
Duane's syndrome H50.81- ☑
Dubin-Johnson disease or syndrome E80.6
Dubois' disease (thymus gland) A50.59 [E35]
Dubowitz' syndrome Q87.1
Duchenne-Aran muscular atrophy G12.21
Duchenne-Griesinger disease G71.01
Duchenne's
  disease or syndrome
    motor neuron disease G12.22
    muscular dystrophy G71.01
  locomotor ataxia (syphilitic) A52.11
  paralysis
    birth injury P14.0
    due to or associated with
      motor neuron disease G12.22
      muscular dystrophy G71.01
Ducrey's chancre A57
Duct, ductus — *see* condition
Duhring's disease (dermatitis herpetiformis) L13.0
Dullness, cardiac (decreased) (increased) R01.2
Dumb ague — *see* Malaria
Dumbness — *see* Aphasia
Dumdum fever B55.0
Dumping syndrome (postgastrectomy) K91.1
Duodenitis (nonspecific) (peptic) K29.80
  with bleeding K29.81
Duodenocholangitis — *see* Cholangitis
Duodenum, duodenal — *see* condition
Duplay's bursitis or periarthritis — *see* Tendinitis, calcific, shoulder
Duplication, duplex (*see also* Accessory)
  alimentary tract Q45.8
  anus Q43.4
  appendix (and cecum) Q43.4
  biliary duct (any) Q44.5
  bladder Q64.79
  cecum (and appendix) Q43.4
  cervix Q51.820
  chromosome NEC
    with complex rearrangements NEC Q92.5
    seen only at prometaphase Q92.8
  cystic duct Q44.5
  digestive organs Q45.8
  esophagus Q39.8
  frontonasal process Q75.8
  intestine (large) (small) Q43.4
  kidney Q63.0
  liver Q44.7
  pancreas Q45.3
  penis Q55.69
  respiratory organs NEC Q34.8
  salivary duct Q38.4
  spinal cord (incomplete) Q06.2
  stomach Q40.2
Dupré's disease (meningism) R29.1
Dupuytren's contraction or disease M72.0
Durand-Nicolas-Favre disease A55
Durotomy (inadvertent) (incidental) G97.41
Duroziez's disease (congenital mitral stenosis) Q23.2
Dutton's relapsing fever (West African) A68.1
Dwarfism E34.3
  achondroplastic Q77.4
  congenital E34.3
  constitutional E34.3
  hypochondroplastic Q77.4
  hypophyseal E23.0
  infantile E34.3
  Laron-type E34.3
  Lorain (-Levi) type E23.0
  metatropic Q77.8
  nephrotic-glycosuric (with hypophosphatemic rickets) E72.09
  nutritional E45
  pancreatic K86.89
  pituitary E23.0
  renal N25.0
  thanatophoric Q77.1
Dyke-Young anemia (secondary) (symptomatic) D59.1
Dysacusis — *see* Abnormal, auditory perception
Dysadrenocortism E27.9

▽ Subterms under main terms may continue to next column or page

Dysadrenocortism — *continued*
  hyperfunction E27.Ø
Dysarthria R47.1
  following
    cerebral infarction I69.322
    cerebrovascular disease I69.922
      specified disease NEC I69.822
    intracerebral hemorrhage I69.122
    nontraumatic intracranial hemorrhage NEC I69.222
    subarachnoid hemorrhage I69.Ø22
Dysautonomia (familial) G90.1
Dysbarism T7Ø.3 ☑
Dysbasia R26.2
  angiosclerotica intermittens I73.9
  hysterical F44.4
  lordotica (progressiva) G24.1
  nonorganic origin F44.4
  psychogenic F44.4
Dysbetalipoproteinemia (familial) E78.2
Dyscalculia R48.8
  developmental F81.2
Dyschezia K59.ØØ
Dyschondroplasia (with hemangiomata) Q78.4
Dyschromia (skin) L81.9
Dyscollagenosis M35.9
Dyscranio-pygo-phalangy Q87.Ø
Dyscrasia
  blood (with) D75.9
    antepartum hemorrhage — *see* Hemorrhage, an-
      tepartum, with coagulation defect
    intrapartum hemorrhage O67.Ø
    newborn P61.9
      specified type NEC P61.8
    puerperal, postpartum O72.3
  polyglandular, pluriglandular E31.9
Dysendocrinism E34.9
Dysentery, dysenteric (catarrhal) (diarrhea) (epidemic)
  (hemorrhagic) (infectious) (sporadic) (tropical) A09
  abscess, liver A06.4
  amebic (*see also* Amebiasis) A06.Ø
    with abscess — *see* Abscess, amebic
    acute A06.Ø
    chronic A06.1
  arthritis (*see also* category MØ1) A09
    bacillary (*see also* category MØ1) A03.9
  bacillary A03.9
    arthritis (*see also* category MØ1) A03.9
    Boyd A03.2
    Flexner A03.1
    Schmitz (-Stutzer) A03.Ø
    Shiga (-Kruse) A03.Ø
    Shigella A03.9
      boydii A03.2
      dysenteriae A03.Ø
      flexneri A03.1
      group A A03.Ø
      group B A03.1
      group C A03.2
      group D A03.3
      sonnei A03.3
      specified type NEC A03.8
    Sonne A03.3
    specified type NEC A03.8
  balantidial A07.Ø
  Balantidium coli A07.Ø
  Boyd's A03.2
  candidal B37.82
  Chilomastix A07.8
  Chinese A03.9
  coccidial A07.3
  Dientamoeba (fragilis) A07.8
  Embadomonas A07.8
  Entamoeba, entamebic — *see* Dysentery, amebic
  Flexner-Boyd A03.2
  Flexner's A03.1
  Giardia lamblia A07.1
  Hiss-Russell A03.1
  Lamblia A07.1
  leishmanial B55.Ø
  malarial — *see* Malaria
  metazoal B82.Ø
  monilial B37.82
  protozoal A07.9
  Salmonella A02.Ø
  schistosomal B65.1
  Schmitz (-Stutzer) A03.Ø
  Shiga (-Kruse) A03.Ø
  Shigella NOS — *see* Dysentery, bacillary

Dysentery, dysenteric — *continued*
  Sonne A03.3
  strongyloidiasis B78.Ø
  trichomonal A07.8
  viral (*see also* Enteritis, viral) A08.4
Dysequilibrium R42
Dysesthesia R20.8
  hysterical F44.6
Dysfibrinogenemia (congenital) D68.2
Dysfunction
  adrenal E27.9
    hyperfunction E27.Ø
  autonomic
    due to alcohol G31.2
    somatoform F45.8
  bladder N31.9
    neurogenic NOS — *see* Dysfunction, bladder, neu-
      romuscular
    neuromuscular NOS N31.9
      atonic (motor) (sensory) N31.2
      autonomous N31.2
      flaccid N31.2
      nonreflex N31.2
      reflex N31.1
      specified NEC N31.8
      uninhibited N31.Ø
  bleeding, uterus N93.8
  cerebral G93.89
  colon K59.9
    psychogenic F45.8
  colostomy K94.03
  cystic duct K82.8
  cystostomy (stoma) — *see* Complications, cystostomy
  ejaculatory N53.19
    anejaculatory orgasm N53.13
    painful N53.12
    premature F52.4
    retarded N53.11
  endocrine NOS E34.9
  endometrium N85.8
  enterostomy K94.13
  erectile — *see* Dysfunction, sexual, male, erectile
  gallbladder K82.8
  gastrostomy (stoma) K94.23
  gland, glandular NOS E34.9
    meibomian, of eyelid — *see* Dysfunction, meibomi-
      an gland
  heart I51.89
  hemoglobin D75.89
  hepatic K76.89
  hypophysis E23.7
  hypothalamic NEC E23.3
  ileostomy (stoma) K94.13
  jejunostomy (stoma) K94.13
  kidney — *see* Disease, renal
  labyrinthine — *see* subcategory H83.2 ☑
  left ventricular, following sudden emotional stress
    I51.81
  liver K76.89
  male — *see* Dysfunction, sexual, male
  meibomian gland, of eyelid H02.889
    left H02.886
      lower H02.885
      upper H02.884
      upper and lower eyelids H02.88B
    right H02.883
      lower H02.882
      upper H02.881
      upper and lower eyelids H02.88A
  orgasmic (female) F52.31
    male F52.32
  ovary E28.9
    specified NEC E28.8
  papillary muscle I51.89
  parathyroid E21.4
  physiological NEC R68.89
    psychogenic F59
  pineal gland E34.8
  pituitary (gland) E23.3
  platelets D69.1
  polyglandular E31.9
    specified NEC E31.8
  psychophysiologic F59
  psychosexual F52.9
    with
      dyspareunia F52.6
      premature ejaculation F52.4
      vaginismus F52.5

Dysfunction — *continued*
  pylorus K31.9
  rectum K59.9
    psychogenic F45.8
  reflex (sympathetic) — *see* Syndrome, pain, complex
    regional I
  segmental — *see* Dysfunction, somatic
  senile R54
  sexual (due to) R37
    alcohol F1Ø.981
    amphetamine F15.981
      in
        abuse F15.181
        dependence F15.281
    anxiolytic F13.981
      in
        abuse F13.181
        dependence F13.281
    cocaine F14.981
      in
        abuse F14.181
        dependence F14.281
    excessive sexual drive F52.8
    failure of genital response (male) F52.21
      female F52.22
    female N94.9
      aversion F52.1
      dyspareunia N94.1Ø
        psychogenic F52.6
      frigidity F52.22
      nymphomania F52.8
      orgasmic F52.31
      psychogenic F52.9
        aversion F52.1
        dyspareunia F52.6
        frigidity F52.22
        nymphomania F52.8
        orgasmic F52.31
        vaginismus F52.5
      vaginismus N94.2
        psychogenic F52.5
    hypnotic F13.981
      in
        abuse F13.181
        dependence F13.281
    inhibited orgasm (female) F52.31
      male F52.32
    lack
      of sexual enjoyment F52.1
      or loss of sexual desire F52.Ø
    male N53.9
      anejaculatory orgasm N53.13
      ejaculatory N53.19
        painful N53.12
        premature F52.4
        retarded N53.11
      erectile N52.9
        drug induced N52.2
        due to
          disease classified elsewhere N52.1
          drug N52.2
        postoperative (postprocedural) N52.39
          following
            cryotherapy N52.37
            interstitial seed therapy N52.36
            prostate ablative therapy N52.37
            prostatectomy N52.34
              radical N52.31
            radiation therapy N52.35
            radical cystectomy N52.32
            ultrasound ablative therapy N52.37
            urethral surgery N52.33
        psychogenic F52.21
        specified cause NEC N52.8
        vasculogenic
          arterial insufficiency N52.Ø1
            with corporo-venous occlusive N52.Ø3
          corporo-venous occlusive N52.Ø2
            with arterial insufficiency N52.Ø3
      impotence — *see* Dysfunction, sexual, male,
        erectile
      psychogenic F52.9
        aversion F52.1
        erectile F52.21
        orgasmic F52.32
        premature ejaculation F52.4
        satyriasis F52.8
        specified type NEC F52.8
      specified type NEC N53.8

▽ **Subterms under main terms may continue to next column or page**   ☑ **Additional Character Required — Refer to the Tabular List for Character Selection**   **123**

Dysadrenocortism — Dysfunction

Dysfunction — *continued*
    sexual — *continued*
        nonorganic F52.9
            specified NEC F52.8
        opioid F11.981
            in
                abuse F11.181
                dependence F11.281
        orgasmic dysfunction (female) F52.31
            male F52.32
        premature ejaculation F52.4
        psychoactive substances NEC F19.981
            in
                abuse F19.181
                dependence F19.281
        psychogenic F52.9
        sedative F13.981
            in
                abuse F13.181
                dependence F13.281
        sexual aversion F52.1
        vaginismus (nonorganic) (psychogenic) F52.5
    sinoatrial node I49.5
    somatic M99.09
        abdomen M99.09
        acromioclavicular M99.07
        cervical region M99.01
        cervicothoracic M99.01
        costochondral M99.08
        costovertebral M99.08
        head region M99.00
        hip M99.05
        lower extremity M99.06
        lumbar region M99.03
        lumbosacral M99.03
        occipitocervical M99.00
        pelvic region M99.05
        pubic M99.05
        rib cage M99.08
        sacral region M99.04
        sacrococcygeal M99.04
        sacroiliac M99.04
        specified NEC M99.09
        sternochondral M99.08
        sternoclavicular M99.07
        thoracic region M99.02
        thoracolumbar M99.02
        upper extremity M99.07
    somatoform autonomic F45.8
    stomach K31.89
        psychogenic F45.8
    suprarenal E27.9
        hyperfunction E27.0
    symbolic R48.9
        specified type NEC R48.8
    temporomandibular (joint) M26.69
        joint-pain syndrome M26.62- ☑
    testicular (endocrine) E29.9
        specified NEC E29.8
    thymus E32.9
    thyroid E07.9
    ureterostomy (stoma) — *see* Complications, stoma, urinary tract
    urethrostomy (stoma) — *see* Complications, stoma, urinary tract
    uterus, complicating delivery O62.9
        hypertonic O62.4
        hypotonic O62.2
            primary O62.0
            secondary O62.1
    ventricular I51.9
        with congestive heart failure (*see also* Failure, heart) I50.9
        left, reversible, following sudden emotional stress I51.81
Dysgenesis
    gonadal (due to chromosomal anomaly) Q96.9
        pure Q99.1
    renal Q60.5
        bilateral Q60.4
        unilateral Q60.3
    reticular D72.0
    tidal platelet D69.3
Dysgerminoma
    specified site — *see* Neoplasm, malignant, by site
    unspecified site
        female C56.9
        male C62.90

Dysgeusia R43.2
Dysgraphia R27.8
Dyshidrosis, dysidrosis L30.1
Dyskaryotic cervical smear R87.619
Dyskeratosis L85.8
    cervix — *see* Dysplasia, cervix
    congenital Q82.8
    uterus NEC N85.8
Dyskinesia G24.9
    biliary (cystic duct or gallbladder) K82.8
    drug induced
        orofacial G24.01
    esophagus K22.4
    hysterical F44.4
    intestinal K59.8
    nonorganic origin F44.4
    orofacial (idiopathic) G24.4
        drug induced G24.01
    psychogenic F44.4
    subacute, drug induced G24.01
    tardive G24.01
        neuroleptic induced G24.01
    trachea J39.8
    tracheobronchial J98.09
Dyslalia (developmental) F80.0
Dyslexia R48.0
    developmental F81.0
Dyslipidemia E78.5
    depressed HDL cholesterol E78.6
    elevated fasting triglycerides E78.1
Dysmaturity (*see also* Light for dates)
    pulmonary (newborn) (Wilson-Mikity) P27.0
Dysmenorrhea (essential) (exfoliative) N94.6
    congestive (syndrome) N94.6
    primary N94.4
    psychogenic F45.8
    secondary N94.5
Dysmetabolic syndrome X E88.81
Dysmetria R27.8
Dysmorphism (due to)
    alcohol Q86.0
    exogenous cause NEC Q86.8
    hydantoin Q86.1
    warfarin Q86.2
Dysmorphophobia (nondelusional) F45.22
    delusional F22
Dysnomia R47.01
Dysorexia R63.0
    psychogenic F50.89
Dysostosis
    cleidocranial, cleidocranialis Q74.0
    craniofacial Q75.1
    Fairbank's (idiopathic familial generalized osteophytosis) Q78.9
    mandibulofacial (incomplete) Q75.4
    multiplex E76.01
    oculomandibular Q75.5
Dyspareunia (female) N94.10
    deep N94.12
    male N53.12
    nonorganic F52.6
    psychogenic F52.6
    secondary N94.19
    specified NEC N94.19
    superficial (introital) N94.11
Dyspepsia R10.13
    atonic K30
    functional (allergic) (congenital) (gastrointestinal) (occupational) (reflex) K30
    intestinal K59.8
    nervous F45.8
    neurotic F45.8
    psychogenic F45.8
Dysphagia R13.10
    cervical R13.19
    following
        cerebral infarction I69.391
        cerebrovascular disease I69.991
            specified NEC I69.891
        intracerebral hemorrhage I69.191
        nontraumatic intracranial hemorrhage NEC I69.291
        specified disease NEC I69.891
        subarachnoid hemorrhage I69.091
    functional (hysterical) F45.8
    hysterical F45.8
    nervous (hysterical) F45.8
    neurogenic R13.19
    oral phase R13.11

Dysphagia — *continued*
    oropharyngeal phase R13.12
    pharyngeal phase R13.13
    pharyngoesophageal phase R13.14
    psychogenic F45.8
    sideropenic D50.1
    spastica K22.4
    specified NEC R13.19
Dysphagocytosis, congenital D71
Dysphasia R47.02
    developmental
        expressive type F80.1
        receptive type F80.2
    following
        cerebrovascular disease I69.921
            cerebral infarction I69.321
            intracerebral hemorrhage I69.121
            nontraumatic intracranial hemorrhage NEC I69.221
            specified disease NEC I69.821
            subarachnoid hemorrhage I69.021
Dysphonia R49.0
    functional F44.4
    hysterical F44.4
    psychogenic F44.4
    spastica J38.3
Dysphoria
    gender F64.9
        in
            adolescence and adulthood F64.0
            children F64.2
        specified NEC F64.8
    postpartal O90.6
Dyspituitarism E23.3
Dysplasia (*see also* Anomaly)
    acetabular, congenital Q65.89
    alveolar capillary, with vein misalignment J84.843
    anus (histologically confirmed) (mild) (moderate) K62.82
        severe D01.3
    arrhythmogenic right ventricular I42.8
    arterial, fibromuscular I77.3
    asphyxiating thoracic (congenital) Q77.2
    brain Q07.9
    bronchopulmonary, perinatal P27.1
    cervix (uteri) N87.9
        mild N87.0
        moderate N87.1
        severe D06.9
    chondroectodermal Q77.6
    colon D12.6
    craniometaphyseal Q78.8
    dentinal K00.5
    diaphyseal, progressive Q78.3
    dystrophic Q77.5
    ectodermal (anhidrotic) (congenital) (hereditary) Q82.4
        hydrotic Q82.8
    epithelial, uterine cervix — *see* Dysplasia, cervix
    eye (congenital) Q11.2
    fibrous
        bone NEC (monostotic) M85.00
            ankle M85.07- ☑
            foot M85.07- ☑
            forearm M85.03- ☑
            hand M85.04- ☑
            lower leg M85.06- ☑
            multiple site M85.09
            neck M85.08
            rib M85.08
            shoulder M85.01- ☑
            skull M85.08
            specified site NEC M85.08
            thigh M85.05- ☑
            toe M85.07- ☑
            upper arm M85.02- ☑
            vertebra M85.08
        diaphyseal, progressive Q78.3
        jaw M27.8
        polyostotic Q78.1
    florid osseous (*see also* Cyst, calcifying odontogenic)
    high grade, focal D12.6
    hip, congenital Q65.89
    joint, congenital Q74.8
    kidney Q61.4
        multicystic Q61.4
    leg Q74.2
    lung, congenital (not associated with short gestation) Q33.6

☑ **Additional Character Required** — Refer to the Tabular List for Character Selection   ▽ **Subterms under main terms may continue to next column or page**

ysplasia — *continued*
  mammary (gland) (benign) N60.9- ☑
    cyst (solitary) — *see* Cyst, breast
    cystic — *see* Mastopathy, cystic
    duct ectasia — *see* Ectasia, mammary duct
    fibroadenosis — *see* Fibroadenosis, breast
    fibrosclerosis — *see* Fibrosclerosis, breast
    specified type NEC N60.8- ☑
  metaphyseal Q78.5
  muscle Q79.8
  oculodentodigital Q87.0
  periapical (cemental) (cemento-osseous) — *see* Cyst,
      calcifying odontogenic
  periosteum — *see* Disorder, bone, specified type NEC
  polyostotic fibrous Q78.1
  prostate (*see also* Neoplasia, intraepithelial, prostate)
      N42.30
    severe D07.5
    specified NEC N42.39
  renal Q61.4
    multicystic Q61.4
  retinal, congenital Q14.1
  right ventricular, arrhythmogenic I42.8
  septo-optic Q04.4
  skin L98.8
  spinal cord Q06.1
  spondyloepiphyseal Q77.7
  thymic, with immunodeficiency D82.1
  vagina N89.3
    mild N89.0
    moderate N89.1
    severe NEC D07.2
  vulva N90.3
    mild N90.0
    moderate N90.1
    severe NEC D07.1
ysplasminogenemia E88.02
yspnea (nocturnal) (paroxysmal) R06.00
  asthmatic (bronchial) J45.909
    with
      bronchitis J45.909
        with
          exacerbation (acute) J45.901
          status asthmaticus J45.902
        chronic J44.9
      exacerbation (acute) J45.901
      status asthmaticus J45.902
  cardiac — *see* Failure, ventricular, left
  cardiac — *see* Failure, ventricular, left
  functional F45.8
  hyperventilation R06.4
  hysterical F45.8
  newborn P28.89
  orthopnea R06.01
  psychogenic F45.8
  shortness of breath R06.02
  specified type NEC R06.09
yspraxia R27.8
  developmental (syndrome) F82
ysproteinemia E88.09
ysreflexia, autonomic G90.4
ysrhythmia
  cardiac I49.9
    newborn
      bradycardia P29.12
      occurring before birth P03.819
        before onset of labor P03.810
        during labor P03.811
      tachycardia P29.11
    postoperative I97.89
  cerebral or cortical — *see* Epilepsy
yssomnia — *see* Disorder, sleep
yssynergia
  biliary K83.8
  bladder sphincter N36.44
  cerebellaris myoclonica (Hunt's ataxia) G11.1
ysthymia F34.1
ysthyroidism E07.9
ystocia O66.9
  affecting newborn P03.1
  cervical (hypotonic) O62.2
    affecting newborn P03.6
    primary O62.0
    secondary O62.1
  contraction ring O62.4
  fetal O66.9
    abnormality NEC O66.3
    conjoined twins O66.3

Dystocia — *continued*
  fetal — *continued*
    oversize O66.2
  maternal O66.9
  positional O64.9 ☑
  shoulder (girdle) O66.0
    causing obstructed labor O66.0
  uterine NEC O62.4
Dystonia G24.9
  cervical G24.3
  deformans progressiva G24.1
  drug induced NEC G24.09
    acute G24.02
    specified NEC G24.09
  familial G24.1
  idiopathic G24.1
    familial G24.1
    nonfamilial G24.2
    orofacial G24.4
  lenticularis G24.8
  musculorum deformans G24.1
  neuroleptic induced (acute) G24.02
  orofacial (idiopathic) G24.4
  oromandibular G24.4
    due to drug G24.01
  specified NEC G24.8
  torsion (familial) (idiopathic) G24.1
    acquired G24.8
    genetic G24.1
    symptomatic (nonfamilial) G24.2
Dystonic movements R25.8
Dystrophy, dystrophia
  adiposogenital E23.6
  autosomal recessive, childhood type, muscular dystro-
      phy resembling Duchenne or Becker G71.01
  Becker's type G71.01
  cervical sympathetic G90.2
  choroid (hereditary) H31.20
    central areolar H31.22
    choroideremia H31.21
    gyrate atrophy H31.23
    specified type NEC H31.29
  cornea (hereditary) H18.50
    endothelial H18.51
    epithelial H18.52
    granular H18.53
    lattice H18.54
    macular H18.55
    specified type NEC H18.59
  Duchenne's type G71.01
  due to malnutrition E45
  Erb's G71.02
  Fuchs' H18.51
  Gower's muscular G71.01
  hair L67.8
  infantile neuraxonal G31.89
  Landouzy-Déjérine G71.02
  Leyden-Möbius G71.09
  muscular G71.00
    autosomal recessive, childhood type, muscular
        dystrophy resembling Duchenne or Becker
        G71.01
    benign (Becker type) G71.01
      scapuloperoneal with early contractures [Emery-
          Dreifuss] G71.09
    congenital (hereditary) (progressive) (with specific
        morphological abnormalities of the muscle
        fiber) G71.09
      myotonic G71.11
    distal G71.09
    Duchenne type G71.01
    Emery-Dreifuss G71.09
    Erb type G71.02
    facioscapulohumeral G71.02
    Gower's G71.01
    hereditary (progressive) G71.09
    Landouzy-Déjérine type G71.02
    limb-girdle G71.09
    myotonic G71.11
    progressive (hereditary) G71.09
      Charcot-Marie (-Tooth) type G60.0
    pseudohypertrophic (infantile) G71.01
    scapulohumeral G71.02
    scapuloperoneal G71.09
    severe (Duchenne type) G71.01
    specified type NEC G71.09
  myocardium, myocardial — *see* Degeneration, myocar-
      dial
  nail L60.3

Dystrophy, dystrophia — *continued*
  nail — *continued*
    congenital Q84.6
  nutritional E45
  ocular G71.09
  oculocerebrorenal E72.03
  oculopharyngeal G71.09
  ovarian N83.8
  polyglandular E31.8
  reflex (neuromuscular) (sympathetic) — *see* Syndrome,
      pain, complex regional I
  retinal (hereditary) H35.50
    in
      lipid storage disorders E75.6 [H36]
      systemic lipidoses E75.6 [H36]
    involving
      pigment epithelium H35.54
      sensory area H35.53
    pigmentary H35.52
    vitreoretinal H35.51
  Salzmann's nodular — *see* Degeneration, cornea,
      nodular
  scapuloperoneal G71.09
  skin NEC L98.8
  sympathetic (reflex) — *see* Syndrome, pain, complex
      regional I
    cervical G90.2
  tapetoretinal H35.54
  thoracic, asphyxiating Q77.2
  unguium L60.3
    congenital Q84.6
  vitreoretinal H35.51
  vulva N90.4
  yellow (liver) — *see* Failure, hepatic
Dysuria R30.0
  psychogenic F45.8

E

Eales' disease H35.06- ☑
Ear (*see also* condition)
  piercing Z41.3
  tropical NEC B36.9 [H62.40]
    in
      aspergillosis B44.89
      candidiasis B37.84
      moniliasis B37.84
  wax (impacted) H61.20
    left H61.22
      with right H61.23
    right H61.21
      with left H61.23
Earache — *see* subcategory H92.0 ☑
Early satiety R68.81
Eaton-Lambert syndrome — *see* Syndrome, Lambert-
    Eaton
Eberth's disease (typhoid fever) A01.00
Ebola virus disease A98.4
Ebstein's anomaly or syndrome (heart) Q22.5
Eccentro-osteochondrodysplasia E76.29
Ecchondroma — *see* Neoplasm, bone, benign
Ecchondrosis D48.0
Ecchymosis R58
  conjunctiva — *see* Hemorrhage, conjunctiva
  eye (traumatic) — *see* Contusion, eyeball
  eyelid (traumatic) — *see* Contusion, eyelid
  newborn P54.5
  spontaneous R23.3
  traumatic — *see* Contusion
Echinococciasis — *see* Echinococcus
Echinococcosis — *see* Echinococcus
Echinococcus (infection) B67.90
  granulosus B67.4
    bone B67.2
    liver B67.0
    lung B67.1
    multiple sites B67.32
    specified site NEC B67.39
    thyroid B67.31
  liver NOS B67.8
    granulosus B67.0
    multilocularis B67.5
  lung NEC B67.99
    granulosus B67.1
    multilocularis B67.69
  multilocularis B67.7
    liver B67.5
    multiple sites B67.61

Echinococcus — *continued*
  multilocularis — *continued*
    specified site NEC B67.69
  specified site NEC B67.99
    granulosus B67.39
    multilocularis B67.69
  thyroid NEC B67.99
    granulosus B67.31
    multilocularis B67.69 [E35]
Echinorhynchiasis B83.8
Echinostomiasis B66.8
Echolalia R48.8
Echovirus, as cause of disease classified elsewhere B97.12
Eclampsia, eclamptic (coma) (convulsions) (delirium) (with hypertension) NEC O15.9
  complicating
    labor and delivery O15.1
    postpartum O15.2
    pregnancy O15.0- ☑
    puerperium O15.2
Economic circumstances affecting care Z59.9
Economo's disease A85.8
Ectasia, ectasis
  annuloaortic I35.8
  aorta I77.819
    with aneurysm — *see* Aneurysm, aorta
    abdominal I77.811
    thoracic I77.810
    thoracoabdominal I77.812
  breast — *see* Ectasia, mammary duct
  capillary I78.8
  cornea H18.71- ☑
  gastric antral vascular (GAVE) K31.819
    with hemorrhage K31.811
    without hemorrhage K31.819
  mammary duct N60.4- ☑
  salivary gland (duct) K11.8
  sclera — *see* Sclerectasia
Ecthyma L08.0
  contagiosum B08.02
  gangrenosum L08.0
  infectiosum B08.02
Ectocardia Q24.8
Ectodermal dysplasia (anhidrotic) Q82.4
Ectodermosis erosiva pluriorificialis L51.1
Ectopic, ectopia (congenital)
  abdominal viscera Q45.8
    due to defect in anterior abdominal wall Q79.59
  ACTH syndrome E24.3
  adrenal gland Q89.1
  anus Q43.5
  atrial beats I49.1
  beats I49.49
    atrial I49.1
    ventricular I49.3
  bladder Q64.10
  bone and cartilage in lung Q33.5
  brain Q04.8
  breast tissue Q83.8
  cardiac Q24.8
  cerebral Q04.8
  cordis Q24.8
  endometrium — *see* Endometriosis
  gastric mucosa Q40.2
  gestation — *see* Pregnancy, by site
  heart Q24.8
  hormone secretion NEC E34.2
  kidney (crossed) (pelvis) Q63.2
  lens, lentis Q12.1
  mole — *see* Pregnancy, by site
  organ or site NEC — *see* Malposition, congenital
  pancreas Q45.3
  pregnancy — *see* Pregnancy, ectopic
  pupil — *see* Abnormality, pupillary
  renal Q63.2
  sebaceous glands of mouth Q38.6
  spleen Q89.09
  testis Q53.00
    bilateral Q53.02
    unilateral Q53.01
  thyroid Q89.2
  tissue in lung Q33.5
  ureter Q62.63
  ventricular beats I49.3
  vesicae Q64.10
Ectromelia Q73.8

Ectromelia — *continued*
  lower limb — *see* Defect, reduction, limb, lower, specified type NEC
  upper limb — *see* Defect, reduction, limb, upper, specified type NEC
Ectropion H02.109
  cervix N86
    with cervicitis N72
  congenital Q10.1
  eyelid H02.109
    cicatricial H02.119
      left H02.116
        lower H02.115
        upper H02.114
      right H02.113
        lower H02.112
        upper H02.111
    congenital Q10.1
    left H02.106
      lower H02.105
      upper H02.104
    mechanical H02.129
      left H02.126
        lower H02.125
        upper H02.124
      right H02.123
        lower H02.122
        upper H02.121
    paralytic H02.159
      left H02.156
        lower H02.155
        upper H02.154
      right H02.153
        lower H02.152
        upper H02.151
    right H02.103
      lower H02.102
      upper H02.101
    senile H02.139
      left H02.136
        lower H02.135
        upper H02.134
      right H02.133
        lower H02.132
        upper H02.131
    spastic H02.149
      left H02.146
        lower H02.145
        upper H02.144
      right H02.143
        lower H02.142
        upper H02.141
  iris H21.89
  lip (acquired) K13.0
    congenital Q38.0
  urethra N36.8
  uvea H21.89
Eczema (acute) (chronic) (erythematous) (fissum) (rubrum) (squamous) (*see also* Dermatitis) L30.9
  contact — *see* Dermatitis, contact
  dyshydrotic L30.1
  external ear — *see* Otitis, externa, acute, eczematoid
  flexural L20.82
  herpeticum B00.0
  hypertrophicum L28.0
  hypostatic — *see* Varix, leg, with, inflammation
  impetiginous L01.1
  infantile (due to any substance) L20.83
    intertriginous L21.1
    seborrheic L21.1
  intertriginous NEC L30.4
    infantile L21.1
  intrinsic (allergic) L20.84
  lichenified NEC L28.0
  marginatum (hebrae) B35.6
  pustular L30.3
  stasis I87.2
    with varicose veins — *see* Varix, leg, with, inflammation
  vaccination, vaccinatum T88.1 ☑
  varicose — *see* Varix, leg, with, inflammation
Eczematid L30.2
Eddowes (-Spurway) **syndrome** Q78.0
Edema, edematous (infectious) (pitting) (toxic) R60.9
  with nephritis — *see* Nephrosis
  allergic T78.3 ☑
  amputation stump (surgical) (sequelae (late effect)) T87.89

Edema, edematous — *continued*
  angioneurotic (allergic) (any site) (with urticaria) T78.3 ☑
    hereditary D84.1
  angiospastic I73.9
  Berlin's (traumatic) S05.8X- ☑
  brain (cytotoxic) (vasogenic) G93.6
    due to birth injury P11.0
      newborn (anoxia or hypoxia) P52.4
        birth injury P11.0
    traumatic — *see* Injury, intracranial, cerebral edema
  cardiac — *see* Failure, heart, congestive
  cardiovascular — *see* Failure, heart, congestive
  cerebral — *see* Edema, brain
  cerebrospinal — *see* Edema, brain
  cervix (uteri) (acute) N88.8
    puerperal, postpartum O90.89
  chronic hereditary Q82.0
  circumscribed, acute T78.3 ☑
    hereditary D84.1
  conjunctiva H11.42- ☑
  cornea H18.2- ☑
    idiopathic H18.22- ☑
    secondary H18.23- ☑
      due to contact lens H18.21- ☑
  due to
    lymphatic obstruction I89.0
    salt retention E87.0
  epiglottis — *see* Edema, glottis
  essential, acute T78.3 ☑
    hereditary D84.1
  extremities, lower — *see* Edema, legs
  eyelid NEC H02.849
    left H02.846
      lower H02.845
      upper H02.844
    right H02.843
      lower H02.842
      upper H02.841
  familial, hereditary Q82.0
  famine — *see* Malnutrition, severe
  generalized R60.1
  glottis, glottic, glottidis (obstructive) (passive) J38.4
    allergic T78.3 ☑
      hereditary D84.1
  heart — *see* Failure, heart, congestive
  heat T67.7 ☑
  hereditary Q82.0
  inanition — *see* Malnutrition, severe
  intracranial G93.6
  iris H21.89
  joint — *see* Effusion, joint
  larynx — *see* Edema, glottis
  legs R60.0
    due to venous obstruction I87.1
    hereditary Q82.0
  localized R60.0
    due to venous obstruction I87.1
  lower limbs — *see* Edema, legs
  lung J81.1
    with heart condition or failure — *see* Failure, ventricular, left
    acute J81.0
    chemical (acute) J68.1
      chronic J68.1
    chronic J81.1
      due to
        chemicals, gases, fumes or vapors (inhalation) J68.1
        external agent J70.9
          specified NEC J70.8
        radiation J70.1
    due to
      chemicals, fumes or vapors (inhalation) J68.1
      external agent J70.9
        specified NEC J70.8
      high altitude T70.29 ☑
      near drowning T75.1 ☑
      radiation J70.0
    meaning failure, left ventricle I50.1
  lymphatic I89.0
    due to mastectomy I97.2
  macula H35.81
    cystoid, following cataract surgery — *see* Complications, postprocedural, following cataract surgery
    diabetic — *see* Diabetes, by type, with, retinopathy with macular edema

☑ **Additional Character Required** — Refer to the Tabular List for Character Selection   ▽ Subterms under main terms may continue to next column or page

Edema, edematous — *continued*
  malignant — *see* Gangrene, gas
  Milroy's Q82.0
  nasopharynx J39.2
  newborn P83.30
    hydrops fetalis — *see* Hydrops, fetalis
    specified NEC P83.39
  nutritional (*see also* Malnutrition, severe)
    with dyspigmentation, skin and hair E40
  optic disc or nerve — *see* Papilledema
  orbit H05.22- ☑
  pancreas K86.89
  papilla, optic — *see* Papilledema
  penis N48.89
  periodic T78.3 ☑
    hereditary D84.1
  pharynx J39.2
  pulmonary — *see* Edema, lung
  Quincke's T78.3 ☑
    hereditary D84.1
  renal — *see* Nephrosis
  retina H35.81
    diabetic — *see* Diabetes, by type, with, retinopathy,
      with macular edema
  salt E87.0
  scrotum N50.89
  seminal vesicle N50.89
  spermatic cord N50.89
  spinal (cord) (vascular) (nontraumatic) G95.19
  starvation — *see* Malnutrition, severe
  stasis — *see* Hypertension, venous, (chronic)
  subglottic — *see* Edema, glottis
  supraglottic — *see* Edema, glottis
  testis N44.8
  tunica vaginalis N50.89
  vas deferens N50.89
  vulva (acute) N90.89
Edentulism — *see* Absence, teeth, acquired
Edsall's disease T67.2 ☑
Educational handicap Z55.9
  specified NEC Z55.8
Edward's syndrome — *see* Trisomy, 18
Effect(s) (of) (from) — *see* Effect, adverse NEC
Effect, adverse
  abnormal gravitational (G) forces or states T75.81 ☑
  abuse — *see* Maltreatment
  air pressure T70.9 ☑
    specified NEC T70.8 ☑
  altitude (high) — *see* Effect, adverse, high altitude
  anesthesia (*see also* Anesthesia) T88.59 ☑
    in labor and delivery O74.9
    local, toxic
      in labor and delivery O74.4
      in pregnancy NEC O29.3- ☑
      postpartum, puerperal O89.3
    postpartum, puerperal O89.9
    specified NEC T88.59 ☑
      in labor and delivery O74.8
      postpartum, puerperal O89.8
    spinal and epidural T88.59 ☑
      headache T88.59 ☑
        in labor and delivery O74.5
        postpartum, puerperal O89.4
      specified NEC
        in labor and delivery O74.6
        postpartum, puerperal O89.5
  antitoxin — *see* Complications, vaccination
  atmospheric pressure T70.9 ☑
    due to explosion T70.8 ☑
    high T70.3 ☑
    low — *see* Effect, adverse, high altitude
    specified effect NEC T70.8 ☑
  biological, correct substance properly administered —
    see Effect, adverse, drug
  blood (derivatives) (serum) (transfusion) — *see* Complications, transfusion
  chemical substance — *see* Table of Drugs and Chemicals
  cold (temperature) (weather) T69.9 ☑
    chilblains T69.1 ☑
    frostbite — *see* Frostbite
    specified effect NEC T69.8 ☑
  drugs and medicaments T88.7 ☑
    specified drug — *see* Table of Drugs and Chemicals,
      by drug, adverse effect
    specified effect — *code to* condition
  electric current, electricity (shock) T75.4 ☑

Effect, adverse — *continued*
  electric current, electricity — *continued*
    burn — *see* Burn
  exertion (excessive) T73.3 ☑
  exposure — *see* Exposure
  external cause NEC T75.89 ☑
  foodstuffs T78.1 ☑
    allergic reaction — *see* Allergy, food
      causing anaphylaxis — *see* Shock, anaphylactic,
        due to food
    noxious — *see* Poisoning, food, noxious
  gases, fumes, or vapors T59.9- ☑
    specified agent — *see* Table of Drugs and Chemicals
  glue (airplane) sniffing
    due to drug abuse — *see* Abuse, drug, inhalant
    due to drug dependence — *see* Dependence, drug,
      inhalant
  heat — *see* Heat
  high altitude NEC T70.29 ☑
    anoxia T70.29 ☑
    on
      ears T70.0 ☑
      sinuses T70.1 ☑
    polycythemia D75.1
  high pressure fluids T70.4 ☑
  hot weather — *see* Heat
  hunger T73.0 ☑
  immersion, foot — *see* Immersion
  immunization — *see* Complications, vaccination
  immunological agents — *see* Complications, vaccination
  infrared (radiation) (rays) NOS T66 ☑
    dermatitis or eczema L59.8
  infusion — *see* Complications, infusion
  lack of care of infants — *see* Maltreatment, child
  lightning — *see* Lightning
  medical care T88.9 ☑
    specified NEC T88.8 ☑
  medicinal substance, correct, properly administered
    — *see* Effect, adverse, drug
  motion T75.3 ☑
  noise, on inner ear — *see* subcategory H83.3 ☑
  overheated places — *see* Heat
  psychosocial, of work environment Z56.5
  radiation (diagnostic) (infrared) (natural source) (therapeutic) (ultraviolet) (X-ray) NOS T66 ☑
    dermatitis or eczema — *see* Dermatitis, due to, radiation
    fibrosis of lung J70.1
    pneumonitis J70.0
    pulmonary manifestations
      acute J70.0
      chronic J70.1
    skin L59.9
  radioactive substance NOS
    dermatitis or eczema — *see* Radiodermatitis
  reduced temperature T69.9 ☑
    immersion foot or hand — *see* Immersion
    specified effect NEC T69.8 ☑
  serum NEC (*see also* Reaction, serum) T80.69 ☑
  specified NEC T78.8 ☑
    external cause NEC T75.89 ☑
  strangulation — *see* Asphyxia, traumatic
  submersion T75.1 ☑
  thirst T73.1 ☑
  toxic — *see* Toxicity
  transfusion — *see* Complications, transfusion
  ultraviolet (radiation) (rays) NOS T66 ☑
    burn — *see* Burn
    dermatitis or eczema — *see* Dermatitis, due to, ultraviolet rays
      acute L56.8
  vaccine (any) — *see* Complications, vaccination
  vibration — *see* Vibration, adverse effects
  water pressure NEC T70.9 ☑
    specified NEC T70.8 ☑
  weightlessness T75.82 ☑
  whole blood — *see* Complications, transfusion
  work environment Z56.5
Effects, late — *see* Sequelae
Effluvium
  anagen L65.1
  telogen L65.0
Effort syndrome (psychogenic) F45.8
Effusion
  amniotic fluid — *see* Pregnancy, complicated by, prematue rupture of membranes

Effusion — *continued*
  brain (serous) G93.6
  bronchial — *see* Bronchitis
  cerebral G93.6
  cerebrospinal (*see also* Meningitis)
    vessel G93.6
  chest — *see* Effusion, pleura
  chylous, chyliform (pleura) J94.0
  intracranial G93.6
  joint M25.40
    ankle M25.47- ☑
    elbow M25.42- ☑
    foot joint M25.47- ☑
    hand joint M25.44- ☑
    hip M25.45- ☑
    knee M25.46- ☑
    shoulder M25.41- ☑
    specified joint NEC M25.48
    wrist M25.43- ☑
  malignant pleural J91.0
  meninges — *see* Meningitis
  pericardium, pericardial (noninflammatory) I31.3
    acute — *see* Pericarditis, acute
  peritoneal (chronic) R18.8
  pleura, pleurisy, pleuritic, pleuropericardial J90
    chylous, chyliform J94.0
    due to systemic lupus erythematosis M32.13
    in conditions classified elsewhere J91.8
    influenzal — *see* Influenza, with, respiratory manifestations NEC
    malignant J91.0
    newborn P28.89
    tuberculous NEC A15.6
      primary (progressive) A15.7
  spinal — *see* Meningitis
  thorax, thoracic — *see* Effusion, pleura
Egg shell nails L60.3
  congenital Q84.6
Egyptian splenomegaly B65.1
Ehlers-Danlos syndrome Q79.6
Ehrlichiosis A77.40
  due to
    E. chafeensis A77.41
    E. sennetsu A79.81
    specified organism NEC A77.49
Eichstedt's disease B36.0
Eisenmenger's
  complex or syndrome I27.83
  defect Q21.8
Ejaculation
  delayed F52.32
  painful N53.12
  premature F52.4
  retarded N53.11
  retrograde N53.14
  semen, painful N53.12
    psychogenic F52.6
Ekbom's syndrome (restless legs) G25.81
Ekman's syndrome (brittle bones and blue sclera) Q78.0
Elastic skin Q82.8
  acquired L57.4
Elastofibroma — *see* Neoplasm, connective tissue, benign
Elastoma (juvenile) Q82.8
  Miescher's L87.2
Elastomyofibrosis I42.4
Elastosis
  actinic, solar L57.8
  atrophicans (senile) L57.4
  perforans serpiginosa L87.2
  senilis L57.4
Elbow — *see* condition
Electric current, electricity, effects (concussion) (fatal)
    (nonfatal) (shock) T75.4 ☑
  burn — *see* Burn
Electric feet syndrome E53.8
Electrocution T75.4 ☑
  from electroshock gun (taser) T75.4 ☑
Electrolyte imbalance E87.8
  with
    abortion — *see* Abortion by type, complicated by,
      electrolyte imbalance
    ectopic pregnancy O08.5
    molar pregnancy O08.5
Elephantiasis (nonfilarial) I89.0
  arabicum — *see* Infestation, filarial
  bancroftian B74.0

Elephantiasis — *continued*
congenital (any site) (hereditary) Q82.0
due to
Brugia (malayi) B74.1
timori B74.2
mastectomy I97.2
Wuchereria (bancrofti) B74.0
eyelid H02.859
left H02.856
lower H02.855
upper H02.854
right H02.853
lower H02.852
upper H02.851
filarial, filariensis — *see* Infestation, filarial
glandular I89.0
graecorum A30.9
lymphangiectatic I89.0
lymphatic vessel I89.0
due to mastectomy I97.2
scrotum (nonfilarial) I89.0
streptococcal I89.0
surgical I97.89
postmastectomy I97.2
telangiectodes I89.0
vulva (nonfilarial) N90.89

Elevated, elevation
antibody titer R76.0
basal metabolic rate R94.8
blood pressure (*see also* Hypertension)
reading (incidental) (isolated) (nonspecific), no diagnosis of hypertension R03.0
blood sugar R73.9
body temperature (of unknown origin) R50.9
cancer antigen 125 [CA 125] R97.1
carcinoembryonic antigen [CEA] R97.0
cholesterol E78.00
with high triglycerides E78.2
conjugate, eye H51.0
C-reactive protein (CRP) R79.82
diaphragm, congenital Q79.1
erythrocyte sedimentation rate R70.0
fasting glucose R73.01
fasting triglycerides E78.1
finding on laboratory examination — *see* Findings, abnormal, inconclusive, without diagnosis, by type of exam
GFR (glomerular filtration rate) — *see* Findings, abnormal, inconclusive, without diagnosis, by type of exam
glucose tolerance (oral) R73.02
immunoglobulin level R76.8
indoleacetic acid R82.5
lactic acid dehydrogenase (LDH) level R74.0
leukocytes D72.829
lipoprotein a (Lp(a)) level E78.41
liver function
study R94.5
test R79.89
alkaline phosphatase R74.8
aminotransferase R74.0
bilirubin R17
hepatic enzyme R74.8
lactate dehydrogenase R74.0
Lp(a) (lipoprotein(a)) E78.41
lymphocytes D72.820
prostate specific antigen [PSA] R97.20
Rh titer — *see* Complication(s), transfusion, incompatibility reaction, Rh (factor)
scapula, congenital Q74.0
sedimentation rate R70.0
SGOT R74.0
SGPT R74.0
transaminase level R74.0
triglycerides E78.1
with high cholesterol E78.2
tumor associated antigens [TAA] NEC R97.8
tumor specific antigens [TSA] NEC R97.8
urine level of
17-ketosteroids R82.5
catecholamine R82.5
indoleacetic acid R82.5
steroids R82.5
vanillylmandelic acid (VMA) R82.5
venous pressure I87.8
white blood cell count D72.829
specified NEC D72.828

Elliptocytosis (congenital) (hereditary) D58.1

Elliptocytosis — *continued*
Hb C (disease) D58.1
hemoglobin disease D58.1
sickle-cell (disease) D57.8- ☑
trait D57.3

Ellison-Zollinger syndrome E16.4

Ellis-van Creveld syndrome (chondroectodermal dysplasia) Q77.6

Elongated, elongation (congenital) (*see also* Distortion)
bone Q79.9
cervix (uteri) Q51.828
acquired N88.4
hypertrophic N88.4
colon Q43.8
common bile duct Q44.5
cystic duct Q44.5
frenulum, penis Q55.69
labia minora (acquired) N90.69
ligamentum patellae Q74.1
petiolus (epiglottidis) Q31.8
tooth, teeth K00.2
uvula Q38.6

Eltor cholera A00.1

Emaciation (due to malnutrition) E41

Embadomoniasis A07.8

Embedded tooth, teeth K01.0
root only K08.3

Embolic — *see* condition

Embolism (multiple) (paradoxical) I74.9
air (any site) (traumatic) T79.0 ☑
following
abortion — *see* Abortion by type complicated by embolism
ectopic pregnancy O08.2
infusion, therapeutic injection or transfusion T80.0 ☑
molar pregnancy O08.2
procedure NEC
artery T81.719 ☑
mesenteric T81.710 ☑
renal T81.711 ☑
specified NEC T81.718 ☑
vein T81.72 ☑
in pregnancy, childbirth or puerperium — *see* Embolism, obstetric
amniotic fluid (pulmonary) (*see also* Embolism, obstetric)
following
abortion — *see* Abortion by type complicated by embolism
ectopic pregnancy O08.2
molar pregnancy O08.2
aorta, aortic I74.10
abdominal I74.09
saddle I74.01
bifurcation I74.09
saddle I74.01
thoracic I74.11
artery I74.9
auditory, internal I65.8
basilar — *see* Occlusion, artery, basilar
carotid (common) (internal) — *see* Occlusion, artery, carotid
cerebellar (anterior inferior) (posterior inferior) (superior) I66.3
cerebral — *see* Occlusion, artery, cerebral
choroidal (anterior) I65.8
communicating posterior I65.8
coronary (*see also* Infarct, myocardium)
not resulting in infarction I24.0
extremity I74.4
lower I74.3
upper I74.2
hypophyseal I65.8
iliac I74.5
limb I74.4
lower I74.3
upper I74.2
mesenteric (with gangrene) (*see also* Ischemia, intestine, acute) K55.059
ophthalmic — *see* Occlusion, artery, retina
peripheral I74.4
pontine I65.8
precerebral — *see* Occlusion, artery, precerebral
pulmonary — *see* Embolism, pulmonary
renal N28.0
retinal — *see* Occlusion, artery, retina
septic I76

Embolism — *continued*
artery — *continued*
specified NEC I74.8
vertebral — *see* Occlusion, artery, vertebral
basilar (artery) I65.1
blood clot
following
abortion — *see* Abortion by type complicated by embolism
ectopic or molar pregnancy O08.2
in pregnancy, childbirth or puerperium — *see* Embolism, obstetric
brain (*see also* Occlusion, artery, cerebral)
following
abortion — *see* Abortion by type complicated by embolism
ectopic or molar pregnancy O08.2
puerperal, postpartum, childbirth — *see* Embolism, obstetric
capillary I78.8
cardiac (*see also* Infarct, myocardium)
not resulting in infarction I51.3
carotid (artery) (common) (internal) — *see* Occlusion, artery, carotid
cavernous sinus (venous) — *see* Embolism, intracranial venous sinus
cerebral — *see* Occlusion, artery, cerebral
cholesterol — *see* Atheroembolism
coronary (artery or vein) (systemic) — *see* Occlusion, coronary
due to device, implant or graft (*see also* Complications, by site and type, specified NEC)
arterial graft NEC T82.818 ☑
breast (implant) T85.818 ☑
catheter NEC T85.818 ☑
dialysis (renal) T82.818 ☑
intraperitoneal T85.818 ☑
infusion NEC T82.818 ☑
spinal (epidural) (subdural) T85.810 ☑
urinary (indwelling) T83.81 ☑
electronic (electrode) (pulse generator) (stimulator)
bone T84.81 ☑
cardiac T82.817 ☑
nervous system (brain) (peripheral nerve) (spinal) T85.810 ☑
urinary T83.81 ☑
fixation, internal (orthopedic) NEC T84.81 ☑
gastrointestinal (bile duct) (esophagus) T85.818 ☑
genital NEC T83.81 ☑
heart (graft) (valve) T82.817 ☑
joint prosthesis T84.81 ☑
ocular (corneal graft) (orbital implant) T85.818 ☑
orthopedic (bone graft) NEC T86.838
specified NEC T85.818 ☑
urinary (graft) NEC T83.81 ☑
vascular NEC T82.818 ☑
ventricular intracranial shunt T85.810 ☑
extremities
lower — *see* Embolism, vein, lower extremity
arterial I74.3
upper I74.2
eye H34.9
fat (cerebral) (pulmonary) (systemic) T79.1 ☑
complicating delivery — *see* Embolism, obstetric
following
abortion — *see* Abortion by type complicated by embolism
ectopic or molar pregnancy O08.2
following
abortion — *see* Abortion by type complicated by embolism
ectopic or molar pregnancy O08.2
infusion, therapeutic injection or transfusion air T80.0 ☑
heart (fatty) (*see also* Infarct, myocardium)
not resulting in infarction I51.3
hepatic (vein) I82.0
in pregnancy, childbirth or puerperium — *see* Embolism, obstetric
intestine (artery) (vein) (with gangrene) (*see also* Ischemia, intestine, acute) K55.039
intracranial (*see also* Occlusion, artery, cerebral)
venous sinus (any) G08
nonpyogenic I67.6
intraspinal venous sinuses or veins G08
nonpyogenic G95.19
kidney (artery) N28.0

☑ Additional Character Required — Refer to the Tabular List for Character Selection

Subterms under main terms may continue to next column or page

Embolism — continued
- lateral sinus (venous) — see Embolism, intracranial, venous sinus
- leg — see Embolism, vein, lower extremity
  - arterial I74.3
- longitudinal sinus (venous) — see Embolism, intracranial, venous sinus
- lung (massive) — see Embolism, pulmonary
- meninges I66.8
- mesenteric (artery) (vein) (with gangrene) (see also Ischemia, intestine, acute) K55.059
- obstetric (in) (pulmonary)
  - childbirth O88.22
    - air O88.02
    - amniotic fluid O88.12
    - blood clot O88.22
    - fat O88.82
    - pyemic O88.32
    - septic O88.32
    - specified type NEC O88.82
  - pregnancy O88.21- ☑
    - air O88.01- ☑
    - amniotic fluid O88.11- ☑
    - blood clot O88.21- ☑
    - fat O88.81- ☑
    - pyemic O88.31- ☑
    - septic O88.31- ☑
    - specified type NEC O88.81- ☑
  - puerperal O88.23
    - air O88.03
    - amniotic fluid O88.13
    - blood clot O88.23
    - fat O88.83
    - pyemic O88.33
    - septic O88.33
    - specified type NEC O88.83
- ophthalmic — see Occlusion, artery, retina
- penis N48.81
- peripheral artery NOS I74.4
- pituitary E23.6
- popliteal (artery) I74.3
- portal (vein) I81
- postoperative, postprocedural
  - artery T81.719 ☑
    - mesenteric T81.710 ☑
    - renal T81.711 ☑
    - specified NEC T81.718 ☑
  - vein T81.72 ☑
- precerebral artery — see Occlusion, artery, precerebral
- puerperal — see Embolism, obstetric
- pulmonary (acute) (artery) (vein) I26.99
  - with acute cor pulmonale I26.09
  - chronic I27.82
  - following
    - abortion — see Abortion by type complicated by embolism
    - ectopic or molar pregnancy O08.2
  - healed or old Z86.711
  - in pregnancy, childbirth or puerperium — see Embolism, obstetric
  - personal history of Z86.711
  - saddle I26.92
    - with acute cor pulmonale I26.02
  - septic I26.90
    - with acute cor pulmonale I26.01
- pyemic (multiple) I76
  - following
    - abortion — see Abortion by type complicated by embolism
    - ectopic or molar pregnancy O08.2
  - Hemophilus influenzae A41.3
  - pneumococcal A40.3
    - with pneumonia J13
  - puerperal, postpartum, childbirth (any organism) — see Embolism, obstetric
  - specified organism NEC A41.89
  - staphylococcal A41.2
  - streptococcal A40.9
- renal (artery) N28.0
  - vein I82.3
- retina, retinal — see Occlusion, artery, retina
- saddle
  - abdominal aorta I74.01
  - pulmonary artery I26.92
    - with acute cor pulmonale I26.02
- septic (arterial) I76
  - complicating abortion — see Abortion, by type, complicated by, embolism

Embolism — continued
- sinus — see Embolism, intracranial, venous sinus
- soap complicating abortion — see Abortion, by type, complicated by, embolism
- spinal cord G95.19
  - pyogenic origin G06.1
- spleen, splenic (artery) I74.8
- upper extremity I74.2
- vein (acute) I82.90
  - antecubital I82.61- ☑
    - chronic I82.71- ☑
  - axillary I82.A1- ☑ (following I82.7)
    - chronic I82.A2- ☑ (following I82.7)
  - basilic I82.61- ☑
    - chronic I82.71- ☑
  - brachial I82.62- ☑
    - chronic I82.72- ☑
  - brachiocephalic (innominate) I82.290
    - chronic I82.291
  - cephalic I82.61- ☑
    - chronic I82.71- ☑
  - chronic I82.91
  - deep (DVT) I82.40- ☑
    - calf I82.4Z- ☑
      - chronic I82.5Z- ☑
    - lower leg I82.4Z- ☑
      - chronic I82.5Z- ☑
    - thigh I82.4Y- ☑
      - chronic I82.5Y- ☑
    - upper leg I82.4Y ☑
      - chronic I82.5Y-
  - femoral I82.41- ☑
    - chronic I82.51- ☑
  - iliac (iliofemoral) I82.42- ☑
    - chronic I82.52- ☑
  - innominate I82.290
    - chronic I82.291
  - internal jugular I82.C1- ☑ (following I82.7)
    - chronic I82.C2- ☑ (following I82.7)
  - lower extremity
    - deep I82.40- ☑
      - chronic I82.50- ☑
      - specified NEC I82.49- ☑
        - chronic NEC I82.59- ☑
    - distal
      - deep I82.4Z- ☑
    - proximal
      - deep I82.4Y- ☑
        - chronic I82.5Y- ☑
    - superficial I82.81- ☑
  - popliteal I82.43- ☑
    - chronic I82.53- ☑
  - radial I82.62- ☑
    - chronic I82.72- ☑
  - renal I82.3
  - saphenous (greater) (lesser) I82.81- ☑
  - specified NEC I82.890
    - chronic NEC I82.891
  - subclavian I82.B1- ☑ (following I82.7)
    - chronic I82.B2- ☑ (following I82.7)
  - thoracic NEC I82.290
    - chronic I82.291
  - tibial I82.44- ☑
    - chronic I82.54- ☑
  - ulnar I82.62- ☑
    - chronic I82.72- ☑
  - upper extremity I82.60- ☑
    - chronic I82.70- ☑
    - deep I82.62- ☑
      - chronic I82.72- ☑
    - superficial I82.61- ☑
      - chronic I82.71- ☑
  - vena cava
    - inferior (acute) I82.220
      - chronic I82.221
    - superior (acute) I82.210
      - chronic I82.211
  - venous sinus G08
- vessels of brain — see Occlusion, artery, cerebral

Embolus — see Embolism

Embryoma (see also Neoplasm, uncertain behavior, by site)
- benign — see Neoplasm, benign, by site
- kidney C64.- ☑
- liver C22.0
- malignant (see also Neoplasm, malignant, by site)

Embryoma — continued
- malignant (see also Neoplasm, malignant, by site) — continued
  - kidney C64.- ☑
  - liver C22.0
  - testis C62.9- ☑
    - descended (scrotal) C62.1- ☑
    - undescended C62.0- ☑
  - testis C62.9- ☑
    - descended (scrotal) C62.1- ☑
    - undescended C62.0- ☑

Embryonic
- circulation Q28.9
- heart Q28.9
- vas deferens Q55.4

Embryopathia NOS Q89.9

Embryotoxon Q13.4

Emesis — see Vomiting

Emotional lability R45.86

Emotionality, pathological F60.3

Emotogenic disease — see Disorder, psychogenic

Emphysema (atrophic) (bullous) (chronic) (interlobular) (lung) (obstructive) (pulmonary) (senile) (vesicular) J43.9
- cellular tissue (traumatic) T79.7 ☑
  - surgical T81.82 ☑
- centrilobular J43.2
- compensatory J98.3
- congenital (interstitial) P25.0
- conjunctiva H11.89
- connective tissue (traumatic) T79.7 ☑
  - surgical T81.82 ☑
- due to chemicals, gases, fumes or vapors J68.4
- eyelid(s) — see Disorder, eyelid, specified type NEC
  - surgical T81.82 ☑
  - traumatic T79.7 ☑
- interstitial J98.2
  - congenital P25.0
  - perinatal period P25.0
- laminated tissue T79.7 ☑
  - surgical T81.82 ☑
- mediastinal J98.2
  - newborn P25.2
- orbit, orbital — see Disorder, orbit, specified type NEC
- panacinar J43.1
- panlobular J43.1
- specified NEC J43.8
- subcutaneous (traumatic) T79.7 ☑
  - nontraumatic J98.2
  - postprocedural T81.82 ☑
  - surgical T81.82 ☑
- surgical T81.82 ☑
- thymus (gland) (congenital) E32.8
- traumatic (subcutaneous) T79.7 ☑
- unilateral J43.0

Empty nest syndrome Z60.0

Empyema (acute) (chest) (double) (pleura) (supradiaphragmatic) (thorax) J86.9
- with fistula J86.0
- accessory sinus (chronic) — see Sinusitis
- antrum (chronic) — see Sinusitis, maxillary
- brain (any part) — see Abscess, brain
- ethmoidal (chronic) (sinus) — see Sinusitis, ethmoidal
- extradural — see Abscess, extradural
- frontal (chronic) (sinus) — see Sinusitis, frontal
- gallbladder K81.0
- mastoid (process) (acute) — see Mastoiditis, acute
- maxilla, maxillary M27.2
  - sinus (chronic) — see Sinusitis, maxillary
- nasal sinus (chronic) — see Sinusitis
- sinus (accessory) (chronic) (nasal) — see Sinusitis
- sphenoidal (sinus) (chronic) — see Sinusitis, sphenoidal
- subarachnoid — see Abscess, extradural
- subdural — see Abscess, subdural
- tuberculous A15.6
- ureter — see Ureteritis
- ventricular — see Abscess, brain

En coup de sabre lesion L94.1

Enamel pearls K00.2

Enameloma K00.2

Enanthema, viral B09

Encephalitis (chronic) (hemorrhagic) (idiopathic) (nonepidemic) (spurious) (subacute) G04.90
- acute (see also Encephalitis, viral) A86
  - disseminated G04.00
    - infectious G04.01
    - noninfectious G04.81

Encephalitis — continued
acute (see also Encephalitis, viral) — continued
  disseminated — continued
    postimmunization (postvaccination) G04.02
    postinfectious G04.01
  inclusion body A85.8
  necrotizing hemorrhagic G04.30
    postimmunization G04.32
    postinfectious G04.31
    specified NEC G04.39
arboviral, arbovirus NEC A85.2
arthropod-borne NEC (viral) A85.2
Australian A83.4
California (virus) A83.5
Central European (tick-borne) A84.1
Czechoslovakian A84.1
Dawson's (inclusion body) A81.1
diffuse sclerosing A81.1
disseminated, acute G04.00
due to
  cat scratch disease A28.1
  human immunodeficiency virus (HIV) disease
    B20 [G05.3]
  malaria — see Malaria
  rickettsiosis — see Rickettsiosis
  smallpox inoculation G04.02
  typhus — see Typhus
Eastern equine A83.2
endemic (viral) A86
epidemic NEC (viral) A86
equine (acute) (infectious) (viral) A83.9
  Eastern A83.2
  Venezuelan A92.2
  Western A83.1
Far Eastern (tick-borne) A84.0
following vaccination or other immunization procedure
  G04.02
herpes zoster B02.0
herpesviral B00.4
  due to herpesvirus 6 B10.01
  due to herpesvirus 7 B10.09
  specified NEC B10.09
Ilheus (virus) A83.8
in (due to)
  actinomycosis A42.82
  adenovirus A85.1
  African trypanosomiasis B56.9 [G05.3]
  Chagas' disease (chronic) B57.42
  cytomegalovirus B25.8
  enterovirus A85.0
  herpes (simplex) virus B00.4
    due to herpesvirus 6 B10.01
    due to herpesvirus 7 B10.09
    specified NEC B10.09
  infectious disease NEC B99 ☑ [G05.3]
  influenza — see Influenza, with, encephalopathy
  listeriosis A32.12
  measles B05.0
  mumps B26.2
  naegleriasis B60.2
  parasitic disease NEC B89 [G05.3]
  poliovirus A80.9 [G05.3]
  rubella B06.01
  syphilis
    congenital A50.42
    late A52.14
  systemic lupus erythematosus M32.19
  toxoplasmosis (acquired) B58.2
    congenital P37.1
  tuberculosis A17.82
  zoster B02.0
inclusion body A81.1
infectious (acute) (virus) NEC A86
Japanese (B type) A83.0
La Crosse A83.5
lead — see Poisoning, lead
lethargica (acute) (infectious) A85.8
louping ill A84.8
lupus erythematosus, systemic M32.19
lymphatica A87.2
Mengo A85.8
meningococcal A39.81
Murray Valley A83.4
otitic NEC H66.40 [G05.3]
parasitic NOS B71.9
periaxial G37.0
periaxialis (concentrica) (diffuse) G37.5
postchickenpox B01.11

Encephalitis — continued
postexanthematous NEC B09
postimmunization G04.02
postinfectious NEC G04.01
postmeasles B05.0
postvaccinal G04.02
postvaricella B01.11
postviral NEC A86
Powassan A84.8
Rasmussen G04.81
Rio Bravo A85.8
Russian
  autumnal A83.0
  spring-summer (taiga) A84.0
saturnine — see Poisoning, lead
specified NEC G04.81
St. Louis A83.3
subacute sclerosing A81.1
summer A83.0
suppurative G04.81
tick-borne A84.9
Torula, torular (cryptococcal) B45.1
toxic NEC G92
trichinosis B75 [G05.3]
type
  B A83.0
  C A83.3
van Bogaert's A81.1
Venezuelan equine A92.2
Vienna A85.8
viral, virus A86
  arthropod-borne NEC A85.2
    mosquito-borne A83.9
      Australian X disease A83.4
      California virus A83.5
      Eastern equine A83.2
      Japanese (B type) A83.0
      Murray Valley A83.4
      specified NEC A83.8
      St. Louis A83.3
      type B A83.0
      type C A83.3
      Western equine A83.1
    tick-borne A84.9
      biundulant A84.1
      central European A84.1
      Czechoslovakian A84.1
      diphasic meningoencephalitis A84.1
      Far Eastern A84.0
      Russian spring-summer (taiga) A84.0
      specified NEC A84.8
  specified type NEC A85.8
Western equine A83.1

Encephalocele Q01.9
frontal Q01.0
nasofrontal Q01.1
occipital Q01.2
specified NEC Q01.8

Encephalocystocele — see Encephalocele
Encephaloduroarteriomyosynangiosis (EDAMS) I67.5
Encephalomalacia (brain) (cerebellar) (cerebral) — see
  Softening, brain
Encephalomeningitis — see Meningoencephalitis
Encephalomeningocele — see Encephalocele
Encephalomeningomyelitis — see Meningoencephalitis
Encephalomyelitis (see also Encephalitis) G04.90
acute disseminated G04.00
  infectious G04.01
  noninfectious G04.81
  postimmunization G04.02
  postinfectious G04.01
acute necrotizing hemorrhagic G04.30
  postimmunization G04.32
  postinfectious G04.31
  specified NEC G04.39
benign myalgic G93.3
equine A83.9
  Eastern A83.2
  Venezuelan A92.2
  Western A83.1
in diseases classified elsewhere G05.3
myalgic, benign G93.3
postchickenpox B01.11
postinfectious NEC G04.01
postmeasles B05.0
postvaccinal G04.02
postvaricella B01.11
rubella B06.01

Encephalomyelitis — continued
specified NEC G04.81
Venezuelan equine A92.2
Encephalomyelocele — see Encephalocele
Encephalomyelomeningitis — see Meningoencephalitis
Encephalomyelopathy G96.9
Encephalomyeloradiculitis (acute) G61.0
Encephalomyeloradiculoneuritis (acute) (Guillain-
  Barré) G61.0
Encephalomyeloradiculopathy G96.9
Encephalopathia hyperbilirubinemica, newborn
  P57.9
due to isoimmunization (conditions in P55) P57.0
Encephalopathy (acute) G93.40
acute necrotizing hemorrhagic G04.30
  postimmunization G04.32
  postinfectious G04.31
  specified NEC G04.39
alcoholic G31.2
anoxic — see Damage, brain, anoxic
arteriosclerotic I67.2
centrolobar progressive (Schilder) G37.0
congenital Q07.9
degenerative, in specified disease NEC G32.89
demyelinating callosal G37.1
due to
  drugs (see also Table of Drugs and Chemicals) G92
hepatic — see Failure, hepatic
hyperbilirubinemic, newborn P57.9
  due to isoimmunization (conditions in P55) P57.0
hypertensive I67.4
hypoglycemic E16.2
hypoxic — see Damage, brain, anoxic
hypoxic ischemic P91.60
  mild P91.61
  moderate P91.62
  severe P91.63
in (due to) (with)
  birth injury P11.1
  hyperinsulinism E16.1 [G94]
  influenza — see Influenza, with, encephalopathy
  lack of vitamin (see also Deficiency, vitamin)
    E56.9 [G32.89]
  neoplastic disease (see also Neoplasm) D49.9 [G13.1]
  serum (see also Reaction, serum) T80.69 ☑
  syphilis A52.17
  trauma (postconcussional) F07.81
    current injury — see Injury, intracranial
  vaccination G04.02
lead — see Poisoning, lead
metabolic G93.41
  drug induced G92
  toxic G92
myoclonic, early, symptomatic — see Epilepsy, generalized, specified NEC
necrotizing, subacute (Leigh) G31.82
neonatal P91.819
  in diseases classified elsewhere P91.811
pellagrous E52 [G32.89]
portosystemic — see Failure, hepatic
postcontusional F07.81
  current injury — see Injury, intracranial, diffuse
posthypoglycemic (coma) E16.1 [G94]
postradiation G93.89
saturnine — see Poisoning, lead
septic G93.41
specified NEC G93.49
spongioform, subacute (viral) A81.09
toxic G92
  metabolic G92
traumatic (postconcussional) F07.81
  current injury — see Injury, intracranial
vitamin B deficiency NEC E53.9 [G32.89]
  vitamin B1 E51.2
Wernicke's E51.2
Encephalorrhagia — see Hemorrhage, intracranial, intracerebral
Encephalosis, posttraumatic F07.81
Enchondroma (see also Neoplasm, bone, benign)
Enchondromatosis (cartilaginous) (multiple) Q78.4
Encopresis R15.9
functional F98.1
nonorganic origin F98.1
psychogenic F98.1
Encounter (with health service) (for) Z76.89
adjustment and management (of)
  breast implant Z45.81 ☑
  implanted device NEC Z45.89

Encounter — *continued*
  adjustment and management — *continued*
    myringotomy device (stent) (tube) Z45.82
  administrative purpose only Z02.9
    examination for
      adoption Z02.82
      armed forces Z02.3
      disability determination Z02.71
      driving license Z02.4
      employment Z02.1
      insurance Z02.6
      medical certificate NEC Z02.79
      paternity testing Z02.81
      residential institution admission Z02.2
      school admission Z02.0
      sports Z02.5
      specified reason NEC Z02.89
  aftercare — *see* Aftercare
  antenatal screening Z36.9
    cervical length Z36.86
    chromosomal anomalies Z36.0
    congenital cardiac abnormalities Z36.83
    elevated maternal serum alphafetoprotein Z36.1
    fetal growth retardation Z36.4
    fetal lung maturity Z36.84
    fetal macrosomia Z36.88
    hydrops fetalis Z36.81
    intrauterine growth restriction (IUGR) /small-for-dates Z36.4
    isoimmunization Z36.5
    large-for-dates Z36.88
    malformations Z36.3
    non-visualized anatomy on a previous scan Z36.2
    nuchal translucency Z36.82
    raised alphafetoprotein level Z36.1
    risk of pre-term labor Z36.86
    specified follow-up NEC Z36.2
    specified genetic defects NEC Z36.8A
    specified type NEC Z36.89
    Streptococcus B Z36.85
    suspected anomaly Z36.3
    uncertain dates Z36.87
  assisted reproductive fertility procedure cycle Z31.83
  blood typing Z01.83
    Rh typing Z01.83
  breast augmentation or reduction Z41.1
  breast implant exchange (different material) (different size) Z45.81 ☑
  breast reconstruction following mastectomy Z42.1
  check-up — *see* Examination
  chemotherapy for neoplasm Z51.11
  colonoscopy, screening Z12.11
  counseling — *see* Counseling
  delivery, full-term, uncomplicated O80
    cesarean, without indication O82
  desensitization to allergens Z51.6
  ear piercing Z41.3
  examination — *see* Examination
  expectant parent(s) (adoptive) pre-birth pediatrician visit Z76.81
  fertility preservation procedure (prior to cancer therapy) (prior to removal of gonads) Z31.84
  fitting (of) — *see* Fitting (and adjustment) (of)
  genetic
    counseling
      nonprocreative Z71.83
      procreative Z31.5
    testing — *see* Test, genetic
  hearing conservation and treatment Z01.12
  immunotherapy for neoplasm Z51.12
  in vitro fertilization cycle Z31.83
  instruction (in)
    child care (postpartal) (prenatal) Z32.3
    childbirth Z32.2
    natural family planning
      procreative Z31.61
      to avoid pregnancy Z30.02
  insulin pump titration Z46.81
  joint prosthesis insertion following prior explantation of joint prosthesis (staged procedure)
    hip Z47.32
    knee Z47.33
    shoulder Z47.31
  laboratory (as part of a general medical examination) Z00.00
    with abnormal findings Z00.01
  mental health services (for)
    abuse NEC

Encounter — *continued*
  mental health services — *continued*
    abuse — *continued*
      perpetrator Z69.82
      victim Z69.81
    child abuse
      nonparental
        perpetrator Z69.021
        victim Z69.020
      parental
        perpetrator Z69.011
        victim Z69.010
    child neglect
      nonparental
        perpetrator Z69.021
        victim Z69.020
      parental
        perpetrator Z69.011
        victim Z69.010
    child psychological abuse
      nonparental
        perpetrator Z69.021
        victim Z69.020
      parental
        perpetrator Z69.011
        victim Z69.010
    child sexual abuse
      nonparental
        perpetrator Z69.021
        victim Z69.020
      parental
        perpetrator Z69.011
        victim Z69.010
    non-spousal adult abuse (perpetrator) (victim) Z69.81
    spousal or partner
      abuse
        perpetrator Z69.12
        victim Z69.11
      neglect
        perpetrator Z69.12
        victim Z69.11
      psychological abuse
        perpetrator Z69.12
        victim Z69.11
      violence
        perpetrator (physical) (sexual) Z69.12
        victim (physical) Z69.11
          sexual Z69.81
  observation (for) (ruled out)
    exposure to (suspected)
      anthrax Z03.810
      biological agent NEC Z03.818
  pediatrician visit, by expectant parent(s) (adoptive) Z76.81
  placental sample (taken vaginally) (*see also* Encounter, antenatal screening) Z36.9
  plastic and reconstructive surgery following medical procedure or healed injury NEC Z42.8
  pregnancy
    supervision of — *see* Pregnancy, supervision of
    test Z32.00
      result negative Z32.02
      result positive Z32.01
  procreative management and counseling for gestational carrier Z31.7
  prophylactic measures Z29.9
    antivenin Z29.12
    fluoride administration Z29.3
    immunotherapy for respiratory syncytial virus (RSV) Z29.11
    rabies immune globin Z29.14
    Rho (D) immune globulin Z29.13
    specified NEC Z29.8
  radiation therapy (antineoplastic) Z51.0
  radiological (as part of a general medical examination) Z00.00
    with abnormal findings Z00.01
  reconstructive surgery following medical procedure or healed injury NEC Z42.8
  removal (of) (*see also* Removal)
    artificial
      arm Z44.00- ☑
        complete Z44.01- ☑
        partial Z44.02- ☑
      eye Z44.2- ☑
      leg Z44.10- ☑
        complete Z44.11- ☑

Encounter — *continued*
  removal (*see also* Removal) — *continued*
    artificial — *continued*
      leg — *continued*
        partial Z44.12- ☑
    breast implant Z45.81 ☑
      tissue expander (without synchronous insertion of permanent implant) Z45.81 ☑
    device Z46.9
      specified NEC Z46.89
    external
      fixation device — *code to* fracture with seventh character D
      prosthesis, prosthetic device Z44.9
        breast Z44.3- ☑
        specified NEC Z44.8
    implanted device NEC Z45.89
    insulin pump Z46.81
    internal fixation device Z47.2
    myringotomy device (stent) (tube) Z45.82
    nervous system device NEC Z46.2
      brain neuropacemaker Z46.2
      visual substitution device Z46.2
        implanted Z45.31
    non-vascular catheter Z46.82
    orthodontic device Z46.4
    stent
      ureteral Z46.6
    urinary device Z46.6
  repeat cervical smear to confirm findings of recent normal smear following initial abnormal smear Z01.42
  respirator [ventilator] use during power failure Z99.12
  Rh typing Z01.83
  screening — *see* Screening
  specified NEC Z76.89
  sterilization Z30.2
  suspected condition, ruled out
    amniotic cavity and membrane Z03.71
    cervical shortening Z03.75
    fetal anomaly Z03.73
    fetal growth Z03.74
    maternal and fetal conditions NEC Z03.79
    oligohydramnios Z03.71
    placental problem Z03.72
    polyhydramnios Z03.71
  suspected exposure (to), ruled out
    anthrax Z03.810
    biological agents NEC Z03.818
  termination of pregnancy, elective Z33.2
  testing — *see* Test
  therapeutic drug level monitoring Z51.81
  titration, insulin pump Z46.81
  to determine fetal viability of pregnancy O36.80 ☑
  training
    insulin pump Z46.81
  X-ray of chest (as part of a general medical examination) Z00.00
    with abnormal findings Z00.01
Encystment — *see* Cyst
Endarteritis (bacterial) (subacute) (infective) I77.6
  brain I67.7
  cerebral or cerebrospinal I67.7
  deformans — *see* Arteriosclerosis
  embolic — *see* Embolism
  obliterans (*see also* Arteriosclerosis)
    pulmonary I28.8
  pulmonary I28.8
  retina — *see* Vasculitis, retina
  senile — *see* Arteriosclerosis
  syphilitic A52.09
    brain or cerebral A52.04
    congenital A50.54 [I79.8]
  tuberculous A18.89
Endemic — *see* condition
Endocarditis (chronic) (marantic) (nonbacterial) (thrombotic) (valvular) I38
  with rheumatic fever (conditions in I00)
    active — *see* Endocarditis, acute, rheumatic
    inactive or quiescent (with chorea) I09.1
  acute or subacute I33.9
    infective I33.0
    rheumatic (aortic) (mitral) (pulmonary) (tricuspid) I01.1
      with chorea (acute) (rheumatic) (Sydenham's) I02.0
  aortic (heart) (nonrheumatic) (valve) I35.8

Endocarditis — *continued*
  aortic — *continued*
    with
      mitral disease I08.0
        with tricuspid (valve) disease I08.3
          active or acute I01.1
            with chorea (acute) (rheumatic) (Sydenham's) I02.0
        rheumatic fever (conditions in I00)
          active — *see* Endocarditis, acute, rheumatic
          inactive or quiescent (with chorea) I06.9
      tricuspid (valve) disease I08.2
        with mitral (valve) disease I08.3
    acute or subacute I33.9
    arteriosclerotic I35.8
    rheumatic I06.9
      with mitral disease I08.0
        with tricuspid (valve) disease I08.3
          active or acute I01.1
            with chorea (acute) (rheumatic) (Sydenham's) I02.0
      active or acute I01.1
        with chorea (acute) (rheumatic) (Sydenham's) I02.0
      specified NEC I06.8
    specified cause NEC I35.8
    syphilitic A52.03
  arteriosclerotic I38
  atypical verrucous (Libman-Sacks) M32.11
  bacterial (any valve) (subacute) I33.0
  candidal B37.6
  congenital Q24.8
  constrictive I33.0
  Coxiella burnetii A78 [I39]
  Coxsackie B33.21
  due to
    prosthetic cardiac valve T82.6 ☑
    Q fever A78 [I39]
    Serratia marcescens I33.0
    typhoid (fever) A01.02
  gonococcal A54.83
  infectious or infective (acute) (any valve) (subacute) I33.0
  lenta (acute) (any valve) (subacute) I33.0
  Libman-Sacks M32.11
  listerial A32.82
  Löffler's I42.3
  malignant (acute) (any valve) (subacute) I33.0
  meningococcal A39.51
  mitral (chronic) (double) (fibroid) (heart) (inactive) (valve) (with chorea) I05.9
    with
      aortic (valve) disease I08.0
        with tricuspid (valve) disease I08.3
          active or acute I01.1
            with chorea (acute) (rheumatic) (Sydenham's) I02.0
        rheumatic fever (conditions in I00)
          active — *see* Endocarditis, acute, rheumatic
          inactive or quiescent (with chorea) I05.9
      tricuspid (valve) disease I08.1
        with aortic (valve) disease I08.3
    active or acute I01.1
      with chorea (acute) (rheumatic) (Sydenham's) I02.0
      bacterial I33.0
    arteriosclerotic I34.8
    nonrheumatic I34.8
      acute or subacute I33.9
    specified NEC I05.8
  monilial B37.6
  multiple valves I08.9
    specified disorders I08.8
  mycotic (acute) (any valve) (subacute) I33.0
  pneumococcal (acute) (any valve) (subacute) I33.0
  pulmonary (chronic) (heart) (valve) I37.8
    with rheumatic fever (conditions in I00)
      active — *see* Endocarditis, acute, rheumatic
      inactive or quiescent (with chorea) I09.89
        with aortic, mitral or tricuspid disease I08.8
    acute or subacute I33.9
      rheumatic I01.1
        with chorea (acute) (rheumatic) (Sydenham's) I02.0
    arteriosclerotic I37.8
    congenital Q22.2
    rheumatic (chronic) (inactive) (with chorea) I09.89
      active or acute I01.1

Endocarditis — *continued*
  pulmonary — *continued*
    rheumatic — *continued*
      active or acute — *continued*
        with chorea (acute) (rheumatic) (Sydenham's) I02.0
    syphilitic A52.03
  purulent (acute) (any valve) (subacute) I33.0
  Q fever A78 [I39]
  rheumatic (chronic) (inactive) (with chorea) I09.1
    active or acute (aortic) (mitral) (pulmonary) (tricuspid) I01.1
      with chorea (acute) (rheumatic) (Sydenham's) I02.0
  rheumatoid — *see* Rheumatoid, carditis
  septic (acute) (any valve) (subacute) I33.0
  streptococcal (acute) (any valve) (subacute) I33.0
  subacute — *see* Endocarditis, acute
  suppurative (acute) (any valve) (subacute) I33.0
  syphilitic A52.03
  toxic I33.9
  tricuspid (chronic) (heart) (inactive) (rheumatic) (valve) (with chorea) I07.9
    with
      aortic (valve) disease I08.2
        mitral (valve) disease I08.3
      mitral (valve) disease I08.1
        aortic (valve) disease I08.3
      rheumatic fever (conditions in I00)
        active — *see* Endocarditis, acute, rheumatic
        inactive or quiescent (with chorea) I07.8
    active or acute I01.1
      with chorea (acute) (rheumatic) (Sydenham's) I02.0
    arteriosclerotic I36.8
    nonrheumatic I36.8
      acute or subacute I33.9
    specified cause, except rheumatic I36.8
  tuberculous — *see* Tuberculosis, endocarditis
  typhoid A01.02
  ulcerative (acute) (any valve) (subacute) I33.0
  vegetative (acute) (any valve) (subacute) I33.0
  verrucous (atypical) (nonbacterial) (nonrheumatic) M32.11

Endocardium, endocardial (*see also* condition)
  cushion defect Q21.2
Endocervicitis (*see also* Cervicitis)
  due to intrauterine (contraceptive) device T83.69 ☑
  hyperplastic N72
Endocrine — *see* condition
Endocrinopathy, pluriglandular E31.9
Endodontic
  overfill M27.52
  underfill M27.53
Endodontitis K04.01
  irreversible K04.02
  reversible K04.01
Endomastoiditis — *see* Mastoiditis
Endometrioma N80.9
Endometriosis N80.9
  appendix N80.5
  bladder N80.8
  bowel N80.5
  broad ligament N80.3
  cervix N80.0
  colon N80.5
  cul-de-sac (Douglas') N80.3
  exocervix N80.0
  fallopian tube N80.2
  female genital organ NEC N80.8
  gallbladder N80.8
  in scar of skin N80.6
  internal N80.0
  intestine N80.5
  lung N80.8
  myometrium N80.0
  ovary N80.1
  parametrium N80.3
  pelvic peritoneum N80.3
  peritoneal (pelvic) N80.3
  rectovaginal septum N80.4
  rectum N80.5
  round ligament N80.3
  skin (scar) N80.6
  specified site NEC N80.8
  stromal D39.0
  thorax N80.8
  umbilicus N80.8

Endometriosis — *continued*
  uterus (internal) N80.0
  vagina N80.4
  vulva N80.8
Endometritis (decidual) (nonspecific) (purulent) (senile) (atrophic) (suppurative) N71.9
  with ectopic pregnancy O08.0
  acute N71.0
  blenorrhagic (gonococcal) (acute) (chronic) A54.24
  cervix, cervical (with erosion or ectropion) (*see also* Cervicitis)
    hyperplastic N72
  chlamydial A56.11
  chronic N71.1
  following
    abortion — *see* Abortion by type complicated by genital infection
    ectopic or molar pregnancy O08.0
  gonococcal, gonorrheal (acute) (chronic) A54.24
  hyperplastic (*see also* Hyperplasia, endometrial) N85.00
    cervix N72
  puerperal, postpartum, childbirth O86.12
  subacute N71.0
  tuberculous A18.17
Endometrium — *see* condition
Endomyocardiopathy, South African I42.3
Endomyocarditis — *see* Endocarditis
Endomyofibrosis I42.3
Endomyometritis — *see* Endometritis
Endopericarditis — *see* Endocarditis
Endoperineuritis — *see* Disorder, nerve
Endophlebitis — *see* Phlebitis
Endophthalmia — *see* Endophthalmitis, purulent
Endophthalmitis (acute) (infective) (metastatic) (subacute) H44.009
  bleb associated (*see also* Bleb, inflamed (infected), postprocedural H59.4 ☑
  gonorrheal A54.39
  in (due to)
    cysticercosis B69.1
    onchocerciasis B73.01
    toxocariasis B83.0
  panuveitis — *see* Panuveitis
  parasitic H44.12- ☑
  purulent H44.00- ☑
    panophthalmitis — *see* Panophthalmitis
    vitreous abscess H44.02- ☑
  specified NEC H44.19
  sympathetic — *see* Uveitis, sympathetic
Endosalpingioma D28.2
Endosalpingiosis N94.89
Endosteitis — *see* Osteomyelitis
Endothelioma, bone — *see* Neoplasm, bone, malignant
Endotheliosis (hemorrhagic infectional) D69.8
Endotoxemia — code to condition
Endotrachelitis — *see* Cervicitis
Engelmann (-Camurati) **syndrome** Q78.3
English disease — *see* Rickets
Engman's disease L30.3
Engorgement
  breast N64.59
    newborn P83.4
    puerperal, postpartum O92.79
  lung (passive) — *see* Edema, lung
  pulmonary (passive) — *see* Edema, lung
  stomach K31.89
  venous, retina — *see* Occlusion, retina, vein, engorgement
Enlargement, enlarged (*see also* Hypertrophy)
  adenoids J35.2
    with tonsils J35.3
  alveolar ridge K08.89
    congenital — *see* Anomaly, alveolar
  apertures of diaphragm (congenital) Q79.1
  gingival K06.1
  heart, cardiac — *see* Hypertrophy, cardiac
  labium majus, childhood asymmetric (CALME) N90.6
  lacrimal gland, chronic H04.03- ☑
  liver — *see* Hypertrophy, liver
  lymph gland or node R59.9
    generalized R59.1
    localized R59.0
  orbit H05.34- ☑
  organ or site, congenital NEC — *see* Anomaly, by site
  parathyroid (gland) E21.0
  pituitary fossa R93.0
  prostate N40.0

☑ **Additional Character Required** — Refer to the Tabular List for Character Selection ▽ **Subterms under main terms may continue to next column or page**

Enlargement, enlarged — *continued*
  prostate — *continued*
    with lower urinary tract symptoms (LUTS) N40.1
    without lower urinary tract symptoms (LUTS) N40.0
  sella turcica R93.0
  spleen — *see* Splenomegaly
  thymus (gland) (congenital) E32.0
  thyroid (gland) — *see* Goiter
  tongue K14.8
  tonsils J35.1
    with adenoids J35.3
  uterus N85.2
  vestibular aqueduct Q16.5
Enophthalmos H05.40- ☑
  due to
    orbital tissue atrophy H05.41- ☑
    trauma or surgery H05.42- ☑
Enostosis M27.8
Entamebic, entamebiasis — *see* Amebiasis
Entanglement
  umbilical cord(s) O69.82 ☑
    with compression O69.2 ☑
    around neck (with compression) O69.81 ☑
      with compression O69.1 ☑
      without compression O69.81 ☑
    of twins in monoamniotic sac O69.2 ☑
    without compression O69.82 ☑
Enteralgia — *see* Pain, abdominal
Enteric — *see* condition
Enteritis (acute) (diarrheal) (hemorrhagic) (noninfective) K52.9
  adenovirus A08.2
  aertrycke infection A02.0
  allergic K52.29
    with
      eosinophilic gastritis or gastroenteritis K52.81
      food protein-induced enterocolitis syndrome K52.21
      food protein-induced enteropathy K52.22
      FPIES K52.21
  amebic (acute) A06.0
    with abscess — *see* Abscess, amebic
    chronic A06.1
      with abscess — *see* Abscess, amebic
      nondysenteric A06.2
    nondysenteric A06.2
  astrovirus A08.32
  bacillary NOS A03.9
  bacterial A04.9
    specified NEC A04.8
  calicivirus A08.31
  candidal B37.82
  Chilomastix A07.8
  choleriformis A00.1
  chronic (noninfectious) K52.9
    ulcerative — *see* Colitis, ulcerative
  cicatrizing (chronic) — *see* Enteritis, regional, small intestine
  Clostridium
    botulinum (food poisoning) A05.1
    difficile
      not specified as recurrent A04.72
      recurrent A04.71
  coccidial A07.3
  coxsackie virus A08.39
  dietetic (*see also* Enteritis, allergic) K52.29
  drug-induced K52.1
  due to
    astrovirus A08.32
    calicivirus A08.31
    coxsackie virus A08.39
    drugs K52.1
    echovirus A08.39
    enterovirus NEC A08.39
    food hypersensitivity (*see also* Enteritis, allergic) K52.29
    infectious organism (bacterial) (viral) — *see* Enteritis, infectious
    torovirus A08.39
    Yersinia enterocolitica A04.6
  echovirus A08.39
  eltor A00.1
  enterovirus NEC A08.39
  eosinophilic K52.81
  epidemic (infectious) A09
  fulminant (*see also* Ischemia, intestine, acute) K55.019
  gangrenous — *see* Enteritis, infectious
  giardial A07.1

Enteritis — *continued*
  infectious NOS A09
    due to
      adenovirus A08.2
      Aerobacter aerogenes A04.8
      Arizona (bacillus) A02.0
      bacteria NOS A04.9
        specified NEC A04.8
      Campylobacter A04.5
      Clostridium difficile
        not specified as recurrent A04.72
        recurrent A04.71
      Clostridium perfringens A04.8
      Enterobacter aerogenes A04.8
      enterovirus A08.39
      Escherichia coli A04.4
        enteroaggregative A04.4
        enterohemorrhagic A04.3
        enteroinvasive A04.2
        enteropathogenic A04.0
        enterotoxigenic A04.1
        specified NEC A04.4
      specified
        bacteria NEC A04.8
        virus NEC A08.39
      Staphylococcus A04.8
      virus NEC A08.4
        specified type NEC A08.39
      Yersinia enterocolitica A04.6
    specified organism NEC A08.8
  influenzal — *see* Influenza, with, digestive manifestations
  ischemic K55.9
    acute (*see also* Ischemia, intestine, acute) K55.019
    chronic K55.1
  microsporidial A07.8
  mucomembranous, myxomembranous — *see* Syndrome, irritable bowel
  mucous — *see* Syndrome, irritable bowel
  necroticans A05.2
  necrotizing of newborn — *see* Enterocolitis, necrotizing, in newborn
  neurogenic — *see* Syndrome, irritable bowel
  newborn necrotizing — *see* Enterocolitis, necrotizing, in newborn
  noninfectious K52.9
  norovirus A08.11
  parasitic NEC B82.9
  paratyphoid (fever) — *see* Fever, paratyphoid
  protozoal A07.9
    specified NEC A07.8
  radiation K52.0
  regional (of) K50.90
    with
      complication K50.919
        abscess K50.914
        fistula K50.913
        intestinal obstruction K50.912
        rectal bleeding K50.911
        specified complication NEC K50.918
    colon — *see* Enteritis, regional, large intestine
    duodenum — *see* Enteritis, regional, small intestine
    ileum — *see* Enteritis, regional, small intestine
    jejunum — *see* Enteritis, regional, small intestine
    large bowel — *see* Enteritis, regional, large intestine
    large intestine (colon) (rectum) K50.10
      with
        complication K50.119
          abscess K50.114
          fistula K50.113
          intestinal obstruction K50.112
          rectal bleeding K50.111
          small intestine (duodenum) (ileum) (jejunum) involvement K50.80
          with
            complication K50.819
              abscess K50.814
              fistula K50.813
              intestinal obstruction K50.812
              rectal bleeding K50.811
              specified complication NEC K50.818
        specified complication NEC K50.118
    rectum — *see* Enteritis, regional, large intestine
    small intestine (duodenum) (ileum) (jejunum) K50.00
      with
        complication K50.019
          abscess K50.014

Enteritis — *continued*
  regional — *continued*
    small intestine — *continued*
      with — *continued*
        complication — *continued*
          fistula K50.013
          intestinal obstruction K50.012
          large intestine (colon) (rectum) involvement K50.80
          with
            complication K50.819
              abscess K50.814
              fistula K50.813
              intestinal obstruction K50.812
              rectal bleeding K50.811
              specified complication NEC K50.818
        rectal bleeding K50.011
        specified complication NEC K50.018
  rotaviral A08.0
  Salmonella, salmonellosis (arizonae) (cholerae-suis) (enteritidis) (typhimurium) A02.0
  segmental — *see* Enteritis, regional
  septic A09
  Shigella — *see* Infection, Shigella
  small round structured NEC A08.19
  spasmodic, spastic — *see* Syndrome, irritable bowel
  staphylococcal A04.8
    due to food A05.0
  torovirus A08.39
  toxic NEC K52.1
    due to Clostridium difficile
      not specified as recurrent A04.72
      recurrent A04.71
  trichomonal A07.8
  tuberculous A18.32
  typhosa A01.00
  ulcerative (chronic) — *see* Colitis, ulcerative
  viral A08.4
    adenovirus A08.2
    enterovirus A08.39
    Rotavirus A08.0
    small round structured NEC A08.19
    specified NEC A08.39
    virus specified NEC A08.39
Enterobiasis B80
Enterobius vermicularis (infection) (infestation) B80
Enterocele (*see also* Hernia, abdomen)
  pelvic, pelvis (acquired) (congenital) N81.5
  vagina, vaginal (acquired) (congenital) NEC N81.5
Enterocolitis (*see also* Enteritis) K52.9
  due to Clostridium difficile
    not specified as recurrent A04.72
    recurrent A04.71
  fulminant ischemic (*see also* Ischemia, intestine, acute) K55.059
  granulomatous — *see* Enteritis, regional
  hemorrhagic (acute) (*see also* Ischemia, intestine, acute) K55.059
    chronic K55.1
  infectious NEC A09
  ischemic K55.9
  necrotizing K55.30
    with
      perforation K55.33
      pneumatosis K55.32
        and perforation K55.33
    due to Clostridium difficile
      not specified as recurrent A04.72
      recurrent A04.71
    in non-newborn K55.30
      stage 1 (without pneumatosis, without perforation) K55.31
      stage 2 (with pneumatosis, without perforation) K55.32
      stage 3 (with pneumatosis, with perforation) K55.33
    in newborn P77.9
      stage 1 (without pneumatosis, without perforation) P77.1
      stage 2 (with pneumatosis, without perforation) P77.2
      stage 3 (with pneumatosis, with perforation) P77.3
    without pneumatosis or perforation K55.31
  noninfectious K52.9
    newborn — *see* Enterocolitis, necrotizing, in newborn

Enterocolitis — continued
  pseudomembranous (newborn)
    not specified as recurrent A04.72
    recurrent A04.71
  radiation K52.0
    newborn — see Enterocolitis, necrotizing, in new-
      born
  ulcerative (chronic) — see Pancolitis, ulcerative
    (chronic)
Enterogastritis — see Enteritis
Enteropathy K63.9
  celiac-gluten-sensitive K90.0
    non-celiac K90.41
  food protein-induced enterocolitis (FPIES) K52.22
  hemorrhagic, terminal (see also Ischemia, intestine,
    acute) K55.059
  protein-losing K90.49
Enteroperitonitis — see Peritonitis
Enteroptosis K63.4
Enterorrhagia K92.2
Enterospasm (see also Syndrome, irritable, bowel)
  psychogenic F45.8
Enterostenosis (see also Obstruction, intestine, specified
  NEC) K56.699
Enterostomy
  complication — see Complication, enterostomy
  status Z93.4
Enterovirus, as cause of disease classified elsewhere
  B97.10
  coxsackievirus B97.11
  echovirus B97.12
  other specified B97.19
Enthesopathy (peripheral) M77.9
  Achilles tendinitis — see Tendinitis, Achilles
  ankle and tarsus M77.9
    specified type NEC — see Enthesopathy, foot,
      specified type NEC
  anterior tibial syndrome M76.81- ☑
  calcaneal spur — see Spur, bone, calcaneal
  elbow region M77.8
    lateral epicondylitis — see Epicondylitis, lateral
    medial epicondylitis — see Epicondylitis, medial
  foot NEC M77.9
    metatarsalgia — see Metatarsalgia
    specified type NEC M77.5- ☑
  forearm M77.9
  gluteal tendinitis — see Tendinitis, gluteal
  hand M77.9
  hip — see Enthesopathy, lower limb, specified type
    NEC
  iliac crest spur — see Spur, bone, iliac crest
  iliotibial band syndrome — see Syndrome, iliotibial
    band
  knee — see Enthesopathy, lower limb, lower leg,
    specified type NEC
  lateral epicondylitis — see Epicondylitis, lateral
  lower limb (excluding foot) M76.9
    Achilles tendinitis — see Tendinitis, Achilles
    anterior tibial syndrome M76.81- ☑
    gluteal tendinitis — see Tendinitis, gluteal
    iliac crest spur — see Spur, bone, iliac crest
    iliotibial band syndrome — see Syndrome, iliotibial
      band
    patellar tendinitis — see Tendinitis, patellar
    pelvic region — see Enthesopathy, lower limb,
      specified type NEC
    peroneal tendinitis — see Tendinitis, peroneal
    posterior tibial syndrome M76.82- ☑
    psoas tendinitis — see Tendinitis, psoas
    shoulder M77.9
    specified type NEC M76.89- ☑
    tibial collateral bursitis — see Bursitis, tibial collater-
      al
  medial epicondylitis — see Epicondylitis, medial
  metatarsalgia — see Metatarsalgia
  multiple sites M77.9
  patellar tendinitis — see Tendinitis, patellar
  pelvis M77.9
  periarthritis of wrist — see Periarthritis, wrist
  peroneal tendinitis — see Tendinitis, peroneal
  posterior tibial syndrome M76.82- ☑
  psoas tendinitis — see Tendinitis, psoas
  shoulder region — see Lesion, shoulder
  specified site NEC M77.9
  specified type NEC M77.8
  spinal M46.00
    cervical region M46.02

Enthesopathy — continued
  spinal — continued
    cervicothoracic region M46.03
    lumbar region M46.06
    lumbosacral region M46.07
    multiple sites M46.09
    occipito-atlanto-axial region M46.01
    sacrococcygeal region M46.08
    thoracic region M46.04
    thoracolumbar region M46.05
  tibial collateral bursitis — see Bursitis, tibial collateral
  upper arm M77.9
  wrist and carpus NEC M77.8
    calcaneal spur — see Spur, bone, calcaneal
    periarthritis of wrist — see Periarthritis, wrist
Entomophobia F40.218
Entomophthoromycosis B46.8
Entrance, air into vein — see Embolism, air
Entrapment, nerve — see Neuropathy, entrapment
Entropion (eyelid) (paralytic) H02.009
  cicatricial H02.019
    left H02.016
      lower H02.015
      upper H02.014
    right H02.013
      lower H02.012
      upper H02.011
  congenital Q10.2
  left H02.006
    lower H02.005
    upper H02.004
  mechanical H02.029
    left H02.026
      lower H02.025
      upper H02.024
    right H02.023
      lower H02.022
      upper H02.021
  right H02.003
    lower H02.002
    upper H02.001
  senile H02.039
    left H02.036
      lower H02.035
      upper H02.034
    right H02.033
      lower H02.032
      upper H02.031
  spastic H02.049
    left H02.046
      lower H02.045
      upper H02.044
    right H02.043
      lower H02.042
      upper H02.041
Enucleated eye (traumatic, current) S05.7- ☑
Enuresis R32
  functional F98.0
  habit disturbance F98.0
  nocturnal N39.44
    psychogenic F98.0
  nonorganic origin F98.0
  psychogenic F98.0
Eosinopenia — see Agranulocytosis
Eosinophilia (allergic) (hereditary) (idiopathic) (secondary) D72.1
  with
    angiolymphoid hyperplasia (ALHE) D18.01
  infiltrative J82
  Löffler's J82
  peritoneal — see Peritonitis, eosinophilic
  pulmonary NEC J82
  tropical (pulmonary) J82
Eosinophilia-myalgia syndrome M35.8
Ependymitis (acute) (cerebral) (chronic) (granular) —
  see Encephalomyelitis
Ependymoblastoma
  specified site — see Neoplasm, malignant, by site
  unspecified site C71.9
Ependymoma (epithelial) (malignant)
  anaplastic
    specified site — see Neoplasm, malignant, by site
    unspecified site C71.9
  benign
    specified site — see Neoplasm, benign, by site
    unspecified site D33.2
  myxopapillary D43.2

Ependymoma — continued
  myxopapillary — continued
    specified site — see Neoplasm, uncertain behavior,
      by site
    unspecified site D43.2
  papillary D43.2
    specified site — see Neoplasm, uncertain behavior,
      by site
    unspecified site D43.2
  specified site — see Neoplasm, malignant, by site
  unspecified site C71.9
Ependymopathy G93.89
Ephelis, ephelides L81.2
Epiblepharon (congenital) Q10.3
Epicanthus, epicanthic fold (eyelid) (congenital) Q10.3
Epicondylitis (elbow)
  lateral M77.1- ☑
  medial M77.0- ☑
Epicystitis — see Cystitis
Epidemic — see condition
Epidermidalization, cervix — see Dysplasia, cervix
Epidermis, epidermal — see condition
Epidermodysplasia verruciformis B07.8
Epidermolysis
  bullosa (congenital) Q81.9
    acquired L12.30
      drug-induced L12.31
        specified cause NEC L12.35
    dystrophica Q81.2
    letalis Q81.1
    simplex Q81.0
    specified NEC Q81.8
  necroticans combustiformis L51.2
    due to drug — see Table of Drugs and Chemicals,
      by drug
Epidermophytid — see Dermatophytosis
Epidermophytosis (infected) — see Dermatophytosis
Epididymis — see condition
Epididymitis (acute) (nonvenereal) (recurrent) (residual
  N45.1
  with orchitis N45.3
  blennorrhagic (gonococcal) A54.23
  caseous (tuberculous) A18.15
  chlamydial A56.19
  filarial (see also Infestation, filarial) B74.9 [N51]
  gonococcal A54.23
  syphilitic A52.76
  tuberculous A18.15
Epididymo-orchitis (see also Epididymitis) N45.3
Epidural — see condition
Epigastrium, epigastric — see condition
Epigastrocele — see Hernia, ventral
Epiglottis — see condition
Epiglottitis, epiglottiditis (acute) J05.10
  with obstruction J05.11
  chronic J37.0
Epignathus Q89.4
Epilepsia partialis continua (see also Kozhevnikof's
  epilepsy) G40.1- ☑
Epilepsy, epileptic, epilepsia (attack) (cerebral) (convul-
  sion) (fit) (seizure) G40.909

*Note: the following terms are to be considered
equivalent to intractable: pharmacoresistant
(pharmacologically resistant), treatment resistant,
refractory (medically) and poorly controlled*

  with
    complex partial seizures — see Epilepsy, localiza-
      tion-related, symptomatic, with complex
      partial seizures
    grand mal seizures on awakening — see Epilepsy,
      generalized, specified NEC
    myoclonic absences — see Epilepsy, generalized,
      specified NEC
    myoclonic-astatic seizures — see Epilepsy, general-
      ized, specified NEC
    simple partial seizures — see Epilepsy, localization-
      related, symptomatic, with simple partial
      seizures
  akinetic — see Epilepsy, generalized, specified NEC
  benign childhood with centrotemporal EEG spikes
    — see Epilepsy, localization-related, idiopathic
  benign myoclonic in infancy G40.80- ☑
  Bravais-jacksonian — see Epilepsy, localization-related
    symptomatic, with simple partial seizures

Epilepsy, epileptic, epilepsia — continued
  childhood
    with occipital EEG paroxysms — see Epilepsy, local-
      ization-related, idiopathic
    absence G40.A09 (following G40.3)
      intractable G40.A19 (following G40.3)
        with status epilepticus G40.A11 (following
          G40.3)
        without status epilepticus G40.A19 (following
          G40.3)
      not intractable G40.A09 (following G40.3)
        with status epilepticus G40.A01 (following
          G40.3)
        without status epilepticus G40.A09 (following
          G40.3)
  climacteric — see Epilepsy, specified NEC
  cysticercosis B69.0
  deterioration (mental) F06.8
  due to syphilis A52.19
  focal — see Epilepsy, localization-related, symptomatic,
    with simple partial seizures
  generalized
    idiopathic G40.309
      intractable G40.319
        with status epilepticus G40.311
        without status epilepticus G40.319
      not intractable G40.309
        with status epilepticus G40.301
        without status epilepticus G40.309
    specified NEC G40.409
      intractable G40.419
        with status epilepticus G40.411
        without status epilepticus G40.419
      not intractable G40.409
        with status epilepticus G40.401
        without status epilepticus G40.409
  impulsive petit mal — see Epilepsy, juvenile myoclonic
  intractable G40.919
    with status epilepticus G40.911
    without status epilepticus G40.919
  juvenile absence G40.A09 (following G40.3)
    intractable G40.A19 (following G40.3)
      with status epilepticus G40.A11 (following G40.3)
      without status epilepticus G40.A19 (following
        G40.3)
    not intractable G40.A09 (following G40.3)
      with status epilepticus G40.A01 (following G40.3)
      without status epilepticus G40.A09 (following
        G40.3)
  juvenile myoclonic G40.B09 (following G40.3)
    intractable G40.B19 (following G40.3)
      with status epilepticus G40.B11 (following G40.3)
      without status epilepticus G40.B19 (following
        G40.3)
    not intractable G40.B09 (following G40.3)
      with status epilepticus G40.B01 (following G40.3)
      without status epilepticus G40.B09 (following
        G40.3)
  localization-related (focal) (partial)
    idiopathic G40.009
      with seizures of localized onset G40.009
        intractable G40.019
          with status epilepticus G40.011
          without status epilepticus G40.019
        not intractable G40.009
          with status epilepticus G40.001
          without status epilepticus G40.009
    symptomatic
      with complex partial seizures G40.209
        intractable G40.219
          with status epilepticus G40.211
          without status epilepticus G40.219
        not intractable G40.209
          with status epilepticus G40.201
          without status epilepticus G40.209
      with simple partial seizures G40.109
        intractable G40.119
          with status epilepticus G40.111
          without status epilepticus G40.119
        not intractable G40.109
          with status epilepticus G40.101
          without status epilepticus G40.109
  myoclonus, myoclonic — see Epilepsy, generalized,
    specified NEC
  progressive — see Epilepsy, generalized, idiopathic
  not intractable G40.909
    with status epilepticus G40.901
    without status epilepticus G40.909

Epilepsy, epileptic, epilepsia — continued
  on awakening — see Epilepsy, generalized, specified
    NEC
  parasitic NOS B71.9 [G94]
  partialis continua (see also Kozhevnikof's epilepsy)
    G40.1- ☑
  peripheral — see Epilepsy, specified NEC
  procursiva — see Epilepsy, localization-related, symp-
    tomatic, with simple partial seizures
  progressive (familial) myoclonic — see Epilepsy, gener-
    alized, idiopathic
  reflex — see Epilepsy, specified NEC
  related to
    alcohol G40.509
      not intractable G40.509
        with status epilepticus G40.501
        without status epilepticus G40.509
    drugs G40.509
      not intractable G40.509
        with status epilepticus G40.501
        without status epilepticus G40.509
    external causes G40.509
      not intractable G40.509
        with status epilepticus G40.501
        without status epilepticus G40.509
    hormonal changes G40.509
      not intractable G40.509
        with status epilepticus G40.501
        without status epilepticus G40.509
    sleep deprivation G40.509
      not intractable G40.509
        with status epilepticus G40.501
        without status epilepticus G40.509
    stress G40.509
      not intractable G40.509
        with status epilepticus G40.501
        without status epliepticus G40.509
  somatomotor — see Epilepsy, localization-related,
    symptomatic, with simple partial seizures
  somatosensory — see Epilepsy, localization-related,
    symptomatic, with simple partial seizures
  spasms G40.822
    intractable G40.824
      with status epilepticus G40.823
      without status epilepticus G40.824
    not intractable G40.822
      with status epilepticus G40.821
      without status epilepticus G40.822
  specified NEC G40.802
    intractable G40.804
      with status epilepticus G40.803
      without status epilepticus G40.804
    not intractable G40.802
      with status epilepticus G40.801
      without status epilepticus G40.802
  syndromes
    generalized
      idiopathic G40.309
        intractable G40.319
          with status epilepticus G40.311
          without status epilepticus G40.319
        not intractable G40.309
          with status epilepticus G40.301
          without status epilepticus G40.309
      specified NEC G40.409
        intractable G40.419
          with status epilepticus G40.411
          without status epilepticus G40.419
        not intractable G40.409
          with status epilepticus G40.401
          without status epilepticus G40.409
    localization-related (focal) (partial)
      idiopathic G40.009
        with seizures of localized onset G40.009
          intractable G40.019
            with status epilepticus G40.011
            without status epilepticus G40.019
          not intractable G40.009
            with status epilepticus G40.001
            without status epilepticus G40.009
      symptomatic
        with complex partial seizures G40.209
          intractable G40.219
            with status epilepticus G40.211
            without status epilepticus G40.219
          not intractable G40.209
            with status epilepticus G40.201
            without status epilepticus G40.209

Epilepsy, epileptic, epilepsia — continued
  syndromes — continued
    localization-related — continued
      symptomatic — continued
        with simple partial seizures G40.109
          intractable G40.119
            with status epilepticus G40.111
            without status epilepticus G40.119
          not intractable G40.109
            with status epilepticus G40.101
            without status epilepticus G40.109
    specified NEC G40.802
      intractable G40.804
        with status epilepticus G40.803
        without status epilepticus G40.804
      not intractable G40.802
        with status epilepticus G40.801
        without status epilepticus G40.802
  tonic (-clonic) — see Epilepsy, generalized, specified
    NEC
  twilight F05
  uncinate (gyrus) — see Epilepsy, localization-related,
    symptomatic, with complex partial seizures
  Unverricht (-Lundborg) (familial myoclonic) — see
    Epilepsy, generalized, idiopathic
  visceral — see Epilepsy, specified NEC
  visual — see Epilepsy, specified NEC
Epiloia Q85.1
Epimenorrhea N92.0
Epipharyngitis — see Nasopharyngitis
Epiphora H04.20- ☑
  due to
    excess lacrimation H04.21- ☑
    insufficient drainage H04.22- ☑
Epiphyseal arrest — see Arrest, epiphyseal
Epiphyseolysis, epiphysiolysis — see Osteochondropathy
Epiphysitis (see also Osteochondropathy)
  juvenile M92.9
  syphilitic (congenital) A50.02
Epiplocele — see Hernia, abdomen
Epiploitis — see Peritonitis
Epiplosarcomphalocele — see Hernia, umbilicus
Episcleritis (suppurative) H15.10- ☑
  in (due to)
    syphilis A52.71
    tuberculosis A18.51
  nodular H15.12- ☑
  periodica fugax H15.11- ☑
    angioneurotic — see Edema, angioneurotic
  syphilitic (late) A52.71
  tuberculous A18.51
Episode
  affective, mixed F39
  depersonalization (in neurotic state) F48.1
  depressive F32.9
    major F32.9
      mild F32.0
      moderate F32.1
      severe (without psychotic symptoms) F32.2
        with psychotic symptoms F32.3
    recurrent F33.9
    brief F33.8
    specified NEC F32.89
  hypomanic F30.8
  manic F30.9
    with
      psychotic symptoms F30.2
      remission (full) F30.4
        partial F30.3
    other specified F30.8
    recurrent F31.89
    without psychotic symptoms F30.10
      mild F30.11
      moderate F30.12
      severe (without psychotic symptoms) F30.13
        with psychotic symptoms F30.2
  psychotic F23
    organic F06.8
  schizophrenic (acute) NEC, brief F23
Epispadias (female) (male) Q64.0
Episplenitis D73.89
Epistaxis (multiple) R04.0
  hereditary I78.0
  vicarious menstruation N94.89
Epithelioma (malignant) (see also Neoplasm, malignant,
  by site)
  adenoides cysticum — see Neoplasm, skin, benign

Epithelioma — continued
  basal cell — see Neoplasm, skin, malignant
  benign — see Neoplasm, benign, by site
  Bowen's — see Neoplasm, skin, in situ
  calcifying, of Malherbe — see Neoplasm, skin, benign
  external site — see Neoplasm, skin, malignant
  intraepidermal, Jadassohn — see Neoplasm, skin, benign
  squamous cell — see Neoplasm, malignant, by site
Epitheliomatosis pigmented Q82.1
Epitheliopathy, multifocal placoid pigment H30.14- ☑
Epithelium, epithelial — see condition
Epituberculosis (with atelectasis) (allergic) A15.7
Eponychia Q84.6
Epstein's
  nephrosis or syndrome — see Nephrosis
  pearl K09.8
Epulis (gingiva) (fibrous) (giant cell) K06.8
Equinia A24.0
Equinovarus (congenital) (talipes) Q66.0
  acquired — see Deformity, limb, clubfoot
Equivalent
  convulsive (abdominal) — see Epilepsy, specified NEC
  epileptic (psychic) — see Epilepsy, localization-related, symptomatic, with complex partial seizures
Erb (-Duchenne) **paralysis** (birth injury) (newborn) P14.0
Erb-Goldflam disease or syndrome G70.00
  with exacerbation (acute) G70.01
  in crisis G70.01
Erb's
  disease G71.02
  palsy, paralysis (brachial) (birth) (newborn) P14.0
    spinal (spastic) syphilitic A52.17
  pseudohypertrophic muscular dystrophy G71.02
Erdheim's syndrome (acromegalic macrospondylitis) E22.0
Erection, painful (persistent) — see Priapism
Ergosterol deficiency (vitamin D) E55.9
  with
    adult osteomalacia M83.8
    rickets — see Rickets
Ergotism (see also Poisoning, food, noxious, plant)
  from ergot used as drug (migraine therapy) — see Table of Drugs and Chemicals
Erosio interdigitalis blastomycetica B37.2
Erosion
  artery I77.2
    without rupture I77.89
  bone — see Disorder, bone, density and structure, specified NEC
  bronchus J98.09
  cartilage (joint) — see Disorder, cartilage, specified type NEC
  cervix (uteri) (acquired) (chronic) (congenital) N86
    with cervicitis N72
  cornea (nontraumatic) — see Ulcer, cornea
    recurrent H18.83- ☑
    traumatic — see Abrasion, cornea
  dental (idiopathic) (occupational) (due to diet, drugs or vomiting) K03.2
  duodenum, postpyloric — see Ulcer, duodenum
  esophagus K22.10
    with bleeding K22.11
  gastric — see Ulcer, stomach
  gastrojejunal — see Ulcer, gastrojejunal
  implanted mesh — see Complications, mesh
  intestine K63.3
  lymphatic vessel I89.8
  pylorus, pyloric (ulcer) — see Ulcer, stomach
  spine, aneurysmal A52.09
  stomach — see Ulcer, stomach
  subcutaneous device pocket
    nervous system prosthetic device, implant, or graft T85.890 ☑
    other internal prosthetic device, implant, or graft T85.898 ☑
  teeth (idiopathic) (occupational) (due to diet, drugs or vomiting) K03.2
  urethra N36.8
  uterus N85.8
Erotomania F52.8
Error
  metabolism, inborn — see Disorder, metabolism
  refractive — see Disorder, refraction
Eructation R14.2
  nervous or psychogenic F45.8

Eruption
  creeping B76.9
  drug (generalized) (taken internally) L27.0
    fixed L27.1
    in contact with skin — see Dermatitis, due to drugs
    localized L27.1
  Hutchinson, summer L56.4
  Kaposi's varicelliform B00.0
  napkin L22
  polymorphous light (sun) L56.4
  recalcitrant pustular L13.8
  ringed R23.8
  skin (nonspecific) R21
    creeping (meaning hookworm) B76.9
    due to inoculation/vaccination (generalized) (see also Dermatitis, due to, vaccine) L27.0
      localized L27.1
    erysipeloid A26.0
    feigned L98.1
    Kaposi's varicelliform B00.0
    lichenoid L28.0
    meaning dermatitis — see Dermatitis
    toxic NEC L53.0
  tooth, teeth, abnormal (incomplete) (late) (premature) (sequence) K00.6
  vesicular R23.8
Erysipelas (gangrenous) (infantile) (newborn) (phlegmonous) (suppurative) A46
  external ear A46 [H62.40]
  puerperal, postpartum O86.89
Erysipeloid A26.9
  cutaneous (Rosenbach's) A26.0
  disseminated A26.8
  sepsis A26.7
  specified NEC A26.8
Erythema, erythematous (infectional) (inflammation) L53.9
  ab igne L59.0
  annulare (centrifugum) (rheumaticum) L53.1
  arthriticum epidemicum A25.1
  brucellum — see Brucellosis
  chronic figurate NEC L53.3
  chronicum migrans (Borrelia burgdorferi) A69.20
  diaper L22
  due to
    chemical NEC L53.0
      in contact with skin L24.5
    drug (internal use) — see Dermatitis, due to, drugs
  elevatum diutinum L95.1
  endemic E52
  epidemic, arthritic A25.1
  figuratum perstans L53.3
  gluteal L22
  heat — code by site under Burn, first degree
  ichthyosiforme congenitum bullous Q80.3
  in diseases classified elsewhere L54
  induratum (nontuberculous) L52
    tuberculous A18.4
  infectiosum B08.3
  intertrigo L30.4
  iris L51.9
  marginatum L53.2
    in (due to) acute rheumatic fever I00
  medicamentosum — see Dermatitis, due to, drugs
  migrans A26.0
    chronicum A69.20
    tongue K14.1
  multiforme (major) (minor) L51.9
    bullous, bullosum L51.1
    conjunctiva L51.1
    nonbullous L51.0
    pemphigoides L12.0
    specified NEC L51.8
  napkin L22
  neonatorum P83.88
    toxic P83.1
  nodosum L52
    tuberculous A18.4
  palmar L53.8
  pernio T69.1 ☑
  rash, newborn P83.88
  scarlatiniform (recurrent) (exfoliative) L53.8
  solare L55.0
  specified NEC L53.8
  toxic, toxicum NEC L53.0
    newborn P83.1
  tuberculous (primary) A18.4
Erythematous, erythematosus — see condition

Erythermalgia (primary) I73.81
Erythralgia I73.81
Erythrasma L08.1
Erythredema (polyneuropathy) — see Poisoning, mercury
Erythremia (acute) C94.0- ☑
  chronic D45
  secondary D75.1
Erythroblastopenia (see also Aplasia, red cell) D60.9
  congenital D61.01
Erythroblastophthisis D61.09
Erythroblastosis (fetalis) (newborn) P55.9
  due to
    ABO (antibodies) (incompatibility) (isoimmunization) P55.1
    Rh (antibodies) (incompatibility) (isoimmunization) P55.0
Erythrocyanosis (crurum) I73.89
Erythrocythemia — see Erythremia
Erythrocytosis (megalosplenic) (secondary) D75.1
  familial D75.0
  oval, hereditary — see Elliptocytosis
  secondary D75.1
  stress D75.1
Erythroderma (secondary) (see also Erythema) L53.9
  bullous ichthyosiform, congenital Q80.3
  desquamativum L21.1
  ichthyosiform, congenital (bullous) Q80.3
  neonatorum P83.88
  psoriaticum L40.8
Erythrodysesthesia, palmar plantar (PPE) L27.1
Erythrogenesis imperfecta D61.09
Erythroleukemia C94.0- ☑
Erythromelalgia I73.81
Erythrophagocytosis D75.89
Erythrophobia F40.298
Erythroplakia, oral epithelium, and tongue K13.29
Erythroplasia (Queyrat) D07.4
  specified site — see Neoplasm, skin, in situ
  unspecified site D07.4
Escherichia coli (E. coli), **as cause of disease classified elsewhere** B96.20
  non-O157 Shiga toxin-producing (with known O group) B96.22
  non-Shiga toxin-producing B96.29
  O157 with confirmation of Shiga toxin when H antigen is unknown, or is not H7 B96.21
  O157:H- (nonmotile) with confirmation of Shiga toxin B96.21
  O157:H7 with or without confirmation of Shiga toxin production B96.21
    specified NEC B96.22-
  Shiga toxin-producing (with unspecified O group) (STEC) B96.23
    O157 B96.21
    specified NEC B96.29
Esophagismus K22.4
Esophagitis (acute) (alkaline) (chemical) (chronic) (infectional) (necrotic) (peptic) (postoperative) K20.9
  candidal B37.81
  due to gastrointestinal reflux disease K21.0
  eosinophilic K20.0
  reflux K21.0
  specified NEC K20.8
  tuberculous A18.83
  ulcerative K22.10
    with bleeding K22.11
Esophagocele K22.5
Esophagomalacia K22.8
Esophagospasm K22.4
Esophagostenosis K22.2
Esophagostomiasis B81.8
Esophagotracheal — see condition
Esophagus — see condition
Esophoria H50.51
  convergence, excess H51.12
  divergence, insufficiency H51.8
Esotropia — see Strabismus, convergent concomitant
Espundia B55.2
Essential — see condition
Esthesioneuroblastoma C30.0
Esthesioneurocytoma C30.0
Esthesioneuroepithelioma C30.0
Esthiomene A55
Estivo-autumnal malaria (fever) B50.9
Estrangement (marital) Z63.5
  parent-child NEC Z62.890

Epithelioma — Estrangement

136   ☑ **Additional Character Required — Refer to the Tabular List for Character Selection**   🔻 **Subterms under main terms may continue to next column or page**

Estriasis — *see* Myiasis
Ethanolism — *see* Alcoholism
Etherism — *see* Dependence, drug, inhalant
Ethmoid, ethmoidal — *see* condition
Ethmoiditis (chronic) (nonpurulent) (purulent) (*see also* Sinusitis, ethmoidal)
  influenzal — *see* Influenza, with, respiratory manifestations NEC
  Woakes' J33.1
Ethylism — *see* Alcoholism
Eulenburg's disease (congenital paramyotonia) G71.19
Eumycetoma B47.0
Eunuchoidism E29.1
  hypogonadotropic E23.0
European blastomycosis — *see* Cryptococcosis
Eustachian — *see* condition
Evaluation (for) (of)
  development state
    adolescent Z00.3
    period of
      delayed growth in childhood Z00.70
        with abnormal findings Z00.71
      rapid growth in childhood Z00.2
      puberty Z00.3
  growth and developmental state (period of rapid growth) Z00.2
    delayed growth Z00.70
      with abnormal findings Z00.71
  mental health (status) Z00.8
    requested by authority Z04.6
  period of
    delayed growth in childhood Z00.70
      with abnormal findings Z00.71
    rapid growth in childhood Z00.2
  suspected condition — *see* Observation
Evans syndrome D69.41
Event
  apparent life threatening in newborn and infant (ALTE) R68.13
  brief resolved unexplained event (BRUE) R68.13
Eventration (*see also* Hernia, ventral)
  colon into chest — *see* Hernia, diaphragm
  diaphragm (congenital) Q79.1
Eversion
  bladder N32.89
  cervix (uteri) N86
    with cervicitis N72
  foot NEC (*see also* Deformity, valgus, ankle)
    congenital Q66.6
  punctum lacrimale (postinfectional) (senile) H04.52- ☑
  ureter (meatus) N28.89
  urethra (meatus) N36.8
  uterus N81.4
Evidence
  cytologic
    of malignancy on anal smear R85.614
    of malignancy on cervical smear R87.614
    of malignancy on vaginal smear R87.624
Evisceration
  birth injury P15.8
  traumatic NEC
    eye — *see* Enucleated eye
Evulsion — *see* Avulsion
Ewing's sarcoma or tumor — *see* Neoplasm, bone, malignant
Examination (for) (following) (general) (of) (routine) Z00.00
  with abnormal findings Z00.01
  abuse, physical (alleged), ruled out
    adult Z04.71
    child Z04.72
  adolescent (development state) Z00.3
  alleged rape or sexual assault (victim), ruled out
    adult Z04.41
    child Z04.42
  allergy Z01.82
  annual (adult) (periodic) (physical) Z00.00
    with abnormal findings Z00.01
    gynecological Z01.419
      with abnormal findings Z01.411
  antibody response Z01.84
  blood — *see* Examination, laboratory
  blood pressure Z01.30
    with abnormal findings Z01.31
  cancer staging — *see* Neoplasm, malignant, by site
  cervical Papanicolaou smear Z12.4
    as part of routine gynecological examination Z01.419

Examination — *continued*
  cervical Papanicolaou smear — *continued*
    as part of routine gynecological examination — *continued*
      with abnormal findings Z01.411
  child (over 28 days old) Z00.129
    with abnormal findings Z00.121
    under 28 days old — *see* Newborn, examination
  clinical research control or normal comparison (control) (participant) Z00.6
  contraceptive (drug) maintenance (routine) Z30.8
    device (intrauterine) Z30.431
  dental Z01.20
    with abnormal findings Z01.21
  developmental — *see* Examination, child
  donor (potential) Z00.5
  ear Z01.10
    with abnormal findings NEC Z01.118
  eye Z01.00
    with abnormal findings Z01.01
  follow-up (routine) (following) Z09
    chemotherapy NEC Z09
      malignant neoplasm Z08
    fracture Z09
    malignant neoplasm Z08
    postpartum Z39.2
    psychotherapy Z09
    radiotherapy NEC Z09
      malignant neoplasm Z08
    surgery NEC Z09
      malignant neoplasm Z08
  following
    accident NEC Z04.3
      transport Z04.1
      work Z04.2
    assault, alleged, ruled out
      adult Z04.71
      child Z04.72
    motor vehicle accident Z04.1
    treatment (for) Z09
      combined NEC Z09
        fracture Z09
        malignant neoplasm Z08
      malignant neoplasm Z08
      mental disorder Z09
      specified condition NEC Z09
  forced sexual exploitation Z04.81
  forced labor exploitation Z04.82
  gynecological Z01.419
    with abnormal findings Z01.411
    for contraceptive maintenance Z30.8
  health — *see* Examination, medical
  hearing Z01.10
    with abnormal findings NEC Z01.118
    following failed hearing screening Z01.110
    infant or child (over 28 days old) Z00.129
      with abnormal findings Z00.121
  immunity status testing Z01.84
  laboratory (as part of a general medical examination) Z00.00
    with abnormal findings Z00.01
    preprocedural Z01.812
  lactating mother Z39.1
  medical (adult) (for) (of) Z00.00
    with abnormal findings Z00.01
    administrative purpose only Z02.9
      specified NEC Z02.89
    admission to
      armed forces Z02.3
      old age home Z02.2
      prison Z02.89
      residential institution Z02.2
      school Z02.0
        following illness or medical treatment Z02.0
      summer camp Z02.89
    adoption Z02.82
    blood alcohol or drug level Z02.83
    camp (summer) Z02.89
    clinical research, normal subject (control) (participant) Z00.6
    control subject in clinical research (normal comparison) (participant) Z00.6
    donor (potential) Z00.5
    driving license Z02.4
    general (adult) Z00.00
      with abnormal findings Z00.01
    immigration Z02.89
    insurance purposes Z02.6
    marriage Z02.89

Examination — *continued*
  medical — *continued*
    medicolegal reasons NEC Z04.89
    naturalization Z02.89
    participation in sport Z02.5
    paternity testing Z02.81
    population survey Z00.8
    pre-employment Z02.1
    pre-operative — *see* Examination, pre-procedural
    pre-procedural
      cardiovascular Z01.810
      respiratory Z01.811
      specified NEC Z01.818
    preschool children
      for admission to school Z02.0
    prisoners
      for entrance into prison Z02.89
    recruitment for armed forces Z02.3
    specified NEC Z00.8
    sport competition Z02.5
  medicolegal reason NEC Z04.89
    following
      forced sexual exploitation Z04.81
      forced labor exploitation Z04.82
  newborn — *see* Newborn, examination
  pelvic (annual) (periodic) Z01.419
    with abnormal findings Z01.411
  period of rapid growth in childhood Z00.2
  periodic (adult) (annual) (routine) Z00.00
    with abnormal findings Z00.01
  physical (adult) (*see also* Examination, medical) Z00.00
    sports Z02.5
  postpartum
    immediately after delivery Z39.0
    routine follow-up Z39.2
  pre-chemotherapy (antineoplastic) Z01.818
  prenatal (normal pregnancy) (*see also* Pregnancy, normal) Z34.9- ☑
  pre-procedural (pre-operative)
    cardiovascular Z01.810
    laboratory Z01.812
    respiratory Z01.811
    specified NEC Z01.818
  prior to chemotherapy (antineoplastic) Z01.818
  psychiatric NEC Z00.8
    follow-up not needing further care Z09
    requested by authority Z04.6
  radiological (as part of a general medical examination) Z00.00
    with abnormal findings Z00.01
  repeat cervical smear to confirm findings of recent normal smear following initial abnormal smear Z01.42
  skin (hypersensitivity) Z01.82
  special (*see also* Examination, by type) Z01.89
    specified type NEC Z01.89
  specified type or reason NEC Z04.89
  teeth Z01.20
    with abnormal findings Z01.21
  urine — *see* Examination, laboratory
  vision Z01.00
    with abnormal findings Z01.01
    infant or child (over 28 days old) Z00.129
      with abnormal findings Z00.121
Exanthem, exanthema (*see also* Rash)
  with enteroviral vesicular stomatitis B08.4
  Boston A88.0
  epidemic with meningitis A88.0 [G02]
  subitum B08.20
    due to human herpesvirus 6 B08.21
    due to human herpesvirus 7 B08.22
  viral, virus B09
    specified type NEC B08.8
Excess, excessive, excessively
  alcohol level in blood R78.0
  androgen (ovarian) E28.1
  attrition, tooth, teeth K03.0
  carotene, carotin (dietary) E67.1
  cold, effects of T69.9 ☑
    specified effect NEC T69.8 ☑
  convergence H51.12
  crying
    in child, adolescent, or adult R45.83
    in infant R68.11
  development, breast N62
  divergence H51.8
  drinking (alcohol) NEC (without dependence) F10.10
    habitual (continual) (without remission) F10.20

Excess, excessive, excessively — continued
eating R63.2
estrogen E28.0
fat (see also Obesity)
  in heart — see Degeneration, myocardial
  localized E65
foreskin N47.8
gas R14.0
glucagon E16.3
heat — see Heat
intermaxillary vertical dimension of fully erupted teeth M26.37
interocclusal distance of fully erupted teeth M26.37
kalium E87.5
large
  colon K59.39
    congenital Q43.8
  infant P08.0
  organ or site, congenital NEC — see Anomaly, by site
long
  organ or site, congenital NEC — see Anomaly, by site
menstruation (with regular cycle) N92.0
  with irregular cycle N92.1
napping Z72.821
natrium E87.0
number of teeth K00.1
nutrient (dietary) NEC R63.2
potassium (K) E87.5
salivation K11.7
secretion (see also Hypersecretion)
  milk O92.6
  sputum R09.3
  sweat R61
sexual drive F52.8
short
  organ or site, congenital NEC — see Anomaly, by site
  umbilical cord in labor or delivery O69.3 ☑
skin L98.7
  and subcutaneous tissue L98.7
  eyelid (acquired) — see Blepharochalasis
    congenital Q10.3
sodium (Na) E87.0
spacing of fully erupted teeth M26.32
sputum R09.3
sweating R61
thirst R63.1
  due to deprivation of water T73.1 ☑
tuberosity of jaw M26.07
vitamin
  A (dietary) E67.0
    administered as drug (prolonged intake) — see Table of Drugs and Chemicals, vitamins, adverse effect
    overdose or wrong substance given or taken — see Table of Drugs and Chemicals, vitamins, poisoning
  D (dietary) E67.3
    administered as drug (prolonged intake) — see Table of Drugs and Chemicals, vitamins, adverse effect
    overdose or wrong substance given or taken — see Table of Drugs and Chemicals, vitamins, poisoning
weight
  gain R63.5
  loss R63.4

Excitability, abnormal, under minor stress (personality disorder) F60.3

Excitation
anomalous atrioventricular I45.6
psychogenic F30.8
reactive (from emotional stress, psychological trauma) F30.8

Excitement
hypomanic F30.8
manic F30.9
mental, reactive (from emotional stress, psychological trauma) F30.8
state, reactive (from emotional stress, psychological trauma) F30.8

Excoriation (traumatic) (see also Abrasion)
neurotic L98.1
skin picking disorder F42.4

Exfoliation
due to erythematous conditions according to extent of body surface involved L49.0
  10-19 percent of body surface L49.1
  20-29 percent of body surface L49.2
  30-39 percent of body surface L49.3
  40-49 percent of body surface L49.4
  50-59 percent of body surface L49.5
  60-69 percent of body surface L49.6
  70-79 percent of body surface L49.7
  80-89 percent of body surface L49.8
  90-99 percent of body surface L49.9
  less than 10 percent of body surface L49.0
teeth, due to systemic causes K08.0

Exfoliative — see condition

Exhaustion, exhaustive (physical NEC) R53.83
battle F43.0
cardiac — see Failure, heart
delirium F43.0
due to
  cold T69.8 ☑
  excessive exertion T73.3 ☑
  exposure T73.2 ☑
  neurasthenia F48.8
heart — see Failure, heart
heat (see also Heat, exhaustion) T67.5 ☑
  due to
    salt depletion T67.4 ☑
    water depletion T67.3 ☑
maternal, complicating delivery O75.81
mental F48.8
myocardium, myocardial — see Failure, heart
nervous F48.8
old age R54
psychogenic F48.8
psychosis F43.0
senile R54
vital NEC Z73.0

Exhibitionism F65.2
Exocervicitis — see Cervicitis
Exomphalos Q79.2
meaning hernia — see Hernia, umbilicus
Exophoria H50.52
convergence, insufficiency H51.11
divergence, excess H51.8
Exophthalmos H05.2- ☑
congenital Q15.8
constant NEC H05.24- ☑
displacement, globe — see Displacement, globe
due to thyrotoxicosis (hyperthyroidism) — see Hyperthyroidism, with, goiter (diffuse)
dysthyroid — see Hyperthyroidism, with, goiter (diffuse)
goiter — see Hyperthyroidism, with, goiter (diffuse)
intermittent NEC H05.25- ☑
malignant — see Hyperthyroidism, with, goiter (diffuse)
orbital
  edema — see Edema, orbit
  hemorrhage — see Hemorrhage, orbit
pulsating NEC H05.26- ☑
thyrotoxic, thyrotropic — see Hyperthyroidism, with, goiter (diffuse)

Exostosis (see also Disorder, bone)
cartilaginous — see Neoplasm, bone, benign
congenital (multiple) Q78.6
external ear canal H61.81- ☑
gonococcal A54.49
jaw (bone) M27.8
multiple, congenital Q78.6
orbit H05.35- ☑
osteocartilaginous — see Neoplasm, bone, benign
syphilitic A52.77

Exotropia — see Strabismus, divergent concomitant
Explanation of
investigation finding Z71.2
medication Z71.89

Exposure (to) (see also Contact, with) T75.89 ☑
acariasis Z20.7
AIDS virus Z20.6
air pollution Z77.110
algae and algae toxins Z77.121
algae bloom Z77.121
anthrax Z20.810
aromatic amines Z77.020
aromatic (hazardous) compounds NEC Z77.028
aromatic dyes NOS Z77.028
arsenic Z77.010

Exposure — continued
asbestos Z77.090
bacterial disease NEC Z20.818
benzene Z77.021
blue-green algae bloom Z77.121
body fluids (potentially hazardous) Z77.21
brown tide Z77.121
chemicals (chiefly nonmedicinal) (hazardous) NEC Z77.098
cholera Z20.09
chromium compounds Z77.018
cold, effects of T69.9 ☑
  specified effect NEC T69.8 ☑
communicable disease Z20.9
  bacterial NEC Z20.818
  specified NEC Z20.89
  viral NEC Z20.828
  Zika virus Z20.821
cyanobacteria bloom Z77.121
disaster Z65.5
discrimination Z60.5
dyes Z77.098
effects of T73.9 ☑
environmental tobacco smoke (acute) (chronic) Z77.22
Escherichia coli (E. coli) Z20.01
exhaustion due to T73.2 ☑
fiberglass — see Table of Drugs and Chemicals, fiberglass
German measles Z20.4
gonorrhea Z20.2
hazardous metals NEC Z77.018
hazardous substances NEC Z77.29
hazards in the physical environment NEC Z77.128
hazards to health NEC Z77.9
human immunodeficiency virus (HIV) Z20.6
human T-lymphotropic virus type-1 (HTLV-1) Z20.89
implanted
  mesh — see Complications, mesh
  prosthetic materials NEC — see Complications, prosthetic materials NEC
infestation (parasitic) NEC Z20.7
intestinal infectious disease NEC Z20.09
  Escherichia coli (E. coli) Z20.01
lead Z77.011
meningococcus Z20.811
mold (toxic) Z77.120
nickel dust Z77.018
noise Z77.122
occupational
  air contaminants NEC Z57.39
  dust Z57.2
  environmental tobacco smoke Z57.31
  extreme temperature Z57.6
  noise Z57.0
  radiation Z57.1
  risk factors Z57.9
    specified NEC Z57.8
  toxic agents (gases) (liquids) (solids) (vapors) in agriculture Z57.4
  toxic agents (gases) (liquids) (solids) (vapors) in industry NEC Z57.5
  vibration Z57.7
parasitic disease NEC Z20.7
pediculosis Z20.7
persecution Z60.5
pfiesteria piscicida Z77.121
poliomyelitis Z20.89
pollution
  air Z77.110
  environmental NEC Z77.118
  soil Z77.112
  water Z77.111
polycyclic aromatic hydrocarbons Z77.028
prenatal (drugs) (toxic chemicals) — see Newborn, affected by, noxious substances transmitted via placenta or breast milk
rabies Z20.3
radiation, naturally occurring NEC Z77.123
radon Z77.123
red tide (Florida) Z77.121
rubella Z20.4
second hand tobacco smoke (acute) (chronic) Z77.22
  in the perinatal period P96.81
sexually-transmitted disease Z20.2
smallpox (laboratory) Z20.89
syphilis Z20.2
terrorism Z65.4
torture Z65.4

Exposure — continued
- tuberculosis Z20.1
- uranium Z77.012
- varicella Z20.820
- venereal disease Z20.2
- viral disease NEC Z20.828
- war Z65.5
- water pollution Z77.111
- Zika virus Z20.821

Exsanguination — see Hemorrhage

Exstrophy
- abdominal contents Q45.8
- bladder Q64.10
  - cloacal Q64.12
  - specified type NEC Q64.19
  - supravesical fissure Q64.11

Extensive — see condition

Extra (see also Accessory)
- marker chromosomes (normal individual) Q92.61
  - in abnormal individual Q92.62
- rib Q76.6
  - cervical Q76.5

Extrasystoles (supraventricular) I49.49
- atrial I49.1
- auricular I49.1
- junctional I49.2
- ventricular I49.3

Extrauterine gestation or pregnancy — see Pregnancy, by site

Extravasation
- blood R58
- chyle into mesentery I89.8
- pelvicalyceal N13.8
- pyelosinus N13.8
- urine (from ureter) R39.0
- vesicant agent
  - antineoplastic chemotherapy T80.810 ☑
  - other agent NEC T80.818 ☑

Extremity — see condition, limb

Extrophy — see Exstrophy

Extroversion
- bladder Q64.19
- uterus N81.4
  - complicating delivery O71.2
  - postpartal (old) N81.4

Extruded tooth (teeth) M26.34

Extrusion
- breast implant (prosthetic) T85.42 ☑
- eye implant (globe) (ball) T85.328 ☑
- intervertebral disc — see Displacement, intervertebral disc
- ocular lens implant (prosthetic) — see Complications, intraocular lens
- vitreous — see Prolapse, vitreous

Exudate
- pleural — see Effusion, pleura
- retina H35.89

Exudative — see condition

Eye, eyeball, eyelid — see condition

Eyestrain — see Disturbance, vision, subjective

Eyeworm disease of Africa B74.3

F

Faber's syndrome (achlorhydric anemia) D50.9

Fabry (-Anderson) **disease** E75.21

Faciocephalalgia, autonomic (see also Neuropathy, peripheral, autonomic) G90.09

Factor(s)
- psychic, associated with diseases classified elsewhere F54
- psychological
  - affecting physical conditions F54
  - or behavioral
    - affecting general medical condition F54
    - associated with disorders or diseases classified elsewhere F54

Fahr disease (of brain) G23.8

Fahr Volhard disease (of kidney) I12.- ☑

Failure, failed
- abortion — see Abortion, attempted
- aortic (valve) I35.8
  - rheumatic I06.8
- attempted abortion — see Abortion, attempted
- biventricular I50.82
  - due to left heart failure I50.814
- bone marrow — see Anemia, aplastic

Failure, failed — continued
- cardiac — see Failure, heart
- cardiorenal (chronic) (see also Failure, renal, and Failure, heart) I50.9
  - hypertensive I13.2
- cardiorespiratory (see also Failure, heart) R09.2
- cardiovascular (chronic) — see Failure, heart
- cerebrovascular I67.9
- cervical dilatation in labor O62.0
- circulation, circulatory (peripheral) R57.9
  - newborn P29.89
- compensation — see Disease, heart
- compliance with medical treatment or regimen — see Noncompliance
- congestive — see Failure, heart, congestive
- dental implant (endosseous) M27.69
  - due to
    - failure of dental prosthesis M27.63
    - lack of attached gingiva M27.62
    - occlusal trauma (poor prosthetic design) M27.62
    - parafunctional habits M27.62
    - periodontal infection (peri-implantitis) M27.62
    - poor oral hygiene M27.62
  - osseointegration M27.61
    - due to
      - complications of systemic disease M27.61
      - poor bone quality M27.61
    - iatrogenic M27.61
  - post-osseointegration
    - biological M27.62
    - due to complications of systemic disease M27.62
    - iatrogenic M27.62
    - mechanical M27.63
  - pre-integration M27.61
  - pre-osseointegration M27.61
  - specified NEC M27.69
- descent of head (at term) of pregnancy (mother) O32.4 ☑
- endosseous dental implant — see Failure, dental implant
- engagement of head (term of pregnancy) (mother) O32.4 ☑
- erection (penile) (see also Dysfunction, sexual, male, erectile) N52.9
  - nonorganic F52.21
- examination(s), anxiety concerning Z55.2
- expansion terminal respiratory units (newborn) (primary) P28.0
- forceps NOS (with subsequent cesarean delivery) O66.5
- gain weight (child over 28 days old) R62.51
  - adult R62.7
  - newborn P92.6
- genital response (male) F52.21
  - female F52.22
- heart (acute) (senile) (sudden) I50.9
  - with
    - acute pulmonary edema — see Failure, ventricular, left
    - decompensation (see also Failure, heart, by type as diastolic or systolic, acute and chronic) I50.9
    - dilatation — see Disease, heart
    - normal ejection fraction — see Failure, heart, diastolic
    - preserved ejection fraction — see Failure, heart, diastolic
    - reduced ejection fraction — see Failure, heart, systolic
  - arteriosclerotic I70.90
  - biventricular I50.82
    - due to left heart failure I50.814
  - combined left-right sided I50.82
    - due to left heart failure I50.814
  - compensated (see also Failure, heart, by type as diastolic or systolic, chronic) I50.9
  - complicating
    - anesthesia (general) (local) or other sedation in labor and delivery O74.2
      - in pregnancy O29.12- ☑
      - postpartum, puerperal O89.1
    - delivery (cesarean) (instrumental) O75.4
  - congestive I50.9
    - with rheumatic fever (conditions in I00)
      - active I01.8
      - inactive or quiescent (with chorea) I09.81
    - newborn P29.0
    - rheumatic (chronic) (inactive) (with chorea) I09.81

Failure, failed — continued
- heart — continued
  - congestive — continued
    - rheumatic — continued
      - active or acute I01.8
        - with chorea I02.0
    - decompensated (see also Failure, heart, by type as diastolic or systolic, acute and chronic) I50.9
    - degenerative — see Degeneration, myocardial
    - diastolic (congestive) (left ventricular) I50.30
      - acute (congestive) I50.31
        - and (on) chronic (congestive) I50.33
      - chronic (congestive) I50.32
        - and (on) acute (congestive) I50.33
      - combined with systolic (congestive) I50.40
        - acute (congestive) I50.41
          - and (on) chronic (congestive) I50.43
        - chronic (congestive) I50.42
          - and (on) acute (congestive) I50.43
    - due to presence of cardiac prosthesis I97.13- ☑
    - end stage (see also Failure, heart, by type as diastolic or systolic, chronic) I50.84
    - following cardiac surgery I97.13- ☑
    - high output NOS I50.83
    - hypertensive — see Hypertension, heart
    - left (ventricular) (see also Failure, ventricular, left)
      - combined diastolic and systolic — see Failure, heart, diastolic, combined with systolic
      - diastolic — see Failure, heart, diastolic
      - systolic — see Failure, heart, systolic
    - low output (syndrome) NOS I50.9
    - newborn P29.0
    - organic — see Disease, heart
    - peripartum O90.3
    - postprocedural I97.13- ☑
    - rheumatic (chronic) (inactive) I09.9
    - right (isolated) (ventricular) I50.810
      - acute I50.811
        - and (on) chronic I50.813
      - chronic I50.812
        - and acute I50.813
      - secondary to left heart failure I50.814
    - specified NEC I50.89

Note: heart failure stages A, B, C, and D are based on the American College of Cardiology and American Heart Association stages of heart failure, which complement and should not be confused with the New York Heart Association Classification of Heart Failure, into Class I, Class II, Class III, and Class IV

- stage A Z91.89
- stage B (see also Failure, heart, by type as diastolic or systolic) I50.9
- stage C (see also Failure, heart, by type as diastolic or systolic) I50.9
- stage D (see also Failure, heart, by type as diastolic or systolic, chronic) I50.84
- systolic (congestive) (left ventricular) I50.20
  - acute (congestive) I50.21
    - and (on) chronic (congestive) I50.23
  - chronic (congestive) I50.22
    - and (on) acute (congestive) I50.23
  - combined with diastolic (congestive) I50.40
    - acute (congestive) I50.41
      - and (on) chronic (congestive) I50.43
    - chronic (congestive) I50.42
      - and (on) acute (congestive) I50.43
- thyrotoxic (see also Thyrotoxicosis) E05.90 [I43]
  - with
    - high output (see also Thyrotoxicosis) I50.83
    - thyroid storm E05.91 [I43]
      - high output (see also Thyrotoxicosis) I50.83
- valvular — see Endocarditis
- hepatic K72.90
  - with coma K72.91
  - acute or subacute K72.00
    - with coma K72.01
    - due to drugs K71.10
      - with coma K71.11
  - alcoholic (acute) (chronic) (subacute) K70.40
    - with coma K70.41
  - chronic K72.10
    - with coma K72.11
    - due to drugs (acute) (subacute) (chronic) K71.10
      - with coma K71.11
  - due to drugs (acute) (subacute) (chronic) K71.10
    - with coma K71.11

Failure, failed — *continued*
hepatic — *continued*
  postprocedural K91.82
hepatorenal K76.7
induction (of labor) O61.9
  abortion — *see* Abortion, attempted
  by
    oxytocic drugs O61.0
    prostaglandins O61.0
  instrumental O61.1
  mechanical O61.1
  medical O61.0
  specified NEC O61.8
  surgical O61.1
intubation during anesthesia T88.4 ☑
  in pregnancy O29.6- ☑
  labor and delivery O74.7
  postpartum, puerperal O89.6
involution, thymus (gland) E32.0
kidney (*see also* Disease, kidney, chronic) N19
  acute (*see also* Failure, renal, acute) N17.9
lactation (complete) O92.3
  partial O92.4
Leydig's cell, adult E29.1
liver — *see* Failure, hepatic
menstruation at puberty N91.0
mitral I05.8
myocardial, myocardium (*see also* Failure, heart) I50.9
  chronic (*see also* Failure, heart, congestive) I50.9
  congestive (*see also* Failure, heart, congestive) I50.9
orgasm (female) (psychogenic) F52.31
  male F52.32
ovarian (primary) E28.39
  iatrogenic E89.40
    asymptomatic E89.40
    symptomatic E89.41
  postprocedural (postablative) (postirradiation)
      (postsurgical) E89.40
    asymptomatic E89.40
    symptomatic E89.41
ovulation causing infertility N97.0
polyglandular, autoimmune E31.0
prosthetic joint implant — *see* Complications, joint
    prosthesis, mechanical, breakdown, by site
renal N19
  with
    tubular necrosis (acute) N17.0
  acute N17.9
    with
      cortical necrosis N17.1
      medullary necrosis N17.2
      tubular necrosis N17.0
    specified NEC N17.8
  chronic N18.9
    hypertensive — *see* Hypertension, kidney
  congenital P96.0
  end stage (chronic) N18.6
    due to hypertension I12.0
  following
    abortion — *see* Abortion by type complicated
        by specified condition NEC
    crushing T79.5 ☑
    ectopic or molar pregnancy O08.4
    labor and delivery (acute) O90.4
  hypertensive — *see* Hypertension, kidney
  postprocedural N99.0
respiration, respiratory J96.90
  with
    hypercapnia J96.92
    hypercarbia J96.02
    hypoxia J96.91
  acute J96.00
    with
      hypercapnia J96.02
      hypercarbia J96.02
      hypoxia J96.01
  center G93.89
  acute and (on) chronic J96.20
    with
      hypercapnia J96.22
      hypercarbia J96.22
      hypoxia J96.21
  chronic J96.10
    with
      hypercapnia J96.12
      hypercarbia J96.12
      hypoxia J96.11
  newborn P28.5

Failure, failed — *continued*
respiration, respiratory — *continued*
  postprocedural (acute) J95.821
    acute and chronic J95.822
  rotation
    cecum Q43.3
    colon Q43.3
    intestine Q43.3
    kidney Q63.2
  sedation (conscious) (moderate) during procedure
      T88.52 ☑
    history of Z92.83
  segmentation (*see also* Fusion)
    fingers — *see* Syndactylism, complex, fingers
    vertebra Q76.49
      with scoliosis Q76.3
  seminiferous tubule, adult E29.1
  senile (general) R54
  sexual arousal (male) F52.21
    female F52.22
  testicular endocrine function E29.1
  to thrive (child over 28 days old) R62.51
    adult R62.7
    newborn P92.6
  transplant T86.92
    bone T86.831
      marrow T86.02
    cornea T86.841
    heart T86.22
      with lung(s) T86.32
    intestine T86.851
    kidney T86.12
    liver T86.42
    lung(s) T86.811
      with heart T86.32
    pancreas T86.891
    skin (allograft) (autograft) T86.821
    specified organ or tissue NEC T86.891
    stem cell (peripheral blood) (umbilical cord) T86.5
  trial of labor (with subsequent cesarean delivery)
      O66.40
    following previous cesarean delivery O66.41
  tubal ligation N99.89
  urinary — *see* Disease, kidney, chronic
  vacuum extraction NOS (with subsequent cesarean
      delivery) O66.5
  vasectomy N99.89
  ventouse NOS (with subsequent cesarean delivery)
      O66.5
  ventricular (*see also* Failure, heart) I50.9
    left (*see also* Failure, heart, left) I50.1
      with rheumatic fever (conditions in I00)
        active I01.8
          with chorea I02.0
        inactive or quiescent (with chorea) I09.81
      rheumatic (chronic) (inactive) (with chorea)
          I09.81
        active or acute I01.8
          with chorea I02.0
    right — *see* Failure, heart, right
  vital centers, newborn P91.88
Fainting (fit) R55
Fallen arches — *see* Deformity, limb, flat foot
Falling, falls (repeated) R29.6
  any organ or part — *see* Prolapse
Fallopian
  insufflation Z31.41
  tube — *see* condition
Fallot's
  pentalogy Q21.8
  tetrad or tetralogy Q21.3
  triad or trilogy Q22.3
False (*see also* condition)
  croup J38.5
  joint — *see* Nonunion, fracture
  labor (pains) O47.9
    at or after 37 completed weeks of gestation O47.1
    before 37 completed weeks of gestation O47.0-
  passage, urethra (prostatic) N36.5
  pregnancy F45.8
Family, familial (*see also* condition)
  disruption Z63.8
    involving divorce or separation Z63.5
  Li-Fraumeni (syndrome) Z15.01
  planning advice Z30.09
  problem Z63.9
    specified NEC Z63.8
  retinoblastoma C69.2- ☑

Famine (effects of) T73.0 ☑
  edema — *see* Malnutrition, severe
Fanconi (-de Toni)(-Debré) **syndrome** E72.09
  with cystinosis E72.04
Fanconi's anemia (congenital pancytopenia) D61.09
Farber's disease or syndrome E75.29
Farcy A24.0
Farmer's
  lung J67.0
  skin L57.8
Farsightedness — *see* Hypermetropia
Fascia — *see* condition
Fasciculation R25.3
Fasciitis M72.9
  diffuse (eosinophilic) M35.4
  infective M72.8
    necrotizing M72.6
  necrotizing M72.6
  nodular M72.4
  perirenal (with ureteral obstruction) N13.5
    with infection N13.6
  plantar M72.2
  specified NEC M72.8
  traumatic (old) M72.8
    current — *code by* site under Sprain
Fascioliasis B66.3
Fasciolopsis, fasciolopsiasis (intestinal) B66.5
Fascioscapulohumeral myopathy G71.02
Fast pulse R00.0
Fat
  embolism — *see* Embolism, fat
  excessive (*see also* Obesity)
    in heart — *see* Degeneration, myocardial
  in stool R19.5
  localized (pad) E65
    heart — *see* Degeneration, myocardial
    knee M79.4
    retropatellar M79.4
  necrosis
    breast N64.1
    mesentery K65.4
    omentum K65.4
  pad E65
    knee M79.4
Fatigue R53.83
  auditory deafness — *see* Deafness
  chronic R53.82
  combat F43.0
  general R53.83
    psychogenic F48.8
  heat (transient) T67.6 ☑
  muscle M62.89
  myocardium — *see* Failure, heart
  neoplasm-related R53.0
  nervous, neurosis F48.8
  operational F48.8
  psychogenic (general) F48.8
  senile R54
  voice R49.8
Fatness — *see* Obesity
Fatty (*see also* condition)
  apron E65
  degeneration — *see* Degeneration, fatty
  heart (enlarged) — *see* Degeneration, myocardial
  liver NEC K76.0
    alcoholic K70.0
    nonalcoholic K76.0
  necrosis — *see* Degeneration, fatty
Fauces — *see* condition
Fauchard's disease (periodontitis) — *see* Periodontit
Faucitis J02.9
Favism (anemia) D55.0
Favus — *see* Dermatophytosis
Fazio-Londe disease or syndrome G12.1
Fear complex or reaction F40.9
Fear of — *see* Phobia
Feared complaint unfounded Z71.1
Febris, febrile (*see also* Fever)
  flava (*see also* Fever, yellow) A95.9
  melitensis A23.0
  pestis — *see* Plague
  recurrens — *see* Fever, relapsing
  rubra A38.9
Fecal
  incontinence R15.9
  smearing R15.1
  soiling R15.1

☑ **Additional Character Required** — **Refer to the Tabular List for Character Selection** ▽ **Subterms under main terms may continue to next column or pag**

Fecal — *continued*
  urgency R15.2
Fecalith (impaction) K56.41
  appendix K38.1
  congenital P76.8
Fede's disease K14.0
Feeble rapid pulse due to shock following injury
  T79.4 ☑
Feeble-minded F70
Feeding
  difficulties R63.3
  problem R63.3
    newborn P92.9
      specified NEC P92.8
    nonorganic (adult) — *see* Disorder, eating
Feeling (of)
  foreign body in throat R09.89
Feer's disease — *see* Poisoning, mercury
Feet — *see* condition
Feigned illness Z76.5
Feil-Klippel syndrome (brevicollis) Q76.1
Feinmesser's (hidrotic) **ectodermal dysplasia** Q82.4
Felinophobia F40.218
Felon (*see also* Cellulitis, digit)
  with lymphangitis — *see* Lymphangitis, acute, digit
Felty's syndrome M05.00
  ankle M05.07- ☑
  elbow M05.02- ☑
  foot joint M05.07- ☑
  hand joint M05.04- ☑
  hip M05.05- ☑
  knee M05.06- ☑
  multiple site M05.09
  shoulder M05.01- ☑
  vertebra — *see* Spondylitis, ankylosing
  wrist M05.03- ☑
Female genital cutting status — *see* Female genital
  mutilation status (FGM)
Female genital mutilation status (FGM) N90.810
  specified NEC N90.818
  type I (clitorectomy status) N90.811
  type II (clitorectomy with excision of labia minora sta-
    tus) N90.812
  type III (infibulation status) N90.813
  type IV N90.818
Femur, femoral — *see* condition
Fenestration, fenestrated (*see also* Imperfect, closure)
  aortico-pulmonary Q21.4
  cusps, heart valve NEC Q24.8
    pulmonary Q22.3
  pulmonic cusps Q22.3
Fernell's disease (aortic aneurysm) I71.9
Fertile eunuch syndrome E23.0
Fetid
  breath R19.6
  sweat L75.0
Fetishism F65.0
  transvestic F65.1
Fetus, fetal (*see also* condition)
  alcohol syndrome (dysmorphic) Q86.0
  compressus O31.0- ☑
  hydantoin syndrome Q86.1
  lung tissue P28.0
  papyraceous O31.0- ☑
Fever (inanition) (of unknown origin) (persistent) (with
  chills) (with rigor) R50.9
  abortus A23.1
  Aden (dengue) A90
  African tick-borne A68.1
  American
    mountain (tick) A93.2
    spotted A77.0
  aphthous B08.8
  arbovirus, arboviral A94
    hemorrhagic A94
    specified NEC A93.8
  Argentinian hemorrhagic A96.0
  Assam B55.0
  Australian Q A78
  Bangkok hemorrhagic A91
  Barmah forest A92.8
  Bartonella A44.0
  bilious, hemoglobinuric B50.8
  blackwater B50.8
  blister B00.1
  Bolivian hemorrhagic A96.1
  Bonvale dam T73.3 ☑

Fever — *continued*
  boutonneuse A77.1
  brain — *see* Encephalitis
  Brazilian purpuric A48.4
  breakbone A90
  Bullis A77.0
  Bunyamwera A92.8
  Burdwan B55.0
  Bwamba A92.8
  Cameroon — *see* Malaria
  Canton A75.9
  catarrhal (acute) J00
    chronic J31.0
  cat-scratch A28.1
  Central Asian hemorrhagic A98.0
  cerebral — *see* Encephalitis
  cerebrospinal meningococcal A39.0
  Chagres B50.9
  Chandipura A92.8
  Changuinola A93.1
  Charcot's (biliary) (hepatic) (intermittent) — *see* Calcu-
    lus, bile duct
  Chikungunya (viral) (hemorrhagic) A92.0
  Chitral A93.1
  Colombo — *see* Fever, paratyphoid
  Colorado tick (virus) A93.2
  congestive (remittent) — *see* Malaria
  Congo virus A98.0
  continued malarial B50.9
  Corsican — *see* Malaria
  Crimean-Congo hemorrhagic A98.0
  Cyprus — *see* Brucellosis
  dandy A90
  deer fly — *see* Tularemia
  dengue (virus) A90
    hemorrhagic A91
    sandfly A93.1
  desert B38.0
  drug induced R50.2
  due to
    conditions classified elsewhere R50.81
    heat T67.0 ☑
  enteric A01.00
  enteroviral exanthematous (Boston exanthem) A88.0
  ephemeral (of unknown origin) R50.9
  epidemic hemorrhagic A98.5
  erysipelatous — *see* Erysipelas
  estivo-autumnal (malarial) B50.9
  famine A75.0
  five day A79.0
  following delivery O86.4
  Fort Bragg A27.89
  gastroenteric A01.00
  gastromalarial — *see* Malaria
  Gibraltar — *see* Brucellosis
  glandular — *see* Mononucleosis, infectious
  Guama (viral) A92.8
  Haverhill A25.1
  hay (allergic) J30.1
    with asthma (bronchial) J45.909
      with
        exacerbation (acute) J45.901
        status asthmaticus J45.902
    due to
      allergen other than pollen J30.89
      pollen, any plant or tree J30.1
  heat (effects) T67.0 ☑
  hematuric, bilious B50.8
  hemoglobinuric (malarial) (bilious) B50.8
  hemorrhagic (arthropod-borne) NOS A94
    with renal syndrome A98.5
    arenaviral A96.9
      specified NEC A96.8
    Argentinian A96.0
    Bangkok A91
    Bolivian A96.1
    Central Asian A98.0
    Chikungunya A92.0
    Crimean-Congo A98.0
    dengue (virus) A91
    epidemic A98.5
    Junin (virus) A96.0
    Korean A98.5
    Kyasanur forest A98.2
    Machupo (virus) A96.1
    mite-borne A93.8
    mosquito-borne A92.8
    Omsk A98.1

Fever — *continued*
  hemorrhagic — *continued*
    Philippine A91
    Russian A98.5
    Singapore A91
    Southeast Asia A91
    Thailand A91
    tick-borne NEC A93.8
    viral A99
      specified NEC A98.8
  hepatic — *see* Cholecystitis
  herpetic — *see* Herpes
  icterohemorrhagic A27.0
  Indiana A93.8
  infective B99.9
    specified NEC B99.8
  intermittent (bilious) (*see also* Malaria)
    of unknown origin R50.9
    pernicious B50.9
  iodide R50.2
  Japanese river A75.3
  jungle (*see also* Malaria)
    yellow A95.0
  Junin (virus) hemorrhagic A96.0
  Katayama B65.2
  kedani A75.3
  Kenya (tick) A77.1
  Kew Garden A79.1
  Korean hemorrhagic A98.5
  Lassa A96.2
  Lone Star A77.0
  Machupo (virus) hemorrhagic A96.1
  malaria, malarial — *see* Malaria
  Malta A23.9
  Marseilles A77.1
  marsh — *see* Malaria
  Mayaro (viral) A92.8
  Mediterranean (*see also* Brucellosis) A23.9
    familial M04.1
    tick A77.1
  meningeal — *see* Meningitis
  Meuse A79.0
  Mexican A75.2
  mianeh A68.1
  miasmatic — *see* Malaria
  mosquito-borne (viral) A92.9
    hemorrhagic A92.8
  mountain (*see also* Brucellosis)
    meaning Rocky Mountain spotted fever A77.0
    tick (American) (Colorado) (viral) A93.2
  Mucambo (viral) A92.8
  mud A27.9
  Neapolitan — *see* Brucellosis
  neutropenic D70.9
  newborn P81.9
    environmental P81.0
  Nine-Mile A78
  non-exanthematous tick A93.2
  North Asian tick-borne A77.2
  Omsk hemorrhagic A98.1
  O'nyong-nyong (viral) A92.1
  Oropouche (viral) A93.0
  Oroya A44.0
  paludal — *see* Malaria
  Panama (malarial) B50.9
  Pappataci A93.1
  paratyphoid A01.4
    A A01.1
    B A01.2
    C A01.3
  parrot A70
  periodic (Mediterranean) M04.1
  persistent (of unknown origin) R50.9
  petechial A39.0
  pharyngoconjunctival B30.2
  Philippine hemorrhagic A91
  phlebotomus A93.1
  Piry (virus) A93.8
  Pixuna (viral) A92.8
  Plasmodium ovale B53.0
  polioviral (nonparalytic) A80.4
  Pontiac A48.2
  postimmunization R50.83
  postoperative R50.82
    due to infection T81.40 ☑
  posttransfusion R50.84
  postvaccination R50.83
  presenting with conditions classified elsewhere R50.81

☞ Subterms under main terms may continue to next column or page ☑ Additional Character Required — Refer to the Tabular List for Character Selection 141

Fecal — Fever

Fever — *continued*
 pretibial A27.89
 puerperal O86.4
 Q A78
 quadrilateral A78
 quartan (malaria) B52.9
 Queensland (coastal) (tick) A77.3
 quintan A79.0
 rabbit — *see* Tularemia
 rat-bite A25.9
  due to
   Spirillum A25.0
   Streptobacillus moniliformis A25.1
 recurrent — *see* Fever, relapsing
 relapsing (Borrelia) A68.9
  Carter's (Asiatic) A68.1
  Dutton's (West African) A68.1
  Koch's A68.9
  louse-borne A68.0
  Novy's
   louse-borne A68.0
   tick-borne A68.1
  Obermeyer's (European) A68.0
  tick-borne A68.1
 remittent (bilious) (congestive) (gastric) — *see* Malaria
 rheumatic (active) (acute) (chronic) (subacute) I00
  with central nervous system involvement I02.9
  active with heart involvement — *see* category I01 ☑
  inactive or quiescent with
   cardiac hypertrophy I09.89
   carditis I09.9
   endocarditis I09.1
    aortic (valve) I06.9
     with mitral (valve) disease I08.0
    mitral (valve) I05.9
     with aortic (valve) disease I08.0
    pulmonary (valve) I09.89
    tricuspid (valve) I07.8
   heart disease NEC I09.89
   heart failure (congestive) (conditions in category I50.) I09.81
   left ventricular failure (conditions in I50.1-I50.4-) I09.81
   myocarditis, myocardial degeneration (conditions in I51.4) I09.0
   pancarditis I09.9
   pericarditis I09.2
 Rift Valley (viral) A92.4
 Rocky Mountain spotted A77.0
 rose J30.1
 Ross River B33.1
 Russian hemorrhagic A98.5
 San Joaquin (Valley) B38.0
 sandfly A93.1
 Sao Paulo A77.0
 scarlet A38.9
 seven day (leptospirosis) (autumnal) (Japanese) A27.89
  dengue A90
 shin-bone A79.0
 Singapore hemorrhagic A91
 solar A90
 Songo A98.5
 sore B00.1
 South African tick-bite A68.1
 Southeast Asia hemorrhagic A91
 spinal — *see* Meningitis
 spirillary A25.0
 splenic — *see* Anthrax
 spotted A77.9
  American A77.0
  Brazilian A77.0
  cerebrospinal meningitis A39.0
  Colombian A77.0
  due to Rickettsia
   australis A77.3
   conorii A77.1
   rickettsii A77.0
   sibirica A77.2
   specified type NEC A77.8
  Ehrlichiosis A77.40
   due to
    E. chafeensis A77.41
    specified organism NEC A77.49
  Rocky Mountain A77.0
 steroid R50.2
 streptobacillary A25.1
 subtertian B50.9
 Sumatran mite A75.3

Fever — *continued*
 sun A90
 swamp A27.9
 swine A02.8
 sylvatic, yellow A95.0
 Tahyna B33.8
 tertian — *see* Malaria, tertian
 Thailand hemorrhagic A91
 thermic T67.0 ☑
 three-day A93.1
 tick
  American mountain A93.2
  Colorado A93.2
  Kemerovo A93.8
  Mediterranean A77.1
  mountain A93.2
  nonexanthematous A93.2
  Quaranfil A93.8
 tick-bite NEC A93.8
 tick-borne (hemorrhagic) NEC A93.8
 trench A79.0
 tsutsugamushi A75.3
 typhogastric A01.00
 typhoid (abortive) (hemorrhagic) (intermittent) (malignant) A01.00
  complicated by
   arthritis A01.04
   heart involvement A01.02
   meningitis A01.01
   osteomyelitis A01.05
   pneumonia A01.03
   specified NEC A01.09
 typhomalarial — *see* Malaria
 typhus — *see* Typhus (fever)
 undulant — *see* Brucellosis
 unknown origin R50.9
 uveoparotid D86.89
 valley B38.0
 Venezuelan equine A92.2
 vesicular stomatitis A93.8
 viral hemorrhagic — *see* Fever, hemorrhagic, by type of virus
 Volhynian A79.0
 Wesselsbron (viral) A92.8
 West
  African B50.8
  Nile (viral) A92.30
   with
    complications NEC A92.39
    cranial nerve disorders A92.32
    encephalitis A92.31
    encephalomyelitis A92.31
    neurologic manifestation NEC A92.32
    optic neuritis A92.32
    polyradiculitis A92.32
 Whitmore's — *see* Melioidosis
 Wolhynian A79.0
 worm B83.9
 yellow A95.9
  jungle A95.0
  sylvatic A95.0
  urban A95.1
 Zika virus A92.5
Fibrillation
 atrial or auricular (established) I48.91
  chronic I48.2
  paroxysmal I48.0
  permanent I48.2
  persistent I48.1
 cardiac I49.8
 heart I49.8
 muscular M62.89
 ventricular I49.01
Fibrin
 ball or bodies, pleural (sac) J94.1
 chamber, anterior (eye) (gelatinous exudate) — *see* Iridocyclitis, acute
Fibrinogenolysis — *see* Fibrinolysis
Fibrinogenopenia D68.8
 acquired D65
 congenital D68.2
Fibrinolysis (hemorrhagic) (acquired) D65
 antepartum hemorrhage — *see* Hemorrhage, antepartum, with coagulation defect
 following
  abortion — *see* Abortion by type complicated by hemorrhage
  ectopic or molar pregnancy O08.1

Fibrinolysis — *continued*
 intrapartum O67.0
 newborn, transient P60
 postpartum O72.3
Fibrinopenia (hereditary) D68.2
 acquired D68.4
Fibrinopurulent — *see* condition
Fibrinous — *see* condition
Fibroadenoma
 cellular intracanalicular D24- ☑
 giant D24- ☑
 intracanalicular
  cellular D24- ☑
  giant D24- ☑
  specified site — *see* Neoplasm, benign, by site
  unspecified site D24- ☑
 juvenile D24- ☑
 pericanalicular
  specified site — *see* Neoplasm, benign, by site
  unspecified site D24- ☑
 phyllodes D24- ☑
 prostate D29.1
 specified site NEC — *see* Neoplasm, benign, by site
 unspecified site D24- ☑
Fibroadenosis, breast (chronic) (cystic) (diffuse) (periodic) (segmental) N60.2- ☑
Fibroangioma (*see also* Neoplasm, benign, by site)
 juvenile
  specified site — *see* Neoplasm, benign, by site
  unspecified site D10.6
Fibrochondrosarcoma — *see* Neoplasm, cartilage, malignant
Fibrocystic
 disease (*see also* Fibrosis, cystic)
  breast — *see* Mastopathy, cystic
  jaw M27.49
  kidney (congenital) Q61.8
  liver Q44.6
  pancreas E84.9
 kidney (congenital) Q61.8
Fibrodysplasia ossificans progressiva — *see* Myositis ossificans, progressiva
Fibroelastosis (cordis) (endocardial) (endomyocardial) I42.4
Fibroid (tumor) (*see also* Neoplasm, connective tissue, benign)
 disease, lung (chronic) — *see* Fibrosis, lung
 heart (disease) — *see* Myocarditis
 in pregnancy or childbirth O34.1- ☑
  causing obstructed labor O65.5
 induration, lung (chronic) — *see* Fibrosis, lung
 lung — *see* Fibrosis, lung
 pneumonia (chronic) — *see* Fibrosis, lung
 uterus (*see also* Leiomyoma, uterus) D25.9
Fibrolipoma — *see* Lipoma
Fibroliposarcoma — *see* Neoplasm, connective tissue, malignant
Fibroma (*see also* Neoplasm, connective tissue, benign)
 ameloblastic — *see* Cyst, calcifying odontogenic
 bone (nonossifying) — *see* Disorder, bone, specified type NEC
  ossifying — *see* Neoplasm, bone, benign
 cementifying — *see* Neoplasm, bone, benign
 chondromyxoid — *see* Neoplasm, bone, benign
 desmoplastic — *see* Neoplasm, connective tissue, uncertain behavior
 durum — *see* Neoplasm, connective tissue, benign
 fascial — *see* Neoplasm, connective tissue, benign
 invasive — *see* Neoplasm, connective tissue, uncertain behavior
 molle — *see* Lipoma
 myxoid — *see* Neoplasm, connective tissue, benign
 nasopharynx, nasopharyngeal (juvenile) D10.6
 nonosteogenic (nonossifying) — *see* Dysplasia, fibrous
 odontogenic (central) — *see* Cyst, calcifying odontogenic
 ossifying — *see* Neoplasm, bone, benign
 periosteal — *see* Neoplasm, bone, benign
 soft — *see* Lipoma
Fibromatosis M72.9
 abdominal — *see* Neoplasm, connective tissue, uncertain behavior
 aggressive — *see* Neoplasm, connective tissue, uncertain behavior
 congenital generalized — *see* Neoplasm, connective tissue, uncertain behavior
 Dupuytren's M72.0

Fibromatosis — *continued*
  gingival K06.1
  palmar (fascial) M72.0
  plantar (fascial) M72.2
  pseudosarcomatous (proliferative) (subcutaneous)
    M72.4
  retroperitoneal D48.3
  specified NEC M72.8
Fibromyalgia M79.7
Fibromyoma (*see also* Neoplasm, connective tissue, benign)
  uterus (corpus) (*see also* Leiomyoma, uterus)
    in pregnancy or childbirth — *see* Fibroid, in preg-
      nancy or childbirth
      causing obstructed labor O65.5
Fibromyositis M79.7
Fibromyxolipoma D17.9
Fibromyxoma — *see* Neoplasm, connective tissue, benign
Fibromyxosarcoma — *see* Neoplasm, connective tissue,
  malignant
Fibro-odontoma, ameloblastic — *see* Cyst, calcifying
  odontogenic
Fibro-osteoma — *see* Neoplasm, bone, benign
Fibroplasia, retrolental H35.17- ☑
Fibropurulent — *see* condition
Fibrosarcoma (*see also* Neoplasm, connective tissue,
  malignant)
  ameloblastic C41.1
    upper jaw (bone) C41.0
  congenital — *see* Neoplasm, connective tissue, malig-
    nant
  fascial — *see* Neoplasm, connective tissue, malignant
  infantile — *see* Neoplasm, connective tissue, malignant
  odontogenic C41.1
    upper jaw (bone) C41.0
  periosteal — *see* Neoplasm, bone, malignant
Fibrosclerosis
  breast N60.3- ☑
  multifocal M35.5
  penis (corpora cavernosa) N48.6
Fibrosis, fibrotic
  adrenal (gland) E27.8
  amnion O41.8X- ☑
  anal papillae K62.89
  arteriocapillary — *see* Arteriosclerosis
  bladder N32.89
    interstitial — *see* Cystitis, chronic, interstitial
    localized submucosal — *see* Cystitis, chronic, inter-
      stitial
    panmural — *see* Cystitis, chronic, interstitial
  breast — *see* Fibrosclerosis, breast
  capillary (*see also* Arteriosclerosis) I70.90
    lung (chronic) — *see* Fibrosis, lung
  cardiac — *see* Myocarditis
  cervix N88.8
  chorion O41.8X- ☑
  corpus cavernosum (sclerosing) N48.6
  cystic (of pancreas) E84.9
    with
      distal intestinal obstruction syndrome E84.19
      fecal impaction E84.19
      intestinal manifestations NEC E84.19
      pulmonary manifestations E84.0
      specified manifestations NEC E84.8
  due to device, implant or graft (*see also* Complications,
    by site and type, specified NEC) T85.828 ☑
    arterial graft NEC T82.828 ☑
    breast (implant) T85.828 ☑
    catheter NEC T85.828 ☑
      dialysis (renal) T82.828 ☑
        intraperitoneal T85.828 ☑
      infusion NEC T82.828 ☑
        spinal (epidural) (subdural) T85.820 ☑
      urinary (indwelling) T83.82 ☑
    electronic (electrode) (pulse generator) (stimulator)
      bone T84.82 ☑
      cardiac T82.827 ☑
      nervous system (brain) (peripheral nerve) (spinal)
        T85.820 ☑
      urinary T83.82 ☑
    fixation, internal (orthopedic) NEC T84.82 ☑
    gastrointestinal (bile duct) (esophagus) T85.828 ☑
    genital NEC T83.82 ☑
    heart NEC T82.827 ☑
    joint prosthesis T84.82 ☑

Fibrosis, fibrotic — *continued*
  due to device, implant or graft (*see also* Complications,
    by site and type, specified) — *continued*
    ocular (corneal graft) (orbital implant) NEC
      T85.828 ☑
    orthopedic NEC T84.82 ☑
    specified NEC T85.828 ☑
    urinary NEC T83.82 ☑
    vascular NEC T82.828 ☑
    ventricular intracranial shunt T85.820 ☑
  ejaculatory duct N50.89
  endocardium — *see* Endocarditis
  endomyocardial (tropical) I42.3
  epididymis N50.89
  eye muscle — *see* Strabismus, mechanical
  heart — *see* Myocarditis
  hepatic — *see* Fibrosis, liver
  hepatolienal (portal hypertension) K76.6
  hepatosplenic (portal hypertension) K76.6
  infrapatellar fat pad M79.4
  intrascrotal N50.89
  kidney N26.9
  liver K74.0
    with sclerosis K74.2
    alcoholic K70.2
  lung (atrophic) (chronic) (confluent) (massive) (perialve-
    olar) (peribronchial) J84.10
    with
      anthracosilicosis J60
      anthracosis J60
      asbestosis J61
      bagassosis J67.1
      bauxite J63.1
      berylliosis J63.2
      byssinosis J66.0
      calcicosis J62.8
      chalicosis J62.8
      dust reticulation J64
      farmer's lung J67.0
      ganister disease J62.8
      graphite J63.3
      pneumoconiosis NOS J64
      siderosis J63.4
      silicosis J62.8
    capillary J84.10
    congenital P27.8
    diffuse (idiopathic) J84.10
      chemicals, gases, fumes or vapors (inhalation)
        J68.4
      interstitial J84.10
        acute J84.114
      talc J62.0
    following radiation J70.1
    idiopathic J84.112
    postinflammatory J84.10
    silicotic J62.8
    tuberculous — *see* Tuberculosis, pulmonary
  lymphatic gland I89.8
  median bar — *see* Hyperplasia, prostate
  mediastinum (idiopathic) J98.59
  meninges G96.19
  myocardium, myocardial — *see* Myocarditis
  ovary N83.8
  oviduct N83.8
  pancreas K86.89
  penis NEC N48.6
  pericardium I31.0
  perineum, in pregnancy or childbirth O34.7- ☑
    causing obstructed labor O65.5
  pleura J94.1
  popliteal fat pad M79.4
  prostate (chronic) — *see* Hyperplasia, prostate
  pulmonary (*see also* Fibrosis, lung) J84.10
    congenital P27.8
    idiopathic J84.112
  rectal sphincter K62.89
  retroperitoneal, idiopathic (with ureteral obstruction)
    N13.5
    with infection N13.6
  sclerosing mesenteric (idiopathic) K65.4
  scrotum N50.89
  seminal vesicle N50.89
  senile R54
  skin L90.5
  spermatic cord N50.89
  spleen D73.89
    in schistosomiasis (bilharziasis) B65.9 [D77]
  subepidermal nodular — *see* Neoplasm, skin, benign

Fibrosis, fibrotic — *continued*
  submucous (oral) (tongue) K13.5
  testis N44.8
    chronic, due to syphilis A52.76
  thymus (gland) E32.8
  tongue, submucous K13.5
  tunica vaginalis N50.89
  uterus (non-neoplastic) N85.8
  vagina N89.8
  valve, heart — *see* Endocarditis
  vas deferens N50.89
  vein I87.8
Fibrositis (periarticular) M79.7
  nodular, chronic (Jaccoud's) (rheumatoid) — *see*
    Arthropathy, postrheumatic, chronic
Fibrothorax J94.1
Fibrotic — *see* Fibrosis
Fibrous — *see* condition
Fibroxanthoma (*see also* Neoplasm, connective tissue,
  benign)
  atypical — *see* Neoplasm, connective tissue, uncertain
    behavior
  malignant — *see* Neoplasm, connective tissue, malig-
    nant
Fibroxanthosarcoma — *see* Neoplasm, connective tissue, malignant
Fiedler's
  disease (icterohemorrhagic leptospirosis) A27.0
  myocarditis (acute) I40.1
Fifth disease B08.3
  venereal A55
Filaria, filarial, filariasis — *see* Infestation, filarial
Filatov's disease — *see* Mononucleosis, infectious
File-cutter's disease — *see* Poisoning, lead
Filling defect
  biliary tract R93.2
  bladder R93.41
  duodenum R93.3
  gallbladder R93.2
  gastrointestinal tract R93.3
  intestine R93.3
  kidney R93.42- ☑
  stomach R93.3
  ureter R93.41
  urinary organs, specified NEC R93.49
Fimbrial cyst Q50.4
Financial problem affecting care NOS Z59.9
  bankruptcy Z59.8
  foreclosure on loan Z59.8
Findings, abnormal, inconclusive, without diagnosis
  (*see also* Abnormal)
  17-ketosteroids, elevated R82.5
  acetonuria R82.4
  alcohol in blood R78.0
  anisocytosis R71.8
  antenatal screening of mother O28.9
    biochemical O28.1
    chromosomal O28.5
    cytological O28.2
    genetic O28.5
    hematological O28.0
    radiological O28.4
    specified NEC O28.8
    ultrasonic O28.3
  antibody titer, elevated R76.0
  anticardiolipin antibody R76.0
  antiphosphatidylglycerol antibody R76.0
  antiphosphatidylinositol antibody R76.0
  antiphosphatidylserine antibody R76.0
  antiphospholipid antibody R76.0
  bacteriuria R82.71
  bicarbonate E87.8
  bile in urine R82.2
  blood sugar R73.09
    high R73.9
    low (transient) E16.2
  body fluid or substance, specified NEC R88.8
  casts, urine R82.998
  catecholamines R82.5
  cells, urine R82.998
  chloride E87.8
  cholesterol E78.9
    high E78.00
      with high triglycerides E78.2
  chyluria R82.0
  cloudy
    dialysis effluent R88.0
    urine R82.90

Findings, abnormal, inconclusive, without diagnosis
— continued
creatinine clearance R94.4
crystals, urine R82.998
culture
  blood R78.81
  positive — see Positive, culture
echocardiogram R93.1
electrolyte level, urinary R82.998
function study NEC R94.8
  bladder R94.8
  endocrine NEC R94.7
    thyroid R94.6
  kidney R94.4
  liver R94.5
  pancreas R94.8
  placenta R94.8
  pulmonary R94.2
  spleen R94.8
gallbladder, nonvisualization R93.2
glucose (tolerance test) (non-fasting) R73.09
glycosuria R81
heart
  shadow R93.1
  sounds R01.2
hematinuria R82.3
hematocrit drop (precipitous) R71.0
hemoglobinuria R82.3
human papillomavirus (HPV) DNA test positive
  cervix
    high risk R87.810
    low risk R87.820
  vagina
    high risk R87.811
    low risk R87.821
  in blood (of substance not normally found in blood)
    R78.9
  addictive drug NEC R78.4
  alcohol (excessive level) R78.0
  cocaine R78.2
  hallucinogen R78.3
  heavy metals (abnormal level) R78.79
  lead R78.71
  lithium (abnormal level) R78.89
  opiate drug R78.1
  psychotropic drug R78.5
  specified substance NEC R78.89
  steroid agent R78.6
indoleacetic acid, elevated R82.5
ketonuria R82.4
lactic acid dehydrogenase (LDH) R74.0
liver function test R79.89
mammogram NEC R92.8
  calcification (calculus) R92.1
  inconclusive result (due to dense breasts) R92.2
  microcalcification R92.0
mediastinal shift R93.89
melanin, urine R82.998
myoglobinuria R82.1
neonatal screening P09
nonvisualization of gallbladder R93.2
odor of urine NOS R82.90
Papanicolaou cervix R87.619
  non-atypical endometrial cells R87.618
pneumoencephalogram R93.0
poikilocytosis R71.8
potassium (deficiency) E87.6
  excess E87.5
PPD R76.11
radiologic (X-ray) R93.89
  abdomen R93.5
  biliary tract R93.2
  breast R92.8
  gastrointestinal tract R93.3
  genitourinary organs R93.89
  head R93.0
  inconclusive due to excess body fat of patient R93.9
  intrathoracic organs NEC R93.1
  placenta R93.89
  retroperitoneum R93.5
  skin R93.89
  skull R93.0
  subcutaneous tissue R93.89
  testis R93.81- ☑
red blood cell (count) (morphology) (sickling) (volume)
    R71.8
scan NEC R94.8
  bladder R94.8
  bone R94.8

Findings, abnormal, inconclusive, without diagnosis
— continued
scan — continued
  kidney R94.4
  liver R93.2
  lung R94.2
  pancreas R94.8
  placental R94.8
  spleen R94.8
  thyroid R94.6
sedimentation rate, elevated R70.0
SGOT R74.0
SGPT R74.0
sodium (deficiency) E87.1
  excess E87.0
specified body fluid NEC R88.8
stress test R94.39
testis R93.81- ☑
thyroid (function) (metabolic rate) (scan) (uptake) R94.6
transaminase (level) R74.0
triglycerides E78.9
  high E78.1
    with high cholesterol E78.2
tuberculin skin test (without active tuberculosis) R76.11
urine R82.90
  acetone R82.4
  bacteria R82.71
  bile R82.2
  casts or cells R82.998
  chyle R82.0
  culture positive R82.79
  glucose R81
  hemoglobin R82.3
  ketone R82.4
  sugar R81
vanillylmandelic acid (VMA), elevated R82.5
vectorcardiogram (VCG) R94.39
ventriculogram R93.0
white blood cell (count) (differential) (morphology)
    D72.9
xerography R92.8
Finger — see condition
Fire, Saint Anthony's — see Erysipelas
Fire-setting
  pathological (compulsive) F63.1
Fish hook stomach K31.89
Fishmeal-worker's lung J67.8
Fissure, fissured
  anus, anal K60.2
    acute K60.0
    chronic K60.1
    congenital Q43.8
  ear, lobule, congenital Q17.8
  epiglottis (congenital) Q31.8
  larynx J38.7
    congenital Q31.8
  lip K13.0
    congenital — see Cleft, lip
  nipple N64.0
    associated with
      lactation O92.13
      pregnancy O92.11- ☑
      puerperium O92.12
  nose Q30.2
  palate (congenital) — see Cleft, palate
  skin R23.4
  spine (congenital) (see also Spina bifida)
    with hydrocephalus — see Spina bifida, by site, with
      hydrocephalus
  tongue (acquired) K14.5
    congenital Q38.3
Fistula (cutaneous) L98.8
  abdomen (wall) K63.2
    bladder N32.2
    intestine NEC K63.2
    ureter N28.89
    uterus N82.5
  abdominorectal K63.2
  abdominosigmoidal K63.2
  abdominothoracic J86.0
  abdominouterine N82.5
    congenital Q51.7
  abdominovesical N32.2
  accessory sinuses — see Sinusitis
  actinomycotic — see Actinomycosis
  alveolar antrum — see Sinusitis, maxillary
  alveolar process K04.6
  anorectal K60.5

Fistula — continued
antrobuccal — see Sinusitis, maxillary
antrum — see Sinusitis, maxillary
anus, anal (recurrent) (infectional) K60.3
  congenital Q43.6
    with absence, atresia and stenosis Q42.2
  tuberculous A18.32
aorta-duodenal I77.2
appendix, appendicular K38.3
arteriovenous (acquired) (nonruptured) I77.0
  brain I67.1
    congenital Q28.2
      ruptured I60.8
    ruptured I60.8
  cerebral — see Fistula, arteriovenous, brain
  congenital (peripheral) (see also Malformation, arte-
    riovenous)
    brain Q28.2
      ruptured I60.8
    coronary Q24.5
    pulmonary Q25.72
  coronary I25.41
    congenital Q24.5
  pulmonary I28.0
    congenital Q25.72
  surgically created (for dialysis) Z99.2
    complication — see Complication, arteriovenous
      fistula, surgically created
  traumatic — see Injury, blood vessel
artery I77.2
aural (mastoid) — see Mastoiditis, chronic
auricle (see also Disorder, pinna, specified type NEC)
  congenital Q18.1
Bartholin's gland N82.8
bile duct (common) (hepatic) K83.3
  with calculus, stones — see Calculus, bile duct
biliary (tract) — see Fistula, bile duct
bladder (sphincter) NEC (see also Fistula, vesico-) N32.2
  into seminal vesicle N32.2
bone (see also Disorder, bone, specified type NEC)
  with osteomyelitis, chronic — see Osteomyelitis,
    chronic, with draining sinus
brain G93.89
  arteriovenous (acquired) I67.1
    congenital Q28.2
branchial (cleft) Q18.0
branchiogenous Q18.0
breast N61.0
  puerperal, postpartum or gestational, due to mastitis
    (purulent) — see Mastitis, obstetric, purulent
bronchial J86.0
bronchocutaneous, bronchomediastinal, bronchopleural, bronchopleuromediastinal (infective) J86.0
  tuberculous NEC A15.5
bronchoesophageal J86.0
  congenital Q39.2
    with atresia of esophagus Q39.1
bronchovisceral J86.0
buccal cavity (infective) K12.2
cecosigmoidal K63.2
cecum K63.2
cerebrospinal (fluid) G96.0
cervical, lateral Q18.1
cervicoaural Q18.1
cervicosigmoidal N82.4
cervicovesical N82.1
cervix N82.8
chest (wall) J86.0
cholecystenteric — see Fistula, gallbladder
cholecystocolic — see Fistula, gallbladder
cholecystocolonic — see Fistula, gallbladder
cholecystoduodenal — see Fistula, gallbladder
cholecystogastric — see Fistula, gallbladder
cholecystointestinal — see Fistula, gallbladder
choledochoduodenal — see Fistula, bile duct
cholocolic K82.3
coccyx — see Sinus, pilonidal
colon K63.2
colostomy K94.09
common duct — see Fistula, bile duct
congenital, site not listed — see Anomaly, by site
coronary, arteriovenous I25.41
  congenital Q24.5
costal region J86.0
cul-de-sac, Douglas' N82.8
cystic duct (see also Fistula, gallbladder)
  congenital Q44.5
dental K04.6

☑ **Additional Character Required — Refer to the Tabular List for Character Selection**
▽ **Subterms under main terms may continue to next column or pag**

Fistula — *continued*
  diaphragm J86.0
  duodenum K31.6
  ear (external) (canal) — *see* Disorder, ear, external,
      specified type NEC
  enterocolic K63.2
  enterocutaneous K63.2
  enterouterine N82.4
      congenital Q51.7
  enterovaginal N82.4
      congenital Q52.2
      large intestine N82.3
      small intestine N82.2
  enterovesical N32.1
  epididymis N50.89
      tuberculous A18.15
  esophagobronchial J86.0
      congenital Q39.2
          with atresia of esophagus Q39.1
  esophagocutaneous K22.8
  esophagopleural-cutaneous J86.0
  esophagotracheal J86.0
      congenital Q39.2
          with atresia of esophagus Q39.1
  esophagus K22.8
      congenital Q39.2
          with atresia of esophagus Q39.1
  ethmoid — *see* Sinusitis, ethmoidal
  eyeball (cornea) (sclera) — *see* Disorder, globe, hy-
      potony
  eyelid H01.8
  fallopian tube, external N82.5
  fecal K63.2
      congenital Q43.6
  from periapical abscess K04.6
  frontal sinus — *see* Sinusitis, frontal
  gallbladder K82.3
      with calculus, cholelithiasis, stones — *see* Calculus,
          gallbladder
  gastric K31.6
  gastrocolic K31.6
      congenital Q40.2
      tuberculous A18.32
  gastroenterocolic K31.6
  gastroesophageal K31.6
  gastrojejunal K31.6
  gastrojejunocolic K31.6
  genital tract (female) N82.9
      specified NEC N82.8
      to intestine NEC N82.4
      to skin N82.5
  hepatic artery-portal vein, congenital Q26.6
  hepatopleural J86.0
  hepatopulmonary J86.0
  ileorectal or ileosigmoidal K63.2
  ileovaginal N82.2
  ileovesical N32.1
  ileum K63.2
  in ano K60.3
      tuberculous A18.32
  inner ear (labyrinth) — *see* subcategory H83.1 ☑
  intestine NEC K63.2
  intestinocolonic (abdominal) K63.2
  intestinoureteral N28.89
  intestinouterine N82.4
  intestinovaginal N82.4
      large intestine N82.3
      small intestine N82.2
  intestinovesical N32.1
  ischiorectal (fossa) K61.39
  jejunum K63.2
  joint M25.10
      ankle M25.17- ☑
      elbow M25.12- ☑
      foot joint M25.17- ☑
      hand joint M25.14- ☑
      hip M25.15- ☑
      knee M25.16- ☑
      shoulder M25.11- ☑
      specified joint NEC M25.18
      tuberculous — *see* Tuberculosis, joint
      vertebrae M25.18
      wrist M25.13- ☑
  kidney N28.89
  labium (majus) (minus) N82.8
  labyrinth — *see* subcategory H83.1 ☑
  lacrimal (gland) (sac) H04.61- ☑
  lacrimonasal duct — *see* Fistula, lacrimal

Fistula — *continued*
  laryngotracheal, congenital Q34.8
  larynx J38.7
  lip K13.0
      congenital Q38.0
  lumbar, tuberculous A18.01
  lung J86.0
  lymphatic I89.8
  mammary (gland) N61.0
  mastoid (process) (region) — *see* Mastoiditis, chronic
  maxillary J32.0
  medial, face and neck Q18.8
  mediastinal J86.0
  mediastinobronchial J86.0
  mediastinocutaneous J86.0
  middle ear — *see* subcategory H74.8 ☑
  mouth K12.2
  nasal J34.89
      sinus — *see* Sinusitis
  nasopharynx J39.2
  nipple N64.0
  nose J34.89
  oral (cutaneous) K12.2
      maxillary J32.0
      nasal (with cleft palate) — *see* Cleft, palate
  orbit, orbital — *see* Disorder, orbit, specified type NEC
  oroantral J32.0
  oviduct, external N82.5
  palate (hard) M27.8
  pancreatic K86.89
  pancreaticoduodenal K86.89
  parotid (gland) K11.4
      region K12.2
  penis N48.89
  perianal K60.3
  pericardium (pleura) (sac) — *see* Pericarditis
  pericecal K63.2
  perineorectal K60.4
  perineosigmoidal K63.2
  perineum, perineal (with urethral involvement) NEC
      N36.0
      tuberculous A18.13
      ureter N28.89
  perirectal K60.4
      tuberculous A18.32
  peritoneum K65.9
  pharyngoesophageal J39.2
  pharynx J39.2
      branchial cleft (congenital) Q18.0
  pilonidal (infected) (rectum) — *see* Sinus, pilonidal
  pleura, pleural, pleurocutaneous, pleuroperitoneal
      J86.0
      tuberculous NEC A15.6
  pleuropericardial I31.8
  portal vein-hepatic artery, congenital Q26.6
  postauricular H70.81- ☑
  postoperative, persistent T81.83 ☑
      specified site — *see* Fistula, by site
  preauricular (congenital) Q18.1
  prostate N42.89
  pulmonary J86.0
      arteriovenous I28.0
          congenital Q25.72
      tuberculous — *see* Tuberculosis, pulmonary
  pulmonoperitoneal J86.0
  rectolabial N82.4
  rectosigmoid (intercommunicating) K63.2
  rectoureteral N28.89
  rectourethral N36.0
      congenital Q64.73
  rectouterine N82.4
      congenital Q51.7
  rectovaginal N82.3
      congenital Q52.2
      tuberculous A18.18
  rectovesical N32.1
      congenital Q64.79
  rectovesicovaginal N82.3
  rectovulval N82.4
      congenital Q52.79
  rectum (to skin) K60.4
      congenital Q43.6
          with absence, atresia and stenosis Q42.0
      tuberculous A18.32
  renal N28.89
  retroauricular — *see* Fistula, postauricular
  salivary duct or gland (any) K11.4
      congenital Q38.4

Fistula — *continued*
  scrotum (urinary) N50.89
      tuberculous A18.15
  semicircular canals — *see* subcategory H83.1 ☑
  sigmoid K63.2
      to bladder N32.1
  sinus — *see* Sinusitis
  skin L98.8
      to genital tract (female) N82.5
  splenocolic D73.89
  stercoral K63.2
  stomach K31.6
  sublingual gland K11.4
  submandibular gland K11.4
  submaxillary (gland) K11.4
      region K12.2
  thoracic J86.0
      duct I89.8
  thoracoabdominal J86.0
  thoracogastric J86.0
  thoracointestinal J86.0
  thorax J86.0
  thyroglossal duct Q89.2
  thyroid E07.89
  trachea, congenital (external) (internal) Q32.1
  tracheoesophageal J86.0
      congenital Q39.2
          with atresia of esophagus Q39.1
      following tracheostomy J95.04
  traumatic arteriovenous — *see* Injury, blood vessel, by
      site
  tuberculous — *code by* site under Tuberculosis
  typhoid A01.09
  umbilicourinary Q64.8
  urachus, congenital Q64.4
  ureter (persistent) N28.89
  ureteroabdominal N28.89
  ureterorectal N28.89
  ureterosigmoido-abdominal N28.89
  ureterovaginal N82.1
  ureterovesical N32.2
  urethra N36.0
      congenital Q64.79
      tuberculous A18.13
  urethroperineal N36.0
  urethroperineovesical N32.2
  urethrorectal N36.0
      congenital Q64.73
  urethroscrotal N50.89
  urethrovaginal N82.1
  urethrovesical N32.2
  urinary (tract) (persistent) (recurrent) N36.0
  uteroabdominal N82.5
      congenital Q51.7
  uteroenteric, uterointestinal N82.4
      congenital Q51.7
  uterorectal N82.4
      congenital Q51.7
  uteroureteric N82.1
  uterourethral Q51.7
  uterovaginal N82.8
  uterovesical N82.1
      congenital Q51.7
  uterus N82.8
  vagina (postpartal) (wall) N82.8
  vaginocutaneous (postpartal) N82.5
  vaginointestinal NEC N82.4
      large intestine N82.3
      small intestine N82.2
  vaginoperineal N82.5
  vasocutaneous, congenital Q55.7
  vesical NEC N32.2
  vesicoabdominal N32.2
  vesicocervicovaginal N82.1
  vesicocolic N32.1
  vesicocutaneous N32.2
  vesicoenteric N32.1
  vesicointestinal N32.1
  vesicometrorectal N82.4
  vesicoperineal N32.2
  vesicorectal N32.1
      congenital Q64.79
  vesicosigmoidal N32.1
  vesicosigmoidovaginal N82.3
  vesicoureteral N32.2
  vesicoureterovaginal N82.1
  vesicourethral N32.2
  vesicourethrorectal N32.1
  vesicouterine N82.1

Fistula — *continued*
  vesicouterine — *continued*
    congenital Q51.7
  vesicovaginal N82.0
  vulvorectal N82.4
    congenital Q52.79
Fit R56.9
  epileptic — *see* Epilepsy
  fainting R55
  hysterical F44.5
  newborn P90
Fitting (and adjustment) (of)
  artificial
    arm — *see* Admission, adjustment, artificial, arm
    breast Z44.3 ☑
    eye Z44.2 ☑
    leg — *see* Admission, adjustment, artificial, leg
  automatic implantable cardiac defibrillator (with synchronous cardiac pacemaker) Z45.02
  brain neuropacemaker Z46.2
    implanted Z45.42
  cardiac defibrillator — *see* Fitting (and adjustment) (of), automatic implantable cardiac defibrillator
  catheter, non-vascular Z46.82
  colostomy belt Z46.89
  contact lenses Z46.0
  CRT-D (resynchronization therapy defibrillator) Z45.02
  CRT-P (cardiac resynchronization therapy pacemaker) Z45.018
    pulse generator Z45.010
  cystostomy device Z46.6
  defibrillator, cardiac — *see* Fitting (and adjustment) (of), automatic implantable cardiac defibrillator
  dentures Z46.3
  device NOS Z46.9
    abdominal Z46.89
    gastrointestinal NEC Z46.59
    implanted NEC Z45.89
    nervous system Z46.2
      implanted — *see* Admission, adjustment, device, implanted, nervous system
    orthodontic Z46.4
    orthoptic Z46.0
    orthotic Z46.89
    prosthetic (external) Z44.9
      breast Z44.3 ☑
      dental Z46.3
      eye Z44.2 ☑
      specified NEC Z44.8
    specified NEC Z46.89
    substitution
      auditory Z46.2
        implanted — *see* Admission, adjustment, device, implanted, hearing device
      nervous system Z46.2
        implanted — *see* Admission, adjustment, device, implanted, nervous system
      visual Z46.2
        implanted Z45.31
    urinary Z46.6
  gastric lap band Z46.51
  gastrointestinal appliance NEC Z46.59
  glasses (reading) Z46.0
  hearing aid Z46.1
  ileostomy device Z46.89
  insulin pump Z46.81
  intestinal appliance NEC Z46.89
  myringotomy device (stent) (tube) Z45.82
  neuropacemaker Z46.2
    implanted Z45.42
  non-vascular catheter Z46.82
  orthodontic device Z46.4
  orthopedic device (brace) (cast) (corset) (shoes) Z46.89
  pacemaker (cardiac) (cardiac resynchronization therapy (CRT-P)) Z45.018
    nervous system (brain) (peripheral nerve) (spinal cord) Z46.2
      implanted Z45.42
    pulse generator Z45.010
  portacath (port-a-cath) Z45.2
  prosthesis (external) Z44.9
    arm — *see* Admission, adjustment, artificial, arm
    breast Z44.3 ☑
    dental Z46.3
    eye Z44.2 ☑
    leg — *see* Admission, adjustment, artificial, leg
    specified NEC Z44.8
  spectacles Z46.0

Fitting — *continued*
  wheelchair Z46.89
Fitzhugh-Curtis syndrome
  due to
    Chlamydia trachomatis A74.81
    Neisseria gonorrhorea (gonococcal peritonitis) A54.85
Fitz's syndrome (acute hemorrhagic pancreatitis) (*see also* Pancreatitis, acute) K85.80
Fixation
  joint — *see* Ankylosis
  larynx J38.7
  stapes — *see* Ankylosis, ear ossicles
    deafness — *see* Deafness, conductive
  uterus (acquired) — *see* Malposition, uterus
  vocal cord J38.3
Flabby ridge K06.8
Flaccid (*see also* condition)
  palate, congenital Q38.5
Flail
  chest S22.5 ☑
    newborn (birth injury) P13.8
  joint (paralytic) M25.20
    ankle M25.27- ☑
    elbow M25.22- ☑
    foot joint M25.27- ☑
    hand joint M25.24- ☑
    hip M25.25- ☑
    knee M25.26- ☑
    shoulder M25.21- ☑
    specified joint NEC M25.28
    wrist M25.23- ☑
Flajani's disease — *see* Hyperthyroidism, with, goiter (diffuse)
Flap, liver K71.3
Flashbacks (residual to hallucinogen use) F16.283
Flat
  chamber (eye) — *see* Disorder, globe, hypotony, flat anterior chamber
  chest, congenital Q67.8
  foot (acquired) (fixed type) (painful) (postural) (*see also* Deformity, limb, flat foot)
    congenital (rigid) (spastic (everted)) Q66.5- ☑
    rachitic sequelae (late effect) E64.3
  organ or site, congenital NEC — *see* Anomaly, by site
  pelvis M95.5
    with disproportion (fetopelvic) O33.0
      causing obstructed labor O65.0
    congenital Q74.2
Flatau-Schilder disease G37.0
Flatback syndrome M40.30
  lumbar region M40.36
  lumbosacral region M40.37
  thoracolumbar region M40.35
Flattening
  head, femur M89.8X5
  hip — *see* Coxa, plana
  lip (congenital) Q18.8
  nose (congenital) Q67.4
    acquired M95.0
Flatulence R14.3
  psychogenic F45.8
Flatus R14.3
  vaginalis N89.8
Flax-dresser's disease J66.1
Flea bite — *see* Injury, bite, by site, superficial, insect
Flecks, glaucomatous (subcapsular) — *see* Cataract, complicated
Fleischer (-Kayser) **ring** (cornea) H18.04- ☑
Fleshy mole O02.0
Flexibilitas cerea — *see* Catalepsy
Flexion
  amputation stump (surgical) T87.89
  cervix — *see* Malposition, uterus
  contracture, joint — *see* Contraction, joint
  deformity, joint (*see also* Deformity, limb, flexion) M21.20
    hip, congenital Q65.89
  uterus (*see also* Malposition, uterus)
    lateral — *see* Lateroversion, uterus
Flexner-Boyd dysentery A03.2
Flexner's dysentery A03.1
Flexure — *see* Flexion
Flint murmur (aortic insufficiency) I35.1
Floater, vitreous — *see* Opacity, vitreous
Floating
  cartilage (joint) (*see also* Loose, body, joint)

Floating — *continued*
  cartilage (*see also* Loose, body, joint) — *continued*
    knee — *see* Derangement, knee, loose body
  gallbladder, congenital Q44.1
  kidney N28.89
    congenital Q63.8
  spleen D73.89
Flooding N92.0
Floor — *see* condition
Floppy
  baby syndrome (nonspecific) P94.2
  iris syndrome (intraoperative) (IFIS) H21.81
  nonrheumatic mitral valve syndrome I34.1
Flu (*see also* Influenza)
  avian (*see also* Influenza, due to, identified novel influenza A virus) J09.X2
  bird (*see also* Influenza, due to, identified novel influenza A virus) J09.X2
  intestinal NEC A08.4
  swine (viruses that normally cause infections in pigs) (*see also* Influenza, due to, identified novel influenza A virus) J09.X2
Fluctuating blood pressure I99.8
Fluid
  abdomen R18.8
  chest J94.8
  heart — *see* Failure, heart, congestive
  joint — *see* Effusion, joint
  loss (acute) E86.9
  lung — *see* Edema, lung
  overload E87.70
    specified NEC E87.79
  peritoneal cavity R18.8
  pleural cavity J94.8
  retention R60.9
Flukes NEC (*see also* Infestation, fluke)
  blood NEC — *see* Schistosomiasis
  liver B66.3
Fluor (vaginalis) N89.8
  trichomonal or due to Trichomonas (vaginalis) A59.00
Fluorosis
  dental K00.3
  skeletal M85.10
    ankle M85.17- ☑
    foot M85.17- ☑
    forearm M85.13- ☑
    hand M85.14- ☑
    lower leg M85.16- ☑
    multiple site M85.19
    neck M85.18
    rib M85.18
    shoulder M85.11- ☑
    skull M85.18
    specified site NEC M85.18
    thigh M85.15- ☑
    toe M85.17- ☑
    upper arm M85.12- ☑
    vertebra M85.18
Flush syndrome E34.0
Flushing R23.2
  menopausal N95.1
Flutter
  atrial or auricular I48.92
    atypical I48.4
      type I I48.3
      type II I48.4
    typical I48.3
  heart I49.8
    atrial or auricular I48.92
      atypical I48.4
        type I I48.3
        type II I48.4
      typical I48.3
    ventricular I49.02
  ventricular I49.02
FNHTR (febrile nonhemolytic transfusion reaction) R50.84
Fochier's abscess — *code by* site under Abscess
Focus, Assmann's — *see* Tuberculosis, pulmonary
Fogo selvagem L10.3
Foix-Alajouanine syndrome G95.19
Fold, folds (anomalous) (*see also* Anomaly, by site)
  Descemet's membrane — *see* Change, corneal membrane, Descemet's, fold
  epicanthic Q10.3
  heart Q24.8
Folie à deux F24

☑ **Additional Character Required** — **Refer to the Tabular List for Character Selection**   ⬙ **Subterms under main terms may continue to next column or page**

Follicle
- cervix (nabothian) (ruptured) N88.8
- graafian, ruptured, with hemorrhage N83.0- ☑
- nabothian N88.8

Follicular — *see* condition

Folliculitis (superficial) L73.9
- abscedens et suffodiens L66.3
- cyst N83.0- ☑
- decalvans L66.2
- deep — *see* Furuncle, by site
- gonococcal (acute) (chronic) A54.01
- keloid, keloidalis L73.0
- pustular L01.02
- ulerythematosa reticulata L66.4

Folliculome lipidique
- specified site — *see* Neoplasm, benign, by site
- unspecified site
  - female D27.9
  - male D29.20

Fölling's disease E70.0

Follow-up — *see* Examination, follow-up

Fong's syndrome (hereditary osteo-onychodysplasia) Q87.2

Food
- allergy L27.2
- asphyxia (from aspiration or inhalation) — *see* Foreign body, by site
- choked on — *see* Foreign body, by site
- deprivation T73.0 ☑
  - specified kind of food NEC E63.8
- intoxication — *see* Poisoning, food
- lack of T73.0 ☑
- poisoning — *see* Poisoning, food
- rejection NEC — *see* Disorder, eating
- strangulation or suffocation — *see* Foreign body, by site
- toxemia — *see* Poisoning, food

Foot — *see* condition

Foramen ovale (nonclosure) (patent) (persistent) Q21.1

Forbes' glycogen storage disease E74.03

Fordyce-Fox disease L75.2

Fordyce's disease (mouth) Q38.6

Forearm — *see* condition

Foreign body
- with
  - laceration — *see* Laceration, by site, with foreign body
  - puncture wound — *see* Puncture, by site, with foreign body
- accidentally left following a procedure T81.509 ☑
  - aspiration T81.506 ☑
    - resulting in
      - adhesions T81.516 ☑
      - obstruction T81.526 ☑
      - perforation T81.536 ☑
      - specified complication NEC T81.596 ☑
  - cardiac catheterization T81.505 ☑
    - resulting in
      - acute reaction T81.60 ☑
        - aseptic peritonitis T81.61 ☑
        - specified NEC T81.69 ☑
      - adhesions T81.515 ☑
      - obstruction T81.525 ☑
      - perforation T81.535 ☑
      - specified complication NEC T81.595 ☑
  - causing
    - acute reaction T81.60 ☑
      - aseptic peritonitis T81.61 ☑
      - specified complication NEC T81.69 ☑
    - adhesions T81.519 ☑
    - aseptic peritonitis T81.61 ☑
    - obstruction T81.529 ☑
    - perforation T81.539 ☑
    - specified complication NEC T81.599 ☑
  - endoscopy T81.504 ☑
    - resulting in
      - adhesions T81.514 ☑
      - obstruction T81.524 ☑
      - perforation T81.534 ☑
      - specified complication NEC T81.594 ☑
  - immunization T81.503 ☑
    - resulting in
      - adhesions T81.513 ☑
      - obstruction T81.523 ☑
      - perforation T81.533 ☑
      - specified complication NEC T81.593 ☑

Foreign body — *continued*
- accidentally left following a procedure — *continued*
  - infusion T81.501 ☑
    - resulting in
      - adhesions T81.511 ☑
      - obstruction T81.521 ☑
      - perforation T81.531 ☑
      - specified complication NEC T81.591 ☑
  - injection T81.503 ☑
    - resulting in
      - adhesions T81.513 ☑
      - obstruction T81.523 ☑
      - perforation T81.533 ☑
      - specified complication NEC T81.593 ☑
  - kidney dialysis T81.502 ☑
    - resulting in
      - adhesions T81.512 ☑
      - obstruction T81.522 ☑
      - perforation T81.532 ☑
      - specified complication NEC T81.592 ☑
  - packing removal T81.507 ☑
    - resulting in
      - acute reaction T81.60 ☑
        - aseptic peritonitis T81.61 ☑
        - specified NEC T81.69 ☑
      - adhesions T81.517 ☑
      - obstruction T81.527 ☑
      - perforation T81.537 ☑
      - specified complication NEC T81.597 ☑
  - puncture T81.506 ☑
    - resulting in
      - adhesions T81.516 ☑
      - obstruction T81.526 ☑
      - perforation T81.536 ☑
      - specified complication NEC T81.596 ☑
  - specified procedure NEC T81.508 ☑
    - resulting in
      - acute reaction T81.60 ☑
        - aseptic peritonitis T81.61 ☑
        - specified NEC T81.69 ☑
      - adhesions T81.518 ☑
      - obstruction T81.528 ☑
      - perforation T81.538 ☑
      - specified complication NEC T81.598 ☑
  - surgical operation T81.500 ☑
    - resulting in
      - acute reaction T81.60 ☑
        - aseptic peritonitis T81.61 ☑
        - specified NEC T81.69 ☑
      - adhesions T81.510 ☑
      - obstruction T81.520 ☑
      - perforation T81.530 ☑
      - specified complication NEC T81.590 ☑
  - transfusion T81.501 ☑
    - resulting in
      - adhesions T81.511 ☑
      - obstruction T81.521 ☑
      - perforation T81.531 ☑
      - specified complication NEC T81.591 ☑
- alimentary tract T18.9 ☑
  - anus T18.5 ☑
  - colon T18.4 ☑
  - esophagus — *see* Foreign body, esophagus
  - mouth T18.0 ☑
  - multiple sites T18.8 ☑
  - rectosigmoid (junction) T18.5 ☑
  - rectum T18.5 ☑
  - small intestine T18.3 ☑
  - specified site NEC T18.8 ☑
  - stomach T18.2 ☑
- anterior chamber (eye) S05.5- ☑
- auditory canal — *see* Foreign body, entering through orifice, ear
- bronchus T17.508 ☑
  - causing
    - asphyxiation T17.500 ☑
      - food (bone) (seed) T17.520 ☑
      - gastric contents (vomitus) T17.510 ☑
      - specified type NEC T17.590 ☑
    - injury NEC T17.508 ☑
      - food (bone) (seed) T17.528 ☑
      - gastric contents (vomitus) T17.518 ☑
      - specified type NEC T17.598 ☑
- canthus — *see* Foreign body, conjunctival sac
- ciliary body (eye) S05.5- ☑
- conjunctival sac T15.1- ☑

Foreign body — *continued*
- cornea T15.0- ☑
- entering through orifice
  - accessory sinus T17.0 ☑
  - alimentary canal T18.9 ☑
    - multiple parts T18.8 ☑
    - specified part NEC T18.8 ☑
  - alveolar process T18.0 ☑
  - antrum (Highmore's) T17.0 ☑
  - anus T18.5 ☑
  - appendix T18.4 ☑
  - auditory canal — *see* Foreign body, entering through orifice, ear
  - auricle — *see* Foreign body, entering through orifice, ear
  - bladder T19.1 ☑
  - bronchioles — *see* Foreign body, respiratory tract, specified site NEC
  - bronchus (main) — *see* Foreign body, bronchus
  - buccal cavity T18.0 ☑
  - canthus (inner) — *see* Foreign body, conjunctival sac
  - cecum T18.4 ☑
  - cervix (canal) (uteri) T19.3 ☑
  - colon T18.4 ☑
  - conjunctival sac — *see* Foreign body, conjunctival sac
  - cornea — *see* Foreign body, cornea
  - digestive organ or tract NOS T18.9 ☑
    - multiple parts T18.8 ☑
    - specified part NEC T18.8 ☑
  - duodenum T18.3 ☑
  - ear (external) T16.- ☑
  - esophagus — *see* Foreign body, esophagus
  - eye (external) NOS T15.9- ☑
    - conjunctival sac — *see* Foreign body, conjunctival sac
    - cornea — *see* Foreign body, cornea
    - specified part NEC T15.8- ☑
  - eyeball (*see also* Foreign body, entering through orifice, eye, specified part NEC)
    - with penetrating wound — *see* Puncture, eyeball
  - eyelid (*see also* Foreign body, conjunctival sac)
    - with
      - laceration — *see* Laceration, eyelid, with foreign body
      - puncture — *see* Puncture, eyelid, with foreign body
      - superficial injury — *see* Foreign body, superficial, eyelid
  - gastrointestinal tract T18.9 ☑
    - multiple parts T18.8 ☑
    - specified part NEC T18.8 ☑
  - genitourinary tract T19.9 ☑
    - multiple parts T19.8 ☑
    - specified part NEC T19.8 ☑
  - globe — *see* Foreign body, entering through orifice, eyeball
  - gum T18.0 ☑
  - Highmore's antrum T17.0 ☑
  - hypopharynx — *see* Foreign body, pharynx
  - ileum T18.3 ☑
  - intestine (small) T18.3 ☑
    - large T18.4 ☑
  - lacrimal apparatus (punctum) — *see* Foreign body, entering through orifice, eye, specified part NEC
  - large intestine T18.4 ☑
  - larynx — *see* Foreign body, larynx
  - lung — *see* Foreign body, respiratory tract, specified site NEC
  - maxillary sinus T17.0 ☑
  - mouth T18.0 ☑
  - nasal sinus T17.0 ☑
  - nasopharynx — *see* Foreign body, pharynx
  - nose (passage) T17.1 ☑
  - nostril T17.1 ☑
  - oral cavity T18.0 ☑
  - palate T18.0 ☑
  - penis T19.4 ☑
  - pharynx — *see* Foreign body, pharynx
  - piriform sinus — *see* Foreign body, pharynx
  - rectosigmoid (junction) T18.5 ☑
  - rectum T18.5 ☑
  - respiratory tract — *see* Foreign body, respiratory tract

Foreign body — *continued*
- entering through orifice — *continued*
  - sinus (accessory) (frontal) (maxillary) (nasal) T17.0 ☑
    - piriform — *see* Foreign body, pharynx
  - small intestine T18.3 ☑
  - stomach T18.2 ☑
  - suffocation by — *see* Foreign body, by site
  - tear ducts or glands — *see* Foreign body, entering through orifice, eye, specified part NEC
  - throat — *see* Foreign body, pharynx
  - tongue T18.0 ☑
  - tonsil, tonsillar (fossa) — *see* Foreign body, pharynx
  - trachea — *see* Foreign body, trachea
  - ureter T19.8 ☑
  - urethra T19.0 ☑
  - uterus (any part) T19.3 ☑
  - vagina T19.2 ☑
  - vulva T19.2 ☑
- esophagus T18.108 ☑
  - causing
    - injury NEC T18.108 ☑
      - food (bone) (seed) T18.128 ☑
      - gastric contents (vomitus) T18.118 ☑
      - specified type NEC T18.198 ☑
    - tracheal compression T18.100 ☑
      - food (bone) (seed) T18.120 ☑
      - gastric contents (vomitus) T18.110 ☑
      - specified type NEC T18.190 ☑
- feeling of, in throat R09.89
- fragment — *see* Retained, foreign body fragments (type of)
- genitourinary tract T19.9 ☑
  - bladder T19.1 ☑
  - multiple parts T19.8 ☑
  - penis T19.4 ☑
  - specified site NEC T19.8 ☑
  - urethra T19.0 ☑
  - uterus T19.3 ☑
    - IUD Z97.5
  - vagina T19.2 ☑
    - contraceptive device Z97.5
  - vulva T19.2 ☑
- granuloma (old) (soft tissue) (*see also* Granuloma, foreign body)
  - skin L92.3
- in
  - laceration — *see* Laceration, by site, with foreign body
  - puncture wound — *see* Puncture, by site, with foreign body
  - soft tissue (residual) M79.5
- inadvertently left in operation wound — *see* Foreign body, accidentally left during a procedure
- ingestion, ingested NOS T18.9 ☑
- inhalation or inspiration — *see* Foreign body, by site
- internal organ, not entering through a natural orifice — code as specific injury with foreign body
- intraocular S05.5- ☑
  - old, retained (nonmagnetic) H44.70- ☑
    - anterior chamber H44.71- ☑
    - ciliary body H44.72- ☑
    - iris H44.72- ☑
    - lens H44.73- ☑
    - magnetic H44.60- ☑
      - anterior chamber H44.61- ☑
      - ciliary body H44.62- ☑
      - iris H44.62- ☑
      - lens H44.63- ☑
      - posterior wall H44.64- ☑
      - specified site NEC H44.69- ☑
      - vitreous body H44.65- ☑
    - posterior wall H44.74- ☑
    - specified site NEC H44.79- ☑
    - vitreous body H44.75- ☑
  - iris — *see* Foreign body, intraocular
- lacrimal punctum — *see* Foreign body, entering through orifice, eye, specified part NEC
- larynx T17.308 ☑
  - causing
    - asphyxiation T17.300 ☑
      - food (bone) (seed) T17.320 ☑
      - gastric contents (vomitus) T17.310 ☑
      - specified type NEC T17.390 ☑
    - injury NEC T17.308 ☑
      - food (bone) (seed) T17.328 ☑
      - gastric contents (vomitus) T17.318 ☑

Foreign body — *continued*
- larynx — *continued*
  - causing — *continued*
    - injury — *continued*
      - specified type NEC T17.398 ☑
- lens — *see* Foreign body, intraocular
- ocular muscle S05.4- ☑
  - old, retained — *see* Foreign body, orbit, old
- old or residual
  - soft tissue (residual) M79.5
- operation wound, left accidentally — *see* Foreign body, accidentally left during a procedure
- orbit S05.4- ☑
  - old, retained H05.5- ☑
- pharynx T17.208 ☑
  - causing
    - asphyxiation T17.200 ☑
      - food (bone) (seed) T17.220 ☑
      - gastric contents (vomitus) T17.210 ☑
      - specified type NEC T17.290 ☑
    - injury NEC T17.208 ☑
      - food (bone) (seed) T17.228 ☑
      - gastric contents (vomitus) T17.218 ☑
      - specified type NEC T17.298 ☑
- respiratory tract T17.908 ☑
  - bronchioles — *see* Foreign body, respiratory tract, specified site NEC
  - bronchus — *see* Foreign body, bronchus
  - causing
    - asphyxiation T17.900 ☑
      - food (bone) (seed) T17.920 ☑
      - gastric contents (vomitus) T17.910 ☑
      - specified type NEC T17.990 ☑
    - injury NEC T17.908 ☑
      - food (bone) (seed) T17.928 ☑
      - gastric contents (vomitus) T17.918 ☑
      - specified type NEC T17.998 ☑
  - larynx — *see* Foreign body, larynx
  - lung — *see* Foreign body, respiratory tract, specified site NEC
  - multiple parts — *see* Foreign body, respiratory tract, specified site NEC
  - nasal sinus T17.0 ☑
  - nasopharynx — *see* Foreign body, pharynx
  - nose T17.1 ☑
  - nostril T17.1 ☑
  - pharynx — *see* Foreign body, pharynx
  - specified site NEC T17.808 ☑
    - causing
      - asphyxiation T17.800 ☑
        - food (bone) (seed) T17.820 ☑
        - gastric contents (vomitus) T17.810 ☑
        - specified type NEC T17.890 ☑
      - injury NEC T17.808 ☑
        - food (bone) (seed) T17.828 ☑
        - gastric contents (vomitus) T17.818 ☑
        - specified type NEC T17.898 ☑
  - throat — *see* Foreign body, pharynx
  - trachea — *see* Foreign body, trachea
- retained (old) (nonmagnetic) (in)
  - anterior chamber (eye) — *see* Foreign body, intraocular, old, retained, anterior chamber
    - magnetic — *see* Foreign body, intraocular, old, retained, magnetic, anterior chamber
  - ciliary body — *see* Foreign body, intraocular, old, retained, ciliary body
    - magnetic — *see* Foreign body, intraocular, old, retained, magnetic, ciliary body
  - eyelid H02.819
    - left H02.816
      - lower H02.815
      - upper H02.814
    - right H02.813
      - lower H02.812
      - upper H02.811
  - fragments — *see* Retained, foreign body fragments (type of)
  - globe — *see* Foreign body, intraocular, old, retained
    - magnetic — *see* Foreign body, intraocular, old, retained, magnetic
  - intraocular — *see* Foreign body, intraocular, old, retained
    - magnetic — *see* Foreign body, intraocular, old, retained, magnetic
  - iris — *see* Foreign body, intraocular, old, retained, iris

Foreign body — *continued*
- retained — *continued*
  - iris — *see* Foreign body, intraocular, old, retained, iris — *continued*
    - magnetic — *see* Foreign body, intraocular, old, retained, magnetic, iris
  - lens — *see* Foreign body, intraocular, old, retained, lens
    - magnetic — *see* Foreign body, intraocular, old, retained, magnetic, lens
  - muscle — *see* Foreign body, retained, soft tissue
  - orbit — *see* Foreign body, orbit, old
  - posterior wall of globe — *see* Foreign body, intraocular, old, retained, posterior wall
    - magnetic — *see* Foreign body, intraocular, old, retained, magnetic, posterior wall
  - retrobulbar — *see* Foreign body, orbit, old, retrobulbar
  - soft tissue M79.5
  - vitreous — *see* Foreign body, intraocular, old, retained, vitreous body
    - magnetic — *see* Foreign body, intraocular, old, retained, magnetic, vitreous body
- retina S05.5- ☑
- superficial, without open wound
  - abdomen, abdominal (wall) S30.851 ☑
  - alveolar process S00.552 ☑
  - ankle S90.55- ☑
  - antecubital space — *see* Foreign body, superficial, forearm
  - anus S30.857 ☑
  - arm (upper) S40.85- ☑
  - auditory canal — *see* Foreign body, superficial, ear
  - auricle — *see* Foreign body, superficial, ear
  - axilla — *see* Foreign body, superficial, arm
  - back, lower S30.850 ☑
  - breast S20.15- ☑
  - brow S00.85 ☑
  - buttock S30.850 ☑
  - calf — *see* Foreign body, superficial, leg
  - canthus — *see* Foreign body, superficial, eyelid
  - cheek S00.85 ☑
    - internal S00.552 ☑
  - chest wall — *see* Foreign body, superficial, thorax
  - chin S00.85 ☑
  - clitoris S30.854 ☑
  - costal region — *see* Foreign body, superficial, thorax
  - digit(s)
    - foot — *see* Foreign body, superficial, toe
    - hand — *see* Foreign body, superficial, finger
  - ear S00.45- ☑
  - elbow S50.35- ☑
  - epididymis S30.853 ☑
  - epigastric region S30.851 ☑
  - epiglottis S10.15 ☑
  - esophagus, cervical S10.15 ☑
  - eyebrow — *see* Foreign body, superficial, eyelid
  - eyelid S00.25- ☑
  - face S00.85 ☑
  - finger(s) S60.459 ☑
    - index S60.45- ☑
    - little S60.45- ☑
    - middle S60.45- ☑
    - ring S60.45- ☑
  - flank S30.851 ☑
  - foot (except toe(s) alone) S90.85- ☑
    - toe — *see* Foreign body, superficial, toe
  - forearm S50.85- ☑
    - elbow only — *see* Foreign body, superficial, elbow
  - forehead S00.85 ☑
  - genital organs, external
    - female S30.856 ☑
    - male S30.855 ☑
  - groin S30.851 ☑
  - gum S00.552 ☑
  - hand S60.55- ☑
  - head S00.95 ☑
    - ear — *see* Foreign body, superficial, ear
    - eyelid — *see* Foreign body, superficial, eyelid
    - lip S00.551 ☑
    - nose S00.35 ☑
    - oral cavity S00.552 ☑
    - scalp S00.05 ☑
    - specified site NEC S00.85 ☑
  - heel — *see* Foreign body, superficial, foot

☑ **Additional Character Required — Refer to the Tabular List for Character Selection**   ▽ **Subterms under main terms may continue to next column or page**

Foreign body — *continued*

superficial, without open wound — *continued*

hip S70.25- ☑
inguinal region S30.851 ☑
interscapular region S20.459 ☑
jaw S00.85 ☑
knee S80.25- ☑
labium (majus) (minus) S30.854 ☑
larynx S10.15 ☑
leg (lower) S80.85- ☑
knee — *see* Foreign body, superficial, knee
upper — *see* Foreign body, superficial, thigh
lip S00.551 ☑
lower back S30.850 ☑
lumbar region S30.850 ☑
malar region S00.85 ☑
mammary — *see* Foreign body, superficial, breast
mastoid region S00.85 ☑
mouth S00.552 ☑
nail
finger — *see* Foreign body, superficial, finger
toe — *see* Foreign body, superficial, toe
nape S10.85 ☑
nasal S00.35 ☑
neck S10.95 ☑
specified site NEC S10.85 ☑
throat S10.15 ☑
nose S00.35 ☑
occipital region S00.05 ☑
oral cavity S00.552 ☑
orbital region — *see* Foreign body, superficial, eyelid
palate S00.552 ☑
palm — *see* Foreign body, superficial, hand
parietal region S00.05 ☑
pelvis S30.850 ☑
penis S30.852 ☑
perineum
female S30.854 ☑
male S30.850 ☑
periocular area — *see* Foreign body, superficial, eyelid
phalanges
finger — *see* Foreign body, superficial, finger
toe — *see* Foreign body, superficial, toe
pharynx S10.15 ☑
pinna — *see* Foreign body, superficial, ear
popliteal space — *see* Foreign body, superficial, knee
prepuce S30.852 ☑
pubic region S30.850 ☑
pudendum
female S30.856 ☑
male S30.855 ☑
sacral region S30.850 ☑
scalp S00.05 ☑
scapular region — *see* Foreign body, superficial, shoulder
scrotum S30.853 ☑
shin — *see* Foreign body, superficial, leg
shoulder S40.25- ☑
sternal region S20.359 ☑
submaxillary region S00.85 ☑
submental region S00.85 ☑
subungual
finger(s) — *see* Foreign body, superficial, finger
toe(s) — *see* Foreign body, superficial, toe
supraclavicular fossa S10.85 ☑
supraorbital S00.85 ☑
temple S00.85 ☑
temporal region S00.85 ☑
testis S30.853 ☑
thigh S70.35- ☑
thorax, thoracic (wall) S20.95 ☑
back S20.45- ☑
front S20.35- ☑
throat S10.15 ☑
thumb S60.35- ☑
toe(s) (lesser) S90.456 ☑
great S90.45- ☑
tongue S00.552 ☑
trachea S10.15 ☑
tunica vaginalis S30.853 ☑
tympanum, tympanic membrane — *see* Foreign body, superficial, ear
uvula S00.552 ☑
vagina S30.854 ☑

Foreign body — *continued*

superficial, without open wound — *continued*

vocal cords S10.15 ☑
vulva S30.854 ☑
wrist S60.85- ☑
swallowed T18.9 ☑
trachea T17.408 ☑
causing
asphyxiation T17.400 ☑
food (bone) (seed) T17.420 ☑
gastric contents (vomitus) T17.410 ☑
specified type NEC T17.490 ☑
injury NEC T17.408 ☑
food (bone) (seed) T17.428 ☑
gastric contents (vomitus) T17.418 ☑
specified type NEC T17.498 ☑
type of fragment — *see* Retained, foreign body fragments (type of)
vitreous (humor) S05.5- ☑
Forestier's disease (rhizomelic pseudopolyarthritis) M35.3
meaning ankylosing hyperostosis — *see* Hyperostosis, ankylosing
Formation
hyalin in cornea — *see* Degeneration, cornea
sequestrum in bone (due to infection) — *see* Osteomyelitis, chronic
valve
colon, congenital Q43.8
ureter (congenital) Q62.39
Formication R20.2
Fort Bragg fever A27.89
Fossa (*see also* condition)
pyriform — *see* condition
Foster-Kennedy syndrome H47.14- ☑
Fothergill's
disease (trigeminal neuralgia) (*see also* Neuralgia, trigeminal)
scarlatina anginosa A38.9
Foul breath R19.6
Foundling Z76.1
Fournier disease or gangrene N49.3
female N76.89
Fourth
cranial nerve — *see* condition
molar K00.1
Foville's (peduncular) **disease or syndrome** G46.3
Fox (-Fordyce) disease (apocrine miliaria) L75.2
FPIES (food protein-induced enteropathy syndrome) K52.21
Fracture, burst — *see* Fracture, traumatic, by site
Fracture, chronic — *see* Fracture, pathological, by site
Fracture, insufficiency — *see* Fracture, pathological, by site
Fracture, nontraumatic, NEC
atypical
femur M84.750- ☑
complete
oblique M84.759 ☑
left side M84.758 ☑
right side M84.757 ☑
transverse M84.756 ☑
left side M84.755 ☑
right side M84.754 ☑
incomplete M84.753 ☑
left side M84.752 ☑
right side M84.751 ☑
Fracture, pathological (pathologic) (*see also* Fracture, traumatic) M84.40 ☑
ankle M84.47- ☑
carpus M84.44- ☑
clavicle M84.41- ☑
compression (not due to trauma) (*see also* Collapse, vertebra) M48.50- ☑
dental implant M27.63
dental restorative material K08.539
with loss of material K08.531
without loss of material K08.530
due to
neoplastic disease NEC (*see also* Neoplasm) M84.50 ☑
ankle M84.57- ☑
carpus M84.54- ☑
clavicle M84.51- ☑
femur M84.55- ☑
fibula M84.56- ☑

Fracture, pathological — *continued*

due to — *continued*
neoplastic disease (*see also* Neoplasm) — *continued*
finger M84.54- ☑
hip M84.559 ☑
humerus M84.52- ☑
ilium M84.550 ☑
ischium M84.550 ☑
metacarpus M84.54- ☑
metatarsus M84.57- ☑
neck M84.58 ☑
pelvis M84.550 ☑
radius M84.53- ☑
rib M84.58 ☑
scapula M84.51- ☑
skull M84.58 ☑
specified site NEC M84.58 ☑
tarsus M84.57- ☑
tibia M84.56- ☑
toe M84.57- ☑
ulna M84.53- ☑
vertebra M84.58 ☑
osteoporosis M80.00 ☑
disuse — *see* Osteoporosis, specified type NEC, with pathological fracture
drug-induced — *see* Osteoporosis, drug induced, with pathological fracture
idiopathic — *see* Osteoporosis, specified type NEC, with pathological fracture
postmenopausal — *see* Osteoporosis, postmenopausal, with pathological fracture
postoophorectomy — *see* Osteoporosis, postoophorectomy, with pathological fracture
postsurgical malabsorption — *see* Osteoporosis, specified type NEC, with pathological fracture
specified cause NEC — *see* Osteoporosis, specified type NEC, with pathological fracture
specified disease NEC M84.60 ☑
ankle M84.67- ☑
carpus M84.64- ☑
clavicle M84.61- ☑
femur M84.65- ☑
fibula M84.66- ☑
finger M84.64- ☑
hip M84.65- ☑
humerus M84.62- ☑
ilium M84.650 ☑
ischium M84.650 ☑
metacarpus M84.64- ☑
metatarsus M84.67- ☑
neck M84.68 ☑
radius M84.63- ☑
rib M84.68 ☑
scapula M84.61- ☑
skull M84.68 ☑
tarsus M84.67- ☑
tibia M84.66- ☑
toe M84.67- ☑
ulna M84.63- ☑
vertebra M84.68 ☑
femur M84.45- ☑
fibula M84.46- ☑
finger M84.44- ☑
hip M84.459 ☑
humerus M84.42- ☑
ilium M84.454 ☑
ischium M84.454 ☑
joint prosthesis — *see* Complications, joint prosthesis, mechanical, breakdown, by site
periprosthetic — *see* Fracture, pathological, periprosthetic
metacarpus M84.44- ☑
metatarsus M84.47- ☑
neck M84.48 ☑
pelvis M84.454 ☑
periprosthetic M97.9 ☑
ankle M97.2- ☑
elbow M97.4- ☑
finger M97.8 ☑
hip M97.0- ☑
knee M97.1- ☑
other specified joint M97.8 ☑
shoulder M97.3- ☑
spinal joint M97.8 ☑

Fracture, pathological — *continued*
  periprosthetic — *continued*
    toe joint M97.8 ☑
    wrist joint M97.8 ☑
  radius M84.43- ☑
  restorative material (dental) K08.539
    with loss of material K08.531
    without loss of material K08.530
  rib M84.48 ☑
  scapula M84.41- ☑
  skull M84.48 ☑
  tarsus M84.47- ☑
  tibia M84.46- ☑
  toe M84.47- ☑
  ulna M84.43- ☑
  vertebra M84.48 ☑

Fracture, traumatic (abduction) (adduction) (separation)
  (*see also* Fracture, pathological) T14.8 ☑
  acetabulum S32.40- ☑
    column
      anterior (displaced) (iliopubic) S32.43- ☑
        nondisplaced S32.436
      posterior (displaced) (ilioischial) S32.443 ☑
        nondisplaced S32.44- ☑
    dome (displaced) S32.48- ☑
      nondisplaced S32.48 ☑
    specified NEC S32.49- ☑
    transverse (displaced) S32.45- ☑
      with associated posterior wall fracture (displaced) S32.46- ☑
        nondisplaced S32.46- ☑
      nondisplaced S32.45- ☑
    wall
      anterior (displaced) S32.41- ☑
        nondisplaced S32.41- ☑
      medial (displaced) S32.47- ☑
        nondisplaced S32.47- ☑
      posterior (displaced) S32.42- ☑
        with associated transverse fracture (displaced) S32.46- ☑
          nondisplaced S32.46- ☑
        nondisplaced S32.42- ☑
  acromion — *see* Fracture, scapula, acromial process
  ankle S82.899 ☑
    bimalleolar (displaced) S82.84- ☑
      nondisplaced S82.84- ☑
    lateral malleolus only (displaced) S82.6- ☑
      nondisplaced S82.6- ☑
    medial malleolus (displaced) S82.5- ☑
      associated with Maisonneuve's fracture — *see* Fracture, Maisonneuve's
      nondisplaced S82.5- ☑
    talus — *see* Fracture, tarsal, talus
    trimalleolar (displaced) S82.85- ☑
      nondisplaced S82.85- ☑
  arm (upper) (*see also* Fracture, humerus, shaft)
    humerus — *see* Fracture, humerus
    radius — *see* Fracture, radius
    ulna — *see* Fracture, ulna
  astragalus — *see* Fracture, tarsal, talus
  atlas — *see* Fracture, neck, cervical vertebra, first
  axis — *see* Fracture, neck, cervical vertebra, second
  back — *see* Fracture, vertebra
  Barton's — *see* Barton's fracture
  base of skull — *see* Fracture, skull, base
  basicervical (basal) (femoral) S72.0 ☑
  Bennett's — *see* Bennett's fracture
  bimalleolar — *see* Fracture, ankle, bimalleolar
  blow-out S02.3- ☑
  bone NEC T14.8 ☑
    birth injury P13.9
    following insertion of orthopedic implant, joint prosthesis or bone plate — *see* Fracture, following insertion of orthopedic implant, joint prosthesis or bone plate
    in (due to) neoplastic disease NEC — *see* Fracture, pathological, due to, neoplastic disease
    pathological (cause unknown) — *see* Fracture, pathological
  breast bone — *see* Fracture, sternum
  bucket handle (semilunar cartilage) — *see* Tear, meniscus
  burst — *see* Fracture, traumatic, by site
  calcaneus — *see* Fracture, tarsal, calcaneus
  carpal bone(s) S62.10- ☑
    capitate (displaced) S62.13- ☑

Fracture, traumatic — *continued*
  carpal bone(s) — *continued*
    capitate — *continued*
      nondisplaced S62.13- ☑
    cuneiform — *see* Fracture, carpal bone, triquetrum
    hamate (body) (displaced) S62.143 ☑
      hook process (displaced) S62.15- ☑
        nondisplaced S62.15- ☑
      nondisplaced S62.14- ☑
    larger multangular — *see* Fracture, carpal bones, trapezium
    lunate (displaced) S62.12- ☑
      nondisplaced S62.12- ☑
    navicular S62.00- ☑
      distal pole (displaced) S62.01- ☑
        nondisplaced S62.01- ☑
      middle third (displaced) S62.02- ☑
        nondisplaced S62.02- ☑
      proximal third (displaced) S62.03- ☑
        nondisplaced S62.03- ☑
      volar tuberosity — *see* Fracture, carpal bones, navicular, distal pole
    os magnum — *see* Fracture, carpal bones, capitate
    pisiform (displaced) S62.16- ☑
      nondisplaced S62.16- ☑
    semilunar — *see* Fracture, carpal bones, lunate
    smaller multangular — *see* Fracture, carpal bones, trapezoid
    trapezium (displaced) S62.17- ☑
      nondisplaced S62.17- ☑
    trapezoid (displaced) S62.18- ☑
      nondisplaced S62.18- ☑
    triquetrum (displaced) S62.11- ☑
      nondisplaced S62.11- ☑
    unciform — *see* Fracture, carpal bones, hamate
  cervical — *see* Fracture, vertebra, cervical
  clavicle S42.00- ☑
    acromial end (displaced) S42.03- ☑
      nondisplaced S42.03- ☑
    birth injury P13.4
    lateral end — *see* Fracture, clavicle, acromial end
    shaft (displaced) S42.02- ☑
      nondisplaced S42.02- ☑
    sternal end (anterior) (displaced) S42.01- ☑
      nondisplaced S42.01- ☑
      posterior S42.01- ☑
  coccyx S32.2 ☑
  collapsed — *see* Collapse, vertebra
  collar bone — *see* Fracture, clavicle
  Colles' — *see* Colles' fracture
  coronoid process — *see* Fracture, ulna, upper end, coronoid process
  corpus cavernosum penis S39.840 ☑
  costochondral cartilage S23.41 ☑
  costochondral, costosternal junction — *see* Fracture, rib
  cranium — *see* Fracture, skull
  cricoid cartilage S12.8 ☑
  cuboid (ankle) — *see* Fracture, tarsal, cuboid
  cuneiform
    foot — *see* Fracture, tarsal, cuneiform
    wrist — *see* Fracture, carpal, triquetrum
  delayed union — *see* Delay, union, fracture
  dental restorative material K08.539
    with loss of material K08.531
    without loss of material K08.530
  due to
    birth injury — *see* Birth, injury, fracture
    osteoporosis — *see* Osteoporosis, with fracture
  Dupuytren's — *see* Fracture, ankle, lateral malleolus
  elbow S42.40- ☑
  ethmoid (bone) (sinus) — *see* Fracture, skull, base
  face bone S02.92 ☑
  fatigue (*see also* Fracture, stress)
    vertebra M48.40 ☑
      cervical region M48.42 ☑
      cervicothoracic region M48.43 ☑
      lumbar region M48.46 ☑
      lumbosacral region M48.47 ☑
      occipito-atlanto-axial region M48.41 ☑
      sacrococcygeal region M48.48 ☑
      thoracic region M48.44 ☑
      thoracolumbar region M48.45 ☑
  femur, femoral S72.9- ☑
    basicervical (basal) S72.0 ☑
    birth injury P13.2

Fracture, traumatic — *continued*
  femur, femoral — *continued*
    capital epiphyseal S79.01- ☑
    condyles, epicondyles — *see* Fracture, femur, lower end
    distal end — *see* Fracture, femur, lower end
    epiphysis
      head — *see* Fracture, femur, upper end, epiphysis
      lower — *see* Fracture, femur, lower end, epiphysis
      upper — *see* Fracture, femur, upper end, epiphysis
    following insertion of implant, prosthesis or plate M96.66- ☑
    head — *see* Fracture, femur, upper end, head
    intertrochanteric — *see* Fracture, femur, trochanteric
    intratrochanteric — *see* Fracture, femur, trochanteric
    lower end S72.40- ☑
      condyle (displaced) S72.41- ☑
        lateral (displaced) S72.42- ☑
          nondisplaced S72.42- ☑
        medial (displaced) S72.43- ☑
          nondisplaced S72.43- ☑
        nondisplaced S72.41- ☑
      epiphysis (displaced) S72.44- ☑
        nondisplaced S72.44- ☑
      physeal S79.10- ☑
        Salter-Harris
          Type I S79.11- ☑
          Type II S79.12- ☑
          Type III S79.13- ☑
          Type IV S79.14- ☑
        specified NEC S79.19- ☑
      specified NEC S72.49- ☑
      supracondylar (displaced) S72.45- ☑
        with intracondylar extension (displaced) S72.46- ☑
          nondisplaced S72.46- ☑
        nondisplaced S72.45- ☑
      torus S72.47- ☑
    neck — *see* Fracture, femur, upper end, neck
    pertrochanteric — *see* Fracture, femur, trochanteric
    shaft (lower third) (middle third) (upper third) S72.30- ☑
      comminuted (displaced) S72.35- ☑
        nondisplaced S72.35- ☑
      oblique (displaced) S72.33- ☑
        nondisplaced S72.33- ☑
      segmental (displaced) S72.36- ☑
        nondisplaced S72.36- ☑
      specified NEC S72.39- ☑
      spiral (displaced) S72.34- ☑
        nondisplaced S72.34- ☑
      transverse (displaced) S72.32- ☑
        nondisplaced S72.32- ☑
    specified site NEC — *see subcategory* S72.8 ☑
    subcapital (displaced) S72.01- ☑
    subtrochanteric (region) (section) (displaced) S72.2- ☑
      nondisplaced S72.2- ☑
    transcervical — *see* Fracture, femur, upper end, neck
    transtrochanteric — *see* Fracture, femur, trochanteric
    trochanteric S72.10- ☑
      apophyseal (displaced) S72.13- ☑
        nondisplaced S72.13- ☑
      greater trochanter (displaced) S72.11- ☑
        nondisplaced S72.11- ☑
      intertrochanteric (displaced) S72.14- ☑
        nondisplaced S72.14- ☑
      lesser trochanter (displaced) S72.12- ☑
        nondisplaced S72.12- ☑
    upper end S72.00- ☑
      apophyseal (displaced) S72.13- ☑
        nondisplaced S72.13- ☑
      cervicotrochanteric — *see* Fracture, femur, upper end, neck, base
      epiphysis (displaced) S72.02- ☑
        nondisplaced S72.02- ☑
      head S72.05- ☑
        articular (displaced) S72.06- ☑
          nondisplaced S72.06- ☑
        specified NEC S72.09- ☑
      intertrochanteric (displaced) S72.14- ☑

Fracture, traumatic — *continued*
  femur, femoral — *continued*
    upper end — *continued*
      intertrochanteric — *continued*
        nondisplaced S72.14- ☑
      intracapsular S72.01- ☑
      midcervical (displaced) S72.03- ☑
        nondisplaced S72.03- ☑
      neck S72.00- ☑
        base (displaced) S72.04- ☑
          nondisplaced S72.04- ☑
        specified NEC S72.09- ☑
      pertrochanteric — *see* Fracture, femur, upper
        end, trochanteric
      physeal S79.00- ☑
        Salter-Harris type I S79.01- ☑
        specified NEC S79.09- ☑
      subcapital (displaced) S72.01- ☑
      subtrochanteric (displaced) S72.2- ☑
        nondisplaced S72.2- ☑
      transcervical — *see* Fracture, femur, upper end,
        midcervical
      trochanteric S72.10- ☑
        greater (displaced) S72.11- ☑
          nondisplaced S72.11- ☑
        lesser (displaced) S72.12- ☑
          nondisplaced S72.12- ☑
  fibula (shaft) (styloid) S82.40- ☑
    comminuted (displaced) S82.45- ☑
      nondisplaced S82.45- ☑
    following insertion of implant, prosthesis or plate
      M96.67- ☑
    involving ankle or malleolus — *see* Fracture, fibula,
      lateral malleolus
    lateral malleolus (displaced) S82.6- ☑
      nondisplaced S82.6- ☑
    lower end
      physeal S89.30- ☑
        Salter-Harris
          Type I S89.31- ☑
          Type II S89.32- ☑
        specified NEC S89.39- ☑
      specified NEC S82.83- ☑
      torus S82.82- ☑
    oblique (displaced) S82.43- ☑
      nondisplaced S82.43- ☑
    segmental (displaced) S82.46- ☑
      nondisplaced S82.46- ☑
    specified NEC S82.49- ☑
    spiral (displaced) S82.44- ☑
      nondisplaced S82.44- ☑
    transverse (displaced) S82.42- ☑
      nondisplaced S82.42- ☑
    upper end
      physeal S89.20- ☑
        Salter-Harris
          Type I S89.21- ☑
          Type II S89.22- ☑
        specified NEC S89.29- ☑
      specified NEC S82.83- ☑
      torus S82.81- ☑
  finger (except thumb) S62.60- ☑
    distal phalanx (displaced) S62.63- ☑
      nondisplaced S62.66- ☑
    index S62.60- ☑
      distal phalanx (displaced) S62.63- ☑
        nondisplaced S62.66- ☑
      middle phalanx (displaced) S62.62- ☑
        nondisplaced S62.65- ☑
      proximal phalanx (displaced) S62.61- ☑
        nondisplaced S62.64- ☑
    little S62.60- ☑
      distal phalanx (displaced) S62.63- ☑
        nondisplaced S62.66- ☑
      middle phalanx (displaced) S62.62- ☑
        nondisplaced S62.65- ☑
      proximal phalanx (displaced) S62.61- ☑
        nondisplaced S62.64- ☑
    middle S62.60- ☑
      distal phalanx (displaced) S62.63- ☑
        nondisplaced S62.66- ☑
      middle phalanx (displaced) S62.62- ☑
        nondisplaced S62.65- ☑
      proximal phalanx (displaced) S62.61- ☑
        nondisplaced S62.64- ☑
    middle phalanx (displaced) S62.62- ☑

Fracture, traumatic — *continued*
  finger — *continued*
    middle phalanx — *continued*
      nondisplaced S62.65- ☑
    proximal phalanx (displaced) S62.61- ☑
      nondisplaced S62.64- ☑
    ring S62.60- ☑
      distal phalanx (displaced) S62.63- ☑
        nondisplaced S62.66- ☑
      middle phalanx (displaced) S62.62- ☑
        nondisplaced S62.65- ☑
      proximal phalanx (displaced) S62.61- ☑
        nondisplaced S62.64- ☑
    thumb — *see* Fracture, thumb
  following insertion (intraoperative) (postoperative) of
    orthopedic implant, joint prosthesis or bone
    plate M96.69
    femur M96.66- ☑
    fibula M96.67- ☑
    humerus M96.62- ☑
    pelvis M96.65
    radius M96.63- ☑
    specified bone NEC M96.69
    tibia M96.67- ☑
    ulna M96.63- ☑
  foot S92.90- ☑
    astragalus — *see* Fracture, tarsal, talus
    calcaneus — *see* Fracture, tarsal, calcaneus
    cuboid — *see* Fracture, tarsal, cuboid
    cuneiform — *see* Fracture, tarsal, cuneiform
    metatarsal — *see* Fracture, metatarsal
    navicular — *see* Fracture, tarsal, navicular
    sesamoid S92.81- ☑
    specified NEC S92.81- ☑
    talus — *see* Fracture, tarsal, talus
    tarsal — *see* Fracture, tarsal
    toe — *see* Fracture, toe
  forearm S52.9- ☑
    radius — *see* Fracture, radius
    ulna — *see* Fracture, ulna
  fossa (anterior) (middle) (posterior) S02.19 ☑
  frontal (bone) (skull) S02.0 ☑
    sinus S02.19
  glenoid (cavity) (scapula) — *see* Fracture, scapula,
    glenoid cavity
  greenstick — *see* Fracture, by site
  hallux — *see* Fracture, toe, great
  hand S62.9- ☑
    carpal — *see* Fracture, carpal bone
    finger (except thumb) — *see* Fracture, finger
    metacarpal — *see* Fracture, metacarpal
    navicular (scaphoid) (hand) — *see* Fracture, carpal
      bone, navicular
    thumb — *see* Fracture, thumb
  healed or old
    with complications — *code by* Nature of the compli-
      cation
  heel bone — *see* Fracture, tarsal, calcaneus
  Hill-Sachs S42.29- ☑
  hip — *see* Fracture, femur, neck
  humerus S42.30- ☑
    anatomical neck — *see* Fracture, humerus, upper
      end
    articular process — *see* Fracture, humerus, lower
      end
    capitellum — *see* Fracture, humerus, lower end,
      condyle, lateral
    distal end — *see* Fracture, humerus, lower end
    epiphysis
      lower — *see* Fracture, humerus, lower end, phy-
        seal
      upper — *see* Fracture, humerus, upper end,
        physeal
    external condyle — *see* Fracture, humerus, lower
      end, condyle, lateral
    following insertion of implant, prosthesis or plate
      M96.62- ☑
    great tuberosity — *see* Fracture, humerus, upper
      end, greater tuberosity
    intercondylar — *see* Fracture, humerus, lower end
    internal epicondyle — *see* Fracture, humerus, lower
      end, epicondyle, medial
    lesser tuberosity — *see* Fracture, humerus, upper
      end, lesser tuberosity
    lower end S42.40- ☑
      condyle
        lateral (displaced) S42.45- ☑

Fracture, traumatic — *continued*
  humerus — *continued*
    lower end — *continued*
      condyle — *continued*
        lateral — *continued*
          nondisplaced S42.45- ☑
        medial (displaced) S42.46- ☑
          nondisplaced S42.46- ☑
      epicondyle
        lateral (displaced) S42.43- ☑
          nondisplaced S42.43- ☑
        medial (displaced) S42.44- ☑
          incarcerated S42.44- ☑
          nondisplaced S42.44- ☑
      physeal S49.10- ☑
        Salter-Harris
          Type I S49.11- ☑
          Type II S49.12- ☑
          Type III S49.13- ☑
          Type IV S49.14- ☑
        specified NEC S49.19- ☑
      specified NEC (displaced) S42.49- ☑
        nondisplaced S42.49- ☑
      supracondylar (simple) (displaced) S42.41- ☑
        with intercondylar fracture — *see* Fracture,
          humerus, lower end
        comminuted (displaced) S42.42- ☑
          nondisplaced S42.42- ☑
        nondisplaced S42.41- ☑
      torus S42.48- ☑
      transcondylar (displaced) S42.47- ☑
        nondisplaced S42.47- ☑
    proximal end — *see* Fracture, humerus, upper end
    shaft S42.30- ☑
      comminuted (displaced) S42.35- ☑
        nondisplaced S42.35- ☑
      greenstick S42.31- ☑
      oblique (displaced) S42.33- ☑
        nondisplaced S42.33- ☑
      segmental (displaced) S42.36- ☑
        nondisplaced S42.36- ☑
      specified NEC S42.39- ☑
      spiral (displaced) S42.34- ☑
        nondisplaced S42.34- ☑
      transverse (displaced) S42.32- ☑
        nondisplaced S42.32- ☑
    supracondylar — *see* Fracture, humerus, lower end
    surgical neck — *see* Fracture, humerus, upper end,
      surgical neck
    trochlea — *see* Fracture, humerus, lower end,
      condyle, medial
    tuberosity — *see* Fracture, humerus, upper end
    upper end S42.20- ☑
      anatomical neck — *see* Fracture, humerus, upper
        end, specified NEC
      articular head — *see* Fracture, humerus, upper
        end, specified NEC
      epiphysis — *see* Fracture, humerus, upper end,
        physeal
      greater tuberosity (displaced) S42.25- ☑
        nondisplaced S42.25- ☑
      lesser tuberosity (displaced) S42.26- ☑
        nondisplaced S42.26- ☑
      physeal S49.00- ☑
        Salter-Harris
          Type I S49.01- ☑
          Type II S49.02- ☑
          Type III S49.03- ☑
          Type IV S49.04- ☑
        specified NEC S49.09- ☑
      specified NEC (displaced) S42.29- ☑
        nondisplaced S42.29- ☑
      surgical neck (displaced) S42.21- ☑
        four-part S42.24- ☑
        nondisplaced S42.21- ☑
        three-part S42.23- ☑
        two-part (displaced) S42.22- ☑
          nondisplaced S42.22- ☑
      torus S42.27- ☑
      transepiphyseal — *see* Fracture, humerus, upper
        end, physeal
  hyoid bone S12.8 ☑
  ilium S32.30- ☑
    with disruption of pelvic ring — *see* Disruption,
      pelvic ring
    avulsion (displaced) S32.31- ☑

▽ Subterms under main terms may continue to next column or page   ☑ Additional Character Required — Refer to the Tabular List for Character Selection   151

Fracture, traumatic — *continued*
ilium — *continued*
  avulsion — *continued*
    nondisplaced S32.31- ☑
  specified NEC S32.39- ☑
  impaction, impacted — *code as* Fracture, by site
  innominate bone — *see* Fracture, ilium
  instep — *see* Fracture, foot
  ischium S32.60- ☑
    with disruption of pelvic ring — *see* Disruption, pelvic ring
    avulsion (displaced) S32.61- ☑
      nondisplaced S32.61- ☑
    specified NEC S32.69- ☑
  jaw (bone) (lower) — *see* Fracture, mandible
    upper — *see* Fracture, maxilla
  joint prosthesis — *see* Complications, joint prosthesis, mechanical, breakdown, by site
    periprosthetic — *see* Fracture, traumatic, periprosthetic
  knee cap — *see* Fracture, patella
  larynx S12.8 ☑
  late effects — *see* Sequelae, fracture
  leg (lower) S82.9- ☑
    ankle — *see* Fracture, ankle
    femur — *see* Fracture, femur
    fibula — *see* Fracture, fibula
    malleolus — *see* Fracture, ankle
    patella — *see* Fracture, patella
    specified site NEC S82.89- ☑
    tibia — *see* Fracture, tibia
  lumbar spine — *see* Fracture, vertebra, lumbar
  lumbosacral spine S32.9 ☑
  Maisonneuve's (displaced) S82.86- ☑
    nondisplaced S82.86- ☑
  malar bone (*see also* Fracture, maxilla) S02.400 ☑
    left side S02.40B ☑
    right side S02.40A ☑
  malleolus — *see* Fracture, ankle
  malunion — *see* Fracture, by site
  mandible (lower jaw (bone)) S02.609 ☑
    alveolus S02.67- ☑
    angle (of jaw) S02.65- ☑
    body, unspecified S02.600 ☑
      left side S02.602 ☑
      right side S02.601 ☑
    condylar process S02.61- ☑
    coronoid process S02.63- ☑
    ramus, unspecified S02.64- ☑
    specified site NEC S02.69 ☑
    subcondylar process S02.62- ☑
    symphysis S02.66 ☑
  manubrium (sterni) S22.21 ☑
    dissociation from sternum S22.23 ☑
  march — *see* Fracture, traumatic, stress, by site
  maxilla, maxillary (bone) (sinus) (superior) (upper jaw) S02.401 ☑
    alveolus S02.42 ☑
    inferior — *see* Fracture, mandible
    LeFort I S02.411 ☑
    LeFort II S02.412 ☑
    LeFort III S02.413 ☑
    left side S02.40D ☑
    right side S02.40C ☑
  metacarpal S62.309 ☑
    base (displaced) S62.319 ☑
      nondisplaced S62.349 ☑
    fifth S62.30- ☑
      base (displaced) S62.31- ☑
        nondisplaced S62.34- ☑
      neck (displaced) S62.33- ☑
        nondisplaced S62.36- ☑
      shaft (displaced) S62.32- ☑
        nondisplaced S62.35- ☑
      specified NEC S62.398 ☑
    first S62.20- ☑
      base NEC (displaced) S62.23- ☑
        nondisplaced S62.23- ☑
      Bennett's — *see* Bennett's fracture
      neck (displaced) S62.25- ☑
        nondisplaced S62.25- ☑
      shaft (displaced) S62.24- ☑
        nondisplaced S62.24- ☑
      specified NEC S62.29- ☑
    fourth S62.30- ☑
      base (displaced) S62.31- ☑

Fracture, traumatic — *continued*
metacarpal — *continued*
  fourth — *continued*
    base — *continued*
      nondisplaced S62.34- ☑
    neck (displaced) S62.33- ☑
      nondisplaced S62.36- ☑
    shaft (displaced) S62.32- ☑
      nondisplaced S62.35- ☑
    specified NEC S62.39- ☑
  neck (displaced) S62.33- ☑
    nondisplaced S62.36- ☑
  Rolando's — *see* Rolando's fracture
  second S62.30- ☑
    base (displaced) S62.31- ☑
      nondisplaced S62.34- ☑
    neck (displaced) S62.33- ☑
      nondisplaced S62.36- ☑
    shaft (displaced) S62.32- ☑
      nondisplaced S62.35- ☑
    specified NEC S62.39- ☑
  shaft (displaced) S62.32- ☑
    nondisplaced S62.35- ☑
  specified NEC S62.399 ☑
  third S62.30- ☑
    base (displaced) S62.31- ☑
      nondisplaced S62.34- ☑
    neck (displaced) S62.33- ☑
      nondisplaced S62.36- ☑
    shaft (displaced) S62.32- ☑
      nondisplaced S62.35- ☑
    specified NEC S62.39- ☑
metastatic — *see* Fracture, pathological, due to, neoplastic disease (*see also* Neoplasm)
metatarsal bone S92.30- ☑
  fifth (displaced) S92.35- ☑
    nondisplaced S92.35- ☑
  first (displaced) S92.31- ☑
    nondisplaced S92.31- ☑
  fourth (displaced) S92.34- ☑
    nondisplaced S92.34- ☑
  physeal S99.10- ☑
    Salter-Harris
      Type I S99.11- ☑
      Type II S99.12- ☑
      Type III S99.13- ☑
      Type IV S99.14- ☑
    specified NEC S99.19- ☑
  second (displaced) S92.32- ☑
    nondisplaced S92.32- ☑
  third (displaced) S92.33- ☑
    nondisplaced S92.33- ☑
Monteggia's — *see* Monteggia's fracture
multiple
  hand (and wrist) NEC — *see* Fracture, by site
  ribs — *see* Fracture, rib, multiple
nasal (bone(s)) S02.2 ☑
navicular (scaphoid) (foot) (*see also* Fracture, tarsal, navicular)
  hand — *see* Fracture, carpal, navicular
neck S12.9 ☑
  cervical vertebra S12.9 ☑
    fifth (displaced) S12.400 ☑
      nondisplaced S12.401 ☑
      specified type NEC (displaced) S12.490 ☑
        nondisplaced S12.491 ☑
    first (displaced) S12.000 ☑
      burst (stable) S12.01 ☑
        unstable S12.02 ☑
      lateral mass (displaced) S12.040 ☑
        nondisplaced S12.041 ☑
      nondisplaced S12.001 ☑
      posterior arch (displaced) S12.030 ☑
        nondisplaced S12.031 ☑
      specified type NEC (displaced) S12.090 ☑
        nondisplaced S12.091 ☑
    fourth (displaced) S12.300 ☑
      nondisplaced S12.301 ☑
      specified type NEC (displaced) S12.390 ☑
        nondisplaced S12.391 ☑
    second (displaced) S12.100 ☑
      dens (anterior) (displaced) (type II) S12.110 ☑
        nondisplaced S12.112 ☑
        posterior S12.111 ☑
        specified type NEC (displaced) S12.120 ☑
          nondisplaced S12.121 ☑

Fracture, traumatic — *continued*
neck — *continued*
  cervical vertebra — *continued*
    second — *continued*
      nondisplaced S12.101 ☑
      specified type NEC (displaced) S12.190 ☑
        nondisplaced S12.191 ☑
    seventh (displaced) S12.600 ☑
      nondisplaced S12.601 ☑
      specified type NEC (displaced) S12.690 ☑
        nondisplaced S12.691 ☑
    sixth (displaced) S12.500 ☑
      nondisplaced S12.501 ☑
      specified type NEC (displaced) S12.590 ☑
        nondisplaced S12.591 ☑
    third (displaced) S12.200 ☑
      nondisplaced S12.201 ☑
      specified type NEC (displaced) S12.290 ☑
        nondisplaced S12.291 ☑
  hyoid bone S12.8 ☑
  larynx S12.8 ☑
  specified site NEC S12.8 ☑
  thyroid cartilage S12.8 ☑
  trachea S12.8 ☑
neoplastic NEC — *see* Fracture, pathological, due to, neoplastic disease
neural arch — *see* Fracture, vertebra
newborn — *see* Birth, injury, fracture
nontraumatic — *see* Fracture, pathological
nonunion — *see* Nonunion, fracture
nose, nasal (bone) (septum) S02.2 ☑
occiput — *see* Fracture, skull, base, occiput
odontoid process — *see* Fracture, neck, cervical vertebra, second
olecranon (process) (ulna) — *see* Fracture, ulna, upper end, olecranon process
orbit, orbital (bone) (region) S02.8- ☑
  floor (blow-out) S02.3- ☑
  roof S02.19 ☑
os
  calcis — *see* Fracture, tarsal, calcaneus
  magnum — *see* Fracture, carpal, capitate
  pubis — *see* Fracture, pubis
palate S02.8- ☑
parietal bone (skull) S02.0 ☑
patella S82.00- ☑
  comminuted (displaced) S82.04- ☑
    nondisplaced S82.04- ☑
  longitudinal (displaced) S82.02- ☑
    nondisplaced S82.02- ☑
  osteochondral (displaced) S82.01- ☑
    nondisplaced S82.01- ☑
  specified NEC S82.09- ☑
  transverse (displaced) S82.03- ☑
    nondisplaced S82.03- ☑
pedicle (of vertebral arch) — *see* Fracture, vertebra
pelvis, pelvic (bone) S32.9 ☑
  acetabulum — *see* Fracture, acetabulum
  circle — *see* Disruption, pelvic ring
  following insertion of implant, prosthesis or plate M96.65
  ilium — *see* Fracture, ilium
  ischium — *see* Fracture, ischium
  multiple
    with disruption of pelvic ring (circle) — *see* Disruption, pelvic ring
    without disruption of pelvic ring (circle) S32.82- ☑
  pubis — *see* Fracture, pubis
  sacrum — *see* Fracture, sacrum
  specified site NEC S32.89 ☑
periprosthetic, around internal prosthetic joint M97.9 ☑
  ankle M97.2- ☑
  elbow M97.4- ☑
  finger M97.8 ☑
  hip M97.0- ☑
  knee M97.1- ☑
  shoulder M97.3- ☑
  specified joint NEC M97.8 ☑
  spine M97.8 ☑
  toe M97.8 ☑
  wrist M97.8 ☑
phalanx
  foot — *see* Fracture, toe
  hand — *see* Fracture, finger

☑ **Additional Character Required** — **Refer to the Tabular List for Character Selection**   ▽ **Subterms under main terms may continue to next column or page**

Fracture, traumatic — *continued*
- pisiform — *see* Fracture, carpal, pisiform
- pond — *see* Fracture, skull
- prosthetic device, internal — *see* Complications, prosthetic device, by site, mechanical
- pubis S32.5Ø- ☑
  - with disruption of pelvic ring — *see* Disruption, pelvic ring
  - specified site NEC S32.59- ☑
  - superior rim S32.51- ☑
- radius S52.9- ☑
  - distal end — *see* Fracture, radius, lower end
  - following insertion of implant, prosthesis or plate M96.63- ☑
  - head — *see* Fracture, radius, upper end, head
  - lower end S52.5Ø- ☑
    - Barton's — *see* Barton's fracture
    - Colles' — *see* Colles' fracture
    - extraarticular NEC S52.55- ☑
    - intraarticular NEC S52.57- ☑
    - physeal S59.2Ø- ☑
      - Salter-Harris
        - Type I S59.21- ☑
        - Type II S59.22- ☑
        - Type III S59.23- ☑
        - Type IV S59.24- ☑
      - specified NEC S59.29- ☑
    - Smith's — *see* Smith's fracture
    - specified NEC S52.59- ☑
    - styloid process (displaced) S52.51- ☑
      - nondisplaced S52.51- ☑
    - torus S52.52- ☑
  - neck — *see* Fracture, radius, upper end
  - proximal end — *see* Fracture, radius, upper end
  - shaft S52.3Ø- ☑
    - bent bone S52.38- ☑
    - comminuted (displaced) S52.35- ☑
      - nondisplaced S52.35- ☑
    - Galeazzi's — *see* Galeazzi's fracture
    - greenstick S52.31- ☑
    - oblique (displaced) S52.33- ☑
      - nondisplaced S52.33- ☑
    - segmental (displaced) S52.36- ☑
      - nondisplaced S52.36- ☑
    - specified NEC S52.39- ☑
    - spiral (displaced) S52.34- ☑
      - nondisplaced S52.34- ☑
    - transverse (displaced) S52.32- ☑
      - nondisplaced S52.32- ☑
  - upper end S52.1Ø- ☑
    - head (displaced) S52.12- ☑
      - nondisplaced S52.12- ☑
    - neck (displaced) S52.13- ☑
      - nondisplaced S52.13- ☑
    - physeal S59.1Ø- ☑
      - Salter-Harris
        - Type I S59.11- ☑
        - Type II S59.12- ☑
        - Type III S59.13- ☑
        - Type IV S59.14- ☑
      - specified NEC S59.19- ☑
    - specified NEC S52.18- ☑
    - torus S52.11- ☑
- ramus
  - inferior or superior, pubis — *see* Fracture, pubis
  - mandible — *see* Fracture, mandible
- restorative material (dental) KØ8.539
  - with loss of material KØ8.531
  - without loss of material KØ8.53Ø
- rib S22.3- ☑
  - with flail chest — *see* Flail, chest
  - multiple S22.4- ☑
    - with flail chest — *see* Flail, chest
- root, tooth — *see* Fracture, tooth
- sacrum S32.1Ø ☑
  - specified NEC S32.19 ☑
  - Type
    - 1 S32.14 ☑
    - 2 S32.15 ☑
    - 3 S32.16 ☑
    - 4 S32.17 ☑
  - Zone
    - I S32.119 ☑
      - displaced (minimally) S32.111 ☑
        - severely S32.112 ☑
      - nondisplaced S32.11Ø ☑

Fracture, traumatic — *continued*
- sacrum — *continued*
  - Zone — *continued*
    - II S32.129 ☑
      - displaced (minimally) S32.121 ☑
        - severely S32.122 ☑
      - nondisplaced S32.12Ø ☑
    - III S32.139 ☑
      - displaced (minimally) S32.131 ☑
        - severely S32.132 ☑
      - nondisplaced S32.13Ø ☑
- scaphoid (hand) (*see also* Fracture, carpal, navicular)
  - foot — *see* Fracture, tarsal, navicular
- scapula S42.1Ø- ☑
  - acromial process (displaced) S42.12- ☑
    - nondisplaced S42.12- ☑
  - body (displaced) S42.11- ☑
    - nondisplaced S42.11- ☑
  - coracoid process (displaced) S42.13- ☑
    - nondisplaced S42.13- ☑
  - glenoid cavity (displaced) S42.14- ☑
    - nondisplaced S42.14- ☑
  - neck (displaced) S42.15- ☑
    - nondisplaced S42.15- ☑
  - specified NEC S42.19- ☑
- semilunar bone, wrist — *see* Fracture, carpal, lunate
- sequelae — *see* Sequelae, fracture
- sesamoid bone
  - foot S92.81- ☑
  - hand — *see* Fracture, carpal
  - other — *see* Fracture, traumatic, by site
- shepherd's — *see* Fracture, tarsal, talus
- shoulder (girdle) S42.9- ☑
  - blade — *see* Fracture, scapula
- sinus (ethmoid) (frontal) SØ2.19 ☑
- skull SØ2.91 ☑
  - base SØ2.1Ø- ☑
    - occiput SØ2.119 ☑
      - condyle SØ2.113 ☑
        - specified NEC SØ2.118 ☑
          - left side SØ2.11H ☑
          - right side SØ2.11G ☑
        - type I SØ2.11Ø ☑
          - left side SØ2.11B ☑
          - right side SØ2.11A ☑
        - type II SØ2.111 ☑
          - left side SØ2.11D ☑
          - right side SØ2.11C ☑
        - type III SØ2.112 ☑
          - left side SØ2.11F ☑
          - right side SØ2.11E ☑
    - specified NEC SØ2.19 ☑
  - birth injury P13.Ø
  - frontal bone SØ2.Ø ☑
  - parietal bone SØ2.Ø ☑
  - specified site NEC SØ2.8- ☑
  - temporal bone SØ2.19 ☑
  - vault SØ2.Ø ☑
- Smith's — *see* Smith's fracture
- sphenoid (bone) (sinus) SØ2.19 ☑
- spine — *see* Fracture, vertebra
- spinous process — *see* Fracture, vertebra
- spontaneous (cause unknown) — *see* Fracture, pathological
- stave (of thumb) — *see* Fracture, metacarpal, first
- sternum S22.2Ø ☑
  - with flail chest — *see* Flail, chest
  - body S22.22 ☑
  - manubrium S22.21 ☑
  - xiphoid (process) S22.24 ☑
- stress M84.3Ø ☑
  - ankle M84.37- ☑
  - carpus M84.34- ☑
  - clavicle M84.31- ☑
  - femoral neck M84.359 ☑
  - femur M84.35- ☑
  - fibula M84.36- ☑
  - finger M84.34- ☑
  - hip M84.359 ☑
  - humerus M84.32- ☑
  - ilium M84.35Ø ☑
  - ischium M84.35Ø ☑
  - metacarpus M84.34- ☑
  - metatarsus M84.37- ☑
  - neck — *see* Fracture, fatigue, vertebra
  - pelvis M84.35Ø ☑

Fracture, traumatic — *continued*
- stress — *continued*
  - radius M84.33- ☑
  - rib M84.38 ☑
  - scapula M84.31- ☑
  - skull M84.38 ☑
  - tarsus M84.37- ☑
  - tibia M84.36- ☑
  - toe M84.37- ☑
  - ulna M84.33- ☑
  - vertebra — *see* Fracture, fatigue, vertebra
- supracondylar, elbow — *see* Fracture, humerus, lower end, supracondylar
- symphysis pubis — *see* Fracture, pubis
- talus (ankle bone) — *see* Fracture, tarsal, talus
- tarsal bone(s) S92.2Ø- ☑
  - astragalus — *see* Fracture, tarsal, talus
  - calcaneus S92.ØØ- ☑
    - anterior process (displaced) S92.Ø2- ☑
      - nondisplaced S92.Ø2- ☑
    - body (displaced) S92.Ø1- ☑
      - nondisplaced S92.Ø1- ☑
    - extraarticular NEC (displaced) S92.Ø5- ☑
      - nondisplaced S92.Ø5- ☑
    - intraarticular (displaced) S92.Ø6- ☑
      - nondisplaced S92.Ø6- ☑
    - physeal S99.ØØ- ☑
      - Salter-Harris
        - Type I S99.Ø1- ☑
        - Type II S99.Ø2- ☑
        - Type III S99.Ø3- ☑
        - Type IV S99.Ø4- ☑
      - specified NEC S99.Ø9- ☑
    - tuberosity (displaced) S92.Ø4- ☑
      - avulsion (displaced) S92.Ø3- ☑
        - nondisplaced S92.Ø3- ☑
      - nondisplaced S92.Ø4- ☑
  - cuboid (displaced) S92.21- ☑
    - nondisplaced S92.21- ☑
  - cuneiform
    - intermediate (displaced) S92.23- ☑
      - nondisplaced S92.23- ☑
    - lateral (displaced) S92.22- ☑
      - nondisplaced S92.22- ☑
    - medial (displaced) S92.24- ☑
      - nondisplaced S92.24- ☑
  - navicular (displaced) S92.25- ☑
    - nondisplaced S92.25- ☑
  - scaphoid — *see* Fracture, tarsal, navicular
  - talus S92.1Ø- ☑
    - avulsion (displaced) S92.15- ☑
      - nondisplaced S92.15- ☑
    - body (displaced) S92.12- ☑
      - nondisplaced S92.12- ☑
    - dome (displaced) S92.14- ☑
      - nondisplaced S92.14- ☑
    - head (displaced) S92.12- ☑
      - nondisplaced S92.12- ☑
    - lateral process (displaced) S92.14- ☑
      - nondisplaced S92.14- ☑
    - neck (displaced) S92.11- ☑
      - nondisplaced S92.11- ☑
    - posterior process (displaced) S92.13- ☑
      - nondisplaced S92.13- ☑
    - specified NEC S92.19- ☑
- temporal bone (styloid) SØ2.19 ☑
- thorax (bony) S22.9 ☑
  - with flail chest — *see* Flail, chest
  - rib S22.3- ☑
    - multiple S22.4- ☑
      - with flail chest — *see* Flail, chest
  - sternum S22.2Ø ☑
    - body S22.22 ☑
    - manubrium S22.21 ☑
    - xiphoid process S22.24 ☑
  - vertebra (displaced) S22.ØØ9 ☑
    - burst (stable) S22.ØØ1 ☑
      - unstable S22.ØØ2 ☑
    - eighth S22.Ø69 ☑
      - burst (stable) S22.Ø61 ☑
        - unstable S22.Ø62 ☑
      - specified type NEC S22.Ø68 ☑
      - wedge compression S22.Ø6Ø ☑
    - eleventh S22.Ø89 ☑
      - burst (stable) S22.Ø81 ☑
        - unstable S22.Ø82 ☑

▽ Subterms under main terms may continue to next column or page   ☑ Additional Character Required — Refer to the Tabular List for Character Selection   153

Fracture, traumatic — Fracture, traumatic

Fracture, traumatic — *continued*
 thorax — *continued*
  vertebra — *continued*
   eleventh — *continued*
    specified type NEC S22.088 ☑
    wedge compression S22.080 ☑
   fifth S22.059 ☑
    burst (stable) S22.051 ☑
     unstable S22.052 ☑
    specified type NEC S22.058 ☑
    wedge compression S22.050 ☑
   first S22.019 ☑
    burst (stable) S22.011 ☑
     unstable S22.012 ☑
    specified type NEC S22.018 ☑
    wedge compression S22.010 ☑
   fourth S22.049 ☑
    burst (stable) S22.041 ☑
     unstable S22.042 ☑
    specified type NEC S22.048 ☑
    wedge compression S22.040 ☑
   ninth S22.079 ☑
    burst (stable) S22.071 ☑
     unstable S22.072 ☑
    specified type NEC S22.078 ☑
    wedge compression S22.070 ☑
   nondisplaced S22.001 ☑
   second S22.029 ☑
    burst (stable) S22.021 ☑
     unstable S22.022 ☑
    specified type NEC S22.028 ☑
    wedge compression S22.020 ☑
   seventh S22.069 ☑
    burst (stable) S22.061 ☑
     unstable S22.062 ☑
    specified type NEC S22.068 ☑
    wedge compression S22.060 ☑
   sixth S22.059 ☑
    burst (stable) S22.051 ☑
     unstable S22.052 ☑
    specified type NEC S22.058 ☑
    wedge compression S22.050 ☑
   specified type NEC S22.008 ☑
   tenth S22.079 ☑
    burst (stable) S22.071 ☑
     unstable S22.072 ☑
    specified type NEC S22.078 ☑
    wedge compression S22.070 ☑
   third S22.039 ☑
    burst (stable) S22.031 ☑
     unstable S22.032 ☑
    specified type NEC S22.038 ☑
    wedge compression S22.030 ☑
   twelfth S22.089 ☑
    burst (stable) S22.081 ☑
     unstable S22.082 ☑
    specified type NEC S22.088 ☑
    wedge compression S22.080 ☑
   wedge compression S22.000 ☑
 thumb S62.50- ☑
  distal phalanx (displaced) S62.52- ☑
   nondisplaced S62.52- ☑
  proximal phalanx (displaced) S62.51- ☑
   nondisplaced S62.51- ☑
 thyroid cartilage S12.8 ☑
 tibia (shaft) S82.20- ☑
  comminuted (displaced) S82.25- ☑
   nondisplaced S82.25- ☑
  condyles — *see* Fracture, tibia, upper end
  distal end — *see* Fracture, tibia, lower end
  epiphysis
   lower — *see* Fracture, tibia, lower end
   upper — *see* Fracture, tibia, upper end
  following insertion of implant, prosthesis or plate
   M96.67- ☑
  head (involving knee joint) — *see* Fracture, tibia,
   upper end
  intercondyloid eminence — *see* Fracture, tibia, upper end
  involving ankle or malleolus — *see* Fracture, ankle,
   medial malleolus
  lower end S82.30- ☑
   physeal S89.10- ☑
    Salter-Harris
     Type I S89.11- ☑
     Type II S89.12- ☑

Fracture, traumatic — *continued*
 tibia — *continued*
  lower end — *continued*
   physeal — *continued*
    Salter-Harris — *continued*
     Type III S89.13- ☑
     Type IV S89.14- ☑
    specified NEC S89.19- ☑
   pilon (displaced) S82.87- ☑
    nondisplaced S82.87- ☑
   specified NEC S82.39- ☑
   torus S82.31- ☑
  malleolus — *see* Fracture, ankle, medial malleolus
  oblique (displaced) S82.23- ☑
   nondisplaced S82.23- ☑
  pilon — *see* Fracture, tibia, lower end, pilon
  proximal end — *see* Fracture, tibia, upper end
  segmental (displaced) S82.26- ☑
   nondisplaced S82.26- ☑
  specified NEC S82.29- ☑
  spine — *see* Fracture, tibia, upper end, spine
  spiral (displaced) S82.24- ☑
   nondisplaced S82.24- ☑
  transverse (displaced) S82.22- ☑
   nondisplaced S82.22- ☑
  tuberosity — *see* Fracture, tibia, upper end,
   tuberosity
  upper end S82.10- ☑
   bicondylar (displaced) S82.14- ☑
    nondisplaced S82.14- ☑
   lateral condyle (displaced) S82.12- ☑
    nondisplaced S82.12- ☑
   medial condyle (displaced) S82.13- ☑
    nondisplaced S82.13- ☑
   physeal S89.00- ☑
    Salter-Harris
     Type I S89.01- ☑
     Type II S89.02- ☑
     Type III S89.03- ☑
     Type IV S89.04- ☑
    specified NEC S89.09- ☑
   plateau — *see* Fracture, tibia, upper end, bicondy-
    lar
   specified NEC S82.19- ☑
   spine (displaced) S82.11- ☑
    nondisplaced S82.11- ☑
   torus S82.16- ☑
   tuberosity (displaced) S82.15- ☑
    nondisplaced S82.15- ☑
 toe S92.91- ☑
  great (displaced) S92.40- ☑
   distal phalanx (displaced) S92.42- ☑
    nondisplaced S92.42- ☑
   nondisplaced S92.40- ☑
   proximal phalanx (displaced) S92.41- ☑
    nondisplaced S92.41- ☑
   specified NEC S92.49- ☑
  lesser (displaced) S92.50- ☑
   distal phalanx (displaced) S92.53- ☑
    nondisplaced S92.53- ☑
   medial phalanx (displaced) S92.52- ☑
    nondisplaced S92.52- ☑
   nondisplaced S92.50- ☑
   proximal phalanx (displaced) S92.51- ☑
    nondisplaced S92.51- ☑
   specified NEC S92.59- ☑
  physeal
   phalanx S99.20- ☑
    Salter-Harris
     Type I S99.21- ☑
     Type II S99.22- ☑
     Type III S99.23- ☑
     Type IV S99.24- ☑
    specified NEC S99.29- ☑
 tooth (root) S02.5 ☑
 trachea (cartilage) S12.8 ☑
 transverse process — *see* Fracture, vertebra
 trapezium or trapezoid bone — *see* Fracture, carpal
 trimalleolar — *see* Fracture, ankle, trimalleolar
 triquetrum (cuneiform of carpus) — *see* Fracture,
  carpal, triquetrum
 trochanter — *see* Fracture, femur, trochanteric
 tuberosity (external) — *see* Fracture, traumatic, by site
 ulna (shaft) S52.20- ☑
  bent bone S52.28- ☑

Fracture, traumatic — *continued*
 ulna — *continued*
  coronoid process — *see* Fracture, ulna, upper end,
   coronoid process
  distal end — *see* Fracture, ulna, lower end
  following insertion of implant, prosthesis or plate
   M96.63- ☑
  head S52.60- ☑
  lower end S52.60- ☑
   physeal S59.00- ☑
    Salter-Harris
     Type I S59.01- ☑
     Type II S59.02- ☑
     Type III S59.03- ☑
     Type IV S59.04- ☑
    specified NEC S59.09- ☑
   specified NEC S52.69- ☑
   styloid process (displaced) S52.61- ☑
    nondisplaced S52.61- ☑
   torus S52.62- ☑
  proximal end — *see* Fracture, ulna, upper end
  shaft S52.20- ☑
   comminuted (displaced) S52.25- ☑
    nondisplaced S52.25- ☑
   greenstick S52.21- ☑
   Monteggia's — *see* Monteggia's fracture
   oblique (displaced) S52.23- ☑
    nondisplaced S52.23- ☑
   segmental (displaced) S52.26- ☑
    nondisplaced S52.26- ☑
   specified NEC S52.29- ☑
   spiral (displaced) S52.24- ☑
    nondisplaced S52.24- ☑
   transverse (displaced) S52.22- ☑
    nondisplaced S52.22- ☑
  upper end S52.00- ☑
   coronoid process (displaced) S52.04- ☑
    nondisplaced S52.04- ☑
   olecranon process (displaced) S52.02- ☑
    with intraarticular extension S52.03- ☑
    nondisplaced S52.02- ☑
     with intraarticular extension S52.03- ☑
   specified NEC S52.09- ☑
   torus S52.01- ☑
 unciform — *see* Fracture, carpal, hamate
 vault of skull S02.0 ☑
 vertebra, vertebral (arch) (body) (column) (neural arch)
  (pedicle) (spinous process) (transverse process
  atlas — *see* Fracture, neck, cervical vertebra, first
  axis — *see* Fracture, neck, cervical vertebra, secon
  cervical (teardrop) S12.9 ☑
   axis — *see* Fracture, neck, cervical vertebra, sec
    ond
   first (atlas) — *see* Fracture, neck, cervical verte
    bra, first
   second (axis) — *see* Fracture, neck, cervical ve
    tebra, second
  chronic M84.48 ☑
  coccyx S32.2 ☑
  dorsal — *see* Fracture, thorax, vertebra
  lumbar S32.009 ☑
   burst (stable) S32.001 ☑
    unstable S32.002 ☑
   fifth S32.059 ☑
    burst (stable) S32.051 ☑
     unstable S32.052 ☑
    specified type NEC S32.058 ☑
    wedge compression S32.050 ☑
   first S32.019 ☑
    burst (stable) S32.011 ☑
     unstable S32.012 ☑
    specified type NEC S32.018 ☑
    wedge compression S32.010 ☑
   fourth S32.049 ☑
    burst (stable) S32.041 ☑
     unstable S32.042 ☑
    specified type NEC S32.048 ☑
    wedge compression S32.040 ☑
   second S32.029 ☑
    burst (stable) S32.021 ☑
     unstable S32.022 ☑
    specified type NEC S32.028 ☑
    wedge compression S32.020 ☑
   specified type NEC S32.008 ☑
   third S32.039 ☑
    burst (stable) S32.031 ☑

☑ **Additional Character Required** — **Refer to the Tabular List for Character Selection**   ▽ **Subterms under main terms may continue to next column or pag**

Fracture, traumatic — *continued*
  vertebra, vertebral — *continued*
    lumbar — *continued*
      third — *continued*
        burst — *continued*
          unstable S32.032 ☑
        specified type NEC S32.038 ☑
        wedge compression S32.030 ☑
      wedge compression S32.000 ☑
    metastatic — *see* Collapse, vertebra, in, specified
      disease NEC (*see also* Neoplasm)
    newborn (birth injury) P11.5
    sacrum S32.10 ☑
      specified NEC S32.19 ☑
      Type
        1 S32.14 ☑
        2 S32.15 ☑
        3 S32.16 ☑
        4 S32.17 ☑
      Zone
        I S32.119 ☑
          displaced (minimally) S32.111 ☑
            severely S32.112 ☑
          nondisplaced S32.110 ☑
        II S32.129 ☑
          displaced (minimally) S32.121 ☑
            severely S32.122 ☑
          nondisplaced S32.120 ☑
        III S32.139 ☑
          displaced (minimally) S32.131 ☑
            severely S32.132 ☑
          nondisplaced S32.130 ☑
    thoracic — *see* Fracture, thorax, vertebra
  vertex S02.0 ☑
  vomer (bone) S02.2 ☑
  wrist S62.10- ☑
    carpal — *see* Fracture, carpal bone
    navicular (scaphoid) (hand) — *see* Fracture, carpal,
      navicular
  xiphisternum, xiphoid (process) S22.24 ☑
  zygoma S02.402 ☑
    left side S02.40F ☑
    right side S02.40E ☑
Fragile, fragility
  autosomal site Q95.5
  bone, congenital (with blue sclera) Q78.0
  capillary (hereditary) D69.8
  hair L67.8
  nails L60.3
  non-sex chromosome site Q95.5
  X chromosome Q99.2
Fragilitas
  crinium L67.8
  ossium (with blue sclerae) (hereditary) Q78.0
  unguium L60.3
    congenital Q84.6
Fragments, cataract (lens), **following cataract surgery**
  H59.02- ☑
  retained foreign body — *see* Retained, foreign body
    fragments (type of)
Frailty (frail) R54
  mental R41.81
Frambesia, frambesial (tropica) (*see also* Yaws)
  initial lesion or ulcer A66.0
  primary A66.0
Frambeside
  gummatous A66.4
  of early yaws A66.2
Frambesioma A66.1
Franceschetti-Klein (-Wildervanck) **disease or syndrome** Q75.4
Francis' disease — *see* Tularemia
Franklin disease C88.2
Frank's essential thrombocytopenia D69.3
Fraser's syndrome Q87.0
Freckle(s) L81.2
  malignant melanoma in — *see* Melanoma
  melanotic (Hutchinson's) — *see* Melanoma, in situ
  retinal D49.81
Frederickson's hyperlipoproteinemia, type
  I and V E78.3
  IIA E78.00
  IIB and III E78.2
  IV E78.1
Freeman Sheldon syndrome Q87.0
Freezing (*see also* Effect, adverse, cold) T69.9 ☑

Freiberg's disease (infraction of metatarsal head or osteochondrosis) — *see* Osteochondrosis, juvenile,
  metatarsus
Frei's disease A55
Fremitus, friction, cardiac R01.2
Frenum, frenulum
  external os Q51.828
  tongue (shortening) (congenital) Q38.1
Frequency micturition (nocturnal) R35.0
  psychogenic F45.8
Frey's syndrome
  auriculotemporal G50.8
  hyperhidrosis L74.52
Friction
  burn — *see* Burn, by site
  fremitus, cardiac R01.2
  precordial R01.2
  sounds, chest R09.89
Friderichsen-Waterhouse syndrome or disease A39.1
Friedländer's B (bacillus) NEC (*see also* condition) A49.8
Friedreich's
  ataxia G11.1
  combined systemic disease G11.1
  facial hemihypertrophy Q67.4
  sclerosis (cerebellum) (spinal cord) G11.1
Frigidity F52.22
Fröhlich's syndrome E23.6
Frontal (*see also* condition)
  lobe syndrome F07.0
Frostbite (superficial) T33.90 ☑
  with
    partial thickness skin loss — *see* Frostbite (superfi-
      cial), by site
    tissue necrosis T34.90 ☑
  abdominal wall T33.3 ☑
    with tissue necrosis T34.3 ☑
  ankle T33.81- ☑
    with tissue necrosis T34.81- ☑
  arm T33.4- ☑
    with tissue necrosis T34.4- ☑
    finger(s) — *see* Frostbite, finger
    hand — *see* Frostbite, hand
    wrist — *see* Frostbite, wrist
  ear T33.01- ☑
    with tissue necrosis T34.01- ☑
  face T33.09 ☑
    with tissue necrosis T34.09 ☑
  finger T33.53- ☑
    with tissue necrosis T34.53- ☑
  foot T33.82- ☑
    with tissue necrosis T34.82- ☑
  hand T33.52- ☑
    with tissue necrosis T34.52- ☑
  head T33.09 ☑
    with tissue necrosis T34.09 ☑
    ear — *see* Frostbite, ear
    nose — *see* Frostbite, nose
  hip (and thigh) T33.6- ☑
    with tissue necrosis T34.6- ☑
  knee T33.7- ☑
    with tissue necrosis T34.7- ☑
  leg T33.9- ☑
    with tissue necrosis T34.9- ☑
    ankle — *see* Frostbite, ankle
    foot — *see* Frostbite, foot
    knee — *see* Frostbite, knee
    lower T33.7- ☑
      with tissue necrosis T34.7- ☑
    thigh — *see* Frostbite, hip
    toe — *see* Frostbite, toe
  limb
    lower T33.99 ☑
      with tissue necrosis T34.99 ☑
    upper — *see* Frostbite, arm
  neck T33.1 ☑
    with tissue necrosis T34.1 ☑
  nose T33.02 ☑
    with tissue necrosis T34.02 ☑
  pelvis T33.3 ☑
    with tissue necrosis T34.3 ☑
  specified site NEC T33.99 ☑
    with tissue necrosis T34.99 ☑
  thigh — *see* Frostbite, hip
  thorax T33.2 ☑
    with tissue necrosis T34.2 ☑
  toes T33.83- ☑

Frostbite — *continued*
  toes — *continued*
    with tissue necrosis T34.83- ☑
  trunk T33.99 ☑
    with tissue necrosis T34.99 ☑
  wrist T33.51- ☑
    with tissue necrosis T34.51- ☑
Frotteurism F65.81
Frozen (*see also* Effect, adverse, cold) T69.9 ☑
  pelvis (female) N94.89
    male K66.8
  shoulder — *see* Capsulitis, adhesive
Fructokinase deficiency E74.11
Fructose 1,6 diphosphatase deficiency E74.19
Fructosemia (benign) (essential) E74.12
Fructosuria (benign) (essential) E74.11
Fuchs'
  black spot (myopic) (*see also* Myopia, degenerative)
    H44.2- ☑
  dystrophy (corneal endothelium) H18.51
  heterochromic cyclitis — *see* Cyclitis, Fuchs' hete-
    rochromic
Fucosidosis E77.1
Fugue R68.89
  dissociative F44.1
  hysterical (dissociative) F44.1
  postictal in epilepsy — *see* Epilepsy
  reaction to exceptional stress (transient) F43.0
Fulminant, fulminating — *see* condition
Functional (*see also* condition)
  bleeding (uterus) N93.8
Functioning, intellectual, borderline R41.83
Fundus — *see* condition
Fungemia NOS B49
Fungus, fungous
  cerebral G93.89
  disease NOS B49
  infection — *see* Infection, fungus
Funiculitis (acute) (chronic) (endemic) N49.1
  gonococcal (acute) (chronic) A54.23
  tuberculous A18.15
Funnel
  breast (acquired) M95.4
    congenital Q67.6
    sequelae (late effect) of rickets E64.3
  chest (acquired) M95.4
    congenital Q67.6
    sequelae (late effect) of rickets E64.3
  pelvis (acquired) M95.5
    with disproportion (fetopelvic) O33.3 ☑
      causing obstructed labor O65.3
    congenital Q74.2
FUO (fever of unknown origin) R50.9
Furfur L21.0
  microsporon B36.0
Furrier's lung J67.8
Furrowed K14.5
  nail(s) (transverse) L60.4
    congenital Q84.6
  tongue K14.5
    congenital Q38.3
Furuncle L02.92
  abdominal wall L02.221
  ankle — *see* Furuncle, lower limb
  antecubital space — *see* Furuncle, upper limb
  anus K61.0
  arm — *see* Furuncle, upper limb
  auditory canal, external — *see* Abscess, ear, external
  auricle (ear) — *see* Abscess, ear, external
  axilla (region) L02.42- ☑
  back (any part) L02.222
  breast N61.1
  buttock L02.32
  cheek (external) L02.02
  chest wall L02.223
  chin L02.02
  corpus cavernosum N48.21
  ear, external — *see* Abscess, ear, external
  external auditory canal — *see* Abscess, ear, external
  eyelid — *see* Abscess, eyelid
  face L02.02
  femoral (region) — *see* Furuncle, lower limb
  finger — *see* Furuncle, hand
  flank L02.221
  foot L02.62- ☑
  forehead L02.02
  gluteal (region) L02.32

▽ **Subterms under main terms may continue to next column or page**   ☑ **Additional Character Required** — **Refer to the Tabular List for Character Selection**   **155**

Fracture, traumatic — Furuncle

Furuncle — *continued*
  groin L02.224
  hand L02.52- ☑
  head L02.821
    face L02.02
  hip — *see* Furuncle, lower limb
  kidney — *see* Abscess, kidney
  knee — *see* Furuncle, lower limb
  labium (majus) (minus) N76.4
  lacrimal
    gland — *see* Dacryoadenitis
    passages (duct) (sac) — *see* Inflammation, lacrimal,
        passages, acute
  leg (any part) — *see* Furuncle, lower limb
  lower limb L02.42- ☑
  malignant A22.0
  mouth K12.2
  navel L02.226
  neck L02.12
  nose J34.0
  orbit, orbital — *see* Abscess, orbit
  palmar (space) — *see* Furuncle, hand
  partes posteriores L02.32
  pectoral region L02.223
  penis N48.21
  perineum L02.225
  pinna — *see* Abscess, ear, external
  popliteal — *see* Furuncle, lower limb
  prepatellar — *see* Furuncle, lower limb
  scalp L02.821
  seminal vesicle N49.0
  shoulder — *see* Furuncle, upper limb
  specified site NEC L02.828
  submandibular K12.2
  temple (region) L02.02
  thumb — *see* Furuncle, hand
  toe — *see* Furuncle, foot
  trunk L02.229
    abdominal wall L02.221
    back L02.222

Furuncle — *continued*
  trunk — *continued*
    chest wall L02.223
    groin L02.224
    perineum L02.225
    umbilicus L02.226
  umbilicus L02.226
  upper limb L02.42- ☑
  vulva N76.4
Furunculosis — *see* Furuncle
Fused — *see* Fusion, fused
Fusion, fused (congenital)
  astragaloscaphoid Q74.2
  atria Q21.1
  auditory canal Q16.1
  auricles, heart Q21.1
  binocular with defective stereopsis H53.32
  bone Q79.8
  cervical spine M43.22
  choanal Q30.0
  commissure, mitral valve Q23.2
  cusps, heart valve NEC Q24.8
    mitral Q23.2
    pulmonary Q22.1
    tricuspid Q22.4
  ear ossicles Q16.3
  fingers Q70.0 ☑
  hymen Q52.3
  joint (acquired) (*see also* Ankylosis)
    congenital Q74.8
  kidneys (incomplete) Q63.1
  labium (majus) (minus) Q52.5
  larynx and trachea Q34.8
  limb, congenital Q74.8
    lower Q74.2
    upper Q74.0
  lobes, lung Q33.8
  lumbosacral (acquired) M43.27
    arthrodesis status Z98.1
    congenital Q76.49

Fusion, fused — *continued*
  lumbosacral — *continued*
    postprocedural status Z98.1
  nares, nose, nasal, nostril(s) Q30.0
  organ or site not listed — *see* Anomaly, by site
  ossicles Q79.9
    auditory Q16.3
  pulmonic cusps Q22.1
  ribs Q76.6
  sacroiliac (joint) (acquired) M43.28
    arthrodesis status Z98.1
    congenital Q74.2
    postprocedural status Z98.1
  spine (acquired) NEC M43.20
    arthrodesis status Z98.1
    cervical region M43.22
    cervicothoracic region M43.23
    congenital Q76.49
    lumbar M43.26
    lumbosacral region M43.27
    occipito-atlanto-axial region M43.21
    postoperative status Z98.1
    sacrococcygeal region M43.28
    thoracic region M43.24
    thoracolumbar region M43.25
  sublingual duct with submaxillary duct at opening in
        mouth Q38.4
  testes Q55.1
  toes Q70.2- ☑
  tooth, teeth K00.2
  trachea and esophagus Q39.8
  twins Q89.4
  vagina Q52.4
  ventricles, heart Q21.0
  vertebra (arch) — *see* Fusion, spine
  vulva Q52.5
Fusospirillosis (mouth) (tongue) (tonsil) A69.1
Fussy baby R68.12

☑ **Additional Character Required** — **Refer to the Tabular List for Character Selection**   ▽ **Subterms under main terms may continue to next column or page**

G

Gain in weight (abnormal) (excessive) (*see also* Weight, gain)
Gaisböck's disease (polycythemia hypertonica) D75.1
Gait abnormality R26.9
　ataxic R26.0
　falling R29.6
　hysterical (ataxic) (staggering) F44.4
　paralytic R26.1
　spastic R26.1
　specified type NEC R26.89
　staggering R26.0
　unsteadiness R26.81
　walking difficulty NEC R26.2
Galactocele (breast) N64.89
　puerperal, postpartum O92.79
Galactokinase deficiency E74.29
Galactophoritis N61.0
　gestational, puerperal, postpartum O91.2- ☑
Galactorrhea O92.6
　not associated with childbirth N64.3
Galactosemia (classic) (congenital) E74.21
Galactosuria E74.29
Galacturia R82.0
　schistosomiasis (bilharziasis) B65.0
GALD (gestational alloimmune liver disease) P78.84
Galeazzi's fracture S52.37- ☑
Galen's vein — *see* condition
Galeophobia F40.218
Gall duct — *see* condition
Gallbladder (*see also* condition)
　acute K81.0
Gallop rhythm R00.8
Gallstone (colic) (cystic duct) (gallbladder) (impacted) (multiple) (*see also* Calculus, gallbladder)
　with
　　cholecystitis — *see* Calculus, gallbladder, with cholecystitis
　bile duct (common) (hepatic) — *see* Calculus, bile duct
　causing intestinal obstruction K56.3
　specified NEC K80.80
　　with obstruction K80.81
Gambling Z72.6
　pathological (compulsive) F63.0
Gammopathy (of undetermined significance [MGUS]) D47.2
　associated with lymphoplasmacytic dyscrasia D47.2
　monoclonal D47.2
　polyclonal D89.0
Gamna's disease (siderotic splenomegaly) D73.1
Gamophobia F40.298
Gampsodactylia (congenital) Q66.7
Gamstorp's disease (adynamia episodica hereditaria) G72.3
Gandy-Nanta disease (siderotic splenomegaly) D73.1
Gang
　membership offenses Z72.810
Gangliocytoma D36.10
Ganglioglioma — *see* Neoplasm, uncertain behavior, by site
Ganglion (compound) (diffuse) (joint) (tendon (sheath)) M67.40
　ankle M67.47- ☑
　foot M67.47- ☑
　forearm M67.43- ☑
　hand M67.44- ☑
　lower leg M67.46- ☑
　multiple sites M67.49
　of yaws (early) (late) A66.6
　pelvic region M67.45- ☑
　periosteal — *see* Periostitis
　shoulder region M67.41- ☑
　specified site NEC M67.48
　thigh region M67.45- ☑
　tuberculous A18.09
　upper arm M67.42- ☑
　wrist M67.43- ☑
Ganglioneuroblastoma — *see* Neoplasm, nerve, malignant
Ganglioneuroma D36.10
　malignant — *see* Neoplasm, nerve, malignant
Ganglioneuromatosis D36.10
Ganglionitis
　fifth nerve — *see* Neuralgia, trigeminal
　gasserian (postherpetic) (postzoster) B02.21

Ganglionitis — *continued*
　geniculate G51.1
　　newborn (birth injury) P11.3
　　postherpetic, postzoster B02.21
　herpes zoster B02.21
　postherpetic geniculate B02.21
Gangliosidosis E75.10
　GM1 E75.19
　GM2 E75.00
　　other specified E75.09
　　Sandhoff disease E75.01
　　Tay-Sachs disease E75.02
　GM3 E75.19
　mucolipidosis IV E75.11
Gangosa A66.5
Gangrene, gangrenous (connective tissue) (dropsical) (dry) (moist) (skin) (ulcer) (*see also* Necrosis) I96
　with diabetes (mellitus) — *see* Diabetes, gangrene
　abdomen (wall) I96
　alveolar M27.3
　appendix K35.80
　　with
　　　peritonitis, localized (*see also* Appendicitis) K35.31
　arteriosclerotic (general) (senile) — *see* Arteriosclerosis, extremities, with, gangrene
　auricle I96
　Bacillus welchii A48.0
　bladder (infectious) — *see* Cystitis, specified type NEC
　bowel, cecum, or colon — *see* Gangrene, intestine
　Clostridium perfringens or welchii A48.0
　cornea H18.89- ☑
　corpora cavernosa N48.29
　　noninfective N48.89
　cutaneous, spreading I96
　decubital — *see* Ulcer, pressure, by site
　diabetic (any site) — *see* Diabetes, gangrene
　emphysematous — *see* Gangrene, gas
　epidemic — *see* Poisoning, food, noxious, plant
　epididymis (infectional) N45.1
　erysipelas — *see* Erysipelas
　extremity (lower) (upper) I96
　Fournier N49.3
　　female N76.89
　fusospirochetal A69.0
　gallbladder — *see* Cholecystitis, acute
　gas (bacillus) A48.0
　　following
　　　abortion — *see* Abortion by type complicated by infection
　　　ectopic or molar pregnancy O08.0
　glossitis K14.0
　hernia — *see* Hernia, by site, with gangrene
　intestine, intestinal (hemorrhagic) (massive) (*see also* Infarct, intestine) K55.069
　　with
　　　mesenteric embolism (*see also* Infarct, intestine) K55.069
　　　obstruction — *see* Obstruction, intestine
　laryngitis J04.0
　limb (lower) (upper) I96
　lung J85.0
　　spirochetal A69.8
　lymphangitis I89.1
　Meleney's (synergistic) — *see* Ulcer, skin
　mesentery (*see also* Infarct, intestine) K55.069
　　with
　　　embolism (*see also* Infarct, intestine) K55.069
　　　intestinal obstruction — *see* Obstruction, intestine
　mouth A69.0
　ovary — *see* Oophoritis
　pancreas — *see* Pancreatitis, acute
　penis N48.29
　　noninfective N48.89
　perineum I96
　pharynx (*see also* Pharyngitis)
　　Vincent's A69.1
　presenile I73.1
　progressive synergistic — *see* Ulcer, skin
　pulmonary J85.0
　pulpal (dental) K04.1
　quinsy J36
　Raynaud's (symmetric gangrene) I73.01
　retropharyngeal J39.2
　scrotum N49.3
　　noninfective N50.89

Gangrene, gangrenous — *continued*
　senile (atherosclerotic) — *see* Arteriosclerosis, extremities, with, gangrene
　spermatic cord N49.1
　　noninfective N50.89
　spine I96
　spirochetal NEC A69.8
　spreading cutaneous I96
　stomatitis A69.0
　symmetrical I73.01
　testis (infectional) N45.2
　　noninfective N44.8
　throat (*see also* Pharyngitis)
　　diphtheritic A36.0
　　Vincent's A69.1
　thyroid (gland) E07.89
　tooth (pulp) K04.1
　tuberculous NEC — *see* Tuberculosis
　tunica vaginalis N49.1
　　noninfective N50.89
　umbilicus I96
　uterus — *see* Endometritis
　uvulitis K12.2
　vas deferens N49.1
　　noninfective N50.89
　vulva N76.89
Ganister disease J62.8
Ganser's syndrome (hysterical) F44.89
Gardner-Diamond syndrome (autoerythrocyte sensitization) D69.2
Gargoylism E76.01
Garré's disease, osteitis (sclerosing), osteomyelitis — *see* Osteomyelitis, specified type NEC
Garrod's pad, knuckle M72.1
Gartner's duct
　cyst Q52.4
　persistent Q50.6
Gas R14.3
　asphyxiation, inhalation, poisoning, suffocation NEC — *see* Table of Drugs and Chemicals
　excessive R14.0
　gangrene A48.0
　　following
　　　abortion — *see* Abortion by type complicated by infection
　　　ectopic or molar pregnancy O08.0
　on stomach R14.0
　pains R14.1
Gastralgia (*see also* Pain, abdominal)
Gastrectasis K31.0
　psychogenic F45.8
Gastric — *see* condition
Gastrinoma
　malignant
　　pancreas C25.4
　　specified site NEC — *see* Neoplasm, malignant, by site
　　unspecified site C25.4
　specified site — *see* Neoplasm, uncertain behavior
　unspecified site D37.9
Gastritis (simple) K29.70
　with bleeding K29.71
　acute (erosive) K29.00
　　with bleeding K29.01
　alcoholic K29.20
　　with bleeding K29.21
　allergic K29.60
　　with bleeding K29.61
　atrophic (chronic) K29.40
　　with bleeding K29.41
　chronic (antral) (fundal) K29.50
　　with bleeding K29.51
　　atrophic K29.40
　　　with bleeding K29.41
　　superficial K29.30
　　　with bleeding K29.31
　dietary counseling and surveillance Z71.3
　due to diet deficiency E63.9
　eosinophilic K52.81
　giant hypertrophic K29.60
　　with bleeding K29.61
　granulomatous K29.60
　　with bleeding K29.61
　hypertrophic (mucosa) K29.60
　　with bleeding K29.61
　nervous F54
　spastic K29.60
　　with bleeding K29.61

Index

Gastritis — *continued*
- specified NEC K29.60
  - with bleeding K29.61
- superficial chronic K29.30
  - with bleeding K29.31
- tuberculous A18.83
- viral NEC A08.4

Gastrocarcinoma — *see* Neoplasm, malignant, stomach

Gastrocolic — *see* condition

Gastrodisciasis, gastrodiscoidiasis B66.8

Gastroduodenitis K29.90
- with bleeding K29.91
- virus, viral A08.4
  - specified type NEC A08.39

Gastrodynia — *see* Pain, abdominal

Gastroenteritis (acute) (chronic) (noninfectious) (*see also* Enteritis) K52.9
- allergic K52.29
  - with
    - eosinophilic gastritis or gastroenteritis K52.81
    - food protein-induced enterocolitis syndrome K52.21
    - food protein-induced enteropathy K52.22
- dietetic (*see also* Gastroenteritis, allergic) K52.29
- drug-induced K52.1
- due to
  - Cryptosporidium A07.2
  - drugs K52.1
  - food poisoning — *see* Intoxication, foodborne
  - radiation K52.0
- eosinophilic K52.81
- epidemic (infectious) A09
- food hypersensitivity (*see also* Gastroenteritis, allergic) K52.29
- infectious — *see* Enteritis, infectious
- influenzal — *see* Influenza, with gastroenteritis
- noninfectious K52.9
  - specified NEC K52.89
- rotaviral A08.0
- Salmonella A02.0
- toxic K52.1
- viral NEC A08.4
  - acute infectious A08.39
    - type Norwalk A08.11
  - infantile (acute) A08.39
  - Norwalk agent A08.11
  - rotaviral A08.0
  - severe of infants A08.39
  - specified type NEC A08.39

Gastroenteropathy (*see also* Gastroenteritis) K52.9
- acute, due to Norovirus A08.11
- acute, due to Norwalk agent A08.11
- infectious A09

Gastroenteroptosis K63.4

Gastroesophageal laceration- hemorrhage syndrome K22.6

Gastrointestinal — *see* condition

Gastrojejunal — *see* condition

Gastrojejunitis (*see also* Enteritis) K52.9

Gastrojejunocolic — *see* condition

Gastroliths K31.89

Gastromalacia K31.89

Gastroparalysis K31.84
- diabetic — *see* Diabetes, gastroparalysis

Gastroparesis K31.84
- diabetic — *see* Diabetes, by type, with gastroparesis

Gastropathy K31.9
- congestive portal K31.89
- erythematous K29.70
- exudative K90.89
- portal hypertensive K31.89

Gastroptosis K31.89

Gastrorrhagia K92.2
- psychogenic F45.8

Gastroschisis (congenital) Q79.3

Gastrospasm (neurogenic) (reflex) K31.89
- neurotic F45.8
- psychogenic F45.8

Gastrostaxis — *see* Gastritis, with bleeding

Gastrostenosis K31.89

Gastrostomy
- attention to Z43.1
- status Z93.1

Gastrosuccorrhea (continuous) (intermittent) K31.89
- neurotic F45.8
- psychogenic F45.8

Gatophobia F40.218

Gaucher's disease or splenomegaly (adult) (infantile) E75.22

Gee (-Herter)(-Thaysen) **disease** (nontropical sprue) K90.0

Gélineau's syndrome G47.419
- with cataplexy G47.411

Gemination, tooth, teeth K00.2

Gemistocytoma
- specified site — *see* Neoplasm, malignant, by site
- unspecified site C71.9

General, generalized — *see* condition

Genetic
- carrier (status)
  - cystic fibrosis Z14.1
  - hemophilia A (asymptomatic) Z14.01
    - symptomatic Z14.02
  - specified NEC Z14.8
- susceptibility to disease NEC Z15.89
  - malignant neoplasm Z15.09
    - breast Z15.01
    - endometrium Z15.04
    - ovary Z15.02
    - prostate Z15.03
    - specified NEC Z15.09
  - multiple endocrine neoplasia Z15.81

Genital — *see* condition

Genito-anorectal syndrome A55

Genitourinary system — *see* condition

Genu
- congenital Q74.1
- extrorsum (acquired) (*see also* Deformity, varus, knee)
  - congenital Q74.1
  - sequelae (late effect) of rickets E64.3
- introrsum (acquired) (*see also* Deformity, valgus, knee)
  - congenital Q74.1
  - sequelae (late effect) of rickets E64.3
- rachitic (old) E64.3
- recurvatum (acquired) (*see also* Deformity, limb, specified type NEC, lower leg)
  - congenital Q68.2
  - sequelae (late effect) of rickets E64.3
- valgum (acquired) (knock-knee) M21.06- ☑
  - congenital Q74.1
  - sequelae (late effect) of rickets E64.3
- varum (acquired) (bowleg) M21.16- ☑
  - congenital Q74.1
  - sequelae (late effect) of rickets E64.3

Geographic tongue K14.1

Geophagia — *see* Pica

Geotrichosis B48.3
- stomatitis B48.3

Gephyrophobia F40.242

Gerbode defect Q21.0

GERD (gastroesophageal reflux disease) K21.9

Gerhardt's
- disease (erythromelalgia) I73.81
- syndrome (vocal cord paralysis) J38.00
  - bilateral J38.02
  - unilateral J38.01

German measles (*see also* Rubella)
- exposure to Z20.4

Germinoblastoma (diffuse) C85.9- ☑
- follicular C82.9- ☑

Germinoma — *see* Neoplasm, malignant, by site

Gerontoxon — *see* Degeneration, cornea, senile

Gerstmann's syndrome R48.8
- developmental F81.2

Gerstmann-Sträussler-Scheinker syndrome (GSS) A81.82

Gestation (period) (*see also* Pregnancy)
- ectopic — *see* Pregnancy, by site
- multiple O30.9- ☑
  - greater than quadruplets — *see* Pregnancy, multiple (gestation), specified NEC
  - specified NEC — *see* Pregnancy, multiple (gestation), specified NEC

Gestational
- mammary abscess O91.11- ☑
- purulent mastitis O91.11- ☑
- subareolar abscess O91.11- ☑

Ghon tubercle, primary infection A15.7

Ghost
- teeth K00.4
- vessels (cornea) H16.41- ☑

Ghoul hand A66.3

Gianotti-Crosti disease L44.4

Giant
- cell
  - epulis K06.8
  - peripheral granuloma K06.8
- esophagus, congenital Q39.5
- kidney, congenital Q63.3
- urticaria T78.3 ☑
  - hereditary D84.1

Giardiasis A07.1

Gibert's disease or pityriasis L42

Giddiness R42
- hysterical F44.89
- psychogenic F45.8

Gierke's disease (glycogenosis I) E74.01

Gigantism (cerebral) (hypophyseal) (pituitary) E22.0
- constitutional E34.4

Gilbert's disease or syndrome E80.4

Gilchrist's disease B40.9

Gilford-Hutchinson disease E34.8

Gilles de la Tourette's disease or syndrome (motor-verbal tic) F95.2

Gingivitis K05.10
- acute (catarrhal) K05.00
  - necrotizing A69.1
  - nonplaque induced K05.01
  - plaque induced K05.00
- chronic (desquamative) (hyperplastic) (simple marginal) (pregnancy associated) (ulcerative) K05.10
  - nonplaque induced K05.11
  - plaque induced K05.10
- expulsiva — *see* Periodontitis
- necrotizing ulcerative (acute) A69.1
- pellagrous E52
  - acute necrotizing A69.1
- Vincent's A69.1

Gingivoglossitis K14.0

Gingivopericementitis — *see* Periodontitis

Gingivosis — *see* Gingivitis, chronic

Gingivostomatitis K05.10
- herpesviral B00.2
- necrotizing ulcerative (acute) A69.1

Gland, glandular — *see* condition

Glanders A24.0

Glanzmann (-Naegeli) **disease or thrombasthenia** D69.1

Glasgow coma scale
- total score
  - 13-15 R40.241 ☑
  - 3-8 R40.243 ☑
  - 9-12 R40.242 ☑

Glass-blower's disease (cataract) — *see* Cataract, specified NEC

Glaucoma H40.9
- with
  - increased episcleral venous pressure H40.81- ☑
  - pseudoexfoliation of lens — *see* Glaucoma, open angle, primary, capsular
- absolute H44.51- ☑
- angle-closure (primary) H40.20- ☑
  - acute (attack) (crisis) H40.21- ☑
  - chronic H40.22- ☑
  - intermittent H40.23- ☑
  - residual stage H40.24- ☑
- borderline H40.00- ☑
- capsular (with pseudoexfoliation of lens) — *see* Glaucoma, open angle, primary, capsular
- childhood Q15.0
- closed angle — *see* Glaucoma, angle-closure
- congenital Q15.0
- corticosteroid-induced — *see* Glaucoma, secondary, drugs
- hypersecretion H40.82- ☑
- in (due to)
  - amyloidosis E85.4 [H42]
  - aniridia Q13.1 [H42]
  - concussion of globe — *see* Glaucoma, secondary, trauma
  - dislocation of lens — *see* Glaucoma, secondary
  - disorder of lens NEC — *see* Glaucoma, secondary
  - drugs — *see* Glaucoma, secondary, drugs
  - endocrine disease NOS E34.9 [H42]
  - eye
    - inflammation — *see* Glaucoma, secondary, inflammation
    - trauma — *see* Glaucoma, secondary, trauma
  - hypermature cataract — *see* Glaucoma, secondary

Glaucoma — *continued*
  in — *continued*
    iridocyclitis — *see* Glaucoma, secondary, inflammation
    lens disorder — *see* Glaucoma, secondary
    Lowe's syndrome E72.03 [H42]
    metabolic disease NOS E88.9 [H42]
    ocular disorders NEC — *see* Glaucoma, secondary
    onchocerciasis B73.02
    pupillary block — *see* Glaucoma, secondary
    retinal vein occlusion — *see* Glaucoma, secondary
    Rieger's anomaly Q13.81 [H42]
    rubeosis of iris — *see* Glaucoma, secondary
    tumor of globe — *see* Glaucoma, secondary
  infantile Q15.0
  low tension — *see* Glaucoma, open angle, primary, low-tension
  malignant H40.83- ☑
  narrow angle — *see* Glaucoma, angle-closure
  newborn Q15.0
  noncongestive (chronic) — *see* Glaucoma, open angle
  nonobstructive — *see* Glaucoma, open angle
  obstructive (*see also* Glaucoma, angle-closure)
    due to lens changes — *see* Glaucoma, secondary
  open angle H40.10- ☑
    primary H40.11- ☑
      capsular (with pseudoexfoliation of lens) H40.14- ☑
      low-tension H40.12- ☑
      pigmentary H40.13- ☑
      residual stage H40.15- ☑
  phacolytic — *see* Glaucoma, secondary
  pigmentary — *see* Glaucoma, open angle, primary, pigmentary
  postinfectious — *see* Glaucoma, secondary, inflammation
  secondary (to) H40.5- ☑
    drugs H40.6- ☑
    inflammation H40.4- ☑
    trauma H40.3- ☑
  simple (chronic) H40.11- ☑
  simplex H40.11- ☑
  specified type NEC H40.89
  suspect H40.00- ☑
  syphilitic A52.71
  traumatic (*see also* Glaucoma, secondary, trauma)
    newborn (birth injury) P15.3
  tuberculous A18.59
Glaucomatous flecks (subcapsular) — *see* Cataract, complicated
Glazed tongue K14.4
Gleet (gonococcal) A54.01
Glénard's disease K63.4
Glioblastoma (multiforme)
  with sarcomatous component
    specified site — *see* Neoplasm, malignant, by site
    unspecified site C71.9
  giant cell
    specified site — *see* Neoplasm, malignant, by site
    unspecified site C71.9
  specified site — *see* Neoplasm, malignant, by site
  unspecified site C71.9
Glioma (malignant)
  astrocytic
    specified site — *see* Neoplasm, malignant, by site
    unspecified site C71.9
  mixed
    specified site — *see* Neoplasm, malignant, by site
    unspecified site C71.9
  nose Q30.8
  specified site NEC — *see* Neoplasm, malignant, by site
  subependymal D43.2
    specified site — *see* Neoplasm, uncertain behavior, by site
    unspecified site D43.2
  unspecified site C71.9
Gliomatosis cerebri C71.0
Glioneuroma — *see* Neoplasm, uncertain behavior, by site
Gliosarcoma
  specified site — *see* Neoplasm, malignant, by site
  unspecified site C71.9
Gliosis (cerebral) G93.89
  spinal G95.89
Glisson's disease — *see* Rickets
Globinuria R82.3
Globus (hystericus) F45.8

Glomangioma D18.00
  intra-abdominal D18.03
  intracranial D18.02
  skin D18.01
  specified site NEC D18.09
Glomangiomyoma D18.00
  intra-abdominal D18.03
  intracranial D18.02
  skin D18.01
  specified site NEC D18.09
Glomangiosarcoma — *see* Neoplasm, connective tissue, malignant
Glomerular
  disease in syphilis A52.75
  nephritis — *see* Glomerulonephritis
Glomerulitis — *see* Glomerulonephritis
Glomerulonephritis (*see also* Nephritis) N05.9
  with
    edema — *see* Nephrosis
    minimal change N05.0
    minor glomerular abnormality N05.0
  acute N00.9
  chronic N03.9
  crescentic (diffuse) NEC (*see also* N00-N07 with fourth character .7) N05.7
  dense deposit (*see also* N00-N07 with fourth character .6) N05.6
  diffuse
    crescentic (*see also* N00-N07 with fourth character .7) N05.7
    endocapillary proliferative (*see also* N00-N07 with fourth character .4) N05.4
    membranous (*see also* N00-N07 with fourth character .2) N05.2
    mesangial proliferative (*see also* N00-N07 with fourth character .3) N05.3
    mesangiocapillary (*see also* N00-N07 with fourth character .5) N05.5
    sclerosing N18.9
  endocapillary proliferative (diffuse) NEC (*see also* N00-N07 with fourth character .4) N05.4
  extracapillary NEC (*see also* N00-N07 with fourth character .7) N05.7
  focal (and segmental) (*see also* N00-N07 with fourth character .1) N05.1
  hypocomplementemic — *see* Glomerulonephritis, membranoproliferative
  IgA — *see* Nephropathy, IgA
  immune complex (circulating) NEC N05.8
  in (due to)
    amyloidosis E85.4 [N08]
    bilharziasis B65.9 [N08]
    cryoglobulinemia D89.1 [N08]
    defibrination syndrome D65 [N08]
    diabetes mellitus — *see* Diabetes, glomerulosclerosis
    disseminated intravascular coagulation D65 [N08]
    Fabry (-Anderson) disease E75.21 [N08]
    Goodpasture's syndrome M31.0
    hemolytic-uremic syndrome D59.3
    Henoch (-Schönlein) purpura D69.0 [N08]
    lecithin cholesterol acyltransferase deficiency E78.6 [N08]
    microscopic polyangiitis M31.7 [N08]
    multiple myeloma C90.0- ☑ [N08]
    Plasmodium malariae B52.0
    schistosomiasis B65.9 [N08]
    sepsis A41.9 [N08]
      streptococcal A40- ☑ [N08]
    sickle-cell disorders D57.- ☑ [N08]
    strongyloidiasis B78.9 [N08]
    subacute bacterial endocarditis I33.0 [N08]
    syphilis (late) congenital A50.59 [N08]
    systemic lupus erythematosus M32.14
    thrombotic thrombocytopenic purpura M31.1 [N08]
    typhoid fever A01.09
    Waldenström macroglobulinemia C88.0 [N08]
    Wegener's granulomatosis M31.31
  latent or quiescent N03.9
  lobular, lobulonodular — *see* Glomerulonephritis, membranoproliferative
  membranoproliferative (diffuse)(type 1 or 3) (*see also* N00-N07 with fourth character .5) N05.5
    dense deposit (type 2) NEC (*see also* N00-N07 with fourth character .6) N05.6
  membranous (diffuse) NEC (*see also* N00-N07 with fourth character .2) N05.2

Glomerulonephritis — *continued*
  mesangial
    IgA/IgG — *see* Nephropathy, IgA
    proliferative (diffuse) NEC (*see also* N00-N07 with fourth character .3) N05.3
  mesangiocapillary (diffuse) NEC (*see also* N00-N07 with fourth character .5) N05.5
  necrotic, necrotizing NEC (*see also* N00-N07 with fourth character .8) N05.8
  nodular — *see* Glomerulonephritis, membranoproliferative
  poststreptococcal NEC N05.9
    acute N00.9
    chronic N03.9
    rapidly progressive N01.9
  proliferative NEC (*see also* N00-N07 with fourth character .8) N05.8
    diffuse (lupus) M32.14
  rapidly progressive N01.9
  sclerosing, diffuse N18.9
  specified pathology NEC (*see also* N00-N07 with fourth character .8) N05.8
  subacute N01.9
Glomerulopathy — *see* Glomerulonephritis
Glomerulosclerosis (*see also* Sclerosis, renal)
  intercapillary (nodular) (with diabetes) — *see* Diabetes, glomerulosclerosis
  intracapillary — *see* Diabetes, glomerulosclerosis
Glossagra K14.6
Glossalgia K14.6
Glossitis (chronic superficial) (gangrenous) (Moeller's) K14.0
  areata exfoliativa K14.1
  atrophic K14.4
  benign migratory K14.1
  cortical superficial, sclerotic K14.0
  Hunter's D51.0
  interstitial, sclerous K14.0
  median rhomboid K14.2
  pellagrous E52
  superficial, chronic K14.0
Glossocele K14.8
Glossodynia K14.6
  exfoliativa K14.4
Glossoncus K14.8
Glossopathy K14.9
Glossophytia K14.3
Glossoplegia K14.8
Glossoptosis K14.8
Glossopyrosis K14.6
Glossotrichia K14.3
Glossy skin L90.8
Glottis — *see* condition
Glottitis (*see also* Laryngitis) J04.0
Glucagonoma
  pancreas
    benign D13.7
    malignant C25.4
    uncertain behavior D37.8
  specified site NEC
    benign — *see* Neoplasm, benign, by site
    malignant — *see* Neoplasm, malignant, by site
    uncertain behavior — *see* Neoplasm, uncertain behavior, by site
  unspecified site
    benign D13.7
    malignant C25.4
    uncertain behavior D37.8
Glucoglycinuria E72.51
Glucose-galactose malabsorption E74.39
Glue
  ear — *see* Otitis, media, nonsuppurative, chronic, mucoid
  sniffing (airplane) — *see* Abuse, drug, inhalant dependence — *see* Dependence, drug, inhalant
Glutaric aciduria E72.3
Glycinemia E72.51
Glycinuria (renal) (with ketosis) E72.09
Glycogen
  infiltration — *see* Disease, glycogen storage
  storage disease — *see* Disease, glycogen storage
Glycogenosis (diffuse) (generalized) (*see also* Disease, glycogen storage)
  cardiac E74.02 [I43]
  diabetic, secondary — *see* Diabetes, glycogenosis, secondary
  pulmonary interstitial J84.842

Subterms under main terms may continue to next column or page   ☑ Additional Character Required — Refer to the Tabular List for Character Selection   159

Glaucoma — Glycogenosis

Glycopenia E16.2
Glycosuria R81
  renal E74.8
Gnathostoma spinigerum (infection) (infestation), **gnathostomiasis** (wandering swelling) B83.1
Goiter (plunging) (substernal) E04.9
  with
    hyperthyroidism (recurrent) — *see* Hyperthyroidism, with, goiter
    thyrotoxicosis — *see* Hyperthyroidism, with, goiter
  adenomatous — *see* Goiter, nodular
  cancerous C73
  congenital (nontoxic) E03.0
    diffuse E03.0
    parenchymatous E03.0
    transitory, with normal functioning P72.0
  cystic E04.2
    due to iodine-deficiency E01.1
  due to
    enzyme defect in synthesis of thyroid hormone E07.1
    iodine-deficiency (endemic) E01.2
  dyshormonogenetic (familial) E07.1
  endemic (iodine-deficiency) E01.2
    diffuse E01.0
    multinodular E01.1
  exophthalmic — *see* Hyperthyroidism, with, goiter
  iodine-deficiency (endemic) E01.2
    diffuse E01.0
    multinodular E01.1
    nodular E01.1
  lingual Q89.2
  lymphadenoid E06.3
  malignant C73
  multinodular (cystic) (nontoxic) E04.2
    toxic or with hyperthyroidism E05.20
      with thyroid storm E05.21
  neonatal NEC P72.0
  nodular (nontoxic) (due to) E04.9
    with
      hyperthyroidism E05.20
        with thyroid storm E05.21
      thyrotoxicosis E05.20
        with thyroid storm E05.21
    endemic E01.1
    iodine-deficiency E01.1
    sporadic E04.9
    toxic E05.20
      with thyroid storm E05.21
  nontoxic E04.9
    diffuse (colloid) E04.0
    multinodular E04.2
    simple E04.0
    specified NEC E04.8
    uninodular E04.1
  simple E04.0
  toxic — *see* Hyperthyroidism, with, goiter
  uninodular (nontoxic) E04.1
    toxic or with hyperthyroidism E05.10
      with thyroid storm E05.11
Goiter-deafness syndrome E07.1
Goldberg syndrome Q89.8
Goldberg-Maxwell syndrome E34.51
Goldblatt's hypertension or kidney I70.1
Goldenhar (-Gorlin) **syndrome** Q87.0
Goldflam-Erb disease or syndrome G70.00
  with exacerbation (acute) G70.01
  in crisis G70.01
Goldscheider's disease Q81.8
Goldstein's disease (familial hemorrhagic telangiectasia) I78.0
Golfer's elbow — *see* Epicondylitis, medial
Gonadoblastoma
  specified site — *see* Neoplasm, uncertain behavior, by site
  unspecified site
    female D39.10
    male D40.10
Gonecystitis — *see* Vesiculitis
Gongylonemiasis B83.8
Goniosynechiae — *see* Adhesions, iris, goniosynechiae
Gonococcemia A54.86
Gonococcus, gonococcal (disease) (infection) (*see also* condition) A54.9
  anus A54.6
  bursa, bursitis A54.49
  conjunctiva, conjunctivitis (neonatorum) A54.31
  endocardium A54.83

Gonococcus, gonococcal — *continued*
  eye A54.30
    conjunctivitis A54.31
    iridocyclitis A54.32
    keratitis A54.33
    newborn A54.31
    other specified A54.39
  fallopian tubes (acute) (chronic) A54.24
  genitourinary (organ) (system) (tract) (acute) A54.00
    lower A54.00
      with abscess (accessory gland) (periurethral) A54.1
    upper (*see also* condition) A54.29
  heart A54.83
  iridocyclitis A54.32
  joint A54.42
  lymphatic (gland) (node) A54.89
  meninges, meningitis A54.81
  musculoskeletal A54.40
    arthritis A54.42
    osteomyelitis A54.43
    other specified A54.49
    spondylopathy A54.41
  pelviperitonitis A54.24
  pelvis (acute) (chronic) A54.24
  pharynx A54.5
  proctitis A54.6
  pyosalpinx (acute) (chronic) A54.24
  rectum A54.6
  skin A54.89
  specified site NEC A54.89
  tendon sheath A54.49
  throat A54.5
  urethra (acute) (chronic) A54.01
    with abscess (accessory gland) (periurethral) A54.1
  vulva (acute) (chronic) A54.02
Gonocytoma
  specified site — *see* Neoplasm, uncertain behavior, by site
  unspecified site
    female D39.10
    male D40.10
Gonorrhea (acute) (chronic) A54.9
  Bartholin's gland (acute) (chronic) (purulent) A54.02
    with abscess (accessory gland) (periurethral) A54.1
  bladder A54.01
  cervix A54.03
  conjunctiva, conjunctivitis (neonatorum) A54.31
  contact Z20.2
  Cowper's gland (with abscess) A54.1
  exposure to Z20.2
  fallopian tube (acute) (chronic) A54.24
  kidney (acute) (chronic) A54.21
  lower genitourinary tract A54.00
    with abscess (accessory gland) (periurethral) A54.1
  ovary (acute) (chronic) A54.24
  pelvis (acute) (chronic) A54.24
    female pelvic inflammatory disease A54.24
  penis A54.09
  prostate (acute) (chronic) A54.22
  seminal vesicle (acute) (chronic) A54.23
  specified site not listed (*see also* Gonococcus) A54.89
  spermatic cord (acute) (chronic) A54.23
  urethra A54.01
    with abscess (accessory gland) (periurethral) A54.1
  vagina A54.02
  vas deferens (acute) (chronic) A54.23
  vulva A54.02
Goodall's disease A08.19
Goodpasture's syndrome M31.0
Gopalan's syndrome (burning feet) E53.0
Gorlin-Chaudry-Moss syndrome Q87.0
Gottron's papules L94.4
Gougerot-Blum syndrome (pigmented purpuric lichenoid dermatitis) L81.7
Gougerot-Carteaud disease or syndrome (confluent reticulate papillomatosis) L83
Gougerot's syndrome (trisymptomatic) L81.7
Gouley's syndrome (constrictive pericarditis) I31.1
Goundou A66.6
Gout, chronic (*see also* Gout, gouty) M1A.9 ☑ (*following* M08)
  drug-induced M1A.20 ☑ (*following* M08)
    ankle M1A.27- ☑ (*following* M08)
    elbow M1A.22- ☑ (*following* M08)
    foot joint M1A.27- ☑ (*following* M08)
    hand joint M1A.24- ☑ (*following* M08)
    hip M1A.25- ☑ (*following* M08)

Gout, chronic — *continued*
  drug-induced — *continued*
    knee M1A.26- ☑ (*following* M08)
    multiple site M1A.29- ☑ (*following* M08)
    shoulder M1A.21- ☑ (*following* M08)
    vertebrae M1A.28 ☑ (*following* M08)
    wrist M1A.23- ☑ (*following* M08)
  idiopathic M1A.00 ☑ (*following* M08)
    ankle M1A.07- ☑ (*following* M08)
    elbow M1A.02- ☑ (*following* M08)
    foot joint M1A.07- ☑ (*following* M08)
    hand joint M1A.04- ☑ (*following* M08)
    hip M1A.05- ☑ (*following* M08)
    knee M1A.06- ☑ (*following* M08)
    multiple site M1A.09 ☑ (*following* M08)
    shoulder M1A.01- ☑ (*following* M08)
    vertebrae M1A.08 ☑ (*following* M08)
    wrist M1A.03- ☑ (*following* M08)
  in (due to) renal impairment M1A.30 ☑ (*following* M08)
    ankle M1A.37- ☑ (*following* M08)
    elbow M1A.32- ☑ (*following* M08)
    foot joint M1A.37- ☑ (*following* M08)
    hand joint M1A.34- ☑ (*following* M08)
    hip M1A.35- ☑ (*following* M08)
    knee M1A.36- ☑ (*following* M08)
    multiple site M1A.39 ☑ (*following* M08)
    shoulder M1A.31- ☑ (*following* M08)
    vertebrae M1A.38 ☑ (*following* M08)
    wrist M1A.33- ☑ (*following* M08)
  lead-induced M1A.10 ☑ (*following* M08)
    ankle M1A.17- ☑ (*following* M08)
    elbow M1A.12- ☑ (*following* M08)
    foot joint M1A.17- ☑ (*following* M08)
    hand joint M1A.14- ☑ (*following* M08)
    hip M1A.15- ☑ (*following* M08)
    knee M1A.16- ☑ (*following* M08)
    multiple site M1A.19 ☑ (*following* M08)
    shoulder M1A.11- ☑ (*following* M08)
    vertebrae M1A.18 ☑ (*following* M08)
    wrist M1A.13- ☑ (*following* M08)
  primary — *see* Gout, chronic, idiopathic
  saturnine — *see* Gout, chronic, lead-induced
  secondary NEC M1A.40 ☑ (*following* M08)
    ankle M1A.47- ☑ (*following* M08)
    elbow M1A.42- ☑ (*following* M08)
    foot joint M1A.47- ☑ (*following* M08)
    hand joint M1A.44- ☑ (*following* M08)
    hip M1A.45- ☑ (*following* M08)
    knee M1A.46- ☑ (*following* M08)
    multiple site M1A.49 ☑ (*following* M08)
    shoulder M1A.41- ☑ (*following* M08)
    vertebrae M1A.48 ☑ (*following* M08)
    wrist M1A.43- ☑ (*following* M08)
  syphilitic (*see also* subcategory M14.8-) A52.77
  tophi M1A.9 ☑ (*following* M08)
Gout, gouty (acute) (attack) (flare) (*see also* Gout, chronic) M10.9
  drug-induced M10.20
    ankle M10.27- ☑
    elbow M10.22- ☑
    foot joint M10.27- ☑
    hand joint M10.24- ☑
    hip M10.25- ☑
    knee M10.26- ☑
    multiple site M10.29
    shoulder M10.21- ☑
    vertebrae M10.28
    wrist M10.23- ☑
  idiopathic M10.00
    ankle M10.07- ☑
    elbow M10.02- ☑
    foot joint M10.07- ☑
    hand joint M10.04- ☑
    hip M10.05- ☑
    knee M10.06- ☑
    multiple site M10.09
    shoulder M10.01- ☑
    vertebrae M10.08
    wrist M10.03- ☑
  in (due to) renal impairment M10.30
    ankle M10.37- ☑
    elbow M10.32- ☑
    foot joint M10.37- ☑
    hand joint M10.34- ☑
    hip M10.35- ☑
    knee M10.36- ☑

Gout, gouty — *continued*
 in renal impairment — *continued*
  multiple site M10.39
  shoulder M10.31- ☑
  vertebrae M10.38
  wrist M10.33- ☑
 lead-induced M10.10
  ankle M10.17- ☑
  elbow M10.12- ☑
  foot joint M10.17- ☑
  hand joint M10.14- ☑
  hip M10.15- ☑
  knee M10.16- ☑
  multiple site M10.19
  shoulder M10.11- ☑
  vertebrae M10.18
  wrist M10.13- ☑
 primary — *see* Gout, idiopathic
 saturnine — *see* Gout, lead-induced
 secondary NEC M10.40
  ankle M10.47- ☑
  elbow M10.42- ☑
  foot joint M10.47- ☑
  hand joint M10.44- ☑
  hip M10.45- ☑
  knee M10.46- ☑
  multiple site M10.49
  shoulder M10.41- ☑
  vertebrae M10.48
  wrist M10.43- ☑
 syphilitic (*see also* subcategory M14.8-) A52.77
 tophi — *see* Gout, chronic
Gower's
 muscular dystrophy G71.01
 syndrome (vasovagal attack) R55
Gradenigo's syndrome — *see* Otitis, media, suppurative, acute
Graefe's disease — *see* Strabismus, paralytic, ophthalmoplegia, progressive
Graft-versus-host disease D89.813
 acute D89.810
 acute on chronic D89.812
 chronic D89.811
Grain mite (itch) B88.0
Grainhandler's disease or lung J67.8
Grand mal — *see* Epilepsy, generalized, specified NEC
Grand multipara status only (not pregnant) Z64.1
 pregnant — *see* Pregnancy, complicated by, grand multiparity
Granite worker's lung J62.8
Granular (*see also* condition)
 inflammation, pharynx J31.2
 kidney (contracting) — *see* Sclerosis, renal
 liver K74.69
Granulation tissue (abnormal) (excessive) L92.9
 postmastoidectomy cavity — *see* Complications, postmastoidectomy, granulation
Granulocytopenia (primary) (malignant) — *see* Agranulocytosis
Granuloma L92.9
 abdomen K66.8
  from residual foreign body L92.3
  pyogenicum L98.0
 actinic L57.5
 annulare (perforating) L92.0
 apical K04.5
 aural — *see* Otitis, externa, specified NEC
 beryllium (skin) L92.3
 bone
  eosinophilic C96.6
  from residual foreign body — *see* Osteomyelitis, specified type NEC
  lung C96.6
 brain (any site) G06.0
  schistosomiasis B65.9 [G07]
 canaliculus lacrimalis — *see* Granuloma, lacrimal
 candidal (cutaneous) B37.2
 cerebral (any site) G06.0
 coccidioidal (primary) (progressive) B38.7
  lung B38.1
  meninges B38.4
 colon K63.89
 conjunctiva H11.22- ☑
 dental K04.5
 ear, middle — *see* Cholesteatoma
 eosinophilic C96.6
  bone C96.6

Granuloma — *continued*
 eosinophilic — *continued*
  lung C96.6
  oral mucosa K13.4
  skin L92.2
 eyelid H01.8
 facial (e) L92.2
 foreign body (in soft tissue) NEC M60.20
  ankle M60.27- ☑
  foot M60.27- ☑
  forearm M60.23- ☑
  hand M60.24- ☑
  in operation wound — *see* Foreign body, accidentally left during a procedure
  lower leg M60.26- ☑
  pelvic region M60.25- ☑
  shoulder region M60.21- ☑
  skin L92.3
  specified site NEC M60.28
  subcutaneous tissue L92.3
  thigh M60.25- ☑
  upper arm M60.22- ☑
 gangraenescens M31.2
 genito-inguinale A58
 giant cell (central) (reparative) (jaw) M27.1
  gingiva (peripheral) K06.8
 gland (lymph) I88.8
 hepatic NEC K75.3
  in (due to)
   berylliosis J63.2 [K77]
   sarcoidosis D86.89
 Hodgkin C81.9 ☑
 ileum K63.89
 infectious B99.9
  specified NEC B99.8
 inguinale (Donovan) (venereal) A58
 intestine NEC K63.89
 intracranial (any site) G06.0
 intraspinal (any part) G06.1
 iridocyclitis — *see* Iridocyclitis, chronic
 jaw (bone) (central) M27.1
  reparative giant cell M27.1
 kidney (*see also* Infection, kidney) N15.8
 lacrimal H04.81- ☑
 larynx J38.7
 lethal midline (faciale(e)) M31.2
 liver NEC — *see* Granuloma, hepatic
 lung (infectious) (*see also* Fibrosis, lung)
  coccidioidal B38.1
  eosinophilic C96.6
 Majocchi's B35.8
 malignant (facial(e)) M31.2
 mandible (central) M27.1
 midline (lethal) M31.2
 monilial (cutaneous) B37.2
 nasal sinus — *see* Sinusitis
 operation wound T81.89 ☑
  foreign body — *see* Foreign body, accidentally left during a procedure
  stitch T81.89 ☑
  talc — *see* Foreign body, accidentally left during a procedure
 oral mucosa K13.4
 orbit, orbital H05.11- ☑
 paracoccidioidal B41.8
 penis, venereal A58
 periapical K04.5
 peritoneum K66.8
  due to ova of helminths NOS (*see also* Helminthiasis) B83.9 [K67]
 postmastoidectomy cavity — *see* Complications, postmastoidectomy, recurrent cholesteatoma
 prostate N42.89
 pudendi (ulcerating) A58
 pulp, internal (tooth) K03.3
 pyogenic, pyogenicum (of) (skin) L98.0
  gingiva K06.8
  maxillary alveolar ridge K04.5
  oral mucosa K13.4
 rectum K62.89
 reticulohistiocytic D76.3
 rubrum nasi L74.8
 Schistosoma — *see* Schistosomiasis
 septic (skin) L98.0
 silica (skin) L92.3
 sinus (accessory) (infective) (nasal) — *see* Sinusitis
 skin L92.9
  from residual foreign body L92.3

Granuloma — *continued*
 skin — *continued*
  pyogenicum L98.0
 spine
  syphilitic (epidural) A52.19
  tuberculous A18.01
 stitch (postoperative) T81.89 ☑
 suppurative (skin) L98.0
 swimming pool A31.1
 talc (*see also* Granuloma, foreign body)
  in operation wound — *see* Foreign body, accidentally left during a procedure
 telangiectaticum (skin) L98.0
 tracheostomy J95.09
 trichophyticum B35.8
 tropicum A66.4
 umbilical P83.81
 umbilicus P83.81
 urethra N36.8
 uveitis — *see* Iridocyclitis, chronic
 vagina A58
 venereum A58
 vocal cord J38.3
Granulomatosis L92.9
 lymphoid C83.8- ☑
 miliary (listerial) A32.89
 necrotizing, respiratory M31.30
 progressive septic D71
 specified NEC L92.8
 Wegener's M31.30
  with renal involvement M31.31
Granulomatous tissue (abnormal) (excessive) L92.9
Granulosis rubra nasi L74.8
Graphite fibrosis (of lung) J63.3
Graphospasm F48.8
 organic G25.89
Grating scapula M89.8X1
Gravel (urinary) — *see* Calculus, urinary
Graves' disease — *see* Hyperthyroidism, with, goiter
Gravis — *see* condition
Grawitz tumor C64.- ☑
Gray syndrome (newborn) P93.0
Grayness, hair (premature) L67.1
 congenital Q84.2
Green sickness D50.8
Greenfield's disease
 meaning
  concentric sclerosis (encephalitis periaxialis concentrica) G37.5
  metachromatic leukodystrophy E75.25
Greenstick fracture — *code as* Fracture, by site
Grey syndrome (newborn) P93.0
Grief F43.21
 prolonged F43.29
 reaction (*see also* Disorder, adjustment) F43.20
Griesinger's disease B76.9
Grinder's lung or pneumoconiosis J62.8
Grinding, teeth
 psychogenic F45.8
 sleep related G47.63
Grip
 Dabney's B33.0
 devil's B33.0
Grippe, grippal (*see also* Influenza)
 Balkan A78
 summer, of Italy A93.1
Grisel's disease M43.6
Groin — *see* condition
Grooved tongue K14.5
Ground itch B76.9
Grover's disease or syndrome L11.1
Growing pains, children R29.898
Growth (fungoid) (neoplastic) (new) (*see also* Neoplasm)
 adenoid (vegetative) J35.8
 benign — *see* Neoplasm, benign, by site
 malignant — *see* Neoplasm, malignant, by site
 rapid, childhood Z00.2
 secondary — *see* Neoplasm, secondary, by site
Gruby's disease B35.0
Gubler-Millard paralysis or syndrome G46.3
Guerin-Stern syndrome Q74.3
Guidance, insufficient anterior (occlusal) M26.54
Guillain-Barré disease or syndrome G61.0
 sequelae G65.0
Guinea worms (infection) (infestation) B72
Guinon's disease (motor-verbal tic) F95.2
Gull's disease E03.4

Gum — see condition
Gumboil K04.7
  with sinus K04.6
Gumma (syphilitic) A52.79
  artery A52.09
    cerebral A52.04
  bone A52.77
    of yaws (late) A66.6
  brain A52.19
  cauda equina A52.19
  central nervous system A52.3
  ciliary body A52.71
  congenital A50.59
  eyelid A52.71
  heart A52.06
  intracranial A52.19
  iris A52.71
  kidney A52.75
  larynx A52.73
  leptomeninges A52.19
  liver A52.74
  meninges A52.19
  myocardium A52.06
  nasopharynx A52.73
  neurosyphilitic A52.3
  nose A52.73
  orbit A52.71
  palate (soft) A52.79
  penis A52.76
  pericardium A52.06
  pharynx A52.73
  pituitary A52.79
  scrofulous (tuberculous) A18.4
  skin A52.79
  specified site NEC A52.79
  spinal cord A52.19
  tongue A52.79
  tonsil A52.73
  trachea A52.73
  tuberculous A18.4
  ulcerative due to yaws A66.4
  ureter A52.75
  yaws A66.4
    bone A66.6
Gunn's syndrome Q07.8
Gunshot wound (see also Wound, open)
  fracture — code as Fracture, by site
  internal organs — see Injury, by site
Gynandrism Q56.0
Gynandroblastoma
  specified site — see Neoplasm, uncertain behavior, by
    site
  unspecified site
    female D39.10
    male D40.10
Gynecological examination (periodic) (routine) Z01.419
  with abnormal findings Z01.411
Gynecomastia N62
Gynephobia F40.291
Gyrate scalp Q82.8

H

H (Hartnup's) **disease** E72.02
Haas' disease or osteochondrosis (juvenile) (head of
  humerus) — see Osteochondrosis, juvenile, humerus
Habit, habituation
  bad sleep Z72.821
  chorea F95.8
  disturbance, child F98.9
  drug — see Dependence, drug
  irregular sleep Z72.821
  laxative F55.2
  spasm — see Tic
  tic — see Tic
Haemophilus (H.) **influenzae, as cause of disease
  classified elsewhere** B96.3
Haff disease — see Poisoning, mercury
Hageman's factor defect, deficiency or disease D68.2
Haglund's disease or osteochondrosis (juvenile) (os
  tibiale externum) — see Osteochondrosis, juvenile,
  tarsus
Hailey-Hailey disease Q82.8
Hair (see also condition)
  plucking F63.3
    in stereotyped movement disorder F98.4
  tourniquet syndrome (see also Constriction, external,
    by site)

Hair — continued
  tourniquet syndrome (see also Constriction, external,
    by site) — continued
    finger S60.44- ☑
    penis S30.842 ☑
    thumb S60.34- ☑
    toe S90.44- ☑
Hairball in stomach T18.2 ☑
Hair-pulling, pathological (compulsive) F63.3
Hairy black tongue K14.3
Half vertebra Q76.49
Halitosis R19.6
Hallerman-Streiff syndrome Q87.0
Hallervorden-Spatz disease G23.0
Hallopeau's acrodermatitis or disease L40.2
Hallucination R44.3
  auditory R44.0
  gustatory R44.2
  olfactory R44.2
  specified NEC R44.2
  tactile R44.2
  visual R44.1
Hallucinosis (chronic) F28
  alcoholic (acute) F10.951
    in
      abuse F10.151
      dependence F10.251
  drug-induced F19.951
    cannabis F12.951
    cocaine F14.951
    hallucinogen F16.151
    in
      abuse F19.151
        cannabis F12.151
        cocaine F14.151
        hallucinogen F16.151
        inhalant F18.151
        opioid F11.151
        sedative, anxiolytic or hypnotic F13.151
        stimulant NEC F15.151
      dependence F19.251
        cannabis F12.251
        cocaine F14.251
        hallucinogen F16.251
        inhalant F18.251
        opioid F11.251
        sedative, anxiolytic or hypnotic F13.251
        stimulant NEC F15.251
    inhalant F18.951
    opioid F11.951
    sedative, anxiolytic or hypnotic F13.951
    stimulant NEC F15.951
  organic F06.0
Hallux
  deformity (acquired) NEC M20.5X- ☑
  limitus M20.5X- ☑
  malleus (acquired) NEC M20.3- ☑
  rigidus (acquired) M20.2- ☑
    congenital Q74.2
    sequelae (late effect) of rickets E64.3
  valgus (acquired) M20.1- ☑
    congenital Q66.6
  varus (acquired) M20.3- ☑
    congenital Q66.3
Halo, visual H53.19
Hamartoma, hamartoblastoma Q85.9
  epithelial (gingival), odontogenic, central or peripheral
    — see Cyst, calcifying odontogenic
Hamartosis Q85.9
Hamman-Rich syndrome J84.114
Hammer toe (acquired) NEC (see also Deformity, toe,
  hammer toe)
  congenital Q66.89
  sequelae (late effect) of rickets E64.3
Hand — see condition
Hand-foot syndrome L27.1
Handicap, handicapped
  educational Z55.9
    specified NEC Z55.8
Hand-Schüller-Christian disease or syndrome C96.5
Hanging (asphyxia) (strangulation) (suffocation) — see
  Asphyxia, traumatic, due to mechanical threat
Hangnail (see also Cellulitis, digit)
  with lymphangitis — see Lymphangitis, acute, digit
Hangover (alcohol) F10.129
Hanhart's syndrome Q87.0
Hanot-Chauffard (-Troisier) **syndrome** E83.19

Hanot's cirrhosis or disease K74.3
Hansen's disease — see Leprosy
Hantaan virus disease (Korean hemorrhagic fever) A98.5
Hantavirus disease (with renal manifestations) (Dobrava)
  (Puumala) (Seoul) A98.5
  with pulmonary manifestations (Andes) (Bayou)
    (Bermejo) (Black Creek Canal) (Choclo) (Juquitiba)
    (Laguna negra) (Lechiguanas) (New York) (Oran)
    (Sin nombre) B33.4
Happy puppet syndrome Q93.51
Harada's disease or syndrome H30.81- ☑
Hardening
  artery — see Arteriosclerosis
  brain G93.89
Harelip (complete) (incomplete) — see Cleft, lip
Harlequin (newborn) Q80.4
Harley's disease D59.6
Harmful use (of)
  alcohol F10.10
  anxiolytics — see Abuse, drug, sedative
  cannabinoids — see Abuse, drug, cannabis
  cocaine — see Abuse, drug, cocaine
  drug — see Abuse, drug
  hallucinogens — see Abuse, drug, hallucinogen
  hypnotics — see Abuse, drug, sedative
  opioids — see Abuse, drug, opioid
  PCP (phencyclidine) — see Abuse, drug, hallucinogen
  sedatives — see Abuse, drug, sedative
  stimulants NEC — see Abuse, drug, stimulant
Harris' lines — see Arrest, epiphyseal
Hartnup's disease E72.02
Harvester's lung J67.0
Harvesting ovum for in vitro fertilization Z31.83
Hashimoto's disease or thyroiditis E06.3
Hashitoxicosis (transient) E06.3
Hassal-Henle bodies or warts (cornea) H18.49
Haut mal — see Epilepsy, generalized, specified NEC
Haverhill fever A25.1
Hay fever (see also Fever, hay) J30.1
Hayem-Widal syndrome D59.8
Haygarth's nodes M15.8
Haymaker's lung J67.0
Hb (abnormal)
  Bart's disease D56.0
  disease — see Disease, hemoglobin
  trait — see Trait
Head — see condition
Headache R51
  allergic NEC G44.89
  associated with sexual activity G44.82
  chronic daily R51
  cluster G44.009
    chronic G44.029
      intractable G44.021
      not intractable G44.029
    episodic G44.019
      intractable G44.011
      not intractable G44.019
    intractable G44.001
    not intractable G44.009
  cough (primary) G44.83
  daily chronic R51
  drug-induced NEC G44.40
    intractable G44.41
    not intractable G44.40
  exertional (primary) G44.84
  histamine G44.009
    intractable G44.001
    not intractable G44.009
  hypnic G44.81
  lumbar puncture G97.1
  medication overuse G44.40
    intractable G44.41
    not intractable G44.40
  menstrual — see Migraine, menstrual
  migraine (type) (see also Migraine) G43.909
  nasal septum R51
  neuralgiform, short lasting unilateral, with conjunctival
    injection and tearing (SUNCT) G44.059
    intractable G44.051
    not intractable G44.059
  new daily persistent (NDPH) G44.52
  orgasmic G44.82
  periodic syndromes in adults and children G43.C0 (fol-
    lowing G43.7)
    with refractory migraine G43.C1 (following G43.7)
    intractable G43.C1 (following G43.7)

☑ Additional Character Required — Refer to the Tabular List for Character Selection   Subterms under main terms may continue to next column or page

Headache — *continued*
  periodic syndromes in adults and children — *continued*
    not intractable G43.C0 (*following* G43.7)
    without refractory migraine G43.C0 (*following* G43.7)
  postspinal puncture G97.1
  post-traumatic G44.309
    acute G44.319
      intractable G44.311
      not intractable G44.319
    chronic G44.329
      intractable G44.321
      not intractable G44.329
    intractable G44.301
    not intractable G44.309
  pre-menstrual — *see* Migraine, menstrual
  preorgasmic G44.82
  primary
    cough G44.83
    exertional G44.84
    stabbing G44.85
    thunderclap G44.53
  rebound G44.40
    intractable G44.41
    not intractable G44.40
  short lasting unilateral neuralgiform, with conjunctival injection and tearing (SUNCT) G44.059
    intractable G44.051
    not intractable G44.059
  specified syndrome NEC G44.89
  spinal and epidural anesthesia - induced T88.59 ☑
    in labor and delivery O74.5
    in pregnancy O29.4-
    postpartum, puerperal O89.4
  spinal fluid loss (from puncture) G97.1
  stabbing (primary) G44.85
  tension (-type) G44.209
    chronic G44.229
      intractable G44.221
      not intractable G44.229
    episodic G44.219
      intractable G44.211
      not intractable G44.219
    intractable G44.201
    not intractable G44.209
  thunderclap (primary) G44.53
  vascular NEC G44.1
Healthy
  infant
    accompanying sick mother Z76.3
    receiving care Z76.2
  person accompanying sick person Z76.3
Hearing examination Z01.10
  with abnormal findings NEC Z01.118
  following failed hearing screening Z01.110
  for hearing conservation and treatment Z01.12
  infant or child (over 28 days old) Z00.129
    with abnormal findings Z00.121
Heart — *see* condition
Heart beat
  abnormality R00.9
    specified NEC R00.8
  awareness R00.2
  rapid R00.0
  slow R00.1
Heartburn R12
  psychogenic F45.8
Heartland virus disease A93.8
Heat (effects) T67.9 ☑
  apoplexy T67.0 ☑
  burn (*see also* Burn) L55.9
  collapse T67.1 ☑
  cramps T67.2 ☑
  dermatitis or eczema L59.0
  edema T67.7 ☑
  erythema — *code by site under* Burn, first degree
  excessive T67.9 ☑
    specified effect NEC T67.8 ☑
  exhaustion T67.5 ☑
    anhydrotic T67.3 ☑
    due to
      salt (and water) depletion T67.4 ☑
      water depletion T67.3 ☑
        with salt depletion T67.4 ☑
  fatigue (transient) T67.6 ☑
  fever T67.0 ☑
  hyperpyrexia T67.0 ☑
  prickly L74.0

Heat — *continued*
  prostration — *see* Heat, exhaustion
  pyrexia T67.0 ☑
  rash L74.0
  specified effect NEC T67.8 ☑
  stroke T67.0 ☑
  sunburn — *see* Sunburn
  syncope T67.1 ☑
Heavy-for-dates NEC (infant) (4000g to 4499g) P08.1
  exceptionally (4500g or more) P08.0
Hebephrenia, hebephrenic (schizophrenia) F20.1
Heberden's disease or nodes (with arthropathy) M15.1
Hebra's
  pityriasis L26
  prurigo L28.2
Heel — *see* condition
Heerfordt's disease D86.89
Hegglin's anomaly or syndrome D72.0
Heilmeyer-Schoner disease D45
Heine-Medin disease A80.9
Heinz body anemia, congenital D58.2
Heliophobia F40.228
Heller's disease or syndrome F84.3
HELLP syndrome (hemolysis, elevated liver enzymes and low platelet count) O14.2- ☑
  complicating
    childbirth O14.24
    puerperium O14.25
Helminthiasis (*see also* Infestation, helminth)
  Ancylostoma B76.0
  intestinal B82.0
    mixed types (types classifiable to more than one of the titles B65.0-B81.3 and B81.8) B81.4
    specified type NEC B81.8
  mixed types (intestinal) (types classifiable to more than one of the titles B65.0-B81.3 and B81.8) B81.4
  Necator (americanus) B76.1
  specified type NEC B83.8
Heloma L84
Hemangioblastoma — *see* Neoplasm, connective tissue, uncertain behavior
  malignant — *see* Neoplasm, connective tissue, malignant
Hemangioendothelioma (*see also* Neoplasm, uncertain behavior, by site)
  benign D18.00
    intra-abdominal D18.03
    intracranial D18.02
    skin D18.01
    specified site NEC D18.09
  bone (diffuse) — *see* Neoplasm, bone, malignant
  epithelioid (*see also* Neoplasm, uncertain behavior, by site)
    malignant — *see* Neoplasm, malignant, by site
  malignant — *see* Neoplasm, connective tissue, malignant
Hemangiofibroma — *see* Neoplasm, benign, by site
Hemangiolipoma — *see* Lipoma
Hemangioma D18.00
  arteriovenous D18.00
    intra-abdominal D18.03
    intracranial D18.02
    skin D18.01
    specified site NEC D18.09
  capillary D18.00
    intra-abdominal D18.03
    intracranial D18.02
    skin D18.01
    specified site NEC D18.09
  cavernous D18.00
    intra-abdominal D18.03
    intracranial D18.02
    skin D18.01
    specified site NEC D18.09
  epithelioid D18.00
    intra-abdominal D18.03
    intracranial D18.02
    skin D18.01
    specified site NEC D18.09
  histiocytoid D18.00
    intra-abdominal D18.03
    intracranial D18.02
    skin D18.01
    specified site NEC D18.09
  infantile D18.00
    intra-abdominal D18.03
    intracranial D18.02
    skin D18.01

Hemangioma — *continued*
  infantile — *continued*
    specified site NEC D18.09
  intra-abdominal D18.03
  intracranial D18.02
  intramuscular D18.00
    intra-abdominal D18.03
    intracranial D18.02
    skin D18.01
    specified site NEC D18.09
  intrathoracic structures D18.09
  juvenile D18.00
  malignant — *see* Neoplasm, connective tissue, malignant
  plexiform D18.00
    intra-abdominal D18.03
    intracranial D18.02
    skin D18.01
    specified site NEC D18.09
  racemose D18.00
    intra-abdominal D18.03
    intracranial D18.02
    skin D18.01
    specified site NEC D18.09
  sclerosing — *see* Neoplasm, skin, benign
  simplex D18.00
    intra-abdominal D18.03
    intracranial D18.02
    skin D18.01
    specified site NEC D18.09
  skin D18.01
  specified site NEC D18.09
  venous D18.00
    intra-abdominal D18.03
    intracranial D18.02
    skin D18.01
    specified site NEC D18.09
  verrucous keratotic D18.00
    intra-abdominal D18.03
    intracranial D18.02
    skin D18.01
    specified site NEC D18.09
Hemangiomatosis (systemic) I78.8
  involving single site — *see* Hemangioma
Hemangiopericytoma (*see also* Neoplasm, connective tissue, uncertain behavior)
  benign — *see* Neoplasm, connective tissue, benign
  malignant — *see* Neoplasm, connective tissue, malignant
Hemangiosarcoma — *see* Neoplasm, connective tissue, malignant
Hemarthrosis (nontraumatic) M25.00
  ankle M25.07- ☑
  elbow M25.02- ☑
  foot joint M25.07- ☑
  hand joint M25.04- ☑
  hip M25.05- ☑
  in hemophilic arthropathy — *see* Arthropathy, hemophilic
  knee M25.06- ☑
  shoulder M25.01- ☑
  specified joint NEC M25.08
  traumatic — *see* Sprain, by site
  vertebrae M25.08
  wrist M25.03- ☑
Hematemesis K92.0
  with ulcer — *code by site under* Ulcer, with hemorrhage K27.4
  newborn, neonatal P54.0
    due to swallowed maternal blood P78.2
Hematidrosis L74.8
Hematinuria (*see also* Hemoglobinuria)
  malarial B50.8
Hematobilia K83.8
Hematocele
  female NEC N94.89
    with ectopic pregnancy O00.90
      with intrauterine pregnancy O00.91
    ovary N83.8
  male N50.1
Hematochezia (*see also* Melena) K92.1
Hematochyluria (*see also* Infestation, filarial)
  schistosomiasis (bilharziasis) B65.0
Hematocolpos (with hematometra or hematosalpinx) N89.7
Hematocornea — *see* Pigmentation, cornea, stromal
Hematogenous — *see* condition

Hematoma (traumatic) (skin surface intact) (see also Contusion)
  with
    injury of internal organs — see Injury, by site
    open wound — see Wound, open
  amputation stump (surgical) (late) T87.89
  aorta, dissecting I71.00
    abdominal I71.02
    thoracic I71.01
    thoracoabdominal I71.03
  aortic intramural — see Dissection, aorta
  arterial (complicating trauma) — see Injury, blood vessel, by site
  auricle — see Contusion, ear
    nontraumatic — see Disorder, pinna, hematoma
  birth injury NEC P15.8
  brain (traumatic)
    with
      cerebral laceration or contusion (diffuse) — see Injury, intracranial, diffuse
      focal — see Injury, intracranial, focal
    cerebellar, traumatic S06.37- ☑
    intracerebral, traumatic — see Injury, intracranial, intracerebral hemorrhage
    newborn NEC P52.4
      birth injury P10.1
    nontraumatic — see Hemorrhage, intracranial
    subarachnoid, arachnoid, traumatic — see Injury, intracranial, subarachnoid hemorrhage
    subdural, traumatic — see Injury, intracranial, subdural hemorrhage
  breast (nontraumatic) N64.89
  broad ligament (nontraumatic) N83.7
    traumatic S37.892 ☑
  cerebellar, traumatic S06.37- ☑
  cerebral — see Hematoma, brain
  cerebrum S06.36- ☑
    left S06.35- ☑
    right S06.34- ☑
  cesarean delivery wound O90.2
  complicating delivery (perineal) (pelvic) (vagina) (vulva) O71.7
  corpus cavernosum (nontraumatic) N48.89
  epididymis (nontraumatic) N50.1
  epidural (traumatic) — see Injury, intracranial, epidural hemorrhage
    spinal — see Injury, spinal cord, by region
  episiotomy O90.2
  face, birth injury P15.4
  genital organ NEC (nontraumatic)
    female (nonobstetric) N94.89
      traumatic S30.202 ☑
    male N50.1
      traumatic S30.201 ☑
  internal organs — see Injury, by site
  intracerebral, traumatic — see Injury, intracranial, intracerebral hemorrhage
  intraoperative — see Complications, intraoperative, hemorrhage
  labia (nontraumatic) (nonobstetric) N90.89
  liver (subcapsular) (nontraumatic) K76.89
    birth injury P15.0
  mediastinum — see Injury, intrathoracic
  mesosalpinx (nontraumatic) N83.7
    traumatic S37.898 ☑
  muscle — code by site under Contusion
  nontraumatic
    muscle M79.81
    soft tissue M79.81
  obstetrical surgical wound O90.2
  orbit, orbital (nontraumatic) (see also Hemorrhage, orbit)
    traumatic — see Contusion, orbit
  pelvis (female) (nontraumatic) (nonobstetric) N94.89
    obstetric O71.7
    traumatic — see Injury, by site
  penis (nontraumatic) N48.89
    birth injury P15.5
  perianal (nontraumatic) K64.5
  perineal S30.23 ☑
    complicating delivery O71.7
  perirenal — see Injury, kidney
  pinna — see Contusion, ear
    nontraumatic — see Disorder, pinna, hematoma
  placenta O43.89- ☑
  postoperative (postprocedural) — see Complication, postprocedural, hematoma

Hematoma — continued
  retroperitoneal (nontraumatic) K66.1
    traumatic S36.892 ☑
  scrotum, superficial S30.22 ☑
    birth injury P15.5
  seminal vesicle (nontraumatic) N50.1
    traumatic S37.892 ☑
  spermatic cord (traumatic) S37.892 ☑
    nontraumatic N50.1
  spinal (cord) (meninges) (see also Injury, spinal cord, by region)
    newborn (birth injury) P11.5
  spleen D73.5
    intraoperative — see Complications, intraoperative, hemorrhage, spleen
    postprocedural (postoperative) — see Complications, postprocedural, hemorrhage, spleen
  sternocleidomastoid, birth injury P15.2
  sternomastoid, birth injury P15.2
  subarachnoid (traumatic) — see Injury, intracranial, subarachnoid hemorrhage
    newborn (nontraumatic) P52.5
      due to birth injury P10.3
    nontraumatic — see Hemorrhage, intracranial, subarachnoid
  subdural (traumatic) — see Injury, intracranial, subdural hemorrhage
    newborn (localized) P52.8
      birth injury P10.0
    nontraumatic — see Hemorrhage, intracranial, subdural
  superficial, newborn P54.5
  testis (nontraumatic) N50.1
    birth injury P15.5
  tunica vaginalis (nontraumatic) N50.1
  umbilical cord, complicating delivery O69.5 ☑
  uterine ligament (broad) (nontraumatic) N83.7
    traumatic S37.892 ☑
  vagina (ruptured) (nontraumatic) N89.8
    complicating delivery O71.7
  vas deferens (nontraumatic) N50.1
    traumatic S37.892 ☑
  vitreous — see Hemorrhage, vitreous
  vulva (nontraumatic) (nonobstetric) N90.89
    complicating delivery O71.7
    newborn (birth injury) P15.5
Hematometra N85.7
  with hematocolpos N89.7
Hematomyelia (central) G95.19
  newborn (birth injury) P11.5
  traumatic T14.8 ☑
Hematomyelitis G04.90
Hematoperitoneum — see Hemoperitoneum
Hematophobia F40.230
Hematopneumothorax (see Hemothorax)
Hematopoiesis, cyclic D70.4
Hematoporphyria — see Porphyria
Hematorachis, hematorrhachis G95.19
  newborn (birth injury) P11.5
Hematosalpinx N83.6
  with
    hematocolpos N89.7
    hematometra N85.7
      with hematocolpos N89.7
  infectional — see Salpingitis
Hematospermia R36.1
Hematothorax (see Hemothorax)
Hematuria R31.9
  benign (familial) (of childhood) (see also Hematuria, idiopathic)
    essential microscopic R31.1
  due to sulphonamide, sulfonamide — see Table of Drugs and Chemicals, by drug
  endemic (see also Schistosomiasis) B65.0
  gross R31.0
  idiopathic N02.9
    with glomerular lesion
      crescentic (diffuse) glomerulonephritis N02.7
      dense deposit disease N02.6
      endocapillary proliferative glomerulonephritis N02.4
      focal and segmental hyalinosis or sclerosis N02.1
      membranoproliferative (diffuse) N02.5
      membranous (diffuse) N02.2
      mesangial proliferative (diffuse) N02.3
      mesangiocapillary (diffuse) N02.5
      minor abnormality N02.0
      proliferative NEC N02.8

Hematuria — continued
  idiopathic — continued
    with glomerular lesion — continued
      specified pathology NEC N02.8
  intermittent — see Hematuria, idiopathic
  malarial B50.8
  microscopic NEC (with symptoms) R31.29
    asymptomatic R31.21
    benign essential R31.1
  paroxysmal (see also Hematuria, idiopathic)
    nocturnal D59.5
  persistent — see Hematuria, idiopathic
  recurrent — see Hematuria, idiopathic
  tropical (see also Schistosomiasis) B65.0
  tuberculous A18.13
Hemeralopia (day blindness) H53.11
  vitamin A deficiency E50.5
Hemi-akinesia R41.4
Hemianalgesia R20.0
Hemianencephaly Q00.0
Hemianesthesia R20.0
Hemianopia, hemianopsia (heteronymous) H53.47
  homonymous H53.46- ☑
  syphilitic A52.71
Hemiathetosis R25.8
Hemiatrophy R68.89
  cerebellar G31.9
  face, facial, progressive (Romberg) G51.8
  tongue K14.8
Hemiballism (us) G25.5
Hemicardia Q24.8
Hemicephalus, hemicephaly Q00.0
Hemichorea G25.5
Hemicolitis, left — see Colitis, left sided
Hemicrania
  congenital malformation Q00.0
  continua G44.51
  meaning migraine (see also Migraine) G43.909
  paroxysmal G44.039
    chronic G44.049
      intractable G44.041
      not intractable G44.049
    episodic G44.039
      intractable G44.031
      not intractable G44.039
    intractable G44.031
    not intractable G44.039
Hemidystrophy — see Hemiatrophy
Hemiectromelia Q73.8
Hemihypalgesia R20.8
Hemihypesthesia R20.1
Hemi-inattention R41.4
Hemimelia Q73.8
  lower limb — see Defect, reduction, lower limb, specified type NEC
  upper limb — see Defect, reduction, upper limb, specified type NEC
Hemiparalysis — see Hemiplegia
Hemiparesis — see Hemiplegia
Hemiparesthesia R20.2
Hemiparkinsonism G20
Hemiplegia G81.9- ☑
  alternans facialis G83.89
  ascending NEC G81.90
    spinal G95.89
  congenital (cerebral) G80.8
    spastic G80.2
  embolic (current episode) I63.4- ☑
  flaccid G81.0- ☑
  following
    cerebrovascular disease I69.959
      cerebral infarction I69.35- ☑
      intracerebral hemorrhage I69.15- ☑
      nontraumatic intracranial hemorrhage NEC I69.25- ☑
      specified disease NEC I69.85- ☑
      stroke NOS I69.35- ☑
      subarachnoid hemorrhage I69.05- ☑
  hysterical F44.4
  newborn NEC P91.88
    birth injury P11.9
  spastic G81.1- ☑
    congenital G80.2
  thrombotic (current episode) I63.3- ☑
Hemisection, spinal cord — see Injury, spinal cord, by region
Hemispasm (facial) R25.2

Hemisporosis B48.8
Hemitremor R25.1
Hemivertebra Q76.49
  failure of segmentation with scoliosis Q76.3
  fusion with scoliosis Q76.3
Hemochromatosis E83.119
  with refractory anemia D46.1
  due to repeated red blood cell transfusion E83.111
  hereditary (primary) E83.110
  neonatal P78.84
  primary E83.110
  specified NEC E83.118
Hemoglobin (*see also* condition)
  abnormal (disease) — *see* Disease, hemoglobin
  AS genotype D57.3
  Constant Spring D58.2
  E-beta thalassemia D56.5
  fetal, hereditary persistence (HPFH) D56.4
  H Constant Spring D56.0
  low NOS D64.9
  S (Hb S), heterozygous D57.3
Hemoglobinemia D59.9
  due to blood transfusion T80.89 ☑
  paroxysmal D59.6
  nocturnal D59.5
Hemoglobinopathy (mixed) D58.2
  with thalassemia D56.8
  sickle-cell D57.1
    with thalassemia D57.40
      with crisis (vasoocclusive pain) D57.419
        with
          acute chest syndrome D57.411
          splenic sequestration D57.412
      without crisis D57.40
Hemoglobinuria R82.3
  with anemia, hemolytic, acquired (chronic) NEC D59.6
  cold (agglutinin) (paroxysmal) (with Raynaud's syndrome) D59.6
  due to exertion or hemolysis NEC D59.6
  intermittent D59.6
  malarial B50.8
  march D59.6
  nocturnal (paroxysmal) D59.5
  paroxysmal (cold) D59.6
    nocturnal D59.5
Hemolymphangioma D18.1
Hemolysis
  intravascular
    with
      abortion — *see* Abortion, by type, complicated by, hemorrhage
      ectopic or molar pregnancy O08.1
      hemorrhage
        antepartum — *see* Hemorrhage, antepartum, with coagulation defect
        intrapartum (*see also* Hemorrhage, complicating, delivery) O67.0
      postpartum O72.3
  neonatal (excessive) P58.9
    specified NEC P58.8
Hemolytic — *see* condition
Hemopericardium I31.2
  following acute myocardial infarction (current complication) I23.0
  newborn P54.8
  traumatic — *see* Injury, heart, with hemopericardium
Hemoperitoneum K66.1
  infectional K65.9
  traumatic S36.899 ☑
    with open wound — *see* Wound, open, with penetration into peritoneal cavity
Hemophilia (classical) (familial) (hereditary) D66
  A D66
  acquired D68.311
  autoimmune D68.311
  B D67
  C D68.1
  calcipriva (*see also* Defect, coagulation) D68.4
  nonfamilial (*see also* Defect, coagulation) D68.4
  secondary D68.311
  vascular D68.0
Hemophthalmos H44.81- ☑
Hemopneumothorax (*see also* Hemothorax)
  traumatic S27.2 ☑
Hemoptysis R04.2
  newborn P26.9
  tuberculous — *see* Tuberculosis, pulmonary
Hemorrhage, hemorrhagic (concealed) R58

Hemorrhage, hemorrhagic — *continued*
  abdomen R58
  accidental antepartum — *see* Hemorrhage, antepartum
  acute idiopathic pulmonary, in infants R04.81
  adenoid J35.8
  adrenal (capsule) (gland) E27.49
    medulla E27.8
    newborn P54.4
  after delivery — *see* Hemorrhage, postpartum
  alveolar
    lung, newborn P26.8
    process K08.89
  alveolus K08.89
  amputation stump (surgical) T87.89
  anemia (chronic) D50.0
    acute D62
  antepartum (with) O46.90
    with coagulation defect O46.00- ☑
      afibrinogenemia O46.01- ☑
      disseminated intravascular coagulation O46.02- ☑
      hypofibrinogenemia O46.01- ☑
      specified defect NEC O46.09- ☑
    before 20 weeks gestation O20.9
      specified type NEC O20.8
      threatened abortion O20.0
    due to
      abruptio placenta (*see also* Abruptio placentae) O45.9-
      leiomyoma, uterus — *see* Hemorrhage, antepartum, specified cause NEC
      placenta previa O44.1- ☑
    specified cause NEC — *see* subcategory O46.8X- ☑
  anus (sphincter) K62.5
  apoplexy (stroke) — *see* Hemorrhage, intracranial, intracerebral
  arachnoid — *see* Hemorrhage, intracranial, subarachnoid
  artery R58
    brain — *see* Hemorrhage, intracranial, intracerebral
  basilar (ganglion) I61.0
  bladder N32.89
  bowel K92.2
    newborn P54.3
  brain (miliary) (nontraumatic) — *see* Hemorrhage, intracranial, intracerebral
    due to
      birth injury P10.1
      syphilis A52.05
    epidural or extradural (traumatic) — *see* Injury, intracranial, epidural hemorrhage
    newborn P52.4
      birth injury P10.1
    subarachnoid — *see* Hemorrhage, intracranial, subarachnoid
    subdural — *see* Hemorrhage, intracranial, subdural
  brainstem (nontraumatic) I61.3
    traumatic S06.38- ☑
  breast N64.59
  bronchial tube — *see* Hemorrhage, lung
  bronchopulmonary — *see* Hemorrhage, lung
  bronchus — *see* Hemorrhage, lung
  bulbar I61.5
  capillary I78.8
    primary D69.8
  cecum K92.2
  cerebellar, cerebellum (nontraumatic) I61.4
    newborn P52.6
    traumatic S06.37- ☑
  cerebral, cerebrum (*see also* Hemorrhage, intracranial, intracerebral)
    lobe I61.1
    newborn (anoxic) P52.4
      birth injury P10.1
  cerebromeningeal I61.8
  cerebrospinal — *see* Hemorrhage, intracranial, intracerebral
  cervix (uteri) (stump) NEC N88.8
  chamber, anterior (eye) — *see* Hyphema
  childbirth — *see* Hemorrhage, complicating, delivery
  choroid H31.30- ☑
    expulsive H31.31- ☑
  ciliary body — *see* Hyphema
  cochlea — *see* subcategory H83.8 ☑
  colon K92.2
  complicating
    abortion — *see* Abortion, by type, complicated by, hemorrhage

Hemorrhage, hemorrhagic — *continued*
  complicating — *continued*
    delivery O67.9
      associated with coagulation defect (afibrinogenemia) (DIC) (hyperfibrinolysis) O67.0
      specified cause NEC O67.8
      surgical procedure — *see* Hemorrhage, intraoperative
  conjunctiva H11.3- ☑
    newborn P54.8
  cord, newborn (stump) P51.9
  corpus luteum (ruptured) cyst N83.1- ☑
  cortical (brain) I61.1
  cranial — *see* Hemorrhage, intracranial
  cutaneous R23.3
    due to autosensitivity, erythrocyte D69.2
    newborn P54.5
  delayed
    following ectopic or molar pregnancy O08.1
    postpartum O72.2
  diathesis (familial) D69.9
  disease D69.9
    newborn P53
    specified type NEC D69.8
  due to or associated with
    afibrinogenemia or other coagulation defect (conditions in categories D65- D69)
      antepartum — *see* Hemorrhage, antepartum, with coagulation defect
      intrapartum O67.0
  dental implant M27.61
  device, implant or graft (*see also* Complications, by site and type, specified NEC) T85.838 ☑
    arterial graft NEC T82.838 ☑
    breast T85.838 ☑
    catheter NEC T85.838 ☑
      dialysis (renal) T82.838 ☑
        intraperitoneal T85.838 ☑
      infusion NEC T82.838 ☑
        spinal (epidural) (subdural) T85.830 ☑
      urinary (indwelling) T83.83 ☑
    electronic (electrode) (pulse generator) (stimulator)
      bone T84.83 ☑
      cardiac T82.837 ☑
      nervous system (brain) (peripheral nerve) (spinal) T85.830 ☑
      urinary T83.83 ☑
    fixation, internal (orthopedic) NEC T84.83 ☑
    gastrointestinal (bile duct) (esophagus) T85.838 ☑
    genital NEC T83.83 ☑
    heart NEC T82.837 ☑
    joint prosthesis T84.83 ☑
    ocular (corneal graft) (orbital implant) NEC T85.838 ☑
    orthopedic NEC T84.83 ☑
      bone graft T86.838 ☑
    specified NEC T85.838 ☑
    urinary NEC T83.83 ☑
    vascular NEC T82.838 ☑
    ventricular intracranial shunt T85.830 ☑
  duodenum, duodenal K92.2
    ulcer — *see* Ulcer, duodenum, with hemorrhage
  dura mater — *see* Hemorrhage, intracranial, subdural
  endotracheal — *see* Hemorrhage, lung
  epicranial subaponeurotic (massive), birth injury P12.2
  epidural (traumatic) (*see also* Injury, intracranial, epidural hemorrhage)
    nontraumatic I62.1
  esophagus K22.8
    varix I85.01
      secondary I85.11
  excessive, following ectopic gestation (subsequent episode) O08.1
  extradural (traumatic) — *see* Injury, intracranial, epidural hemorrhage
    birth injury P10.8
    newborn (anoxic) (nontraumatic) P52.8
    nontraumatic I62.1
  eye NEC H57.89
    fundus — *see* Hemorrhage, retina
    lid — *see* Disorder, eyelid, specified type NEC
  fallopian tube N83.6
  fibrinogenolysis — *see* Fibrinolysis
  fibrinolytic (acquired) — *see* Fibrinolysis

Hemorrhage, hemorrhagic — *continued*
from
  ear (nontraumatic) — *see* Otorrhagia
  tracheostomy stoma J95.01
fundus, eye — *see* Hemorrhage, retina
funis — *see* Hemorrhage, umbilicus, cord
gastric — *see* Hemorrhage, stomach
gastroenteric K92.2
  newborn P54.3
gastrointestinal (tract) K92.2
  newborn P54.3
genital organ, male N50.1
genitourinary (tract) NOS R31.9
gingiva K06.8
globe (eye) — *see* Hemophthalmos
graafian follicle cyst (ruptured) N83.0- ☑
gum K06.8
heart I51.89
hypopharyngeal (throat) R04.1
intermenstrual (regular) N92.3
  irregular N92.1
internal (organs) NEC R58
  capsule I61.0
  ear — *see* subcategory H83.8 ☑
  newborn P54.8
intestine K92.2
  newborn P54.3
intra-abdominal R58
intra-alveolar (lung), newborn P26.8
intracerebral (nontraumatic) — *see* Hemorrhage, intracranial, intracerebral
intracranial (nontraumatic) I62.9
  birth injury P10.9
  epidural, nontraumatic I62.1
  extradural, nontraumatic I62.1
  intracerebral (nontraumatic) (in) I61.9
    brain stem I61.3
    cerebellum I61.4
    hemisphere I61.2
      cortical (superficial) I61.1
      subcortical (deep) I61.0
    intraoperative
      during a nervous system procedure G97.31
      during other procedure G97.32
    intraventricular I61.5
    multiple localized I61.6
    newborn P52.4
      birth injury P10.1
    postprocedural
      following a nervous system procedure G97.51
      following other procedure G97.52
    specified NEC I61.8
    superficial I61.1
    traumatic (diffuse) — *see* Injury, intracranial, diffuse
      focal — *see* Injury, intracranial, focal
  newborn P52.9
    specified NEC P52.8
  subarachnoid (nontraumatic) (from) I60.9
    intracranial (cerebral) artery I60.7
      anterior communicating I60.2
      basilar I60.4
      carotid siphon and bifurcation I60.0- ☑
      communicating I60.7
        anterior I60.2
        posterior I60.3- ☑
      middle cerebral I60.1- ☑
      posterior communicating I60.3- ☑
      specified artery NEC I60.6
      vertebral I60.5- ☑
    newborn P52.5
      birth injury P10.3
    specified NEC I60.8
    traumatic S06.6X- ☑
  subdural (nontraumatic) I62.00
    acute I62.01
    birth injury P10.0
    chronic I62.03
    newborn (anoxic) (hypoxic) P52.8
      birth injury P10.0
    spinal G95.19
    subacute I62.02
    traumatic — *see* Injury, intracranial, subdural hemorrhage
  traumatic — *see* Injury, intracranial, focal brain injury
intramedullary NEC G95.19
intraocular — *see* Hemophthalmos

Hemorrhage, hemorrhagic — *continued*
intraoperative, intraprocedural — *see* Complication, hemorrhage (hematoma), intraoperative (intraprocedural), by site
intrapartum — *see* Hemorrhage, complicating, delivery
intrapelvic
  female N94.89
  male K66.1
intraperitoneal K66.1
intrapontine I61.3
intraprocedural — *see* Complication, hemorrhage (hematoma), intraoperative (intraprocedural), by site
intrauterine N85.7
  complicating delivery (*see also* Hemorrhage, complicating, delivery) O67.9
  postpartum — *see* Hemorrhage, postpartum
intraventricular I61.5
  newborn (nontraumatic) (*see also* Newborn, affected by, hemorrhage) P52.3
    due to birth injury P10.2
    grade
      1 P52.0
      2 P52.1
      3 P52.21
      4 P52.22
intravesical N32.89
iris (postinfectional) (postinflammatory) (toxic) — *see* Hyphema
joint (nontraumatic) — *see* Hemarthrosis
kidney N28.89
knee (joint) (nontraumatic) — *see* Hemarthrosis, knee
labyrinth — *see* subcategory H83.8 ☑
lenticular striate artery I61.0
ligature, vessel — *see* Hemorrhage, postoperative
liver K76.89
lung R04.89
  newborn P26.9
    massive P26.1
    specified NEC P26.8
  tuberculous — *see* Tuberculosis, pulmonary
massive umbilical, newborn P51.0
mediastinum — *see* Hemorrhage, lung
medulla I61.3
membrane (brain) I60.8
  spinal cord — *see* Hemorrhage, spinal cord
meninges, meningeal (brain) (middle) I60.8
  spinal cord — *see* Hemorrhage, spinal cord
mesentery K66.1
metritis — *see* Endometritis
mouth K13.79
mucous membrane NEC R58
  newborn P54.8
muscle M62.89
nail (subungual) L60.8
nasal turbinate R04.0
  newborn P54.8
navel, newborn P51.9
newborn P54.9
  specified NEC P54.8
nipple N64.59
nose R04.0
  newborn P54.8
omentum K66.1
optic nerve (sheath) H47.02- ☑
orbit, orbital H05.23- ☑
ovary NEC N83.8
oviduct N83.6
pancreas K86.89
parathyroid (gland) (spontaneous) E21.4
parturition — *see* Hemorrhage, complicating, delivery
penis N48.89
pericardium, pericarditis I31.2
peritoneum, peritoneal K66.1
peritonsillar tissue J35.8
  due to infection J36
petechial R23.3
  due to autosensitivity, erythrocyte D69.2
pituitary (gland) E23.6
pleura — *see* Hemorrhage, lung
polioencephalitis, superior E51.2
polymyositis — *see* Polymyositis
pons, pontine I61.3
posterior fossa (nontraumatic) I61.8
  newborn P52.6
postmenopausal N95.0
postnasal R04.0

Hemorrhage, hemorrhagic — *continued*
postoperative — *see* Complications, postprocedural, hemorrhage, by site
postpartum NEC (following delivery of placenta) O72.1
  delayed or secondary O72.2
    retained placenta O72.0
    third stage O72.0
pregnancy — *see* Hemorrhage, antepartum
preretinal — *see* Hemorrhage, retina
prostate N42.1
puerperal — *see* Hemorrhage, postpartum
  delayed or secondary O72.2
pulmonary R04.89
  newborn P26.9
    massive P26.1
    specified NEC P26.8
  tuberculous — *see* Tuberculosis, pulmonary
purpura (primary) D69.3
rectum (sphincter) K62.5
  newborn P54.2
recurring, following initial hemorrhage at time of injury T79.2 ☑
renal N28.89
respiratory passage or tract R04.9
  specified NEC R04.89
retina, retinal (vessels) H35.6- ☑
  diabetic — *see* Diabetes, retinal, hemorrhage
retroperitoneal R58
scalp R58
scrotum N50.1
secondary (nontraumatic) R58
  following initial hemorrhage at time of injury T79.2 ☑
seminal vesicle N50.1
skin R23.3
  newborn P54.5
slipped umbilical ligature P51.8
spermatic cord N50.1
spinal (cord) G95.19
  newborn (birth injury) P11.5
spleen D73.5
  intraoperative — *see* Complications, intraoperative hemorrhage, spleen
  postprocedural — *see* Complications, postprocedural, hemorrhage, spleen
stomach K92.2
  newborn P54.3
  ulcer — *see* Ulcer, stomach, with hemorrhage
subarachnoid (nontraumatic) — *see* Hemorrhage, in tracranial, subarachnoid
subconjunctival (*see also* Hemorrhage, conjunctiva)
  birth injury P15.3
subcortical (brain) I61.0
subcutaneous R23.3
subdiaphragmatic R58
subdural (acute) (nontraumatic) — *see* Hemorrhage, intracranial, subdural
subependymal
  newborn P52.0
    with intraventricular extension P52.1
      and intracerebral extension P52.22
subgaleal P12.2
subhyaloid — *see* Hemorrhage, retina
subperiosteal — *see* Disorder, bone, specified type NE
subretinal — *see* Hemorrhage, retina
subtentorial — *see* Hemorrhage, intracranial, subdura
subtentorial L60.8
suprarenal (capsule) (gland) E27.49
  newborn P54.4
tentorium (traumatic) NEC — *see* Hemorrhage, brai
  newborn (birth injury) P10.4
testis N50.1
third stage (postpartum) O72.0
thorax — *see* Hemorrhage, lung
throat R04.1
thymus (gland) E32.8
thyroid (cyst) (gland) E07.89
tongue K14.8
tonsil J35.8
trachea — *see* Hemorrhage, lung
tracheobronchial R04.89
  newborn P26.0
traumatic — *code to* specific injury
  cerebellar — *see* Hemorrhage, brain
  intracranial — *see* Hemorrhage, brain
  recurring or secondary (following initial hemorrhag at time of injury) T79.2 ☑

Hemorrhage, hemorrhagic — *continued*
 tuberculous NEC (*see also* Tuberculosis, pulmonary)
  A15.0
 tunica vaginalis N50.1
 ulcer — *code by* site under Ulcer, with hemorrhage
  K27.4
 umbilicus, umbilical
  cord
   after birth, newborn P51.9
   complicating delivery O69.5 ☑
  newborn P51.9
   massive P51.0
   slipped ligature P51.8
  stump P51.9
 urethra (idiopathic) N36.8
 uterus, uterine (abnormal) N93.9
  climacteric N92.4
  complicating delivery — *see* Hemorrhage, complicating, delivery
  dysfunctional or functional N93.8
  intermenstrual (regular) N92.3
   irregular N92.1
  postmenopausal N95.0
  postpartum — *see* Hemorrhage, postpartum
  preclimacteric or premenopausal N92.4
  prepubertal N93.8
  pubertal N92.2
 vagina (abnormal) N93.9
  newborn P54.6
 vas deferens N50.1
 vasa previa O69.4 ☑
 ventricular I61.5
 vesical N32.89
 viscera NEC R58
  newborn P54.8
 vitreous (humor) (intraocular) H43.1- ☑
 vulva N90.89
Hemorrhoids (bleeding) (without mention of degree)
  K64.9
 1st degree (grade/stage I) (without prolapse outside
  of anal canal) K64.0
 2nd degree (grade/stage II) (that prolapse with straining but retract spontaneously) K64.1
 3rd degree (grade/stage III) (that prolapse with straining and require manual replacement back inside
  anal canal) K64.2
 4th degree (grade/stage IV) (with prolapsed tissue that
  cannot be manually replaced) K64.3
 complicating
  pregnancy O22.4 ☑
  puerperium O87.2
 external K64.4
  with
   thrombosis K64.5
 internal (without mention of degree) K64.8
  prolapsed K64.8
 skin tags
  anus K64.4
  residual K64.4
 specified NEC K64.8
 strangulated (*see also* Hemorrhoids, by degree) K64.8
 thrombosed (*see also* Hemorrhoids, by degree) K64.5
 ulcerated (*see also* Hemorrhoids, by degree) K64.8
Hemosalpinx N83.6
 with
  hematocolpos N89.7
  hematometra N85.7
   with hematocolpos N89.7
Hemosiderosis (dietary) E83.19
 pulmonary, idiopathic E83.1- ☑ [J84.03]
 transfusion T80.89 ☑
Hemothorax (bacterial) (nontuberculous) J94.2
 newborn P54.8
 traumatic S27.1 ☑
  with pneumothorax S27.2 ☑
 tuberculous NEC A15.6
Henoch (-Schönlein) **disease or syndrome** (purpura)
  D69.0
Henpue, henpuye A66.6
Hepar lobatum (syphilitic) A52.74
Hepatalgia K76.89
Hepatitis K75.9
 acute B17.9
  with coma K72.01
   with hepatic failure — *see* Failure, hepatic
  alcoholic — *see* Hepatitis, alcoholic
  infectious B17.9
  non-viral K72.0 ☑

Hepatitis — *continued*
 acute — *continued*
  viral B17.9
  alcoholic (acute) (chronic) K70.10
   with ascites K70.11
  amebic — *see* Abscess, liver, amebic
  anicteric, (viral) — *see* Hepatitis, viral
  antigen-associated (HAA) — *see* Hepatitis, B
  Australia-antigen (positive) — *see* Hepatitis, B
  autoimmune K75.4
  B B19.10
   with hepatic coma B19.11
   acute B16.9
    with
     delta-agent (coinfection) (without hepatic
      coma) B16.1
      with hepatic coma B16.0
     hepatic coma (without delta-agent coinfec-
      tion) B16.2
   chronic B18.1
    with delta-agent B18.0
  bacterial NEC K75.89
  C (viral) B19.20
   with hepatic coma B19.21
   acute B17.10
    with hepatic coma B17.11
   chronic B18.2
  catarrhal (acute) B15.9
   with hepatic coma B15.0
  cholangiolitic K75.89
  cholestatic K75.89
  chronic K73.9
   active NEC K73.2
   lobular NEC K73.1
   persistent NEC K73.0
   specified NEC K73.8
  cytomegaloviral B25.1
  due to ethanol (acute) (chronic) — *see* Hepatitis, alcoholic
  epidemic B15.9
   with hepatic coma B15.0
  fulminant NEC (viral) — *see* Hepatitis, viral
  granulomatous NEC K75.3
  herpesviral B00.81
  history of
   B Z86.19
   C Z86.19
  homologous serum — *see* Hepatitis, viral, type B
  in (due to)
   mumps B26.81
   toxoplasmosis (acquired) B58.1
    congenital (active) P37.1 [K77]
  infectious, infective B15.9
   acute (subacute) B17.9
   chronic B18.9
  inoculation — *see* Hepatitis, viral, type B
  interstitial (chronic) K74.69
  lupoid NEC K75.4
  malignant NEC (with hepatic failure) K72.90
   with coma K72.91
  neonatal (idiopathic) (toxic) P59.29
  neonatal giant cell P59.29
  newborn P59.29
  non-viral K72.0 ☑
  postimmunization — *see* Hepatitis, viral, type B
  post-transfusion — *see* Hepatitis, viral, type B
  reactive, nonspecific K75.2
  serum — *see* Hepatitis, viral, type B
  specified type NEC
   with hepatic failure — *see* Failure, hepatic
  syphilitic (late) A52.74
   congenital (early) A50.08 [K77]
    late A50.59 [K77]
   secondary A51.45
  toxic (*see also* Disease, liver, toxic) K71.6
  tuberculous A18.83
  viral, virus B19.9
   with hepatic coma B19.0
   acute B17.9
   chronic B18.9
    specified NEC B18.8
    type
     B B18.1
      with delta-agent B18.0
     C B18.2
   congenital P35.3
   coxsackie B33.8 [K77]
   cytomegalic inclusion B25.1

Hepatitis — *continued*
 viral, virus — *continued*
  in remission, any type — *code to* Hepatitis, chronic,
   by type
  non-A, non-B B17.8
  specified type NEC (with or without coma) B17.8
  type
   A B15.9
    with hepatic coma B15.0
   B B19.10
    with hepatic coma B19.11
    acute B16.9
     with
      delta-agent (coinfection) (without
       hepatic coma) B16.1
       with hepatic coma B16.0
      hepatic coma (without delta-agent
       coinfection) B16.2
    chronic B18.1
     with delta-agent B18.0
   C B19.20
    with hepatic coma B19.21
    acute B17.10
     with hepatic coma B17.11
    chronic B18.2
   E B17.2
  non-A, non-B B17.8
Hepatization lung (acute) — *see* Pneumonia, lobar
Hepatoblastoma C22.2
Hepatocarcinoma C22.0
Hepatocholangiocarcinoma C22.0
Hepatocholangioma, benign D13.4
Hepatocholangitis K75.89
Hepatolenticular degeneration E83.01
Hepatoma (malignant) C22.0
 benign D13.4
 embryonal C22.0
Hepatomegaly (*see also* Hypertrophy, liver)
 with splenomegaly R16.2
 congenital Q44.7
 in mononucleosis
  gammaherpesviral B27.09
  infectious specified NEC B27.89
Hepatoptosis K76.89
Hepatorenal syndrome following labor and delivery
  O90.4
Hepatosis K76.89
Hepatosplenomegaly R16.2
 hyperlipemic (Bürger-Grütz type) E78.3 [K77]
Hereditary — *see* condition
Heredodegeneration, macular — *see* Dystrophy, retina
Heredopathia atactica polyneuritiformis G60.1
Heredosyphilis — *see* Syphilis, congenital
Herlitz' syndrome Q81.1
Hermansky-Pudlak syndrome E70.331
Hermaphrodite, hermaphroditism (true) Q56.0
 46,XX with streak gonads Q99.1
 46,XX/46,XY Q99.0
 46,XY with streak gonads Q99.1
 chimera 46,XX/46,XY Q99.0
Hernia, hernial (acquired) (recurrent) K46.9
 with
  gangrene — *see* Hernia, by site, with, gangrene
  incarceration — *see* Hernia, by site, with, obstruction
  irreducible — *see* Hernia, by site, with, obstruction
  obstruction — *see* Hernia, by site, with, obstruction
  strangulation — *see* Hernia, by site, with, obstruction
 abdomen, abdominal K46.9
  with
   gangrene (and obstruction) K46.1
   obstruction K46.0
  femoral — *see* Hernia, femoral
  incisional — *see* Hernia, incisional
  inguinal — *see* Hernia, inguinal
  specified site NEC K45.8
   with
    gangrene (and obstruction) K45.1
    obstruction K45.0
  umbilical — *see* Hernia, umbilical
  wall — *see* Hernia, ventral
 appendix — *see* Hernia, abdomen
 bladder (mucosa) (sphincter)
  congenital (female) (male) Q79.51
  female Cystocele
  male N32.89
 brain, congenital — *see* Encephalocele

Hernia, hernial — *continued*

cartilage, vertebra — *see* Displacement, intervertebral disc
cerebral, congenital (*see also* Encephalocele)
  endaural Q01.8
ciliary body (traumatic) S05.2- ☑
colon — *see* Hernia, abdomen
Cooper's — *see* Hernia, abdomen, specified site NEC
crural — *see* Hernia, femoral
diaphragm, diaphragmatic K44.9
  with
    gangrene (and obstruction) K44.1
    obstruction K44.0
  congenital Q79.0
direct (inguinal) — *see* Hernia, inguinal
diverticulum, intestine — *see* Hernia, abdomen
double (inguinal) — *see* Hernia, inguinal, bilateral
due to adhesions (with obstruction) K56.50
epigastric (*see also* Hernia, ventral) K43.9
esophageal hiatus — *see* Hernia, hiatal
external (inguinal) — *see* Hernia, inguinal
fallopian tube N83.4- ☑
fascia M62.89
femoral K41.90
  with
    gangrene (and obstruction) K41.40
      not specified as recurrent K41.40
      recurrent K41.41
    obstruction K41.30
      not specified as recurrent K41.30
      recurrent K41.31
  not specified as recurrent K41.90
  recurrent K41.91
  bilateral K41.20
    with
      gangrene (and obstruction) K41.10
        not specified as recurrent K41.10
        recurrent K41.11
      obstruction K41.00
        not specified as recurrent K41.00
        recurrent K41.01
    not specified as recurrent K41.20
    recurrent K41.21
  unilateral K41.90
    with
      gangrene (and obstruction) K41.40
        not specified as recurrent K41.40
        recurrent K41.41
      obstruction K41.30
        not specified as recurrent K41.30
        recurrent K41.31
    not specified as recurrent K41.90
    recurrent K41.91
foramen magnum G93.5
  congenital Q01.8
funicular (umbilical) (*see also* Hernia, umbilicus)
  spermatic (cord) — *see* Hernia, inguinal
gastrointestinal tract — *see* Hernia, abdomen
Hesselbach's — *see* Hernia, femoral, specified site NEC
hiatal (esophageal) (sliding) K44.9
  with
    gangrene (and obstruction) K44.1
    obstruction K44.0
  congenital Q40.1
hypogastric — *see* Hernia, ventral
incarcerated (*see also* Hernia, by site, with obstruction)
  with gangrene — *see* Hernia, by site, with gangrene
incisional K43.2
  with
    gangrene (and obstruction) K43.1
    obstruction K43.0
indirect (inguinal) — *see* Hernia, inguinal
inguinal (direct) (external) (funicular) (indirect) (internal) (oblique) (scrotal) (sliding) K40.90
  with
    gangrene (and obstruction) K40.40
      not specified as recurrent K40.40
      recurrent K40.41
    obstruction K40.30
      not specified as recurrent K40.30
      recurrent K40.31
  not specified as recurrent K40.90
  recurrent K40.91
  bilateral K40.20
    with
      gangrene (and obstruction) K40.10
        not specified as recurrent K40.10
        recurrent K40.11

Hernia, hernial — *continued*

inguinal — *continued*
  bilateral — *continued*
    with — *continued*
      obstruction K40.00
        not specified as recurrent K40.00
        recurrent K40.01
    not specified as recurrent K40.20
    recurrent K40.21
  unilateral K40.90
    with
      gangrene (and obstruction) K40.40
        not specified as recurrent K40.40
        recurrent K40.41
      obstruction K40.30
        not specified as recurrent K40.30
        recurrent K40.31
    not specified as recurrent K40.90
    recurrent K40.91
internal (*see also* Hernia, abdomen)
  inguinal — *see* Hernia, inguinal
interstitial — *see* Hernia, abdomen
intervertebral cartilage or disc — *see* Displacement, intervertebral disc
intestine, intestinal — *see* Hernia, by site
intra-abdominal — *see* Hernia, abdomen
iris (traumatic) S05.2- ☑
irreducible (*see also* Hernia, by site, with obstruction)
  with gangrene — *see* Hernia, by site, with gangrene
ischiatic — *see* Hernia, abdomen, specified site NEC
ischiorectal — *see* Hernia, abdomen, specified site NEC
lens (traumatic) S05.2- ☑
linea (alba) (semilunaris) — *see* Hernia, ventral
Littre's — *see* Hernia, abdomen
lumbar — *see* Hernia, abdomen, specified site NEC
lung (subcutaneous) J98.4
mediastinum J98.59
mesenteric (internal) — *see* Hernia, abdomen
midline — *see* Hernia, ventral
muscle (sheath) M62.89
nucleus pulposus — *see* Displacement, intervertebral disc
oblique (inguinal) — *see* Hernia, inguinal
obstructive (*see also* Hernia, by site, with obstruction)
  with gangrene — *see* Hernia, by site, with gangrene
obturator — *see* Hernia, abdomen, specified site NEC
omental — *see* Hernia, abdomen
ovary N83.4- ☑
oviduct N83.4- ☑
paraesophageal (*see also* Hernia, diaphragm)
  congenital Q40.1
parastomal K43.5
  with
    gangrene (and obstruction) K43.4
    obstruction K43.3
paraumbilical — *see* Hernia, umbilicus
perineal — *see* Hernia, abdomen, specified site NEC
Petit's — *see* Hernia, abdomen, specified site NEC
postoperative — *see* Hernia, incisional
pregnant uterus — *see* Abnormal, uterus in pregnancy or childbirth
prevesical N32.89
properitoneal — *see* Hernia, abdomen, specified site NEC
pudendal — *see* Hernia, abdomen, specified site NEC
rectovaginal N81.6
retroperitoneal — *see* Hernia, abdomen, specified site NEC
Richter's — *see* Hernia, abdomen, with obstruction
Rieux's, Riex's — *see* Hernia, abdomen, specified site NEC
sac condition (adhesion) (dropsy) (inflammation) (laceration) (suppuration) — *code by site under* Hernia
sciatic — *see* Hernia, abdomen, specified site NEC
scrotum, scrotal — *see* Hernia, inguinal
sliding (inguinal) (*see also* Hernia, inguinal)
  hiatus — *see* Hernia, hiatal
spigelian — *see* Hernia, ventral
spinal — *see* Spina bifida
strangulated (*see also* Hernia, by site, with obstruction)
  with gangrene — *see* Hernia, by site, with gangrene
subxiphoid — *see* Hernia, ventral
supra-umbilicus — *see* Hernia, ventral
tendon — *see* Disorder, tendon, specified type NEC
Treitz's (fossa) — *see* Hernia, abdomen, specified site NEC

Hernia, hernial — *continued*

tunica vaginalis Q55.29
umbilicus, umbilical K42.9
  with
    gangrene (and obstruction) K42.1
    obstruction K42.0
ureter N28.89
urethra, congenital Q64.79
urinary meatus, congenital Q64.79
uterus N81.4
  pregnant — *see* Abnormal, uterus in pregnancy or childbirth
vaginal (anterior) (wall) — *see* Cystocele
Velpeau's — *see* Hernia, femoral
ventral K43.9
  with
    gangrene (and obstruction) K43.7
    obstruction K43.6
  incisional K43.2
    with
      gangrene (and obstruction) K43.1
      obstruction K43.0
    recurrent — *see* Hernia, incisional
  specified NEC K43.9
    with
      gangrene (and obstruction) K43.7
      obstruction K43.6
vesical
  congenital (female) (male) Q79.51
  female — *see* Cystocele
  male N32.89
vitreous (into wound) S05.2- ☑
  into anterior chamber — *see* Prolapse, vitreous
Herniation (*see also* Hernia)
brain (stem) G93.5
cerebral G93.5
mediastinum J98.59
nucleus pulposus — *see* Displacement, intervertebral disc
Herpangina B08.5
Herpes, herpesvirus, herpetic B00.9
anogenital A60.9
  perianal skin A60.1
  rectum A60.1
  urogenital tract A60.00
    cervix A60.03
    male genital organ NEC A60.02
    penis A60.01
    specified site NEC A60.09
    vagina A60.04
    vulva A60.04
blepharitis (zoster) B02.39
  simplex B00.59
circinatus B35.4
  bullosus L12.0
conjunctivitis (simplex) B00.53
  zoster B02.31
cornea B02.33
encephalitis B00.4
  due to herpesvirus 6 B10.01
  due to herpesvirus 7 B10.09
  specified NEC B10.09
eye (zoster) B02.30
  simplex B00.50
eyelid (zoster) B02.39
  simplex B00.59
facialis B00.1
febrilis B00.1
geniculate ganglionitis B02.21
genital, genitalis A60.00
  female A60.09
  male A60.02
gestational, gestationis O26.4- ☑
gingivostomatitis B00.2
human B00.9
  1 — *see* Herpes, simplex
  2 — *see* Herpes, simplex
  3 — *see* Varicella
  4 — *see* Mononucleosis, Epstein-Barr (virus)
  5 — *see* Disease, cytomegalic inclusion (generalized)
  6
    encephalitis B10.01
    specified NEC B10.81
  7
    encephalitis B10.09
    specified NEC B10.82
  8 B10.89
infection NEC B10.89

☑ **Additional Character Required** — Refer to the Tabular List for Character Selection   ▽ **Subterms under main terms may continue to next column or page**

Herpes, herpesvirus, herpetic — continued
infection — continued
Kaposi's sarcoma associated B10.89
iridocyclitis (simplex) B00.51
zoster B02.32
iris (vesicular erythema multiforme) L51.9
iritis (simplex) B00.51
Kaposi's sarcoma associated B10.89
keratitis (simplex) (dendritic) (disciform) (interstitial) B00.52
zoster (interstitial) B02.33
keratoconjunctivitis (simplex) B00.52
zoster B02.33
labialis B00.1
lip B00.1
meningitis (simplex) B00.3
zoster B02.1
ophthalmicus (zoster) NEC B02.30
simplex B00.50
penis A60.01
perianal skin A60.1
pharyngitis, pharyngotonsillitis B00.2
rectum A60.1
scrotum A60.02
sepsis B00.7
simplex B00.9
complicated NEC B00.89
congenital P35.2
conjunctivitis B00.53
external ear B00.1
eyelid B00.59
hepatitis B00.81
keratitis (interstitial) B00.52
myelitis B00.82
specified complication NEC B00.89
visceral B00.89
stomatitis B00.2
tonsurans B35.0
visceral B00.89
vulva A60.04
whitlow B00.89
zoster (see also condition) B02.9
auricularis B02.21
complicated NEC B02.8
conjunctivitis B02.31
disseminated B02.7
encephalitis B02.0
eye (lid) B02.39
geniculate ganglionitis B02.21
keratitis (interstitial) B02.33
meningitis B02.1
myelitis B02.24
neuritis, neuralgia B02.29
ophthalmicus NEC B02.30
oticus B02.21
polyneuropathy B02.23
specified complication NEC B02.8
trigeminal neuralgia B02.22
Herpesvirus (human) — see Herpes
Herpetophobia F40.218
Herrick's anemia — see Disease, sickle-cell
Hers' disease E74.09
Herter-Gee syndrome K90.0
Herxheimer's reaction R68.89
Hesitancy
of micturition R39.11
urinary R39.11
Hesselbach's hernia — see Hernia, femoral, specified site NEC
Heterochromia (congenital) Q13.2
cataract — see Cataract, complicated
cyclitis (Fuchs) — see Cyclitis, Fuchs' heterochromic
hair L67.1
iritis — see Cyclitis, Fuchs' heterochromic
retained metallic foreign body (nonmagnetic) — see Foreign body, intraocular, old, retained
magnetic — see Foreign body, intraocular, old, retained, magnetic
uveitis — see Cyclitis, Fuchs' heterochromic
Heterophoria — see Strabismus, heterophoria
Heterophyes, heterophyiasis (small intestine) B66.8
Heterotopia, heterotopic (see also Malposition, congenital)
cerebralis Q04.8
Heterotropia — see Strabismus
Heubner-Herter disease K90.0
Hexadactylism Q69.9

HGSIL (cytology finding) (high grade squamous intraepithelial lesion on cytologic smear) (Pap smear finding)
anus R85.613
cervix R87.613
biopsy (histology) finding — see Neoplasia, intraepithelial, cervix, grade II or grade III
vagina R87.623
biopsy (histology) finding — see Neoplasia, intraepithelial, cervix, grade II or grade III
Hibernoma — see Lipoma
Hiccup, hiccough R06.6
epidemic B33.0
psychogenic F45.8
Hidden penis (congenital) Q55.64
acquired N48.83
Hidradenitis (axillaris) (suppurative) L73.2
Hidradenoma (nodular) (see also Neoplasm, skin, benign)
clear cell — see Neoplasm, skin, benign
papillary — see Neoplasm, skin, benign
Hidrocystoma — see Neoplasm, skin, benign
High
altitude effects T70.20 ☑
anoxia T70.29 ☑
on
ears T70.0 ☑
sinuses T70.1 ☑
polycythemia D75.1
arch
foot Q66.7
palate, congenital Q38.5
arterial tension — see Hypertension
basal metabolic rate R94.8
blood pressure (see also Hypertension)
borderline R03.0
reading (incidental) (isolated) (nonspecific), without diagnosis of hypertension R03.0
cholesterol E78.00
with high triglycerides E78.2
diaphragm (congenital) Q79.1
expressed emotional level within family Z63.8
head at term O32.4 ☑
palate, congenital Q38.5
risk
infant NEC Z76.2
sexual behavior (heterosexual) Z72.51
bisexual Z72.53
homosexual Z72.52
scrotal testis, testes
bilateral Q53.23
unilateral Q53.13
temperature (of unknown origin) R50.9
thoracic rib Q76.6
triglycerides E78.1
with high cholesterol E78.2
Hildenbrand's disease A75.0
Hilum — see condition
Hip — see condition
Hippel's disease Q85.8
Hippophobia F40.218
Hippus H57.09
Hirschsprung's disease or megacolon Q43.1
Hirsutism, hirsuties L68.0
Hirudiniasis
external B88.3
internal B83.4
Hiss-Russell dysentery A03.1
Histidinemia, histidinuria E70.41
Histiocytoma (see also Neoplasm, skin, benign)
fibrous (see also Neoplasm, skin, benign)
atypical — see Neoplasm, connective tissue, uncertain behavior
malignant — see Neoplasm, connective tissue, malignant
Histiocytosis D76.3
acute differentiated progressive C96.0
Langerhans' cell NEC C96.6
multifocal X
multisystemic (disseminated) C96.0
unisystemic C96.5
pulmonary, adult (adult PLCH) J84.82
unifocal (X) C96.6
lipid, lipoid D76.3
essential E75.29
malignant C96.A (following C96.6)
mononuclear phagocytes NEC D76.1
Langerhans' cells C96.6
non-Langerhans cell D76.3

Histiocytosis — continued
polyostotic sclerosing D76.3
sinus, with massive lymphadenopathy D76.3
syndrome NEC D76.3
X NEC C96.6
acute (progressive) C96.0
chronic C96.6
multifocal C96.5
multisystemic C96.0
unifocal C96.6
Histoplasmosis B39.9
with pneumonia NEC B39.2
African B39.5
American — see Histoplasmosis, capsulati
capsulati B39.4
disseminated B39.3
generalized B39.3
pulmonary B39.2
acute B39.0
chronic B39.1
Darling's B39.4
duboisii B39.5
lung NEC B39.2
History
family (of) (see also History, personal (of))
alcohol abuse Z81.1
allergy NEC Z84.89
anemia Z83.2
arthritis Z82.61
asthma Z82.5
blindness Z82.1
cardiac death (sudden) Z82.41
carrier of genetic disease Z84.81
chromosomal anomaly Z82.79
chronic
disabling disease NEC Z82.8
lower respiratory disease Z82.5
colonic polyps Z83.71
congenital malformations and deformations Z82.79
polycystic kidney Z82.71
consanguinity Z84.3
deafness Z82.2
diabetes mellitus Z83.3
disability NEC Z82.8
disease or disorder (of)
allergic NEC Z84.89
behavioral NEC Z81.8
blood and blood-forming organs Z83.2
cardiovascular NEC Z82.49
chronic disabling NEC Z82.8
digestive Z83.79
ear NEC Z83.52
elevated lipoprotein(a) (Lp(a)) Z83.430
endocrine NEC Z83.49
eye NEC Z83.518
glaucoma Z83.511
familial hypercholesterolemia Z83.42
genitourinary NEC Z84.2
glaucoma Z83.511
hematological Z83.2
immune mechanism Z83.2
infectious NEC Z83.1
ischemic heart Z82.49
kidney Z84.1
lipoprotein metabolism Z83.438
mental NEC Z81.8
metabolic Z83.49
musculoskeletal NEC Z82.69
neurological NEC Z82.0
nutritional Z83.49
parasitic NEC Z83.1
psychiatric NEC Z81.8
respiratory NEC Z83.6
skin and subcutaneous tissue NEC Z84.0
specified NEC Z84.89
drug abuse NEC Z81.3
elevated lipoprotein(a) (Lp(a)) Z83.430
epilepsy Z82.0
familial hypercholesterolemia Z83.42
genetic disease carrier Z84.81
glaucoma Z83.511
hearing loss Z82.2
human immunodeficiency virus (HIV) infection Z83.0
Huntington's chorea Z82.0
hyperlipidemia, familial combined Z83.438
intellectual disability Z81.0
leukemia Z80.6
lipidemia NEC Z83.438
malignant neoplasm (of) NOS Z80.9

Index

History — continued
  family (see also History, personal) — continued
    malignant neoplasm — continued
      bladder Z80.52
      breast Z80.3
      bronchus Z80.1
      digestive organ Z80.0
      gastrointestinal tract Z80.0
      genital organ Z80.49
        ovary Z80.41
        prostate Z80.42
        specified organ NEC Z80.49
        testis Z80.43
      hematopoietic NEC Z80.7
      intrathoracic organ NEC Z80.2
      kidney Z80.51
      lung Z80.1
      lymphatic NEC Z80.7
      ovary Z80.41
      prostate Z80.42
      respiratory organ NEC Z80.2
      specified site NEC Z80.8
      testis Z80.43
      trachea Z80.1
      urinary organ or tract Z80.59
        bladder Z80.52
        kidney Z80.51
    mental
      disorder NEC Z81.8
    multiple endocrine neoplasia (MEN) syndrome
        Z83.41
    osteoporosis Z82.62
    polycystic kidney Z82.71
    polyps (colon) Z83.71
    psychiatric disorder Z81.8
    psychoactive substance abuse NEC Z81.3
    respiratory condition NEC Z83.6
      asthma and other lower respiratory conditions
          Z82.5
    self-harmful behavior Z81.8
    SIDS (sudden infant death syndrome) Z84.82
    skin condition Z84.0
    specified condition NEC Z84.89
    stroke (cerebrovascular) Z82.3
    substance abuse NEC Z81.4
      alcohol Z81.1
      drug NEC Z81.3
      psychoactive NEC Z81.3
      tobacco Z81.2
    sudden
      cardiac death Z82.41
      infant death syndrome (SIDS) Z84.82
    tobacco abuse Z81.2
    violence, violent behavior Z81.8
    visual loss Z82.1
  personal (of) (see also History, family (of))
    abuse
      adult Z91.419
        forced labor or sexual exploitation Z91.42
        physical and sexual Z91.410
        psychological Z91.411
      childhood Z62.819
        forced labor or sexual exploitation in child-
            hood Z62.813
        physical Z62.810
        psychological Z62.811
        sexual Z62.810
    alcohol dependence F10.21
    allergy (to) Z88.9
      analgesic agent NEC Z88.6
      anesthetic Z88.4
      antibiotic agent NEC Z88.1
      anti-infective agent NEC Z88.3
      contrast media Z91.041
      drugs, medicaments and biological substances
          Z88.9
        specified NEC Z88.8
      food Z91.018
        additives Z91.02
        eggs Z91.012
        milk products Z91.011
        peanuts Z91.010
        seafood Z91.013
        specified food NEC Z91.018
      insect Z91.038
        bee Z91.030
      latex Z91.040
      medicinal agents Z88.9
        specified NEC Z88.8

History — continued
  personal (see also History, family) — continued
    allergy — continued
      narcotic agent NEC Z88.5
      nonmedicinal agents Z91.048
      penicillin Z88.0
      serum Z88.7
      specified NEC Z91.09
      sulfonamides Z88.2
      vaccine Z88.7
    anaphylactic shock Z87.892
    anaphylaxis Z87.892
    behavioral disorders Z86.59
    benign carcinoid tumor Z86.012
    benign neoplasm Z86.018
      brain Z86.011
      carcinoid Z86.012
      colonic polyps Z86.010
    brain injury (traumatic) Z87.820
    breast implant removal Z98.86
    calculi, renal Z87.442
    cancer — see History, personal (of), malignant
        neoplasm (of)
    cardiac arrest (death), successfully resuscitated
        Z86.74
    cerebral infarction without residual deficit Z86.73
    cervical dysplasia Z87.410
    chemotherapy for neoplastic condition Z92.21
    childhood abuse — see History, personal (of), abuse
    cleft lip (corrected) Z87.730
    cleft palate (corrected) Z87.730
    collapsed vertebra (healed) Z87.311
      due to osteoporosis Z87.310
    combat and operational stress reaction Z86.51
    congenital malformation (corrected) Z87.798
      circulatory system (corrected) Z87.74
      digestive system (corrected) NEC Z87.738
      ear (corrected) Z87.721
      eye (corrected) Z87.720
      face and neck (corrected) Z87.790
      genitourinary system (corrected) NEC Z87.718
      heart (corrected) Z87.74
      integument (corrected) Z87.76
      limb(s) (corrected) Z87.76
      musculoskeletal system (corrected) Z87.76
      neck (corrected) Z87.790
      nervous system (corrected) NEC Z87.728
      respiratory system (corrected) Z87.75
      sense organs (corrected) NEC Z87.728
      specified NEC Z87.798
    contraception Z92.0
    deployment (military) Z91.82
    diabetic foot ulcer Z86.31
    disease or disorder (of) Z87.898
      anaphylaxis Z87.892
      blood and blood-forming organs Z86.2
      circulatory system Z86.79
        specified condition NEC Z86.79
      connective tissue Z87.39
      digestive system Z87.19
        colonic polyp Z86.010
        peptic ulcer disease Z87.11
        specified condition NEC Z87.19
      ear Z86.69
      endocrine Z86.39
        diabetic foot ulcer Z86.31
        gestational diabetes Z86.32
        specified type NEC Z86.39
      eye Z86.69
      genital (track) system NEC
        female Z87.42
        male Z87.438
      hematological Z86.2
      Hodgkin Z85.71
      immune mechanism Z86.2
      infectious Z86.19
        malaria Z86.13
        Methicillin resistant Staphylococcus aureus
            (MRSA) Z86.14
        poliomyelitis Z86.12
        specified NEC Z86.19
        tuberculosis Z86.11
      mental NEC Z86.59
      metabolic Z86.39
        diabetic foot ulcer Z86.31
        gestational diabetes Z86.32
        specified type NEC Z86.39
      musculoskeletal NEC Z87.39
      nervous system Z86.69

History — continued
  personal (see also History, family) — continued
    disease or disorder — continued
      nutritional Z86.39
      parasitic Z86.19
      respiratory system NEC Z87.09
      sense organs Z86.69
      skin Z87.2
      specified site or type NEC Z87.898
      subcutaneous tissue Z87.2
      trophoblastic Z87.59
      urinary system NEC Z87.448
    drug dependence — see Dependence, drug, by
        type, in remission
    drug therapy
      antineoplastic chemotherapy Z92.21
      estrogen Z92.23
      immunosupression Z92.25
      inhaled steroids Z92.240
      monoclonal drug Z92.22
      specified NEC Z92.29
      steroid Z92.241
      systemic steroids Z92.241
    dysplasia
      cervical (mild) (moderate) Z87.410
        severe (grade III) Z86.001
      prostatic Z87.430
      vaginal (mild) (moderate) Z87.411
        severe (grade III) Z86.008
      vulvar (mild) (moderate) Z87.412
        severe (grade III) Z86.008
    embolism (venous) Z86.718
      pulmonary Z86.711
    encephalitis Z86.61
    estrogen therapy Z92.23
    extracorporeal membrane oxygenation (ECMO)
        Z92.81
    failed conscious sedation Z92.83
    failed moderate sedation Z92.83
    fall, falling Z91.81
    forced labor or sexual exploitation Z91.42
      in childhood Z62.813
    fracture (healed)
      fatigue Z87.312
      fragility Z87.310
      osteoporosis Z87.310
      pathological NEC Z87.311
      stress Z87.312
      traumatic Z87.81
    gestational diabetes Z86.32
    hepatitis
      B Z86.19
      C Z86.19
    Hodgkin disease Z85.71
    hyperthermia, malignant Z88.4
    hypospadias (corrected) Z87.710
    hysterectomy Z90.710
    immunosupression therapy Z92.25
    in situ neoplasm
      breast Z86.000
      cervix uteri Z86.001
      specified NEC Z86.008
    in utero procedure during pregnancy Z98.870
    in utero procedure while a fetus Z98.871
    infection NEC Z86.19
      central nervous system Z86.61
      Methicillin resistant Staphylococcus aureus
          (MRSA) Z86.14
      urinary (recurrent) (tract) Z87.440
    injury NEC Z87.828
    irradiation Z92.3
    kidney stones Z87.442
    leukemia Z85.6
    lymphoma (non-Hodgkin) Z85.72
    malignant melanoma (skin) Z85.820
    malignant neoplasm (of) Z85.9
      accessory sinuses Z85.22
      anus NEC Z85.048
        carcinoid Z85.040
      bladder Z85.51
      bone Z85.830
      brain Z85.841
      breast Z85.3
      bronchus NEC Z85.118
        carcinoid Z85.110
      carcinoid — see History, personal (of), maligna
          neoplasm, by site, carcinioid
      cervix Z85.41
      colon NEC Z85.038

History — *continued*
personal (*see also* History, family) — *continued*
  malignant neoplasm — *continued*
    colon — *continued*
      carcinoid Z85.030
    digestive organ Z85.00
      specified NEC Z85.09
    endocrine gland NEC Z85.858
    epididymis Z85.48
    esophagus Z85.01
    eye Z85.840
    gastrointestinal tract — *see* History, malignant neoplasm, digestive organ
    genital organ
      female Z85.40
        specified NEC Z85.44
      male Z85.45
        specified NEC Z85.49
    hematopoietic NEC Z85.79
    intrathoracic organ Z85.20
    kidney NEC Z85.528
      carcinoid Z85.520
    large intestine NEC Z85.038
      carcinoid Z85.030
    larynx Z85.21
    liver Z85.05
    lung NEC Z85.118
      carcinoid Z85.110
    mediastinum Z85.29
    Merkel cell Z85.821
    middle ear Z85.22
    nasal cavities Z85.22
    nervous system NEC Z85.848
    oral cavity Z85.819
      specified site NEC Z85.818
    ovary Z85.43
    pancreas Z85.07
    pelvis Z85.53
    pharynx Z85.819
      specified site NEC Z85.818
    pleura Z85.29
    prostate Z85.46
    rectosigmoid junction NEC Z85.048
      carcinoid Z85.040
    rectum NEC Z85.048
      carcinoid Z85.040
    respiratory organ Z85.20
    sinuses, accessory Z85.22
    skin NEC Z85.828
      melanoma Z85.820
      Merkel cell Z85.821
    small intestine NEC Z85.068
      carcinoid Z85.060
    soft tissue Z85.831
    specified site NEC Z85.89
    stomach NEC Z85.028
      carcinoid Z85.020
    testis Z85.47
    thymus NEC Z85.238
      carcinoid Z85.230
    thyroid Z85.850
    tongue Z85.810
    trachea Z85.12
    urinary organ or tract Z85.50
      specified NEC Z85.59
    uterus Z85.42
  maltreatment Z91.89
  medical treatment NEC Z92.89
  melanoma (malignant) (skin) Z85.820
  meningitis Z86.61
  mental disorder Z86.59
  Merkel cell carcinoma (skin) Z85.821
  Methicillin resistant Staphylococcus aureus (MRSA) Z86.14
  military deployment Z91.82
  military war, peacekeeping and humanitarian deployment (current or past conflict) Z91.82
  myocardial infarction (old) I25.2
  neglect (in)
    adult Z91.412
    childhood Z62.812
  neoplasm
    benign Z86.018
      brain Z86.011
      colon polyp Z86.010
    in situ
      breast Z86.000
      cervix uteri Z86.001
      specified NEC Z86.008

History — *continued*
personal (*see also* History, family) — *continued*
  neoplasm — *continued*
    malignant — *see* History of, malignant neoplasm
    uncertain behavior Z86.03
  nephrotic syndrome Z87.441
  nicotine dependence Z87.891
  noncompliance with medical treatment or regimen — *see* Noncompliance
  nutritional deficiency Z86.39
  obstetric complications Z87.59
    childbirth Z87.59
    pregnancy Z87.59
    pre-term labor Z87.51
    puerperium Z87.59
  osteoporosis fractures Z87.31 ☑
  parasuicide (attempt) Z91.5
  physical trauma NEC Z87.828
    self-harm or suicide attempt Z91.5
  pneumonia (recurrent) Z87.01
  poisoning NEC Z91.89
    self-harm or suicide attempt Z91.5
  poor personal hygiene Z91.89
  preterm labor Z87.51
  procedure during pregnancy Z98.870
  procedure while a fetus Z98.871
  prolonged reversible ischemic neurologic deficit (PRIND) Z86.73
  prostatic dysplasia Z87.430
  psychological
    abuse
      adult Z91.411
      child Z62.811
    trauma, specified NEC Z91.49
  radiation therapy Z92.3
  removal
    implant
      breast Z98.86
  renal calculi Z87.442
  respiratory condition NEC Z87.09
  retained foreign body fully removed Z87.821
  risk factors NEC Z91.89
  self-harm Z91.5
  self-poisoning attempt Z91.5
  sex reassignment Z87.890
  sleep-wake cycle problem Z72.821
  specified NEC Z87.898
  steroid therapy (systemic) Z92.241
    inhaled Z92.240
  stroke without residual deficits Z86.73
  substance abuse NEC F10-F19
  sudden cardiac arrest Z86.74
  sudden cardiac death successfully resuscitated Z86.74
  suicide attempt Z91.5
  surgery NEC Z98.890
    with uterine scar Z98.891
    sex reassignment Z87.890
    transplant — *see* Transplant
  thrombophlebitis Z86.72
  thrombosis (venous) Z86.718
    pulmonary Z86.711
  tobacco dependence Z87.891
  transient ischemic attack (TIA) without residual deficits Z86.73
  trauma (physical) NEC Z87.828
    psychological NEC Z91.49
    self-harm Z91.5
  traumatic brain injury Z87.820
  unhealthy sleep-wake cycle Z72.821
  unintended awareness under general anesthesia Z92.84
  urinary calculi Z87.442
  urinary (recurrent) (tract) infection(s) Z87.440
  uterine scar from previous surgery Z98.891
  vaginal dysplasia Z87.411
  venous thrombosis or embolism Z86.718
    pulmonary Z86.711
  vulvar dysplasia Z87.412
His-Werner disease A79.0
HIV (*see also* Human, immunodeficiency virus) B20
  laboratory evidence (nonconclusive) R75
  nonconclusive test (in infants) R75
  positive, seropositive Z21
Hives (bold) — *see* Urticaria
Hoarseness R49.0
Hobo Z59.0
Hodgkin disease — *see* Lymphoma, Hodgkin

Hodgson's disease I71.2
  ruptured I71.1
Hoffa-Kastert disease E88.89
Hoffa's disease E88.89
Hoffmann-Bouveret syndrome I47.9
Hoffmann's syndrome E03.9 [G73.7]
Hole (round)
  macula H35.34- ☑
  retina (without detachment) — *see* Break, retina, round hole
    with detachment — *see* Detachment, retina, with retinal, break
Holiday relief care Z75.5
Hollenhorst's plaque — *see* Occlusion, artery, retina
Hollow foot (congenital) Q66.7
  acquired — *see* Deformity, limb, foot, specified NEC
Holoprosencephaly Q04.2
Holt-Oram syndrome Q87.2
Homelessness Z59.0
Homesickness — *see* Disorder, adjustment
Homocystinemia, homocystinuria E72.11
Homogentisate 1,2-dioxygenase deficiency E70.29
Homologous serum hepatitis (prophylactic) (therapeutic) — *see* Hepatitis, viral, type B
Honeycomb lung J98.4
  congenital Q33.0
Hooded
  clitoris Q52.6
  penis Q55.69
Hookworm (anemia) (disease) (infection) (infestation) B76.9
  specified NEC B76.8
Hordeolum (eyelid) (externum) (recurrent) H00.019
  internum H00.029
    left H00.026
      lower H00.025
      upper H00.024
    right H00.023
      lower H00.022
      upper H00.021
  left H00.016
    lower H00.015
    upper H00.014
  right H00.013
    lower H00.012
    upper H00.011
Horn
  cutaneous L85.8
  nail L60.2
    congenital Q84.6
Horner (-Claude Bernard) **syndrome** G90.2
  traumatic — *see* Injury, nerve, cervical sympathetic
Horseshoe kidney (congenital) Q63.1
Horton's headache or neuralgia G44.099
  intractable G44.091
  not intractable G44.099
Hospital hopper syndrome — *see* Disorder, factitious
Hospitalism in children — *see* Disorder, adjustment
Hostility R45.5
  towards child Z62.3
Hot flashes
  menopausal N95.1
Hourglass (contracture) (*see also* Contraction, hourglass)
  stomach K31.89
    congenital Q40.2
    stricture K31.2
Household, housing circumstance affecting care Z59.9
  specified NEC Z59.8
Housemaid's knee — *see* Bursitis, prepatellar
Hudson (-Stähli) **line** (cornea) — *see* Pigmentation, cornea, anterior
Human
  bite (open wound) (*see also* Bite)
    intact skin surface — *see* Bite, superficial
  herpesvirus — *see* Herpes
  immunodeficiency virus (HIV) disease (infection) B20
    asymptomatic status Z21
    contact Z20.6
    counseling Z71.7
    dementia B20 [F02.80]
      with behavioral disturbance B20 [F02.81]
    exposure to Z20.6
    laboratory evidence R75
    type-2 (HIV 2) as cause of disease classified elsewhere B97.35

Human — continued
 papillomavirus (HPV)
  DNA test positive
   high risk
    cervix R87.810
    vagina R87.811
   low risk
    cervix R87.820
    vagina R87.821
  screening for Z11.51
  T-cell lymphotropic virus
   type-1 (HTLV-I) infection B33.3
    as cause of disease classified elsewhere B97.33
    carrier Z22.6
   type-2 (HTLV-II) as cause of disease classified elsewhere B97.34
Humidifier lung or pneumonitis J67.7
Humiliation (experience) **in childhood** Z62.898
Humpback (acquired) — see Kyphosis
Hunchback (acquired) — see Kyphosis
Hunger T73.0 ☑
 air, psychogenic F45.8
Hungry bone syndrome E83.81
Hunner's ulcer — see Cystitis, chronic, interstitial
Hunter's
 glossitis D51.0
 syndrome E76.1
Huntington's disease or chorea G10
 with dementia G10 [F02.80]
  with behavioral disturbance G10 [F02.81]
Hunt's
 disease or syndrome (herpetic geniculate ganglionitis) B02.21
 dyssynergia cerebellaris myoclonica G11.1
 neuralgia B02.21
Hurler (-Scheie) **disease or syndrome** E76.02
Hurst's disease G36.1
Hurthle cell
 adenocarcinoma C73
 adenoma D34
 carcinoma C73
 tumor D34
Hutchinson-Boeck disease or syndrome — see Sarcoidosis
Hutchinson-Gilford disease or syndrome E34.8
Hutchinson's
 disease, meaning
  angioma serpiginosum L81.7
  pompholyx (cheiropompholyx) L30.1
  prurigo estivalis L56.4
  summer eruption or summer prurigo L56.4
 melanotic freckle — see Melanoma, in situ
  malignant melanoma in — see Melanoma
 teeth or incisors (congenital syphilis) A50.52
 triad (congenital syphilis) A50.53
Hyalin plaque, sclera, senile H15.89
Hyaline membrane (disease) (lung) (pulmonary) (newborn) P22.0
Hyalinosis
 cutis (et mucosae) E78.89
 focal and segmental (glomerular) (see also N00-N07 with fourth character .1) N05.1
Hyalitis, hyalosis, asteroid (see also Deposit, crystalline)
 syphilitic (late) A52.71
Hydatid
 cyst or tumor — see Echinococcus
 mole — see Hydatidiform mole
 Morgagni
  female Q50.5
  male (epididymal) Q55.4
   testicular Q55.29
Hydatidiform mole (benign) (complicating pregnancy) (delivered) (undelivered) O01.9
 classical O01.0
 complete O01.0
 incomplete O01.1
 invasive D39.2
 malignant D39.2
 partial O01.1
Hydatidosis — see Echinococcus
Hydradenitis (axillaris) (suppurative) L73.2
Hydradenoma — see Hidradenoma
Hydramnios O40.- ☑
Hydranencephaly, hydranencephaly Q04.3
 with spina bifida — see Spina bifida, with hydrocephalus
Hydrargyrism NEC — see Poisoning, mercury
Hydrarthrosis (see also Effusion, joint)

Hydrarthrosis — continued
 gonococcal A54.42
 intermittent M12.40
  ankle M12.47- ☑
  elbow M12.42- ☑
  foot joint M12.47- ☑
  hand joint M12.44- ☑
  hip M12.45- ☑
  knee M12.46- ☑
  multiple site M12.49
  shoulder M12.41- ☑
  specified joint NEC M12.48
  wrist M12.43- ☑
 of yaws (early) (late) (see also subcategory M14.8-) A66.6
 syphilitic (late) A52.77
  congenital A50.55 [M12.80]
Hydremia D64.89
Hydrencephalocele (congenital) — see Encephalocele
Hydrencephalomeningocele (congenital) — see Encephalocele
Hydroa R23.8
 aestivale L56.4
 vacciniforme L56.4
Hydroadenitis (axillaris) (suppurative) L73.2
Hydrocalycosis — see Hydronephrosis
Hydrocele (spermatic cord) (testis) (tunica vaginalis) N43.3
 canal of Nuck N94.89
 communicating N43.2
  congenital P83.5
 congenital P83.5
 encysted N43.0
 female NEC N94.89
 infected N43.1
 newborn P83.5
 round ligament N94.89
 specified NEC N43.2
 spinalis — see Spina bifida
 vulva N90.89
Hydrocephalus (acquired) (external) (internal) (malignant) (recurrent) G91.9
 aqueduct Sylvius stricture Q03.0
 causing disproportion O33.6 ☑
  with obstructed labor O66.3
 communicating G91.0
 congenital (external) (internal) Q03.9
  with spina bifida Q05.4
   cervical Q05.0
   dorsal Q05.1
   lumbar Q05.2
   lumbosacral Q05.2
   sacral Q05.3
   thoracic Q05.1
   thoracolumbar Q05.1
  specified NEC Q03.8
 due to toxoplasmosis (congenital) P37.1
 foramen Magendie block (acquired) G91.1
  congenital (see also Hydrocephalus, congenital) Q03.1
 in (due to)
  infectious disease NEC B89 [G91.4]
  neoplastic disease NEC (see also Neoplasm) G91.4
  parasitic disease B89 [G91.4]
 newborn Q03.9
  with spina bifida — see Spina bifida, with hydrocephalus
 noncommunicating G91.1
 normal pressure G91.2
  secondary G91.0
 obstructive G91.1
 otitic G93.2
 post-traumatic NEC G91.3
 secondary G91.4
  post-traumatic G91.3
 specified NEC G91.8
 syphilitic, congenital A50.49
Hydrocolpos (congenital) N89.8
Hydrocystoma — see Neoplasm, skin, benign
Hydroencephalocele (congenital) — see Encephalocele
Hydroencephalomeningocele (congenital) — see Encephalocele
Hydrohematopneumothorax — see Hemothorax
Hydromeningitis — see Meningitis
Hydromeningocele (spinal) (see also Spina bifida)
 cranial — see Encephalocele
Hydrometra N85.8
Hydrometrocolpos N89.8

Hydromicrocephaly Q02
Hydromphalos (since birth) Q45.8
Hydromyelia Q06.4
Hydromyelocele — see Spina bifida
Hydronephrosis (atrophic) (early) (functionless) (intermittent) (primary) (secondary) NEC N13.30
 with
  infection N13.6
  obstruction (by) (of)
   renal calculus N13.2
    with infection N13.6
   ureteral NEC N13.1
    with infection N13.6
    calculus N13.2
     with infection N13.6
   ureteropelvic junction (congenital) Q62.11
    acquired N13.0
     with infection N13.6
   ureteral stricture NEC N13.1
    with infection N13.6
 congenital Q62.0
  due to acquired occlusion of ureteropelvic junction N13.0
 specified type NEC N13.39
 tuberculous A18.11
Hydropericarditis — see Pericarditis
Hydropericardium — see Pericarditis
Hydroperitoneum R18.8
Hydrophobia — see Rabies
Hydrophthalmos Q15.0
Hydropneumohemothorax — see Hemothorax
Hydropneumopericarditis — see Pericarditis
Hydropneumopericardium — see Pericarditis
Hydropneumothorax J94.8
 traumatic — see Injury, intrathoracic, lung
 tuberculous NEC A15.6
Hydrops R60.9
 abdominis R18.8
 articulorum intermittens — see Hydrarthrosis, intermittent
 cardiac — see Failure, heart, congestive
 causing obstructed labor (mother) O66.3
 endolymphatic H81.0- ☑
 fetal — see Pregnancy, complicated by, hydrops, fetalis
 fetalis P83.2
  due to
   ABO isoimmunization P56.0
   alpha thalassemia D56.0
   hemolytic disease P56.90
    specified NEC P56.99
   isoimmunization (ABO) (Rh) P56.0
   other specified nonhemolytic disease NEC P83.2
   Rh incompatibility P56.0
  during pregnancy — see Pregnancy, complicated by, hydrops, fetalis
 gallbladder K82.1
 joint — see Effusion, joint
 labyrinth H81.0- ☑
 newborn (idiopathic) P83.2
  due to
   ABO isoimmunization P56.0
   alpha thalassemia D56.0
   hemolytic disease P56.90
    specified NEC P56.99
   isoimmunization (ABO) (Rh) P56.0
   Rh incompatibility P56.0
 nutritional — see Malnutrition, severe
 pericardium — see Pericarditis
 pleura — see Hydrothorax
 spermatic cord — see Hydrocele
Hydropyonephrosis N13.6
Hydrorachis Q06.4
Hydrorrhea (nasal) J34.89
 pregnancy — see Rupture, membranes, premature
Hydrosadenitis (axillaris) (suppurative) L73.2
Hydrosalpinx (fallopian tube) (follicularis) N70.11
Hydrothorax (double) (pleura) J94.8
 chylous (nonfilarial) I89.8
  filarial (see also Infestation, filarial) B74.9 [J91.8]
 traumatic — see Injury, intrathoracic
 tuberculous NEC (non primary) A15.6
Hydroureter (see also Hydronephrosis) N13.4
 with infection N13.6
 congenital Q62.39
Hydroureteronephrosis — see Hydronephrosis
Hydrourethra N36.8
Hydroxykynureninuria E70.8

172

☑ Additional Character Required — Refer to the Tabular List for Character Selection   ▽ Subterms under main terms may continue to next column or page

Hydroxylysinemia E72.3
Hydroxyprolinemia E72.59
Hygiene, sleep
  abuse Z72.821
  inadequate Z72.821
  poor Z72.821
Hygroma (congenital) (cystic) D18.1
  praepatellare, prepatellar — see Bursitis, prepatellar
Hymen — see condition
Hymenolepis, hymenolepiasis (diminuta) (infection)
  (infestation) (nana) B71.0
Hypalgesia R20.8
Hyperacidity (gastric) K31.89
  psychogenic F45.8
Hyperactive, hyperactivity F90.9
  basal cell, uterine cervix — see Dysplasia, cervix
  bowel sounds R19.12
  cervix epithelial (basal) — see Dysplasia, cervix
  child F90.9
    attention deficit — see Disorder, attention-deficit
      hyperactivity
  detrusor muscle N32.81
  gastrointestinal K31.89
    psychogenic F45.8
  nasal mucous membrane J34.3
  stomach K31.89
  thyroid (gland) — see Hyperthyroidism
Hyperacusis H93.23- ☑
Hyperadrenalism E27.5
Hyperadrenocorticism E24.9
  congenital E25.0
  iatrogenic E24.2
    correct substance properly administered — see Table of Drugs and Chemicals, by drug, adverse effect
    overdose or wrong substance given or taken — see Table of Drugs and Chemicals, by drug, poisoning
  not associated with Cushing's syndrome E27.0
  pituitary-dependent E24.0
Hyperaldosteronism E26.9
  familial (type I) E26.02
  glucocorticoid-remediable E26.02
  primary (due to (bilateral) adrenal hyperplasia) E26.09
  primary NEC E26.09
  secondary E26.1
  specified NEC E26.89
Hyperalgesia R20.8
Hyperalimentation R63.2
  carotene, carotin E67.1
  specified NEC E67.8
  vitamin
    A E67.0
    D E67.3
Hyperaminoaciduria
  arginine E72.21
  cystine E72.01
  lysine E72.3
  ornithine E72.4
Hyperammonemia (congenital) E72.20
Hyperazotemia — see Uremia
Hyperbetalipoproteinemia (familial) E78.00
  with prebetalipoproteinemia E78.2
Hyperbicarbonatemia P74.41
Hyperbilirubinemia
  constitutional E80.6
  familial conjugated E80.6
  neonatal (transient) — see Jaundice, newborn
Hypercalcemia, hypocalciuric, familial E83.52
Hypercalciuria, idiopathic R82.994
Hypercapnia R06.89
  newborn P84
Hypercarotenemia (dietary) E67.1
Hypercementosis K03.4
Hyperchloremia E87.8
Hyperchlorhydria K31.89
  neurotic F45.8
  psychogenic F45.8
Hypercholesterinemia — see Hypercholesterolemia
Hypercholesterolemia (essential) (primary) (pure) E78.00
  with hyperglyceridemia, endogenous E78.2
  dietary counseling and surveillance Z71.3
  familial E78.01
  hereditary E78.01
Hyperchylia gastrica, psychogenic F45.8
Hyperchylomicronemia (familial) (primary) E78.3
  with hyperbetalipoproteinemia E78.3

Hypercoagulable (state) D68.59
  activated protein C resistance D68.51
  antithrombin (III) deficiency D68.59
  factor V Leiden mutation D68.51
  primary NEC D68.59
  protein C deficiency D68.59
  protein S deficiency D68.59
  prothrombin gene mutation D68.52
  secondary D68.69
  specified NEC D68.69
Hypercoagulation (state) D68.59
Hypercorticalism, pituitary-dependent E24.0
Hypercorticosolism — see Cushing's, syndrome
Hypercorticosteronism E24.2
  correct substance properly administered — see Table of Drugs and Chemicals, by drug, adverse effect
  overdose or wrong substance given or taken — see Table of Drugs and Chemicals, by drug, poisoning
Hypercortisonism E24.2
  correct substance properly administered — see Table of Drugs and Chemicals, by drug, adverse effect
  overdose or wrong substance given or taken — see Table of Drugs and Chemicals, by drug, poisoning
Hyperekplexia Q89.8
Hyperelectrolytemia E87.8
Hyperemesis R11.10
  with nausea R11.2
  gravidarum (mild) O21.0
    with
      carbohydrate depletion O21.1
      dehydration O21.1
      electrolyte imbalance O21.1
      metabolic disturbance O21.1
      severe (with metabolic disturbance) O21.1
  projectile R11.12
  psychogenic F45.8
Hyperemia (acute) (passive) R68.89
  anal mucosa K62.89
  bladder N32.89
  cerebral I67.89
  conjunctiva H11.43- ☑
  ear internal, acute — see subcategory H83.0 ☑
  enteric K59.8
  eye — see Hyperemia, conjunctiva
  eyelid (active) (passive) — see Disorder, eyelid, specified type NEC
  intestine K59.8
  iris — see Disorder, iris, vascular
  kidney N28.89
  labyrinth — see subcategory H83.0 ☑
  liver (active) K76.89
  lung (passive) — see Edema, lung
  pulmonary (passive) — see Edema, lung
  renal N28.89
  retina H35.89
  stomach K31.89
Hyperesthesia (body surface) R20.3
  larynx (reflex) J38.7
    hysterical F44.89
  pharynx (reflex) J39.2
    hysterical F44.89
Hyperestrogenism (drug-induced) (iatrogenic) E28.0
Hyperexplexia Q89.8
Hyperfibrinolysis — see Fibrinolysis
Hyperfructosemia E74.19
Hyperfunction
  adrenal cortex, not associated with Cushing's syndrome E27.0
    medulla E27.5
      adrenomedullary E27.5
    virilism E25.9
      congenital E25.0
  ovarian E28.8
  pancreas K86.89
  parathyroid (gland) E21.3
  pituitary (gland) (anterior) E22.9
    specified NEC E22.8
  polyglandular E31.1
  testicular E29.0
Hypergammaglobulinemia D89.2
  polyclonal D89.0
  Waldenström D89.0
Hypergastrinemia E16.4
Hyperglobulinemia R77.1
Hyperglycemia, hyperglycemic (transient) R73.9
  coma — see Diabetes, by type, with coma
  postpancreatectomy E89.1

Hyperglyceridemia (endogenous) (essential) (familial) (hereditary) (pure) E78.1
  mixed E78.3
Hyperglycinemia (non-ketotic) E72.51
Hypergonadism
  ovarian E28.8
  testicular (primary) (infantile) E29.0
Hyperheparinemia D68.32
Hyperhidrosis, hyperidrosis R61
  focal
    primary L74.519
      axilla L74.510
      face L74.511
      palms L74.512
      soles L74.513
    secondary L74.52
  generalized R61
  localized
    primary L74.519
      axilla L74.510
      face L74.511
      palms L74.512
      soles L74.513
    secondary L74.52
  psychogenic F45.8
  secondary R61
    focal L74.52
Hyperhistidinemia E70.41
Hyperhomocysteinemia E72.11
Hyperhydroxyprolinemia E72.59
Hyperinsulinism (functional) E16.1
  with
    coma (hypoglycemic) E15
    encephalopathy E16.1 [G94]
  ectopic E16.1
  therapeutic misadventure (from administration of insulin) — see subcategory T38.3 ☑
Hyperkalemia E87.5
Hyperkeratosis (see also Keratosis) L85.9
  cervix N88.0
  due to yaws (early) (late) (palmar or plantar) A66.3
  follicularis Q82.8
    penetrans (in cutem) L87.0
  palmoplantaris climacterica L85.1
  pinta A67.1
  senile (with pruritus) L57.0
  universalis congenita Q80.8
  vocal cord J38.3
  vulva N90.4
Hyperkinesia, hyperkinetic (disease) (reaction) (syndrome) (childhood) (adolescence) (see also Disorder, attention-deficit hyperactivity)
  heart I51.89
Hyperleucine-isoleucinemia E71.19
Hyperlipemia, hyperlipidemia E78.5
  combined E78.2
    familial E78.49
  group
    A E78.00
    B E78.1
    C E78.2
    D E78.3
  mixed E78.2
  specified NEC E78.49
Hyperlipidosis E75.6
  hereditary NEC E75.5
Hyperlipoproteinemia E78.5
  Fredrickson's type
    I E78.3
    IIa E78.00
    IIb E78.2
    III E78.2
    IV E78.1
    V E78.3
  low-density-lipoprotein-type (LDL) E78.00
  very-low-density-lipoprotein-type (VLDL) E78.1
Hyperlucent lung, unilateral J43.0
Hyperlysinemia E72.3
Hypermagnesemia E83.41
  neonatal P71.8
Hypermenorrhea N92.0
Hypermethioninemia E72.19
Hypermetropia (congenital) H52.0- ☑
Hypermobility, hypermotility
  cecum — see Syndrome, irritable bowel
  coccyx — see subcategory M53.2 ☑
  colon — see Syndrome, irritable bowel
    psychogenic F45.8

Hypermobility, hypermotility — *continued*
　ileum K58.9
　intestine (*see also* Syndrome, irritable bowel) K58.9
　　psychogenic F45.8
　meniscus (knee) — *see* Derangement, knee, meniscus
　scapula — *see* Instability, joint, shoulder
　stomach K31.89
　　psychogenic F45.8
　syndrome M35.7
　urethra N36.41
　　with intrinsic sphincter deficiency N36.43
Hypernasality R49.21
Hypernatremia E87.0
Hypernephroma C64.- ☑
Hyperopia — *see* Hypermetropia
Hyperorexia nervosa F50.2
Hyperornithinemia E72.4
Hyperosmia R43.1
Hyperosmolality E87.0
Hyperostosis (monomelic) (*see also* Disorder, bone, density and structure, specified NEC)
　ankylosing (spine) M48.10
　　cervical region M48.12
　　cervicothoracic region M48.13
　　lumbar region M48.16
　　lumbosacral region M48.17
　　multiple sites M48.19
　　occipito-atlanto-axial region M48.11
　　sacrococcygeal region M48.18
　　thoracic region M48.14
　　thoracolumbar region M48.15
　cortical (skull) M85.2
　　infantile M89.8X- ☑
　frontal, internal of skull M85.2
　interna frontalis M85.2
　skeletal, diffuse idiopathic — *see* Hyperostosis, ankylosing
　skull M85.2
　　congenital Q75.8
　vertebral, ankylosing — *see* Hyperostosis, ankylosing
Hyperovarism E28.8
Hyperoxaluria R82.992
　primary E72.53
Hyperparathyroidism E21.3
　primary E21.0
　secondary (renal) N25.81
　　non-renal E21.1
　specified NEC E21.2
　tertiary E21.2
Hyperpathia R20.8
Hyperperistalsis R19.2
　psychogenic F45.8
Hyperpermeability, capillary I78.8
Hyperphagia R63.2
Hyperphenylalaninemia NEC E70.1
Hyperphoria (alternating) H50.53
Hyperphosphatemia E83.39
Hyperpiesis, hyperpiesia — *see* Hypertension
Hyperpigmentation (*see also* Pigmentation)
　melanin NEC L81.4
　postinflammatory L81.0
Hyperpinealism E34.8
Hyperpituitarism E22.9
Hyperplasia, hyperplastic
　adenoids J35.2
　adrenal (capsule) (cortex) (gland) E27.8
　　with
　　　sexual precocity (male) E25.9
　　　　congenital E25.0
　　　virilism, adrenal E25.9
　　　　congenital E25.0
　　　virilization (female) E25.9
　　　　congenital E25.0
　　congenital E25.0
　　salt-losing E25.0
　adrenomedullary E27.5
　angiolymphoid, eosinophilia (ALHE) D18.01
　appendix (lymphoid) K38.0
　artery, fibromuscular I77.3
　bone (*see also* Hypertrophy, bone)
　　marrow D75.89
　breast (*see also* Hypertrophy, breast)
　　ductal (atypical) N60.9- ☑
　C-cell, thyroid E07.0
　cementation (tooth) (teeth) K03.4
　cervical gland R59.0
　cervix (uteri) (basal cell) (endometrium) (polypoid) (*see also* Dysplasia, cervix)

Hyperplasia, hyperplastic — *continued*
　cervix (*see also* Dysplasia, cervix) — *continued*
　　congenital Q51.828
　clitoris, congenital Q52.6
　denture K06.2
　endocervicitis N72
　endometrium, endometrial (adenomatous) (benign) (cystic) (glandular) (glandular-cystic) (polypoid) N85.00
　　with atypia N85.02
　　cervix — *see* Dysplasia, cervix
　　complex (without atypia) N85.01
　　simple (without atypia) N85.01
　epithelial L85.9
　　focal, oral, including tongue K13.29
　　nipple N62
　　skin L85.9
　　tongue K13.29
　　vaginal wall N89.3
　erythroid D75.89
　fibromuscular of artery (carotid) (renal) I77.3
　genital
　　female NEC N94.89
　　male N50.89
　gingiva K06.1
　glandularis cystica uteri (interstitialis) (*see also* Hyperplasia, endometrial) N85.00
　gum K06.1
　hymen, congenital Q52.4
　irritative, edentulous (alveolar) K06.2
　jaw M26.09
　　alveolar M26.79
　　lower M26.03
　　　alveolar M26.72
　　upper M26.01
　　　alveolar M26.71
　kidney (congenital) Q63.3
　labia N90.69
　　epithelial N90.3
　liver (congenital) Q44.7
　　nodular, focal K76.89
　lymph gland or node R59.9
　mandible, mandibular M26.03
　　alveolar M26.72
　　unilateral condylar M27.8
　maxilla, maxillary M26.01
　　alveolar M26.71
　myometrium, myometrial N85.2
　neuroendocrine cell, of infancy J84.841
　nose
　　lymphoid J34.89
　　polypoid J33.9
　oral mucosa (irritative) K13.6
　organ or site, congenital NEC — *see* Anomaly, by site
　ovary N83.8
　palate, papillary (irritative) K13.6
　pancreatic islet cells E16.9
　　alpha E16.8
　　　with excess
　　　　gastrin E16.4
　　　　glucagon E16.3
　　beta E16.1
　parathyroid (gland) E21.0
　pharynx (lymphoid) J39.2
　prostate (adenofibromatous) (nodular) N40.0
　　with lower urinary tract symptoms (LUTS) N40.1
　　without lower urinary tract symtpoms (LUTS) N40.0
　renal artery I77.89
　reticulo-endothelial (cell) D75.89
　salivary gland (any) K11.1
　Schimmelbusch's — *see* Mastopathy, cystic
　suprarenal capsule (gland) E27.8
　thymus (gland) (persistent) E32.0
　thyroid (gland) — *see* Goiter
　tonsils (faucial) (infective) (lingual) (lymphoid) J35.1
　　with adenoids J35.3
　unilateral condylar M27.8
　uterus, uterine N85.2
　　endometrium (glandular) (*see also* Hyperplasia, endometrial) N85.00
　vulva N90.69
　　epithelial N90.3
Hyperpnea — *see* Hyperventilation
Hyperpotassemia E87.5
Hyperprebetalipoproteinemia (familial) E78.1
Hyperprolactinemia E22.1
Hyperprolinemia (type I) (type II) E72.59
Hyperproteinemia E88.09

Hyperprothrombinemia, causing coagulation factor deficiency D68.4
Hyperpyrexia R50.9
　heat (effects) T67.0 ☑
　malignant, due to anesthetic T88.3 ☑
　rheumatic — *see* Fever, rheumatic
　unknown origin R50.9
Hyper-reflexia R29.2
Hypersalivation K11.7
Hypersecretion
　ACTH (not associated with Cushing's syndrome) E27.0
　　pituitary E24.0
　adrenaline E27.5
　adrenomedullary E27.5
　androgen (testicular) E29.0
　　ovarian (drug-induced) (iatrogenic) E28.1
　calcitonin E07.0
　catecholamine E27.5
　corticoadrenal E24.9
　cortisol E24.9
　epinephrine E27.5
　estrogen E28.0
　gastric K31.89
　　psychogenic F45.8
　gastrin E16.4
　glucagon E16.3
　hormone(s)
　　ACTH (not associated with Cushing's syndrome) E27.0
　　　pituitary E24.0
　　antidiuretic E22.2
　　growth E22.0
　　intestinal NEC E34.1
　　ovarian androgen E28.1
　　pituitary E22.9
　　testicular E29.0
　　thyroid stimulating E05.80
　　　with thyroid storm E05.81
　insulin — *see* Hyperinsulinism
　lacrimal glands — *see* Epiphora
　medulloadrenal E27.5
　milk O92.6
　ovarian androgens E28.1
　salivary gland (any) K11.7
　thyrocalcitonin E07.0
　upper respiratory J39.8
Hypersegmentation, leukocytic, hereditary D72.0
Hypersensitive, hypersensitiveness, hypersensitivity
　(*see also* Allergy)
　carotid sinus G90.01
　colon — *see* Irritable, colon
　drug T88.7 ☑
　gastrointestinal K52.29
　　immediate K52.29
　　psychogenic F45.8
　labyrinth — *see* subcategory H83.2 ☑
　pain R20.8
　pneumonitis — *see* Pneumonitis, allergic
　reaction T78.40 ☑
　　upper respiratory tract NEC J39.3
Hypersomnia (organic) G47.10
　due to
　　alcohol
　　　abuse F10.182
　　　dependence F10.282
　　　use F10.982
　　amphetamines
　　　abuse F15.182
　　　dependence F15.282
　　　use F15.982
　　caffeine
　　　abuse F15.182
　　　dependence F15.282
　　　use F15.982
　　cocaine
　　　abuse F14.182
　　　dependence F14.282
　　　use F14.982
　　drug NEC
　　　abuse F19.182
　　　dependence F19.282
　　　use F19.982
　　medical condition G47.14
　　mental disorder F51.13
　　opioid
　　　abuse F11.182
　　　dependence F11.282
　　　use F11.982

☑ Additional Character Required — Refer to the Tabular List for Character Selection　　　▽ Subterms under main terms may continue to next column or page

ypersomnia — *continued*
  due to — *continued*
    psychoactive substance NEC
      abuse F19.182
      dependence F19.282
      use F19.982
    sedative, hypnotic, or anxiolytic
      abuse F13.182
      dependence F13.282
      use F13.982
    stimulant NEC
      abuse F15.182
      dependence F15.282
      use F15.982
  idiopathic G47.11
    with long sleep time G47.11
    without long sleep time G47.12
  menstrual related G47.13
  nonorganic origin F51.11
    specified NEC F51.19
  not due to a substance or known physiological condition F51.11
    specified NEC F51.19
  primary F51.11
  recurrent G47.13
  specified NEC G47.19

ypersplenia, hypersplenism D73.1

yperstimulation, ovaries (associated with induced ovulation) N98.1

ypersusceptibility — *see* Allergy

ypertelorism (ocular) (orbital) Q75.2

ypertension, hypertensive (accelerated) (benign) (essential) (idiopathic) (malignant) (systemic) I10
  with
    heart failure (congestive) I11.0
    heart involvement (conditions in I50.-, I51.4- I51.9 due to hypertension) — *see* Hypertension, heart
    kidney involvement — *see* Hypertension, kidney
  benign, intracranial G93.2
  borderline R03.0
  cardiorenal (disease) I13.10
    with heart failure I13.0
      with stage 1 through stage 4 chronic kidney disease I13.0
      with stage 5 or end stage renal disease I13.2
    without heart failure I13.10
      with stage 1 through stage 4 chronic kidney disease I13.10
      with stage 5 or end stage renal disease I13.11
  cardiovascular
    disease (arteriosclerotic) (sclerotic) — *see* Hypertension, heart
    renal (disease) — *see* Hypertension, cardiorenal
  chronic venous — *see* Hypertension, venous (chronic)
  complicating
    childbirth (labor) O16.4
      pre-existing O10.92
        with
          heart disease O10.12
            with renal disease O10.32
          pre-eclampsia O11.4
          renal disease O10.22
            with heart disease O10.32
        essential O10.02
      secondary O10.42
    pregnancy O16.- ☑
      with edema (*see also* Pre-eclampsia) O14.9- ☑
      gestational (pregnancy induced) (without proteinuria) O13.- ☑
        with proteinuria O14.9- ☑
          mild pre-eclampsia O14.0- ☑
          moderate pre-eclampsia O14.0- ☑
          severe pre-eclampsia O14.1- ☑
            with hemolysis, elevated liver enzymes and low platelet count (HELLP) O14.2- ☑
      pre-existing O10.91- ☑
        with
          heart disease O10.11- ☑
            with renal disease O10.31- ☑
          pre-eclampsia — *see* category O11
          renal disease O10.21- ☑
            with heart disease O10.31- ☑
        essential O10.01- ☑
        secondary O10.41- ☑
      transient O13- ☑
    puerperium, pre-existing O16.5

Hypertension, hypertensive — *continued*
  complicating — *continued*
    puerperium, pre-existing — *continued*
      pre-existing
        with
          heart disease O10.13
            with renal disease O10.33
          pre-eclampsia O11.5
          renal disease O10.23
            with heart disease O10.33
        essential O10.03
      pregnancy-induced O13.9
      secondary O10.43
  crisis I16.9
  due to
    endocrine disorders I15.2
    pheochromocytoma I15.2
    renal disorders NEC I15.1
      arterial I15.0
    renovascular disorders I15.0
    specified disease NEC I15.8
  emergency I16.1
  encephalopathy I67.4
  gestational (without significant proteinuria) (pregnancy-induced) (transient) O13.- ☑
    with significant proteinuria — *see* Pre-eclampsia
    complicating
      delivery O13.4
      puerperium O13.5
  Goldblatt's I70.1
  heart (disease) (conditions in I51.4-I51.9 due to hypertension) I11.9
    with
      heart failure (congestive) I11.0
      kidney disease (chronic) — *see* Hypertension, cardiorenal
  intracranial (benign) G93.2
  kidney I12.9
    with
      heart disease — *see* Hypertension, cardiorenal
      stage 1 through stage 4 chronic kidney disease I12.9
      stage 5 chronic kidney disease (CKD) or end stage renal disease (ESRD) I12.0
  lesser circulation I27.0
  maternal O16- ☑
  newborn P29.2
    pulmonary (persistent) P29.30
  ocular H40.05- ☑
  pancreatic duct — *code to* underlying condition
    with chronic pancreatitis K86.1
  portal (due to chronic liver disease) (idiopathic) K76.6
    gastropathy K31.89
    in (due to) schistosomiasis (bilharziasis) B65.9 [K77]
  postoperative I97.3
  psychogenic F45.8
  pulmonary I27.20
    with
      cor pulmonale (chronic) I27.29
        acute I26.09
      right heart ventricular strain/failure I27.29
        acute I26.09
      right to left shunt related to congenital heart disease I27.83
      unclear multifactorial mechanisms I27.29
    arterial (associated) (drug-induced) (toxin-induced) I27.21
    chronic thromboembolic I27.24
    due to
      hematologic disorders I27.29
      left heart disease I27.22
      lung diseases and hypoxia I27.23
      metabolic disorders I27.29
      specified systemic disorders I27.29
    group 1 (associated) (drug-induced) (toxin-induced) I27.21
    group 2 I27.22
    group 3 I27.23
    group 4 I27.24
    group 5 I27.29
    of newborn (persistent) P29.30
    primary (idiopathic) I27.0
    secondary
      arterial I27.21
      specified NEC I27.29
  renal — *see* Hypertension, kidney
  renovascular I15.0
  secondary NEC I15.9

Hypertension, hypertensive — *continued*
  secondary — *continued*
    due to
      endocrine disorders I15.2
      pheochromocytoma I15.2
      renal disorders NEC I15.1
        arterial I15.0
      renovascular disorders I15.0
    specified NEC I15.8
  transient R03.0
    of pregnancy O13.- ☑
  urgency I16.0
  venous (chronic)
    due to
      deep vein thrombosis — *see* Syndrome, post-thrombotic
    idiopathic I87.309
      with
        inflammation I87.32- ☑
          with ulcer I87.33- ☑
        specified complication NEC I87.39- ☑
        ulcer I87.31- ☑
          with inflammation I87.33- ☑
      asymptomatic I87.30- ☑

Hypertensive urgency — *see* Hypertension

Hyperthecosis ovary E28.8

Hyperthermia (of unknown origin) (*see also* Hyperpyrexia)
  malignant, due to anesthesia T88.3 ☑
  newborn P81.9
    environmental P81.0

Hyperthyroid (recurrent) — *see* Hyperthyroidism

Hyperthyroidism (latent) (pre-adult) (recurrent) E05.90
  with
    goiter (diffuse) E05.00
      with thyroid storm E05.01
      nodular (multinodular) E05.20
        with thyroid storm E05.21
        uninodular E05.10
          with thyroid storm E05.11
    storm E05.91
  due to ectopic thyroid tissue E05.30
    with thyroid storm E05.31
  neonatal, transitory P72.1
  specified NEC E05.80
    with thyroid storm E05.81

Hypertony, hypertonia, hypertonicity
  bladder N31.8
  congenital P94.1
  stomach K31.89
    psychogenic F45.8
  uterus, uterine (contractions) (complicating delivery) O62.4

Hypertrichosis L68.9
  congenital Q84.2
  eyelid H02.869
    left H02.866
      lower H02.865
      upper H02.864
    right H02.863
      lower H02.862
      upper H02.861
  lanuginosa Q84.2
    acquired L68.1
  localized L68.2
  specified NEC L68.8

Hypertriglyceridemia, essential E78.1

Hypertrophy, hypertrophic
  adenofibromatous, prostate — *see* Enlargement, enlarged, prostate
  adenoids (infective) J35.2
    with tonsils J35.3
  adrenal cortex E27.8
  alveolar process or ridge — *see* Anomaly, alveolar
  anal papillae K62.89
  artery I77.89
    congenital NEC Q27.8
      digestive system Q27.8
      lower limb Q27.8
      specified site NEC Q27.8
      upper limb Q27.8
  auricular — *see* Hypertrophy, cardiac
  Bartholin's gland N75.8
  bile duct (common) (hepatic) K83.8
  bladder (sphincter) (trigone) N32.89
  bone M89.30
    carpus M89.34- ☑
    clavicle M89.31- ☑

Hypertrophy, hypertrophic — continued
bone — continued
femur M89.35- ☑
fibula M89.36-
finger M89.34- ☑
humerus M89.32- ☑
ilium M89.359
ischium M89.359
metacarpus M89.34- ☑
metatarsus M89.37- ☑
multiple sites M89.39
neck M89.38
radius M89.33- ☑
rib M89.38
scapula M89.31- ☑
skull M89.38
tarsus M89.37- ☑
tibia M89.36- ☑
toe M89.37- ☑
ulna M89.33- ☑
vertebra M89.38
brain G93.89
breast N62
cystic — see Mastopathy, cystic
newborn P83.4
pubertal, massive N62
puerperal, postpartum — see Disorder, breast,
specified type NEC
senile (parenchymatous) N62
cardiac (chronic) (idiopathic) I51.7
with rheumatic fever (conditions in I00)
active I01.8
inactive or quiescent (with chorea) I09.89
congenital NEC Q24.8
fatty — see Degeneration, myocardial
hypertensive — see Hypertension, heart
rheumatic (with chorea) I09.89
active or acute I01.8
with chorea I02.0
valve — see Endocarditis
cartilage — see Disorder, cartilage, specified type NEC
cecum — see Megacolon
cervix (uteri) N88.8
congenital Q51.828
elongation N88.4
clitoris (cirrhotic) N90.89
congenital Q52.6
colon (see also Megacolon)
congenital Q43.2
conjunctiva, lymphoid H11.89
corpora cavernosa N48.89
cystic duct K82.8
duodenum K31.89
endometrium (glandular) (see also Hyperplasia, endometrial) N85.00
cervix N88.8
epididymis N50.89
esophageal hiatus (congenital) Q79.1
with hernia — see Hernia, hiatal
eyelid — see Disorder, eyelid, specified type NEC
fat pad E65
knee (infrapatellar) (popliteal) (prepatellar) (retropatellar) M79.4
foot (congenital) Q74.2
frenulum, frenum (tongue) K14.8
lip K13.0
gallbladder K82.8
gastric mucosa K29.60
with bleeding K29.61
gland, glandular R59.9
generalized R59.1
localized R59.0
gum (mucous membrane) K06.1
heart (idiopathic) (see also Hypertrophy, cardiac)
valve (see also Endocarditis) I38
hemifacial Q67.4
hepatic — see Hypertrophy, liver
hiatus (esophageal) Q79.1
hilus gland R59.0
hymen, congenital Q52.4
ileum K63.89
intestine NEC K63.89
jejunum K63.89
kidney (compensatory) N28.81
congenital Q63.3
labium (majus) (minus) N90.60
ligament — see Disorder, ligament
lingual tonsil (infective) J35.1

Hypertrophy, hypertrophic — continued
lingual tonsil — continued
with adenoids J35.3
lip K13.0
congenital Q18.6
liver R16.0
acute K76.89
cirrhotic — see Cirrhosis, liver
congenital Q44.7
fatty — see Fatty, liver
lymph, lymphatic gland R59.9
generalized R59.1
localized R59.0
tuberculous — see Tuberculosis, lymph gland
mammary gland — see Hypertrophy, breast
Meckel's diverticulum (congenital) Q43.0
malignant — see Table of Neoplasms, small intestine, malignant
median bar — see Hyperplasia, prostate
meibomian gland — see Chalazion
meniscus, knee, congenital Q74.1
metatarsal head — see Hypertrophy, bone, metatarsus
metatarsus — see Hypertrophy, bone, metatarsus
mucous membrane
alveolar ridge K06.2
gum K06.1
nose (turbinate) J34.3
muscle M62.89
muscular coat, artery I77.89
myocardium (see also Hypertrophy, cardiac)
idiopathic I42.2
myometrium N85.2
nail L60.2
congenital Q84.5
nasal J34.89
alae J34.89
bone J34.89
cartilage J34.89
mucous membrane (septum) J34.3
sinus J34.89
turbinate J34.3
nasopharynx, lymphoid (infectional) (tissue) (wall) J35.2
nipple N62
organ or site, congenital NEC — see Anomaly, by site
ovary N83.8
palate (hard) M27.8
soft K13.79
pancreas, congenital Q45.3
parathyroid (gland) E21.0
parotid gland K11.1
penis N48.89
pharyngeal tonsil J35.2
pharynx J39.2
lymphoid (infectional) (tissue) (wall) J35.2
pituitary (anterior) (fossa) (gland) E23.6
prepuce (congenital) N47.8
female N90.89
prostate — see Enlargement, enlarged, prostate
congenital Q55.4
pseudomuscular G71.09
pylorus (adult) (muscle) (sphincter) K31.1
congenital or infantile Q40.0
rectal, rectum (sphincter) K62.89
rhinitis (turbinate) J31.0
salivary gland (any) K11.1
congenital Q38.4
scaphoid (tarsal) — see Hypertrophy, bone, tarsus
scar L91.0
scrotum N50.89
seminal vesicle N50.89
sigmoid — see Megacolon
skin L91.9
specified NEC L91.8
spermatic cord N50.89
spleen — see Splenomegaly
spondylitis — see Spondylosis
stomach K31.89
sublingual gland K11.1
submandibular gland K11.1
suprarenal cortex (gland) E27.8
synovial NEC M67.20
acromioclavicular M67.21- ☑
ankle M67.27- ☑
elbow M67.22- ☑
foot M67.27- ☑
hand M67.24- ☑
hip M67.25- ☑
knee M67.26- ☑

Hypertrophy, hypertrophic — continued
synovial — continued
multiple sites M67.29
specified site NEC M67.28
wrist M67.23- ☑
tendon — see Disorder, tendon, specified type NEC
testis N44.8
congenital Q55.29
thymic, thymus (gland) (congenital) E32.0
thyroid (gland) — see Goiter
toe (congenital) Q74.2
acquired (see also Deformity, toe, specified NEC)
tongue K14.8
congenital Q38.2
papillae (foliate) K14.3
tonsils (faucial) (infective) (lingual) (lymphoid) J35.1
with adenoids J35.3
tunica vaginalis N50.89
ureter N28.89
urethra N36.8
uterus N85.2
neck (with elongation) N88.4
puerperal O90.89
uvula K13.79
vagina N89.8
vas deferens N50.89
vein I87.8
ventricle, ventricular (heart) (see also Hypertrophy, cardiac)
congenital Q24.8
in tetralogy of Fallot Q21.3
verumontanum N36.8
vocal cord J38.3
vulva N90.60
stasis (nonfilarial) N90.69
Hypertropia H50.2- ☑
Hypertyrosinemia E70.21
Hyperuricemia (asymptomatic) E79.0
Hyperuricosuria R82.993
Hypervalinemia E71.19
Hyperventilation (tetany) R06.4
hysterical F45.8
psychogenic F45.8
syndrome F45.8
Hypervitaminosis (dietary) NEC E67.8
A E67.0
administered as drug (prolonged intake) — see Table of Drugs and Chemicals, vitamins, adverse effect
overdose or wrong substance given or taken — see Table of Drugs and Chemicals, vitamins, poisoning
B6 E67.2
D E67.3
administered as drug (prolonged intake) — see Table of Drugs and Chemicals, vitamins, adverse effect
overdose or wrong substance given or taken — see Table of Drugs and Chemicals, vitamins, poisoning
K E67.1
administered as drug (prolonged intake) — see Table of Drugs and Chemicals, vitamins, adverse effect
overdose or wrong substance given or taken — see Table of Drugs and Chemicals, vitamins, poisoning
Hypervolemia E87.70
specified NEC E87.79
Hypesthesia R20.1
cornea — see Anesthesia, cornea
Hyphema H21.0- ☑
traumatic S05.1- ☑
Hypoacidity, gastric K31.89
psychogenic F45.8
Hypoadrenalism, hypoadrenia E27.40
primary E27.1
tuberculous A18.7
Hypoadrenocorticism E27.40
pituitary E23.0
primary E27.1
Hypoalbuminemia E88.09
Hypoaldosteronism E27.40
Hypoalphalipoproteinemia E78.6
Hypobarism T70.29 ☑
Hypobaropathy T70.29 ☑
Hypobetalipoproteinemia (familial) E78.6
Hypocalcemia E83.51

☑ Additional Character Required — Refer to the Tabular List for Character Selection   ▽ Subterms under main terms may continue to next column or page

Hypocalcemia — continued
  dietary E58
  neonatal P71.1
    due to cow's milk P71.0
  phosphate-loading (newborn) P71.1
Hypochloremia E87.8
Hypochlorhydria K31.89
  neurotic F45.8
  psychogenic F45.8
Hypochondria, hypochondriac, hypochondriasis
  (reaction) F45.21
  sleep F51.03
Hypochondrogenesis Q77.0
Hypochondroplasia Q77.4
Hypochromasia, blood cells D50.8
Hypocitraturia R82.991
Hypodontia — see Anodontia
Hypoeosinophilia D72.89
Hypoesthesia R20.1
Hypofibrinogenemia D68.8
  acquired D65
  congenital (hereditary) D68.2
Hypofunction
  adrenocortical E27.40
    drug-induced E27.3
    postprocedural E89.6
    primary E27.1
  adrenomedullary, postprocedural E89.6
  cerebral R29.818
  corticoadrenal NEC E27.40
  intestinal K59.8
  labyrinth — see subcategory H83.2 ☑
  ovary E28.39
  pituitary (gland) (anterior) E23.0
  testicular E29.1
    postprocedural (postsurgical) (postirradiation) (iatrogenic) E89.5
Hypogalactia O92.4
Hypogammaglobulinemia (see also Agammaglobulinemia) D80.1
  hereditary D80.0
  nonfamilial D80.1
  transient, of infancy D80.7
Hypogenitalism (congenital) — see Hypogonadism
Hypoglossia Q38.3
Hypoglycemia (spontaneous) E16.2
  coma E15
    diabetic — see Diabetes, by type, with hypoglycemia, with coma
  diabetic — see Diabetes, hypoglycemia
  dietary counseling and surveillance Z71.3
  drug-induced E16.0
    with coma (nondiabetic) E15
  due to insulin E16.0
    with coma (nondiabetic) E15
    therapeutic misadventure — see subcategory T38.3 ☑
  functional, nonhyperinsulinemic E16.1
  iatrogenic E16.0
    with coma (nondiabetic) E15
  in infant of diabetic mother P70.1
    gestational diabetes P70.0
  infantile E16.1
  leucine-induced E71.19
  neonatal (transitory) P70.4
    iatrogenic P70.3
  reactive (not drug-induced) E16.1
  transitory neonatal P70.4
Hypogonadism
  female E28.39
  hypogonadotropic E23.0
  male E29.1
  ovarian (primary) E28.39
  pituitary E23.0
  testicular (primary) E29.1
Hypohidrosis, hypoidrosis L74.4
Hypoinsulinemia, postprocedural E89.1
Hypokalemia E87.6
Hypoleukocytosis — see Agranulocytosis
Hypolipoproteinemia (alpha) (beta) E78.6
Hypomagnesemia E83.42
  neonatal P71.2
Hypomania, hypomanic reaction F30.8
Hypomenorrhea — see Oligomenorrhea
Hypometabolism R63.8
Hypomotility
  gastrointestinal (tract) K31.89
    psychogenic F45.8

Hypomotility — continued
  intestine K59.8
    psychogenic F45.8
  stomach K31.89
    psychogenic F45.8
Hyponasality R49.22
Hyponatremia E87.1
Hypo-osmolality E87.1
Hypo-ovarianism, hypo-ovarism E28.39
Hypoparathyroidism E20.9
  familial E20.8
  idiopathic E20.0
  neonatal, transitory P71.4
  postprocedural E89.2
  specified NEC E20.8
Hypoperfusion (in)
  newborn P96.89
Hypopharyngitis — see Laryngopharyngitis
Hypophoria H50.53
Hypophosphatemia, hypophosphatasia (acquired) (congenital) (renal) E83.39
  familial E83.31
Hypophyseal, hypophysis (see also condition)
  dwarfism E23.0
  gigantism E22.0
Hypopiesis — see Hypotension
Hypopinealism E34.8
Hypopituitarism (juvenile) E23.0
  drug-induced E23.1
  due to
    hypophysectomy E89.3
    radiotherapy E89.3
  iatrogenic NEC E23.1
  postirradiation E89.3
  postpartum O99.285
  postprocedural E89.3
Hypoplasia, hypoplastic
  adrenal (gland), congenital Q89.1
  alimentary tract, congenital Q45.8
    upper Q40.8
  anus, anal (canal) Q42.3
    with fistula Q42.2
  aorta, aortic Q25.42
    ascending, in hypoplastic left heart syndrome Q23.4
    valve Q23.1
      in hypoplastic left heart syndrome Q23.4
  areola, congenital Q83.8
  arm (congenital) — see Defect, reduction, upper limb
  artery (peripheral) Q27.8
    brain (congenital) Q28.3
    coronary Q24.5
    digestive system Q27.8
    lower limb Q27.8
    pulmonary Q25.79
      functional, unilateral J43.0
    retinal (congenital) Q14.1
    specified site NEC Q27.8
    umbilical Q27.0
    upper limb Q27.8
  auditory canal Q17.8
    causing impairment of hearing Q16.9
  biliary duct or passage Q44.5
  bone NOS Q79.9
    face Q75.8
    marrow D61.9
      megakaryocytic D69.49
    skull — see Hypoplasia, skull
  brain Q02
    gyri Q04.3
    part of Q04.3
  breast (areola) N64.82
  bronchus Q32.4
  cardiac Q24.8
  carpus — see Defect, reduction, upper limb, specified type NEC
  cartilage hair Q78.8
  cecum Q42.8
  cementum K00.4
  cephalic Q02
  cerebellum Q04.3
  cervix (uteri), congenital Q51.821
  clavicle (congenital) Q74.0
  coccyx Q76.49
  colon Q42.9
    specified NEC Q42.8
  corpus callosum Q04.0
  cricoid cartilage Q31.2
  digestive organ(s) or tract NEC Q45.8

Hypoplasia, hypoplastic — continued
  digestive organ(s) or tract — continued
    upper (congenital) Q40.8
  ear (auricle) (lobe) Q17.2
    middle Q16.4
  enamel of teeth (neonatal) (postnatal) (prenatal) K00.4
  endocrine (gland) NEC Q89.2
  endometrium N85.8
  epididymis (congenital) Q55.4
  epiglottis Q31.2
  erythroid, congenital D61.01
  esophagus (congenital) Q39.8
  eustachian tube Q17.8
  eye Q11.2
  eyelid (congenital) Q10.3
  face Q18.8
    bone(s) Q75.8
  femur (congenital) — see Defect, reduction, lower limb, specified type NEC
  fibula (congenital) — see Defect, reduction, lower limb, specified type NEC
  finger (congenital) — see Defect, reduction, upper limb, specified type NEC
  focal dermal Q82.8
  foot — see Defect, reduction, lower limb, specified type NEC
  gallbladder Q44.0
  genitalia, genital organ(s)
    female, congenital Q52.8
      external Q52.79
      internal NEC Q52.8
    in adiposogenital dystrophy E23.6
  glottis Q31.2
  hair Q84.2
  hand (congenital) — see Defect, reduction, upper limb, specified type NEC
  heart Q24.8
  humerus (congenital) — see Defect, reduction, upper limb, specified type NEC
  intestine (small) Q41.9
    large Q42.9
      specified NEC Q42.8
  jaw M26.09
    alveolar M26.79
    lower M26.04
      alveolar M26.74
    upper M26.02
      alveolar M26.73
  kidney(s) Q60.5
    bilateral Q60.4
    unilateral Q60.3
  labium (majus) (minus), congenital Q52.79
  larynx Q31.2
  left heart syndrome Q23.4
  leg (congenital) — see Defect, reduction, lower limb
  limb Q73.8
    lower (congenital) — see Defect, reduction, lower limb
    upper (congenital) — see Defect, reduction, upper limb
  liver Q44.7
  lung (lobe) (not associated with short gestation) Q33.6
    associated with immaturity, low birth weight, prematurity, or short gestation P28.0
  mammary (areola), congenital Q83.8
  mandible, mandibular M26.04
    alveolar M26.74
    unilateral condylar M27.8
  maxillary M26.02
    alveolar M26.73
  medullary D61.9
  megakaryocytic D69.49
  metacarpus — see Defect, reduction, upper limb, specified type NEC
  metatarsus — see Defect, reduction, lower limb, specified type NEC
  muscle Q79.8
  nail(s) Q84.6
  nose, nasal Q30.1
  optic nerve H47.03- ☑
  osseous meatus (ear) Q17.8
  ovary, congenital Q50.39
  pancreas Q45.0
  parathyroid (gland) Q89.2
  parotid gland Q38.4
  patella Q74.1
  pelvis, pelvic girdle Q74.2
  penis (congenital) Q55.62

Hypoplasia, hypoplastic — *continued*
  peripheral vascular system Q27.8
    digestive system Q27.8
    lower limb Q27.8
    specified site NEC Q27.8
    upper limb Q27.8
  pituitary (gland) (congenital) Q89.2
  pulmonary (not associated with short gestation) Q33.6
    artery, functional J43.0
    associated with short gestation P28.0
  radioulnar — *see* Defect, reduction, upper limb, specified type NEC
  radius — *see* Defect, reduction, upper limb
  rectum Q42.1
    with fistula Q42.0
  respiratory system NEC Q34.8
  rib Q76.6
  right heart syndrome Q22.6
  sacrum Q76.49
  scapula Q74.0
  scrotum Q55.1
  shoulder girdle Q74.0
  skin Q82.8
  skull (bone) Q75.8
    with
      anencephaly Q00.0
      encephalocele — *see* Encephalocele
      hydrocephalus Q03.9
        with spina bifida — *see* Spina bifida, by site, with hydrocephalus
      microcephaly Q02
  spinal (cord) (ventral horn cell) Q06.1
  spine Q76.49
  sternum Q76.7
  tarsus — *see* Defect, reduction, lower limb, specified type NEC
  testis Q55.1
  thymic, with immunodeficiency D82.1
  thymus (gland) Q89.2
    with immunodeficiency D82.1
  thyroid (gland) E03.1
    cartilage Q31.2
  tibiofibular (congenital) — *see* Defect, reduction, lower limb, specified type NEC
  toe — *see* Defect, reduction, lower limb, specified type NEC
  tongue Q38.3
  Turner's K00.4
  ulna (congenital) — *see* Defect, reduction, upper limb
  umbilical artery Q27.0
  unilateral condylar M27.8
  ureter Q62.8
  uterus, congenital Q51.811
  vagina Q52.4
  vascular NEC peripheral Q27.8
    brain Q28.3
    digestive system Q27.8
    lower limb Q27.8
    specified site NEC Q27.8
    upper limb Q27.8
  vein(s) (peripheral) Q27.8
    brain Q28.3
    digestive system Q27.8
    great Q26.8
    lower limb Q27.8
    specified site NEC Q27.8
    upper limb Q27.8
  vena cava (inferior) (superior) Q26.8
  vertebra Q76.49
  vulva, congenital Q52.79
  zonule (ciliary) Q12.8
Hypoplasminogenemia E88.02
Hypopnea, obstructive sleep apnea G47.33
Hypopotassemia E87.6
Hypoproconvertinemia, congenital (hereditary) D68.2
Hypoproteinemia E77.8
Hypoprothrombinemia (congenital) (hereditary) (idiopathic) D68.2
  acquired D68.4
  newborn, transient P61.6
Hypoptyalism K11.7
Hypopyon (eye) (anterior chamber) — *see* Iridocyclitis, acute, hypopyon
Hypopyrexia R68.0
Hyporeflexia R29.2
Hyposecretion
  ACTH E23.0
  antidiuretic hormone E23.2

Hyposecretion — *continued*
  ovary E28.39
  salivary gland (any) K11.7
  vasopressin E23.2
Hyposegmentation, leukocytic, hereditary D72.0
Hyposiderinemia D50.9
Hypospadias Q54.9
  balanic Q54.0
  coronal Q54.0
  glandular Q54.0
  penile Q54.1
  penoscrotal Q54.2
  perineal Q54.3
  specified NEC Q54.8
Hypospermatogenesis — *see* Oligospermia
Hyposplenism D73.0
Hypostasis pulmonary, passive — *see* Edema, lung
Hypostatic — *see* condition
Hyposthenuria N28.89
Hypotension (arterial) (constitutional) I95.9
  chronic I95.89
  due to (of) hemodialysis I95.3
  drug-induced I95.2
  iatrogenic I95.89
  idiopathic (permanent) I95.0
  intracranial, following ventricular shunting (ventriculostomy) G97.2
  intra-dialytic I95.3
  maternal, syndrome (following labor and delivery) O26.5- ☑
  neurogenic, orthostatic G90.3
  orthostatic (chronic) I95.1
    due to drugs I95.2
    neurogenic G90.3
  postoperative I95.81
  postural I95.1
  specified NEC I95.89
Hypothermia (accidental) T68 ☑
  due to anesthesia, anesthetic T88.51 ☑
  low environmental temperature T68 ☑
  neonatal P80.9
    environmental (mild) NEC P80.8
    mild P80.8
    severe (chronic) (cold injury syndrome) P80.0
    specified NEC P80.8
  not associated with low environmental temperature R68.0
Hypothyroidism (acquired) E03.9
  autoimmune — *see* Thyroiditis, autoimmune
  congenital (without goiter) E03.1
    with goiter (diffuse) E03.0
  due to
    exogenous substance NEC E03.2
    iodine-deficiency, acquired E01.8
      subclinical E02
    irradiation therapy E89.0
    medicament NEC E03.2
    P-aminosalicylic acid (PAS) E03.2
    phenylbutazone E03.2
    resorcinol E03.2
    sulfonamide E03.2
    surgery E89.0
    thiourea group drugs E03.2
  iatrogenic NEC E03.2
  iodine-deficiency (acquired) E01.8
    congenital — *see* Syndrome, iodine- deficiency, congenital
    subclinical E02
  neonatal, transitory P72.2
  postinfectious E03.3
  postirradiation E89.0
  postprocedural E89.0
  postsurgical E89.0
  specified NEC E03.8
  subclinical, iodine-deficiency related E02
Hypotonia, hypotonicity, hypotony
  bladder N31.2
  congenital (benign) P94.2
  eye — *see* Disorder, globe, hypotony
Hypotrichosis — *see* Alopecia
Hypotropia H50.2- ☑
Hypoventilation R06.89
  congenital central alveolar G47.35
  sleep related
    idiopathic nonobstructive alveolar G47.34
    in conditions classified elsewhere G47.36
Hypovitaminosis — *see* Deficiency, vitamin
Hypovolemia E86.1

Hypovolemia — *continued*
  surgical shock T81.19 ☑
  traumatic (shock) T79.4 ☑
Hypoxemia R09.02
  newborn P84
  sleep related, in conditions classified elsewhere G47.36
Hypoxia (*see also* Anoxia) R09.02
  cerebral, during a procedure NEC G97.81
    postprocedural NEC G97.82
  intrauterine P84
  myocardial — *see* Insufficiency, coronary
  newborn P84
  sleep-related G47.34
Hypsarrhythmia — *see* Epilepsy, generalized, specified NEC
Hysteralgia, pregnant uterus O26.89- ☑
Hysteria, hysterical (conversion) (dissociative state) F44.9
  anxiety F41.8
  convulsions F44.5
  psychosis, acute F44.9
Hysteroepilepsy F44.5

I

IBDU (colonic inflammatory bowel dissease unclassified) K52.3
Ichthyoparasitism due to Vandellia cirrhosa B88.8
Ichthyosis (congenital) Q80.9
  acquired L85.0
  fetalis Q80.4
  hystrix Q80.8
  lamellar Q80.2
  lingual K13.29
  palmaris and plantaris Q82.8
  simplex Q80.0
  vera Q80.8
  vulgaris Q80.0
  X-linked Q80.1
Ichthyotoxism — *see* Poisoning, fish
  bacterial — *see* Intoxication, foodborne
Icteroanemia, hemolytic (acquired) D59.9
  congenital — *see* Spherocytosis
Icterus (*see also* Jaundice)
  conjunctiva R17
  gravis, newborn P55.0
  hematogenous (acquired) D59.9
  hemolytic (acquired) D59.9
    congenital — *see* Spherocytosis
  hemorrhagic (acute) (leptospiral) (spirochetal) A27.0
    newborn P53
  infectious B15.9
    with hepatic coma B15.0
    leptospiral A27.0
    spirochetal A27.0
  neonatorum — *see* Jaundice, newborn
  newborn P59.9
  spirochetal A27.0
Ictus solaris, solis T67.0 ☑
Id reaction (due to bacteria) L30.2
Ideation
  homicidal R45.850
  suicidal R45.851
Identity disorder (child) F64.9
  gender role F64.2
  psychosexual F64.2
Idioglossia F80.0
Idiopathic — *see* condition
Idiot, idiocy (congenital) F73
  amaurotic (Bielschowsky(-Jansky)) (family) (infantile (late)) (juvenile (late)) (Vogt-Spielmeyer) E75.4
  microcephalic Q02
IgE asthma J45.909
IIAC (idiopathic infantile arterial calcification) Q28.8
Ileitis (chronic) (noninfectious) (*see also* Enteritis) K52.9
  backwash — *see* Pancolitis, ulcerative (chronic)
  infectious A09
  regional (ulcerative) — *see* Enteritis, regional, small intestine
  segmental — *see* Enteritis, regional
  terminal (ulcerative) — *see* Enteritis, regional, small intestine
Ileocolitis (*see also* Enteritis) K52.9
  infectious A09
  regional — *see* Enteritis, regional
  ulcerative K51.0- ☑

leostomy
attention to Z43.2
malfunctioning K94.13
status Z93.2
with complication — *see* Complications, enterostomy
leotyphus — *see* Typhoid
leum — *see* condition
leus (bowel) (colon) (inhibitory) (intestine) K56.7
adynamic K56.0
due to gallstone (in intestine) K56.3
duodenal (chronic) K31.5
gallstone K56.3
mechanical NEC (*see also* Obstruction, intestine, specified NEC) K56.699
meconium P76.0
in cystic fibrosis E84.11
meaning meconium plug (without cystic fibrosis) P76.0
myxedema K59.8
neurogenic K56.0
Hirschsprung's disease or megacolon Q43.1
newborn
due to meconium P76.0
in cystic fibrosis E84.11
meaning meconium plug (without cystic fibrosis) P76.0
transitory P76.1
obstructive (*see also* Obstruction, intestine, specified NEC) K56.699
paralytic K56.0
postoperative K91.89
liac — *see* condition
liotibial band syndrome M76.3- ☑
literacy Z55.0
llness (*see also* Disease) R69
manic-depressive — *see* Disorder, bipolar
mbalance R26.89
autonomic G90.8
constituents of food intake E63.1
electrolyte E87.8
with
abortion — *see* Abortion by type, complicated by, electrolyte imbalance
molar pregnancy O08.5
due to hyperemesis gravidarum O21.1
following ectopic or molar pregnancy O08.5
neonatal, transitory NEC P74.49
potassium
hyperkalemia P74.31
hypokalemia P74.32
sodium
hypernatremia P74.21
hyponatremia P74.22
endocrine E34.9
eye muscle NOS H50.9
hormone E34.9
hysterical F44.4
labyrinth — *see* subcategory H83.2 ☑
posture R29.3
protein-energy — *see* Malnutrition
sympathetic G90.8
mbecile, imbecility (I.Q. 35-49) F71
mbedding, intrauterine device T83.39 ☑
mbibition, cholesterol (gallbladder) K82.4
mbrication, teeth,, fully erupted M26.30
merslund (-Gräsbeck) **syndrome** D51.1
mmature (*see also* Immaturity)
birth (less than 37 completed weeks) — *see* Preterm, newborn
extremely (less than 28 completed weeks) — *see* Immaturity, extreme
personality F60.89
mmaturity (less than 37 completed weeks) (*see also* Preterm, newborn)
extreme of newborn (less than 28 completed weeks of gestation) (less than 196 completed days of gestation) (unspecified weeks of gestation) P07.20
gestational age
23 completed weeks (23 weeks, 0 days through 23 weeks, 6 days) P07.22
24 completed weeks (24 weeks, 0 days through 24 weeks, 6 days) P07.23
25 completed weeks (25 weeks, 0 days through 25 weeks, 6 days) P07.24
26 completed weeks (26 weeks, 0 days through 26 weeks, 6 days) P07.25

Immaturity — *continued*
extreme of newborn — *continued*
gestational age — *continued*
27 completed weeks (27 weeks, 0 days through 27 weeks, 6 days) P07.26
less than 23 completed weeks P07.21
fetus or infant light-for-dates — *see* Light-for-dates
lung, newborn P28.0
organ or site NEC — *see* Hypoplasia
pulmonary, newborn P28.0
reaction F60.89
sexual (female) (male), after puberty E30.0
Immersion T75.1 ☑
foot T69.02- ☑
hand T69.01- ☑
Immobile, immobility
complete, due to severe physical disability or frailty R53.2
intestine K59.8
syndrome (paraplegic) M62.3
Immune reconstitution (inflammatory) syndrome [IRIS] D89.3
Immunization (*see also* Vaccination)
ABO — *see* Incompatibility, ABO
in newborn P55.1
appropriate for age
child (over 28 days old) Z00.129
with abnormal findings Z00.121
complication — *see* Complications, vaccination
encounter for Z23
not done (not carried out) Z28.9
because (of)
acute illness of patient Z28.01
allergy to vaccine (or component) Z28.04
caregiver refusal Z28.82
chronic illness of patient Z28.02
contraindication NEC Z28.09
delay in delivery of vaccine Z28.83
group pressure Z28.1
guardian refusal Z28.82
immune compromised state of patient Z28.03
lack of availability of vaccine Z28.83
manufacturer delay of vaccine Z28.83
parent refusal Z28.82
patient had disease being vaccinated against Z28.81
patient refusal Z28.21
patient's belief Z28.1
religious beliefs of patient Z28.1
specified reason NEC Z28.89
of patient Z28.29
unavailability of vaccine Z28.83
unspecified patient reason Z28.20
Rh factor
affecting management of pregnancy NEC O36.09- ☑
anti-D antibody O36.01- ☑
from transfusion — *see* Complication(s), transfusion, incompatibility reaction, Rh (factor)
Immunocytoma C83.0- ☑
Immunodeficiency D84.9
with
adenosine-deaminase deficiency D81.3
antibody defects D80.9
specified type NEC D80.8
hyperimmunoglobulinemia D80.6
increased immunoglobulin M (IgM) D80.5
major defect D82.9
specified type NEC D82.8
partial albinism D82.8
short-limbed stature D82.2
thrombocytopenia and eczema D82.0
antibody with
hyperimmunoglobulinemia D80.6
near-normal immunoglobulins D80.6
autosomal recessive, Swiss type D80.0
combined D81.9
biotin-dependent carboxylase D81.819
biotinidase D81.810
holocarboxylase synthetase D81.818
specified type NEC D81.818
severe (SCID) D81.9
with
low or normal B-cell numbers D81.2
low T- and B-cell numbers D81.1
reticular dysgenesis D81.0
specified type NEC D81.89
common variable D83.9

Immunodeficiency — *continued*
common variable — *continued*
with
abnormalities of B-cell numbers and function D83.0
autoantibodies to B- or T-cells D83.2
immunoregulatory T-cell disorders D83.1
specified type NEC D83.8
following hereditary defective response to Epstein-Barr virus (EBV) D82.3
selective, immunoglobulin
A (IgA) D80.2
G (IgG) (subclasses) D80.3
M (IgM) D80.4
severe combined (SCID) D81.9
specified type NEC D84.8
X-linked, with increased IgM D80.5
Immunotherapy (encounter for)
antineoplastic Z51.12
Impaction, impacted
bowel, colon, rectum (*see also* Impaction, fecal) K56.49
by gallstone K56.3
calculus — *see* Calculus
cerumen (ear) (external) H61.2- ☑
cuspid — *see* Impaction, tooth
dental (same or adjacent tooth) K01.1
fecal, feces K56.41
fracture — *see* Fracture, by site
gallbladder — *see* Calculus, gallbladder
gallstone(s) — *see* Calculus, gallbladder
bile duct (common) (hepatic) — *see* Calculus, bile duct
cystic duct — *see* Calculus, gallbladder
in intestine, with obstruction (any part) K56.3
intestine (calculous) NEC (*see also* Impaction, fecal) K56.49
gallstone, with ileus K56.3
intrauterine device (IUD) T83.39 ☑
molar — *see* Impaction, tooth
shoulder, causing obstructed labor O66.0
tooth, teeth K01.1
turbinate J34.89
Impaired, impairment (function)
auditory discrimination — *see* Abnormal, auditory perception
cognitive, mild, so stated G31.84
dual sensory Z73.82
fasting glucose R73.01
glucose tolerance (oral) R73.02
hearing — *see* Deafness
heart — *see* Disease, heart
kidney N28.9
disorder resulting from N25.9
specified NEC N25.89
liver K72.90
with coma K72.91
mastication K08.89
mild cognitive, so stated G31.84
mobility
ear ossicles — *see* Ankylosis, ear ossicles
requiring care provider Z74.09
myocardium, myocardial — *see* Insufficiency, myocardial
rectal sphincter R19.8
renal (acute) (chronic) N28.9
disorder resulting from N25.9
specified NEC N25.89
vision NEC H54.7
both eyes H54.3
Impediment, speech R47.9
psychogenic (childhood) F98.8
slurring R47.81
specified NEC R47.89
Impending
coronary syndrome I20.0
delirium tremens F10.239
myocardial infarction I20.0
Imperception auditory (acquired) (*see also* Deafness)
congenital H93.25
Imperfect
aeration, lung (newborn) NEC — *see* Atelectasis
closure (congenital)
alimentary tract NEC Q45.8
lower Q43.8
upper Q40.8
atrioventricular ostium Q21.2
atrium (secundum) Q21.1
branchial cleft NOS Q18.2

Imperfect — *continued*
  closure — *continued*
    branchial cleft — *continued*
      cyst Q18.0
      fistula Q18.0
      sinus Q18.0
    choroid Q14.3
    cricoid cartilage Q31.8
    cusps, heart valve NEC Q24.8
      pulmonary Q22.3
    ductus
      arteriosus Q25.0
      Botalli Q25.0
    ear drum (causing impairment of hearing) Q16.4
    esophagus with communication to bronchus or trachea Q39.1
    eyelid Q10.3
    foramen
      botalli Q21.1
      ovale Q21.1
    genitalia, genital organ(s) or system
      female Q52.8
        external Q52.79
        internal NEC Q52.8
      male Q55.8
    glottis Q31.8
    interatrial ostium or septum Q21.1
    interauricular ostium or septum Q21.1
    interventricular ostium or septum Q21.0
    larynx Q31.8
    lip — *see* Cleft, lip
    nasal septum Q30.3
    nose Q30.2
    omphalomesenteric duct Q43.0
    optic nerve entry Q14.2
    organ or site not listed — *see* Anomaly, by site
    ostium
      interatrial Q21.1
      interauricular Q21.1
      interventricular Q21.0
    palate — *see* Cleft, palate
    preauricular sinus Q18.1
    retina Q14.1
    roof of orbit Q75.8
    sclera Q13.5
    septum
      aorticopulmonary Q21.4
      atrial (secundum) Q21.1
      between aorta and pulmonary artery Q21.4
      heart Q21.9
      interatrial (secundum) Q21.1
      interauricular (secundum) Q21.1
      interventricular Q21.0
        in tetralogy of Fallot Q21.3
      nasal Q30.3
      ventricular Q21.0
        with pulmonary stenosis or atresia, dextraposition of aorta, and hypertrophy of right ventricle Q21.3
        in tetralogy of Fallot Q21.3
    skull Q75.0
      with
        anencephaly Q00.0
        encephalocele — *see* Encephalocele
        hydrocephalus Q03.9
          with spina bifida — *see* Spina bifida, by site, with hydrocephalus
        microcephaly Q02
    spine (with meningocele) — *see* Spina bifida
    trachea Q32.1
    tympanic membrane (causing impairment of hearing) Q16.4
    uterus Q51.818
    vitelline duct Q43.0
  erection — *see* Dysfunction, sexual, male, erectile
  fusion — *see* Imperfect, closure
  inflation, lung (newborn) — *see* Atelectasis
  posture R29.3
  rotation, intestine Q43.3
  septum, ventricular Q21.0
Imperfectly descended testis — *see* Cryptorchid
Imperforate (congenital) (*see also* Atresia)
  anus Q42.3
    with fistula Q42.2
  cervix (uteri) Q51.828
  esophagus Q39.0
    with tracheoesophageal fistula Q39.1
  hymen Q52.3

Imperforate — *continued*
  jejunum Q41.1
  pharynx Q38.8
  rectum Q42.1
    with fistula Q42.0
  urethra Q64.39
  vagina Q52.4
Impervious (congenital) (*see also* Atresia)
  anus Q42.3
    with fistula Q42.2
  bile duct Q44.2
  esophagus Q39.0
    with tracheoesophageal fistula Q39.1
  intestine (small) Q41.9
    large Q42.9
      specified NEC Q42.8
  rectum Q42.1
    with fistula Q42.0
  ureter — *see* Atresia, ureter
  urethra Q64.39
Impetiginization of dermatoses L01.1
Impetigo (any organism) (any site) (circinate) (contagiosa) (simplex) (vulgaris) L01.00
  Bockhart's L01.02
  bullous, bullosa L01.03
  external ear L01.00 [H62.40]
  follicularis L01.02
  furfuracea L30.5
  herpetiformis L40.1
    nonobstetrical L40.1
  neonatorum L01.03
  nonbullous L01.01
  specified type NEC L01.09
  ulcerative L01.09
Impingement (on teeth)
  soft tissue
    anterior M26.81
    posterior M26.82
Implant, endometrial N80.9
Implantation
  anomalous — *see* Anomaly, by site
    ureter Q62.63
  cyst
    external area or site (skin) NEC L72.0
    iris — *see* Cyst, iris, implantation
    vagina N89.8
    vulva N90.7
  dermoid (cyst) — *see* Implantation, cyst
Impotence (sexual) N52.9
  counseling Z70.1
  organic origin (*see also* Dysfunction, sexual, male, erectile) N52.9
  psychogenic F52.21
Impression, basilar Q75.8
Imprisonment, anxiety concerning Z65.1
Improper care (child) (newborn) — *see* Maltreatment
Improperly tied umbilical cord (causing hemorrhage) P51.8
Impulsiveness (impulsive) R45.87
Inability to swallow — *see* Aphagia
Inaccessible, inaccessibility
  health care NEC Z75.3
    due to
      waiting period Z75.2
        for admission to facility elsewhere Z75.1
    other helping agencies Z75.4
Inactive — *see* condition
Inadequate, inadequacy
  aesthetics of dental restoration K08.56
  biologic, constitutional, functional, or social F60.7
  development
    child R62.50
    genitalia
      after puberty NEC E30.0
      congenital
        female Q52.8
          external Q52.79
          internal Q52.8
        male Q55.8
    lungs Q33.6
      associated with short gestation P28.0
    organ or site not listed — *see* Anomaly, by site
  diet (causing nutritional deficiency) E63.9
  eating habits Z72.4
  environment, household Z59.1
  family support Z63.8
  food (supply) NEC Z59.4
    hunger effects T73.0 ☑

Inadequate, inadequacy — *continued*
  functional F60.7
  household care, due to
    family member
      handicapped or ill Z74.2
      on vacation Z75.5
      temporarily away from home Z74.2
    technical defects in home Z59.1
    temporary absence from home of person rendering care Z74.2
  housing (heating) (space) Z59.1
  income (financial) Z59.6
  intrafamilial communication Z63.8
  material resources Z59.9
  mental — *see* Disability, intellectual
  parental supervision or control of child Z62.0
  personality F60.7
  pulmonary
    function R06.89
      newborn P28.5
    ventilation, newborn P28.5
  sample of cytologic smear
    anus R85.615
    cervix R87.615
    vagina R87.625
  social F60.7
    insurance Z59.7
    skills NEC Z73.4
  supervision of child by parent Z62.0
  teaching affecting education Z55.8
  welfare support Z59.7
Inanition R64
  with edema — *see* Malnutrition, severe
  due to
    deprivation of food T73.0 ☑
    malnutrition — *see* Malnutrition
  fever R50.9
Inappropriate
  change in quantitative human chorionic gonadotropin (hCG) in early pregnancy O02.81
  diet or eating habits Z72.4
  level of quantitative human chorionic gonadotropin (hCG) for gestational age in early pregnancy O02.81
  secretion
    antidiuretic hormone (ADH) (excessive) E22.2
      deficiency E23.2
    pituitary (posterior) E22.2
Inattention at or after birth — *see* Neglect
Incarceration, incarcerated
  enterocele K46.0
    gangrenous K46.1
  epiplocele K46.0
    gangrenous K46.1
  exomphalos K42.0
    gangrenous K42.1
  hernia (*see also* Hernia, by site, with obstruction)
    with gangrene — *see* Hernia, by site, with gangrene
  iris, in wound — *see* Injury, eye, laceration, with prolapse
  lens, in wound — *see* Injury, eye, laceration, with prolapse
  omphalocele K42.0
  prison, anxiety concerning Z65.1
  rupture — *see* Hernia, by site
  sarcoepiplocele K46.0
    gangrenous K46.1
  sarcoepiplomphalocele K42.0
    with gangrene K42.1
  uterus N85.8
    gravid O34.51- ☑
      causing obstructed labor O65.5
Incised wound
  external — *see* Laceration
  internal organs — *see* Injury, by site
Incision, incisional
  hernia K43.2
    with
      gangrene (and obstruction) K43.1
      obstruction K43.0
  surgical, complication — *see* Complications, surgical procedure
  traumatic
    external — *see* Laceration
    internal organs — *see* Injury, by site
Inclusion
  azurophilic leukocytic D72.0
  blennorrhea (neonatal) (newborn) P39.1

☑ **Additional Character Required — Refer to the Tabular List for Character Selection**   ▽ **Subterms under main terms may continue to next column or page**

Inclusion — *continued*
  gallbladder in liver (congenital) Q44.1
Incompatibility
  ABO
    affecting management of pregnancy O36.11- ☑
      anti-A sensitization O36.11- ☑
      anti-B sensitization O36.19- ☑
      specified NEC O36.19- ☑
    infusion or transfusion reaction — *see* Complication(s), transfusion, incompatibility reaction, ABO
    newborn P55.1
  blood (group) (Duffy) (K) (Kell) (Kidd) (Lewis) (M) (S) NEC
    affecting management of pregnancy O36.11- ☑
      anti-A sensitization O36.11- ☑
      anti-B sensitization O36.19- ☑
    infusion or transfusion reaction T80.89 ☑
    newborn P55.8
  divorce or estrangement Z63.5
  Rh (blood group) (factor) Z31.82
    affecting management of pregnancy NEC O36.09- ☑
      anti-D antibody O36.01- ☑
    infusion or transfusion reaction — *see* Complication(s), transfusion, incompatibility reaction, Rh (factor)
    newborn P55.0
  rhesus — *see* Incompatibility, Rh
Incompetency, incompetent, incompetence
  annular
    aortic (valve) — *see* Insufficiency, aortic
    mitral (valve) I34.0
    pulmonary valve (heart) I37.1
  aortic (valve) — *see* Insufficiency, aortic
  cardiac valve — *see* Endocarditis
  cervix, cervical (os) N88.3
    in pregnancy O34.3- ☑
  chronotropic I45.89
    with
      autonomic dysfunction G90.8
      ischemic heart disease I25.89
      left ventricular dysfunction I51.89
      sinus node dysfunction I49.8
  esophagogastric (junction) (sphincter) K22.0
  mitral (valve) — *see* Insufficiency, mitral
  pelvic fundus N81.89
  pubocervical tissue N81.82
  pulmonary valve (heart) I37.1
    congenital Q22.3
  rectovaginal tissue N81.83
  tricuspid (annular) (valve) — *see* Insufficiency, tricuspid
  valvular — *see* Endocarditis
    congenital Q24.8
  vein, venous (saphenous) (varicose) — *see* Varix, leg
Incomplete (*see also* condition)
  bladder, emptying R33.9
  defecation R15.0
  expansion lungs (newborn) NEC — *see* Atelectasis
  rotation, intestine Q43.3
Inconclusive
  diagnostic imaging due to excess body fat of patient R93.9
  findings on diagnostic imaging of breast NEC R92.8
  mammogram (due to dense breasts) R92.2
Incontinence R32
  anal sphincter R15.9
  coital N39.491
  feces R15.9
    nonorganic origin F98.1
  insensible (urinary) N39.42
  overflow N39.490
  postural (urinary) N39.492
  psychogenic F45.8
  rectal R15.9
  reflex N39.498
  stress (female) (male) N39.3
    and urge N39.46
  urethral sphincter R32
  urge N39.41
    and stress (female) (male) N39.46
  urine (urinary) R32
    continuous N39.45
    due to cognitive impairment, or severe physical disability or immobility R39.81
    functional R39.81
    insensible N39.42
    mixed (stress and urge) N39.46
    nocturnal N39.44

Incontinence — *continued*
  urine — *continued*
    nonorganic origin F98.0
    overflow N39.490
    post dribbling N39.43
    postural N39.492
    reflex N39.498
    specified NEC N39.498
    stress (female) (male) N39.3
      and urge N39.46
    total N39.498
    unaware N39.42
    urge N39.41
      and stress (female) (male) N39.46
Incontinentia pigmenti Q82.3
Incoordinate, incoordination
  esophageal-pharyngeal (newborn) — *see* Dysphagia
  muscular R27.8
  uterus (action) (contractions) (complicating delivery) O62.4
Increase, increased
  abnormal, in development R63.8
  androgens (ovarian) E28.1
  anticoagulants (antithrombin) (anti-VIIIa) (anti-IXa) (anti-Xa) (anti-XIa) — *see* Circulating anticoagulants
  cold sense R20.8
  estrogen E28.0
  function
    adrenal
      cortex — *see* Cushing's, syndrome
      medulla E27.5
    pituitary (gland) (anterior) (lobe) E22.9
      posterior E22.2
  heat sense R20.8
  intracranial pressure (benign) G93.2
  permeability, capillaries I78.8
  pressure, intracranial G93.2
  secretion
    gastrin E16.4
    glucagon E16.3
    pancreas, endocrine E16.9
      growth hormone-releasing hormone E16.8
      pancreatic polypeptide E16.8
      somatostatin E16.8
      vasoactive-intestinal polypeptide E16.8
  sphericity, lens Q12.4
  splenic activity D73.1
  venous pressure I87.8
    portal K76.6
Increta placenta O43.22- ☑
Incrustation, cornea, foreign body (lead)(zinc) — *see* Foreign body, cornea
Incyclophoria H50.54
Incyclotropia — *see* Cyclotropia
Indeterminate sex Q56.4
India rubber skin Q82.8
Indigestion (acid) (bilious) (functional) K30
  catarrhal K31.89
  due to decomposed food NOS A05.9
  nervous F45.8
  psychogenic F45.8
Indirect — *see* condition
Induratio penis plastica N48.6
Induration, indurated
  brain G93.89
  breast (fibrous) N64.51
    puerperal, postpartum O92.29
  broad ligament N83.8
  chancre
    anus A51.1
    congenital A50.07
    extragenital NEC A51.2
  corpora cavernosa (penis) (plastic) N48.6
  liver (chronic) K76.89
  lung (black) (chronic) (fibroid) (*see also* Fibrosis, lung) J84.10
    essential brown J84.03
  penile (plastic) N48.6
  phlebitic — *see* Phlebitis
  skin R23.4
Inebriety (without dependence) — *see* Alcohol, intoxication
Inefficiency, kidney N28.9
Inelasticity, skin R23.4
Inequality, leg (length) (acquired) (*see also* Deformity, limb, unequal length)
  congenital — *see* Defect, reduction, lower limb

Inequality, leg — *continued*
  lower leg — *see* Deformity, limb, unequal length
Inertia
  bladder (neurogenic) N31.2
  stomach K31.89
    psychogenic F45.8
  uterus, uterine during labor O62.2
    during latent phase of labor O62.0
    primary O62.0
    secondary O62.1
  vesical (neurogenic) N31.2
Infancy, infantile, infantilism (*see also* condition)
  celiac K90.0
  genitalia, genitals (after puberty) E30.0
  Herter's (nontropical sprue) K90.0
  intestinal K90.0
  Lorain E23.0
  pancreatic K86.89
  pelvis M95.5
    with disproportion (fetopelvic) O33.1
      causing obstructed labor O65.1
  pituitary E23.0
  renal N25.0
  uterus — *see* Infantile, genitalia
Infant(s) (*see also* Infancy)
  excessive crying R68.11
  irritable child R68.12
  lack of care — *see* Neglect
  liveborn (singleton) Z38.2
    born in hospital Z38.00
      by cesarean Z38.01
    born outside hospital Z38.1
    multiple NEC Z38.8
      born in hospital Z38.68
        by cesarean Z38.69
      born outside hospital Z38.7
    quadruplet Z38.8
      born in hospital Z38.63
        by cesarean Z38.64
      born outside hospital Z38.7
    quintuplet Z38.8
      born in hospital Z38.65
        by cesarean Z38.66
      born outside hospital Z38.7
    triplet Z38.8
      born in hospital Z38.61
        by cesarean Z38.62
      born outside hospital Z38.7
    twin Z38.5
      born in hospital Z38.30
        by cesarean Z38.31
      born outside hospital Z38.4
  of diabetic mother (syndrome of) P70.1
    gestational diabetes P70.0
Infantile (*see also* condition)
  genitalia, genitals E30.0
  os, uterine E30.0
  penis E30.0
  testis E29.1
  uterus E30.0
Infantilism — *see* Infancy
Infarct, infarction
  adrenal (capsule) (gland) E27.49
  appendices epiploicae (*see also* Infarct, intestine) K55.069
  bowel (*see also* Infarct, intestine) K55.069
  brain (stem) — *see* Infarct, cerebral
  breast N64.89
  brewer's (kidney) N28.0
  cardiac — *see* Infarct, myocardium
  cerebellar — *see* Infarct, cerebral
  cerebral (*see also* Occlusion, artery cerebral or precerebral, with infarction) I63.9
    aborted I63.9
    cortical I63.9
    due to
      cerebral venous thrombosis, nonpyogenic I63.6
      embolism
        cerebral arteries I63.4- ☑
        precerebral arteries I63.1- ☑
      occlusion NEC
        cerebral arteries I63.5- ☑
        precerebral arteries I63.2- ☑
        small artery I63.81
      stenosis NEC
        cerebral arteries I63.5- ☑
        precerebral arteries I63.2- ☑
        small artery I63.81

Index

Infarct, infarction — *continued*
  cerebral (*see also* Occlusion, artery cerebral or precere-
    bral, with infarction) — *continued*
    due to — *continued*
      thrombosis
        cerebral artery I63.3- ☑
        precerebral artery I63.0- ☑
      intraoperative
        during cardiac surgery I97.810
        during other surgery I97.811
      postprocedural
        following cardiac surgery I97.820
        following other surgery I97.821
      specified NEC I63.89
  colon (acute) (agnogenic) (embolic) (hemorrhagic)
    (nonocclusive) (nonthrombotic) (occlusive)
    (segmental) (thrombotic) (with gangrene) (*see
    also* Infarct, intestine) K55.049
  coronary artery — *see* Infarct, myocardium
  embolic — *see* Embolism
  fallopian tube N83.8
  gallbladder K82.8
  heart — *see* Infarct, myocardium
  hepatic K76.3
  hypophysis (anterior lobe) E23.6
  impending (myocardium) I20.0
  intestine (acute) (agnogenic) (embolic) (hemorrhagic)
    (nonocclusive) (nonthrombotic) (occlusive)
    (thrombotic) (with gangrene) K55.069
    diffuse K55.062
    focal K55.061
    large K55.049
      diffuse K55.042
      focal K55.041
    small K55.029
      diffuse K55.022
      focal K55.021
  kidney N28.0
  lacunar I63.81
  liver K76.3
  lung (embolic) (thrombotic) — *see* Embolism, pul-
    monary
  lymph node I89.8
  mesentery, mesenteric (embolic) (thrombotic) (with
    gangrene) (*see also* Infarct, intestine) K55.069
  muscle (ischemic) M62.20
    ankle M62.27- ☑
    foot M62.27- ☑
    forearm M62.23- ☑
    hand M62.24- ☑
    lower leg M62.26- ☑
    pelvic region M62.25- ☑
    shoulder region M62.21- ☑
    specified site NEC M62.28
    thigh M62.25- ☑
    upper arm M62.22- ☑
  myocardium, myocardial (acute) (with stated duration
    of 4 weeks or less) I21.9
    associated with revascularization procedure I21.A9
    diagnosed on ECG, but presenting no symptoms
      I25.2
    due to
      demand ischemia I21.A1
      ischemic imbalance I21.A1
    healed or old I25.2
    intraoperative (*see also* Infarct, myocardium, associ-
      ated with revascularization procedure)
      during cardiac surgery I97.790
      during other surgery I97.791
    non-Q wave I21.4
    non-ST elevation (NSTEMI) I21.4
      subsequent I22.2
    nontransmural I21.4
    past (diagnosed on ECG or other investigation, but
      currently presenting no symptoms) I25.2
    postprocedural (*see also* Infarct, myocardium, asso-
      ciated with revascularization procedure)
      following cardiac surgery (*see also* Infarct, my-
        ocardium, type 4 or type 5) I97.190
      following other surgery I97.191
    Q wave (see also, Infarct, myocardium, by site) I21.3
    secondary to
      demand ischemia I21.A1
      ischemic imbalance I21.A1
    ST elevation (STEMI) I21.3
      anterior (anteroapical) (anterolateral) (anteroseptal) (Q wave) (wall) I21.09
        · subsequent I22.0

Infarct, infarction — *continued*
  myocardium, myocardial — *continued*
    ST elevation — *continued*
      inferior (diaphragmatic) (inferolateral) (inferopos-
        terior) (wall) NEC I21.19
        subsequent I22.1
      inferoposterior transmural (Q wave) I21.11
      involving
        coronary artery of anterior wall NEC I21.09
        coronary artery of inferior wall NEC I21.19
        diagonal coronary artery I21.02
        left anterior descending coronary artery I21.02
        left circumflex coronary artery I21.21
        left main coronary artery I21.01
        oblique marginal coronary artery I21.21
        right coronary artery I21.11
      lateral (apical-lateral) (basal-lateral) (high) I21.29
        subsequent I22.8
      posterior (posterobasal) (posterolateral) (pos-
        teroseptal) (true) I21.29
        subsequent I22.8
      septal I21.29
        subsequent I22.8
      specified NEC I21.29
        subsequent I22.8
      subsequent I22.9
    subsequent (recurrent) (reinfarction) I22.9
      anterior (anteroapical) (anterolateral) (anteroseptal) (wall) I22.0
      diaphragmatic (wall) I22.1
      inferior (diaphragmatic) (inferolateral) (inferopos-
        terior) (wall) I22.1
      lateral (apical-lateral) (basal-lateral) (high) I22.8
      non-ST elevation (NSTEMI) I22.2
      posterior (posterobasal) (posterolateral) (pos-
        teroseptal) (true) I22.8
      septal I22.8
      specified NEC I22.8
      ST elevation I22.9
        anterior (anteroapical) (anterolateral) (an-
          teroseptal) (wall) I22.0
        inferior (diaphragmatic) (inferolateral) (infer-
          oposterior) (wall) I22.1
        specified NEC I22.8
      subendocardial I22.2
      transmural I22.9
        anterior (anteroapical) (anterolateral) (an-
          teroseptal) (wall) I22.0
        diaphragmatic (wall) I22.1
        inferior (diaphragmatic) (inferolateral) (infer-
          oposterior) (wall) I22.1
        lateral (apical-lateral) (basal-lateral) (high)
          I22.8
        posterior (posterobasal) (posterolateral)
          (posteroseptal) (true) I22.8
        specified NEC I22.8
      type 1 (*see also* Infarction, myocardial, subse-
        quent, by site, or by ST elevation or non-
        ST elevation) I22.9
      type 2 I21.A1
      type 3 I21.A9
      type 4 I21.A9
      type 5 I21.A9
    syphilitic A52.06
    transmural I21.9
      anterior (anteroapical) (anterolateral) (anteroseptal) (Q wave) (wall) NEC I21.09
      inferior (diaphragmatic) (inferolateral) (inferopos-
        terior) (Q wave) (wall) NEC I21.19
      inferoposterior (Q wave) I21.11
      lateral (apical-lateral) (basal-lateral) (high) NEC
        I21.29
      posterior (posterobasal) (posterolateral) (pos-
        teroseptal) (true) NEC I21.29
      septal NEC I21.29
      specified NEC I21.29
    type 1 (*see also* Infarction, myocardial, by site, or by
      ST elevation or non-ST elevation) I21.9
    type 2 I21.A1
    type 3 I21.A9
    type 4 (a) (b) (c) I21.A9
    type 5 I21.A9
  nontransmural I21.4
  omentum (*see also* Infarct, intestine) K55.069
  ovary N83.8
  pancreas K86.89
  papillary muscle — *see* Infarct, myocardium
  parathyroid gland E21.4
  pituitary (gland) E23.6

Infarct, infarction — *continued*
  placenta O43.81- ☑
  prostate N42.89
  pulmonary (artery) (vein) (hemorrhagic) — *see* Em-
    bolism, pulmonary
  renal (embolic) (thrombotic) N28.0
  retina, retinal (artery) — *see* Occlusion, artery, retina
  spinal (cord) (acute) (embolic) (nonembolic) G95.11
  spleen D73.5
    embolic or thrombotic I74.8
  subendocardial (acute) (nontransmural) I21.4
  suprarenal (capsule) (gland) E27.49
  testis N50.1
  thrombotic (*see also* Thrombosis)
    artery, arterial — *see* Embolism
  thyroid (gland) E07.89
  ventricle (heart) — *see* Infarct, myocardium
Infecting — *see* condition
Infection, infected, infective (opportunistic) B99.9
  with
      drug resistant organism — *see* Resistance (to), dru
        (*see also* specific organism)
      lymphangitis — *see* Lymphangitis
      organ dysfunction (acute) R65.20
        with septic shock R65.21
  abscess (skin) — *code by* site under Abscess
  Absidia — *see* Mucormycosis
  Acanthamoeba — *see* Acanthamebiasis
  Acanthocheilonema (perstans) (streptocerca) B74.4
  accessory sinus (chronic) — *see* Sinusitis
  achorion — *see* Dermatophytosis
  Acremonium falciforme B47.0
  acromioclavicular M00.9
  Actinobacillus (actinomycetem-comitans) A28.8
    mallei A24.0
    muris A25.1
  Actinomadura B47.1
  Actinomyces (israelii) (*see also* Actinomycosis) A42.9
  Actinomycetales — *see* Actinomycosis
  actinomycotic NOS — *see* Actinomycosis
  adenoid (and tonsil) J03.90
    chronic J35.02
  adenovirus NEC
    as cause of disease classified elsewhere B97.0
    unspecified nature or site B34.0
  aerogenes capsulatus A48.0
  aertrycke — *see* Infection, salmonella
  alimentary canal NOS — *see* Enteritis, infectious
  Allescheria boydii B48.2
  Alternaria B48.8
  alveolus, alveolar (process) K04.7
  Ameba, amebic (histolytica) — *see* Amebiasis
  amniotic fluid, sac or cavity O41.10- ☑
    chorioamnionitis O41.12- ☑
    placentitis O41.14- ☑
  amputation stump (surgical) — *see* Complication,
    amputation stump, infection
  Ancylostoma (duodenalis) B76.0
  Anisakiasis, Anisakis larvae B81.0
  anthrax — *see* Anthrax
  antrum (chronic) — *see* Sinusitis, maxillary
  anus, anal (papillae) (sphincter) K62.89
  arbovirus (arbor virus) A94
    specified type NEC A93.8
  artificial insemination N98.0
  Ascaris lumbricoides — *see* Ascariasis
  Ascomycetes B47.0
  Aspergillus (flavus) (fumigatus) (terreus) — *see* As-
    pergillosis
  atypical
    acid-fast (bacilli) — *see* Mycobacterium, atypical
    mycobacteria — *see* Mycobacterium, atypical
    virus A81.9
      specified type NEC A81.89
  auditory meatus (external) — *see* Otitis, externa, infe
    tive
  auricle (ear) — *see* Otitis, externa, infective
  axillary gland (lymph) L04.2
  Bacillus A49.9
    abortus A23.1
    anthracis — *see* Anthrax
    Ducrey's (any location) A57
    Flexner's A03.1
    Friedländer's NEC A49.8
    gas (gangrene) A48.0
    mallei A24.0
    melitensis A23.0
    paratyphoid, paratyphosus A01.4

Infarct, infarction — Infection, infected, infective

☑ **Additional Character Required** — Refer to the Tabular List for Character Selection   ▽ **Subterms under main terms may continue to next column or pag**

Infection, infected, infective — *continued*
- Bacillus — *continued*
  - paratyphoid, paratyphosus — *continued*
    - A A01.1
    - B A01.2
    - C A01.3
  - Shiga (-Kruse) A03.0
  - suipestifer — *see* Infection, salmonella
  - swimming pool A31.1
  - typhosa A01.00
  - welchii — *see* Gangrene, gas
- bacterial NOS A49.9
  - as cause of disease classified elsewhere B96.89
    - Bacteroides fragilis [B. fragilis] B96.6
    - Clostridium perfringens [C. perfringens] B96.7
    - Enterobacter sakazakii B96.89
    - Enterococcus B95.2
    - Escherichia coli [E. coli] (*see also* Escherichia coli) B96.20
    - Helicobacter pylori [H.pylori] B96.81
    - Hemophilus influenzae [H. influenzae] B96.3
    - Klebsiella pneumoniae [K. pneumoniae] B96.1
    - Mycoplasma pneumoniae [M. pneumoniae] B96.0
    - Proteus (mirabilis) (morganii) B96.4
    - Pseudomonas (aeruginosa) (mallei) (pseudomallei) B96.5
    - Staphylococcus B95.8
      - aureus (methicillin susceptible) (MSSA) B95.61
        - methicillin resistant (MRSA) B95.62
      - specified NEC B95.7
    - Streptococcus B95.5
      - group A B95.0
      - group B B95.1
      - pneumoniae B95.3
      - specified NEC B95.4
    - Vibrio vulnificus B96.82
  - specified NEC A48.8
- Bacterium
  - paratyphosum A01.4
    - A A01.1
    - B A01.2
    - C A01.3
  - typhosum A01.00
- Bacteroides NEC A49.8
  - fragilis, as cause of disease classified elsewhere B96.6
- Balantidium coli A07.0
- Bartholin's gland N75.8
- Basidiobolus B46.8
- bile duct (common) (hepatic) — *see* Cholangitis
- bladder — *see* Cystitis
- Blastomyces, blastomycotic (*see also* Blastomycosis)
  - brasiliensis — *see* Paracoccidioidomycosis
  - dermatitidis — *see* Blastomycosis
  - European — *see* Cryptococcosis
  - Loboi B48.0
  - North American B40.9
  - South American — *see* Paracoccidioidomycosis
- bleb, postprocedure — *see* Blebitis
- bone — *see* Osteomyelitis
- Bordetella — *see* Whooping cough
- Borrelia bergdorfi A69.20
- brain (*see also* Encephalitis) G04.90
  - membranes — *see* Meningitis
  - septic G06.0
    - meninges — *see* Meningitis, bacterial
- branchial cyst Q18.0
- breast — *see* Mastitis
- bronchus — *see* Bronchitis
- Brucella A23.9
  - abortus A23.1
  - canis A23.3
  - melitensis A23.0
  - mixed A23.8
  - specified NEC A23.8
  - suis A23.2
- Brugia (malayi) B74.1
  - timori B74.2
- bursa — *see* Bursitis, infective
- buttocks (skin) L08.9
- Campylobacter, intestinal A04.5
  - as cause of disease classified elsewhere B96.81
- Candida (albicans) (tropicalis) — *see* Candidiasis
- candiru B88.8
- Capillaria (intestinal) B81.1
  - hepatica B83.8
  - philippinensis B81.1

Infection, infected, infective — *continued*
- cartilage — *see* Disorder, cartilage, specified type NEC
- cat liver fluke B66.0
- catheter-related bloodstream (CRBSI) T80.211 ☑
- cellulitis — *code by* site under Cellulitis
- central line-associated T80.219 ☑
  - bloodstream (CLABSI) T80.211 ☑
  - specified NEC T80.218 ☑
- Cephalosporium falciforme B47.0
- cerebrospinal — *see* Meningitis
- cervical gland (lymph) L04.0
- cervix — *see* Cervicitis
- cesarean delivery wound (puerperal) O86.00
- cestodes — *see* Infestation, cestodes
- chest J22
- Chilomastix (intestinal) A07.8
- Chlamydia, chlamydial A74.9
  - anus A56.3
  - genitourinary tract A56.2
    - lower A56.00
    - specified NEC A56.19
  - lymphogranuloma A55
  - pharynx A56.4
  - psittaci A70
  - rectum A56.3
  - sexually transmitted NEC A56.8
- cholera — *see* Cholera
- Cladosporium
  - bantianum (brain abscess) B43.1
  - carrionii B43.0
  - castellanii B36.1
  - trichoides (brain abscess) B43.1
  - werneckii B36.1
- Clonorchis (sinensis) (liver) B66.1
- Clostridium NEC
  - bifermentans A48.0
  - botulinum (food poisoning) A05.1
    - infant A48.51
    - wound A48.52
  - difficile
    - as cause of disease classified elsewhere B96.89
    - foodborne (disease)
      - not specified as recurrent A04.72
      - recurrent A04.71
    - gas gangrene A48.0
    - necrotizing enterocolitis
      - not specified as recurrent A04.72
      - recurrent A04.71
    - sepsis A41.4
  - gas-forming NEC A48.0
  - histolyticum A48.0
  - novyi, causing gas gangrene A48.0
  - oedematiens A48.0
  - perfringens
    - as cause of disease classified elsewhere B96.7
    - due to food A05.2
    - foodborne (disease) A05.2
    - gas gangrene A48.0
    - sepsis A41.4
  - septicum, causing gas gangrene A48.0
  - sordellii, causing gas gangrene A48.0
  - welchii
    - as cause of disease classified elsewhere B96.7
    - foodborne (disease) A05.2
    - gas gangrene A48.0
    - necrotizing enteritis A05.2
    - sepsis A41.4
- Coccidioides (immitis) — *see* Coccidioidomycosis
- colon — *see* Enteritis, infectious
- colostomy K94.02
- common duct — *see* Cholangitis
- congenital P39.9
  - Candida (albicans) P37.5
  - cytomegalovirus P35.1
  - hepatitis, viral P35.3
  - herpes simplex P35.2
  - infectious or parasitic disease P37.9
    - specified NEC P37.8
  - listeriosis (disseminated) P37.2
  - malaria NEC P37.4
    - falciparum P37.3
  - Plasmodium falciparum P37.3
  - poliomyelitis P35.8
  - rubella P35.0
  - skin P39.4
  - toxoplasmosis (acute) (subacute) (chronic) P37.1
  - tuberculosis P37.0
  - urinary (tract) P39.3

Infection, infected, infective — *continued*
- congenital — *continued*
  - vaccinia P35.8
  - virus P35.9
    - specified type NEC P35.8
- Conidiobolus B46.8
- coronavirus B34.2
  - as cause of disease classified elsewhere B97.29
  - severe acute respiratory syndrome (SARS associated) B97.21
- corpus luteum — *see* Salpingo-oophoritis
- Corynebacterium diphtheriae — *see* Diphtheria
- cotia virus B08.8
- Coxiella burnetii A78
- coxsackie — *see* Coxsackie
- Cryptococcus neoformans — *see* Cryptococcosis
- Cryptosporidium A07.2
- Cunninghamella — *see* Mucormycosis
- cyst — *see* Cyst
- cystic duct (*see also* Cholecystitis) K81.9
- Cysticercus cellulosae — *see* Cysticercosis
- cytomegalovirus, cytomegaloviral B25.9
  - congenital P35.1
  - maternal, maternal care for (suspected) damage to fetus O35.3 ☑
  - mononucleosis B27.10
    - with
      - complication NEC B27.19
      - meningitis B27.12
      - polyneuropathy B27.11
- delta-agent (acute), in hepatitis B carrier B17.0
- dental (pulpal origin) K04.7
- Deuteromycetes B47.0
- Dicrocoelium dendriticum B66.2
- Dipetalonema (perstans) (streptocerca) B74.4
- diphtherial — *see* Diphtheria
- Diphyllobothrium (adult) (latum) (pacificum) B70.0
  - larval B70.1
- Diplogonoporus (grandis) B71.8
- Dipylidium caninum B67.4
- Dirofilaria B74.8
- Dracunculus medinensis B72
- Drechslera (hawaiiensis) B43.8
- Ducrey Haemophilus (any location) A57
- due to or resulting from
  - artificial insemination N98.0
  - central venous catheter T80.219 ☑
    - bloodstream T80.211 ☑
    - exit or insertion site T80.212 ☑
    - localized T80.212 ☑
    - port or reservoir T80.212 ☑
    - specified NEC T80.218 ☑
    - tunnel T80.212 ☑
  - device, implant or graft (*see also* Complications, by site and type, infection or inflammation) T85.79 ☑
    - arterial graft NEC T82.7 ☑
    - breast (implant) T85.79 ☑
    - catheter NEC T85.79 ☑
      - dialysis (renal) T82.7 ☑
        - intraperitoneal T85.71 ☑
      - infusion NEC T82.7 ☑
        - cranial T85.735 ☑
        - intrathecal T85.735 ☑
        - spinal (epidural) (subdural) T85.735 ☑
        - subarachnoid T85.735 ☑
      - urinary T83.518 ☑
        - cystostomy T83.510 ☑
        - Hopkins T83.518 ☑
        - ileostomy T83.518 ☑
        - nephrostomy T83.512 ☑
        - specified NEC T83.518 ☑
        - urethral indwelling T83.511 ☑
        - urostomy T83.518 ☑
    - electronic (electrode) (pulse generator) (stimulator)
      - bone T84.7 ☑
      - cardiac T82.7 ☑
      - nervous system T85.738 ☑
        - brain T85.731 ☑
        - cranial nerve T85.732 ☑
        - gastric nerve T85.732 ☑
        - generator pocket T85.734 ☑
        - neurostimulator generator T85.734 ☑
        - peripheral nerve T85.732 ☑
        - sacral nerve T85.732 ☑
        - spinal cord T85.733 ☑

Infection, infected, infective — *continued*
  due to or resulting from — *continued*
    device, implant or graft (*see also* Complications, by site and type, infection or inflammation) — *continued*
      electronic — *continued*
        nervous system — *continued*
          vagal nerve T85.732 ☑
          urinary (indwelling) T83.51 ☑
      fixation, internal (orthopedic) NEC — *see* Complication, fixation device, infection
      gastrointestinal (bile duct) (esophagus) T85.79 ☑
        neurostimulator electrode (lead) T85.732 ☑
      genital NEC T83.69 ☑
      heart NEC T82.7 ☑
        valve (prosthesis) T82.6 ☑
          graft T82.7 ☑
      joint prosthesis — *see* Complication, joint prosthesis, infection
      ocular (corneal graft) (orbital implant) NEC T85.79 ☑
      orthopedic NEC T84.7 ☑
      penile (cylinder) (pump) (resevoir) T83.61 ☑
      specified NEC T85.79 ☑
      testicular T83.62 ☑
      urinary NEC T83.598 ☑
        ileal conduit stent T83.593 ☑
        implanted neurostimulation T83.590 ☑
        implanted sphincter T83.591 ☑
        indwelling ureteral stent T83.592 ☑
        nephroureteral stent T83.593 ☑
        specified stent NEC T83.593 ☑
      vascular NEC T82.7 ☑
      ventricular intracranial (communicating) shunt T85.730 ☑
    Hickman catheter T80.219 ☑
      bloodstream T80.211 ☑
      localized T80.212 ☑
      specified NEC T80.218 ☑
    immunization or vaccination T88.0 ☑
    infusion, injection or transfusion NEC T80.29 ☑
    injury NEC — *code by* site under Wound, open
    peripherally inserted central catheter (PICC) T80.219 ☑
      bloodstream T80.211 ☑
      localized T80.212 ☑
      specified NEC T80.218 ☑
    portacath (port-a-cath) T80.219 ☑
      bloodstream T80.211 ☑
      localized T80.212 ☑
      specified NEC T80.218 ☑
    pulmonary artery catheter — *see* Infection, due to or resulting from, central venous catheter
    surgery T81.40 ☑
    Swan Ganz catheter — *see* Infection, due to or resulting from, central venous catheter
    triple lumen catheter T80.219 ☑
      bloodstream T80.211 ☑
      localized T80.212 ☑
      specified NEC T80.218 ☑
    umbilical venous catheter T80.219 ☑
      bloodstream T80.211 ☑
      localized T80.212 ☑
      specified NEC T80.218 ☑
  during labor NEC O75.3
  ear (middle) (*see also* Otitis media)
    external — *see* Otitis, externa, infective
    inner — *see* subcategory H83.0 ☑
  Eberthella typhosa A01.00
  Echinococcus — *see* Echinococcus
  echovirus
    as cause of disease classified elsewhere B97.12
    unspecified nature or site B34.1
  endocardium I33.0
  endocervix — *see* Cervicitis
  Entamoeba — *see* Amebiasis
  enteric — *see* Enteritis, infectious
  Enterobacter sakazakii B96.89
  Enterobius vermicularis B80
  enterostomy K94.12
  enterovirus B34.1
    as cause of disease classified elsewhere B97.10
      coxsackievirus B97.11
      echovirus B97.12
      specified NEC B97.19
  Entomophthora B46.8

Infection, infected, infective — *continued*
  Epidermophyton — *see* Dermatophytosis
  epididymis — *see* Epididymitis
  episiotomy (puerperal) O86.09
  Erysipelothrix (insidiosa) (rhusiopathiae) — *see* Erysipeloid
  erythema infectiosum B08.3
  Escherichia (E.) coli NEC A49.8
    as cause of disease classified elsewhere (*see also* Escherichia coli) B96.20
    congenital P39.8
      sepsis P36.4
    generalized A41.51
    intestinal — *see* Enteritis, infectious, due to, Escherichia coli
  ethmoidal (chronic) (sinus) — *see* Sinusitis, ethmoidal
  eustachian tube (ear) — *see* Salpingitis, eustachian
  external auditory canal (meatus) NEC — *see* Otitis, externa, infective
  eye (purulent) — *see* Endophthalmitis, purulent
  eyelid — *see* Inflammation, eyelid
  fallopian tube — *see* Salpingo-oophoritis
  Fasciola (gigantica) (hepatica) (indica) B66.3
  Fasciolopsis (buski) B66.5
  filarial — *see* Infestation, filarial
  finger (skin) L08.9
    nail L03.01- ☑
      fungus B35.1
  fish tapeworm B70.0
    larval B70.1
  flagellate, intestinal A07.9
  fluke — *see* Infestation, fluke
  focal
    teeth (pulpal origin) K04.7
    tonsils J35.01
  Fonsecaea (compactum) (pedrosoi) B43.0
  food — *see* Intoxication, foodborne
  foot (skin) L08.9
    dermatophytic fungus B35.3
  Francisella tularensis — *see* Tularemia
  frontal (sinus) (chronic) — *see* Sinusitis, frontal
  fungus NOS B49
    beard B35.0
    dermatophytic — *see* Dermatophytosis
    foot B35.3
    groin B35.6
    hand B35.2
    nail B35.1
    pathogenic to compromised host only B48.8
    perianal (area) B35.6
    scalp B35.0
    skin B36.9
      foot B35.3
      hand B35.2
      toenails B35.1
  Fusarium B48.8
  gallbladder — *see* Cholecystitis
  gas bacillus — *see* Gangrene, gas
  gastrointestinal — *see* Enteritis, infectious
  generalized NEC — *see* Sepsis
  generator pocket, implanted electronic neurostimulator T85.734 ☑
  genital organ or tract
    female — *see* Disease, pelvis, inflammatory
    male N49.9
      multiple sites N49.8
      specified NEC N49.8
  Ghon tubercle, primary A15.7
  Giardia lamblia A07.1
  gingiva (chronic) K05.10
    acute K05.00
      nonplaque induced K05.01
      plaque induced K05.00
    nonplaque induced K05.11
    plaque induced K05.10
  glanders A24.0
  glenosporopsis B48.0
  Gnathostoma (spinigerum) B83.1
  Gongylonema B83.8
  gonococcal — *see* Gonococcus
  gram-negative bacilli NOS A49.9
  guinea worm B72
  gum (chronic) K05.10
    acute K05.00
      nonplaque induced K05.01
      plaque induced K05.00
    nonplaque induced K05.11
    plaque induced K05.10

Infection, infected, infective — *continued*
  Haemophilus — *see* Infection, Hemophilus
  heart — *see* Carditis
  Helicobacter pylori A04.8
    as cause of disease classified elsewhere B96.81
  helminths B83.9
    intestinal B82.0
      mixed (types classifiable to more than one of the titles B65.0-B81.3 and B81.8) B81.4
      specified type NEC B81.8
    specified type NEC B83.8
  Hemophilus
    aegyptius, systemic A48.4
    ducrey (any location) A57
    generalized A41.3
    influenzae NEC A49.2
      as cause of disease classified elsewhere B96.3
  herpes (simplex) (*see also* Herpes)
    congenital P35.2
    disseminated B00.7
    zoster B02.9
  herpesvirus, herpesviral — *see* Herpes
  Heterophyes (heterophyes) B66.8
  hip (joint) NEC M00.9
    due to internal joint prosthesis
      left T84.52 ☑
      right T84.51 ☑
    skin NEC L08.9
  Histoplasma — *see* Histoplasmosis
    American B39.4
    capsulatum B39.4
  hookworm B76.9
  human
    papilloma virus A63.0
    T-cell lymphotropic virus type-1 (HTLV-1) B33.3
  hydrocele N43.0
  Hymenolepis B71.0
  hypopharynx — *see* Pharyngitis
  inguinal (lymph) glands L04.1
    due to soft chancre A57
  intervertebral disc, pyogenic M46.30
    cervical region M46.32
    cervicothoracic region M46.33
    lumbar region M46.36
    lumbosacral region M46.37
    multiple sites M46.39
    occipito-atlanto-axial region M46.31
    sacrococcygeal region M46.38
    thoracic region M46.34
    thoracolumbar region M46.35
  intestine, intestinal — *see* Enteritis, infectious
    specified NEC A08.8
  intra-amniotic affecting newborn NEC P39.2
  Isospora belli or hominis A07.3
  Japanese B encephalitis A83.0
  jaw (bone) (lower) (upper) M27.2
  joint NEC M00.9
    due to internal joint prosthesis T84.50 ☑
  kidney (cortex) (hematogenous) N15.9
    with calculus N20.0
      with hydronephrosis N13.6
    following ectopic gestation O08.83
    pelvis and ureter (cystic) N28.85
    puerperal (postpartum) O86.21
    specified NEC N15.8
  Klebsiella (K.) pneumoniae NEC A49.8
    as cause of disease classified elsewhere B96.1
  knee (joint) NEC M00.9
    joint M00.9
    due to internal joint prosthesis
      left T84.54 ☑
      right T84.53 ☑
    skin L08.9
  Koch's — *see* Tuberculosis
  labia (majora) (minora) (acute) — *see* Vulvitis
  lacrimal
    gland — *see* Dacryoadenitis
    passages (duct) (sac) — *see* Inflammation, lacrimal passages
  lancet fluke B66.2
  larynx NEC J38.7
  leg (skin) NOS L08.9
  Legionella pneumophila A48.1
    nonpneumonic A48.2
  Leishmania (*see also* Leishmaniasis)
    aethiopica B55.1
    braziliensis B55.2
    chagasi B55.0

Infection, infected, infective — *continued*
  Leishmania (*see also* Leishmaniasis) — *continued*
    donovani B55.Ø
    infantum B55.Ø
    major B55.1
    mexicana B55.1
    tropica B55.1
  lentivirus, as cause of disease classified elsewhere
    B97.31
  Leptosphaeria senegalensis B47.Ø
  Leptospira interrogans A27.9
    autumnalis A27.89
    canicola A27.89
    hebdomadis A27.89
    icterohaemorrhagiae A27.Ø
    pomona A27.89
    specified type NEC A27.89
  leptospirochetal NEC — *see* Leptospirosis
  Listeria monocytogenes (*see also* Listeriosis)
    congenital P37.2
  Loa loa B74.3
    with conjunctival infestation B74.3
    eyelid B74.3
  Loboa loboi B48.Ø
  local, skin (staphylococcal) (streptococcal) LØ8.9
    abscess — *code by* site under Abscess
    cellulitis — *code by* site under Cellulitis
    specified NEC LØ8.89
    ulcer — *see* Ulcer, skin
  Loefflerella mallei A24.Ø
  lung (*see also* Pneumonia) J18.9
    atypical Mycobacterium A31.Ø
    spirochetal A69.8
    tuberculous — *see* Tuberculosis, pulmonary
    virus — *see* Pneumonia, viral
  lymph gland (*see also* Lymphadenitis, acute)
    mesenteric I88.Ø
  lymphoid tissue, base of tongue or posterior pharynx,
    NEC (chronic) J35.Ø3
  Madurella (grisea) (mycetomii) B47.Ø
  major
    following ectopic or molar pregnancy OØ8.Ø
    puerperal, postpartum, childbirth O85
  Malassezia furfur B36.Ø
  Malleomyces
    mallei A24.Ø
    pseudomallei (whitmori) — *see* Melioidosis
  mammary gland N61.Ø
  Mansonella (ozzardi) (perstans) (streptocerca) B74.4
  mastoid — *see* Mastoiditis
  maxilla, maxillary M27.2
    sinus (chronic) — *see* Sinusitis, maxillary
  mediastinum J98.51
  Medina (worm) B72
  meibomian cyst or gland — *see* Hordeolum
  meninges — *see* Meningitis, bacterial
  meningococcal (*see also* condition) A39.9
    adrenals A39.1
    brain A39.81
    cerebrospinal A39.Ø
    conjunctiva A39.89
    endocardium A39.51
    heart A39.5Ø
      endocardium A39.51
      myocardium A39.52
      pericardium A39.53
    joint A39.83
    meninges A39.Ø
    meningococcemia A39.4
      acute A39.2
      chronic A39.3
    myocardium A39.52
    pericardium A39.53
    retrobulbar neuritis A39.82
    specified site NEC A39.89
  mesenteric lymph nodes or glands NEC I88.Ø
  Metagonimus B66.8
  metatarsophalangeal MØØ.9
  methicillin
    resistant Staphylococcus aureus (MRSA) A49.Ø2
    susceptible Staphylococcus aureus (MSSA) A49.Ø1
  Microsporum, microsporic — *see* Dermatophytosis
  mixed flora (bacterial) NEC A49.8
  Monilia — *see* Candidiasis
  Monosporium apiospermum B48.2
  mouth, parasitic B37.Ø
  Mucor — *see* Mucormycosis
  muscle NEC — *see* Myositis, infective

Infection, infected, infective — *continued*
  mycelium NOS B49
  mycetoma B47.9
    actinomycotic NEC B47.1
    mycotic NEC B47.Ø
  Mycobacterium, mycobacterial — *see* Mycobacterium
  Mycoplasma NEC A49.3
    pneumoniae, as cause of disease classified else-
      where B96.Ø
  mycotic NOS B49
    pathogenic to compromised host only B48.8
    skin NOS B36.9
  myocardium NEC I4Ø.Ø
  nail (chronic)
    with lymphangitis — *see* Lymphangitis, acute, digit
    finger LØ3.Ø1- ☑
      fungus B35.1
    ingrowing L6Ø.Ø
    toe LØ3.Ø3- ☑
      fungus B35.1
  nasal sinus (chronic) — *see* Sinusitis
  nasopharynx — *see* Nasopharyngitis
  navel LØ8.82
  Necator americanus B76.1
  Neisseria — *see* Gonococcus
  Neotestudina rosatii B47.Ø
  newborn P39.9
    intra-amniotic NEC P39.2
    skin P39.4
    specified type NEC P39.8
  nipple N61.Ø
    associated with
      lactation O91.Ø3
      pregnancy O91.Ø1- ☑
      puerperium O91.Ø2
  Nocardia — *see* Nocardiosis
  obstetrical surgical wound (puerperal) O86.ØØ
    incisional site
      deep O86.Ø2
      superficial O86.Ø1
    organ and space site O86.Ø3
    surgical site specified NEC O86.Ø9
  Oesophagostomum (apiostomum) B81.8
  Oestrus ovis — *see* Myiasis
  Oidium albicans B37.9
  Onchocerca (volvulus) — *see* Onchocerciasis
  oncovirus, as cause of disease classified elsewhere
    B97.32
  operation wound T81.49 ☑
  Opisthorchis (felineus) (viverrini) B66.Ø
  orbit, orbital — *see* Inflammation, orbit
  orthopoxvirus NEC BØ8.Ø9
  ovary — *see* Salpingo-oophoritis
  Oxyuris vermicularis B8Ø
  pancreas (acute) — *see* Pancreatitis, acute
    abscess — *see* Pancreatitis, acute
    specified NEC (*see also* Pancreatitis, acute) K85.8Ø
  papillomavirus, as cause of disease classified elsewhere
    B97.7
  papovavirus NEC B34.4
  Paracoccidioides brasiliensis — *see* Paracoccidioidomy-
    cosis
  Paragonimus (westermani) B66.4
  parainfluenza virus B34.8
  parameningococcus NOS A39.9
  parapoxvirus BØ8.6Ø
    specified NEC BØ8.69
  parasitic B89
  Parastrongylus
    cantonensis B83.2
    costaricensis B81.3
    paratyphoid AØ1.4
      Type A AØ1.1
      Type B AØ1.2
      Type C AØ1.3
  paraurethral ducts N34.2
  parotid gland — *see* Sialoadenitis
  parvovirus NEC B34.3
    as cause of disease classified elsewhere B97.6
  Pasteurella NEC A28.Ø
    multocida A28.Ø
    pestis — *see* Plague
    pseudotuberculosis A28.Ø
    septica (cat bite) (dog bite) A28.Ø
    tularensis — *see* Tularemia
  pelvic, female — *see* Disease, pelvis, inflammatory
  Penicillium (marneffei) B48.4
  penis (glans) (retention) NEC N48.29

Infection, infected, infective — *continued*
  periapical KØ4.5
  peridental, periodontal KØ5.2Ø
    generalized — *see* Peridontitis, aggressive, general-
      ized
    localized — *see* Peridontitis, aggressive, localized
  perinatal period P39.9
    specified type NEC P39.8
  perineal repair (puerperal) O86.Ø9
  periorbital — *see* Inflammation, orbit
  perirectal K62.89
  perirenal — *see* Infection, kidney
  peritoneal — *see* Peritonitis
  periureteral N28.89
  Petriellidium boydii B48.2
  pharynx (*see also* Pharyngitis)
    coxsackievirus BØ8.5
    posterior, lymphoid (chronic) J35.Ø3
  Phialophora
    gougerotii (subcutaneous abscess or cyst) B43.2
    jeanselmei (subcutaneous abscess or cyst) B43.2
    verrucosa (skin) B43.Ø
  Piedraia hortae B36.3
  pinta A67.9
    intermediate A67.1
    late A67.2
    mixed A67.3
    primary A67.Ø
  pinworm B8Ø
  pityrosporum furfur B36.Ø
  pleuro-pneumonia-like organism (PPLO) NEC A49.3
    as cause of disease classified elsewhere B96.Ø
  pneumococcus, pneumococcal NEC A49.1
    as cause of disease classified elsewhere B95.3
    generalized (purulent) A4Ø.3
      with pneumonia J13
  Pneumocystis carinii (pneumonia) B59
  Pneumocystis jiroveci (pneumonia) B59
  port or reservoir T8Ø.212 ☑
  postoperative T81.4Ø ☑
  postoperative wound T81.49 ☑
    surgical site
      deep incisional T81.42 ☑
      organ and space T81.43 ☑
      specified NEC T81.49 ☑
      superficial incisional T81.41 ☑
  postprocedural T81.4Ø ☑
  postvaccinal T88.Ø ☑
  prepuce NEC N47.7
    with penile inflammation N47.6
  prion — *see* Disease, prion, central nervous system
  prostate (capsule) — *see* Prostatitis
  Proteus (mirabilis) (morganii) (vulgaris) NEC A49.8
    as cause of disease classified elsewhere B96.4
  protozoal NEC B64
    intestinal AØ7.9
      specified NEC AØ7.8
    specified NEC B6Ø.8
  Pseudoallescheria boydii B48.2
  Pseudomonas NEC A49.8
    as cause of disease classified elsewhere B96.5
    mallei A24.Ø
    pneumonia J15.1
    pseudomallei — *see* Melioidosis
  puerperal O86.4
    genitourinary tract NEC O86.89
    major or generalized O85
    minor O86.4
    specified NEC O86.89
  pulmonary — *see* Infection, lung
  purulent — *see* Abscess
  Pyrenochaeta romeroi B47.Ø
  Q fever A78
  rectum (sphincter) K62.89
  renal (*see also* Infection, kidney)
    pelvis and ureter (cystic) N28.85
  reovirus, as cause of disease classified elsewhere B97.5
  respiratory (tract) NEC J98.8
    acute J22
    chronic J98.8
    influenzal (upper) (acute) — *see* Influenza, with,
      respiratory manifestations NEC
    lower (acute) J22
      chronic — *see* Bronchitis, chronic
    rhinovirus JØØ
    syncytial virus, as cause of disease classified else-
      where B97.4
    upper (acute) NOS JØ6.9

Infection, infected, infective — *continued*
 respiratory — *continued*
  upper — *continued*
   chronic J39.8
   streptococcal J06.9
   viral NOS J06.9
 resulting from
  presence of internal prosthesis, implant, graft —
   see Complications, by site and type, infection
 retortamoniasis A07.8
 retroperitoneal NEC K68.9
 retrovirus B33.3
  as cause of disease classified elsewhere B97.30
   human
    immunodeficiency, type 2 (HIV 2) B97.35
    T-cell lymphotropic
     type I (HTLV-I) B97.33
     type II (HTLV-II) B97.34
   lentivirus B97.31
   oncovirus B97.32
   specified NEC B97.39
 Rhinosporidium (seeberi) B48.1
 rhinovirus
  as cause of disease classified elsewhere B97.89
  unspecified nature or site B34.8
 Rhizopus — *see* Mucormycosis
 rickettsial NOS A79.9
 roundworm (large) NEC B82.0
  Ascariasis (*see also* Ascariasis) B77.9
 rubella — *see* Rubella
 Saccharomyces — *see* Candidiasis
 salivary duct or gland (any) — *see* Sialoadenitis
 Salmonella (aertrycke) (arizonae) (callinarum) (cholerae-
  suis) (enteritidis) (suipestifer) (typhimurium)
  A02.9
  with
   (gastro)enteritis A02.0
   sepsis A02.1
   specified manifestation NEC A02.8
  due to food (poisoning) A02.9
  hirschfeldii A01.3
  localized A02.20
   arthritis A02.23
   meningitis A02.21
   osteomyelitis A02.24
   pneumonia A02.22
   pyelonephritis A02.25
   specified NEC A02.29
  paratyphi A01.4
   A A01.1
   B A01.2
   C A01.3
  schottmuelleri A01.2
  typhi, typhosa — *see* Typhoid
 Sarcocystis A07.8
 scabies B86
 Schistosoma — *see* Infestation, Schistosoma
 scrotum (acute) NEC N49.2
 seminal vesicle — *see* Vesiculitis
 septic
  localized, skin — *see* Abscess
 sheep liver fluke B66.3
 Shigella A03.9
  boydii A03.2
  dysenteriae A03.0
  flexneri A03.1
  group
   A A03.0
   B A03.1
   C A03.2
   D A03.3
  Schmitz (-Stutzer) A03.0
  schmitzii A03.0
  shigae A03.0
  sonnei A03.3
  specified NEC A03.8
 shoulder (joint) NEC M00.9
  due to internal joint prosthesis T84.59 ☑
  skin NEC L08.9
 sinus (accessory) (chronic) (nasal) (*see also* Sinusitis)
  pilonidal — *see* Sinus, pilonidal
  skin NEC L08.89
 Skene's duct or gland — *see* Urethritis
 skin (local) (staphylococcal) (streptococcal) L08.9
  abscess — *code by* site under Abscess
  cellulitis — *code by* site under Cellulitis
  due to fungus B36.9
   specified type NEC B36.8

 skin — *continued*
  mycotic B36.9
   specified type NEC B36.8
  newborn P39.4
  ulcer — *see* Ulcer, skin
 slow virus A81.9
  specified NEC A81.89
 Sparganum (mansoni) (proliferum) (baxteri) B70.1
 specific (*see also* Syphilis)
  to perinatal period — *see* Infection, congenital
 specified NEC B99.8
 spermatic cord NEC N49.1
 sphenoidal (sinus) — *see* Sinusitis, sphenoidal
 spinal cord NOS (*see also* Myelitis) G04.91
  abscess G06.1
  meninges — *see* Meningitis
  streptococcal G04.89
 Spirillum A25.0
 spirochetal NOS A69.9
  lung A69.8
  specified NEC A69.8
 Spirometra larvae B70.1
 spleen D73.89
 Sporotrichum, Sporothrix (schenckii) — *see* Sporotrichosis
 staphylococcal, unspecified site
  as cause of disease classified elsewhere B95.8
   aureus (methicillin susceptible) (MSSA) B95.61
    methicillin resistant (MRSA) B95.62
   specified NEC B95.7
  aureus (methicillin susceptible) (MSSA) A49.01
   methicillin resistant (MRSA) A49.02
  food poisoning A05.0
  generalized (purulent) A41.2
  pneumonia — *see* Pneumonia, staphylococcal
 Stellantchasmus falcatus B66.8
 streptobacillus moniliformis A25.1
 streptococcal NEC A49.1
  as cause of disease classified elsewhere B95.5
  B genitourinary complicating
   childbirth O98.82
   pregnancy O98.81- ☑
   puerperium O98.83
  congenital
   sepsis P36.10
    group B P36.0
    specified NEC P36.19
  generalized (purulent) A40.9
 Streptomyces B47.1
 Strongyloides (stercoralis) — *see* Strongyloidiasis
 stump (amputation) (surgical) — *see* Complication,
  amputation stump, infection
 subcutaneous tissue, local L08.9
 suipestifer — *see* Infection, salmonella
 swimming pool bacillus A31.1
 Taenia — *see* Infestation, Taenia
 Taeniarhynchus saginatus B68.1
 tapeworm — *see* Infestation, tapeworm
 tendon (sheath) — *see* Tenosynovitis, infective NEC
 Ternidens diminutus B81.8
 testis — *see* Orchitis
 threadworm B80
 throat — *see* Pharyngitis
 thyroglossal duct K14.8
 toe (skin) L08.9
  cellulitis L03.03- ☑
   fungus B35.1
  nail L03.03- ☑
   fungus B35.1
 tongue NEC K14.0
  parasitic B37.0
 tonsil (and adenoid) (faucial) (lingual) (pharyngeal) —
  see Tonsillitis
 tooth, teeth K04.7
  periapical K04.7
  peridental, periodontal K05.20
   generalized — *see* Peridontitis, aggressive, gen-
    eralized
   localized — *see* Peridontitis, aggressive, localized
  pulp K04.01
   irreversible K04.02
   reversible K04.01
  socket M27.3
 TORCH — *see* Infection, congenital
  without active infection P00.2
 Torula histolytica — *see* Cryptococcosis
 Toxocara (canis) (cati) (felis) B83.0

 Toxoplasma gondii — *see* Toxoplasma
 trachea, chronic J42
 trematode NEC — *see* Infestation, fluke
 trench fever A79.0
 Treponema pallidum — *see* Syphilis
 Trichinella (spiralis) B75
 Trichomonas A59.9
  cervix A59.09
  intestine A07.8
  prostate A59.02
  specified site NEC A59.8
  urethra A59.03
  urogenitalis A59.00
  vagina A59.01
  vulva A59.01
 Trichophyton, trichophytic — *see* Dermatophytosis
 Trichosporon (beigelii) cutaneum B36.2
 Trichostrongylus B81.2
 Trichuris (trichiura) B79
 Trombicula (irritans) B88.0
 Trypanosoma
  brucei
   gambiense B56.0
   rhodesiense B56.1
  cruzi — *see* Chagas' disease
 tubal — *see* Salpingo-oophoritis
 tuberculous NEC — *see* Tuberculosis
 tubo-ovarian — *see* Salpingo-oophoritis
 tunica vaginalis N49.1
 tunnel T80.212 ☑
 tympanic membrane NEC — *see* Myringitis
 typhoid (abortive) (ambulant) (bacillus) — *see* Typho-
 typhus A75.9
  flea-borne A75.2
  mite-borne A75.3
  recrudescent A75.1
  tick-borne A77.9
   African A77.1
   North Asian A77.2
 umbilicus L08.82
 ureter N28.86
 urethra — *see* Urethritis
 urinary (tract) N39.0
  bladder — *see* Cystitis
  complicating
   pregnancy O23.4- ☑
    specified type NEC O23.3- ☑
  kidney — *see* Infection, kidney
  newborn P39.3
  puerperal (postpartum) O86.20
  tuberculous A18.13
  urethra — *see* Urethritis
 uterus, uterine — *see* Endometritis
 vaccination T88.0 ☑
 vaccinia not from vaccination B08.011
 vagina (acute) — *see* Vaginitis
 varicella B01.9
 varicose veins — *see* Varix
 vas deferens NEC N49.1
 vesical — *see* Cystitis
 Vibrio
  cholerae A00.0
   El Tor A00.1
  parahaemolyticus (food poisoning) A05.3
  vulnificus
   as cause of disease classified elsewhere B96.
   foodborne intoxication A05.5
 Vincent's (gum) (mouth) (tonsil) A69.1
 virus, viral NOS B34.9
  adenovirus
   as cause of disease classified elsewhere B97.
   unspecified nature or site B34.0
  arborvirus, arbovirus arthropod-borne A94
  as cause of disease classified elsewhere B97.89
   adenovirus B97.0
   coronavirus B97.29
    SARS-associated B97.21
   coxsackievirus B97.11
   echovirus B97.12
   enterovirus B97.10
    coxsackievirus B97.11
    echovirus B97.12
    specified NEC B97.19
  human
   immunodeficiency, type 2 (HIV 2) B97.35
   metapneumovirus B97.81

☑ **Additional Character Required** — **Refer to the Tabular List for Character Selection**

▽ **Subterms under main terms may continue to next column or p**

Infection, infected, infective — continued
  virus, viral — continued
    as cause of disease classified elsewhere — contin-
        ued
      human — continued
        T-cell lymphotropic,
          type I (HTLV-I) B97.33
          type II (HTLV-II) B97.34
      papillomavirus B97.7
      parvovirus B97.6
      reovirus B97.5
      respiratory syncytial B97.4
      retrovirus B97.30
        human
          immunodeficiency, type 2 (HIV 2) B97.35
          T-cell lymphotropic,
            type I (HTLV-I) B97.33
            type II (HTLV-II) B97.34
        lentivirus B97.31
        oncovirus B97.32
        specified NEC B97.39
      specified NEC B97.89
    central nervous system A89
      atypical A81.9
        specified NEC A81.89
      enterovirus NEC A88.8
        meningitis A87.0
      slow virus A81.9
        specified NEC A81.89
      specified NEC A88.8
    chest J98.8
    cotia B08.8
    coxsackie (see also Infection, coxsackie) B34.1
      as cause of disease classified elsewhere B97.11
    ECHO
      as cause of disease classified elsewhere B97.12
      unspecified nature or site B34.1
    encephalitis, tick-borne A84.9
    enterovirus, as cause of disease classified elsewhere
        B97.10
      coxsackievirus B97.11
      echovirus B97.12
      specified NEC B97.19
    exanthem NOS B09
    human metapneumovirus as cause of disease clas-
        sified elsewhere B97.81
    human papilloma as cause of disease classified
        elsewhere B97.7
    intestine — see Enteritis, viral
    respiratory syncytial
      as cause of disease classified elsewhere B97.4
      bronchopneumonia J12.1
      common cold syndrome J00
      nasopharyngitis (acute) J00
    rhinovirus
      as cause of disease classified elsewhere B97.89
      unspecified nature or site B34.8
    slow A81.9
      specified NEC A81.89
    specified type NEC B33.8
      as cause of disease classified elsewhere B97.89
      unspecified nature or site B34.8
    unspecified nature or site B34.9
    West Nile — see Virus, West Nile
  vulva (acute) — see Vulvitis
  West Nile — see Virus, West Nile
  whipworm B79
  worms B83.9
    specified type NEC B83.8
  Wuchereria (bancrofti) B74.0
    malayi B74.1
  yatapoxvirus B08.70
    specified NEC B08.79
  yeast (see also Candidiasis) B37.9
  yellow fever — see Fever, yellow
  Yersinia
    enterocolitica (intestinal) A04.6
    pestis — see Plague
    pseudotuberculosis A28.2
  Zeis' gland — see Hordeolum
  Zika virus A92.5
    congenital P35.4
  zoonotic bacterial NOS A28.9
  Zopfia senegalensis B47.0
Infective, infectious — see condition
Infertility
  female N97.9
    age-related N97.8

Infertility — continued
  female — continued
    associated with
      anovulation N97.0
      cervical (mucus) disease or anomaly N88.3
      congenital anomaly
        cervix N88.3
        fallopian tube N97.1
        uterus N97.2
        vagina N97.8
      dysmucorrhea N88.3
      fallopian tube disease or anomaly N97.1
      pituitary-hypothalamic origin E23.0
      specified origin NEC N97.8
      Stein-Leventhal syndrome E28.2
      uterine disease or anomaly N97.2
      vaginal disease or anomaly N97.8
    due to
      cervical anomaly N88.3
      fallopian tube anomaly N97.1
      ovarian failure E28.39
      Stein-Leventhal syndrome E28.2
      uterine anomaly N97.2
      vaginal anomaly N97.8
    nonimplantation N97.2
    origin
      cervical N88.3
      tubal (block) (occlusion) (stenosis) N97.1
      uterine N97.2
      vaginal N97.8
  male N46.9
    azoospermia N46.01
      extratesticular cause N46.029
        drug therapy N46.021
        efferent duct obstruction N46.023
        infection N46.022
        radiation N46.024
        specified cause NEC N46.029
        systemic disease N46.025
    oligospermia N46.11
      extratesticular cause N46.129
        drug therapy N46.121
        efferent duct obstruction N46.123
        infection N46.122
        radiation N46.124
        specified cause NEC N46.129
        systemic disease N46.125
    specified type NEC N46.8
Infestation B88.9
  Acanthocheilonema (perstans) (streptocerca) B74.4
  Acariasis B88.0
    demodex folliculorum B88.0
    sarcoptes scabiei B86
    trombiculae B88.0
  Agamofilaria streptocerca B74.4
  Ancylostoma, ankylostoma (braziliense) (caninum)
      (ceylanicum) (duodenale) B76.0
    americanum B76.1
    new world B76.1
  Anisakis larvae, anisakiasis B81.0
  arthropod NEC B88.2
  Ascaris lumbricoides — see Ascariasis
  Balantidium coli A07.0
  beef tapeworm B68.1
  Bothriocephalus (latus) B70.0
    larval B70.1
  broad tapeworm B70.0
    larval B70.1
  Brugia (malayi) B74.1
    timori B74.2
  candiru B88.8
  Capillaria
    hepatica B83.8
    philippinensis B81.1
  cat liver fluke B66.0
  cestodes B71.9
    diphyllobothrium — see Infestation, diphyllobotho-
        rium
    dipylidiasis B71.1
    hymenolepiasis B71.0
    specified type NEC B71.8
  chigger B88.0
  chigo, chigoe B88.1
  Clonorchis (sinensis) (liver) B66.1
  coccidial A07.3
  crab-lice B85.3
  Cysticercus cellulosae — see Cysticercosis
  Demodex (folliculorum) B88.0
  Dermanyssus gallinae B88.0

Infestation — continued
  Dermatobia (hominis) — see Myiasis
  Dibothriocephalus (latus) B70.0
    larval B70.1
  Dicrocoelium dendriticum B66.2
  Diphyllobothrium (adult) (latum) (intestinal) (pacificum)
      B70.0
    larval B70.1
  Diplogonoporus (grandis) B71.8
  Dipylidium caninum B67.4
  Distoma hepaticum B66.3
  dog tapeworm B67.4
  Dracunculus medinensis B72
  dragon worm B72
  dwarf tapeworm B71.0
  Echinococcus — see Echinococcus
  Echinostomum ilocanum B66.8
  Entamoeba (histolytica) — see Infection, Ameba
  Enterobius vermicularis B80
  eyelid
    in (due to)
      leishmaniasis B55.1
      loiasis B74.3
      onchocerciasis B73.09
      phthiriasis B85.3
    parasitic NOS B89
  eyeworm B74.3
  Fasciola (gigantica) (hepatica) (indica) B66.3
  Fasciolopsis (buski) (intestine) B66.5
  filarial B74.9
    bancroftian B74.0
    conjunctiva B74.9
    due to
      Acanthocheilonema (perstans) (streptocerca)
          B74.4
      Brugia (malayi) B74.1
        timori B74.2
      Dracunculus medinensis B72
      guinea worm B72
      loa loa B74.3
      Mansonella (ozzardi) (perstans) (streptocerca)
          B74.4
      Onchocerca volvulus B73.00
        eye B73.00
        eyelid B73.09
      Wuchereria (bancrofti) B74.0
    Malayan B74.1
    ozzardi B74.4
    specified type NEC B74.8
  fish tapeworm B70.0
    larval B70.1
  fluke B66.9
    blood NOS — see Schistosomiasis
    cat liver B66.0
    intestinal B66.5
    lancet B66.2
    liver (sheep) B66.3
      cat B66.0
      Chinese B66.1
      due to clonorchiasis B66.1
      oriental B66.1
    lung (oriental) B66.4
    sheep liver B66.3
    specified type NEC B66.8
  fly larvae — see Myiasis
  Gasterophilus (intestinalis) — see Myiasis
  Gastrodiscoides hominis B66.8
  Giardia lamblia A07.1
  Gnathostoma (spinigerum) B83.1
  Gongylonema B83.8
  guinea worm B72
  helminth B83.9
    angiostrongyliasis B83.2
      intestinal B81.3
    gnathostomiasis B83.1
    hirudiniasis, internal B83.4
    intestinal B82.0
      angiostrongyliasis B81.3
      anisakiasis B81.0
      ascariasis — see Ascariasis
      capillariasis B81.1
      cysticercosis — see Cysticercosis
      diphyllobothriasis — see Infestation, diphyl-
          lobothriasis
      dracunculiasis B72
      echinococcus — see Echinococcosis
      enterobiasis B80
      filariasis — see Infestation, filarial

Infestation — *continued*
  helminth — *continued*
    intestinal — *continued*
      fluke — *see* Infestation, fluke
      hookworm — *see* Infestation, hookworm
      mixed (types classifiable to more than one of the titles B65.Ø-B81.3 and B81.8) B81.4
      onchocerciasis — *see* Onchocerciasis
      schistosomiasis — *see* Infestation, schistosoma
      specified
        cestode NEC — *see* Infestation, cestode
        type NEC B81.8
      strongyloidiasis — *see* Strongyloidiasis
      taenia — *see* Infestation, taenia
      trichinellosis B75
      trichostrongyliasis B81.2
      trichuriasis B79
    specified type NEC B83.8
    syngamiasis B83.3
    visceral larva migrans B83.Ø
  Heterophyes (heterophyes) B66.8
  hookworm B76.9
    ancylostomiasis B76.Ø
    necatoriasis B76.1
    specified type NEC B76.8
  Hymenolepis (diminuta) (nana) B71.Ø
  intestinal NEC B82.9
  leeches (aquatic) (land) — *see* Hirudiniasis
  Leishmania — *see* Leishmaniasis
  lice, louse — *see* Infestation, Pediculus
  Linguatula B88.8
  Liponyssoides sanguineus B88.Ø
  Loa loa B74.3
    conjunctival B74.3
    eyelid B74.3
  louse — *see* Infestation, Pediculus
  maggots — *see* Myiasis
  Mansonella (ozzardi) (perstans) (streptocerca) B74.4
  Medina (worm) B72
  Metagonimus (yokogawai) B66.8
  microfilaria streptocerca — *see* Onchocerciasis
    eye B73.ØØ
    eyelid B73.Ø9
  mites B88.9
    scabic B86
  Monilia (albicans) — *see* Candidiasis
  mouth B37.Ø
  Necator americanus B76.1
  nematode NEC (intestinal) B82.Ø
    Ancylostoma B76.Ø
    conjunctiva NEC B83.9
    Enterobius vermicularis B8Ø
    Gnathostoma spinigerum B83.1
    physaloptera B8Ø
    specified NEC B81.8
    trichostrongylus B81.2
    trichuris (trichuria) B79
  Oesophagostomum (apiostomum) B81.8
  Oestrus ovis (*see also* Myiasis) B87.9
  Onchocerca (volvulus) — *see* Onchocerciasis
  Opisthorchis (felineus) (viverrini) B66.Ø
  orbit, parasitic NOS B89
  Oxyuris vermicularis B8Ø
  Paragonimus (westermani) B66.4
  parasite, parasitic B89
    eyelid B89
    intestinal NOS B82.9
    mouth B37.Ø
    skin B88.9
    tongue B37.Ø
  Parastrongylus
    cantonensis B83.2
    costaricensis B81.3
  Pediculus B85.2
    body B85.1
    capitis (humanus) (any site) B85.Ø
    corporis (humanus) (any site) B85.1
    head B85.Ø
    mixed (classifiable to more than one of the titles B85.Ø - B85.3) B85.4
    pubis (any site) B85.3
  Pentastoma B88.8
  Phthirus (pubis) (any site) B85.3
    with any infestation classifiable to B85.Ø - B85.2 B85.4
  pinworm B8Ø
  pork tapeworm (adult) B68.Ø
  protozoal NEC B64

Infestation — *continued*
  protozoal — *continued*
    intestinal AØ7.9
      specified NEC AØ7.8
    specified NEC B6Ø.8
  pubic, louse B85.3
  rat tapeworm B71.Ø
  red bug B88.Ø
  roundworm (large) NEC B82.Ø
    Ascariasis (*see also* Ascariasis) B77.9
  sandflea B88.1
  Sarcoptes scabiei B86
  scabies B86
  Schistosoma B65.9
    bovis B65.8
    cercariae B65.3
    haematobium B65.Ø
    intercalatum B65.8
    japonicum B65.2
    mansoni B65.1
    mattheei B65.8
    mekongi B65.8
    specified type NEC B65.8
    spindale B65.8
  screw worms — *see* Myiasis
  skin NOS B88.9
  Sparganum (mansoni) (proliferum) (baxteri) B7Ø.1
    larval B7Ø.1
  specified type NEC B88.8
  Spirometra larvae B7Ø.1
  Stellantchasmus falcatus B66.8
  Strongyloides stercoralis — *see* Strongyloidiasis
  Taenia B68.9
    diminuta B71.Ø
    echinococcus — *see* Echinococcus
    mediocanellata B68.1
    nana B71.Ø
    saginata B68.1
    solium (intestinal form) B68.Ø
      larval form — *see* Cysticercosis
  Taeniarhynchus saginatus B68.1
  tapeworm B71.9
    beef B68.1
    broad B7Ø.Ø
      larval B7Ø.1
    dog B67.4
    dwarf B71.Ø
    fish B7Ø.Ø
      larval B7Ø.1
    pork B68.Ø
    rat B71.Ø
  Ternidens diminutus B81.8
  Tetranychus molestissimus B88.Ø
  threadworm B8Ø
  tongue B37.Ø
  Toxocara (canis) (cati) (felis) B83.Ø
  trematode(s) NEC — *see* Infestation, fluke
  Trichinella (spiralis) B75
  Trichocephalus B79
  Trichomonas — *see* Trichomoniasis
  Trichostrongylus B81.2
  Trichuris (trichiura) B79
  Trombicula (irritans) B88.Ø
  Tunga penetrans B88.1
  Uncinaria americana B76.1
  Vandellia cirrhosa B88.8
  whipworm B79
  worms B83.9
    intestinal B82.Ø
  Wuchereria (bancrofti) B74.Ø

Infiltrate, infiltration
  amyloid (generalized) (localized) — *see* Amyloidosis
  calcareous NEC R89.7
    localized — *see* Degeneration, by site
  calcium salt R89.7
  cardiac
    fatty — *see* Degeneration, myocardial
    glycogenic E74.Ø2 [I43]
  corneal — *see* Edema, cornea
  eyelid — *see* Inflammation, eyelid
  glycogen, glycogenic — *see* Disease, glycogen storage
  heart, cardiac
    fatty — *see* Degeneration, myocardial
    glycogenic E74.Ø2 [I43]
  inflammatory in vitreous H43.89
  kidney N28.89
  leukemic — *see* Leukemia
  liver K76.89

Infiltrate, infiltration — *continued*
  liver — *continued*
    fatty — *see* Fatty, liver NEC
    glycogen (*see also* Disease, glycogen storage) E74.Ø3 [K77]
  lung R91.8
    eosinophilic J82
  lymphatic (*see also* Leukemia, lymphatic) C91.9- ✓
    gland I88.9
  muscle, fatty M62.89
  myocardium, myocardial
    fatty — *see* Degeneration, myocardial
    glycogenic E74.Ø2 [I43]
  on chest x-ray R91.8
  pulmonary R91.8
    with eosinophilia J82
  skin (lymphocytic) L98.6
  thymus (gland) (fatty) E32.8
  urine R39.Ø
  vesicant agent
    antineoplastic chemotherapy T8Ø.81Ø ✓
    other agent NEC T8Ø.818 ✓
  vitreous body H43.89
Infirmity R68.89
  senile R54
Inflammation, inflamed, inflammatory (with exudation)
  abducent (nerve) — *see* Strabismus, paralytic, sixth nerve
  accessory sinus (chronic) — *see* Sinusitis
  adrenal (gland) E27.8
  alveoli, teeth M27.3
    scorbutic E54
  anal canal, anus K62.89
  antrum (chronic) — *see* Sinusitis, maxillary
  appendix — *see* Appendicitis
  arachnoid — *see* Meningitis
  areola N61.Ø
    puerperal, postpartum or gestational — *see* Infection, nipple
  areolar tissue NOS LØ8.9
  artery — *see* Arteritis
  auditory meatus (external) — *see* Otitis, externa
  Bartholin's gland N75.8
  bile duct (common) (hepatic) or passage — *see* Cholangitis
  bladder — *see* Cystitis
  bone — *see* Osteomyelitis
  brain (*see also* Encephalitis)
    membrane — *see* Meningitis
  breast N61.Ø
    puerperal, postpartum, gestational — *see* Mastitis, obstetric
  broad ligament — *see* Disease, pelvis, inflammatory
  bronchi — *see* Bronchitis
  catarrhal JØØ
  cecum — *see* Appendicitis
  cerebral (*see also* Encephalitis)
    membrane — *see* Meningitis
  cerebrospinal
    meningococcal A39.Ø
  cervix (uteri) — *see* Cervicitis
  chest J98.8
  chorioretinal H3Ø.9- ✓
    cyclitis — *see* Cyclitis
    disseminated H3Ø.1Ø- ✓
      generalized H3Ø.13- ✓
      peripheral H3Ø.12- ✓
      posterior pole H3Ø.11- ✓
    epitheliopathy — *see* Epitheliopathy
    focal H3Ø.ØØ- ✓
      juxtapapillary H3Ø.Ø1- ✓
      macular H3Ø.Ø4- ✓
      paramacular — *see* Inflammation, chorioretinal, focal, macular
      peripheral H3Ø.Ø3- ✓
      posterior pole H3Ø.Ø2- ✓
    specified type NEC H3Ø.89- ✓
  choroid — *see* Inflammation, chorioretinal
  chronic, postmastoidectomy cavity — *see* Complications, postmastoidectomy, inflammation
  colon — *see* Enteritis
  connective tissue (diffuse) NEC — *see* Disorder, soft tissue, specified type NEC
  cornea — *see* Keratitis
  corpora cavernosa N48.29
  cranial nerve — *see* Disorder, nerve, cranial

✓ **Additional Character Required** — Refer to the Tabular List for Character Selection   ⬏ Subterms under main terms may continue to next column or page

nflammation, inflamed, inflammatory —
continued
Douglas' cul-de-sac or pouch (chronic) N73.0
due to device, implant or graft (*see also* Complications,
by site and type, infection or inflammation)
arterial graft T82.7 ☑
breast (implant) T85.79 ☑
catheter T85.79 ☑
dialysis (renal) T82.7 ☑
intraperitoneal T85.71 ☑
infusion T82.7 ☑
cranial T85.735 ☑
intrathecal T85.735 ☑
spinal (epidural) (subdural) T85.735 ☑
subarachnoid T85.735 ☑
urinary T83.518 ☑
cystostomy T83.510 ☑
Hopkins T83.518 ☑
ileostomy T83.518 ☑
nephrostomy T83.512 ☑
specified NEC T83.518 ☑
urethral indwelling T83.511 ☑
urostomy T83.518 ☑
electronic (electrode) (pulse generator) (stimulator)
bone T84.7 ☑
cardiac T82.7 ☑
nervous system T85.738 ☑
brain T85.731 ☑
cranial nerve T85.732 ☑
gastric nerve T85.732 ☑
neurostimulator generator T85.734 ☑
peripheral nerve T85.732 ☑
sacral nerve T85.732 ☑
spinal cord T85.733 ☑
vagal nerve T85.732 ☑
urinary T83.590 ☑
fixation, internal (orthopedic) NEC — *see* Complication, fixation device, infection
gastrointestinal (bile duct) (esophagus) T85.79 ☑
neurostimulator electrode (lead) T85.732 ☑
genital NEC T83.69 ☑
heart NEC T82.7 ☑
valve (prosthesis) T82.6 ☑
graft T82.7 ☑
joint prosthesis — *see* Complication, joint prosthesis, infection
ocular (corneal graft) (orbital implant) NEC T85.79 ☑
orthopedic NEC T84.7 ☑
penile (cylinder) (pump) (resevoir) T83.61 ☑
specified NEC T85.79 ☑
testicular T83.62 ☑
urinary NEC T83.598 ☑
ileal conduit stent T83.593 ☑
implanted neurostimulation T83.590 ☑
implanted sphincter T83.591 ☑
indwelling ureteral stent T83.592 ☑
nephroureteral stent T83.593 ☑
specified stent NEC T83.593 ☑
vascular NEC T82.7 ☑
ventricular intracranial (communicating) shunt
T85.730 ☑
duodenum K29.80
with bleeding K29.81
dura mater — *see* Meningitis
ear (middle) (*see also* Otitis, media)
external — *see* Otitis, externa
inner — *see* subcategory H83.0 ☑
epididymis — *see* Epididymitis
esophagus K20.9
ethmoidal (sinus) (chronic) — *see* Sinusitis, ethmoidal
eustachian tube (catarrhal) — *see* Salpingitis, eustachian
eyelid H01.9
abscess — *see* Abscess, eyelid
blepharitis — *see* Blepharitis
chalazion — *see* Chalazion
dermatosis (noninfectious) — *see* Dermatosis, eyelid
hordeolum — *see* Hordeolum
specified NEC H01.8
fallopian tube — *see* Salpingo-oophoritis
fascia — *see* Myositis
follicular, pharynx J31.2
frontal (sinus) (chronic) — *see* Sinusitis, frontal
gallbladder — *see* Cholecystitis
gastric — *see* Gastritis
gastrointestinal — *see* Enteritis

Inflammation, inflamed, inflammatory —
continued
genital organ (internal) (diffuse)
female — *see* Disease, pelvis, inflammatory
male N49.9
multiple sites N49.8
specified NEC N49.8
gland (lymph) — *see* Lymphadenitis
glottis — *see* Laryngitis
granular, pharynx J31.2
gum K05.10
nonplaque induced K05.11
plaque induced K05.10
heart — *see* Carditis
hepatic duct — *see* Cholangitis
ileoanal (internal) pouch K91.850
ileum (*see also* Enteritis)
regional or terminal — *see* Enteritis, regional
intestinal pouch K91.850
intestine (any part) — *see* Enteritis
jaw (acute) (bone) (chronic) (lower) (suppurative) (upper) M27.2
joint NEC — *see* Arthritis
sacroiliac M46.1
kidney — *see* Nephritis
knee (joint) M13.169
tuberculous A18.02
labium (majus) (minus) — *see* Vulvitis
lacrimal
gland — *see* Dacryoadenitis
passages (duct) (sac) (*see also* Dacryocystitis)
canaliculitis — *see* Canaliculitis, lacrimal
larynx — *see* Laryngitis
leg NOS L08.9
lip K13.0
liver (capsule) (*see also* Hepatitis)
chronic K73.9
suppurative K75.0
lung (acute) (*see also* Pneumonia)
chronic J98.4
lymph gland or node — *see* Lymphadenitis
lymphatic vessel — *see* Lymphangitis
maxilla, maxillary M27.2
sinus (chronic) — *see* Sinusitis, maxillary
membranes of brain or spinal cord — *see* Meningitis
meninges — *see* Meningitis
mouth K12.1
muscle — *see* Myositis
myocardium — *see* Myocarditis
nasal sinus (chronic) — *see* Sinusitis
nasopharynx — *see* Nasopharyngitis
navel L08.82
nerve NEC — *see* Neuralgia
nipple N61.0
puerperal, postpartum or gestational — *see* Infection, nipple
nose — *see* Rhinitis
oculomotor (nerve) — *see* Strabismus, paralytic, third
nerve
optic nerve — *see* Neuritis, optic
orbit (chronic) H05.10
acute H05.00
abscess — *see* Abscess, orbit
cellulitis — *see* Cellulitis, orbit
osteomyelitis — *see* Osteomyelitis, orbit
periostitis — *see* Periostitis, orbital
tenonitis — *see* Tenonitis, eye
granuloma — *see* Granuloma, orbit
myositis — *see* Myositis, orbital
ovary — *see* Salpingo-oophoritis
oviduct — *see* Salpingo-oophoritis
pancreas (acute) — *see* Pancreatitis
parametrium N73.0
parotid region L08.9
pelvis, female — *see* Disease, pelvis, inflammatory
penis (corpora cavernosa) N48.29
perianal K62.89
pericardium — *see* Pericarditis
perineum (female) (male) L08.9
perirectal K62.89
peritoneum — *see* Peritonitis
periuterine — *see* Disease, pelvis, inflammatory
perivesical — *see* Cystitis
petrous bone (acute) (chronic) — *see* Petrositis
pharynx (acute) — *see* Pharyngitis
pia mater — *see* Meningitis
pleura — *see* Pleurisy

Inflammation, inflamed, inflammatory —
continued
polyp, colon (*see also* Polyp, colon, inflammatory)
K51.40
prostate (*see also* Prostatitis)
specified type NEC N41.8
rectosigmoid — *see* Rectosigmoiditis
rectum (*see also* Proctitis) K62.89
respiratory, upper (*see also* Infection, respiratory, upper)
J06.9
acute, due to radiation J70.0
chronic, due to external agent — *see* condition,
respiratory, chronic, due to
due to
chemicals, gases, fumes or vapors (inhalation)
J68.2
radiation J70.1
retina — *see* Chorioretinitis
retrocecal — *see* Appendicitis
retroperitoneal — *see* Peritonitis
salivary duct or gland (any) (suppurative) — *see*
Sialoadenitis
scorbutic, alveoli, teeth E54
scrotum N49.2
seminal vesicle — *see* Vesiculitis
sigmoid — *see* Enteritis
sinus — *see* Sinusitis
Skene's duct or gland — *see* Urethritis
skin L08.9
spermatic cord N49.1
sphenoidal (sinus) — *see* Sinusitis, sphenoidal
spinal
cord — *see* Encephalitis
membrane — *see* Meningitis
nerve — *see* Disorder, nerve
spine — *see* Spondylopathy, inflammatory
spleen (capsule) D73.89
stomach — *see* Gastritis
subcutaneous tissue L08.9
suprarenal (gland) E27.8
synovial — *see* Tenosynovitis
tendon (sheath) NEC — *see* Tenosynovitis
testis — *see* Orchitis
throat (acute) — *see* Pharyngitis
thymus (gland) E32.8
thyroid (gland) — *see* Thyroiditis
tongue K14.0
tonsil — *see* Tonsillitis
trachea — *see* Tracheitis
trochlear (nerve) — *see* Strabismus, paralytic, fourth
nerve
tubal — *see* Salpingo-oophoritis
tuberculous NEC — *see* Tuberculosis
tubo-ovarian — *see* Salpingo-oophoritis
tunica vaginalis N49.1
tympanic membrane — *see* Tympanitis
umbilicus, umbilical L08.82
uterine ligament — *see* Disease, pelvis, inflammatory
uterus (catarrhal) — *see* Endometritis
uveal tract (anterior) NOS (*see also* Iridocyclitis)
posterior — *see* Chorioretinitis
vagina — *see* Vaginitis
vas deferens N49.1
vein (*see also* Phlebitis)
intracranial or intraspinal (septic) G08
thrombotic I80.9
leg — *see* Phlebitis, leg
lower extremity — *see* Phlebitis, leg
vocal cord J38.3
vulva — *see* Vulvitis
Wharton's duct (suppurative) — *see* Sialoadenitis
Inflation, lung, imperfect (newborn) — *see* Atelectasis
Influenza (bronchial) (epidemic) (respiratory (upper))
(unidentified influenza virus) J11.1
with
digestive manifestations J11.2
encephalopathy J11.81
enteritis J11.2
gastroenteritis J11.2
gastrointestinal manifestations J11.2
laryngitis J11.1
myocarditis J11.82
otitis media J11.83
pharyngitis J11.1
pneumonia J11.00
specified type J11.08
respiratory manifestations NEC J11.1

Influenza — *continued*
- with — *continued*
  - specified manifestation NEC J11.89
- A/H5N1 (*see also* Influenza, due to, identified novel influenza A virus) J09.X2
- avian (*see also* Influenza, due to, identified novel influenza A virus) J09.X2
- bird (*see also* Influenza, due to, identified novel influenza A virus) J09.X2
- novel (2009) H1N1 influenza (*see also* Influenza, due to, identified influenza virus NEC) J10.1
- novel influenza A/H1N1 (*see also* Influenza, due to, identified influenza virus NEC) J10.1
- due to
  - avian (*see also* Influenza, due to, identified novel influenza A virus) J09.X2
  - identified influenza virus NEC J10.1
    - with
      - digestive manifestations J10.2
      - encephalopathy J10.81
      - enteritis J10.2
      - gastroenteritis J10.2
      - gastrointestinal manifestations J10.2
      - laryngitis J10.1
      - myocarditis J10.82
      - otitis media J10.83
      - pharyngitis J10.1
      - pneumonia (unspecified type) J10.00
        - with same identified influenza virus J10.01
        - specified type NEC J10.08
      - respiratory manifestations NEC J10.1
      - specified manifestation NEC J10.89
  - identified novel influenza A virus J09.X2
    - with
      - digestive manifestations J09.X3
      - encephalopathy J09.X9
      - enteritis J09.X3
      - gastroenteritis J09.X3
      - gastrointestinal manifestations J09.X3
      - laryngitis J09.X2
      - myocarditis J09.X9
      - otitis media J09.X9
      - pharyngitis J09.X2
      - pneumonia J09.X1
      - respiratory manifestations NEC J09.X2
      - specified manifestation NEC J09.X9
      - upper respiratory symptoms J09.X2
  - of other animal origin, not bird or swine (*see also* Influenza, due to, identified novel influenza A virus) J09.X2
  - swine (viruses that normally cause infections in pigs) (*see also* Influenza, due to, identified novel influenza A virus) J09.X2
Influenzal — *see* Influenza
Influenza-like disease — *see* Influenza
Infraction, Freiberg's (metatarsal head) — *see* Osteochondrosis, juvenile, metatarsus
Infraeruption of tooth (teeth) M26.34
Infusion complication, misadventure, or reaction — *see* Complications, infusion
Ingestion
- chemical — *see* Table of Drugs and Chemicals, by substance, poisoning
- drug or medicament
  - correct substance properly administered — *see* Table of Drugs and Chemicals, by drug, adverse effect
  - overdose or wrong substance given or taken — *see* Table of Drugs and Chemicals, by drug, poisoning
- foreign body — *see* Foreign body, alimentary tract
- tularemia A21.3
Ingrowing
- hair (beard) L73.1
- nail (finger) (toe) L60.0
Inguinal (*see also* condition)
- testicle Q53.9
  - bilateral Q53.212
  - unilateral Q53.112
Inhalant-induced
- anxiety disorder F18.980
- depressive disorder F18.94
- major neurocognitive disorder F18.97
- mild neurocognitive disorder F18.988
- psychotic disorder F18.959
Inhalation
- anthrax A22.1

Inhalation — *continued*
- flame T27.3
- food or foreign body — *see* Foreign body, by site
- gases, fumes, or vapors NEC T59.9- ☑
  - specified agent — *see* Table of Drugs and Chemicals, by substance
- liquid or vomitus — *see* Asphyxia
- meconium (newborn) P24.00
  - with
    - with respiratory symptoms P24.01
    - pneumonia (pneumonitis) P24.01
- mucus — *see* Asphyxia, mucus
- oil or gasoline (causing suffocation) — *see* Foreign body, by site
- smoke J70.5
  - due to chemicals, gases, fumes and vapors J68.9
- steam — *see* Toxicity, vapors
- stomach contents or secretions — *see* Foreign body, by site
  - due to anesthesia (general) (local) or other sedation T88.59 ☑
    - in labor and delivery O74.0
    - in pregnancy O29.01- ☑
    - postpartum, puerperal O89.01
Inhibition, orgasm
- female F52.31
- male F52.32
Inhibitor, systemic lupus erythematosus (presence of) D68.62
Iniencephalus, iniencephaly Q00.2
Injection, traumatic jet (air) (industrial) (water) (paint or dye) T70.4 ☑
Injury (*see also* specified injury type) T14.90 ☑
- abdomen, abdominal S39.91
  - blood vessel — *see* Injury, blood vessel, abdomen
  - cavity — *see* Injury, intra-abdominal
  - contusion S30.1 ☑
  - internal — *see* Injury, intra-abdominal
  - intra-abdominal organ — *see* Injury, intra-abdominal
  - nerve — *see* Injury, nerve, abdomen
  - open — *see* Wound, open, abdomen
  - specified NEC S39.81 ☑
  - superficial — *see* Injury, superficial, abdomen
- Achilles tendon S86.00- ☑
  - laceration S86.02- ☑
  - specified type NEC S86.09- ☑
  - strain S86.01- ☑
- acoustic, resulting in deafness — *see* Injury, nerve, acoustic
- adrenal (gland) S37.819 ☑
  - contusion S37.812 ☑
  - laceration S37.813 ☑
  - specified type NEC S37.818 ☑
- alveolar (process) S09.93 ☑
- ankle S99.91- ☑
  - contusion — *see* Contusion, ankle
  - dislocation — *see* Dislocation, ankle
  - fracture — *see* Fracture, ankle
  - nerve — *see* Injury, nerve, ankle
  - open — *see* Wound, open, ankle
  - specified type NEC S99.81- ☑
  - sprain — *see* Sprain, ankle
  - superficial — *see* Injury, superficial, ankle
- anterior chamber, eye — *see* Injury, eye, specified site NEC
- anus — *see* Injury, abdomen
- aorta (thoracic) S25.00 ☑
  - abdominal S35.00 ☑
    - laceration (minor) (superficial) S35.01 ☑
      - major S35.02 ☑
    - specified type NEC S35.09 ☑
  - laceration (minor) (superficial) S25.01 ☑
    - major S25.02 ☑
  - specified type NEC S25.09 ☑
- arm (upper) S49.9- ☑
  - blood vessel — *see* Injury, blood vessel, arm
  - contusion — *see* Contusion, arm, upper
  - fracture — *see* Fracture, humerus
  - lower — *see* Injury, forearm
  - muscle — *see* Injury, muscle, shoulder
  - nerve — *see* Injury, nerve, arm
  - open — *see* Wound, open, arm
  - specified type NEC S49.8- ☑
  - superficial — *see* Injury, superficial, arm

Injury — *continued*
- artery (complicating trauma) (*see also* Injury, blood vessel, by site)
  - cerebral or meningeal — *see* Injury, intracranial
- auditory canal (external) (meatus) S09.91 ☑
- auricle, auris, ear S09.91 ☑
- axilla — *see* Injury, shoulder
- back — *see* Injury, back, lower
- bile duct S36.13 ☑
- birth (*see also* Birth, injury) P15.9
- bladder (sphincter) S37.20 ☑
  - at delivery O71.5
  - contusion S37.22 ☑
  - laceration S37.23 ☑
  - obstetrical trauma O71.5
  - specified type NEC S37.29 ☑
- blast (air) (hydraulic) (immersion) (underwater) NEC T14.8 ☑
  - acoustic nerve trauma — *see* Injury, nerve, acoustic
  - bladder — *see* Injury, bladder
  - brain — *see* Concussion
  - colon — *see* Injury, intestine, large
  - ear (primary) S09.31- ☑
    - secondary S09.39- ☑
  - generalized T70.8 ☑
  - lung — *see* Injury, intrathoracic, lung
  - multiple body organs T70.8 ☑
  - peritoneum S36.81 ☑
  - rectum S36.61 ☑
  - retroperitoneum S36.898 ☑
  - small intestine S36.419 ☑
    - duodenum S36.410 ☑
    - specified site NEC S36.418 ☑
  - specified
    - intra-abdominal organ NEC S36.898 ☑
    - pelvic organ NEC S37.899 ☑
- blood vessel NEC T14.8 ☑
  - abdomen S35.9 ☑
    - aorta — *see* Injury, aorta, abdominal
    - celiac artery — *see* Injury, blood vessel, celiac artery
    - iliac vessel — *see* Injury, blood vessel, iliac
    - laceration S35.91 ☑
    - mesenteric vessel — *see* Injury, mesenteric
    - portal vein — *see* Injury, blood vessel, portal vein
    - renal vessel — *see* Injury, blood vessel, renal
    - specified vessel NEC S35.8X- ☑
    - splenic vessel — *see* Injury, blood vessel, splenic
    - vena cava — *see* Injury, vena cava, inferior
  - ankle — *see* Injury, blood vessel, foot
  - aorta (abdominal) (thoracic) — *see* Injury, aorta
  - arm (upper) NEC S45.90- ☑
    - forearm — *see* Injury, blood vessel, forearm
    - laceration S45.91- ☑
    - specified
      - site NEC S45.80- ☑
        - laceration S45.81- ☑
        - specified type NEC S45.89- ☑
      - type NEC S45.99- ☑
    - superficial vein S45.30- ☑
      - laceration S45.31- ☑
      - specified type NEC S45.39- ☑
  - axillary
    - artery S45.00- ☑
      - laceration S45.01- ☑
      - specified type NEC S45.09- ☑
    - vein S45.20- ☑
      - laceration S45.21- ☑
      - specified type NEC S45.29- ☑
  - azygos vein — *see* Injury, blood vessel, thoracic, specified site NEC
  - brachial
    - artery S45.10- ☑
      - laceration S45.11- ☑
      - specified type NEC S45.19- ☑
    - vein S45.20- ☑
      - laceration S45.219 ☑
      - specified type NEC S45.29- ☑
  - carotid artery (common) (external) (internal, extracranial) S15.00- ☑
    - internal, intracranial S06.8- ☑
    - laceration (minor) (superficial) S15.01- ☑
      - major S15.02- ☑
    - specified type NEC S15.09- ☑
  - celiac artery S35.219 ☑
    - branch S35.299 ☑

☑ **Additional Character Required** — Refer to the Tabular List for Character Selection ▽ Subterms under main terms may continue to next column or page

Injury — *continued*
blood vessel — *continued*
  celiac artery — *continued*
    branch — *continued*
      laceration (minor) (superficial) S35.291 ☑
        major S35.292 ☑
        specified NEC S35.298 ☑
    laceration (minor) (superficial) S35.211 ☑
      major S35.212 ☑
    specified type NEC S35.218 ☑
  cerebral — *see* Injury, intracranial
  deep plantar — *see* Injury, blood vessel, plantar artery
  digital (hand) — *see* Injury, blood vessel, finger
  dorsal
    artery (foot) S95.00- ☑
      laceration S95.01- ☑
      specified type NEC S95.09- ☑
    vein (foot) S95.20- ☑
      laceration S95.21- ☑
      specified type NEC S95.29- ☑
  due to accidental laceration during procedure — *see* Laceration, accidental complicating surgery
  extremity — *see* Injury, blood vessel, limb
  femoral
    artery (common) (superficial) S75.00- ☑
      laceration (minor) (superficial) S75.01- ☑
        major S75.02- ☑
      specified type NEC S75.09- ☑
    vein (hip level) (thigh level) S75.10- ☑
      laceration (minor) (superficial) S75.11- ☑
        major S75.12- ☑
      specified type NEC S75.19- ☑
  finger S65.50- ☑
    index S65.50- ☑
      laceration S65.51- ☑
      specified type NEC S65.59- ☑
    laceration S65.51- ☑
    little S65.50- ☑
      laceration S65.51- ☑
      specified type NEC S65.59- ☑
    middle S65.50- ☑
      laceration S65.51- ☑
      specified type NEC S65.59- ☑
    specified type NEC S65.59- ☑
    thumb — *see* Injury, blood vessel, thumb
  foot S95.90- ☑
    dorsal
      artery — *see* Injury, blood vessel, dorsal, artery
      vein — *see* Injury, blood vessel, dorsal, vein
    laceration S95.91- ☑
    plantar artery — *see* Injury, blood vessel, plantar artery
    specified
      site NEC S95.80- ☑
        laceration S95.81- ☑
        specified type NEC S95.89- ☑
      specified type NEC S95.99- ☑
  forearm S55.90- ☑
    laceration S55.91- ☑
    radial artery — *see* Injury, blood vessel, radial artery
    specified
      site NEC S55.80- ☑
        laceration S55.81- ☑
        specified type NEC S55.89- ☑
      type NEC S55.99- ☑
    ulnar artery — *see* Injury, blood vessel, ulnar artery
    vein S55.20- ☑
      laceration S55.21- ☑
      specified type NEC S55.29- ☑
  gastric
    artery — *see* Injury, mesenteric, artery, branch
    vein — *see* Injury, blood vessel, abdomen
  gastroduodenal artery — *see* Injury, mesenteric, artery, branch
  greater saphenous vein (lower leg level) S85.30- ☑
    hip (and thigh) level S75.20- ☑
      laceration (minor) (superficial) S75.21- ☑
        major S75.22- ☑
      specified type NEC S75.29- ☑
    laceration S85.31- ☑
    specified type NEC S85.39- ☑

Injury — *continued*
blood vessel — *continued*
  hand (level) S65.90- ☑
    finger — *see* Injury, blood vessel, finger
    laceration S65.91- ☑
    palmar arch — *see* Injury, blood vessel, palmar arch
    radial artery — *see* Injury, blood vessel, radial artery, hand
    specified
      site NEC S65.80- ☑
        laceration S65.81- ☑
        specified type NEC S65.89- ☑
      type NEC S65.99- ☑
    thumb — *see* Injury, blood vessel, thumb
    ulnar artery — *see* Injury, blood vessel, ulnar artery, hand
  head S09.0 ☑
    intracranial — *see* Injury, intracranial
    multiple S09.0 ☑
  hepatic
    artery — *see* Injury, mesenteric, artery
    vein — *see* Injury, vena cava, inferior
  hip S75.90- ☑
    femoral artery — *see* Injury, blood vessel, femoral, artery
    femoral vein — *see* Injury, blood vessel, femoral, vein
    greater saphenous vein — *see* Injury, blood vessel, greater saphenous, hip level
    laceration S75.91- ☑
    specified
      site NEC S75.80- ☑
        laceration S75.81- ☑
        specified type NEC S75.89- ☑
      type NEC S75.99- ☑
  hypogastric (artery) (vein) — *see* Injury, blood vessel, iliac
  iliac S35.5- ☑
    artery S35.51- ☑
    specified vessel NEC S35.5- ☑
    uterine vessel — *see* Injury, blood vessel, uterine
    vein S35.51- ☑
  innominate — *see* Injury, blood vessel, thoracic, innominate
  intercostal (artery) (vein) — *see* Injury, blood vessel, thoracic, intercostal
  jugular vein (external) S15.20- ☑
    internal S15.30- ☑
      laceration (minor) (superficial) S15.31- ☑
        major S15.32- ☑
      specified type NEC S15.39- ☑
    laceration (minor) (superficial) S15.21- ☑
      major S15.22- ☑
    specified type NEC S15.29- ☑
  leg (level) (lower) S85.90- ☑
    greater saphenous — *see* Injury, blood vessel, greater saphenous
    laceration S85.91- ☑
    lesser saphenous — *see* Injury, blood vessel, lesser saphenous
    peroneal artery — *see* Injury, blood vessel, peroneal artery
    popliteal
      artery — *see* Injury, blood vessel, popliteal, artery
      vein — *see* Injury, blood vessel, popliteal, vein
    specified
      site NEC S85.80- ☑
        laceration S85.81- ☑
        specified type NEC S85.89- ☑
      type NEC S85.99- ☑
    thigh — *see* Injury, blood vessel, hip
    tibial artery — *see* Injury, blood vessel, tibial artery
  lesser saphenous vein (lower leg level) S85.40- ☑
    laceration S85.41- ☑
    specified type NEC S85.49- ☑
  limb
    lower — *see* Injury, blood vessel, leg
    upper — *see* Injury, blood vessel, arm
  lower back — *see* Injury, blood vessel, abdomen
    specified NEC — *see* Injury, blood vessel, abdomen, specified, site NEC
  mammary (artery) (vein) — *see* Injury, blood vessel, thoracic, specified site NEC

Injury — *continued*
blood vessel — *continued*
  mesenteric (inferior) (superior)
    artery — *see* Injury, mesenteric, artery
    vein — *see* Injury, blood vessel, mesenteric, vein
  neck S15.9 ☑
    specified site NEC S15.8 ☑
  ovarian (artery) (vein) — *see* subcategory S35.8 ☑
  palmar arch (superficial) S65.20- ☑
    deep S65.30- ☑
      laceration S65.31- ☑
      specified type NEC S65.39- ☑
    laceration S65.21- ☑
    specified type NEC S65.29- ☑
  pelvis — *see* Injury, blood vessel, abdomen
    specified NEC — *see* Injury, blood vessel, abdomen, specified, site NEC
  peroneal artery S85.20- ☑
    laceration S85.21- ☑
    specified type NEC S85.29- ☑
  plantar artery (deep) (foot) S95.10- ☑
    laceration S95.11- ☑
    specified type NEC S95.19- ☑
  popliteal
    artery S85.00- ☑
      laceration S85.01- ☑
      specified type NEC S85.09- ☑
    vein S85.50- ☑
      laceration S85.51- ☑
      specified type NEC S85.59- ☑
  portal vein S35.319 ☑
    laceration S35.311 ☑
    specified type NEC S35.318 ☑
  precerebral — *see* Injury, blood vessel, neck
  pulmonary (artery) (vein) — *see* Injury, blood vessel, thoracic, pulmonary
  radial artery (forearm level) S55.10- ☑
    hand and wrist (level) S65.10- ☑
      laceration S65.11- ☑
      specified type NEC S65.19- ☑
    laceration S55.11- ☑
    specified type NEC S55.19- ☑
  renal
    artery S35.40- ☑
      laceration S35.41- ☑
      specified S35.49- ☑
    vein S35.40- ☑
      laceration S35.41- ☑
      specified NEC S35.49- ☑
  saphenous vein (greater) (lower leg level) — *see* Injury, blood vessel, greater saphenous
    hip and thigh level — *see* Injury, blood vessel, greater saphenous, hip level
    lesser — *see* Injury, blood vessel, lesser saphenous
  shoulder
    specified NEC — *see* Injury, blood vessel, arm, specified site NEC
    superficial vein — *see* Injury, blood vessel, arm, superficial vein
  specified NEC T14.8 ☑
  splenic
    artery — *see* Injury, blood vessel, celiac artery, branch
    vein S35.329 ☑
      laceration S35.321 ☑
      specified NEC S35.328 ☑
  subclavian — *see* Injury, blood vessel, thoracic, innominate
  thigh — *see* Injury, blood vessel, hip
  thoracic S25.90 ☑
    aorta S25.00 ☑
      laceration (minor) (superficial) S25.01 ☑
        major S25.02 ☑
      specified type NEC S25.09 ☑
    azygos vein — *see* Injury, blood vessel, thoracic, specified, site NEC
    innominate
      artery S25.10- ☑
        laceration (minor) (superficial) S25.11- ☑
          major S25.12- ☑
        specified type NEC S25.19- ☑
      vein S25.30- ☑
        laceration (minor) (superficial) S25.31- ☑
          major S25.32- ☑
        specified type NEC S25.39- ☑

Injury — *continued*
  blood vessel — *continued*
    thoracic — *continued*
      intercostal S25.50- ☑
        laceration S25.51- ☑
        specified type NEC S25.59- ☑
      laceration S25.91 ☑
      mammary vessel — *see* Injury, blood vessel, thoracic, specified, site NEC
      pulmonary S25.40- ☑
        laceration (minor) (superficial) S25.41- ☑
          major S25.42- ☑
        specified type NEC S25.49- ☑
      specified
        site NEC S25.80- ☑
          laceration S25.81 ☑
          specified type NEC S25.89 ☑
        type NEC S25.99 ☑
      subclavian — *see* Injury, blood vessel, thoracic, innominate
      vena cava (superior) S25.20 ☑
        laceration (minor) (superficial) S25.21 ☑
          major S25.22 ☑
        specified type NEC S25.29 ☑
    thumb S65.40- ☑
      laceration S65.41- ☑
      specified type NEC S65.49- ☑
    tibial artery S85.10- ☑
      anterior S85.13- ☑
        laceration S85.14- ☑
        specified injury NEC S85.15- ☑
      laceration S85.11- ☑
      posterior S85.16- ☑
        laceration S85.17- ☑
        specified injury NEC S85.18- ☑
      specified injury NEC S85.12- ☑
    ulnar artery (forearm level) S55.00- ☑
      hand and wrist (level) S65.00- ☑
        laceration S65.01- ☑
        specified type NEC S65.09- ☑
      laceration S55.01- ☑
      specified type NEC S55.09- ☑
    upper arm (level) — *see* Injury, blood vessel, arm
      superficial vein — *see* Injury, blood vessel, arm, superficial vein
    uterine S35.5- ☑
      artery S35.53- ☑
      vein S35.53- ☑
    vena cava — *see* Injury, vena cava
    vertebral artery S15.10- ☑
      laceration (minor) (superficial) S15.11- ☑
        major S15.12- ☑
      specified type NEC S15.19- ☑
    wrist (level) — *see* Injury, blood vessel, hand
  brachial plexus S14.3 ☑
    newborn P14.3
  brain (traumatic) S06.9- ☑
    diffuse (axonal) S06.2X- ☑
    focal S06.30- ☑
  brainstem S06.38- ☑
  breast NOS S29.9 ☑
  broad ligament — *see* Injury, pelvic organ, specified site NEC
  bronchus, bronchi — *see* Injury, intrathoracic, bronchus
  brow S09.90 ☑
  buttock S39.92 ☑
  canthus, eye S05.90 ☑
  cardiac plexus — *see* Injury, nerve, thorax, sympathetic
  cauda equina S34.3 ☑
  cavernous sinus — *see* Injury, intracranial
  cecum — *see* Injury, colon
  celiac ganglion or plexus — *see* Injury, nerve, lumbosacral, sympathetic
  cerebellum — *see* Injury, intracranial
  cerebral — *see* Injury, intracranial
  cervix (uteri) — *see* Injury, uterus
  cheek (wall) S09.93 ☑
  chest — *see* Injury, thorax
  childbirth (newborn) (*see also* Birth, injury)
    maternal NEC O71.9
  chin S09.93 ☑
  choroid (eye) — *see* Injury, eye, specified site NEC
  clitoris S39.94 ☑
  coccyx (*see also* Injury, back, lower)
    complicating delivery O71.6
  colon — *see* Injury, intestine, large

Injury — *continued*
  common bile duct — *see* Injury, liver
  conjunctiva (superficial) — *see* Injury, eye, conjunctiva
  conus medullaris — *see* Injury, spinal, sacral
  cord
    spermatic (pelvic region) S37.898 ☑
      scrotal region S39.848 ☑
    spinal — *see* Injury, spinal cord, by region
  cornea — *see* Injury, eye, specified site NEC
    abrasion — *see* Injury, eye, cornea, abrasion
  cortex (cerebral) (*see also* Injury, intracranial)
    visual — *see* Injury, nerve, optic
  costal region NEC S29.9 ☑
  costochondral NEC S29.9 ☑
  cranial
    cavity — *see* Injury, intracranial
    nerve — *see* Injury, nerve, cranial
  crushing — *see* Crush
  cutaneous sensory nerve
  cystic duct — *see* Injury, liver
  deep tissue — *see* Contusion, by site
    meaning pressure ulcer — *see* Ulcer, pressure, unstageable, by site
  delivery (newborn) P15.9
    maternal NEC O71.9
  Descemet's membrane — *see* Injury, eyeball, penetrating
  diaphragm — *see* Injury, intrathoracic, diaphragm
  duodenum — *see* Injury, intestine, small, duodenum
  ear (auricle) (external) (canal) S09.91 ☑
    abrasion — *see* Abrasion, ear
    bite — *see* Bite, ear
    blister — *see* Blister, ear
    bruise — *see* Contusion, ear
    contusion — *see* Contusion, ear
    external constriction — *see* Constriction, external, ear
    hematoma — *see* Hematoma, ear
    inner — *see* Injury, ear, middle
    laceration — *see* Laceration, ear
    middle S09.30- ☑
      blast — *see* Injury, blast, ear
      specified NEC S09.39- ☑
    puncture — *see* Puncture, ear
    superficial — *see* Injury, superficial, ear
  eighth cranial nerve (acoustic or auditory) — *see* Injury, nerve, acoustic
  elbow S59.90- ☑
    contusion — *see* Contusion, elbow
    dislocation — *see* Dislocation, elbow
    fracture — *see* Fracture, ulna, upper end
    open — *see* Wound, open, elbow
    specified NEC S59.80- ☑
    sprain — *see* Sprain, elbow
    superficial — *see* Injury, superficial, elbow
  eleventh cranial nerve (accessory) — *see* Injury, nerve, accessory
  epididymis S39.94 ☑
  epigastric region S39.91 ☑
  epiglottis NEC S19.89 ☑
  esophageal plexus — *see* Injury, nerve, thorax, sympathetic
  esophagus (thoracic part) (*see also* Injury, intrathoracic, esophagus)
    cervical NEC S19.85 ☑
  eustachian tube S09.30 ☑
  eye S05.9- ☑
    avulsion S05.7- ☑
    ball — *see* Injury, eyeball
    conjunctiva S05.0- ☑
    cornea
      abrasion S05.0- ☑
      laceration S05.3- ☑
        with prolapse S05.2- ☑
    lacrimal apparatus S05.8X- ☑
    orbit penetration S05.4- ☑
    specified site NEC S05.8X- ☑
  eyeball S05.8X- ☑
    contusion S05.1- ☑
    penetrating S05.6- ☑
      with
        foreign body S05.5- ☑
        prolapse or loss of intraocular tissue S05.2- ☑
      without prolapse or loss of intraocular tissue S05.3- ☑
    specified type NEC S05.8- ☑

Injury — *continued*
  eyebrow S09.93 ☑
  eyelid S09.93 ☑
    abrasion — *see* Abrasion, eyelid
    contusion — *see* Contusion, eyelid
    open — *see* Wound, open, eyelid
  face S09.93 ☑
  fallopian tube S37.509 ☑
    bilateral S37.502 ☑
      blast injury S37.512 ☑
      contusion S37.522 ☑
      laceration S37.532 ☑
      specified type NEC S37.592 ☑
    blast injury (primary) S37.519 ☑
      bilateral S37.512 ☑
      secondary — *see* Injury, fallopian tube, specified type NEC
      unilateral S37.511 ☑
    contusion S37.529 ☑
      bilateral S37.522 ☑
      unilateral S37.521 ☑
    laceration S37.539 ☑
      bilateral S37.532 ☑
      unilateral S37.531 ☑
    specified type NEC S37.599 ☑
      bilateral S37.592 ☑
      unilateral S37.591 ☑
    unilateral S37.501 ☑
      blast injury S37.511 ☑
      contusion S37.521 ☑
      laceration S37.531 ☑
      specified type NEC S37.591 ☑
  fascia — *see* Injury, muscle
  fifth cranial nerve (trigeminal) — *see* Injury, nerve, trigeminal
  finger (nail) S69.9- ☑
    blood vessel — *see* Injury, blood vessel, finger
    contusion — *see* Contusion, finger
    dislocation — *see* Dislocation, finger
    fracture — *see* Fracture, finger
    muscle — *see* Injury, muscle, finger
    nerve — *see* Injury, nerve, digital, finger
    open — *see* Wound, open, finger
    specified NEC S69.8- ☑
    sprain — *see* Sprain, finger
    superficial — *see* Injury, superficial, finger
  first cranial nerve (olfactory) — *see* Injury, nerve, olfactory
  flank — *see* Injury, abdomen
  foot S99.92- ☑
    blood vessel — *see* Injury, blood vessel, foot
    contusion — *see* Contusion, foot
    dislocation — *see* Dislocation, foot
    fracture — *see* Fracture, foot
    muscle — *see* Injury, muscle, foot
    open — *see* Wound, open, foot
    specified type NEC S99.82- ☑
    sprain — *see* Sprain, foot
    superficial — *see* Injury, superficial, foot
  forceps NOS P15.9
  forearm S59.91- ☑
    blood vessel — *see* Injury, blood vessel, forearm
    contusion — *see* Contusion, forearm
    fracture — *see* Fracture, forearm
    muscle — *see* Injury, muscle, forearm
    nerve — *see* Injury, nerve, forearm
    open — *see* Wound, open, forearm
    specified NEC S59.81- ☑
    superficial — *see* Injury, superficial, forearm
  forehead S09.90 ☑
  fourth cranial nerve (trochlear) — *see* Injury, nerve, trochlear
  gallbladder S36.129 ☑
    contusion S36.122 ☑
    laceration S36.123 ☑
    specified NEC S36.128 ☑
  ganglion
    celiac, coeliac — *see* Injury, nerve, lumbosacral, sympathetic
    gasserian — *see* Injury, nerve, trigeminal
    stellate — *see* Injury, nerve, thorax, sympathetic
    thoracic sympathetic — *see* Injury, nerve, thorax, sympathetic
  gasserian ganglion — *see* Injury, nerve, trigeminal
  gastric artery — *see* Injury, blood vessel, celiac artery branch

Injury — *continued*
  gastroduodenal artery — *see* Injury, blood vessel, celiac
    artery, branch
  gastrointestinal tract — *see* Injury, intra-abdominal
    with open wound into abdominal cavity — *see*
      Wound, open, with penetration into peri-
      toneal cavity
    colon — *see* Injury, intestine, large
    rectum — *see* Injury, intestine, large, rectum
      with open wound into abdominal cavity
      S36.61 ☑
    small intestine — *see* Injury, intestine, small
    specified site NEC — *see* Injury, intra-abdominal,
      specified, site NEC
    stomach — *see* Injury, stomach
  genital organ(s)
    external S39.94 ☑
      specified NEC S39.848 ☑
    internal S37.90 ☑
      fallopian tube — *see* Injury, fallopian tube
      ovary — *see* Injury, ovary
      prostate — *see* Injury, prostate
      seminal vesicle — *see* Injury, pelvis, organ,
        specified site NEC
      uterus — *see* Injury, uterus
      vas deferens — *see* Injury, pelvis, organ, specified
        site NEC
    obstetrical trauma O71.9
  gland
    lacrimal laceration — *see* Injury, eye, specified site
      NEC
    salivary S09.93 ☑
    thyroid NEC S19.84 ☑
  globe (eye) S05.90 ☑
    specified NEC S05.8X- ☑
  groin — *see* Injury, abdomen
  gum S09.90 ☑
  hand S69.9- ☑
    blood vessel — *see* Injury, blood vessel, hand
    contusion — *see* Contusion, hand
    fracture — *see* Fracture, hand
    muscle — *see* Injury, muscle, hand
    nerve — *see* Injury, nerve, hand
    open — *see* Wound, open, hand
    specified NEC S69.8- ☑
    sprain — *see* Sprain, hand
    superficial — *see* Injury, superficial, hand
  head S09.90 ☑
    with loss of consciousness S06.9- ☑
    specified NEC S09.8 ☑
  heart S26.90 ☑
    with hemopericardium S26.00 ☑
      contusion S26.01 ☑
      laceration (mild) S26.020 ☑
        major S26.022 ☑
        moderate S26.021 ☑
      specified type NEC S26.09 ☑
    contusion S26.91 ☑
    laceration S26.92 ☑
    specified type NEC S26.99 ☑
    without hemopericardium S26.10 ☑
      contusion S26.11 ☑
      laceration S26.12 ☑
      specified type NEC S26.19 ☑
  heel — *see* Injury, foot
  hepatic
    artery — *see* Injury, blood vessel, celiac artery,
      branch
    duct — *see* Injury, liver
    vein — *see* Injury, vena cava, inferior
  hip S79.91- ☑
    blood vessel — *see* Injury, blood vessel, hip
    contusion — *see* Contusion, hip
    dislocation — *see* Dislocation, hip
    fracture — *see* Fracture, femur, neck
    muscle — *see* Injury, muscle, hip
    nerve — *see* Injury, nerve, hip
    open — *see* Wound, open, hip
    specified NEC S79.81- ☑
    sprain — *see* Sprain, hip
    superficial — *see* Injury, superficial, hip
  hymen S39.94 ☑
  hypogastric
    blood vessel — *see* Injury, blood vessel, iliac
    plexus — *see* Injury, nerve, lumbosacral, sympathet-
      ic

Injury — *continued*
  ileum — *see* Injury, intestine, small
  iliac region S39.91 ☑
  instrumental (during surgery) — *see* Laceration, acci-
    dental complicating surgery
    birth injury — *see* Birth, injury
    nonsurgical — *see* Injury, by site
    obstetrical O71.9
      bladder O71.5
      cervix O71.3
      high vaginal O71.4
      perineal NOS O70.9
      urethra O71.5
      uterus O71.5
        with rupture or perforation O71.1
  internal T14.8 ☑
    aorta — *see* Injury, aorta
    bladder (sphincter) — *see* Injury, bladder
      with
        ectopic or molar pregnancy O08.6
        following ectopic or molar pregnancy O08.6
        obstetrical trauma O71.5
    bronchus, bronchi — *see* Injury, intrathoracic,
      bronchus
    cecum — *see* Injury, intestine, large
    cervix (uteri) (*see also* Injury, uterus)
      with ectopic or molar pregnancy O08.6
      following ectopic or molar pregnancy O08.6
      obstetrical trauma O71.3
    chest — *see* Injury, intrathoracic
    gastrointestinal tract — *see* Injury, intra-abdominal
    heart — *see* Injury, heart
    intestine NEC — *see* Injury, intestine
    intrauterine — *see* Injury, uterus
    mesentery — *see* Injury, intra-abdominal, specified,
      site NEC
    pelvis, pelvic (organ) S37.90 ☑
      following ectopic or molar pregnancy (subse-
        quent episode) O08.6
      obstetrical trauma NEC O71.5
        rupture or perforation O71.1
      specified NEC S39.83 ☑
    rectum — *see* Injury, intestine, large, rectum
    stomach — *see* Injury, stomach
    ureter — *see* Injury, ureter
    urethra (sphincter) following ectopic or molar
      pregnancy O08.6
    uterus — *see* Injury, uterus
  interscapular area — *see* Injury, thorax
  intestine
    large S36.509 ☑
      ascending (right) S36.500 ☑
        blast injury (primary) S36.510 ☑
          secondary S36.590 ☑
        contusion S36.520 ☑
        laceration S36.530 ☑
        specified type NEC S36.590 ☑
      blast injury (primary) S36.519 ☑
        ascending (right) S36.510 ☑
        descending (left) S36.512 ☑
        rectum S36.61 ☑
        sigmoid S36.513 ☑
        specified site NEC S36.518 ☑
        transverse S36.511 ☑
      contusion S36.529 ☑
        ascending (right) S36.520 ☑
        descending (left) S36.522 ☑
        rectum S36.62 ☑
        sigmoid S36.523 ☑
        specified site NEC S36.528 ☑
        transverse S36.521 ☑
      descending (left) S36.502 ☑
        blast injury (primary) S36.512 ☑
          secondary S36.592 ☑
        contusion S36.522 ☑
        laceration S36.532 ☑
        specified type NEC S36.592 ☑
      laceration S36.539 ☑
        ascending (right) S36.530 ☑
        descending (left) S36.532 ☑
        rectum S36.63 ☑
        sigmoid S36.533 ☑
        specified site NEC S36.538 ☑
        transverse S36.531 ☑
      rectum S36.60 ☑
        blast injury (primary) S36.61 ☑
          secondary S36.69 ☑

Injury — *continued*
  intestine — *continued*
    large — *continued*
      rectum — *continued*
        contusion S36.62 ☑
        laceration S36.63 ☑
        specified type NEC S36.69 ☑
      sigmoid S36.503 ☑
        blast injury (primary) S36.513 ☑
          secondary S36.593 ☑
        contusion S36.523 ☑
        laceration S36.533 ☑
        specified type NEC S36.593 ☑
      specified
        site NEC S36.508 ☑
          blast injury (primary) S36.518 ☑
            secondary S36.598 ☑
          contusion S36.528 ☑
          laceration S36.538 ☑
          specified type NEC S36.598 ☑
        type NEC S36.599 ☑
          ascending (right) S36.590 ☑
          descending (left) S36.592 ☑
          rectum S36.69 ☑
          sigmoid S36.593 ☑
          specified site NEC S36.598 ☑
          transverse S36.591 ☑
      transverse S36.501 ☑
        blast injury (primary) S36.511 ☑
          secondary S36.591 ☑
        contusion S36.521 ☑
        laceration S36.531 ☑
        specified type NEC S36.591 ☑
    small S36.409 ☑
      blast injury (primary) S36.419 ☑
        duodenum S36.410 ☑
        secondary S36.499 ☑
          duodenum S36.490 ☑
          specified site NEC S36.498 ☑
        specified site NEC S36.418 ☑
      contusion S36.429 ☑
        duodenum S36.420 ☑
        specified site NEC S36.428 ☑
      duodenum S36.400 ☑
        blast injury (primary) S36.410 ☑
          secondary S36.490 ☑
        contusion S36.420 ☑
        laceration S36.430 ☑
        specified NEC S36.490 ☑
      laceration S36.439 ☑
        duodenum S36.430 ☑
        specified site NEC S36.438 ☑
      specified
        site NEC S36.408 ☑
        type NEC S36.499 ☑
          duodenum S36.490 ☑
          specified site NEC S36.498 ☑
  intra-abdominal S36.90 ☑
    adrenal gland — *see* Injury, adrenal gland
    bladder — *see* Injury, bladder
    colon — *see* Injury, intestine, large
    contusion S36.92 ☑
    fallopian tube — *see* Injury, fallopian tube
    gallbladder — *see* Injury, gallbladder
    intestine — *see* Injury, intestine
    kidney — *see* Injury, kidney
    laceration S36.93 ☑
    liver — *see* Injury, liver
    ovary — *see* Injury, ovary
    pancreas — *see* Injury, pancreas
    pelvic NOS S37.90 ☑
    peritoneum — *see* Injury, intra-abdominal, specified,
      site NEC
    prostate — *see* Injury, prostate
    rectum — *see* Injury, intestine, large, rectum
    retroperitoneum — *see* Injury, intra-abdominal,
      specified, site NEC
    seminal vesicle — *see* Injury, pelvis, organ, specified
      site NEC
    small intestine — *see* Injury, intestine, small
    specified
      pelvic S37.90 ☑
      specified
        site NEC S37.899 ☑
          specified type NEC S37.898 ☑
        type NEC S37.99 ☑

Injury — *continued*
  intra-abdominal — *continued*
    specified — *continued*
      site NEC S36.899 ☑
        contusion S36.892 ☑
        laceration S36.893 ☑
        specified type NEC S36.898 ☑
      type NEC S36.99 ☑
    spleen — *see* Injury, spleen
    stomach — *see* Injury, stomach
    ureter — *see* Injury, ureter
    urethra — *see* Injury, urethra
    uterus — *see* Injury, uterus
    vas deferens — *see* Injury, pelvis, organ, specified site NEC
  intracranial (traumatic) S06.9- ☑
    cerebellar hemorrhage, traumatic — *see* Injury, intracranial, focal
    cerebral edema, traumatic S06.1X- ☑
      diffuse S06.1X- ☑
      focal S06.1X- ☑
    diffuse (axonal) S06.2X- ☑
    epidural hemorrhage (traumatic) S06.4X- ☑
    focal brain injury S06.30- ☑
      contusion — *see* Contusion, cerebral
      laceration — *see* Laceration, cerebral
    intracerebral hemorrhage, traumatic S06.36- ☑
      left side S06.35- ☑
      right side S06.34- ☑
    subarachnoid hemorrhage, traumatic S06.6X- ☑
    subdural hemorrhage, traumatic S06.5X- ☑
  intraocular — *see* Injury, eyeball, penetrating
  intrathoracic S27.9 ☑
    bronchus S27.409 ☑
      bilateral S27.402 ☑
      blast injury (primary) S27.419 ☑
        bilateral S27.412 ☑
        secondary — *see* Injury, intrathoracic, bronchus, specified type NEC
        unilateral S27.411 ☑
      contusion S27.429 ☑
        bilateral S27.422 ☑
        unilateral S27.421 ☑
      laceration S27.439 ☑
        bilateral S27.432 ☑
        unilateral S27.431 ☑
      specified type NEC S27.499 ☑
        bilateral S27.492 ☑
        unilateral S27.491 ☑
      unilateral S27.401 ☑
    diaphragm S27.809 ☑
      contusion S27.802 ☑
      laceration S27.803 ☑
      specified type NEC S27.808 ☑
    esophagus (thoracic) S27.819 ☑
      contusion S27.812 ☑
      laceration S27.813 ☑
      specified type NEC S27.818 ☑
    heart — *see* Injury, heart
    hemopneumothorax S27.2 ☑
    hemothorax S27.1 ☑
    lung S27.309 ☑
      aspiration J69.0
      bilateral S27.302 ☑
      blast injury (primary) S27.319 ☑
        bilateral S27.312 ☑
        secondary — *see* Injury, intrathoracic, lung, specified type NEC
        unilateral S27.311 ☑
      contusion S27.329 ☑
        bilateral S27.322 ☑
        unilateral S27.321 ☑
      laceration S27.339 ☑
        bilateral S27.332 ☑
        unilateral S27.331 ☑
      specified type NEC S27.399 ☑
        bilateral S27.392 ☑
        unilateral S27.391 ☑
      unilateral S27.301 ☑
    pleura S27.60 ☑
      laceration S27.63 ☑
      specified type NEC S27.69 ☑
    pneumothorax S27.0 ☑
    specified organ NEC S27.899 ☑
      contusion S27.892 ☑
      laceration S27.893 ☑

Injury — *continued*
  intrathoracic — *continued*
    specified organ — *continued*
      specified type NEC S27.898 ☑
    thoracic duct — *see* Injury, intrathoracic, specified organ NEC
    thymus gland — *see* Injury, intrathoracic, specified organ NEC
    trachea, thoracic S27.50 ☑
      blast (primary) S27.51 ☑
      contusion S27.52 ☑
      laceration S27.53 ☑
      specified type NEC S27.59 ☑
  iris — *see* Injury, eye, specified site NEC
    penetrating — *see* Injury, eyeball, penetrating
  jaw S09.93 ☑
  jejunum — *see* Injury, intestine, small
  joint NOS T14.8 ☑
    old or residual — *see* Disorder, joint, specified type NEC
  kidney S37.00- ☑
    acute (nontraumatic) N17.9
    contusion — *see* Contusion, kidney
    laceration — *see* Laceration, kidney
    specified NEC S37.09- ☑
  knee S89.9- ☑
    contusion — *see* Contusion, knee
    dislocation — *see* Dislocation, knee
    meniscus (lateral) (medial) — *see* Sprain, knee, specified site NEC
      old injury or tear — *see* Derangement, knee, meniscus, due to old injury
    open — *see* Wound, open, knee
    specified NEC S89.8- ☑
    sprain — *see* Sprain, knee
    superficial — *see* Injury, superficial, knee
  labium (majus) (minus) S39.94 ☑
  labyrinth, ear S09.30- ☑
  lacrimal apparatus, duct, gland, or sac — *see* Injury, eye, specified site NEC
  larynx NEC S19.81 ☑
  leg (lower) S89.9- ☑
    blood vessel — *see* Injury, blood vessel, leg
    contusion — *see* Contusion, leg
    fracture — *see* Fracture, leg
    muscle — *see* Injury, muscle, leg
    nerve — *see* Injury, nerve, leg
    open — *see* Wound, open, leg
    specified NEC S89.8- ☑
    superficial — *see* Injury, superficial, leg
  lens, eye — *see* Injury, eye, specified site NEC
    penetrating — *see* Injury, eyeball, penetrating
  limb NEC T14.8 ☑
  lip S09.93 ☑
  liver S36.119 ☑
    contusion S36.112 ☑
    laceration S36.113 ☑
      major (stellate) S36.116 ☑
      minor S36.114 ☑
      moderate S36.115 ☑
    specified NEC S36.118 ☑
  lower back S39.92 ☑
    specified NEC S39.82 ☑
  lumbar, lumbosacral (region) S39.92 ☑
    plexus — *see* Injury, lumbosacral plexus
  lumbosacral plexus S34.4 ☑
  lung (*see also* Injury, intrathoracic, lung)
    aspiration J69.0
    transfusion-related (TRALI) J95.84
  lymphatic thoracic duct — *see* Injury, intrathoracic, specified organ NEC
  malar region S09.93 ☑
  mastoid region S09.90 ☑
  maxilla S09.93 ☑
  mediastinum — *see* Injury, intrathoracic, specified organ NEC
  membrane, brain — *see* Injury, intracranial
  meningeal artery — *see* Injury, intracranial, subdural hemorrhage
  meninges (cerebral) — *see* Injury, intracranial
  mesenteric
    artery
      branch S35.299 ☑
        laceration (minor) (superficial) S35.291 ☑
        major S35.292 ☑
        specified NEC S35.298 ☑

Injury — *continued*
  mesenteric — *continued*
    artery — *continued*
      inferior S35.239 ☑
        laceration (minor) (superficial) S35.231 ☑
        major S35.232 ☑
        specified NEC S35.238 ☑
      superior S35.229 ☑
        laceration (minor) (superficial) S35.221 ☑
        major S35.222 ☑
        specified NEC S35.228 ☑
      plexus (inferior) (superior) — *see* Injury, nerve, lumbosacral, sympathetic
    vein
      inferior S35.349 ☑
        laceration S35.341 ☑
        specified NEC S35.348 ☑
      superior S35.339 ☑
        laceration S35.331 ☑
        specified NEC S35.338 ☑
  mesentery — *see* Injury, intra-abdominal, specified site NEC
  mesosalpinx — *see* Injury, pelvic organ, specified site NEC
  middle ear S09.30- ☑
  midthoracic region NOS S29.9 ☑
  mouth S09.93 ☑
  multiple NOS T07 ☑
  muscle (and fascia) (and tendon)
    abdomen S39.001 ☑
      laceration S39.021 ☑
      specified type NEC S39.091 ☑
      strain S39.011 ☑
    abductor
      thumb, forearm level — *see* Injury, muscle, thumb, abductor
    adductor
      thigh S76.20- ☑
        laceration S76.22- ☑
        specified type NEC S76.29- ☑
        strain S76.21- ☑
    ankle — *see* Injury, muscle, foot
    anterior muscle group, at leg level (lower) S86.20- ☑
      laceration S86.22- ☑
      specified type NEC S86.29- ☑
      strain S86.21- ☑
    arm (upper) — *see* Injury, muscle, shoulder
    biceps (parts NEC) S46.20- ☑
      laceration S46.22- ☑
      long head S46.10- ☑
        laceration S46.12- ☑
        specified type NEC S46.19- ☑
        strain S46.11- ☑
      specified type NEC S46.29- ☑
      strain S46.21- ☑
    extensor
      finger(s) (other than thumb) — *see* Injury, muscle, finger by site, extensor
      forearm level, specified NEC — *see* Injury, muscle, forearm, extensor
      thumb — *see* Injury, muscle, thumb, extensor
      toe (large) (ankle level) (foot level) — *see* Injury, muscle, toe, extensor
    finger
      extensor (forearm level) S56.40- ☑
        hand level S66.309 ☑
          laceration S66.329 ☑
          specified type NEC S66.399 ☑
          strain S66.319 ☑
        laceration S56.429 ☑
        specified type NEC S56.499 ☑
        strain S56.419 ☑
      flexor (forearm level) S56.10- ☑
        hand level S66.109 ☑
          laceration S66.129 ☑
          specified type NEC S66.199 ☑
          strain S66.119 ☑
        laceration S56.129 ☑
        specified type NEC S56.199 ☑
        strain S56.119 ☑
      index
        extensor (forearm level)
          hand level S66.308 ☑
            laceration S66.32- ☑
            specified type NEC S66.39- ☑
            strain S66.31- ☑

☑ **Additional Character Required — Refer to the Tabular List for Character Selection**

▽ Subterms under main terms may continue to next column or page

Injury — *continued*
  muscle — *continued*
    finger — *continued*
      index — *continued*
        extensor — *continued*
          specified type NEC S56.492- ☑
        flexor (forearm level)
          hand level S66.108 ☑
            laceration S66.12- ☑
              specified type NEC S66.19- ☑
              strain S66.11- ☑
          specified type NEC S56.19- ☑
          strain S56.11- ☑
        intrinsic S66.50- ☑
          laceration S66.52- ☑
          specified type NEC S66.59- ☑
          strain S66.51- ☑
      intrinsic S66.509 ☑
        laceration S66.529 ☑
        specified type NEC S66.599 ☑
        strain S66.519 ☑
      little
        extensor (forearm level)
          hand level S66.30- ☑
            laceration S66.32- ☑
              specified type NEC S66.39- ☑
              strain S66.31- ☑
          laceration S56.42- ☑
          specified type NEC S56.49- ☑
          strain S56.41- ☑
        flexor (forearm level)
          hand level S66.10- ☑
            laceration S66.12- ☑
              specified type NEC S66.19- ☑
              strain S66.11- ☑
          laceration S56.12- ☑
          specified type NEC S56.19- ☑
          strain S56.11- ☑
        intrinsic S66.50- ☑
          laceration S66.52- ☑
          specified type NEC S66.59- ☑
          strain S66.51- ☑
      middle
        extensor (forearm level)
          hand level S66.30- ☑
            laceration S66.32- ☑
              specified type NEC S66.39- ☑
              strain S66.31- ☑
          laceration S56.42- ☑
          specified type NEC S56.49- ☑
          strain S56.41- ☑
        flexor (forearm level)
          hand level S66.10- ☑
            laceration S66.12- ☑
              specified type NEC S66.19- ☑
              strain S66.11- ☑
          laceration S56.12- ☑
          specified type NEC S56.19- ☑
          strain S56.11- ☑
        intrinsic S66.50- ☑
          laceration S66.52- ☑
          specified type NEC S66.59- ☑
          strain S66.51- ☑
      ring
        extensor (forearm level)
          hand level S66.30- ☑
            laceration S66.32- ☑
              specified type NEC S66.39- ☑
              strain S66.31- ☑
          laceration S56.42- ☑
          specified type NEC S56.49- ☑
          strain S56.41- ☑
        flexor (forearm level)
          hand level S66.10- ☑
            laceration S66.12- ☑
              specified type NEC S66.19- ☑
              strain S66.11- ☑
          laceration S56.12- ☑
          specified type NEC S56.19- ☑
          strain S56.11- ☑
        intrinsic S66.50- ☑
          laceration S66.52- ☑
          specified type NEC S66.59- ☑
          strain S66.51- ☑

Injury — *continued*
  muscle — *continued*
    flexor
      finger(s) (other than thumb) — *see* Injury, muscle, finger
      forearm level, specified NEC — *see* Injury, muscle, forearm, flexor
      thumb — *see* Injury, muscle, thumb, flexor
      toe (long) (ankle level) (foot level) — *see* Injury, muscle, toe, flexor
    foot S96.90- ☑
      intrinsic S96.20- ☑
        laceration S96.22- ☑
        specified type NEC S96.29- ☑
        strain S96.21- ☑
      laceration S96.92- ☑
      long extensor, toe — *see* Injury, muscle, toe, extensor
      long flexor, toe — *see* Injury, muscle, toe, flexor
      specified
        site NEC S96.80- ☑
          laceration S96.82- ☑
          specified type NEC S96.89- ☑
          strain S96.81- ☑
        type S96.99- ☑
      strain S96.91- ☑
    forearm (level) S56.90- ☑
      extensor S56.50- ☑
        laceration S56.52- ☑
        specified type NEC S56.59- ☑
        strain S56.51- ☑
      flexor S56.20- ☑
        laceration S56.22- ☑
        specified type NEC S56.29- ☑
        strain S56.21- ☑
      laceration S56.92- ☑
      specified S56.99- ☑
        site NEC S56.80- ☑
          laceration S56.82- ☑
          strain S56.81- ☑
          type NEC S56.89- ☑
      strain S56.91- ☑
    hand (level) S66.90- ☑
      laceration S66.92- ☑
      specified
        site NEC S66.80- ☑
          laceration S66.82- ☑
          specified type NEC S66.89- ☑
          strain S66.81- ☑
        type NEC S66.99- ☑
      strain S66.91- ☑
    head S09.10 ☑
      laceration S09.12 ☑
      specified type NEC S09.19 ☑
      strain S09.11 ☑
    hip NEC S76.00- ☑
      laceration S76.02- ☑
      specified type NEC S76.09- ☑
      strain S76.01- ☑
    intrinsic
      ankle and foot level — *see* Injury, muscle, foot, intrinsic
      finger (other than thumb) — *see* Injury, muscle, finger by site, intrinsic
      foot (level) — *see* Injury, muscle, foot, intrinsic
      thumb — *see* Injury, muscle, thumb, intrinsic
    leg (level) (lower) S86.90- ☑
      Achilles tendon — *see* Injury, Achilles tendon
      anterior muscle group — *see* Injury, muscle, anterior muscle group
      laceration S86.92- ☑
      peroneal muscle group — *see* Injury, muscle, peroneal muscle group
      posterior muscle group — *see* Injury, muscle, posterior muscle group, leg level
      specified
        site NEC S86.80- ☑
          laceration S86.82- ☑
          specified type NEC S86.89- ☑
          strain S86.81- ☑
        type NEC S86.99- ☑
      strain S86.91- ☑
    long
      extensor toe, at ankle and foot level — *see* Injury, muscle, toe, extensor

Injury — *continued*
  muscle — *continued*
    long — *continued*
      flexor, toe, at ankle and foot level — *see* Injury, muscle, toe, flexor
      head, biceps — *see* Injury, muscle, biceps, long head
    lower back S39.002 ☑
      laceration S39.022 ☑
      specified type NEC S39.092 ☑
      strain S39.012 ☑
    neck (level) S16.9 ☑
      laceration S16.2 ☑
      specified type NEC S16.8 ☑
      strain S16.1 ☑
    pelvis S39.003 ☑
      laceration S39.023 ☑
      specified type NEC S39.093 ☑
      strain S39.013 ☑
    peroneal muscle group, at leg level (lower) S86.30- ☑
      laceration S86.32- ☑
      specified type NEC S86.39- ☑
      strain S86.31- ☑
    posterior muscle (group)
      leg level (lower) S86.10- ☑
        laceration S86.12- ☑
        specified type NEC S86.19- ☑
        strain S86.11- ☑
      thigh level S76.30- ☑
        laceration S76.32- ☑
        specified type NEC S76.39- ☑
        strain S76.31- ☑
    quadriceps (thigh) S76.10- ☑
      laceration S76.12- ☑
      specified type NEC S76.19- ☑
      strain S76.11- ☑
    shoulder S46.90- ☑
      laceration S46.92- ☑
      rotator cuff — *see* Injury, rotator cuff
      specified site NEC S46.80- ☑
        laceration S46.82- ☑
        specified type NEC S46.89- ☑
        strain S46.81- ☑
      specified type NEC S46.99- ☑
      strain S46.91- ☑
    thigh NEC (level) S76.90- ☑
      adductor — *see* Injury, muscle, adductor, thigh
      laceration S76.92- ☑
      posterior muscle (group) — *see* Injury, muscle, posterior muscle, thigh level
      quadriceps — *see* Injury, muscle, quadriceps
      specified
        site NEC S76.80- ☑
          laceration S76.82- ☑
          specified type NEC S76.89- ☑
          strain S76.81- ☑
        type NEC S76.99- ☑
      strain S76.91- ☑
    thorax (level) S29.009 ☑
      back wall S29.002 ☑
      front wall S29.001 ☑
      laceration S29.029 ☑
        back wall S29.022 ☑
        front wall S29.021 ☑
      specified type NEC S29.099 ☑
        back wall S29.092 ☑
        front wall S29.091 ☑
      strain S29.019 ☑
        back wall S29.012 ☑
        front wall S29.011 ☑
    thumb
      abductor (forearm level) S56.30- ☑
        laceration S56.32- ☑
        specified type NEC S56.39- ☑
        strain S56.31- ☑
      extensor (forearm level) S56.30- ☑
        hand level S66.20- ☑
          laceration S66.22- ☑
          specified type NEC S66.29- ☑
          strain S66.21- ☑
        laceration S56.32- ☑
        specified type NEC S56.39- ☑
        strain S56.31- ☑
      flexor (forearm level) S56.00- ☑
        hand level S66.00- ☑

Injury — continued
  muscle — continued
    thumb — continued
      flexor — continued
        hand level — continued
          laceration S66.02- ☑
          specified type NEC S66.09- ☑
          strain S66.01- ☑
        laceration S56.02- ☑
        specified type NEC S56.09- ☑
        strain S56.01- ☑
        wrist level — see Injury, muscle, thumb, flexor, hand level
      intrinsic S66.40- ☑
        laceration S66.42- ☑
        specified type NEC S66.49- ☑
        strain S66.41- ☑
    toe (see also Injury, muscle, foot)
      extensor, long S96.10- ☑
        laceration S96.12- ☑
        specified type NEC S96.19- ☑
        strain S96.11- ☑
      flexor, long S96.00- ☑
        laceration S96.02- ☑
        specified type NEC S96.09- ☑
        strain S96.01- ☑
    triceps S46.30- ☑
      laceration S46.32- ☑
      specified type NEC S46.39- ☑
      strain S46.31- ☑
    wrist (and hand) level — see Injury, muscle, hand
  musculocutaneous nerve — see Injury, nerve, musculocutaneous
  myocardium — see Injury, heart
  nape — see Injury, neck
  nasal (septum) (sinus) S09.92 ☑
  nasopharynx S09.92 ☑
  neck S19.9 ☑
    specified NEC S19.80 ☑
    specified site NEC S19.89 ☑
  nerve NEC T14.8 ☑
    abdomen S34.9 ☑
      peripheral S34.6 ☑
      specified site NEC S34.8 ☑
    abducens S04.4- ☑
      contusion S04.4- ☑
      laceration S04.4- ☑
      specified type NEC S04.4- ☑
    abducent — see Injury, nerve, abducens
    accessory S04.7- ☑
      contusion S04.7- ☑
      laceration S04.7- ☑
      specified type NEC S04.7- ☑
    acoustic S04.6- ☑
      contusion S04.6- ☑
      laceration S04.6- ☑
      specified type NEC S04.6- ☑
    ankle S94.9- ☑
      cutaneous sensory S94.3- ☑
      specified site NEC — see subcategory S94.8 ☑
    anterior crural, femoral — see Injury, nerve, femoral
    arm (upper) S44.9- ☑
      axillary — see Injury, nerve, axillary
      cutaneous — see Injury, nerve, cutaneous, arm
      median — see Injury, nerve, median, upper arm
      musculocutaneous — see Injury, nerve, musculocutaneous
      radial — see Injury, nerve, radial, upper arm
      specified site NEC — see subcategory S44.8 ☑
      ulnar — see Injury, nerve, ulnar, arm
    auditory — see Injury, nerve, acoustic
    axillary S44.3- ☑
    brachial plexus — see Injury, brachial plexus
    cervical sympathetic S14.5 ☑
    cranial S04.9 ☑
      contusion S04.9 ☑
      eighth (acoustic or auditory) — see Injury, nerve, acoustic
      eleventh (accessory) — see Injury, nerve, accessory
      fifth (trigeminal) — see Injury, nerve, trigeminal
      first (olfactory) — see Injury, nerve, olfactory
      fourth (trochlear) — see Injury, nerve, trochlear
      laceration S04.9
      ninth (glossopharyngeal) — see Injury, nerve, glossopharyngeal

Injury — continued
  nerve — continued
    cranial — continued
      second (optic) — see Injury, nerve, optic
      seventh (facial) — see Injury, nerve, facial
      sixth (abducent) — see Injury, nerve, abducens
      specified
        nerve NEC S04.89- ☑
          contusion S04.89- ☑
          laceration S04.89- ☑
          specified type NEC S04.89- ☑
        type NEC S04.9 ☑
      tenth (pneumogastric or vagus) — see Injury, nerve, vagus
      third (oculomotor) — see Injury, nerve, oculomotor
      twelfth (hypoglossal) — see Injury, nerve, hypoglossal
    cutaneous sensory
      ankle (level) S94.3- ☑
      arm (upper) (level) S44.5- ☑
      foot (level) — see Injury, nerve, cutaneous sensory, ankle
      forearm (level) S54.3- ☑
      hip (level) S74.2- ☑
      leg (lower level) S84.2- ☑
      shoulder (level) — see Injury, nerve, cutaneous sensory, arm
      thigh (level) — see Injury, nerve, cutaneous sensory, hip
    deep peroneal — see Injury, nerve, peroneal, foot
    digital
      finger S64.4- ☑
        index S64.49- ☑
        little S64.49- ☑
        middle S64.49- ☑
        ring S64.49- ☑
      thumb S64.3- ☑
      toe — see Injury, nerve, ankle, specified site NEC
    eighth cranial (acoustic or auditory) — see Injury, nerve, acoustic
    eleventh cranial (accessory) — see Injury, nerve, accessory
    facial S04.5- ☑
      contusion S04.5- ☑
      laceration S04.5- ☑
      newborn P11.3
      specified type NEC S04.5- ☑
    femoral (hip level) (thigh level) S74.1- ☑
    fifth cranial (trigeminal) — see Injury, nerve, trigeminal
    finger (digital) — see Injury, nerve, digital, finger
    first cranial (olfactory) — see Injury, nerve, olfactory
    foot S94.9- ☑
      cutaneous sensory S94.3- ☑
      deep peroneal S94.2- ☑
      lateral plantar S94.0- ☑
      medial plantar S94.1- ☑
      specified site NEC — see subcategory S94.8 ☑
    forearm (level) S54.9- ☑
      cutaneous sensory — see Injury, nerve, cutaneous sensory, forearm
      median — see Injury, nerve, median
      radial — see Injury, nerve, radial
      specified site NEC — see subcategory S54.8 ☑
      ulnar — see Injury, nerve, ulnar
    fourth cranial (trochlear) — see Injury, nerve, trochlear
    glossopharyngeal S04.89- ☑
      specified type NEC S04.89- ☑
    hand S64.9- ☑
      median — see Injury, nerve, median, hand
      radial — see Injury, nerve, radial, hand
      specified NEC — see subcategory S64.8 ☑
      ulnar — see Injury, nerve, ulnar, hand
    hip (level) S74.9- ☑
      cutaneous sensory — see Injury, nerve, cutaneous sensory, hip
      femoral — see Injury, nerve, femoral
      sciatic — see Injury, nerve, sciatic
      specified site NEC — see subcategory S74.8 ☑
    hypoglossal S04.89- ☑
      specified type NEC S04.89- ☑
    lateral plantar S94.0- ☑
    leg (lower) S84.9- ☑

Injury — continued
  nerve — continued
    leg — continued
      cutaneous sensory — see Injury, nerve, cutaneous sensory, leg
      peroneal — see Injury, nerve, peroneal
      specified site NEC — see subcategory S84.8 ☑
      tibial — see Injury, nerve, tibial
      upper — see Injury, nerve, thigh
    lower
      back — see Injury, nerve, abdomen, specified site NEC
        peripheral — see Injury, nerve, abdomen, peripheral
      limb — see Injury, nerve, leg
    lumbar plexus — see Injury, nerve, lumbosacral, sympathetic
    lumbar spinal — see Injury, nerve, spinal, lumbar
    lumbosacral
      plexus — see Injury, nerve, lumbosacral, sympathetic
      sympathetic S34.5 ☑
    medial plantar S94.1- ☑
    median (forearm level) S54.1- ☑
      hand (level) S64.1- ☑
      upper arm (level) S44.1- ☑
      wrist (level) — see Injury, nerve, median, hand
    musculocutaneous S44.4- ☑
    musculospiral (upper arm level) — see Injury, nerve, radial, upper arm
    neck S14.9 ☑
      peripheral S14.4 ☑
      specified site NEC S14.8 ☑
      sympathetic S14.5 ☑
    ninth cranial (glossopharyngeal) — see Injury, nerve, glossopharyngeal
    oculomotor S04.1- ☑
      contusion S04.1- ☑
      laceration S04.1- ☑
      specified type NEC S04.1- ☑
    olfactory S04.81- ☑
      specified type NEC S04.81- ☑
    optic S04.01- ☑
      contusion S04.01- ☑
      laceration S04.01- ☑
      specified type NEC S04.01- ☑
    pelvic girdle — see Injury, nerve, hip
    pelvis — see Injury, nerve, abdomen, specified site NEC
      peripheral — see Injury, nerve, abdomen, peripheral
    peripheral NEC T14.8 ☑
      abdomen — see Injury, nerve, abdomen, peripheral
      lower back — see Injury, nerve, abdomen, peripheral
      neck — see Injury, nerve, neck, peripheral
      pelvis — see Injury, nerve, abdomen, peripheral
      specified NEC T14.8 ☑
    peroneal (lower leg level) S84.1- ☑
      foot S94.2- ☑
    plexus
      brachial — see Injury, brachial plexus
      celiac, coeliac — see Injury, nerve, lumbosacral, sympathetic
      mesenteric, inferior — see Injury, nerve, lumbosacral, sympathetic
      sacral — see Injury, lumbosacral plexus
      spinal
        brachial — see Injury, brachial plexus
        lumbosacral — see Injury, lumbosacral plexus
    pneumogastric — see Injury, nerve, vagus
    radial (forearm level) S54.2- ☑
      hand (level) S64.2- ☑
      upper arm (level) S44.2- ☑
      wrist (level) — see Injury, nerve, radial, hand
    root — see Injury, nerve, spinal, root
    sacral plexus — see Injury, lumbosacral plexus
    sacral spinal — see Injury, nerve, spinal, sacral
    sciatic (hip level) (thigh level) S74.0- ☑
    second cranial (optic) — see Injury, nerve, optic
    seventh cranial (facial) — see Injury, nerve, facial
    shoulder — see Injury, nerve, arm
    sixth cranial (abducent) — see Injury, nerve, abducens

Injury — continued
  nerve — continued
    spinal
      plexus — see Injury, nerve, plexus, spinal
      root
        cervical S14.2 ☑
        dorsal S24.2 ☑
        lumbar S34.21 ☑
        sacral S34.22 ☑
        thoracic — see Injury, nerve, spinal, root, dorsal
      splanchnic — see Injury, nerve, lumbosacral, sympathetic
      sympathetic NEC — see Injury, nerve, lumbosacral, sympathetic
        cervical — see Injury, nerve, cervical sympathetic
      tenth cranial (pneumogastric or vagus) — see Injury, nerve, vagus
      thigh (level) — see Injury, nerve, hip
        cutaneous sensory — see Injury, nerve, cutaneous sensory, hip
        femoral — see Injury, nerve, femoral
        sciatic — see Injury, nerve, sciatic
        specified NEC — see Injury, nerve, hip
      third cranial (oculomotor) — see Injury, nerve, oculomotor
      thorax S24.9 ☑
        peripheral S24.3 ☑
        specified site NEC S24.8 ☑
        sympathetic S24.4 ☑
      thumb, digital — see Injury, nerve, digital, thumb
      tibial (lower leg level) (posterior) S84.0- ☑
      toe — see Injury, nerve, ankle
      trigeminal S04.3- ☑
        contusion S04.3- ☑
        laceration S04.3- ☑
        specified type NEC S04.3- ☑
      trochlear S04.2- ☑
        contusion S04.2- ☑
        laceration S04.2- ☑
        specified type NEC S04.2- ☑
      twelfth cranial (hypoglossal) — see Injury, nerve, hypoglossal
      ulnar (forearm level) S54.0- ☑
        arm (upper) (level) S44.0- ☑
        hand (level) S64.0- ☑
        wrist (level) — see Injury, nerve, ulnar, hand
      vagus S04.89- ☑
        specified type NEC S04.89- ☑
      wrist (level) — see Injury, nerve, hand
    ninth cranial nerve (glossopharyngeal) — see Injury, nerve, glossopharyngeal
  nose (septum) S09.92 ☑
  obstetrical O71.9
    specified NEC O71.89
  occipital (region) (scalp) S09.90 ☑
    lobe — see Injury, intracranial
  optic chiasm S04.02 ☑
  optic radiation S04.03- ☑
  optic tract and pathways S04.03- ☑
  orbit, orbital (region) — see Injury, eye
    penetrating (with foreign body) — see Injury, eye, orbit, penetrating
    specified NEC — see Injury, eye, specified site NEC
  ovary, ovarian S37.409 ☑
    bilateral S37.402 ☑
      contusion S37.422 ☑
      laceration S37.432 ☑
      specified type NEC S37.492 ☑
    blood vessel — see Injury, blood vessel, ovarian
    contusion S37.429 ☑
      bilateral S37.422 ☑
      unilateral S37.421 ☑
    laceration S37.439 ☑
      bilateral S37.432 ☑
      unilateral S37.431 ☑
    specified type NEC S37.499 ☑
      bilateral S37.492 ☑
      unilateral S37.491 ☑
    unilateral S37.401 ☑
      contusion S37.421 ☑
      laceration S37.431 ☑
      specified type NEC S37.491 ☑
  palate (hard) (soft) S09.93 ☑
  pancreas S36.209 ☑
    body S36.201 ☑

Injury — continued
  pancreas — continued
    body — continued
      contusion S36.221 ☑
      laceration S36.231 ☑
        major S36.261 ☑
        minor S36.241 ☑
        moderate S36.251 ☑
      specified type NEC S36.291 ☑
    contusion S36.229 ☑
    head S36.200 ☑
      contusion S36.220 ☑
      laceration S36.230 ☑
        major S36.260 ☑
        minor S36.240 ☑
        moderate S36.250 ☑
      specified type NEC S36.290 ☑
    laceration S36.239 ☑
      major S36.269 ☑
      minor S36.249 ☑
      moderate S36.259 ☑
    specified type NEC S36.299 ☑
    tail S36.202 ☑
      contusion S36.222 ☑
      laceration S36.232 ☑
        major S36.262 ☑
        minor S36.242 ☑
        moderate S36.252 ☑
      specified type NEC S36.292 ☑
  parietal (region) (scalp) S09.90 ☑
    lobe — see Injury, intracranial
  patellar ligament (tendon) S76.10- ☑
    laceration S76.12- ☑
    specified NEC S76.19- ☑
    strain S76.11- ☑
  pelvis, pelvic (floor) S39.93 ☑
    complicating delivery O70.1
    joint or ligament, complicating delivery O71.6
    organ S37.90 ☑
      with ectopic or molar pregnancy O08.6
      complication of abortion — see Abortion
      contusion S37.92 ☑
      following ectopic or molar pregnancy O08.6
      laceration S37.93 ☑
      obstetrical trauma NEC O71.5
      specified
        site NEC S37.899 ☑
          contusion S37.892 ☑
          laceration S37.893 ☑
          specified type NEC S37.898 ☑
        type NEC S37.99 ☑
    specified NEC S39.83 ☑
  penis S39.94 ☑
  perineum S39.94 ☑
  peritoneum S36.81 ☑
    laceration S36.893 ☑
  periurethral tissue — see Injury, urethra
    complicating delivery O71.82
  phalanges
    foot — see Injury, foot
    hand — see Injury, hand
  pharynx NEC S19.85 ☑
  pleura — see Injury, intrathoracic, pleura
  plexus
    brachial — see Injury, brachial plexus
    cardiac — see Injury, nerve, thorax, sympathetic
    celiac, coeliac — see Injury, nerve, lumbosacral, sympathetic
    esophageal — see Injury, nerve, thorax, sympathetic
    hypogastric — see Injury, nerve, lumbosacral, sympathetic
    lumbar, lumbosacral — see Injury, lumbosacral plexus
    mesenteric — see Injury, nerve, lumbosacral, sympathetic
    pulmonary — see Injury, nerve, thorax, sympathetic
  postcardiac surgery (syndrome) I97.0
  prepuce S39.94 ☑
  prostate S37.829 ☑
    contusion S37.822 ☑
    laceration S37.823 ☑
    specified type NEC S37.828 ☑
  pubic region S39.94 ☑
  pudendum S39.94 ☑
  pulmonary plexus — see Injury, nerve, thorax, sympathetic

Injury — continued
  rectovaginal septum NEC S39.83 ☑
  rectum — see Injury, intestine, large, rectum
  retina — see Injury, eye, specified site NEC
    penetrating — see Injury, eyeball, penetrating
  retroperitoneal — see Injury, intra-abdominal, specified site NEC
  rotator cuff (muscle(s)) (tendon(s)) S46.00- ☑
    laceration S46.02- ☑
    specified type NEC S46.09- ☑
    strain S46.01- ☑
  round ligament — see Injury, pelvic organ, specified site NEC
  sacral plexus — see Injury, lumbosacral plexus
  salivary duct or gland S09.93 ☑
  scalp S09.90 ☑
    newborn (birth injury) P12.9
      due to monitoring (electrode) (sampling incision) P12.4
      specified NEC P12.89
        caput succedaneum P12.81
  scapular region — see Injury, shoulder
  sclera — see Injury, eye, specified site NEC
    penetrating — see Injury, eyeball, penetrating
  scrotum S39.94 ☑
  second cranial nerve (optic) — see Injury, nerve, optic
  seminal vesicle — see Injury, pelvic organ, specified site NEC
  seventh cranial nerve (facial) — see Injury, nerve, facial
  shoulder S49.9- ☑
    blood vessel — see Injury, blood vessel, arm
    contusion — see Contusion, shoulder
    dislocation — see Dislocation, shoulder
    fracture — see Fracture, shoulder
    muscle — see Injury, muscle, shoulder
    nerve — see Injury, nerve, shoulder
    open — see Wound, open, shoulder
    specified type NEC S49.8- ☑
    sprain — see Sprain, shoulder girdle
    superficial — see Injury, superficial, shoulder
  sinus
    cavernous — see Injury, intracranial
    nasal S09.92 ☑
  sixth cranial nerve (abducent) — see Injury, nerve, abducens
  skeleton, birth injury P13.9
    specified part NEC P13.8
  skin NEC T14.8 ☑
    surface intact — see Injury, superficial
  skull NEC S09.90 ☑
  specified NEC T14.8 ☑
  spermatic cord (pelvic region) S37.898 ☑
    scrotal region S39.848 ☑
  spinal (cord)
    cervical (neck) S14.109 ☑
      anterior cord syndrome S14.139 ☑
        C1 level S14.131 ☑
        C2 level S14.132 ☑
        C3 level S14.133 ☑
        C4 level S14.134 ☑
        C5 level S14.135 ☑
        C6 level S14.136 ☑
        C7 level S14.137 ☑
        C8 level S14.138 ☑
      Brown-Séquard syndrome S14.149 ☑
        C1 level S14.141 ☑
        C2 level S14.142 ☑
        C3 level S14.143 ☑
        C4 level S14.144 ☑
        C5 level S14.145 ☑
        C6 level S14.146 ☑
        C7 level S14.147 ☑
        C8 level S14.148 ☑
      C1 level S14.101 ☑
      C2 level S14.102 ☑
      C3 level S14.103 ☑
      C4 level S14.104 ☑
      C5 level S14.105 ☑
      C6 level S14.106 ☑
      C7 level S14.107 ☑
      C8 level S14.108 ☑
      central cord syndrome S14.129 ☑
        C1 level S14.121 ☑
        C2 level S14.122 ☑
        C3 level S14.123 ☑
        C4 level S14.124 ☑

Injury — *continued*
  spinal — *continued*
    cervical — *continued*
      central cord syndrome — *continued*
        C5 level S14.125 ☑
        C6 level S14.126 ☑
        C7 level S14.127 ☑
        C8 level S14.128 ☑
      complete lesion S14.119 ☑
        C1 level S14.111 ☑
        C2 level S14.112 ☑
        C3 level S14.113 ☑
        C4 level S14.114 ☑
        C5 level S14.115 ☑
        C6 level S14.116 ☑
        C7 level S14.117 ☑
        C8 level S14.118 ☑
      concussion S14.0 ☑
      edema S14.0 ☑
      incomplete lesion specified NEC S14.159 ☑
        C1 level S14.151 ☑
        C2 level S14.152 ☑
        C3 level S14.153 ☑
        C4 level S14.154 ☑
        C5 level S14.155 ☑
        C6 level S14.156 ☑
        C7 level S14.157 ☑
        C8 level S14.158 ☑
      posterior cord syndrome S14.159 ☑
        C1 level S14.151 ☑
        C2 level S14.152 ☑
        C3 level S14.153 ☑
        C4 level S14.154 ☑
        C5 level S14.155 ☑
        C6 level S14.156 ☑
        C7 level S14.157 ☑
        C8 level S14.158 ☑
    dorsal — *see* Injury, spinal, thoracic
    lumbar S34.109 ☑
      complete lesion S34.119 ☑
        L1 level S34.111 ☑
        L2 level S34.112 ☑
        L3 level S34.113 ☑
        L4 level S34.114 ☑
        L5 level S34.115 ☑
      concussion S34.01 ☑
      edema S34.01 ☑
      incomplete lesion S34.129 ☑
        L1 level S34.121 ☑
        L2 level S34.122 ☑
        L3 level S34.123 ☑
        L4 level S34.124 ☑
        L5 level S34.125 ☑
      L1 level S34.101 ☑
      L2 level S34.102 ☑
      L3 level S34.103 ☑
      L4 level S34.104 ☑
      L5 level S34.105 ☑
    nerve root NEC
      cervical — *see* Injury, nerve, spinal, root, cervical
      dorsal — *see* Injury, nerve, spinal, root, dorsal
      lumbar S34.21 ☑
      sacral S34.22 ☑
      thoracic — *see* Injury, nerve, spinal, root, dorsal
    plexus
      brachial — *see* Injury, brachial plexus
      lumbosacral — *see* Injury, lumbosacral plexus
    sacral S34.139 ☑
      complete lesion S34.131 ☑
      incomplete lesion S34.132 ☑
    thoracic S24.109 ☑
      anterior cord syndrome S24.139 ☑
        T1 level S24.131 ☑
        T2-T6 level S24.132 ☑
        T7-T10 level S24.133 ☑
        T11-T12 level S24.134 ☑
      Brown-Séquard syndrome S24.149 ☑
        T1 level S24.141 ☑
        T2-T6 level S24.142 ☑
        T7-T10 level S24.143 ☑
        T11-T12 level S24.144 ☑
      complete lesion S24.119 ☑
        T1 level S24.111 ☑
        T2-T6 level S24.112 ☑
        T7-T10 level S24.113 ☑
        T11-T12 level S24.114 ☑

Injury — *continued*
  spinal — *continued*
    thoracic — *continued*
      concussion S24.0 ☑
      edema S24.0 ☑
      incomplete lesion specified NEC S24.159 ☑
        T1 level S24.151 ☑
        T2-T6 level S24.152 ☑
        T7-T10 level S24.153 ☑
        T11-T12 level S24.154 ☑
      posterior cord syndrome S24.159 ☑
        T1 level S24.151 ☑
        T2-T6 level S24.152 ☑
        T7-T10 level S24.153 ☑
        T11-T12 level S24.154 ☑
      T1 level S24.101 ☑
      T2-T6 level S24.102 ☑
      T7-T10 level S24.103 ☑
      T11-T12 level S24.104 ☑
    splanchnic nerve — *see* Injury, nerve, lumbosacral, sympathetic
  spleen S36.00 ☑
    contusion S36.029 ☑
      major S36.021 ☑
      minor S36.020 ☑
    laceration S36.039 ☑
      major (massive) (stellate) S36.032 ☑
      moderate S36.031 ☑
      superficial (capsular) (minor) S36.030 ☑
    specified type NEC S36.09 ☑
  splenic artery — *see* Injury, blood vessel, celiac artery, branch
  stellate ganglion — *see* Injury, nerve, thorax, sympathetic
  sternal region S29.9 ☑
  stomach S36.30 ☑
    contusion S36.32 ☑
    laceration S36.33 ☑
    specified type NEC S36.39 ☑
  subconjunctival — *see* Injury, eye, conjunctiva
  subcutaneous NEC T14.8 ☑
  submaxillary region S09.93 ☑
  submental region S09.93 ☑
  subungual
    fingers — *see* Injury, hand
    toes — *see* Injury, foot
  superficial NEC T14.8 ☑
    abdomen, abdominal (wall) S30.92 ☑
      abrasion S30.811 ☑
      bite S30.871 ☑
        insect S30.861 ☑
      contusion S30.1 ☑
      external constriction S30.841 ☑
      foreign body S30.851 ☑
    abrasion — *see* Abrasion, by site
    adnexa, eye NEC — *see* Injury, eye, specified site NEC
    alveolar process — *see* Injury, superficial, oral cavity
    ankle S90.91- ☑
      abrasion — *see* Abrasion, ankle
      bite — *see* Bite, ankle
      blister — *see* Blister, ankle
      contusion — *see* Contusion, ankle
      external constriction — *see* Constriction, external, ankle
      foreign body — *see* Foreign body, superficial, ankle
    anus S30.98 ☑
    arm (upper) S40.92- ☑
      abrasion — *see* Abrasion, arm
      bite — *see* Bite, superficial, arm
      blister — *see* Blister, arm (upper)
      contusion — *see* Contusion, arm
      external constriction — *see* Constriction, external, arm
      foreign body — *see* Foreign body, superficial, arm
    auditory canal (external) (meatus) — *see* Injury, superficial, ear
    auricle — *see* Injury, superficial, ear
    axilla — *see* Injury, superficial, arm
    back (*see also* Injury, superficial, thorax, back)
      lower S30.91 ☑
        abrasion S30.810 ☑
        contusion S30.0 ☑
        external constriction S30.840 ☑

Injury — *continued*
  superficial — *continued*
    back (*see also* Injury, superficial, thorax, back) — *continued*
      lower — *continued*
        superficial
          bite NEC S30.870 ☑
            insect S30.860 ☑
          foreign body S30.850 ☑
    bite NEC — *see* Bite, superficial NEC, by site
    blister — *see* Blister, by site
    breast S20.10- ☑
      abrasion — *see* Abrasion, breast
      bite — *see* Bite, superficial, breast
      contusion — *see* Contusion, breast
      external constriction — *see* Constriction, external, breast
      foreign body — *see* Foreign body, superficial, breast
    brow — *see* Injury, superficial, head, specified NEC
    buttock S30.91 ☑
    calf — *see* Injury, superficial, leg
    canthus, eye — *see* Injury, superficial, periocular area
    cheek (external) — *see* Injury, superficial, head, specified NEC
      internal — *see* Injury, superficial, oral cavity
    chest wall — *see* Injury, superficial, thorax
    chin — *see* Injury, superficial, head NEC
    clitoris S30.95 ☑
    conjunctiva — *see* Injury, eye, conjunctiva
      with foreign body (in conjunctival sac) — *see* Foreign body, conjunctival sac
    contusion — *see* Contusion, by site
    costal region — *see* Injury, superficial, thorax
    digit(s)
      hand — *see* Injury, superficial, finger
    ear (auricle) (canal) (external) S00.40- ☑
      abrasion — *see* Abrasion, ear
      bite — *see* Bite, superficial, ear
      contusion — *see* Contusion, ear
      external constriction — *see* Constriction, external, ear
      foreign body — *see* Foreign body, superficial, ear
    elbow S50.90- ☑
      abrasion — *see* Abrasion, elbow
      bite — *see* Bite, superficial, elbow
      blister — *see* Blister, elbow
      contusion — *see* Contusion, elbow
      external constriction — *see* Constriction, external, elbow
      foreign body — *see* Foreign body, superficial, elbow
    epididymis S30.94 ☑
    epigastric region S30.92 ☑
    epiglottis — *see* Injury, superficial, throat
    esophagus
      cervical — *see* Injury, superficial, throat
    external constriction — *see* Constriction, external, by site
    extremity NEC T14.8 ☑
    eyeball NEC — *see* Injury, eye, specified site NEC
    eyebrow — *see* Injury, superficial, periocular area
    eyelid S00.20- ☑
      abrasion — *see* Abrasion, eyelid
      bite — *see* Bite, superficial, eyelid
      contusion — *see* Contusion, eyelid
      external constriction — *see* Constriction, external, eyelid
      foreign body — *see* Foreign body, superficial, eyelid
    face NEC — *see* Injury, superficial, head, specified NEC
    finger(s) S60.949 ☑
      abrasion — *see* Abrasion, finger
      bite — *see* Bite, superficial, finger
      blister — *see* Blister, finger
      contusion — *see* Contusion, finger
      external constriction — *see* Constriction, external, finger
      foreign body — *see* Foreign body, superficial, finger
      index S60.94- ☑
      insect bite — *see* Bite, by site, superficial, insect
      little S60.94- ☑
      middle S60.94- ☑

☑ **Additional Character Required — Refer to the Tabular List for Character Selection**

▽ **Subterms under main terms may continue to next column or page**

Injury —continued
superficial —continued
finger(s) —continued
ring S60.94- ☑
flank S30.92 ☑
foot S90.92- ☑
abrasion —see Abrasion, foot
bite —see Bite, foot
blister —see Blister, foot
contusion —see Contusion, foot
external constriction —see Constriction, external, foot
foreign body —see Foreign body, superficial, foot
forearm S50.91- ☑
abrasion —see Abrasion, forearm
bite —see Bite, forearm, superficial
blister —see Blister, forearm
contusion —see Contusion, forearm
elbow only —see Injury, superficial, elbow
external constriction —see Constriction, external, forearm
foreign body —see Foreign body, superficial, forearm
forehead —see Injury, superficial, head NEC
foreign body —see Foreign body, superficial
genital organs, external
female S30.97 ☑
male S30.96 ☑
globe (eye) —see Injury, eye, specified site NEC
groin S30.92 ☑
gum —see Injury, superficial, oral cavity
hand S60.92- ☑
abrasion —see Abrasion, hand
bite —see Bite, superficial, hand
contusion —see Contusion, hand
external constriction —see Constriction, external, hand
foreign body —see Foreign body, superficial, hand
head S00.90 ☑
ear —see Injury, superficial, ear
eyelid —see Injury, superficial, eyelid
nose S00.30 ☑
oral cavity S00.502 ☑
scalp S00.00 ☑
specified site NEC S00.80 ☑
heel —see Injury, superficial, foot
hip S70.91- ☑
abrasion —see Abrasion, hip
bite —see Bite, superficial, hip
blister —see Blister, hip
contusion —see Contusion, hip
external constriction —see Constriction, external, hip
foreign body —see Foreign body, superficial, hip
iliac region —see Injury, superficial, abdomen
inguinal region —see Injury, superficial, abdomen
insect bite —see Bite, by site, superficial, insect
interscapular region —see Injury, superficial, thorax, back
jaw —see Injury, superficial, head, specified NEC
knee S80.91- ☑
abrasion —see Abrasion, knee
bite —see Bite, superficial, knee
blister —see Blister, knee
contusion —see Contusion, knee
external constriction —see Constriction, external, knee
foreign body —see Foreign body, superficial, knee
labium (majus) (minus) S30.95 ☑
lacrimal (apparatus) (gland) (sac) —see Injury, eye, specified site NEC
larynx —see Injury, superficial, throat
leg (lower) S80.92- ☑
abrasion —see Abrasion, leg
bite —see Bite, superficial, leg
contusion —see Contusion, leg
external constriction —see Constriction, external, leg
foreign body —see Foreign body, superficial, leg
knee —see Injury, superficial, knee
limb NEC T14.8 ☑

Injury —continued
superficial —continued
lip S00.501 ☑
lower back S30.91 ☑
lumbar region S30.91 ☑
malar region —see Injury, superficial, head, specified NEC
mammary —see Injury, superficial, breast
mastoid region —see Injury, superficial, head, specified NEC
mouth —see Injury, superficial, oral cavity
muscle NEC T14.8 ☑
nail NEC T14.8 ☑
finger —see Injury, superficial, finger
toe —see Injury, superficial, toe
nasal (septum) —see Injury, superficial, nose
neck S10.90 ☑
specified site NEC S10.80 ☑
nose (septum) S00.30 ☑
occipital region —see Injury, superficial, scalp
oral cavity S00.502 ☑
orbital region —see Injury, superficial, periocular area
palate —see Injury, superficial, oral cavity
palm —see Injury, superficial, hand
parietal region —see Injury, superficial, scalp
pelvis S30.91 ☑
girdle —see Injury, superficial, hip
penis S30.93 ☑
perineum
female S30.95 ☑
male S30.91 ☑
periocular area S00.20- ☑
abrasion —see Abrasion, eyelid
bite —see Bite, superficial, eyelid
contusion —see Contusion, eyelid
external constriction —see Constriction, external, eyelid
foreign body —see Foreign body, superficial, eyelid
phalanges
finger —see Injury, superficial, finger
toe —see Injury, superficial, toe
pharynx —see Injury, superficial, throat
pinna —see Injury, superficial, ear
popliteal space —see Injury, superficial, knee
prepuce S30.93 ☑
pubic region S30.91 ☑
pudendum
female S30.97 ☑
male S30.96 ☑
sacral region S30.91 ☑
scalp S00.00 ☑
scapular region —see Injury, superficial, shoulder
sclera —see Injury, eye, specified site NEC
scrotum S30.94 ☑
shin —see Injury, superficial, leg
shoulder S40.91- ☑
abrasion —see Abrasion, shoulder
bite —see Bite, superficial, shoulder
blister —see Blister, shoulder
contusion —see Contusion, shoulder
external constriction —see Constriction, external, shoulder
foreign body —see Foreign body, superficial, shoulder
skin NEC T14.8 ☑
sternal region —see Injury, superficial, thorax, front
subconjunctival —see Injury, eye, specified site NEC
subcutaneous NEC T14.8 ☑
submaxillary region —see Injury, superficial, head, specified NEC
submental region —see Injury, superficial, head, specified NEC
subungual
finger(s) —see Injury, superficial, finger
toe(s) —see Injury, superficial, toe
supraclavicular fossa —see Injury, superficial, neck
supraorbital —see Injury, superficial, head, specified NEC
temple —see Injury, superficial, head, specified NEC
temporal region —see Injury, superficial, head, specified NEC
testis S30.94 ☑
thigh S70.92- ☑
abrasion —see Abrasion, thigh

Injury —continued
superficial —continued
thigh —continued
bite —see Bite, superficial, thigh
blister —see Blister, thigh
contusion —see Contusion, thigh
external constriction —see Constriction, external, thigh
foreign body —see Foreign body, superficial, thigh
thorax, thoracic (wall) S20.90 ☑
abrasion —see Abrasion, thorax
back S20.40- ☑
bite —see Bite, thorax, superficial
blister —see Blister, thorax
contusion —see Contusion, thorax
external constriction —see Constriction, external, thorax
foreign body —see Foreign body, superficial, thorax
front S20.30- ☑
throat S10.10 ☑
abrasion S10.11 ☑
bite S10.17 ☑
insect S10.16 ☑
blister S10.12 ☑
contusion S10.0 ☑
external constriction S10.14 ☑
foreign body S10.15 ☑
thumb S60.93- ☑
abrasion —see Abrasion, thumb
bite —see Bite, superficial, thumb
blister —see Blister, thumb
contusion —see Contusion, thumb
external constriction —see Constriction, external, thumb
foreign body —see Foreign body, superficial, thumb
insect bite —see Bite, by site, superficial, insect
specified type NEC S60.39 ☑
toe(s) S90.93- ☑
abrasion —see Abrasion, toe
bite —see Bite, toe
blister —see Blister, toe
contusion —see Contusion, toe
external constriction —see Constriction, external, toe
foreign body —see Foreign body, superficial, toe
great S90.93- ☑
tongue —see Injury, superficial, oral cavity
tooth, teeth —see Injury, superficial, oral cavity
trachea S10.10 ☑
tunica vaginalis S30.94 ☑
tympanum, tympanic membrane —see Injury, superficial, ear
uvula —see Injury, superficial, oral cavity
vagina S30.95 ☑
vocal cords —see Injury, superficial, throat
vulva S30.95 ☑
wrist S60.91- ☑
supraclavicular region —see Injury, neck
supraorbital S09.93 ☑
suprarenal gland (multiple) —see Injury, adrenal
surgical complication (external or internal site) —see Laceration, accidental complicating surgery
temple S09.90 ☑
temporal region S09.90 ☑
tendon (see also Injury, muscle, by site)
abdomen —see Injury, muscle, abdomen
Achilles —see Injury, Achilles tendon
lower back —see Injury, muscle, lower back
pelvic organs —see Injury, muscle, pelvis
tenth cranial nerve (pneumogastric or vagus) —see Injury, nerve, vagus
testis S39.94 ☑
thigh S79.92- ☑
blood vessel —see Injury, blood vessel, hip
contusion —see Contusion, thigh
fracture —see Fracture, femur
muscle —see Injury, muscle, thigh
nerve —see Injury, nerve, thigh
open —see Wound, open, thigh
specified NEC S79.82- ☑
superficial —see Injury, superficial, thigh

Injury — *continued*
- third cranial nerve (oculomotor) — *see* Injury, nerve, oculomotor
- thorax, thoracic S29.9 ☑
  - blood vessel — *see* Injury, blood vessel, thorax
  - cavity — *see* Injury, intrathoracic
  - dislocation — *see* Dislocation, thorax
  - external (wall) S29.9 ☑
    - contusion — *see* Contusion, thorax
    - nerve — *see* Injury, nerve, thorax
    - open — *see* Wound, open, thorax
    - specified NEC S29.8 ☑
    - sprain — *see* Sprain, thorax
    - superficial — *see* Injury, superficial, thorax
  - fracture — *see* Fracture, thorax
  - internal — *see* Injury, intrathoracic
  - intrathoracic organ — *see* Injury, intrathoracic
  - sympathetic ganglion — *see* Injury, nerve, thorax, sympathetic
- throat (*see also* Injury, neck) S19.9 ☑
- thumb S69.9- ☑
  - blood vessel — *see* Injury, blood vessel, thumb
  - contusion — *see* Contusion, thumb
  - dislocation — *see* Dislocation, thumb
  - fracture — *see* Fracture, thumb
  - muscle — *see* Injury, muscle, thumb
  - nerve — *see* Injury, nerve, digital, thumb
  - open — *see* Wound, open, thumb
  - specified NEC S69.8- ☑
  - sprain — *see* Sprain, thumb
  - superficial — *see* Injury, superficial, thumb
- thymus (gland) — *see* Injury, intrathoracic, specified organ NEC
- thyroid (gland) NEC S19.84 ☑
- toe S99.92- ☑
  - contusion — *see* Contusion, toe
  - dislocation — *see* Dislocation, toe
  - fracture — *see* Fracture, toe
  - muscle — *see* Injury, muscle, toe
  - open — *see* Wound, open, toe
  - specified type NEC S99.82- ☑
  - sprain — *see* Sprain, toe
  - superficial — *see* Injury, superficial, toe
- tongue S09.93 ☑
- tonsil S09.93 ☑
- tooth S09.93 ☑
- trachea (cervical) NEC S19.82 ☑
  - thoracic — *see* Injury, intrathoracic, trachea, thoracic
- transfusion-related acute lung (TRALI) J95.84
- tunica vaginalis S39.94 ☑
- twelfth cranial nerve (hypoglossal) — *see* Injury, nerve, hypoglossal
- ureter S37.10 ☑
  - contusion S37.12 ☑
  - laceration S37.13 ☑
  - specified type NEC S37.19 ☑
- urethra (sphincter) S37.30 ☑
  - at delivery O71.5
  - contusion S37.32 ☑
  - laceration S37.33 ☑
  - specified type NEC S37.39 ☑
- urinary organ S37.90 ☑
  - contusion S37.92 ☑
  - laceration S37.93 ☑
  - specified
    - site NEC S37.899 ☑
      - contusion S37.892 ☑
      - laceration S37.893 ☑
      - specified type NEC S37.898 ☑
    - type NEC S37.99 ☑
- uterus, uterine S37.60 ☑
  - with ectopic or molar pregnancy O08.6
  - blood vessel — *see* Injury, blood vessel, iliac
  - contusion S37.62 ☑
  - laceration S37.63 ☑
    - cervix at delivery O71.3
  - rupture associated with obstetrics — *see* Rupture, uterus
  - specified type NEC S37.69 ☑
- uvula S09.93 ☑
- vagina S39.93 ☑
  - abrasion S30.814 ☑
  - bite S31.45 ☑
    - insect S30.864 ☑
    - superficial NEC S30.874 ☑
  - contusion S30.23 ☑

Injury — *continued*
- vagina — *continued*
  - crush S38.03 ☑
  - during delivery — *see* Laceration, vagina, during delivery
  - external constriction S30.844 ☑
  - insect bite S30.864 ☑
  - laceration S31.41 ☑
    - with foreign body S31.42 ☑
  - open wound S31.40 ☑
  - puncture S31.43 ☑
    - with foreign body S31.44 ☑
  - superficial S30.95 ☑
    - foreign body S30.854 ☑
- vas deferens — *see* Injury, pelvic organ, specified site NEC
- vascular NEC T14.8 ☑
- vein — *see* Injury, blood vessel
- vena cava (superior) S25.20 ☑
  - inferior S35.10 ☑
    - laceration (minor) (superficial) S35.11 ☑
      - major S35.12 ☑
    - specified type NEC S35.19 ☑
  - laceration (minor) (superficial) S25.21 ☑
    - major S25.22 ☑
  - specified type NEC S25.29 ☑
- vesical (sphincter) — *see* Injury, bladder
- visual cortex S04.04- ☑
- vitreous (humor) S05.90 ☑
  - specified NEC S05.8X- ☑
- vocal cord NEC S19.83 ☑
- vulva S39.94 ☑
  - abrasion S30.814 ☑
  - bite S31.45 ☑
    - insect S30.864 ☑
    - superficial NEC S30.874 ☑
  - contusion S30.23 ☑
  - crush S38.03 ☑
  - during delivery — *see* Laceration, perineum, female, during delivery
  - external constriction S30.844 ☑
  - insect bite S30.864 ☑
  - laceration S31.41 ☑
    - with foreign body S31.42 ☑
  - open wound S31.40 ☑
  - puncture S31.43 ☑
    - with foreign body S31.44 ☑
  - superficial S30.95 ☑
    - foreign body S30.854 ☑
- whiplash (cervical spine) S13.4 ☑
- wrist S69.9- ☑
  - blood vessel — *see* Injury, blood vessel, hand
  - contusion — *see* Contusion, wrist
  - dislocation — *see* Dislocation, wrist
  - fracture — *see* Fracture, wrist
  - muscle — *see* Injury, muscle, hand
  - nerve — *see* Injury, nerve, hand
  - open — *see* Wound, open, wrist
  - specified NEC S69.8- ☑
  - sprain — *see* Sprain, wrist
  - superficial — *see* Injury, superficial, wrist

Inoculation (*see also* Vaccination)
- complication or reaction — *see* Complications, vaccination

Insanity, insane (*see also* Psychosis)
- adolescent — *see* Schizophrenia
- confusional F28
  - acute or subacute F05
- delusional F22
- senile F03 ☑

Insect
- bite — *see* Bite, by site, superficial, insect
- venomous, poisoning NEC (by) — *see* Venom, arthropod

Insensitivity
- adrenocorticotropin hormone (ACTH) E27.49
- androgen E34.50
  - complete E34.51
  - partial E34.52

Insertion
- cord (umbilical) lateral or velamentous O43.12- ☑
- intrauterine contraceptive device (encounter for) — *see* Intrauterine contraceptive device

Insolation (sunstroke) T67.0 ☑
Insomnia (organic) G47.00
- adjustment F51.02

Insomnia — *continued*
- adjustment disorder F51.02
- behavioral, of childhood Z73.819
  - combined type Z73.812
  - limit setting type Z73.811
  - sleep-onset association type Z73.810
- childhood Z73.819
- chronic F51.04
  - somatized tension F51.04
- conditioned F51.04
- due to
  - alcohol
    - abuse F10.182
    - dependence F10.282
    - use F10.982
  - amphetamines
    - abuse F15.182
    - dependence F15.282
    - use F15.982
  - anxiety disorder F51.05
  - caffeine
    - abuse F15.182
    - dependence F15.282
    - use F15.982
  - cocaine
    - abuse F14.182
    - dependence F14.282
    - use F14.982
  - depression F51.05
  - drug NEC
    - abuse F19.182
    - dependence F19.282
    - use F19.982
  - medical condition G47.01
  - mental disorder NEC F51.05
  - opioid
    - abuse F11.182
    - dependence F11.282
    - use F11.982
  - psychoactive substance NEC
    - abuse F19.182
    - dependence F19.182
    - use F19.982
  - sedative, hypnotic, or anxiolytic
    - abuse F13.182
    - dependence F13.282
    - use F13.982
  - stimulant NEC
    - abuse F15.182
    - dependence F15.282
    - use F15.982
- fatal familial (FFI) A81.83
- idiopathic F51.01
- learned F51.3
- nonorganic origin F51.01
- not due to a substance or known physiological condition F51.01
- specified NEC F51.09
- paradoxical F51.03
- primary F51.01
- psychiatric F51.05
- psychophysiologic F51.04
- related to psychopathology F51.05
- short-term F51.02
- specified NEC G47.09
- stress-related F51.02
- transient F51.02
- without objective findings F51.02
Inspiration
- food or foreign body — *see* Foreign body, by site
- mucus — *see* Asphyxia, mucus
Inspissated bile syndrome (newborn) P59.1
Instability
- emotional (excessive) F60.3
- joint (post-traumatic) M25.30
  - ankle M25.37- ☑
  - due to old ligament injury — *see* Disorder, ligament
  - elbow M25.32- ☑
  - flail — *see* Flail, joint
  - foot M25.37- ☑
  - hand M25.34- ☑
  - hip M25.35- ☑
  - knee M25.36- ☑
  - lumbosacral — *see* subcategory M53.2 ☑
  - prosthesis — *see* Complications, joint prosthesis, mechanical, displacement, by site
  - sacroiliac — *see* subcategory M53.2 ☑

☑ Additional Character Required — Refer to the Tabular List for Character Selection ▽ Subterms under main terms may continue to next column or page

Instability — *continued*
　joint — *continued*
　　secondary to
　　　old ligament injury — *see* Disorder, ligament
　　　removal of joint prosthesis M96.89
　　shoulder (region) M25.31- ☑
　　spine — *see* subcategory M53.2 ☑
　　wrist M25.33- ☑
　knee (chronic) M23.5- ☑
　lumbosacral — *see* subcategory M53.2 ☑
　nervous F48.8
　personality (emotional) F60.3
　spine — *see* Instability, joint, spine
　vasomotor R55
Institutional syndrome (childhood) F94.2
Institutionalization, affecting child Z62.22
　disinhibited attachment F94.2
Insufficiency, insufficient
　accommodation, old age H52.4
　adrenal (gland) E27.40
　　primary E27.1
　adrenocortical E27.40
　　drug-induced E27.3
　　iatrogenic E27.3
　　primary E27.1
　anatomic crown height K08.89
　anterior (occlusal) guidance M26.54
　anus K62.89
　aortic (valve) I35.1
　　with
　　　mitral (valve) disease I08.0
　　　　with tricuspid (valve) disease I08.3
　　　stenosis I35.2
　　　tricuspid (valve) disease I08.2
　　　　with mitral (valve) disease I08.3
　　congenital Q23.1
　　rheumatic I06.1
　　　with
　　　　mitral (valve) disease I08.0
　　　　　with tricuspid (valve) disease I08.3
　　　　stenosis I06.2
　　　　　with mitral (valve) disease I08.0
　　　　　　with tricuspid (valve) disease I08.3
　　　　tricuspid (valve) disease I08.2
　　　　　with mitral (valve) disease I08.3
　　specified cause NEC I35.1
　　syphilitic A52.03
　arterial I77.1
　　basilar G45.0
　　carotid (hemispheric) G45.1
　　cerebral I67.81
　　coronary (acute or subacute) I24.8
　　mesenteric K55.1
　　peripheral I73.9
　　precerebral (multiple) (bilateral) G45.2
　　vertebral G45.0
　arteriovenous I99.8
　biliary K83.8
　cardiac (*see also* Insufficiency, myocardial)
　　due to presence of (cardiac) prosthesis I97.11- ☑
　　postprocedural I97.11- ☑
　cardiorenal, hypertensive I13.2
　cardiovascular — *see* Disease, cardiovascular
　cerebrovascular (acute) I67.81
　　with transient focal neurological signs and symptoms G45.8
　circulatory NEC I99.8
　　newborn P29.89
　clinical crown length K08.89
　convergence H51.11
　coronary (acute or subacute) I24.8
　　chronic or with a stated duration of over 4 weeks I25.89
　corticoadrenal E27.40
　　primary E27.1
　dietary E63.9
　divergence H51.8
　food T73.0 ☑
　gastroesophageal K22.8
　gonadal
　　ovary E28.39
　　testis E29.1
　heart (*see also* Insufficiency, myocardial)
　　newborn P29.0
　　valve — *see* Endocarditis
　hepatic — *see* Failure, hepatic
　idiopathic autonomic G90.09

Insufficiency, insufficient — *continued*
　interocclusal distance of fully erupted teeth (ridge) M26.36
　kidney N28.9
　　acute N28.9
　　chronic N18.9
　lacrimal (secretion) H04.12- ☑
　　passages — *see* Stenosis, lacrimal
　liver — *see* Failure, hepatic
　lung — *see* Insufficiency, pulmonary
　mental (congenital) — *see* Disability, intellectual
　mesenteric K55.1
　mitral (valve) I34.0
　　with
　　　aortic valve disease I08.0
　　　　with tricuspid (valve) disease I08.3
　　　obstruction or stenosis I05.2
　　　　with aortic valve disease I08.0
　　　tricuspid (valve) disease I08.1
　　　　with aortic (valve) disease I08.3
　　congenital Q23.3
　　rheumatic I05.1
　　　with
　　　　aortic valve disease I08.0
　　　　　with tricuspid (valve) disease I08.3
　　　　obstruction or stenosis I05.2
　　　　　with aortic valve disease I08.0
　　　　　　with tricuspid (valve) disease I08.3
　　　　tricuspid (valve) disease I08.1
　　　　　with aortic (valve) disease I08.3
　　　active or acute I01.1
　　　　with chorea, rheumatic (Sydenham's) I02.0
　　specified cause, except rheumatic I34.0
　muscle (*see also* Disease, muscle)
　　heart — *see* Insufficiency, myocardial
　　ocular NEC H50.9
　myocardial, myocardium (with arteriosclerosis) (*see also* Failure, heart) I50.9
　　with
　　　rheumatic fever (conditions in I00) I09.0
　　　　active, acute or subacute I01.2
　　　　　with chorea I02.0
　　　　inactive or quiescent (with chorea) I09.0
　　congenital Q24.8
　　hypertensive — *see* Hypertension, heart
　　newborn P29.0
　　rheumatic I09.9
　　　active, acute, or subacute I01.2
　　syphilitic A52.06
　nourishment T73.0 ☑
　pancreatic K86.89
　　exocrine K86.81
　parathyroid (gland) E20.9
　peripheral vascular (arterial) I73.9
　pituitary E23.0
　placental (mother) O36.51- ☑
　platelets D69.6
　prenatal care affecting management of pregnancy O09.3- ☑
　progressive pluriglandular E31.0
　pulmonary J98.4
　　acute, following surgery (nonthoracic) J95.2
　　　thoracic J95.1
　　chronic, following surgery J95.3
　　following
　　　shock J98.4
　　　trauma J98.4
　　newborn P28.5
　　valve I37.1
　　　with stenosis I37.2
　　　congenital Q22.2
　　　rheumatic I09.89
　　　　with aortic, mitral or tricuspid (valve) disease I08.8
　pyloric K31.89
　renal (acute) N28.9
　　chronic N18.9
　respiratory R06.89
　　newborn P28.5
　rotation — *see* Malrotation
　sleep syndrome F51.12
　social insurance Z59.7
　suprarenal E27.40
　　primary E27.1
　tarso-orbital fascia, congenital Q10.3
　testis E29.1
　thyroid (gland) (acquired) E03.9
　　congenital E03.1

Insufficiency, insufficient — *continued*
　tricuspid (valve) (rheumatic) I07.1
　　with
　　　aortic (valve) disease I08.2
　　　　with mitral (valve) disease I08.3
　　　mitral (valve) disease I08.1
　　　　with aortic (valve) disease I08.3
　　　obstruction or stenosis I07.2
　　　　with aortic (valve) disease I08.2
　　　　　with mitral (valve) disease I08.3
　　congenital Q22.8
　　nonrheumatic I36.1
　　　with stenosis I36.2
　urethral sphincter R32
　valve, valvular (heart) I38
　　aortic — *see* Insufficiency, aortic (valve)
　　congenital Q24.8
　　mitral — *see* Insufficiency, mitral (valve)
　　pulmonary — *see* Insufficiency, pulmonary, valve
　　tricuspid — *see* Insufficiency, tricuspid (valve)
　vascular I99.9
　　intestine K55.9
　　　acute (*see also* Ischemia, intestine, acute) K55.059
　　mesenteric K55.1
　　peripheral I73.9
　　renal — *see* Hypertension, kidney
　velopharyngeal
　　acquired K13.79
　　congenital Q38.8
　venous (chronic) (peripheral) I87.2
　ventricular — *see* Insufficiency, myocardial
　welfare support Z59.7
Insufflation, fallopian Z31.41
Insular — *see* condition
Insulinoma
　pancreas
　　benign D13.7
　　malignant C25.4
　　uncertain behavior D37.8
　specified site
　　benign — *see* Neoplasm, by site, benign
　　malignant — *see* Neoplasm, by site, malignant
　　uncertain behavior — *see* Neoplasm, by site, uncertain behavior
　unspecified site
　　benign D13.7
　　malignant C25.4
　　uncertain behavior D37.8
Insuloma — *see* Insulinoma
Interference
　balancing side M26.56
　non-working side M26.56
Intermenstrual — *see* condition
Intermittent — *see* condition
Internal — *see* condition
Interrogation
　cardiac defibrillator (automatic) (implantable) Z45.02
　cardiac pacemaker Z45.018
　cardiac (event) (loop) recorder Z45.09
　infusion pump (implanted) (intrathecal) Z45.1
　neurostimulator Z46.2
Interruption
　aortic arch Q25.21
　bundle of His I44.30
　phase-shift, sleep cycle — *see* Disorder, sleep, circadian rhythm
　sleep phase-shift, or 24 hour sleep-wake cycle — *see* Disorder, sleep, circadian rhythm
Interstitial — *see* condition
Intertrigo L30.4
　labialis K13.0
Intervertebral disc — *see* condition
Intestine, intestinal — *see* condition
Intolerance
　carbohydrate K90.49
　disaccharide, hereditary E73.0
　fat NEC K90.49
　　pancreatic K90.3
　food K90.49
　　dietary counseling and surveillance Z71.3
　fructose E74.10
　　hereditary E74.12
　glucose (-galactose) E74.39
　gluten K90.41
　lactose E73.9
　　specified NEC E73.8
　lysine E72.3
　milk NEC K90.49

Intolerance — *continued*
  milk — *continued*
    lactose E73.9
  protein K90.49
  starch NEC K90.49
  sucrose (-isomaltose) E74.31
Intoxicated NEC (without dependence) — *see* Alcohol, intoxication
Intoxication
  acid E87.2
  alcoholic (acute) (without dependence) — *see* Alcohol, intoxication
  alimentary canal K52.1
  amphetamine (without dependence) — *see* Abuse, drug, stimulant, with intoxication
    with dependence — *see* Dependence, drug, stimulant, with intoxication
  anxiolytic (acute) (without dependence) — *see* Abuse, drug, sedative, with intoxication
    with dependence — *see* Dependence, drug, sedative, with intoxication
  caffeine F15.929
    with dependence — *see* Dependence, drug, stimulant, with intoxication
  cannabinoids (acute) (without dependence) — *see* Use, cannabis, with intoxication
    with
      abuse — *see* Abuse, drug, cannabis, with intoxication
      dependence — *see* Dependence, drug, cannabis, with intoxication
  chemical — *see* Table of Drugs and Chemicals
    via placenta or breast milk — *see* - Absorption, chemical, through placenta
  cocaine (acute) (without dependence) — *see* Abuse, drug, cocaine, with intoxication
    with dependence — *see* Dependence, drug, cocaine, with intoxication
  drug
    acute (without dependence) — *see* Abuse, drug, by type with intoxication
      with dependence — *see* Dependence, drug, by type with intoxication
    addictive
      via placenta or breast milk — *see* Absorption, drug, addictive, through placenta
    newborn P93.8
      gray baby syndrome P93.0
    overdose or wrong substance given or taken — *see* Table of Drugs and Chemicals, by drug, poisoning
  enteric K52.1
  foodborne A05.9
    bacterial A05.9
    classical (Clostridium botulinum) A05.1
    due to
      Bacillus cereus A05.4
      bacterium A05.9
        specified NEC A05.8
      Clostridium
        botulinum A05.1
        perfringens A05.2
        welchii A05.2
      Salmonella A02.9
        with
          (gastro)enteritis A02.0
          localized infection(s) A02.20
            arthritis A02.23
            meningitis A02.21
            osteomyelitis A02.24
            pneumonia A02.22
            pyelonephritis A02.25
            specified NEC A02.29
          sepsis A02.1
          specified manifestation NEC A02.8
      Staphylococcus A05.0
      Vibrio
        parahaemolyticus A05.3
        vulnificus A05.5
    enterotoxin, staphylococcal A05.0
    noxious — *see* Poisoning, food, noxious
  gastrointestinal K52.1
  hallucinogenic (without dependence) — *see* Abuse, drug, hallucinogen, with intoxication
    with dependence — *see* Dependence, drug, hallucinogen, with intoxication
  hypnotic (acute) (without dependence) — *see* Abuse, drug, sedative, with intoxication

Intoxication — *continued*
  hypnotic — *see* Abuse, drug, sedative, with intoxication — *continued*
    with dependence — *see* Dependence, drug, sedative, with intoxication
  inhalant (acute) (without dependence) — *see* Abuse, drug, inhalant, with intoxication
    with dependence — *see* Dependence, drug, inhalant, with intoxication
  meaning
    inebriation — *see* category F10 ☑
    poisoning — *see* Table of Drugs and Chemicals
  methyl alcohol (acute) (without dependence) — *see* Alcohol, intoxication
  opioid (acute) (without dependence) — *see* Abuse, drug, opioid, with intoxication
    with dependence — *see* Dependence, drug, opioid, with intoxication
  pathologic NEC (without dependence) — *see* Alcohol, intoxication
  phencyclidine (without dependence) — *see* Abuse, drug, hallucinogen, with intoxication
    with dependence — *see* Dependence, drug, hallucinogen, with intoxication
  potassium (K) E87.5
  psychoactive substance NEC (without dependence) — *see* Abuse, drug, psychoactive NEC, with intoxication
    with dependence — *see* Dependence, drug, psychoactive NEC, with intoxication
  sedative (acute) (without dependence) — *see* Abuse, drug, sedative, with intoxication
    with dependence — *see* Dependence, drug, sedative, with intoxication
  serum (*see also* Reaction, serum) T80.69 ☑
  uremic — *see* Uremia
  volatile solvents (acute) (without dependence) — *see* Abuse, drug, inhalant, with intoxication
    with dependence — *see* Dependence, drug, inhalant, with intoxication
  water E87.79
Intraabdominal testis, testes
  bilateral Q53.211
  unilateral Q53.111
Intracranial — *see* condition
Intrahepatic gallbladder Q44.1
Intraligamentous — *see* condition
Intrathoracic (*see also* condition)
  kidney Q63.2
Intrauterine contraceptive device
  checking Z30.431
  in situ Z97.5
  insertion Z30.430
    immediately following removal Z30.433
  management Z30.431
  reinsertion Z30.433
  removal Z30.432
  replacement Z30.433
  retention in pregnancy O26.3- ☑
Intraventricular — *see* condition
Intrinsic deformity — *see* Deformity
Intubation, difficult or failed T88.4 ☑
Intumescence, lens (eye) (cataract) — *see* Cataract
Intussusception (bowel) (colon) (enteric) (ileocecal) (ileocolic) (intestine) (rectum) K56.1
  appendix K38.8
  congenital Q43.8
  ureter (with obstruction) N13.5
Invagination (bowel, colon, intestine or rectum) K56.1
Inversion
  albumin-globulin (A-G) ratio E88.09
  bladder N32.89
  cecum — *see* Intussusception
  cervix N88.8
  chromosome in normal individual Q95.1
  circadian rhythm — *see* Disorder, sleep, circadian rhythm
  nipple N64.59
    congenital Q83.8
    gestational — *see* Retraction, nipple
    puerperal, postpartum — *see* Retraction, nipple
  nyctohemeral rhythm — *see* Disorder, sleep, circadian rhythm
  optic papilla Q14.2
  organ or site, congenital NEC — *see* Anomaly, by site
  sleep rhythm — *see* Disorder, sleep, circadian rhythm
  testis (congenital) Q55.29

Inversion — *continued*
  uterus (chronic) (postinfectional) (postpartal, old) N85.5
    postpartum O71.2
  vagina (posthysterectomy) N99.3
  ventricular Q20.5
Investigation (*see also* Examination) Z04.9
  clinical research subject (control) (normal comparison) (participant) Z00.6
Involuntary movement, abnormal R25.9
Involution, involutional (*see also* condition)
  breast, cystic — *see* Dysplasia, mammary, specified type NEC
  depression (single episode) F32.89
    recurrent episode F33.9
  melancholia (single episode) F32.89
    recurrent episode F33.8
  ovary, senile — *see* Atrophy, ovary
  thymus failure E32.8
I.Q.
  20-34 F72
  35-49 F71
  50-69 F70
  under 20 F73
IRDS (type I) P22.0
  type II P22.1
Irideremia Q13.1
Iridis rubeosis — *see* Disorder, iris, vascular
Iridochoroiditis (panuveitis) — *see* Panuveitis
Iridocyclitis H20.9
  acute H20.0- ☑
    hypopyon H20.05- ☑
    primary H20.01- ☑
    recurrent H20.02- ☑
    secondary (noninfectious) H20.04- ☑
      infectious H20.03- ☑
  chronic H20.1- ☑
  due to allergy — *see* Iridocyclitis, acute, secondary
  endogenous — *see* Iridocyclitis, acute, primary
  Fuchs' — *see* Cyclitis, Fuchs' heterochromic
  gonococcal A54.32
  granulomatous — *see* Iridocyclitis, chronic
  herpes, herpetic (simplex) B00.51
    zoster B02.32
  hypopyon — *see* Iridocyclitis, acute, hypopyon
  in (due to)
    ankylosing spondylitis M45.9
    gonococcal infection A54.32
    herpes (simplex) virus B00.51
      zoster B02.32
    infectious disease NOS B99 ☑
    parasitic disease NOS B89 [H22]
    sarcoidosis D86.83
    syphilis A51.43
    tuberculosis A18.54
    zoster B02.32
  lens-induced H20.2- ☑
  nongranulomatous — *see* Iridocyclitis, acute
  recurrent — *see* Iridocyclitis, acute, recurrent
  rheumatic — *see* Iridocyclitis, chronic
  subacute — *see* Iridocyclitis, acute
  sympathetic — *see* Uveitis, sympathetic
  syphilitic (secondary) A51.43
  tuberculous (chronic) A18.54
  Vogt-Koyanagi H20.82- ☑
Iridocyclochoroiditis (panuveitis) — *see* Panuveitis
Iridodialysis H21.53- ☑
Iridodonesis H21.89
Iridoplegia (complete) (partial) (reflex) H57.09
Iridoschisis H21.25- ☑
Iris (*see also* condition)
  bombé — *see* Membrane, pupillary
Iritis (*see also* Iridocyclitis)
  chronic — *see* Iridocyclitis, chronic
  diabetic — *see* E08-E13 with .39
  due to
    herpes simplex B00.51
    leprosy A30.9 [H22]
  gonococcal A54.32
  gouty (*see also* Gout, by type) M10.9 [H22]
  granulomatous — *see* Iridocyclitis, chronic
  lens induced — *see* Iridocyclitis, lens-induced
  papulosa (syphilitic) A52.71
  rheumatic — *see* Iridocyclitis, chronic
  syphilitic (secondary) A51.43
    congenital (early) A50.01
    late A52.71
  tuberculous A18.54

Iron — *see* condition
Iron-miner's lung J63.4
Irradiated enamel (tooth, teeth) K03.89
Irradiation effects, adverse T66 ☑
Irreducible, irreducibility — *see* condition
Irregular, irregularity
  action, heart I49.9
  alveolar process K08.89
  bleeding N92.6
  breathing R06.89
  contour of cornea (acquired) — *see* Deformity, cornea
    congenital Q13.4
  contour, reconstructed breast N65.0
  dentin (in pulp) K04.3
  eye movements H55.89
    nystagmus — *see* Nystagmus
    saccadic H55.81
  labor O62.2
  menstruation (cause unknown) N92.6
  periods N92.6
  prostate N42.9
  pupil — *see* Abnormality, pupillary
  reconstructed breast N65.0
  respiratory R06.89
  septum (nasal) J34.2
  shape, organ or site, congenital NEC — *see* Distortion
  sleep-wake pattern (rhythm) G47.23
Irritable, irritability R45.4
  bladder N32.89
  bowel (syndrome) K58.9
    with
      constipation K58.1
      diarrhea K58.0
    mixed K58.2
    psychogenic F45.8
    specified NEC K58.8
  bronchial — *see* Bronchitis
  cerebral, in newborn P91.3
  colon (*see also* Irritable, bowel) K58.9
    with diarrhea K58.0
    psychogenic F45.8
  duodenum K59.8
  heart (psychogenic) F45.8
  hip — *see* Derangement, joint, specified type NEC, hip
  ileum K59.8
  infant R68.12
  jejunum K59.8
  rectum K59.8
  stomach K31.89
    psychogenic F45.8
  sympathetic G90.8
  urethra N36.8
Irritation
  anus K62.89
  axillary nerve G54.0
  bladder N32.89
  brachial plexus G54.0
  bronchial — *see* Bronchitis
  cervical plexus G54.2
  cervix — *see* Cervicitis
  choroid, sympathetic — *see* Endophthalmitis
  cranial nerve — *see* Disorder, nerve, cranial
  gastric K31.89
    psychogenic F45.8
  globe, sympathetic — *see* Uveitis, sympathetic
  labyrinth — *see* subcategory H83.2 ☑
  lumbosacral plexus G54.1
  meninges (traumatic) — *see* Injury, intracranial
    nontraumatic — *see* Meningismus
  nerve — *see* Disorder, nerve
  nervous R45.0
  penis N48.89
  perineum NEC L29.3
  peripheral autonomic nervous system G90.8
  peritoneum — *see* Peritonitis
  pharynx J39.2
  plantar nerve — *see* Lesion, nerve, plantar
  spinal (cord) (traumatic) (*see also* Injury, spinal cord, by region)
    nerve G58.9
      root NEC — *see* Radiculopathy
      nontraumatic — *see* Myelopathy
  stomach K31.89
    psychogenic F45.8
  sympathetic nerve NEC G90.8
  ulnar nerve — *see* Lesion, nerve, ulnar
  vagina N89.8
Ischemia, ischemic I99.8

Ischemia, ischemic — *continued*
  bowel (transient)
    acute (*see also* Ischemia, intestine, acute) K55.059
    chronic K55.1
    due to mesenteric artery insufficiency K55.1
  brain — *see* Ischemia, cerebral
  cardiac (see Disease, heart, ischemic)
  cardiomyopathy I25.5
  cerebral (chronic) (generalized) I67.82
    arteriosclerotic I67.2
    intermittent G45.9
    newborn P91.0
    recurrent focal G45.8
    transient G45.9
  colon chronic (due to mesenteric artery insufficiency) K55.1
  coronary — *see* Disease, heart, ischemic
  demand (coronary) (*see also* Angina) I24.8
    with myocardial infarction I21.A1
    resulting in myocardial infarction I21.A1
  heart (chronic or with a stated duration of over 4 weeks) I25.9
    acute or with a stated duration of 4 weeks or less I24.9
    subacute I24.9
  infarction, muscle — *see* Infarct, muscle
  intestine (large) (small) (transient) K55.9
    acute K55.059
      diffuse K55.052
      focal K55.051
      large K55.039
        diffuse K55.032
        focal K55.031
      small K55.019
        diffuse K55.012
        focal K55.011
    chronic K55.1
    due to mesenteric artery insufficiency K55.1
  kidney N28.0
  mesenteric, acute (*see also* Ischemia, intestine, acute) K55.059
  muscle, traumatic T79.6 ☑
  myocardium, myocardial (chronic or with a stated duration of over 4 weeks) I25.9
    acute, without myocardial infarction I51.3
    silent (asymptomatic) I25.6
    transient of newborn P29.4
  renal N28.0
  retina, retinal — *see* Occlusion, artery, retina
  small bowel
    acute K55.019
      diffuse K55.012
      focal K55.011
    chronic K55.1
    due to mesenteric artery insufficiency K55.1
  spinal cord G95.11
  subendocardial — *see* Insufficiency, coronary
  supply (coronary) (*see also* Angina) I25.9
    due to vasospasm I20.1
Ischial spine — *see* condition
Ischialgia — *see* Sciatica
Ischiopagus Q89.4
Ischium, ischial — *see* condition
Ischuria R34
Iselin's disease or osteochondrosis — *see* Osteochondrosis, juvenile, metatarsus
Islands of
  parotid tissue in
    lymph nodes Q38.6
    neck structures Q38.6
  submaxillary glands in
    fascia Q38.6
    lymph nodes Q38.6
    neck muscles Q38.6
Islet cell tumor, pancreas D13.7
Isoimmunization NEC (*see also* Incompatibility)
  affecting management of pregnancy (ABO) (with hydrops fetalis) O36.11- ☑
    anti-A sensitization O36.11- ☑
    anti-B sensitization O36.19- ☑
    anti-c sensitization O36.09- ☑
    anti-C sensitization O36.09- ☑
    anti-e sensitization O36.09- ☑
    anti-E sensitization O36.09- ☑
    Rh NEC O36.09- ☑
      anti-D antibody O36.01- ☑
    specified NEC O36.19- ☑
  newborn P55.9

Isoimmunization — *continued*
  newborn — *continued*
    with
      hydrops fetalis P56.0
      kernicterus P57.0
    ABO (blood groups) P55.1
    Rhesus (Rh) factor P55.0
    specified type NEC P55.8
Isolation, isolated
  dwelling Z59.8
  family Z63.79
  social Z60.4
Isoleucinosis E71.19
Isomerism atrial appendages (with asplenia or polysplenia) Q20.6
Isosporiasis, isosporosis A07.3
Isovaleric acidemia E71.110
Issue of
  medical certificate Z02.79
    for disability determination Z02.71
  repeat prescription (appliance) (glasses) (medicinal substance, medicament, medicine) Z76.0
    contraception — *see* Contraception
Itch, itching (*see also* Pruritus)
  baker's L23.6
  barber's B35.0
  bricklayer's L24.5
  cheese B88.0
  clam digger's B65.3
  coolie B76.9
  copra B88.0
  dew B76.9
  dhobi B35.6
  filarial — *see* Infestation, filarial
  grain B88.0
  grocer's B88.0
  ground B76.9
  harvest B88.0
  jock B35.6
  Malabar B35.5
    beard B35.0
    foot B35.3
    scalp B35.0
  meaning scabies B86
  Norwegian B86
  perianal L29.0
  poultrymen's B88.0
  sarcoptic B86
  scabies B86
  scrub B88.0
  straw B88.0
  swimmer's B65.3
  water B76.9
  winter L29.8
Ivemark's syndrome (asplenia with congenital heart disease) Q89.01
Ivory bones Q78.2
Ixodiasis NEC B88.8

J

Jaccoud's syndrome — *see* Arthropathy, postrheumatic, chronic
Jackson's
  membrane Q43.3
  paralysis or syndrome G83.89
  veil Q43.3
Jacquet's dermatitis (diaper dermatitis) L22
Jadassohn-Pellizari's disease or anetoderma L90.2
Jadassohn's
  blue nevus — *see* Nevus
  intraepidermal epithelioma — *see* Neoplasm, skin, benign
Jaffe-Lichtenstein (-Uehlinger) **syndrome** — *see* Dysplasia, fibrous, bone NEC
Jakob-Creutzfeldt disease or syndrome — *see* Creutzfeldt-Jakob disease or syndrome
Jaksch-Luzet disease D64.89
Jamaican
  neuropathy G92
  paraplegic tropical ataxic-spastic syndrome G92
Janet's disease F48.8
Janiceps Q89.4
Jansky-Bielschowsky amaurotic idiocy E75.4
Japanese
  B-type encephalitis A83.0
  river fever A75.3
Jaundice (yellow) R17

Jaundice — *continued*
  acholuric (familial) (splenomegalic) (*see also* Spherocytosis)
    acquired D59.8
  breast-milk (inhibitor) P59.3
  catarrhal (acute) B15.9
    with hepatic coma B15.0
  cholestatic (benign) R17
  due to or associated with
    delayed conjugation P59.8
      associated with (due to) preterm delivery P59.0
    preterm delivery P59.0
  epidemic (catarrhal) B15.9
    with hepatic coma B15.0
    leptospiral A27.0
    spirochetal A27.0
  familial nonhemolytic (congenital) (Gilbert) E80.4
    Crigler-Najjar E80.5
  febrile (acute) B15.9
    with hepatic coma B15.0
    leptospiral A27.0
    spirochetal A27.0
  hematogenous D59.9
  hemolytic (acquired) D59.9
    congenital — *see* Spherocytosis
  hemorrhagic (acute) (leptospiral) (spirochetal) A27.0
  infectious (acute) (subacute) B15.9
    with hepatic coma B15.0
    leptospiral A27.0
    spirochetal A27.0
  leptospiral (hemorrhagic) A27.0
  malignant (without coma) K72.90
    with coma K72.91
  neonatal — *see* Jaundice, newborn
  newborn P59.9
    due to or associated with
      ABO
        antibodies P55.1
        incompatibility, maternal/fetal P55.1
        isoimmunization P55.1
      absence or deficiency of enzyme system for bilirubin conjugation (congenital) P59.8
      bleeding P58.1
      breast milk inhibitors to conjugation P59.3
        associated with preterm delivery P59.0
      bruising P58.0
      Crigler-Najjar syndrome E80.5
      delayed conjugation P59.8
        associated with preterm delivery P59.0
      drugs or toxins
        given to newborn P58.42
        transmitted from mother P58.41
      excessive hemolysis P58.9
        due to
          bleeding P58.1
          bruising P58.0
          drugs or toxins
            given to newborn P58.42
            transmitted from mother P58.41
          infection P58.2
          polycythemia P58.3
          swallowed maternal blood P58.5
        specified type NEC P58.8
      galactosemia E74.21
      Gilbert syndrome E80.4
      hemolytic disease P55.9
        ABO isoimmunization P55.1
        Rh isoimmunization P55.0
        specified NEC P55.8
      hepatocellular damage P59.20
        specified NEC P59.29
      hereditary hemolytic anemia P58.8
      hypothyroidism, congenital E03.1
      incompatibility, maternal/fetal NOS P55.9
      infection P58.2
      inspissated bile syndrome P59.1
      isoimmunization NOS P55.9
      mucoviscidosis E84.9
      polycythemia P58.3
      preterm delivery P59.0
      Rh
        antibodies P55.0
        incompatibility, maternal/fetal P55.0
        isoimmunization P55.0
      specified cause NEC P59.8
      swallowed maternal blood P58.5
    spherocytosis (congenital) D58.0
    nonhemolytic congenital familial (Gilbert) E80.4

Jaundice — *continued*
  nuclear, newborn (*see also* Kernicterus of newborn) P57.9
  obstructive (*see also* Obstruction, bile duct) K83.1
  post-immunization — *see* Hepatitis, viral, type, B
  post-transfusion — *see* Hepatitis, viral, type, B
  regurgitation (*see also* Obstruction, bile duct) K83.1
  serum (homologous) (prophylactic) (therapeutic) — *see* Hepatitis, viral, type, B
  spirochetal (hemorrhagic) A27.0
  symptomatic R17
    newborn P59.9
Jaw — *see* condition
Jaw-winking phenomenon or syndrome Q07.8
Jealousy
  alcoholic F10.988
  childhood F93.8
  sibling F93.8
Jejunitis — *see* Enteritis
Jejunostomy status Z93.4
Jejunum, jejunal — *see* condition
Jensen's disease — *see* Inflammation, chorioretinal, focal, juxtapapillary
Jerks, myoclonic G25.3
Jervell-Lange-Nielsen syndrome I45.81
Jeune's disease Q77.2
Jigger disease B88.1
Job's syndrome (chronic granulomatous disease) D71
Joint (*see also* condition)
  mice — *see* Loose, body, joint
    knee M23.4- ☑
Jordan's anomaly or syndrome D72.0
Joseph-Diamond-Blackfan anemia (congenital hypoplastic) D61.01
Jungle yellow fever A95.0
Jüngling's disease — *see* Sarcoidosis
Juvenile — *see* condition

K

Kahler's disease C90.0- ☑
Kakke E51.11
Kala-azar B55.0
Kallmann's syndrome E23.0
Kanner's syndrome (autism) — *see* Psychosis, childhood
Kaposi's
  dermatosis (xeroderma pigmentosum) Q82.1
  lichen ruber L44.0
    acuminatus L44.0
  sarcoma
    colon C46.4
    connective tissue C46.1
    gastrointestinal organ C46.4
    lung C46.5- ☑
    lymph node (multiple) C46.3
    palate (hard) (soft) C46.2
    rectum C46.4
    skin (multiple sites) C46.0
    specified site NEC C46.7
    stomach C46.4
    unspecified site C46.9
  varicelliform eruption B00.0
    vaccinia T88.1 ☑
Kartagener's syndrome or triad (sinusitis, bronchiectasis, situs inversus) Q89.3
Karyotype
  with abnormality except iso (Xq) Q96.2
  45,X Q96.0
  46,X
    iso (Xq) Q96.1
  46,XX Q98.3
    with streak gonads Q50.32
    hermaphrodite (true) Q99.1
    male Q98.3
  46,XY
    with streak gonads Q56.1
    female Q97.3
    hermaphrodite (true) Q99.1
  47,XXX Q97.0
  47,XXY Q98.0
  47,XYY Q98.5
Kaschin-Beck disease — *see* Disease, Kaschin-Beck
Katayama's disease or fever B65.2
Kawasaki's syndrome M30.3
Kayser-Fleischer ring (cornea) (pseudosclerosis) H18.04- ☑

Kaznelson's syndrome (congenital hypoplastic anemia) D61.01
Kearns-Sayre syndrome H49.81- ☑
Kedani fever A75.3
Kelis L91.0
Kelly (-Patterson) **syndrome** (sideropenic dysphagia) D50.1
Keloid, cheloid L91.0
  acne L73.0
  Addison's L94.0
  cornea — *see* Opacity, cornea
  Hawkin's L91.0
  scar L91.0
Keloma L91.0
Kenya fever A77.1
Keratectasia (*see also* Ectasia, cornea)
  congenital Q13.4
Keratinization of alveolar ridge mucosa
  excessive K13.23
  minimal K13.22
Keratinized residual ridge mucosa
  excessive K13.23
  minimal K13.22
Keratitis (nodular) (nonulcerative) (simple) (zonular) H16.9
  with ulceration (central) (marginal) (perforated) (ring) — *see* Ulcer, cornea
  actinic — *see* Photokeratitis
  arborescens (herpes simplex) B00.52
  areolar H16.11- ☑
  bullosa H16.8
  deep H16.309
    specified type NEC H16.399
  dendritic (a) (herpes simplex) B00.52
  disciform (is) (herpes simplex) B00.52
    varicella B01.81
  filamentary H16.12- ☑
  gonococcal (congenital or prenatal) A54.33
  herpes, herpetic (simplex) B00.52
    zoster B02.33
  in (due to)
    acanthamebiasis B60.13
    adenovirus B30.0
    exanthema (*see also* Exanthem) B09
    herpes (simplex) virus B00.52
    measles B05.81
    syphilis A50.31
    tuberculosis A18.52
    zoster B02.33
  interstitial (nonsyphilitic) H16.30- ☑
    diffuse H16.32- ☑
    herpes, herpetic (simplex) B00.52
      zoster B02.33
    sclerosing H16.33- ☑
    specified type NEC H16.39- ☑
    syphilitic (congenital) (late) A50.31
    tuberculous A18.52
  macular H16.11- ☑
  nummular H16.11- ☑
  oyster shuckers' H16.8
  parenchymatous — *see* Keratitis, interstitial
  petrificans H16.8
  postmeasles B05.81
  punctata
    leprosa A30.9 [H16.14-] ☑
    syphilitic (profunda) A50.31
  punctate H16.14- ☑
  purulent H16.8
  rosacea L71.8
  sclerosing H16.33- ☑
  specified type NEC H16.8
  stellate H16.11- ☑
  striate H16.11- ☑
  superficial H16.10- ☑
    with conjunctivitis — *see* Keratoconjunctivitis
    due to light — *see* Photokeratitis
  suppurative H16.8
  syphilitic (congenital) (prenatal) A50.31
  trachomatous A71.1
    sequelae B94.0
  tuberculous A18.52
  vesicular H16.8
  xerotic (*see also* Keratomalacia) H16.8
    vitamin A deficiency E50.4
Keratoacanthoma L85.8
Keratocele — *see* Descemetocele
Keratoconjunctivitis H16.20- ☑

Keratoconjunctivitis — *continued*
Acanthamoeba B60.13
adenoviral B30.0
epidemic B30.0
exposure H16.21- ☑
herpes, herpetic (simplex) B00.52
zoster B02.33
in exanthema (*see also* Exanthem) B09
infectious B30.0
lagophthalmic — *see* Keratoconjunctivitis, specified type NEC
neurotrophic H16.23- ☑
phlyctenular H16.25- ☑
postmeasles B05.81
shipyard B30.0
sicca (Sjogren's) M35.0- ☑
not Sjogren's H16.22- ☑
specified type NEC H16.29- ☑
tuberculous (phlyctenular) A18.52
vernal H16.26- ☑
Keratoconus H18.60- ☑
congenital Q13.4
stable H18.61- ☑
unstable H18.62- ☑
Keratocyst (dental) (odontogenic) — *see* Cyst, calcifying odontogenic
Keratoderma, keratodermia (congenital) (palmaris et plantaris) (symmetrical) Q82.8
acquired L85.1
in diseases classified elsewhere L86
climactericum L85.1
gonococcal A54.89
gonorrheal A54.89
punctata L85.2
Reiter's — *see* Reiter's disease
Keratodermatocele — *see* Descemetocele
Keratoglobus H18.79 ☑
congenital Q15.8
with glaucoma Q15.0
Keratohemia — *see* Pigmentation, cornea, stromal
Keratoiritis (*see also* Iridocyclitis)
syphilitic A50.39
tuberculous A18.54
Keratoma L57.0
palmaris and plantaris hereditarium Q82.8
senile L57.0
Keratomalacia H18.44- ☑
vitamin A deficiency E50.4
Keratomegaly Q13.4
Keratomycosis B49
nigrans, nigricans (palmaris) B36.1
Keratopathy H18.9
band H18.42- ☑
bullous (aphakic), following cataract surgery H59.01- ☑
bullous H18.1- ☑
Keratoscleritis, tuberculous A18.52
Keratosis L57.0
actinic L57.0
arsenical L85.8
congenital, specified NEC Q80.8
female genital NEC N94.89
follicularis Q82.8
acquired L11.0
congenita Q82.8
et parafollicularis in cutem penetrans L87.0
spinulosa (decalvans) Q82.8
vitamin A deficiency E50.8
gonococcal A54.89
male genital (external) N50.89
nigricans L83
obturans, external ear (canal) — *see* Cholesteatoma, external ear
palmaris et plantaris (inherited) (symmetrical) Q82.8
acquired L85.1
penile N48.89
pharynx J39.2
pilaris, acquired L85.8
punctata (palmaris et plantaris) L85.2
scrotal N50.89
seborrheic L82.1
inflamed L82.0
senile L57.0
solar L57.0
tonsillaris J35.8
vagina N89.4
vegetans Q82.8
vitamin A deficiency E50.8
vocal cord J38.3

Kerato-uveitis — *see* Iridocyclitis
Kerion (celsi) B35.0
Kernicterus of newborn (not due to isoimmunization) P57.9
due to isoimmunization (conditions in P55.0-P55.9) P57.0
specified type NEC P57.8
Kerunoparalysis T75.09 ☑
Keshan disease E59
Ketoacidosis E87.2
diabetic — *see* Diabetes, by type, with ketoacidosis
Ketonuria R82.4
Ketosis NEC E88.89
diabetic — *see* Diabetes, by type, with with ketoacidosis
Kew Garden fever A79.1
Kidney — *see* condition
Kienböck's disease (*see also* Osteochondrosis, juvenile, hand, carpal lunate)
adult M93.1
Kimmelstiel (-Wilson) **disease** — *see* Diabetes, Kimmelstiel (-Wilson) disease
Kink, kinking
artery I77.1
hair (acquired) L67.8
ileum or intestine — *see* Obstruction, intestine
Lane's — *see* Obstruction, intestine
organ or site, congenital NEC — *see* Anomaly, by site
ureter (pelvic junction) N13.5
with
hydronephrosis N13.1
with infection N13.6
pyelonephritis (chronic) N11.1
congenital Q62.39
vein(s) I87.8
caval I87.1
peripheral I87.1
Kinnier Wilson's disease (hepatolenticular degeneration) E83.01
Kissing spine M48.20
cervical region M48.22
cervicothoracic region M48.23
lumbar region M48.26
lumbosacral region M48.27
occipito-atlanto-axial region M48.21
thoracic region M48.24
thoracolumbar region M48.25
Klatskin's tumor C22.1
Klauder's disease A26.8
Klebs' disease (*see also* Glomerulonephritis) N05- ☑
Klebsiella (K.) **pneumoniae, as cause of disease classified elsewhere** B96.1
Klein (e)-**Levin syndrome** G47.13
Kleptomania F63.2
Klinefelter's syndrome Q98.4
karyotype 47,XXY Q98.0
male with more than two X chromosomes Q98.1
Klippel-Feil deficiency, disease, or syndrome (brevicollis) Q76.1
Klippel's disease I67.2
Klippel-Trenaunay (-Weber) **syndrome** Q87.2
Klumpke (-Déjerine) **palsy, paralysis** (birth) (newborn) P14.1
Knee — *see* condition
Knock knee (acquired) M21.06- ☑
congenital Q74.1
Knot(s)
intestinal, syndrome (volvulus) K56.2
surfer S89.8- ☑
umbilical cord (true) O69.2 ☑
Knotting (of)
hair L67.8
intestine K56.2
Knuckle pad (Garrod's) M72.1
Koch's
infection — *see* Tuberculosis
relapsing fever A68.9
Koch-Weeks' conjunctivitis — *see* Conjunctivitis, acute, mucopurulent
Köebner's syndrome Q81.8
Köenig's disease (osteochondritis dissecans) — *see* Osteochondritis, dissecans
Köhler-Pellegrini-Steida disease or syndrome (calcification, knee joint) — *see* Bursitis, tibial collateral
Köhler's disease
patellar — *see* Osteochondrosis, juvenile, patella
tarsal navicular — *see* Osteochondrosis, juvenile, tarsus

Koilonychia L60.3
congenital Q84.6
Kojevnikof's, epilepsy — *see* Kozhevnikof's epilepsy
Koplik's spots B05.9
Kopp's asthma E32.8
Korsakoff's (Wernicke) **disease, psychosis or syndrome** (alcoholic) F10.96
with dependence F10.26
drug-induced
due to drug abuse — *see* Abuse, drug, by type, with amnestic disorder
due to drug dependence — *see* Dependence, drug, by type, with amnestic disorder
nonalcoholic F04
Korsakov's disease, psychosis or syndrome — *see* Korsakoff's disease
Korsakow's disease, psychosis or syndrome — *see* Korsakoff's disease
Kostmann's disease or syndrome (infantile genetic agranulocytosis) — *see* Agranulocytosis
Kozhevnikof's epilepsy G40.109
intractable G40.119
with status epilepticus G40.111
without status epilepticus G40.119
not intractable G40.109
with status epilepticus G40.101
without status epilepticus G40.109
Krabbe's
disease E75.23
syndrome, congenital muscle hypoplasia Q79.8
Kraepelin-Morel disease — *see* Schizophrenia
Kraft-Weber-Dimitri disease Q85.8
Kraurosis
ani K62.89
penis N48.0
vagina N89.8
vulva N90.4
Kreotoxism A05.9
Krukenberg's
spindle — *see* Pigmentation, cornea, posterior
tumor C79.6- ☑
Kufs' disease E75.4
Kugelberg-Welander disease G12.1
Kuhnt-Junius degeneration (*see also* Degeneration, macula) H35.32- ☑
Kümmell's disease or spondylitis — *see* Spondylopathy, traumatic
Kupffer cell sarcoma C22.3
Kuru A81.81
Kussmaul's
disease M30.0
respiration E87.2
in diabetic acidosis — *see* Diabetes, by type, with ketoacidosis
Kwashiorkor E40
marasmic, marasmus type E42
Kyasanur Forest disease A98.2
Kyphoscoliosis, kyphoscoliotic (acquired) (*see also* Scoliosis) M41.9
congenital Q67.5
heart (disease) I27.1
sequelae of rickets E64.3
tuberculous A18.01
Kyphosis, kyphotic (acquired) M40.209
cervical region M40.202
cervicothoracic region M40.203
congenital Q76.419
cervical region Q76.412
cervicothoracic region Q76.413
occipito-atlanto-axial region Q76.411
thoracic region Q76.414
thoracolumbar region Q76.415
Morquio-Brailsford type (spinal) (*see also* subcategory M49.8) E76.219
postlaminectomy M96.3
postradiation therapy M96.2
postural (adolescent) M40.00
cervicothoracic region M40.03
thoracic region M40.04
thoracolumbar region M40.05
secondary NEC M40.10
cervical region M40.12
cervicothoracic region M40.13
thoracic region M40.14
thoracolumbar region M40.15
sequelae of rickets E64.3
specified type NEC M40.299
cervical region M40.292

Subterms under main terms may continue to next column or page   ☑ Additional Character Required — Refer to the Tabular List for Character Selection   205

Keratoconjunctivitis — Kyphosis, kyphotic

Kyphosis, kyphotic — *continued*
  specified type — *continued*
    cervicothoracic region M40.293
    thoracic region M40.294
    thoracolumbar region M40.295
  syphilitic, congenital A50.56
  thoracic region M40.204
  thoracolumbar region M40.205
  tuberculous A18.01
Kyrle disease L87.0

L

Labia, labium — *see* condition
Labile
  blood pressure R09.89
  vasomotor system I73.9
Labioglossal paralysis G12.29
Labium leporinum — *see* Cleft, lip
Labor — *see* Delivery
Labored breathing — *see* Hyperventilation
Labyrinthitis (circumscribed) (destructive) (diffuse) (inner ear) (latent) (purulent) (suppurative) (*see also* subcategory) H83.0 ☑
  syphilitic A52.79
Laceration
  with abortion — *see* Abortion, by type, complicated by laceration of pelvic organs
  abdomen, abdominal
    wall S31.119 ☑
      with
        foreign body S31.129 ☑
        penetration into peritoneal cavity S31.619 ☑
          with foreign body S31.629 ☑
      epigastric region S31.112 ☑
        with
          foreign body S31.122 ☑
          penetration into peritoneal cavity S31.612 ☑
            with foreign body S31.622 ☑
      left
        lower quadrant S31.114 ☑
          with
            foreign body S31.124 ☑
            penetration into peritoneal cavity S31.614 ☑
              with foreign body S31.624 ☑
        upper quadrant S31.111 ☑
          with
            foreign body S31.121 ☑
            penetration into peritoneal cavity S31.611 ☑
              with foreign body S31.621 ☑
      periumbilic region S31.115 ☑
        with
          foreign body S31.125 ☑
          penetration into peritoneal cavity S31.615 ☑
            with foreign body S31.625 ☑
      right
        lower quadrant S31.113 ☑
          with
            foreign body S31.123 ☑
            penetration into peritoneal cavity S31.613 ☑
              with foreign body S31.623 ☑
        upper quadrant S31.110 ☑
          with
            foreign body S31.120 ☑
            penetration into peritoneal cavity S31.610 ☑
              with foreign body S31.620 ☑
  accidental, complicating surgery — *see* Complications, surgical, accidental puncture or laceration
  Achilles tendon S86.02- ☑
  adrenal gland S37.813 ☑
  alveolar (process) — *see* Laceration, oral cavity
  ankle S91.01- ☑
    with
      foreign body S91.02- ☑
  antecubital space — *see* Laceration, elbow
  anus (sphincter) S31.831 ☑
    with
      ectopic or molar pregnancy O08.6
      foreign body S31.832 ☑
    complicating delivery — *see* Delivery, complicated, by, laceration, anus (sphincter)

Laceration — *continued*
  anus — *continued*
    following ectopic or molar pregnancy O08.6
    nontraumatic, nonpuerperal — *see* Fissure, anus
  arm (upper) S41.11- ☑
    with foreign body S41.12- ☑
    lower — *see* Laceration, forearm
  auditory canal (external) (meatus) — *see* Laceration, ear
  auricle, ear — *see* Laceration, ear
  axilla — *see* Laceration, arm
  back (*see also* Laceration, thorax, back)
    lower S31.010 ☑
      with
        foreign body S31.020 ☑
          with penetration into retroperitoneal space S31.021 ☑
        penetration into retroperitoneal space S31.011 ☑
  bile duct S36.13 ☑
  bladder S37.23 ☑
    with ectopic or molar pregnancy O08.6
    following ectopic or molar pregnancy O08.6
    obstetrical trauma O71.5
  blood vessel — *see* Injury, blood vessel
  bowel (*see also* Laceration, intestine)
    with ectopic or molar pregnancy O08.6
    complicating abortion — *see* Abortion, by type, complicated by, specified condition NEC
    following ectopic or molar pregnancy O08.6
    obstetrical trauma O71.5
  brain (any part) (cortex) (diffuse) (membrane) (*see also* Injury, intracranial, diffuse)
    during birth P10.8
      with hemorrhage P10.1
    focal — *see* Injury, intracranial, focal brain injury
  brainstem S06.38- ☑
  breast S21.01- ☑
    with foreign body S21.02- ☑
  broad ligament S37.893 ☑
    with ectopic or molar pregnancy O08.6
    following ectopic or molar pregnancy O08.6
    laceration syndrome N83.8
    obstetrical trauma O71.6
    syndrome (laceration) N83.8
  buttock S31.801 ☑
    with foreign body S31.802 ☑
    left S31.821 ☑
      with foreign body S31.822 ☑
    right S31.811 ☑
      with foreign body S31.812 ☑
  calf — *see* Laceration, leg
  canaliculus lacrimalis — *see* Laceration, eyelid
  canthus, eye — *see* Laceration, eyelid
  capsule, joint — *see* Sprain
  causing eversion of cervix uteri (old) N86
  central (perineal), complicating delivery O70.9
  cerebellum, traumatic S06.37- ☑
  cerebral S06.33- ☑
    during birth P10.8
      with hemorrhage P10.1
    left side S06.32- ☑
    right side S06.31- ☑
  cervix (uteri)
    with ectopic or molar pregnancy O08.6
    following ectopic or molar pregnancy O08.6
    nonpuerperal, nontraumatic N88.1
    obstetrical trauma (current) O71.3
    old (postpartal) N88.1
    traumatic S37.63 ☑
  cheek (external) S01.41- ☑
    with foreign body S01.42- ☑
    internal — *see* Laceration, oral cavity
  chest wall — *see* Laceration, thorax
  chin — *see* Laceration, head, specified site NEC
  chordae tendinae NEC I51.1
    concurrent with acute myocardial infarction — *see* Infarct, myocardium
    following acute myocardial infarction (current complication) I23.4
  clitoris — *see* Laceration, vulva
  colon — *see* Laceration, intestine, large, colon
  common bile duct S36.13 ☑
  cortex (cerebral) — *see* Injury, intracranial, diffuse
  costal region — *see* Laceration, thorax
  cystic duct S36.13 ☑
  diaphragm S27.803 ☑

Laceration — *continued*
  digit(s)
    foot — *see* Laceration, toe
    hand — *see* Laceration, finger
  duodenum S36.430 ☑
  ear (canal) (external) S01.31- ☑
    with foreign body S01.32- ☑
    drum S09.2- ☑
  elbow S51.01- ☑
    with
      foreign body S51.02- ☑
  epididymis — *see* Laceration, testis
  epigastric region — *see* Laceration, abdomen, wall, epigastric region
  esophagus K22.8
    traumatic
      cervical S11.21 ☑
        with foreign body S11.22 ☑
      thoracic S27.813 ☑
  eye (ball) S05.3- ☑
    with prolapse or loss of intraocular tissue S05.2- ☑
    penetrating S05.6- ☑
  eyebrow — *see* Laceration, eyelid
  eyelid S01.11- ☑
    with foreign body S01.12- ☑
  face NEC — *see* Laceration, head, specified site NEC
  fallopian tube S37.539 ☑
    bilateral S37.532 ☑
    unilateral S37.531 ☑
  finger(s) S61.219 ☑
    with
      damage to nail S61.319 ☑
        with
          foreign body S61.329 ☑
      foreign body S61.229 ☑
    index S61.218 ☑
      with
        damage to nail S61.318 ☑
          with
            foreign body S61.328 ☑
        foreign body S61.228 ☑
      left S61.211 ☑
        with
          damage to nail S61.311 ☑
            with
              foreign body S61.321 ☑
          foreign body S61.221 ☑
      right S61.210 ☑
        with
          damage to nail S61.310 ☑
            with
              foreign body S61.320 ☑
          foreign body S61.220 ☑
    little S61.218 ☑
      with
        damage to nail S61.318 ☑
          with
            foreign body S61.328 ☑
        foreign body S61.228 ☑
      left S61.217 ☑
        with
          damage to nail S61.317 ☑
            with
              foreign body S61.327 ☑
          foreign body S61.227 ☑
      right S61.216 ☑
        with
          damage to nail S61.316 ☑
            with
              foreign body S61.326 ☑
          foreign body S61.226 ☑
    middle S61.218 ☑
      with
        damage to nail S61.318 ☑
          with
            foreign body S61.328 ☑
        foreign body S61.228 ☑
      left S61.213 ☑
        with
          damage to nail S61.313 ☑
            with
              foreign body S61.323 ☑
          foreign body S61.223 ☑
      right S61.212 ☑
        with
          damage to nail S61.312 ☑

206

☑ **Additional Character Required** — Refer to the Tabular List for Character Selection   ▽ **Subterms under main terms may continue to next column or page**

Laceration — *continued*
  finger(s) — *continued*
    middle — *continued*
      right — *continued*
        with — *continued*
          damage to nail — *continued*
            with
              foreign body S61.322 ☑
          foreign body S61.222 ☑
    ring S61.218 ☑
      with
        damage to nail S61.318 ☑
          with
            foreign body S61.328 ☑
        foreign body S61.228 ☑
      left S61.215 ☑
        with
          damage to nail S61.315 ☑
            with
              foreign body S61.325 ☑
          foreign body S61.225 ☑
      right S61.214 ☑
        with
          damage to nail S61.314 ☑
            with
              foreign body S61.324 ☑
          foreign body S61.224 ☑
  flank S31.119 ☑
    with foreign body S31.129 ☑
  foot (except toe(s) alone) S91.319 ☑
    with foreign body S91.329 ☑
    left S91.312 ☑
      with foreign body S91.322 ☑
    right S91.311 ☑
      with foreign body S91.321 ☑
    toe — *see* Laceration, toe
  forearm S51.819 ☑
    with
      foreign body S51.829 ☑
    elbow only — *see* Laceration, elbow
    left S51.812 ☑
      with
        foreign body S51.822 ☑
    right S51.811 ☑
      with
        foreign body S51.821 ☑
  forehead S01.81 ☑
    with foreign body S01.82 ☑
  fourchette O70.0
    with ectopic or molar pregnancy O08.6
    complicating delivery O70.0
    following ectopic or molar pregnancy O08.6
  gallbladder S36.123 ☑
  genital organs, external
    female S31.512 ☑
      with foreign body S31.522 ☑
      vagina — *see* Laceration, vagina
      vulva — *see* Laceration, vulva
    male S31.511 ☑
      with foreign body S31.521 ☑
      penis — *see* Laceration, penis
      scrotum — *see* Laceration, scrotum
      testis — *see* Laceration, testis
  groin — *see* Laceration, abdomen, wall
  gum — *see* Laceration, oral cavity
  hand S61.419 ☑
    with
      foreign body S61.429 ☑
    finger — *see* Laceration, finger
    left S61.412 ☑
      with
        foreign body S61.422 ☑
    right S61.411 ☑
      with
        foreign body S61.421 ☑
    thumb — *see* Laceration, thumb
  head S01.91 ☑
    with foreign body S01.92 ☑
    cheek — *see* Laceration, cheek
    ear — *see* Laceration, ear
    eyelid — *see* Laceration, eyelid
    lip — *see* Laceration, lip
    nose — *see* Laceration, nose
    oral cavity — *see* Laceration, oral cavity
    scalp S01.01 ☑
      with foreign body S01.02 ☑

Laceration — *continued*
  head — *continued*
    specified site NEC S01.81 ☑
      with foreign body S01.82 ☑
    temporomandibular area — *see* Laceration, cheek
  heart — *see* Injury, heart, laceration
  heel — *see* Laceration, foot
  hepatic duct S36.13 ☑
  hip S71.019 ☑
    with foreign body S71.029 ☑
    left S71.012 ☑
      with foreign body S71.022 ☑
    right S71.011 ☑
      with foreign body S71.021 ☑
  hymen — *see* Laceration, vagina
  hypochondrium — *see* Laceration, abdomen, wall
  hypogastric region — *see* Laceration, abdomen, wall
  ileum S36.438 ☑
  inguinal region — *see* Laceration, abdomen, wall
  instep — *see* Laceration, foot
  internal organ — *see* Injury, by site
  interscapular region — *see* Laceration, thorax, back
  intestine
    large
      colon S36.539 ☑
        ascending S36.530 ☑
        descending S36.532 ☑
        sigmoid S36.533 ☑
        specified site NEC S36.538 ☑
      rectum S36.63 ☑
      transverse S36.531 ☑
    small S36.439 ☑
      duodenum S36.430 ☑
      specified site NEC S36.438 ☑
  intra-abdominal organ S36.93 ☑
    intestine — *see* Laceration, intestine
    liver — *see* Laceration, liver
    pancreas — *see* Laceration, pancreas
    peritoneum S36.81 ☑
    specified site NEC S36.893 ☑
    spleen — *see* Laceration, spleen
    stomach — *see* Laceration, stomach
  intracranial NEC (*see also* Injury, intracranial, diffuse)
    birth injury P10.9
  jaw — *see* Laceration, head, specified site NEC
  jejunum S36.438 ☑
  joint capsule — *see* Sprain, by site
  kidney S37.03- ☑
    major (greater than 3 cm) (massive) (stellate) S37.06- ☑
    minor (less than 1 cm) S37.04- ☑
    moderate (1 to 3 cm) S37.05- ☑
      multiple S37.06- ☑
  knee S81.01- ☑
    with foreign body S81.02- ☑
  labium (majus) (minus) — *see* Laceration, vulva
  lacrimal duct — *see* Laceration, eyelid
  large intestine — *see* Laceration, intestine, large
  larynx S11.011 ☑
    with foreign body S11.012 ☑
  leg (lower) S81.819 ☑
    with foreign body S81.829 ☑
    foot — *see* Laceration, foot
    knee — *see* Laceration, knee
    left S81.812 ☑
      with foreign body S81.822 ☑
    right S81.811 ☑
      with foreign body S81.821 ☑
    upper — *see* Laceration, thigh
  ligament — *see* Sprain
  lip S01.511 ☑
    with foreign body S01.521 ☑
  liver S36.113 ☑
    major (stellate) S36.116 ☑
    minor S36.114 ☑
    moderate S36.115 ☑
  loin — *see* Laceration, abdomen, wall
  lower back — *see* Laceration, back, lower
  lumbar region — *see* Laceration, back, lower
  lung S27.339 ☑
    bilateral S27.332 ☑
    unilateral S27.331 ☑
  malar region — *see* Laceration, head, specified site NEC
  mammary — *see* Laceration, breast
  mastoid region — *see* Laceration, head, specified site NEC

Laceration — *continued*
  meninges — *see* Injury, intracranial, diffuse
  meniscus — *see* Tear, meniscus
  mesentery S36.893 ☑
  mesosalpinx S37.893 ☑
  mouth — *see* Laceration, oral cavity
  muscle — *see* Injury, muscle, by site, laceration
  nail
    finger — *see* Laceration, finger, with damage to nail
    toe — *see* Laceration, toe, with damage to nail
  nasal (septum) (sinus) — *see* Laceration, nose
  nasopharynx — *see* Laceration, head, specified site NEC
  neck S11.91 ☑
    with foreign body S11.92 ☑
    involving
      cervical esophagus S11.21 ☑
        with foreign body S11.22 ☑
      larynx — *see* Laceration, larynx
      pharynx — *see* Laceration, pharynx
      thyroid gland — *see* Laceration, thyroid gland
      trachea — *see* Laceration, trachea
    specified site NEC S11.81 ☑
      with foreign body S11.82 ☑
  nerve — *see* Injury, nerve
  nose (septum) (sinus) S01.21 ☑
    with foreign body S01.22 ☑
  ocular NOS S05.3- ☑
    adnexa NOS S01.11- ☑
  oral cavity S01.512 ☑
    with foreign body S01.522 ☑
  orbit (eye) — *see* Wound, open, ocular, orbit
  ovary S37.439 ☑
    bilateral S37.432 ☑
    unilateral S37.431 ☑
  palate — *see* Laceration, oral cavity
  palm — *see* Laceration, hand
  pancreas S36.239 ☑
  pelvic S31.010 ☑
    with
      foreign body S31.020 ☑
        penetration into retroperitoneal cavity S31.021 ☑
      penetration into retroperitoneal cavity S31.011 ☑
    floor (*see also* Laceration, back, lower)
      with ectopic or molar pregnancy O08.6
      complicating delivery O70.1
      following ectopic or molar pregnancy O08.6
      old (postpartal) N81.89
    organ S37.93 ☑
  penis S31.21 ☑
    with foreign body S31.22 ☑
  perineum
    female S31.41 ☑
      with
        ectopic or molar pregnancy O08.6
        foreign body S31.42 ☑
      during delivery O70.9
        first degree O70.0
        fourth degree O70.3
        second degree O70.1
        third degree (*see also* Delivery, complicated, by, laceration, perineum, third degree) O70.20
      old (postpartal) N81.89
      postpartal N81.89
      secondary (postpartal) O90.1
    male S31.119 ☑
      with foreign body S31.129 ☑
  periocular area (with or without lacrimal passages) — *see* Laceration, eyelid
  peritoneum S36.893 ☑
  periumbilic region — *see* Laceration, abdomen, wall, periumbilic
  periurethral tissue — *see* Laceration, urethra
  phalanges
    finger — *see* Laceration, finger
    toe — *see* Laceration, toe
  pharynx S11.21 ☑
    with foreign body S11.22 ☑
  pinna — *see* Laceration, ear
  popliteal space — *see* Laceration, knee
  prepuce — *see* Laceration, penis
  prostate S37.823 ☑
  pubic region S31.119 ☑
    with foreign body S31.129 ☑

Laceration — *continued*
- pudendum — *see* Laceration, genital organs, external
- rectovaginal septum — *see* Laceration, vagina
- rectum S36.63
- retroperitoneum S36.893 ☑
- round ligament S37.893 ☑
- sacral region — *see* Laceration, back, lower
- sacroiliac region — *see* Laceration, back, lower
- salivary gland — *see* Laceration, oral cavity
- scalp S01.01 ☑
  - with foreign body S01.02 ☑
- scapular region — *see* Laceration, shoulder
- scrotum S31.31 ☑
  - with foreign body S31.32 ☑
- seminal vesicle S37.893 ☑
- shin — *see* Laceration, leg
- shoulder S41.019 ☑
  - with foreign body S41.029 ☑
  - left S41.012 ☑
    - with foreign body S41.022 ☑
  - right S41.011 ☑
    - with foreign body S41.021 ☑
- small intestine — *see* Laceration, intestine, small
- spermatic cord — *see* Laceration, testis
- spinal cord (meninges) (*see also* Injury, spinal cord, by region)
  - due to injury at birth P11.5
  - newborn (birth injury) P11.5
- spleen S36.039 ☑
  - major (massive) (stellate) S36.032 ☑
  - moderate S36.031 ☑
  - superficial (minor) S36.030 ☑
- sternal region — *see* Laceration, thorax, front
- stomach S36.33 ☑
- submaxillary region — *see* Laceration, head, specified site NEC
- submental region — *see* Laceration, head, specified site NEC
- subungual
  - finger(s) — *see* Laceration, finger, with damage to nail
  - toe(s) — *see* Laceration, toe, with damage to nail
- suprarenal gland — *see* Laceration, adrenal gland
- temple, temporal region — *see* Laceration, head, specified site NEC
- temporomandibular area — *see* Laceration, cheek
- tendon — *see* Injury, muscle, by site, laceration
  - Achilles S86.02-
- tentorium cerebelli — *see* Injury, intracranial, diffuse
- testis S31.31 ☑
  - with foreign body S31.32 ☑
- thigh S71.11-
  - with foreign body S71.12-
- thorax, thoracic (wall) S21.91 ☑
  - with foreign body S21.92 ☑
    - back S21.22-
      - with penetration into thoracic cavity S21.42-
    - front S21.12-
      - with penetration into thoracic cavity S21.32-
    - back S21.21-
      - with
        - foreign body S21.22-
          - with penetration into thoracic cavity S21.42-
        - penetration into thoracic cavity S21.41-
    - breast — *see* Laceration, breast
    - front S21.11-
      - with
        - foreign body S21.12-
          - with penetration into thoracic cavity S21.32-
        - penetration into thoracic cavity S21.31-
- thumb S61.019 ☑
  - with
    - damage to nail S61.119 ☑
      - with
        - foreign body S61.129 ☑
    - foreign body S61.029 ☑
  - left S61.012 ☑
    - with
      - damage to nail S61.112 ☑
        - with
          - foreign body S61.122 ☑
      - foreign body S61.022 ☑

Laceration — *continued*
- thumb — *continued*
  - right S61.011 ☑
    - with
      - damage to nail S61.111 ☑
        - with
          - foreign body S61.121 ☑
      - foreign body S61.021 ☑
- thyroid gland S11.11 ☑
  - with foreign body S11.12 ☑
- toe(s) S91.119 ☑
  - with
    - damage to nail S91.219 ☑
      - with
        - foreign body S91.229 ☑
    - foreign body S91.129 ☑
  - great S91.113 ☑
    - with
      - damage to nail S91.213 ☑
        - with
          - foreign body S91.223 ☑
      - foreign body S91.123 ☑
    - left S91.112 ☑
      - with
        - damage to nail S91.212 ☑
          - with
            - foreign body S91.222 ☑
        - foreign body S91.122 ☑
    - right S91.111 ☑
      - with
        - damage to nail S91.211 ☑
          - with
            - foreign body S91.221 ☑
        - foreign body S91.121 ☑
  - lesser S91.116 ☑
    - with
      - damage to nail S91.216 ☑
        - with
          - foreign body S91.226 ☑
      - foreign body S91.126 ☑
    - left S91.115 ☑
      - with
        - damage to nail S91.215 ☑
          - with
            - foreign body S91.225 ☑
        - foreign body S91.125 ☑
    - right S91.114 ☑
      - with
        - damage to nail S91.214 ☑
          - with
            - foreign body S91.224 ☑
        - foreign body S91.124 ☑
- tongue — *see* Laceration, oral cavity
- trachea S11.021 ☑
  - with foreign body S11.022 ☑
- tunica vaginalis — *see* Laceration, testis
- tympanum, tympanic membrane — *see* Laceration, ear, drum
- umbilical region S31.115 ☑
  - with foreign body S31.125 ☑
- ureter S37.13 ☑
- urethra S37.33 ☑
  - with or following ectopic or molar pregnancy O08.6
  - obstetrical trauma O71.5
- urinary organ NEC S37.893 ☑
- uterus S37.63 ☑
  - with ectopic or molar pregnancy O08.6
  - following ectopic or molar pregnancy O08.6
  - nonpuerperal, nontraumatic N85.8
  - obstetrical trauma NEC O71.81
  - old (postpartal) N85.8
- uvula — *see* Laceration, oral cavity
- vagina S31.41 ☑
  - with
    - ectopic or molar pregnancy O08.6
    - foreign body S31.42 ☑
  - during delivery O71.4
    - with perineal laceration — *see* Laceration, perineum, female, during delivery
  - following ectopic or molar pregnancy O08.6
  - nonpuerperal, nontraumatic N89.8
  - old (postpartal) N89.8
- vas deferens S37.893 ☑
- vesical — *see* Laceration, bladder
- vocal cords S11.031 ☑
  - with foreign body S11.032 ☑
- vulva S31.41 ☑

Laceration — *continued*
- vulva — *continued*
  - with
    - ectopic or molar pregnancy O08.6
    - foreign body S31.42 ☑
  - complicating delivery O70.0
  - following ectopic or molar pregnancy O08.6
  - nonpuerperal, nontraumatic N90.89
  - old (postpartal) N90.89
- wrist S61.519 ☑
  - with
    - foreign body S61.529 ☑
  - left S61.512 ☑
    - with
      - foreign body S61.522 ☑
  - right S61.511 ☑
    - with
      - foreign body S61.521 ☑

Lack of
- achievement in school Z55.3
- adequate
  - food Z59.4
  - intermaxillary vertical dimension of fully erupted teeth M26.36
  - sleep Z72.820
- appetite (*see* Anorexia) R63.0
- awareness R41.9
- care
  - in home Z74.2
  - of infant (at or after birth) T76.02 ☑
    - confirmed T74.02 ☑
- cognitive functions R41.9
- coordination R27.9
  - ataxia R27.0
  - specified type NEC R27.8
- development (physiological) R62.50
  - failure to thrive (child over 28 days old) R62.51
    - adult R62.7
    - newborn P92.6
  - short stature R62.52
  - specified type NEC R62.59
- energy R53.83
- financial resources Z59.6
- food T73.0 ☑
- growth R62.52
- heating Z59.1
- housing (permanent) (temporary) Z59.0
  - adequate Z59.1
- learning experiences in childhood Z62.898
- leisure time (affecting life-style) Z73.2
- material resources Z59.9
- memory (*see also* Amnesia)
  - mild, following organic brain damage F06.8
- ovulation N97.0
- parental supervision or control of child Z62.0
- person able to render necessary care Z74.2
- physical exercise Z72.3
- play experience in childhood Z62.898
- posterior occlusal support M26.57
- relaxation (affecting life-style) Z73.2
- sexual
  - desire F52.0
  - enjoyment F52.1
- shelter Z59.0
- sleep (adequate) Z72.820
- supervision of child by parent Z62.0
- support, posterior occlusal M26.57
- water T73.1 ☑

Lacrimal — *see* condition
Lacrimation, abnormal — *see* Epiphora
Lacrimonasal duct — *see* condition
Lactation, lactating (breast) (puerperal, postpartum)
- associated
  - cracked nipple O92.13
  - retracted nipple O92.03
- defective O92.4
- disorder NEC O92.79
- excessive O92.6
- failed (complete) O92.3
  - partial O92.4
- mastitis NEC — *see* Mastitis, obstetric
- mother (care and/or examination) Z39.1
- nonpuerperal N64.3
Lacticemia, excessive E87.2
Lacunar skull Q75.8
Laennec's cirrhosis K70.30
- with ascites K70.31
- nonalcoholic K74.69

208

☑ **Additional Character Required** — Refer to the Tabular List for Character Selection   ▽ Subterms under main terms may continue to next column or page

Lafora's disease — see Epilepsy, generalized, idiopathic
Lag, lid (nervous) — see Retraction, lid
Lagophthalmos (eyelid) (nervous) H02.209
  bilateral, upper and lower eyelids H02.20C
  cicatricial H02.219
    bilateral, upper and lower eyelids H02.21C
    left H02.216
      lower H02.215
      upper H02.214
      upper and lower eyelids H02.21B
    right H02.213
      lower H02.212
      upper H02.211
      upper and lower eyelids H02.21A
  keratoconjunctivitis — see Keratoconjunctivitis
  left H02.206
    lower H02.205
    upper H02.204
    upper and lower eyelids H02.20B
  mechanical H02.229
    bilateral, upper and lower eyelids H02.22C
    left H02.226
      lower H02.225
      upper H02.224
      upper and lower eyelids H02.22B
    right H02.223
      lower H02.222
      upper H02.221
      upper and lower eyelids H02.22A
  paralytic H02.239
    bilateral, upper and lower eyelids H02.23C
    left H02.236
      lower H02.235
      upper H02.234
      upper and lower eyelids H02.23B
    right H02.233
      lower H02.232
      upper H02.231
      upper and lower eyelids H02.23A
  right H02.203
    lower H02.202
    upper H02.201
    upper and lower eyelids H02.20A
Laki-Lorand factor deficiency — see Defect, coagulation, specified type NEC
Lalling F80.0
Lambert-Eaton syndrome — see Syndrome, Lambert-Eaton
Lambliasis, lambliosis A07.1
Landau-Kleffner syndrome — see Epilepsy, specified NEC
Landouzy-Déjérine dystrophy or facioscapulohumeral atrophy G71.02
Landouzy's disease (icterohemorrhagic leptospirosis) A27.0
Landry-Guillain-Barré, syndrome or paralysis G61.0
Landry's disease or paralysis G61.0
Lane's
  band Q43.3
  kink — see Obstruction, intestine
  syndrome K90.2
Langdon Down syndrome — see Trisomy, 21
Lapsed immunization schedule status Z28.3
Large
  baby (regardless of gestational age) (4000g to 4499g) P08.1
  ear, congenital Q17.1
  physiological cup Q14.2
  stature R68.89
Large-for-dates NEC (infant) (4000g to 4499g) P08.1
  affecting management of pregnancy O36.6- ☑
  exceptionally (4500g or more) P08.0
Larsen-Johansson disease orosteochondrosis — see Osteochondrosis, juvenile, patella
Larsen's syndrome (flattened facies and multiple congenital dislocations) Q74.8
Larva migrans
  cutaneous B76.9
    Ancylostoma B76.0
  visceral B83.0
Laryngeal — see condition
Laryngismus (stridulus) J38.5
  congenital P28.89
  diphtheritic A36.2
Laryngitis (acute) (edematous) (fibrinous) (infective) (infiltrative) (malignant) (membranous) (phlegmonous) (pneumococcal) (pseudomembranous) (septic) (subglottic) (suppurative) (ulcerative) J04.0

Laryngitis — continued
  with
    influenza, flu, or grippe — see Influenza, with, laryngitis
    tracheitis (acute) — see Laryngotracheitis
  atrophic J37.0
  catarrhal J37.0
  chronic J37.0
    with tracheitis (chronic) J37.1
  diphtheritic A36.2
  due to external agent — see Inflammation, respiratory, upper, due to
  H. influenzae J04.0
  Hemophilus influenzae J04.0
  hypertrophic J37.0
  influenzal — see Influenza, with, respiratory manifestations NEC
  obstructive J05.0
  sicca J37.0
  spasmodic J05.0
    acute J04.0
  streptococcal J04.0
  stridulous J05.0
  syphilitic (late) A52.73
    congenital A50.59 [J99]
      early A50.03 [J99]
  tuberculous A15.5
  Vincent's A69.1
Laryngocele (congenital) (ventricular) Q31.3
Laryngofissure J38.7
  congenital Q31.8
Laryngomalacia (congenital) Q31.5
Laryngopharyngitis (acute) J06.0
  chronic J37.0
  due to external agent — see Inflammation, respiratory, upper, due to
Laryngoplegia J38.00
  bilateral J38.02
  unilateral J38.01
Laryngoptosis J38.7
Laryngospasm J38.5
Laryngostenosis J38.6
Laryngotracheitis (acute) (Infectional) (infective) (viral) J04.2
  atrophic J37.1
  catarrhal J37.1
  chronic J37.1
  diphtheritic A36.2
  due to external agent — see Inflammation, respiratory, upper, due to
  Hemophilus influenzae J04.2
  hypertrophic J37.1
  influenzal — see Influenza, with, respiratory manifestations NEC
  pachydermic J38.7
  sicca J37.1
  spasmodic J38.5
    acute J05.0
  streptococcal J04.2
  stridulous J38.5
  syphilitic (late) A52.73
    congenital A50.59 [J99]
      early A50.03 [J99]
  tuberculous A15.5
  Vincent's A69.1
Laryngotracheobronchitis — see Bronchitis
Larynx, laryngeal — see condition
Lassa fever A96.2
Lassitude — see Weakness
Late
  talker R62.0
  walker R62.0
Late effect(s) — See Sequelae
Latent — see condition
Laterocession — see Lateroversion
Lateroflexion — see Lateroversion
Lateroversion
  cervix — see Lateroversion, uterus
  uterus, uterine (cervix) (postinfectional) (postpartal, old) N85.4
    congenital Q51.818
    in pregnancy or childbirth O34.59- ☑
Lathyrism — see Poisoning, food, noxious, plant
Launois' syndrome (pituitary gigantism) E22.0
Launois-Bensaude adenolipomatosis E88.89
Laurence-Moon (-Bardet)-**Biedl syndrome** Q87.89
Lax, laxity (see also Relaxation)
  ligament (ous) (see also Disorder, ligament)

Lax, laxity — continued
  ligament (see also Disorder, ligament) — continued
    familial M35.7
    knee — see Derangement, knee
  skin (acquired) L57.4
    congenital Q82.8
Laxative habit F55.2
Lazy leukocyte syndrome D70.8
Lead miner's lung J63.6
Leak, leakage
  air NEC J93.82
    postprocedural J95.812
  amniotic fluid — see Rupture, membranes, premature
  blood (microscopic), fetal, into maternal circulation affecting management of pregnancy — see Pregnancy, complicated by
  cerebrospinal fluid G96.0
    from spinal (lumbar) puncture G97.0
  device, implant or graft (see also Complications, by site and type, mechanical)
    arterial graft NEC — see Complication, cardiovascular device, mechanical, vascular
    breast (implant) T85.43 ☑
    catheter NEC T85.638 ☑
      dialysis (renal) T82.43 ☑
        intraperitoneal T85.631 ☑
      infusion NEC T82.534 ☑
        spinal (epidural) (subdural) T85.630 ☑
      urinary T83.038 ☑
        cystostomy T83.030 ☑
        Hopkins T83.038 ☑
        ileostomy T83.038 ☑
        indwelling T83.031 ☑
        nephrostomy T83.032 ☑
        specified T83.038 ☑
        urostomy T83.038 ☑
    gastrointestinal — see Complications, prosthetic device, mechanical, gastrointestinal device
    genital NEC T83.498 ☑
      penile prosthesis (cylinder) (implanted) (pump) (reservoir) T83.490 ☑
      testicular prosthesis T83.491 ☑
    heart NEC — see Complication, cardiovascular device, mechanical
    joint prosthesis — see Complications, joint prosthesis, mechanical, specified NEC, by site
    ocular NEC — see Complications, prosthetic device, mechanical, ocular device
    orthopedic NEC — see Complication, orthopedic, device, mechanical
    persistent air J93.82
    specified NEC T85.638 ☑
    urinary NEC (see also Complication, genitourinary, device, urinary, mechanical)
      graft T83.23 ☑
    vascular NEC — see Complication, cardiovascular device, mechanical
    ventricular intracranial shunt T85.03 ☑
  urine — see Incontinence
Leaky heart — see Endocarditis
Learning defect (specific) F81.9
Leather bottle stomach C16.9
Leber's
  congenital amaurosis H35.50
  optic atrophy (hereditary) H47.22
Lederer's anemia D59.1
Leeches (external) — see Hirudiniasis
Leg — see condition
Legg (-Calvé)-**Perthes disease, syndrome or osteochondrosis** M91.1- ☑
Legionellosis A48.1
  nonpneumonic A48.2
Legionnaires'
  disease A48.1
    nonpneumonic A48.2
  pneumonia A48.1
Leigh's disease G31.82
Leiner's disease L21.1
Leiofibromyoma — see Leiomyoma
Leiomyoblastoma — see Neoplasm, connective tissue, benign
Leiomyofibroma (see also Neoplasm, connective tissue, benign)
  uterus (cervix) (corpus) D25.9
Leiomyoma (see also Neoplasm, connective tissue, benign)

Leiomyoma — *continued*
  bizarre — *see* Neoplasm, connective tissue, benign
  cellular — *see* Neoplasm, connective tissue, benign
  epithelioid — *see* Neoplasm, connective tissue, benign
  uterus (cervix) (corpus) D25.9
    intramural D25.1
    submucous D25.0
    subserosal D25.2
  vascular — *see* Neoplasm, connective tissue, benign
Leiomyoma, leiomyomatosis (intravascular) — *see* Neoplasm, connective tissue, uncertain behavior
Leiomyosarcoma (*see also* Neoplasm, connective tissue, malignant)
  epithelioid — *see* Neoplasm, connective tissue, malignant
  myxoid — *see* Neoplasm, connective tissue, malignant
Leishmaniasis B55.9
  American (mucocutaneous) B55.2
    cutaneous B55.1
  Asian Desert B55.1
  Brazilian B55.2
  cutaneous (any type) B55.1
  dermal (*see also* Leishmaniasis, cutaneous)
    post-kala-azar B55.0
  eyelid B55.1
  infantile B55.0
  Mediterranean B55.0
  mucocutaneous (American) (New World) B55.2
  naso-oral B55.2
  nasopharyngeal B55.2
  old world B55.1
  tegumentaria diffusa B55.1
  visceral B55.0
Leishmanoid, dermal (*see also* Leishmaniasis, cutaneous)
  post-kala-azar B55.0
Lenegre's disease I44.2
Lengthening, leg — *see* Deformity, limb, unequal length
Lennert's lymphoma — *see* Lymphoma, Lennert's
Lennox-Gastaut syndrome G40.812
  intractable G40.814
    with status epilepticus G40.813
    without status epilepticus G40.814
  not intractable G40.812
    with status epilepticus G40.811
    without status epilepticus G40.812
Lens — *see* condition
Lenticonus (anterior) (posterior) (congenital) Q12.8
Lenticular degeneration, progressive E83.01
Lentiglobus (posterior) (congenital) Q12.8
Lentigo (congenital) L81.4
  maligna (*see also* Melanoma, in situ)
    melanoma — *see* Melanoma
Lentivirus, as cause of disease classified elsewhere B97.31
Leontiasis
  ossium M85.2
  syphilitic (late) A52.78
    congenital A50.59
Lepothrix A48.8
Lepra — *see* Leprosy
Leprechaunism E34.8
Leprosy A30.- ☑
  with muscle disorder A30.9 [M63.80]
    ankle A30.9 [M63.87-] ☑
    foot A30.9 [M63.87-] ☑
    forearm A30.9 [M63.83-] ☑
    hand A30.9 [M63.84-] ☑
    lower leg A30.9 [M63.86-] ☑
    multiple sites A30.9 [M63.89]
    pelvic region A30.9 [M63.85-] ☑
    shoulder region A30.9 [M63.81-] ☑
    specified site NEC A30.9 [M63.88]
    thigh A30.9 [M63.85-] ☑
    upper arm A30.9 [M63.82-] ☑
  anesthetic A30.9
  BB A30.3
  BL A30.4
  borderline (infiltrated) (neuritic) A30.3
    lepromatous A30.4
    tuberculoid A30.2
  BT A30.2
  dimorphous (infiltrated) (neuritic) A30.3
  I A30.0
  indeterminate (macular) (neuritic) A30.0
  lepromatous (diffuse) (infiltrated) (macular) (neuritic) (nodular) A30.5

Leprosy — *continued*
  LL A30.5
  macular (early) (neuritic) (simple) A30.9
  maculoanesthetic A30.9
  mixed A30.3
  neural A30.9
  nodular A30.5
  primary neuritic A30.3
  specified type NEC A30.8
  TT A30.1
  tuberculoid (major) (minor) A30.1
Leptocytosis, hereditary D56.9
Leptomeningitis (chronic) (circumscribed) (hemorrhagic) (nonsuppurative) — *see* Meningitis
Leptomeningopathy G96.19
Leptospiral — *see* condition
Leptospirochetal — *see* condition
Leptospirosis A27.9
  canicola A27.89
  due to Leptospira interrogans serovar icterohaemorrhagiae A27.0
  icterohemorrhagica A27.0
  pomona A27.89
  Weil's disease A27.0
Leptus dermatitis B88.0
Leriche's syndrome (aortic bifurcation occlusion) I74.09
Leri's pleonosteosis Q78.8
Leri-Weill syndrome Q77.8
Lermoyez' syndrome — *see* Vertigo, peripheral NEC
Lesch-Nyhan syndrome E79.1
Leser-Trélat disease L82.1
  inflamed L82.0
Lesion(s) (nontraumatic)
  abducens nerve — *see* Strabismus, paralytic, sixth nerve
  alveolar process K08.9
  angiocentric immunoproliferative D47.Z9 (*following* D47.4)
  anorectal K62.9
  aortic (valve) I35.9
  auditory nerve — *see* subcategory H93.3 ☑
  basal ganglion G25.9
  bile duct — *see* Disease, bile duct
  biomechanical M99.9
    specified type NEC M99.89
      abdomen M99.89
      acromioclavicular M99.87
      cervical region M99.81
      cervicothoracic M99.81
      costochondral M99.88
      costovertebral M99.88
      head region M99.80
      hip M99.85
      lower extremity M99.86
      lumbar region M99.83
      lumbosacral M99.83
      occipitocervical M99.80
      pelvic region M99.85
      pubic M99.85
      rib cage M99.88
      sacral region M99.84
      sacrococcygeal M99.84
      sacroiliac M99.84
      specified NEC M99.89
      sternochondral M99.88
      sternoclavicular M99.87
      thoracic region M99.82
      thoracolumbar M99.82
      upper extremity M99.87
  bladder N32.9
  bone — *see* Disorder, bone
  brachial plexus G54.0
  brain G93.9
    congenital Q04.9
    vascular I67.9
      degenerative I67.9
      hypertensive I67.4
  buccal cavity K13.79
  calcified — *see* Calcification
  canthus — *see* Disorder, eyelid
  carate — *see* Pinta, lesions
  cardia K31.9
  cardiac (*see also* Disease, heart) I51.9
    congenital Q24.9
    valvular — *see* Endocarditis
  cauda equina G83.4
  cecum K63.9
  cerebral — *see* Lesion, brain
  cerebrovascular I67.9

Lesion(s) — *continued*
  cerebrovascular — *continued*
    degenerative I67.9
    hypertensive I67.4
  cervical (nerve) root NEC G54.2
  chiasmal — *see* Disorder, optic, chiasm
  chorda tympani G51.8
  coin, lung R91.1
  colon K63.9
  combined periodontic - endodontic K05.5
  congenital — *see* Anomaly, by site
  conjunctiva H11.9
  conus medullaris — *see* Injury, conus medullaris
  coronary artery — *see* Ischemia, heart
  cranial nerve G52.9
    eighth — *see* Disorder, ear
    eleventh G52.9
    fifth G50.9
    first G52.0
    fourth — *see* Strabismus, paralytic, fourth nerve
    seventh G51.9
    sixth — *see* Strabismus, paralytic, sixth nerve
    tenth G52.2
    twelfth G52.3
  cystic — *see* Cyst
  degenerative — *see* Degeneration
  duodenum K31.9
  edentulous (alveolar) ridge, associated with trauma, due to traumatic occlusion K06.2
  en coup de sabre L94.1
  eyelid — *see* Disorder, eyelid
  gasserian ganglion G50.8
  gastric K31.9
  gastroduodenal K31.9
  gastrointestinal K63.9
  gingiva, associated with trauma K06.2
  glomerular
    focal and segmental (*see also* N00-N07 with fourth character .1) N05.1
    minimal change (*see also* N00-N07 with fourth character .0) N05.0
  heart (organic) — *see* Disease, heart
  hyperchromic, due to pinta (carate) A67.1
  hyperkeratotic — *see* Hyperkeratosis
  hypothalamic E23.7
  ileocecal K63.9
  ileum K63.9
  iliohypogastric nerve G57.8- ☑
  inflammatory — *see* Inflammation
  intestine K63.9
  intracerebral — *see* Lesion, brain
  intrachiasmal (optic) — *see* Disorder, optic, chiasm
  intracranial, space-occupying R90.0
  joint — *see* Disorder, joint
    sacroiliac (old) M53.3
  keratotic — *see* Keratosis
  kidney — *see* Disease, renal
  laryngeal nerve (recurrent) G52.2
  lip K13.0
  liver K76.9
  lumbosacral
    plexus G54.1
    root (nerve) NEC G54.4
  lung (coin) R91.1
  maxillary sinus J32.0
  mitral I05.9
  Morel-Lavallée — *see* Hematoma, by site
  motor cortex NEC G93.89
  mouth K13.79
  nerve G58.9
    femoral G57.2- ☑
    median G56.1- ☑
      carpal tunnel syndrome — *see* Syndrome, carpal tunnel
    plantar G57.6- ☑
    popliteal (lateral) G57.3- ☑
      medial G57.4- ☑
    radial G56.3- ☑
    sciatic G57.0- ☑
    spinal — *see* Injury, nerve, spinal
    ulnar G56.2- ☑
  nervous system, congenital Q07.9
  nonallopathic — *see* Lesion, biomechanical
  nose (internal) J34.89
  obstructive — *see* Obstruction
  obturator nerve G57.8- ☑
  oral mucosa K13.70

Lesion(s) — *continued*
organ or site NEC — *see* Disease, by site
osteolytic — *see* Osteolysis
peptic K27.9
periodontal, due to traumatic occlusion K05.5
pharynx J39.2
pigment, pigmented (skin) L81.9
pinta — *see* Pinta, lesions
polypoid — *see* Polyp
prechiasmal (optic) — *see* Disorder, optic, chiasm
primary (*see also* Syphilis, primary) A51.0
carate A67.0
pinta A67.0
yaws A66.0
pulmonary J98.4
valve I37.9
pylorus K31.9
rectosigmoid K63.9
retina, retinal H35.9
sacroiliac (joint) (old) M53.3
salivary gland K11.9
benign lymphoepithelial K11.8
saphenous nerve G57.8- ☑
sciatic nerve G57.0- ☑
secondary — *see* Syphilis, secondary
shoulder (region) M75.9- ☑
specified NEC M75.8- ☑
sigmoid K63.9
sinus (accessory) (nasal) J34.89
skin L98.9
suppurative L08.0
SLAP S43.43- ☑
spinal cord G95.9
congenital Q06.9
spleen D73.89
stomach K31.9
superior glenoid labrum S43.43- ☑
syphilitic — *see* Syphilis
tertiary — *see* Syphilis, tertiary
thoracic root (nerve) NEC G54.3
tonsillar fossa J35.9
tooth, teeth K08.9
white spot
chewing surface K02.51
pit and fissure surface K02.51
smooth surface K02.61
traumatic — *see* specific type of injury by site
tricuspid (valve) I07.9
nonrheumatic I36.9
trigeminal nerve G50.9
ulcerated or ulcerative — *see* Ulcer, skin
uterus N85.9
vagina N89.8
vagus nerve G52.2
valvular — *see* Endocarditis
vascular I99.9
affecting central nervous system I67.9
following trauma NEC T14.8 ☑
umbilical cord, complicating delivery O69.5 ☑
vulva N90.89
warty — *see* Verruca
white spot (tooth)
chewing surface K02.51
pit and fissure surface K02.51
smooth surface K02.61
Lethargic — *see* condition
Lethargy R53.83
Letterer-Siwe's disease C96.0
Leukemia, leukemic C95.9- ☑
acute basophilic C94.8- ☑
acute bilineal C95.0- ☑
acute erythroid C94.0- ☑
acute lymphoblastic C91.0- ☑
acute megakaryoblastic C94.2- ☑
acute megakaryocytic C94.2- ☑
acute mixed lineage C95.0- ☑
acute monoblastic (monoblastic/monocytic) C93.0- ☑
acute monocytic (monoblastic/monocytic) C93.0- ☑
acute myeloblastic (minimal differentiation) (with
maturation) C92.0- ☑
acute myeloid, NOS C92.0- ☑
with
11q23-abnormality C92.6- ☑
dysplasia of remaining hematopoesis and/or
myelodysplastic disease in its history
C92.A- ☑ (*following* C92.6)

Leukemia, leukemic — *continued*
acute myeloid, — *continued*
with — *continued*
multilineage dysplasia C92.A- ☑ (*following*
C92.6)
variation of MLL-gene C92.6- ☑
M6 (a)(b) C94.0- ☑
M7 C94.2- ☑
acute myelomonocytic C92.5- ☑
acute promyelocytic C92.4- ☑
adult T-cell (HTLV-1-associated) (acute variant)
(chronic variant) (lymphomatoid variant)
(smouldering variant) C91.5- ☑
aggressive NK-cell C94.8- ☑
AML (1/ETO) (M0) (M1) (M2) (without a FAB classification) C92.0- ☑
AML M3 C92.4- ☑
AML M4 (Eo with inv(16) or t(16;16)) C92.5- ☑
AML M5 C93.0- ☑
AML M5a C93.0- ☑
AML M5b C93.0- ☑
AML Me with t (15;17) and variants C92.4- ☑
atypical chronic myeloid, BCR/ABL-negative C92.2- ☑
biphenotypic acute C95.0- ☑
blast cell C95.0- ☑
Burkitt-type, mature B-cell C91.A- ☑ (*following* C91.6)
chronic lymphocytic, of B-cell type C91.1- ☑
chronic monocytic C93.1- ☑
chronic myelogenous (Philadelphia chromosome (Ph1)
positive) (t(9;22)) (q34;q11) (with crisis of blast
cells) C92.1- ☑
chronic myeloid, BCR/ABL-positive C92.1- ☑
atypical, BCR/ABL-negative C92.2- ☑
chronic myelomonocytic C93.1- ☑
chronic neutrophilic D47.1
CMML (-1) (-2) (with eosinophilia) C93.1- ☑
granulocytic (*see also* Category C92) C92.9- ☑
hairy cell C91.4- ☑
juvenile myelomonocytic C93.3- ☑
lymphoid C91.9- ☑
specified NEC C91.Z- ☑ (*following* C91.6)
mast cell C94.3- ☑
mature B-cell, Burkitt-type C91.A- ☑ (*following* C91.6)
monocytic (subacute) C93.9- ☑
specified NEC C93.Z- ☑ (*following* C93.3)
myelogenous (*see also* Category C92) C92.9- ☑
myeloid C92.9- ☑
specified NEC C92.Z- ☑ (*following* C92.6)
plasma cell C90.1- ☑
plasmacytic C90.1- ☑
prolymphocytic
of B-cell type C91.3- ☑
of T-cell type C91.6- ☑
specified NEC C94.8- ☑
stem cell, of unclear lineage C95.0- ☑
subacute lymphocytic C91.9- ☑
T-cell large granular lymphocytic C91.Z- ☑ (*following*
C91.6)
unspecified cell type C95.9- ☑
acute C95.0- ☑
chronic C95.1- ☑
Leukemoid reaction (*see also* Reaction, leukemoid)
D72.823
Leukoaraiosis (hypertensive) I67.81
Leukoariosis — *see* Leukoaraiosis
Leukocoria — *see* Disorder, globe, degenerated condition, leucocoria
Leukocytopenia D72.819
Leukocytosis D72.829
eosinophilic D72.1
Leukoderma, leukodermia NEC L81.5
syphilitic A51.39
late A52.79
Leukodystrophy E75.29
Leukoedema, oral epithelium K13.29
Leukoencephalitis G04.81
acute (subacute) hemorrhagic G36.1
postimmunization or postvaccinal G04.02
postinfectious G04.01
subacute sclerosing A81.1
van Bogaert's (sclerosing) A81.1
Leukoencephalopathy (*see also* Encephalopathy) G93.49
Binswanger's I67.3
heroin vapor G92
metachromatic E75.25
multifocal (progressive) A81.2

Leukoencephalopathy — *continued*
postimmunization and postvaccinal G04.02
progressive multifocal A81.2
reversible, posterior G93.6
van Bogaert's (sclerosing) A81.1
vascular, progressive I67.3
Leukoerythroblastosis D75.9
Leukokeratosis (*see also* Leukoplakia)
mouth K13.21
nicotina palati K13.24
oral mucosa K13.21
tongue K13.21
vocal cord J38.3
Leukokraurosis vulva (e) N90.4
Leukoma (cornea) (*see also* Opacity, cornea)
adherent H17.0- ☑
interfering with central vision — *see* Opacity, cornea,
central
Leukomalacia, cerebral, newborn P91.2
periventricular P91.2
Leukomelanopathy, hereditary D72.0
Leukonychia (punctata) (striata) L60.8
congenital Q84.4
Leukopathia unguium L60.8
congenital Q84.4
Leukopenia D72.819
basophilic D72.818
chemotherapy (cancer) induced D70.1
congenital D70.0
cyclic D70.0
drug induced NEC D70.2
due to cytoreductive cancer chemotherapy D70.1
eosinophilic D72.818
familial D70.0
infantile genetic D70.0
malignant D70.9
periodic D70.0
transitory neonatal P61.5
Leukopenic — *see* condition
Leukoplakia
anus K62.89
bladder (postinfectional) N32.89
buccal K13.21
cervix (uteri) N88.0
esophagus K22.8
gingiva K13.21
hairy (oral mucosa) (tongue) K13.3
kidney (pelvis) N28.89
larynx J38.7
lip K13.21
mouth K13.21
oral epithelium, including tongue (mucosa) K13.21
palate K13.21
pelvis (kidney) N28.89
penis (infectional) N48.0
rectum K62.89
syphilitic (late) A52.79
tongue K13.21
ureter (postinfectional) N28.89
urethra (postinfectional) N36.8
uterus N85.8
vagina N89.4
vocal cord J38.3
vulva N90.4
Leukorrhea N89.8
due to Trichomonas (vaginalis) A59.00
trichomonal A59.00
Leukosarcoma C85.9- ☑
Levocardia (isolated) Q24.1
with situs inversus Q89.3
Levotransposition Q20.5
Lev's disease or syndrome (acquired complete heart
block) I44.2
Levulosuria — *see* Fructosuria
Levulrid L30.2
Lewy body (ies) (dementia) (disease) G31.83
Leyden-Moebius dystrophy G71.09.
Leydig cell
carcinoma
specified site — *see* Neoplasm, malignant, by site
unspecified site
female C56.9
male C62.9- ☑
tumor
benign
specified site — *see* Neoplasm, benign, by site
unspecified site
female D27.- ☑

Leydig cell — *continued*
  tumor — *continued*
    benign — *continued*
      unspecified site — *continued*
        male D29.2- ☑
      malignant
        specified site — *see* Neoplasm, malignant, by site
        unspecified site
          female C56.- ☑
          male C62.9- ☑
      specified site — *see* Neoplasm, uncertain behavior, by site
      unspecified site
        female D39.1- ☑
        male D40.1- ☑
Leydig-Sertoli cell tumor
  specified site — *see* Neoplasm, benign, by site
  unspecified site
    female D27.- ☑
    male D29.2- ☑
LGSIL (Low grade squamous intraepithelial lesion on cytologic smear of)
  anus R85.612
  cervix R87.612
  vagina R87.622
Liar, pathologic F60.2
Libido
  decreased R68.82
Libman-Sacks disease M32.11
Lice (infestation) B85.2
  body (Pediculus corporis) B85.1
  crab B85.3
  head (Pediculus capitis) B85.0
  mixed (classifiable to more than one of the titles B85.0-B85.3) B85.4
  pubic (Phthirus pubis) B85.3
Lichen L28.0
  albus L90.0
    penis N48.0
    vulva N90.4
  amyloidosis E85.4 [L99]
  atrophicus L90.0
    penis N48.0
    vulva N90.4
  congenital Q82.8
  myxedematosus L98.5
  nitidus L44.1
  pilaris Q82.8
    acquired L85.8
  planopilaris L66.1
  planus (chronicus) L43.9
    annularis L43.8
    bullous L43.1
    follicular L66.1
    hypertrophic L43.0
    moniliformis L44.3
    of Wilson L43.9
    specified NEC L43.8
    subacute (active) L43.3
    tropicus L43.3
  ruber
    acuminatus L44.0
    moniliformis L44.3
    planus L43.9
  sclerosus (et atrophicus) L90.0
    penis N48.0
    vulva N90.4
  scrofulosus (primary) (tuberculous) A18.4
  simplex (chronicus) (circumscriptus) L28.0
  striatus L44.2
  urticatus L28.2
Lichenification L28.0
Lichenoides tuberculosis (primary) A18.4
Lichtheim's disease or syndrome — *see* Degeneration, combined
Lien migrans D73.89
Ligament — *see* condition
Light
  for gestational age — *see* Light for dates
  headedness R42
Light-for-dates (infant) P05.00
  with weight of
    499 grams or less P05.01
    500-749 grams P05.02
    750-999 grams P05.03
    1000-1249 grams P05.04
    1250-1499 grams P05.05

Light-for-dates — *continued*
  with weight of — *continued*
    1500-1749 grams P05.06
    1750-1999 grams P05.07
    2000-2499 grams P05.08
    2500 grams and over P05.09
  affecting management of pregnancy O36.59- ☑
  and small-for-dates — *see* Small for dates
  specified NEC P05.09
Lightning (effects) (stroke) (struck by) T75.00 ☑
  burn — *see* Burn
  foot E53.8
  shock T75.01 ☑
  specified effect NEC T75.09 ☑
Lightwood-Albright syndrome N25.89
Lightwood's disease or syndrome (renal tubular acidosis) N25.89
Lignac (-de Toni) (-Fanconi) (-Debré) **disease or syndrome** E72.09
  with cystinosis E72.04
Ligneous thyroiditis E06.5
Likoff's syndrome I20.8
Limb — *see* condition
Limbic epilepsy personality syndrome F07.0
Limitation, limited
  activities due to disability Z73.6
  cardiac reserve — *see* Disease, heart
  eye muscle duction, traumatic — *see* Strabismus, mechanical
  mandibular range of motion M26.52
Lindau (-von Hippel) **disease** Q85.8
Line(s)
  Beau's L60.4
  Harris' — *see* Arrest, epiphyseal
  Hudson's (cornea) — *see* Pigmentation, cornea, anterior
  Stähli's (cornea) — *see* Pigmentation, cornea, anterior
Linea corneae senilis — *see* Change, cornea, senile
Lingua
  geographica K14.1
  nigra (villosa) K14.3
  plicata K14.5
  tylosis K13.29
Lingual — *see* condition
Linguatulosis B88.8
Linitis (gastric) **plastica** C16.9
Lip — *see* condition
Lipedema — *see* Edema
Lipemia (*see also* Hyperlipidemia)
  retina, retinalis E78.3
Lipidosis E75.6
  cerebral (infantile) (juvenile) (late) E75.4
  cerebroretinal E75.4
  cerebroside E75.22
  cholesterol (cerebral) E75.5
  glycolipid E75.21
  hepatosplenomegalic E78.3
  sphingomyelin — *see* Niemann-Pick disease or syndrome
  sulfatide E75.29
Lipoadenoma — *see* Neoplasm, benign, by site
Lipoblastoma — *see* Lipoma
Lipoblastomatosis — *see* Lipoma
Lipochondrodystrophy E76.01
Lipochrome histiocytosis (familial) D71
Lipodermatosclerosis — *see* Varix, leg, with, inflammation
  ulcerated — *see* Varix, leg, with, ulcer, with inflammation by site
Lipodystrophia progressiva E88.1
Lipodystrophy (progressive) E88.1
  insulin E88.1
  intestinal K90.81
  mesenteric K65.4
Lipofibroma — *see* Lipoma
Lipofuscinosis, neuronal (with ceroidosis) E75.4
Lipogranuloma, sclerosing L92.8
Lipogranulomatosis E78.89
Lipoid (*see also* condition)
  histiocytosis D76.3
    essential E75.29
  nephrosis N04.9
  proteinosis of Urbach E78.89
Lipoidemia — *see* Hyperlipidemia
Lipoidosis — *see* Lipidosis
Lipoma D17.9
  fetal D17.9
    fat cell D17.9

Lipoma — *continued*
  infiltrating D17.9
  intramuscular D17.9
  pleomorphic D17.9
  site classification
    arms (skin) (subcutaneous) D17.2- ☑
    connective tissue D17.30
      intra-abdominal D17.5
      intrathoracic D17.4
      peritoneum D17.79
      retroperitoneum D17.79
      specified site NEC D17.39
      spermatic cord D17.6
    face (skin) (subcutaneous) D17.0
    genitourinary organ NEC D17.72
    head (skin) (subcutaneous) D17.0
    intra-abdominal D17.5
    intrathoracic D17.4
    kidney D17.71
    legs (skin) (subcutaneous) D17.2- ☑
    neck (skin) (subcutaneous) D17.0
    peritoneum D17.79
    retroperitoneum D17.79
    skin D17.30
      specified site NEC D17.39
    specified site NEC D17.79
    spermatic cord D17.6
    subcutaneous D17.30
      specified site NEC D17.39
    trunk (skin) (subcutaneous) D17.1
    unspecified D17.9
  spindle cell D17.9
Lipomatosis E88.2
  dolorosa (Dercum) E88.2
  fetal — *see* Lipoma
  Launois-Bensaude E88.89
Lipomyoma — *see* Lipoma
Lipomyxoma — *see* Lipoma
Lipomyxosarcoma — *see* Neoplasm, connective tissue, malignant
Lipoprotein metabolism disorder E78.9
Lipoproteinemia E78.5
  broad-beta E78.2
  floating-beta E78.2
  hyper-pre-beta E78.1
Liposarcoma (*see also* Neoplasm, connective tissue, malignant)
  dedifferentiated — *see* Neoplasm, connective tissue, malignant
  differentiated type — *see* Neoplasm, connective tissue, malignant
  embryonal — *see* Neoplasm, connective tissue, malignant
  mixed type — *see* Neoplasm, connective tissue, malignant
  myxoid — *see* Neoplasm, connective tissue, malignant
  pleomorphic — *see* Neoplasm, connective tissue, malignant
  round cell — *see* Neoplasm, connective tissue, malignant
  well differentiated type — *see* Neoplasm, connective tissue, malignant
Liposynovitis prepatellaris E88.89
Lipping, cervix N86
Lipschütz disease or ulcer N76.6
Lipuria R82.0
  schistosomiasis (bilharziasis) B65.0
Lisping F80.0
Lissauer's paralysis A52.17
Lissencephalia, lissencephaly Q04.3
Listeriosis, listerellosis A32.9
  congenital (disseminated) P37.2
  cutaneous A32.0
  neonatal, newborn (disseminated) P37.2
  oculoglandular A32.81
  specified NEC A32.89
Lithemia E79.0
Lithiasis — *see* Calculus
Lithosis J62.8
Lithuria R82.998
Litigation, anxiety concerning Z65.3
Little leaguer's elbow — *see* Epicondylitis, medial
Little's disease G80.9
Littre's
  gland — *see* condition
  hernia — *see* Hernia, abdomen
Littritis — *see* Urethritis

Livedo (annularis) (racemosa) (reticularis) R23.1
Liver — *see* condition
Living alone (problems with) Z60.2
    with handicapped person Z74.2
Lloyd's syndrome — *see* Adenomatosis, endocrine
Loa loa, loaiasis, loasis B74.3
Lobar — *see* condition
Lobomycosis B48.0
Lobo's disease B48.0
Lobotomy syndrome F07.0
Lobstein (-Ekman) **disease or syndrome** Q78.0
Lobster-claw hand Q71.6- ☑
Lobulation (congenital) (*see also* Anomaly, by site)
    kidney, Q63.1
    liver, abnormal Q44.7
    spleen Q89.09
Lobule, lobular — *see* condition
Local, localized — *see* condition
Locked twins causing obstructed labor O66.1
Locked-in state G83.5
Locking
    joint — *see* Derangement, joint, specified type NEC
        knee — *see* Derangement, knee
Lockjaw — *see* Tetanus
Löffler's
    endocarditis I42.3
    eosinophilia J82
    pneumonia J82
    syndrome (eosinophilic pneumonitis) J82
Loiasis (with conjunctival infestation) (eyelid) B74.3
Lone Star fever A77.0
Long
    labor O63.9
        first stage O63.0
        second stage O63.1
    QT syndrome I45.81
Longitudinal stripes or grooves, nails L60.8
    congenital Q84.6
Long-term (current) (prophylactic) **drug therapy** (use of)
    agents affecting estrogen receptors and estrogen levels NEC Z79.818
    anastrozole (Arimidex) Z79.811
    antibiotics Z79.2
        short-term use — *omit code*
    anticoagulants Z79.01
    anti-inflammatory, non-steroidal (NSAID) Z79.1
    antiplatelet Z79.02
    antithrombotics Z79.02
    aromatase inhibitors Z79.811
    aspirin Z79.82
    birth control pill or patch Z79.3
    bisphosphonates Z79.83
    contraceptive, oral Z79.3
    drug, specified NEC Z79.899
    estrogen receptor downregulators Z79.818
    Evista Z79.810
    exemestane (Aromasin) Z79.811
    Fareston Z79.810
    fulvestrant (Faslodex) Z79.818
    gonadotropin-releasing hormone (GnRH) agonist Z79.818
    goserelin acetate (Zoladex) Z79.818
    hormone replacement Z79.890
    insulin Z79.4
    letrozole (Femara) Z79.811
    leuprolide acetate (leuprorelin) (Lupron) Z79.818
    megestrol acetate (Megace) Z79.818
    methadone for pain management Z79.891
    Nolvadex Z79.810
    non-steroidal anti-inflammatories (NSAID) Z79.1
    opiate analgesic Z79.891
    oral
        antidiabetic Z79.84
        contraceptive Z79.3
        hypoglycemic Z79.84
    raloxifene (Evista) Z79.810
    selective estrogen receptor modulators (SERMs) Z79.810
    steroids
        inhaled Z79.51
        systemic Z79.52
    tamoxifen (Nolvadex) Z79.810
    toremifene (Fareston) Z79.810
Loop
    intestine — *see* Volvulus
    vascular on papilla (optic) Q14.2
Loose (*see also* condition)

Loose — *continued*
    body
        joint M24.00
            ankle M24.07- ☑
            elbow M24.02- ☑
            hand M24.04- ☑
            hip M24.05- ☑
            knee M23.4- ☑
            shoulder (region) M24.01- ☑
            specified site NEC M24.08
            toe M24.07- ☑
            vertebra M24.08
            wrist M24.03- ☑
        knee M23.4- ☑
        sheath, tendon — *see* Disorder, tendon, specified type NEC
    cartilage — *see* Loose, body, joint
    skin and subcutaneous tissue (following bariatric surgery weight loss) (following dietary weight loss) L98.7
    tooth, teeth K08.89
Loosening
    aseptic
        joint prosthesis — *see* Complications, joint prosthesis, mechanical, loosening, by site
        epiphysis — *see* Osteochondropathy
    mechanical
        joint prosthesis — *see* Complications, joint prosthesis, mechanical, loosening, by site
Looser-Milkman (-Debray) **syndrome** M83.8
Lop ear (deformity) Q17.3
Lorain (-Levi) **short stature syndrome** E23.0
Lordosis M40.50
    acquired — *see* Lordosis, specified type NEC
    congenital Q76.429
        lumbar region Q76.426
        lumbosacral region Q76.427
        sacral region Q76.428
        sacrococcygeal region Q76.428
        thoracolumbar region Q76.425
    lumbar region M40.56
    lumbosacral region M40.57
    postsurgical M96.4
    postural — *see* Lordosis, specified type NEC
    rachitic (late effect) (sequelae) E64.3
    sequelae of rickets E64.3
    specified type NEC M40.40
        lumbar region M40.46
        lumbosacral region M40.47
        thoracolumbar region M40.45
    thoracolumbar region M40.55
    tuberculous A18.01
Loss (of)
    appetite (*see also* Anorexia) R63.0
        hysterical F50.89
        nonorganic origin F50.89
        psychogenic F50.89
    blood — *see* Hemorrhage
    bone — *see* Loss, substance of, bone
    consciousness, transient R55
        traumatic — *see* Injury, intracranial
    control, sphincter, rectum R15.9
        nonorganic origin F98.1
    elasticity, skin R23.4
    family (member) in childhood Z62.898
    fluid (acute) E86.9
    function of labyrinth — *see* subcategory H83.2 ☑
    hair, nonscarring — *see* Alopecia
    hearing (*see also* Deafness)
        central NOS H90.5
        conductive H90.2
            bilateral H90.0
            unilateral
                with
                    restricted hearing on the contralateral side H90.A1- ☑
                    unrestricted hearing on the contralateral side H90.1- ☑
        mixed conductive and sensorineural hearing loss H90.8
            bilateral H90.6
            unilateral
                with
                    restricted hearing on the contralateral side H90.A3- ☑
                    unrestricted hearing on the contralateral side H90.7- ☑
        neural NOS H90.5

Loss — *continued*
    hearing (*see also* Deafness) — *continued*
        perceptive NOS H90.5
        sensorineural NOS H90.5
            bilateral H90.3
            unilateral
                with
                    restricted hearing on the contralateral side H90.A2- ☑
                    unrestricted hearing on the contralateral side H90.4- ☑
        sensory NOS H90.5
    height R29.890
    limb or member, traumatic, current — *see* Amputation, traumatic
    love relationship in childhood Z62.898
    memory (*see also* Amnesia)
        mild, following organic brain damage F06.8
    mind — *see* Psychosis
    occlusal vertical dimension of fully erupted teeth M26.37
    organ or part — *see* Absence, by site, acquired
    ossicles, ear (partial) H74.32- ☑
    parent in childhood Z63.4
    pregnancy, recurrent N96
        care in current pregnancy O26.2- ☑
        without current pregnancy N96
    recurrent pregnancy — *see* Loss, pregnancy, recurrent
    self-esteem, in childhood Z62.898
    sense of
        smell — *see* Disturbance, sensation, smell
        taste — *see* Disturbance, sensation, taste
        touch R20.8
    sensory R44.9
        dissociative F44.6
    sexual desire F52.0
    sight (acquired) (complete) (congenital) — *see* Blindness
    substance of
        bone — *see* Disorder, bone, density and structure, specified NEC
            horizontal alveolar K06.3
        cartilage — *see* Disorder, cartilage, specified type NEC
            auricle (ear) — *see* Disorder, pinna, specified type NEC
        vitreous (humor) H15.89
    tooth, teeth — *see* Absence, teeth, acquired
    vision, visual H54.7
        both eyes H54.3
        one eye H54.60
            left (normal vision on right) H54.62
            right (normal vision on left) H54.61
        specified as blindness — *see* Blindness
        subjective
            sudden H53.13- ☑
            transient H53.12- ☑
    vitreous — *see* Prolapse, vitreous
    voice — *see* Aphonia
    weight (abnormal) (cause unknown) R63.4
Louis-Bar syndrome (ataxia-telangiectasia) G11.3
Louping ill (encephalitis) A84.8
Louse, lousiness — *see* Lice
Low
    achiever, school Z55.3
    back syndrome M54.5
    basal metabolic rate R94.8
    birthweight (2499 grams or less) P07.10
        with weight of
            1000-1249 grams P07.14
            1250-1499 grams P07.15
            1500-1749 grams P07.16
            1750-1999 grams P07.17
            2000-2499 grams P07.18
        extreme (999 grams or less) P07.00
            with weight of
                499 grams or less P07.01
                500-749 grams P07.02
                750-999 grams P07.03
        for gestational age — *see* Light for dates
    blood pressure (*see also* Hypotension)
        reading (incidental) (isolated) (nonspecific) R03.1
    cardiac reserve — *see* Disease, heart
    function (*see also* Hypofunction)
        kidney N28.9
    hematocrit D64.9
    hemoglobin D64.9
    income Z59.6

Low — *continued*
  level of literacy Z55.Ø
  lying
    kidney N28.89
    organ or site, congenital — *see* Malposition, congenital
  output syndrome (cardiac) — *see* Failure, heart
  platelets (blood) — *see* Thrombocytopenia
  reserve, kidney N28.89
  salt syndrome E87.1
  self esteem R45.81
  set ears Q17.4
  vision H54.2X- ☑
    one eye (other eye normal) H54.5Ø
      left (normal vision on right) H54.52A- ☑
      other eye blind — *see* Blindness
      right (normal vision on left) H54.511- ☑
Low-density-lipoprotein-type (LDL) **hyperlipoproteinemia** E78.ØØ
Lowe's syndrome E72.Ø3
Lown-Ganong-Levine syndrome I45.6
LSD reaction (acute) (without dependence) F16.9Ø
  with dependence F16.2Ø
L-shaped kidney Q63.8
Ludwig's angina or disease K12.2
Lues (venerea), **luetic** — *see* Syphilis
Luetscher's syndrome (dehydration) E86.Ø
Lumbago, lumbalgia M54.5
  with sciatica M54.4- ☑
    due to intervertebral disc disorder M51.17
  due to displacement, intervertebral disc M51.27
    with sciatica M51.17
Lumbar — *see* condition
Lumbarization, vertebra, congenital Q76.49
Lumbermen's itch B88.Ø
Lump (*see also* Mass)
  breast N63.Ø
    axillary tail
      left N63.32
      right N63.31
    left
      lower inner quadrant N63.24
      lower outer quadrant N63.23
      unspecified quadrant N63.2Ø
      upper inner quadrant N63.22
      upper outer quadrant N63.21
    right
      lower inner quadrant N63.14
      lower outer quadrant N63.13
      unspecified quadrant N63.1Ø
      upper inner quadrant N63.12
      upper outer quadrant N63.11
    subareolar
      left N63.42
      right N63.41
Lunacy — *see* Psychosis
Lung — *see* condition
Lupoid (miliary) **of Boeck** D86.3
Lupus
  anticoagulant D68.62
    with
      hemorrhagic disorder D68.312
      hypercoagulable state D68.62
    finding without diagnosis R76.Ø
  discoid (local) L93.Ø
  erythematosus (discoid) (local) L93.Ø
    disseminated — *see* Lupus, erythematosus, systemic
    eyelid HØ1.129
      left HØ1.126
        lower HØ1.125
        upper HØ1.124
      right HØ1.123
        lower HØ1.122
        upper HØ1.121
    profundus L93.2
    specified NEC L93.2
    subacute cutaneous L93.1
    systemic M32.9
      with organ or system involvement M32.1Ø
        endocarditis M32.11
        lung M32.13
        pericarditis M32.12
        renal (glomerular) M32.14
          tubulo-interstitial M32.15
        specified organ or system NEC M32.19
      drug-induced M32.Ø
      inhibitor (presence of) D68.62

Lupus — *continued*
  erythematosus — *continued*
    systemic — *continued*
      inhibitor — *continued*
        with
          hemorrhagic disorder D68.312
          hypercoagulable state D68.62
        finding without diagnosis R76.Ø
      specified NEC M32.8
  exedens A18.4
  hydralazine M32.Ø
    correct substance properly administered — *see* Table of Drugs and Chemicals, by drug, adverse effect
    overdose or wrong substance given or taken — *see* Table of Drugs and Chemicals, by drug, poisoning
  nephritis (chronic) M32.14
  nontuberculous, not disseminated L93.Ø
  panniculitis L93.2
  pernio (Besnier) D86.3
  systemic — *see* Lupus, erythematosus, systemic
  tuberculous A18.4
    eyelid A18.4
  vulgaris A18.4
    eyelid A18.4
Luteinoma D27.- ☑
Lutembacher's disease or syndrome (atrial septal defect with mitral stenosis) Q21.1
Luteoma D27.- ☑
Lutz (-Splendore-de Almeida) **disease** — *see* Paracoccidioidomycosis
Luxation (*see also* Dislocation)
  eyeball (nontraumatic) — *see* Luxation, globe
    birth injury P15.3
  globe, nontraumatic H44.82- ☑
  lacrimal gland — *see* Dislocation, lacrimal gland
  lens (old) (partial) (spontaneous)
    congenital Q12.1
    syphilitic A5Ø.39
Lycanthropy F22
Lyell's syndrome L51.2
  due to drug L51.2
    correct substance properly administered — *see* Table of Drugs and Chemicals, by drug, adverse effect
    overdose or wrong substance given or taken — *see* Table of Drugs and Chemicals, by drug, poisoning
Lyme disease A69.2Ø
Lymph
  gland or node — *see* condition
  scrotum — *see* Infestation, filarial
Lymphadenitis I88.9
  with ectopic or molar pregnancy OØ8.Ø
  acute LØ4.9
    axilla LØ4.2
    face LØ4.Ø
    head LØ4.Ø
    hip LØ4.3
    limb
      lower LØ4.3
      upper LØ4.2
    neck LØ4.Ø
    shoulder LØ4.2
    specified site NEC LØ4.8
    trunk LØ4.1
  anthracosis (occupational) J6Ø
  any site, except mesenteric I88.9
    chronic I88.1
    subacute I88.1
  breast
    gestational — *see* Mastitis, obstetric
    puerperal, postpartum (nonpurulent) O91.22
  chancroidal (congenital) A57
  chronic I88.1
    mesenteric I88.Ø
  due to
    Brugia (malayi) B74.1
      timori B74.2
    chlamydial lymphogranuloma A55
    diphtheria (toxin) A36.89
    lymphogranuloma venereum A55
    Wuchereria bancrofti B74.Ø
  following ectopic or molar pregnancy OØ8.Ø
  gonorrheal A54.89
  infective — *see* Lymphadenitis, acute

Lymphadenitis — *continued*
  mesenteric (acute) (chronic) (nonspecific) (subacute) I88.Ø
    due to Salmonella typhi AØ1.Ø9
    tuberculous A18.39
  mycobacterial A31.8
  purulent — *see* Lymphadenitis, acute
  pyogenic — *see* Lymphadenitis, acute
  regional, nonbacterial I88.8
  septic — *see* Lymphadenitis, acute
  subacute, unspecified site I88.1
  suppurative — *see* Lymphadenitis, acute
  syphilitic (early) (secondary) A51.49
    late A52.79
  tuberculous — *see* Tuberculosis, lymph gland
  venereal (chlamydial) A55
Lymphadenoid goiter E06.3
Lymphadenopathy (generalized) R59.1
  angioimmunoblastic, with dysproteinemia (AILD) C86.5
  due to toxoplasmosis (acquired) B58.89
    congenital (acute) (subacute) (chronic) P37.1
  localized R59.Ø
  syphilitic (early) (secondary) A51.49
Lymphadenosis R59.1
Lymphangiectasis I89.Ø
  conjunctiva H11.89
  postinfectional I89.Ø
  scrotum I89.Ø
Lymphangiectatic elephantiasis, nonfilarial I89.Ø
Lymphangioendothelioma D18.1
  malignant — *see* Neoplasm, connective tissue, malignant
Lymphangioleiomyomatosis J84.81
Lymphangioma D18.1
  capillary D18.1
  cavernous D18.1
  cystic D18.1
  malignant — *see* Neoplasm, connective tissue, malignant
Lymphangiomyoma D18.1
Lymphangiomyomatosis J84.81
Lymphangiosarcoma — *see* Neoplasm, connective tissue, malignant
Lymphangitis I89.1
  with
    abscess — *code by* site under Abscess
    cellulitis — *code by* site under Cellulitis
    ectopic or molar pregnancy OØ8.Ø
  acute LØ3.91
    abdominal wall LØ3.321
    ankle — *see* Lymphangitis, acute, lower limb
    arm — *see* Lymphangitis, acute, upper limb
    auricle (ear) — *see* Lymphangitis, acute, ear
    axilla LØ3.12- ☑
    back (any part) LØ3.322
    buttock LØ3.327
    cervical (meaning neck) LØ3.222
    cheek (external) LØ3.212
    chest wall LØ3.323
    digit
      finger — *see* Lymphangitis, acute, finger
      toe — *see* Lymphangitis, acute, toe
    ear (external) H60.1- ☑
    external auditory canal — *see* Lymphangitis, acute, ear
    eyelid — *see* Abscess, eyelid
    face NEC LØ3.212
    finger (intrathecal) (periosteal) (subcutaneous) (subcuticular) LØ3.Ø2- ☑
    foot — *see* Lymphangitis, acute, lower limb
    gluteal (region) LØ3.327
    groin LØ3.324
    hand — *see* Lymphangitis, acute, upper limb
    head NEC LØ3.891
      face (any part, except ear, eye and nose) LØ3.21
    heel — *see* Lymphangitis, acute, lower limb
    hip — *see* Lymphangitis, acute, lower limb
    jaw (region) LØ3.212
    knee — *see* Lymphangitis, acute, lower limb
    leg — *see* Lymphangitis, acute, lower limb
    lower limb LØ3.12- ☑
      toe — *see* Lymphangitis, acute, toe
    navel LØ3.326
    neck (region) LØ3.222
    orbit, orbital — *see* Cellulitis, orbit
    pectoral (region) LØ3.323
    perineal, perineum LØ3.325

☑ **Additional Character Required** — **Refer to the Tabular List for Character Selection**   ▽ **Subterms under main terms may continue to next column or page**

Lymphangitis — *continued*
  acute — *continued*
    scalp (any part) LØ3.891
    shoulder — *see* Lymphangitis, acute, upper limb
    specified site NEC LØ3.898
    thigh — *see* Lymphangitis, acute, lower limb
    thumb (intrathecal) (periosteal) (subcutaneous)
      (subcuticular) — *see* Lymphangitis, acute,
      finger
    toe (intrathecal) (periosteal) (subcutaneous) (subcu-
      ticular) LØ3.Ø4- ☑
    trunk LØ3.329
      abdominal wall LØ3.321
      back (any part) LØ3.322
      buttock LØ3.327
      chest wall LØ3.323
      groin LØ3.324
      perineal, perineum LØ3.325
      umbilicus LØ3.326
    umbilicus LØ3.326
    upper limb LØ3.12- ☑
      axilla — *see* Lymphangitis, acute, axilla
      finger — *see* Lymphangitis, acute, finger
      thumb — *see* Lymphangitis, acute, finger
    wrist — *see* Lymphangitis, acute, upper limb
  breast
    gestational — *see* Mastitis, obstetric
  chancroidal A57
  chronic (any site) I89.1
  due to
    Brugia (malayi) B74.1
      timori B74.2
    Wuchereria bancrofti B74.Ø
  following ectopic or molar pregnancy OØ8.89
  penis
    acute N48.29
    gonococcal (acute) (chronic) A54.Ø9
  puerperal, postpartum, childbirth O86.89
  strumous, tuberculous A18.2
  subacute (any site) I89.1
  tuberculous — *see* Tuberculosis, lymph gland
.ymphatic (vessel) — *see* condition
.ymphatism E32.8
.ymphectasia I89.Ø
.ymphedema (acquired) (*see also* Elephantiasis)
  congenital Q82.Ø
  hereditary (chronic) (idiopathic) Q82.Ø
  postmastectomy I97.2
  praecox I89.Ø
  secondary I89.Ø
  surgical NEC I97.89
    postmastectomy (syndrome) I97.2
.ymphoblastic — *see* condition
.ymphoblastoma (diffuse) — *see* Lymphoma, lymphoblastic (diffuse)
  giant follicular — *see* Lymphoma, lymphoblastic (dif-
    fuse)
  macrofollicular — *see* Lymphoma, lymphoblastic (dif-
    fuse)
.ymphocele I89.8
.ymphocytic
  chorioencephalitis (acute) (serous) A87.2
  choriomeningitis (acute) (serous) A87.2
  meningoencephalitis A87.2
.ymphocytoma, benign cutis L98.8
.ymphocytopenia D72.81Ø
.ymphocytosis (symptomatic) D72.82Ø
  infectious (acute) B33.8
.ymphoepithelioma — *see* Neoplasm, malignant, by
  site
.ymphogranuloma (malignant) (*see also* Lymphoma,
  Hodgkin)
  chlamydial A55
  inguinale A55
  venereum (any site) (chlamydial) (with stricture of rec-
    tum) A55
.ymphogranulomatosis (malignant) (*see also* Lymphoma, Hodgkin)
  benign (Boeck's sarcoid) (Schaumann's) D86.1
.ymphohistiocytosis, hemophagocytic (familial) D76.1
.ymphoid — *see* condition
.ymphoma (of) (malignant) C85.9Ø
  adult T-cell (HTLV-1-associated) (acute variant)
    (chronic variant) (lymphomatoid variant)
    (smouldering variant) C91.5- ☑
  anaplastic large cell
    ALK-negative C84.7- ☑
    ALK-positive C84.6- ☑

Lymphoma — *continued*
  anaplastic large cell — *continued*
    CD3Ø-positive C84.6- ☑
    primary cutaneous C86.6
  angioimmunoblastic T-cell C86.5
  BALT C88.4
  B-cell C85.1- ☑
  blastic NK-cell C86.4
  blastic plasmacytoid dendritic cell neoplasm (BPDCN)
    C86.4
  B-precursor C83.5- ☑
  bronchial-associated lymphoid tissue [BALT-lymphoma]
    C88.4
  Burkitt (atypical) C83.7- ☑
  Burkitt-like C83.7- ☑
  centrocytic C83.1- ☑
  cutaneous follicle center C82.6- ☑
  cutaneous T-cell C84.A- ☑ (*following* C84.7)
  diffuse follicle center C82.5- ☑
  diffuse large cell C83.3- ☑
    anaplastic C83.3- ☑
    B-cell C83.3- ☑
    CD3Ø-positive C83.3- ☑
    centroblastic C83.3- ☑
    immunoblastic C83.3- ☑
    plasmablastic C83.3- ☑
    subtype not specified C83.3- ☑
    T-cell rich C83.3- ☑
  enteropathy-type (associated) (intestinal) T-cell C86.2
  extranodal marginal zone B-cell lymphoma of mucosa-
    associated lymphoid tissue [MALT-lymphoma]
    C88.4
  extranodal NK/T-cell, nasal type C86.Ø
  follicular C82.9- ☑
    grade
      I C82.Ø- ☑
      II C82.1- ☑
      III C82.2- ☑
      IIIa C82.3- ☑
      IIIb C82.4- ☑
    specified NEC C82.8- ☑
  hepatosplenic T-cell (alpha-beta) (gamma-delta) C86.1
  histiocytic C85.9- ☑
    true C96.A (*following* C96.6)
  Hodgkin C81.9 ☑
    lymphocyte depleted (classical) C81.3- ☑
    lymphocyte-rich (classical) C81.4- ☑
    mixed cellularity (classical) C81.2- ☑
    nodular
      lymphocyte predominant C81.Ø- ☑
      sclerosis (classical) C81.1- ☑
    nodular sclerosis (classical) C81.1- ☑
    specified NEC (classical) C81.7- ☑
  intravascular large B-cell C83.8- ☑
  Lennert's C84.4- ☑
  lymphoblastic (diffuse) C83.5- ☑
  lymphoblastic B-cell C83.5- ☑
  lymphoblastic T-cell C83.5- ☑
  lymphoepithelioid C84.4- ☑
  lymphoplasmacytic C83.Ø- ☑
    with IgM-production C88.Ø
  MALT C88.4
  mantle cell C83.1- ☑
  mature T-cell NEC C84.4- ☑
  mature T/NK-cell C84.9- ☑
    specified NEC C84.Z- ☑ (*following* C84.7)
  mediastinal (thymic) large B-cell C85.2- ☑
  Mediterranean C88.3
  mucosa-associated lymphoid tissue [MALT-lymphoma]
    C88.4
  NK/T cell C84.9- ☑
  nodal marginal zone C83.Ø- ☑
  non-follicular (diffuse) C83.9- ☑
    specified NEC C83.8- ☑
  non-Hodgkin (*see also* Lymphoma, by type) C85.9- ☑
    specified NEC C85.8- ☑
  non-leukemic variant of B-CLL C83.Ø- ☑
  peripheral T-cell, not classified C84.4- ☑
  primary cutaneous
    anaplastic large cell C86.6
    CD3Ø-positive large T-cell C86.6
  primary effusion B-cell C83.8- ☑
  SALT C88.4
  skin-associated lymphoid tissue [SALT-lymphoma]
    C88.4
  small cell B-cell C83.Ø- ☑

Lymphoma — *continued*
  splenic marginal zone C83.Ø- ☑
  subcutaneous panniculitis-like T-cell C86.3
  T-precursor C83.5- ☑
  true histiocytic C96.A (*following* C96.6)
Lymphomatosis — *see* Lymphoma
Lymphopathia venereum, veneris A55
Lymphopenia D72.81Ø
Lymphoplasmacytic leukemia — *see* Leukemia,
  chronic lymphocytic, B-cell type
Lymphoproliferation, X-linked disease D82.3
Lymphoreticulosis, benign (of inoculation) A28.1
Lymphorrhea I89.8
Lymphosarcoma (diffuse) (*see also* Lymphoma) C85.9- ☑
Lymphostasis I89.8
Lypemania — *see* Melancholia
Lysine and hydroxylysine metabolism disorder E72.3
Lyssa — *see* Rabies

M

Macacus ear Q17.3
Maceration, wet feet, tropical (syndrome) T69.Ø2- ☑
MacLeod's syndrome J43.Ø
Macrocephalia, macrocephaly Q75.3
Macrocheilia, macrochilia (congenital) Q18.6
Macrocolon (*see also* Megacolon) Q43.1
Macrocornea Q15.8
  with glaucoma Q15.Ø
Macrocytic — *see* condition
Macrocytosis D75.89
Macrodactylia, macrodactylism (fingers) (thumbs)
  Q74.Ø
  toes Q74.2
Macrodontia KØØ.2
Macrogenia M26.Ø5
Macrogenitosomia (adrenal) (male) (praecox) E25.9
  congenital E25.Ø
Macroglobulinemia (idiopathic) (primary) C88.Ø
  monoclonal (essential) D47.2
  Waldenström C88.Ø
Macroglossia (congenital) Q38.2
  acquired K14.8
Macrognathia, macrognathism (congenital)
  (mandibular) (maxillary) M26.Ø9
Macrogyria (congenital) QØ4.8
Macrohydrocephalus — *see* Hydrocephalus
Macromastia — *see* Hypertrophy, breast
Macrophthalmos Q11.3
  in congenital glaucoma Q15.Ø
Macropsia H53.15
Macrosigmoid K59.39
  congenital Q43.2
Macrospondylitis , acromegalic E22.Ø
Macrostomia (congenital) Q18.4
Macrotia (external ear) (congenital) Q17.1
Macula
  cornea, corneal — *see* Opacity, cornea
  degeneration (atrophic) (exudative) (senile) (*see also*
    Degeneration, macula)
    hereditary — *see* Dystrophy, retina
Maculae ceruleae B85.1
Maculopathy, toxic — *see* Degeneration, macula, toxic
Madarosis (eyelid) HØ2.729
  left HØ2.726
    lower HØ2.725
    upper HØ2.724
  right HØ2.723
    lower HØ2.722
    upper HØ2.721
Madelung's
  deformity (radius) Q74.Ø
  disease
    radial deformity Q74.Ø
    symmetrical lipomas, neck E88.89
Madness — *see* Psychosis
Madura
  foot B47.9
    actinomycotic B47.1
    mycotic B47.Ø
Maduromycosis B47.Ø
Maffucci's syndrome Q78.4
Magnesium metabolism disorder — *see* Disorder,
  metabolism, magnesium
Main en griffe (acquired) (*see also* Deformity, limb,
  clawhand)
  congenital Q74.Ø

Maintenance (encounter for)
  antineoplastic chemotherapy Z51.11
  antineoplastic radiation therapy Z51.0
  methadone F11.20
Majocchi's
  disease L81.7
  granuloma B35.8
Major — *see* condition
Mal de los pintos — *see* Pinta
Mal de mer T75.3 ☑
Malabar itch (any site) B35.5
Malabsorption K90.9
  calcium K90.89
  carbohydrate K90.49
  disaccharide E73.9
  fat K90.49
  galactose E74.20
  glucose (-galactose) E74.39
  intestinal K90.9
    specified NEC K90.89
  isomaltose E74.31
  lactose E73.9
  methionine E72.19
  monosaccharide E74.39
  postgastrectomy K91.2
  postsurgical K91.2
  protein K90.49
  starch K90.49
  sucrose E74.39
  syndrome K90.9
    postsurgical K91.2
Malacia, bone (adult) M83.9
  juvenile — *see* Rickets
Malacoplakia
  bladder N32.89
  pelvis (kidney) N28.89
  ureter N28.89
  urethra N36.8
Malacosteon, juvenile — *see* Rickets
Maladaptation — *see* Maladjustment
Maladie de Roger Q21.0
Maladjustment
  conjugal Z63.0
    involving divorce or estrangement Z63.5
  educational Z55.4
  family Z63.9
  marital Z63.0
    involving divorce or estrangement Z63.5
  occupational NEC Z56.89
  simple, adult — *see* Disorder, adjustment
  situational — *see* Disorder, adjustment
  social Z60.9
    due to
      acculturation difficulty Z60.3
      discrimination and persecution (perceived) Z60.5
      exclusion and isolation Z60.4
      life-cycle (phase of life) transition Z60.0
      rejection Z60.4
      specified reason NEC Z60.8
Malaise R53.81
Malakoplakia — *see* Malacoplakia
Malaria, malarial (fever) B54
  with
    blackwater fever B50.8
      hemoglobinuric (bilious) B50.8
    hemoglobinuria B50.8
  accidentally induced (therapeutically) — *code by* type
    under Malaria
  algid B50.9
  cerebral B50.0 [G94]
  clinically diagnosed (without parasitological confirmation) B54
  congenital NEC P37.4
    falciparum P37.3
  congestion, congestive B54
  continued (fever) B50.9
  estivo-autumnal B50.9
  falciparum B50.9
    with complications NEC B50.8
      cerebral B50.0 [G94]
      severe B50.8
  hemorrhagic B54
  malariae B52.9
    with
      complications NEC B52.8
      glomerular disorder B52.0
  malignant (tertian) — *see* Malaria, falciparum

Malaria, malarial — *continued*
  mixed infections — *code to* first listed type in B50-B53
  ovale B53.0
  parasitologically confirmed NEC B53.8
  pernicious, acute — *see* Malaria, falciparum
  Plasmodium (P.)
    falciparum NEC — *see* Malaria, falciparum
    malariae NEC B52.9
      with Plasmodium
        falciparum (and or vivax) — *see* Malaria, falciparum
        vivax (*see also* Malaria, vivax)
          and falciparum — *see* Malaria, falciparum
    ovale B53.0
      with Plasmodium malariae (*see also* Malaria, malariae)
        and vivax (*see also* Malaria, vivax)
          and falciparum — *see* Malaria, falciparum
    simian B53.1
      with Plasmodium malariae (*see also* Malaria, malariae)
        and vivax (*see also* Malaria, vivax)
          and falciparum — *see* Malaria, falciparum
    vivax NEC B51.9
      with Plasmodium falciparum — *see* Malaria, falciparum
  quartan — *see* Malaria, malariae
  quotidian — *see* Malaria, falciparum
  recurrent B54
  remittent B54
  specified type NEC (parasitologically confirmed) B53.8
  spleen B54
  subtertian (fever) — *see* Malaria, falciparum
  tertian (benign) (*see also* Malaria, vivax)
    malignant B50.9
  tropical B50.9
  typhoid B54
  vivax B51.9
    with
      complications NEC B51.8
      ruptured spleen B51.0
Malassez's disease (cystic) N50.89
Malassimilation K90.9
Maldescent, testis Q53.9
  bilateral Q53.20
    abdominal Q53.211
    perineal Q53.22
  unilateral Q53.10
    abdominal Q53.111
    perineal Q53.12
Maldevelopment (*see also* Anomaly)
  brain Q07.9
  colon Q43.9
  hip Q74.2
    congenital dislocation Q65.2
      bilateral Q65.1
      unilateral Q65.0- ☑
  mastoid process Q75.8
  middle ear Q16.4
    except ossicles Q16.4
    ossicles Q16.3
  ossicles Q16.3
  spine Q76.49
  toe Q74.2
Male type pelvis Q74.2
  with disproportion (fetopelvic) O33.3 ☑
    causing obstructed labor O65.3
Malformation (congenital) (*see also* Anomaly)
  adrenal gland Q89.1
  affecting multiple systems with skeletal changes NEC Q87.5
  alimentary tract Q45.9
    specified type NEC Q45.8
    upper Q40.9
      specified type NEC Q40.8
  aorta Q25.40
    absence Q25.41
    aneurysm, congenital Q25.43
    aplasia Q25.41
    atresia Q25.29
      aortic arch Q25.21
    coarctation (preductal) (postductal) Q25.1
    dilatation, congenital Q25.44
    hypoplasia Q25.42
    patent ductus arteriosus Q25.0
    specified type NEC Q25.49
    stenosis Q25.1
      supravalvular Q25.3

Malformation — *continued*
  aortic valve Q23.9
    specified NEC Q23.8
  arteriovenous, aneurysmatic (congenital) Q27.30
    brain Q28.2
    cerebral Q28.2
    peripheral Q27.30
      digestive system Q27.33
      lower limb Q27.32
      other specified site Q27.39
      renal vessel Q27.34
      upper limb Q27.31
    precerebral vessels (nonruptured) Q28.0
  auricle
    ear (congenital) Q17.3
      acquired H61.119
        left H61.112
          with right H61.113
        right H61.111
          with left H61.113
  bile duct Q44.5
  bladder Q64.79
    aplasia Q64.5
    diverticulum Q64.6
    exstrophy — *see* Exstrophy, bladder
    neck obstruction Q64.31
  bone Q79.9
    face Q75.9
      specified type NEC Q75.8
    skull Q75.9
      specified type NEC Q75.8
  brain (multiple) Q04.9
    arteriovenous Q28.2
    specified type NEC Q04.8
  branchial cleft Q18.2
  breast Q83.9
    specified type NEC Q83.8
  broad ligament Q50.6
  bronchus Q32.4
  bursa Q79.9
  cardiac
    chambers Q20.9
      specified type NEC Q20.8
    septum Q21.9
      specified type NEC Q21.8
  cerebral Q04.9
    vessels Q28.3
  cervix uteri Q51.9
    specified type NEC Q51.828
  Chiari
    Type I G93.5
    Type II Q07.01
  choroid (congenital) Q14.3
    plexus Q07.8
  circulatory system Q28.9
  cochlea Q16.5
  cornea Q13.4
  coronary vessels Q24.5
  corpus callosum (congenital) Q04.0
  diaphragm Q79.1
  digestive system NEC, specified type NEC Q45.8
  dura Q07.9
    brain Q04.9
    spinal Q06.9
  ear Q17.9
    causing impairment of hearing Q16.9
    external Q17.9
      accessory auricle Q17.0
      causing impairment of hearing Q16.9
        absence of
          auditory canal Q16.1
          auricle Q16.0
      macrotia Q17.1
      microtia Q17.2
      misplacement Q17.4
      misshapen NEC Q17.3
      prominence Q17.5
      specified type NEC Q17.8
    inner Q16.5
    middle Q16.4
      absence of eustachian tube Q16.2
      ossicles (fusion) Q16.3
    ossicles Q16.3
    specified type NEC Q17.8
  epididymis Q55.4
  esophagus Q39.9
    specified type NEC Q39.8
  eye Q15.9
    lid Q10.3

Malformation — *continued*

eye — *continued*
    specified NEC Q15.8
fallopian tube Q50.6
genital organ — *see* Anomaly, genitalia
great
    artery Q25.9
        aorta — *see* Malformation, aorta
        pulmonary artery — *see* Malformation, pulmonary, artery
        specified type NEC Q25.8
    vein Q26.9
        anomalous
            portal venous connection Q26.5
            pulmonary venous connection Q26.4
                partial Q26.3
                total Q26.2
        persistent left superior vena cava Q26.1
        portal vein-hepatic artery fistula Q26.6
        specified type NEC Q26.8
        vena cava stenosis, congenital Q26.0
gum Q38.6
hair Q84.2
heart Q24.9
    specified type NEC Q24.8
integument Q84.9
    specified type NEC Q84.8
internal ear Q16.5
intestine Q43.9
    specified type NEC Q43.8
iris Q13.2
joint Q74.9
    ankle Q74.2
    lumbosacral Q76.49
    sacroiliac Q74.2
    specified type NEC Q74.8
kidney Q63.9
    accessory Q63.0
    giant Q63.3
    horseshoe Q63.1
    hydronephrosis Q62.0
    malposition Q63.2
    specified type NEC Q63.8
lacrimal apparatus Q10.6
lingual Q38.3
lip Q38.0
liver Q44.7
lung Q33.9
meninges or membrane (congenital) Q07.9
    cerebral Q04.8
    spinal (cord) Q06.9
middle ear Q16.4
    ossicles Q16.3
mitral valve Q23.9
    specified NEC Q23.8
Mondini's (congenital) (malformation, cochlea) Q16.5
mouth (congenital) Q38.6
multiple types NEC Q89.7
musculoskeletal system Q79.9
myocardium Q24.8
nail Q84.6
nervous system (central) Q07.9
nose Q30.9
    specified type NEC Q30.8
optic disc Q14.2
orbit Q10.7
ovary Q50.39
palate Q38.5
parathyroid gland Q89.2
pelvic organs or tissues NEC
    in pregnancy or childbirth O34.8- ☑
        causing obstructed labor O65.5
penis Q55.69
    aplasia Q55.5
    curvature (lateral) Q55.61
    hypoplasia Q55.62
pericardium Q24.8
peripheral vascular system Q27.9
    specified type NEC Q27.8
pharynx Q38.8
precerebral vessels Q28.1
prostate Q55.4
pulmonary
    arteriovenous Q25.72
    artery Q25.9
        atresia Q25.5
        specified type NEC Q25.79
        stenosis Q25.6
    valve Q22.3

Malformation — *continued*

renal artery Q27.2
respiratory system Q34.9
retina Q14.1
scrotum — *see* Malformation, testis and scrotum
seminal vesicles Q55.4
sense organs NEC Q07.9
skin Q82.9
specified NEC Q89.8
spinal
    cord Q06.9
    nerve root Q07.8
spine Q76.49
    kyphosis — *see* Kyphosis, congenital
    lordosis — *see* Lordosis, congenital
spleen Q89.09
stomach Q40.3
    specified type NEC Q40.2
teeth, tooth K00.9
tendon Q79.9
testis and scrotum Q55.20
    aplasia Q55.0
    hypoplasia Q55.1
    polyorchism Q55.21
    retractile testis Q55.22
    scrotal transposition Q55.23
    specified NEC Q55.29
thorax, bony Q76.9
throat Q38.8
thyroid gland Q89.2
tongue (congenital) Q38.3
    hypertrophy Q38.2
    tie Q38.1
trachea Q32.1
tricuspid valve Q22.9
    specified type NEC Q22.8
umbilical cord NEC (complicating delivery) O69.89 ☑
umbilicus Q89.9
ureter Q62.8
    agenesis Q62.4
    duplication Q62.5
    malposition — *see* Malposition, congenital, ureter
    obstructive defect — *see* Defect, obstructive, ureter
    vesico-uretero-renal reflux Q62.7
urethra Q64.79
    aplasia Q64.5
    duplication Q64.74
    posterior valves Q64.2
    prolapse Q64.71
    stricture Q64.32
urinary system Q64.9
uterus Q51.9
    specified type NEC Q51.818
vagina Q52.4
vas deferens Q55.4
    atresia Q55.3
vascular system, peripheral Q27.9
venous — *see* Anomaly, vein(s)
vulva Q52.70

Malfunction (*see also* Dysfunction)

cardiac electronic device T82.119 ☑
    electrode T82.110 ☑
    pulse generator T82.111 ☑
    specified type NEC T82.118 ☑
catheter device NEC T85.618 ☑
    cystostomy T83.010 ☑
    dialysis (renal) (vascular) T82.41 ☑
        intraperitoneal T85.611 ☑
    infusion NEC T82.514 ☑
        cranial T85.610 ☑
        epidural T85.610 ☑
        intrathecal T85.610 ☑
        spinal T85.610 ☑
        subarachnoid T85.610 ☑
        subdural T85.610 ☑
    urinary (*see also* Breakdown, device, catheter) T83.018 ☑
colostomy K94.03
    valve K94.03
cystostomy (stoma) N99.512
    catheter T83.010 ☑
enteric stoma K94.13
enterostomy K94.13
esophagostomy K94.33
gastroenteric K31.89
gastrostomy K94.23
ileostomy K94.13
    valve K94.13

Malfunction — *continued*

intrathecal infusion pump T85.615 ☑
jejunostomy K94.13
nervous system device, implant or graft, specified NEC T85.615 ☑
pacemaker — *see* Malfunction, cardiac electronic device
prosthetic device, internal — *see* Complications, prosthetic device, by site, mechanical
tracheostomy J95.03
urinary device NEC — *see* Complication, genitourinary, device, urinary, mechanical
valve
    colostomy K94.03
    heart T82.09 ☑
    ileostomy K94.13
vascular graft or shunt NEC — *see* Complication, cardiovascular device, mechanical, vascular
ventricular (communicating shunt) T85.01 ☑
Malherbe's tumor — *see* Neoplasm, skin, benign
Malibu disease L98.8
Malignancy (*see also* Neoplasm, malignant, by site)
    unspecified site (primary) C80.1
Malignant — *see* condition
Malingerer, malingering Z76.5
Mallet finger (acquired) — *see* Deformity, finger, mallet finger
    congenital Q74.0
    sequelae of rickets E64.3
Malleus A24.0
Mallory's bodies R89.7
Mallory-Weiss syndrome K22.6
Malnutrition E46
    degree
        first E44.1
        mild (protein) E44.1
        moderate (protein) E44.0
        second E44.0
        severe (protein-energy) E43
            intermediate form E42
                with
                    kwashiorkor (and marasmus) E42
                    marasmus E41
        third E43
    following gastrointestinal surgery K91.2
    intrauterine
        light-for-dates — *see* Light for dates
        small-for-dates — *see* Small for dates
    lack of care, or neglect (child) (infant) T76.02 ☑
        confirmed T74.02 ☑
    malignant E40
    protein E46
        calorie E46
            mild E44.1
            moderate E44.0
            severe E43
                intermediate form E42
                    with
                        kwashiorkor (and marasmus) E42
                        marasmus E41
        energy E46
            mild E44.1
            moderate E44.0
            severe E43
                intermediate form E42
                    with
                        kwashiorkor (and marasmus) E42
                        marasmus E41
    severe (protein-energy) E43
        with
            kwashiorkor (and marasmus) E42
            marasmus E41
Malocclusion (teeth) M26.4
    Angle's M26.219
        class I M26.211
        class II M26.212
        class III M26.213
    due to
        abnormal swallowing M26.59
        mouth breathing M26.59
        tongue, lip or finger habits M26.59
    temporomandibular (joint) M26.69
Malposition
    cervix — *see* Malposition, uterus
    congenital
        adrenal (gland) Q89.1
        alimentary tract Q45.8
            lower Q43.8

Malposition — *continued*
  congenital — *continued*
    alimentary tract — *continued*
      upper Q40.8
    aorta Q25.49
    appendix Q43.8
    arterial trunk Q20.0
    artery (peripheral) Q27.8
      coronary Q24.5
      digestive system Q27.8
      lower limb Q27.8
      pulmonary Q25.79
      specified site NEC Q27.8
      upper limb Q27.8
    auditory canal Q17.8
      causing impairment of hearing Q16.9
    auricle (ear) Q17.4
      causing impairment of hearing Q16.9
      cervical Q18.2
    biliary duct or passage Q44.5
    bladder (mucosa) — *see* Exstrophy, bladder
    brachial plexus Q07.8
    brain tissue Q04.8
    breast Q83.8
    bronchus Q32.4
    cecum Q43.8
    clavicle Q74.0
    colon Q43.8
    digestive organ or tract NEC Q45.8
      lower Q43.8
      upper Q40.8
    ear (auricle) (external) Q17.4
      ossicles Q16.3
    endocrine (gland) NEC Q89.2
    epiglottis Q31.8
    eustachian tube Q17.8
    eye Q15.8
    facial features Q18.8
    fallopian tube Q50.6
    finger(s) Q68.1
      supernumerary Q69.0
    foot Q66.9
    gallbladder Q44.1
    gastrointestinal tract Q45.8
    genitalia, genital organ(s) or tract
      female Q52.8
        external Q52.79
        internal NEC Q52.8
      male Q55.8
    glottis Q31.8
    hand Q68.1
    heart Q24.8
      dextrocardia Q24.0
        with complete transposition of viscera Q89.3
    hepatic duct Q44.5
    hip (joint) Q65.89
    intestine (large) (small) Q43.8
      with anomalous adhesions, fixation or malrotation Q43.3
    joint NEC Q68.8
    kidney Q63.2
    larynx Q31.8
    limb Q68.8
      lower Q68.8
      upper Q68.8
    liver Q44.7
    lung (lobe) Q33.8
    nail(s) Q84.6
    nerve Q07.8
    nervous system NEC Q07.8
    nose, nasal (septum) Q30.8
    organ or site not listed — *see* Anomaly, by site
    ovary Q50.39
    pancreas Q45.3
    parathyroid (gland) Q89.2
    patella Q74.1
    peripheral vascular system Q27.8
    pituitary (gland) Q89.2
    respiratory organ or system NEC Q34.8
    rib (cage) Q76.6
      supernumerary in cervical region Q76.5
    scapula Q74.0
    shoulder Q74.0
    spinal cord Q06.8
    spleen Q89.09
    sternum NEC Q76.7
    stomach Q40.2
    symphysis pubis Q74.2
    thymus (gland) Q89.2

Malposition — *continued*
  congenital — *continued*
    thyroid (gland) (tissue) Q89.2
      cartilage Q31.8
    toe(s) Q66.9
      supernumerary Q69.2
    tongue Q38.3
    trachea Q32.1
    ureter Q62.60
      deviation Q62.61
      displacement Q62.62
      ectopia Q62.63
      specified type NEC Q62.69
    uterus Q51.818
    vein(s) (peripheral) Q27.8
      great Q26.8
    vena cava (inferior) (superior) Q26.8
  device, implant or graft (*see also* Complications, by site and type, mechanical) T85.628 ☑
    arterial graft NEC — *see* Complication, cardiovascular device, mechanical, vascular
    breast (implant) T85.42 ☑
    catheter NEC T85.628 ☑
      cystostomy T83.020 ☑
      dialysis (renal) T82.42 ☑
        intraperitoneal T85.621 ☑
      infusion NEC T82.524 ☑
        spinal (epidural) (subdural) T85.620 ☑
      urinary (*see also* Displacement, device, catheter, urinary) T83.028 ☑
    electronic (electrode) (pulse generator) (stimulator)
      bone T84.320 ☑
      cardiac T82.129 ☑
        electrode T82.120 ☑
        pulse generator T82.121 ☑
        specified type NEC T82.128 ☑
      nervous system — *see* Complication, prosthetic device, mechanical, electronic nervous system stimulator
      urinary — *see* Complication, genitourinary, device, urinary, mechanical
    fixation, internal (orthopedic) NEC — *see* Complication, fixation device, mechanical
    gastrointestinal — *see* Complications, prosthetic device, mechanical, gastrointestinal device
    genital NEC T83.428 ☑
      intrauterine contraceptive device (string) T83.32 ☑
      penile prosthesis (cylinder) (implanted) (pump) (reservoir) T83.420 ☑
      testicular prosthesis T83.421 ☑
    heart NEC — *see* Complication, cardiovascular device, mechanical
    joint prosthesis — *see* Complication, joint prosthesis, mechanical
    ocular NEC — *see* Complications, prosthetic device, mechanical, ocular device
    orthopedic NEC — *see* Complication, orthopedic, device, mechanical
    specified NEC T85.628 ☑
    urinary NEC (*see also* Complication, genitourinary, device, urinary, mechanical)
      graft T83.22 ☑
    vascular NEC — *see* Complication, cardiovascular device, mechanical
    ventricular intracranial shunt T85.02 ☑
  fetus — *see* Pregnancy, complicated by (management affected by), presentation, fetal
  gallbladder K82.8
  gastrointestinal tract, congenital Q45.8
  heart, congenital NEC Q24.8
  joint prosthesis — *see* Complications, joint prosthesis, mechanical, displacement, by site
  stomach K31.89
    congenital Q40.2
  tooth, teeth, fully erupted M26.30
  uterus (acute) (acquired) (adherent) (asymptomatic) (postinfectional) (postpartal, old) N85.4
    anteflexion or anteversion N85.4
      congenital Q51.818
    flexion N85.4
      lateral — *see* Lateroversion, uterus
    inversion N85.5
    lateral (flexion) (version) — *see* Lateroversion, uterus
      in pregnancy or childbirth — *see* subcategory O34.5 ☑

Malposition — *continued*
  uterus — *continued*
    retroflexion or retroversion — *see* Retroversion, uterus
Malposture R29.3
Malrotation
  cecum Q43.3
  colon Q43.3
  intestine Q43.3
  kidney Q63.2
Malta fever — *see* Brucellosis
Maltreatment
  adult
    abandonment
      confirmed T74.01 ☑
      suspected T76.01 ☑
    bullying
      confirmed T74.31 ☑
      suspected T76.31 ☑
    confirmed T74.91 ☑
    history of Z91.419
    intimidation (through social media)
      confirmed T74.31 ☑
      suspected T76.31 ☑
    neglect
      confirmed T74.01 ☑
      suspected T76.01 ☑
    physical abuse
      confirmed T74.11 ☑
      suspected T76.11 ☑
    psychological abuse
      confirmed T74.31 ☑
      history of Z91.411
      suspected T76.31 ☑
    sexual abuse
      confirmed T74.21 ☑
      suspected T76.21 ☑
    suspected T76.91 ☑
  child
    abandonment
      confirmed T74.02 ☑
      suspected T76.02 ☑
    bullying
      confirmed T74.32 ☑
      suspected T76.32 ☑
    confirmed T74.92 ☑
    history of — *see* History, personal (of), abuse
    intimidation (through social media)
      confirmed T74.32 ☑
      suspected T76.32 ☑
    neglect
      confirmed T74.02 ☑
      history of — *see* History, personal (of), abuse
      suspected T76.02 ☑
    physical abuse
      confirmed T74.12 ☑
      history of — *see* History, personal (of), abuse
      suspected T76.12 ☑
    psychological abuse
      confirmed T74.32 ☑
      history of — *see* History, personal (of), abuse
      suspected T76.32 ☑
    sexual abuse
      confirmed T74.22 ☑
      history of — *see* History, personal (of), abuse
      suspected T76.22 ☑
    suspected T76.92 ☑
  personal history of Z91.89
Maltworker's lung J67.4
Malunion, fracture — *see* Fracture, by site
Mammillitis N61.0
  puerperal, postpartum O91.02
Mammitis — *see* Mastitis
Mammogram (examination) Z12.39
  routine Z12.31
Mammoplasia N62
Management (of)
  bone conduction hearing device (implanted) Z45.32
  cardiac pacemaker NEC Z45.018
  cerebrospinal fluid drainage device Z45.41
  cochlear device (implanted) Z45.321
  contraceptive Z30.9
    specified NEC Z30.8
  implanted device Z45.9
    specified NEC Z45.89
  infusion pump Z45.1
  procreative Z31.9

☑ **Additional Character Required** — Refer to the Tabular List for Character Selection

▽ **Subterms under main terms may continue to next column or page**

Management — *continued*
  procreative — *continued*
    male factor infertility in female Z31.81
    specified NEC Z31.89
  prosthesis (external) (*see also* Fitting) Z44.9
    implanted Z45.9
      specified NEC Z45.89
  renal dialysis catheter Z49.01
  vascular access device Z45.2
Mangled — *see* specified injury by site
Mania (monopolar) (*see also* Disorder, mood, manic episode)
  with psychotic symptoms F30.2
  without psychotic symptoms F30.10
    mild F30.11
    moderate F30.12
    severe F30.13
  Bell's F30.8
  chronic (recurrent) F31.89
  hysterical F44.89
  puerperal F30.8
  recurrent F31.89
Manic depression F31.9
Manic-depressive insanity, psychosis, or syndrome — *see* Disorder, bipolar
Mannosidosis E77.1
Mansonelliasis, mansonellosis B74.4
Manson's
  disease B65.1
  schistosomiasis B65.1
Manual — *see* condition
Maple-bark-stripper's lung (disease) J67.6
Maple-syrup-urine disease E71.0
Marable's syndrome (celiac artery compression) I77.4
Marasmus E41
  due to malnutrition E41
  intestinal E41
  nutritional E41
  senile R54
  tuberculous NEC — *see* Tuberculosis
Marble
  bones Q78.2
  skin R23.8
Marburg virus disease A98.3
March
  fracture — *see* Fracture, traumatic, stress, by site
  hemoglobinuria D59.6
Marchesani (-Weill) **syndrome** Q87.0
Marchiafava (-Bignami) **syndrome or disease** G37.1
Marchiafava-Micheli syndrome D59.5
Marcus Gunn's syndrome Q07.8
Marfan's syndrome — *see* Syndrome, Marfan's
Marie-Bamberger disease — *see* Osteoarthropathy, hypertrophic, specified NEC
Marie-Charcot-Tooth neuropathic muscular atrophy G60.0
Marie's
  cerebellar ataxia (late-onset) G11.2
  disease or syndrome (acromegaly) E22.0
Marie-Strümpell arthritis, disease or spondylitis — *see* Spondylitis, ankylosing
Marion's disease (bladder neck obstruction) N32.0
Marital conflict Z63.0
Mark
  port wine Q82.5
  raspberry Q82.5
  strawberry Q82.5
  stretch L90.6
  tattoo L81.8
Marker heterochromatin — *see* Extra, marker chromosomes
Maroteaux-Lamy syndrome (mild) (severe) E76.29
Marrow (bone)
  arrest D61.9
  poor function D75.89
Marseilles fever A77.1
Marsh fever — *see* Malaria
Marshall's (hidrotic) **ectodermal dysplasia** Q82.4
Marsh's disease (exophthalmic goiter) E05.00
  with storm E05.01
Masculinization (female) **with adrenal hyperplasia** E25.9
  congenital E25.0
Masculinovoblastoma D27.- ☑
Masochism (sexual) F65.51
Mason's lung J62.8

Mass
  abdominal R19.00
    epigastric R19.06
    generalized R19.07
    left lower quadrant R19.04
    left upper quadrant R19.02
    periumbilic R19.05
    right lower quadrant R19.03
    right upper quadrant R19.01
    specified site NEC R19.09
  breast (*see also* Lump, breast) N63.0
  chest R22.2
  cystic — *see* Cyst
  ear H93.8- ☑
  head R22.0
  intra-abdominal (diffuse) (generalized) — *see* Mass, abdominal
  kidney N28.89
  liver R16.0
  localized (skin) R22.9
    chest R22.2
    head R22.0
    limb
      lower R22.4- ☑
      upper R22.3- ☑
    neck R22.1
    trunk R22.2
  lung R91.8
  malignant — *see* Neoplasm, malignant, by site
  neck R22.1
  pelvic (diffuse) (generalized) — *see* Mass, abdominal
  specified organ NEC — *see* Disease, by site
  splenic R16.1
  substernal thyroid — *see* Goiter
  superficial (localized) R22.9
  umbilical (diffuse) (generalized) R19.09
Massive — *see* condition
Mast cell
  disease, systemic tissue D47.02
  leukemia C94.3- ☑
  neoplasm
    malignant C96.20
      specified type NEC C96.29
    of uncertain behavior NEC D47.09
  sarcoma C96.22
  tumor D47.09
Mastalgia N64.4
Masters-Allen syndrome N83.8
Mastitis (acute) (diffuse) (nonpuerperal) (subacute) N61.0
  with abscess N61.1
  chronic (cystic) — *see* Mastopathy, cystic
  cystic (Schimmelbusch's type) — *see* Mastopathy, cystic
  fibrocystic — *see* Mastopathy, cystic
  infective N61.0
    newborn P39.0
  interstitial, gestational or puerperal — *see* Mastitis, obstetric
  neonatal (noninfective) P83.4
    infective P39.0
  obstetric (interstitial) (nonpurulent)
    associated with
      lactation O91.23
      pregnancy O91.21- ☑
      puerperium O91.22
    purulent
      associated with
        lactation O91.13
        pregnancy O91.11- ☑
        puerperium O91.12
  periductal — *see* Ectasia, mammary duct
  phlegmonous — *see* Mastopathy, cystic
  plasma cell — *see* Ectasia, mammary duct
  without abscess N61.0
Mastocytoma (extracutaneous) D47.09
  malignant C96.29
  solitary D47.01
Mastocytosis D47.09
  aggressive systemic C96.21
  cutaneous (diffuse) (maculopapular) D47.01
    congenital Q82.2
    of neonatal onset Q82.2
    of newborn onset Q82.2
  indolent systemic D47.02
  isolated bone marrow D47.02
  malignant C96.29
  systemic (indolent) (smoldering)
    with an associated hematological non-mast cell lineage disease (SM-AHNMD) D47.02

Mastodynia N64.4
Mastoid — *see* condition
Mastoidalgia — *see* subcategory H92.0 ☑
Mastoiditis (coalescent) (hemorrhagic) (suppurative) H70.9- ☑
  acute, subacute H70.00- ☑
    complicated NEC H70.09- ☑
    subperiosteal H70.01- ☑
  chronic (necrotic) (recurrent) H70.1- ☑
  in (due to)
    infectious disease NEC B99 ☑ [H75.0-] ☑
    parasitic disease NEC B89 [H75.0-] ☑
    tuberculosis A18.03
  petrositis — *see* Petrositis
  postauricular fistula — *see* Fistula, postauricular
  specified NEC H70.89- ☑
  tuberculous A18.03
Mastopathy, mastopathia N64.9
  chronica cystica — *see* Mastopathy, cystic
  cystic (chronic) (diffuse) N60.1- ☑
    with epithelial proliferation N60.3- ☑
  diffuse cystic — *see* Mastopathy, cystic
  estrogenic, oestrogenica N64.89
  ovarian origin N64.89
Mastoplasia, mastoplastia N62
Masturbation (excessive) F98.8
Maternal care (for) — *see* Pregnancy (complicated by) (management affected by)
Matheiu's disease (leptospiral jaundice) A27.0
Mauclaire's disease or osteochondrosis — *see* Osteochondrosis, juvenile, hand, metacarpal
Maxcy's disease A75.2
Maxilla, maxillary — *see* condition
May (-Hegglin) **anomaly or syndrome** D72.0
McArdle (-Schmid)(-Pearson) **disease** (glycogen storage) E74.04
McCune-Albright syndrome Q78.1
McQuarrie's syndrome (idiopathic familial hypoglycemia) E16.2
Meadow's syndrome Q86.1
Measles (black) (hemorrhagic) (suppressed) B05.9
  with
    complications NEC B05.89
    encephalitis B05.0
    intestinal complications B05.4
    keratitis (keratoconjunctivitis) B05.81
    meningitis B05.1
    otitis media B05.3
    pneumonia B05.2
  French — *see* Rubella
  German — *see* Rubella
  Liberty — *see* Rubella
Meatitis, urethral — *see* Urethritis
Meatus, meatal — *see* condition
Meat-wrappers' asthma J68.9
Meckel-Gruber syndrome Q61.9
Meckel's diverticulitis, diverticulum (displaced) (hypertrophic) Q43.0
  malignant — *see* Table of Neoplasms, small intestine, malignant
Meconium
  ileus, newborn P76.0
    in cystic fibrosis E84.11
    meaning meconium plug (without cystic fibrosis) P76.0
  obstruction, newborn P76.0
    due to fecaliths P76.0
    in mucoviscidosis E84.11
  peritonitis P78.0
  plug syndrome (newborn) NEC P76.0
Median (*see also* condition)
  arcuate ligament syndrome I77.4
  bar (prostate) (vesical orifice) — *see* Hyperplasia, prostate
  rhomboid glossitis K14.2
Mediastinal shift R93.89
Mediastinitis (acute) (chronic) J98.51
  syphilitic A52.73
  tuberculous A15.8
Mediastinopericarditis (*see also* Pericarditis)
  acute I30.9
  adhesive I31.0
  chronic I31.8
    rheumatic I09.2
Mediastinum, mediastinal — *see* condition
Medicine poisoning — *see* Table of Drugs and Chemicals, by drug, poisoning

Mediterranean
  fever — *see* Brucellosis
    familial M04.1
    tick A77.1
  kala-azar B55.0
  leishmaniasis B55.0
  tick fever A77.1
Medulla — *see* condition
Medullary cystic kidney Q61.5
Medullated fibers
  optic (nerve) Q14.8
  retina Q14.1
Medulloblastoma
  desmoplastic C71.6
  specified site — *see* Neoplasm, malignant, by site
  unspecified site C71.6
Medulloepithelioma (*see also* Neoplasm, malignant, by
    site)
  teratoid — *see* Neoplasm, malignant, by site
Medullomyoblastoma
  specified site — *see* Neoplasm, malignant, by site
  unspecified site C71.6
Meekeren-Ehlers-Danlos syndrome Q79.6
Megacolon (acquired) (functional) (not Hirschsprung's
    disease) (in) K59.39
  Chagas' disease B57.32
  congenital, congenitum (aganglionic) Q43.1
  Hirschsprung's (disease) Q43.1
  toxic NEC K59.31
    due to Clostridium difficile
      not specified as recurrent A04.72
      recurrent A04.71
Megaesophagus (functional) K22.0
  congenital Q39.5
  in (due to) Chagas' disease B57.31
Megalencephaly Q04.5
Megalerythema (epidemic) B08.3
Megaloappendix Q43.8
Megalocephalus, megalocephaly NEC Q75.3
Megalocornea Q15.8
  with glaucoma Q15.0
Megalocytic anemia D53.1
Megalodactylia (fingers) (thumbs) (congenital) Q74.0
  toes Q74.2
Megaloduodenum Q43.8
Megaloesophagus (functional) K22.0
  congenital Q39.5
Megalogastria (acquired) K31.89
  congenital Q40.2
Megalophthalmos Q11.3
Megalopsia H53.15
Megalosplenia — *see* Splenomegaly
Megaloureter N28.82
  congenital Q62.2
Megarectum K62.89
Megasigmoid K59.39
  congenital Q43.2
Megaureter N28.82
  congenital Q62.2
Megavitamin-B6 syndrome E67.2
Megrim — *see* Migraine
Meibomian
  cyst, infected — *see* Hordeolum
  gland — *see* condition
  sty, stye — *see* Hordeolum
Meibomitis — *see* Hordeolum
Meige-Milroy disease (chronic hereditary edema) Q82.0
Meige's syndrome Q82.0
Melalgia, nutritional E53.8
Melancholia F32.9
  climacteric (single episode) F32.89
    recurrent episode F33.8
  hypochondriac F45.29
  intermittent (single episode) F32.89
    recurrent episode F33.8
  involutional (single episode) F32.89
    recurrent episode F33.8
  menopausal (single episode) F32.89
    recurrent episode F33.8
  puerperal F32.89
  reactive (emotional stress or trauma) F32.3
  recurrent F33.9
  senile F03 ☑
  stuporous (single episode) F32.89
    recurrent episode F33.8
Melanemia R79.89
Melanoameloblastoma — *see* Neoplasm, bone, benign

Melanoblastoma — *see* Melanoma
Melanocarcinoma — *see* Melanoma
Melanocytoma, eyeball D31.9- ☑
Melanocytosis, neurocutaneous Q82.8
Melanoderma, melanodermia L81.4
Melanodontia, infantile K03.89
Melanodontoclasia K03.89
Melanoepithelioma — *see* Melanoma
Melanoma (malignant) C43.9
  acral lentiginous, malignant — *see* Melanoma, skin, by
    site
  amelanotic — *see* Melanoma, skin, by site
  balloon cell — *see* Melanoma, skin, by site
  benign — *see* Nevus
  desmoplastic, malignant — *see* Melanoma, skin, by
    site
  epithelioid cell — *see* Melanoma, skin, by site
    with spindle cell, mixed — *see* Melanoma, skin, by
      site
  in
    giant pigmented nevus — *see* Melanoma, skin, by
      site
    Hutchinson's melanotic freckle — *see* Melanoma,
      skin, by site
    junctional nevus — *see* Melanoma, skin, by site
    precancerous melanosis — *see* Melanoma, skin, by
      site
  in situ D03.9
    abdominal wall D03.59
    ala nasi D03.39
    ankle D03.7- ☑
    anus, anal (margin) (skin) D03.51
    arm D03.6- ☑
    auditory canal D03.2- ☑
    auricle (ear) D03.2- ☑
    auricular canal (external) D03.2- ☑
    axilla, axillary fold D03.59
    back D03.59
    breast D03.52
    brow D03.39
    buttock D03.59
    canthus (eye) D03.1- ☑
    cheek (external) D03.39
    chest wall D03.59
    chin D03.39
    choroid D03.8
    conjunctiva D03.8
    ear (external) D03.2- ☑
    external meatus (ear) D03.2- ☑
    eye D03.8
    eyebrow D03.39
    eyelid (lower) (upper) D03.1- ☑
    face D03.30
      specified NEC D03.39
    female genital organ (external) NEC D03.8
    finger D03.6- ☑
    flank D03.59
    foot D03.7- ☑
    forearm D03.6- ☑
    forehead D03.39
    foreskin D03.8
    gluteal region D03.59
    groin D03.59
    hand D03.6- ☑
    heel D03.7- ☑
    helix D03.2- ☑
    hip D03.7- ☑
    interscapular region D03.59
    iris D03.8
    jaw D03.39
    knee D03.7- ☑
    labium (majus) (minus) D03.8
    lacrimal gland D03.8
    leg D03.7- ☑
    lip (lower) (upper) D03.0
    lower limb NEC D03.7- ☑
    male genital organ (external) NEC D03.8
    nail D03.9
      finger D03.6- ☑
      toe D03.7- ☑
    neck D03.4
    nose (external) D03.39
    orbit D03.8
    penis D03.8
    perianal skin D03.51
    perineum D03.51
    pinna D03.2- ☑

Melanoma — *continued*
  in situ — *continued*
    popliteal fossa or space D03.7- ☑
    prepuce D03.8
    pudendum D03.8
    retina D03.8
    retrobulbar D03.8
    scalp D03.4
    scrotum D03.8
    shoulder D03.6- ☑
    specified site NEC D03.8
    submammary fold D03.52
    temple D03.39
    thigh D03.7- ☑
    toe D03.7- ☑
    trunk NEC D03.59
    umbilicus D03.59
    upper limb NEC D03.6- ☑
    vulva D03.8
  juvenile — *see* Nevus
  malignant, of soft parts except skin — *see* Neoplasm,
      connective tissue, malignant
  metastatic
    breast C79.81
    genital organ C79.82
    specified site NEC C79.89
  neurotropic, malignant — *see* Melanoma, skin, by site
  nodular — *see* Melanoma, skin, by site
  regressing, malignant — *see* Melanoma, skin, by site
  skin C43.9
    abdominal wall C43.59
    ala nasi C43.31
    ankle C43.7- ☑
    anus, anal (skin) C43.51
    arm C43.6- ☑
    auditory canal (external) C43.2- ☑
    auricle (ear) C43.2- ☑
    auricular canal (external) C43.2- ☑
    axilla, axillary fold C43.59
    back C43.59
    breast (female) (male) C43.52
    brow C43.39
    buttock C43.59
    canthus (eye) C43.1- ☑
    cheek (external) C43.39
    chest wall C43.59
    chin C43.39
    ear (external) C43.2- ☑
    elbow C43.6- ☑
    external meatus (ear) C43.2- ☑
    eyebrow C43.39
    eyelid (lower) (upper) C43.1- ☑
    face C43.30
      specified NEC C43.39
    female genital organ (external) NEC C51.9
    finger C43.6- ☑
    flank C43.59
    foot C43.7- ☑
    forearm C43.6- ☑
    forehead C43.39
    foreskin C60.0
    glabella C43.39
    gluteal region C43.59
    groin C43.59
    hand C43.6- ☑
    heel C43.7- ☑
    helix C43.2- ☑
    hip C43.7- ☑
    interscapular region C43.59
    jaw (external) C43.39
    knee C43.7- ☑
    labium C51.9
      majus C51.0
      minus C51.1
    leg C43.7- ☑
    lip (lower) (upper) C43.0
    lower limb NEC C43.7- ☑
    male genital organ (external) NEC C63.9
    nail
      finger C43.6- ☑
      toe C43.7- ☑
    nasolabial groove C43.39
    nates C43.59
    neck C43.4
    nose (external) C43.31
    overlapping site C43.8
    palpebra C43.1- ☑

☑ **Additional Character Required** — Refer to the Tabular List for Character Selection   ⩔ **Subterms under main terms may continue to next column or page**

Melanoma — *continued*
  skin — *continued*
    penis C60.9
    perianal skin C43.51
    perineum C43.51
    pinna C43.2- ☑
    popliteal fossa or space C43.7- ☑
    prepuce C60.0
    pudendum C51.9
    scalp C43.4
    scrotum C63.2
    shoulder C43.6- ☑
    skin NEC C43.9
    submammary fold C43.52
    temple C43.39
    thigh C43.7- ☑
    toe C43.7- ☑
    trunk NEC C43.59
    umbilicus C43.59
    upper limb NEC C43.6- ☑
    vulva C51.9
      overlapping sites C51.8
  spindle cell
    with epithelioid, mixed — *see* Melanoma, skin, by site
    type A C69.4- ☑
    type B C69.4- ☑
  superficial spreading — *see* Melanoma, skin, by site
Melanosarcoma (*see also* Melanoma)
  epithelioid cell — *see* Melanoma
Melanosis L81.4
  addisonian E27.1
    tuberculous A18.7
  adrenal E27.1
  colon K63.89
  conjunctiva — *see* Pigmentation, conjunctiva
    congenital Q13.89
  cornea (presenile) (senile) (*see also* Pigmentation, cornea)
    congenital Q13.4
  eye NEC H57.89
    congenital Q15.8
  lenticularis progressiva Q82.1
  liver K76.89
  precancerous (*see also* Melanoma, in situ)
    malignant melanoma in — *see* Melanoma
  Riehl's L81.4
  sclera H15.89
    congenital Q13.89
  suprarenal E27.1
  tar L81.4
  toxic L81.4
Melanuria R82.998
MELAS syndrome E88.41
Melasma L81.1
  adrenal (gland) E27.1
  suprarenal (gland) E27.1
Melena K92.1
  with ulcer — *code by* site under Ulcer, with hemorrhage K27.4
  due to swallowed maternal blood P78.2
  newborn, neonatal P54.1
    due to swallowed maternal blood P78.2
Meleney's
  gangrene (cutaneous) — *see* Ulcer, skin
  ulcer (chronic undermining) — *see* Ulcer, skin
Melioidosis A24.9
  acute A24.1
  chronic A24.2
  fulminating A24.1
  pneumonia A24.1
  pulmonary (chronic) A24.2
    acute A24.1
    subacute A24.2
  sepsis A24.1
  specified NEC A24.3
  subacute A24.2
Melitensis, febris A23.0
Melkersson (-Rosenthal) **syndrome** G51.2
Mellitus, diabetes — *see* Diabetes
Melorheostosis (bone) — *see* Disorder, bone, density and structure, specified NEC
Meloschisis Q18.4
Melotia Q17.4
Membrana
  capsularis lentis posterior Q13.89
  epipapillaris Q14.2
Membranacea placenta O43.19- ☑

Membranaceous uterus N85.8
Membrane(s), membranous (*see also* condition)
  cyclitic — *see* Membrane, pupillary
  folds, congenital — *see* Web
  Jackson's Q43.3
  over face of newborn P28.9
  premature rupture — *see* Rupture, membranes, premature
  pupillary H21.4- ☑
    persistent Q13.89
  retained (with hemorrhage) (complicating delivery) O72.2
    without hemorrhage O73.1
  secondary cataract — *see* Cataract, secondary
  unruptured (causing asphyxia) — *see* Asphyxia, newborn
  vitreous — *see* Opacity, vitreous, membranes and strands
Membranitis — *see* Chorioamnionitis
Memory disturbance, lack or loss (*see also* Amnesia)
  mild, following organic brain damage F06.8
Menadione deficiency E56.1
Menarche
  delayed E30.0
  precocious E30.1
Mendacity, pathologic F60.2
Mendelson's syndrome (due to anesthesia) J95.4
  in labor and delivery O74.0
  in pregnancy O29.01- ☑
  obstetric O74.0
  postpartum, puerperal O89.01
Ménétrier's disease or syndrome K29.60
  with bleeding K29.61
Ménière's disease, syndrome or vertigo H81.0- ☑
Meninges, meningeal — *see* condition
Meningioma (*see also* Neoplasm, meninges, benign)
  angioblastic — *see* Neoplasm, meninges, benign
  angiomatous — *see* Neoplasm, meninges, benign
  endotheliomatous — *see* Neoplasm, meninges, benign
  fibroblastic — *see* Neoplasm, meninges, benign
  fibrous — *see* Neoplasm, meninges, benign
  hemangioblastic — *see* Neoplasm, meninges, benign
  hemangiopericytic — *see* Neoplasm, meninges, benign
  malignant — *see* Neoplasm, meninges, malignant
  meningiothelial — *see* Neoplasm, meninges, benign
  meningotheliomatous — *see* Neoplasm, meninges, benign
  mixed — *see* Neoplasm, meninges, benign
  multiple — *see* Neoplasm, meninges, uncertain behavior
  papillary — *see* Neoplasm, meninges, uncertain behavior
  psammomatous — *see* Neoplasm, meninges, benign
  syncytial — *see* Neoplasm, meninges, benign
  transitional — *see* Neoplasm, meninges, benign
Meningiomatosis (diffuse) — *see* Neoplasm, meninges, uncertain behavior
Meningism — *see* Meningismus
Meningismus (infectional) (pneumococcal) R29.1
  due to serum or vaccine R29.1
  influenzal — *see* Influenza, with, manifestations NEC
Meningitis (basal) (basic) (brain) (cerebral) (cervical) (congestive) (diffuse) (hemorrhagic) (infantile) (membranous) (metastatic) (nonspecific) (pontine) (progressive) (simple) (spinal) (subacute) (sympathetic) (toxic) G03.9
  abacterial G03.0
  actinomycotic A42.81
  adenoviral A87.1
  arbovirus A87.8
  aseptic (acute) G03.0
  bacterial G00.9
    Escherichia coli (E. coli) G00.8
    Friedländer (bacillus) G00.8
    gram-negative G00.9
    H. influenzae G00.0
    Klebsiella G00.8
    pneumococcal G00.1
    specified organism NEC G00.8
    staphylococcal G00.3
    streptococcal (acute) G00.2
  benign recurrent (Mollaret) G03.2
  candidal B37.5
  caseous (tuberculous) A17.0
  cerebrospinal A39.0
  chronic NEC G03.1
  clear cerebrospinal fluid NEC G03.0

Meningitis — *continued*
  coxsackievirus A87.0
  cryptococcal B45.1
  diplococcal (gram positive) A39.0
  echovirus A87.0
  enteroviral A87.0
  eosinophilic B83.2
  epidemic NEC A39.0
  Escherichia coli (E. coli) G00.8
  fibrinopurulent G00.9
    specified organism NEC G00.8
  Friedländer (bacillus) G00.8
  gonococcal A54.81
  gram-negative cocci G00.9
  gram-positive cocci G00.9
  H. influenzae G00.0
  Haemophilus (influenzae) G00.0
  in (due to)
    adenovirus A87.1
    African trypanosomiasis B56.9 [G02]
    anthrax A22.8
    bacterial disease NEC A48.8 [G01]
    Chagas' disease (chronic) B57.41
    chickenpox B01.0
    coccidioidomycosis B38.4
    Diplococcus pneumoniae G00.1
    enterovirus A87.0
    herpes (simplex) virus B00.3
      zoster B02.1
    infectious mononucleosis B27.92
    leptospirosis A27.81
    Listeria monocytogenes A32.11
    Lyme disease A69.21
    measles B05.1
    mumps (virus) B26.1
    neurosyphilis (late) A52.13
    parasitic disease NEC B89 [G02]
    poliovirus A80.9 [G02]
    preventive immunization, inoculation or vaccination G03.8
    rubella B06.02
    Salmonella infection A02.21
    specified cause NEC G03.8
    Streptococcal pneumoniae G00.1
    typhoid fever A01.01
    varicella B01.0
    viral disease NEC A87.8
    whooping cough A37.90
    zoster B02.1
  infectious G00.9
  influenzal (H. influenzae) G00.0
  Klebsiella G00.8
  leptospiral (aseptic) A27.81
  lymphocytic (acute) (benign) (serous) A87.2
  meningococcal A39.0
  Mima polymorpha G00.8
  Mollaret (benign recurrent) G03.2
  monilial B37.5
  mycotic NEC B49 [G02]
  Neisseria A39.0
  nonbacterial G03.0
  nonpyogenic NEC G03.0
  ossificans G96.19
  pneumococcal streptococcus pneumoniae G00.1
  poliovirus A80.9 [G02]
  postmeasles B05.1
  purulent G00.9
    specified organism NEC G00.8
  pyogenic G00.9
    specified organism NEC G00.8
  Salmonella (arizonae) (Cholerae-Suis) (enteritidis) (typhimurium) A02.21
  septic G00.9
    specified organism NEC G00.8
  serosa circumscripta NEC G03.0
  serous NEC G93.2
  specified organism NEC G00.8
  sporotrichosis B42.81
  staphylococcal G00.3
  sterile G03.0
  Streptococcal (acute) G00.2
    pneumoniae G00.1
  suppurative G00.9
    specified organism NEC G00.8
  syphilitic (late) (tertiary) A52.13
    acute A51.41
    congenital A50.41
    secondary A51.41
  Torula histolytica (cryptococcal) B45.1

▽ Subterms under main terms may continue to next column or page   ☑ Additional Character Required — Refer to the Tabular List for Character Selection   221

Melanoma — Meningitis

Meningitis — *continued*
  traumatic (complication of injury) T79.8 ☑
  tuberculous A17.0
  typhoid A01.01
  viral NEC A87.9
  Yersinia pestis A20.3
Meningocele (spinal) (*see also* Spina bifida)
  with hydrocephalus — *see* Spina bifida, by site, with
    hydrocephalus
  acquired (traumatic) G96.19
  cerebral — *see* Encephalocele
Meningocerebritis — *see* Meningoencephalitis
Meningococcemia A39.4
  acute A39.2
  chronic A39.3
Meningococcus, meningococcal (*see also* condition)
  A39.9
  adrenalitis, hemorrhagic A39.1
  carrier (suspected) of Z22.31
  meningitis (cerebrospinal) A39.0
Meningoencephalitis (*see also* Encephalitis) G04.90
  acute NEC (*see also* Encephalitis, viral) A86
  bacterial NEC G04.2
  California A83.5
  diphasic A84.1
  eosinophilic B83.2
  epidemic A39.81
  herpesviral, herpetic B00.4
    due to herpesvirus 6 B10.01
    due to herpesvirus 7 B10.09
    specified NEC B10.09
  in (due to)
    blastomycosis NEC B40.81
    diseases classified elsewhere G05.3
    free-living amebae B60.2
    H. influenzae G00.0
    Hemophilus influenzae (H .influenzae) G00.0
    herpes B00.4
      due to herpesvirus 6 B10.01
      due to herpesvirus 7 B10.09
      specified NEC B10.09
    Lyme disease A69.22
    mercury — *see* subcategory T56.1 ☑
    mumps B26.2
    Naegleria (amebae) (organisms) (fowleri) B60.2
    Parastrongylus cantonensis B83.2
    toxoplasmosis (acquired) B58.2
      congenital P37.1
  infectious (acute) (viral) A86
  influenzal (H. influenzae) G00.0
  Listeria monocytogenes A32.12
  lymphocytic (serous) A87.2
  mumps B26.2
  parasitic NEC B89 [G05.3]
  pneumococcal G04.2
  primary amebic B60.2
  specific (syphilitic) A52.14
  specified organism NEC G04.81
  staphylococcal G04.2
  streptococcal G04.2
  syphilitic A52.14
  toxic NEC G92
    due to mercury — *see* subcategory T56.1 ☑
  tuberculous A17.82
  virus NEC A86
Meningoencephalocele (*see also* Encephalocele)
  syphilitic A52.19
    congenital A50.49
Meningoencephalomyelitis (*see also* Meningoencephalitis)
  acute NEC (viral) A86
    disseminated G04.00
      postimmunization or postvaccination G04.02
      postinfectious G04.01
  due to
    actinomycosis A42.82
    Torula B45.1
    Toxoplasma or toxoplasmosis (acquired) B58.2
      congenital P37.1
  postimmunization or postvaccination G04.02
Meningoencephalomyelopathy G96.9
Meningoencephalopathy G96.9
Meningomyelitis (*see also* Meningoencephalitis)
  bacterial NEC G04.2
  blastomycotic NEC B40.81
  cryptococcal B45.1
  in diseases classified elsewhere G05.4
  meningococcal A39.81

Meningomyelitis — *continued*
  syphilitic A52.14
  tuberculous A17.82
Meningomyelocele (*see also* Spina bifida)
  syphilitic A52.19
Meningomyeloneuritis — *see* Meningoencephalitis
Meningoradiculitis — *see* Meningitis
Meningovascular — *see* condition
Menkes' disease or syndrome E83.09
  meaning maple-syrup-urine disease E71.0
Menometrorrhagia N92.1
Menopause, menopausal (asymptomatic) (state) Z78.0
  arthritis (any site) NEC — *see* Arthritis, specified form
    NEC
  bleeding N92.4
  depression (single episode) F32.89
    agitated (single episode) F32.2
      recurrent episode F33.9
    psychotic (single episode) F32.89
      recurrent episode F33.9
    recurrent episode F33.8
  melancholia (single episode) F32.89
    recurrent episode F33.8
  paranoid state F22
  premature E28.319
    asymptomatic E28.319
      postirradiation E89.40
      postsurgical E89.40
    symptomatic E28.310
      postirradiation E89.41
      postsurgical E89.41
  psychosis NEC F28
  symptomatic N95.1
  toxic polyarthritis NEC — *see* Arthritis, specified form
    NEC
Menorrhagia (primary) N92.0
  climacteric N92.4
    menopausal N92.4
  menopausal N92.4
  postclimacteric N95.0
  postmenopausal N95.0
  preclimacteric or premenopausal N92.4
  pubertal (menses retained) N92.2
Menostaxis N92.0
Menses, retention N94.89
Menstrual — *see* Menstruation
Menstruation
  absent — *see* Amenorrhea
  anovulatory N97.0
  cycle, irregular N92.6
  delayed N91.0
  disorder N93.9
    psychogenic F45.8
  during pregnancy O20.8
  excessive (with regular cycle) N92.0
    with irregular cycle N92.1
    at puberty N92.2
  frequent N92.0
  infrequent — *see* Oligomenorrhea
  irregular N92.6
    specified NEC N92.5
  latent N92.5
  membranous N92.5
  painful (*see also* Dysmenorrhea) N94.6
    primary N94.4
    psychogenic F45.8
    secondary N94.5
  passage of clots N92.0
  precocious E30.1
  protracted N92.5
  rare — *see* Oligomenorrhea
  retained N94.89
  retrograde N92.5
  scanty — *see* Oligomenorrhea
  suppression N94.89
  vicarious (nasal) N94.89
Mental (*see also* condition)
  deficiency — *see* Disability, intellectual
  deterioration — *see* Psychosis
  disorder — *see* Disorder, mental
  exhaustion F48.8
  insufficiency (congenital) — *see* Disability, intellectual
  observation without need for further medical care
    Z03.89
  retardation — *see* Disability, intellectual
  subnormality — *see* Disability, intellectuall
  upset — *see* Disorder, mental
Meralgia paresthetica G57.1- ☑

Mercurial — *see* condition
Mercurialism — *see* subcategory T56.1 ☑
Merkel cell tumor — *see* Carcinoma, Merkel cell
Merocele — *see* Hernia, femoral
Meromelia
  lower limb — *see* Defect, reduction, lower limb
    intercalary
      femur — *see* Defect, reduction, lower limb,
        specified type NEC
        tibiofibular (complete) (incomplete) — *see*
          Defect, reduction, lower limb
  upper limb — *see* Defect, reduction, upper limb
    intercalary, humeral, radioulnar — *see* Agenesis,
      arm, with hand present
MERRF syndrome (myoclonic epilepsy associated with
  ragged-red fiber) E88.42
Merzbacher-Pelizaeus disease E75.29
Mesaortitis — *see* Aortitis
Mesarteritis — *see* Arteritis
Mesencephalitis — *see* Encephalitis
Mesenchymoma (*see also* Neoplasm, connective tissue,
  uncertain behavior)
  benign — *see* Neoplasm, connective tissue, benign
  malignant — *see* Neoplasm, connective tissue, malig-
    nant
Mesenteritis
  retractile K65.4
  sclerosing K65.4
Mesentery, mesenteric — *see* condition
Mesiodens, mesiodentes K00.1
Mesio-occlusion M26.213
Mesocolon — *see* condition
Mesonephroma (malignant) — *see* Neoplasm, malig-
  nant, by site
  benign — *see* Neoplasm, benign, by site
Mesophlebitis — *see* Phlebitis
Mesostromal dysgenesia Q13.89
Mesothelioma (malignant) C45.9
  benign
    mesentery D19.1
    mesocolon D19.1
    omentum D19.1
    peritoneum D19.1
    pleura D19.0
    specified site NEC D19.7
    unspecified site D19.9
  biphasic C45.9
    benign
      mesentery D19.1
      mesocolon D19.1
      omentum D19.1
      peritoneum D19.1
      pleura D19.0
      specified site NEC D19.7
      unspecified site D19.9
  cystic D48.4
  epithelioid C45.9
    benign
      mesentery D19.1
      mesocolon D19.1
      omentum D19.1
      peritoneum D19.1
      pleura D19.0
      specified site NEC D19.7
      unspecified site D19.9
  fibrous C45.9
    benign
      mesentery D19.1
      mesocolon D19.1
      omentum D19.1
      peritoneum D19.1
      pleura D19.0
      specified site NEC D19.7
      unspecified site D19.9
  site classification
    liver C45.7
    lung C45.7
    mediastinum C45.7
    mesentery C45.1
    mesocolon C45.1
    omentum C45.1
    pericardium C45.2
    peritoneum C45.1
    pleura C45.0
      parietal C45.0
    retroperitoneum C45.7
    specified site NEC C45.7
    unspecified C45.9

☑ **Additional Character Required** — Refer to the Tabular List for Character Selection
▽ **Subterms under main terms may continue to next column or page**

Metabolic syndrome E88.81
Metagonimiasis B66.8
Metagonimus infestation (intestine) B66.8
Metal
  pigmentation L81.8
  polisher's disease J62.8
Metamorphopsia H53.15
Metaplasia
  apocrine (breast) — *see* Dysplasia, mammary, specified
    type NEC
  cervix (squamous) — *see* Dysplasia, cervix
  endometrium (squamous) (uterus) N85.8
  esophagus K22.7- ☑
  kidney (pelvis) (squamous) N28.89
  myelogenous D73.1
  myeloid (agnogenic) (megakaryocytic) D73.1
  spleen D73.1
  squamous cell, bladder N32.89
Metastasis, metastatic
  abscess — *see* Abscess
  calcification E83.59
  cancer
    from specified site — *see* Neoplasm, malignant, by
     site
    to specified site — *see* Neoplasm, secondary, by site
  deposits (in) — *see* Neoplasm, secondary, by site
  disease (*see also* Neoplasm, secondary, by site) C79.9
  spread (to) — *see* Neoplasm, secondary, by site
Metastrongyliasis B83.8
Metatarsalgia M77.4- ☑
  anterior G57.6- ☑
  Morton's G57.6- ☑
Metatarsus, metatarsal (*see also* condition)
  adductus, congenital Q66.22
  valgus (abductus), congenital Q66.6
  varus (congenital) Q66.22
    primus Q66.21
Methadone use — *see* Use, opioid
Methemoglobinemia D74.9
  acquired (with sulfhemoglobinemia) D74.8
  congenital D74.0
  enzymatic (congenital) D74.0
  Hb M disease D74.0
  hereditary D74.0
  toxic D74.8
Methemoglobinuria — *see* Hemoglobinuria
Methioninemia E72.19
Methylmalonic acidemia E71.120
Metritis (catarrhal) (hemorrhagic) (septic) (suppurative)
  (*see also* Endometritis)
  cervical — *see* Cervicitis
Metropathia hemorrhagica N93.8
Metroperitonitis — *see* Peritonitis, pelvic, female
Metrorrhagia N92.1
  climacteric N92.4
  menopausal N92.4
  postpartum NEC (atonic) (following delivery of placen-
    ta) O72.1
    delayed or secondary O72.2
  preclimacteric or premenopausal N92.4
  psychogenic F45.8
Metrorrhexis — *see* Rupture, uterus
Metrosalpingitis N70.91
Metrostaxis N93.8
Metrovaginitis — *see* Endometritis
Meyer-Schwickerath and Weyers syndrome Q87.0
Meynert's amentia (nonalcoholic) F04
  alcoholic F10.96
    with dependence F10.26
Mibelli's disease (porokeratosis) Q82.8
Mice, joint — *see* Loose, body, joint
  knee M23.4- ☑
Micrencephalon, micrencephaly Q02
Microalbuminuria R80.9
Microaneurysm, retinal (*see also* Disorder, retina, mi-
  croaneurysms)
  diabetic — *see* E08-E13 with .31
Microangiopathy (peripheral) I73.9
  thrombotic M31.1
Microcalcifications, breast R92.0
Microcephalus, microcephalic, microcephaly Q02
  due to toxoplasmosis (congenital) P37.1
Microcheilia Q18.7
Microcolon (congenital) Q43.8
Microcornea (congenital) Q13.4
Microcytic — *see* condition
Microdeletions NEC Q93.88

Microdontia K00.2
Microdrepanocytosis D57.40
  with crisis (vasoocclusive pain) D57.419
    with
      acute chest syndrome D57.411
      splenic sequestration D57.412
Microembolism
  atherothrombotic — *see* Atheroembolism
  retinal — *see* Occlusion, artery, retina
Microencephalon Q02
Microfilaria streptocerca infestation — *see* Onchocer-
  ciasis
Microgastria (congenital) Q40.2
Microgenia M26.06
Microgenitalia, congenital
  female Q52.8
  male Q55.8
Microglioma — *see* Lymphoma, non-Hodgkin, specified
  NEC
Microglossia (congenital) Q38.3
Micrognathia, micrognathism (congenital) (mandibu-
  lar) (maxillary) M26.09
Microgyria (congenital) Q04.3
Microinfarct of heart — *see* Insufficiency, coronary
Microlentia (congenital) Q12.8
Microlithiasis, alveolar, pulmonary J84.02
Micromastia N64.82
Micromyelia (congenital) Q06.8
Micropenis Q55.62
Microphakia (congenital) Q12.8
Microphthalmos, microphthalmia (congenital) Q11.2
  due to toxoplasmosis P37.1
Micropsia H53.15
Microscopic polyangiitis (polyarteritis) M31.7
Microsporidiosis B60.8
  intestinal A07.8
Microsporon furfur infestation B36.0
Microsporosis (*see also* Dermatophytosis)
  nigra B36.1
Microstomia (congenital) Q18.5
Microtia (congenital) (external ear) Q17.2
Microtropia H50.40
Microvillus inclusion disease (MVD) (MVID) Q43.8
Micturition
  disorder NEC (*see also* Difficulty, micturition) R39.198
    psychogenic F45.8
  frequency R35.0
    psychogenic F45.8
  hesitancy R39.11
  incomplete emptying R39.14
  nocturnal R35.1
  painful R30.9
    dysuria R30.0
    psychogenic F45.8
    tenesmus R30.1
  poor stream R39.12
  position dependent R39.192
  split stream R39.13
  straining R39.16
  urgency R39.15
Mid plane — *see* condition
Middle
  ear — *see* condition
  lobe (right) syndrome J98.19
Miescher's elastoma L87.2
Mietens' syndrome Q87.2
Migraine (idiopathic) G43.909
  with refractory migraine G43.919
    with status migrainosus G43.911
    without status migrainosus G43.919
  with aura (acute-onset) (prolonged) (typical) (without
    headache) G43.109
    with refractory migraine G43.119
      with status migrainosus G43.111
      without status migrainosus G43.119
    intractable G43.119
      with status migrainosus G43.111
      without status migrainosus G43.119
    not intractable G43.109
      with status migrainosus G43.101
      without status migrainosus G43.109
    persistent G43.509
      with cerebral infarction G43.609
        with refractory migraine G43.619
          with status migrainosus G43.611
          without status migrainosus G43.619
        intractable G43.619
          with status migrainosus G43.611

Migraine — *continued*
  with aura — *continued*
    persistent — *continued*
      with cerebral infarction — *continued*
        intractable — *continued*
          without status migrainosus G43.619
        not intractable G43.609
          with status migrainosus G43.601
          without status migrainosus G43.609
        without refractory migraine G43.609
          with status migrainosus G43.601
          without status migrainosus G43.609
      without cerebral infarction G43.509
        with refractory migraine G43.519
          with status migrainosus G43.511
          without status migrainosus G43.519
        intractable G43.519
          with status migrainosus G43.511
          without status migrainosus G43.519
        not intractable G43.509
          with status migrainosus G43.501
          without status migrainosus G43.509
        without refractory migraine G43.509
          with status migrainosus G43.501
          without status migrainosus G43.509
    without mention of refractory migraine G43.109
      with status migrainosus G43.101
      without status migrainosus G43.109
  abdominal G43.D0 (*following* G43.7)
    with refractory migraine G43.D1 (*following* G43.7)
    intractable G43.D1 (*following* G43.7)
    not intractable G43.D0 (*following* G43.7)
    without refractory migraine G43.D0 (*following* G43.7)
  basilar — *see* Migraine, with aura
  classical — *see* Migraine, with aura
  common — *see* Migraine, without aura
  complicated G43.109
  equivalents — *see* Migraine, with aura
  familiar — *see* Migraine, hemiplegic
  hemiplegic G43.409
    with refractory migraine G43.419
      with status migrainosus G43.411
      without status migrainosus G43.419
    intractable G43.419
      with status migrainosus G43.411
      without status migrainosus G43.419
    not intractable G43.409
      with status migrainosus G43.401
      without status migrainosus G43.409
    without refractory migraine G43.409
      with status migrainosus G43.401
      without status migrainosus G43.409
  intractable G43.919
    with status migrainosus G43.911
    without status migrainosus G43.919
  menstrual G43.829
    with refractory migraine G43.839
      with status migrainosus G43.831
      without status migrainosus G43.839
    intractable G43.839
      with status migrainosus G43.831
      without status migrainosus G43.839
    not intractable 4G43.829
      with status migrainosus G43.821
      without status migrainosus G43.829
    without refractory migraine G43.829
      with status migrainosus G43.821
      without status migrainosus G43.829
  menstrually related — *see* Migraine, menstrual
  not intractable G43.909
    with status migrainosus G43.901
    without status migrainosus G43.919
  ophthalmoplegic G43.B0 (*following* G43.7)
    with refractory migraine G43.B1 (*following* G43.7)
    intractable G43.B1 (*following* G43.7)
    not intractable G43.B0 (*following* G43.7)
    without refractory migraine G43.B0 (*following* G43.7)
  persistent aura (with, without) cerebral infarction —
    see Migraine, with aura, persistent
  preceded or accompanied by transient focal neurolog-
    ical phenomena — *see* Migraine, with aura
  pre-menstrual — *see* Migraine, menstrual
  pure menstrual — *see* Migraine, menstrual
  retinal — *see* Migraine, with aura
  specified NEC G43.809
    intractable G43.819
      with status migrainosus G43.811
      without status migrainosus G43.819

Subterms under main terms may continue to next column or page   ☑ Additional Character Required — Refer to the Tabular List for Character Selection   223

Metabolic syndrome — Migraine

Migraine — continued
  specified — continued
    not intractable G43.809
      with status migrainosus G43.801
      without status migrainosus G43.809
  sporadic — see Migraine, hemiplegic
  transformed — see Migraine, without aura, chronic
  triggered seizures — see Migraine, with aura
  without aura G43.009
    with refractory migraine G43.019
      with status migrainosus G43.011
      without status migrainosus G43.019
    chronic G43.709
      with refractory migraine G43.719
        with status migrainosus G43.711
        without status migrainosus G43.719
      intractable
        with status migrainosus G43.711
        without status migrainosus G43.719
      not intractable
        with status migrainosus G43.701
        without status migrainosus G43.709
      without refractory migraine G43.709
        with status migrainosus G43.701
        without status migrainosus G43.709
    intractable
      with status migrainosus G43.011
      without status migrainosus G43.019
    not intractable
      with status migrainosus G43.001
      without status migrainosus G43.009
    without mention of refractory migraine G43.009
      with status migrainosus G43.001
      without status migrainosus G43.009
    without refractory migraine G43.909
      with status migrainosus G43.901
      without status migrainosus G43.919
Migrant, social Z59.0
Migration, anxiety concerning Z60.3
Migratory, migrating (see also condition)
  person Z59.0
  testis Q55.29
Mikity-Wilson disease or syndrome P27.0
Mikulicz' disease or syndrome K11.8
Miliaria L74.3
  alba L74.1
  apocrine L75.2
  crystallina L74.1
  profunda L74.2
  rubra L74.0
  tropicalis L74.2
Miliary — see condition
Milium L72.0
  colloid L57.8
Milk
  crust L21.0
  excessive secretion O92.6
  poisoning — see Poisoning, food, noxious
  retention O92.79
  sickness — see Poisoning, food, noxious
  spots I31.0
Milk-alkali disease or syndrome E83.52
Milk-leg (deep vessels) (nonpuerperal) — see Embolism, vein, lower extremity
  complicating pregnancy O22.3- ☑
  puerperal, postpartum, childbirth O87.1
Milkman's disease or syndrome M83.8
Milky urine — see Chyluria
Millard-Gubler (-Foville) **paralysis or syndrome** G46.3
Millar's asthma J38.5
Miller Fisher syndrome G61.0
Mills' disease — see Hemiplegia
Millstone maker's pneumoconiosis J62.8
Milroy's disease (chronic hereditary edema) Q82.0
Minamata disease T56.1 ☑
Miners' asthma or lung J60
Minkowski-Chauffard syndrome — see Spherocytosis
Minor — see condition
Minor's disease (hematomyelia) G95.19
Minot's disease (hemorrhagic disease), newborn P53
Minot-von Willebrand-Jurgens disease or syndrome (angiohemophilia) D68.0
Minus (and plus) **hand** (intrinsic) — see Deformity, limb, specified type NEC, forearm
Miosis (pupil) H57.03
Mirizzi's syndrome (hepatic duct stenosis) K83.1
Mirror writing F81.0

Misadventure (of) (prophylactic) (therapeutic) (see also Complications) T88.9 ☑
  administration of insulin (by accident) — see subcategory T38.3
  infusion — see Complications, infusion
  local applications (of fomentations, plasters, etc.) T88.9 ☑
    burn or scald — see Burn
    specified NEC T88.8 ☑
  medical care (early) (late) T88.9 ☑
    adverse effect of drugs or chemicals — see Table of Drugs and Chemicals
    burn or scald — see Burn
    specified NEC T88.8 ☑
  specified NEC T88.8 ☑
  surgical procedure (early) (late) — see Complications, surgical procedure
  transfusion — see Complications, transfusion
  vaccination or other immunological procedure — see Complications, vaccination
Miscarriage O03.9
Misdirection, aqueous H40.83- ☑
Misperception, sleep state F51.02
Misplaced, misplacement
  ear Q17.4
  kidney (acquired) N28.89
    congenital Q63.2
  organ or site, congenital NEC — see Malposition, congenital
Missed
  abortion O02.1
  delivery O36.4 ☑
Missing (see also Absence)
  string of intrauterine contraceptive device T83.32- ☑
Misuse of drugs F19.99
Mitchell's disease (erythromelalgia) I73.81
Mite(s) (infestation) B88.9
  diarrhea B88.0
  grain (itch) B88.0
  hair follicle (itch) B88.0
  in sputum B88.0
Mitral — see condition
Mittelschmerz N94.0
Mixed — see condition
MMN (multifocal motor neuropathy) G61.82
MNGIE (Mitochondrial Neurogastrointestinal Encephalopathy) **syndrome** E88.49
Mobile, mobility
  cecum Q43.3
  excessive — see Hypermobility
  gallbladder, congenital Q44.1
  kidney N28.89
  organ or site, congenital NEC — see Malposition, congenital
Mobitz heart block (atrioventricular) I44.1
Moebius, Möbius
  disease (ophthalmoplegic migraine) — see Migraine, ophthalmoplegic
  syndrome Q87.0
    congenital oculofacial paralysis (with other anomalies) Q87.0
    ophthalmoplegic migraine — see Migraine, ophthalmoplegic
Moeller's glossitis K14.0
Mohr's syndrome (Types I and II) Q87.0
Mola destruens D39.2
Molar pregnancy O02.0
Molarization of premolars K00.2
Molding, head (during birth) — omit code
Mole (pigmented) (see also Nevus)
  blood O02.0
  Breus' O02.0
  cancerous — see Melanoma
  carneous O02.0
  destructive D39.2
  fleshy O02.0
  hydatid, hydatidiform (benign) (complicating pregnancy) (delivered) (undelivered) O01.9
    classical O01.0
    complete O01.0
    incomplete O01.1
    invasive D39.2
    malignant D39.2
    partial O01.1
  intrauterine O02.0
  invasive (hydatidiform) D39.2

Mole — continued
  malignant
    meaning
      malignant hydatidiform mole D39.2
      melanoma — see Melanoma
  nonhydatidiform O02.0
  nonpigmented — see Nevus
  pregnancy NEC O02.0
  skin — see Nevus
  tubal O00.10- ☑
    with intrauterine pregnancy O00.11- ☑
  vesicular — see Mole, hydatidiform
Molimen, molimina (menstrual) N94.3
Molluscum contagiosum (epitheliale) B08.1
Mönckeberg's arteriosclerosis, disease, or sclerosis — see Arteriosclerosis, extremities
Mondini's malformation (cochlea) Q16.5
Mondor's disease I80.8
Monge's disease T70.29 ☑
Monilethrix (congenital) Q84.1
Moniliasis (see also Candidiasis) B37.9
  neonatal P37.5
Monitoring (encounter for)
  therapeutic drug level Z51.81
Monkey malaria B53.1
Monkeypox B04
Monoarthritis M13.10
  ankle M13.17- ☑
  elbow M13.12- ☑
  foot joint M13.17- ☑
  hand joint M13.14- ☑
  hip M13.15- ☑
  knee M13.16- ☑
  shoulder M13.11- ☑
  wrist M13.13- ☑
Monoblastic — see condition
Monochromat (ism), monochromatopsia (acquired) (congenital) H53.51
Monocytic — see condition
Monocytopenia D72.818
Monocytosis (symptomatic) D72.821
Monomania — see Psychosis
Mononeuritis G58.9
  cranial nerve — see Disorder, nerve, cranial
  femoral nerve G57.2- ☑
  lateral
    cutaneous nerve of thigh G57.1- ☑
    popliteal nerve G57.3- ☑
  lower limb G57.9- ☑
    specified nerve NEC G57.8- ☑
  medial popliteal nerve G57.4- ☑
  median nerve G56.1- ☑
  multiplex G58.7
  plantar nerve G57.6- ☑
  posterior tibial nerve G57.5- ☑
  radial nerve G56.3- ☑
  sciatic nerve G57.0- ☑
  specified NEC G58.8
  tibial nerve G57.4- ☑
  ulnar nerve G56.2- ☑
  upper limb G56.9- ☑
    specified nerve NEC G56.8- ☑
  vestibular — see subcategory H93.3 ☑
Mononeuropathy G58.9
  carpal tunnel syndrome — see Syndrome, carpal tunnel
  diabetic NEC — see E08-E13 with .41
  femoral nerve — see Lesion, nerve, femoral
  ilioinguinal nerve G57.8- ☑
  in diseases classified elsewhere — see category G59
  intercostal G58.0
  lower limb G57.9- ☑
    causalgia — see Causalgia, lower limb
    femoral nerve — see Lesion, nerve, femoral
    meralgia paresthetica G57.1- ☑
    plantar nerve — see Lesion, nerve, plantar
    popliteal nerve — see Lesion, nerve, popliteal
    sciatic nerve — see Lesion, nerve, sciatic
    specified NEC G57.8- ☑
    tarsal tunnel syndrome — see Syndrome, tarsal tunnel
  median nerve — see Lesion, nerve, median
  multiplex G58.7
  obturator nerve G57.8- ☑
  popliteal nerve — see Lesion, nerve, popliteal
  radial nerve — see Lesion, nerve, radial
  saphenous nerve G57.8- ☑

224

☑ Additional Character Required — Refer to the Tabular List for Character Selection   ⬇ Subterms under main terms may continue to next column or page

Mononeuropathy — *continued*
  specified NEC G58.8
  tarsal tunnel syndrome — *see* Syndrome, tarsal tunnel
  tuberculous A17.83
  ulnar nerve — *see* Lesion, nerve, ulnar
  upper limb G56.9- ☑
    carpal tunnel syndrome — *see* Syndrome, carpal tunnel
    causalgia — *see* Causalgia
    median nerve — *see* Lesion, nerve, median
    radial nerve — *see* Lesion, nerve, radial
    specified site NEC G56.8- ☑
    ulnar nerve — *see* Lesion, nerve, ulnar
Mononucleosis, infectious B27.90
  with
    complication NEC B27.99
    meningitis B27.92
    polyneuropathy B27.91
  cytomegaloviral B27.10
    with
      complication NEC B27.19
      meningitis B27.12
      polyneuropathy B27.11
  Epstein-Barr (virus) B27.00
    with
      complication NEC B27.09
      meningitis B27.02
      polyneuropathy B27.01
  gammaherpesviral B27.00
    with
      complication NEC B27.09
      meningitis B27.02
      polyneuropathy B27.01
  specified NEC B27.80
    with
      complication NEC B27.89
      meningitis B27.82
      polyneuropathy B27.81
Monoplegia G83.3- ☑
  congenital (cerebral) G80.8
    spastic G80.1
  embolic (current episode) I63.4- ☑
  following
    cerebrovascular disease
      cerebral infarction
        lower limb I69.34- ☑
        upper limb I69.33- ☑
      intracerebral hemorrhage
        lower limb I69.14- ☑
        upper limb I69.13- ☑
      lower limb I69.94- ☑
      nontraumatic intracranial hemorrhage NEC
        lower limb I69.24- ☑
        upper limb I69.23- ☑
      specified disease NEC
        lower limb I69.84- ☑
        upper limb I69.83- ☑
      stroke NOS
        lower limb I69.34- ☑
        upper limb I69.33- ☑
      subarachnoid hemorrhage
        lower limb I69.04- ☑
        upper limb I69.03- ☑
      upper limb I69.93- ☑
  hysterical (transient) F44.4
  lower limb G83.1- ☑
  psychogenic (conversion reaction) F44.4
  thrombotic (current episode) I63.3- ☑
  transient R29.818
  upper limb G83.2- ☑
Monorchism, monorchidism Q55.0
Monosomy (*see also* Deletion, chromosome) Q93.9
  specified NEC Q93.89
  whole chromosome
    meiotic nondisjunction Q93.0
    mitotic nondisjunction Q93.1
    mosaicism Q93.1
  X Q96.9
Monster, monstrosity (single) Q89.7
  acephalic Q00.0
  twin Q89.4
Monteggia's fracture (-dislocation) S52.27- ☑
Mooren's ulcer (cornea) — *see* Ulcer, cornea, Mooren's
Moore's syndrome — *see* Epilepsy, specified NEC
Mooser-Neill reaction A75.2
Mooser's bodies A75.2
Morbidity not stated or unknown R69

Morbilli — *see* Measles
Morbus (*see also* Disease)
  angelicus, anglorum E55.0
  Beigel B36.2
  caducus — *see* Epilepsy
  celiacus K90.0
  comitialis — *see* Epilepsy
  cordis (*see also* Disease, heart) I51.9
    valvulorum — *see* Endocarditis
  coxae senilis M16.9
    tuberculous A18.02
  hemorrhagicus neonatorum P53
  maculosus neonatorum P54.5
Morel (-Stewart)(-Morgagni) **syndrome** M85.2
Morel-Kraepelin disease — *see* Schizophrenia
Morel-Moore syndrome M85.2
Morgagni's
  cyst, organ, hydatid, or appendage
    female Q50.5
    male (epididymal) Q55.4
      testicular Q55.29
  syndrome M85.2
Morgagni-Stewart-Morel syndrome M85.2
Morgagni-Stokes-Adams syndrome I45.9
Morgagni-Turner (-Albright) **syndrome** Q96.9
Moria F07.0
Moron (I.Q. 50-69) F70
Morphea L94.0
Morphinism (without remission) F11.20
  with remission F11.21
Morphinomania (without remission) F11.20
  with remission F11.21
Morquio (-Ullrich)(-Brailsford) **disease or syndrome** — *see* Mucopolysaccharidosis
Mortification (dry) (moist) — *see* Gangrene
Morton's metatarsalgia (neuralgia)(neuroma) (syndrome) G57.6- ☑
Morvan's disease or syndrome G60.8
Mosaicism, mosaic (autosomal) (chromosomal)
  45,X/46,XX Q96.3
  45,X/other cell lines NEC with abnormal sex chromosome Q96.4
  sex chromosome
    female Q97.8
    lines with various numbers of X chromosomes Q97.2
    male Q98.7
  XY Q96.3
Moschowitz' disease M31.1
Mother yaw A66.0
Motion sickness (from travel, any vehicle) (from round-abouts or swings) T75.3 ☑
Mottled, mottling, teeth (enamel) (endemic) (nonendemic) K00.3
Mounier-Kuhn syndrome Q32.4
  with bronchiectasis J47.9
    exacerbation (acute) J47.1
    lower respiratory infection J47.0
  acquired J98.09
    with bronchiectasis J47.9
      with
        exacerbation (acute) J47.1
        lower respiratory infection J47.0
Mountain
  sickness T70.29 ☑
    with polycythemia , acquired (acute) D75.1
  tick fever A93.2
Mouse, joint — *see* Loose, body, joint
  knee M23.4- ☑
Mouth — *see* condition
Movable
  coccyx — *see* subcategory M53.2 ☑
  kidney N28.89
    congenital Q63.8
  spleen D73.89
Movements, dystonic R25.8
Moyamoya disease I67.5
MRSA (Methicillin resistant Staphylococcus aureus)
  infection A49.02
    as the cause of diseases classified elsewhere B95.62
  sepsis A41.02
MSD (multiple sulfatase deficiency) E75.26
MSSA (Methicillin susceptible Staphylococcus aureus)
  infection A49.01
    as the cause of diseases classified elsewhere B95.61
  sepsis A41.01
Mucha-Habermann disease L41.0
Mucinosis (cutaneous) (focal) (papular) (skin) L98.5

Mucinosis — *continued*
  oral K13.79
Mucocele
  appendix K38.8
  buccal cavity K13.79
  gallbladder K82.1
  lacrimal sac, chronic H04.43- ☑
  nasal sinus J34.1
  nose J34.1
  salivary gland (any) K11.6
  sinus (accessory) (nasal) J34.1
  turbinate (bone) (middle) (nasal) J34.1
  uterus N85.8
Mucolipidosis
  I E77.1
  II, III E77.0
  IV E75.11
Mucopolysaccharidosis E76.3
  beta-gluduronidase deficiency E76.29
  cardiopathy E76.3 [I52]
  Hunter's syndrome E76.1
  Hurler's syndrome E76.01
  Hurler-Scheie syndrome E76.02
  Maroteaux-Lamy syndrome E76.29
  Morquio syndrome E76.219
    A E76.210
    B E76.211
    classic E76.210
  Sanfilippo syndrome E76.22
  Scheie's syndrome E76.03
  specified NEC E76.29
  type
    I
      Hurler's syndrome E76.01
      Hurler-Scheie syndrome E76.02
      Scheie's syndrome E76.03
    II E76.1
    III E76.22
    IV E76.219
    IVA E76.210
    IVB E76.211
    VI E76.29
    VII E76.29
Mucormycosis B46.5
  cutaneous B46.3
  disseminated B46.4
  gastrointestinal B46.2
  generalized B46.4
  pulmonary B46.0
  rhinocerebral B46.1
  skin B46.3
  subcutaneous B46.3
Mucositis (ulcerative) K12.30
  due to drugs NEC K12.32
  gastrointestinal K92.81
  mouth (oral) (oropharyngeal) K12.30
    due to antineoplastic therapy K12.31
    due to drugs NEC K12.32
    due to radiation K12.33
    specified NEC K12.39
    viral K12.39
  nasal J34.81
  oral cavity — *see* Mucositis, mouth
  oral soft tissues — *see* Mucositis, mouth
  vagina and vulva N76.81
Mucositis necroticans agranulocytica — *see* Agranulocytosis
Mucous (*see also* condition)
  patches (syphilitic) A51.39
    congenital A50.07
Mucoviscidosis E84.9
  with meconium obstruction E84.11
Mucus
  asphyxia or suffocation — *see* Asphyxia, mucus
  in stool R19.5
  plug — *see* Asphyxia, mucus
Muguet B37.0
Mulberry molars (congenital syphilis) A50.52
Müllerian mixed tumor
  specified site — *see* Neoplasm, malignant, by site
  unspecified site C54.9
Multicystic kidney (development) Q61.4
Multiparity (grand) Z64.1
  affecting management of pregnancy, labor and delivery (supervision only) O09.4- ☑
  requiring contraceptive management — *see* Contraception
Multipartita placenta O43.19- ☑

Multiple, multiplex (*see also* condition)
digits (congenital) Q69.9
endocrine neoplasia — *see* Neoplasia, endocrine, multiple (MEN)
personality F44.81
Mumps B26.9
arthritis B26.85
complication NEC B26.89
encephalitis B26.2
hepatitis B26.81
meningitis (aseptic) B26.1
meningoencephalitis B26.2
myocarditis B26.82
oophoritis B26.89
orchitis B26.0
pancreatitis B26.3
polyneuropathy B26.84
Mumu (*see also* Infestation, filarial) B74.9 [N51]
Münchhausen's syndrome — *see* Disorder, factitious
Münchmeyer's syndrome — *see* Myositis, ossificans, progressiva
Mural — *see* condition
Murmur (cardiac) (heart) (organic) R01.1
abdominal R19.15
aortic (valve) — *see* Endocarditis, aortic
benign R01.0
diastolic — *see* Endocarditis
Flint I35.1
functional R01.0
Graham Steell I37.1
innocent R01.0
mitral (valve) — *see* Insufficiency, mitral
nonorganic R01.0
presystolic, mitral — *see* Insufficiency, mitral
pulmonic (valve) I37.8
systolic R01.1
tricuspid (valve) I07.9
valvular — *see* Endocarditis
Murri's disease (intermittent hemoglobinuria) D59.6
Muscle, muscular (*see also* condition)
carnitine (palmityltransferase) deficiency E71.314
Musculoneuralgia — *see* Neuralgia
Mushrooming hip — *see* Derangement, joint, specified NEC, hip
Mushroom-workers' (pickers') **disease or lung** J67.5
Mutation(s)
factor V Leiden D68.51
prothrombin gene D68.52
surfactant, of lung J84.83
Mutism (*see also* Aphasia)
deaf (acquired) (congenital) NEC H91.3
elective (adjustment reaction) (childhood) F94.0
hysterical F44.4
selective (childhood) F94.0
MVD (microvillus inclusion disease) Q43.8
MVID (microvillus inclusion disease) Q43.8
Myalgia M79.10
auxiliary muscles, head and neck M79.12
epidemic (cervical) B33.0
mastication muscle M79.11
site specified NEC M79.18
traumatic NEC T14.8 ☑
Myasthenia G70.9
congenital G70.2
cordis — *see* Failure, heart
developmental G70.2
gravis G70.00
with exacerbation (acute) G70.01
in crisis G70.01
neonatal, transient P94.0
pseudoparalytica G70.00
with exacerbation (acute) G70.01
in crisis G70.01
stomach, psychogenic F45.8
syndrome
in
diabetes mellitus — *see* E08-E13 with .44
neoplastic disease (*see also* Neoplasm) D49.9 [G73.3]
pernicious anemia D51.0 [G73.3]
thyrotoxicosis E05.90 [G73.3]
with thyroid storm E05.91 [G73.3]
Myasthenic M62.81
Mycelium infection B49
Mycetismus — *see* Poisoning, food, noxious, mushroom
Mycetoma B47.9
actinomycotic B47.1
bone (mycotic) B47.9 [M90.80]

Mycetoma — *continued*
eumycotic B47.0
foot B47.9
actinomycotic B47.1
mycotic B47.0
madurae NEC B47.9
mycotic B47.0
maduromycotic B47.0
mycotic B47.0
nocardial B47.1
Mycobacteriosis — *see* Mycobacterium
Mycobacterium, mycobacterial (infection) A31.9
anonymous A31.9
atypical A31.9
cutaneous A31.1
pulmonary A31.0
tuberculous — *see* Tuberculosis, pulmonary
specified site NEC A31.8
avium (intracellulare complex) A31.0
balnei A31.1
Battey A31.0
chelonei A31.8
cutaneous A31.1
extrapulmonary systemic A31.8
fortuitum A31.8
intracellulare (Battey bacillus) A31.0
kakaferifu A31.8
kansasii (yellow bacillus) A31.0
kasongo A31.8
leprae (*see also* Leprosy) A30.9
luciflavum A31.1
marinum (M. balnei) A31.1
nonspecific — *see* Mycobacterium, atypical
pulmonary (atypical) A31.0
tuberculous — *see* Tuberculosis, pulmonary
scrofulaceum A31.8
simiae A31.8
systemic, extrapulmonary A31.8
szulgai A31.8
terrae A31.8
triviale A31.8
tuberculosis (human, bovine) — *see* Tuberculosis
ulcerans A31.1
xenopi A31.8
Mycoplasma (M.) **pneumoniae, as cause of disease classified elsewhere** B96.0
Mycosis, mycotic B49
cutaneous NEC B36.9
ear B36.9
in
aspergillosis B44.89
candidiasis B37.84
moniliasis B37.84
fungoides (extranodal) (solid organ) C84.0- ☑
mouth B37.0
nails B35.1
opportunistic B48.8
skin NEC B36.9
specified NEC B48.8
stomatitis B37.0
vagina, vaginitis (candidal) B37.3
Mydriasis (pupil) H57.04
Myelatelia Q06.1
Myelinolysis, pontine, central G37.2
Myelitis (acute) (ascending) (childhood) (chronic) (descending) (diffuse) (disseminated) (idiopathic) (pressure) (progressive) (spinal cord) (subacute) (*see also* Encephalitis) G04.91
herpes simplex B00.82
herpes zoster B02.24
in diseases classified elsewhere G05.4
necrotizing, subacute G37.4
optic neuritis in G36.0
postchickenpox B01.12
postherpetic B02.24
postimmunization G04.02
postinfectious NEC G04.89
postvaccinal G04.02
specified NEC G04.89
syphilitic (transverse) A52.14
toxic G92
transverse (in demyelinating diseases of central nervous system) G37.3
tuberculous A17.82
varicella B01.12
Myeloblastic — *see* condition
Myeloblastoma
granular cell (*see also* Neoplasm, connective tissue)

Myeloblastoma — *continued*
granular cell (*see also* Neoplasm, connective tissue) — *continued*
malignant — *see* Neoplasm, connective tissue, malignant
tongue D10.1
Myelocele — *see* Spina bifida
Myelocystocele — *see* Spina bifida
Myelocytic — *see* condition
Myelodysplasia D46.9
specified NEC D46.Z (*following* D46.4)
spinal cord (congenital) Q06.1
Myelodysplastic syndrome D46.9
with
5q deletion D46.C (*following* D46.2)
isolated del (5q) chromosomal abnormality D46.C (*following* D46.2)
specified NEC D46.Z (*following* D46.4)
Myeloencephalitis — *see* Encephalitis
Myelofibrosis D75.81
with myeloid metaplasia D47.4
acute C94.4- ☑
idiopathic (chronic) D47.4
primary D47.1
secondary D75.81
in myeloproliferative disease D47.4
Myelogenous — *see* condition
Myeloid — *see* condition
Myelokathexis D70.9
Myeloleukodystrophy E75.29
Myelolipoma — *see* Lipoma
Myeloma (multiple) C90.0- ☑
monostotic C90.3 ☑
plasma cell C90.0- ☑
plasma cell C90.0- ☑
solitary (*see also* Plasmacytoma, solitary) C90.3- ☑
Myelomalacia G95.89
Myelomatosis C90.0- ☑
Myelomeningitis — *see* Meningoencephalitis
Myelomeningocele (spinal cord) — *see* Spina bifida
Myelo-osteo-musculodysplasia hereditaria Q79.8
Myelopathic
anemia D64.89
muscle atrophy — *see* Atrophy, muscle, spinal
pain syndrome G89.0
Myelopathy (spinal cord) G95.9
drug-induced G95.89
in (due to)
degeneration or displacement, intervertebral disc NEC — *see* Disorder, disc, with, myelopathy
infection — *see* Encephalitis
intervertebral disc disorder (*see also* Disorder, disc, with, myelopathy)
mercury — *see* subcategory T56.1 ☑
neoplastic disease (*see also* Neoplasm) D49.9 [G99.2]
pernicious anemia D51.0 [G99.2]
spondylosis — *see* Spondylosis, with myelopathy NEC
necrotic (subacute) (vascular) G95.19
radiation-induced G95.89
spondylogenic NEC — *see* Spondylosis, with myelopathy NEC
toxic G95.89
transverse, acute G37.3
vascular G95.19
vitamin B12 E53.8 [G32.0]
Myelophthisis D61.82
Myeloradiculitis G04.91
Myeloradiculodysplasia (spinal) Q06.1
Myelosarcoma C92.3- ☑
Myelosclerosis D75.89
with myeloid metaplasia D47.4
disseminated, of nervous system G35
megakaryocytic D47.4
with myeloid metaplasia D47.4
Myelosis
acute C92.0- ☑
aleukemic C92.9- ☑
chronic D47.1
erythremic (acute) C94.0- ☑
megakaryocytic C94.2- ☑
nonleukemic D72.828
subacute C92.9- ☑
Myiasis (cavernous) B87.9
aural B87.4
creeping B87.0
cutaneous B87.0

Myiasis — *continued*
 dermal B87.0
 ear (external) (middle) B87.4
 eye B87.2
 genitourinary B87.81
 intestinal B87.82
 laryngeal B87.3
 nasopharyngeal B87.3
 ocular B87.2
 orbit B87.2
 skin B87.0
 specified site NEC B87.89
 traumatic B87.1
 wound B87.1
Myoadenoma, prostate — *see* Hyperplasia, prostate
Myoblastoma
 granular cell (*see also* Neoplasm, connective tissue, benign)
  malignant — *see* Neoplasm, connective tissue, malignant
 tongue D10.1
Myocardial — *see* condition
Myocardiopathy (congestive) (constrictive) (familial) (hypertrophic nonobstructive) (idiopathic) (infiltrative) (obstructive) (primary) (restrictive) (sporadic) (*see also* Cardiomyopathy) I42.9
 alcoholic I42.6
 cobalt-beer I42.6
 glycogen storage E74.02 [I43]
 hypertrophic obstructive I42.1
 in (due to)
  beriberi E51.12
  cardiac glycogenosis E74.02 [I43]
  Friedreich's ataxia G11.1 [I43]
  myotonia atrophica G71.11 [I43]
  progressive muscular dystrophy G71.09 [I43]
 obscure (African) I42.8
 secondary I42.9
 thyrotoxic E05.90 [I43]
  with storm E05.91 [I43]
 toxic NEC I42.7
Myocarditis (with arteriosclerosis)(chronic)(fibroid) (interstitial) (old) (progressive) (senile) I51.4
 with
  rheumatic fever (conditions in I00) I09.0
   active — *see* Myocarditis, acute, rheumatic
   inactive or quiescent (with chorea) I09.0
 active I40.9
  rheumatic I01.2
   with chorea (acute) (rheumatic) (Sydenham's) I02.0
 acute or subacute (interstitial) I40.9
  due to
   streptococcus (beta-hemolytic) I01.2
  idiopathic I40.1
  rheumatic I01.2
   with chorea (acute) (rheumatic) (Sydenham's) I02.0
  specified NEC I40.8
 aseptic of newborn B33.22
 bacterial (acute) I40.0
 Coxsackie (virus) B33.22
 diphtheritic A36.81
 eosinophilic I40.1
 epidemic of newborn (Coxsackie) B33.22
 Fiedler's (acute) (isolated) I40.1
 giant cell (acute) (subacute) I40.1
 gonococcal A54.83
 granulomatous (idiopathic) (isolated) (nonspecific) I40.1
 hypertensive — *see* Hypertension, heart
 idiopathic (granulomatous) I40.1
 in (due to)
  diphtheria A36.81
  epidemic louse-borne typhus A75.0 [I41]
  Lyme disease A69.29
  sarcoidosis D86.85
  scarlet fever A38.1
  toxoplasmosis (acquired) B58.81
  typhoid A01.02
  typhus NEC A75.9 [I41]
 infective I40.0
 influenzal — *see* Influenza, with, myocarditis
 isolated (acute) I40.1
 meningococcal A39.52
 mumps B26.82
 nonrheumatic, active I40.9
 parenchymatous I40.9
 pneumococcal I40.0

Myocarditis — *continued*
 rheumatic (chronic) (inactive) (with chorea) I09.0
  active or acute I01.2
   with chorea (acute) (rheumatic) (Sydenham's) I02.0
 rheumatoid — *see* Rheumatoid, carditis
 septic I40.0
 staphylococcal I40.0
 suppurative I40.0
 syphilitic (chronic) A52.06
 toxic I40.8
  rheumatic — *see* Myocarditis, acute, rheumatic
 tuberculous A18.84
 typhoid A01.02
 valvular — *see* Endocarditis
 virus, viral I40.0
  of newborn (Coxsackie) B33.22
Myocardium, myocardial — *see* condition
Myocardosis — *see* Cardiomyopathy
Myoclonus, myoclonic, myoclonia (familial) (essential) (multifocal) (simplex) G25.3
 drug-induced G25.3
 epilepsy (*see also* Epilepsy, generalized, specified NEC) G40.4- ☑
  familial (progressive) G25.3
 epileptica G40.409
  with status epilepticus G40.401
 facial G51.3- ☑
 familial progressive G25.3
 Friedreich's G25.3
 jerks G25.3
 massive G25.3
 palatal G25.3
 pharyngeal G25.3
Myocytolysis I51.5
Myodiastasis — *see* Diastasis, muscle
Myoendocarditis — *see* Endocarditis
Myoepithelioma — *see* Neoplasm, benign, by site
Myofasciitis (acute) — *see* Myositis
Myofibroma (*see also* Neoplasm, connective tissue, benign)
 uterus (cervix) (corpus) — *see* Leiomyoma
Myofibromatosis D48.1
 infantile Q89.8
Myofibrosis M62.89
 heart — *see* Myocarditis
 scapulohumeral — *see* Lesion, shoulder, specified NEC
Myofibrositis M79.7
 scapulohumeral — *see* Lesion, shoulder, specified NEC
Myoglobulinuria, myoglobinuria (primary) R82.1
Myokymia, facial G51.4
Myolipoma — *see* Lipoma
Myoma (*see also* Neoplasm, connective tissue, benign)
 malignant — *see* Neoplasm, connective tissue, malignant
 prostate D29.1
 uterus (cervix) (corpus) — *see* Leiomyoma
Myomalacia M62.89
Myometritis — *see* Endometritis
Myometrium — *see* condition
Myonecrosis, clostridial A48.0
Myopathy G72.9
 acute
  necrotizing G72.81
  quadriplegic G72.81
 alcoholic G72.1
 benign congenital G71.2
 central core G71.2
 centronuclear G71.2
 congenital (benign) G71.2
 critical illness G72.81
 distal G71.09
 drug-induced G72.0
 endocrine NEC E34.9 [G73.7]
 extraocular muscles H05.82- ☑
 facioscapulohumeral G71.02
 hereditary G71.9
  specified NEC G71.8
 immune NEC G72.49
 in (due to)
  Addison's disease E27.1 [G73.7]
  alcohol G72.1
  amyloidosis E85.0 [G73.7]
  cretinism E00.9 [G73.7]
  Cushing's syndrome E24.9 [G73.7]
  drugs G72.0
  endocrine disease NEC E34.9 [G73.7]
  giant cell arteritis M31.6 [G73.7]

Myopathy — *continued*
 in — *continued*
  glycogen storage disease E74.00 [G73.7]
  hyperadrenocorticism E24.9 [G73.7]
  hyperparathyroidism NEC E21.3 [G73.7]
  hypoparathyroidism E20.9 [G73.7]
  hypopituitarism E23.0 [G73.7]
  hypothyroidism E03.9 [G73.7]
  infectious disease NEC B99 ☑ [G73.7]
  lipid storage disease E75.6 [G73.7]
  metabolic disease NEC E88.9 [G73.7]
  myxedema E03.9 [G73.7]
  parasitic disease NEC B89 [G73.7]
  polyarteritis nodosa M30.0 [G73.7]
  rheumatoid arthritis — *see* Rheumatoid, myopathy
  sarcoidosis D86.87
  scleroderma M34.82
  sicca syndrome M35.03
  Sjögren's syndrome M35.03
  systemic lupus erythematosus M32.19
  thyrotoxicosis (hyperthyroidism) E05.90 [G73.7]
   with thyroid storm E05.91 [G73.7]
  toxic agent NEC G72.2
 inflammatory NEC G72.49
 intensive care (ICU) G72.81
 limb-girdle G71.09
 mitochondrial NEC G71.3
 myotubular G71.2
 myotonic, proximal (PROMM) G71.11
 nemaline G71.2
 ocular G71.09
 oculopharyngeal G71.09
 of critical illness G72.81
 primary G71.9
  specified NEC G71.8
 progressive NEC G72.89
 proximal myotonic (PROMM) G71.11
 rod G71.2
 scapulohumeral G71.02
 specified NEC G72.89
 toxic G72.2
Myopericarditis (*see also* Pericarditis)
 chronic rheumatic I09.2
Myopia (axial) (congenital) H52.1- ☑
 degenerative (malignant) H44.20
  with
   choroidal neovascularization H44.2A- ☑
   foveoschisis H44.2D- ☑
   macular hole H44.2B- ☑
   retinal detachment H44.2C- ☑
   specified maculopathy NEC H44.2E- ☑
  bilateral H44.23
  left eye H44.22
  right eye H44.21
 malignant (*see also* Myopia, degenerative) H44.2- ☑
 pernicious (*see also* Myopia, degenerative) H44.2- ☑
 progressive high (degenerative) (*see also* Myopia, degenerative) H44.2- ☑
Myosarcoma — *see* Neoplasm, connective tissue, malignant
Myosis (pupil) H57.03
 stromal (endolymphatic) D39.0
Myositis M60.9
 clostridial A48.0
 due to posture — *see* Myositis, specified type NEC
 epidemic B33.0
 fibrosa or fibrous (chronic), Volkmann's T79.6 ☑
 foreign body granuloma — *see* Granuloma, foreign body
 in (due to)
  bilharziasis B65.9 [M63.8-] ☑
  cysticercosis B69.81
  leprosy A30.9 [M63.8-] ☑
  mycosis B49 [M63.8-] ☑
  sarcoidosis D86.87
  schistosomiasis B65.9 [M63.8-] ☑
  syphilis
   late A52.78
   secondary A51.49
  toxoplasmosis (acquired) B58.82
  trichinellosis B75 [M63.8-] ☑
  tuberculosis A18.09
 inclusion body [IBM] G72.41
 infective M60.009
  arm M60.002
   left M60.001
   right M60.000
  leg M60.005

Myositis — *continued*
  infective — *continued*
    leg — *continued*
      left M60.004
      right M60.003
    lower limb M60.005
      ankle M60.07- ☑
      foot M60.07- ☑
      lower leg M60.06- ☑
      thigh M60.05- ☑
      toe M60.07- ☑
    multiple sites M60.09
    specified site NEC M60.08
    upper limb M60.002
      finger M60.04- ☑
      forearm M60.03- ☑
      hand M60.04- ☑
      shoulder region M60.01- ☑
      upper arm M60.02- ☑
  interstitial M60.10
    ankle M60.17- ☑
    foot M60.17- ☑
    forearm M60.13- ☑
    hand M60.14- ☑
    lower leg M60.16- ☑
    multiple sites M60.19
    shoulder region M60.11- ☑
    specified site NEC M60.18
    thigh M60.15- ☑
    upper arm M60.12- ☑
  mycotic B49 [M63.8-] ☑
  orbital, chronic H05.12- ☑
  ossificans or ossifying (circumscripta) (*see also* Ossification, muscle, specified NEC)
    in (due to)
      burns M61.30
        ankle M61.37- ☑
        foot M61.37- ☑
        forearm M61.33- ☑
        hand M61.34- ☑
        lower leg M61.36- ☑
        multiple sites M61.39
        pelvic region M61.35- ☑
        shoulder region M61.31- ☑
        specified site NEC M61.38
        thigh M61.35- ☑
        upper arm M61.32- ☑
      quadriplegia or paraplegia M61.20
        ankle M61.27- ☑
        foot M61.27- ☑
        forearm M61.23- ☑
        hand M61.24- ☑

Myositis — *continued*
  ossificans or ossifying (*see also* Ossification, muscle, specified) — *continued*
    in — *continued*
      quadriplegia or paraplegia — *continued*
        lower leg M61.26- ☑
        multiple sites M61.29
        pelvic region M61.25- ☑
        shoulder region M61.21- ☑
        specified site NEC M61.28
        thigh M61.25- ☑
        upper arm M61.22- ☑
    progressiva M61.10
      ankle M61.17- ☑
      finger M61.14- ☑
      foot M61.17- ☑
      forearm M61.13- ☑
      hand M61.14- ☑
      lower leg M61.16- ☑
      multiple sites M61.19
      pelvic region M61.15- ☑
      shoulder region M61.11- ☑
      specified site NEC M61.18
      thigh M61.15- ☑
      toe M61.17- ☑
      upper arm M61.12- ☑
    traumatica M61.00
      ankle M61.07- ☑
      foot M61.07- ☑
      forearm M61.03- ☑
      hand M61.04- ☑
      lower leg M61.06- ☑
      multiple sites M61.09
      pelvic region M61.05- ☑
      shoulder region M61.01- ☑
      specified site NEC M61.08
      thigh M61.05- ☑
      upper arm M61.02- ☑
  purulent — *see* Myositis, infective
  specified type NEC M60.80
    ankle M60.87- ☑
    foot M60.87- ☑
    forearm M60.83- ☑
    hand M60.84- ☑
    lower leg M60.86- ☑
    multiple sites M60.89
    pelvic region M60.85- ☑
    shoulder region M60.81- ☑
    specified site NEC M60.88
    thigh M60.85- ☑
    upper arm M60.82- ☑
  suppurative — *see* Myositis, infective

Myositis — *continued*
  traumatic (old) — *see* Myositis, specified type NEC
Myospasia impulsiva F95.2
Myotonia (acquisita) (intermittens) M62.89
  atrophica G71.11
  chondrodystrophic G71.13
  congenita (acetazolamide responsive) (dominant) (recessive) G71.12
  drug-induced G71.14
  dystrophica G71.11
  fluctuans G71.19
  levior G71.12
  permanens G71.19
  symptomatic G71.19
Myotonic pupil — *see* Anomaly, pupil, function, tonic pupil
Myriapodiasis B88.2
Myringitis H73.2- ☑
  with otitis media — *see* Otitis, media
  acute H73.00- ☑
    bullous H73.01- ☑
    specified NEC H73.09- ☑
  bullous — *see* Myringitis, acute, bullous
  chronic H73.1- ☑
Mysophobia F40.228
Mytilotoxism — *see* Poisoning, fish
Myxadenitis labialis K13.0
Myxedema (adult) (idiocy) (infantile) (juvenile) (*see also* Hypothyroidism) E03.9
  circumscribed E05.90
    with storm E05.91
  coma E03.5
  congenital E00.1
  cutis L98.5
  localized (pretibial) E05.90
    with storm E05.91
  papular L98.5
Myxochondrosarcoma — *see* Neoplasm, cartilage, malignant
Myxofibroma — *see* Neoplasm, connective tissue, benign
  odontogenic — *see* Cyst, calcifying odontogenic
Myxofibrosarcoma — *see* Neoplasm, connective tissue, malignant
Myxolipoma D17.9
Myxoliposarcoma — *see* Neoplasm, connective tissue, malignant
Myxoma (*see also* Neoplasm, connective tissue, benign)
  nerve sheath — *see* Neoplasm, nerve, benign
  odontogenic — *see* Cyst, calcifying odontogenic
Myxosarcoma — *see* Neoplasm, connective tissue, malignant

N

Naegeli's
  disease Q82.8
  leukemia, monocytic C93.1- ☑
Naegleriasis (with meningoencephalitis) B60.2
Naffziger's syndrome G54.0
Naga sore — *see* Ulcer, skin
Nägele's pelvis M95.5
  with disproportion (fetopelvic) O33.0
    causing obstructed labor O65.0
Nail (*see also* condition)
  biting F98.8
  patella syndrome Q87.2
Nanism, nanosomia — *see* Dwarfism
Nanophyetiasis B66.8
Nanukayami A27.89
Napkin rash L22
Narcolepsy G47.419
  with cataplexy G47.411
  in conditions classified elsewhere G47.429
    with cataplexy G47.421
Narcosis R06.89
Narcotism — *see* Dependence
NARP (Neuropathy, Ataxia and Retinitis pigmentosa)
  syndrome E88.49
Narrow
  anterior chamber angle H40.03- ☑
  gingival width (of periodontal soft tissue) K05.5
  pelvis — *see* Contraction, pelvis
Narrowing (*see also* Stenosis)
  artery I77.1
    auditory, internal I65.8
    basilar — *see* Occlusion, artery, basilar
    carotid — *see* Occlusion, artery, carotid
    cerebellar — *see* Occlusion, artery, cerebellar
    cerebral — *see* Occlusion artery, cerebral
    choroidal — *see* Occlusion, artery, cerebral, specified NEC
    communicating posterior — *see* Occlusion, artery, cerebral, specified NEC
    coronary (*see also* Disease, heart, ischemic, atherosclerotic)
      congenital Q24.5
        syphilitic A50.54 [I52]
      due to syphilis NEC A52.06
    hypophyseal — *see* Occlusion, artery, cerebral, specified NEC
    pontine — *see* Occlusion, artery, cerebral, specified NEC
    precerebral — *see* Occlusion, artery, precerebral
    vertebral — *see* Occlusion, artery, vertebral
  auditory canal (external) — *see* Stenosis, external ear canal
  eustachian tube — *see* Obstruction, eustachian tube
  eyelid — *see* Disorder, eyelid function
  larynx J38.6
  mesenteric artery (*see also* Ischemia, intestine, acute) K55.059
  palate M26.89
  palpebral fissure — *see* Disorder, eyelid function
  ureter N13.5
    with infection N13.6
  urethra — *see* Stricture, urethra
Narrowness, abnormal, eyelid Q10.3
Nasal — *see* condition
Nasolachrymal, nasolacrimal — *see* condition
Nasopharyngeal (*see also* condition)
  pituitary gland Q89.2
  torticollis M43.6
Nasopharyngitis (acute) (infective) (streptococcal) (subacute) J00
  chronic (suppurative) (ulcerative) J31.1
Nasopharynx, nasopharyngeal — *see* condition
Natal tooth, teeth K00.6
Nausea (without vomiting) R11.0
  with vomiting R11.2
  gravidarum — *see* Hyperemesis, gravidarum
  marina T75.3 ☑
  navalis T75.3 ☑
Navel — *see* condition
Neapolitan fever — *see* Brucellosis
Near drowning T75.1 ☑
Nearsightedness — *see* Myopia
Near-syncope R55
Nebula, cornea — *see* Opacity, cornea

Necator americanus infestation B76.1
Necatoriasis B76.1
Neck — *see* condition
Necrobiosis R68.89
  lipoidica NEC L92.1
    with diabetes — *see* E08-E13 with .620
Necrolysis, toxic epidermal L51.2
  due to drug
    correct substance properly administered — *see* Table of Drugs and Chemicals, by drug, adverse effect
    overdose or wrong substance given or taken — *see* Table of Drugs and Chemicals, by drug, poisoning
Necrophilia F65.89
Necrosis, necrotic (ischemic) (*see also* Gangrene)
  adrenal (capsule) (gland) E27.49
  amputation stump (surgical) (late) T87.50
    arm T87.5- ☑
    leg T87.5- ☑
  antrum J32.0
  aorta (hyaline) (*see also* Aneurysm, aorta)
    cystic medial — *see* Dissection, aorta
  artery I77.5
  bladder (aseptic) (sphincter) N32.89
  bone (*see also* Osteonecrosis) M87.9
    aseptic or avascular — *see* Osteonecrosis
      idiopathic M87.00
    ethmoid J32.2
    jaw M27.2
    tuberculous — *see* Tuberculosis, bone
  brain I67.89
  breast (aseptic) (fat) (segmental) N64.1
  bronchus J98.09
  central nervous system NEC I67.89
  cerebellar I67.89
  cerebral I67.89
  colon (*see also* Infarct, intestine) K55.049
  cornea H18.89- ☑
  cortical (acute) (renal) N17.1
  cystic medial (aorta) — *see* Dissection, aorta
  dental pulp K04.1
  esophagus K22.8
  ethmoid (bone) J32.2
  eyelid — *see* Disorder, eyelid, degenerative
  fat, fatty (generalized) (*see also* Disorder, soft tissue, specified type NEC)
    abdominal wall K65.4
    breast (aseptic) (segmental) N64.1
    localized — *see* Degeneration, by site, fatty
    mesentery K65.4
    omentum K65.4
    pancreas K86.89
    peritoneum K65.4
    skin (subcutaneous), newborn P83.0
    subcutaneous, due to birth injury P15.6
  gallbladder — *see* Cholecystitis, acute
  heart — *see* Infarct, myocardium
  hip, aseptic or avascular — *see* Osteonecrosis, by type, femur
  intestine (acute) (hemorrhagic) (massive) (*see also* Infarct, intestine) K55.069
  jaw M27.2
  kidney (bilateral) N28.0
    acute N17.9
    cortical (acute) (bilateral) N17.1
      with ectopic or molar pregnancy O08.4
    medullary (bilateral) (in acute renal failure) (papillary) N17.2
    papillary (bilateral) (in acute renal failure) N17.2
    tubular N17.0
      with ectopic or molar pregnancy O08.4
      complicating
        abortion — *see* Abortion, by type, complicated by, tubular necrosis
        ectopic or molar pregnancy O08.4
        pregnancy — *see* Pregnancy, complicated by, diseases of, specified type or system NEC
      following ectopic or molar pregnancy O08.4
      traumatic T79.5 ☑
  larynx J38.7
  liver (with hepatic failure) (cell) — *see* Failure, hepatic
    hemorrhagic, central K76.2
  lung J85.0
  lymphatic gland — *see* Lymphadenitis, acute
  mammary gland (fat) (segmental) N64.1
  mastoid (chronic) — *see* Mastoiditis, chronic

Necrosis, necrotic — *continued*
  medullary (acute) (renal) N17.2
  mesentery (*see also* Infarct, intestine) K55.069
    fat K65.4
  mitral valve — *see* Insufficiency, mitral
  myocardium, myocardial — *see* Infarct, myocardium
  nose J34.0
  omentum (with mesenteric infarction) (*see also* Infarct, intestine) K55.069
    fat K65.4
  orbit, orbital — *see* Osteomyelitis, orbit
  ossicles, ear — *see* Abnormal, ear ossicles
  ovary N70.92
  pancreas (aseptic) (duct) (fat) K86.89
    acute (infective) — *see* Pancreatitis, acute
    infective — *see* Pancreatitis, acute
  papillary (acute) (renal) N17.2
  perineum N90.89
  peritoneum (with mesenteric infarction) (*see also* Infarct, intestine) K55.069
    fat K65.4
  pharynx J02.9
    in granulocytopenia — *see* Neutropenia
    Vincent's A69.1
  phosphorus — *see* subcategory T54.2 ☑
  pituitary (gland) E23.0
    postpartum O99.285
    Sheehan O99.285
  pressure — *see* Ulcer, pressure, by site
  pulmonary J85.0
  pulp (dental) K04.1
  radiation — *see* Necrosis, by site
  radium — *see* Necrosis, by site
  renal — *see* Necrosis, kidney
  sclera H15.89
  scrotum N50.89
  skin or subcutaneous tissue NEC I96
  spine, spinal (column) (*see also* Osteonecrosis, by type, vertebra)
    cord G95.19
  spleen D73.5
  stomach K31.89
  stomatitis (ulcerative) A69.0
  subcutaneous fat, newborn P83.88
  subendocardial (acute) I21.4
    chronic I25.89
  suprarenal (capsule) (gland) E27.49
  testis N50.89
  thymus (gland) E32.8
  tonsil J35.8
  trachea J39.8
  tuberculous NEC — *see* Tuberculosis
  tubular (acute) (anoxic) (renal) (toxic) N17.0
    postprocedural N99.0
  vagina N89.8
  vertebra (*see also* Osteonecrosis, by type, vertebra)
    tuberculous A18.01
  vulva N90.89
  X-ray — *see* Necrosis, by site
Necrospermia — *see* Infertility, male
Need (for)
  care provider because (of)
    assistance with personal care Z74.1
    continuous supervision required Z74.3
    impaired mobility Z74.09
    no other household member able to render care Z74.2
    specified reason NEC Z74.8
  immunization — *see* Vaccination
  vaccination — *see* Vaccination
Neglect
  adult
    confirmed T74.01 ☑
    history of Z91.412
    suspected T76.01 ☑
  child (childhood)
    confirmed T74.02 ☑
    history of Z62.812
    suspected T76.02 ☑
  emotional, in childhood Z62.898
  hemispatial R41.4
  left-sided R41.4
  sensory R41.4
  visuospatial R41.4
Neisserian infection NEC — *see* Gonococcus
Nelaton's syndrome G60.8
Nelson's syndrome E24.1
Nematodiasis (intestinal) B82.0

Index

Naegeli's — Nematodiasis

Index

Nematodiasis — Nephropathy

Nematodiasis — continued
 Ancylostoma B76.0
Neonatal (see also Newborn)
 acne L70.4
 bradycardia P29.12
 screening, abnormal findings on P09
 tachycardia P29.11
 tooth, teeth K00.6
Neonatorum — see condition
Neoplasia
 endocrine, multiple (MEN) E31.20
  type I E31.21
  type IIA E31.22
  type IIB E31.23
 intraepithelial (histologically confirmed)
  anal (AIN) (histologically confirmed) K62.82
   grade I K62.82
   grade II K62.82
   severe D01.3
  cervical glandular (histologically confirmed) D06.9
  cervix (uteri) (CIN) (histologically confirmed) N87.9
   glandular D06.9
   grade I N87.0
   grade II N87.1
   grade III (severe dysplasia) (see also Carcinoma,
    cervix uteri, in situ) D06.9
  prostate (histologically confirmed) (PIN) N42.31
   grade I N42.31
   grade II N42.31
   grade III (severe dysplasia) D07.5
  vagina (histologically confirmed) (VAIN) N89.3
   grade I N89.0
   grade II N89.1
   grade III (severe dysplasia) D07.2
  vulva (histologically confirmed) (VIN) N90.3
   grade I N90.0
   grade II N90.1
   grade III (severe dysplasia) D07.1
Neoplasm, neoplastic (see also Table of Neoplasms)
 lipomatous, benign — see Lipoma
 malignant mast cell C96.20
  specified type NEC C96.29
 mast cell, of uncertain behavior NEC D47.09
Neovascularization
 ciliary body — see Disorder, iris, vascular
 cornea H16.40- ☑
  deep H16.44- ☑
  ghost vessels — see Ghost, vessels
  localized H16.43- ☑
  pannus — see Pannus
 iris — see Disorder, iris, vascular
 retina H35.05- ☑
Nephralgia N23
Nephritis, nephritic (albuminuric) (azotemic) (congenital) (disseminated) (epithelial) (familial) (focal)
  (granulomatous) (hemorrhagic) (infantile) (nonsuppurative, excretory) (uremic) N05.9
 with
  dense deposit disease N05.6
  diffuse
   crescentic glomerulonephritis N05.7
   endocapillary proliferative glomerulonephritis
    N05.4
   membranous glomerulonephritis N05.2
   mesangial proliferative glomerulonephritis N05.3
   mesangiocapillary glomerulonephritis N05.5
  edema — see Nephrosis
  focal and segmental glomerular lesions N05.1
  foot process disease N04.9
  glomerular lesion
   diffuse sclerosing N05.8
   hypocomplementemic — see Nephritis, membra-
    noproliferative
   IgA — see Nephropathy, IgA
   lobular, lobulonodular — see Nephritis, membra-
    noproliferative
   nodular — see Nephritis, membranoproliferative
  lesion of
   glomerulonephritis, proliferative N05.8
   renal necrosis N05.9
  minor glomerular abnormality N05.0
  specified morphological changes NEC N05.8
 acute N00.9
  with
   dense deposit disease N00.6
   diffuse
    crescentic glomerulonephritis N00.7

Nephritis, nephritic — continued
 acute — continued
  with — continued
   diffuse — continued
    endocapillary proliferative glomerulonephritis
     N00.4
    membranous glomerulonephritis N00.2
    mesangial proliferative glomerulonephritis
     N00.3
    mesangiocapillary glomerulonephritis N00.5
   focal and segmental glomerular lesions N00.1
   minor glomerular abnormality N00.0
   specified morphological changes NEC N00.8
  amyloid E85.4 [N08]
  antiglomerular basement membrane (anti-GBM) antibody NEC
   in Goodpasture's syndrome M31.0
  antitubular basement membrane (tubulo-interstitial)
   NEC N12
   toxic — see Nephropathy, toxic
  arteriolar — see Hypertension, kidney
  arteriosclerotic — see Hypertension, kidney
  ascending — see Nephritis, tubulo-interstitial
  atrophic N03.9
  Balkan (endemic) N15.0
  calculous, calculus — see Calculus, kidney
  cardiac — see Hypertension, kidney
  cardiovascular — see Hypertension, kidney
  chronic N03.9
   with
    dense deposit disease N03.6
    diffuse
     crescentic glomerulonephritis N03.7
     endocapillary proliferative glomerulonephritis
      N03.4
     membranous glomerulonephritis N03.2
     mesangial proliferative glomerulonephritis
      N03.3
     mesangiocapillary glomerulonephritis N03.5
    focal and segmental glomerular lesions N03.1
    minor glomerular abnormality N03.0
    specified morphological changes NEC N03.8
   arteriosclerotic — see Hypertension, kidney
  cirrhotic N26.9
  complicating pregnancy O26.83- ☑
  croupous N00.9
  degenerative — see Nephrosis
  diffuse sclerosing N05.8
  due to
   diabetes mellitus — see E08-E13 with .21
   subacute bacterial endocarditis I33.0
   systemic lupus erythematosus (chronic) M32.14
   typhoid fever A01.09
  gonococcal (acute) (chronic) A54.21
  hypocomplementemic — see Nephritis, membranoproliferative
  IgA — see Nephropathy, IgA
  immune complex (circulating) NEC N05.8
  infective — see Nephritis, tubulo-interstitial
  interstitial — see Nephritis, tubulo-interstitial
  lead N14.3
  membranoproliferative (diffuse) (type 1 or 3) (see also
   N00-N07 with fourth character .5) N05.5
   type 2 (see also N00-N07 with fourth character .6)
    N05.6
  minimal change N05.0
  necrotic, necrotizing NEC (see also N00-N07 with fourth
   character .8) N05.8
  nephrotic — see Nephrosis
  nodular — see Nephritis, membranoproliferative
  polycystic Q61.3
   adult type Q61.2
   autosomal
    dominant Q61.2
    recessive NEC Q61.19
   childhood type NEC Q61.19
   infantile type NEC Q61.19
  poststreptococcal N05.9
   acute N00.9
   chronic N03.9
   rapidly progressive N01.9
  proliferative NEC (see also N00-N07 with fourth character .8) N05.8
  purulent — see Nephritis, tubulo-interstitial
  rapidly progressive N01.9
   with
    dense deposit disease N01.6
    diffuse

Nephritis, nephritic — continued
 rapidly progressive — continued
  with — continued
   diffuse — continued
    crescentic glomerulonephritis N01.7
    endocapillary proliferative glomerulonephritis
     N01.4
    membranous glomerulonephritis N01.2
    mesangial proliferative glomerulonephritis
     N01.3
    mesangiocapillary glomerulonephritis N01.5
   focal and segmental glomerular lesions N01.1
   minor glomerular abnormality N01.0
   specified morphological changes NEC N01.8
 salt losing or wasting NEC N28.89
 saturnine N14.3
 sclerosing, diffuse N05.8
 septic — see Nephritis, tubulo-interstitial
 specified pathology NEC (see also N00-N07 with fourth
  character .8) N05.8
 subacute N01.9
 suppurative — see Nephritis, tubulo-interstitial
 syphilitic (late) A52.75
  congenital A50.59 [N08]
  early (secondary) A51.44
 toxic — see Nephropathy, toxic
 tubal, tubular — see Nephritis, tubulo-interstitial
 tuberculous A18.11
 tubulo-interstitial (in) N12
  acute (infectious) N10
  chronic (infectious) N11.9
   nonobstructive N11.8
    reflux-associated N11.0
   obstructive N11.1
   specified NEC N11.8
  due to
   brucellosis A23.9 [N16]
   cryoglobulinemia D89.1 [N16]
   glycogen storage disease E74.00 [N16]
  Sjögren's syndrome M35.04
 vascular — see Hypertension, kidney
 war N00.9
Nephroblastoma (epithelial) (mesenchymal) C64- ☑
Nephrocalcinosis E83.59 [N29]
Nephrocystitis, pustular — see Nephritis, tubulo-interstitial
Nephrolithiasis (congenital) (pelvis) (recurrent) (see also
  Calculus, kidney)
Nephroma C64- ☑
 mesoblastic D41.0- ☑
Nephronephritis — see Nephrosis
Nephronophthisis Q61.5
Nephropathia epidemica A98.5
Nephropathy (see also Nephritis) N28.9
 with
  edema — see Nephrosis
  glomerular lesion — see Glomerulonephritis
 amyloid, hereditary E85.0
 analgesic N14.0
  with medullary necrosis, acute N17.2
 Balkan (endemic) N15.0
 chemical — see Nephropathy, toxic
 diabetic — see E08-E13 with .21
 drug-induced N14.2
  specified NEC N14.1
 focal and segmental hyalinosis or sclerosis N02.1
 heavy metal-induced N14.3
 hereditary NEC N07.9
  with
   dense deposit disease N07.6
   diffuse
    crescentic glomerulonephritis N07.7
    endocapillary proliferative glomerulonephri
     N07.4
    membranous glomerulonephritis N07.2
    mesangial proliferative glomerulonephriti
     N07.3
    mesangiocapillary glomerulonephritis N07
   focal and segmental glomerular lesions N07.1
   minor glomerular abnormality N07.0
   specified morphological changes NEC N07.8
 hypercalcemic N25.89
 hypertensive — see Hypertension, kidney
 hypokalemic (vacuolar) N25.89
 IgA N02.8
  with glomerular lesion N02.9
   focal and segmental hyalinosis or sclerosis N02
   membranoproliferative (diffuse) N02.5

☑ Additional Character Required — Refer to the Tabular List for Character Selection
Subterms under main terms may continue to next column or pag

Nephropathy — *continued*
  IgA — *continued*
    with glomerular lesion — *continued*
      membranous (diffuse) N02.2
      mesangial proliferative (diffuse) N02.3
      mesangiocapillary (diffuse) N02.5
      proliferative NEC N02.8
      specified pathology NEC N02.8
  lead N14.3
  membranoproliferative (diffuse) N02.5
  membranous (diffuse) N02.2
  mesangial (IgA/IgG) — *see* Nephropathy, IgA
    proliferative (diffuse) N02.3
  mesangiocapillary (diffuse) N02.5
  obstructive N13.8
  phenacetin N17.2
  phosphate-losing N25.0
  potassium depletion N25.89
  pregnancy-related O26.83- ☑
  proliferative NEC (*see also* N00-N07 with fourth character .8) N05.8
  protein-losing N25.89
  saturnine N14.3
  sickle-cell D57.- ☑ [N08]
  toxic NEC N14.4
    due to
      drugs N14.2
        analgesic N14.0
          specified NEC N14.1
      heavy metals N14.3
  vasomotor N17.0
  water-losing N25.89
Nephroptosis N28.83
Nephropyosis — *see* Abscess, kidney
Nephrorrhagia N28.89
Nephrosclerosis (arteriolar)(arteriosclerotic) (chronic) (hyaline) (*see also* Hypertension, kidney)
  hyperplastic — *see* Hypertension, kidney
  senile N26.9
Nephrosis, nephrotic (Epstein's) (syndrome) (congenital) N04.9
  with
    foot process disease N04.9
    glomerular lesion N04.1
    hypocomplementemic N04.5
  acute N04.9
  anoxic — *see* Nephrosis, tubular
  chemical — *see* Nephrosis, tubular
  cholemic K76.7
  diabetic — *see* E08-E13 with .21
  Finnish type (congenital) Q89.8
  hemoglobin N10
  hemoglobinuric — *see* Nephrosis, tubular
  in
    amyloidosis E85.4 [N08]
    diabetes mellitus — *see* E08-E13 with .21
    epidemic hemorrhagic fever A98.5
    malaria (malariae) B52.0
  ischemic — *see* Nephrosis, tubular
  lipoid N04.9
  lower nephron — *see* Nephrosis, tubular
  malarial (malariae) B52.0
  minimal change N04.0
  myoglobin N10
  necrotizing — *see* Nephrosis, tubular
  osmotic (sucrose) N25.89
  radiation N04.9
  syphilitic (late) A52.75
  toxic — *see* Nephrosis, tubular
  tubular (acute) N17.0
    postprocedural N99.0
    radiation N04.9
Nephrosonephritis, hemorrhagic (endemic) A98.5
Nephrostomy
  attention to Z43.6
  status Z93.6
Nerve (*see also* condition)
  injury — *see* Injury, nerve, by body site
Nerves R45.0
Nervous (*see also* condition) R45.0
  heart F45.8
  stomach F45.8
  tension R45.0
Nervousness R45.0
Nesidioblastoma
  pancreas D13.7
  specified site NEC — *see* Neoplasm, benign, by site
  unspecified site D13.7

Nettleship's syndrome — *see* Urticaria pigmentosa
Neumann's disease or syndrome L10.1
Neuralgia, neuralgic (acute) M79.2
  accessory (nerve) G52.8
  acoustic (nerve) — *see* subcategory H93.3 ☑
  auditory (nerve) — *see* subcategory H93.3 ☑
  ciliary G44.009
    intractable G44.001
    not intractable G44.009
  cranial
    nerve (*see also* Disorder, nerve, cranial)
      fifth or trigeminal — *see* Neuralgia, trigeminal
    postherpetic, postzoster B02.29
  ear — *see* subcategory H92.0 ☑
  facialis vera G51.1
  Fothergill's — *see* Neuralgia, trigeminal
  glossopharyngeal (nerve) G52.1
  Horton's G44.099
    intractable G44.091
    not intractable G44.099
  Hunt's B02.21
  hypoglossal (nerve) G52.3
  infraorbital — *see* Neuralgia, trigeminal
  malarial — *see* Malaria
  migrainous G44.009
    intractable G44.001
    not intractable G44.009
  Morton's G57.6- ☑
  nerve, cranial — *see* Disorder, nerve, cranial
  nose G52.0
  occipital M54.81
  olfactory G52.0
  penis N48.9
  perineum R10.2
  postherpetic NEC B02.29
    trigeminal B02.22
  pubic region R10.2
  scrotum R10.2
  Sluder's G44.89
  specified nerve NEC G58.8
  spermatic cord R10.2
  sphenopalatine (ganglion) G90.09
  trifacial — *see* Neuralgia, trigeminal
  trigeminal G50.0
    postherpetic, postzoster B02.22
  vagus (nerve) G52.2
  writer's F48.8
    organic G25.89
Neurapraxia — *see* Injury, nerve
Neurasthenia F48.8
  cardiac F45.8
  gastric F45.8
  heart F45.8
Neurilemmoma (*see also* Neoplasm, nerve, benign)
  acoustic (nerve) D33.3
  malignant (*see also* Neoplasm, nerve, malignant)
    acoustic (nerve) C72.4- ☑
Neurilemmosarcoma — *see* Neoplasm, nerve, malignant
Neurinoma — *see* Neoplasm, nerve, benign
Neurinomatosis — *see* Neoplasm, nerve, uncertain behavior
Neuritis (rheumatoid) M79.2
  abducens (nerve) — *see* Strabismus, paralytic, sixth nerve
  accessory (nerve) G52.8
  acoustic (nerve) (*see also* subcategory) H93.3 ☑
    in (due to)
      infectious disease NEC B99 ☑ [H94.0-] ☑
      parasitic disease NEC B89 [H94.0-] ☑
    syphilitic A52.15
  alcoholic G62.1
    with psychosis — *see* Psychosis, alcoholic
  amyloid, any site E85.4 [G63]
  auditory (nerve) — *see* subcategory H93.3 ☑
  brachial — *see* Radiculopathy
    due to displacement, intervertebral disc — *see* Disorder, disc, cervical, with neuritis
  cranial nerve
    due to Lyme disease A69.22
    eighth or acoustic or auditory — *see* subcategory H93.3 ☑
    eleventh or accessory G52.8
    fifth or trigeminal G51.0
    first or olfactory G52.0
    fourth or trochlear — *see* Strabismus, paralytic, fourth nerve
    second or optic — *see* Neuritis, optic
    seventh or facial G51.8

Neuritis — *continued*
  cranial nerve — *continued*
    seventh or facial — *continued*
      newborn (birth injury) P11.3
    sixth or abducent — *see* Strabismus, paralytic, sixth nerve
    tenth or vagus G52.2
    third or oculomotor — *see* Strabismus, paralytic, third nerve
    twelfth or hypoglossal G52.3
  Déjérine-Sottas G60.0
  diabetic (mononeuropathy) — *see* E08-E13 with .41
    polyneuropathy — *see* E08-E13 with .42
  due to
    beriberi E51.11
    displacement, prolapse or rupture, intervertebral disc — *see* Disorder, disc, with, radiculopathy
    herniation, nucleus pulposus M51.9 [G55]
  endemic E51.11
  facial G51.8
    newborn (birth injury) P11.3
  general — *see* Polyneuropathy
  geniculate ganglion G51.1
    due to herpes (zoster) B02.21
  gouty (*see also* Gout, by type) M10.9 [G63]
  hypoglossal (nerve) G52.3
  ilioinguinal (nerve) G57.9- ☑
  infectious (multiple) NEC G61.0
  interstitial hypertrophic progressive G60.0
  lumbar M54.16
  lumbosacral M54.17
  multiple (*see also* Polyneuropathy)
    endemic E51.11
    infective, acute G61.0
  multiplex endemica E51.11
  nerve root — *see* Radiculopathy
  oculomotor (nerve) — *see* Strabismus, paralytic, third nerve
  olfactory nerve G52.0
  optic (nerve) (hereditary) (sympathetic) H46.9
    with demyelination G36.0
    in myelitis G36.0
    nutritional H46.2
    papillitis — *see* Papillitis, optic
    retrobulbar H46.1- ☑
    specified type NEC H46.8
    toxic H46.3
  peripheral (nerve) G62.9
    multiple — *see* Polyneuropathy
    single — *see* Mononeuritis
  pneumogastric (nerve) G52.2
  postherpetic, postzoster B02.29
  progressive hypertrophic interstitial G60.0
  retrobulbar (*see also* Neuritis, optic, retrobulbar)
    in (due to)
      late syphilis A52.15
      meningococcal infection A39.82
    meningococcal A39.82
    syphilitic A52.15
  sciatic (nerve) (*see also* Sciatica)
    due to displacement of intervertebral disc — *see* Disorder, disc, with, radiculopathy
  serum (*see also* Reaction, serum) T80.69 ☑
  shoulder-girdle G54.5
  specified nerve NEC G58.8
  spinal (nerve) root — *see* Radiculopathy
  syphilitic A52.15
  thenar (median) G56.1- ☑
  thoracic M54.14
  toxic NEC G62.2
  trochlear (nerve) — *see* Strabismus, paralytic, fourth nerve
  vagus (nerve) G52.2
Neuroastrocytoma — *see* Neoplasm, uncertain behavior, by site
Neuroavitaminosis E56.9 [G99.8]
Neuroblastoma
  olfactory C30.0
  specified site — *see* Neoplasm, malignant, by site
  unspecified site C74.90
Neurochorioretinitis — *see* Chorioretinitis
Neurocirculatory asthenia F45.8
Neurocysticercosis B69.0
Neurocytoma — *see* Neoplasm, benign, by site
Neurodermatitis (circumscribed) (circumscripta) (local) L28.0
  atopic L20.81
  diffuse (Brocq) L20.81

Neurodermatitis — *continued*
disseminated L20.81
Neuroencephalomyelopathy, optic G36.0
Neuroepithelioma (*see also* Neoplasm, malignant, by site)
olfactory C30.0
Neurofibroma (*see also* Neoplasm, nerve, benign)
melanotic — *see* Neoplasm, nerve, benign
multiple — *see* Neurofibromatosis
plexiform — *see* Neoplasm, nerve, benign
Neurofibromatosis (multiple) (nonmalignant) Q85.00
acoustic Q85.02
malignant — *see* Neoplasm, nerve, malignant
specified NEC Q85.09
type 1 (von Recklinghausen) Q85.01
type 2 Q85.02
Neurofibrosarcoma — *see* Neoplasm, nerve, malignant
Neurogenic (*see also* condition)
bladder (*see also* Dysfunction, bladder, neuromuscular) N31.9
cauda equina syndrome G83.4
bowel NEC K59.2
heart F45.8
Neuroglioma — *see* Neoplasm, uncertain behavior, by site
Neurolabyrinthitis (of Dix and Hallpike) — *see* Neuronitis, vestibular
Neurolathyrism — *see* Poisoning, food, noxious, plant
Neuroleprosy A30.9
Neuroma (*see also* Neoplasm, nerve, benign)
acoustic (nerve) D33.3
amputation (stump) (traumatic) (surgical complication) (late) T87.3- ☑
arm T87.3- ☑
leg T87.3- ☑
digital (toe) G57.6- ☑
interdigital G58.8
lower limb (toe) G57.8- ☑
upper limb G56.8- ☑
intermetatarsal G57.8- ☑
Morton's G57.6- ☑
nonneoplastic
arm G56.9- ☑
leg G57.9- ☑
lower extremity G57.9- ☑
upper extremity G56.9- ☑
optic (nerve) D33.3
plantar G57.6- ☑
plexiform — *see* Neoplasm, nerve, benign
surgical (nonneoplastic)
arm G56.9- ☑
leg G57.9- ☑
lower extremity G57.9- ☑
upper extremity G56.9- ☑
Neuromyalgia — *see* Neuralgia
Neuromyasthenia (epidemic) (postinfectious) G93.3
Neuromyelitis G36.9
ascending G61.0
optica G36.0
Neuromyopathy G70.9
paraneoplastic D49.9 [G13.0]
Neuromyotonia (Isaacs) G71.19
Neuronevus — *see* Nevus
Neuronitis G58.9
ascending (acute) G57.2- ☑
vestibular H81.2- ☑
Neuroparalytic — *see* condition
Neuropathy, neuropathic G62.9
acute motor G62.81
alcoholic G62.1
with psychosis — *see* Psychosis, alcoholic
arm G56.9- ☑
autonomic, peripheral — *see* Neuropathy, peripheral, autonomic
axillary G56.9- ☑
bladder N31.9
atonic (motor) (sensory) N31.2
autonomous N31.2
flaccid N31.2
nonreflex N31.2
reflex N31.1
uninhibited N31.0
brachial plexus G54.0
cervical plexus G54.2
chronic
progressive segmentally demyelinating G62.89
relapsing demyelinating G62.89

Neuropathy, neuropathic — *continued*
Déjérine-Sottas G60.0
diabetic — *see* E08-E13 with .40
mononeuropathy — *see* E08-E13 with .41
polyneuropathy — *see* E08-E13 with .42
entrapment G58.9
iliohypogastric nerve G57.8- ☑
ilioinguinal nerve G57.8- ☑
lateral cutaneous nerve of thigh G57.1- ☑
median nerve G56.0- ☑
obturator nerve G57.8- ☑
peroneal nerve G57.3- ☑
posterior tibial nerve G57.5- ☑
saphenous nerve G57.8- ☑
ulnar nerve G56.2- ☑
facial nerve G51.9
hereditary G60.9
motor and sensory (types I-IV) G60.0
sensory G60.8
specified NEC G60.8
hypertrophic G60.0
Charcot-Marie-Tooth G60.0
Déjérine-Sottas G60.0
interstitial progressive G60.0
of infancy G60.0
Refsum G60.1
idiopathic G60.9
progressive G60.3
specified NEC G60.8
in association with hereditary ataxia G60.2
intercostal G58.0
ischemic — *see* Disorder, nerve
Jamaica (ginger) G62.2
leg NEC G57.9- ☑
lower extremity G57.9- ☑
lumbar plexus G54.1
median nerve G56.1- ☑
motor and sensory (*see also* Polyneuropathy)
hereditary (types I-IV) G60.0
multifocal motor (MMN) G61.82
multiple (acute) (chronic) — *see* Polyneuropathy
optic (nerve) (*see also* Neuritis, optic)
ischemic H47.01- ☑
paraneoplastic (sensorial) (Denny Brown) D49.9 [G13.0]
peripheral (nerve) (*see also* Polyneuropathy) G62.9
autonomic G90.9
idiopathic G90.09
in (due to)
amyloidosis E85.4 [G99.0]
diabetes mellitus — *see* E08-E13 with .43
endocrine disease NEC E34.9 [G99.0]
gout M10.00 [G99.0]
hyperthyroidism E05.90 [G99.0]
with thyroid storm E05.91 [G99.0]
metabolic disease NEC E88.9 [G99.0]
idiopathic G60.9
progressive G60.3
in (due to)
antitetanus serum G62.0
arsenic G62.2
drugs NEC G62.0
lead G62.2
organophosphate compounds G62.2
toxic agent NEC G62.2
plantar nerves G57.6- ☑
progressive
hypertrophic interstitial G60.0
inflammatory G62.81
radicular NEC — *see* Radiculopathy
sacral plexus G54.1
sciatic G57.0- ☑
serum G61.1
toxic NEC G62.2
trigeminal sensory G50.8
ulnar nerve G56.2- ☑
uremic N18.9 [G63]
vitamin B12 E53.8 [G63]
with anemia (pernicious) D51.0 [G63]
due to dietary deficiency D51.3 [G63]
Neurophthisis (*see also* Disorder, nerve)
peripheral, diabetic — *see* E08-E13 with .42
Neuroretinitis — *see* Chorioretinitis
Neuroretinopathy, hereditary optic H47.22
Neurosarcoma — *see* Neoplasm, nerve, malignant
Neurosclerosis — *see* Disorder, nerve
Neurosis, neurotic F48.9
anankastic F42.8
anxiety (state) F41.1

Neurosis, neurotic — *continued*
anxiety — *continued*
panic type F41.0
asthenic F48.8
bladder F45.8
cardiac (reflex) F45.8
cardiovascular F45.8
character F60.9
colon F45.8
compensation F68.10
compulsive, compulsion F42.8
conversion F44.9
craft F48.8
cutaneous F45.8
depersonalization F48.1
depressive (reaction) (type) F34.1
environmental F48.8
excoriation L98.1
fatigue F48.8
functional — *see* Disorder, somatoform
gastric F45.8
gastrointestinal F45.8
heart F45.8
hypochondriacal F45.21
hysterical F44.9
incoordination F45.8
larynx F45.8
vocal cord F45.8
intestine F45.8
larynx (sensory) F45.8
hysterical F44.4
mixed NEC F48.8
musculoskeletal F45.8
obsessional F42.8
obsessive-compulsive F42.8
occupational F48.8
ocular NEC F45.8
organ — *see* Disorder, somatoform
pharynx F45.8
phobic F40.9
posttraumatic (situational) F43.10
acute F43.11
chronic F43.12
psychasthenic (type) F48.8
railroad F48.8
rectum F45.8
respiratory F45.8
rumination F45.8
sexual F65.9
situational F48.8
social F40.10
generalized F40.11
specified type NEC F48.8
state F48.9
with depersonalization episode F48.1
stomach F45.8
traumatic F43.10
acute F43.11
chronic F43.12
vasomotor F45.8
visceral F45.8
war F48.8
Neurospongioblastosis diffusa Q85.1
Neurosyphilis (arrested) (early) (gumma) (late) (latent) (recurrent) (relapse) A52.3
with ataxia (cerebellar) (locomotor) (spastic) (spinal) A52.19
aneurysm (cerebral) A52.05
arachnoid (adhesive) A52.13
arteritis (any artery) (cerebral) A52.04
asymptomatic A52.2
congenital A50.40
dura (mater) A52.13
general paresis A52.17
hemorrhagic A52.05
juvenile (asymptomatic) (meningeal) A50.40
leptomeninges (aseptic) A52.13
meningeal, meninges (adhesive) A52.13
meningitis A52.13
meningovascular (diffuse) A52.13
optic atrophy A52.15
parenchymatous (degenerative) A52.19
paresis, paretic A52.17
juvenile A50.45
remission in (sustained) A52.3
serological (without symptoms) A52.2
specified nature or site NEC A52.19
tabes, tabetic (dorsalis) A52.11
juvenile A50.45

☑ **Additional Character Required** — **Refer to the Tabular List for Character Selection** ▽ Subterms under main terms may continue to next column or page

Neurosyphilis — continued
  taboparesis A52.17
    juvenile A50.45
  thrombosis (cerebral) A52.05
  vascular (cerebral) NEC A52.05
Neurothekeoma — see Neoplasm, nerve, benign
Neurotic — see Neurosis
Neurotoxemia — see Toxemia
Neutroclusion M26.211
Neutropenia, neutropenic (chronic) (genetic) (idiopathic) (immune) (infantile) (malignant) (pernicious)
  (splenic) D70.9
  congenital (primary) D70.0
  cyclic D70.4
  cytoreductive cancer chemotherapy sequela D70.1
  drug-induced D70.2
    due to cytoreductive cancer chemotherapy D70.1
  due to infection D70.3
  fever D70.9
  neonatal, transitory (isoimmune) (maternal transfer)
    P61.5
  periodic D70.4
  secondary (cyclic) (periodic) (splenic) D70.4
    drug-induced D70.2
      due to cytoreductive cancer chemotherapy D70.1
  toxic D70.8
Neutrophilia, hereditary giant D72.0
Nevocarcinoma — see Melanoma
Nevus D22.9
  achromic — see Neoplasm, skin, benign
  amelanotic — see Neoplasm, skin, benign
  angiomatous D18.00
    intra-abdominal D18.03
    intracranial D18.02
    skin D18.01
    specified site NEC D18.09
  araneus I78.1
  balloon cell — see Neoplasm, skin, benign
  bathing trunk D48.5
  blue — see Neoplasm, skin, benign
    cellular — see Neoplasm, skin, benign
    giant — see Neoplasm, skin, benign
    Jadassohn's — see Neoplasm, skin, benign
    malignant — see Melanoma
  capillary D18.00
    intra-abdominal D18.03
    intracranial D18.02
    skin D18.01
    specified site NEC D18.09
  cavernous D18.00
    intra-abdominal D18.03
    intracranial D18.02
    skin D18.01
    specified site NEC D18.09
  cellular — see Neoplasm, skin, benign
    blue — see Neoplasm, skin, benign
  choroid D31.3- ☑
  comedonicus Q82.5
  conjunctiva D31.0- ☑
  dermal — see Neoplasm, skin, benign
    with epidermal nevus — see Neoplasm, skin, benign
  dysplastic — see Neoplasm, skin, benign
  eye D31.9- ☑
  flammeus Q82.5
  hemangiomatous D18.00
    intra-abdominal D18.03
    intracranial D18.02
    skin D18.01
    specified site NEC D18.09
  iris D31.4- ☑
  lacrimal gland D31.5- ☑
  lymphatic D18.1
  magnocellular
    specified site — see Neoplasm, benign, by site
    unspecified site D31.40
  malignant — see Melanoma
  meaning hemangioma D18.00
    intra-abdominal D18.03
    intracranial D18.02
    skin D18.01
    specified site NEC D18.09
  mouth (mucosa) D10.30
    specified site NEC D10.39
    white sponge Q38.6
  multiplex Q85.1
  non-neoplastic I78.1
  oral mucosa D10.30
    specified site NEC D10.39

Nevus — continued
  oral mucosa — continued
    white sponge Q38.6
  orbit D31.6- ☑
  pigmented
    giant (see also Neoplasm, skin, uncertain behavior)
      D48.5
    malignant melanoma in — see Melanoma
  portwine Q82.5
  retina D31.2- ☑
  retrobulbar D31.6- ☑
  sanguineous Q82.5
  senile I78.1
  skin D22.9
    abdominal wall D22.5
    ala nasi D22.39
    ankle D22.7- ☑
    anus, anal D22.5
    arm D22.6- ☑
    auditory canal (external) D22.2- ☑
    auricle (ear) D22.2- ☑
    auricular canal (external) D22.2- ☑
    axilla, axillary fold D22.5
    back D22.5
    breast D22.5
    brow D22.39
    buttock D22.5
    canthus (eye) D22.1- ☑
    cheek (external) D22.39
    chest wall D22.5
    chin D22.39
    ear (external) D22.2- ☑
    external meatus (ear) D22.2- ☑
    eyebrow D22.39
    eyelid (lower) (upper) D22.1- ☑
    face D22.30
      specified NEC D22.39
    female genital organ (external) NEC D28.0
    finger D22.6- ☑
    flank D22.5
    foot D22.7- ☑
    forearm D22.6- ☑
    forehead D22.39
    foreskin D29.0
    genital organ (external) NEC
      female D28.0
      male D29.9
    gluteal region D22.5
    groin D22.5
    hand D22.6- ☑
    heel D22.7- ☑
    helix D22.2- ☑
    hip D22.7- ☑
    interscapular region D22.5
    jaw D22.39
    knee D22.7- ☑
    labium (majus) (minus) D28.0
    leg D22.7- ☑
    lip (lower) (upper) D22.0
    lower limb D22.7- ☑
    male genital organ (external) D29.9
    nail D22.9
      finger D22.6- ☑
      toe D22.7- ☑
    nasolabial groove D22.39
    nates D22.5
    neck D22.4
    nose (external) D22.39
    palpebra D22.1- ☑
    penis D29.0
    perianal skin D22.5
    perineum D22.5
    pinna D22.2- ☑
    popliteal fossa or space D22.7- ☑
    prepuce D29.0
    pudendum D28.0
    scalp D22.4
    scrotum D29.4
    shoulder D22.6- ☑
    submammary fold D22.5
    temple D22.39
    thigh D22.7- ☑
    toe D22.7- ☑
    trunk NEC D22.5
    umbilicus D22.5
    upper limb D22.6- ☑
    vulva D28.0

Nevus — continued
  specified site NEC — see Neoplasm, by site, benign
  spider I78.1
  stellar I78.1
  strawberry Q82.5
  Sutton's benign D22.9
  unius lateris Q82.5
  Unna's Q82.5
  vascular Q82.5
  verrucous Q82.5
Newborn (infant) (liveborn) (singleton) Z38.2
  abstinence syndrome P96.1
  acne L70.4
  affected by
    abnormalities of membranes P02.9
      specified NEC P02.8
    abruptio placenta P02.1
    amino-acid metabolic disorder, transitory P74.8
    amniocentesis (while in utero) P00.6
    amnionitis P02.78
    apparent life threatening event (ALTE) R68.13
    bleeding (into)
      cerebral cortex P52.22
      germinal matrix P52.0
      ventricles P52.1
    breech delivery P03.0
    cardiac arrest P29.81
    cardiomyopathy I42.8
      congenital I42.4
    cerebral ischemia P91.0
    Cesarean delivery P03.4
    chemotherapy agents P04.11
    chorioamnionitis P02.78
    cocaine (crack) P04.41
    complications of labor and delivery P03.9
      specified NEC P03.89
    compression of umbilical cord NEC P02.5
    contracted pelvis P03.1
    delivery P03.9
      Cesarean P03.4
      forceps P03.2
      vacuum extractor P03.3
    drugs of addiction P04.40
      cocaine P04.41
      hallucinogens P04.42
      specified drug NEC P04.49
    entanglement (knot) in umbilical cord P02.5
    environmental chemicals P04.6
    fetal (intrauterine)
      growth retardation P05.9
      inflammatory response syndrome (FIRS) P02.70
      malnutrition not light or small for gestational
        age P05.2
    FIRS (fetal inflammatory response syndrome) P02.70
    forceps delivery P03.2
    heart rate abnormalities
      bradycardia P29.12
      intrauterine P03.819
        before onset of labor P03.810
        during labor P03.811
      tachycardia P29.11
    hemorrhage (antepartum) P02.1
      cerebellar (nontraumatic) P52.6
      intracerebral (nontraumatic) P52.4
      intracranial (nontraumatic) P52.9
        specified NEC P52.8
      intraventricular (nontraumatic) P52.3
        grade 1 P52.0
        grade 2 P52.1
        grade 3 P52.21
        grade 4 P52.22
      posterior fossa (nontraumatic) P52.6
      subarachnoid (nontraumatic) P52.5
      subependymal P52.0
        with intracerebral extension P52.22
        with intraventricular extension P52.1
          with enlargment of ventricles P52.21
        without intraventricular extension P52.0
    hypoxic ischemic encephalopathy [HIE] P91.60
      mild P91.61
      moderate P91.62
      severe P91.63
    induction of labor P03.89
    intestinal perforation P78.0
    intrauterine (fetal) blood loss P50.9
      due to (from)
        cut end of co-twin cord P50.5
        hemorrhage into
          co-twin P50.3

Newborn — continued
  affected by — continued
    intrauterine blood loss — continued
      due to — continued
        hemorrhage into — continued
          maternal circulation P50.4
        placenta P50.2
        ruptured cord blood P50.1
        vasa previa P50.0
      specified NEC P50.8
    intrauterine (fetal) hemorrhage P50.9
    intrauterine (in utero) procedure P96.5
    malpresentation (malposition) NEC P03.1
    maternal (complication of) (use of)
      alcohol P04.3
      amphetamines P04.16
      analgesia (maternal) P04.0
      anesthesia (maternal) P04.0
      anticonvulsants P04.13
      antidepressants P04.15
      antineoplastic chemotherapy P04.11
      anxiolytics P04.1A
      blood loss P02.1
      cannabis P04.81
      circulatory disease P00.3
      condition P00.9
        specified NEC P00.89
      cytotoxic drugs P04.12
      delivery P03.9
        Cesarean P03.4
        forceps P03.2
        vacuum extractor P03.3
      diabetes mellitus (pre-existing) P70.1
      disorder P00.9
        specified NEC P00.89
      drugs (addictive) (illegal) NEC P04.49
      ectopic pregnancy P01.4
      gestational diabetes P70.0
      hemorrhage P02.1
      hypertensive disorder P00.0
      incompetent cervix P01.0
      infectious disease P00.2
      injury P00.5
      labor and delivery P03.9
      malpresentation before labor P01.7
      maternal death P01.6
      medical procedure P00.7
      medication P04.19
        specified type NEC P04.18
      multiple pregnancy P01.5
      nutritional disorder P00.4
      oligohydramnios P01.2
      opiates P04.14
        administered for procedures during pregnan-
          cy or labor and delivery P04.0
      parasitic disease P00.2
      periodontal disease P00.81
      placenta previa P02.0
      polyhydramnios P01.3
      precipitate delivery P03.5
      pregnancy P01.9
        specified P01.8
      premature rupture of membranes P01.1
      renal disease P00.1
      respiratory disease P00.3
      sedative-hypnotics P04.17
      surgical procedure P00.6
      tranquilizers administered for procedures during
        pregnancy or labor and delivery P04.0
      urinary tract disease P00.1
      uterine contraction (abnormal) P03.6
    meconium peritonitis P78.0
    medication (legal) (maternal use) (prescribed)
      P04.19
    membrane abnormalities P02.9
      specified NEC P02.8
    membranitis P02.78
    methamphetamine(s) P04.49
    mixed metabolic and respiratory acidosis P84
    neonatal abstinence syndrome P96.1
    noxious substances transmitted via placenta or
      breast milk P04.9
      cannabis P04.81
      specified NEC P04.89
    nutritional supplements P04.5
    placenta previa P02.0
    placental
      abnormality (functional) (morphological) P02.20
        specified NEC P02.29

Newborn — continued
  affected by — continued
    placental — continued
      dysfunction P02.29
      infarction P02.29
      insufficiency P02.29
      separation NEC P02.1
      transfusion syndromes P02.3
    placentitis P02.78
    precipitate delivery P03.5
    prolapsed cord P02.4
    respiratory arrest P28.81
    slow intrauterine growth P05.9
    tobacco P04.2
    twin to twin transplacental transfusion P02.3
    umbilical cord (tightly) around neck P02.5
    umbilical cord condition P02.60
      short cord P02.69
      specified NEC P02.69
    uterine contractions (abnormal) P03.6
    vasa previa P02.69
      from intrauterine blood loss P50.0
  apnea P28.4
    obstructive P28.4
    primary P28.3
    sleep (central) (obstructive) (primary) P28.3
  born in hospital Z38.00
    by cesarean Z38.01
  born outside hospital Z38.1
  breast buds P96.89
  breast engorgement P83.4
  check-up — see Newborn, examination
  convulsion P90
  dehydration P74.1
  examination
    8 to 28 days old Z00.111
    under 8 days old Z00.110
  fever P81.9
    environmentally-induced P81.0
  hyperbilirubinemia P59.9
    of prematurity P59.0
  hypernatremia P74.21
  hyponatremia P74.22
  infection P39.9
    candidal P37.5
    specified NEC P39.8
    urinary tract P39.3
  jaundice P59.9
    due to
      breast milk inhibitor P59.3
      hepatocellular damage P59.20
        specified NEC P59.29
      preterm delivery P59.0
    of prematurity P59.0
    specified NEC P59.8
  late metabolic acidosis P74.0
  mastitis P39.0
    infective P39.0
    noninfective P83.4
  multiple born NEC Z38.8
    born in hospital Z38.68
      by cesarean Z38.69
    born outside hospital Z38.7
  omphalitis P38.9
    with mild hemorrhage P38.1
    without hemorrhage P38.9
  post-term P08.21
  prolonged gestation (over 42 completed weeks) P08.22
  quadruplet Z38.8
    born in hospital Z38.63
      by cesarean Z38.64
    born outside hospital Z38.7
  quintuplet Z38.8
    born in hospital Z38.65
      by cesarean Z38.66
    born outside hospital Z38.7
  seizure P90
  sepsis (congenital) P36.9
    due to
      anaerobes NEC P36.5
      Escherichia coli P36.4
      Staphylococcus P36.30
        aureus P36.2
        specified NEC P36.39
      Streptococcus P36.10
        group B P36.0
        specified NEC P36.19
    specified NEC P36.8
  triplet Z38.8

Newborn — continued
  triplet — continued
    born in hospital Z38.61
      by cesarean Z38.62
    born outside hospital Z38.7
  twin Z38.5
    born in hospital Z38.30
      by cesarean Z38.31
    born outside hospital Z38.4
  vomiting P92.09
    bilious P92.01
  weight check Z00.111
Newcastle conjunctivitis or disease B30.8
Nezelof's syndrome (pure alymphocytosis) D81.4
Niacin (amide) **deficiency** E52
Nicolas (-Durand)-**Favre disease** A55
Nicotine — see Tobacco
Nicotinic acid deficiency E52
Niemann-Pick disease or syndrome E75.249
  specified NEC E75.248
  type
    A E75.240
    B E75.241
    C E75.242
    D E75.243
Night
  blindness — see Blindness, night
  sweats R61
  terrors (child) F51.4
Nightmares (REM sleep type) F51.5
NIHSS (National Institutes of Health Stroke Scale) **score**
  R29.7- ☑
Nipple — see condition
Nisbet's chancre A57
Nishimoto (-Takeuchi) **disease** I67.5
Nitritoid crisis or reaction — see Crisis, nitritoid
Nitrosohemoglobinemia D74.8
Njovera A65
Nocardiosis, nocardiasis A43.9
  cutaneous A43.1
  lung A43.0
  pneumonia A43.0
  pulmonary A43.0
  specified site NEC A43.8
Nocturia R35.1
  psychogenic F45.8
Nocturnal — see condition
Nodal rhythm I49.8
Node(s) (see also Nodule)
  Bouchard's (with arthropathy) M15.2
  Haygarth's M15.8
  Heberden's (with arthropathy) M15.1
  larynx J38.7
  lymph — see condition
  milker's B08.03
  Osler's I33.0
  Schmorl's — see Schmorl's disease
  singer's J38.2
  teacher's J38.2
  tuberculous — see Tuberculosis, lymph gland
  vocal cord J38.2
Nodule(s), **nodular**
  actinomycotic — see Actinomycosis
  breast NEC (see also Lump, breast) N63.0
  colloid (cystic), thyroid E04.1
  cutaneous — see Swelling, localized
  endometrial (stromal) D26.1
  Haygarth's M15.8
  inflammatory — see Inflammation
  juxta-articular
    syphilitic A52.77
    yaws A66.7
  larynx J38.7
  lung, solitary (subsegmental branch of the bronchial
    tree) R91.1
    multiple R91.8
  milker's B08.03
  prostate N40.2
    with lower urinary tract symptoms (LUTS) N40.3
    without lower urinary tract symtpoms (LUTS) N40
  pulmonary, solitary (subsegmental branch of the
    bronchial tree) R91.1
  retrocardiac R09.89
  rheumatoid M06.30
    ankle M06.37- ☑
    elbow M06.32- ☑
    foot joint M06.37- ☑
    hand joint M06.34- ☑

Nodule(s), **nodular** — *continued*
  rheumatoid — *continued*
    hip M06.35- ☑
    knee M06.36- ☑
    multiple site M06.39
    shoulder M06.31- ☑
    vertebra M06.38
    wrist M06.33- ☑
  scrotum (inflammatory) N49.2
  singer's J38.2
  solitary, lung (subsegmental branch of the bronchial tree) R91.1
    multiple R91.8
  subcutaneous — *see* Swelling, localized
  teacher's J38.2
  thyroid (cold) (gland) (nontoxic) E04.1
    with thyrotoxicosis E05.20
      with thyroid storm E05.21
    toxic or with hyperthyroidism E05.20
      with thyroid storm E05.21
  vocal cord J38.2
Noma (gangrenous) (hospital) (infective) A69.0
  auricle I96
  mouth A69.0
  pudendi N76.89
  vulvae N76.89
Nomad, nomadism Z59.0
NOMID (neonatal onset multisystemic inflammatory disorder) M04.2
Nonadherence to medical treatment Z91.19
Nonautoimmune hemolytic anemia D59.4
  drug-induced D59.2
Nonclosure (*see also* Imperfect, closure)
  ductus arteriosus (Botallo's) Q25.0
  foramen
    botalli Q21.1
    ovale Q21.1
Noncompliance Z91.19
  with
    dialysis Z91.15
    dietary regimen Z91.11
    medical treatment Z91.19
    medication regimen NEC Z91.14
      underdosing (*see also* Table of Drugs and Chemicals, categories T36-T50, with final character 6) Z91.14
        intentional NEC Z91.128
          due to financial hardship of patient Z91.120
        unintentional NEC Z91.138
          due to patient's age related debility Z91.130
    renal dialysis Z91.15
Nondescent (congenital) (*see also* Malposition, congenital)
  cecum Q43.3
  colon Q43.3
  testicle Q53.9
    bilateral Q53.20
      abdominal Q53.211
      perineal Q53.22
    unilateral Q53.10
      abdominal Q53.111
      perineal Q53.12
Nondevelopment
  brain Q02
    part of Q04.3
  heart Q24.8
  organ or site, congenital NEC — *see* Hypoplasia
Nonengagement
  head NEC O32.4 ☑
    in labor, causing obstructed labor O64.8 ☑
Nonexanthematous tick fever A93.2
Nonexpansion, lung (newborn) P28.0
Nonfunctioning
  cystic duct (*see also* Disease, gallbladder) K82.8
  gallbladder (*see also* Disease, gallbladder) K82.8
  kidney N28.9
  labyrinth — *see* subcategory H83.2 ☑
Non-Hodgkin lymphoma NEC — *see* Lymphoma, non-Hodgkin
Nonimplantation, ovum N97.2
Noninsufflation, fallopian tube N97.1
Non-ketotic hyperglycinemia E72.51
Nonne-Milroy syndrome Q82.0
Non-palpable testicle(s)
  bilateral R39.84

Non-palpable testicle(s) — *continued*
  unilateral R39.83
Nonpatent fallopian tube N97.1
Nonpneumatization, lung NEC P28.0
Nonrotation — *see* Malrotation
Nonsecretion, urine — *see* Anuria
Nonunion
  fracture — *see* Fracture, by site
  joint, following fusion or arthrodesis M96.0
  organ or site, congenital NEC — *see* Imperfect, closure
  symphysis pubis, congenital Q74.2
Nonvisualization, gallbladder R93.2
Nonvital, nonvitalized tooth K04.99
Non-working side interference M26.56
Noonan's syndrome Q87.1
Normocytic anemia (infectional) due to blood loss (chronic) D50.0
  acute D62
Norrie's disease (congenital) Q15.8
North American blastomycosis B40.9
Norwegian itch B86
Nose, nasal — *see* condition
Nosebleed R04.0
Nose-picking F98.8
Nosomania F45.21
Nosophobia F45.22
Nostalgia F43.20
Notch of iris Q13.2
Notching nose, congenital (tip) Q30.2
Nothnagel's
  syndrome — *see* Strabismus, paralytic, third nerve
  vasomotor acroparesthesia I73.89
Novy's relapsing fever A68.9
  louse-borne A68.0
  tick-borne A68.1
Noxious
  foodstuffs, poisoning by — *see* Poisoning, food, noxious, plant
  substances transmitted through placenta or breast milk P04.9
Nucleus pulposus — *see* condition
Numbness R20.0
Nuns' knee — *see* Bursitis, prepatellar
Nursemaid's elbow S53.03- ☑
Nutcracker esophagus K22.4
Nutmeg liver K76.1
Nutrient element deficiency E61.9
  specified NEC E61.8
Nutrition deficient or insufficient (*see also* Malnutrition) E46
  due to
    insufficient food T73.0 ☑
    lack of
      care (child) T76.02 ☑
        adult T76.01 ☑
      food T73.0 ☑
Nutritional stunting E45
Nyctalopia (night blindness) — *see* Blindness, night
Nycturia R35.1
  psychogenic F45.8
Nymphomania F52.8
Nystagmus H55.00
  benign paroxysmal — *see* Vertigo, benign paroxysmal
  central positional H81.4- ☑
  congenital H55.01
  dissociated H55.04
  latent H55.02
  miners' H55.09
  positional
    benign paroxysmal H81.4- ☑
    central H81.4- ☑
  specified form NEC H55.09
  visual deprivation H55.03

O

Obermeyer's relapsing fever (European) A68.0
Obesity E66.9
  with alveolar hypoventilation E66.2
  adrenal E27.8
  complicating
    childbirth O99.214
    pregnancy O99.21- ☑
    puerperium O99.215
  constitutional E66.8
  dietary counseling and surveillance Z71.3
  drug-induced E66.1

Obesity — *continued*
  due to
    drug E66.1
    excess calories E66.09
      morbid E66.01
      severe E66.01
  endocrine E66.8
  endogenous E66.8
  exogenous E66.09
  familial E66.8
  glandular E66.8
  hypothyroid — *see* Hypothyroidism
  hypoventilation syndrome (OHS) E66.2
  morbid E66.01
    with
      alveolar hypoventilation E66.2
      obesity hypoventilation syndrome (OHS) E66.2
    due to excess calories E66.01
  nutritional E66.09
  pituitary E23.6
  severe E66.01
  specified type NEC E66.8
Oblique — *see* condition
Obliteration
  appendix (lumen) K38.8
  artery I77.1
  bile duct (noncalculous) K83.1
  common duct (noncalculous) K83.1
  cystic duct — *see* Obstruction, gallbladder
  disease, arteriolar I77.1
  endometrium N85.8
  eye, anterior chamber — *see* Disorder, globe, hypotony
  fallopian tube N97.1
  lymphatic vessel I89.0
    due to mastectomy I97.2
  organ or site, congenital NEC — *see* Atresia, by site
  ureter N13.5
    with infection N13.6
  urethra — *see* Stricture, urethra
  vein I87.8
  vestibule (oral) K08.89
Observation (following) (for) (without need for further medical care) Z04.9
  accident NEC Z04.3
    at work Z04.2
    transport Z04.1
  adverse effect of drug Z03.6
  alleged rape or sexual assault (victim), ruled out
    adult Z04.41
    child Z04.42
  criminal assault Z04.89
  development state
    adolescent Z00.3
    period of rapid growth in childhood Z00.2
    puberty Z00.3
  disease, specified NEC Z03.89
  following work accident Z04.2
  forced sexual exploitation Z04.81
  forced labor exploitation Z04.82
  growth and development state — *see* Observation, development state
  injuries (accidental) NEC (*see also* Observation, accident)
  newborn (for)
    suspected condition, related to exposure from the mother or birth process — *see* Newborn, affected by, maternal
      ruled out Z05.9
        cardiac Z05.0
        connective tissue Z05.73
        gastrointestinal Z05.5
        genetic Z05.41
        genitourinary Z05.6
        immunologic Z05.43
        infectious Z05.1
        metabolic Z05.42
        musculoskeletal Z05.72
        neurological Z05.2
        respiratory Z05.3
        skin and subcutaneous tissue Z05.71
        specified condition NEC Z05.8
  postpartum
    immediately after delivery Z39.0
    routine follow-up Z39.2
  pregnancy (normal) (without complication) Z34.9- ☑
    high risk O09.9- ☑
  suicide attempt, alleged NEC Z03.89
    self-poisoning Z03.6

Observation — continued
- suspected, ruled out (*see also* Suspected condition, ruled out)
  - abuse, physical
    - adult Z04.71
    - child Z04.72
  - accident at work Z04.2
  - adult battering victim Z04.71
  - child battering victim Z04.72
  - condition NEC Z03.89
    - newborn (*see also* Observation, newborn (for), suspected condition, ruled out) Z05.9
  - drug poisoning or adverse effect Z03.6
  - exposure (to)
    - anthrax Z03.810
    - biological agent NEC Z03.818
  - inflicted injury NEC Z04.89
  - suicide attempt, alleged Z03.89
    - self-poisoning Z03.6
  - toxic effects from ingested substance (drug) (poison) Z03.6
  - toxic effects from ingested substance (drug) (poison) Z03.6

Obsession, obsessional state F42.8
- mixed thoughts and acts F42.2

Obsessive-compulsive neurosis or reaction F42.8

Obstetric embolism, septic — *see* Embolism, obstetric, septic

Obstetrical trauma (complicating delivery) O71.9
- with or following ectopic or molar pregnancy O08.6
- specified type NEC O71.89

Obstipation — *see* Constipation

Obstruction, obstructed, obstructive
- airway J98.8
  - with
    - allergic alveolitis J67.9
    - asthma J45.909
      - with
        - exacerbation (acute) J45.901
        - status asthmaticus J45.902
    - bronchiectasis J47.9
      - with
        - exacerbation (acute) J47.1
        - lower respiratory infection J47.0
    - bronchitis (chronic) J44.9
    - emphysema J43.9
    - chronic J44.9
      - with
        - allergic alveolitis — *see* Pneumonitis, hypersensitivity
        - bronchiectasis J47.9
          - with
            - exacerbation (acute) J47.1
            - lower respiratory infection J47.0
  - due to
    - foreign body — *see* Foreign body, by site, causing asphyxia
    - inhalation of fumes or vapors J68.9
    - laryngospasm J38.5
- ampulla of Vater K83.1
- aortic (heart) (valve) — *see* Stenosis, aortic
- aortoiliac I74.09
- aqueduct of Sylvius G91.1
  - congenital Q03.0
    - with spina bifida — *see* Spina bifida, by site, with hydrocephalus
- Arnold-Chiari — *see* Arnold-Chiari disease
- artery (*see also* Atherosclerosis, artery) I70.9 ☑
  - basilar (complete) (partial) — *see* Occlusion, artery, basilar
  - carotid (complete) (partial) — *see* Occlusion, artery, carotid
  - cerebellar — *see* Occlusion, artery, cerebellar
  - cerebral (anterior) (middle) (posterior) — *see* Occlusion, artery, cerebral
  - precerebral — *see* Occlusion, artery, precerebral
  - renal N28.0
  - retinal NEC — *see* Occlusion, artery, retina
  - stent — *see* Restenosis, stent
  - vertebral (complete) (partial) — *see* Occlusion, artery, vertebral
- band (intestinal) (*see also* Obstruction, intestine, specified NEC) K56.699
- bile duct or passage (common) (hepatic) (noncalculous) K83.1
  - with calculus K80.51
  - congenital (causing jaundice) Q44.3
- biliary (duct) (tract) K83.1

Obstruction, obstructed, obstructive — continued
- biliary — continued
  - gallbladder K82.0
- bladder-neck (acquired) N32.0
  - congenital Q64.31
  - due to hyperplasia (hypertrophy) of prostate — *see* Hyperplasia, prostate
- bowel — *see* Obstruction, intestine
- bronchus J98.09
- canal, ear — *see* Stenosis, external ear canal
- cardia K22.2
- caval veins (inferior) (superior) I87.1
- cecum — *see* Obstruction, intestine
- circulatory I99.8
- colon — *see* Obstruction, intestine
- common duct (noncalculous) K83.1
- coronary (artery) — *see* Occlusion, coronary
- cystic duct (*see also* Obstruction, gallbladder)
  - with calculus K80.21
- device, implant or graft (*see also* Complications, by site and type, mechanical) T85.698 ☑
  - arterial graft NEC — *see* Complication, cardiovascular device, mechanical, vascular
  - catheter NEC T85.628 ☑
    - cystostomy T83.090 ☑
    - dialysis (renal) T82.49 ☑
      - intraperitoneal T85.691 ☑
    - Hopkins T83.098 ☑
    - ileostomy T83.098 ☑
    - infusion NEC T82.594 ☑
      - spinal (epidural) (subdural) T85.690 ☑
    - nephrostomy T83.092 ☑
    - urethral indwelling T83.091 ☑
    - urinary T83.098 ☑
    - urostomy T83.098 ☑
  - due to infection T85.79 ☑
  - gastrointestinal — *see* Complications, prosthetic device, mechanical, gastrointestinal device
  - genital NEC T83.498 ☑
    - intrauterine contraceptive device T83.39 ☑
    - penile prosthesis (cylinder) (implanted) (pump) (resevoir) T83.490 ☑
    - testicular prosthesis T83.491 ☑
  - heart NEC — *see* Complication, cardiovascular device, mechanical
  - joint prosthesis — *see* Complications, joint prosthesis, mechanical, specified NEC, by site
  - orthopedic NEC — *see* Complication, orthopedic, device, mechanical
  - specified NEC T85.628 ☑
  - urinary NEC (*see also* Complication, genitourinary, device, urinary, mechanical)
    - graft T83.29 ☑
  - vascular NEC — *see* Complication, cardiovascular device, mechanical
  - ventricular intracranial shunt T85.09 ☑
- due to foreign body accidentally left in operative wound T81.529 ☑
- duodenum K31.5
- ejaculatory duct N50.89
- esophagus K22.2
- eustachian tube (complete) (partial) H68.10- ☑
  - cartilagenous (extrinsic) H68.13- ☑
    - intrinsic H68.12- ☑
  - osseous H68.11- ☑
- fallopian tube (bilateral) N97.1
- fecal K56.41
  - with hernia — *see* Hernia, by site, with obstruction
- foramen of Monro (congenital) Q03.8
  - with spina bifida — *see* Spina bifida, by site, with hydrocephalus
- foreign body — *see* Foreign body
- gallbladder K82.0
  - with calculus, stones K80.21
  - congenital Q44.1
- gastric outlet K31.1
- gastrointestinal — *see* Obstruction, intestine
- hepatic K76.89
  - duct (noncalculous) K83.1
- ileum — *see* Obstruction, intestine
- iliofemoral (artery) I74.5
- intestine K56.609
  - with
    - adhesions (intestinal) (peritoneal) K56.50
      - complete K56.52
      - incomplete K56.51
      - partial K56.51

Obstruction, obstructed, obstructive — continued
- intestine — continued
  - adynamic K56.0
  - by gallstone K56.3
  - complete K56.601
  - congenital (small) Q41.9
    - large Q42.9
      - specified part NEC Q42.8
  - incomplete K56.600
  - neurogenic K56.0
    - Hirschsprung's disease or megacolon Q43.1
  - newborn P76.9
    - due to
      - fecaliths P76.8
      - inspissated milk P76.2
      - meconium (plug) P76.0
        - in mucoviscidosis E84.11
    - specified NEC P76.8
  - partial K56.600
  - postoperative K91.30
    - complete K91.32
    - incomplete K91.31
    - partial K91.31
  - reflex K56.0
  - specified NEC K56.699
    - complete K56.691
    - incomplete K56.690
    - partial K56.690
  - volvulus K56.2
- intracardiac ball valve prosthesis T82.09 ☑
- jejunum — *see* Obstruction, intestine
- joint prosthesis — *see* Complications, joint prosthesis mechanical, specified NEC, by site
- kidney (calices) N28.89
- labor — *see* Delivery
- lacrimal (passages) (duct)
  - by
    - dacryolith — *see* Dacryolith
    - stenosis — *see* Stenosis, lacrimal
  - congenital Q10.5
  - neonatal H04.53- ☑
- lacrimonasal duct — *see* Obstruction, lacrimal
- lacteal, with steatorrhea K90.2
- laryngitis — *see* Laryngitis
- larynx J38.6
  - congenital Q31.8
- lung J98.4
  - disease, chronic J44.9
- lymphatic I89.0
- meconium (plug)
  - newborn P76.0
    - due to fecaliths P76.0
    - in mucoviscidosis E84.11
- mitral — *see* Stenosis, mitral
- nasal J34.89
- nasolacrimal duct (*see also* Obstruction, lacrimal)
  - congenital Q10.5
- nasopharynx J39.2
- nose J34.89
- organ or site, congenital NEC — *see* Atresia, by site
- pancreatic duct K86.89
- parotid duct or gland K11.8
- pelviureteral junction N13.5
  - with hydronephrosis N13.0
  - congenital Q62.39
- pharynx J39.2
- portal (circulation) (vein) I81
- prostate (*see also* Hyperplasia, prostate)
  - valve (urinary) N32.0
- pulmonary valve (heart) I37.0
- pyelonephritis (chronic) N11.1
- pylorus
  - adult K31.1
  - congenital or infantile Q40.0
- rectosigmoid — *see* Obstruction, intestine
- rectum K62.4
- renal N28.89
  - outflow N13.8
  - pelvis, congenital Q62.39
- respiratory J98.8
  - chronic J44.9
- retinal (vessels) H34.9
- salivary duct (any) K11.8
  - with calculus K11.5
- sigmoid — *see* Obstruction, intestine
- sinus (accessory) (nasal) J34.89
- Stensen's duct K11.8
- stomach NEC K31.89

☑ **Additional Character Required** — **Refer to the Tabular List for Character Selection**   Subterms under main terms may continue to next column or page

Obstruction, obstructed, obstructive — *continued*
  stomach — *continued*
    acute K31.0
    congenital Q40.2
    due to pylorospasm K31.3
  submandibular duct K11.8
  submaxillary gland K11.8
    with calculus K11.5
  thoracic duct I89.0
  thrombotic — *see* Thrombosis
  trachea J39.8
  tracheostomy airway J95.03
  tricuspid (valve) — *see* Stenosis, tricuspid
  upper respiratory, congenital Q34.8
  ureter (functional) (pelvic junction) NEC N13.5
    with
      hydronephrosis N13.1
        with infection N13.6
      pyelonephritis (chronic) N11.1
      congenital Q62.39
    due to calculus — *see* Calculus, ureter
  urethra NEC N36.8
    congenital Q64.39
  urinary (moderate) N13.9
    due to hyperplasia (hypertrophy) of prostate — *see* Hyperplasia, prostate
    organ or tract (lower) N13.9
    prostatic valve N32.0
    specified NEC N13.8
  uropathy N13.9
  uterus N85.8
  vagina N89.5
  valvular — *see* Endocarditis
  vein, venous I87.1
    caval (inferior) (superior) I87.1
    thrombotic — *see* Thrombosis
  vena cava (inferior) (superior) I87.1
  vesical NEC N32.0
  vesicourethral orifice N32.0
    congenital Q64.31
  vessel NEC I99.8
    stent — *see* Restenosis, stent
Obturator — *see* condition
Occlusal wear, teeth K03.0
Occlusio pupillae — *see* Membrane, pupillary
Occlusion, occluded
  anus K62.4
    congenital Q42.3
      with fistula Q42.2
  aortoiliac (chronic) I74.09
  aqueduct of Sylvius G91.1
    congenital Q03.0
      with spina bifida — *see* Spina bifida, by site, with hydrocephalus
  artery (*see also* Atherosclerosis, artery) I70.9 ☑
    auditory, internal I65.8
    basilar I65.1
      with
        infarction I63.22
          due to
            embolism I63.12
            thrombosis I63.02
    brain or cerebral I66.9
      with infarction (due to) I63.5- ☑
        embolism I63.4- ☑
        thrombosis I63.3- ☑
    carotid I65.2- ☑
      with
        infarction I63.23- ☑
          due to
            embolism I63.13- ☑
            thrombosis I63.03- ☑
    cerebellar (anterior inferior) (posterior inferior) (superior) I66.3
      with infarction I63.54- ☑
        due to
          embolism I63.44- ☑
          thrombosis I63.34- ☑
    cerebral I66.9
      with infarction I63.50
        due to
          embolism I63.40
            specified NEC I63.49
          thrombosis I63.30
            specified NEC I63.39
      anterior I66.1- ☑
        with infarction I63.52- ☑

Occlusion, occluded — *continued*
  artery (*see also* Atherosclerosis, artery) — *continued*
    cerebral — *continued*
      anterior — *continued*
        with infarction — *continued*
          due to
            embolism I63.42- ☑
            thrombosis I63.32- ☑
      middle I66.0- ☑
        with infarction I63.51- ☑
          due to
            embolism I63.41- ☑
            thrombosis I63.31- ☑
      posterior I66.2- ☑
        with infarction I63.53- ☑
          due to
            embolism I63.43- ☑
            thrombosis I63.33- ☑
      specified NEC I66.8
        with infarction I63.59
          due to
            embolism I63.4- ☑
            thrombosis I63.3- ☑
    choroidal (anterior) — *see* Occlusion, artery, precerebral, specified NEC
    communicating posterior — *see* Occlusion, artery, precerebral, specified NEC
    complete
      coronary I25.82
      extremities I70.92
    coronary (acute) (thrombotic) (without myocardial infarction) I24.0
      with myocardial infarction — *see* Infarction, myocardium
      chronic total I25.82
      complete I25.82
      healed or old I25.2
      total (chronic) I25.82
    hypophyseal — *see* Occlusion, artery, precerebral, specified NEC
    iliac I74.5
    lower extremities due to stenosis or stricture I77.1
    mesenteric (embolic) (thrombotic) (*see also* Infarct, intestine) K55.069
    perforating — *see* Occlusion, artery, cerebral, specified NEC
    peripheral I77.9
      thrombotic or embolic I74.4
    pontine — *see* Occlusion, artery, precerebral, specified NEC
    precerebral I65.9
      with infarction I63.20
        specified NEC I63.29
          due to
            embolism I63.10
              specified NEC I63.19
            thrombosis I63.00
              specified NEC I63.09
      basilar — *see* Occlusion, artery, basilar
      carotid — *see* Occlusion, artery, carotid
      puerperal O88.23
      specified NEC I65.8
        with infarction I63.29
          due to
            embolism I63.19
            thrombosis I63.09
      vertebral — *see* Occlusion, artery, vertebral
    renal N28.0
    retinal
      branch H34.23- ☑
      central H34.1- ☑
      partial H34.21- ☑
      transient H34.0- ☑
    spinal — *see* Occlusion, artery, precerebral, vertebral
    total (chronic)
      coronary I25.82
      extremities I70.92
    vertebral I65.0- ☑
      with
        infarction I63.21- ☑
          due to
            embolism I63.11- ☑
            thrombosis I63.01- ☑
  basilar artery — *see* Occlusion, artery, basilar
  bile duct (common) (hepatic) (noncalculous) K83.1
  bowel — *see* Obstruction, intestine

Occlusion, occluded — *continued*
  carotid (artery) (common) (internal) — *see* Occlusion, artery, carotid
  centric (of teeth) M26.59
    maximum intercuspation discrepancy M26.55
  cerebellar (artery) — *see* Occlusion, artery, cerebellar
  cerebral (artery) — *see* Occlusion, artery, cerebral
  cerebrovascular (*see also* Occlusion, artery, cerebral)
    with infarction I63.5- ☑
  cervical canal — *see* Stricture, cervix
  cervix (uteri) — *see* Stricture, cervix
  choanal Q30.0
  choroidal (artery) — *see* Occlusion, artery, precerebral, specified NEC
  colon — *see* Obstruction, intestine
  communicating posterior artery — *see* Occlusion, artery, precerebral, specified NEC
  coronary (artery) (vein) (thrombotic) (*see also* Infarct, myocardium)
    chronic total I25.82
    healed or old I25.2
    not resulting in infarction I24.0
    total (chronic) I25.82
  cystic duct — *see* Obstruction, gallbladder
  embolic — *see* Embolism
  fallopian tube N97.1
    congenital Q50.6
  gallbladder (*see also* Obstruction, gallbladder)
    congenital (causing jaundice) Q44.1
  gingiva, traumatic K06.2
  hymen N89.6
    congenital Q52.3
  hypophyseal (artery) — *see* Occlusion, artery, precerebral, specified NEC
  iliac artery I74.5
  intestine — *see* Obstruction, intestine
  lacrimal passages — *see* Obstruction, lacrimal
  lung J98.4
  lymph or lymphatic channel I89.0
  mammary duct N64.89
  mesenteric artery (embolic) (thrombotic) (*see also* Infarct, intestine) K55.069
  nose J34.89
    congenital Q30.0
  organ or site, congenital NEC — *see* Atresia, by site
  oviduct N97.1
    congenital Q50.6
  peripheral arteries
    due to stricture or stenosis I77.1
    upper extremity I74.2
  pontine (artery) — *see* Occlusion, artery, precerebral, specified NEC
  posterior lingual, of mandibular teeth M26.29
  precerebral artery — *see* Occlusion, artery, precerebral
  punctum lacrimale — *see* Obstruction, lacrimal
  pupil — *see* Membrane, pupillary
  pylorus, adult (*see also* Stricture, pylorus) K31.1
  renal artery N28.0
  retina, retinal
    artery — *see* Occlusion, artery, retinal
    vein (central) H34.81- ☑
      engorgement H34.82- ☑
      tributary H34.83- ☑
    vessels H34.9
  spinal artery — *see* Occlusion, artery, precerebral, vertebral
  teeth (mandibular) (posterior lingual) M26.29
  thoracic duct I89.0
  thrombotic — *see* Thrombosis, artery
  traumatic
    edentulous (alveolar) ridge K06.2
    gingiva K06.2
    periodontal K05.5
  tubal N97.1
  ureter (complete) (partial) N13.5
    congenital Q62.10
  ureteropelvic junction N13.5
    congenital Q62.11
  ureterovesical orifice N13.5
    congenital Q62.12
  urethra — *see* Stricture, urethra
  uterus N85.8
  vagina N89.5
  vascular NEC I99.8
  vein — *see* Thrombosis
    retinal — *see* Occlusion, retinal, vein
  vena cava (inferior) (superior) — *see* Embolism, vena cava

Occlusion, occluded — *continued*
  ventricle (brain) NEC G91.1
  vertebral (artery) — *see* Occlusion, artery, vertebral
  vessel (blood) I99.8
  vulva N90.5
Occult
  blood in feces (stools) R19.5
Occupational
  problems NEC Z56.89
Ochlophobia — *see* Agoraphobia
Ochronosis (endogenous) E70.29
Ocular muscle — *see* condition
Oculogyric crisis or disturbance H51.8
  psychogenic F45.8
Oculomotor syndrome H51.9
Oculopathy
  syphilitic NEC A52.71
    congenital
      early A50.01
      late A50.30
    early (secondary) A51.43
    late A52.71
Oddi's sphincter spasm K83.4
Odontalgia K08.89
Odontoameloblastoma — *see* Cyst, calcifying odonto-genic
Odontoclasia K03.89
Odontodysplasia, regional K00.4
Odontogenesis imperfecta K00.5
Odontoma (ameloblastic) (complex) (compound) (fibroameloblastic) — *see* Cyst, calcifying odontogenic
Odontomyelitis (closed) (open) K04.01
  irreversible K04.02
  reversible K04.01
Odontorrhagia K08.89
Odontosarcoma, ameloblastic C41.1
  upper jaw (bone) C41.0
Oestriasis — *see* Myiasis
Oguchi's disease H53.63
Ohara's disease — *see* Tularemia
OHS (obesity hypoventilation syndrome) E66.2
Oidiomycosis — *see* Candidiasis
Oidium albicans infection — *see* Candidiasis
Old age (without mention of debility) R54
  dementia F03 ☑
Old (previous) **myocardial infarction** I25.2
Olfactory — *see* condition
Oligemia — *see* Anemia
Oligoastrocytoma
  specified site — *see* Neoplasm, malignant, by site
  unspecified site C71.9
Oligocythemia D64.9
Oligodendroblastoma
  specified site — *see* Neoplasm, malignant
  unspecified site C71.9
Oligodendroglioma
  anaplastic type
    specified site — *see* Neoplasm, malignant, by site
    unspecified site C71.9
  specified site — *see* Neoplasm, malignant, by site
  unspecified site C71.9
Oligodontia — *see* Anodontia
Oligoencephalon Q02
Oligohidrosis L74.4
Oligohydramnios O41.0- ☑
Oligohydrosis L74.4
Oligomenorrhea N91.5
  primary N91.3
  secondary N91.4
Oligophrenia (*see also* Disability, intellectual)
  phenylpyruvic E70.0
Oligospermia N46.11
  due to
    drug therapy N46.121
    efferent duct obstruction N46.123
    infection N46.122
    radiation N46.124
    specified cause NEC N46.129
    systemic disease N46.125
Oligotrichia — *see* Alopecia
Oliguria R34
  with, complicating or following ectopic or molar pregnancy O08.4
  postprocedural N99.0
Ollier's disease Q78.4
Omenotocele — *see* Hernia, abdomen, specified site NEC
Omentitis — *see* Peritonitis

Omentum, omental — *see* condition
Omphalitis (congenital) (newborn) P38.9
  with mild hemorrhage P38.1
  without hemorrhage P38.9
  not of newborn L08.82
  tetanus A33
Omphalocele Q79.2
Omphalomesenteric duct, persistent Q43.0
Omphalorrhagia, newborn P51.9
Omsk hemorrhagic fever A98.1
Onanism (excessive) F98.8
Onchocerciasis, onchocercosis B73.1
  with
    eye disease B73.00
      endophthalmitis B73.01
      eyelid B73.09
      glaucoma B73.02
      specified NEC B73.09
  eyelid B73.09
  eye NEC B73.00
Oncocytoma — *see* Neoplasm, benign, by site
Oncovirus, as cause of disease classified elsewhere B97.32
Ondine's curse — *see* Apnea, sleep
Oneirophrenia F23
Onychauxis L60.2
  congenital Q84.5
Onychia (*see also* Cellulitis, digit)
  with lymphangitis — *see* Lymphangitis, acute, digit
  candidal B37.2
  dermatophytic B35.1
Onychitis (*see also* Cellulitis, digit)
  with lymphangitis — *see* Lymphangitis, acute, digit
Onychocryptosis L60.0
Onychodystrophy L60.3
  congenital Q84.6
Onychogryphosis, onychogryposis L60.2
Onycholysis L60.1
Onychomadesis L60.8
Onychomalacia L60.3
Onychomycosis (finger) (toe) B35.1
Onycho-osteodysplasia Q87.2
Onychophagia F98.8
Onychophosis L60.8
Onychoptosis L60.8
Onychorrhexis L60.3
  congenital Q84.6
Onychoschizia L60.3
Onyxis (finger) (toe) L60.0
Onyxitis (*see also* Cellulitis, digit)
  with lymphangitis — *see* Lymphangitis, acute, digit
Oophoritis (cystic) (infectional) (interstitial) N70.92
  with salpingitis N70.93
  acute N70.02
    with salpingitis N70.03
  chronic N70.12
    with salpingitis N70.13
  complicating abortion — *see* Abortion, by type, complicated by, oophoritis
Oophorocele N83.4- ☑
Opacity, opacities
  cornea H17.- ☑
    central H17.1- ☑
    congenital Q13.3
    degenerative — *see* Degeneration, cornea
    hereditary — *see* Dystrophy, cornea
    inflammatory — *see* Keratitis
    minor H17.81- ☑
    peripheral H17.82- ☑
    sequelae of trachoma (healed) B94.0
    specified NEC H17.89
  enamel (teeth) (fluoride) (nonfluoride) K00.3
  lens — *see* Cataract
  snowball — *see* Deposit, crystalline
  vitreous (humor) NEC H43.39- ☑
    congenital Q14.0
    membranes and strands H43.31- ☑
Opalescent dentin (hereditary) K00.5
Open, opening
  abnormal, organ or site, congenital — *see* Imperfect, closure
  angle with
    borderline
      findings
        high risk H40.02- ☑
        low risk H40.01- ☑
      intraocular pressure H40.00- ☑

Open, opening — *continued*
  angle with — *continued*
    cupping of discs H40.01- ☑
    glaucoma (primary) — *see* Glaucoma, open angle
  bite
    anterior M26.220
    posterior M26.221
  false — *see* Imperfect, closure
  margin on tooth restoration K08.51
  restoration margins of tooth K08.51
  wound — *see* Wound, open
Operational fatigue F48.8
Operative — *see* condition
Operculitis — *see* Periodontitis
Operculum — *see* Break, retina
Ophiasis L63.2
Ophthalmia (*see also* Conjunctivitis) H10.9
  actinic rays — *see* Photokeratitis
  allergic (acute) — *see* Conjunctivitis, acute, atopic
  blennorrhagic (gonococcal) (neonatorum) A54.31
  diphtheritic A36.86
  Egyptian A71.1
  electrica — *see* Photokeratitis
  gonococcal (neonatorum) A54.31
  metastatic — *see* Endophthalmitis, purulent
  migraine — *see* Migraine, ophthalmoplegic
  neonatorum, newborn P39.1
    gonococcal A54.31
  nodosa H16.24- ☑
  purulent — *see* Conjunctivitis, acute, mucopurulent
  spring — *see* Conjunctivitis, acute, atopic
  sympathetic — *see* Uveitis, sympathetic
Ophthalmitis — *see* Ophthalmia
Ophthalmocele (congenital) Q15.8
Ophthalmoneuromyelitis G36.0
Ophthalmoplegia (*see also* Strabismus, paralytic)
  anterior internuclear — *see* Ophthalmoplegia, internuclear
  ataxia-areflexia G61.0
  diabetic — *see* E08-E13 with .39
  exophthalmic E05.00
    with thyroid storm E05.01
  external H49.88- ☑
    progressive H49.4- ☑
      with pigmentary retinopathy — *see* Kearns-Sayre syndrome
    total H49.3- ☑
  internal (complete) (total) H52.51- ☑
  internuclear H51.2- ☑
  migraine — *see* Migraine, ophthalmoplegic
  Parinaud's H49.88- ☑
  progressive external — *see* Ophthalmoplegia, external, progressive
  supranuclear, progressive G23.1
  total (external) — *see* Ophthalmoplegia, external, total
Opioid(s)
  abuse — *see* Abuse, drug, opioids
  dependence — *see* Dependence, drug, opioids
  induced, without use disorder
    anxiety disorder F11.988
    delirium F11.921
    depressive disorder F11.94
    sexual dysfunction F11.981
    sleep disorder F11.982
Opisthognathism M26.09
Opisthorchiasis (felineus) (viverrini) B66.0
Opitz' disease D73.2
Opiumism — *see* Dependence, drug, opioid
Oppenheim's disease G70.2
Oppenheim-Urbach disease (necrobiosis lipoidica diabeticorum) — *see* E08-E13 with .620
Optic nerve — *see* condition
Orbit — *see* condition
Orchioblastoma C62.9- ☑
Orchitis (gangrenous) (nonspecific) (septic) (suppurative) N45.2
  blennorrhagic (gonococcal) (acute) (chronic) A54.23
  chlamydial A56.19
  filarial (*see also* Infestation, filarial) B74.9 [N51]
  gonococcal (acute) (chronic) A54.23
  mumps B26.0
  syphilitic A52.76
  tuberculous A18.15
Orf (virus disease) B08.02
Organic (*see also* condition)
  brain syndrome F09
  heart — *see* Disease, heart

Organic — *continued*
  mental disorder F09
  psychosis F09
Orgasm
  anejaculatory N53.13
Oriental
  bilharziasis B65.2
  schistosomiasis B65.2
Orifice — *see* condition
Origin of both great vessels from right ventricle Q20.1
Ormond's disease (with ureteral obstruction) N13.5
  with infection N13.6
Ornithine metabolism disorder E72.4
Ornithinemia (Type I) (Type II) E72.4
Ornithosis A70
Orotaciduria, oroticaciduria (congenital) (hereditary) (pyrimidine deficiency) E79.8
  anemia D53.0
Orthodontics
  adjustment Z46.4
  fitting Z46.4
Orthopnea R06.01
Orthopoxvirus B08.09
  specified NEC B08.09
Os, uterus — *see* condition
Osgood-Schlatter disease or osteochondrosis — *see* Osteochondrosis, juvenile, tibia
Osler (-Weber)-Rendu disease I78.0
Osler's nodes I33.0
Osmidrosis L75.0
Osseous — *see* condition
Ossification
  artery — *see* Arteriosclerosis
  auricle (ear) — *see* Disorder, pinna, specified type NEC
  bronchial J98.09
  cardiac — *see* Degeneration, myocardial
  cartilage (senile) — *see* Disorder, cartilage, specified type NEC
  coronary (artery) — *see* Disease, heart, ischemic, atherosclerotic
  diaphragm J98.6
  ear, middle — *see* Otosclerosis
  falx cerebri G96.19
  fontanel, premature Q75.0
  heart (*see also* Degeneration, myocardial)
    valve — *see* Endocarditis
  larynx J38.7
  ligament — *see* Disorder, tendon, specified type NEC
    posterior longitudinal — *see* Spondylopathy, specified NEC
  meninges (cerebral) (spinal) G96.19
  multiple, eccentric centers — *see* Disorder, bone, development or growth
  muscle (*see also* Calcification, muscle)
    due to burns — *see* Myositis, ossificans, in, burns
    paralytic — *see* Myositis, ossificans, in, quadriplegia
    progressive — *see* Myositis, ossificans, progressiva
    specified NEC M61.50
      ankle M61.57- ☑
      foot M61.57- ☑
      forearm M61.53- ☑
      hand M61.54- ☑
      lower leg M61.56- ☑
      multiple sites M61.59
      pelvic region M61.55- ☑
      shoulder region M61.51- ☑
      specified site NEC M61.58
      thigh M61.55- ☑
      upper arm M61.52- ☑
    traumatic — *see* Myositis, ossificans, traumatica
  myocardium, myocardial — *see* Degeneration, myocardial
  penis N48.89
  periarticular — *see* Disorder, joint, specified type NEC
  pinna — *see* Disorder, pinna, specified type NEC
  rider's bone — *see* Ossification, muscle, specified NEC
  sclera H15.89
  subperiosteal, post-traumatic M89.8X- ☑
  tendon — *see* Disorder, tendon, specified type NEC
  trachea J39.8
  tympanic membrane — *see* Disorder, tympanic membrane, specified NEC
  vitreous (humor) — *see* Deposit, crystalline
Osteitis (*see also* Osteomyelitis)
  alveolar M27.3
  condensans M85.30

Osteitis — *continued*
  condensans — *continued*
    ankle M85.37- ☑
    foot M85.37- ☑
    forearm M85.33- ☑
    hand M85.34- ☑
    lower leg M85.36- ☑
    multiple site M85.39
    neck M85.38
    rib M85.38
    shoulder M85.31- ☑
    skull M85.38
    specified site NEC M85.38
    thigh M85.35- ☑
    toe M85.37- ☑
    upper arm M85.32- ☑
    vertebra M85.38
  deformans M88.9
    in (due to)
      malignant neoplasm of bone C41.9 [M90.60]
      neoplastic disease (*see also* Neoplasm) D49.9 [M90.60]
        carpus D49.9 [M90.64-] ☑
        clavicle D49.9 [M90.61-] ☑
        femur D49.9 [M90.65-] ☑
        fibula D49.9 [M90.66-] ☑
        finger D49.9 [M90.64-] ☑
        humerus D49.9 [M90.62-] ☑
        ilium D49.9 [M90.65-] ☑
        ischium D49.9 [M90.65-] ☑
        metacarpus D49.9 [M90.64-] ☑
        metatarsus D49.9 [M90.67-] ☑
        multiple sites D49.9 [M90.69]
        neck D49.9 [M90.68]
        radius D49.9 [M90.63-] ☑
        rib D49.9 [M90.68]
        scapula D49.9 [M90.61-] ☑
        skull D49.9 [M90.68]
        tarsus D49.9 [M90.67-] ☑
        tibia D49.9 [M90.66-] ☑
        toe D49.9 [M90.67-] ☑
        ulna D49.9 [M90.63-] ☑
        vertebra D49.9 [M90.68]
    skull M88.0
    specified NEC — *see* Paget's disease, bone, by site
    vertebra M88.1
  due to yaws A66.6
  fibrosa NEC — *see* Cyst, bone, by site
    circumscripta — *see* Dysplasia, fibrous, bone NEC
    cystica (generalisata) E21.0
    disseminata Q78.1
    osteoplastica E21.0
  fragilitans Q78.0
  Garr's (sclerosing) — *see* Osteomyelitis, specified type NEC
  jaw (acute) (chronic) (lower) (suppurative) (upper) M27.2
  parathyroid E21.0
  petrous bone (acute) (chronic) — *see* Petrositis
  sclerotic, nonsuppurative — *see* Osteomyelitis, specified type NEC
  tuberculosa A18.09
    cystica D86.89
    multiplex cystoides D86.89
Osteoarthritis M19.90
  ankle M19.07- ☑
  elbow M19.02- ☑
  foot joint M19.07- ☑
  generalized M15.9
    erosive M15.4
    primary M15.0
    specified NEC M15.8
  hand joint M19.04- ☑
    first carpometacarpal joint M18.9
  hip M16.1- ☑
    bilateral M16.0
    due to hip dysplasia (unilateral) M16.3- ☑
      bilateral M16.2
  interphalangeal
    distal (Heberden) M15.1
    proximal (Bouchard) M15.2
  knee M17.1- ☑
    bilateral M17.0
  post-traumatic NEC M19.92
    ankle M19.17- ☑
    elbow M19.12- ☑
    foot joint M19.17- ☑

Osteoarthritis — *continued*
  post-traumatic — *continued*
    hand joint M19.14- ☑
      first carpometacarpal joint M18.3- ☑
        bilateral M18.2
    hip M16.5- ☑
      bilateral M16.4
    knee M17.3- ☑
      bilateral M17.2
    shoulder M19.11- ☑
    wrist M19.13- ☑
  primary M19.91
    ankle M19.07- ☑
    elbow M19.02- ☑
    foot joint M19.07- ☑
    hand joint M19.04- ☑
      first carpometacarpal joint M18.1- ☑
        bilateral M18.0
    hip M16.1- ☑
      bilateral M16.0
    knee M17.1- ☑
      bilateral M17.0
    shoulder M19.01- ☑
    spine — *see* Spondylosis
    wrist M19.03- ☑
  secondary M19.93
    ankle M19.27- ☑
    elbow M19.22- ☑
    foot joint M19.27- ☑
    hand joint M19.24- ☑
      first carpometacarpal joint M18.5- ☑
        bilateral M18.4
    hip M16.7
      bilateral M16.6
    knee M17.5
      bilateral M17.4
    multiple M15.3
    shoulder M19.21- ☑
    spine — *see* Spondylosis
    wrist M19.23- ☑
  shoulder M19.01- ☑
  spine — *see* Spondylosis
  wrist M19.03- ☑
Osteoarthropathy (hypertrophic) M19.90
  ankle — *see* Osteoarthritis, primary, ankle
  elbow — *see* Osteoarthritis, primary, elbow
  foot joint — *see* Osteoarthritis, primary, foot
  hand joint — *see* Osteoarthritis, primary, hand joint
  knee joint — *see* Osteoarthritis, primary, knee
  multiple site — *see* Osteoarthritis, primary, multiple joint
  pulmonary (*see also* Osteoarthropathy, specified type NEC)
    hypertrophic — *see* Osteoarthropathy, hypertrophic, specified type NEC
  secondary — *see* Osteoarthropathy, specified type NEC
  secondary hypertrophic — *see* Osteoarthropathy, specified type NEC
  shoulder — *see* Osteoarthritis, primary, shoulder
  specified joint NEC — *see* Osteoarthritis, primary, specified joint NEC
  specified type NEC M89.40
    carpus M89.44- ☑
    clavicle M89.41- ☑
    femur M89.45- ☑
    fibula M89.46- ☑
    finger M89.44- ☑
    humerus M89.42- ☑
    ilium M89.459
    ischium M89.459
    metacarpus M89.44- ☑
    metatarsus M89.47- ☑
    multiple sites M89.49
    neck M89.48
    radius M89.43- ☑
    rib M89.48
    scapula M89.41- ☑
    skull M89.48
    tarsus M89.47- ☑
    tibia M89.46- ☑
    toe M89.47- ☑
    ulna M89.43- ☑
    vertebra M89.48
  spine — *see* Spondylosis
  wrist — *see* Osteoarthritis, primary, wrist
Osteoarthrosis (degenerative) (hypertrophic) (joint) (*see also* Osteoarthritis)

Osteoarthrosis — *continued*
  deformans alkaptonurica E70.29 [M36.8]
  erosive M15.4
  generalized M15.9
    primary M15.0
  polyarticular M15.9
  spine — *see* Spondylosis
Osteoblastoma — *see* Neoplasm, bone, benign
  aggressive — *see* Neoplasm, bone, uncertain behavior
Osteochondritis (*see also* Osteochondropathy, by site)
  Brailsford's — *see* Osteochondrosis, juvenile, radius
  dissecans M93.20
    ankle M93.27- ☑
    elbow M93.22- ☑
    foot M93.27- ☑
    hand M93.24- ☑
    hip M93.25- ☑
    knee M93.26- ☑
    multiple sites M93.29
    shoulder joint M93.21- ☑
    specified site NEC M93.28
    wrist M93.23- ☑
  juvenile M92.9
    patellar — *see* Osteochondrosis, juvenile, patella
  syphilitic (congenital) (early) A50.02 [M90.80]
    ankle A50.02 [M90.87-] ☑
    elbow A50.02 [M90.82-] ☑
    foot A50.02 [M90.87-] ☑
    forearm A50.02 [M90.83-] ☑
    hand A50.02 [M90.84-] ☑
    hip A50.02 [M90.85-] ☑
    knee A50.02 [M90.86-] ☑
    multiple sites A50.02 [M90.89]
    shoulder joint A50.02 [M90.81-] ☑
    specified site NEC A50.02 [M90.88]
Osteochondroarthrosis deformans endemica — *see* Disease, Kaschin-Beck
Osteochondrodysplasia Q78.9
  with defects of growth of tubular bones and spine Q77.9
    specified NEC Q77.8
  specified NEC Q78.8
Osteochondrodystrophy E78.9
Osteochondrolysis — *see* Osteochondritis, dissecans
Osteochondroma — *see* Neoplasm, bone, benign
Osteochondromatosis D48.0
  syndrome Q78.4
Osteochondromyxosarcoma — *see* Neoplasm, bone, malignant
Osteochondropathy M93.90
  ankle M93.97- ☑
  elbow M93.92- ☑
  foot M93.97- ☑
  hand M93.94- ☑
  hip M93.95- ☑
  Kienböck's disease of adults M93.1
  knee M93.96- ☑
  multiple joints M93.99
  osteochondritis dissecans — *see* Osteochondritis, dissecans
  osteochondrosis — *see* Osteochondrosis
  shoulder region M93.91- ☑
  slipped upper femoral epiphysis — *see* Slipped, epiphysis, upper femoral
  specified joint NEC M93.98
  specified type NEC M93.80
    ankle M93.87- ☑
    elbow M93.82- ☑
    foot M93.87- ☑
    hand M93.84- ☑
    hip M93.85- ☑
    knee M93.86- ☑
    multiple joints M93.89
    shoulder region M93.81- ☑
    specified joint NEC M93.88
    wrist M93.83- ☑
  syphilitic, congenital
    early A50.02 [M90.80]
    late A50.56 [M90.80]
  wrist M93.93- ☑
Osteochondrosarcoma — *see* Neoplasm, bone, malignant
Osteochondrosis (*see also* Osteochondropathy, by site)
  acetabulum (juvenile) M91.0
  adult — *see* Osteochondropathy, specified type NEC, by site

Osteochondrosis — *continued*
  astragalus (juvenile) — *see* Osteochondrosis, juvenile, tarsus
  Blount's — *see* Osteochondrosis, juvenile, tibia
  Buchanan's M91.0
  Burns' — *see* Osteochondrosis, juvenile, ulna
  calcaneus (juvenile) — *see* Osteochondrosis, juvenile, tarsus
  capitular epiphysis (femur) (juvenile) — *see* Legg-Calvé-Perthes disease
  carpal (juvenile) (lunate) (scaphoid) — *see* Osteochondrosis, juvenile, hand, carpal lunate
    adult M93.1
  coxae juvenilis — *see* Legg-Calvé-Perthes disease
  deformans juvenilis, coxae — *see* Legg-Calvé-Perthes disease
  Diaz's — *see* Osteochondrosis, juvenile, tarsus
  dissecans (knee) (shoulder) — *see* Osteochondritis, dissecans
  femoral capital epiphysis (juvenile) — *see* Legg-Calvé-Perthes disease
  femur (head), juvenile — *see* Legg-Calvé-Perthes disease
  fibula (juvenile) — *see* Osteochondrosis, juvenile, fibula
  foot NEC (juvenile) M92.8
  Freiberg's — *see* Osteochondrosis, juvenile, metatarsus
  Haas' (juvenile) — *see* Osteochondrosis, juvenile, humerus
  Haglund's — *see* Osteochondrosis, juvenile, tarsus
  hip (juvenile) — *see* Legg-Calvé-Perthes disease
  humerus (capitulum) (head) (juvenile) — *see* Osteochondrosis, juvenile, humerus
  ilium, iliac crest (juvenile) M91.0
  ischiopubic synchondrosis M91.0
  Iselin's — *see* Osteochondrosis, juvenile, metatarsus
  juvenile, juvenilis M92.9
    after congenital dislocation of hip reduction — *see* Osteochondrosis, juvenile, hip, specified NEC
    arm — *see* Osteochondrosis, juvenile, upper limb NEC
    capitular epiphysis (femur) — *see* Legg-Calvé-Perthes disease
    clavicle, sternal epiphysis — *see* Osteochondrosis, juvenile, upper limb NEC
    coxae — *see* Legg-Calvé-Perthes disease
    deformans M92.9
    fibula M92.5- ☑
    foot NEC M92.8
    hand M92.20- ☑
      carpal lunate M92.21- ☑
      metacarpal head M92.22- ☑
      specified site NEC M92.29- ☑
    head of femur — *see* Legg-Calvé-Perthes disease
    hip and pelvis M91.9- ☑
      coxa plana — *see* Coxa, plana
      femoral head — *see* Legg-Calvé-Perthes disease
      pelvis M91.0
      pseudocoxalgia — *see* Pseudocoxalgia
      specified NEC M91.8- ☑
    humerus M92.0- ☑
    limb
      lower NEC M92.8
      upper NEC — *see* Osteochondrosis, juvenile, upper limb NEC
    medial cuneiform bone — *see* Osteochondrosis, juvenile, tarsus
    metatarsus M92.7- ☑
    patella M92.4- ☑
    radius M92.1- ☑
    specified site NEC M92.8
    spine M42.00
      cervical region M42.02
      cervicothoracic region M42.03
      lumbar region M42.06
      lumbosacral region M42.07
      multiple sites M42.09
      occipito-atlanto-axial region M42.01
      sacrococcygeal region M42.08
      thoracic region M42.04
      thoracolumbar region M42.05
    tarsus M92.6- ☑
    tibia M92.5- ☑
    ulna M92.1- ☑
    upper limb NEC M92.3- ☑

Osteochondrosis — *continued*
  juvenile, juvenilis — *continued*
    vertebra (body) (epiphyseal plates) (Calvé's) (Scheuermann's) — *see* Osteochondrosis, juvenile, spine
  Kienböck's — *see* Osteochondrosis, juvenile, hand, carpal lunate
    adult M93.1
  Köhler's
    patellar — *see* Osteochondrosis, juvenile, patella
    tarsal navicular — *see* Osteochondrosis, juvenile, tarsus
  Legg-Perthes (-Calvé)(-Waldenström) — *see* Legg-Calvé-Perthes disease
  limb
    lower NEC (juvenile) M92.8
    upper NEC (juvenile) — *see* Osteochondrosis, juvenile, upper limb NEC
  lunate bone (carpal) (juvenile) (*see also* Osteochondrosis, juvenile, hand, carpal lunate)
    adult M93.1
  Mauclaire's — *see* Osteochondrosis, juvenile, hand, metacarpal
  metacarpal (head) (juvenile) — *see* Osteochondrosis, juvenile, hand, metacarpal
  metatarsus (fifth) (head) (juvenile) (second) — *see* Osteochondrosis, juvenile, metatarsus
  navicular (juvenile) — *see* Osteochondrosis, juvenile, tarsus
  os
    calcis (juvenile) — *see* Osteochondrosis, juvenile, tarsus
    tibiale externum (juvenile) — *see* Osteochondrosis, juvenile, tarsus
  Osgood-Schlatter — *see* Osteochondrosis, juvenile, tibia
  Panner's — *see* Osteochondrosis, juvenile, humerus
  patellar center (juvenile) (primary) (secondary) — *see* Osteochondrosis, juvenile, patella
  pelvis (juvenile) M91.0
  Pierson's M91.0
  radius (head) (juvenile) — *see* Osteochondrosis, juvenile, radius
  Scheuermann's — *see* Osteochondrosis, juvenile, spine
  Sever's — *see* Osteochondrosis, juvenile, tarsus
  Sinding-Larsen — *see* Osteochondrosis, juvenile, patella
  spine M42.9
    adult M42.10
      cervical region M42.12
      cervicothoracic region M42.13
      lumbar region M42.16
      lumbosacral region M42.17
      multiple sites M42.19
      occipito-atlanto-axial region M42.11
      sacrococcygeal region M42.18
      thoracic region M42.14
      thoracolumbar region M42.15
    juvenile — *see* Osteochondrosis, juvenile, spine
  symphysis pubis (juvenile) M91.0
  syphilitic (congenital) A50.02
  talus (juvenile) — *see* Osteochondrosis, juvenile, tarsus
  tarsus (navicular) (juvenile) — *see* Osteochondrosis, juvenile, tarsus
  tibia (proximal) (tubercle) (juvenile) — *see* Osteochondrosis, juvenile, tibia
  tuberculous — *see* Tuberculosis, bone
  ulna (lower) (juvenile) — *see* Osteochondrosis, juvenile, ulna
  van Neck's M91.0
  vertebral — *see* Osteochondrosis, spine
Osteoclastoma D48.0
  malignant — *see* Neoplasm, bone, malignant
Osteodynia — *see* Disorder, bone, specified type NEC
Osteodystrophy Q78.9
  azotemic N25.0
  congenital Q78.9
  parathyroid, secondary E21.1
  renal N25.0
Osteofibroma — *see* Neoplasm, bone, benign
Osteofibrosarcoma — *see* Neoplasm, bone, maligna
Osteogenesis imperfecta Q78.0
Osteogenic — *see* condition
Osteolysis M89.50
  carpus M89.54- ☑
  clavicle M89.51- ☑
  femur M89.55- ☑

☑ **Additional Character Required** — **Refer to the Tabular List for Character Selection**   ▽ **Subterms under main terms may continue to next column or page**

Osteolysis — continued
- fibula M89.56- ☑
- finger M89.54- ☑
- humerus M89.52- ☑
- ilium M89.559
- ischium M89.559
- joint prosthesis (periprosthetic) — see Complications, joint prosthesis, mechanical, periprosthetic, osteolysis, by site
- metacarpus M89.54- ☑
- metatarsus M89.57- ☑
- multiple sites M89.59
- neck M89.58
- periprosthetic — see Complications, joint prosthesis, mechanical, periprosthetic, osteolysis, by site
- radius M89.53- ☑
- rib M89.58
- scapula M89.51- ☑
- skull M89.58
- tarsus M89.57- ☑
- tibia M89.56- ☑
- toe M89.57- ☑
- ulna M89.53- ☑
- vertebra M89.58

Osteoma (see also Neoplasm, bone, benign)
- osteoid (see also Neoplasm, bone, benign)
  - giant — see Neoplasm, bone, benign

Osteomalacia M83.9
- adult M83.9
  - drug-induced NEC M83.5
  - due to
    - malabsorption (postsurgical) M83.2
    - malnutrition M83.3
  - specified NEC M83.8
- aluminium-induced M83.4
- infantile — see Rickets
- juvenile — see Rickets
- oncogenic E83.89
- pelvis M83.8
- puerperal M83.0
- senile M83.1
- vitamin-D-resistant in adults E83.31 [M90.8-] ☑
  - carpus E83.31 [M90.84-] ☑
  - clavicle E83.31 [M90.81-] ☑
  - femur E83.31 [M90.85-] ☑
  - fibula E83.31 [M90.86-] ☑
  - finger E83.31 [M90.84-] ☑
  - humerus E83.31 [M90.82-] ☑
  - ilium E83.31 [M90.859]
  - ischium E83.31 [M90.859]
  - metacarpus E83.31 [M90.84-] ☑
  - metatarsus E83.31 [M90.87-] ☑
  - multiple sites E83.31 [M90.89]
  - neck E83.31 [M90.88]
  - radius E83.31 [M90.83-] ☑
  - rib E83.31 [M90.88]
  - scapula E83.31 [M90.819]
  - skull E83.31 [M90.88]
  - tarsus E83.31 [M90.879]
  - tibia E83.31 [M90.869]
  - toe E83.31 [M90.879]
  - ulna E83.31 [M90.839]
  - vertebra E83.31 [M90.88]

Osteomyelitis (general) (infective) (localized) (neonatal) (purulent) (septic) (staphylococcal) (streptococcal) (suppurative) (with periostitis) M86.9
- acute M86.10
  - carpus M86.14- ☑
  - clavicle M86.11- ☑
  - femur M86.15- ☑
  - fibula M86.16- ☑
  - finger M86.14- ☑
  - hematogenous M86.00
    - carpus M86.04- ☑
    - clavicle M86.01- ☑
    - femur M86.05- ☑
    - fibula M86.06- ☑
    - finger M86.04- ☑
    - humerus M86.02- ☑
    - ilium M86.059
    - ischium M86.059
    - mandible M27.2
    - metacarpus M86.04- ☑
    - metatarsus M86.07- ☑
    - multiple sites M86.09
    - neck M86.08
    - orbit H05.02- ☑

Osteomyelitis — continued
- acute — continued
  - hematogenous — continued
    - petrous bone — see Petrositis
    - radius M86.03- ☑
    - rib M86.08
    - scapula M86.01- ☑
    - skull M86.08
    - tarsus M86.07- ☑
    - tibia M86.06- ☑
    - toe M86.07- ☑
    - ulna M86.03- ☑
    - vertebra — see Osteomyelitis, vertebra
  - humerus M86.12- ☑
  - ilium M86.159
  - ischium M86.159
  - mandible M27.2
  - metacarpus M86.14- ☑
  - metatarsus M86.17- ☑
  - multiple sites M86.19
  - neck M86.18
  - orbit H05.02- ☑
  - petrous bone — see Petrositis
  - radius M86.13- ☑
  - rib M86.18
  - scapula M86.11- ☑
  - skull M86.18
  - tarsus M86.17- ☑
  - tibia M86.16- ☑
  - toe M86.17- ☑
  - ulna M86.13- ☑
  - vertebra — see Osteomyelitis, vertebra
- chronic (or old) M86.60
  - with draining sinus M86.40
    - carpus M86.44- ☑
    - clavicle M86.41- ☑
    - femur M86.45- ☑
    - fibula M86.46- ☑
    - finger M86.44- ☑
    - humerus M86.42- ☑
    - ilium M86.459
    - ischium M86.459
    - mandible M27.2
    - metacarpus M86.44- ☑
    - metatarsus M86.47- ☑
    - multiple sites M86.49
    - neck M86.48
    - orbit H05.02- ☑
    - petrous bone — see Petrositis
    - radius M86.43- ☑
    - rib M86.48
    - scapula M86.41- ☑
    - skull M86.48
    - tarsus M86.47- ☑
    - tibia M86.46- ☑
    - toe M86.47- ☑
    - ulna M86.43- ☑
    - vertebra — see Osteomyelitis, vertebra
  - carpus M86.64- ☑
  - clavicle M86.61- ☑
  - femur M86.65- ☑
  - fibula M86.66- ☑
  - finger M86.64- ☑
  - hematogenous NEC M86.50
    - carpus M86.54- ☑
    - clavicle M86.51- ☑
    - femur M86.55- ☑
    - fibula M86.56- ☑
    - finger M86.54- ☑
    - humerus M86.52- ☑
    - ilium M86.559
    - ischium M86.559
    - mandible M27.2
    - metacarpus M86.54- ☑
    - metatarsus M86.57- ☑
    - multifocal M86.30
      - carpus M86.34- ☑
      - clavicle M86.31- ☑
      - femur M86.35- ☑
      - fibula M86.36- ☑
      - finger M86.34- ☑
      - humerus M86.32- ☑
      - ilium M86.359
      - ischium M86.359
      - metacarpus M86.34- ☑
      - metatarsus M86.37- ☑

Osteomyelitis — continued
- chronic — continued
  - hematogenous — continued
    - multifocal — continued
      - multiple sites M86.39
      - neck M86.38
      - radius M86.33- ☑
      - rib M86.38
      - scapula M86.31- ☑
      - skull M86.38
      - tarsus M86.37- ☑
      - tibia M86.36- ☑
      - toe M86.37- ☑
      - ulna M86.33- ☑
      - vertebra — see Osteomyelitis, vertebra
    - multiple sites M86.59
    - neck M86.58
    - orbit H05.02- ☑
    - petrous bone — see Petrositis
    - radius M86.53- ☑
    - rib M86.58
    - scapula M86.51- ☑
    - skull M86.58
    - tarsus M86.57- ☑
    - tibia M86.56- ☑
    - toe M86.57- ☑
    - ulna M86.53- ☑
    - vertebra — see Osteomyelitis, vertebra
  - humerus M86.62- ☑
  - ilium M86.659
  - ischium M86.659
  - mandible M27.2
  - metacarpus M86.64- ☑
  - metatarsus M86.67- ☑
  - multifocal — see Osteomyelitis, chronic, hematogenous, multifocal
  - multiple sites M86.69
  - neck M86.68
  - orbit H05.02- ☑
  - petrous bone — see Petrositis
  - radius M86.63- ☑
  - rib M86.68
  - scapula M86.61- ☑
  - skull M86.68
  - tarsus M86.67- ☑
  - tibia M86.66- ☑
  - toe M86.67- ☑
  - ulna M86.63- ☑
  - vertebra — see Osteomyelitis, vertebra
- echinococcal B67.2
- Garr's — see Osteomyelitis, specified type NEC
- in diabetes mellitus — see E08-E13 with .69
- jaw (acute) (chronic) (lower) (neonatal) (suppurative) (upper) M27.2
- nonsuppurating — see Osteomyelitis, specified type NEC
- orbit H05.02- ☑
- petrous bone — see Petrositis
- Salmonella (arizonae) (cholerae-suis) (enteritidis) (typhimurium) A02.24
- sclerosing, nonsuppurative — see Osteomyelitis, specified type NEC
- specified type NEC (see also subcategory) M86.8X- ☑
  - mandible M27.2
  - orbit H05.02- ☑
  - petrous bone — see Petrositis
  - vertebra — see Osteomyelitis, vertebra
- subacute M86.20
  - carpus M86.24- ☑
  - clavicle M86.21- ☑
  - femur M86.25- ☑
  - fibula M86.26- ☑
  - finger M86.24- ☑
  - humerus M86.22- ☑
  - mandible M27.2
  - metacarpus M86.24- ☑
  - metatarsus M86.27- ☑
  - multiple sites M86.29
  - neck M86.28
  - orbit H05.02- ☑
  - petrous bone — see Petrositis
  - radius M86.23- ☑
  - rib M86.28
  - scapula M86.21- ☑
  - skull M86.28
  - tarsus M86.27- ☑
  - tibia M86.26- ☑

Osteomyelitis — continued
  subacute — continued
    toe M86.27- ☑
    ulna M86.23- ☑
    vertebra — see Osteomyelitis, vertebra
  syphilitic A52.77
    congenital (early) A50.02 [M90.80]
  tuberculous — see Tuberculosis, bone
  typhoid A01.05
  vertebra M46.20
    cervical region M46.22
    cervicothoracic region M46.23
    lumbar region M46.26
    lumbosacral region M46.27
    occipito-atlanto-axial region M46.21
    sacrococcygeal region M46.28
    thoracic region M46.24
    thoracolumbar region M46.25
Osteomyelofibrosis D47.4
Osteomyelosclerosis D75.89
Osteonecrosis M87.9
  due to
    drugs — see Osteonecrosis, secondary, due to, drugs
    trauma — see Osteonecrosis, secondary, due to, trauma
  idiopathic aseptic M87.00
    ankle M87.07- ☑
    carpus M87.03- ☑
    clavicle M87.01- ☑
    femur M87.05- ☑
    fibula M87.06- ☑
    finger M87.04- ☑
    humerus M87.02- ☑
    ilium M87.050
    ischium M87.050
    metacarpus M87.04- ☑
    metatarsus M87.07- ☑
    multiple sites M87.09
    neck M87.08
    pelvis M87.050
    radius M87.03- ☑
    rib M87.08
    scapula M87.01- ☑
    skull M87.08
    tarsus M87.07- ☑
    tibia M87.06- ☑
    toe M87.07- ☑
    ulna M87.03- ☑
    vertebra M87.08
  secondary NEC M87.30
    carpus M87.33- ☑
    clavicle M87.31- ☑
    due to
      drugs M87.10
        carpus M87.13- ☑
        clavicle M87.11- ☑
        femur M87.15- ☑
        fibula M87.16- ☑
        finger M87.14- ☑
        humerus M87.12- ☑
        ilium M87.159
        ischium M87.159
        jaw M87.180
        metacarpus M87.14- ☑
        metatarsus M87.17- ☑
        multiple sites M87.19
        neck M87.18
        radius M87.13- ☑
        rib M87.18 ☑
        scapula M87.11- ☑
        skull M87.18 ☑
        tarsus M87.17- ☑
        tibia M87.16- ☑
        toe M87.17- ☑
        ulna M87.13- ☑
        vertebra M87.18 ☑
      hemoglobinopathy NEC D58.2 [M90.50]
        carpus D58.2 [M90.54-] ☑
        clavicle D58.2 [M90.51-] ☑
        femur D58.2 [M90.55-] ☑
        fibula D58.2 [M90.56-] ☑
        finger D58.2 [M90.54-] ☑
        humerus D58.2 [M90.52-] ☑
        ilium D58.2 [M90.55-] ☑
        ischium D58.2 [M90.55-] ☑
        metacarpus D58.2 [M90.54-] ☑
        metatarsus D58.2 [M90.57-] ☑

Osteonecrosis — continued
  secondary — continued
    due to — continued
      hemoglobinopathy — continued
        multiple sites D58.2 [M90.58]
        neck D58.2 [M90.58]
        radius D58.2 [M90.53-] ☑
        rib D58.2 [M90.58]
        scapula D58.2 [M90.51-] ☑
        skull D58.2 [M90.58]
        tarsus D58.2 [M90.57-] ☑
        tibia D58.2 [M90.56-] ☑
        toe D58.2 [M90.57-] ☑
        ulna D58.2 [M90.53-] ☑
        vertebra D58.2 [M90.58]
      trauma (previous) M87.20
        carpus M87.23- ☑
        clavicle M87.21- ☑
        femur M87.25- ☑
        fibula M87.26- ☑
        finger M87.24- ☑
        humerus M87.22- ☑
        ilium M87.25- ☑
        ischium M87.25- ☑
        metacarpus M87.24- ☑
        metatarsus M87.27- ☑
        multiple sites M87.29
        neck M87.28
        radius M87.23- ☑
        rib M87.28
        scapula M87.21- ☑
        skull M87.28
        tarsus M87.27- ☑
        tibia M87.26- ☑
        toe M87.27- ☑
        ulna M87.23- ☑
        vertebra M87.28
    femur M87.35- ☑
    fibula M87.36- ☑
    finger M87.34- ☑
    humerus M87.32- ☑
    ilium M87.350
    in
      caisson disease T70.3 ☑ [M90.50]
        carpus T70.3 ☑ [M90.54-] ☑
        clavicle T70.3 ☑ [M90.51-] ☑
        femur T70.3 ☑ [M90.55-] ☑
        fibula T70.3 ☑ [M90.56-] ☑
        finger T70.3 ☑ [M90.54-] ☑
        humerus T70.3 ☑ [M90.52-] ☑
        ilium T70.3 ☑ [M90.55-] ☑
        ischium T70.3 ☑ [M90.55-] ☑
        metacarpus T70.3 ☑ [M90.54-] ☑
        metatarsus T70.3 ☑ [M90.57-] ☑
        multiple sites T70.3 ☑ [M90.59]
        neck T70.3 ☑ [M90.58]
        radius T70.3 ☑ [M90.53-] ☑
        rib T70.3 ☑ [M90.58]
        scapula T70.3 ☑ [M90.51-] ☑
        skull T70.3 ☑ [M90.58]
        tarsus T70.3 ☑ [M90.57-] ☑
        tibia T70.3 ☑ [M90.56-] ☑
        toe T70.3 ☑ [M90.57-] ☑
        ulna T70.3 ☑ [M90.53-] ☑
        vertebra T70.3 ☑ [M90.58]
    ischium M87.350
    metacarpus M87.34- ☑
    metatarsus M87.37- ☑
    multiple site M87.39
    neck M87.38
    radius M87.33- ☑
    rib M87.38
    scapula M87.319
    skull M87.38
    tarsus M87.379
    tibia M87.366
    toe M87.379
    ulna M87.33- ☑
    vertebra M87.38
  specified type NEC M87.80
    carpus M87.83- ☑
    clavicle M87.81- ☑
    femur M87.85- ☑
    fibula M87.86- ☑
    finger M87.84- ☑
    humerus M87.82- ☑

Osteonecrosis — continued
  specified type — continued
    ilium M87.85- ☑
    ischium M87.85- ☑
    metacarpus M87.84- ☑
    metatarsus M87.87- ☑
    multiple sites M87.89
    neck M87.88
    radius M87.83- ☑
    rib M87.88
    scapula M87.81- ☑
    skull M87.88
    tarsus M87.87- ☑
    tibia M87.86- ☑
    toe M87.87- ☑
    ulna M87.83- ☑
    vertebra M87.88
Osteo-onycho-arthro-dysplasia Q87.2
Osteo-onychodysplasia, hereditary Q87.2
Osteopathia condensans disseminata Q78.8
Osteopathy (see also Osteomyelitis, Osteonecrosis, Osteoporosis)
  after poliomyelitis M89.60
    carpus M89.64- ☑
    clavicle M89.61- ☑
    femur M89.65- ☑
    fibula M89.66- ☑
    finger M89.64- ☑
    humerus M89.62- ☑
    ilium M89.659
    ischium M89.659
    metacarpus M89.64- ☑
    metatarsus M89.67- ☑
    multiple sites M89.69
    neck M89.68
    radius M89.63- ☑
    rib M89.68
    scapula M89.61- ☑
    skull M89.68
    tarsus M89.67- ☑
    tibia M89.66- ☑
    toe M89.67- ☑
    ulna M89.63- ☑
    vertebra M89.68
  in (due to)
    renal osteodystrophy N25.0
    specified diseases classified elsewhere — see subcategory M90.8 ☑
Osteopenia M85.8- ☑
  borderline M85.8- ☑
Osteoperiostitis — see Osteomyelitis, specified type NEC
Osteopetrosis (familial) Q78.2
Osteophyte M25.70
  ankle M25.77- ☑
  elbow M25.72- ☑
  foot joint M25.77- ☑
  hand joint M25.74- ☑
  hip M25.75- ☑
  knee M25.76- ☑
  shoulder M25.71- ☑
  spine M25.78
  vertebrae M25.78
  wrist M25.73- ☑
Osteopoikilosis Q78.8
Osteoporosis (female) (male) M81.0
  with current pathological fracture M80.00 ☑
  age-related M81.0
    with current pathologic fracture M80.00 ☑
      carpus M80.04- ☑
      clavicle M80.01- ☑
      fibula M80.06- ☑
      finger M80.04- ☑
      humerus M80.02- ☑
      ilium M80.05- ☑
      ischium M80.05- ☑
      metacarpus M80.04- ☑
      metatarsus M80.07- ☑
      pelvis M80.05- ☑
      radius M80.03- ☑
      scapula M80.01- ☑
      tarsus M80.07- ☑
      tibia M80.06- ☑
      toe M80.07- ☑
      ulna M80.03- ☑
      vertebra M80.08 ☑

☑ Additional Character Required — Refer to the Tabular List for Character Selection

ᴺᴱᵂ Subterms under main terms may continue to next column or page

Osteoporosis — *continued*
  disuse M81.8
    with current pathological fracture M80.80 ☑
      carpus M80.84- ☑
      clavicle M80.81- ☑
      fibula M80.86- ☑
      finger M80.84- ☑
      humerus M80.82- ☑
      ilium M80.85- ☑
      ischium M80.85- ☑
      metacarpus M80.84- ☑
      metatarsus M80.87- ☑
      pelvis M80.85- ☑
      radius M80.83- ☑
      scapula M80.81- ☑
      tarsus M80.87- ☑
      tibia M80.86- ☑
      toe M80.87- ☑
      ulna M80.83- ☑
      vertebra M80.88 ☑
  drug-induced — *see* Osteoporosis, specified type NEC
  idiopathic — *see* Osteoporosis, specified type NEC
  involutional — *see* Osteoporosis, age-related
  Lequesne M81.6
  localized M81.6
  postmenopausal M81.0
    with pathological fracture M80.00 ☑
      carpus M80.04- ☑
      clavicle M80.01- ☑
      fibula M80.06- ☑
      finger M80.04- ☑
      humerus M80.02- ☑
      ilium M80.05- ☑
      ischium M80.05- ☑
      metacarpus M80.04- ☑
      metatarsus M80.07- ☑
      pelvis M80.05- ☑
      radius M80.03- ☑
      scapula M80.01- ☑
      tarsus M80.07- ☑
      tibia M80.06- ☑
      toe M80.07- ☑
      ulna M80.03- ☑
      vertebra M80.08 ☑
  postoophorectomy — *see* Osteoporosis, specified type NEC
  postsurgical malabsorption — *see* Osteoporosis, specified type NEC
  post-traumatic — *see* Osteoporosis, specified type NEC
  senile — *see* Osteoporosis, age-related
  specified type NEC M81.8
    with pathological fracture M80.80 ☑
      carpus M80.84- ☑
      clavicle M80.81- ☑
      fibula M80.86- ☑
      finger M80.84- ☑
      humerus M80.82- ☑
      ilium M80.85- ☑
      ischium M80.85- ☑
      metacarpus M80.84- ☑
      metatarsus M80.87- ☑
      pelvis M80.85- ☑
      radius M80.83- ☑
      scapula M80.81- ☑
      tarsus M80.87- ☑
      tibia M80.86- ☑
      toe M80.87- ☑
      ulna M80.83- ☑
      vertebra M80.88 ☑
Osteopsathyrosis (idiopathica) Q78.0
Osteoradionecrosis, jaw (acute) (chronic) (lower) (suppurative) (upper) M27.2
Osteosarcoma (any form) — *see* Neoplasm, bone, malignant
Osteosclerosis Q78.2
  acquired M85.8- ☑
  congenita Q77.4
  fragilitas (generalisata) Q78.2
  myelofibrosis D75.81
Osteosclerotic anemia D64.89
Osteosis
  cutis L94.2
  renal fibrocystic N25.0
Osterreicher-Turner syndrome Q87.2
Ostium
  atrioventriculare commune Q21.2

Ostium — *continued*
  primum (arteriosum) (defect) (persistent) Q21.2
  secundum (arteriosum) (defect) (patent) (persistent) Q21.1
Ostrum-Furst syndrome Q75.8
Otalgia H92.0
Otitis (acute) H66.90
  with effusion (*see also* Otitis, media, nonsuppurative)
    purulent — *see* Otitis, media, suppurative
  adhesive — *see* subcategory H74.1
  chronic (*see also* Otitis, media, chronic)
    with effusion (*see also* Otitis, media, nonsuppurative, chronic)
  externa H60.9-
    abscess — *see* Abscess, ear, external
    acute (noninfective) H60.50- ☑
      actinic H60.51- ☑
      chemical H60.52- ☑
      contact H60.53- ☑
      eczematoid H60.54- ☑
      infective — *see* Otitis, externa, infective
      reactive H60.55- ☑
      specified NEC H60.59- ☑
    cellulitis — *see* Cellulitis, ear
    chronic H60.6- ☑
    diffuse — *see* Otitis, externa, infective, diffuse
    hemorrhagic — *see* Otitis, externa, infective, hemorrhagic
    in (due to)
      aspergillosis B44.89
      candidiasis B37.84
      erysipelas A46 [H62.40]
      herpes (simplex) virus infection B00.1
        zoster B02.8
      impetigo L01.00 [H62.40]
      infectious disease NEC B99 [H62.4-] ☑
      mycosis NEC B36.9 [H62.40]
      parasitic disease NEC B89 [H62.40]
      viral disease NEC B34.9 [H62.40]
      zoster B02.8
    infective NEC H60.39- ☑
      abscess — *see* Abscess, ear, external
      cellulitis — *see* Cellulitis, ear
      diffuse H60.31- ☑
      hemorrhagic H60.32- ☑
      swimmer's ear — *see* Swimmer's, ear
    malignant H60.2- ☑
    mycotic NEC B36.9 [H62.40]
      in
        aspergillosis B44.89
        candidiasis B37.84
        moniliasis B37.84
    necrotizing — *see* Otitis, externa, malignant
    Pseudomonas aeruginosa — *see* Otitis, externa, malignant
    reactive — *see* Otitis, externa, acute, reactive
    specified NEC — *see* subcategory H60.8 ☑
    tropical NEC B36.9 [H62.40]

        aspergillosis B44.89
        candidiasis B37.84
        moniliasis B37.84
  insidiosa — *see* Otosclerosis
  interna H83.0 ☑
  media (hemorrhagic) (staphylococcal) (streptococcal) H66.9-
    with effusion (nonpurulent) — *see* Otitis, media, nonsuppurative
    acute, subacute H66.90
      allergic — *see* Otitis, media, nonsuppurative, acute, allergic
      exudative — *see* Otitis, media, suppurative, acute
      mucoid — *see* Otitis, media, nonsuppurative, acute
      necrotizing (*see also* Otitis, media, suppurative, acute)
        in
          measles B05.3
          scarlet fever A38.0
      nonsuppurative NEC — *see* Otitis, media, nonsuppurative, acute
      purulent — *see* Otitis, media, suppurative, acute
      sanguinous — *see* Otitis, media, nonsuppurative, acute
      secretory — *see* Otitis, media, nonsuppurative, acute, serous
      seromucinous — *see* Otitis, media, nonsuppurative, acute

Otitis — *continued*
  media — *continued*
    acute, subacute — *continued*
      serous — *see* Otitis, media, nonsuppurative, acute, serous
      suppurative — *see* Otitis, media, suppurative, acute
    allergic — *see* Otitis, media, nonsuppurative
    catarrhal — *see* Otitis, media, nonsuppurative
    chronic H66.90
      with effusion (nonpurulent) — *see* Otitis, media, nonsuppurative, chronic
      allergic — *see* Otitis, media, nonsuppurative, chronic, allergic
      benign suppurative — *see* Otitis, media, suppurative, chronic, tubotympanic
      catarrhal — *see* Otitis, media, nonsuppurative, chronic, serous
      exudative — *see* Otitis, media, nonsuppurative, chronic
      mucinous — *see* Otitis, media, nonsuppurative, chronic, mucoid
      mucoid — *see* Otitis, media, nonsuppurative, chronic, mucoid
      nonsuppurative NEC — *see* Otitis, media, nonsuppurative, chronic
      purulent — *see* Otitis, media, suppurative, chronic
      secretory — *see* Otitis, media, nonsuppurative, chronic, mucoid
      seromucinous — *see* Otitis, media, nonsuppurative, chronic
      serous — *see* Otitis, media, nonsuppurative, chronic, serous
      suppurative — *see* Otitis, media, suppurative, chronic
      transudative — *see* Otitis, media, nonsuppurative, chronic, mucoid
    exudative — *see* Otitis, media, suppurative
    in (due to) (with)
      influenza — *see* Influenza, with, otitis media
      measles B05.3
      scarlet fever A38.0
      tuberculosis A18.6
      viral disease NEC B34.- ☑ [H67.-] ☑
    mucoid — *see* Otitis, media, nonsuppurative
    nonsuppurative H65.9- ☑
      acute or subacute NEC H65.19- ☑
        allergic H65.11- ☑
          recurrent H65.11- ☑
        recurrent H65.19- ☑
        secretory — *see* Otitis, media, nonsuppurative, serous
        serous H65.0- ☑
          recurrent H65.0- ☑
      chronic H65.49- ☑
        allergic H65.41- ☑
        mucoid H65.3- ☑
        serous H65.2- ☑
    postmeasles B05.3
    purulent — *see* Otitis, media, suppurative
    secretory — *see* Otitis, media, nonsuppurative
    seromucinous — *see* Otitis, media, nonsuppurative
    serous — *see* Otitis, media, nonsuppurative
    suppurative H66.4- ☑
      acute H66.00- ☑
        with rupture of ear drum H66.01- ☑
        recurrent H66.00- ☑
          with rupture of ear drum H66.01- ☑
      chronic (*see also* subcategory) H66.3 ☑
        atticoantral H66.2- ☑
        benign — *see* Otitis, media, suppurative, chronic, tubotympanic
        tubotympanic H66.1- ☑
    transudative — *see* Otitis, media, nonsuppurative
    tuberculous A18.6
Otocephaly Q18.2
Otolith syndrome — *see* subcategory H81.8 ☑
Otomycosis (diffuse) **NEC** B36.9 [H62.40]
  in
    aspergillosis B44.89
    candidiasis B37.84
    moniliasis B37.84
Otoporosis — *see* Otosclerosis
Otorrhagia (nontraumatic) H92.2- ☑
  traumatic — *code by* Type of injury
Otorrhea H92.1- ☑

Otorrhea — *continued*
  cerebrospinal G96.0
Otosclerosis (general) H80.9- ☑
  cochlear (endosteal) H80.2- ☑
  involving
    otic capsule — *see* Otosclerosis, cochlear
    oval window
      nonobliterative H80.0- ☑
      obliterative H80.1- ☑
    round window — *see* Otosclerosis, cochlear
  nonobliterative — *see* Otosclerosis, involving, oval window, nonobliterative
  obliterative — *see* Otosclerosis, involving, oval window, obliterative
  specified NEC H80.8- ☑
Otospongiosis — *see* Otosclerosis
Otto's disease or pelvis M24.7
Outcome of delivery Z37.9
  multiple births Z37.9
    all liveborn Z37.50
      quadruplets Z37.52
      quintuplets Z37.53
      sextuplets Z37.54
      specified number NEC Z37.59
      triplets Z37.51
    all stillborn Z37.7
    some liveborn Z37.60
      quadruplets Z37.62
      quintuplets Z37.63
      sextuplets Z37.64
      specified number NEC Z37.69
      triplets Z37.61
  single NEC Z37.9
    liveborn Z37.0
    stillborn Z37.1
  twins NEC Z37.9
    both liveborn Z37.2
    both stillborn Z37.4
    one liveborn, one stillborn Z37.3
Outlet — *see* condition
Ovalocytosis (congenital) (hereditary) — *see* Elliptocytosis
Ovarian — *see* Condition
Ovariocele N83.4- ☑
Ovaritis (cystic) — *see* Oophoritis
Ovary, ovarian (*see also* condition)
  resistant syndrome E28.39
  vein syndrome N13.8
Overactive (*see also* Hyperfunction)
  adrenal cortex NEC E27.0
  bladder N32.81
  hypothalamus E23.3
  thyroid — *see* Hyperthyroidism
Overactivity R46.3
  child — *see* Disorder, attention-deficit hyperactivity
Overbite (deep) (excessive) (horizontal) (vertical) M26.29
Overbreathing — *see* Hyperventilation
Overconscientious personality F60.5
Overdevelopment — *see* Hypertrophy
Overdistension — *see* Distension
Overdose, overdosage (drug) — *see* Table of Drugs and Chemicals, by drug, poisoning
Overeating R63.2
  nonorganic origin F50.89
  psychogenic F50.89
Overexertion (effects) (exhaustion) T73.3 ☑
Overexposure (effects) T73.9 ☑
  exhaustion T73.2 ☑
Overfeeding — *see* Overeating
  newborn P92.4
Overfill, endodontic M27.52
Overgrowth, bone — *see* Hypertrophy, bone
Overhanging of dental restorative material (unrepairable) K08.52
Overheated (places) (effects) — *see* Heat
Overjet (excessive horizontal) M26.23
Overlaid, overlying (suffocation) — *see* Asphyxia, traumatic, due to mechanical threat
Overlap, excessive horizontal (teeth) M26.23
Overlapping toe (acquired) (*see also* Deformity, toe, specified NEC)
  congenital (fifth toe) Q66.89
Overload
  circulatory, due to transfusion (blood) (blood components) (TACO) E87.71
  fluid E87.70

Overload — *continued*
  fluid — *continued*
    due to transfusion (blood) (blood components) E87.71
    specified NEC E87.79
  iron, due to repeated red blood cell transfusions E83.111
  potassium (K) E87.5
  sodium (Na) E87.0
Overnutrition — *see* Hyperalimentation
Overproduction (*see also* Hypersecretion)
  ACTH E27.0
  catecholamine E27.5
  growth hormone E22.0
Overprotection, child by parent Z62.1
Overriding
  aorta Q25.49
  finger (acquired) — *see* Deformity, finger
    congenital Q68.1
  toe (acquired) (*see also* Deformity, toe, specified NEC)
    congenital Q66.89
Overstrained R53.83
  heart — *see* Hypertrophy, cardiac
Overuse, muscle NEC M70.8- ☑
Overweight E66.3
Overworked R53.83
Oviduct — *see* condition
Ovotestis Q56.0
Ovulation (cycle)
  failure or lack of N97.0
  pain N94.0
Ovum — *see* condition
Owren's disease or syndrome (parahemophilia) D68.2
Ox heart — *see* Hypertrophy, cardiac
Oxalosis E72.53
Oxaluria E72.53
Oxycephaly, oxycephalic Q75.0
  syphilitic, congenital A50.02
Oxyuriasis B80
Oxyuris vermicularis (infestation) B80
Ozena J31.0

P

Pachyderma, pachydermia L85.9
  larynx (verrucosa) J38.7
Pachydermatocele (congenital) Q82.8
Pachydermoperiostosis (*see also* Osteoarthropathy, hypertrophic, specified type NEC)
  clubbed nail M89.40 [L62]
Pachygyria Q04.3
Pachymeningitis (adhesive) (basal) (brain) (cervical) (chronic)(circumscribed) (external) (fibrous) (hemorrhagic) (hypertrophic) (internal) (purulent) (spinal) (suppurative) — *see* Meningitis
Pachyonychia (congenital) Q84.5
Pacinian tumor — *see* Neoplasm, skin, benign
Pad, knuckle or Garrod's M72.1
Paget's disease
  with infiltrating duct carcinoma — *see* Neoplasm, breast, malignant
  bone M88.9
    carpus M88.84- ☑
    clavicle M88.81- ☑
    femur M88.85- ☑
    fibula M88.86- ☑
    finger M88.84- ☑
    humerus M88.82- ☑
    ilium M88.85- ☑
    in neoplastic disease — *see* Osteitis, deformans, in neoplastic disease
    ischium M88.85- ☑
    metacarpus M88.84- ☑
    metatarsus M88.87- ☑
    multiple sites M88.89
    neck M88.88
    radius M88.83- ☑
    rib M88.88
    scapula M88.81- ☑
    skull M88.0
    tarsus M88.87- ☑
    tibia M88.86- ☑
    toe M88.87- ☑
    ulna M88.83- ☑
    vertebra M88.88
  breast (female) C50.01- ☑

Paget's disease — *continued*
  breast — *continued*
    male C50.02- ☑
  extramammary (*see also* Neoplasm, skin, malignant)
    anus C21.0
    margin C44.590
    skin C44.590
  intraductal carcinoma — *see* Neoplasm, breast, malignant
  malignant — *see* Neoplasm, skin, malignant
    breast (female) C50.01- ☑
      male C50.02- ☑
    unspecified site (female) C50.01- ☑
      male C50.02- ☑
  mammary — *see* Paget's disease, breast
  nipple — *see* Paget's disease, breast
  osteitis deformans — *see* Paget's disease, bone
Paget-Schroetter syndrome I82.890
Pain(s) (*see also* Painful) R52
  abdominal R10.9
    colic R10.83
    generalized R10.84
      with acute abdomen R10.0
    lower R10.30
      left quadrant R10.32
      pelvic or perineal R10.2
      periumbilical R10.33
      right quadrant R10.31
    rebound — *see* Tenderness, abdominal, rebound
    severe with abdominal rigidity R10.0
    tenderness — *see* Tenderness, abdominal
    upper R10.10
      epigastric R10.13
      left quadrant R10.12
      right quadrant R10.11
  acute R52
    due to trauma G89.11
    neoplasm related G89.3
    postprocedural NEC G89.18
    post-thoracotomy G89.12
    specified by site — *code to* Pain, by site
  adnexa (uteri) R10.2
  anginoid — *see* Pain, precordial
  anus K62.89
  arm — *see* Pain, limb, upper
  axillary (axilla) M79.62- ☑
  back (postural) M54.9
  bladder R39.89
    associated with micturition — *see* Micturition, painful
    chronic R39.82
  bone — *see* Disorder, bone, specified type NEC
  breast N64.4
  broad ligament R10.2
  cancer associated (acute) (chronic) G89.3
  cecum — *see* Pain, abdominal
  cervicobrachial M53.1
  chest (central) R07.9
    anterior wall R07.89
    atypical R07.89
    ischemic I20.9
    musculoskeletal R07.89
    non-cardiac R07.89
    on breathing R07.1
    pleurodynia R07.81
    precordial R07.2
    wall (anterior) R07.89
  chronic G89.29
    associated with significant psychosocial dysfunction G89.4
    due to trauma G89.21
    neoplasm related G89.3
    postoperative NEC G89.28
    postprocedural NEC G89.28
    post-thoracotomy G89.22
    specified NEC G89.29
  coccyx M53.3
  colon — *see* Pain, abdominal
  coronary — *see* Angina
  costochondral R07.1
  diaphragm R07.1
  due to cancer G89.3
  due to device, implant or graft (*see also* Complication, by site and type, specified NEC) T85.848 ☑
    arterial graft NEC T82.848 ☑
    breast (implant) T85.848 ☑
    catheter NEC T85.848 ☑
    dialysis (renal) T82.848 ☑

☑ **Additional Character Required** — **Refer to the Tabular List for Character Selection**   Subterms under main terms may continue to next column or pag

Otorrhea — Pain

Pain(s) — *continued*
  due to device, implant or graft (*see also* Complications, by site and type, specified) — *continued*
    catheter — *continued*
      dialysis — *continued*
        intraperitoneal T85.848 ☑
      infusion NEC T82.848 ☑
        spinal (epidural) (subdural) T85.840 ☑
      urinary (indwelling) T83.84 ☑
    electronic (electrode) (pulse generator) (stimulator)
      bone T85.840 ☑
      cardiac T82.847 ☑
      nervous system (brain) (peripheral nerve) (spinal) T85.84 ☑
      urinary T83.84 ☑
    fixation, internal (orthopedic) NEC T84.84 ☑
    gastrointestinal (bile duct) (esophagus) T85.848 ☑
    genital NEC T83.84 ☑
    heart NEC T82.847 ☑
    infusion NEC T85.848 ☑
    joint prosthesis T84.84 ☑
    ocular (corneal graft) (orbital implant) NEC T85.848 ☑
    orthopedic NEC T84.84 ☑
    specified NEC T85.848 ☑
    urinary NEC T83.84 ☑
    vascular NEC T82.848 ☑
    ventricular intracranial shunt T85.840 ☑
  due to malignancy (primary) (secondary) G89.3
  ear — *see* subcategory H92.0 ☑
  epigastric, epigastrium R10.13
  eye — *see* Pain, ocular
  face, facial R51
    atypical G50.1
  female genital organs NEC N94.89
  finger — *see* Pain, limb, upper
  flank — *see* Pain, abdominal
  foot — *see* Pain, limb, lower
  gallbladder K82.9
  gas (intestinal) R14.1
  gastric — *see* Pain, abdominal
  generalized NOS R52
  genital organ
    female N94.89
    male N50.89
  groin — *see* Pain, abdominal, lower
  hand — *see* Pain, limb, upper
  head — *see* Headache
  heart — *see* Pain, precordial
  infra-orbital — *see* Neuralgia, trigeminal
  intercostal R07.82
  intermenstrual N94.0
  jaw R68.84
  joint M25.50
    ankle M25.57- ☑
    elbow M25.52- ☑
    finger M25.54- ☑
    foot M25.57- ☑
    hand M25.54- ☑
    hip M25.55- ☑
    knee M25.56- ☑
    shoulder M25.51- ☑
    toe M25.57- ☑
    wrist M25.53- ☑
  kidney N23
  laryngeal R07.0
  leg — *see* Pain, limb, lower
  limb M79.609
    lower M79.60- ☑
      foot M79.67- ☑
      lower leg M79.66- ☑
      thigh M79.65- ☑
      toe M79.67- ☑
    upper M79.60- ☑
      axilla M79.62- ☑
      finger M79.64- ☑
      forearm M79.63- ☑
      hand M79.64- ☑
      upper arm M79.62- ☑
  loin M54.5
  low back M54.5
  lumbar region M54.5
  mandibular R68.84
  mastoid — *see* subcategory H92.0 ☑
  maxilla R68.84
  menstrual (*see also* Dysmenorrhea) N94.6
  metacarpophalangeal (joint) — *see* Pain, joint, hand

Pain(s) — *continued*
  metatarsophalangeal (joint) — *see* Pain, joint, foot
  mouth K13.79
  muscle — *see* Myalgia
  musculoskeletal (*see also* Pain, by site) M79.18
  myofascial M79.18
  nasal J34.89
  nasopharynx J39.2
  neck NEC M54.2
  nerve NEC — *see* Neuralgia
  neuromuscular — *see* Neuralgia
  nose J34.89
  ocular H57.1- ☑
  ophthalmic — *see* Pain, ocular
  orbital region — *see* Pain, ocular
  ovary N94.89
  over heart — *see* Pain, precordial
  ovulation N94.0
  pelvic (female) R10.2
  penis N48.89
  pericardial — *see* Pain, precordial
  perineal, perineum R10.2
  pharynx J39.2
  pleura, pleural, pleuritic R07.81
  postoperative NOS G89.18
  postprocedural NOS G89.18
  post-thoracotomy G89.12
  precordial (region) R07.2
  premenstrual N94.3
  psychogenic (persistent) (any site) F45.41
  radicular (spinal) — *see* Radiculopathy
  rectum K62.89
  respiration R07.1
  retrosternal R07.2
  rheumatoid, muscular — *see* Myalgia
  rib R07.81
  root (spinal) — *see* Radiculopathy
  round ligament (stretch) R10.2
  sacroiliac M53.3
  sciatic — *see* Sciatica
  scrotum N50.82
  seminal vesicle N50.89
  shoulder M25.51- ☑
  spermatic cord N50.89
  spinal root — *see* Radiculopathy
  spine M54.9
    cervical M54.2
    low back M54.5
      with sciatica M54.4- ☑
    thoracic M54.6
  stomach — *see* Pain, abdominal
  substernal R07.2
  temporomandibular (joint) M26.62- ☑
  testis N50.81- ☑
  thoracic spine M54.6
    with radicular and visceral pain M54.14
  throat R07.0
  tibia — *see* Pain, limb, lower
  toe — *see* Pain, limb, lower
  tongue K14.6
  tooth K08.89
  trigeminal — *see* Neuralgia, trigeminal
  tumor associated G89.3
  ureter N23
  urinary (organ) (system) N23
  uterus NEC N94.89
  vagina R10.2
  vertebrogenic (syndrome) M54.89
  vesical R39.89
    associated with micturition — *see* Micturition, painful
  vulva R10.2
Painful (*see also* Pain)
  coitus
    female N94.10
    male N53.12
    psychogenic F52.6
  ejaculation (semen) N53.12
    psychogenic F52.6
  erection — *see* Priapism
  feet syndrome E53.8
  joint replacement (hip) (knee) T84.84 ☑
  menstruation — *see* Dysmenorrhea
    psychogenic F45.8
  micturition — *see* Micturition, painful
  respiration R07.1
  scar NEC L90.5
  wire sutures T81.89 ☑

Painter's colic — *see* subcategory T56.0 ☑
Palate — *see* condition
Palatoplegia K13.79
Palatoschisis — *see* Cleft, palate
Palilalia R48.8
Palliative care Z51.5
Pallor R23.1
  optic disc, temporal — *see* Atrophy, optic
Palmar (*see also* condition)
  fascia — *see* condition
Palpable
  cecum K63.89
  kidney N28.89
  ovary N83.8
  prostate N42.9
  spleen — *see* Splenomegaly
Palpitations (heart) R00.2
  psychogenic F45.8
Palsy (*see also* Paralysis) G83.9
  atrophic diffuse (progressive) G12.22
  Bell's (*see also* Palsy, facial)
    newborn P11.3
  brachial plexus NEC G54.0
    newborn (birth injury) P14.3
  brain — *see* Palsy, cerebral
  bulbar (progressive) (chronic) G12.22
    of childhood (Fazio-Londe) G12.1
    pseudo NEC G12.29
    supranuclear (progressive) G23.1
  cerebral (congenital) G80.9
    ataxic G80.4
    athetoid G80.3
    choreathetoid G80.3
    diplegic G80.8
      spastic G80.1
    dyskinetic G80.3
      athetoid G80.3
      choreathetoid G80.3
      distonic G80.3
    dystonic G80.3
    hemiplegic G80.8
      spastic G80.2
    mixed G80.8
    monoplegic G80.8
      spastic G80.1
    paraplegic G80.8
      spastic G80.1
    quadriplegic G80.8
      spastic G80.0
    spastic G80.1
      diplegic G80.1
      hemiplegic G80.2
      monoplegic G80.1
      quadriplegic G80.0
      specified NEC G80.1
      tetrapelgic G80.0
    specified NEC G80.8
    syphilitic A52.12
      congenital A50.49
    tetrapelgic G80.8
      spastic G80.0
  cranial nerve (*see also* Disorder, nerve, cranial)
    multiple G52.7
      in
        infectious disease B99 ☑ [G53]
        neoplastic disease (*see also* Neoplasm) D49.9 [G53]
        parasitic disease B89 [G53]
        sarcoidosis D86.82
  creeping G12.22
  diver's T70.3 ☑
  Erb's P14.0
  facial G51.0
    newborn (birth injury) P11.3
  glossopharyngeal G52.1
  Klumpke (-Déjérine) P14.1
  lead — *see* subcategory T56.0 ☑
  median nerve (tardy) G56.1- ☑
  nerve G58.9
    specified NEC G58.8
  peroneal nerve (acute) (tardy) G57.3- ☑
  progressive supranuclear G23.1
  pseudobulbar NEC G12.29
  radial nerve (acute) G56.3- ☑
  seventh nerve (*see also* Palsy, facial)
    newborn P11.3
  shaking — *see* Parkinsonism
  spastic (cerebral) (spinal) G80.1

Palsy — *continued*
ulnar nerve (tardy) G56.2- ☑
wasting G12.29
Paludism — *see* Malaria
Panangiitis M30.0
Panaris, panaritium (*see also* Cellulitis, digit)
with lymphangitis — *see* Lymphangitis, acute, digit
Panarteritis nodosa M30.0
brain or cerebral I67.7
Pancake heart R93.1
with cor pulmonale (chronic) I27.81
Pancarditis (acute) (chronic) I51.89
rheumatic I09.89
active or acute I01.8
Pancoast's syndrome or tumor C34.1- ☑
Pancolitis, ulcerative (chronic) K51.00
with
abscess K51.014
complication K51.019
fistula K51.013
obstruction K51.012
rectal bleeding K51.011
specified complication NEC K51.018
Pancreas, pancreatic — *see* condition
Pancreatitis (annular) (apoplectic) (calcareous) (edematous) (hemorrhagic) (malignant) (recurrent) (subacute) (suppurative) K85.90
with necrosis (uninfected) K85.91
infected K85.92
acute (without necrosis or infection) K85.90
with necrosis (uninfected) K85.91
infected K85.92
alcohol induced (without necrosis or infection) K85.20
with necrosis (uninfected) K85.21
infected K85.22
biliary (without necrosis or infection) K85.10
with necrosis (uninfected) K85.11
infected K85.12
drug induced (without necrosis or infection) K85.30
with necrosis (uninfected) K85.31
infected K85.32
gallstone (without necrosis or infection) K85.10
with necrosis (uninfected) K85.11
infected K85.12
idiopathic (without necrosis or infection) K85.00
with necrosis (uninfected) K85.01
infected K85.02
specified NEC (without necrosis or infection) K85.80
with necrosis (uninfected) K85.81
infected K85.82
chronic (infectious) K86.1
alcohol-induced K86.0
recurrent K86.1
relapsing K86.1
cystic (chronic) K86.1
cytomegaloviral B25.2
fibrous (chronic) K86.1
gallstone (without necrosis or infection) K85.10
with necrosis (uninfected) K85.11
infected K85.12
gangrenous — *see* Pancreatitis, acute
interstitial (chronic) K86.1
acute (*see also* Pancreatitis, acute) K85.80
mumps B26.3
recurrent (chronic) K86.1
relapsing, chronic K86.1
syphilitic A52.74
Pancreatoblastoma — *see* Neoplasm, pancreas, malignant
Pancreolithiasis K86.89
Pancytolysis D75.89
Pancytopenia (acquired) D61.818
with
malformations D61.09
myelodysplastic syndrome — *see* Syndrome, myelodysplastic
antineoplastic chemotherapy induced D61.810
congenital D61.09
drug-induced NEC D61.811
PANDAS (pediatric autoimmune neuropsychiatric disorders associated with streptococcal infections syndrome) D89.89
Panencephalitis, subacute, sclerosing A81.1
Panhematopenia D61.9
congenital D61.09
constitutional D61.09
splenic, primary D73.1

Panhemocytopenia D61.9
congenital D61.09
constitutional D61.09
Panhypogonadism E29.1
Panhypopituitarism E23.0
prepubertal E23.0
Panic (attack) (state) F41.0
reaction to exceptional stress (transient) F43.0
Panmyelopathy, familial, constitutional D61.09
Panmyelophthisis D61.82
congenital D61.09
Panmyelosis (acute) (with myelofibrosis) C94.4- ☑
Panner's disease — *see* Osteochondrosis, juvenile, humerus
Panneuritis endemica E51.11
Panniculitis (nodular) (nonsuppurative) M79.3
back M54.00
cervical region M54.02
cervicothoracic region M54.03
lumbar region M54.06
lumbosacral region M54.07
multiple sites M54.09
occipito-atlanto-axial region M54.01
sacrococcygeal region M54.08
thoracic region M54.04
thoracolumbar region M54.05
lupus L93.2
mesenteric K65.4
neck M54.02
cervicothoracic region M54.03
occipito-atlanto-axial region M54.01
relapsing M35.6
Panniculus adiposus (abdominal) E65
Pannus (allergic) (cornea) (degenerativus) (keratic) H16.42- ☑
abdominal (symptomatic) E65
trachomatosus, trachomatous (active) A71.1
Panophthalmitis H44.01- ☑
Pansinusitis (chronic) (hyperplastic) (nonpurulent) (purulent) J32.4
acute J01.40
recurrent J01.41
tuberculous A15.8
Panuveitis (sympathetic) H44.11- ☑
Panvalvular disease I08.9
specified NEC I08.8
PAPA (pyogenic arthritis, pyoderma gangrenosum, and acne syndrome) M04.8
Papanicolaou smear, cervix Z12.4
as part of routine gynecological examination Z01.419
with abnormal findings Z01.411
for suspected neoplasm Z12.4
nonspecific abnormal finding R87.619
routine Z01.419
with abnormal findings Z01.411
Papilledema (choked disc) H47.10
associated with
decreased ocular pressure H47.12
increased intracranial pressure H47.11
retinal disorder H47.13
Foster-Kennedy syndrome H47.14- ☑
Papillitis H46.00
anus K62.89
chronic lingual K14.4
necrotizing, kidney N17.2
optic H46.0- ☑
rectum K62.89
renal, necrotizing N17.2
tongue K14.0
Papilloma (*see also* Neoplasm, benign, by site)
acuminatum (female) (male) (anogenital) A63.0
basal cell L82.1
inflamed L82.0
benign pinta (primary) A67.0
bladder (urinary) (transitional cell) D41.4
choroid plexus (lateral ventricle) (third ventricle) D33.0
anaplastic C71.5
fourth ventricle D33.1
malignant C71.5
renal pelvis (transitional cell) D41.1- ☑
benign D30.1- ☑
Schneiderian
specified site — *see* Neoplasm, benign, by site
unspecified site D14.0
serous surface
borderline malignancy
specified site — *see* Neoplasm, uncertain behavior, by site

Papilloma — *continued*
serous surface — *continued*
borderline malignancy — *continued*
unspecified site D39.10
specified site — *see* Neoplasm, benign, by site
unspecified site D27.9
transitional (cell)
bladder (urinary) D41.4
inverted type — *see* Neoplasm, uncertain behavior, by site
renal pelvis D41.1- ☑
ureter D41.2- ☑
ureter (transitional cell) D41.2- ☑
benign D30.2- ☑
urothelial — *see* Neoplasm, uncertain behavior, by site
villous — *see* Neoplasm, uncertain behavior, by site
adenocarcinoma in — *see* Neoplasm, malignant, by site
in situ — *see* Neoplasm, in situ
yaws, plantar or palmar A66.1
Papillomata, multiple, of yaws A66.1
Papillomatosis (*see also* Neoplasm, benign, by site)
confluent and reticulated L83
cystic, breast — *see* Mastopathy, cystic
ductal, breast — *see* Mastopathy, cystic
intraductal (diffuse) — *see* Neoplasm, benign, by site
subareolar duct D24- ☑
Papillomavirus, as cause of disease classified elsewhere B97.7
Papillon-Léage and Psaume syndrome Q87.0
Papule(s) R23.8
carate (primary) A67.0
fibrous, of nose D22.39
Gottron's L94.4
pinta (primary) A67.0
Papulosis
lymphomatoid C86.6
malignant I77.89
Papyraceous fetus O31.0- ☑
Para-albuminemia E88.09
Paracephalus Q89.7
Parachute mitral valve Q23.2
Paracoccidioidomycosis B41.9
disseminated B41.7
generalized B41.7
mucocutaneous-lymphangitic B41.8
pulmonary B41.0
specified NEC B41.8
visceral B41.8
Paradentosis K05.4
Paraffinoma T88.8 ☑
Paraganglioma D44.7
adrenal D35.0- ☑
malignant C74.1- ☑
aortic body D44.7
malignant C75.5
carotid body D44.6
malignant C75.4
chromaffin (*see also* Neoplasm, benign, by site)
malignant — *see* Neoplasm, malignant, by site
extra-adrenal D44.7
malignant C75.5
specified site — *see* Neoplasm, malignant, by site
unspecified site C75.5
specified site — *see* Neoplasm, uncertain behavior, by site
unspecified site D44.7
gangliocytic D13.2
specified site — *see* Neoplasm, benign, by site
unspecified site D13.2
glomus jugulare D44.7
malignant C75.5
jugular D44.7
malignant C75.5
specified site — *see* Neoplasm, malignant, by site
unspecified site C75.5
nonchromaffin D44.7
malignant C75.5
specified site — *see* Neoplasm, malignant, by site
unspecified site C75.5
specified site — *see* Neoplasm, uncertain behavior, by site
unspecified site D44.7
parasympathetic D44.7

Paraganglioma — *continued*
  parasympathetic — *continued*
    specified site — *see* Neoplasm, uncertain behavior, by site
    unspecified site D44.7
  specified site — *see* Neoplasm, uncertain behavior, by site
  sympathetic D44.7
    specified site — *see* Neoplasm, uncertain behavior, by site
    unspecified site D44.7
  unspecified site D44.7
Parageusia R43.2
  psychogenic F45.8
Paragonimiasis B66.4
Paragranuloma, Hodgkin — *see* Lymphoma, Hodgkin, specified NEC
Parahemophilia (*see also* Defect, coagulation) D68.2
Parakeratosis R23.4
  variegata L41.0
Paralysis, paralytic (complete) (incomplete) G83.9
  with
    syphilis A52.17
  abducens, abducent (nerve) — *see* Strabismus, paralytic, sixth nerve
  abductor, lower extremity G57.9- ☑
  accessory nerve G52.8
  accommodation (*see also* Paresis, of accommodation)
    hysterical F44.89
  acoustic nerve (except Deafness) H93.3 ☑
  agitans (*see also* Parkinsonism) G20
    arteriosclerotic G21.4
  alternating (oculomotor) G83.89
  amyotrophic G12.21
  ankle G57.9- ☑
  anus (sphincter) K62.89
  arm — *see* Monoplegia, upper limb
  ascending (spinal), acute G61.0
  association G12.29
  asthenic bulbar G70.00
    with exacerbation (acute) G70.01
    in crisis G70.01
  ataxic (hereditary) G11.9
    general (syphilitic) A52.17
  atrophic G58.9
    infantile, acute — *see* Poliomyelitis, paralytic
    progressive G12.22
    spinal (acute) — *see* Poliomyelitis, paralytic
  axillary G54.0
  Babinski-Nageotte's G83.89
  Bell's G51.0
    newborn P11.3
  Benedikt's G46.3
  birth injury P14.9
    spinal cord P11.5
  bladder (neurogenic) (sphincter) N31.2
  bowel, colon or intestine K56.0
  brachial plexus G54.0
    birth injury P14.3
    newborn (birth injury) P14.3
  brain G83.9
    diplegia G83.0
    triplegia G83.89
  bronchial J98.09
  Brown-Séquard G83.81
  bulbar (chronic) (progressive) G12.22
    infantile — *see* Poliomyelitis, paralytic
    poliomyelitic — *see* Poliomyelitis, paralytic
    pseudo G12.29
  bulbospinal G70.00
    with exacerbation (acute) G70.01
    in crisis G70.01
  cardiac (*see also* Failure, heart) I50.9
  cerebrocerebellar, diplegic G80.1
  cervical
    plexus G54.2
    sympathetic G90.09
  Céstan-Chenais G46.3
  Charcot-Marie-Tooth type G60.0
  Clark's G80.9
  colon K56.0
  compressed air T70.3 ☑
  compression
    arm G56.9- ☑
    leg G57.9- ☑
    lower extremity G57.9- ☑
    upper extremity G56.9- ☑
  congenital (cerebral) — *see* Palsy, cerebral

Paralysis, paralytic — *continued*
  conjugate movement (gaze) (of eye) H51.0
    cortical (nuclear) (supranuclear) H51.0
  cordis — *see* Failure, heart
  cranial or cerebral nerve G52.9
  creeping G12.22
  crossed leg G83.89
  crutch — *see* Injury, brachial plexus
  deglutition R13.0
    hysterical F44.4
  dementia A52.17
  descending (spinal) NEC G12.29
  diaphragm (flaccid) J98.6
    due to accidental dissection of phrenic nerve during procedure — *see* Puncture, accidental complicating surgery
  digestive organs NEC K59.8
  diplegic — *see* Diplegia
  divergence (nuclear) H51.8
  diver's T70.3 ☑
  Duchenne's
    birth injury P14.0
    due to or associated with
      motor neuron disease G12.22
      muscular dystrophy G71.01
  due to intracranial or spinal birth injury — *see* Palsy, cerebral
  embolic (current episode) I63.4- ☑
  Erb (-Duchenne) (birth) (newborn) P14.0
  Erb's syphilitic spastic spinal A52.17
  esophagus K22.8
  eye muscle (extrinsic) H49.9
    intrinsic (*see also* Paresis, of accommodation)
  facial (nerve) G51.0
    birth injury P11.3
    congenital P11.3
    following operation NEC — *see* Puncture, accidental complicating surgery
    newborn (birth injury) P11.3
  familial (recurrent) (periodic) G72.3
    spastic G11.4
  fauces J39.2
  finger G56.9- ☑
  gait R26.1
  gastric nerve (nondiabetic) G52.2
  gaze, conjugate H51.0
  general (progressive) (syphilitic) A52.17
    juvenile A50.45
  glottis J38.00
    bilateral J38.02
    unilateral J38.01
  gluteal G54.1
  Gubler (-Millard) G46.3
  hand — *see* Monoplegia, upper limb
  heart — *see* Arrest, cardiac
  hemiplegic — *see* Hemiplegia
  hyperkalemic periodic (familial) G72.3
  hypoglossal (nerve) G52.3
  hypokalemic periodic G72.3
  hysterical F44.4
  ileus K56.0
  infantile (*see also* Poliomyelitis, paralytic) A80.30
    bulbar — *see* Poliomyelitis, paralytic
    cerebral — *see* Palsy, cerebral
    spastic — *see* Palsy, cerebral, spastic
  infective — *see* Poliomyelitis, paralytic
  inferior nuclear G83.9
  internuclear — *see* Ophthalmoplegia, internuclear
  intestine K56.0
  iris H57.09
    due to diphtheria (toxin) A36.89
  ischemic, Volkmann's (complicating trauma) T79.6 ☑
  Jackson's G83.89
  jake — *see* Poisoning, food, noxious, plant
  Jamaica ginger (jake) G62.2
  juvenile general A50.45
  Klumpke (-Déjérine) (birth) (newborn) P14.1
  labioglossal (laryngeal) (pharyngeal) G12.29
  Landry's G61.0
  laryngeal nerve (recurrent) (superior) (unilateral) J38.00
    bilateral J38.02
    unilateral J38.01
  larynx J38.00
    bilateral J38.02
    due to diphtheria (toxin) A36.2
    unilateral J38.01
  lateral G12.23
  lead T56.0 ☑

Paralysis, paralytic — *continued*
  left side — *see* Hemiplegia
  leg G83.1- ☑
    both — *see* Paraplegia
    crossed G83.89
    hysterical F44.4
    psychogenic F44.4
    transient or transitory R29.818
      traumatic NEC — *see* Injury, nerve, leg
  levator palpebrae superioris — *see* Blepharoptosis, paralytic
  limb — *see* Monoplegia
  lip K13.0
  Lissauer's A52.17
  lower limb — *see* Monoplegia, lower limb
    both — *see* Paraplegia
  lung J98.4
  median nerve G56.1- ☑
  medullary (tegmental) G83.89
  mesencephalic NEC G83.89
    tegmental G83.89
  middle alternating G83.89
  Millard-Gubler-Foville G46.3
  monoplegic — *see* Monoplegia
  motor G83.9
  muscle, muscular NEC G72.89
    due to nerve lesion G58.9
    eye (extrinsic) H49.9
      intrinsic — *see* Paresis, of accommodation
      oblique — *see* Strabismus, paralytic, fourth nerve
    iris sphincter H21.9
    ischemic (Volkmann's) (complicating trauma) T79.6 ☑
    progressive G12.21
    pseudohypertrophic G71.02
  musculocutaneous nerve G56.9- ☑
  musculospiral G56.9- ☑
  nerve (*see also* Disorder, nerve)
    abducent — *see* Strabismus, paralytic, sixth nerve
    accessory G52.8
    auditory (except Deafness) H93.3 ☑
    birth injury P14.9
    cranial or cerebral G52.9
    facial G51.0
      birth injury P11.3
      congenital P11.3
      newborn (birth injury) P11.3
    fourth or trochlear — *see* Strabismus, paralytic, fourth nerve
    newborn (birth injury) P14.9
    oculomotor — *see* Strabismus, paralytic, third nerve
    phrenic (birth injury) P14.2
    radial G56.3- ☑
    seventh or facial G51.0
      newborn (birth injury) P11.3
    sixth or abducent — *see* Strabismus, paralytic, sixth nerve
    syphilitic A52.15
    third or oculomotor — *see* Strabismus, paralytic, third nerve
    trigeminal G50.9
    trochlear — *see* Strabismus, paralytic, fourth nerve
    ulnar G56.2- ☑
  normokalemic periodic G72.3
  ocular H49.9
    alternating G83.89
  oculofacial, congenital (Moebius) Q87.0
  oculomotor (external bilateral) (nerve) — *see* Strabismus, paralytic, third nerve
  palate (soft) K13.79
  paratrigeminal G50.9
  periodic (familial) (hyperkalemic) (hypokalemic) (myotonic) (normokalemic) (potassium sensitive) (secondary) G72.3
  peripheral autonomic nervous system — *see* Neuropathy, peripheral, autonomic
  peroneal (nerve) G57.3- ☑
  pharynx J39.2
  phrenic nerve G56.8- ☑
  plantar nerve(s) G57.6- ☑
  pneumogastric nerve G52.2
  poliomyelitis (current) — *see* Poliomyelitis, paralytic
  popliteal nerve G57.3- ☑
  postepileptic transitory G83.84
  progressive (atrophic) (bulbar) (spinal) G12.22
    general A52.17
    infantile acute — *see* Poliomyelitis, paralytic
    supranuclear G23.1

▽ Subterms under main terms may continue to next column or page   ☑ Additional Character Required — Refer to the Tabular List for Character Selection   247

Paraganglioma — Paralysis, paralytic

Paralysis, paralytic — *continued*
- pseudobulbar G12.29
- pseudohypertrophic (muscle) G71.09
- psychogenic F44.4
- quadriceps G57.9- ☑
- quadriplegic — *see* Tetraplegia
- radial nerve G56.3- ☑
- rectus muscle (eye) H49.9
- recurrent isolated sleep G47.53
- respiratory (muscle) (system) (tract) R06.81
  - center NEC G93.89
  - congenital P28.89
  - newborn P28.89
- right side — *see* Hemiplegia
- saturnine T56.0 ☑
- sciatic nerve G57.0- ☑
- senile G83.9
- shaking — *see* Parkinsonism
- shoulder G56.9- ☑
- sleep, recurrent isolated G47.53
- spastic G83.9
  - cerebral — *see* Palsy, cerebral, spastic
  - congenital (cerebral) — *see* Palsy, cerebral, spastic
  - familial G11.4
  - hereditary G11.4
  - quadriplegic G80.0
  - syphilitic (spinal) A52.17
- sphincter, bladder — *see* Paralysis, bladder
- spinal (cord) G83.9
  - accessory nerve G52.8
  - acute — *see* Poliomyelitis, paralytic
  - ascending acute G61.0
  - atrophic (acute) (*see also* Poliomyelitis, paralytic)
    - spastic, syphilitic A52.17
  - congenital NEC — *see* Palsy, cerebral
  - hereditary G95.89
  - infantile — *see* Poliomyelitis, paralytic
  - progressive G12.21
  - sequelae NEC G83.89
- sternomastoid G52.8
- stomach K31.84
  - diabetic — *see* Diabetes, by type, with gastroparesis
  - nerve G52.2
    - diabetic — *see* Diabetes, by type, with gastroparesis
- stroke — *see* Infarct, brain
- subcapsularis G56.8- ☑
- supranuclear (progressive) G23.1
- sympathetic G90.8
  - cervical G90.09
  - nervous system — *see* Neuropathy, peripheral, autonomic
- syndrome G83.9
  - specified NEC G83.89
- syphilitic spastic spinal (Erb's) A52.17
- thigh G57.9- ☑
- throat J39.2
  - diphtheritic A36.0
  - muscle J39.2
- thrombotic (current episode) I63.3- ☑
- thumb G56.9- ☑
- tick — *see* Toxicity, venom, arthropod, specified NEC
- Todd's (postepileptic transitory paralysis) G83.84
- toe G57.6- ☑
- tongue K14.8
- transient R29.5
  - arm or leg NEC R29.818
  - traumatic NEC — *see* Injury, nerve
- trapezius G52.8
- traumatic, transient NEC — *see* Injury, nerve
- trembling — *see* Parkinsonism
- triceps brachii G56.9- ☑
- trigeminal nerve G50.9
- trochlear (nerve) — *see* Strabismus, paralytic, fourth nerve
- ulnar nerve G56.2- ☑
- upper limb — *see* Monoplegia, upper limb
- uremic N18.9 [G99.8]
- uveoparotitic D86.89
- uvula K13.79
  - postdiphtheritic A36.0
- vagus nerve G52.2
- vasomotor NEC G90.8
- velum palati K13.79
- vesical — *see* Paralysis, bladder
- vestibular nerve (except Vertigo) H93.3 ☑
- vocal cords J38.00
  - bilateral J38.02

Paralysis, paralytic — *continued*
- vocal cords — *continued*
  - unilateral J38.01
- Volkmann's (complicating trauma) T79.6 ☑
- wasting G12.29
- Weber's G46.3
- wrist G56.9- ☑
- **Paramedial urethrovesical orifice** Q64.79
- **Paramenia** N92.6
- **Parametritis** (*see also* Disease, pelvis, inflammatory) N73.2
  - acute N73.0
  - complicating abortion — *see* Abortion, by type, complicated by, parametritis
- **Parametrium, parametric** — *see* condition
- **Paramnesia** — *see* Amnesia
- **Paramolar** K00.1
- **Paramyloidosis** E85.89
- **Paramyoclonus multiplex** G25.3
- **Paramyotonia** (congenita) G71.19
- **Parangi** — *see* Yaws
- **Paranoia** (querulans) F22
  - senile F03 ☑
- **Paranoid**
  - dementia (senile) F03 ☑
    - praecox — *see* Schizophrenia
  - personality F60.0
  - psychosis (climacteric) (involutional) (menopausal) F22
    - psychogenic (acute) F23
    - senile F03 ☑
  - reaction (acute) F23
    - chronic F22
  - schizophrenia F20.0
  - state (climacteric) (involutional) (menopausal) (simple) F22
    - senile F03 ☑
  - tendencies F60.0
  - traits F60.0
  - trends F60.0
  - type, psychopathic personality F60.0
- **Paraparesis** — *see* Paraplegia
- **Paraphasia** R47.02
- **Paraphilia** F65.9
- **Paraphimosis** (congenital) N47.2
  - chancroidal A57
- **Paraphrenia, paraphrenic** (late) F22
  - schizophrenia F20.0
- **Paraplegia** (lower) G82.20
  - ataxic — *see* Degeneration, combined, spinal cord
  - complete G82.21
  - congenital (cerebral) G80.8
    - spastic G80.1
  - familial spastic G11.4
  - functional (hysterical) F44.4
  - hereditary, spastic G11.4
  - hysterical F44.4
  - incomplete G82.22
  - Pott's A18.01
  - psychogenic F44.4
  - spastic
    - Erb's spinal, syphilitic A52.17
    - hereditary G11.4
    - tropical G04.1
  - syphilitic (spastic) A52.17
  - traumatic
    - current injury — code to injury with seventh character A
    - sequela of previous injury — code to injury with seventh character S
  - tropical spastic G04.1
- **Parapoxvirus** B08.60
  - specified NEC B08.69
- **Paraproteinemia** D89.2
  - benign (familial) D89.2
  - monoclonal D47.2
  - secondary to malignant disease D47.2
- **Parapsoriasis** L41.9
  - en plaques L41.4
  - guttata L41.1
  - large plaque L41.4
  - retiform, retiformis L41.5
  - small plaque L41.3
  - specified NEC L41.8
  - varioliformis (acuta) L41.0
- **Parasitic** (*see also* condition)
  - disease NEC B89
  - stomatitis B37.0
  - sycosis (beard) (scalp) B35.0

Parasitic — *continued*
- twin Q89.4
- **Parasitism** B89
  - intestinal B82.9
  - skin B88.9
  - specified — *see* Infestation
- **Parasitophobia** F40.218
- **Parasomnia** G47.50
  - due to
    - alcohol
      - abuse F10.182
      - dependence F10.282
      - use F10.982
    - amphetamines
      - abuse F15.182
      - dependence F15.282
      - use F15.982
    - caffeine
      - abuse F15.182
      - dependence F15.282
      - use F15.982
    - cocaine
      - abuse F14.182
      - dependence F14.282
      - use F14.982
    - drug NEC
      - abuse F19.182
      - dependence F19.282
      - use F19.982
    - opioid
      - abuse F11.182
      - dependence F11.282
      - use F11.982
    - psychoactive substance NEC
      - abuse F19.182
      - dependence F19.282
      - use F19.982
    - sedative, hypnotic, or anxiolytic
      - abuse F13.182
      - dependence F13.282
      - use F13.982
    - stimulant NEC
      - abuse F15.182
      - dependence F15.282
      - use F15.982
  - in conditions classified elsewhere G47.54
  - nonorganic origin F51.8
  - organic G47.50
  - specified NEC G47.59
- **Paraspadias** Q54.9
- **Paraspasmus facialis** G51.8
- **Parasuicide** (attempt)
  - history of (personal) Z91.5
    - in family Z81.8
- **Parathyroid gland** — *see* condition
- **Parathyroid tetany** E20.9
- **Paratrachoma** A74.0
- **Paratyphilitis** — *see* Appendicitis
- **Paratyphoid** (fever) — *see* Fever, paratyphoid
- **Paratyphus** — *see* Fever, paratyphoid
- **Paraurethral duct** Q64.79
  - nonorganic origin F51.5
- **Paraurethritis** (*see also* Urethritis)
  - gonococcal (acute) (chronic) (with abscess) A54.1
- **Paravaccinia NEC** B08.04
- **Paravaginitis** — *see* Vaginitis
- **Parencephalitis** (*see also* Encephalitis)
  - sequelae G09
- **Parent-child conflict** — *see* Conflict, parent-child
  - estrangement NEC Z62.890
- **Paresis** (*see also* Paralysis)
  - accommodation — *see* Paresis, of accommodation
  - Bernhardt's G57.1- ☑
  - bladder (sphincter) (*see also* Paralysis, bladder)
    - tabetic A52.17
  - bowel, colon or intestine K56.0
  - extrinsic muscle, eye H49.9
  - general (progressive) (syphilitic) A52.17
    - juvenile A50.45
  - heart — *see* Failure, heart
  - insane (syphilitic) A52.17
  - juvenile (general) A50.45
  - of accommodation H52.52- ☑
  - peripheral progressive (idiopathic) G60.3
  - pseudohypertrophic G71.09
  - senile G83.9
  - syphilitic (general) A52.17
    - congenital A50.45

Paresis — *continued*
vesical NEC N31.2
Paresthesia (*see also* Disturbance, sensation, skin) R20.2
Bernhardt G57.1- ☑
Paretic — *see* condition
Parinaud's
conjunctivitis H10.89
oculoglandular syndrome H10.89
ophthalmoplegia H49.88- ☑
Parkinsonism (idiopathic) (primary) G20
with neurogenic orthostatic hypotension (symptomatic) G90.3
arteriosclerotic G21.4
dementia G31.83 [F02.80]
with behavioral disturbance G31.83 [F02.81]
due to
drugs NEC G21.19
neuroleptic G21.11
medication-induced NEC G21.19
neuroleptic induced G21.11
postencephalitic G21.3
secondary G21.9
due to
arteriosclerosis G21.4
drugs NEC G21.19
neuroleptic G21.11
encephalitis G21.3
external agents NEC G21.2
syphilis A52.19
specified NEC G21.8
syphilitic A52.19
treatment-induced NEC G21.19
vascular G21.4
Parkinson's disease, syndrome or tremor — *see* Parkinsonism
Parodontitis — *see* Periodontitis
Parodontosis K05.4
Paronychia (*see also* Cellulitis, digit)
with lymphangitis — *see* Lymphangitis, acute, digit
candidal (chronic) B37.2
tuberculous (primary) A18.4
Parorexia (psychogenic) F50.89
Parosmia R43.1
psychogenic F45.8
Parotid gland — *see* condition
Parotitis, parotiditis (allergic)(nonspecific toxic) (purulent) (septic) (suppurative) (*see also* Sialoadenitis)
epidemic — *see* Mumps
infectious — *see* Mumps
postoperative K91.89
surgical K91.89
Parrot fever A70
Parrot's disease (early congenital syphilitic pseudoparalysis) A50.02
Parry-Romberg syndrome G51.8
Parry's disease or syndrome E05.00
with thyroid storm E05.01
Pars planitis — *see* Cyclitis
Parsonage (-Aldren)-**Turner syndrome** G54.5
Parson's disease (exophthalmic goiter) E05.00
with thyroid storm E05.01
Particolored infant Q82.8
Parturition — *see* Delivery
Parulis K04.7
with sinus K04.6
Parvovirus, as cause of disease classified elsewhere B97.6
Pasini and Pierini's atrophoderma L90.3
Passage
false, urethra N36.5
meconium (newborn) during delivery P03.82
of sounds or bougies — *see* Attention to, artificial, opening
Passive — *see also* condition
smoking Z77.22
Pasteurella septica A28.0
Pasteurellosis — *see* Infection, Pasteurella
PAT (paroxysmal atrial tachycardia) I47.1
Patau's syndrome — *see* Trisomy, 13
Patches
mucous (syphilitic) A51.39
congenital A50.07
smokers' (mouth) K13.24
Patellar — *see* condition
Patent (*see also* Imperfect, closure)
canal of Nuck Q52.4
cervix N88.3

Patent — *continued*
ductus arteriosus or Botallo's Q25.0
foramen
botalli Q21.1
ovale Q21.1
interauricular septum Q21.1
interventricular septum Q21.0
omphalomesenteric duct Q43.0
os (uteri) — *see* Patent, cervix
ostium secundum Q21.1
urachus Q64.4
vitelline duct Q43.0
Paterson (-Brown)(-Kelly) **syndrome or web** D50.1
Pathologic, pathological (*see also* condition)
asphyxia R09.01
fire-setting F63.1
gambling F63.0
ovum O02.0
resorption, tooth K03.3
stealing F63.2
Pathology (of) — *see* Disease
periradicular, associated with previous endodontic treatment NEC M27.59
Pattern, sleep-wake, irregular G47.23
Patulous (*see also* Imperfect, closure (congenital))
alimentary tract Q45.8
lower Q43.8
upper Q40.8
eustachian tube H69.0- ☑
Pause, sinoatrial I49.5
Paxton's disease B36.2
Pearl(s)
enamel K00.2
Epstein's K09.8
Pearl-worker's disease — *see* Osteomyelitis, specified type NEC
Pectenosis K62.4
Pectoral — *see* condition
Pectus
carinatum (congenital) Q67.7
acquired M95.4
rachitic sequelae (late effect) E64.3
excavatum (congenital) Q67.6
acquired M95.4
rachitic sequelae (late effect) E64.3
recurvatum (congenital) Q67.6
Pedatrophia E41
Pederosis F65.4
Pediculosis (infestation) B85.2
capitis (head-louse) (any site) B85.0
corporis (body-louse) (any site) B85.1
eyelid B85.0
mixed (classifiable to more than one of the titles B85.0-B85.3) B85.4
pubis (pubic louse) (any site) B85.3
vestimenti B85.1
vulvae B85.3
Pediculus (infestation) — *see* Pediculosis
Pedophilia F65.4
Peg-shaped teeth K00.2
Pelade — *see* Alopecia, areata
Pelger-Huët anomaly or syndrome D72.0
Peliosis (rheumatica) D69.0
hepatis K76.4
with toxic liver disease K71.8
Pelizaeus-Merzbacher disease E75.29
Pellagra (alcoholic) (with polyneuropathy) E52
Pellagra-cerebellar-ataxia-renal aminoaciduria syndrome E72.02
Pellegrini (-Stieda) **disease or syndrome** — *see* Bursitis, tibial collateral
Pellizzi's syndrome E34.8
Pel's crisis A52.11
Pelvic (*see also* condition)
examination (periodic) (routine) Z01.419
with abnormal findings Z01.411
kidney, congenital Q63.2
Pelviolithiasis — *see* Calculus, kidney
Pelviperitonitis (*see also* Peritonitis, pelvic)
gonococcal A54.24
puerperal O85
Pelvis — *see* condition or type
Pemphigoid L12.9
benign, mucous membrane L12.1
bullous L12.0
cicatricial L12.1
juvenile L12.2
ocular L12.1

Pemphigoid — *continued*
specified NEC L12.8
Pemphigus L10.9
benign familial (chronic) Q82.8
Brazilian L10.3
circinatus L13.0
conjunctiva L12.1
drug-induced L10.5
erythematosus L10.4
foliaceous L10.2
gangrenous — *see* Gangrene
neonatorum L01.03
ocular L12.1
paraneoplastic L10.81
specified NEC L10.89
syphilitic (congenital) A50.06
vegetans L10.1
vulgaris L10.0
wildfire L10.3
Pendred's syndrome E07.1
Pendulous
abdomen, in pregnancy — *see* Pregnancy, complicated by, abnormal, pelvic organs or tissues NEC
breast N64.89
Penetrating wound (*see also* Puncture)
with internal injury — *see* Injury, by site
eyeball — *see* Puncture, eyeball
orbit (with or without foreign body) — *see* Puncture, orbit
uterus by instrument with or following ectopic or molar pregnancy O08.6
Penicillosis B48.4
Penis — *see* condition
Penitis N48.29
Pentalogy of Fallot Q21.8
Pentasomy X syndrome Q97.1
Pentosuria (essential) E74.8
Percreta placenta - O43.23 ☑
Peregrinating patient — *see* Disorder, factitious
Perforation, perforated (nontraumatic) (of)
accidental during procedure (blood vessel) (nerve) (organ) — *see* Complication, accidental puncture or laceration
antrum — *see* Sinusitis, maxillary
appendix K35.32
with localized peritonitis K35.32
atrial septum, multiple Q21.1
attic, ear — *see* Perforation, tympanum, attic
bile duct (common) (hepatic) K83.2
cystic K82.2
bladder (urinary)
with or following ectopic or molar pregnancy O08.6
obstetrical trauma O71.5
traumatic S37.29 ☑
at delivery O71.5
bowel K63.1
with or following ectopic or molar pregnancy O08.6
newborn P78.0
obstetrical trauma O71.5
traumatic — *see* Laceration, intestine
broad ligament N83.8
with or following ectopic or molar pregnancy O08.6
obstetrical trauma O71.6
by
device, implant or graft (*see also* Complications, by site and type, mechanical) T85.628 ☑
arterial graft NEC — *see* Complication, cardiovascular device, mechanical, vascular
breast (implant) T85.49 ☑
catheter NEC T85.698 ☑
cystostomy T83.090 ☑
dialysis (renal) T82.49 ☑
intraperitoneal T85.691 ☑
infusion NEC T82.594 ☑
spinal (epidural) (subdural) T85.690 ☑
urinary (*see also* Complications, catheter, urinary T83.098 ☑
electronic (electrode) (pulse generator) (stimulator)
bone T84.390 ☑
cardiac T82.199 ☑
electrode T82.190 ☑
pulse generator T82.191 ☑
specified type NEC T82.198 ☑
nervous system — *see* Complication, prosthetic device, mechanical, electronic nervous system stimulator

Perforation, perforated — *continued*
  by — *continued*
    device, implant or graft (*see also* Complications, by
        site and type, mechanical) — *continued*
      electronic — *continued*
        urinary — *see* Complication, genitourinary,
            device, urinary, mechanical
      fixation, internal (orthopedic) NEC — *see* Compli-
          cation, fixation device, mechanical
      gastrointestinal — *see* Complications, prosthetic
          device, mechanical, gastrointestinal device
      genital NEC T83.498 ☑
        intrauterine contraceptive device T83.39 ☑
        penile prosthesis T83.490 ☑
      heart NEC — *see* Complication, cardiovascular
          device, mechanical
      joint prosthesis — *see* Complications, joint
          prosthesis, mechanical, specified NEC, by
          site
      ocular NEC — *see* Complications, prosthetic de-
          vice, mechanical, ocular device
      orthopedic NEC — *see* Complication, orthopedic,
          device, mechanical
      specified NEC T85.628 ☑
      urinary NEC (*see also* Complication, genitouri-
          nary, device, urinary, mechanical)
        graft T83.29 ☑
      vascular NEC — *see* Complication, cardiovascular
          device, mechanical
      ventricular intracranial shunt T85.09 ☑
    foreign body left accidentally in operative wound
        T81.539 ☑
    instrument (any) during a procedure, accidental —
        see Puncture, accidental complicating surgery
  cecum K35.32
    with localized peritonitis K35.32
  cervix (uteri) N88.8
    with or following ectopic or molar pregnancy O08.6
    obstetrical trauma O71.3
  colon K63.1
    newborn P78.0
    obstetrical trauma O71.5
    traumatic — *see* Laceration, intestine, large
  common duct (bile) K83.2
  cornea (due to ulceration) — *see* Ulcer, cornea, perfo-
      rated
  cystic duct K82.2
  diverticulum (intestine) K57.80
    with bleeding K57.81
    large intestine K57.20
      with
        bleeding K57.21
        small intestine K57.40
          with bleeding K57.41
    small intestine K57.00
      with
        bleeding K57.01
        large intestine K57.40
          with bleeding K57.41
  ear drum — *see* Perforation, tympanum
  esophagus K22.3
  ethmoidal sinus — *see* Sinusitis, ethmoidal
  frontal sinus — *see* Sinusitis, frontal
  gallbladder K82.2
  heart valve — *see* Endocarditis
  ileum K63.1
    newborn P78.0
    obstetrical trauma O71.5
    traumatic — *see* Laceration, intestine, small
  instrumental, surgical (accidental) (blood vessel) (nerve)
      (organ) — *see* Puncture, accidental complicating
      surgery
  intestine NEC K63.1
    with ectopic or molar pregnancy O08.6
    newborn P78.0
    obstetrical trauma O71.5
    traumatic — *see* Laceration, intestine
    ulcerative NEC K63.1
      newborn P78.0
  jejunum, jejunal K63.1
    obstetrical trauma O71.5
    traumatic — *see* Laceration, intestine, small
    ulcer — *see* Ulcer, gastrojejunal, with perforation
  joint prosthesis — *see* Complications, joint prosthesis,
      mechanical, specified NEC, by site
  mastoid (antrum) (cell) — *see* Disorder, mastoid,
      specified NEC
  maxillary sinus — *see* Sinusitis, maxillary

Perforation, perforated — *continued*
  membrana tympani — *see* Perforation, tympanum
  nasal
    septum J34.89
      congenital Q30.3
      syphilitic A52.73
    sinus J34.89
      congenital Q30.8
      due to sinusitis — *see* Sinusitis
  palate (*see also* Cleft, palate) Q35.9
    syphilitic A52.79
  palatine vault (*see also* Cleft, palate, hard) Q35.1
    syphilitic A52.79
    congenital A50.59
  pars flaccida (ear drum) — *see* Perforation, tympanum,
      attic
  pelvic
    floor S31.030 ☑
      with
        ectopic or molar pregnancy O08.6
        penetration into retroperitoneal space
            S31.031 ☑
        retained foreign body S31.040 ☑
          with penetration into retroperitoneal
              space S31.041 ☑
      following ectopic or molar pregnancy O08.6
      obstetrical trauma O70.1
    organ S37.99 ☑
      adrenal gland S37.818 ☑
      bladder — *see* Perforation, bladder
      fallopian tube S37.599 ☑
        bilateral S37.592 ☑
        unilateral S37.591 ☑
      kidney S37.09- ☑
      obstetrical trauma O71.5
      ovary S37.499 ☑
        bilateral S37.492 ☑
        unilateral S37.491 ☑
      prostate S37.828 ☑
      specified organ NEC S37.898 ☑
      ureter — *see* Perforation, ureter
      urethra — *see* Perforation, urethra
      uterus — *see* Perforation, uterus
  perineum — *see* Laceration, perineum
  pharynx J39.2
  rectum K63.1
    newborn P78.0
    obstetrical trauma O71.5
    traumatic S36.63 ☑
  root canal space due to endodontic treatment M27.51
  sigmoid K63.1
    newborn P78.0
    obstetrical trauma O71.5
    traumatic S36.533 ☑
  sinus (accessory) (chronic) (nasal) J34.89
  sphenoidal sinus — *see* Sinusitis, sphenoidal
  surgical (accidental) (by instrument) (blood vessel)
      (nerve) (organ) — *see* Puncture, accidental
      complicating surgery
  traumatic
    external — *see* Puncture
    eye — *see* Puncture, eyeball
    internal organ — *see* Injury, by site
  tympanum, tympanic (membrane) (persistent post-
      traumatic) (postinflammatory) H72.9- ☑
    attic H72.1- ☑
      multiple — *see* Perforation, tympanum, multiple
      total — *see* Perforation, tympanum, total
    central H72.0- ☑
      multiple — *see* Perforation, tympanum, multiple
      total — *see* Perforation, tympanum, total
    marginal NEC — *see* subcategory H72.2 ☑
    multiple H72.81- ☑
    pars flaccida — *see* Perforation, tympanum, attic
    total H72.82- ☑
    traumatic, current episode S09.2- ☑
  typhoid, gastrointestinal — *see* Typhoid
  ulcer — *see* Ulcer, by site, with perforation
  ureter N28.89
    traumatic S37.19 ☑
  urethra N36.8
    with ectopic or molar pregnancy O08.6
    following ectopic or molar pregnancy O08.6
    obstetrical trauma O71.5
    traumatic S37.39 ☑
      at delivery O71.5

Perforation, perforated — *continued*
  uterus
    with ectopic or molar pregnancy O08.6
    by intrauterine contraceptive device T83.39 ☑
    following ectopic or molar pregnancy O08.6
    obstetrical trauma O71.1
    traumatic S37.69 ☑
      obstetric O71.1
  uvula K13.79
    syphilitic A52.79
  vagina N71.4
    obstetrical trauma O71.4
    other trauma — *see* Puncture, vagina
Periadenitis mucosa necrotica recurrens K12.0
Periappendicitis (acute) — *see* Appendicitis
Periarteritis nodosa (disseminated) (infectious) (necro-
    tizing) M30.0
Periarthritis (joint) (*see also* Enthesopathy)
  Duplay's M75.0- ☑
  gonococcal A54.42
  humeroscapularis — *see* Capsulitis, adhesive
  scapulohumeral — *see* Capsulitis, adhesive
  shoulder — *see* Capsulitis, adhesive
  wrist M77.2- ☑
Periarthrosis (angioneural) — *see* Enthesopathy
Pericapsulitis, adhesive (shoulder) — *see* Capsulitis,
    adhesive
Pericarditis (with decompensation) (with effusion) I31.9
  with rheumatic fever (conditions in I00)
    active — *see* Pericarditis, rheumatic
    inactive or quiescent I09.2
  acute (hemorrhagic) (nonrheumatic) (Sicca) I30.9
    with chorea (acute) (rheumatic) (Sydenham's) I02.0
    benign I30.8
    nonspecific I30.0
    rheumatic I01.0
      with chorea (acute) (Sydenham's) I02.0
  adhesive or adherent (chronic) (external) (internal) I31.0
    acute — *see* Pericarditis, acute
    rheumatic I09.2
  bacterial (acute) (subacute) (with serous or seropuru-
      lent effusion) I30.1
  calcareous I31.1
  cholesterol (chronic) I31.8
    acute I30.9
  chronic (nonrheumatic) I31.9
    rheumatic I09.2
  constrictive (chronic) I31.1
  coxsackie B33.23
  fibrinocaseous (tuberculous) A18.84
  fibrinopurulent I30.1
  fibrinous I30.8
  fibrous I31.0
  gonococcal A54.83
  idiopathic I30.0
  in systemic lupus erythematosus M32.12
  infective I30.1
  meningococcal A39.53
  neoplastic (chronic) I31.8
    acute I30.9
  obliterans, obliterating I31.0
  plastic I31.0
  pneumococcal I30.1
  postinfarction I24.1
  purulent I30.1
  rheumatic (active) (acute) (with effusion) (with pneu-
      monia) I01.0
    with chorea (acute) (rheumatic) (Sydenham's) I02.0
    chronic or inactive (with chorea) I09.2
  rheumatoid — *see* Rheumatoid, carditis
  septic I30.1
  serofibrinous I30.8
  staphylococcal I30.1
  streptococcal I30.1
  suppurative I30.1
  syphilitic A52.06
  tuberculous A18.84
  uremic N18.9 [I32]
  viral I30.1
Pericardium, pericardial — *see* condition
Pericellulitis — *see* Cellulitis
Pericementitis (chronic) (suppurative) (*see also* Periodon-
    titis)
  acute K05.20
    generalized — *see* Peridontitis, aggressive, general-
        ized
    localized — *see* Peridontitis, aggressive, localized

Perichondritis
 auricle — see Perichondritis, ear
 bronchus J98.09
 ear (external) H61.00- ☑
  acute H61.01- ☑
  chronic H61.02- ☑
 external auditory canal — see Perichondritis, ear
 larynx J38.7
  syphilitic A52.73
  typhoid A01.09
 nose J34.89
 pinna — see Perichondritis, ear
 trachea J39.8
Periclasia K05.4
Pericoronitis — see Periodontitis
Pericystitis N30.90
 with hematuria N30.91
Peridiverticulitis (intestine) K57.92
 cecum — see Diverticulitis, intestine, large
 colon — see Diverticulitis, intestine, large
 duodenum — see Diverticulitis, intestine, small
 intestine — see Diverticulitis, intestine
 jejunum — see Diverticulitis, intestine, small
 rectosigmoid — see Diverticulitis, intestine, large
 rectum — see Diverticulitis, intestine, large
 sigmoid — see Diverticulitis, intestine, large
Periendocarditis — see Endocarditis
Periepididymitis N45.1
Perifolliculitis L01.02
 abscedens, caput, scalp L66.3
 capitis, abscedens (et suffodiens) L66.3
 superficial pustular L01.02
Perihepatitis K65.8
Perilabyrinthitis (acute) — see subcategory H83.0 ☑
Perimeningitis — see Meningitis
Perimetritis — see Endometritis
Perimetrosalpingitis — see Salpingo-oophoritis
Perineocele N81.81
Perinephric, perinephritic — see condition
Perinephritis (see also Infection, kidney)
 purulent — see Abscess, kidney
Perineum, perineal — see condition
Perineuritis NEC — see Neuralgia
Periodic — see condition
Periodontitis (chronic) (complex) (compound) (local)
  (simplex) K05.30
 acute K05.20
  generalized K05.229
   moderate K05.222
   severe K05.223
   slight K05.221
  localized K05.219
   moderate K05.212
   severe K05.213
   slight K05.211
 apical K04.5
  acute (pulpal origin) K04.4
 generalized K05.329
  moderate K05.322
  severe K05.323
  slight K05.321
 localized K05.319
  moderate K05.312
  severe K05.313
  slight K05.311
Periodontoclasia K05.4
Periodontosis (juvenile) K05.4
Periods (see also Menstruation)
 heavy N92.0
 irregular N92.6
 shortened intervals (irregular) N92.1
Perionychia (see also Cellulitis, digit)
 with lymphangitis — see Lymphangitis, acute, digit
Perioophoritis — see Salpingo-oophoritis
Periorchitis N45.2
Periosteum, periosteal — see condition
Periostitis (albuminosa) (circumscribed) (diffuse) (infective) (monomelic) (see also Osteomyelitis)
 alveolar M27.3
 alveolodental M27.3
 dental M27.3
 gonorrheal A54.43
 jaw (lower) (upper) M27.2
 orbit H05.03- ☑
 syphilitic A52.77
  congenital (early) A50.02 [M90.80]
  secondary A51.46

Periostitis — continued
 tuberculous — see Tuberculosis, bone
 yaws (hypertrophic) (early) (late) A66.6 [M90.80]
Periostosis (hyperplastic) (see also Disorder, bone, specified type NEC)
 with osteomyelitis — see Osteomyelitis, specified type
  NEC
Peripartum
 cardiomyopathy O90.3
Periphlebitis — see Phlebitis
Periproctitis K62.89
Periprostatitis — see Prostatitis
Perirectal — see condition
Perirenal — see condition
Perisalpingitis — see Salpingo-oophoritis
Perisplenitis (infectional) D73.89
Peristalsis, visible or reversed R19.2
Peritendinitis — see Enthesopathy
Peritoneum, peritoneal — see condition
Peritonitis (adhesive) (bacterial) (fibrinous) (hemorrhagic)
  (idiopathic) (localized) (perforative) (primary) (with
  adhesions) (with effusion) K65.9
 with or following
  abscess K65.1
  appendicitis
   with perforation or rupture K35.32
   generalized (see also Appendicitis) K35.20
   localized (see also Appendicitis) K35.30
  diverticular disease (intestine) K57.80
   with bleeding K57.81
   ectopic or molar pregnancy O08.0
   large intestine K57.20
    with
     bleeding K57.21
     small intestine K57.40
      with bleeding K57.41
    small intestine K57.00
     with
      bleeding K57.01
      large intestine K57.40
       with bleeding K57.41
 acute (generalized) K65.0
 aseptic T81.61 ☑
 bile, biliary K65.3
 chemical T81.61 ☑
 chlamydial A74.81
 chronic proliferative K65.8
 complicating abortion — see Abortion, by type, complicated by, pelvic peritonitis
 congenital P78.1
 diaphragmatic K65.0
 diffuse K65.0
 diphtheritic A36.89
 disseminated K65.0
 due to
  bile K65.3
  foreign
   body or object accidentally left during a procedure (instrument) (sponge) (swab)
    T81.599 ☑
   substance accidentally left during a procedure
    (chemical) (powder) (talc) T81.61 ☑
  talc T81.61 ☑
  urine K65.8
 eosinophilic K65.8
  acute K65.0
 fibrocaseous (tuberculous) A18.31
 fibropurulent K65.0
 following ectopic or molar pregnancy O08.0
 general (ized) K65.0
 gonococcal A54.85
 meconium (newborn) P78.0
 neonatal P78.1
  meconium P78.0
 pancreatic K65.0
 paroxysmal, familial E85.0
  benign E85.0
 pelvic
  female N73.5
   acute N73.3
   chronic N73.4
    with adhesions N73.6
  male K65.0
 periodic, familial E85.0
 proliferative, chronic K65.8
 puerperal, postpartum, childbirth O85
 purulent K65.0
 septic K65.0

Peritonitis — continued
 specified NEC K65.8
 spontaneous bacterial K65.2
 subdiaphragmatic K65.0
 subphrenic K65.0
 suppurative K65.0
 syphilitic A52.74
  congenital (early) A50.08 [K67]
 talc T81.61 ☑
 tuberculous A18.31
 urine K65.8
Peritonsillar — see condition
Peritonsillitis J36
Perityphlitis K37
Periureteritis N28.89
Periurethral — see condition
Periurethritis (gangrenous) — see Urethritis
Periuterine — see condition
Perivaginitis — see Vaginitis
Perivasculitis, retinal H35.06- ☑
Perivasitis (chronic) N49.1
Perivesiculitis (seminal) — see Vesiculitis
Perlèche NEC K13.0
 due to
  candidiasis B37.83
  moniliasis B37.83
  riboflavin deficiency E53.0
  vitamin B2 (riboflavin) deficiency E53.0
Pernicious — see condition
Pernio, perniosis T69.1 ☑
Perpetrator (of abuse) — see Index to External Causes
  of Injury, Perpetrator
Persecution
 delusion F22
 social Z60.5
Perseveration (tonic) R48.8
Persistence, persistent (congenital)
 anal membrane Q42.3
  with fistula Q42.2
 arteria stapedia Q16.3
 atrioventricular canal Q21.2
 branchial cleft NOS Q18.2
  cyst Q18.0
  fistula Q18.0
  sinus Q18.0
 bulbus cordis in left ventricle Q21.8
 canal of Cloquet Q14.0
 capsule (opaque) Q12.8
 cilioretinal artery or vein Q14.8
 cloaca Q43.7
 communication — see Fistula, congenital
 convolutions
  aortic arch Q25.46
  fallopian tube Q50.6
  oviduct Q50.6
  uterine tube Q50.6
 double aortic arch Q25.45
 ductus arteriosus (Botalli) Q25.0
 fetal
  circulation P29.38
  form of cervix (uteri) Q51.828
  hemoglobin, hereditary (HPFH) D56.4
 foramen
  Botalli Q21.1
  ovale Q21.1
 Gartner's duct Q52.4
 hemoglobin, fetal (hereditary) (HPFH) D56.4
 hyaloid
  artery (generally incomplete) Q14.0
  system Q14.8
 hymen, in pregnancy or childbirth — see Pregnancy,
   complicated by, abnormal, vulva
 lanugo Q84.2
 left
  posterior cardinal vein Q26.8
  root with right arch of aorta Q25.49
  superior vena cava Q26.1
 Meckel's diverticulum Q43.0
  malignant — see Table of Neoplasms, small intestine, malignant
 mucosal disease (middle ear) — see Otitis, media,
   suppurative, chronic, tubotympanic
 nail(s), anomalous Q84.6
 omphalomesenteric duct Q43.0
 organ or site not listed — see Anomaly, by site
 ostium
  atrioventriculare commune Q21.2
  primum Q21.2

Persistence, persistent — *continued*
- ostium — *continued*
  - secundum Q21.1
- ovarian rests in fallopian tube Q50.6
- pancreatic tissue in intestinal tract Q43.8
- primary (deciduous)
  - teeth K00.6
  - vitreous hyperplasia Q14.0
- pupillary membrane Q13.89
- rhesus (Rh) titer — *see* Complication(s), transfusion, incompatibility reaction, Rh (factor)
- right aortic arch Q25.47
- sinus
  - urogenitalis
    - female Q52.8
    - male Q55.8
  - venosus with imperfect incorporation in right auricle Q26.8
- thymus (gland) (hyperplasia) E32.0
- thyroglossal duct Q89.2
- thyrolingual duct Q89.2
- truncus arteriosus or communis Q20.0
- tunica vasculosa lentis Q12.2
- umbilical sinus Q64.4
- urachus Q64.4
- vitelline duct Q43.0

Person (with)
- admitted for clinical research, as a control subject (normal comparison) (participant) Z00.6
- awaiting admission to adequate facility elsewhere Z75.1
- concern (normal) about sick person in family Z63.6
- consulting on behalf of another Z71.0
- feigning illness Z76.5
- living (in)
  - alone Z60.2
  - boarding school Z59.3
  - residential institution Z59.3
  - without
    - adequate housing (heating) (space) Z59.1
    - housing (permanent) (temporary) Z59.0
    - person able to render necessary care Z74.2
    - shelter Z59.0
- on waiting list Z75.1
- sick or handicapped in family Z63.6

Personality (disorder) F60.9
- accentuation of traits (type A pattern) Z73.1
- affective F34.0
- aggressive F60.3
- amoral F60.2
- anacastic, anankastic F60.5
- antisocial F60.2
- anxious F60.6
- asocial F60.2
- asthenic F60.7
- avoidant F60.6
- borderline F60.3
- change due to organic condition (enduring) F07.0
- compulsive F60.5
- cycloid F34.0
- cyclothymic F34.0
- dependent F60.7
- depressive F34.1
- dissocial F60.2
- dual F44.81
- eccentric F60.89
- emotionally unstable F60.3
- expansive paranoid F60.0
- explosive F60.3
- fanatic F60.0
- haltlose type F60.89
- histrionic F60.4
- hyperthymic F34.0
- hypothymic F34.1
- hysterical F60.4
- immature F60.89
- inadequate F60.7
- labile (emotional) F60.3
- mixed (nonspecific) F60.89
- morally defective F60.2
- multiple F44.81
- narcissistic F60.81
- obsessional F60.5
- obsessive (-compulsive) F60.5
- organic F07.0
- overconscientious F60.5
- paranoid F60.0
- passive (-dependent) F60.7
- passive-aggressive F60.89

Personality — *continued*
- pathologic F60.9
- pattern defect or disturbance F60.9
- pseudopsychopathic (organic) F07.0
- pseudoretarded (organic) F07.0
- psychoinfantile F60.4
- psychoneurotic NEC F60.89
- psychopathic F60.2
- querulant F60.0
- sadistic F60.89
- schizoid F60.1
- self-defeating F60.7
- sensitive paranoid F60.0
- sociopathic (amoral) (antisocial) (asocial) (dissocial) F60.2
- specified NEC F60.89
- type A Z73.1
- unstable (emotional) F60.3

Perthes' disease — *see* Legg-Calvé-Perthes disease

Pertussis (*see also* Whooping cough) A37.90

Perversion, perverted
- appetite F50.89
  - psychogenic F50.89
- function
  - pituitary gland E23.2
    - posterior lobe E22.2
- sense of smell and taste R43.8
  - psychogenic F45.8
- sexual — *see* Deviation, sexual

Pervious, congenital (*see also* Imperfect, closure)
- ductus arteriosus Q25.0

Pes (congenital) (*see also* Talipes)
- acquired (*see also* Deformity, limb, foot, specified NEC)
  - planus — *see* Deformity, limb, flat foot
- adductus Q66.89
- cavus Q66.7
- deformity NEC, acquired — *see* Deformity, limb, foot, specified NEC
- planus (acquired) (any degree) (*see also* Deformity, limb, flat foot)
  - rachitic sequelae (late effect) E64.3
- valgus Q66.6

Pest, pestis — *see* Plague

Petechia, petechiae R23.3
- newborn P54.5

Petechial typhus A75.1

Peter's anomaly Q13.4

Petit mal seizure — *see* Epilepsy, generalized, specified NEC

Petit's hernia — *see* Hernia, abdomen, specified site NEC

Petrellidosis B48.2

Petrositis H70.20- ☑
- acute H70.21- ☑
- chronic H70.22- ☑

Peutz-Jeghers disease or syndrome Q85.8

Peyronie's disease N48.6

PFAPA (periodic fever, aphthous stomatitis, pharyngitis, and adenopathy syndrome) M04.8

Pfeiffer's disease — *see* Mononucleosis, infectious

Phagedena (dry) (moist) (sloughing) (*see also* Gangrene)
- geometric L88
- penis N48.29
- tropical — *see* Ulcer, skin
- vulva N76.6

Phagedenic — *see* condition

Phakoma H35.89

Phakomatosis (*see also* specific eponymous syndromes) Q85.9
- Bourneville's Q85.1
- specified NEC Q85.8

Phantom limb syndrome (without pain) G54.7
- with pain G54.6

Pharyngeal pouch syndrome D82.1

Pharyngitis (acute) (catarrhal) (gangrenous) (infective) (malignant) (membranous) (phlegmonous) (pseudomembranous) (simple) (subacute) (suppurative) (ulcerative) (viral) J02.9
- with influenza, flu, or grippe — *see* Influenza, with, pharyngitis
- aphthous B08.5
- atrophic J31.2
- chlamydial A56.4
- chronic (atrophic) (granular) (hypertrophic) J31.2
- coxsackievirus B08.5
- diphtheritic A36.0
- enteroviral vesicular B08.5
- follicular (chronic) J31.2
- fusospirochetal A69.1

Pharyngitis — *continued*
- gonococcal A54.5
- granular (chronic) J31.2
- herpesviral B00.2
- hypertrophic J31.2
- infectional, chronic J31.2
- influenzal — *see* Influenza, with, respiratory manifestations NEC
- lymphonodular, acute (enteroviral) B08.8
- pneumococcal J02.8
- purulent J02.9
- putrid J02.9
- septic J02.0
- sicca J31.2
- specified organism NEC J02.8
- staphylococcal J02.8
- streptococcal J02.0
- syphilitic, congenital (early) A50.03
- tuberculous A15.8
- vesicular, enteroviral B08.5
- viral NEC J02.8

Pharyngoconjunctivitis, viral B30.2

Pharyngolaryngitis (acute) J06.0
- chronic J37.0

Pharyngoplegia J39.2

Pharyngotonsillitis, herpesviral B00.2

Pharyngotracheitis, chronic J42

Pharynx, pharyngeal — *see* condition

Phencyclidine-induced
- anxiety disorder F16.980
- bipolar and related disorder F16.94
- depressive disorder F16.94
- psychotic disorder F16.959

Phenomenon
- Arthus' — *see* Arthus' phenomenon
- jaw-winking Q07.8
- lupus erythematosus (LE) cell M32.9
- Raynaud's (secondary) I73.00
  - with gangrene I73.01
- vasomotor R55
- vasospastic I73.9
- vasovagal R55
- Wenckebach's I44.1

Phenylketonuria E70.1
- classical E70.0
- maternal E70.1

Pheochromoblastoma
- specified site — *see* Neoplasm, malignant, by site
- unspecified site C74.10

Pheochromocytoma
- malignant
  - specified site — *see* Neoplasm, malignant, by site
  - unspecified site C74.10
- specified site — *see* Neoplasm, benign, by site
- unspecified site D35.00

Pheohyphomycosis — *see* Chromomycosis

Pheomycosis — *see* Chromomycosis

Phimosis (congenital) (due to infection) N47.1
- chancroidal A57

Phlebectasia (*see also* Varix)
- congenital Q27.4

Phlebitis (infective) (pyemic) (septic) (suppurative) I80.9
- antepartum — *see* Thrombophlebitis, antepartum
- blue — *see* Phlebitis, leg, deep
- breast, superficial I80.8
- cavernous (venous) sinus — *see* Phlebitis, intracranial (venous) sinus
- cerebral (venous) sinus — *see* Phlebitis, intracranial (venous) sinus
- chest wall, superficial I80.8
- cranial (venous) sinus — *see* Phlebitis, intracranial (venous) sinus
- deep (vessels) — *see* Phlebitis, leg, deep
- due to implanted device — *see* Complications, by site and type, specified NEC
- during or resulting from a procedure T81.72 ☑
- femoral vein (superficial) I80.1- ☑
- femoropopliteal vein I80.0- ☑
- gestational — *see* Phlebopathy, gestational
- hepatic veins I80.8
- iliofemoral — *see* Phlebitis, femoral vein
- intracranial (venous) sinus (any) G08
  - nonpyogenic I67.6
- intraspinal venous sinuses and veins G08
  - nonpyogenic G95.19
- lateral (venous) sinus — *see* Phlebitis, intracranial (venous) sinus
- leg I80.3

☑ **Additional Character Required** — Refer to the Tabular List for Character Selection   ◗ **Subterms under main terms may continue to next column or page**

Phlebitis — continued
  leg — continued
    antepartum — see Thrombophlebitis, antepartum
    deep (vessels) NEC I80.20- ☑
      iliac I80.21- ☑
      popliteal vein I80.22- ☑
      specified vessel NEC I80.29- ☑
      tibial vein I80.23- ☑
    femoral vein (superficial) I80.1- ☑
    superficial (vessels) I80.0- ☑
  longitudinal sinus — see Phlebitis, intracranial (venous) sinus
  lower limb — see Phlebitis, leg
  migrans, migrating (superficial) I82.1
  pelvic
    with ectopic or molar pregnancy O08.0
    following ectopic or molar pregnancy O08.0
    puerperal, postpartum O87.1
  popliteal vein — see Phlebitis, leg, deep, popliteal
  portal (vein) K75.1
  postoperative T81.72 ☑
  pregnancy — see Thrombophlebitis, antepartum
  puerperal, postpartum, childbirth O87.0
    deep O87.1
    pelvic O87.1
    superficial O87.0
  retina — see Vasculitis, retina
  saphenous (accessory) (great) (long) (small) — see Phlebitis, leg, superficial
  sinus (meninges) — see Phlebitis, intracranial (venous) sinus
  specified site NEC I80.8
  syphilitic A52.09
  tibial vein — see Phlebitis, leg, deep, tibial
  ulcerative I80.9
    leg — see Phlebitis, leg
  umbilicus I80.8
  uterus (septic) — see Endometritis
  varicose (leg) (lower limb) — see Varix, leg, with, inflammation
Phlebofibrosis I87.8
Phleboliths I87.8
Phlebopathy,
  gestational O22.9- ☑
  puerperal O87.9
Phlebosclerosis I87.8
Phlebothrombosis (see also Thrombosis)
  antepartum — see Thrombophlebitis, antepartum
  pregnancy — see Thrombophlebitis, antepartum
  puerperal — see Thrombophlebitis, puerperal
Phlebotomus fever A93.1
Phlegmasia
  alba dolens O87.1
    nonpuerperal — see Phlebitis, femoral vein
  cerulea dolens — see Phlebitis, leg, deep
Phlegmon — see Abscess
Phlegmonous — see condition
Phlyctenulosis (allergic) (keratoconjunctivitis) (nontuberculous) (see also Keratoconjunctivitis)
  cornea — see Keratoconjunctivitis
  tuberculous A18.52
Phobia, phobic F40.9
  animal F40.218
    spiders F40.210
  examination F40.298
  reaction F40.9
  simple F40.298
  social F40.10
    generalized F40.11
  specific (isolated) F40.298
    animal F40.218
      spiders F40.210
    blood F40.230
    injection F40.231
    injury F40.233
    men F40.290
    natural environment F40.228
      thunderstorms F40.220
    situational F40.248
      bridges F40.242
      closed in spaces F40.240
      flying F40.243
      heights F40.241
    specified focus NEC F40.298
    transfusion F40.231
    women F40.291
  specified NEC F40.8

Phobia, phobic — continued
  specified — continued
    medical care NEC F40.232
  state F40.9
Phocas' disease — see Mastopathy, cystic
Phocomelia Q73.1
  lower limb — see Agenesis, leg, with foot present
  upper limb — see Agenesis, arm, with hand present
Phoria H50.50
Phosphate-losing tubular disorder N25.0
Phosphatemia E83.39
Phosphaturia E83.39
Photodermatitis (sun) L56.8
  chronic L57.8
  due to drug L56.8
  light other than sun L59.8
Photokeratitis H16.13- ☑
Photophobia H53.14- ☑
Photophthalmia — see Photokeratitis
Photopsia H53.19
Photoretinitis — see Retinopathy, solar
Photosensitivity, photosensitization (sun) skin L56.8
  light other than sun L59.8
Phrenitis — see Encephalitis
Phrynoderma (vitamin A deficiency) E50.8
Phthiriasis (pubis) B85.3
  with any infestation classifiable to B85.0-B85.2 B85.4
Phthirus infestation — see Phthiriasis
Phthisis (see also Tuberculosis)
  bulbi (infectional) — see Disorder, globe, degenerated condition, atrophy
  eyeball (due to infection) — see Disorder, globe, degenerated condition, atrophy
Phycomycosis — see Zygomycosis
Physalopteriasis B81.8
Physical restraint status Z78.1
Phytobezoar T18.9 ☑
  intestine T18.3 ☑
  stomach T18.2 ☑
Pian — see Yaws
Pianoma A66.1
Pica F50.89
  in adults F50.89
  infant or child F98.3
Picking, nose F98.8
Pick-Niemann disease — see Niemann-Pick disease or syndrome
Pick's
  cerebral atrophy G31.01 [F02.80]
    with behavioral disturbance G31.01 [F02.81]
  disease or syndrome (brain) G31.01 [F02.80]
    with behavioral disturbance G31.01 [F02.81]
    brain G31.01 [F02.80]
      with behavioral disturbance G31.01 [F02.81]
    pericardium (pericardial pseudocirrhosis of liver) I31.1
  syndrome
    brain G31.01 [F02.80]
      with behavioral disturbance G31.01 [F02.81]
    of heart (pericardial pseudocirrhosis of liver) I31.1
Pickwickian syndrome E66.2
Piebaldism E70.39
Piedra (beard) (scalp) B36.8
  black B36.3
  white B36.2
Pierre Robin deformity or syndrome Q87.0
Pierson's disease or osteochondrosis M91.0
Pig-bel A05.2
Pigeon
  breast or chest (acquired) M95.4
    congenital Q67.7
      rachitic sequelae (late effect) E64.3
  breeder's disease or lung J67.2
  fancier's disease or lung J67.2
  toe — see Deformity, toe, specified NEC
Pigmentation (abnormal) (anomaly) L81.9
  conjunctiva H11.13- ☑
  cornea (anterior) H18.01- ☑
    posterior H18.05- ☑
    stromal H18.06- ☑
  diminished melanin formation NEC L81.6
  iron L81.8
  lids, congenital Q82.8
  limbus corneae — see Pigmentation, cornea
  metals L81.8
  optic papilla, congenital Q14.2
  retina, congenital (grouped) (nevoid) Q14.1

Pigmentation — continued
  scrotum, congenital Q82.8
  tattoo L81.8
Piles (see also Hemorrhoids) K64.9
Pili
  annulati or torti (congenital) Q84.1
  incarnati L73.1
Pill roller hand (intrinsic) — see Parkinsonism
Pilomatrixoma — see Neoplasm, skin, benign
  malignant — see Neoplasm, skin, malignant
Pilonidal — see condition
Pimple R23.8
PIN — see Neoplasia, intraepithelial, prostate
Pinched nerve — see Neuropathy, entrapment
Pindborg tumor — see Cyst, calcifying odontogenic
Pineal body or gland — see condition
Pinealoblastoma C75.3
Pinealoma D44.5
  malignant C75.3
Pineoblastoma C75.3
Pineocytoma D44.5
Pinguecula H11.15- ☑
Pingueculitis H10.81- ☑
Pinhole meatus (see also Stricture, urethra) N35.919
Pink
  disease — see subcategory T56.1 ☑
  eye — see Conjunctivitis, acute, mucopurulent
Pinkus' disease (lichen nitidus) L44.1
Pinpoint
  meatus — see Stricture, urethra
  os (uteri) — see Stricture, cervix
Pins and needles R20.2
Pinta A67.9
  cardiovascular lesions A67.2
  chancre (primary) A67.0
  erythematous plaques A67.1
  hyperchromic lesions A67.1
  hyperkeratosis A67.1
  lesions A67.9
    cardiovascular A67.2
    hyperchromic A67.1
    intermediate A67.1
    late A67.2
    mixed A67.3
    primary A67.0
    skin (achromic) (cicatricial) (dyschromic) A67.2
      hyperchromic A67.1
      mixed (achromic and hyperchromic) A67.3
  papule (primary) A67.0
  skin lesions (achromic) (cicatricial) (dyschromic) A67.2
    hyperchromic A67.1
    mixed (achromic and hyperchromic) A67.3
  vitiligo A67.2
Pintids A67.1
Pinworm (disease) (infection) (infestation) B80
Piroplasmosis B60.0
Pistol wound — see Gunshot wound
Pitchers' elbow — see Derangement, joint, specified type NEC, elbow
Pithecoid pelvis Q74.2
  with disproportion (fetopelvic) O33.0
    causing obstructed labor O65.0
Pithiatism F48.8
Pitted — see Pitting
Pitting (see also Edema) R60.9
  lip R60.0
  nail L60.8
  teeth K00.4
Pituitary gland — see condition
Pituitary-snuff-taker's disease J67.8
Pityriasis (capitis) L21.0
  alba L30.5
  circinata (et maculata) L42
  furfuracea L21.0
  Hebra's L26
  lichenoides L41.0
    chronica L41.1
    et varioliformis (acuta) L41.0
  maculata (et circinata) L30.5
  nigra B36.1
  pilaris, Hebra's L44.0
  rosea L42
  rotunda L44.8
  rubra (Hebra) pilaris L44.0
  simplex L30.5
  specified type NEC L30.5
  streptogenes L30.5

▼ **Subterms under main terms may continue to next column or page**   ☑ **Additional Character Required — Refer to the Tabular List for Character Selection**   **253**

Phlebitis — Pityriasis

Pityriasis — *continued*
versicolor (scrotal) B36.0
Placenta, placental — *see* Pregnancy, complicated by (care of) (management affected by), specified condition
Placentitis O41.14- ☑
Plagiocephaly Q67.3
Plague A20.9
abortive A20.8
ambulatory A20.8
asymptomatic A20.8
bubonic A20.0
cellulocutaneous A20.1
cutaneobubonic A20.1
lymphatic gland A20.0
meningitis A20.3
pharyngeal A20.8
pneumonic (primary) (secondary) A20.2
pulmonary, pulmonic A20.2
septicemic A20.7
tonsillar A20.8
septicemic A20.7
Planning, family
contraception Z30.9
procreation Z31.69
Plaque(s)
artery, arterial — *see* Arteriosclerosis
calcareous — *see* Calcification
coronary, lipid rich I25.83
epicardial I31.8
erythematous, of pinta A67.1
Hollenhorst's — *see* Occlusion, artery, retina
lipid rich, coronary I25.83
pleural (without asbestos) J92.9
with asbestos J92.0
tongue K13.29
Plasmacytoma C90.3- ☑
extramedullary C90.2- ☑
medullary C90.0- ☑
solitary C90.3- ☑
Plasmacytopenia D72.818
Plasmacytosis D72.822
Plaster ulcer — *see* Ulcer, pressure, by site
Plateau iris syndrome (post-iridectomy) (postprocedural) (without glaucoma) H21.82
with glaucoma H40.22- ☑
Platybasia Q75.8
Platyonychia (congenital) Q84.6
acquired L60.8
Platypelloid pelvis M95.5
with disproportion (fetopelvic) O33.0
causing obstructed labor O65.0
congenital Q74.2
Platyspondylisis Q76.49
Plaut (-Vincent) **disease** (*see also* Vincent's) A69.1
Plethora R23.2
newborn P61.1
Pleura, pleural — *see* condition
Pleuralgia R07.81
Pleurisy (acute) (adhesive) (chronic) (costal) (diaphragmatic) (double) (dry) (fibrinous) (fibrous) (interlobar) (latent) (plastic) (primary) (residual) (sicca) (sterile) (subacute) (unresolved) R09.1
with
adherent pleura J86.0
effusion J90
chylous, chyliform J94.0
tuberculous (non primary) A15.6
primary (progressive) A15.7
tuberculosis — *see* Pleurisy, tuberculous (non primary)
encysted — *see* Pleurisy, with effusion
exudative — *see* Pleurisy, with effusion
fibrinopurulent, fibropurulent — *see* Pyothorax
hemorrhagic — *see* Hemothorax
pneumococcal J90
purulent — *see* Pyothorax
septic — *see* Pyothorax
serofibrinous — *see* Pleurisy, with effusion
seropurulent — *see* Pyothorax
serous — *see* Pleurisy, with effusion
staphylococcal J86.9
streptococcal J90
suppurative — *see* Pyothorax
traumatic (post) (current) — *see* Injury, intrathoracic, pleura
tuberculous (with effusion) (non primary) A15.6

Pleurisy — *continued*
tuberculous — *continued*
primary (progressive) A15.7
Pleuritis sicca — *see* Pleurisy
Pleurobronchopneumonia — *see* Pneumonia, broncho-
Pleurodynia R07.81
epidemic B33.0
viral B33.0
Pleuropericarditis (*see also* Pericarditis)
acute I30.9
Pleuropneumonia (acute) (bilateral) (double) (septic) (*see also* Pneumonia) J18.8
chronic — *see* Fibrosis, lung
Pleuro-pneumonia-like-organism (PPLO), as cause of disease classified elsewhere B96.0
Pleurorrhea — *see* Pleurisy, with effusion
Plexitis, brachial G54.0
Plica
polonica B85.0
syndrome, knee M67.5- ☑
tonsil J35.8
Plicated tongue K14.5
Plug
bronchus NEC J98.09
meconium (newborn) NEC syndrome P76.0
mucus — *see* Asphyxia, mucus
Plumbism — *see* subcategory T56.0 ☑
Plummer's disease E05.20
with thyroid storm E05.21
Plummer-Vinson syndrome D50.1
Pluricarential syndrome of infancy E40
Plus (and minus) **hand** (intrinsic) — *see* Deformity, limb, specified type NEC, forearm
Pneumathemia — *see* Air, embolism
Pneumatic hammer (drill) syndrome T75.21 ☑
Pneumatocele (lung) J98.4
intracranial G93.89
tension J44.9
Pneumatosis
cystoides intestinalis K63.89
intestinalis K63.89
peritonei K66.8
Pneumaturia R39.89
Pneumoblastoma — *see* Neoplasm, lung, malignant
Pneumocephalus G93.89
Pneumococcemia A40.3
Pneumococcus, pneumococcal — *see* condition
Pneumoconiosis (due to) (inhalation of) J64
with tuberculosis (any type in A15) J65
aluminum J63.0
asbestos J61
bagasse, bagassosis J67.1
bauxite J63.1
beryllium J63.2
coal miners' (simple) J60
coalworkers' (simple) J60
collier's J60
cotton dust J66.0
diatomite (diatomaceous earth) J62.8
dust
inorganic NEC J63.6
lime J62.8
marble J62.8
organic NEC J66.8
fumes or vapors (from silo) J68.9
graphite J63.3
grinder's J62.8
kaolin J62.8
mica J62.8
millstone maker's J62.8
mineral fibers NEC J61
miner's J60
moldy hay J67.0
potter's J62.8
rheumatoid — *see* Rheumatoid, lung
sandblaster's J62.8
silica, silicate NEC J62.8
with carbon J60
stonemason's J62.8
talc (dust) J62.0
Pneumocystis carinii pneumonia B59
Pneumocystis jiroveci (pneumonia) B59
Pneumocystosis (with pneumonia) B59
Pneumohemopericardium I31.2
Pneumohemothorax J94.2
traumatic S27.2 ☑
Pneumohydropericardium — *see* Pericarditis

Pneumohydrothorax — *see* Hydrothorax
Pneumomediastinum J98.2
congenital or perinatal P25.2
Pneumomycosis B49 [J99]
Pneumonia (acute) (double) (migratory) (purulent) (septic) (unresolved) J18.9
with
influenza — *see* Influenza, with, pneumonia
lung abscess J85.1
due to specified organism — *see* Pneumonia, in (due to)
adenoviral J12.0
adynamic J18.2
alba A50.04
allergic (eosinophilic) J82
alveolar — *see* Pneumonia, lobar
anaerobes J15.8
anthrax A22.1
apex, apical — *see* Pneumonia, lobar
Ascaris B77.81
aspiration J69.0
due to
aspiration of microorganisms
bacterial J15.9
viral J12.9
food (regurgitated) J69.0
gastric secretions J69.0
milk (regurgitated) J69.0
oils, essences J69.1
solids, liquids NEC J69.8
vomitus J69.0
newborn P24.81
amniotic fluid (clear) P24.11
blood P24.21
food (regurgitated) P24.31
liquor (amnii) P24.11
meconium P24.01
milk P24.31
mucus P24.11
specified NEC P24.81
stomach contents P24.31
postprocedural J95.4
atypical NEC J18.9
bacillus J15.9
specified NEC J15.8
bacterial J15.9
specified NEC J15.8
Bacteroides (fragilis) (oralis) (melaninogenicus) J15.8
basal, basic, basilar — *see* Pneumonia, by type
bronchiolitis obliterans organized (BOOP) J84.89
broncho-, bronchial (confluent) (croupous) (diffuse) (disseminated) (hemorrhagic) (involving lobes) (lobar) (terminal) J18.0
allergic (eosinophilic) J82
aspiration — *see* Pneumonia, aspiration
bacterial J15.9
specified NEC J15.8
chronic — *see* Fibrosis, lung
diplococcal J13
Eaton's agent J15.7
Escherichia coli (E. coli) J15.5
Friedländer's bacillus J15.0
Hemophilus influenzae J14
hypostatic J18.2
inhalation (*see also* Pneumonia, aspiration)
due to fumes or vapors (chemical) J68.0
of oils or essences J69.1
Klebsiella (pneumoniae) J15.0
lipid, lipoid J69.1
endogenous J84.89
Mycoplasma (pneumoniae) J15.7
pleuro-pneumonia-like-organisms (PPLO) J15.7
pneumococcal J13
Proteus J15.6
Pseudomonas J15.1
Serratia marcescens J15.6
specified organism NEC J16.8
staphylococcal — *see* Pneumonia, staphylococcal
streptococcal NEC J15.4
group B J15.3
pneumoniae J13
viral, virus — *see* Pneumonia, viral
Butyrivibrio (fibriosolvens) J15.8
Candida B37.1
caseous — *see* Tuberculosis, pulmonary
catarrhal — *see* Pneumonia, broncho
chlamydial J16.0
congenital P23.1

☑ **Additional Character Required** — **Refer to the Tabular List for Character Selection**   ▽ **Subterms under main terms may continue to next column or page**

Pneumonia — *continued*
  cholesterol J84.89
  cirrhotic (chronic) — *see* Fibrosis, lung
  Clostridium (haemolyticum) (novyi) J15.8
  confluent — *see* Pneumonia, broncho
  congenital (infective) P23.9
    due to
      bacterium NEC P23.6
      Chlamydia P23.1
      Escherichia coli P23.4
      Haemophilus influenzae P23.6
      infective organism NEC P23.8
      Klebsiella pneumoniae P23.6
      Mycoplasma P23.6
      Pseudomonas P23.5
      Staphylococcus P23.2
      Streptococcus (except group B) P23.6
        group B P23.3
      viral agent P23.0
    specified NEC P23.8
  croupous — *see* Pneumonia, lobar
  cryptogenic organizing J84.116
  cytomegalic inclusion B25.0
  cytomegaloviral B25.0
  deglutition — *see* Pneumonia, aspiration
  desquamative interstitial J84.117
  diffuse — *see* Pneumonia, broncho
  diplococcal, diplococcus (broncho-) (lobar) J13
  disseminated (focal) — *see* Pneumonia, broncho
  Eaton's agent J15.7
  embolic, embolism — *see* Embolism, pulmonary
  Enterobacter J15.6
  eosinophilic J82
  Escherichia coli (E. coli) J15.5
  Eubacterium J15.8
  fibrinous — *see* Pneumonia, lobar
  fibroid, fibrous (chronic) — *see* Fibrosis, lung
  Friedländer's bacillus J15.0
  Fusobacterium (nucleatum) J15.8
  gangrenous J85.0
  giant cell (measles) B05.2
  gonococcal A54.84
  gram-negative bacteria NEC J15.6
    anaerobic J15.8
  Hemophilus influenzae (broncho) (lobar) J14
  human metapneumovirus J12.3
  hypostatic (broncho) (lobar) J18.2
  in (due to)
    actinomycosis A42.0
    adenovirus J12.0
    anthrax A22.1
    ascariasis B77.81
    aspergillosis B44.9
    Bacillus anthracis A22.1
    Bacterium anitratum J15.6
    candidiasis B37.1
    chickenpox B01.2
    Chlamydia J16.0
      neonatal P23.1
    coccidioidomycosis B38.2
      acute B38.0
      chronic B38.1
    cytomegalovirus disease B25.0
    Diplococcus (pneumoniae) J13
    Eaton's agent J15.7
    Enterobacter J15.6
    Escherichia coli (E. coli) J15.5
    Friedländer's bacillus J15.0
    fumes and vapors (chemical) (inhalation) J68.0
    gonorrhea A54.84
    Hemophilus influenzae (H. influenzae) J14
    Herellea J15.6
    histoplasmosis B39.2
      acute B39.0
      chronic B39.1
    human metapneumovirus J12.3
    Klebsiella (pneumoniae) J15.0
    measles B05.2
    Mycoplasma (pneumoniae) J15.7
    nocardiosis, nocardiasis A43.0
    ornithosis A70
    parainfluenza virus J12.2
    pleuro-pneumonia-like-organism (PPLO) J15.7
    pneumococcus J13
    pneumocystosis (Pneumocystis carinii) (Pneumocystis jiroveci) B59
    Proteus J15.6
    Pseudomonas NEC J15.1

Pneumonia — *continued*
  in — *continued*
    Pseudomonas — *continued*
      pseudomallei A24.1
    psittacosis A70
    Q fever A78
    respiratory syncytial virus J12.1
    rheumatic fever I00 [J17]
    rubella B06.81
    Salmonella (infection) A02.22
      typhi A01.03
    schistosomiasis B65.9 [J17]
    Serratia marcescens J15.6
    specified
      bacterium NEC J15.8
      organism NEC J16.8
    spirochetal NEC A69.8
    Staphylococcus J15.20
      aureus (methicillin susceptible) (MSSA) J15.211
        methicillin resistant (MRSA) J15.212
      specified NEC J15.29
    Streptococcus J15.4
      group B J15.3
      pneumoniae J13
      specified NEC J15.4
    toxoplasmosis B58.3
    tularemia A21.2
    typhoid (fever) A01.03
    varicella B01.2
    virus — *see* Pneumonia, viral
    whooping cough A37.91
      due to
        Bordetella parapertussis A37.11
        Bordetella pertussis A37.01
        specified NEC A37.81
    Yersinia pestis A20.2
  inhalation of food or vomit — *see* Pneumonia, aspiration
  interstitial J84.9
    chronic J84.111
    desquamative J84.117
    due to
      collagen vascular disease J84.17
      known underlying cause J84.17
    idiopathic NOS J84.111
    in disease classified elsewhere J84.17
    lymphocytic (due to collagen vascular disease) (in diseases classified elsewhere) J84.17
    lymphoid J84.2
    non-specific J84.89
      due to
        collagen vascular disease J84.17
        known underlying cause J84.17
      idiopathic J84.113
      in diseases classified elsewhere J84.17
    plasma cell B59
    pseudomonas J15.1
    usual J84.112
      due to collagen vascular disease J84.17
      idiopathic J84.112
      in diseases classified elsewhere J84.17
  Klebsiella (pneumoniae) J15.0
  lipid, lipoid (exogenous) J69.1
    endogenous J84.89
  lobar (disseminated) (double) (interstitial) J18.1
    bacterial J15.9
      specified NEC J15.8
    chronic — *see* Fibrosis, lung
    Escherichia coli (E. coli) J15.5
    Friedländer's bacillus J15.0
    Hemophilus influenzae J14
    hypostatic J18.2
    Klebsiella (pneumoniae) J15.0
    pneumococcal J13
    Proteus J15.6
    Pseudomonas J15.1
    specified organism NEC J16.8
    staphylococcal — *see* Pneumonia, staphylococcal
    streptococcal NEC J15.4
    Streptococcus pneumoniae J13
    viral, virus — *see* Pneumonia, viral
  lobular — *see* Pneumonia, broncho
  Löffler's J82
  lymphoid interstitial J84.2
  massive — *see* Pneumonia, lobar
  meconium P24.01
  MRSA (methicillin resistant Staphylococcus aureus) J15.212

Pneumonia — *continued*
  MSSA (methicillin susceptible Staphylococcus aureus) J15.211
  multilobar — *see* Pneumonia, by type
  Mycoplasma (pneumoniae) J15.7
  necrotic J85.0
  neonatal P23.9
    aspiration — *see* Aspiration, by substance, with pneumonia
  nitrogen dioxide J68.0
  organizing J84.89
    due to
      collagen vascular disease J84.17
      known underlying cause J84.17
    in diseases classified elsewhere J84.17
  orthostatic J18.2
  parainfluenza virus J12.2
  parenchymatous — *see* Fibrosis, lung
  passive J18.2
  patchy — *see* Pneumonia, broncho
  Peptococcus J15.8
  Peptostreptococcus J15.8
  plasma cell (of infants) B59
  pleurolobar — *see* Pneumonia, lobar
  pleuro-pneumonia-like organism (PPLO) J15.7
  pneumococcal (broncho) (lobar) J13
  Pneumocystis (carinii) (jiroveci) B59
  postinfectional NEC B99 ☑ [J17]
  postmeasles B05.2
  Proteus J15.6
  Pseudomonas J15.1
  psittacosis A70
  radiation J70.0
  respiratory syncytial virus J12.1
  resulting from a procedure J95.89
  rheumatic I00 [J17]
  Salmonella (arizonae) (cholerae-suis) (enteritidis) (typhimurium) A02.22
    typhi A01.03
    typhoid fever A01.03
  SARS-associated coronavirus J12.81
  segmented, segmental — *see* Pneumonia, broncho-
  Serratia marcescens J15.6
  specified NEC J18.8
    bacterium NEC J15.8
    organism NEC J16.8
    virus NEC J12.89
  spirochetal NEC A69.8
  staphylococcal (broncho) (lobar) J15.20
    aureus (methicillin susceptible) (MSSA) J15.211
      methicillin resistant (MRSA) J15.212
    specified NEC J15.29
  static, stasis J18.2
  streptococcal NEC (broncho) (lobar) J15.4
    group
      A J15.4
      B J15.3
      specified NEC J15.4
  Streptococcus pneumoniae J13
  syphilitic, congenital (early) A50.04
  traumatic (complication) (early) (secondary) T79.8 ☑
  tuberculous (any) — *see* Tuberculosis, pulmonary
  tularemic A21.2
  varicella B01.2
  Veillonella J15.8
  ventilator associated J95.851
  viral, virus (broncho) (interstitial) (lobar) J12.9
    adenoviral J12.0
    congenital P23.0
    human metapneumovirus J12.3
    parainfluenza J12.2
    respiratory syncytial J12.1
    SARS-associated coronavirus J12.81
    specified NEC J12.89
  white (congenital) A50.04
Pneumonic — *see* condition
Pneumonitis (acute) (primary) (*see also* Pneumonia)
  air-conditioner J67.7
  allergic (due to) J67.9
    organic dust NEC J67.8
    red cedar dust J67.8
    sequoiosis J67.8
    wood dust J67.8
  aspiration J69.0
    due to
      anesthesia J95.4
        during
          labor and delivery O74.0

⬚ Subterms under main terms may continue to next column or page   ☑ Additional Character Required — Refer to the Tabular List for Character Selection   255

Pneumonia — Pneumonitis

Pneumonitis — *continued*
  aspiration — *continued*
    due to — *continued*
      anesthesia — *continued*
        during — *continued*
          pregnancy O29.01- ☑
          puerperium O89.01
      fumes or gases J68.0
      obstetric O74.0
  chemical (due to gases, fumes or vapors) (inhalation) J68.0
    due to anesthesia J95.4
  cholesterol J84.89
  chronic — *see* Fibrosis, lung
  congenital rubella P35.0
  crack (cocaine) J68.0
  due to
    beryllium J68.0
    cadmium J68.0
    crack (cocaine) J68.0
    detergent J69.8
    fluorocarbon-polymer J68.0
    food, vomit (aspiration) J69.0
    fumes or vapors J68.0
    gases, fumes or vapors (inhalation) J68.0
    inhalation
      blood J69.8
      essences J69.1
      food (regurgitated), milk, vomit J69.0
      oils, essences J69.1
      saliva J69.0
      solids, liquids NEC J69.8
    manganese J68.0
    nitrogen dioxide J68.0
    oils, essences J69.1
    solids, liquids NEC J69.8
    toxoplasmosis (acquired) B58.3
      congenital P37.1
    vanadium J68.0
    ventilator J95.851
  eosinophilic J82
  hypersensitivity J67.9
    air conditioner lung J67.7
    bagassosis J67.1
    bird fancier's lung J67.2
    farmer's lung J67.0
    maltworker's lung J67.4
    maple bark-stripper's lung J67.6
    mushroom worker's lung J67.5
    specified organic dust NEC J67.8
    suberosis J67.3
  interstitial (chronic) J84.89
    acute J84.114
    lymphoid J84.2
    non-specific J84.89
      idiopathic J84.113
  lymphoid, interstitial J84.2
  meconium P24.01
  postanesthetic J95.4
    correct substance properly administered — *see* Table of Drugs and Chemicals, by drug, adverse effect
    in labor and delivery O74.0
    in pregnancy O29.01- ☑
    obstetric O74.0
    overdose or wrong substance given or taken (by accident) — *see* Table of Drugs and Chemicals, by drug, poisoning
    postpartum, puerperal O89.01
  postoperative J95.4
    obstetric O74.0
  radiation J70.0
  rubella, congenital P35.0
  ventilation (air-conditioning) J67.7
  ventilator associated J95.851
  wood-dust J67.8
Pneumonoconiosis — *see* Pneumoconiosis
Pneumoparotid K11.8
Pneumopathy NEC J98.4
  alveolar J84.09
  due to organic dust NEC J66.8
  parietoalveolar J84.09
Pneumopericarditis (*see also* Pericarditis)
  acute I30.9
Pneumopericardium (*see also* Pericarditis)
  congenital P25.3
  newborn P25.3
  traumatic (post) — *see* Injury, heart

Pneumophagia (psychogenic) F45.8
Pneumopleurisy, pneumopleuritis (*see also* Pneumonia) J18.8
Pneumopyopericardium I30.1
Pneumopyothorax — *see* Pyopneumothorax
  with fistula J86.0
Pneumorrhagia (*see also* Hemorrhage, lung)
  tuberculous — *see* Tuberculosis, pulmonary
Pneumothorax NOS J93.9
  acute J93.83
  chronic J93.81
  congenital P25.1
  perinatal period P25.1
  postprocedural J95.811
  specified NEC J93.83
  spontaneous NOS J93.83
    newborn P25.1
    primary J93.11
    secondary J93.12
    tension J93.0
  tense valvular, infectional J93.0
  tension (spontaneous) J93.0
  traumatic S27.0 ☑
    with hemothorax S27.2 ☑
  tuberculous — *see* Tuberculosis, pulmonary
Podagra (*see also* Gout) M10.9
Podencephalus Q01.9
Poikilocytosis R71.8
Poikiloderma L81.6
  Civatte's L57.3
  congenital Q82.8
  vasculare atrophicans L94.5
Poikilodermatomyositis M33.10
  with
    myopathy M33.12
    respiratory involvement M33.11
    specified organ involvement NEC M33.19
Pointed ear (congenital) Q17.3
Poison ivy, oak, sumac or other plant dermatitis (allergic) (contact) L23.7
Poisoning (acute) (*see also* Table of Drugs and Chemicals)
  algae and toxins T65.82- ☑
  Bacillus B (aertrycke) (cholerae (suis)) (paratyphosus) (suipestifer) A02.9
    botulinus A05.1
  bacterial toxins A05.9
  berries, noxious — *see* Poisoning, food, noxious, berries
  botulism A05.1
  ciguatera fish T61.0- ☑
  Clostridium botulinum A05.1
  death-cap (Amanita phalloides) (Amanita verna) — *see* Poisoning, food, noxious, mushrooms
  drug — *see* Table of Drugs and Chemicals, by drug, poisoning
  epidemic, fish (noxious) — *see* Poisoning, seafood
    bacterial A05.9
  fava bean D55.0
  fish (noxious) T61.9- ☑
    bacterial — *see* Intoxication, foodborne, by agent
    ciguatera fish — *see* Poisoning, ciguatera fish
    scombroid fish — *see* Poisoning, scombroid fish
    specified type NEC T61.77- ☑
  food (acute) (diseased) (infected) (noxious) NEC T62.9- ☑
    bacterial — *see* Intoxication, foodborne, by agent
    due to
      Bacillus (aertrycke) (choleraesuis) (paratyphosus) (suipestifer) A02.9
        botulinus A05.1
      Clostridium (perfringens) (Welchii) A05.2
      salmonella (aertrycke) (callinarum) (choleraesuis) (enteritidis) (paratyphi) (suipestifer) A02.9
        with
          gastroenteritis A02.0
          sepsis A02.1
      staphylococcus A05.0
      Vibrio
        parahaemolyticus A05.3
        vulnificus A05.5
    noxious or naturally toxic T62.9- ☑
      berries — *see* subcategory T62.1 ☑
      fish — *see* Poisoning, seafood
      mushrooms — *see* subcategory T62.0X ☑
      plants NEC — *see* subcategory T62.2X ☑
      seafood — *see* Poisoning, seafood
      specified NEC — *see* subcategory T62.8X ☑
  ichthyotoxism — *see* Poisoning, seafood

Poisoning — *continued*
  kreotoxism, food A05.9
  latex T65.81- ☑
  lead T56.0- ☑
  mushroom — *see* Poisoning, food, noxious, mushroom
  mussels (*see also* Poisoning, shellfish)
    bacterial — *see* Intoxication, foodborne, by agent
  nicotine (tobacco) T65.2- ☑
  noxious foodstuffs — *see* Poisoning, food, noxious
  plants, noxious — *see* Poisoning, food, noxious, plants NEC
  ptomaine — *see* Poisoning, food
  radiation J70.0
  Salmonella (arizonae) (cholerae-suis) (enteritidis) (typhimurium) A02.9
  scombroid fish T61.1- ☑
  seafood (noxious) T61.9- ☑
    bacterial — *see* Intoxication, foodborne, by agent
    fish — *see* Poisoning, fish
    shellfish — *see* Poisoning, shellfish
    specified NEC — *see* subcategory T61.8X ☑
  shellfish (amnesic) (azaspiracid) (diarrheic) (neurotoxic) (noxious) (paralytic) T61.78- ☑
    bacterial — *see* Intoxication, foodborne, by agent
    ciguatera mollusk — *see* Poisoning, ciguatera fish
  specified substance NEC T65.891 ☑
  Staphylococcus, food A05.0
  tobacco (nicotine) T65.2- ☑
  water E87.79
Poker spine — *see* Spondylitis, ankylosing
Poland syndrome Q79.8
Polioencephalitis (acute) (bulbar) A80.9
  inferior G12.22
  influenzal — *see* Influenza, with, encephalopathy
  superior hemorrhagic (acute) (Wernicke's) E51.2
  Wernicke's E51.2
Polioencephalomyelitis (acute) (anterior) A80.9
  with beriberi E51.2
Polioencephalopathy, superior hemorrhagic E51.2
  with
    beriberi E51.11
    pellagra E52
Poliomeningoencephalitis — *see* Meningoencephalitis
Poliomyelitis (acute) (anterior) (epidemic) A80.9
  with paralysis (bulbar) — *see* Poliomyelitis, paralytic
  abortive A80.4
  ascending (progressive) — *see* Poliomyelitis, paralytic
  bulbar (paralytic) — *see* Poliomyelitis, paralytic
  congenital P35.8
  nonepidemic A80.9
  nonparalytic A80.4
  paralytic A80.30
    specified NEC A80.39
    vaccine-associated A80.0
    wild virus
      imported A80.1
      indigenous A80.2
  spinal, acute A80.9
Poliosis (eyebrow) (eyelashes) L67.1
  circumscripta, acquired L67.1
Pollakiuria R35.0
  psychogenic F45.8
Pollinosis J30.1
Pollitzer's disease L73.2
Polyadenitis (*see also* Lymphadenitis)
  malignant A20.0
Polyalgia M79.89
Polyangiitis M30.0
  microscopic M31.7
  overlap syndrome M30.8
Polyarteritis
  microscopic M31.7
  nodosa M30.0
    with lung involvement M30.1
    juvenile M30.2
    related condition NEC M30.8
Polyarthralgia — *see* Pain, joint
Polyarthritis, polyarthropathy (*see also* Arthritis) M13.0
  due to or associated with other specified conditions — *see* Arthritis
  epidemic (Australian) (with exanthema) B33.1
  infective — *see* Arthritis, pyogenic or pyemic
  inflammatory M06.4
  juvenile (chronic) (seronegative) M08.3
  migratory — *see* Fever, rheumatic
  rheumatic, acute — *see* Fever, rheumatic
Polyarthrosis M15.9

Polyarthrosis — *continued*
  post-traumatic M15.3
  primary M15.0
  specified NEC M15.8
Polycarential syndrome of infancy E40
Polychondritis (atrophic) (chronic) (*see also* Disorder,
  cartilage, specified type NEC)
  relapsing M94.1
Polycoria Q13.2
Polycystic (disease)
  degeneration, kidney Q61.3
    autosomal dominant (adult type) Q61.2
    autosomal recessive (infantile type) NEC Q61.19
  kidney Q61.3
    autosomal
      dominant Q61.2
      recessive NEC Q61.19
    autosomal dominant (adult type) Q61.2
    autosomal recessive (childhood type) NEC Q61.19
    infantile type NEC Q61.19
  liver Q44.6
  lung J98.4
    congenital Q33.0
  ovary, ovaries E28.2
  spleen Q89.09
Polycythemia (secondary) D75.1
  acquired D75.1
  benign (familial) D75.0
  due to
    donor twin P61.1
    erythropoietin D75.1
    fall in plasma volume D75.1
    high altitude D75.1
    maternal-fetal transfusion P61.1
    stress D75.1
  emotional D75.1
  erythropoietin D75.1
  familial (benign) D75.0
  Gaisböck's (hypertonica) D75.1
  high altitude D75.1
  hypertonica D75.1
  hypoxemic D75.1
  neonatorum P61.1
  nephrogenous D75.1
  relative D75.1
  secondary D75.1
  spurious D75.1
  stress D75.1
  vera D45
Polycytosis cryptogenica D75.1
Polydactylism, polydactyly Q69.9
  toes Q69.2
Polydipsia R63.1
Polydystrophy, pseudo-Hurler E77.0
Polyembryoma — *see* Neoplasm, malignant, by site
Polyglandular
  deficiency E31.0
  dyscrasia E31.9
  dysfunction E31.9
  syndrome E31.8
Polyhydramnios O40.- ☑
Polymastia Q83.1
Polymenorrhea N92.0
Polymyalgia M35.3
  arteritica, giant cell M31.5
  rheumatica M35.3
    with giant cell arteritis M31.5
Polymyositis (acute) (chronic) (hemorrhagic) M33.20
  with
    myopathy M33.22
    respiratory involvement M33.21
    skin involvement — *see* Dermatopolymyositis
    specified organ involvement NEC M33.29
  ossificans (generalisata) (progressiva) — *see* Myositis,
    ossificans, progressiva
Polyneuritis, polyneuritic (*see also* Polyneuropathy)
  acute (post-)infective G61.0
  alcoholic G62.1
  cranialis G52.7
  demyelinating, chronic inflammatory (CIDP) G61.81
  diabetic — *see* Diabetes, polyneuropathy
  diphtheritic A36.83
  due to lack of vitamin NEC E56.9 [G63]
  endemic E51.11
  erythredema — *see* subcategory T56.1 ☑
  febrile, acute G61.0
  hereditary ataxic G60.1
  idiopathic, acute G61.0

Polyneuritis, polyneuritic — *continued*
  infective (acute) G61.0
  inflammatory, chronic demyelinating (CIDP) G61.81
  nutritional E63.9 [G63]
  postinfective (acute) G61.0
  specified NEC G62.89
Polyneuropathy (peripheral) G62.9
  alcoholic G62.1
  amyloid (Portuguese) E85.1 [G63]
    transthyretin-related (ATTR) familial E85.1
  arsenical G62.2
  critical illness G62.81
  demyelinating, chronic inflammatory (CIDP) G61.81
  diabetic — *see* Diabetes, polyneuropathy
  drug-induced G62.0
  hereditary G60.9
    specified NEC G60.8
  idiopathic G60.9
    progressive G60.3
  in (due to)
    alcohol G62.1
      sequelae G65.2
    amyloidosis, familial (Portuguese) E85.1 [G63]
    antitetanus serum G61.1
    arsenic G62.2
      sequelae G65.2
    avitaminosis NEC E56.9 [G63]
    beriberi E51.11
    collagen vascular disease NEC M35.9 [G63]
    deficiency (of)
      B (-complex) vitamins E53.9 [G63]
      vitamin B6 E53.1 [G63]
    diabetes — *see* Diabetes, polyneuropathy
    diphtheria A36.83
    drug or medicament G62.0
      correct substance properly administered — *see*
        Table of Drugs and Chemicals, by drug,
        adverse effect
      overdose or wrong substance given or taken —
        see Table of Drugs and Chemicals, by drug,
        poisoning
    endocrine disease NEC E34.9 [G63]
    herpes zoster B02.23
    hypoglycemia E16.2 [G63]
    infectious
      disease NEC B99 ☑ [G63]
      mononucleosis B27.91
    lack of vitamin NEC E56.9 [G63]
    lead G62.2
      sequelae G65.2
    leprosy A30.9 [G63]
    Lyme disease A69.22
    metabolic disease NEC E88.9 [G63]
    microscopic polyangiitis M31.7 [G63]
    mumps B26.84
    neoplastic disease (*see also* Neoplasm) D49.9 [G63]
    nutritional deficiency NEC E63.9 [G63]
    organophosphate compounds G62.2
      sequelae G65.2
    parasitic disease NEC B89 [G63]
    pellagra E52 [G63]
    polyarteritis nodosa M30.0
    porphyria E80.20 [G63]
    radiation G62.82
    rheumatoid arthritis — *see* Rheumatoid, polyneu-
      ropathy
    sarcoidosis D86.89
    serum G61.1
    syphilis (late) A52.15
      congenital A50.43
    systemic
      connective tissue disorder M35.9 [G63]
      lupus erythematosus M32.19
    toxic agent NEC G62.2
      sequelae G65.2
  inflammatory G61.9
    chronic demyelinating (CIDP) G61.81
    sequelae G65.1
    specified NEC G61.89
  lead G62.2
    sequelae G65.2
  nutritional NEC E63.9 [G63]
  postherpetic (zoster) B02.23
  progressive G60.3
  radiation-induced G62.82
  sensory (hereditary) (idiopathic) G60.8
  specified NEC G62.89
  syphilitic (late) A52.15

Polyneuropathy — *continued*
  syphilitic — *continued*
    congenital A50.43
  transthyretin-related (ATTR) familial amyloid E85.1
    triorthocresyl phosphate G62.2
      sequelae G65.2
    tuberculosis A17.89
    uremia N18.9 [G63]
    vitamin B12 deficiency E53.8 [G63]
      with anemia (pernicious) D51.0 [G63]
        due to dietary deficiency D51.3 [G63]
    zoster B02.23
Polyopia H53.8
Polyorchism, polyorchidism Q55.21
Polyosteoarthritis (*see also* Osteoarthritis, generalized)
  M15.9
  post-traumatic M15.3
  specified NEC M15.8
Polyostotic fibrous dysplasia Q78.1
Polyotia Q17.0
Polyp, polypus
  accessory sinus J33.8
  adenocarcinoma in — *see* Neoplasm, malignant, by
    site
  adenocarcinoma in situ in — *see* Neoplasm, in situ, by
    site
  adenoid tissue J33.0
  adenomatous (*see also* Neoplasm, benign, by site)
    adenocarcinoma in — *see* Neoplasm, malignant, by
      site
    adenocarcinoma in situ in — *see* Neoplasm, in situ,
      by site
    carcinoma in — *see* Neoplasm, malignant, by site
    carcinoma in situ in — *see* Neoplasm, in situ, by site
    multiple — *see* Neoplasm, benign
      adenocarcinoma in — *see* Neoplasm, malignant,
        by site
      adenocarcinoma in situ in — *see* Neoplasm, in
        situ, by site
  antrum J33.8
  anus, anal (canal) K62.0
  Bartholin's gland N84.3
  bladder D41.4
  carcinoma in — *see* Neoplasm, malignant, by site
  carcinoma in situ in — *see* Neoplasm, in situ, by site
  cecum D12.0
  cervix (uteri) N84.1
    in pregnancy or childbirth — *see* Pregnancy, com-
      plicated by, abnormal, cervix
    mucous N84.1
    nonneoplastic N84.1
  choanal J33.0
  cholesterol K82.4
  clitoris N84.3
  colon K63.5
    adenomatous D12.6
    ascending D12.2
    cecum D12.0
    descending D12.4
    inflammatory K51.40
      with
        abscess K51.414
        complication K51.419
          specified NEC K51.418
        fistula K51.413
        intestinal obstruction K51.412
        rectal bleeding K51.411
    sigmoid D12.5
    transverse D12.3
  corpus uteri N84.0
  dental K04.01
    irreversible K04.02
    reversible K04.01
  duodenum K31.7
  ear (middle) H74.4- ☑
  endometrium N84.0
  ethmoidal (sinus) J33.8
  fallopian tube N84.8
  female genital tract N84.9
    specified NEC N84.8
  frontal (sinus) J33.8
  gallbladder K82.4
  gingiva, gum K06.8
  labia, labium (majus) (minus) N84.3
  larynx (mucous) J38.1
    adenomatous D14.1
  malignant — *see* Neoplasm, malignant, by site
  maxillary (sinus) J33.8

Polyp, polypus — *continued*
   middle ear — *see* Polyp, ear (middle)
   myometrium N84.0
   nares
      anterior J33.9
      posterior J33.0
   nasal (mucous) J33.9
      cavity J33.0
      septum J33.0
   nasopharyngeal J33.0
   nose (mucous) J33.9
   oviduct N84.8
   pharynx J39.2
   placenta O90.89
   prostate — *see* Enlargement, enlarged, prostate
   pudenda, pudendum N84.3
   pulpal (dental) K04.01
      irreversible K04.02
      reversible K04.01
   rectum (nonadenomatous) K62.1
      adenomatous — *see* Polyp, adenomatous
   septum (nasal) J33.0
   sinus (accessory) (ethmoidal) (frontal) (maxillary)
      (sphenoidal) J33.8
   sphenoidal (sinus) J33.8
   stomach K31.7
      adenomatous D13.1
   tube, fallopian N84.8
   turbinate, mucous membrane J33.8
   umbilical, newborn P83.6
   ureter N28.89
   urethra N36.2
   uterus (body) (corpus) (mucous) N84.0
      cervix N84.1
      in pregnancy or childbirth — *see* Pregnancy, com-
         plicated by, tumor, uterus
   vagina N84.2
   vocal cord (mucous) J38.1
   vulva N84.3
Polyphagia R63.2
Polyploidy Q92.7
Polypoid — *see* condition
Polyposis (*see also* Polyp)
   coli (adenomatous) D12.6
      adenocarcinoma in C18.9
      adenocarcinoma in situ in — *see* Neoplasm, in situ,
         by site
      carcinoma in C18.9
   colon (adenomatous) D12.6
   familial D12.6
      adenocarcinoma in situ in — *see* Neoplasm, in situ,
         by site
   intestinal (adenomatous) D12.6
   malignant lymphomatous C83.1- ☑
   multiple, adenomatous (*see also* Neoplasm, benign)
      D36.9
Polyradiculitis — *see* Polyneuropathy
Polyradiculoneuropathy (acute) (postinfective) (seg-
     mentally demyelinating) G61.0
Polyserositis
   due to pericarditis I31.1
   pericardial I31.1
   periodic, familial E85.0
   tuberculous A19.9
      acute A19.1
      chronic A19.8
Polysplenia syndrome Q89.09
Polysyndactyly (*see also* Syndactylism, syndactyly) Q70.4
Polytrichia L68.3
Polyunguia Q84.6
Polyuria R35.8
   nocturnal R35.1
   psychogenic F45.8
Pompe's disease (glycogen storage) E74.02
Pompholyx L30.1
Poncet's disease (tuberculous rheumatism) A18.09
Pond fracture — *see* Fracture, skull
Ponos B55.0
Pons, pontine — *see* condition
Poor
   aesthetic of existing restoration of tooth K08.56
   contractions, labor O62.2
   gingival margin to tooth restoration K08.51
   personal hygiene R46.0
   prenatal care, affecting management of pregnancy —
     see Pregnancy, complicated by, insufficient,
     prenatal care
   sucking reflex (newborn) R29.2

Poor — *continued*
   urinary stream R39.12
   vision NEC H54.7
Poradenitis, nostras inguinalis or venerea A55
Porencephaly (congenital) (developmental) (true) Q04.6
   acquired G93.0
   nondevelopmental G93.0
   traumatic (post) F07.89
Porocephaliasis B88.8
Porokeratosis Q82.8
Poroma, eccrine — *see* Neoplasm, skin, benign
Porphyria (South African) E80.20
   acquired E80.20
   acute intermittent (hepatic) (Swedish) E80.21
   cutanea tarda (hereditary) (symptomatic) E80.1
   due to drugs E80.20
      correct substance properly administered — *see* Ta-
         ble of Drugs and Chemicals, by drug, adverse
         effect
      overdose or wrong substance given or taken — *see*
         Table of Drugs and Chemicals, by drug, poi-
         soning
   erythropoietic (congenital) (hereditary) E80.0
   hepatocutaneous type E80.1
   secondary E80.20
   toxic NEC E80.20
   variegata E80.20
Porphyrinuria — *see* Porphyria
Porphyruria — *see* Porphyria
Port wine nevus, mark, or stain Q82.5
Portal — *see* condition
Posadas-Wernicke disease B38.9
Positive
   culture (nonspecific)
      blood R78.81
      bronchial washings R84.5
      cerebrospinal fluid R83.5
      cervix R87.5
      nasal secretions R84.5
      nipple discharge R89.5
      nose R84.5
         staphylococcus (Methicillin susceptible) Z22.321
            Methicillin resistant Z22.322
      peritoneal fluid R85.5
      pleural fluid R84.5
      prostatic secretions R86.5
      saliva R85.5
      seminal fluid R86.5
      sputum R84.5
      synovial fluid R89.5
      throat scrapings R84.5
      urine R82.79
      vagina R87.5
      vulva R87.5
      wound secretions R89.5
   PPD (skin test) R76.11
   serology for syphilis A53.0
      false R76.8
      with signs or symptoms — *code as* Syphilis, by site
         and stage
   skin test, tuberculin (without active tuberculosis) R76.11
   test, human immunodeficiency virus (HIV) R75
   VDRL A53.0
      with signs or symptoms — *code by* site and stage
         under Syphilis A53.9
   Wassermann reaction A53.0
Postcardiotomy syndrome I97.0
Postcaval ureter Q62.62
Postcholecystectomy syndrome K91.5
Postclimacteric bleeding N95.0
Postcommissurotomy syndrome I97.0
Postconcussional syndrome F07.81
Postconcussion syndrome F07.81
Postcontusional syndrome F07.81
Postcricoid region — *see* condition
Post-dates (40-42 weeks) (pregnancy) (mother) O48.0
   more than 42 weeks gestation O48.1
Postencephalitic syndrome F07.89
Posterior — *see* condition
Posterolateral sclerosis (spinal cord) — *see* Degenera-
   tion, combined
Postexanthematous — *see* condition
Postfebrile — *see* condition
Postgastrectomy dumping syndrome K91.1
Posthemiplegic chorea — *see* Monoplegia
Posthemorrhagic anemia (chronic) D50.0
   acute D62
   newborn P61.3
Postherpetic neuralgia (zoster) B02.29

Postherpetic neuralgia — *continued*
   trigeminal B02.22
Posthitis N47.7
Postimmunization complication or reaction — *see*
   Complications, vaccination
Postinfectious — *see* condition
Postlaminectomy syndrome NEC M96.1
Postleukotomy syndrome F07.0
Postmastectomy lymphedema (syndrome) I97.2
Postmaturity, postmature (over 42 weeks)
   maternal (over 42 weeks gestation) O48.1
   newborn P08.22
Postmeasles complication NEC (*see also* condition)
   B05.89
Postmenopausal
   endometrium (atrophic) N95.8
      suppurative (*see also* Endometritis) N71.9
   osteoporosis — *see* Osteoporosis, postmenopausal
Postnasal drip R09.82
   due to
      allergic rhinitis — *see* Rhinitis, allergic
      common cold J00
      gastroesophageal reflux — *see* Reflux, gastroe-
         sophageal
      nasopharyngitis — *see* Nasopharyngitis
      other known condition — *code to* condition
      sinusitis — *see* Sinusitis
Postnatal — *see* condition
Postoperative (postprocedural) — *see* Complication,
   postoperative
   pneumothorax, therapeutic Z98.3
   state NEC Z98.890
Postpancreatectomy hyperglycemia E89.1
Postpartum — *see* Puerperal
Postphlebitic syndrome — *see* Syndrome, postthrom-
   botic
Postpolio (myelitic) **syndrome** G14
Postpoliomyelitic (*see also* condition)
   osteopathy — *see* Osteopathy, after poliomyelitis
Postprocedural (*see also* Postoperative)
   hypoinsulinemia E89.1
Postschizophrenic depression F32.89
Postsurgery status (*see also* Status (post))
   pneumothorax, therapeutic Z98.3
Post-term (40-42 weeks) (pregnancy) (mother) O48.0
   infant P08.21
   more than 42 weeks gestation (mother) O48.1
Post-traumatic brain syndrome, nonpsychotic F07.81
Post-typhoid abscess A01.09
Postures, hysterical F44.2
Postvaccinal reaction or complication — *see* Complications, vaccination
Postvalvulotomy syndrome I97.0
Potain's
   disease (pulmonary edema) — *see* Edema, lung
   syndrome (gastrectasis with dyspepsia) K31.0
Potter's
   asthma J62.8
   facies Q60.6
   lung J62.8
   syndrome (with renal agenesis) Q60.6
Pott's
   curvature (spinal) A18.01
   disease or paraplegia A18.01
   spinal curvature A18.01
   tumor, puffy — *see* Osteomyelitis, specified type NEC
Pouch
   bronchus Q32.4
   Douglas' — *see* condition
   esophagus, esophageal, congenital Q39.6
      acquired K22.5
   gastric K31.4
   Hartmann's K82.8
   pharynx, pharyngeal (congenital) Q38.7
Pouchitis K91.850
Poultrymen's itch B88.0
Poverty NEC Z59.6
   extreme Z59.5
Poxvirus NEC B08.8
Prader-Willi syndrome Q87.1
Preauricular appendage or tag Q17.0
Prebetalipoproteinemia (acquired) (essential) (familial)
   (hereditary) (primary) (secondary) E78.1
   with chylomicronemia E78.3
Precipitate labor or delivery O62.3
Preclimacteric bleeding (menorrhagia) N92.4

Precocious
- adrenarche E30.1
- menarche E30.1
- menstruation E30.1
- pubarche E30.1
- puberty E30.1
  - central E22.8
- sexual development NEC E30.1
- thelarche E30.8

Precocity, sexual (constitutional) (cryptogenic) (female) (idiopathic) (male) E30.1
- with adrenal hyperplasia E25.9
- congenital E25.0

Precordial pain R07.2

Prediciduous teeth K00.2

Prediabetes, prediabetic R73.03
- complicating
  - pregnancy — *see* Pregnancy, complicated by, diseases of, specified type or system NEC
  - puerperium O99.89

Predislocation status of hip at birth Q65.6

Pre-eclampsia O14.9- ☑
- with pre-existing hypertension — *see* Hypertension, complicating pregnancy, pre-existing, with, pre-eclampsia
- complicating
  - childbirth O14.94
  - puerperium O14.95
- mild O14.0- ☑
  - complicating
    - childbirth O14.04
    - puerperium O14.05
- moderate O14.0- ☑
  - complicating
    - childbirth O14.04
    - puerperium O14.05
- severe O14.1- ☑
  - with hemolysis, elevated liver enzymes and low platelet count (HELLP) O14.2- ☑
    - complicating
      - childbirth O14.24
      - puerperium O14.25
  - complicating
    - childbirth O14.14
    - puerperium O14.15

Pre-eruptive color change, teeth, tooth K00.8

Pre-excitation atrioventricular conduction I45.6

Preglaucoma H40.00- ☑

Pregnancy (single) (uterine) (*see also* Delivery and Puerperal)

> Note: The Tabular must be reviewed for assignment of appropriate seventh character for multiple gestation codes in Chapter 15

> Note: The Tabular must be reviewed for assignment of the appropriate character indicating the trimester of the pregnancy

- abdominal (ectopic) O00.00
  - with intrauterine pregnancy O00.01
    - with viable fetus O36.7- ☑
- ampullar O00.10- ☑
  - with intrauterine pregnancy O00.11- ☑
- biochemical O02.81
- broad ligament O00.80
  - with intrauterine pregnancy O00.81
- cervical O00.8
  - with intrauterine pregnancy O00.81
- chemical O02.81
- complicated by (care of) (management affected by)
  - abnormal, abnormality
    - cervix O34.4-
      - causing obstructed labor O65.5
    - cord (umbilical) O69.9 ☑
    - fetal heart rate or rhythm O36.83- ☑
    - findings on antenatal screening of mother O28.9
      - biochemical O28.1
      - chromosomal O28.5
      - cytological O28.2
      - genetic O28.5
      - hematological O28.0
      - radiological O28.4
      - specified NEC O28.8
      - ultrasonic O28.3
    - glucose (tolerance) NEC O99.810
    - pelvic organs O34.9-
      - specified NEC O34.8- ☑
        - causing obstructed labor O65.5

Pregnancy — *continued*
- complicated by — *continued*
  - abnormal, abnormality — *continued*
    - pelvis (bony) (major) NEC O33.0
    - perineum O34.7- ☑
    - position
      - placenta O44.0- ☑
        - with hemorrhage O44.1- ☑
      - uterus O34.59- ☑
    - uterus O34.59- ☑
      - causing obstructed labor O65.5
      - congenital O34.0- ☑
    - vagina O34.6- ☑
      - causing obstructed labor O65.5
    - vulva O34.7- ☑
      - causing obstructed labor O65.5
  - abruptio placentae — *see* Abruptio placentae
  - abscess or cellulitis
    - bladder O23.1- ☑
    - breast O91.11- ☑
    - genital organ or tract O23.9- ☑
  - abuse
    - physical O9A.31 ☑ (*following* O99)
    - psychological O9A.51 ☑ (*following* O99)
    - sexual O9A.41 ☑ (*following* O99)
  - adverse effect anesthesia O29.9- ☑
    - aspiration pneumonitis O29.01- ☑
    - cardiac arrest O29.11- ☑
    - cardiac complication NEC O29.19- ☑
    - cardiac failure O29.12- ☑
    - central nervous system complication NEC O29.29- ☑
    - cerebral anoxia O29.21- ☑
    - failed or difficult intubation O29.6- ☑
    - inhalation of stomach contents or secretions NOS O29.01- ☑
    - local, toxic reaction O29.3X ☑
    - Mendelson's syndrome O29.01- ☑
    - pressure collapse of lung O29.02- ☑
    - pulmonary complications NEC O29.09- ☑
    - specified NEC O29.8X- ☑
    - spinal and epidural type NEC O29.5X ☑
      - induced headache O29.4- ☑
  - albuminuria (*see also* Proteinuria, gestational) O12.1- ☑
  - alcohol use O99.31- ☑
  - amnionitis O41.12- ☑
  - anaphylactoid syndrome of pregnancy O88.01- ☑
  - anemia (conditions in D50-D64) (pre-existing) O99.01- ☑
    - complicating the puerperium O99.03
  - antepartum hemorrhage O46.9- ☑
    - with coagulation defect — *see* Hemorrhage, antepartum, with coagulation defect
    - specified NEC O46.8X- ☑
  - appendicitis O99.61- ☑
  - atrophy (yellow) (acute) liver (subacute) O26.61- ☑
  - bariatric surgery status O99.84- ☑
  - bicornis or bicornuate uterus O34.0- ☑
  - biliary tract problems O26.61- ☑
  - breech presentation O32.1 ☑
  - cardiovascular diseases (conditions in I00-I09, I20-I52, I70-I99) O99.41- ☑
  - cerebrovascular disorders (conditions in I60-I69) O99.41- ☑
  - cervical shortening O26.87- ☑
  - cervicitis O23.51- ☑
  - chloasma (gravidarum) O26.89- ☑
  - cholecystitis O99.61- ☑
  - cholestasis (intrahepatic) O26.61- ☑
  - chorioamnionitis O41.12- ☑
  - circulatory system disorder (conditions in I00-I09, I20-I99, O99.41-)
  - compound presentation O32.6 ☑
  - conjoined twins O30.02- ☑
  - connective system disorders (conditions in M00-M99) O99.89
  - contracted pelvis (general) O33.1
    - inlet O33.2
    - outlet O33.3 ☑
  - convulsions (eclamptic) (uremic) (*see also* Eclampsia) O15.9
  - cracked nipple O92.11- ☑
  - cystitis O23.1- ☑
  - cystocele O34.8- ☑
  - death of fetus (near term) O36.4 ☑

Pregnancy — *continued*
- complicated by — *continued*
  - death of fetus — *continued*
    - early pregnancy O02.1
    - of one fetus or more in multiple gestation O31.2- ☑
  - deciduitis O41.14- ☑
  - decreased fetal movement O36.81- ☑
  - dental problems O99.61- ☑
  - diabetes (mellitus) O24.91- ☑
    - gestational (pregnancy induced) — *see* Diabetes, gestational
    - pre-existing O24.31- ☑
      - specified NEC O24.81- ☑
      - type 1 O24.01- ☑
      - type 2 O24.11- ☑
  - digestive system disorders (conditions in K00-K93) O99.61- ☑
  - diseases of — *see* Pregnancy, complicated by, specified body system disease
    - biliary tract O26.61- ☑
    - blood NEC (conditions in D65-D77) O99.11- ☑
    - liver O26.61- ☑
    - specified NEC O99.89
  - disorders of — *see* Pregnancy, complicated by, specified body system disorder
    - amniotic fluid and membranes O41.9- ☑
      - specified NEC O41.8X- ☑
    - biliary tract O26.61- ☑
    - ear and mastoid process (conditions in H60-H95) O99.89
    - eye and adnexa (conditions in H00-H59) O99.89
    - liver O26.61- ☑
    - skin (conditions in L00-L99) O99.71- ☑
    - specified NEC O99.89
  - displacement, uterus NEC O34.59- ☑
    - causing obstructed labor O65.5
  - disproportion (due to) O33.9
    - fetal (ascites) (hydrops) (meningomyelocele) (sacral teratoma) (tumor) deformities NEC O33.7 ☑
    - generally contracted pelvis O33.1
    - hydrocephalic fetus O33.6 ☑
    - inlet contraction of pelvis O33.2
    - mixed maternal and fetal origin O33.4 ☑
    - specified NEC O33.8
  - double uterus O34.0- ☑
    - causing obstructed labor O65.5
  - drug use (conditions in F11-F19) O99.32- ☑
  - eclampsia, eclamptic (coma) (convulsions) (delirium) (nephritis) (uremia) (*see also* Eclampsia) O15.- ☑
  - ectopic pregnancy — *see* Pregnancy, ectopic
  - edema O12.0- ☑
    - with
      - gestational hypertension, mild (*see also* Pre-eclampsia) O14.0- ☑
      - proteinuria O12.2- ☑
  - effusion, amniotic fluid — *see* Pregnancy, complicated by, premature rupture of membranes
  - elderly
    - multigravida O09.52- ☑
    - primigravida O09.51- ☑
  - embolism (*see also* Embolism, obstetric, pregnancy) O88.- ☑
  - endocrine diseases NEC O99.28- ☑
  - endometritis O86.12
  - excessive weight gain O26.0- ☑
  - exhaustion O26.81- ☑
    - during labor and delivery O75.81
  - face presentation O32.3 ☑
  - failed induction of labor O61.9
    - instrumental O61.1
    - mechanical O61.1
    - medical O61.0
    - specified NEC O61.8
    - surgical O61.1
  - failed or difficult intubation for anesthesia O29.6- ☑
  - false labor (pains) O47.9
    - at or after 37 completed weeks of pregnancy O47.1
    - before 37 completed weeks of pregnancy O47.0- ☑
  - fatigue O26.81- ☑
    - during labor and delivery O75.81
  - fatty metamorphosis of liver O26.61- ☑
  - female genital mutilation O34.8- ☑ [N90.81-] ☑

Index

Pregnancy — Pregnancy

Pregnancy — *continued*
  complicated by — *continued*
    fetal (maternal care for)
      abnormality or damage O35.9 ☑
        acid-base balance O68
        specified type NEC O35.8 ☑
      acidemia O68
      acidosis O68
      alkalosis O68
      anemia and thrombocytopenia O36.82- ☑
      anencephaly O35.0 ☑
      chromosomal abnormality (conditions in Q90-Q99) O35.1 ☑
      conjoined twins O30.02- ☑
      damage from
        amniocentesis O35.7 ☑
        biopsy procedures O35.7 ☑
        drug addiction O35.5 ☑
        hematological investigation O35.7 ☑
        intrauterine contraceptive device O35.7 ☑
        maternal
          alcohol addiction O35.4 ☑
          cytomegalovirus infection O35.3 ☑
          disease NEC O35.8 ☑
          drug addiction O35.5 ☑
          listeriosis O35.8 ☑
          rubella O35.3 ☑
          toxoplasmosis O35.8 ☑
          viral infection O35.3 ☑
        medical procedure NEC O35.7 ☑
        radiation O35.6 ☑
      death (near term) O36.4 ☑
        early pregnancy O02.1
      decreased movement O36.81- ☑
      disproportion due to deformity (fetal) O33.7 ☑
      excessive growth (large for dates) O36.6- ☑
      growth retardation O36.59- ☑
        light for dates O36.59- ☑
        small for dates O36.59- ☑
      heart rate irregularity (bradycardia) (decelerations) (tachycardia) O76
      hereditary disease O35.2 ☑
      hydrocephalus O35.0 ☑
      intrauterine death O36.4 ☑
      poor growth O36.59- ☑
        light for dates O36.59- ☑
        small for dates O36.59- ☑
      problem O36.9- ☑
        specified NEC O36.89- ☑
      reduction (elective) O31.3- ☑
      selective termination O31.3- ☑
      spina bifida O35.0 ☑
      thrombocytopenia O36.82- ☑
    fibroid (tumor) (uterus) O34.1- ☑
    fissure of nipple O92.11- ☑
    gallstones O99.61- ☑
    gastric banding status O99.84- ☑
    gastric bypass status O99.84- ☑
    genital herpes (asymptomatic) (history of) (inactive) O98.3- ☑
    genital tract infection O23.9- ☑
    glomerular diseases (conditions in N00-N07) O26.83- ☑
      with hypertension, pre-existing — *see* Hypertension, complicating, pregnancy, pre-existing, with, renal disease
    gonorrhea O98.21- ☑
    grand multiparity O09.4 ☑
    habitual aborter — *see* Pregnancy, complicated by, recurrent pregnancy loss
    HELLP syndrome (hemolysis, elevated liver enzymes and low platelet count) O14.2- ☑
    hemorrhage
      antepartum — *see* Hemorrhage, antepartum
      before 20 completed weeks gestation O20.9
        specified NEC O20.8
      due to premature separation, placenta (*see also* Abruptio placentae) O45.9- ☑
      early O20.9
        specified NEC O20.8
      threatened abortion O20.0
    hemorrhoids O22.4- ☑
    hepatitis (viral) O98.41- ☑
    herniation of uterus O34.59- ☑
    high
      head at term O32.4 ☑

Pregnancy — *continued*
  complicated by — *continued*
    high — *continued*
      risk — *see* Supervision (of) (for), high-risk
    history of in utero procedure during previous pregnancy O09.82- ☑
    HIV O98.71- ☑
    human immunodeficiency virus (HIV) disease O98.71- ☑
    hydatidiform mole (*see also* Mole, hydatidiform) O01.9
    hydramnios O40.- ☑
    hydrocephalic fetus (disproportion) O33.6 ☑
    hydrops
      amnii O40.- ☑
      fetalis O36.2- ☑
        associated with isoimmunization (*see also* Pregnancy, complicated by, isoimmunization) O36.11- ☑
    hydrorrhea O42.90
    hyperemesis (gravidarum) (mild) (*see also* Hyperemesis, gravidarum) O21.0
    hypertension — *see* Hypertension, complicating pregnancy
    hypertensive
      heart and renal disease, pre-existing — *see* Hypertension, complicating, pregnancy, pre-existing, with, heart disease, with renal disease
      heart disease, pre-existing — *see* Hypertension, complicating, pregnancy, pre-existing, with, heart disease
      renal disease, pre-existing — *see* Hypertension, complicating, pregnancy, pre-existing, with, renal disease
    hypotension O26.5- ☑
    immune disorders NEC (conditions in D80-D89) O99.11- ☑
    incarceration, uterus O34.51- ☑
    incompetent cervix O34.3- ☑
    inconclusive fetal viability O36.80 ☑
    infection(s) O98.91- ☑
      amniotic fluid or sac O41.10- ☑
      bladder O23.1- ☑
      carrier state NEC O99.830
        streptococcus B O99.820
      genital organ or tract O23.9- ☑
        specified NEC O23.59- ☑
      genitourinary tract O23.9- ☑
      gonorrhea O98.21- ☑
      hepatitis (viral) O98.41- ☑
      HIV O98.71- ☑
      human immunodeficiency virus (HIV) O98.71- ☑
      kidney O23.0- ☑
      nipple O91.01- ☑
      parasitic disease O98.91- ☑
        specified NEC O98.81- ☑
      protozoal disease O98.61- ☑
      sexually transmitted NEC O98.31- ☑
      specified type NEC O98.81- ☑
      syphilis O98.11- ☑
      tuberculosis O98.01- ☑
      urethra O23.2- ☑
      urinary (tract) O23.4- ☑
        specified NEC O23.3- ☑
      viral disease O98.51- ☑
    injury or poisoning (conditions in S00-T88) O9A.21- ☑ (*following* O99)
      due to abuse
        physical O9A.31- ☑ (*following* O99)
        psychological O9A.51- ☑ (*following* O99)
        sexual O9A.41- ☑ (*following* O99)
    insufficient
      prenatal care O09.3- ☑
      weight gain O26.1- ☑
    insulin resistance O26.89 ☑
    intrauterine fetal death (near term) O36.4 ☑
      early pregnancy O02.1
      multiple gestation (one fetus or more) O31.2- ☑
    isoimmunization O36.11- ☑
      anti-A sensitization O36.11- ☑
      anti-B sensitization O36.19- ☑
      Rh O36.09- ☑
        anti-D antibody O36.01- ☑
      specified NEC O36.19- ☑
    laceration of uterus NEC O71.81

Pregnancy — *continued*
  complicated by — *continued*
    malformation
      placenta, placental (vessel) O43.10- ☑
        specified NEC O43.19- ☑
      uterus (congenital) O34.0- ☑
    malnutrition (conditions in E40-E46) O25.1- ☑
    maternal hypotension syndrome O26.5- ☑
    mental disorders (conditions in F01-F09, F20-F99) O99.34- ☑
      alcohol use O99.31- ☑
      drug use O99.32- ☑
      smoking O99.33- ☑
    mentum presentation O32.3 ☑
    metabolic disorders O99.28- ☑
    missed
      abortion O02.1
      delivery O36.4
    multiple gestations O30.9- ☑
      conjoined twins O30.02- ☑
      quadruplet — *see* Pregnancy, quadruplet
      specified complication NEC O31.8X- ☑
      specified number of multiples NEC — *see* Pregnancy, multiple (gestation), specified NEC
      triplet — *see* Pregnancy, triplet
      twin — *see* Pregnancy, twin
    musculoskeletal condition (conditions is M00-M99) O99.89
    necrosis, liver (conditions in K72) O26.61- ☑
    neoplasm
      benign
        cervix O34.4- ☑
        corpus uteri O34.1- ☑
        uterus O34.1- ☑
      malignant O9A.11- ☑ (*following* O99)
    nephropathy NEC O26.83- ☑
    nervous system condition (conditions in G00-G99) O99.35- ☑
    nutritional diseases NEC O99.28- ☑
    obesity (pre-existing) O99.21- ☑
    obesity surgery status O99.84- ☑
    oblique lie or presentation O32.2 ☑
    older mother — *see* Pregnancy, complicated by, elderly
    oligohydramnios O41.0- ☑
      with premature rupture of membranes (*see also* Pregnancy, complicated by, premature rupture of membranes) O42.- ☑
    onset (spontaneous) of labor after 37 completed weeks of gestation but before 39 completed weeks gestation, with delivery by (planned) cesarean section O75.82
    oophoritis O23.52- ☑
    overdose, drug (*see also* Table of Drugs and Chemicals, by drug, poisoning) O9A.21- ☑ (*following* O99)
    oversize fetus O33.5 ☑
    papyraceous fetus O31.0- ☑
    pelvic inflammatory disease O99.89
    periodontal disease O99.61- ☑
    peripheral neuritis O26.82- ☑
    peritoneal (pelvic) adhesions O99.89
    phlebitis O22.9- ☑
    phlebopathy O22.9- ☑
    phlebothrombosis (superficial) O22.2- ☑
      deep O22.3- ☑
    placenta accreta O43.21- ☑
    placenta increta O43.22- ☑
    placenta percreta O43.23- ☑
    placenta previa O44.0- ☑
      complete O44.0- ☑
        with hemorrhage O44.1- ☑
      marginal O44.2- ☑
        with hemorrhage O44.3- ☑
      partial O44.2- ☑
        with hemorrhage O44.3- ☑
    placental disorder O43.9- ☑
      specified NEC O43.89- ☑
    placental dysfunction O43.89- ☑
    placental infarction O43.81- ☑
    placental insufficiency O36.51- ☑
    placental transfusion syndromes
      fetomaternal O43.01- ☑
      fetus to fetus O43.02- ☑
      maternofetal O43.01- ☑
    placentitis O41.14- ☑

☑ Additional Character Required — Refer to the Tabular List for Character Selection   ▽ Subterms under main terms may continue to next column or page

Pregnancy — *continued*
  complicated by — *continued*
    pneumonia O99.51- ☑
    poisoning (*see also* Table of Drugs and Chemicals)
      O9A.21 ☑ (*following* O99)
    polyhydramnios O40- ☑
    polymorphic eruption of pregnancy O26.86
    poor obstetric history NEC O09.29- ☑
    postmaturity (post-term) (40 to 42 weeks) O48.0
      more than 42 completed weeks gestation (prolonged) O48.1
    pre-eclampsia O14.9- ☑
      mild O14.0- ☑
      moderate O14.0- ☑
      severe O14.1- ☑
        with hemolysis, elevated liver enzymes and low platelet count (HELLP) O14.2- ☑
    premature labor — *see* Pregnancy, complicated by, preterm labor
    premature rupture of membranes O42.90
      with onset of labor
        within 24 hours O42.00
          at or after 37 weeks gestation, onset of labor within 24 hours of rupture O42.02
          pre-term (before 37 completed weeks of gestation) O42.01- ☑
        after 24 hours O42.10
          at or after 37 weeks gestation, onset of labor more than 24 hours following rupture O42.12
          pre-term (before 37 completed weeks of gestation) O42.11- ☑
      at or after 37 weeks gestation, unspecified as to length of time between rupture and onset of labor O42.92
      full-term, unspecified as to length of time between rupture and onset of labor O42.92
      pre-term (before 37 completed weeks of gestation) O42.91- ☑
    premature separation of placenta (*see also* Abruptio placentae) O45.9- ☑
    presentation, fetal — *see* Delivery, complicated by, malposition
    preterm delivery O60.10 ☑
    preterm labor
      with delivery O60.10 ☑
        preterm O60.10 ☑
        term O60.20 ☑
      second trimester
        with term delivery O60.22 ☑
        without delivery O60.02
        with preterm delivery
          second trimester O60.12 ☑
          third trimester O60.13 ☑
      third trimester
        with term delivery O60.23 ☑
        without delivery O60.03
        with third trimester preterm delivery O60.14 ☑
      without delivery O60.00
        second trimester O60.02
        third trimester O60.03
    previous history of — *see* Pregnancy, supervision of, high-risk
    prolapse, uterus O34.52- ☑
    proteinuria (gestational) (*see also* Proteinuria, gestational) O12.1- ☑
      with edema O12.2- ☑
    pruritic urticarial papules and plaques of pregnancy (PUPPP) O26.86
    pruritus (neurogenic) O26.89- ☑
    psychosis or psychoneurosis (puerperal) F53.1
    ptyalism O26.89- ☑
    PUPPP (pruritic urticarial papules and plaques of pregnancy) O26.86
    pyelitis O23.0- ☑
    recurrent pregnancy loss O26.2- ☑
    renal disease or failure NEC O26.83- ☑
      with secondary hypertension, pre-existing — *see* Hypertension, complicating, pregnancy, pre-existing, secondary
      hypertensive, pre-existing — *see* Hypertension, complicating, pregnancy, pre-existing, with, renal disease
    respiratory condition (conditions in J00-J99) O99.51- ☑

Pregnancy — *continued*
  complicated by — *continued*
    retained, retention
      dead ovum O02.0
      intrauterine contraceptive device O26.3- ☑
    retroversion, uterus O34.53- ☑
    Rh immunization, incompatibility or sensitization NEC O36.09- ☑
      anti-D antibody O36.01- ☑
    rupture
      amnion (premature) (*see also* Pregnancy, complicated by, premature rupture of membranes) O42- ☑
      membranes (premature) (*see also* Pregnancy, complicated by, premature rupture of membranes) O42- ☑
      uterus (during labor) O71.1
        before onset of labor O71.0- ☑
    salivation (excessive) O26.89- ☑
    salpingitis O23.52- ☑
    salpingo-oophoritis O23.52- ☑
    sepsis (conditions in A40, A41) O98.81- ☑
    size date discrepancy (uterine) O26.84- ☑
    skin condition (conditions in L00-L99) O99.71- ☑
    smoking (tobacco) O99.33- ☑
    social problem O09.7- ☑
    specified condition NEC O26.89- ☑
    spotting O26.85- ☑
    streptococcus group B (GBS) carrier state O99.820
    subluxation of symphysis (pubis) O26.71- ☑
    syphilis (conditions in A50-A53) O98.11- ☑
    threatened
      abortion O20.0
      labor O47.9
        at or after 37 completed weeks of gestation O47.1
        before 37 completed weeks of gestation O47.0- ☑
    thrombophlebitis (superficial) O22.2- ☑
    thrombosis O22.9- ☑
      cerebral venous O22.5- ☑
      cerebrovenous sinus O22.5- ☑
      deep O22.3- ☑
    tobacco use disorder (smoking) O99.33- ☑
    torsion of uterus O34.59- ☑
    toxemia O14.9- ☑
    transverse lie or presentation O32.2 ☑
    tuberculosis (conditions in A15-A19) O98.01- ☑
    tumor (benign)
      cervix O34.4- ☑
      malignant O9A.11- ☑ (*following* O99)
      uterus O34.1- ☑
    unstable lie O32.0 ☑
    upper respiratory infection O99.51- ☑
    urethritis O23.2- ☑
    uterine size date discrepancy O26.84- ☑
    vaginitis or vulvitis O23.59- ☑
    varicose veins (lower extremities) O22.0- ☑
      genitals O22.1- ☑
      legs O22.0- ☑
      perineal O22.1- ☑
      vaginal or vulval O22.1- ☑
    venereal disease NEC (conditions in A63.8) O98.31- ☑
    venous disorders O22.9- ☑
      specified NEC O22.8X- ☑
    very young mother — *see* Pregnancy, complicated by, young mother
    viral diseases (conditions in A80-B09, B25-B34) O98.51- ☑
    vomiting O21.9
      due to diseases classified elsewhere O21.8
      hyperemesis gravidarum (mild) (*see also* Hyperemesis, gravidarum) O21.0
      late (occurring after 20 weeks of gestation) O21.2
    young mother
      multigravida O09.62- ☑
      primigravida O09.61- ☑
  complicated NOS O26.9- ☑
  concealed O09.3- ☑
  continuing following
    elective fetal reduction of one or more fetus O31.3- ☑
    intrauterine death of one or more fetus O31.2- ☑
    spontaneous abortion of one or more fetus O31.1- ☑
  cornual O00.80

Pregnancy — *continued*
  cornual — *continued*
    with intrauterine pregnancy O00.81
  ectopic (ruptured) O00.90
    with intrauterine pregnancy O00.91
    abdominal O00.00
      with
        intrauterine pregnancy O00.01
        viable fetus O36.7- ☑
    cervical O00.80
      with intrauterine pregnancy O00.81
    complicated (by) O08.9
      afibrinogenemia O08.1
      cardiac arrest O08.81
      chemical damage of pelvic organ(s) O08.6
      circulatory collapse O08.3
      defibrination syndrome O08.1
      electrolyte imbalance O08.5
      embolism (amniotic fluid) (blood clot) (pulmonary) (septic) O08.2
      endometritis O08.0
      genital tract and pelvic infection O08.0
      hemorrhage (delayed) (excessive) O08.1
      infection
        genital tract or pelvic O08.0
        kidney O08.83
        urinary tract O08.3
      intravascular coagulation O08.1
      laceration of pelvic organ(s) O08.6
      metabolic disorder O08.5
      oliguria O08.4
      oophoritis O08.0
      parametritis O08.0
      pelvic peritonitis O08.0
      perforation of pelvic organ(s) O08.6
      renal failure or shutdown O08.4
      salpingitis or salpingo-oophoritis O08.0
      sepsis O08.82
      shock O08.83
        septic O08.82
      specified condition NEC O08.89
      tubular necrosis (renal) O08.4
      uremia O08.4
      urinary infection O08.83
      venous complication NEC O08.7
        embolism O08.2
    cornual O00.80
      with intrauterine pregnancy O00.81
    intraligamentous O00.80
      with intrauterine pregnancy O00.81
    mural O00.80
      with intrauterine pregnancy O00.81
    ovarian O00.20- ☑
      with intrauterine pregnancy O00.21- ☑
    specified site NEC O00.80
      with intrauterine pregnancy O00.81
    tubal (ruptured) O00.10- ☑
      with intrauterine pregnancy O00.11- ☑
  examination (normal) Z34.9- ☑
    first Z34.0- ☑
    high-risk — *see* Pregnancy, supervision of, high-risk
    specified Z34.8- ☑
  extrauterine — *see* Pregnancy, ectopic
  fallopian O00.10- ☑
    with intrauterine pregnancy O00.11- ☑
  false F45.8
  gestational carrier Z33.3
  heptachorionic, hepta-amniotic (septuplets) O30.83- ☑
  hexachorionic, hexa-amniotic (sextuplets) O30.83- ☑
  hidden O09.3- ☑
  high-risk — *see* Pregnancy, supervision of, high-risk
  incidental finding Z33.1
  interstitial O00.80
    with intrauterine pregnancy O00.81
  intraligamentous O00.80
    with intrauterine pregnancy O00.81
  intramural O00.80
    with intrauterine pregnancy O00.81
  intraperitoneal O00.00
    with intrauterine pregnancy O00.01
  isthmian O00.10- ☑
    with intrauterine pregnancy O00.11- ☑
  mesometric (mural) O00.80
    with intrauterine pregnancy O00.81
  molar NEC O02.0
    complicated (by) O08.9
      afibrinogenemia O08.1
      cardiac arrest O08.81

Pregnancy — *continued*
  molar — *continued*
    complicated — *continued*
      chemical damage of pelvic organ(s) O08.6
      circulatory collapse O08.3
      defibrination syndrome O08.1
      electrolyte imbalance O08.5
      embolism (amniotic fluid) (blood clot) (pulmonary) (septic) O08.2
      endometritis O08.0
      genital tract and pelvic infection O08.0
      hemorrhage (delayed) (excessive) O08.1
      infection
        genital tract or pelvic O08.0
        kidney O08.83
        urinary tract O08.83
      intravascular coagulation O08.1
      laceration of pelvic organ(s) O08.6
      metabolic disorder O08.5
      oliguria O08.4
      oophoritis O08.0
      parametritis O08.0
      pelvic peritonitis O08.0
      perforation of pelvic organ(s) O08.6
      renal failure or shutdown O08.4
      salpingitis or salpingo-oophoritis O08.0
      sepsis O08.82
      shock O08.3
        septic O08.82
      specified condition NEC O08.89
      tubular necrosis (renal) O08.4
      uremia O08.4
      urinary infection O08.83
      venous complication NEC O08.7
        embolism O08.2
    hydatidiform (*see also* Mole, hydatidiform) O01.9
  multiple (gestation) O30.9- ☑
    greater than quadruplets — *see* Pregnancy, multiple (gestation), specified NEC
    specified NEC O30.80- ☑
      with
        two or more monoamniotic fetuses O30.82- ☑
        two or more monochorionic fetuses O30.81- ☑
        number of chorions and amnions are both equal to the number of fetuses O30.83- ☑
        two or more monoamniotic fetuses O30.82- ☑
        two or more monochorionic fetuses O30.81- ☑
        unable to determine number of placenta and number of amniotic sacs O30.89- ☑
        unspecified number of placenta and unspecified number of amniotic sacs O30.80- ☑
  mural O00.80
    with intrauterine pregnancy O00.81
  normal (supervision of) Z34.9- ☑
    first Z34.0- ☑
    high-risk — *see* Pregnancy, supervision of, high-risk
    specified Z34.8- ☑
  ovarian O00.20- ☑
    with intrauterine pregnancy O00.21- ☑
  pentachorionic, penta-amniotic (quintuplets) O30.83- ☑
  postmature (40 to 42 weeks) O48.0
    more than 42 weeks gestation O48.1
  post-term (40 to 42 weeks) O48.0
  prenatal care only Z34.9- ☑
    first Z34.0- ☑
    high-risk — *see* Pregnancy, supervision of, high-risk
    specified Z34.8- ☑
  prolonged (more than 42 weeks gestation) O48.1
  quadruplet O30.20- ☑
    with
      two or more monoamniotic fetuses O30.22- ☑
      two or more monochorionic fetuses O30.21- ☑
    quadrachorionic/quadra-amniotic O30.23- ☑
    two or more monoamniotic fetuses O30.22- ☑
    two or more monochorionic fetuses O30.21- ☑
    unable to determine number of placenta and number of amniotic sacs O30.29- ☑
    unspecified number of placenta and unspecified number of amniotic sacs O30.20- ☑
  quintuplet — *see* Pregnancy, multiple (gestation), specified NEC
  sextuplet — *see* Pregnancy, multiple (gestation), specified NEC

Pregnancy — *continued*
  supervision of
    concealed pregnancy O09.3- ☑
    elderly mother
      multigravida O09.52- ☑
      primigravida O09.51- ☑
    hidden pregnancy O09.3- ☑
    high-risk O09.9- ☑
      due to (history of)
        ectopic pregnancy O09.1- ☑
        elderly — *see* Pregnancy, supervision, elderly mother
        grand multiparity O09.4 ☑
        in utero procedure during previous pregnancy O09.82- ☑
        in vitro fertilization O09.81- ☑
        infertility O09.0- ☑
        insufficient prenatal care O09.3- ☑
        molar pregnancy O09.A- ☑
        multiple previous pregnancies O09.4- ☑
        older mother — *see* Pregnancy, supervision of, elderly mother
        poor reproductive or obstetric history NEC O09.29- ☑
        pre-term labor O09.21- ☑
        previous
          neonatal death O09.29- ☑
        social problems O09.7- ☑
        specified NEC O09.89- ☑
        very young mother — *see* Pregnancy, supervision, young mother
      resulting from in vitro fertilization O09.81- ☑
    normal Z34.9- ☑
      first Z34.0- ☑
      specified NEC Z34.8- ☑
    young mother
      multigravida O09.62- ☑
      primigravida O09.61- ☑
  triplet O30.10- ☑
    with
      two or more monoamniotic fetuses O30.12- ☑
      two or more monochorionic fetuses O30.11- ☑
    trichorionic/triamniotic O30.13- ☑
    two or more monoamniotic fetuses O30.12- ☑
    two or more monochorionic fetuses O30.11- ☑
    unable to determine number of placenta and number of amniotic sacs O30.19- ☑
    unspecified number of placenta and unspecified number of amniotic sacs O30.10- ☑
  tubal (with abortion) (with rupture) O00.10- ☑
    with intrauterine pregnancy O00.11- ☑
  twin O30.00- ☑
    conjoined O30.02- ☑
    dichorionic/diamniotic (two placenta, two amniotic sacs) O30.04- ☑
    monochorionic/diamniotic (one placenta, two amniotic sacs) O30.03- ☑
    monochorionic/monoamniotic (one placenta, one amniotic sac) O30.01- ☑
    unable to determine number of placenta and number of amniotic sacs O30.09- ☑
    unspecified number of placenta and unspecified number of amniotic sacs O30.00- ☑
  unwanted Z64.0
  weeks of gestation
    8 weeks Z3A.08 (*following* Z36)
    9 weeks Z3A.09 (*following* Z36)
    10 weeks Z3A.10 (*following* Z36)
    11 weeks Z3A.11 (*following* Z36)
    12 weeks Z3A.12 (*following* Z36)
    13 weeks Z3A.13 (*following* Z36)
    14 weeks Z3A.14 (*following* Z36)
    15 weeks Z3A.15 (*following* Z36)
    16 weeks Z3A.16 (*following* Z36)
    17 weeks Z3A.17 (*following* Z36)
    18 weeks Z3A.18 (*following* Z36)
    19 weeks Z3A.19 (*following* Z36)
    20 weeks Z3A.20 (*following* Z36)
    21 weeks Z3A.21 (*following* Z36)
    22 weeks Z3A.22 (*following* Z36)
    23 weeks Z3A.23 (*following* Z36)
    24 weeks Z3A.24 (*following* Z36)
    25 weeks Z3A.25 (*following* Z36)
    26 weeks Z3A.26 (*following* Z36)
    27 weeks Z3A.27 (*following* Z36)
    28 weeks Z3A.28 (*following* Z36)
    29 weeks Z3A.29 (*following* Z36)

Pregnancy — *continued*
  weeks of gestation — *continued*
    30 weeks Z3A.30 (*following* Z36)
    31 weeks Z3A.31 (*following* Z36)
    32 weeks Z3A.32 (*following* Z36)
    33 weeks Z3A.33 (*following* Z36)
    34 weeks Z3A.34 (*following* Z36)
    35 weeks Z3A.35 (*following* Z36)
    36 weeks Z3A.36 (*following* Z36)
    37 weeks Z3A.37 (*following* Z36)
    38 weeks Z3A.38 (*following* Z36)
    39 weeks Z3A.39 (*following* Z36)
    40 weeks Z3A.40 (*following* Z36)
    41 weeks Z3A.41 (*following* Z36)
    42 weeks Z3A.42 (*following* Z36)
    greater than 42 weeks Z3A.49 (*following* Z36)
    less than 8 weeks Z3A.01 (*following* Z36)
    not specified Z3A.00 (*following* Z36)
Preiser's disease — *see* Osteonecrosis, secondary, due to, trauma, metacarpus
Pre-kwashiorkor — *see* Malnutrition, severe
Preleukemia (syndrome) D46.9
Preluxation, hip, congenital Q65.6
Premature (*see also* condition)
  adrenarche E27.0
  aging E34.8
  beats I49.40
    atrial I49.1
    auricular I49.1
    supraventricular I49.1
  birth NEC — *see* Preterm, newborn
  closure, foramen ovale Q21.8
  contraction
    atrial I49.1
    atrioventricular I49.2
    auricular I49.1
    auriculoventricular I49.49
    heart (extrasystole) I49.49
    junctional I49.2
    ventricular I49.3
  delivery (*see also* Pregnancy, complicated by, preterm labor) O60.10 ☑
  ejaculation F52.4
  infant NEC — *see* Preterm, newborn
    light-for-dates — *see* Light for dates
  labor — *see* Pregnancy, complicated by, preterm labor
  lungs P28.0
  menopause E28.319
    asymptomatic E28.319
    symptomatic E28.310
  newborn
    extreme (less than 28 completed weeks) — *see* Immaturity, extreme
    less than 37 completed weeks — *see* Preterm, newborn
  puberty E30.1
  rupture membranes or amnion — *see* Pregnancy, complicated by, premature rupture of membranes
  senility E34.8
  thelarche E30.8
  ventricular systole I49.3
Prematurity NEC (less than 37 completed weeks) — *see* Preterm, newborn
  extreme (less than 28 completed weeks) — *see* Immaturity, extreme
Premenstrual
  dysphoric disorder (PMDD) F32.81
  tension (syndrome) N94.3
Premolarization, cuspids K00.2
Prenatal
  care, normal pregnancy — *see* Pregnancy, normal
  screening of mother (*see also* Encounter, antenatal screening) Z36.9
  teeth K00.6
Preparatory care for subsequent treatment NEC
  for dialysis Z49.01
    peritoneal Z49.02
Prepartum — *see* condition
Preponderance, left or right ventricular I51.7
Prepuce — *see* condition
PRES (posterior reversible encephalopathy syndrome) I67.83
Presbycardia R54
Presbycusis, presbyacusia H91.1- ☑
Presbyesophagus K22.8
Presbyophrenia F03 ☑
Presbyopia H52.4

Prescription of contraceptives (initial) Z30.019
  barrier Z30.018
  diaphragm Z30.018
  emergency (postcoital) Z30.012
  implantable subdermal Z30.017
  injectable Z30.013
  intrauterine contraceptive device Z30.014
  pills Z30.011
  postcoital (emergency) Z30.012
  repeat Z30.40
    barrier Z30.49
    diaphragm Z30.49
    implantable subdermal Z30.46
    injectable Z30.42
    pills Z30.41
    specified type NEC Z30.49
    transdermal patch hormonal Z30.45
    vaginal ring hormonal Z30.44
  specified type NEC Z30.018
    transdermal patch hormonal Z30.016
    vaginal ring hormonal Z30.015
Presence (of)
  ankle-joint implant (functional) (prosthesis) Z96.66- ☑
  aortocoronary (bypass) graft Z95.1
  arterial-venous shunt (dialysis) Z99.2
  artificial
    eye (globe) Z97.0
    heart (fully implantable) (mechanical) Z95.812
      valve Z95.2
    larynx Z96.3
    lens (intraocular) Z96.1
    limb (complete) (partial) Z97.1- ☑
      arm Z97.1-
        bilateral Z97.15
      leg Z97.1- ☑
        bilateral Z97.16
  audiological implant (functional) Z96.29
  bladder implant (functional) Z96.0
  bone
    conduction hearing device Z96.29
    implant (functional) NEC Z96.7
    joint (prosthesis) — see Presence, joint implant
  cardiac
    defibrillator (functional) (with synchronous cardiac pacemaker) Z95.810
    implant or graft Z95.9
      specified type NEC Z95.818
    pacemaker Z95.0
    resynchronization therapy
      defibrillator Z95.810
      pacemaker Z95.0
  cardioverter-defibrillator (ICD) Z95.810
  cerebrospinal fluid drainage device Z98.2
  cochlear implant (functional) Z96.21
  contact lens (es) Z97.3
  coronary artery graft or prosthesis Z95.5
  CRT-D (cardiac resynchronization therapy defibrillator) Z95.810
  CRT-P (cardiac resynchronization therapy pacemaker) Z95.0
  CSF shunt Z98.2
  dental prosthesis device Z97.2
  dentures Z97.2
  device (external) NEC Z97.8
    cardiac NEC Z95.818
    heart assist Z95.811
    implanted (functional) Z96.9
      specified NEC Z96.89
    prosthetic Z97.8
  ear implant Z96.20
    cochlear implant Z96.21
    myringotomy tube Z96.22
    specified type NEC Z96.29
  elbow-joint implant (functional) (prosthesis) Z96.62- ☑
  endocrine implant (functional) NEC Z96.49
  eustachian tube stent or device (functional) Z96.29
  external hearing-aid or device Z97.4
  finger-joint implant (functional) (prosthetic) Z96.69- ☑
  functional implant Z96.9
    specified NEC Z96.89
  graft
    cardiac NEC Z95.818
    vascular NEC Z95.828
  hearing-aid or device (external) Z97.4
    implant (bone) (cochlear) (functional) Z96.21
  heart assist device Z95.811
  heart valve implant (functional) Z95.2
    prosthetic Z95.2

Presence — continued
  heart valve implant — continued
    specified type NEC Z95.4
    xenogenic Z95.3
  hip-joint implant (functional) (prosthesis) Z96.64- ☑
  ICD (cardioverter-defibrillator) Z95.810
  implanted device (artificial) (functional) (prosthetic) Z96.9
    automatic cardiac defibrillator (with synchronous cardiac pacemaker) Z95.810
    cardiac pacemaker Z95.0
    cochlear Z96.21
    dental Z96.5
    heart Z95.812
    heart valve Z95.2
      prosthetic Z95.2
      specified NEC Z95.4
      xenogenic Z95.3
    insulin pump Z96.41
    intraocular lens Z96.1
    joint Z96.60
      ankle Z96.66- ☑
      elbow Z96.62- ☑
      finger Z96.69- ☑
      hip Z96.64- ☑
      knee Z96.65- ☑
      shoulder Z96.61- ☑
      specified NEC Z96.698
      wrist Z96.63- ☑
    larynx Z96.3
    myringotomy tube Z96.22
    otological Z96.20
      cochlear Z96.21
      eustachian stent Z96.29
      myringotomy Z96.22
      specified NEC Z96.29
      stapes Z96.29
    skin Z96.81
    skull plate Z96.7
    specified NEC Z96.89
    urogenital Z96.0
  insulin pump (functional) Z96.41
  intestinal bypass or anastomosis Z98.0
  intraocular lens (functional) Z96.1
  intrauterine contraceptive device (IUD) Z97.5
  intravascular implant (functional) (prosthetic) NEC Z95.9
    coronary artery Z95.5
    defibrillator (with synchronous cardiac pacemaker) Z95.810
    peripheral vessel (with angioplasty) Z95.820
  joint implant (prosthetic) (any) Z96.60
    ankle — see Presence, ankle joint implant
    elbow — see Presence, elbow joint implant
    finger — see Presence, finger joint implant
    hip — see Presence, hip joint implant
    knee — see Presence, knee joint implant
    shoulder — see Presence, shoulder joint implant
    specified joint NEC Z96.698
    wrist — see Presence, wrist joint implant
  knee-joint implant (functional) (prosthesis) Z96.65- ☑
  laryngeal implant (functional) Z96.3
  mandibular implant (dental) Z96.5
  myringotomy tube(s) Z96.22
  orthopedic-joint implant (prosthetic) (any) — see Presence, joint implant
  otological implant (functional) Z96.29
  shoulder-joint implant (functional) (prosthesis) Z96.61- ☑
  skull-plate implant Z96.7
  spectacles Z97.3
  stapes implant (functional) Z96.29
  systemic lupus erythematosus [SLE] inhibitor D68.62
  tendon implant (functional) (graft) Z96.7
  tooth root(s) implant Z96.5
  ureteral stent Z96.0
  urethral stent Z96.0
  urogenital implant (functional) Z96.0
  vascular implant or device Z95.9
    access port device Z95.828
    specified type NEC Z95.828
  wrist-joint implant (functional) (prosthesis) Z96.63- ☑
Presenile (see also condition)
  dementia F03 ☑
  premature aging E34.8
Presentation, fetal — see Delivery, complicated by, malposition
Prespondylolisthesis (congenital) Q76.2

Pressure
  area, skin — see Ulcer, pressure, by site
  brachial plexus G54.0
  brain G93.5
    injury at birth NEC P11.1
  cerebral — see Pressure, brain
  chest R07.89
  cone, tentorial G93.5
  hyposystolic (see also Hypotension)
    incidental reading, without diagnosis of hypotension R03.1
  increased
    intracranial (benign) G93.2
      injury at birth P11.0
    intraocular H40.05- ☑
  lumbosacral plexus G54.1
  mediastinum J98.59
  necrosis (chronic) — see Ulcer, pressure, by site
  parental, inappropriate (excessive) Z62.6
  sore (chronic) — see Ulcer, pressure, by site
  spinal cord G95.20
  ulcer (chronic) — see Ulcer, pressure, by site
  venous, increased I87.8
Pre-syncope R55
Preterm
  delivery (see also Pregnancy, complicated by, preterm labor) O60.10 ☑
  labor — see Pregnancy, complicated by, preterm labor
  newborn (infant) P07.30
    gestational age
      28 completed weeks (28 weeks, 0 days through 28 weeks, 6 days) P07.31
      29 completed weeks (29 weeks, 0 days through 29 weeks, 6 days) P07.32
      30 completed weeks (30 weeks, 0 days through 30 weeks, 6 days) P07.33
      31 completed weeks (31 weeks, 0 days through 31 weeks, 6 days) P07.34
      32 completed weeks (32 weeks, 0 days through 32 weeks, 6 days) P07.35
      33 completed weeks (33 weeks, 0 days through 33 weeks, 6 days) P07.36
      34 completed weeks (34 weeks, 0 days through 34 weeks, 6 days) P07.37
      35 completed weeks (35 weeks, 0 days through 35 weeks, 6 days) P07.38
      36 completed weeks (36 weeks, 0 days through 36 weeks, 6 days) P07.39
Previa
  placenta (total) (without hemorrhage) O44.0- ☑
    with hemorrhage O44.1- ☑
    complete O44.0- ☑
      with hemorrhage O44.1- ☑
    low (see also Delivery, complicated, by, placenta, low) O44.4- ☑
      with hemorrhage O44.5- ☑
    marginal O44.2- ☑
      with hemorrhage O44.3- ☑
    partial O44.2- ☑
      with hemorrhage O44.3- ☑
  vasa O69.4 ☑
Priapism N48.30
  due to
    disease classified elsewhere N48.32
    drug N48.33
    specified cause NEC N48.39
    trauma N48.31
Prickling sensation (skin) R20.2
Prickly heat L74.0
Primary — see condition
Primigravida
  elderly, affecting management of pregnancy, labor and delivery (supervision only) — see Pregnancy, complicated by, elderly, primigravida
  older, affecting management of pregnancy, labor and delivery (supervision only) — see Pregnancy, complicated by, elderly, primigravida
  very young, affecting management of pregnancy, labor and delivery (supervision only) — see Pregnancy, complicated by, young mother, primigravida
Primipara
  elderly, affecting management of pregnancy, labor and delivery (supervision only) — see Pregnancy, complicated by, elderly, primigravida
  older, affecting management of pregnancy, labor and delivery (supervision only) — see Pregnancy, complicated by, elderly, primigravida

Primipara — continued
  very young, affecting management of pregnancy, labor and delivery (supervision only) — see Pregnancy, complicated by, young mother, primigravida
Primus varus (bilateral) Q66.2 ☑
PRIND (Prolonged reversible ischemic neurologic deficit) I63.9
Pringle's disease (tuberous sclerosis) Q85.1
Prinzmetal angina I20.1
Prizefighter ear — see Cauliflower ear
Problem (with) (related to)
  academic Z55.8
  acculturation Z60.3
  adjustment (to)
    change of job Z56.1
    life-cycle transition Z60.0
    pension Z60.0
    retirement Z60.0
  adopted child Z62.821
  alcoholism in family Z63.72
  atypical parenting situation Z62.9
  bankruptcy Z59.8
  behavioral (adult) F69
    drug seeking Z76.5
  birth of sibling affecting child Z62.898
  care (of)
    provider dependency Z74.9
      specified NEC Z74.8
    sick or handicapped person in family or household Z63.6
  child
    abuse (affecting the child) — see Maltreatment, child
    custody or support proceedings Z65.3
    in care of non-parental family member Z62.21
    in foster care Z62.21
    in welfare custody Z62.21
    living in orphanage or group home Z62.22
  child-rearing Z62.9
    specified NEC Z62.898
  communication (developmental) F80.9
  conflict or discord (with)
    boss Z56.4
    classmates Z55.4
    counselor Z64.4
    employer Z56.4
    family Z63.9
      specified NEC Z63.8
    probation officer Z64.4
    social worker Z64.4
    teachers Z55.4
    workmates Z56.4
  conviction in legal proceedings Z65.0
    with imprisonment Z65.1
  counselor Z64.4
  creditors Z59.8
  digestive K92.9
  drug addict in family Z63.72
  ear — see Disorder, ear
  economic Z59.9
    affecting care Z59.9
    specified NEC Z59.8
  education Z55.9
    specified NEC Z55.8
  employment Z56.9
    change of job Z56.1
    discord Z56.4
    environment Z56.5
    sexual harassment Z56.81
    specified NEC Z56.89
    stressful schedule Z56.3
    stress NEC Z56.6
    threat of job loss Z56.2
    unemployment Z56.0
  enuresis, child F98.0
  eye H57.9
  failed examinations (school) Z55.2
  falling Z91.81
  family (see also Disruption, family) Z63.9
    specified NEC Z63.8
  feeding (elderly) (infant) R63.3
    newborn P92.9
      breast P92.5
      overfeeding P92.4
      slow P92.2
      specified NEC P92.8
      underfeeding P92.3
    nonorganic F50.89

Problem — continued
  finance Z59.9
    specified NEC Z59.8
  foreclosure on loan Z59.8
  foster child Z62.822
  frightening experience(s) in childhood Z62.898
  genital NEC
    female N94.9
    male N50.9
  health care Z75.9
    specified NEC Z75.8
  hearing — see Deafness
  homelessness Z59.0
  housing Z59.9
    inadequate Z59.1
    isolated Z59.8
    specified NEC Z59.8
  identity (of childhood) F93.8
  illegitimate pregnancy (unwanted) Z64.0
  illiteracy Z55.0
  impaired mobility Z74.09
  imprisonment or incarceration Z65.1
  inadequate teaching affecting education Z55.8
  inappropriate (excessive) parental pressure Z62.6
  influencing health status NEC Z78.9
  in-law Z63.1
  institutionalization, affecting child Z62.22
  intrafamilial communication Z63.8
  jealousy, child F93.8
  landlord Z59.2
  language (developmental) F80.9
  learning (developmental) F81.9
  legal Z65.3
    conviction without imprisonment Z65.0
    imprisonment Z65.1
    release from prison Z65.2
  life-management Z73.9
    specified NEC Z73.89
  life-style Z72.9
    gambling Z72.6
    high-risk sexual behavior (heterosexual) Z72.51
      bisexual Z72.53
      homosexual Z72.52
    inappropriate eating habits Z72.4
    self-damaging behavior NEC Z72.89
    specified NEC Z72.89
    tobacco use Z72.0
  literacy Z55.9
    low level Z55.0
    specified NEC Z55.8
  living alone Z60.2
  lodgers Z59.2
  loss of love relationship in childhood Z62.898
  marital Z63.0
    involving
      divorce Z63.5
      estrangement Z63.5
      gender identity F66
  mastication K08.89
  medical
    care, within family Z63.6
    facilities Z75.9
      specified NEC Z75.8
  mental F48.9
  multiparity Z64.1
  negative life events in childhood Z62.9
    altered pattern of family relationships Z62.898
    frightening experience Z62.898
    loss of
      love relationship Z62.898
      self-esteem Z62.898
    physical abuse (alleged) — see Maltreatment, child
    removal from home Z62.29
    specified event NEC Z62.898
  neighbor Z59.2
  neurological NEC R29.818
  new step-parent affecting child Z62.898
  none (feared complaint unfounded) Z71.1
  occupational NEC Z56.89
  parent-child — see Conflict, parent-child
  personal hygiene Z91.89
  personality F69
  phase-of-life transition, adjustment Z60.0
  presence of sick or disabled person in family or household Z63.79
    needing care Z63.6
  primary support group (family) Z63.9
    specified NEC Z63.8
  probation officer Z64.4

Problem — continued
  psychiatric F99
  psychosexual (development) F66
  psychosocial Z65.9
    religious or spiritual Z65.8
    specified NEC Z65.8
  relationship Z63.9
    childhood F93.8
  release from prison Z65.2
    religious or spiritual Z65.8
  removal from home affecting child Z62.29
  seeking and accepting known hazardous and harmful behavioral or psychological interventions Z65.8
    chemical, nutritional or physical interventions Z65.8
  sexual function (nonorganic) F52.9
  sight H54.7
  sleep disorder, child F51.9
  smell — see Disturbance, sensation, smell
  social
    environment Z60.9
      specified NEC Z60.8
    exclusion and rejection Z60.4
    worker Z64.4
  speech R47.9
    developmental F80.9
    specified NEC R47.89
  swallowing — see Dysphagia
  taste — see Disturbance, sensation, taste
  tic, child F95.0
  underachievement in school Z55.3
  unemployment Z56.0
    threatened Z56.2
  unwanted pregnancy Z64.0
  upbringing Z62.9
    specified NEC Z62.898
  urinary N39.9
  voice production R47.89
  work schedule (stressful) Z56.3
Procedure (surgical)
  converted
    arthroscopic to open Z53.33
    laparoscopic to open Z53.31
    specified procedure NEC to open Z53.39
    thoracoscopic to open Z53.32
  for purpose other than remedying health state Z41.9
    specified NEC Z41.8
  not done Z53.9
    because of
      administrative reasons Z53.8
      contraindication Z53.09
        smoking Z53.01
      patient's decision Z53.20
        for reasons of belief or group pressure Z53.1
        left against medical advice (AMA) Z53.21
        specified reason NEC Z53.29
    specified reason NEC Z53.8
Procidentia (uteri) N81.3
Proctalgia K62.89
  fugax K59.4
  spasmodic K59.4
Proctitis K62.89
  amebic (acute) A06.0
  chlamydial A56.3
  gonococcal A54.6
  granulomatous — see Enteritis, regional, large intestine
  herpetic A60.1
  radiation K62.7
  tuberculous A18.32
  ulcerative (chronic) K51.20
    with
      complication K51.219
        abscess K51.214
        fistula K51.213
        obstruction K51.212
        rectal bleeding K51.211
        specified NEC K51.218
Proctocele
  female (without uterine prolapse) N81.6
    with uterine prolapse N81.2
      complete N81.3
  male K62.3
Proctocolitis
  food protein-induced K52.82
  food-induced eosinophilic K52.82
  milk protein-induced K52.82
  mucosal — see Rectosigmoiditis, ulcerative
Proctoptosis K62.3
Proctorrhagia K62.5

☑ **Additional Character Required** — Refer to the Tabular List for Character Selection   ▽ **Subterms under main terms may continue to next column or page**

Proctosigmoiditis K63.89
  ulcerative (chronic) — *see* Rectosigmoiditis, ulcerative
Proctospasm K59.4
  psychogenic F45.8
Profichet's disease — *see* Disorder, soft tissue, specified type NEC
Progeria E34.8
Prognathism (mandibular) (maxillary) M26.19
Progonoma (melanotic) — *see* Neoplasm, benign, by site
Progressive — *see* condition
Prolactinoma
  specified site — *see* Neoplasm, benign, by site
  unspecified site D35.2
Prolapse, prolapsed
  anus, anal (canal) (sphincter) K62.2
  arm or hand O32.2 ☑
    causing obstructed labor O64.4 ☑
  bladder (mucosa) (sphincter) (acquired)
    congenital Q79.4
    female — *see* Cystocele
    male N32.89
  breast implant (prosthetic) T85.49 ☑
  cecostomy K94.09
  cecum K63.4
  cervix, cervical (hypertrophied) N81.2
    anterior lip, obstructing labor O65.5
    congenital Q51.828
    postpartal, old N81.2
    stump N81.85
  ciliary body (traumatic) — *see* Laceration, eye(ball), with prolapse or loss of interocular tissue
  colon (pedunculated) K63.4
  colostomy K94.09
  disc (intervertebral) — *see* Displacement, intervertebral disc
  eye implant (orbital) T85.398 ☑
    lens (ocular) — *see* Complications, intraocular lens
  fallopian tube N83.4- ☑
  gastric (mucosa) K31.89
  genital, female N81.9
    specified NEC N81.89
  globe, nontraumatic — *see* Luxation, globe
  ileostomy bud K94.19
  intervertebral disc — *see* Displacement, intervertebral disc
  intestine (small) K63.4
  iris (traumatic) — *see* Laceration, eye(ball), with prolapse or loss of interocular tissue
    nontraumatic H21.89
  kidney N28.83
    congenital Q63.2
  laryngeal muscles or ventricle J38.7
  liver K76.89
  meatus urinarius N36.8
  mitral (valve) I34.1
  ocular lens implant — *see* Complications, intraocular lens
  organ or site, congenital NEC — *see* Malposition, congenital
  ovary N83.4- ☑
  pelvic floor, female N81.89
  perineum, female N81.89
  rectum (mucosa) (sphincter) K62.3
    due to trichuris trichuria B79
  spleen D73.89
  stomach K31.89
  umbilical cord
    complicating delivery O69.0 ☑
  urachus, congenital Q64.4
  ureter N28.89
    with obstruction N13.5
      with infection N13.6
  ureterovesical orifice N28.89
  urethra (acquired) (infected) (mucosa) N36.8
    congenital Q64.71
  urinary meatus N36.8
    congenital Q64.72
  uterovaginal N81.4
    complete N81.3
    incomplete N81.2
  uterus (with prolapse of vagina) N81.4
    complete N81.3
    congenital Q51.818
    first degree N81.2
    in pregnancy or childbirth — *see* Pregnancy, complicated by, abnormal, uterus
    incomplete N81.2

Prolapse, prolapsed — *continued*
  uterus — *continued*
    postpartal (old) N81.4
    second degree N81.2
    third degree N81.3
  uveal (traumatic) — *see* Laceration, eye(ball), with prolapse or loss of interocular tissue
  vagina (anterior) (wall) — *see* Cystocele
    with prolapse of uterus N81.4
      complete N81.3
      incomplete N81.2
    posterior wall N81.6
    posthysterectomy N99.3
  vitreous (humor) H43.0- ☑
    in wound — *see* Laceration, eye(ball), with prolapse or loss of interocular tissue
  womb — *see* Prolapse, uterus
Prolapsus, female N81.9
  specified NEC N81.89
Proliferation(s)
  primary cutaneous CD30-positive large T-cell C86.6
  prostate, atypical small acinar N42.32
Proliferative — *see* condition
Prolonged, prolongation (of)
  bleeding (time) (idiopathic) R79.1
  coagulation (time) R79.1
  gestation (over 42 completed weeks)
    mother O48.1
    newborn P08.22
  interval I44.0
  labor O63.9
    first stage O63.0
    second stage O63.1
  partial thromboplastin time (PTT) R79.1
  pregnancy (more than 42 weeks gestation) O48.1
  prothrombin time R79.1
  QT interval I45.81
  uterine contractions in labor O62.4
Prominence, prominent
  auricle (congenital) (ear) Q17.5
  ischial spine or sacral promontory with disproportion (fetopelvic)
    with disproportion (fetopelvic) O33.0
      causing obstructed labor O65.0
  nose (congenital) acquired M95.0
Promiscuity — *see* High, risk, sexual behavior
Pronation
  ankle — *see* Deformity, limb, foot, specified NEC
  foot (*see also* Deformity, limb, foot, specified NEC)
    congenital Q74.2
Prophylactic
  administration of
    antibiotics, long-term Z79.2
      short-term use — *omit code*
    drug (*see also* Long-term (current) drug therapy (use of)) Z79.899
  medication Z79.899
  organ removal (for neoplasia management) Z40.00
    breast Z40.01
    fallopian tube(s) Z40.03
      with ovary(s) Z40.02
    ovary(s) Z40.02
    specified site NEC Z40.09
  surgery Z40.9
    for risk factors related to malignant neoplasm — *see* Prophylactic, organ removal
    specified NEC Z40.8
  vaccination Z23
Propionic acidemia E71.121
Proptosis (ocular) (*see also* Exophthalmos)
  thyroid — *see* Hyperthyroidism, with goiter
Prosecution, anxiety concerning Z65.3
Prosopagnosia R48.3
Prostadynia N42.81
Prostate, prostatic — *see* condition
Prostatism — *see* Hyperplasia, prostate
Prostatitis (congestive) (suppurative) (with cystitis) N41.9
  acute N41.0
  cavitary N41.8
  chronic N41.1
  diverticular N41.8
  due to Trichomonas (vaginalis) A59.02
  fibrous N41.1
  gonococcal (acute) (chronic) A54.22
  granulomatous N41.4
  hypertrophic N41.1
  subacute N41.1
  trichomonal A59.02

Prostatitis — *continued*
  tuberculous A18.14
Prostatocystitis N41.3
Prostatorrhea N42.89
Prostatosis N42.82
Prostration R53.83
  heat (*see also* Heat, exhaustion)
    anhydrotic T67.3 ☑
    due to
      salt (and water) depletion T67.4 ☑
      water depletion T67.3 ☑
  nervous F48.8
  senile R54
Protanomaly (anomalous trichromat) H53.54
Protanopia (complete) (incomplete) H53.54
Protection (against) (from) — *see* Prophylactic
Protein
  deficiency NEC — *see* Malnutrition
  malnutrition — *see* Malnutrition
  sickness (*see also* Reaction, serum) T80.69 ☑
Proteinemia R77.9
Proteinosis
  alveolar (pulmonary) J84.01
  lipid or lipoid (of Urbach) E78.89
Proteinuria R80.9
  Bence Jones R80.3
  complicating pregnancy — *see* Proteinuria, gestational
  gestational
    complicating
      childbirth O12.14
      pregnancy O12.1- ☑
        with edema O12.2- ☑
      puerperium O12.15
  idiopathic R80.0
  isolated R80.0
    with glomerular lesion N06.9
      dense deposit disease N06.6
      diffuse
        crescentic glomerulonephritis N06.7
        endocapillary proliferative glomerulonephritis N06.4
        mesangiocapillary glomerulonephritis N06.5
      focal and segmental hyalinosis or sclerosis N06.1
      membranous (diffuse) N06.2
      mesangial proliferative (diffuse) N06.3
      minimal change N06.0
      specified pathology NEC N06.8
  orthostatic R80.2
    with glomerular lesion — *see* Proteinuria, isolated, with glomerular lesion
  persistent R80.1
    with glomerular lesion — *see* Proteinuria, isolated, with glomerular lesion
  postural R80.2
    with glomerular lesion — *see* Proteinuria, isolated, with glomerular lesion
  pre-eclamptic — *see* Pre-eclampsia
  puerperal O12.15
  specified type NEC R80.8
Proteolysis, pathologic D65
Proteus (mirabilis) (morganii), **as cause of disease classified elsewhere** B96.4
Prothrombin gene mutation D68.52
Protoporphyria, erythropoietic E80.0
Protozoal (*see also* condition)
  disease B64
    specified NEC B60.8
Protrusion, protrusio
  acetabuli M24.7
  acetabulum (into pelvis) M24.7
  device, implant or graft (*see also* Complications, by site and type, mechanical) T85.698 ☑
    arterial graft NEC — *see* Complication, cardiovascular device, mechanical, vascular
    breast (implant) T85.49 ☑
    catheter NEC T85.698 ☑
      cystostomy T83.090 ☑
      dialysis (renal) T82.49 ☑
        intraperitoneal T85.691 ☑
      infusion NEC T82.594 ☑
        spinal (epidural) (subdural) T85.690 ☑
      urinary (*see also* Complications, catheter, urinary) T83.098 ☑
    electronic (electrode) (pulse generator) (stimulator)
      bone T84.390 ☑

Subterms under main terms may continue to next column or page   ☑ Additional Character Required — Refer to the Tabular List for Character Selection   265

Proctosigmoiditis — Protrusion, protrusio

Protrusion, protrusio — *continued*
  device, implant or graft (*see also* Complications, by site and type, mechanical) — *continued*
    electronic — *continued*
      nervous system — *see* Complication, prosthetic device, mechanical, electronic nervous system stimulator
    fixation, internal (orthopedic) NEC — *see* Complication, fixation device, mechanical
    gastrointestinal — *see* Complications, prosthetic device, mechanical, gastrointestinal device
    genital NEC T83.498 ☑
      intrauterine contraceptive device T83.39 ☑
      penile prosthesis (cylinder) (implanted) (pump) (resevoir) T83.490 ☑
      testicular prosthesis T83.491 ☑
    heart NEC — *see* Complication, cardiovascular device, mechanical
    joint prosthesis — *see* Complications, joint prosthesis, mechanical, specified NEC, by site
    ocular NEC — *see* Complications, prosthetic device, mechanical, ocular device
    orthopedic NEC — *see* Complication, orthopedic, device, mechanical
    specified NEC T85.628 ☑
    urinary NEC (*see also* Complication, genitourinary, device, urinary, mechanical)
      graft T83.29 ☑
    vascular NEC — *see* Complication, cardiovascular device, mechanical
    ventricular intracranial shunt T85.09 ☑
  intervertebral disc — *see* Displacement, intervertebral disc
  joint prosthesis — *see* Complications, joint prosthesis, mechanical, specified NEC, by site
  nucleus pulposus — *see* Displacement, intervertebral disc
Prune belly (syndrome) Q79.4
Prurigo (ferox) (gravis) (Hebrae) (Hebra's) (mitis) (simplex) L28.2
  Besnier's L20.0
  estivalis L56.4
  nodularis L28.1
  psychogenic F45.8
Pruritus, pruritic (essential) L29.9
  ani, anus L29.0
    psychogenic F45.8
  anogenital L29.3
    psychogenic F45.8
  due to onchocerca volvulus B73.1
  gravidarum — *see* Pregnancy, complicated by, specified pregnancy-related condition NEC
  hiemalis L29.8
  neurogenic (any site) F45.8
  perianal L29.0
  psychogenic (any site) F45.8
  scroti, scrotum L29.1
    psychogenic F45.8
  senile, senilis L29.8
  specified NEC L29.8
    psychogenic F45.8
  Trichomonas A59.9
  vulva, vulvae L29.2
    psychogenic F45.8
Pseudarthrosis, pseudoarthrosis (bone) — *see* Nonunion, fracture
  clavicle, congenital Q74.0
  joint, following fusion or arthrodesis M96.0
Pseudoaneurysm — *see* Aneurysm
Pseudoangina (pectoris) — *see* Angina
Pseudoangioma I81
Pseudoarteriosus Q28.8
Pseudoarthrosis — *see* Pseudarthrosis
Pseudobulbar affect (PBA) F48.2
Pseudochromhidrosis L67.8
Pseudocirrhosis, liver, pericardial I31.1
Pseudocowpox B08.03
Pseudocoxalgia M91.3- ☑
Pseudocroup J38.5
Pseudo-Cushing's syndrome, alcohol-induced E24.4
Pseudocyesis F45.8
Pseudocyst
  lung J98.4
  pancreas K86.3
  retina — *see* Cyst, retina
Pseudoelephantiasis neuroarthritica Q82.0

Pseudoexfoliation, capsule (lens) — *see* Cataract, specified NEC
Pseudofolliculitis barbae L73.1
Pseudoglioma H44.89
Pseudohemophilia (Bernuth's) (hereditary) (type B) D68.0
  Type A D69.8
  vascular D69.8
Pseudohermaphroditism Q56.3
  adrenal E25.8
  female Q56.2
    with adrenocortical disorder E25.8
    without adrenocortical disorder Q56.2
      adrenal (congenital) E25.0
      unspecified E25.9
  male Q56.1
    with
      5-alpha-reductase deficiency E29.1
      adrenocortical disorder E25.8
      androgen resistance E34.51
      cleft scrotum Q56.1
      feminizing testis E34.51
    without gonadal disorder Q56.1
    adrenal E25.8
    unspecified E25.9
Pseudo-Hurler's polydystrophy E77.0
Pseudohydrocephalus G93.2
Pseudohypertrophic muscular dystrophy (Erb's) G71.02
Pseudohypertrophy, muscle G71.09
Pseudohypoparathyroidism E20.1
Pseudoinsomnia F51.03
Pseudoleukemia, infantile D64.89
Pseudomembranous — *see* condition
Pseudomeningocele (cerebral) (infective) (post-traumatic) G96.19
  postprocedural (spinal) G97.82
Pseudomenses (newborn) P54.6
Pseudomenstruation (newborn) P54.6
Pseudomonas
  aeruginosa, as cause of disease classified elsewhere B96.5
  mallei infection A24.0
    as cause of disease classified elsewhere B96.5
  pseudomallei, as cause of disease classified elsewhere B96.5
Pseudomyotonia G71.19
Pseudomyxoma peritonei C78.6
Pseudoneuritis, optic (nerve) (disc) (papilla), **congenital** Q14.2
Pseudo-obstruction intestine (acute) (chronic) (idiopathic) (intermittent secondary) (primary) K59.8
Pseudopapilledema H47.33- ☑
  congenital Q14.2
Pseudoparalysis
  arm or leg R29.818
  atonic, congenital P94.2
Pseudopelade L66.0
Pseudophakia Z96.1
Pseudopolyarthritis, rhizomelic M35.3
Pseudopolycythemia D75.1
Pseudopseudohypoparathyroidism E20.1
Pseudopterygium H11.81- ☑
Pseudoptosis (eyelid) — *see* Blepharochalasis
Pseudopuberty, precocious
  female heterosexual E25.8
  male isosexual E25.8
Pseudorickets (renal) N25.0
Pseudorubella B08.20
Pseudosclerema, newborn P83.88
Pseudosclerosis (brain)
  Jakob's — *see* Creutzfeldt-Jakob disease or syndrome of Westphal (Strümpell) E83.01
  spastic — *see* Creutzfeldt-Jakob disease or syndrome
Pseudotetanus — *see* Convulsions
Pseudotetany R29.0
  hysterical F44.5
Pseudotruncus arteriosus Q25.49
Pseudotuberculosis A28.2
  enterocolitis A04.8
  pasteurella (infection) A28.0
Pseudotumor
  cerebri G93.2
  orbital H05.11 ☑
Pseudoxanthoma elasticum Q82.8
Psilosis (sprue) (tropical) K90.1
  nontropical K90.0

Psittacosis A70
Psoitis M60.88
Psoriasis L40.9
  arthropathic L40.50
    arthritis mutilans L40.52
    distal interphalangeal L40.51
    juvenile L40.54
    other specified L40.59
    spondylitis L40.53
  buccal K13.29
  flexural L40.8
  guttate L40.4
  mouth K13.29
  nummular L40.0
  plaque L40.0
  psychogenic F54
  pustular (generalized) L40.1
    palmaris et plantaris L40.3
  specified NEC L40.8
  vulgaris L40.0
Psychasthenia F48.8
Psychiatric disorder or problem F99
Psychogenic (*see also* condition)
  factors associated with physical conditions F54
Psychological and behavioral factors affecting medical condition F59
Psychoneurosis, psychoneurotic (*see also* Neurosis)
  anxiety (state) F41.1
  depersonalization F48.1
  hypochondriacal F45.21
  hysteria F44.9
  neurasthenic F48.8
  personality NEC F60.89
Psychopathy, psychopathic
  affectionless F94.2
  autistic F84.5
  constitution, post-traumatic F07.81
  personality — *see* Disorder, personality
  sexual — *see* Deviation, sexual
  state F60.2
Psychosexual identity disorder of childhood F64.2
Psychosis, psychotic F29
  acute (transient) F23
    hysterical F44.9
  affective — *see* Disorder, mood
  alcoholic F10.959
    with
      abuse F10.159
      anxiety disorder F10.980
        with
          abuse F10.180
          dependence F10.280
      delirium tremens F10.231
      delusions F10.950
        with
          abuse F10.150
          dependence F10.250
      dementia F10.97
        with dependence F10.27
      dependence F10.259
      hallucinosis F10.951
        with
          abuse F10.151
          dependence F10.251
      mood disorder F10.94
        with
          abuse F10.14
          dependence F10.24
      paranoia F10.950
        with
          abuse F10.150
          dependence F10.250
      persisting amnesia F10.96
        with dependence F10.26
    amnestic confabulatory F10.96
      with dependence F10.26
    delirium tremens F10.231
    Korsakoff's, Korsakov's, Korsakow's F10.26
    paranoid type F10.950
      with
        abuse F10.150
        dependence F10.250
  anergastic — *see* Psychosis, organic
  arteriosclerotic (simple type) (uncomplicated) F01.50
    with behavioral disturbance F01.51
  childhood F84.0
    atypical F84.8
  climacteric — *see* Psychosis, involutional

☑ **Additional Character Required** — Refer to the Tabular List for Character Selection   ▽ **Subterms under main terms may continue to next column or page**

Psychosis, psychotic — *continued*
confusional F29
  acute or subacute F05
  reactive F23
cycloid F23
depressive — *see* Disorder, depressive
disintegrative (childhood) F84.3
drug-induced — *see* F11-F19 with .X59
  paranoid and hallucinatory states — *see* F11-F19
    with .X50 or .X51
due to or associated with
  addiction, drug — *see* F11-F19 with .X59
  dependence
    alcohol F10.259
    drug — *see* F11-F19 with .X59
  epilepsy F06.8
  Huntington's chorea F06.8
  ischemia, cerebrovascular (generalized) F06.8
  multiple sclerosis F06.8
  physical disease F06.8
  presenile dementia F03 ☑
  senile dementia F03 ☑
  vascular disease (arteriosclerotic) (cerebral) F01.50
    with behavioral disturbance F01.51
epileptic F06.8
episode F23
  due to or associated with physical condition F06.8
exhaustive F43.0
hallucinatory, chronic F28
hypomanic F30.8
hysterical (acute) F44.9
induced F24
infantile F84.0
  atypical F84.8
infective (acute) (subacute) F05
involutional F28
  depressive — *see* Disorder, depressive
  melancholic — *see* Disorder, depressive
  paranoid (state) F22
Korsakoff's, Korsakov's, Korsakow's (nonalcoholic) F04
  alcoholic F10.96
    in dependence F10.26
  induced by other psychoactive substance — *see*
    categories F11-F19 with .X5X
mania, manic (single episode) F30.2
  recurrent type F31.89
manic-depressive — *see* Disorder, bipolar
menopausal — *see* Psychosis, involutional
mixed schizophrenic and affective F25.8
multi-infarct (cerebrovascular) F01.50
  with behavioral disturbance F01.51
nonorganic F29
  specified NEC F28
organic F09
  due to or associated with
    arteriosclerosis (cerebral) — *see* Psychosis, arte-
      riosclerotic
    cerebrovascular disease, arteriosclerotic — *see*
      Psychosis, arteriosclerotic
    childbirth — *see* Psychosis, puerperal
    Creutzfeldt-Jakob disease or syndrome — *see*
      Creutzfeldt-Jakob disease or syndrome
    dependence, alcohol F10.259
    disease
      alcoholic liver F10.259
      brain, arteriosclerotic — *see* Psychosis, arte-
        riosclerotic
      cerebrovascular F01.50
        with behavioral disturbance F01.51
      Creutzfeldt-Jakob — *see* Creutzfeldt-Jakob
        disease or syndrome
      endocrine or metabolic F06.8
        acute or subacute F05
      liver, alcoholic F10.259
    epilepsy transient (acute) F05
    infection
      brain (intracranial) F06.8
        acute or subacute F05
    intoxication
      alcoholic (acute) F10.259
      drug F11-F19 with .x59
    ischemia, cerebrovascular (generalized) — *see*
      Psychosis, arteriosclerotic
    puerperium — *see* Psychosis, puerperal
    trauma, brain (birth) (from electric current) (sur-
      gical) F06.8
      acute or subacute F05
    infective F06.8

Psychosis, psychotic — *continued*
organic — *continued*
  infective — *continued*
    acute or subacute F05
    post-traumatic F06.8
      acute or subacute F05
paranoiac F22
paranoid (climacteric) (involutional) (menopausal) F22
  psychogenic (acute) F23
  schizophrenic F20.0
  senile F03 ☑
postpartum (NOS) F53.1
presbyophrenic (type) F03 ☑
presenile F03 ☑
psychogenic (paranoid) F23
  depressive F32.3
puerperal (NOS) F53.1
  specified type — *see* Psychosis, by type
reactive (brief) (transient) (emotional stress) (psychological trauma) F23
  depressive F32.3
    recurrent F33.3
  excitative type F30.8
schizoaffective F25.9
  depressive type F25.1
  manic type F25.0
schizophrenia, schizophrenic — *see* Schizophrenia
schizophrenia-like, in epilepsy F06.2
schizophreniform F20.81
  affective type F25.9
  brief F23
  confusional type F23
  mixed type F25.0
senile NEC F03 ☑
  depressed or paranoid type F03 ☑
  simple deterioration F03 ☑
  specified type — *code to* condition
shared F24
situational (reactive) F23
symbiotic (childhood) F84.3
symptomatic F09
Psychosomatic — *see* Disorder, psychosomatic
Psychosyndrome, organic F07.9
**Psychotic episode due to or associated with physical
  condition** F06.8-
Pterygium (eye) H11.00- ☑
  amyloid H11.01- ☑
  central H11.02- ☑
  colli Q18.3
  double H11.03- ☑
  peripheral
    progressive H11.05- ☑
    stationary H11.04- ☑
  recurrent H11.06- ☑
Ptilosis (eyelid) — *see* Madarosis
Ptomaine (poisoning) — *see* Poisoning, food
Ptosis (*see also* Blepharoptosis)
  adipose (false) — *see* Blepharoptosis
  breast N64.81-
  brow H57.81- ☑
  cecum K63.4
  colon K63.4
  congenital (eyelid) Q10.0
    specified site NEC — *see* Anomaly, by site
  eyebrow H57.81- ☑
  eyelid — *see* Blepharoptosis
    congenital Q10.0
  gastric K31.89
  intestine K63.4
  kidney N28.83
  liver K76.89
  renal N28.83
  splanchnic K63.4
  spleen D73.89
  stomach K31.89
  viscera K63.4
PTP D69.51
Ptyalism (periodic) K11.7
  hysterical F45.8
  pregnancy — *see* Pregnancy, complicated by, specified
    pregnancy-related condition NEC
  psychogenic F45.8
Ptyalolithiasis K11.5
Pubarche, precocious E30.1
Pubertas praecox E30.1
Puberty (development state) Z00.3
  bleeding (excessive) N92.2

Puberty — *continued*
delayed E30.0
precocious (constitutional) (cryptogenic) (idiopathic)
  E30.1
  central E22.8
  due to
    ovarian hyperfunction E28.1
      estrogen E28.0
    testicular hyperfunction E29.0
  premature E30.1
  due to
    adrenal cortical hyperfunction E25.8
    pineal tumor E34.8
    pituitary (anterior) hyperfunction E22.8
Puckering, macula — *see* Degeneration, macula, puckering
Pudenda, pudendum — *see* condition
Puente's disease (simple glandular cheilitis) K13.0
Puerperal, puerperium (complicated by, complications)
abnormal glucose (tolerance test) O99.815
abscess
  areola O91.02
    associated with lactation O91.03
  Bartholin's gland O86.19
  breast O91.12
    associated with lactation O91.13
  cervix (uteri) O86.11
  genital organ NEC O86.19
  kidney O86.21
  mammary O91.12
    associated with lactation O91.13
  nipple O91.02
    associated with lactation O91.03
  peritoneum O85
  subareolar O91.12
    associated with lactation O91.13
  urinary tract — *see* Puerperal, infection, urinary
  uterus O86.12
  vagina (wall) O86.13
  vaginorectal O86.13
  vulvovaginal gland O86.13
adnexitis O86.19
afibrinogenemia, or other coagulation defect O72.3
albuminuria (acute) (subacute) — *see* Proteinuria,
  gestational
alcohol use O99.315
anemia O90.81
  pre-existing (pre-pregnancy) O99.03
anesthetic death O89.8
apoplexy O99.43
bariatric surgery status O99.845
blood disorder NEC O99.13
blood dyscrasia O72.3
cardiomyopathy O90.3
cerebrovascular disorder (conditions in I60-I69) O99.43
cervicitis O86.11
circulatory system disorder O99.43
coagulopathy (any) O99.13
  with hemorrhage O72.3
complications O90.9
  specified NEC O90.89
convulsions — *see* Eclampsia
cystitis O86.22
cystopyelitis O86.29
delirium NEC F05
diabetes O24.93
  gestational — *see* Puerperal, gestational diabetes
  pre-existing O24.33
    specified NEC O24.83
    type 1 O24.03
    type 2 O24.13
digestive system disorder O99.63
disease O90.9
  breast NEC O92.29
  cerebrovascular (acute) O99.43
  nonobstetric NEC O99.89
  tubo-ovarian O86.19
  Valsuani's O99.03
disorder O90.9
  biliary tract O26.63
  lactation O92.70
  liver O26.63
  nonobstetric NEC O99.89
disruption
  cesarean wound O90.0
  episiotomy wound O90.1
  perineal laceration wound O90.1
drug use O99.325

Puerperal, puerperium — *continued*
eclampsia (with pre-existing hypertension) O15.2
embolism (pulmonary) (blood clot) — *see* Embolism, obstetric, puerperal
endocrine, nutritional or metabolic disease NEC O99.285
endophlebitis — *see* Puerperal, phlebitis
endotrachelitis O86.11
failure
  lactation (complete) O92.3
    partial O92.4
  renal, acute O90.4
fever (of unknown origin) O86.4
  septic O85
fissure, nipple O92.12
  associated with lactation O92.13
fistula
  breast (due to mastitis) O91.12
    associated with lactation O91.13
  nipple O91.02
    associated with lactation O91.03
galactophoritis O91.22
  associated with lactation O91.23
galactorrhea O92.6
gastric banding status O99.845
gastric bypass status O99.845
gastrointestinal disease NEC O99.63
gestational
  diabetes O24.439
    diet controlled O24.430
    insulin (and diet) controlled O24.434
    oral drug controlled (antidiabetic) (hypoglycemic) O24.435
  edema O12.05
    with proteinuria O12.25
  proteinuria O12.15
gonorrhea O98.23
hematoma, subdural O99.43
hemiplegia, cerebral O99.355
  due to cerbrovascular disorder O99.43
hemorrhage O72.1
  brain O99.43
  bulbar O99.43
  cerebellar O99.43
  cerebral O99.43
  cortical O99.43
  delayed or secondary O72.2
  extradural O99.43
  internal capsule O99.43
  intracranial O99.43
  intrapontine O99.43
  meningeal O99.43
  pontine O99.43
  retained placenta O72.0
  subarachnoid O99.43
  subcortical O99.43
  subdural O99.43
  third stage O72.0
  uterine, delayed O72.2
  ventricular O99.43
hemorrhoids O87.2
hepatorenal syndrome O90.4
hypertension — *see* Hypertension, complicating, puerperium
hypertrophy, breast O92.29
induration breast (fibrous) O92.29
infection O86.4
  cervix O86.11
  generalized O85
  genital tract NEC O86.19
    obstetric surgical wound O86.09
  kidney (bacillus coli) O86.21
  maternal O98.93
    carrier state NEC O99.835
    gonorrhea O98.23
    human immunodeficiency virus (HIV) O98.73
    protozoal O98.63
    sexually transmitted NEC O98.33
    specified NEC O98.83
    streptococcus group B (GBS) carrier state O99.825
    syphilis O98.13
    tuberculosis O98.03
    viral hepatitis O98.43
    viral NEC O98.53
  nipple O91.02
    associated with lactation O91.03
  peritoneum O85
  renal O86.21
  specified NEC O86.89

Puerperal, puerperium — *continued*
infection — *continued*
  urinary (asymptomatic) (tract) NEC O86.20
    bladder O86.22
    kidney O86.21
    specified site NEC O86.29
    urethra O86.22
  vagina O86.13
  vein — *see* Puerperal, phlebitis
ischemia, cerebral O99.43
lymphangitis O86.89
  breast O91.22
    associated with lactation O91.23
malignancy O9A.13 (*following* O99)
malnutrition O25.3
mammillitis O91.02
  associated with lactation O91.03
mammitis O91.22
  associated with lactation O91.23
mania F30.8
mastitis O91.22
  associated with lactation O91.23
  purulent O91.12
    associated with lactation O91.13
melancholia — *see* Disorder, depressive
mental disorder NEC O99.345
metroperitonitis O85
metrorrhagia — *see* Hemorrhage, postpartum
metrosalpingitis O86.19
metrovaginitis O86.13
milk leg O87.1
monoplegia, cerebral O99.43
mood disturbance O90.6
necrosis, liver (acute) (subacute) (conditions in subcategory K72.0) O26.63
  with renal failure O90.4
nervous system disorder O99.355
obesity (pre-existing prior to pregnancy) O99.215
obesity surgery status O99.845
occlusion, precerebral artery O99.43
paralysis
  bladder (sphincter) O90.89
  cerebral O99.43
paralytic stroke O99.43
parametritis O85
paravaginitis O86.13
pelviperitonitis O85
perimetritis O86.12
perimetrosalpingitis O86.19
perinephritis O86.21
periphlebitis — *see* Puerperal phlebitis
peritoneal infection O85
peritonitis (pelvic) O85
perivaginitis O86.13
phlebitis O87.0
  deep O87.1
  pelvic O87.1
  superficial O87.0
phlebothrombosis, deep O87.1
phlegmasia alba dolens O87.1
placental polyp O90.89
pneumonia, embolic — *see* Embolism, obstetric, puerperal
pre-eclampsia — *see* Pre-eclampsia
psychosis (NOS) F53.1
pyelitis O86.21
pyelocystitis O86.29
pyelonephritis O86.21
pyelonephrosis O86.21
pyemia O85
pyocystitis O86.29
pyohemia O85
pyometra O86.12
pyonephritis O86.21
pyosalpingitis O86.19
pyrexia (of unknown origin) O86.4
renal
  disease NEC O90.89
  failure O90.4
respiratory disease NEC O99.53
retention
  decidua — *see* Retention, decidua
  placenta O72.0
  secundines — *see* Retention, secundines
retrated nipple O92.02
salpingo-ovaritis O86.19
salpingoperitonitis O85
secondary perineal tear O90.1

Puerperal, puerperium — *continued*
sepsis (pelvic) O85
sepsis O85
septic thrombophlebitis O86.81
skin disorder NEC O99.73
specified condition NEC O99.89
stroke O99.43
subinvolution (uterus) O90.89
subluxation of symphysis (pubis) O26.73
suppuration — *see* Puerperal, abscess
tetanus A34
thelitis O91.02
  associated with lactation O91.03
thrombocytopenia O72.3
thrombophlebitis (superficial) O87.0
  deep O87.1
  pelvic O87.1
  septic O86.81
thrombosis (venous) — *see* Thrombosis, puerperal
thyroiditis O90.5
toxemia (eclamptic) (pre-eclamptic) (with convulsions) O15.2
trauma, non-obstetric O9A.23 (*following* O99)
  caused by abuse (physical) (suspected) O9A.33 (*following* O99)
    confirmed O9A.33 (*following* O99)
    psychological (suspected) O9A.53 (*following* O99)
      confirmed O9A.53 (*following* O99)
    sexual (suspected) O9A.43 (*following* O99)
      confirmed O9A.43 (*following* O99)
uremia (due to renal failure) O90.4
urethritis O86.22
vaginitis O86.13
varicose veins (legs) O87.4
  vulva or perineum O87.8
venous O87.9
vulvitis O86.19
vulvovaginitis O86.13
white leg O87.1
Puerperium — *see* Puerperal
Pulmolithiasis J98.4
Pulmonary — *see* condition
Pulpitis (acute) (anachoretic) (chronic) (hyperplastic) (putrescent) (suppurative) (ulcerative) K04.01
irreversible K04.02
reversible K04.01
Pulpless tooth K04.99
Pulse
alternating R00.8
bigeminal R00.8
fast R00.0
feeble, rapid due to shock following injury T79.4 ☑
rapid R00.0
weak R09.89
Pulsus alternans or trigeminus R00.8
Punch drunk F07.81
Punctum lacrimale occlusion — *see* Obstruction, lacrimal
Puncture
abdomen, abdominal
  wall S31.139 ☑
    with
      foreign body S31.149 ☑
      penetration into peritoneal cavity S31.639 ☑
        with foreign body S31.649 ☑
      epigastric region S31.132 ☑
        with
          foreign body S31.142 ☑
          penetration into peritoneal cavity S31.632 ☑
            with foreign body S31.642 ☑
    left
      lower quadrant S31.134 ☑
        with
          foreign body S31.144 ☑
          penetration into peritoneal cavity S31.634 ☑
            with foreign body S31.644 ☑
      upper quadrant S31.131 ☑
        with
          foreign body S31.141 ☑
          penetration into peritoneal cavity S31.631 ☑
            with foreign body S31.641 ☑
    periumbilic region S31.135 ☑
      with
        foreign body S31.145 ☑

Puncture — *continued*
 abdomen, abdominal — *continued*
  wall — *continued*
   periumbilic region — *continued*
    with — *continued*
     penetration into peritoneal cavity
      S31.635 ☑
      with foreign body S31.645 ☑
    right
     lower quadrant S31.133 ☑
      with
       foreign body S31.143 ☑
       penetration into peritoneal cavity
        S31.633 ☑
        with foreign body S31.643 ☑
     upper quadrant S31.130 ☑
      with
       foreign body S31.140 ☑
       penetration into peritoneal cavity
        S31.630 ☑
        with foreign body S31.640 ☑
 accidental, complicating surgery — *see* Complication,
  accidental puncture or laceration
 alveolar (process) — *see* Puncture, oral cavity
 ankle S91.039 ☑
  with
   foreign body S91.049 ☑
  left S91.032 ☑
   with
    foreign body S91.042 ☑
  right S91.031 ☑
   with
    foreign body S91.041 ☑
 anus S31.833 ☑
  with foreign body S31.834 ☑
 arm (upper) S41.139 ☑
  with foreign body S41.149 ☑
  left S41.132 ☑
   with foreign body S41.142 ☑
  lower — *see* Puncture, forearm
  right S41.131 ☑
   with foreign body S41.141 ☑
 auditory canal (external) (meatus) — *see* Puncture, ear
 auricle, ear — *see* Puncture, ear
 axilla — *see* Puncture, arm
 back (*see also* Puncture, thorax, back)
  lower S31.030 ☑
   with
    foreign body S31.040 ☑
     with penetration into retroperitoneal
      space S31.041 ☑
     penetration into retroperitoneal space
      S31.031 ☑
 bladder (traumatic) S37.29 ☑
  nontraumatic N32.89
 breast S21.039 ☑
  with foreign body S21.049 ☑
  left S21.032 ☑
   with foreign body S21.042 ☑
  right S21.031 ☑
   with foreign body S21.041 ☑
 buttock S31.803 ☑
  with foreign body S31.804 ☑
  left S31.823 ☑
   with foreign body S31.824 ☑
  right S31.813 ☑
   with foreign body S31.814 ☑
 by
  device, implant or graft — *see* Complications, by
   site and type, mechanical
  foreign body left accidentally in operative wound
   T81.539 ☑
  instrument (any) during a procedure, accidental —
   see Puncture, accidental complicating surgery
 calf — *see* Puncture, leg
 canaliculus lacrimalis — *see* Puncture, eyelid
 canthus, eye — *see* Puncture, eyelid
 cervical esophagus S11.23 ☑
  with foreign body S11.24 ☑
 cheek (external) S01.439 ☑
  with foreign body S01.449 ☑
  internal — *see* Puncture, oral cavity
  left S01.432 ☑
   with foreign body S01.442 ☑
  right S01.431 ☑
   with foreign body S01.441 ☑

Puncture — *continued*
 chest wall — *see* Puncture, thorax
 chin — *see* Puncture, head, specified site NEC
 clitoris — *see* Puncture, vulva
 costal region — *see* Puncture, thorax
 digit(s)
  foot — *see* Puncture, toe
  hand — *see* Puncture, finger
 ear (canal) (external) S01.339 ☑
  with foreign body S01.349 ☑
  drum S09.2- ☑
  left S01.332 ☑
   with foreign body S01.342 ☑
  right S01.331 ☑
   with foreign body S01.341 ☑
 elbow S51.039 ☑
  with
   foreign body S51.049 ☑
  left S51.032 ☑
   with
    foreign body S51.042 ☑
  right S51.031 ☑
   with
    foreign body S51.041 ☑
 epididymis — *see* Puncture, testis
 epigastric region — *see* Puncture, abdomen, wall, epigastric
 epiglottis S11.83 ☑
  with foreign body S11.84 ☑
 esophagus
  cervical S11.23 ☑
   with foreign body S11.24 ☑
  thoracic S27.818 ☑
 eyeball S05.6- ☑
  with foreign body S05.5- ☑
 eyebrow — *see* Puncture, eyelid
 eyelid S01.13- ☑
  with foreign body S01.14- ☑
  left S01.132 ☑
   with foreign body S01.142 ☑
  right S01.131 ☑
   with foreign body S01.141 ☑
 face NEC — *see* Puncture, head, specified site NEC
 finger(s) S61.239 ☑
  with
   damage to nail S61.339 ☑
    with
     foreign body S61.349 ☑
   foreign body S61.249 ☑
  index S61.238 ☑
   with
    damage to nail S61.338 ☑
     with
      foreign body S61.348 ☑
    foreign body S61.248 ☑
   left S61.231 ☑
    with
     damage to nail S61.331 ☑
      with
       foreign body S61.341 ☑
     foreign body S61.241 ☑
   right S61.230 ☑
    with
     damage to nail S61.330 ☑
      with
       foreign body S61.340 ☑
     foreign body S61.240 ☑
  little S61.238 ☑
   with
    damage to nail S61.338 ☑
     with
      foreign body S61.348 ☑
    foreign body S61.248 ☑
   left S61.237 ☑
    with
     damage to nail S61.337 ☑
      with
       foreign body S61.347 ☑
     foreign body S61.247 ☑
   right S61.236 ☑
    with
     damage to nail S61.336 ☑
      with
       foreign body S61.346 ☑
     foreign body S61.246 ☑
  middle S61.238 ☑

Puncture — *continued*
 finger(s) — *continued*
  middle — *continued*
   with
    damage to nail S61.338 ☑
     with
      foreign body S61.348 ☑
    foreign body S61.248 ☑
   left S61.233 ☑
    with
     damage to nail S61.333 ☑
      with
       foreign body S61.343 ☑
     foreign body S61.243 ☑
   right S61.232 ☑
    with
     damage to nail S61.332 ☑
      with
       foreign body S61.342 ☑
     foreign body S61.242 ☑
  ring S61.238 ☑
   with
    damage to nail S61.338 ☑
     with
      foreign body S61.348 ☑
    foreign body S61.248 ☑
   left S61.235 ☑
    with
     damage to nail S61.335 ☑
      with
       foreign body S61.345 ☑
     foreign body S61.245 ☑
   right S61.234 ☑
    with
     damage to nail S61.334 ☑
      with
       foreign body S61.344 ☑
     foreign body S61.244 ☑
 flank S31.139 ☑
  with foreign body S31.149 ☑
 foot (except toe(s) alone) S91.339 ☑
  with foreign body S91.349 ☑
  left S91.332 ☑
   with foreign body S91.342 ☑
  right S91.331 ☑
   with foreign body S91.341 ☑
  toe — *see* Puncture, toe
 forearm S51.839 ☑
  with
   foreign body S51.849 ☑
  elbow only — *see* Puncture, elbow
  left S51.832 ☑
   with
    foreign body S51.842 ☑
  right S51.831 ☑
   with
    foreign body S51.841 ☑
 forehead — *see* Puncture, head, specified site NEC
 genital organs, external
  female S31.532 ☑
   with foreign body S31.542 ☑
   vagina — *see* Puncture, vagina
   vulva — *see* Puncture, vulva
  male S31.531 ☑
   with foreign body S31.541 ☑
   penis — *see* Puncture, penis
   scrotum — *see* Puncture, scrotum
   testis — *see* Puncture, testis
 groin — *see* Puncture, abdomen, wall
 gum — *see* Puncture, oral cavity
 hand S61.439 ☑
  with
   foreign body S61.449 ☑
  finger — *see* Puncture, finger
  left S61.432 ☑
   with
    foreign body S61.442 ☑
  right S61.431 ☑
   with
    foreign body S61.441 ☑
  thumb — *see* Puncture, thumb
 head S01.93 ☑
  with foreign body S01.94 ☑
  cheek — *see* Puncture, cheek
  ear — *see* Puncture, ear
  eyelid — *see* Puncture, eyelid

Puncture — *continued*
head — *continued*
lip — *see* Puncture, oral cavity
nose — *see* Puncture, nose
oral cavity — *see* Puncture, oral cavity
scalp S01.03 ☑
with foreign body S01.04 ☑
specified site NEC S01.83 ☑
with foreign body S01.84 ☑
temporomandibular area — *see* Puncture, cheek
heart S26.99 ☑
with hemopericardium S26.09 ☑
without hemopericardium S26.19 ☑
heel — *see* Puncture, foot
hip S71.039 ☑
with foreign body S71.049 ☑
left S71.032 ☑
with foreign body S71.042 ☑
right S71.031 ☑
with foreign body S71.041 ☑
hymen — *see* Puncture, vagina
hypochondrium — *see* Puncture, abdomen, wall
hypogastric region — *see* Puncture, abdomen, wall
inguinal region — *see* Puncture, abdomen, wall
instep — *see* Puncture, foot
internal organs — *see* Injury, by site
interscapular region — *see* Puncture, thorax, back
intestine
large
colon S36.599 ☑
ascending S36.590 ☑
descending S36.592 ☑
sigmoid S36.593 ☑
specified site NEC S36.598 ☑
transverse S36.591 ☑
rectum S36.69 ☑
small S36.499 ☑
duodenum S36.490 ☑
specified site NEC S36.498 ☑
intra-abdominal organ S36.99 ☑
gallbladder S36.128 ☑
intestine — *see* Puncture, intestine
liver S36.118 ☑
pancreas — *see* Puncture, pancreas
peritoneum S36.81 ☑
specified site NEC S36.898 ☑
spleen S36.09 ☑
stomach S36.39 ☑
jaw — *see* Puncture, head, specified site NEC
knee S81.039 ☑
with foreign body S81.049 ☑
left S81.032 ☑
with foreign body S81.042 ☑
right S81.031 ☑
with foreign body S81.041 ☑
labium (majus) (minus) — *see* Puncture, vulva
lacrimal duct — *see* Puncture, eyelid
larynx S11.013 ☑
with foreign body S11.014 ☑
leg (lower) S81.839 ☑
with foreign body S81.849 ☑
foot — *see* Puncture, foot
knee — *see* Puncture, knee
left S81.832 ☑
with foreign body S81.842 ☑
right S81.831 ☑
with foreign body S81.841 ☑
upper — *see* Puncture, thigh
lip S01.531 ☑
with foreign body S01.541 ☑
loin — *see* Puncture, abdomen, wall
lower back — *see* Puncture, back, lower
lumbar region — *see* Puncture, back, lower
malar region — *see* Puncture, head, specified site NEC
mammary — *see* Puncture, breast
mastoid region — *see* Puncture, head, specified site NEC
mouth — *see* Puncture, oral cavity
nail
finger — *see* Puncture, finger, with damage to nail
toe — *see* Puncture, toe, with damage to nail
nasal (septum) (sinus) — *see* Puncture, nose
nasopharynx — *see* Puncture, head, specified site NEC
neck S11.93 ☑
with foreign body S11.94 ☑

Puncture — *continued*
neck — *continued*
involving
cervical esophagus — *see* Puncture, cervical esophagus
larynx — *see* Puncture, larynx
pharynx — *see* Puncture, pharynx
thyroid gland — *see* Puncture, thyroid gland
trachea — *see* Puncture, trachea
specified site NEC S11.83 ☑
with foreign body S11.84 ☑
nose (septum) (sinus) S01.23 ☑
with foreign body S01.24 ☑
ocular — *see* Puncture, eyeball
oral cavity S01.532 ☑
with foreign body S01.542 ☑
orbit S05.4- ☑
palate — *see* Puncture, oral cavity
palm — *see* Puncture, hand
pancreas S36.299 ☑
body S36.291 ☑
head S36.290 ☑
tail S36.292 ☑
pelvis — *see* Puncture, back, lower
penis S31.23 ☑
with foreign body S31.24 ☑
perineum
female S31.43 ☑
with foreign body S31.44 ☑
male S31.139 ☑
with foreign body S31.149 ☑
periocular area (with or without lacrimal passages) — *see* Puncture, eyelid
phalanges
finger — *see* Puncture, finger
toe — *see* Puncture, toe
pharynx S11.23 ☑
with foreign body S11.24 ☑
pinna — *see* Puncture, ear
popliteal space — *see* Puncture, knee
prepuce — *see* Puncture, penis
pubic region S31.139 ☑
with foreign body S31.149 ☑
pudendum — *see* Puncture, genital organs, external
rectovaginal septum — *see* Puncture, vagina
sacral region — *see* Puncture, back, lower
sacroiliac region — *see* Puncture, back, lower
salivary gland — *see* Puncture, oral cavity
scalp S01.03 ☑
with foreign body S01.04 ☑
scapular region — *see* Puncture, shoulder
scrotum S31.33 ☑
with foreign body S31.34 ☑
shin — *see* Puncture, leg
shoulder S41.039 ☑
with foreign body S41.049 ☑
left S41.032 ☑
with foreign body S41.042 ☑
right S41.031 ☑
with foreign body S41.041 ☑
spermatic cord — *see* Puncture, testis
sternal region — *see* Puncture, thorax, front
submaxillary region — *see* Puncture, head, specified site NEC
submental region — *see* Puncture, head, specified site NEC
subungual
finger(s) — *see* Puncture, finger, with damage to nail
toe — *see* Puncture, toe, with damage to nail
supraclavicular fossa — *see* Puncture, neck, specified site NEC
temple, temporal region — *see* Puncture, head, specified site NEC
temporomandibular area — *see* Puncture, cheek
testis S31.33 ☑
with foreign body S31.34 ☑
thigh S71.139 ☑
with foreign body S71.149 ☑
left S71.132 ☑
with foreign body S71.142 ☑
right S71.131 ☑
with foreign body S71.141 ☑
thorax, thoracic (wall) S21.93 ☑
with foreign body S21.94 ☑
back S21.23- ☑

Puncture — *continued*
thorax, thoracic — *continued*
back — *continued*
with
foreign body S21.24- ☑
with penetration S21.44 ☑
penetration S21.43 ☑
breast — *see* Puncture, breast
front S21.13- ☑
with
foreign body S21.14- ☑
with penetration S21.34 ☑
penetration S21.33 ☑
throat — *see* Puncture, neck
thumb S61.039 ☑
with
damage to nail S61.139 ☑
with
foreign body S61.149 ☑
foreign body S61.049 ☑
left S61.032 ☑
with
damage to nail S61.132 ☑
with
foreign body S61.142 ☑
foreign body S61.042 ☑
right S61.031 ☑
with
damage to nail S61.131 ☑
with
foreign body S61.141 ☑
foreign body S61.041 ☑
thyroid gland S11.13 ☑
with foreign body S11.14 ☑
toe(s) S91.139 ☑
with
damage to nail S91.239 ☑
with
foreign body S91.249 ☑
foreign body S91.149 ☑
great S91.133 ☑
with
damage to nail S91.233 ☑
with
foreign body S91.243 ☑
foreign body S91.143 ☑
left S91.132 ☑
with
damage to nail S91.232 ☑
with
foreign body S91.242 ☑
foreign body S91.142 ☑
right S91.131 ☑
with
damage to nail S91.231 ☑
with
foreign body S91.241 ☑
foreign body S91.141 ☑
lesser S91.136 ☑
with
damage to nail S91.236 ☑
with
foreign body S91.246 ☑
foreign body S91.146 ☑
left S91.135 ☑
with
damage to nail S91.235 ☑
with
foreign body S91.245 ☑
foreign body S91.145 ☑
right S91.134 ☑
with
damage to nail S91.234 ☑
with
foreign body S91.244 ☑
foreign body S91.144 ☑
tongue — *see* Puncture, oral cavity
trachea S11.023 ☑
with foreign body S11.024 ☑
tunica vaginalis — *see* Puncture, testis
tympanum, tympanic membrane S09.2- ☑
umbilical region S31.135 ☑
with foreign body S31.145 ☑
uvula — *see* Puncture, oral cavity
vagina S31.43 ☑
with foreign body S31.44 ☑

☑ Additional Character Required — Refer to the Tabular List for Character Selection

🔻 Subterms under main terms may continue to next column or page

Puncture — *continued*
  vocal cords S11.033 ☑
    with foreign body S11.034 ☑
  vulva S31.43 ☑
    with foreign body S31.44 ☑
  wrist S61.539 ☑
    with
      foreign body S61.549 ☑
    left S61.532 ☑
      with
        foreign body S61.542 ☑
    right S61.531 ☑
      with
        foreign body S61.541 ☑
PUO (pyrexia of unknown origin) R50.9
Pupillary membrane (persistent) Q13.89
Pupillotonia — *see* Anomaly, pupil, function, tonic pupil
Purpura D69.2
  abdominal D69.0
  allergic D69.0
  anaphylactoid D69.0
  annularis telangiectodes L81.7
  arthritic D69.0
  autoerythrocyte sensitization D69.2
  autoimmune D69.0
  bacterial D69.0
  Bateman's (senile) D69.2
  capillary fragility (hereditary) (idiopathic) D69.8
  cryoglobulinemic D89.1
  Devil's pinches D69.2
  fibrinolytic — *see* Fibrinolysis
  fulminans, fulminous D65
  gangrenous D65
  hemorrhagic, hemorrhagica D69.3
    not due to thrombocytopenia D69.0
  Henoch (-Schönlein) (allergic) D69.0
  hypergammaglobulinemic (benign) (Waldenström)
    D89.0
  idiopathic (thrombocytopenic) D69.3
    nonthrombocytopenic D69.0
  immune thrombocytopenic D69.3
  infectious D69.0
  malignant D69.0
  neonatorum P54.5
  nervosa D69.0
  newborn P54.5
  nonthrombocytopenic D69.2
    hemorrhagic D69.0
    idiopathic D69.0
  nonthrombopenic D69.2
  peliosis rheumatica D69.0
  posttransfusion (post-transfusion) (from (fresh) whole
    blood or blood products) D69.51
  primary D69.49
  red cell membrane sensitivity D69.2
  rheumatica D69.0
  Schönlein (-Henoch) (allergic) D69.0
  scorbutic E54 [D77]
  senile D69.2
  simplex D69.2
  symptomatica D69.0
  telangiectasia annularis L81.7
  thrombocytopenic D69.49
    congenital D69.42
    hemorrhagic D69.3
    hereditary D69.42
    idiopathic D69.3
    immune D69.3
    neonatal, transitory P61.0
    thrombotic M31.1
  thrombohemolytic — *see* Fibrinolysis
  thrombolytic — *see* Fibrinolysis
  thrombopenic D69.49
  thrombotic, thrombocytopenic M31.1
  toxic D69.0
  vascular D69.0
  visceral symptoms D69.0
Purpuric spots R23.3
Purulent — *see* condition
Pus
  in
    stool R19.5
    urine N39.0
  tube (rupture) — *see* Salpingo-oophoritis
Pustular rash L08.0
Pustule (nonmalignant) L08.9
  malignant A22.0
Pustulosis palmaris et plantaris L40.3

Putnam (-Dana) **disease or syndrome** — *see* Degeneration, combined
Putrescent pulp (dental) K04.1
Pyarthritis, pyarthrosis — *see* Arthritis, pyogenic or pyemic
  tuberculous — *see* Tuberculosis, joint
Pyelectasis — *see* Hydronephrosis
Pyelitis (congenital) (uremic) (*see also* Pyelonephritis)
  with
    calculus — *see* category N20 ☑
      with hydronephrosis N13.2
    contracted kidney N11.9
  acute N10
  chronic N11.9
    with calculus — *see* category N20 ☑
      with hydronephrosis N13.2
  cystica N28.84
  puerperal (postpartum) O86.21
  tuberculous A18.11
Pyelocystitis — *see* Pyelonephritis
Pyelonephritis (*see also* Nephritis, tubulo-interstitial)
  with
    calculus — *see* category N20 ☑
      with hydronephrosis N13.2
    contracted kidney N11.9
  acute N10
  calculous — *see* category N20 ☑
    with hydronephrosis N13.2
  chronic N11.9
    with calculus — *see* category N20 ☑
      with hydronephrosis N13.2
    associated with ureteral obstruction or stricture
      N11.1
    nonobstructive N11.8
      with reflux (vesicoureteral) N11.0
    obstructive N11.1
    specified NEC N11.8
  in (due to)
    brucellosis A23.9 [N16]
    cryoglobulinemia (mixed) D89.1 [N16]
    cystinosis E72.04
    diphtheria A36.84
    glycogen storage disease E74.09 [N16]
    leukemia NEC C95.9- ☑ [N16]
    lymphoma NEC C85.90 [N16]
    multiple myeloma C90.0- ☑ [N16]
    obstruction N11.1
    Salmonella infection A02.25
    sarcoidosis D86.84
    sepsis A41.9 [N16]
    Sjögren's disease M35.04
    toxoplasmosis B58.83
    transplant rejection T86.91 [N16]
    Wilson's disease E83.01 [N16]
  nonobstructive N12
    with reflux (vesicoureteral) N11.0
    chronic N11.8
  syphilitic A52.75
Pyelonephrosis (obstructive) N11.1
  chronic N11.9
Pyelophlebitis I80.8
Pyeloureteritis cystica N28.85
Pyemia, pyemic (fever) (infection) (purulent) (*see also* Sepsis)
  joint — *see* Arthritis, pyogenic or pyemic
  liver K75.1
  pneumococcal A40.3
  portal K75.1
  postvaccinal T88.0 ☑
  puerperal, postpartum, childbirth O85
  specified organism NEC A41.89
  tuberculous — *see* Tuberculosis, miliary
Pygopagus Q89.4
Pyknoepilepsy (idiopathic) — *see* Pyknolepsy
Pyknolepsy G40.A09 (*following* G40.3)
  intractable G40.A19 (*following* G40.3)
    with status epilepticus G40.A11 (*following* G40.3)
    without status epilepticus G40.A19 (*following* G40.3)
  not intractable G40.A09 (*following* G40.3)
    with status epilepticus G40.A01 (*following* G40.3)
    without status epilepticus G40.A09 (*following* G40.3)
Pylephlebitis K75.1
Pyle's syndrome Q78.5
Pylethrombophlebitis K75.1
Pylethrombosis K75.1
Pyloritis K29.90
  with bleeding K29.91
Pylorospasm (reflex) **NEC** K31.3

Pylorospasm (reflex) **NEC** — *continued*
  congenital or infantile Q40.0
  neurotic F45.8
  newborn Q40.0
  psychogenic F45.8
Pylorus, pyloric — *see* condition
Pyoarthrosis — *see* Arthritis, pyogenic or pyemic
Pyocele
  mastoid — *see* Mastoiditis, acute
  sinus (accessory) — *see* Sinusitis
  turbinate (bone) J32.9
  urethra (*see also* Urethritis) N34.0
Pyocolpos — *see* Vaginitis
Pyocystitis N30.80
  with hematuria N30.81
Pyoderma, pyodermia L08.0
  gangrenosum L88
  newborn P39.4
  phagedenic L88
  vegetans L08.81
Pyodermatitis L08.0
  vegetans L08.81
Pyogenic — *see* condition
Pyohydronephrosis N13.6
Pyometra, pyometrium, pyometritis — *see* Endometritis
Pyomyositis (tropical) — *see* Myositis, infective
Pyonephritis N12
Pyonephrosis N13.6
  tuberculous A18.11
Pyo-oophoritis — *see* Salpingo-oophoritis
Pyo-ovarium — *see* Salpingo-oophoritis
Pyopericarditis, pyopericardium I30.1
Pyophlebitis — *see* Phlebitis
Pyopneumopericardium I30.1
Pyopneumothorax (infective) J86.9
  with fistula J86.0
  tuberculous NEC A15.6
Pyosalpinx, pyosalpingitis (*see also* Salpingo-oophoritis)
Pyothorax J86.9
  with fistula J86.0
  tuberculous NEC A15.6
Pyoureter N28.89
  tuberculous A18.11
Pyramidopallidonigral syndrome G20
Pyrexia (of unknown origin) R50.9
  atmospheric T67.0 ☑
  during labor NEC O75.2
  heat T67.0 ☑
  newborn P81.9
    environmentally-induced P81.0
  persistent R50.9
  puerperal O86.4
Pyroglobulinemia NEC E88.09
Pyromania F63.1
Pyrosis R12
Pyuria (bacterial) N39.0

Q

Q fever A78
  with pneumonia A78
Quadricuspid aortic valve Q23.8
Quadrilateral fever A78
Quadriparesis — *see* Quadriplegia
  meaning muscle weakness M62.81
Quadriplegia G82.50
  complete
    C1-C4 level G82.51
    C5-C7 level G82.53
  congenital (cerebral) (spinal) G80.8
    spastic G80.0
  embolic (current episode) I63.4- ☑
  functional R53.2
  incomplete
    C1-C4 level G82.52
    C5-C7 level G82.54
  thrombotic (current episode) I63.3- ☑
  traumatic — *code to* injury with seventh character S
    current episode — *see* Injury, spinal (cord), cervical
Quadruplet, pregnancy — *see* Pregnancy, quadruplet
Quarrelsomeness F60.3
Queensland fever A77.3
Quervain's disease M65.4
  thyroid E06.1
Queyrat's erythroplasia D07.4

Queyrat's erythroplasia — *continued*
  penis DØ7.4
  specified site — *see* Neoplasm, skin, in situ
  unspecified site DØ7.4
Quincke's disease or edema T78.3 ☑
  hereditary D84.1
Quinsy (gangrenous) J36
Quintan fever A79.Ø
Quintuplet, pregnancy — *see* Pregnancy, quintuplet

R

Rabbit fever — *see* Tularemia
Rabies A82.9
  contact Z2Ø.3
  exposure to Z2Ø.3
  inoculation reaction — *see* Complications, vaccination
  sylvatic A82.Ø
  urban A82.1
Rachischisis — *see* Spina bifida
Rachitic (*see also* condition)
  deformities of spine (late effect) (sequelae) E64.3
  pelvis (late effect) (sequelae) E64.3
    with disproportion (fetopelvic) O33.Ø
      causing obstructed labor O65.Ø
Rachitis, rachitism (acute) (tarda) (*see also* Rickets)
  renalis N25.Ø
  sequelae E64.3
Radial nerve — *see* condition
Radiation
  burn — *see* Burn
  effects NOS T66 ☑
  sickness NOS T66 ☑
  therapy, encounter for Z51.Ø
Radiculitis (pressure) (vertebrogenic) — *see* Radiculopathy
Radiculomyelitis (*see also* Encephalitis)
  toxic, due to
    Clostridium tetani A35
    Corynebacterium diphtheriae A36.82
Radiculopathy M54.1Ø
  cervical region M54.12
  cervicothoracic region M54.13
  due to
    disc disorder
      C3 M5Ø.11
      C4 M5Ø.11
      C5 M5Ø.121
      C6 M5Ø.122
      C7 M5Ø.123
    displacement of intervertebral disc — *see* Disorder, disc, with, radiculopathy
  leg M54.1- ☑
  lumbar region M54.16
  lumbosacral region M54.17
  occipito-atlanto-axial region M54.11
  postherpetic BØ2.29
  sacrococcygeal region M54.18
  syphilitic A52.11
  thoracic region (with visceral pain) M54.14
  thoracolumbar region M54.15
Radiodermal burns (acute, chronic, or occupational) — *see* Burn
Radiodermatitis L58.9
  acute L58.Ø
  chronic L58.1
Radiotherapy session Z51.Ø
RAEB (refractory anemia with excess blasts) D46.2- ☑
Rage, meaning rabies — *see* Rabies
Ragpicker's disease A22.1
Ragsorter's disease A22.1
Raillietiniasis B71.8
Railroad neurosis F48.8
Railway spine F48.8
Raised (*see also* Elevated)
  antibody titer R76.Ø
Rake teeth, tooth M26.39
Rales RØ9.89
Ramifying renal pelvis Q63.8
Ramsay-Hunt disease or syndrome (*see also* Hunt's disease) BØ2.21
  meaning dyssynergia cerebellaris myoclonica G11.1
Ranula K11.6
  congenital Q38.4
Rape
  adult
    confirmed T74.21 ☑

Rape — *continued*
  adult — *continued*
    suspected T76.21 ☑
  alleged, observation or examination, ruled out
    adult ZØ4.41
    child ZØ4.42
  child
    confirmed T74.22 ☑
    suspected T76.22 ☑
Rapid
  feeble pulse, due to shock, following injury T79.4 ☑
  heart (beat) RØØ.Ø
    psychogenic F45.8
  second stage (delivery) O62.3
  time-zone change syndrome G47.25
Rarefaction, bone — *see* Disorder, bone, density and structure, specified NEC
Rash (toxic) R21
  canker A38.9
  diaper L22
  drug (internal use) L27.Ø
    contact (*see also* Dermatitis, due to, drugs, external) L25.1
  following immunization T88.1 ☑
  food — *see* Dermatitis, due to, food
  heat L74.Ø
  napkin (psoriasiform) L22
  nettle — *see* Urticaria
  pustular LØ8.Ø
  rose R21
    epidemic BØ6.9
  scarlet A38.9
  serum (*see also* Reaction, serum) T8Ø.69 ☑
  wandering tongue K14.1
Rasmussen aneurysm — *see* Tuberculosis, pulmonary
Rasmussen encephalitis GØ4.81
Rat-bite fever A25.9
  due to Streptobacillus moniliformis A25.1
  spirochetal (morsus muris) A25.Ø
Rathke's pouch tumor D44.3
Raymond (-Céstan) syndrome I65.8
Raynaud's disease, phenomenon or syndrome (secondary) I73.ØØ
  with gangrene (symmetric) I73.Ø1
RDS (newborn) (type I) P22.Ø
  type II P22.1
Reaction (*see also* Disorder)
  withdrawing, child or adolescent F93.8
  adaptation — *see* Disorder, adjustment
  adjustment (anxiety) (conduct disorder) (depressiveness) (distress) — *see* Disorder, adjustment
    with
      mutism, elective (child) (adolescent) F94.Ø
  adverse
    food (any) (ingested) NEC T78.1 ☑
      anaphylactic — *see* Shock, anaphylactic, due to food
  affective — *see* Disorder, mood
  allergic — *see* Allergy
  anaphylactic — *see* Shock, anaphylactic
  anaphylactoid — *see* Shock, anaphylactic
  anesthesia — *see* Anesthesia, complication
  antitoxin (prophylactic) (therapeutic) — *see* Complications, vaccination
  anxiety F41.1
  Arthus — *see* Arthus' phenomenon
  asthenic F48.8
  combat and operational stress F43.Ø
  compulsive F42.8
  conversion F44.9
  crisis, acute F43.Ø
  deoxyribonuclease (DNA) (DNase) hypersensitivity D69.2
  depressive (single episode) F32.9
    affective (single episode) F31.4
      recurrent episode F33.9
    neurotic F34.1
    psychoneurotic F34.1
    psychotic F32.3
    recurrent — *see* Disorder, depressive, recurrent
  dissociative F44.9
  drug NEC T88.7 ☑
    addictive — *see* Dependence, drug
      transmitted via placenta or breast milk — *see* Absorption, drug, addictive, through placenta
    allergic — *see* Allergy, drug
    lichenoid L43.2

Reaction — *continued*
  drug — *continued*
    newborn P93.8
      gray baby syndrome P93.Ø
    overdose or poisoning (by accident) — *see* Table of Drugs and Chemicals, by drug, poisoning
    photoallergic L56.1
    phototoxic L56.Ø
    withdrawal — *see* Dependence, by drug, with, withdrawal
      infant of dependent mother P96.1
      newborn P96.1
    wrong substance given or taken (by accident) — *see* Table of Drugs and Chemicals, by drug, poisoning
  fear F4Ø.9
    child (abnormal) F93.8
  febrile nonhemolytic transfusion (FNHTR) R5Ø.84
  fluid loss, cerebrospinal G97.1
  foreign
    body NEC — *see* Granuloma, foreign body
      in operative wound (inadvertently left) — *see* Foreign body, accidentally left during a procedure
    substance accidentally left during a procedure (chemical) (powder) (talc) T81.6Ø ☑
      aseptic peritonitis T81.61 ☑
      body or object (instrument) (sponge) (swab) — *see* Foreign body, accidentally left during a procedure
      specified reaction NEC T81.69 ☑
  grief — *see* Disorder, adjustment
  Herxheimer's R68.89
  hyperkinetic — *see* Hyperkinesia
  hypochondriacal F45.2Ø
  hypoglycemic, due to insulin E16.Ø
    with coma (diabetic) — *see* Diabetes, coma
      nondiabetic E15
    therapeutic misadventure — *see* subcategory T38.3 ☑
  hypomanic F3Ø.8
  hysterical F44.9
  immunization — *see* Complications, vaccination
  incompatibility
    ABO blood group (infusion) (transfusion) — *see* Complication(s), transfusion, incompatibility reaction, ABO
    delayed serologic T8Ø.39 ☑
    minor blood group (Duffy) (E) (K) (Kell) (Kidd) (Lewis) (M) (N) (P) (S) T8Ø.89 ☑
    Rh (factor) (infusion) (transfusion) — *see* Complication(s), transfusion, incompatibility reaction, Rh (factor)
  inflammatory — *see* Infection
  infusion — *see* Complications, infusion
  inoculation (immune serum) — *see* Complications, vaccination
  insulin T38.3- ☑
  involutional psychotic — *see* Disorder, depressive
  leukemoid D72.823
    basophilic D72.823
    lymphocytic D72.823
    monocytic D72.823
    myelocytic D72.823
    neutrophilic D72.823
  LSD (acute)
    due to drug abuse — *see* Abuse, drug, hallucinogen
    due to drug dependence — *see* Dependence, drug, hallucinogen
  lumbar puncture G97.1
  manic-depressive — *see* Disorder, bipolar
  neurasthenic F48.8
  neurogenic — *see* Neurosis
  neurotic F48.9
  neurotic-depressive F34.1
  nitritoid — *see* Crisis, nitritoid
  nonspecific
    to
      cell mediated immunity measurement of gamma interferon antigen response without active tuberculosis R76.12
      QuantiFERON-TB test (QFT) without active tuberculosis R76.12
      tuberculin test (*see also* Reaction, tuberculin skin test) R76.11
  obsessive-compulsive F42.8
  organic, acute or subacute — *see* Delirium
  paranoid (acute) F23

☑ Additional Character Required — Refer to the Tabular List for Character Selection   ▽ Subterms under main terms may continue to next column or page

Reaction — *continued*
  paranoid — *continued*
    chronic F22
    senile F03 ☑
  passive dependency F60.7
  phobic F40.9
  post-traumatic stress, uncomplicated Z73.3
  psychogenic F99
  psychoneurotic (*see also* Neurosis)
    compulsive F42.8
    depersonalization F48.1
    depressive F34.1
    hypochondriacal F45.20
    neurasthenic F48.8
    obsessive F42.8
  psychophysiologic — *see* Disorder, somatoform
  psychosomatic — *see* Disorder, somatoform
  psychotic — *see* Psychosis
  scarlet fever toxin — *see* Complications, vaccination
  schizophrenic F23
    acute (brief) (undifferentiated) F23
    latent F21
    undifferentiated (acute) (brief) F23
  serological for syphilis — *see* Serology for syphilis
  serum T80.69 ☑
    anaphylactic (immediate) (*see also* Shock, anaphylactic) T80.59 ☑
    specified reaction NEC
      due to
        administration of blood and blood products T80.61 ☑
        immunization T80.62 ☑
        serum specified NEC T80.69 ☑
        vaccination T80.62 ☑
  situational — *see* Disorder, adjustment
  somatization — *see* Disorder, somatoform
  spinal puncture G97.1
  stress (severe) F43.9
    acute (agitation) ("daze") (disorientation) (disturbance of consciousness) (flight reaction) (fugue) F43.0
    specified NEC F43.8
  surgical procedure — *see* Complications, surgical procedure
  tetanus antitoxin — *see* Complications, vaccination
  toxic, to local anesthesia T88.59 ☑
    in labor and delivery O74.4
    in pregnancy O29.3X- ☑
    postpartum, puerperal O89.3
  toxin-antitoxin — *see* Complications, vaccination
  transfusion (blood) (bone marrow) (lymphocytes) (allergic) — *see* Complications, transfusion
  tuberculin skin test, abnormal R76.11
  vaccination (any) — *see* Complications, vaccination
Reactive airway disease — *see* Asthma
Reactive depression — *see* Reaction, depressive
Rearrangement
  chromosomal
    balanced (in) Q95.9
      abnormal individual (autosomal) Q95.2
      non-sex (autosomal) chromosomes Q95.2
      sex/non-sex chromosomes Q95.3
      specified NEC Q95.8
Recalcitrant patient — *see* Noncompliance
Recanalization, thrombus — *see* Thrombosis
Recession, receding
  chamber angle (eye) H21.55- ☑
  chin M26.09
  gingival (postinfective) (postoperative)
    generalized K06.020
      minimal K06.021
      moderate K06.022
      severe K06.023
    localized K06.010
      minimal K06.011
      moderate K06.012
      severe K06.013
Recklinghausen disease Q85.01
  bones E21.0
Reclus' disease (cystic) — *see* Mastopathy, cystic
Recrudescent typhus (fever) A75.1
Recruitment, auditory H93.21- ☑
Rectalgia K62.89
Rectitis K62.89
Rectocele
  female (without uterine prolapse) N81.6
    with uterine prolapse N81.4

Rectocele — *continued*
  female — *continued*
    with uterine prolapse — *continued*
      incomplete N81.2
    in pregnancy — *see* Pregnancy, complicated by, abnormal, pelvic organs or tissues NEC
  male K62.3
Rectosigmoid junction — *see* condition
Rectosigmoiditis K63.89
  ulcerative (chronic) K51.30
    with
      complication K51.319
        abscess K51.314
        fistula K51.313
        obstruction K51.312
        rectal bleeding K51.311
        specified NEC K51.318
Rectourethral — *see* condition
Rectovaginal — *see* condition
Rectovesical — *see* condition
Rectum, rectal — *see* condition
Recurrent — *see* condition
  pregnancy loss — *see* Loss (of), pregnancy, recurrent
Red bugs B88.0
Red tide (*see also* Table of Drugs and Chemicals) T65.82- ☑
Red-cedar lung or pneumonitis J67.8
Reduced
  mobility Z74.09
  ventilatory or vital capacity R94.2
Redundant, redundancy
  anus (congenital) Q43.8
  clitoris N90.89
  colon (congenital) Q43.8
  foreskin (congenital) N47.8
  intestine (congenital) Q43.8
  labia N90.69
  organ or site, congenital NEC — *see* Accessory
  panniculus (abdominal) E65
  prepuce (congenital) N47.8
  pylorus K31.89
  rectum (congenital) Q43.8
  scrotum N50.89
  sigmoid (congenital) Q43.8
  skin L98.7
    and subcutaneous tissue L98.7
    of face L57.4
      eyelids — *see* Blepharochalasis
  stomach K31.89
Reduplication — *see* Duplication
Reflex R29.2
  hyperactive gag J39.2
  pupillary, abnormal — *see* Anomaly, pupil, function
  vasoconstriction I73.9
  vasovagal R55
Reflux K21.9
  acid K21.9
  esophageal K21.9
    with esophagitis K21.0
    newborn P78.83
  gastroesophageal K21.9
    with esophagitis K21.0
  mitral — *see* Insufficiency, mitral
  ureteral — *see* Reflux, vesicoureteral
  vesicoureteral (with scarring) N13.70
    with
      nephropathy N13.729
        with hydroureter N13.739
          bilateral N13.732
          unilateral N13.731
        bilateral N13.722
        unilateral N13.721
        without hydroureter N13.729
          bilateral N13.722
          unilateral N13.721
      pyelonephritis (chronic) N11.0
    congenital Q62.7
    without nephropathy N13.71
Reforming, artificial openings — *see* Attention to, artificial, opening
Refractive error — *see* Disorder, refraction
Refsum's disease or syndrome G60.1
Refusal of
  food, psychogenic F50.89
  treatment (because of) Z53.20
    left against medical advice (AMA) Z53.21
    patient's decision NEC Z53.29
    reasons of belief or group pressure Z53.1

Regional — *see* condition
Regurgitation R11.10
  aortic (valve) — *see* Insufficiency, aortic
  food (*see also* Vomiting)
    with reswallowing — *see* Rumination
    newborn P92.1
  gastric contents — *see* Vomiting
  heart — *see* Endocarditis
  mitral (valve) — *see* Insufficiency, mitral
    congenital Q23.3
  myocardial — *see* Endocarditis
  pulmonary (valve) (heart) I37.1
    congenital Q22.2
    syphilitic A52.03
  tricuspid — *see* Insufficiency, tricuspid
  valve, valvular — *see* Endocarditis
    congenital Q24.8
  vesicoureteral — *see* Reflux, vesicoureteral
Reichmann's disease or syndrome K31.89
Reifenstein syndrome E34.52
Reinsertion
  implantable subdermal contraceptive Z30.46
  intrauterine contraceptive device Z30.433
Reiter's disease, syndrome, or urethritis M02.30
  ankle M02.37- ☑
  elbow M02.32- ☑
  foot joint M02.37- ☑
  hand joint M02.34- ☑
  hip M02.35- ☑
  knee M02.36- ☑
  multiple site M02.39
  shoulder M02.31- ☑
  vertebra M02.38
  wrist M02.33- ☑
Rejection
  food, psychogenic F50.89
  transplant T86.91
    bone T86.830
      marrow T86.01
    cornea T86.840
    heart T86.21
      with lung(s) T86.31
    intestine T86.850
    kidney T86.11
    liver T86.41
    lung(s) T86.810
      with heart T86.31
    organ (immune or nonimmune cause) T86.91
    pancreas T86.890
    skin (allograft) (autograft) T86.820
    specified NEC T86.890
    stem cell (peripheral blood) (umbilical cord) T86.5
Relapsing fever A68.9
  Carter's (Asiatic) A68.1
  Dutton's (West African) A68.1
  Koch's A68.9
  louse-borne (epidemic) A68.0
  Novy's (American) A68.1
  Obermeyers's (European) A68.0
  Spirillum A68.9
  tick-borne (endemic) A68.1
Relationship
  occlusal
    open anterior M26.220
    open posterior M26.221
Relaxation
  anus (sphincter) K62.89
    psychogenic F45.8
  arch (foot) (*see also* Deformity, limb, flat foot)
  back ligaments — *see* Instability, joint, spine
  bladder (sphincter) N31.2
  cardioesophageal K21.9
  cervix — *see* Incompetency, cervix
  diaphragm J98.6
  joint (capsule) (ligament) (paralytic) — *see* Flail, joint
    congenital NEC Q74.8
  lumbosacral (joint) — *see* subcategory M53.2 ☑
  pelvic floor N81.89
  perineum N81.89
  posture R29.3
  rectum (sphincter) K62.89
  sacroiliac (joint) — *see* subcategory M53.2 ☑
  scrotum N50.89
  urethra (sphincter) N36.44
  vesical N31.2
Release from prison, anxiety concerning Z65.2
Remains
  canal of Cloquet Q14.0

Remains — continued
  capsule (opaque) Q14.8
Remittent fever (malarial) B54
Remnant
  canal of Cloquet Q14.0
  capsule (opaque) Q14.8
  cervix, cervical stump (acquired) (postoperative) N88.8
  cystic duct, postcholecystectomy K91.5
  fingernail L60.8
    congenital Q84.6
  meniscus, knee — see Derangement, knee, meniscus,
    specified NEC
  thyroglossal duct Q89.2
  tonsil J35.8
    infected (chronic) J35.01
  urachus Q64.4
Removal (from) (of)
  artificial
    arm Z44.00- ☑
      complete Z44.01- ☑
      partial Z44.02- ☑
    eye Z44.2- ☑
    leg Z44.10- ☑
      complete Z44.11- ☑
      partial Z44.12- ☑
  breast implant Z45.81
  cardiac pulse generator (battery) (end-of-life) Z45.010
  catheter (urinary) (indwelling) Z46.6
    from artificial opening — see Attention to, artificial,
      opening
    non-vascular Z46.82
    vascular NEC Z45.2
  device Z46.9
    contraceptive Z30.432
      implantable subdermal Z30.46
    implanted NEC Z45.89
    specified NEC Z46.89
  drains Z48.03
  dressing (nonsurgical) Z48.00
    surgical Z48.01
  external
    fixation device — code to fracture with seventh
      character D
    prosthesis, prosthetic device Z44.9
      breast Z44.3- ☑
      specified NEC Z44.8
  home in childhood (to foster home or institution)
    Z62.29
  ileostomy Z43.2
  insulin pump Z46.81
  myringotomy device (stent) (tube) Z45.82
  nervous system device NEC Z46.2
    brain neuropacemaker Z46.2
    visual substitution device Z46.2
      implanted Z45.31
  non-vascular catheter Z46.82
  organ, prophylactic (for neoplasia management) —
    see Prophylactic, organ removal
  orthodontic device Z46.4
  staples Z48.02
  stent
    ureteral Z46.6
  suture Z48.02
  urinary device Z46.6
  vascular access device or catheter Z45.2
Ren
  arcuatus Q63.1
  mobile, mobilis N28.89
    congenital Q63.8
  unguliformis Q63.1
Renal — see condition
Rendu-Osler-Weber disease or syndrome I78.0
Reninoma D41.0- ☑
Renon-Delille syndrome E23.3
Reovirus, as cause of disease classified elsewhere
  B97.5
Repeated falls NEC R29.6
Replaced chromosome by dicentric ring Q93.2
Replacement by artificial or mechanical device or
  prosthesis of
  bladder Z96.0
  blood vessel NEC Z95.828
  bone NEC Z96.7
  cochlea Z96.21
  coronary artery Z95.5
  eustachian tube Z96.29
  eye globe Z97.0
  heart Z95.812

Replacement by artificial or mechanical device or
  prosthesis of — continued
  heart — continued
    valve Z95.2
      prosthetic Z95.2
      specified NEC Z95.4
      xenogenic Z95.3
  intestine Z96.89
  joint Z96.60
    hip — see Presence, hip joint implant
    knee — see Presence, knee joint implant
    specified site NEC Z96.698
  larynx Z96.3
  lens Z96.1
  limb(s) — see Presence, artificial, limb
  mandible NEC (for tooth root implant(s)) Z96.5
  organ NEC Z96.89
  peripheral vessel NEC Z95.828
  stapes Z96.29
  teeth Z97.2
  tendon Z96.7
  tissue NEC Z96.89
  tooth root(s) Z96.5
  vessel NEC Z95.828
    coronary (artery) Z95.5
Request for expert evidence Z04.89
Reserve, decreased or low
  cardiac — see Disease, heart
  kidney N28.89
Residual (see also condition)
  ovary syndrome N99.83
  state, schizophrenic F20.5
  urine R39.198
Resistance, resistant (to)
  activated protein C D68.51
  complicating pregnancy O26.89 ☑
  insulin E88.81
  organism(s)
    to
      drug Z16.30
        aminoglycosides Z16.29
        amoxicillin Z16.11
        ampicillin Z16.11
        antibiotic(s) Z16.20
          multiple Z16.24
          specified NEC Z16.29
        antifungal Z16.32
        antimicrobial (single) Z16.30
          multiple Z16.35
          specified NEC Z16.39
        antimycobacterial (single) Z16.341
          multiple Z16.342
        antiparasitic Z16.31
        antiviral Z16.33
        beta lactam antibiotics Z16.10
          specified NEC Z16.19
        cephalosporins Z16.19
        extended beta lactamase (ESBL) Z16.12
        fluoroquinolones Z16.23
        macrolides Z16.29
        methicillin — see MRSA
        multiple drugs (MDRO)
          antibiotics Z16.24
          antimicrobial Z16.35
          antimycobacterials Z16.342
        penicillins Z16.11
        quinine (and related compounds) Z16.31
        quinolones Z16.23
        sulfonamides Z16.29
        tetracyclines Z16.29
        tuberculostatics (single) Z16.341
          multiple Z16.342
        vancomycin Z16.21
          related antibiotics Z16.22
  thyroid hormone E07.89
Resorption
  dental (roots) K03.3
    alveoli M26.79
  teeth (external) (internal) (pathological) (roots) K03.3
Respiration
  Cheyne-Stokes R06.3
  decreased due to shock, following injury T79.4 ☑
  disorder of, psychogenic F45.8
  insufficient, or poor R06.89
    newborn P28.5
  painful R07.1
  sighing, psychogenic F45.8
Respiratory (see also condition)

Respiratory — continued
  distress syndrome (newborn) (type I) P22.0
    type II P22.1
  syncytial virus, as cause of disease classified elsewhere
    B97.4
Respite care Z75.5
Response (drug)
  photoallergic L56.1
  phototoxic L56.0
Restenosis
  stent
    vascular
      end stent
        adjacent to stent — see Arteriosclerosis
        within the stent
          coronary T82.855 ☑
          peripheral T82.856 ☑
      in stent
        coronary vessel T82.855 ☑
        peripheral vessel T82.856 ☑
Restless legs (syndrome) G25.81
Restlessness R45.1
Restoration (of)
  dental
    aesthetically inadequate or displeasing K08.56
    defective K08.50
      specified NEC K08.59
    failure of marginal integrity K08.51
    failure of periodontal anatomical intergrity K08.54
  organ continuity from previous sterilization (tuboplas-
    ty) (vasoplasty) Z31.0
    aftercare Z31.42
  tooth (existing)
    contours biologically incompatible with oral health
      K08.54
    open margins K08.51
    overhanging K08.52
    poor aesthetic K08.56
    poor gingival margins K08.51
  unsatisfactory, of tooth K08.50
    specified NEC K08.59
Restorative material (dental)
  allergy to K08.55
  fractured K08.539
    with loss of material K08.531
    without loss of material K08.530
  unrepairable overhanging of K08.52
Restriction of housing space Z59.1
Rests, ovarian, in fallopian tube Q50.6
Restzustand (schizophrenic) F20.5
Retained (see also Retention)
  cholelithiasis following cholecystectomy K91.86
  foreign body fragments (type of) Z18.9
    acrylics Z18.2
    animal quill(s) or spines Z18.31
    cement Z18.83
    concrete Z18.83
    crystalline Z18.83
    depleted isotope Z18.09
    depleted uranium Z18.01
    diethylhexyl phthalates Z18.2
    glass Z18.81
    isocyanate Z18.2
    magnetic metal Z18.11
    metal Z18.10
    nonmagnectic metal Z18.12
    nontherapeutic radioactive Z18.09
    organic NEC Z18.39
    plastic Z18.2
    quill(s) (animal) Z18.31
    radioactive (nontherapeutic) NEC Z18.09
    specified NEC Z18.89
    spine(s) (animal) Z18.31
    stone Z18.83
    tooth (teeth) Z18.32
    wood Z18.33
  fragments (type of) Z18.9
    acrylics Z18.2
    animal quill(s) or spines Z18.31
    cement Z18.83
    concrete Z18.83
    crystalline Z18.83
    depleted isotope Z18.09
    depleted uranium Z18.01
    diethylhexyl phthalates Z18.2
    glass Z18.81
    isocyanate Z18.2
    magnetic metal Z18.11

☑ Additional Character Required — Refer to the Tabular List for Character Selection   ▽ Subterms under main terms may continue to next column or page

Retained — *continued*
  fragments — *continued*
    metal Z18.10
    nonmagnetic metal Z18.12
    nontherapeutic radioactive Z18.09
    organic NEC Z18.39
    plastic Z18.2
    quill(s) (animal) Z18.31
    radioactive (nontherapeutic) NEC Z18.09
    specified NEC Z18.89
    spine(s) (animal) Z18.31
    stone Z18.83
    tooth (teeth) Z18.32
    wood Z18.33
  gallstones, following cholecystectomy K91.86
Retardation
  development, developmental, specific — *see* Disorder, developmental
  endochondral bone growth — *see* Disorder, bone, development or growth
  growth R62.50
    due to malnutrition E45
  mental — *see* Disability, intellectual
  motor function, specific F82
  physical (child) R62.52
    due to malnutrition E45
  reading (specific) F81.0
  spelling (specific) (without reading disorder) F81.81
Retching — *see* Vomiting
Retention (*see also* Retained)
  bladder — *see* Retention, urine
  carbon dioxide E87.2
  cholelithiasis following cholecystectomy K91.86
  cyst — *see* Cyst
  dead
    fetus (at or near term) (mother) O36.4 ☑
      early fetal death O02.1
    ovum O02.0
  decidua (fragments) (following delivery) (with hemorrhage) O72.2
    without hemorrhage O73.1
  deciduous tooth K00.6
  dental root K08.3
  fecal — *see* Constipation
  fetus
    dead O36.4 ☑
      early O02.1
  fluid R60.9
  foreign body (*see also* Foreign body, retained)
    current trauma — *code as* Foreign body, by site or type
  gallstones, following cholecystectomy K91.86
  gastric K31.89
  intrauterine contraceptive device, in pregnancy — *see* Pregnancy, complicated by, retention, intrauterine device
  membranes (complicating delivery) (with hemorrhage) O72.2
    with abortion — *see* Abortion, by type
    without hemorrhage O73.1
  meniscus — *see* Derangement, meniscus
  menses N94.89
  milk (puerperal, postpartum) O92.79
  nitrogen, extrarenal R39.2
  ovary syndrome N99.83
  placenta (total) (with hemorrhage) O72.0
    without hemorrhage O73.0
    portions or fragments (with hemorrhage) O72.2
      without hemorrhage O73.1
  products of conception
    early pregnancy (dead fetus) O02.1
    following
      delivery (with hemorrhage) O72.2
        without hemorrhage O73.1
  secundines (following delivery) (with hemorrhage) O72.0
    without hemorrhage O73.0
    complicating puerperium (delayed hemorrhage) O72.2
    partial O72.2
      without hemorrhage O73.1
  smegma, clitoris N90.89
  urine R33.9
    due to hyperplasia (hypertrophy) of prostate — *see* Hyperplasia, prostate
    drug-induced R33.0
    organic R33.8
      drug-induced R33.0

Retention — *continued*
  urine — *continued*
    psychogenic F45.8
    specified NEC R33.8
  water (in tissues) — *see* Edema
Reticulation, dust — *see* Pneumoconiosis
Reticulocytosis R70.1
Reticuloendotheliosis
  acute infantile C96.0
  leukemic C91.4- ☑
  nonlipid C96.0
Reticulohistiocytoma (giant-cell) D76.3
Reticuloid, actinic L57.1
Reticulosis (skin)
  acute of infancy C96.0
  hemophagocytic, familial D76.1
  histiocytic medullary C96.A (*following* C96.6)
  lipomelanotic I89.8
  malignant (midline) C86.0
  polymorphic C83.8- ☑
  Sézary — *see* Sézary disease
Retina, retinal (*see also* condition)
  dark area D49.81
Retinitis (*see also* Inflammation, chorioretinal)
  albuminurica N18.9 [H32]
  diabetic — *see* Diabetes, retinitis
  disciformis — *see* Degeneration, macula
  focal — *see* Inflammation, chorioretinal, focal
  gravidarum — *see* Pregnancy, complicated by, specified pregnancy-related condition NEC
  juxtapapillaris — *see* Inflammation, chorioretinal, focal, juxtapapillary
  luetic — *see* Retinitis, syphilitic
  pigmentosa H35.52
  proliferans — *see* Disorder, globe, degenerative, specified type NEC
  proliferating — *see* Disorder, globe, degenerative, specified type NEC
  renal N18.9 [H32]
  syphilitic (early) (secondary) A51.43
    central, recurrent A52.71
    congenital (early) A50.01 [H32]
    late A52.71
  tuberculous A18.53
Retinoblastoma C69.2- ☑
  differentiated C69.2- ☑
  undifferentiated C69.2- ☑
Retinochoroiditis (*see also* Inflammation, chorioretinal)
  disseminated — *see* Inflammation, chorioretinal, disseminated
    syphilitic A52.71
  focal — *see* Inflammation, chorioretinal
  juxtapapillaris — *see* Inflammation, chorioretinal, focal, juxtapapillary
Retinopathy (background) H35.00
  arteriosclerotic I70.8 [H35.0-] ☑
  atherosclerotic I70.8 [H35.0-] ☑
  central serous — *see* Chorioretinopathy, central serous
  Coats H35.02- ☑
  diabetic — *see* Diabetes, retinopathy
  exudative H35.02- ☑
  hypertensive H35.03- ☑
  in (due to)
    diabetes — *see* Diabetes, retinopathy
    sickle-cell disorders D57.- ☑ [H36]
  of prematurity H35.10- ☑
    stage 0 H35.11- ☑
    stage 1 H35.12- ☑
    stage 2 H35.13- ☑
    stage 3 H35.14- ☑
    stage 4 H35.15- ☑
    stage 5 H35.16- ☑
  pigmentary, congenital — *see* Dystrophy, retina
  proliferative NEC H35.2- ☑
    diabetic — *see* Diabetes, retinopathy, proliferative
    sickle-cell D57.- ☑ [H36]
  solar H31.02- ☑
Retinoschisis H33.10- ☑
  congenital Q14.1
  specified type NEC H33.19- ☑
Retortamoniasis A07.8
Retractile testis Q55.22
Retraction
  cervix — *see* Retroversion, uterus
  drum (membrane) — *see* Disorder, tympanic membrane, specified NEC
  finger — *see* Deformity, finger

Retraction — *continued*
  lid H02.539
    left H02.536
      lower H02.535
      upper H02.534
    right H02.533
      lower H02.532
      upper H02.531
  lung J98.4
  mediastinum J98.59
  nipple N64.53
    associated with
      lactation O92.03
      pregnancy O92.01- ☑
      puerperium O92.02
    congenital Q83.8
  palmar fascia M72.0
  pleura — *see* Pleurisy
  ring, uterus (Bandl's) (pathological) O62.4
  sternum (congenital) Q76.7
    acquired M95.4
  uterus — *see* Retroversion, uterus
  valve (heart) — *see* Endocarditis
Retrobulbar — *see* condition
Retrocecal — *see* condition
Retrocession — *see* Retroversion
Retrodisplacement — *see* Retroversion
Retroflection, retroflexion — *see* Retroversion
Retrognathia, retrognathism (mandibular) (maxillary) M26.19
Retrograde menstruation N92.5
Retroperineal — *see* condition
Retroperitoneal — *see* condition
Retroperitonitis K68.9
Retropharyngeal — *see* condition
Retroplacental — *see* condition
Retroposition — *see* Retroversion
Retroprosthetic membrane T85.398 ☑
Retrosternal thyroid (congenital) Q89.2
Retroversion, retroverted
  cervix — *see* Retroversion, uterus
  female NEC — *see* Retroversion, uterus
  iris H21.89
  testis (congenital) Q55.29
  uterus (acquired) (acute) (any degree) (asymptomatic) (cervix) (postinfectional) (postpartal, old) N85.4
    congenital Q51.818
    in pregnancy O34.53- ☑
Retrovirus, as cause of disease classified elsewhere B97.30
  human
    immunodeficiency, type 2 (HIV 2) B97.35
    T-cell lymphotropic
      type I (HTLV-I) B97.33
      type II (HTLV-II) B97.34
  lentivirus B97.31
  oncovirus B97.32
  specified NEC B97.39
Retrusion, premaxilla (developmental) M26.09
Rett's disease or syndrome F84.2
Reverse peristalsis R19.2
Reye's syndrome G93.7
Rh (factor)
  hemolytic disease (newborn) P55.0
  incompatibility, immunization or sensitization
    affecting management of pregnancy NEC O36.09- ☑
      anti-D antibody O36.01- ☑
    newborn P55.0
    transfusion reaction — *see* Complication(s), transfusion, incompatibility reaction, Rh (factor)
  negative mother affecting newborn P55.0
  titer elevated — *see* Complication(s), transfusion, incompatibility reaction, Rh (factor)
  transfusion reaction — *see* Complication(s), transfusion, incompatibility reaction, Rh (factor)
Rhabdomyolysis (idiopathic) NEC M62.82
  traumatic T79.6 ☑
Rhabdomyoma (*see also* Neoplasm, connective tissue, benign)
  adult — *see* Neoplasm, connective tissue, benign
  fetal — *see* Neoplasm, connective tissue, benign
  glycogenic — *see* Neoplasm, connective tissue, benign
Rhabdomyosarcoma (any type) — *see* Neoplasm, connective tissue, malignant
Rhabdosarcoma — *see* Rhabdomyosarcoma
Rhesus (factor) **incompatibility** — *see* Rh, incompatibility

Rheumatic (acute) (subacute) (chronic)
  adherent pericardium I09.2
  coronary arteritis I01.9
  degeneration, myocardium I09.0
  fever (acute) — see Fever, rheumatic
  heart — see Disease, heart, rheumatic
  myocardial degeneration — see Degeneration, myocardium
  myocarditis (chronic) (inactive) (with chorea) I09.0
    active or acute I01.2
      with chorea (acute) (rheumatic) (Sydenham's) I02.0
  pancarditis, acute I01.8
    with chorea (acute (rheumatic) Sydenham's) I02.0
  pericarditis (active) (acute) (with effusion) (with pneumonia) I01.0
    with chorea (acute) (rheumatic) (Sydenham's) I02.0
    chronic or inactive I09.2
  pneumonia I00 [J17]
  torticollis M43.6
  typhoid fever A01.09
Rheumatism (articular) (neuralgic) (nonarticular) M79.0
  gout — see Arthritis, rheumatoid
  intercostal, meaning Tietze's disease M94.0
  palindromic (any site) M12.30
    ankle M12.37- ☑
    elbow M12.32- ☑
    foot joint M12.37- ☑
    hand joint M12.34- ☑
    hip M12.35- ☑
    knee M12.36- ☑
    multiple site M12.39
    shoulder M12.31- ☑
    specified joint NEC M12.38
    vertebrae M12.38
    wrist M12.33- ☑
  sciatic M54.4- ☑
Rheumatoid (see also condition)
  arthritis (see also Arthritis, rheumatoid)
    with involvement of organs NEC M05.60
      ankle M05.67- ☑
      elbow M05.62- ☑
      foot joint M05.67- ☑
      hand joint M05.64- ☑
      hip M05.65- ☑
      knee M05.66- ☑
      multiple site M05.69
      shoulder M05.61- ☑
      vertebra — see Spondylitis, ankylosing
      wrist M05.63- ☑
    seronegative — see Arthritis, rheumatoid, seronegative
    seropositive — see Arthritis, rheumatoid, seropositive
  carditis M05.30
    ankle M05.37- ☑
    elbow M05.32- ☑
    foot joint M05.37- ☑
    hand joint M05.34- ☑
    hip M05.35- ☑
    knee M05.36- ☑
    multiple site M05.39
    shoulder M05.31- ☑
    vertebra — see Spondylitis, ankylosing
    wrist M05.33- ☑
  endocarditis — see Rheumatoid, carditis
  lung (disease) M05.10
    ankle M05.17- ☑
    elbow M05.12- ☑
    foot joint M05.17- ☑
    hand joint M05.14- ☑
    hip M05.15- ☑
    knee M05.16- ☑
    multiple site M05.19
    shoulder M05.11- ☑
    vertebra — see Spondylitis, ankylosing
    wrist M05.13- ☑
  myocarditis — see Rheumatoid, carditis
  myopathy M05.40
    ankle M05.47- ☑
    elbow M05.42- ☑
    foot joint M05.47- ☑
    hand joint M05.44- ☑
    hip M05.45- ☑
    knee M05.46- ☑
    multiple site M05.49
    shoulder M05.41- ☑
    vertebra — see Spondylitis, ankylosing

Rheumatoid — continued
  myopathy — continued
    wrist M05.43- ☑
  pericarditis — see Rheumatoid, carditis
  polyarthritis — see Arthritis, rheumatoid
  polyneuropathy M05.50
    ankle M05.57- ☑
    elbow M05.52- ☑
    foot joint M05.57- ☑
    hand joint M05.54- ☑
    hip M05.55- ☑
    knee M05.56- ☑
    multiple site M05.59
    shoulder M05.51- ☑
    vertebra — see Spondylitis, ankylosing
    wrist M05.53- ☑
  vasculitis M05.20
    ankle M05.27- ☑
    elbow M05.22- ☑
    foot joint M05.27- ☑
    hand joint M05.24- ☑
    hip M05.25- ☑
    knee M05.26- ☑
    multiple site M05.29
    shoulder M05.21- ☑
    vertebra — see Spondylitis, ankylosing
    wrist M05.23- ☑
Rhinitis (atrophic) (catarrhal) (chronic) (croupous) (fibrinous) (granulomatous) (hyperplastic) (hypertrophic) (membranous) (obstructive) (purulent) (suppurative) (ulcerative) J31.0
  with
    sore throat — see Nasopharyngitis
  acute J00
  allergic J30.9
    with asthma J45.909
      with
        exacerbation (acute) J45.901
        status asthmaticus J45.902
    due to
      food J30.5
      pollen J30.1
    nonseasonal J30.89
    perennial J30.89
    seasonal NEC J30.2
    specified NEC J30.89
  infective J00
  pneumococcal J00
  syphilitic A52.73
    congenital A50.05 [J99]
  tuberculous A15.8
  vasomotor J30.0
Rhinoantritis (chronic) — see Sinusitis, maxillary
Rhinodacryolith — see Dacryolith
Rhinolith (nasal sinus) J34.89
Rhinomegaly J34.89
Rhinopharyngitis (acute) (subacute) (see also Nasopharyngitis)
  chronic J31.1
  destructive ulcerating A66.5
  mutilans A66.5
Rhinophyma L71.1
Rhinorrhea J34.89
  cerebrospinal (fluid) G96.0
  paroxysmal — see Rhinitis, allergic
  spasmodic — see Rhinitis, allergic
Rhinosalpingitis — see Salpingitis, eustachian
Rhinoscleroma A48.8
Rhinosporidiosis B48.1
Rhinovirus infection NEC B34.8
Rhizomelic chondrodysplasia punctata E71.540
Rhythm
  atrioventricular nodal I49.8
  disorder I49.9
    coronary sinus I49.8
    ectopic I49.8
    nodal I49.8
  escape I49.9
  heart, abnormal I49.9
  idioventricular I44.2
  nodal I49.8
  sleep, inversion G47.2- ☑
    nonorganic origin — see Disorder, sleep, circadian rhythm, psychogenic
Rhytidosis facialis L98.8
Rib (see also condition)
  cervical Q76.5

Riboflavin deficiency E53.0
Rice bodies (see also Loose, body, joint)
  knee M23.4- ☑
Richter syndrome — see Leukemia, chronic lymphocytic, B-cell type
Richter's hernia — see Hernia, abdomen, with obstruction
Ricinism — see Poisoning, food, noxious, plant
Rickets (active) (acute) (adolescent) (chest wall) (congenital) (current) (infantile) (intestinal) E55.0
  adult — see Osteomalacia
  celiac K90.0
  hypophosphatemic with nephrotic-glycosuric dwarfism E72.09
  inactive E64.3
  kidney N25.0
  renal N25.0
  sequelae, any E64.3
  vitamin-D-resistant E83.31 [M90.80]
Rickettsial disease A79.9
  specified type NEC A79.89
Rickettsialpox (Rickettsia akari) A79.1
Rickettsiosis A79.9
  due to
    Ehrlichia sennetsu A79.81
    Rickettsia akari (rickettsialpox) A79.1
  specified type NEC A79.89
  tick-borne A77.9
  vesicular A79.1
Rider's bone — see Ossification, muscle, specified NEC
Ridge, alveolus (see also condition)
  flabby K06.8
Ridged ear, congenital Q17.3
Riedel's
  lobe, liver Q44.7
  struma, thyroiditis or disease E06.5
Rieger's anomaly or syndrome Q13.81
Riehl's melanosis L81.4
Rietti-Greppi-Micheli anemia D56.9
Rieux's hernia — see Hernia, abdomen, specified site NEC
Riga (-Fede) **disease** K14.0
Riggs' disease — see Periodontitis
Right aortic arch Q25.47
Right middle lobe syndrome J98.11
Rigid, rigidity (see also condition)
  abdominal R19.30
    with severe abdominal pain R10.0
    epigastric R19.36
    generalized R19.37
    left lower quadrant R19.34
    left upper quadrant R19.32
    periumbilic R19.35
    right lower quadrant R19.33
    right upper quadrant R19.31
  articular, multiple, congenital Q68.8
  cervix (uteri) in pregnancy — see Pregnancy, complicated by, abnormal, cervix
  hymen (acquired) (congenital) N89.6
  nuchal R29.1
  pelvic floor in pregnancy — see Pregnancy, complicated by, abnormal, pelvic organs or tissues NEC
  perineum or vulva in pregnancy — see Pregnancy, complicated by, abnormal, vulva
  spine — see Dorsopathy, specified NEC
  vagina in pregnancy — see Pregnancy, complicated by, abnormal, vagina
Rigors R68.89
  with fever R50.9
Riley-Day syndrome G90.1
RIND (reversible ischemic neurologic deficit) I63.9
Ring(s)
  aorta (vascular) Q25.45
  Bandl's O62.4
  contraction, complicating delivery O62.4
  esophageal, lower (muscular) K22.2
  Fleischer's (cornea) H18.04- ☑
  hymenal, tight (acquired) (congenital) N89.6
  Kayser-Fleischer (cornea) H18.04- ☑
  retraction, uterus, pathological O62.4
  Schatzki's (esophagus) (lower) K22.2
    congenital Q39.3
  Soemmerring's — see Cataract, secondary
  vascular (congenital) Q25.8
    aorta Q25.45
Ringed hair (congenital) Q84.1
Ringworm B35.9
  beard B35.0

☑ Additional Character Required — Refer to the Tabular List for Character Selection
▽ Subterms under main terms may continue to next column or page

Ringworm — *continued*
  black dot B35.Ø
  body B35.4
  Burmese B35.5
  corporeal B35.4
  foot B35.3
  groin B35.6
  hand B35.2
  honeycomb B35.Ø
  nails B35.1
  perianal (area) B35.6
  scalp B35.Ø
  specified NEC B35.8
  Tokelau B35.5
Rise, venous pressure I87.8
Rising, PSA following treatment for malignant neoplasm of prostate R97.21
Risk
  for
    dental caries Z91.849
      high Z91.843
      low Z91.841
      moderate Z91.842
    suicidal
      meaning personal history of attempted suicide Z91.5
      meaning suicidal ideation — *see* Ideation, suicidal
Ritter's disease LØØ
Rivalry, sibling Z62.891
Rivalta's disease A42.2
River blindness B73.Ø1
Robert's pelvis Q74.2
  with disproportion (fetopelvic) O33.Ø
    causing obstructed labor O65.Ø
Robin (-Pierre) **syndrome** Q87.Ø
Robinow-Silvermann-Smith syndrome Q87.1
Robinson's (hidrotic) **ectodermal dysplasia or syndrome** Q82.4
Robles' disease B73.Ø1
Rocky Mountain (spotted) **fever** A77.Ø
Roetheln — *see* Rubella
Roger's disease Q21.Ø
Rokitansky-Aschoff sinuses (gallbladder) K82.8
Rolando's fracture (displaced) S62.22- ☑
  nondisplaced S62.22- ☑
Romano-Ward (prolonged QT interval) **syndrome** I45.81
Romberg's disease or syndrome G51.8
Roof, mouth — *see* condition
Rosacea L71.9
  acne L71.9
  keratitis L71.8
  specified NEC L71.8
Rosary, rachitic E55.Ø
Rose
  cold J3Ø.1
  fever J3Ø.1
  rash R21
    epidemic BØ6.9
Rosenbach's erysipeloid A26.Ø
Rosenthal's disease or syndrome D68.1
Roseola BØ9
  infantum BØ8.2Ø
    due to human herpesvirus 6 BØ8.21
    due to human herpesvirus 7 BØ8.22
Ross River disease or fever B33.1
Rossbach's disease K31.89
  psychogenic F45.8
Rostan's asthma (cardiac) — *see* Failure, ventricular, left
Rotation
  anomalous, incomplete or insufficient, intestine Q43.3
  cecum (congenital) Q43.3
  colon (congenital) Q43.3
  spine, incomplete or insufficient — *see* Dorsopathy, deforming, specified NEC
  tooth, teeth, fully erupted M26.35
  vertebra, incomplete or insufficient — *see* Dorsopathy, deforming, specified NEC
Rotes Quérol disease or syndrome — *see* Hyperostosis, ankylosing
Roth (-Bernhardt) **disease or syndrome** — *see* Meralgia paraesthetica
Rothmund (-Thomson) **syndrome** Q82.8
Rotor's disease or syndrome E8Ø.6
Round
  back (with wedging of vertebrae) — *see* Kyphosis
    sequelae (late effect) of rickets E64.3
  worms (large) (infestation) NEC B82.Ø
    Ascariasis (*see also* Ascariasis) B77.9

Roussy-Lévy syndrome G6Ø.Ø
Rubella (German measles) BØ6.9
  complication NEC BØ6.Ø9
    neurological BØ6.ØØ
  congenital P35.Ø
  contact Z2Ø.4
  exposure to Z2Ø.4
  maternal
    care for (suspected) damage to fetus O35.3 ☑
    manifest rubella in infant P35.Ø
    suspected damage to fetus affecting management of pregnancy O35.3 ☑
  specified complications NEC BØ6.89
Rubeola (meaning measles) — *see* Measles
  meaning rubella — *see* Rubella
Rubeosis, iris — *see* Disorder, iris, vascular
Rubinstein-Taybi syndrome Q87.2
Rudimentary (congenital) (*see also* Agenesis)
  arm — *see* Defect, reduction, upper limb
  bone Q79.9
  cervix uteri Q51.828
  eye Q11.2
  lobule of ear Q17.3
  patella Q74.1
  respiratory organs in thoracopagus Q89.4
  tracheal bronchus Q32.4
  uterus Q51.818
    in male Q56.1
  vagina Q52.Ø
Ruled out condition — *see* Observation, suspected
Rumination R11.1Ø
  with nausea R11.2
  disorder of infancy F98.21
  neurotic F42.8
  newborn P92.1
  obsessional F42.8
  psychogenic F42.8
Runeberg's disease D51.Ø
Runny nose RØ9.89
Rupia (syphilitic) A51.39
  congenital A5Ø.Ø6
  tertiary A52.79
Rupture, ruptured
  abscess (spontaneous) — *code by* site under Abscess
  aneurysm — *see* Aneurysm
  anus (sphincter) — *see* Laceration, anus
  aorta, aortic I71.8
    abdominal I71.3
    arch I71.1
    ascending I71.1
    descending I71.8
      abdominal I71.3
      thoracic I71.1
    syphilitic A52.Ø1
    thoracoabdominal I71.5
    thorax, thoracic I71.1
    transverse I71.1
    traumatic — *see* Injury, aorta, laceration, major
    valve or cusp (*see also* Endocarditis, aortic) I35.8
  appendix (with peritonitis) (*see also* Appendicitis) K35.32
    with localized peritonitis (*see also* Appendicitis) K35.32
  arteriovenous fistula, brain I6Ø.8
  artery I77.2
    brain — *see* Hemorrhage, intracranial, intracerebral
    coronary — *see* Infarct, myocardium
    heart — *see* Infarct, myocardium
    pulmonary I28.8
    traumatic (complication) — *see* Injury, blood vessel
  bile duct (common) (hepatic) K83.2
    cystic K82.2
  bladder (sphincter) (nontraumatic) (spontaneous) N32.89
    following ectopic or molar pregnancy OØ8.6
    obstetrical trauma O71.5
    traumatic S37.29 ☑
  blood vessel (*see also* Hemorrhage)
    brain — *see* Hemorrhage, intracranial, intracerebral
    heart — *see* Infarct, myocardium
    traumatic (complication) — *see* Injury, blood vessel, laceration, major, by site
  bone — *see* Fracture
  bowel (nontraumatic) K63.1
  brain
    aneurysm (congenital) (*see also* Hemorrhage, intracranial, subarachnoid)
      syphilitic A52.Ø5

Rupture, ruptured — *continued*
  brain — *continued*
    hemorrhagic — *see* Hemorrhage, intracranial, intracerebral
  capillaries I78.8
  cardiac (auricle) (ventricle) (wall) I23.3
    with hemopericardium I23.Ø
    infectional I4Ø.9
    traumatic — *see* Injury, heart
  cartilage (articular) (current) (*see also* Sprain)
    knee S83.3- ☑
    semilunar — *see* Tear, meniscus
  cecum (with peritonitis) K65.Ø
    with peritoneal abscess K35.33
    traumatic S36.598 ☑
  celiac artery, traumatic — *see* Injury, blood vessel, celiac artery, laceration, major
  cerebral aneurysm (congenital) (*see* Hemorrhage, intracranial, subarachnoid)
  cervix (uteri)
    with ectopic or molar pregnancy OØ8.6
    following ectopic or molar pregnancy OØ8.6
    obstetrical trauma O71.3
    traumatic S37.69 ☑
  chordae tendineae NEC I51.1
    concurrent with acute myocardial infarction — *see* Infarct, myocardium
    following acute myocardial infarction (current complication) I23.4
  choroid (direct) (indirect) (traumatic) H31.32- ☑
  circle of Willis I6Ø.6
  colon (nontraumatic) K63.1
    traumatic — *see* Injury, intestine, large
  cornea (traumatic) — *see* Injury, eye, laceration
  coronary (artery) (thrombotic) — *see* Infarct, myocardium
  corpus luteum (infected) (ovary) N83.1- ☑
  cyst — *see* Cyst
  cystic duct K82.2
  Descemet's membrane — *see* Change, corneal membrane, Descemet's, rupture
    traumatic — *see* Injury, eye, laceration
  diaphragm, traumatic — *see* Injury, intrathoracic, diaphragm
  disc — *see* Rupture, intervertebral disc
  diverticulum (intestine) K57.8Ø
    with K57.81
    bladder N32.3
    large intestine K57.2Ø
      with
        bleeding K57.21
        small intestine K57.4Ø
          with bleeding K57.41
      small intestine K57.ØØ
        with
          bleeding K57.Ø1
          large intestine K57.4Ø
            with bleeding K57.41
  duodenal stump K31.89
  ear drum (nontraumatic) (*see also* Perforation, tympanum)
    traumatic SØ9.2- ☑
    due to blast injury — *see* Injury, blast, ear
  esophagus K22.3
  eye (without prolapse or loss of intraocular tissue) — *see* Injury, eye, laceration
  fallopian tube NEC (nonobstetric) (nontraumatic) N83.8
    due to pregnancy OØØ.1Ø- ☑
    with intrauterine pregnancy OØØ.11- ☑
  fontanel P13.1
  gallbladder K82.2
    traumatic S36.128 ☑
  gastric (*see also* Rupture, stomach)
    vessel K92.2
  globe (eye) (traumatic) — *see* Injury, eye, laceration
  graafian follicle (hematoma) N83.Ø- ☑
  heart — *see* Rupture, cardiac
  hymen (nontraumatic) (nonintentional) N89.8
  internal organ, traumatic — *see* Injury, by site
  intervertebral disc — *see* Displacement, intervertebral disc
    traumatic — *see* Rupture, traumatic, intervertebral disc
  intestine NEC (nontraumatic) K63.1
    traumatic — *see* Injury, intestine
  iris (*see also* Abnormality, pupillary)
    traumatic — *see* Injury, eye, laceration

Rupture, ruptured — *continued*

joint capsule, traumatic — *see* Sprain

kidney (traumatic) S37.06- ☑
- birth injury P15.8
- nontraumatic N28.89

lacrimal duct (traumatic) — *see* Injury, eye, specified site NEC

lens (cataract) (traumatic) — *see* Cataract, traumatic

ligament, traumatic — *see* Rupture, traumatic, ligament, by site

liver S36.116 ☑
- birth injury P15.0

lymphatic vessel I89.8

marginal sinus (placental) (with hemorrhage) — *see* Hemorrhage, antepartum, specified cause NEC

membrana tympani (nontraumatic) — *see* Perforation, tympanum

membranes (spontaneous)
- artificial
  - delayed delivery following O75.5
  - delayed delivery following — *see* Pregnancy, complicated by, premature rupture of membranes

meningeal artery I60.8

meniscus (knee) (*see also* Tear, meniscus)
- old — *see* Derangement, meniscus
- site other than knee — *code as* Sprain

mesenteric artery, traumatic — *see* Injury, mesenteric, artery, laceration, major

mesentery (nontraumatic) K66.8
- traumatic — *see* Injury, intra-abdominal, specified, site NEC

mitral (valve) I34.8

muscle (traumatic) (*see also* Strain)
- diastasis — *see* Diastasis, muscle
- nontraumatic M62.10
  - ankle M62.17- ☑
  - foot M62.17- ☑
  - forearm M62.13- ☑
  - hand M62.14- ☑
  - lower leg M62.16- ☑
  - pelvic region M62.15- ☑
  - shoulder region M62.11- ☑
  - specified site NEC M62.18
  - thigh M62.15- ☑
  - upper arm M62.12- ☑
- traumatic — *see* Strain, by site

musculotendinous junction NEC, nontraumatic — *see* Rupture, tendon, spontaneous

mycotic aneurysm causing cerebral hemorrhage — *see* Hemorrhage, intracranial, subarachnoid

myocardium, myocardial — *see* Rupture, cardiac
- traumatic — *see* Injury, heart

nontraumatic, meaning hernia — *see* Hernia

obstructed — *see* Hernia, by site, obstructed

operation wound — *see* Disruption, wound, operation

ovary, ovarian N83.8
- corpus luteum cyst N83.1- ☑
- follicle (graafian) N83.0- ☑

oviduct (nonobstetric) (nontraumatic) N83.8
- due to pregnancy O00.10- ☑
  - with intrauterine pregnancy O00.11- ☑

pancreas (nontraumatic) K86.89
- traumatic S36.299 ☑

papillary muscle NEC I51.2
- following acute myocardial infarction (current complication) I23.5

pelvic
- floor, complicating delivery O70.1
- organ NEC, obstetrical trauma O71.5

perineum (nonobstetric) (nontraumatic) N90.89
- complicating delivery — *see* Delivery, complicated, by, laceration, anus (sphincter)

postoperative wound — *see* Disruption, wound, operation

prostate (traumatic) S37.828 ☑

pulmonary
- artery I28.8
- valve (heart) I37.8
- vein I28.8
- vessel I28.8

pus tube — *see* Salpingitis

pyosalpinx — *see* Salpingitis

rectum (nontraumatic) K63.1
- traumatic S36.69 ☑

retina, retinal (traumatic) (without detachment) (*see also* Break, retina)

Rupture, ruptured — *continued*

retina, retinal (*see also* Break, retina) — *continued*
- with detachment — *see* Detachment, retina, with retinal, break

rotator cuff (nontraumatic) M75.10- ☑
- complete M75.12- ☑
- incomplete M75.11- ☑

sclera — *see* Injury, eye, laceration

sigmoid (nontraumatic) K63.1
- traumatic S36.593 ☑

spinal cord (*see also* Injury, spinal cord, by region)
- due to injury at birth P11.5
- newborn (birth injury) P11.5

spleen (traumatic) S36.09 ☑
- birth injury P15.1
- congenital (birth injury) P15.1
- due to P. vivax malaria B51.0
- nontraumatic D73.5
- spontaneous D73.5

splenic vein R58
- traumatic — *see* Injury, blood vessel, splenic vein

stomach (nontraumatic) (spontaneous) K31.89
- traumatic S36.39 ☑

supraspinatus (complete) (incomplete) (nontraumatic) — *see* Tear, rotator cuff

symphysis pubis
- obstetric O71.6
- traumatic S33.4 ☑

synovium (cyst) M66.10
- ankle M66.17- ☑
- elbow M66.12- ☑
- finger M66.14- ☑
- foot M66.17- ☑
- forearm M66.13- ☑
- hand M66.14- ☑
- pelvic region M66.15- ☑
- shoulder region M66.11- ☑
- specified site NEC M66.18
- thigh M66.15- ☑
- toe M66.17- ☑
- upper arm M66.12- ☑
- wrist M66.13- ☑

tendon (traumatic) — *see* Strain
- nontraumatic (spontaneous) M66.9
  - ankle M66.87- ☑
  - extensor M66.20
    - ankle M66.27- ☑
    - foot M66.27- ☑
    - forearm M66.23- ☑
    - hand M66.24- ☑
    - lower leg M66.26- ☑
    - multiple sites M66.29
    - pelvic region M66.25- ☑
    - shoulder region M66.21- ☑
    - specified site NEC M66.28
    - thigh M66.25- ☑
    - upper arm M66.22- ☑
  - flexor M66.30
    - ankle M66.37- ☑
    - foot M66.37- ☑
    - forearm M66.33- ☑
    - hand M66.34- ☑
    - lower leg M66.36- ☑
    - multiple sites M66.39
    - pelvic region M66.35- ☑
    - shoulder region M66.31- ☑
    - specified site NEC M66.38
    - thigh M66.35- ☑
    - upper arm M66.32- ☑
  - foot M66.87- ☑
  - forearm M66.83- ☑
  - hand M66.84- ☑
  - lower leg M66.86- ☑
  - multiple sites M66.89
  - pelvic region M66.85- ☑
  - shoulder region M66.81- ☑
  - specified
    - site NEC M66.88
    - tendon M66.80
  - thigh M66.85- ☑
  - upper arm M66.82- ☑

thoracic duct I89.8

tonsil J35.8

traumatic
- aorta — *see* Injury, aorta, laceration, major
- diaphragm — *see* Injury, intrathoracic, diaphragm
- external site — *see* Wound, open, by site

Rupture, ruptured — *continued*

traumatic — *continued*
- eye — *see* Injury, eye, laceration
- internal organ — *see* Injury, by site
- intervertebral disc
  - cervical S13.0 ☑
  - lumbar S33.0 ☑
  - thoracic S23.0 ☑
- kidney S37.06- ☑
- ligament (*see also* Sprain)
  - ankle — *see* Sprain, ankle
  - carpus — *see* Rupture, traumatic, ligament, wrist
  - collateral (hand) — *see* Rupture, traumatic, ligament, finger, collateral
  - finger (metacarpophalangeal) (interphalangeal) S63.40- ☑
    - collateral S63.41- ☑
      - index S63.41- ☑
      - little S63.41- ☑
      - middle S63.41- ☑
      - ring S63.41- ☑
    - index S63.40- ☑
    - little S63.40- ☑
    - middle S63.40- ☑
    - palmar S63.42- ☑
      - index S63.42- ☑
      - little S63.42- ☑
      - middle S63.42- ☑
      - ring S63.42- ☑
    - ring S63.40- ☑
    - specified site NEC S63.499 ☑
      - index S63.49- ☑
      - little S63.49- ☑
      - middle S63.49- ☑
      - ring S63.49- ☑
    - volar plate S63.43- ☑
      - index S63.43- ☑
      - little S63.43- ☑
      - middle S63.43- ☑
      - ring S63.43- ☑
  - foot — *see* Sprain, foot
  - radial collateral S53.2- ☑
  - radiocarpal — *see* Rupture, traumatic, ligament, wrist, radiocarpal
  - ulnar collateral S53.3- ☑
  - ulnocarpal — *see* Rupture, traumatic, ligament, wrist, ulnocarpal
  - wrist S63.30- ☑
    - collateral S63.31- ☑
    - radiocarpal S63.32- ☑
    - specified site NEC S63.39- ☑
    - ulnocarpal (palmar) S63.33- ☑
- liver S36.116 ☑
- membrana tympani — *see* Rupture, ear drum, traumatic
- muscle or tendon — *see* Strain
- myocardium — *see* Injury, heart
- pancreas S36.299 ☑
- rectum S36.69 ☑
- sigmoid S36.593 ☑
- spleen S36.09 ☑
- stomach S36.39 ☑
- symphysis pubis S33.4 ☑
- tympanum, tympanic (membrane) — *see* Rupture, ear drum, traumatic
- ureter S37.19 ☑
- uterus S37.69 ☑
- vagina — *see* Injury, vagina
- vena cava — *see* Injury, vena cava, laceration, major

tricuspid (heart) (valve) I07.8

tube, tubal (nonobstetric) (nontraumatic) N83.8
- abscess — *see* Salpingitis
- due to pregnancy O00.10- ☑
  - with intrauterine pregnancy O00.11- ☑

tympanum, tympanic (membrane) (nontraumatic) (*see also* Perforation, tympanic membrane) H72.9- ☑
- traumatic — *see* Rupture, ear drum, traumatic

umbilical cord, complicating delivery O69.89 ☑

ureter (traumatic) S37.19 ☑
- nontraumatic N28.89

urethra (nontraumatic) N36.8
- with ectopic or molar pregnancy O08.6
- following ectopic or molar pregnancy O08.6
- obstetrical trauma O71.5
- traumatic S37.39 ☑

Rupture, ruptured — continued
  uterosacral ligament (nonobstetric) (nontraumatic)
    N83.8
  uterus (traumatic) S37.69 ☑
    before labor O71.0- ☑
    during or after labor O71.1
    nonpuerperal, nontraumatic N85.8
    pregnant (during labor) O71.1
      before labor O71.0- ☑
  vagina — see Injury, vagina
  valve, valvular (heart) — see Endocarditis
  varicose vein — see Varix
  varix — see Varix
  vena cava R58
    traumatic — see Injury, vena cava, laceration, major
  vesical (urinary) N32.89
  vessel (blood) R58
    pulmonary I28.8
    traumatic — see Injury, blood vessel
  viscus R19.8
  vulva complicating delivery O70.0
Russell-Silver syndrome Q87.1
Russian spring-summer type encephalitis A84.0
Rust's disease (tuberculous cervical spondylitis) A18.01
Ruvalcaba-Myhre-Smith syndrome E71.440
Rytand-Lipsitch syndrome I44.2

S

Saber, sabre shin or tibia (syphilitic) A50.56 [M90.8-] ☑
Sac lacrimal — see condition
Saccharomyces infection B37.9
Saccharopinuria E72.3
Saccular — see condition
Sacculation
  aorta (nonsyphilitic) — see Aneurysm, aorta
  bladder N32.3
  intralaryngeal (congenital) (ventricular) Q31.3
  larynx (congenital) (ventricular) Q31.3
  organ or site, congenital — see Distortion
  pregnant uterus — see Pregnancy, complicated by,
    abnormal, uterus
  ureter N28.89
  urethra N36.1
  vesical N32.3
Sachs' amaurotic familial idiocy or disease E75.02
Sachs-Tay disease E75.02
Sacks-Libman disease M32.11
Sacralgia M53.3
Sacralization Q76.49
Sacrodynia M53.3
Sacroiliac joint — see condition
Sacroiliitis NEC M46.1
Sacrum — see condition
Saddle
  back — see Lordosis
  embolus
    abdominal aorta I74.01
    pulmonary artery I26.92
      with acute cor pulmonale I26.02
  injury — code to condition
  nose M95.0
    due to syphilis A50.57
Sadism (sexual) F65.52
Sadness, postpartal O90.6
Sadomasochism F65.50
Saemisch's ulcer (cornea) — see Ulcer, cornea, central
Sagging
  skin and subcutaneous tissue (following bariatric
    surgery weight loss) (following dietary weight
    loss) L98.7
Sahib disease B55.0
Sailors' skin L57.8
Saint
  Anthony's fire — see Erysipelas
  triad — see Hernia, diaphragm
  Vitus' dance — see Chorea, Sydenham's
Salaam
  attack(s) — see Epilepsy, spasms
  tic R25.8
Salicylism
  abuse F55.8
  overdose or wrong substance given — see Table of
    Drugs and Chemicals, by drug, poisoning
Salivary duct or gland — see condition
Salivation, excessive K11.7
Salmonella — see Infection, Salmonella

Salmonellosis A02.0
Salpingitis (catarrhal) (fallopian tube) (nodular) (pseud-
    ofollicular) (purulent) (septic) N70.91
  with oophoritis N70.93
  acute N70.01
    with oophoritis N70.03
  chlamydial A56.11
  chronic N70.11
    with oophoritis N70.13
  complicating abortion — see Abortion, by type, com-
    plicated by, salpingitis
  ear — see Salpingitis, eustachian
  eustachian (tube) H68.00- ☑
    acute H68.01- ☑
    chronic H68.02- ☑
  follicularis N70.11
    with oophoritis N70.13
  gonococcal (acute) (chronic) A54.24
  interstitial, chronic N70.11
    with oophoritis N70.13
  isthmica nodosa N70.11
    with oophoritis N70.13
  specific (gonococcal) (acute) (chronic) A54.24
  tuberculous (acute) (chronic) A18.17
  venereal (gonococcal) (acute) (chronic) A54.24
Salpingocele N83.4- ☑
Salpingo-oophoritis (catarrhal) (purulent) (ruptured)
    (septic) (suppurative) N70.93
  acute N70.03
    with ectopic or molar pregnancy O08.0
    following ectopic or molar pregnancy O08.0
    gonococcal A54.24
  chronic N70.13
  following ectopic or molar pregnancy O08.0
  gonococcal (acute) (chronic) A54.24
  puerperal O86.19
  specific (gonococcal) (acute) (chronic) A54.24
  subacute N70.03
  tuberculous (acute) (chronic) A18.17
  venereal (gonococcal) (acute) (chronic) A54.24
Salpingo-ovaritis — see Salpingo-oophoritis
Salpingoperitonitis — see Salpingo-oophoritis
Salzmann's nodular dystrophy — see Degeneration,
    cornea, nodular
Sampson's cyst or tumor N80.1
San Joaquin (Valley) **fever** B38.0
Sandblaster's asthma, lung or pneumoconiosis J62.8
Sander's disease (paranoia) F22
Sandfly fever A93.1
Sandhoff's disease E75.01
Sanfilippo (Type B) (Type C) (Type D) **syndrome** E76.22
Sanger-Brown ataxia G11.2
Sao Paulo fever or typhus A77.0
Saponification, mesenteric K65.8
Sarcocele (benign)
  syphilitic A52.76
    congenital A50.59
Sarcocystosis A07.8
Sarcoepiplocele — see Hernia
Sarcoepiplomphalocele Q79.2
Sarcoid (see also Sarcoidosis)
  arthropathy D86.86
  Boeck's D86.9
  Darier-Roussy D86.3
  iridocyclitis D86.83
  meningitis D86.81
  myocarditis D86.85
  myositis D86.87
  pyelonephritis D86.84
  Spiegler-Fendt L08.89
Sarcoidosis D86.9
  with
    cranial nerve palsies D86.82
    hepatic granuloma D86.89
    polyarthritis D86.86
    tubulo-interstitial nephropathy D86.84
  combined sites NEC D86.89
  lung D86.0
    and lymph nodes D86.2
  lymph nodes D86.1
    and lung D86.2
  meninges D86.81
  skin D86.3
  specified type NEC D86.89
Sarcoma (of) (see also Neoplasm, connective tissue, ma-
    lignant)
  alveolar soft part — see Neoplasm, connective tissue,
    malignant

Sarcoma — continued
  ameloblastic C41.1
    upper jaw (bone) C41.0
  botryoid — see Neoplasm, connective tissue, malignant
  botryoides — see Neoplasm, connective tissue, malig-
    nant
  cerebellar C71.6
    circumscribed (arachnoidal) C71.6
  circumscribed (arachnoidal) cerebellar C71.6
  clear cell (see also Neoplasm, connective tissue, malig-
    nant)
    kidney C64.- ☑
  dendritic cells (accessory cells) C96.4
  embryonal — see Neoplasm, connective tissue, malig-
    nant
  endometrial (stromal) C54.1
    isthmus C54.0
  epithelioid (cell) — see Neoplasm, connective tissue,
    malignant
  Ewing's — see Neoplasm, bone, malignant
  follicular dendritic cell C96.4
  germinoblastic (diffuse) — see Lymphoma, diffuse
    large cell
  follicular — see Lymphoma, follicular, specified NEC
  giant cell (except of bone) (see also Neoplasm, connec-
    tive tissue, malignant)
    bone — see Neoplasm, bone, malignant
  glomoid — see Neoplasm, connective tissue, malignant
  granulocytic C92.3- ☑
  hemangioendothelial — see Neoplasm, connective
    tissue, malignant
  hemorrhagic, multiple — see Sarcoma, Kaposi's
  histiocytic C96.A (following C96.6)
  Hodgkin — see Lymphoma, Hodgkin
  immunoblastic (diffuse) — see Lymphoma, diffuse
    large cell
  interdigitating dendritic cell C96.4
  Kaposi's
    colon C46.4
    connective tissue C46.1
    gastrointestinal organ C46.4
    lung C46.5- ☑
    lymph node(s) C46.3
    palate (hard) (soft) C46.2
    rectum C46.4
    skin C46.0
    specified site NEC C46.7
    stomach C46.4
    unspecified site C46.9
  Kupffer cell C22.3
  Langerhans cell C96.4
  leptomeningeal — see Neoplasm, meninges, malignant
  liver NEC C22.4
  lymphangioendothelial — see Neoplasm, connective
    tissue, malignant
  lymphoblastic — see Lymphoma, lymphoblastic (dif-
    fuse)
  lymphocytic — see Lymphoma, small cell B-cell
  mast cell C96.22
  melanotic — see Melanoma
  meningeal — see Neoplasm, meninges, malignant
  meningothelial — see Neoplasm, meninges, malignant
  mesenchymal (see also Neoplasm, connective tissue,
    malignant)
    mixed — see Neoplasm, connective tissue, malig-
      nant
  mesothelial — see Mesothelioma
  monstrocellular
    specified site — see Neoplasm, malignant, by site
    unspecified site C71.9
  myeloid C92.3- ☑
  neurogenic — see Neoplasm, nerve, malignant
  odontogenic C41.1
    upper jaw (bone) C41.0
  osteoblastic — see Neoplasm, bone, malignant
  osteogenic (see also Neoplasm, bone, malignant)
    juxtacortical — see Neoplasm, bone, malignant
    periosteal — see Neoplasm, bone, malignant
  periosteal (see also Neoplasm, bone, malignant)
    osteogenic — see Neoplasm, bone, malignant
  pleomorphic cell — see Neoplasm, connective tissue,
    malignant
  reticulum cell (diffuse) — see Lymphoma, diffuse large
    cell
    nodular — see Lymphoma, follicular
    pleomorphic cell type — see Lymphoma, diffuse
      large cell

Sarcoma — *continued*
  rhabdoid — *see* Neoplasm, malignant, by site
  round cell — *see* Neoplasm, connective tissue, malignant
  small cell — *see* Neoplasm, connective tissue, malignant
  soft tissue — *see* Neoplasm, connective tissue, malignant
  spindle cell — *see* Neoplasm, connective tissue, malignant
  stromal (endometrial) C54.1
    isthmus C54.0
  synovial (*see also* Neoplasm, connective tissue, malignant)
    biphasic — *see* Neoplasm, connective tissue, malignant
    epithelioid cell — *see* Neoplasm, connective tissue, malignant
    spindle cell — *see* Neoplasm, connective tissue, malignant
Sarcomatosis
  meningeal — *see* Neoplasm, meninges, malignant
  specified site NEC — *see* Neoplasm, connective tissue, malignant
  unspecified site C80.1
Sarcopenia (age-related) M62.84
Sarcosinemia E72.59
Sarcosporidiosis (intestinal) A07.8
Satiety, early R68.81
Saturnine — *see* condition
Saturnism
  overdose or wrong substance given or taken — *see* Table of Drugs and Chemicals, by drug, poisoning
Satyriasis F52.8
Sauriasis — *see* Ichthyosis
SBE (subacute bacterial endocarditis) I33.0
Scabies (any site) B86
Scabs R23.4
Scaglietti-Dagnini syndrome E22.0
Scald — *see* Burn
Scalenus anticus (anterior) **syndrome** G54.0
Scales R23.4
Scaling, skin R23.4
Scalp — *see* condition
Scapegoating affecting child Z62.3
Scaphocephaly Q75.0
Scapulalgia M89.8X1
Scapulohumeral myopathy G71.02
Scar, scarring (*see also* Cicatrix) L90.5
  adherent L90.5
  atrophic L90.5
  cervix
    in pregnancy or childbirth — *see* Pregnancy, complicated by, abnormal cervix
  cheloid L91.0
  chorioretinal H31.00- ☑
    posterior pole macula H31.01- ☑
    postsurgical H59.81- ☑
    solar retinopathy H31.02- ☑
    specified type NEC H31.09- ☑
  choroid — *see* Scar, chorioretinal
  conjunctiva H11.24- ☑
  cornea H17.9
    xerophthalmic (*see also* Opacity, cornea)
      vitamin A deficiency E50.6
  duodenum, obstructive K31.5
  hypertrophic L91.0
  keloid L91.0
  labia N90.89
  lung (base) J98.4
  macula — *see* Scar, chorioretinal, posterior pole
  muscle M62.89
  myocardium, myocardial I25.2
  painful L90.5
  posterior pole (eye) — *see* Scar, chorioretinal, posterior pole
  retina — *see* Scar, chorioretinal
  trachea J39.8
  transmural uterine, in pregnancy O34.29
  uterus N85.8
    in pregnancy O34.29
  vagina N89.8
    postoperative N99.2
  vulva N90.89
Scarabiasis B88.2
Scarlatina (anginosa) (maligna) A38.9
  myocarditis (acute) A38.1

Scarlatina — *continued*
  myocarditis — *continued*
    old — *see* Myocarditis
  otitis media A38.0
  ulcerosa A38.8
Scarlet fever (albuminuria) (angina) A38.9
Schamberg's disease (progressive pigmentary dermatosis) L81.7
Schatzki's ring (acquired) (esophagus) (lower) K22.2
  congenital Q39.3
Schaufenster krankheit I20.8
Schaumann's
  benign lymphogranulomatosis D86.1
  disease or syndrome — *see* Sarcoidosis
Scheie's syndrome E76.03
Schenck's disease B42.1
Scheuermann's disease or osteochondrosis — *see* Osteochondrosis, juvenile, spine
Schilder (-Flatau) **disease** G37.0
Schilling-type monocytic leukemia C93.0- ☑
Schimmelbusch's disease, cystic mastitis, or hyperplasia — *see* Mastopathy, cystic
Schistosoma infestation — *see* Infestation, Schistosoma
Schistosomiasis B65.9
  with muscle disorder B65.9 [M63.80]
    ankle B65.9 [M63.87-] ☑
    foot B65.9 [M63.87-] ☑
    forearm B65.9 [M63.83-] ☑
    hand B65.9 [M63.84-] ☑
    lower leg B65.9 [M63.86-] ☑
    multiple sites B65.9 [M63.89]
    pelvic region B65.9 [M63.85-] ☑
    shoulder region B65.9 [M63.81-] ☑
    specified site NEC B65.9 [M63.88]
    thigh B65.9 [M63.85-] ☑
    upper arm B65.9 [M63.82-] ☑
  Asiatic B65.2
  bladder B65.0
  chestermani B65.8
  colon B65.1
  cutaneous B65.3
  due to
    S. haematobium B65.0
    S. japonicum B65.2
    S. mansoni B65.1
    S. mattheii B65.8
  Eastern B65.2
  genitourinary tract B65.0
  intestinal B65.1
  lung NEC B65.9 [J99]
    pneumonia B65.9 [J17]
  Manson's (intestinal) B65.1
  oriental B65.2
  pulmonary NEC B65.9 [J99]
    pneumonia B65.9
  Schistosoma
    haematobium B65.0
    japonicum B65.2
    mansoni B65.1
  specified type NEC B65.8
  urinary B65.0
  vesical B65.0
Schizencephaly Q04.6
Schizoaffective psychosis F25.9
Schizodontia K00.2
Schizoid personality F60.1
Schizophrenia, schizophrenic F20.9
  acute (brief) (undifferentiated) F23
  atypical (form) F20.3
  borderline F21
  catalepsy F20.2
  catatonic (type) (excited) (withdrawn) F20.2
  cenesthopathic, cenesthesiopathic F20.89
  childhood type F84.5
  chronic undifferentiated F20.5
  cyclic F25.0
  disorganized (type) F20.1
  flexibilitas cerea F20.2
  hebephrenic (type) F20.1
  incipient F21
  latent F21
  negative type F20.5
  paranoid (type) F20.0
  paraphrenic F20.0
  post-psychotic depression F32.89
  prepsychotic F21
  prodromal F21
  pseudoneurotic F21

Schizophrenia, schizophrenic — *continued*
  pseudopsychopathic F21
  reaction F23
  residual (state) (type) F20.5
  restzustand F20.5
  schizoaffective (type) — *see* Psychosis, schizoaffective
  simple (type) F20.89
  simplex F20.89
  specified type NEC F20.89
  spectrum and other psychotic disorder F29
    specified NEC F28
  stupor F20.2
  syndrome of childhood F84.5
  undifferentiated (type) F20.3
    chronic F20.5
Schizothymia (persistent) F60.1
Schlatter-Osgood disease or osteochondrosis — *see* Osteochondrosis, juvenile, tibia
Schlatter's tibia — *see* Osteochondrosis, juvenile, tibia
Schmidt's syndrome (polyglandular, autoimmune) E31.0
Schmincke's carcinoma or tumor — *see* Neoplasm, nasopharynx, malignant
Schmitz (-Stutzer) **dysentery** A03.0
Schmorl's disease or nodes
  lumbar region M51.46
  lumbosacral region M51.47
  sacrococcygeal region M53.3
  thoracic region M51.44
  thoracolumbar region M51.45
Schneiderian
  papilloma — *see* Neoplasm, nasopharynx, benign
    specified site — *see* Neoplasm, benign, by site
    unspecified site D14.0
  specified site — *see* Neoplasm, malignant, by site
    unspecified site C30.0
Scholte's syndrome (malignant carcinoid) E34.0
Scholz (-Bielchowsky-Henneberg) **disease or syndrome** E75.25
Schönlein (-Henoch) disease or purpura (primary) (rheumatic) D69.0
Schottmuller's disease A01.4
Schroeder's syndrome (endocrine hypertensive) E27.0
Schüller-Christian disease or syndrome C96.5
Schultze's type acroparesthesia, simple I73.89
Schultz's disease or syndrome — *see* Agranulocytosis
Schwalbe-Ziehen-Oppenheim disease G24.1
Schwannoma (*see also* Neoplasm, nerve, benign)
  malignant (*see also* Neoplasm, nerve, malignant)
    with rhabdomyoblastic differentiation — *see* Neoplasm, nerve, malignant
  melanocytic — *see* Neoplasm, nerve, benign
  pigmented — *see* Neoplasm, nerve, benign
Schwannomatosis Q85.03
Schwartz (-Jampel) **syndrome** G71.13
Schwartz-Bartter syndrome E22.2
Schweniger-Buzzi anetoderma L90.1
Sciatic — *see* condition
Sciatica (infective)
  with lumbago M54.4- ☑
    due to intervertebral disc disorder — *see* Disorder, disc, with, radiculopathy
  due to displacement of intervertebral disc (with lumbago) — *see* Disorder, disc, with, radiculopathy
  wallet M54.3- ☑
Scimitar syndrome Q26.8
Sclera — *see* condition
Sclerectasia H15.84- ☑
Scleredema
  adultorum — *see* Sclerosis, systemic
  Buschke's — *see* Sclerosis, systemic
  newborn P83.0
Sclerema (adiposum) (edematosum) (neonatorum) (newborn) P83.0
  adultorum — *see* Sclerosis, systemic
Scleriasis — *see* Scleroderma
Scleritis H15.00- ☑
  with corneal involvement H15.04- ☑
  anterior H15.01- ☑
  brawny H15.02- ☑
  in (due to) zoster B02.34
  posterior H15.03- ☑
  specified type NEC H15.09- ☑
  syphilitic A52.71
  tuberculous (nodular) A18.51
Sclerochoroiditis H31.8
Scleroconjunctivitis — *see* Scleritis
Sclerocystic ovary syndrome E28.2

Sclerodactyly, sclerodactylia L94.3
Scleroderma, sclerodermia (acrosclerotic) (diffuse)
    (generalized) (progressive) (pulmonary) (see also
    Sclerosis, systemic) M34.9
  circumscribed L94.Ø
  linear L94.1
  localized L94.Ø
  newborn P83.88
  systemic M34.9
Sclerokeratitis H16.8
  tuberculous A18.52
Scleroma nasi A48.8
Scleromalacia (perforans) H15.Ø5- ☑
Scleromyxedema L98.5
Sclérose en plaques G35
Sclerosis, sclerotic
  adrenal (gland) E27.8
  Alzheimer's — see Disease, Alzheimer's
  amyotrophic (lateral) G12.21
  aorta, aortic I7Ø.Ø
      valve — see Endocarditis, aortic
  artery, arterial, arteriolar, arteriovascular — see Arte-
      riosclerosis
  ascending multiple G35
  brain (generalized) (lobular) G37.9
      artery, arterial I67.2
      diffuse G37.Ø
      disseminated G35
      insular G35
      Krabbe's E75.23
      miliary G35
      multiple G35
      presenile (Alzheimer's) — see Disease, Alzheimer's,
          early onset
      senile (arteriosclerotic) I67.2
      stem, multiple G35
      tuberous Q85.1
  bulbar, multiple G35
  bundle of His I44.39
  cardiac — see Disease, heart, ischemic, atherosclerotic
  cardiorenal — see Hypertension, cardiorenal
  cardiovascular (see also Disease, cardiovascular)
      renal — see Hypertension, cardiorenal
  cerebellar — see Sclerosis, brain
  cerebral — see Sclerosis, brain
  cerebrospinal (disseminated) (multiple) G35
  cerebrovascular I67.2
  choroid — see Degeneration, choroid
  combined (spinal cord) (see also Degeneration, com-
      bined)
      multiple G35
  concentric (Balo) G37.5
  cornea — see Opacity, cornea
  coronary (artery) I25.1Ø
      with angina pectoris — see Arteriosclerosis, coro-
          nary (artery),
  corpus cavernosum
      female N9Ø.89
      male N48.6
  diffuse (brain) (spinal cord) G37.Ø
  disseminated G35
  dorsal G35
  dorsolateral (spinal cord) — see Degeneration, com-
      bined
  endometrium N85.5
  extrapyramidal G25.9
  eye, nuclear (senile) — see Cataract, senile, nuclear
  focal and segmental (glomerular) (see also NØØ-NØ7
      with fourth character .1) NØ5.1
  Friedreich's (spinal cord) G11.1
  funicular (spermatic cord) N5Ø.89
  general (vascular) — see Arteriosclerosis
  gland (lymphatic) I89.8
  hepatic K74.1
      alcoholic K7Ø.2
  hereditary
      cerebellar G11.9
      spinal (Friedreich's ataxia) G11.1
  hippocampal G93.81
  insular G35
  kidney — see Sclerosis, renal
  larynx J38.7
  lateral (amyotrophic) (descending) (spinal) G12.21
      primary G12.23
  lens, senile nuclear — see Cataract, senile, nuclear
  liver K74.1
      with fibrosis K74.2
          alcoholic K7Ø.2

Sclerosis, sclerotic — continued
  liver — continued
      alcoholic K7Ø.2
      cardiac K76.1
  lung — see Fibrosis, lung
  mastoid — see Mastoiditis, chronic
  mesial temporal G93.81
  mitral IØ5.8
  Mönckeberg's (medial) — see Arteriosclerosis, extrem-
      ities
  multiple (brain stem) (cerebral) (generalized) (spinal
      cord) G35
  myocardium, myocardial — see Disease, heart, is-
      chemic, atherosclerotic
  nuclear (senile), eye — see Cataract, senile, nuclear
  ovary N83.8
  pancreas K86.89
  penis N48.6
  peripheral arteries — see Arteriosclerosis, extremities
  plaques G35
  pluriglandular E31.8
  polyglandular E31.8
  posterolateral (spinal cord) — see Degeneration,
      combined
  presenile (Alzheimer's) — see Disease, Alzheimer's,
      early onset
  primary, lateral G12.23
  progressive, systemic M34.Ø
  pulmonary — see Fibrosis, lung
      artery I27.Ø
      valve (heart) — see Endocarditis, pulmonary
  renal N26.9
      with
          cystine storage disease E72.Ø9
          hypertensive heart disease (conditions in I11) —
              see Hypertension, cardiorenal
          arteriolar (hyaline) (hyperplastic) — see Hyperten-
              sion, kidney
  retina (senile) (vascular) H35.ØØ
  senile (vascular) — see Arteriosclerosis
  spinal (cord) (progressive) G95.89
      ascending G61.Ø
      combined (see also Degeneration, combined)
          multiple G35
          syphilitic A52.11
      disseminated G35
      dorsolateral — see Degeneration, combined
      hereditary (Friedreich's) (mixed form) G11.1
      lateral (amyotrophic) G12.23
      multiple G35
      posterior (syphilitic) A52.11
  stomach K31.89
  subendocardial, congenital I42.4
  systemic M34.9
      with
          lung involvement M34.81
          myopathy M34.82
          polyneuropathy M34.83
      drug-induced M34.2
      due to chemicals NEC M34.2
      progressive M34.Ø
      specified NEC M34.89
  temporal (mesial) G93.81
  tricuspid (heart) (valve) IØ7.8
  tuberous (brain) Q85.1
  tympanic membrane — see Disorder, tympanic mem-
      brane, specified NEC
  valve, valvular (heart) — see Endocarditis
  vascular — see Arteriosclerosis
  vein I87.8
Scoliosis (acquired) (postural) M41.9
  adolescent (idiopathic) — see Scoliosis, idiopathic,
      adolescent
  congenital Q67.5
      due to bony malformation Q76.3
      failure of segmentation (hemivertebra) Q76.3
      hemivertebra fusion Q76.3
      postural Q67.5
  idiopathic M41.2Ø
      adolescent M41.129
          cervical region M41.122
          cervicothoracic region M41.123
          lumbar region M41.126
          lumbosacral region M41.127
          thoracic region M41.124
          thoracolumbar region M41.125
      cervical region M41.22
      cervicothoracic region M41.23

Scoliosis — continued
  idiopathic — continued
      infantile M41.ØØ
          cervical region M41.Ø2
          cervicothoracic region M41.Ø3
          lumbar region M41.Ø6
          lumbosacral region M41.Ø7
          sacrococcygeal region M41.Ø8
          thoracic region M41.Ø4
          thoracolumbar region M41.Ø5
      juvenile M41.119
          cervical region M41.112
          cervicothoracic region M41.113
          lumbar region M41.116
          lumbosacral region M41.117
          thoracic region M41.114
          thoracolumbar region M41.115
      lumbar region M41.26
      lumbosacral region M41.27
      thoracic region M41.24
      thoracolumbar region M41.25
  infantile — see Scoliosis, idiopathic, infantile
  neuromuscular M41.4Ø
      cervical region M41.42
      cervicothoracic region M41.43
      lumbar region M41.46
      lumbosacral region M41.47
      occipito-atlanto-axial region M41.41
      thoracic region M41.44
      thoracolumbar region M41.45
  paralytic — see Scoliosis, neuromuscular
  postradiation therapy M96.5
  rachitic (late effect or sequelae) E64.3 [M49.8Ø]
      cervical region E64.3 [M49.82]
      cervicothoracic region E64.3 [M49.83]
      lumbar region E64.3 [M49.86]
      lumbosacral region E64.3 [M49.87]
      multiple sites E64.3 [M49.89]
      occipito-atlanto-axial region E64.3 [M49.81]
      sacrococcygeal region E64.3 [M49.88]
      thoracic region E64.3 [M49.84]
      thoracolumbar region E64.3 [M49.85]
  sciatic M54.4- ☑
  secondary (to) NEC M41.5Ø
      cerebral palsy, Friedreich's ataxia, poliomyelitis,
          neuromuscular disorders — see Scoliosis,
          neuromuscular
      cervical region M41.52
      cervicothoracic region M41.53
      lumbar region M41.56
      lumbosacral region M41.57
      thoracic region M41.54
      thoracolumbar region M41.55
  specified form NEC M41.8Ø
      cervical region M41.82
      cervicothoracic region M41.83
      lumbar region M41.86
      lumbosacral region M41.87
      thoracic region M41.84
      thoracolumbar region M41.85
  thoracogenic M41.3Ø
      thoracic region M41.34
      thoracolumbar region M41.35
  tuberculous A18.Ø1
Scoliotic pelvis
  with disproportion (fetopelvic) O33.Ø
      causing obstructed labor O65.Ø
Scorbutus, scorbutic (see also Scurvy)
  anemia D53.2
Score, NIHSS (National Institutes of Health Stroke Scale)
  R29.7- ☑
Scotoma (arcuate) (Bjerrum) (central) (ring) (see also Defect, visual field, localized, scotoma)
  scintillating H53.19
Scratch — see Abrasion
Scratchy throat RØ9.89
Screening (for) Z13.9
  alcoholism Z13.39
  anemia Z13.Ø
  anomaly, congenital Z13.89
  antenatal, of mother (see also Encounter, antenatal
      screening) Z36.9
  arterial hypertension Z13.6
  arthropod-borne viral disease NEC Z11.59
  autism Z13.41
  bacteriuria, asymptomatic Z13.89
  behavioral disorder Z13.3Ø
      specified NEC Z13.39

Screening — continued
- brain injury, traumatic Z13.850
- bronchitis, chronic Z13.83
- brucellosis Z11.2
- cardiovascular disorder Z13.6
- cataract Z13.5
- chlamydial diseases Z11.8
- cholera Z11.0
- chromosomal abnormalities (nonprocreative) NEC Z13.79
- colonoscopy Z12.11
- congenital
  - dislocation of hip Z13.89
  - eye disorder Z13.5
  - malformation or deformation Z13.89
- contamination NEC Z13.88
- cystic fibrosis Z13.228
- dengue fever Z11.59
- dental disorder Z13.84
- depression (adult) (adolescent) (child) Z13.31
  - maternal Z13.32
  - perinatal Z13.32
- developmental
  - delays Z13.40
    - global (milestones) Z13.42
    - specified NEC Z13.49
  - handicap Z13.42
    - in early childhood Z13.42
- diabetes mellitus Z13.1
- diphtheria Z11.2
- disability, intellectual Z13.39
- disease or disorder Z13.9
  - bacterial NEC Z11.2
    - intestinal infectious Z11.0
    - respiratory tuberculosis Z11.1
  - behavioral Z13.30
    - specified NEC Z13.39
  - blood or blood-forming organ Z13.0
  - cardiovascular Z13.6
  - Chagas' Z11.6
  - chlamydial Z11.8
  - dental Z13.89
  - developmental delays Z13.40
    - global (milestones) Z13.42
    - specified NEC Z13.49
  - digestive tract NEC Z13.818
    - lower GI Z13.811
    - upper GI Z13.810
  - ear Z13.5
  - endocrine Z13.29
  - eye Z13.5
  - genitourinary Z13.89
  - heart Z13.6
  - human immunodeficiency virus (HIV) infection Z11.4
  - immunity Z13.0
  - infection
    - intestinal Z11.0
      - specified NEC Z11.6
  - infectious Z11.9
  - mental health and behavioral Z13.30
    - specified NEC Z13.39
  - metabolic Z13.228
  - neurological Z13.89
  - nutritional Z13.21
    - metabolic Z13.228
      - lipoid disorders Z13.220
  - protozoal Z11.6
    - intestinal Z11.0
  - respiratory Z13.83
  - rheumatic Z13.828
  - rickettsial Z11.8
  - sexually-transmitted NEC Z11.3
    - human immunodeficiency virus (HIV) Z11.4
  - sickle-cell (trait) Z13.0
  - skin Z13.89
  - specified NEC Z13.89
  - spirochetal Z11.8
  - thyroid Z13.29
  - vascular Z13.6
  - venereal Z11.3
  - viral NEC Z11.59
    - human immunodeficiency virus (HIV) Z11.4
    - intestinal Z11.0
- elevated titer Z13.89
- emphysema Z13.83
- encephalitis, viral (mosquito- or tick-borne) Z11.59
- exposure to contaminants (toxic) Z13.88
- fever
  - dengue Z11.59

Screening — continued
- fever — continued
  - hemorrhagic Z11.59
  - yellow Z11.59
- filariasis Z11.6
- galactosemia Z13.228
- gastrointestinal condition Z13.818
- genetic (nonprocreative) - for procreative management — see Testing, genetic, for procreative management
  - disease carrier status (nonprocreative) Z13.71
  - specified NEC (nonprocreative) Z13.79
- genitourinary condition Z13.89
- glaucoma Z13.5
- gonorrhea Z11.3
- gout Z13.89
- helminthiasis (intestinal) Z11.6
- hematopoietic malignancy Z12.89
- hemoglobinopathies NEC Z13.0
- hemorrhagic fever Z11.59
- Hodgkin disease Z12.89
- human immunodeficiency virus (HIV) Z11.4
- human papillomavirus Z11.51
- hypertension Z13.6
- immunity disorders Z13.0
- infant or child (over 28 days old) Z00.129
  - with abnormal findings Z00.121
- infection
  - mycotic Z11.8
  - parasitic Z11.8
- ingestion of radioactive substance Z13.88
- intellectual disability Z13.39
- intestinal
  - helminthiasis Z11.6
  - infectious disease Z11.0
- leishmaniasis Z11.6
- leprosy Z11.2
- leptospirosis Z11.8
- leukemia Z12.89
- lymphoma Z12.89
- malaria Z11.6
- malnutrition Z13.29
  - metabolic Z13.228
  - nutritional Z13.21
- measles Z11.59
- mental health disorder Z13.30
  - specified NEC Z13.39
- metabolic errors, inborn Z13.228
- multiphasic Z13.89
- musculoskeletal disorder Z13.828
  - osteoporosis Z13.820
- mycoses Z11.8
- myocardial infarction (acute) Z13.6
- neoplasm (malignant) (of) Z12.9
  - bladder Z12.6
  - blood Z12.89
  - breast Z12.39
    - routine mammogram Z12.31
  - cervix Z12.4
  - colon Z12.11
  - genitourinary organs NEC Z12.79
    - bladder Z12.6
    - cervix Z12.4
    - ovary Z12.73
    - prostate Z12.5
    - testis Z12.71
    - vagina Z12.72
  - hematopoietic system Z12.89
  - intestinal tract Z12.10
    - colon Z12.11
    - rectum Z12.12
    - small intestine Z12.13
  - lung Z12.2
  - lymph (glands) Z12.89
  - nervous system Z12.82
  - oral cavity Z12.81
  - prostate Z12.5
  - rectum Z12.12
  - respiratory organs Z12.2
  - skin Z12.83
  - small intestine Z12.13
  - specified site NEC Z12.89
  - stomach Z12.0
- nephropathy Z13.89
- nervous system disorders NEC Z13.858
- neurological condition Z13.89
- osteoporosis Z13.820
- parasitic infestation Z11.9
  - specified NEC Z11.8

Screening — continued
- phenylketonuria Z13.228
- plague Z11.2
- poisoning (chemical) (heavy metal) Z13.88
- poliomyelitis Z11.59
- postnatal, chromosomal abnormalities Z13.89
- prenatal, of mother (see also Encounter, antenatal screening) Z36.9
- protozoal disease Z11.6
  - intestinal Z11.0
- pulmonary tuberculosis Z11.1
- radiation exposure Z13.88
- respiratory condition Z13.83
- respiratory tuberculosis Z11.1
- rheumatoid arthritis Z13.828
- rubella Z11.59
- schistosomiasis Z11.6
- sexually-transmitted disease NEC Z11.3
  - human immunodeficiency virus (HIV) Z11.4
- sickle-cell disease or trait Z13.0
- skin condition Z13.89
- sleeping sickness Z11.6
- special Z13.9
  - specified NEC Z13.89
- syphilis Z11.3
- tetanus Z11.2
- trachoma Z11.8
- traumatic brain injury Z13.850
- trypanosomiasis Z11.6
- tuberculosis, respiratory Z11.1
- venereal disease Z11.3
- viral encephalitis (mosquito- or tick-borne) Z11.59
- whooping cough Z11.2
- worms, intestinal Z11.6
- yaws Z11.8
- yellow fever Z11.59

Scrofula, scrofulosis (tuberculosis of cervical lymph glands) A18.2

Scrofulide (primary) (tuberculous) A18.4

Scrofuloderma, scrofulodermia (any site) (primary) A18.4

Scrofulosus lichen (primary) (tuberculous) A18.4

Scrofulous — see condition

Scrotal tongue K14.5

Scrotum — see condition

Scurvy, scorbutic E54
- anemia D53.2
- gum E54
- infantile E54
- rickets E55.0 [M90.80]

Sealpox B08.62

Seasickness T75.3 ☑

Seatworm (infection) (infestation) B80

Sebaceous (see also condition)
- cyst — see Cyst, sebaceous

Seborrhea, seborrheic L21.9
- capillitii R23.8
- capitis L21.0
- dermatitis L21.9
  - infantile L21.1
- eczema L21.9
  - infantile L21.1
- sicca L21.0

Seckel's syndrome Q87.1

Seclusion, pupil — see Membrane, pupillary

Second hand tobacco smoke exposure (acute) (chronic) Z77.22
- in the perinatal period P96.81

Secondary
- dentin (in pulp) K04.3
- neoplasm, secondaries — see Table of Neoplasms, secondary

Secretion
- antidiuretic hormone, inappropriate E22.2
- catecholamine, by pheochromocytoma E27.5
- hormone
  - antidiuretic, inappropriate (syndrome) E22.2
  - by
    - carcinoid tumor E34.0
    - pheochromocytoma E27.5
  - ectopic NEC E34.2
- urinary
  - excessive R35.8
  - suppression R34

Section
- nerve, traumatic — see Injury, nerve

Sedative, hypnotic, or anxiolytic-induced
- anxiety disorder F13.980

☑ Additional Character Required — Refer to the Tabular List for Character Selection   ⩔ Subterms under main terms may continue to next column or pag

Sedative, hypnotic, or anxiolytic-induced — *continued*
  bipolar and related disorder F13.94
  delirium F13.921
  depressive disorder F13.94
  major neurocognitive disorder F13.97
  mild neurocognitive disorder F13.988
  psychotic disorder F13.959
  sexual dysfunction F13.981
  sleep disorder F13.982
Segmentation, incomplete (congenital) (*see also* Fusion)
  bone NEC Q78.8
  lumbosacral (joint) (vertebra) Q76.49
Seitelberger's syndrome (infantile neuraxonal dystrophy) G31.89
Seizure(s) (*see also* Convulsions) R56.9
  akinetic — *see* Epilepsy, generalized, specified NEC
  atonic — *see* Epilepsy, generalized, specified NEC
  autonomic (hysterical) F44.5
  convulsive — *see* Convulsions
  cortical (focal) (motor) — *see* Epilepsy, localization-related, symptomatic, with simple partial seizures
  disorder (*see also* Epilepsy) G40.909
  due to stroke — *see* Sequelae (of), disease, cerebrovascular, by type, specified NEC
  epileptic — *see* Epilepsy
  febrile (simple) R56.00
    with status epilepticus G40.901
    complex (atypical) (complicated) R56.01
      with status epilepticus G40.901
  grand mal G40.409
    intractable G40.419
      with status epilepticus G40.411
      without status epilepticus G40.419
    not intractable G40.409
      with status epilepticus G40.401
      without status epilepticus G40.409
  heart — *see* Disease, heart
  hysterical F44.5
  intractable G40.919
    with status epilepticus G40.911
  Jacksonian (focal) (motor type) (sensory type) — *see* Epilepsy, localization-related, symptomatic, with simple partial seizures
  newborn P90
  nonspecific epileptic
    atonic — *see* Epilepsy, generalized, specified NEC
    clonic — *see* Epilepsy, generalized, specified NEC
    myoclonic — *see* Epilepsy, generalized, specified NEC
    tonic — *see* Epilepsy, generalized, specified NEC
    tonic-clonic — *see* Epilepsy, generalized, specified NEC
  partial, developing into secondarily generalized seizures
    complex — *see* Epilepsy, localization-related, symptomatic, with complex partial seizures
    simple — *see* Epilepsy, localization-related, symptomatic, with simple partial seizures
  petit mal G40.409
    intractable G40.419
      with status epilepticus G40.411
      without status epilepticus G40.419
    not intractable G40.409
      with status epilepticus G40.401
      without status epilepticus G40.409
  post traumatic R56.1
  recurrent G40.909
  specified NEC G40.89
  uncinate — *see* Epilepsy, localization-related, symptomatic, with complex partial seizures
Selenium deficiency, dietary E59
Self-damaging behavior (life-style) Z72.89
Self-harm (attempted)
  history (personal) Z91.5
    in family Z81.8
Self-mutilation (attempted)
  history (personal) Z91.5
    in family Z81.8
Self-poisoning
  history (personal) Z91.5
    in family Z81.8
  observation following (alleged) attempt Z03.6
Semicoma R40.1
Seminal vesiculitis N49.0
Seminoma C62.9- ☑
  specified site — *see* Neoplasm, malignant, by site

Senear-Usher disease or syndrome L10.4
Senectus R54
Senescence (without mention of psychosis) R54
Senile, senility (*see also* condition) R41.81
  with
    acute confusional state F05
    mental changes NOS F03 ☑
    psychosis NEC — *see* Psychosis, senile
  asthenia R54
  cervix (atrophic) N88.8
  debility R54
  endometrium (atrophic) N85.8
  fallopian tube (atrophic) — *see* Atrophy, fallopian tube
  heart (failure) R54
  ovary (atrophic) — *see* Atrophy, ovary
  premature E34.8
  vagina, vaginitis (atrophic) N95.2
  wart L82.1
Sensation
  burning (skin) R20.8
    tongue K14.6
  loss of R20.8
  prickling (skin) R20.2
  tingling (skin) R20.2
Sense loss
  smell — *see* Disturbance, sensation, smell
  taste — *see* Disturbance, sensation, taste
  touch R20.8
Sensibility disturbance (cortical) (deep) (vibratory) R20.9
Sensitive, sensitivity (*see also* Allergy)
  carotid sinus G90.01
  child (excessive) F93.8
  cold, autoimmune D59.1
  dentin K03.89
  gluten (non-celiac) K90.41
  latex Z91.040
  methemoglobin D74.8
  tuberculin, without clinical or radiological symptoms R76.11
  visual
    glare H53.71
    impaired contrast H53.72
Sensitiver Beziehungswahn F22
Sensitization, auto-erythrocytic D69.2
Separation
  anxiety, abnormal (of childhood) F93.0
  apophysis, traumatic — *code as* Fracture, by site
  choroid — *see* Detachment, choroid
  epiphysis, epiphyseal
    nontraumatic (*see also* Osteochondropathy, specified type NEC)
      upper femoral — *see* Slipped, epiphysis, upper femoral
    traumatic — *code as* Fracture, by site
  fracture — *see* Fracture
  infundibulum cardiac from right ventricle by a partition Q24.3
  joint (traumatic) (current) — *code by* site under Dislocation
  pubic bone, obstetrical trauma O71.6
  retina, retinal — *see* Detachment, retina
  symphysis pubis, obstetrical trauma O71.6
  tracheal ring, incomplete, congenital Q32.1
Sepsis (generalized) (unspecified organism) A41.9
  with
    organ dysfunction (acute) (multiple) R65.20
      with septic shock R65.21
  actinomycotic A42.7
  adrenal hemorrhage syndrome (meningococcal) A39.1
  anaerobic A41.4
  Bacillus anthracis A22.7
  Brucella (*see also* Brucellosis) A23.9
  candidal B37.7
  cryptogenic A41.9
  due to device, implant or graft T85.79 ☑
    arterial graft NEC T82.7 ☑
    breast (implant) T85.79 ☑
    catheter NEC T85.79 ☑
      dialysis (renal) T82.7 ☑
        intraperitoneal T85.71 ☑
      infusion NEC T82.7 ☑
        spinal (cranial) (epidural) (intrathecal) (spinal) (subarachnoid) (subdural) T85.735 ☑
      urethral indwelling T83.511 ☑
      urinary T83.518 ☑
  ectopic or molar pregnancy O08.82

Sepsis — *continued*
  due to device, implant or graft — *continued*
    electronic (electrode) (pulse generator) (stimulator)
      bone T84.7 ☑
      cardiac T82.7 ☑
      nervous system T85.738 ☑
        brain T85.731 ☑
        neurostimulator generator T85.734 ☑
        peripheral nerve T85.732 ☑
        spinal cord T85.733 ☑
      urinary T83.590 ☑
    fixation, internal (orthopedic) — *see* Complication, fixation device, infection
    gastrointestinal (bile duct) (esophagus) T85.79 ☑
      neurostimulator electrode (lead) T85.732 ☑
    genital T83.69 ☑
    heart NEC T82.7 ☑
      valve (prosthesis) T82.6 ☑
      graft T82.7 ☑
    joint prosthesis — *see* Complication, joint prosthesis, infection
    ocular (corneal graft) (orbital implant) T85.79 ☑
    orthopedic NEC T84.7 ☑
      fixation device, internal — *see* Complication, fixation device, infection
    specified NEC T85.79 ☑
    vascular T82.7 ☑
    ventricular intracranial (communicating) shunt T85.730 ☑
  during labor O75.3
  Enterococcus A41.81
  Erysipelothrix (rhusiopathiae) (erysipeloid) A26.7
  Escherichia coli (E. coli) A41.5 ☑
  extraintestinal yersiniosis A28.2
  following
    abortion (subsequent episode) O08.0
      current episode — *see* Abortion
    ectopic or molar pregnancy O08.82
    immunization T88.0 ☑
    infusion, therapeutic injection or transfusion NEC T80.29 ☑
    obstetrical procedure O86.04
  gangrenous A41.9
  gonococcal A54.86
  Gram-negative (organism) A41.5 ☑
    anaerobic A41.4
  Haemophilus influenzae A41.3
  herpesviral B00.7
  intra-abdominal K65.1
  intraocular — *see* Endophthalmitis, purulent
  Listeria monocytogenes A32.7
  localized — *code to* specific localized infection
    in operation wound T81.49 ☑
    skin — *see* Abscess
  malleus A24.0
  melioidosis A24.1
  meningeal — *see* Meningitis
  meningococcal A39.4
    acute A39.2
    chronic A39.3
  MSSA (Methicillin susceptible Staphylococcus aureus) A41.01
  newborn P36.9
    due to
      anaerobes NEC P36.5
      Escherichia coli P36.4
      Staphylococcus P36.30
        aureus P36.2
        specified NEC P36.39
      Streptococcus P36.10
        group B P36.0
        specified NEC P36.19
    specified NEC P36.8
  Pasteurella multocida A28.0
  pelvic, puerperal, postpartum, childbirth O85
  pneumococcal A40.3
  postprocedural T81.44 ☑
  puerperal, postpartum, childbirth (pelvic) O85
  Salmonella (arizonae) (cholerae-suis) (enteritidis) (typhimurium) A02.1
  severe R65.20
    with septic shock R65.21
  Shigella (*see also* Dysentery, bacillary) A03.9
  skin, localized — *see* Abscess
  specified organism NEC A41.89
  Staphylococcus, staphylococcal A41.2
    aureus (methicillin susceptible) (MSSA) A41.01

Sepsis

Sepsis — *continued*
  Staphylococcus, staphylococcal — *continued*
    aureus — *continued*
      methicillin resistant (MRSA) A41.02
    coagulase-negative A41.1
    specified NEC A41.1
  Streptococcus, streptococcal A40.9
    agalactiae A40.1
    group
      A A40.0
      B A40.1
      D A41.81
    neonatal P36.10
      group B P36.0
      specified NEC P36.19
    pneumoniae A40.3
    pyogenes A40.0
    specified NEC A40.8
  tracheostomy stoma J95.02
  tularemic A21.7
  umbilical, umbilical cord (newborn) — *see* Sepsis, newborn
  Yersinia pestis A20.7
Septate — *see* Septum
Septic — *see* condition
  arm — *see* Cellulitis, upper limb
    with lymphangitis — *see* Lymphangitis, acute, upper limb
  embolus — *see* Embolism
  finger — *see* Cellulitis, digit
    with lymphangitis — *see* Lymphangitis, acute, digit
  foot — *see* Cellulitis, lower limb
    with lymphangitis — *see* Lymphangitis, acute, lower limb
  gallbladder (acute) K81.0
  hand — *see* Cellulitis, upper limb
    with lymphangitis — *see* Lymphangitis, acute, upper limb
  joint — *see* Arthritis, pyogenic or pyemic
  leg — *see* Cellulitis, lower limb
    with lymphangitis — *see* Lymphangitis, acute, lower limb
  nail (*see also* Cellulitis, digit)
    with lymphangitis — *see* Lymphangitis, acute, digit
  sore (*see also* Abscess)
    throat J02.0
      streptococcal J02.0
  spleen (acute) D73.89
  teeth, tooth (pulpal origin) K04.4
  throat — *see* Pharyngitis
  thrombus — *see* Thrombosis
  toe — *see* Cellulitis, digit
    with lymphangitis — *see* Lymphangitis, acute, digit
  tonsils, chronic J35.01
    with adenoiditis J35.03
  uterus — *see* Endometritis
Septicemia A41.9
  meaning sepsis — *see* Sepsis
Septum, septate (congenital) (*see also* Anomaly, by site)
  anal Q42.3
    with fistula Q42.2
  aqueduct of Sylvius Q03.0
    with spina bifida — *see* Spina bifida, by site, with hydrocephalus
  uterus Q51.20
    complete Q51.21
    partial Q51.22
    specified NEC Q51.28
  vagina Q52.10
    in pregnancy — *see* Pregnancy, complicated by, abnormal vagina
      causing obstructed labor O65.5
    longitudinal Q52.129
      microperforate
        left side Q52.124
        right side Q52.123
      nonobstruction Q52.120
      obstructing Q52.129
        left side Q52.122
        right side Q52.121
    transverse Q52.11
Sequelae (of) (*see also* condition)
  abscess, intracranial or intraspinal (conditions in G06) G09

Sequelae — *continued*
  amputation — *code to* injury with seventh character S
  burn and corrosion — *code to* injury with seventh character S
  calcium deficiency E64.8
  cerebrovascular disease — *see* Sequelae, disease, cerebrovascular
  childbirth O94
  contusion — *code to* injury with seventh character S
  corrosion — *see* Sequelae, burn and corrosion
  crushing injury — *code to* injury with seventh character S
  disease
    cerebrovascular I69.90
      alteration of sensation I69.998
      aphasia I69.920
      apraxia I69.990
      ataxia I69.993
      cognitive deficits I69.91 ☑
      disturbance of vision I69.998
      dysarthria I69.922
      dysphagia I69.991
      dysphasia I69.921
      facial droop I69.992
      facial weakness I69.992
      fluency disorder I69.923
      hemiplegia I69.95- ☑
      hemorrhage
        intracerebral — *see* Sequelae, hemorrhage, intracerebral
        intracranial, nontraumatic NEC — *see* Sequelae, hemorrhage, intracranial, nontraumatic
        subarachnoid — *see* Sequelae, hemorrhage, subarachnoid
      language deficit I69.928
      monoplegia
        lower limb I69.94- ☑
        upper limb I69.93- ☑
      paralytic syndrome I69.96- ☑
      specified effect NEC I69.998
      specified type NEC I69.80
        alteration of sensation I69.898
        aphasia I69.820
        apraxia I69.890
        ataxia I69.893
        cognitive deficits I69.81 ☑
        disturbance of vision I69.898
        dysarthria I69.822
        dysphagia I69.891
        dysphasia I69.821
        facial droop I69.892
        facial weakness I69.892
        fluency disorder I69.823
        hemiplegia I69.85- ☑
        language deficit I69.828
        monoplegia
          lower limb I69.84- ☑
          upper limb I69.83- ☑
        paralytic syndrome I69.86- ☑
        specified effect NEC I69.898
      speech deficit I69.928
      speech deficit I69.828
    stroke NOS — *see* Sequelae, stroke NOS
  dislocation — *code to* injury with seventh character S
  encephalitis or encephalomyelitis (conditions in G04) G09
    in infectious disease NEC B94.8
    viral B94.1
  external cause — *code to* injury with seventh character S
  foreign body entering natural orifice — *code to* injury with seventh character S
  fracture — *code to* injury with seventh character S
  frostbite — *code to* injury with seventh character S
  Hansen's disease B92
  hemorrhage
    intracerebral I69.10
      alteration of sensation I69.198
      aphasia I69.120
      apraxia I69.190
      ataxia I69.193
      cognitive deficits I69.11 ☑
      disturbance of vision I69.198
      dysarthria I69.122
      dysphagia I69.191
      dysphasia I69.121

Sequelae — *continued*
  hemorrhage — *continued*
    intracerebral — *continued*
      facial droop I69.192
      facial weakness I69.192
      fluency disorder I69.123
      hemiplegia I69.15- ☑
      language deficit NEC I69.128
      monoplegia
        lower limb I69.14- ☑
        upper limb I69.13- ☑
      paralytic syndrome I69.16- ☑
      specified effect NEC I69.198
      speech deficit NEC I69.128
    intracranial, nontraumatic NEC I69.20
      alteration of sensation I69.298
      aphasia I69.220
      apraxia I69.290
      ataxia I69.293
      cognitive deficits I69.21 ☑
      disturbance of vision I69.298
      dysarthria I69.222
      dysphagia I69.291
      dysphasia I69.221
      facial droop I69.292
      facial weakness I69.292
      fluency disorder I69.223
      hemiplegia I69.25- ☑
      language deficit NEC I69.228
      monoplegia
        lower limb I69.24- ☑
        upper limb I69.23- ☑
      paralytic syndrome I69.26- ☑
      specified effect NEC I69.298
      speech deficit NEC I69.228
    subarachnoid I69.00
      alteration of sensation I69.098
      aphasia I69.020
      apraxia I69.090
      ataxia I69.093
      cognitive deficits — *see* subcategory I69.01- ☑
      disturbance of vision I69.098
      dysarthria I69.022
      dysphagia I69.091
      dysphasia I69.021
      facial droop I69.092
      facial weakness I69.092
      fluency disorder I69.023
      hemiplegia I69.05- ☑
      language deficit NEC I69.028
      monoplegia
        lower limb I69.04- ☑
        upper limb I69.03- ☑
      paralytic syndrome I69.06- ☑
      specified effect NEC I69.098
      speech deficit NEC I69.028
  hepatitis, viral B94.2
  hyperalimentation E68
  infarction
    cerebral I69.30
      alteration of sensation I69.398
      aphasia I69.320
      apraxia I69.390
      ataxia I69.393
      cognitive deficits I69.31 ☑
      disturbance of vision I69.398
      dysarthria I69.322
      dysphagia I69.391
      dysphasia I69.321
      facial droop I69.392
      facial weakness I69.392
      fluency disorder I69.323
      hemiplegia I69.35- ☑
      language deficit NEC I69.328
      monoplegia
        lower limb I69.34- ☑
        upper limb I69.33- ☑
      paralytic syndrome I69.36- ☑
      specified effect NEC I69.398
      speech deficit NEC I69.328
  infection, pyogenic, intracranial or intraspinal G09
  infectious disease B94.9
    specified NEC B94.8
  injury — *code to* injury with seventh character S
  leprosy B92
  meningitis
    bacterial (conditions in G00) G09
    other or unspecified cause (conditions in G03) G09

☑ Additional Character Required — Refer to the Tabular List for Character Selection   ▽ Subterms under main terms may continue to next column or page

Sequelae — *continued*
  muscle (and tendon) injury — *code to* injury with seventh character S
  myelitis — *see* Sequelae, encephalitis
  niacin deficiency E64.8
  nutritional deficiency E64.9
    specified NEC E64.8
  obstetrical condition O94
  parasitic disease B94.9
  phlebitis or thrombophlebitis of intracranial or intraspinal venous sinuses and veins (conditions in G08) G09
  poisoning — *code to* poisoning with seventh character S
    nonmedicinal substance — *see* Sequelae, toxic effect, nonmedicinal substance
  poliomyelitis (acute) B91
  pregnancy O94
  protein-energy malnutrition E64.0
  puerperium O94
  rickets E64.3
  selenium deficiency E64.8
  sprain and strain — *code to* injury with seventh character S
  stroke NOS I69.30
    alteration in sensation I69.398
    aphasia I69.320
    apraxia I69.390
    ataxia I69.393
    cognitive deficits I69.31 ☑
    disturbance of vision I69.398
    dysarthria I69.322
    dysphagia I69.391
    dysphasia I69.321
    facial droop I69.392
    facial weakness I69.392
    hemiplegia I69.35-
    language deficit NEC I69.328
    monoplegia
      lower limb I69.34- ☑
      upper limb I69.33- ☑
    paralytic syndrome I69.36- ☑
    specified effect NEC I69.398
    speech deficit NEC I69.328
  tendon and muscle injury — *code to* injury with seventh character S
  thiamine deficiency E64.8
  trachoma B94.0
  tuberculosis B90.9
    bones and joints B90.2
    central nervous system B90.0
    genitourinary B90.1
    pulmonary (respiratory) B90.9
    specified organs NEC B90.8
  viral
    encephalitis B94.1
    hepatitis B94.2
  vitamin deficiency NEC E64.8
    A E64.1
    B E64.8
    C E64.2
  wound, open — *code to* injury with seventh character S
Sequestration (*see also* Sequestrum)
  disk — *see* Displacement, intervertebral disk
  lung, congenital Q33.2
Sequestrum
  bone — *see* Osteomyelitis, chronic
  dental M27.2
  jaw bone M27.2
  orbit — *see* Osteomyelitis, orbit
  sinus (accessory) (nasal) — *see* Sinusitis
Sequoiosis lung or pneumonitis J67.8
Serology for syphilis
  doubtful
    with signs or symptoms — *code by* site and stage under Syphilis
    follow-up of latent syphilis — *see* Syphilis, latent
  negative, with signs or symptoms — *code by* site and stage under Syphilis
  positive A53.0
    with signs or symptoms — *code by* site and stage under Syphilis
  reactivated A53.0
Seroma (*see also* Hematoma)
  postprocedural — *see* Complication, postprocedural, seroma
  traumatic, secondary and recurrent T79.2 ☑

Seropurulent — *see* condition
Serositis, multiple K65.8
  pericardial I31.1
  peritoneal K65.8
Serous — *see* condition
Sertoli cell
  adenoma
    specified site — *see* Neoplasm, benign, by site
    unspecified site
      female D27.9
      male D29.20
  carcinoma
    specified site — *see* Neoplasm, malignant, by site
    unspecified site (male) C62.9- ☑
      female C56.9
  tumor
    with lipid storage
      specified site — *see* Neoplasm, benign, by site
      unspecified site
        female D27.9
        male D29.20
    specified site — *see* Neoplasm, benign, by site
    unspecified site
      female D27.9
      male D29.20
Sertoli-Leydig cell tumor — *see* Neoplasm, benign, by site
  specified site — *see* Neoplasm, benign, by site
  unspecified site
    female D27.9
    male D29.20
Serum
  allergy, allergic reaction (*see also* Reaction, serum) T80.69 ☑
    shock (*see also* Shock, anaphylactic) T80.59
  arthritis (*see also* Reaction, serum) T80.69
  complication or reaction NEC (*see also* Reaction, serum) T80.69 ☑
  disease NEC (*see also* Reaction, serum) T80.69 ☑
  hepatitis (*see also* Hepatitis, viral, type B)
    carrier (suspected) of B18.1
  intoxication (*see also* Reaction, serum) T80.69 ☑
  neuritis (*see also* Reaction, serum) T80.69 ☑
  neuropathy G61.1
  poisoning NEC (*see also* Reaction, serum) T80.69 ☑
  rash NEC (*see also* Reaction, serum) T80.69 ☑
  reaction NEC (*see also* Reaction, serum) T80.69 ☑
  sickness NEC (*see also* Reaction, serum) T80.69 ☑
  urticaria (*see also* Reaction, serum) T80.69 ☑
Sesamoiditis M25.8- ☑
Severe sepsis R65.20
  with septic shock R65.21
Sever's disease or osteochondrosis — *see* Osteochondrosis, juvenile, tarsus
Sex
  chromosome mosaics Q97.8
    lines with various numbers of X chromosomes Q97.2
  education Z70.8
  reassignment surgery status Z87.890
Sextuplet pregnancy — *see* Pregnancy, sextuplet
Sexual
  function, disorder of (psychogenic) F52.9
  immaturity (female) (male) E30.0
  impotence (psychogenic) organic origin NEC — *see* Dysfunction, sexual, male
  precocity (constitutional) (cryptogenic) (female) (idiopathic) (male) E30.1
Sexuality, pathologic — *see* Deviation, sexual
Sézary disease C84.1- ☑
Shadow, lung R91.8
Shaking palsy or paralysis — *see* Parkinsonism
Shallowness, acetabulum — *see* Derangement, joint, specified type NEC, hip
Shaver's disease J63.1
Sheath (tendon) — *see* condition
Sheathing, retinal vessels H35.01- ☑
Shedding
  nail L60.8
  premature, primary (deciduous) teeth K00.6
Sheehan's disease or syndrome E23.0
Shelf, rectal K62.89
Shell teeth K00.5
Shellshock (current) F43.0
  lasting state — *see* Disorder, post-traumatic stress
Shield kidney Q63.1
Shift
  auditory threshold (temporary) H93.24- ☑

Shift — *continued*
  mediastinal R93.89
Shifting sleep-work schedule (affecting sleep) G47.26
Shiga (-Kruse) **dysentery** A03.0
Shiga's bacillus A03.0
Shigella (dysentery) — *see* Dysentery, bacillary
Shigellosis A03.9
  Group A A03.0
  Group B A03.1
  Group C A03.2
  Group D A03.3
Shin splints S86.89- ☑
Shingles — *see* Herpes, zoster
Shipyard disease or eye B30.0
Shirodkar suture, in pregnancy — *see* Pregnancy, complicated by, incompetent cervix
Shock R57.9
  with ectopic or molar pregnancy O08.3
  adrenal (cortical) (Addisonian) E27.2
  adverse food reaction (anaphylactic) — *see* Shock, anaphylactic, due to food
  allergic — *see* Shock, anaphylactic
  anaphylactic T78.2 ☑
    chemical — *see* Table of Drugs and Chemicals
    due to drug or medicinal substance
      correct substance properly administered T88.6 ☑
      overdose or wrong substance given or taken (by accident) — *see* Table of Drugs and Chemicals, by drug, poisoning
    due to food (nonpoisonous) T78.00 ☑
      additives T78.06 ☑
      dairy products T78.07 ☑
      eggs T78.08 ☑
      fish T78.03 ☑
        shellfish T78.02 ☑
      fruit T78.04 ☑
      milk T78.07 ☑
      nuts T78.05 ☑
        multiple types T78.05 ☑
        peanuts T78.01 ☑
      peanuts T78.01 ☑
      seeds T78.05 ☑
      specified type NEC T78.09 ☑
      vegetable T78.04 ☑
    following sting(s) — *see* Venom
    immunization T80.52 ☑
    serum T80.59 ☑
      blood and blood products T80.51 ☑
      immunization T80.52 ☑
      specified NEC T80.59 ☑
      vaccination T80.52 ☑
  anaphylactoid — *see* Shock, anaphylactic
  anesthetic
    correct substance properly administered T88.2 ☑
    overdose or wrong substance given or taken — *see* Table of Drugs and Chemicals, by drug, poisoning
      specified anesthetic — *see* Table of Drugs and Chemicals, by drug, poisoning
  cardiogenic R57.0
  chemical substance — *see* Table of Drugs and Chemicals
  complicating ectopic or molar pregnancy O08.3
  culture — *see* Disorder, adjustment
  drug
    due to correct substance properly administered T88.6 ☑
    overdose or wrong substance given or taken (by accident) — *see* Table of Drugs and Chemicals, by drug, poisoning
  during or after labor and delivery O75.1
  electric T75.4 ☑
    (taser) T75.4 ☑
  endotoxic R65.21
    postprocedural (resulting from a procedure, not elsewhere classified) T81.12 ☑
  following
    ectopic or molar pregnancy O08.3
    injury (immediate) (delayed) T79.4 ☑
    labor and delivery O75.1
  food (anaphylactic) — *see* Shock, anaphylactic, due to food
  from electroshock gun (taser) T75.4 ☑
  gram-negative R65.21
    postprocedural (resulting from a procedure, not elsewhere classified) T81.12 ☑
  hematologic R57.8

Subterms under main terms may continue to next column or page   ☑ Additional Character Required — Refer to the Tabular List for Character Selection   285

Sequelae — Shock

Shock — *continued*
hemorrhagic R57.8
  surgery (intraoperative) (postoperative) T81.19 ☑
  trauma T79.4 ☑
hypovolemic R57.1
  surgical T81.19 ☑
  traumatic T79.4 ☑
insulin E15
  therapeutic misadventure — *see* subcategory
   T38.3 ☑
kidney N17.0
  traumatic (following crushing) T79.5 ☑
lightning T75.01 ☑
liver K72.00
lung J80
obstetric O75.1
  with ectopic or molar pregnancy O08.3
  following ectopic or molar pregnancy O08.3
pleural (surgical) T81.19 ☑
  due to trauma T79.4 ☑
postprocedural (postoperative) T81.10 ☑
  with ectopic or molar pregnancy O08.3
  cardiogenic T81.11 ☑
  endotoxic T81.12 ☑
  following ectopic or molar pregnancy O08.3
  gram-negative T81.12 ☑
  hypovolemic T81.19 ☑
  septic T81.12 ☑
  specified type NEC T81.19 ☑
psychic F43.0
septic (due to severe sepsis) R65.21
specified NEC R57.8
surgical T81.10 ☑
taser gun (taser) T75.4 ☑
therapeutic misadventure NEC T81.10 ☑
thyroxin
  overdose or wrong substance given or taken — *see*
   Table of Drugs and Chemicals, by drug, poisoning
toxic, syndrome A48.3
transfusion — *see* Complications, transfusion
traumatic (immediate) (delayed) T79.4 ☑
Shoemaker's chest M95.4
Short, shortening, shortness
arm (acquired) (*see also* Deformity, limb, unequal
  length)
  congenital Q71.81- ☑
  forearm — *see* Deformity, limb, unequal length
bowel syndrome K91.2
breath R06.02
cervical (complicating pregnancy) O26.87- ☑
  non-gravid uterus N88.3
common bile duct, congenital Q44.5
cord (umbilical), complicating delivery O69.3 ☑
cystic duct, congenital Q44.5
esophagus (congenital) Q39.8
femur (acquired) — *see* Deformity, limb, unequal
  length, femur
  congenital — *see* Defect, reduction, lower limb,
   longitudinal, femur
frenum, frenulum, linguae (congenital) Q38.1
hip (acquired) (*see also* Deformity, limb, unequal
  length)
  congenital Q65.89
leg (acquired) (*see also* Deformity, limb, unequal
  length)
  congenital Q72.81- ☑
  lower leg (*see also* Deformity, limb, unequal length)
limbed stature, with immunodeficiency D82.2
lower limb (acquired) (*see also* Deformity, limb, unequal
  length)
  congenital Q72.81- ☑
organ or site, congenital NEC — *see* Distortion
palate, congenital Q38.5
radius (acquired) (*see also* Deformity, limb, unequal
  length)
  congenital — *see* Defect, reduction, upper limb,
   longitudinal, radius
rib syndrome Q77.2
stature (child) (hereditary) (idiopathic) NEC R62.52
  constitutional E34.3
  due to endocrine disorder E34.3
  Laron-type E34.3
tendon (*see also* Contraction, tendon)
  with contracture of joint — *see* Contraction, joint
  Achilles (acquired) M67.0- ☑
   congenital Q66.89

Short, shortening, shortness — *continued*
tendon (*see also* Contraction, tendon) — *continued*
  congenital Q79.8
thigh (acquired) (*see also* Deformity, limb, unequal
  length, femur)
  congenital — *see* Defect, reduction, lower limb,
   longitudinal, femur
tibialis anterior (tendon) — *see* Contraction, tendon
umbilical cord
  complicating delivery O69.3 ☑
upper limb, congenital — *see* Defect, reduction, upper
  limb, specified type NEC
urethra N36.8
uvula, congenital Q38.5
vagina (congenital) Q52.4
Shortsightedness — *see* Myopia
Shoshin (acute fulminating beriberi) E51.11
Shoulder — *see* condition
Shovel-shaped incisors K00.2
Shower, thromboembolic — *see* Embolism
Shunt
arterial-venous (dialysis) Z99.2
arteriovenous, pulmonary (acquired) I28.0
  congenital Q25.72
cerebral ventricle (communicating) in situ Z98.2
surgical, prosthetic, with complications —*see* Compli-
  cations, cardiovascular, device or implant
Shutdown, renal N28.9
Shy-Drager syndrome G90.3
Sialadenitis, sialadenosis (any gland) (chronic) (period-
  ic) (suppurative) — *see* Sialoadenitis
Sialectasia K11.8
Sialidosis E77.1
Sialitis, silitis (any gland) (chronic) (suppurative) — *see*
  Sialoadenitis
Sialoadenitis (any gland) (periodic) (suppurative) K11.20 ☑
  acute K11.21
   recurrent K11.22
  chronic K11.23
Sialoadenopathy K11.9
Sialoangitis — *see* Sialoadenitis
Sialodochitis (fibrinosa) — *see* Sialoadenitis
Sialodocholithiasis K11.5
Sialolithiasis K11.5
Sialometaplasia, necrotizing K11.8
Sialorrhea (*see also* Ptyalism)
  periodic — *see* Sialoadenitis
Sialosis K11.7
Siamese twin Q89.4
Sibling rivalry Z62.891
Sicard's syndrome G52.7
Sicca syndrome M35.00
  with
   keratoconjunctivitis M35.01
   lung involvement M35.02
   myopathy M35.03
   renal tubulo-interstitial disorders M35.04
   specified organ involvement NEC M35.09
Sick R69
  or handicapped person in family Z63.79
   needing care at home Z63.6
  sinus (syndrome) I49.5
Sick-euthyroid syndrome E07.81
Sickle-cell
  anemia — *see* Disease, sickle-cell
  trait D57.3
Sicklemia (*see also* Disease, sickle-cell)
  trait D57.3
Sickness
air (travel) T75.3 ☑
airplane T75.3 ☑
alpine T70.29 ☑
altitude T70.20 ☑
Andes T70.29 ☑
aviator's T70.29 ☑
balloon T70.29 ☑
car T75.3 ☑
compressed air T70.3 ☑
decompression T70.3 ☑
green D50.8
milk — *see* Poisoning, food, noxious
motion T75.3 ☑
mountain T70.29 ☑
  acute D75.1
protein (*see also* Reaction, serum) T80.69 ☑
radiation T66
roundabout (motion) T75.3 ☑

Sickness — *continued*
sea T75.3 ☑
serum NEC (*see also* Reaction, serum) T80.69 ☑
sleeping (African) B56.9
  by Trypanosoma B56.9
   brucei
    gambiense B56.0
    rhodesiense B56.1
  East African B56.1
  Gambian B56.0
  Rhodesian B56.1
  West African B56.0
swing (motion) T75.3 ☑
train (railway) (travel) T75.3 ☑
travel (any vehicle) T75.3 ☑
Sideropenia — *see* Anemia, iron deficiency
Siderosilicosis J62.8
Siderosis (lung) J63.4
  eye (globe) — *see* Disorder, globe, degenerative,
   siderosis
Siemens' syndrome (ectodermal dysplasia) Q82.8
Sighing R06.89
  psychogenic F45.8
Sigmoid (*see also* condition)
  flexure — *see* condition
  kidney Q63.1
Sigmoiditis (*see also* Enteritis) K52.9
  infectious A09
  noninfectious K52.9
Silfversköld's syndrome Q78.9
Silicosiderosis J62.8
Silicosis, silicotic (simple) (complicated) J62.8
  with tuberculosis J65
Silicotuberculosis J65
Silo-fillers' disease J68.8
  bronchitis J68.0
  pneumonitis J68.0
  pulmonary edema J68.1
Silver's syndrome Q87.1
Simian malaria B53.1
Simmonds' cachexia or disease E23.0
Simons' disease or syndrome (progressive lipodystro-
  phy) E88.1
Simple, simplex — *see* condition
Simulation, conscious (of illness) Z76.5
Simultanagnosia (asimultagnosia) R48.3
Sin Nombre virus disease (Hantavirus) (cardio)-pul-
  monary syndrome) B33.4
Sinding-Larsen disease or osteochondrosis — *see*
  Osteochondrosis, juvenile, patella
Singapore hemorrhagic fever A91
Singer's node or nodule J38.2
Single
atrium Q21.2
coronary artery Q24.5
umbilical artery Q27.0
ventricle Q20.4
Singultus R06.6
  epidemicus B33.0
Sinus (*see also* Fistula)
abdominal K63.89
arrest I45.5
arrhythmia I49.8
bradycardia R00.1
branchial cleft (internal) (external) Q18.0
coccygeal — *see* Sinus, pilonidal
dental K04.6
dermal (congenital) Q06.8
  with abscess Q06.8
  coccygeal, pilonidal — *see* Sinus, coccygeal
infected, skin NEC L08.89
marginal, ruptured or bleeding — *see* Hemorrhage,
  antepartum, specified cause NEC
medial, face and neck Q18.8
pause I45.5
pericranii Q01.9
pilonidal (infected) (rectum) L05.92
  with abscess L05.02
preauricular Q18.1
rectovaginal N82.3
Rokitansky-Aschoff (gallbladder) K82.8
sacrococcygeal (dermoid) (infected) — *see* Sinus, pilonidal
tachycardia R00.0
  paroxysmal I47.1
tarsi syndrome M25.57- ☑
testis N50.89

☑ **Additional Character Required** — Refer to the Tabular List for Character Selection   ▽ **Subterms under main terms may continue to next column or page**

Sinus — continued
   tract (postinfective) — see Fistula
   urachus Q64.4
Sinusitis (accessory) (chronic) (hyperplastic) (nasal)
      (nonpurulent) (purulent) J32.9
   acute J01.90
      ethmoidal J01.20
         recurrent J01.21
      frontal J01.10
         recurrent J01.11
      involving more than one sinus, other than pansinusi-
         tis J01.80
         recurrent J01.81
      maxillary J01.00
         recurrent J01.01
      pansinusitis J01.40
         recurrent J01.41
      recurrent J01.91
      specified NEC J01.80
         recurrent J01.81
      sphenoidal J01.30
         recurrent J01.31
   allergic — see Rhinitis, allergic
   due to high altitude T70.1 ☑
   ethmoidal J32.2
      acute J01.20
         recurrent J01.21
   frontal J32.1
      acute J01.10
         recurrent J01.11
   influenzal — see Influenza, with, respiratory manifesta-
      tions NEC
   involving more than one sinus but not pansinusitis
      J32.8
      acute J01.80
         recurrent J01.81
   maxillary J32.0
      acute J01.00
         recurrent J01.01
   sphenoidal J32.3
      acute J01.30
         recurrent J01.31
   tuberculous, any sinus A15.8
Sinusitis-bronchiectasis-situs inversus (syndrome)
   (triad) Q89.3
Sipple's syndrome E31.22
Sirenomelia (syndrome) Q87.2
Siriasis T67.0 ☑
Sirkari's disease B55.0
Siti A65
Situation, psychiatric F99
Situational
   disturbance (transient) — see Disorder, adjustment
      acute F43.0
   maladjustment — see Disorder, adjustment
   reaction — see Disorder, adjustment
      acute F43.0
Situs inversus or transversus (abdominalis) (thoracis)
   Q89.3
Sixth disease B08.20
   due to human herpesvirus 6 B08.21
   due to human herpesvirus 7 B08.22
Sjögren-Larsson syndrome Q87.1
Sjögren's syndrome or disease — see Sicca syndrome
Skeletal — see condition
Skene's gland — see condition
Skenitis — see Urethritis
Skerljevo A65
Skevas-Zerfus disease — see Toxicity, venom, marine
   animal, sea anemone
Skin (see also condition)
   clammy R23.1
   donor — see Donor, skin
   hidebound M35.9
Slate-dressers' or slate-miners' lung J62.8
Sleep
   apnea — see Apnea, sleep
   deprivation Z72.820
   disorder or disturbance G47.9
      child F51.9
         nonorganic origin F51.9
         specified NEC G47.8
   disturbance G47.9
      nonorganic origin F51.9
   drunkenness F51.9
   rhythm inversion G47.2- ☑
   terrors F51.4
   walking F51.3

Sleep — continued
   walking — continued
      hysterical F44.89
Sleep hygiene
   abuse Z72.821
   inadequate Z72.821
   poor Z72.821
Sleeping sickness — see Sickness, sleeping
Sleeplessness — see Insomnia
   menopausal N95.1
Sleep-wake schedule disorder G47.20
Slim disease (in HIV infection) B20
Slipped, slipping
   epiphysis (traumatic) (see also Osteochondropathy,
         specified type NEC)
      capital femoral (traumatic)
         acute (on chronic) S79.01- ☑
         current traumatic — code as Fracture, by site
      upper femoral (nontraumatic) M93.00- ☑
         acute M93.01- ☑
            on chronic M93.03- ☑
         chronic M93.02- ☑
   intervertebral disc — see Displacement, intervertebral
      disc
   ligature, umbilical P51.8
   patella — see Disorder, patella, derangement NEC
   rib M89.8X8
   sacroiliac joint — see subcategory M53.2 ☑
   tendon — see Disorder, tendon
   ulnar nerve, nontraumatic — see Lesion, nerve, ulnar
   vertebra NEC — see Spondylolisthesis
Slocumb's syndrome E27.0
Sloughing (multiple) (phagedena) (skin) (see also Gan-
      grene)
   abscess — see Abscess
   appendix K38.8
   fascia — see Disorder, soft tissue, specified type NEC
   scrotum N50.89
   tendon — see Disorder, tendon
   transplanted organ — see Rejection, transplant
   ulcer — see Ulcer, skin
Slow
   feeding, newborn P92.2
   flow syndrome, coronary I20.8
   heart (beat) R00.1
Slowing, urinary stream R39.198
Sluder's neuralgia (syndrome) G44.89
Slurred, slurring speech R47.81
Small (ness)
   for gestational age — see Small for dates
   introitus, vagina N89.6
   kidney (unknown cause) N27.9
      bilateral N27.1
      unilateral N27.0
   ovary (congenital) Q50.39
   pelvis
      with disproportion (fetopelvic) O33.1
         causing obstructed labor O65.1
   uterus N85.8
   white kidney N03.9
Small-and-light-for-dates — see Small for dates
Small-for-dates (infant) P05.10
   with weight of
      499 grams or less P05.11
      500-749 grams P05.12
      750-999 grams P05.13
      1000-1249 grams P05.14
      1250-1499 grams P05.15
      1500-1749 grams P05.16
      1750-1999 grams P05.17
      2000-2499 grams P05.18
      2500 grams and over P05.19
   specified NEC P05.19
Smallpox B03
Smearing, fecal R15.1
Smith-Lemli-Opitz syndrome E78.72
Smith's fracture S52.54- ☑
Smoker — see Dependence, drug, nicotine
Smoker's
   bronchitis J41.0
   cough J41.0
   palate K13.24
   throat J31.2
   tongue K13.24
Smoking
   passive Z77.22
Smothering spells R06.81

Snaggle teeth, tooth M26.39
Snapping
   finger — see Trigger finger
   hip — see Derangement, joint, specified type NEC, hip
      involving the iliotibial band M76.3- ☑
   knee — see Derangement, knee
      involving the iliotiblial band M76.3- ☑
Sneddon-Wilkinson disease or syndrome (sub-corneal
   pustular dermatosis) L13.1
Sneezing (intractable) R06.7
Sniffing
   cocaine
      abuse — see Abuse, drug, cocaine
      dependence — see Dependence, drug, cocaine
   gasoline
      abuse — see Abuse, drug, inhalant
      dependence — see Dependence, drug, inhalant
   glue (airplane)
      abuse — see Abuse, drug, inhalant
      drug dependence — see Dependence, drug, in-
         halant
Sniffles
   newborn P28.89
Snoring R06.83
Snow blindness — see Photokeratitis
Snuffles (non-syphilitic) R06.5
   newborn P28.89
   syphilitic (infant) A50.05 [J99]
Social
   exclusion Z60.4
      due to discrimination or persecution (perceived)
         Z60.5
   migrant Z59.0
      acculturation difficulty Z60.3
   rejection Z60.4
      due to discrimination or persecution Z60.5
   role conflict NEC Z73.5
   skills inadequacy NEC Z73.4
   transplantation Z60.3
Sodoku A25.0
Soemmerring's ring — see Cataract, secondary
Soft (see also condition)
   nails L60.3
Softening
   bone — see Osteomalacia
   brain (necrotic) (progressive) G93.89
      congenital Q04.8
      embolic I63.4- ☑
         hemorrhagic — see Hemorrhage, intracranial, intrac-
            erebral
         occlusive I63.5- ☑
         thrombotic I63.3- ☑
   cartilage M94.2- ☑
      patella M22.4- ☑
   cerebellar — see Softening, brain
   cerebral — see Softening, brain
   cerebrospinal — see Softening, brain
   myocardial, heart — see Degeneration, myocardial
   spinal cord G95.89
   stomach K31.89
Soldier's
   heart F45.8
   patches I31.0
Solitary
   cyst, kidney N28.1
   kidney, congenital Q60.0
Solvent abuse — see Abuse, drug, inhalant
   dependence — see Dependence, drug, inhalant
Somatization reaction, somatic reaction — see Disorder, somatoform
Somnambulism F51.3
   hysterical F44.89
Somnolence R40.0
   nonorganic origin F51.11
Sonne dysentery A03.3
Soor B37.0
Sore
   bed — see Ulcer, pressure, by site
   chiclero B55.1
   Delhi B55.1
   desert — see Ulcer, skin
   eye H57.1- ☑
   Lahore B55.1
   mouth K13.79
      canker K12.0
   muscle M79.10
   Naga — see Ulcer, skin

Sore — *continued*
- of skin — *see* Ulcer, skin
- oriental B55.1
- pressure — *see* Ulcer, pressure, by site
- skin L98.9
- soft A57
- throat (acute) (*see also* Pharyngitis)
  - with influenza, flu, or grippe — *see* Influenza, with, respiratory manifestations NEC
  - chronic J31.2
  - coxsackie (virus) B08.5
  - diphtheritic A36.0
  - herpesviral B00.2
  - influenzal — *see* Influenza, with, respiratory manifestations NEC
  - septic J02.0
  - streptococcal (ulcerative) J02.0
  - viral NEC J02.8
    - coxsackie B08.5
- tropical — *see* Ulcer, skin
- veldt — *see* Ulcer, skin

Soto's syndrome (cerebral gigantism) Q87.3
South African cardiomyopathy syndrome I42.8
Southeast Asian hemorrhagic fever A91
Spacing
- abnormal, tooth, teeth, fully erupted M26.30
- excessive, tooth, fully erupted M26.32

Spade-like hand (congenital) Q68.1
Spading nail L60.8
- congenital Q84.6

Spanish collar N47.1
Sparganosis B70.1
Spasm(s), spastic, spasticity (*see also* condition) R25.2
- accommodation — *see* Spasm, of accommodation
- ampulla of Vater K83.4
- anus, ani (sphincter) (reflex) K59.4
  - psychogenic F45.8
- artery I73.9
  - cerebral G45.9
- Bell's G51.3- ☑
- bladder (sphincter, external or internal) N32.89
  - psychogenic F45.8
- bronchus, bronchiole J98.01
- cardia K22.0
- cardiac I20.1
- carpopedal — *see* Tetany
- cerebral (arteries) (vascular) G45.9
- cervix, complicating delivery O62.4
- ciliary body (of accommodation) — *see* Spasm, of accommodation
- colon (*see also* Irritable, bowel) K58.9
  - with diarrhea K58.0
  - psychogenic F45.8
- common duct K83.8
- compulsive — *see* Tic
- conjugate H51.8
- coronary (artery) I20.1
- diaphragm (reflex) R06.6
  - epidemic B33.0
  - psychogenic F45.8
- duodenum K59.8
- epidemic diaphragmatic (transient) B33.0
- esophagus (diffuse) K22.4
  - psychogenic F45.8
- facial G51.3- ☑
- fallopian tube N83.8
- gastrointestinal (tract) K31.89
  - psychogenic F45.8
- glottis J38.5
  - hysterical F44.4
  - psychogenic F45.8
    - conversion reaction F44.4
  - reflex through recurrent laryngeal nerve J38.5
- habit — *see* Tic
- heart I20.1
- hemifacial (clonic) G51.3- ☑
- hourglass — *see* Contraction, hourglass
- hysterical F44.4
- infantile — *see* Epilepsy, spasms
- inferior oblique, eye H51.8
- intestinal (*see also* Syndrome, irritable bowel) K58.9
  - psychogenic F45.8
- larynx, laryngeal J38.5
  - hysterical F44.4
  - psychogenic F45.8
    - conversion reaction F44.4
- levator palpebrae superioris — *see* Disorder, eyelid function

Spasm(s), spastic, spasticity — *continued*
- muscle NEC M62.838
  - back M62.830
- nerve, trigeminal G51.0
- nervous F45.8
- nodding F98.4
- occupational F48.8
- oculogyric H51.8
  - psychogenic F45.8
- of accommodation H52.53- ☑
- ophthalmic artery — *see* Occlusion, artery, retina
- perineal, female N94.89
- peroneo-extensor (*see also* Deformity, limb, flat foot)
- pharynx (reflex) J39.2
  - hysterical F45.8
  - psychogenic F45.8
- psychogenic F45.8
- pylorus NEC K31.3
  - adult hypertrophic K31.89
  - congenital or infantile Q40.0
  - psychogenic F45.8
- rectum (sphincter) K59.4
  - psychogenic F45.8
- retinal (artery) — *see* Occlusion, artery, retina
- sigmoid (*see also* Syndrome, irritable bowel) K58.9
  - psychogenic F45.8
- sphincter of Oddi K83.4
- stomach K31.89
  - neurotic F45.8
- throat J39.2
  - hysterical F45.8
  - psychogenic F45.8
- tic F95.9
  - chronic F95.1
  - transient of childhood F95.0
- tongue K14.8
- torsion (progressive) G24.1
- trigeminal nerve — *see* Neuralgia, trigeminal
- ureter N13.5
- urethra (sphincter) N35.919
- uterus N85.8
  - complicating labor O62.4
- vagina N94.2
  - psychogenic F52.5
- vascular I73.9
- vasomotor I73.9
- vein NEC I87.8
- viscera — *see* Pain, abdominal

Spasmodic — *see* condition
Spasmophilia — *see* Tetany
Spasmus nutans F98.4
Spastic, spasticity (*see also* Spasm)
- child (cerebral) (congenital) (paralysis) G80.1

Speaker's throat R49.8
Specific, specified — *see* condition
Speech
- defect, disorder, disturbance, impediment R47.9
  - psychogenic, in childhood and adolescence F98.8
  - slurring R47.81
  - specified NEC R47.89

Spencer's disease A08.19
Spens' syndrome (syncope with heart block) I45.9
Sperm counts (fertility testing) Z31.41
- postvasectomy Z30.8
- reversal Z31.42

Spermatic cord — *see* condition
Spermatocele N43.40
- congenital Q55.4
- multiple N43.42
- single N43.41

Spermatocystitis N49.0
Spermatocytoma C62.9- ☑
- specified site — *see* Neoplasm, malignant, by site

Spermatorrhea N50.89
Sphacelus — *see* Gangrene
Sphenoidal — *see* condition
Sphenoiditis (chronic) — *see* Sinusitis, sphenoidal
Sphenopalatine ganglion neuralgia G90.09
Sphericity, increased, lens (congenital) Q12.4
Spherocytosis (congenital) (familial) (hereditary) D58.0
- hemoglobin disease D58.0
- sickle-cell (disease) D57.8- ☑

Spherophakia Q12.4
Sphincter — *see* condition
Sphincteritis, sphincter of Oddi — *see* Cholangitis
Sphingolipidosis E75.3
- specified NEC E75.29

Sphingomyelinosis E75.3

Spicule tooth K00.2
Spider
- bite — *see* Toxicity, venom, spider
- fingers — *see* Syndrome, Marfan's
- nevus I78.1
- toes — *see* Syndrome, Marfan's
- vascular I78.1

Spiegler-Fendt
- benign lymphocytoma L98.8
- sarcoid L08.89

Spielmeyer-Vogt disease E75.4
Spina bifida (aperta) Q05.9
- with hydrocephalus NEC Q05.4
- cervical Q05.5
  - with hydrocephalus Q05.0
- dorsal Q05.6
  - with hydrocephalus Q05.1
- lumbar Q05.7
  - with hydrocephalus Q05.2
- lumbosacral Q05.7
  - with hydrocephalus Q05.2
- occulta Q76.0
- sacral Q05.8
  - with hydrocephalus Q05.3
- thoracic Q05.6
  - with hydrocephalus Q05.1
- thoracolumbar Q05.6
  - with hydrocephalus Q05.1

Spindle, Krukenberg's — *see* Pigmentation, cornea, posterior
Spine, spinal — *see* condition
Spiradenoma (eccrine) — *see* Neoplasm, skin, benign
Spirillosis A25.0
Spirillum
- minus A25.0
- obermeieri infection A68.0

Spirochetal — *see* condition
Spirochetosis A69.9
- arthritic, arthritica A69.9
- bronchopulmonary A69.8
- icterohemorrhagic A27.0
- lung A69.8

Spirometrosis B70.1
Spitting blood — *see* Hemoptysis
Splanchnoptosis K63.4
Spleen, splenic — *see* condition
Splenectasis — *see* Splenomegaly
Splenitis (interstitial) (malignant) (nonspecific) D73.89
- malarial (*see also* Malaria) B54 [D77]
- tuberculous A18.85

Splenocele D73.89
Splenomegaly, splenomegalia (Bengal) (cryptogenic) (idiopathic) (tropical) R16.1
- with hepatomegaly R16.2
- cirrhotic D73.2
- congenital Q89.09
- congestive, chronic D73.2
- Egyptian B65.1
- Gaucher's E75.22
- malarial (*see also* Malaria) B54 [D77]
- neutropenic D73.81
- Niemann-Pick — *see* Niemann-Pick disease or syndrome
- siderotic D73.2
- syphilitic A52.79
  - congenital (early) A50.08 [D77]

Splenopathy D73.9
Splenoptosis D73.89
Splenosis D73.89
Splinter — *see* Foreign body, superficial, by site
Split, splitting
- foot Q72.7- ☑
- hand Q71.6 ☑
- heart sounds R01.2
- lip, congenital — *see* Cleft, lip
- nails L60.3
- urinary stream R39.13

Spondylarthrosis — *see* Spondylosis
Spondylitis (chronic) (*see also* Spondylopathy, inflammatory)
- ankylopoietica — *see* Spondylitis, ankylosing
- ankylosing (chronic) M45.9
  - with lung involvement M45.9 [J99]
  - cervical region M45.2
  - cervicothoracic region M45.3
  - juvenile M08.1
  - lumbar region M45.6
  - lumbosacral region M45.7

☑ **Additional Character Required** — Refer to the Tabular List for Character Selection   ▽ **Subterms under main terms may continue to next column or page**

Spondylitis — *continued*
  ankylosing — *continued*
    multiple sites M45.0
    occipito-atlanto-axial region M45.1
    sacrococcygeal region M45.8
    thoracic region M45.4
    thoracolumbar region M45.5
  atrophic (ligamentous) — *see* Spondylitis, ankylosing
  deformans (chronic) — *see* Spondylosis
  gonococcal A54.41
  gouty (*see also* Gout, by type, vertebrae) M10.08
  in (due to)
    brucellosis A23.9 [M49.80]
      cervical region A23.9 [M49.82]
      cervicothoracic region A23.9 [M49.83]
      lumbar region A23.9 [M49.86]
      lumbosacral region A23.9 [M49.87]
      multiple sites A23.9 [M49.89]
      occipito-atlanto-axial region A23.9 [M49.81]
      sacrococcygeal region A23.9 [M49.88]
      thoracic region A23.9 [M49.84]
      thoracolumbar region A23.9 [M49.85]
    enterobacteria (*see also* subcategory M49.8) A04.9
    tuberculosis A18.01
  infectious NEC — *see* Spondylopathy, infective
  juvenile ankylosing (chronic) M08.1
  Kümmell's — *see* Spondylopathy, traumatic
  Marie-Strümpell — *see* Spondylitis, ankylosing
  muscularis — *see* Spondylopathy, specified NEC
  psoriatic L40.53
  rheumatoid — *see* Spondylitis, ankylosing
  rhizomelica — *see* Spondylitis, ankylosing
  sacroiliac NEC M46.1
  senescent, senile — *see* Spondylosis
  traumatic (chronic) or post-traumatic — *see* Spondylopathy, traumatic
  tuberculous A18.01
  typhosa A01.05
Spondylolisthesis (acquired) (degenerative) M43.10
  with disproportion (fetopelvic) O33.0
    causing obstructed labor O65.0
  cervical region M43.12
  cervicothoracic region M43.13
  congenital Q76.2
  lumbar region M43.16
  lumbosacral region M43.17
  multiple sites M43.19
  occipito-atlanto-axial region M43.11
  sacrococcygeal region M43.18
  thoracic region M43.14
  thoracolumbar region M43.15
  traumatic (old) M43.10
    acute
      fifth cervical (displaced) S12.430 ☑
        nondisplaced S12.431 ☑
        specified type NEC (displaced) S12.450 ☑
          nondisplaced S12.451 ☑
        type III S12.44 ☑
      fourth cervical (displaced) S12.330 ☑
        nondisplaced S12.331 ☑
        specified type NEC (displaced) S12.350 ☑
          nondisplaced S12.351 ☑
        type III S12.34 ☑
      second cervical (displaced) S12.130 ☑
        nondisplaced S12.131 ☑
        specified type NEC (displaced) S12.150 ☑
          nondisplaced S12.151 ☑
        type III S12.14 ☑
      seventh cervical (displaced) S12.630 ☑
        nondisplaced S12.631 ☑
        specified type NEC (displaced) S12.650 ☑
          nondisplaced S12.651 ☑
        type III S12.64 ☑
      sixth cervical (displaced) S12.530 ☑
        nondisplaced S12.531 ☑
        specified type NEC (displaced) S12.550 ☑
          nondisplaced S12.551 ☑
        type III S12.54 ☑
      third cervical (displaced) S12.230 ☑
        nondisplaced S12.231 ☑
        specified type NEC (displaced) S12.250 ☑
          nondisplaced S12.251 ☑
        type III S12.24 ☑
Spondylolysis (acquired) M43.00
  cervical region M43.02
  cervicothoracic region M43.03
  congenital Q76.2

Spondylolysis — *continued*
  lumbar region M43.06
  lumbosacral region M43.07
    with disproportion (fetopelvic) O33.0
      causing obstructed labor O65.8
  multiple sites M43.09
  occipito-atlanto-axial region M43.01
  sacrococcygeal region M43.08
  thoracic region M43.04
  thoracolumbar region M43.05
Spondylopathy M48.9
  infective NEC M46.50
    cervical region M46.52
    cervicothoracic region M46.53
    lumbar region M46.56
    lumbosacral region M46.57
    multiple sites M46.59
    occipito-atlanto-axial region M46.51
    sacrococcygeal region M46.58
    thoracic region M46.54
    thoracolumbar region M46.55
  inflammatory M46.90
    cervical region M46.92
    cervicothoracic region M46.93
    lumbar region M46.96
    lumbosacral region M46.97
    multiple sites M46.99
    occipito-atlanto-axial region M46.91
    sacrococcygeal region M46.98
    specified type NEC M46.80
      cervical region M46.82
      cervicothoracic region M46.83
      lumbar region M46.86
      lumbosacral region M46.87
      multiple sites M46.89
      occipito-atlanto-axial region M46.81
      sacrococcygeal region M46.88
      thoracic region M46.84
      thoracolumbar region M46.85
    thoracic region M46.94
    thoracolumbar region M46.95
  neuropathic, in
    syringomyelia and syringobulbia G95.0
    tabes dorsalis A52.11
  specified NEC — *see* subcategory M48.8 ☑
  traumatic M48.30
    cervical region M48.32
    cervicothoracic region M48.33
    lumbar region M48.36
    lumbosacral region M48.37
    occipito-atlanto-axial region M48.31
    sacrococcygeal region M48.38
    thoracic region M48.34
    thoracolumbar region M48.35
Spondylosis M47.9
  with
    disproportion (fetopelvic) O33.0
      causing obstructed labor O65.0
    myelopathy NEC M47.10
      cervical region M47.12
      cervicothoracic region M47.13
      lumbar region M47.16
      occipito-atlanto-axial region M47.11
      thoracic region M47.14
      thoracolumbar region M47.15
    radiculopathy M47.20
      cervical region M47.22
      cervicothoracic region M47.23
      lumbar region M47.26
      lumbosacral region M47.27
      occipito-atlanto-axial region M47.21
      sacrococcygeal region M47.28
      thoracic region M47.24
      thoracolumbar region M47.25
  specified NEC M47.899
    cervical region M47.892
    cervicothoracic region M47.893
    lumbar region M47.896
    lumbosacral region M47.897
    occipito-atlanto-axial region M47.891
    sacrococcygeal region M47.898
    thoracic region M47.894
    thoracolumbar region M47.895
  traumatic — *see* Spondylopathy, traumatic
  without myelopathy or radiculopathy M47.819
    cervical region M47.812
    cervicothoracic region M47.813
    lumbar region M47.816
    lumbosacral region M47.817

Spondylosis — *continued*
  without myelopathy or radiculopathy — *continued*
    occipito-atlanto-axial region M47.811
    sacrococcygeal region M47.818
    thoracic region M47.814
    thoracolumbar region M47.815
Sponge
  inadvertently left in operation wound — *see* Foreign body, accidentally left during a procedure
  kidney (medullary) Q61.5
Sponge-diver's disease — *see* Toxicity, venom, marine animal, sea anemone
Spongioblastoma (any type) — *see* Neoplasm, malignant, by site
  specified site — *see* Neoplasm, malignant, by site
  unspecified site C71.9
Spongioneuroblastoma — *see* Neoplasm, malignant, by site
Spontaneous (*see also* condition)
  fracture (cause unknown) — *see* Fracture, pathological
Spoon nail L60.3
  congenital Q84.6
Sporadic — *see* condition
Sporothrix schenckii infection — *see* Sporotrichosis
Sporotrichosis B42.9
  arthritis B42.82
  disseminated B42.7
  generalized B42.7
  lymphocutaneous (fixed) (progressive) B42.1
  pulmonary B42.0
  specified NEC B42.89
Spots, spotting (in) (of)
  Bitot's (*see also* Pigmentation, conjunctiva)
    in the young child E50.1
      vitamin A deficiency E50.1
  café, au lait L81.3
  Cayenne pepper I78.1
  cotton wool, retina — *see* Occlusion, artery, retina
  de Morgan's (senile angiomas) I78.1
  Fuchs' black (myopic) (*see also* Myopia, degenerative) H44.2- ☑
  intermenstrual (regular) N92.0
    irregular N92.1
  Koplik's B05.9
  liver L81.4
  pregnancy O26.85- ☑
  purpuric R23.3
  ruby I78.1
Spotted fever — *see* Fever, spotted N92.3
Sprain (joint) (ligament)
  acromioclavicular joint or ligament S43.5- ☑
  ankle S93.40- ☑
    calcaneofibular ligament S93.41- ☑
    deltoid ligament S93.42- ☑
    internal collateral ligament — *see* Sprain, ankle, specified ligament NEC
    specified ligament NEC S93.49- ☑
    talofibular ligament — *see* Sprain, ankle, specified ligament NEC
    tibiofibular ligament S93.43- ☑
  anterior longitudinal, cervical S13.4 ☑
  atlas, atlanto-axial, atlanto-occipital S13.4 ☑
  breast bone — *see* Sprain, sternum
  calcaneofibular — *see* Sprain, ankle
  carpal — *see* Sprain, wrist
  carpometacarpal — *see* Sprain, hand, specified site NEC
  cartilage
    costal S23.41 ☑
    semilunar (knee) — *see* Sprain, knee, specified site NEC
      with current tear — *see* Tear, meniscus
    thyroid region S13.5 ☑
    xiphoid — *see* Sprain, sternum
  cervical, cervicodorsal, cervicothoracic S13.4 ☑
  chondrosternal S23.421 ☑
  coracoclavicular S43.8- ☑
  coracohumeral S43.41- ☑
  coronary, knee — *see* Sprain, knee, specified site NEC
  costal cartilage S23.41 ☑
  cricoarytenoid articulation or ligament S13.5 ☑
  cricothyroid articulation S13.5 ☑
  cruciate, knee — *see* Sprain, knee, cruciate
  deltoid, ankle — *see* Sprain, ankle
  dorsal (spine) S23.3 ☑
  elbow S53.40- ☑

☟ Subterms under main terms may continue to next column or page   ☑ Additional Character Required — Refer to the Tabular List for Character Selection   289

Spondylitis — Sprain

Sprain — continued
  elbow — continued
    radial collateral ligament S53.43- ☑
    radiohumeral S53.41- ☑
    rupture
      radial collateral ligament — see Rupture, traumatic, ligament, radial collateral
      ulnar collateral ligament — see Rupture, traumatic, ligament, ulnar collateral
    specified type NEC S53.49- ☑
    ulnar collateral ligament S53.44- ☑
    ulnohumeral S53.42- ☑
  femur, head — see Sprain, hip
  fibular collateral, knee — see Sprain, knee, collateral
  fibulocalcaneal — see Sprain, ankle
  finger(s) S63.61- ☑
    index S63.61- ☑
    interphalangeal (joint) S63.63- ☑
      index S63.63- ☑
      little S63.63- ☑
      middle S63.63- ☑
      ring S63.63- ☑
    little S63.61- ☑
    metacarpophalangeal (joint) S63.65- ☑
    middle S63.61- ☑
    ring S63.61- ☑
    specified site NEC S63.69- ☑
      index S63.69- ☑
      little S63.69- ☑
      middle S63.69- ☑
      ring S63.69- ☑
  foot S93.60- ☑
    specified ligament NEC S93.69- ☑
    tarsal ligament S93.61- ☑
    tarsometatarsal ligament S93.62- ☑
    toe — see Sprain, toe
  hand S63.9- ☑
    finger — see Sprain, finger
    specified site NEC — see subcategory S63.8 ☑
    thumb — see Sprain, thumb
  head S03.9 ☑
  hip S73.10- ☑
    iliofemoral ligament S73.11- ☑
    ischiocapsular (ligament) S73.12- ☑
    specified NEC S73.19- ☑
  iliofemoral — see Sprain, hip
  innominate
    acetabulum — see Sprain, hip
    sacral junction S33.6 ☑
  internal
    collateral, ankle — see Sprain, ankle
    semilunar cartilage — see Sprain, knee, specified site NEC
  interphalangeal
    finger — see Sprain, finger, interphalangeal (joint)
    toe — see Sprain, toe, interphalangeal joint
  ischiocapsular — see Sprain, hip
  ischiofemoral — see Sprain, hip
  jaw (articular disc) (cartilage) (meniscus) S03.4- ☑
    old M26.69
  knee S83.9- ☑
    collateral ligament S83.40- ☑
      lateral (fibular) S83.42- ☑
      medial (tibial) S83.41- ☑
    cruciate ligament S83.50- ☑
      anterior S83.51- ☑
      posterior S83.52- ☑
    lateral (fibular) collateral ligament S83.42- ☑
    medial (tibial) collateral ligament S83.41- ☑
    patellar ligament S76.11- ☑
    specified site NEC S83.8X- ☑
    superior tibiofibular joint (ligament) S83.6- ☑
  lateral collateral, knee — see Sprain, knee, collateral
  lumbar (spine) S33.5 ☑
  lumbosacral S33.9 ☑
  mandible (articular disc) S03.4- ☑
    old M26.69
  medial collateral, knee — see Sprain, knee, collateral
  meniscus
    jaw S03.4- ☑
      old M26.69
    knee — see Sprain, knee, specified site NEC
      with current tear — see Tear, meniscus
      old — see Derangement, knee, meniscus, due to old tear
    mandible S03.4- ☑

Sprain — continued
  meniscus — continued
    mandible — continued
      old M26.69
  metacarpal (distal) (proximal) — see Sprain, hand, specified site NEC
  metacarpophalangeal — see Sprain, finger, metacarpophalangeal (joint)
  metatarsophalangeal — see Sprain, toe, metatarsophalangeal joint
  midcarpal — see Sprain, hand, specified site NEC
  midtarsal — see Sprain, foot, specified site NEC
  neck S13.9 ☑
    anterior longitudinal cervical ligament S13.4 ☑
    atlanto-axial joint S13.4 ☑
    atlanto-occipital joint S13.4 ☑
    cervical spine S13.4 ☑
    cricoarytenoid ligament S13.5 ☑
    cricothyroid ligament S13.5 ☑
    specified site NEC S13.8 ☑
    thyroid region (cartilage) S13.5 ☑
  nose S03.8 ☑
  orbicular, hip — see Sprain, hip
  patella — see Sprain, knee, specified site NEC
  patellar ligament S76.11- ☑
  pelvis NEC S33.8 ☑
  phalanx
    finger — see Sprain, finger
    toe — see Sprain, toe
  pubofemoral — see Sprain, hip
  radiocarpal — see Sprain, wrist
  radiohumeral — see Sprain, elbow
  radius, collateral — see Rupture, traumatic, ligament, radial collateral
  rib (cage) S23.41 ☑
  rotator cuff (capsule) S43.42- ☑
  sacroiliac (region)
    chronic or old — see subcategory M53.2 ☑
    joint S33.6 ☑
  scaphoid (hand) — see Sprain, hand, specified site NEC
  scapula (r) — see Sprain, shoulder girdle, specified site NEC
  semilunar cartilage (knee) — see Sprain, knee, specified site NEC
    with current tear — see Tear, meniscus
    old — see Derangement, knee, meniscus, due to old tear
  shoulder joint S43.40- ☑
    acromioclavicular joint (ligament) — see Sprain, acromioclavicular joint
    blade — see Sprain, shoulder, girdle, specified site NEC
    coracoclavicular joint (ligament) — see Sprain, coracoclavicular joint
    coracohumeral ligament — see Sprain, coracohumeral joint
    girdle S43.9- ☑
      specified site NEC S43.8- ☑
    rotator cuff — see Sprain, rotator cuff
    specified site NEC S43.49- ☑
    sternoclavicular joint (ligament) — see Sprain, sternoclavicular joint
  spine
    cervical S13.4 ☑
    lumbar S33.5 ☑
    thoracic S23.3 ☑
  sternoclavicular joint S43.6- ☑
  sternum S23.429 ☑
    chondrosternal joint S23.421 ☑
    specified site NEC S23.428 ☑
    sternoclavicular (joint) (ligament) S23.420 ☑
  symphysis
    jaw S03.4- ☑
      old M26.69
    mandibular S03.4- ☑
      old M26.69
  talofibular — see Sprain, ankle
  tarsal — see Sprain, foot, specified site NEC
  tarsometatarsal — see Sprain, foot, specified site NEC
  temporomandibular S03.4- ☑
    old M26.69
  thorax S23.9 ☑
    ribs S23.41 ☑
    specified site NEC S23.8 ☑
    spine S23.3 ☑
    sternum — see Sprain, sternum

Sprain — continued
  thumb S63.60- ☑
    interphalangeal (joint) S63.62- ☑
    metacarpophalangeal (joint) S63.64- ☑
    specified site NEC S63.68- ☑
  thyroid cartilage or region S13.5 ☑
  tibia (proximal end) — see Sprain, knee, specified site NEC
  tibial collateral, knee — see Sprain, knee, collateral
  tibiofibular
    distal — see Sprain, ankle
    superior — see Sprain, knee, specified site NEC
  toe(s) S93.50- ☑
    great S93.50- ☑
    interphalangeal joint S93.51- ☑
      great S93.51- ☑
      lesser S93.51- ☑
    lesser S93.50- ☑
    metatarsophalangeal joint S93.52- ☑
      great S93.52- ☑
      lesser S93.52- ☑
  ulna, collateral — see Rupture, traumatic, ligament, ulnar collateral
  ulnohumeral — see Sprain, elbow
  wrist S63.50- ☑
    carpal S63.51- ☑
    radiocarpal S63.52- ☑
    specified site NEC S63.59- ☑
  xiphoid cartilage — see Sprain, sternum
Sprengel's deformity (congenital) Q74.0
Sprue (tropical) K90.1
  celiac K90.0
  idiopathic K90.49
  meaning thrush B37.0
  nontropical K90.0
Spur, bone (see also Enthesopathy)
  calcaneal M77.3- ☑
  iliac crest M76.2- ☑
  nose (septum) J34.89
Spurway's syndrome Q78.0
Sputum
  abnormal (amount) (color) (odor) (purulent) R09.3
  blood-stained R04.2
  excessive (cause unknown) R09.3
Squamous (see also condition)
  epithelium in
    cervical canal (congenital) Q51.828
    uterine mucosa (congenital) Q51.818
Squashed nose M95.0
  congenital Q67.4
Squeeze, diver's T70.3 ☑
Squint (see also Strabismus)
  accommodative — see Strabismus, convergent concomitant
SSADHD (succinic semialdehyde dehydrogenase deficiency) E72.81
St. Hubert's disease A82.9
Stab (see also Laceration)
  internal organs — see Injury, by site
Stafne's cyst or cavity M27.0
Staggering gait R26.0
  hysterical F44.4
Staghorn calculus — see Calculus, kidney
Stähli's line (cornea) (pigment) — see Pigmentation, cornea, anterior
Stain, staining
  meconium (newborn) P96.83
  port wine Q82.5
  tooth, teeth (hard tissues) (extrinsic) K03.6
    due to
      accretions K03.6
      deposits (betel) (black) (green) (materia alba) (orange) (soft) (tobacco) K03.6
      metals (copper) (silver) K03.7
      nicotine K03.6
      pulpal bleeding K03.7
      tobacco K03.6
    intrinsic K00.8
Stammering (see also Disorder, fluency) F80.81
Standstill
  auricular I45.5
  cardiac — see Arrest, cardiac
  sinoatrial I45.5
  ventricular — see Arrest, cardiac
Stannosis J63.5
Stanton's disease — see Melioidosis

☑ Additional Character Required — Refer to the Tabular List for Character Selection   ▽ Subterms under main terms may continue to next column or page

Staphylitis (acute) (catarrhal) (chronic) (gangrenous) (membranous) (suppurative) (ulcerative) K12.2
Staphylococcal scalded skin syndrome L00
Staphylococcemia A41.2
Staphylococcus, staphylococcal (see also condition)
  as cause of disease classified elsewhere B95.8
    aureus (methicillin susceptible) (MSSA) B95.61
      methicillin resistant (MRSA) B95.62
    specified NEC, as cause of disease classified elsewhere B95.7
Staphyloma (sclera)
  cornea H18.72- ☑
  equatorial H15.81- ☑
  localized (anterior) H15.82- ☑
  posticum H15.83- ☑
  ring H15.85- ☑
Stargardt's disease — see Dystrophy, retina
Starvation (inanition) (due to lack of food) T73.0 ☑
  edema — see Malnutrition, severe
Stasis
  bile (noncalculous) K83.1
  bronchus J98.09
    with infection — see Bronchitis
  cardiac — see Failure, heart, congestive
  cecum K59.8
  colon K59.8
  dermatitis I87.2
    with
      varicose ulcer — see Varix, leg, with ulcer, with inflammation
      varicose veins — see Varix, leg, with, inflammation
      due to postthrombotic syndrome — see Syndrome, postthrombotic
  duodenal K31.5
  eczema — see Varix, leg, with, inflammation
  edema — see Hypertension, venous (chronic), idiopathic
  foot T69.0- ☑
  ileocecal coil K59.8
  ileum K59.8
  intestinal K59.8
  jejunum K59.8
  kidney N19
  liver (cirrhotic) K76.1
  lymphatic I89.8
  pneumonia J18.2
  pulmonary — see Edema, lung
  rectal K59.8
  renal N19
    tubular N17.0
  ulcer — see Varix, leg, with, ulcer
    without varicose veins I87.2
  urine — see Retention, urine
  venous I87.8
State (of)
  affective and paranoid, mixed, organic psychotic F06.8
  agitated R45.1
    acute reaction to stress F43.0
  anxiety (neurotic) F41.1
  apprehension F41.1
  burn-out Z73.0
  climacteric, female Z78.0
    symptomatic N95.1
  compulsive F42.8
    mixed with obsessional thoughts F42.2
  confusional (psychogenic) F44.89
    acute (see also Delirium)
      with
        arteriosclerotic dementia F01.50
          with behavioral disturbance F01.51
        senility or dementia F05
          alcoholic F10.231
      epileptic F05
      reactive (from emotional stress, psychological trauma) F44.89
    subacute — see Delirium
  convulsive — see Convulsions
  crisis F43.0
  depressive F32.9
    neurotic F34.1
  dissociative F44.9
  emotional shock (stress) R45.7
  hypercoagulation — see Hypercoagulable
  locked-in G83.5
  menopausal Z78.0
    symptomatic N95.1
  neurotic F48.9

State — continued
  neurotic — continued
    with depersonalization F48.1
    obsessional F42.8
  oneiroid (schizophrenia-like) F23
  organic
    hallucinatory (nonalcoholic) F06.0
    paranoid (-hallucinatory) F06.2
  panic F41.0
  paranoid F22
    climacteric F22
    involutional F22
    menopausal F22
    organic F06.2
    senile F03 ☑
    simple F22
  persistent vegetative R40.3
  phobic F40.9
  postleukotomy F07.0
  pregnant
    gestational carrier Z33.3
    incidental Z33.1
  psychogenic, twilight F44.89
  psychopathic (constitutional) F60.2
  psychotic, organic (see also Psychosis, organic)
    mixed paranoid and affective F06.8
    senile or presenile F03 ☑
    transient NEC F06.8
      with
        depression F06.31
        hallucinations F06.0
  residual schizophrenic F20.5
  restlessness R45.1
  stress (emotional) R45.7
  tension (mental) F48.9
    specified NEC F48.8
  transient organic psychotic NEC F06.8
    depressive type F06.31
    hallucinatory type F06.0
  twilight
    epileptic F05
    psychogenic F44.89
  vegetative, persistent R40.3
  vital exhaustion Z73.0
  withdrawal, — see Withdrawal, state
Status (post) (see also Presence (of))
  absence, epileptic — see Epilepsy, by type, with status epilepticus
  administration of tPA (rtPA) in a different facility within the last 24 hours prior to admission to current facility Z92.82
  adrenalectomy (unilateral) (bilateral) E89.6
  anastomosis Z98.0
  anginosus I20.9
  angioplasty (peripheral) Z98.62
    with implant Z95.820
    coronary artery Z98.61
      with implant Z95.5
  aortocoronary bypass Z95.1
  arthrodesis Z98.1
  artificial opening (of) Z93.9
    gastrointestinal tract Z93.4
    specified NEC Z93.8
    urinary tract Z93.6
    vagina Z93.8
  asthmaticus — see Asthma, by type, with status asthmaticus
  awaiting organ transplant Z76.82
  bariatric surgery Z98.84
  bed confinement Z74.01
  bleb, filtering (vitreous), after glaucoma surgery Z98.83
  breast implant Z98.82
    removal Z98.86
  cataract extraction Z98.4- ☑
  cholecystectomy Z90.49
  clitorectomy N90.811
    with excision of labia minora N90.812
  colectomy (complete) (partial) Z90.49
  colonization — see Carrier (suspected) of
  colostomy Z93.3
  convulsivus idiopathicus — see Epilepsy, by type, with status epilepticus
  coronary artery angioplasty — see Status, angioplasty, coronary artery
  coronary artery bypass graft Z95.1
  cystectomy (urinary bladder) Z90.6
  cystostomy Z93.50
    appendico-vesicostomy Z93.52

Status — continued
  cystostomy — continued
    cutaneous Z93.51
    specified NEC Z93.59
  delinquent immunization Z28.3
  dental Z98.818
    crown Z98.811
    fillings Z98.811
    restoration Z98.811
    sealant Z98.810
    specified NEC Z98.818
  deployment (current) (military) Z56.82
  dialysis (hemodialysis) (peritoneal) Z99.2
  do not resuscitate (DNR) Z66
  donor — see Donor
  embedded fragments — see Retained, foreign body fragments (type of)
  embedded splinter — see Retained, foreign body fragments (type of)
  enterostomy Z93.4
  epileptic, epilepticus (see also Epilepsy, by type, with status epilepticus) G40.901
  estrogen receptor
    negative Z17.1
    positive Z17.0
  female genital cutting — see Female genital mutilation status
  female genital mutilation — see Female genital mutilation status
  filtering (vitreous) bleb after glaucoma surgery Z98.83
  gastrectomy (complete) (partial) Z90.3
  gastric banding Z98.84
  gastric bypass for obesity Z98.84
  gastrostomy Z93.1
  human immunodeficiency virus (HIV) infection, asymptomatic Z21
  hysterectomy (complete) (total) Z90.710
    partial (with remaining cervial stump) Z90.711
  ileostomy Z93.2
  implant
    breast Z98.82
  infibulation N90.813
  intestinal bypass Z98.0
  jejunostomy Z93.4
  lapsed immunization schedule Z28.3
  laryngectomy Z90.02
  lymphaticus E32.8
  malignancy
    castrate resistant prostate Z19.2
    hormone resistant Z19.2
    hormone sensitive Z19.1
  marmoratus G80.3
  mastectomy (unilateral) (bilateral) Z90.1- ☑
  military deployment status (current) Z56.82
    in theater or in support of military war, peacekeeping and humanitarian operations Z56.82
  nephrectomy (unilateral) (bilateral) Z90.5
  nephrostomy Z93.6
  obesity surgery Z98.84
  oophorectomy
    bilateral Z90.722
    unilateral Z90.721
  organ replacement
    by artificial or mechanical device or prosthesis of
      artery Z95.828
      bladder Z96.0
      blood vessel Z95.828
      breast Z97.8
      eye globe Z97.0
      heart Z95.812
        valve Z95.2
      intestine Z97.8
      joint Z96.60
        hip — see Presence, hip joint implant
        knee — see Presence, knee joint implant
        specified site NEC Z96.698
      kidney Z97.8
      larynx Z96.3
      lens Z96.1
      limbs — see Presence, artificial, limb
      liver Z97.8
      lung Z97.8
      pancreas Z97.8
    by organ transplant (heterologous)(homologous) — see Transplant
  pacemaker
    brain Z96.89
    cardiac Z95.0

⬇ Subterms under main terms may continue to next column or page   ☑ Additional Character Required — Refer to the Tabular List for Character Selection   291

Staphylitis — Status

Status — *continued*
  pacemaker — *continued*
    specified NEC Z96.89
  pancreatectomy Z90.410
    complete Z90.410
    partial Z90.411
    total Z90.410
  physical restraint Z78.1
  pneumonectomy (complete) (partial) Z90.2
  pneumothorax, therapeutic Z98.3
  postcommotio cerebri F07.81
  postoperative (postprocedural) NEC Z98.890
    breast implant Z98.82
    dental Z98.818
      crown Z98.811
      fillings Z98.811
      restoration Z98.811
      sealant Z98.810
      specified NEC Z98.818
    pneumothorax, therapeutic Z98.3
    uterine scar Z98.891
  postpartum (routine follow-up) Z39.2
    care immediately after delivery Z39.0
  postsurgical (postprocedural) NEC Z98.890
    pneumothorax, therapeutic Z98.3
  pregnancy, incidental Z33.1
  prosthesis coronary angioplasty Z95.5
  pseudophakia Z96.1
  renal dialysis (hemodialysis) (peritoneal) Z99.2
  retained foreign body — *see* Retained, foreign body fragments (type of)
  reversed jejunal transposition (for bypass) Z98.0
  salpingo-oophorectomy
    bilateral Z90.722
    unilateral Z90.721
  sex reassignment surgery status Z87.890
  shunt
    arteriovenous (for dialysis) Z99.2
    cerebrospinal fluid Z98.2
    ventricular (communicating) (for drainage) Z98.2
  splenectomy Z90.81
  thymicolymphaticus E32.8
  thymicus E32.8
  thymolymphaticus E32.8
  thyroidectomy (hypothyroidism) E89.0
  tooth (teeth) extraction (*see also* Absence, teeth, acquired) K08.409
  tPA (rtPA) administration in a different facility within the last 24 hours prior to admission to current facility Z92.82
  tracheostomy Z93.0
  transplant — *see* Transplant
    organ removed Z98.85
  tubal ligation Z98.51
  underimmunization Z28.3
  ureterostomy Z93.6
  urethrostomy Z93.6
  vagina, artificial Z93.8
  vasectomy Z98.52
  wheelchair confinement Z99.3
Stealing
  child problem F91.8
    in company with others Z72.810
  pathological (compulsive) F63.2
Steam burn — *see* Burn
Steatocystoma multiplex L72.2
Steatohepatitis (nonalcoholic) (NASH) K75.81
Steatoma L72.3
  eyelid (cystic) — *see* Dermatosis, eyelid
    infected — *see* Hordeolum
Steatorrhea (chronic) K90.9
  with lacteal obstruction K90.2
  idiopathic (adult) (infantile) K90.9
  pancreatic K90.3
  primary K90.0
  tropical K90.1
Steatosis E88.89
  heart — *see* Degeneration, myocardial
  kidney N28.89
  liver NEC K76.0
Steele-Richardson-Olszewski disease or syndrome G23.1
Steinbrocker's syndrome G90.8
Steinert's disease G71.11
Stein-Leventhal syndrome E28.2
Stein's syndrome E28.2
STEMI (*see also* Infarct, myocardium, ST elevation) I21.3
Stenocardia I20.8

Stenocephaly Q75.8
Stenosis, stenotic (cicatricial) (*see also* Stricture)
  ampulla of Vater K83.1
  anus, anal (canal) (sphincter) K62.4
    and rectum K62.4
    congenital Q42.3
      with fistula Q42.2
  aorta (ascending) (supraventricular) (congenital) Q25.1
    arteriosclerotic I70.0
    calcified I70.0
    supravalvular Q25.3
  aortic (valve) I35.0
    with insufficiency I35.2
    congenital Q23.0
    rheumatic I06.0
      with
        incompetency, insufficiency or regurgitation I06.2
          with mitral (valve) disease I08.0
            with tricuspid (valve) disease I08.3
        mitral (valve) disease I08.0
          with tricuspid (valve) disease I08.3
        tricuspid (valve) disease I08.2
          with mitral (valve) disease I08.3
    specified cause NEC I35.0
    syphilitic A52.03
  aqueduct of Sylvius (congenital) Q03.0
    with spina bifida — *see* Spina bifida, by site, with hydrocephalus
    acquired G91.1
  artery NEC (*see also* Arteriosclerosis) I77.1
    celiac I77.4
    cerebral — *see* Occlusion, artery, cerebral
    extremities — *see* Arteriosclerosis, extremities
    precerebral — *see* Occlusion, artery, precerebral
    pulmonary (congenital) Q25.6
      acquired I28.8
    renal I70.1
    stent
      coronary T82.855 ☑
      peripheral T82.856 ☑
  bile duct (common) (hepatic) K83.1
    congenital Q44.3
  bladder-neck (acquired) N32.0
    congenital Q64.31
  brain G93.89
  bronchus J98.09
    congenital Q32.3
    syphilitic A52.72
  cardia (stomach) K22.2
    congenital Q39.3
  cardiovascular — *see* Disease, cardiovascular
  caudal M48.08
  cervix, cervical (canal) N88.2
    congenital Q51.828
    in pregnancy or childbirth — *see* Pregnancy, complicated by, abnormal cervix
  colon (*see also* Obstruction, intestine)
    congenital Q42.9
      specified NEC Q42.8
  colostomy K94.03
  common (bile) duct K83.1
    congenital Q44.3
  coronary (artery) — *see* Disease, heart, ischemic, atherosclerotic
  cystic duct — *see* Obstruction, gallbladder
  due to presence of device, implant or graft (*see also* Complications, by site and type, specified NEC) T85.858 ☑
    arterial graft NEC T82.858 ☑
    breast (implant) T85.858 ☑
    catheter T85.858 ☑
      dialysis (renal) T82.858 ☑
        intraperitoneal T85.858 ☑
      infusion NEC T82.858 ☑
        spinal (epidural) (subdural) T85.850 ☑
      urinary (indwelling) T83.85 ☑
    fixation, internal (orthopedic) NEC T84.85 ☑
    gastrointestinal (bile duct) (esophagus) T85.858 ☑
    genital NEC T83.85 ☑
    heart NEC T82.857 ☑
    joint prosthesis T84.85 ☑
    ocular (corneal graft) (orbital implant) NEC T85.858 ☑
    orthopedic NEC T84.85 ☑
    specified NEC T85.858 ☑
    urinary NEC T83.85 ☑
    vascular NEC T82.858 ☑

Stenosis, stenotic — *continued*
  due to presence of device, implant or graft (*see also* Complications, by site and type, specified) — *continued*
    ventricular intracranial shunt T85.850 ☑
  duodenum K31.5
    congenital Q41.0
  ejaculatory duct NEC N50.89
    stent
      vascular
        end stent
          adjacent to stent — *see* Arteriosclerosis
          within the stent
            coronary T82.855 ☑
            peripheral T82.856 ☑
        in stent
          coronary vessel T82.855 ☑
          peripheral vessel T82.856 ☑
  endocervical os — *see* Stenosis, cervix
  enterostomy K94.13
  esophagus K22.2
    congenital Q39.3
    syphilitic A52.79
      congenital A50.59 [K23]
  eustachian tube — *see* Obstruction, eustachian tube
  external ear canal (acquired) H61.30- ☑
    congenital Q16.1
    due to
      inflammation H61.32- ☑
      trauma H61.31- ☑
    postprocedural H95.81- ☑
    specified cause NEC H61.39- ☑
  gallbladder — *see* Obstruction, gallbladder
  glottis J38.6
  heart valve (congenital) Q24.8
    aortic Q23.0
    mitral Q23.2
    pulmonary Q22.1
    tricuspid Q22.4
  hepatic duct K83.1
  hymen N89.6
  hypertrophic subaortic (idiopathic) I42.1
  ileum (*see also* Obstruction, intestine, specified NEC) K56.699
    congenital Q41.2
  infundibulum cardia Q24.3
  intervertebral foramina (*see also* Lesion, biomechanical, specified NEC)
    connective tissue M99.79
      abdomen M99.79
      cervical region M99.71
      cervicothoracic M99.71
      head region M99.70
      lumbar region M99.73
      lumbosacral M99.73
      occipitocervical M99.70
      sacral region M99.74
      sacrococcygeal M99.74
      sacroiliac M99.74
      specified NEC M99.79
      thoracic region M99.72
      thoracolumbar M99.72
    disc M99.79
      abdomen M99.79
      cervical region M99.71
      cervicothoracic M99.71
      head region M99.70
      lower extremity M99.76
      lumbar region M99.73
      lumbosacral M99.73
      occipitocervical M99.70
      pelvic M99.75
      rib cage M99.78
      sacral region M99.74
      sacrococcygeal M99.74
      sacroiliac M99.74
      specified NEC M99.79
      thoracic region M99.72
      thoracolumbar M99.72
      upper extremity M99.77
    osseous M99.69
      abdomen M99.69
      cervical region M99.61
      cervicothoracic M99.61
      head region M99.60
      lower extremity M99.66
      lumbar region M99.63
      lumbosacral M99.63

☑ **Additional Character Required** — Refer to the Tabular List for Character Selection   ▽ **Subterms under main terms may continue to next column or page**

Stenosis, stenotic — *continued*
  intervertebral foramina (*see also* Lesion, biomechanical, specified) — *continued*
    osseous — *continued*
      occipitocervical M99.60
      pelvic M99.65
      rib cage M99.68
      sacral region M99.64
      sacrococcygeal M99.64
      sacroiliac M99.64
      specified NEC M99.69
      thoracic region M99.62
      thoracolumbar M99.62
      upper extremity M99.67
    subluxation — *see* Stenosis, intervertebral foramina, osseous
  intestine (*see also* Obstruction, intestine)
    congenital (small) Q41.9
      large Q42.9
        specified NEC Q42.8
      specified NEC Q41.8
    jejunum (*see also* Obstruction, intestine, specified NEC) K56.699
      congenital Q41.1
  lacrimal (passage)
    canaliculi H04.54- ☑
    congenital Q10.5
    duct H04.55- ☑
    punctum H04.56- ☑
    sac H04.57- ☑
  lacrimonasal duct — *see* Stenosis, lacrimal, duct
    congenital Q10.5
  larynx J38.6
    congenital NEC Q31.8
      subglottic Q31.1
    syphilitic A52.73
      congenital A50.59 [J99]
  mitral (chronic) (inactive) (valve) I05.0
    with
      aortic valve disease I08.0
      incompetency, insufficiency or regurgitation I05.2
    active or acute I01.1
      with rheumatic or Sydenham's chorea I02.0
    congenital Q23.2
    specified cause, except rheumatic I34.2
    syphilitic A52.03
  myocardium, myocardial (*see also* Degeneration, myocardial)
    hypertrophic subaortic (idiopathic) I42.1
  nares (anterior) (posterior) J34.89
    congenital Q30.0
  nasal duct (*see also* Stenosis, lacrimal, duct)
    congenital Q10.5
  nasolacrimal duct (*see also* Stenosis, lacrimal, duct)
    congenital Q10.5
  neural canal (*see also* Lesion, biomechanical, specified NEC)
    connective tissue M99.49
      abdomen M99.49
      cervical region M99.41
      cervicothoracic M99.41
      head region M99.40
      lower extremity M99.46
      lumbar region M99.43
      lumbosacral M99.43
      occipitocervical M99.40
      pelvic M99.45
      rib cage M99.48
      sacral region M99.44
      sacrococcygeal M99.44
      sacroiliac M99.44
      specified NEC M99.49
      thoracic region M99.42
      thoracolumbar M99.42
      upper extremity M99.47
    intervertebral disc M99.59
      abdomen M99.59
      cervical region M99.51
      cervicothoracic M99.51
      head region M99.50
      lower extremity M99.56
      lumbar region M99.53
      lumbosacral M99.53
      occipitocervical M99.50
      pelvic M99.55
      rib cage M99.58
      sacral region M99.54

Stenosis, stenotic — *continued*
  neural canal (*see also* Lesion, biomechanical, specified) — *continued*
    intervertebral disc — *continued*
      sacrococcygeal M99.54
      sacroiliac M99.54
      specified NEC M99.59
      thoracic region M99.52
      thoracolumbar M99.52
      upper extremity M99.57
    osseous M99.39
      abdomen M99.39
      cervical region M99.31
      cervicothoracic M99.31
      head region M99.30
      lower extremity M99.36
      lumbar region M99.33
      lumbosacral M99.33
      occipitocervical M99.30
      pelvic M99.35
      rib cage M99.38
      sacral region M99.34
      sacrococcygeal M99.34
      sacroiliac M99.34
      specified NEC M99.39
      thoracic region M99.32
      thoracolumbar M99.32
      upper extremity M99.37
    subluxation M99.29
      cervical region M99.21
      cervicothoracic M99.21
      head region M99.20
      lower extremity M99.26
      lumbar region M99.23
      lumbosacral M99.23
      occipitocervical M99.20
      pelvic M99.25
      rib cage M99.28
      sacral region M99.24
      sacrococcygeal M99.24
      sacroiliac M99.24
      specified NEC M99.29
      thoracic region M99.22
      thoracolumbar M99.22
      upper extremity M99.27
  organ or site, congenital NEC — *see* Atresia, by site
  papilla of Vater K83.1
  pulmonary (artery) (congenital) Q25.6
    with ventricular septal defect, transposition of aorta, and hypertrophy of right ventricle Q21.3
    acquired I28.8
    in tetralogy of Fallot Q21.3
    infundibular Q24.3
    subvalvular Q24.3
    supravalvular Q25.6
    valve I37.0
      with insufficiency I37.2
      congenital Q22.1
      rheumatic I09.89
        with aortic, mitral or tricuspid (valve) disease I08.8
    vein, acquired I28.8
    vessel NEC I28.8
  pulmonic (congenital) Q22.1
    infundibular Q24.3
    subvalvular Q24.3
  pylorus (hypertrophic) (acquired) K31.1
    adult K31.1
    congenital Q40.0
    infantile Q40.0
  rectum (sphincter) — *see* Stricture, rectum
  renal artery I70.1
    congenital Q27.1
  salivary duct (any) K11.8
  sphincter of Oddi K83.1
  spinal M48.00
    cervical region M48.02
    cervicothoracic region M48.03
    lumbar region (NOS) (without neurogenic claudication) M48.061
      with neurogenic claudication M48.062
    lumbosacral region M48.07
    occipito-atlanto-axial region M48.01
    sacrococcygeal region M48.08
    thoracic region M48.04
    thoracolumbar region M48.05
  stomach, hourglass K31.2
  subaortic (congenital) Q24.4
    hypertrophic (idiopathic) I42.1

Stenosis, stenotic — *continued*
  subglottic J38.6
    congenital Q31.1
    postprocedural J95.5
  trachea J39.8
    congenital Q32.1
    syphilitic A52.73
    tuberculous NEC A15.5
  tracheostomy J95.03
  tricuspid (valve) I07.0
    with
      aortic (valve) disease I08.2
      incompetency, insufficiency or regurgitation I07.2
        with aortic (valve) disease I08.2
          with mitral (valve) disease I08.3
      mitral (valve) disease I08.1
        with aortic (valve) disease I08.3
    congenital Q22.4
    nonrheumatic I36.0
      with insufficiency I36.2
  tubal N97.1
  ureter — *see* Atresia, ureter
  ureteropelvic junction, congenital Q62.11
  ureterovesical orifice, congenital Q62.12
  urethra (valve) (*see also* Stricture, urethra)
    congenital Q64.32
  urinary meatus, congenital Q64.33
  vagina N89.5
    congenital Q52.4
    in pregnancy — *see* Pregnancy, complicated by, abnormal vagina
    causing obstructed labor O65.5
  valve (cardiac) (heart) (*see also* Endocarditis) I38
    congenital Q24.8
      aortic Q23.0
      mitral Q23.2
      pulmonary Q22.1
      tricuspid Q22.4
  vena cava (inferior) (superior) I87.1
    congenital Q26.0
  vesicourethral orifice Q64.31
  vulva N90.5

Stent jail T82.897 ☑
Stercolith (impaction) K56.41
  appendix K38.1
Stercoraceous, stercoral ulcer K63.3
  anus or rectum K62.6
Stereotypies NEC F98.4
Sterility — *see* Infertility
Sterilization — *see* Encounter (for), sterilization
Sternalgia — *see* Angina
Sternopagus Q89.4
Sternum bifidum Q76.7
Steroid
  effects (adverse) (adrenocortical) (iatrogenic)
    cushingoid E24.2
      correct substance properly administered — *see* Table of Drugs and Chemicals, by drug, adverse effect
      overdose or wrong substance given or taken — *see* Table of Drugs and Chemicals, by drug, poisoning
    diabetes — *see* subcategory E09 ☑
      correct substance properly administered — *see* Table of Drugs and Chemicals, by drug, adverse effect
      overdose or wrong substance given or taken — *see* Table of Drugs and Chemicals, by drug, poisoning
    fever R50.2
    insufficiency E27.3
      correct substance properly administered — *see* Table of Drugs and Chemicals, by drug, adverse effect
      overdose or wrong substance given or taken — *see* Table of Drugs and Chemicals, by drug, poisoning
  responder H40.04- ☑
Stevens-Johnson disease or syndrome L51.1
  toxic epidermal necrolysis overlap L51.3
Stewart-Morel syndrome M85.2
Sticker's disease B08.3
Sticky eye — *see* Conjunctivitis, acute, mucopurulent
Stieda's disease — *see* Bursitis, tibial collateral
Stiff neck — *see* Torticollis
Stiff-man syndrome G25.82
Stiffness, joint NEC M25.60

Stiffness, joint — *continued*
    ankle M25.67- ☑
    ankylosis — *see* Ankylosis, joint
    contracture — *see* Contraction, joint
    elbow M25.62- ☑
    foot M25.67- ☑
    hand M25.64- ☑
    hip M25.65- ☑
    knee M25.66- ☑
    shoulder M25.61- ☑
    wrist M25.63- ☑
Stigmata congenital syphilis A50.59
Stillbirth P95
Still-Felty syndrome — *see* Felty's syndrome
Still's disease or syndrome (juvenile) M08.20
    adult-onset M06.1
    ankle M08.27- ☑
    elbow M08.22- ☑
    foot joint M08.27- ☑
    hand joint M08.24- ☑
    hip M08.25- ☑
    knee M08.26- ☑
    multiple site M08.29
    shoulder M08.21- ☑
    vertebra M08.28
    wrist M08.23- ☑
Stimulation, ovary E28.1
Sting (venomous) (with allergic or anaphylactic shock)
        — *see* Table of Drugs and Chemicals, by animal or
        substance, poisoning
Stippled epiphyses Q78.8
Stitch
    abscess T81.41 ☑
    burst (in operation wound) — *see* Disruption, wound,
        operation
Stokes' disease E05.00
    with thyroid storm E05.01
Stokes-Adams disease or syndrome I45.9
Stokvis (-Talma) **disease** D74.8
Stoma malfunction
    colostomy K94.03
    enterostomy K94.13
    gastrostomy K94.23
    ileostomy K94.13
    tracheostomy J95.03
Stomach — *see* condition
Stomatitis (denture) (ulcerative) K12.1
    angular K13.0
        due to dietary or vitamin deficiency E53.0
    aphthous K12.0
    bovine B08.61
    candidal B37.0
    catarrhal K12.1
    diphtheritic A36.89
    due to
        dietary deficiency E53.0
        thrush B37.0
        vitamin deficiency
            B group NEC E53.9
            B2 (riboflavin) E53.0
    epidemic B08.8
    epizootic B08.8
    follicular K12.1
    gangrenous A69.0
    Geotrichum B48.3
    herpesviral, herpetic B00.2
    herpetiformis K12.0
    malignant K12.1
    membranous acute K12.1
    monilial B37.0
    mycotic B37.0
    necrotizing ulcerative A69.0
    parasitic B37.0
    septic K12.1
    spirochetal A69.1
    suppurative (acute) K12.2
    ulceromembranous A69.1
    vesicular K12.1
        with exanthem (enteroviral) B08.4
        virus disease A93.8
    Vincent's A69.1
Stomatocytosis D58.8
Stomatomycosis B37.0
Stomatorrhagia K13.79
Stone(s) (*see also* Calculus)
    bladder (diverticulum) N21.0
    cystine E72.09

Stone(s) — *continued*
    heart syndrome I50.1
    kidney N20.0
    prostate N42.0
    pulpal (dental) K04.2
    renal N20.0
    salivary gland or duct (any) K11.5
    urethra (impacted) N21.1
    urinary (duct) (impacted) (passage) N20.9
        bladder (diverticulum) N21.0
        lower tract N21.9
        specified NEC N21.8
    xanthine E79.8 [N22]
Stonecutter's lung J62.8
**Stonemason's asthma, disease, lung or pneumoco-
        niosis** J62.8
Stoppage
    heart — *see* Arrest, cardiac
    urine — *see* Retention, urine
Storm, thyroid — *see* Thyrotoxicosis
Strabismus (congenital) (nonparalytic) H50.9
    concomitant H50.40
        convergent — *see* Strabismus, convergent concomi-
            tant
        divergent — *see* Strabismus, divergent concomitant
    convergent concomitant H50.00
        accommodative component H50.43
        alternating H50.05
            with
                A pattern H50.06
                specified nonconcomitances NEC H50.08
                V pattern H50.07
        monocular H50.01- ☑
            with
                A pattern H50.02- ☑
                specified nonconcomitances NEC H50.04- ☑
                V pattern H50.03- ☑
            intermittent H50.31- ☑
                alternating H50.32
    cyclotropia H50.41 ☑
    divergent concomitant H50.10
        alternating H50.15
            with
                A pattern H50.16
                specified noncomitances NEC H50.18
                V pattern H50.17
        monocular H50.11- ☑
            with
                A pattern H50.12- ☑
                specified noncomitances NEC H50.14- ☑
                V pattern H50.13- ☑
            intermittent H50.33 ☑
                alternating H50.34
    Duane's syndrome H50.81- ☑
    due to adhesions, scars H50.69
    heterophoria H50.50
        alternating H50.55
        cyclophoria H50.54
        esophoria H50.51
        exophoria H50.52
        vertical H50.53
    heterotropia H50.40
        intermittent H50.30
    hypertropia H50.2- ☑
    hypotropia — *see* Hypertropia
    latent H50.50
    mechanical H50.60
        Brown's sheath syndrome H50.61- ☑
        specified type NEC H50.69
    monofixation syndrome H50.42
    paralytic H49.9
        abducens nerve H49.2- ☑
        fourth nerve H49.1- ☑
        Kearns-Sayre syndrome H49.81- ☑
        ophthalmoplegia (external)
            progressive H49.4- ☑
                with pigmentary retinopathy H49.81- ☑
            total H49.3- ☑
        sixth nerve H49.2- ☑
        specified type NEC H49.88- ☑
        third nerve H49.0- ☑
        trochlear nerve H49.1- ☑
    specified type NEC H50.89
    vertical H50.2- ☑
Strain
    back S39.012 ☑
    cervical S16.1 ☑

Strain — *continued*
    eye NEC — *see* Disturbance, vision, subjective
    heart — *see* Disease, heart
    low back S39.012 ☑
    mental NOS Z73.3
        work-related Z56.6
    muscle (tendon) — *see* Injury, muscle, by site, strain
    neck S16.1 ☑
    physical NOS Z73.3
        work-related Z56.6
    postural (*see also* Disorder, soft tissue, due to use)
    psychological NEC Z73.3
    tendon — *see* Injury, muscle, by site, strain
Straining, on urination R39.16
Strand, vitreous — *see* Opacity, vitreous, membranes
        and strands
Strangulation, strangulated (*see also* Asphyxia, trau-
        matic)
    appendix K38.8
    bladder-neck N32.0
    bowel or colon K56.2
    food or foreign body — *see* Foreign body, by site
    hemorrhoids — *see* Hemorrhoids, with complication
    hernia (*see also* Hernia, by site, with obstruction)
        with gangrene — *see* Hernia, by site, with gangrene
    intestine (large) (small) K56.2
        with hernia (*see also* Hernia, by site, with obstruc-
            tion)
            with gangrene — *see* Hernia, by site, with gan-
                grene
    mesentery K56.2
    mucus — *see* Asphyxia, mucus
    omentum K56.2
    organ or site, congenital NEC — *see* Atresia, by site
    ovary — *see* Torsion, ovary
    penis N48.89
        foreign body T19.4 ☑
    rupture — *see* Hernia, by site, with obstruction
    stomach due to hernia (*see also* Hernia, by site, with
        obstruction)
        with gangrene — *see* Hernia, by site, with gangrene
    vesicourethral orifice N32.0
Strangury R30.0
Straw itch B88.0
Strawberry
    gallbladder K82.4
    mark Q82.5
    tongue (red) (white) K14.3
Streak(s)
    macula, angioid H35.33
    ovarian Q50.32
Strephosymbolia F81.0
    secondary to organic lesion R48.8
Streptobacillary fever A25.1
Streptobacillosis A25.1
Streptobacillus moniliformis A25.1
Streptococcus, streptococcal (*see also* condition)
    as cause of disease classified elsewhere B95.5
    group
        A, as cause of disease classified elsewhere B95.0
        B, as cause of disease classified elsewhere B95.1
        D, as cause of disease classified elsewhere B95.2
    pneumoniae, as cause of disease classified elsewhere
        B95.3
    specified NEC, as cause of disease classified elsewhere
        B95.4
Streptomycosis B47.1
Streptotrichosis A48.8
Stress F43.9
    family — *see* Disruption, family
    fetal P84
        complicating pregnancy O77.9
            due to drug administration O77.1
    mental NEC Z73.3
        work-related Z56.6
    physical NEC Z73.3
        work-related Z56.6
    polycythemia D75.1
    reaction (*see also* Reaction, stress) F43.9
    work schedule Z56.3
Stretching, nerve — *see* Injury, nerve
Striae albicantes, atrophicae or distensae (cutis) L90.6
Stricture (*see also* Stenosis)
    ampulla of Vater K83.1
    anus (sphincter) K62.4
        congenital Q42.3
            with fistula Q42.2

Stricture — *continued*
 anus — *continued*
  infantile Q42.3
   with fistula Q42.2
 aorta (ascending) (congenital) Q25.1
  arteriosclerotic I70.0
  calcified I70.0
  supravalvular, congenital Q25.3
 aortic (valve) — *see* Stenosis, aortic
 aqueduct of Sylvius (congenital) Q03.0
  with spina bifida — *see* Spina bifida, by site, with hydrocephalus
  acquired G91.1
 artery I77.1
  basilar — *see* Occlusion, artery, basilar
  carotid — *see* Occlusion, artery, carotid
  celiac I77.4
  congenital (peripheral) Q27.8
   cerebral Q28.3
   coronary Q24.5
   digestive system Q27.8
   lower limb Q27.8
   retinal Q14.1
   specified site NEC Q27.8
   umbilical Q27.0
   upper limb Q27.8
  coronary — *see* Disease, heart, ischemic, atherosclerotic
   congenital Q24.5
  precerebral — *see* Occlusion, artery, precerebral
  pulmonary (congenital) Q25.6
   acquired I28.8
  renal I70.1
  vertebral — *see* Occlusion, artery, vertebral
 auditory canal (external) (congenital)
  acquired — *see* Stenosis, external ear canal
 bile duct (common) (hepatic) K83.1
  congenital Q44.3
  postoperative K91.89
 bladder N32.89
  neck N32.0
 bowel — *see* Obstruction, intestine
 brain G93.89
 bronchus J98.09
  congenital Q32.3
  syphilitic A52.72
 cardia (stomach) K22.2
  congenital Q39.3
 cardiac (*see also* Disease, heart)
  orifice (stomach) K22.2
 cecum — *see* Obstruction, intestine
 cervix, cervical (canal) N88.2
  congenital Q51.828
  in pregnancy — *see* Pregnancy, complicated by, abnormal cervix
   causing obstructed labor O65.5
 colon (*see also* Obstruction, intestine)
  congenital Q42.9
   specified NEC Q42.8
 colostomy K94.03
 common (bile) duct K83.1
 coronary (artery) — *see* Disease, heart, ischemic, atherosclerotic
 cystic duct — *see* Obstruction, gallbladder
 digestive organs NEC, congenital Q45.8
 duodenum K31.5
  congenital Q41.0
 ear canal (external) (congenital) Q16.1
  acquired — *see* Stricture, auditory canal, acquired
 ejaculatory duct N50.89
 enterostomy K94.13
 esophagus K22.2
  congenital Q39.3
  syphilitic A52.79
   congenital A50.59 [K23]
 eustachian tube (*see also* Obstruction, eustachian tube)
  congenital Q17.8
 fallopian tube N97.1
  gonococcal A54.24
  tuberculous A18.17
 gallbladder — *see* Obstruction, gallbladder
 glottis J38.6
 heart (*see also* Disease, heart)
  valve (*see also* Endocarditis) I38
   aortic Q23.0
   mitral Q23.2
   pulmonary Q22.1
   tricuspid Q22.4

Stricture — *continued*
 hepatic duct K83.1
 hourglass, of stomach K31.2
 hymen N89.6
 hypopharynx J39.2
 ileum (*see also* Obstruction, intestine, specified NEC) K56.699
  congenital Q41.2
 intestine (*see also* Obstruction, intestine)
  congenital (small) Q41.9
   large Q42.9
    specified NEC Q42.8
   specified NEC Q41.8
  ischemic K55.1
 jejunum (*see also* Obstruction, intestine, specified NEC) K56.699
  congenital Q41.1
 lacrimal passages (*see also* Stenosis, lacrimal)
  congenital Q10.5
 larynx J38.6
  congenital NEC Q31.8
   subglottic Q31.1
  syphilitic A52.73
   congenital A50.59 [J99]
 meatus
  ear (congenital) Q16.1
   acquired — *see* Stricture, auditory canal, acquired
  osseous (ear) (congenital) Q16.1
   acquired — *see* Stricture, auditory canal, acquired
  urinarius (*see also* Stricture, urethra)
   congenital Q64.33
 mitral (valve) — *see* Stenosis, mitral
 myocardium, myocardial I51.5
  hypertrophic subaortic (idiopathic) I42.1
 nares (anterior) (posterior) J34.89
  congenital Q30.0
 nasal duct (*see also* Stenosis, lacrimal, duct)
  congenital Q10.5
 nasolacrimal duct (*see also* Stenosis, lacrimal, duct)
  congenital Q10.5
 nasopharynx J39.2
  syphilitic A52.73
 nose J34.89
  congenital Q30.0
 nostril (anterior) (posterior) J34.89
  congenital Q30.0
  syphilitic A52.73
   congenital A50.59 [J99]
 organ or site, congenital NEC — *see* Atresia, by site
 os uteri — *see* Stricture, cervix
 osseous meatus (ear) (congenital) Q16.1
  acquired — *see* Stricture, auditory canal, acquired
 oviduct — *see* Stricture, fallopian tube
 pelviureteric junction (congenital) Q62.11
  acquired, with hydronephrosis N13.0
 penis, by foreign body T19.4 ☑
 pharynx J39.2
 prostate N42.89
 pulmonary, pulmonic
  artery (congenital) Q25.6
   acquired I28.8
   noncongenital I28.8
  infundibulum (congenital) Q24.3
  valve I37.0
   congenital Q22.1
  vein, acquired I28.8
  vessel NEC I28.8
 punctum lacrimale (*see also* Stenosis, lacrimal, punctum)
  congenital Q10.5
 pylorus (hypertrophic) K31.1
  adult K31.1
  congenital Q40.0
  infantile Q40.0
 rectosigmoid (*see also* Obstruction, intestine, specified NEC) K56.699
 rectum (sphincter) K62.4
  congenital Q42.1
   with fistula Q42.0
  due to
   chlamydial lymphogranuloma A55
   irradiation K91.89
   lymphogranuloma venereum A55
  gonococcal A54.6
  inflammatory (chlamydial) A55
  syphilitic A52.74

Stricture — *continued*
 rectum — *continued*
  tuberculous A18.32
 renal artery I70.1
  congenital Q27.1
 salivary duct or gland (any) K11.8
 sigmoid (flexure) — *see* Obstruction, intestine
 spermatic cord N50.89
 stoma (following) (of)
  colostomy K94.03
  enterostomy K94.13
  gastrostomy K94.23
  ileostomy K94.13
  tracheostomy J95.03
 stomach K31.89
  congenital Q40.2
  hourglass K31.2
 subaortic Q24.4
  hypertrophic (acquired) (idiopathic) I42.1
 subglottic J38.6
 syphilitic NEC A52.79
 trachea J39.8
  congenital Q32.1
  syphilitic A52.73
  tuberculous NEC A15.5
 tracheostomy J95.03
 tricuspid (valve) — *see* Stenosis, tricuspid
 tunica vaginalis N50.89
 ureter (postoperative) N13.5
  with
   hydronephrosis N13.1
    with infection N13.6
   pyelonephritis (chronic) N11.1
  congenital — *see* Atresia, ureter
  tuberculous A18.11
 ureteropelvic junction (congenital) Q62.11
  acquired, with hydronephrosis N13.0
 ureterovesical orifice N13.5
  with infection N13.6
 urethra (organic) (spasmodic) (*see also* Stricture, urethra, male) N35.919
  associated with schistosomiasis B65.0 [N37]
  congenital Q64.39
   valvular (posterior) Q64.2
  due to
   infection — *see* Stricture, urethra, postinfective
   trauma — *see* Stricture, urethra, post-traumatic
  female N35.92
  gonococcal, gonorrheal A54.01
  infective NEC — *see* Stricture, urethra, postinfective
  late effect (sequelae) of injury — *see* Stricture, urethra, post-traumatic
  male N35.919
   anterior urethra N35.914
   bulbous urethra N35.912
   meatal N35.911
   membranous urethra N35.913
   overlapping sites N35.916
  postcatheterization — *see* Stricture, urethra, postprocedural
  postinfective NEC
   female N35.12
   male N35.119
    anterior urethra N35.114
    bulbous urethra N35.112
    meatal N35.111
    membranous urethra N35.113
    overlapping sites N35.116
  postobstetric N35.021
  postoperative — *see* Stricture, urethra, postprocedural
  postprocedural
   female N99.12
   male N99.114
    anterior bulbous urethra N99.113
    bulbous urethra N99.111
    fossa navicularis N99.115
    meatal N99.110
    membranous urethra N99.112
    overlapping sites N99.116
  post-traumatic
   female N35.028
    due to childbirth N35.021
   male N35.014
    anterior urethra N35.013
    bulbous urethra N35.011
    meatal N35.010
    membranous urethra N35.012

Stricture — *continued*
  urethra (*see also* Stricture, urethra, male) — *continued*
    post-traumatic — *continued*
      male — *continued*
        overlapping sites N35.016
      sequela (late effect) of
        childbirth N35.021
        injury — *see* Stricture, urethra, post-traumatic
      specified cause NEC
        female N35.82
        male N35.819
          anterior urethra N35.814
          bulbous urethra N35.812
          meatal N35.811
          membranous urethra N35.813
          overlapping sites N35.816
    syphilitic A52.76
    traumatic — *see* Stricture, urethra, post-traumatic
    valvular (posterior), congenital Q64.2
  urinary meatus — *see* Stricture, urethra
  uterus, uterine (synechiae) N85.6
    os (external) (internal) — *see* Stricture, cervix
  vagina (outlet) — *see* Stenosis, vagina
  valve (cardiac) (heart) (*see also* Endocarditis)
    congenital
      aortic Q23.0
      mitral Q23.2
      pulmonary Q22.1
      tricuspid Q22.4
  vas deferens N50.89
    congenital Q55.4
  vein I87.1
  vena cava (inferior) (superior) NEC I87.1
    congenital Q26.0
  vesicourethral orifice N32.0
    congenital Q64.31
  vulva (acquired) N90.5
Stridor R06.1
  congenital (larynx) P28.89
Stridulous — *see* condition
Stroke (apoplectic) (brain) (embolic) (ischemic) (paralytic) (thrombotic) I63.9
  cryptogenic (*see also* infarction, cerebral) I63.9
  epileptic — *see* Epilepsy
  heat T67.0 ☑
  in evolution I63.9
  intraoperative
    during cardiac surgery I97.810
    during other surgery I97.811
  lightning — *see* Lightning
  meaning
    cerebral hemorrhage — *code to* Hemorrhage, intracranial
    cerebral infarction — *code to* Infarction, cerebral
  postprocedural
    following cardiac surgery I97.820
    following other surgery I97.821
  unspecified (NOS) I63.9
Stromatosis, endometrial D39.0
Strongyloidiasis, strongyloidosis B78.9
  cutaneous B78.1
  disseminated B78.7
  intestinal B78.0
Strophulus pruriginosus L28.2
Struck by lightning — *see* Lightning
Struma (*see also* Goiter)
  Hashimoto E06.3
  lymphomatosa E06.3
  nodosa (simplex) E04.9
    endemic E01.2
      multinodular E01.1
    multinodular E04.2
      iodine-deficiency related E01.1
    toxic or with hyperthyroidism E05.20
      with thyroid storm E05.21
      multinodular E05.20
        with thyroid storm E05.21
      uninodular E05.10
        with thyroid storm E05.11
    toxicosa E05.20
      with thyroid storm E05.21
      multinodular E05.20
        with thyroid storm E05.21
      uninodular E05.10
        with thyroid storm E05.11
    uninodular E04.1
  ovarii D27.- ☑

Struma — *continued*
  Riedel's E06.5
Strumipriva cachexia E03.4
Strümpell-Marie spine — *see* Spondylitis, ankylosing
Strümpell-Westphal pseudosclerosis E83.01
Stuart deficiency disease (factor X) D68.2
Stuart-Prower factor deficiency (factor X) D68.2
Student's elbow — *see* Bursitis, elbow, olecranon
Stump — *see* Amputation
Stunting, nutritional E45
Stupor (catatonic) R40.1
  depressive (single episode) F32.89
    recurrent episode F33.8
  dissociative F44.2
  manic F30.2
  manic-depressive F31.89
  psychogenic (anergic) F44.2
  reaction to exceptional stress (transient) F43.0
Sturge (-Weber) (-Dimitri) (-Kalischer) **disease or syndrome** Q85.8
Stuttering F80.81
  adult onset F98.5
  childhood onset F80.81
  following cerebrovascular disease — *see* Disorder, fluency. following cerebrovascular disease
  in conditions classified elsewhere R47.82
Sty, stye (external) (internal) (meibomian) (zeisian) — *see* Hordeolum
Subacidity, gastric K31.89
  psychogenic F45.8
Subacute — *see* condition
Subarachnoid — *see* condition
Subcortical — *see* condition
Subcostal syndrome, nerve compression — *see* Mononeuropathy, upper limb, specified site NEC
Subcutaneous, subcuticular — *see* condition
Subdural — *see* condition
Subendocardium — *see* condition
Subependymoma
  specified site — *see* Neoplasm, uncertain behavior, by site
  unspecified site D43.2
Suberosis J67.3
Subglossitis — *see* Glossitis
Subhemophilia D66
Subinvolution
  breast (postlactational) (postpuerperal) N64.89
  puerperal O90.89
  uterus (chronic) (nonpuerperal) N85.3
    puerperal O90.89
Sublingual — *see* condition
Sublinguitis — *see* Sialoadenitis
Subluxatable hip Q65.6
Subluxation (*see also* Dislocation)
  acromioclavicular S43.11- ☑
  ankle S93.0- ☑
  atlantoaxial, recurrent M43.4
    with myelopathy M43.3
  carpometacarpal (joint) NEC S63.05- ☑
    thumb S63.04- ☑
  complex, vertebral — *see* Complex, subluxation
  congenital (*see also* Malposition, congenital)
    hip — *see* Dislocation, hip, congenital, partial
    joint (excluding hip)
      lower limb Q68.8
      shoulder Q68.8
      upper limb Q68.8
  elbow (traumatic) S53.10- ☑
    anterior S53.11- ☑
    lateral S53.14- ☑
    medial S53.13- ☑
    posterior S53.12- ☑
    specified type NEC S53.19- ☑
  finger S63.20- ☑
    index S63.20- ☑
    interphalangeal S63.22- ☑
      distal S63.24- ☑
        index S63.24- ☑
        little S63.24- ☑
        middle S63.24- ☑
        ring S63.24- ☑
      index S63.22- ☑
      little S63.22- ☑
      middle S63.22- ☑
      proximal S63.23- ☑
        index S63.23- ☑
        little S63.23- ☑

Subluxation — *continued*
  finger — *continued*
    interphalangeal — *continued*
      proximal — *continued*
        middle S63.23- ☑
        ring S63.23- ☑
      ring S63.22- ☑
      little S63.20- ☑
    metacarpophalangeal S63.21- ☑
      index S63.21- ☑
      little S63.21- ☑
      middle S63.21- ☑
      ring S63.21- ☑
    middle S63.20- ☑
    ring S63.20- ☑
  foot S93.30- ☑
    specified site NEC S93.33- ☑
    tarsal joint S93.31- ☑
    tarsometatarsal joint S93.32- ☑
    toe — *see* Subluxation, toe
  hip S73.00- ☑
    anterior S73.03- ☑
      obturator S73.02- ☑
    central S73.04- ☑
    posterior S73.01- ☑
  interphalangeal (joint)
    finger S63.22- ☑
      distal joint S63.24- ☑
        index S63.24- ☑
        little S63.24- ☑
        middle S63.24- ☑
        ring S63.24- ☑
      index S63.22- ☑
      little S63.22- ☑
      middle S63.22- ☑
      proximal joint S63.23- ☑
        index S63.23- ☑
        little S63.23- ☑
        middle S63.23- ☑
        ring S63.23- ☑
      ring S63.22- ☑
    thumb S63.12- ☑
    toe S93.13- ☑
      great S93.13- ☑
      lesser S93.13- ☑
  joint prosthesis — *see* Complications, joint prosthesis, mechanical, displacement, by site
  knee S83.10- ☑
    cap — *see* Subluxation, patella
    patella — *see* Subluxation, patella
    proximal tibia
      anteriorly S83.11- ☑
      laterally S83.14- ☑
      medially S83.13- ☑
      posteriorly S83.12- ☑
    specified type NEC S83.19- ☑
  lens — *see* Dislocation, lens, partial
  ligament, traumatic — *see* Sprain, by site
  metacarpal (bone)
    proximal end S63.06- ☑
  metacarpophalangeal (joint)
    finger S63.21- ☑
      index S63.21- ☑
      little S63.21- ☑
      middle S63.21- ☑
      ring S63.21- ☑
    thumb S63.11- ☑
  metatarsophalangeal joint S93.14- ☑
    great toe S93.14- ☑
    lesser toe S93.14- ☑
  midcarpal (joint) S63.03- ☑
  patella S83.00- ☑
    lateral S83.01- ☑
    recurrent (nontraumatic) — *see* Dislocation, patella, recurrent, incomplete
    specified type NEC S83.09- ☑
  pathological — *see* Dislocation, pathological
  radial head S53.00- ☑
    anterior S53.01- ☑
    nursemaid's elbow S53.03- ☑
    posterior S53.02- ☑
    specified type NEC S53.09- ☑
  radiocarpal (joint) S63.02- ☑
  radioulnar (joint)
    distal S63.01- ☑
    proximal — *see* Subluxation, elbow

☑ **Additional Character Required** — Refer to the Tabular List for Character Selection   ▽ **Subterms under main terms may continue to next column or page**

Subluxation — *continued*
  shoulder
    congenital Q68.8
    girdle S43.30- ☑
      scapula S43.31- ☑
      specified site NEC S43.39- ☑
    traumatic S43.00- ☑
      anterior S43.01- ☑
      inferior S43.03- ☑
      posterior S43.02- ☑
      specified type NEC S43.08- ☑
  sternoclavicular (joint) S43.20- ☑
    anterior S43.21- ☑
    posterior S43.22- ☑
  symphysis (pubis)
  thumb S63.103 ☑
    interphalangeal joint — *see* Subluxation, interphalangeal (joint), thumb
    metacarpophalangeal joint — *see* Subluxation, metacarpophalangeal (joint), thumb
  toe(s) S93.10- ☑
    great S93.10- ☑
      interphalangeal joint S93.13- ☑
      metatarsophalangeal joint S93.14- ☑
    interphalangeal joint S93.13- ☑
    lesser S93.10- ☑
      interphalangeal joint S93.13- ☑
      metatarsophalangeal joint S93.14- ☑
    metatarsophalangeal joint S93.149 ☑
  ulna
    distal end S63.07- ☑
    proximal end — *see* Subluxation, elbow
  ulnohumeral joint — *see* Subluxation, elbow
  vertebral
    recurrent NEC — *see* subcategory M43.5 ☑
    traumatic
      cervical S13.100 ☑
        atlantoaxial joint S13.120 ☑
        atlantooccipital joint S13.110 ☑
        atloidooccipital joint S13.110 ☑
        joint between
          C0 and C1 S13.110 ☑
          C1 and C2 S13.120 ☑
          C2 and C3 S13.130 ☑
          C3 and C4 S13.140 ☑
          C4 and C5 S13.150 ☑
          C5 and C6 S13.160 ☑
          C6 and C7 S13.170 ☑
          C7 and T1 S13.180 ☑
        occipitoatloid joint S13.110 ☑
      lumbar S33.100 ☑
        joint between
          L1 and L2 S33.110 ☑
          L2 and L3 S33.120 ☑
          L3 and L4 S33.130 ☑
          L4 and L5 S33.140 ☑
      thoracic S23.100 ☑
        joint between
          T1 and T2 S23.110 ☑
          T2 and T3 S23.120 ☑
          T3 and T4 S23.122 ☑
          T4 and T5 S23.130 ☑
          T5 and T6 S23.132 ☑
          T6 and T7 S23.140 ☑
          T7 and T8 S23.142 ☑
          T8 and T9 S23.150 ☑
          T9 and T10 S23.152 ☑
          T10 and T11 S23.160 ☑
          T11 and T12 S23.162 ☑
          T12 and L1 S23.170 ☑
  wrist (carpal bone) S63.00- ☑
    carpometacarpal joint — *see* Subluxation, carpometacarpal (joint)
    distal radioulnar joint — *see* Subluxation, radioulnar (joint), distal
    metacarpal bone, proximal — *see* Subluxation, metacarpal (bone), proximal end
    midcarpal — *see* Subluxation, midcarpal (joint)
    radiocarpal joint — *see* Subluxation, radiocarpal (joint)
    recurrent — *see* Dislocation, recurrent, wrist
    specified site NEC S63.09- ☑
    ulna — *see* Subluxation, ulna, distal end
Submaxillary — *see* condition
Submersion (fatal) (nonfatal) T75.1 ☑
Submucous — *see* condition

Subnormal, subnormality
  accommodation (old age) H52.4
  mental — *see* Disability, intellectual
  temperature (accidental) T68 ☑
Subphrenic — *see* condition
Subscapular nerve — *see* condition
Subseptus uterus Q51.28
Subsiding appendicitis K36
Substance (other psychoactive) **-induced**
  anxiety disorder F19.980
  bipolar and related disorder F19.94
  delirium F19.921
  depressive disorder F19.94
  major neurocognitive disorder F19.97
  mild neurocognitive disorder F19.988
  obsessive-compulsive and related disorder F19.988
  psychotic disorder F19.959
  sexual dysfunction F19.981
  sleep disorder F19.982
Substernal thyroid E04.9
  congenital Q89.2
Substitution disorder F44.9
Subtentorial — *see* condition
Subthyroidism (acquired) (*see also* Hypothyroidism)
  congenital E03.1
Succenturiate placenta O43.19- ☑
Sucking thumb, child (excessive) F98.8
Sudamen, sudamina L74.1
Sudanese kala-azar B55.0
Sudden
  hearing loss — *see* Deafness, sudden
  heart failure — *see* Failure, heart
Sudeck's atrophy, disease, or syndrome — *see* Algoneurodystrophy
Suffocation — *see* Asphyxia, traumatic
Sugar
  blood
    high (transient) R73.9
    low (transient) E16.2
  in urine R81
Suicide, suicidal (attempted) T14.91 ☑
  by poisoning — *see* Table of Drugs and Chemicals
  history of (personal) Z91.5
    in family Z81.8
  ideation — *see* Ideation, suicidal
  risk
    meaning personal history of attempted suicide Z91.5
    meaning suicidal ideation — *see* Ideation, suicidal
  tendencies
    meaning personal history of attempted suicide Z91.5
    meaning suicidal ideation — *see* Ideation, suicidal
  trauma — *see* nature of injury by site
Suipestifer infection — *see* Infection, salmonella
Sulfhemoglobinemia, sulphemoglobinemia (acquired) (with methemoglobinemia) D74.8
Sumatran mite fever A75.3
Summer — *see* condition
Sunburn L55.9
  due to
    tanning bed (acute) L56.8
      chronic L57.8
    ultraviolet radiation (acute) L56.8
      chronic L57.8
  first degree L55.0
  second degree L55.1
  third degree L55.2
SUNCT (short lasting unilateral neuralgiform headache with conjunctival injection and tearing) G44.059
  intractable G44.051
  not intractable G44.059
Sundowning F05
Sunken acetabulum — *see* Derangement, joint, specified type NEC, hip
Sunstroke T67.0 ☑
Superfecundation — *see* Pregnancy, multiple
Superfetation — *see* Pregnancy, multiple
Superinvolution (uterus) N85.8
Supernumerary (congenital)
  aortic cusps Q23.8
  auditory ossicles Q16.3
  bone Q79.8
  breast Q83.1
  carpal bones Q74.0
  cusps, heart valve NEC Q24.8
    aortic Q23.8
    mitral Q23.2
    pulmonary Q22.3

Supernumerary — *continued*
  digit(s) Q69.9
  ear (lobule) Q17.0
  fallopian tube Q50.6
  finger Q69.0
  hymen Q52.4
  kidney Q63.0
  lacrimonasal duct Q10.6
  lobule (ear) Q17.0
  mitral cusps Q23.2
  muscle Q79.8
  nipple(s) Q83.3
  organ or site not listed — *see* Accessory
  ossicles, auditory Q16.3
  ovary Q50.31
  oviduct Q50.6
  pulmonary, pulmonic cusps Q22.3
  rib Q76.6
    cervical or first (syndrome) Q76.5
  roots (of teeth) K00.2
  spleen Q89.09
  tarsal bones Q74.2
  teeth K00.1
  testis Q55.29
  thumb Q69.1
  toe Q69.2
  uterus Q51.28
  vagina Q52.1 ☑
  vertebra Q76.49
Supervision (of)
  contraceptive — *see* Prescription, contraceptives
  dietary (for) Z71.3
    allergy (food) Z71.3
    colitis Z71.3
    diabetes mellitus Z71.3
    food allergy or intolerance Z71.3
    gastritis Z71.3
    hypercholesterolemia Z71.3
    hypoglycemia Z71.3
    intolerance (food) Z71.3
    obesity Z71.3
    specified NEC Z71.3
  healthy infant or child Z76.2
    foundling Z76.1
  high-risk pregnancy — *see* Pregnancy, complicated by, high, risk
  lactation Z39.1
  pregnancy — *see* Pregnancy, supervision of
Supplemental teeth K00.1
Suppression
  binocular vision H53.34
  lactation O92.5
  menstruation N94.89
  ovarian secretion E28.39
  renal N28.9
  urine, urinary secretion R34
Suppuration, suppurative (*see also* condition)
  accessory sinus (chronic) — *see* Sinusitis
  adrenal gland
  antrum (chronic) — *see* Sinusitis, maxillary
  bladder — *see* Cystitis
  brain G06.0
    sequelae G09
  breast N61.1
    puerperal, postpartum or gestational — *see* Mastitis, obstetric, purulent
  dental periosteum M27.3
  ear (middle) (*see also* Otitis, media)
    external NEC — *see* Otitis, externa, infective
    internal — *see* subcategory H83.0 ☑
  ethmoidal (chronic) (sinus) — *see* Sinusitis, ethmoidal
  fallopian tube — *see* Salpingo-oophoritis
  frontal (chronic) (sinus) — *see* Sinusitis, frontal
  gallbladder (acute) K81.0
  gum K05.20
    generalized — *see* Peridontitis, aggressive, generalized
    localized — *see* Peridontitis, aggressive, localized
  intracranial G06.0
  joint — *see* Arthritis, pyogenic or pyemic
  labyrinthine — *see* subcategory H83.0 ☑
  lung — *see* Abscess, lung
  mammary gland N61.1
    puerperal, postpartum O91.12
      associated with lactation O91.13
  maxilla, maxillary M27.2
    sinus (chronic) — *see* Sinusitis, maxillary
  muscle — *see* Myositis, infective

Suppuration, suppurative — continued
nasal sinus (chronic) — see Sinusitis
pancreas, acute (see also Pancreatitis, acute) K85.8Ø
parotid gland — see Sialoadenitis
pelvic
female — see Disease, pelvis, inflammatory
male K65.Ø
pericranial — see Osteomyelitis
salivary duct or gland (any) — see Sialoadenitis
sinus (accessory) (chronic) (nasal) — see Sinusitis
sphenoidal sinus (chronic) — see Sinusitis, sphenoidal
thymus (gland) E32.1
thyroid (gland) EØ6.Ø
tonsil — see Tonsillitis
uterus — see Endometritis
Supraeruption of tooth (teeth) M26.34
Supraglottitis JØ4.3Ø
with obstruction JØ4.31
Suprarenal (gland) — see condition
Suprascapular nerve — see condition
Suprasellar — see condition
Surfer's knots or nodules S89.8- ☑
Surgical
emphysema T81.82 ☑
procedures, complication or misadventure — see
Complications, surgical procedures
shock T81.1Ø ☑
Surveillance (of) (for) (see also Observation)
alcohol abuse Z71.41
contraceptive — see Prescription, contraceptives
dietary Z71.3
drug abuse Z71.51
Susceptibility to disease, genetic Z15.89
malignant neoplasm Z15.Ø9
breast Z15.Ø1
endometrium Z15.Ø4
ovary Z15.Ø2
prostate Z15.Ø3
specified NEC Z15.Ø9
multiple endocrine neoplasia Z15.81
Suspected condition, ruled out (see also Observation, suspected)
amniotic cavity and membrane ZØ3.71
cervical shortening ZØ3.75
fetal anomaly ZØ3.73
fetal growth ZØ3.74
maternal and fetal conditions NEC ZØ3.79
newborn (see also Observation, newborn, suspected condition ruled out) ZØ5.9
oligohydramnios ZØ3.71
placental problem ZØ3.72
polyhydramnios ZØ3.71
Suspended uterus
in pregnancy or childbirth — see Pregnancy, complicated by, abnormal uterus
Sutton's nevus D22.9
Suture
burst (in operation wound) T81.31 ☑
external operation wound T81.31 ☑
internal operation wound T81.32 ☑
inadvertently left in operation wound — see Foreign body, accidentally left during a procedure
removal Z48.Ø2
Swab inadvertently left in operation wound — see Foreign body, accidentally left during a procedure
Swallowed, swallowing
difficulty — see Dysphagia
foreign body — see Foreign body, alimentary tract
Swan-neck deformity (finger) — see Deformity, finger, swan-neck
Swearing, compulsive F42.8
in Gilles de la Tourette's syndrome F95.2
Sweat, sweats
fetid L75.Ø
night R61
Sweating, excessive R61
Sweeley-Klionsky disease E75.21
Sweet's disease or dermatosis L98.2
Swelling (of) R6Ø.9
abdomen, abdominal (not referable to any particular organ) — see Mass, abdominal
ankle — see Effusion, joint, ankle
arm M79.89
forearm M79.89
breast (see also Lump, breast) N63.Ø
Calabar B74.3
cervical gland R59.Ø

Swelling — continued
chest, localized R22.2
ear H93.8- ☑
extremity (lower) (upper) — see Disorder, soft tissue, specified type NEC
finger M79.89
foot M79.89
glands R59.9
generalized R59.1
localized R59.Ø
hand M79.89
head (localized) R22.Ø
inflammatory — see Inflammation
intra-abdominal — see Mass, abdominal
joint — see Effusion, joint
leg M79.89
lower M79.89
limb — see Disorder, soft tissue, specified type NEC
localized (skin) R22.9
chest R22.2
head R22.Ø
limb
lower — see Mass, localized, limb, lower
upper — see Mass, localized, limb, upper
neck R22.1
trunk R22.2
neck (localized) R22.1
pelvic — see Mass, abdominal
scrotum N5Ø.89
splenic — see Splenomegaly
testis N5Ø.89
toe M79.89
umbilical R19.Ø9
wandering, due to Gnathostoma (spinigerum) B83.1
white — see Tuberculosis, arthritis
Swift (-Feer) **disease**
overdose or wrong substance given or taken — see Table of Drugs and Chemicals, by drug, poisoning
Swimmer's
cramp T75.1 ☑
ear H6Ø.33- ☑
itch B65.3
Swimming in the head R42
Swollen — see Swelling
Swyer syndrome Q99.1
Sycosis L73.8
barbae (not parasitic) L73.8
contagiosa (mycotic) B35.Ø
lupoides L73.8
mycotic B35.Ø
parasitic B35.Ø
vulgaris L73.8
Sydenham's chorea — see Chorea, Sydenham's
Sylvatic yellow fever A95.Ø
Sylvest's disease B33.Ø
Symblepharon H11.23- ☑
congenital Q1Ø.3
Symond's syndrome G93.2
Sympathetic — see condition
Sympatheticotonia G9Ø.8
Sympathicoblastoma
specified site — see Neoplasm, malignant, by site
unspecified site C74.9Ø
Sympathogonioma — see Sympathicoblastoma
Symphalangy (fingers) (toes) Q7Ø.9
Symptoms NEC R68.89
breast NEC N64.59
cold JØØ
development NEC R63.8
factitious, self-induced — see Disorder, factitious
genital organs, female R1Ø.2
involving
abdomen NEC R19.8
appearance NEC R46.89
awareness R41.9
altered mental status R41.82
amnesia — see Amnesia
borderline intellectual functioning R41.83
coma — see Coma
disorientation R41.Ø
neurologic neglect syndrome R41.4
senile cognitive decline R41.81
specified symptom NEC R41.89
behavior NEC R46.89
cardiovascular system NEC RØ9.89
chest NEC RØ9.89
circulatory system NEC RØ9.89
cognitive functions R41.9

Symptoms — continued
involving — continued
cognitive functions — continued
altered mental status R41.82
amnesia — see Amnesia
borderline intellectual functioning R41.83
coma — see Coma
disorientation R41.Ø
neurologic neglect syndrome R41.4
senile cognitive decline R41.81
specified symptom NEC R41.89
development NEC R62.5Ø
digestive system NEC R19.8
emotional state NEC R45.89
emotional lability R45.86
food and fluid intake R63.8
general perceptions and sensations R44.9
specified NEC R44.8
musculoskeletal system R29.91
specified NEC R29.898
nervous system R29.9Ø
specified NEC R29.818
pelvis NEC R19.8
respiratory system NEC RØ9.89
skin and integument R23.9
urinary system R39.9
menopausal N95.1
metabolism NEC R63.8
neurotic F48.8
of infancy R68.19
pelvis NEC, female R1Ø.2
skin and integument NEC R23.9
subcutaneous tissue NEC R23.9
viral cold JØØ
Sympus Q74.2
Syncephalus Q89.4
Synchondrosis
abnormal (congenital) Q78.8
ischiopubic M91.Ø
Synchysis (scintillans) (senile) (vitreous body) H43.89
Syncope (near) (pre-) R55
anginosa I2Ø.8
bradycardia RØØ.1
cardiac R55
carotid sinus G9Ø.Ø1
due to spinal (lumbar) puncture G97.1
heart R55
heat T67.1 ☑
laryngeal RØ5
psychogenic F48.8
tussive RØ5
vasoconstriction R55
vasodepressor R55
vasomotor R55
vasovagal R55
Syndactylism, syndactyly Q7Ø.9
complex (with synostosis)
fingers Q7Ø.Ø- ☑
toes Q7Ø.2- ☑
simple (without synostosis)
fingers Q7Ø.1- ☑
toes Q7Ø.3- ☑
Syndrome (see also Disease)
5q minus NOS D46.C (following D46.2)
48,XXXX Q97.1
49,XXXXX Q97.1
abdominal
acute R1Ø.Ø
muscle deficiency Q79.4
abnormal innervation HØ2.519
left HØ2.516
lower HØ2.515
upper HØ2.514
right HØ2.513
lower HØ2.512
upper HØ2.511
abstinence, neonatal P96.1
acid pulmonary aspiration, obstetric O74.Ø
acquired immunodeficiency — see Human, immunodeficiency virus (HIV) disease
acute abdominal R1Ø.Ø
acute respiratory distress (adult) (child) J8Ø
idiopathic J84.114
Adair-Dighton Q78.Ø
Adams-Stokes (-Morgagni) I45.9
adiposogenital E23.6
adrenal
hemorrhage (meningococcal) A39.1

298

☑ Additional Character Required — Refer to the Tabular List for Character Selection ▽ Subterms under main terms may continue to next column or page

Syndrome — *continued*
  adrenal — *continued*
    meningococcic A39.1
  adrenocortical — *see* Cushing's, syndrome
  adrenogenital E25.9
    congenital, associated with enzyme deficiency E25.0
  afferent loop NEC K91.89
  Alagille's Q44.7
  alcohol withdrawal (without convulsions) — *see* Dependence, alcohol, with, withdrawal
  Alder's D72.0
  Aldrich (-Wiskott) D82.0
  alien hand R41.4
  Alport Q87.81
  alveolar hypoventilation E66.2
  alveolocapillary block J84.10
  amnesic, amnestic (confabulatory) (due to) — *see* Disorder, amnesic
  amyostatic (Wilson's disease) E83.01
  androgen insensitivity E34.50
    complete E34.51
    partial E34.52
  androgen resistance (*see also* Syndrome, androgen insensitivity) E34.50
  Angelman Q93.51
  anginal — *see* Angina
  ankyloglossia superior Q38.1
  anterior
    chest wall R07.89
    cord G83.82
    spinal artery G95.19
      compression M47.019
        cervical region M47.012
        cervicothoracic region M47.013
        lumbar region M47.016
        occipito-atlanto-axial region M47.011
        thoracic region M47.014
        thoracolumbar region M47.015
    tibial M76.81- ☑
  antibody deficiency D80.9
    agammaglobulinemic D80.1
      hereditary D80.0
    congenital D80.0
    hypogammaglobulinemic D80.1
      hereditary D80.0
  anticardiolipin (-antibody) D68.61
  antidepressant discontinuation T43.205 ☑
  antiphospholipid (-antibody) D68.61
  aortic
    arch M31.4
    bifurcation I74.09
  aortomesenteric duodenum occlusion K31.5
  apical ballooning (transient left ventricular) I51.81
  arcuate ligament I77.4
  argentaffin, argintaffinoma E34.0
  Arnold-Chiari — *see* Arnold-Chiari disease
  Arrillaga-Ayerza I27.0
  arterial tortuosity Q87.82
  arteriovenous steal T82.898- ☑
  Asherman's N85.6
  aspiration, of newborn — *see* Aspiration, by substance, with pneumonia
    meconium P24.01
  ataxia-telangiectasia G11.3
  auriculotemporal G50.8
  autoerythrocyte sensitization (Gardner-Diamond) D69.2
  autoimmune lymphoproliferative [ALPS] D89.82
  autoimmune polyglandular E31.0
  autoinflammatory M04.9
    specified type NEC M04.8
  autosomal — *see* Abnormal, autosomes
  Avellis' G46.8
  Ayerza (-Arrillaga) I27.0
  Babinski-Nageotte G83.89
  Bakwin-Krida Q78.5
  bare lymphocyte D81.6
  Barré-Guillain G61.0
  Barré-Liéou M53.0
  Barrett's — *see* Barrett's, esophagus
  Barsony-Polgar K22.4
  Bársony-Teschendorf K22.4
  Barth E78.71
  Bartter's E26.81
  basal cell nevus Q87.89
  Basedow's E05.00
    with thyroid storm E05.01
  basilar artery G45.0
  Batten-Steinert G71.11

Syndrome — *continued*
  battered
    baby or child — *see* Maltreatment, child, physical abuse
    spouse — *see* Maltreatment, adult, physical abuse
  Beals Q87.40
  Beau's I51.5
  Beck's I65.8
  Benedikt's G46.3
  Béquez César (-Steinbrinck-Chédiak-Higashi) E70.330
  Bernhardt-Roth — *see* Meralgia paresthetica
  Bernheim's — *see* Failure, heart, right
  big spleen D73.1
  bilateral polycystic ovarian E28.2
  Bing-Horton's — *see* Horton's headache
  Birt-Hogg-Dube syndrome Q87.89
  Björck (-Thorsen) E34.0
  black
    lung J60
    widow spider bite — *see* Toxicity, venom, spider, black widow
  Blackfan-Diamond D61.01
  Blau M04.8
  blind loop K90.2
    congenital Q43.8
    postsurgical K91.2
  blue sclera Q78.0
  blue toe I75.02- ☑
  Boder-Sedgewick G11.3
  Boerhaave's K22.3
  Borjeson Forssman Lehmann Q89.8
  Bouillaud's I01.9
  Bourneville (-Pringle) Q85.1
  Bouveret (-Hoffman) I47.9
  brachial plexus G54.0
  bradycardia-tachycardia I49.5
  brain (nonpsychotic) F09
    with psychosis, psychotic reaction F09
    acute or subacute — *see* Delirium
    congenital — *see* Disability, intellectual
    organic F09
      post-traumatic (nonpsychotic) F07.81
        psychotic F09
      personality change F07.0
      postcontusional F07.81
      post-traumatic, nonpsychotic F07.81
      psycho-organic F09
      psychotic F06.8
  brain stem stroke G46.3
  Brandt's (acrodermatitis enteropathica) E83.2
  broad ligament laceration N83.8
  Brock's J98.11
  bronze baby P83.88
  Brown-Sequard G83.81
  Brugada I49.8
  bubbly lung P27.0
  Buchem's M85.2
  Budd-Chiari I82.0
  bulbar (progressive) G12.22
  Bürger-Grütz E78.3
  Burke's K86.89
  Burnett's (milk-alkali) E83.52
  burning feet E53.9
  Bywaters' T79.5 ☑
  Call-Fleming I67.841
  carbohydrate-deficient glycoprotein (CDGS) E77.8
  carcinogenic thrombophlebitis I82.1
  carcinoid E34.0
  cardiac asthma I50.1
  cardiacos negros I27.0
  cardiofaciocutaneous Q87.89
  cardiopulmonary-obesity E66.2
  cardiorenal — *see* Hypertension, cardiorenal
  cardiorespiratory distress (idiopathic), newborn P22.0
  cardiovascular renal — *see* Hypertension, cardiorenal
  carotid
    artery (hemispheric) (internal) G45.1
      body G90.01
      sinus G90.01
  carpal tunnel G56.0- ☑
  Cassidy (-Scholte) E34.0
  cat cry Q93.4
  cat eye Q92.8
  cauda equina G83.4
  causalgia — *see* Causalgia
  celiac K90.0
    artery compression I77.4
    axis I77.4

Syndrome — *continued*
  central pain G89.0
  cerebellar
    hereditary G11.9
    stroke G46.4
  cerebellomedullary malformation — *see* Spina bifida
  cerebral
    artery
      anterior G46.1
      middle G46.0
      posterior G46.2
    gigantism E22.0
  cervical (root) M53.1
    disc — *see* Disorder, disc, cervical, with neuritis
    fusion Q76.1
    posterior, sympathicus M53.0
    rib Q76.5
    sympathetic paralysis G90.2
  cervicobrachial (diffuse) M53.1
  cervicocranial M53.0
  cervicodorsal outlet G54.2
  cervicothoracic outlet G54.0
  Céstan (-Raymond) I65.8
  Charcot's (angina cruris) (intermittent claudication) I73.9
  Charcot-Weiss-Baker G90.09
  CHARGE Q89.8
  Chédiak-Higashi (-Steinbrinck) E70.330
  chest wall R07.1
  Chiari's (hepatic vein thrombosis) I82.0
  Chilaiditi's Q43.3
  child maltreatment — *see* Maltreatment, child
  chondrocostal junction M94.0
  chondroectodermal dysplasia Q77.6
  chromosome 4 short arm deletion Q93.3
  chromosome 5 short arm deletion Q93.4
  chronic
    infantile neurological, cutaneous and articular (CINCA) M04.2
    pain G89.4
      personality F68.8
  Clarke-Hadfield K86.89
  Clerambault's automatism G93.89
  Clouston's (hidrotic ectodermal dysplasia) Q82.4
  clumsiness, clumsy child F82
  cluster headache G44.009
    intractable G44.001
    not intractable G44.009
  Coffin-Lowry Q89.8
  cold injury (newborn) P80.0
  combined immunity deficiency D81.9
  compartment (deep) (posterior) (traumatic) T79.A0 ☑ (*following* T79.7)
    abdomen T79.A3 ☑ (*following* T79.7)
    lower extremity (hip, buttock, thigh, leg, foot, toes) T79.A2 ☑ (*following* T79.7)
    nontraumatic
      abdomen M79.A3 (*following* M79.7)
      lower extremity (hip, buttock, thigh, leg, foot, toes) M79.A2- ☑ (*following* M79.7)
      specified site NEC M79.A9 (*following* M79.7)
      upper extremity (shoulder, arm, forearm, wrist, hand, fingers) M79.A1- ☑ (*following* M79.7)
    postprocedural — *see* Syndrome, compartment, nontraumatic
    specified site NEC T79.A9 ☑ (*following* T79.7)
    upper extremity (shoulder, arm, forearm, wrist, hand, fingers) T79.A1 ☑ (*following* T79.7)
  complex regional pain — *see* Syndrome, pain, complex regional
  compression T79.5 ☑
    anterior spinal — *see* Syndrome, anterior, spinal artery, compression
    cauda equina G83.4
    celiac artery I77.4
    vertebral artery M47.029
      cervical region M47.022
      occipito-atlanto-axial region M47.021
  concussion F07.81
  congenital
    affecting multiple systems NEC Q87.89
    central alveolar hypoventilation G47.35
    facial diplegia Q87.0
    muscular hypertrophy-cerebral Q87.89
    oculo-auriculovertebral Q87.89
    oculofacial diplegia (Moebius) Q87.0
    rubella (manifest) P35.0

▽ Subterms under main terms may continue to next column or page   ☑ Additional Character Required — Refer to the Tabular List for Character Selection   **299**

Syndrome — Syndrome

Syndrome — *continued*

congestion-fibrosis (pelvic), female N94.89
congestive dysmenorrhea N94.6
connective tissue M35.9
  overlap NEC M35.1
Conn's E26.01
conus medullaris G95.81
cord
  anterior G83.82
  posterior G83.83
coronary
  acute NEC I24.9
  insufficiency or intermediate I20.0
  slow flow I20.8
Costen's (complex) M26.69
costochondral junction M94.0
costoclavicular G54.0
costovertebral E22.0
Cowden Q85.8
craniovertebral M53.0
Creutzfeldt-Jakob — *see* Creutzfeldt-Jakob disease or
  syndrome
crib death R99
cricopharyngeal — *see* Dysphagia
cri-du-chat Q93.4
croup J05.0
CRPS I — *see* Syndrome, pain, complex regional I
crush T79.5 ☑
cryopyrin-associated perodic M04.2
cryptophthalmos Q87.0
cubital tunnel — *see* Lesion, nerve, ulnar
Curschmann (-Batten) (-Steinert) G71.11
Cushing's E24.9
  alcohol-induced E24.4
  due to
    alcohol
      drugs E24.2
    ectopic ACTH E24.3
    overproduction of pituitary ACTH E24.0
  drug-induced E24.2
  overdose or wrong substance given or taken — *see*
    Table of Drugs and Chemicals, by drug, poi-
    soning
  pituitary-dependent E24.0
  specified type NEC E24.8
cystic duct stump K91.5
Dana-Putnam D51.0
Danbolt (-Cross) (acrodermatitis enteropathica) E83.2
Dandy-Walker Q03.1
  with spina bifida Q07.01
Danlos' Q79.6
De Quervain E34.51
de Toni-Fanconi (-Debré) E72.09
  with cystinosis E72.04
defibrination (*see also* Fibrinolysis)
  with
    antepartum hemorrhage — *see* Hemorrhage,
      antepartum, with coagulation defect
    intrapartum hemorrhage — *see* Hemorrhage,
      complicating, delivery
    newborn P60
    postpartum O72.3
Degos' I77.89
Déjérine-Roussy G89.0
delayed sleep phase G47.21
demyelinating G37.9
dependence — *see* F10-F19 with fourth character .2
depersonalization (-derealization) F48.1
di George's D82.1
diabetes mellitus in newborn infant P70.2
diabetes mellitus-hypertension-nephrosis — *see* Diabetes, nephrosis
diabetes-nephrosis — *see* Diabetes, nephrosis
diabetic amyotrophy — *see* Diabetes, amyotrophy
dialysis associated steal T82.898- ☑
Diamond-Blackfan D61.01
Diamond-Gardener D69.2
DIC (diffuse or disseminated intravascular coagulopathy) D65
Dighton's Q78.0
disequilibrium E87.8
Döhle body-panmyelopathic D72.0
dorsolateral medullary G46.4
double athetosis G80.3
Down (*see also* Down syndrome) Q90.9
Dresbach's (elliptocytosis) D58.1
Dressler's (postmyocardial infarction) I24.1
  postcardiotomy I97.0

Syndrome — *continued*

drug withdrawal, infant of dependent mother P96.1
dry eye H04.12- ☑
due to abnormality
  chromosomal Q99.9
    sex
      female phenotype Q97.9
      male phenotype Q98.9
      specified NEC Q99.8
dumping (postgastrectomy) K91.1
  nonsurgical K31.89
Dupré's (meningism) R29.1
dysmetabolic X E88.81
dyspraxia, developmental F82
Eagle-Barrett Q79.4
Eaton-Lambert — *see* Syndrome, Lambert-Eaton
Ebstein's Q22.5
ectopic ACTH E24.3
eczema-thrombocytopenia D82.0
Eddowes' Q78.0
effort (psychogenic) F45.8
Ehlers-Danlos Q79.6
Eisenmenger's I27.83
Ekman's Q78.0
electric feet E53.8
Ellis-van Creveld Q77.6
empty nest Z60.0
endocrine-hypertensive E27.0
entrapment — *see* Neuropathy, entrapment
eosinophilia-myalgia M35.8
epileptic (*see also* Epilepsy, by type)
  absence G40.A09 (*following* G40.3)
    intractable G40.A19 (*following* G40.3)
      with status epilepticus G40.A11 (*following*
        G40.3)
      without status epilepticus G40.A19 (*following*
        G40.3)
    not intractable G40.A09 (*following* G40.3)
      with status epilepticus G40.A01 (*following*
        G40.3)
      without status epilepticus G40.A09 (*following*
        G40.3)
Erdheim-Chester (ECD) E88.89
Erdheim's E22.0
erythrocyte fragmentation D59.4
Evans D69.41
exhaustion F48.8
extrapyramidal G25.9
  specified NEC G25.89
eye retraction — *see* Strabismus
eyelid-malar-mandible Q87.0
Faber's D50.9
facial pain, paroxysmal G50.0
Fallot's Q21.3
familial cold autoinflammatory M04.2
familial eczema-thrombocytopenia (Wiskott-Aldrich)
  D82.0
Fanconi (-de Toni) (-Debré) E72.09
  with cystinosis E72.04
Fanconi's (anemia) (congenital pancytopenia) D61.09
fatigue
  chronic R53.82
  psychogenic F48.8
faulty bowel habit K59.39
Feil-Klippel (brevicollis) Q76.1
Felty's — *see* Felty's syndrome
fertile eunuch E23.0
fetal
  alcohol (dysmorphic) Q86.0
  hydantoin Q86.1
Fiedler's I40.1
first arch Q87.0
fish odor E72.89
Fisher's G61.0
Fitzhugh-Curtis
  due to
    Chlamydia trachomatis A74.81
    Neisseria gonorrhorea (gonococcal peritonitis)
      A54.85
Fitz's (*see also* Pancreatitis, acute) K85.80
Flajani (-Basedow) E05.00
  with thyroid storm E05.01
flatback — *see* Flatback syndrome
floppy
  baby P94.2
  iris (intraoeprative) (IFIS) H21.81
  mitral valve I34.1
flush E34.0

Syndrome — *continued*

Foix-Alajouanine G95.19
Fong's Q87.2
food protein-induced enterocolitis (FPIES) K52.21
foramen magnum G93.5
Foster-Kennedy H47.14- ☑
Foville's (peduncular) G46.3
fragile X Q99.2
Franceschetti Q75.4
Frey's
  auriculotemporal G50.8
  hyperhidrosis L74.52
Friderichsen-Waterhouse A39.1
Froin's G95.89
frontal lobe F07.0
Fukuhara E88.49
functional
  bowel K59.9
  prepubertal castrate E29.1
Gaisböck's D75.1
ganglion (basal ganglia brain) G25.9
  geniculi G51.1
Gardner-Diamond D69.2
gastroesophageal
  junction K22.0
  laceration-hemorrhage K22.6
gastrojejunal loop obstruction K91.89
Gee-Herter-Heubner K90.0
Gelineau's G47.419
  with cataplexy G47.411
genito-anorectal A55
Gerstmann-Sträussler-Scheinker (GSS) A81.82
Gianotti-Crosti L44.4
giant platelet (Bernard-Soulier) D69.1
Gilles de la Tourette's F95.2
goiter-deafness E07.1
Goldberg Q89.8
Goldberg-Maxwell E34.51
Good's D83.8
Gopalan' (burning feet) E53.8
Gorlin's Q87.89
Gougerot-Blum L81.7
Gouley's I31.1
Gower's R55
gray or grey (newborn) P93.0
  platelet D69.1
Gubler-Millard G46.3
Guillain-Barré (-Strohl) G61.0
gustatory sweating G50.8
Hadfield-Clarke K86.89
hair tourniquet — *see* Constriction, external, by site
Hamman's J98.19
hand-foot L27.1
hand-shoulder G90.8
hantavirus (cardio)-pulmonary (HPS) (HCPS) B33.4
happy puppet Q93.51
Harada's H30.81- ☑
Hayem-Faber D50.9
headache NEC G44.89
  complicated NEC G44.59
Heberden's I20.8
Hedinger's E34.0
Hegglin's D72.0
HELLP (hemolysis, elevated liver enzymes and low
  platelet count) O14.2- ☑
  complicating
    childbirth O14.24
    puerperium O14.25
hemolytic-uremic D59.3
hemophagocytic, infection-associated D76.2
Henoch-Schönlein D69.0
hepatic flexure K59.8
hepatopulmonary K76.81
hepatorenal K76.7
  following delivery O90.4
  postoperative or postprocedural K91.83
  postpartum, puerperal O90.4
hepatourologic K76.7
Herter (-Gee) (nontropical sprue) K90.0
Heubner-Herter K90.0
Heyd's K76.7
Hilger's G90.09
histamine-like (fish poisoning) — *see* Poisoning, fish
histiocytic D76.3
histiocytosis NEC D76.3
HIV infection, acute B20
Hoffmann-Werdnig G12.0
Hollander-Simons E88.1
Hoppe-Goldflam G70.00

Syndrome — *continued*
  Hoppe-Goldflam — *continued*
    with exacerbation (acute) G70.01
    in crisis G70.01
  Horner's G90.2
  hungry bone E83.81
  hunterian glossitis D51.0
  Hutchinson's triad A50.53
  hyperabduction G54.0
  hyperammonemia-hyperornithinemia-homocitrulline-
    mia E72.4
  hypereosinophilic (idiopathic) D72.1
  hyperimmunoglobulin D M04.1
  hyperimmunoglobulin E (IgE) D82.4
  hyperkalemic E87.5
  hyperkinetic — *see* Hyperkinesia
  hypermobility M35.7
  hypernatremia E87.0
  hyperosmolarity E87.0
  hyperperfusion G97.82
  hypersplenic D73.1
  hypertransfusion, newborn P61.1
  hyperventilation F45.8
  hyperviscosity (of serum)
    polycythemic D75.1
    sclerothymic D58.8
  hypoglycemic (familial) (neonatal) E16.2
  hypokalemic E87.6
  hyponatremic E87.1
  hypopituitarism E23.0
  hypoplastic left-heart Q23.4
  hypopotassemia E87.6
  hyposmolality E87.1
  hypotension, maternal O26.5- ☑
  hypothenar hammer I73.89
  hypoventilation, obesity (OHS) E66.2
  ICF (intravascular coagulation-fibrinolysis) D65
  idiopathic
    cardiorespiratory distress, newborn P22.0
    nephrotic (infantile) N04.9
  iliotibial band M76.3- ☑
  immobility, immobilization (paraplegic) M62.3
  immune reconstitution D89.3
  immune reconstitution inflammatory [IRIS] D89.3
  immunity deficiency, combined D81.9
  immunodeficiency
    acquired — *see* Human, immunodeficiency virus
      (HIV) disease
    combined D81.9
  impending coronary I20.0
  impingement, shoulder M75.4- ☑
  inappropriate secretion of antidiuretic hormone E22.2
  infant
    gestational diabetes P70.0
    of diabetic mother P70.1
  infantilism (pituitary) E23.0
  inferior vena cava I87.1
  inspissated bile (newborn) P59.1
  institutional (childhood) F94.2
  insufficient sleep F51.12
  intermediate coronary (artery) I20.0
  interspinous ligament — *see* Spondylopathy, specified
    NEC
  intestinal
    carcinoid E34.0
    knot K56.2
  intravascular coagulation-fibrinolysis (ICF) D65
  iodine-deficiency, congenital E00.9
    type
      mixed E00.2
      myxedematous E00.1
      neurological E00.0
  IRDS (idiopathic respiratory distress, newborn) P22.0
  irritable
    bowel K58.9
      with
        constipation K58.1
        diarrhea K58.0
      mixed K58.2
      psychogenic F45.8
      specified NEC K58.8
    heart (psychogenic) F45.8
    weakness F48.8
  ischemic
    bowel (transient) K55.9
      chronic K55.1
      due to mesenteric artery insufficiency K55.1
    steal T82.898 ☑

Syndrome — *continued*
  IVC (intravascular coagulopathy) D65
  Ivemark's Q89.01
  Jaccoud's — *see* Arthropathy, postrheumatic, chronic
  Jackson's G83.89
  Jakob-Creutzfeldt — *see* Creutzfeldt-Jakob disease or
    syndrome
  jaw-winking Q07.8
  Jervell-Lange-Nielsen I45.81
  jet lag G47.25
  Job's D71
  Joseph-Diamond-Blackfan D61.01
  jugular foramen G52.7
  Kabuki Q89.8
  Kanner's (autism) F84.0
  Kartagener's Q89.3
  Kelly's D50.1
  Kimmelstiel-Wilson — *see* Diabetes, specified type,
    with Kimmelstiel-Wilson disease
  Klein (e)-Levine G47.13
  Klippel-Feil (brevicollis) Q76.1
  Köhler-Pellegrini-Steida — *see* Bursitis, tibial collateral
  König's K59.8
  Korsakoff (-Wernicke) (nonalcoholic) F04
    alcoholic F10.26
  Kostmann's D70.0
  Krabbe's congenital muscle hypoplasia Q79.8
  labyrinthine — *see* subcategory H83.2 ☑
  lacunar NEC G46.7
  Lambert-Eaton G70.80
    in
      neoplastic disease G73.1
      specified disease NEC G70.81
  Landau-Kleffner — *see* Epilepsy, specified NEC
  Larsen's Q74.8
  lateral
    cutaneous nerve of thigh G57.1- ☑
    medullary G46.4
  Launois' E22.0
  lazy
    leukocyte D70.8
    posture M62.3
  Lemiere I80.8
  Lennox-Gastaut G40.812
    intractable G40.814
      with status epilepticus G40.813
      without status epilepticus G40.814
    not intractable G40.812
      with status epilepticus G40.811
      without status epilepticus G40.812
  lenticular, progressive E83.01
  Leopold-Levi's E05.90
  Lev's I44.2
  Lichtheim's D51.0
  Li-Fraumeni Z15.01
  Lightwood's N25.89
  Lignac (de Toni) (-Fanconi) (-Debré) E72.09
    with cystinosis E72.04
  Likoff's I20.8
  limbic epilepsy personality F07.0
  liver-kidney K76.7
  lobotomy F07.0
  Loffler's J82
  long arm 18 or 21 deletion Q93.89
  long QT I45.81
  Louis-Barré G11.3
  low
    atmospheric pressure T70.29 ☑
    back M54.5
    output (cardiac) I50.9
  lower radicular, newborn (birth injury) P14.8
  Luetscher's (dehydration) E86.0
  Lupus anticoagulant D68.62
  Lutembacher's Q21.1
  macrophage activation D76.1
    due to infection D76.2
  magnesium-deficiency R29.0
  Majeed M04.8
  Mal de Debarquement R42
  malabsorption K90.9
    postsurgical K91.2
  malformation, congenital, due to
    alcohol Q86.0
    exogenous cause NEC Q86.8
    hydantoin Q86.1
    warfarin Q86.2
  malignant
    carcinoid E34.0

Syndrome — *continued*
  malignant — *continued*
    neuroleptic G21.0
  Mallory-Weiss K22.6
  mandibulofacial dysostosis Q75.4
  manic-depressive — *see* Disorder, bipolar
  maple-syrup-urine E71.0
  Marable's I77.4
  Marfan's Q87.40
    with
      cardiovascular manifestations Q87.418
        aortic dilation Q87.410
      ocular manifestations Q87.42
      skeletal manifestations Q87.43
  Marie's (acromegaly) E22.0
  mast cell activation — *see* Activation, mast cell
  maternal hypotension — *see* Syndrome, hypotension,
    maternal
  May (-Hegglin) D72.0
  McArdle (-Schmidt) (-Pearson) E74.04
  McQuarrie's E16.2
  meconium plug (newborn) P76.0
  median arcuate ligament I77.4
  Meekeren-Ehlers-Danlos Q79.6
  megavitamin-B6 E67.2
  Meige G24.4
  MELAS E88.41
  Mendelson's O74.0
  MERRF (myoclonic epilepsy associated with ragged-
    red fibers) E88.42
  mesenteric
    artery (superior) K55.1
    vascular insufficiency K55.1
  metabolic E88.81
  metastatic carcinoid E34.0
  micrognathia-glossoptosis Q87.0
  midbrain NEC G93.89
  middle lobe (lung) J98.19
  middle radicular G54.0
  migraine (*see also* Migraine) G43.909
  Mikulicz' K11.8
  milk-alkali E83.52
  Millard-Gubler G46.3
  Miller-Dieker Q93.88
  Miller-Fisher G61.0
  Minkowski-Chauffard D58.0
  Mirizzi's K83.1
  MNGIE (Mitochondrial Neurogastrointestinal En-
    cephalopathy) E88.49
  Möbius, ophthalmoplegic migraine — *see* Migraine,
    ophthalmoplegic
  monofixation H50.42
  Morel-Moore M85.2
  Morel-Morgagni M85.2
  Morgagni (-Morel) (-Stewart) M85.2
  Morgagni-Adams-Stokes I45.9
  Mounier-Kuhn Q32.4
    with bronchiectasis J47.9
      with
        exacerbation (acute) J47.1
        lower respiratory infection J47.0
    acquired J98.09
      with bronchiectasis J47.9
        with
          exacerbation (acute) J47.1
          lower respiratory infection J47.0
  Muckle-Wells M04.2
  mucocutaneous lymph node (acute febrile) (MCLS)
    M30.3
  multiple endocrine neoplasia (MEN) — *see* Neoplasia,
    endocrine, multiple (MEN)
  multiple operations — *see* Disorder, factitious
  myasthenic G70.9
    in
      diabetes mellitus — *see* Diabetes, amyotrophy
      endocrine disease NEC E34.9 [G73.3]
      neoplastic disease (*see also* Neoplasm)
        D49.9 [G73.3]
      thyrotoxicosis (hyperthyroidism) E05.90 [G73.3]
        with thyroid storm E05.91 [G73.3]
  myelodysplastic D46.9
    with
      5q deletion D46.C (*following* D46.2)
      isolated del (5q) chromosomal abnormality D46.C
        (*following* D46.2)
    lesions, low grade D46.20
    specified NEC D46.Z (*following* D46.4)
  myelopathic pain G89.0

Syndrome — *continued*

myeloproliferative (chronic) D47.1

myofascial pain M79.18

Naffziger's G54.0

nail patella Q87.2

NARP (Neuropathy, Ataxia and Retinitis pigmentosa) E88.49

neonatal abstinence P96.1

nephritic (*see also* Nephritis)

  with edema — *see* Nephrosis

  acute N00.9

  chronic N03.9

  rapidly progressive N01.9

nephrotic (congenital) (*see also* Nephrosis) N04.9

  with

    dense deposit disease N04.6

    diffuse

      crescentic glomerulonephritis N04.7

      endocapillary proliferative glomerulonephritis N04.4

      membranous glomerulonephritis N04.2

      mesangial proliferative glomerulonephritis N04.3

      mesangiocapillary glomerulonephritis N04.5

    focal and segmental glomerular lesions N04.1

    minor glomerular abnormality N04.0

    specified morphological changes NEC N04.8

  diabetic — *see* Diabetes, nephrosis

neurologic neglect R41.4

Nezelof's D81.4

Nonne-Milroy-Meige Q82.0

Nothnagel's vasomotor acroparesthesia I73.89

obesity hypoventilation (OHS) E66.2

oculomotor H51.9

ophthalmoplegia-cerebellar ataxia — *see* Strabismus, paralytic, third nerve

oral allergy T78.1 ☑

oral-facial-digital Q87.0

organic

  affective F06.30

  amnesic (not alcohol- or drug-induced) F04

  brain F09

  depressive F06.31

  hallucinosis F06.0

  personality F07.0

Ormond's N13.5

oro-facial-digital Q87.0

os trigonum Q68.8

Osler-Weber-Rendu I78.0

osteoporosis-osteomalacia M83.8

Osterreicher-Turner Q87.2

otolith — *see* subcategory H81.8 ☑

oto-palatal-digital Q87.0

outlet (thoracic) G54.0

ovary

  polycystic E28.2

  resistant E28.39

  sclerocystic E28.2

Owren's D68.2

Paget-Schroetter I82.890

pain (*see also* Pain)

  complex regional I G90.50

    lower limb G90.52- ☑

    specified site NEC G90.59

    upper limb G90.51- ☑

  complex regional II — *see* Causalgia

painful

  bruising D69.2

  feet E53.8

  prostate N42.81

paralysis agitans — *see* Parkinsonism

paralytic G83.9

  specified NEC G83.89

Parinaud's H51.0

parkinsonian — *see* Parkinsonism

Parkinson's — *see* Parkinsonism

paroxysmal facial pain G50.0

Parry's E05.00

  with thyroid storm E05.01

Parsonage (-Aldren)-Turner G54.5

patella clunk M25.86- ☑

Paterson (-Brown) (-Kelly) D50.1

pectoral girdle I77.89

pectoralis minor I77.89

pediatric autoimmune neuropsychiatric disorders associated with streptococcal infections (PANDAS) D89.89

Pelger-Huet D72.0

Syndrome — *continued*

pellagra-cerebellar ataxia-renal aminoaciduria E72.02

pellagroid E52

Pellegrini-Stieda — *see* Bursitis, tibial collateral

pelvic congestion-fibrosis, female N94.89

penta X Q97.1

peptic ulcer — *see* Ulcer, peptic

perabduction I77.89

periodic fever M04.1

periodic fever, aphthous stomatitis, pharyngitis, and adenopathy [PFAPA] M04.8

periodic headache, in adults and children — *see* Headache, periodic syndromes in adults and children

periurethral fibrosis N13.5

phantom limb (without pain) G54.7

  with pain G54.6

pharyngeal pouch D82.1

Pick's — *see* Disease, Pick's

Pickwickian E66.2

PIE (pulmonary infiltration with eosinophilia) J82

pigmentary pallidal degeneration (progressive) G23.0

pineal E34.8

pituitary E22.0

placental transfusion — *see* Pregnancy, complicated by, placental transfusion syndromes

plantar fascia M72.2

plateau iris (post-iridectomy) (postprocedural) H21.82

Plummer-Vinson D50.1

pluricarential of infancy E40

plurideficiency E40

pluriglandular (compensatory) E31.8

  autoimmune E31.0

polyangiitis overlap M30.8

polycarential of infancy E40

polyglandular E31.8

  autoimmune E31.0

polysplenia Q89.09

pontine NEC G93.89

popliteal

  artery entrapment I77.89

  web Q87.89

post chemoembolization — *code to* associated conditions

postcardiac injury

  postcardiotomy I97.0

  postmyocardial infarction I24.1

postcardiotomy I97.0

postcholecystectomy K91.5

postcommissurotomy I97.0

postconcussional F07.81

postcontusional F07.81

postencephalitic F07.89

posterior

  cervical sympathetic M53.0

  cord G83.83

  fossa compression G93.5

  reversible encephalopathy (PRES) I67.83

postgastrectomy (dumping) K91.1

postgastric surgery K91.1

postinfarction I24.1

postlaminectomy NEC M96.1

postleukotomy F07.0

postmastectomy lymphedema I97.2

postmyocardial infarction I24.1

postoperative NEC T81.9 ☑

  blind loop K90.2

postpartum panhypopituitary (Sheehan) E23.0

postpolio (myelitic) G14

postthrombotic I87.009

  with

    inflammation I87.02- ☑

      with ulcer I87.03- ☑

    specified complication NEC I87.09- ☑

    ulcer I87.01- ☑

      with inflammation I87.03- ☑

  asymptomatic I87.00- ☑

postvagotomy K91.1

postvalvulotomy I97.0

postviral NEC G93.3

  fatigue G93.3

Potain's K31.0

potassium intoxication E87.5

precerebral artery (multiple) (bilateral) G45.2

preinfarction I20.0

preleukemic D46.9

premature senility E34.8

Syndrome — *continued*

premenstrual dysphoric F32.89

premenstrual tension N94.3

Prinzmetal-Massumi R07.1

prune belly Q79.4

pseudo -Turner's Q87.1

pseudocarpal tunnel (sublimis) — *see* Syndrome, carpal tunnel

pseudoparalytica G70.00

  with exacerbation (acute) G70.01

  in crisis G70.01

psycho-organic (nonpsychotic severity) F07.9

  acute or subacute F05

  depressive type F06.31

  hallucinatory type F06.0

  nonpsychotic severity F07.0

  specified NEC F07.89

pulmonary

  arteriosclerosis I27.0

  dysmaturity (Wilson-Mikity) P27.0

  hypoperfusion (idiopathic) P22.0

  renal (hemorrhagic) (Goodpasture's) M31.0

pure

  motor lacunar G46.5

  sensory lacunar G46.6

Putnam-Dana D51.0

pyogenic arthritis, pyoderma gangrenosum, and acne [PAPA] M04.8

pyramidopallidonigral G20

pyriformis — *see* Lesion, nerve, sciatic

QT interval prolongation I45.81

radicular NEC — *see* Radiculopathy

  upper limbs, newborn (birth injury) P14.3

rapid time-zone change G47.25

Rasmussen G04.81

Raymond (-Céstan) I65.8

Raynaud's I73.00

  with gangrene I73.01

RDS (respiratory distress syndrome, newborn) P22.0

reactive airways dysfunction J68.3

Refsum's G60.1

Reifenstein E34.52

renal glomerulohyalinosis-diabetic — *see* Diabetes, nephrosis

Rendu-Osler-Weber I78.0

residual ovary N99.83

resistant ovary E28.39

respiratory

  distress

    acute J80

      adult J80

      child J80

      idiopathic J84.114

    newborn (idiopathic) (type I) P22.0

      type II P22.1

restless legs G25.81

retinoblastoma (familial) C69.2 ☑

retroperitoneal fibrosis N13.5

retroviral seroconversion (acute) Z21

Reye's G93.7

Richter — *see* Leukemia, chronic lymphocytic, B-cell type

Ridley's I50.1

right

  heart, hypoplastic Q22.6

  ventricular obstruction — *see* Failure, heart, congestive

Romano-Ward (prolonged QT interval) I45.81

rotator cuff, shoulder (*see also* Tear, rotator cuff) M75.10- ☑

Rotes Quérol — *see* Hyperostosis, ankylosing

Roth — *see* Meralgia paresthetica

rubella (congenital) P35.0

Ruvalcaba-Myhre-Smith E71.440

Rytand-Lipsitch I44.2

salt

  depletion E87.1

    due to heat NEC T67.8 ☑

      causing heat exhaustion or prostration T67.4 ☑

  low E87.1

salt-losing N28.89

Scaglietti-Dagnini E22.0

scalenus anticus (anterior) G54.0

scapulocostal — *see* Mononeuropathy, upper limb, specified site NEC

scapuloperoneal G71.09

schizophrenic, of childhood NEC F84.5

Syndrome — *continued*
- Schnitzler D47.2
- Scholte's E34.0
- Schroeder's E27.0
- Schüller-Christian C96.5
- Schwachman's — *see* Syndrome, Shwachman's
- Schwartz (-Jampel) G71.13
- Schwartz-Bartter E22.2
- scimitar Q26.8
- sclerocystic ovary E28.2
- Seitelberger's G31.89
- septicemic adrenal hemorrhage A39.1
- seroconversion, retroviral (acute) Z21
- serous meningitis G93.2
- severe acute respiratory (SARS) J12.81
- shaken infant T74.4 ☑
- shock (traumatic) T79.4 ☑
  - kidney N17.0
    - following crush injury T79.5 ☑
  - toxic A48.3
- shock-lung J80
- Shone's — *code to* specific anomalies
- short
  - bowel K91.2
  - rib Q77.2
- shoulder-hand — *see* Algoneurodystrophy
- Shwachman's D70.4
- sicca — *see* Sicca syndrome
- sick
  - cell E87.1
  - sinus I49.5
- sick-euthyroid E07.81
- sideropenic D50.1
- Siemens' ectodermal dysplasia Q82.4
- Silfversköld's Q78.9
- Simons' E88.1
- sinus tarsi M25.57- ☑
- sinusitis-bronchiectasis-situs inversus Q89.3
- Sipple's E31.22
- sirenomelia Q87.2
- Slocumb's E27.0
- slow flow, coronary I20.8
- Sluder's G44.89
- Smith-Magenis Q93.88
- Sneddon-Wilkinson L13.1
- Sotos' Q87.3
- South African cardiomyopathy I42.8
- spasmodic
  - upward movement, eyes H51.8
  - winking F95.8
- Spen's I45.9
- splenic
  - agenesis Q89.01
  - flexure K59.8
  - neutropenia D73.81
- Spurway's Q78.0
- staphylococcal scalded skin L00
- steal
  - arteriovenous T82.898- ☑
  - ischemic T82.898- ☑
  - subclavian G45.8
- Stein-Leventhal E28.2
- Stein's E28.2
- Stevens-Johnson syndrome L51.1
  - toxic epidermal necrolysis overlap L51.3
- Stewart-Morel M85.2
- Stickler Q89.8
- stiff baby Q89.8
- stiff man G25.82
- Still-Felty — *see* Felty's syndrome
- Stokes (-Adams) I45.9
- stone heart I50.1
- straight back, congenital Q76.49
- subclavian steal G45.8
- subcoracoid-pectoralis minor G54.0
- subcostal nerve compression I77.89
- subphrenic interposition Q43.3
- superior
  - cerebellar artery I63.89
  - mesenteric artery K55.1
  - semi-circular canal dehiscence H83.8X- ☑
  - vena cava I87.1
- supine hypotensive (maternal) — *see* Syndrome, hypotension, maternal
- suprarenal cortical E27.0
- supraspinatus (*see also* Tear, rotator cuff) M75.10- ☑
- Susac G93.49
- swallowed blood P78.2

Syndrome — *continued*
- sweat retention L74.0
- Swyer Q99.1
- Symond's G93.2
- sympathetic
  - cervical paralysis G90.2
  - pelvic, female N94.89
- systemic inflammatory response (SIRS), of non-infectious origin (without organ dysfunction) R65.10
  - with acute organ dysfunction R65.11
- tachycardia-bradycardia I49.5
- takotsubo I51.81
- TAR (thrombocytopenia with absent radius) Q87.2
- tarsal tunnel G57.5- ☑
- teething K00.7
- tegmental G93.89
- telangiectasic-pigmentation-cataract Q82.8
- temporal pyramidal apex — *see* Otitis, media, suppurative, acute
- temporomandibular joint-pain-dysfunction M26.62- ☑
- Terry's (*see also* Myopia, degenerative) H44.2- ☑
- testicular feminization (*see also* Syndrome, androgen insensitivity) E34.51
- thalamic pain (hyperesthetic) G89.0
- thoracic outlet (compression) G54.0
- Thorson-Björck E34.0
- thrombocytopenia with absent radius (TAR) Q87.2
- thyroid-adrenocortical insufficiency E31.0
- tibial
  - anterior M76.81- ☑
  - posterior M76.82- ☑
- Tietze's M94.0
- time-zone (rapid) G47.25
- Toni-Fanconi E72.09
  - with cystinosis E72.04
- Touraine's Q79.8
- tourniquet — *see* Constriction, external, by site
- toxic shock A48.3
- transient left ventricular apical ballooning I51.81
- traumatic vasospastic T75.22 ☑
- Treacher Collins Q75.4
- triple X, female Q97.0
- trisomy Q92.9
  - 13 Q91.7
    - meiotic nondisjunction Q91.4
    - mitotic nondisjunction Q91.5
    - mosaicism Q91.5
    - translocation Q91.6
  - 18 Q91.3
    - meiotic nondisjunction Q91.0
    - mitotic nondisjunction Q91.1
    - mosaicism Q91.1
    - translocation Q91.2
  - 20 (q)(p) Q92.8
  - 21 Q90.9
    - meiotic nondisjunction Q90.0
    - mitotic nondisjunction Q90.1
    - mosaicism Q90.1
    - translocation Q90.2
  - 22 Q92.8
- tropical wet feet T69.0- ☑
- Trousseau's I82.1
- tumor lysis (following antineoplastic chemotherapy) (spontaneous) NEC E88.3
- tumor necrosis factor receptor associated periodic (TRAPS) M04.1
- Twiddler's (due to)
  - automatic implantable defibrillator T82.198 ☑
  - cardiac pacemaker T82.198 ☑
- Unverricht (-Lundborg) — *see* Epilepsy, generalized, idiopathic
- upward gaze H51.8
- uremia, chronic (*see also* Disease, kidney, chronic) N18.9
- urethral N34.3
- urethro-oculo-articular — *see* Reiter's disease
- urohepatic K76.7
- vago-hypoglossal G52.7
- van Buchem's M85.2
- van der Hoeve's Q78.0
- vascular NEC in cerebrovascular disease G46.8
- vasoconstriction, reversible cerebrovascular I67.841
- vasomotor I73.9
- vasospastic (traumatic) T75.22 ☑
- vasovagal R55
- VATER Q87.2
- velo-cardio-facial Q93.81
- vena cava (inferior) (superior) (obstruction) I87.1

Syndrome — *continued*
- vertebral
  - artery G45.0
    - compression — *see* Syndrome, anterior, spinal artery, compression
  - steal G45.0
- vertebro-basilar artery G45.0
- vertebrogenic (pain) M54.89
- vertiginous — *see* Disorder, vestibular function
- Vinson-Plummer D50.1
- virus B34.9
- visceral larva migrans B83.0
- visual disorientation H53.8
- vitamin B6 deficiency E53.1
- vitreal corneal H59.01- ☑
- vitreous (touch) H59.01- ☑
- Vogt-Koyanagi H20.82- ☑
- Volkmann's T79.6 ☑
- von Schroetter's I82.890
- von Willebrand (-Jürgen) D68.0
- Waldenström-Kjellberg D50.1
- Wallenberg's G46.3
- water retention E87.79
- Waterhouse (-Friderichsen) A39.1
- Weber-Gubler G46.3
- Weber-Leyden G46.3
- Weber's G46.3
- Wegener's M31.30
  - with
    - kidney involvement M31.31
    - lung involvement M31.30
      - with kidney involvement M31.31
- Weingarten's (tropical eosinophilia) J82
- Weiss-Baker G90.09
- Werdnig-Hoffman G12.0
- Wermer's E31.21
- Werner's E34.8
- Wernicke-Korsakoff (nonalcoholic) F04
  - alcoholic F10.26
- Westphal-Strümpell E83.01
- West's — *see* Epilepsy, spasms
- wet
  - feet (maceration) (tropical) T69.0- ☑
  - lung, newborn P22.1
- whiplash S13.4 ☑
- whistling face Q87.0
- Wilkie's K55.1
- Wilkinson-Sneddon L13.1
- Willebrand (-Jürgens) D68.0
- Williams Q93.82
- Wilson's (hepatolenticular degeneration) E83.01
- Wiskott-Aldrich D82.0
- withdrawal — *see* Withdrawal, state
  - drug
    - infant of dependent mother P96.1
    - therapeutic use, newborn P96.2
- Woakes' (ethmoiditis) J33.1
- Wright's (hyperabduction) G54.0
- X I20.9
- XXXX Q97.1
- XXXXX Q97.1
- XXXXY Q98.1
- XXY Q98.0
- Yao M04.8
- yellow nail L60.5
- Zahorsky's B08.5
- Zellweger syndrome E71.510
- Zellweger-like syndrome E71.541

Synechia (anterior) (iris) (posterior) (pupil) (*see also* Adhesions, iris)
- intra-uterine (traumatic) N85.6

Synesthesia R20.8

Syngamiasis, syngamosis B83.3

Synodontia K00.2

Synorchidism, synorchism Q55.1

Synostosis (congenital) Q78.8
- astragalo-scaphoid Q74.2
- radioulnar Q74.0

Synovial sarcoma — *see* Neoplasm, connective tissue, malignant

Synovioma (malignant) (*see also* Neoplasm, connective tissue, malignant)
- benign — *see* Neoplasm, connective tissue, benign

Synoviosarcoma — *see* Neoplasm, connective tissue, malignant

Synovitis (*see also* Tenosynovitis) M65.9
- crepitant
  - hand M70.0- ☑

☁ **Subterms under main terms may continue to next column or page** ☑ **Additional Character Required — Refer to the Tabular List for Character Selection** 303

Syndrome — Synovitis

Synovitis — *continued*
  crepitant — *continued*
    wrist M70.03-☑
  gonococcal A54.49
  gouty — *see* Gout
  in (due to)
    crystals M65.8-☑
    gonorrhea A54.49
    syphilis (late) A52.78
    use, overuse, pressure — *see* Disorder, soft tissue, due to use
  infective NEC — *see* Tenosynovitis, infective NEC
  specified NEC — *see* Tenosynovitis, specified type NEC
  syphilitic A52.78
    congenital (early) A50.02
  toxic — *see* Synovitis, transient
  transient M67.3-☑
    ankle M67.37-☑
    elbow M67.32-☑
    foot joint M67.37-☑
    hand joint M67.34-☑
    hip M67.35-☑
    knee M67.36-☑
    multiple site M67.39
    pelvic region M67.35-☑
    shoulder M67.31-☑
    specified joint NEC M67.38
    wrist M67.33-☑
  traumatic, current — *see* Sprain
  tuberculous — *see* Tuberculosis, synovitis
  villonodular (pigmented) M12.2-☑
    ankle M12.27-☑
    elbow M12.22-☑
    foot joint M12.27-☑
    hand joint M12.24-☑
    hip M12.25-☑
    knee M12.26-☑
    multiple site M12.29
    pelvic region M12.25-☑
    shoulder M12.21-☑
    specified joint NEC M12.28
    vertebrae M12.28
    wrist M12.23-☑

Syphilid A51.39
  congenital A50.06
  newborn A50.06
  tubercular (late) A52.79

Syphilis, syphilitic (acquired) A53.9
  abdomen (late) A52.79
  acoustic nerve A52.15
  adenopathy (secondary) A51.49
  adrenal (gland) (with cortical hypofunction) A52.79
  age under 2 years NOS (*see also* Syphilis, congenital, early)
    acquired A51.9
  alopecia (secondary) A51.32
  anemia (late) A52.79 [D63.8]
  aneurysm (aorta) (ruptured) A52.01
    central nervous system A52.05
    congenital A50.54 [I79.0]
  anus (late) A52.74
    primary A51.1
    secondary A51.39
  aorta (arch) (abdominal) (thoracic) A52.02
    aneurysm A52.01
  aortic (insufficiency) (regurgitation) (stenosis) A52.03
    aneurysm A52.01
  arachnoid (adhesive) (cerebral) (spinal) A52.13
  asymptomatic — *see* Syphilis, latent
  ataxia (locomotor) A52.11
  atrophoderma maculatum A51.39
  auricular fibrillation A52.06
  bladder (late) A52.76
  bone A52.77
    secondary A51.46
  brain A52.17
  breast (late) A52.79
  bronchus (late) A52.72
  bubo (primary) A51.0
  bulbar palsy A52.19
  bursa (late) A52.78
  cardiac decompensation A52.06
  cardiovascular A52.00
  central nervous system (late) (recurrent) (relapse) (tertiary) A52.3
    with
      ataxia A52.11
      general paralysis A52.17

Syphilis, syphilitic — *continued*
  central nervous system — *continued*
    with — *continued*
      general paralysis — *continued*
        juvenile A50.45
      paresis (general) A52.17
        juvenile A50.45
      tabes (dorsalis) A52.11
        juvenile A50.45
      taboparesis A52.17
        juvenile A50.45
    aneurysm A52.05
    congenital A50.40
    juvenile A50.40
    remission (in sustained) A52.3
    serology doubtful, negative, or positive A52.3
    specified nature or site NEC A52.19
    vascular A52.05
  cerebral A52.17
    meningovascular A52.13
    nerves (multiple palsies) A52.15
    sclerosis A52.17
    thrombosis A52.05
  cerebrospinal (tabetic type) A52.12
  cerebrovascular A52.05
  cervix (late) A52.76
  chancre (multiple) A51.0
    extragenital A51.2
    Rollet's A51.0
  Charcot's joint A52.16
  chorioretinitis A51.43
    congenital A50.01
    late A52.71
    prenatal A50.01
  choroiditis — *see* Syphilitic chorioretinitis
  choroidoretinitis — *see* Syphilitic chorioretinitis
  ciliary body (secondary) A51.43
    late A52.71
  colon (late) A52.74
  combined spinal sclerosis A52.11
  condyloma (latum) A51.31
  congenital A50.9
    with
      paresis (general) A50.45
      tabes (dorsalis) A50.45
      taboparesis A50.45
    chorioretinitis, choroiditis A50.01 [H32]
    early, or less than 2 years after birth NEC A50.2
      with manifestations — *see* Syphilis, congenital, early, symptomatic
      latent (without manifestations) A50.1
        negative spinal fluid test A50.1
        serology positive A50.1
      symptomatic A50.09
        cutaneous A50.06
        mucocutaneous A50.07
        oculopathy A50.01
        osteochondropathy A50.02
        pharyngitis A50.03
        pneumonia A50.04
        rhinitis A50.05
        visceral A50.08
    interstitial keratitis A50.31
    juvenile neurosyphilis A50.45
    late, or 2 years or more after birth NEC A50.7
      chorioretinitis, choroiditis A50.32
      interstitial keratitis A50.31
      juvenile neurosyphilis A50.45
      latent (without manifestations) A50.6
        negative spinal fluid test A50.6
        serology positive A50.6
      symptomatic or with manifestations NEC A50.59
        arthropathy A50.55
        cardiovascular A50.54
        Clutton's joints A50.51
        Hutchinson's teeth A50.52
        Hutchinson's triad A50.53
        osteochondropathy A50.56
        saddle nose A50.57
  conjugal A53.9
    tabes A52.11
  conjunctiva (late) A52.71
  contact Z20.2
  cord bladder A52.19
  cornea, late A52.71
  coronary (artery) (sclerosis) A52.06
  coryza, congenital A50.05
  cranial nerve A52.15
    multiple palsies A52.15

Syphilis, syphilitic — *continued*
  cutaneous — *see* Syphilis, skin
  dacryocystitis (late) A52.71
  degeneration, spinal cord A52.12
  dementia paralytica A52.17
    juvenilis A50.45
  destruction of bone A52.77
  dilatation, aorta A52.01
  due to blood transfusion A53.9
  dura mater A52.13
  ear A52.79
    inner A52.79
      nerve (eighth) A52.15
      neurorecurrence A52.15
  early A51.9
    cardiovascular A52.00
    central nervous system A52.3
    latent (without manifestations) (less than 2 years after infection) A51.5
      negative spinal fluid test A51.5
      serological relapse after treatment A51.5
      serology positive A51.5
    relapse (treated, untreated) A51.9
    skin A51.39
    symptomatic A51.9
      extragenital chancre A51.2
      primary, except extragenital chancre A51.0
      secondary (*see also* Syphilis, secondary) A51.39
        relapse (treated, untreated) A51.49
    ulcer A51.39
  eighth nerve (neuritis) A52.15
  endemic A65
  endocarditis A52.03
    aortic A52.03
    pulmonary A52.03
  epididymis (late) A52.76
  epiglottis (late) A52.73
  epiphysitis (congenital) (early) A50.02
  episcleritis (late) A52.71
  esophagus A52.79
  eustachian tube A52.73
  exposure to Z20.2
  eye A52.71
  eyelid (late) (with gumma) A52.71
  fallopian tube (late) A52.76
  fracture A52.77
  gallbladder (late) A52.74
  gastric (polyposis) (late) A52.74
  general A53.9
    paralysis A52.17
      juvenile A50.45
  genital (primary) A51.0
  glaucoma A52.71
  gumma NEC A52.79
    cardiovascular system A52.00
    central nervous system A52.3
    congenital A50.59
  heart (block) (decompensation) (disease) (failure) A52.06 [I52]
    valve NEC A52.03
  hemianesthesia A52.19
  hemianopsia A52.71
  hemiparesis A52.17
  hemiplegia A52.17
  hepatic artery A52.09
  hepatis A52.74
  hepatomegaly, congenital A50.08
  hereditaria tarda — *see* Syphilis, congenital, late
  hereditary — *see* Syphilis, congenital
  Hutchinson's teeth A50.52
  hyalitis A52.71
  inactive — *see* Syphilis, latent
  infantum — *see* Syphilis, congenital
  inherited — *see* Syphilis, congenital
  internal ear A52.79
  intestine (late) A52.74
  iris, iritis (secondary) A51.43
    late A52.71
  joint (late) A52.77
  keratitis (congenital) (interstitial) (late) A50.31
  kidney (late) A52.75
  lacrimal passages (late) A52.71
  larynx (late) A52.73
  late A52.9
    cardiovascular A52.00
    central nervous system A52.3
    kidney A52.75

☑ **Additional Character Required** — Refer to the Tabular List for Character Selection   ▽ **Subterms under main terms may continue to next column or page**

Subterms under main terms may continue to next column or page   ☑ Additional Character Required — Refer to the Tabular List for Character Selection   305

Syphilis, syphilitic — Syringobulbia

Syringocystadenoma — *see* Neoplasm, skin, benign
  papillary — *see* Neoplasm, skin, benign
Syringoma (*see also* Neoplasm, skin, benign)
  chondroid — *see* Neoplasm, skin, benign

Syringomyelia G95.Ø
Syringomyelitis — *see* Encephalitis
Syringomyelocele — *see* Spina bifida
Syringopontia G95.Ø

System, systemic (*see also* condition)
  disease, combined — *see* Degeneration, combined
  inflammatory response syndrome (SIRS) of non-infectious origin (without organ dysfunction) R65.1Ø
  lupus erythematosus M32.9
    with acute organ dysfunction R65.11
    inhibitor present D68.62

☑ **Additional Character Required — Refer to the Tabular List for Character Selection**   ▽ **Subterms under main terms may continue to next column or page**

T

Tabacism, tabacosis, tabagism (*see also* Poisoning, tobacco)
  meaning dependence (without remission) F17.200
    with
      disorder F17.299
        in remission F17.211
        specified disorder NEC F17.298
        withdrawal F17.203
Tabardillo A75.9
  flea-borne A75.2
  louse-borne A75.0
Tabes, tabetic A52.10
  with
    central nervous system syphilis A52.10
    Charcot's joint A52.16
    cord bladder A52.19
    crisis, viscera (any) A52.19
    paralysis, general A52.17
    paresis (general) A52.17
    perforating ulcer (foot) A52.19
  arthropathy (Charcot) A52.16
  bladder A52.19
  bone A52.11
  cerebrospinal A52.12
  congenital A50.45
  conjugal A52.10
  dorsalis A52.11
    juvenile A50.49
  juvenile A50.49
  latent A52.19
  mesenterica A18.39
  paralysis, insane, general A52.17
  spasmodic A52.17
  syphilis (cerebrospinal) A52.12
Taboparalysis A52.17
Taboparesis (remission) A52.17
  juvenile A50.45
TAC (trigeminal autonomic cephalgia) **NEC** G44.099
  intractable G44.091
  not intractable G44.099
Tache noir S60.22- ☑
Tachyalimentation K91.2
Tachyarrhythmia, tachyrhythmia — *see* Tachycardia
Tachycardia R00.0
  atrial (paroxysmal) I47.1
  auricular I47.1
  AV nodal re-entry (re-entrant) I47.1
  junctional (paroxysmal) I47.1
  newborn P29.11
  nodal (paroxysmal) I47.1
  non-paroxysmal AV nodal I45.89
  paroxysmal (sustained) (nonsustained) I47.9
    with sinus bradycardia I49.5
    atrial (PAT) I47.1
    atrioventricular (AV) (re-entrant) I47.1
      psychogenic F54
    junctional I47.1
      ectopic I47.1
    nodal I47.1
    psychogenic (atrial) (supraventricular) (ventricular) F54
    supraventricular (sustained) I47.1
      psychogenic F54
    ventricular I47.2
      psychogenic F54
  psychogenic F45.8
  sick sinus I49.5
  sinoauricular NOS R00.0
    paroxysmal I47.1
  sinus [sinusal] NOS R00.0
    paroxysmal I47.1
  supraventricular I47.1
  ventricular (paroxysmal) (sustained) I47.2
    psychogenic F54
Tachygastria K31.89
Tachypnea R06.82
  hysterical F45.8
  newborn (idiopathic) (transitory) P22.1
  psychogenic F45.8
  transitory, of newborn P22.1
TACO (transfusion associated circulatory overload) E87.71
Taenia (infection) (infestation) B68.9
  diminuta B71.0
  echinococcal infestation B67.90
  mediocanellata B68.1

Taenia — *continued*
  nana B71.0
  saginata B68.1
  solium (intestinal form) B68.0
    larval form — *see* Cysticercosis
Taeniasis (intestine) — *see* Taenia
Tag (hypertrophied skin) (infected) L91.8
  adenoid J35.8
  anus K64.4
  hemorrhoidal K64.4
  hymen N89.8
  perineal N90.89
  preauricular Q17.0
  sentinel K64.4
  skin L91.8
    accessory (congenital) Q82.8
    anus K64.4
    congenital Q82.8
    preauricular Q17.0
  tonsil J35.8
  urethra, urethral N36.8
  vulva N90.89
Tahyna fever B33.8
Takahara's disease E80.3
Takayasu's disease or syndrome M31.4
Talcosis (pulmonary) J62.0
Talipes (congenital) Q66.89
  acquired, planus — *see* Deformity, limb, flat foot
  asymmetric Q66.89
  calcaneovalgus Q66.4
  calcaneovarus Q66.1
  calcaneus Q66.89
  cavus Q66.7
  equinovalgus Q66.6
  equinovarus Q66.0
  equinus Q66.89
  percavus Q66.7
  planovalgus Q66.6
  planus (acquired) (any degree) (*see also* Deformity, limb, flat foot)
    congenital Q66.5- ☑
    due to rickets (sequelae) E64.3
  valgus Q66.6
  varus Q66.3
Tall stature, constitutional E34.4
Talma's disease M62.89
Talon noir S90.3- ☑
  hand S60.22- ☑
  heel S90.3- ☑
  toe S90.1- ☑
Tamponade, heart I31.4
Tanapox (virus disease) B08.71
Tangier disease E78.6
Tantrum, child problem F91.8
Tapeworm (infection) (infestation) — *see* Infestation, tapeworm
Tapia's syndrome G52.7
TAR (thrombocytopenia with absent radius) **syndrome** Q87.2
Tarral-Besnier disease L44.0
Tarsal tunnel syndrome — *see* Syndrome, tarsal tunnel
Tarsalgia — *see* Pain, limb, lower
Tarsitis (eyelid) H01.8
  syphilitic A52.71
  tuberculous A18.4
Tartar (teeth) (dental calculus) K03.6
Tattoo (mark) L81.8
Tauri's disease E74.09
Taurodontism K00.2
Taussig-Bing syndrome Q20.1
Taybi's syndrome Q87.2
Tay-Sachs amaurotic familial idiocy or disease E75.02
TBI (traumatic brain injury) S06.9 ☑
Teacher's node or nodule J38.2
Tear, torn (traumatic) (*see also* Laceration)
  with abortion — *see* Abortion
  annular fibrosis M51.35
  anus, anal (sphincter) S31.831 ☑
    complicating delivery
      with third degree perineal laceration (*see also* Delivery, complicated, by, laceration, perineum, third degree) O70.20
        with mucosa O70.3
      without third degree perineal laceration O70.4
    nontraumatic (healed) (old) K62.81
  articular cartilage, old — *see* Derangement, joint, articular cartilage, by site

Tear, torn — *continued*
  bladder
    with ectopic or molar pregnancy O08.6
    following ectopic or molar pregnancy O08.6
    obstetrical O71.5
    traumatic — *see* Injury, bladder
  bowel
    with ectopic or molar pregnancy O08.6
    following ectopic or molar pregnancy O08.6
    obstetrical trauma O71.5
  broad ligament
    with ectopic or molar pregnancy O08.6
    following ectopic or molar pregnancy O08.6
    obstetrical trauma O71.6
  bucket handle (knee) (meniscus) — *see* Tear, meniscus
  capsule, joint — *see* Sprain
  cartilage (*see also* Sprain)
    articular, old — *see* Derangement, joint, articular cartilage, by site
  cervix
    with ectopic or molar pregnancy O08.6
    following ectopic or molar pregnancy O08.6
    obstetrical trauma (current) O71.3
    old N88.1
    traumatic — *see* Injury, uterus
  dural G97.41
    nontraumatic G96.11
  internal organ — *see* Injury, by site
  knee cartilage
    articular (current) S83.3- ☑
    old — *see* Derangement, knee, meniscus, due to old tear
  ligament — *see* Sprain
  meniscus (knee) (current injury) S83.209 ☑
    bucket-handle S83.20- ☑
    lateral
      bucket-handle S83.25- ☑
      complex S83.27- ☑
      peripheral S83.26- ☑
      specified type NEC S83.28- ☑
    medial
      bucket-handle S83.21- ☑
      complex S83.23- ☑
      peripheral S83.22- ☑
      specified type NEC S83.24- ☑
    old — *see* Derangement, knee, meniscus, due to old tear
    site other than knee — *code as* Sprain
    specified type NEC S83.20- ☑
  muscle — *see* Strain
  pelvic
    floor, complicating delivery O70.1
    organ NEC, obstetrical trauma O71.5
      with ectopic or molar pregnancy O08.6
      following ectopic or molar pregnancy O08.6
  perineal, secondary O90.1
  periurethral tissue, obstetrical trauma O71.82
    with ectopic or molar pregnancy O08.6
    following ectopic or molar pregnancy O08.6
  rectovaginal septum — *see* Laceration, vagina
  retina, retinal (without detachment) (horseshoe) (*see also* Break, retina, horseshoe)
    with detachment — *see* Detachment, retina, with retinal, break
  rotator cuff (nontraumatic) M75.10- ☑
    complete M75.12- ☑
    incomplete M75.11- ☑
    traumatic S46.01- ☑
      capsule S43.42- ☑
  semilunar cartilage, knee — *see* Tear, meniscus
  supraspinatus (complete) (incomplete) (nontraumatic) (*see also* Tear, rotator cuff) M75.10- ☑
  tendon — *see* Strain
  tentorial, at birth P10.4
  umbilical cord
    complicating delivery O69.89 ☑
  urethra
    with ectopic or molar pregnancy O08.6
    following ectopic or molar pregnancy O08.6
    obstetrical trauma O71.5
  uterus — *see* Injury, uterus
  vagina — *see* Laceration, vagina
  vessel, from catheter — *see* Puncture, accidental complicating surgery
  vulva, complicating delivery O70.0
Tear-stone — *see* Dacryolith
Teeth (*see also* condition)

Teeth — *continued*
  grinding
    psychogenic F45.8
    sleep related G47.63
Teething (syndrome) K00.7
Telangiectasia, telangiectasis (verrucous) I78.1
  ataxic (cerebellar) (Louis-Bar) G11.3
  familial I78.0
  hemorrhagic, hereditary (congenital) (senile) I78.0
  hereditary, hemorrhagic (congenital) (senile) I78.0
  juxtafoveal H35.07- ☑
  macular H35.07- ☑
  macularis eruptiva perstans D47.01
  parafoveal H35.07- ☑
  retinal (idiopathic) (juxtafoveal) (macular) (parafoveal) H35.07- ☑
  spider I78.1
Telephone scatologia F65.89
Telescoped bowel or intestine K56.1
  congenital Q43.8
Temperature
  body, high (of unknown origin) R50.9
  cold, trauma from T69.9 ☑
    newborn P80.0
    specified effect NEC T69.8 ☑
Temple — *see* condition
Temporal — *see* condition
Temporomandibular joint pain-dysfunction syndrome M26.62- ☑
Temporosphenoidal — *see* condition
Tendency
  bleeding — *see* Defect, coagulation
  suicide
    meaning personal history of attempted suicide Z91.5
    meaning suicidal ideation — *see* Ideation, suicidal
  to fall R29.6
Tenderness, abdominal R10.819
  epigastric R10.816
  generalized R10.817
  left lower quadrant R10.814
  left upper quadrant R10.812
  periumbilic R10.815
  rebound R10.829
    epigastric R10.826
    generalized R10.827
    left lower quadrant R10.824
    left upper quadrant R10.822
    periumbilic R10.825
    right lower quadrant R10.823
    right upper quadrant R10.821
  right lower quadrant R10.813
  right upper quadrant R10.811
Tendinitis, tendonitis (*see also* Enthesopathy)
  Achilles M76.6- ☑
  adhesive — *see* Tenosynovitis, specified type NEC
    shoulder — *see* Capsulitis, adhesive
  bicipital M75.2- ☑
  calcific M65.2- ☑
    ankle M65.27- ☑
    foot M65.27- ☑
    forearm M65.23- ☑
    hand M65.24- ☑
    lower leg M65.26- ☑
    multiple sites M65.29
    pelvic region M65.25- ☑
    shoulder M75.3- ☑
    specified site NEC M65.28
    thigh M65.25- ☑
    upper arm M65.22- ☑
  due to use, overuse, pressure (*see also* Disorder, soft tissue, due to use)
    specified NEC — *see* Disorder, soft tissue, due to use, specified NEC
  gluteal M76.0- ☑
  patellar M76.5- ☑
  peroneal M76.7- ☑
  psoas M76.1- ☑
  tibial (posterior) M76.82- ☑
    anterior M76.81- ☑
  trochanteric — *see* Bursitis, hip, trochanteric
Tendon — *see* condition
Tendosynovitis — *see* Tenosynovitis
Tenesmus (rectal) R19.8
  vesical R30.1
Tennis elbow — *see* Epicondylitis, lateral
Tenonitis (*see also* Tenosynovitis)
  eye (capsule) H05.04- ☑

Tenontosynovitis — *see* Tenosynovitis
Tenontothecitis — *see* Tenosynovitis
Tenophyte — *see* Disorder, synovium, specified type NEC
Tenosynovitis (*see also* Synovitis) M65.9
  adhesive — *see* Tenosynovitis, specified type NEC
    shoulder — *see* Capsulitis, adhesive
  bicipital (calcifying) — *see* Tendinitis, bicipital
  gonococcal A54.49
  in (due to)
    crystals M65.8- ☑
    gonorrhea A54.49
    syphilis (late) A52.78
    use, overuse, pressure (*see also* Disorder, soft tissue, due to use)
      specified NEC — *see* Disorder, soft tissue, due to use, specified NEC
  infective NEC M65.1- ☑
    ankle M65.17- ☑
    foot M65.17- ☑
    forearm M65.13- ☑
    hand M65.14- ☑
    lower leg M65.16- ☑
    multiple sites M65.19
    pelvic region M65.15- ☑
    shoulder region M65.11- ☑
    specified site NEC M65.18
    thigh M65.15- ☑
    upper arm M65.12- ☑
  radial styloid M65.4
  shoulder region M65.81- ☑
    adhesive — *see* Capsulitis, adhesive
  specified type NEC M65.88
    ankle M65.87- ☑
    foot M65.87- ☑
    forearm M65.83- ☑
    hand M65.84- ☑
    lower leg M65.86- ☑
    multiple sites M65.89
    pelvic region M65.85- ☑
    shoulder region M65.81- ☑
    specified site NEC M65.88
    thigh M65.85- ☑
    upper arm M65.82- ☑
  tuberculous — *see* Tuberculosis, tenosynovitis
Tenovaginitis — *see* Tenosynovitis
Tension
  arterial, high (*see also* Hypertension)
    without diagnosis of hypertension R03.0
  headache G44.209
    intractable G44.201
    not intractable G44.209
  nervous R45.0
  pneumothorax J93.0
  premenstrual N94.3
  state (mental) F48.9
Tentorium — *see* condition
Teratencephalus Q89.8
Teratism Q89.7
Teratoblastoma (malignant) — *see* Neoplasm, malignant, by site
Teratocarcinoma (*see also* Neoplasm, malignant, by site)
  liver C22.7
Teratoma (solid) (*see also* Neoplasm, uncertain behavior, by site)
  with embryonal carcinoma, mixed — *see* Neoplasm, malignant, by site
  with malignant transformation — *see* Neoplasm, malignant, by site
  adult (cystic) — *see* Neoplasm, benign, by site
  benign — *see* Neoplasm, benign, by site
  combined with choriocarcinoma — *see* Neoplasm, malignant, by site
  cystic (adult) — *see* Neoplasm, benign, by site
  differentiated — *see* Neoplasm, benign, by site
  embryonal (*see also* Neoplasm, malignant, by site)
    liver C22.7
  immature — *see* Neoplasm, malignant, by site
  liver C22.7
    adult, benign, cystic, differentiated type or mature D13.4
  malignant (*see also* Neoplasm, malignant, by site)
    anaplastic — *see* Neoplasm, malignant, by site
    intermediate — *see* Neoplasm, malignant, by site
      specified site — *see* Neoplasm, malignant, by site
    unspecified site C62.90

Teratoma — *continued*
  malignant (*see also* Neoplasm, malignant, by site) — *continued*
    undifferentiated — *see* Neoplasm, malignant, by site
  mature — *see* Neoplasm, uncertain behavior, by site
    malignant — *see* Neoplasm, by site, malignant, by site
  ovary D27.- ☑
    embryonal, immature or malignant C56- ☑
  solid — *see* Neoplasm, uncertain behavior, by site
  testis C62.9- ☑
    adult, benign, cystic, differentiated type or mature D29.2- ☑
    scrotal C62.1- ☑
    undescended C62.0- ☑
Termination
  anomalous (*see also* Malposition, congenital)
    right pulmonary vein Q26.3
  pregnancy, elective Z33.2
Ternidens diminutus infestation B81.8
Ternidensiasis B81.8
Terror(s) night (child) F51.4
Terrorism, victim of Z65.4
Terry's syndrome (*see also* Myopia, degenerative) H44.2- ☑
Tertiary — *see* condition
Test, tests, testing (for)
  adequacy (for dialysis)
    hemodialysis Z49.31
    peritoneal Z49.32
  blood pressure Z01.30
    abnormal reading — *see* Blood, pressure
  blood typing Z01.83
    Rh typing Z01.83
  blood-alcohol Z04.89
    positive — *see* Findings, abnormal, in blood
  blood-drug Z04.89
    positive — *see* Findings, abnormal, in blood
  cardiac pulse generator (battery) Z45.010
  fertility Z31.41
  genetic
    disease carrier status for procreative management
      female Z31.430
      male Z31.440
    male partner of patient with recurrent pregnancy loss Z31.441
    procreative management NEC
      female Z31.438
      male Z31.448
  hearing Z01.10
    with abnormal findings NEC Z01.118
    infant or child (over 28 days old) Z00.129
      with abnormal findings Z00.121
  HIV (human immunodeficiency virus)
    nonconclusive (in infants) R75
    positive Z21
    seropositive Z21
  immunity status Z01.84
  intelligence NEC Z01.89
  laboratory (as part of a general medical examination) Z00.00
    with abnormal finding Z00.01
  for medicolegal reason NEC Z04.89
  male partner of patient with recurrent pregnancy loss Z31.441
  Mantoux (for tuberculosis) Z11.1
    abnormal result R76.11
  pregnancy, positive first pregnancy — *see* Pregnancy, normal, first
  procreative Z31.49
    fertility Z31.41
  skin, diagnostic
    allergy Z01.82
      special screening examination — *see* Screening, by name of disease
    Mantoux Z11.1
    tuberculin Z11.1
  specified NEC Z01.89
  tuberculin Z11.1
    abnormal result R76.11
  vision Z01.00
    with abnormal findings Z01.01
    infant or child (over 28 days old) Z00.129
      with abnormal findings Z00.121
  Wassermann Z11.3
    positive — *see* Serology for syphilis, positive
Testicle, testicular, testis (*see also* condition)

308
☑ Additional Character Required — Refer to the Tabular List for Character Selection
🔺 Subterms under main terms may continue to next column or page

Testicle, testicular, testis — *continued*
  feminization syndrome (*see also* Syndrome, androgen insensitivity) E34.51
  migrans Q55.29
Tetanus, tetanic (cephalic) (convulsions) A35
  with
    abortion A34
    ectopic or molar pregnancy O08.0
  following ectopic or molar pregnancy O08.0
  inoculation reaction (due to serum) — *see* Complications, vaccination
  neonatorum A33
  obstetrical A34
  puerperal, postpartum, childbirth A34
Tetany (due to) R29.0
  alkalosis E87.3
  associated with rickets E55.0
  convulsions R29.0
    hysterical F44.5
  functional (hysterical) F44.5
  hyperkinetic R29.0
    hysterical F44.5
  hyperpnea R06.4
    hysterical F44.5
    psychogenic F45.8
  hyperventilation (*see also* Hyperventilation) R06.4
    hysterical F44.5
  neonatal (without calcium or magnesium deficiency) P71.3
  parathyroid (gland) E20.9
  parathyroprival E89.2
  post- (para)thyroidectomy E89.2
  postoperative E89.2
  pseudotetany R29.0
  psychogenic (conversion reaction) F44.5
Tetralogy of Fallot Q21.3
Tetraplegia (chronic) (*see also* Quadriplegia) G82.50
Thailand hemorrhagic fever A91
Thalassanemia — *see* Thalassemia
Thalassemia (anemia) (disease) D56.9
  with other hemoglobinopathy D56.8
  alpha (major) (severe) (triple gene defect) D56.0
    minor D56.3
    silent carrier D56.3
    trait D56.3
  beta (severe) D56.1
    homozygous D56.1
    major D56.1
    minor D56.3
    trait D56.3
  delta-beta (homozygous) D56.2
    minor D56.3
    trait D56.3
  dominant D56.8
  hemoglobin
    C D56.8
    E-beta D56.5
  intermedia D56.1
  major D56.1
  minor D56.3
  mixed D56.8
  sickle-cell — *see* Disease, sickle-cell, thalassemia
  specified type NEC D56.8
  trait D56.3
  variants D56.8
Thanatophoric dwarfism or short stature Q77.1
Thaysen-Gee disease (nontropical sprue) K90.0
Thaysen's disease K90.0
Thecoma D27- ☑
  luteinized D27- ☑
  malignant C56- ☑
Thelarche, premature E30.8
Thelaziasis B83.8
Thelitis N61.0
  puerperal, postpartum or gestational — *see* Infection, nipple
Therapeutic — *see* condition
Therapy
  drug, long-term (current) (prophylactic)
    agents affecting estrogen receptors and estrogen levels NEC Z79.818
    anastrozole (Arimidex) Z79.811
    antibiotics Z79.2
      short-term use — *omit code*
    anticoagulants Z79.01
    anti-inflammatory Z79.1
    antiplatelet Z79.02
    antithrombotics Z79.02

Therapy — *continued*
  drug, long-term — *continued*
    aromatase inhibitors Z79.811
    aspirin Z79.82
    birth control pill or patch Z79.3
    bisphosphonates Z79.83
    contraceptive, oral Z79.3
    drug, specified NEC Z79.899
    estrogen receptor downregulators Z79.818
    Evista Z79.810
    exemestane (Aromasin) Z79.811
    Fareston Z79.810
    fulvestrant (Faslodex) Z79.818
    gonadotropin-releasing hormone (GnRH) agonist Z79.818
    goserelin acetate (Zoladex) Z79.818
    hormone replacement Z79.890
    insulin Z79.4
    letrozole (Femara) Z79.811
    leuprolide acetate (leuprorelin) (Lupron) Z79.818
    megestrol acetate (Megace) Z79.818
    methadone
      for pain management Z79.891
      maintenance therapy F11.20
    Nolvadex Z79.810
    opiate analgesic Z79.891
    oral contraceptive Z79.3
    raloxifene (Evista) Z79.810
    selective estrogen receptor modulators (SERMs) Z79.810
    short term — *omit code*
    steroids
      inhaled Z79.51
      systemic Z79.52
    tamoxifen (Nolvadex) Z79.810
    toremifene (Fareston) Z79.810
Thermic — *see* condition
Thermography (abnormal) (*see also* Abnormal, diagnostic imaging) R93.89
  breast R92.8
Thermoplegia T67.0 ☑
Thesaurismosis, glycogen — *see* Disease, glycogen storage
Thiamin deficiency E51.9
  specified NEC E51.8
Thiaminic deficiency with beriberi E51.11
Thibierge-Weissenbach syndrome — *see* Sclerosis, systemic
Thickening
  bone — *see* Hypertrophy, bone
  breast N64.59
  endometrium R93.89
  epidermal L85.9
    specified NEC L85.8
  hymen N89.6
  larynx J38.7
  nail L60.2
    congenital Q84.5
  periosteal — *see* Hypertrophy, bone
  pleura J92.9
    with asbestos J92.0
  skin R23.4
  subepiglottic J38.7
  tongue K14.8
  valve, heart — *see* Endocarditis
Thigh — *see* condition
Thinning vertebra — *see* Spondylopathy, specified NEC
Thirst, excessive R63.1
  due to deprivation of water T73.1 ☑
Thomsen disease G71.12
Thoracic (*see also* condition)
  kidney Q63.2
  outlet syndrome G54.0
Thoracogastroschisis (congenital) Q79.8
Thoracopagus Q89.4
Thorax — *see* condition
Thorn's syndrome N28.89
Thorson-Björck syndrome E34.0
Threadworm (infection) (infestation) B80
Threatened
  abortion O20.0
    with subsequent abortion O03.9
  job loss, anxiety concerning Z56.2
  labor (without delivery) O47.9
    at or after 37 completed weeks of gestation O47.1
    before 37 completed weeks of gestation O47.0- ☑
  loss of job, anxiety concerning Z56.2
  miscarriage O20.0

Threatened — *continued*
  unemployment, anxiety concerning Z56.2
Three-day fever A93.1
Threshers' lung J67.0
Thrix annulata (congenital) Q84.1
Throat — *see* condition
Thrombasthenia (Glanzmann) (hemorrhagic) (hereditary) D69.1
Thromboangiitis I73.1
  obliterans (general) I73.1
    cerebral I67.89
    vessels
      brain I67.89
      spinal cord I67.89
Thromboarteritis — *see* Arteritis
Thromboasthenia (Glanzmann) (hemorrhagic) (hereditary) D69.1
Thrombocytasthenia (Glanzmann) D69.1
Thrombocythemia (essential) (hemorrhagic) (idiopathic) (primary) D47.3
Thrombocytopathy (dystrophic) (granulopenic) D69.1
Thrombocytopenia, thrombocytopenic D69.6
  with absent radius (TAR) Q87.2
  congenital D69.42
  dilutional D69.59
  due to
    (massive) blood transfusion D69.59
    drugs D69.59
    extracorporeal circulation of blood D69.59
    platelet alloimmunization D69.59
  essential D69.3
  heparin induced (HIT) D75.82
  hereditary D69.42
  idiopathic D69.3
  neonatal, transitory P61.0
    due to
      exchange transfusion P61.0
      idiopathic maternal thrombocytopenia P61.0
      isoimmunization P61.0
  primary NEC D69.49
    idiopathic D69.3
  puerperal, postpartum O72.3
  secondary D69.59
  transient neonatal P61.0
Thrombocytosis, essential D47.3
  primary D47.3
Thromboembolism — *see* Embolism
Thrombopathy (Bernard-Soulier) D69.1
  constitutional D68.0
  Willebrand-Jurgens D68.0
Thrombopenia — *see* Thrombocytopenia
Thrombophilia D68.59
  primary NEC D68.59
  secondary NEC D68.69
  specified NEC D68.69
Thrombophlebitis I80.9
  antepartum O22.2- ☑
    deep O22.3- ☑
    superficial O22.2- ☑
  cavernous (venous) sinus G08
    complicating pregnancy O22.5- ☑
    nonpyogenic I67.6
  cerebral (sinus) (vein) G08
    nonpyogenic I67.6
    sequelae G09
  due to implanted device — *see* Complications, by site and type, specified NEC
  during or resulting from a procedure NEC T81.72 ☑
  femoral vein (superficial) I80.1- ☑
  femoropopliteal vein I80.0- ☑
  hepatic (vein) I80.8
  idiopathic, recurrent I82.1
  iliofemoral I80.1- ☑
  intracranial venous sinus (any) G08
    nonpyogenic I67.6
    sequelae G09
  intraspinal venous sinuses and veins G08
    nonpyogenic G95.19
  lateral (venous) sinus G08
    nonpyogenic I67.6
  leg I80.3
    superficial I80.0- ☑
  longitudinal (venous) sinus G08
    nonpyogenic I67.6
  lower extremity I80.299
  migrans, migrating I82.1
  pelvic
    with ectopic or molar pregnancy O08.0

Thrombophlebitis — *continued*
- pelvic — *continued*
  - following ectopic or molar pregnancy O08.0
  - puerperal O87.1
- popliteal vein — *see* Phlebitis, leg, deep, popliteal
- portal (vein) K75.1
- postoperative T81.72 ☑
- pregnancy — *see* Thrombophlebitis, antepartum
- puerperal, postpartum, childbirth O87.0
  - deep O87.1
  - pelvic O87.1
  - septic O86.81
  - superficial O87.0
- saphenous (greater) (lesser) I80.0- ☑
- sinus (intracranial) G08
  - nonpyogenic I67.6
- specified site NEC I80.8
- tibial vein I80.23- ☑

Thrombosis, thrombotic (bland) (multiple) (progressive) (silent) (vessel) I82.90
- anal K64.5
- antepartum — *see* Thrombophlebitis, antepartum
- aorta, aortic I74.10
  - abdominal I74.09
    - saddle I74.01
  - bifurcation I74.09
  - saddle I74.01
  - specified site NEC I74.19
  - terminal I74.09
  - thoracic I74.11
  - valve — *see* Endocarditis, aortic
- apoplexy I63.3- ☑
- artery, arteries (postinfectional) I74.9
  - auditory, internal — *see* Occlusion, artery, precerebral, specified NEC
  - basilar — *see* Occlusion, artery, basilar
  - carotid (common) (internal) — *see* Occlusion, artery, carotid
  - cerebellar (anterior inferior) (posterior inferior) (superior) — *see* Occlusion, artery, cerebellar
  - cerebral — *see* Occlusion, artery, cerebral
  - choroidal (anterior) — *see* Occlusion, artery, precerebral, specified NEC
  - communicating, posterior — *see* Occlusion, artery, precerebral, specified NEC
  - coronary (*see also* Infarct, myocardium)
    - not resulting in infarction I24.0
  - hepatic I74.8
  - hypophyseal — *see* Occlusion, artery, precerebral, specified NEC
  - iliac I74.5
  - limb I74.4
    - lower I74.3
    - upper I74.2
  - meningeal, anterior or posterior — *see* Occlusion, artery, cerebral, specified NEC
  - mesenteric (with gangrene) (*see also* Infarct, intestine) K55.069
  - ophthalmic — *see* Occlusion, artery, retina
  - pontine — *see* Occlusion, artery, precerebral, specified NEC
  - precerebral — *see* Occlusion, artery, precerebral
  - pulmonary (iatrogenic) — *see* Embolism, pulmonary
  - renal N28.0
  - retinal — *see* Occlusion, artery, retina
  - spinal, anterior or posterior G95.11
  - traumatic NEC T14.8 ☑
  - vertebral — *see* Occlusion, artery, vertebral
- atrium, auricular (*see also* Infarct, myocardium)
  - following acute myocardial infarction (current complication) I23.6
  - not resulting in infarction I51.3
  - old I51.3
- basilar (artery) — *see* Occlusion, artery, basilar
- brain (artery) (stem) (*see also* Occlusion, artery, cerebral)
  - due to syphilis A52.05
  - puerperal O99.43
  - sinus — *see* Thrombosis, intracranial venous sinus
- capillary I78.8
- cardiac (*see also* Infarct, myocardium)
  - not resulting in infarction I51.3
  - old I51.3
  - valve — *see* Endocarditis
- carotid (artery) (common) (internal) — *see* Occlusion, artery, carotid
- cavernous (venous) sinus — *see* Thrombosis, intracranial venous sinus

Thrombosis, thrombotic — *continued*
- cerebellar artery (anterior inferior) (posterior inferior) (superior) I66.3
- cerebral (artery) — *see* Occlusion, artery, cerebral
- cerebrovenous sinus (*see also* Thrombosis, intracranial venous sinus)
  - puerperium O87.3
- chronic I82.91
- coronary (artery) (vein) (*see also* Infarct, myocardium)
  - not resulting in infarction I24.0
- corpus cavernosum N48.89
- cortical I66.9
- deep — *see* Embolism, vein, lower extremity
- due to device, implant or graft (*see also* Complications, by site and type, specified NEC) T85.868 ☑
  - arterial graft NEC T82.868 ☑
  - breast (implant) T85.868 ☑
  - catheter NEC T85.868 ☑
    - dialysis (renal) T82.868 ☑
      - intraperitoneal T85.868 ☑
    - infusion NEC T82.868 ☑
      - spinal (epidural) (subdural) T85.860 ☑
    - urinary (indwelling) T83.86 ☑
  - electronic (electrode) (pulse generator) (stimulator)
    - bone T84.86 ☑
    - cardiac T82.867 ☑
    - nervous system (brain) (peripheral nerve) (spinal) T85.860 ☑
    - urinary T83.86 ☑
  - fixation, internal (orthopedic) NEC T84.86 ☑
  - gastrointestinal (bile duct) (esophagus) T85.868 ☑
  - genital NEC T83.86 ☑
  - heart T82.867 ☑
  - joint prosthesis T84.86 ☑
  - ocular (corneal graft) (orbital implant) NEC T85.868 ☑
  - orthopedic NEC T84.86 ☑
  - specified NEC T85.868 ☑
  - urinary NEC T83.86 ☑
  - vascular NEC T82.868 ☑
  - ventricular intracranial shunt T85.860 ☑
- during the puerperium — *see* Thrombosis, puerperal
- endocardial (*see also* Infarct, myocardium)
  - not resulting in infarction I51.3
- eye — *see* Occlusion, retina
- genital organ
  - female NEC N94.89
    - pregnancy — *see* Thrombophlebitis, antepartum
  - male N50.1
- gestational — *see* Phlebopathy, gestational
- heart (chamber) (*see also* Infarct, myocardium)
  - not resulting in infarction I51.3
  - old I51.3
- hepatic (vein) I82.0
  - artery I74.8
- history (of) Z86.718
- intestine (with gangrene) (*see also* Infarct, intestine) K55.069
- intracardiac NEC (apical) (atrial) (auricular) (ventricular) (old) I51.3
- intracranial (arterial) I66.9
  - venous sinus (any) G08
    - nonpyogenic origin I67.6
    - puerperium O87.3
- intramural (*see also* Infarct, myocardium)
  - not resulting in infarction I51.3
  - old I51.3
- intraspinal venous sinuses and veins G08
  - nonpyogenic G95.19
- kidney (artery) N28.0
- lateral (venous) sinus — *see* Thrombosis, intracranial venous sinus
- leg — *see* Thrombosis, vein, lower extremity
  - arterial I74.3
- liver (venous) I82.0
  - artery I74.8
  - portal vein I81
- longitudinal (venous) sinus — *see* Thrombosis, intracranial venous sinus
- lower limb — *see* Thrombosis, vein, lower extremity
- lung (iatrogenic) (postoperative) — *see* Embolism, pulmonary
- meninges (brain) (arterial) I66.8
- mesenteric (artery) (with gangrene) (*see also* Infarct, intestine) K55.069
  - vein (inferior) (superior) I81
- mitral I34.8

Thrombosis, thrombotic — *continued*
- mural (*see also* Infarct, myocardium)
  - due to syphilis A52.06
  - not resulting in infarction I51.3
  - old I51.3
- omentum (with gangrene) (*see also* Infarct, intestine) K55.069
- ophthalmic — *see* Occlusion, retina
- pampiniform plexus (male) N50.1
- parietal (*see also* Infarct, myocardium)
  - not resulting in infarction I24.0
- penis, superficial vein N48.81
- perianal venous K64.5
- peripheral arteries I74.4
  - upper I74.2
- personal history (of) Z86.718
- portal I81
  - due to syphilis A52.09
- precerebral artery — *see* Occlusion, artery, precerebral
- puerperal, postpartum O87.0
  - brain (artery) O99.43
    - venous (sinus) O87.3
  - cardiac O99.43
  - cerebral (artery) O99.43
    - venous (sinus) O87.3
  - superficial O87.0
- pulmonary (artery) (iatrogenic) (postoperative) (vein) — *see* Embolism, pulmonary
- renal (artery) N28.0
  - vein I82.3
- resulting from presence of device, implant or graft — *see* Complications, by site and type, specified NEC
- retina, retinal — *see* Occlusion, retina
- scrotum N50.1
- seminal vesicle N50.1
- sigmoid (venous) sinus — *see* Thrombosis, intracranial venous sinus
- sinus, intracranial (any) — *see* Thrombosis, intracranial venous sinus
- specified site NEC I82.890
  - chronic I82.891
- spermatic cord N50.1
- spinal cord (arterial) G95.11
  - due to syphilis A52.09
  - pyogenic origin G06.1
- spleen, splenic D73.5
  - artery I74.8
- testis N50.1
- traumatic NEC T14.8 ☑
- tricuspid I07.8
- tumor — *see* Neoplasm, unspecified behavior, by site
- tunica vaginalis N50.1
- umbilical cord (vessels), complicating delivery O69.5 ☑
- vas deferens N50.1
- vein (acute) I82.90
  - antecubital I82.61- ☑
    - chronic I82.71- ☑
  - axillary I82.A1- ☑ (*following* I82.7)
    - chronic I82.A2- ☑ (*following* I82.7)
  - basilic I82.61- ☑
    - chronic I82.71- ☑
  - brachial I82.62- ☑
    - chronic I82.72- ☑
  - brachiocephalic (innominate) I82.290
    - chronic I82.291
  - cephalic I82.61- ☑
    - chronic I82.71- ☑
  - cerebral, nonpyogenic I67.6
  - chronic I82.91
  - deep (DVT) I82.40- ☑
    - calf I82.4Z- ☑
      - chronic I82.5Z- ☑
    - lower leg I82.4Z- ☑
      - chronic I82.5Z- ☑
    - thigh I82.4Y- ☑
      - chronic I82.5Y- ☑
    - upper leg I82.4Y ☑
      - chronic I82.5Y- ☑
  - femoral I82.41- ☑
    - chronic I82.51- ☑
  - iliac (iliofemoral) I82.42- ☑
    - chronic I82.52- ☑
  - innominate I82.290
    - chronic I82.291
  - internal jugular I82.C1- ☑ (*following* I82.7)
    - chronic I82.C2- ☑ (*following* I82.7)

☑ Additional Character Required — Refer to the Tabular List for Character Selection   ▽ Subterms under main terms may continue to next column or page

Thrombosis, thrombotic — *continued*
  vein — *continued*
    lower extremity
      deep I82.40- ☑
        chronic I82.50- ☑
          specified NEC I82.49- ☑
            chronic NEC I82.59- ☑
      distal
        deep I82.4Z- ☑
      proximal
        deep I82.4Y- ☑
          chronic I82.5Y- ☑
      superficial I82.81- ☑
    perianal K64.5
    popliteal I82.43- ☑
      chronic I82.53- ☑
    radial I82.62- ☑
      chronic I82.72- ☑
    renal I82.3
    saphenous (greater) (lesser) I82.81- ☑
    specified NEC I82.890
      chronic NEC I82.891
    subclavian I82.B1- ☑ (*following* I82.7)
      chronic I82.B2- ☑ (*following* I82.7)
    thoracic NEC I82.290
      chronic I82.291
    tibial I82.44- ☑
      chronic I82.54- ☑
    ulnar I82.62- ☑
      chronic I82.72- ☑
    upper extremity I82.60- ☑
      chronic I82.70- ☑
      deep I82.62- ☑
        chronic I82.72- ☑
      superficial I82.61- ☑
        chronic I82.71- ☑
  vena cava
    inferior I82.220
      chronic I82.221
    superior I82.210
      chronic I82.211
  venous, perianal K64.5
  ventricle (*see also* Infarct, myocardium)
    following acute myocardial infarction (current complication) I23.6
    not resulting in infarction I24.0
    old I51.3
Thrombus — *see* Thrombosis
Thrush (*see also* Candidiasis)
  newborn P37.5
  oral B37.0
  vaginal B37.3
Thumb (*see also* condition)
  sucking (child problem) F98.8
Thymitis E32.8
Thymoma (benign) D15.0
  malignant C37
Thymus, thymic (gland) — *see* condition
Thyrocele — *see* Goiter
Thyroglossal (*see also* condition)
  cyst Q89.2
  duct, persistent Q89.2
Thyroid (gland) (body) (*see also* condition)
  hormone resistance E07.89
  lingual Q89.2
  nodule (cystic) (nontoxic) (single) E04.1
Thyroiditis E06.9
  acute (nonsuppurative) (pyogenic) (suppurative) E06.0
  autoimmune E06.3
  chronic (nonspecific) (sclerosing) E06.5
    with thyrotoxicosis, transient E06.2
    fibrous E06.5
    lymphadenoid E06.3
    lymphocytic E06.3
    lymphoid E06.3
  de Quervain's E06.1
  drug-induced E06.4
  fibrous (chronic) E06.5
  giant-cell (follicular) E06.1
  granulomatous (de Quervain) (subacute) E06.1
  Hashimoto's (struma lymphomatosa) E06.3
  iatrogenic E06.4
  ligneous E06.5
  lymphocytic (chronic) E06.3
  lymphoid E06.3
  lymphomatous E06.3
  nonsuppurative E06.1

Thyroiditis — *continued*
  postpartum, puerperal O90.5
  pseudotuberculous E06.1
  pyogenic E06.0
  radiation E06.4
  Riedel's E06.5
  subacute (granulomatous) E06.1
  suppurative E06.0
  tuberculous A18.81
  viral E06.1
  woody E06.5
Thyrolingual duct, persistent Q89.2
Thyromegaly E01.0
Thyrotoxic
  crisis — *see* Thyrotoxicosis
  heart disease or failure (*see also* Thyrotoxicosis) E05.90 [I43]
    with thyroid storm E05.91 [I43]
  storm — *see* Thyrotoxicosis
Thyrotoxicosis (recurrent) E05.90
  with
    goiter (diffuse) E05.00
      with thyroid storm E05.01
      adenomatous uninodular E05.10
        with thyroid storm E05.11
      multinodular E05.20
        with thyroid storm E05.21
      nodular E05.20
        with thyroid storm E05.21
      uninodular E05.10
        with thyroid storm E05.11
    infiltrative
      dermopathy E05.00
        with thyroid storm E05.01
      ophthalmopathy E05.00
        with thyroid storm E05.01
    single thyroid nodule E05.10
      with thyroid storm E05.11
    thyroid storm E05.91
  due to
    ectopic thyroid nodule or tissue E05.30
      with thyroid storm E05.31
    ingestion of (excessive) thyroid material E05.40
      with thyroid storm E05.41
    overproduction of thyroid-stimulating hormone E05.80
      with thyroid storm E05.81
    specified cause NEC E05.80
      with thyroid storm E05.81
  factitia E05.40
    with thyroid storm E05.41
  heart (*see also* Failure, heart, high-output) E05.90 [I43]
    with thyroid storm (*see also* Failure, heart, high-output) E05.91 [I43]
  failure (*see also* Failure, heart, high-output) E05.90 [I43]
  neonatal (transient) P72.1
  transient with chronic thyroiditis E06.2
Tibia vara — *see* Osteochondrosis, juvenile, tibia
Tic (disorder) F95.9
  breathing F95.8
  child problem F95.0
  compulsive F95.1
  de la Tourette F95.2
  degenerative (generalized) (localized) G25.69
    facial G25.69
  disorder
    chronic
      motor F95.1
      vocal F95.1
    combined vocal and multiple motor F95.2
    transient F95.0
  douloureux G50.0
    atypical G50.1
    postherpetic, postzoster B02.22
  drug-induced G25.61
  eyelid F95.8
  habit F95.9
    chronic F95.1
    transient of childhood F95.0
  lid, transient of childhood F95.0
  motor-verbal F95.2
  occupational F48.8
  orbicularis F95.8
    transient of childhood F95.0
  organic origin G25.69
  postchoreic G25.69
  provisional F95.0

Tic — *continued*
  psychogenic, compulsive F95.1
  salaam R25.8
  spasm (motor or vocal) F95.9
    chronic F95.1
    transient of childhood F95.0
  specified NEC F95.8
Tick-borne — *see* condition
Tietze's disease or syndrome M94.0
Tight, tightness
  anus K62.89
  chest R07.89
  fascia (lata) M62.89
  foreskin (congenital) N47.1
  hymen, hymenal ring N89.6
  introitus (acquired) (congenital) N89.6
  rectal sphincter K62.89
  tendon — *see* Short, tendon
  urethral sphincter N35.919
Tilting vertebra — *see* Dorsopathy, deforming, specified NEC
Timidity, child F93.8
Tinea (intersecta) (tarsi) B35.9
  amiantacea L44.8
  asbestina B35.0
  barbae B35.0
  beard B35.0
  black dot B35.0
  blanca B36.2
  capitis B35.0
  corporis B35.4
  cruris B35.6
  flava B36.0
  foot B35.3
  furfuracea B36.0
  imbricata (Tokelau) B35.5
  kerion B35.0
  manuum B35.2
  microsporic — *see* Dermatophytosis
  nigra B36.1
  nodosa — *see* Piedra
  pedis B35.3
  scalp B35.0
  specified NEC B35.8
  sycosis B35.0
  tonsurans B35.0
  trichophytic — *see* Dermatophytosis
  unguium B35.1
  versicolor B36.0
Tingling sensation (skin) R20.2
Tin-miner's lung J63.5
Tinnitus NOS H93.1- ☑
  audible H93.1- ☑
  aurium H93.1- ☑
  pulsatile H93.A- ☑
  subjective H93.1- ☑
Tipped tooth (teeth) M26.33
Tipping
  pelvis M95.5
    with disproportion (fetopelvic) O33.0
      causing obstructed labor O65.0
  tooth (teeth), fully erupted M26.33
Tiredness R53.83
Tissue — *see* condition
Tobacco (nicotine)
  abuse — *see* Tobacco, use
  dependence — *see* Dependence, drug, nicotine
  harmful use Z72.0
  heart — *see* Tobacco, toxic effect
  maternal use, affecting newborn P04.2
  toxic effect — *see* Table of Drugs and Chemicals, by substance, poisoning
    chewing tobacco — *see* Table of Drugs and Chemicals, by substance, poisoning
    cigarettes — *see* Table of Drugs and Chemicals, by substance, poisoning
  use Z72.0
    complicating
      childbirth O99.334
      pregnancy O99.33- ☑
      puerperium O99.335
    counseling and surveillance Z71.6
    history Z87.891
  withdrawal state (*see also* Dependence, drug, nicotine) F17.203
Tocopherol deficiency E56.0
Todd's
  cirrhosis K74.3

Todd's — continued
  paralysis (postepileptic) (transitory) G83.84
Toe — see condition
Toilet, artificial opening — see Attention to, artificial, opening
Tokelau (ringworm) B35.5
Tollwut — see Rabies
Tommaselli's disease R31.9
  correct substance properly administered — see Table of Drugs and Chemicals, by drug, adverse effect
  overdose or wrong substance given or taken — see Table of Drugs and Chemicals, by drug, poisoning
Tongue (see also condition)
  tie Q38.1
Tonic pupil — see Anomaly, pupil, function, tonic pupil
Toni-Fanconi syndrome (cystinosis) E72.09
  with cystinosis E72.04
Tonsil — see condition
Tonsillitis (acute) (catarrhal) (croupous) (follicular) (gangrenous) (infective) (lacunar) (lingual) (malignant) (membranous) (parenchymatous) (phlegmonous) (pseudomembranous) (purulent) (septic) (subacute) (suppurative) (toxic) (ulcerative) (vesicular) (viral) J03.90
  chronic J35.01
    with adenoiditis J35.03
  diphtheritic A36.0
  hypertrophic J35.01
    with adenoiditis J35.03
  recurrent J03.91
  specified organism NEC J03.80
    recurrent J03.81
  staphylococcal J03.80
    recurrent J03.81
  streptococcal J03.00
    recurrent J03.01
  tuberculous A15.8
  Vincent's A69.1
Tooth, teeth — see condition
Toothache K08.89
Topagnosis R20.8
Tophi — see Gout, chronic
TORCH infection — see Infection, congenital
  without active infection P00.2
Torn — see Tear
Tornwaldt's cyst or disease J39.2
Torsion
  accessory tube — see Torsion, fallopian tube
  adnexa (female) — see Torsion, fallopian tube
  aorta, acquired I77.1
  appendix epididymis N44.04
  appendix testis N44.03
  bile duct (common) (hepatic) K83.8
    congenital Q44.5
  bowel, colon or intestine K56.2
  cervix — see Malposition, uterus
  cystic duct K82.8
  dystonia — see Dystonia, torsion
  epididymis (appendix) N44.04
  fallopian tube N83.52- ☑
    with ovary N83.53
  gallbladder K82.8
    congenital Q44.1
  hydatid of Morgagni
    female N83.52- ☑
    male N44.03
  kidney (pedicle) (leading to infarction) N28.0
  Meckel's diverticulum (congenital) Q43.0
    malignant — see Table of Neoplasms, small intestine, malignant
  mesentery K56.2
  omentum K56.2
  organ or site, congenital NEC — see Anomaly, by site
  ovary (pedicle) N83.51- ☑
    with fallopian tube N83.53
    congenital Q50.2
  oviduct — see Torsion, fallopian tube
  penis (acquired) N48.82
    congenital Q55.63
  spasm — see Dystonia, torsion
  spermatic cord N44.02
    extravaginal N44.01
    intravaginal N44.02
  spleen D73.5
  testis, testicle N44.00
    appendix N44.03
  tibia — see Deformity, limb, specified type NEC, lower leg

Torsion — continued
  uterus — see Malposition, uterus
Torticollis (intermittent) (spastic) M43.6
  congenital (sternomastoid) Q68.0
  due to birth injury P15.8
  hysterical F44.4
  ocular R29.891
  psychogenic F45.8
    conversion reaction F44.4
  rheumatic M43.6
  rheumatoid M06.88
  spasmodic G24.3
  traumatic, current S13.4 ☑
Tortipelvis G24.1
Tortuous
  aortic arch Q25.46
  artery I77.1
  organ or site, congenital NEC — see Distortion
  retinal vessel, congenital Q14.1
  ureter N13.8
  urethra N36.8
  vein — see Varix
Torture, victim of Z65.4
Torula, torular (histolytica) (infection) — see Cryptococcosis
Torulosis — see Cryptococcosis
Torus (mandibularis) (palatinus) M27.0
  fracture — see Fracture, by site, torus
Touraine's syndrome Q79.8
Tourette's syndrome F95.2
Tourniquet syndrome — see Constriction, external, by site
Tower skull Q75.0
  with exophthalmos Q87.0
Toxemia R68.89
  bacterial — see Sepsis
  burn — see Burn
  eclamptic (with pre-existing hypertension) — see Eclampsia
  erysipelatous — see Erysipelas
  fatigue R68.89
  food — see Poisoning, food
  gastrointestinal K52.1
  intestinal K52.1
  kidney — see Uremia
  malarial — see Malaria
  myocardial — see Myocarditis, toxic
  of pregnancy — see Pre-eclampsia
  pre-eclamptic — see Pre-eclampsia
  small intestine K52.1
  staphylococcal, due to food A05.0
  stasis R68.89
  uremic — see Uremia
  urinary — see Uremia
Toxemica cerebropathia psychica (nonalcoholic) F04
  alcoholic — see Alcohol, amnestic disorder
Toxic (poisoning) (see also condition) T65.91 ☑
  effect — see Table of Drugs and Chemicals, by substance, poisoning
  shock syndrome A48.3
  thyroid (gland) — see Thyrotoxicosis
Toxicemia — see Toxemia
Toxicity — see Table of Drugs and Chemicals, by substance, poisoning
  fava bean D55.0
  food, noxious — see Poisoning, food
  from drug or nonmedicinal substance — see Table of Drugs and Chemicals, by drug
Toxicosis (see also Toxemia)
  capillary, hemorrhagic D69.0
Toxinfection, gastrointestinal K52.1
Toxocariasis B83.0
Toxoplasma, toxoplasmosis (acquired) B58.9
  with
    hepatitis B58.1
    meningoencephalitis B58.2
    ocular involvement B58.00
    other organ involvement B58.89
    pneumonia, pneumonitis B58.3
  congenital (acute) (subacute) (chronic) P37.1
  maternal, manifest toxoplasmosis in infant (acute) (subacute) (chronic) P37.1
tPA (rtPA) **administration in a different facility within the last 24 hours prior to admission to current facility** Z92.82
Trabeculation, bladder N32.89
Trachea — see condition

Tracheitis (catarrhal) (infantile) (membranous) (plastic) (septal) (suppurative) (viral) J04.10
  with
    bronchitis (15 years of age and above) J40
      acute or subacute — see Bronchitis, acute
      chronic J42
      tuberculous NEC A15.5
      under 15 years of age J20.9
    laryngitis (acute) J04.2
      chronic J37.1
      tuberculous NEC A15.5
  acute J04.10
    with obstruction J04.11
  chronic J42
    with
      bronchitis (chronic) J42
      laryngitis (chronic) J37.1
  diphtheritic (membranous) A36.89
  due to external agent — see Inflammation, respiratory, upper, due to
  syphilitic A52.73
  tuberculous A15.5
Trachelitis (nonvenereal) — see Cervicitis
Tracheobronchial — see condition
Tracheobronchitis (15 years of age and above) (see also Bronchitis)
  due to
    Bordetella bronchiseptica A37.80
      with pneumonia A37.81
    Francisella tularensis A21.8
Tracheobronchomegaly Q32.4
  with bronchiectasis J47.9
    with
      exacerbation (acute) J47.1
      lower respiratory infection J47.0
  acquired J98.09
    with bronchiectasis J47.9
      with
        exacerbation (acute) J47.1
        lower respiratory infection J47.0
Tracheobronchopneumonitis — see Pneumonia, broncho-
Tracheocele (external) (internal) J39.8
  congenital Q32.1
Tracheomalacia J39.8
  congenital Q32.0
Tracheopharyngitis (acute) J06.9
  chronic J42
  due to external agent — see Inflammation, respiratory, upper, due to
Tracheostenosis J39.8
Tracheostomy
  complication — see Complication, tracheostomy
  status Z93.0
    attention to Z43.0
    malfunctioning J95.03
Trachoma, trachomatous A71.9
  active (stage) A71.1
  contraction of conjunctiva A71.1
  dubium A71.0
  healed or sequelae B94.0
  initial (stage) A71.0
  pannus A71.1
  Türck's J37.0
Traction, vitreomacular H43.82- ☑
Train sickness T75.3 ☑
Trait(s)
  Hb-S D57.3
  hemoglobin
    abnormal NEC D58.2
      with thalassemia D56.3
    C — see Disease, hemoglobin C
    S (Hb-S) D57.3
  Lepore D56.3
  personality, accentuated Z73.1
  sickle-cell D57.3
    with elliptocytosis or spherocytosis D57.3
  type A personality Z73.1
Tramp Z59.0
Trance R41.89
  hysterical F44.89
Transaminasemia R74.0
Transection
  abdomen (partial) S38.3 ☑
  aorta (incomplete) (see also Injury, aorta)
    complete — see Injury, aorta, laceration, major
  carotid artery (incomplete) (see also Injury, blood vessel, carotid, laceration)

Transection — continued
carotid artery (see also Injury, blood vessel, carotid, laceration) — continued
  complete — see Injury, blood vessel, carotid, laceration, major
celiac artery (incomplete) S35.211 ☑
  branch (incomplete) S35.291 ☑
    complete S35.292 ☑
  complete S35.212 ☑
innominate
  artery (incomplete) (see also Injury, blood vessel, thoracic, innominate, artery, laceration)
    complete — see Injury, blood vessel, thoracic, innominate, artery, laceration, major
  vein (incomplete) (see also Injury, blood vessel, thoracic, innominate, vein, laceration)
    complete — see Injury, blood vessel, thoracic, innominate, vein, laceration, major
jugular vein (external) (incomplete) (see also Injury, blood vessel, jugular vein, laceration)
  complete — see Injury, blood vessel, jugular vein, laceration, major
  internal (incomplete) (see also Injury, blood vessel, jugular vein, internal, laceration)
    complete — see Injury, blood vessel, jugular vein, internal, laceration, major
mesenteric artery (incomplete) (see also Injury, mesenteric, artery, laceration)
  complete — see Injury, mesenteric artery, laceration, major
pulmonary vessel (incomplete) (see also Injury, blood vessel, thoracic, pulmonary, laceration)
  complete — see Injury, blood vessel, thoracic, pulmonary, laceration, major
subclavian — see Transection, innominate
vena cava (incomplete) (see also Injury, vena cava)
  complete — see Injury, vena cava, laceration, major
vertebral artery (incomplete) (see also Injury, blood vessel, vertebral, laceration)
  complete — see Injury, blood vessel, vertebral, laceration, major

Transfusion
associated (red blood cell) hemochromatosis E83.111
blood
  ABO incompatible — see Complication(s), transfusion, incompatibility reaction, ABO
  minor blood group (Duffy) (E) (K) (Kell) (Kidd) (Lewis) (M) (N) (P) (S) T80.89 ☑
  reaction or complication — see Complications, transfusion
fetomaternal (mother) — see Pregnancy, complicated by, placenta, transfusion syndrome
maternofetal (mother) — see Pregnancy, complicated by, placenta, transfusion syndrome
placental (syndrome) (mother) — see Pregnancy, complicated by, placenta, transfusion syndrome
reaction (adverse) — see Complications, transfusion
related acute lung injury (TRALI) J95.84
twin-to-twin — see Pregnancy, complicated by, placenta, transfusion syndrome, fetus to fetus
Transient (meaning homeless) (see also condition) Z59.0
Translocation
balanced autosomal Q95.9
  in normal individual Q95.0
chromosomes NEC Q99.8
  balanced and insertion in normal individual Q95.0
Down syndrome Q90.2
trisomy
  13 Q91.6
  18 Q91.2
  21 Q90.2
Translucency, iris — see Degeneration, iris
Transmission of chemical substances through the placenta — see Absorption, chemical, through placenta
Transparency, lung, unilateral J43.0
Transplant (ed) (status) Z94.9
awaiting organ Z76.82
bone Z94.6
  marrow Z94.81
candidate Z76.82
complication — see Complication, transplant
cornea Z94.7
heart Z94.1
  and lung(s) Z94.3
  valve Z95.2
    prosthetic Z95.2

Transplant — continued
heart — continued
  valve — continued
    specified NEC Z95.4
    xenogenic Z95.3
intestine Z94.82
kidney Z94.0
liver Z94.4
lung(s) Z94.2
  and heart Z94.3
organ (failure) (infection) (rejection) Z94.9
  removal status Z98.85
pancreas Z94.83
skin Z94.5
social Z60.3
specified organ or tissue NEC Z94.89
stem cells Z94.84
tissue Z94.9
Transplants, ovarian, endometrial N80.1
Transposed — see Transposition
Transposition (congenital) (see also Malposition, congenital)
abdominal viscera Q89.3
aorta (dextra) Q20.3
appendix Q43.8
colon Q43.8
corrected Q20.5
great vessels (complete) (partial) Q20.3
heart Q24.0
  with complete transposition of viscera Q89.3
intestine (large) (small) Q43.8
reversed jejunal (for bypass) (status) Z98.0
scrotum Q55.23
stomach Q40.2
  with general transposition of viscera Q89.3
tooth, teeth, fully erupted M26.30
vessels, great (complete) (partial) Q20.3
viscera (abdominal) (thoracic) Q89.3
Transsexualism F64.0
Transverse (see also condition)
arrest (deep), in labor O64.0 ☑
lie (mother) O32.2 ☑
  causing obstructed labor O64.8 ☑
Transvestism, transvestitism (dual-role) F64.1
fetishistic F65.1
Trapped placenta (with hemorrhage) O72.0
without hemorrhage O73.0
TRAPS (tumor necrosis factor receptor associated periodic syndrome) M04.1
Trauma, traumatism (see also Injury)
acoustic — see subcategory H83.3 ☑
birth — see Birth, injury
complicating ectopic or molar pregnancy O08.6
during delivery O71.9
following ectopic or molar pregnancy O08.6
obstetric O71.9
  specified NEC O71.89
occlusal
  primary K08.81
  secondary K08.82
Traumatic (see also condition)
brain injury S06.9 ☑
Treacher Collins syndrome Q75.4
Treitz's hernia — see Hernia, abdomen, specified site NEC
Trematode infestation — see Infestation, fluke
Trematodiasis — see Infestation, fluke
Trembling paralysis — see Parkinsonism
Tremor(s) R25.1
drug induced G25.1
essential (benign) G25.0
familial G25.0
hereditary G25.0
hysterical F44.4
intention G25.2
medication induced postural G25.1
mercurial — see subcategory T56.1 ☑
Parkinson's — see Parkinsonism
psychogenic (conversion reaction) F44.4
senilis R54
specified type NEC G25.2
Trench
fever A79.0
foot — see Immersion, foot
mouth A69.1
Treponema pallidum infection — see Syphilis

Treponematosis
due to
  T. pallidum — see Syphilis
  T. pertenue — see Yaws
Triad
Hutchinson's (congenital syphilis) A50.53
Kartagener's Q89.3
Saint's — see Hernia, diaphragm
Trichiasis (eyelid) H02.059
with entropion — see Entropion
left H02.056
  lower H02.055
  upper H02.054
right H02.053
  lower H02.052
  upper H02.051
Trichinella spiralis (infection) (infestation) B75
Trichinellosis, trichiniasis, trichinelliasis, trichinosis B75
with muscle disorder B75 [M63.80]
  ankle B75 [M63.87-] ☑
  foot B75 [M63.87-] ☑
  forearm B75 [M63.83-] ☑
  hand B75 [M63.84-] ☑
  lower leg B75 [M63.86-] ☑
  multiple sites B75 [M63.89]
  pelvic region B75 [M63.85-] ☑
  shoulder region B75 [M63.81-] ☑
  specified site NEC B75 [M63.88]
  thigh B75 [M63.85-] ☑
  upper arm B75 [M63.82-] ☑
Trichobezoar T18.9 ☑
intestine T18.3 ☑
stomach T18.2 ☑
Trichocephaliasis, trichocephalosis B79
Trichocephalus infestation B79
Trichoclasis L67.8
Trichoepithelioma (see also Neoplasm, skin, benign)
malignant — see Neoplasm, skin, malignant
Trichofolliculoma — see Neoplasm, skin, benign
Tricholemmoma — see Neoplasm, skin, benign
Trichomoniasis A59.9
bladder A59.03
cervix A59.09
intestinal A07.8
prostate A59.02
seminal vesicles A59.09
specified site NEC A59.8
urethra A59.03
urogenitalis A59.00
vagina A59.01
vulva A59.01
Trichomycosis
axillaris A48.8
nodosa, nodularis B36.8
Trichonodosis L67.8
Trichophytid, trichophyton infection — see Dermatophytosis
Trichophytobezoar T18.9 ☑
intestine T18.3 ☑
stomach T18.2 ☑
Trichophytosis — see Dermatophytosis
Trichoptilosis L67.8
Trichorrhexis (nodosa) (invaginata) L67.0
Trichosis axillaris A48.8
Trichosporosis nodosa B36.2
Trichostasis spinulosa (congenital) Q84.1
Trichostrongyliasis, trichostrongylosis (small intestine) B81.2
Trichostrongylus infection B81.2
Trichotillomania F63.3
Trichromat, trichromatopsia, anomalous (congenital) H53.55
Trichuriasis B79
Trichuris trichiura (infection) (infestation) (any site) B79
Tricuspid (valve) — see condition
Trifid (see also Accessory)
kidney (pelvis) Q63.8
tongue Q38.3
Trigeminal neuralgia — see Neuralgia, trigeminal
Trigeminy R00.8
Trigger finger (acquired) M65.30
congenital Q74.0
index finger M65.32- ☑
little finger M65.35- ☑
middle finger M65.33- ☑
ring finger M65.34- ☑

▽ Subterms under main terms may continue to next column or page | ☑ Additional Character Required — Refer to the Tabular List for Character Selection | 313

Transection — Trigger finger

Trigger finger — continued
thumb M65.31- ☑
Trigonitis (bladder) (chronic) (pseudomembranous) N30.30
with hematuria N30.31
Trigonocephaly Q75.0
Trilocular heart — see Cor triloculare
Trimethylaminuria E72.52
Tripartite placenta O43.19- ☑
Triphalangeal thumb Q74.0
Triple (see also Accessory)
kidneys Q63.0
uteri Q51.818
X, female Q97.0
Triplegia G83.89
congenital G80.8
Triplet (newborn) (see also Newborn, triplet)
complicating pregnancy — see Pregnancy, triplet
Triplication — see Accessory
Triploidy Q92.7
Trismus R25.2
neonatorum A33
newborn A33
Trisomy (syndrome) Q92.9
13 (partial) Q91.7
meiotic nondisjunction Q91.4
mitotic nondisjunction Q91.5
mosaicism Q91.5
translocation Q91.6
18 (partial) Q91.3
meiotic nondisjunction Q91.0
mitotic nondisjunction Q91.1
mosaicism Q91.1
translocation Q91.2
20 Q92.8
21 (partial) Q90.9
meiotic nondisjunction Q90.0
mitotic nondisjunction Q90.1
mosaicism Q90.1
translocation Q90.2
22 Q92.8
autosomes Q92.9
chromosome specified NEC Q92.8
partial Q92.2
due to unbalanced translocation Q92.5
specified NEC Q92.8
whole (nonsex chromosome)
meiotic nondisjunction Q92.0
mitotic nondisjunction Q92.1
mosaicism Q92.1
due to
dicentrics — see Extra, marker chromosomes
extra rings — see Extra, marker chromosomes
isochromosomes — see Extra, marker chromosomes
specified NEC Q92.8
whole chromosome Q92.9
meiotic nondisjunction Q92.0
mitotic nondisjunction Q92.1
mosaicism Q92.1
partial Q92.9
specified NEC Q92.8
Tritanomaly, tritanopia H53.55
Trombiculosis, trombiculiasis, trombidiosis B88.0
Trophedema (congenital) (hereditary) Q82.0
Trophoblastic disease (see also Mole, hydatidiform) O01.9
Tropholymphedema Q82.0
Trophoneurosis NEC G96.8
disseminated M34.9
Tropical — see condition
Trouble (see also Disease)
heart — see Disease, heart
kidney — see Disease, renal
nervous R45.0
sinus — see Sinusitis
Trousseau's syndrome (thrombophlebitis migrans) I82.1
Truancy, childhood
from school Z72.810
Truncus
arteriosus (persistent) Q20.0
communis Q20.0
Trunk — see condition
Trypanosomiasis
African B56.9
by Trypanosoma brucei
gambiense B56.0
rhodesiense B56.1
American — see Chagas' disease

Trypanosomiasis — continued
Brazilian — see Chagas' disease
by Trypanosoma
brucei gambiense B56.0
brucei rhodesiense B56.1
cruzi — see Chagas' disease
gambiensis, Gambian B56.0
rhodesiensis, Rhodesian B56.1
South American — see Chagas' disease
where
African trypanosomiasis is prevalent B56.9
Chagas' disease is prevalent B57.2
T-shaped incisors K00.2
Tsutsugamushi (disease) (fever) A75.3
Tube, tubal, tubular — see condition
Tubercle (see also Tuberculosis)
brain, solitary A17.81
Darwin's Q17.8
Ghon, primary infection A15.7
Tuberculid, tuberculide (indurating, subcutaneous) (lichenoid) (miliary) (papulonecrotic) (primary) (skin) A18.4
Tuberculoma (see also Tuberculosis)
brain A17.81
meninges (cerebral) (spinal) A17.1
spinal cord A17.81
Tuberculosis, tubercular, tuberculous (calcification) (calcified) (caseous) (chromogenic acid-fast bacilli) (degeneration) (fibrocaseous) (fistula) (interstitial) (isolated circumscribed lesions) (necrosis) (parenchymatous) (ulcerative) A15.9
with pneumoconiosis (any condition in J60-J64) J65
abdomen (lymph gland) A18.39
abscess (respiratory) A15.9
bone A18.03
hip A18.02
knee A18.02
sacrum A18.01
specified site NEC A18.03
spinal A18.01
vertebra A18.01
brain A17.81
breast A18.89
Cowper's gland A18.15
dura (mater) (cerebral) (spinal) A17.81
epidural (cerebral) (spinal) A17.81
female pelvis A18.17
frontal sinus A15.8
genital organs NEC A18.10
genitourinary A18.10
gland (lymphatic) — see Tuberculosis, lymph gland
hip A18.02
intestine A18.32
ischiorectal A18.32
joint NEC A18.02
hip A18.02
knee A18.02
specified NEC A18.02
vertebral A18.01
kidney A18.11
knee A18.02
latent R76.11
lumbar (spine) A18.01
lung — see Tuberculosis, pulmonary
meninges (cerebral) (spinal) A17.0
muscle A18.09
perianal (fistula) A18.32
perinephritic A18.11
perirectal A18.32
rectum A18.32
retropharyngeal A15.8
sacrum A18.01
scrofulous A18.2
scrotum A18.15
skin (primary) A18.4
spinal cord A17.81
spine or vertebra (column) A18.01
subdiaphragmatic A18.31
testis A18.15
urinary A18.13
uterus A18.17
accessory sinus — see Tuberculosis, sinus
Addison's disease A18.7
adenitis — see Tuberculosis, lymph gland
adenoids A15.8
adenopathy — see Tuberculosis, lymph gland
adherent pericardium A18.84
adnexa (uteri) A18.17

Tuberculosis, tubercular, tuberculous — continued
adrenal (capsule) (gland) A18.7
alimentary canal A18.32
anemia A18.89
ankle (joint) (bone) A18.02
anus A18.32
apex, apical — see Tuberculosis, pulmonary
appendicitis, appendix A18.32
arachnoid A17.0
artery, arteritis A18.89
cerebral A18.89
arthritis (chronic) (synovial) A18.02
spine or vertebra (column) A18.01
articular — see Tuberculosis, joint
ascites A18.31
asthma — see Tuberculosis, pulmonary
axilla, axillary (gland) A18.2
bladder A18.12
bone A18.03
hip A18.02
knee A18.02
limb NEC A18.03
sacrum A18.01
spine or vertebral column A18.01
bowel (miliary) A18.32
brain A17.81
breast A18.89
broad ligament A18.17
bronchi, bronchial, bronchus A15.5
ectasia, ectasis (bronchiectasis) — see Tuberculosis, pulmonary
fistula A15.5
primary (progressive) A15.7
gland or node A15.4
primary (progressive) A15.7
lymph gland or node A15.4
primary (progressive) A15.7
bronchiectasis — see Tuberculosis, pulmonary
bronchitis A15.5
bronchopleural A15.6
bronchopneumonia, bronchopneumonic — see Tuberculosis, pulmonary
bronchorrhagia A15.5
bronchotracheal A15.5
bronze disease A18.7
buccal cavity A18.83
bulbourethral gland A18.15
bursa A18.09
cachexia A15.9
cardiomyopathy A18.84
caries — see Tuberculosis, bone
cartilage A18.02
intervertebral A18.01
catarrhal — see Tuberculosis, respiratory
cecum A18.32
cellulitis (primary) A18.4
cerebellum A17.81
cerebral, cerebrum A17.81
cerebrospinal A17.81
meninges A17.0
cervical (lymph gland or node) A18.2
cervicitis, cervix (uteri) A18.16
chest — see Tuberculosis, respiratory
chorioretinitis A18.53
choroid, choroiditis A18.53
ciliary body A18.54
colitis A18.32
collier's J65
colliquativa (primary) A18.4
colon A18.32
complex, primary A15.7
congenital P37.0
conjunctiva A18.59
connective tissue (systemic) A18.89
contact Z20.1
cornea (ulcer) A18.52
Cowper's gland A18.15
coxae A18.02
coxalgia A18.02
cul-de-sac of Douglas A18.17
curvature, spine A18.01
cutis (colliquativa) (primary) A18.4
cyst, ovary A18.18
cystitis A18.12
dactylitis A18.03
diarrhea A18.32
diffuse — see Tuberculosis, miliary
digestive tract A18.32

Tuberculosis, tubercular, tuberculous — *continued*
  disseminated — *see* Tuberculosis, miliary
  duodenum A18.32
  dura (mater) (cerebral) (spinal) A17.0
    abscess (cerebral) (spinal) A17.81
  dysentery A18.32
  ear (inner) (middle) A18.6
    bone A18.03
    external (primary) A18.4
    skin (primary) A18.4
  elbow A18.02
  emphysema — *see* Tuberculosis, pulmonary
  empyema A15.6
  encephalitis A17.82
  endarteritis A18.89
  endocarditis A18.84
      aortic A18.84
      mitral A18.84
      pulmonary A18.84
      tricuspid A18.84
  endocrine glands NEC A18.82
  endometrium A18.17
  enteric, enterica, enteritis A18.32
  enterocolitis A18.32
  epididymis, epididymitis A18.15
  epidural abscess (cerebral) (spinal) A17.81
  epiglottis A15.5
  episcleritis A18.51
  erythema (induratum) (nodosum) (primary) A18.4
  esophagus A18.83
  eustachian tube A18.6
  exposure (to) Z20.1
  exudative — *see* Tuberculosis, pulmonary
  eye A18.50
  eyelid (primary) (lupus) A18.4
  fallopian tube (acute) (chronic) A18.17
  fascia A18.09
  fauces A15.8
  female pelvic inflammatory disease A18.17
  finger A18.03
  first infection A15.7
  gallbladder A18.83
  ganglion A18.09
  gastritis A18.83
  gastrocolic fistula A18.32
  gastroenteritis A18.32
  gastrointestinal tract A18.32
  general, generalized — *see* Tuberculosis, miliary
  genital organs A18.10
  genitourinary A18.10
  genu A18.02
  glandula suprarenalis A18.7
  glandular, general A18.2
  glottis A15.5
  grinder's J65
  gum A18.83
  hand A18.03
  heart A18.84
  hematogenous — *see* Tuberculosis, miliary
  hemoptysis — *see* Tuberculosis, pulmonary
  hemorrhage NEC — *see* Tuberculosis, pulmonary
  hemothorax A15.6
  hepatitis A18.83
  hilar lymph nodes A15.4
    primary (progressive) A15.7
  hip (joint) (disease) (bone) A18.02
  hydropneumothorax A15.6
  hydrothorax A15.6
  hypoadrenalism A18.7
  hypopharynx A15.8
  ileocecal (hyperplastic) A18.32
  ileocolitis A18.32
  ileum A18.32
  iliac spine (superior) A18.03
  immunological findings only A15.7
  indurativa (primary) A18.4
  infantile A15.7
  infection A15.9
    without clinical manifestations A15.7
  infraclavicular gland A18.2
  inguinal gland A18.2
  inguinalis A18.2
  intestine (any part) A18.32
  iridocyclitis A18.54
  iris, iritis A18.54
  ischiorectal A18.32
  jaw A18.03
  jejunum A18.32

Tuberculosis, tubercular, tuberculous — *continued*
  joint A18.02
      vertebral A18.01
  keratitis (interstitial) A18.52
  keratoconjunctivitis A18.52
  kidney A18.11
  knee (joint) A18.02
  kyphosis, kyphoscoliosis A18.01
  laryngitis A15.5
  larynx A15.5
  latent R76.11
  leptomeninges, leptomeningitis (cerebral) (spinal)
      A17.0
  lichenoides (primary) A18.4
  linguae A18.83
  lip A18.83
  liver A18.83
  lordosis A18.01
  lung — *see* Tuberculosis, pulmonary
  lupus vulgaris A18.4
  lymph gland or node (peripheral) A18.2
      abdomen A18.39
      bronchial A15.4
          primary (progressive) A15.7
      cervical A18.2
      hilar A15.4
          primary (progressive) A15.7
      intrathoracic A15.4
          primary (progressive) A15.7
      mediastinal A15.4
          primary (progressive) A15.7
      mesenteric A18.39
      retroperitoneal A18.39
      tracheobronchial A15.4
          primary (progressive) A15.7
  lymphadenitis — *see* Tuberculosis, lymph gland
  lymphangitis — *see* Tuberculosis, lymph gland
  lymphatic (gland) (vessel) — *see* Tuberculosis, lymph
      gland
  mammary gland A18.89
  marasmus A15.9
  mastoiditis A18.03
  mediastinal lymph gland or node A15.4
      primary (progressive) A15.7
  mediastinitis A15.8
      primary (progressive) A15.7
  mediastinum A15.8
      primary (progressive) A15.7
  medulla A17.81
  melanosis, Addisonian A18.7
  meninges, meningitis (basilar) (cerebral) (cerebrospinal)
      (spinal) A17.0
  meningoencephalitis A17.82
  mesentery, mesenteric (gland or node) A18.39
  miliary A19.9
      acute A19.2
          multiple sites A19.1
          single specified site A19.0
      chronic A19.8
      specified NEC A19.8
  millstone makers' J65
  miner's J65
  molder's J65
  mouth A18.83
  multiple A19.9
      acute A19.1
      chronic A19.8
  muscle A18.09
  myelitis A17.82
  myocardium, myocarditis A18.84
  nasal (passage) (sinus) A15.8
  nasopharynx A15.8
  neck gland A18.2
  nephritis A18.11
  nerve (mononeuropathy) A17.83
  nervous system A17.9
  nose (septum) A15.8
  ocular A18.50
  omentum A18.31
  oophoritis (acute) (chronic) A18.17
  optic (nerve trunk) (papilla) A18.59
  orbit A18.59
  orchitis A18.15
  organ, specified NEC A18.89
  osseous — *see* Tuberculosis, bone
  osteitis — *see* Tuberculosis, bone
  osteomyelitis — *see* Tuberculosis, bone
  otitis media A18.6

Tuberculosis, tubercular, tuberculous — *continued*
  ovary, ovaritis (acute) (chronic) A18.17
  oviduct (acute) (chronic) A18.17
  pachymeningitis A17.0
  palate (soft) A18.83
  pancreas A18.83
  papulonecrotic (a) (primary) A18.4
  parathyroid glands A18.82
  paronychia (primary) A18.4
  parotid gland or region A18.83
  pelvis (bony) A18.03
  penis A18.15
  peribronchitis A15.5
  pericardium, pericarditis A18.84
  perichondritis, larynx A15.5
  periostitis — *see* Tuberculosis, bone
  perirectal fistula A18.32
  peritoneum NEC A18.31
  peritonitis A18.31
  pharynx, pharyngitis A15.8
  phlyctenulosis (keratoconjunctivitis) A18.52
  phthisis NEC — *see* Tuberculosis, pulmonary
  pituitary gland A18.82
  pleura, pleural, pleurisy, pleuritis (fibrinous) (oblitera-
      tive) (purulent) (simple plastic) (with effusion)
      A15.6
      primary (progressive) A15.7
  pneumonia, pneumonic — *see* Tuberculosis, pul-
      monary
  pneumothorax (spontaneous) (tense valvular) — *see*
      Tuberculosis, pulmonary
  polyneuropathy A17.89
  polyserositis A19.9
      acute A19.1
      chronic A19.8
  potter's J65
  prepuce A18.15
  primary (complex) A15.7
  proctitis A18.32
  prostate, prostatitis A18.14
  pulmonalis — *see* Tuberculosis, pulmonary
  pulmonary (cavitated) (fibrotic) (infiltrative) (nodular)
      A15.0
      childhood type or first infection A15.7
      primary (complex) A15.7
  pyelitis A18.11
  pyelonephritis A18.11
  pyemia — *see* Tuberculosis, miliary
  pyonephrosis A18.11
  pyopneumothorax A15.6
  pyothorax A15.6
  rectum (fistula) (with abscess) A18.32
  reinfection stage — *see* Tuberculosis, pulmonary
  renal A18.11
  renis A18.11
  respiratory A15.9
      primary A15.7
      specified site NEC A15.8
  retina, retinitis A18.53
  retroperitoneal (lymph gland or node) A18.39
  rheumatism NEC A18.09
  rhinitis A15.8
  sacroiliac (joint) A18.01
  sacrum A18.01
  salivary gland A18.83
  salpingitis (acute) (chronic) A18.17
  sandblaster's J65
  sclera A18.51
  scoliosis A18.01
  scrofulous A18.2
  scrotum A18.15
  seminal tract or vesicle A18.15
  senile A15.9
  septic — *see* Tuberculosis, miliary
  shoulder (joint) A18.02
      blade A18.03
  sigmoid A18.32
  sinus (any nasal) A15.8
      bone A18.03
      epididymis A18.15
  skeletal NEC A18.03
  skin (any site) (primary) A18.4
  small intestine A18.32
  soft palate A18.83
  spermatic cord A18.15
  spine, spinal (column) A18.01
      cord A17.81
      medulla A17.81

Index

Tuberculosis, tubercular, tuberculous — Tuberculosis, tubercular, tuberculous

Tuberculosis, tubercular, tuberculous — *continued*
- spine, spinal — *continued*
  - membrane A17.0
  - meninges A17.0
- spleen, splenitis A18.85
- spondylitis A18.01
- sternoclavicular joint A18.02
- stomach A18.83
- stonemason's J65
- subcutaneous tissue (cellular) (primary) A18.4
- subcutis (primary) A18.4
- subdeltoid bursa A18.83
- submaxillary (region) A18.83
- supraclavicular gland A18.2
- suprarenal (capsule) (gland) A18.7
- swelling, joint (*see also* category M01) (*see also* Tuberculosis, joint) A18.02
- symphysis pubis A18.02
- synovitis A18.09
  - articular A18.02
  - spine or vertebra A18.01
- systemic — *see* Tuberculosis, miliary
- tarsitis A18.4
- tendon (sheath) — *see* Tuberculosis, tenosynovitis
- tenosynovitis A18.09
  - spine or vertebra A18.01
- testis A18.15
- throat A15.8
- thymus gland A18.82
- thyroid gland A18.81
- tongue A18.83
- tonsil, tonsillitis A15.8
- trachea, tracheal A15.5
  - lymph gland or node A15.4
    - primary (progressive) A15.7
- tracheobronchial A15.5
  - lymph gland or node A15.4
    - primary (progressive) A15.7
- tubal (acute) (chronic) A18.17
- tunica vaginalis A18.15
- ulcer (skin) (primary) A18.4
  - bowel or intestine A18.32
  - specified NEC — *see* Tuberculosis, by site
- unspecified site A15.9
- ureter A18.11
- urethra, urethral (gland) A18.13
- urinary organ or tract A18.13
- uterus A18.17
- uveal tract A18.54
- uvula A18.83
- vagina A18.18
- vas deferens A18.15
- verruca, verrucosa (cutis) (primary) A18.4
- vertebra (column) A18.01
- vesiculitis A18.15
- vulva A18.18
- wrist (joint) A18.02

Tuberculum
- Carabelli — *see* Excludes Note at K00.2
- occlusal — *see* Excludes Note at K00.2
- paramolare K00.2

Tuberosity, enitre maxillary M26.07
Tuberous sclerosis (brain) Q85.1
Tubo-ovarian — *see* condition
Tuboplasty, after previous sterilization Z31.0
- aftercare Z31.42
Tubotympanitis, catarrhal (chronic) — *see* Otitis, media, nonsuppurative, chronic, serous
Tularemia A21.9
- with
  - conjunctivitis A21.1
  - pneumonia A21.2
- abdominal A21.3
- bronchopneumonic A21.2
- conjunctivitis A21.1
- cryptogenic A21.3
- enteric A21.3
- gastrointestinal A21.3
- generalized A21.7
- ingestion A21.3
- intestinal A21.3
- oculoglandular A21.1
- ophthalmic A21.1
- pneumonia (any), pneumonic A21.2
- pulmonary A21.2
- sepsis A21.7
- specified NEC A21.8
- typhoidal A21.7

Tularemia — *continued*
- ulceroglandular A21.0
Tularensis conjunctivitis A21.1
Tumefaction (*see also* Swelling)
- liver — *see* Hypertrophy, liver
Tumor (*see also* Neoplasm, unspecified behavior, by site)
- acinar cell — *see* Neoplasm, uncertain behavior, by site
- acinic cell — *see* Neoplasm, uncertain behavior, by site
- adenocarcinoid — *see* Neoplasm, malignant, by site
- adenomatoid (*see also* Neoplasm, benign, by site)
  - odontogenic — *see* Cyst, calcifying odontogenic
- adnexal (skin) — *see* Neoplasm, skin, benign, by site
- adrenal
  - cortical (benign) D35.0- ☑
    - malignant C74.0- ☑
  - rest — *see* Neoplasm, benign, by site
- alpha-cell
  - malignant
    - pancreas C25.4
    - specified site NEC — *see* Neoplasm, malignant, by site
    - unspecified site C25.4
  - pancreas D13.7
  - specified site NEC — *see* Neoplasm, benign, by site
  - unspecified site D13.7
- aneurysmal — *see* Aneurysm
- aortic body D44.7
  - malignant C75.5
- Askin's — *see* Neoplasm, connective tissue, malignant
- basal cell (*see also* Neoplasm, skin, uncertain behavior) D48.5
- Bednar — *see* Neoplasm, skin, malignant
- benign (unclassified) — *see* Neoplasm, benign, by site
- beta-cell
  - malignant
    - pancreas C25.4
    - specified site NEC — *see* Neoplasm, malignant, by site
    - unspecified site C25.4
  - pancreas D13.7
  - specified site NEC — *see* Neoplasm, benign, by site
  - unspecified site D13.7
- Brenner D27.9
  - borderline malignancy D39.1- ☑
  - malignant C56- ☑
  - proliferating D39.1- ☑
- bronchial alveolar, intravascular D38.1
- Brooke's — *see* Neoplasm, skin, benign
- brown fat — *see* Lipoma
- Burkitt — *see* Lymphoma, Burkitt
- calcifying epithelial odontogenic — *see* Cyst, calcifying odontogenic
- carcinoid
  - benign D3A.00 (*following* D36)
    - appendix D3A.020 (*following* D36)
    - ascending colon D3A.022 (*following* D36)
    - bronchus (lung) D3A.090 (*following* D36)
    - cecum D3A.021 (*following* D36)
    - colon D3A.029 (*following* D36)
    - descending colon D3A.024 (*following* D36)
    - duodenum D3A.010 (*following* D36)
    - foregut NOS D3A.094 (*following* D36)
    - hindgut NOS D3A.096 (*following* D36)
    - ileum D3A.012 (*following* D36)
    - jejunum D3A.011 (*following* D36)
    - kidney D3A.093 (*following* D36)
    - large intestine D3A.029 (*following* D36)
    - lung (bronchus) D3A.090 (*following* D36)
    - midgut NOS D3A.095 (*following* D36)
    - rectum D3A.026 (*following* D36)
    - sigmoid colon D3A.025 (*following* D36)
    - small intestine D3A.019 (*following* D36)
    - specified NEC D3A.098 (*following* D36)
    - stomach D3A.092 (*following* D36)
    - thymus D3A.091 (*following* D36)
    - transverse colon D3A.023 (*following* D36)
  - malignant C7A.00 (*following* C75)
    - appendix C7A.020 (*following* C75)
    - ascending colon C7A.022 (*following* C75)
    - bronchus (lung) C7A.090 (*following* C75)
    - cecum C7A.021 (*following* C75)
    - colon C7A.029 (*following* C75)
    - descending colon C7A.024 (*following* C75)
    - duodenum C7A.010 (*following* C75)
    - foregut NOS C7A.094 (*following* C75)
    - hindgut NOS C7A.096 (*following* C75)
    - ileum C7A.012 (*following* C75)
    - jejunum C7A.011 (*following* C75)

Tumor — *continued*
- carcinoid — *continued*
  - malignant — *continued*
    - kidney C7A.093 (*following* C75)
    - large intestine C7A.029 (*following* C75)
    - lung (bronchus) C7A.090 (*following* C75)
    - midgut NOS C7A.095 (*following* C75)
    - rectum C7A.026 (*following* C75)
    - sigmoid colon C7A.025 (*following* C75)
    - small intestine C7A.019 (*following* C75)
    - specified NEC C7A.098 (*following* C75)
    - stomach C7A.092 (*following* C75)
    - thymus C7A.091 (*following* C75)
    - transverse colon C7A.023 (*following* C75)
  - mesentary metastasis C7B.04 (*following* C75)
  - secondary C7B.00 (*following* C75)
    - bone C7B.03 (*following* C75)
    - distant lymph nodes C7B.01 (*following* C75)
    - liver C7B.02 (*following* C75)
    - peritoneum C7B.04 (*following* C75)
    - specified NEC C7B.09 (*following* C75)
- carotid body D44.6
  - malignant C75.4
- cells (*see also* Neoplasm, unspecified behavior, by site)
  - benign — *see* Neoplasm, benign, by site
  - malignant — *see* Neoplasm, malignant, by site
  - uncertain whether benign or malignant — *see* Neoplasm, uncertain behavior, by site
- cervix, in pregnancy or childbirth — *see* Pregnancy, complicated by, tumor, cervix
- chondromatous giant cell — *see* Neoplasm, bone, benign
- chromaffin (*see also* Neoplasm, benign, by site)
  - malignant — *see* Neoplasm, malignant, by site
- Cock's peculiar L72.3
- Codman's — *see* Neoplasm, bone, benign
- dentigerous, mixed — *see* Cyst, calcifying odontogenic
- dermoid — *see* Neoplasm, benign, by site
  - with malignant transformation C56- ☑
- desmoid (extra-abdominal) (*see also* Neoplasm, connective tissue, uncertain behavior)
  - abdominal — *see* Neoplasm, connective tissue, uncertain behavior
- embolus — *see* Neoplasm, secondary, by site
- embryonal (mixed) (*see also* Neoplasm, uncertain behavior, by site)
  - liver C22.7
- endodermal sinus
  - specified site — *see* Neoplasm, malignant, by site
  - unspecified site
    - female C56.- ☑
    - male C62.90
- epithelial
  - benign — *see* Neoplasm, benign, by site
  - malignant — *see* Neoplasm, malignant, by site
- Ewing's — *see* Neoplasm, bone, malignant, by site
- fatty — *see* Lipoma
- fibroid — *see* Leiomyoma
- G cell
  - malignant
    - pancreas C25.4
    - specified site NEC — *see* Neoplasm, malignant, by site
    - unspecified site C25.4
  - specified site — *see* Neoplasm, uncertain behavior, by site
  - unspecified site D37.8
- germ cell (*see also* Neoplasm, malignant, by site)
  - mixed — *see* Neoplasm, malignant, by site
- ghost cell, odontogenic — *see* Cyst, calcifying odontogenic
- giant cell (*see also* Neoplasm, uncertain behavior, by site)
  - bone D48.0
    - malignant — *see* Neoplasm, bone, malignant
    - chondromatous — *see* Neoplasm, bone, benign
    - malignant — *see* Neoplasm, malignant, by site
    - soft parts — *see* Neoplasm, connective tissue, uncertain behavior
      - malignant — *see* Neoplasm, connective tissue, malignant
- glomus D18.00
  - intra-abdominal D18.03
  - intracranial D18.02
  - jugulare D44.7
    - malignant C75.5
  - skin D18.01
  - specified site NEC D18.09

☑ **Additional Character Required — Refer to the Tabular List for Character Selection**   ⩔ **Subterms under main terms may continue to next column or page**

Tumor — *continued*
- gonadal stromal — *see* Neoplasm, uncertain behavior, by site
- granular cell (*see also* Neoplasm, connective tissue, benign)
  - malignant — *see* Neoplasm, connective tissue, malignant
- granulosa cell D39.1- ☑
  - juvenile D39.1- ☑
  - malignant C56- ☑
- granulosa cell-theca cell D39.1- ☑
  - malignant C56- ☑
- Grawitz's C64- ☑
- hemorrhoidal — *see* Hemorrhoids
- hilar cell D27- ☑
- hilus cell D27- ☑
- Hurthle cell (benign) D34
  - malignant C73
- hydatid — *see* Echinococcus
- hypernephroid (*see also* Neoplasm, uncertain behavior, by site)
- interstitial cell (*see also* Neoplasm, uncertain behavior, by site)
  - benign — *see* Neoplasm, benign, by site
  - malignant — *see* Neoplasm, malignant, by site
- intravascular bronchial alveolar D38.1
- islet cell — *see* Neoplasm, benign, by site
  - malignant — *see* Neoplasm, malignant, by site
    - pancreas C25.4
    - specified site NEC — *see* Neoplasm, malignant, by site
    - unspecified site C25.4
  - pancreas D13.7
  - specified site NEC — *see* Neoplasm, benign, by site
  - unspecified site D13.7
- juxtaglomerular D41.0- ☑
- Klatskin's C22.1
- Krukenberg's C79.6- ☑
- Leydig cell — *see* Neoplasm, uncertain behavior, by site
  - benign — *see* Neoplasm, benign, by site
    - specified site — *see* Neoplasm, benign, by site
    - unspecified site
      - female D27.9
      - male D29.20
  - malignant — *see* Neoplasm, malignant, by site
    - specified site — *see* Neoplasm, malignant, by site
    - unspecified site
      - female C56.9
      - male C62.90
  - specified site — *see* Neoplasm, uncertain behavior, by site
  - unspecified site
    - female D39.10
    - male D40.10
- lipid cell, ovary D27- ☑
- lipoid cell, ovary D27- ☑
- malignant (*see also* Neoplasm, malignant, by site) C80.1
  - fusiform cell (type) C80.1
  - giant cell (type) C80.1
  - localized, plasma cell — *see* Plasmacytoma, solitary
  - mixed NEC C80.1
  - small cell (type) C80.1
  - spindle cell (type) C80.1
  - unclassified C80.1
- mast cell D47.09
- melanotic, neuroectodermal — *see* Neoplasm, benign, by site
- Merkel cell — *see* Carcinoma, Merkel cell
- mesenchymal
  - malignant — *see* Neoplasm, connective tissue, malignant
  - mixed — *see* Neoplasm, connective tissue, uncertain behavior
- mesodermal, mixed (*see also* Neoplasm, malignant, by site)
  - liver C22.4
- mesonephric (*see also* Neoplasm, uncertain behavior, by site)
  - malignant — *see* Neoplasm, malignant, by site
- metastatic
  - from specified site — *see* Neoplasm, malignant, by site
  - of specified site — *see* Neoplasm, malignant, by site
  - to specified site — *see* Neoplasm, secondary, by site
- mixed NEC (*see also* Neoplasm, benign, by site)

Tumor — *continued*
- mixed (*see also* Neoplasm, benign, by site) — *continued*
  - malignant — *see* Neoplasm, malignant, by site
- mucinous of low malignant potential
  - specified site — *see* Neoplasm, malignant, by site
  - unspecified site C56.9
- mucocarcinoid
  - specified site — *see* Neoplasm, malignant, by site
  - unspecified site C18.1
- mucoepidermoid — *see* Neoplasm, uncertain behavior, by site
- Müllerian, mixed
  - specified site — *see* Neoplasm, malignant, by site
  - unspecified site C54.9
- myoepithelial — *see* Neoplasm, benign, by site
- neuroectodermal (peripheral) — *see* Neoplasm, malignant, by site
  - primitive
    - specified site — *see* Neoplasm, malignant, by site
    - unspecified site C71.9
- neuroendocrine D3A.8 (*following* D36)
  - malignant poorly differentiated C7A.1 (*following* C75)
  - secondary NEC C7B.8 (*following* C75)
  - specified NEC C7A.8 (*following* C75)
- neurogenic olfactory C30.0
- nonencapsulated sclerosing C73
- odontogenic (adenomatoid) (benign) (calcifying epithelial) (keratocystic) (squamous) — *see* Cyst, calcifying odontogenic
  - malignant C41.1
    - upper jaw (bone) C41.0
- ovarian stromal D39.1- ☑
- ovary, in pregnancy — *see* Pregnancy, complicated by
- pacinian — *see* Neoplasm, skin, benign
- Pancoast's — *see* Pancoast's syndrome
- papillary (*see also* Papilloma)
  - cystic D37.9
  - mucinous of low malignant potential C56- ☑
    - specified site — *see* Neoplasm, malignant, by site
    - unspecified site C56.9
  - serous of low malignant potential
    - specified site — *see* Neoplasm, malignant, by site
    - unspecified site C56.9
- pelvic, in pregnancy or childbirth — *see* Pregnancy, complicated by
- phantom F45.8
- phyllodes D48.6- ☑
  - benign D24- ☑
  - malignant — *see* Neoplasm, breast, malignant
- Pindborg — *see* Cyst, calcifying odontogenic
- placental site trophoblastic D39.2
- plasma cell (malignant) (localized) — *see* Plasmacytoma, solitary
- polyvesicular vitelline
  - specified site — *see* Neoplasm, malignant, by site
  - unspecified site
    - female C56.9
    - male C62.90
- Pott's puffy — *see* Osteomyelitis, specified NEC
- Rathke's pouch D44.3
- retinal anlage — *see* Neoplasm, benign, by site
- salivary gland type, mixed — *see* Neoplasm, salivary gland, benign
  - malignant — *see* Neoplasm, salivary gland, malignant
- Sampson's N80.1
- Schmincke's — *see* Neoplasm, nasopharynx, malignant
- sclerosing stromal D27- ☑
- sebaceous — *see* Cyst, sebaceous
- secondary — *see* Neoplasm, secondary, by site
  - carcinoid C7B.00 (*following* C75)
    - bone C7B.03 (*following* C75)
    - distant lymph nodes C7B.01 (*following* C75)
    - liver C7B.02 (*following* C75)
    - peritoneum C7B.04 (*following* C75)
    - specified NEC C7B.09 (*following* C75)
  - neuroendocrine NEC C7B.8 (*following* C75)
- serous of low malignant potential
  - specified site — *see* Neoplasm, malignant, by site
  - unspecified site C56.9
- Sertoli cell — *see* Neoplasm, benign, by site
  - with lipid storage
    - specified site — *see* Neoplasm, benign, by site

Tumor — *continued*
- Sertoli cell — *see* Neoplasm, benign, by site — *continued*
  - with lipid storage — *continued*
    - unspecified site
      - female D27.9
      - male D29.20
    - specified site — *see* Neoplasm, benign, by site
    - unspecified site
      - female D27.9
      - male D29.20
- Sertoli-Leydig cell — *see* Neoplasm, benign, by site
  - specified site — *see* Neoplasm, benign, by site
  - unspecified site
    - female D27.9
    - male D29.20
- sex cord (-stromal) — *see* Neoplasm, uncertain behavior, by site
  - with annular tubules D39.1- ☑
- skin appendage — *see* Neoplasm, skin, benign
- smooth muscle — *see* Neoplasm, connective tissue, uncertain behavior
- soft tissue
  - benign — *see* Neoplasm, connective tissue, benign
  - malignant — *see* Neoplasm, connective tissue, malignant
- sternomastoid (congenital) Q68.0
- stromal
  - endometrial D39.0
  - gastric D48.1
    - benign D21.4
    - malignant C16.9
    - uncertain behavior D48.1
  - gastrointestinal C49.A- ☑
    - benign D21.4
    - esophagus C49.A1
    - malignant C49.A0
      - colon C49.A4
      - duodenum C49.A3
      - esophagus C49.A1
      - ileum C49.A3
      - jejunum C49.A3
      - large intestine C49.A4
      - Meckel diverticulum C49.A3
      - omentum C49.A9
      - peritoneum C49.A9
      - rectum C49.A5
      - small intestine C49.A3
      - specified site NEC C49.A9
      - stomach C49.A2
    - rectum C49.A5
    - small intestine C49.A3
    - specified site NEC C49.A9
    - stomach C49.A2
    - uncertain behavior D48.1
  - intestine
    - benign D21.4
    - malignant
      - large C49.A4
      - small C49.A3
    - uncertain behavior D48.1
  - ovarian D39.1- ☑
  - stomach C49.A2
    - benign D21.4
    - malignant C49.A2
    - uncertain behavior D48.1
- sweat gland (*see also* Neoplasm, skin, uncertain behavior)
  - benign — *see* Neoplasm, skin, benign
  - malignant — *see* Neoplasm, skin, malignant
- syphilitic, brain A52.17
- testicular D40.10
- testicular stromal D40.1- ☑
- theca cell D27- ☑
- theca cell-granulosa cell D39.1- ☑
- Triton, malignant — *see* Neoplasm, nerve, malignant
- trophoblastic, placental site D39.2
- turban D23.4
- uterus (body), in pregnancy or childbirth — *see* Pregnancy, complicated by, tumor, uterus
- vagina, in pregnancy or childbirth — *see* Pregnancy, complicated by
- varicose — *see* Varix
- von Recklinghausen's — *see* Neurofibromatosis
- vulva or perineum, in pregnancy or childbirth — *see* Pregnancy, complicated by
  - causing obstructed labor O65.5
- Warthin's — *see* Neoplasm, salivary gland, benign

Index

Tumor — *continued*
 Wilms' C64-
 yolk sac — *see* Neoplasm, malignant, by site
  specified site — *see* Neoplasm, malignant, by site
  unspecified site
   female C56.9
   male C62.90
Tumor lysis syndrome (following antineoplastic chemotherapy) (spontaneous) NEC E88.3
Tumorlet — *see* Neoplasm, uncertain behavior, by site
Tungiasis B88.1
Tunica vasculosa lentis Q12.2
Turban tumor D23.4
Türck's trachoma J37.0
Turner-Kieser syndrome Q87.2
Turner-like syndrome Q87.1
Turner's
 hypoplasia (tooth) K00.4
 syndrome Q96.9
  specified NEC Q96.8
 tooth K00.4
Turner-Ullrich syndrome Q96.9
Tussis convulsiva — *see* Whooping cough
Twiddler's syndrome (due to)
 automatic implantable defibrillatorT82.198
 cardiac pacemaker T82.198 ☑
Twilight state
 epileptic F05
 psychogenic F44.89
Twin (newborn) (*see also* Newborn, twin)
 conjoined Q89.4
 pregnancy — *see* Pregnancy, twin
Twinning, teeth K00.2
Twist, twisted
 bowel, colon or intestine K56.2
 hair (congenital) Q84.1
 mesentery K56.2
 omentum K56.2
 organ or site, congenital NEC — *see* Anomaly, by site
 ovarian pedicle — *see* Torsion, ovary
Twitching R25.3
Tylosis (acquired) L84
 buccalis K13.29
 linguae K13.29
 palmaris et plantaris (congenital) (inherited) Q82.8
  acquired L85.1
Tympanism R14.0
Tympanites (abdominal) (intestinal) R14.0
Tympanitis — *see* Myringitis
Tympanosclerosis H74.0 ☑
Tympanum — *see* condition
Tympany
 abdomen R14.0
 chest R09.89
Type A behavior pattern Z73.1
Typhlitis — *see* Appendicitis
Typhoenteritis — *see* Typhoid
Typhoid (abortive) (ambulant) (any site) (clinical) (fever) (hemorrhagic) (infection) (intermittent) (malignant) (rheumatic) (Widal negative) A01.00
 with pneumonia A01.03
 abdominal A01.09
 arthritis A01.04
 carrier (suspected) of Z22.0
 cholecystitis (current) A01.09
 endocarditis A01.02
 heart involvement A01.02
 inoculation reaction — *see* Complications, vaccination
 meningitis A01.01
 mesenteric lymph nodes A01.09
 myocarditis A01.02
 osteomyelitis A01.05
 perichondritis, larynx A01.09
 pneumonia A01.03
 specified NEC A01.09
 spine A01.05
 ulcer (perforating) A01.09
Typhomalaria (fever) — *see* Malaria
Typhomania A01.00
Typhoperitonitis A01.09
Typhus (fever) A75.9
 abdominal, abdominalis — *see* Typhoid
 African tick A77.1
 amarillic A95.9
 brain A75.9 [G94]
 cerebral A75.9 [G94]
 classical A75.0

Typhus — *continued*
 due to Rickettsia
  prowazekii A75.0
   recrudescent A75.1
  tsutsugamushi A75.3
  typhi A75.2
 endemic (flea-borne) A75.2
 epidemic (louse-borne) A75.0
 exanthematicus SAI A75.0
  brillii SAI A75.1
  mexicanus SAI A75.2
  typhus murinus A75.2
 exanthematic NEC A75.0
 flea-borne A75.2
 India tick A77.1
 Kenya (tick) A77.1
 louse-borne A75.0
 Mexican A75.2
 mite-borne A75.3
 murine A75.2
 North Asian tick-borne A77.2
 petechial A75.9
 Queensland tick A77.3
 rat A75.2
 recrudescent A75.1
 recurrens — *see* Fever, relapsing
 Sao Paulo A77.0
 scrub (China) (India) (Malaysia) (New Guinea) A75.3
 shop (of Malaysia) A75.2
 Siberian tick A77.2
 tick-borne A77.9
 tropical (mite-borne) A75.3
Tyrosinemia E70.21
 newborn, transitory P74.5
Tyrosinosis E70.21
Tyrosinuria E70.29

U

Uhl's anomaly or disease Q24.8
Ulcer, ulcerated, ulcerating, ulceration, ulcerative
 alveolar process M27.3
 amebic (intestine) A06.1
  skin A06.7
 anastomotic — *see* Ulcer, gastrojejunal
 anorectal K62.6
 antral — *see* Ulcer, stomach
 anus (sphincter) (solitary) K62.6
 aorta — *see* Aneurysm
 aphthous (oral) (recurrent) K12.0
  genital organ(s)
   female N76.6
   male N50.89
 artery I77.2
 atrophic — *see* Ulcer, skin
  decubitus — *see* Ulcer, pressure, by site
 back L98.429
  with
   bone involvement without evidence of necrosis L98.426
   bone necrosis L98.424
   exposed fat layer L98.422
   muscle involvement without evidence of necrosis L98.425
   muscle necrosis L98.423
   skin breakdown only L98.421
   specified severity NEC L98.428
 Barrett's (esophagus) K22.10
  with bleeding K22.11
 bile duct (common) (hepatic) K83.8
 bladder (solitary) (sphincter) NEC N32.89
  bilharzial B65.9 [N33]
  in schistosomiasis (bilharzial) B65.9 [N33]
  submucosal — *see* Cystitis, interstitial
  tuberculous A18.12
 bleeding K27.4
 bone — *see* Osteomyelitis, specified type NEC
 bowel — *see* Ulcer, intestine
 breast N61.1
 bronchus J98.09
 buccal (cavity) (traumatic) K12.1
 Buruli A31.1
 buttock L98.419
  with
   bone involvement without evidence of necrosis L98.416
   bone necrosis L98.414
   exposed fat layer L98.412

Ulcer, ulcerated, ulcerating, ulceration, ulcerative — *continued*
 buttock — *continued*
  with — *continued*
   muscle involvement without evidence of necrosis L98.415
   muscle necrosis L98.413
   skin breakdown only L98.411
   specified severity NEC L98.418
 cancerous — *see* Neoplasm, malignant, by site
 cardia K22.10
  with bleeding K22.11
 cardioesophageal (peptic) K22.10
  with bleeding K22.11
 cecum — *see* Ulcer, intestine
 cervix (uteri) (decubitus) (trophic) N86
  with cervicitis N72
 chancroidal A57
 chiclero B55.1
 chronic (cause unknown) — *see* Ulcer, skin
 Cochin-China B55.1
 colon — *see* Ulcer, intestine
 conjunctiva H10.89
 cornea H16.00- ☑
  with hypopyon H16.03- ☑
  central H16.01- ☑
  dendritic (herpes simplex) B00.52
  marginal H16.04- ☑
  Mooren's H16.05- ☑
  mycotic H16.06- ☑
  perforated H16.07- ☑
  ring H16.02- ☑
  tuberculous (phlyctenular) A18.52
 corpus cavernosum (chronic) N48.5
 crural — *see* Ulcer, lower limb
 Curling's — *see* Ulcer, peptic, acute
 Cushing's — *see* Ulcer, peptic, acute
 cystic duct K82.8
 cystitis (interstitial) — *see* Cystitis, interstitial
 decubitus — *see* Ulcer, pressure, by site
 dendritic, cornea (herpes simplex) B00.52
 diabetes, diabetic — *see* Diabetes, ulcer
 Dieulafoy's K25.0
 due to
  infection NEC — *see* Ulcer, skin
  radiation NEC L59.8
  trophic disturbance (any region) — *see* Ulcer, skin
  X-ray L58.1
 duodenum, duodenal (eroded) (peptic) K26.9
  with
   hemorrhage K26.4
    and perforation K26.6
   perforation K26.5
  acute K26.3
   with
    hemorrhage K26.0
     and perforation K26.2
    perforation K26.1
  chronic K26.7
   with
    hemorrhage K26.4
     and perforation K26.6
    perforation K26.5
 dysenteric A09
 elusive — *see* Cystitis, interstitial
 endocarditis (acute) (chronic) (subacute) I28.8
 epiglottis J38.7
 esophagus (peptic) K22.10
  with bleeding K22.11
  due to
   aspirin K22.10
    with bleeding K22.11
   gastrointestinal reflux disease K21.0
   ingestion of chemical or medicament K22.10
    with bleeding K22.11
  fungal K22.10
   with bleeding K22.11
  infective K22.10
   with bleeding K22.11
  varicose — *see* Varix, esophagus
 eyelid (region) H01.8
 fauces J39.2
 Fenwick (-Hunner) (solitary) — *see* Cystitis, interstitial
 fistulous — *see* Ulcer, skin
 foot (indolent) (trophic) — *see* Ulcer, lower limb
 frambesial, initial A66.0
 frenum (tongue) K14.0
 gallbladder or duct K82.8

☑ **Additional Character Required** — Refer to the Tabular List for Character Selection 🔁 **Subterms under main terms may continue to next column or page**

Tumor — Ulcer, ulcerated, ulcerating, ulceration, ulcerative

Ulcer, ulcerated, ulcerating, ulceration, ulcerative
— continued
gangrenous — see Gangrene
gastric — see Ulcer, stomach
gastrocolic — see Ulcer, gastrojejunal
gastroduodenal — see Ulcer, peptic
gastroesophageal — see Ulcer, stomach
gastrointestinal — see Ulcer, gastrojejunal
gastrojejunal (peptic) K28.9
　with
　　hemorrhage K28.4
　　　and perforation K28.6
　　perforation K28.5
　acute K28.3
　　with
　　　hemorrhage K28.0
　　　　and perforation K28.2
　　　perforation K28.1
　chronic K28.7
　　with
　　　hemorrhage K28.4
　　　　and perforation K28.6
　　　perforation K28.5
gastrojejunocolic — see Ulcer, gastrojejunal
gingiva K06.8
gingivitis K05.10
　nonplaque induced K05.11
　plaque induced K05.10
glottis J38.7
granuloma of pudenda A58
gum K06.8
gumma, due to yaws A66.4
heel — see Ulcer, lower limb
hemorrhoid (see also Hemorrhoids, by degree) K64.8
Hunner's — see Cystitis, interstitial
hypopharynx J39.2
hypopyon (chronic) (subacute) — see Ulcer, cornea, with hypopyon
hypostaticum — see Ulcer, varicose
ileum — see Ulcer, intestine
intestine, intestinal K63.3
　with perforation K63.1
　amebic A06.1
　duodenal — see Ulcer, duodenum
　granulocytopenic (with hemorrhage) — see Neutropenia
　marginal — see Ulcer, gastrojejunal
　perforating K63.1
　　newborn P78.0
　primary, small intestine K63.3
　rectum K62.6
　stercoraceous, stercoral K63.3
　tuberculous A18.32
　typhoid (fever) — see Typhoid
　varicose I86.8
jejunum, jejunal — see Ulcer, gastrojejunal
keratitis — see Ulcer, cornea
knee — see Ulcer, lower limb
labium (majus) (minus) N76.6
laryngitis — see Laryngitis
larynx (aphthous) (contact) J38.7
　diphtheritic A36.2
leg — see Ulcer, lower limb
lip K13.0
Lipschütz's N76.6
lower limb (atrophic) (chronic) (neurogenic) (perforating) (pyogenic) (trophic) (tropical) L97.909
　with
　　bone involvement without evidence of necrosis L97.906
　　bone necrosis L97.904
　　exposed fat layer L97.902
　　muscle involvement without evidence of necrosis L97.905
　　muscle necrosis L97.903
　　skin breakdown only L97.901
　　specified severity NEC L97.908
　ankle L97.309
　　with
　　　bone involvement without evidence of necrosis L97.306
　　　bone necrosis L97.304
　　　exposed fat layer L97.302
　　　muscle involvement without evidence of necrosis L97.305
　　　muscle necrosis L97.303
　　　skin breakdown only L97.301
　　　specified severity NEC L97.308

Ulcer, ulcerated, ulcerating, ulceration, ulcerative
— continued
lower limb — continued
　ankle — continued
　　left L97.329
　　　with
　　　　bone involvement without evidence of necrosis L97.326
　　　　bone necrosis L97.324
　　　　exposed fat layer L97.322
　　　　muscle involvement without evidence of necrosis L97.325
　　　　muscle necrosis L97.323
　　　　skin breakdown only L97.321
　　　　specified severity NEC L97.328
　　right L97.319
　　　with
　　　　bone involvement without evidence of necrosis L97.316
　　　　bone necrosis L97.314
　　　　exposed fat layer L97.312
　　　　muscle involvement without evidence of necrosis L97.315
　　　　muscle necrosis L97.313
　　　　skin breakdown only L97.311
　　　　specified severity NEC L97.318
　calf L97.209
　　with
　　　bone involvement without evidence of necrosis L97.206
　　　bone necrosis L97.204
　　　exposed fat layer L97.202
　　　muscle involvement without evidence of necrosis L97.205
　　　muscle necrosis L97.203
　　　skin breakdown only L97.201
　　　specified severity NEC L97.208
　　left L97.229
　　　with
　　　　bone involvement without evidence of necrosis L97.226
　　　　bone necrosis L97.224
　　　　exposed fat layer L97.222
　　　　muscle involvement without evidence of necrosis L97.225
　　　　muscle necrosis L97.223
　　　　skin breakdown only L97.221
　　　　specified severity NEC L97.228
　　right L97.219
　　　with
　　　　bone involvement without evidence of necrosis L97.216
　　　　bone necrosis L97.214
　　　　exposed fat layer L97.212
　　　　muscle involvement without evidence of necrosis L97.215
　　　　muscle necrosis L97.213
　　　　skin breakdown only L97.211
　　　　specified severity NEC L97.218
　decubitus — see Ulcer, pressure, by site
　foot specified NEC L97.509
　　with
　　　bone involvement without evidence of necrosis L97.506
　　　bone necrosis L97.504
　　　exposed fat layer L97.502
　　　muscle involvement without evidence of necrosis L97.505
　　　muscle necrosis L97.503
　　　skin breakdown only L97.501
　　　specified severity NEC L97.508
　　left L97.529
　　　with
　　　　bone involvement without evidence of necrosis L97.526
　　　　bone necrosis L97.524
　　　　exposed fat layer L97.522
　　　　muscle involvement without evidence of necrosis L97.525
　　　　muscle necrosis L97.523
　　　　skin breakdown only L97.521
　　　　specified severity NEC L97.528
　　right L97.519
　　　with
　　　　bone involvement without evidence of necrosis L97.516
　　　　bone necrosis L97.514
　　　　exposed fat layer L97.512

Ulcer, ulcerated, ulcerating, ulceration, ulcerative
— continued
lower limb — continued
　foot specified — continued
　　right — continued
　　　with — continued
　　　　muscle involvement without evidence of necrosis L97.515
　　　　muscle necrosis L97.513
　　　　skin breakdown only L97.511
　　　　specified severity NEC L97.518
　　heel L97.409
　　　with
　　　　bone involvement without evidence of necrosis L97.406
　　　　bone necrosis L97.404
　　　　exposed fat layer L97.402
　　　　muscle involvement without evidence of necrosis L97.405
　　　　muscle necrosis L97.403
　　　　skin breakdown only L97.401
　　　　specified severity NEC L97.408
　　　left L97.429
　　　　with
　　　　　bone involvement without evidence of necrosis L97.426
　　　　　bone necrosis L97.424
　　　　　exposed fat layer L97.422
　　　　　muscle involvement without evidence of necrosis L97.425
　　　　　muscle necrosis L97.423
　　　　　skin breakdown only L97.421
　　　　　specified severity NEC L97.428
　　　right L97.419
　　　　with
　　　　　bone involvement without evidence of necrosis L97.416
　　　　　bone necrosis L97.414
　　　　　exposed fat layer L97.412
　　　　　muscle involvement without evidence of necrosis L97.415
　　　　　muscle necrosis L97.413
　　　　　skin breakdown only L97.411
　　　　　specified severity NEC L97.418
　　left L97.929
　　　with
　　　　bone involvement without evidence of necrosis L97.926
　　　　bone necrosis L97.924
　　　　exposed fat layer L97.922
　　　　muscle involvement without evidence of necrosis L97.925
　　　　muscle necrosis L97.923
　　　　skin breakdown only L97.921
　　　　specified severity NEC L97.928
　leprous A30.1
　lower leg NOS L97.909
　　with
　　　bone involvement without evidence of necrosis L97.906
　　　bone necrosis L97.904
　　　exposed fat layer L97.902
　　　muscle involvement without evidence of necrosis L97.905
　　　muscle necrosis L97.903
　　　skin breakdown only L97.901
　　　specified severity NEC L97.908
　　left L97.929
　　　with
　　　　bone involvement without evidence of necrosis L97.926
　　　　bone necrosis L97.924
　　　　exposed fat layer L97.922
　　　　muscle involvement without evidence of necrosis L97.925
　　　　muscle necrosis L97.923
　　　　skin breakdown only L97.921
　　　　specified severity NEC L97.928
　　right L97.919
　　　with
　　　　bone involvement without evidence of necrosis L97.916
　　　　bone necrosis L97.914
　　　　exposed fat layer L97.912
　　　　muscle involvement without evidence of necrosis L97.915
　　　　muscle necrosis L97.913
　　　　skin breakdown only L97.911
　　　　specified severity NEC L97.918

Ulcer, ulcerated, ulcerating, ulceration, ulcerative
— *continued*
  lower limb — *continued*
    lower leg — *continued*
      specified site NEC L97.809
        with
          bone involvement without evidence of necrosis L97.806
          bone necrosis L97.804
          exposed fat layer L97.802
          muscle involvement without evidence of necrosis L97.805
          muscle necrosis L97.803
          skin breakdown only L97.801
          specified severity NEC L97.808
      left L97.829
        with
          bone involvement without evidence of necrosis L97.826
          bone necrosis L97.824
          exposed fat layer L97.822
          muscle involvement without evidence of necrosis L97.825
          muscle necrosis L97.823
          skin breakdown only L97.821
          specified severity NEC L97.828
      right L97.819
        with
          bone involvement without evidence of necrosis L97.816
          bone necrosis L97.814
          exposed fat layer L97.812
          muscle involvement without evidence of necrosis L97.815
          muscle necrosis L97.813
          skin breakdown only L97.811
          specified severity NEC L97.818
    midfoot L97.409
      with
        bone involvement without evidence of necrosis L97.406
        bone necrosis L97.404
        exposed fat layer L97.402
        muscle involvement without evidence of necrosis L97.405
        muscle necrosis L97.403
        skin breakdown only L97.401
        specified severity NEC L97.408
      left L97.429
        with
          bone involvement without evidence of necrosis L97.426
          bone necrosis L97.424
          exposed fat layer L97.422
          muscle involvement without evidence of necrosis L97.425
          muscle necrosis L97.423
          skin breakdown only L97.421
          specified severity NEC L97.428
      right L97.419
        with
          bone involvement without evidence of necrosis L97.416
          bone necrosis L97.414
          exposed fat layer L97.412
          muscle involvement without evidence of necrosis L97.415
          muscle necrosis L97.413
          skin breakdown only L97.411
          specified severity NEC L97.418
    syphilitic A52.19
    thigh L97.109
      with
        bone involvement without evidence of necrosis L97.106
        bone necrosis L97.104
        exposed fat layer L97.102
  right L97.919
    with
      bone involvement without evidence of necrosis L97.916
      bone necrosis L97.914
      exposed fat layer L97.912
      muscle involvement without evidence of necrosis L97.915
      muscle necrosis L97.913
      skin breakdown only L97.911
      specified severity NEC L97.918

Ulcer, ulcerated, ulcerating, ulceration, ulcerative
— *continued*
  lower limb — *continued*
    thigh — *continued*
      with — *continued*
        muscle involvement without evidence of necrosis L97.105
        muscle necrosis L97.103
        skin breakdown only L97.101
        specified severity NEC L97.108
      left L97.129
        with
          bone involvement without evidence of necrosis L97.126
          bone necrosis L97.124
          exposed fat layer L97.122
          muscle involvement without evidence of necrosis L97.125
          muscle necrosis L97.123
          skin breakdown only L97.121
          specified severity NEC L97.128
      right L97.119
        with
          bone involvement without evidence of necrosis L97.116
          bone necrosis L97.114
          exposed fat layer L97.112
          muscle involvement without evidence of necrosis L97.115
          muscle necrosis L97.113
          skin breakdown only L97.111
          specified severity NEC L97.118
    toe L97.509
      with
        bone involvement without evidence of necrosis L97.506
        bone necrosis L97.504
        exposed fat layer L97.502
        muscle involvement without evidence of necrosis L97.505
        muscle necrosis L97.503
        skin breakdown only L97.501
        specified severity NEC L97.508
      left L97.529
        with
          bone involvement without evidence of necrosis L97.526
          bone necrosis L97.524
          exposed fat layer L97.522
          muscle involvement without evidence of necrosis L97.525
          muscle necrosis L97.523
          skin breakdown only L97.521
          specified severity NEC L97.528
      right L97.519
        with
          bone involvement without evidence of necrosis L97.516
          bone necrosis L97.514
          exposed fat layer L97.512
          muscle involvement without evidence of necrosis L97.515
          muscle necrosis L97.513
          skin breakdown only L97.511
          specified severity NEC L97.518
    varicose — *see* Varix, leg, with, ulcer
  luetic — *see* Ulcer, syphilitic
  lung J98.4
    tuberculous — *see* Tuberculosis, pulmonary
  malignant — *see* Neoplasm, malignant, by site
  marginal NEC — *see* Ulcer, gastrojejunal
  meatus (urinarius) N34.2
  Meckel's diverticulum Q43.0
    malignant — *see* Table of Neoplasms, small intestine, malignant
  Meleney's (chronic undermining) — *see* Ulcer, skin
  Mooren's (cornea) — *see* Ulcer, cornea, Mooren's
  mycobacterial (skin) A31.1
  nasopharynx J39.2
  neck, uterus N86
  neurogenic NEC — *see* Ulcer, skin
  nose, nasal (passage) (infective) (septum) J34.0
    skin — *see* Ulcer, skin
    spirochetal A69.8
    varicose (bleeding) I86.8
  oral mucosa (traumatic) K12.1
  palate (soft) K12.1
  penis (chronic) N48.5

Ulcer, ulcerated, ulcerating, ulceration, ulcerative
— *continued*
  peptic (site unspecified) K27.9
    with
      hemorrhage K27.4
        and perforation K27.6
      perforation K27.5
    acute K27.3
      with
        hemorrhage K27.0
          and perforation K27.2
        perforation K27.1
    chronic K27.7
      with
        hemorrhage K27.4
          and perforation K27.6
        perforation K27.5
    esophagus K22.10
      with bleeding K22.11
    newborn P78.82
  perforating K27.5
    skin — *see* Ulcer, skin
  peritonsillar J35.8
  phagedenic (tropical) — *see* Ulcer, skin
  pharynx J39.2
  phlebitis — *see* Phlebitis
  plaster — *see* Ulcer, pressure, by site
  popliteal space — *see* Ulcer, lower limb
  postpyloric — *see* Ulcer, duodenum
  prepuce N47.7
  prepyloric — *see* Ulcer, stomach
  pressure (pressure area) L89.9- ☑
    ankle L89.5- ☑
    back L89.1- ☑
    buttock L89.3- ☑
    coccyx L89.15- ☑
    contiguous site of back, buttock, hip L89.4- ☑
    elbow L89.0- ☑
    face L89.81- ☑
    head L89.81- ☑
    heel L89.6- ☑
    hip L89.2- ☑
    sacral region (tailbone) L89.15- ☑
    specified site NEC L89.89- ☑
    stage 1 (healing) (pre-ulcer skin changes limited to persistent focal edema)
      ankle L89.5- ☑
      back L89.1- ☑
      buttock L89.3- ☑
      coccyx L89.15- ☑
      contiguous site of back, buttock, hip L89.4- ☑
      elbow L89.0- ☑
      face L89.81- ☑
      head L89.81- ☑
      heel L89.6- ☑
      hip L89.2- ☑
      sacral region (tailbone) L89.15- ☑
      specified site NEC L89.89- ☑
    stage 2 (healing) (abrasion, blister, partial thickness skin loss involving epidermis and/or dermis)
      ankle L89.5- ☑
      back L89.1- ☑
      buttock L89.3- ☑
      coccyx L89.15- ☑
      contiguous site of back, buttock, hip L89.4- ☑
      elbow L89.0- ☑
      face L89.81- ☑
      head L89.81- ☑
      heel L89.6- ☑
      hip L89.2- ☑
      sacral region (tailbone) L89.15- ☑
      specified site NEC L89.89- ☑
    stage 3 (healing) (full thickness skin loss involving damage or necrosis of subcutaneous tissue)
      ankle L89.5- ☑
      back L89.1- ☑
      buttock L89.3- ☑
      coccyx L89.15- ☑
      contiguous site of back, buttock, hip L89.4- ☑
      elbow L89.0- ☑
      face L89.81- ☑
      head L89.81- ☑
      heel L89.6- ☑
      hip L89.2- ☑
      sacral region (tailbone) L89.15- ☑
      specified site NEC L89.89- ☑

☑ Additional Character Required — Refer to the Tabular List for Character Selection   ▽ Subterms under main terms may continue to next column or page

Unsatisfactory
- restoration of tooth K08.50
  - specified NEC K08.59
- sample of cytologic smear
  - anus R85.615
  - cervix R87.615
  - vagina R87.625
- surroundings Z59.1
- work Z56.5

Unsoundness of mind — *see* Psychosis

Unstable
- back NEC — *see* Instability, joint, spine
- hip (congenital) Q65.6
  - acquired — *see* Derangement, joint, specified type NEC, hip
- joint — *see* Instability, joint
  - secondary to removal of joint prosthesis M96.89
- lie (mother) O32.0 ☑
- lumbosacral joint (congenital)
  - acquired — *see* subcategory M53.2 ☑
- sacroiliac — *see* subcategory M53.2 ☑
- spine NEC — *see* Instability, joint, spine

Unsteadiness on feet R26.81

Untruthfulness, child problem F91.8

Unverricht (-Lundborg) **disease or epilepsy** — *see* Epilepsy, generalized, idiopathic

Unwanted pregnancy Z64.0

Upbringing, institutional Z62.22
- away from parents NEC Z62.29
- in care of non-parental family member Z62.21
- in foster care Z62.21
- in orphanage or group home Z62.22
- in welfare custody Z62.21

Upper respiratory — *see* condition

Upset
- gastric K30
- gastrointestinal K30
  - psychogenic F45.8
- intestinal (large) (small) K59.9
  - psychogenic F45.8
- menstruation N93.9
- mental F48.9
- stomach K30
  - psychogenic F45.8

Urachus (*see also* condition)
- patent or persistent Q64.4

Urbach-Oppenheim disease (necrobiosis lipoidica diabeticorum) — *see* E08-E13 with .620

Urbach's lipoid proteinosis E78.89

Urbach-Wiethe disease E78.89

Urban yellow fever A95.1

Urea
- blood, high — *see* Uremia
- cycle metabolism disorder — *see* Disorder, urea cycle metabolism

Uremia, uremic N19
- with
  - ectopic or molar pregnancy O08.4
  - polyneuropathy N18.9 [G63]
- chronic NOS (*see also* Disease, kidney, chronic) N18.9
  - due to hypertension — *see* Hypertensive, kidney
- complicating
  - ectopic or molar pregnancy O08.4
- congenital P96.0
- extrarenal R39.2
- following ectopic or molar pregnancy O08.4
- newborn P96.0
- prerenal R39.2

Ureter, ureteral — *see* condition

Ureteralgia N23

Ureterectasis — *see* Hydroureter

Ureteritis N28.89
- cystica N28.86
- due to calculus N20.1
  - with calculus, kidney N20.2
    - with hydronephrosis N13.2
- gonococcal (acute) (chronic) A54.21
- nonspecific N28.89

Ureterocele N28.89
- congenital (orthotopic) Q62.31
  - ectopic Q62.32

Ureterolith, ureterolithiasis — *see* Calculus, ureter

Ureterostomy
- attention to Z43.6
- status Z93.6

Urethra, urethral — *see* condition

Urethralgia R39.89

Urethritis (anterior) (posterior) N34.2
- calculous N21.1
- candidal B37.41
- chlamydial A56.01
- diplococcal (gonococcal) A54.01
  - with abscess (accessory gland) (periurethral) A54.1
- gonococcal A54.01
  - with abscess (accessory gland) (periurethral) A54.1
- nongonococcal N34.1
  - Reiter's — *see* Reiter's disease
- nonspecific N34.1
- nonvenereal N34.1
- postmenopausal N34.2
- puerperal O86.22
- Reiter's — *see* Reiter's disease
- specified NEC N34.2
- trichomonal or due to Trichomonas (vaginalis) A59.03

Urethrocele N81.0
- with
  - cystocele — *see* Cystocele
  - prolapse of uterus — *see* Prolapse, uterus

Urethrolithiasis (with colic or infection) N21.1

Urethrorectal — *see* condition

Urethrorrhagia N36.8

Urethrorrhea R36.9

Urethrostomy
- attention to Z43.6
- status Z93.6

Urethrotrigonitis — *see* Trigonitis

Urethrovaginal — *see* condition

Urgency
- fecal R15.2
- hypertensive — *see* Hypertension
- urinary R39.15

Urhidrosis, uridrosis L74.8

Uric acid in blood (increased) E79.0

Uricacidemia (asymptomatic) E79.0

Uricemia (asymptomatic) E79.0

Uricosuria R82.998

Urinary — *see* condition

Urination
- frequent R35.0
- painful R30.9

Urine
- blood in — *see* Hematuria
- discharge, excessive R35.8
- enuresis, nonorganic origin F98.0
- extravasation R39.0
- frequency R35.0
- incontinence R32
  - nonorganic origin F98.0
- intermittent stream R39.198
- pus in N39.0
- retention or stasis R33.9
  - organic R33.8
    - candidal R33.0
    - drug-induced R33.0
  - psychogenic F45.8
- secretion
  - deficient R34
  - excessive R35.8
  - frequency R35.0
- stream
  - intermittent R39.198
  - slowing R39.198
  - splitting R39.13
  - weak R39.12

Urinemia — *see* Uremia

Urinoma, urethra N36.8

Uroarthritis, infectious (Reiter's) — *see* Reiter's disease

Urodialysis R34

Urolithiasis — *see* Calculus, urinary

Uronephrosis — *see* Hydronephrosis

Uropathy N39.9
- obstructive N13.9
  - specified NEC N13.8
- reflux N13.9
  - specified NEC N13.8
- vesicoureteral reflux-associated — *see* Reflux, vesicoureteral

Urosepsis — *code to* condition

Urticaria L50.9
- with angioneurotic edema T78.3 ☑
  - hereditary D84.1
- allergic L50.0
- cholinergic L50.5
- chronic L50.8
- cold, familial L50.2
- contact L50.6

Urticaria — *continued*
- dermatographic L50.3
- due to
  - cold or heat L50.2
  - drugs L50.0
  - food L50.0
  - inhalants L50.0
  - plants L50.6
  - serum (*see also* Reaction, serum) T80.69 ☑
- factitial L50.3
- familial cold M04.2
- giant T78.3 ☑
  - hereditary D84.1
- gigantea T78.3 ☑
- idiopathic L50.1
- larynx T78.3 ☑
  - hereditary D84.1
- neonatorum P83.88
- nonallergic L50.1
- papulosa (Hebra) L28.2
- pigmentosa D47.01
  - congenital Q82.2
  - of neonatal onset Q82.2
  - of newborn onset Q82.2
- recurrent periodic L50.8
- serum (*see also* Reaction, serum) T80.69 ☑
- solar L56.3
- specified type NEC L50.8
- thermal (cold) (heat) L50.2
- vibratory L50.4
- xanthelasmoidea — *see* Urticaria pigmentosa

Use (of)
- alcohol Z72.89
  - with
    - intoxication F10.929
    - sleep disorder F10.982
  - harmful — *see* Abuse, alcohol
- amphetamines — *see* Use, stimulant NEC
- caffeine — *see* Use, stimulant NEC
- cannabis F12.90
  - with
    - anxiety disorder F12.980
    - intoxication F12.929
      - with
        - delirium F12.921
        - perceptual disturbance F12.922
      - uncomplicated F12.920
    - other specified disorder F12.988
    - psychosis F12.959
      - delusions F12.950
      - hallucinations F12.951
    - unspecified disorder F12.99
    - withdrawal F12.93
- cocaine F14.90
  - with
    - anxiety disorder F14.980
    - intoxication F14.929
      - with
        - delirium F14.921
        - perceptual disturbance F14.922
      - uncomplicated F14.920
    - other specified disorder F14.988
    - psychosis F14.959
      - delusions F14.950
      - hallucinations F14.951
    - sexual dysfunction F14.981
    - sleep disorder F14.982
    - unspecified disorder F14.99
  - harmful — *see* Abuse, drug, cocaine
- drug(s) NEC F19.90
  - with sleep disorder F19.982
  - harmful — *see* Abuse, drug, by type
- hallucinogen NEC F16.90
  - with
    - anxiety disorder F16.980
    - intoxication F16.929
      - with
        - delirium F16.921
      - uncomplicated F16.920
    - mood disorder F16.94
    - other specified disorder F16.988
    - perception disorder (flashbacks) F16.983
    - psychosis F16.959
      - delusions F16.950
      - hallucinations F16.951
    - unspecified disorder F16.99
  - harmful — *see* Abuse, drug, hallucinogen NEC
- inhalants F18.90

Jse — *continued*
  inhalants — *continued*
    with
      anxiety disorder F18.98Ø
      intoxication F18.929
        with delirium F18.921
        uncomplicated F18.92Ø
      mood disorder F18.94
      other specified disorder F18.988
      persisting dementia F18.97
      psychosis F18.959
        delusions F18.95Ø
        hallucinations F18.951
      unspecified disorder F18.99
    harmful — *see* Abuse, drug, inhalant
  methadone — *see* Use, opioid
  nonprescribed drugs F19.9Ø
    harmful — *see* Abuse, non-psychoactive substance
  opioid F11.9Ø
    with
      disorder F11.99
        mood F11.94
        sleep F11.982
        specified type NEC F11.988
      intoxication F11.929
        with
          delirium F11.921
          perceptual disturbance F11.922
        uncomplicated F11.92Ø
      withdrawal F11.93
    harmful — *see* Abuse, drug, opioid
  patent medicines F19.9Ø
    harmful — *see* Abuse, non-psychoactive substance
  psychoactive drug NEC F19.9Ø
    with
      anxiety disorder F19.98Ø
      intoxication F19.929
        with
          delirium F19.921
          perceptual disturbance F19.922
        uncomplicated F19.92Ø
      mood disorder F19.94
      other specified disorder F19.988
      persisting
        amnestic disorder F19.96
        dementia F19.97
      psychosis F19.959
        delusions F19.95Ø
        hallucinations F19.951
      sexual dysfunction F19.981
      sleep disorder F19.982
      unspecified disorder F19.99
      withdrawal F19.939
        with
          delirium F19.931
          perceptual disturbance F19.932
        uncomplicated F19.93Ø
    harmful — *see* Abuse, drug NEC, psychoactive NEC
  sedative, hypnotic, or anxiolytic F13.9Ø
    with
      anxiety disorder F13.98Ø
      intoxication F13.929
        with
          delirium F13.921
        uncomplicated F13.92Ø
      other specified disorder F13.988
      persisting
        amnestic disorder F13.96
        dementia F13.97
      psychosis F13.959
        delusions F13.95Ø
        hallucinations F13.951
      sexual dysfunction F13.981
      sleep disorder F13.982
      unspecified disorder F13.99
    harmful — *see* Abuse, drug, sedative, hypnotic, or
      anxiolytic
  stimulant NEC F15.9Ø
    with
      anxiety disorder F15.98Ø
      intoxication F15.929
        with
          delirium F15.921
          perceptual disturbance F15.922
        uncomplicated F15.92Ø
      mood disorder F15.94
      other specified disorder F15.988
      psychosis F15.959

Use — *continued*
  stimulant — *continued*
    with — *continued*
      psychosis — *continued*
        delusions F15.95Ø
        hallucinations F15.951
      sexual dysfunction F15.981
      sleep disorder F15.982
      unspecified disorder F15.99
      withdrawal F15.93
    harmful — *see* Abuse, drug, stimulant NEC
  tobacco Z72.Ø
    with dependence — *see* Dependence, drug, nicotine
  volatile solvents (*see also* Use, inhalant) F18.9Ø
    harmful — *see* Abuse, drug, inhalant
Usher-Senear disease or syndrome L1Ø.4
Uta B55.1
Uteromegaly N85.2
Uterovaginal — *see* condition
Uterovesical — *see* condition
Uveal — *see* condition
Uveitis (anterior) (*see also* Iridocyclitis)
  acute — *see* Iridocyclitis, acute
  chronic — *see* Iridocyclitis, chronic
  due to toxoplasmosis (acquired) B58.Ø9
    congenital P37.1
  granulomatous — *see* Iridocyclitis, chronic
  heterochromic — *see* Cyclitis, Fuchs' heterochromic
  lens-induced — *see* Iridocyclitis, lens-induced
  posterior — *see* Chorioretinitis
  sympathetic H44.13- ☑
  syphilitic (secondary) A51.43
    congenital (early) A5Ø.Ø1
    late A52.71
  tuberculous A18.54
Uveoencephalitis — *see* Inflammation, chorioretinal
Uveokeratitis — *see* Iridocyclitis
Uveoparotitis D86.89
Uvula — *see* condition
Uvulitis (acute) (catarrhal) (chronic) (membranous)
  (suppurative) (ulcerative) K12.2

V

Vaccination (prophylactic)
  complication or reaction — *see* Complications, vacci-
    nation
  delayed Z28.9
  encounter for Z23
  not done — *see* Immunization, not done, because (of)
Vaccinia (generalized) (localized) T88.1 ☑
  congenital P35.8
  without vaccination BØ8.Ø11
Vacuum, in sinus (accessory) (nasal) J34.89
Vagabond, vagabondage Z59.Ø
Vagabond's disease B85.1
Vagina, vaginal — *see* condition
Vaginalitis (tunica) (testis) N49.1
Vaginismus (reflex) N94.2
  functional F52.5
  nonorganic F52.5
  psychogenic F52.5
  secondary N94.2
Vaginitis (acute) (circumscribed) (diffuse) (emphysematous) (nonvenereal) (ulcerative) N76.Ø
  with ectopic or molar pregnancy OØ8.Ø
  amebic AØ6.82
  atrophic, postmenopausal N95.2
  bacterial N76.Ø
  blennorrhagic (gonococcal) A54.Ø2
  candidal B37.3
  chlamydial A56.Ø2
  chronic N76.1
  due to Trichomonas (vaginalis) A59.Ø1
  following ectopic or molar pregnancy OØ8.Ø
  gonococcal A54.Ø2
    with abscess (accessory gland) (periurethral) A54.1
  granuloma A58
  in (due to)
    candidiasis B37.3
    herpesviral (herpes simplex) infection A6Ø.Ø4
    pinworm infection B8Ø [N77.1]
  monilial B37.3
  mycotic (candidal) B37.3
  postmenopausal atrophic N95.2
  puerperal (postpartum) O86.13
  senile (atrophic) N95.2

Vaginitis — *continued*
  subacute or chronic N76.1
  syphilitic (early) A51.Ø
    late A52.76
  trichomonal A59.Ø1
  tuberculous A18.18
Vaginosis — *see* Vaginitis
Vagotonia G52.2
Vagrancy Z59.Ø
VAIN — *see* Neoplasia, intraepithelial, vagina
Vallecula — *see* condition
Valley fever B38.Ø
Valsuani's disease — *see* Anemia, obstetric
Valve, valvular (formation) (*see also* condition)
  cerebral ventricle (communicating) in situ Z98.2
  cervix, internal os Q51.828
  congenital NEC — *see* Atresia, by site
  ureter (pelvic junction) (vesical orifice) Q62.39
  urethra (congenital) (posterior) Q64.2
Valvulitis (chronic) — *see* Endocarditis
Valvulopathy — *see* Endocarditis
Van Bogaert's leukoencephalopathy (sclerosing)
  (subacute) A81.1
Van Bogaert-Scherer-Epstein disease or syndrome
  E75.5
Van Buchem's syndrome M85.2
Van Creveld-von Gierke disease E74.Ø1
Van der Hoeve (-de Kleyn) **syndrome** Q78.Ø
Van der Woude's syndrome Q38.Ø
Van Neck's disease or osteochondrosis M91.Ø
Vanishing lung J44.9
Vapor asphyxia or suffocation T59.9 ☑
  specified agent — *see* Table of Drugs and Chemicals
Variance, lethal ball, prosthetic heart valve T82.Ø9 ☑
Variants, thalassemic D56.8
Variations in hair color L67.1
Varicella BØ1.9
  with
    complications NEC BØ1.89
    encephalitis BØ1.11
    encephalomyelitis BØ1.11
    meningitis BØ1.Ø
    myelitis BØ1.12
    pneumonia BØ1.2
  congenital P35.8
Varices — *see* Varix
Varicocele (scrotum) (thrombosed) I86.1
  ovary I86.2
  perineum I86.3
  spermatic cord (ulcerated) I86.1
Varicose
  aneurysm (ruptured) I77.Ø
  dermatitis — *see* Varix, leg, with, inflammation
  eczema — *see* Varix, leg, with, inflammation
  phlebitis — *see* Varix, with, inflammation
  tumor — *see* Varix
  ulcer (lower limb, any part) (*see also* Varix, leg, with,
    ulcer)
    anus (*see also* Hemorrhoids) K64.8
    esophagus — *see* Varix, esophagus
    inflamed or infected — *see* Varix, leg, with ulcer,
      with inflammation
    nasal septum I86.8
    perineum I86.3
    scrotum I86.1
    specified site NEC I86.8
  vein — *see* Varix
  vessel — *see* Varix, leg
Varicosis, varicosities, varicosity — *see* Varix
Variola (major) (minor) BØ3
Varioloid BØ3
Varix (lower limb) (ruptured) I83.9Ø
  with
    edema I83.899
    inflammation I83.1Ø
      with ulcer (venous) I83.2Ø9
    pain I83.819
    specified complication NEC I83.899
    stasis dermatitis I83.1Ø
      with ulcer (venous) I83.2Ø9
    swelling I83.899
    ulcer I83.ØØ9
      with inflammation I83.2Ø9
  aneurysmal I77.Ø
  asymptomatic I83.9- ☑
  bladder I86.2
  broad ligament I86.2

Index

Varix — Vertigo

Varix — *continued*
  complicating
    childbirth (lower extremity) O87.4
      anus or rectum O87.2
      genital (vagina, vulva or perineum) O87.8
    pregnancy (lower extremity) O22.0- ☑
      anus or rectum O22.4- ☑
      genital (vagina, vulva or perineum) O22.1- ☑
    puerperium (lower extremity) O87.4
      anus or rectum O87.2
      genital (vagina, vulva, perineum) O87.8
  congenital (any site) Q27.8
  esophagus (idiopathic) (primary) (ulcerated) I85.00
    bleeding I85.01
    congenital Q27.8
    in (due to)
      alcoholic liver disease I85.10
        bleeding I85.11
      cirrhosis of liver I85.10
        bleeding I85.11
      portal hypertension I85.10
        bleeding I85.11
      schistosomiasis I85.10
        bleeding I85.11
      toxic liver disease I85.10
        bleeding I85.11
    secondary I85.10
      bleeding I85.11
  gastric I86.4
  inflamed or infected I83.10
    ulcerated I83.209
  labia (majora) I86.3
  leg (asymptomatic) I83.90
    with
      edema I83.899
      inflammation I83.10
        with ulcer — *see* Varix, leg, with, ulcer, with inflammation by site
      pain I83.819
      specified complication NEC I83.899
      swelling I83.899
      ulcer I83.009
        with inflammation I83.209
        ankle I83.003
          with inflammation I83.203
        calf I83.002
          with inflammation I83.202
        foot NEC I83.005
          with inflammation I83.205
        heel I83.004
          with inflammation I83.204
        lower leg NEC I83.008
          with inflammation I83.208
        midfoot I83.004
          with inflammation I83.204
        thigh I83.001
          with inflammation I83.201
    bilateral (asymptomatic) I83.93
      with
        edema I83.893
        pain I83.813
        specified complication NEC I83.893
        swelling I83.893
        ulcer I83.0- ☑
          with inflammation I83.209
    left (asymptomatic) I83.92
      with
        edema I83.892
        inflammation I83.12
          with ulcer — *see* Varix, leg, with, ulcer, with inflammation by site
        pain I83.812
        specified complication NEC I83.892
        swelling I83.892
        ulcer I83.029
          with inflammation I83.229
          ankle I83.023
            with inflammation I83.223
          calf I83.022
            with inflammation I83.222
          foot NEC I83.025
            with inflammation I83.225
          heel I83.024
            with inflammation I83.224
          lower leg NEC I83.028
            with inflammation I83.228
          midfoot I83.024
            with inflammation I83.224

Varix — *continued*
  leg — *continued*
    left — *continued*
      with — *continued*
        ulcer — *continued*
          thigh I83.021
            with inflammation I83.221
    right (asymptomatic) I83.91
      with
        edema I83.891
        inflammation I83.11
          with ulcer — *see* Varix, leg, with, ulcer, with inflammation by site
        pain I83.811
        specified complication NEC I83.891
        swelling I83.891
        ulcer I83.019
          with inflammation I83.219
          ankle I83.013
            with inflammation I83.213
          calf I83.012
            with inflammation I83.212
          foot NEC I83.015
            with inflammation I83.215
          heel I83.014
            with inflammation I83.214
          lower leg NEC I83.018
            with inflammation I83.218
          midfoot I83.014
            with inflammation I83.214
          thigh I83.011
            with inflammation I83.211
  nasal septum I86.8
  orbit I86.8
    congenital Q27.8
  ovary I86.2
  papillary I78.1
  pelvis I86.2
  perineum I86.3
  pharynx I86.8
  placenta O43.89- ☑
  renal papilla I86.8
  retina H35.09
  scrotum (ulcerated) I86.1
  sigmoid colon I86.8
  specified site NEC I86.8
  spinal (cord) (vessels) I86.8
  spleen, splenic (vein) (with phlebolith) I86.8
  stomach I86.4
  sublingual I86.0
  ulcerated I83.009
    inflamed or infected I83.209
  uterine ligament I86.2
  vagina I86.8
  vocal cord I86.8
  vulva I86.3
Vas deferens — *see* condition
Vas deferentitis N49.1
Vasa previa O69.4 ☑
  hemorrhage from, affecting newborn P50.0
Vascular (*see also* condition)
  loop on optic papilla Q14.2
  spasm I73.9
  spider I78.1
Vascularization, cornea — *see* Neovascularization, cornea
Vasculitis I77.6
  allergic D69.0
  cryoglobulinemic D89.1
  disseminated I77.6
  hypocomplementemic M31.8
  kidney I77.89
  livedoid L95.0
  nodular L95.8
  retina H35.06- ☑
  rheumatic — *see* Fever, rheumatic
  rheumatoid — *see* Rheumatoid, vasculitis
  skin (limited to) L95.9
    specified NEC L95.8
  systemic M31.8
Vasculopathy, necrotizing M31.9
  cardiac allograft T86.290
  specified NEC M31.8
Vasitis (nodosa) N49.1
  tuberculous A18.15
Vasodilation I73.9
Vasomotor — *see* condition
Vasoplasty, after previous sterilization Z31.0

Vasoplasty, after previous sterilization — *continued*
  aftercare Z31.42
Vasospasm (vasoconstriction) I73.9
  cerebral (cerebrovascular) (artery) I67.848
    reversible I67.841
  coronary I20.1
  nerve
    arm — *see* Mononeuropathy, upper limb
    brachial plexus G54.0
    cervical plexus G54.2
    leg — *see* Mononeuropathy, lower limb
  peripheral NOS I73.9
  retina (artery) — *see* Occlusion, artery, retina
Vasospastic — *see* condition
Vasovagal attack (paroxysmal) R55
  psychogenic F45.8
VATER syndrome Q87.2
Vater's ampulla — *see* condition
Vegetation, vegetative
  adenoid (nasal fossa) J35.8
  endocarditis (acute) (any valve) (subacute) I33.0
  heart (mycotic) (valve) I33.0
Veil
  Jackson's Q43.3
Vein, venous — *see* condition
Veldt sore — *see* Ulcer, skin
Velpeau's hernia — *see* Hernia, femoral
Venereal
  bubo A55
  disease A64
  granuloma inguinale A58
  lymphogranuloma (Durand-Nicolas-Favre) A55
Venofibrosis I87.8
Venom, venomous — *see* Table of Drugs and Chemicals, by animal or substance, poisoning
Venous — *see* condition
Ventilator lung, newborn P27.8
Ventral — *see* condition
Ventricle, ventricular (*see also* condition)
  escape I49.3
  inversion Q20.5
Ventriculitis (cerebral) (*see also* Encephalitis) G04.90
Ventriculostomy status Z98.2
Vernet's syndrome G52.7
Verneuil's disease (syphilitic bursitis) A52.78
Verruca (due to HPV) (filiformis) (simplex) (viral) (vulgaris) B07.9
  acuminata A63.0
  necrogenica (primary) (tuberculosa) A18.4
  plana B07.8
  plantaris B07.0
  seborrheica L82.1
    inflamed L82.0
  senile (seborrheic) L82.1
    inflamed L82.0
  tuberculosa (primary) A18.4
  venereal A63.0
Verrucosities — *see* Verruca
Verruga peruana, peruviana A44.1
Version
  with extraction
  cervix — *see* Malposition, uterus
  uterus (postinfectional) (postpartal, old) — *see* Malposition, uterus
Vertebra, vertebral — *see* condition
Vertical talus (congenital) Q66.80
  left foot Q66.82
  right foot Q66.81
Vertigo R42
  auditory — *see* Vertigo, aural
  aural H81.31- ☑
  benign paroxysmal (positional) H81.1- ☑
  central (origin) H81.4- ☑
  cerebral H81.4- ☑
  Dix and Hallpike (epidemic) — *see* Neuronitis, vestibular
  due to infrasound T75.23 ☑
  epidemic A88.1
    Dix and Hallpike — *see* Neuronitis, vestibular
    Pedersen's — *see* Neuronitis, vestibular
    vestibular neuronitis — *see* Neuronitis, vestibular
  hysterical F44.89
  infrasound T75.23 ☑
  labyrinthine — *see* subcategory H81.0 ☑
  laryngeal R05
  malignant positional H81.4- ☑

☑ **Additional Character Required** — Refer to the Tabular List for Character Selection   ▽ Subterms under main terms may continue to next column or page

Vertigo — *continued*
  Ménière's — *see* subcategory H81.0 ☑
  menopausal N95.1
  otogenic — *see* Vertigo, aural
  paroxysmal positional, benign — *see* Vertigo, benign paroxysmal
  Pedersen's (epidemic) — *see* Neuronitis, vestibular
  peripheral NEC H81.39- ☑
  positional
    benign paroxysmal — *see* Vertigo, benign paroxysmal
    malignant H81.4- ☑
Very-low-density-lipoprotein-type (VLDL) **hyperlipoproteinemia** E78.1
Vesania — *see* Psychosis
Vesical — *see* condition
Vesicle
  cutaneous R23.8
  seminal — *see* condition
  skin R23.8
Vesicocolic — *see* condition
Vesicoperineal — *see* condition
Vesicorectal — *see* condition
Vesicourethrorectal — *see* condition
Vesicovaginal — *see* condition
Vesicular — *see* condition
Vesiculitis (seminal) N49.0
  amebic A06.82
  gonorrheal (acute) (chronic) A54.23
  trichomonal A59.09
  tuberculous A18.15
Vestibulitis (ear) (*see also* subcategory) H83.0 ☑
  nose (external) J34.89
  vulvar N94.810
Vestibulopathy , acute peripheral (recurrent) — *see* Neuronitis, vestibular
Vestige, vestigial (*see also* Persistence)
  branchial Q18.0
  structures in vitreous Q14.0
Vibration
  adverse effects T75.20 ☑
    pneumatic hammer syndrome T75.21 ☑
    specified effect NEC T75.29 ☑
    vasospastic syndrome T75.22 ☑
    vertigo from infrasound T75.23 ☑
  exposure (occupational) Z57.7
  vertigo T75.23 ☑
Vibriosis A28.9
Victim (of)
  crime Z65.4
  disaster Z65.5
  terrorism Z65.4
  torture Z65.4
  war Z65.5
Vidal's disease L28.0
Villaret's syndrome G52.7
Villous — *see* condition
VIN — *see* Neoplasia, intraepithelial, vulva
Vincent's infection (angina) (gingivitis) A69.1
  stomatitis NEC A69.1
Vinson-Plummer syndrome D50.1
Violence, physical R45.6
Viosterol deficiency — *see* Deficiency, calciferol
Vipoma — *see* Neoplasm, malignant, by site
Viremia B34.9
Virilism (adrenal) E25.9
  congenital E25.0
Virilization (female) (suprarenal) E25.9
  congenital E25.0
  isosexual E28.2
Virulent bubo A57
Virus, viral (*see also* condition)
  as cause of disease classified elsewhere B97.89
  cytomegalovirus B25.9
  human immunodeficiency (HIV) — *see* Human, immunodeficiency virus (HIV) disease
  infection — *see* Infection, virus
  specified NEC B34.8
  swine influenza (viruses that normally cause infections in pigs) (*see also* Influenza, due to, identified novel influenza A virus) J09.X2
  West Nile (fever) A92.30
    with
      complications NEC A92.39
      cranial nerve disorders A92.32
      encephalitis A92.31
      encephalomyelitis A92.31

Virus, viral — *continued*
  West Nile — *continued*
    with — *continued*
      neurologic manifestation NEC A92.32
      optic neuritis A92.32
      polyradiculitis A92.32
Viscera, visceral — *see* condition
Visceroptosis K63.4
Visible peristalsis R19.2
Vision, visual
  binocular, suppression H53.34
  blurred, blurring H53.8
    hysterical F44.6
  defect, defective NEC H54.7
  disorientation (syndrome) H53.8
  disturbance H53.9
    hysterical F44.6
  double H53.2
  examination Z01.00
    with abnormal findings Z01.01
  field, limitation (defect) — *see* Defect, visual field
  hallucinations R44.1
  halos H53.19
  loss — *see* Loss, vision
    sudden — *see* Disturbance, vision, subjective, loss, sudden
  low (both eyes) — *see* Low, vision
  perception, simultaneous without fusion H53.33
Vitality, lack or want of R53.83
  newborn P96.89
Vitamin deficiency — *see* Deficiency, vitamin
Vitelline duct, persistent Q43.0
Vitiligo L80
  eyelid H02.739
    left H02.736
      lower H02.735
      upper H02.734
    right H02.733
      lower H02.732
      upper H02.731
  pinta A67.2
  vulva N90.89
Vitreal corneal syndrome H59.01- ☑
Vitreoretinopathy, proliferative (*see also* Retinopathy, proliferative)
  with retinal detachment — *see* Detachment, retina, traction
Vitreous (*see also* condition)
  touch syndrome — *see* Complication, postprocedural, following cataract surgery
Vocal cord — *see* condition
Vogt-Koyanagi syndrome H20.82- ☑
Vogt's disease or syndrome G80.3
Vogt-Spielmeyer amaurotic idiocy or disease E75.4
Voice
  change R49.9
    specified NEC R49.8
  loss — *see* Aphonia
Volhynian fever A79.0
Volkmann's ischemic contracture or paralysis (complicating trauma) T79.6 ☑
Volvulus (bowel) (colon) (intestine) K56.2
  with perforation K56.2
  congenital Q43.8
  duodenum K31.5
  fallopian tube — *see* Torsion, fallopian tube
  oviduct — *see* Torsion, fallopian tube
  stomach (due to absence of gastrocolic ligament) K31.89
Vomiting R11.10
  with nausea R11.2
  asphyxia — *see* Foreign body, by site, causing asphyxia, gastric contents
  bilious (cause unknown) R11.14
    following gastro-intestinal surgery K91.0
    in newborn P92.01
  blood — *see* Hematemesis
  causing asphyxia, choking, or suffocation — *see* Foreign body, by site
  cyclical G43.A0 (*following* G43.7)
    with refractory migraine G43.A1 (*following* G43.7)
    intractable G43.A1 (*following* G43.7)
    not intractable G43.A0 (*following* G43.7)
    psychogenic F50.89
    without refractory migraine G43.A0 (*following* G43.7)
  fecal mater R11.13
  following gastrointestinal surgery K91.0
    psychogenic F50.89

Vomiting — *continued*
  functional K31.89
  hysterical F50.89
  nervous F50.89
  neurotic F50.89
  newborn NEC P92.09
    bilious P92.01
  periodic R11.10
    psychogenic F50.89
  projectile R11.12
  psychogenic F50.89
  uremic — *see* Uremia
  without nausea R11.11
Vomito negro — *see* Fever, yellow
Von Bezold's abscess — *see* Mastoiditis, acute
Von Economo-Cruchet disease A85.8
Von Eulenburg's disease G71.19
Von Gierke's disease E74.01
Von Hippel (-Lindau) **disease or syndrome** Q85.8
Von Jaksch's anemia or disease D64.89
Von Recklinghausen
  disease (neurofibromatosis) Q85.01
    bones E21.0
Von Schroetter's syndrome I82.890
Von Willebrand (-Jurgens)(-Minot) **disease or syndrome** D68.0
Von Zumbusch's disease L40.1
Voyeurism F65.3
Vrolik's disease Q78.0
Vulva — *see* condition
Vulvismus N94.2
Vulvitis (acute) (allergic) (atrophic) (hypertrophic) (intertriginous) (senile) N76.2
  with ectopic or molar pregnancy O08.0
  adhesive, congenital Q52.79
  blennorrhagic (gonococcal) A54.02
  candidal B37.3
  chlamydial A56.02
  due to Haemophilus ducreyi A57
  following ectopic or molar pregnancy O08.0
  gonococcal A54.02
    with abscess (accessory gland) (periurethral) A54.1
  herpesviral A60.04
  leukoplakic N90.4
  monilial B37.3
  puerperal (postpartum) O86.19
  subacute or chronic N76.3
  syphilitic (early) A51.0
    late A52.76
  trichomonal A59.01
  tuberculous A18.18
Vulvodynia N94.819
  specified NEC N94.818
Vulvorectal — *see* condition
Vulvovaginitis (acute) — *see* Vaginitis

W

Waiting list, person on Z75.1
  for organ transplant Z76.82
  undergoing social agency investigation Z75.2
Waldenström
  hypergammaglobulinemia D89.0
  syndrome or macroglobulinemia C88.0
Waldenström-Kjellberg syndrome D50.1
Walking
  difficulty R26.2
    psychogenic F44.4
  sleep F51.3
    hysterical F44.89
Wall, abdominal — *see* condition
Wallenberg's disease or syndrome G46.3
Wallgren's disease I87.8
Wandering
  gallbladder, congenital Q44.1
  in diseases classified elsewhere Z91.83
  kidney, congenital Q63.8
  organ or site, congenital NEC — *see* Malposition, congenital, by site
  pacemaker (heart) I49.8
  spleen D73.89
War neurosis F48.8
Wart (due to HPV) (filiform) (infectious) (viral) B07.9
  anogenital region (venereal) A63.0
  common B07.8
  external genital organs (venereal) A63.0
  flat B07.8
  Hassal-Henle's (of cornea) H18.49

↵ Subterms under main terms may continue to next column or page   ☑ Additional Character Required — Refer to the Tabular List for Character Selection   325

Vertigo — Wart

Wart — *continued*
Peruvian A44.1
plantar B07.0
prosector (tuberculous) A18.4
seborrheic L82.1
inflamed L82.0
senile (seborrheic) L82.1
inflamed L82.0
tuberculous A18.4
venereal A63.0
Warthin's tumor — *see* Neoplasm, salivary gland, benign
Wassilieff's disease A27.0
Wasting
disease R64
due to malnutrition E41
extreme (due to malnutrition) E41
muscle NEC — *see* Atrophy, muscle
Water
clefts (senile cataract) — *see* Cataract, senile, incipient
deprivation of T73.1 ☑
intoxication E87.79
itch B76.9
lack of T73.1 ☑
loading E87.70
on
brain — *see* Hydrocephalus
chest J94.8
poisoning E87.79
Waterbrash R12
Waterhouse (-Friderichsen) **syndrome or disease** (meningococcal) A39.1
Water-losing nephritis N25.89
Watermelon stomach K31.819
with hemorrhage K31.811
without hemorrhage K31.819
Watsoniasis B66.8
Wax in ear — *see* Impaction, cerumen
Weak, weakening, weakness (generalized) R53.1
arches (acquired) (*see also* Deformity, limb, flat foot) R32
bladder (sphincter) R32
facial R29.810
following
cerebrovascular disease I69.992
cerebral infarction I69.392
intracerebral hemorrhage I69.192
nontraumatic intracranial hemorrhage NEC I69.292
specified disease NEC I69.892
stroke I69.392
subarachnoid hemorrhage I69.092
foot (double) — *see* Weak, arches
heart, cardiac — *see* Failure, heart
mind F70
muscle M62.81
myocardium — *see* Failure, heart
newborn P96.89
pelvic fundus N81.89
pubocervical tissue N81.82
rectovaginal tissue N81.83
senile R54
urinary stream R39.12
valvular — *see* Endocarditis
Wear, worn (with normal or routine use)
articular bearing surface of internal joint prosthesis — *see* Complications, joint prosthesis, mechanical, wear of articular bearing surfaces, by site
device, implant or graft — *see* Complications, by site, mechanical complication
tooth, teeth (approximal) (hard tissues) (interproximal) (occlusal) K03.0
Weather, weathered
effects of
cold T69.9 ☑
specified effect NEC T69.8 ☑
hot — *see* Heat
skin L57.8
Weaver's syndrome Q87.3
Web, webbed (congenital)
duodenal Q43.8
esophagus Q39.4
fingers Q70.1- ☑
larynx (glottic) (subglottic) Q31.0
neck (pterygium colli) Q18.3
Paterson-Kelly D50.1
popliteal syndrome Q87.89
toes Q70.3- ☑
Weber-Christian disease M35.6

Weber-Cockayne syndrome (epidermolysis bullosa) Q81.8
Weber-Gubler syndrome G46.3
Weber-Leyden syndrome G46.3
Weber-Osler syndrome I78.0
Weber's paralysis or syndrome G46.3
Wedge-shaped or wedging vertebra — *see* Collapse, vertebra NEC
Wegener's granulomatosis or syndrome M31.30
with
kidney involvement M31.31
lung involvement M31.30
with kidney involvement M31.31
Wegner's disease A50.02
Weight
1000-2499 grams at birth (low) — *see* Low, birthweight
999 grams or less at birth (extremely low) — *see* Low, birthweight, extreme
and length below 10th percentile for gestational age P05.1- ☑
below but length above 10th percentile for gestational age P05.0- ☑
gain (abnormal) (excessive) R63.5
in pregnancy — *see* Pregnancy, complicated by, excessive weight gain
low — *see* Pregnancy, complicated by, insufficient, weight gain
loss (abnormal) (cause unknown) R63.4
Weightlessness (effect of) T75.82 ☑
Weil (l)**-Marchesani syndrome** Q87.1
Weil's disease A27.0
Weingarten's syndrome J82
Weir Mitchell's disease I73.81
Weiss-Baker syndrome G90.09
Wells' disease L98.3
Wen — *see* Cyst, sebaceous
Wenckebach's block or phenomenon I44.1
Werdnig-Hoffmann syndrome (muscular atrophy) G12.0
Werlhof's disease D69.3
Wermer's disease or syndrome E31.21
Werner-His disease A79.0
Werner's disease or syndrome E34.8
Wernicke-Korsakoff's syndrome or psychosis (alcoholic) F10.96
with dependence F10.26
drug-induced
due to drug abuse — *see* Abuse, drug, by type, with amnestic disorder
due to drug dependence — *see* Dependence, drug, by type, with amnestic disorder
nonalcoholic F04
Wernicke-Posadas disease B38.9
Wernicke's
developmental aphasia F80.2
disease or syndrome E51.2
encephalopathy E51.2
polioencephalitis, superior E51.2
West African fever B50.8
Westphal-Strümpell syndrome E83.01
West's syndrome — *see* Epilepsy, spasms
Wet
feet, tropical (maceration) (syndrome) — *see* Immersion, foot
lung (syndrome), newborn P22.1
Wharton's duct — *see* condition
Wheal — *see* Urticaria
Wheezing R06.2
Whiplash injury S13.4 ☑
Whipple's disease (*see also* subcategory M14.8-) K90.81
Whipworm (disease) (infection) (infestation) B79
Whistling face Q87.0
White (*see also* condition)
kidney, small N03.9
leg, puerperal, postpartum, childbirth O87.1
mouth B37.0
patches of mouth K13.29
spot lesions, teeth
chewing surface K02.51
pit and fissure surface K02.51
smooth surface K02.61
Whitehead L70.0
Whitlow (*see also* Cellulitis, digit)
with lymphangitis — *see* Lymphangitis, acute, digit
herpesviral B00.89
Whitmore's disease or fever — *see* Melioidosis
Whooping cough A37.90

Whooping cough — *continued*
with pneumonia A37.91
due to Bordetella
bronchiseptica A37.81
parapertussis A37.11
pertussis A37.01
specified organism NEC A37.81
due to
Bordetella
bronchiseptica A37.80
with pneumonia A37.81
parapertussis A37.10
with pneumonia A37.11
pertussis A37.00
with pneumonia A37.01
specified NEC A37.80
with pneumonia A37.81
Wichman's asthma J38.5
Wide cranial sutures, newborn P96.3
Widening aorta — *see* Ectasia, aorta
with aneurysm — *see* Aneurysm, aorta
Wilkie's disease or syndrome K55.1
Wilkinson-Sneddon disease or syndrome L13.1
Willebrand (-Jürgens) **thrombopathy** D68.0
Williams syndrome Q93.82
Willige-Hunt disease or syndrome G23.1
Wilms' tumor C64- ☑
Wilson-Mikity syndrome P27.0
Wilson's
disease or syndrome E83.01
hepatolenticular degeneration E83.01
lichen ruber L43.9
Window (*see also* Imperfect, closure)
aorticopulmonary Q21.4
Winter — *see* condition
Wiskott-Aldrich syndrome D82.0
Withdrawal state (*see also* Dependence, drug by type with withdrawal)
alcohol
with perceptual disturbances F10.232
without perceptual disturbances F10.239
caffeine F15.93
cannabis F12.23
newborn
correct therapeutic substance properly administere⬛ P96.2
infant of dependent mother P96.1
therapeutic substance, neonatal P96.2
Witts' anemia D50.8
Witzelsucht F07.0
Woakes' ethmoiditis or syndrome J33.1
Wolff-Hirschorn syndrome Q93.3
Wolff-Parkinson-White syndrome I45.6
Wolhynian fever A79.0
Wolman's disease E75.5
Wood lung or pneumonitis J67.8
Woolly, wooly hair (congenital) (nevus) Q84.1
Woolsorter's disease A22.1
Word
blindness (congenital) (developmental) F81.0
deafness (congenital) (developmental) H93.25
Worm(s) (infection) (infestation) (*see also* Infestation, helminth)
guinea B72
in intestine NEC B82.0
Worm-eaten soles A66.3
Worn out — *see* Exhaustion
cardiac
defibrillator (with synchronous cardiace pacemake⬛ Z45.02
pacemaker
battery Z45.010
lead Z45.018
device, implant or graft — *see* Complications, by si⬛ mechanical
Worried well Z71.1
Worries R45.82
Wound check Z48.0- ☑
due to injury — *code to* Injury, by site, using approp⬛ ate seventh character for subsequent encount⬛
Wound, open T14.8- ☑
abdomen, abdominal
wall S31.109 ☑
with penetration into peritoneal cavity S31.609 ☑
bite — *see* Bite, abdomen, wall
epigastric region S31.102 ☑

☑ **Additional Character Required — Refer to the Tabular List for Character Selection**   ⬛ **Subterms under main terms may continue to next column or pag⬛**

Wound, open — *continued*
  abdomen, abdominal — *continued*
    wall — *continued*
      epigastric region — *continued*
        with penetration into peritoneal cavity S31.602 ☑
        bite — *see* Bite, abdomen, wall, epigastric region
        laceration — *see* Laceration, abdomen, wall, epigastric region
        puncture — *see* Puncture, abdomen, wall, epigastric region
      laceration — *see* Laceration, abdomen, wall
      left
        lower quadrant S31.104 ☑
          with penetration into peritoneal cavity S31.604 ☑
          bite — *see* Bite, abdomen, wall, left, lower quadrant
          laceration — *see* Laceration, abdomen, wall, left, lower quadrant
          puncture — *see* Puncture, abdomen, wall, left, lower quadrant
        upper quadrant S31.101 ☑
          with penetration into peritoneal cavity S31.601 ☑
          bite — *see* Bite, abdomen, wall, left, upper quadrant
          laceration — *see* Laceration, abdomen, wall, left, upper quadrant
          puncture — *see* Puncture, abdomen, wall, left, upper quadrant
      periumbilic region S31.105 ☑
        with penetration into peritoneal cavity S31.605 ☑
        bite — *see* Bite, abdomen, wall, periumbilic region
        laceration — *see* Laceration, abdomen, wall, periumbilic region
        puncture — *see* Puncture, abdomen, wall, periumbilic region
      puncture — *see* Puncture, abdomen, wall
      right
        lower quadrant S31.103 ☑
          with penetration into peritoneal cavity S31.603 ☑
          bite — *see* Bite, abdomen, wall, right, lower quadrant
          laceration — *see* Laceration, abdomen, wall, right, lower quadrant
          puncture — *see* Puncture, abdomen, wall, right, lower quadrant
        upper quadrant S31.100 ☑
          with penetration into peritoneal cavity S31.600 ☑
          bite — *see* Bite, abdomen, wall, right, upper quadrant
          laceration — *see* Laceration, abdomen, wall, right, upper quadrant
          puncture — *see* Puncture, abdomen, wall, right, upper quadrant
  alveolar (process) — *see* Wound, open, oral cavity
  ankle S91.00- ☑
    bite — *see* Bite, ankle
    laceration — *see* Laceration, ankle
    puncture — *see* Puncture, ankle
  antecubital space — *see* Wound, open, elbow
  anterior chamber, eye — *see* Wound, open, ocular
  anus S31.839 ☑
    bite S31.835 ☑
    laceration — *see* Laceration, anus
    puncture — *see* Puncture, anus
  arm (upper) S41.10- ☑
    with amputation — *see* Amputation, traumatic, arm
    bite — *see* Bite, arm
    forearm — *see* Wound, open, forearm
    laceration — *see* Laceration, arm
    puncture — *see* Puncture, arm
  auditory canal (external) (meatus) — *see* Wound, open, ear
  auricle, ear — *see* Wound, open, ear
  axilla — *see* Wound, open, arm
  back (*see also* Wound, open, thorax, back)
    lower S31.000 ☑
      with penetration into retroperitoneal space S31.001 ☑
      bite — *see* Bite, back, lower

Wound, open — *continued*
  back (*see also* Wound, open, thorax, back) — *continued*
    lower — *continued*
      laceration — *see* Laceration, back, lower
      puncture — *see* Puncture, back, lower
  bite — *see* Bite
  blood vessel — *see* Injury, blood vessel
  breast S21.00- ☑
    with amputation — *see* Amputation, traumatic, breast
    bite — *see* Bite, breast
    laceration — *see* Laceration, breast
    puncture — *see* Puncture, breast
  buttock S31.809 ☑
    bite — *see* Bite, buttock
    laceration — *see* Laceration, buttock
    left S31.829 ☑
    puncture — *see* Puncture, buttock
    right S31.819 ☑
  calf — *see* Wound, open, leg
  canaliculus lacrimalis — *see* Wound, open, eyelid
  canthus, eye — *see* Wound, open, eyelid
  cervical esophagus S11.20 ☑
    bite S11.25 ☑
    laceration — *see* Laceration, esophagus, traumatic, cervical
    puncture — *see* Puncture, cervical esophagus
  cheek (external) S01.40- ☑
    bite — *see* Bite, cheek
    internal — *see* Wound, open, oral cavity
    laceration — *see* Laceration, cheek
    puncture — *see* Puncture, cheek
  chest wall — *see* Wound, open, thorax
  chin — *see* Wound, open, head, specified site NEC
  choroid — *see* Wound, open, ocular
  ciliary body (eye) — *see* Wound, open, ocular
  clitoris S31.40 ☑
    with amputation — *see* Amputation, traumatic, clitoris
    bite S31.45 ☑
    laceration — *see* Laceration, vulva
    puncture — *see* Puncture, vulva
  conjunctiva — *see* Wound, open, ocular
  cornea — *see* Wound, open, ocular
  costal region — *see* Wound, open, thorax
  Descemet's membrane — *see* Wound, open, ocular
  digit(s)
    foot — *see* Wound, open, toe
    hand — *see* Wound, open, finger
  ear (canal) (external) S01.30- ☑
    with amputation — *see* Amputation, traumatic, ear
    bite — *see* Bite, ear
    drum S09.2- ☑
    laceration — *see* Laceration, ear
    puncture — *see* Puncture, ear
  elbow S51.00- ☑
    bite — *see* Bite, elbow
    laceration — *see* Laceration, elbow
    puncture — *see* Puncture, elbow
  epididymis — *see* Wound, open, testis
  epigastric region S31.102 ☑
    with penetration into peritoneal cavity S31.602 ☑
    bite — *see* Bite, abdomen, wall, epigastric region
    laceration — *see* Laceration, abdomen, wall, epigastric region
    puncture — *see* Puncture, abdomen, wall, epigastric region
  epiglottis — *see* Wound, open, neck, specified site NEC
  esophagus (thoracic) S27.819 ☑
    cervical — *see* Wound, open, cervical esophagus
    laceration S27.813 ☑
    specified type NEC S27.818 ☑
  eye — *see* Wound, open, ocular
  eyeball — *see* Wound, open, ocular
  eyebrow — *see* Wound, open, eyelid
  eyelid S01.10- ☑
    bite — *see* Bite, eyelid
    laceration — *see* Laceration, eyelid
    puncture — *see* Puncture, eyelid
  face NEC — *see* Wound, open, head, specified site NEC
  finger(s) S61.209 ☑
    with
      amputation — *see* Amputation, traumatic, finger
      damage to nail S61.309 ☑
    bite — *see* Bite, finger

Wound, open — *continued*
  finger(s) — *continued*
    index S61.208 ☑
      with
        damage to nail S61.308 ☑
      left S61.201 ☑
        with
          damage to nail S61.301 ☑
      right S61.200 ☑
        with
          damage to nail S61.300 ☑
    laceration — *see* Laceration, finger
    little S61.208 ☑
      with
        damage to nail S61.308 ☑
      left S61.207 ☑
        with damage to nail S61.307 ☑
      right S61.206 ☑
        with damage to nail S61.306 ☑
    middle S61.208 ☑
      with
        damage to nail S61.308 ☑
      left S61.203 ☑
        with damage to nail S61.303 ☑
      right S61.202 ☑
        with damage to nail S61.302 ☑
    puncture — *see* Puncture, finger
    ring S61.208 ☑
      with
        damage to nail S61.308 ☑
      left S61.205 ☑
        with damage to nail S61.305 ☑
      right S61.204 ☑
        with damage to nail S61.304 ☑
  flank — *see* Wound, open, abdomen, wall
  foot (except toe(s) alone) S91.30- ☑
    with amputation — *see* Amputation, traumatic, foot
    bite — *see* Bite, foot
    laceration — *see* Laceration, foot
    puncture — *see* Puncture, foot
    toe — *see* Wound, open, toe
  forearm S51.80- ☑
    with
      amputation — *see* Amputation, traumatic, forearm
    bite — *see* Bite, forearm
    elbow only — *see* Wound, open, elbow
    laceration — *see* Laceration, forearm
    puncture — *see* Puncture, forearm
  forehead — *see* Wound, open, head, specified site NEC
  genital organs, external
    with amputation — *see* Amputation, traumatic, genital organs
    bite — *see* Bite, genital organ
    female S31.502 ☑
      vagina S31.40 ☑
      vulva S31.40 ☑
    laceration — *see* Laceration, genital organ
    male S31.501 ☑
      penis S31.20 ☑
      scrotum S31.30 ☑
      testes S31.30 ☑
    puncture — *see* Puncture, genital organ
  globe (eye) — *see* Wound, open, ocular
  groin — *see* Wound, open, abdomen, wall
  gum — *see* Wound, open, oral cavity
  hand S61.40- ☑
    with
      amputation — *see* Amputation, traumatic, hand
    bite — *see* Bite, hand
    finger(s) — *see* Wound, open, finger
    laceration — *see* Laceration, hand
    puncture — *see* Puncture, hand
    thumb — *see* Wound, open, thumb
  head S01.90 ☑
    bite — *see* Bite, head
    cheek — *see* Wound, open, cheek
    ear — *see* Wound, open, ear
    eyelid — *see* Wound, open, eyelid
    laceration — *see* Laceration, head
    lip — *see* Wound, open, lip
    nose S01.20 ☑
    oral cavity — *see* Wound, open, oral cavity
    puncture — *see* Puncture, head
    scalp — *see* Wound, open, scalp
    specified site NEC S01.80 ☑

☑ Additional Character Required — Refer to the Tabular List for Character Selection

▽ Subterms under main terms may continue to next column or page

Note: The list below gives the code number for neoplasms by anatomical site. For each site there are six possible code numbers according to whether the neoplasm in question is malignant, benign, in situ, of uncertain behavior, or of unspecified nature. The description of the neoplasm will often indicate which of the six columns is appropriate; e.g., malignant melanoma of skin, benign fibroadenoma of breast, carcinoma in situ of cervix uteri. Where such descriptors are not present, the remainder of the Index should be consulted where guidance is given to the appropriate column for each morphological (histological) variety listed; e.g., Mesonephroma – see Neoplasm, malignant; Embryoma (see also Neoplasm, uncertain behavior); Disease, Bowen's – see Neoplasm, skin, in situ. However, the guidance in the Index can be overridden if one of the descriptors mentioned above is present; e.g., malignant adenoma of colon is coded to C18.9 and not to D12.6 as the adjective "malignant" overrides the Index entry "Adenoma (see also Neoplasm, benign, by site)." Codes listed with a dash -, following the code have a required additional character for laterality. The tabular list must be reviewed for the complete code.

	Malignant Primary	Malignant Secondary	Ca in situ	Benign	Uncertain	Unspecified Behavior
Neoplasm, neoplastic	C80.1	C79.9	D09.9	D36.9	D48.9	D49.9
abdomen,						
abdominal	C76.2	C79.8-✓	D09.8	D36.7	D48.7	D49.89
cavity	C76.2	C79.8-✓	D09.8	D36.7	D48.7	D49.89
organ	C76.2	C79.8-✓	D09.8	D36.7	D48.7	D49.89
viscera	C76.2	C79.8-✓	D09.8	D36.7	D48.7	D49.89
wall — *see also* Neoplasm, abdomen, wall, skin	C44.509	C79.2	D04.5	D23.5	D48.5	D49.2
connective tissue	C49.4	C79.8-✓	—	D21.4	D48.1	D49.2
skin	C44.509					
basal cell carcinoma	C44.519					
specified type NEC	C44.599		—	—	—	—
squamous cell carcinoma	C44.529					
abdominopelvic	C76.8	C79.8-✓		D36.7	D48.7	D49.89
accessory sinus — *see* Neoplasm, sinus						
acoustic nerve	C72.4-✓	C79.49	—	D33.3	D43.3	D49.7
adenoid (pharynx) (tissue)	C11.1	C79.89	D00.08	D10.6	D37.05	D49.0
adipose tissue — *see also* Neoplasm, connective tissue	C49.4	C79.89	—	D21.9	D48.1	D49.2
adnexa (uterine)	C57.4	C79.89	D07.39	D28.7	D39.8	D49.59
adrenal	C74.9-✓	C79.7-✓	D09.3	D35.0-✓	D44.1-✓	D49.7
capsule	C74.9-✓	C79.7-✓	D09.3	D35.0-✓	D44.1-✓	D49.7
cortex	C74.0-✓	C79.7-✓	D09.3	D35.0-✓	D44.1-✓	D49.7
gland	C74.9-✓	C79.7-✓	D09.3	D35.0-✓	D44.1-✓	D49.7
medulla	C74.1-✓	C79.7-✓	D09.3	D35.0-✓	D44.1-✓	D49.7
ala nasi (external) — *see also* Neoplasm, skin, nose	C44.301	C79.2	D04.39	D23.39	D48.5	D49.2
alimentary canal or tract NEC	C26.9	C78.80	D01.9	D13.9	D37.9	D49.0
alveolar	C03.9	C79.89	D00.03	D10.39	D37.09	D49.0
mucosa	C03.9	C79.89	D00.03	D10.39	D37.09	D49.0
lower	C03.1	C79.89	D00.03	D10.39	D37.09	D49.0
upper	C03.0	C79.89	D00.03	D10.39	D37.09	D49.0
ridge or process	C41.1	C79.51	—	D16.5	D48.0	D49.2
carcinoma	C03.9	C79.8-✓	—	—	—	—
lower	C03.1	C79.8-✓	—	—	—	—
upper	C03.0	C79.8-✓	—	—	—	—
lower	C41.1	C79.51	—	D16.5	D48.0	D49.2
mucosa	C03.9	C79.89	D00.03	D10.39	D37.09	D49.0
lower	C03.1	C79.89	D00.03	D10.39	D37.09	D49.0
upper	C03.0	C79.89	D00.03	D10.39	D37.09	D49.0
upper	C41.0	C79.51	—	D16.4	D48.0	D49.2
sulcus	C06.1	C79.89	D00.02	D10.39	D37.09	D49.0
alveolus	C03.9	C79.89	D00.03	D10.39	D37.09	D49.0
lower	C03.1	C79.89	D00.03	D10.39	D37.09	D49.0
upper	C03.0	C79.89	D00.03	D10.39	D37.09	D49.0
ampulla of Vater	C24.1	C78.89	D01.5	D13.5	D37.6	D49.0
ankle NEC	C76.5-✓	C79.89	D04.7-✓	D36.7	D48.7	D49.89
anorectum, anorectal (junction)	C21.8	C78.5	D01.3	D12.9	D37.8	D49.0
antecubital fossa or space	C76.4-✓	C79.89	D04.6-✓	D36.7	D48.7	D49.89

	Malignant Primary	Malignant Secondary	Ca in situ	Benign	Uncertain	Unspecified Behavior
Neoplasm, neoplastic						
— continued						
antrum (Highmore) (maxillary)	C31.0	C78.39	D02.3	D14.0	D38.5	D49.1
pyloric	C16.3	C78.89	D00.2	D13.1	D37.1	D49.0
tympanicum	C30.1	C78.39	D02.3	D14.0	D38.5	D49.1
anus, anal	C21.0	C78.5	D01.3	D12.9	D37.8	D49.0
canal	C21.1	C78.5	D01.3	D12.9	D37.8	D49.0
cloacogenic zone	C21.2	C78.5	D01.3	D12.9	D37.8	D49.0
margin — *see also* Neoplasm, anus, skin	C44.500	C79.2	D04.5	D23.5	D48.5	D49.2
overlapping lesion with rectosigmoid junction or rectum	C21.8	—	—	—	—	—
skin	C44.500	C79.2	D04.5	D23.5	D48.5	D49.2
basal cell carcinoma	C44.510	—	—	—	—	—
specified type NEC	C44.590	—	—	—	—	—
squamous cell carcinoma	C44.520	—	—	—	—	—
sphincter	C21.1	C78.5	D01.3	D12.9	D37.8	D49.0
aorta (thoracic)	C49.3	C79.89	—	D21.3	D48.1	D49.2
abdominal	C49.4	C79.89	—	D21.4	D48.1	D49.2
aortic body	C75.5	C79.89	—	D35.6	D44.7	D49.7
aponeurosis	C49.9	C79.89	—	D21.9	D48.1	D49.2
palmar	C49.1-✓	C79.89	—	D21.1-✓	D48.1	D49.2
plantar	C49.2-✓	C79.89	—	D21.2-✓	D48.1	D49.2
appendix	C18.1	C78.5	D01.0	D12.1	D37.3	D49.0
arachnoid	C70.9	C79.49	—	D32.9	D42.9	D49.7
cerebral	C70.0	C79.32	—	D32.0	D42.0	D49.7
spinal	C70.1	C79.49	—	D32.1	D42.1	D49.7
areola	C50.0-✓	C79.81	D05-✓	D24-✓	D48.6-✓	D49.3
arm NEC	C76.4-✓	C79.89	D04.6-✓	D36.7	D48.7	D49.89
artery — *see* Neoplasm, connective tissue						
aryepiglottic fold	C13.1	C79.89	D00.08	D10.7	D37.05	D49.0
hypopharyngeal aspect	C13.1	C79.89	D00.08	D10.7	D37.05	D49.0
laryngeal aspect	C32.1	C78.39	D02.0	D14.1	D38.0	D49.1
marginal zone	C13.1	C79.89	D00.08	D10.7	D37.05	D49.0
arytenoid (cartilage)	C32.3	C78.39	D02.0	D14.1	D38.0	D49.1
fold — *see* Neoplasm, aryepiglottic						
associated with transplanted organ	C80.2	—	—	—	—	—
atlas	C41.2	C79.51	—	D16.6	D48.0	D49.2
atrium, cardiac	C38.0	C79.89	—	D15.1	D48.7	D49.89
auditory						
canal (external) (skin)	C44.20-✓	C79.2	D04.2-✓	D23.2-✓	D48.5	D49.2
internal	C30.1	C78.39	D02.3	D14.0	D38.5	D49.1
nerve	C72.4-✓	C79.49	—	D33.3	D43.3	D49.7
tube	C30.1	C78.39	D02.3	D14.0	D38.5	D49.1
opening	C11.2	C79.89	D00.08	D10.6	D37.05	D49.0
auricle, ear — *see also* Neoplasm, skin, ear	C44.20-✓	C79.2	D04.2-✓	D23.2-✓	D48.5	D49.2
auricular canal (external) — *see also* Neoplasm, skin, ear	C44.20-✓	C79.2	D04.2-✓	D23.2-✓	D48.5	D49.2
internal	C30.1	C78.39	D02.3	D14.0	D38.5	D49.2
autonomic nerve or nervous system NEC (see Neoplasm, nerve, peripheral)						
axilla, axillary	C76.1	C79.89	D09.8	D36.7	D48.7	D49.89
fold — *see also* Neoplasm, skin, trunk	C44.509	C79.2	D04.5	D23.5	D48.5	D49.2
back NEC	C76.8	C79.89	D04.5	D36.7	D48.7	D49.89
Bartholin's gland	C51.0	C79.82	D07.1	D28.0	D39.8	D49.59
basal ganglia	C71.0	C79.31	—	D33.0	D43.0	D49.6
basis pedunculi	C71.7	C79.31	—	D33.1	D43.1	D49.6
bile or biliary (tract)	C24.9	C78.89	D01.5	D13.5	D37.6	D49.0

Neoplasm, neoplastic — continued

bile or biliary — continued

	Malignant Primary	Malignant Secondary	Ca in situ	Benign	Uncertain	Unspecified Behavior
canaliculi (biliferi) (intrahepatic)	C22.1	C78.7	D01.5	D13.4	D37.6	D49.0
canals, interlobular	C22.1	C78.89	D01.5	D13.4	D37.6	D49.0
duct or passage (common) (cystic) (extrahepatic)	C24.0	C78.89	D01.5	D13.5	D37.6	D49.0
interlobular	C22.1	C78.89	D01.5	D13.4	D37.6	D49.0
intrahepatic	C22.1	C78.7	D01.5	D13.4	D37.6	D49.0
and extrahepatic	C24.8	C78.89	D01.5	D13.5	D37.6	D49.0
bladder (urinary)	C67.9	C79.11	D09.0	D30.3	D41.4	D49.4
dome	C67.1	C79.11	D09.0	D30.3	D41.4	D49.4
neck	C67.5	C79.11	D09.0	D30.3	D41.4	D49.4
orifice	C67.9	C79.11	D09.0	D30.3	D41.4	D49.4
ureteric	C67.6	C79.11	D09.0	D30.3	D41.4	D49.4
urethral	C67.5	C79.11	D09.0	D30.3	D41.4	D49.4
overlapping lesion	C67.8	—	—	—	—	—
sphincter	C67.8	C79.11	D09.0	D30.3	D41.4	D49.4
trigone	C67.0	C79.11	D09.0	D30.3	D41.4	D49.4
urachus	C67.7	C79.11	D09.0	D30.3	D41.4	D49.4
wall	C67.9	C79.11	D09.0	D30.3	D41.4	D49.4
anterior	C67.3	C79.11	D09.0	D30.3	D41.4	D49.4
lateral	C67.2	C79.11	D09.0	D30.3	D41.4	D49.4
posterior	C67.4	C79.11	D09.0	D30.3		
blood vessel — *see* Neoplasm, connective tissue						
bone (periosteum)	C41.9	C79.51	—	D16.9	D48.0	D49.2
acetabulum	C41.4	C79.51	—	D16.8	D48.0	D49.2
ankle	C40.3-✓	C79.51	—	D16.3-✓	—	—
arm NEC	C40.0-✓	C79.51	—	D16.0-✓	—	—
astragalus	C40.3-✓	C79.51	—	D16.3-✓	—	—
atlas	C41.2	C79.51	—	D16.6	D48.0	D49.2
axis	C41.2	C79.51	—	D16.6	D48.0	D49.2
back NEC	C41.2	C79.51	—	D16.6	D48.0	D49.2
calcaneus	C40.3-✓	C79.51	—	D16.3-✓	—	—
calvarium	C41.0	C79.51	—	D16.4	D48.0	D49.2
carpus (any)	C40.1-✓	C79.51	—	D16.1-✓	—	—
cartilage NEC	C41.9	C79.51	—	D16.9	D48.0	D49.2
clavicle	C41.3	C79.51	—	D16.7	D48.0	D49.2
clivus	C41.0	C79.51	—	D16.4	D48.0	D49.2
coccygeal vertebra	C41.4	C79.51	—	D16.8	D48.0	D49.2
coccyx	C41.4	C79.51	—	D16.8	D48.0	D49.2
costal cartilage	C41.3	C79.51	—	D16.7	D48.0	D49.2
costovertebral joint	C41.3	C79.51	—	D16.7	D48.0	D49.2
cranial	C41.0	C79.51	—	D16.4	D48.0	D49.2
cuboid	C40.3-✓	C79.51	—	D16.3-✓	—	—
cuneiform	C41.9	C79.51	—	D16.9	D48.0	D49.2
elbow	C40.0-✓	C79.51	—	D16.0-✓	—	—
ethmoid (labyrinth)	C41.0	C79.51	—	D16.4	D48.0	D49.2
face	C41.0	C79.51	—	D16.4	D48.0	D49.2
femur (any part)	C40.2-✓	C79.51	—	D16.2-✓	—	—
fibula (any part)	C40.2-✓	C79.51	—	D16.2-✓	—	—
finger (any)	C40.1-✓	C79.51	—	D16.1-✓	—	—
foot	C40.3-✓	C79.51	—	D16.3-✓	—	—
forearm	C40.0-✓	C79.51	—	D16.0-✓	—	—
frontal	C41.0	C79.51	—	D16.4	D48.0	
hand	C40.1-✓	C79.51	—	D16.1-✓	—	—
heel	C40.3-✓	C79.51	—	D16.3-✓	—	—.
hip	C41.4	C79.51	—	D16.8	D48.0	D49.2
humerus (any part)	C40.0-✓	C79.51	—	D16.0-✓	—	—
hyoid	C41.0	C79.51	—	D16.4	D48.0	D49.2
ilium	C41.4	C79.51	—	D16.8	D48.0	D49.2
innominate	C41.4	C79.51	—	D16.8	D48.0	D49.2
intervertebral cartilage or disc	C41.2	C79.51	—	D16.6	D48.0	D49.2
ischium	C41.4	C79.51	—	D16.8	D48.0	D49.2
jaw (lower)	C41.1	C79.51	—	D16.5	D48.0	D49.2
knee	C40.2-✓	C79.51	—	D16.2-✓	—	—
leg NEC	C40.2-✓	C79.51	—	D16.2-✓	—	—
limb NEC	C40.9-✓	C79.51	—	D16.9	—	—

Neoplasm, neoplastic — continued

bone — continued

limb — continued

	Malignant Primary	Malignant Secondary	Ca in situ	Benign	Uncertain	Unspecified Behavior
lower (long bones)	C40.2-✓	C79.51	—	D16.2-✓	—	—
short bones	C40.3-✓	C79.51	—	D16.3-✓	—	—
upper (long bones)	C40.0-✓	C79.51	—	D16.0-✓	—	—
short bones	C40.1-✓	C79.51	—	D16.1-✓	—	—
malar	C41.0	C79.51	—	D16.4	D48.0	D49.2
mandible	C41.1	C79.51	—	D16.5	D48.0	D49.2
marrow NEC (any bone)	C96.9	C79.52	—	—	D47.9	D49.89
mastoid	C41.0	C79.51	—	D16.4	D48.0	D49.2
maxilla, maxillary (superior)	C41.0	C79.51	—	D16.4	D48.0	D49.2
inferior	C41.1	C79.51	—	D16.5	D48.0	D49.2
metacarpus (any)	C40.1-✓	C79.51	—	D16.1-✓	—	—
metatarsus (any)	C40.3-✓	C79.51	—	D16.3-✓	—	—
navicular ankle	C40.3-✓	C79.51	—	—	—	—
hand	C40.1-✓	C79.51	—	—	—	—
nose, nasal	C41.0	C79.51	—	D16.4	D48.0	D49.2
occipital	C41.0	C79.51	—	D16.4	D48.0	D49.2
orbit	C41.0	C79.51	—	D16.4	D48.0	D49.2
overlapping sites	C40.8-✓	—	—	—	—	—
parietal	C41.0	C79.51	—	D16.4	D48.0	D49.2
patella	C40.2-✓	C79.51	—	—	—	—
pelvic	C41.4	C79.51	—	D16.8	D48.0	D49.2
phalanges foot	C40.3-✓	C79.51	—	—	—	—
hand	C40.1-✓	C79.51	—	—	—	—
pubic	C41.4	C79.51	—	D16.8	D48.0	D49.2
radius (any part)	C40.0-✓	C79.51	—	D16.0-✓	—	—
rib	C41.3	C79.51	—	D16.7	D48.0	D49.2
sacral vertebra	C41.4	C79.51	—	D16.8	D48.0	D49.2
sacrum	C41.4	C79.51	—	D16.8	D48.0	D49.2
scaphoid of ankle	C40.3-✓	C79.51	—	—	—	—
of hand	C40.1-✓	C79.51	—	—	—	—
scapula (any part)	C40.0-✓	C79.51	—	D16.0-✓	—	—
sella turcica	C41.0	C79.51	—	D16.4	D48.0	D49.2
shoulder	C40.0-✓	C79.51	—	D16.0-✓	—	—
skull	C41.0	C79.51	—	D16.4	D48.0	D49.2
sphenoid	C41.0	C79.51	—	D16.4	D48.0	D49.2
spine, spinal (column)	C41.2	C79.51	—	D16.6	D48.0	D49.2
coccyx	C41.4	C79.51	—	D16.8	D48.0	D49.2
sacrum	C41.4	C79.51	—	D16.8	D48.0	D49.2
sternum	C41.3	C79.51	—	D16.7	D48.0	D49.2
tarsus (any)	C40.3-✓	C79.51	—	—	—	—
temporal	C41.0	C79.51	—	D16.4	D48.0	D49.2
thumb	C40.1-✓	C79.51	—	—	—	—
tibia (any part)	C40.2-✓	C79.51	—	—	—	—
toe (any)	C40.3-✓	C79.51	—	—	—	—
trapezium	C40.1-✓	C79.51	—	—	—	—
trapezoid	C40.1-✓	C79.51	—	—	—	—
turbinate	C41.0	C79.51	—	D16.4	D48.0	D49.2
ulna (any part)	C40.0-✓	C79.51	—	D16.0-✓	—	—
unciform	C40.1-✓	C79.51	—	—	—	—
vertebra (column)	C41.2	C79.51	—	D16.6	D48.0	D49.2
coccyx	C41.4	C79.51	—	D16.8	D48.0	D49.2
sacrum	C41.4	C79.51	—	D16.8	D48.0	D49.2
vomer	C41.0	C79.51	—	D16.4	D48.0	D49.2
wrist	C40.1-✓	C79.51	—	—	—	—
xiphoid process	C41.3	C79.51	—	D16.7	D48.0	D49.2
zygomatic	C41.0	C79.51	—	D16.4	D48.0	D49.2
book-leaf (mouth) — *ventral surface of tongue and floor of mouth*	C06.89	C79.89	D00.00	D10.39	D37.09	D49.0
bowel — *see* Neoplasm, intestine						
brachial plexus	C47.1-✓	C79.89	—	D36.12	D48.2	D49.2
brain NEC	C71.9	C79.31	—	D33.2	D43.2	D49.6

✓ **Additional Character Required** — Refer to the Tabular List for Character Selection   ▽ Subterms under main terms may continue to next column or page

Neoplasm, neoplastic — continued

	Malignant Primary	Malignant Secondary	Ca in situ	Benign	Uncertain	Unspecified Behavior
brain — continued						
basal ganglia	C71.0	C79.31	—	D33.0	D43.0	D49.6
cerebellopontine angle	C71.6	C79.31	—	D33.1	D43.1	D49.6
cerebellum NOS	C71.6	C79.31	—	D33.1	D43.1	D49.6
cerebrum	C71.0	C79.31	—	D33.0	D43.0	D49.6
choroid plexus	C71.7	C79.31	—	D33.1	D43.1	D49.6
corpus callosum	C71.8	C79.31	—	D33.2	D43.2	D49.6
corpus striatum	C71.0	C79.31	—	D33.0	D43.0	D49.6
cortex (cerebral)	C71.0	C79.31	—	D33.0	D43.0	D49.6
frontal lobe	C71.1	C79.31	—	D33.0	D43.0	D49.6
globus pallidus	C71.0	C79.31	—	D33.0	D43.0	D49.6
hippocampus	C71.2	C79.31	—	D33.0	D43.0	D49.6
hypothalamus	C71.0	C79.31	—	D33.0	D43.0	D49.6
internal capsule	C71.0	C79.31	—	D33.0	D43.0	D49.6
medulla oblongata	C71.7	C79.31	—	D33.1	D43.1	D49.6
meninges	C70.0	C79.32	—	D32.0	D42.0	D49.7
midbrain	C71.7	C79.31	—	D33.1	D43.1	D49.6
occipital lobe	C71.4	C79.31	—	D33.0	D43.0	D49.6
overlapping lesion	C71.8	C79.31	—	—	—	—
parietal lobe	C71.3	C79.31	—	D33.0	D43.0	D49.6
peduncle	C71.7	C79.31	—	D33.1	D43.1	D49.6
pons	C71.7	C79.31	—	D33.1	D43.1	D49.6
stem	C71.7	C79.31	—	D33.1	D43.1	D49.6
tapetum	C71.8	C79.31	—	D33.2	D43.2	D49.6
temporal lobe	C71.2	C79.31	—	D33.0	D43.0	D49.6
thalamus	C71.0	C79.31	—	D33.0	D43.0	D49.6
uncus	C71.2	C79.31	—	D33.0	D43.0	D49.6
ventricle (floor)	C71.5	C79.31	—	D33.0	D43.0	D49.6
fourth	C71.7	C79.31	—	D33.1	D43.1	D49.6
branchial (cleft) (cyst) (vestiges)	C10.4	C79.89	D00.08	D10.5	D37.05	D49.0
breast (connective tissue) (glandular tissue) (soft parts)	C50.9-✓	C79.81	D05.-✓	D24.-✓	D48.6-✓	D49.3
areola	C50.0-✓	C79.81	D05.-✓	D24.-✓	D48.6-✓	D49.3
axillary tail	C50.6-✓	C79.81	D05.-✓	D24.-✓	D48.6-✓	D49.3
central portion	C50.1-✓	C79.81	D05.-✓	D24.-✓	D48.6-✓	D49.3
inner	C50.8-✓	C79.81	D05.-✓	D24.-✓	D48.6-✓	D49.3
lower	C50.8-✓	C79.81	D05.-✓	D24.-✓	D48.6-✓	D49.3
lower-inner quadrant	C50.3-✓	C79.81	D05.-✓	D24.-✓	D48.6-✓	D49.3
lower-outer quadrant	C50.5-✓	C79.81	D05.-✓	D24.-✓	D48.6-✓	D49.3
mastectomy site (skin) — see also Neoplasm, breast, skin	C44.501	C79.2	—	—	—	—
specified as breast tissue	C50.8-✓	C79.81	—	—	—	—
midline	C50.8-✓	C79.81	D05.-✓	D24.-✓	D48.6-✓	D49.3
nipple	C50.0-✓	C79.81	D05.-✓	D24.-✓	D48.6-✓	D49.3
outer	C50.8-✓	C79.81	D05.-✓	D24.-✓	D48.6-✓	D49.3
overlapping lesion	C50.8-✓	—	—	—	—	—
skin	C44.501	C79.2	D04.5	D23.5	D48.5	D49.2
basal cell carcinoma	C44.511	—	—	—	—	—
specified type NEC	C44.591	—	—	—	—	—
squamous cell carcinoma	C44.521	—	—	—	—	—
tail (axillary)	C50.6-✓	C79.81	D05.-✓	D24.-✓	D48.6-✓	D49.3
upper	C50.8-✓	C79.81	D05.-✓	D24.-✓	D48.6-✓	D49.3
upper-inner quadrant	C50.2-✓	C79.81	D05.-✓	D24.-✓	D48.6-✓	D49.3
upper-outer quadrant	C50.4-✓	C79.81	D05.-✓	D24.-✓	D48.6-✓	D49.3
broad ligament	C57.1-✓	C79.82	D07.39	D28.2	D39.8	D49.59
bronchiogenic, bronchogenic (lung)	C34.9-✓	C78.0-✓	D02.2-✓	D14.3-✓	D38.1	D49.1
bronchiole	C34.9-✓	C78.0-✓	D02.2-✓	D14.3-✓	D38.1	D49.1
bronchus	C34.9-✓	C78.0-✓	D02.2-✓	D14.3-✓	D38.1	D49.1
carina	C34.0-✓	C78.0-✓	D02.2-✓	D14.3-✓	D38.1	D49.1
lower lobe of lung	C34.3-✓	C78.0-✓	D02.2-✓	D14.3-✓	D38.1	D49.1

Neoplasm, neoplastic — continued

	Malignant Primary	Malignant Secondary	Ca in situ	Benign	Uncertain	Unspecified Behavior
bronchus — continued						
main	C34.0-✓	C78.0-✓	D02.2-✓	D14.3-✓	D38.1	D49.1
middle lobe of lung	C34.2	C78.0-✓	D02.21	D14.31	D38.1	D49.1
overlapping lesion	C34.8-✓	—	—	—	—	—
upper lobe of lung	C34.1-✓	C78.0-✓	D02.2-✓	D14.3-✓	D38.1	D49.1
brow	C44.309	C79.2	D04.39	D23.39	D48.5	D49.2
basal cell carcinoma	C44.319					
specified type NEC	C44.399	—	—	—	—	—
squamous cell carcinoma	C44.329					
buccal (cavity)	C06.9	C79.89	D00.00	D10.39	D37.09	D49.0
commissure	C06.0	C79.89	D00.02	D10.39	D37.09	D49.0
groove (lower) (upper)	C06.1	C79.89	D00.02	D10.39	D37.09	D49.0
mucosa	C06.0	C79.89	D00.02	D10.39	D37.09	D49.0
sulcus (lower) (upper)	C06.1	C79.89	D00.02	D10.39	D37.09	D49.0
bulbourethral gland	C68.0	C79.19	D09.19	D30.4	D41.3	D49.59
bursa — see Neoplasm, connective tissue						
buttock NEC	C76.3	C79.89	D04.5	D36.7	D48.7	D49.89
calf	C76.5-✓	C79.89	D04.7-✓	D36.7	D48.7	D49.89
calvarium	C41.0	C79.51	—	D16.4	D48.0	D49.2
calyx, renal	C65.-✓	C79.0-✓	D09.19	D30.1-✓	D41.1-✓	D49.51-✓
canal						
anal	C21.1	C78.5	D01.3	D12.9	D37.8	D49.0
auditory (external) — see also Neoplasm, skin, ear	C44.20-✓	C79.2	D04.2-✓	D23.2-✓	D48.5	D49.2
auricular (external) — see also Neoplasm, skin, ear	C44.20-✓	C79.2	D04.2-✓	D23.2-✓	D48.5	D49.2
canaliculi, biliary (biliferi) (intrahepatic)	C22.1	C78.7	D01.5	D13.4	D37.6	D49.0
canthus (eye) (inner) (outer)	C44.10-✓	C79.2	D04.1-✓	D23.1-✓	D48.5	D49.2
basal cell carcinoma	C44.11-✓	—	—	—	—	—
sebaceous cell	C44.13-✓	—	—	—	—	—
specified type NEC	C44.19-✓	—	—	—	—	—
squamous cell carcinoma	C44.12-✓					
capillary — see Neoplasm, connective tissue						
caput coli	C18.0	C78.5	D01.0	D12.0	D37.4	D49.0
carcinoid — see Tumor, carcinoid						
cardia (gastric)	C16.0	C78.89	D00.2	D13.1	D37.1	D49.0
cardiac orifice (stomach)	C16.0	C78.89	D00.2	D13.1	D37.1	D49.0
cardio-esophageal junction	C16.0	C78.89	D00.2	D13.1	D37.1	D49.0
cardio-esophagus	C16.0	C78.89	D00.2	D13.1	D37.1	D49.0
carina (bronchus)	C34.0-✓	C78.0-✓	D02.2-✓	D14.3-✓	D38.1	D49.1
carotid (artery)	C49.0	C79.89	—	D21.0	D48.1	D49.2
body	C75.4	C79.89	—	D35.5	D44.6	D49.7
carpus (any bone)	C40.1-✓	C79.51	—	D16.1-✓	—	—
cartilage (articular) (joint) NEC — see also Neoplasm, bone	C41.9	C79.51	—	D16.9	D48.0	D49.2
arytenoid	C32.3	C78.39	D02.0	D14.1	D38.0	D49.1
auricular	C49.0	C79.89	—	D21.0	D48.1	D49.2
bronchi	C34.0-✓	C78.39	—	D14.3-✓	D38.1	D49.1
costal	C41.3	C79.51	—	D16.7	D48.0	D49.2
cricoid	C32.3	C78.39	D02.0	D14.1	D38.0	D49.1
cuneiform	C32.3	C78.39	D02.0	D14.1	D38.0	D49.1
ear (external)	C49.0	C79.89	—	D21.0	D48.1	D49.2
ensiform	C41.3	C79.51	—	D16.7	D48.0	D49.2
epiglottis	C32.1	C78.39	D02.0	D14.1	D38.0	D49.1

Neoplasm, neoplastic — continued

	Malignant Primary	Malignant Secondary	Ca in situ	Benign	Uncertain	Unspecified Behavior
cartilage — see also Neoplasm, bone — continued						
epiglottis — continued						
anterior						
surface	C10.1	C79.89	D00.08	D10.5	D37.05	D49.0
eyelid	C49.0	C79.89	—	D21.0	D48.1	D49.2
intervertebral	C41.2	C79.51	—	D16.6	D48.0	D49.2
larynx, laryngeal	C32.3	C78.39	D02.0	D14.1	D38.0	D49.1
nose, nasal	C30.0	C78.39	D02.3	D14.0	D38.5	D49.1
pinna	C49.0	C79.89	—	D21.0	D48.1	D49.2
rib	C41.3	C79.51	—	D16.7	D48.0	D49.2
semilunar (knee)	C40.2-☑	C79.51	—	D16.2-☑	D48.0	D49.2
thyroid	C32.3	C78.39	D02.0	D14.1	D38.0	D49.1
trachea	C33	C78.39	D02.1	D14.2	D38.1	D49.1
cauda equina	C72.1	C79.49	—	D33.4	D43.4	D49.7
cavity						
buccal	C06.9	C79.89	D00.00	D10.30	D37.09	D49.0
nasal	C30.0	C78.39	D02.3	D14.0	D38.5	D49.1
oral	C06.9	C79.89	D00.00	D10.30	D37.09	D49.0
peritoneal	C48.2	C78.6	—	D20.1	D48.4	D49.0
tympanic	C30.1	C78.39	D02.3	D14.0	D38.5	D49.1
cecum	C18.0	C78.5	D01.0	D12.0	D37.4	D49.0
central nervous system	C72.9	C79.40	—	—	—	—
cerebellopontine (angle)	C71.6	C79.31	—	D33.1	D43.1	D49.6
cerebellum, cerebellar	C71.6	C79.31	—	D33.1	D43.1	D49.6
cerebrum, cerebral (cortex) (hemisphere) (white matter)	C71.0	C79.31	—	D33.0	D43.0	D49.6
meninges	C70.0	C79.32	—	D32.0	D42.0	D49.7
peduncle	C71.7	C79.31	—	D33.1	D43.1	D49.6
ventricle	C71.5	C79.31	—	D33.0	D43.0	D49.6
fourth	C71.7	C79.31	—	D33.1	D43.1	D49.6
cervical region	C76.0	C79.89	D09.8	D36.7	D48.7	D49.89
cervix (cervical) (uteri) (uterus)	C53.9	C79.82	D06.9	D26.0	D39.0	D49.59
canal	C53.0	C79.82	D06.0	D26.0	D39.0	D49.59
endocervix (canal) (gland)	C53.0	C79.82	D06.0	D26.0	D39.0	D49.59
exocervix	C53.1	C79.82	D06.1	D26.0	D39.0	D49.59
external os	C53.1	C79.82	D06.1	D26.0	D39.0	D49.59
internal os	C53.0	C79.82	D06.0	D26.0	D39.0	D49.59
nabothian gland	C53.0	C79.82	D06.0	D26.0	D39.0	D49.59
overlapping lesion	C53.8	—	—	—	—	—
squamocolumnar junction	C53.8	C79.82	D06.7	D26.0	D39.0	D49.59
stump	C53.8	C79.82	D06.7	D26.0	D39.0	D49.59
cheek	C76.0	C79.89	D09.8	D36.7	D48.7	D49.89
external	C44.309	C79.2	D04.39	D23.39	D48.5	D49.2
basal cell carcinoma	C44.319	—	—	—	—	—
specified type NEC	C44.399	—	—	—	—	—
squamous cell carcinoma	C44.329	—	—	—	—	—
inner aspect	C06.0	C79.89	D00.02	D10.39	D37.09	D49.0
internal	C06.0	C79.89	D00.02	D10.39	D37.09	D49.0
mucosa	C06.0	C79.89	D00.02	D10.39	D37.09	D49.0
chest (wall) NEC	C76.1	C79.89	D09.8	D36.7	D48.7	D49.89
chiasma opticum	C72.3-☑	C79.49	—	D33.3	D43.3	D49.7
chin	C44.309	C79.2	D04.39	D23.39	D48.5	D49.2
basal cell carcinoma	C44.319	—	—	—	—	—
specified type NEC	C44.399	—	—	—	—	—
squamous cell carcinoma	C44.329	—	—	—	—	—
choana	C11.3	C79.89	D00.08	D10.6	D37.05	D49.0
cholangiole	C22.1	C78.89	D01.5	D13.4	D37.6	D49.0
choledochal duct	C24.0	C78.89	D01.5	D13.5	D37.6	D49.0
choroid	C69.3-☑	C79.49	D09.2-☑	D31.3-☑	D48.7	D49.81
plexus	C71.5	C79.31	—	D33.0	D43.0	D49.6
ciliary body	C69.4-☑	C79.49	D09.2-☑	D31.4-☑	D48.7	D49.89
clavicle	C41.3	C79.51	—	D16.7	D48.0	D49.2

Neoplasm, neoplastic — continued

	Malignant Primary	Malignant Secondary	Ca in situ	Benign	Uncertain	Unspecified Behavior
clitoris	C51.2	C79.82	D07.1	D28.0	D39.8	D49.59
clivus	C41.0	C79.51	—	D16.4	D48.0	D49.2
cloacogenic zone	C21.2	C78.5	D01.3	D12.9	D37.8	D49.0
coccygeal						
body or glomus	C49.5	C79.89	—	D21.5	D48.1	D49.2
vertebra	C41.4	C79.51	—	D16.8	D48.0	D49.2
coccyx	C41.4	C79.51	—	D16.8	D48.0	D49.2
colon — see also Neoplasm, intestine, large	C18.9	C78.5	—	—	—	—
with rectum	C19	C78.5	D01.1	D12.7	D37.5	D49.0
columnella — see also Neoplasm, skin, face	C44.390	C79.2	D04.39	D23.39	D48.5	D49.2
column, spinal — see Neoplasm, spine						
commissure						
labial, lip	C00.6	C79.89	D00.01	D10.39	D37.01	D49.0
laryngeal	C32.0	C78.39	D02.0	D14.1	D38.0	D49.1
common (bile) duct	C24.0	C78.89	D01.5	D13.5	D37.6	D49.0
concha — see also Neoplasm, skin, ear	C44.20-☑	C79.2	D04.2-☑	D23.2-☑	D48.5	D49.2
nose	C30.0	C78.39	D02.3	D14.0	D38.5	D49.1
conjunctiva	C69.0-☑	C79.49	D09.2-☑	D31.0-☑	D48.7	D49.89
connective tissue NEC	C49.9	C79.89	—	D21.9	D48.1	D49.2

Note: For neoplasms of connective tissue (blood vessel, bursa, fascia, ligament, muscle, peripheral nerves, sympathetic and parasympathetic nerves and ganglia, synovia, tendon, etc.) or of morphological types that indicate connective tissue, code according to the list under "Neoplasm, connective tissue". For sites that do not appear in this list, code to neoplasm of that site; e.g., fibrosarcoma, pancreas (C25.9)

Note: Morphological types that indicate connective tissue appear in their proper place in the alphabetic index with the instruction "see Neoplasm, connective tissue ...."

	Malignant Primary	Malignant Secondary	Ca in situ	Benign	Uncertain	Unspecified Behavior
abdomen	C49.4	C79.89	—	D21.4	D48.1	D49.2
abdominal wall	C49.4	C79.89	—	D21.4	D48.1	D49.2
ankle	C49.2-☑	C79.89	—	D21.2-☑	D48.1	D49.2
antecubital fossa or space	C49.1-☑	C79.89	—	D21.1-☑	D48.1	D49.2
arm	C49.1-☑	C79.89	—	D21.1-☑	D48.1	D49.2
auricle (ear)	C49.0	C79.89	—	D21.0	D48.1	D49.2
axilla	C49.3	C79.89	—	D21.3	D48.1	D49.2
back	C49.6	C79.89	—	D21.6	D48.1	D49.2
breast — see Neoplasm, breast						
buttock	C49.5	C79.89	—	D21.5	D48.1	D49.2
calf	C49.2-☑	C79.89	—	D21.2-☑	D48.1	D49.2
cervical region	C49.0	C79.89	—	D21.0	D48.1	D49.2
cheek	C49.0	C79.89	—	D21.0	D48.1	D49.2
chest (wall)	C49.3	C79.89	—	D21.3	D48.1	D49.2
chin	C49.0	C79.89	—	D21.0	D48.1	D49.2
diaphragm	C49.3	C79.89	—	D21.3	D48.1	D49.2
ear (external)	C49.0	C79.89	—	D21.0	D48.1	D49.2
elbow	C49.1-☑	C79.89	—	D21.1-☑	D48.1	D49.2
extrarectal	C49.5	C79.89	—	D21.5	D48.1	D49.2
extremity	C49.9	C79.89	—	D21.9	D48.1	D49.2
lower	C49.2-☑	C79.89	—	D21.2-☑	D48.1	D49.2
upper	C49.1-☑	C79.89	—	D21.1-☑	D48.1	D49.2
eyelid	C49.0	C79.89	—	D21.0	D48.1	D49.2
face	C49.0	C79.89	—	D21.0	D48.1	D49.2
finger	C49.1-☑	C79.89	—	D21.1-☑	D48.1	D49.2
flank	C49.6	C79.89	—	D21.6	D48.1	D49.2
foot	C49.2-☑	C79.89	—	D21.2-☑	D48.1	D49.2
forearm	C49.1-☑	C79.89	—	D21.1-☑	D48.1	D49.2
forehead	C49.0	C79.89	—	D21.0	D48.1	D49.2
gastric	C49.4	C79.89	—	D21.4	D48.1	D49.2
gastrointestinal	C49.4	C79.89	—	D21.4	D48.1	D49.2
gluteal region	C49.5	C79.89	—	D21.5	D48.1	D49.2
great vessels NEC	C49.3	C79.89	—	D21.3	D48.1	D49.2
groin	C49.5	C79.89	—	D21.5	D48.1	D49.2
hand	C49.1-☑	C79.89	—	D21.1-☑	D48.1	D49.2
head	C49.0	C79.89	—	D21.0	D48.1	D49.2

☑ Additional Character Required — Refer to the Tabular List for Character Selection   ▽ Subterms under main terms may continue to next column or page

Neoplasm, neoplastic
— *continued*
connective tissue — *continued*

	Malignant Primary	Malignant Secondary	Ca in situ	Benign	Uncertain	Unspecified Behavior
heel	C49.2-✓	C79.89	—	D21.2-✓	D48.1	D49.2
hip	C49.2-✓	C79.89	—	D21.2-✓	D48.1	D49.2
hypochondrium	C49.4	C79.89	—	D21.4	D48.1	D49.2
iliopsoas muscle	C49.5	C79.89	—	D21.5	D48.1	D49.2
infraclavicular region	C49.3	C79.89	—	D21.3	D48.1	D49.2
inguinal (canal) (region)	C49.5	C79.89	—	D21.5	D48.1	D49.2
intestinal	C49.4	C79.89	—	D21.4	D48.1	D49.2
intrathoracic	C49.3	C79.89	—	D21.3	D48.1	D49.2
ischiorectal fossa	C49.5	C79.89	—	D21.5	D48.1	D49.2
jaw	C03.9	C79.89	D00.03	D10.39	D48.1	D49.0
knee	C49.2-✓	C79.89	—	D21.2-✓	D48.1	D49.2
leg	C49.2-✓	C79.89	—	D21.2-✓	D48.1	D49.2
limb NEC	C49.9	C79.89	—	D21.9	D48.1	D49.2
lower	C49.2-✓	C79.89	—	D21.2-✓	D48.1	D49.2
upper	C49.1-✓	C79.89	—	D21.1-✓	D48.1	D49.2
nates	C49.5	C79.89	—	D21.5	D48.1	D49.2
neck	C49.0	C79.89	—	D21.0	D48.1	D49.2
orbit	C69.6-✓	C79.49	D09.2-✓	D31.6-✓	D48.1	D49.89
overlapping lesion	C49.8	—	—	—	—	—
pararectal	C49.5	C79.89	—	D21.5	D48.1	D49.2
para-urethral	C49.5	C79.89	—	D21.5	D48.1	D49.2
paravaginal	C49.5	C79.89	—	D21.5	D48.1	D49.2
pelvis (floor)	C49.5	C79.89	—	D21.5	D48.1	D49.2
pelvo-abdominal	C49.8	C79.89	—	D21.6	D48.1	D49.2
perineum	C49.5	C79.89	—	D21.5	D48.1	D49.2
perirectal (tissue)	C49.5	C79.89	—	D21.5	D48.1	D49.2
periurethral (tissue)	C49.5	C79.89	—	D21.5	D48.1	D49.2
popliteal fossa or space	C49.2-✓	C79.89	—	D21.2-✓	D48.1	D49.2
presacral	C49.5	C79.89	—	D21.5	D48.1	D49.2
psoas muscle	C49.4	C79.89	—	D21.4	D48.1	D49.2
pterygoid fossa	C49.0	C79.89	—	D21.0	D48.1	D49.2
rectovaginal septum or wall	C49.5	C79.89	—	D21.5	D48.1	D49.2
rectovesical	C49.5	C79.89	—	D21.5	D48.1	D49.2
retroperitoneum	C48.0	C78.6	—	D20.0	D48.3	D49.0
sacrococcygeal region	C49.5	C79.89	—	D21.5	D48.1	D49.2
scalp	C49.0	C79.89	—	D21.0	D48.1	D49.2
scapular region	C49.3	C79.89	—	D21.3	D48.1	D49.2
shoulder	C49.1-✓	C79.89	—	D21.1-✓	D48.1	D49.2
skin (dermis) NEC — *see also* Neoplasm, skin, by site	C44.90	C79.2	D04.9	D23.9	D48.5	D49.2
stomach	C49.4	C79.89	—	D21.4	D48.1	D49.2
submental	C49.0	C79.89	—	D21.0	D48.1	D49.2
supraclavicular region	C49.0	C79.89	—	D21.0	D48.1	D49.2
temple	C49.0	C79.89	—	D21.0	D48.1	D49.2
temporal region	C49.0	C79.89	—	D21.0	D48.1	D49.2
thigh	C49.2-✓	C79.89	—	D21.2-✓	D48.1	D49.2
thoracic (duct) (wall)	C49.3	C79.89	—	D21.3	D48.1	D49.2
thorax	C49.3	C79.89	—	D21.3	D48.1	D49.2
thumb	C49.1-✓	C79.89	—	D21.1-✓	D48.1	D49.2
toe	C49.2-✓	C79.89	—	D21.2-✓	D48.1	D49.2
trunk	C49.6	C79.89	—	D21.6	D48.1	D49.2
umbilicus	C49.4	C79.89	—	D21.4	D48.1	D49.2
vesicorectal	C49.5	C79.89	—	D21.5	D48.1	D49.2
wrist	C49.1-✓	C79.89	—	D21.1-✓	D48.1	D49.2
conus medullaris	C72.0	C79.49	—	D33.4	D43.4	D49.7
cord (true) (vocal)	C32.0	C78.39	D02.0	D14.1	D38.0	D49.1
false	C32.1	C78.39	D02.0	D14.1	D38.0	D49.1
spermatic	C63.1-✓	C79.82	D07.69	D29.8	D40.8	D49.59
spinal (cervical) (lumbar) (thoracic)	C72.0	C79.49	—	D33.4	D43.4	D49.7
cornea (limbus)	C69.1-✓	C79.49	D09.2-✓	D31.1-✓	D48.7	D49.89
corpus						
albicans	C56.-✓	C79.6-✓	D07.39	D27.-✓	D39.1-✓	D49.59
callosum, brain	C71.0	C79.31	—	D33.2	D43.2	D49.6

Neoplasm, neoplastic
— *continued*
corpus — *continued*

	Malignant Primary	Malignant Secondary	Ca in situ	Benign	Uncertain	Unspecified Behavior
cavernosum	C60.2	C79.82	D07.4	D29.0	D40.8	D49.59
gastric	C16.2	C78.89	D00.2	D13.1	D37.1	D49.0
overlapping sites	C54.8	—	—	—	—	—
penis	C60.2	C79.82	D07.4	D29.0	D40.8	D49.59
striatum, cerebrum	C71.0	C79.31	—	D33.0	D43.0	D49.6
uteri	C54.9	C79.82	D07.0	D26.1	D39.0	D49.59
isthmus	C54.0	C79.82	D07.0	D26.1	D39.0	D49.59
cortex						
adrenal	C74.0-✓	C79.7-✓	D09.3	D35.0-✓	D44.1-✓	D49.7
cerebral	C71.0	C79.31	—	D33.0	D43.0	D49.6
costal cartilage	C41.3	C79.51	—	D16.7	D48.0	D49.2
costovertebral joint	C41.3	C79.51	—	D16.7	D48.0	D49.2
Cowper's gland	C68.0	C79.19	D09.19	D30.4	D41.3	D49.59
cranial (fossa, any)	C71.9	C79.31	—	D33.2	D43.2	D49.6
meninges	C70.0	C79.32	—	D32.0	D42.0	D49.7
nerve	C72.50	C79.49	—	D33.3	D43.3	D49.7
specified NEC	C72.59	C79.49	—	D33.3	D43.3	D49.7
craniobuccal pouch	C75.2	C79.89	D09.3	D35.2	D44.3	D49.7
craniopharyngeal (duct) (pouch)	C75.2	C79.89	D09.3	D35.3	D44.4	D49.7
cricoid	C13.0	C79.89	D00.08	D10.7	D37.05	D49.0
cartilage	C32.3	C78.39	D02.0	D14.1	D38.0	D49.1
cricopharynx	C13.0	C79.89	D00.08	D10.7	D37.05	D49.0
crypt of Morgagni	C21.8	C78.5	D01.3	D12.9	D37.8	D49.0
crystalline lens	C69.4-✓	C79.49	D09.2-✓	D31.4-✓	D48.7	D49.89
cul-de-sac (Douglas')	C48.1	C78.6	—	D20.1	D48.4	D49.0
cuneiform cartilage	C32.3	C78.39	D02.0	D14.1	D38.0	D49.1
cutaneous — *see* Neoplasm, skin						
cutis — *see* Neoplasm, skin						
cystic (bile) duct (common)	C24.0	C78.89	D01.5	D13.5	D37.6	D49.0
dermis — *see* Neoplasm, skin						
diaphragm	C49.3	C79.89	—	D21.3	D48.1	D49.2
digestive organs, system, tube, or tract NEC	C26.9	C78.89	D01.9	D13.9	D37.9	D49.0
disc, intervertebral	C41.2	C79.51	—	D16.6	D48.0	D49.2
disease, generalized	C80.0	—	—	—	—	—
disseminated	C80.0	—	—	—	—	—
Douglas' cul-de-sac or pouch	C48.1	C78.6	—	D20.1	D48.4	D49.0
duodenojejunal junction	C17.8	C78.4	D01.49	D13.39	D37.2	D49.0
duodenum	C17.0	C78.4	D01.49	D13.2	D37.2	D49.0
dura (cranial) (mater)	C70.9	C79.49	—	D32.9	D42.9	D49.7
cerebral	C70.0	C79.32	—	D32.0	D42.0	D49.7
spinal	C70.1	C79.49	—	D32.1	D42.1	D49.7
ear (external) — *see also* Neoplasm, skin, ear	C44.20-✓	C79.2	D04.2-✓	D23.2-✓	D48.5	D49.2
auricle or auris — *see also* Neoplasm, skin, ear	C44.20-✓	C79.2	D04.2-✓	D23.2-✓	D48.5	D49.2
canal, external — *see also* Neoplasm, skin, ear	C44.20-✓	C79.2	D04.2-✓	D23.2-✓	D48.5	D49.2
cartilage	C49.0	C79.89	—	D21.0	D48.1	D49.2
external meatus — *see also* Neoplasm, skin, ear	C44.20-✓	C79.2	D04.2-✓	D23.2-✓	D48.5	D49.2
inner	C30.1	C78.39	D02.3	D14.0	D38.5	D49.1
lobule — *see also* Neoplasm, skin, ear	C44.20-✓	C79.2	D04.2-✓	D23.2-✓	D48.5	D49.2
middle	C30.1	C78.39	D02.3	D14.0	D38.5	D49.1
overlapping lesion with accessory sinuses	C31.8	—	—	—	—	—

Neoplasm Table

Neoplasm, ear — Neoplasm, frenulum

Neoplasm, neoplastic	Malignant Primary	Malignant Secondary	Ca in situ	Benign	Uncertain	Unspecified Behavior
— continued						
ear — see also Neoplasm, skin, ear — continued						
skin	C44.20-☑	C79.2	D04.2-☑	D23.2-☑	D48.5	D49.2
basal cell carcinoma	C44.21-☑	—	—	—	—	—
specified type NEC	C44.29-☑	—	—	—	—	—
squamous cell carcinoma	C44.22-☑	—	—	—	—	—
earlobe	C44.20-☑	C79.2	D04.2-☑	D23.2-☑	D48.5	D49.2
basal cell carcinoma	C44.21-☑	—	—	—	—	—
specified type NEC	C44.29-☑	—	—	—	—	—
squamous cell carcinoma	C44.22-☑	—	—	—	—	—
ejaculatory duct	C63.7	C79.82	D07.69	D29.8	D40.8	D49.59
elbow NEC	C76.4-☑	C79.89	D04.6-☑	D36.7	D48.7	D49.89
endocardium	C38.0	C79.89	—	D15.1	D48.7	D49.89
endocervix (canal) (gland)	C53.0	C79.82	D06.0	D26.0	D39.0	D49.59
endocrine gland NEC	C75.9	C79.89	D09.3	D35.9	D44.9	D49.7
pluriglandular	C75.8	C79.89	D09.3	D35.7	D44.9	D49.7
endometrium (gland) (stroma)	C54.1	C79.82	D07.0	D26.1	D39.0	D49.59
ensiform cartilage	C41.3	C79.51	—	D16.7	D48.0	D49.2
enteric — see Neoplasm, intestine						
ependyma (brain)	C71.5	C79.31	—	D33.0	D43.0	D49.6
fourth ventricle	C71.7	C79.31	—	D33.1	D43.1	D49.6
epicardium	C38.0	C79.89	—	D15.1	D48.7	D49.89
epididymis	C63.0-☑	C79.82	D07.69	D29.3-☑	D40.8	D49.59
epidural	C72.9	C79.49	—	D33.9	D43.9	D49.7
epiglottis	C32.1	C78.39	D02.0	D14.1	D38.0	D49.1
anterior aspect or surface	C10.1	C79.89	D00.08	D10.5	D37.05	D49.0
cartilage	C32.3	C78.39	D02.0	D14.1	D38.0	D49.1
free border (margin)	C10.1	C79.89	D00.08	D10.5	D37.05	D49.0
junctional region	C10.8	C79.89	D00.08	D10.5	D37.05	D49.0
posterior (laryngeal) surface	C32.1	C78.39	D02.0	D14.1	D38.0	D49.1
suprahyoid portion	C32.1	C78.39	D02.0	D14.1	D38.0	D49.1
esophagogastric junction	C16.0	C78.89	D00.2	D13.1	D37.1	D49.0
esophagus	C15.9	C78.89	D00.1	D13.0	D37.8	D49.0
abdominal	C15.5	C78.89	D00.1	D13.0	D37.8	D49.0
cervical	C15.3	C78.89	D00.1	D13.0	D37.8	D49.0
distal (third)	C15.5	C78.89	D00.1	D13.0	D37.8	D49.0
lower (third)	C15.5	C78.89	D00.1	D13.0	D37.8	D49.0
middle (third)	C15.4	C78.89	D00.1	D13.0	D37.8	D49.0
overlapping lesion	C15.8	—	—	—	—	—
proximal (third)	C15.3	C78.89	D00.1	D13.0	D37.8	D49.0
thoracic	C15.4	C78.89	D00.1	D13.0	D37.8	D49.0
upper (third)	C15.3	C78.89	D00.1	D13.0	D37.8	D49.0
ethmoid (sinus)	C31.1	C78.39	D02.3	D14.0	D38.5	D49.1
bone or labyrinth	C41.0	C79.51	—	D16.4	D48.0	D49.2
eustachian tube	C30.1	C78.39	D02.3	D14.0	D38.5	D49.1
exocervix	C53.1	C79.82	D06.1	D26.0	D39.0	D49.59
external						
meatus (ear) — see also Neoplasm, skin, ear	C44.20-☑	C79.2	D04.2-☑	D23.2-☑	D48.5	D49.2
os, cervix uteri	C53.1	C79.82	D06.1	D26.0	D39.0	D49.59
extradural	C72.9	C79.49	—	D33.9	D43.9	D49.7
extrahepatic (bile) duct	C24.0	C78.89	D01.5	D13.5	D37.6	D49.0
overlapping lesion with gallbladder	C24.8	—	—	—	—	—
extraocular muscle	C69.6-☑	C79.49	D09.2-☑	D31.6-☑	D48.7	D49.89
extrarectal	C76.3	C79.89	D09.8	D36.7	D48.7	D49.89
extremity	C76.8	C79.89	D04.8	D36.7	D48.7	D49.89

Neoplasm, neoplastic	Malignant Primary	Malignant Secondary	Ca in situ	Benign	Uncertain	Unspecified Behavior
— continued						
extremity — continued						
lower	C76.5-☑	C79.89	D04.7-☑	D36.7	D48.7	D49.89
upper	C76.4-☑	C79.89	D04.6-☑	D36.7	D48.7	D49.89
eyeball	C69.9-☑	C79.49	D09.2-☑	D31.9-☑	D48.7	D49.89
eyebrow	C44.309	C79.2	D04.39	D23.39	D48.5	D49.2
basal cell carcinoma	C44.319	—	—	—	—	—
specified type NEC	C44.399	—	—	—	—	—
squamous cell carcinoma	C44.329	—	—	—	—	—
eyelid (lower) (skin) (upper)	C44.10-☑	—	—	—	—	—
basal cell carcinoma	C44.11-☑	—	—	—	—	—
cartilage	C49.0	C79.89	—	D21.0	D48.1	D49.2
sebaceous cell	C44.13-☑	—	—	—	—	—
specified type NEC	C44.19-☑	—	—	—	—	—
squamous cell carcinoma	C44.12-☑	—	—	—	—	—
eye NEC	C69.9-☑	C79.49	D09.2-☑	D31.9-☑	D48.7	D49.89
overlapping sites	C69.8-☑	—	—	—	—	—
face NEC	C76.0	C79.89	D04.39	D36.7	D48.7	D49.89
fallopian tube (accessory)	C57.0-☑	C79.82	D07.39	D28.2	D39.8	D49.59
falx (cerebella) (cerebri)	C70.0	C79.32	—	D32.0	D42.0	D49.7
fascia — see also Neoplasm, connective tissue						
palmar	C49.1-☑	C79.89	—	D21.1-☑	D48.1	D49.2
plantar	C49.2-☑	C79.89	—	D21.2-☑	D48.1	D49.2
fatty tissue — see Neoplasm, connective tissue						
fauces, faucial NEC	C10.9	C79.89	D00.08	D10.5	D37.05	D49.0
pillars	C09.1	C79.89	D00.08	D10.5	D37.05	D49.0
tonsil	C09.9	C79.89	D00.08	D10.4	D37.05	D49.0
femur (any part)	C40.2-☑	—	—	D16.2-☑	—	—
fetal membrane	C58	C79.82	D07.0	D26.7	D39.2	D49.59
fibrous tissue — see Neoplasm, connective tissue						
fibula (any part)	C40.2-☑	C79.51	—	D16.2-☑	—	—
filum terminale	C72.0	C79.49	—	D33.4	D43.4	D49.7
finger NEC	C76.4-☑	C79.89	D04.6-☑	D36.7	D48.7	D49.89
flank NEC	C76.8	C79.89	D04.5	D36.7	D48.7	D49.89
follicle, nabothian	C53.0	C79.82	D06.0	D26.0	D39.0	D49.59
foot NEC	C76.5-☑	C79.89	D04.7-☑	D36.7	D48.7	D49.89
forearm NEC	C76.4-☑	C79.89	D04.6-☑	D36.7	D48.7	D49.89
forehead (skin)	C44.309	C79.2	D04.39	D23.39	D48.5	D49.2
basal cell carcinoma	C44.319	—	—	—	—	—
specified type NEC	C44.399	—	—	—	—	—
squamous cell carcinoma	C44.329	—	—	—	—	—
foreskin	C60.0	C79.82	D07.4	D29.0	D40.8	D49.59
fornix						
pharyngeal	C11.3	C79.89	D00.08	D10.6	D37.05	D49.0
vagina	C52	C79.82	D07.2	D28.1	D39.8	D49.59
fossa (of)						
anterior (cranial)	C71.9	C79.31	—	D33.2	D43.2	D49.6
cranial	C71.9	C79.31	—	D33.2	D43.2	D49.6
ischiorectal	C76.3	C79.89	D09.8	D36.7	D48.7	D49.89
middle (cranial)	C71.9	C79.31	—	D33.2	D43.2	D49.6
piriform	C12	C79.89	D00.08	D10.7	D37.05	D49.0
pituitary	C75.1	C79.89	D09.3	D35.2	D44.3	D49.7
posterior (cranial)	C71.9	C79.31	—	D33.2	D43.2	D49.6
pterygoid	C49.0	C79.89	—	D21.0	D48.1	D49.2
pyriform	C12	C79.89	D00.08	D10.7	D37.05	D49.0
Rosenmuller	C11.2	C79.89	D00.08	D10.6	D37.05	D49.0
tonsillar	C09.0	C79.89	D00.08	D10.5	D37.05	D49.0
fourchette	C51.9	C79.82	D07.1	D28.0	D39.8	D49.59
frenulum						
labii — see Neoplasm, lip, internal						

	Malignant Primary	Malignant Secondary	Ca in situ	Benign	Uncertain	Unspecified Behavior
Neoplasm, neoplastic						
— continued						
frenulum — continued						
linguae	C02.2	C79.89	D00.07	D10.1	D37.02	D49.0
frontal						
bone	C41.0	C79.51	—	D16.4	D48.0	D49.2
lobe, brain	C71.1	C79.31	—	D33.0	D43.0	D49.6
pole	C71.1	C79.31	—	D33.0	D43.0	D49.6
sinus	C31.2	C78.39	D02.3	D14.0	D38.5	D49.1
fundus						
stomach	C16.1	C78.89	D00.2	D13.1	D37.1	D49.0
uterus	C54.3	C79.82	D07.0	D26.1	D39.0	D49.59
gallbladder	C23	C78.89	D01.5	D13.5	D37.6	D49.0
overlapping lesion with extrahepatic bile ducts	C24.8	—	—	—	—	—
gall duct (extrahepatic)	C24.0	C78.89	D01.5	D13.5	D37.6	D49.0
intrahepatic	C22.1	C78.7	D01.5	D13.4	D37.6	D49.0
ganglia — see also Neoplasm, nerve, peripheral	C47.9	C79.89	—	D36.10	D48.2	D49.2
basal	C71.0	C79.31	—	D33.0	D43.0	D49.6
cranial nerve	C72.50	C79.49	—	D33.3	D43.3	D49.7
Gartner's duct	C52	C79.82	D07.2	D28.1	D39.8	D49.59
gastric — see Neoplasm, stomach						
gastrocolic	C26.9	C78.89	D01.9	D13.9	D37.9	D49.0
gastroesophageal junction	C16.0	C78.89	D00.2	D13.1	D37.1	D49.0
gastrointestinal (tract) NEC	C26.9	C78.89	D01.9	D13.9	D37.9	D49.0
generalized	C80.0	—	—	—	—	—
genital organ or tract						
female NEC	C57.9	C79.82	D07.30	D28.9	D39.9	D49.59
overlapping lesion	C57.8	—	—	—	—	—
specified site NEC	C57.7	C79.82	D07.39	D28.7	D39.8	D49.59
male NEC	C63.9	C79.82	D07.60	D29.9	D40.9	D49.59
overlapping lesion	C63.8	—	—	—	—	—
specified site NEC	C63.7	C79.82	D07.69	D29.8	D40.8	D49.59
genitourinary tract						
female	C57.9	C79.82	D07.30	D28.9	D39.9	D49.59
male	C63.9	C79.82	D07.60	D29.9	D40.9	D49.59
gingiva (alveolar) (marginal)	C03.9	C79.89	D00.03	D10.39	D37.09	D49.0
lower	C03.1	C79.89	D00.03	D10.39	D37.09	D49.0
mandibular	C03.1	C79.89	D00.03	D10.39	D37.09	D49.0
maxillary	C03.0	C79.89	D00.03	D10.39	D37.09	D49.0
upper	C03.0	C79.89	D00.03	D10.39	D37.09	D49.0
gland, glandular (lymphatic) (system) — see also Neoplasm, lymph gland						
endocrine NEC	C75.9	C79.89	D09.3	D35.9	D44.9	D49.7
salivary — see Neoplasm, salivary gland						
glans penis	C60.1	C79.82	D07.4	D29.0	D40.8	D49.59
globus pallidus	C71.0	C79.31	—	D33.0	D43.0	D49.6
glomus						
coccygeal	C49.5	C79.89	—	D21.5	D48.1	D49.2
jugularis	C75.5	C79.89	—	D35.6	D44.7	D49.7
glosso-epiglottic fold(s)	C10.1	C79.89	D00.08	D10.5	D37.05	D49.0
glossopalatine fold	C09.1	C79.89	D00.08	D10.5	D37.05	D49.0
glossopharyngeal sulcus	C09.0	C79.89	D00.08	D10.5	D37.05	D49.0
glottis	C32.0	C78.39	D02.0	D14.1	D38.0	D49.1
gluteal region	C76.3	C79.89	D04.5	D36.7	D48.7	D49.89
great vessels NEC	C49.3	C79.89	—	D21.3	D48.1	D49.2
groin NEC	C76.3	C79.89	D04.5	D36.7	D48.7	D49.89
gum	C03.9	C79.89	D00.03	D10.39	D37.09	D49.0
lower	C03.1	C79.89	D00.03	D10.39	D37.09	D49.0
upper	C03.0	C79.89	D00.03	D10.39	D37.09	D49.0
hand NEC	C76.4-☑	C79.89	D04.6-☑	D36.7	D48.7	D49.89
head NEC	C76.0	C79.89	D04.4	D36.7	D48.7	D49.89
heart	C38.0	C79.89		D15.1	D48.7	D49.89
Neoplasm, neoplastic						
— continued						
heel NEC	C76.5-☑	C79.89	D04.7-☑	D36.7	D48.7	D49.89
helix — see also Neoplasm, skin, ear	C44.20-☑	C79.2	D04.2-☑	D23.2-☑	D48.5	D49.2
hematopoietic, hemopoietic tissue NEC	C96.9	—	—	—	—	—
specified NEC	C96.Z	—	—	—	—	—
hemisphere, cerebral	C71.0	C79.31		D33.0	D43.0	D49.6
hemorrhoidal zone	C21.1	C78.5	D01.3	D12.9	D37.8	D49.0
hepatic — see also Index to disease, by histology	C22.9	C78.7	D01.5	D13.4	D37.6	D49.0
duct (bile)	C24.0	C78.89	D01.5	D13.5	D37.6	D49.0
flexure (colon)	C18.3	C78.5	D01.0	D12.3	D37.4	D49.0
primary	C22.8	C78.7	D01.5	D13.4	D37.6	D49.0
hepatobiliary	C24.9	C78.89	D01.5	D13.5	D37.6	D49.0
hepatoblastoma	C22.2	C78.7	D01.5	D13.4	D37.6	D49.0
hepatoma	C22.0	C78.7	D01.5	D13.4	D37.6	D49.0
hilus of lung	C34.0-☑	C78.0-☑	D02.2-☑	D14.3-☑	D38.1	D49.1
hippocampus, brain	C71.2	C79.31	—	D33.0	D43.0	D49.6
hip NEC	C76.5-☑	C79.89	D04.7-☑	D36.7	D48.7	D49.89
humerus (any part)	C40.0-☑	C79.51		D16.0-☑		—
hymen	C52	C79.82	D07.2	D28.1	D39.8	D49.59
hypopharynx, hypopharyngeal NEC	C13.9	C79.89	D00.08	D10.7	D37.05	D49.0
overlapping lesion	C13.8	—	—	—	—	—
postcricoid region	C13.0	C79.89	D00.08	D10.7	D37.05	D49.0
posterior wall	C13.2	C79.89	D00.08	D10.7	D37.05	D49.0
pyriform fossa (sinus)	C12	C79.89	D00.08	D10.7	D37.05	D49.0
hypophysis	C75.1	C79.89	D09.3	D35.2	D44.3	D49.7
hypothalamus	C71.0	C79.31	—	D33.0	D43.0	D49.6
ileocecum, ileocecal (coil) (junction) (valve)	C18.0	C78.5	D01.0	D12.0	D37.4	D49.0
ileum	C17.2	C78.4	D01.49	D13.39	D37.2	D49.0
ilium	C41.4	C79.51	—	D16.8	D48.0	D49.2
immunoproliferative NEC	C88.9	—	—	—	—	—
infraclavicular (region)	C76.1	C79.89	D04.5	D36.7	D48.7	D49.89
inguinal (region)	C76.3	C79.89	D04.5	D36.7	D48.7	D49.89
insula	C71.0	C79.31	—	D33.0	D43.0	D49.6
insular tissue (pancreas)	C25.4	C78.89	D01.7	D13.7	D37.8	D49.0
brain	C71.0	C79.31	—	D33.0	D43.0	D49.6
interarytenoid fold	C13.1	C78.39	D00.08	D10.7	D37.05	D49.0
hypopharyngeal aspect	C13.1	C79.89	D00.08	D10.7	D37.05	D49.0
laryngeal aspect	C32.1	C78.39	D02.0	D14.1	D38.0	D49.1
marginal zone	C13.1	C79.89	D00.08	D10.7	D37.05	D49.0
interdental papillae	C03.9	C79.89	D00.03	D10.39	D37.09	D49.0
lower	C03.1	C79.89	D00.03	D10.39	D37.09	D49.0
upper	C03.0	C79.89	D00.03	D10.39	D37.09	D49.0
internal						
capsule	C71.0	C79.31	—	D33.0	D43.0	D49.6
os (cervix)	C53.0	C79.82	D06.0	D26.0	D39.0	D49.59
intervertebral cartilage or disc	C41.2	C79.51	—	D16.6	D48.0	D49.2
intestine, intestinal	C26.0	C78.80	D01.40	D13.9	D37.8	D49.0
large	C18.9	C78.5	D01.0	D12.6	D37.4	D49.0
appendix	C18.1	C78.5	D01.0	D12.1	D37.3	D49.0
caput coli	C18.0	C78.5	D01.0	D12.0	D37.4	D49.0
cecum	C18.0	C78.5	D01.0	D12.0	D37.4	D49.0
colon	C18.9	C78.5	D01.0	D12.6	D37.4	D49.0
and rectum	C19	C78.5	D01.1	D12.7	D37.5	D49.0
ascending	C18.2	C78.5	D01.0	D12.2	D37.4	D49.0
caput	C18.0	C78.5	D01.0	D12.0	D37.4	D49.0
descending	C18.6	C78.5	D01.0	D12.4	D37.4	D49.0
distal	C18.6	C78.5	D01.0	D12.4	D37.4	D49.0

▽ **Subterms under main terms may continue to next column or page**   ☑ **Additional Character Required — Refer to the Tabular List for Character Selection**

	Malignant Primary	Malignant Secondary	Ca in situ	Benign	Uncertain	Unspecified Behavior
Neoplasm, neoplastic						
— *continued*						
intestine, intestinal — *continued*						
large — *continued*						
colon — *continued*						
left	C18.6	C78.5	D01.0	D12.4	D37.4	D49.0
overlapping lesion	C18.8	—	—	—	—	—
pelvic	C18.7	C78.5	D01.0	D12.5	D37.4	D49.0
right	C18.2	C78.5	D01.0	D12.2	D37.4	D49.0
sigmoid (flexure)	C18.7	C78.5	D01.0	D12.5	D37.4	D49.0
transverse	C18.4	C78.5	D01.0	D12.3	D37.4	D49.0
hepatic flexure	C18.3	C78.5	D01.0	D12.3	D37.4	D49.0
ileocecum, ileocecal (coil) (valve)	C18.0	C78.5	D01.0	D12.0	D37.4	D49.0
overlapping lesion	C18.8	—	—	—	—	—
sigmoid flexure (lower) (upper)	C18.7	C78.5	D01.0	D12.5	D37.4	D49.0
splenic flexure	C18.5	C78.5	D01.0	D12.3	D37.4	D49.0
small	C17.9	C78.4	D01.40	D13.30	D37.2	D49.0
duodenum	C17.0	C78.4	D01.49	D13.2	D37.2	D49.0
ileum	C17.2	C78.4	D01.49	D13.39	D37.2	D49.0
jejunum	C17.1	C78.4	D01.49	D13.39	D37.2	D49.0
overlapping lesion	C17.8					
tract NEC	C26.0	C78.89	D01.40	D13.9	D37.8	D49.0
intra-abdominal	C76.2	C79.89	D09.8	D36.7	D48.7	D49.89
intracranial NEC	C71.9	C79.31	—	D33.2	D43.2	D49.6
intrahepatic (bile) duct	C22.1	C78.7	D01.5	D13.4	D37.6	D49.0
intraocular	C69.9-✓	C79.49	D09.2-✓	D31.9-✓	D48.7	D49.89
intraorbital	C69.6-✓	C79.49	D09.2-✓	D31.6-✓	D48.7	D49.89
intrasellar	C75.1	C79.89	D09.3	D35.2	D44.3	D49.7
intrathoracic (cavity) (organs)	C76.1	C79.89	D09.8	D15.9	D48.7	D49.89
specified NEC	C76.1	C79.89	D09.8	D15.7	—	—
iris	C69.4-✓	C79.49	D09.2-✓	D31.4-✓	D48.7	D49.89
ischiorectal (fossa)	C76.3	C79.89	D09.8	D36.7	D48.7	D49.89
ischium	C41.4	C79.51	—	D16.8	D48.0	D49.2
island of Reil	C71.0	C79.31	—	D33.0	D43.0	D49.6
islands or islets of Langerhans	C25.4	C78.89	D01.7	D13.7	D37.8	D49.0
isthmus uteri	C54.0	C79.82	D07.0	D26.1	D39.0	D49.59
jaw	C76.0	C79.89	D09.8	D36.7	D48.7	D49.89
bone	C41.1	C79.51	—	D16.5	D48.0	D49.2
lower	C41.1	C79.51	—	D16.5	—	—
upper	C41.0	C79.51	—	D16.4	—	—
carcinoma (any type) (lower) (upper)	C76.0	C79.89	—	—	—	—
skin — *see also* Neoplasm, skin, face	C44.309	C79.2	D04.39	D23.39	D48.5	D49.2
soft tissues	C03.9	C79.89	D00.03	D10.39	D37.09	D49.0
lower	C03.1	C79.89	D00.03	D10.39	D37.09	D49.0
upper	C03.0	C79.89	D00.03	D10.39	D37.09	D49.0
jejunum	C17.1	C78.4	D01.49	D13.39	D37.2	D49.0
joint NEC — *see also* Neoplasm, bone	C41.9	C79.51	—	D16.9	D48.0	D49.2
acromioclavicular	C40.0-✓	C79.51	—	D16.0-✓	—	—
bursa or synovial membrane — *see* Neoplasm, connective tissue						
costovertebral	C41.3	C79.51	—	D16.7	D48.0	D49.2
sternocostal	C41.3	C79.51	—	D16.7	D48.0	D49.2
temporomandibular	C41.1	C79.51	—	D16.5	D48.0	D49.2
junction						
anorectal	C21.8	C78.5	D01.3	D12.9	D37.8	D49.0
cardioesophageal	C16.0	C78.89	D00.2	D13.1	D37.1	D49.0
esophagogastric	C16.0	C78.89	D00.2	D13.1	D37.1	D49.0
gastroesophageal	C16.0	C78.89	D00.2	D13.1	D37.1	D49.0
hard and soft palate	C05.9	C79.89	D00.00	D10.39	D37.09	D49.0
ileocecal	C18.0	C78.5	D01.0	D12.0	D37.4	D49.0

	Malignant Primary	Malignant Secondary	Ca in situ	Benign	Uncertain	Unspecified Behavior
Neoplasm, neoplastic						
— *continued*						
junction — *continued*						
pelvirectal	C19	C78.5	D01.1	D12.7	D37.5	D49.0
pelviureteric	C65.-✓	C79.0-✓	D09.19	D30.1-✓	D41.1-✓	D49.59
rectosigmoid	C19	C78.5	D01.1	D12.7	D37.5	D49.0
squamocolumnar, of cervix	C53.8	C79.82	D06.7	D26.0	D39.0	D49.59
Kaposi's sarcoma — *see* Kaposi's, sarcoma						
kidney (parenchymal)	C64.-✓	C79.0-✓	D09.19	D30.0-✓	D41.0-✓	D49.51-✓
calyx	C65.-✓	C79.0-✓	D09.19	D30.1-✓	D41.1-✓	D49.51-✓
hilus	C65.-✓	C79.0-✓	D09.19	D30.1-✓	D41.1-✓	D49.51-✓
pelvis	C65.-✓	C79.0-✓	D09.19	D30.1-✓	D41.1-✓	D49.51-✓
knee NEC	C76.5-✓	C79.89	D04.7-✓	D36.7	D48.7	D49.89
labia (skin)	C51.9	C79.82	D07.1	D28.0	D39.8	D49.59
majora	C51.0	C79.82	D07.1	D28.0	D39.8	D49.59
minora	C51.1	C79.82	D07.1	D28.0	D39.8	D49.59
labial — *see also* Neoplasm, lip	C00.9	C79.89	D00.01	D10.0	D37.01	D49.0
sulcus (lower) (upper)	C06.1	C79.89	D00.02	D10.39	D37.09	D49.0
labium (skin)	C51.9	C79.82	D07.1	D28.0	D39.8	D49.59
majus	C51.0	C79.82	D07.1	D28.0	D39.8	D49.59
minus	C51.1	C79.82	D07.1	D28.0	D39.8	D49.59
lacrimal						
canaliculi	C69.5-✓	C79.49	D09.2-✓	D31.5-✓	D48.7	D49.89
duct (nasal)	C69.5-✓	C79.49	D09.2-✓	D31.5-✓	D48.7	D49.89
gland	C69.5-✓	C79.49	D09.2-✓	D31.5-✓	D48.7	D49.89
punctum	C69.5-✓	C79.49	D09.2-✓	D31.5-✓	D48.7	D49.89
sac	C69.5-✓	C79.49	D09.2-✓	D31.5-✓	D48.7	D49.89
Langerhans, islands or islets	C25.4	C78.89	D01.7	D13.7	D37.8	D49.0
laryngopharynx	C13.9	C79.89	D00.08	D10.7	D37.05	D49.0
larynx, laryngeal NEC	C32.9	C78.39	D02.0	D14.1	D38.0	D49.1
aryepiglottic fold	C32.1	C78.39	D02.0	D14.1	D38.0	D49.1
cartilage (arytenoid) (cricoid) (cuneiform) (thyroid)	C32.3	C78.39	D02.0	D14.1	D38.0	D49.1
commissure (anterior) (posterior)	C32.0	C78.39	D02.0	D14.1	D38.0	D49.1
extrinsic NEC	C32.1	C78.39	D02.0	D14.1	D38.0	D49.1
meaning hypopharynx	C13.9	C79.89	D00.08	D10.7	D37.05	D49.0
interarytenoid fold	C32.1	C78.39	D02.0	D14.1	D38.0	D49.1
intrinsic	C32.0	C78.39	D02.0	D14.1	D38.0	D49.1
overlapping lesion	C32.8	—	—	—	—	—
ventricular band	C32.1	C78.39	D02.0	D14.1	D38.0	D49.1
leg NEC	C76.5-✓	C79.89	D04.7-✓	D36.7	D48.7	D49.89
lens, crystalline	C69.4-✓	C79.49	D09.2-✓	D31.4-✓	D48.7	D49.89
lid (lower) (upper)	C44.10-✓	C79.2	D04.1-✓	D23.1-✓	D48.5	D49.2
basal cell carcinoma	C44.11-✓	—	—	—	—	—
sebaceous cell	C44.13-✓	—	—	—	—	—
specified type NEC	C44.19-✓	—	—	—	—	—
squamous cell carcinoma	C44.12-✓	—	—	—	—	—
ligament — *see also* Neoplasm, connective tissue						
broad	C57.1-✓	C79.82	D07.39	D28.2	D39.8	D49.59
Mackenrodt's	C57.7	C79.82	D07.39	D28.7	D39.8	D49.59
non-uterine — *see* Neoplasm, connective tissue						
round	C57.2-✓	C79.82	—	D28.2	D39.8	D49.59
sacro-uterine	C57.3	C79.82	—	D28.2	D39.8	D49.59
uterine	C57.3	C79.82	—	D28.2	D39.8	D49.59
utero-ovarian	C57.7	C79.82	D07.39	D28.2	D39.8	D49.59
uterosacral	C57.3	C79.82	—	D28.2	D39.8	D49.59
limb	C76.8	C79.89	D04.8	D36.7	D48.7	D49.89
lower	C76.5-✓	C79.89	D04.7-✓	D36.7	D48.7	D49.89
upper	C76.4-✓	C79.89	D04.6-✓	D36.7	D48.7	D49.89
limbus of cornea	C69.1-✓	C79.49	D09.2-✓	D31.1-✓	D48.7	D49.89

✓ Additional Character Required — Refer to the Tabular List for Character Selection   ▽ Subterms under main terms may continue to next column or page

Neoplasm, neoplastic	Malignant Primary	Malignant Secondary	Ca in situ	Benign	Uncertain	Unspecified Behavior
— *continued*						
lingual NEC — *see also* Neoplasm, tongue	C02.9	C79.89	D00.07	D10.1	D37.02	D49.0
lingula, lung	C34.1-☑	C78.0-☑	D02.2-☑	D14.3-☑	D38.1	D49.1
lip	C00.9	C79.89	D00.01	D10.0	D37.01	D49.0
buccal aspect — *see* Neoplasm, lip, internal						
commissure	C00.6	C79.89	D00.01	D10.0	D37.01	D49.0
external	C00.2	C79.89	D00.01	D10.0	D37.01	D49.0
lower	C00.1	C79.89	D00.01	D10.0	D37.01	D49.0
upper	C00.0	C79.89	D00.01	D10.0	D37.01	D49.0
frenulum — *see* Neoplasm, lip, internal						
inner aspect — *see* Neoplasm, lip, internal						
internal	C00.5	C79.89	D00.01	D10.0	D37.01	D49.0
lower	C00.4	C79.89	D00.01	D10.0	D37.01	D49.0
upper	C00.3	C79.89	D00.01	D10.0	D37.01	D49.0
lipstick area	C00.2	C79.89	D00.01	D10.0	D37.01	D49.0
lower	C00.1	C79.89	D00.01	D10.0	D37.01	D49.0
upper	C00.0	C79.89	D00.01	D10.0	D37.01	D49.0
lower	C00.1	C79.89	D00.01	D10.0	D37.01	D49.0
internal	C00.4	C79.89	D00.01	D10.0	D37.01	D49.0
mucosa — *see* Neoplasm, lip, internal						
oral aspect — *see* Neoplasm, lip, internal						
overlapping lesion	C00.8	—	—	—	—	—
with oral cavity or pharynx	C14.8	—	—	—	—	—
skin (commissure) (lower) (upper)	C44.00	C79.2	D04.0	D23.0	D48.5	D49.2
basal cell carcinoma	C44.01	—	—	—	—	—
specified type NEC	C44.09	—	—	—	—	—
squamous cell carcinoma	C44.02	—	—	—	—	—
upper	C00.0	C79.89	D00.01	D10.0	D37.01	D49.0
internal	C00.3	C79.89	D00.01	D10.0	D37.01	D49.0
vermilion border	C00.2	C79.89	D00.01	D10.0	D37.01	D49.0
lower	C00.1	C79.89	D00.01	D10.0	D37.01	D49.0
upper	C00.0	C79.89	D00.01	D10.0	D37.01	D49.0
lipomatous — *see* Lipoma, by site						
liver — *see also* Index to disease, by histology	C22.9	C78.7	D01.5	D13.4	D37.6	D49.0
primary	C22.8	C78.7	D01.5	D13.4	D37.6	D49.0
lumbosacral plexus	C47.5	C79.89	—	D36.16	D48.2	D49.2
lung	C34.9-☑	C78.0-☑	D02.2-☑	D14.3-☑	D38.1	D49.1
azygos lobe	C34.1-☑	C78.0-☑	D02.2-☑	D14.3-☑	D38.1	D49.1
carina	C34.0-☑	C78.0-☑	D02.2-☑	D14.3-☑	D38.1	D49.1
hilus	C34.0-☑	C78.0-☑	D02.2-☑	D14.3-☑	D38.1	D49.1
linqula	C34.1-☑	C78.0-☑	D02.2-☑	D14.3-☑	D38.1	D49.1
lobe NEC	C34.9-☑	C78.0-☑	D02.2-☑	D14.3-☑	D38.1	D49.1
lower lobe	C34.3-☑	C78.0-☑	D02.2-☑	D14.3-☑	D38.1	D49.1
main bronchus	C34.0-☑	C78.0-☑	D02.2-☑	D14.3-☑	D38.1	D49.1
mesothelioma — *see* Mesothelioma						
middle lobe	C34.2	C78.0-☑	D02.21	D14.31	D38.1	D49.1
overlapping lesion	C34.8-☑	—	—	—	—	—
upper lobe	C34.1-☑	C78.0-☑	D02.2-☑	D14.3-☑	D38.1	D49.1
lymph, lymphatic channel NEC	C49.9	C79.89	—	D21.9	D48.1	D49.2
gland (secondary)	—	C77.9	—	D36.0	D48.7	D49.89
abdominal	—	C77.2	—	D36.0	D48.7	D49.89
aortic	—	C77.2	—	D36.0	D48.7	D49.89
arm	—	C77.3	—	D36.0	D48.7	D49.89

Neoplasm, neoplastic	Malignant Primary	Malignant Secondary	Ca in situ	Benign	Uncertain	Unspecified Behavior
— *continued*						
lymph, lymphatic channel — *continued*						
gland — *continued*						
auricular (anterior) (posterior)	—	C77.0	—	D36.0	D48.7	D49.89
axilla, axillary	—	C77.3	—	D36.0	D48.7	D49.89
brachial	—	C77.3	—	D36.0	D48.7	D49.89
bronchial	—	C77.1	—	D36.0	D48.7	D49.89
bronchopulmonary	—	C77.1	—	D36.0	D48.7	D49.89
celiac	—	C77.2	—	D36.0	D48.7	D49.89
cervical	—	C77.0	—	D36.0	D48.7	D49.89
cervicofacial	—	C77.0	—	D36.0	D48.7	D49.89
Cloquet	—	C77.4	—	D36.0	D48.7	D49.89
colic	—	C77.2	—	D36.0	D48.7	D49.89
common duct	—	C77.2	—	D36.0	D48.7	D49.89
cubital	—	C77.3	—	D36.0	D48.7	D49.89
diaphragmatic	—	C77.1	—	D36.0	D48.7	
epigastric, inferior	—	C77.1	—	D36.0	D48.7	D49.89
epitrochlear	—	C77.3	—	D36.0	D48.7	D49.89
esophageal	—	C77.1	—	D36.0	D48.7	D49.89
face	—	C77.0	—	D36.0	D48.7	D49.89
femoral	—	C77.4	—	D36.0	D48.7	D49.89
gastric	—	C77.2	—	D36.0	D48.7	D49.89
groin	—	C77.4	—	D36.0	D48.7	D49.89
head	—	C77.0	—	D36.0	D48.7	D49.89
hepatic	—	C77.2	—	D36.0	D48.7	D49.89
hilar (pulmonary)	—	C77.1	—	D36.0	D48.7	D49.89
splenic	—	C77.2	—	D36.0	D48.7	D49.89
hypogastric	—	C77.5	—	D36.0	D48.7	D49.89
ileocolic	—	C77.2	—	D36.0	D48.7	D49.89
iliac	—	C77.5	—	D36.0	D48.7	D49.89
infraclavicular	—	C77.3	—	D36.0	D48.7	D49.89
inguina, inguinal	—	C77.4	—	D36.0	D48.7	D49.89
innominate	—	C77.1	—	D36.0	D48.7	D49.89
intercostal	—	C77.1	—	D36.0	D48.7	D49.89
intestinal	—	C77.2	—	D36.0	D48.7	D49.89
intrabdominal	—	C77.2	—	D36.0	D48.7	D49.89
intrapelvic	—	C77.5	—	D36.0	D48.7	D49.89
intrathoracic	—	C77.1	—	D36.0	D48.7	D49.89
jugular	—	C77.0	—	D36.0	D48.7	D49.89
leg	—	C77.4	—	D36.0	D48.7	D49.89
limb						
lower	—	C77.4	—	D36.0	D48.7	D49.89
upper	—	C77.3	—	D36.0	D48.7	D49.89
lower limb	—	C77.4	—	D36.0	D48.7	D49.89
lumbar	—	C77.2	—	D36.0	D48.7	D49.89
mandibular	—	C77.0	—	D36.0	D48.7	D49.89
mediastinal	—	C77.1	—	D36.0	D48.7	D49.89
mesenteric (inferior) (superior)	—	C77.2	—	D36.0	D48.7	D49.89
midcolic	—	C77.2	—	D36.0	D48.7	
multiple sites in categories C77.0 - C77.5	—	C77.8	—	D36.0	D48.7	D49.89
neck	—	C77.0	—	D36.0	D48.7	D49.89
obturator	—	C77.5	—	D36.0	D48.7	D49.89
occipital	—	C77.0	—	D36.0	D48.7	D49.89
pancreatic	—	C77.2	—	D36.0	D48.7	D49.89
para-aortic	—	C77.2	—	D36.0	D48.7	D49.89
paracervical	—	C77.5	—	D36.0	D48.7	D49.89
parametrial	—	C77.5	—	D36.0	D48.7	D49.89
parasternal	—	C77.1	—	D36.0	D48.7	D49.89
parotid	—	C77.0	—	D36.0	D48.7	D49.89
pectoral	—	C77.3	—	D36.0	D48.7	D49.89
pelvic	—	C77.5	—	D36.0	D48.7	D49.89
peri-aortic	—	C77.2	—	D36.0	D48.7	D49.89
peripancreatic	—	C77.2	—	D36.0	D48.7	D49.89
popliteal	—	C77.4	—	D36.0	D48.7	D49.89
porta hepatis	—	C77.2	—	D36.0	D48.7	D49.89
portal	—	C77.2	—	D36.0	D48.7	D49.89
preauricular	—	C77.0	—	D36.0	D48.7	D49.89
prelaryngeal	—	C77.0	—	D36.0	D48.7	D49.89
presymphysial	—	C77.5	—	D36.0	D48.7	D49.89
pretracheal	—	C77.0	—	D36.0	D48.7	D49.89
primary (any site) NEC	C96.9	—	—	—	—	—

Neoplasm

	Malignant Primary	Malignant Secondary	Ca in situ	Benign	Uncertain	Unspecified Behavior
Neoplasm, neoplastic						
— *continued*						
lymph, lymphatic						
channel —						
continued						
gland — *continued*						
pulmonary						
(hiler)	—	C77.1	—	D36.0	D48.7	D49.89
pyloric	—	C77.2	—	D36.0	D48.7	D49.89
retroperitoneal	—	C77.2	—	D36.0	D48.7	D49.89
retropharyngeal	—	C77.0	—	D36.0	D48.7	D49.89
Rosenmuller's	—	C77.4	—	D36.0	D48.7	D49.89
sacral	—	C77.5	—	D36.0	D48.7	D49.89
scalene	—	C77.0	—	D36.0	D48.7	D49.89
site NEC	—	C77.9	—	D36.0	D48.7	D49.89
splenic (hilar)	—	C77.2	—	D36.0	D48.7	D49.89
subclavicular	—	C77.3	—	D36.0	D48.7	D49.89
subinguinal	—	C77.4	—	D36.0	D48.7	D49.89
sublingual	—	C77.0	—	D36.0	D48.7	D49.89
submandibular	—	C77.0	—	D36.0	D48.7	D49.89
submaxillary	—	C77.0	—	D36.0	D48.7	D49.89
submental	—	C77.0	—	D36.0	D48.7	D49.89
subscapular	—	C77.3	—	D36.0	D48.7	D49.89
supraclavicular	—	C77.0	—	D36.0	D48.7	D49.89
thoracic	—	C77.1	—	D36.0	D48.7	D49.89
tibial	—	C77.4	—	D36.0	D48.7	D49.89
tracheal	—	C77.1	—	D36.0	D48.7	D49.89
tracheobronchial	—	C77.1	—	D36.0	D48.7	D49.89
upper limb	—	C77.3	—	D36.0	D48.7	D49.89
Virchow's	—	C77.0	—	D36.0	D48.7	D49.89
node — *see also*						
Neoplasm, lymph						
gland						
primary NEC	C96.9	—		—	—	—
vessel — *see also*						
Neoplasm,						
connective						
tissue	C49.9	C79.89	—	D21.9	D48.1	D49.2
Mackenrodt's						
ligament	C57.7	C79.82	D07.39	D28.7	D39.8	D49.59
malar	C41.0	C79.51	—	D16.4	D48.0	D49.2
region — *see*						
Neoplasm, cheek						
mammary gland — *see*						
Neoplasm, breast						
mandible	C41.1	C79.51	—	D16.5	D48.0	D49.2
alveolar						
mucosa						
(carcinoma)	C03.1	C79.89	D00.03	D10.39	D37.09	D49.0
ridge or						
process	C41.1	C79.51	—	D16.5	D48.0	D49.2
marrow (bone)						
NEC	C96.9	C79.52	—	—	D47.9	D49.89
mastectomy site (skin)						
— *see also*						
Neoplasm, breast,						
skin	C44.501	C79.2	—	—	—	—
specified as breast						
tissue	C50.8-☑	C79.81	—	—	—	—
mastoid (air cells)						
(antrum)						
(cavity)	C30.1	C78.39	D02.3	D14.0	D38.5	D49.1
bone or process	C41.0	C79.51	—	D16.4	D48.0	D49.2
maxilla, maxillary						
(superior)	C41.0	C79.51	—	D16.4	D48.0	D49.2
alveolar						
mucosa	C03.0	C79.89	D00.03	D10.39	D37.09	D49.0
ridge or process						
(carcinoma)	C41.0	C79.51	—	D16.4	D48.0	D49.2
antrum	C31.0	C78.39	D02.3	D14.0	D38.5	D49.1
carcinoma	C03.0	C79.51	—	—	—	—
inferior — *see*						
Neoplasm,						
mandible						
sinus	C31.0	C78.39	D02.3	D14.0	D38.5	D49.1
meatus external (ear)						
— *see also*						
Neoplasm, skin,						
ear	C44.20-☑	C79.2	D04.2-☑	D23.2-☑	D48.5	D49.2
Meckel diverticulum,						
malignant	C17.3	C78.4	D01.49	D13.39	D37.2	D49.0
mediastinum,						
mediastinal	C38.3	C78.1	—	D15.2	D38.3	D49.89
anterior	C38.1	C78.1	—	D15.2	D38.3	D49.89

	Malignant Primary	Malignant Secondary	Ca in situ	Benign	Uncertain	Unspecified Behavior
Neoplasm, neoplastic						
— *continued*						
mediastinum,						
mediastinal —						
continued						
posterior	C38.2	C78.1	—	D15.2	D38.3	D49.89
medulla						
adrenal	C74.1-☑	C79.7-☑	D09.3	D35.0-☑	D44.1-☑	D49.7
oblongata	C71.7	C79.31	—	D33.1	D43.1	D49.6
meibomian gland	C44.10-☑	C79.2	D04.1-☑	D23.1-☑	D48.5	D49.2
basal cell						
carcinoma	C44.11-☑	—	—	—	—	—
sebaceous cell	C44.13-☑	—	—	—	—	—
specified type						
NEC	C44.19-☑	—	—	—	—	—
squamous cell						
carcinoma	C44.12-☑	—	—	—	—	—
melanoma — *see*						
Melanoma						
meninges	C70.9	C79.49	—	D32.9	D42.9	D49.7
brain	C70.0	C79.32	—	D32.0	D42.0	D49.7
cerebral	C70.0	C79.32	—	D32.0	D42.0	D49.7
crainial	C70.0	C79.32	—	D32.0	D42.0	D49.7
intracranial	C70.0	C79.32	—	D32.0	D42.0	D49.7
spinal (cord)	C70.1	C79.49	—	D32.1	D42.1	D49.7
meniscus, knee joint						
(lateral)						
(medial)	C40.2-☑	C79.51	—	D16.2-☑	D48.0	D49.2
Merkel cell — *see*						
Carcinoma, Merkel						
cell						
mesentery,						
mesenteric	C48.1	C78.6	—	D20.1	D48.4	D49.0
mesoappendix	C48.1	C78.6	—	D20.1	D48.4	D49.0
mesocolon	C48.1	C78.6	—	D20.1	D48.4	D49.0
mesopharynx — *see*						
Neoplasm,						
oropharynx						
mesosalpinx	C57.1-☑	C79.82	D07.39	D28.2	D39.8	D49.59
mesothelial tissue —						
see Mesothelioma						
mesothelioma — *see*						
Mesothelioma						
mesovarium	C57.1-☑	C79.82	D07.39	D28.2	D39.8	D49.59
metacarpus (any						
bone)	C40.1-☑	C79.51	—	D16.1-☑	—	—
metastatic NEC — *see*						
also Neoplasm, by						
site,						
secondary	—	C79.9		—	—	—
metatarsus (any						
bone)	C40.3-☑	C79.51	—	D16.3-☑	—	—
midbrain	C71.7	C79.31	—	D33.1	D43.1	D49.6
milk duct — *see*						
Neoplasm, breast						
mons						
pubis	C51.9	C79.82	D07.1	D28.0	D39.8	D49.59
veneris	C51.9	C79.82	D07.1	D28.0	D39.8	D49.59
motor tract	C72.9	C79.49	—	D33.9	D43.9	D49.7
brain	C71.9	C79.31	—	D33.2	D43.2	D49.6
cauda equina	C72.1	C79.49	—	D33.4	D43.4	D49.7
spinal	C72.0	C79.49	—	D33.4	D43.4	D49.7
mouth	C06.9	C79.89	D00.00	D10.30	D37.09	D49.0
book-leaf	C06.89	C79.89	—	—	—	—
floor	C04.9	C79.89	D00.06	D10.2	D37.09	D49.0
anterior						
portion	C04.0	C79.89	D00.06	D10.2	D37.09	D49.0
lateral portion	C04.1	C79.89	D00.06	D10.2	D37.09	D49.0
overlapping						
lesion	C04.8	—	—	—	—	—
overlapping						
NEC	C06.80	—	—	—	—	—
roof	C05.9	C79.89	D00.00	D10.39	D37.09	D49.0
specified part						
NEC	C06.89	C79.89	D00.00	D10.39	D37.09	D49.0
vestibule	C06.1	C79.89	D00.00	D10.39	D37.09	D49.0
mucosa						
alveolar (ridge or						
process)	C03.9	C79.89	D00.03	D10.39	D37.09	D49.0
lower	C03.1	C79.89	D00.03	D10.39	D37.09	D49.0
upper	C03.0	C79.89	D00.03	D10.39	D37.09	D49.0
buccal	C06.0	C79.89	D00.02	D10.39	D37.09	D49.0
cheek	C06.0	C79.89	D00.02	D10.39	D37.09	D49.0

☑ Additional Character Required — Refer to the Tabular List for Character Selection   ▽ Subterms under main terms may continue to next column or page

Neoplasm, neoplastic — continued

	Malignant Primary	Malignant Secondary	Ca in situ	Benign	Uncertain	Unspecified Behavior
mucosa — continued						
lip — see Neoplasm, lip, internal						
nasal	C30.0	C78.39	D02.3	D14.0	D38.5	D49.1
oral	C06.0	C79.89	D00.02	D10.39	D37.09	D49.0
Mullerian duct						
female	C57.7	C79.82	D07.39	D28.7	D39.8	D49.59
male	C63.7	C79.82	D07.69	D29.8	D40.8	D49.59
muscle — see also Neoplasm, connective tissue						
extraocular	C69.6-✓	C79.49	D09.2-✓	D31.6-✓	D48.7	D49.89
myocardium	C38.0	C79.49	—	D15.1	D48.7	D49.89
myometrium	C54.2	C79.82	D07.0	D26.1	D39.0	D49.59
myopericardium	C38.0	C79.89	—	D15.1	D48.7	D49.89
nabothian gland (follicle)	C53.0	C79.82	D06.0	D26.0	D39.0	D49.59
nail — see also Neoplasm, skin, limb	C44.90	C79.2	D04.9	D23.9	D48.5	D49.2
finger — see also Neoplasm, skin, limb, upper	C44.60-✓	C79.2	D04.6-✓	D23.6-✓	D48.5	D49.2
toe — see also Neoplasm, skin, limb, lower	C44.70-✓	C79.2	D04.7-✓	D23.7-✓	D48.5	D49.2
nares, naris (anterior) (posterior)	C30.0	C78.39	D02.3	D14.0	D38.5	D49.1
nasal — see Neoplasm, nose						
nasolabial groove — see also Neoplasm, skin, face	C44.309	C79.2	D04.39	D23.39	D48.5	D49.2
nasolacrimal duct	C69.5-✓	C79.49	D09.2-✓	D31.5-✓	D48.7	D49.89
nasopharynx, nasopharyngeal	C11.9	C79.89	D00.08	D10.6	D37.05	D49.0
floor	C11.3	C79.89	D00.08	D10.6	D37.05	D49.0
overlapping lesion	C11.8	—	—	—	—	—
roof	C11.0	C79.89	D00.08	D10.6	D37.05	D49.0
wall	C11.9	C79.89	D00.08	D10.6	D37.05	D49.0
anterior	C11.3	C79.89	D00.08	D10.6	D37.05	D49.0
lateral	C11.2	C79.89	D00.08	D10.6	D37.05	D49.0
posterior	C11.1	C79.89	D00.08	D10.6	D37.05	D49.0
superior	C11.0	C79.89	D00.08	D10.6	D37.05	D49.0
nates — see also Neoplasm, skin, trunk	C44.509	C79.2	D04.5	D23.5	D48.5	D49.2
neck NEC	C76.0	C79.89	D09.8	D36.7	D48.7	D49.89
skin	C44.40	—	—	—	—	—
basal cell carcinoma	C44.41	—	—	—	—	—
specified type NEC	C44.49	—	—	—	—	—
squamous cell carcinoma	C44.42	—	—	—	—	—
nerve (ganglion)	C47.9	C79.89	—	D36.10	D48.2	D49.2
abducens	C72.59	C79.49	—	D33.3	D43.3	D49.7
accessory (spinal)	C72.59	C79.49	—	D33.3	D43.3	D49.7
acoustic	C72.4-✓	C79.49	—	D33.3	D43.3	D49.7
auditory	C72.4-✓	C79.49	—	D33.3	D43.3	D49.7
autonomic NEC — see also Neoplasm, nerve, peripheral	C47.9	C79.89	—	D36.10	D48.2	D49.2
brachial	C47.1-✓	C79.89	—	D36.12	D48.2	D49.2
cranial	C72.50	C79.49	—	D33.3	D43.3	D49.7
specified NEC	C72.59	C79.49	—	D33.3	D43.3	D49.7
facial	C72.59	C79.49	—	D33.3	D43.3	D49.7
femoral	C47.2-✓	C79.89	—	D36.13	D48.2	D49.2
ganglion NEC — see also Neoplasm, nerve, peripheral	C47.9	C79.89	—	D36.10	D48.2	D49.2
glossopharyngeal	C72.59	C79.49	—	D33.3	D43.3	D49.7
hypoglossal	C72.59	C79.49	—	D33.3	D43.3	D49.7
intercostal	C47.3	C79.89	—	D36.14	D48.2	D49.2
lumbar	C47.6	C79.89	—	D36.17	D48.2	D49.2
median	C47.1-✓	C79.89	—	D36.12	D48.2	D49.2
obturator	C47.2-✓	C79.89	—	D36.13	D48.2	D49.2

Neoplasm, neoplastic — continued

	Malignant Primary	Malignant Secondary	Ca in situ	Benign	Uncertain	Unspecified Behavior
nerve — continued						
oculomotor	C72.59	C79.49	—	D33.3	D43.3	D49.7
olfactory	C47.2-✓	C79.49	—	D33.3	D43.3	D49.7
optic	C72.3-✓	C79.49	—	D33.3	D43.3	D49.7
parasympathetic NEC	C47.9	C79.89	—	D36.10	D48.2	D49.2
peripheral NEC	C47.9	C79.89	—	D36.10	D48.2	D49.2
abdomen	C47.4	C79.89	—	D36.15	D48.2	D49.2
abdominal wall	C47.4	C79.89	—	D36.15	D48.2	D49.2
ankle	C47.2-✓	C79.89	—	D36.13	D48.2	D49.2
antecubital fossa or space	C47.1-✓	C79.89	—	D36.12	D48.2	D49.2
arm	C47.1-✓	C79.89	—	D36.12	D48.2	D49.2
auricle (ear)	C47.0	C79.89	—	D36.11	D48.2	D49.2
axilla	C47.3	C79.89	—	D36.12	D48.2	D49.2
back	C47.6	C79.89	—	D36.17	D48.2	D49.2
buttock	C47.5	C79.89	—	D36.16	D48.2	D49.2
calf	C47.2-✓	C79.89	—	D36.13	D48.2	D49.2
cervical region	C47.0	C79.89	—	D36.11	D48.2	D49.2
cheek	C47.0	C79.89	—	D36.11	D48.2	D49.2
chest (wall)	C47.3	C79.89	—	D36.14	D48.2	D49.2
chin	C47.0	C79.89	—	D36.11	D48.2	D49.2
ear (external)	C47.0	C79.89	—	D36.11	D48.2	D49.2
elbow	C47.1-✓	C79.89	—	D36.12	D48.2	D49.2
extrarectal	C47.5	C79.89	—	D36.16	D48.2	D49.2
extremity	C47.9	C79.89	—	D36.10	D48.2	D49.2
lower	C47.2-✓	C79.89	—	D36.13	D48.2	D49.2
upper	C47.1-✓	C79.89	—	D36.12	D48.2	D49.2
eyelid	C47.0	C79.89	—	D36.11	D48.2	D49.2
face	C47.0	C79.89	—	D36.11	D48.2	D49.2
finger	C47.1-✓	C79.89	—	D36.12	D48.2	D49.2
flank	C47.6	C79.89	—	D36.17	D48.2	D49.2
foot	C47.2-✓	C79.89	—	D36.13	D48.2	D49.2
forearm	C47.1-✓	C79.89	—	D36.12	D48.2	D49.2
forehead	C47.0	C79.89	—	D36.11	D48.2	D49.2
gluteal region	C47.5	C79.89	—	D36.16	D48.2	D49.2
groin	C47.5	C79.89	—	D36.16	D48.2	D49.2
hand	C47.1-✓	C79.89	—	D36.12	D48.2	D49.2
head	C47.0	C79.89	—	D36.11	D48.2	D49.2
heel	C47.2-✓	C79.89	—	D36.13	D48.2	D49.2
hip	C47.2-✓	C79.89	—	D36.13	D48.2	D49.2
infraclavicular region	C47.3	C79.89	—	D36.14	D48.2	D49.2
inguinal (canal) (region)	C47.5	C79.89	—	D36.16	D48.2	D49.2
intrathoracic	C47.3	C79.89	—	D36.14	D48.2	D49.2
ischiorectal fossa	C47.5	C79.89	—	D36.16	D48.2	D49.2
knee	C47.2-✓	C79.89	—	D36.13	D48.2	D49.2
leg	C47.2-✓	C79.89	—	D36.13	D48.2	D49.2
limb NEC	C47.9	C79.89	—	D36.10	D48.2	D49.2
lower	C47.2-✓	C79.89	—	D36.13	D48.2	D49.2
upper	C47.1-✓	C79.89	—	D36.12	D48.2	D49.2
nates	C47.5	C79.89	—	D36.16	D48.2	D49.2
neck	C47.0	C79.89	—	D36.11	D48.2	D49.2
orbit	C69.6-✓	C79.49	—	D31.6-✓	D48.7	D49.2
pararectal	C47.5	C79.89	—	D36.16	D48.2	D49.2
paraurethral	C47.5	C79.89	—	D36.16	D48.2	D49.2
paravaginal	C47.5	C79.89	—	D36.16	D48.2	D49.2
pelvis (floor)	C47.5	C79.89	—	D36.16	D48.2	D49.2
pelvoabdominal	C47.8	C79.89	—	D36.17	D48.2	D49.2
perineum	C47.5	C79.89	—	D36.16	D48.2	D49.2
perirectal (tissue)	C47.5	C79.89	—	D36.16	D48.2	D49.2
periurethral (tissue)	C47.5	C79.89	—	D36.16	D48.2	D49.2
popliteal fossa or space	C47.2-✓	C79.89	—	D36.13	D48.2	D49.2
presacral	C47.5	C79.89	—	D36.16	D48.2	D49.2
pterygoid fossa	C47.0	C79.89	—	D36.11	D48.2	D49.2
rectovaginal septum or wall	C47.5	C79.89	—	D36.16	D48.2	D49.2
rectovesical	C47.5	C79.89	—	D36.16	D48.2	D49.2
sacrococcygeal region	C47.5	C79.89	—	D36.16	D48.2	D49.2
scalp	C47.0	C79.89	—	D36.11	D48.2	D49.2

Neoplasm, neoplastic — continued

	Malignant Primary	Malignant Secondary	Ca in situ	Benign	Uncertain	Unspecified Behavior
nerve — continued						
peripheral — continued						
scapular region	C47.3	C79.89	—	D36.14	D48.2	D49.2
shoulder	C47.1-☑	C79.89	—	D36.12	D48.2	D49.2
submental	C47.0	C79.89	—	D36.11	D48.2	D49.2
supraclavicular region	C47.0	C79.89	—	D36.11	D48.2	D49.2
temple	C47.0	C79.89	—	D36.11	D48.2	D49.2
temporal region	C47.0	C79.89	—	D36.11	D48.2	D49.2
thigh	C47.2-☑	C79.89	—	D36.13	D48.2	D49.2
thoracic (duct) (wall)	C47.3	C79.89	—	D36.14	D48.2	D49.2
thorax	C47.3	C79.89	—	D36.14	D48.2	D49.2
thumb	C47.1-☑	C79.89	—	D36.12	D48.2	D49.2
toe	C47.2-☑	C79.89	—	D36.13	D48.2	D49.2
trunk	C47.6	C79.89	—	D36.17	D48.2	D49.2
umbilicus	C47.4	C79.89	—	D36.15	D48.2	D49.2
vesicorectal	C47.5	C79.89	—	D36.16	D48.2	D49.2
wrist	C47.1-☑	C79.89	—	D36.12	D48.2	D49.2
radial	C47.1-☑	C79.89	—	D36.12	D48.2	D49.2
sacral	C47.5	C79.89	—	D36.16	D48.2	D49.2
sciatic	C47.2-☑	C79.89	—	D36.13	D48.2	D49.2
spinal NEC	C47.9	C79.89	—	D36.10	D48.2	D49.2
accessory	C72.59	C79.49	—	D33.3	D43.3	D49.7
sympathetic NEC — see also Neoplasm, nerve, peripheral	C47.9	C79.89	—	D36.10	D48.2	D49.2
trigeminal	C72.59	C79.49	—	D33.3	D43.3	D49.7
trochlear	C72.59	C79.49	—	D33.3	D43.3	D49.7
ulnar	C47.1-☑	C79.89	—	D36.12	D48.2	D49.2
vagus	C72.59	C79.49	—	D33.3	D43.3	D49.7
nervous system (central)	C72.9	C79.40	—	D33.9	D43.9	D49.7
autonomic — see Neoplasm, nerve, peripheral						
parasympathetic — see Neoplasm, nerve, peripheral						
specified site NEC	—	C79.49	—	D33.7	D43.8	—
sympathetic — see Neoplasm, nerve, peripheral						
nevus — see Nevus						
nipple	C50.0-☑	C79.81	D05.-☑	D24.-☑		
nose, nasal	C76.0	C79.89	D09.8	D36.7	D48.7	D49.89
ala (external) (nasi) — see also Neoplasm, nose, skin						
skin	C44.301	C79.2	D04.39	D23.39	D48.5	D49.2
bone	C41.0	C79.51	—	D16.4	D48.0	D49.2
cartilage	C30.0	C78.39	D02.3	D14.0	D38.5	D49.1
cavity	C30.0	C78.39	D02.3	D14.0	D38.5	D49.1
choana	C11.3	C79.89	D00.08	D10.6	D37.05	D49.0
external (skin) — see also Neoplasm, nose, skin						
fossa	C30.0	C78.39	D02.3	D14.0	D38.5	D49.1
internal	C30.0	C78.39	D02.3	D14.0	D38.5	D49.1
mucosa	C30.0	C78.39	D02.3	D14.0	D38.5	D49.1
septum	C30.0	C78.39	D02.3	D14.0	D38.5	D49.1
posterior margin	C11.3	C79.89	D00.08	D10.6	D37.05	D49.0
sinus — see Neoplasm, sinus						
skin	C44.301	C79.2	D04.39	D23.39	D48.5	D49.2
basal cell carcinoma	C44.311	—	—	—	—	—
specified type NEC	C44.391	—	—	—	—	—
squamous cell carcinoma	C44.321	—	—	—	—	—
turbinate (mucosa)	C30.0	C78.39	D02.3	D14.0	D38.5	D49.1
bone	C41.0	C79.51	—	D16.4	D48.0	D49.2
vestibule	C30.0	C78.39	D02.3	D14.0	D38.5	D49.1

Neoplasm, neoplastic — continued

	Malignant Primary	Malignant Secondary	Ca in situ	Benign	Uncertain	Unspecified Behavior
nostril	C30.0	C78.39	D02.3	D14.0	D38.5	D49.1
nucleus pulposus	C41.2	C79.51	—	D16.6	D48.0	D49.2
occipital bone	C41.0	C79.51	—	D16.4	D48.0	D49.2
lobe or pole, brain	C71.4	C79.31	—	D33.0	D43.0	D49.6
odontogenic — see Neoplasm, jaw bone						
olfactory nerve or bulb	C72.2-☑	C79.49	—	D33.3	D43.3	D49.7
olive (brain)	C71.7	C79.31	—	D33.1	D43.1	D49.6
omentum	C48.1	C78.6	—	D20.1	D48.4	D49.0
operculum (brain)	C71.0	C79.31	—	D33.0	D43.0	D49.6
optic nerve, chiasm, or tract	C72.3-☑	C79.49	—	D33.3	D43.3	D49.7
oral (cavity)	C06.9	C79.89	D00.00	D10.30	D37.09	D49.0
ill-defined	C14.8	C79.89	D00.00	D10.30	D37.09	D49.0
mucosa	C06.0	C79.89	D00.02	D10.39	D37.09	D49.0
orbit	C69.6-☑	C79.49	D09.2-☑	D31.6-☑	D48.7	D49.89
autonomic nerve	C69.6-☑	C79.49	—	D31.6-☑	D48.7	D49.2
bone	C41.0	C79.51	—	D16.4	D48.0	D49.2
eye	C69.6-☑	C79.49	D09.2-☑	D31.6-☑	D48.7	D49.89
peripheral nerves	C69.6-☑	C79.49	—	D31.6-☑	D48.7	D49.2
soft parts	C69.6-☑	C79.49	D09.2-☑	D31.6-☑	D48.7	D49.89
organ of Zuckerkandl	C75.5	C79.89	—	D35.6	D44.7	D49.7
oropharynx	C10.9	C79.89	D00.08	D10.5	D37.05	D49.0
branchial cleft (vestige)	C10.4	C79.89	D00.08	D10.5	D37.05	D49.0
junctional region	C10.8	C79.89	D00.08	D10.5	D37.05	D49.0
lateral wall	C10.2	C79.89	D00.08	D10.5	D37.05	D49.0
overlapping lesion	C10.8	—	—	—	—	—
pillars or fauces	C09.1	C79.89	D00.08	D10.5	D37.05	D49.0
posterior wall	C10.3	C79.89	D00.08	D10.5	D37.05	D49.0
vallecula	C10.0	C79.89	D00.08	D10.5	D37.05	D49.0
os						
external	C53.1	C79.82	D06.1	D26.0	D39.0	D49.59
internal	C53.0	C79.82	D06.0	D26.0	D39.0	D49.59
ovary	C56.-☑	C79.6-☑	D07.39	D27.-☑	D39.1-☑	D49.59
oviduct	C57.0-☑	C79.82	D07.39	D28.2	D39.8	D49.59
palate	C05.9	C79.89	D00.00	D10.39	D37.09	D49.0
hard	C05.0	C79.89	D00.05	D10.39	D37.09	D49.0
junction of hard and soft palate	C05.9	C79.89	D00.00	D10.39	D37.09	D49.0
overlapping lesions	C05.8	—	—	—	—	—
soft	C05.1	C79.89	D00.04	D10.39	D37.09	D49.0
nasopharyngeal surface	C11.3	C79.89	D00.08	D10.6	D37.05	D49.0
posterior surface	C11.3	C79.89	D00.08	D10.6	D37.05	D49.0
superior surface	C11.3	C79.89	D00.08	D10.6	D37.05	D49.0
palatoglossal arch	C09.1	C79.89	D00.00	D10.5	D37.09	D49.0
palatopharyngeal arch	C09.1	C79.89	D00.00	D10.5	D37.09	D49.0
pallium	C71.0	C79.31	—	D33.0	D43.0	D49.6
palpebra	C44.10-☑	C79.2	D04.1-☑	D23.1-☑	D48.5	D49.2
basal cell carcinoma	C44.11-☑	—	—	—	—	—
sebaceous cell	C44.13-☑	—	—	—	—	—
specified type NEC	C44.19-☑	—	—	—	—	—
squamous cell carcinoma	C44.12-☑	—	—	—	—	—
pancreas	C25.9	C78.89	D01.7	D13.6	D37.8	D49.0
body	C25.1	C78.89	D01.7	D13.6	D37.8	D49.0
duct (of Santorini) (of Wirsung)	C25.3	C78.89	D01.7	D13.6	D37.8	D49.0
ectopic tissue	C25.7	C78.89	—	D13.6	D37.8	D49.0
head	C25.0	C78.89	D01.7	D13.6	D37.8	D49.0
islet cells	C25.4	C78.89	D01.7	D13.7	D37.8	D49.0
neck	C25.7	C78.89	D01.7	D13.6	D37.8	D49.0
overlapping lesion	C25.8	—	—	—	—	—
tail	C25.2	C78.89	D01.7	D13.6	D37.8	D49.0

Neoplasm, neoplastic — continued (left column)

	Malignant Primary	Malignant Secondary	Ca in situ	Benign	Uncertain	Unspecified Behavior
— *continued*						
para-aortic body	C75.5	C79.89	—	D35.6	D44.7	D49.7
paraganglion NEC	C75.5	C79.89	—	D35.6	D44.7	D49.7
parametrium	C57.3	C79.82	—	D28.2	D39.8	D49.59
paranephric	C48.0	C78.6	—	D20.0	D48.3	D49.0
pararectal	C76.3	C79.89	—	D36.7	D48.7	D49.89
parasagittal (region)	C76.0	C79.89	D09.8	D36.7	D48.7	D49.89
parasellar	C72.9	C79.49	—	D33.9	D43.8	D49.7
parathyroid (gland)	C75.0	C79.89	D09.3	D35.1	D44.2	D49.7
paraurethral	C76.3	C79.89	—	D36.7	D48.7	D49.89
gland	C68.1	C79.19	D09.19	D30.8	D41.8	D49.59
paravaginal	C76.3	C79.89	—	D36.7	D48.7	D49.89
parenchyma, kidney	C64.-☑	C79.0-☑	D09.19	D30.0-☑	D41.0-☑	D49.51-☑
parietal						
bone	C41.0	C79.51	—	D16.4	D48.0	D49.2
lobe, brain	C71.3	C79.31	—	D33.0	D43.0	D49.6
paroophoron	C57.1-☑	C79.82	D07.39	D28.2	D39.8	D49.59
parotid (duct) (gland)	C07	C79.89	D00.00	D11.0	D37.030	D49.0
parovarium	C57.1-☑	C79.82	D07.39	D28.2	D39.8	D49.59
patella	C40.20	C79.51	—	—	—	—
peduncle, cerebral	C71.7	C79.31	—	D33.1	D43.1	D49.6
pelvirectal junction	C19	C78.5	D01.1	D12.7	D37.5	D49.0
pelvis, pelvic	C76.3	C79.89	D09.8	D36.7	D48.7	D49.89
bone	C41.4	C79.51	—	D16.8	D48.0	D49.2
floor	C76.3	C79.89	D09.8	D36.7	D48.7	D49.89
renal	C65.-☑	C79.0-☑	D09.19	D30.1-☑	D41.1-☑	D49.51-☑
viscera	C76.3	C79.89	D09.8	D36.7	D48.7	D49.89
wall	C76.3	C79.89	D09.8	D36.7	D48.7	D49.89
pelvo-abdominal	C76.8	C79.89	D09.8	D36.7	D48.7	D49.89
penis	C60.9	C79.82	D07.4	D29.0	D40.8	D49.59
body	C60.2	C79.82	D07.4	D29.0	D40.8	D49.59
corpus (cavernosum)	C60.2	C79.82	D07.4	D29.0	D40.8	D49.59
glans	C60.1	C79.82	D07.4	D29.0	D40.8	D49.59
overlapping sites	C60.8	—	—	—	—	—
skin NEC	C60.9	C79.82	D07.4	D29.0	D40.8	D49.59
periadrenal (tissue)	C48.0	C78.6	—	D20.0	D48.3	D49.0
perianal (skin) — *see also* Neoplasm, anus, skin	C44.500	C79.2	D04.5	D23.5	D48.5	D49.2
pericardium	C38.0	C79.89	—	D15.1	D48.7	D49.89
perinephric	C48.0	C78.6	—	D20.0	D48.3	D49.0
perineum	C76.3	C79.89	D09.8	D36.7	D48.7	D49.89
periodontal tissue NEC	C03.9	C79.89	D00.03	D10.39	D37.09	D49.0
periosteum — *see* Neoplasm, bone						
peripancreatic	C48.0	C78.6	—	D20.0	D48.3	D49.0
peripheral nerve NEC	C47.9	C79.89	—	D36.10	D48.2	D49.2
perirectal (tissue)	C76.3	C79.89	—	D36.7	D48.7	D49.89
perirenal (tissue)	C48.0	C78.6	—	D20.0	D48.3	D49.0
peritoneum, peritoneal (cavity)	C48.2	C78.6	—	D20.1	D48.4	D49.0
benign mesothelial tissue — *see* Mesothelioma, benign						
overlapping lesion with digestive organs	C48.8 / C26.9	—	—	—	—	—
parietal	C48.1	C78.6	—	D20.1	D48.4	D49.0
pelvic	C48.1	C78.6	—	D20.1	D48.4	D49.0
specified part NEC	C48.1	C78.6	—	D20.1	D48.4	D49.0
peritonsillar (tissue)	C76.0	C79.89	D09.8	D36.7	D48.7	D49.89
periurethral tissue	C76.3	C79.89	—	D36.7	D48.7	D49.89
phalanges						
foot	C40.3-☑	C79.51	—	D16.3-☑	—	—
hand	C40.1-☑	C79.51	—	D16.1-☑	—	—
pharynx, pharyngeal	C14.0	C79.89	D00.08	D10.9	D37.05	D49.0
bursa	C11.1	C79.89	D00.08	D10.6	D37.05	D49.0

Neoplasm, neoplastic — continued (right column)

	Malignant Primary	Malignant Secondary	Ca in situ	Benign	Uncertain	Unspecified Behavior
— *continued*						
pharynx, pharyngeal — *continued*						
fornix	C11.3	C79.89	D00.08	D10.6	D37.05	D49.0
recess	C11.2	C79.89	D00.08	D10.6	D37.05	D49.0
region	C14.0	C79.89	D00.08	D10.9	D37.05	D49.0
tonsil	C11.1	C79.89	D00.08	D10.6	D37.05	D49.0
wall (lateral) (posterior)	C14.0	C79.89	D00.08	D10.9	D37.05	D49.0
pia mater	C70.9	C79.40	—	D32.9	D42.9	D49.7
cerebral	C70.0	C79.32	—	D32.0	D42.0	D49.7
cranial	C70.0	C79.32	—	D32.0	D42.0	D49.7
spinal	C70.1	C79.49	—	D32.1	D42.1	D49.7
pillars of fauces	C09.1	C79.89	D00.08	D10.5	D37.05	D49.0
pineal (body) (gland)	C75.3	C79.89	D09.3	D35.4	D44.5	D49.7
pinna (ear) NEC — *see also* Neoplasm, skin, ear	C44.20-☑	C79.2	D04.2-☑	D23.2-☑	D48.5	D49.2
piriform fossa or sinus	C12	C79.89	D00.08	D10.7	D37.05	D49.0
pituitary (body) (fossa) (gland) (lobe)	C75.1	C79.89	D09.3	D35.2	D44.3	D49.7
placenta	C58	C79.82	D07.0	D26.7	D39.2	D49.59
pleura, pleural (cavity)	C38.4	C78.2	—	D19.0	D38.2	D49.1
overlapping lesion with heart or mediastinum	C38.8	—	—	—	—	—
parietal	C38.4	C78.2	—	D19.0	D38.2	D49.1
visceral	C38.4	C78.2	—	D19.0	D38.2	D49.1
plexus						
brachial	C47.1-☑	C79.89	—	D36.12	D48.2	D49.2
cervical	C47.0	C79.89	—	D36.11	D48.2	D49.2
choroid	C71.5	C79.31	—	D33.0	D43.0	D49.6
lumbosacral	C47.5	C79.89	—	D36.16	D48.2	D49.2
sacral	C47.5	C79.89	—	D36.16	D48.2	D49.2
pluriendocrine	C75.8	C79.89	D09.3	D35.7	D44.9	D49.7
pole						
frontal	C71.1	C79.31	—	D33.0	D43.0	D49.6
occipital	C71.4	C79.31	—	D33.0	D43.0	D49.6
pons (varolii)	C71.7	C79.31	—	D33.1	D43.1	D49.6
popliteal fossa or space	C76.5-☑	C79.89	D04.7-☑	D36.7	D48.7	D49.89
postcricoid (region)	C13.0	C79.89	D00.08	D10.7	D37.05	D49.0
posterior fossa (cranial)	C71.9	C79.31	—	D33.2	D43.2	D49.6
postnasal space	C11.9	C79.89	D00.08	D10.6	D37.05	D49.0
prepuce	C60.0	C79.82	D07.4	D29.0	D40.8	D49.59
prepylorus	C16.4	C78.89	D00.2	D13.1	D37.1	D49.0
presacral (region)	C76.3	C79.89	—	D36.7	D48.7	D49.89
prostate (gland)	C61	C79.82	D07.5	D29.1	D40.0	D49.59
utricle	C68.0	C79.19	D09.19	D30.4	D41.3	D49.59
pterygoid fossa	C49.0	C79.89	—	D21.0	D48.1	D49.2
pubic bone	C41.4	C79.51	—	D16.8	D48.0	D49.2
pudenda, pudendum (female)	C51.9	C79.82	D07.1	D28.0	D39.8	D49.59
pulmonary — *see also* Neoplasm, lung	C34.9-☑	C78.0-☑	D02.2-☑	D14.3-☑	D38.1	D49.1
putamen	C71.0	C79.31	—	D33.0	D43.0	D49.6
pyloric						
antrum	C16.3	C78.89	D00.2	D13.1	D37.1	D49.0
canal	C16.4	C78.89	D00.2	D13.1	D37.1	D49.0
pylorus	C16.4	C78.89	D00.2	D13.1	D37.1	D49.0
pyramid (brain)	C71.7	C79.31	—	D33.1	D43.1	D49.6
pyriform fossa or sinus	C12	C79.89	D00.08	D10.7	D37.05	D49.0
radius (any part)	C40.0-☑	C79.51	—	D16.0-☑	—	—
Rathke's pouch	C75.1	C79.89	D09.3	D35.2	D44.3	D49.7
rectosigmoid (junction)	C19	C78.5	D01.1	D12.7	D37.5	D49.0
overlapping lesion with anus or rectum	C21.8	—	—	—	—	—
rectouterine pouch	C48.1	C78.6	—	D20.1	D48.4	D49.0
rectovaginal septum or wall	C76.3	C79.89	D09.8	D36.7	D48.7	D49.89
rectovesical septum	C76.3	C79.89	D09.8	D36.7	D48.7	D49.89
rectum (ampulla)	C20	C78.5	D01.2	D12.8	D37.5	D49.0

Neoplasm, neoplastic — continued

	Malignant Primary	Malignant Secondary	Ca in situ	Benign	Uncertain	Unspecified Behavior
rectum — continued						
and colon	C19	C78.5	D01.1	D12.7	D37.5	D49.0
overlapping lesion with anus or rectosigmoid junction	C21.8	—	—	—	—	—
renal	C64.-☑	C79.0-☑	D09.19	D30.0-☑	D41.0-☑	D49.51-☑
calyx	C65.-☑	C79.0-☑	D09.19	D30.1-☑	D41.1-☑	D49.51-☑
hilus	C65.-☑	C79.0-☑	D09.19	D30.1-☑	D41.1-☑	D49.51-☑
parenchyma	C64.-☑	C79.0-☑	D09.19	D30.0-☑	D41.0-☑	D49.51-☑
pelvis	C65.-☑	C79.0-☑	D09.19	D30.1-☑	D41.1-☑	D49.51-☑
respiratory						
organs or system NEC	C39.9	C78.30	D02.4	D14.4	D38.6	D49.1
tract NEC	C39.9	C78.30	D02.4	D14.4	D38.5	D49.1
upper	C39.0	C78.30	D02.4	D14.4	D38.5	D49.1
retina	C69.2-☑	C79.49	D09.2-☑	D31.2-☑	D48.7	D49.81
retrobulbar	C69.6-☑	C79.49	—	D31.6-☑	D48.7	D49.89
retrocecal	C48.0	C78.6	—	D20.0	D48.3	D49.0
retromolar (area) (triangle) (trigone)	C06.2	C79.89	D00.00	D10.39	D37.09	D49.0
retro-orbital	C76.0	C79.89	D09.8	D36.7	D48.7	D49.89
retroperitoneal (space) (tissue)	C48.0	C78.6	—	D20.0	D48.3	D49.0
retroperitoneum	C48.0	C78.6	—	D20.0	D48.3	D49.0
retropharyngeal	C14.0	C79.89	D00.08	D10.9	D37.05	D49.0
retrovesical (septum)	C76.3	C79.89	D09.8	D36.7	D48.7	D49.89
rhinencephalon	C71.0	C79.31	—	D33.0	D43.0	D49.6
rib	C41.3	C79.51	—	D16.7	D48.0	D49.2
Rosenmuller's fossa	C11.2	C79.89	D00.08	D10.6	D37.05	D49.0
round ligament	C57.2-☑	C79.82	—	D28.2	D39.8	D49.59
sacrococcyx, sacrococcygeal	C41.4	C79.51	—	D16.8	D48.0	D49.2
region	C76.3	C79.89	D09.8	D36.7	D48.7	D49.89
sacrouterine ligament	C57.3	C79.82	—	D28.2	D39.8	D49.59
sacrum, sacral (vertebra)	C41.4	C79.51	—	D16.8	D48.0	D49.2
salivary gland or duct (major)	C08.9	C79.89	D00.00	D11.9	D37.039	D49.0
minor NEC	C06.9	C79.89	D00.00	D10.39	D37.04	D49.0
overlapping lesion	C08.9	—	—	—	—	—
parotid	C07	C79.89	D00.00	D11.0	D37.030	D49.0
pluriglandular	C08.9	C79.89	D00.00	D11.9	D37.039	D49.0
sublingual	C08.1	C79.89	D00.00	D11.7	D37.031	D49.0
submandibular	C08.0	C79.89	D00.00	D11.7	D37.032	D49.0
submaxillary	C08.0	C79.89	D00.00	D11.7	D37.032	D49.0
salpinx (uterine)	C57.0-☑	C79.82	D07.39	D28.2	D39.8	D49.59
Santorini's duct	C25.3	C78.89	D01.7	D13.6	D37.8	D49.0
scalp	C44.40	C79.2	D04.4	D23.4	D48.5	D49.2
basal cell carcinoma	C44.41	—	—	—	—	—
specified type NEC	C44.49	—	—	—	—	—
squamous cell carcinoma	C44.42	—	—	—	—	—
scapula (any part)	C40.0-☑	C79.51	—	D16.0-☑	—	—
scapular region	C76.1	C79.89	D09.8	D36.7	D48.7	D49.89
scar NEC — see also Neoplasm, skin, by site	C44.90	C79.2	D04.9	D23.9	D48.5	D49.2
sciatic nerve	C47.2-☑	C79.89	—	D36.13	D48.2	D49.2
sclera	C69.4-☑	C79.49	D09.2-☑	D31.4-☑	D48.7	D49.89
scrotum (skin)	C63.2	C79.82	D07.61	D29.4	D40.8	D49.59
sebaceous gland — see Neoplasm, skin						
sella turcica	C75.1	C79.89	D09.3	D35.2	D44.3	D49.7
bone	C41.0	C79.51	—	D16.4	D48.0	D49.2
semilunar cartilage (knee)	C40.2-☑	C79.51	—	D16.2-☑	D48.0	D49.2
seminal vesicle	C63.7	C79.82	D07.69	D29.8	D40.8	D49.59
septum						
nasal	C30.0	C78.39	D02.3	D14.0	D38.5	D49.1
posterior margin	C11.3	C79.89	D00.08	D10.6	D37.05	D49.0
rectovaginal	C76.3	C79.89	D09.8	D36.7	D48.7	D49.89
rectovesical	C76.3	C79.89	D09.8	D36.7	D48.7	D49.89

Neoplasm, neoplastic — continued

	Malignant Primary	Malignant Secondary	Ca in situ	Benign	Uncertain	Unspecified Behavior
septum — continued						
urethrovaginal	C57.9	C79.82	D07.30	D28.9	D39.9	D49.59
vesicovaginal	C57.9	C79.82	D07.30	D28.9	D39.9	D49.59
shoulder NEC	C76.4-☑	C79.89	D04.6-☑	D36.7	D48.7	D49.89
sigmoid flexure (lower) (upper)	C18.7	C78.5	D01.0	D12.5	D37.4	D49.0
sinus (accessory)	C31.9	C78.39	D02.3	D14.0	D38.5	D49.1
bone (any)	C41.0	C79.51	—	D16.4	D48.0	D49.2
ethmoidal	C31.1	C78.39	D02.3	D14.0	D38.5	D49.1
frontal	C31.2	C78.39	D02.3	D14.0	D38.5	D49.1
maxillary	C31.0	C78.39	D02.3	D14.0	D38.5	D49.1
nasal, paranasal NEC	C31.9	C78.39	D02.3	D14.0	D38.5	D49.1
overlapping lesion	C31.8	—	—	—	—	—
pyriform	C12	C79.89	D00.08	D10.7	D37.05	D49.0
sphenoid	C31.3	C78.39	D02.3	D14.0	D38.5	D49.1
skeleton, skeletal NEC	C41.9	C79.51	—	D16.9	D48.0	D49.2
Skene's gland	C68.1	C79.19	D09.19	D30.8	D41.8	D49.59
skin NOS	C44.90	C79.2	D04.9	D23.9	D48.5	D49.2
abdominal wall	C44.509	C79.2	D04.5	D23.5	D48.5	D49.2
basal cell carcinoma	C44.519	—	—	—	—	—
specified type NEC	C44.599	—	—	—	—	—
squamous cell carcinoma	C44.529	—	—	—	—	—
ala nasi — see also Neoplasm, nose, skin	C44.301	C79.2	D04.39	D23.39	D48.5	D49.2
ankle — see also Neoplasm, skin, limb, lower	C44.70-☑	C79.2	D04.7-☑	D23.7-☑	D48.5	D49.2
antecubital space — see also Neoplasm, skin, limb, upper	C44.60-☑	C79.2	D04.6-☑	D23.6-☑	D48.5	D49.2
anus	C44.500	C79.2	D04.5	D23.5	D48.5	D49.2
basal cell carcinoma	C44.510	—	—	—	—	—
specified type NEC	C44.590	—	—	—	—	—
squamous cell carcinoma	C44.520	—	—	—	—	—
arm — see also Neoplasm, skin, limb, upper	C44.60-☑	C79.2	D04.6-☑	D23.6-☑	D48.5	D49.2
auditory canal (external) — see also Neoplasm, skin, ear	C44.20-☑	C79.2	D04.2-☑	D23.2-☑	D48.5	D49.2
auricle (ear) — see also Neoplasm, skin, ear	C44.20-☑	C79.2	D04.2-☑	D23.2-☑	D48.5	D49.2
auricular canal (external) — see also Neoplasm, skin, ear	C44.20-☑	C79.2	D04.2-☑	D23.2-☑	D48.5	D49.2
axilla, axillary fold — see also Neoplasm, skin, trunk	C44.509	C79.2	D04.5	D23.5	D48.5	D49.2
back — see also Neoplasm, skin, trunk	C44.509	C79.2	D04.5	D23.5	D48.5	D49.2
basal cell carcinoma	C44.91	—	—	—	—	—
breast	C44.501	C79.2	D04.5	D23.5	D48.5	D49.2
basal cell carcinoma	C44.511	—	—	—	—	—
specified type NEC	C44.591	—	—	—	—	—
squamous cell carcinoma	C44.521	—	—	—	—	—
brow — see also Neoplasm, skin, face	C44.309	C79.2	D04.39	D23.39	D48.5	D49.2
buttock — see also Neoplasm, skin, trunk	C44.509	C79.2	D04.5	D23.5	D48.5	D49.2

☑ Additional Character Required — Refer to the Tabular List for Character Selection

Subterms under main terms may continue to next column or page

	Malignant Primary	Malignant Secondary	Ca in situ	Benign	Uncertain	Unspecified Behavior
Neoplasm, neoplastic						
— *continued*						
skin — *continued*						
calf — *see also Neoplasm, skin, limb, lower*	C44.70-☑	C79.2	D04.7-☑	D23.7-☑	D48.5	D49.2
canthus (eye) (inner) (outer)	C44.10-☑	C79.2	D04.1-☑	D23.1-☑	D48.5	D49.2
basal cell carcinoma	C44.11-☑	—	—	—	—	—
sebaceous cell	C44.13-☑	—	—	—	—	—
specified type NEC	C44.19-☑	—	—	—	—	—
squamous cell carcinoma	C44.12-☑	—	—	—	—	—
cervical region — *see also Neoplasm, skin, neck*	C44.40	C79.2	D04.4	D23.4	D48.5	D49.2
cheek (external) — *see also Neoplasm, skin, face*	C44.309	C79.2	D04.39	D23.39	D48.5	D49.2
chest (wall) — *see also Neoplasm, skin, trunk*	C44.509	C79.2	D04.5	D23.5	D48.5	D49.2
chin — *see also Neoplasm, skin, face*	C44.309	C79.2	D04.39	D23.39	D48.5	D49.2
clavicular area — *see also Neoplasm, skin, trunk*	C44.509	C79.2	D04.5	D23.5	D48.5	D49.2
clitoris	C51.2	C79.82	D07.1	D28.0	D39.8	D49.59
columnella — *see also Neoplasm, skin, face*	C44.309	C79.2	D04.39	D23.39	D48.5	D49.2
concha — *see also Neoplasm, skin, ear*	C44.20-☑	C79.2	D04.2-☑	D23.2-☑	D48.5	D49.2
ear (external)	C44.20-☑	C79.2	D04.2-☑	D23.2-☑	D48.5	D49.2
basal cell carcinoma	C44.21-☑	—	—	—	—	—
specified type NEC	C44.29-☑	—	—	—	—	—
squamous cell carcinoma	C44.22-☑	—	—	—	—	—
elbow — *see also Neoplasm, skin, limb, upper*	C44.60-☑	C79.2	D04.6-☑	D23.6-☑	D48.5	D49.2
eyebrow — *see also Neoplasm, skin, face*	C44.309	C79.2	D04.39	D23.39	D48.5	D49.2
eyelid	C44.10-☑	C79.2	D04.1-☑	D23.1-☑	D48.5	D49.2
basal cell carcinoma	C44.11-☑	—	—	—	—	—
sebaceous cell	C44.13-☑	—	—	—	—	—
specified type NEC	C44.19-☑	—	—	—	—	—
squamous cell carcinoma	C44.12-☑	—	—	—	—	—
face NOS	C44.300	C79.2	D04.30	D23.30	D48.5	D49.2
basal cell carcinoma	C44.310	—	—	—	—	—
specified type NEC	C44.390	—	—	—	—	—
squamous cell carcinoma	C44.320	—	—	—	—	—
female genital organs (external)	C51.9	C79.82	D07.1	D28.0	D39.8	D49.59
clitoris	C51.2	C79.82	D07.1	D28.0	D39.8	D49.59
labium NEC	C51.9	C79.82	D07.1	D28.0	D39.8	D49.59
majus	C51.0	C79.82	D07.1	D28.0	D39.8	D49.59
minus	C51.1	C79.82	D07.1	D28.0	D39.8	D49.59
pudendum	C51.9	C79.82	D07.1	D28.0	D39.8	D49.59
vulva	C51.9	C79.82	D07.1	D28.0	D39.8	D49.59
finger — *see also Neoplasm, skin, limb, upper*	C44.60-☑	C79.2	D04.6-☑	D23.6-☑	D48.5	D49.2
flank — *see also Neoplasm, skin, trunk*	C44.509	C79.2	D04.5	D23.5	D48.5	D49.2
foot — *see also Neoplasm, skin, limb, lower*	C44.70-☑	C79.2	D04.7-☑	D23.7-☑	D48.5	D49.2
forearm — *see also Neoplasm, skin, limb, upper*	C44.60-☑	C79.2	D04.6-☑	D23.6-☑	D48.5	D49.2
forehead — *see also Neoplasm, skin, face*	C44.309	C79.2	D04.39	D23.39	D48.5	D49.2
glabella — *see also Neoplasm, skin, face*	C44.309	C79.2	D04.39	D23.39	D48.5	D49.2
gluteal region — *see also Neoplasm, skin, trunk*	C44.509	C79.2	D04.5	D23.5	D48.5	D49.2
groin — *see also Neoplasm, skin, trunk*	C44.509	C79.2	D04.5	D23.5	D48.5	D49.2
hand — *see also Neoplasm, skin, limb, upper*	C44.60-☑	C79.2	D04.6-☑	D23.6-☑	D48.5	D49.2
head NEC — *see also Neoplasm, skin, scalp*	C44.40	C79.2	D04.4	D23.4	D48.5	D49.2
heel — *see also Neoplasm, skin, limb, lower*	C44.70-☑	C79.2	D04.7-☑	D23.7-☑	D48.5	D49.2
helix — *see also Neoplasm, skin, ear*	C44.20-☑	C79.2	D04.2-☑	D23.2-☑	D48.5	D49.2
hip — *see also Neoplasm, skin, limb, lower*	C44.70-☑	C79.2	D04.7-☑	D23.7-☑	D48.5	D49.2
infraclavicular region — *see also Neoplasm, skin, trunk*	C44.509	C79.2	D04.5	D23.5	D48.5	D49.2
inguinal region — *see also Neoplasm, skin, trunk*	C44.509	C79.2	D04.5	D23.5	D48.5	D49.2
jaw — *see also Neoplasm, skin, face*	C44.309	C79.2	D04.39	D23.39	D48.5	D49.2
Kaposi's sarcoma — *see Kaposi's, sarcoma, skin*						
knee — *see also Neoplasm, skin, limb, lower*	C44.70-☑	C79.2	D04.7-☑	D23.7-☑	D48.5	D49.2
labia						
majora	C51.0	C79.82	D07.1	D28.0	D39.8	D49.59
minora	C51.1	C79.82	D07.1	D28.0	D39.8	D49.59
leg — *see also Neoplasm, skin, limb, lower*	C44.70-☑	C79.2	D04.7-☑	D23.7-☑	D48.5	D49.2
lid (lower) (upper)	C44.10-☑	C79.2	D04.1-☑	D23.1-☑	D48.5	D49.2
basal cell carcinoma	C44.11-☑	—	—	—	—	—
sebaceous cell	C44.13-☑	—	—	—	—	—
specified type NEC	C44.19-☑	—	—	—	—	—
squamous cell carcinoma	C44.12-☑	—	—	—	—	—
limb NEC	C44.90	C79.2	D04.9	D23.9	D48.5	D49.2
basal cell carcinoma	C44.91	—	—	—	—	—
lower	C44.70-☑	C79.2	D04.7-☑	D23.7-☑	D48.5	D49.2
basal cell carcinoma	C44.71-☑	—	—	—	—	—
specified type NEC	C44.79-☑	—	—	—	—	—
squamous cell carcinoma	C44.72-☑	—	—	—	—	—
upper	C44.60-☑	C79.2	D04.6-☑	D23.6-☑	D48.5	D49.2
basal cell carcinoma	C44.61-☑	—	—	—	—	—
specified type NEC	C44.69-☑	—	—	—	—	—
squamous cell carcinoma	C44.62-☑	—	—	—	—	—
lip (lower) (upper)	C44.00	C79.2	D04.0	D23.0	D48.5	D49.2

Neoplasm, neoplastic	Malignant Primary	Malignant Secondary	Ca in situ	Benign	Uncertain	Unspecified Behavior
— continued						
skin — continued						
lip — continued						
basal cell carcinoma	C44.01	—	—	—	—	—
specified type NEC	C44.09	—	—	—	—	—
squamous cell carcinoma	C44.02	—	—	—	—	—
male genital organs	C63.9	C79.82	D07.60	D29.9	D40.8	D49.59
penis	C60.9	C79.82	D07.4	D29.0	D40.8	D49.59
prepuce	C60.0	C79.82	D07.4	D29.0	D40.8	D49.59
scrotum	C63.2	C79.82	D07.61	D29.4	D40.8	D49.59
mastectomy site (skin) — see also Neoplasm, skin, breast	C44.501	C79.2	—	—	—	—
specified as breast tissue	C50.8-✓	C79.81	—	—	—	—
meatus, acoustic (external) — see also Neoplasm, skin, ear	C44.20-✓	C79.2	D04.2-✓	D23.2-✓	D48.5	D49.2
melanotic — see Melanoma						
Merkel cell — see Carcinoma, Merkel cell						
nates — see also Neoplasm, skin, trunk	C44.509	C79.2	D04.5	D23.5	D48.5	D49.2
neck	C44.40	C79.2	D04.4	D23.4	D48.5	D49.2
basal cell carcinoma	C44.41	—	—	—	—	—
specified type NEC	C44.49	—	—	—	—	—
squamous cell carcinoma	C44.42	—	—	—	—	—
nevus — see Nevus, skin						
nose (external) — see also Neoplasm, nose, skin	C44.301	C79.2	D04.39	D23.39	D48.5	D49.2
overlapping lesion	C44.80	—	—	—	—	—
basal cell carcinoma	C44.81	—	—	—	—	—
specified type NEC	C44.89	—	—	—	—	—
squamous cell carcinoma	C44.82	—	—	—	—	—
palm — see also Neoplasm, skin, limb, upper	C44.60-✓	C79.2	D04.6-✓	D23.6-✓	D48.5	D49.2
palpebra	C44.10-✓	C79.2	D04.1-✓	D23.1-✓	D48.5	D49.2
basal cell carcinoma	C44.11-✓	—	—	—	—	—
sebaceous cell	C44.13-✓	—	—	—	—	—
specified type NEC	C44.19-✓	—	—	—	—	—
squamous cell carcinoma	C44.12-✓	—	—	—	—	—
penis NEC	C60.9	C79.82	D07.4	D29.0	D40.8	D49.59
perianal — see also Neoplasm, skin, anus	C44.500	C79.2	D04.5	D23.5	D48.5	D49.2
perineum — see also Neoplasm, skin, anus	C44.500	C79.2	D04.5	D23.5	D48.5	D49.2
pinna — see also Neoplasm, skin, ear	C44.20-✓	C79.2	D04.2-✓	D23.2-✓	D48.5	D49.2
plantar — see also Neoplasm, skin, limb, lower	C44.70-✓	C79.2	D04.7-✓	D23.7-✓	D48.5	D49.2
popliteal fossa or space — see also Neoplasm, skin, limb, lower	C44.70-✓	C79.2	D04.7-✓	D23.7-✓	D48.5	D49.2
prepuce	C60.0	C79.82	D07.4	D29.0	D40.8	D49.59
pubes — see also Neoplasm, skin, trunk	C44.509	C79.2	D04.5	D23.5	D48.5	D49.2
sacrococcygeal region — see also Neoplasm, skin, trunk	C44.509	C79.2	D04.5	D23.5	D48.5	D49.2
scalp	C44.40	C79.2	D04.4	D23.4	D48.5	D49.2
basal cell carcinoma	C44.41	—	—	—	—	—
specified type NEC	C44.49	—	—	—	—	—
squamous cell carcinoma	C44.42	—	—	—	—	—
scapular region — see also Neoplasm, skin, trunk	C44.509	C79.2	D04.5	D23.5	D48.5	D49.2
scrotum	C63.2	C79.82	D07.61	D29.4	D40.8	D49.59
shoulder — see also Neoplasm, skin, limb, upper	C44.60-✓	C79.2	D04.6-✓	D23.6-✓	D48.5	D49.2
sole (foot) — see also Neoplasm, skin, limb, lower	C44.70-✓	C79.2	D04.7-✓	D23.7-✓	D48.5	D49.2
specified sites NEC	C44.80	C79.2	D04.8	D23.9	D48.5	D49.2
basal cell carcinoma	C44.81	—	—	—	—	—
specified type NEC	C44.89	—	—	—	—	—
squamous cell carcinoma	C44.82	—	—	—	—	—
specified type NEC	C44.99	—	—	—	—	—
squamous cell carcinoma	C44.92	—	—	—	—	—
submammary fold — see also Neoplasm, skin, trunk	C44.509	C79.2	D04.5	D23.5	D48.5	D49.2
supraclavicular region — see also Neoplasm, skin, neck	C44.40	C79.2	D04.4	D23.4	D48.5	D49.2
temple — see also Neoplasm, skin, face	C44.309	C79.2	D04.39	D23.39	D48.5	D49.2
thigh — see also Neoplasm, skin, limb, lower	C44.70-✓	C79.2	D04.7-✓	D23.7-✓	D48.5	D49.2
thoracic wall — see also Neoplasm, skin, trunk	C44.509	C79.2	D04.5	D23.5	D48.5	D49.2
thumb — see also Neoplasm, skin, limb, upper	C44.60-✓	C79.2	D04.6-✓	D23.6-✓	D48.5	D49.2
toe — see also Neoplasm, skin, limb, lower	C44.70-✓	C79.2	D04.7-✓	D23.7-✓	D48.5	D49.2
tragus — see also Neoplasm, skin, ear	C44.20-✓	C79.2	D04.2-✓	D23.2-✓	D48.5	D49.2
trunk	C44.509	C79.2	D04.5	D23.5	D48.5	D49.2
basal cell carcinoma	C44.519	—	—	—	—	—
specified type NEC	C44.599	—	—	—	—	—
squamous cell carcinoma	C44.529	—	—	—	—	—
umbilicus — see also Neoplasm, skin, trunk	C44.509	C79.2	D04.5	D23.5	D48.5	D49.2
vulva	C51.9	C79.82	D07.1	D28.0	D39.8	D49.59
overlapping lesion	C51.8					
wrist — see also Neoplasm, skin, limb, upper	C44.60-✓	C79.2	D04.6-✓	D23.6-✓	D48.5	D49.2
skull	C41.0	C79.51	—	D16.4	D48.0	D49.2

✓ Additional Character Required — Refer to the Tabular List for Character Selection   ▽ Subterms under main terms may continue to next column or page

Neoplasm, neoplastic	Malignant Primary	Malignant Secondary	Ca in situ	Benign	Uncertain	Unspecified Behavior
— continued						
soft parts or tissues — see Neoplasm, connective tissue						
specified site NEC	C76.8	C79.89	D09.8	D36.7	D48.7	D49.89
spermatic cord	C63.1-✓	C79.82	D07.69	D29.8	D40.8	D49.59
sphenoid	C31.3	C78.39	D02.3	D14.0	D38.5	D49.1
bone	C41.0	C79.51	—	D16.4	D48.0	D49.2
sinus	C31.3	C78.39	D02.3	D14.0	D38.5	D49.1
sphincter						
anal	C21.1	C78.5	D01.3	D12.9	D37.8	D49.0
of Oddi	C24.0	C78.89	D01.5	D13.5	D37.6	D49.0
spine, spinal						
(column)	C41.2	C79.51	—	D16.6	D48.0	D49.2
bulb	C71.7	C79.31	—	D33.1	D43.1	D49.6
coccyx	C41.4	C79.51	—	D16.8	D48.0	D49.2
cord (cervical) (lumbar) (sacral) (thoracic)	C72.0	C79.49	—	D33.4	D43.4	D49.7
dura mater	C70.1	C79.49	—	D32.1	D42.1	D49.7
lumbosacral	C41.2	C79.51	—	D16.6	D48.0	D49.2
marrow NEC	C96.9	C79.52	—	—	D47.9	D49.89
membrane	C70.1	C79.49	—	D32.1	D42.1	D49.7
meninges	C70.1	C79.49	—	D32.1	D42.1	D49.7
nerve (root)	C47.9	C79.89	—	D36.10	D48.2	D49.2
pia mater	C70.1	C79.49	—	D32.1	D42.1	D49.7
root	C47.9	C79.89	—	D36.10	D48.2	D49.2
sacrum	C41.4	C79.51	—	D16.8	D48.0	D49.2
spleen, splenic						
NEC	C26.1	C78.89	D01.7	D13.9	D37.8	D49.0
flexure (colon)	C18.5	C78.5	D01.0	D12.3	D37.4	D49.0
stem, brain	C71.7	C79.31	—	D33.1	D43.1	D49.6
Stensen's duct	C07	C79.89	D00.00	D11.0	D37.030	D49.0
sternum	C41.3	C79.51	—	D16.7	D48.0	D49.2
stomach	C16.9	C78.89	D00.2	D13.1	D37.1	D49.0
antrum (pyloric)	C16.3	C78.89	D00.2	D13.1	D37.1	D49.0
body	C16.2	C78.89	D00.2	D13.1	D37.1	D49.0
cardia	C16.0	C78.89	D00.2	D13.1	D37.1	D49.0
cardiac orifice	C16.0	C78.89	D00.2	D13.1	D37.1	D49.0
corpus	C16.2	C78.89	D00.2	D13.1	D37.1	D49.0
fundus	C16.1	C78.89	D00.2	D13.1	D37.1	D49.0
greater curvature NEC	C16.6	C78.89	D00.2	D13.1	D37.1	D49.0
lesser curvature NEC	C16.5	C78.89	D00.2	D13.1	D37.1	D49.0
overlapping lesion	C16.8	—	—	—	—	—
prepylorus	C16.4	C78.89	D00.2	D13.1	D37.1	D49.0
pylorus	C16.4	C78.89	D00.2	D13.1	D37.1	D49.0
wall NEC	C16.9	C78.89	D00.2	D13.1	D37.1	D49.0
anterior NEC	C16.8	C78.89	D00.2	D13.1	D37.1	D49.0
posterior NEC	C16.8	C78.89	D00.2	D13.1	D37.1	D49.0
stroma, endometrial	C54.1	C79.82	D07.0	D26.1	D39.0	D49.59
stump, cervical	C53.8	C79.82	D06.7	D26.0	D39.0	D49.59
subcutaneous (nodule) (tissue) NEC — see Neoplasm, connective tissue						
subdural	C70.9	C79.32	—	D32.9	D42.9	D49.7
subglottis, subglottic	C32.2	C78.39	D02.0	D14.1	D38.0	D49.1
sublingual	C04.9	C79.89	D00.06	D10.2	D37.09	D49.0
gland or duct	C08.1	C79.89	D00.00	D11.7	D37.031	D49.0
submandibular gland	C08.0	C79.89	D00.00	D11.7	D37.032	D49.0
submaxillary gland or duct	C08.0	C79.89	D00.00	D11.7	D37.032	D49.0
submental	C76.0	C79.89	D09.8	D36.7	D48.7	D49.89
subpleural	C34.9-✓	C78.0-✓	D02.2-✓	D14.3-✓	D38.1	D49.1
substernal	C38.1	C78.1	—	D15.2	D38.3	D49.89
sudoriferous, sudoriparous gland, site unspecified	C44.90	C79.2	D04.9	D23.9	D48.5	D49.2
specified site — see Neoplasm, skin						
supraclavicular region	C76.0	C79.89	D09.8	D36.7	D48.7	D49.89
supraglottis	C32.1	C78.39	D02.0	D14.1	D38.0	D49.1
suprarenal	C74.9-✓	C79.7-✓	D09.3	D35.0-✓	D44.1-✓	D49.7
capsule	C74.9-✓	C79.7-✓	D09.3	D35.0-✓	D44.1-✓	D49.7

Neoplasm, neoplastic	Malignant Primary	Malignant Secondary	Ca in situ	Benign	Uncertain	Unspecified Behavior
— continued						
suprarenal — continued						
cortex	C74.0-✓	C79.7-✓	D09.3	D35.0-✓	D44.1-✓	D49.7
gland	C74.9-✓	C79.7-✓	D09.3	D35.0-✓	D44.1-✓	D49.7
medulla	C74.1-✓	C79.7-✓	D09.3	D35.0-✓	D44.1-✓	D49.7
suprasellar (region)	C71.9	C79.31	—	D33.2	D43.2	D49.6
NEC	C71.0	C79.31	—	D33.0	D43.0	D49.6
sweat gland (apocrine) (eccrine), site unspecified	C44.90	C79.2	D04.9	D23.9	D48.5	D49.2
specified site — see Neoplasm, skin						
sympathetic nerve or nervous system NEC	C47.9	C79.89	—	D36.10	D48.2	D49.2
symphysis pubis	C41.4	C79.51	—	D16.8	D48.0	D49.2
synovial membrane — see Neoplasm, connective tissue						
tapetum, brain	C71.8	C79.31	—	D33.2	D43.2	D49.6
tarsus (any bone)	C40.3-✓	C79.51	—	D16.3-✓	—	—
temple (skin) — see also Neoplasm, skin, face	C44.309	C79.2	D04.39	D23.39	D48.5	D49.2
temporal						
bone	C41.0	C79.51	—	D16.4	D48.0	D49.2
lobe or pole	C71.2	C79.31	—	D33.0	D43.0	D49.6
region	C76.0	C79.89	D09.8	D36.7	D48.7	D49.89
skin — see also Neoplasm, skin, face	C44.309	C79.2	D04.39	D23.39	D48.5	D49.2
tendon (sheath) — see Neoplasm, connective tissue						
tentorium (cerebelli)	C70.0	C79.32	—	D32.0	D42.0	D49.7
testis, testes	C62.9-✓	C79.82	D07.69	D29.2-✓	D40.1-✓	D49.59
descended	C62.1-✓	C79.82	D07.69	D29.2-✓	D40.1-✓	D49.59
ectopic	C62.0-✓	C79.82	D07.69	D29.2-✓	D40.1-✓	D49.59
retained	C62.0-✓	C79.82	D07.69	D29.2-✓	D40.1-✓	D49.59
scrotal	C62.1-✓	C79.82	D07.69	D29.2-✓	D40.1-✓	D49.59
undescended	C62.0-✓	C79.82	D07.69	D29.2-✓	D40.1-✓	D49.59
unspecified whether descended or undescended	C62.9-✓	C79.82	D07.69	D29.2-✓	D40.1-✓	D49.59
thalamus	C71.0	C79.31	—	D33.0	D43.0	D49.6
thigh NEC	C76.5-✓	C79.89	D04.7-✓	D36.7	D48.7	D49.89
thorax, thoracic (cavity) (organs NEC)	C76.1	C79.89	D09.8	D36.7	D48.7	D49.89
duct	C49.3	C79.89	—	D21.3	D48.1	D49.2
wall NEC	C76.1	C79.89	D09.8	D36.7	D48.7	D49.89
throat	C14.0	C79.89	D00.08	D10.9	D37.05	D49.0
thumb NEC	C76.4-✓	C79.89	D04.6-✓	D36.7	D48.7	D49.89
thymus (gland)	C37	C79.89	D09.3	D15.0	D38.4	D49.89
thyroglossal duct	C73	C79.89	D09.3	D34	D44.0	D49.7
thyroid (gland)	C73	C79.89	D09.3	D34	D44.0	D49.7
cartilage	C32.3	C78.39	D02.0	D14.1	D38.0	D49.1
tibia (any part)	C40.2-✓	C79.51	—	D16.2-✓	—	—
toe NEC	C76.5-✓	C79.89	D04.7-✓	D36.7	D48.7	D49.89
tongue	C02.9	C79.89	D00.07	D10.1	D37.02	D49.0
anterior (two-thirds) NEC	C02.3	C79.89	D00.07	D10.1	D37.02	D49.0
dorsal surface	C02.0	C79.89	D00.07	D10.1	D37.02	D49.0
ventral surface	C02.2	C79.89	D00.07	D10.1	D37.02	D49.0
base (dorsal surface)	C01	C79.89	D00.07	D10.1	D37.02	D49.0
border (lateral)	C02.1	C79.89	D00.07	D10.1	D37.02	D49.0
dorsal surface NEC	C02.0	C79.89	D00.07	D10.1	D37.02	D49.0
fixed part NEC	C01	C79.89	D00.07	D10.1	D37.02	D49.0
foramen cecum	C02.0	C79.89	D00.07	D10.1	D37.02	D49.0
frenulum linguae	C02.2	C79.89	D00.07	D10.1	D37.02	D49.0
junctional zone	C02.8	C79.89	D00.07	D10.1	D37.02	D49.0
margin (lateral)	C02.1	C79.89	D00.07	D10.1	D37.02	D49.0
midline NEC	C02.0	C79.89	D00.07	D10.1	D37.02	D49.0
mobile part NEC	C02.3	C79.89	D00.07	D10.1	D37.02	D49.0

Neoplasm, neoplastic	Malignant Primary	Malignant Secondary	Ca in situ	Benign	Uncertain	Unspecified Behavior
— continued						
tongue — continued						
overlapping						
lesion	C02.8	—	—	—	—	—
posterior (third)	C01	C79.89	D00.07	D10.1	D37.02	D49.0
root	C01	C79.89	D00.07	D10.1	D37.02	D49.0
surface (dorsal)	C02.0	C79.89	D00.07	D10.1	D37.02	D49.0
base	C01	C79.89	D00.07	D10.1	D37.02	D49.0
ventral	C02.2	C79.89	D00.07	D10.1	D37.02	D49.0
tip	C02.1	C79.89	D00.07	D10.1	D37.02	D49.0
tonsil	C02.4	C79.89	D00.07	D10.1	D37.02	D49.0
tonsil	C09.9	C79.89	D00.08	D10.4	D37.05	D49.0
fauces, faucial	C09.9	C79.89	D00.08	D10.4	D37.05	D49.0
lingual	C02.4	C79.89	D00.07	D10.1	D37.02	D49.0
overlapping						
sites	C09.8	—	—	—	—	—
palatine	C09.9	C79.89	D00.08	D10.4	D37.05	D49.0
pharyngeal	C11.1	C79.89	D00.08	D10.6	D37.05	D49.0
pillar (anterior)						
(posterior)	C09.1	C79.89	D00.08	D10.5	D37.05	D49.0
tonsillar fossa	C09.0	C79.89	D00.08	D10.5	D37.05	D49.0
tooth socket NEC	C03.9	C79.89	D00.03	D10.39	D37.09	D49.0
trachea (cartilage)						
(mucosa)	C33	C78.39	D02.1	D14.2	D38.1	D49.1
overlapping lesion						
with bronchus or						
lung	C34.8-✓	—	—	—	—	—
tracheobronchial	C34.8-✓	C78.39	D02.1	D14.2	D38.1	D49.1
overlapping lesion						
with lung	C34.8-✓	—	—	—	—	—
tragus — see also						
Neoplasm, skin,						
ear	C44.20-✓	C79.2	D04.2-✓	D23.2-✓	D48.5	D49.2
trunk NEC	C76.8	C79.89	D04.5	D36.7	D48.7	D49.89
tubo-ovarian	C57.8	C79.82	D07.39	D28.7	D39.8	D49.59
tunica vaginalis	C63.7	C79.82	D07.69	D29.8	D40.8	D49.59
turbinate (bone)	C41.0	C79.51	—	D16.4	D48.0	D49.2
nasal	C30.0	C78.39	D02.3	D14.0	D38.5	D49.1
tympanic cavity	C30.1	C78.39	D02.3	D14.0	D38.5	D49.1
ulna (any part)	C40.0-✓	C79.51	—	D16.0-✓	—	—
umbilicus, umbilical —						
see also Neoplasm,						
skin, trunk	C44.509	C79.2	D04.5	D23.5	D48.5	D49.2
uncus, brain	C71.2	C79.31	—	D33.0	D43.0	D49.6
unknown site or						
unspecified	C80.1	C79.9	D09.9	D36.9	D48.9	D49.9
urachus	C67.7	C79.11	D09.0	D30.3	D41.4	D49.4
ureter-bladder						
(junction)	C67.6	C79.11	D09.0	D30.3	D41.4	D49.4
ureter, ureteral	C66.-✓	C79.19	D09.19	D30.2-✓	D41.2-✓	D49.59
orifice (bladder)	C67.6	C79.11	D09.0	D30.3	D41.4	D49.4
urethra, urethral						
(gland)	C68.0	C79.19	D09.19	D30.4	D41.3	D49.59
orifice, internal	C67.5	C79.11	D09.0	D30.3	D41.4	D49.4
urethrovaginal						
(septum)	C57.9	C79.82	D07.30	D28.9	D39.8	D49.59
urinary organ or						
system	C68.9	C79.10	D09.10	D30.9	D41.9	D49.59
bladder — see						
Neoplasm,						
bladder						
overlapping						
lesion	C68.8	—	—	—	—	—
specified sites						
NEC	C68.8	C79.19	D09.19	D30.8	D41.8	D49.59
utero-ovarian	C57.8	C79.82	D07.39	D28.7	D39.8	D49.59
ligament	C57.1-✓	C79.82	D07.39	D28.2	D39.8	D49.59
uterosacral						
ligament	C57.3	C79.82	—	D28.2	D39.8	D49.59
uterus, uteri,						
uterine	C55	C79.82	D07.0	D26.9	D39.0	D49.59
adnexa NEC	C57.4	C79.82	D07.39	D28.7	D39.8	D49.59
body	C54.9	C79.82	D07.0	D26.1	D39.0	D49.59
cervix	C53.9	C79.82	D06.9	D26.0	D39.0	D49.59
cornu	C54.9	C79.82	D07.0	D26.1	D39.0	D49.59
corpus	C54.9	C79.82	D07.0	D26.1	D39.0	D49.59
endocervix (canal)						
(gland)	C53.0	C79.82	D06.0	D26.0	D39.0	D49.59
endometrium	C54.1	C79.82	D07.0	D26.1	D39.0	D49.59
exocervix	C53.1	C79.82	D06.1	D26.0	D39.0	D49.59
external os	C53.1	C79.82	D06.1	D26.0	D39.0	D49.59
fundus	C54.3	C79.82	D07.0	D26.1	D39.0	D49.59

Neoplasm, neoplastic	Malignant Primary	Malignant Secondary	Ca in situ	Benign	Uncertain	Unspecified Behavior
— continued						
uterus, uteri, uterine						
— continued						
internal os	C53.0	C79.82	D06.0	D26.0	D39.0	D49.59
isthmus	C54.0	C79.82	D07.0	D26.1	D39.0	D49.59
ligament	C57.3	C79.82	—	D28.2	D39.8	D49.59
broad	C57.1-✓	C79.82	D07.39	D28.2	D39.8	D49.59
round	C57.2-✓	C79.82	—	D28.2	D39.8	D49.59
lower segment	C54.0	C79.82	D07.0	D26.1	D39.0	D49.59
myometrium	C54.2	C79.82	D07.0	D26.1	D39.0	D49.59
overlapping						
sites	C54.8	—	—	—	—	—
squamocolumnar						
junction	C53.8	C79.82	D06.7	D26.0	D39.0	D49.59
tube	C57.0-✓	C79.82	D07.39	D28.2	D39.8	D49.59
utricle, prostatic	C68.0	C79.19	D09.19	D30.4	D41.3	D49.59
uveal tract	C69.4-✓	C79.49	D09.2-✓	D31.4-✓	D48.7	D49.89
uvula	C05.2	C79.89	D00.04	D10.39	D37.09	D49.0
vagina, vaginal (fornix)						
(vault) (wall)	C52	C79.82	D07.2	D28.1	D39.8	D49.59
vaginovesical	C57.9	C79.82	D07.30	D28.9	D39.9	D49.59
septum	C57.9	C79.82	D07.30	D28.9	D39.9	D49.59
vallecula						
(epiglottis)	C10.0	C79.89	D00.08	D10.5	D37.05	D49.0
vascular — see						
Neoplasm,						
connective tissue						
vas deferens	C63.1-✓	C79.82	D07.69	D29.8	D40.8	D49.59
Vater's ampulla	C24.1	C78.89	D01.5	D13.5	D37.6	D49.0
vein, venous — see						
Neoplasm,						
connective tissue						
vena cava (abdominal)						
(inferior)	C49.4	C79.89	—	D21.4	D48.1	D49.2
superior	C49.3	C79.89	—	D21.3	D48.1	D49.2
ventricle (cerebral)						
(floor) (lateral)						
(third)	C71.5	C79.31	—	D33.0	D43.0	D49.6
cardiac (left)						
(right)	C38.0	C79.89	—	D15.1	D48.7	D49.89
fourth	C71.7	C79.31	—	D33.1	D43.1	D49.6
ventricular band of						
larynx	C32.1	C78.39	D02.0	D14.1	D38.0	D49.1
ventriculus — see						
Neoplasm,						
stomach						
vermillion border —						
see Neoplasm, lip						
vermis,						
cerebellum	C71.6	C79.31	—	D33.1	D43.1	D49.6
vertebra (column)	C41.2	C79.51	—	D16.6	D48.0	D49.2
coccyx	C41.4	C79.51	—	D16.8	D48.0	D49.2
marrow NEC	C96.9	C79.52	—	—	D47.9	D49.89
sacrum	C41.4	C79.51	—	D16.8	D48.0	D49.2
vesical — see						
Neoplasm, bladder						
vesicle, seminal	C63.7	C79.82	D07.69	D29.8	D40.8	D49.59
vesicocervical						
tissue	C57.9	C79.82	D07.30	D28.9	D39.9	D49.59
vesicorectal	C76.3	C79.82	D09.8	D36.7	D48.7	D49.89
vesicovaginal	C57.9	C79.82	D07.30	D28.9	D39.9	D49.59
septum	C57.9	C79.82	D07.30	D28.9	D39.9	D49.59
vessel (blood) — see						
Neoplasm,						
connective tissue						
vestibular gland,						
greater	C51.0	C79.82	D07.1	D28.0	D39.8	D49.59
vestibule						
mouth	C06.1	C79.89	D00.00	D10.39	D37.09	D49.0
nose	C30.0	C78.39	D02.3	D14.0	D38.5	D49.1
Virchow's gland	C77.0	C77.0	—	D36.0	D48.7	D49.89
viscera NEC	C76.8	C79.89	D09.8	D36.7	D48.7	D49.89
vocal cords (true)	C32.0	C78.39	D02.0	D14.1	D38.0	D49.1
false	C32.1	C78.39	D02.0	D14.1	D38.0	D49.1
vomer	C41.0	C79.51	—	D16.4	D48.0	D49.2
vulva	C51.9	C79.82	D07.1	D28.0	D39.8	D49.59
vulvovaginal						
gland	C51.0	C79.82	D07.1	D28.0	D39.8	D49.59
Waldeyer's ring	C14.2	C79.89	D00.08	D10.9	D37.05	D49.0
Wharton's duct	C08.0	C79.89	D00.00	D11.7	D37.032	D49.0
white matter (central)						
(cerebral)	C71.0	C79.31	—	D33.0	D43.0	D49.6

	Malignant Primary	Malignant Secondary	Ca in situ	Benign	Uncertain	Unspecified Behavior
Neoplasm, neoplastic						
— continued						
windpipe	C33	C78.39	D02.1	D14.2	D38.1	D49.1
Wirsung's duct	C25.3	C78.89	D01.7	D13.6	D37.8	D49.0
wolffian (body) (duct)						
female	C57.7	C79.82	D07.39	D28.7	D39.8	D49.59
male	C63.7	C79.82	D07.69	D29.8	D40.8	D49.59
womb — see						
Neoplasm, uterus						
wrist NEC	C76.4-☑	C79.89	D04.6-☑	D36.7	D48.7	D49.89
xiphoid process	C41.3	C79.51	—	D16.7	D48.0	D49.2
Zuckerkandl						
organ	C75.5	C79.89	—	D35.6	D44.7	D49.7

Substance	Poisoning, Accidental (unintentional)	Poisoning, Intentional Self-harm	Poisoning, Assault	Poisoning, Undetermined	Adverse Effect	Under-dosing
14-Hydroxydihydromorphinone	T40.2X1	T40.2X2	T40.2X3	T40.2X4	T40.2X5	T40.2X6
1-Propanol	T51.3X1	T51.3X2	T51.3X3	T51.3X4	—	—
2,3,7,8-Tetrachlorodibenzo-p-dioxin	T53.7X1	T53.7X2	T53.7X3	T53.7X4	—	—
2,4,5-T (trichlorophenoxyacetic acid)	T60.1X1	T60.1X2	T60.1X3	T60.1X4	—	—
2,4,5-Trichlorophenoxyacetic acid	T60.3X1	T60.3X2	T60.3X3	T60.3X4	—	—
2,4-D (dichlorophenoxyacetic acid)	T60.3X1	T60.3X2	T60.3X3	T60.3X4	—	—
2,4-Toluene diisocyanate	T65.0X1	T65.0X2	T65.0X3	T65.0X4	—	—
2-Deoxy-5-fluorouridine	T45.1X1	T45.1X2	T45.1X3	T45.1X4	T45.1X5	T45.1X6
2-Ethoxyethanol	T52.3X1	T52.3X2	T52.3X3	T52.3X4	—	—
2-Methoxyethanol	T52.3X1	T52.3X2	T52.3X3	T52.3X4	—	—
2-Propanol	T51.2X1	T51.2X2	T51.2X3	T51.2X4	—	—
3,4-methylenedioxymeth-amphetamine	T43.641	T43.642	T43.643	T43.644	—	—
4-Aminobutyric acid	T43.8X1	T43.8X2	T43.8X3	T43.8X4	T43.8X5	T43.8X6
4-Aminophenol derivatives	T39.1X1	T39.1X2	T39.1X3	T39.1X4	T39.1X5	T39.1X6
5-Deoxy-5-fluorouridine	T45.1X1	T45.1X2	T45.1X3	T45.1X4	T45.1X5	T45.1X6
5-Methoxypsoralen (5-MOP)	T50.991	T50.992	T50.993	T50.994	T50.995	T50.996
8-Aminoquinoline drugs	T37.2X1	T37.2X2	T37.2X3	T37.2X4	T37.2X5	T37.2X6
8-Methoxypsoralen (8-MOP)	T50.991	T50.992	T50.993	T50.994	T50.995	T50.996
ABOB	T37.5X1	T37.5X2	T37.5X3	T37.5X4	T37.5X5	T37.5X6
Abrine	T62.2X1	T62.2X2	T62.2X3	T62.2X4	—	—
Abrus (seed)	T62.2X1	T62.2X2	T62.2X3	T62.2X4	—	—
Absinthe	T51.0X1	T51.0X2	T51.0X3	T51.0X4	—	—
beverage	T51.0X1	T51.0X2	T51.0X3	T51.0X4	—	—
Acaricide	T60.8X1	T60.8X2	T60.8X3	T60.8X4	—	—
Acebutolol	T44.7X1	T44.7X2	T44.7X3	T44.7X4	T44.7X5	T44.7X6
Acecarbromal	T42.6X1	T42.6X2	T42.6X3	T42.6X4	T42.6X5	T42.6X6
Aceclidine	T44.1X1	T44.1X2	T44.1X3	T44.1X4	T44.1X5	T44.1X6
Acedapsone	T37.0X1	T37.0X2	T37.0X3	T37.0X4	T37.0X5	T37.0X6
Acefylline piperazine	T48.6X1	T48.6X2	T48.6X3	T48.6X4	T48.6X5	T48.6X6
Acemorphan	T40.2X1	T40.2X2	T40.2X3	T40.2X4	T40.2X5	T40.2X6
Acenocoumarin	T45.511	T45.512	T45.513	T45.514	T45.515	T45.516
Acenocoumarol	T45.511	T45.512	T45.513	T45.514	T45.515	T45.516
Acepifylline	T48.6X1	T48.6X2	T48.6X3	T48.6X4	T48.6X5	T48.6X6
Acepromazine	T43.3X1	T43.3X2	T43.3X3	T43.3X4	T43.3X5	T43.3X6
Acesulfamethoxypyridazine	T37.0X1	T37.0X2	T37.0X3	T37.0X4	T37.0X5	T37.0X6
Acetal	T52.8X1	T52.8X2	T52.8X3	T52.8X4	—	—
Acetaldehyde (vapor)	T52.8X1	T52.8X2	T52.8X3	T52.8X4	—	—
liquid	T65.891	T65.892	T65.893	T65.894	—	—
Acetaminophen	T39.1X1	T39.1X2	T39.1X3	T39.1X4	T39.1X5	T39.1X6
Acetaminosalol	T39.1X1	T39.1X2	T39.1X3	T39.1X4	T39.1X5	T39.1X6
Acetanilide	T39.1X1	T39.1X2	T39.1X3	T39.1X4	T39.1X5	T39.1X6
Acetarsol	T37.3X1	T37.3X2	T37.3X3	T37.3X4	T37.3X5	T37.3X6
Acetazolamide	T50.2X1	T50.2X2	T50.2X3	T50.2X4	T50.2X5	T50.2X6
Acetiamine	T45.2X1	T45.2X2	T45.2X3	T45.2X4	T45.2X5	T45.2X6
Acetic						
acid	T54.2X1	T54.2X2	T54.2X3	T54.2X4	—	—
with sodium acetate (ointment)	T49.3X1	T49.3X2	T49.3X3	T49.3X4	T49.3X5	T49.3X6
ester (solvent)(vapor)	T52.8X1	T52.8X2	T52.8X3	T52.8X4	—	—
irrigating solution	T50.3X1	T50.3X2	T50.3X3	T50.3X4	T50.3X5	T50.3X6
medicinal (lotion)	T49.2X1	T49.2X2	T49.2X3	T49.2X4	T49.2X5	T49.2X6
anhydride	T65.891	T65.892	T65.893	T65.894	—	—
ether (vapor)	T52.8X1	T52.8X2	T52.8X3	T52.8X4	—	—
Acetohexamide	T38.3X1	T38.3X2	T38.3X3	T38.3X4	T38.3X5	T38.3X6
Acetohydroxamic acid	T50.991	T50.992	T50.993	T50.994	T50.995	T50.996
Acetomenaphthone	T45.7X1	T45.7X2	T45.7X3	T45.7X4	T45.7X5	T45.7X6
Acetomorphine	T40.1X1	T40.1X2	T40.1X3	T40.1X4	—	—
Acetone (oils)	T52.4X1	T52.4X2	T52.4X3	T52.4X4	—	—
chlorinated	T52.4X1	T52.4X2	T52.4X3	T52.4X4	—	—
vapor	T52.4X1	T52.4X2	T52.4X3	T52.4X4	—	—
Acetonitrile	T52.8X1	T52.8X2	T52.8X3	T52.8X4	—	—
Acetophenazine	T43.3X1	T43.3X2	T43.3X3	T43.3X4	T43.3X5	T43.3X6
Acetophenetedin	T39.1X1	T39.1X2	T39.1X3	T39.1X4	T39.1X5	T39.1X6
Acetophenone	T52.4X1	T52.4X2	T52.4X3	T52.4X4	—	—
Acetorphine	T40.2X1	T40.2X2	T40.2X3	T40.2X4	—	—
Acetosulfone (sodium)	T37.1X1	T37.1X2	T37.1X3	T37.1X4	T37.1X5	T37.1X6
Acetrizoate (sodium)	T50.8X1	T50.8X2	T50.8X3	T50.8X4	T50.8X5	T50.8X6
Acetrizoic acid	T50.8X1	T50.8X2	T50.8X3	T50.8X4	T50.8X5	T50.8X6
Acetyl						
bromide	T53.6X1	T53.6X2	T53.6X3	T53.6X4	—	—
Acetyl — continued						
chloride	T53.6X1	T53.6X2	T53.6X3	T53.6X4	—	—
Acetylcarbromal	T42.6X1	T42.6X2	T42.6X3	T42.6X4	T42.6X5	T42.6X6
Acetylcholine						
chloride	T44.1X1	T44.1X2	T44.1X3	T44.1X4	T44.1X5	T44.1X6
derivative	T44.1X1	T44.1X2	T44.1X3	T44.1X4	T44.1X5	T44.1X6
Acetylcysteine	T48.4X1	T48.4X2	T48.4X3	T48.4X4	T48.4X5	T48.4X6
Acetyldigitoxin	T46.0X1	T46.0X2	T46.0X3	T46.0X4	T46.0X5	T46.0X6
Acetyldigoxin	T46.0X1	T46.0X2	T46.0X3	T46.0X4	T46.0X5	T46.0X6
Acetyldihydrocodeine	T40.2X1	T40.2X2	T40.2X3	T40.2X4	—	—
Acetyldihydrocodeinone	T40.2X1	T40.2X2	T40.2X3	T40.2X4	—	—
Acetylene (gas)	T59.891	T59.892	T59.893	T59.894	—	—
dichloride	T53.6X1	T53.6X2	T53.6X3	T53.6X4	—	—
incomplete combustion of	T58.12	T58.13		T58.14	—	—
industrial	T59.891	T59.892	T59.893	T59.894	—	—
tetrachloride	T53.6X1	T53.6X2	T53.6X3	T53.6X4	—	—
vapor	T53.6X1	T53.6X2	T53.6X3	T53.6X4	—	—
Acetylpheneturide	T42.6X1	T42.6X2	T42.6X3	T42.6X4	T42.6X5	T42.6X6
Acetylphenylhydrazine	T39.8X1	T39.8X2	T39.8X3	T39.8X4	T39.8X5	T39.8X6
Acetylsalicylic acid (salts)	T39.011	T39.012	T39.013	T39.014	T39.015	T39.016
enteric coated	T39.011	T39.012	T39.013	T39.014	T39.015	T39.016
Acetylsulfamethoxypyridazine	T37.0X1	T37.0X2	T37.0X3	T37.0X4	T37.0X5	T37.0X6
Achromycin	T36.4X1	T36.4X2	T36.4X3	T36.4X4	T36.4X5	T36.4X6
ophthalmic preparation	T49.5X1	T49.5X2	T49.5X3	T49.5X4	T49.5X5	T49.5X6
topical NEC	T49.0X1	T49.0X2	T49.0X3	T49.0X4	T49.0X5	T49.0X6
Aciclovir	T37.5X1	T37.5X2	T37.5X3	T37.5X4	T37.5X5	T37.5X6
Acidifying agent NEC	T50.901	T50.902	T50.903	T50.904	T50.905	T50.906
Acid (corrosive) NEC	T54.2X1	T54.2X2	T54.2X3	T54.2X4	—	—
Acipimox	T46.6X1	T46.6X2	T46.6X3	T46.6X4	T46.6X5	T46.6X6
Acitretin	T50.991	T50.992	T50.993	T50.994	T50.995	T50.996
Aclarubicin	T45.1X1	T45.1X2	T45.1X3	T45.1X4	T45.1X5	T45.1X6
Aclatonium napadisilate	T48.1X1	T48.1X2	T48.1X3	T48.1X4	T48.1X5	T48.1X6
Aconite (wild)	T46.991	T46.992	T46.993	T46.994	T46.995	T46.996
Aconitine	T46.991	T46.992	T46.993	T46.994	T46.995	T46.996
Aconitum ferox	T46.991	T46.992	T46.993	T46.994	T46.995	T46.996
Acridine	T65.6X1	T65.6X2	T65.6X3	T65.6X4	—	—
vapor	T59.891	T59.892	T59.893	T59.894	—	—
Acriflavine	T37.91	T37.92	T37.93	T37.94	T37.95	T37.96
Acriflavinium chloride	T49.0X1	T49.0X2	T49.0X3	T49.0X4	T49.0X5	T49.0X6
Acrinol	T49.0X1	T49.0X2	T49.0X3	T49.0X4	T49.0X5	T49.0X6
Acrisorcin	T49.0X1	T49.0X2	T49.0X3	T49.0X4	T49.0X5	T49.0X6
Acrivastine	T45.0X1	T45.0X2	T45.0X3	T45.0X4	T45.0X5	T45.0X6
Acrolein (gas)	T59.891	T59.892	T59.893	T59.894	—	—
liquid	T54.1X1	T54.1X2	T54.1X3	T54.1X4	—	—
Acrylamide	T65.891	T65.892	T65.893	T65.894	—	—
Acrylic resin	T49.3X1	T49.3X2	T49.3X3	T49.3X4	T49.3X5	T49.3X6
Acrylonitrile	T65.891	T65.892	T65.893	T65.894	—	—
Actaea spicata	T62.2X1	T62.2X2	T62.2X3	T62.2X4	—	—
berry	T62.1X1	T62.1X2	T62.1X3	T62.1X4	—	—
Acterol	T37.3X1	T37.3X2	T37.3X3	T37.3X4	T37.3X5	T37.3X6
ACTH	T38.811	T38.812	T38.813	T38.814	T38.815	T38.816
Actinomycin C	T45.1X1	T45.1X2	T45.1X3	T45.1X4	T45.1X5	T45.1X6
Actinomycin D	T45.1X1	T45.1X2	T45.1X3	T45.1X4	T45.1X5	T45.1X6
Activated charcoal — see also Charcoal, medicinal	T47.6X1	T47.6X2	T47.6X3	T47.6X4	T47.6X5	T47.6X6
Acyclovir	T37.5X1	T37.5X2	T37.5X3	T37.5X4	T37.5X5	T37.5X6
Adenine	T45.2X1	T45.2X2	T45.2X3	T45.2X4	T45.2X5	T45.2X6
arabinoside	T37.5X1	T37.5X2	T37.5X3	T37.5X4	T37.5X5	T37.5X6
Adenosine (phosphate)	T46.2X1	T46.2X2	T46.2X3	T46.2X4	T46.2X5	T46.2X6
ADH	T38.891	T38.892	T38.893	T38.894	T38.895	T38.896
Adhesive NEC	T65.891	T65.892	T65.893	T65.894	—	—
Adicillin	T36.0X1	T36.0X2	T36.0X3	T36.0X4	T36.0X5	T36.0X6
Adiphenine	T44.3X1	T44.3X2	T44.3X3	T44.3X4	T44.3X5	T44.3X6
Adipiodone	T50.8X1	T50.8X2	T50.8X3	T50.8X4	T50.8X5	T50.8X6
Adjunct, pharmaceutical	T50.901	T50.902	T50.903	T50.904	T50.905	T50.906
Adrenal (extract, cortex or medulla) (glucocorticoids) (hormones) (mineralocorticoids)	T38.0X1	T38.0X2	T38.0X3	T38.0X4	T38.0X5	T38.0X6
ENT agent	T49.6X1	T49.6X2	T49.6X3	T49.6X4	T49.6X5	T49.6X6
ophthalmic preparation	T49.5X1	T49.5X2	T49.5X3	T49.5X4	T49.5X5	T49.5X6
topical NEC	T49.0X1	T49.0X2	T49.0X3	T49.0X4	T49.0X5	T49.0X6
Adrenalin — see Adrenaline						
Adrenaline	T44.5X1	T44.5X2	T44.5X3	T44.5X4	T44.5X5	T44.5X6
Adrenergic NEC	T44.901	T44.902	T44.903	T44.904	T44.905	T44.906
blocking agent NEC	T44.8X1	T44.8X2	T44.8X3	T44.8X4	T44.8X5	T44.8X6
beta, heart	T44.7X1	T44.7X2	T44.7X3	T44.7X4	T44.7X5	T44.7X6
specified NEC	T44.991	T44.992	T44.993	T44.994	T44.995	T44.996

350

Additional Character May Be Required — Refer to the Tabular List for Character Selection ▽ Subterms under main terms may continue to next column or page

Substance	Poisoning, Accidental (unintentional)	Poisoning, Intentional Self-harm	Poisoning, Assault	Poisoning, Undetermined	Adverse Effect	Under-dosing
Adrenochrome						
derivative	T46.991	T46.992	T46.993	T46.994	T46.995	T46.996
(mono) semicarbazone	T46.991	T46.992	T46.993	T46.994	T46.995	T46.996
Adrenocorticotrophic hormone	T38.811	T38.812	T38.813	T38.814	T38.815	T38.816
Adrenocorticotrophin	T38.811	T38.812	T38.813	T38.814	T38.815	T38.816
Adriamycin	T45.1X1	T45.1X2	T45.1X3	T45.1X4	T45.1X5	T45.1X6
Aerosol spray NEC	T65.91	T65.92	T65.93	T65.94	—	—
Aerosporin	T36.8X1	T36.8X2	T36.8X3	T36.8X4	T36.8X5	T36.8X6
ENT agent	T49.6X1	T49.6X2	T49.6X3	T49.6X4	T49.6X5	T49.6X6
ophthalmic preparation	T49.5X1	T49.5X2	T49.5X3	T49.5X4	T49.5X5	T49.5X6
topical NEC	T49.0X1	T49.0X2	T49.0X3	T49.0X4	T49.0X5	T49.0X6
Aethusa cynapium	T62.2X1	T62.2X2	T62.2X3	T62.2X4	—	—
Afghanistan black	T40.7X1	T40.7X2	T40.7X3	T40.7X4	T40.7X5	T40.7X6
Aflatoxin	T64.01	T64.02	T64.03	T64.04		
Afloqualone	T42.8X1	T42.8X2	T42.8X3	T42.8X4	T42.8X5	T42.8X6
African boxwood	T62.2X1	T62.2X2	T62.2X3	T62.2X4	—	—
Agar	T47.4X1	T47.4X2	T47.4X3	T47.4X4	T47.4X5	T47.4X6
Agonist						
predominantly						
alpha-adrenoreceptor	T44.4X1	T44.4X2	T44.4X3	T44.4X4	T44.4X5	T44.4X6
beta-adrenoreceptor	T44.5X1	T44.5X2	T44.5X3	T44.5X4	T44.5X5	T44.5X6
Agricultural agent NEC	T65.91	T65.92	T65.93	T65.94	—	—
Agrypnal	T42.3X1	T42.3X2	T42.3X3	T42.3X4	T42.3X5	T42.3X6
AHLG	T50.Z11	T50.Z12	T50.Z13	T50.Z14	T50.Z15	T50.Z16
Air contaminant(s), source/type NOS	T65.91	T65.92	T65.93	T65.94	—	—
Ajmaline	T46.2X1	T46.2X2	T46.2X3	T46.2X4	T46.2X5	T46.2X6
Akee	T62.1X1	T62.1X2	T62.1X3	T62.1X4	—	—
Akrinol	T49.0X1	T49.0X2	T49.0X3	T49.0X4	T49.0X5	T49.0X6
Akritoin	T37.8X1	T37.8X2	T37.8X3	T37.8X4	T37.8X5	T37.8X6
Alacepril	T46.4X1	T46.4X2	T46.4X3	T46.4X4	T46.4X5	T46.4X6
Alantolactone	T37.4X1	T37.4X2	T37.4X3	T37.4X4	T37.4X5	T37.4X6
Albamycin	T36.8X1	T36.8X2	T36.8X3	T36.8X4	T36.8X5	T36.8X6
Albendazole	T37.4X1	T37.4X2	T37.4X3	T37.4X4	T37.4X5	T37.4X6
Albumin						
bovine	T45.8X1	T45.8X2	T45.8X3	T45.8X4	T45.8X5	T45.8X6
human serum	T45.8X1	T45.8X2	T45.8X3	T45.8X4	T45.8X5	T45.8X6
salt-poor	T45.8X1	T45.8X2	T45.8X3	T45.8X4	T45.8X5	T45.8X6
normal human serum	T45.8X1	T45.8X2	T45.8X3	T45.8X4	T45.8X5	T45.8X6
Albuterol	T48.6X1	T48.6X2	T48.6X3	T48.6X4	T48.6X5	T48.6X6
Albutoin	T42.0X1	T42.0X2	T42.0X3	T42.0X4	T42.0X5	T42.0X6
Alclometasone	T49.0X1	T49.0X2	T49.0X3	T49.0X4	T49.0X5	T49.0X6
Alcohol	T51.91	T51.92	T51.93	T51.94	—	—
absolute	T51.0X1	T51.0X2	T51.0X3	T51.0X4	—	—
beverage	T51.0X1	T51.0X2	T51.0X3	T51.0X4	—	—
allyl	T51.8X1	T51.8X2	T51.8X3	T51.8X4	—	—
amyl	T51.3X1	T51.3X2	T51.3X3	T51.3X4	—	—
antifreeze	T51.1X1	T51.1X2	T51.1X3	T51.1X4	—	—
beverage	T51.0X1	T51.0X2	T51.0X3	T51.0X4	—	—
butyl	T51.3X1	T51.3X2	T51.3X3	T51.3X4	—	—
dehydrated	T51.0X1	T51.0X2	T51.0X3	T51.0X4	—	—
beverage	T51.0X1	T51.0X2	T51.0X3	T51.0X4	—	—
denatured	T51.0X1	T51.0X2	T51.0X3	T51.0X4	—	—
deterrent NEC	T50.6X1	T50.6X2	T50.6X3	T50.6X4	T50.6X5	T50.6X6
diagnostic (gastric function)	T50.8X1	T50.8X2	T50.8X3	T50.8X4	T50.8X5	T50.8X6
ethyl	T51.0X1	T51.0X2	T51.0X3	T51.0X4	—	—
beverage	T51.0X1	T51.0X2	T51.0X3	T51.0X4	—	—
grain	T51.0X1	T51.0X2	T51.0X3	T51.0X4	—	—
beverage	T51.0X1	T51.0X2	T51.0X3	T51.0X4	—	—
industrial	T51.0X1	T51.0X2	T51.0X3	T51.0X4	—	—
isopropyl	T51.2X1	T51.2X2	T51.2X3	T51.2X4	—	—
methyl	T51.1X1	T51.1X2	T51.1X3	T51.1X4	—	—
preparation for consumption	T51.0X1	T51.0X2	T51.0X3	T51.0X4	—	—
propyl	T51.3X1	T51.3X2	T51.3X3	T51.3X4		
secondary	T51.2X1	T51.2X2	T51.2X3	T51.2X4	—	—
radiator	T51.1X1	T51.1X2	T51.1X3	T51.1X4	—	—
rubbing	T51.2X1	T51.2X2	T51.2X3	T51.2X4	—	—
specified type NEC	T51.8X1	T51.8X2	T51.8X3	T51.8X4	—	—
surgical	T51.0X1	T51.0X2	T51.0X3	T51.0X4	—	—
vapor (from any type of Alcohol)	T59.891	T59.892	T59.893	T59.894	—	—
wood	T51.1X1	T51.1X2	T51.1X3	T51.1X4	—	—
Alcuronium (chloride)	T48.1X1	T48.1X2	T48.1X3	T48.1X4	T48.1X5	T48.1X6
Aldactone	T50.0X1	T50.0X2	T50.0X3	T50.0X4	T50.0X5	T50.0X6
Aldesulfone sodium	T37.1X1	T37.1X2	T37.1X3	T37.1X4	T37.1X5	T37.1X6
Aldicarb	T60.0X1	T60.0X2	T60.0X3	T60.0X4	—	—
Aldomet	T46.5X1	T46.5X2	T46.5X3	T46.5X4	T46.5X5	T46.5X6
Aldosterone	T50.0X1	T50.0X2	T50.0X3	T50.0X4	T50.0X5	T50.0X6
Aldrin (dust)	T60.1X1	T60.1X2	T60.1X3	T60.1X4	—	—
Aleve — see Naproxen						
Alexitol sodium	T47.1X1	T47.1X2	T47.1X3	T47.1X4	T47.1X5	T47.1X6
Alfacalcidol	T45.2X1	T45.2X2	T45.2X3	T45.2X4	T45.2X5	T45.2X6
Alfadolone	T41.1X1	T41.1X2	T41.1X3	T41.1X4	T41.1X5	T41.1X6
Alfaxalone	T41.1X1	T41.1X2	T41.1X3	T41.1X4	T41.1X5	T41.1X6
Alfentanil	T40.4X1	T40.4X2	T40.4X3	T40.4X4	T40.4X5	T40.4X6
Alfuzosin (hydrochloride)	T44.8X1	T44.8X2	T44.8X3	T44.8X4	T44.8X5	T44.8X6
Algae (harmful) (toxin)	T65.821	T65.822	T65.823	T65.824		
Algeldrate	T47.1X1	T47.1X2	T47.1X3	T47.1X4	T47.1X5	T47.1X6
Algin	T47.8X1	T47.8X2	T47.8X3	T47.8X4	T47.8X5	T47.8X6
Alglucerase	T45.3X1	T45.3X2	T45.3X3	T45.3X4	T45.3X5	T45.3X6
Alidase	T45.3X1	T45.3X2	T45.3X3	T45.3X4	T45.3X5	T45.3X6
Alimemazine	T43.3X1	T43.3X2	T43.3X3	T43.3X4	T43.3X5	T43.3X6
Aliphatic thiocyanates	T65.0X1	T65.0X2	T65.0X3	T65.0X4		
Alizapride	T45.0X1	T45.0X2	T45.0X3	T45.0X4	T45.0X5	T45.0X6
Alkali (caustic)	T54.3X1	T54.3X2	T54.3X3	T54.3X4		
Alkaline antiseptic solution (aromatic)	T49.6X1	T49.6X2	T49.6X3	T49.6X4	T49.6X5	T49.6X6
Alkalinizing agents (medicinal)	T50.901	T50.902	T50.903	T50.904	T50.905	T50.906
Alkalizing agent NEC	T50.901	T50.902	T50.903	T50.904	T50.905	T50.906
Alka-seltzer	T39.011	T39.012	T39.013	T39.014	T39.015	T39.016
Alkavervir	T46.5X1	T46.5X2	T46.5X3	T46.5X4	T46.5X5	T46.5X6
Alkonium (bromide)	T49.0X1	T49.0X2	T49.0X3	T49.0X4	T49.0X5	T49.0X6
Alkylating drug NEC	T45.1X1	T45.1X2	T45.1X3	T45.1X4	T45.1X5	T45.1X6
antimyeloproliferative	T45.1X1	T45.1X2	T45.1X3	T45.1X4	T45.1X5	T45.1X6
lymphatic	T45.1X1	T45.1X2	T45.1X3	T45.1X4	T45.1X5	T45.1X6
Alkylisocyanate	T65.0X1	T65.0X2	T65.0X3	T65.0X4		
Allantoin	T49.4X1	T49.4X2	T49.4X3	T49.4X4	T49.4X5	T49.4X6
Allegron	T43.011	T43.012	T43.013	T43.014	T43.015	T43.016
Allethrin	T49.0X1	T49.0X2	T49.0X3	T49.0X4	T49.0X5	T49.0X6
Allobarbital	T42.3X1	T42.3X2	T42.3X3	T42.3X4	T42.3X5	T42.3X6
Allopurinol	T50.4X1	T50.4X2	T50.4X3	T50.4X4	T50.4X5	T50.4X6
Allyl						
alcohol	T51.8X1	T51.8X2	T51.8X3	T51.8X4		
disulfide	T46.6X1	T46.6X2	T46.6X3	T46.6X4	T46.6X5	T46.6X6
Allylestrenol	T38.5X1	T38.5X2	T38.5X3	T38.5X4	T38.5X5	T38.5X6
Allylisopropylacetylurea	T42.6X1	T42.6X2	T42.6X3	T42.6X4	T42.6X5	T42.6X6
Allylisopropylmalonylurea	T42.3X1	T42.3X2	T42.3X3	T42.3X4	T42.3X5	T42.3X6
Allylthiourea	T49.3X1	T49.3X2	T49.3X3	T49.3X4	T49.3X5	T49.3X6
Allyltribromide	T42.6X1	T42.6X2	T42.6X3	T42.6X4	T42.6X5	T42.6X6
Allypropymal	T42.3X1	T42.3X2	T42.3X3	T42.3X4	T42.3X5	T42.3X6
Almagate	T47.1X1	T47.1X2	T47.1X3	T47.1X4	T47.1X5	T47.1X6
Almasilate	T47.1X1	T47.1X2	T47.1X3	T47.1X4	T47.1X5	T47.1X6
Almitrine	T50.7X1	T50.7X2	T50.7X3	T50.7X4	T50.7X5	T50.7X6
Aloes	T47.2X1	T47.2X2	T47.2X3	T47.2X4	T47.2X5	T47.2X6
Aloglutamol	T47.1X1	T47.1X2	T47.1X3	T47.1X4	T47.1X5	T47.1X6
Aloin	T47.2X1	T47.2X2	T47.2X3	T47.2X4	T47.2X5	T47.2X6
Aloxidone	T42.2X1	T42.2X2	T42.2X3	T42.2X4	T42.2X5	T42.2X6
Alpha						
acetyldigoxin	T46.0X1	T46.0X2	T46.0X3	T46.0X4	T46.0X5	T46.0X6
adrenergic blocking drug	T44.6X1	T44.6X2	T44.6X3	T44.6X4	T44.6X5	T44.6X6
amylase	T45.3X1	T45.3X2	T45.3X3	T45.3X4	T45.3X5	T45.3X6
tocoferol (acetate)	T45.2X1	T45.2X2	T45.2X3	T45.2X4	T45.2X5	T45.2X6
tocopherol	T45.2X1	T45.2X2	T45.2X3	T45.2X4	T45.2X5	T45.2X6
Alphadolone	T41.1X1	T41.1X2	T41.1X3	T41.1X4	T41.1X5	T41.1X6
Alphaprodine	T40.4X1	T40.4X2	T40.4X3	T40.4X4	T40.4X5	T40.4X6
Alphaxalone	T41.1X1	T41.1X2	T41.1X3	T41.1X4	T41.1X5	T41.1X6
Alprazolam	T42.4X1	T42.4X2	T42.4X3	T42.4X4	T42.4X5	T42.4X6
Alprenolol	T44.7X1	T44.7X2	T44.7X3	T44.7X4	T44.7X5	T44.7X6
Alprostadil	T46.7X1	T46.7X2	T46.7X3	T46.7X4	T46.7X5	T46.7X6
Alsactide	T38.811	T38.812	T38.813	T38.814	T38.815	T38.816
Alseroxylon	T46.5X1	T46.5X2	T46.5X3	T46.5X4	T46.5X5	T46.5X6
Alteplase	T45.611	T45.612	T45.613	T45.614	T45.615	T45.616
Altizide	T50.2X1	T50.2X2	T50.2X3	T50.2X4	T50.2X5	T50.2X6
Altretamine	T45.1X1	T45.1X2	T45.1X3	T45.1X4	T45.1X5	T45.1X6
Alum (medicinal)	T49.4X1	T49.4X2	T49.4X3	T49.4X4	T49.4X5	T49.4X6
nonmedicinal (ammonium) (potassium)	T56.891	T56.892	T56.893	T56.894	—	—
Aluminium, aluminum						
acetate	T49.2X1	T49.2X2	T49.2X3	T49.2X4	T49.2X5	T49.2X6
solution	T49.0X1	T49.0X2	T49.0X3	T49.0X4	T49.0X5	T49.0X6
aspirin	T39.011	T39.012	T39.013	T39.014	T39.015	T39.016
bis (acetylsalicylate)	T39.011	T39.012	T39.013	T39.014	T39.015	T39.016
carbonate (gel, basic)	T47.1X1	T47.1X2	T47.1X3	T47.1X4	T47.1X5	T47.1X6
chlorhydroxide-complex	T47.1X1	T47.1X2	T47.1X3	T47.1X4	T47.1X5	T47.1X6
chloride	T49.2X1	T49.2X2	T49.2X3	T49.2X4	T49.2X5	T49.2X6
clofibrate	T46.6X1	T46.6X2	T46.6X3	T46.6X4	T46.6X5	T46.6X6
diacetate	T49.2X1	T49.2X2	T49.2X3	T49.2X4	T49.2X5	T49.2X6
glycinate	T47.1X1	T47.1X2	T47.1X3	T47.1X4	T47.1X5	T47.1X6
hydroxide (gel)	T47.1X1	T47.1X2	T47.1X3	T47.1X4	T47.1X5	T47.1X6
hydroxide-magnesium carb. gel	T47.1X1	T47.1X2	T47.1X3	T47.1X4	T47.1X5	T47.1X6
magnesium silicate	T47.1X1	T47.1X2	T47.1X3	T47.1X4	T47.1X5	T47.1X6

Substance	Poisoning, Accidental (unintentional)	Poisoning, Intentional Self-harm	Poisoning, Assault	Poisoning, Undetermined	Adverse Effect	Under-dosing
Aluminium, aluminum — continued						
nicotinate	T46.7X1	T46.7X2	T46.7X3	T46.7X4	T46.7X5	T46.7X6
ointment (surgical) (topical)	T49.3X1	T49.3X2	T49.3X3	T49.3X4	T49.3X5	T49.3X6
phosphate	T47.1X1	T47.1X2	T47.1X3	T47.1X4	T47.1X5	T47.1X6
salicylate	T39.091	T39.092	T39.093	T39.094	T39.095	T39.096
silicate	T47.1X1	T47.1X2	T47.1X3	T47.1X4	T47.1X5	T47.1X6
sodium silicate	T47.1X1	T47.1X2	T47.1X3	T47.1X4	T47.1X5	T47.1X6
subacetate	T49.2X1	T49.2X2	T49.2X3	T49.2X4	T49.2X5	T49.2X6
sulfate	T49.0X1	T49.0X2	T49.0X3	T49.0X4	T49.0X5	T49.0X6
tannate	T47.6X1	T47.6X2	T47.6X3	T47.6X4	T47.6X5	T47.6X6
topical NEC	T49.3X1	T49.3X2	T49.3X3	T49.3X4	T49.3X5	T49.3X6
Alurate	T42.3X1	T42.3X2	T42.3X3	T42.3X4	T42.3X5	T42.3X6
Alverine	T44.3X1	T44.3X2	T44.3X3	T44.3X4	T44.3X5	T44.3X6
Alvodine	T40.2X1	T40.2X2	T40.2X3	T40.2X4	T40.2X5	T40.2X6
Amanita phalloides	T62.0X1	T62.0X2	T62.0X3	T62.0X4	—	—
Amanitine	T62.0X1	T62.0X2	T62.0X3	T62.0X4	—	—
Amantadine	T42.8X1	T42.8X2	T42.8X3	T42.8X4	T42.8X5	T42.8X6
Ambazone	T49.6X1	T49.6X2	T49.6X3	T49.6X4	T49.6X5	T49.6X6
Ambenonium (chloride)	T44.0X1	T44.0X2	T44.0X3	T44.0X4	T44.0X5	T44.0X6
Ambroxol	T48.4X1	T48.4X2	T48.4X3	T48.4X4	T48.4X5	T48.4X6
Ambuphylline	T48.6X1	T48.6X2	T48.6X3	T48.6X4	T48.6X5	T48.6X6
Ambutonium bromide	T44.3X1	T44.3X2	T44.3X3	T44.3X4	T44.3X5	T44.3X6
Amcinonide	T49.0X1	T49.0X2	T49.0X3	T49.0X4	T49.0X5	T49.0X6
Amdinocilline	T36.0X1	T36.0X2	T36.0X3	T36.0X4	T36.0X5	T36.0X6
Ametazole	T50.8X1	T50.8X2	T50.8X3	T50.8X4	T50.8X5	T50.8X6
Amethocaine	T41.3X1	T41.3X2	T41.3X3	T41.3X4	T41.3X5	T41.3X6
regional	T41.3X1	T41.3X2	T41.3X3	T41.3X4	T41.3X5	T41.3X6
spinal	T41.3X1	T41.3X2	T41.3X3	T41.3X4	T41.3X5	T41.3X6
Amethopterin	T45.1X1	T45.1X2	T45.1X3	T45.1X4	T45.1X5	T45.1X6
Amezinium metilsulfate	T44.991	T44.992	T44.993	T44.994	T44.995	T44.996
Amfebutamone	T43.291	T43.292	T43.293	T43.294	T43.295	T43.296
Amfepramone	T50.5X1	T50.5X2	T50.5X3	T50.5X4	T50.5X5	T50.5X6
Amfetamine	T43.621	T43.622	T43.623	T43.624	T43.625	T43.626
Amfetaminil	T43.621	T43.622	T43.623	T43.624	T43.625	T43.626
Amfomycin	T36.8X1	T36.8X2	T36.8X3	T36.8X4	T36.8X5	T36.8X6
Amidefrine mesilate	T48.5X1	T48.5X2	T48.5X3	T48.5X4	T48.5X5	T48.5X6
Amidone	T40.3X1	T40.3X2	T40.3X3	T40.3X4	T40.3X5	T40.3X6
Amidopyrine	T39.2X1	T39.2X2	T39.2X3	T39.2X4	T39.2X5	T39.2X6
Amidotrizoate	T50.8X1	T50.8X2	T50.8X3	T50.8X4	T50.8X5	T50.8X6
Amiflamine	T43.1X1	T43.1X2	T43.1X3	T43.1X4	T43.1X5	T43.1X6
Amikacin	T36.5X1	T36.5X2	T36.5X3	T36.5X4	T36.5X5	T36.5X6
Amikhelline	T46.3X1	T46.3X2	T46.3X3	T46.3X4	T46.3X5	T46.3X6
Amiloride	T50.2X1	T50.2X2	T50.2X3	T50.2X4	T50.2X5	T50.2X6
Aminacrine	T49.0X1	T49.0X2	T49.0X3	T49.0X4	T49.0X5	T49.0X6
Amineptine	T43.011	T43.012	T43.013	T43.014	T43.015	T43.016
Aminitrozole	T37.3X1	T37.3X2	T37.3X3	T37.3X4	T37.3X5	T37.3X6
Aminoacetic acid (derivatives)	T50.3X1	T50.3X2	T50.3X3	T50.3X4	T50.3X5	T50.3X6
Amino acids	T50.3X1	T50.3X2	T50.3X3	T50.3X4	T50.3X5	T50.3X6
Aminoacridine	T49.0X1	T49.0X2	T49.0X3	T49.0X4	T49.0X5	T49.0X6
Aminobenzoic acid (-p)	T49.3X1	T49.3X2	T49.3X3	T49.3X4	T49.3X5	T49.3X6
Aminocaproic acid	T45.621	T45.622	T45.623	T45.624	T45.625	T45.626
Aminoethylisothiourium	T45.8X1	T45.8X2	T45.8X3	T45.8X4	T45.8X5	T45.8X6
Aminofenazone	T39.2X1	T39.2X2	T39.2X3	T39.2X4	T39.2X5	T39.2X6
Aminoglutethimide	T45.1X1	T45.1X2	T45.1X3	T45.1X4	T45.1X5	T45.1X6
Aminohippuric acid	T50.8X1	T50.8X2	T50.8X3	T50.8X4	T50.8X5	T50.8X6
Aminomethylbenzoic acid	T45.691	T45.692	T45.693	T45.694	T45.695	T45.696
Aminometradine	T50.2X1	T50.2X2	T50.2X3	T50.2X4	T50.2X5	T50.2X6
Aminopentamide	T44.3X1	T44.3X2	T44.3X3	T44.3X4	T44.3X5	T44.3X6
Aminophenazone	T39.2X1	T39.2X2	T39.2X3	T39.2X4	T39.2X5	T39.2X6
Aminophenol	T54.0X1	T54.0X2	T54.0X3	T54.0X4	—	—
Aminophenylpyridone	T43.591	T43.592	T43.593	T43.594	T43.595	T43.596
Aminophylline	T48.6X1	T48.6X2	T48.6X3	T48.6X4	T48.6X5	T48.6X6
Aminopterin sodium	T45.1X1	T45.1X2	T45.1X3	T45.1X4	T45.1X5	T45.1X6
Aminopyrine	T39.2X1	T39.2X2	T39.2X3	T39.2X4	T39.2X5	T39.2X6
Aminorex	T50.5X1	T50.5X2	T50.5X3	T50.5X4	T50.5X5	T50.5X6
Aminosalicylic acid	T37.1X1	T37.1X2	T37.1X3	T37.1X4	T37.1X5	T37.1X6
Aminosalylum	T37.1X1	T37.1X2	T37.1X3	T37.1X4	T37.1X5	T37.1X6
Amiodarone	T46.2X1	T46.2X2	T46.2X3	T46.2X4	T46.2X5	T46.2X6
Amiphenazole	T50.7X1	T50.7X2	T50.7X3	T50.7X4	T50.7X5	T50.7X6
Amiquinsin	T46.5X1	T46.5X2	T46.5X3	T46.5X4	T46.5X5	T46.5X6
Amisometradine	T50.2X1	T50.2X2	T50.2X3	T50.2X4	T50.2X5	T50.2X6
Amisulpride	T43.591	T43.592	T43.593	T43.594	T43.595	T43.596
Amitriptyline	T43.011	T43.012	T43.013	T43.014	T43.015	T43.016
Amitriptylinoxide	T43.011	T43.012	T43.013	T43.014	T43.015	T43.016
Amlexanox	T48.6X1	T48.6X2	T48.6X3	T48.6X4	T48.6X5	T48.6X6
Ammonia (fumes) (gas) (vapor)	T59.891	T59.892	T59.893	T59.894	—	—
aromatic spirit	T48.991	T48.992	T48.993	T48.994	T48.995	T48.996
liquid (household)	T54.3X1	T54.3X2	T54.3X3	T54.3X4	—	—
Ammoniated mercury	T49.0X1	T49.0X2	T49.0X3	T49.0X4	T49.0X5	T49.0X6
Ammonium						
acid tartrate	T49.5X1	T49.5X2	T49.5X3	T49.5X4	T49.5X5	T49.5X6
bromide	T42.6X1	T42.6X2	T42.6X3	T42.6X4	T42.6X5	T42.6X6
carbonate	T54.3X1	T54.3X2	T54.3X3	T54.3X4	—	—
chloride	T50.991	T50.992	T50.993	T50.994	T50.995	T50.996
expectorant	T48.4X1	T48.4X2	T48.4X3	T48.4X4	T48.4X5	T48.4X6
compounds (household) NEC	T54.3X1	T54.3X2	T54.3X3	T54.3X4	—	—
fumes (any usage)	T59.891	T59.892	T59.893	T59.894	—	—
industrial	T54.3X1	T54.3X2	T54.3X3	T54.3X4	—	—
ichthyosulronate	T49.4X1	T49.4X2	T49.4X3	T49.4X4	T49.4X5	T49.4X6
mandelate	T37.91	T37.92	T37.93	T37.94	T37.95	T37.96
sulfamate	T60.3X1	T60.3X2	T60.3X3	T60.3X4	—	—
sulfonate resin	T47.8X1	T47.8X2	T47.8X3	T47.8X4	T47.8X5	T47.8X6
Amobarbital (sodium)	T42.3X1	T42.3X2	T42.3X3	T42.3X4	T42.3X5	T42.3X6
Amodiaquine	T37.2X1	T37.2X2	T37.2X3	T37.2X4	T37.2X5	T37.2X6
Amopyroquin (e)	T37.2X1	T37.2X2	T37.2X3	T37.2X4	T37.2X5	T37.2X6
Amoxapine	T43.011	T43.012	T43.013	T43.014	T43.015	T43.016
Amoxicillin	T36.0X1	T36.0X2	T36.0X3	T36.0X4	T36.0X5	T36.0X6
Amperozide	T43.591	T43.592	T43.593	T43.594	T43.595	T43.596
Amphenidone	T43.591	T43.592	T43.593	T43.594	T43.595	T43.596
Amphetamine NEC	T43.621	T43.622	T43.623	T43.624	T43.625	T43.626
Amphomycin	T36.8X1	T36.8X2	T36.8X3	T36.8X4	T36.8X5	T36.8X6
Amphotalide	T37.4X1	T37.4X2	T37.4X3	T37.4X4	T37.4X5	T37.4X6
Amphotericin B	T36.7X1	T36.7X2	T36.7X3	T36.7X4	T36.7X5	T36.7X6
topical	T49.0X1	T49.0X2	T49.0X3	T49.0X4	T49.0X5	T49.0X6
Ampicillin	T36.0X1	T36.0X2	T36.0X3	T36.0X4	T36.0X5	T36.0X6
Amprotropine	T44.3X1	T44.3X2	T44.3X3	T44.3X4	T44.3X5	T44.3X6
Amsacrine	T45.1X1	T45.1X2	T45.1X3	T45.1X4	T45.1X5	T45.1X6
Amygdaline	T62.2X1	T62.2X2	T62.2X3	T62.2X4	—	—
Amyl						
acetate	T52.8X1	T52.8X2	T52.8X3	T52.8X4	—	—
vapor	T59.891	T59.892	T59.893	T59.894	—	—
alcohol	T51.3X1	T51.3X2	T51.3X3	T51.3X4	—	—
chloride	T53.6X1	T53.6X2	T53.6X3	T53.6X4	—	—
formate	T52.8X1	T52.8X2	T52.8X3	T52.8X4	—	—
nitrite	T46.3X1	T46.3X2	T46.3X3	T46.3X4	T46.3X5	T46.3X6
propionate	T47.5X1	T47.5X2	T47.5X3	T47.5X4	T47.5X5	T47.5X6
Amylase	T41.3X1	T41.3X2	T41.3X3	T41.3X4	T41.3X5	T41.3X6
Amyleine, regional	T41.3X1	T41.3X2	T41.3X3	T41.3X4	T41.3X5	T41.3X6
Amylene						
dichloride	T53.6X1	T53.6X2	T53.6X3	T53.6X4	—	—
hydrate	T51.3X1	T51.3X2	T51.3X3	T51.3X4	—	—
Amylmetacresol	T49.6X1	T49.6X2	T49.6X3	T49.6X4	T49.6X5	T49.6X6
Amylobarbitone	T42.3X1	T42.3X2	T42.3X3	T42.3X4	T42.3X5	T42.3X6
Amylocaine, regional	T41.3X1	T41.3X2	T41.3X3	T41.3X4	T41.3X5	T41.3X6
infiltration (subcutaneous)	T41.3X1	T41.3X2	T41.3X3	T41.3X4	T41.3X5	T41.3X6
nerve block (peripheral) (plexus)	T41.3X1	T41.3X2	T41.3X3	T41.3X4	T41.3X5	T41.3X6
spinal	T41.3X1	T41.3X2	T41.3X3	T41.3X4	T41.3X5	T41.3X6
topical (surface)	T41.3X1	T41.3X2	T41.3X3	T41.3X4	T41.3X5	T41.3X6
Amylopectin	T47.6X1	T47.6X2	T47.6X3	T47.6X4	T47.6X5	T47.6X6
Amytal (sodium)	T42.3X1	T42.3X2	T42.3X3	T42.3X4	T42.3X5	T42.3X6
Anabolic steroid	T38.7X1	T38.7X2	T38.7X3	T38.7X4	T38.7X5	T38.7X6
Analeptic NEC	T50.7X1	T50.7X2	T50.7X3	T50.7X4	T50.7X5	T50.7X6
Analgesic	T39.91	T39.92	T39.93	T39.94	T39.95	T39.96
anti-inflammatory NEC	T39.91	T39.92	T39.93	T39.94	T39.95	T39.96
propionic acid derivative	T39.311	T39.312	T39.313	T39.314	T39.315	T39.316
antirheumatic NEC	T39.4X1	T39.4X2	T39.4X3	T39.4X4	T39.4X5	T39.4X6
aromatic NEC	T39.1X1	T39.1X2	T39.1X3	T39.1X4	T39.1X5	T39.1X6
narcotic NEC	T40.601	T40.602	T40.603	T40.604	T40.605	T40.606
combination	T40.601	T40.602	T40.603	T40.604	T40.605	T40.606
obstetric	T40.601	T40.602	T40.603	T40.604	T40.605	T40.606
non-narcotic NEC	T39.91	T39.92	T39.93	T39.94	T39.95	T39.96
combination	T39.91	T39.92	T39.93	T39.94	T39.95	T39.96
pyrazole	T39.2X1	T39.2X2	T39.2X3	T39.2X4	T39.2X5	T39.2X6
specified NEC	T39.8X1	T39.8X2	T39.8X3	T39.8X4	T39.8X5	T39.8X6
Analgin	T39.2X1	T39.2X2	T39.2X3	T39.2X4	T39.2X5	T39.2X6
Anamirta cocculus	T62.1X1	T62.1X2	T62.1X3	T62.1X4	—	—
Ancillin	T36.0X1	T36.0X2	T36.0X3	T36.0X4	T36.0X5	T36.0X6
Ancrod	T45.691	T45.692	T45.693	T45.694	T45.695	T45.696
Androgen	T38.7X1	T38.7X2	T38.7X3	T38.7X4	T38.7X5	T38.7X6
Androgen-estrogen mixture	T38.7X1	T38.7X2	T38.7X3	T38.7X4	T38.7X5	T38.7X6
Androstalone	T38.7X1	T38.7X2	T38.7X3	T38.7X4	T38.7X5	T38.7X6
Androstanolone	T38.7X1	T38.7X2	T38.7X3	T38.7X4	T38.7X5	T38.7X6
Androsterone	T38.7X1	T38.7X2	T38.7X3	T38.7X4	T38.7X5	T38.7X6
Anemone pulsatilla	T62.2X1	T62.2X2	T62.2X3	T62.2X4	—	—
Anesthesia						
caudal	T41.3X1	T41.3X2	T41.3X3	T41.3X4	T41.3X5	T41.3X6
endotracheal	T41.0X1	T41.0X2	T41.0X3	T41.0X4	T41.0X5	T41.0X6
epidural	T41.3X1	T41.3X2	T41.3X3	T41.3X4	T41.3X5	T41.3X6
inhalation	T41.0X1	T41.0X2	T41.0X3	T41.0X4	T41.0X5	T41.0X6

Substance	Poisoning, Accidental (unintentional)	Poisoning, Intentional Self-harm	Poisoning, Assault	Poisoning, Undetermined	Adverse Effect	Under-dosing
Anesthesia — *continued*						
local	T41.3X1	T41.3X2	T41.3X3	T41.3X4	T41.3X5	T41.3X6
mucosal	T41.3X1	T41.3X2	T41.3X3	T41.3X4	T41.3X5	T41.3X6
muscle relaxation	T48.1X1	T48.1X2	T48.1X3	T48.1X4	T48.1X5	T48.1X6
nerve blocking	T41.3X1	T41.3X2	T41.3X3	T41.3X4	T41.3X5	T41.3X6
plexus blocking	T41.3X1	T41.3X2	T41.3X3	T41.3X4	T41.3X5	T41.3X6
potentiated	T41.201	T41.202	T41.203	T41.204	T41.205	T41.206
rectal	T41.201	T41.202	T41.203	T41.204	T41.205	T41.206
general	T41.201	T41.202	T41.203	T41.204	T41.205	T41.206
local	T41.3X1	T41.3X2	T41.3X3	T41.3X4	T41.3X5	T41.3X6
regional	T41.3X1	T41.3X2	T41.3X3	T41.3X4	T41.3X5	T41.3X6
surface	T41.3X1	T41.3X2	T41.3X3	T41.3X4	T41.3X5	T41.3X6
Anesthetic NEC — *see also*	T41.41	T41.42	T41.43	T41.44	T41.45	T41.46
Anesthesia						
with muscle relaxant	T41.201	T41.202	T41.203	T41.204	T41.205	T41.206
general	T41.201	T41.202	T41.203	T41.204	T41.205	T41.206
local	T41.3X1	T41.3X2	T41.3X3	T41.3X4	T41.3X5	T41.3X6
gaseous NEC	T41.0X1	T41.0X2	T41.0X3	T41.0X4	T41.0X5	T41.0X6
general NEC	T41.201	T41.202	T41.203	T41.204	T41.205	T41.206
halogenated hydrocarbon derivatives NEC	T41.0X1	T41.0X2	T41.0X3	T41.0X4	T41.0X5	T41.0X6
infiltration NEC	T41.3X1	T41.3X2	T41.3X3	T41.3X4	T41.3X5	T41.3X6
intravenous NEC	T41.1X1	T41.1X2	T41.1X3	T41.1X4	T41.1X5	T41.1X6
local NEC	T41.3X1	T41.3X2	T41.3X3	T41.3X4	T41.3X5	T41.3X6
rectal	T41.201	T41.202	T41.203	T41.204	T41.205	T41.206
general	T41.201	T41.202	T41.203	T41.204	T41.205	T41.206
local	T41.3X1	T41.3X2	T41.3X3	T41.3X4	T41.3X5	T41.3X6
regional NEC	T41.3X1	T41.3X2	T41.3X3	T41.3X4	T41.3X5	T41.3X6
spinal NEC	T41.3X1	T41.3X2	T41.3X3	T41.3X4	T41.3X5	T41.3X6
thiobarbiturate	T41.1X1	T41.1X2	T41.1X3	T41.1X4	T41.1X5	T41.1X6
topical	T41.3X1	T41.3X2	T41.3X3	T41.3X4	T41.3X5	T41.3X6
Aneurine	T45.2X1	T45.2X2	T45.2X3	T45.2X4	T45.2X5	T45.2X6
Angio-Conray	T50.8X1	T50.8X2	T50.8X3	T50.8X4	T50.8X5	T50.8X6
Angiotensin	T44.5X1	T44.5X2	T44.5X3	T44.5X4	T44.5X5	T44.5X6
Angiotensinamide	T44.991	T44.992	T44.993	T44.994	T44.995	T44.996
Anhydrohydroxy-progesterone	T38.5X1	T38.5X2	T38.5X3	T38.5X4	T38.5X5	T38.5X6
Anhydron	T50.2X1	T50.2X2	T50.2X3	T50.2X4	T50.2X5	T50.2X6
Anileridine	T40.4X1	T40.4X2	T40.4X3	T40.4X4	T40.4X5	T40.4X6
Aniline (dye) (liquid)	T65.3X1	T65.3X2	T65.3X3	T65.3X4	—	—
analgesic	T39.1X1	T39.1X2	T39.1X3	T39.1X4	T39.1X5	T39.1X6
derivatives, therapeutic NEC	T39.1X1	T39.1X2	T39.1X3	T39.1X4	T39.1X5	T39.1X6
vapor	T65.3X1	T65.3X2	T65.3X3	T65.3X4	—	—
Aniscoropine	T44.3X1	T44.3X2	T44.3X3	T44.3X4	T44.3X5	T44.3X6
Anise oil	T47.5X1	T47.5X2	T47.5X3	T47.5X4	T47.5X5	T47.5X6
Anisidine	T65.3X1	T65.3X2	T65.3X3	T65.3X4	—	—
Anisindione	T45.511	T45.512	T45.513	T45.514	T45.515	T45.516
Anisotropine	T44.3X1	T44.3X2	T44.3X3	T44.3X4	T44.3X5	T44.3X6
methyl-bromide						
Anistreplase	T45.611	T45.612	T45.613	T45.614	T45.615	T45.616
Anorexiant (central)	T50.5X1	T50.5X2	T50.5X3	T50.5X4	T50.5X5	T50.5X6
Anorexic agents	T50.5X1	T50.5X2	T50.5X3	T50.5X4	T50.5X5	T50.5X6
Ansamycin	T36.6X1	T36.6X2	T36.6X3	T36.6X4	T36.6X5	T36.6X6
Ant (bite) (sting)	T63.421	T63.422	T63.423	T63.424	—	—
Antabuse	T50.6X1	T50.6X2	T50.6X3	T50.6X4	T50.6X5	T50.6X6
Antacid NEC	T47.1X1	T47.1X2	T47.1X3	T47.1X4	T47.1X5	T47.1X6
Antagonist						
Aldosterone	T50.0X1	T50.0X2	T50.0X3	T50.0X4	T50.0X5	T50.0X6
alpha-adrenoreceptor	T44.6X1	T44.6X2	T44.6X3	T44.6X4	T44.6X5	T44.6X6
anticoagulant	T45.7X1	T45.7X2	T45.7X3	T45.7X4	T45.7X5	T45.7X6
beta-adrenoreceptor	T44.7X1	T44.7X2	T44.7X3	T44.7X4	T44.7X5	T44.7X6
extrapyramidal NEC	T44.3X1	T44.3X2	T44.3X3	T44.3X4	T44.3X5	T44.3X6
folic acid	T45.1X1	T45.1X2	T45.1X3	T45.1X4	T45.1X5	T45.1X6
H2 receptor	T47.0X1	T47.0X2	T47.0X3	T47.0X4	T47.0X5	T47.0X6
heavy metal	T45.8X1	T45.8X2	T45.8X3	T45.8X4	T45.8X5	T45.8X6
narcotic analgesic	T50.7X1	T50.7X2	T50.7X3	T50.7X4	T50.7X5	T50.7X6
opiate	T50.7X1	T50.7X2	T50.7X3	T50.7X4	T50.7X5	T50.7X6
pyrimidine	T45.1X1	T45.1X2	T45.1X3	T45.1X4	T45.1X5	T45.1X6
serotonin	T46.5X1	T46.5X2	T46.5X3	T46.5X4	T46.5X5	T46.5X6
Antazolin (e)	T45.0X1	T45.0X2	T45.0X3	T45.0X4	T45.0X5	T45.0X6
Anterior pituitary hormone NEC	T38.811	T38.812	T38.813	T38.814	T38.815	T38.816
Anthelmintic NEC	T37.4X1	T37.4X2	T37.4X3	T37.4X4	T37.4X5	T37.4X6
Anthiolimine	T37.4X1	T37.4X2	T37.4X3	T37.4X4	T37.4X5	T37.4X6
Anthralin	T49.4X1	T49.4X2	T49.4X3	T49.4X4	T49.4X5	T49.4X6
Anthramycin	T45.1X1	T45.1X2	T45.1X3	T45.1X4	T45.1X5	T45.1X6
Antiadrenergic NEC	T44.8X1	T44.8X2	T44.8X3	T44.8X4	T44.8X5	T44.8X6
Antiallergic NEC	T45.0X1	T45.0X2	T45.0X3	T45.0X4	T45.0X5	T45.0X6
Antiandrogen NEC	T38.6X1	T38.6X2	T38.6X3	T38.6X4	T38.6X5	T38.6X6
Anti-anemic (drug) (preparation)	T45.8X1	T45.8X2	T45.8X3	T45.8X4	T45.8X5	T45.8X6
Antianxiety drug NEC	T43.501	T43.502	T43.503	T43.504	T43.505	T43.506
Antiaris toxicaria	T65.891	T65.892	T65.893	T65.894	—	—
Antiarteriosclerotic drug	T46.6X1	T46.6X2	T46.6X3	T46.6X4	T46.6X5	T46.6X6
Antiasthmatic drug NEC	T48.6X1	T48.6X2	T48.6X3	T48.6X4	T48.6X5	T48.6X6
Antibiotic NEC	T36.91	T36.92	T36.93	T36.94	T36.95	T36.96
aminoglycoside	T36.5X1	T36.5X2	T36.5X3	T36.5X4	T36.5X5	T36.5X6
anticancer	T45.1X1	T45.1X2	T45.1X3	T45.1X4	T45.1X5	T45.1X6
antifungal	T36.7X1	T36.7X2	T36.7X3	T36.7X4	T36.7X5	T36.7X6
antimycobacterial	T36.5X1	T36.5X2	T36.5X3	T36.5X4	T36.5X5	T36.5X6
antineoplastic	T45.1X1	T45.1X2	T45.1X3	T45.1X4	T45.1X5	T45.1X6
b-lactam NEC	T36.1X1	T36.1X2	T36.1X3	T36.1X4	T36.1X5	T36.1X6
cephalosporin (group)	T36.1X1	T36.1X2	T36.1X3	T36.1X4	T36.1X5	T36.1X6
chloramphenicol (group)	T36.2X1	T36.2X2	T36.2X3	T36.2X4	T36.2X5	T36.2X6
ENT	T49.6X1	T49.6X2	T49.6X3	T49.6X4	T49.6X5	T49.6X6
eye	T49.5X1	T49.5X2	T49.5X3	T49.5X4	T49.5X5	T49.5X6
fungicidal (local)	T49.0X1	T49.0X2	T49.0X3	T49.0X4	T49.0X5	T49.0X6
intestinal	T36.8X1	T36.8X2	T36.8X3	T36.8X4	T36.8X5	T36.8X6
local	T49.0X1	T49.0X2	T49.0X3	T49.0X4	T49.0X5	T49.0X6
macrolides	T36.3X1	T36.3X2	T36.3X3	T36.3X4	T36.3X5	T36.3X6
polypeptide	T36.8X1	T36.8X2	T36.8X3	T36.8X4	T36.8X5	T36.8X6
specified NEC	T36.8X1	T36.8X2	T36.8X3	T36.8X4	T36.8X5	T36.8X6
tetracycline (group)	T36.4X1	T36.4X2	T36.4X3	T36.4X4	T36.4X5	T36.4X6
throat	T49.6X1	T49.6X2	T49.6X3	T49.6X4	T49.6X5	T49.6X6
Anticancer agents NEC	T45.1X1	T45.1X2	T45.1X3	T45.1X4	T45.1X5	T45.1X6
Anticholesterolemic drug NEC	T46.6X1	T46.6X2	T46.6X3	T46.6X4	T46.6X5	T46.6X6
Anticholinergic NEC	T44.3X1	T44.3X2	T44.3X3	T44.3X4	T44.3X5	T44.3X6
Anticholinesterase	T44.0X1	T44.0X2	T44.0X3	T44.0X4	T44.0X5	T44.0X6
organophosphorus	T44.0X1	T44.0X2	T44.0X3	T44.0X4	T44.0X5	T44.0X6
insecticide	T60.0X1	T60.0X2	T60.0X3	T60.0X4	—	—
nerve gas	T59.891	T59.892	T59.893	T59.894	—	—
reversible	T44.0X1	T44.0X2	T44.0X3	T44.0X4	T44.0X5	T44.0X6
ophthalmological	T49.5X1	T49.5X2	T49.5X3	T49.5X4	T49.5X5	T49.5X6
Anticoagulant NEC	T45.511	T45.512	T45.513	T45.514	T45.515	T45.516
Antagonist	T45.7X1	T45.7X2	T45.7X3	T45.7X4	T45.7X5	T45.7X6
Anti-common-cold drug NEC	T48.5X1	T48.5X2	T48.5X3	T48.5X4	T48.5X5	T48.5X6
Anticonvulsant	T42.71	T42.72	T42.73	T42.74	T42.75	T42.76
barbiturate	T42.3X1	T42.3X2	T42.3X3	T42.3X4	T42.3X5	T42.3X6
combination (with barbiturate)	T42.3X1	T42.3X2	T42.3X3	T42.3X4	T42.3X5	T42.3X6
hydantoin	T42.0X1	T42.0X2	T42.0X3	T42.0X4	T42.0X5	T42.0X6
hypnotic NEC	T42.6X1	T42.6X2	T42.6X3	T42.6X4	T42.6X5	T42.6X6
oxazolidinedione	T42.2X1	T42.2X2	T42.2X3	T42.2X4	T42.2X5	T42.2X6
pyrimidinedione	T42.6X1	T42.6X2	T42.6X3	T42.6X4	T42.6X5	T42.6X6
specified NEC	T42.6X1	T42.6X2	T42.6X3	T42.6X4	T42.6X5	T42.6X6
succinimide	T42.2X1	T42.2X2	T42.2X3	T42.2X4	T42.2X5	T42.2X6
Antidepressant	T43.201	T43.202	T43.203	T43.204	T43.205	T43.206
monoamine oxidase inhibitor	T43.1X1	T43.1X2	T43.1X3	T43.1X4	T43.1X5	T43.1X6
selective serotonin norepinephrine reuptake inhibitor	T43.211	T43.212	T43.213	T43.214	T43.215	T43.216
selective serotonin reuptake inhibitor	T43.221	T43.222	T43.223	T43.224	T43.225	T43.226
specified NEC	T43.291	T43.292	T43.293	T43.294	T43.295	T43.296
tetracyclic	T43.021	T43.022	T43.023	T43.024	T43.025	T43.026
triazolopyridine	T43.211	T43.212	T43.213	T43.214	T43.215	T43.216
tricyclic	T43.011	T43.012	T43.013	T43.014	T43.015	T43.016
Antidiabetic NEC	T38.3X1	T38.3X2	T38.3X3	T38.3X4	T38.3X5	T38.3X6
biguanide	T38.3X1	T38.3X2	T38.3X3	T38.3X4	T38.3X5	T38.3X6
and sulfonyl combined	T38.3X1	T38.3X2	T38.3X3	T38.3X4	T38.3X5	T38.3X6
combined	T38.3X1	T38.3X2	T38.3X3	T38.3X4	T38.3X5	T38.3X6
sulfonylurea	T38.3X1	T38.3X2	T38.3X3	T38.3X4	T38.3X5	T38.3X6
Antidiarrheal drug NEC	T47.6X1	T47.6X2	T47.6X3	T47.6X4	T47.6X5	T47.6X6
absorbent	T47.6X1	T47.6X2	T47.6X3	T47.6X4	T47.6X5	T47.6X6
Anti-D immunoglobulin (human)	T50.Z11	T50.Z12	T50.Z13	T50.Z14	T50.Z15	T50.Z16
Antidiphtheria serum	T50.Z11	T50.Z12	T50.Z13	T50.Z14	T50.Z15	T50.Z16
Antidiuretic hormone	T38.891	T38.892	T38.893	T38.894	T38.895	T38.896
Antidote NEC	T50.6X1	T50.6X2	T50.6X3	T50.6X4	T50.6X5	T50.6X6
heavy metal	T45.8X1	T45.8X2	T45.8X3	T45.8X4	T45.8X5	T45.8X6
Antidysrhythmic NEC	T46.2X1	T46.2X2	T46.2X3	T46.2X4	T46.2X5	T46.2X6
Antiemetic drug	T45.0X1	T45.0X2	T45.0X3	T45.0X4	T45.0X5	T45.0X6
Antiepilepsy agent	T42.71	T42.72	T42.73	T42.74	T42.75	T42.76
combination	T42.5X1	T42.5X2	T42.5X3	T42.5X4	T42.5X5	T42.5X6
mixed	T42.5X1	T42.5X2	T42.5X3	T42.5X4	T42.5X5	T42.5X6
specified, NEC	T42.6X1	T42.6X2	T42.6X3	T42.6X4	T42.6X5	T42.6X6
Antiestrogen NEC	T38.6X1	T38.6X2	T38.6X3	T38.6X4	T38.6X5	T38.6X6
Antifertility pill	T38.4X1	T38.4X2	T38.4X3	T38.4X4	T38.4X5	T38.4X6
Antifibrinolytic drug	T45.621	T45.622	T45.623	T45.624	T45.625	T45.626
Antifilarial drug	T37.4X1	T37.4X2	T37.4X3	T37.4X4	T37.4X5	T37.4X6
Antiflatulent	T47.5X1	T47.5X2	T47.5X3	T47.5X4	T47.5X5	T47.5X6
Antifreeze	T65.91	T65.92	T65.93	T65.94	—	—
alcohol	T51.1X1	T51.1X2	T51.1X3	T51.1X4	—	—

Table of Drugs and Chemicals

Antifreeze — Aralen

Substance	Poisoning, Accidental (unintentional)	Poisoning, Intentional Self-harm	Poisoning, Assault	Poisoning, Undetermined	Adverse Effect	Under-dosing
Antifreeze — *continued*						
ethylene glycol	T51.8X1	T51.8X2	T51.8X3	T51.8X4	—	—
Antifungal						
antibiotic (systemic)	T36.7X1	T36.7X2	T36.7X3	T36.7X4	T36.7X5	T36.7X6
anti-infective NEC	T37.91	T37.92	T37.93	T37.94	T37.95	T37.96
disinfectant, local	T49.0X1	T49.0X2	T49.0X3	T49.0X4	T49.0X5	T49.0X6
nonmedicinal (spray)	T60.3X1	T60.3X2	T60.3X3	T60.3X4	—	—
topical	T49.0X1	T49.0X2	T49.0X3	T49.0X4	T49.0X5	T49.0X6
Anti-gastric-secretion drug NEC	T47.1X1	T47.1X2	T47.1X3	T47.1X4	T47.1X5	T47.1X6
Antigonadotrophin NEC	T38.6X1	T38.6X2	T38.6X3	T38.6X4	T38.6X5	T38.6X6
Antihallucinogen	T43.501	T43.502	T43.503	T43.504	T43.505	T43.506
Antihelmintics	T37.4X1	T37.4X2	T37.4X3	T37.4X4	T37.4X5	T37.4X6
Antihemophilic						
factor	T45.8X1	T45.8X2	T45.8X3	T45.8X4	T45.8X5	T45.8X6
fraction	T45.8X1	T45.8X2	T45.8X3	T45.8X4	T45.8X5	T45.8X6
globulin concentrate	T45.7X1	T45.7X2	T45.7X3	T45.7X4	T45.7X5	T45.7X6
human plasma	T45.8X1	T45.8X2	T45.8X3	T45.8X4	T45.8X5	T45.8X6
plasma, dried	T45.7X1	T45.7X2	T45.7X3	T45.7X4	T45.7X5	T45.7X6
Antihemorrhoidal preparation	T49.2X1	T49.2X2	T49.2X3	T49.2X4	T49.2X5	T49.2X6
Antiheparin drug	T45.7X1	T45.7X2	T45.7X3	T45.7X4	T45.7X5	T45.7X6
Antihistamine	T45.0X1	T45.0X2	T45.0X3	T45.0X4	T45.0X5	T45.0X6
Antihookworm drug	T37.4X1	T37.4X2	T37.4X3	T37.4X4	T37.4X5	T37.4X6
Anti-human lymphocytic globulin	T50.Z11	T50.Z12	T50.Z13	T50.Z14	T50.Z15	T50.Z16
Antihyperlipidemic drug	T46.6X1	T46.6X2	T46.6X3	T46.6X4	T46.6X5	T46.6X6
Antihypertensive drug NEC	T46.5X1	T46.5X2	T46.5X3	T46.5X4	T46.5X5	T46.5X6
Anti-infective NEC	T37.91	T37.92	T37.93	T37.94	T37.95	T37.96
anthelmintic	T37.4X1	T37.4X2	T37.4X3	T37.4X4	T37.4X5	T37.4X6
antibiotics	T36.91	T36.92	T36.93	T36.94	T36.95	T36.96
specified NEC	T36.8X1	T36.8X2	T36.8X3	T36.8X4	T36.8X5	T36.8X6
antimalarial	T37.2X1	T37.2X2	T37.2X3	T37.2X4	T37.2X5	T37.2X6
antimycobacterial NEC	T37.1X1	T37.1X2	T37.1X3	T37.1X4	T37.1X5	T37.1X6
antibiotics	T36.5X1	T36.5X2	T36.5X3	T36.5X4	T36.5X5	T36.5X6
antiprotozoal NEC	T37.3X1	T37.3X2	T37.3X3	T37.3X4	T37.3X5	T37.3X6
blood	T37.2X1	T37.2X2	T37.2X3	T37.2X4	T37.2X5	T37.2X6
antiviral	T37.5X1	T37.5X2	T37.5X3	T37.5X4	T37.5X5	T37.5X6
arsenical	T37.8X1	T37.8X2	T37.8X3	T37.8X4	T37.8X5	T37.8X6
bismuth, local	T49.0X1	T49.0X2	T49.0X3	T49.0X4	T49.0X5	T49.0X6
ENT	T49.6X1	T49.6X2	T49.6X3	T49.6X4	T49.6X5	T49.6X6
eye NEC	T49.5X1	T49.5X2	T49.5X3	T49.5X4	T49.5X5	T49.5X6
heavy metals NEC	T37.8X1	T37.8X2	T37.8X3	T37.8X4	T37.8X5	T37.8X6
local NEC	T49.0X1	T49.0X2	T49.0X3	T49.0X4	T49.0X5	T49.0X6
specified NEC	T49.0X1	T49.0X2	T49.0X3	T49.0X4	T49.0X5	T49.0X6
mixed	T37.91	T37.92	T37.93	T37.94	T37.95	T37.96
ophthalmic preparation	T49.5X1	T49.5X2	T49.5X3	T49.5X4	T49.5X5	T49.5X6
topical NEC	T49.0X1	T49.0X2	T49.0X3	T49.0X4	T49.0X5	T49.0X6
Anti-inflammatory drug NEC	T39.391	T39.392	T39.393	T39.394	T39.395	T39.396
local	T49.0X1	T49.0X2	T49.0X3	T49.0X4	T49.0X5	T49.0X6
nonsteroidal NEC	T39.391	T39.392	T39.393	T39.394	T39.395	T39.396
propionic acid derivative	T39.311	T39.312	T39.313	T39.314	T39.315	T39.316
specified NEC	T39.391	T39.392	T39.393	T39.394	T39.395	T39.396
Antikaluretic	T50.3X1	T50.3X2	T50.3X3	T50.3X4	T50.3X5	T50.3X6
Antiknock (tetraethyl lead)	T56.0X1	T56.0X2	T56.0X3	T56.0X4	—	—
Antilipemic drug NEC	T46.6X1	T46.6X2	T46.6X3	T46.6X4	T46.6X5	T46.6X6
Antimalarial	T37.2X1	T37.2X2	T37.2X3	T37.2X4	T37.2X5	T37.2X6
prophylactic NEC	T37.2X1	T37.2X2	T37.2X3	T37.2X4	T37.2X5	T37.2X6
pyrimidine derivative	T37.2X1	T37.2X2	T37.2X3	T37.2X4	T37.2X5	T37.2X6
Antimetabolite	T45.1X1	T45.1X2	T45.1X3	T45.1X4	T45.1X5	T45.1X6
Antimitotic agent	T45.1X1	T45.1X2	T45.1X3	T45.1X4	T45.1X5	T45.1X6
Antimony (compounds) (vapor) NEC	T56.891	T56.892	T56.893	T56.894	—	—
anti-infectives	T37.8X1	T37.8X2	T37.8X3	T37.8X4	T37.8X5	T37.8X6
dimercaptosuccinate	T37.3X1	T37.3X2	T37.3X3	T37.3X4	T37.3X5	T37.3X6
hydride	T56.891	T56.892	T56.893	T56.894	—	—
pesticide (vapor)	T60.8X1	T60.8X2	T60.8X3	T60.8X4	—	—
potassium (sodium) tartrate	T37.8X1	T37.8X2	T37.8X3	T37.8X4	T37.8X5	T37.8X6
sodium dimercaptosuccinate	T37.3X1	T37.3X2	T37.3X3	T37.3X4	T37.3X5	T37.3X6
tartrated	T37.8X1	T37.8X2	T37.8X3	T37.8X4	T37.8X5	T37.8X6
Antimuscarinic NEC	T44.3X1	T44.3X2	T44.3X3	T44.3X4	T44.3X5	T44.3X6
Antimycobacterial drug NEC	T37.1X1	T37.1X2	T37.1X3	T37.1X4	T37.1X5	T37.1X6
antibiotics	T36.5X1	T36.5X2	T36.5X3	T36.5X4	T36.5X5	T36.5X6
combination	T37.1X1	T37.1X2	T37.1X3	T37.1X4	T37.1X5	T37.1X6
Antinausea drug	T45.0X1	T45.0X2	T45.0X3	T45.0X4	T45.0X5	T45.0X6
Antinematode drug	T37.4X1	T37.4X2	T37.4X3	T37.4X4	T37.4X5	T37.4X6
Antineoplastic NEC	T45.1X1	T45.1X2	T45.1X3	T45.1X4	T45.1X5	T45.1X6
alkaloidal	T45.1X1	T45.1X2	T45.1X3	T45.1X4	T45.1X5	T45.1X6
Antineoplastic — *continued*						
antibiotics	T45.1X1	T45.1X2	T45.1X3	T45.1X4	T45.1X5	T45.1X6
combination	T45.1X1	T45.1X2	T45.1X3	T45.1X4	T45.1X5	T45.1X6
estrogen	T38.5X1	T38.5X2	T38.5X3	T38.5X4	T38.5X5	T38.5X6
steroid	T38.7X1	T38.7X2	T38.7X3	T38.7X4	T38.7X5	T38.7X6
Antiparasitic drug (systemic)	T37.91	T37.92	T37.93	T37.94	T37.95	T37.96
local	T49.0X1	T49.0X2	T49.0X3	T49.0X4	T49.0X5	T49.0X6
specified NEC	T37.8X1	T37.8X2	T37.8X3	T37.8X4	T37.8X5	T37.8X6
Antiparkinsonism drug NEC	T42.8X1	T42.8X2	T42.8X3	T42.8X4	T42.8X5	T42.8X6
Antiperspirant NEC	T49.2X1	T49.2X2	T49.2X3	T49.2X4	T49.2X5	T49.2X6
Antiphlogistic NEC	T39.4X1	T39.4X2	T39.4X3	T39.4X4	T39.4X5	T39.4X6
Antiplatyhelmintic drug	T37.4X1	T37.4X2	T37.4X3	T37.4X4	T37.4X5	T37.4X6
Antiprotozoal drug NEC	T37.3X1	T37.3X2	T37.3X3	T37.3X4	T37.3X5	T37.3X6
blood	T37.2X1	T37.2X2	T37.2X3	T37.2X4	T37.2X5	T37.2X6
local	T49.0X1	T49.0X2	T49.0X3	T49.0X4	T49.0X5	T49.0X6
Antipruritic drug NEC	T49.1X1	T49.1X2	T49.1X3	T49.1X4	T49.1X5	T49.1X6
Antipsychotic drug	T43.501	T43.502	T43.503	T43.504	T43.505	T43.506
specified NEC	T43.591	T43.592	T43.593	T43.594	T43.595	T43.596
Antipyretic	T39.93	T39.92	T39.93	T39.94	T39.95	T39.96
specified NEC	T39.8X1	T39.8X2	T39.8X3	T39.8X4	T39.8X5	T39.8X6
Antipyrine	T39.2X1	T39.2X2	T39.2X3	T39.2X4	T39.2X5	T39.2X6
Antirabies hyperimmune serum	T50.Z11	T50.Z12	T50.Z13	T50.Z14	T50.Z15	T50.Z16
Antirheumatic NEC	T39.4X1	T39.4X2	T39.4X3	T39.4X4	T39.4X5	T39.4X6
Antirigidity drug NEC	T42.8X1	T42.8X2	T42.8X3	T42.8X4	T42.8X5	T42.8X6
Antischistosomal drug	T37.4X1	T37.4X2	T37.4X3	T37.4X4	T37.4X5	T37.4X6
Antiscorpion sera	T50.Z11	T50.Z12	T50.Z13	T50.Z14	T50.Z15	T50.Z16
Antiseborrheics	T49.4X1	T49.4X2	T49.4X3	T49.4X4	T49.4X5	T49.4X6
Antiseptics (external) (medicinal)	T49.0X1	T49.0X2	T49.0X3	T49.0X4	T49.0X5	T49.0X6
Antistine	T45.0X1	T45.0X2	T45.0X3	T45.0X4	T45.0X5	T45.0X6
Antitapeworm drug	T37.4X1	T37.4X2	T37.4X3	T37.4X4	T37.4X5	T37.4X6
Antitetanus immunoglobulin	T50.Z11	T50.Z12	T50.Z13	T50.Z14	T50.Z15	T50.Z16
Antithrombotic	T45.521	T45.522	T45.523	T45.524	T45.525	T45.526
Antithyroid drug NEC	T38.2X1	T38.2X2	T38.2X3	T38.2X4	T38.2X5	T38.2X6
Antitoxin	T50.Z11	T50.Z12	T50.Z13	T50.Z14	T50.Z15	T50.Z16
diphtheria	T50.Z11	T50.Z12	T50.Z13	T50.Z14	T50.Z15	T50.Z16
gas gangrene	T50.Z11	T50.Z12	T50.Z13	T50.Z14	T50.Z15	T50.Z16
tetanus	T50.Z11	T50.Z12	T50.Z13	T50.Z14	T50.Z15	T50.Z16
Antitrichomonal drug	T37.3X1	T37.3X2	T37.3X3	T37.3X4	T37.3X5	T37.3X6
Antituberculars	T37.1X1	T37.1X2	T37.1X3	T37.1X4	T37.1X5	T37.1X6
antibiotics	T36.5X1	T36.5X2	T36.5X3	T36.5X4	T36.5X5	T36.5X6
Antitussive NEC	T48.3X1	T48.3X2	T48.3X3	T48.3X4	T48.3X5	T48.3X6
codeine mixture	T40.2X1	T40.2X2	T40.2X3	T40.2X4	T40.2X5	T40.2X6
opiate	T40.2X1	T40.2X2	T40.2X3	T40.2X4	T40.2X5	T40.2X6
Antivaricose drug	T46.8X1	T46.8X2	T46.8X3	T46.8X4	T46.8X5	T46.8X6
Antivenin, antivenom (sera)	T50.Z11	T50.Z12	T50.Z13	T50.Z14	T50.Z15	T50.Z16
crotaline	T50.Z11	T50.Z12	T50.Z13	T50.Z14	T50.Z15	T50.Z16
spider bite	T50.Z11	T50.Z12	T50.Z13	T50.Z14	T50.Z15	T50.Z16
Antivertigo drug	T45.0X1	T45.0X2	T45.0X3	T45.0X4	T45.0X5	T45.0X6
Antiviral drug NEC	T37.5X1	T37.5X2	T37.5X3	T37.5X4	T37.5X5	T37.5X6
eye	T49.5X1	T49.5X2	T49.5X3	T49.5X4	T49.5X5	T49.5X6
Antiwhipworm drug	T37.4X1	T37.4X2	T37.4X3	T37.4X4	T37.4X5	T37.4X6
Ant poison — *see* Insecticide						
Antrol — *see also* by specific chemical substance	T60.91	T60.92	T60.93	T60.94		
fungicide	T60.91	T60.92	T60.93	T60.94	—	—
ANTU (alpha naphthylthiourea)	T60.4X1	T60.4X2	T60.4X3	T60.4X4	—	—
Apalcillin	T36.0X1	T36.0X2	T36.0X3	T36.0X4	T36.0X5	T36.0X6
APC	T48.5X1	T48.5X2	T48.5X3	T48.5X4	T48.5X5	T48.5X6
Aplonidine	T44.4X1	T44.4X2	T44.4X3	T44.4X4	T44.4X5	T44.4X6
Apomorphine	T47.7X1	T47.7X2	T47.7X3	T47.7X4	T47.7X5	T47.7X6
Appetite depressants, central	T50.5X1	T50.5X2	T50.5X3	T50.5X4	T50.5X5	T50.5X6
Apraclonidine (hydrochloride)	T44.4X1	T44.4X2	T44.4X3	T44.4X4	T44.4X5	T44.4X6
Apresoline	T46.5X1	T46.5X2	T46.5X3	T46.5X4	T46.5X5	T46.5X6
Aprindine	T46.2X1	T46.2X2	T46.2X3	T46.2X4	T46.2X5	T46.2X6
Aprobarbital	T42.3X1	T42.3X2	T42.3X3	T42.3X4	T42.3X5	T42.3X6
Apronalide	T42.6X1	T42.6X2	T42.6X3	T42.6X4	T42.6X5	T42.6X6
Aprotinin	T45.621	T45.622	T45.623	T45.624	T45.625	T45.626
Aptocaine	T41.3X1	T41.3X2	T41.3X3	T41.3X4	T41.3X5	T41.3X6
Aqua fortis	T54.2X1	T54.2X2	T54.2X3	T54.2X4	—	—
Ara-A	T37.5X1	T37.5X2	T37.5X3	T37.5X4	T37.5X5	T37.5X6
Ara-C	T45.1X1	T45.1X2	T45.1X3	T45.1X4	T45.1X5	T45.1X6
Arachis oil	T49.3X1	T49.3X2	T49.3X3	T49.3X4	T49.3X5	T49.3X6
cathartic	T47.4X1	T47.4X2	T47.4X3	T47.4X4	T47.4X5	T47.4X6
Aralen	T37.2X1	T37.2X2	T37.2X3	T37.2X4	T37.2X5	T37.2X6

Additional Character May Be Required — Refer to the Tabular List for Character Selection

▽ Subterms under main terms may continue to next column or page

Table of Drugs and Chemicals

Substance	Poisoning, Accidental (unintentional)	Poisoning, Intentional Self-harm	Poisoning, Assault	Poisoning, Undetermined	Adverse Effect	Under-dosing
Arecoline	T44.1X1	T44.1X2	T44.1X3	T44.1X4	T44.1X5	T44.1X6
Arginine	T50.991	T50.992	T50.993	T50.994	T50.995	T50.996
glutamate	T50.991	T50.992	T50.993	T50.994	T50.995	T50.996
Argyrol	T49.0X1	T49.0X2	T49.0X3	T49.0X4	T49.0X5	T49.0X6
ENT agent	T49.6X1	T49.6X2	T49.6X3	T49.6X4	T49.6X5	T49.6X6
ophthalmic preparation	T49.5X1	T49.5X2	T49.5X3	T49.5X4	T49.5X5	T49.5X6
Aristocort	T38.0X1	T38.0X2	T38.0X3	T38.0X4	T38.0X5	T38.0X6
ENT agent	T49.6X1	T49.6X2	T49.6X3	T49.6X4	T49.6X5	T49.6X6
ophthalmic preparation	T49.5X1	T49.5X2	T49.5X3	T49.5X4	T49.5X5	T49.5X6
topical NEC	T49.0X1	T49.0X2	T49.0X3	T49.0X4	T49.0X5	T49.0X6
Aromatics, corrosive	T54.1X1	T54.1X2	T54.1X3	T54.1X4	—	—
disinfectants	T54.1X1	T54.1X2	T54.1X3	T54.1X4	—	—
Arsenate of lead	T57.0X1	T57.0X2	T57.0X3	T57.0X4	—	—
herbicide	T57.0X1	T57.0X2	T57.0X3	T57.0X4	—	—
Arsenic, arsenicals (compounds) (dust) (vapor) **NEC**	T57.0X1	T57.0X2	T57.0X3	T57.0X4	—	—
anti-infectives	T37.8X1	T37.8X2	T37.8X3	T37.8X4	T37.8X5	T37.8X6
pesticide (dust) (fumes)	T57.0X1	T57.0X2	T57.0X3	T57.0X4	—	—
Arsine (gas)	T57.0X1	T57.0X2	T57.0X3	T57.0X4	—	—
Arsphenamine (silver)	T37.8X1	T37.8X2	T37.8X3	T37.8X4	T37.8X5	T37.8X6
Arsthinol	T37.3X1	T37.3X2	T37.3X3	T37.3X4	T37.3X5	T37.3X6
Artane	T44.3X1	T44.3X2	T44.3X3	T44.3X4	T44.3X5	T44.3X6
Arthropod (venomous) **NEC**	T63.481	T63.482	T63.483	T63.484	—	—
Articaine	T41.3X1	T41.3X2	T41.3X3	T41.3X4	T41.3X5	T41.3X6
Asbestos	T57.8X1	T57.8X2	T57.8X3	T57.8X4	—	—
Ascaridole	T37.4X1	T37.4X2	T37.4X3	T37.4X4	T37.4X5	T37.4X6
Ascorbic acid	T45.2X1	T45.2X2	T45.2X3	T45.2X4	T45.2X5	T45.2X6
Asiaticoside	T49.0X1	T49.0X2	T49.0X3	T49.0X4	T49.0X5	T49.0X6
Asparaginase	T45.1X1	T45.1X2	T45.1X3	T45.1X4	T45.1X5	T45.1X6
Aspidium (oleoresin)	T37.4X1	T37.4X2	T37.4X3	T37.4X4	T37.4X5	T37.4X6
Aspirin (aluminum) (soluble)	T39.011	T39.012	T39.013	T39.014	T39.015	T39.016
Aspoxicillin	T36.0X1	T36.0X2	T36.0X3	T36.0X4	T36.0X5	T36.0X6
Astemizole	T45.0X1	T45.0X2	T45.0X3	T45.0X4	T45.0X5	T45.0X6
Astringent (local)	T49.2X1	T49.2X2	T49.2X3	T49.2X4	T49.2X5	T49.2X6
specified NEC	T49.2X1	T49.2X2	T49.2X3	T49.2X4	T49.2X5	T49.2X6
Astromicin	T36.5X1	T36.5X2	T36.5X3	T36.5X4	T36.5X5	T36.5X6
Ataractic drug NEC	T43.501	T43.502	T43.503	T43.504	T43.505	T43.506
Atenolol	T44.7X1	T44.7X2	T44.7X3	T44.7X4	T44.7X5	T44.7X6
Atonia drug, intestinal	T47.4X1	T47.4X2	T47.4X3	T47.4X4	T47.4X5	T47.4X6
Atophan	T50.4X1	T50.4X2	T50.4X3	T50.4X4	T50.4X5	T50.4X6
Atracurium besilate	T48.1X1	T48.1X2	T48.1X3	T48.1X4	T48.1X5	T48.1X6
Atropine	T44.3X1	T44.3X2	T44.3X3	T44.3X4	T44.3X5	T44.3X6
derivative	T44.3X1	T44.3X2	T44.3X3	T44.3X4	T44.3X5	T44.3X6
methonitrate	T44.3X1	T44.3X2	T44.3X3	T44.3X4	T44.3X5	T44.3X6
Attapulgite	T47.6X1	T47.6X2	T47.6X3	T47.6X4	T47.6X5	T47.6X6
Auramine	T65.891	T65.892	T65.893	T65.894	—	—
dye	T65.6X1	T65.6X2	T65.6X3	T65.6X4	—	—
fungicide	T60.3X1	T60.3X2	T60.3X3	T60.3X4	—	—
Auranofin	T39.4X1	T39.4X2	T39.4X3	T39.4X4	T39.4X5	T39.4X6
Aurantiin	T46.991	T46.992	T46.993	T46.994	T46.995	T46.996
Aureomycin	T36.4X1	T36.4X2	T36.4X3	T36.4X4	T36.4X5	T36.4X6
ophthalmic preparation	T49.5X1	T49.5X2	T49.5X3	T49.5X4	T49.5X5	T49.5X6
topical NEC	T49.0X1	T49.0X2	T49.0X3	T49.0X4	T49.0X5	T49.0X6
Aurothioglucose	T39.4X1	T39.4X2	T39.4X3	T39.4X4	T39.4X5	T39.4X6
Aurothioglycanide	T39.4X1	T39.4X2	T39.4X3	T39.4X4	T39.4X5	T39.4X6
Aurothiomalate sodium	T39.4X1	T39.4X2	T39.4X3	T39.4X4	T39.4X5	T39.4X6
Aurotioprol	T39.4X1	T39.4X2	T39.4X3	T39.4X4	T39.4X5	T39.4X6
Automobile fuel	T52.0X1	T52.0X2	T52.0X3	T52.0X4	—	—
Autonomic nervous system agent NEC	T44.901	T44.902	T44.903	T44.904	T44.905	T44.906
Avlosulfon	T37.1X1	T37.1X2	T37.1X3	T37.1X4	T37.1X5	T37.1X6
Avomine	T42.6X1	T42.6X2	T42.6X3	T42.6X4	T42.6X5	T42.6X6
Axerophthol	T45.2X1	T45.2X2	T45.2X3	T45.2X4	T45.2X5	T45.2X6
Azacitidine	T45.1X1	T45.1X2	T45.1X3	T45.1X4	T45.1X5	T45.1X6
Azacyclonol	T43.591	T43.592	T43.593	T43.594	T43.595	T43.596
Azadirachta	T60.2X1	T60.2X2	T60.2X3	T60.2X4	—	—
Azanidazole	T37.3X1	T37.3X2	T37.3X3	T37.3X4	T37.3X5	T37.3X6
Azapetine	T46.7X1	T46.7X2	T46.7X3	T46.7X4	T46.7X5	T46.7X6
Azapropazone	T39.2X1	T39.2X2	T39.2X3	T39.2X4	T39.2X5	T39.2X6
Azaribine	T45.1X1	T45.1X2	T45.1X3	T45.1X4	T45.1X5	T45.1X6
Azaserine	T45.1X1	T45.1X2	T45.1X3	T45.1X4	T45.1X5	T45.1X6
Azatadine	T45.0X1	T45.0X2	T45.0X3	T45.0X4	T45.0X5	T45.0X6
Azatepa	T45.1X1	T45.1X2	T45.1X3	T45.1X4	T45.1X5	T45.1X6
Azathioprine	T45.1X1	T45.1X2	T45.1X3	T45.1X4	T45.1X5	T45.1X6
Azelaic acid	T49.0X1	T49.0X2	T49.0X3	T49.0X4	T49.0X5	T49.0X6
Azelastine	T45.0X1	T45.0X2	T45.0X3	T45.0X4	T45.0X5	T45.0X6
Azidocillin	T36.0X1	T36.0X2	T36.0X3	T36.0X4	T36.0X5	T36.0X6
Azidothymidine	T37.5X1	T37.5X2	T37.5X3	T37.5X4	T37.5X5	T37.5X6
Azinphos (ethyl) (methyl)	T60.0X1	T60.0X2	T60.0X3	T60.0X4	—	—
Aziridine (chelating)	T54.1X1	T54.1X2	T54.1X3	T54.1X4	—	—
Azithromycin	T36.3X1	T36.3X2	T36.3X3	T36.3X4	T36.3X5	T36.3X6
Azlocillin	T36.0X1	T36.0X2	T36.0X3	T36.0X4	T36.0X5	T36.0X6
Azobenzene smoke	T65.3X1	T65.3X2	T65.3X3	T65.3X4	—	—
acaricide	T60.8X1	T60.8X2	T60.8X3	T60.8X4	—	—
Azosulfamide	T37.0X1	T37.0X2	T37.0X3	T37.0X4	T37.0X5	T37.0X6
AZT	T37.5X1	T37.5X2	T37.5X3	T37.5X4	T37.5X5	T37.5X6
Aztreonam	T36.1X1	T36.1X2	T36.1X3	T36.1X4	T36.1X5	T36.1X6
Azulfidine	T37.0X1	T37.0X2	T37.0X3	T37.0X4	T37.0X5	T37.0X6
Azuresin	T50.8X1	T50.8X2	T50.8X3	T50.8X4	T50.8X5	T50.8X6
b-acetyldigoxin	T46.0X1	T46.0X2	T46.0X3	T46.0X4	T46.0X5	T46.0X6
P-Acetamidophenol	T39.1X1	T39.1X2	T39.1X3	T39.1X4	T39.1X5	T39.1X6
Bacampicillin	T36.0X1	T36.0X2	T36.0X3	T36.0X4	T36.0X5	T36.0X6
Bacillus						
lactobacillus	T47.8X1	T47.8X2	T47.8X3	T47.8X4	T47.8X5	T47.8X6
subtilis	T47.6X1	T47.6X2	T47.6X3	T47.6X4	T47.6X5	T47.6X6
Bacimycin	T49.0X1	T49.0X2	T49.0X3	T49.0X4	T49.0X5	T49.0X6
ophthalmic preparation	T49.5X1	T49.5X2	T49.5X3	T49.5X4	T49.5X5	T49.5X6
Bacitracin zinc	T49.0X1	T49.0X2	T49.0X3	T49.0X4	T49.0X5	T49.0X6
with neomycin	T49.0X1	T49.0X2	T49.0X3	T49.0X4	T49.0X5	T49.0X6
ENT agent	T49.6X1	T49.6X2	T49.6X3	T49.6X4	T49.6X5	T49.6X6
ophthalmic preparation	T49.5X1	T49.5X2	T49.5X3	T49.5X4	T49.5X5	T49.5X6
topical NEC	T49.0X1	T49.0X2	T49.0X3	T49.0X4	T49.0X5	T49.0X6
Baclofen	T42.8X1	T42.8X2	T42.8X3	T42.8X4	T42.8X5	T42.8X6
Baking soda	T50.991	T50.992	T50.993	T50.994	T50.995	T50.996
BAL	T45.8X1	T45.8X2	T45.8X3	T45.8X4	T45.8X5	T45.8X6
Bambuterol	T48.6X1	T48.6X2	T48.6X3	T48.6X4	T48.6X5	T48.6X6
Bamethan (sulfate)	T46.7X1	T46.7X2	T46.7X3	T46.7X4	T46.7X5	T46.7X6
Bamifylline	T48.6X1	T48.6X2	T48.6X3	T48.6X4	T48.6X5	T48.6X6
Bamipine	T45.0X1	T45.0X2	T45.0X3	T45.0X4	T45.0X5	T45.0X6
Baneberry — see Actaea spicata						
Banewort — see Belladonna						
Barbenyl	T42.3X1	T42.3X2	T42.3X3	T42.3X4	T42.3X5	T42.3X6
Barbexaclone	T42.6X1	T42.6X2	T42.6X3	T42.6X4	T42.6X5	T42.6X6
Barbital	T42.3X1	T42.3X2	T42.3X3	T42.3X4	T42.3X5	T42.3X6
sodium	T42.3X1	T42.3X2	T42.3X3	T42.3X4	T42.3X5	T42.3X6
Barbitone	T42.3X1	T42.3X2	T42.3X3	T42.3X4	T42.3X5	T42.3X6
Barbiturate NEC	T42.3X1	T42.3X2	T42.3X3	T42.3X4	T42.3X5	T42.3X6
with tranquilizer	T42.3X1	T42.3X2	T42.3X3	T42.3X4	T42.3X5	T42.3X6
anesthetic (intravenous)	T41.1X1	T41.1X2	T41.1X3	T41.1X4	T41.1X5	T41.1X6
Barium (carbonate) (chloride) (sulfite)	T57.8X1	T57.8X2	T57.8X3	T57.8X4	—	—
diagnostic agent	T50.8X1	T50.8X2	T50.8X3	T50.8X4	T50.8X5	T50.8X6
pesticide	T60.4X1	T60.4X2	T60.4X3	T60.4X4	—	—
rodenticide	T60.4X1	T60.4X2	T60.4X3	T60.4X4	—	—
sulfate (medicinal)	T50.8X1	T50.8X2	T50.8X3	T50.8X4	T50.8X5	T50.8X6
Barrier cream	T49.3X1	T49.3X2	T49.3X3	T49.3X4	T49.3X5	T49.3X6
Basic fuchsin	T49.0X1	T49.0X2	T49.0X3	T49.0X4	T49.0X5	T49.0X6
Battery acid or fluid	T54.2X1	T54.2X2	T54.2X3	T54.2X4	—	—
Bay rum	T51.8X1	T51.8X2	T51.8X3	T51.8X4	—	—
b-benzalbutyramide	T46.6X1	T46.6X2	T46.6X3	T46.6X4	T46.6X5	T46.6X6
BCG (vaccine)	T50.A91	T50.A92	T50.A93	T50.A94	T50.A95	T50.A96
BCNU	T45.1X1	T45.1X2	T45.1X3	T45.1X4	T45.1X5	T45.1X6
Bearsfoot	T62.2X1	T62.2X2	T62.2X3	T62.2X4	—	—
Beclamide	T42.6X1	T42.6X2	T42.6X3	T42.6X4	T42.6X5	T42.6X6
Beclomethasone	T44.5X1	T44.5X2	T44.5X3	T44.5X4	T44.5X5	T44.5X6
Bee (sting) (venom)	T63.441	T63.442	T63.443	T63.444	—	—
Befunolol	T49.5X1	T49.5X2	T49.5X3	T49.5X4	T49.5X5	T49.5X6
Bekanamycin	T36.5X1	T36.5X2	T36.5X3	T36.5X4	T36.5X5	T36.5X6
Belladonna — see also Nightshade						
alkaloids	T44.3X1	T44.3X2	T44.3X3	T44.3X4	T44.3X5	T44.3X6
extract	T44.3X1	T44.3X2	T44.3X3	T44.3X4	T44.3X5	T44.3X6
herb	T44.3X1	T44.3X2	T44.3X3	T44.3X4	T44.3X5	T44.3X6
Bemegride	T50.7X1	T50.7X2	T50.7X3	T50.7X4	T50.7X5	T50.7X6
Benactyzine	T44.3X1	T44.3X2	T44.3X3	T44.3X4	T44.3X5	T44.3X6
Benadryl	T45.0X1	T45.0X2	T45.0X3	T45.0X4	T45.0X5	T45.0X6
Benaprizine	T44.3X1	T44.3X2	T44.3X3	T44.3X4	T44.3X5	T44.3X6
Benazepril	T46.4X1	T46.4X2	T46.4X3	T46.4X4	T46.4X5	T46.4X6
Bencyclane	T46.7X1	T46.7X2	T46.7X3	T46.7X4	T46.7X5	T46.7X6
Bendazol	T46.3X1	T46.3X2	T46.3X3	T46.3X4	T46.3X5	T46.3X6
Bendrofluazide	T50.2X1	T50.2X2	T50.2X3	T50.2X4	T50.2X5	T50.2X6
Bendroflumethiazide	T50.2X1	T50.2X2	T50.2X3	T50.2X4	T50.2X5	T50.2X6
Benemid	T50.4X1	T50.4X2	T50.4X3	T50.4X4	T50.4X5	T50.4X6
Benethamine penicillin	T36.0X1	T36.0X2	T36.0X3	T36.0X4	T36.0X5	T36.0X6
Benexate	T47.1X1	T47.1X2	T47.1X3	T47.1X4	T47.1X5	T47.1X6
Benfluorex	T46.6X1	T46.6X2	T46.6X3	T46.6X4	T46.6X5	T46.6X6
Benfotiamine	T45.2X1	T45.2X2	T45.2X3	T45.2X4	T45.2X5	T45.2X6
Benisone	T49.0X1	T49.0X2	T49.0X3	T49.0X4	T49.0X5	T49.0X6
Benomyl	T60.0X1	T60.0X2	T60.0X3	T60.0X4	—	—
Benoquin	T49.8X1	T49.8X2	T49.8X3	T49.8X4	T49.8X5	T49.8X6
Benoxinate	T41.3X1	T41.3X2	T41.3X3	T41.3X4	T41.3X5	T41.3X6
Benperidol	T43.4X1	T43.4X2	T43.4X3	T43.4X4	T43.4X5	T43.4X6
Benproperine	T48.3X1	T48.3X2	T48.3X3	T48.3X4	T48.3X5	T48.3X6
Benserazide	T42.8X1	T42.8X2	T42.8X3	T42.8X4	T42.8X5	T42.8X6
Bentazepam	T42.4X1	T42.4X2	T42.4X3	T42.4X4	T42.4X5	T42.4X6

▽ **Subterms under main terms may continue to next column or page**   **Additional Character May Be Required — Refer to the Tabular List for Character Selection**

Table of Drugs and Chemicals

Bentiromide — Blockain

Substance	Poisoning, Accidental (unintentional)	Poisoning, Intentional Self-harm	Poisoning, Assault	Poisoning, Undetermined	Adverse Effect	Under-dosing
Bentiromide	T50.8X1	T50.8X2	T50.8X3	T50.8X4	T50.8X5	T50.8X6
Bentonite	T49.3X1	T49.3X2	T49.3X3	T49.3X4	T49.3X5	T49.3X6
Benzalbutyramide	T46.6X1	T46.6X2	T46.6X3	T46.6X4	T46.6X5	T46.6X6
Benzalkonium (chloride)	T49.0X1	T49.0X2	T49.0X3	T49.0X4	T49.0X5	T49.0X6
ophthalmic preparation	T49.5X1	T49.5X2	T49.5X3	T49.5X4	T49.5X5	T49.5X6
Benzamidosalicylate (calcium)	T37.1X1	T37.1X2	T37.1X3	T37.1X4	T37.1X5	T37.1X6
Benzamine	T41.3X1	T41.3X2	T41.3X3	T41.3X4	T41.3X5	T41.3X6
lactate	T49.1X1	T49.1X2	T49.1X3	T49.1X4	T49.1X5	T49.1X6
Benzamphetamine	T50.5X1	T50.5X2	T50.5X3	T50.5X4	T50.5X5	T50.5X6
Benzapril hydrochloride	T46.5X1	T46.5X2	T46.5X3	T46.5X4	T46.5X5	T46.5X6
Benzathine benzylpenicillin	T36.0X1	T36.0X2	T36.0X3	T36.0X4	T36.0X5	T36.0X6
Benzathine penicillin	T36.0X1	T36.0X2	T36.0X3	T36.0X4	T36.0X5	T36.0X6
Benzatropine	T42.8X1	T42.8X2	T42.8X3	T42.8X4	T42.8X5	T42.8X6
Benzbromarone	T50.4X1	T50.4X2	T50.4X3	T50.4X4	T50.4X5	T50.4X6
Benzcarbimine	T45.1X1	T45.1X2	T45.1X3	T45.1X4	T45.1X5	T45.1X6
Benzedrex	T44.991	T44.992	T44.993	T44.994	T44.995	T44.996
Benzedrine (amphetamine)	T43.621	T43.622	T43.623	T43.624	T43.625	T43.626
Benzenamine	T65.3X1	T65.3X2	T65.3X3	T65.3X4	—	—
Benzene	T52.1X1	T52.1X2	T52.1X3	T52.1X4	—	—
homologues (acetyl) (dimethyl) (methyl) (solvent)	T52.2X1	T52.2X2	T52.2X3	T52.2X4	—	—
Benzethonium (chloride)	T49.0X1	T49.0X2	T49.0X3	T49.0X4	T49.0X5	T49.0X6
Benzfetamine	T50.5X1	T50.5X2	T50.5X3	T50.5X4	T50.5X5	T50.5X6
Benzhexol	T44.3X1	T44.3X2	T44.3X3	T44.3X4	T44.3X5	T44.3X6
Benzhydramine (chloride)	T45.0X1	T45.0X2	T45.0X3	T45.0X4	T45.0X5	T45.0X6
Benzidine	T65.891	T65.892	T65.893	T65.894	—	—
Benzilonium bromide	T44.3X1	T44.3X2	T44.3X3	T44.3X4	T44.3X5	T44.3X6
Benzimidazole	T60.3X1	T60.3X2	T60.3X3	T60.3X4	—	—
Benzin (e) — see Ligroin						
Benziodarone	T46.3X1	T46.3X2	T46.3X3	T46.3X4	T46.3X5	T46.3X6
Benznidazole	T37.3X1	T37.3X2	T37.3X3	T37.3X4	T37.3X5	T37.3X6
Benzocaine	T41.3X1	T41.3X2	T41.3X3	T41.3X4	T41.3X5	T41.3X6
Benzodiapin	T42.4X1	T42.4X2	T42.4X3	T42.4X4	T42.4X5	T42.4X6
Benzodiazepine NEC	T42.4X1	T42.4X2	T42.4X3	T42.4X4	T42.4X5	T42.4X6
Benzoic acid	T49.0X1	T49.0X2	T49.0X3	T49.0X4	T49.0X5	T49.0X6
with salicylic acid	T49.0X1	T49.0X2	T49.0X3	T49.0X4	T49.0X5	T49.0X6
Benzoin (tincture)	T48.5X1	T48.5X2	T48.5X3	T48.5X4	T48.5X5	T48.5X6
Benzol (benzene)	T52.1X1	T52.1X2	T52.1X3	T52.1X4	—	—
vapor	T52.0X1	T52.0X2	T52.0X3	T52.0X4	—	—
Benzomorphan	T40.2X1	T40.2X2	T40.2X3	T40.2X4	T40.2X5	T40.2X6
Benzonatate	T48.3X1	T48.3X2	T48.3X3	T48.3X4	T48.3X5	T48.3X6
Benzophenones	T49.3X1	T49.3X2	T49.3X3	T49.3X4	T49.3X5	T49.3X6
Benzopyrone	T46.991	T46.992	T46.993	T46.994	T46.995	T46.996
Benzothiadiazides	T50.2X1	T50.2X2	T50.2X3	T50.2X4	T50.2X5	T50.2X6
Benzoxonium chloride	T49.0X1	T49.0X2	T49.0X3	T49.0X4	T49.0X5	T49.0X6
Benzoylpas calcium	T37.1X1	T37.1X2	T37.1X3	T37.1X4	T37.1X5	T37.1X6
Benzoyl peroxide	T49.0X1	T49.0X2	T49.0X3	T49.0X4	T49.0X5	T49.0X6
Benzperidin	T43.591	T43.592	T43.593	T43.594	T43.595	T43.596
Benzperidol	T43.591	T43.592	T43.593	T43.594	T43.595	T43.596
Benzphetamine	T50.5X1	T50.5X2	T50.5X3	T50.5X4	T50.5X5	T50.5X6
Benzpyrinium bromide	T44.1X1	T44.1X2	T44.1X3	T44.1X4	T44.1X5	T44.1X6
Benzquinamide	T45.0X1	T45.0X2	T45.0X3	T45.0X4	T45.0X5	T45.0X6
Benzthiazide	T50.2X1	T50.2X2	T50.2X3	T50.2X4	T50.2X5	T50.2X6
Benztropine						
anticholinergic	T44.3X1	T44.3X2	T44.3X3	T44.3X4	T44.3X5	T44.3X6
antiparkinson	T42.8X1	T42.8X2	T42.8X3	T42.8X4	T42.8X5	T42.8X6
Benzydamine	T49.0X1	T49.0X2	T49.0X3	T49.0X4	T49.0X5	T49.0X6
Benzyl						
acetate	T52.8X1	T52.8X2	T52.8X3	T52.8X4	—	—
alcohol	T49.0X1	T49.0X2	T49.0X3	T49.0X4	T49.0X5	T49.0X6
benzoate	T49.0X1	T49.0X2	T49.0X3	T49.0X4	T49.0X5	T49.0X6
Benzoic acid	T49.0X1	T49.0X2	T49.0X3	T49.0X4	T49.0X5	T49.0X6
morphine	T40.2X1	T40.2X2	T40.2X3	T40.2X4	—	—
nicotinate	T46.6X1	T46.6X2	T46.6X3	T46.6X4	T46.6X5	T46.6X6
penicillin	T36.0X1	T36.0X2	T36.0X3	T36.0X4	T36.0X5	T36.0X6
Benzylhydrochlorthiazide	T50.2X1	T50.2X2	T50.2X3	T50.2X4	T50.2X5	T50.2X6
Benzylpenicillin	T36.0X1	T36.0X2	T36.0X3	T36.0X4	T36.0X5	T36.0X6
Benzylthiouracil	T38.2X1	T38.2X2	T38.2X3	T38.2X4	T38.2X5	T38.2X6
Bephenium hydroxynaphthoate	T37.4X1	T37.4X2	T37.4X3	T37.4X4	T37.4X5	T37.4X6
Bepridil	T46.1X1	T46.1X2	T46.1X3	T46.1X4	T46.1X5	T46.1X6
Bergamot oil	T65.891	T65.892	T65.893	T65.894	—	—
Bergapten	T50.991	T50.992	T50.993	T50.994	T50.995	T50.996
Berries, poisonous	T62.1X1	T62.1X2	T62.1X3	T62.1X4	—	—
Beryllium (compounds)	T56.7X1	T56.7X2	T56.7X3	T56.7X4	—	—
beta adrenergic blocking agent, heart	T44.7X1	T44.7X2	T44.7X3	T44.7X4	T44.7X5	T44.7X6
Betacarotene	T45.2X1	T45.2X2	T45.2X3	T45.2X4	T45.2X5	T45.2X6
Beta-Chlor	T42.6X1	T42.6X2	T42.6X3	T42.6X4	T42.6X5	T42.6X6
Betahistine	T46.7X1	T46.7X2	T46.7X3	T46.7X4	T46.7X5	T46.7X6
Betaine	T47.5X1	T47.5X2	T47.5X3	T47.5X4	T47.5X5	T47.5X6

Substance	Poisoning, Accidental (unintentional)	Poisoning, Intentional Self-harm	Poisoning, Assault	Poisoning, Undetermined	Adverse Effect	Under-dosing
Betamethasone	T49.0X1	T49.0X2	T49.0X3	T49.0X4	T49.0X5	T49.0X6
topical	T49.0X1	T49.0X2	T49.0X3	T49.0X4	T49.0X5	T49.0X6
Betamicin	T36.8X1	T36.8X2	T36.8X3	T36.8X4	T36.8X5	T36.8X6
Betanidine	T46.5X1	T46.5X2	T46.5X3	T46.5X4	T46.5X5	T46.5X6
Betaxolol	T44.7X1	T44.7X2	T44.7X3	T44.7X4	T44.7X5	T44.7X6
Betazole	T50.8X1	T50.8X2	T50.8X3	T50.8X4	T50.8X5	T50.8X6
Bethanechol	T44.1X1	T44.1X2	T44.1X3	T44.1X4	T44.1X5	T44.1X6
chloride	T44.1X1	T44.1X2	T44.1X3	T44.1X4	T44.1X5	T44.1X6
Bethanidine	T46.5X1	T46.5X2	T46.5X3	T46.5X4	T46.5X5	T46.5X6
Betoxycaine	T41.3X1	T41.3X2	T41.3X3	T41.3X4	T41.3X5	T41.3X6
Betula oil	T49.3X1	T49.3X2	T49.3X3	T49.3X4	T49.3X5	T49.3X6
Bevantolol	T44.7X1	T44.7X2	T44.7X3	T44.7X4	T44.7X5	T44.7X6
Bevonium metilsulfate	T44.3X1	T44.3X2	T44.3X3	T44.3X4	T44.3X5	T44.3X6
Bezafibrate	T46.6X1	T46.6X2	T46.6X3	T46.6X4	T46.6X5	T46.6X6
Bezitramide	T40.4X1	T40.4X2	T40.4X3	T40.4X4	T40.4X5	T40.4X6
BHA	T50.991	T50.992	T50.993	T50.994	T50.995	T50.996
Bhang	T40.7X1	T40.7X2	T40.7X3	T40.7X4	T40.7X5	T40.7X6
BHC (medicinal)	T49.0X1	T49.0X2	T49.0X3	T49.0X4	T49.0X5	T49.0X6
nonmedicinal (vapor)	T53.6X1	T53.6X2	T53.6X3	T53.6X4	—	—
Bialamicol	T37.3X1	T37.3X2	T37.3X3	T37.3X4	T37.3X5	T37.3X6
Bibenzonium bromide	T48.3X1	T48.3X2	T48.3X3	T48.3X4	T48.3X5	T48.3X6
Bibrocathol	T49.5X1	T49.5X2	T49.5X3	T49.5X4	T49.5X5	T49.5X6
Bichloride of mercury — see Mercury, chloride						
Bichromates (calcium) (potassium)(sodium) (crystals)	T57.8X1	T57.8X2	T57.8X3	T57.8X4		
fumes	T56.2X1	T56.2X2	T56.2X3	T56.2X4		
Biclotymol	T49.6X1	T49.6X2	T49.6X3	T49.6X4	T49.6X5	T49.6X6
Bicucculine	T50.7X1	T50.7X2	T50.7X3	T50.7X4	T50.7X5	T50.7X6
Bifemelane	T43.291	T43.292	T43.293	T43.294	T43.295	T43.296
Biguanide derivatives, oral	T38.3X1	T38.3X2	T38.3X3	T38.3X4	T38.3X5	T38.3X6
Bile salts	T47.5X1	T47.5X2	T47.5X3	T47.5X4	T47.5X5	T47.5X6
Biligrafin	T50.8X1	T50.8X2	T50.8X3	T50.8X4	T50.8X5	T50.8X6
Bilopaque	T50.8X1	T50.8X2	T50.8X3	T50.8X4	T50.8X5	T50.8X6
Binifibrate	T46.6X1	T46.6X2	T46.6X3	T46.6X4	T46.6X5	T46.6X6
Binitrobenzol	T65.3X1	T65.3X2	T65.3X3	T65.3X4		
Bioflavonoid(s)	T46.991	T46.992	T46.993	T46.994	T46.995	T46.996
Biological substance NEC	T50.901	T50.902	T50.903	T50.904	T50.905	T50.906
Biotin	T45.2X1	T45.2X2	T45.2X3	T45.2X4	T45.2X5	T45.2X6
Biperiden	T44.3X1	T44.3X2	T44.3X3	T44.3X4	T44.3X5	T44.3X6
Bisacodyl	T47.2X1	T47.2X2	T47.2X3	T47.2X4	T47.2X5	T47.2X6
Bisbentiamine	T45.2X1	T45.2X2	T45.2X3	T45.2X4	T45.2X5	T45.2X6
Bisbutiamine	T45.2X1	T45.2X2	T45.2X3	T45.2X4	T45.2X5	T45.2X6
Bisdequalinium (salts) (diacetate)	T49.6X1	T49.6X2	T49.6X3	T49.6X4	T49.6X5	T49.6X6
Bishydroxycoumarin	T45.511	T45.512	T45.513	T45.514	T45.515	T45.516
Bismarsen	T37.8X1	T37.8X2	T37.8X3	T37.8X4	T37.8X5	T37.8X6
Bismuth salts	T47.6X1	T47.6X2	T47.6X3	T47.6X4	T47.6X5	T47.6X6
aluminate	T47.1X1	T47.1X2	T47.1X3	T47.1X4	T47.1X5	T47.1X6
anti-infectives	T37.8X1	T37.8X2	T37.8X3	T37.8X4	T37.8X5	T37.8X6
formic iodide	T49.0X1	T49.0X2	T49.0X3	T49.0X4	T49.0X5	T49.0X6
glycolylarsenate	T49.0X1	T49.0X2	T49.0X3	T49.0X4	T49.0X5	T49.0X6
nonmedicinal (compounds) NEC	T65.91	T65.92	T65.93	T65.94	—	—
subcarbonate	T47.6X1	T47.6X2	T47.6X3	T47.6X4	T47.6X5	T47.6X6
subsalicylate	T37.8X1	T37.8X2	T37.8X3	T37.8X4	T37.8X5	T37.8X6
sulfarsphenamine	T37.8X1	T37.8X2	T37.8X3	T37.8X4	T37.8X5	T37.8X6
Bisoprolol	T44.7X1	T44.7X2	T44.7X3	T44.7X4	T44.7X5	T44.7X6
Bisoxatin	T47.2X1	T47.2X2	T47.2X3	T47.2X4	T47.2X5	T47.2X6
Bisulepin (hydrochloride)	T45.0X1	T45.0X2	T45.0X3	T45.0X4	T45.0X5	T45.0X6
Bithionol	T37.8X1	T37.8X2	T37.8X3	T37.8X4	T37.8X5	T37.8X6
anthelminthic	T37.4X1	T37.4X2	T37.4X3	T37.4X4	T37.4X5	T37.4X6
Bitolterol	T48.6X1	T48.6X2	T48.6X3	T48.6X4	T48.6X5	T48.6X6
Bitoscanate	T37.4X1	T37.4X2	T37.4X3	T37.4X4	T37.4X5	T37.4X6
Bitter almond oil	T62.8X1	T62.8X2	T62.8X3	T62.8X4	—	—
Bittersweet	T62.2X1	T62.2X2	T62.2X3	T62.2X4	—	—
Black						
flag	T60.91	T60.92	T60.93	T60.94	—	—
henbane	T62.2X1	T62.2X2	T62.2X3	T62.2X4	—	—
leaf (40)	T60.91	T60.92	T60.93	T60.94	—	—
widow spider (bite)	T63.311	T63.312	T63.313	T63.314	—	—
antivenin	T50.Z11	T50.Z12	T50.Z13	T50.Z14	T50.Z15	T50.Z16
Blast furnace gas (carbon monoxide from)	T58.8X1	T58.8X2	T58.8X3	T58.8X4	—	—
Bleach	T54.91	T54.92	T54.93	T54.94	—	—
Bleaching agent (medicinal)	T49.4X1	T49.4X2	T49.4X3	T49.4X4	T49.4X5	T49.4X6
Bleomycin	T45.1X1	T45.1X2	T45.1X3	T45.1X4	T45.1X5	T45.1X6
Blockain	T41.3X1	T41.3X2	T41.3X3	T41.3X4	T41.3X5	T41.3X6
infiltration (subcutaneous)	T41.3X1	T41.3X2	T41.3X3	T41.3X4	T41.3X5	T41.3X6

Additional Character May Be Required — Refer to the Tabular List for Character Selection   Subterms under main terms may continue to next column or page

Substance	Poisoning, Accidental (unintentional)	Poisoning, Intentional Self-harm	Poisoning, Assault	Poisoning, Undetermined	Adverse Effect	Under-dosing
Blockain — continued						
nerve block (peripheral) (plexus)	T41.3X1	T41.3X2	T41.3X3	T41.3X4	T41.3X5	T41.3X6
topical (surface)	T41.3X1	T41.3X2	T41.3X3	T41.3X4	T41.3X5	T41.3X6
Blockers, calcium channel	T46.1X1	T46.1X2	T46.1X3	T46.1X4	T46.1X5	T46.1X6
Blood (derivatives) (natural) (plasma) (whole)	T45.8X1	T45.8X2	T45.8X3	T45.8X4	T45.8X5	T45.8X6
dried	T45.8X1	T45.8X2	T45.8X3	T45.8X4	T45.8X5	T45.8X6
drug affecting NEC	T45.91	T45.92	T45.93	T45.94	T45.95	T45.96
expander NEC	T45.8X1	T45.8X2	T45.8X3	T45.8X4	T45.8X5	T45.8X6
fraction NEC	T45.8X1	T45.8X2	T45.8X3	T45.8X4	T45.8X5	T45.8X6
substitute (macromolecular)	T45.8X1	T45.8X2	T45.8X3	T45.8X4	T45.8X5	T45.8X6
Blue velvet	T40.2X1	T40.2X2	T40.2X3	T40.2X4	—	—
Bone meal	T62.8X1	T62.8X2	T62.8X3	T62.8X4	—	—
Bonine	T45.0X1	T45.0X2	T45.0X3	T45.0X4	T45.0X5	T45.0X6
Bopindolol	T44.7X1	T44.7X2	T44.7X3	T44.7X4	T44.7X5	T44.7X6
Boracic acid	T49.0X1	T49.0X2	T49.0X3	T49.0X4	T49.0X5	T49.0X6
ENT agent	T49.6X1	T49.6X2	T49.6X3	T49.6X4	T49.6X5	T49.6X6
ophthalmic preparation	T49.5X1	T49.5X2	T49.5X3	T49.5X4	T49.5X5	T49.5X6
Borane complex	T57.8X1	T57.8X2	T57.8X3	T57.8X4	—	—
Borate(s)	T57.8X1	T57.8X2	T57.8X3	T57.8X4	—	—
buffer	T50.991	T50.992	T50.993	T50.994	T50.995	T50.996
cleanser	T54.91	T54.92	T54.93	T54.94	—	—
sodium	T57.8X1	T57.8X2	T57.8X3	T57.8X4	—	—
Borax (cleanser)	T54.91	T54.92	T54.93	T54.94	—	—
Bordeaux mixture	T60.3X1	T60.3X2	T60.3X3	T60.3X4	—	—
Boric acid	T49.0X1	T49.0X2	T49.0X3	T49.0X4	T49.0X5	T49.0X6
ENT agent	T49.6X1	T49.6X2	T49.6X3	T49.6X4	T49.6X5	T49.6X6
ophthalmic preparation	T49.5X1	T49.5X2	T49.5X3	T49.5X4	T49.5X5	T49.5X6
Bornaprine	T44.3X1	T44.3X2	T44.3X3	T44.3X4	T44.3X5	T44.3X6
Boron	T57.8X1	T57.8X2	T57.8X3	T57.8X4	—	—
hydride NEC	T57.8X1	T57.8X2	T57.8X3	T57.8X4	—	—
fumes or gas	T57.8X1	T57.8X2	T57.8X3	T57.8X4	—	—
trifluoride	T59.891	T59.892	T59.893	T59.894	—	—
Botox	T48.291	T48.292	T48.293	T48.294	T48.295	T48.296
Botulinus anti-toxin (type A, B)	T50.Z11	T50.Z12	T50.Z13	T50.Z14	T50.Z15	T50.Z16
Brake fluid vapor	T59.891	T59.892	T59.893	T59.894	—	—
Brallobarbital	T42.3X1	T42.3X2	T42.3X3	T42.3X4	T42.3X5	T42.3X6
Bran (wheat)	T47.4X1	T47.4X2	T47.4X3	T47.4X4	T47.4X5	T47.4X6
Brass (fumes)	T56.891	T56.892	T56.893	T56.894	—	—
Brasso	T52.0X1	T52.0X2	T52.0X3	T52.0X4	—	—
Bretylium tosilate	T46.2X1	T46.2X2	T46.2X3	T46.2X4	T46.2X5	T46.2X6
Brevital (sodium)	T41.1X1	T41.1X2	T41.1X3	T41.1X4	T41.1X5	T41.1X6
Brinase	T45.3X1	T45.3X2	T45.3X3	T45.3X4	T45.3X5	T45.3X6
British antilewisite	T45.8X1	T45.8X2	T45.8X3	T45.8X4	T45.8X5	T45.8X6
Brodifacoum	T60.4X1	T60.4X2	T60.4X3	T60.4X4	—	—
Bromal (hydrate)	T42.6X1	T42.6X2	T42.6X3	T42.6X4	T42.6X5	T42.6X6
Bromazepam	T42.4X1	T42.4X2	T42.4X3	T42.4X4	T42.4X5	T42.4X6
Bromazine	T45.0X1	T45.0X2	T45.0X3	T45.0X4	T45.0X5	T45.0X6
Brombenzylcyanide	T59.3X1	T59.3X2	T59.3X3	T59.3X4	—	—
Bromelains	T45.3X1	T45.3X2	T45.3X3	T45.3X4	T45.3X5	T45.3X6
Bromethalin	T60.4X1	T60.4X2	T60.4X3	T60.4X4	—	—
Bromhexine	T48.4X1	T48.4X2	T48.4X3	T48.4X4	T48.4X5	T48.4X6
Bromide salts	T42.6X1	T42.6X2	T42.6X3	T42.6X4	T42.6X5	T42.6X6
Bromindione	T45.511	T45.512	T45.513	T45.514	T45.515	T45.516
Bromine						
compounds (medicinal)	T42.6X1	T42.6X2	T42.6X3	T42.6X4	T42.6X5	T42.6X6
sedative	T42.6X1	T42.6X2	T42.6X3	T42.6X4	T42.6X5	T42.6X6
vapor	T59.891	T59.892	T59.893	T59.894	—	—
Bromisoval	T42.6X1	T42.6X2	T42.6X3	T42.6X4	T42.6X5	T42.6X6
Bromisovalum	T42.6X1	T42.6X2	T42.6X3	T42.6X4	T42.6X5	T42.6X6
Bromobenzylcyanide	T59.3X1	T59.3X2	T59.3X3	T59.3X4	—	—
Bromochlorosalicylani-lide	T49.0X1	T49.0X2	T49.0X3	T49.0X4	T49.0X5	T49.0X6
Bromocriptine	T42.8X1	T42.8X2	T42.8X3	T42.8X4	T42.8X5	T42.8X6
Bromodiphenhydramine	T45.0X1	T45.0X2	T45.0X3	T45.0X4	T45.0X5	T45.0X6
Bromoform	T42.6X1	T42.6X2	T42.6X3	T42.6X4	T42.6X5	T42.6X6
Bromophenol blue reagent	T50.991	T50.992	T50.993	T50.994	T50.995	T50.996
Bromopride	T47.8X1	T47.8X2	T47.8X3	T47.8X4	T47.8X5	T47.8X6
Bromosalicylchloranitide	T49.0X1	T49.0X2	T49.0X3	T49.0X4	T49.0X5	T49.0X6
Bromosalicylhydroxamic acid	T37.1X1	T37.1X2	T37.1X3	T37.1X4	T37.1X5	T37.1X6
Bromo-seltzer	T39.1X1	T39.1X2	T39.1X3	T39.1X4	T39.1X5	T39.1X6
Bromoxynil	T60.3X1	T60.3X2	T60.3X3	T60.3X4	—	—
Bromperidol	T43.4X1	T43.4X2	T43.4X3	T43.4X4	T43.4X5	T43.4X6
Brompheniramine	T45.0X1	T45.0X2	T45.0X3	T45.0X4	T45.0X5	T45.0X6
Bromsulfophthalein	T50.8X1	T50.8X2	T50.8X3	T50.8X4	T50.8X5	T50.8X6
Bromural	T42.6X1	T42.6X2	T42.6X3	T42.6X4	T42.6X5	T42.6X6
Bromvaletone	T42.6X1	T42.6X2	T42.6X3	T42.6X4	T42.6X5	T42.6X6
Bronchodilator NEC	T48.6X1	T48.6X2	T48.6X3	T48.6X4	T48.6X5	T48.6X6
Brotizolam	T42.4X1	T42.4X2	T42.4X3	T42.4X4	T42.4X5	T42.4X6
Brovincamine	T46.7X1	T46.7X2	T46.7X3	T46.7X4	T46.7X5	T46.7X6
Brown recluse spider (bite) (venom)	T63.331	T63.332	T63.333	T63.334	—	—
Brown spider (bite) (venom)	T63.391	T63.392	T63.393	T63.394	—	—
Broxaterol	T48.6X1	T48.6X2	T48.6X3	T48.6X4	T48.6X5	T48.6X6
Broxuridine	T45.1X1	T45.1X2	T45.1X3	T45.1X4	T45.1X5	T45.1X6
Broxyquinoline	T37.8X1	T37.8X2	T37.8X3	T37.8X4	T37.8X5	T37.8X6
Bruceine	T48.291	T48.292	T48.293	T48.294	T48.295	T48.296
Brucia	T62.2X1	T62.2X2	T62.2X3	T62.2X4	—	—
Brucine	T65.1X1	T65.1X2	T65.1X3	T65.1X4	—	—
Brunswick green — see Copper						
Bruten — see Ibuprofen						
Bryonia	T47.2X1	T47.2X2	T47.2X3	T47.2X4	T47.2X5	T47.2X6
Buclizine	T45.0X1	T45.0X2	T45.0X3	T45.0X4	T45.0X5	T45.0X6
Buclosamide	T49.0X1	T49.0X2	T49.0X3	T49.0X4	T49.0X5	T49.0X6
Budesonide	T44.5X1	T44.5X2	T44.5X3	T44.5X4	T44.5X5	T44.5X6
Budralazine	T46.5X1	T46.5X2	T46.5X3	T46.5X4	T46.5X5	T46.5X6
Bufferin	T39.011	T39.012	T39.013	T39.014	T39.015	T39.016
Buflomedil	T46.7X1	T46.7X2	T46.7X3	T46.7X4	T46.7X5	T46.7X6
Buformin	T38.3X1	T38.3X2	T38.3X3	T38.3X4	T38.3X5	T38.3X6
Bufotenine	T40.991	T40.992	T40.993	T40.994	—	—
Bufrolin	T48.6X1	T48.6X2	T48.6X3	T48.6X4	T48.6X5	T48.6X6
Bufylline	T48.6X1	T48.6X2	T48.6X3	T48.6X4	T48.6X5	T48.6X6
Bulk filler	T50.5X1	T50.5X2	T50.5X3	T50.5X4	T50.5X5	T50.5X6
cathartic	T47.4X1	T47.4X2	T47.4X3	T47.4X4	T47.4X5	T47.4X6
Bumetanide	T50.1X1	T50.1X2	T50.1X3	T50.1X4	T50.1X5	T50.1X6
Bunaftine	T46.2X1	T46.2X2	T46.2X3	T46.2X4	T46.2X5	T46.2X6
Bunamiodyl	T50.8X1	T50.8X2	T50.8X3	T50.8X4	T50.8X5	T50.8X6
Bunazosin	T44.6X1	T44.6X2	T44.6X3	T44.6X4	T44.6X5	T44.6X6
Bunitrolol	T44.7X1	T44.7X2	T44.7X3	T44.7X4	T44.7X5	T44.7X6
Buphenine	T46.7X1	T46.7X2	T46.7X3	T46.7X4	T46.7X5	T46.7X6
Bupivacaine	T41.3X1	T41.3X2	T41.3X3	T41.3X4	T41.3X5	T41.3X6
infiltration (subcutaneous)	T41.3X1	T41.3X2	T41.3X3	T41.3X4	T41.3X5	T41.3X6
nerve block (peripheral) (plexus)	T41.3X1	T41.3X2	T41.3X3	T41.3X4	T41.3X5	T41.3X6
spinal	T41.3X1	T41.3X2	T41.3X3	T41.3X4	T41.3X5	T41.3X6
Bupranolol	T44.7X1	T44.7X2	T44.7X3	T44.7X4	T44.7X5	T44.7X6
Buprenorphine	T40.4X1	T40.4X2	T40.4X3	T40.4X4	T40.4X5	T40.4X6
Bupropion	T43.291	T43.292	T43.293	T43.294	T43.295	T43.296
Burimamide	T47.1X1	T47.1X2	T47.1X3	T47.1X4	T47.1X5	T47.1X6
Buserelin	T38.892	T38.892	T38.893	T38.894	T38.895	T38.896
Buspirone	T43.591	T43.592	T43.593	T43.594	T43.595	T43.596
Busulfan, busulphan	T45.1X1	T45.1X2	T45.1X3	T45.1X4	T45.1X5	T45.1X6
Butabarbital (sodium)	T42.3X1	T42.3X2	T42.3X3	T42.3X4	T42.3X5	T42.3X6
Butabarbitone	T42.3X1	T42.3X2	T42.3X3	T42.3X4	T42.3X5	T42.3X6
Butabarpal	T42.3X1	T42.3X2	T42.3X3	T42.3X4	T42.3X5	T42.3X6
Butacaine	T41.3X1	T41.3X2	T41.3X3	T41.3X4	T41.3X5	T41.3X6
Butalamine	T46.7X1	T46.7X2	T46.7X3	T46.7X4	T46.7X5	T46.7X6
Butalbital	T42.3X1	T42.3X2	T42.3X3	T42.3X4	T42.3X5	T42.3X6
Butallylonal	T42.3X1	T42.3X2	T42.3X3	T42.3X4	T42.3X5	T42.3X6
Butamben	T41.3X1	T41.3X2	T41.3X3	T41.3X4	T41.3X5	T41.3X6
Butamirate	T48.3X1	T48.3X2	T48.3X3	T48.3X4	T48.3X5	T48.3X6
Butane (distributed in mobile container)	T59.891	T59.892	T59.893	T59.894	—	—
distributed through pipes	T59.891	T59.892	T59.893	T59.894	—	—
incomplete combustion	T58.11	T58.12	T58.13	T58.14	—	—
Butanilicaine	T41.3X1	T41.3X2	T41.3X3	T41.3X4	T41.3X5	T41.3X6
Butanol	T51.3X1	T51.3X2	T51.3X3	T51.3X4	—	—
Butanone, 2-butanone	T52.4X1	T52.4X2	T52.4X3	T52.4X4	—	—
Butantrone	T49.4X1	T49.4X2	T49.4X3	T49.4X4	T49.4X5	T49.4X6
Butaperazine	T43.3X1	T43.3X2	T43.3X3	T43.3X4	T43.3X5	T43.3X6
Butazolidin	T39.2X1	T39.2X2	T39.2X3	T39.2X4	T39.2X5	T39.2X6
Butetamate	T48.6X1	T48.6X2	T48.6X3	T48.6X4	T48.6X5	T48.6X6
Butethal	T42.3X1	T42.3X2	T42.3X3	T42.3X4	T42.3X5	T42.3X6
Butethamate	T44.3X1	T44.3X2	T44.3X3	T44.3X4	T44.3X5	T44.3X6
Buthalitone (sodium)	T41.1X1	T41.1X2	T41.1X3	T41.1X4	T41.1X5	T41.1X6
Butisol (sodium)	T42.3X1	T42.3X2	T42.3X3	T42.3X4	T42.3X5	T42.3X6
Butizide	T50.2X1	T50.2X2	T50.2X3	T50.2X4	T50.2X5	T50.2X6
Butobarbital	T42.3X1	T42.3X2	T42.3X3	T42.3X4	T42.3X5	T42.3X6
sodium	T42.3X1	T42.3X2	T42.3X3	T42.3X4	T42.3X5	T42.3X6
Butobarbitone	T42.3X1	T42.3X2	T42.3X3	T42.3X4	T42.3X5	T42.3X6
Butoconazole (nitrate)	T49.0X1	T49.0X2	T49.0X3	T49.0X4	T49.0X5	T49.0X6
Butorphanol	T40.4X1	T40.4X2	T40.4X3	T40.4X4	T40.4X5	T40.4X6
Butriptyline	T43.011	T43.012	T43.013	T43.014	T43.015	T43.016
Butropium bromide	T44.3X1	T44.3X2	T44.3X3	T44.3X4	T44.3X5	T44.3X6
Buttercups	T62.2X1	T62.2X2	T62.2X3	T62.2X4	—	—
Butter of antimony — see Antimony						
Butyl						
acetate (secondary)	T52.8X1	T52.8X2	T52.8X3	T52.8X4	—	—
alcohol	T51.3X1	T51.3X2	T51.3X3	T51.3X4	—	—
aminobenzoate	T41.3X1	T41.3X2	T41.3X3	T41.3X4	T41.3X5	T41.3X6

Substance	Poisoning, Accidental (unintentional)	Poisoning, Intentional Self-harm	Poisoning, Assault	Poisoning, Undetermined	Adverse Effect	Under-dosing
Butyl — continued						
butyrate	T52.8X1	T52.8X2	T52.8X3	T52.8X4	—	—
carbinol	T51.3X1	T51.3X2	T51.3X3	T51.3X4	—	—
carbitol	T52.3X1	T52.3X2	T52.3X3	T52.3X4	—	—
cellosolve	T52.3X1	T52.3X2	T52.3X3	T52.3X4	—	—
chloral (hydrate)	T42.6X1	T42.6X2	T42.6X3	T42.6X4	T42.6X5	T42.6X6
formate	T52.8X1	T52.8X2	T52.8X3	T52.8X4	—	—
lactate	T52.8X1	T52.8X2	T52.8X3	T52.8X4	—	—
propionate	T52.8X1	T52.8X2	T52.8X3	T52.8X4	—	—
scopolamine bromide	T44.3X1	T44.3X2	T44.3X3	T44.3X4	T44.3X5	T44.3X6
thiobarbital sodium	T41.1X1	T41.1X2	T41.1X3	T41.1X4	T41.1X5	T41.1X6
Butylated hydroxyanisole	T50.991	T50.992	T50.993	T50.994	T50.995	T50.996
Butylchloral hydrate	T42.6X1	T42.6X2	T42.6X3	T42.6X4	T42.6X5	T42.6X6
Butyltoluene	T52.2X1	T52.2X2	T52.2X3	T52.2X4	—	—
Butyn	T41.3X1	T41.3X2	T41.3X3	T41.3X4	T41.3X5	T41.3X6
Butyrophenone (-based tranquilizers)	T43.4X1	T43.4X2	T43.4X3	T43.4X4	T43.4X5	T43.4X6
Cabergoline	T42.8X1	T42.8X2	T42.8X3	T42.8X4	T42.8X5	T42.8X6
Cacodyl, cacodylic acid	T57.0X1	T57.0X2	T57.0X3	T57.0X4	—	—
Cactinomycin	T45.1X1	T45.1X2	T45.1X3	T45.1X4	T45.1X5	T45.1X6
Cade oil	T49.4X1	T49.4X2	T49.4X3	T49.4X4	T49.4X5	T49.4X6
Cadexomer iodine	T49.0X1	T49.0X2	T49.0X3	T49.0X4	T49.0X5	T49.0X6
Cadmium (chloride) (fumes) (oxide)	T56.3X1	T56.3X2	T56.3X3	T56.3X4		
sulfide (medicinal) NEC	T49.4X1	T49.4X2	T49.4X3	T49.4X4	T49.4X5	T49.4X6
Cadralazine	T46.5X1	T46.5X2	T46.5X3	T46.5X4	T46.5X5	T46.5X6
Caffeine	T43.611	T43.612	T43.613	T43.614	T43.615	T43.616
Calabar bean	T62.2X1	T62.2X2	T62.2X3	T62.2X4	—	—
Caladium seguinum	T62.2X1	T62.2X2	T62.2X3	T62.2X4	—	—
Calamine (lotion)	T49.3X1	T49.3X2	T49.3X3	T49.3X4	T49.3X5	T49.3X6
Calcifediol	T45.2X1	T45.2X2	T45.2X3	T45.2X4	T45.2X5	T45.2X6
Calciferol	T45.2X1	T45.2X2	T45.2X3	T45.2X4	T45.2X5	T45.2X6
Calcitonin	T50.991	T50.992	T50.993	T50.994	T50.995	T50.996
Calcitriol	T45.2X1	T45.2X2	T45.2X3	T45.2X4	T45.2X5	T45.2X6
Calcium	T50.3X1	T50.3X2	T50.3X3	T50.3X4	T50.3X5	T50.3X6
actylsalicylate	T39.011	T39.012	T39.013	T39.014	T39.015	T39.016
benzamidosalicylate	T37.1X1	T37.1X2	T37.1X3	T37.1X4	T37.1X5	T37.1X6
bromide	T42.6X1	T42.6X2	T42.6X3	T42.6X4	T42.6X5	T42.6X6
bromolactobionate	T42.6X1	T42.6X2	T42.6X3	T42.6X4	T42.6X5	T42.6X6
carbaspirin	T39.011	T39.012	T39.013	T39.014	T39.015	T39.016
carbimide	T50.6X1	T50.6X2	T50.6X3	T50.6X4	T50.6X5	T50.6X6
carbonate	T47.1X1	T47.1X2	T47.1X3	T47.1X4	T47.1X5	T47.1X6
chloride	T50.991	T50.992	T50.993	T50.994	T50.995	T50.996
anhydrous	T50.991	T50.992	T50.993	T50.994	T50.995	T50.996
cyanide	T57.8X1	T57.8X2	T57.8X3	T57.8X4	—	—
dioctyl sulfosuccinate	T47.4X1	T47.4X2	T47.4X3	T47.4X4	T47.4X5	T47.4X6
disodium edathamil	T45.8X1	T45.8X2	T45.8X3	T45.8X4	T45.8X5	T45.8X6
disodium edetate	T45.8X1	T45.8X2	T45.8X3	T45.8X4	T45.8X5	T45.8X6
dobesilate	T46.991	T46.992	T46.993	T46.994	T46.995	T46.996
EDTA	T45.8X1	T45.8X2	T45.8X3	T45.8X4	T45.8X5	T45.8X6
ferrous citrate	T45.4X1	T45.4X2	T45.4X3	T45.4X4	T45.4X5	T45.4X6
folinate	T45.8X1	T45.8X2	T45.8X3	T45.8X4	T45.8X5	T45.8X6
glubionate	T50.3X1	T50.3X2	T50.3X3	T50.3X4	T50.3X5	T50.3X6
gluconate	T50.3X1	T50.3X2	T50.3X3	T50.3X4	T50.3X5	T50.3X6
gluconogalactogluconate	T50.3X1	T50.3X2	T50.3X3	T50.3X4	T50.3X5	T50.3X6
hydrate, hydroxide	T54.3X1	T54.3X2	T54.3X3	T54.3X4	—	—
hypochlorite	T54.3X1	T54.3X2	T54.3X3	T54.3X4	—	—
iodide	T48.4X1	T48.4X2	T48.4X3	T48.4X4	T48.4X5	T48.4X6
ipodate	T50.8X1	T50.8X2	T50.8X3	T50.8X4	T50.8X5	T50.8X6
lactate	T50.3X1	T50.3X2	T50.3X3	T50.3X4	T50.3X5	T50.3X6
leucovorin	T45.8X1	T45.8X2	T45.8X3	T45.8X4	T45.8X5	T45.8X6
mandelate	T37.91	T37.92	T37.93	T37.94	T37.95	T37.96
oxide	T54.3X1	T54.3X2	T54.3X3	T54.3X4	—	—
pantothenate	T45.2X1	T45.2X2	T45.2X3	T45.2X4	T45.2X5	T45.2X6
phosphate	T50.3X1	T50.3X2	T50.3X3	T50.3X4	T50.3X5	T50.3X6
salicylate	T39.091	T39.092	T39.093	T39.094	T39.095	T39.096
salts	T50.3X1	T50.3X2	T50.3X3	T50.3X4	T50.3X5	T50.3X6
Calculus-dissolving drug	T50.991	T50.992	T50.993	T50.994	T50.995	T50.996
Calomel	T49.0X1	T49.0X2	T49.0X3	T49.0X4	T49.0X5	T49.0X6
Caloric agent	T50.3X1	T50.3X2	T50.3X3	T50.3X4	T50.3X5	T50.3X6
Calusterone	T38.7X1	T38.7X2	T38.7X3	T38.7X4	T38.7X5	T38.7X6
Camazepam	T42.4X1	T42.4X2	T42.4X3	T42.4X4	T42.4X5	T42.4X6
Camomile	T49.0X1	T49.0X2	T49.0X3	T49.0X4	T49.0X5	T49.0X6
Camoquin	T37.2X1	T37.2X2	T37.2X3	T37.2X4	T37.2X5	T37.2X6
Camphor						
insecticide	T60.2X1	T60.2X2	T60.2X3	T60.2X4	—	—
medicinal	T49.8X1	T49.8X2	T49.8X3	T49.8X4	T49.8X5	T49.8X6
Camylofin	T44.3X1	T44.3X2	T44.3X3	T44.3X4	T44.3X5	T44.3X6
Cancer chemotherapy drug regimen	T45.1X1	T45.1X2	T45.1X3	T45.1X4	T45.1X5	T45.1X6
Candeptin	T49.0X1	T49.0X2	T49.0X3	T49.0X4	T49.0X5	T49.0X6
Candicidin	T49.0X1	T49.0X2	T49.0X3	T49.0X4	T49.0X5	T49.0X6
Cannabinol	T40.7X1	T40.7X2	T40.7X3	T40.7X4	T40.7X5	T40.7X6
Cannabis (derivatives)	T40.7X1	T40.7X2	T40.7X3	T40.7X4	T40.7X5	T40.7X6
Canned heat	T51.1X1	T51.1X2	T51.1X3	T51.1X4	—	—
Canrenoic acid	T50.0X1	T50.0X2	T50.0X3	T50.0X4	T50.0X5	T50.0X6
Canrenone	T50.0X1	T50.0X2	T50.0X3	T50.0X4	T50.0X5	T50.0X6
Cantharides, cantharidin, cantharis	T49.8X1	T49.8X2	T49.8X3	T49.8X4	T49.8X5	T49.8X6
Canthaxanthin	T50.991	T50.992	T50.993	T50.994	T50.995	T50.996
Capillary-active drug NEC	T46.901	T46.902	T46.903	T46.904	T46.905	T46.906
Capreomycin	T36.8X1	T36.8X2	T36.8X3	T36.8X4	T36.8X5	T36.8X6
Capsicum	T49.4X1	T49.4X2	T49.4X3	T49.4X4	T49.4X5	T49.4X6
Captafol	T60.3X1	T60.3X2	T60.3X3	T60.3X4	—	—
Captan	T60.3X1	T60.3X2	T60.3X3	T60.3X4	—	—
Captodiame, captodiamine	T43.591	T43.592	T43.593	T43.594	T43.595	T43.596
Captopril	T46.4X1	T46.4X2	T46.4X3	T46.4X4	T46.4X5	T46.4X6
Caramiphen	T44.3X1	T44.3X2	T44.3X3	T44.3X4	T44.3X5	T44.3X6
Carazolol	T44.7X1	T44.7X2	T44.7X3	T44.7X4	T44.7X5	T44.7X6
Carbachol	T44.1X1	T44.1X2	T44.1X3	T44.1X4	T44.1X5	T44.1X6
Carbacrylamine (resin)	T50.3X1	T50.3X2	T50.3X3	T50.3X4	T50.3X5	T50.3X6
Carbamate (insecticide)	T60.0X1	T60.0X2	T60.0X3	T60.0X4	—	—
Carbamate (sedative)	T42.6X1	T42.6X2	T42.6X3	T42.6X4	T42.6X5	T42.6X6
herbicide	T60.0X1	T60.0X2	T60.0X3	T60.0X4	—	—
insecticide	T60.0X1	T60.0X2	T60.0X3	T60.0X4	—	—
Carbamazepine	T42.1X1	T42.1X2	T42.1X3	T42.1X4	T42.1X5	T42.1X6
Carbamide	T47.3X1	T47.3X2	T47.3X3	T47.3X4	T47.3X5	T47.3X6
peroxide	T49.0X1	T49.0X2	T49.0X3	T49.0X4	T49.0X5	T49.0X6
topical	T49.8X1	T49.8X2	T49.8X3	T49.8X4	T49.8X5	T49.8X6
Carbamylcholine chloride	T44.1X1	T44.1X2	T44.1X3	T44.1X4	T44.1X5	T44.1X6
Carbaril	T60.0X1	T60.0X2	T60.0X3	T60.0X4	—	—
Carbarsone	T37.3X1	T37.3X2	T37.3X3	T37.3X4	T37.3X5	T37.3X6
Carbaryl	T60.0X1	T60.0X2	T60.0X3	T60.0X4	—	—
Carbaspirin	T39.011	T39.012	T39.013	T39.014	T39.015	T39.016
Carbazochrome (salicylate) (sodium sulfonate)	T49.4X1	T49.4X2	T49.4X3	T49.4X4	T49.4X5	T49.4X6
Carbenicillin	T36.0X1	T36.0X2	T36.0X3	T36.0X4	T36.0X5	T36.0X6
Carbenoxolone	T47.1X1	T47.1X2	T47.1X3	T47.1X4	T47.1X5	T47.1X6
Carbetapentane	T48.3X1	T48.3X2	T48.3X3	T48.3X4	T48.3X5	T48.3X6
Carbethyl salicylate	T39.091	T39.092	T39.093	T39.094	T39.095	T39.096
Carbidopa (with levodopa)	T42.8X1	T42.8X2	T42.8X3	T42.8X4	T42.8X5	T42.8X6
Carbimazole	T38.2X1	T38.2X2	T38.2X3	T38.2X4	T38.2X5	T38.2X6
Carbinol	T51.1X1	T51.1X2	T51.1X3	T51.1X4	—	—
Carbinoxamine	T45.0X1	T45.0X2	T45.0X3	T45.0X4	T45.0X5	T45.0X6
Carbiphene	T39.8X1	T39.8X2	T39.8X3	T39.8X4	T39.8X5	T39.8X6
Carbitol	T52.3X1	T52.3X2	T52.3X3	T52.3X4	—	—
Carbocaine						
infiltration (subcutaneous)	T41.3X1	T41.3X2	T41.3X3	T41.3X4	T41.3X5	T41.3X6
nerve block (peripheral) (plexus)	T41.3X1	T41.3X2	T41.3X3	T41.3X4	T41.3X5	T41.3X6
topical (surface)	T41.3X1	T41.3X2	T41.3X3	T41.3X4	T41.3X5	T41.3X6
Carbocisteine	T48.4X1	T48.4X2	T48.4X3	T48.4X4	T48.4X5	T48.4X6
Carbocromen	T46.3X1	T46.3X2	T46.3X3	T46.3X4	T46.3X5	T46.3X6
Carbol fuchsin	T49.0X1	T49.0X2	T49.0X3	T49.0X4	T49.0X5	T49.0X6
Carbolic acid — see also Phenol	T54.0X1	T54.0X2	T54.0X3	T54.0X4	—	—
Carbolonium (bromide)	T48.1X1	T48.1X2	T48.1X3	T48.1X4	T48.1X5	T48.1X6
Carbo medicinalis	T47.6X1	T47.6X2	T47.6X3	T47.6X4	T47.6X5	T47.6X6
Carbomycin	T36.8X1	T36.8X2	T36.8X3	T36.8X4	T36.8X5	T36.8X6
Carbon						
bisulfide (liquid)	T65.4X1	T65.4X2	T65.4X3	T65.4X4	—	—
vapor	T65.4X1	T65.4X2	T65.4X3	T65.4X4	—	—
dioxide (gas)	T59.7X1	T59.7X2	T59.7X3	T59.7X4	—	—
medicinal	T41.5X1	T41.5X2	T41.5X3	T41.5X4	T41.5X5	T41.5X6
nonmedicinal	T59.7X1	T59.7X2	T59.7X3	T59.7X4	—	—
snow	T49.4X1	T49.4X2	T49.4X3	T49.4X4	T49.4X5	T49.4X6
disulfide (liquid)	T65.4X1	T65.4X2	T65.4X3	T65.4X4	—	—
vapor	T65.4X1	T65.4X2	T65.4X3	T65.4X4	—	—
monoxide (from incomplete combustion)	T58.91	T58.92	T58.93	T58.94	—	—
blast furnace gas	T58.8X1	T58.8X2	T58.8X3	T58.8X4	—	—
butane (distributed in mobile container)	T58.11	T58.12	T58.13	T58.14	—	—
distributed through pipes	T58.11	T58.12	T58.13	T58.14	—	—
charcoal fumes	T58.2X1	T58.2X2	T58.2X3	T58.2X4	—	—
coal	T58.2X1	T58.2X2	T58.2X3	T58.2X4	—	—
coke (in domestic stoves, fireplaces)	T58.2X1	T58.2X2	T58.2X3	T58.2X4	—	—
exhaust gas (motor) not in transit	T58.01	T58.02	T58.03	T58.04	—	—
combustion engine, any not in watercraft	T58.01	T58.02	T58.03	T58.04	—	—
farm tractor, not in transit	T58.01	T58.02	T58.03	T58.04	—	—

Additional Character May Be Required — Refer to the Tabular List for Character Selection   ▽ Subterms under main terms may continue to next column or page

Table of Drugs and Chemicals

Substance	Poisoning, Accidental (unintentional)	Poisoning, Intentional Self-harm	Poisoning, Assault	Poisoning, Undetermined	Adverse Effect	Under-dosing
Carbon — *continued*						
monoxide — *continued*						
exhaust gas not in transit — *continued*						
gas engine	T58.Ø1	T58.Ø2	T58.Ø3	T58.Ø4	—	—
motor pump	T58.Ø1	T58.Ø2	T58.Ø3	T58.Ø4	—	—
motor vehicle, not in transit	T58.Ø1	T58.Ø2	T58.Ø3	T58.Ø4	—	—
fuel (in domestic use)	T58.2X1	T58.2X2	T58.2X3	T58.2X4	—	—
gas (piped)	T58.11	T58.12	T58.13	T58.14	—	—
in mobile container	T58.11	T58.12	T58.13	T58.14	—	—
piped (natural)	T58.11	T58.12	T58.13	T58.14	—	—
utility	T58.11	T58.12	T58.13	T58.14	—	—
in mobile container	T58.11	T58.12	T58.13	T58.14	—	—
gas (piped)	T58.11	T58.12	T58.13	T58.14	—	—
illuminating gas	T58.11	T58.12	T58.13	T58.14	—	—
industrial fuels or gases, any	T58.8X1	T58.8X2	T58.8X3	T58.8X4	—	—
kerosene (in domestic stoves, fireplaces)	T58.2X1	T58.2X2	T58.2X3	T58.2X4	—	—
kiln gas or vapor	T58.8X1	T58.8X2	T58.8X3	T58.8X4	—	—
motor exhaust gas, not in transit	T58.Ø1	T58.Ø2	T58.Ø3	T58.Ø4	—	—
piped gas (manufactured) (natural)	T58.11	T58.12	T58.13	T58.14	—	—
producer gas	T58.8X1	T58.8X2	T58.8X3	T58.8X4	—	—
propane (distributed in mobile container)	T58.11	T58.12	T58.13	T58.14	—	—
distributed through pipes	T58.11	T58.12	T58.13	T58.14	—	—
solid (in domestic stoves, fireplaces)	T58.2X1	T58.2X2	T58.2X3	T58.2X4	—	—
specified source NEC	T58.8X1	T58.8X2	T58.8X3	T58.8X4	—	—
stove gas	T58.11	T58.12	T58.13	T58.14	—	—
piped	T58.11	T58.12	T58.13	T58.14	—	—
utility gas	T58.11	T58.12	T58.13	T58.14	—	—
piped	T58.11	T58.12	T58.13	T58.14	—	—
water gas	T58.11	T58.12	T58.13	T58.14	—	—
wood (in domestic stoves, fireplaces)	T58.2X1	T58.2X2	T58.2X3	T58.2X4	—	—
tetrachloride (vapor) NEC	T53.ØX1	T53.ØX2	T53.ØX3	T53.ØX4	—	—
liquid (cleansing agent) NEC	T53.ØX1	T53.ØX2	T53.ØX3	T53.ØX4	—	—
solvent	T53.ØX1	T53.ØX2	T53.ØX3	T53.ØX4	—	—
Carbonic acid gas	T59.7X1	T59.7X2	T59.7X3	T59.7X4	—	—
anhydrase inhibitor NEC	T50.2X1	T50.2X2	T50.2X3	T50.2X4	T50.2X5	T50.2X6
Carbophenothion	T60.ØX1	T60.ØX2	T60.ØX3	T60.ØX4	—	—
Carboplatin	T45.1X1	T45.1X2	T45.1X3	T45.1X4	T45.1X5	T45.1X6
Carboprost	T48.ØX1	T48.ØX2	T48.ØX3	T48.ØX4	T48.ØX5	T48.ØX6
Carboquone	T45.1X1	T45.1X2	T45.1X3	T45.1X4	T45.1X5	T45.1X6
Carbowax	T49.3X1	T49.3X2	T49.3X3	T49.3X4	T49.3X5	T49.3X6
Carboxymethylcellulose	T47.4X1	T47.4X2	T47.4X3	T47.4X4	T47.4X5	T47.4X6
Carbrital	T42.3X1	T42.3X2	T42.3X3	T42.3X4	T42.3X5	T42.3X6
Carbromal	T42.6X1	T42.6X2	T42.6X3	T42.6X4	T42.6X5	T42.6X6
Carbutamide	T38.3X1	T38.3X2	T38.3X3	T38.3X4	T38.3X5	T38.3X6
Carbuterol	T48.6X1	T48.6X2	T48.6X3	T48.6X4	T48.6X5	T48.6X6
Cardiac						
depressants	T46.2X1	T46.2X2	T46.2X3	T46.2X4	T46.2X5	T46.2X6
rhythm regulator	T46.2X1	T46.2X2	T46.2X3	T46.2X4	T46.2X5	T46.2X6
specified NEC	T46.2X1	T46.2X2	T46.2X3	T46.2X4	T46.2X5	T46.2X6
Cardiografin	T50.8X1	T50.8X2	T50.8X3	T50.8X4	T50.8X5	T50.8X6
Cardiogreen	T50.8X1	T50.8X2	T50.8X3	T50.8X4	T50.8X5	T50.8X6
Cardiotonic (glycoside) NEC	T46.ØX1	T46.ØX2	T46.ØX3	T46.ØX4	T46.ØX5	T46.ØX6
Cardiovascular drug NEC	T46.9Ø1	T46.9Ø2	T46.9Ø3	T46.9Ø4	T46.9Ø5	T46.9Ø6
Cardrase	T50.2X1	T50.2X2	T50.2X3	T50.2X4	T50.2X5	T50.2X6
Carfecillin	T36.ØX1	T36.ØX2	T36.ØX3	T36.ØX4	T36.ØX5	T36.ØX6
Carfenazine	T43.3X1	T43.3X2	T43.3X3	T43.3X4	T43.3X5	T43.3X6
Carfusin	T49.ØX1	T49.ØX2	T49.ØX3	T49.ØX4	T49.ØX5	T49.ØX6
Carindacillin	T36.ØX1	T36.ØX2	T36.ØX3	T36.ØX4	T36.ØX5	T36.ØX6
Carisoprodol	T42.8X1	T42.8X2	T42.8X3	T42.8X4	T42.8X5	T42.8X6
Carmellose	T47.4X1	T47.4X2	T47.4X3	T47.4X4	T47.4X5	T47.4X6
Carminative	T47.5X1	T47.5X2	T47.5X3	T47.5X4	T47.5X5	T47.5X6
Carmofur	T45.1X1	T45.1X2	T45.1X3	T45.1X4	T45.1X5	T45.1X6
Carmustine	T45.1X1	T45.1X2	T45.1X3	T45.1X4	T45.1X5	T45.1X6
Carotene	T45.2X1	T45.2X2	T45.2X3	T45.2X4	T45.2X5	T45.2X6
Carphenazine	T43.3X1	T43.3X2	T43.3X3	T43.3X4	T43.3X5	T43.3X6
Carpipramine	T42.4X1	T42.4X2	T42.4X3	T42.4X4	T42.4X5	T42.4X6
Carprofen	T39.311	T39.312	T39.313	T39.314	T39.315	T39.316
Carpronium chloride	T44.3X1	T44.3X2	T44.3X3	T44.3X4	T44.3X5	T44.3X6
Carrageenan	T47.8X1	T47.8X2	T47.8X3	T47.8X4	T47.8X5	T47.8X6
Carteolol	T44.7X1	T44.7X2	T44.7X3	T44.7X4	T44.7X5	T44.7X6
Carter's Little Pills	T47.2X1	T47.2X2	T47.2X3	T47.2X4	T47.2X5	T47.2X6
Cascara (sagrada)	T47.2X1	T47.2X2	T47.2X3	T47.2X4	T47.2X5	T47.2X6

Substance	Poisoning, Accidental (unintentional)	Poisoning, Intentional Self-harm	Poisoning, Assault	Poisoning, Undetermined	Adverse Effect	Under-dosing
Cassava	T62.2X1	T62.2X2	T62.2X3	T62.2X4		
Castellani's paint	T49.ØX1	T49.ØX2	T49.ØX3	T49.ØX4	T49.ØX5	T49.ØX6
Castor						
bean	T62.2X1	T62.2X2	T62.2X3	T62.2X4	—	—
oil	T47.2X1	T47.2X2	T47.2X3	T47.2X4	T47.2X5	T47.2X6
Catalase	T45.3X1	T45.3X2	T45.3X3	T45.3X4	T45.3X5	T45.3X6
Caterpillar (sting)	T63.431	T63.432	T63.433	T63.434		
Catha (edulis) (tea)	T43.691	T43.692	T43.693	T43.694	—	—
Cathartic NEC	T47.4X1	T47.4X2	T47.4X3	T47.4X4	T47.4X5	T47.4X6
anthracene derivative	T47.2X1	T47.2X2	T47.2X3	T47.2X4	T47.2X5	T47.2X6
bulk	T47.4X1	T47.4X2	T47.4X3	T47.4X4	T47.4X5	T47.4X6
contact	T47.2X1	T47.2X2	T47.2X3	T47.2X4	T47.2X5	T47.2X6
emollient NEC	T47.4X1	T47.4X2	T47.4X3	T47.4X4	T47.4X5	T47.4X6
irritant NEC	T47.2X1	T47.2X2	T47.2X3	T47.2X4	T47.2X5	T47.2X6
mucilage	T47.4X1	T47.4X2	T47.4X3	T47.4X4	T47.4X5	T47.4X6
saline	T47.3X1	T47.3X2	T47.3X3	T47.3X4	T47.3X5	T47.3X6
vegetable	T47.2X1	T47.2X2	T47.2X3	T47.2X4	T47.2X5	T47.2X6
Cathine	T50.5X1	T50.5X2	T50.5X3	T50.5X4	T50.5X5	T50.5X6
Cathomycin	T36.8X1	T36.8X2	T36.8X3	T36.8X4	T36.8X5	T36.8X6
Cation exchange resin	T50.3X1	T50.3X2	T50.3X3	T50.3X4	T50.3X5	T50.3X6
Caustic(s) NEC	T54.91	T54.92	T54.93	T54.94	—	—
alkali	T54.3X1	T54.3X2	T54.3X3	T54.3X4	—	—
hydroxide	T54.3X1	T54.3X2	T54.3X3	T54.3X4	—	—
potash	T54.3X1	T54.3X2	T54.3X3	T54.3X4	—	—
soda	T54.3X1	T54.3X2	T54.3X3	T54.3X4	—	—
specified NEC	T54.91	T54.92	T54.93	T54.94	—	—
Ceepryn	T49.ØX1	T49.ØX2	T49.ØX3	T49.ØX4	T49.ØX5	T49.ØX6
ENT agent	T49.6X1	T49.6X2	T49.6X3	T49.6X4	T49.6X5	T49.6X6
lozenges	T49.6X1	T49.6X2	T49.6X3	T49.6X4	T49.6X5	T49.6X6
Cefacetrile	T36.1X1	T36.1X2	T36.1X3	T36.1X4	T36.1X5	T36.1X6
Cefaclor	T36.1X1	T36.1X2	T36.1X3	T36.1X4	T36.1X5	T36.1X6
Cefadroxil	T36.1X1	T36.1X2	T36.1X3	T36.1X4	T36.1X5	T36.1X6
Cefalexin	T36.1X1	T36.1X2	T36.1X3	T36.1X4	T36.1X5	T36.1X6
Cefaloglycin	T36.1X1	T36.1X2	T36.1X3	T36.1X4	T36.1X5	T36.1X6
Cefaloridine	T36.1X1	T36.1X2	T36.1X3	T36.1X4	T36.1X5	T36.1X6
Cefalosporins	T36.1X1	T36.1X2	T36.1X3	T36.1X4	T36.1X5	T36.1X6
Cefalotin	T36.1X1	T36.1X2	T36.1X3	T36.1X4	T36.1X5	T36.1X6
Cefamandole	T36.1X1	T36.1X2	T36.1X3	T36.1X4	T36.1X5	T36.1X6
Cefamycin antibiotic	T36.1X1	T36.1X2	T36.1X3	T36.1X4	T36.1X5	T36.1X6
Cefapirin	T36.1X1	T36.1X2	T36.1X3	T36.1X4	T36.1X5	T36.1X6
Cefatrizine	T36.1X1	T36.1X2	T36.1X3	T36.1X4	T36.1X5	T36.1X6
Cefazedone	T36.1X1	T36.1X2	T36.1X3	T36.1X4	T36.1X5	T36.1X6
Cefazolin	T36.1X1	T36.1X2	T36.1X3	T36.1X4	T36.1X5	T36.1X6
Cefbuperazone	T36.1X1	T36.1X2	T36.1X3	T36.1X4	T36.1X5	T36.1X6
Cefetamet	T36.1X1	T36.1X2	T36.1X3	T36.1X4	T36.1X5	T36.1X6
Cefixime	T36.1X1	T36.1X2	T36.1X3	T36.1X4	T36.1X5	T36.1X6
Cefmenoxime	T36.1X1	T36.1X2	T36.1X3	T36.1X4	T36.1X5	T36.1X6
Cefmetazole	T36.1X1	T36.1X2	T36.1X3	T36.1X4	T36.1X5	T36.1X6
Cefminox	T36.1X1	T36.1X2	T36.1X3	T36.1X4	T36.1X5	T36.1X6
Cefonicid	T36.1X1	T36.1X2	T36.1X3	T36.1X4	T36.1X5	T36.1X6
Cefoperazone	T36.1X1	T36.1X2	T36.1X3	T36.1X4	T36.1X5	T36.1X6
Ceforanide	T36.1X1	T36.1X2	T36.1X3	T36.1X4	T36.1X5	T36.1X6
Cefotaxime	T36.1X1	T36.1X2	T36.1X3	T36.1X4	T36.1X5	T36.1X6
Cefotetan	T36.1X1	T36.1X2	T36.1X3	T36.1X4	T36.1X5	T36.1X6
Cefotiam	T36.1X1	T36.1X2	T36.1X3	T36.1X4	T36.1X5	T36.1X6
Cefoxitin	T36.1X1	T36.1X2	T36.1X3	T36.1X4	T36.1X5	T36.1X6
Cefpimizole	T36.1X1	T36.1X2	T36.1X3	T36.1X4	T36.1X5	T36.1X6
Cefpiramide	T36.1X1	T36.1X2	T36.1X3	T36.1X4	T36.1X5	T36.1X6
Cefradine	T36.1X1	T36.1X2	T36.1X3	T36.1X4	T36.1X5	T36.1X6
Cefroxadine	T36.1X1	T36.1X2	T36.1X3	T36.1X4	T36.1X5	T36.1X6
Cefsulodin	T36.1X1	T36.1X2	T36.1X3	T36.1X4	T36.1X5	T36.1X6
Ceftazidime	T36.1X1	T36.1X2	T36.1X3	T36.1X4	T36.1X5	T36.1X6
Cefteram	T36.1X1	T36.1X2	T36.1X3	T36.1X4	T36.1X5	T36.1X6
Ceftezole	T36.1X1	T36.1X2	T36.1X3	T36.1X4	T36.1X5	T36.1X6
Ceftizoxime	T36.1X1	T36.1X2	T36.1X3	T36.1X4	T36.1X5	T36.1X6
Ceftriaxone	T36.1X1	T36.1X2	T36.1X3	T36.1X4	T36.1X5	T36.1X6
Cefuroxime	T36.1X1	T36.1X2	T36.1X3	T36.1X4	T36.1X5	T36.1X6
Cefuzonam	T36.1X1	T36.1X2	T36.1X3	T36.1X4	T36.1X5	T36.1X6
Celestone	T38.ØX1	T38.ØX2	T38.ØX3	T38.ØX4	T38.ØX5	T38.ØX6
topical	T49.ØX1	T49.ØX2	T49.ØX3	T49.ØX4	T49.ØX5	T49.ØX6
Celiprolol	T44.7X1	T44.7X2	T44.7X3	T44.7X4	T44.7X5	T44.7X6
Cellosolve	T52.91	T52.92	T52.93	T52.94	—	—
Cell stimulants and proliferants	T49.8X1	T49.8X2	T49.8X3	T49.8X4	T49.8X5	T49.8X6
Cellulose						
cathartic	T47.4X1	T47.4X2	T47.4X3	T47.4X4	T47.4X5	T47.4X6
hydroxyethyl	T47.4X1	T47.4X2	T47.4X3	T47.4X4	T47.4X5	T47.4X6
nitrates (topical)	T49.3X1	T49.3X2	T49.3X3	T49.3X4	T49.3X5	T49.3X6
oxidized	T49.4X1	T49.4X2	T49.4X3	T49.4X4	T49.4X5	T49.4X6
Centipede (bite)	T63.411	T63.412	T63.413	T63.414		
Central nervous system						
depressants	T42.71	T42.72	T42.73	T42.74	T42.75	T42.76
anesthetic (general) NEC	T41.2Ø1	T41.2Ø2	T41.2Ø3	T41.2Ø4	T41.2Ø5	T41.2Ø6

Carbon — Central nervous system

Substance	Poisoning, Accidental (unintentional)	Poisoning, Intentional Self-harm	Poisoning, Assault	Poisoning, Undetermined	Adverse Effect	Under-dosing
Central nervous system — continued						
depressants — continued						
anesthetic — continued						
gases NEC	T41.0X1	T41.0X2	T41.0X3	T41.0X4	T41.0X5	T41.0X6
intravenous	T41.1X1	T41.1X2	T41.1X3	T41.1X4	T41.1X5	T41.1X6
barbiturates	T42.3X1	T42.3X2	T42.3X3	T42.3X4	T42.3X5	T42.3X6
benzodiazepines	T42.4X1	T42.4X2	T42.4X3	T42.4X4	T42.4X5	T42.4X6
bromides	T42.6X1	T42.6X2	T42.6X3	T42.6X4	T42.6X5	T42.6X6
cannabis sativa	T40.7X1	T40.7X2	T40.7X3	T40.7X4	T40.7X5	T40.7X6
chloral hydrate	T42.6X1	T42.6X2	T42.6X3	T42.6X4	T42.6X5	T42.6X6
ethanol	T51.0X1	T51.0X2	T51.0X3	T51.0X4		
hallucinogens	T40.901	T40.902	T40.903	T40.904	T40.905	T40.906
hypnotics	T42.71	T42.72	T42.73	T42.74	T42.75	T42.76
specified NEC	T42.6X1	T42.6X2	T42.6X3	T42.6X4	T42.6X5	T42.6X6
muscle relaxants	T42.8X1	T42.8X2	T42.8X3	T42.8X4	T42.8X5	T42.8X6
paraldehyde	T42.6X1	T42.6X2	T42.6X3	T42.6X4	T42.6X5	T42.6X6
sedatives;	T42.71	T42.72	T42.73	T42.74	T42.75	T42.76
sedative-hypnotics						
mixed NEC	T42.6X1	T42.6X2	T42.6X3	T42.6X4	T42.6X5	T42.6X6
specified NEC	T42.6X1	T42.6X2	T42.6X3	T42.6X4	T42.6X5	T42.6X6
muscle-tone depressants	T42.8X1	T42.8X2	T42.8X3	T42.8X4	T42.8X5	T42.8X6
stimulants	T43.601	T43.602	T43.603	T43.604	T43.605	T43.606
amphetamines	T43.621	T43.622	T43.623	T43.624	T43.625	T43.626
analeptics	T50.7X1	T50.7X2	T50.7X3	T50.7X4	T50.7X5	T50.7X6
antidepressants	T43.201	T43.202	T43.203	T43.204	T43.205	T43.206
opiate antagonists	T50.7X1	T50.7X2	T50.7X3	T50.7X4	T50.7X5	T50.7X6
specified NEC	T43.691	T43.692	T43.693	T43.694	T43.695	T43.696
Cephalexin	T36.1X1	T36.1X2	T36.1X3	T36.1X4	T36.1X5	T36.1X6
Cephaloglycin	T36.1X1	T36.1X2	T36.1X3	T36.1X4	T36.1X5	T36.1X6
Cephaloridine	T36.1X1	T36.1X2	T36.1X3	T36.1X4	T36.1X5	T36.1X6
Cephalosporins	T36.1X1	T36.1X2	T36.1X3	T36.1X4	T36.1X5	T36.1X6
N (adicillin)	T36.0X1	T36.0X2	T36.0X3	T36.0X4	T36.0X5	T36.0X6
Cephalothin	T36.1X1	T36.1X2	T36.1X3	T36.1X4	T36.1X5	T36.1X6
Cephalotin	T36.1X1	T36.1X2	T36.1X3	T36.1X4	T36.1X5	T36.1X6
Cephradine	T36.1X1	T36.1X2	T36.1X3	T36.1X4	T36.1X5	T36.1X6
Cerbera (odollam)	T62.2X1	T62.2X2	T62.2X3	T62.2X4	—	—
Cerberin	T46.0X1	T46.0X2	T46.0X3	T46.0X4	T46.0X5	T46.0X6
Cerebral stimulants	T43.601	T43.602	T43.603	T43.604	T43.605	T43.606
psychotherapeutic	T43.601	T43.602	T43.603	T43.604	T43.605	T43.606
specified NEC	T43.691	T43.692	T43.693	T43.694	T43.695	T43.696
Cerium oxalate	T45.0X1	T45.0X2	T45.0X3	T45.0X4	T45.0X5	T45.0X6
Cerous oxalate	T45.0X1	T45.0X2	T45.0X3	T45.0X4	T45.0X5	T45.0X6
Ceruletide	T50.8X1	T50.8X2	T50.8X3	T50.8X4	T50.8X5	T50.8X6
Cetalkonium (chloride)	T49.0X1	T49.0X2	T49.0X3	T49.0X4	T49.0X5	T49.0X6
Cethexonium chloride	T49.0X1	T49.0X2	T49.0X3	T49.0X4	T49.0X5	T49.0X6
Cetiedil	T46.7X1	T46.7X2	T46.7X3	T46.7X4	T46.7X5	T46.7X6
Cetirizine	T45.0X1	T45.0X2	T45.0X3	T45.0X4	T45.0X5	T45.0X6
Cetomacrogol	T50.991	T50.992	T50.993	T50.994	T50.995	T50.996
Cetotiamine	T45.2X1	T45.2X2	T45.2X3	T45.2X4	T45.2X5	T45.2X6
Cetoxime	T45.0X1	T45.0X2	T45.0X3	T45.0X4	T45.0X5	T45.0X6
Cetraxate	T47.1X1	T47.1X2	T47.1X3	T47.1X4	T47.1X5	T47.1X6
Cetrimide	T49.0X1	T49.0X2	T49.0X3	T49.0X4	T49.0X5	T49.0X6
Cetrimonium (bromide)	T49.0X1	T49.0X2	T49.0X3	T49.0X4	T49.0X5	T49.0X6
Cetylpyridinium chloride	T49.0X1	T49.0X2	T49.0X3	T49.0X4	T49.0X5	T49.0X6
ENT agent	T49.6X1	T49.6X2	T49.6X3	T49.6X4	T49.6X5	T49.6X6
lozenges	T49.6X1	T49.6X2	T49.6X3	T49.6X4	T49.6X5	T49.6X6
Cevadilla — see Sabadilla						
Cevitamic acid	T45.2X1	T45.2X2	T45.2X3	T45.2X4	T45.2X5	T45.2X6
Chalk, precipitated	T47.1X1	T47.1X2	T47.1X3	T47.1X4	T47.1X5	T47.1X6
Chamomile	T49.0X1	T49.0X2	T49.0X3	T49.0X4	T49.0X5	T49.0X6
Ch'an su	T46.0X1	T46.0X2	T46.0X3	T46.0X4	T46.0X5	T46.0X6
Charcoal	T47.6X1	T47.6X2	T47.6X3	T47.6X4	T47.6X5	T47.6X6
activated — see also Charcoal, medicinal	T47.6X1	T47.6X2	T47.6X3	T47.6X4	T47.6X5	T47.6X6
fumes (Carbon monoxide)	T58.2X1	T58.2X2	T58.2X3	T58.2X4	—	—
industrial	T58.8X1	T58.8X2	T58.8X3	T58.8X4	—	—
medicinal (activated)	T47.6X1	T47.6X2	T47.6X3	T47.6X4	T47.6X5	T47.6X6
antidiarrheal	T47.6X1	T47.6X2	T47.6X3	T47.6X4	T47.6X5	T47.6X6
poison control	T47.8X1	T47.8X2	T47.8X3	T47.8X4	T47.8X5	T47.8X6
specified use other than for diarrhea	T47.8X1	T47.8X2	T47.8X3	T47.8X4	T47.8X5	T47.8X6
topical	T49.8X1	T49.8X2	T49.8X3	T49.8X4	T49.8X5	T49.8X6
Chaulmosulfone	T37.1X1	T37.1X2	T37.1X3	T37.1X4	T37.1X5	T37.1X6
Chelating agent NEC	T50.6X1	T50.6X2	T50.6X3	T50.6X4	T50.6X5	T50.6X6
Chelidonium majus	T62.2X1	T62.2X2	T62.2X3	T62.2X4	—	—
Chemical substance NEC	T65.91	T65.92	T65.93	T65.94	—	—
Chenodeoxycholic acid	T47.5X1	T47.5X2	T47.5X3	T47.5X4	T47.5X5	T47.5X6
Chenodiol	T47.5X1	T47.5X2	T47.5X3	T47.5X4	T47.5X5	T47.5X6
Chenopodium	T37.4X1	T37.4X2	T37.4X3	T37.4X4	T37.4X5	T37.4X6
Cherry laurel	T62.2X1	T62.2X2	T62.2X3	T62.2X4	—	—
Chinidin (e)	T46.2X1	T46.2X2	T46.2X3	T46.2X4	T46.2X5	T46.2X6
Chiniofon	T37.8X1	T37.8X2	T37.8X3	T37.8X4	T37.8X5	T37.8X6

Substance	Poisoning, Accidental (unintentional)	Poisoning, Intentional Self-harm	Poisoning, Assault	Poisoning, Undetermined	Adverse Effect	Under-dosing
Chlophedianol	T48.3X1	T48.3X2	T48.3X3	T48.3X4	T48.3X5	T48.3X6
Chloral	T42.6X1	T42.6X2	T42.6X3	T42.6X4	T42.6X5	T42.6X6
derivative	T42.6X1	T42.6X2	T42.6X3	T42.6X4	T42.6X5	T42.6X6
hydrate	T42.6X1	T42.6X2	T42.6X3	T42.6X4	T42.6X5	T42.6X6
Chloralamide	T42.6X1	T42.6X2	T42.6X3	T42.6X4	T42.6X5	T42.6X6
Chloralodol	T42.6X1	T42.6X2	T42.6X3	T42.6X4	T42.6X5	T42.6X6
Chloralose	T60.4X1	T60.4X2	T60.4X3	T60.4X4		
Chlorambucil	T45.1X1	T45.1X2	T45.1X3	T45.1X4	T45.1X5	T45.1X6
Chloramine	T57.8X1	T57.8X2	T57.8X3	T57.8X4		
T	T49.0X1	T49.0X2	T49.0X3	T49.0X4	T49.0X5	T49.0X6
topical	T49.0X1	T49.0X2	T49.0X3	T49.0X4	T49.0X5	T49.0X6
Chloramphenicol	T36.2X1	T36.2X2	T36.2X3	T36.2X4	T36.2X5	T36.2X6
ENT agent	T49.6X1	T49.6X2	T49.6X3	T49.6X4	T49.6X5	T49.6X6
ophthalmic preparation	T49.5X1	T49.5X2	T49.5X3	T49.5X4	T49.5X5	T49.5X6
topical NEC	T49.0X1	T49.0X2	T49.0X3	T49.0X4	T49.0X5	T49.0X6
Chlorate (potassium) (sodium) NEC	T60.3X1	T60.3X2	T60.3X3	T60.3X4		
herbicide	T60.3X1	T60.3X2	T60.3X3	T60.3X4		
Chlorazanil	T50.2X1	T50.2X2	T50.2X3	T50.2X4	T50.2X5	T50.2X6
Chlorbenzene, chlorbenzol	T53.7X1	T53.7X2	T53.7X3	T53.7X4	—	—
Chlorbenzoxamine	T44.3X1	T44.3X2	T44.3X3	T44.3X4	T44.3X5	T44.3X6
Chlorbutol	T42.6X1	T42.6X2	T42.6X3	T42.6X4	T42.6X5	T42.6X6
Chlorcyclizine	T45.0X1	T45.0X2	T45.0X3	T45.0X4	T45.0X5	T45.0X6
Chlordan (e) (dust)	T60.1X1	T60.1X2	T60.1X3	T60.1X4	—	—
Chlordantoin	T49.0X1	T49.0X2	T49.0X3	T49.0X4	T49.0X5	T49.0X6
Chlordiazepoxide	T42.4X1	T42.4X2	T42.4X3	T42.4X4	T42.4X5	T42.4X6
Chlordiethyl benzamide	T49.3X1	T49.3X2	T49.3X3	T49.3X4	T49.3X5	T49.3X6
Chloresium	T49.8X1	T49.8X2	T49.8X3	T49.8X4	T49.8X5	T49.8X6
Chlorethiazol	T42.6X1	T42.6X2	T42.6X3	T42.6X4	T42.6X5	T42.6X6
Chlorethyl — see Ethyl chloride						
Chloretone	T42.6X1	T42.6X2	T42.6X3	T42.6X4	T42.6X5	T42.6X6
Chlorex	T53.6X1	T53.6X2	T53.6X3	T53.6X4	—	—
insecticide	T60.1X1	T60.1X2	T60.1X3	T60.1X4	—	—
Chlorfenvinphos	T60.0X1	T60.0X2	T60.0X3	T60.0X4	—	—
Chlorhexadol	T42.6X1	T42.6X2	T42.6X3	T42.6X4	T42.6X5	T42.6X6
Chlorhexamide	T45.1X1	T45.1X2	T45.1X3	T45.1X4	T45.1X5	T45.1X6
Chlorhexidine	T49.0X1	T49.0X2	T49.0X3	T49.0X4	T49.0X5	T49.0X6
Chlorhydroxyquinolin	T49.0X1	T49.0X2	T49.0X3	T49.0X4	T49.0X5	T49.0X6
Chloride of lime (bleach)	T54.3X1	T54.3X2	T54.3X3	T54.3X4	—	—
Chlorimipramine	T43.011	T43.012	T43.013	T43.014	T43.015	T43.016
Chlorinated						
camphene	T53.6X1	T53.6X2	T53.6X3	T53.6X4	—	—
diphenyl	T53.7X1	T53.7X2	T53.7X3	T53.7X4	—	—
hydrocarbons NEC	T53.91	T53.92	T53.93	T53.94	—	—
solvents	T53.91	T53.92	T53.93	T53.94	—	—
lime (bleach)	T54.3X1	T54.3X2	T54.3X3	T54.3X4	—	—
and boric acid solution	T49.0X1	T49.0X2	T49.0X3	T49.0X4	T49.0X5	T49.0X6
naphthalene (insecticide)	T60.1X1	T60.1X2	T60.1X3	T60.1X4	—	—
industrial (non-pesticide)	T53.7X1	T53.7X2	T53.7X3	T53.7X4	—	—
pesticide NEC	T60.8X1	T60.8X2	T60.8X3	T60.8X4	—	—
soda — see also sodium hypochlorite						
solution	T49.0X1	T49.0X2	T49.0X3	T49.0X4	T49.0X5	T49.0X6
Chlorine (fumes) (gas)	T59.4X1	T59.4X2	T59.4X3	T59.4X4	—	—
bleach	T54.3X1	T54.3X2	T54.3X3	T54.3X4	—	—
compound gas NEC	T59.4X1	T59.4X2	T59.4X3	T59.4X4	—	—
disinfectant	T59.4X1	T59.4X2	T59.4X3	T59.4X4	—	—
releasing agents NEC	T59.4X1	T59.4X2	T59.4X3	T59.4X4	—	—
Chlorisondamine chloride	T46.991	T46.992	T46.993	T46.994	T46.995	T46.996
Chlormadinone	T38.5X1	T38.5X2	T38.5X3	T38.5X4	T38.5X5	T38.5X6
Chlormephos	T60.0X1	T60.0X2	T60.0X3	T60.0X4	—	—
Chlormerodrin	T50.2X1	T50.2X2	T50.2X3	T50.2X4	T50.2X5	T50.2X6
Chlormethiazole	T42.6X1	T42.6X2	T42.6X3	T42.6X4	T42.6X5	T42.6X6
Chlormethine	T45.1X1	T45.1X2	T45.1X3	T45.1X4	T45.1X5	T45.1X6
Chlormethylenecycline	T36.4X1	T36.4X2	T36.4X3	T36.4X4	T36.4X5	T36.4X6
Chlormezanone	T42.6X1	T42.6X2	T42.6X3	T42.6X4	T42.6X5	T42.6X6
Chloroacetic acid	T60.3X1	T60.3X2	T60.3X3	T60.3X4	—	—
Chloroacetone	T59.3X1	T59.3X2	T59.3X3	T59.3X4	—	—
Chloroacetophenone	T59.3X1	T59.3X2	T59.3X3	T59.3X4	—	—
Chloroaniline	T53.7X1	T53.7X2	T53.7X3	T53.7X4	—	—
Chlorobenzene, chlorobenzol	T53.7X1	T53.7X2	T53.7X3	T53.7X4	—	—
Chlorobromomethane (fire extinguisher)	T53.6X1	T53.6X2	T53.6X3	T53.6X4	—	—
Chlorobutanol	T49.0X1	T49.0X2	T49.0X3	T49.0X4	T49.0X5	T49.0X6
Chlorocresol	T49.0X1	T49.0X2	T49.0X3	T49.0X4	T49.0X5	T49.0X6
Chlorodehydromethyltestosterone	T38.7X1	T38.7X2	T38.7X3	T38.7X4	T38.7X5	T38.7X6
Chlorodinitrobenzene	T53.7X1	T53.7X2	T53.7X3	T53.7X4	—	—
dust or vapor	T53.7X1	T53.7X2	T53.7X3	T53.7X4	—	—
Chlorodiphenyl	T53.7X1	T53.7X2	T53.7X3	T53.7X4	—	—

Additional Character May Be Required — Refer to the Tabular List for Character Selection   ▽ Subterms under main terms may continue to next column or page

Substance	Poisoning, Accidental (unintentional)	Poisoning, Intentional Self-harm	Poisoning, Assault	Poisoning, Undetermined	Adverse Effect	Under-dosing
Chloroethane — see Ethyl chloride						
Chloroethylene	T53.6X1	T53.6X2	T53.6X3	T53.6X4	—	—
Chlorofluorocarbons	T53.5X1	T53.5X2	T53.5X3	T53.5X4	—	—
Chloroform (fumes) (vapor)	T53.1X1	T53.1X2	T53.1X3	T53.1X4	—	—
anesthetic	T41.0X1	T41.0X2	T41.0X3	T41.0X4	T41.0X5	T41.0X6
solvent	T53.1X1	T53.1X2	T53.1X3	T53.1X4	—	—
water, concentrated	T41.0X1	T41.0X2	T41.0X3	T41.0X4	T41.0X5	T41.0X6
Chloroguanide	T37.2X1	T37.2X2	T37.2X3	T37.2X4	T37.2X5	T37.2X6
Chloromycetin	T36.2X1	T36.2X2	T36.2X3	T36.2X4	T36.2X5	T36.2X6
ENT agent	T49.6X1	T49.6X2	T49.6X3	T49.6X4	T49.6X5	T49.6X6
ophthalmic preparation	T49.5X1	T49.5X2	T49.5X3	T49.5X4	T49.5X5	T49.5X6
otic solution	T49.6X1	T49.6X2	T49.6X3	T49.6X4	T49.6X5	T49.6X6
topical NEC	T49.0X1	T49.0X2	T49.0X3	T49.0X4	T49.0X5	T49.0X6
Chloronitrobenzene	T53.7X1	T53.7X2	T53.7X3	T53.7X4	—	—
dust or vapor	T53.7X1	T53.7X2	T53.7X3	T53.7X4	—	—
Chlorophacinone	T60.4X1	T60.4X2	T60.4X3	T60.4X4	—	—
Chlorophenol	T53.7X1	T53.7X2	T53.7X3	T53.7X4	—	—
Chlorophenothane	T60.1X1	T60.1X2	T60.1X3	T60.1X4	—	—
Chlorophyll	T50.991	T50.992	T50.993	T50.994	T50.995	T50.996
Chloropicrin (fumes)	T53.6X1	T53.6X2	T53.6X3	T53.6X4	—	—
fumigant	T60.8X1	T60.8X2	T60.8X3	T60.8X4	—	—
fungicide	T60.3X1	T60.3X2	T60.3X3	T60.3X4	—	—
pesticide	T60.8X1	T60.8X2	T60.8X3	T60.8X4	—	—
Chloroprocaine	T41.3X1	T41.3X2	T41.3X3	T41.3X4	T41.3X5	T41.3X6
infiltration (subcutaneous)	T41.3X1	T41.3X2	T41.3X3	T41.3X4	T41.3X5	T41.3X6
nerve block (peripheral) (plexus)	T41.3X1	T41.3X2	T41.3X3	T41.3X4	T41.3X5	T41.3X6
spinal	T41.3X1	T41.3X2	T41.3X3	T41.3X4	T41.3X5	T41.3X6
Chloroptic	T49.5X1	T49.5X2	T49.5X3	T49.5X4	T49.5X5	T49.5X6
Chloropurine	T45.1X1	T45.1X2	T45.1X3	T45.1X4	T45.1X5	T45.1X6
Chloropyramine	T45.0X1	T45.0X2	T45.0X3	T45.0X4	T45.0X5	T45.0X6
Chloropyrifos	T60.0X1	T60.0X2	T60.0X3	T60.0X4	—	—
Chloropyrilene	T45.0X1	T45.0X2	T45.0X3	T45.0X4	T45.0X5	T45.0X6
Chloroquine	T37.2X1	T37.2X2	T37.2X3	T37.2X4	T37.2X5	T37.2X6
Chlorothalonil	T60.3X1	T60.3X2	T60.3X3	T60.3X4	—	—
Chlorothen	T45.0X1	T45.0X2	T45.0X3	T45.0X4	T45.0X5	T45.0X6
Chlorothiazide	T50.2X1	T50.2X2	T50.2X3	T50.2X4	T50.2X5	T50.2X6
Chlorothymol	T49.4X1	T49.4X2	T49.4X3	T49.4X4	T49.4X5	T49.4X6
Chlorotrianisene	T38.5X1	T38.5X2	T38.5X3	T38.5X4	T38.5X5	T38.5X6
Chlorovinyldichloroarsine, not in war	T57.0X1	T57.0X2	T57.0X3	T57.0X4	—	—
Chloroxine	T49.4X1	T49.4X2	T49.4X3	T49.4X4	T49.4X5	T49.4X6
Chloroxylenol	T49.0X1	T49.0X2	T49.0X3	T49.0X4	T49.0X5	T49.0X6
Chlorphenamine	T45.0X1	T45.0X2	T45.0X3	T45.0X4	T45.0X5	T45.0X6
Chlorphenesin	T42.8X1	T42.8X2	T42.8X3	T42.8X4	T42.8X5	T42.8X6
topical (antifungal)	T49.0X1	T49.0X2	T49.0X3	T49.0X4	T49.0X5	T49.0X6
Chlorpheniramine	T45.0X1	T45.0X2	T45.0X3	T45.0X4	T45.0X5	T45.0X6
Chlorphenoxamine	T45.0X1	T45.0X2	T45.0X3	T45.0X4	T45.0X5	T45.0X6
Chlorphentermine	T50.5X1	T50.5X2	T50.5X3	T50.5X4	T50.5X5	T50.5X6
Chlorprocaine — see Chloroprocaine						
Chlorproguanil	T37.2X1	T37.2X2	T37.2X3	T37.2X4	T37.2X5	T37.2X6
Chlorpromazine	T43.3X1	T43.3X2	T43.3X3	T43.3X4	T43.3X5	T43.3X6
Chlorpropamide	T38.3X1	T38.3X2	T38.3X3	T38.3X4	T38.3X5	T38.3X6
Chlorprothixene	T43.4X1	T43.4X2	T43.4X3	T43.4X4	T43.4X5	T43.4X6
Chlorquinaldol	T49.0X1	T49.0X2	T49.0X3	T49.0X4	T49.0X5	T49.0X6
Chlorquinol	T49.0X1	T49.0X2	T49.0X3	T49.0X4	T49.0X5	T49.0X6
Chlortalidone	T50.2X1	T50.2X2	T50.2X3	T50.2X4	T50.2X5	T50.2X6
Chlortetracycline	T36.4X1	T36.4X2	T36.4X3	T36.4X4	T36.4X5	T36.4X6
Chlorthalidone	T50.2X1	T50.2X2	T50.2X3	T50.2X4	T50.2X5	T50.2X6
Chlorthion	T60.0X1	T60.0X2	T60.0X3	T60.0X4	—	—
Chlorthiophos	T60.0X1	T60.0X2	T60.0X3	T60.0X4	—	—
Chlortrianisene	T38.5X1	T38.5X2	T38.5X3	T38.5X4	T38.5X5	T38.5X6
Chlor-Trimeton	T45.0X1	T45.0X2	T45.0X3	T45.0X4	T45.0X5	T45.0X6
Chlorzoxazone	T42.8X1	T42.8X2	T42.8X3	T42.8X4	T42.8X5	T42.8X6
Choke damp	T59.7X1	T59.7X2	T59.7X3	T59.7X4		
Cholagogues	T47.5X1	T47.5X2	T47.5X3	T47.5X4	T47.5X5	T47.5X6
Cholebrine	T50.8X1	T50.8X2	T50.8X3	T50.8X4	T50.8X5	T50.8X6
Cholecalciferol	T45.2X1	T45.2X2	T45.2X3	T45.2X4	T45.2X5	T45.2X6
Cholecystokinin	T50.8X1	T50.8X2	T50.8X3	T50.8X4	T50.8X5	T50.8X6
Cholera vaccine	T50.A91	T50.A92	T50.A93	T50.A94	T50.A95	T50.A96
Choleretic	T47.5X1	T47.5X2	T47.5X3	T47.5X4	T47.5X5	T47.5X6
Cholesterol-lowering agents	T46.6X1	T46.6X2	T46.6X3	T46.6X4	T46.6X5	T46.6X6
Cholestyramine (resin)	T46.6X1	T46.6X2	T46.6X3	T46.6X4	T46.6X5	T46.6X6
Cholic acid	T47.5X1	T47.5X2	T47.5X3	T47.5X4	T47.5X5	T47.5X6
Choline	T48.6X1	T48.6X2	T48.6X3	T48.6X4	T48.6X5	T48.6X6
chloride	T50.991	T50.992	T50.993	T50.994	T50.995	T50.996
dihydrogen citrate	T50.991	T50.992	T50.993	T50.994	T50.995	T50.996
salicylate	T39.091	T39.092	T39.093	T39.094	T39.095	T39.096
theophyllinate	T48.6X1	T48.6X2	T48.6X3	T48.6X4	T48.6X5	T48.6X6
Cholinergic (drug) NEC	T44.1X1	T44.1X2	T44.1X3	T44.1X4	T44.1X5	T44.1X6

Substance	Poisoning, Accidental (unintentional)	Poisoning, Intentional Self-harm	Poisoning, Assault	Poisoning, Undetermined	Adverse Effect	Under-dosing
Cholinergic (drug) NEC — continued						
muscle tone enhancer	T44.1X1	T44.1X2	T44.1X3	T44.1X4	T44.1X5	T44.1X6
organophosphorus	T44.0X1	T44.0X2	T44.0X3	T44.0X4	T44.0X5	T44.0X6
insecticide	T60.0X1	T60.0X2	T60.0X3	T60.0X4	—	—
nerve gas	T59.891	T59.892	T59.893	T59.894	—	—
trimethyl ammonium propanediol	T44.1X1	T44.1X2	T44.1X3	T44.1X4	T44.1X5	T44.1X6
Cholinesterase reactivator	T50.6X1	T50.6X2	T50.6X3	T50.6X4	T50.6X5	T50.6X6
Cholografin	T50.8X1	T50.8X2	T50.8X3	T50.8X4	T50.8X5	T50.8X6
Chorionic gonadotropin	T38.891	T38.892	T38.893	T38.894	T38.895	T38.896
Chromate	T56.2X1	T56.2X2	T56.2X3	T56.2X4	—	—
dust or mist	T56.2X1	T56.2X2	T56.2X3	T56.2X4	—	—
lead — see also lead	T56.0X1	T56.0X2	T56.0X3	T56.0X4	—	—
paint	T56.0X1	T56.0X2	T56.0X3	T56.0X4	—	—
Chromic						
acid	T56.2X1	T56.2X2	T56.2X3	T56.2X4	—	—
dust or mist	T56.2X1	T56.2X2	T56.2X3	T56.2X4	—	—
phosphate 32P	T45.1X1	T45.1X2	T45.1X3	T45.1X4	T45.1X5	T45.1X6
Chromium	T56.2X1	T56.2X2	T56.2X3	T56.2X4	—	—
compounds — see Chromate						
sesquioxide	T50.8X1	T50.8X2	T50.8X3	T50.8X4	T50.8X5	T50.8X6
Chromomycin A3	T45.1X1	T45.1X2	T45.1X3	T45.1X4	T45.1X5	T45.1X6
Chromonar	T46.3X1	T46.3X2	T46.3X3	T46.3X4	T46.3X5	T46.3X6
Chromyl chloride	T56.2X1	T56.2X2	T56.2X3	T56.2X4	—	—
Chrysarobin	T49.4X1	T49.4X2	T49.4X3	T49.4X4	T49.4X5	T49.4X6
Chrysazin	T47.2X1	T47.2X2	T47.2X3	T47.2X4	T47.2X5	T47.2X6
Chymar	T45.3X1	T45.3X2	T45.3X3	T45.3X4	T45.3X5	T45.3X6
ophthalmic preparation	T49.5X1	T49.5X2	T49.5X3	T49.5X4	T49.5X5	T49.5X6
Chymopapain	T45.3X1	T45.3X2	T45.3X3	T45.3X4	T45.3X5	T45.3X6
Chymotrypsin	T45.3X1	T45.3X2	T45.3X3	T45.3X4	T45.3X5	T45.3X6
ophthalmic preparation	T49.5X1	T49.5X2	T49.5X3	T49.5X4	T49.5X5	T49.5X6
Cianidanol	T50.991	T50.992	T50.993	T50.994	T50.995	T50.996
Cianopramine	T43.011	T43.012	T43.013	T43.014	T43.015	T43.016
Cibenzoline	T46.2X1	T46.2X2	T46.2X3	T46.2X4	T46.2X5	T46.2X6
Ciclacillin	T36.0X1	T36.0X2	T36.0X3	T36.0X4	T36.0X5	T36.0X6
Ciclobarbital — see Hexobarbital						
Ciclonicate	T46.7X1	T46.7X2	T46.7X3	T46.7X4	T46.7X5	T46.7X6
Ciclopirox (olamine)	T49.0X1	T49.0X2	T49.0X3	T49.0X4	T49.0X5	T49.0X6
Ciclosporin	T45.1X1	T45.1X2	T45.1X3	T45.1X4	T45.1X5	T45.1X6
Cicuta maculata or virosa	T62.2X1	T62.2X2	T62.2X3	T62.2X4	—	—
Cicutoxin	T62.2X1	T62.2X2	T62.2X3	T62.2X4	—	—
Cigarette lighter fluid	T52.0X1	T52.0X2	T52.0X3	T52.0X4	—	—
Cigarettes (tobacco)	T65.221	T65.222	T65.223	T65.224	—	—
Ciguatoxin	T61.01	T61.02	T61.03	T61.04	—	—
Cilazapril	T46.4X1	T46.4X2	T46.4X3	T46.4X4	T46.4X5	T46.4X6
Cimetidine	T47.0X1	T47.0X2	T47.0X3	T47.0X4	T47.0X5	T47.0X6
Cimetropium bromide	T44.3X1	T44.3X2	T44.3X3	T44.3X4	T44.3X5	T44.3X6
Cinchocaine	T41.3X1	T41.3X2	T41.3X3	T41.3X4	T41.3X5	T41.3X6
topical (surface)	T41.3X1	T41.3X2	T41.3X3	T41.3X4	T41.3X5	T41.3X6
Cinchona	T37.2X1	T37.2X2	T37.2X3	T37.2X4	T37.2X5	T37.2X6
Cinchonine alkaloids	T37.2X1	T37.2X2	T37.2X3	T37.2X4	T37.2X5	T37.2X6
Cinchophen	T50.4X1	T50.4X2	T50.4X3	T50.4X4	T50.4X5	T50.4X6
Cinepazide	T46.7X1	T46.7X2	T46.7X3	T46.7X4	T46.7X5	T46.7X6
Cinnamedrine	T48.5X1	T48.5X2	T48.5X3	T48.5X4	T48.5X5	T48.5X6
Cinnarizine	T45.0X1	T45.0X2	T45.0X3	T45.0X4	T45.0X5	T45.0X6
Cinoxacin	T37.8X1	T37.8X2	T37.8X3	T37.8X4	T37.8X5	T37.8X6
Ciprofibrate	T46.6X1	T46.6X2	T46.6X3	T46.6X4	T46.6X5	T46.6X6
Ciprofloxacin	T36.8X1	T36.8X2	T36.8X3	T36.8X4	T36.8X5	T36.8X6
Cisapride	T47.8X1	T47.8X2	T47.8X3	T47.8X4	T47.8X5	T47.8X6
Cisplatin	T45.1X1	T45.1X2	T45.1X3	T45.1X4	T45.1X5	T45.1X6
Citalopram	T43.221	T43.222	T43.223	T43.224	T43.225	T43.226
Citanest	T41.3X1	T41.3X2	T41.3X3	T41.3X4	T41.3X5	T41.3X6
infiltration (subcutaneous)	T41.3X1	T41.3X2	T41.3X3	T41.3X4	T41.3X5	T41.3X6
nerve block (peripheral) (plexus)	T41.3X1	T41.3X2	T41.3X3	T41.3X4	T41.3X5	T41.3X6
Citric acid	T47.5X1	T47.5X2	T47.5X3	T47.5X4	T47.5X5	T47.5X6
Citrovorum (factor)	T45.8X1	T45.8X2	T45.8X3	T45.8X4	T45.8X5	T45.8X6
Claviceps purpurea	T62.2X1	T62.2X2	T62.2X3	T62.2X4	—	—
Clavulanic acid	T36.1X1	T36.1X2	T36.1X3	T36.1X4	T36.1X5	T36.1X6
Cleaner, cleansing agent, type not specified	T65.891	T65.892	T65.893	T65.894	—	—
of paint or varnish	T52.91	T52.92	T52.93	T52.94	—	—
specified type NEC	T65.891	T65.892	T65.893	T65.894	—	—
Clebopride	T47.8X1	T47.8X2	T47.8X3	T47.8X4	T47.8X5	T47.8X6
Clefamide	T37.3X1	T37.3X2	T37.3X3	T37.3X4	T37.3X5	T37.3X6
Clemastine	T45.0X1	T45.0X2	T45.0X3	T45.0X4	T45.0X5	T45.0X6
Clematis vitalba	T62.2X1	T62.2X2	T62.2X3	T62.2X4	—	—
Clemizole	T45.0X1	T45.0X2	T45.0X3	T45.0X4	T45.0X5	T45.0X6
penicillin	T36.0X1	T36.0X2	T36.0X3	T36.0X4	T36.0X5	T36.0X6
Clenbuterol	T48.6X1	T48.6X2	T48.6X3	T48.6X4	T48.6X5	T48.6X6
Clidinium bromide	T44.3X1	T44.3X2	T44.3X3	T44.3X4	T44.3X5	T44.3X6

Table of Drugs and Chemicals

Substance	Poisoning, Accidental (unintentional)	Poisoning, Intentional Self-harm	Poisoning, Assault	Poisoning, Undetermined	Adverse Effect	Under-dosing
Clindamycin	T36.8X1	T36.8X2	T36.8X3	T36.8X4	T36.8X5	T36.8X6
Clinofibrate	T46.6X1	T46.6X2	T46.6X3	T46.6X4	T46.6X5	T46.6X6
Clioquinol	T37.8X1	T37.8X2	T37.8X3	T37.8X4	T37.8X5	T37.8X6
Cliradon	T40.2X1	T40.2X2	T40.2X3	T40.2X4	—	—
Clobazam	T42.4X1	T42.4X2	T42.4X3	T42.4X4	T42.4X5	T42.4X6
Clobenzorex	T50.5X1	T50.5X2	T50.5X3	T50.5X4	T50.5X5	T50.5X6
Clobetasol	T49.0X1	T49.0X2	T49.0X3	T49.0X4	T49.0X5	T49.0X6
Clobetasone	T49.0X1	T49.0X2	T49.0X3	T49.0X4	T49.0X5	T49.0X6
Clobutinol	T48.3X1	T48.3X2	T48.3X3	T48.3X4	T48.3X5	T48.3X6
Clocortolone	T38.0X1	T38.0X2	T38.0X3	T38.0X4	T38.0X5	T38.0X6
Clodantoin	T49.0X1	T49.0X2	T49.0X3	T49.0X4	T49.0X5	T49.0X6
Clodronic acid	T50.991	T50.992	T50.993	T50.994	T50.995	T50.996
Clofazimine	T37.1X1	T37.1X2	T37.1X3	T37.1X4	T37.1X5	T37.1X6
Clofedanol	T48.3X1	T48.3X2	T48.3X3	T48.3X4	T48.3X5	T48.3X6
Clofenamide	T50.2X1	T50.2X2	T50.2X3	T50.2X4	T50.2X5	T50.2X6
Clofenotane	T49.0X1	T49.0X2	T49.0X3	T49.0X4	T49.0X5	T49.0X6
Clofezone	T39.2X1	T39.2X2	T39.2X3	T39.2X4	T39.2X5	T39.2X6
Clofibrate	T46.6X1	T46.6X2	T46.6X3	T46.6X4	T46.6X5	T46.6X6
Clofibride	T46.6X1	T46.6X2	T46.6X3	T46.6X4	T46.6X5	T46.6X6
Cloforex	T50.5X1	T50.5X2	T50.5X3	T50.5X4	T50.5X5	T50.5X6
Clomethiazole	T42.6X1	T42.6X2	T42.6X3	T42.6X4	T42.6X5	T42.6X6
Clometocillin	T36.0X1	T36.0X2	T36.0X3	T36.0X4	T36.0X5	T36.0X6
Clomifene	T38.5X1	T38.5X2	T38.5X3	T38.5X4	T38.5X5	T38.5X6
Clomiphene	T38.5X1	T38.5X2	T38.5X3	T38.5X4	T38.5X5	T38.5X6
Clomipramine	T43.011	T43.012	T43.013	T43.014	T43.015	T43.016
Clomocycline	T36.4X1	T36.4X2	T36.4X3	T36.4X4	T36.4X5	T36.4X6
Clonazepam	T42.4X1	T42.4X2	T42.4X3	T42.4X4	T42.4X5	T42.4X6
Clonidine	T46.5X1	T46.5X2	T46.5X3	T46.5X4	T46.5X5	T46.5X6
Clonixin	T39.8X1	T39.8X2	T39.8X3	T39.8X4	T39.8X5	T39.8X6
Clopamide	T50.2X1	T50.2X2	T50.2X3	T50.2X4	T50.2X5	T50.2X6
Clopenthixol	T43.4X1	T43.4X2	T43.4X3	T43.4X4	T43.4X5	T43.4X6
Cloperastine	T48.3X1	T48.3X2	T48.3X3	T48.3X4	T48.3X5	T48.3X6
Clophedianol	T48.3X1	T48.3X2	T48.3X3	T48.3X4	T48.3X5	T48.3X6
Cloponone	T36.2X1	T36.2X2	T36.2X3	T36.2X4	T36.2X5	T36.2X6
Cloprednol	T38.0X1	T38.0X2	T38.0X4	T38.0X4	T38.0X5	T38.0X6
Cloral betaine	T42.6X1	T42.6X2	T42.6X3	T42.6X4	T42.6X5	T42.6X6
Cloramfenicol	T36.2X1	T36.2X2	T36.2X3	T36.2X4	T36.2X5	T36.2X6
Clorazepate (dipotassium)	T42.4X1	T42.4X2	T42.4X3	T42.4X4	T42.4X5	T42.4X6
Clorexolone	T50.2X1	T50.2X2	T50.2X3	T50.2X4	T50.2X5	T50.2X6
Clorfenamine	T45.0X1	T45.0X2	T45.0X3	T45.0X4	T45.0X5	T45.0X6
Clorgiline	T43.1X1	T43.1X2	T43.1X3	T43.1X4	T43.1X5	T43.1X6
Clorotepine	T44.3X1	T44.3X2	T44.3X3	T44.3X4	T44.3X5	T44.3X6
Clorox (bleach)	T54.91	T54.92	T54.93	T54.94	—	—
Clorprenaline	T48.6X1	T48.6X2	T48.6X3	T48.6X4	T48.6X5	T48.6X6
Clortermine	T50.5X1	T50.5X2	T50.5X3	T50.5X4	T50.5X5	T50.5X6
Clotiapine	T43.591	T43.592	T43.593	T43.594	T43.595	T43.596
Clotiazepam	T42.4X1	T42.4X2	T42.4X3	T42.4X4	T42.4X5	T42.4X6
Clotibric acid	T46.6X1	T46.6X2	T46.6X3	T46.6X4	T46.6X5	T46.6X6
Clotrimazole	T49.0X1	T49.0X2	T49.0X3	T49.0X4	T49.0X5	T49.0X6
Cloxacillin	T36.0X1	T36.0X2	T36.0X3	T36.0X4	T36.0X5	T36.0X6
Cloxazolam	T42.4X1	T42.4X2	T42.4X3	T42.4X4	T42.4X5	T42.4X6
Cloxiquine	T49.0X1	T49.0X2	T49.0X3	T49.0X4	T49.0X5	T49.0X6
Clozapine	T42.4X1	T42.4X2	T42.4X3	T42.4X4	T42.4X5	T42.4X6
Coagulant NEC	T45.7X1	T45.7X2	T45.7X3	T45.7X4	T45.7X5	T45.7X6
Coal (carbon monoxide from) — see also Carbon, monoxide, coal	T58.2X1	T58.2X2	T58.2X3	T58.2X4	—	—
oil — see Kerosene						
tar	T49.1X1	T49.1X2	T49.1X3	T49.1X4	T49.1X5	T49.1X6
fumes	T59.891	T59.892	T59.893	T59.894	—	—
medicinal (ointment)	T49.4X1	T49.4X2	T49.4X3	T49.4X4	T49.4X5	T49.4X6
analgesics NEC	T39.2X1	T39.2X2	T39.2X3	T39.2X4	T39.2X5	T39.2X6
naphtha (solvent)	T52.0X1	T52.0X2	T52.0X3	T52.0X4	—	—
Cobalamine	T45.2X1	T45.2X2	T45.2X3	T45.2X4	T45.2X5	T45.2X6
Cobalt (nonmedicinal) (fumes) (industrial)	T56.891	T56.892	T56.893	T56.894	—	—
medicinal (trace) (chloride)	T45.8X1	T45.8X2	T45.8X3	T45.8X4	T45.8X5	T45.8X6
Cobra (venom)	T63.041	T63.042	T63.043	T63.044	—	—
Coca (leaf)	T40.5X1	T40.5X2	T40.5X3	T40.5X4	T40.5X5	T40.5X6
Cocaine	T40.5X1	T40.5X2	T40.5X3	T40.5X4	T40.5X5	T40.5X6
topical anesthetic	T41.3X1	T41.3X2	T41.3X3	T41.3X4	T41.3X5	T41.3X6
Cocarboxylase	T45.3X1	T45.3X2	T45.3X3	T45.3X4	T45.3X5	T45.3X6
Coccidioidin	T50.8X1	T50.8X2	T50.8X3	T50.8X4	T50.8X5	T50.8X6
Cocculus indicus	T62.1X1	T62.1X2	T62.1X3	T62.1X4	—	—
Cochineal	T65.6X1	T65.6X2	T65.6X3	T65.6X4	—	—
medicinal products	T50.991	T50.992	T50.993	T50.994	T50.995	T50.996
Codeine	T40.2X1	T40.2X2	T40.2X3	T40.2X4	T40.2X5	T40.2X6
Cod-liver oil	T45.2X1	T45.2X2	T45.2X3	T45.2X4	T45.2X5	T45.2X6
Coenzyme A	T50.991	T50.992	T50.993	T50.994	T50.995	T50.996
Coffee	T62.8X1	T62.8X2	T62.8X3	T62.8X4	—	—
Cogalactoisomerase	T50.991	T50.992	T50.993	T50.994	T50.995	T50.996
Cogentin	T44.3X1	T44.3X2	T44.3X3	T44.3X4	T44.3X5	T44.3X6

Substance	Poisoning, Accidental (unintentional)	Poisoning, Intentional Self-harm	Poisoning, Assault	Poisoning, Undetermined	Adverse Effect	Under-dosing
Coke fumes or gas (carbon monoxide)	T58.2X1	T58.2X2	T58.2X3	T58.2X4	—	—
industrial use	T58.8X1	T58.8X2	T58.8X3	T58.8X4	—	—
Colace	T47.4X1	T47.4X2	T47.4X3	T47.4X4	T47.4X5	T47.4X6
Colaspase	T45.1X1	T45.1X2	T45.1X3	T45.1X4	T45.1X5	T45.1X6
Colchicine	T50.4X1	T50.4X2	T50.4X3	T50.4X4	T50.4X5	T50.4X6
Colchicum	T62.2X1	T62.2X2	T62.2X3	T62.2X4	—	—
Cold cream	T49.3X1	T49.3X2	T49.3X3	T49.3X4	T49.3X5	T49.3X6
Colecalciferol	T45.2X1	T45.2X2	T45.2X3	T45.2X4	T45.2X5	T45.2X6
Colestipol	T46.6X1	T46.6X2	T46.6X3	T46.6X4	T46.6X5	T46.6X6
Colestyramine	T46.6X1	T46.6X2	T46.6X3	T46.6X4	T46.6X5	T46.6X6
Colimycin	T36.8X1	T36.8X2	T36.8X3	T36.8X4	T36.8X5	T36.8X6
Colistimethate	T36.8X1	T36.8X2	T36.8X3	T36.8X4	T36.8X5	T36.8X6
Colistin	T36.8X1	T36.8X2	T36.8X3	T36.8X4	T36.8X5	T36.8X6
sulfate (eye preparation)	T49.5X1	T49.5X2	T49.5X3	T49.5X4	T49.5X5	T49.5X6
Collagen	T50.991	T50.992	T50.993	T50.994	T50.995	T50.996
Collagenase	T49.4X1	T49.4X2	T49.4X3	T49.4X4	T49.4X5	T49.4X6
Collodion	T49.3X1	T49.3X2	T49.3X3	T49.3X4	T49.3X5	T49.3X6
Colocynth	T47.2X1	T47.2X2	T47.2X3	T47.2X4	T47.2X5	T47.2X6
Colophony adhesive	T49.3X1	T49.3X2	T49.3X3	T49.3X4	T49.3X5	T49.3X6
Colorant — see also Dye	T50.991	T50.992	T50.993	T50.994	T50.995	T50.996
Coloring matter — see Dye(s)						
Combustion gas (after combustion) — see Carbon, monoxide						
prior to combustion	T59.891	T59.892	T59.893	T59.894	—	—
Compazine	T43.3X1	T43.3X2	T43.3X3	T43.3X4	T43.3X5	T43.3X6
Compound						
1080 (sodium fluoroacetate)	T60.4X1	T60.4X2	T60.4X3	T60.4X4	—	—
269 (endrin)	T60.1X1	T60.1X2	T60.1X3	T60.1X4	—	—
3422 (parathion)	T60.0X1	T60.0X2	T60.0X3	T60.0X4	—	—
3911 (phorate)	T60.0X1	T60.0X2	T60.0X3	T60.0X4	—	—
3956 (toxaphene)	T60.1X1	T60.1X2	T60.1X3	T60.1X4	—	—
4049 (malathion)	T60.0X1	T60.0X2	T60.0X3	T60.0X4	—	—
4069 (malathion)	T60.0X1	T60.0X2	T60.0X3	T60.0X4	—	—
4124 (dicapthon)	T60.0X1	T60.0X2	T60.0X3	T60.0X4	—	—
42 (warfarin)	T60.4X1	T60.4X2	T60.4X3	T60.4X4	—	—
497 (dieldrin)	T60.1X1	T60.1X2	T60.1X3	T60.1X4	—	—
E (cortisone)	T38.0X1	T38.0X2	T38.0X3	T38.0X4	T38.0X5	T38.0X6
F (hydrocortisone)	T38.0X1	T38.0X2	T38.0X3	T38.0X4	T38.0X5	T38.0X6
Congener, anabolic	T38.7X1	T38.7X2	T38.7X3	T38.7X4	T38.7X5	T38.7X6
Congo red	T50.8X1	T50.8X2	T50.8X3	T50.8X4	T50.8X5	T50.8X6
Coniine, conine	T62.2X1	T62.2X2	T62.2X3	T62.2X4	—	—
Conium (maculatum)	T62.2X1	T62.2X2	T62.2X3	T62.2X4	—	—
Conjugated estrogenic substances	T38.5X1	T38.5X2	T38.5X3	T38.5X4	T38.5X5	T38.5X6
Contac	T48.5X1	T48.5X2	T48.5X3	T48.5X4	T48.5X5	T48.5X6
Contact lens solution	T49.5X1	T49.5X2	T49.5X3	T49.5X4	T49.5X5	T49.5X6
Contraceptive (oral)	T38.4X1	T38.4X2	T38.4X3	T38.4X4	T38.4X5	T38.4X6
vaginal	T49.8X1	T49.8X2	T49.8X3	T49.8X4	T49.8X5	T49.8X6
Contrast medium, radiography	T50.8X1	T50.8X2	T50.8X3	T50.8X4	T50.8X5	T50.8X6
Convallaria glycosides	T46.0X1	T46.0X2	T46.0X3	T46.0X4	T46.0X5	T46.0X6
Convallaria majalis	T62.2X1	T62.2X2	T62.2X3	T62.2X4	—	—
berry	T62.1X1	T62.1X2	T62.1X3	T62.1X4	—	—
Copperhead snake (bite) (venom)	T63.061	T63.062	T63.063	T63.064	—	—
Copper (dust) (fumes) (nonmedicinal) NEC	T56.4X1	T56.4X2	T56.4X3	T56.4X4	—	—
arsenate, arsenite	T57.0X1	T57.0X2	T57.0X3	T57.0X4	—	—
insecticide	T60.2X1	T60.2X2	T60.2X3	T60.2X4	—	—
emetic	T47.7X1	T47.7X2	T47.7X3	T47.7X4	T47.7X5	T47.7X
fungicide	T60.3X1	T60.3X2	T60.3X3	T60.3X4	—	—
gluconate	T49.0X1	T49.0X2	T49.0X3	T49.0X4	T49.0X5	T49.0X
insecticide	T60.2X1	T60.2X2	T60.2X3	T60.2X4	—	—
medicinal (trace)	T45.8X1	T45.8X2	T45.8X3	T45.8X4	T45.8X5	T45.8X
oleate	T49.0X1	T49.0X2	T49.0X3	T49.0X4	T49.0X5	T49.0X
sulfate	T56.4X1	T56.4X2	T56.4X3	T56.4X4	—	—
cupric	T56.4X1	T56.4X2	T56.4X3	T56.4X4	—	—
fungicide	T60.3X1	T60.3X2	T60.3X3	T60.3X4	—	—
medicinal						
ear	T49.6X1	T49.6X2	T49.6X3	T49.6X4	T49.6X5	T49.6X
emetic	T47.7X1	T47.7X2	T47.7X3	T47.7X4	T47.7X5	T47.7X
eye	T49.5X1	T49.5X2	T49.5X3	T49.5X4	T49.5X5	T49.5X
cuprous	T56.4X1	T56.4X2	T56.4X3	T56.4X4	—	—
fungicide	T60.3X1	T60.3X2	T60.3X3	T60.3X4	—	—
medicinal						
ear	T49.6X1	T49.6X2	T49.6X3	T49.6X4	T49.6X5	T49.6X
emetic	T47.7X1	T47.7X2	T47.7X3	T47.7X4	T47.7X5	T47.7X
eye	T49.5X1	T49.5X2	T49.5X3	T49.5X4	T49.5X5	T49.5X
Coral (sting)	T63.691	T63.692	T63.693	T63.694	—	—
snake (bite) (venom)	T63.021	T63.022	T63.023	T63.024	—	—

Additional Character May Be Required — Refer to the Tabular List for Character Selection   ⬇ Subterms under main terms may continue to next column or page

Substance	Poisoning, Accidental (unintentional)	Poisoning, Intentional Self-harm	Poisoning, Assault	Poisoning, Undetermined	Adverse Effect	Under-dosing
Corbadrine	T49.6X1	T49.6X2	T49.6X3	T49.6X4	T49.6X5	T49.6X6
Cordite	T65.891	T65.892	T65.893	T65.894	—	—
vapor	T59.891	T59.892	T59.893	T59.894	—	—
Cordran	T49.0X1	T49.0X2	T49.0X3	T49.0X4	T49.0X5	T49.0X6
Corn cures	T49.4X1	T49.4X2	T49.4X3	T49.4X4	T49.4X5	T49.4X6
Cornhusker's lotion	T49.3X1	T49.3X2	T49.3X3	T49.3X4	T49.3X5	T49.3X6
Corn starch	T49.3X1	T49.3X2	T49.3X3	T49.3X4	T49.3X5	T49.3X6
Coronary vasodilator NEC	T46.3X1	T46.3X2	T46.3X3	T46.3X4	T46.3X5	T46.3X6
Corrosive NEC	T54.91	T54.92	T54.93	T54.94	—	—
acid NEC	T54.2X1	T54.2X2	T54.2X3	T54.2X4	—	—
aromatics	T54.1X1	T54.1X2	T54.1X3	T54.1X4	—	—
disinfectant	T54.1X1	T54.1X2	T54.1X3	T54.1X4	—	—
fumes NEC	T54.91	T54.92	T54.93	T54.94	—	—
specified NEC	T54.91	T54.92	T54.93	T54.94	—	—
sublimate	T56.1X1	T56.1X2	T56.1X3	T56.1X4	—	—
Cortate	T38.0X1	T38.0X2	T38.0X3	T38.0X4	T38.0X5	T38.0X6
Cort-Dome	T38.0X1	T38.0X2	T38.0X3	T38.0X4	T38.0X5	T38.0X6
ENT agent	T49.6X1	T49.6X2	T49.6X3	T49.6X4	T49.6X5	T49.6X6
ophthalmic preparation	T49.5X1	T49.5X2	T49.5X3	T49.5X4	T49.5X5	T49.5X6
topical NEC	T49.0X1	T49.0X2	T49.0X3	T49.0X4	T49.0X5	T49.0X6
Cortef	T38.0X1	T38.0X2	T38.0X3	T38.0X4	T38.0X5	T38.0X6
ENT agent	T49.6X1	T49.6X2	T49.6X3	T49.6X4	T49.6X5	T49.6X6
ophthalmic preparation	T49.5X1	T49.5X2	T49.5X3	T49.5X4	T49.5X5	T49.5X6
topical NEC	T49.0X1	T49.0X2	T49.0X3	T49.0X4	T49.0X5	T49.0X6
Corticosteroid	T38.0X1	T38.0X2	T38.0X3	T38.0X4	T38.0X5	T38.0X6
ENT agent	T49.6X1	T49.6X2	T49.6X3	T49.6X4	T49.6X5	T49.6X6
mineral	T50.0X1	T50.0X2	T50.0X3	T50.0X4	T50.0X5	T50.0X6
ophthalmic	T49.5X1	T49.5X2	T49.5X3	T49.5X4	T49.5X5	T49.5X6
topical NEC	T49.0X1	T49.0X2	T49.0X3	T49.0X4	T49.0X5	T49.0X6
Corticotropin	T38.811	T38.812	T38.813	T38.814	T38.815	T38.816
Cortisol	T49.0X1	T49.0X2	T49.0X3	T49.0X4	T49.0X5	T49.0X6
ENT agent	T49.6X1	T49.6X2	T49.6X3	T49.6X4	T49.6X5	T49.6X6
ophthalmic preparation	T49.5X1	T49.5X2	T49.5X3	T49.5X4	T49.5X5	T49.5X6
topical NEC	T49.0X1	T49.0X2	T49.0X3	T49.0X4	T49.0X5	T49.0X6
Cortisone (acetate)	T38.0X1	T38.0X2	T38.0X3	T38.0X4	T38.0X5	T38.0X6
ENT agent	T49.6X1	T49.6X2	T49.6X3	T49.6X4	T49.6X5	T49.6X6
ophthalmic preparation	T49.5X1	T49.5X2	T49.5X3	T49.5X4	T49.5X5	T49.5X6
topical NEC	T49.0X1	T49.0X2	T49.0X3	T49.0X4	T49.0X5	T49.0X6
Cortivazol	T38.0X1	T38.0X2	T38.0X3	T38.0X4	T38.0X5	T38.0X6
Cortogen	T38.0X1	T38.0X2	T38.0X3	T38.0X4	T38.0X5	T38.0X6
ENT agent	T49.6X1	T49.6X2	T49.6X3	T49.6X4	T49.6X5	T49.6X6
ophthalmic preparation	T49.5X1	T49.5X2	T49.5X3	T49.5X4	T49.5X5	T49.5X6
Cortone	T38.0X1	T38.0X2	T38.0X3	T38.0X4	T38.0X5	T38.0X6
ENT agent	T49.6X1	T49.6X2	T49.6X3	T49.6X4	T49.6X5	T49.6X6
ophthalmic preparation	T49.5X1	T49.5X2	T49.5X3	T49.5X4	T49.5X5	T49.5X6
Cortril	T38.0X1	T38.0X2	T38.0X3	T38.0X4	T38.0X5	T38.0X6
ENT agent	T49.6X1	T49.6X2	T49.6X3	T49.6X4	T49.6X5	T49.6X6
ophthalmic preparation	T49.5X1	T49.5X2	T49.5X3	T49.5X4	T49.5X5	T49.5X6
topical NEC	T49.0X1	T49.0X2	T49.0X3	T49.0X4	T49.0X5	T49.0X6
Corynebacterium parvum	T45.1X1	T45.1X2	T45.1X3	T45.1X4	T45.1X5	T45.1X6
Cosmetic preparation	T49.8X1	T49.8X2	T49.8X3	T49.8X4	T49.8X5	T49.8X6
Cosmetics	T49.8X1	T49.8X2	T49.8X3	T49.8X4	T49.8X5	T49.8X6
Cosyntropin	T38.811	T38.812	T38.813	T38.814	T38.815	T38.816
Cotarnine	T45.7X1	T45.7X2	T45.7X3	T45.7X4	T45.7X5	T45.7X6
Co-trimoxazole	T36.8X1	T36.8X2	T36.8X3	T36.8X4	T36.8X5	T36.8X6
Cottonseed oil	T49.3X1	T49.3X2	T49.3X3	T49.3X4	T49.3X5	T49.3X6
Cough mixture (syrup)	T48.4X1	T48.4X2	T48.4X3	T48.4X4	T48.4X5	T48.4X6
containing opiates	T40.2X1	T40.2X2	T40.2X3	T40.2X4	T40.2X5	T40.2X6
expectorants	T48.4X1	T48.4X2	T48.4X3	T48.4X4	T48.4X5	T48.4X6
Coumadin	T45.511	T45.512	T45.513	T45.514	T45.515	T45.516
rodenticide	T60.4X1	T60.4X2	T60.4X3	T60.4X4	—	—
Coumaphos	T60.0X1	T60.0X2	T60.0X3	T60.0X4	—	—
Coumarin	T45.511	T45.512	T45.513	T45.514	T45.515	T45.516
Coumetarol	T45.511	T45.512	T45.513	T45.514	T45.515	T45.516
Cowbane	T62.2X1	T62.2X2	T62.2X3	T62.2X4	—	—
Cozyme	T45.2X1	T45.2X2	T45.2X3	T45.2X4	T45.2X5	T45.2X6
Crack	T40.5X1	T40.5X2	T40.5X3	T40.5X4	—	—
Crataegus extract	T46.0X1	T46.0X2	T46.0X3	T46.0X4	T46.0X5	T46.0X6
Creolin	T54.1X1	T54.1X2	T54.1X3	T54.1X4	—	—
disinfectant	T54.1X1	T54.1X2	T54.1X3	T54.1X4	—	—
Creosol (compound)	T49.0X1	T49.0X2	T49.0X3	T49.0X4	T49.0X5	T49.0X6
Creosote (coal tar) (beechwood)	T49.0X1	T49.0X2	T49.0X3	T49.0X4	T49.0X5	T49.0X6
medicinal (expectorant)	T48.4X1	T48.4X2	T48.4X3	T48.4X4	T48.4X5	T48.4X6
syrup	T48.4X1	T48.4X2	T48.4X3	T48.4X4	T48.4X5	T48.4X6
Cresol(s)	T49.0X1	T49.0X2	T49.0X3	T49.0X4	T49.0X5	T49.0X6
and soap solution	T49.0X1	T49.0X2	T49.0X3	T49.0X4	T49.0X5	T49.0X6
Cresyl acetate	T49.0X1	T49.0X2	T49.0X3	T49.0X4	T49.0X5	T49.0X6
Cresylic acid	T49.0X1	T49.0X2	T49.0X3	T49.0X4	T49.0X5	T49.0X6
Crimidine	T60.4X1	T60.4X2	T60.4X3	T60.4X4	—	—
Croconazole	T37.8X1	T37.8X2	T37.8X3	T37.8X4	T37.8X5	T37.8X6
Cromoglicic acid	T48.6X1	T48.6X2	T48.6X3	T48.6X4	T48.6X5	T48.6X6
Cromolyn	T48.6X1	T48.6X2	T48.6X3	T48.6X4	T48.6X5	T48.6X6

Substance	Poisoning, Accidental (unintentional)	Poisoning, Intentional Self-harm	Poisoning, Assault	Poisoning, Undetermined	Adverse Effect	Under-dosing
Cromonar	T46.3X1	T46.3X2	T46.3X3	T46.3X4	T46.3X5	T46.3X6
Cropropamide	T39.8X1	T39.8X2	T39.8X3	T39.8X4	T39.8X5	T39.8X6
with crotethamide	T50.7X1	T50.7X2	T50.7X3	T50.7X4	T50.7X5	T50.7X6
Crotamiton	T49.0X1	T49.0X2	T49.0X3	T49.0X4	T49.0X5	T49.0X6
Crotethamide	T39.8X1	T39.8X2	T39.8X3	T39.8X4	T39.8X5	T39.8X6
with cropropamide	T50.7X1	T50.7X2	T50.7X3	T50.7X4	T50.7X5	T50.7X6
Croton (oil)	T47.2X1	T47.2X2	T47.2X3	T47.2X4	T47.2X5	T47.2X6
chloral	T42.6X1	T42.6X2	T42.6X3	T42.6X4	T42.6X5	T42.6X6
Crude oil	T52.0X1	T52.0X2	T52.0X3	T52.0X4	—	—
Cryogenine	T39.8X1	T39.8X2	T39.8X3	T39.8X4	T39.8X5	T39.8X6
Cryolite (vapor)	T60.1X1	T60.1X2	T60.1X3	T60.1X4	—	—
insecticide	T60.1X1	T60.1X2	T60.1X3	T60.1X4	—	—
Cryptenamine (tannates)	T46.5X1	T46.5X2	T46.5X3	T46.5X4	T46.5X5	T46.5X6
Crystal violet	T49.0X1	T49.0X2	T49.0X3	T49.0X4	T49.0X5	T49.0X6
Cuckoopint	T62.2X1	T62.2X2	T62.2X3	T62.2X4	—	—
Cumetharol	T45.511	T45.512	T45.513	T45.514	T45.515	T45.516
Cupric						
acetate	T60.3X1	T60.3X2	T60.3X3	T60.3X4	—	—
acetoarsenite	T57.0X1	T57.0X2	T57.0X3	T57.0X4	—	—
arsenate	T57.0X1	T57.0X2	T57.0X3	T57.0X4	—	—
gluconate	T49.0X1	T49.0X2	T49.0X3	T49.0X4	T49.0X5	T49.0X6
oleate	T49.0X1	T49.0X2	T49.0X3	T49.0X4	T49.0X5	T49.0X6
sulfate	T56.4X1	T56.4X2	T56.4X3	T56.4X4	—	—
Cuprous sulfate — see also Copper sulfate	T56.4X1	T56.4X2	T56.4X3	T56.4X4	—	—
Curare, curarine	T48.1X1	T48.1X2	T48.1X3	T48.1X4	T48.1X5	T48.1X6
Cyamemazine	T43.3X1	T43.3X2	T43.3X3	T43.3X4	T43.3X5	T43.3X6
Cyamopsis tetragonoloba	T46.6X1	T46.6X2	T46.6X3	T46.6X4	T46.6X5	T46.6X6
Cyanacetyl hydrazide	T37.1X1	T37.1X2	T37.1X3	T37.1X4	T37.1X5	T37.1X6
Cyanic acid (gas)	T59.891	T59.892	T59.893	T59.894	—	—
Cyanide(s) (compounds) (potassium) (sodium) NEC	T65.0X1	T65.0X2	T65.0X3	T65.0X4	—	—
dust or gas (inhalation) NEC	T57.3X1	T57.3X2	T57.3X3	T57.3X4	—	—
fumigant	T65.0X1	T65.0X2	T65.0X3	T65.0X4	—	—
hydrogen	T57.3X1	T57.3X2	T57.3X3	T57.3X4	—	—
mercuric — see Mercury						
pesticide (dust) (fumes)	T65.0X1	T65.0X2	T65.0X3	T65.0X4	—	—
Cyanoacrylate adhesive	T49.3X1	T49.3X2	T49.3X3	T49.3X4	T49.3X5	T49.3X6
Cyanocobalamin	T45.8X1	T45.8X2	T45.8X3	T45.8X4	T45.8X5	T45.8X6
Cyanogen (chloride) (gas) NEC	T59.891	T59.892	T59.893	T59.894	—	—
Cyclacillin	T36.0X1	T36.0X2	T36.0X3	T36.0X4	T36.0X5	T36.0X6
Cyclaine	T41.3X1	T41.3X2	T41.3X3	T41.3X4	T41.3X5	T41.3X6
Cyclamate	T50.991	T50.992	T50.993	T50.994	T50.995	T50.996
Cyclamen europaeum	T62.2X1	T62.2X2	T62.2X3	T62.2X4	—	—
Cyclandelate	T46.7X1	T46.7X2	T46.7X3	T46.7X4	T46.7X5	T46.7X6
Cyclazocine	T50.7X1	T50.7X2	T50.7X3	T50.7X4	T50.7X5	T50.7X6
Cyclizine	T45.0X1	T45.0X2	T45.0X3	T45.0X4	T45.0X5	T45.0X6
Cyclobarbital	T42.3X1	T42.3X2	T42.3X3	T42.3X4	T42.3X5	T42.3X6
Cyclobarbitone	T42.3X1	T42.3X2	T42.3X3	T42.3X4	T42.3X5	T42.3X6
Cyclobenzaprine	T48.1X1	T48.1X2	T48.1X3	T48.1X4	T48.1X5	T48.1X6
Cyclodrine	T44.3X1	T44.3X2	T44.3X3	T44.3X4	T44.3X5	T44.3X6
Cycloguanil embonate	T37.2X1	T37.2X2	T37.2X3	T37.2X4	T37.2X5	T37.2X6
Cyclohexane	T52.8X1	T52.8X2	T52.8X3	T52.8X4	—	—
Cyclohexanol	T51.8X1	T51.8X2	T51.8X3	T51.8X4	—	—
Cyclohexanone	T52.4X1	T52.4X2	T52.4X3	T52.4X4	—	—
Cycloheximide	T60.3X1	T60.3X2	T60.3X3	T60.3X4	—	—
Cyclohexyl acetate	T52.8X1	T52.8X2	T52.8X3	T52.8X4	—	—
Cycloleucin	T45.1X1	T45.1X2	T45.1X3	T45.1X4	T45.1X5	T45.1X6
Cyclomethycaine	T41.3X1	T41.3X2	T41.3X3	T41.3X4	T41.3X5	T41.3X6
Cyclopentamine	T44.4X1	T44.4X2	T44.4X3	T44.4X4	T44.4X5	T44.4X6
Cyclopenthiazide	T50.2X1	T50.2X2	T50.2X3	T50.2X4	T50.2X5	T50.2X6
Cyclopentolate	T44.3X1	T44.3X2	T44.3X3	T44.3X4	T44.3X5	T44.3X6
Cyclophosphamide	T45.1X1	T45.1X2	T45.1X3	T45.1X4	T45.1X5	T45.1X6
Cycloplegic drug	T49.5X1	T49.5X2	T49.5X3	T49.5X4	T49.5X5	T49.5X6
Cyclopropane	T41.291	T41.292	T41.293	T41.294	T41.295	T41.296
Cyclopyrabital	T39.8X1	T39.8X2	T39.8X3	T39.8X4	T39.8X5	T39.8X6
Cycloserine	T37.1X1	T37.1X2	T37.1X3	T37.1X4	T37.1X5	T37.1X6
Cyclosporin	T45.1X1	T45.1X2	T45.1X3	T45.1X4	T45.1X5	T45.1X6
Cyclothiazide	T50.2X1	T50.2X2	T50.2X3	T50.2X4	T50.2X5	T50.2X6
Cycrimine	T44.3X1	T44.3X2	T44.3X3	T44.3X4	T44.3X5	T44.3X6
Cyhalothrin	T60.1X1	T60.1X2	T60.1X3	T60.1X4	—	—
Cymarin	T46.0X1	T46.0X2	T46.0X3	T46.0X4	T46.0X5	T46.0X6
Cypermethrin	T60.1X1	T60.1X2	T60.1X3	T60.1X4	—	—
Cyphenothrin	T60.2X1	T60.2X2	T60.2X3	T60.2X4	—	—
Cyproheptadine	T45.0X1	T45.0X2	T45.0X3	T45.0X4	T45.0X5	T45.0X6
Cyproterone	T38.6X1	T38.6X2	T38.6X3	T38.6X4	T38.6X5	T38.6X6
Cysteamine	T50.6X1	T50.6X2	T50.6X3	T50.6X4	T50.6X5	T50.6X6
Cytarabine	T45.1X1	T45.1X2	T45.1X3	T45.1X4	T45.1X5	T45.1X6
Cytisus						
laburnum	T62.2X1	T62.2X2	T62.2X3	T62.2X4	—	—

Substance	Poisoning, Accidental (unintentional)	Poisoning, Intentional Self-harm	Poisoning, Assault	Poisoning, Undetermined	Adverse Effect	Under-dosing
Cytisus — continued						
scoparius	T62.2X1	T62.2X2	T62.2X3	T62.2X4	—	—
Cytochrome C	T47.5X1	T47.5X2	T47.5X3	T47.5X4	T47.5X5	T47.5X6
Cytomel	T38.1X1	T38.1X2	T38.1X3	T38.1X4	T38.1X5	T38.1X6
Cytosine arabinoside	T45.1X1	T45.1X2	T45.1X3	T45.1X4	T45.1X5	T45.1X6
Cytoxan	T45.1X1	T45.1X2	T45.1X3	T45.1X4	T45.1X5	T45.1X6
Cytozyme	T45.7X1	T45.7X2	T45.7X3	T45.7X4	T45.7X5	T45.7X6
S-Carboxymethylcysteine	T48.4X1	T48.4X2	T48.4X3	T48.4X4	T48.4X5	T48.4X6
Dacarbazine	T45.1X1	T45.1X2	T45.1X3	T45.1X4	T45.1X5	T45.1X6
Dactinomycin	T45.1X1	T45.1X2	T45.1X3	T45.1X4	T45.1X5	T45.1X6
DADPS	T37.1X1	T37.1X2	T37.1X3	T37.1X4	T37.1X5	T37.1X6
Dakin's solution	T49.0X1	T49.0X2	T49.0X3	T49.0X4	T49.0X5	T49.0X6
Dalapon (sodium)	T60.3X1	T60.3X2	T60.3X3	T60.3X4	—	—
Dalmane	T42.4X1	T42.4X2	T42.4X3	T42.4X4	T42.4X5	T42.4X6
Danazol	T38.6X1	T38.6X2	T38.6X3	T38.6X4	T38.6X5	T38.6X6
Danilone	T45.511	T45.512	T45.513	T45.514	T45.515	T45.516
Danthron	T47.2X1	T47.2X2	T47.2X3	T47.2X4	T47.2X5	T47.2X6
Dantrolene	T42.8X1	T42.8X2	T42.8X3	T42.8X4	T42.8X5	T42.8X6
Dantron	T47.2X1	T47.2X2	T47.2X3	T47.2X4	T47.2X5	T47.2X6
Daphne (gnidium) (mezereum)	T62.2X1	T62.2X2	T62.2X3	T62.2X4	—	—
berry	T62.1X1	T62.1X2	T62.1X3	T62.1X4	—	—
Dapsone	T37.1X1	T37.1X2	T37.1X3	T37.1X4	T37.1X5	T37.1X6
Daraprim	T37.2X1	T37.2X2	T37.2X3	T37.2X4	T37.2X5	T37.2X6
Darnel	T62.2X1	T62.2X2	T62.2X3	T62.2X4	—	—
Darvon	T39.8X1	T39.8X2	T39.8X3	T39.8X4	T39.8X5	T39.8X6
Daunomycin	T45.1X1	T45.1X2	T45.1X3	T45.1X4	T45.1X5	T45.1X6
Daunorubicin	T45.1X1	T45.1X2	T45.1X3	T45.1X4	T45.1X5	T45.1X6
DBI	T38.3X1	T38.3X2	T38.3X3	T38.3X4	T38.3X5	T38.3X6
D-Con	T60.91	T60.92	T60.93	T60.94	—	—
insecticide	T60.2X1	T60.2X2	T60.2X3	T60.2X4	—	—
rodenticide	T60.4X1	T60.4X2	T60.4X3	T60.4X4	—	—
DDAVP	T38.891	T38.892	T38.893	T38.894	T38.895	T38.896
DDE (bis(chlorophenyl)-dichloroethylene)	T60.2X1	T60.2X2	T60.2X3	T60.2X4	—	—
DDS	T37.1X1	T37.1X2	T37.1X3	T37.1X4	T37.1X5	T37.1X6
DDT (dust)	T60.1X1	T60.1X2	T60.1X3	T60.1X4	—	—
Deadly nightshade — see also Belladonna	T62.2X1	T62.2X2	T62.2X3	T62.2X4	—	—
berry	T62.1X1	T62.1X2	T62.1X3	T62.1X4	—	—
Deamino-D-arginine vasopressin	T38.891	T38.892	T38.893	T38.894	T38.895	T38.896
Deanol (aceglumate)	T50.991	T50.992	T50.993	T50.994	T50.995	T50.996
Debrisoquine	T46.5X1	T46.5X2	T46.5X3	T46.5X4	T46.5X5	T46.5X6
Decaborane	T57.8X1	T57.8X2	T57.8X3	T57.8X4	—	—
fumes	T59.891	T59.892	T59.893	T59.894	—	—
Decadron	T38.0X1	T38.0X2	T38.0X3	T38.0X4	T38.0X5	T38.0X6
ENT agent	T49.6X1	T49.6X2	T49.6X3	T49.6X4	T49.6X5	T49.6X6
ophthalmic preparation	T49.5X1	T49.5X2	T49.5X3	T49.5X4	T49.5X5	T49.5X6
topical NEC	T49.0X1	T49.0X2	T49.0X3	T49.0X4	T49.0X5	T49.0X6
Decahydronaphthalene	T52.8X1	T52.8X2	T52.8X3	T52.8X4	—	—
Decalin	T52.8X1	T52.8X2	T52.8X3	T52.8X4	—	—
Decamethonium (bromide)	T48.1X1	T48.1X2	T48.1X3	T48.1X4	T48.1X5	T48.1X6
Decholin	T47.5X1	T47.5X2	T47.5X3	T47.5X4	T47.5X5	T47.5X6
Declomycin	T36.4X1	T36.4X2	T36.4X3	T36.4X4	T36.4X5	T36.4X6
Decongestant, nasal (mucosa)	T48.5X1	T48.5X2	T48.5X3	T48.5X4	T48.5X5	T48.5X6
combination	T48.5X1	T48.5X2	T48.5X3	T48.5X4	T48.5X5	T48.5X6
Deet	T60.8X1	T60.8X2	T60.8X3	T60.8X4	—	—
Deferoxamine	T45.8X1	T45.8X2	T45.8X3	T45.8X4	T45.8X5	T45.8X6
Deflazacort	T38.0X1	T38.0X2	T38.0X3	T38.0X4	T38.0X5	T38.0X6
Deglycyrrhizinized extract of licorice	T48.4X1	T48.4X2	T48.4X3	T48.4X4	T48.4X5	T48.4X6
Dehydrocholic acid	T47.5X1	T47.5X2	T47.5X3	T47.5X4	T47.5X5	T47.5X6
Dehydroemetine	T37.3X1	T37.3X2	T37.3X3	T37.3X4	T37.3X5	T37.3X6
Dekalin	T52.8X1	T52.8X2	T52.8X3	T52.8X4	—	—
Delalutin	T38.5X1	T38.5X2	T38.5X3	T38.5X4	T38.5X5	T38.5X6
Delorazepam	T42.4X1	T42.4X2	T42.4X3	T42.4X4	T42.4X5	T42.4X6
Delphinium	T62.2X1	T62.2X2	T62.2X3	T62.2X4	—	—
Deltamethrin	T60.1X1	T60.1X2	T60.1X3	T60.1X4	—	—
Deltasone	T38.0X1	T38.0X2	T38.0X3	T38.0X4	T38.0X5	T38.0X6
Deltra	T38.0X1	T38.0X2	T38.0X3	T38.0X4	T38.0X5	T38.0X6
Delvinal	T42.3X1	T42.3X2	T42.3X3	T42.3X4	T42.3X5	T42.3X6
Demecarium (bromide)	T49.5X1	T49.5X2	T49.5X3	T49.5X4	T49.5X5	T49.5X6
Demeclocycline	T36.4X1	T36.4X2	T36.4X3	T36.4X4	T36.4X5	T36.4X6
Demecolcine	T45.1X1	T45.1X2	T45.1X3	T45.1X4	T45.1X5	T45.1X6
Demegestone	T38.5X1	T38.5X2	T38.5X3	T38.5X4	T38.5X5	T38.5X6
Demelanizing agents	T49.8X1	T49.8X2	T49.8X3	T49.8X4	T49.8X5	T49.8X6
Demephion -O and -S	T60.0X1	T60.0X2	T60.0X3	T60.0X4	—	—
Demerol	T40.2X1	T40.2X2	T40.2X3	T40.2X4	T40.2X5	T40.2X6
Demethylchlortetracycline	T36.4X1	T36.4X2	T36.4X3	T36.4X4	T36.4X5	T36.4X6
Demethyltetracycline	T36.4X1	T36.4X2	T36.4X3	T36.4X4	T36.4X5	T36.4X6
Demeton -O and -S	T60.0X1	T60.0X2	T60.0X3	T60.0X4	—	—

Substance	Poisoning, Accidental (unintentional)	Poisoning, Intentional Self-harm	Poisoning, Assault	Poisoning, Undetermined	Adverse Effect	Under-dosing
Demulcent (external)	T49.3X1	T49.3X2	T49.3X3	T49.3X4	T49.3X5	T49.3X6
specified NEC	T49.3X1	T49.3X2	T49.3X3	T49.3X4	T49.3X5	T49.3X6
Demulen	T38.4X1	T38.4X2	T38.4X3	T38.4X4	T38.4X5	T38.4X6
Denatured alcohol	T51.0X1	T51.0X2	T51.0X3	T51.0X4	—	—
Dendrid	T49.5X1	T49.5X2	T49.5X3	T49.5X4	T49.5X5	T49.5X6
Dental drug, topical application NEC	T49.7X1	T49.7X2	T49.7X3	T49.7X4	T49.7X5	T49.7X6
Dentifrice	T49.7X1	T49.7X2	T49.7X3	T49.7X4	T49.7X5	T49.7X6
Deodorant spray (feminine hygiene)	T49.8X1	T49.8X2	T49.8X3	T49.8X4	T49.8X5	T49.8X6
Deoxycortone	T50.0X1	T50.0X2	T50.0X3	T50.0X4	T50.0X5	T50.0X6
Deoxyribonuclease (pancreatic)	T45.3X1	T45.3X2	T45.3X3	T45.3X4	T45.3X5	T45.3X6
Depilatory	T49.4X1	T49.4X2	T49.4X3	T49.4X4	T49.4X5	T49.4X6
Deprenalin	T42.8X1	T42.8X2	T42.8X3	T42.8X4	T42.8X5	T42.8X6
Deprenyl	T42.8X1	T42.8X2	T42.8X3	T42.8X4	T42.8X5	T42.8X6
Depressant						
appetite (central)	T50.5X1	T50.5X2	T50.5X3	T50.5X4	T50.5X5	T50.5X6
cardiac	T46.2X1	T46.2X2	T46.2X3	T46.2X4	T46.2X5	T46.2X6
central nervous system (anesthetic) — see also Central nervous system, depressants	T42.71	T42.72	T42.73	T42.74	T42.75	T42.76
general anesthetic	T41.201	T41.202	T41.203	T41.204	T41.205	T41.206
muscle tone	T42.8X1	T42.8X2	T42.8X3	T42.8X4	T42.8X5	T42.8X6
muscle tone, central	T42.8X1	T42.8X2	T42.8X3	T42.8X4	T42.8X5	T42.8X6
psychotherapeutic	T43.501	T43.502	T43.503	T43.504	T43.505	T43.506
Depressant, appetite	T50.5X1	T50.5X2	T50.5X3	T50.5X4	T50.5X5	T50.5X6
Deptropine	T45.0X1	T45.0X2	T45.0X3	T45.0X4	T45.0X5	T45.0X6
Dequalinium (chloride)	T49.0X1	T49.0X2	T49.0X3	T49.0X4	T49.0X5	T49.0X6
Derris root	T60.2X1	T60.2X2	T60.2X3	T60.2X4	—	—
Deserpidine	T46.5X1	T46.5X2	T46.5X3	T46.5X4	T46.5X5	T46.5X6
Desferrioxamine	T45.8X1	T45.8X2	T45.8X3	T45.8X4	T45.8X5	T45.8X6
Desipramine	T43.011	T43.012	T43.013	T43.014	T43.015	T43.016
Deslanoside	T46.0X1	T46.0X2	T46.0X3	T46.0X4	T46.0X5	T46.0X6
Desloughing agent	T49.4X1	T49.4X2	T49.4X3	T49.4X4	T49.4X5	T49.4X6
Desmethylimipramine	T43.011	T43.012	T43.013	T43.014	T43.015	T43.016
Desmopressin	T38.891	T38.892	T38.893	T38.894	T38.895	T38.896
Desocodeine	T40.2X1	T40.2X2	T40.2X3	T40.2X4	T40.2X5	T40.2X6
Desogestrel	T38.5X1	T38.5X2	T38.5X3	T38.5X4	T38.5X5	T38.5X6
Desomorphine	T40.2X1	T40.2X2	T40.2X3	T40.2X4	—	—
Desonide	T49.0X1	T49.0X2	T49.0X3	T49.0X4	T49.0X5	T49.0X6
Desoximetasone	T49.0X1	T49.0X2	T49.0X3	T49.0X4	T49.0X5	T49.0X6
Desoxycorticosteroid	T50.0X1	T50.0X2	T50.0X3	T50.0X4	T50.0X5	T50.0X6
Desoxycortone	T50.0X1	T50.0X2	T50.0X3	T50.0X4	T50.0X5	T50.0X6
Desoxyephedrine	T43.621	T43.622	T43.623	T43.624	T43.625	T43.626
Detaxtran	T46.6X1	T46.6X2	T46.6X3	T46.6X4	T46.6X5	T46.6X6
Detergent	T49.2X1	T49.2X2	T49.2X3	T49.2X4	T49.2X5	T49.2X6
external medication	T49.2X1	T49.2X2	T49.2X3	T49.2X4	T49.2X5	T49.2X6
local	T49.2X1	T49.2X2	T49.2X3	T49.2X4	T49.2X5	T49.2X6
medicinal	T49.2X1	T49.2X2	T49.2X3	T49.2X4	T49.2X5	T49.2X6
nonmedicinal	T55.1X1	T55.1X2	T55.1X3	T55.1X4	—	—
specified NEC	T55.1X1	T55.1X2	T55.1X3	T55.1X4	—	—
Deterrent, alcohol	T50.6X1	T50.6X2	T50.6X3	T50.6X4	T50.6X5	T50.6X6
Detoxifying agent	T50.6X1	T50.6X2	T50.6X3	T50.6X4	T50.6X5	T50.6X6
Detrothyronine	T38.1X1	T38.1X2	T38.1X3	T38.1X4	T38.1X5	T38.1X6
Dettol (external medication)	T49.0X1	T49.0X2	T49.0X3	T49.0X4	T49.0X5	T49.0X6
Dexamethasone	T38.0X1	T38.0X2	T38.0X3	T38.0X4	T38.0X5	T38.0X6
ENT agent	T49.6X1	T49.6X2	T49.6X3	T49.6X4	T49.6X5	T49.6X6
ophthalmic preparation	T49.5X1	T49.5X2	T49.5X3	T49.5X4	T49.5X5	T49.5X6
topical NEC	T49.0X1	T49.0X2	T49.0X3	T49.0X4	T49.0X5	T49.0X6
Dexamfetamine	T43.621	T43.622	T43.623	T43.624	T43.625	T43.626
Dexampfetamine	T43.621	T43.622	T43.623	T43.624	T43.625	T43.626
Dexbrompheniramine	T45.0X1	T45.0X2	T45.0X3	T45.0X4	T45.0X5	T45.0X6
Dexchlorpheniramine	T45.0X1	T45.0X2	T45.0X3	T45.0X4	T45.0X5	T45.0X6
Dexedrine	T43.621	T43.622	T43.623	T43.624	T43.625	T43.626
Dexetimide	T44.3X1	T44.3X2	T44.3X3	T44.3X4	T44.3X5	T44.3X6
Dexfenfluramine	T50.5X1	T50.5X2	T50.5X3	T50.5X4	T50.5X5	T50.5X6
Dexpanthenol	T45.2X1	T45.2X2	T45.2X3	T45.2X4	T45.2X5	T45.2X6
Dextran (40) (70) (150)	T45.8X1	T45.8X2	T45.8X3	T45.8X4	T45.8X5	T45.8X6
Dextriferron	T45.4X1	T45.4X2	T45.4X3	T45.4X4	T45.4X5	T45.4X6
Dextroamphetamine	T43.621	T43.622	T43.623	T43.624	T43.625	T43.626
Dextro calcium pantothenate	T45.2X1	T45.2X2	T45.2X3	T45.2X4	T45.2X5	T45.2X6
Dextromethorphan	T48.3X1	T48.3X2	T48.3X3	T48.3X4	T48.3X5	T48.3X6
Dextromoramide	T40.4X1	T40.4X2	T40.4X3	T40.4X4	—	—
topical	T49.8X1	T49.8X2	T49.8X3	T49.8X4	T49.8X5	T49.8X6
Dextro pantothenyl alcohol	T45.2X1	T45.2X2	T45.2X3	T45.2X4	T45.2X5	T45.2X6
Dextropropoxyphene	T40.4X1	T40.4X2	T40.4X3	T40.4X4	T40.4X5	T40.4X6
Dextrorphan	T40.2X1	T40.2X2	T40.2X3	T40.2X4	T40.2X5	T40.2X6
Dextrose	T50.3X1	T50.3X2	T50.3X3	T50.3X4	T50.3X5	T50.3X6

Additional Character May Be Required — Refer to the Tabular List for Character Selection ▽ Subterms under main terms may continue to next column or page

Substance	Poisoning, Accidental (unintentional)	Poisoning, Intentional Self-harm	Poisoning, Assault	Poisoning, Undetermined	Adverse Effect	Under-dosing
Dextrose — *continued*						
concentrated solution, intravenous	T46.8X1	T46.8X2	T46.8X3	T46.8X4	T46.8X5	T46.8X6
Dextrothyroxin	T38.1X1	T38.1X2	T38.1X3	T38.1X4	T38.1X5	T38.1X6
Dextrothyroxine sodium	T38.1X1	T38.1X2	T38.1X3	T38.1X4	T38.1X5	T38.1X6
DFP	T44.0X1	T44.0X2	T44.0X3	T44.0X4	T44.0X5	T44.0X6
DHE	T37.3X1	T37.3X2	T37.3X3	T37.3X4	T37.3X5	T37.3X6
45	T46.5X1	T46.5X2	T46.5X3	T46.5X4	T46.5X5	T46.5X6
Diabinese	T38.3X1	T38.3X2	T38.3X3	T38.3X4	T38.3X5	T38.3X6
Diacetone alcohol	T52.4X1	T52.4X2	T52.4X3	T52.4X4	—	—
Diacetyl monoxime	T50.991	T50.992	T50.993	T50.994	—	—
Diacetylmorphine	T40.1X1	T40.1X2	T40.1X3	T40.1X4	—	—
Diachylon plaster	T49.4X1	T49.4X2	T49.4X3	T49.4X4	T49.4X5	T49.4X6
Diaethylstilboestrolum	T38.5X1	T38.5X2	T38.5X3	T38.5X4	T38.5X5	T38.5X6
Diagnostic agent NEC	T50.8X1	T50.8X2	T50.8X3	T50.8X4	T50.8X5	T50.8X6
Dial (soap)	T49.2X1	T49.2X2	T49.2X3	T49.2X4	T49.2X5	T49.2X6
sedative	T42.3X1	T42.3X2	T42.3X3	T42.3X4	T42.3X5	T42.3X6
Dialkyl carbonate	T52.91	T52.92	T52.93	T52.94	—	—
Diallylbarbituric acid	T42.3X1	T42.3X2	T42.3X3	T42.3X4	T42.3X5	T42.3X6
Diallymal	T42.3X1	T42.3X2	T42.3X3	T42.3X4	T42.3X5	T42.3X6
Dialysis solution (intraperitoneal)	T50.3X1	T50.3X2	T50.3X3	T50.3X4	T50.3X5	T50.3X6
Diaminodiphenylsulfone	T37.1X1	T37.1X2	T37.1X3	T37.1X4	T37.1X5	T37.1X6
Diamorphine	T40.1X1	T40.1X2	T40.1X3	T40.1X4	—	—
Diamox	T50.2X1	T50.2X2	T50.2X3	T50.2X4	T50.2X5	T50.2X6
Diamthazole	T49.0X1	T49.0X2	T49.0X3	T49.0X4	T49.0X5	T49.0X6
Dianthone	T47.2X1	T47.2X2	T47.2X3	T47.2X4	T47.2X5	T47.2X6
Diaphenylsulfone	T37.0X1	T37.0X2	T37.0X3	T37.0X4	T37.0X5	T37.0X6
Diasone (sodium)	T37.1X1	T37.1X2	T37.1X3	T37.1X4	T37.1X5	T37.1X6
Diastase	T47.5X1	T47.5X2	T47.5X3	T47.5X4	T47.5X5	T47.5X6
Diatrizoate	T50.8X1	T50.8X2	T50.8X3	T50.8X4	T50.8X5	T50.8X6
Diazepam	T42.4X1	T42.4X2	T42.4X3	T42.4X4	T42.4X5	T42.4X6
Diazinon	T60.0X1	T60.0X2	T60.0X3	T60.0X4	—	—
Diazomethane (gas)	T59.891	T59.892	T59.893	T59.894	—	—
Diazoxide	T46.5X1	T46.5X2	T46.5X3	T46.5X4	T46.5X5	T46.5X6
Dibekacin	T36.5X1	T36.5X2	T36.5X3	T36.5X4	T36.5X5	T36.5X6
Dibenamine	T44.6X1	T44.6X2	T44.6X3	T44.6X4	T44.6X5	T44.6X6
Dibenzepin	T43.011	T43.012	T43.013	T43.014	T43.015	T43.016
Dibenzheptropine	T45.0X1	T45.0X2	T45.0X3	T45.0X4	T45.0X5	T45.0X6
Dibenzyline	T44.6X1	T44.6X2	T44.6X3	T44.6X4	T44.6X5	T44.6X6
Diborane (gas)	T59.891	T59.892	T59.893	T59.894	—	—
Dibromochloropropane	T60.8X1	T60.8X2	T60.8X3	T60.8X4	—	—
Dibromodulcitol	T45.1X1	T45.1X2	T45.1X3	T45.1X4	T45.1X5	T45.1X6
Dibromoethane	T53.6X1	T53.6X2	T53.6X3	T53.6X4	—	—
Dibromomannitol	T45.1X1	T45.1X2	T45.1X3	T45.1X4	T45.1X5	T45.1X6
Dibromopropamidine isethionate	T49.0X1	T49.0X2	T49.0X3	T49.0X4	T49.0X5	T49.0X6
Dibrompropamidine	T49.0X1	T49.0X2	T49.0X3	T49.0X4	T49.0X5	T49.0X6
Dibucaine	T41.3X1	T41.3X2	T41.3X3	T41.3X4	T41.3X5	T41.3X6
topical (surface)	T41.3X1	T41.3X2	T41.3X3	T41.3X4	T41.3X5	T41.3X6
Dibunate sodium	T48.3X1	T48.3X2	T48.3X3	T48.3X4	T48.3X5	T48.3X6
Dibutoline sulfate	T44.3X1	T44.3X2	T44.3X3	T44.3X4	T44.3X5	T44.3X6
Dicamba	T60.3X1	T60.3X2	T60.3X3	T60.3X4	—	—
Dicapthon	T60.0X1	T60.0X2	T60.0X3	T60.0X4	—	—
Dichlobenil	T60.3X1	T60.3X2	T60.3X3	T60.3X4	—	—
Dichlone	T60.3X1	T60.3X2	T60.3X3	T60.3X4	—	—
Dichloralphenozone	T42.6X1	T42.6X2	T42.6X3	T42.6X4	T42.6X5	T42.6X6
Dichlorbenzidine	T65.3X1	T65.3X2	T65.3X3	T65.3X4	—	—
Dichlorhydrin	T52.8X1	T52.8X2	T52.8X3	T52.8X4	—	—
Dichlorhydroxyquinoline	T37.8X1	T37.8X2	T37.8X3	T37.8X4	T37.8X5	T37.8X6
Dichlorobenzene	T53.7X1	T53.7X2	T53.7X3	T53.7X4	—	—
Dichlorobenzyl alcohol	T49.6X1	T49.6X2	T49.6X3	T49.6X4	T49.6X5	T49.6X6
Dichlorodifluoromethane	T53.5X1	T53.5X2	T53.5X3	T53.5X4	—	—
Dichloroethane	T52.8X1	T52.8X2	T52.8X3	T52.8X4	—	—
Dichloroethylene	T53.6X1	T53.6X2	T53.6X3	T53.6X4	—	—
Dichloroethyl sulfide, not in war	T59.891	T59.892	T59.893	T59.894		
Dichloroformoxine, not in war	T59.891	T59.892	T59.893	T59.894		
Dichlorohydrin, alpha-dichlorohydrin	T52.8X1	T52.8X2	T52.8X3	T52.8X4	—	
Dichloromethane (solvent)	T53.4X1	T53.4X2	T53.4X3	T53.4X4	—	—
vapor	T53.4X1	T53.4X2	T53.4X3	T53.4X4	—	—
Dichloronaphthoquinone	T60.3X1	T60.3X2	T60.3X3	T60.3X4	—	—
Dichlorophen	T37.4X1	T37.4X2	T37.4X3	T37.4X4	T37.4X5	T37.4X6
Dichloropropene	T60.3X1	T60.3X2	T60.3X3	T60.3X4	—	—
Dichloropropionic acid	T60.3X1	T60.3X2	T60.3X3	T60.3X4	—	—
Dichlorphenamide	T50.2X1	T50.2X2	T50.2X3	T50.2X4	T50.2X5	T50.2X6
Dichlorvos	T60.0X1	T60.0X2	T60.0X3	T60.0X4	—	—
Diclofenac	T39.391	T39.392	T39.393	T39.394	T39.395	T39.396
Diclofenamide	T50.2X1	T50.2X2	T50.2X3	T50.2X4	T50.2X5	T50.2X6
Diclofensine	T43.291	T43.292	T43.293	T43.294	T43.295	T43.296
Diclonixine	T39.8X1	T39.8X2	T39.8X3	T39.8X4	T39.8X5	T39.8X6

Substance	Poisoning, Accidental (unintentional)	Poisoning, Intentional Self-harm	Poisoning, Assault	Poisoning, Undetermined	Adverse Effect	Under-dosing
Dicloxacillin	T36.0X1	T36.0X2	T36.0X3	T36.0X4	T36.0X5	T36.0X6
Dicophane	T49.0X1	T49.0X2	T49.0X3	T49.0X4	T49.0X5	T49.0X6
Dicoumarol, dicoumarin, dicumarol	T45.511	T45.512	T45.513	T45.514	T45.515	T45.516
Dicrotophos	T60.0X1	T60.0X2	T60.0X3	T60.0X4	—	—
Dicyanogen (gas)	T65.0X1	T65.0X2	T65.0X3	T65.0X4	—	—
Dicyclomine	T44.3X1	T44.3X2	T44.3X3	T44.3X4	T44.3X5	T44.3X6
Dicycloverine	T44.3X1	T44.3X2	T44.3X3	T44.3X4	T44.3X5	T44.3X6
Dideoxycytidine	T37.5X1	T37.5X2	T37.5X3	T37.5X4	T37.5X5	T37.5X6
Dideoxyinosine	T37.5X1	T37.5X2	T37.5X3	T37.5X4	T37.5X5	T37.5X6
Dieldrin (vapor)	T60.1X1	T60.1X2	T60.1X3	T60.1X4	—	—
Diemal	T42.3X1	T42.3X2	T42.3X3	T42.3X4	T42.3X5	T42.3X6
Dienestrol	T38.5X1	T38.5X2	T38.5X3	T38.5X4	T38.5X5	T38.5X6
Dienoestrol	T38.5X1	T38.5X2	T38.5X3	T38.5X4	T38.5X5	T38.5X6
Dietetic drug NEC	T50.901	T50.902	T50.903	T50.904	T50.905	T50.906
Diethazine	T42.8X1	T42.8X2	T42.8X3	T42.8X4	T42.8X5	T42.8X6
Diethyl						
barbituric acid	T42.3X1	T42.3X2	T42.3X3	T42.3X4	T42.3X5	T42.3X6
carbamazine	T37.4X1	T37.4X2	T37.4X3	T37.4X4	T37.4X5	T37.4X6
carbinol	T51.3X1	T51.3X2	T51.3X3	T51.3X4	—	—
carbonate	T52.8X1	T52.8X2	T52.8X3	T52.8X4	—	—
ether (vapor) — *see also* ether	T41.0X1	T41.0X2	T41.0X3	T41.0X4	T41.0X5	T41.0X6
oxide	T52.8X1	T52.8X2	T52.8X3	T52.8X4	—	—
propion	T50.5X1	T50.5X2	T50.5X3	T50.5X4	T50.5X5	T50.5X6
stilbestrol	T38.5X1	T38.5X2	T38.5X3	T38.5X4	T38.5X5	T38.5X6
toluamide (nonmedicinal)	T60.8X1	T60.8X2	T60.8X3	T60.8X4	—	—
medicinal	T49.3X1	T49.3X2	T49.3X3	T49.3X4	T49.3X5	T49.3X6
Diethylcarbamazine	T37.4X1	T37.4X2	T37.4X3	T37.4X4	T37.4X5	T37.4X6
Diethylene						
dioxide	T52.8X1	T52.8X2	T52.8X3	T52.8X4	—	—
glycol (monoacetate) (monobutyl ether) (monoethyl ether)	T52.3X1	T52.3X2	T52.3X3	T52.3X4	—	—
Diethylhexylphthalate	T65.891	T65.892	T65.893	T65.894	—	—
Diethylpropion	T50.5X1	T50.5X2	T50.5X3	T50.5X4	T50.5X5	T50.5X6
Diethylstilbestrol	T38.5X1	T38.5X2	T38.5X3	T38.5X4	T38.5X5	T38.5X6
Diethylstilboestrol	T38.5X1	T38.5X2	T38.5X3	T38.5X4	T38.5X5	T38.5X6
Diethylsulfone-diethylmethane	T42.6X1	T42.6X2	T42.6X3	T42.6X4	T42.6X5	T42.6X6
Diethyltoluamide	T49.0X1	T49.0X2	T49.0X3	T49.0X4	T49.0X5	T49.0X6
Diethyltryptamine (DET)	T40.991	T40.992	T40.993	T40.994	—	—
Difebarbamate	T42.3X1	T42.3X2	T42.3X3	T42.3X4	T42.3X5	T42.3X6
Difencloxazine	T40.2X1	T40.2X2	T40.2X3	T40.2X4	T40.2X5	T40.2X6
Difenidol	T45.0X1	T45.0X2	T45.0X3	T45.0X4	T45.0X5	T45.0X6
Difenoxin	T47.6X1	T47.6X2	T47.6X3	T47.6X4	T47.6X5	T47.6X6
Difetarsone	T37.3X1	T37.3X2	T37.3X3	T37.3X4	T37.3X5	T37.3X6
Diffusin	T45.3X1	T45.3X2	T45.3X3	T45.3X4	T45.3X5	T45.3X6
Diflorasone	T49.0X1	T49.0X2	T49.0X3	T49.0X4	T49.0X5	T49.0X6
Diflos	T44.0X1	T44.0X2	T44.0X3	T44.0X4	T44.0X5	T44.0X6
Diflubenzuron	T60.1X1	T60.1X2	T60.1X3	T60.1X4	—	—
Diflucortolone	T49.0X1	T49.0X2	T49.0X3	T49.0X4	T49.0X5	T49.0X6
Diflunisal	T39.091	T39.092	T39.093	T39.094	T39.095	T39.096
Difluoromethyldopa	T42.8X1	T42.8X2	T42.8X3	T42.8X4	T42.8X5	T42.8X6
Difluorophate	T44.0X1	T44.0X2	T44.0X3	T44.0X4	T44.0X5	T44.0X6
Digestant NEC	T47.5X1	T47.5X2	T47.5X3	T47.5X4	T47.5X5	T47.5X6
Digitalin (e)	T46.0X1	T46.0X2	T46.0X3	T46.0X4	T46.0X5	T46.0X6
Digitalis (leaf)(glycoside)	T46.0X1	T46.0X2	T46.0X3	T46.0X4	T46.0X5	T46.0X6
lanata	T46.0X1	T46.0X2	T46.0X3	T46.0X4	T46.0X5	T46.0X6
purpurea	T46.0X1	T46.0X2	T46.0X3	T46.0X4	T46.0X5	T46.0X6
Digitoxin	T46.0X1	T46.0X2	T46.0X3	T46.0X4	T46.0X5	T46.0X6
Digitoxose	T46.0X1	T46.0X2	T46.0X3	T46.0X4	T46.0X5	T46.0X6
Digoxin	T46.0X1	T46.0X2	T46.0X3	T46.0X4	T46.0X5	T46.0X6
Digoxine	T46.0X1	T46.0X2	T46.0X3	T46.0X4	T46.0X5	T46.0X6
Dihydralazine	T46.5X1	T46.5X2	T46.5X3	T46.5X4	T46.5X5	T46.5X6
Dihydrazine	T46.5X1	T46.5X2	T46.5X3	T46.5X4	T46.5X5	T46.5X6
Dihydrocodeine	T40.2X1	T40.2X2	T40.2X3	T40.2X4	T40.2X5	T40.2X6
Dihydrocodeinone	T40.2X1	T40.2X2	T40.2X3	T40.2X4	T40.2X5	T40.2X6
Dihydroergocornine	T46.7X1	T46.7X2	T46.7X3	T46.7X4	T46.7X5	T46.7X6
Dihydroergocristine (mesilate)	T46.7X1	T46.7X2	T46.7X3	T46.7X4	T46.7X5	T46.7X6
Dihydroergokryptine	T46.7X1	T46.7X2	T46.7X3	T46.7X4	T46.7X5	T46.7X6
Dihydroergotamine	T46.5X1	T46.5X2	T46.5X3	T46.5X4	T46.5X5	T46.5X6
Dihydroergotoxine	T46.7X1	T46.7X2	T46.7X3	T46.7X4	T46.7X5	T46.7X6
mesilate	T46.7X1	T46.7X2	T46.7X3	T46.7X4	T46.7X5	T46.7X6
Dihydrohydroxycodeinone	T40.2X1	T40.2X2	T40.2X3	T40.2X4	T40.2X5	T40.2X6
Dihydrohydroxymorphinone	T40.2X1	T40.2X2	T40.2X3	T40.2X4	T40.2X5	T40.2X6
Dihydroisocodeine	T40.2X1	T40.2X2	T40.2X3	T40.2X4	T40.2X5	T40.2X6
Dihydromorphine	T40.2X1	T40.2X2	T40.2X3	T40.2X4	—	—
Dihydromorphinone	T40.2X1	T40.2X2	T40.2X3	T40.2X4	T40.2X5	T40.2X6
Dihydrostreptomycin	T36.5X1	T36.5X2	T36.5X3	T36.5X4	T36.5X5	T36.5X6
Dihydrotachysterol	T45.2X1	T45.2X2	T45.2X3	T45.2X4	T45.2X5	T45.2X6
Dihydroxyaluminum aminoacetate	T47.1X1	T47.1X2	T47.1X3	T47.1X4	T47.1X5	T47.1X6

Subterms under main terms may continue to next column or page　　　Additional Character May Be Required — Refer to the Tabular List for Character Selection　　　365

Dextrose — Dihydroxyaluminum aminoacetate

Table of Drugs and Chemicals

Dihydroxyaluminum sodium carbonate — DNOC

Substance	Poisoning, Accidental (unintentional)	Poisoning, Intentional Self-harm	Poisoning, Assault	Poisoning, Undetermined	Adverse Effect	Under-dosing
Dihydroxyaluminum sodium carbonate	T47.1X1	T47.1X2	T47.1X3	T47.1X4	T47.1X5	T47.1X6
Dihydroxyanthraquinone	T47.2X1	T47.2X2	T47.2X3	T47.2X4	T47.2X5	T47.2X6
Dihydroxycodeinone	T40.2X1	T40.2X2	T40.2X3	T40.2X4	T40.2X5	T40.2X6
Dihydroxypropyl theophylline	T50.2X1	T50.2X2	T50.2X3	T50.2X4	T50.2X5	T50.2X6
Diiodohydroxyquin	T37.8X1	T37.8X2	T37.8X3	T37.8X4	T37.8X5	T37.8X6
topical	T49.0X1	T49.0X2	T49.0X3	T49.0X4	T49.0X5	T49.0X6
Diiodohydroxyquinoline	T37.8X1	T37.8X2	T37.8X3	T37.8X4	T37.8X5	T37.8X6
Diiodotyrosine	T38.2X1	T38.2X2	T38.2X3	T38.2X4	T38.2X5	T38.2X6
Diisopromine	T44.3X1	T44.3X2	T44.3X3	T44.3X4	T44.3X5	T44.3X6
Diisopropylamine	T46.3X1	T46.3X2	T46.3X3	T46.3X4	T46.3X5	T46.3X6
Diisopropylfluorophosphonate	T44.0X1	T44.0X2	T44.0X3	T44.0X4	T44.0X5	T44.0X6
Dilantin	T42.0X1	T42.0X2	T42.0X3	T42.0X4	T42.0X5	T42.0X6
Dilaudid	T40.2X1	T40.2X2	T40.2X3	T40.2X4	T40.2X5	T40.2X6
Dilazep	T46.3X1	T46.3X2	T46.3X3	T46.3X4	T46.3X5	T46.3X6
Dill	T47.5X1	T47.5X2	T47.5X3	T47.5X4	T47.5X5	T47.5X6
Diloxanide	T37.3X1	T37.3X2	T37.3X3	T37.3X4	T37.3X5	T37.3X6
Diltiazem	T46.1X1	T46.1X2	T46.1X3	T46.1X4	T46.1X5	T46.1X6
Dimazole	T49.0X1	T49.0X2	T49.0X3	T49.0X4	T49.0X5	T49.0X6
Dimefline	T50.7X1	T50.7X2	T50.7X3	T50.7X4	T50.7X5	T50.7X6
Dimefox	T60.0X1	T60.0X2	T60.0X3	T60.0X4	—	—
Dimemorfan	T48.3X1	T48.3X2	T48.3X3	T48.3X4	T48.3X5	T48.3X6
Dimenhydrinate	T45.0X1	T45.0X2	T45.0X3	T45.0X4	T45.0X5	T45.0X6
Dimercaprol (British anti-lewisite)	T45.8X1	T45.8X2	T45.8X3	T45.8X4	T45.8X5	T45.8X6
Dimercaptopropanol	T45.8X1	T45.8X2	T45.8X3	T45.8X4	T45.8X5	T45.8X6
Dimestrol	T38.5X1	T38.5X2	T38.5X3	T38.5X4	T38.5X5	T38.5X6
Dimetane	T45.0X1	T45.0X2	T45.0X3	T45.0X4	T45.0X5	T45.0X6
Dimethicone	T47.1X1	T47.1X2	T47.1X3	T47.1X4	T47.1X5	T47.1X6
Dimethindene	T45.0X1	T45.0X2	T45.0X3	T45.0X4	T45.0X5	T45.0X6
Dimethisoquin	T49.1X1	T49.1X2	T49.1X3	T49.1X4	T49.1X5	T49.1X6
Dimethisterone	T38.5X1	T38.5X2	T38.5X3	T38.5X4	T38.5X5	T38.5X6
Dimethoate	T60.0X1	T60.0X2	T60.0X3	T60.0X4	—	—
Dimethocaine	T41.3X1	T41.3X2	T41.3X3	T41.3X4	T41.3X5	T41.3X6
Dimethoxanate	T48.3X1	T48.3X2	T48.3X3	T48.3X4	T48.3X5	T48.3X6
Dimethyl						
arsine, arsinic acid	T57.0X1	T57.0X2	T57.0X3	T57.0X4	—	—
carbinol	T51.2X1	T51.2X2	T51.2X3	T51.2X4	—	—
carbonate	T52.8X1	T52.8X2	T52.8X3	T52.8X4	—	—
diguanide	T38.3X1	T38.3X2	T38.3X3	T38.3X4	T38.3X5	T38.3X6
ketone	T52.4X1	T52.4X2	T52.4X3	T52.4X4	—	—
vapor	T52.4X1	T52.4X2	T52.4X3	T52.4X4	—	—
meperidine	T40.2X1	T40.2X2	T40.2X3	T40.2X4	T40.2X5	T40.2X6
parathion	T60.0X1	T60.0X2	T60.0X3	T60.0X4	—	—
phthlate	T49.3X1	T49.3X2	T49.3X3	T49.3X4	T49.3X5	T49.3X6
polysiloxane	T47.8X1	T47.8X2	T47.8X3	T47.8X4	T47.8X5	T47.8X6
sulfate (fumes)	T59.891	T59.892	T59.893	T59.894	—	—
liquid	T65.891	T65.892	T65.893	T65.894	—	—
sulfoxide (nonmedicinal)	T52.8X1	T52.8X2	T52.8X3	T52.8X4	—	—
medicinal	T49.4X1	T49.4X2	T49.4X3	T49.4X4	T49.4X5	T49.4X6
tryptamine	T40.991	T40.992	T40.993	T40.994	—	—
tubocurarine	T48.1X1	T48.1X2	T48.1X3	T48.1X4	T48.1X5	T48.1X6
Dimethylamine sulfate	T49.4X1	T49.4X2	T49.4X3	T49.4X4	T49.4X5	T49.4X6
Dimethylformamide	T52.8X1	T52.8X2	T52.8X3	T52.8X4	—	—
Dimethyltubocurarinium chloride	T48.1X1	T48.1X2	T48.1X3	T48.1X4	T48.1X5	T48.1X6
Dimeticone	T47.1X1	T47.1X2	T47.1X3	T47.1X4	T47.1X5	T47.1X6
Dimetilan	T60.0X1	T60.0X2	T60.0X3	T60.0X4	—	—
Dimetindene	T45.0X1	T45.0X2	T45.0X3	T45.0X4	T45.0X5	T45.0X6
Dimetotiazine	T43.3X1	T43.3X2	T43.3X3	T43.3X4	T43.3X5	T43.3X6
Dimorpholamine	T50.7X1	T50.7X2	T50.7X3	T50.7X4	T50.7X5	T50.7X6
Dimoxyline	T46.3X1	T46.3X2	T46.3X3	T46.3X4	T46.3X5	T46.3X6
Dinitrobenzene	T65.3X1	T65.3X2	T65.3X3	T65.3X4	—	—
vapor	T59.891	T59.892	T59.893	T59.894	—	—
Dinitrobenzol	T65.3X1	T65.3X2	T65.3X3	T65.3X4	—	—
vapor	T59.891	T59.892	T59.893	T59.894	—	—
Dinitrobutylphenol	T65.3X1	T65.3X2	T65.3X3	T65.3X4	—	—
Dinitro (-ortho-)cresol (pesticide) (spray)	T65.3X1	T65.3X2	T65.3X3	T65.3X4	—	—
Dinitrocyclohexylphenol	T65.3X1	T65.3X2	T65.3X3	T65.3X4	—	—
Dinitrophenol	T65.3X1	T65.3X2	T65.3X3	T65.3X4	—	—
Dinoprost	T48.0X1	T48.0X2	T48.0X3	T48.0X4	T48.0X5	T48.0X6
Dinoprostone	T48.0X1	T48.0X2	T48.0X3	T48.0X4	T48.0X5	T48.0X6
Dinoseb	T60.3X1	T60.3X2	T60.3X3	T60.3X4	—	—
Dioctyl sulfosuccinate (calcium) (sodium)	T47.4X1	T47.4X2	T47.4X3	T47.4X4	T47.4X5	T47.4X6
Diodone	T50.8X1	T50.8X2	T50.8X3	T50.8X4	T50.8X5	T50.8X6
Diodoquin	T37.8X1	T37.8X2	T37.8X3	T37.8X4	T37.8X5	T37.8X6
Dionin	T40.2X1	T40.2X2	T40.2X3	T40.2X4	T40.2X5	T40.2X6
Diosmin	T46.991	T46.992	T46.993	T46.994	T46.995	T46.996
Dioxane	T52.8X1	T52.8X2	T52.8X3	T52.8X4	—	—
Dioxathion	T60.0X1	T60.0X2	T60.0X3	T60.0X4	—	—

Substance	Poisoning, Accidental (unintentional)	Poisoning, Intentional Self-harm	Poisoning, Assault	Poisoning, Undetermined	Adverse Effect	Under-dosing
Dioxin	T53.7X1	T53.7X2	T53.7X3	T53.7X4	—	—
Dioxopromethazine	T43.3X1	T43.3X2	T43.3X3	T43.3X4	T43.3X5	T43.3X6
Dioxyline	T46.3X1	T46.3X2	T46.3X3	T46.3X4	T46.3X5	T46.3X6
Dipentene	T52.8X1	T52.8X2	T52.8X3	T52.8X4	—	—
Diperodon	T41.3X1	T41.3X2	T41.3X3	T41.3X4	T41.3X5	T41.3X6
Diphacinone	T60.4X1	T60.4X2	T60.4X3	T60.4X4	—	—
Diphemanil	T44.3X1	T44.3X2	T44.3X3	T44.3X4	T44.3X5	T44.3X6
metilsulfate	T44.3X1	T44.3X2	T44.3X3	T44.3X4	T44.3X5	T44.3X6
Diphenadione	T45.511	T45.512	T45.513	T45.514	T45.515	T45.516
rodenticide	T60.4X1	T60.4X2	T60.4X3	T60.4X4	—	—
Diphenhydramine	T45.0X1	T45.0X2	T45.0X3	T45.0X4	T45.0X5	T45.0X6
Diphenidol	T45.0X1	T45.0X2	T45.0X3	T45.0X4	T45.0X5	T45.0X6
Diphenoxylate	T47.6X1	T47.6X2	T47.6X3	T47.6X4	T47.6X5	T47.6X6
Diphenylamine	T65.3X1	T65.3X2	T65.3X3	T65.3X4	—	—
Diphenylbutazone	T39.2X1	T39.2X2	T39.2X3	T39.2X4	T39.2X5	T39.2X6
Diphenylchloroarsine, not in war	T57.0X1	T57.0X2	T57.0X3	T57.0X4	—	—
Diphenylhydantoin	T42.0X1	T42.0X2	T42.0X3	T42.0X4	T42.0X5	T42.0X6
Diphenylmethane dye	T52.1X1	T52.1X2	T52.1X3	T52.1X4	—	—
Diphenylpyraline	T45.0X1	T45.0X2	T45.0X3	T45.0X4	T45.0X5	T45.0X6
Diphtheria						
antitoxin	T50.Z11	T50.Z12	T50.Z13	T50.Z14	T50.Z15	T50.Z16
toxoid	T50.A91	T50.A92	T50.A93	T50.A94	T50.A95	T50.A96
with tetanus toxoid	T50.A21	T50.A22	T50.A23	T50.A24	T50.A25	T50.A26
with pertussis component	T50.A11	T50.A12	T50.A13	T50.A14	T50.A15	T50.A16
vaccine	T50.A91	T50.A92	T50.A93	T50.A94	T50.A95	T50.A96
combination						
without pertussis	T50.A21	T50.A22	T50.A23	T50.A24	T50.A25	T50.A26
including pertussis	T50.A11	T50.A12	T50.A13	T50.A14	T50.A15	T50.A16
Diphylline	T50.2X1	T50.2X2	T50.2X3	T50.2X4	T50.2X5	T50.2X6
Dipipanone	T40.4X1	T40.4X2	T40.4X3	T40.4X4	—	—
Dipivefrine	T49.5X1	T49.5X2	T49.5X3	T49.5X4	T49.5X5	T49.5X6
Diplovax	T50.B91	T50.B92	T50.B93	T50.B94	T50.B95	T50.B96
Diprophylline	T50.2X1	T50.2X2	T50.2X3	T50.2X4	T50.2X5	T50.2X6
Dipropyline	T48.291	T48.292	T48.293	T48.294	T48.295	T48.296
Dipyridamole	T46.3X1	T46.3X2	T46.3X3	T46.3X4	T46.3X5	T46.3X6
Dipyrone	T39.2X1	T39.2X2	T39.2X3	T39.2X4	T39.2X5	T39.2X6
Diquat (dibromide)	T60.3X1	T60.3X2	T60.3X3	T60.3X4	—	—
Disinfectant	T65.891	T65.892	T65.893	T65.894	—	—
alkaline	T54.3X1	T54.3X2	T54.3X3	T54.3X4	—	—
aromatic	T54.1X1	T54.1X2	T54.1X3	T54.1X4	—	—
intestinal	T37.8X1	T37.8X2	T37.8X3	T37.8X4	T37.8X5	T37.8X6
Disipal	T42.8X1	T42.8X2	T42.8X3	T42.8X4	T42.8X5	T42.8X6
Disodium edetate	T50.6X1	T50.6X2	T50.6X3	T50.6X4	T50.6X5	T50.6X6
Disoprofol	T41.291	T41.292	T41.293	T41.294	T41.295	T41.296
Disopyramide	T46.2X1	T46.2X2	T46.2X3	T46.2X4	T46.2X5	T46.2X6
Distigmine (bromide)	T44.0X1	T44.0X2	T44.0X3	T44.0X4	T44.0X5	T44.0X6
Disulfamide	T50.2X1	T50.2X2	T50.2X3	T50.2X4	T50.2X5	T50.2X6
Disulfanilamide	T37.0X1	T37.0X2	T37.0X3	T37.0X4	T37.0X5	T37.0X6
Disulfiram	T50.6X1	T50.6X2	T50.6X3	T50.6X4	T50.6X5	T50.6X6
Disulfoton	T60.0X1	T60.0X2	T60.0X3	T60.0X4	—	—
Dithiazanine iodide	T37.4X1	T37.4X2	T37.4X3	T37.4X4	T37.4X5	T37.4X6
Dithiocarbamate	T60.0X1	T60.0X2	T60.0X3	T60.0X4	—	—
Dithranol	T49.4X1	T49.4X2	T49.4X3	T49.4X4	T49.4X5	T49.4X6
Diucardin	T50.2X1	T50.2X2	T50.2X3	T50.2X4	T50.2X5	T50.2X6
Diupres	T50.2X1	T50.2X2	T50.2X3	T50.2X4	T50.2X5	T50.2X6
Diuretic NEC	T50.2X1	T50.2X2	T50.2X3	T50.2X4	T50.2X5	T50.2X6
benzothiadiazine	T50.2X1	T50.2X2	T50.2X3	T50.2X4	T50.2X5	T50.2X6
carbonic acid anhydrase inhibitors	T50.2X1	T50.2X2	T50.2X3	T50.2X4	T50.2X5	T50.2X6
furfuryl NEC	T50.2X1	T50.2X2	T50.2X3	T50.2X4	T50.2X5	T50.2X6
loop (high-ceiling)	T50.1X1	T50.1X2	T50.1X3	T50.1X4	T50.1X5	T50.1X6
mercurial NEC	T50.2X1	T50.2X2	T50.2X3	T50.2X4	T50.2X5	T50.2X6
osmotic	T50.2X1	T50.2X2	T50.2X3	T50.2X4	T50.2X5	T50.2X6
purine NEC	T50.2X1	T50.2X2	T50.2X3	T50.2X4	T50.2X5	T50.2X6
saluretic NEC	T50.2X1	T50.2X2	T50.2X3	T50.2X4	T50.2X5	T50.2X6
sulfonamide	T50.2X1	T50.2X2	T50.2X3	T50.2X4	T50.2X5	T50.2X6
thiazide NEC	T50.2X1	T50.2X2	T50.2X3	T50.2X4	T50.2X5	T50.2X6
xanthine	T50.2X1	T50.2X2	T50.2X3	T50.2X4	T50.2X5	T50.2X6
Diurgin	T50.2X1	T50.2X2	T50.2X3	T50.2X4	T50.2X5	T50.2X6
Diuril	T50.2X1	T50.2X2	T50.2X3	T50.2X4	T50.2X5	T50.2X6
Diuron	T60.3X1	T60.3X2	T60.3X3	T60.3X4	—	—
Divalproex	T42.6X1	T42.6X2	T42.6X3	T42.6X4	T42.6X5	T42.6X6
Divinyl ether	T41.0X1	T41.0X2	T41.0X3	T41.0X4	T41.0X5	T41.0X6
Dixanthogen	T49.0X1	T49.0X2	T49.0X3	T49.0X4	T49.0X5	T49.0X6
Dixyrazine	T43.3X1	T43.3X2	T43.3X3	T43.3X4	T43.3X5	T43.3X6
D-lysergic acid diethylamide	T40.8X1	T40.8X2	T40.8X3	T40.8X4		
DMCT	T36.4X1	T36.4X2	T36.4X3	T36.4X4	T36.4X5	T36.4X6
DMSO — see Dimethyl sulfoxide						
DNBP	T60.3X1	T60.3X2	T60.3X3	T60.3X4	—	—
DNOC	T65.3X1	T65.3X2	T65.3X3	T65.3X4	—	—

Additional Character May Be Required — Refer to the Tabular List for Character Selection ▽ **Subterms under main terms may continue to next column or page**

Substance	Poisoning, Accidental (unintentional)	Poisoning, Intentional Self-harm	Poisoning, Assault	Poisoning, Undetermined	Adverse Effect	Under-dosing
Dobutamine	T44.5X1	T44.5X2	T44.5X3	T44.5X4	T44.5X5	T44.5X6
DOCA	T38.0X1	T38.0X2	T38.0X3	T38.0X4	T38.0X5	T38.0X6
Docusate sodium	T47.4X1	T47.4X2	T47.4X3	T47.4X4	T47.4X5	T47.4X6
Dodicin	T49.0X1	T49.0X2	T49.0X3	T49.0X4	T49.0X5	T49.0X6
Dofamium chloride	T49.0X1	T49.0X2	T49.0X3	T49.0X4	T49.0X5	T49.0X6
Dolophine	T40.3X1	T40.3X2	T40.3X3	T40.3X4	T40.3X5	T40.3X6
Doloxene	T39.8X1	T39.8X2	T39.8X3	T39.8X4	T39.8X5	T39.8X6
Domestic gas (after combustion) — see Gas, utility						
prior to combustion	T59.891	T59.892	T59.893	T59.894	—	—
Domiodol	T48.4X1	T48.4X2	T48.4X3	T48.4X4	T48.4X5	T48.4X6
Domiphen (bromide)	T49.0X1	T49.0X2	T49.0X3	T49.0X4	T49.0X5	T49.0X6
Domperidone	T45.0X1	T45.0X2	T45.0X3	T45.0X4	T45.0X5	T45.0X6
Dopa	T42.8X1	T42.8X2	T42.8X3	T42.8X4	T42.8X5	T42.8X6
Dopamine	T44.991	T44.992	T44.993	T44.994	T44.995	T44.996
Doriden	T42.6X1	T42.6X2	T42.6X3	T42.6X4	T42.6X5	T42.6X6
Dormiral	T42.3X1	T42.3X2	T42.3X3	T42.3X4	T42.3X5	T42.3X6
Dormison	T42.6X1	T42.6X2	T42.6X3	T42.6X4	T42.6X5	T42.6X6
Dornase	T48.4X1	T48.4X2	T48.4X3	T48.4X4	T48.4X5	T48.4X6
Dorsacaine	T41.3X1	T41.3X2	T41.3X3	T41.3X4	T41.3X5	T41.3X6
Dosulepin	T43.011	T43.012	T43.013	T43.014	T43.015	T43.016
Dothiepin	T43.011	T43.012	T43.013	T43.014	T43.015	T43.016
Doxantrazole	T48.6X1	T48.6X2	T48.6X3	T48.6X4	T48.6X5	T48.6X6
Doxapram	T50.7X1	T50.7X2	T50.7X3	T50.7X4	T50.7X5	T50.7X6
Doxazosin	T44.6X1	T44.6X2	T44.6X3	T44.6X4	T44.6X5	T44.6X6
Doxepin	T43.011	T43.012	T43.013	T43.014	T43.015	T43.016
Doxifluridine	T45.1X1	T45.1X2	T45.1X3	T45.1X4	T45.1X5	T45.1X6
Doxorubicin	T45.1X1	T45.1X2	T45.1X3	T45.1X4	T45.1X5	T45.1X6
Doxycycline	T36.4X1	T36.4X2	T36.4X3	T36.4X4	T36.4X5	T36.4X6
Doxylamine	T45.0X1	T45.0X2	T45.0X3	T45.0X4	T45.0X5	T45.0X6
Dramamine	T45.0X1	T45.0X2	T45.0X3	T45.0X4	T45.0X5	T45.0X6
Drano (drain cleaner)	T54.3X1	T54.3X2	T54.3X3	T54.3X4	—	—
Dressing, live pulp	T49.7X1	T49.7X2	T49.7X3	T49.7X4	T49.7X5	T49.7X6
Drocode	T40.2X1	T40.2X2	T40.2X3	T40.2X4	T40.2X5	T40.2X6
Dromoran	T40.2X1	T40.2X2	T40.2X3	T40.2X4	T40.2X5	T40.2X6
Dromostanolone	T38.7X1	T38.7X2	T38.7X3	T38.7X4	T38.7X5	T38.7X6
Dronabinol	T40.7X1	T40.7X2	T40.7X3	T40.7X4	T40.7X5	T40.7X6
Droperidol	T43.591	T43.592	T43.593	T43.594	T43.595	T43.596
Dropropizine	T48.3X1	T48.3X2	T48.3X3	T48.3X4	T48.3X5	T48.3X6
Drostanolone	T38.7X1	T38.7X2	T38.7X3	T38.7X4	T38.7X5	T38.7X6
Drotaverine	T44.3X1	T44.3X2	T44.3X3	T44.3X4	T44.3X5	T44.3X6
Drotrecogin alfa	T45.511	T45.512	T45.513	T45.514	T45.515	T45.516
Drug NEC	T50.901	T50.902	T50.903	T50.904	T50.905	T50.906
specified NEC	T50.991	T50.992	T50.993	T50.994	T50.995	T50.996
DTIC	T45.1X1	T45.1X2	T45.1X3	T45.1X4	T45.1X5	T45.1X6
Duboisine	T44.3X1	T44.3X2	T44.3X3	T44.3X4	T44.3X5	T44.3X6
Dulcolax	T47.2X1	T47.2X2	T47.2X3	T47.2X4	T47.2X5	T47.2X6
Duponol (C) (EP)	T49.2X1	T49.2X2	T49.2X3	T49.2X4	T49.2X5	T49.2X6
Durabolin	T38.7X1	T38.7X2	T38.7X3	T38.7X4	T38.7X5	T38.7X6
Dyclone	T41.3X1	T41.3X2	T41.3X3	T41.3X4	T41.3X5	T41.3X6
Dyclonine	T41.3X1	T41.3X2	T41.3X3	T41.3X4	T41.3X5	T41.3X6
Dydrogesterone	T38.5X1	T38.5X2	T38.5X3	T38.5X4	T38.5X5	T38.5X6
Dye NEC	T65.6X1	T65.6X2	T65.6X3	T65.6X4	—	—
antiseptic	T49.0X1	T49.0X2	T49.0X3	T49.0X4	T49.0X5	T49.0X6
diagnostic agents	T50.8X1	T50.8X2	T50.8X3	T50.8X4	T50.8X5	T50.8X6
pharmaceutical NEC	T50.901	T50.902	T50.903	T50.904	T50.905	T50.906
Dyflos	T44.0X1	T44.0X2	T44.0X3	T44.0X4	T44.0X5	T44.0X6
Dymelor	T38.3X1	T38.3X2	T38.3X3	T38.3X4	T38.3X5	T38.3X6
Dynamite	T65.3X1	T65.3X2	T65.3X3	T65.3X4	—	—
fumes	T59.891	T59.892	T59.893	T59.894	—	—
Dyphylline	T44.3X1	T44.3X2	T44.3X3	T44.3X4	T44.3X5	T44.3X6
b-eucaine	T49.1X1	T49.1X2	T49.1X3	T49.1X4	T49.1X5	T49.1X6
Ear drug NEC	T49.6X1	T49.6X2	T49.6X3	T49.6X4	T49.6X5	T49.6X6
Ear preparations	T49.6X1	T49.6X2	T49.6X3	T49.6X4	T49.6X5	T49.6X6
Echothiophate, echothiopate, ecothiopate	T49.5X1	T49.5X2	T49.5X3	T49.5X4	T49.5X5	T49.5X6
Econazole	T49.0X1	T49.0X2	T49.0X3	T49.0X4	T49.0X5	T49.0X6
Ecothiopate iodide	T49.5X1	T49.5X2	T49.5X3	T49.5X4	T49.5X5	T49.5X6
Ecstasy	T43.641	T43.642	T43.643	T43.644	—	—
Ectylurea	T42.6X1	T42.6X2	T42.6X3	T42.6X4	T42.6X5	T42.6X6
Edathamil disodium	T45.8X1	T45.8X2	T45.8X3	T45.8X4	T45.8X5	T45.8X6
Edecrin	T50.1X1	T50.1X2	T50.1X3	T50.1X4	T50.1X5	T50.1X6
Edetate, disodium (calcium)	T45.8X1	T45.8X2	T45.8X3	T45.8X4	T45.8X5	T45.8X6
Edoxudine	T49.5X1	T49.5X2	T49.5X3	T49.5X4	T49.5X5	T49.5X6
Edrophonium	T44.0X1	T44.0X2	T44.0X3	T44.0X4	T44.0X5	T44.0X6
chloride	T44.0X1	T44.0X2	T44.0X3	T44.0X4	T44.0X5	T44.0X6
EDTA	T50.6X1	T50.6X2	T50.6X3	T50.6X4	T50.6X5	T50.6X6
Eflornithine	T37.2X1	T37.2X2	T37.2X3	T37.2X4	T37.2X5	T37.2X6
Efloxate	T46.3X1	T46.3X2	T46.3X3	T46.3X4	T46.3X5	T46.3X6
Elase	T49.8X1	T49.8X2	T49.8X3	T49.8X4	T49.8X5	T49.8X6
Elastase	T47.5X1	T47.5X2	T47.5X3	T47.5X4	T47.5X5	T47.5X6
Elaterium	T47.2X1	T47.2X2	T47.2X3	T47.2X4	T47.2X5	T47.2X6
Elcatonin	T50.991	T50.992	T50.993	T50.994	T50.995	T50.996
Elder	T62.2X1	T62.2X2	T62.2X3	T62.2X4	—	—
berry, (unripe)	T62.1X1	T62.1X2	T62.1X3	T62.1X4	—	—
Electrolyte balance drug	T50.3X1	T50.3X2	T50.3X3	T50.3X4	T50.3X5	T50.3X6
Electrolytes NEC	T50.3X1	T50.3X2	T50.3X3	T50.3X4	T50.3X5	T50.3X6
Electrolytic agent NEC	T50.3X1	T50.3X2	T50.3X3	T50.3X4	T50.3X5	T50.3X6
Elemental diet	T50.901	T50.902	T50.903	T50.904	T50.905	T50.906
Elliptinium acetate	T45.1X1	T45.1X2	T45.1X3	T45.1X4	T45.1X5	T45.1X6
Embramine	T45.0X1	T45.0X2	T45.0X3	T45.0X4	T45.0X5	T45.0X6
Emepronium (salts)	T44.3X1	T44.3X2	T44.3X3	T44.3X4	T44.3X5	T44.3X6
bromide	T44.3X1	T44.3X2	T44.3X3	T44.3X4	T44.3X5	T44.3X6
Emetic NEC	T47.7X1	T47.7X2	T47.7X3	T47.7X4	T47.7X5	T47.7X6
Emetine	T37.3X1	T37.3X2	T37.3X3	T37.3X4	T37.3X5	T37.3X6
Emollient NEC	T49.3X1	T49.3X2	T49.3X3	T49.3X4	T49.3X5	T49.3X6
Emorfazone	T39.8X1	T39.8X2	T39.8X3	T39.8X4	T39.8X5	T39.8X6
Emylcamate	T43.591	T43.592	T43.593	T43.594	T43.595	T43.596
Enalapril	T46.4X1	T46.4X2	T46.4X3	T46.4X4	T46.4X5	T46.4X6
Enalaprilat	T46.4X1	T46.4X2	T46.4X3	T46.4X4	T46.4X5	T46.4X6
Encainide	T46.2X1	T46.2X2	T46.2X3	T46.2X4	T46.2X5	T46.2X6
Endocaine	T41.3X1	T41.3X2	T41.3X3	T41.3X4	T41.3X5	T41.3X6
Endosulfan	T60.2X1	T60.2X2	T60.2X3	T60.2X4	—	—
Endothall	T60.3X1	T60.3X2	T60.3X3	T60.3X4	—	—
Endralazine	T46.5X1	T46.5X2	T46.5X3	T46.5X4	T46.5X5	T46.5X6
Endrin	T60.1X1	T60.1X2	T60.1X3	T60.1X4	—	—
Enflurane	T41.0X1	T41.0X2	T41.0X3	T41.0X4	T41.0X5	T41.0X6
Enhexymal	T42.3X1	T42.3X2	T42.3X3	T42.3X4	T42.3X5	T42.3X6
Enocitabine	T45.1X1	T45.1X2	T45.1X3	T45.1X4	T45.1X5	T45.1X6
Enovid	T38.4X1	T38.4X2	T38.4X3	T38.4X4	T38.4X5	T38.4X6
Enoxacin	T36.8X1	T36.8X2	T36.8X3	T36.8X4	T36.8X5	T36.8X6
Enoxaparin (sodium)	T45.511	T45.512	T45.513	T45.514	T45.515	T45.516
Enpiprazole	T43.591	T43.592	T43.593	T43.594	T43.595	T43.596
Enprofylline	T48.6X1	T48.6X2	T48.6X3	T48.6X4	T48.6X5	T48.6X6
Enprostil	T47.1X1	T47.1X2	T47.1X3	T47.1X4	T47.1X5	T47.1X6
Enterogastrone	T38.891	T38.892	T38.893	T38.894	T38.895	T38.896
ENT preparations (anti-infectives)	T49.6X1	T49.6X2	T49.6X3	T49.6X4	T49.6X5	T49.6X6
Enviomycin	T36.8X1	T36.8X2	T36.8X3	T36.8X4	T36.8X5	T36.8X6
Enzodase	T45.3X1	T45.3X2	T45.3X3	T45.3X4	T45.3X5	T45.3X6
Enzyme NEC	T45.3X1	T45.3X2	T45.3X3	T45.3X4	T45.3X5	T45.3X6
depolymerizing	T49.8X1	T49.8X2	T49.8X3	T49.8X4	T49.8X5	T49.8X6
fibrolytic	T45.3X1	T45.3X2	T45.3X3	T45.3X4	T45.3X5	T45.3X6
gastric	T47.5X1	T47.5X2	T47.5X3	T47.5X4	T47.5X5	T47.5X6
intestinal	T47.5X1	T47.5X2	T47.5X3	T47.5X4	T47.5X5	T47.5X6
local action	T49.4X1	T49.4X2	T49.4X3	T49.4X4	T49.4X5	T49.4X6
proteolytic	T49.4X1	T49.4X2	T49.4X3	T49.4X4	T49.4X5	T49.4X6
thrombolytic	T45.3X1	T45.3X2	T45.3X3	T45.3X4	T45.3X5	T45.3X6
EPAB	T41.3X1	T41.3X2	T41.3X3	T41.3X4	T41.3X5	T41.3X6
Epanutin	T42.0X1	T42.0X2	T42.0X3	T42.0X4	T42.0X5	T42.0X6
Ephedra	T44.991	T44.992	T44.993	T44.994	T44.995	T44.996
Ephedrine	T44.991	T44.992	T44.993	T44.994	T44.995	T44.996
Epichlorhydrin, epichlorohydrin	T52.8X1	T52.8X2	T52.8X3	T52.8X4	—	—
Epicillin	T36.0X1	T36.0X2	T36.0X3	T36.0X4	T36.0X5	T36.0X6
Epiestriol	T38.5X1	T38.5X2	T38.5X3	T38.5X4	T38.5X5	T38.5X6
Epilim — see Sodium valproate						
Epimestrol	T38.5X1	T38.5X2	T38.5X3	T38.5X4	T38.5X5	T38.5X6
Epinephrine	T44.5X1	T44.5X2	T44.5X3	T44.5X4	T44.5X5	T44.5X6
Epirubicin	T45.1X1	T45.1X2	T45.1X3	T45.1X4	T45.1X5	T45.1X6
Epitiostanol	T38.7X1	T38.7X2	T38.7X3	T38.7X4	T38.7X5	T38.7X6
Epitizide	T50.2X1	T50.2X2	T50.2X3	T50.2X4	T50.2X5	T50.2X6
EPN	T60.0X1	T60.0X2	T60.0X3	T60.0X4	—	—
EPO	T45.8X1	T45.8X2	T45.8X3	T45.8X4	T45.8X5	T45.8X6
Epoetin alpha	T45.8X1	T45.8X2	T45.8X3	T45.8X4	T45.8X5	T45.8X6
Epomediol	T50.991	T50.992	T50.993	T50.994	T50.995	T50.996
Epoprostenol	T45.521	T45.522	T45.523	T45.524	T45.525	T45.526
Epoxy resin	T65.891	T65.892	T65.893	T65.894	—	—
Eprazinone	T48.4X1	T48.4X2	T48.4X3	T48.4X4	T48.4X5	T48.4X6
Epsilon aminocaproic acid	T45.621	T45.622	T45.623	T45.624	T45.625	T45.626
Epsom salt	T47.3X1	T47.3X2	T47.3X3	T47.3X4	T47.3X5	T47.3X6
Eptazocine	T40.4X1	T40.4X2	T40.4X3	T40.4X4	T40.4X5	T40.4X6
Equanil	T43.591	T43.592	T43.593	T43.594	T43.595	T43.596
Equisetum	T62.2X1	T62.2X2	T62.2X3	T62.2X4	—	—
diuretic	T50.2X1	T50.2X2	T50.2X3	T50.2X4	T50.2X5	T50.2X6
Ergobasine	T48.0X1	T48.0X2	T48.0X3	T48.0X4	T48.0X5	T48.0X6
Ergocalciferol	T45.2X1	T45.2X2	T45.2X3	T45.2X4	T45.2X5	T45.2X6
Ergoloid mesylates	T46.7X1	T46.7X2	T46.7X3	T46.7X4	T46.7X5	T46.7X6
Ergometrine	T48.0X1	T48.0X2	T48.0X3	T48.0X4	T48.0X5	T48.0X6
Ergonovine	T48.0X1	T48.0X2	T48.0X3	T48.0X4	T48.0X5	T48.0X6
Ergotamine	T46.5X1	T46.5X2	T46.5X3	T46.5X4	T46.5X5	T46.5X6
Ergotocine	T48.0X1	T48.0X2	T48.0X3	T48.0X4	T48.0X5	T48.0X6
Ergotrate	T48.0X1	T48.0X2	T48.0X3	T48.0X4	T48.0X5	T48.0X6
Ergot NEC	T64.81	T64.82	T64.83	T64.84	—	—
derivative	T48.0X1	T48.0X2	T48.0X3	T48.0X4	T48.0X5	T48.0X6

Substance	Poisoning, Accidental (unintentional)	Poisoning, Intentional Self-harm	Poisoning, Assault	Poisoning, Undetermined	Adverse Effect	Under-dosing
Ergot — *continued*						
medicinal (alkaloids)	T48.0X1	T48.0X2	T48.0X3	T48.0X4	T48.0X5	T48.0X6
prepared	T48.0X1	T48.0X2	T48.0X3	T48.0X4	T48.0X5	T48.0X6
Eritrityl tetranitrate	T46.3X1	T46.3X2	T46.3X3	T46.3X4	T46.3X5	T46.3X6
Erythrityl tetranitrate	T46.3X1	T46.3X2	T46.3X3	T46.3X4	T46.3X5	T46.3X6
Erythrol tetranitrate	T46.3X1	T46.3X2	T46.3X3	T46.3X4	T46.3X5	T46.3X6
Erythromycin (salts)	T36.3X1	T36.3X2	T36.3X3	T36.3X4	T36.3X5	T36.3X6
ophthalmic preparation	T49.5X1	T49.5X2	T49.5X3	T49.5X4	T49.5X5	T49.5X6
topical NEC	T49.0X1	T49.0X2	T49.0X3	T49.0X4	T49.0X5	T49.0X6
Erythropoietin	T45.8X1	T45.8X2	T45.8X3	T45.8X4	T45.8X5	T45.8X6
human	T45.8X1	T45.8X2	T45.8X3	T45.8X4	T45.8X5	T45.8X6
Escin	T46.991	T46.992	T46.993	T46.994	T46.995	T46.996
Esculin	T45.2X1	T45.2X2	T45.2X3	T45.2X4	T45.2X5	T45.2X6
Esculoside	T45.2X1	T45.2X2	T45.2X3	T45.2X4	T45.2X5	T45.2X6
ESDT (ether-soluble tar distillate)	T49.1X1	T49.1X2	T49.1X3	T49.1X4	T49.1X5	T49.1X6
Eserine	T49.5X1	T49.5X2	T49.5X3	T49.5X4	T49.5X5	T49.5X6
Esflurbiprofen	T39.311	T39.312	T39.313	T39.314	T39.315	T39.316
Eskabarb	T42.3X1	T42.3X2	T42.3X3	T42.3X4	T42.3X5	T42.3X6
Eskalith	T43.8X1	T43.8X2	T43.8X3	T43.8X4	T43.8X5	T43.8X6
Esmolol	T44.7X1	T44.7X2	T44.7X3	T44.7X4	T44.7X5	T44.7X6
Estanozolol	T38.7X1	T38.7X2	T38.7X3	T38.7X4	T38.7X5	T38.7X6
Estazolam	T42.4X1	T42.4X2	T42.4X3	T42.4X4	T42.4X5	T42.4X6
Estradiol	T38.5X1	T38.5X2	T38.5X3	T38.5X4	T38.5X5	T38.5X6
with testosterone	T38.7X1	T38.7X2	T38.7X3	T38.7X4	T38.7X5	T38.7X6
benzoate	T38.5X1	T38.5X2	T38.5X3	T38.5X4	T38.5X5	T38.5X6
Estramustine	T45.1X1	T45.1X2	T45.1X3	T45.1X4	T45.1X5	T45.1X6
Estriol	T38.5X1	T38.5X2	T38.5X3	T38.5X4	T38.5X5	T38.5X6
Estrogen	T38.5X1	T38.5X2	T38.5X3	T38.5X4	T38.5X5	T38.5X6
with progesterone	T38.5X1	T38.5X2	T38.5X3	T38.5X4	T38.5X5	T38.5X6
conjugated	T38.5X1	T38.5X2	T38.5X3	T38.5X4	T38.5X5	T38.5X6
Estrone	T38.5X1	T38.5X2	T38.5X3	T38.5X4	T38.5X5	T38.5X6
Estropipate	T38.5X1	T38.5X2	T38.5X3	T38.5X4	T38.5X5	T38.5X6
Etacrynate sodium	T50.1X1	T50.1X2	T50.1X3	T50.1X4	T50.1X5	T50.1X6
Etacrynic acid	T50.1X1	T50.1X2	T50.1X3	T50.1X4	T50.1X5	T50.1X6
Etafedrine	T48.6X1	T48.6X2	T48.6X3	T48.6X4	T48.6X5	T48.6X6
Etafenone	T46.3X1	T46.3X2	T46.3X3	T46.3X4	T46.3X5	T46.3X6
Etambutol	T37.1X1	T37.1X2	T37.1X3	T37.1X4	T37.1X5	T37.1X6
Etamiphyllin	T48.6X1	T48.6X2	T48.6X3	T48.6X4	T48.6X5	T48.6X6
Etamivan	T50.7X1	T50.7X2	T50.7X3	T50.7X4	T50.7X5	T50.7X6
Etamsylate	T45.7X1	T45.7X2	T45.7X3	T45.7X4	T45.7X5	T45.7X6
Etebenecid	T50.4X1	T50.4X2	T50.4X3	T50.4X4	T50.4X5	T50.4X6
Ethacridine	T49.0X1	T49.0X2	T49.0X3	T49.0X4	T49.0X5	T49.0X6
Ethacrynic acid	T50.1X1	T50.1X2	T50.1X3	T50.1X4	T50.1X5	T50.1X6
Ethadione	T42.2X1	T42.2X2	T42.2X3	T42.2X4	T42.2X5	T42.2X6
Ethambutol	T37.1X1	T37.1X2	T37.1X3	T37.1X4	T37.1X5	T37.1X6
Ethamide	T50.2X1	T50.2X2	T50.2X3	T50.2X4	T50.2X5	T50.2X6
Ethamivan	T50.7X1	T50.7X2	T50.7X3	T50.7X4	T50.7X5	T50.7X6
Ethamsylate	T45.7X1	T45.7X2	T45.7X3	T45.7X4	T45.7X5	T45.7X6
Ethanol	T51.0X1	T51.0X2	T51.0X3	T51.0X4	—	—
beverage	T51.0X1	T51.0X2	T51.0X3	T51.0X4	—	—
Ethanolamine oleate	T46.8X1	T46.8X2	T46.8X3	T46.8X4	T46.8X5	T46.8X6
Ethaverine	T44.3X1	T44.3X2	T44.3X3	T44.3X4	T44.3X5	T44.3X6
Ethchlorvynol	T42.6X1	T42.6X2	T42.6X3	T42.6X4	T42.6X5	T42.6X6
Ethebenecid	T50.4X1	T50.4X2	T50.4X3	T50.4X4	T50.4X5	T50.4X6
Ether (vapor)	T41.0X1	T41.0X2	T41.0X3	T41.0X4	T41.0X5	T41.0X6
anesthetic	T41.0X1	T41.0X2	T41.0X3	T41.0X4	T41.0X5	T41.0X6
divinyl	T41.0X1	T41.0X2	T41.0X3	T41.0X4	T41.0X5	T41.0X6
ethyl (medicinal)	T41.0X1	T41.0X2	T41.0X3	T41.0X4	T41.0X5	T41.0X6
nonmedicinal	T52.8X1	T52.8X2	T52.8X3	T52.8X4	—	—
petroleum — *see* Ligroin						
solvent	T52.8X1	T52.8X2	T52.8X3	T52.8X4	—	—
Ethiazide	T50.2X1	T50.2X2	T50.2X3	T50.2X4	T50.2X5	T50.2X6
Ethidium chloride (vapor)	T59.891	T59.892	T59.893	T59.894	—	—
Ethinamate	T42.6X1	T42.6X2	T42.6X3	T42.6X4	T42.6X5	T42.6X6
Ethinylestradiol, ethinyloestradiol	T38.5X1	T38.5X2	T38.5X3	T38.5X4	T38.5X5	T38.5X6
with						
levonorgestrel	T38.4X1	T38.4X2	T38.4X3	T38.4X4	T38.4X5	T38.4X6
norethisterone	T38.4X1	T38.4X2	T38.4X3	T38.4X4	T38.4X5	T38.4X6
Ethiodized oil (131 I)	T50.8X1	T50.8X2	T50.8X3	T50.8X4	T50.8X5	T50.8X6
Ethion	T60.0X1	T60.0X2	T60.0X3	T60.0X4	—	—
Ethionamide	T37.1X1	T37.1X2	T37.1X3	T37.1X4	T37.1X5	T37.1X6
Ethioniamide	T37.1X1	T37.1X2	T37.1X3	T37.1X4	T37.1X5	T37.1X6
Ethisterone	T38.5X1	T38.5X2	T38.5X3	T38.5X4	T38.5X5	T38.5X6
Ethobral	T42.3X1	T42.3X2	T42.3X3	T42.3X4	T42.3X5	T42.3X6
Ethocaine (infiltration) (topical)	T41.3X1	T41.3X2	T41.3X3	T41.3X4	T41.3X5	T41.3X6
nerve block (peripheral) (plexus)	T41.3X1	T41.3X2	T41.3X3	T41.3X4	T41.3X5	T41.3X6
spinal	T41.3X1	T41.3X2	T41.3X3	T41.3X4	T41.3X5	T41.3X6
Ethoheptazine	T40.4X1	T40.4X2	T40.4X3	T40.4X4	T40.4X5	T40.4X6
Ethopropazine	T44.3X1	T44.3X2	T44.3X3	T44.3X4	T44.3X5	T44.3X6

Substance	Poisoning, Accidental (unintentional)	Poisoning, Intentional Self-harm	Poisoning, Assault	Poisoning, Undetermined	Adverse Effect	Under-dosing
Ethosuximide	T42.2X1	T42.2X2	T42.2X3	T42.2X4	T42.2X5	T42.2X6
Ethotoin	T42.0X1	T42.0X2	T42.0X3	T42.0X4	T42.0X5	T42.0X6
Ethoxazene	T37.91	T37.92	T37.93	T37.94	T37.95	T37.96
Ethoxazorutoside	T46.991	T46.992	T46.993	T46.994	T46.995	T46.996
Ethoxzolamide	T50.2X1	T50.2X2	T50.2X3	T50.2X4	T50.2X5	T50.2X6
Ethyl						
acetate	T52.8X1	T52.8X2	T52.8X3	T52.8X4	—	—
alcohol	T51.0X1	T51.0X2	T51.0X3	T51.0X4	—	—
beverage	T51.0X1	T51.0X2	T51.0X3	T51.0X4	—	—
aldehyde (vapor)	T59.891	T59.892	T59.893	T59.894	—	—
liquid	T52.8X1	T52.8X2	T52.8X3	T52.8X4	—	—
aminobenzoate	T41.3X1	T41.3X2	T41.3X3	T41.3X4	T41.3X5	T41.3X6
aminophenothiazine	T43.3X1	T43.3X2	T43.3X3	T43.3X4	T43.3X5	T43.3X6
benzoate	T52.8X1	T52.8X2	T52.8X3	T52.8X4	—	—
biscoumacetate	T45.511	T45.512	T45.513	T45.514	T45.515	T45.516
bromide (anesthetic)	T41.0X1	T41.0X2	T41.0X3	T41.0X4	T41.0X5	T41.0X6
carbamate	T45.1X1	T45.1X2	T45.1X3	T45.1X4	T45.1X5	T45.1X6
carbinol	T51.3X1	T51.3X2	T51.3X3	T51.3X4	—	—
carbonate	T52.8X1	T52.8X2	T52.8X3	T52.8X4	—	—
chaulmoograte	T37.1X1	T37.1X2	T37.1X3	T37.1X4	T37.1X5	T37.1X6
chloride (anesthetic)	T41.0X1	T41.0X2	T41.0X3	T41.0X4	T41.0X5	T41.0X6
anesthetic (local)	T41.3X1	T41.3X2	T41.3X3	T41.3X4	T41.3X5	T41.3X6
inhaled	T41.0X1	T41.0X2	T41.0X3	T41.0X4	T41.0X5	T41.0X6
local	T49.4X1	T49.4X2	T49.4X3	T49.4X4	T49.4X5	T49.4X6
solvent	T53.6X1	T53.6X2	T53.6X3	T53.6X4	—	—
dibunate	T48.3X1	T48.3X2	T48.3X3	T48.3X4	T48.3X5	T48.3X6
dichloroarsine (vapor)	T57.0X1	T57.0X2	T57.0X3	T57.0X4	—	—
estranol	T38.7X1	T38.7X2	T38.7X3	T38.7X4	T38.7X5	T38.7X6
ether — *see also* ether	T52.8X1	T52.8X2	T52.8X3	T52.8X4	—	—
formate NEC (solvent)	T52.0X1	T52.0X2	T52.0X3	T52.0X4	—	—
fumarate	T49.4X1	T49.4X2	T49.4X3	T49.4X4	T49.4X5	T49.4X6
hydroxyisobutyrate NEC (solvent)	T52.8X1	T52.8X2	T52.8X3	T52.8X4	—	—
iodoacetate	T59.3X1	T59.3X2	T59.3X3	T59.3X4	—	—
lactate NEC (solvent)	T52.8X1	T52.8X2	T52.8X3	T52.8X4	—	—
loflazepate	T42.4X1	T42.4X2	T42.4X3	T42.4X4	T42.4X5	T42.4X6
mercuric chloride	T56.1X1	T56.1X2	T56.1X3	T56.1X4	—	—
methylcarbinol	T51.8X1	T51.8X2	T51.8X3	T51.8X4	—	—
morphine	T40.2X1	T40.2X2	T40.2X3	T40.2X4	T40.2X5	T40.2X6
noradrenaline	T48.6X1	T48.6X2	T48.6X3	T48.6X4	T48.6X5	T48.6X6
oxybutyrate NEC (solvent)	T52.8X1	T52.8X2	T52.8X3	T52.8X4	—	—
Ethylene (gas)	T59.891	T59.892	T59.893	T59.894	—	—
anesthetic (general)	T41.0X1	T41.0X2	T41.0X3	T41.0X4	T41.0X5	T41.0X6
chlorohydrin	T52.8X1	T52.8X2	T52.8X3	T52.8X4	—	—
vapor	T53.6X1	T53.6X2	T53.6X3	T53.6X4	—	—
dichloride	T52.8X1	T52.8X2	T52.8X3	T52.8X4	—	—
vapor	T53.6X1	T53.6X2	T53.6X3	T53.6X4	—	—
dinitrate	T52.3X1	T52.3X2	T52.3X3	T52.3X4	—	—
glycol(s)	T52.8X1	T52.8X2	T52.8X3	T52.8X4	—	—
dinitrate	T52.3X1	T52.3X2	T52.3X3	T52.3X4	—	—
monobutyl ether	T52.3X1	T52.3X2	T52.3X3	T52.3X4	—	—
imine	T54.1X1	T54.1X2	T54.1X3	T54.1X4	—	—
oxide (fumigant) (nonmedicinal)	T59.891	T59.892	T59.893	T59.894	—	—
medicinal	T49.0X1	T49.0X2	T49.0X3	T49.0X4	T49.0X5	T49.0X6
Ethylenediaminetetra-acetic acid	T50.6X1	T50.6X2	T50.6X3	T50.6X4	T50.6X5	T50.6X6
Ethylenediamine theophylline	T48.6X1	T48.6X2	T48.6X3	T48.6X4	T48.6X5	T48.6X6
Ethylenedinitrilotetra-acetate	T50.6X1	T50.6X2	T50.6X3	T50.6X4	T50.6X5	T50.6X6
Ethylestrenol	T38.7X1	T38.7X2	T38.7X3	T38.7X4	T38.7X5	T38.7X6
Ethylhydroxycellulose	T47.4X1	T47.4X2	T47.4X3	T47.4X4	T47.4X5	T47.4X6
Ethylidene						
chloride NEC	T53.6X1	T53.6X2	T53.6X3	T53.6X4	—	—
diacetate	T60.3X1	T60.3X2	T60.3X3	T60.3X4	—	—
dicoumarin	T45.511	T45.512	T45.513	T45.514	T45.515	T45.51...
dicoumarol	T45.511	T45.512	T45.513	T45.514	T45.515	T45.51...
diethyl ether	T52.0X1	T52.0X2	T52.0X3	T52.0X4	—	—
Ethylmorphine	T40.2X1	T40.2X2	T40.2X3	T40.2X4	T40.2X5	T40.2X...
Ethylnorepinephrine	T48.6X1	T48.6X2	T48.6X3	T48.6X4	T48.6X5	T48.6...
Ethylparachlorophen-oxyisobutyrate	T46.6X1	T46.6X2	T46.6X3	T46.6X4	T46.6X5	T46.6...
Ethynodiol	T38.4X1	T38.4X2	T38.4X3	T38.4X4	T38.4X5	T38.4...
with mestranol diacetate	T38.4X1	T38.4X2	T38.4X3	T38.4X4	T38.4X5	T38.4...
Etidocaine	T41.3X1	T41.3X2	T41.3X3	T41.3X4	T41.3X5	T41.3...
infiltration (subcutaneous)	T41.3X1	T41.3X2	T41.3X3	T41.3X4	T41.3X5	T41.3...
nerve (peripheral) (plexus)	T41.3X1	T41.3X2	T41.3X3	T41.3X4	T41.3X5	T41.3...
Etidronate	T50.991	T50.992	T50.993	T50.994	T50.995	T50.9...
Etidronic acid (disodium salt)	T50.991	T50.992	T50.993	T50.994	T50.995	T50.9...
Etifoxine	T42.6X1	T42.6X2	T42.6X3	T42.6X4	T42.6X5	T42.6...
Etilefrine	T44.4X1	T44.4X2	T44.4X3	T44.4X4	T44.4X5	T44.4...
Etilfen	T42.3X1	T42.3X2	T42.3X3	T42.3X4	T42.3X5	T42.3...

Substance	Poisoning, Accidental (unintentional)	Poisoning, Intentional Self-harm	Poisoning, Assault	Poisoning, Undetermined	Adverse Effect	Under-dosing
Etinodiol	T38.4X1	T38.4X2	T38.4X3	T38.4X4	T38.4X5	T38.4X6
Etiroxate	T46.6X1	T46.6X2	T46.6X3	T46.6X4	T46.6X5	T46.6X6
Etizolam	T42.4X1	T42.4X2	T42.4X3	T42.4X4	T42.4X5	T42.4X6
Etodolac	T39.391	T39.392	T39.393	T39.394	T39.395	T39.396
Etofamide	T37.3X1	T37.3X2	T37.3X3	T37.3X4	T37.3X5	T37.3X6
Etofibrate	T46.6X1	T46.6X2	T46.6X3	T46.6X4	T46.6X5	T46.6X6
Etofylline	T46.7X1	T46.7X2	T46.7X3	T46.7X4	T46.7X5	T46.7X6
clofibrate	T46.6X1	T46.6X2	T46.6X3	T46.6X4	T46.6X5	T46.6X6
Etoglucid	T45.1X1	T45.1X2	T45.1X3	T45.1X4	T45.1X5	T45.1X6
Etomidate	T41.1X1	T41.1X2	T41.1X3	T41.1X4	T41.1X5	T41.1X6
Etomide	T39.8X1	T39.8X2	T39.8X3	T39.8X4	T39.8X5	T39.8X6
Etomidoline	T44.3X1	T44.3X2	T44.3X3	T44.3X4	T44.3X5	T44.3X6
Etoposide	T45.1X1	T45.1X2	T45.1X3	T45.1X4	T45.1X5	T45.1X6
Etorphine	T40.2X1	T40.2X2	T40.2X3	T40.2X4	T40.2X5	T40.2X6
Etoval	T42.3X1	T42.3X2	T42.3X3	T42.3X4	T42.3X5	T42.3X6
Etozolin	T50.1X1	T50.1X2	T50.1X3	T50.1X4	T50.1X5	T50.1X6
Etretinate	T50.991	T50.992	T50.993	T50.994	T50.995	T50.996
Etryptamine	T43.691	T43.692	T43.693	T43.694	T43.695	T43.696
Etybenzatropine	T44.3X1	T44.3X2	T44.3X3	T44.3X4	T44.3X5	T44.3X6
Etynodiol	T38.4X1	T38.4X2	T38.4X3	T38.4X4	T38.4X5	T38.4X6
Eucaine	T41.3X1	T41.3X2	T41.3X3	T41.3X4	T41.3X5	T41.3X6
Eucalyptus oil	T49.7X1	T49.7X2	T49.7X3	T49.7X4	T49.7X5	T49.7X6
Eucatropine	T49.5X1	T49.5X2	T49.5X3	T49.5X4	T49.5X5	T49.5X6
Eucodal	T40.2X1	T40.2X2	T40.2X3	T40.2X4	T40.2X5	T40.2X6
Euneryl	T42.3X1	T42.3X2	T42.3X3	T42.3X4	T42.3X5	T42.3X6
Euphthalmine	T44.3X1	T44.3X2	T44.3X3	T44.3X4	T44.3X5	T44.3X6
Eurax	T49.0X1	T49.0X2	T49.0X3	T49.0X4	T49.0X5	T49.0X6
Euresol	T49.4X1	T49.4X2	T49.4X3	T49.4X4	T49.4X5	T49.4X6
Euthroid	T38.1X1	T38.1X2	T38.1X3	T38.1X4	T38.1X5	T38.1X6
Evans blue	T50.8X1	T50.8X2	T50.8X3	T50.8X4	T50.8X5	T50.8X6
Evipal	T42.3X1	T42.3X2	T42.3X3	T42.3X4	T42.3X5	T42.3X6
sodium	T41.1X1	T41.1X2	T41.1X3	T41.1X4	T41.1X5	T41.1X6
Evipan	T42.3X1	T42.3X2	T42.3X3	T42.3X4	T42.3X5	T42.3X6
sodium	T41.1X1	T41.1X2	T41.1X3	T41.1X4	T41.1X5	T41.1X6
Exalamide	T49.0X1	T49.0X2	T49.0X3	T49.0X4	T49.0X5	T49.0X6
Exalgin	T39.1X1	T39.1X2	T39.1X3	T39.1X4	T39.1X5	T39.1X6
Excipients, pharmaceutical	T50.901	T50.902	T50.903	T50.904	T50.905	T50.906
Exhaust gas (engine) (motor vehicle)	T58.01	T58.02	T58.03	T58.04	—	—
Ex-Lax (phenolphthalein)	T47.2X1	T47.2X2	T47.2X3	T47.2X4	T47.2X5	T47.2X6
Expectorant NEC	T48.4X1	T48.4X2	T48.4X3	T48.4X4	T48.4X5	T48.4X6
Extended insulin zinc suspension	T38.3X1	T38.3X2	T38.3X3	T38.3X4	T38.3X5	T38.3X6
External medications (skin) (mucous membrane)	T49.91	T49.92	T49.93	T49.94	T49.95	T49.96
dental agent	T49.7X1	T49.7X2	T49.7X3	T49.7X4	T49.7X5	T49.7X6
ENT agent	T49.6X1	T49.6X2	T49.6X3	T49.6X4	T49.6X5	T49.6X6
ophthalmic preparation	T49.5X1	T49.5X2	T49.5X3	T49.5X4	T49.5X5	T49.5X6
specified NEC	T49.8X1	T49.8X2	T49.8X3	T49.8X4	T49.8X5	T49.8X6
Extrapyramidal antagonist NEC	T44.3X1	T44.3X2	T44.3X3	T44.3X4	T44.3X5	T44.3X6
Eye agents (anti-infective)	T49.5X1	T49.5X2	T49.5X3	T49.5X4	T49.5X5	T49.5X6
Eye drug NEC	T49.5X1	T49.5X2	T49.5X3	T49.5X4	T49.5X5	T49.5X6
FAC (fluorouracil + doxorubicin + cyclophosphamide)	T45.1X1	T45.1X2	T45.1X3	T45.1X4	T45.1X5	T45.1X6
Factor						
I (fibrinogen)	T45.8X1	T45.8X2	T45.8X3	T45.8X4	T45.8X5	T45.8X6
III (thromboplastin)	T45.8X1	T45.8X2	T45.8X3	T45.8X4	T45.8X5	T45.8X6
IX complex	T45.7X1	T45.7X2	T45.7X3	T45.7X4	T45.7X5	T45.7X6
human	T45.8X1	T45.8X2	T45.8X3	T45.8X4	T45.8X5	T45.8X6
VIII (antihemophilic Factor) (concentrate)	T45.8X1	T45.8X2	T45.8X3	T45.8X4	T45.8X5	T45.8X6
Famotidine	T47.0X1	T47.0X2	T47.0X3	T47.0X4	T47.0X5	T47.0X6
Fat suspension, intravenous	T50.991	T50.992	T50.993	T50.994	T50.995	T50.996
Fazadinium bromide	T48.1X1	T48.1X2	T48.1X3	T48.1X4	T48.1X5	T48.1X6
Febarbamate	T42.3X1	T42.3X2	T42.3X3	T42.3X4	T42.3X5	T42.3X6
Fecal softener	T47.4X1	T47.4X2	T47.4X3	T47.4X4	T47.4X5	T47.4X6
Fedrilate	T48.3X1	T48.3X2	T48.3X3	T48.3X4	T48.3X5	T48.3X6
Felodipine	T46.1X1	T46.1X2	T46.1X3	T46.1X4	T46.1X5	T46.1X6
Felypressin	T38.891	T38.892	T38.893	T38.894	T38.895	T38.896
Femoxetine	T43.221	T43.222	T43.223	T43.224	T43.225	T43.226
Fenalcomine	T46.3X1	T46.3X2	T46.3X3	T46.3X4	T46.3X5	T46.3X6
Fenamisal	T37.1X1	T37.1X2	T37.1X3	T37.1X4	T37.1X5	T37.1X6
Fenazone	T39.2X1	T39.2X2	T39.2X3	T39.2X4	T39.2X5	T39.2X6
Fenbendazole	T37.4X1	T37.4X2	T37.4X3	T37.4X4	T37.4X5	T37.4X6
Fenbutrazate	T50.5X1	T50.5X2	T50.5X3	T50.5X4	T50.5X5	T50.5X6
Fencamfamine	T43.691	T43.692	T43.693	T43.694	T43.695	T43.696
Fendiline	T46.1X1	T46.1X2	T46.1X3	T46.1X4	T46.1X5	T46.1X6
Fenetylline	T43.691	T43.692	T43.693	T43.694	T43.695	T43.696
Fenflumizole	T39.391	T39.392	T39.393	T39.394	T39.395	T39.396
Fenfluramine	T50.5X1	T50.5X2	T50.5X3	T50.5X4	T50.5X5	T50.5X6
Fenobarbital	T42.3X1	T42.3X2	T42.3X3	T42.3X4	T42.3X5	T42.3X6
Fenofibrate	T46.6X1	T46.6X2	T46.6X3	T46.6X4	T46.6X5	T46.6X6
Fenoprofen	T39.311	T39.312	T39.313	T39.314	T39.315	T39.316
Fenoterol	T48.6X1	T48.6X2	T48.6X3	T48.6X4	T48.6X5	T48.6X6
Fenoverine	T44.3X1	T44.3X2	T44.3X3	T44.3X4	T44.3X5	T44.3X6
Fenoxazoline	T48.5X1	T48.5X2	T48.5X3	T48.5X4	T48.5X5	T48.5X6
Fenproporex	T50.5X1	T50.5X2	T50.5X3	T50.5X4	T50.5X5	T50.5X6
Fenquizone	T50.2X1	T50.2X2	T50.2X3	T50.2X4	T50.2X5	T50.2X6
Fentanyl	T40.4X1	T40.4X2	T40.4X3	T40.4X4	T40.4X5	T40.4X6
Fentazin	T43.3X1	T43.3X2	T43.3X3	T43.3X4	T43.3X5	T43.3X6
Fenthion	T60.0X1	T60.0X2	T60.0X3	T60.0X4	—	—
Fenticlor	T49.0X1	T49.0X2	T49.0X3	T49.0X4	T49.0X5	T49.0X6
Fenylbutazone	T39.2X1	T39.2X2	T39.2X3	T39.2X4	T39.2X5	T39.2X6
Feprazone	T39.2X1	T39.2X2	T39.2X3	T39.2X4	T39.2X5	T39.2X6
Fer de lance (bite) (venom)	T63.061	T63.062	T63.063	T63.064	—	—
Ferric — *see also* Iron						
chloride	T45.4X1	T45.4X2	T45.4X3	T45.4X4	T45.4X5	T45.4X6
citrate	T45.4X1	T45.4X2	T45.4X3	T45.4X4	T45.4X5	T45.4X6
hydroxide						
colloidal	T45.4X1	T45.4X2	T45.4X3	T45.4X4	T45.4X5	T45.4X6
polymaltose	T45.4X1	T45.4X2	T45.4X3	T45.4X4	T45.4X5	T45.4X6
pyrophosphate	T45.4X1	T45.4X2	T45.4X3	T45.4X4	T45.4X5	T45.4X6
Ferritin	T45.4X1	T45.4X2	T45.4X3	T45.4X4	T45.4X5	T45.4X6
Ferrocholinate	T45.4X1	T45.4X2	T45.4X3	T45.4X4	T45.4X5	T45.4X6
Ferrodextrane	T45.4X1	T45.4X2	T45.4X3	T45.4X4	T45.4X5	T45.4X6
Ferropolimaler	T45.4X1	T45.4X2	T45.4X3	T45.4X4	T45.4X5	T45.4X6
Ferrous — *see also* Iron						
phosphate	T45.4X1	T45.4X2	T45.4X3	T45.4X4	T45.4X5	T45.4X6
salt	T45.4X1	T45.4X2	T45.4X3	T45.4X4	T45.4X5	T45.4X6
with folic acid	T45.4X1	T45.4X2	T45.4X3	T45.4X4	T45.4X5	T45.4X6
Ferrous fumarate, gluconate, lactate, salt NEC, sulfate (medicinal)	T45.4X1	T45.4X2	T45.4X3	T45.4X4	T45.4X5	T45.4X6
Ferrovanadium (fumes)	T59.891	T59.892	T59.893	T59.894	—	—
Ferrum — *see* Iron						
Fertilizers NEC	T65.891	T65.892	T65.893	T65.894	—	—
with herbicide mixture	T60.3X1	T60.3X2	T60.3X3	T60.3X4	—	—
Fetoxilate	T47.6X1	T47.6X2	T47.6X3	T47.6X4	T47.6X5	T47.6X6
Fiber, dietary	T47.4X1	T47.4X2	T47.4X3	T47.4X4	T47.4X5	T47.4X6
Fiberglass	T65.831	T65.832	T65.833	T65.834	—	—
Fibrinogen (human)	T45.8X1	T45.8X2	T45.8X3	T45.8X4	T45.8X5	T45.8X6
Fibrinolysin (human)	T45.691	T45.692	T45.693	T45.694	T45.695	T45.696
Fibrinolysis						
affecting drug	T45.601	T45.602	T45.603	T45.604	T45.605	T45.606
inhibitor NEC	T45.621	T45.622	T45.623	T45.624	T45.625	T45.626
Fibrinolytic drug	T45.611	T45.612	T45.613	T45.614	T45.615	T45.616
Filix mas	T37.4X1	T37.4X2	T37.4X3	T37.4X4	T37.4X5	T37.4X6
Filtering cream	T49.3X1	T49.3X2	T49.3X3	T49.3X4	T49.3X5	T49.3X6
Fiorinal	T39.011	T39.012	T39.013	T39.014	T39.015	T39.016
Firedamp	T59.891	T59.892	T59.893	T59.894	—	—
Fish, noxious, nonbacterial	T61.91	T61.92	T61.93	T61.94	—	—
ciguatera	T61.01	T61.02	T61.03	T61.04	—	—
scombroid	T61.11	T61.12	T61.13	T61.14	—	—
shell	T61.781	T61.782	T61.783	T61.784	—	—
specified NEC	T61.771	T61.772	T61.773	T61.774	—	—
Flagyl	T37.3X1	T37.3X2	T37.3X3	T37.3X4	T37.3X5	T37.3X6
Flavine adenine dinucleotide	T45.2X1	T45.2X2	T45.2X3	T45.2X4	T45.2X5	T45.2X6
Flavodic acid	T46.991	T46.992	T46.993	T46.994	T46.995	T46.996
Flavoxate	T44.3X1	T44.3X2	T44.3X3	T44.3X4	T44.3X5	T44.3X6
Flaxedil	T48.1X1	T48.1X2	T48.1X3	T48.1X4	T48.1X5	T48.1X6
Flaxseed (medicinal)	T49.3X1	T49.3X2	T49.3X3	T49.3X4	T49.3X5	T49.3X6
Flecainide	T46.2X1	T46.2X2	T46.2X3	T46.2X4	T46.2X5	T46.2X6
Fleroxacin	T36.8X1	T36.8X2	T36.8X3	T36.8X4	T36.8X5	T36.8X6
Floctafenine	T39.8X1	T39.8X2	T39.8X3	T39.8X4	T39.8X5	T39.8X6
Flomax	T44.6X1	T44.6X2	T44.6X3	T44.6X4	T44.6X5	T44.6X6
Flomoxef	T36.1X1	T36.1X2	T36.1X3	T36.1X4	T36.1X5	T36.1X6
Flopropione	T44.3X1	T44.3X2	T44.3X3	T44.3X4	T44.3X5	T44.3X6
Florantyrone	T47.5X1	T47.5X2	T47.5X3	T47.5X4	T47.5X5	T47.5X6
Floraquin	T37.8X1	T37.8X2	T37.8X3	T37.8X4	T37.8X5	T37.8X6
Florinef	T38.0X1	T38.0X2	T38.0X3	T38.0X4	T38.0X5	T38.0X6
ENT agent	T49.6X1	T49.6X2	T49.6X3	T49.6X4	T49.6X5	T49.6X6
ophthalmic preparation	T49.5X1	T49.5X2	T49.5X3	T49.5X4	T49.5X5	T49.5X6
topical NEC	T49.0X1	T49.0X2	T49.0X3	T49.0X4	T49.0X5	T49.0X6
Flowers of sulfur	T49.4X1	T49.4X2	T49.4X3	T49.4X4	T49.4X5	T49.4X6
Floxuridine	T45.1X1	T45.1X2	T45.1X3	T45.1X4	T45.1X5	T45.1X6
Fluanisone	T43.4X1	T43.4X2	T43.4X3	T43.4X4	T43.4X5	T43.4X6
Flubendazole	T37.4X1	T37.4X2	T37.4X3	T37.4X4	T37.4X5	T37.4X6
Fluclorolone acetonide	T49.0X1	T49.0X2	T49.0X3	T49.0X4	T49.0X5	T49.0X6
Flucloxacillin	T36.0X1	T36.0X2	T36.0X3	T36.0X4	T36.0X5	T36.0X6
Fluconazole	T37.8X1	T37.8X2	T37.8X3	T37.8X4	T37.8X5	T37.8X6
Flucytosine	T37.8X1	T37.8X2	T37.8X3	T37.8X4	T37.8X5	T37.8X6

Subterms under main terms may continue to next column or page   Additional Character May Be Required — Refer to the Tabular List for Character Selection   369

Etinodiol — Flucytosine

Substance	Poisoning, Accidental (unintentional)	Poisoning, Intentional Self-harm	Poisoning, Assault	Poisoning, Undetermined	Adverse Effect	Under-dosing
Fludeoxyglucose (18F)	T50.8X1	T50.8X2	T50.8X3	T50.8X4	T50.8X5	T50.8X6
Fludiazepam	T42.4X1	T42.4X2	T42.4X3	T42.4X4	T42.4X5	T42.4X6
Fludrocortisone	T50.0X1	T50.0X2	T50.0X3	T50.0X4	T50.0X5	T50.0X6
ENT agent	T49.6X1	T49.6X2	T49.6X3	T49.6X4	T49.6X5	T49.6X6
ophthalmic preparation	T49.5X1	T49.5X2	T49.5X3	T49.5X4	T49.5X5	T49.5X6
topical NEC	T49.0X1	T49.0X2	T49.0X3	T49.0X4	T49.0X5	T49.0X6
Fludroxycortide	T49.0X1	T49.0X2	T49.0X3	T49.0X4	T49.0X5	T49.0X6
Flufenamic acid	T39.391	T39.392	T39.393	T39.394	T39.395	T39.396
Fluindione	T45.511	T45.512	T45.513	T45.514	T45.515	T45.516
Flumequine	T37.8X1	T37.8X2	T37.8X3	T37.8X4	T37.8X5	T37.8X6
Flumethasone	T49.0X1	T49.0X2	T49.0X3	T49.0X4	T49.0X5	T49.0X6
Flumethiazide	T50.2X1	T50.2X2	T50.2X3	T50.2X4	T50.2X5	T50.2X6
Flumidin	T37.5X1	T37.5X2	T37.5X3	T37.5X4	T37.5X5	T37.5X6
Flunarizine	T46.7X1	T46.7X2	T46.7X3	T46.7X4	T46.7X5	T46.7X6
Flunidazole	T37.8X1	T37.8X2	T37.8X3	T37.8X4	T37.8X5	T37.8X6
Flunisolide	T48.6X1	T48.6X2	T48.6X3	T48.6X4	T48.6X5	T48.6X6
Flunitrazepam	T42.4X1	T42.4X2	T42.4X3	T42.4X4	T42.4X5	T42.4X6
Fluocinolone (acetonide)	T49.0X1	T49.0X2	T49.0X3	T49.0X4	T49.0X5	T49.0X6
Fluocinonide	T49.0X1	T49.0X2	T49.0X3	T49.0X4	T49.0X5	T49.0X6
Fluocortin (butyl)	T49.0X1	T49.0X2	T49.0X3	T49.0X4	T49.0X5	T49.0X6
Fluocortolone	T49.0X1	T49.0X2	T49.0X3	T49.0X4	T49.0X5	T49.0X6
Fluohydrocortisone	T38.0X1	T38.0X2	T38.0X3	T38.0X4	T38.0X5	T38.0X6
ENT agent	T49.6X1	T49.6X2	T49.6X3	T49.6X4	T49.6X5	T49.6X6
ophthalmic preparation	T49.5X1	T49.5X2	T49.5X3	T49.5X4	T49.5X5	T49.5X6
topical NEC	T49.0X1	T49.0X2	T49.0X3	T49.0X4	T49.0X5	T49.0X6
Fluonid	T49.0X1	T49.0X2	T49.0X3	T49.0X4	T49.0X5	T49.0X6
Fluopromazine	T43.3X1	T43.3X2	T43.3X3	T43.3X4	T43.3X5	T43.3X6
Fluoracetate	T60.8X1	T60.8X2	T60.8X3	T60.8X4	—	—
Fluorescein	T50.8X1	T50.8X2	T50.8X3	T50.8X4	T50.8X5	T50.8X6
Fluorhydrocortisone	T50.0X1	T50.0X2	T50.0X3	T50.0X4	T50.0X5	T50.0X6
Fluoride (nonmedicinal) (pesticide) (sodium) NEC	T60.8X1	T60.8X2	T60.8X3	T60.8X4	—	—
hydrogen — see Hydrofluoric acid						
medicinal NEC	T50.991	T50.992	T50.993	T50.994	T50.995	T50.996
dental use	T49.7X1	T49.7X2	T49.7X3	T49.7X4	T49.7X5	T49.7X6
not pesticide NEC	T54.91	T54.92	T54.93	T54.94	—	—
stannous	T49.7X1	T49.7X2	T49.7X3	T49.7X4	T49.7X5	T49.7X6
Fluorinated corticosteroids	T38.0X1	T38.0X2	T38.0X3	T38.0X4	T38.0X5	T38.0X6
Fluorine (gas)	T59.5X1	T59.5X2	T59.5X3	T59.5X4	—	—
salt — see Fluoride(s)						
Fluoristan	T49.7X1	T49.7X2	T49.7X3	T49.7X4	T49.7X5	T49.7X6
Fluormetholone	T49.0X1	T49.0X2	T49.0X3	T49.0X4	T49.0X5	T49.0X6
Fluoroacetate	T60.8X1	T60.8X2	T60.8X3	T60.8X4	—	—
Fluorocarbon monomer	T53.6X1	T53.6X2	T53.6X3	T53.6X4	—	—
Fluorocytosine	T37.8X1	T37.8X2	T37.8X3	T37.8X4	T37.8X5	T37.8X6
Fluorodeoxyuridine	T45.1X1	T45.1X2	T45.1X3	T45.1X4	T45.1X5	T45.1X6
Fluorometholone	T49.0X1	T49.0X2	T49.0X3	T49.0X4	T49.0X5	T49.0X6
ophthalmic preparation	T49.5X1	T49.5X2	T49.5X3	T49.5X4	T49.5X5	T49.5X6
Fluorophosphate insecticide	T60.0X1	T60.0X2	T60.0X3	T60.0X4	—	—
Fluorosol	T46.3X1	T46.3X2	T46.3X3	T46.3X4	T46.3X5	T46.3X6
Fluorouracil	T45.1X1	T45.1X2	T45.1X3	T45.1X4	T45.1X5	T45.1X6
Fluorphenylalanine	T49.5X1	T49.5X2	T49.5X3	T49.5X4	T49.5X5	T49.5X6
Fluothane	T41.0X1	T41.0X2	T41.0X3	T41.0X4	T41.0X5	T41.0X6
Fluoxetine	T43.221	T43.222	T43.223	T43.224	T43.225	T43.226
Fluoxymesterone	T38.7X1	T38.7X2	T38.7X3	T38.7X4	T38.7X5	T38.7X6
Flupenthixol	T43.4X1	T43.4X2	T43.4X3	T43.4X4	T43.4X5	T43.4X6
Flupentixol	T43.4X1	T43.4X2	T43.4X3	T43.4X4	T43.4X5	T43.4X6
Fluphenazine	T43.3X1	T43.3X2	T43.3X3	T43.3X4	T43.3X5	T43.3X6
Fluprednidene	T49.0X1	T49.0X2	T49.0X3	T49.0X4	T49.0X5	T49.0X6
Fluprednisolone	T38.0X1	T38.0X2	T38.0X3	T38.0X4	T38.0X5	T38.0X6
Fluradoline	T39.8X1	T39.8X2	T39.8X3	T39.8X4	T39.8X5	T39.8X6
Flurandrenolide	T49.0X1	T49.0X2	T49.0X3	T49.0X4	T49.0X5	T49.0X6
Flurandrenolone	T49.0X1	T49.0X2	T49.0X3	T49.0X4	T49.0X5	T49.0X6
Flurazepam	T42.4X1	T42.4X2	T42.4X3	T42.4X4	T42.4X5	T42.4X6
Flurbiprofen	T39.311	T39.312	T39.313	T39.314	T39.315	T39.316
Flurobate	T49.0X1	T49.0X2	T49.0X3	T49.0X4	T49.0X5	T49.0X6
Fluroxene	T41.0X1	T41.0X2	T41.0X3	T41.0X4	T41.0X5	T41.0X6
Fluspirilene	T43.591	T43.592	T43.593	T43.594	T43.595	T43.596
Flutamide	T38.6X1	T38.6X2	T38.6X3	T38.6X4	T38.6X5	T38.6X6
Flutazolam	T38.0X1	T38.0X2	T38.0X3	T38.0X4	T38.0X5	T38.0X6
Fluticasone propionate	T38.0X1	T38.0X2	T38.0X3	T38.0X4	T38.0X5	T38.0X6
Flutoprazepam	T42.4X1	T42.4X2	T42.4X3	T42.4X4	T42.4X5	T42.4X6
Flutropium bromide	T48.6X1	T48.6X2	T48.6X3	T48.6X4	T48.6X5	T48.6X6
Fluvoxamine	T43.221	T43.222	T43.223	T43.224	T43.225	T43.226
Folacin	T45.8X1	T45.8X2	T45.8X3	T45.8X4	T45.8X5	T45.8X6
Folic acid	T45.8X1	T45.8X2	T45.8X3	T45.8X4	T45.8X5	T45.8X6
with ferrous salt	T45.2X1	T45.2X2	T45.2X3	T45.2X4	T45.2X5	T45.2X6
antagonist	T45.1X1	T45.1X2	T45.1X3	T45.1X4	T45.1X5	T45.1X6
Folinic acid	T45.8X1	T45.8X2	T45.8X3	T45.8X4	T45.8X5	T45.8X6
Folium stramoniae	T48.6X1	T48.6X2	T48.6X3	T48.6X4	T48.6X5	T48.6X6

Substance	Poisoning, Accidental (unintentional)	Poisoning, Intentional Self-harm	Poisoning, Assault	Poisoning, Undetermined	Adverse Effect	Under-dosing
Follicle-stimulating hormone, human	T38.811	T38.812	T38.813	T38.814	T38.815	T38.816
Folpet	T60.3X1	T60.3X2	T60.3X3	T60.3X4	—	—
Fominoben	T48.3X1	T48.3X2	T48.3X3	T48.3X4	T48.3X5	T48.3X6
Food, foodstuffs, noxious, nonbacterial, NEC	T62.91	T62.92	T62.93	T62.94	—	—
berries	T62.1X1	T62.1X2	T62.1X3	T62.1X4	—	—
fish — see also Fish	T62.0X1	T62.0X2	T62.0X3	T62.0X4	—	—
mushrooms	T62.0X1	T62.0X2	T62.0X3	T62.0X4	—	—
plants	T62.2X1	T62.2X2	T62.2X3	T62.2X4	—	—
seafood	T61.91	T61.92	T61.93	T61.94	—	—
specified NEC	T61.8X1	T61.8X2	T61.8X3	T61.8X4	—	—
seeds	T62.2X1	T62.2X2	T62.2X3	T62.2X4	—	—
shellfish	T61.781	T61.782	T61.783	T61.784	—	—
specified NEC	T62.8X1	T62.8X2	T62.8X3	T62.8X4	—	—
Fool's parsley	T62.2X1	T62.2X2	T62.2X3	T62.2X4	—	—
Formaldehyde (solution), gas or vapor	T59.2X1	T59.2X2	T59.2X3	T59.2X4	—	—
fungicide	T60.3X1	T60.3X2	T60.3X3	T60.3X4	—	—
Formalin	T59.2X1	T59.2X2	T59.2X3	T59.2X4	—	—
fungicide	T60.3X1	T60.3X2	T60.3X3	T60.3X4	—	—
vapor	T59.2X1	T59.2X2	T59.2X3	T59.2X4	—	—
Formic acid	T54.2X1	T54.2X2	T54.2X3	T54.2X4	—	—
vapor	T59.891	T59.892	T59.893	T59.894	—	—
Foscarnet sodium	T37.5X1	T37.5X2	T37.5X3	T37.5X4	T37.5X5	T37.5X6
Fosfestrol	T38.5X1	T38.5X2	T38.5X3	T38.5X4	T38.5X5	T38.5X6
Fosfomycin	T36.8X1	T36.8X2	T36.8X3	T36.8X4	T36.8X5	T36.8X6
Fosfonet sodium	T37.5X1	T37.5X2	T37.5X3	T37.5X4	T37.5X5	T37.5X6
Fosinopril	T46.4X1	T46.4X2	T46.4X3	T46.4X4	T46.4X5	T46.4X6
sodium	T46.4X1	T46.4X2	T46.4X3	T46.4X4	T46.4X5	T46.4X6
Fowler's solution	T57.0X1	T57.0X2	T57.0X3	T57.0X4	—	—
Foxglove	T62.2X1	T62.2X2	T62.2X3	T62.2X4	—	—
Framycetin	T36.5X1	T36.5X2	T36.5X3	T36.5X4	T36.5X5	T36.5X6
Frangula	T47.2X1	T47.2X2	T47.2X3	T47.2X4	T47.2X5	T47.2X6
extract	T47.2X1	T47.2X2	T47.2X3	T47.2X4	T47.2X5	T47.2X6
Frei antigen	T50.8X1	T50.8X2	T50.8X3	T50.8X4	T50.8X5	T50.8X6
Freon	T53.5X1	T53.5X2	T53.5X3	T53.5X4	—	—
Fructose	T50.3X1	T50.3X2	T50.3X3	T50.3X4	T50.3X5	T50.3X6
Frusemide	T50.1X1	T50.1X2	T50.1X3	T50.1X4	T50.1X5	T50.1X6
FSH	T38.811	T38.812	T38.813	T38.814	T38.815	T38.816
Ftorafur	T45.1X1	T45.1X2	T45.1X3	T45.1X4	T45.1X5	T45.1X6
Fuel						
automobile	T52.0X1	T52.0X2	T52.0X3	T52.0X4	—	—
exhaust gas, not in transit	T58.01	T58.02	T58.03	T58.04		
vapor NEC	T52.0X1	T52.0X2	T52.0X3	T52.0X4	—	—
gas (domestic use) — see also Carbon, monoxide, fuel, utility	T59.891	T59.892	T59.893	T59.894		
utility	T59.891	T59.892	T59.893	T59.894		
incomplete combustion of — see Carbon, monoxide, fuel, utility						
in mobile container	T59.891	T59.892	T59.893	T59.894		
piped (natural)	T59.891	T59.892	T59.893	T59.894		
industrial, incomplete combustion	T58.8X1	T58.8X2	T58.8X3	T58.8X4		
Fugillin	T36.8X1	T36.8X2	T36.8X3	T36.8X4	T36.8X5	T36.8X6
Fulminate of mercury	T56.1X1	T56.1X2	T56.1X3	T56.1X4		
Fulvicin	T36.7X1	T36.7X2	T36.7X3	T36.7X4	T36.7X5	T36.7X6
Fumadil	T36.8X1	T36.8X2	T36.8X3	T36.8X4	T36.8X5	T36.8X6
Fumagillin	T36.8X1	T36.8X2	T36.8X3	T36.8X4	T36.8X5	T36.8X6
Fumaric acid	T49.4X1	T49.4X2	T49.4X3	T49.4X4	T49.4X5	T49.4X6
Fumes (from)	T59.91	T59.92	T59.93	T59.94	—	—
carbon monoxide — see Carbon, monoxide						
charcoal (domestic use) — see Charcoal, fumes						
chloroform — see Chloroform						
coke (in domestic stoves, fireplaces) — see Coke fumes						
corrosive NEC	T54.91	T54.92	T54.93	T54.94	—	—
ether — see ether						
freons	T53.5X1	T53.5X2	T53.5X3	T53.5X4	—	—
hydrocarbons	T59.891	T59.892	T59.893	T59.894	—	—
petroleum (liquefied)	T59.891	T59.892	T59.893	T59.894	—	—
distributed through pipes (pure or mixed with air)	T59.891	T59.892	T59.893	T59.894	—	—
lead — see lead						
metal — see Metals, or the specified metal						

Additional Character May Be Required — Refer to the Tabular List for Character Selection ▽ Subterms under main terms may continue to next column or page

Substance	Poisoning, Accidental (unintentional)	Poisoning, Intentional Self-harm	Poisoning, Assault	Poisoning, Undetermined	Adverse Effect	Under-dosing
Fumes — continued						
nitrogen dioxide	T59.0X1	T59.0X2	T59.0X3	T59.0X4	—	—
pesticides — see Pesticides						
petroleum (liquefied)	T59.891	T59.892	T59.893	T59.894	—	—
distributed through pipes (pure or mixed with air)	T59.891	T59.892	T59.893	T59.894	—	—
polyester	T59.891	T59.892	T59.893	T59.894	—	—
specified source NEC — see also substance specified	T59.891	T59.892	T59.893	T59.894	—	—
sulfur dioxide	T59.1X1	T59.1X2	T59.1X3	T59.1X4	—	—
Fumigant NEC	T60.91	T60.92	T60.93	T60.94	—	—
Fungicide NEC (nonmedicinal)	T60.3X1	T60.3X2	T60.3X3	T60.3X4	—	—
Fungi, noxious, used as food	T62.0X1	T62.0X2	T62.0X3	T62.0X4	—	—
Fungizone	T36.7X1	T36.7X2	T36.7X3	T36.7X4	T36.7X5	T36.7X6
topical	T49.0X1	T49.0X2	T49.0X3	T49.0X4	T49.0X5	T49.0X6
Furacin	T49.0X1	T49.0X2	T49.0X3	T49.0X4	T49.0X5	T49.0X6
Furadantin	T37.91	T37.92	T37.93	T37.94	T37.95	T37.96
Furazolidone	T37.8X1	T37.8X2	T37.8X3	T37.8X4	T37.8X5	T37.8X6
Furazolium chloride	T49.0X1	T49.0X2	T49.0X3	T49.0X4	T49.0X5	T49.0X6
Furfural	T52.8X1	T52.8X2	T52.8X3	T52.8X4	—	—
Furnace (coal burning) (domestic), gas from	T58.2X1	T58.2X2	T58.2X3	T58.2X4	—	—
industrial	T58.8X1	T58.8X2	T58.8X3	T58.8X4	—	—
Furniture polish	T65.891	T65.892	T65.893	T65.894	—	—
Furosemide	T50.1X1	T50.1X2	T50.1X3	T50.1X4	T50.1X5	T50.1X6
Furoxone	T37.91	T37.92	T37.93	T37.94	T37.95	T37.96
Fursultiamine	T45.2X1	T45.2X2	T45.2X3	T45.2X4	T45.2X5	T45.2X6
Fusafungine	T36.8X1	T36.8X2	T36.8X3	T36.8X4	T36.8X5	T36.8X6
Fusel oil (any) (amyl) (butyl) (propyl), vapor	T51.3X1	T51.3X2	T51.3X3	T51.3X4	—	—
Fusidate (ethanolamine) (sodium)	T36.8X1	T36.8X2	T36.8X3	T36.8X4	T36.8X5	T36.8X6
Fusidic acid	T36.8X1	T36.8X2	T36.8X3	T36.8X4	T36.8X5	T36.8X6
Fytic acid, nonasodium	T50.6X1	T50.6X2	T50.6X3	T50.6X4	T50.6X5	T50.6X6
b-Galactosidase	T47.5X1	T47.5X2	T47.5X3	T47.5X4	T47.5X5	T47.5X6
GABA	T43.8X1	T43.8X2	T43.8X3	T43.8X4	T43.8X5	T43.8X6
Gadopentetic acid	T50.8X1	T50.8X2	T50.8X3	T50.8X4	T50.8X5	T50.8X6
Galactose	T50.3X1	T50.3X2	T50.3X3	T50.3X4	T50.3X5	T50.3X6
Galantamine	T44.0X1	T44.0X2	T44.0X3	T44.0X4	T44.0X5	T44.0X6
Gallamine (triethiodide)	T48.1X1	T48.1X2	T48.1X3	T48.1X4	T48.1X5	T48.1X6
Gallium citrate	T50.991	T50.992	T50.993	T50.994	T50.995	T50.996
Gallopamil	T46.1X1	T46.1X2	T46.1X3	T46.1X4	T46.1X5	T46.1X6
Gamboge	T47.2X1	T47.2X2	T47.2X3	T47.2X4	T47.2X5	T47.2X6
Gamimune	T50.Z11	T50.Z12	T50.Z13	T50.Z14	T50.Z15	T50.Z16
Gamma-aminobutyric acid	T43.8X1	T43.8X2	T43.8X3	T43.8X4	T43.8X5	T43.8X6
Gamma-benzene hexachloride (medicinal)	T49.0X1	T49.0X2	T49.0X3	T49.0X4	T49.0X5	T49.0X6
nonmedicinal, vapor	T53.6X1	T53.6X2	T53.6X3	T53.6X4	—	—
Gamma-BHC (medicinal) — see also Gamma-benzene hexachloride	T49.0X1	T49.0X2	T49.0X3	T49.0X4	T49.0X5	T49.0X6
Gamma globulin	T50.Z11	T50.Z12	T50.Z13	T50.Z14	T50.Z15	T50.Z16
Gamulin	T50.Z11	T50.Z12	T50.Z13	T50.Z14	T50.Z15	T50.Z16
Ganciclovir (sodium)	T37.5X1	T37.5X2	T37.5X3	T37.5X4	T37.5X5	T37.5X6
Ganglionic blocking drug NEC	T44.2X1	T44.2X2	T44.2X3	T44.2X4	T44.2X5	T44.2X6
specified NEC	T44.2X1	T44.2X2	T44.2X3	T44.2X4	T44.2X5	T44.2X6
Ganja	T40.7X1	T40.7X2	T40.7X3	T40.7X4	T40.7X5	T40.7X6
Garamycin	T36.5X1	T36.5X2	T36.5X3	T36.5X4	T36.5X5	T36.5X6
ophthalmic preparation	T49.5X1	T49.5X2	T49.5X3	T49.5X4	T49.5X5	T49.5X6
topical NEC	T49.0X1	T49.0X2	T49.0X3	T49.0X4	T49.0X5	T49.0X6
Gardenal	T42.3X1	T42.3X2	T42.3X3	T42.3X4	T42.3X5	T42.3X6
Gardepanyl	T42.3X1	T42.3X2	T42.3X3	T42.3X4	T42.3X5	T42.3X6
Gaseous substance — see Gas						
Gasoline	T52.0X1	T52.0X2	T52.0X3	T52.0X4	—	—
vapor	T52.0X1	T52.0X2	T52.0X3	T52.0X4	—	—
Gastric enzymes	T47.5X1	T47.5X2	T47.5X3	T47.5X4	T47.5X5	T47.5X6
Gastrografin	T50.8X1	T50.8X2	T50.8X3	T50.8X4	T50.8X5	T50.8X6
Gastrointestinal drug	T47.91	T47.92	T47.93	T47.94	T47.95	T47.96
biological	T47.8X1	T47.8X2	T47.8X3	T47.8X4	T47.8X5	T47.8X6
specified NEC	T47.8X1	T47.8X2	T47.8X3	T47.8X4	T47.8X5	T47.8X6
Gas NEC	T59.91	T59.92	T59.93	T59.94	—	—
acetylene	T59.891	T59.892	T59.893	T59.894	—	—
incomplete combustion of	T58.11	T58.12	T58.13	T58.14	—	—
air contaminants, source or type not specified	T59.91	T59.92	T59.93	T59.94	—	—
anesthetic	T41.0X1	T41.0X2	T41.0X3	T41.0X4	T41.0X5	T41.0X6
blast furnace	T58.8X1	T58.8X2	T58.8X3	T58.8X4	—	—
butane — see butane						
Gas — continued						
carbon monoxide — see Carbon, monoxide						
chlorine	T59.4X1	T59.4X2	T59.4X3	T59.4X4	—	—
coal	T58.2X1	T58.2X2	T58.2X3	T58.2X4	—	—
cyanide	T57.3X1	T57.3X2	T57.3X3	T57.3X4	—	—
dicyanogen	T65.0X1	T65.0X2	T65.0X3	T65.0X4	—	—
domestic — see Domestic gas						
exhaust	T58.01	T58.02	T58.03	T58.04	—	—
from utility (for cooking, heating, or lighting) (after combustion) — see Carbon, monoxide, fuel, utility						
prior to combustion	T59.891	T59.892	T59.893	T59.894	—	—
from wood- or coal-burning stove or fireplace	T58.2X1	T58.2X2	T58.2X3	T58.2X4	—	—
fuel (domestic use) (after combustion) — see also Carbon, monoxide, fuel						
industrial use	T58.8X1	T58.8X2	T58.8X3	T58.8X4	—	—
prior to combustion	T59.891	T59.892	T59.893	T59.894	—	—
utility	T59.891	T59.892	T59.893	T59.894	—	—
incomplete combustion of — see Carbon, monoxide, fuel, utility						
in mobile container	T59.891	T59.892	T59.893	T59.894	—	—
piped (natural)	T59.891	T59.892	T59.893	T59.894	—	—
garage	T58.01	T58.02	T58.03	T58.04	—	—
hydrocarbon NEC	T59.891	T59.892	T59.893	T59.894	—	—
incomplete combustion of — see Carbon, monoxide, fuel, utility						
liquefied — see butane						
piped	T59.891	T59.892	T59.893	T59.894	—	—
hydrocyanic acid	T65.0X1	T65.0X2	T65.0X3	T65.0X4	—	—
illuminating (after combustion)	T58.11	T58.12	T58.13	T58.14	—	—
prior to combustion	T59.891	T59.892	T59.893	T59.894	—	—
incomplete combustion, any — see Carbon, monoxide						
kiln	T58.8X1	T58.8X2	T58.8X3	T58.8X4	—	—
lacrimogenic	T59.3X1	T59.3X2	T59.3X3	T59.3X4	—	—
liquefied petroleum — see butane						
marsh	T59.891	T59.892	T59.893	T59.894	—	—
motor exhaust, not in transit	T58.01	T58.02	T58.03	T58.04	—	—
mustard, not in war	T59.891	T59.892	T59.893	T59.894	—	—
natural	T59.891	T59.892	T59.893	T59.894	—	—
nerve, not in war	T59.91	T59.92	T59.93	T59.94	—	—
oil	T52.0X1	T52.0X2	T52.0X3	T52.0X4	—	—
petroleum (liquefied) (distributed in mobile containers)	T59.891	T59.892	T59.893	T59.894	—	—
piped (pure or mixed with air)	T59.891	T59.892	T59.893	T59.894	—	—
piped (manufactured) (natural) NEC	T59.891	T59.892	T59.893	T59.894	—	—
producer	T58.8X1	T58.8X2	T58.8X3	T58.8X4	—	—
propane — see propane						
refrigerant (chlorofluoro-carbon)	T53.5X1	T53.5X2	T53.5X3	T53.5X4	—	—
not chlorofluoro-carbon	T59.891	T59.892	T59.893	T59.894	—	—
sewer	T59.91	T59.92	T59.93	T59.94	—	—
specified source NEC	T59.91	T59.92	T59.93	T59.94	—	—
stove (after combustion)	T58.11	T58.12	T58.13	T58.14	—	—
prior to combustion	T59.891	T59.892	T59.893	T59.894	—	—
tear	T59.3X1	T59.3X2	T59.3X3	T59.3X4	—	—
therapeutic	T41.5X1	T41.5X2	T41.5X3	T41.5X4	T41.5X5	T41.5X6
utility (for cooking, heating, or lighting) (piped) NEC	T59.891	T59.892	T59.893	T59.894	—	—
incomplete combustion of — see Carbon, monoxide, fuel, utilty						
in mobile container	T59.891	T59.892	T59.893	T59.894	—	—
piped (natural)	T59.891	T59.892	T59.893	T59.894	—	—
water	T58.11	T58.12	T58.13	T58.14	—	—
incomplete combustion of — see Carbon, monoxide, fuel, utility						
Gaultheria procumbens	T62.2X1	T62.2X2	T62.2X3	T62.2X4	—	—
Gefarnate	T44.3X1	T44.3X2	T44.3X3	T44.3X4	T44.3X5	T44.3X6
Gelatin (intravenous)	T45.8X1	T45.8X2	T45.8X3	T45.8X4	T45.8X5	T45.8X6

Subterms under main terms may continue to next column or page

Additional Character May Be Required — Refer to the Tabular List for Character Selection

Table of Drugs and Chemicals

Gelatin — Hedaquinium

Substance	Poisoning, Accidental (unintentional)	Poisoning, Intentional Self-harm	Poisoning, Assault	Poisoning, Undetermined	Adverse Effect	Under-dosing
Gelatin — continued						
absorbable (sponge)	T45.7X1	T45.7X2	T45.7X3	T45.7X4	T45.7X5	T45.7X6
Gelfilm	T49.8X1	T49.8X2	T49.8X3	T49.8X4	T49.8X5	T49.8X6
Gelfoam	T45.7X1	T45.7X2	T45.7X3	T45.7X4	T45.7X5	T45.7X6
Gelsemine	T50.991	T50.992	T50.993	T50.994	T50.995	T50.996
Gelsemium (sempervirens)	T62.2X1	T62.2X2	T62.2X3	T62.2X4		
Gemeprost	T48.0X1	T48.0X2	T48.0X3	T48.0X4	T48.0X5	T48.0X6
Gemfibrozil	T46.6X1	T46.6X2	T46.6X3	T46.6X4	T46.6X5	T46.6X6
Gemonil	T42.3X1	T42.3X2	T42.3X3	T42.3X4	T42.3X5	T42.3X6
Gentamicin	T36.5X1	T36.5X2	T36.5X3	T36.5X4	T36.5X5	T36.5X6
ophthalmic preparation	T49.5X1	T49.5X2	T49.5X3	T49.5X4	T49.5X5	T49.5X6
topical NEC	T49.0X1	T49.0X2	T49.0X3	T49.0X4	T49.0X5	T49.0X6
Gentian	T47.5X1	T47.5X2	T47.5X3	T47.5X4	T47.5X5	T47.5X6
violet	T49.0X1	T49.0X2	T49.0X3	T49.0X4	T49.0X5	T49.0X6
Gepefrine	T44.4X1	T44.4X2	T44.4X3	T44.4X4	T44.4X5	T44.4X6
Gestonorone caproate	T38.5X1	T38.5X2	T38.5X3	T38.5X4	T38.5X5	T38.5X6
Gexane	T49.0X1	T49.0X2	T49.0X3	T49.0X4	T49.0X5	T49.0X6
Gila monster (venom)	T63.111	T63.112	T63.113	T63.114	—	—
Ginger	T47.5X1	T47.5X2	T47.5X3	T47.5X4	T47.5X5	T47.5X6
Jamaica — see Jamaica, ginger						
Gitalin	T46.0X1	T46.0X2	T46.0X3	T46.0X4	T46.0X5	T46.0X6
amorphous	T46.0X1	T46.0X2	T46.0X3	T46.0X4	T46.0X5	T46.0X6
Gitaloxin	T46.0X1	T46.0X2	T46.0X3	T46.0X4	T46.0X5	T46.0X6
Gitoxin	T46.0X1	T46.0X2	T46.0X3	T46.0X4	T46.0X5	T46.0X6
Glafenine	T39.8X1	T39.8X2	T39.8X3	T39.8X4	T39.8X5	T39.8X6
Glandular extract (medicinal) NEC	T50.Z91	T50.Z92	T50.Z93	T50.Z94	T50.Z95	T50.Z96
Glaucarubin	T37.3X1	T37.3X2	T37.3X3	T37.3X4	T37.3X5	T37.3X6
Glibenclamide	T38.3X1	T38.3X2	T38.3X3	T38.3X4	T38.3X5	T38.3X6
Glibornuride	T38.3X1	T38.3X2	T38.3X3	T38.3X4	T38.3X5	T38.3X6
Gliclazide	T38.3X1	T38.3X2	T38.3X3	T38.3X4	T38.3X5	T38.3X6
Glimidine	T38.3X1	T38.3X2	T38.3X3	T38.3X4	T38.3X5	T38.3X6
Glipizide	T38.3X1	T38.3X2	T38.3X3	T38.3X4	T38.3X5	T38.3X6
Gliquidone	T38.3X1	T38.3X2	T38.3X3	T38.3X4	T38.3X5	T38.3X6
Glisolamide	T38.3X1	T38.3X2	T38.3X3	T38.3X4	T38.3X5	T38.3X6
Glisoxepide	T38.3X1	T38.3X2	T38.3X3	T38.3X4	T38.3X5	T38.3X6
Globin zinc insulin	T38.3X1	T38.3X2	T38.3X3	T38.3X4	T38.3X5	T38.3X6
Globulin						
antilymphocytic	T50.Z11	T50.Z12	T50.Z13	T50.Z14	T50.Z15	T50.Z16
antirhesus	T50.Z11	T50.Z12	T50.Z13	T50.Z14	T50.Z15	T50.Z16
antivenin	T50.Z11	T50.Z12	T50.Z13	T50.Z14	T50.Z15	T50.Z16
antiviral	T50.Z11	T50.Z12	T50.Z13	T50.Z14	T50.Z15	T50.Z16
Glucagon	T38.3X1	T38.3X2	T38.3X3	T38.3X4	T38.3X5	T38.3X6
Glucocorticoids	T38.0X1	T38.0X2	T38.0X3	T38.0X4	T38.0X5	T38.0X6
Glucocorticosteroid	T38.0X1	T38.0X2	T38.0X3	T38.0X4	T38.0X5	T38.0X6
Gluconic acid	T50.991	T50.992	T50.993	T50.994	T50.995	T50.996
Glucosamine sulfate	T39.4X1	T39.4X2	T39.4X3	T39.4X4	T39.4X5	T39.4X6
Glucose	T50.3X1	T50.3X2	T50.3X3	T50.3X4	T50.3X5	T50.3X6
with sodium chloride	T50.3X1	T50.3X2	T50.3X3	T50.3X4	T50.3X5	T50.3X6
Glucosulfone sodium	T37.1X1	T37.1X2	T37.1X3	T37.1X4	T37.1X5	T37.1X6
Glucurolactone	T47.8X1	T47.8X2	T47.8X3	T47.8X4	T47.8X5	T47.8X6
Glue NEC	T52.8X1	T52.8X2	T52.8X3	T52.8X4	—	—
Glutamic acid	T47.5X1	T47.5X2	T47.5X3	T47.5X4	T47.5X5	T47.5X6
Glutaral (medicinal)	T49.0X1	T49.0X2	T49.0X3	T49.0X4	T49.0X5	T49.0X6
nonmedicinal	T65.891	T65.892	T65.893	T65.894	—	—
Glutaraldehyde (nonmedicinal)	T65.891	T65.892	T65.893	T65.894	—	—
medicinal	T49.0X1	T49.0X2	T49.0X3	T49.0X4	T49.0X5	T49.0X6
Glutathione	T50.6X1	T50.6X2	T50.6X3	T50.6X4	T50.6X5	T50.6X6
Glutethimide	T42.6X1	T42.6X2	T42.6X3	T42.6X4	T42.6X5	T42.6X6
Glyburide	T38.3X1	T38.3X2	T38.3X3	T38.3X4	T38.3X5	T38.3X6
Glycerin	T47.4X1	T47.4X2	T47.4X3	T47.4X4	T47.4X5	T47.4X6
Glycerol	T47.4X1	T47.4X2	T47.4X3	T47.4X4	T47.4X5	T47.4X6
borax	T49.6X1	T49.6X2	T49.6X3	T49.6X4	T49.6X5	T49.6X6
intravenous	T50.3X1	T50.3X2	T50.3X3	T50.3X4	T50.3X5	T50.3X6
iodinated	T48.4X1	T48.4X2	T48.4X3	T48.4X4	T48.4X5	T48.4X6
Glycerophosphate	T50.991	T50.992	T50.993	T50.994	T50.995	T50.996
Glyceryl						
gualacolate	T48.4X1	T48.4X2	T48.4X3	T48.4X4	T48.4X5	T48.4X6
nitrate	T46.3X1	T46.3X2	T46.3X3	T46.3X4	T46.3X5	T46.3X6
triacetate (topical)	T49.0X1	T49.0X2	T49.0X3	T49.0X4	T49.0X5	T49.0X6
trinitrate	T46.3X1	T46.3X2	T46.3X3	T46.3X4	T46.3X5	T46.3X6
Glycine	T50.3X1	T50.3X2	T50.3X3	T50.3X4	T50.3X5	T50.3X6
Glyclopyramide	T38.3X1	T38.3X2	T38.3X3	T38.3X4	T38.3X5	T38.3X6
Glycobiarsol	T37.3X1	T37.3X2	T37.3X3	T37.3X4	T37.3X5	T37.3X6
Glycols (ether)	T52.3X1	T52.3X2	T52.3X3	T52.3X4	—	—
Glyconiazide	T37.1X1	T37.1X2	T37.1X3	T37.1X4	T37.1X5	T37.1X6
Glycopyrrolate	T44.3X1	T44.3X2	T44.3X3	T44.3X4	T44.3X5	T44.3X6
Glycopyrronium	T44.3X1	T44.3X2	T44.3X3	T44.3X4	T44.3X5	T44.3X6
bromide	T44.3X1	T44.3X2	T44.3X3	T44.3X4	T44.3X5	T44.3X6
Glycoside, cardiac (stimulant)	T46.0X1	T46.0X2	T46.0X3	T46.0X4	T46.0X5	T46.0X6
Glycyclamide	T38.3X1	T38.3X2	T38.3X3	T38.3X4	T38.3X5	T38.3X6

Substance	Poisoning, Accidental (unintentional)	Poisoning, Intentional Self-harm	Poisoning, Assault	Poisoning, Undetermined	Adverse Effect	Under-dosing
Glycyrrhiza extract	T48.4X1	T48.4X2	T48.4X3	T48.4X4	T48.4X5	T48.4X6
Glycyrrhizic acid	T48.4X1	T48.4X2	T48.4X3	T48.4X4	T48.4X5	T48.4X6
Glycyrrhizinate potassium	T48.4X1	T48.4X2	T48.4X3	T48.4X4	T48.4X5	T48.4X6
Glymidine sodium	T38.3X1	T38.3X2	T38.3X3	T38.3X4	T38.3X5	T38.3X6
Glyphosate	T60.3X1	T60.3X2	T60.3X3	T60.3X4	—	—
Glyphylline	T48.6X1	T48.6X2	T48.6X3	T48.6X4	T48.6X5	T48.6X6
Gold						
colloidal (I98Au)	T45.1X1	T45.1X2	T45.1X3	T45.1X4	T45.1X5	T45.1X6
salts	T39.4X1	T39.4X2	T39.4X3	T39.4X4	T39.4X5	T39.4X6
Golden sulfide of antimony	T56.891	T56.892	T56.893	T56.894	—	—
Goldylocks	T62.2X1	T62.2X2	T62.2X3	T62.2X4	—	—
Gonadal tissue extract	T38.901	T38.902	T38.903	T38.904	T38.905	T38.906
female	T38.5X1	T38.5X2	T38.5X3	T38.5X4	T38.5X5	T38.5X6
male	T38.7X1	T38.7X2	T38.7X3	T38.7X4	T38.7X5	T38.7X6
Gonadorelin	T38.891	T38.892	T38.893	T38.894	T38.895	T38.896
Gonadotropin	T38.891	T38.892	T38.893	T38.894	T38.895	T38.896
chorionic	T38.891	T38.892	T38.893	T38.894	T38.895	T38.896
pituitary	T38.811	T38.812	T38.813	T38.814	T38.815	T38.816
Goserelin	T45.1X1	T45.1X2	T45.1X3	T45.1X4	T45.1X5	T45.1X6
Grain alcohol	T51.0X1	T51.0X2	T51.0X3	T51.0X4	—	—
Gramicidin	T49.0X1	T49.0X2	T49.0X3	T49.0X4	T49.0X5	T49.0X6
Granisetron	T45.0X1	T45.0X2	T45.0X3	T45.0X4	T45.0X5	T45.0X6
Gratiola officinalis	T62.2X1	T62.2X2	T62.2X3	T62.2X4	—	—
Grease	T65.891	T65.892	T65.893	T65.894	—	—
Green hellebore	T62.2X1	T62.2X2	T62.2X3	T62.2X4	—	—
Green soap	T49.2X1	T49.2X2	T49.2X3	T49.2X4	T49.2X5	T49.2X6
Grifulvin	T36.7X1	T36.7X2	T36.7X3	T36.7X4	T36.7X5	T36.7X6
Griseofulvin	T36.7X1	T36.7X2	T36.7X3	T36.7X4	T36.7X5	T36.7X6
Growth hormone	T38.811	T38.812	T38.813	T38.814	T38.815	T38.816
Guaiacol derivatives	T48.4X1	T48.4X2	T48.4X3	T48.4X4	T48.4X5	T48.4X6
Guaiac reagent	T50.991	T50.992	T50.993	T50.994	T50.995	T50.996
Guaifenesin	T48.4X1	T48.4X2	T48.4X3	T48.4X4	T48.4X5	T48.4X6
Guaimesal	T48.4X1	T48.4X2	T48.4X3	T48.4X4	T48.4X5	T48.4X6
Guaiphenesin	T48.4X1	T48.4X2	T48.4X3	T48.4X4	T48.4X5	T48.4X6
Guamecycline	T36.4X1	T36.4X2	T36.4X3	T36.4X4	T36.4X5	T36.4X6
Guanabenz	T46.5X1	T46.5X2	T46.5X3	T46.5X4	T46.5X5	T46.5X6
Guanacline	T46.5X1	T46.5X2	T46.5X3	T46.5X4	T46.5X5	T46.5X6
Guanadrel	T46.5X1	T46.5X2	T46.5X3	T46.5X4	T46.5X5	T46.5X6
Guanatol	T37.2X1	T37.2X2	T37.2X3	T37.2X4	T37.2X5	T37.2X6
Guanethidine	T46.5X1	T46.5X2	T46.5X3	T46.5X4	T46.5X5	T46.5X6
Guanfacine	T46.5X1	T46.5X2	T46.5X3	T46.5X4	T46.5X5	T46.5X6
Guano	T65.891	T65.892	T65.893	T65.894	—	—
Guanochlor	T46.5X1	T46.5X2	T46.5X3	T46.5X4	T46.5X5	T46.5X6
Guanoclor	T46.5X1	T46.5X2	T46.5X3	T46.5X4	T46.5X5	T46.5X6
Guanoctine	T46.5X1	T46.5X2	T46.5X3	T46.5X4	T46.5X5	T46.5X6
Guanoxabenz	T46.5X1	T46.5X2	T46.5X3	T46.5X4	T46.5X5	T46.5X6
Guanoxan	T46.5X1	T46.5X2	T46.5X3	T46.5X4	T46.5X5	T46.5X6
Guar gum (medicinal)	T46.6X1	T46.6X2	T46.6X3	T46.6X4	T46.6X5	T46.6X6
Hachimycin	T36.7X1	T36.7X2	T36.7X3	T36.7X4	T36.7X5	T36.7X6
Hair						
dye	T49.4X1	T49.4X2	T49.4X3	T49.4X4	T49.4X5	T49.4X6
preparation NEC	T49.4X1	T49.4X2	T49.4X3	T49.4X4	T49.4X5	T49.4X6
Halazepam	T42.4X1	T42.4X2	T42.4X3	T42.4X4	T42.4X5	T42.4X6
Halcinolone	T49.0X1	T49.0X2	T49.0X3	T49.0X4	T49.0X5	T49.0X6
Halcinonide	T49.0X1	T49.0X2	T49.0X3	T49.0X4	T49.0X5	T49.0X6
Halethazole	T49.0X1	T49.0X2	T49.0X3	T49.0X4	T49.0X5	T49.0X6
Hallucinogen NEC	T40.901	T40.902	T40.903	T40.904	T40.905	T40.906
Halofantrine	T37.2X1	T37.2X2	T37.2X3	T37.2X4	T37.2X5	T37.2X6
Halofenate	T46.6X1	T46.6X2	T46.6X3	T46.6X4	T46.6X5	T46.6X6
Halometasone	T49.0X1	T49.0X2	T49.0X3	T49.0X4	T49.0X5	T49.0X6
Haloperidol	T43.4X1	T43.4X2	T43.4X3	T43.4X4	T43.4X5	T43.4X6
Haloprogin	T49.0X1	T49.0X2	T49.0X3	T49.0X4	T49.0X5	T49.0X6
Halotex	T49.0X1	T49.0X2	T49.0X3	T49.0X4	T49.0X5	T49.0X6
Halothane	T41.0X1	T41.0X2	T41.0X3	T41.0X4	T41.0X5	T41.0X6
Haloxazolam	T42.4X1	T42.4X2	T42.4X3	T42.4X4	T42.4X5	T42.4X6
Halquinols	T49.0X1	T49.0X2	T49.0X3	T49.0X4	T49.0X5	T49.0X6
Hamamelis	T49.2X1	T49.2X2	T49.2X3	T49.2X4	T49.2X5	T49.2X6
Haptendextran	T45.8X1	T45.8X2	T45.8X3	T45.8X4	T45.8X5	T45.8X6
Harmonyl	T46.5X1	T46.5X2	T46.5X3	T46.5X4	T46.5X5	T46.5X6
Hartmann's solution	T50.3X1	T50.3X2	T50.3X3	T50.3X4	T50.3X5	T50.3X6
Hashish	T40.7X1	T40.7X2	T40.7X3	T40.7X4	T40.7X5	T40.7X6
Hawaiian Woodrose seeds	T40.991	T40.992	T40.993	T40.994	—	—
HCB	T60.3X1	T60.3X2	T60.3X3	T60.3X4	—	—
HCH	T53.6X1	T53.6X2	T53.6X3	T53.6X4	—	—
medicinal	T49.0X1	T49.0X2	T49.0X3	T49.0X4	T49.0X5	T49.0X6
HCN	T57.3X1	T57.3X2	T57.3X3	T57.3X4	—	—
Headache cures, drugs, powders NEC	T50.901	T50.902	T50.903	T50.904	T50.905	T50.906
Heavenly Blue (morning glory)	T40.991	T40.992	T40.993	T40.994	—	—
Heavy metal antidote	T45.8X1	T45.8X2	T45.8X3	T45.8X4	T45.8X5	T45.8X6
Hedaquinium	T49.0X1	T49.0X2	T49.0X3	T49.0X4	T49.0X5	T49.0X6

Additional Character May Be Required — Refer to the Tabular List for Character Selection

Subterms under main terms may continue to next column or page

Substance	Poisoning, Accidental (unintentional)	Poisoning, Intentional Self-harm	Poisoning, Assault	Poisoning, Undetermined	Adverse Effect	Under-dosing
Hedge hyssop	T62.2X1	T62.2X2	T62.2X3	T62.2X4		
Heet	T49.8X1	T49.8X2	T49.8X3	T49.8X4	T49.8X5	T49.8X6
Helenin	T37.4X1	T37.4X2	T37.4X3	T37.4X4	T37.4X5	T37.4X6
Helium (nonmedicinal) **NEC**	T59.891	T59.892	T59.893	T59.894		
medicinal	T48.991	T48.992	T48.993	T48.994	T48.995	T48.996
Hellebore (black) (green)	T62.2X1	T62.2X2	T62.2X3	T62.2X4		
(white)						
Hematin	T45.8X1	T45.8X2	T45.8X3	T45.8X4	T45.8X5	T45.8X6
Hematinic preparation	T45.8X1	T45.8X2	T45.8X3	T45.8X4	T45.8X5	T45.8X6
Hematological agent	T45.91	T45.92	T45.93	T45.94	T45.95	T45.96
specified NEC	T45.8X1	T45.8X2	T45.8X3	T45.8X4	T45.8X5	T45.8X6
Hemlock	T62.2X1	T62.2X2	T62.2X3	T62.2X4		
Hemostatic	T45.621	T45.622	T45.623	T45.624	T45.625	T45.626
drug, systemic	T45.621	T45.622	T45.623	T45.624	T45.625	T45.626
Hemostyptic	T49.4X1	T49.4X2	T49.4X3	T49.4X4	T49.4X5	T49.4X6
Henbane	T62.2X1	T62.2X2	T62.2X3	T62.2X4		
Heparin (sodium)	T45.511	T45.512	T45.513	T45.514	T45.515	T45.516
action reverser	T45.7X1	T45.7X2	T45.7X3	T45.7X4	T45.7X5	T45.7X6
Heparin-fraction	T45.511	T45.512	T45.513	T45.514	T45.515	T45.516
Heparinoid (systemic)	T45.511	T45.512	T45.513	T45.514	T45.515	T45.516
Hepatic secretion stimulant	T47.8X1	T47.8X2	T47.8X3	T47.8X4	T47.8X5	T47.8X6
Hepatitis B						
immune globulin	T50.Z11	T50.Z12	T50.Z13	T50.Z14	T50.Z15	T50.Z16
vaccine	T50.B91	T50.B92	T50.B93	T50.B94	T50.B95	T50.B96
Hepronicate	T46.7X1	T46.7X2	T46.7X3	T46.7X4	T46.7X5	T46.7X6
Heptabarb	T42.3X1	T42.3X2	T42.3X3	T42.3X4	T42.3X5	T42.3X6
Heptabarbital	T42.3X1	T42.3X2	T42.3X3	T42.3X4	T42.3X5	T42.3X6
Heptabarbitone	T42.3X1	T42.3X2	T42.3X3	T42.3X4	T42.3X5	T42.3X6
Heptachlor	T60.1X1	T60.1X2	T60.1X3	T60.1X4		
Heptalgin	T40.2X1	T40.2X2	T40.2X3	T40.2X4	T40.2X5	T40.2X6
Heptaminol	T46.3X1	T46.3X2	T46.3X3	T46.3X4	T46.3X5	T46.3X6
Herbicide NEC	T60.3X1	T60.3X2	T60.3X3	T60.3X4		
Heroin	T40.1X1	T40.1X2	T40.1X3	T40.1X4		
Herplex	T49.5X1	T49.5X2	T49.5X3	T49.5X4	T49.5X5	T49.5X6
HES	T45.8X1	T45.8X2	T45.8X3	T45.8X4	T45.8X5	T45.8X6
Hesperidin	T46.991	T46.992	T46.993	T46.994	T46.995	T46.996
Hetacillin	T36.0X1	T36.0X2	T36.0X3	T36.0X4	T36.0X5	T36.0X6
Hetastarch	T45.8X1	T45.8X2	T45.8X3	T45.8X4	T45.8X5	T45.8X6
HETP	T60.0X1	T60.0X2	T60.0X3	T60.0X4		
Hexachlorobenzene (vapor)	T60.3X1	T60.3X2	T60.3X3	T60.3X4		
Hexachlorocyclohexane	T53.6X1	T53.6X2	T53.6X3	T53.6X4		
Hexachlorophene	T49.0X1	T49.0X2	T49.0X3	T49.0X4	T49.0X5	T49.0X6
Hexadiline	T46.3X1	T46.3X2	T46.3X3	T46.3X4	T46.3X5	T46.3X6
Hexadimethrine (bromide)	T45.7X1	T45.7X2	T45.7X3	T45.7X4	T45.7X5	T45.7X6
Hexadylamine	T46.3X1	T46.3X2	T46.3X3	T46.3X4	T46.3X5	T46.3X6
Hexaethyl tetraphosphate	T60.0X1	T60.0X2	T60.0X3	T60.0X4		
Hexafluorenium bromide	T48.1X1	T48.1X2	T48.1X3	T48.1X4	T48.1X5	T48.1X6
Hexafluronium (bromide)	T48.1X1	T48.1X2	T48.1X3	T48.1X4	T48.1X5	T48.1X6
Hexa-germ	T49.2X1	T49.2X2	T49.2X3	T49.2X4	T49.2X5	T49.2X6
Hexahydrobenzol	T52.8X1	T52.8X2	T52.8X3	T52.8X4		
Hexahydrocresol(s)	T51.8X1	T51.8X2	T51.8X3	T51.8X4		
arsenide	T57.0X1	T57.0X2	T57.0X3	T57.0X4		
arseniurated	T57.0X1	T57.0X2	T57.0X3	T57.0X4		
cyanide	T57.3X1	T57.3X2	T57.3X3	T57.3X4		
gas	T59.891	T59.892	T59.893	T59.894		
Fluoride (liquid)	T57.8X1	T57.8X2	T57.8X3	T57.8X4		
vapor	T59.891	T59.892	T59.893	T59.894		
phophorated	T60.0X1	T60.0X2	T60.0X3	T60.0X4		
sulfate	T57.8X1	T57.8X2	T57.8X3	T57.8X4		
sulfide (gas)	T59.6X1	T59.6X2	T59.6X3	T59.6X4		
arseniurated	T57.0X1	T57.0X2	T57.0X3	T57.0X4		
sulfurated	T57.8X1	T57.8X2	T57.8X3	T57.8X4		
Hexahydrophenol	T51.8X1	T51.8X2	T51.8X3	T51.8X4		
Hexalen	T51.8X1	T51.8X2	T51.8X3	T51.8X4		
Hexamethonium bromide	T44.2X1	T44.2X2	T44.2X3	T44.2X4	T44.2X5	T44.2X6
Hexamethylene	T52.8X1	T52.8X2	T52.8X3	T52.8X4		
Hexamethylmelamine	T45.1X1	T45.1X2	T45.1X3	T45.1X4	T45.1X5	T45.1X6
Hexamidine	T49.0X1	T49.0X2	T49.0X3	T49.0X4	T49.0X5	T49.0X6
Hexamine (mandelate)	T37.8X1	T37.8X2	T37.8X3	T37.8X4	T37.8X5	T37.8X6
Hexanone, 2-hexanone	T52.4X1	T52.4X2	T52.4X3	T52.4X4		
Hexanuorenium	T48.1X1	T48.1X2	T48.1X3	T48.1X4	T48.1X5	T48.1X6
Hexapropymate	T42.6X1	T42.6X2	T42.6X3	T42.6X4	T42.6X5	T42.6X6
Hexasonium iodide	T44.3X1	T44.3X2	T44.3X3	T44.3X4	T44.3X5	T44.3X6
Hexcarbacholine bromide	T48.1X1	T48.1X2	T48.1X3	T48.1X4	T48.1X5	T48.1X6
Hexemal	T42.3X1	T42.3X2	T42.3X3	T42.3X4	T42.3X5	T42.3X6
Hexestrol	T38.5X1	T38.5X2	T38.5X3	T38.5X4	T38.5X5	T38.5X6
Hexethal (sodium)	T42.3X1	T42.3X2	T42.3X3	T42.3X4	T42.3X5	T42.3X6
Hexetidine	T37.8X1	T37.8X2	T37.8X3	T37.8X4	T37.8X5	T37.8X6
Hexobarbital	T42.3X1	T42.3X2	T42.3X3	T42.3X4	T42.3X5	T42.3X6
rectal	T41.291	T41.292	T41.293	T41.294	T41.295	T41.296
sodium	T41.1X1	T41.1X2	T41.1X3	T41.1X4	T41.1X5	T41.1X6

Substance	Poisoning, Accidental (unintentional)	Poisoning, Intentional Self-harm	Poisoning, Assault	Poisoning, Undetermined	Adverse Effect	Under-dosing
Hexobendine	T46.3X1	T46.3X2	T46.3X3	T46.3X4	T46.3X5	T46.3X6
Hexocyclium	T44.3X1	T44.3X2	T44.3X3	T44.3X4	T44.3X5	T44.3X6
metilsulfate	T44.3X1	T44.3X2	T44.3X3	T44.3X4	T44.3X5	T44.3X6
Hexoestrol	T38.5X1	T38.5X2	T38.5X3	T38.5X4	T38.5X5	T38.5X6
Hexone	T52.4X1	T52.4X2	T52.4X3	T52.4X4		
Hexoprenaline	T48.6X1	T48.6X2	T48.6X3	T48.6X4	T48.6X5	T48.6X6
Hexylcaine	T41.3X1	T41.3X2	T41.3X3	T41.3X4	T41.3X5	T41.3X6
Hexylresorcinol	T52.2X1	T52.2X2	T52.2X3	T52.2X4		
HGH (human growth hormone)	T38.811	T38.812	T38.813	T38.814	T38.815	T38.816
Hinkle's pills	T47.2X1	T47.2X2	T47.2X3	T47.2X4	T47.2X5	T47.2X6
Histalog	T50.8X1	T50.8X2	T50.8X3	T50.8X4	T50.8X5	T50.8X6
Histamine (phosphate)	T50.8X1	T50.8X2	T50.8X3	T50.8X4	T50.8X5	T50.8X6
Histoplasmin	T50.8X1	T50.8X2	T50.8X3	T50.8X4	T50.8X5	T50.8X6
Holly berries	T62.2X1	T62.2X2	T62.2X3	T62.2X4		
Homatropine	T44.3X1	T44.3X2	T44.3X3	T44.3X4	T44.3X5	T44.3X6
methylbromide	T44.3X1	T44.3X2	T44.3X3	T44.3X4	T44.3X5	T44.3X6
Homochlorcyclizine	T45.0X1	T45.0X2	T45.0X3	T45.0X4	T45.0X5	T45.0X6
Homosalate	T49.3X1	T49.3X2	T49.3X3	T49.3X4	T49.3X5	T49.3X6
Homo-tet	T50.Z11	T50.Z12	T50.Z13	T50.Z14	T50.Z15	T50.Z16
Hormone	T38.801	T38.802	T38.803	T38.804	T38.805	T38.806
adrenal cortical steroids	T38.0X1	T38.0X2	T38.0X3	T38.0X4	T38.0X5	T38.0X6
androgenic	T38.7X1	T38.7X2	T38.7X3	T38.7X4	T38.7X5	T38.7X6
anterior pituitary NEC	T38.811	T38.812	T38.813	T38.814	T38.815	T38.816
antidiabetic agents	T38.3X1	T38.3X2	T38.3X3	T38.3X4	T38.3X5	T38.3X6
antidiuretic	T38.891	T38.892	T38.893	T38.894	T38.895	T38.896
cancer therapy	T45.1X1	T45.1X2	T45.1X3	T45.1X4	T45.1X5	T45.1X6
follicle stimulating	T38.811	T38.812	T38.813	T38.814	T38.815	T38.816
gonadotropic	T38.891	T38.892	T38.893	T38.894	T38.895	T38.896
pituitary	T38.811	T38.812	T38.813	T38.814	T38.815	T38.816
growth	T38.811	T38.812	T38.813	T38.814	T38.815	T38.816
luteinizing	T38.811	T38.812	T38.813	T38.814	T38.815	T38.816
ovarian	T38.5X1	T38.5X2	T38.5X3	T38.5X4	T38.5X5	T38.5X6
oxytocic	T48.0X1	T48.0X2	T48.0X3	T48.0X4	T48.0X5	T48.0X6
parathyroid (derivatives)	T50.991	T50.992	T50.993	T50.994	T50.995	T50.996
pituitary (posterior) NEC	T38.891	T38.892	T38.893	T38.894	T38.895	T38.896
anterior	T38.811	T38.812	T38.813	T38.814	T38.815	T38.816
specified, NEC	T38.891	T38.892	T38.893	T38.894	T38.895	T38.896
thyroid	T38.1X1	T38.1X2	T38.1X3	T38.1X4	T38.1X5	T38.1X6
Hornet (sting)	T63.451	T63.452	T63.453	T63.454		
Horse anti-human lymphocytic serum	T50.Z11	T50.Z12	T50.Z13	T50.Z14	T50.Z15	T50.Z16
Horticulture agent NEC	T65.91	T65.92	T65.93	T65.94		
with pesticide	T60.91	T60.92	T60.93	T60.94		
Human						
albumin	T45.8X1	T45.8X2	T45.8X3	T45.8X4	T45.8X5	T45.8X6
growth hormone (HGH)	T38.811	T38.812	T38.813	T38.814	T38.815	T38.816
immune serum	T50.Z11	T50.Z12	T50.Z13	T50.Z14	T50.Z15	T50.Z16
Hyaluronidase	T45.3X1	T45.3X2	T45.3X3	T45.3X4	T45.3X5	T45.3X6
Hyazyme	T45.3X1	T45.3X2	T45.3X3	T45.3X4	T45.3X5	T45.3X6
Hycodan	T40.2X1	T40.2X2	T40.2X3	T40.2X4	T40.2X5	T40.2X6
Hydantoin derivative NEC	T42.0X1	T42.0X2	T42.0X3	T42.0X4	T42.0X5	T42.0X6
Hydeltra	T38.0X1	T38.0X2	T38.0X3	T38.0X4	T38.0X5	T38.0X6
Hydergine	T44.6X1	T44.6X2	T44.6X3	T44.6X4	T44.6X5	T44.6X6
Hydrabamine penicillin	T36.0X1	T36.0X2	T36.0X3	T36.0X4	T36.0X5	T36.0X6
Hydralazine	T46.5X1	T46.5X2	T46.5X3	T46.5X4	T46.5X5	T46.5X6
Hydrargaphen	T49.0X1	T49.0X2	T49.0X3	T49.0X4	T49.0X5	T49.0X6
Hydrargyri aminochloridum	T49.0X1	T49.0X2	T49.0X3	T49.0X4	T49.0X5	T49.0X6
Hydrastine	T48.291	T48.292	T48.293	T48.294	T48.295	T48.296
Hydrazine	T54.1X1	T54.1X2	T54.1X3	T54.1X4		
monoamine oxidase inhibitors	T43.1X1	T43.1X2	T43.1X3	T43.1X4	T43.1X5	T43.1X6
Hydrazoic acid, azides	T54.2X1	T54.2X2	T54.2X3	T54.2X4		
Hydriodic acid	T48.4X1	T48.4X2	T48.4X3	T48.4X4	T48.4X5	T48.4X6
Hydrocarbon gas	T59.891	T59.892	T59.893	T59.894		
incomplete combustion of — *see* Carbon, monoxide, fuel, utility						
liquefied (mobile container)	T59.891	T59.892	T59.893	T59.894		
piped (natural)	T59.891	T59.892	T59.893	T59.894		
Hydrochloric acid (liquid)	T54.2X1	T54.2X2	T54.2X3	T54.2X4		
medicinal (digestant)	T47.5X1	T47.5X2	T47.5X3	T47.5X4	T47.5X5	T47.5X6
vapor	T59.891	T59.892	T59.893	T59.894		
Hydrochlorothiazide	T50.2X1	T50.2X2	T50.2X3	T50.2X4	T50.2X5	T50.2X6
Hydrocodone	T40.2X1	T40.2X2	T40.2X3	T40.2X4	T40.2X5	T40.2X6
Hydrocortisone	T38.0X1	T38.0X2	T38.0X3	T38.0X4	T38.0X5	T38.0X6
(derivatives)						
aceponate	T49.0X1	T49.0X2	T49.0X3	T49.0X4	T49.0X5	T49.0X6
ENT agent	T49.6X1	T49.6X2	T49.6X3	T49.6X4	T49.6X5	T49.6X6
ophthalmic preparation	T49.5X1	T49.5X2	T49.5X3	T49.5X4	T49.5X5	T49.5X6
topical NEC	T49.0X1	T49.0X2	T49.0X3	T49.0X4	T49.0X5	T49.0X6

Substance	Poisoning, Accidental (unintentional)	Poisoning, Intentional Self-harm	Poisoning, Assault	Poisoning, Undetermined	Adverse Effect	Under-dosing
Hydrocortone	T38.0X1	T38.0X2	T38.0X3	T38.0X4	T38.0X5	T38.0X6
ENT agent	T49.6X1	T49.6X2	T49.6X3	T49.6X4	T49.6X5	T49.6X6
ophthalmic preparation	T49.5X1	T49.5X2	T49.5X3	T49.5X4	T49.5X5	T49.5X6
topical NEC	T49.0X1	T49.0X2	T49.0X3	T49.0X4	T49.0X5	T49.0X6
Hydrocyanic acid (liquid)	T57.3X1	T57.3X2	T57.3X3	T57.3X4	—	—
gas	T65.0X1	T65.0X2	T65.0X3	T65.0X4	—	—
Hydroflumethiazide	T50.2X1	T50.2X2	T50.2X3	T50.2X4	T50.2X5	T50.2X6
Hydrofluoric acid (liquid)	T54.2X1	T54.2X2	T54.2X3	T54.2X4	—	—
vapor	T59.891	T59.892	T59.893	T59.894	—	—
Hydrogen	T59.891	T59.892	T59.893	T59.894	—	—
arsenide	T57.0X1	T57.0X2	T57.0X3	T57.0X4	—	—
arseniureted	T57.0X1	T57.0X2	T57.0X3	T57.0X4	—	—
chloride	T57.8X1	T57.8X2	T57.8X3	T57.8X4	—	—
cyanide (salts)	T57.3X1	T57.3X2	T57.3X3	T57.3X4	—	—
gas	T57.3X1	T57.3X2	T57.3X3	T57.3X4	—	—
Fluoride	T59.5X1	T59.5X2	T59.5X3	T59.5X4	—	—
vapor	T59.5X1	T59.5X2	T59.5X3	T59.5X4	—	—
peroxide	T49.0X1	T49.0X2	T49.0X3	T49.0X4	T49.0X5	T49.0X6
phosphureted	T57.1X1	T57.1X2	T57.1X3	T57.1X4	—	—
sulfide	T59.6X1	T59.6X2	T59.6X3	T59.6X4	—	—
arseniureted	T57.0X1	T57.0X2	T57.0X3	T57.0X4	—	—
sulfureted	T59.6X1	T59.6X2	T59.6X3	T59.6X4	—	—
Hydromethylpyridine	T46.7X1	T46.7X2	T46.7X3	T46.7X4	T46.7X5	T46.7X6
Hydromorphinol	T40.2X1	T40.2X2	T40.2X3	T40.2X4		
Hydromorphinone	T40.2X1	T40.2X2	T40.2X3	T40.2X4	T40.2X5	T40.2X6
Hydromorphone	T40.2X1	T40.2X2	T40.2X3	T40.2X4	T40.2X5	T40.2X6
Hydromox	T50.2X1	T50.2X2	T50.2X3	T50.2X4	T50.2X5	T50.2X6
Hydrophilic lotion	T49.3X1	T49.3X2	T49.3X3	T49.3X4	T49.3X5	T49.3X6
Hydroquinidine	T46.2X1	T46.2X2	T46.2X3	T46.2X4	T46.2X5	T46.2X6
Hydroquinone	T52.2X1	T52.2X2	T52.2X3	T52.2X4	—	—
vapor	T59.891	T59.892	T59.893	T59.894	—	—
Hydrosulfuric acid (gas)	T59.6X1	T59.6X2	T59.6X3	T59.6X4	—	—
Hydrotalcite	T47.1X1	T47.1X2	T47.1X3	T47.1X4	T47.1X5	T47.1X6
Hydrous wool fat	T49.3X1	T49.3X2	T49.3X3	T49.3X4	T49.3X5	T49.3X6
Hydroxide, caustic	T54.3X1	T54.3X2	T54.3X3	T54.3X4	—	—
Hydroxocobalamin	T45.8X1	T45.8X2	T45.8X3	T45.8X4	T45.8X5	T45.8X6
Hydroxyamphetamine	T49.5X1	T49.5X2	T49.5X3	T49.5X4	T49.5X5	T49.5X6
Hydroxycarbamide	T45.1X1	T45.1X2	T45.1X3	T45.1X4	T45.1X5	T45.1X6
Hydroxychloroquine	T37.8X1	T37.8X2	T37.8X3	T37.8X4	T37.8X5	T37.8X6
Hydroxydihydrocodeinone	T40.2X1	T40.2X2	T40.2X3	T40.2X4	T40.2X5	T40.2X6
Hydroxyestrone	T38.5X1	T38.5X2	T38.5X3	T38.5X4	T38.5X5	T38.5X6
Hydroxyethyl starch	T45.8X1	T45.8X2	T45.8X3	T45.8X4	T45.8X5	T45.8X6
Hydroxymethylpentanone	T52.4X1	T52.4X2	T52.4X3	T52.4X4	—	—
Hydroxyphenamate	T43.591	T43.592	T43.593	T43.594	T43.595	T43.596
Hydroxyphenylbutazone	T39.2X1	T39.2X2	T39.2X3	T39.2X4	T39.2X5	T39.2X6
Hydroxyprogesterone	T38.5X1	T38.5X2	T38.5X3	T38.5X4	T38.5X5	T38.5X6
caproate	T38.5X1	T38.5X2	T38.5X3	T38.5X4	T38.5X5	T38.5X6
Hydroxyquinoline (derivatives) NEC	T37.8X1	T37.8X2	T37.8X3	T37.8X4	T37.8X5	T37.8X6
Hydroxystilbamidine	T37.3X1	T37.3X2	T37.3X3	T37.3X4	T37.3X5	T37.3X6
Hydroxytoluene (nonmedicinal)	T54.0X1	T54.0X2	T54.0X3	T54.0X4	—	—
medicinal	T49.0X1	T49.0X2	T49.0X3	T49.0X4	T49.0X5	T49.0X6
Hydroxyurea	T45.1X1	T45.1X2	T45.1X3	T45.1X4	T45.1X5	T45.1X6
Hydroxyzine	T43.591	T43.592	T43.593	T43.594	T43.595	T43.596
Hyoscine	T44.3X1	T44.3X2	T44.3X3	T44.3X4	T44.3X5	T44.3X6
Hyoscyamine	T44.3X1	T44.3X2	T44.3X3	T44.3X4	T44.3X5	T44.3X6
Hyoscyamus	T44.3X1	T44.3X2	T44.3X3	T44.3X4	T44.3X5	T44.3X6
dry extract	T44.3X1	T44.3X2	T44.3X3	T44.3X4	T44.3X5	T44.3X6
Hypaque	T50.8X1	T50.8X2	T50.8X3	T50.8X4	T50.8X5	T50.8X6
Hypertussis	T50.Z11	T50.Z12	T50.Z13	T50.Z14	T50.Z15	T50.Z16
Hypnotic	T42.71	T42.72	T42.73	T42.74	T42.75	T42.76
anticonvulsant	T42.71	T42.72	T42.73	T42.74	T42.75	T42.76
specified NEC	T42.6X1	T42.6X2	T42.6X3	T42.6X4	T42.6X5	T42.6X6
Hypochlorite	T49.0X1	T49.0X2	T49.0X3	T49.0X4	T49.0X5	T49.0X6
Hypophysis, posterior	T38.891	T38.892	T38.893	T38.894	T38.895	T38.896
Hypotensive NEC	T46.5X1	T46.5X2	T46.5X3	T46.5X4	T46.5X5	T46.5X6
Hypromellose	T49.5X1	T49.5X2	T49.5X3	T49.5X4	T49.5X5	T49.5X6
Ibacitabine	T37.5X1	T37.5X2	T37.5X3	T37.5X4	T37.5X5	T37.5X6
Ibopamine	T44.991	T44.992	T44.993	T44.994	T44.995	T44.996
Ibufenac	T39.311	T39.312	T39.313	T39.314	T39.315	T39.316
Ibuprofen	T39.311	T39.312	T39.313	T39.314	T39.315	T39.316
Ibuproxam	T39.311	T39.312	T39.313	T39.314	T39.315	T39.316
Ibuterol	T48.6X1	T48.6X2	T48.6X3	T48.6X4	T48.6X5	T48.6X6
Ichthammol	T49.0X1	T49.0X2	T49.0X3	T49.0X4	T49.0X5	T49.0X6
Ichthyol	T49.4X1	T49.4X2	T49.4X3	T49.4X4	T49.4X5	T49.4X6
Idarubicin	T45.1X1	T45.1X2	T45.1X3	T45.1X4	T45.1X5	T45.1X6
Idrocilamide	T42.8X1	T42.8X2	T42.8X3	T42.8X4	T42.8X5	T42.8X6
Ifenprodil	T46.7X1	T46.7X2	T46.7X3	T46.7X4	T46.7X5	T46.7X6
Ifosfamide	T45.1X1	T45.1X2	T45.1X3	T45.1X4	T45.1X5	T45.1X6
Iletin	T38.3X1	T38.3X2	T38.3X3	T38.3X4	T38.3X5	T38.3X6
Ilex	T62.2X1	T62.2X2	T62.2X3	T62.2X4	—	—

Substance	Poisoning, Accidental (unintentional)	Poisoning, Intentional Self-harm	Poisoning, Assault	Poisoning, Undetermined	Adverse Effect	Under-dosing
Illuminating gas (after combustion)	T58.11	T58.12	T58.13	T58.14	—	—
prior to combustion	T59.891	T59.892	T59.893	T59.894		
Ilopan	T45.2X1	T45.2X2	T45.2X3	T45.2X4	T45.2X5	T45.2X6
Iloprost	T46.7X1	T46.7X2	T46.7X3	T46.7X4	T46.7X5	T46.7X6
Ilotycin	T36.3X1	T36.3X2	T36.3X3	T36.3X4	T36.3X5	T36.3X6
ophthalmic preparation	T49.5X1	T49.5X2	T49.5X3	T49.5X4	T49.5X5	T49.5X6
topical NEC	T49.0X1	T49.0X2	T49.0X3	T49.0X4	T49.0X5	T49.0X6
Imidazole-4-carboxamide	T45.1X1	T45.1X2	T45.1X3	T45.1X4	T45.1X5	T45.1X6
Iminostilbene	T42.1X1	T42.1X2	T42.1X3	T42.1X4	T42.1X5	T42.1X6
Imipenem	T36.0X1	T36.0X2	T36.0X3	T36.0X4	T36.0X5	T36.0X6
Imipramine	T43.011	T43.012	T43.013	T43.014	T43.015	T43.016
Immu-G	T50.Z11	T50.Z12	T50.Z13	T50.Z14	T50.Z15	T50.Z16
Immuglobin	T50.Z11	T50.Z12	T50.Z13	T50.Z14	T50.Z15	T50.Z16
Immune						
globulin	T50.Z11	T50.Z12	T50.Z13	T50.Z14	T50.Z15	T50.Z16
serum globulin	T50.Z11	T50.Z12	T50.Z13	T50.Z14	T50.Z15	T50.Z16
Immunoglobin human (intravenous) (normal)						
unmodified	T50.Z11	T50.Z12	T50.Z13	T50.Z14	T50.Z15	T50.Z16
Immunosuppressive drug	T45.1X1	T45.1X2	T45.1X3	T45.1X4	T45.1X5	T45.1X6
Immu-tetanus	T50.Z11	T50.Z12	T50.Z13	T50.Z14	T50.Z15	T50.Z16
Indalpine	T43.221	T43.222	T43.223	T43.224	T43.225	T43.226
Indanazoline	T48.5X1	T48.5X2	T48.5X3	T48.5X4	T48.5X5	T48.5X6
Indandione (derivatives)	T45.511	T45.512	T45.513	T45.514	T45.515	T45.516
Indapamide	T46.5X1	T46.5X2	T46.5X3	T46.5X4	T46.5X5	T46.5X6
Indendione (derivatives)	T45.511	T45.512	T45.513	T45.514	T45.515	T45.516
Indenolol	T44.7X1	T44.7X2	T44.7X3	T44.7X4	T44.7X5	T44.7X6
Inderal	T44.7X1	T44.7X2	T44.7X3	T44.7X4	T44.7X5	T44.7X6
Indian						
hemp	T40.7X1	T40.7X2	T40.7X3	T40.7X4	T40.7X5	T40.7X6
tobacco	T62.2X1	T62.2X2	T62.2X3	T62.2X4	—	—
Indigo carmine	T50.8X1	T50.8X2	T50.8X3	T50.8X4	T50.8X5	T50.8X6
Indobufen	T45.521	T45.522	T45.523	T45.524	T45.525	T45.526
Indocin	T39.2X1	T39.2X2	T39.2X3	T39.2X4	T39.2X5	T39.2X6
Indocyanine green	T50.8X1	T50.8X2	T50.8X3	T50.8X4	T50.8X5	T50.8X6
Indometacin	T39.391	T39.392	T39.393	T39.394	T39.395	T39.396
Indomethacin	T39.391	T39.392	T39.393	T39.394	T39.395	T39.396
farnesil	T39.4X1	T39.4X2	T39.4X3	T39.4X4	T39.4X5	T39.4X6
Indoramin	T44.6X1	T44.6X2	T44.6X3	T44.6X4	T44.6X5	T44.6X6
Industrial						
alcohol	T51.0X1	T51.0X2	T51.0X3	T51.0X4	—	—
fumes	T59.891	T59.892	T59.893	T59.894	—	—
solvents (fumes) (vapors)	T52.91	T52.92	T52.93	T52.94	—	—
Influenza vaccine	T50.B91	T50.B92	T50.B93	T50.B94	T50.B95	T50.B96
Ingested substance NEC	T65.91	T65.92	T65.93	T65.94	—	—
INH	T37.1X1	T37.1X2	T37.1X3	T37.1X4	T37.1X5	T37.1X6
Inhalation, gas (noxious) — see Gas						
Inhibitor						
angiotensin-converting enzyme	T46.4X1	T46.4X2	T46.4X3	T46.4X4	T46.4X5	T46.4X6
carbonic anhydrase	T50.2X1	T50.2X2	T50.2X3	T50.2X4	T50.2X5	T50.2X6
fibrinolysis	T45.621	T45.622	T45.623	T45.624	T45.625	T45.626
monoamine oxidase NEC	T43.1X1	T43.1X2	T43.1X3	T43.1X4	T43.1X5	T43.1X6
hydrazine	T43.1X1	T43.1X2	T43.1X3	T43.1X4	T43.1X5	T43.1X6
postsynaptic	T43.8X1	T43.8X2	T43.8X3	T43.8X4	T43.8X5	T43.8X6
prothrombin synthesis	T45.511	T45.512	T45.513	T45.514	T45.515	T45.516
Ink	T65.891	T65.892	T65.893	T65.894	—	—
Inorganic substance NEC	T57.91	T57.92	T57.93	T57.94	—	—
Inosine pranobex	T37.5X1	T37.5X2	T37.5X3	T37.5X4	T37.5X5	T37.5X6
Inositol	T50.991	T50.992	T50.993	T50.994	T50.995	T50.996
nicotinate	T46.7X1	T46.7X2	T46.7X3	T46.7X4	T46.7X5	T46.7X6
Inproquone	T45.1X1	T45.1X2	T45.1X3	T45.1X4	T45.1X5	T45.1X6
Insecticide NEC	T60.91	T60.92	T60.93	T60.94	—	—
carbamate	T60.0X1	T60.0X2	T60.0X3	T60.0X4	—	—
chlorinated	T60.1X1	T60.1X2	T60.1X3	T60.1X4	—	—
mixed	T60.91	T60.92	T60.93	T60.94	—	—
organochlorine	T60.1X1	T60.1X2	T60.1X3	T60.1X4	—	—
organophosphorus	T60.0X1	T60.0X2	T60.0X3	T60.0X4	—	—
Insect (sting), venomous	T63.481	T63.482	T63.483	T63.484	—	—
ant	T63.421	T63.422	T63.423	T63.424	—	—
bee	T63.441	T63.442	T63.443	T63.444	—	—
caterpillar	T63.431	T63.432	T63.433	T63.434	—	—
hornet	T63.451	T63.452	T63.453	T63.454	—	—
wasp	T63.461	T63.462	T63.463	T63.464	—	—
Insular tissue extract	T38.3X1	T38.3X2	T38.3X3	T38.3X4	T38.3X5	T38.3X6
Insulin (amorphous) (globin) (isophane) (Lente) (NPH) (Semilente) (Ultralente)						
defalan	T38.3X1	T38.3X2	T38.3X3	T38.3X4	T38.3X5	T38.3X6
human	T38.3X1	T38.3X2	T38.3X3	T38.3X4	T38.3X5	T38.3X6
injection, soluble	T38.3X1	T38.3X2	T38.3X3	T38.3X4	T38.3X5	T38.3X6

Additional Character May Be Required — Refer to the Tabular List for Character Selection

▽ **Subterms under main terms may continue to next column or page**

Substance	Poisoning, Accidental (unintentional)	Poisoning, Intentional Self-harm	Poisoning, Assault	Poisoning, Undetermined	Adverse Effect	Under-dosing
Insulin — *continued*						
injection, soluble — *continued*						
biphasic	T38.3X1	T38.3X2	T38.3X3	T38.3X4	T38.3X5	T38.3X6
intermediate acting	T38.3X1	T38.3X2	T38.3X3	T38.3X4	T38.3X5	T38.3X6
protamine zinc	T38.3X1	T38.3X2	T38.3X3	T38.3X4	T38.3X5	T38.3X6
slow acting	T38.3X1	T38.3X2	T38.3X3	T38.3X4	T38.3X5	T38.3X6
zinc						
protamine injection	T38.3X1	T38.3X2	T38.3X3	T38.3X4	T38.3X5	T38.3X6
suspension (amorphous) (crystalline)	T38.3X1	T38.3X2	T38.3X3	T38.3X4	T38.3X5	T38.3X6
Interferon (alpha) (beta) (gamma)	T37.5X1	T37.5X2	T37.5X3	T37.5X4	T37.5X5	T37.5X6
Intestinal motility control drug	T47.6X1	T47.6X2	T47.6X3	T47.6X4	T47.6X5	T47.6X6
biological	T47.8X1	T47.8X2	T47.8X3	T47.8X4	T47.8X5	T47.8X6
Intranarcon	T41.1X1	T41.1X2	T41.1X3	T41.1X4	T41.1X5	T41.1X6
Intravenous						
amino acids	T50.991	T50.992	T50.993	T50.994	T50.995	T50.996
fat suspension	T50.991	T50.992	T50.993	T50.994	T50.995	T50.996
Inulin	T50.8X1	T50.8X2	T50.8X3	T50.8X4	T50.8X5	T50.8X6
Invert sugar	T50.3X1	T50.3X2	T50.3X3	T50.3X4	T50.3X5	T50.3X6
Inza — *see* Naproxen						
Iobenzamic acid	T50.8X1	T50.8X2	T50.8X3	T50.8X4	T50.8X5	T50.8X6
Iocarmic acid	T50.8X1	T50.8X2	T50.8X3	T50.8X4	T50.8X5	T50.8X6
Iocetamic acid	T50.8X1	T50.8X2	T50.8X3	T50.8X4	T50.8X5	T50.8X6
Iodamide	T50.8X1	T50.8X2	T50.8X3	T50.8X4	T50.8X5	T50.8X6
Iodide NEC — *see also* Iodine	T49.0X1	T49.0X2	T49.0X3	T49.0X4	T49.0X5	T49.0X6
mercury (ointment)	T49.0X1	T49.0X2	T49.0X3	T49.0X4	T49.0X5	T49.0X6
methylate	T49.0X1	T49.0X2	T49.0X3	T49.0X4	T49.0X5	T49.0X6
potassium (expectorant) NEC	T48.4X1	T48.4X2	T48.4X3	T48.4X4	T48.4X5	T48.4X6
Iodinated						
contrast medium	T50.8X1	T50.8X2	T50.8X3	T50.8X4	T50.8X5	T50.8X6
glycerol	T48.4X1	T48.4X2	T48.4X3	T48.4X4	T48.4X5	T48.4X6
human serum albumin (131I)	T50.8X1	T50.8X2	T50.8X3	T50.8X4	T50.8X5	T50.8X6
Iodine (antiseptic, external) (tincture) **NEC**	T49.0X1	T49.0X2	T49.0X3	T49.0X4	T49.0X5	T49.0X6
125 — *see also* Radiation sickness, and Exposure to radioactivce isotopes	T50.8X1	T50.8X2	T50.8X3	T50.8X4	T50.8X5	T50.8X6
therapeutic	T50.991	T50.992	T50.993	T50.994	T50.995	T50.996
131 — *see also* Radiation sickness, and Exposure to radioactivce isotopes	T50.8X1	T50.8X2	T50.8X3	T50.8X4	T50.8X5	T50.8X6
therapeutic	T38.2X1	T38.2X2	T38.2X3	T38.2X4	T38.2X5	T38.2X6
diagnostic	T50.8X1	T50.8X2	T50.8X3	T50.8X4	T50.8X5	T50.8X6
for thyroid conditions (antithyroid)	T38.2X1	T38.2X2	T38.2X3	T38.2X4	T38.2X5	T38.2X6
solution	T49.0X1	T49.0X2	T49.0X3	T49.0X4	T49.0X5	T49.0X6
vapor	T59.891	T59.892	T59.893	T59.894	—	—
Iodipamide	T50.8X1	T50.8X2	T50.8X3	T50.8X4	T50.8X5	T50.8X6
Iodized (poppy seed) oil	T50.8X1	T50.8X2	T50.8X3	T50.8X4	T50.8X5	T50.8X6
Iodobismitol	T37.8X1	T37.8X2	T37.8X3	T37.8X4	T37.8X5	T37.8X6
Iodochlorhydroxyquin	T37.8X1	T37.8X2	T37.8X3	T37.8X4	T37.8X5	T37.8X6
topical	T49.0X1	T49.0X2	T49.0X3	T49.0X4	T49.0X5	T49.0X6
Iodochlorhydroxyquinoline	T37.8X1	T37.8X2	T37.8X3	T37.8X4	T37.8X5	T37.8X6
Iodocholesterol (131I)	T50.8X1	T50.8X2	T50.8X3	T50.8X4	T50.8X5	T50.8X6
Iodoform	T49.0X1	T49.0X2	T49.0X3	T49.0X4	T49.0X5	T49.0X6
Iodohippuric acid	T50.8X1	T50.8X2	T50.8X3	T50.8X4	T50.8X5	T50.8X6
Iodopanoic acid	T50.8X1	T50.8X2	T50.8X3	T50.8X4	T50.8X5	T50.8X6
Iodophthalein (sodium)	T50.8X1	T50.8X2	T50.8X3	T50.8X4	T50.8X5	T50.8X6
Iodopyracet	T50.8X1	T50.8X2	T50.8X3	T50.8X4	T50.8X5	T50.8X6
Iodoquinol	T37.8X1	T37.8X2	T37.8X3	T37.8X4	T37.8X5	T37.8X6
Iodoxamic acid	T50.8X1	T50.8X2	T50.8X3	T50.8X4	T50.8X5	T50.8X6
Iofendylate	T50.8X1	T50.8X2	T50.8X3	T50.8X4	T50.8X5	T50.8X6
Ioglycamic acid	T50.8X1	T50.8X2	T50.8X3	T50.8X4	T50.8X5	T50.8X6
Iohexol	T50.8X1	T50.8X2	T50.8X3	T50.8X4	T50.8X5	T50.8X6
Ion exchange resin						
anion	T47.8X1	T47.8X2	T47.8X3	T47.8X4	T47.8X5	T47.8X6
cation	T50.3X1	T50.3X2	T50.3X3	T50.3X4	T50.3X5	T50.3X6
cholestyramine	T46.6X1	T46.6X2	T46.6X3	T46.6X4	T46.6X5	T46.6X6
intestinal	T47.8X1	T47.8X2	T47.8X3	T47.8X4	T47.8X5	T47.8X6
Iopamidol	T50.8X1	T50.8X2	T50.8X3	T50.8X4	T50.8X5	T50.8X6
Iopanoic acid	T50.8X1	T50.8X2	T50.8X3	T50.8X4	T50.8X5	T50.8X6
Iophenoic acid	T50.8X1	T50.8X2	T50.8X3	T50.8X4	T50.8X5	T50.8X6
Iopodate, sodium	T50.8X1	T50.8X2	T50.8X3	T50.8X4	T50.8X5	T50.8X6
Iopodic acid	T50.8X1	T50.8X2	T50.8X3	T50.8X4	T50.8X5	T50.8X6
Iopromide	T50.8X1	T50.8X2	T50.8X3	T50.8X4	T50.8X5	T50.8X6
Iopydol	T50.8X1	T50.8X2	T50.8X3	T50.8X4	T50.8X5	T50.8X6
Iotalamic acid	T50.8X1	T50.8X2	T50.8X3	T50.8X4	T50.8X5	T50.8X6
Iothalamate	T50.8X1	T50.8X2	T50.8X3	T50.8X4	T50.8X5	T50.8X6
Iothiouracil	T38.2X1	T38.2X2	T38.2X3	T38.2X4	T38.2X5	T38.2X6
Iotrol	T50.8X1	T50.8X2	T50.8X3	T50.8X4	T50.8X5	T50.8X6
Iotrolan	T50.8X1	T50.8X2	T50.8X3	T50.8X4	T50.8X5	T50.8X6
Iotroxate	T50.8X1	T50.8X2	T50.8X3	T50.8X4	T50.8X5	T50.8X6
Iotroxic acid	T50.8X1	T50.8X2	T50.8X3	T50.8X4	T50.8X5	T50.8X6
Ioversol	T50.8X1	T50.8X2	T50.8X3	T50.8X4	T50.8X5	T50.8X6
Ioxaglate	T50.8X1	T50.8X2	T50.8X3	T50.8X4	T50.8X5	T50.8X6
Ioxaglic acid	T50.8X1	T50.8X2	T50.8X3	T50.8X4	T50.8X5	T50.8X6
Ioxitalamic acid	T50.8X1	T50.8X2	T50.8X3	T50.8X4	T50.8X5	T50.8X6
Ipecac	T47.7X1	T47.7X2	T47.7X3	T47.7X4	T47.7X5	T47.7X6
Ipecacuanha	T48.4X1	T48.4X2	T48.4X3	T48.4X4	T48.4X5	T48.4X6
Ipodate, calcium	T50.8X1	T50.8X2	T50.8X3	T50.8X4	T50.8X5	T50.8X6
Ipral	T42.3X1	T42.3X2	T42.3X3	T42.3X4	T42.3X5	T42.3X6
Ipratropium (bromide)	T48.6X1	T48.6X2	T48.6X3	T48.6X4	T48.6X5	T48.6X6
Ipriflavone	T46.3X1	T46.3X2	T46.3X3	T46.3X4	T46.3X5	T46.3X6
Iprindole	T43.011	T43.012	T43.013	T43.014	T43.015	T43.016
Iproclozide	T43.1X1	T43.1X2	T43.1X3	T43.1X4	T43.1X5	T43.1X6
Iprofenin	T50.8X1	T50.8X2	T50.8X3	T50.8X4	T50.8X5	T50.8X6
Iproheptine	T49.2X1	T49.2X2	T49.2X3	T49.2X4	T49.2X5	T49.2X6
Iproniazid	T43.1X1	T43.1X2	T43.1X3	T43.1X4	T43.1X5	T43.1X6
Iproplatin	T45.1X1	T45.1X2	T45.1X3	T45.1X4	T45.1X5	T45.1X6
Iproveratril	T46.1X1	T46.1X2	T46.1X3	T46.1X4	T46.1X5	T46.1X6
Iron (compounds) (medicinal) **NEC**	T45.4X1	T45.4X2	T45.4X3	T45.4X4	T45.4X5	T45.4X6
ammonium	T45.4X1	T45.4X2	T45.4X3	T45.4X4	T45.4X5	T45.4X6
dextran injection	T45.4X1	T45.4X2	T45.4X3	T45.4X4	T45.4X5	T45.4X6
nonmedicinal	T56.891	T56.892	T56.893	T56.894	—	—
salts	T45.4X1	T45.4X2	T45.4X3	T45.4X4	T45.4X5	T45.4X6
sorbitex	T45.4X1	T45.4X2	T45.4X3	T45.4X4	T45.4X5	T45.4X6
sorbitol citric acid complex	T45.4X1	T45.4X2	T45.4X3	T45.4X4	T45.4X5	T45.4X6
Irrigating fluid (vaginal)	T49.8X1	T49.8X2	T49.8X3	T49.8X4	T49.8X5	T49.8X6
eye	T49.5X1	T49.5X2	T49.5X3	T49.5X4	T49.5X5	T49.5X6
Isepamicin	T36.5X1	T36.5X2	T36.5X3	T36.5X4	T36.5X5	T36.5X6
Isoaminile (citrate)	T48.3X1	T48.3X2	T48.3X3	T48.3X4	T48.3X5	T48.3X6
Isoamyl nitrite	T46.3X1	T46.3X2	T46.3X3	T46.3X4	T46.3X5	T46.3X6
Isobenzan	T60.1X1	T60.1X2	T60.1X3	T60.1X4	—	—
Isobutyl acetate	T52.8X1	T52.8X2	T52.8X3	T52.8X4	—	—
Isocarboxazid	T43.1X1	T43.1X2	T43.1X3	T43.1X4	T43.1X5	T43.1X6
Isoconazole	T49.0X1	T49.0X2	T49.0X3	T49.0X4	T49.0X5	T49.0X6
Isocyanate	T65.0X1	T65.0X2	T65.0X3	T65.0X4	—	—
Isoephedrine	T44.991	T44.992	T44.993	T44.994	T44.995	T44.996
Isoetarine	T48.6X1	T48.6X2	T48.6X3	T48.6X4	T48.6X5	T48.6X6
Isoethadione	T42.2X1	T42.2X2	T42.2X3	T42.2X4	T42.2X5	T42.2X6
Isoetharine	T44.5X1	T44.5X2	T44.5X3	T44.5X4	T44.5X5	T44.5X6
Isoflurane	T41.0X1	T41.0X2	T41.0X3	T41.0X4	T41.0X5	T41.0X6
Isoflurophate	T44.0X1	T44.0X2	T44.0X3	T44.0X4	T44.0X5	T44.0X6
Isomaltose, ferric complex	T45.4X1	T45.4X2	T45.4X3	T45.4X4	T45.4X5	T45.4X6
Isometheptene	T44.3X1	T44.3X2	T44.3X3	T44.3X4	T44.3X5	T44.3X6
Isoniazid	T37.1X1	T37.1X2	T37.1X3	T37.1X4	T37.1X5	T37.1X6
with						
rifampicin	T36.6X1	T36.6X2	T36.6X3	T36.6X4	T36.6X5	T36.6X6
thioacetazone	T37.1X1	T37.1X2	T37.1X3	T37.1X4	T37.1X5	T37.1X6
Isonicotinic acid hydrazide	T37.1X1	T37.1X2	T37.1X3	T37.1X4	T37.1X5	T37.1X6
Isonipecaine	T40.4X1	T40.4X2	T40.4X3	T40.4X4	T40.4X5	T40.4X6
Isopentaquine	T37.2X1	T37.2X2	T37.2X3	T37.2X4	T37.2X5	T37.2X6
Isophane insulin	T38.3X1	T38.3X2	T38.3X3	T38.3X4	T38.3X5	T38.3X6
Isophorone	T65.891	T65.892	T65.893	T65.894	—	—
Isophosphamide	T45.1X1	T45.1X2	T45.1X3	T45.1X4	T45.1X5	T45.1X6
Isopregnenone	T38.5X1	T38.5X2	T38.5X3	T38.5X4	T38.5X5	T38.5X6
Isoprenaline	T48.6X1	T48.6X2	T48.6X3	T48.6X4	T48.6X5	T48.6X6
Isopromethazine	T43.3X1	T43.3X2	T43.3X3	T43.3X4	T43.3X5	T43.3X6
Isopropamide	T44.3X1	T44.3X2	T44.3X3	T44.3X4	T44.3X5	T44.3X6
iodide	T44.3X1	T44.3X2	T44.3X3	T44.3X4	T44.3X5	T44.3X6
Isopropanol	T51.2X1	T51.2X2	T51.2X3	T51.2X4	—	—
Isopropyl						
acetate	T52.8X1	T52.8X2	T52.8X3	T52.8X4	—	—
alcohol	T51.2X1	T51.2X2	T51.2X3	T51.2X4	—	—
medicinal	T49.4X1	T49.4X2	T49.4X3	T49.4X4	T49.4X5	T49.4X6
ether	T52.8X1	T52.8X2	T52.8X3	T52.8X4	—	—
Isopropylaminophenazone	T39.2X1	T39.2X2	T39.2X3	T39.2X4	T39.2X5	T39.2X6
Isoproterenol	T48.6X1	T48.6X2	T48.6X3	T48.6X4	T48.6X5	T48.6X6
Isosorbide dinitrate	T46.3X1	T46.3X2	T46.3X3	T46.3X4	T46.3X5	T46.3X6
Isothipendyl	T45.0X1	T45.0X2	T45.0X3	T45.0X4	T45.0X5	T45.0X6
Isotretinoin	T50.991	T50.992	T50.993	T50.994	T50.995	T50.996
Isoxazolyl penicillin	T36.0X1	T36.0X2	T36.0X3	T36.0X4	T36.0X5	T36.0X6
Isoxicam	T39.391	T39.392	T39.393	T39.394	T39.395	T39.396
Isoxsuprine	T46.7X1	T46.7X2	T46.7X3	T46.7X4	T46.7X5	T46.7X6
Ispagula	T47.4X1	T47.4X2	T47.4X3	T47.4X4	T47.4X5	T47.4X6
husk	T47.4X1	T47.4X2	T47.4X3	T47.4X4	T47.4X5	T47.4X6
Isradipine	T46.1X1	T46.1X2	T46.1X3	T46.1X4	T46.1X5	T46.1X6
I-thyroxine sodium	T38.1X1	T38.1X2	T38.1X3	T38.1X4	T38.1X5	T38.1X6
Itraconazole	T37.8X1	T37.8X2	T37.8X3	T37.8X4	T37.8X5	T37.8X6
Itramin tosilate	T46.3X1	T46.3X2	T46.3X3	T46.3X4	T46.3X5	T46.3X6

Substance	Poisoning, Accidental (unintentional)	Poisoning, Intentional Self-harm	Poisoning, Assault	Poisoning, Undetermined	Adverse Effect	Under-dosing
Ivermectin	T37.4X1	T37.4X2	T37.4X3	T37.4X4	T37.4X5	T37.4X6
Izoniazid	T37.1X1	T37.1X2	T37.1X3	T37.1X4	T37.1X5	T37.1X6
with thioacetazone	T37.1X1	T37.1X2	T37.1X3	T37.1X4	T37.1X5	T37.1X6
Jalap	T47.2X1	T47.2X2	T47.2X3	T47.2X4	T47.2X5	T47.2X6
Jamaica						
dogwood (bark)	T39.8X1	T39.8X2	T39.8X3	T39.8X4	T39.8X5	T39.8X6
ginger	T65.891	T65.892	T65.893	T65.894	—	—
root	T62.2X1	T62.2X2	T62.2X3	T62.2X4	—	—
Jatropha	T62.2X1	T62.2X2	T62.2X3	T62.2X4	—	—
curcas	T62.2X1	T62.2X2	T62.2X3	T62.2X4	—	—
Jectofer	T45.4X1	T45.4X2	T45.4X3	T45.4X4	T45.4X5	T45.4X6
Jellyfish (sting)	T63.621	T63.622	T63.623	T63.624	—	—
Jequirity (bean)	T62.2X1	T62.2X2	T62.2X3	T62.2X4	—	—
Jimson weed (stramonium)	T62.2X1	T62.2X2	T62.2X3	T62.2X4	—	—
seeds	T62.2X1	T62.2X2	T62.2X3	T62.2X4	—	—
Josamycin	T36.3X1	T36.3X2	T36.3X3	T36.3X4	T36.3X5	T36.3X6
Juniper tar	T49.1X1	T49.1X2	T49.1X3	T49.1X4	T49.1X5	T49.1X6
Kallidinogenase	T46.7X1	T46.7X2	T46.7X3	T46.7X4	T46.7X5	T46.7X6
Kallikrein	T46.7X1	T46.7X2	T46.7X3	T46.7X4	T46.7X5	T46.7X6
Kanamycin	T36.5X1	T36.5X2	T36.5X3	T36.5X4	T36.5X5	T36.5X6
Kantrex	T36.5X1	T36.5X2	T36.5X3	T36.5X4	T36.5X5	T36.5X6
Kaolin	T47.6X1	T47.6X2	T47.6X3	T47.6X4	T47.6X5	T47.6X6
light	T47.6X1	T47.6X2	T47.6X3	T47.6X4	T47.6X5	T47.6X6
Karaya (gum)	T47.4X1	T47.4X2	T47.4X3	T47.4X4	T47.4X5	T47.4X6
Kebuzone	T39.2X1	T39.2X2	T39.2X3	T39.2X4	T39.2X5	T39.2X6
Kelevan	T60.1X1	T60.1X2	T60.1X3	T60.1X4	—	—
Kemithal	T41.1X1	T41.1X2	T41.1X3	T41.1X4	T41.1X5	T41.1X6
Kenacort	T38.0X1	T38.0X2	T38.0X3	T38.0X4	T38.0X5	T38.0X6
Keratolytic drug NEC	T49.4X1	T49.4X2	T49.4X3	T49.4X4	T49.4X5	T49.4X6
anthracene	T49.4X1	T49.4X2	T49.4X3	T49.4X4	T49.4X5	T49.4X6
Keratoplastic NEC	T49.4X1	T49.4X2	T49.4X3	T49.4X4	T49.4X5	T49.4X6
Kerosene, kerosine (fuel) (solvent) NEC	T52.0X1	T52.0X2	T52.0X3	T52.0X4		
insecticide	T52.0X1	T52.0X2	T52.0X3	T52.0X4	—	—
vapor	T52.0X1	T52.0X2	T52.0X3	T52.0X4	—	—
Ketamine	T41.291	T41.292	T41.293	T41.294	T41.295	T41.296
Ketazolam	T42.4X1	T42.4X2	T42.4X3	T42.4X4	T42.4X5	T42.4X6
Ketazon	T39.2X1	T39.2X2	T39.2X3	T39.2X4	T39.2X5	T39.2X6
Ketobemidone	T40.4X1	T40.4X2	T40.4X3	T40.4X4	—	—
Ketoconazole	T49.0X1	T49.0X2	T49.0X3	T49.0X4	T49.0X5	T49.0X6
Ketols	T52.4X1	T52.4X2	T52.4X3	T52.4X4	—	—
Ketone oils	T52.4X1	T52.4X2	T52.4X3	T52.4X4	—	—
Ketoprofen	T39.311	T39.312	T39.313	T39.314	T39.315	T39.316
Ketorolac	T39.8X1	T39.8X2	T39.8X3	T39.8X4	T39.8X5	T39.8X6
Ketotifen	T45.0X1	T45.0X2	T45.0X3	T45.0X4	T45.0X5	T45.0X6
Khat	T43.691	T43.692	T43.693	T43.694	—	—
Khellin	T46.3X1	T46.3X2	T46.3X3	T46.3X4	T46.3X5	T46.3X6
Khelloside	T46.3X1	T46.3X2	T46.3X3	T46.3X4	T46.3X5	T46.3X6
Kiln gas or vapor (carbon monoxide)	T58.8X1	T58.8X2	T58.8X3	T58.8X4	—	—
Kitasamycin	T36.3X1	T36.3X2	T36.3X3	T36.3X4	T36.3X5	T36.3X6
Konsyl	T47.4X1	T47.4X2	T47.4X3	T47.4X4	T47.4X5	T47.4X6
Kosam seed	T62.2X1	T62.2X2	T62.2X3	T62.2X4	—	—
Krait (venom)	T63.091	T63.092	T63.093	T63.094	—	—
Kwell (insecticide)	T60.1X1	T60.1X2	T60.1X3	T60.1X4	—	—
anti-infective (topical)	T49.0X1	T49.0X2	T49.0X3	T49.0X4	T49.0X5	T49.0X6
Labetalol	T44.8X1	T44.8X2	T44.8X3	T44.8X4	T44.8X5	T44.8X6
Laburnum (seeds)	T62.2X1	T62.2X2	T62.2X3	T62.2X4	—	—
leaves	T62.2X1	T62.2X2	T62.2X3	T62.2X4	—	—
Lachesine	T49.5X1	T49.5X2	T49.5X3	T49.5X4	T49.5X5	T49.5X6
Lacidipine	T46.5X1	T46.5X2	T46.5X3	T46.5X4	T46.5X5	T46.5X6
Lacquer	T65.6X1	T65.6X2	T65.6X3	T65.6X4	—	—
Lacrimogenic gas	T59.3X1	T59.3X2	T59.3X3	T59.3X4	—	—
Lactated potassic saline	T50.3X1	T50.3X2	T50.3X3	T50.3X4	T50.3X5	T50.3X6
Lactic acid	T49.8X1	T49.8X2	T49.8X3	T49.8X4	T49.8X5	T49.8X6
Lactobacillus						
acidophilus	T47.6X1	T47.6X2	T47.6X3	T47.6X4	T47.6X5	T47.6X6
compound	T47.6X1	T47.6X2	T47.6X3	T47.6X4	T47.6X5	T47.6X6
bifidus, lyophilized	T47.6X1	T47.6X2	T47.6X3	T47.6X4	T47.6X5	T47.6X6
bulgaricus	T47.6X1	T47.6X2	T47.6X3	T47.6X4	T47.6X5	T47.6X6
sporogenes	T47.6X1	T47.6X2	T47.6X3	T47.6X4	T47.6X5	T47.6X6
Lactoflavin	T45.2X1	T45.2X2	T45.2X3	T45.2X4	T45.2X5	T45.2X6
Lactose (as excipient)	T50.901	T50.902	T50.903	T50.904	T50.905	T50.906
Lactuca (virosa) (extract)	T42.6X1	T42.6X2	T42.6X3	T42.6X4	T42.6X5	T42.6X6
Lactucarium	T42.6X1	T42.6X2	T42.6X3	T42.6X4	T42.6X5	T42.6X6
Lactulose	T47.3X1	T47.3X2	T47.3X3	T47.3X4	T47.3X5	T47.3X6
Laevo — see Levo-						
Lanatosides	T46.0X1	T46.0X2	T46.0X3	T46.0X4	T46.0X5	T46.0X6
Lanolin	T49.3X1	T49.3X2	T49.3X3	T49.3X4	T49.3X5	T49.3X6
Largactil	T43.3X1	T43.3X2	T43.3X3	T43.3X4	T43.3X5	T43.3X6
Larkspur	T62.2X1	T62.2X2	T62.2X3	T62.2X4	—	—
Laroxyl	T43.011	T43.012	T43.013	T43.014	T43.015	T43.016
Lasix	T50.1X1	T50.1X2	T50.1X3	T50.1X4	T50.1X5	T50.1X6

Substance	Poisoning, Accidental (unintentional)	Poisoning, Intentional Self-harm	Poisoning, Assault	Poisoning, Undetermined	Adverse Effect	Under-dosing
Lassar's paste	T49.4X1	T49.4X2	T49.4X3	T49.4X4	T49.4X5	T49.4X6
Latamoxef	T36.1X1	T36.1X2	T36.1X3	T36.1X4	T36.1X5	T36.1X6
Latex	T65.811	T65.812	T65.813	T65.814	—	—
Lathyrus (seed)	T62.2X1	T62.2X2	T62.2X3	T62.2X4	—	—
Laudanum	T40.0X1	T40.0X2	T40.0X3	T40.0X4	T40.0X5	T40.0X6
Laudexium	T48.1X1	T48.1X2	T48.1X3	T48.1X4	T48.1X5	T48.1X6
Laughing gas	T41.0X1	T41.0X2	T41.0X3	T41.0X4	T41.0X5	T41.0X6
Laurel, black or cherry	T62.2X1	T62.2X2	T62.2X3	T62.2X4	—	—
Laurolinium	T49.0X1	T49.0X2	T49.0X3	T49.0X4	T49.0X5	T49.0X6
Lauryl sulfoacetate	T49.2X1	T49.2X2	T49.2X3	T49.2X4	T49.2X5	T49.2X6
Laxative NEC	T47.4X1	T47.4X2	T47.4X3	T47.4X4	T47.4X5	T47.4X6
osmotic	T47.3X1	T47.3X2	T47.3X3	T47.3X4	T47.3X5	T47.3X6
saline	T47.3X1	T47.3X2	T47.3X3	T47.3X4	T47.3X5	T47.3X6
stimulant	T47.2X1	T47.2X2	T47.2X3	T47.2X4	T47.2X5	T47.2X6
L-dopa	T42.8X1	T42.8X2	T42.8X3	T42.8X4	T42.8X5	T42.8X6
Lead (dust) (fumes) (vapor)	T56.0X1	T56.0X2	T56.0X3	T56.0X4	—	—
NEC	T56.0X1	T56.0X2	T56.0X3	T56.0X4	—	—
acetate	T49.2X1	T49.2X2	T49.2X3	T49.2X4	T49.2X5	T49.2X6
alkyl (fuel additive)	T56.0X1	T56.0X2	T56.0X3	T56.0X4	—	—
anti-infectives	T37.8X1	T37.8X2	T37.8X3	T37.8X4	T37.8X5	T37.8X6
antiknock compound (tetraethyl)	T56.0X1	T56.0X2	T56.0X3	T56.0X4	—	—
arsenate, arsenite (dust)(herbicide) (insecticide) (vapor)	T57.0X1	T57.0X2	T57.0X3	T57.0X4	—	—
carbonate	T56.0X1	T56.0X2	T56.0X3	T56.0X4	—	—
paint	T56.0X1	T56.0X2	T56.0X3	T56.0X4	—	—
chromate	T56.0X1	T56.0X2	T56.0X3	T56.0X4	—	—
paint	T56.0X1	T56.0X2	T56.0X3	T56.0X4	—	—
dioxide	T56.0X1	T56.0X2	T56.0X3	T56.0X4	—	—
inorganic	T56.0X1	T56.0X2	T56.0X3	T56.0X4	—	—
iodide	T56.0X1	T56.0X2	T56.0X3	T56.0X4	—	—
pigment (paint)	T56.0X1	T56.0X2	T56.0X3	T56.0X4	—	—
monoxide (dust)	T56.0X1	T56.0X2	T56.0X3	T56.0X4	—	—
paint	T56.0X1	T56.0X2	T56.0X3	T56.0X4	—	—
organic	T56.0X1	T56.0X2	T56.0X3	T56.0X4	—	—
oxide	T56.0X1	T56.0X2	T56.0X3	T56.0X4	—	—
paint	T56.0X1	T56.0X2	T56.0X3	T56.0X4	—	—
paint	T56.0X1	T56.0X2	T56.0X3	T56.0X4	—	—
salts	T56.0X1	T56.0X2	T56.0X3	T56.0X4	—	—
specified compound NEC	T56.0X1	T56.0X2	T56.0X3	T56.0X4	—	—
tetra-ethyl	T56.0X1	T56.0X2	T56.0X3	T56.0X4	—	—
Lebanese red	T40.7X1	T40.7X2	T40.7X3	T40.7X4	T40.7X5	T40.7X6
Lefetamine	T39.8X1	T39.8X2	T39.8X3	T39.8X4	T39.8X5	T39.8X6
Lenperone	T43.4X1	T43.4X2	T43.4X3	T43.4X4	T43.4X5	T43.4X6
Lente lietin (insulin)	T38.3X1	T38.3X2	T38.3X3	T38.3X4	T38.3X5	T38.3X6
Leptazol	T50.7X1	T50.7X2	T50.7X3	T50.7X4	T50.7X5	T50.7X6
Leptophos	T60.0X1	T60.0X2	T60.0X3	T60.0X4	—	—
Leritine	T40.2X1	T40.2X2	T40.2X3	T40.2X4	T40.2X5	T40.2X6
Letosteine	T48.4X1	T48.4X2	T48.4X3	T48.4X4	T48.4X5	T48.4X6
Letter	T38.1X1	T38.1X2	T38.1X3	T38.1X4	T38.1X5	T38.1X6
Lettuce opium	T42.6X1	T42.6X2	T42.6X3	T42.6X4	T42.6X5	T42.6X6
Leucinocaine	T41.3X1	T41.3X2	T41.3X3	T41.3X4	T41.3X5	T41.3X6
Leucocianidol	T46.991	T46.992	T46.993	T46.994	T46.995	T46.996
Leucovorin (factor)	T45.8X1	T45.8X2	T45.8X3	T45.8X4	T45.8X5	T45.8X6
Leukeran	T45.1X1	T45.1X2	T45.1X3	T45.1X4	T45.1X5	T45.1X6
Leuprolide	T38.891	T38.892	T38.893	T38.894	T38.895	T38.896
Levalbuterol	T48.6X1	T48.6X2	T48.6X3	T48.6X4	T48.6X5	T48.6X6
Levallorphan	T50.7X1	T50.7X2	T50.7X3	T50.7X4	T50.7X5	T50.7X6
Levamisole	T37.4X1	T37.4X2	T37.4X3	T37.4X4	T37.4X5	T37.4X6
Levanil	T42.6X1	T42.6X2	T42.6X3	T42.6X4	T42.6X5	T42.6X6
Levarterenol	T44.4X1	T44.4X2	T44.4X3	T44.4X4	T44.4X5	T44.4X6
Levdropropizine	T48.3X1	T48.3X2	T48.3X3	T48.3X4	T48.3X5	T48.3X6
Levobunolol	T49.5X1	T49.5X2	T49.5X3	T49.5X4	T49.5X5	T49.5X6
Levocabastine (hydrochloride)	T45.0X1	T45.0X2	T45.0X3	T45.0X4	T45.0X5	T45.0X6
Levocarnitine	T50.991	T50.992	T50.993	T50.994	T50.995	T50.996
Levodopa	T42.8X1	T42.8X2	T42.8X3	T42.8X4	T42.8X5	T42.8X6
with carbidopa	T42.8X1	T42.8X2	T42.8X3	T42.8X4	T42.8X5	T42.8X6
Levo-dromoran	T40.2X1	T40.2X2	T40.2X3	T40.2X4	T40.2X5	T40.2X6
Levoglutamide	T50.991	T50.992	T50.993	T50.994	T50.995	T50.996
Levoid	T38.1X1	T38.1X2	T38.1X3	T38.1X4	T38.1X5	T38.1X6
Levo-isomethadone	T40.3X1	T40.3X2	T40.3X3	T40.3X4	T40.3X5	T40.3X6
Levomepromazine	T43.3X1	T43.3X2	T43.3X3	T43.3X4	T43.3X5	T43.3X6
Levonordefrin	T49.6X1	T49.6X2	T49.6X3	T49.6X4	T49.6X5	T49.6X6
Levonorgestrel	T38.4X1	T38.4X2	T38.4X3	T38.4X4	T38.4X5	T38.4X6
with ethinylestradiol	T38.5X1	T38.5X2	T38.5X3	T38.5X4	T38.5X5	T38.5X6
Levopromazine	T43.3X1	T43.3X2	T43.3X3	T43.3X4	T43.3X5	T43.3X6
Levoprome	T42.6X1	T42.6X2	T42.6X3	T42.6X4	T42.6X5	T42.6X6
Levopropoxyphene	T40.4X1	T40.4X2	T40.4X3	T40.4X4	T40.4X5	T40.4X6
Levopropylhexedrine	T50.5X1	T50.5X2	T50.5X3	T50.5X4	T50.5X5	T50.5X6
Levoproxyphylline	T48.6X1	T48.6X2	T48.6X3	T48.6X4	T48.6X5	T48.6X6
Levorphanol	T40.4X1	T40.4X2	T40.4X3	T40.4X4	T40.4X5	T40.4X6

Additional Character May Be Required — Refer to the Tabular List for Character Selection   ▽ Subterms under main terms may continue to next column or page

Substance	Poisoning, Accidental (unintentional)	Poisoning, Intentional Self-harm	Poisoning, Assault	Poisoning, Undetermined	Adverse Effect	Under-dosing
Levothyroxine	T38.1X1	T38.1X2	T38.1X3	T38.1X4	T38.1X5	T38.1X6
sodium	T38.1X1	T38.1X2	T38.1X3	T38.1X4	T38.1X5	T38.1X6
Levsin	T44.3X1	T44.3X2	T44.3X3	T44.3X4	T44.3X5	T44.3X6
Levulose	T50.3X1	T50.3X2	T50.3X3	T50.3X4	T50.3X5	T50.3X6
Lewisite (gas), not in war	T57.0X1	T57.0X2	T57.0X3	T57.0X4	—	—
Librium	T42.4X1	T42.4X2	T42.4X3	T42.4X4	T42.4X5	T42.4X6
Lidex	T49.0X1	T49.0X2	T49.0X3	T49.0X4	T49.0X5	T49.0X6
Lidocaine	T41.3X1	T41.3X2	T41.3X3	T41.3X4	T41.3X5	T41.3X6
regional	T41.3X1	T41.3X2	T41.3X3	T41.3X4	T41.3X5	T41.3X6
spinal	T41.3X1	T41.3X2	T41.3X3	T41.3X4	T41.3X5	T41.3X6
Lidofenin	T50.8X1	T50.8X2	T50.8X3	T50.8X4	T50.8X5	T50.8X6
Lidoflazine	T46.1X1	T46.1X2	T46.1X3	T46.1X4	T46.1X5	T46.1X6
Lighter fluid	T52.0X1	T52.0X2	T52.0X3	T52.0X4	—	—
Lignin hemicellulose	T47.6X1	T47.6X2	T47.6X3	T47.6X4	T47.6X5	T47.6X6
Lignocaine	T41.3X1	T41.3X2	T41.3X3	T41.3X4	T41.3X5	T41.3X6
regional	T41.3X1	T41.3X2	T41.3X3	T41.3X4	T41.3X5	T41.3X6
spinal	T41.3X1	T41.3X2	T41.3X3	T41.3X4	T41.3X5	T41.3X6
Ligroin (e) (solvent)	T52.0X1	T52.0X2	T52.0X3	T52.0X4	—	—
vapor	T59.891	T59.892	T59.893	T59.894	—	—
Ligustrum vulgare	T62.2X1	T62.2X2	T62.2X3	T62.2X4	—	—
Lily of the valley	T62.2X1	T62.2X2	T62.2X3	T62.2X4	—	—
Lime (chloride)	T54.3X1	T54.3X2	T54.3X3	T54.3X4	—	—
Limonene	T52.8X1	T52.8X2	T52.8X3	T52.8X4	—	—
Lincomycin	T36.8X1	T36.8X2	T36.8X3	T36.8X4	T36.8X5	T36.8X6
Lindane (insecticide) (nonmedicinal) (vapor)	T53.6X1	T53.6X2	T53.6X3	T53.6X4	—	—
medicinal	T49.0X1	T49.0X2	T49.0X3	T49.0X4	T49.0X5	T49.0X6
Liniments NEC	T49.91	T49.92	T49.93	T49.94	T49.95	T49.96
Linoleic acid	T46.6X1	T46.6X2	T46.6X3	T46.6X4	T46.6X5	T46.6X6
Linolenic acid	T46.6X1	T46.6X2	T46.6X3	T46.6X4	T46.6X5	T46.6X6
Linseed	T47.4X1	T47.4X2	T47.4X3	T47.4X4	T47.4X5	T47.4X6
Liothyronine	T38.1X1	T38.1X2	T38.1X3	T38.1X4	T38.1X5	T38.1X6
Liotrix	T38.1X1	T38.1X2	T38.1X3	T38.1X4	T38.1X5	T38.1X6
Lipancreatin	T47.5X1	T47.5X2	T47.5X3	T47.5X4	T47.5X5	T47.5X6
Lipo-alprostadil	T46.7X1	T46.7X2	T46.7X3	T46.7X4	T46.7X5	T46.7X6
Lipo-Lutin	T38.5X1	T38.5X2	T38.5X3	T38.5X4	T38.5X5	T38.5X6
Lipotropic drug NEC	T50.901	T50.902	T50.903	T50.904	T50.905	T50.906
Liquefied petroleum gases	T59.891	T59.892	T59.893	T59.894	—	—
piped (pure or mixed with air)	T59.891	T59.892	T59.893	T59.894	—	—
Liquid						
paraffin	T47.4X1	T47.4X2	T47.4X3	T47.4X4	T47.4X5	T47.4X6
petrolatum	T47.4X1	T47.4X2	T47.4X3	T47.4X4	T47.4X5	T47.4X6
topical	T49.3X1	T49.3X2	T49.3X3	T49.3X4	T49.3X5	T49.3X6
specified NEC	T65.891	T65.892	T65.893	T65.894	—	—
substance	T65.91	T65.92	T65.93	T65.94	—	—
Liquor creosolis compositus	T65.891	T65.892	T65.893	T65.894	—	—
Liquorice	T48.4X1	T48.4X2	T48.4X3	T48.4X4	T48.4X5	T48.4X6
extract	T47.8X1	T47.8X2	T47.8X3	T47.8X4	T47.8X5	T47.8X6
Lisinopril	T46.4X1	T46.4X2	T46.4X3	T46.4X4	T46.4X5	T46.4X6
Lisuride	T42.8X1	T42.8X2	T42.8X3	T42.8X4	T42.8X5	T42.8X6
Lithane	T43.8X1	T43.8X2	T43.8X3	T43.8X4	T43.8X5	T43.8X6
Lithium	T56.891	T56.892	T56.893	T56.894	—	—
gluconate	T43.591	T43.592	T43.593	T43.594	T43.595	T43.596
salts (carbonate)	T43.591	T43.592	T43.593	T43.594	T43.595	T43.596
Lithonate	T43.8X1	T43.8X2	T43.8X3	T43.8X4	T43.8X5	T43.8X6
Liver						
extract	T45.8X1	T45.8X2	T45.8X3	T45.8X4	T45.8X5	T45.8X6
for parenteral use	T45.8X1	T45.8X2	T45.8X3	T45.8X4	T45.8X5	T45.8X6
fraction 1	T45.8X1	T45.8X2	T45.8X3	T45.8X4	T45.8X5	T45.8X6
hydrolysate	T45.8X1	T45.8X2	T45.8X3	T45.8X4	T45.8X5	T45.8X6
Lizard (bite) (venom)	T63.121	T63.122	T63.123	T63.124	—	—
LMD	T45.8X1	T45.8X2	T45.8X3	T45.8X4	T45.8X5	T45.8X6
Lobelia	T62.2X1	T62.2X2	T62.2X3	T62.2X4	—	—
Lobeline	T50.7X1	T50.7X2	T50.7X3	T50.7X4	T50.7X5	T50.7X6
Local action drug NEC	T49.8X1	T49.8X2	T49.8X3	T49.8X4	T49.8X5	T49.8X6
Locorten	T49.0X1	T49.0X2	T49.0X3	T49.0X4	T49.0X5	T49.0X6
Lofepramine	T43.011	T43.012	T43.013	T43.014	T43.015	T43.016
Lolium temulentum	T62.2X1	T62.2X2	T62.2X3	T62.2X4	—	—
Lomotil	T47.6X1	T47.6X2	T47.6X3	T47.6X4	T47.6X5	T47.6X6
Lomustine	T45.1X1	T45.1X2	T45.1X3	T45.1X4	T45.1X5	T45.1X6
Lonidamine	T45.1X1	T45.1X2	T45.1X3	T45.1X4	T45.1X5	T45.1X6
Loperamide	T47.6X1	T47.6X2	T47.6X3	T47.6X4	T47.6X5	T47.6X6
Loprazolam	T42.4X1	T42.4X2	T42.4X3	T42.4X4	T42.4X5	T42.4X6
Lorajmine	T46.2X1	T46.2X2	T46.2X3	T46.2X4	T46.2X5	T46.2X6
Loratadine	T45.0X1	T45.0X2	T45.0X3	T45.0X4	T45.0X5	T45.0X6
Lorazepam	T42.4X1	T42.4X2	T42.4X3	T42.4X4	T42.4X5	T42.4X6
Lorcainide	T46.2X1	T46.2X2	T46.2X3	T46.2X4	T46.2X5	T46.2X6
Lormetazepam	T42.4X1	T42.4X2	T42.4X3	T42.4X4	T42.4X5	T42.4X6
Lotions NEC	T49.91	T49.92	T49.93	T49.94	T49.95	T49.96
Lotusate	T42.3X1	T42.3X2	T42.3X3	T42.3X4	T42.3X5	T42.3X6
Lovastatin	T46.6X1	T46.6X2	T46.6X3	T46.6X4	T46.6X5	T46.6X6
Lowila	T49.2X1	T49.2X2	T49.2X3	T49.2X4	T49.2X5	T49.2X6
Loxapine	T43.591	T43.592	T43.593	T43.594	T43.595	T43.596
Lozenges (throat)	T49.6X1	T49.6X2	T49.6X3	T49.6X4	T49.6X5	T49.6X6
LSD	T40.8X1	T40.8X2	T40.8X3	T40.8X4	—	—
L-Tryptophan — see amino acid						
Lubricant, eye	T49.5X1	T49.5X2	T49.5X3	T49.5X4	T49.5X5	T49.5X6
Lubricating oil NEC	T52.0X1	T52.0X2	T52.0X3	T52.0X4	—	—
Lucanthone	T37.4X1	T37.4X2	T37.4X3	T37.4X4	T37.4X5	T37.4X6
Luminal	T42.3X1	T42.3X2	T42.3X3	T42.3X4	T42.3X5	T42.3X6
Lung irritant (gas) NEC	T59.91	T59.92	T59.93	T59.94	—	—
Luteinizing hormone	T38.811	T38.812	T38.813	T38.814	T38.815	T38.816
Lutocylol	T38.5X1	T38.5X2	T38.5X3	T38.5X4	T38.5X5	T38.5X6
Lutromone	T38.5X1	T38.5X2	T38.5X3	T38.5X4	T38.5X5	T38.5X6
Lututrin	T48.291	T48.292	T48.293	T48.294	T48.295	T48.296
Lye (concentrated)	T54.3X1	T54.3X2	T54.3X3	T54.3X4	—	—
Lygranum (skin test)	T50.8X1	T50.8X2	T50.8X3	T50.8X4	T50.8X5	T50.8X6
Lymecycline	T36.4X1	T36.4X2	T36.4X3	T36.4X4	T36.4X5	T36.4X6
Lymphogranuloma venereum antigen	T50.8X1	T50.8X2	T50.8X3	T50.8X4	T50.8X5	T50.8X6
Lynestrenol	T38.4X1	T38.4X2	T38.4X3	T38.4X4	T38.4X5	T38.4X6
Lyovac Sodium Edecrin	T50.1X1	T50.1X2	T50.1X3	T50.1X4	T50.1X5	T50.1X6
Lypressin	T38.891	T38.892	T38.893	T38.894	T38.895	T38.896
Lysergic acid diethylamide	T40.8X1	T40.8X2	T40.8X3	T40.8X4	—	—
Lysergide	T40.8X1	T40.8X2	T40.8X3	T40.8X4	—	—
Lysine vasopressin	T38.891	T38.892	T38.893	T38.894	T38.895	T38.896
Lysol	T54.1X1	T54.1X2	T54.1X3	T54.1X4	—	—
Lysozyme	T49.0X1	T49.0X2	T49.0X3	T49.0X4	T49.0X5	T49.0X6
Lytta (vitatta)	T49.8X1	T49.8X2	T49.8X3	T49.8X4	T49.8X5	T49.8X6
Mace	T59.3X1	T59.3X2	T59.3X3	T59.3X4	—	—
Macrogol	T50.991	T50.992	T50.993	T50.994	T50.995	T50.996
Macrolide						
anabolic drug	T38.7X1	T38.7X2	T38.7X3	T38.7X4	T38.7X5	T38.7X6
antibiotic	T36.3X1	T36.3X2	T36.3X3	T36.3X4	T36.3X5	T36.3X6
Mafenide	T49.0X1	T49.0X2	T49.0X3	T49.0X4	T49.0X5	T49.0X6
Magaldrate	T47.1X1	T47.1X2	T47.1X3	T47.1X4	T47.1X5	T47.1X6
Magic mushroom	T40.991	T40.992	T40.993	T40.994	—	—
Magnamycin	T36.8X1	T36.8X2	T36.8X3	T36.8X4	T36.8X5	T36.8X6
Magnesia magma	T47.1X1	T47.1X2	T47.1X3	T47.1X4	T47.1X5	T47.1X6
Magnesium NEC	T56.891	T56.892	T56.893	T56.894	—	—
carbonate	T47.1X1	T47.1X2	T47.1X3	T47.1X4	T47.1X5	T47.1X6
citrate	T47.4X1	T47.4X2	T47.4X3	T47.4X4	T47.4X5	T47.4X6
hydroxide	T47.1X1	T47.1X2	T47.1X3	T47.1X4	T47.1X5	T47.1X6
oxide	T47.1X1	T47.1X2	T47.1X3	T47.1X4	T47.1X5	T47.1X6
peroxide	T49.0X1	T49.0X2	T49.0X3	T49.0X4	T49.0X5	T49.0X6
salicylate	T39.091	T39.092	T39.093	T39.094	T39.095	T39.096
silicofluoride	T50.3X1	T50.3X2	T50.3X3	T50.3X4	T50.3X5	T50.3X6
sulfate	T47.4X1	T47.4X2	T47.4X3	T47.4X4	T47.4X5	T47.4X6
thiosulfate	T45.0X1	T45.0X2	T45.0X3	T45.0X4	T45.0X5	T45.0X6
trisilicate	T47.1X1	T47.1X2	T47.1X3	T47.1X4	T47.1X5	T47.1X6
Malathion (medicinal)	T49.0X1	T49.0X2	T49.0X3	T49.0X4	T49.0X5	T49.0X6
insecticide	T60.0X1	T60.0X2	T60.0X3	T60.0X4	—	—
Male fern extract	T37.4X1	T37.4X2	T37.4X3	T37.4X4	T37.4X5	T37.4X6
M-AMSA	T45.1X1	T45.1X2	T45.1X3	T45.1X4	T45.1X5	T45.1X6
Mandelic acid	T37.8X1	T37.8X2	T37.8X3	T37.8X4	T37.8X5	T37.8X6
Manganese (dioxide) (salts)	T57.2X1	T57.2X2	T57.2X3	T57.2X4	—	—
medicinal	T50.991	T50.992	T50.993	T50.994	T50.995	T50.996
Mannitol	T47.3X1	T47.3X2	T47.3X3	T47.3X4	T47.3X5	T47.3X6
hexanitrate	T46.3X1	T46.3X2	T46.3X3	T46.3X4	T46.3X5	T46.3X6
Mannomustine	T45.1X1	T45.1X2	T45.1X3	T45.1X4	T45.1X5	T45.1X6
MAO inhibitors	T43.1X1	T43.1X2	T43.1X3	T43.1X4	T43.1X5	T43.1X6
Mapharsen	T37.8X1	T37.8X2	T37.8X3	T37.8X4	T37.8X5	T37.8X6
Maphenide	T49.0X1	T49.0X2	T49.0X3	T49.0X4	T49.0X5	T49.0X6
Maprotiline	T43.021	T43.022	T43.023	T43.024	T43.025	T43.026
Marcaine	T41.3X1	T41.3X2	T41.3X3	T41.3X4	T41.3X5	T41.3X6
infiltration (subcutaneous)	T41.3X1	T41.3X2	T41.3X3	T41.3X4	T41.3X5	T41.3X6
nerve block (peripheral) (plexus)	T41.3X1	T41.3X2	T41.3X3	T41.3X4	T41.3X5	T41.3X6
Marezine	T45.0X1	T45.0X2	T45.0X3	T45.0X4	T45.0X5	T45.0X6
Marihuana	T40.7X1	T40.7X2	T40.7X3	T40.7X4	T40.7X5	T40.7X6
Marijuana	T40.7X1	T40.7X2	T40.7X3	T40.7X4	T40.7X5	T40.7X6
Marine (sting)	T63.691	T63.692	T63.693	T63.694	—	—
animals (sting)	T63.691	T63.692	T63.693	T63.694	—	—
plants (sting)	T63.711	T63.712	T63.713	T63.714	—	—
Marplan	T43.1X1	T43.1X2	T43.1X3	T43.1X4	T43.1X5	T43.1X6
Marsh gas	T59.891	T59.892	T59.893	T59.894	—	—
Marsilid	T43.1X1	T43.1X2	T43.1X3	T43.1X4	T43.1X5	T43.1X6
Matulane	T45.1X1	T45.1X2	T45.1X3	T45.1X4	T45.1X5	T45.1X6
Mazindol	T50.5X1	T50.5X2	T50.5X3	T50.5X4	T50.5X5	T50.5X6
MCPA	T60.3X1	T60.3X2	T60.3X3	T60.3X4	—	—
MDMA	T43.641	T43.642	T43.643	T43.644	—	—
Meadow saffron	T62.2X1	T62.2X2	T62.2X3	T62.2X4	—	—
Measles virus vaccine (attenuated)	T50.B91	T50.B92	T50.B93	T50.B94	T50.B95	T50.B96

Substance	Poisoning, Accidental (unintentional)	Poisoning, Intentional Self-harm	Poisoning, Assault	Poisoning, Undetermined	Adverse Effect	Under-dosing
Meat, noxious	T62.8X1	T62.8X2	T62.8X3	T62.8X4	—	—
Meballymal	T42.3X1	T42.3X2	T42.3X3	T42.3X4	T42.3X5	T42.3X6
Mebanazine	T43.1X1	T43.1X2	T43.1X3	T43.1X4	T43.1X5	T43.1X6
Mebaral	T42.3X1	T42.3X2	T42.3X3	T42.3X4	T42.3X5	T42.3X6
Mebendazole	T37.4X1	T37.4X2	T37.4X3	T37.4X4	T37.4X5	T37.4X6
Mebeverine	T44.3X1	T44.3X2	T44.3X3	T44.3X4	T44.3X5	T44.3X6
Mebhydrolin	T45.0X1	T45.0X2	T45.0X3	T45.0X4	T45.0X5	T45.0X6
Mebumal	T42.3X1	T42.3X2	T42.3X3	T42.3X4	T42.3X5	T42.3X6
Mebutamate	T44.2X1	T44.2X2	T44.2X3	T44.2X4	T44.2X5	T44.2X6
Mecamylamine	T44.2X1	T44.2X2	T44.2X3	T44.2X4	T44.2X5	T44.2X6
Mechlorethamine	T45.1X1	T45.1X2	T45.1X3	T45.1X4	T45.1X5	T45.1X6
Mecillinam	T36.0X1	T36.0X2	T36.0X3	T36.0X4	T36.0X5	T36.0X6
Meclizine (hydrochloride)	T45.0X1	T45.0X2	T45.0X3	T45.0X4	T45.0X5	T45.0X6
Meclocycline	T36.4X1	T36.4X2	T36.4X3	T36.4X4	T36.4X5	T36.4X6
Meclofenamate	T39.391	T39.392	T39.393	T39.394	T39.395	T39.396
Meclofenamic acid	T39.391	T39.392	T39.393	T39.394	T39.395	T39.396
Meclofenoxate	T43.691	T43.692	T43.693	T43.694	T43.695	T43.696
Meclozine	T45.0X1	T45.0X2	T45.0X3	T45.0X4	T45.0X5	T45.0X6
Mecobalamin	T45.8X1	T45.8X2	T45.8X3	T45.8X4	T45.8X5	T45.8X6
Mecoprop	T60.3X1	T60.3X2	T60.3X3	T60.3X4	—	—
Mecrilate	T49.3X1	T49.3X2	T49.3X3	T49.3X4	T49.3X5	T49.3X6
Mecysteine	T48.4X1	T48.4X2	T48.4X3	T48.4X4	T48.4X5	T48.4X6
Medazepam	T42.4X1	T42.4X2	T42.4X3	T42.4X4	T42.4X5	T42.4X6
Medicament NEC	T50.901	T50.902	T50.903	T50.904	T50.905	T50.906
Medinal	T42.3X1	T42.3X2	T42.3X3	T42.3X4	T42.3X5	T42.3X6
Medomin	T42.3X1	T42.3X2	T42.3X3	T42.3X4	T42.3X5	T42.3X6
Medrogestone	T38.5X1	T38.5X2	T38.5X3	T38.5X4	T38.5X5	T38.5X6
Medroxalol	T44.8X1	T44.8X2	T44.8X3	T44.8X4	T44.8X5	T44.8X6
Medroxyprogesterone acetate (depot)	T38.5X1	T38.5X2	T38.5X3	T38.5X4	T38.5X5	T38.5X6
Medrysone	T49.0X1	T49.0X2	T49.0X3	T49.0X4	T49.0X5	T49.0X6
Mefenamic acid	T39.391	T39.392	T39.393	T39.394	T39.395	T39.396
Mefenorex	T50.5X1	T50.5X2	T50.5X3	T50.5X4	T50.5X5	T50.5X6
Mefloquine	T37.2X1	T37.2X2	T37.2X3	T37.2X4	T37.2X5	T37.2X6
Mefruside	T50.2X1	T50.2X2	T50.2X3	T50.2X4	T50.2X5	T50.2X6
Megahallucinogen	T40.901	T40.902	T40.903	T40.904	T40.905	T40.906
Megestrol	T38.5X1	T38.5X2	T38.5X3	T38.5X4	T38.5X5	T38.5X6
Meglumine						
antimoniate	T37.8X1	T37.8X2	T37.8X3	T37.8X4	T37.8X5	T37.8X6
diatrizoate	T50.8X1	T50.8X2	T50.8X3	T50.8X4	T50.8X5	T50.8X6
iodipamide	T50.8X1	T50.8X2	T50.8X3	T50.8X4	T50.8X5	T50.8X6
iotroxate	T50.8X1	T50.8X2	T50.8X3	T50.8X4	T50.8X5	T50.8X6
MEK (methyl ethyl ketone)	T52.4X1	T52.4X2	T52.4X3	T52.4X4	—	—
Meladinin	T49.3X1	T49.3X2	T49.3X3	T49.3X4	T49.3X5	T49.3X6
Meladrazine	T44.3X1	T44.3X2	T44.3X3	T44.3X4	T44.3X5	T44.3X6
Melaleuca alternifolia oil	T49.0X1	T49.0X2	T49.0X3	T49.0X4	T49.0X5	T49.0X6
Melanizing agents	T49.3X1	T49.3X2	T49.3X3	T49.3X4	T49.3X5	T49.3X6
Melanocyte-stimulating hormone	T38.891	T38.892	T38.893	T38.894	T38.895	T38.896
Melarsonyl potassium	T37.3X1	T37.3X2	T37.3X3	T37.3X4	T37.3X5	T37.3X6
Melarsoprol	T37.3X1	T37.3X2	T37.3X3	T37.3X4	T37.3X5	T37.3X6
Melia azedarach	T62.2X1	T62.2X2	T62.2X3	T62.2X4	—	—
Melitracen	T43.011	T43.012	T43.013	T43.014	T43.015	T43.016
Mellaril	T43.3X1	T43.3X2	T43.3X3	T43.3X4	T43.3X5	T43.3X6
Meloxine	T49.3X1	T49.3X2	T49.3X3	T49.3X4	T49.3X5	T49.3X6
Melperone	T43.4X1	T43.4X2	T43.4X3	T43.4X4	T43.4X5	T43.4X6
Melphalan	T45.1X1	T45.1X2	T45.1X3	T45.1X4	T45.1X5	T45.1X6
Memantine	T43.8X1	T43.8X2	T43.8X3	T43.8X4	T43.8X5	T43.8X6
Menadiol	T45.7X1	T45.7X2	T45.7X3	T45.7X4	T45.7X5	T45.7X6
sodium sulfate	T45.7X1	T45.7X2	T45.7X3	T45.7X4	T45.7X5	T45.7X6
Menadione	T45.7X1	T45.7X2	T45.7X3	T45.7X4	T45.7X5	T45.7X6
sodium bisulfite	T45.7X1	T45.7X2	T45.7X3	T45.7X4	T45.7X5	T45.7X6
Menaphthone	T45.7X1	T45.7X2	T45.7X3	T45.7X4	T45.7X5	T45.7X6
Menaquinone	T45.7X1	T45.7X2	T45.7X3	T45.7X4	T45.7X5	T45.7X6
Menatetrenone	T45.7X1	T45.7X2	T45.7X3	T45.7X4	T45.7X5	T45.7X6
Meningococcal vaccine	T50.A91	T50.A92	T50.A93	T50.A94	T50.A95	T50.A96
Menningovax (-AC) (-C)	T50.A91	T50.A92	T50.A93	T50.A94	T50.A95	T50.A96
Menotropins	T38.811	T38.812	T38.813	T38.814	T38.815	T38.816
Menthol	T48.5X1	T48.5X2	T48.5X3	T48.5X4	T48.5X5	T48.5X6
Mepacrine	T37.2X1	T37.2X2	T37.2X3	T37.2X4	T37.2X5	T37.2X6
Meparfynol	T42.6X1	T42.6X2	T42.6X3	T42.6X4	T42.6X5	T42.6X6
Mepartricin	T36.7X1	T36.7X2	T36.7X3	T36.7X4	T36.7X5	T36.7X6
Mepazine	T43.3X1	T43.3X2	T43.3X3	T43.3X4	T43.3X5	T43.3X6
Mepenzolate	T44.3X1	T44.3X2	T44.3X3	T44.3X4	T44.3X5	T44.3X6
bromide	T44.3X1	T44.3X2	T44.3X3	T44.3X4	T44.3X5	T44.3X6
Meperidine	T40.4X1	T40.4X2	T40.4X3	T40.4X4	T40.4X5	T40.4X6
Mephebarbital	T42.3X1	T42.3X2	T42.3X3	T42.3X4	T42.3X5	T42.3X6
Mephenamin (e)	T42.8X1	T42.8X2	T42.8X3	T42.8X4	T42.8X5	T42.8X6
Mephenesin	T42.8X1	T42.8X2	T42.8X3	T42.8X4	T42.8X5	T42.8X6
Mephenhydramine	T45.0X1	T45.0X2	T45.0X3	T45.0X4	T45.0X5	T45.0X6
Mephenoxalone	T42.8X1	T42.8X2	T42.8X3	T42.8X4	T42.8X5	T42.8X6
Mephentermine	T44.991	T44.992	T44.993	T44.994	T44.995	T44.996
Mephenytoin	T42.0X1	T42.0X2	T42.0X3	T42.0X4	T42.0X5	T42.0X6

Substance	Poisoning, Accidental (unintentional)	Poisoning, Intentional Self-harm	Poisoning, Assault	Poisoning, Undetermined	Adverse Effect	Under-dosing
Mephenytoin — continued						
with phenobarbital	T42.3X1	T42.3X2	T42.3X3	T42.3X4	T42.3X5	T42.3X6
Mephobarbital	T42.3X1	T42.3X2	T42.3X3	T42.3X4	T42.3X5	T42.3X6
Mephosfolan	T60.0X1	T60.0X2	T60.0X3	T60.0X4	—	—
Mepindolol	T44.7X1	T44.7X2	T44.7X3	T44.7X4	T44.7X5	T44.7X6
Mepiperphenidol	T44.3X1	T44.3X2	T44.3X3	T44.3X4	T44.3X5	T44.3X6
Mepitiostane	T38.7X1	T38.7X2	T38.7X3	T38.7X4	T38.7X5	T38.7X6
Mepivacaine	T41.3X1	T41.3X2	T41.3X3	T41.3X4	T41.3X5	T41.3X6
epidural	T41.3X1	T41.3X2	T41.3X3	T41.3X4	T41.3X5	T41.3X6
Meprednisone	T38.0X1	T38.0X2	T38.0X3	T38.0X4	T38.0X5	T38.0X6
Meprobam	T43.591	T43.592	T43.593	T43.594	T43.595	T43.596
Meprobamate	T43.591	T43.592	T43.593	T43.594	T43.595	T43.596
Meproscillarin	T46.0X1	T46.0X2	T46.0X3	T46.0X4	T46.0X5	T46.0X6
Meprylcaine	T41.3X1	T41.3X2	T41.3X3	T41.3X4	T41.3X5	T41.3X6
Meptazinol	T39.8X1	T39.8X2	T39.8X3	T39.8X4	T39.8X5	T39.8X6
Mepyramine	T45.0X1	T45.0X2	T45.0X3	T45.0X4	T45.0X5	T45.0X6
Mequitazine	T43.3X1	T43.3X2	T43.3X3	T43.3X4	T43.3X5	T43.3X6
Meralluride	T50.2X1	T50.2X2	T50.2X3	T50.2X4	T50.2X5	T50.2X6
Merbaphen	T50.2X1	T50.2X2	T50.2X3	T50.2X4	T50.2X5	T50.2X6
Merbromin	T49.0X1	T49.0X2	T49.0X3	T49.0X4	T49.0X5	T49.0X6
Mercaptobenzothiazole salts	T49.0X1	T49.0X2	T49.0X3	T49.0X4	T49.0X5	T49.0X6
Mercaptomerin	T50.2X1	T50.2X2	T50.2X3	T50.2X4	T50.2X5	T50.2X6
Mercaptopurine	T45.1X1	T45.1X2	T45.1X3	T45.1X4	T45.1X5	T45.1X6
Mercumatilin	T50.2X1	T50.2X2	T50.2X3	T50.2X4	T50.2X5	T50.2X6
Mercuramide	T50.2X1	T50.2X2	T50.2X3	T50.2X4	T50.2X5	T50.2X6
Mercurochrome	T49.0X1	T49.0X2	T49.0X3	T49.0X4	T49.0X5	T49.0X6
Mercurophylline	T50.2X1	T50.2X2	T50.2X3	T50.2X4	T50.2X5	T50.2X6
Mercury, mercurial, mercuric, mercurous (compounds) (cyanide) (fumes) (nonmedicinal) (vapor) NEC	T56.1X1	T56.1X2	T56.1X3	T56.1X4	—	—
ammoniated	T49.0X1	T49.0X2	T49.0X3	T49.0X4	T49.0X5	T49.0X6
anti-infective						
local	T49.0X1	T49.0X2	T49.0X3	T49.0X4	T49.0X5	T49.0X6
systemic	T37.8X1	T37.8X2	T37.8X3	T37.8X4	T37.8X5	T37.8X6
topical	T49.0X1	T49.0X2	T49.0X3	T49.0X4	T49.0X5	T49.0X6
chloride (ammoniated)	T49.0X1	T49.0X2	T49.0X3	T49.0X4	T49.0X5	T49.0X6
fungicide	T56.1X1	T56.1X2	T56.1X3	T56.1X4	—	—
diuretic NEC	T50.2X1	T50.2X2	T50.2X3	T50.2X4	T50.2X5	T50.2X6
fungicide	T56.1X1	T56.1X2	T56.1X3	T56.1X4	—	—
organic (fungicide)	T56.1X1	T56.1X2	T56.1X3	T56.1X4	—	—
oxide, yellow	T49.0X1	T49.0X2	T49.0X3	T49.0X4	T49.0X5	T49.0X6
Mersalyl	T50.2X1	T50.2X2	T50.2X3	T50.2X4	T50.2X5	T50.2X6
Merthiolate	T49.0X1	T49.0X2	T49.0X3	T49.0X4	T49.0X5	T49.0X6
ophthalmic preparation	T49.5X1	T49.5X2	T49.5X3	T49.5X4	T49.5X5	T49.5X6
Meruvax	T50.B91	T50.B92	T50.B93	T50.B94	T50.B95	T50.B96
Mesalazine	T47.8X1	T47.8X2	T47.8X3	T47.8X4	T47.8X5	T47.8X6
Mescal buttons	T40.991	T40.992	T40.993	T40.994	—	—
Mescaline	T40.991	T40.992	T40.993	T40.994	—	—
Mesna	T48.4X1	T48.4X2	T48.4X3	T48.4X4	T48.4X5	T48.4X6
Mesoglycan	T46.6X1	T46.6X2	T46.6X3	T46.6X4	T46.6X5	T46.6X6
Mesoridazine	T43.3X1	T43.3X2	T43.3X3	T43.3X4	T43.3X5	T43.3X6
Mestanolone	T38.7X1	T38.7X2	T38.7X3	T38.7X4	T38.7X5	T38.7X6
Mesterolone	T38.7X1	T38.7X2	T38.7X3	T38.7X4	T38.7X5	T38.7X6
Mestranol	T38.5X1	T38.5X2	T38.5X3	T38.5X4	T38.5X5	T38.5X6
Mesulergine	T42.8X1	T42.8X2	T42.8X3	T42.8X4	T42.8X5	T42.8X6
Mesulfen	T49.0X1	T49.0X2	T49.0X3	T49.0X4	T49.0X5	T49.0X6
Mesuximide	T42.2X1	T42.2X2	T42.2X3	T42.2X4	T42.2X5	T42.2X6
Metabutethamine	T41.3X1	T41.3X2	T41.3X3	T41.3X4	T41.3X5	T41.3X6
Metactesylacetate	T49.0X1	T49.0X2	T49.0X3	T49.0X4	T49.0X5	T49.0X6
Metacycline	T36.4X1	T36.4X2	T36.4X3	T36.4X4	T36.4X5	T36.4X6
Metaldehyde (snail killer) NEC	T60.8X1	T60.8X2	T60.8X3	T60.8X4	—	—
Metals (heavy) (nonmedicinal)	T56.91	T56.92	T56.93	T56.94	—	—
dust, fumes, or vapor NEC	T56.91	T56.92	T56.93	T56.94	—	—
light NEC	T56.91	T56.92	T56.93	T56.94	—	—
dust, fumes, or vapor NEC	T56.91	T56.92	T56.93	T56.94	—	—
specified NEC	T56.891	T56.892	T56.893	T56.894	—	—
thallium	T56.811	T56.812	T56.813	T56.814	—	—
Metamfetamine	T43.621	T43.622	T43.623	T43.624	T43.625	T43.626
Metamizole sodium	T39.2X1	T39.2X2	T39.2X3	T39.2X4	T39.2X5	T39.2X6
Metampicillin	T36.0X1	T36.0X2	T36.0X3	T36.0X4	T36.0X5	T36.0X6
Metamucil	T47.4X1	T47.4X2	T47.4X3	T47.4X4	T47.4X5	T47.4X6
Metandienone	T38.7X1	T38.7X2	T38.7X3	T38.7X4	T38.7X5	T38.7X6
Metandrostenolone	T38.7X1	T38.7X2	T38.7X3	T38.7X4	T38.7X5	T38.7X6
Metaphen	T49.0X1	T49.0X2	T49.0X3	T49.0X4	T49.0X5	T49.0X6
Metaphos	T60.0X1	T60.0X2	T60.0X3	T60.0X4	—	—
Metapramine	T43.011	T43.012	T43.013	T43.014	T43.015	T43.016
Metaproterenol	T48.291	T48.292	T48.293	T48.294	T48.295	T48.296

Substance	Poisoning, Accidental (unintentional)	Poisoning, Intentional Self-harm	Poisoning, Assault	Poisoning, Undetermined	Adverse Effect	Under-dosing
Metaraminol	T44.4X1	T44.4X2	T44.4X3	T44.4X4	T44.4X5	T44.4X6
Metaxalone	T42.8X1	T42.8X2	T42.8X3	T42.8X4	T42.8X5	T42.8X6
Metenolone	T38.7X1	T38.7X2	T38.7X3	T38.7X4	T38.7X5	T38.7X6
Metergoline	T42.8X1	T42.8X2	T42.8X3	T42.8X4	T42.8X5	T42.8X6
Metescufylline	T46.991	T46.992	T46.993	T46.994	T46.995	T46.996
Metetoin	T42.0X1	T42.0X2	T42.0X3	T42.0X4	T42.0X5	T42.0X6
Metformin	T38.3X1	T38.3X2	T38.3X3	T38.3X4	T38.3X5	T38.3X6
Methacholine	T44.1X1	T44.1X2	T44.1X3	T44.1X4	T44.1X5	T44.1X6
Methacycline	T36.4X1	T36.4X2	T36.4X3	T36.4X4	T36.4X5	T36.4X6
Methadone	T40.3X1	T40.3X2	T40.3X3	T40.3X4	T40.3X5	T40.3X6
Methallenestril	T38.5X1	T38.5X2	T38.5X3	T38.5X4	T38.5X5	T38.5X6
Methallenoestril	T38.5X1	T38.5X2	T38.5X3	T38.5X4	T38.5X5	T38.5X6
Methamphetamine	T43.621	T43.622	T43.623	T43.624	T43.625	T43.626
Methampyrone	T39.2X1	T39.2X2	T39.2X3	T39.2X4	T39.2X5	T39.2X6
Methandienone	T38.7X1	T38.7X2	T38.7X3	T38.7X4	T38.7X5	T38.7X6
Methandriol	T38.7X1	T38.7X2	T38.7X3	T38.7X4	T38.7X5	T38.7X6
Methandrostenolone	T38.7X1	T38.7X2	T38.7X3	T38.7X4	T38.7X5	T38.7X6
Methane	T59.891	T59.892	T59.893	T59.894	—	—
Methanethiol	T59.891	T59.892	T59.893	T59.894	—	—
Methaniazide	T37.1X1	T37.1X2	T37.1X3	T37.1X4	T37.1X5	T37.1X6
Methanol (vapor)	T51.1X1	T51.1X2	T51.1X3	T51.1X4	—	—
Methantheline	T44.3X1	T44.3X2	T44.3X3	T44.3X4	T44.3X5	T44.3X6
Methanthelinium bromide	T44.3X1	T44.3X2	T44.3X3	T44.3X4	T44.3X5	T44.3X6
Methaphenilene	T45.0X1	T45.0X2	T45.0X3	T45.0X4	T45.0X5	T45.0X6
Methapyrilene	T45.0X1	T45.0X2	T45.0X3	T45.0X4	T45.0X5	T45.0X6
Methaqualone (compound)	T42.6X1	T42.6X2	T42.6X3	T42.6X4	T42.6X5	T42.6X6
Metharbital	T42.3X1	T42.3X2	T42.3X3	T42.3X4	T42.3X5	T42.3X6
Methazolamide	T50.2X1	T50.2X2	T50.2X3	T50.2X4	T50.2X5	T50.2X6
Methdilazine	T43.3X1	T43.3X2	T43.3X3	T43.3X4	T43.3X5	T43.3X6
Methedrine	T43.621	T43.622	T43.623	T43.624	T43.625	T43.626
Methenamine (mandelate)	T37.8X1	T37.8X2	T37.8X3	T37.8X4	T37.8X5	T37.8X6
Methenolone	T38.7X1	T38.7X2	T38.7X3	T38.7X4	T38.7X5	T38.7X6
Methergine	T48.0X1	T48.0X2	T48.0X3	T48.0X4	T48.0X5	T48.0X6
Methetoin	T42.0X1	T42.0X2	T42.0X3	T42.0X4	T42.0X5	T42.0X6
Methiacil	T38.2X1	T38.2X2	T38.2X3	T38.2X4	T38.2X5	T38.2X6
Methicillin	T36.0X1	T36.0X2	T36.0X3	T36.0X4	T36.0X5	T36.0X6
Methimazole	T38.2X1	T38.2X2	T38.2X3	T38.2X4	T38.2X5	T38.2X6
Methiodal sodium	T50.8X1	T50.8X2	T50.8X3	T50.8X4	T50.8X5	T50.8X6
Methionine	T50.991	T50.992	T50.993	T50.994	T50.995	T50.996
Methisazone	T37.5X1	T37.5X2	T37.5X3	T37.5X4	T37.5X5	T37.5X6
Methisoprinol	T37.5X1	T37.5X2	T37.5X3	T37.5X4	T37.5X5	T37.5X6
Methitural	T42.3X1	T42.3X2	T42.3X3	T42.3X4	T42.3X5	T42.3X6
Methixene	T44.3X1	T44.3X2	T44.3X3	T44.3X4	T44.3X5	T44.3X6
Methobarbital, methobarbitone	T42.3X1	T42.3X2	T42.3X3	T42.3X4	T42.3X5	T42.3X6
Methocarbamol	T42.8X1	T42.8X2	T42.8X3	T42.8X4	T42.8X5	T42.8X6
skeletal muscle relaxant	T48.1X1	T48.1X2	T48.1X3	T48.1X4	T48.1X5	T48.1X6
Methohexital	T41.1X1	T41.1X2	T41.1X3	T41.1X4	T41.1X5	T41.1X6
Methohexitone	T41.1X1	T41.1X2	T41.1X3	T41.1X4	T41.1X5	T41.1X6
Methoin	T42.0X1	T42.0X2	T42.0X3	T42.0X4	T42.0X5	T42.0X6
Methopholine	T39.8X1	T39.8X2	T39.8X3	T39.8X4	T39.8X5	T39.8X6
Methopromazine	T43.3X1	T43.3X2	T43.3X3	T43.3X4	T43.3X5	T43.3X6
Methorate	T48.3X1	T48.3X2	T48.3X3	T48.3X4	T48.3X5	T48.3X6
Methoserpidine	T46.5X1	T46.5X2	T46.5X3	T46.5X4	T46.5X5	T46.5X6
Methotrexate	T45.1X1	T45.1X2	T45.1X3	T45.1X4	T45.1X5	T45.1X6
Methotrimeprazine	T43.3X1	T43.3X2	T43.3X3	T43.3X4	T43.3X5	T43.3X6
Methoxa-Dome	T49.3X1	T49.3X2	T49.3X3	T49.3X4	T49.3X5	T49.3X6
Methoxamine	T44.4X1	T44.4X2	T44.4X3	T44.4X4	T44.4X5	T44.4X6
Methoxsalen	T50.991	T50.992	T50.993	T50.994	T50.995	T50.996
Methoxyaniline	T65.3X1	T65.3X2	T65.3X3	T65.3X4	—	—
Methoxybenzyl penicillin	T36.0X1	T36.0X2	T36.0X3	T36.0X4	T36.0X5	T36.0X6
Methoxychlor	T53.7X1	T53.7X2	T53.7X3	T53.7X4	—	—
Methoxy-DDT	T53.7X1	T53.7X2	T53.7X3	T53.7X4	—	—
Methoxyflurane	T41.0X1	T41.0X2	T41.0X3	T41.0X4	T41.0X5	T41.0X6
Methoxyphenamine	T48.6X1	T48.6X2	T48.6X3	T48.6X4	T48.6X5	T48.6X6
Methoxypromazine	T43.3X1	T43.3X2	T43.3X3	T43.3X4	T43.3X5	T43.3X6
Methscopolamine bromide	T44.3X1	T44.3X2	T44.3X3	T44.3X4	T44.3X5	T44.3X6
Methsuximide	T42.2X1	T42.2X2	T42.2X3	T42.2X4	T42.2X5	T42.2X6
Methyclothiazide	T50.2X1	T50.2X2	T50.2X3	T50.2X4	T50.2X5	T50.2X6
Methyl						
acetate	T52.4X1	T52.4X2	T52.4X3	T52.4X4	—	—
acetone	T52.4X1	T52.4X2	T52.4X3	T52.4X4	—	—
acrylate	T65.891	T65.892	T65.893	T65.894	—	—
alcohol	T51.1X1	T51.1X2	T51.1X3	T51.1X4	—	—
aminophenol	T65.3X1	T65.3X2	T65.3X3	T65.3X4	—	—
amphetamine	T43.621	T43.622	T43.623	T43.624	T43.625	T43.626
androstanolone	T38.7X1	T38.7X2	T38.7X3	T38.7X4	T38.7X5	T38.7X6
atropine	T44.3X1	T44.3X2	T44.3X3	T44.3X4	T44.3X5	T44.3X6
benzene	T52.2X1	T52.2X2	T52.2X3	T52.2X4	—	—
benzoate	T52.8X1	T52.8X2	T52.8X3	T52.8X4	—	—
benzol	T52.2X1	T52.2X2	T52.2X3	T52.2X4	—	—
bromide (gas)	T59.891	T59.892	T59.893	T59.894	—	—

Substance	Poisoning, Accidental (unintentional)	Poisoning, Intentional Self-harm	Poisoning, Assault	Poisoning, Undetermined	Adverse Effect	Under-dosing
Methyl — continued						
bromide — continued						
fumigant	T60.8X1	T60.8X2	T60.8X3	T60.8X4	—	—
butanol	T51.3X1	T51.3X2	T51.3X3	T51.3X4	—	—
carbinol	T51.1X1	T51.1X2	T51.1X3	T51.1X4	—	—
carbonate	T52.8X1	T52.8X2	T52.8X3	T52.8X4	—	—
CCNU	T45.1X1	T45.1X2	T45.1X3	T45.1X4	T45.1X5	T45.1X6
cellosolve	T52.91	T52.92	T52.93	T52.94	—	—
cellulose	T47.4X1	T47.4X2	T47.4X3	T47.4X4	T47.4X5	T47.4X6
chloride (gas)	T59.891	T59.892	T59.893	T59.894	—	—
chloroformate	T59.3X1	T59.3X2	T59.3X3	T59.3X4	—	—
cyclohexane	T52.8X1	T52.8X2	T52.8X3	T52.8X4	—	—
cyclohexanol	T51.8X1	T51.8X2	T51.8X3	T51.8X4	—	—
cyclohexanone	T52.8X1	T52.8X2	T52.8X3	T52.8X4	—	—
cyclohexyl acetate	T52.8X1	T52.8X2	T52.8X3	T52.8X4	—	—
demeton	T60.0X1	T60.0X2	T60.0X3	T60.0X4	—	—
dihydromorphinone	T40.2X1	T40.2X2	T40.2X3	T40.2X4	T40.2X5	T40.2X6
ergometrine	T48.0X1	T48.0X2	T48.0X3	T48.0X4	T48.0X5	T48.0X6
ergonovine	T48.0X1	T48.0X2	T48.0X3	T48.0X4	T48.0X5	T48.0X6
ethyl ketone	T52.4X1	T52.4X2	T52.4X3	T52.4X4	—	—
glucamine antimonate	T37.8X1	T37.8X2	T37.8X3	T37.8X4	T37.8X5	T37.8X6
hydrazine	T65.891	T65.892	T65.893	T65.894	—	—
iodide	T65.891	T65.892	T65.893	T65.894	—	—
isobutyl ketone	T52.4X1	T52.4X2	T52.4X3	T52.4X4	—	—
isothiocyanate	T60.3X1	T60.3X2	T60.3X3	T60.3X4	—	—
mercaptan	T59.891	T59.892	T59.893	T59.894	—	—
morphine NEC	T40.2X1	T40.2X2	T40.2X3	T40.2X4	T40.2X5	T40.2X6
nicotinate	T49.4X1	T49.4X2	T49.4X3	T49.4X4	T49.4X5	T49.4X6
paraben	T49.0X1	T49.0X2	T49.0X3	T49.0X4	T49.0X5	T49.0X6
parafynol	T42.6X1	T42.6X2	T42.6X3	T42.6X4	T42.6X5	T42.6X6
parathion	T60.0X1	T60.0X2	T60.0X3	T60.0X4	—	—
peridol	T43.4X1	T43.4X2	T43.4X3	T43.4X4	T43.4X5	T43.4X6
phenidate	T43.631	T43.632	T43.633	T43.634	T43.635	T43.636
prednisolone	T38.0X1	T38.0X2	T38.0X3	T38.0X4	T38.0X5	T38.0X6
ENT agent	T49.6X1	T49.6X2	T49.6X3	T49.6X4	T49.6X5	T49.6X6
ophthalmic preparation	T49.5X1	T49.5X2	T49.5X3	T49.5X4	T49.5X5	T49.5X6
topical NEC	T49.0X1	T49.0X2	T49.0X3	T49.0X4	T49.0X5	T49.0X6
propylcarbinol	T51.3X1	T51.3X2	T51.3X3	T51.3X4	—	—
rosaniline NEC	T49.0X1	T49.0X2	T49.0X3	T49.0X4	T49.0X5	T49.0X6
salicylate	T49.2X1	T49.2X2	T49.2X3	T49.2X4	T49.2X5	T49.2X6
sulfate (fumes)	T59.891	T59.892	T59.893	T59.894	—	—
liquid	T52.8X1	T52.8X2	T52.8X3	T52.8X4	—	—
sulfonal	T42.6X1	T42.6X2	T42.6X3	T42.6X4	T42.6X5	T42.6X6
testosterone	T38.7X1	T38.7X2	T38.7X3	T38.7X4	T38.7X5	T38.7X6
thiouracil	T38.2X1	T38.2X2	T38.2X3	T38.2X4	T38.2X5	T38.2X6
Methylamphetamine	T43.621	T43.622	T43.623	T43.624	T43.625	T43.626
Methylated spirit	T51.1X1	T51.1X2	T51.1X3	T51.1X4	—	—
Methylatropine nitrate	T44.3X1	T44.3X2	T44.3X3	T44.3X4	T44.3X5	T44.3X6
Methylbenactyzium bromide	T44.3X1	T44.3X2	T44.3X3	T44.3X4	T44.3X5	T44.3X6
Methylbenzethonium chloride	T49.0X1	T49.0X2	T49.0X3	T49.0X4	T49.0X5	T49.0X6
Methylcellulose	T47.4X1	T47.4X2	T47.4X3	T47.4X4	T47.4X5	T47.4X6
laxative	T47.4X1	T47.4X2	T47.4X3	T47.4X4	T47.4X5	T47.4X6
Methylchlorophenoxyacetic acid	T60.3X1	T60.3X2	T60.3X3	T60.3X4	—	—
Methyldopa	T46.5X1	T46.5X2	T46.5X3	T46.5X4	T46.5X5	T46.5X6
Methyldopate	T46.5X1	T46.5X2	T46.5X3	T46.5X4	T46.5X5	T46.5X6
Methylene						
blue	T50.6X1	T50.6X2	T50.6X3	T50.6X4	T50.6X5	T50.6X6
chloride or dichloride (solvent) NEC	T53.4X1	T53.4X2	T53.4X3	T53.4X4	—	—
Methylenedioxyamphetamine	T43.621	T43.622	T43.623	T43.624	T43.625	T43.626
Methylenedioxymeth-amphetamine	T43.641	T43.642	T43.643	T43.644	—	—
Methylergometrine	T48.0X1	T48.0X2	T48.0X3	T48.0X4	T48.0X5	T48.0X6
Methylergonovine	T48.0X1	T48.0X2	T48.0X3	T48.0X4	T48.0X5	T48.0X6
Methylestrenolone	T38.5X1	T38.5X2	T38.5X3	T38.5X4	T38.5X5	T38.5X6
Methylethyl cellulose	T50.991	T50.992	T50.993	T50.994	T50.995	T50.996
Methylhexabital	T42.3X1	T42.3X2	T42.3X3	T42.3X4	T42.3X5	T42.3X6
Methylmorphine	T40.2X1	T40.2X2	T40.2X3	T40.2X4	T40.2X5	T40.2X6
Methylparaben (ophthalmic)	T49.5X1	T49.5X2	T49.5X3	T49.5X4	T49.5X5	T49.5X6
Methylparafynol	T42.6X1	T42.6X2	T42.6X3	T42.6X4	T42.6X5	T42.6X6
Methylpentynol, methylpenthynol	T42.6X1	T42.6X2	T42.6X3	T42.6X4	T42.6X5	T42.6X6
Methylphenidate	T43.631	T43.632	T43.633	T43.634	T43.635	T43.636
Methylphenobarbital	T42.3X1	T42.3X2	T42.3X3	T42.3X4	T42.3X5	T42.3X6
Methylpolysiloxane	T47.1X1	T47.1X2	T47.1X3	T47.1X4	T47.1X5	T47.1X6
Methylprednisolone — see Methyl, prednisolone						
Methylrosaniline	T49.0X1	T49.0X2	T49.0X3	T49.0X4	T49.0X5	T49.0X6

Subterms under main terms may continue to next column or page   Additional Character May Be Required — Refer to the Tabular List for Character Selection

Substance	Poisoning, Accidental (unintentional)	Poisoning, Intentional Self-harm	Poisoning, Assault	Poisoning, Undetermined	Adverse Effect	Under-dosing
Methylrosanilinium chloride	T49.0X1	T49.0X2	T49.0X3	T49.0X4	T49.0X5	T49.0X6
Methyltestosterone	T38.7X1	T38.7X2	T38.7X3	T38.7X4	T38.7X5	T38.7X6
Methylthionine chloride	T50.6X1	T50.6X2	T50.6X3	T50.6X4	T50.6X5	T50.6X6
Methylthioninium chloride	T50.6X1	T50.6X2	T50.6X3	T50.6X4	T50.6X5	T50.6X6
Methylthiouracil	T38.2X1	T38.2X2	T38.2X3	T38.2X4	T38.2X5	T38.2X6
Methyprylon	T42.6X1	T42.6X2	T42.6X3	T42.6X4	T42.6X5	T42.6X6
Methysergide	T46.5X1	T46.5X2	T46.5X3	T46.5X4	T46.5X5	T46.5X6
Metiamide	T47.1X1	T47.1X2	T47.1X3	T47.1X4	T47.1X5	T47.1X6
Meticillin	T36.0X1	T36.0X2	T36.0X3	T36.0X4	T36.0X5	T36.0X6
Meticrane	T50.2X1	T50.2X2	T50.2X3	T50.2X4	T50.2X5	T50.2X6
Metildigoxin	T46.0X1	T46.0X2	T46.0X3	T46.0X4	T46.0X5	T46.0X6
Metipranolol	T49.5X1	T49.5X2	T49.5X3	T49.5X4	T49.5X5	T49.5X6
Metirosine	T46.5X1	T46.5X2	T46.5X3	T46.5X4	T46.5X5	T46.5X6
Metisazone	T37.5X1	T37.5X2	T37.5X3	T37.5X4	T37.5X5	T37.5X6
Metixene	T44.3X1	T44.3X2	T44.3X3	T44.3X4	T44.3X5	T44.3X6
Metizoline	T48.5X1	T48.5X2	T48.5X3	T48.5X4	T48.5X5	T48.5X6
Metoclopramide	T45.0X1	T45.0X2	T45.0X3	T45.0X4	T45.0X5	T45.0X6
Metofenazate	T43.3X1	T43.3X2	T43.3X3	T43.3X4	T43.3X5	T43.3X6
Metofoline	T39.8X1	T39.8X2	T39.8X3	T39.8X4	T39.8X5	T39.8X6
Metolazone	T50.2X1	T50.2X2	T50.2X3	T50.2X4	T50.2X5	T50.2X6
Metopon	T40.2X1	T40.2X2	T40.2X3	T40.2X4	T40.2X5	T40.2X6
Metoprine	T45.1X1	T45.1X2	T45.1X3	T45.1X4	T45.1X5	T45.1X6
Metoprolol	T44.7X1	T44.7X2	T44.7X3	T44.7X4	T44.7X5	T44.7X6
Metrifonate	T60.0X1	T60.0X2	T60.0X3	T60.0X4	—	—
Metrizamide	T50.8X1	T50.8X2	T50.8X3	T50.8X4	T50.8X5	T50.8X6
Metrizoic acid	T50.8X1	T50.8X2	T50.8X3	T50.8X4	T50.8X5	T50.8X6
Metronidazole	T37.8X1	T37.8X2	T37.8X3	T37.8X4	T37.8X5	T37.8X6
Metycaine	T41.3X1	T41.3X2	T41.3X3	T41.3X4	T41.3X5	T41.3X6
infiltration (subcutaneous)	T41.3X1	T41.3X2	T41.3X3	T41.3X4	T41.3X5	T41.3X6
nerve block (peripheral) (plexus)	T41.3X1	T41.3X2	T41.3X3	T41.3X4	T41.3X5	T41.3X6
topical (surface)	T41.3X1	T41.3X2	T41.3X3	T41.3X4	T41.3X5	T41.3X6
Metyrapone	T50.8X1	T50.8X2	T50.8X3	T50.8X4	T50.8X5	T50.8X6
Mevinphos	T60.0X1	T60.0X2	T60.0X3	T60.0X4	—	—
Mexazolam	T42.4X1	T42.4X2	T42.4X3	T42.4X4	T42.4X5	T42.4X6
Mexenone	T49.3X1	T49.3X2	T49.3X3	T49.3X4	T49.3X5	T49.3X6
Mexiletine	T46.2X1	T46.2X2	T46.2X3	T46.2X4	T46.2X5	T46.2X6
Mezereon	T62.2X1	T62.2X2	T62.2X3	T62.2X4	—	—
berries	T62.1X1	T62.1X2	T62.1X3	T62.1X4	—	—
Mezlocillin	T36.0X1	T36.0X2	T36.0X3	T36.0X4	T36.0X5	T36.0X6
Mianserin	T43.021	T43.022	T43.023	T43.024	T43.025	T43.026
Micatin	T49.0X1	T49.0X2	T49.0X3	T49.0X4	T49.0X5	T49.0X6
Miconazole	T49.0X1	T49.0X2	T49.0X3	T49.0X4	T49.0X5	T49.0X6
Micronomicin	T36.5X1	T36.5X2	T36.5X3	T36.5X4	T36.5X5	T36.5X6
Midazolam	T42.4X1	T42.4X2	T42.4X3	T42.4X4	T42.4X5	T42.4X6
Midecamycin	T36.3X1	T36.3X2	T36.3X3	T36.3X4	T36.3X5	T36.3X6
Mifepristone	T38.6X1	T38.6X2	T38.6X3	T38.6X4	T38.6X5	T38.6X6
Milk of magnesia	T47.1X1	T47.1X2	T47.1X3	T47.1X4	T47.1X5	T47.1X6
Millipede (tropical)	T63.411	T63.412	T63.413	T63.414	—	—
(venomous)						
Miltown	T43.591	T43.592	T43.593	T43.594	T43.595	T43.596
Milverine	T44.3X1	T44.3X2	T44.3X3	T44.3X4	T44.3X5	T44.3X6
Minaprine	T43.291	T43.292	T43.293	T43.294	T43.295	T43.296
Minaxolone	T41.291	T41.292	T41.293	T41.294	T41.295	T41.296
Mineral						
acids	T54.2X1	T54.2X2	T54.2X3	T54.2X4	—	—
oil (laxative)(medicinal)	T47.4X1	T47.4X2	T47.4X3	T47.4X4	T47.4X5	T47.4X6
emulsion	T47.2X1	T47.2X2	T47.2X3	T47.2X4	T47.2X5	T47.2X6
nonmedicinal	T52.0X1	T52.0X2	T52.0X3	T52.0X4	—	—
topical	T49.3X1	T49.3X2	T49.3X3	T49.3X4	T49.3X5	T49.3X6
salt NEC	T50.3X1	T50.3X2	T50.3X3	T50.3X4	T50.3X5	T50.3X6
spirits	T52.0X1	T52.0X2	T52.0X3	T52.0X4	—	—
Mineralocorticosteroid	T50.0X1	T50.0X2	T50.0X3	T50.0X4	T50.0X5	T50.0X6
Minocycline	T36.4X1	T36.4X2	T36.4X3	T36.4X4	T36.4X5	T36.4X6
Minoxidil	T46.7X1	T46.7X2	T46.7X3	T46.7X4	T46.7X5	T46.7X6
Miokamycin	T36.3X1	T36.3X2	T36.3X3	T36.3X4	T36.3X5	T36.3X6
Miotic drug	T49.5X1	T49.5X2	T49.5X3	T49.5X4	T49.5X5	T49.5X6
Mipafox	T60.0X1	T60.0X2	T60.0X3	T60.0X4	—	—
Mirex	T60.1X1	T60.1X2	T60.1X3	T60.1X4	—	—
Mirtazapine	T43.021	T43.022	T43.023	T43.024	T43.025	T43.026
Misonidazole	T37.3X1	T37.3X2	T37.3X3	T37.3X4	T37.3X5	T37.3X6
Misoprostol	T47.1X1	T47.1X2	T47.1X3	T47.1X4	T47.1X5	T47.1X6
Mithramycin	T45.1X1	T45.1X2	T45.1X3	T45.1X4	T45.1X5	T45.1X6
Mitobronitol	T45.1X1	T45.1X2	T45.1X3	T45.1X4	T45.1X5	T45.1X6
Mitoguazone	T45.1X1	T45.1X2	T45.1X3	T45.1X4	T45.1X5	T45.1X6
Mitolactol	T45.1X1	T45.1X2	T45.1X3	T45.1X4	T45.1X5	T45.1X6
Mitomycin	T45.1X1	T45.1X2	T45.1X3	T45.1X4	T45.1X5	T45.1X6
Mitopodozide	T45.1X1	T45.1X2	T45.1X3	T45.1X4	T45.1X5	T45.1X6
Mitotane	T45.1X1	T45.1X2	T45.1X3	T45.1X4	T45.1X5	T45.1X6
Mitoxantrone	T45.1X1	T45.1X2	T45.1X3	T45.1X4	T45.1X5	T45.1X6
Mivacurium chloride	T48.1X1	T48.1X2	T48.1X3	T48.1X4	T48.1X5	T48.1X6

Substance	Poisoning, Accidental (unintentional)	Poisoning, Intentional Self-harm	Poisoning, Assault	Poisoning, Undetermined	Adverse Effect	Under-dosing
Miyari bacteria	T47.6X1	T47.6X2	T47.6X3	T47.6X4	T47.6X5	T47.6X6
Moclobemide	T43.1X1	T43.1X2	T43.1X3	T43.1X4	T43.1X5	T43.1X6
Moderil	T46.5X1	T46.5X2	T46.5X3	T46.5X4	T46.5X5	T46.5X6
Mofebutazone	T39.2X1	T39.2X2	T39.2X3	T39.2X4	T39.2X5	T39.2X6
Mogadon — see Nitrazepam						
Molindone	T43.591	T43.592	T43.593	T43.594	T43.595	T43.596
Molsidomine	T46.3X1	T46.3X2	T46.3X3	T46.3X4	T46.3X5	T46.3X6
Mometasone	T49.0X1	T49.0X2	T49.0X3	T49.0X4	T49.0X5	T49.0X6
Monistat	T49.0X1	T49.0X2	T49.0X3	T49.0X4	T49.0X5	T49.0X6
Monkshood	T62.2X1	T62.2X2	T62.2X3	T62.2X4	—	—
Monoamine oxidase inhibitor NEC	T43.1X1	T43.1X2	T43.1X3	T43.1X4	T43.1X5	T43.1X6
hydrazine	T43.1X1	T43.1X2	T43.1X3	T43.1X4	T43.1X5	T43.1X6
Monobenzone	T49.4X1	T49.4X2	T49.4X3	T49.4X4	T49.4X5	T49.4X6
Monochloroacetic acid	T60.3X1	T60.3X2	T60.3X3	T60.3X4	—	—
Monochlorobenzene	T53.7X1	T53.7X2	T53.7X3	T53.7X4	—	—
Monoethanolamine	T46.8X1	T46.8X2	T46.8X3	T46.8X4	T46.8X5	T46.8X6
oleate	T46.8X1	T46.8X2	T46.8X3	T46.8X4	T46.8X5	T46.8X6
Monooctanoin	T50.991	T50.992	T50.993	T50.994	T50.995	T50.996
Monophenylbutazone	T39.2X1	T39.2X2	T39.2X3	T39.2X4	T39.2X5	T39.2X6
Monosodium glutamate	T65.891	T65.892	T65.893	T65.894	—	—
Monosulfiram	T49.0X1	T49.0X2	T49.0X3	T49.0X4	T49.0X5	T49.0X6
Monoxide, carbon — see Carbon, monoxide						
Monoxidine hydrochloride	T46.1X1	T46.1X2	T46.1X3	T46.1X4	T46.1X5	T46.1X6
Monuron	T60.3X1	T60.3X2	T60.3X3	T60.3X4	—	—
Moperone	T43.4X1	T43.4X2	T43.4X3	T43.4X4	T43.4X5	T43.4X6
Mopidamol	T45.1X1	T45.1X2	T45.1X3	T45.1X4	T45.1X5	T45.1X6
MOPP (mechloreth-amine + vincristine + prednisone + procarba-zine)	T45.1X1	T45.1X2	T45.1X3	T45.1X4	T45.1X5	T45.1X6
Morfin	T40.2X1	T40.2X2	T40.2X3	T40.2X4	T40.2X5	T40.2X6
Morinamide	T37.1X1	T37.1X2	T37.1X3	T37.1X4	T37.1X5	T37.1X6
Morning glory seeds	T40.991	T40.992	T40.993	T40.994	—	—
Moroxydine	T37.5X1	T37.5X2	T37.5X3	T37.5X4	T37.5X5	T37.5X6
Morphazinamide	T37.1X1	T37.1X2	T37.1X3	T37.1X4	T37.1X5	T37.1X6
Morphine	T40.2X1	T40.2X2	T40.2X3	T40.2X4	T40.2X5	T40.2X6
antagonist	T50.7X1	T50.7X2	T50.7X3	T50.7X4	T50.7X5	T50.7X6
Morpholinylethylmorphine	T40.2X1	T40.2X2	T40.2X3	T40.2X4	—	—
Morsuximide	T42.2X1	T42.2X2	T42.2X3	T42.2X4	T42.2X5	T42.2X6
Mosapramine	T43.591	T43.592	T43.593	T43.594	T43.595	T43.596
Moth balls — see also Pesticides	T60.2X1	T60.2X2	T60.2X3	T60.2X4	—	—
naphthalene	T60.2X1	T60.2X2	T60.2X3	T60.2X4	—	—
paradichlorobenzene	T60.1X1	T60.1X2	T60.1X3	T60.1X4	—	—
Motor exhaust gas	T58.01	T58.02	T58.03	T58.04	—	—
Mouthwash (antiseptic) (zinc chloride)	T49.6X1	T49.6X2	T49.6X3	T49.6X4	T49.6X5	T49.6X6
Moxastine	T45.0X1	T45.0X2	T45.0X3	T45.0X4	T45.0X5	T45.0X6
Moxaverine	T44.3X1	T44.3X2	T44.3X3	T44.3X4	T44.3X5	T44.3X6
Moxisylyte	T46.7X1	T46.7X2	T46.7X3	T46.7X4	T46.7X5	T46.7X6
Mucilage, plant	T47.4X1	T47.4X2	T47.4X3	T47.4X4	T47.4X5	T47.4X6
Mucolytic drug	T48.4X1	T48.4X2	T48.4X3	T48.4X4	T48.4X5	T48.4X6
Mucomyst	T48.4X1	T48.4X2	T48.4X3	T48.4X4	T48.4X5	T48.4X6
Mucous membrane agents (external)	T49.91	T49.92	T49.93	T49.94	T49.95	T49.96
specified NEC	T49.8X1	T49.8X2	T49.8X3	T49.8X4	T49.8X5	T49.8X6
Mumps						
immune globulin (human)	T50.Z11	T50.Z12	T50.Z13	T50.Z14	T50.Z15	T50.Z16
skin test antigen	T50.8X1	T50.8X2	T50.8X3	T50.8X4	T50.8X5	T50.8X6
vaccine	T50.B91	T50.B92	T50.B93	T50.B94	T50.B95	T50.B96
Mumpsvax	T50.B91	T50.B92	T50.B93	T50.B94	T50.B95	T50.B96
Mupirocin	T49.0X1	T49.0X2	T49.0X3	T49.0X4	T49.0X5	T49.0X6
Muriatic acid — see Hydrochloric acid						
Muromonab-CD3	T45.1X1	T45.1X2	T45.1X3	T45.1X4	T45.1X5	T45.1X6
Muscle-action drug NEC	T48.201	T48.202	T48.203	T48.204	T48.205	T48.206
Muscle affecting agents NEC	T48.201	T48.202	T48.203	T48.204	T48.205	T48.206
oxytocic	T48.0X1	T48.0X2	T48.0X3	T48.0X4	T48.0X5	T48.0X6
relaxants	T48.201	T48.202	T48.203	T48.204	T48.205	T48.206
central nervous system	T42.8X1	T42.8X2	T42.8X3	T42.8X4	T42.8X5	T42.8X6
skeletal	T48.1X1	T48.1X2	T48.1X3	T48.1X4	T48.1X5	T48.1X6
smooth	T44.3X1	T44.3X2	T44.3X3	T44.3X4	T44.3X5	T44.3X6
Muscle relaxant — see Relaxant, muscle						
Muscle-tone depressant, central NEC	T42.8X1	T42.8X2	T42.8X3	T42.8X4	T42.8X5	T42.8X6
specified NEC	T42.8X1	T42.8X2	T42.8X3	T42.8X4	T42.8X5	T42.8X6
Mushroom, noxious	T62.0X1	T62.0X2	T62.0X3	T62.0X4	—	—
Mussel, noxious	T61.781	T61.782	T61.783	T61.784	—	—
Mustard (emetic)	T47.7X1	T47.7X2	T47.7X3	T47.7X4	T47.7X5	T47.7X6
black	T47.7X1	T47.7X2	T47.7X3	T47.7X4	T47.7X5	T47.7X6

Additional Character May Be Required — Refer to the Tabular List for Character Selection   ▽ Subterms under main terms may continue to next column or page

Substance	Poisoning, Accidental (unintentional)	Poisoning, Intentional Self-harm	Poisoning, Assault	Poisoning, Undetermined	Adverse Effect	Under-dosing
Mustard — continued						
gas, not in war	T59.91	T59.92	T59.93	T59.94	—	—
nitrogen	T45.1X1	T45.1X2	T45.1X3	T45.1X4	T45.1X5	T45.1X6
Mustine	T45.1X1	T45.1X2	T45.1X3	T45.1X4	T45.1X5	T45.1X6
M-vac	T45.1X1	T45.1X2	T45.1X3	T45.1X4	T45.1X5	T45.1X6
Mycifradin	T36.5X1	T36.5X2	T36.5X3	T36.5X4	T36.5X5	T36.5X6
topical	T49.0X1	T49.0X2	T49.0X3	T49.0X4	T49.0X5	T49.0X6
Mycitracin	T36.8X1	T36.8X2	T36.8X3	T36.8X4	T36.8X5	T36.8X6
ophthalmic preparation	T49.5X1	T49.5X2	T49.5X3	T49.5X4	T49.5X5	T49.5X6
Mycostatin	T36.7X1	T36.7X2	T36.7X3	T36.7X4	T36.7X5	T36.7X6
topical	T49.0X1	T49.0X2	T49.0X3	T49.0X4	T49.0X5	T49.0X6
Mycotoxins	T64.81	T64.82	T64.83	T64.84	—	—
aflatoxin	T64.01	T64.02	T64.03	T64.04	—	—
specified NEC	T64.81	T64.82	T64.83	T64.84	—	—
Mydriacyl	T44.3X1	T44.3X2	T44.3X3	T44.3X4	T44.3X5	T44.3X6
Mydriatic drug	T49.5X1	T49.5X2	T49.5X3	T49.5X4	T49.5X5	T49.5X6
Myelobromal	T45.1X1	T45.1X2	T45.1X3	T45.1X4	T45.1X5	T45.1X6
Myleran	T45.1X1	T45.1X2	T45.1X3	T45.1X4	T45.1X5	T45.1X6
Myochrysin (e)	T39.2X1	T39.2X2	T39.2X3	T39.2X4	T39.2X5	T39.2X6
Myoneural blocking agents	T48.1X1	T48.1X2	T48.1X3	T48.1X4	T48.1X5	T48.1X6
Myralact	T49.0X1	T49.0X2	T49.0X3	T49.0X4	T49.0X5	T49.0X6
Myristica fragrans	T62.2X1	T62.2X2	T62.2X3	T62.2X4	—	—
Myristicin	T65.891	T65.892	T65.893	T65.894	—	—
Mysoline	T42.3X1	T42.3X2	T42.3X3	T42.3X4	T42.3X5	T42.3X6
Nabilone	T40.7X1	T40.7X2	T40.7X3	T40.7X4	T40.7X5	T40.7X6
Nabumetone	T39.391	T39.392	T39.393	T39.394	T39.395	T39.396
Nadolol	T44.7X1	T44.7X2	T44.7X3	T44.7X4	T44.7X5	T44.7X6
Nafcillin	T36.0X1	T36.0X2	T36.0X3	T36.0X4	T36.0X5	T36.0X6
Nafoxidine	T38.6X1	T38.6X2	T38.6X3	T38.6X4	T38.6X5	T38.6X6
Naftazone	T46.991	T46.992	T46.993	T46.994	T46.995	T46.996
Naftidrofuryl (oxalate)	T46.7X1	T46.7X2	T46.7X3	T46.7X4	T46.7X5	T46.7X6
Naftifine	T49.0X1	T49.0X2	T49.0X3	T49.0X4	T49.0X5	T49.0X6
Nail polish remover	T52.91	T52.92	T52.93	T52.94	—	—
Nalbuphine	T40.4X1	T40.4X2	T40.4X3	T40.4X4	T40.4X5	T40.4X6
Naled	T60.0X1	T60.0X2	T60.0X3	T60.0X4	—	—
Nalidixic acid	T37.8X1	T37.8X2	T37.8X3	T37.8X4	T37.8X5	T37.8X6
Nalorphine	T50.7X1	T50.7X2	T50.7X3	T50.7X4	T50.7X5	T50.7X6
Naloxone	T50.7X1	T50.7X2	T50.7X3	T50.7X4	T50.7X5	T50.7X6
Naltrexone	T50.7X1	T50.7X2	T50.7X3	T50.7X4	T50.7X5	T50.7X6
Namenda	T43.8X1	T43.8X2	T43.8X3	T43.8X4	T43.8X5	T43.8X6
Nandrolone	T38.7X1	T38.7X2	T38.7X3	T38.7X4	T38.7X5	T38.7X6
Naphazoline	T48.5X1	T48.5X2	T48.5X3	T48.5X4	T48.5X5	T48.5X6
Naphtha (painters') (petroleum)	T52.0X1	T52.0X2	T52.0X3	T52.0X4		
solvent	T52.0X1	T52.0X2	T52.0X3	T52.0X4	—	—
vapor	T52.0X1	T52.0X2	T52.0X3	T52.0X4	—	—
Naphthalene (non-chlorinated)	T60.2X1	T60.2X2	T60.2X3	T60.2X4	—	—
chlorinated	T60.1X1	T60.1X2	T60.1X3	T60.1X4	—	—
vapor	T60.1X1	T60.1X2	T60.1X3	T60.1X4	—	—
insecticide or moth repellent	T60.2X1	T60.2X2	T60.2X3	T60.2X4	—	—
chlorinated	T60.1X1	T60.1X2	T60.1X3	T60.1X4	—	—
vapor	T60.2X1	T60.2X2	T60.2X3	T60.2X4	—	—
chlorinated	T60.1X1	T60.1X2	T60.1X3	T60.1X4	—	—
Naphthol	T65.891	T65.892	T65.893	T65.894	—	—
Naphthylamine	T65.891	T65.892	T65.893	T65.894	—	—
Naphthylthiourea (ANTU)	T60.4X1	T60.4X2	T60.4X3	T60.4X4	—	—
Naprosyn — see Naproxen						
Naproxen	T39.311	T39.312	T39.313	T39.314	T39.315	T39.316
Narcotic (drug)	T40.601	T40.602	T40.603	T40.604	T40.605	T40.606
analgesic NEC	T40.601	T40.602	T40.603	T40.604	T40.605	T40.606
antagonist	T50.7X1	T50.7X2	T50.7X3	T50.7X4	T50.7X5	T50.7X6
specified NEC	T40.691	T40.692	T40.693	T40.694	T40.695	T40.696
synthetic	T40.4X1	T40.4X2	T40.4X3	T40.4X4	T40.4X5	T40.4X6
Narcotine	T48.3X1	T48.3X2	T48.3X3	T48.3X4	T48.3X5	T48.3X6
Nardil	T43.1X1	T43.1X2	T43.1X3	T43.1X4	T43.1X5	T43.1X6
Nasal drug NEC	T49.6X1	T49.6X2	T49.6X3	T49.6X4	T49.6X5	T49.6X6
Natamycin	T49.0X1	T49.0X2	T49.0X3	T49.0X4	T49.0X5	T49.0X6
Natrium cyanide — see Cyanide(s)						
Natural						
blood (product)	T45.8X1	T45.8X2	T45.8X3	T45.8X4	T45.8X5	T45.8X6
gas (piped)	T59.891	T59.892	T59.893	T59.894		
incomplete combustion	T58.11	T58.12	T58.13	T58.14	—	—
Nealbarbital	T42.3X1	T42.3X2	T42.3X3	T42.3X4	T42.3X5	T42.3X6
Nectadon	T48.3X1	T48.3X2	T48.3X3	T48.3X4	T48.3X5	T48.3X6
Nedocromil	T48.6X1	T48.6X2	T48.6X3	T48.6X4	T48.6X5	T48.6X6
Nefopam	T39.8X1	T39.8X2	T39.8X3	T39.8X4	T39.8X5	T39.8X6
Nematocyst (sting)	T63.691	T63.692	T63.693	T63.694		
Nembutal	T42.3X1	T42.3X2	T42.3X3	T42.3X4	T42.3X5	T42.3X6
Nemonapride	T43.591	T43.592	T43.593	T43.594	T43.595	T43.596

Substance	Poisoning, Accidental (unintentional)	Poisoning, Intentional Self-harm	Poisoning, Assault	Poisoning, Undetermined	Adverse Effect	Under-dosing
Neoarsphenamine	T37.8X1	T37.8X2	T37.8X3	T37.8X4	T37.8X5	T37.8X6
Neocinchophen	T50.4X1	T50.4X2	T50.4X3	T50.4X4	T50.4X5	T50.4X6
Neomycin (derivatives)	T36.5X1	T36.5X2	T36.5X3	T36.5X4	T36.5X5	T36.5X6
with						
bacitracin	T49.0X1	T49.0X2	T49.0X3	T49.0X4	T49.0X5	T49.0X6
neostigmine	T44.0X1	T44.0X2	T44.0X3	T44.0X4	T44.0X5	T44.0X6
ENT agent	T49.6X1	T49.6X2	T49.6X3	T49.6X4	T49.6X5	T49.6X6
ophthalmic preparation	T49.5X1	T49.5X2	T49.5X3	T49.5X4	T49.5X5	T49.5X6
topical NEC	T49.0X1	T49.0X2	T49.0X3	T49.0X4	T49.0X5	T49.0X6
Neonal	T42.3X1	T42.3X2	T42.3X3	T42.3X4	T42.3X5	T42.3X6
Neoprontosil	T37.0X1	T37.0X2	T37.0X3	T37.0X4	T37.0X5	T37.0X6
Neosalvarsan	T37.8X1	T37.8X2	T37.8X3	T37.8X4	T37.8X5	T37.8X6
Neosilversalvarsan	T37.8X1	T37.8X2	T37.8X3	T37.8X4	T37.8X5	T37.8X6
Neosporin	T36.8X1	T36.8X2	T36.8X3	T36.8X4	T36.8X5	T36.8X6
ENT agent	T49.6X1	T49.6X2	T49.6X3	T49.6X4	T49.6X5	T49.6X6
opthalmic preparation	T49.5X1	T49.5X2	T49.5X3	T49.5X4	T49.5X5	T49.5X6
topical NEC	T49.0X1	T49.0X2	T49.0X3	T49.0X4	T49.0X5	T49.0X6
Neostigmine bromide	T44.0X1	T44.0X2	T44.0X3	T44.0X4	T44.0X5	T44.0X6
Neraval	T42.3X1	T42.3X2	T42.3X3	T42.3X4	T42.3X5	T42.3X6
Neravan	T42.3X1	T42.3X2	T42.3X3	T42.3X4	T42.3X5	T42.3X6
Nerium oleander	T62.2X1	T62.2X2	T62.2X3	T62.2X4	—	—
Nerve gas, not in war	T59.91	T59.92	T59.93	T59.94	—	—
Nesacaine	T41.3X1	T41.3X2	T41.3X3	T41.3X4	T41.3X5	T41.3X6
infiltration (subcutaneous)	T41.3X1	T41.3X2	T41.3X3	T41.3X4	T41.3X5	T41.3X6
nerve block (peripheral) (plexus)	T41.3X1	T41.3X2	T41.3X3	T41.3X4	T41.3X5	T41.3X6
Netilmicin	T36.5X1	T36.5X2	T36.5X3	T36.5X4	T36.5X5	T36.5X6
Neurobarb	T42.3X1	T42.3X2	T42.3X3	T42.3X4	T42.3X5	T42.3X6
Neuroleptic drug NEC	T43.501	T43.502	T43.503	T43.504	T43.505	T43.506
Neuromuscular blocking drug	T48.1X1	T48.1X2	T48.1X3	T48.1X4	T48.1X5	T48.1X6
Neutral insulin injection	T38.3X1	T38.3X2	T38.3X3	T38.3X4	T38.3X5	T38.3X6
Neutral spirits	T51.0X1	T51.0X2	T51.0X3	T51.0X4	—	—
beverage	T51.0X1	T51.0X2	T51.0X3	T51.0X4	—	—
Niacin	T46.7X1	T46.7X2	T46.7X3	T46.7X4	T46.7X5	T46.7X6
Niacinamide	T45.2X1	T45.2X2	T45.2X3	T45.2X4	T45.2X5	T45.2X6
Nialamide	T43.1X1	T43.1X2	T43.1X3	T43.1X4	T43.1X5	T43.1X6
Niaprazine	T42.6X1	T42.6X2	T42.6X3	T42.6X4	T42.6X5	T42.6X6
Nicametate	T46.7X1	T46.7X2	T46.7X3	T46.7X4	T46.7X5	T46.7X6
Nicardipine	T46.1X1	T46.1X2	T46.1X3	T46.1X4	T46.1X5	T46.1X6
Nicergoline	T46.7X1	T46.7X2	T46.7X3	T46.7X4	T46.7X5	T46.7X6
Nickel (carbonyl) (tetra-carbonyl) (fumes) (vapor)	T56.891	T56.892	T56.893	T56.894	—	—
Nickelocene	T56.891	T56.892	T56.893	T56.894	—	—
Niclosamide	T37.4X1	T37.4X2	T37.4X3	T37.4X4	T37.4X5	T37.4X6
Nicofuranose	T46.7X1	T46.7X2	T46.7X3	T46.7X4	T46.7X5	T46.7X6
Nicomorphine	T40.2X1	T40.2X2	T40.2X3	T40.2X4	—	—
Nicorandil	T46.3X1	T46.3X2	T46.3X3	T46.3X4	T46.3X5	T46.3X6
Nicotiana (plant)	T62.2X1	T62.2X2	T62.2X3	T62.2X4	—	—
Nicotinamide	T45.2X1	T45.2X2	T45.2X3	T45.2X4	T45.2X5	T45.2X6
Nicotine (insecticide) (spray) (sulfate) NEC	T60.2X1	T60.2X2	T60.2X3	T60.2X4	—	—
from tobacco	T65.291	T65.292	T65.293	T65.294	—	—
cigarettes	T65.221	T65.222	T65.223	T65.224	—	—
not insecticide	T65.291	T65.292	T65.293	T65.294	—	—
Nicotinic acid	T46.7X1	T46.7X2	T46.7X3	T46.7X4	T46.7X5	T46.7X6
Nicotinyl alcohol	T46.7X1	T46.7X2	T46.7X3	T46.7X4	T46.7X5	T46.7X6
Nicoumalone	T45.511	T45.512	T45.513	T45.514	T45.515	T45.516
Nifedipine	T46.1X1	T46.1X2	T46.1X3	T46.1X4	T46.1X5	T46.1X6
Nifenazone	T39.2X1	T39.2X2	T39.2X3	T39.2X4	T39.2X5	T39.2X6
Nifuraldezone	T37.91	T37.92	T37.93	T37.94	T37.95	T37.96
Nifuratel	T37.8X1	T37.8X2	T37.8X3	T37.8X4	T37.8X5	T37.8X6
Nifurtimox	T37.3X1	T37.3X2	T37.3X3	T37.3X4	T37.3X5	T37.3X6
Nifurtoinol	T37.8X1	T37.8X2	T37.8X3	T37.8X4	T37.8X5	T37.8X6
Nightshade, deadly (solanum) — see also Belladonna	T62.2X1	T62.2X2	T62.2X3	T62.2X4		
berry	T62.1X1	T62.1X2	T62.1X3	T62.1X4	—	—
Nikethamide	T50.7X1	T50.7X2	T50.7X3	T50.7X4	T50.7X5	T50.7X6
Nilstat	T36.7X1	T36.7X2	T36.7X3	T36.7X4	T36.7X5	T36.7X6
topical	T49.0X1	T49.0X2	T49.0X3	T49.0X4	T49.0X5	T49.0X6
Nilutamide	T38.6X1	T38.6X2	T38.6X3	T38.6X4	T38.6X5	T38.6X6
Nimesulide	T39.391	T39.392	T39.393	T39.394	T39.395	T39.396
Nimetazepam	T42.4X1	T42.4X2	T42.4X3	T42.4X4	T42.4X5	T42.4X6
Nimodipine	T46.1X1	T46.1X2	T46.1X3	T46.1X4	T46.1X5	T46.1X6
Nimorazole	T37.3X1	T37.3X2	T37.3X3	T37.3X4	T37.3X5	T37.3X6
Nimustine	T45.1X1	T45.1X2	T45.1X3	T45.1X4	T45.1X5	T45.1X6
Niridazole	T37.4X1	T37.4X2	T37.4X3	T37.4X4	T37.4X5	T37.4X6
Nisentil	T40.2X1	T40.2X2	T40.2X3	T40.2X4	T40.2X5	T40.2X6
Nisoldipine	T46.1X1	T46.1X2	T46.1X3	T46.1X4	T46.1X5	T46.1X6
Nitramine	T65.3X1	T65.3X2	T65.3X3	T65.3X4	—	—
Nitrate, organic	T46.3X1	T46.3X2	T46.3X3	T46.3X4	T46.3X5	T46.3X6
Nitrazepam	T42.4X1	T42.4X2	T42.4X3	T42.4X4	T42.4X5	T42.4X6
Nitrefazole	T50.6X1	T50.6X2	T50.6X3	T50.6X4	T50.6X5	T50.6X6

Substance	Poisoning, Accidental (unintentional)	Poisoning, Intentional Self-harm	Poisoning, Assault	Poisoning, Undetermined	Adverse Effect	Under-dosing
Nitrendipine	T46.1X1	T46.1X2	T46.1X3	T46.1X4	T46.1X5	T46.1X6
Nitric						
acid (liquid)	T54.2X1	T54.2X2	T54.2X3	T54.2X4	—	—
vapor	T59.891	T59.892	T59.893	T59.894	—	—
oxide (gas)	T59.0X1	T59.0X2	T59.0X3	T59.0X4	—	—
Nitrimidazine	T37.3X1	T37.3X2	T37.3X3	T37.3X4	T37.3X5	T37.3X6
Nitrite, amyl (medicinal)	T46.3X1	T46.3X2	T46.3X3	T46.3X4	T46.3X5	T46.3X6
(vapor)						
Nitroaniline	T65.3X1	T65.3X2	T65.3X3	T65.3X4	—	—
vapor	T59.891	T59.892	T59.893	T59.894	—	—
Nitrobenzene, nitrobenzol	T65.3X1	T65.3X2	T65.3X3	T65.3X4	—	—
vapor	T65.3X1	T65.3X2	T65.3X3	T65.3X4	—	—
Nitrocellulose	T65.891	T65.892	T65.893	T65.894	—	—
lacquer	T65.891	T65.892	T65.893	T65.894	—	—
Nitrodiphenyl	T65.3X1	T65.3X2	T65.3X3	T65.3X4	—	—
Nitrofural	T49.0X1	T49.0X2	T49.0X3	T49.0X4	T49.0X5	T49.0X6
Nitrofurantoin	T37.8X1	T37.8X2	T37.8X3	T37.8X4	T37.8X5	T37.8X6
Nitrofurazone	T49.0X1	T49.0X2	T49.0X3	T49.0X4	T49.0X5	T49.0X6
Nitrogen	T59.0X1	T59.0X2	T59.0X3	T59.0X4	—	—
mustard	T45.1X1	T45.1X2	T45.1X3	T45.1X4	T45.1X5	T45.1X6
Nitroglycerin, nitroglycerol (medicinal)	T46.3X1	T46.3X2	T46.3X3	T46.3X4	T46.3X5	T46.3X6
nonmedicinal	T65.5X1	T65.5X2	T65.5X3	T65.5X4	—	—
fumes	T65.5X1	T65.5X2	T65.5X3	T65.5X4	—	—
Nitroglycol	T52.3X1	T52.3X2	T52.3X3	T52.3X4	—	—
Nitrohydrochloric acid	T54.2X1	T54.2X2	T54.2X3	T54.2X4	—	—
Nitromersol	T49.0X1	T49.0X2	T49.0X3	T49.0X4	T49.0X5	T49.0X6
Nitronaphthalene	T65.891	T65.892	T65.893	T65.894	—	—
Nitrophenol	T54.0X1	T54.0X2	T54.0X3	T54.0X4	—	—
Nitropropane	T52.8X1	T52.8X2	T52.8X3	T52.8X4	—	—
Nitroprusside	T46.5X1	T46.5X2	T46.5X3	T46.5X4	T46.5X5	T46.5X6
Nitrosodimethylamine	T65.3X1	T65.3X2	T65.3X3	T65.3X4	—	—
Nitrothiazol	T37.4X1	T37.4X2	T37.4X3	T37.4X4	T37.4X5	T37.4X6
Nitrotoluene, nitrotoluol	T65.3X1	T65.3X2	T65.3X3	T65.3X4	—	—
vapor	T65.3X1	T65.3X2	T65.3X3	T65.3X4	—	—
Nitrous						
acid (liquid)	T54.2X1	T54.2X2	T54.2X3	T54.2X4	—	—
fumes	T59.891	T59.892	T59.893	T59.894	—	—
ether spirit	T46.3X1	T46.3X2	T46.3X3	T46.3X4	T46.3X5	T46.3X6
oxide	T41.0X1	T41.0X2	T41.0X3	T41.0X4	T41.0X5	T41.0X6
Nitroxoline	T37.8X1	T37.8X2	T37.8X3	T37.8X4	T37.8X5	T37.8X6
Nitrozone	T49.0X1	T49.0X2	T49.0X3	T49.0X4	T49.0X5	T49.0X6
Nizatidine	T47.0X1	T47.0X2	T47.0X3	T47.0X4	T47.0X5	T47.0X6
Nizofenone	T43.8X1	T43.8X2	T43.8X3	T43.8X4	T43.8X5	T43.8X6
Noctec	T42.6X1	T42.6X2	T42.6X3	T42.6X4	T42.6X5	T42.6X6
Noludar	T42.6X1	T42.6X2	T42.6X3	T42.6X4	T42.6X5	T42.6X6
Nomegestrol	T38.5X1	T38.5X2	T38.5X3	T38.5X4	T38.5X5	T38.5X6
Nomifensine	T43.291	T43.292	T43.293	T43.294	T43.295	T43.296
Nonoxinol	T49.8X1	T49.8X2	T49.8X3	T49.8X4	T49.8X5	T49.8X6
Nonylphenoxy (polyethoxyethanol)	T49.8X1	T49.8X2	T49.8X3	T49.8X4	T49.8X5	T49.8X6
Noptil	T42.3X1	T42.3X2	T42.3X3	T42.3X4	T42.3X5	T42.3X6
Noradrenaline	T44.4X1	T44.4X2	T44.4X3	T44.4X4	T44.4X5	T44.4X6
Noramidopyrine	T39.2X1	T39.2X2	T39.2X3	T39.2X4	T39.2X5	T39.2X6
methanesulfonate sodium	T39.2X1	T39.2X2	T39.2X3	T39.2X4	T39.2X5	T39.2X6
Norbormide	T60.4X1	T60.4X2	T60.4X3	T60.4X4	—	—
Nordazepam	T42.4X1	T42.4X2	T42.4X3	T42.4X4	T42.4X5	T42.4X6
Norepinephrine	T44.4X1	T44.4X2	T44.4X3	T44.4X4	T44.4X5	T44.4X6
Norethandrolone	T38.7X1	T38.7X2	T38.7X3	T38.7X4	T38.7X5	T38.7X6
Norethindrone	T38.4X1	T38.4X2	T38.4X3	T38.4X4	T38.4X5	T38.4X6
Norethisterone (acetate)	T38.4X1	T38.4X2	T38.4X3	T38.4X4	T38.4X5	T38.4X6
(enantate)						
with ethinylestradiol	T38.5X1	T38.5X2	T38.5X3	T38.5X4	T38.5X5	T38.5X6
Noretynodrel	T38.5X1	T38.5X2	T38.5X3	T38.5X4	T38.5X5	T38.5X6
Norfenefrine	T44.4X1	T44.4X2	T44.4X3	T44.4X4	T44.4X5	T44.4X6
Norfloxacin	T36.8X1	T36.8X2	T36.8X3	T36.8X4	T36.8X5	T36.8X6
Norgestrel	T38.4X1	T38.4X2	T38.4X3	T38.4X4	T38.4X5	T38.4X6
Norgestrienone	T38.4X1	T38.4X2	T38.4X3	T38.4X4	T38.4X5	T38.4X6
Norlestrin	T38.4X1	T38.4X2	T38.4X3	T38.4X4	T38.4X5	T38.4X6
Norlutin	T38.4X1	T38.4X2	T38.4X3	T38.4X4	T38.4X5	T38.4X6
Normal serum albumin (human), salt-poor	T45.8X1	T45.8X2	T45.8X3	T45.8X4	T45.8X5	T45.8X6
Normethandrone	T38.5X1	T38.5X2	T38.5X3	T38.5X4	T38.5X5	T38.5X6
Normison — see Benzodiazepines						
Normorphine	T40.2X1	T40.2X2	T40.2X3	T40.2X4	—	—
Norpseudoephedrine	T50.5X1	T50.5X2	T50.5X3	T50.5X4	T50.5X5	T50.5X6
Nortestosterone (furanpropionate)	T38.7X1	T38.7X2	T38.7X3	T38.7X4	T38.7X5	T38.7X6
Nortriptyline	T43.011	T43.012	T43.013	T43.014	T43.015	T43.016
Noscapine	T48.3X1	T48.3X2	T48.3X3	T48.3X4	T48.3X5	T48.3X6
Nose preparations	T49.6X1	T49.6X2	T49.6X3	T49.6X4	T49.6X5	T49.6X6
Novobiocin	T36.5X1	T36.5X2	T36.5X3	T36.5X4	T36.5X5	T36.5X6

Substance	Poisoning, Accidental (unintentional)	Poisoning, Intentional Self-harm	Poisoning, Assault	Poisoning, Undetermined	Adverse Effect	Under-dosing
Novocain (infiltration) (topical)	T41.3X1	T41.3X2	T41.3X3	T41.3X4	T41.3X5	T41.3X6
nerve block (peripheral) (plexus)	T41.3X1	T41.3X2	T41.3X3	T41.3X4	T41.3X5	T41.3X6
spinal	T41.3X1	T41.3X2	T41.3X3	T41.3X4	T41.3X5	T41.3X6
Noxious foodstuff	T62.91	T62.92	T62.93	T62.94	—	—
specified NEC	T62.8X1	T62.8X2	T62.8X3	T62.8X4	—	—
Noxiptiline	T43.011	T43.012	T43.013	T43.014	T43.015	T43.016
Noxytiolin	T49.0X1	T49.0X2	T49.0X3	T49.0X4	T49.0X5	T49.0X6
NPH Iletin (insulin)	T38.3X1	T38.3X2	T38.3X3	T38.3X4	T38.3X5	T38.3X6
Numorphan	T40.2X1	T40.2X2	T40.2X3	T40.2X4	T40.2X5	T40.2X6
Nunol	T42.3X1	T42.3X2	T42.3X3	T42.3X4	T42.3X5	T42.3X6
Nupercaine (spinal anesthetic)	T41.3X1	T41.3X2	T41.3X3	T41.3X4	T41.3X5	T41.3X6
topical (surface)	T41.3X1	T41.3X2	T41.3X3	T41.3X4	T41.3X5	T41.3X6
Nutmeg oil (liniment)	T49.3X1	T49.3X2	T49.3X3	T49.3X4	T49.3X5	T49.3X6
Nutritional supplement	T50.901	T50.902	T50.903	T50.904	T50.905	T50.906
Nux vomica	T65.1X1	T65.1X2	T65.1X3	T65.1X4	—	—
Nydrazid	T37.1X1	T37.1X2	T37.1X3	T37.1X4	T37.1X5	T37.1X6
Nylidrin	T46.7X1	T46.7X2	T46.7X3	T46.7X4	T46.7X5	T46.7X6
Nystatin	T36.7X1	T36.7X2	T36.7X3	T36.7X4	T36.7X5	T36.7X6
topical	T49.0X1	T49.0X2	T49.0X3	T49.0X4	T49.0X5	T49.0X6
Nytol	T45.0X1	T45.0X2	T45.0X3	T45.0X4	T45.0X5	T45.0X6
Obidoxime chloride	T50.6X1	T50.6X2	T50.6X3	T50.6X4	T50.6X5	T50.6X6
Octafonium (chloride)	T49.3X1	T49.3X2	T49.3X3	T49.3X4	T49.3X5	T49.3X6
Octamethyl pyrophosphoramide	T60.0X1	T60.0X2	T60.0X3	T60.0X4	—	—
Octanoin	T50.991	T50.992	T50.993	T50.994	T50.995	T50.99…
Octatropine methylbromide	T44.3X1	T44.3X2	T44.3X3	T44.3X4	T44.3X5	T44.3X…
Octotiamine	T45.2X1	T45.2X2	T45.2X3	T45.2X4	T45.2X5	T45.2X…
Octoxinol (9)	T49.8X1	T49.8X2	T49.8X3	T49.8X4	T49.8X5	T49.8X…
Octreotide	T38.991	T38.992	T38.993	T38.994	T38.995	T38.99…
Octyl nitrite	T46.3X1	T46.3X2	T46.3X3	T46.3X4	T46.3X5	T46.3X…
Oestradiol	T38.5X1	T38.5X2	T38.5X3	T38.5X4	T38.5X5	T38.5X…
Oestriol	T38.5X1	T38.5X2	T38.5X3	T38.5X4	T38.5X5	T38.5X…
Oestrogen	T38.5X1	T38.5X2	T38.5X3	T38.5X4	T38.5X5	T38.5X…
Oestrone	T38.5X1	T38.5X2	T38.5X3	T38.5X4	T38.5X5	T38.5X…
Ofloxacin	T36.8X1	T36.8X2	T36.8X3	T36.8X4	T36.8X5	T36.8X…
Oil (of)	T65.891	T65.892	T65.893	T65.894	—	—
bitter almond	T62.8X1	T62.8X2	T62.8X3	T62.8X4	—	—
cloves	T49.7X1	T49.7X2	T49.7X3	T49.7X4	T49.7X5	T49.7X…
colors	T65.6X1	T65.6X2	T65.6X3	T65.6X4	—	—
fumes	T59.891	T59.892	T59.893	T59.894	—	—
lubricating	T52.0X1	T52.0X2	T52.0X3	T52.0X4	—	—
Niobe	T52.8X1	T52.8X2	T52.8X3	T52.8X4	—	—
vitriol (liquid)	T54.2X1	T54.2X2	T54.2X3	T54.2X4	—	—
fumes	T54.2X1	T54.2X2	T54.2X3	T54.2X4	—	—
wintergreen (bitter) NEC	T49.3X1	T49.3X2	T49.3X3	T49.3X4	T49.3X5	T49.3…
Oily preparation (for skin)	T49.3X1	T49.3X2	T49.3X3	T49.3X4	T49.3X5	T49.3…
Ointment NEC	T49.3X1	T49.3X2	T49.3X3	T49.3X4	T49.3X5	T49.3…
Olanzapine	T43.591	T43.592	T43.593	T43.594	T43.595	T43.5…
Oleander	T62.2X1	T62.2X2	T62.2X3	T62.2X4	—	—
Oleandomycin	T36.3X1	T36.3X2	T36.3X3	T36.3X4	T36.3X5	T36.3…
Oleandrin	T46.0X1	T46.0X2	T46.0X3	T46.0X4	T46.0X5	T46.0…
Oleic acid	T46.6X1	T46.6X2	T46.6X3	T46.6X4	T46.6X5	T46.6…
Oleovitamin A	T45.2X1	T45.2X2	T45.2X3	T45.2X4	T45.2X5	T45.2…
Oleum ricini	T47.2X1	T47.2X2	T47.2X3	T47.2X4	T47.2X5	T47.2…
Olive oil (medicinal) NEC	T47.4X1	T47.4X2	T47.4X3	T47.4X4	T47.4X5	T47.4…
Olivomycin	T45.1X1	T45.1X2	T45.1X3	T45.1X4	T45.1X5	T45.1…
Olsalazine	T47.8X1	T47.8X2	T47.8X3	T47.8X4	T47.8X5	T47.8…
Omeprazole	T47.1X1	T47.1X2	T47.1X3	T47.1X4	T47.1X5	T47.1…
OMPA	T60.0X1	T60.0X2	T60.0X3	T60.0X4	—	—
Oncovin	T45.1X1	T45.1X2	T45.1X3	T45.1X4	T45.1X5	T45.1…
Ondansetron	T45.0X1	T45.0X2	T45.0X3	T45.0X4	T45.0X5	T45.0…
Ophthaine	T41.3X1	T41.3X2	T41.3X3	T41.3X4	T41.3X5	T41.3…
Ophthetic	T41.3X1	T41.3X2	T41.3X3	T41.3X4	T41.3X5	T41.3…
Opiate NEC	T40.601	T40.602	T40.603	T40.604	T40.605	T40.6…
antagonists	T50.7X1	T50.7X2	T50.7X3	T50.7X4	T50.7X5	T50.7…
Opioid NEC	T40.2X1	T40.2X2	T40.2X3	T40.2X4	T40.2X5	T40.2…
Opipramol	T43.011	T43.012	T43.013	T43.014	T43.015	T43.0…
Opium alkaloids (total)	T40.0X1	T40.0X2	T40.0X3	T40.0X4	T40.0X5	T40.0…
standardized powdered	T40.0X1	T40.0X2	T40.0X3	T40.0X4	T40.0X5	T40.0…
tincture (camphorated)	T40.0X1	T40.0X2	T40.0X3	T40.0X4	T40.0X5	T40.0…
Oracon	T38.4X1	T38.4X2	T38.4X3	T38.4X4	T38.4X5	T38.4…
Oragrafin	T50.8X1	T50.8X2	T50.8X3	T50.8X4	T50.8X5	T50.…
Oral contraceptives	T38.4X1	T38.4X2	T38.4X3	T38.4X4	T38.4X5	T38.4…
Oral rehydration salts	T50.3X1	T50.3X2	T50.3X3	T50.3X4	T50.3X5	T50.…
Orazamide	T50.991	T50.992	T50.993	T50.994	T50.995	T50.…
Orciprenaline	T48.291	T48.292	T48.293	T48.294	T48.295	T48.…
Organidin	T48.4X1	T48.4X2	T48.4X3	T48.4X4	T48.4X5	T48.…
Organonitrate NEC	T46.3X1	T46.3X2	T46.3X3	T46.3X4	T46.3X5	T46.…
Organophosphates	T60.0X1	T60.0X2	T60.0X3	T60.0X4	—	—

Substance	Poisoning, Accidental (unintentional)	Poisoning, Intentional Self-harm	Poisoning, Assault	Poisoning, Undetermined	Adverse Effect	Under-dosing
Orimune	T50.B91	T50.B92	T50.B93	T50.B94	T50.B95	T50.B96
Orinase	T38.3X1	T38.3X2	T38.3X3	T38.3X4	T38.3X5	T38.3X6
Ormeloxifene	T38.6X1	T38.6X2	T38.6X3	T38.6X4	T38.6X5	T38.6X6
Ornidazole	T37.3X1	T37.3X2	T37.3X3	T37.3X4	T37.3X5	T37.3X6
Ornithine aspartate	T50.991	T50.992	T50.993	T50.994	T50.995	T50.996
Ornoprostil	T47.1X1	T47.1X2	T47.1X3	T47.1X4	T47.1X5	T47.1X6
Orphenadrine	T42.8X1	T42.8X2	T42.8X3	T42.8X4	T42.8X5	T42.8X6
(hydrochloride)						
Ortal (sodium)	T42.3X1	T42.3X2	T42.3X3	T42.3X4	T42.3X5	T42.3X6
Orthoboric acid	T49.0X1	T49.0X2	T49.0X3	T49.0X4	T49.0X5	T49.0X6
ENT agent	T49.6X1	T49.6X2	T49.6X3	T49.6X4	T49.6X5	T49.6X6
ophthalmic preparation	T49.5X1	T49.5X2	T49.5X3	T49.5X4	T49.5X5	T49.5X6
Orthocaine	T41.3X1	T41.3X2	T41.3X3	T41.3X4	T41.3X5	T41.3X6
Orthodichlorobenzene	T53.7X1	T53.7X2	T53.7X3	T53.7X4	—	—
Ortho-Novum	T38.4X1	T38.4X2	T38.4X3	T38.4X4	T38.4X5	T38.4X6
Orthotolidine (reagent)	T54.2X1	T54.2X2	T54.2X3	T54.2X4	—	—
Osmic acid (liquid)	T54.2X1	T54.2X2	T54.2X3	T54.2X4	—	—
fumes	T54.2X1	T54.2X2	T54.2X3	T54.2X4	—	—
Osmotic diuretics	T50.2X1	T50.2X2	T50.2X3	T50.2X4	T50.2X5	T50.2X6
Otilonium bromide	T44.3X1	T44.3X2	T44.3X3	T44.3X4	T44.3X5	T44.3X6
Otorhinolaryngological drug NEC	T49.6X1	T49.6X2	T49.6X3	T49.6X4	T49.6X5	T49.6X6
Ouabain (e)	T46.0X1	T46.0X2	T46.0X3	T46.0X4	T46.0X5	T46.0X6
Ovarian						
hormone	T38.5X1	T38.5X2	T38.5X3	T38.5X4	T38.5X5	T38.5X6
stimulant	T38.5X1	T38.5X2	T38.5X3	T38.5X4	T38.5X5	T38.5X6
Ovral	T38.4X1	T38.4X2	T38.4X3	T38.4X4	T38.4X5	T38.4X6
Ovulen	T38.4X1	T38.4X2	T38.4X3	T38.4X4	T38.4X5	T38.4X6
Oxacillin	T36.0X1	T36.0X2	T36.0X3	T36.0X4	T36.0X5	T36.0X6
Oxalic acid	T54.2X1	T54.2X2	T54.2X3	T54.2X4	—	—
ammonium salt	T50.991	T50.992	T50.993	T50.994	T50.995	T50.996
Oxamniquine	T37.4X1	T37.4X2	T37.4X3	T37.4X4	T37.4X5	T37.4X6
Oxanamide	T43.591	T43.592	T43.593	T43.594	T43.595	T43.596
Oxandrolone	T38.7X1	T38.7X2	T38.7X3	T38.7X4	T38.7X5	T38.7X6
Oxantel	T37.4X1	T37.4X2	T37.4X3	T37.4X4	T37.4X5	T37.4X6
Oxapium iodide	T44.3X1	T44.3X2	T44.3X3	T44.3X4	T44.3X5	T44.3X6
Oxaprotiline	T43.021	T43.022	T43.023	T43.024	T43.025	T43.026
Oxaprozin	T39.311	T39.312	T39.313	T39.314	T39.315	T39.316
Oxatomide	T45.0X1	T45.0X2	T45.0X3	T45.0X4	T45.0X5	T45.0X6
Oxazepam	T42.4X1	T42.4X2	T42.4X3	T42.4X4	T42.4X5	T42.4X6
Oxazimedrine	T50.5X1	T50.5X2	T50.5X3	T50.5X4	T50.5X5	T50.5X6
Oxazolam	T42.4X1	T42.4X2	T42.4X3	T42.4X4	T42.4X5	T42.4X6
Oxazolidine derivatives	T42.2X1	T42.2X2	T42.2X3	T42.2X4	T42.2X5	T42.2X6
Oxazolidinedione	T42.2X1	T42.2X2	T42.2X3	T42.2X4	T42.2X5	T42.2X6
(derivative)						
Ox bile extract	T47.5X1	T47.5X2	T47.5X3	T47.5X4	T47.5X5	T47.5X6
Oxcarbazepine	T42.1X1	T42.1X2	T42.1X3	T42.1X4	T42.1X5	T42.1X6
Oxedrine	T44.4X1	T44.4X2	T44.4X3	T44.4X4	T44.4X5	T44.4X6
Oxeladin (citrate)	T48.3X1	T48.3X2	T48.3X3	T48.3X4	T48.3X5	T48.3X6
Oxendolone	T38.5X1	T38.5X2	T38.5X3	T38.5X4	T38.5X5	T38.5X6
Oxetacaine	T41.3X1	T41.3X2	T41.3X3	T41.3X4	T41.3X5	T41.3X6
Oxethazine	T41.3X1	T41.3X2	T41.3X3	T41.3X4	T41.3X5	T41.3X6
Oxetorone	T39.8X1	T39.8X2	T39.8X3	T39.8X4	T39.8X5	T39.8X6
Oxiconazole	T49.0X1	T49.0X2	T49.0X3	T49.0X4	T49.0X5	T49.0X6
Oxidizing agent NEC	T54.91	T54.92	T54.93	T54.94	—	—
Oxipurinol	T50.4X1	T50.4X2	T50.4X3	T50.4X4	T50.4X5	T50.4X6
Oxitriptan	T43.291	T43.292	T43.293	T43.294	T43.295	T43.296
Oxitropium bromide	T48.6X1	T48.6X2	T48.6X3	T48.6X4	T48.6X5	T48.6X6
Oxodipine	T46.1X1	T46.1X2	T46.1X3	T46.1X4	T46.1X5	T46.1X6
Oxolamine	T48.3X1	T48.3X2	T48.3X3	T48.3X4	T48.3X5	T48.3X6
Oxolinic acid	T37.8X1	T37.8X2	T37.8X3	T37.8X4	T37.8X5	T37.8X6
Oxomemazine	T43.3X1	T43.3X2	T43.3X3	T43.3X4	T43.3X5	T43.3X6
Oxophenarsine	T37.3X1	T37.3X2	T37.3X3	T37.3X4	T37.3X5	T37.3X6
Oxprenolol	T44.7X1	T44.7X2	T44.7X3	T44.7X4	T44.7X5	T44.7X6
Oxsoralen	T49.3X1	T49.3X2	T49.3X3	T49.3X4	T49.3X5	T49.3X6
Oxtriphylline	T48.6X1	T48.6X2	T48.6X3	T48.6X4	T48.6X5	T48.6X6
Oxybate sodium	T41.291	T41.292	T41.293	T41.294	T41.295	T41.296
Oxybuprocaine	T41.3X1	T41.3X2	T41.3X3	T41.3X4	T41.3X5	T41.3X6
Oxybutynin	T44.3X1	T44.3X2	T44.3X3	T44.3X4	T44.3X5	T44.3X6
Oxychlorosene	T49.0X1	T49.0X2	T49.0X3	T49.0X4	T49.0X5	T49.0X6
Oxycodone	T40.2X1	T40.2X2	T40.2X3	T40.2X4	T40.2X5	T40.2X6
Oxyfedrine	T46.3X1	T46.3X2	T46.3X3	T46.3X4	T46.3X5	T46.3X6
Oxygen	T41.5X1	T41.5X2	T41.5X3	T41.5X4	T41.5X5	T41.5X6
Oxylone	T49.0X1	T49.0X2	T49.0X3	T49.0X4	T49.0X5	T49.0X6
ophthalmic preparation	T49.5X1	T49.5X2	T49.5X3	T49.5X4	T49.5X5	T49.5X6
Oxymesterone	T38.7X1	T38.7X2	T38.7X3	T38.7X4	T38.7X5	T38.7X6
Oxymetazoline	T48.5X1	T48.5X2	T48.5X3	T48.5X4	T48.5X5	T48.5X6
Oxymetholone	T38.7X1	T38.7X2	T38.7X3	T38.7X4	T38.7X5	T38.7X6
Oxymorphone	T40.2X1	T40.2X2	T40.2X3	T40.2X4	T40.2X5	T40.2X6
Oxypertine	T43.591	T43.592	T43.593	T43.594	T43.595	T43.596
Oxyphenbutazone	T39.2X1	T39.2X2	T39.2X3	T39.2X4	T39.2X5	T39.2X6
Oxyphencyclimine	T44.3X1	T44.3X2	T44.3X3	T44.3X4	T44.3X5	T44.3X6
Oxyphenisatine	T47.2X1	T47.2X2	T47.2X3	T47.2X4	T47.2X5	T47.2X6
Oxyphenonium bromide	T44.3X1	T44.3X2	T44.3X3	T44.3X4	T44.3X5	T44.3X6
Oxypolygelatin	T45.8X1	T45.8X2	T45.8X3	T45.8X4	T45.8X5	T45.8X6
Oxyquinoline (derivatives)	T37.8X1	T37.8X2	T37.8X3	T37.8X4	T37.8X5	T37.8X6
Oxytetracycline	T36.4X1	T36.4X2	T36.4X3	T36.4X4	T36.4X5	T36.4X6
Oxytocic drug NEC	T48.0X1	T48.0X2	T48.0X3	T48.0X4	T48.0X5	T48.0X6
Oxytocin (synthetic)	T48.0X1	T48.0X2	T48.0X3	T48.0X4	T48.0X5	T48.0X6
Ozone	T59.891	T59.892	T59.893	T59.894	—	—
PABA	T49.3X1	T49.3X2	T49.3X3	T49.3X4	T49.3X5	T49.3X6
Packed red cells	T45.8X1	T45.8X2	T45.8X3	T45.8X4	T45.8X5	T45.8X6
Padimate	T49.3X1	T49.3X2	T49.3X3	T49.3X4	T49.3X5	T49.3X6
Paint NEC	T65.6X1	T65.6X2	T65.6X3	T65.6X4	—	—
cleaner	T52.91	T52.92	T52.93	T52.94	—	—
fumes NEC	T59.891	T59.892	T59.893	T59.894	—	—
lead (fumes)	T56.0X1	T56.0X2	T56.0X3	T56.0X4	—	—
solvent NEC	T52.8X1	T52.8X2	T52.8X3	T52.8X4	—	—
stripper	T52.8X1	T52.8X2	T52.8X3	T52.8X4	—	—
Palfium	T40.2X1	T40.2X2	T40.2X3	T40.2X4	—	—
Palm kernel oil	T50.991	T50.992	T50.993	T50.994	T50.995	T50.996
Paludrine	T37.2X1	T37.2X2	T37.2X3	T37.2X4	T37.2X5	T37.2X6
PAM (pralidoxime)	T50.6X1	T50.6X2	T50.6X3	T50.6X4	T50.6X5	T50.6X6
Pamaquine (naphthoute)	T37.2X1	T37.2X2	T37.2X3	T37.2X4	T37.2X5	T37.2X6
Panadol	T39.1X1	T39.1X2	T39.1X3	T39.1X4	T39.1X5	T39.1X6
Pancreatic						
digestive secretion stimulant	T47.8X1	T47.8X2	T47.8X3	T47.8X4	T47.8X5	T47.8X6
dornase	T45.3X1	T45.3X2	T45.3X3	T45.3X4	T45.3X5	T45.3X6
Pancreatin	T47.5X1	T47.5X2	T47.5X3	T47.5X4	T47.5X5	T47.5X6
Pancrelipase	T47.5X1	T47.5X2	T47.5X3	T47.5X4	T47.5X5	T47.5X6
Pancuronium (bromide)	T48.1X1	T48.1X2	T48.1X3	T48.1X4	T48.1X5	T48.1X6
Pangamic acid	T45.2X1	T45.2X2	T45.2X3	T45.2X4	T45.2X5	T45.2X6
Panthenol	T45.2X1	T45.2X2	T45.2X3	T45.2X4	T45.2X5	T45.2X6
topical	T49.8X1	T49.8X2	T49.8X3	T49.8X4	T49.8X5	T49.8X6
Pantopon	T40.0X1	T40.0X2	T40.0X3	T40.0X4	T40.0X5	T40.0X6
Pantothenic acid	T45.2X1	T45.2X2	T45.2X3	T45.2X4	T45.2X5	T45.2X6
Panwarfin	T45.511	T45.512	T45.513	T45.514	T45.515	T45.516
Papain	T47.5X1	T47.5X2	T47.5X3	T47.5X4	T47.5X5	T47.5X6
digestant	T47.5X1	T47.5X2	T47.5X3	T47.5X4	T47.5X5	T47.5X6
Papaveretum	T40.0X1	T40.0X2	T40.0X3	T40.0X4	T40.0X5	T40.0X6
Papaverine	T44.3X1	T44.3X2	T44.3X3	T44.3X4	T44.3X5	T44.3X6
Para-acetamidophenol	T39.1X1	T39.1X2	T39.1X3	T39.1X4	T39.1X5	T39.1X6
Para-aminobenzoic acid	T49.3X1	T49.3X2	T49.3X3	T49.3X4	T49.3X5	T49.3X6
Para-aminophenol derivatives	T39.1X1	T39.1X2	T39.1X3	T39.1X4	T39.1X5	T39.1X6
Para-aminosalicylic acid	T37.1X1	T37.1X2	T37.1X3	T37.1X4	T37.1X5	T37.1X6
Paracetaldehyde	T42.6X1	T42.6X2	T42.6X3	T42.6X4	T42.6X5	T42.6X6
Paracetamol	T39.1X1	T39.1X2	T39.1X3	T39.1X4	T39.1X5	T39.1X6
Parachlorophenol (camphorated)	T49.0X1	T49.0X2	T49.0X3	T49.0X4	T49.0X5	T49.0X6
Paracodin	T40.2X1	T40.2X2	T40.2X3	T40.2X4	T40.2X5	T40.2X6
Paradione	T42.2X1	T42.2X2	T42.2X3	T42.2X4	T42.2X5	T42.2X6
Paraffin(s) (wax)	T52.0X1	T52.0X2	T52.0X3	T52.0X4	—	—
liquid (medicinal)	T47.4X1	T47.4X2	T47.4X3	T47.4X4	T47.4X5	T47.4X6
nonmedicinal	T52.0X1	T52.0X2	T52.0X3	T52.0X4	—	—
Paraformaldehyde	T60.3X1	T60.3X2	T60.3X3	T60.3X4	—	—
Paraldehyde	T42.6X1	T42.6X2	T42.6X3	T42.6X4	T42.6X5	T42.6X6
Paramethadione	T42.2X1	T42.2X2	T42.2X3	T42.2X4	T42.2X5	T42.2X6
Paramethasone	T38.0X1	T38.0X2	T38.0X3	T38.0X4	T38.0X5	T38.0X6
acetate	T49.0X1	T49.0X2	T49.0X3	T49.0X4	T49.0X5	T49.0X6
Paraoxon	T60.0X1	T60.0X2	T60.0X3	T60.0X4	—	—
Paraquat	T60.3X1	T60.3X2	T60.3X3	T60.3X4	—	—
Parasympatholytic NEC	T44.3X1	T44.3X2	T44.3X3	T44.3X4	T44.3X5	T44.3X6
Parasympathomimetic drug NEC	T44.1X1	T44.1X2	T44.1X3	T44.1X4	T44.1X5	T44.1X6
Parathion	T60.0X1	T60.0X2	T60.0X3	T60.0X4	—	—
Parathormone	T50.991	T50.992	T50.993	T50.994	T50.995	T50.996
Parathyroid extract	T50.991	T50.992	T50.993	T50.994	T50.995	T50.996
Paratyphoid vaccine	T50.A91	T50.A92	T50.A93	T50.A94	T50.A95	T50.A96
Paredrine	T44.4X1	T44.4X2	T44.4X3	T44.4X4	T44.4X5	T44.4X6
Paregoric	T40.0X1	T40.0X2	T40.0X3	T40.0X4	T40.0X5	T40.0X6
Pargyline	T46.5X1	T46.5X2	T46.5X3	T46.5X4	T46.5X5	T46.5X6
Paris green	T57.0X1	T57.0X2	T57.0X3	T57.0X4	—	—
insecticide	T57.0X1	T57.0X2	T57.0X3	T57.0X4	—	—
Parnate	T43.1X1	T43.1X2	T43.1X3	T43.1X4	T43.1X5	T43.1X6
Paromomycin	T36.5X1	T36.5X2	T36.5X3	T36.5X4	T36.5X5	T36.5X6
Paroxypropione	T45.1X1	T45.1X2	T45.1X3	T45.1X4	T45.1X5	T45.1X6
Parzone	T40.2X1	T40.2X2	T40.2X3	T40.2X4	T40.2X5	T40.2X6
PAS	T37.1X1	T37.1X2	T37.1X3	T37.1X4	T37.1X5	T37.1X6
Pasiniazid	T37.1X1	T37.1X2	T37.1X3	T37.1X4	T37.1X5	T37.1X6
PBB (polybrominated biphenyls)	T65.891	T65.892	T65.893	T65.894	—	—
PCB	T65.891	T65.892	T65.893	T65.894	—	—
PCP						

Subterms under main terms may continue to next column or page   Additional Character May Be Required — Refer to the Tabular List for Character Selection   383

Orimune — PCP

Substance	Poisoning, Accidental (unintentional)	Poisoning, Intentional Self-harm	Poisoning, Assault	Poisoning, Undetermined	Adverse Effect	Under-dosing
PCP — *continued*						
meaning	T60.1X1	T60.1X2	T60.1X3	T60.1X4	—	—
pentachlorophenol						
fungicide	T60.3X1	T60.3X2	T60.3X3	T60.3X4	—	—
herbicide	T60.3X1	T60.3X2	T60.3X3	T60.3X4	—	—
insecticide	T60.1X1	T60.1X2	T60.1X3	T60.1X4	—	—
meaning phencyclidine	T40.991	T40.992	T40.993	T40.994	—	—
Peach kernel oil (emulsion)	T47.4X1	T47.4X2	T47.4X3	T47.4X4	T47.4X5	T47.4X6
Peanut oil (emulsion) **NEC**	T47.4X1	T47.4X2	T47.4X3	T47.4X4	T47.4X5	T47.4X6
topical	T49.3X1	T49.3X2	T49.3X3	T49.3X4	T49.3X5	T49.3X6
Pearly Gates (morning glory seeds)	T40.991	T40.992	T40.993	T40.994	—	—
Pecazine	T43.3X1	T43.3X2	T43.3X3	T43.3X4	T43.3X5	T43.3X6
Pectin	T47.6X1	T47.6X2	T47.6X3	T47.6X4	T47.6X5	T47.6X6
Pefloxacin	T37.8X1	T37.8X2	T37.8X3	T37.8X4	T37.8X5	T37.8X6
Pegademase, bovine	T50.Z91	T50.Z92	T50.Z93	T50.Z94	T50.Z95	T50.Z96
Pelletierine tannate	T37.4X1	T37.4X2	T37.4X3	T37.4X4	T37.4X5	T37.4X6
Pemirolast (potassium)	T48.6X1	T48.6X2	T48.6X3	T48.6X4	T48.6X5	T48.6X6
Pemoline	T50.7X1	T50.7X2	T50.7X3	T50.7X4	T50.7X5	T50.7X6
Pempidine	T44.2X1	T44.2X2	T44.2X3	T44.2X4	T44.2X5	T44.2X6
Penamecillin	T36.0X1	T36.0X2	T36.0X3	T36.0X4	T36.0X5	T36.0X6
Penbutolol	T44.7X1	T44.7X2	T44.7X3	T44.7X4	T44.7X5	T44.7X6
Penethamate	T36.0X1	T36.0X2	T36.0X3	T36.0X4	T36.0X5	T36.0X6
Penfluridol	T43.591	T43.592	T43.593	T43.594	T43.595	T43.596
Penflutizide	T50.2X1	T50.2X2	T50.2X3	T50.2X4	T50.2X5	T50.2X6
Pengitoxin	T46.0X1	T46.0X2	T46.0X3	T46.0X4	T46.0X5	T46.0X6
Penicillamine	T50.6X1	T50.6X2	T50.6X3	T50.6X4	T50.6X5	T50.6X6
Penicillin (any)	T36.0X1	T36.0X2	T36.0X3	T36.0X4	T36.0X5	T36.0X6
Penicillinase	T45.3X1	T45.3X2	T45.3X3	T45.3X4	T45.3X5	T45.3X6
Penicilloyl polylysine	T50.8X1	T50.8X2	T50.8X3	T50.8X4	T50.8X5	T50.8X6
Penimepicycline	T36.4X1	T36.4X2	T36.4X3	T36.4X4	T36.4X5	T36.4X6
Pentachloroethane	T53.6X1	T53.6X2	T53.6X3	T53.6X4	—	—
Pentachloronaphthalene	T53.7X1	T53.7X2	T53.7X3	T53.7X4	—	—
Pentachlorophenol	T60.1X1	T60.1X2	T60.1X3	T60.1X4	—	—
(pesticide)						
fungicide	T60.3X1	T60.3X2	T60.3X3	T60.3X4	—	—
herbicide	T60.3X1	T60.3X2	T60.3X3	T60.3X4	—	—
insecticide	T60.1X1	T60.1X2	T60.1X3	T60.1X4	—	—
Pentaerythritol	T46.3X1	T46.3X2	T46.3X3	T46.3X4	T46.3X5	T46.3X6
chloral	T42.6X1	T42.6X2	T42.6X3	T42.6X4	T42.6X5	T42.6X6
tetranitrate NEC	T46.3X1	T46.3X2	T46.3X3	T46.3X4	T46.3X5	T46.3X6
Pentaerythrityl tetranitrate	T46.3X1	T46.3X2	T46.3X3	T46.3X4	T46.3X5	T46.3X6
Pentagastrin	T50.8X1	T50.8X2	T50.8X3	T50.8X4	T50.8X5	T50.8X6
Pentalin	T53.6X1	T53.6X2	T53.6X3	T53.6X4	—	—
Pentamethonium bromide	T44.2X1	T44.2X2	T44.2X3	T44.2X4	T44.2X5	T44.2X6
Pentamidine	T37.3X1	T37.3X2	T37.3X3	T37.3X4	T37.3X5	T37.3X6
Pentanol	T51.3X1	T51.3X2	T51.3X3	T51.3X4	—	—
Pentapyrrolinium (bitartrate)	T44.2X1	T44.2X2	T44.2X3	T44.2X4	T44.2X5	T44.2X6
Pentaquine	T37.2X1	T37.2X2	T37.2X3	T37.2X4	T37.2X5	T37.2X6
Pentazocine	T40.4X1	T40.4X2	T40.4X3	T40.4X4	T40.4X5	T40.4X6
Pentetrazole	T50.7X1	T50.7X2	T50.7X3	T50.7X4	T50.7X5	T50.7X6
Penthienate bromide	T44.3X1	T44.3X2	T44.3X3	T44.3X4	T44.3X5	T44.3X6
Pentifylline	T46.7X1	T46.7X2	T46.7X3	T46.7X4	T46.7X5	T46.7X6
Pentobarbital	T42.3X1	T42.3X2	T42.3X3	T42.3X4	T42.3X5	T42.3X6
sodium	T42.3X1	T42.3X2	T42.3X3	T42.3X4	T42.3X5	T42.3X6
Pentobarbitone	T42.3X1	T42.3X2	T42.3X3	T42.3X4	T42.3X5	T42.3X6
Pentolonium tartrate	T44.2X1	T44.2X2	T44.2X3	T44.2X4	T44.2X5	T44.2X6
Pentosan polysulfate (sodium)	T39.8X1	T39.8X2	T39.8X3	T39.8X4	T39.8X5	T39.8X6
Pentostatin	T45.1X1	T45.1X2	T45.1X3	T45.1X4	T45.1X5	T45.1X6
Pentothal	T41.1X1	T41.1X2	T41.1X3	T41.1X4	T41.1X5	T41.1X6
Pentoxifylline	T46.7X1	T46.7X2	T46.7X3	T46.7X4	T46.7X5	T46.7X6
Pentoxyverine	T48.3X1	T48.3X2	T48.3X3	T48.3X4	T48.3X5	T48.3X6
Pentrinat	T46.3X1	T46.3X2	T46.3X3	T46.3X4	T46.3X5	T46.3X6
Pentylenetetrazole	T50.7X1	T50.7X2	T50.7X3	T50.7X4	T50.7X5	T50.7X6
Pentylsalicylamide	T37.1X1	T37.1X2	T37.1X3	T37.1X4	T37.1X5	T37.1X6
Pentymal	T42.3X1	T42.3X2	T42.3X3	T42.3X4	T42.3X5	T42.3X6
Peplomycin	T45.1X1	T45.1X2	T45.1X3	T45.1X4	T45.1X5	T45.1X6
Peppermint (oil)	T47.5X1	T47.5X2	T47.5X3	T47.5X4	T47.5X5	T47.5X6
Pepsin	T47.5X1	T47.5X2	T47.5X3	T47.5X4	T47.5X5	T47.5X6
digestant	T47.5X1	T47.5X2	T47.5X3	T47.5X4	T47.5X5	T47.5X6
Pepstatin	T47.1X1	T47.1X2	T47.1X3	T47.1X4	T47.1X5	T47.1X6
Peptavlon	T50.8X1	T50.8X2	T50.8X3	T50.8X4	T50.8X5	T50.8X6
Perazine	T43.3X1	T43.3X2	T43.3X3	T43.3X4	T43.3X5	T43.3X6
Percaine (spinal)	T41.3X1	T41.3X2	T41.3X3	T41.3X4	T41.3X5	T41.3X6
topical (surface)	T41.3X1	T41.3X2	T41.3X3	T41.3X4	T41.3X5	T41.3X6
Perchloroethylene	T53.3X1	T53.3X2	T53.3X3	T53.3X4	—	—
medicinal	T37.4X1	T37.4X2	T37.4X3	T37.4X4	T37.4X5	T37.4X6
vapor	T53.3X1	T53.3X2	T53.3X3	T53.3X4	—	—
Percodan	T40.2X1	T40.2X2	T40.2X3	T40.2X4	T40.2X5	T40.2X6

Substance	Poisoning, Accidental (unintentional)	Poisoning, Intentional Self-harm	Poisoning, Assault	Poisoning, Undetermined	Adverse Effect	Under-dosing
Percogesic — *see also* acetaminophen	T45.0X1	T45.0X2	T45.0X3	T45.0X4	T45.0X5	T45.0X6
Percorten	T38.0X1	T38.0X2	T38.0X3	T38.0X4	T38.0X5	T38.0X6
Pergolide	T42.8X1	T42.8X2	T42.8X3	T42.8X4	T42.8X5	T42.8X6
Pergonal	T38.811	T38.812	T38.813	T38.814	T38.815	T38.816
Perhexilene	T46.3X1	T46.3X2	T46.3X3	T46.3X4	T46.3X5	T46.3X6
Perhexiline (maleate)	T46.3X1	T46.3X2	T46.3X3	T46.3X4	T46.3X5	T46.3X6
Periactin	T45.0X1	T45.0X2	T45.0X3	T45.0X4	T45.0X5	T45.0X6
Periciazine	T43.3X1	T43.3X2	T43.3X3	T43.3X4	T43.3X5	T43.3X6
Periclor	T42.6X1	T42.6X2	T42.6X3	T42.6X4	T42.6X5	T42.6X6
Perindopril	T46.4X1	T46.4X2	T46.4X3	T46.4X4	T46.4X5	T46.4X6
Perisoxal	T39.8X1	T39.8X2	T39.8X3	T39.8X4	T39.8X5	T39.8X6
Peritoneal dialysis solution	T50.3X1	T50.3X2	T50.3X3	T50.3X4	T50.3X5	T50.3X6
Peritrate	T46.3X1	T46.3X2	T46.3X3	T46.3X4	T46.3X5	T46.3X6
Perlapine	T42.4X1	T42.4X2	T42.4X3	T42.4X4	T42.4X5	T42.4X6
Permanganate	T65.891	T65.892	T65.893	T65.894	—	—
Permethrin	T60.1X1	T60.1X2	T60.1X3	T60.1X4	—	—
Pernocton	T42.3X1	T42.3X2	T42.3X3	T42.3X4	T42.3X5	T42.3X6
Pernoston	T42.3X1	T42.3X2	T42.3X3	T42.3X4	T42.3X5	T42.3X6
Peronine	T40.2X1	T40.2X2	T40.2X3	T40.2X4	—	—
Perphenazine	T43.3X1	T43.3X2	T43.3X3	T43.3X4	T43.3X5	T43.3X6
Pertofrane	T43.011	T43.012	T43.013	T43.014	T43.015	T43.016
Pertussis						
immune serum (human)	T50.Z11	T50.Z12	T50.Z13	T50.Z14	T50.Z15	T50.Z16
vaccine (with diphtheria toxoid) (with tetanus toxoid)	T50.A11	T50.A12	T50.A13	T50.A14	T50.A15	T50.A16
Peruvian balsam	T49.0X1	T49.0X2	T49.0X3	T49.0X4	T49.0X5	T49.0X6
Peruvoside	T46.0X1	T46.0X2	T46.0X3	T46.0X4	T46.0X5	T46.0X6
Pesticide (dust) (fumes) (vapor) **NEC**	T60.91	T60.92	T60.93	T60.94	—	—
arsenic	T57.0X1	T57.0X2	T57.0X3	T57.0X4	—	—
chlorinated	T60.1X1	T60.1X2	T60.1X3	T60.1X4	—	—
cyanide	T65.0X1	T65.0X2	T65.0X3	T65.0X4	—	—
kerosene	T52.0X1	T52.0X2	T52.0X3	T52.0X4	—	—
mixture (of compounds)	T60.91	T60.92	T60.93	T60.94	—	—
naphthalene	T60.2X1	T60.2X2	T60.2X3	T60.2X4	—	—
organochlorine (compounds)	T60.1X1	T60.1X2	T60.1X3	T60.1X4	—	—
petroleum (distillate) (products) NEC	T60.8X1	T60.8X2	T60.8X3	T60.8X4	—	—
specified ingredient NEC	T60.8X1	T60.8X2	T60.8X3	T60.8X4	—	—
strychnine	T65.1X1	T65.1X2	T65.1X3	T65.1X4	—	—
thallium	T60.4X1	T60.4X2	T60.4X3	T60.4X4	—	—
Pethidine	T40.4X1	T40.4X2	T40.4X3	T40.4X4	T40.4X5	T40.4X6
Petrichloral	T42.6X1	T42.6X2	T42.6X3	T42.6X4	T42.6X5	T42.6X6
Petrol	T52.0X1	T52.0X2	T52.0X3	T52.0X4	—	—
vapor	T52.0X1	T52.0X2	T52.0X3	T52.0X4	—	—
Petrolatum	T49.3X1	T49.3X2	T49.3X3	T49.3X4	T49.3X5	T49.3X6
hydrophilic	T49.3X1	T49.3X2	T49.3X3	T49.3X4	T49.3X5	T49.3X6
liquid	T47.4X1	T47.4X2	T47.4X3	T47.4X4	T47.4X5	T47.4X6
topical	T49.3X1	T49.3X2	T49.3X3	T49.3X4	T49.3X5	T49.3X6
nonmedicinal	T52.0X1	T52.0X2	T52.0X3	T52.0X4	—	—
red veterinary	T49.3X1	T49.3X2	T49.3X3	T49.3X4	T49.3X5	T49.3X6
white	T49.3X1	T49.3X2	T49.3X3	T49.3X4	T49.3X5	T49.3X6
Petroleum (products) **NEC**	T52.0X1	T52.0X2	T52.0X3	T52.0X4	—	—
benzine(s) — *see* Ligroin						
ether — *see* Ligroin						
jelly — *see* Petrolatum						
naphtha — *see* Ligroin						
pesticide	T60.8X1	T60.8X2	T60.8X3	T60.8X4	—	—
solids	T52.0X1	T52.0X2	T52.0X3	T52.0X4	—	—
solvents	T52.0X1	T52.0X2	T52.0X3	T52.0X4	—	—
vapor	T52.0X1	T52.0X2	T52.0X3	T52.0X4	—	—
Peyote	T40.991	T40.992	T40.993	T40.994	—	—
Phanodorm, phanodorn	T42.3X1	T42.3X2	T42.3X3	T42.3X4	T42.3X5	T42.3X6
Phanquinone	T37.3X1	T37.3X2	T37.3X3	T37.3X4	T37.3X5	T37.3X6
Phanquone	T37.3X1	T37.3X2	T37.3X3	T37.3X4	T37.3X5	T37.3X6
Pharmaceutical						
adjunct NEC	T50.901	T50.902	T50.903	T50.904	T50.905	T50.906
excipient NEC	T50.901	T50.902	T50.903	T50.904	T50.905	T50.906
sweetener	T50.901	T50.902	T50.903	T50.904	T50.905	T50.906
viscous agent	T50.901	T50.902	T50.903	T50.904	T50.905	T50.906
Phemitone	T42.3X1	T42.3X2	T42.3X3	T42.3X4	T42.3X5	T42.3X6
Phenacaine	T41.3X1	T41.3X2	T41.3X3	T41.3X4	T41.3X5	T41.3X6
Phenacemide	T42.6X1	T42.6X2	T42.6X3	T42.6X4	T42.6X5	T42.6X6
Phenacetin	T39.1X1	T39.1X2	T39.1X3	T39.1X4	T39.1X5	T39.1X6
Phenadoxone	T40.2X1	T40.2X2	T40.2X3	T40.2X4	—	—
Phenaglycodol	T43.591	T43.592	T43.593	T43.594	T43.595	T43.596
Phenantoin	T42.0X1	T42.0X2	T42.0X3	T42.0X4	T42.0X5	T42.0X6
Phenaphthazine reagent	T50.991	T50.992	T50.993	T50.994	T50.995	T50.996
Phenazocine	T40.4X1	T40.4X2	T40.4X3	T40.4X4	T40.4X5	T40.4X6
Phenazone	T39.2X1	T39.2X2	T39.2X3	T39.2X4	T39.2X5	T39.2X6

Substance	Poisoning, Accidental (unintentional)	Poisoning, Intentional Self-harm	Poisoning, Assault	Poisoning, Undetermined	Adverse Effect	Under-dosing
Phenazopyridine	T39.8X1	T39.8X2	T39.8X3	T39.8X4	T39.8X5	T39.8X6
Phenbenicillin	T36.0X1	T36.0X2	T36.0X3	T36.0X4	T36.0X5	T36.0X6
Phenbutrazate	T50.5X1	T50.5X2	T50.5X3	T50.5X4	T50.5X5	T50.5X6
Phencyclidine	T40.991	T40.992	T40.993	T40.994	T40.995	T40.996
Phendimetrazine	T50.5X1	T50.5X2	T50.5X3	T50.5X4	T50.5X5	T50.5X6
Phenelzine	T43.1X1	T43.1X2	T43.1X3	T43.1X4	T43.1X5	T43.1X6
Phenemal	T42.3X1	T42.3X2	T42.3X3	T42.3X4	T42.3X5	T42.3X6
Phenergan	T42.6X1	T42.6X2	T42.6X3	T42.6X4	T42.6X5	T42.6X6
Pheneticillin	T36.0X1	T36.0X2	T36.0X3	T36.0X4	T36.0X5	T36.0X6
Pheneturide	T42.6X1	T42.6X2	T42.6X3	T42.6X4	T42.6X5	T42.6X6
Phenformin	T38.3X1	T38.3X2	T38.3X3	T38.3X4	T38.3X5	T38.3X6
Phenglutarimide	T44.3X1	T44.3X2	T44.3X3	T44.3X4	T44.3X5	T44.3X6
Phenicarbazide	T39.8X1	T39.8X2	T39.8X3	T39.8X4	T39.8X5	T39.8X6
Phenindamine	T45.0X1	T45.0X2	T45.0X3	T45.0X4	T45.0X5	T45.0X6
Phenindione	T45.511	T45.512	T45.513	T45.514	T45.515	T45.516
Pheniprazine	T43.1X1	T43.1X2	T43.1X3	T43.1X4	T43.1X5	T43.1X6
Pheniramine	T45.0X1	T45.0X2	T45.0X3	T45.0X4	T45.0X5	T45.0X6
Phenisatin	T47.2X1	T47.2X2	T47.2X3	T47.2X4	T47.2X5	T47.2X6
Phenmetrazine	T50.5X1	T50.5X2	T50.5X3	T50.5X4	T50.5X5	T50.5X6
Phenobal	T42.3X1	T42.3X2	T42.3X3	T42.3X4	T42.3X5	T42.3X6
Phenobarbital	T42.3X1	T42.3X2	T42.3X3	T42.3X4	T42.3X5	T42.3X6
with						
mephenytoin	T42.3X1	T42.3X2	T42.3X3	T42.3X4	T42.3X5	T42.3X6
phenytoin	T42.3X1	T42.3X2	T42.3X3	T42.3X4	T42.3X5	T42.3X6
sodium	T42.3X1	T42.3X2	T42.3X3	T42.3X4	T42.3X5	T42.3X6
Phenobarbitone	T42.3X1	T42.3X2	T42.3X3	T42.3X4	T42.3X5	T42.3X6
Phenobutiodil	T50.8X1	T50.8X2	T50.8X3	T50.8X4	T50.8X5	T50.8X6
Phenoctide	T49.0X1	T49.0X2	T49.0X3	T49.0X4	T49.0X5	T49.0X6
Phenol	T49.0X1	T49.0X2	T49.0X3	T49.0X4	T49.0X5	T49.0X6
disinfectant	T54.0X1	T54.0X2	T54.0X3	T54.0X4	—	—
in oil injection	T46.8X1	T46.8X2	T46.8X3	T46.8X4	T46.8X5	T46.8X6
medicinal	T49.1X1	T49.1X2	T49.1X3	T49.1X4	T49.1X5	T49.1X6
nonmedicinal NEC	T54.0X1	T54.0X2	T54.0X3	T54.0X4	—	—
pesticide	T60.8X1	T60.8X2	T60.8X3	T60.8X4	—	—
red	T50.8X1	T50.8X2	T50.8X3	T50.8X4	T50.8X5	T50.8X6
Phenolic preparation	T49.1X1	T49.1X2	T49.1X3	T49.1X4	T49.1X5	T49.1X6
Phenolphthalein	T47.2X1	T47.2X2	T47.2X3	T47.2X4	T47.2X5	T47.2X6
Phenolsulfonphthalein	T50.8X1	T50.8X2	T50.8X3	T50.8X4	T50.8X5	T50.8X6
Phenomorphan	T40.2X1	T40.2X2	T40.2X3	T40.2X4		
Phenonyl	T42.3X1	T42.3X2	T42.3X3	T42.3X4	T42.3X5	T42.3X6
Phenoperidine	T40.4X1	T40.4X2	T40.4X3	T40.4X4		
Phenopyrazone	T46.991	T46.992	T46.993	T46.994	T46.995	T46.996
Phenoquin	T50.4X1	T50.4X2	T50.4X3	T50.4X4	T50.4X5	T50.4X6
Phenothiazine (psychotropic) NEC	T43.3X1	T43.3X2	T43.3X3	T43.3X4	T43.3X5	T43.3X6
insecticide	T60.2X1	T60.2X2	T60.2X3	T60.2X4	—	—
Phenothrin	T49.0X1	T49.0X2	T49.0X3	T49.0X4	T49.0X5	T49.0X6
Phenoxybenzamine	T46.7X1	T46.7X2	T46.7X3	T46.7X4	T46.7X5	T46.7X6
Phenoxyethanol	T49.0X1	T49.0X2	T49.0X3	T49.0X4	T49.0X5	T49.0X6
Phenoxymethyl penicillin	T36.0X1	T36.0X2	T36.0X3	T36.0X4	T36.0X5	T36.0X6
Phenprobamate	T42.8X1	T42.8X2	T42.8X3	T42.8X4	T42.8X5	T42.8X6
Phenprocoumon	T45.511	T45.512	T45.513	T45.514	T45.515	T45.516
Phensuximide	T42.2X1	T42.2X2	T42.2X3	T42.2X4	T42.2X5	T42.2X6
Phentermine	T50.5X1	T50.5X2	T50.5X3	T50.5X4	T50.5X5	T50.5X6
Phenthicillin	T36.0X1	T36.0X2	T36.0X3	T36.0X4	T36.0X5	T36.0X6
Phentolamine	T46.7X1	T46.7X2	T46.7X3	T46.7X4	T46.7X5	T46.7X6
Phenyl						
butazone	T39.2X1	T39.2X2	T39.2X3	T39.2X4	T39.2X5	T39.2X6
enediamine	T65.3X1	T65.3X2	T65.3X3	T65.3X4	—	—
hydrazine	T65.3X1	T65.3X2	T65.3X3	T65.3X4	—	—
antineoplastic	T45.1X1	T45.1X2	T45.1X3	T45.1X4	T45.1X5	T45.1X6
mercuric compounds — see Mercury						
salicylate	T49.3X1	T49.3X2	T49.3X3	T49.3X4	T49.3X5	T49.3X6
Phenylalanine mustard	T45.1X1	T45.1X2	T45.1X3	T45.1X4	T45.1X5	T45.1X6
Phenylbutazone	T39.2X1	T39.2X2	T39.2X3	T39.2X4	T39.2X5	T39.2X6
Phenylenediamine	T65.3X1	T65.3X2	T65.3X3	T65.3X4	—	—
Phenylephrine	T44.4X1	T44.4X2	T44.4X3	T44.4X4	T44.4X5	T44.4X6
Phenylethylbiguanide	T38.3X1	T38.3X2	T38.3X3	T38.3X4	T38.3X5	T38.3X6
Phenylmercuric						
acetate	T49.0X1	T49.0X2	T49.0X3	T49.0X4	T49.0X5	T49.0X6
borate	T49.0X1	T49.0X2	T49.0X3	T49.0X4	T49.0X5	T49.0X6
nitrate	T49.0X1	T49.0X2	T49.0X3	T49.0X4	T49.0X5	T49.0X6
Phenylmethylbarbitone	T42.3X1	T42.3X2	T42.3X3	T42.3X4	T42.3X5	T42.3X6
Phenylpropanol	T47.5X1	T47.5X2	T47.5X3	T47.5X4	T47.5X5	T47.5X6
Phenylpropanolamine	T44.991	T44.992	T44.993	T44.994	T44.995	T44.996
Phenylsulfthion	T60.0X1	T60.0X2	T60.0X3	T60.0X4	—	—
Phenyltoloxamine	T45.0X1	T45.0X2	T45.0X3	T45.0X4	T45.0X5	T45.0X6
Phenyramidol, phenyramidon	T39.8X1	T39.8X2	T39.8X3	T39.8X4	T39.8X5	T39.8X6
Phenytoin	T42.0X1	T42.0X2	T42.0X3	T42.0X4	T42.0X5	T42.0X6
with Phenobarbital	T42.3X1	T42.3X2	T42.3X3	T42.3X4	T42.3X5	T42.3X6
pHisoHex	T49.2X1	T49.2X2	T49.2X3	T49.2X4	T49.2X5	T49.2X6

Substance	Poisoning, Accidental (unintentional)	Poisoning, Intentional Self-harm	Poisoning, Assault	Poisoning, Undetermined	Adverse Effect	Under-dosing
Pholcodine	T48.3X1	T48.3X2	T48.3X3	T48.3X4	T48.3X5	T48.3X6
Pholedrine	T46.991	T46.992	T46.993	T46.994	T46.995	T46.996
Phorate	T60.0X1	T60.0X2	T60.0X3	T60.0X4	—	—
Phosdrin	T60.0X1	T60.0X2	T60.0X3	T60.0X4	—	—
Phosfolan	T60.0X1	T60.0X2	T60.0X3	T60.0X4	—	—
Phosgene (gas)	T59.891	T59.892	T59.893	T59.894	—	—
Phosphamidon	T60.0X1	T60.0X2	T60.0X3	T60.0X4	—	—
Phosphate	T65.891	T65.892	T65.893	T65.894	—	—
laxative	T47.4X1	T47.4X2	T47.4X3	T47.4X4	T47.4X5	T47.4X6
organic	T60.0X1	T60.0X2	T60.0X3	T60.0X4	—	—
solvent	T52.91	T52.92	T52.93	T52.94	—	—
tricresyl	T65.891	T65.892	T65.893	T65.894	—	—
Phosphine	T57.1X1	T57.1X2	T57.1X3	T57.1X4	—	—
fumigant	T57.1X1	T57.1X2	T57.1X3	T57.1X4	—	—
Phospholine	T49.5X1	T49.5X2	T49.5X3	T49.5X4	T49.5X5	T49.5X6
Phosphoric acid	T54.2X1	T54.2X2	T54.2X3	T54.2X4	—	—
Phosphorus (compound) NEC	T57.1X1	T57.1X2	T57.1X3	T57.1X4	—	—
pesticide	T60.0X1	T60.0X2	T60.0X3	T60.0X4	—	—
Phthalates	T65.891	T65.892	T65.893	T65.894	—	—
Phthalic anhydride	T65.891	T65.892	T65.893	T65.894	—	—
Phthalimidoglutarimide	T42.6X1	T42.6X2	T42.6X3	T42.6X4	T42.6X5	T42.6X6
Phthalylsulfathiazole	T37.0X1	T37.0X2	T37.0X3	T37.0X4	T37.0X5	T37.0X6
Phylloquinone	T45.7X1	T45.7X2	T45.7X3	T45.7X4	T45.7X5	T45.7X6
Physeptone	T40.3X1	T40.3X2	T40.3X3	T40.3X4	T40.3X5	T40.3X6
Physostigma venenosum	T62.2X1	T62.2X2	T62.2X3	T62.2X4		
Physostigmine	T49.5X1	T49.5X2	T49.5X3	T49.5X4	T49.5X5	T49.5X6
Phytolacca decandra	T62.2X1	T62.2X2	T62.2X3	T62.2X4	—	—
berries	T62.1X1	T62.1X2	T62.1X3	T62.1X4	—	—
Phytomenadione	T45.7X1	T45.7X2	T45.7X3	T45.7X4	T45.7X5	T45.7X6
Phytonadione	T45.7X1	T45.7X2	T45.7X3	T45.7X4	T45.7X5	T45.7X6
Picoperine	T48.3X1	T48.3X2	T48.3X3	T48.3X4	T48.3X5	T48.3X6
Picosulfate (sodium)	T47.2X1	T47.2X2	T47.2X3	T47.2X4	T47.2X5	T47.2X6
Picric (acid)	T54.2X1	T54.2X2	T54.2X3	T54.2X4	—	—
Picrotoxin	T50.7X1	T50.7X2	T50.7X3	T50.7X4	T50.7X5	T50.7X6
Piketoprofen	T49.0X1	T49.0X2	T49.0X3	T49.0X4	T49.0X5	T49.0X6
Pilocarpine	T44.1X1	T44.1X2	T44.1X3	T44.1X4	T44.1X5	T44.1X6
Pilocarpus (jaborandi)	T44.1X1	T44.1X2	T44.1X3	T44.1X4	T44.1X5	T44.1X6
extract						
Pilsicainide (hydrochloride)	T46.2X1	T46.2X2	T46.2X3	T46.2X4	T46.2X5	T46.2X6
Pimaricin	T36.7X1	T36.7X2	T36.7X3	T36.7X4	T36.7X5	T36.7X6
Pimeclone	T50.7X1	T50.7X2	T50.7X3	T50.7X4	T50.7X5	T50.7X6
Pimelic ketone	T52.8X1	T52.8X2	T52.8X3	T52.8X4		
Pimethixene	T45.0X1	T45.0X2	T45.0X3	T45.0X4	T45.0X5	T45.0X6
Piminodine	T40.2X1	T40.2X2	T40.2X3	T40.2X4	T40.2X5	T40.2X6
Pimozide	T43.591	T43.592	T43.593	T43.594	T43.595	T43.596
Pinacidil	T46.5X1	T46.5X2	T46.5X3	T46.5X4	T46.5X5	T46.5X6
Pinaverium bromide	T44.3X1	T44.3X2	T44.3X3	T44.3X4	T44.3X5	T44.3X6
Pinazepam	T42.4X1	T42.4X2	T42.4X3	T42.4X4	T42.4X5	T42.4X6
Pindolol	T44.7X1	T44.7X2	T44.7X3	T44.7X4	T44.7X5	T44.7X6
Pindone	T60.4X1	T60.4X2	T60.4X3	T60.4X4	—	—
Pine oil (disinfectant)	T65.891	T65.892	T65.893	T65.894	—	—
Pinkroot	T37.4X1	T37.4X2	T37.4X3	T37.4X4	T37.4X5	T37.4X6
Pipadone	T40.2X1	T40.2X2	T40.2X3	T40.2X4	—	—
Pipamazine	T45.0X1	T45.0X2	T45.0X3	T45.0X4	T45.0X5	T45.0X6
Pipamperone	T43.4X1	T43.4X2	T43.4X3	T43.4X4	T43.4X5	T43.4X6
Pipazetate	T48.3X1	T48.3X2	T48.3X3	T48.3X4	T48.3X5	T48.3X6
Pipemidic acid	T37.8X1	T37.8X2	T37.8X3	T37.8X4	T37.8X5	T37.8X6
Pipenzolate bromide	T44.3X1	T44.3X2	T44.3X3	T44.3X4	T44.3X5	T44.3X6
Piperacetazine	T43.3X1	T43.3X2	T43.3X3	T43.3X4	T43.3X5	T43.3X6
Piperacillin	T36.0X1	T36.0X2	T36.0X3	T36.0X4	T36.0X5	T36.0X6
Piperazine	T37.4X1	T37.4X2	T37.4X3	T37.4X4	T37.4X5	T37.4X6
estrone sulfate	T38.5X1	T38.5X2	T38.5X3	T38.5X4	T38.5X5	T38.5X6
Piper cubeba	T62.2X1	T62.2X2	T62.2X3	T62.2X4		
Piperidione	T48.3X1	T48.3X2	T48.3X3	T48.3X4	T48.3X5	T48.3X6
Piperidolate	T44.3X1	T44.3X2	T44.3X3	T44.3X4	T44.3X5	T44.3X6
Piperocaine	T41.3X1	T41.3X2	T41.3X3	T41.3X4	T41.3X5	T41.3X6
infiltration (subcutaneous)	T41.3X1	T41.3X2	T41.3X3	T41.3X4	T41.3X5	T41.3X6
nerve block (peripheral) (plexus)	T41.3X1	T41.3X2	T41.3X3	T41.3X4	T41.3X5	T41.3X6
topical (surface)	T41.3X1	T41.3X2	T41.3X3	T41.3X4	T41.3X5	T41.3X6
Piperonyl butoxide	T60.8X1	T60.8X2	T60.8X3	T60.8X4	—	—
Pipethanate	T44.3X1	T44.3X2	T44.3X3	T44.3X4	T44.3X5	T44.3X6
Pipobroman	T45.1X1	T45.1X2	T45.1X3	T45.1X4	T45.1X5	T45.1X6
Pipotiazine	T43.3X1	T43.3X2	T43.3X3	T43.3X4	T43.3X5	T43.3X6
Pipoxizine	T45.0X1	T45.0X2	T45.0X3	T45.0X4	T45.0X5	T45.0X6
Pipradrol	T43.691	T43.692	T43.693	T43.694	T43.695	T43.696
Piprinhydrinate	T45.0X1	T45.0X2	T45.0X3	T45.0X4	T45.0X5	T45.0X6
Pirarubicin	T45.1X1	T45.1X2	T45.1X3	T45.1X4	T45.1X5	T45.1X6
Pirazinamide	T37.1X1	T37.1X2	T37.1X3	T37.1X4	T37.1X5	T37.1X6
Pirbuterol	T48.6X1	T48.6X2	T48.6X3	T48.6X4	T48.6X5	T48.6X6
Pirenzepine	T47.1X1	T47.1X2	T47.1X3	T47.1X4	T47.1X5	T47.1X6
Piretanide	T50.1X1	T50.1X2	T50.1X3	T50.1X4	T50.1X5	T50.1X6

Substance	Poisoning, Accidental (unintentional)	Poisoning, Intentional Self-harm	Poisoning, Assault	Poisoning, Undetermined	Adverse Effect	Under-dosing
Piribedil	T42.8X1	T42.8X2	T42.8X3	T42.8X4	T42.8X5	T42.8X6
Piridoxilate	T46.3X1	T46.3X2	T46.3X3	T46.3X4	T46.3X5	T46.3X6
Piritramide	T40.4X1	T40.4X2	T40.4X3	T40.4X4	—	—
Piromidic acid	T37.8X1	T37.8X2	T37.8X3	T37.8X4	T37.8X5	T37.8X6
Piroxicam	T39.391	T39.392	T39.393	T39.394	T39.395	T39.396
beta-cyclodextrin complex	T39.8X1	T39.8X2	T39.8X3	T39.8X4	T39.8X5	T39.8X6
Pirozadil	T46.6X1	T46.6X2	T46.6X3	T46.6X4	T46.6X5	T46.6X6
Piscidia (bark) (erythrina)	T39.8X1	T39.8X2	T39.8X3	T39.8X4	T39.8X5	T39.8X6
Pitch	T65.891	T65.892	T65.893	T65.894	—	—
Pitkin's solution	T41.3X1	T41.3X2	T41.3X3	T41.3X4	T41.3X5	T41.3X6
Pitocin	T48.0X1	T48.0X2	T48.0X3	T48.0X4	T48.0X5	T48.0X6
Pitressin (tannate)	T38.891	T38.892	T38.893	T38.894	T38.895	T38.896
Pituitary extracts	T38.891	T38.892	T38.893	T38.894	T38.895	T38.896
(posterior)						
anterior	T38.811	T38.812	T38.813	T38.814	T38.815	T38.816
Pituitrin	T38.891	T38.892	T38.893	T38.894	T38.895	T38.896
Pivampicillin	T36.0X1	T36.0X2	T36.0X3	T36.0X4	T36.0X5	T36.0X6
Pivmecillinam	T36.0X1	T36.0X2	T36.0X3	T36.0X4	T36.0X5	T36.0X6
Placental hormone	T38.891	T38.892	T38.893	T38.894	T38.895	T38.896
Placidyl	T42.6X1	T42.6X2	T42.6X3	T42.6X4	T42.6X5	T42.6X6
Plague vaccine	T50.A91	T50.A92	T50.A93	T50.A94	T50.A95	T50.A96
Plant						
food or fertilizer NEC	T65.891	T65.892	T65.893	T65.894	—	—
containing herbicide	T60.3X1	T60.3X2	T60.3X3	T60.3X4	—	—
noxious, used as food	T62.2X1	T62.2X2	T62.2X3	T62.2X4	—	—
berries	T62.1X1	T62.1X2	T62.1X3	T62.1X4	—	—
seeds	T62.2X1	T62.2X2	T62.2X3	T62.2X4	—	—
specified type NEC	T62.2X1	T62.2X2	T62.2X3	T62.2X4	—	—
Plasma	T45.8X1	T45.8X2	T45.8X3	T45.8X4	T45.8X5	T45.8X6
expander NEC	T45.8X1	T45.8X2	T45.8X3	T45.8X4	T45.8X5	T45.8X6
protein fraction (human)	T45.8X1	T45.8X2	T45.8X3	T45.8X4	T45.8X5	T45.8X6
Plasmanate	T45.8X1	T45.8X2	T45.8X3	T45.8X4	T45.8X5	T45.8X6
Plasminogen (tissue)	T45.611	T45.612	T45.613	T45.614	T45.615	T45.616
activator						
Plaster dressing	T49.3X1	T49.3X2	T49.3X3	T49.3X4	T49.3X5	T49.3X6
Plastic dressing	T49.3X1	T49.3X2	T49.3X3	T49.3X4	T49.3X5	T49.3X6
Plegicil	T43.3X1	T43.3X2	T43.3X3	T43.3X4	T43.3X5	T43.3X6
Plicamycin	T45.1X1	T45.1X2	T45.1X3	T45.1X4	T45.1X5	T45.1X6
Podophyllotoxin	T49.8X1	T49.8X2	T49.8X3	T49.8X4	T49.8X5	T49.8X6
Podophyllum (resin)	T49.4X1	T49.4X2	T49.4X3	T49.4X4	T49.4X5	T49.4X6
Poisonous berries	T62.1X1	T62.1X2	T62.1X3	T62.1X4	—	—
Poison NEC	T65.91	T65.92	T65.93	T65.94	—	—
Pokeweed (any part)	T62.2X1	T62.2X2	T62.2X3	T62.2X4	—	—
Poldine metilsulfate	T44.3X1	T44.3X2	T44.3X3	T44.3X4	T44.3X5	T44.3X6
Polidexide (sulfate)	T46.6X1	T46.6X2	T46.6X3	T46.6X4	T46.6X5	T46.6X6
Polidocanol	T46.8X1	T46.8X2	T46.8X3	T46.8X4	T46.8X5	T46.8X6
Poliomyelitis vaccine	T50.B91	T50.B92	T50.B93	T50.B94	T50.B95	T50.B96
Polish (car) (floor) (furniture)	T65.891	T65.892	T65.893	T65.894	—	—
(metal) (porcelain)						
(silver)						
abrasive	T65.891	T65.892	T65.893	T65.894	—	—
porcelain	T65.891	T65.892	T65.893	T65.894	—	—
Poloxalkol	T47.4X1	T47.4X2	T47.4X3	T47.4X4	T47.4X5	T47.4X6
Poloxamer	T47.4X1	T47.4X2	T47.4X3	T47.4X4	T47.4X5	T47.4X6
Polyaminostyrene resins	T50.3X1	T50.3X2	T50.3X3	T50.3X4	T50.3X5	T50.3X6
Polycarbophil	T47.4X1	T47.4X2	T47.4X3	T47.4X4	T47.4X5	T47.4X6
Polychlorinated biphenyl	T65.891	T65.892	T65.893	T65.894	—	—
Polycycline	T36.4X1	T36.4X2	T36.4X3	T36.4X4	T36.4X5	T36.4X6
Polyester fumes	T59.891	T59.892	T59.893	T59.894	—	—
Polyester resin hardener	T52.91	T52.92	T52.93	T52.94	—	—
fumes	T59.891	T59.892	T59.893	T59.894	—	—
Polyestradiol phosphate	T38.5X1	T38.5X2	T38.5X3	T38.5X4	T38.5X5	T38.5X6
Polyethanolamine alkyl sulfate	T49.2X1	T49.2X2	T49.2X3	T49.2X4	T49.2X5	T49.2X6
Polyethylene adhesive	T49.3X1	T49.3X2	T49.3X3	T49.3X4	T49.3X5	T49.3X6
Polyferose	T45.4X1	T45.4X2	T45.4X3	T45.4X4	T45.4X5	T45.4X6
Polygeline	T45.8X1	T45.8X2	T45.8X3	T45.8X4	T45.8X5	T45.8X6
Polymyxin	T36.8X1	T36.8X2	T36.8X3	T36.8X4	T36.8X5	T36.8X6
B	T36.8X1	T36.8X2	T36.8X3	T36.8X4	T36.8X5	T36.8X6
ENT agent	T49.6X1	T49.6X2	T49.6X3	T49.6X4	T49.6X5	T49.6X6
ophthalmic preparation	T49.5X1	T49.5X2	T49.5X3	T49.5X4	T49.5X5	T49.5X6
topical NEC	T49.0X1	T49.0X2	T49.0X3	T49.0X4	T49.0X5	T49.0X6
E sulfate (eye preparation)	T49.5X1	T49.5X2	T49.5X3	T49.5X4	T49.5X5	T49.5X6
Polynoxylin	T49.0X1	T49.0X2	T49.0X3	T49.0X4	T49.0X5	T49.0X6
Polyoestradiol phosphate	T38.5X1	T38.5X2	T38.5X3	T38.5X4	T38.5X5	T38.5X6
Polyoxymethyleneurea	T49.0X1	T49.0X2	T49.0X3	T49.0X4	T49.0X5	T49.0X6
Polysilane	T47.8X1	T47.8X2	T47.8X3	T47.8X4	T47.8X5	T47.8X6
Polytetrafluoroethylene (inhaled)	T59.891	T59.892	T59.893	T59.894	—	—
Polythiazide	T50.2X1	T50.2X2	T50.2X3	T50.2X4	T50.2X5	T50.2X6
Polyvidone	T45.8X1	T45.8X2	T45.8X3	T45.8X4	T45.8X5	T45.8X6
Polyvinylpyrrolidone	T45.8X1	T45.8X2	T45.8X3	T45.8X4	T45.8X5	T45.8X6

Substance	Poisoning, Accidental (unintentional)	Poisoning, Intentional Self-harm	Poisoning, Assault	Poisoning, Undetermined	Adverse Effect	Under-dosing
Pontocaine (hydrochloride) (infiltration) (topical)	T41.3X1	T41.3X2	T41.3X3	T41.3X4	T41.3X5	T41.3X6
nerve block (peripheral) (plexus)	T41.3X1	T41.3X2	T41.3X3	T41.3X4	T41.3X5	T41.3X6
spinal	T41.3X1	T41.3X2	T41.3X3	T41.3X4	T41.3X5	T41.3X6
Porfiromycin	T45.1X1	T45.1X2	T45.1X3	T45.1X4	T45.1X5	T45.1X6
Posterior pituitary hormone NEC	T38.891	T38.892	T38.893	T38.894	T38.895	T38.896
Pot	T40.7X1	T40.7X2	T40.7X3	T40.7X4	T40.7X5	T40.7X6
Potash (caustic)	T54.3X1	T54.3X2	T54.3X3	T54.3X4	—	—
Potassic saline injection (lactated)	T50.3X1	T50.3X2	T50.3X3	T50.3X4	T50.3X5	T50.3X6
Potassium (salts) NEC	T50.3X1	T50.3X2	T50.3X3	T50.3X4	T50.3X5	T50.3X6
aminobenzoate	T45.8X1	T45.8X2	T45.8X3	T45.8X4	T45.8X5	T45.8X6
aminosalicylate	T37.1X1	T37.1X2	T37.1X3	T37.1X4	T37.1X5	T37.1X6
antimony ' tartrate'	T37.8X1	T37.8X2	T37.8X3	T37.8X4	T37.8X5	T37.8X6
arsenite (solution)	T57.0X1	T57.0X2	T57.0X3	T57.0X4	—	—
bichromate	T56.2X1	T56.2X2	T56.2X3	T56.2X4	—	—
bisulfate	T47.3X1	T47.3X2	T47.3X3	T47.3X4	T47.3X5	T47.3X6
bromide	T42.6X1	T42.6X2	T42.6X3	T42.6X4	T42.6X5	T42.6X6
canrenoate	T50.0X1	T50.0X2	T50.0X3	T50.0X4	T50.0X5	T50.0X6
carbonate	T54.3X1	T54.3X2	T54.3X3	T54.3X4	—	—
chlorate NEC	T65.891	T65.892	T65.893	T65.894	—	—
chloride	T50.3X1	T50.3X2	T50.3X3	T50.3X4	T50.3X5	T50.3X6
citrate	T50.991	T50.992	T50.993	T50.994	T50.995	T50.996
cyanide	T65.0X1	T65.0X2	T65.0X3	T65.0X4	—	—
ferric hexacyanoferrate (medicinal)	T50.6X1	T50.6X2	T50.6X3	T50.6X4	T50.6X5	T50.6X6
nonmedicinal	T65.891	T65.892	T65.893	T65.894	—	—
Fluoride	T57.8X1	T57.8X2	T57.8X3	T57.8X4	—	—
glucaldrate	T47.1X1	T47.1X2	T47.1X3	T47.1X4	T47.1X5	T47.1X6
hydroxide	T54.3X1	T54.3X2	T54.3X3	T54.3X4	—	—
iodate	T49.0X1	T49.0X2	T49.0X3	T49.0X4	T49.0X5	T49.0X6
iodide	T48.4X1	T48.4X2	T48.4X3	T48.4X4	T48.4X5	T48.4X6
nitrate	T57.8X1	T57.8X2	T57.8X3	T57.8X4	—	—
oxalate	T65.891	T65.892	T65.893	T65.894	—	—
perchlorate (nonmedicinal) NEC	T65.891	T65.892	T65.893	T65.894	—	—
antithyroid	T38.2X1	T38.2X2	T38.2X3	T38.2X4	T38.2X5	T38.2X6
medicinal	T38.2X1	T38.2X2	T38.2X3	T38.2X4	T38.2X5	T38.2X6
Permanganate (nonmedicinal)	T65.891	T65.892	T65.893	T65.894	—	—
medicinal	T49.0X1	T49.0X2	T49.0X3	T49.0X4	T49.0X5	T49.0X6
sulfate	T47.2X1	T47.2X2	T47.2X3	T47.2X4	T47.2X5	T47.2X6
Potassium-removing resin	T50.3X1	T50.3X2	T50.3X3	T50.3X4	T50.3X5	T50.3X6
Potassium-retaining drug	T50.3X1	T50.3X2	T50.3X3	T50.3X4	T50.3X5	T50.3X6
Povidone	T45.8X1	T45.8X2	T45.8X3	T45.8X4	T45.8X5	T45.8X6
iodine	T49.0X1	T49.0X2	T49.0X3	T49.0X4	T49.0X5	T49.0X6
Practolol	T44.7X1	T44.7X2	T44.7X3	T44.7X4	T44.7X5	T44.7X6
Prajmalium bitartrate	T46.2X1	T46.2X2	T46.2X3	T46.2X4	T46.2X5	T46.2X6
Pralidoxime (iodide)	T50.6X1	T50.6X2	T50.6X3	T50.6X4	T50.6X5	T50.6X6
chloride	T50.6X1	T50.6X2	T50.6X3	T50.6X4	T50.6X5	T50.6X6
Pramiverine	T44.3X1	T44.3X2	T44.3X3	T44.3X4	T44.3X5	T44.3X6
Pramocaine	T49.1X1	T49.1X2	T49.1X3	T49.1X4	T49.1X5	T49.1X6
Pramoxine	T49.1X1	T49.1X2	T49.1X3	T49.1X4	T49.1X5	T49.1X6
Prasterone	T38.7X1	T38.7X2	T38.7X3	T38.7X4	T38.7X5	T38.7X6
Pravastatin	T46.6X1	T46.6X2	T46.6X3	T46.6X4	T46.6X5	T46.6X6
Prazepam	T42.4X1	T42.4X2	T42.4X3	T42.4X4	T42.4X5	T42.4X6
Praziquantel	T37.4X1	T37.4X2	T37.4X3	T37.4X4	T37.4X5	T37.4X6
Prazitone	T43.291	T43.292	T43.293	T43.294	T43.295	T43.296
Prazosin	T44.6X1	T44.6X2	T44.6X3	T44.6X4	T44.6X5	T44.6X6
Prednicarbate	T49.0X1	T49.0X2	T49.0X3	T49.0X4	T49.0X5	T49.0X6
Prednimustine	T45.1X1	T45.1X2	T45.1X3	T45.1X4	T45.1X5	T45.1X6
Prednisolone	T38.0X1	T38.0X2	T38.0X3	T38.0X4	T38.0X5	T38.0X6
ENT agent	T49.6X1	T49.6X2	T49.6X3	T49.6X4	T49.6X5	T49.6X6
ophthalmic preparation	T49.5X1	T49.5X2	T49.5X3	T49.5X4	T49.5X5	T49.5X6
steaglate	T49.0X1	T49.0X2	T49.0X3	T49.0X4	T49.0X5	T49.0X6
topical NEC	T49.0X1	T49.0X2	T49.0X3	T49.0X4	T49.0X5	T49.0X6
Prednisone	T38.0X1	T38.0X2	T38.0X3	T38.0X4	T38.0X5	T38.0X6
Prednylidene	T38.0X1	T38.0X2	T38.0X3	T38.0X4	T38.0X5	T38.0X6
Pregnandiol	T38.5X1	T38.5X2	T38.5X3	T38.5X4	T38.5X5	T38.5X6
Pregneninolone	T38.5X1	T38.5X2	T38.5X3	T38.5X4	T38.5X5	T38.5X6
Preludin	T43.691	T43.692	T43.693	T43.694	T43.695	T43.696
Premarin	T38.5X1	T38.5X2	T38.5X3	T38.5X4	T38.5X5	T38.5X6
Premedication anesthetic	T41.201	T41.202	T41.203	T41.204	T41.205	T41.206
Prenalterol	T44.5X1	T44.5X2	T44.5X3	T44.5X4	T44.5X5	T44.5X6
Prenoxdiazine	T48.3X1	T48.3X2	T48.3X3	T48.3X4	T48.3X5	T48.3X6
Prenylamine	T46.3X1	T46.3X2	T46.3X3	T46.3X4	T46.3X5	T46.3X6
Preparation H	T49.8X1	T49.8X2	T49.8X3	T49.8X4	T49.8X5	T49.8X6
Preparation, local	T49.4X1	T49.4X2	T49.4X3	T49.4X4	T49.4X5	T49.4X6
Preservative	T65.891	T65.892	T65.893	T65.894	—	—
(nonmedicinal)						
medicinal	T50.901	T50.902	T50.903	T50.904	T50.905	T50.906

Additional Character May Be Required — Refer to the Tabular List for Character Selection

▼ Subterms under main terms may continue to next column or page

Substance	Poisoning, Accidental (unintentional)	Poisoning, Intentional Self-harm	Poisoning, Assault	Poisoning, Undetermined	Adverse Effect	Underdosing
Preservative — continued						
wood	T60.91	T60.92	T60.93	T60.94	—	—
Prethcamide	T50.7X1	T50.7X2	T50.7X3	T50.7X4	T50.7X5	T50.7X6
Pride of China	T62.2X1	T62.2X2	T62.2X3	T62.2X4	—	—
Pridinol	T44.3X1	T44.3X2	T44.3X3	T44.3X4	T44.3X5	T44.3X6
Prifinium bromide	T44.3X1	T44.3X2	T44.3X3	T44.3X4	T44.3X5	T44.3X6
Prilocaine	T41.3X1	T41.3X2	T41.3X3	T41.3X4	T41.3X5	T41.3X6
infiltration (subcutaneous)	T41.3X1	T41.3X2	T41.3X3	T41.3X4	T41.3X5	T41.3X6
nerve block (peripheral) (plexus)	T41.3X1	T41.3X2	T41.3X3	T41.3X4	T41.3X5	T41.3X6
regional	T41.3X1	T41.3X2	T41.3X3	T41.3X4	T41.3X5	T41.3X6
Primaquine	T37.2X1	T37.2X2	T37.2X3	T37.2X4	T37.2X5	T37.2X6
Primidone	T42.6X1	T42.6X2	T42.6X3	T42.6X4	T42.6X5	T42.6X6
Primula (veris)	T62.2X1	T62.2X2	T62.2X3	T62.2X4	—	—
Prinadol	T40.2X1	T40.2X2	T40.2X3	T40.2X4	T40.2X5	T40.2X6
Priscol, Priscoline	T44.6X1	T44.6X2	T44.6X3	T44.6X4	T44.6X5	T44.6X6
Pristinamycin	T36.3X1	T36.3X2	T36.3X3	T36.3X4	T36.3X5	T36.3X6
Privet	T62.2X1	T62.2X2	T62.2X3	T62.2X4	—	—
berries	T62.1X1	T62.1X2	T62.1X3	T62.1X4	—	—
Privine	T44.4X1	T44.4X2	T44.4X3	T44.4X4	T44.4X5	T44.4X6
Pro-Banthine	T44.3X1	T44.3X2	T44.3X3	T44.3X4	T44.3X5	T44.3X6
Probarbital	T42.3X1	T42.3X2	T42.3X3	T42.3X4	T42.3X5	T42.3X6
Probenecid	T50.4X1	T50.4X2	T50.4X3	T50.4X4	T50.4X5	T50.4X6
Probucol	T46.6X1	T46.6X2	T46.6X3	T46.6X4	T46.6X5	T46.6X6
Procainamide	T46.2X1	T46.2X2	T46.2X3	T46.2X4	T46.2X5	T46.2X6
Procaine	T41.3X1	T41.3X2	T41.3X3	T41.3X4	T41.3X5	T41.3X6
benzylpenicillin	T36.0X1	T36.0X2	T36.0X3	T36.0X4	T36.0X5	T36.0X6
nerve block (periphreal) (plexus)	T41.3X1	T41.3X2	T41.3X3	T41.3X4	T41.3X5	T41.3X6
penicillin G	T36.0X1	T36.0X2	T36.0X3	T36.0X4	T36.0X5	T36.0X6
regional	T41.3X1	T41.3X2	T41.3X3	T41.3X4	T41.3X5	T41.3X6
spinal	T41.3X1	T41.3X2	T41.3X3	T41.3X4	T41.3X5	T41.3X6
Procalmidol	T43.591	T43.592	T43.593	T43.594	T43.595	T43.596
Procarbazine	T45.1X1	T45.1X2	T45.1X3	T45.1X4	T45.1X5	T45.1X6
Procaterol	T44.5X1	T44.5X2	T44.5X3	T44.5X4	T44.5X5	T44.5X6
Prochlorperazine	T43.3X1	T43.3X2	T43.3X3	T43.3X4	T43.3X5	T43.3X6
Procyclidine	T44.3X1	T44.3X2	T44.3X3	T44.3X4	T44.3X5	T44.3X6
Producer gas	T58.8X1	T58.8X2	T58.8X3	T58.8X4	—	—
Profadol	T40.4X1	T40.4X2	T40.4X3	T40.4X4	T40.4X5	T40.4X6
Profenamine	T44.3X1	T44.3X2	T44.3X3	T44.3X4	T44.3X5	T44.3X6
Profenil	T44.3X1	T44.3X2	T44.3X3	T44.3X4	T44.3X5	T44.3X6
Proflavine	T49.0X1	T49.0X2	T49.0X3	T49.0X4	T49.0X5	T49.0X6
Progabide	T42.6X1	T42.6X2	T42.6X3	T42.6X4	T42.6X5	T42.6X6
Progesterone	T38.5X1	T38.5X2	T38.5X3	T38.5X4	T38.5X5	T38.5X6
Progestin	T38.5X1	T38.5X2	T38.5X3	T38.5X4	T38.5X5	T38.5X6
oral contraceptive	T38.4X1	T38.4X2	T38.4X3	T38.4X4	T38.4X5	T38.4X6
Progestogen NEC	T38.5X1	T38.5X2	T38.5X3	T38.5X4	T38.5X5	T38.5X6
Progestone	T38.5X1	T38.5X2	T38.5X3	T38.5X4	T38.5X5	T38.5X6
Proglumide	T47.1X1	T47.1X2	T47.1X3	T47.1X4	T47.1X5	T47.1X6
Proguanil	T37.2X1	T37.2X2	T37.2X3	T37.2X4	T37.2X5	T37.2X6
Prolactin	T38.811	T38.812	T38.813	T38.814	T38.815	T38.816
Prolintane	T43.691	T43.692	T43.693	T43.694	T43.695	T43.696
Proloid	T38.1X1	T38.1X2	T38.1X3	T38.1X4	T38.1X5	T38.1X6
Proluton	T38.5X1	T38.5X2	T38.5X3	T38.5X4	T38.5X5	T38.5X6
Promacetin	T37.1X1	T37.1X2	T37.1X3	T37.1X4	T37.1X5	T37.1X6
Promazine	T43.3X1	T43.3X2	T43.3X3	T43.3X4	T43.3X5	T43.3X6
Promedol	T40.2X1	T40.2X2	T40.2X3	T40.2X4	—	—
Promegestone	T38.5X1	T38.5X2	T38.5X3	T38.5X4	T38.5X5	T38.5X6
Promethazine (teoclate)	T43.3X1	T43.3X2	T43.3X3	T43.3X4	T43.3X5	T43.3X6
Promin	T37.1X1	T37.1X2	T37.1X3	T37.1X4	T37.1X5	T37.1X6
Pronase	T45.3X1	T45.3X2	T45.3X3	T45.3X4	T45.3X5	T45.3X6
Pronestyl (hydrochloride)	T46.2X1	T46.2X2	T46.2X3	T46.2X4	T46.2X5	T46.2X6
Pronetalol	T44.7X1	T44.7X2	T44.7X3	T44.7X4	T44.7X5	T44.7X6
Prontosil	T37.0X1	T37.0X2	T37.0X3	T37.0X4	T37.0X5	T37.0X6
Propachlor	T60.3X1	T60.3X2	T60.3X3	T60.3X4	—	—
Propafenone	T46.2X1	T46.2X2	T46.2X3	T46.2X4	T46.2X5	T46.2X6
Propallylonal	T42.3X1	T42.3X2	T42.3X3	T42.3X4	T42.3X5	T42.3X6
Propamidine	T49.0X1	T49.0X2	T49.0X3	T49.0X4	T49.0X5	T49.0X6
Propane (distributed in mobile container)	T59.891	T59.892	T59.893	T59.894	—	—
distributed through pipes	T59.891	T59.892	T59.893	T59.894	—	—
incomplete combustion	T58.11	T58.12	T58.13	T58.14	—	—
Propanidid	T41.291	T41.292	T41.293	T41.294	T41.295	T41.296
Propanil	T60.3X1	T60.3X2	T60.3X3	T60.3X4	—	—
Propantheline	T44.3X1	T44.3X2	T44.3X3	T44.3X4	T44.3X5	T44.3X6
bromide	T44.3X1	T44.3X2	T44.3X3	T44.3X4	T44.3X5	T44.3X6
Proparacaine	T41.3X1	T41.3X2	T41.3X3	T41.3X4	T41.3X5	T41.3X6
Propatylnitrate	T46.3X1	T46.3X2	T46.3X3	T46.3X4	T46.3X5	T46.3X6
Propicillin	T36.0X1	T36.0X2	T36.0X3	T36.0X4	T36.0X5	T36.0X6
Propiolactone	T49.0X1	T49.0X2	T49.0X3	T49.0X4	T49.0X5	T49.0X6
Propiomazine	T45.0X1	T45.0X2	T45.0X3	T45.0X4	T45.0X5	T45.0X6
Propionaldehyde (medicinal)	T42.6X1	T42.6X2	T42.6X3	T42.6X4	T42.6X5	T42.6X6

Substance	Poisoning, Accidental (unintentional)	Poisoning, Intentional Self-harm	Poisoning, Assault	Poisoning, Undetermined	Adverse Effect	Underdosing
Propionate (calcium) (sodium)	T49.0X1	T49.0X2	T49.0X3	T49.0X4	T49.0X5	T49.0X6
Propion gel	T49.0X1	T49.0X2	T49.0X3	T49.0X4	T49.0X5	T49.0X6
Propitocaine	T41.3X1	T41.3X2	T41.3X3	T41.3X4	T41.3X5	T41.3X6
infiltration (subcutaneous)	T41.3X1	T41.3X2	T41.3X3	T41.3X4	T41.3X5	T41.3X6
nerve block (peripheral) (plexus)	T41.3X1	T41.3X2	T41.3X3	T41.3X4	T41.3X5	T41.3X6
Propofol	T41.291	T41.292	T41.293	T41.294	T41.295	T41.296
Propoxur	T60.0X1	T60.0X2	T60.0X3	T60.0X4	—	—
Propoxycaine						
infiltration (subcutaneous)	T41.3X1	T41.3X2	T41.3X3	T41.3X4	T41.3X5	T41.3X6
nerve block (peripheral) (plexus)	T41.3X1	T41.3X2	T41.3X3	T41.3X4	T41.3X5	T41.3X6
topical (surface)	T41.3X1	T41.3X2	T41.3X3	T41.3X4	T41.3X5	T41.3X6
Propoxyphene	T40.4X1	T40.4X2	T40.4X3	T40.4X4	T40.4X5	T40.4X6
Propranolol	T44.7X1	T44.7X2	T44.7X3	T44.7X4	T44.7X5	T44.7X6
Propyl						
alcohol	T51.3X1	T51.3X2	T51.3X3	T51.3X4	—	—
carbinol	T51.3X1	T51.3X2	T51.3X3	T51.3X4	—	—
hexadrine	T44.4X1	T44.4X2	T44.4X3	T44.4X4	T44.4X5	T44.4X6
iodone	T50.8X1	T50.8X2	T50.8X3	T50.8X4	T50.8X5	T50.8X6
thiouracil	T38.2X1	T38.2X2	T38.2X3	T38.2X4	T38.2X5	T38.2X6
Propylaminophenothiazine	T43.3X1	T43.3X2	T43.3X3	T43.3X4	T43.3X5	T43.3X6
Propylene	T59.891	T59.892	T59.893	T59.894	—	—
Propylhexedrine	T48.5X1	T48.5X2	T48.5X3	T48.5X4	T48.5X5	T48.5X6
Propyliodone	T50.8X1	T50.8X2	T50.8X3	T50.8X4	T50.8X5	T50.8X6
Propylparaben (ophthalmic)	T49.5X1	T49.5X2	T49.5X3	T49.5X4	T49.5X5	T49.5X6
Propylthiouracil	T38.2X1	T38.2X2	T38.2X3	T38.2X4	T38.2X5	T38.2X6
Propyphenazone	T39.2X1	T39.2X2	T39.2X3	T39.2X4	T39.2X5	T39.2X6
Proquazone	T39.391	T39.392	T39.393	T39.394	T39.395	T39.396
Proscillaridin	T46.0X1	T46.0X2	T46.0X3	T46.0X4	T46.0X5	T46.0X6
Prostacyclin	T45.521	T45.522	T45.523	T45.524	T45.525	T45.526
Prostaglandin (I2)	T45.521	T45.522	T45.523	T45.524	T45.525	T45.526
E1	T46.7X1	T46.7X2	T46.7X3	T46.7X4	T46.7X5	T46.7X6
E2	T48.0X1	T48.0X2	T48.0X3	T48.0X4	T48.0X5	T48.0X6
F2 alpha	T48.0X1	T48.0X2	T48.0X3	T48.0X4	T48.0X5	T48.0X6
Prostigmin	T44.0X1	T44.0X2	T44.0X3	T44.0X4	T44.0X5	T44.0X6
Prosultiamine	T45.2X1	T45.2X2	T45.2X3	T45.2X4	T45.2X5	T45.2X6
Protamine sulfate	T45.7X1	T45.7X2	T45.7X3	T45.7X4	T45.7X5	T45.7X6
zinc insulin	T38.3X1	T38.3X2	T38.3X3	T38.3X4	T38.3X5	T38.3X6
Protease	T47.5X1	T47.5X2	T47.5X3	T47.5X4	T47.5X5	T47.5X6
Protectant, skin NEC	T49.3X1	T49.3X2	T49.3X3	T49.3X4	T49.3X5	T49.3X6
Protein hydrolysate	T50.991	T50.992	T50.993	T50.994	T50.995	T50.996
Prothiaden — see Dothiepin hydrochloride						
Prothionamide	T37.1X1	T37.1X2	T37.1X3	T37.1X4	T37.1X5	T37.1X6
Prothipendyl	T43.591	T43.592	T43.593	T43.594	T43.595	T43.596
Prothoate	T60.0X1	T60.0X2	T60.0X3	T60.0X4	—	—
Prothrombin						
activator	T45.7X1	T45.7X2	T45.7X3	T45.7X4	T45.7X5	T45.7X6
synthesis inhibitor	T45.511	T45.512	T45.513	T45.514	T45.515	T45.516
Protionamide	T37.1X1	T37.1X2	T37.1X3	T37.1X4	T37.1X5	T37.1X6
Protirelin	T38.891	T38.892	T38.893	T38.894	T38.895	T38.896
Protokylol	T48.6X1	T48.6X2	T48.6X3	T48.6X4	T48.6X5	T48.6X6
Protopam	T50.6X1	T50.6X2	T50.6X3	T50.6X4	T50.6X5	T50.6X6
Protoveratrine(s) (A) (B)	T46.5X1	T46.5X2	T46.5X3	T46.5X4	T46.5X5	T46.5X6
Protriptyline	T43.011	T43.012	T43.013	T43.014	T43.015	T43.016
Provera	T38.5X1	T38.5X2	T38.5X3	T38.5X4	T38.5X5	T38.5X6
Provitamin A	T45.2X1	T45.2X2	T45.2X3	T45.2X4	T45.2X5	T45.2X6
Proxibarbal	T42.3X1	T42.3X2	T42.3X3	T42.3X4	T42.3X5	T42.3X6
Proxymetacaine	T41.3X1	T41.3X2	T41.3X3	T41.3X4	T41.3X5	T41.3X6
Proxyphylline	T48.6X1	T48.6X2	T48.6X3	T48.6X4	T48.6X5	T48.6X6
Prozac — see Fluoxetine hydrochloride						
Prunus						
laurocerasus	T62.2X1	T62.2X2	T62.2X3	T62.2X4	—	—
virginiana	T62.2X1	T62.2X2	T62.2X3	T62.2X4	—	—
Prussian blue						
commercial	T65.891	T65.892	T65.893	T65.894	—	—
therapeutic	T50.6X1	T50.6X2	T50.6X3	T50.6X4	T50.6X5	T50.6X6
Prussic acid	T65.0X1	T65.0X2	T65.0X3	T65.0X4	—	—
vapor	T57.3X1	T57.3X2	T57.3X3	T57.3X4	—	—
Pseudoephedrine	T44.991	T44.992	T44.993	T44.994	T44.995	T44.996
Psilocin	T40.991	T40.992	T40.993	T40.994	—	—
Psilocybin	T40.991	T40.992	T40.993	T40.994	—	—
Psilocybine	T40.991	T40.992	T40.993	T40.994	—	—
Psoralene (nonmedicinal)	T65.891	T65.892	T65.893	T65.894	—	—
Psoralens (medicinal)	T50.991	T50.992	T50.993	T50.994	T50.995	T50.996
PSP (phenolsulfonphthalein)	T50.8X1	T50.8X2	T50.8X3		T50.8X5	T50.8X6
Psychodysleptic drug NEC	T40.901	T40.902	T40.903	T40.904	T40.905	T40.906
Psychostimulant	T43.601	T43.602	T43.603	T43.604	T43.605	T43.606

Substance	Poisoning, Accidental (unintentional)	Poisoning, Intentional Self-harm	Poisoning, Assault	Poisoning, Undetermined	Adverse Effect	Under-dosing
Psychostimulant — *continued*						
amphetamine	T43.621	T43.622	T43.623	T43.624	T43.625	T43.626
caffeine	T43.611	T43.612	T43.613	T43.614	T43.615	T43.616
methylphenidate	T43.631	T43.632	T43.633	T43.634	T43.635	T43.636
specified NEC	T43.691	T43.692	T43.693	T43.694	T43.695	T43.696
Psychotherapeutic drug NEC	T43.91	T43.92	T43.93	T43.94	T43.95	T43.96
antidepressants — *see also* Antidepressant	T43.201	T43.202	T43.203	T43.204	T43.205	T43.206
specified NEC	T43.8X1	T43.8X2	T43.8X3	T43.8X4	T43.8X5	T43.8X6
tranquilizers NEC	T43.501	T43.502	T43.503	T43.504	T43.505	T43.506
Psychotomimetic agents	T40.901	T40.902	T40.903	T40.904	T40.905	T40.906
Psychotropic drug NEC	T43.91	T43.92	T43.93	T43.94	T43.95	T43.96
specified NEC	T43.8X1	T43.8X2	T43.8X3	T43.8X4	T43.8X5	T43.8X6
Psyllium hydrophilic mucilloid	T47.4X1	T47.4X2	T47.4X3	T47.4X4	T47.4X5	T47.4X6
Pteroylglutamic acid	T45.8X1	T45.8X2	T45.8X3	T45.8X4	T45.8X5	T45.8X6
Pteroyltriglutamate	T45.1X1	T45.1X2	T45.1X3	T45.1X4	T45.1X5	T45.1X6
PTFE — *see* Polytetrafluoroethylene						
Pulp						
devitalizing paste	T49.7X1	T49.7X2	T49.7X3	T49.7X4	T49.7X5	T49.7X6
dressing	T49.7X1	T49.7X2	T49.7X3	T49.7X4	T49.7X5	T49.7X6
Pulsatilla	T62.2X1	T62.2X2	T62.2X3	T62.2X4	—	—
Pumpkin seed extract	T37.4X1	T37.4X2	T37.4X3	T37.4X4	T37.4X5	T37.4X6
Purex (bleach)	T54.91	T54.92	T54.93	T54.94	—	—
Purgative NEC — *see also* Cathartic	T47.4X1	T47.4X2	T47.4X3	T47.4X4	T47.4X5	T47.4X6
Purine analogue (antineoplastic)	T45.1X1	T45.1X2	T45.1X3	T45.1X4	T45.1X5	T45.1X6
Purine diuretics	T50.2X1	T50.2X2	T50.2X3	T50.2X4	T50.2X5	T50.2X6
Purinethol	T45.1X1	T45.1X2	T45.1X3	T45.1X4	T45.1X5	T45.1X6
PVP	T45.8X1	T45.8X2	T45.8X3	T45.8X4	T45.8X5	T45.8X6
Pyrabital	T39.8X1	T39.8X2	T39.8X3	T39.8X4	T39.8X5	T39.8X6
Pyramidon	T39.2X1	T39.2X2	T39.2X3	T39.2X4	T39.2X5	T39.2X6
Pyrantel	T37.4X1	T37.4X2	T37.4X3	T37.4X4	T37.4X5	T37.4X6
Pyrathiazine	T45.0X1	T45.0X2	T45.0X3	T45.0X4	T45.0X5	T45.0X6
Pyrazinamide	T37.1X1	T37.1X2	T37.1X3	T37.1X4	T37.1X5	T37.1X6
Pyrazinoic acid (amide)	T37.1X1	T37.1X2	T37.1X3	T37.1X4	T37.1X5	T37.1X6
Pyrazole (derivatives)	T39.2X1	T39.2X2	T39.2X3	T39.2X4	T39.2X5	T39.2X6
Pyrazolone analgesic NEC	T39.2X1	T39.2X2	T39.2X3	T39.2X4	T39.2X5	T39.2X6
Pyrethrin, pyrethrum (nonmedicinal)	T60.2X1	T60.2X2	T60.2X3	T60.2X4	—	—
Pyrethrum extract	T49.0X1	T49.0X2	T49.0X3	T49.0X4	T49.0X5	T49.0X6
Pyribenzamine	T45.0X1	T45.0X2	T45.0X3	T45.0X4	T45.0X5	T45.0X6
Pyridine	T52.8X1	T52.8X2	T52.8X3	T52.8X4	—	—
aldoxime methiodide	T50.6X1	T50.6X2	T50.6X3	T50.6X4	T50.6X5	T50.6X6
aldoxime methyl chloride	T50.6X1	T50.6X2	T50.6X3	T50.6X4	T50.6X5	T50.6X6
vapor	T59.891	T59.892	T59.893	T59.894	—	—
Pyridium	T39.8X1	T39.8X2	T39.8X3	T39.8X4	T39.8X5	T39.8X6
Pyridostigmine bromide	T44.0X1	T44.0X2	T44.0X3	T44.0X4	T44.0X5	T44.0X6
Pyridoxal phosphate	T45.2X1	T45.2X2	T45.2X3	T45.2X4	T45.2X5	T45.2X6
Pyridoxine	T45.2X1	T45.2X2	T45.2X3	T45.2X4	T45.2X5	T45.2X6
Pyrilamine	T45.0X1	T45.0X2	T45.0X3	T45.0X4	T45.0X5	T45.0X6
Pyrimethamine	T37.2X1	T37.2X2	T37.2X3	T37.2X4	T37.2X5	T37.2X6
with sulfadoxine	T37.2X1	T37.2X2	T37.2X3	T37.2X4	T37.2X5	T37.2X6
Pyrimidine antagonist	T45.1X1	T45.1X2	T45.1X3	T45.1X4	T45.1X5	T45.1X6
Pyriminil	T60.4X1	T60.4X2	T60.4X3	T60.4X4	—	—
Pyrithione zinc	T49.4X1	T49.4X2	T49.4X3	T49.4X4	T49.4X5	T49.4X6
Pyrithyldione	T42.6X1	T42.6X2	T42.6X3	T42.6X4	T42.6X5	T42.6X6
Pyrogallic acid	T49.0X1	T49.0X2	T49.0X3	T49.0X4	T49.0X5	T49.0X6
Pyrogallol	T49.0X1	T49.0X2	T49.0X3	T49.0X4	T49.0X5	T49.0X6
Pyroxylin	T49.3X1	T49.3X2	T49.3X3	T49.3X4	T49.3X5	T49.3X6
Pyrrobutamine	T45.0X1	T45.0X2	T45.0X3	T45.0X4	T45.0X5	T45.0X6
Pyrrolizidine alkaloids	T62.8X1	T62.8X2	T62.8X3	T62.8X4	—	—
Pyrvinium chloride	T37.4X1	T37.4X2	T37.4X3	T37.4X4	T37.4X5	T37.4X6
PZI	T38.3X1	T38.3X2	T38.3X3	T38.3X4	T38.3X5	T38.3X6
Quaalude	T42.6X1	T42.6X2	T42.6X3	T42.6X4	T42.6X5	T42.6X6
Quarternary ammonium						
anti-infective	T49.0X1	T49.0X2	T49.0X3	T49.0X4	T49.0X5	T49.0X6
ganglion blocking	T44.2X1	T44.2X2	T44.2X3	T44.2X4	T44.2X5	T44.2X6
parasympatholytic	T44.3X1	T44.3X2	T44.3X3	T44.3X4	T44.3X5	T44.3X6
Quazepam	T42.4X1	T42.4X2	T42.4X3	T42.4X4	T42.4X5	T42.4X6
Quicklime	T54.3X1	T54.3X2	T54.3X3	T54.3X4	—	—
Quillaja extract	T48.4X1	T48.4X2	T48.4X3	T48.4X4	T48.4X5	T48.4X6
Quinacrine	T37.2X1	T37.2X2	T37.2X3	T37.2X4	T37.2X5	T37.2X6
Quinaglute	T46.2X1	T46.2X2	T46.2X3	T46.2X4	T46.2X5	T46.2X6
Quinalbarbital	T42.3X1	T42.3X2	T42.3X3	T42.3X4	T42.3X5	T42.3X6
Quinalbarbitone sodium	T42.3X1	T42.3X2	T42.3X3	T42.3X4	T42.3X5	T42.3X6
Quinalphos	T60.0X1	T60.0X2	T60.0X3	T60.0X4	—	—
Quinapril	T46.4X1	T46.4X2	T46.4X3	T46.4X4	T46.4X5	T46.4X6
Quinestradiol	T38.5X1	T38.5X2	T38.5X3	T38.5X4	T38.5X5	T38.5X6
Quinestradol	T38.5X1	T38.5X2	T38.5X3	T38.5X4	T38.5X5	T38.5X6

Substance	Poisoning, Accidental (unintentional)	Poisoning, Intentional Self-harm	Poisoning, Assault	Poisoning, Undetermined	Adverse Effect	Under-dosing
Quinestrol	T38.5X1	T38.5X2	T38.5X3	T38.5X4	T38.5X5	T38.5X6
Quinethazone	T50.2X1	T50.2X2	T50.2X3	T50.2X4	T50.2X5	T50.2X6
Quingestanol	T38.4X1	T38.4X2	T38.4X3	T38.4X4	T38.4X5	T38.4X6
Quinidine	T46.2X1	T46.2X2	T46.2X3	T46.2X4	T46.2X5	T46.2X6
Quinine	T37.2X1	T37.2X2	T37.2X3	T37.2X4	T37.2X5	T37.2X6
Quiniobine	T37.8X1	T37.8X2	T37.8X3	T37.8X4	T37.8X5	T37.8X6
Quinisocaine	T49.1X1	T49.1X2	T49.1X3	T49.1X4	T49.1X5	T49.1X6
Quinocide	T37.2X1	T37.2X2	T37.2X3	T37.2X4	T37.2X5	T37.2X6
Quinoline (derivatives) **NEC**	T37.8X1	T37.8X2	T37.8X3	T37.8X4	T37.8X5	T37.8X6
Quinupramine	T43.011	T43.012	T43.013	T43.014	T43.015	T43.016
Quotane	T41.3X1	T41.3X2	T41.3X3	T41.3X4	T41.3X5	T41.3X6
Rabies						
immune globulin (human)	T50.Z11	T50.Z12	T50.Z13	T50.Z14	T50.Z15	T50.Z16
vaccine	T50.B91	T50.B92	T50.B93	T50.B94	T50.B95	T50.B96
Racemoramide	T40.2X1	T40.2X2	T40.2X3	T40.2X4	—	—
Racemorphan	T40.2X1	T40.2X2	T40.2X3	T40.2X4	T40.2X5	T40.2X6
Racepinefrin	T44.5X1	T44.5X2	T44.5X3	T44.5X4	T44.5X5	T44.5X6
Raclopride	T43.591	T43.592	T43.593	T43.594	T43.595	T43.596
Radiator alcohol	T51.1X1	T51.1X2	T51.1X3	T51.1X4	—	—
Radioactive drug NEC	T50.8X1	T50.8X2	T50.8X3	T50.8X4	T50.8X5	T50.8X6
Radio-opaque (drugs) (materials)	T50.8X1	T50.8X2	T50.8X3	T50.8X4	T50.8X5	T50.8X6
Ramifenazone	T39.2X1	T39.2X2	T39.2X3	T39.2X4	T39.2X5	T39.2X6
Ramipril	T46.4X1	T46.4X2	T46.4X3	T46.4X4	T46.4X5	T46.4X6
Ranitidine	T47.0X1	T47.0X2	T47.0X3	T47.0X4	T47.0X5	T47.0X6
Ranunculus	T62.2X1	T62.2X2	T62.2X3	T62.2X4	—	—
Rat poison NEC	T60.4X1	T60.4X2	T60.4X3	T60.4X4	—	—
Rattlesnake (venom)	T63.011	T63.012	T63.013	T63.014	—	—
Raubasine	T46.7X1	T46.7X2	T46.7X3	T46.7X4	T46.7X5	T46.7X6
Raudixin	T46.5X1	T46.5X2	T46.5X3	T46.5X4	T46.5X5	T46.5X6
Rautensin	T46.5X1	T46.5X2	T46.5X3	T46.5X4	T46.5X5	T46.5X6
Rautina	T46.5X1	T46.5X2	T46.5X3	T46.5X4	T46.5X5	T46.5X6
Rautotal	T46.5X1	T46.5X2	T46.5X3	T46.5X4	T46.5X5	T46.5X6
Rauwiloid	T46.5X1	T46.5X2	T46.5X3	T46.5X4	T46.5X5	T46.5X6
Rauwoldin	T46.5X1	T46.5X2	T46.5X3	T46.5X4	T46.5X5	T46.5X6
Rauwolfia (alkaloids)	T46.5X1	T46.5X2	T46.5X3	T46.5X4	T46.5X5	T46.5X6
Razoxane	T45.1X1	T45.1X2	T45.1X3	T45.1X4	T45.1X5	T45.1X6
Realgar	T57.0X1	T57.0X2	T57.0X3	T57.0X4	—	—
Recombinant (R) — *see* specific protein						
Red blood cells, packed	T45.8X1	T45.8X2	T45.8X3	T45.8X4	—	T45.8X6
Red squill (scilliroside)	T60.4X1	T60.4X2	T60.4X3	T60.4X4	—	—
Reducing agent, industrial NEC	T65.891	T65.892	T65.893	T65.894	—	—
Refrigerant gas (chlorofluorocarbon)	T53.5X1	T53.5X2	T53.5X3	T53.5X4	—	—
not chlorofluorocarbon	T59.891	T59.892	T59.893	T59.894	—	—
Regroton	T50.2X1	T50.2X2	T50.2X3	T50.2X4	T50.2X5	T50.2X6
Rehydration salts (oral)	T50.3X1	T50.3X2	T50.3X3	T50.3X4	T50.3X5	T50.3X6
Rela	T42.8X1	T42.8X2	T42.8X3	T42.8X4	T42.8X5	T42.8X6
Relaxant, muscle						
anesthetic	T48.1X1	T48.1X2	T48.1X3	T48.1X4	T48.1X5	T48.1X6
central nervous system	T42.8X1	T42.8X2	T42.8X3	T42.8X4	T42.8X5	T42.8X6
skeletal NEC	T48.1X1	T48.1X2	T48.1X3	T48.1X4	T48.1X5	T48.1X6
smooth NEC	T44.3X1	T44.3X2	T44.3X3	T44.3X4	T44.3X5	T44.3X6
Remoxipride	T43.591	T43.592	T43.593	T43.594	T43.595	T43.596
Renese	T50.2X1	T50.2X2	T50.2X3	T50.2X4	T50.2X5	T50.2X6
Renografin	T50.8X1	T50.8X2	T50.8X3	T50.8X4	T50.8X5	T50.8X6
Replacement solution	T50.3X1	T50.3X2	T50.3X3	T50.3X4	T50.3X5	T50.3X6
Reproterol	T48.6X1	T48.6X2	T48.6X3	T48.6X4	T48.6X5	T48.6X6
Rescinnamine	T46.5X1	T46.5X2	T46.5X3	T46.5X4	T46.5X5	T46.5X6
Reserpin (e)	T46.5X1	T46.5X2	T46.5X3	T46.5X4	T46.5X5	T46.5X6
Resorcin, resorcinol (nonmedicinal)	T65.891	T65.892	T65.893	T65.894	—	—
medicinal	T49.4X1	T49.4X2	T49.4X3	T49.4X4	T49.4X5	T49.4X6
Respaire	T48.4X1	T48.4X2	T48.4X3	T48.4X4	T48.4X5	T48.4X6
Respiratory drug NEC	T48.901	T48.902	T48.903	T48.904	T48.905	T48.906
antiasthmatic NEC	T48.6X1	T48.6X2	T48.6X3	T48.6X4	T48.6X5	T48.6X6
anti-common-cold NEC	T48.5X1	T48.5X2	T48.5X3	T48.5X4	T48.5X5	T48.5X6
expectorant NEC	T48.4X1	T48.4X2	T48.4X3	T48.4X4	T48.4X5	T48.4X6
stimulant	T48.901	T48.902	T48.903	T48.904	T48.905	T48.906
Retinoic acid	T49.0X1	T49.0X2	T49.0X3	T49.0X4	T49.0X5	T49.0X6
Retinol	T45.2X1	T45.2X2	T45.2X3	T45.2X4	T45.2X5	T45.2X6
Rh (D) immune globulin (human)	T50.Z11	T50.Z12	T50.Z13	T50.Z14	T50.Z15	T50.Z16
Rhodine	T39.011	T39.012	T39.013	T39.014	T39.015	T39.016
RhoGAM	T50.Z11	T50.Z12	T50.Z13	T50.Z14	T50.Z15	T50.Z16
Rhubarb						
dry extract	T47.2X1	T47.2X2	T47.2X3	T47.2X4	T47.2X5	T47.2X6
tincture, compound	T47.2X1	T47.2X2	T47.2X3	T47.2X4	T47.2X5	T47.2X6
Ribavirin	T37.5X1	T37.5X2	T37.5X3	T37.5X4	T37.5X5	T37.5X6
Riboflavin	T45.2X1	T45.2X2	T45.2X3	T45.2X4	T45.2X5	T45.2X6
Ribostamycin	T36.5X1	T36.5X2	T36.5X3	T36.5X4	T36.5X5	T36.5X6

Substance	Poisoning, Accidental (unintentional)	Poisoning, Intentional Self-harm	Poisoning, Assault	Poisoning, Undetermined	Adverse Effect	Under-dosing
Ricin	T62.2X1	T62.2X2	T62.2X3	T62.2X4	—	—
Ricinus communis	T62.2X1	T62.2X2	T62.2X3	T62.2X4	—	—
Rickettsial vaccine NEC	T50.A91	T50.A92	T50.A93	T50.A94	T50.A95	T50.A96
Rifabutin	T36.6X1	T36.6X2	T36.6X3	T36.6X4	T36.6X5	T36.6X6
Rifamide	T36.6X1	T36.6X2	T36.6X3	T36.6X4	T36.6X5	T36.6X6
Rifampicin	T36.6X1	T36.6X2	T36.6X3	T36.6X4	T36.6X5	T36.6X6
with isoniazid	T37.1X1	T37.1X2	T37.1X3	T37.1X4	T37.1X5	T37.1X6
Rifampin	T36.6X1	T36.6X2	T36.6X3	T36.6X4	T36.6X5	T36.6X6
Rifamycin	T36.6X1	T36.6X2	T36.6X3	T36.6X4	T36.6X5	T36.6X6
Rifaximin	T36.6X1	T36.6X2	T36.6X3	T36.6X4	T36.6X5	T36.6X6
Rimantadine	T37.5X1	T37.5X2	T37.5X3	T37.5X4	T37.5X5	T37.5X6
Rimazolium metilsulfate	T39.8X1	T39.8X2	T39.8X3	T39.8X4	T39.8X5	T39.8X6
Rimifon	T37.1X1	T37.1X2	T37.1X3	T37.1X4	T37.1X5	T37.1X6
Rimiterol	T48.6X1	T48.6X2	T48.6X3	T48.6X4	T48.6X5	T48.6X6
Ringer (lactate) **solution**	T50.3X1	T50.3X2	T50.3X3	T50.3X4	T50.3X5	T50.3X6
Ristocetin	T36.8X1	T36.8X2	T36.8X3	T36.8X4	T36.8X5	T36.8X6
Ritalin	T43.631	T43.632	T43.633	T43.634	T43.635	T43.636
Ritodrine	T44.5X1	T44.5X2	T44.5X3	T44.5X4	T44.5X5	T44.5X6
Roach killer — *see* Insecticide						
Rociverine	T44.3X1	T44.3X2	T44.3X3	T44.3X4	T44.3X5	T44.3X6
Rocky Mountain spotted fever vaccine	T50.A91	T50.A92	T50.A93	T50.A94	T50.A95	T50.A96
Rodenticide NEC	T60.4X1	T60.4X2	T60.4X3	T60.4X4	—	—
Rohypnol	T42.4X1	T42.4X2	T42.4X3	T42.4X4	T42.4X5	T42.4X6
Rokitamycin	T36.3X1	T36.3X2	T36.3X3	T36.3X4	T36.3X5	T36.3X6
Rolaids	T47.1X1	T47.1X2	T47.1X3	T47.1X4	T47.1X5	T47.1X6
Rolitetracycline	T36.4X1	T36.4X2	T36.4X3	T36.4X4	T36.4X5	T36.4X6
Romilar	T48.3X1	T48.3X2	T48.3X3	T48.3X4	T48.3X5	T48.3X6
Ronifibrate	T46.6X1	T46.6X2	T46.6X3	T46.6X4	T46.6X5	T46.6X6
Rosaprostol	T47.1X1	T47.1X2	T47.1X3	T47.1X4	T47.1X5	T47.1X6
Rose bengal sodium (131I)	T50.8X1	T50.8X2	T50.8X3	T50.8X4	T50.8X5	T50.8X6
Rose water ointment	T49.3X1	T49.3X2	T49.3X3	T49.3X4	T49.3X5	T49.3X6
Rosoxacin	T37.8X1	T37.8X2	T37.8X3	T37.8X4	T37.8X5	T37.8X6
Rotenone	T60.2X1	T60.2X2	T60.2X3	T60.2X4	—	—
Rotoxamine	T45.0X1	T45.0X2	T45.0X3	T45.0X4	T45.0X5	T45.0X6
Rough-on-rats	T60.4X1	T60.4X2	T60.4X3	T60.4X4	—	—
Roxatidine	T47.0X1	T47.0X2	T47.0X3	T47.0X4	T47.0X5	T47.0X6
Roxithromycin	T36.3X1	T36.3X2	T36.3X3	T36.3X4	T36.3X5	T36.3X6
Rt-PA	T45.611	T45.612	T45.613	T45.614	T45.615	T45.616
Rubbing alcohol	T51.2X1	T51.2X2	T51.2X3	T51.2X4	—	—
Rubefacient	T49.4X1	T49.4X2	T49.4X3	T49.4X4	T49.4X5	T49.4X6
Rubella vaccine	T50.B91	T50.B92	T50.B93	T50.B94	T50.B95	T50.B96
Rubeola vaccine	T50.B91	T50.B92	T50.B93	T50.B94	T50.B95	T50.B96
Rubidium chloride Rb82	T50.8X1	T50.8X2	T50.8X3	T50.8X4	T50.8X5	T50.8X6
Rubidomycin	T45.1X1	T45.1X2	T45.1X3	T45.1X4	T45.1X5	T45.1X6
Rue	T62.2X1	T62.2X2	T62.2X3	T62.2X4	—	—
Rufocromomycin	T45.1X1	T45.1X2	T45.1X3	T45.1X4	T45.1X5	T45.1X6
Russel's viper venin	T45.7X1	T45.7X2	T45.7X3	T45.7X4	T45.7X5	T45.7X6
Ruta (graveolens)	T62.2X1	T62.2X2	T62.2X3	T62.2X4	—	—
Rutinum	T46.991	T46.992	T46.993	T46.994	T46.995	T46.996
Rutoside	T46.991	T46.992	T46.993	T46.994	T46.995	T46.996
b-sitosterol(s)	T46.6X1	T46.6X2	T46.6X3	T46.6X4	T46.6X5	T46.6X6
Sabadilla (plant)	T62.2X1	T62.2X2	T62.2X3	T62.2X4	—	—
pesticide	T60.2X1	T60.2X2	T60.2X3	T60.2X4	—	—
Saccharated iron oxide	T45.8X1	T45.8X2	T45.8X3	T45.8X4	T45.8X5	T45.8X6
Saccharin	T50.901	T50.902	T50.903	T50.904	T50.905	T50.906
Saccharomyces boulardii	T47.6X1	T47.6X2	T47.6X3	T47.6X4	T47.6X5	T47.6X6
Safflower oil	T46.6X1	T46.6X2	T46.6X3	T46.6X4	T46.6X5	T46.6X6
Safrazine	T43.1X1	T43.1X2	T43.1X3	T43.1X4	T43.1X5	T43.1X6
Salazosulfapyridine	T37.0X1	T37.0X2	T37.0X3	T37.0X4	T37.0X5	T37.0X6
Salbutamol	T48.6X1	T48.6X2	T48.6X3	T48.6X4	T48.6X5	T48.6X6
Salicylamide	T39.091	T39.092	T39.093	T39.094	T39.095	T39.096
Salicylate NEC	T39.091	T39.092	T39.093	T39.094	T39.095	T39.096
methyl	T49.3X1	T49.3X2	T49.3X3	T49.3X4	T49.3X5	T49.3X6
theobromine calcium	T50.2X1	T50.2X2	T50.2X3	T50.2X4	T50.2X5	T50.2X6
Salicylazosulfapyridine	T37.0X1	T37.0X2	T37.0X3	T37.0X4	T37.0X5	T37.0X6
Salicylhydroxamic acid	T49.0X1	T49.0X2	T49.0X3	T49.0X4	T49.0X5	T49.0X6
Salicylic acid	T49.4X1	T49.4X2	T49.4X3	T49.4X4	T49.4X5	T49.4X6
with benzoic acid	T49.4X1	T49.4X2	T49.4X3	T49.4X4	T49.4X5	T49.4X6
congeners	T39.091	T39.092	T39.093	T39.094	T39.095	T39.096
derivative	T39.091	T39.092	T39.093	T39.094	T39.095	T39.096
salts	T39.091	T39.092	T39.093	T39.094	T39.095	T39.096
Salinazid	T37.1X1	T37.1X2	T37.1X3	T37.1X4	T37.1X5	T37.1X6
Salmeterol	T48.6X1	T48.6X2	T48.6X3	T48.6X4	T48.6X5	T48.6X6
Salol	T49.3X1	T49.3X2	T49.3X3	T49.3X4	T49.3X5	T49.3X6
Salsalate	T39.091	T39.092	T39.093	T39.094	T39.095	T39.096
Salt-replacing drug	T50.901	T50.902	T50.903	T50.904	T50.905	T50.906
Salt-retaining mineralocorticoid	T50.0X1	T50.0X2	T50.0X3	T50.0X4	T50.0X5	T50.0X6
Salt substitute	T50.901	T50.902	T50.903	T50.904	T50.905	T50.906
Saluretic NEC	T50.2X1	T50.2X2	T50.2X3	T50.2X4	T50.2X5	T50.2X6
Saluron	T50.2X1	T50.2X2	T50.2X3	T50.2X4	T50.2X5	T50.2X6
Salvarsan 606 (neosilver) (silver)	T37.8X1	T37.8X2	T37.8X3	T37.8X4	T37.8X5	T37.8X6
Sambucus canadensis	T62.2X1	T62.2X2	T62.2X3	T62.2X4	—	—
berry	T62.1X1	T62.1X2	T62.1X3	T62.1X4	—	—
Sandril	T46.5X1	T46.5X2	T46.5X3	T46.5X4	T46.5X5	T46.5X6
Sanguinaria canadensis	T62.2X1	T62.2X2	T62.2X3	T62.2X4	—	—
Saniflush (cleaner)	T54.2X1	T54.2X2	T54.2X3	T54.2X4	—	—
Santonin	T37.4X1	T37.4X2	T37.4X3	T37.4X4	T37.4X5	T37.4X6
Santyl	T49.8X1	T49.8X2	T49.8X3	T49.8X4	T49.8X5	T49.8X6
Saralasin	T46.5X1	T46.5X2	T46.5X3	T46.5X4	T46.5X5	T46.5X6
Sarcolysin	T45.1X1	T45.1X2	T45.1X3	T45.1X4	T45.1X5	T45.1X6
Sarkomycin	T45.1X1	T45.1X2	T45.1X3	T45.1X4	T45.1X5	T45.1X6
Saroten	T43.011	T43.012	T43.013	T43.014	T43.015	T43.016
Saturnine — *see* Lead						
Savin (oil)	T49.4X1	T49.4X2	T49.4X3	T49.4X4	T49.4X5	T49.4X6
Scammony	T47.2X1	T47.2X2	T47.2X3	T47.2X4	T47.2X5	T47.2X6
Scarlet red	T49.8X1	T49.8X2	T49.8X3	T49.8X4	T49.8X5	T49.8X6
Scheele's green	T57.0X1	T57.0X2	T57.0X3	T57.0X4	—	—
insecticide	T57.0X1	T57.0X2	T57.0X3	T57.0X4	—	—
Schizontozide (blood) (tissue)	T37.2X1	T37.2X2	T37.2X3	T37.2X4	T37.2X5	T37.2X6
Schradan	T60.0X1	T60.0X2	T60.0X3	T60.0X4	—	—
Schweinfurth green	T57.0X1	T57.0X2	T57.0X3	T57.0X4	—	—
insecticide	T57.0X1	T57.0X2	T57.0X3	T57.0X4	—	—
Scilla, rat poison	T60.4X1	T60.4X2	T60.4X3	T60.4X4	—	—
Scillaren	T60.4X1	T60.4X2	T60.4X3	T60.4X4	—	—
Sclerosing agent	T46.8X1	T46.8X2	T46.8X3	T46.8X4	T46.8X5	T46.8X6
Scombrotoxin	T61.11	T61.12	T61.13	T61.14	—	—
Scopolamine	T44.3X1	T44.3X2	T44.3X3	T44.3X4	T44.3X5	T44.3X6
Scopolia extract	T44.3X1	T44.3X2	T44.3X3	T44.3X4	T44.3X5	T44.3X6
Scouring powder	T65.891	T65.892	T65.893	T65.894	—	—
Sea						
anemone (sting)	T63.631	T63.632	T63.633	T63.634	—	—
cucumber (sting)	T63.691	T63.692	T63.693	T63.694	—	—
snake (bite) (venom)	T63.091	T63.092	T63.093	T63.094	—	—
urchin spine (puncture)	T63.691	T63.692	T63.693	T63.694	—	—
Seafood	T61.91	T61.92	T61.93	T61.94	—	—
specified NEC	T61.8X1	T61.8X2	T61.8X3	T61.8X4	—	—
Secbutabarbital	T42.3X1	T42.3X2	T42.3X3	T42.3X4	T42.3X5	T42.3X6
Secbutabarbitone	T42.3X1	T42.3X2	T42.3X3	T42.3X4	T42.3X5	T42.3X6
Secnidazole	T37.3X1	T37.3X2	T37.3X3	T37.3X4	T37.3X5	T37.3X6
Secobarbital	T42.3X1	T42.3X2	T42.3X3	T42.3X4	T42.3X5	T42.3X6
Seconal	T42.3X1	T42.3X2	T42.3X3	T42.3X4	T42.3X5	T42.3X6
Secretin	T50.8X1	T50.8X2	T50.8X3	T50.8X4	T50.8X5	T50.8X6
Sedative NEC	T42.71	T42.72	T42.73	T42.74	T42.75	T42.76
mixed NEC	T42.6X1	T42.6X2	T42.6X3	T42.6X4	T42.6X5	T42.6X6
Sedormid	T42.6X1	T42.6X2	T42.6X3	T42.6X4	T42.6X5	T42.6X6
Seed disinfectant or dressing	T60.8X1	T60.8X2	T60.8X3	T60.8X4	—	—
Seeds (poisonous)	T62.2X1	T62.2X2	T62.2X3	T62.2X4	—	—
Selegiline	T42.8X1	T42.8X2	T42.8X3	T42.8X4	T42.8X5	T42.8X6
Selenium NEC	T56.891	T56.892	T56.893	T56.894	—	—
disulfide or sulfide	T49.4X1	T49.4X2	T49.4X3	T49.4X4	T49.4X5	T49.4X6
fumes	T59.891	T59.892	T59.893	T59.894	—	—
sulfide	T49.4X1	T49.4X2	T49.4X3	T49.4X4	T49.4X5	T49.4X6
Selenomethionine (75Se)	T50.8X1	T50.8X2	T50.8X3	T50.8X4	T50.8X5	T50.8X6
Selsun	T49.4X1	T49.4X2	T49.4X3	T49.4X4	T49.4X5	T49.4X6
Semustine	T45.1X1	T45.1X2	T45.1X3	T45.1X4	T45.1X5	T45.1X6
Senega syrup	T48.4X1	T48.4X2	T48.4X3	T48.4X4	T48.4X5	T48.4X6
Senna	T47.2X1	T47.2X2	T47.2X3	T47.2X4	T47.2X5	T47.2X6
Sennoside A+B	T47.2X1	T47.2X2	T47.2X3	T47.2X4	T47.2X5	T47.2X6
Septisol	T49.2X1	T49.2X2	T49.2X3	T49.2X4	T49.2X5	T49.2X6
Seractide	T38.811	T38.812	T38.813	T38.814	T38.815	T38.816
Serax	T42.4X1	T42.4X2	T42.4X3	T42.4X4	T42.4X5	T42.4X6
Serenesil	T42.6X1	T42.6X2	T42.6X3	T42.6X4	T42.6X5	T42.6X6
Serenium (hydrochloride)	T37.91	T37.92	T37.93	T37.94	T37.95	T37.96
Serepax — *see* Oxazepam						
Sermorelin	T38.891	T38.892	T38.893	T38.894	T38.895	T38.896
Sernyl	T41.1X1	T41.1X2	T41.1X3	T41.1X4	T41.1X5	T41.1X6
Serotonin	T50.991	T50.992	T50.993	T50.994	T50.995	T50.996
Serpasil	T46.5X1	T46.5X2	T46.5X3	T46.5X4	T46.5X5	T46.5X6
Serrapeptase	T45.3X1	T45.3X2	T45.3X3	T45.3X4	T45.3X5	T45.3X6
Serum						
antibotulinus	T50.Z11	T50.Z12	T50.Z13	T50.Z14	T50.Z15	T50.Z16
anticytotoxic	T50.Z11	T50.Z12	T50.Z13	T50.Z14	T50.Z15	T50.Z16
antidiphtheria	T50.Z11	T50.Z12	T50.Z13	T50.Z14	T50.Z15	T50.Z16
antimeningococcus	T50.Z11	T50.Z12	T50.Z13	T50.Z14	T50.Z15	T50.Z16
anti-Rh	T50.Z11	T50.Z12	T50.Z13	T50.Z14	T50.Z15	T50.Z16
anti-snake-bite	T50.Z11	T50.Z12	T50.Z13	T50.Z14	T50.Z15	T50.Z16
antitetanic	T50.Z11	T50.Z12	T50.Z13	T50.Z14	T50.Z15	T50.Z16
antitoxic	T50.Z11	T50.Z12	T50.Z13	T50.Z14	T50.Z15	T50.Z16
complement (inhibitor)	T45.8X1	T45.8X2	T45.8X3	T45.8X4	T45.8X5	T45.8X6
convalescent	T50.Z11	T50.Z12	T50.Z13	T50.Z14	T50.Z15	T50.Z16

▽ Subterms under main terms may continue to next column or page   Additional Character May Be Required — Refer to the Tabular List for Character Selection   389

Ricin — Serum

Table of Drugs and Chemicals

Substance	Poisoning, Accidental (unintentional)	Poisoning, Intentional Self-harm	Poisoning, Assault	Poisoning, Undetermined	Adverse Effect	Under-dosing
Serum — continued						
hemolytic complement	T45.8X1	T45.8X2	T45.8X3	T45.8X4	T45.8X5	T45.8X6
immune (human)	T50.Z11	T50.Z12	T50.Z13	T50.Z14	T50.Z15	T50.Z16
protective NEC	T50.Z11	T50.Z12	T50.Z13	T50.Z14	T50.Z15	T50.Z16
Setastine	T45.0X1	T45.0X2	T45.0X3	T45.0X4	T45.0X5	T45.0X6
Setoperone	T43.591	T43.592	T43.593	T43.594	T43.595	T43.596
Sewer gas	T59.91	T59.92	T59.93	T59.94	—	—
Shampoo	T55.0X1	T55.0X2	T55.0X3	T55.0X4	—	—
Shellfish, noxious, nonbacterial	T61.781	T61.782	T61.783	T61.784		
Sildenafil	T46.7X1	T46.7X2	T46.7X3	T46.7X4	T46.7X5	T46.7X6
Silibinin	T50.991	T50.992	T50.993	T50.994	T50.995	T50.996
Silicone NEC	T65.891	T65.892	T65.893	T65.894		
medicinal	T49.3X1	T49.3X2	T49.3X3	T49.3X4	T49.3X5	T49.3X6
Silvadene	T49.0X1	T49.0X2	T49.0X3	T49.0X4	T49.0X5	T49.0X6
Silver	T49.0X1	T49.0X2	T49.0X3	T49.0X4	T49.0X5	T49.0X6
anti-infectives	T49.0X1	T49.0X2	T49.0X3	T49.0X4	T49.0X5	T49.0X6
arsphenamine	T37.8X1	T37.8X2	T37.8X3	T37.8X4	T37.8X5	T37.8X6
colloidal	T49.0X1	T49.0X2	T49.0X3	T49.0X4	T49.0X5	T49.0X6
nitrate	T49.0X1	T49.0X2	T49.0X3	T49.0X4	T49.0X5	T49.0X6
ophthalmic preparation	T49.5X1	T49.5X2	T49.5X3	T49.5X4	T49.5X5	T49.5X6
toughened (keratolytic)	T49.4X1	T49.4X2	T49.4X3	T49.4X4	T49.4X5	T49.4X6
nonmedicinal (dust)	T56.891	T56.892	T56.893	T56.894	—	—
protein	T49.5X1	T49.5X2	T49.5X3	T49.5X4	T49.5X5	T49.5X6
salvarsan	T37.8X1	T37.8X2	T37.8X3	T37.8X4	T37.8X5	T37.8X6
sulfadiazine	T49.4X1	T49.4X2	T49.4X3	T49.4X4	T49.4X5	T49.4X6
Silymarin	T50.991	T50.992	T50.993	T50.994	T50.995	T50.996
Simaldrate	T47.1X1	T47.1X2	T47.1X3	T47.1X4	T47.1X5	T47.1X6
Simazine	T60.3X1	T60.3X2	T60.3X3	T60.3X4	—	—
Simethicone	T47.1X1	T47.1X2	T47.1X3	T47.1X4	T47.1X5	T47.1X6
Simfibrate	T46.6X1	T46.6X2	T46.6X3	T46.6X4	T46.6X5	T46.6X6
Simvastatin	T46.6X1	T46.6X2	T46.6X3	T46.6X4	T46.6X5	T46.6X6
Sincalide	T50.8X1	T50.8X2	T50.8X3	T50.8X4	T50.8X5	T50.8X6
Sinequan	T43.011	T43.012	T43.013	T43.014	T43.015	T43.016
Singoserp	T46.5X1	T46.5X2	T46.5X3	T46.5X4	T46.5X5	T46.5X6
Sintrom	T45.511	T45.512	T45.513	T45.514	T45.515	T45.516
Sisomicin	T36.5X1	T36.5X2	T36.5X3	T36.5X4	T36.5X5	T36.5X6
Sitosterols	T46.6X1	T46.6X2	T46.6X3	T46.6X4	T46.6X5	T46.6X6
Skeletal muscle relaxants	T48.1X1	T48.1X2	T48.1X3	T48.1X4	T48.1X5	T48.1X6
Skin						
agents (external)	T49.91	T49.92	T49.93	T49.94	T49.95	T49.96
specified NEC	T49.8X1	T49.8X2	T49.8X3	T49.8X4	T49.8X5	T49.8X6
test antigen	T50.8X1	T50.8X2	T50.8X3	T50.8X4	T50.8X5	T50.8X6
Sleep-eze	T45.0X1	T45.0X2	T45.0X3	T45.0X4	T45.0X5	T45.0X6
Sleeping draught, pill	T42.71	T42.72	T42.73	T42.74	T42.75	T42.76
Smallpox vaccine	T50.B11	T50.B12	T50.B13	T50.B14	T50.B15	T50.B16
Smelter fumes NEC	T56.91	T56.92	T56.93	T56.94	—	—
Smog	T59.1X1	T59.1X2	T59.1X3	T59.1X4	—	—
Smoke NEC	T59.811	T59.812	T59.813	T59.814	—	—
Smooth muscle relaxant	T44.3X1	T44.3X2	T44.3X3	T44.3X4	T44.3X5	T44.3X6
Snail killer NEC	T60.8X1	T60.8X2	T60.8X3	T60.8X4	—	—
Snake venom or bite	T63.001	T63.002	T63.003	T63.004	—	—
hemocoagulase	T45.7X1	T45.7X2	T45.7X3	T45.7X4	T45.7X5	T45.7X6
Snuff	T65.211	T65.212	T65.213	T65.214	—	—
Soap (powder) (product)	T55.0X1	T55.0X2	T55.0X3	T55.0X4	—	—
enema	T47.4X1	T47.4X2	T47.4X3	T47.4X4	T47.4X5	T47.4X6
medicinal, soft	T49.2X1	T49.2X2	T49.2X3	T49.2X4	T49.2X5	T49.2X6
superfatted	T49.2X1	T49.2X2	T49.2X3	T49.2X4	T49.2X5	T49.2X6
Sobrerol	T48.4X1	T48.4X2	T48.4X3	T48.4X4	T48.4X5	T48.4X6
Soda (caustic)	T54.3X1	T54.3X2	T54.3X3	T54.3X4	—	—
bicarb	T47.1X1	T47.1X2	T47.1X3	T47.1X4	T47.1X5	T47.1X6
chlorinated — see Sodium, hypochlorite						
Sodium						
acetosulfone	T37.1X1	T37.1X2	T37.1X3	T37.1X4	T37.1X5	T37.1X6
acetrizoate	T50.8X1	T50.8X2	T50.8X3	T50.8X4	T50.8X5	T50.8X6
acid phosphate	T50.3X1	T50.3X2	T50.3X3	T50.3X4	T50.3X5	T50.3X6
alginate	T47.8X1	T47.8X2	T47.8X3	T47.8X4	T47.8X5	T47.8X6
amidotrizoate	T50.8X1	T50.8X2	T50.8X3	T50.8X4	T50.8X5	T50.8X6
aminopterin	T45.1X1	T45.1X2	T45.1X3	T45.1X4	T45.1X5	T45.1X6
amylosulfate	T47.8X1	T47.8X2	T47.8X3	T47.8X4	T47.8X5	T47.8X6
amytal	T42.3X1	T42.3X2	T42.3X3	T42.3X4	T42.3X5	T42.3X6
antimony gluconate	T37.3X1	T37.3X2	T37.3X3	T37.3X4	T37.3X5	T37.3X6
arsenate	T57.0X1	T57.0X2	T57.0X3	T57.0X4	—	—
aurothiomalate	T39.4X1	T39.4X2	T39.4X3	T39.4X4	T39.4X5	T39.4X6
aurothiosulfate	T39.4X1	T39.4X2	T39.4X3	T39.4X4	T39.4X5	T39.4X6
barbiturate	T42.3X1	T42.3X2	T42.3X3	T42.3X4	T42.3X5	T42.3X6
basic phosphate	T47.4X1	T47.4X2	T47.4X3	T47.4X4	T47.4X5	T47.4X6
bicarbonate	T47.1X1	T47.1X2	T47.1X3	T47.1X4	T47.1X5	T47.1X6
bichromate	T57.8X1	T57.8X2	T57.8X3	T57.8X4	—	—
biphosphate	T50.3X1	T50.3X2	T50.3X3	T50.3X4	T50.3X5	T50.3X6
bisulfate	T65.891	T65.892	T65.893	T65.894	—	—
borate						
Sodium — continued						
borate — continued						
cleanser	T57.8X1	T57.8X2	T57.8X3	T57.8X4	—	—
eye	T49.5X1	T49.5X2	T49.5X3	T49.5X4	T49.5X5	T49.5X6
therapeutic	T49.8X1	T49.8X2	T49.8X3	T49.8X4	T49.8X5	T49.8X6
bromide	T42.6X1	T42.6X2	T42.6X3	T42.6X4	T42.6X5	T42.6X6
cacodylate (nonmedicinal)	T50.8X1	T50.8X2	T50.8X3	T50.8X4	T50.8X5	T50.8X6
NEC						
anti-infective	T37.8X1	T37.8X2	T37.8X3	T37.8X4	T37.8X5	T37.8X6
herbicide	T60.3X1	T60.3X2	T60.3X3	T60.3X4	—	—
calcium edetate	T45.8X1	T45.8X2	T45.8X3	T45.8X4	T45.8X5	T45.8X6
carbonate NEC	T54.3X1	T54.3X2	T54.3X3	T54.3X4		
chlorate NEC	T65.891	T65.892	T65.893	T65.894		
herbicide	T54.91	T54.92	T54.93	T54.94		
chloride	T50.3X1	T50.3X2	T50.3X3	T50.3X4	T50.3X5	T50.3X6
with glucose	T50.3X1	T50.3X2	T50.3X3	T50.3X4	T50.3X5	T50.3X6
chromate	T65.891	T65.892	T65.893	T65.894		
citrate	T50.991	T50.992	T50.993	T50.994	T50.995	T50.996
cromoglicate	T48.6X1	T48.6X2	T48.6X3	T48.6X4	T48.6X5	T48.6X6
cyanide	T65.0X1	T65.0X2	T65.0X3	T65.0X4		
cyclamate	T50.3X1	T50.3X2	T50.3X3	T50.3X4	T50.3X5	T50.3X6
dehydrocholate	T45.8X1	T45.8X2	T45.8X3	T45.8X4	T45.8X5	T45.8X6
diatrizoate	T50.8X1	T50.8X2	T50.8X3	T50.8X4	T50.8X5	T50.8X6
dibunate	T48.4X1	T48.4X2	T48.4X3	T48.4X4	T48.4X5	T48.4X6
dioctyl sulfosuccinate	T47.4X1	T47.4X2	T47.4X3	T47.4X4	T47.4X5	T47.4X6
dipantoyl ferrate	T45.8X1	T45.8X2	T45.8X3	T45.8X4	T45.8X5	T45.8X6
edetate	T45.8X1	T45.8X2	T45.8X3	T45.8X4	T45.8X5	T45.8X6
ethacrynate	T50.1X1	T50.1X2	T50.1X3	T50.1X4	T50.1X5	T50.1X6
feredetate	T45.8X1	T45.8X2	T45.8X3	T45.8X4	T45.8X5	T45.8X6
Fluoride — see Fluoride						
fluoroacetate (dust) (pesticide)	T60.4X1	T60.4X2	T60.4X3	T60.4X4		
free salt	T50.3X1	T50.3X2	T50.3X3	T50.3X4	T50.3X5	T50.3X6
fusidate	T36.8X1	T36.8X2	T36.8X3	T36.8X4	T36.8X5	T36.8X6
glucaldrate	T47.1X1	T47.1X2	T47.1X3	T47.1X4	T47.1X5	T47.1X6
glucosulfone	T37.1X1	T37.1X2	T37.1X3	T37.1X4	T37.1X5	T37.1X6
glutamate	T45.8X1	T45.8X2	T45.8X3	T45.8X4	T45.8X5	T45.8X6
hydrogen carbonate	T50.3X1	T50.3X2	T50.3X3	T50.3X4	T50.3X5	T50.3X6
hydroxide	T54.3X1	T54.3X2	T54.3X3	T54.3X4		
hypochlorite (bleach) NEC	T54.3X1	T54.3X2	T54.3X3	T54.3X4		
disinfectant	T54.3X1	T54.3X2	T54.3X3	T54.3X4	—	—
medicinal (anti-infective) (external)	T49.0X1	T49.0X2	T49.0X3	T49.0X4	T49.0X5	T49.0X6
vapor	T54.3X1	T54.3X2	T54.3X3	T54.3X4	—	—
hyposulfite	T49.0X1	T49.0X2	T49.0X3	T49.0X4	T49.0X5	T49.0X6
indigotin disulfonate	T50.8X1	T50.8X2	T50.8X3	T50.8X4	T50.8X5	T50.8X6
iodide	T50.991	T50.992	T50.993	T50.994	T50.995	T50.996
I-131	T50.8X1	T50.8X2	T50.8X3	T50.8X4	T50.8X5	T50.8X6
therapeutic	T38.2X1	T38.2X2	T38.2X3	T38.2X4	T38.2X5	T38.2X6
iodohippurate (131I)	T50.8X1	T50.8X2	T50.8X3	T50.8X4	T50.8X5	T50.8X6
iopodate	T50.8X1	T50.8X2	T50.8X3	T50.8X4	T50.8X5	T50.8X6
iothalamate	T50.8X1	T50.8X2	T50.8X3	T50.8X4	T50.8X5	T50.8X6
iron edetate	T45.4X1	T45.4X2	T45.4X3	T45.4X4	T45.4X5	T45.4X6
lactate (compound solution)	T45.8X1	T45.8X2	T45.8X3	T45.8X4	T45.8X5	T45.8X6
lauryl (sulfate)	T49.2X1	T49.2X2	T49.2X3	T49.2X4	T49.2X5	T49.2X6
L-triiodothyronine	T38.1X1	T38.1X2	T38.1X3	T38.1X4	T38.1X5	T38.1X6
magnesium citrate	T50.991	T50.992	T50.993	T50.994	T50.995	T50.996
mersalate	T50.2X1	T50.2X2	T50.2X3	T50.2X4	T50.2X5	T50.2X6
metasilicate	T65.891	T65.892	T65.893	T65.894	—	—
metrizoate	T50.8X1	T50.8X2	T50.8X3	T50.8X4	T50.8X5	T50.8X6
monofluoroacetate (pesticide)	T60.1X1	T60.1X2	T60.1X3	T60.1X4	—	—
morrhuate	T46.8X1	T46.8X2	T46.8X3	T46.8X4	T46.8X5	T46.8X6
nafcillin	T36.0X1	T36.0X2	T36.0X3	T36.0X4	T36.0X5	T36.0X6
nitrate (oxidizing agent)	T65.891	T65.892	T65.893	T65.894		
nitrite	T50.6X1	T50.6X2	T50.6X3	T50.6X4	T50.6X5	T50.6X6
nitroferricyanide	T46.5X1	T46.5X2	T46.5X3	T46.5X4	T46.5X5	T46.5X6
nitroprusside	T46.5X1	T46.5X2	T46.5X3	T46.5X4	T46.5X5	T46.5X6
oxalate	T65.891	T65.892	T65.893	T65.894	—	—
oxide/peroxide	T65.891	T65.892	T65.893	T65.894	—	—
oxybate	T41.291	T41.292	T41.293	T41.294	T41.295	T41.296
para-aminohippurate	T50.8X1	T50.8X2	T50.8X3	T50.8X4	T50.8X5	T50.8X6
perborate (nonmedicinal) NEC	T65.891	T65.892	T65.893	T65.894		
medicinal	T49.0X1	T49.0X2	T49.0X3	T49.0X4	T49.0X5	T49.0X6
soap	T55.0X1	T55.0X2	T55.0X3	T55.0X4	—	—
percarbonate — see Sodium, perborate						
pertechnetate Tc99m	T50.8X1	T50.8X2	T50.8X3	T50.8X4	T50.8X5	T50.8X6
phosphate						
cellulose	T45.8X1	T45.8X2	T45.8X3	T45.8X4	T45.8X5	T45.8X
dibasic	T47.2X1	T47.2X2	T47.2X3	T47.2X4	T47.2X5	T47.2X

Serum — Sodium

Substance	Poisoning, Accidental (unintentional)	Poisoning, Intentional Self-harm	Poisoning, Assault	Poisoning, Undetermined	Adverse Effect	Under-dosing
Sodium — *continued*						
phosphate — *continued*						
monobasic	T47.2X1	T47.2X2	T47.2X3	T47.2X4	T47.2X5	T47.2X6
phytate	T50.6X1	T50.6X2	T50.6X3	T50.6X4	T50.6X5	T50.6X6
picosulfate	T47.2X1	T47.2X2	T47.2X3	T47.2X4	T47.2X5	T47.2X6
polyhydroxyaluminium monocarbonate	T47.1X1	T47.1X2	T47.1X3	T47.1X4	T47.1X5	T47.1X6
polystyrene sulfonate	T50.3X1	T50.3X2	T50.3X3	T50.3X4	T50.3X5	T50.3X6
propionate	T49.0X1	T49.0X2	T49.0X3	T49.0X4	T49.0X5	T49.0X6
propyl hydroxybenzoate	T50.991	T50.992	T50.993	T50.994	T50.995	T50.996
psylliate	T46.8X1	T46.8X2	T46.8X3	T46.8X4	T46.8X5	T46.8X6
removing resins	T50.3X1	T50.3X2	T50.3X3	T50.3X4	T50.3X5	T50.3X6
salicylate	T39.091	T39.092	T39.093	T39.094	T39.095	T39.096
salt NEC	T50.3X1	T50.3X2	T50.3X3	T50.3X4	T50.3X5	T50.3X6
selenate	T60.2X1	T60.2X2	T60.2X3	T60.2X4	—	—
stibogluconate	T37.3X1	T37.3X2	T37.3X3	T37.3X4	T37.3X5	T37.3X6
sulfate	T47.4X1	T47.4X2	T47.4X3	T47.4X4	T47.4X5	T47.4X6
sulfoxone	T37.1X1	T37.1X2	T37.1X3	T37.1X4	T37.1X5	T37.1X6
tetradecyl sulfate	T46.8X1	T46.8X2	T46.8X3	T46.8X4	T46.8X5	T46.8X6
thiopental	T41.1X1	T41.1X2	T41.1X3	T41.1X4	T41.1X5	T41.1X6
thiosalicylate	T39.091	T39.092	T39.093	T39.094	T39.095	T39.096
thiosulfate	T50.6X1	T50.6X2	T50.6X3	T50.6X4	T50.6X5	T50.6X6
tolbutamide	T38.3X1	T38.3X2	T38.3X3	T38.3X4	T38.3X5	T38.3X6
(L)-triiodothyronine	T38.1X1	T38.1X2	T38.1X3	T38.1X4	T38.1X5	T38.1X6
tyropanoate	T50.8X1	T50.8X2	T50.8X3	T50.8X4	T50.8X5	T50.8X6
valproate	T42.6X1	T42.6X2	T42.6X3	T42.6X4	T42.6X5	T42.6X6
versenate	T50.6X1	T50.6X2	T50.6X3	T50.6X4	T50.6X5	T50.6X6
Sodium-free salt	T50.901	T50.902	T50.903	T50.904	T50.905	T50.906
Sodium-removing resin	T50.3X1	T50.3X2	T50.3X3	T50.3X4	T50.3X5	T50.3X6
Soft soap	T55.0X1	T55.0X2	T55.0X3	T55.0X4	—	—
Solanine	T62.2X1	T62.2X2	T62.2X3	T62.2X4	—	—
berries	T62.1X1	T62.1X2	T62.1X3	T62.1X4	—	—
Solanum dulcamara	T62.2X1	T62.2X2	T62.2X3	T62.2X4	—	—
berries	T62.1X1	T62.1X2	T62.1X3	T62.1X4	—	—
Solapsone	T37.1X1	T37.1X2	T37.1X3	T37.1X4	T37.1X5	T37.1X6
Solar lotion	T49.3X1	T49.3X2	T49.3X3	T49.3X4	T49.3X5	T49.3X6
Solasulfone	T37.1X1	T37.1X2	T37.1X3	T37.1X4	T37.1X5	T37.1X6
Soldering fluid	T65.891	T65.892	T65.893	T65.894	—	—
Solid substance	T65.91	T65.92	T65.93	T65.94	—	—
specified NEC	T65.891	T65.892	T65.893	T65.894	—	—
Solvent, industrial NEC	T52.91	T52.92	T52.93	T52.94	—	—
naphtha	T52.0X1	T52.0X2	T52.0X3	T52.0X4	—	—
petroleum	T52.0X1	T52.0X2	T52.0X3	T52.0X4	—	—
specified NEC	T52.8X1	T52.8X2	T52.8X3	T52.8X4	—	—
Soma	T42.8X1	T42.8X2	T42.8X3	T42.8X4	T42.8X5	T42.8X6
Somatorelin	T38.891	T38.892	T38.893	T38.894	T38.895	T38.896
Somatostatin	T38.991	T38.992	T38.993	T38.994	T38.995	T38.996
Somatotropin	T38.811	T38.812	T38.813	T38.814	T38.815	T38.816
Somatrem	T38.811	T38.812	T38.813	T38.814	T38.815	T38.816
Somatropin	T38.811	T38.812	T38.813	T38.814	T38.815	T38.816
Sominex	T45.0X1	T45.0X2	T45.0X3	T45.0X4	T45.0X5	T45.0X6
Somnos	T42.6X1	T42.6X2	T42.6X3	T42.6X4	T42.6X5	T42.6X6
Somonal	T42.3X1	T42.3X2	T42.3X3	T42.3X4	T42.3X5	T42.3X6
Soneryl	T42.3X1	T42.3X2	T42.3X3	T42.3X4	T42.3X5	T42.3X6
Soothing syrup	T50.901	T50.902	T50.903	T50.904	T50.905	T50.906
Sopor	T42.6X1	T42.6X2	T42.6X3	T42.6X4	T42.6X5	T42.6X6
Soporific	T42.71	T42.72	T42.73	T42.74	T42.75	T42.76
Soporific drug	T42.71	T42.72	T42.73	T42.74	T42.75	T42.76
specified type NEC	T42.6X1	T42.6X2	T42.6X3	T42.6X4	T42.6X5	T42.6X6
Sorbide nitrate	T46.3X1	T46.3X2	T46.3X3	T46.3X4	T46.3X5	T46.3X6
Sorbitol	T47.4X1	T47.4X2	T47.4X3	T47.4X4	T47.4X5	T47.4X6
Sotalol	T44.7X1	T44.7X2	T44.7X3	T44.7X4	T44.7X5	T44.7X6
Sotradecol	T46.8X1	T46.8X2	T46.8X3	T46.8X4	T46.8X5	T46.8X6
Soysterol	T46.6X1	T46.6X2	T46.6X3	T46.6X4	T46.6X5	T46.6X6
Spacoline	T44.3X1	T44.3X2	T44.3X3	T44.3X4	T44.3X5	T44.3X6
Spanish fly	T49.8X1	T49.8X2	T49.8X3	T49.8X4	T49.8X5	T49.8X6
Sparine	T43.3X1	T43.3X2	T43.3X3	T43.3X4	T43.3X5	T43.3X6
Sparteine	T48.0X1	T48.0X2	T48.0X3	T48.0X4	T48.0X5	T48.0X6
Spasmolytic						
anticholinergics	T44.3X1	T44.3X2	T44.3X3	T44.3X4	T44.3X5	T44.3X6
autonomic	T44.3X1	T44.3X2	T44.3X3	T44.3X4	T44.3X5	T44.3X6
bronchial NEC	T48.6X1	T48.6X2	T48.6X3	T48.6X4	T48.6X5	T48.6X6
quaternary ammonium	T44.3X1	T44.3X2	T44.3X3	T44.3X4	T44.3X5	T44.3X6
skeletal muscle NEC	T48.1X1	T48.1X2	T48.1X3	T48.1X4	T48.1X5	T48.1X6
Spectinomycin	T36.5X1	T36.5X2	T36.5X3	T36.5X4	T36.5X5	T36.5X6
Speed	T43.621	T43.622	T43.623	T43.624	T43.625	T43.626
Spermicide	T49.8X1	T49.8X2	T49.8X3	T49.8X4	T49.8X5	T49.8X6
Spider (bite) (venom)	T63.391	T63.392	T63.393	T63.394	—	—
antivenin	T50.Z11	T50.Z12	T50.Z13	T50.Z14	T50.Z15	T50.Z16
Spigelia (root)	T37.4X1	T37.4X2	T37.4X3	T37.4X4	T37.4X5	T37.4X6
Spindle inactivator	T50.4X1	T50.4X2	T50.4X3	T50.4X4	T50.4X5	T50.4X6
Spiperone	T43.4X1	T43.4X2	T43.4X3	T43.4X4	T43.4X5	T43.4X6
Spiramycin	T36.3X1	T36.3X2	T36.3X3	T36.3X4	T36.3X5	T36.3X6

Substance	Poisoning, Accidental (unintentional)	Poisoning, Intentional Self-harm	Poisoning, Assault	Poisoning, Undetermined	Adverse Effect	Under-dosing
Spirapril	T46.4X1	T46.4X2	T46.4X3	T46.4X4	T46.4X5	T46.4X6
Spirilene	T43.591	T43.592	T43.593	T43.594	T43.595	T43.596
Spirit(s) (neutral) **NEC**	T51.0X1	T51.0X2	T51.0X3	T51.0X4	—	—
beverage	T51.0X1	T51.0X2	T51.0X3	T51.0X4	—	—
industrial	T51.0X1	T51.0X2	T51.0X3	T51.0X4	—	—
mineral	T52.0X1	T52.0X2	T52.0X3	T52.0X4	—	—
of salt — *see* Hydrochloric acid						
surgical	T51.0X1	T51.0X2	T51.0X3	T51.0X4	—	—
Spironolactone	T50.0X1	T50.0X2	T50.0X3	T50.0X4	T50.0X5	T50.0X6
Spiroperidol	T43.4X1	T43.4X2	T43.4X3	T43.4X4	T43.4X5	T43.4X6
Sponge, absorbable (gelatin)	T45.7X1	T45.7X2	T45.7X3	T45.7X4	T45.7X5	T45.7X6
Sporostacin	T49.0X1	T49.0X2	T49.0X3	T49.0X4	T49.0X5	T49.0X6
Spray (aerosol)	T65.91	T65.92	T65.93	T65.94	—	—
cosmetic	T65.891	T65.892	T65.893	T65.894	—	—
medicinal NEC	T50.901	T50.902	T50.903	T50.904	T50.905	T50.906
pesticides — *see* Pesticides						
specified content — *see* specific substance						
Spurge flax	T62.2X1	T62.2X2	T62.2X3	T62.2X4	—	—
Spurges	T62.2X1	T62.2X2	T62.2X3	T62.2X4	—	—
Sputum viscosity-lowering drug	T48.4X1	T48.4X2	T48.4X3	T48.4X4	T48.4X5	T48.4X6
Squill	T46.0X1	T46.0X2	T46.0X3	T46.0X4	T46.0X5	T46.0X6
rat poison	T60.4X1	T60.4X2	T60.4X3	T60.4X4	—	—
Squirting cucumber (cathartic)	T47.2X1	T47.2X2	T47.2X3	T47.2X4	T47.2X5	T47.2X6
Stains	T65.6X1	T65.6X2	T65.6X3	T65.6X4	—	—
Stannous fluoride	T49.7X1	T49.7X2	T49.7X3	T49.7X4	T49.7X5	T49.7X6
Stanolone	T38.7X1	T38.7X2	T38.7X3	T38.7X4	T38.7X5	T38.7X6
Stanozolol	T38.7X1	T38.7X2	T38.7X3	T38.7X4	T38.7X5	T38.7X6
Staphisagria or stavesacre (pediculicide)	T49.0X1	T49.0X2	T49.0X3	T49.0X4	T49.0X5	T49.0X6
Starch	T50.901	T50.902	T50.903	T50.904	T50.905	T50.906
Stelazine	T43.3X1	T43.3X2	T43.3X3	T43.3X4	T43.3X5	T43.3X6
Stemetil	T43.3X1	T43.3X2	T43.3X3	T43.3X4	T43.3X5	T43.3X6
Stepronin	T48.4X1	T48.4X2	T48.4X3	T48.4X4	T48.4X5	T48.4X6
Sterculia	T47.4X1	T47.4X2	T47.4X3	T47.4X4	T47.4X5	T47.4X6
Sternutator gas	T59.891	T59.892	T59.893	T59.894	—	—
Steroid	T38.0X1	T38.0X2	T38.0X3	T38.0X4	T38.0X5	T38.0X6
anabolic	T38.7X1	T38.7X2	T38.7X3	T38.7X4	T38.7X5	T38.7X6
androgenic	T38.7X1	T38.7X2	T38.7X3	T38.7X4	T38.7X5	T38.7X6
antineoplastic, hormone	T38.7X1	T38.7X2	T38.7X3	T38.7X4	T38.7X5	T38.7X6
estrogen	T38.5X1	T38.5X2	T38.5X3	T38.5X4	T38.5X5	T38.5X6
ENT agent	T49.6X1	T49.6X2	T49.6X3	T49.6X4	T49.6X5	T49.6X6
ophthalmic preparation	T49.5X1	T49.5X2	T49.5X3	T49.5X4	T49.5X5	T49.5X6
topical NEC	T49.0X1	T49.0X2	T49.0X3	T49.0X4	T49.0X5	T49.0X6
Stibine	T56.891	T56.892	T56.893	T56.894	—	—
Stibogluconate	T37.3X1	T37.3X2	T37.3X3	T37.3X4	T37.3X5	T37.3X6
Stibophen	T37.4X1	T37.4X2	T37.4X3	T37.4X4	T37.4X5	T37.4X6
Stilbamidine (isetionate)	T37.3X1	T37.3X2	T37.3X3	T37.3X4	T37.3X5	T37.3X6
Stilbestrol	T38.5X1	T38.5X2	T38.5X3	T38.5X4	T38.5X5	T38.5X6
Stilboestrol	T38.5X1	T38.5X2	T38.5X3	T38.5X4	T38.5X5	T38.5X6
Stimulant						
central nervous system — *see also* Psychostimulant	T43.601	T43.602	T43.603	T43.604	T43.605	T43.606
analeptics	T50.7X1	T50.7X2	T50.7X3	T50.7X4	T50.7X5	T50.7X6
opiate antagonist	T50.7X1	T50.7X2	T50.7X3	T50.7X4	T50.7X5	T50.7X6
psychotherapeutic NEC — *see also* Psychotherapeutic drug	T43.601	T43.602	T43.603	T43.604	T43.605	T43.606
specified NEC	T43.691	T43.692	T43.693	T43.694	T43.695	T43.696
respiratory	T48.901	T48.902	T48.903	T48.904	T48.905	T48.906
Stone-dissolving drug	T50.901	T50.902	T50.903	T50.904	T50.905	T50.906
Storage battery (cells) (acid)	T54.2X1	T54.2X2	T54.2X3	T54.2X4	—	—
Stovaine	T41.3X1	T41.3X2	T41.3X3	T41.3X4	T41.3X5	T41.3X6
infiltration (subcutaneous)	T41.3X1	T41.3X2	T41.3X3	T41.3X4	T41.3X5	T41.3X6
nerve block (peripheral) (plexus)	T41.3X1	T41.3X2	T41.3X3	T41.3X4	T41.3X5	T41.3X6
spinal	T41.3X1	T41.3X2	T41.3X3	T41.3X4	T41.3X5	T41.3X6
topical (surface)	T41.3X1	T41.3X2	T41.3X3	T41.3X4	T41.3X5	T41.3X6
Stovarsal	T37.8X1	T37.8X2	T37.8X3	T37.8X4	T37.8X5	T37.8X6
Stove gas — *see* Gas, stove						
Stoxil	T49.5X1	T49.5X2	T49.5X3	T49.5X4	T49.5X5	T49.5X6
Stramonium	T48.6X1	T48.6X2	T48.6X3	T48.6X4	T48.6X5	T48.6X6
natural state	T62.2X1	T62.2X2	T62.2X3	T62.2X4	—	—
Streptodornase	T45.3X1	T45.3X2	T45.3X3	T45.3X4	T45.3X5	T45.3X6
Streptoduocin	T36.5X1	T36.5X2	T36.5X3	T36.5X4	T36.5X5	T36.5X6
Streptokinase	T45.611	T45.612	T45.613	T45.614	T45.615	T45.616
Streptomycin (derivative)	T36.5X1	T36.5X2	T36.5X3	T36.5X4	T36.5X5	T36.5X6
Streptonivicin	T36.5X1	T36.5X2	T36.5X3	T36.5X4	T36.5X5	T36.5X6
Streptovarycin	T36.5X1	T36.5X2	T36.5X3	T36.5X4	T36.5X5	T36.5X6

▽ Subterms under main terms may continue to next column or page — Additional Character May Be Required — Refer to the Tabular List for Character Selection

Substance	Poisoning, Accidental (unintentional)	Poisoning, Intentional Self-harm	Poisoning, Assault	Poisoning, Undetermined	Adverse Effect	Under-dosing
Streptozocin	T45.1X1	T45.1X2	T45.1X3	T45.1X4	T45.1X5	T45.1X6
Streptozotocin	T45.1X1	T45.1X2	T45.1X3	T45.1X4	T45.1X5	T45.1X6
Stripper (paint) (solvent)	T52.8X1	T52.8X2	T52.8X3	T52.8X4	—	—
Strobane	T60.1X1	T60.1X2	T60.1X3	T60.1X4	—	—
Strofantina	T46.0X1	T46.0X2	T46.0X3	T46.0X4	T46.0X5	T46.0X6
Strophanthin (g) (k)	T46.0X1	T46.0X2	T46.0X3	T46.0X4	T46.0X5	T46.0X6
Strophanthus	T46.0X1	T46.0X2	T46.0X3	T46.0X4	T46.0X5	T46.0X6
Strophantin	T46.0X1	T46.0X2	T46.0X3	T46.0X4	T46.0X5	T46.0X6
Strophantin-g	T46.0X1	T46.0X2	T46.0X3	T46.0X4	T46.0X5	T46.0X6
Strychnine (nonmedicinal) (pesticide) (salts)	T65.1X1	T65.1X2	T65.1X3	T65.1X4	—	—
medicinal	T48.291	T48.292	T48.293	T48.294	T48.295	T48.296
Strychnos (ignatii) — see Strychnine						
Styramate	T42.8X1	T42.8X2	T42.8X3	T42.8X4	T42.8X5	T42.8X6
Styrene	T65.891	T65.892	T65.893	T65.894	—	—
Succinimide, antiepileptic or anticonvulsant	T42.2X1	T42.2X2	T42.2X3	T42.2X4	T42.2X5	T42.2X6
mercuric — see Mercury						
Succinylcholine	T48.1X1	T48.1X2	T48.1X3	T48.1X4	T48.1X5	T48.1X6
Succinylsulfathiazole	T37.0X1	T37.0X2	T37.0X3	T37.0X4	T37.0X5	T37.0X6
Sucralfate	T47.1X1	T47.1X2	T47.1X3	T47.1X4	T47.1X5	T47.1X6
Sucrose	T50.3X1	T50.3X2	T50.3X3	T50.3X4	T50.3X5	T50.3X6
Sufentanil	T40.4X1	T40.4X2	T40.4X3	T40.4X4	T40.4X5	T40.4X6
Sulbactam	T36.0X1	T36.0X2	T36.0X3	T36.0X4	T36.0X5	T36.0X6
Sulbenicillin	T36.0X1	T36.0X2	T36.0X3	T36.0X4	T36.0X5	T36.0X6
Sulbentine	T49.0X1	T49.0X2	T49.0X3	T49.0X4	T49.0X5	T49.0X6
Sulfacetamide	T49.0X1	T49.0X2	T49.0X3	T49.0X4	T49.0X5	T49.0X6
ophthalmic preparation	T49.5X1	T49.5X2	T49.5X3	T49.5X4	T49.5X5	T49.5X6
Sulfachlorpyridazine	T37.0X1	T37.0X2	T37.0X3	T37.0X4	T37.0X5	T37.0X6
Sulfacitine	T37.0X1	T37.0X2	T37.0X3	T37.0X4	T37.0X5	T37.0X6
Sulfadiasulfone sodium	T37.1X1	T37.1X2	T37.1X3	T37.1X4	T37.1X5	T37.1X6
Sulfadiazine	T37.0X1	T37.0X2	T37.0X3	T37.0X4	T37.0X5	T37.0X6
silver (topical)	T49.0X1	T49.0X2	T49.0X3	T49.0X4	T49.0X5	T49.0X6
Sulfadimethoxine	T37.0X1	T37.0X2	T37.0X3	T37.0X4	T37.0X5	T37.0X6
Sulfadimidine	T37.0X1	T37.0X2	T37.0X3	T37.0X4	T37.0X5	T37.0X6
Sulfadoxine	T37.0X1	T37.0X2	T37.0X3	T37.0X4	T37.0X5	T37.0X6
with pyrimethamine	T37.2X1	T37.2X2	T37.2X3	T37.2X4	T37.2X5	T37.2X6
Sulfaethidole	T37.0X1	T37.0X2	T37.0X3	T37.0X4	T37.0X5	T37.0X6
Sulfafurazole	T37.0X1	T37.0X2	T37.0X3	T37.0X4	T37.0X5	T37.0X6
Sulfaguanidine	T37.0X1	T37.0X2	T37.0X3	T37.0X4	T37.0X5	T37.0X6
Sulfalene	T37.0X1	T37.0X2	T37.0X3	T37.0X4	T37.0X5	T37.0X6
Sulfaloxate	T37.0X1	T37.0X2	T37.0X3	T37.0X4	T37.0X5	T37.0X6
Sulfaloxic acid	T37.0X1	T37.0X2	T37.0X3	T37.0X4	T37.0X5	T37.0X6
Sulfamazone	T39.2X1	T39.2X2	T39.2X3	T39.2X4	T39.2X5	T39.2X6
Sulfamerazine	T37.0X1	T37.0X2	T37.0X3	T37.0X4	T37.0X5	T37.0X6
Sulfameter	T37.0X1	T37.0X2	T37.0X3	T37.0X4	T37.0X5	T37.0X6
Sulfamethazine	T37.0X1	T37.0X2	T37.0X3	T37.0X4	T37.0X5	T37.0X6
Sulfamethizole	T37.0X1	T37.0X2	T37.0X3	T37.0X4	T37.0X5	T37.0X6
Sulfamethoxazole	T37.0X1	T37.0X2	T37.0X3	T37.0X4	T37.0X5	T37.0X6
with trimethoprim	T36.8X1	T36.8X2	T36.8X3	T36.8X4	T36.8X5	T36.8X6
Sulfamethoxydiazine	T37.0X1	T37.0X2	T37.0X3	T37.0X4	T37.0X5	T37.0X6
Sulfamethoxypyridazine	T37.0X1	T37.0X2	T37.0X3	T37.0X4	T37.0X5	T37.0X6
Sulfamethylthiazole	T37.0X1	T37.0X2	T37.0X3	T37.0X4	T37.0X5	T37.0X6
Sulfametoxydiazine	T37.0X1	T37.0X2	T37.0X3	T37.0X4	T37.0X5	T37.0X6
Sulfamidopyrine	T39.2X1	T39.2X2	T39.2X3	T39.2X4	T39.2X5	T39.2X6
Sulfamonomethoxine	T37.0X1	T37.0X2	T37.0X3	T37.0X4	T37.0X5	T37.0X6
Sulfamoxole	T37.0X1	T37.0X2	T37.0X3	T37.0X4	T37.0X5	T37.0X6
Sulfamylon	T49.0X1	T49.0X2	T49.0X3	T49.0X4	T49.0X5	T49.0X6
Sulfan blue (diagnostic dye)	T50.8X1	T50.8X2	T50.8X3	T50.8X4	T50.8X5	T50.8X6
Sulfanilamide	T37.0X1	T37.0X2	T37.0X3	T37.0X4	T37.0X5	T37.0X6
Sulfanilylguanidine	T37.0X1	T37.0X2	T37.0X3	T37.0X4	T37.0X5	T37.0X6
Sulfaperin	T37.0X1	T37.0X2	T37.0X3	T37.0X4	T37.0X5	T37.0X6
Sulfaphenazole	T37.0X1	T37.0X2	T37.0X3	T37.0X4	T37.0X5	T37.0X6
Sulfaphenylthiazole	T37.0X1	T37.0X2	T37.0X3	T37.0X4	T37.0X5	T37.0X6
Sulfaproxyline	T37.0X1	T37.0X2	T37.0X3	T37.0X4	T37.0X5	T37.0X6
Sulfapyridine	T37.0X1	T37.0X2	T37.0X3	T37.0X4	T37.0X5	T37.0X6
Sulfapyrimidine	T37.0X1	T37.0X2	T37.0X3	T37.0X4	T37.0X5	T37.0X6
Sulfarsphenamine	T37.8X1	T37.8X2	T37.8X3	T37.8X4	T37.8X5	T37.8X6
Sulfasalazine	T37.0X1	T37.0X2	T37.0X3	T37.0X4	T37.0X5	T37.0X6
Sulfasuxidine	T37.0X1	T37.0X2	T37.0X3	T37.0X4	T37.0X5	T37.0X6
Sulfasymazine	T37.0X1	T37.0X2	T37.0X3	T37.0X4	T37.0X5	T37.0X6
Sulfated amylopectin	T47.8X1	T47.8X2	T47.8X3	T47.8X4	T47.8X5	T47.8X6
Sulfathiazole	T37.0X1	T37.0X2	T37.0X3	T37.0X4	T37.0X5	T37.0X6
Sulfatostearate	T49.2X1	T49.2X2	T49.2X3	T49.2X4	T49.2X5	T49.2X6
Sulfinpyrazone	T50.4X1	T50.4X2	T50.4X3	T50.4X4	T50.4X5	T50.4X6
Sulfiram	T49.0X1	T49.0X2	T49.0X3	T49.0X4	T49.0X5	T49.0X6
Sulfisomidine	T37.0X1	T37.0X2	T37.0X3	T37.0X4	T37.0X5	T37.0X6
Sulfisoxazole	T37.0X1	T37.0X2	T37.0X3	T37.0X4	T37.0X5	T37.0X6
ophthalmic preparation	T49.5X1	T49.5X2	T49.5X3	T49.5X4	T49.5X5	T49.5X6
Sulfobromophthalein (sodium)	T50.8X1	T50.8X2	T50.8X3	T50.8X4	T50.8X5	T50.8X6
Sulfobromphthalein	T50.8X1	T50.8X2	T50.8X3	T50.8X4	T50.8X5	T50.8X6

Substance	Poisoning, Accidental (unintentional)	Poisoning, Intentional Self-harm	Poisoning, Assault	Poisoning, Undetermined	Adverse Effect	Under-dosing
Sulfogaiacol	T48.4X1	T48.4X2	T48.4X3	T48.4X4	T48.4X5	T48.4X6
Sulfomyxin	T36.8X1	T36.8X2	T36.8X3	T36.8X4	T36.8X5	T36.8X6
Sulfonal	T42.6X1	T42.6X2	T42.6X3	T42.6X4	T42.6X5	T42.6X6
Sulfonamide NEC	T37.0X1	T37.0X2	T37.0X3	T37.0X4	T37.0X5	T37.0X6
eye	T49.5X1	T49.5X2	T49.5X3	T49.5X4	T49.5X5	T49.5X6
Sulfonazide	T37.1X1	T37.1X2	T37.1X3	T37.1X4	T37.1X5	T37.1X6
Sulfones	T37.1X1	T37.1X2	T37.1X3	T37.1X4	T37.1X5	T37.1X6
Sulfonethylmethane	T42.6X1	T42.6X2	T42.6X3	T42.6X4	T42.6X5	T42.6X6
Sulfonmethane	T42.6X1	T42.6X2	T42.6X3	T42.6X4	T42.6X5	T42.6X6
Sulfonphthal, sulfonphthol	T50.8X1	T50.8X2	T50.8X3	T50.8X4	T50.8X5	T50.8X6
Sulfonylurea derivatives, oral	T38.3X1	T38.3X2	T38.3X3	T38.3X4	T38.3X5	T38.3X6
Sulforidazine	T43.3X1	T43.3X2	T43.3X3	T43.3X4	T43.3X5	T43.3X6
Sulfoxone	T37.1X1	T37.1X2	T37.1X3	T37.1X4	T37.1X5	T37.1X6
Sulfuric acid	T54.2X1	T54.2X2	T54.2X3	T54.2X4	—	—
Sulfur, sulfurated, sulfuric, sulfurous, sulfuryl (compounds NEC) (medicinal)	T49.4X1	T49.4X2	T49.4X3	T49.4X4	T49.4X5	T49.4X6
acid	T54.2X1	T54.2X2	T54.2X3	T54.2X4	—	—
dioxide (gas)	T59.1X1	T59.1X2	T59.1X3	T59.1X4	—	—
ether — see Ether(s)						
hydrogen	T59.6X1	T59.6X2	T59.6X3	T59.6X4	—	—
medicinal (keratolytic) (ointment) NEC	T49.4X1	T49.4X2	T49.4X3	T49.4X4	T49.4X5	T49.4X6
ointment	T49.0X1	T49.0X2	T49.0X3	T49.0X4	T49.0X5	T49.0X6
pesticide (vapor)	T60.91	T60.92	T60.93	T60.94	—	—
vapor NEC	T59.891	T59.892	T59.893	T59.894	—	—
Sulglicotide	T47.1X1	T47.1X2	T47.1X3	T47.1X4	T47.1X5	T47.1X6
Sulindac	T39.391	T39.392	T39.393	T39.394	T39.395	T39.396
Sulisatin	T47.2X1	T47.2X2	T47.2X3	T47.2X4	T47.2X5	T47.2X6
Sulisobenzone	T49.3X1	T49.3X2	T49.3X3	T49.3X4	T49.3X5	T49.3X6
Sulkowitch's reagent	T50.8X1	T50.8X2	T50.8X3	T50.8X4	T50.8X5	T50.8X6
Sulmetozine	T44.3X1	T44.3X2	T44.3X3	T44.3X4	T44.3X5	T44.3X6
Suloctidil	T46.7X1	T46.7X2	T46.7X3	T46.7X4	T46.7X5	T46.7X6
Sulph- — see also Sulf-						
Sulphadiazine	T37.0X1	T37.0X2	T37.0X3	T37.0X4	T37.0X5	T37.0X6
Sulphadimethoxine	T37.0X1	T37.0X2	T37.0X3	T37.0X4	T37.0X5	T37.0X6
Sulphadimidine	T37.0X1	T37.0X2	T37.0X3	T37.0X4	T37.0X5	T37.0X6
Sulphadione	T37.1X1	T37.1X2	T37.1X3	T37.1X4	T37.1X5	T37.1X6
Sulphafurazole	T37.0X1	T37.0X2	T37.0X3	T37.0X4	T37.0X5	T37.0X6
Sulphamethizole	T37.0X1	T37.0X2	T37.0X3	T37.0X4	T37.0X5	T37.0X6
Sulphamethoxazole	T37.0X1	T37.0X2	T37.0X3	T37.0X4	T37.0X5	T37.0X6
Sulphan blue	T50.8X1	T50.8X2	T50.8X3	T50.8X4	T50.8X5	T50.8X6
Sulphaphenazole	T37.0X1	T37.0X2	T37.0X3	T37.0X4	T37.0X5	T37.0X6
Sulphapyridine	T37.0X1	T37.0X2	T37.0X3	T37.0X4	T37.0X5	T37.0X6
Sulphasalazine	T37.0X1	T37.0X2	T37.0X3	T37.0X4	T37.0X5	T37.0X6
Sulphinpyrazone	T50.4X1	T50.4X2	T50.4X3	T50.4X4	T50.4X5	T50.4X6
Sulpiride	T43.591	T43.592	T43.593	T43.594	T43.595	T43.596
Sulprostone	T48.0X1	T48.0X2	T48.0X3	T48.0X4	T48.0X5	T48.0X6
Sulpyrine	T39.2X1	T39.2X2	T39.2X3	T39.2X4	T39.2X5	T39.2X6
Sultamicillin	T36.0X1	T36.0X2	T36.0X3	T36.0X4	T36.0X5	T36.0X6
Sulthiame	T42.6X1	T42.6X2	T42.6X3	T42.6X4	T42.6X5	T42.6X6
Sultiame	T42.6X1	T42.6X2	T42.6X3	T42.6X4	T42.6X5	T42.6X6
Sultopride	T43.591	T43.592	T43.593	T43.594	T43.595	T43.596
Sumatriptan	T39.8X1	T39.8X2	T39.8X3	T39.8X4	T39.8X5	T39.8X6
Sunflower seed oil	T46.6X1	T46.6X2	T46.6X3	T46.6X4	T46.6X5	T46.6X6
Superinone	T48.4X1	T48.4X2	T48.4X3	T48.4X4	T48.4X5	T48.4X6
Suprofen	T39.311	T39.312	T39.313	T39.314	T39.315	T39.316
Suramin (sodium)	T37.4X1	T37.4X2	T37.4X3	T37.4X4	T37.4X5	T37.4X6
Surfacaine	T41.3X1	T41.3X2	T41.3X3	T41.3X4	T41.3X5	T41.3X6
Surital	T41.1X1	T41.1X2	T41.1X3	T41.1X4	T41.1X5	T41.1X6
Sutilains	T45.3X1	T45.3X2	T45.3X3	T45.3X4	T45.3X5	T45.3X6
Suxamethonium (chloride)	T48.1X1	T48.1X2	T48.1X3	T48.1X4	T48.1X5	T48.1X6
Suxethonium (chloride)	T48.1X1	T48.1X2	T48.1X3	T48.1X4	T48.1X5	T48.1X6
Suxibuzone	T39.2X1	T39.2X2	T39.2X3	T39.2X4	T39.2X5	T39.2X6
Sweetener	T50.901	T50.902	T50.903	T50.904	T50.905	T50.906
Sweet niter spirit	T46.3X1	T46.3X2	T46.3X3	T46.3X4	T46.3X5	T46.3X6
Sweet oil (birch)	T49.3X1	T49.3X2	T49.3X3	T49.3X4	T49.3X5	T49.3X6
Sym-dichloroethyl ether	T53.6X1	T53.6X2	T53.6X3	T53.6X4	—	—
Sympatholytic NEC	T44.8X1	T44.8X2	T44.8X3	T44.8X4	T44.8X5	T44.8X6
haloalkylamine	T44.8X1	T44.8X2	T44.8X3	T44.8X4	T44.8X5	T44.8X6
Sympathomimetic NEC	T44.901	T44.902	T44.903	T44.904	T44.905	T44.906
anti-common-cold	T48.5X1	T48.5X2	T48.5X3	T48.5X4	T48.5X5	T48.5X6
bronchodilator	T48.6X1	T48.6X2	T48.6X3	T48.6X4	T48.6X5	T48.6X6
specified NEC	T44.991	T44.992	T44.993	T44.994	T44.995	T44.996
Synagis	T50.B91	T50.B92	T50.B93	T50.B94	T50.B95	T50.B96
Synalar	T49.0X1	T49.0X2	T49.0X3	T49.0X4	T49.0X5	T49.0X6
Synthroid	T38.1X1	T38.1X2	T38.1X3	T38.1X4	T38.1X5	T38.1X6
Syntocinon	T48.0X1	T48.0X2	T48.0X3	T48.0X4	T48.0X5	T48.0X6
Syrosingopine	T46.5X1	T46.5X2	T46.5X3	T46.5X4	T46.5X5	T46.5X6
Systemic drug	T45.91	T45.92	T45.93	T45.94	T45.95	T45.96

Substance	Poisoning, Accidental (unintentional)	Poisoning, Intentional Self-harm	Poisoning, Assault	Poisoning, Undetermined	Adverse Effect	Under-dosing
Systemic drug — continued						
specified NEC	T45.8X1	T45.8X2	T45.8X3	T45.8X4	T45.8X5	T45.8X6
Tablets — see also specified substance	T50.901	T50.902	T50.903	T50.904	T50.905	T50.906
Tace	T38.5X1	T38.5X2	T38.5X3	T38.5X4	T38.5X5	T38.5X6
Tacrine	T44.0X1	T44.0X2	T44.0X3	T44.0X4	T44.0X5	T44.0X6
Tadalafil	T46.7X1	T46.7X2	T46.7X3	T46.7X4	T46.7X5	T46.7X6
Talampicillin	T36.0X1	T36.0X2	T36.0X3	T36.0X4	T36.0X5	T36.0X6
Talbutal	T42.3X1	T42.3X2	T42.3X3	T42.3X4	T42.3X5	T42.3X6
Talc powder	T49.3X1	T49.3X2	T49.3X3	T49.3X4	T49.3X5	T49.3X6
Talcum	T49.3X1	T49.3X2	T49.3X3	T49.3X4	T49.3X5	T49.3X6
Taleranol	T38.6X1	T38.6X2	T38.6X3	T38.6X4	T38.6X5	T38.6X6
Tamoxifen	T38.6X1	T38.6X2	T38.6X3	T38.6X4	T38.6X5	T38.6X6
Tamsulosin	T44.6X1	T44.6X2	T44.6X3	T44.6X4	T44.6X5	T44.6X6
Tandearil, tanderil	T39.2X1	T39.2X2	T39.2X3	T39.2X4	T39.2X5	T39.2X6
Tannic acid	T49.2X1	T49.2X2	T49.2X3	T49.2X4	T49.2X5	T49.2X6
medicinal (astringent)	T49.2X1	T49.2X2	T49.2X3	T49.2X4	T49.2X5	T49.2X6
Tannin — see Tannic acid						
Tansy	T62.2X1	T62.2X2	T62.2X3	T62.2X4	—	—
TAO	T36.3X1	T36.3X2	T36.3X3	T36.3X4	T36.3X5	T36.3X6
Tapazole	T38.2X1	T38.2X2	T38.2X3	T38.2X4	T38.2X5	T38.2X6
Taractan	T43.591	T43.592	T43.593	T43.594	T43.595	T43.596
Tarantula (venomous)	T63.321	T63.322	T63.323	T63.324	—	—
Tartar emetic	T37.8X1	T37.8X2	T37.8X3	T37.8X4	T37.8X5	T37.8X6
Tartaric acid	T65.891	T65.892	T65.893	T65.894	—	—
Tartrated antimony (anti-infective)	T37.8X1	T37.8X2	T37.8X3	T37.8X4	T37.8X5	T37.8X6
Tartrate, laxative	T47.4X1	T47.4X2	T47.4X3	T47.4X4	T47.4X5	T47.4X6
Tar NEC	T52.0X1	T52.0X2	T52.0X3	T52.0X4	—	—
camphor	T60.1X1	T60.1X2	T60.1X3	T60.1X4	—	—
distillate	T49.1X1	T49.1X2	T49.1X3	T49.1X4	T49.1X5	T49.1X6
fumes	T59.891	T59.892	T59.893	T59.894	—	—
medicinal	T49.1X1	T49.1X2	T49.1X3	T49.1X4	T49.1X5	T49.1X6
ointment	T49.1X1	T49.1X2	T49.1X3	T49.1X4	T49.1X5	T49.1X6
Tauromustine	T45.1X1	T45.1X2	T45.1X3	T45.1X4	T45.1X5	T45.1X6
TCA — see Trichloroacetic acid						
TCDD	T53.7X1	T53.7X2	T53.7X3	T53.7X4	—	—
TDI (vapor)	T65.0X1	T65.0X2	T65.0X3	T65.0X4	—	—
Tear						
gas	T59.3X1	T59.3X2	T59.3X3	T59.3X4	—	—
solution	T49.5X1	T49.5X2	T49.5X3	T49.5X4	T49.5X5	T49.5X6
Teclothiazide	T50.2X1	T50.2X2	T50.2X3	T50.2X4	T50.2X5	T50.2X6
Teclozan	T37.3X1	T37.3X2	T37.3X3	T37.3X4	T37.3X5	T37.3X6
Tegafur	T45.1X1	T45.1X2	T45.1X3	T45.1X4	T45.1X5	T45.1X6
Tegretol	T42.1X1	T42.1X2	T42.1X3	T42.1X4	T42.1X5	T42.1X6
Teicoplanin	T36.8X1	T36.8X2	T36.8X3	T36.8X4	T36.8X5	T36.8X6
Telepaque	T50.8X1	T50.8X2	T50.8X3	T50.8X4	T50.8X5	T50.8X6
Tellurium	T56.891	T56.892	T56.893	T56.894	—	—
fumes	T56.891	T56.892	T56.893	T56.894	—	—
TEM	T45.1X1	T45.1X2	T45.1X3	T45.1X4	T45.1X5	T45.1X6
Temazepam	T42.4X1	T42.4X2	T42.4X3	T42.4X4	T42.4X5	T42.4X6
Temocillin	T36.0X1	T36.0X2	T36.0X3	T36.0X4	T36.0X5	T36.0X6
Tenamfetamine	T43.621	T43.622	T43.623	T43.624	T43.625	T43.626
Teniposide	T45.1X1	T45.1X2	T45.1X3	T45.1X4	T45.1X5	T45.1X6
Tenitramine	T46.3X1	T46.3X2	T46.3X3	T46.3X4	T46.3X5	T46.3X6
Tenoglicin	T48.4X1	T48.4X2	T48.4X3	T48.4X4	T48.4X5	T48.4X6
Tenonitrozole	T37.3X1	T37.3X2	T37.3X3	T37.3X4	T37.3X5	T37.3X6
Tenoxicam	T39.391	T39.392	T39.393	T39.394	T39.395	T39.396
TEPA	T45.1X1	T45.1X2	T45.1X3	T45.1X4	T45.1X5	T45.1X6
TEPP	T60.0X1	T60.0X2	T60.0X3	T60.0X4	—	—
Teprotide	T46.5X1	T46.5X2	T46.5X3	T46.5X4	T46.5X5	T46.5X6
Terazosin	T44.6X1	T44.6X2	T44.6X3	T44.6X4	T44.6X5	T44.6X6
Terbufos	T60.0X1	T60.0X2	T60.0X3	T60.0X4	—	—
Terbutaline	T48.6X1	T48.6X2	T48.6X3	T48.6X4	T48.6X5	T48.6X6
Terconazole	T49.0X1	T49.0X2	T49.0X3	T49.0X4	T49.0X5	T49.0X6
Terfenadine	T45.0X1	T45.0X2	T45.0X3	T45.0X4	T45.0X5	T45.0X6
Teriparatide (acetate)	T50.991	T50.992	T50.993	T50.994	T50.995	T50.996
Terizidone	T37.1X1	T37.1X2	T37.1X3	T37.1X4	T37.1X5	T37.1X6
Terlipressin	T38.891	T38.892	T38.893	T38.894	T38.895	T38.896
Terodiline	T46.3X1	T46.3X2	T46.3X3	T46.3X4	T46.3X5	T46.3X6
Teroxalene	T37.4X1	T37.4X2	T37.4X3	T37.4X4	T37.4X5	T37.4X6
Terpin (cis) hydrate	T48.4X1	T48.4X2	T48.4X3	T48.4X4	T48.4X5	T48.4X6
Terramycin	T36.4X1	T36.4X2	T36.4X3	T36.4X4	T36.4X5	T36.4X6
Tertatolol	T44.7X1	T44.7X2	T44.7X3	T44.7X4	T44.7X5	T44.7X6
Tessalon	T48.3X1	T48.3X2	T48.3X3	T48.3X4	T48.3X5	T48.3X6
Testolactone	T38.7X1	T38.7X2	T38.7X3	T38.7X4	T38.7X5	T38.7X6
Testosterone	T38.7X1	T38.7X2	T38.7X3	T38.7X4	T38.7X5	T38.7X6
Tetanus toxoid or vaccine	T50.A91	T50.A92	T50.A93	T50.A94	T50.A95	T50.A96
antitoxin	T50.Z11	T50.Z12	T50.Z13	T50.Z14	T50.Z15	T50.Z16
immune globulin (human)	T50.Z11	T50.Z12	T50.Z13	T50.Z14	T50.Z15	T50.Z16
toxoid	T50.A91	T50.A92	T50.A93	T50.A94	T50.A95	T50.A96
with diphtheria toxoid	T50.A21	T50.A22	T50.A23	T50.A24	T50.A25	T50.A26
with pertussis	T50.A11	T50.A12	T50.A13	T50.A14	T50.A15	T50.A16

Substance	Poisoning, Accidental (unintentional)	Poisoning, Intentional Self-harm	Poisoning, Assault	Poisoning, Undetermined	Adverse Effect	Under-dosing
Tetrabenazine	T43.591	T43.592	T43.593	T43.594	T43.595	T43.596
Tetracaine	T41.3X1	T41.3X2	T41.3X3	T41.3X4	T41.3X5	T41.3X6
nerve block (peripheral) (plexus)	T41.3X1	T41.3X2	T41.3X3	T41.3X4	T41.3X5	T41.3X6
regional	T41.3X1	T41.3X2	T41.3X3	T41.3X4	T41.3X5	T41.3X6
spinal	T41.3X1	T41.3X2	T41.3X3	T41.3X4	T41.3X5	T41.3X6
Tetrachlorethylene — see Tetrachloroethylene						
Tetrachlormethiazide	T50.2X1	T50.2X2	T50.2X3	T50.2X4	T50.2X5	T50.2X6
Tetrachloroethane	T53.6X1	T53.6X2	T53.6X3	T53.6X4	—	—
vapor	T53.6X1	T53.6X2	T53.6X3	T53.6X4	—	—
paint or varnish	T53.6X1	T53.6X2	T53.6X3	T53.6X4	—	—
Tetrachloroethylene (liquid)	T53.3X1	T53.3X2	T53.3X3	T53.3X4	—	—
medicinal	T37.4X1	T37.4X2	T37.4X3	T37.4X4	T37.4X5	T37.4X6
vapor	T53.3X1	T53.3X2	T53.3X3	T53.3X4	—	—
Tetrachloromethane — see Carbon tetrachloride						
Tetracosactide	T38.811	T38.812	T38.813	T38.814	T38.815	T38.816
Tetracosactrin	T38.811	T38.812	T38.813	T38.814	T38.815	T38.816
Tetracycline	T36.4X1	T36.4X2	T36.4X3	T36.4X4	T36.4X5	T36.4X6
ophthalmic preparation	T49.5X1	T49.5X2	T49.5X3	T49.5X4	T49.5X5	T49.5X6
topical NEC	T49.0X1	T49.0X2	T49.0X3	T49.0X4	T49.0X5	T49.0X6
Tetradifon	T60.8X1	T60.8X2	T60.8X3	T60.8X4	—	—
Tetradotoxin	T61.771	T61.772	T61.773	T61.774	—	—
Tetraethyl						
lead	T56.0X1	T56.0X2	T56.0X3	T56.0X4	—	—
pyrophosphate	T60.0X1	T60.0X2	T60.0X3	T60.0X4	—	—
Tetraethylammonium chloride	T44.2X1	T44.2X2	T44.2X3	T44.2X4	T44.2X5	T44.2X6
Tetraethylthiuram disulfide	T50.6X1	T50.6X2	T50.6X3	T50.6X4	T50.6X5	T50.6X6
Tetrahydroaminoacridine	T44.0X1	T44.0X2	T44.0X3	T44.0X4	T44.0X5	T44.0X6
Tetrahydrocannabinol	T40.7X1	T40.7X2	T40.7X3	T40.7X4	T40.7X5	T40.7X6
Tetrahydrofuran	T52.8X1	T52.8X2	T52.8X3	T52.8X4	—	—
Tetrahydronaphthalene	T52.8X1	T52.8X2	T52.8X3	T52.8X4	—	—
Tetrahydrozoline	T49.5X1	T49.5X2	T49.5X3	T49.5X4	T49.5X5	T49.5X6
Tetralin	T52.8X1	T52.8X2	T52.8X3	T52.8X4	—	—
Tetramethrin	T60.2X1	T60.2X2	T60.2X3	T60.2X4	—	—
Tetramethylthiuram (disulfide) NEC	T60.3X1	T60.3X2	T60.3X3	T60.3X4	—	—
medicinal	T49.0X1	T49.0X2	T49.0X3	T49.0X4	T49.0X5	T49.0X6
Tetramisole	T37.4X1	T37.4X2	T37.4X3	T37.4X4	T37.4X5	T37.4X6
Tetranicotinoyl fructose	T46.7X1	T46.7X2	T46.7X3	T46.7X4	T46.7X5	T46.7X6
Tetrazepam	T42.4X1	T42.4X2	T42.4X3	T42.4X4	T42.4X5	T42.4X6
Tetronal	T42.6X1	T42.6X2	T42.6X3	T42.6X4	T42.6X5	T42.6X6
Tetryl	T65.3X1	T65.3X2	T65.3X3	T65.3X4	—	—
Tetrylammonium chloride	T44.2X1	T44.2X2	T44.2X3	T44.2X4	T44.2X5	T44.2X6
Tetryzoline	T49.5X1	T49.5X2	T49.5X3	T49.5X4	T49.5X5	T49.5X6
Thalidomide	T45.1X1	T45.1X2	T45.1X3	T45.1X4	T45.1X5	T45.1X6
Thallium (compounds) (dust) NEC	T56.811	T56.812	T56.813	T56.814	—	—
pesticide	T60.4X1	T60.4X2	T60.4X3	T60.4X4	—	—
THC	T40.7X1	T40.7X2	T40.7X3	T40.7X4	T40.7X5	T40.7X6
Thebacon	T48.3X1	T48.3X2	T48.3X3	T48.3X4	T48.3X5	T48.3X6
Thebaine	T40.2X1	T40.2X2	T40.2X3	T40.2X4	T40.2X5	T40.2X6
Thenoic acid	T49.6X1	T49.6X2	T49.6X3	T49.6X4	T49.6X5	T49.6X6
Thenyldiamine	T45.0X1	T45.0X2	T45.0X3	T45.0X4	T45.0X5	T45.0X6
Theobromine (calcium salicylate)	T48.6X1	T48.6X2	T48.6X3	T48.6X4	T48.6X5	T48.6X6
sodium salicylate	T48.6X1	T48.6X2	T48.6X3	T48.6X4	T48.6X5	T48.6X6
Theophyllamine	T48.6X1	T48.6X2	T48.6X3	T48.6X4	T48.6X5	T48.6X6
Theophylline	T48.6X1	T48.6X2	T48.6X3	T48.6X4	T48.6X5	T48.6X6
aminobenzoic acid	T48.6X1	T48.6X2	T48.6X3	T48.6X4	T48.6X5	T48.6X6
ethylenediamine	T48.6X1	T48.6X2	T48.6X3	T48.6X4	T48.6X5	T48.6X6
piperazine	T48.6X1	T48.6X2	T48.6X3	T48.6X4	T48.6X5	T48.6X6
p-amino-benzoate						
Thiabendazole	T37.4X1	T37.4X2	T37.4X3	T37.4X4	T37.4X5	T37.4X6
Thialbarbital	T41.1X1	T41.1X2	T41.1X3	T41.1X4	T41.1X5	T41.1X6
Thiamazole	T38.2X1	T38.2X2	T38.2X3	T38.2X4	T38.2X5	T38.2X6
Thiambutosine	T37.1X1	T37.1X2	T37.1X3	T37.1X4	T37.1X5	T37.1X6
Thiamine	T45.2X1	T45.2X2	T45.2X3	T45.2X4	T45.2X5	T45.2X6
Thiamphenicol	T36.2X1	T36.2X2	T36.2X3	T36.2X4	T36.2X5	T36.2X6
Thiamylal	T41.1X1	T41.1X2	T41.1X3	T41.1X4	T41.1X5	T41.1X6
sodium	T41.1X1	T41.1X2	T41.1X3	T41.1X4	T41.1X5	T41.1X6
Thiazesim	T43.291	T43.292	T43.293	T43.294	T43.295	T43.296
Thiazides (diuretics)	T50.2X1	T50.2X2	T50.2X3	T50.2X4	T50.2X5	T50.2X6
Thiazinamium metilsulfate	T43.3X1	T43.3X2	T43.3X3	T43.3X4	T43.3X5	T43.3X6
Thiethylperazine	T43.3X1	T43.3X2	T43.3X3	T43.3X4	T43.3X5	T43.3X6
Thimerosal	T49.0X1	T49.0X2	T49.0X3	T49.0X4	T49.0X5	T49.0X6
ophthalmic preparation	T49.5X1	T49.5X2	T49.5X3	T49.5X4	T49.5X5	T49.5X6
Thioacetazone	T37.1X1	T37.1X2	T37.1X3	T37.1X4	T37.1X5	T37.1X6

Substance	Poisoning, Accidental (unintentional)	Poisoning, Intentional Self-harm	Poisoning, Assault	Poisoning, Undetermined	Adverse Effect	Under-dosing
Thioacetazone — continued						
with isoniazid	T37.1X1	T37.1X2	T37.1X3	T37.1X4	T37.1X5	T37.1X6
Thiobarbital sodium	T41.1X1	T41.1X2	T41.1X3	T41.1X4	T41.1X5	T41.1X6
Thiobarbiturate anesthetic	T41.1X1	T41.1X2	T41.1X3	T41.1X4	T41.1X5	T41.1X6
Thiobismol	T37.8X1	T37.8X2	T37.8X3	T37.8X4	T37.8X5	T37.8X6
Thiobutabarbital sodium	T41.1X1	T41.1X2	T41.1X3	T41.1X4	T41.1X5	T41.1X6
Thiocarbamate (insecticide)	T60.0X1	T60.0X2	T60.0X3	T60.0X4	—	—
Thiocarbamide	T38.2X1	T38.2X2	T38.2X3	T38.2X4	T38.2X5	T38.2X6
Thiocarbarsone	T37.8X1	T37.8X2	T37.8X3	T37.8X4	T37.8X5	T37.8X6
Thiocarlide	T37.1X1	T37.1X2	T37.1X3	T37.1X4	T37.1X5	T37.1X6
Thioctamide	T50.991	T50.992	T50.993	T50.994	T50.995	T50.996
Thioctic acid	T50.991	T50.992	T50.993	T50.994	T50.995	T50.996
Thiofos	T60.0X1	T60.0X2	T60.0X3	T60.0X4	—	—
Thioglycolate	T49.4X1	T49.4X2	T49.4X3	T49.4X4	T49.4X5	T49.4X6
Thioglycolic acid	T65.891	T65.892	T65.893	T65.894	—	—
Thioguanine	T45.1X1	T45.1X2	T45.1X3	T45.1X4	T45.1X5	T45.1X6
Thiomercaptomerin	T50.2X1	T50.2X2	T50.2X3	T50.2X4	T50.2X5	T50.2X6
Thiomerin	T50.2X1	T50.2X2	T50.2X3	T50.2X4	T50.2X5	T50.2X6
Thiomersal	T49.0X1	T49.0X2	T49.0X3	T49.0X4	T49.0X5	T49.0X6
Thionazin	T60.0X1	T60.0X2	T60.0X3	T60.0X4	—	—
Thiopental (sodium)	T41.1X1	T41.1X2	T41.1X3	T41.1X4	T41.1X5	T41.1X6
Thiopentone (sodium)	T41.1X1	T41.1X2	T41.1X3	T41.1X4	T41.1X5	T41.1X6
Thiopropazate	T43.3X1	T43.3X2	T43.3X3	T43.3X4	T43.3X5	T43.3X6
Thioproperazine	T43.3X1	T43.3X2	T43.3X3	T43.3X4	T43.3X5	T43.3X6
Thioridazine	T43.3X1	T43.3X2	T43.3X3	T43.3X4	T43.3X5	T43.3X6
Thiosinamine	T49.3X1	T49.3X2	T49.3X3	T49.3X4	T49.3X5	T49.3X6
Thiotepa	T45.1X1	T45.1X2	T45.1X3	T45.1X4	T45.1X5	T45.1X6
Thiothixene	T43.4X1	T43.4X2	T43.4X3	T43.4X4	T43.4X5	T43.4X6
Thiouracil (benzyl) (methyl) (propyl)	T38.2X1	T38.2X2	T38.2X3	T38.2X4	T38.2X5	T38.2X6
Thiourea	T38.2X1	T38.2X2	T38.2X3	T38.2X4	T38.2X5	T38.2X6
Thiphenamil	T44.3X1	T44.3X2	T44.3X3	T44.3X4	T44.3X5	T44.3X6
Thiram	T60.3X1	T60.3X2	T60.3X3	T60.3X4	—	—
medicinal	T49.2X1	T49.2X2	T49.2X3	T49.2X4	T49.2X5	T49.2X6
Thonzylamine (systemic)	T45.0X1	T45.0X2	T45.0X3	T45.0X4	T45.0X5	T45.0X6
mucosal decongestant	T48.5X1	T48.5X2	T48.5X3	T48.5X4	T48.5X5	T48.5X6
Thorazine	T43.3X1	T43.3X2	T43.3X3	T43.3X4	T43.3X5	T43.3X6
Thorium dioxide suspension	T50.8X1	T50.8X2	T50.8X3	T50.8X4	T50.8X5	T50.8X6
Thornapple	T62.2X1	T62.2X2	T62.2X3	T62.2X4	—	—
Throat drug NEC	T49.6X1	T49.6X2	T49.6X3	T49.6X4	T49.6X5	T49.6X6
Thrombin	T45.7X1	T45.7X2	T45.7X3	T45.7X4	T45.7X5	T45.7X6
Thrombolysin	T45.611	T45.612	T45.613	T45.614	T45.615	T45.616
Thromboplastin	T45.7X1	T45.7X2	T45.7X3	T45.7X4	T45.7X5	T45.7X6
Thurfyl nicotinate	T46.7X1	T46.7X2	T46.7X3	T46.7X4	T46.7X5	T46.7X6
Thymol	T49.0X1	T49.0X2	T49.0X3	T49.0X4	T49.0X5	T49.0X6
Thymopentin	T37.5X1	T37.5X2	T37.5X3	T37.5X4	T37.5X5	T37.5X6
Thymoxamine	T46.7X1	T46.7X2	T46.7X3	T46.7X4	T46.7X5	T46.7X6
Thymus extract	T38.891	T38.892	T38.893	T38.894	T38.895	T38.896
Thyreotrophic hormone	T38.811	T38.812	T38.813	T38.814	T38.815	T38.816
Thyroglobulin	T38.1X1	T38.1X2	T38.1X3	T38.1X4	T38.1X5	T38.1X6
Thyroid (hormone)	T38.1X1	T38.1X2	T38.1X3	T38.1X4	T38.1X5	T38.1X6
Thyrolar	T38.1X1	T38.1X2	T38.1X3	T38.1X4	T38.1X5	T38.1X6
Thyrotrophin	T38.811	T38.812	T38.813	T38.814	T38.815	T38.816
Thyrotropic hormone	T38.811	T38.812	T38.813	T38.814	T38.815	T38.816
Thyroxine	T38.1X1	T38.1X2	T38.1X3	T38.1X4	T38.1X5	T38.1X6
Tiabendazole	T37.4X1	T37.4X2	T37.4X3	T37.4X4	T37.4X5	T37.4X6
Tiamizide	T50.2X1	T50.2X2	T50.2X3	T50.2X4	T50.2X5	T50.2X6
Tianeptine	T43.291	T43.292	T43.293	T43.294	T43.295	T43.296
Tiapamil	T46.1X1	T46.1X2	T46.1X3	T46.1X4	T46.1X5	T46.1X6
Tiapride	T43.591	T43.592	T43.593	T43.594	T43.595	T43.596
Tiaprofenic acid	T39.311	T39.312	T39.313	T39.314	T39.315	T39.316
Tiaramide	T39.8X1	T39.8X2	T39.8X3	T39.8X4	T39.8X5	T39.8X6
Ticarcillin	T36.0X1	T36.0X2	T36.0X3	T36.0X4	T36.0X5	T36.0X6
Ticlatone	T49.0X1	T49.0X2	T49.0X3	T49.0X4	T49.0X5	T49.0X6
Ticlopidine	T45.521	T45.522	T45.523	T45.524	T45.525	T45.526
Ticrynafen	T50.1X1	T50.1X2	T50.1X3	T50.1X4	T50.1X5	T50.1X6
Tidiacic	T50.991	T50.992	T50.993	T50.994	T50.995	T50.996
Tiemonium	T44.3X1	T44.3X2	T44.3X3	T44.3X4	T44.3X5	T44.3X6
iodide	T44.3X1	T44.3X2	T44.3X3	T44.3X4	T44.3X5	T44.3X6
Tienilic acid	T50.1X1	T50.1X2	T50.1X3	T50.1X4	T50.1X5	T50.1X6
Tifenamil	T44.3X1	T44.3X2	T44.3X3	T44.3X4	T44.3X5	T44.3X6
Tigan	T45.0X1	T45.0X2	T45.0X3	T45.0X4	T45.0X5	T45.0X6
Tigloidine	T44.3X1	T44.3X2	T44.3X3	T44.3X4	T44.3X5	T44.3X6
Tilactase	T47.5X1	T47.5X2	T47.5X3	T47.5X4	T47.5X5	T47.5X6
Tiletamine	T41.291	T41.292	T41.293	T41.294	T41.295	T41.296
Tilidine	T40.4X1	T40.4X2	T40.4X3	T40.4X4	—	—
Timepidium bromide	T44.3X1	T44.3X2	T44.3X3	T44.3X4	T44.3X5	T44.3X6
Timiperone	T43.4X1	T43.4X2	T43.4X3	T43.4X4	T43.4X5	T43.4X6
Timolol	T44.7X1	T44.7X2	T44.7X3	T44.7X4	T44.7X5	T44.7X6
Tincture, iodine — see Iodine						

Substance	Poisoning, Accidental (unintentional)	Poisoning, Intentional Self-harm	Poisoning, Assault	Poisoning, Undetermined	Adverse Effect	Under-dosing
Tindal	T43.3X1	T43.3X2	T43.3X3	T43.3X4	T43.3X5	T43.3X6
Tinidazole	T37.3X1	T37.3X2	T37.3X3	T37.3X4	T37.3X5	T37.3X6
Tin (chloride) (dust) (oxide)	T56.6X1	T56.6X2	T56.6X3	T56.6X4	—	—
NEC						
anti-infectives	T37.8X1	T37.8X2	T37.8X3	T37.8X4	T37.8X5	T37.8X6
Tinoridine	T39.8X1	T39.8X2	T39.8X3	T39.8X4	T39.8X5	T39.8X6
Tiocarlide	T37.1X1	T37.1X2	T37.1X3	T37.1X4	T37.1X5	T37.1X6
Tioclomarol	T45.511	T45.512	T45.513	T45.514	T45.515	T45.516
Tioconazole	T49.0X1	T49.0X2	T49.0X3	T49.0X4	T49.0X5	T49.0X6
Tioguanine	T45.1X1	T45.1X2	T45.1X3	T45.1X4	T45.1X5	T45.1X6
Tiopronin	T50.991	T50.992	T50.993	T50.994	T50.995	T50.996
Tiotixene	T43.4X1	T43.4X2	T43.4X3	T43.4X4	T43.4X5	T43.4X6
Tioxolone	T49.4X1	T49.4X2	T49.4X3	T49.4X4	T49.4X5	T49.4X6
Tipepidine	T48.3X1	T48.3X2	T48.3X3	T48.3X4	T48.3X5	T48.3X6
Tiquizium bromide	T44.3X1	T44.3X2	T44.3X3	T44.3X4	T44.3X5	T44.3X6
Tiratricol	T38.1X1	T38.1X2	T38.1X3	T38.1X4	T38.1X5	T38.1X6
Tisopurine	T50.4X1	T50.4X2	T50.4X3	T50.4X4	T50.4X5	T50.4X6
Titanium (compounds) (vapor)	T56.891	T56.892	T56.893	T56.894		
dioxide	T49.3X1	T49.3X2	T49.3X3	T49.3X4	T49.3X5	T49.3X6
ointment	T49.3X1	T49.3X2	T49.3X3	T49.3X4	T49.3X5	T49.3X6
oxide	T49.3X1	T49.3X2	T49.3X3	T49.3X4	T49.3X5	T49.3X6
tetrachloride	T56.891	T56.892	T56.893	T56.894	—	—
Titanocene	T56.891	T56.892	T56.893	T56.894	—	—
Titroid	T38.1X1	T38.1X2	T38.1X3	T38.1X4	T38.1X5	T38.1X6
Tizanidine	T42.8X1	T42.8X2	T42.8X3	T42.8X4	T42.8X5	T42.8X6
TMTD	T60.3X1	T60.3X2	T60.3X3	T60.3X4	—	—
TNT (fumes)	T65.3X1	T65.3X2	T65.3X3	T65.3X4		
Toadstool	T62.0X1	T62.0X2	T62.0X3	T62.0X4	—	—
Tobacco NEC	T65.291	T65.292	T65.293	T65.294	—	—
cigarettes	T65.221	T65.222	T65.223	T65.224	—	—
Indian	T62.2X1	T62.2X2	T62.2X3	T62.2X4	—	—
smoke, second-hand	T65.221	T65.222	T65.223	T65.224	—	—
Tobramycin	T36.5X1	T36.5X2	T36.5X3	T36.5X4	T36.5X5	T36.5X6
Tocainide	T46.2X1	T46.2X2	T46.2X3	T46.2X4	T46.2X5	T46.2X6
Tocoferol	T45.2X1	T45.2X2	T45.2X3	T45.2X4	T45.2X5	T45.2X6
Tocopherol	T45.2X1	T45.2X2	T45.2X3	T45.2X4	T45.2X5	T45.2X6
acetate	T45.2X1	T45.2X2	T45.2X3	T45.2X4	T45.2X5	T45.2X6
Tocosamine	T48.0X1	T48.0X2	T48.0X3	T48.0X4	T48.0X5	T48.0X6
Todralazine	T46.5X1	T46.5X2	T46.5X3	T46.5X4	T46.5X5	T46.5X6
Tofisopam	T42.4X1	T42.4X2	T42.4X3	T42.4X4	T42.4X5	T42.4X6
Tofranil	T43.011	T43.012	T43.013	T43.014	T43.015	T43.016
Toilet deodorizer	T65.891	T65.892	T65.893	T65.894	—	—
Tolamolol	T44.7X1	T44.7X2	T44.7X3	T44.7X4	T44.7X5	T44.7X6
Tolazamide	T38.3X1	T38.3X2	T38.3X3	T38.3X4	T38.3X5	T38.3X6
Tolazoline	T46.7X1	T46.7X2	T46.7X3	T46.7X4	T46.7X5	T46.7X6
Tolbutamide (sodium)	T38.3X1	T38.3X2	T38.3X3	T38.3X4	T38.3X5	T38.3X6
Tolciclate	T49.0X1	T49.0X2	T49.0X3	T49.0X4	T49.0X5	T49.0X6
Tolmetin	T39.391	T39.392	T39.393	T39.394	T39.395	T39.396
Tolnaftate	T49.0X1	T49.0X2	T49.0X3	T49.0X4	T49.0X5	T49.0X6
Tolonidine	T46.5X1	T46.5X2	T46.5X3	T46.5X4	T46.5X5	T46.5X6
Toloxatone	T42.6X1	T42.6X2	T42.6X3	T42.6X4	T42.6X5	T42.6X6
Tolperisone	T44.3X1	T44.3X2	T44.3X3	T44.3X4	T44.3X5	T44.3X6
Tolserol	T42.8X1	T42.8X2	T42.8X3	T42.8X4	T42.8X5	T42.8X6
Toluene (liquid)	T52.2X1	T52.2X2	T52.2X3	T52.2X4		
diisocyanate	T65.0X1	T65.0X2	T65.0X3	T65.0X4	—	—
Toluidine	T65.891	T65.892	T65.893	T65.894	—	—
vapor	T59.891	T59.892	T59.893	T59.894	—	—
Toluol (liquid)	T52.2X1	T52.2X2	T52.2X3	T52.2X4		
vapor	T52.2X1	T52.2X2	T52.2X3	T52.2X4		
Toluylenediamine	T65.3X1	T65.3X2	T65.3X3	T65.3X4	—	—
Tolylene-2,4-diisocyanate	T65.0X1	T65.0X2	T65.0X3	T65.0X4	—	—
Tonic NEC	T50.901	T50.902	T50.903	T50.904	T50.905	T50.906
Topical action drug NEC	T49.91	T49.92	T49.93	T49.94	T49.95	T49.96
ear, nose or throat	T49.6X1	T49.6X2	T49.6X3	T49.6X4	T49.6X5	T49.6X6
eye	T49.5X1	T49.5X2	T49.5X3	T49.5X4	T49.5X5	T49.5X6
skin	T49.91	T49.92	T49.93	T49.94	T49.95	T49.96
specified NEC	T49.8X1	T49.8X2	T49.8X3	T49.8X4	T49.8X5	T49.8X6
Toquizine	T44.3X1	T44.3X2	T44.3X3	T44.3X4	T44.3X5	T44.3X6
Toremifene	T38.6X1	T38.6X2	T38.6X3	T38.6X4	T38.6X5	T38.6X6
Tosylchloramide sodium	T49.8X1	T49.8X2	T49.8X3	T49.8X4	T49.8X5	T49.8X6
Toxaphene (dust) (spray)	T60.1X1	T60.1X2	T60.1X3	T60.1X4	—	—
Toxin, diphtheria (Schick Test)	T50.8X1	T50.8X2	T50.8X3	T50.8X4	T50.8X5	T50.8X6
Toxoid						
combined	T50.A21	T50.A22	T50.A23	T50.A24	T50.A25	T50.A26
diphtheria	T50.A91	T50.A92	T50.A93	T50.A94	T50.A95	T50.A96
tetanus	T50.A91	T50.A92	T50.A93	T50.A94	T50.A95	T50.A96
Trace element NEC	T45.8X1	T45.8X2	T45.8X3	T45.8X4	T45.8X5	T45.8X6
Tractor fuel NEC	T52.0X1	T52.0X2	T52.0X3	T52.0X4	—	—
Tragacanth	T50.991	T50.992	T50.993	T50.994	T50.995	T50.996
Tramadol	T40.4X1	T40.4X2	T40.4X3	T40.4X4	T40.4X5	T40.4X6
Tramazoline	T48.5X1	T48.5X2	T48.5X3	T48.5X4	T48.5X5	T48.5X6

Additional Character May Be Required — Refer to the Tabular List for Character Selection   ▽ Subterms under main terms may continue to next column or page

Substance	Poisoning, Accidental (unintentional)	Poisoning, Intentional Self-harm	Poisoning, Assault	Poisoning, Undetermined	Adverse Effect	Underdosing
Tranexamic acid	T45.621	T45.622	T45.623	T45.624	T45.625	T45.626
Tranilast	T45.0X1	T45.0X2	T45.0X3	T45.0X4	T45.0X5	T45.0X6
Tranquilizer NEC	T43.501	T43.502	T43.503	T43.504	T43.505	T43.506
with hypnotic or sedative	T42.6X1	T42.6X2	T42.6X3	T42.6X4	T42.6X5	T42.6X6
benzodiazepine NEC	T42.4X1	T42.4X2	T42.4X3	T42.4X4	T42.4X5	T42.4X6
butyrophenone NEC	T43.4X1	T43.4X2	T43.4X3	T43.4X4	T43.4X5	T43.4X6
carbamate	T43.591	T43.592	T43.593	T43.594	T43.595	T43.596
dimethylamine	T43.3X1	T43.3X2	T43.3X3	T43.3X4	T43.3X5	T43.3X6
ethylamine	T43.3X1	T43.3X2	T43.3X3	T43.3X4	T43.3X5	T43.3X6
hydroxyzine	T43.591	T43.592	T43.593	T43.594	T43.595	T43.596
major NEC	T43.501	T43.502	T43.503	T43.504	T43.505	T43.506
penothiazine NEC	T43.3X1	T43.3X2	T43.3X3	T43.3X4	T43.3X5	T43.3X6
phenothiazine-based	T43.3X1	T43.3X2	T43.3X3	T43.3X4	T43.3X5	T43.3X6
piperazine NEC	T43.3X1	T43.3X2	T43.3X3	T43.3X4	T43.3X5	T43.3X6
piperidine	T43.3X1	T43.3X2	T43.3X3	T43.3X4	T43.3X5	T43.3X6
propylamine	T43.3X1	T43.3X2	T43.3X3	T43.3X4	T43.3X5	T43.3X6
specified NEC	T43.591	T43.592	T43.593	T43.594	T43.595	T43.596
thioxanthene NEC	T43.591	T43.592	T43.593	T43.594	T43.595	T43.596
Tranxene	T42.4X1	T42.4X2	T42.4X3	T42.4X4	T42.4X5	T42.4X6
Tranylcypromine	T43.1X1	T43.1X2	T43.1X3	T43.1X4	T43.1X5	T43.1X6
Trapidil	T46.3X1	T46.3X2	T46.3X3	T46.3X4	T46.3X5	T46.3X6
Trasentine	T44.3X1	T44.3X2	T44.3X3	T44.3X4	T44.3X5	T44.3X6
Travert	T50.3X1	T50.3X2	T50.3X3	T50.3X4	T50.3X5	T50.3X6
Trazodone	T43.211	T43.212	T43.213	T43.214	T43.215	T43.216
Trecator	T37.1X1	T37.1X2	T37.1X3	T37.1X4	T37.1X5	T37.1X6
Treosulfan	T45.1X1	T45.1X2	T45.1X3	T45.1X4	T45.1X5	T45.1X6
Tretamine	T45.1X1	T45.1X2	T45.1X3	T45.1X4	T45.1X5	T45.1X6
Tretinoin	T49.0X1	T49.0X2	T49.0X3	T49.0X4	T49.0X5	T49.0X6
Tretoquinol	T48.6X1	T48.6X2	T48.6X3	T48.6X4	T48.6X5	T48.6X6
Triacetin	T49.0X1	T49.0X2	T49.0X3	T49.0X4	T49.0X5	T49.0X6
Triacetoxyanthracene	T49.4X1	T49.4X2	T49.4X3	T49.4X4	T49.4X5	T49.4X6
Triacetyloleandomycin	T36.3X1	T36.3X2	T36.3X3	T36.3X4	T36.3X5	T36.3X6
Triamcinolone	T38.0X1	T38.0X2	T38.0X3	T38.0X4	T38.0X5	T38.0X6
ENT agent	T49.6X1	T49.6X2	T49.6X3	T49.6X4	T49.6X5	T49.6X6
hexacetonide	T49.0X1	T49.0X2	T49.0X3	T49.0X4	T49.0X5	T49.0X6
ophthalmic preparation	T49.5X1	T49.5X2	T49.5X3	T49.5X4	T49.5X5	T49.5X6
topical NEC	T49.0X1	T49.0X2	T49.0X3	T49.0X4	T49.0X5	T49.0X6
Triampyzine	T44.3X1	T44.3X2	T44.3X3	T44.3X4	T44.3X5	T44.3X6
Triamterene	T50.2X1	T50.2X2	T50.2X3	T50.2X4	T50.2X5	T50.2X6
Triazine (herbicide)	T60.3X1	T60.3X2	T60.3X3	T60.3X4	—	—
Triaziquone	T45.1X1	T45.1X2	T45.1X3	T45.1X4	T45.1X5	T45.1X6
Triazolam	T42.4X1	T42.4X2	T42.4X3	T42.4X4	T42.4X5	T42.4X6
Triazole (herbicide)	T60.3X1	T60.3X2	T60.3X3	T60.3X4	—	—
Tribenoside	T46.991	T46.992	T46.993	T46.994	T46.995	T46.996
Tribromacetaldehyde	T42.6X1	T42.6X2	T42.6X3	T42.6X4	T42.6X5	T42.6X6
Tribromoethanol, rectal	T41.291	T41.292	T41.293	T41.294	T41.295	T41.296
Tribromomethane	T42.6X1	T42.6X2	T42.6X3	T42.6X4	T42.6X5	T42.6X6
Trichlorethane	T53.2X1	T53.2X2	T53.2X3	T53.2X4	—	—
Trichlorethylene	T53.2X1	T53.2X2	T53.2X3	T53.2X4	—	—
Trichlorfon	T60.0X1	T60.0X2	T60.0X3	T60.0X4	—	—
Trichlormethiazide	T50.2X1	T50.2X2	T50.2X3	T50.2X4	T50.2X5	T50.2X6
Trichlormethine	T45.1X1	T45.1X2	T45.1X3	T45.1X4	T45.1X5	T45.1X6
Trichloroacetic acid, Trichloracetic acid	T54.2X1	T54.2X2	T54.2X3	T54.2X4	—	—
medicinal	T49.4X1	T49.4X2	T49.4X3	T49.4X4	T49.4X5	T49.4X6
Trichloroethane	T53.2X1	T53.2X2	T53.2X3	T53.2X4	—	—
Trichloroethanol	T42.6X1	T42.6X2	T42.6X3	T42.6X4	T42.6X5	T42.6X6
Trichloroethylene (liquid)	T53.2X1	T53.2X2	T53.2X3	T53.2X4	—	—
(vapor)						
anesthetic (gas)	T41.0X1	T41.0X2	T41.0X3	T41.0X4	T41.0X5	T41.0X6
vapor NEC	T53.2X1	T53.2X2	T53.2X3	T53.2X4	—	—
Trichloroethyl phosphate	T42.6X1	T42.6X2	T42.6X3	T42.6X4	T42.6X5	T42.6X6
Trichlorofluoromethane NEC	T53.5X1	T53.5X2	T53.5X3	T53.5X4	—	—
Trichloronate	T60.0X1	T60.0X2	T60.0X3	T60.0X4	—	—
Trichloropropane	T53.6X1	T53.6X2	T53.6X3	T53.6X4	—	—
Trichlorotriethylamine	T45.1X1	T45.1X2	T45.1X3	T45.1X4	T45.1X5	T45.1X6
Trichomonacides NEC	T37.3X1	T37.3X2	T37.3X3	T37.3X4	T37.3X5	T37.3X6
Trichomycin	T36.7X1	T36.7X2	T36.7X3	T36.7X4	T36.7X5	T36.7X6
Triclobisonium chloride	T49.0X1	T49.0X2	T49.0X3	T49.0X4	T49.0X5	T49.0X6
Triclocarban	T49.0X1	T49.0X2	T49.0X3	T49.0X4	T49.0X5	T49.0X6
Triclofos	T42.6X1	T42.6X2	T42.6X3	T42.6X4	T42.6X5	T42.6X6
Triclosan	T49.0X1	T49.0X2	T49.0X3	T49.0X4	T49.0X5	T49.0X6
Tricresyl phosphate	T65.891	T65.892	T65.893	T65.894	—	—
solvent	T52.91	T52.92	T52.93	T52.94	—	—
Tricyclamol chloride	T44.3X1	T44.3X2	T44.3X3	T44.3X4	T44.3X5	T44.3X6
Tridesilon	T49.0X1	T49.0X2	T49.0X3	T49.0X4	T49.0X5	T49.0X6
Tridihexethyl iodide	T44.3X1	T44.3X2	T44.3X3	T44.3X4	T44.3X5	T44.3X6
Tridione	T42.2X1	T42.2X2	T42.2X3	T42.2X4	T42.2X5	T42.2X6
Trientine	T45.8X1	T45.8X2	T45.8X3	T45.8X4	T45.8X5	T45.8X6
Triethanolamine NEC	T54.3X1	T54.3X2	T54.3X3	T54.3X4	—	—
detergent	T54.3X1	T54.3X2	T54.3X3	T54.3X4	—	—
trinitrate (biphosphate)	T46.3X1	T46.3X2	T46.3X3	T46.3X4	T46.3X5	T46.3X6

Substance	Poisoning, Accidental (unintentional)	Poisoning, Intentional Self-harm	Poisoning, Assault	Poisoning, Undetermined	Adverse Effect	Underdosing
Triethanomelamine	T45.1X1	T45.1X2	T45.1X3	T45.1X4	T45.1X5	T45.1X6
Triethylenemelamine	T45.1X1	T45.1X2	T45.1X3	T45.1X4	T45.1X5	T45.1X6
Triethylenephosphoramide	T45.1X1	T45.1X2	T45.1X3	T45.1X4	T45.1X5	T45.1X6
Triethylenethiophosphoramide	T45.1X1	T45.1X2	T45.1X3	T45.1X4	T45.1X5	T45.1X6
Trifluoperazine	T43.3X1	T43.3X2	T43.3X3	T43.3X4	T43.3X5	T43.3X6
Trifluoroethyl vinyl ether	T41.0X1	T41.0X2	T41.0X3	T41.0X4	T41.0X5	T41.0X6
Trifluperidol	T43.4X1	T43.4X2	T43.4X3	T43.4X4	T43.4X5	T43.4X6
Triflupromazine	T43.3X1	T43.3X2	T43.3X3	T43.3X4	T43.3X5	T43.3X6
Trifluridine	T37.5X1	T37.5X2	T37.5X3	T37.5X4	T37.5X5	T37.5X6
Triflusal	T45.521	T45.522	T45.523	T45.524	T45.525	T45.526
Trihexyphenidyl	T44.3X1	T44.3X2	T44.3X3	T44.3X4	T44.3X5	T44.3X6
Triiodothyronine	T38.1X1	T38.1X2	T38.1X3	T38.1X4	T38.1X5	T38.1X6
Trilene	T41.0X1	T41.0X2	T41.0X3	T41.0X4	T41.0X5	T41.0X6
Trilostane	T38.991	T38.992	T38.993	T38.994	T38.995	T38.996
Trimebutine	T44.3X1	T44.3X2	T44.3X3	T44.3X4	T44.3X5	T44.3X6
Trimecaine	T41.3X1	T41.3X2	T41.3X3	T41.3X4	T41.3X5	T41.3X6
Trimeprazine (tartrate)	T44.3X1	T44.3X2	T44.3X3	T44.3X4	T44.3X5	T44.3X6
Trimetaphan camsilate	T44.2X1	T44.2X2	T44.2X3	T44.2X4	T44.2X5	T44.2X6
Trimetazidine	T46.7X1	T46.7X2	T46.7X3	T46.7X4	T46.7X5	T46.7X6
Trimethadione	T42.2X1	T42.2X2	T42.2X3	T42.2X4	T42.2X5	T42.2X6
Trimethaphan	T44.2X1	T44.2X2	T44.2X3	T44.2X4	T44.2X5	T44.2X6
Trimethidinium	T44.2X1	T44.2X2	T44.2X3	T44.2X4	T44.2X5	T44.2X6
Trimethobenzamide	T45.0X1	T45.0X2	T45.0X3	T45.0X4	T45.0X5	T45.0X6
Trimethoprim	T37.8X1	T37.8X2	T37.8X3	T37.8X4	T37.8X5	T37.8X6
with sulfamethoxazole	T36.8X1	T36.8X2	T36.8X3	T36.8X4	T36.8X5	T36.8X6
Trimethylcarbinol	T51.3X1	T51.3X2	T51.3X3	T51.3X4	—	—
Trimethylpsoralen	T49.3X1	T49.3X2	T49.3X3	T49.3X4	T49.3X5	T49.3X6
Trimeton	T45.0X1	T45.0X2	T45.0X3	T45.0X4	T45.0X5	T45.0X6
Trimetrexate	T45.1X1	T45.1X2	T45.1X3	T45.1X4	T45.1X5	T45.1X6
Trimipramine	T43.011	T43.012	T43.013	T43.014	T43.015	T43.016
Trimustine	T45.1X1	T45.1X2	T45.1X3	T45.1X4	T45.1X5	T45.1X6
Trinitrine	T46.3X1	T46.3X2	T46.3X3	T46.3X4	T46.3X5	T46.3X6
Trinitrobenzol	T65.3X1	T65.3X2	T65.3X3	T65.3X4	—	—
Trinitrophenol	T65.3X1	T65.3X2	T65.3X3	T65.3X4	—	—
Trinitrotoluene (fumes)	T65.3X1	T65.3X2	T65.3X3	T65.3X4	—	—
Trional	T42.6X1	T42.6X2	T42.6X3	T42.6X4	T42.6X5	T42.6X6
Triorthocresyl phosphate	T65.891	T65.892	T65.893	T65.894	—	—
Trioxide of arsenic	T57.0X1	T57.0X2	T57.0X3	T57.0X4	—	—
Trioxysalen	T49.4X1	T49.4X2	T49.4X3	T49.4X4	T49.4X5	T49.4X6
Tripamide	T50.2X1	T50.2X2	T50.2X3	T50.2X4	T50.2X5	T50.2X6
Triparanol	T46.6X1	T46.6X2	T46.6X3	T46.6X4	T46.6X5	T46.6X6
Tripelennamine	T45.0X1	T45.0X2	T45.0X3	T45.0X4	T45.0X5	T45.0X6
Triperiden	T44.3X1	T44.3X2	T44.3X3	T44.3X4	T44.3X5	T44.3X6
Triperidol	T43.4X1	T43.4X2	T43.4X3	T43.4X4	T43.4X5	T43.4X6
Triphenylphosphate	T65.891	T65.892	T65.893	T65.894	—	—
Triple						
bromides	T42.6X1	T42.6X2	T42.6X3	T42.6X4	T42.6X5	T42.6X6
carbonate	T47.1X1	T47.1X2	T47.1X3	T47.1X4	T47.1X5	T47.1X6
vaccine						
DPT	T50.A11	T50.A12	T50.A13	T50.A14	T50.A15	T50.A16
including pertussis	T50.A11	T50.A12	T50.A13	T50.A14	T50.A15	T50.A16
MMR	T50.B91	T50.B92	T50.B93	T50.B94	T50.B95	T50.B96
Triprolidine	T45.0X1	T45.0X2	T45.0X3	T45.0X4	T45.0X5	T45.0X6
Trisodium hydrogen edetate	T50.6X1	T50.6X2	T50.6X3	T50.6X4	T50.6X5	T50.6X6
Trisoralen	T49.3X1	T49.3X2	T49.3X3	T49.3X4	T49.3X5	T49.3X6
Trisulfapyrimidines	T37.0X1	T37.0X2	T37.0X3	T37.0X4	T37.0X5	T37.0X6
Trithiozine	T44.3X1	T44.3X2	T44.3X3	T44.3X4	T44.3X5	T44.3X6
Tritiozine	T44.3X1	T44.3X2	T44.3X3	T44.3X4	T44.3X5	T44.3X6
Tritoqualine	T45.0X1	T45.0X2	T45.0X3	T45.0X4	T45.0X5	T45.0X6
Trofosfamide	T45.1X1	T45.1X2	T45.1X3	T45.1X4	T45.1X5	T45.1X6
Troleandomycin	T36.3X1	T36.3X2	T36.3X3	T36.3X4	T36.3X5	T36.3X6
Trolnitrate (phosphate)	T46.3X1	T46.3X2	T46.3X3	T46.3X4	T46.3X5	T46.3X6
Tromantadine	T37.5X1	T37.5X2	T37.5X3	T37.5X4	T37.5X5	T37.5X6
Trometamol	T50.2X1	T50.2X2	T50.2X3	T50.2X4	T50.2X5	T50.2X6
Tromethamine	T50.2X1	T50.2X2	T50.2X3	T50.2X4	T50.2X5	T50.2X6
Tronothane	T41.3X1	T41.3X2	T41.3X3	T41.3X4	T41.3X5	T41.3X6
Tropacine	T44.3X1	T44.3X2	T44.3X3	T44.3X4	T44.3X5	T44.3X6
Tropatepine	T44.3X1	T44.3X2	T44.3X3	T44.3X4	T44.3X5	T44.3X6
Tropicamide	T44.3X1	T44.3X2	T44.3X3	T44.3X4	T44.3X5	T44.3X6
Trospium chloride	T44.3X1	T44.3X2	T44.3X3	T44.3X4	T44.3X5	T44.3X6
Troxerutin	T46.991	T46.992	T46.993	T46.994	T46.995	T46.996
Troxidone	T42.2X1	T42.2X2	T42.2X3	T42.2X4	T42.2X5	T42.2X6
Tryparsamide	T37.3X1	T37.3X2	T37.3X3	T37.3X4	T37.3X5	T37.3X6
Trypsin	T45.3X1	T45.3X2	T45.3X3	T45.3X4	T45.3X5	T45.3X6
Tryptizol	T43.011	T43.012	T43.013	T43.014	T43.015	T43.016
TSH	T38.811	T38.812	T38.813	T38.814	T38.815	T38.816
Tuaminoheptane	T48.5X1	T48.5X2	T48.5X3	T48.5X4	T48.5X5	T48.5X6
Tuberculin, purified protein derivative (PPD)	T50.8X1	T50.8X2	T50.8X3	T50.8X4	T50.8X5	T50.8X6
Tubocurare	T48.1X1	T48.1X2	T48.1X3	T48.1X4	T48.1X5	T48.1X6
Tubocurarine (chloride)	T48.1X1	T48.1X2	T48.1X3	T48.1X4	T48.1X5	T48.1X6
Tulobuterol	T48.6X1	T48.6X2	T48.6X3	T48.6X4	T48.6X5	T48.6X6

Table of Drugs and Chemicals

Tranexamic acid — Tulobuterol

Substance	Poisoning, Accidental (unintentional)	Poisoning, Intentional Self-harm	Poisoning, Assault	Poisoning, Undetermined	Adverse Effect	Under-dosing
Turpentine (spirits of)	T52.8X1	T52.8X2	T52.8X3	T52.8X4	—	—
vapor	T52.8X1	T52.8X2	T52.8X3	T52.8X4	—	—
Tybamate	T43.591	T43.592	T43.593	T43.594	T43.595	T43.596
Tyloxapol	T48.4X1	T48.4X2	T48.4X3	T48.4X4	T48.4X5	T48.4X6
Tymazoline	T48.5X1	T48.5X2	T48.5X3	T48.5X4	T48.5X5	T48.5X6
Typhoid-paratyphoid vaccine	T50.A91	T50.A92	T50.A93	T50.A94	T50.A95	T50.A96
Typhus vaccine	T50.A91	T50.A92	T50.A93	T50.A94	T50.A95	T50.A96
Tyropanoate	T50.8X1	T50.8X2	T50.8X3	T50.8X4	T50.8X5	T50.8X6
Tyrothricin	T49.6X1	T49.6X2	T49.6X3	T49.6X4	T49.6X5	T49.6X6
ENT agent	T49.6X1	T49.6X2	T49.6X3	T49.6X4	T49.6X5	T49.6X6
ophthalmic preparation	T49.5X1	T49.5X2	T49.5X3	T49.5X4	T49.5X5	T49.5X6
Ufenamate	T39.391	T39.392	T39.393	T39.394	T39.395	T39.396
Ultraviolet light protectant	T49.3X1	T49.3X2	T49.3X3	T49.3X4	T49.3X5	T49.3X6
Undecenoic acid	T49.0X1	T49.0X2	T49.0X3	T49.0X4	T49.0X5	T49.0X6
Undecoylium	T49.0X1	T49.0X2	T49.0X3	T49.0X4	T49.0X5	T49.0X6
Undecylenic acid (derivatives)	T49.0X1	T49.0X2	T49.0X3	T49.0X4	T49.0X5	T49.0X6
Unna's boot	T49.3X1	T49.3X2	T49.3X3	T49.3X4	T49.3X5	T49.3X6
Unsaturated fatty acid	T46.6X1	T46.6X2	T46.6X3	T46.6X4	T46.6X5	T46.6X6
Uracil mustard	T45.1X1	T45.1X2	T45.1X3	T45.1X4	T45.1X5	T45.1X6
Uramustine	T45.1X1	T45.1X2	T45.1X3	T45.1X4	T45.1X5	T45.1X6
Urapidil	T46.5X1	T46.5X2	T46.5X3	T46.5X4	T46.5X5	T46.5X6
Urari	T48.1X1	T48.1X2	T48.1X3	T48.1X4	T48.1X5	T48.1X6
Urate oxidase	T50.4X1	T50.4X2	T50.4X3	T50.4X4	T50.4X5	T50.4X6
Urea	T47.3X1	T47.3X2	T47.3X3	T47.3X4	T47.3X5	T47.3X6
peroxide	T49.0X1	T49.0X2	T49.0X3	T49.0X4	T49.0X5	T49.0X6
stibamine	T37.4X1	T37.4X2	T37.4X3	T37.4X4	T37.4X5	T37.4X6
topical	T49.8X1	T49.8X2	T49.8X3	T49.8X4	T49.8X5	T49.8X6
Urethane	T45.1X1	T45.1X2	T45.1X3	T45.1X4	T45.1X5	T45.1X6
Urginea (maritima) (scilla) — see Squill						
Uric acid metabolism drug NEC	T50.4X1	T50.4X2	T50.4X3	T50.4X4	T50.4X5	T50.4X6
Uricosuric agent	T50.4X1	T50.4X2	T50.4X3	T50.4X4	T50.4X5	T50.4X6
Urinary anti-infective	T37.8X1	T37.8X2	T37.8X3	T37.8X4	T37.8X5	T37.8X6
Urofollitropin	T38.811	T38.812	T38.813	T38.814	T38.815	T38.816
Urokinase	T45.611	T45.612	T45.613	T45.614	T45.615	T45.616
Urokon	T50.8X1	T50.8X2	T50.8X3	T50.8X4	T50.8X5	T50.8X6
Ursodeoxycholic acid	T50.991	T50.992	T50.993	T50.994	T50.995	T50.996
Ursodiol	T50.991	T50.992	T50.993	T50.994	T50.995	T50.996
Urtica	T62.2X1	T62.2X2	T62.2X3	T62.2X4	—	—
Utility gas — see Gas, utility						
Vaccine NEC	T50.Z91	T50.Z92	T50.Z93	T50.Z94	T50.Z95	T50.Z96
antineoplastic	T50.Z91	T50.Z92	T50.Z93	T50.Z94	T50.Z95	T50.Z96
bacterial NEC	T50.A91	T50.A92	T50.A93	T50.A94	T50.A95	T50.A96
with						
other bacterial component	T50.A21	T50.A22	T50.A23	T50.A24	T50.A25	T50.A26
pertussis component	T50.A11	T50.A12	T50.A13	T50.A14	T50.A15	T50.A16
viral-rickettsial component	T50.A21	T50.A22	T50.A23	T50.A24	T50.A25	T50.A26
mixed NEC	T50.A21	T50.A22	T50.A23	T50.A24	T50.A25	T50.A26
BCG	T50.A91	T50.A92	T50.A93	T50.A94	T50.A95	T50.A96
cholera	T50.A91	T50.A92	T50.A93	T50.A94	T50.A95	T50.A96
diphtheria	T50.A91	T50.A92	T50.A93	T50.A94	T50.A95	T50.A96
with tetanus	T50.A21	T50.A22	T50.A23	T50.A24	T50.A25	T50.A26
and pertussis	T50.A11	T50.A12	T50.A13	T50.A14	T50.A15	T50.A16
influenza	T50.B91	T50.B92	T50.B93	T50.B94	T50.B95	T50.B96
measles	T50.B91	T50.B92	T50.B93	T50.B94	T50.B95	T50.B96
with mumps and rubella	T50.B91	T50.B92	T50.B93	T50.B94	T50.B95	T50.B96
meningococcal	T50.A91	T50.A92	T50.A93	T50.A94	T50.A95	T50.A96
mumps	T50.B91	T50.B92	T50.B93	T50.B94	T50.B95	T50.B96
paratyphoid	T50.A91	T50.A92	T50.A93	T50.A94	T50.A95	T50.A96
pertussis	T50.A11	T50.A12	T50.A13	T50.A14	T50.A15	T50.A16
with diphtheria	T50.A11	T50.A12	T50.A13	T50.A14	T50.A15	T50.A16
and tetanus	T50.A11	T50.A12	T50.A13	T50.A14	T50.A15	T50.A16
with other component	T50.A11	T50.A12	T50.A13	T50.A14	T50.A15	T50.A16
plague	T50.A91	T50.A92	T50.A93	T50.A94	T50.A95	T50.A96
poliomyelitis	T50.B91	T50.B92	T50.B93	T50.B94	T50.B95	T50.B96
poliovirus	T50.B91	T50.B92	T50.B93	T50.B94	T50.B95	T50.B96
rabies	T50.B91	T50.B92	T50.B93	T50.B94	T50.B95	T50.B96
respiratory syncytial virus	T50.B91	T50.B92	T50.B93	T50.B94	T50.B95	T50.B96
rickettsial NEC	T50.A91	T50.A92	T50.A93	T50.A94	T50.A95	T50.A96
with bacterial component	T50.A21	T50.A22	T50.A23	T50.A24	T50.A25	T50.A26
Rocky Mountain spotted fever	T50.A91	T50.A92	T50.A93	T50.A94	T50.A95	T50.A96
rubella	T50.B91	T50.B92	T50.B93	T50.B94	T50.B95	T50.B96
sabin oral	T50.B91	T50.B92	T50.B93	T50.B94	T50.B95	T50.B96
smallpox	T50.B11	T50.B12	T50.B13	T50.B14	T50.B15	T50.B16
TAB	T50.A91	T50.A92	T50.A93	T50.A94	T50.A95	T50.A96

Substance	Poisoning, Accidental (unintentional)	Poisoning, Intentional Self-harm	Poisoning, Assault	Poisoning, Undetermined	Adverse Effect	Under-dosing
Vaccine — continued						
tetanus	T50.A91	T50.A92	T50.A93	T50.A94	T50.A95	T50.A96
typhoid	T50.A91	T50.A92	T50.A93	T50.A94	T50.A95	T50.A96
typhus	T50.A91	T50.A92	T50.A93	T50.A94	T50.A95	T50.A96
viral NEC	T50.B91	T50.B92	T50.B93	T50.B94	T50.B95	T50.B96
yellow fever	T50.B91	T50.B92	T50.B93	T50.B94	T50.B95	T50.B96
Vaccinia immune globulin	T50.Z11	T50.Z12	T50.Z13	T50.Z14	T50.Z15	T50.Z16
Vaginal contraceptives	T49.8X1	T49.8X2	T49.8X3	T49.8X4	T49.8X5	T49.8X6
Valerian						
root	T42.6X1	T42.6X2	T42.6X3	T42.6X4	T42.6X5	T42.6X6
tincture	T42.6X1	T42.6X2	T42.6X3	T42.6X4	T42.6X5	T42.6X6
Valethamate bromide	T44.3X1	T44.3X2	T44.3X3	T44.3X4	T44.3X5	T44.3X6
Valisone	T49.0X1	T49.0X2	T49.0X3	T49.0X4	T49.0X5	T49.0X6
Valium	T42.4X1	T42.4X2	T42.4X3	T42.4X4	T42.4X5	T42.4X6
Valmid	T42.6X1	T42.6X2	T42.6X3	T42.6X4	T42.6X5	T42.6X6
Valnoctamide	T42.6X1	T42.6X2	T42.6X3	T42.6X4	T42.6X5	T42.6X6
Valproate (sodium)	T42.6X1	T42.6X2	T42.6X3	T42.6X4	T42.6X5	T42.6X6
Valproic acid	T42.6X1	T42.6X2	T42.6X3	T42.6X4	T42.6X5	T42.6X6
Valpromide	T42.6X1	T42.6X2	T42.6X3	T42.6X4	T42.6X5	T42.6X6
Vanadium	T56.891	T56.892	T56.893	T56.894	—	—
Vancomycin	T36.8X1	T36.8X2	T36.8X3	T36.8X4	T36.8X5	T36.8X6
Vapor — see also Gas	T59.91	T59.92	T59.93	T59.94	—	—
kiln (carbon monoxide)	T58.8X1	T58.8X2	T58.8X3	T58.8X4	—	—
lead — see lead						
specified source NEC	T59.891	T59.892	T59.893	T59.894	—	—
Vardenafil	T46.7X1	T46.7X2	T46.7X3	T46.7X4	T46.7X5	T46.7X6
Varicose reduction drug	T46.8X1	T46.8X2	T46.8X3	T46.8X4	T46.8X5	T46.8X6
Varnish	T65.4X1	T65.4X2	T65.4X3	T65.4X4	—	—
cleaner	T52.91	T52.92	T52.93	T52.94	—	—
Vaseline	T49.3X1	T49.3X2	T49.3X3	T49.3X4	T49.3X5	T49.3X6
Vasodilan	T46.7X1	T46.7X2	T46.7X3	T46.7X4	T46.7X5	T46.7X6
Vasodilator						
coronary NEC	T46.3X1	T46.3X2	T46.3X3	T46.3X4	T46.3X5	T46.3X6
peripheral NEC	T46.7X1	T46.7X2	T46.7X3	T46.7X4	T46.7X5	T46.7X6
Vasopressin	T38.891	T38.892	T38.893	T38.894	T38.895	T38.896
Vasopressor drugs	T38.891	T38.892	T38.893	T38.894	T38.895	T38.896
Vecuronium bromide	T48.1X1	T48.1X2	T48.1X3	T48.1X4	T48.1X5	T48.1X6
Vegetable extract, astringent	T49.2X1	T49.2X2	T49.2X3	T49.2X4	T49.2X5	T49.2X6
Venlafaxine	T43.211	T43.212	T43.213	T43.214	T43.215	T43.216
Venom, venomous (bite) (sting)	T63.91	T63.92	T63.93	T63.94	—	—
amphibian NEC	T63.831	T63.832	T63.833	T63.834	—	—
animal NEC	T63.891	T63.892	T63.893	T63.894	—	—
ant	T63.421	T63.422	T63.423	T63.424	—	—
arthropod NEC	T63.481	T63.482	T63.483	T63.484	—	—
bee	T63.441	T63.442	T63.443	T63.444	—	—
centipede	T63.411	T63.412	T63.413	T63.414	—	—
fish	T63.591	T63.592	T63.593	T63.594	—	—
frog	T63.811	T63.812	T63.813	T63.814	—	—
hornet	T63.451	T63.452	T63.453	T63.454	—	—
insect NEC	T63.481	T63.482	T63.483	T63.484	—	—
lizard	T63.121	T63.122	T63.123	T63.124	—	—
marine						
animals	T63.691	T63.692	T63.693	T63.694	—	—
bluebottle	T63.611	T63.612	T63.613	T63.614	—	—
jellyfish NEC	T63.621	T63.622	T63.623	T63.624	—	—
Portugese Man-o-war	T63.611	T63.612	T63.613	T63.614	—	—
sea anemone	T63.631	T63.632	T63.633	T63.634	—	—
specified NEC	T63.691	T63.692	T63.693	T63.694	—	—
fish	T63.591	T63.592	T63.593	T63.594	—	—
plants	T63.711	T63.712	T63.713	T63.714	—	—
sting ray	T63.511	T63.512	T63.513	T63.514	—	—
millipede (tropical)	T63.411	T63.412	T63.413	T63.414	—	—
plant NEC	T63.791	T63.792	T63.793	T63.794	—	—
marine	T63.711	T63.712	T63.713	T63.714	—	—
reptile	T63.191	T63.192	T63.193	T63.194	—	—
gila monster	T63.111	T63.112	T63.113	T63.114	—	—
lizard NEC	T63.121	T63.122	T63.123	T63.124	—	—
scorpion	T63.2X1	T63.2X2	T63.2X3	T63.2X4	—	—
snake	T63.001	T63.002	T63.003	T63.004	—	—
African NEC	T63.081	T63.082	T63.083	T63.084	—	—
American (North) (South) NEC	T63.061	T63.062	T63.063	T63.064	—	—
Asian	T63.081	T63.082	T63.083	T63.084	—	—
Australian	T63.071	T63.072	T63.073	T63.074	—	—
cobra	T63.041	T63.042	T63.043	T63.044	—	—
coral snake	T63.021	T63.022	T63.023	T63.024	—	—
rattlesnake	T63.011	T63.012	T63.013	T63.014	—	—
specified NEC	T63.091	T63.092	T63.093	T63.094	—	—
taipan	T63.031	T63.032	T63.033	T63.034	—	—
specified NEC	T63.891	T63.892	T63.893	T63.894	—	—
spider	T63.301	T63.302	T63.303	T63.304	—	—

Additional Character May Be Required — Refer to the Tabular List for Character Selection   ▽ Subterms under main terms may continue to next column or page

Substance	Poisoning, Accidental (unintentional)	Poisoning, Intentional Self-harm	Poisoning, Assault	Poisoning, Undetermined	Adverse Effect	Under-dosing
Venom, venomous — continued						
spider — continued						
black widow	T63.311	T63.312	T63.313	T63.314	—	—
brown recluse	T63.331	T63.332	T63.333	T63.334	—	—
specified NEC	T63.391	T63.392	T63.393	T63.394	—	—
tarantula	T63.321	T63.322	T63.323	T63.324	—	—
sting ray	T63.511	T63.512	T63.513	T63.514	—	—
toad	T63.821	T63.822	T63.823	T63.824	—	—
wasp	T63.461	T63.462	T63.463	T63.464	—	—
Venous sclerosing drug NEC	T46.8X1	T46.8X2	T46.8X3	T46.8X4	T46.8X5	T46.8X6
Ventolin — see Albuterol						
Veramon	T42.3X1	T42.3X2	T42.3X3	T42.3X4	T42.3X5	T42.3X6
Verapamil	T46.1X1	T46.1X2	T46.1X3	T46.1X4	T46.1X5	T46.1X6
Veratrine	T46.5X1	T46.5X2	T46.5X3	T46.5X4	T46.5X5	T46.5X6
Veratrum						
album	T62.2X1	T62.2X2	T62.2X3	T62.2X4	—	—
alkaloids	T46.5X1	T46.5X2	T46.5X3	T46.5X4	T46.5X5	T46.5X6
viride	T62.2X1	T62.2X2	T62.2X3	T62.2X4	—	—
Verdigris	T60.3X1	T60.3X2	T60.3X3	T60.3X4	—	—
Veronal	T42.3X1	T42.3X2	T42.3X3	T42.3X4	T42.3X5	T42.3X6
Veroxil	T37.4X1	T37.4X2	T37.4X3	T37.4X4	T37.4X5	T37.4X6
Versenate	T50.6X1	T50.6X2	T50.6X3	T50.6X4	T50.6X5	T50.6X6
Versidyne	T39.8X1	T39.8X2	T39.8X3	T39.8X4	T39.8X5	T39.8X6
Vetrabutine	T48.0X1	T48.0X2	T48.0X3	T48.0X4	T48.0X5	T48.0X6
Vidarabine	T37.5X1	T37.5X2	T37.5X3	T37.5X4	T37.5X5	T37.5X6
Vienna						
green	T57.0X1	T57.0X2	T57.0X3	T57.0X4	—	—
insecticide	T60.2X1	T60.2X2	T60.2X3	T60.2X4	—	—
red	T57.0X1	T57.0X2	T57.0X3	T57.0X4	—	—
pharmaceutical dye	T50.991	T50.992	T50.993	T50.994	T50.995	T50.996
Vigabatrin	T42.6X1	T42.6X2	T42.6X3	T42.6X4	T42.6X5	T42.6X6
Viloxazine	T43.291	T43.292	T43.293	T43.294	T43.295	T43.296
Viminol	T39.8X1	T39.8X2	T39.8X3	T39.8X4	T39.8X5	T39.8X6
Vinbarbital, vinbarbitone	T42.3X1	T42.3X2	T42.3X3	T42.3X4	T42.3X5	T42.3X6
Vinblastine	T45.1X1	T45.1X2	T45.1X3	T45.1X4	T45.1X5	T45.1X6
Vinburnine	T46.7X1	T46.7X2	T46.7X3	T46.7X4	T46.7X5	T46.7X6
Vincamine	T45.1X1	T45.1X2	T45.1X3	T45.1X4	T45.1X5	T45.1X6
Vincristine	T45.1X1	T45.1X2	T45.1X3	T45.1X4	T45.1X5	T45.1X6
Vindesine	T45.1X1	T45.1X2	T45.1X3	T45.1X4	T45.1X5	T45.1X6
Vinesthene, vinethene	T41.0X1	T41.0X2	T41.0X3	T41.0X4	T41.0X5	T41.0X6
Vinorelbine tartrate	T45.1X1	T45.1X2	T45.1X3	T45.1X4	T45.1X5	T45.1X6
Vinpocetine	T46.7X1	T46.7X2	T46.7X3	T46.7X4	T46.7X5	T46.7X6
Vinyl						
acetate	T65.891	T65.892	T65.893	T65.894	—	—
bital	T42.3X1	T42.3X2	T42.3X3	T42.3X4	T42.3X5	T42.3X6
bromide	T65.891	T65.892	T65.893	T65.894	—	—
chloride	T59.891	T59.892	T59.893	T59.894	—	—
ether	T41.0X1	T41.0X2	T41.0X3	T41.0X4	T41.0X5	T41.0X6
Vinylbital	T42.3X1	T42.3X2	T42.3X3	T42.3X4	T42.3X5	T42.3X6
Vinylidene chloride	T65.891	T65.892	T65.893	T65.894	—	—
Vioform	T37.8X1	T37.8X2	T37.8X3	T37.8X4	T37.8X5	T37.8X6
topical	T49.0X1	T49.0X2	T49.0X3	T49.0X4	T49.0X5	T49.0X6
Viomycin	T36.8X1	T36.8X2	T36.8X3	T36.8X4	T36.8X5	T36.8X6
Viosterol	T45.2X1	T45.2X2	T45.2X3	T45.2X4	T45.2X5	T45.2X6
Viper (venom)	T63.091	T63.092	T63.093	T63.094	—	—
Viprynium	T37.4X1	T37.4X2	T37.4X3	T37.4X4	T37.4X5	T37.4X6
Viquidil	T46.7X1	T46.7X2	T46.7X3	T46.7X4	T46.7X5	T46.7X6
Viral vaccine NEC	T50.B91	T50.B92	T50.B93	T50.B94	T50.B95	T50.B96
Virginiamycin	T36.8X1	T36.8X2	T36.8X3	T36.8X4	T36.8X5	T36.8X6
Virugon	T37.5X1	T37.5X2	T37.5X3	T37.5X4	T37.5X5	T37.5X6
Viscous agent	T50.901	T50.902	T50.903	T50.904	T50.905	T50.906
Visine	T49.5X1	T49.5X2	T49.5X3	T49.5X4	T49.5X5	T49.5X6
Visnadine	T46.3X1	T46.3X2	T46.3X3	T46.3X4	T46.3X5	T46.3X6
Vitamin NEC	T45.2X1	T45.2X2	T45.2X3	T45.2X4	T45.2X5	T45.2X6
A	T45.2X1	T45.2X2	T45.2X3	T45.2X4	T45.2X5	T45.2X6
B1	T45.2X1	T45.2X2	T45.2X3	T45.2X4	T45.2X5	T45.2X6
B2	T45.2X1	T45.2X2	T45.2X3	T45.2X4	T45.2X5	T45.2X6
B6	T45.2X1	T45.2X2	T45.2X3	T45.2X4	T45.2X5	T45.2X6
B12	T45.2X1	T45.2X2	T45.2X3	T45.2X4	T45.2X5	T45.2X6
B15	T45.2X1	T45.2X2	T45.2X3	T45.2X4	T45.2X5	T45.2X6
B NEC	T45.2X1	T45.2X2	T45.2X3	T45.2X4	T45.2X5	T45.2X6
nicotinic acid	T46.7X1	T46.7X2	T46.7X3	T46.7X4	T46.7X5	T46.7X6
C	T45.2X1	T45.2X2	T45.2X3	T45.2X4	T45.2X5	T45.2X6
D	T45.2X1	T45.2X2	T45.2X3	T45.2X4	T45.2X5	T45.2X6
D2	T45.2X1	T45.2X2	T45.2X3	T45.2X4	T45.2X5	T45.2X6
D3	T45.2X1	T45.2X2	T45.2X3	T45.2X4	T45.2X5	T45.2X6
E	T45.2X1	T45.2X2	T45.2X3	T45.2X4	T45.2X5	T45.2X6
E acetate	T45.2X1	T45.2X2	T45.2X3	T45.2X4	T45.2X5	T45.2X6
hematopoietic	T45.8X1	T45.8X2	T45.8X3	T45.8X4	T45.8X5	T45.8X6
K1	T45.7X1	T45.7X2	T45.7X3	T45.7X4	T45.7X5	T45.7X6
K2	T45.7X1	T45.7X2	T45.7X3	T45.7X4	T45.7X5	T45.7X6
K NEC	T45.7X1	T45.7X2	T45.7X3	T45.7X4	T45.7X5	T45.7X6
Vitamin — continued						
PP	T45.2X1	T45.2X2	T45.2X3	T45.2X4	T45.2X5	T45.2X6
ulceroprotectant	T47.1X1	T47.1X2	T47.1X3	T47.1X4	T47.1X5	T47.1X6
Vleminckx's solution	T49.4X1	T49.4X2	T49.4X3	T49.4X4	T49.4X5	T49.4X6
Voltaren — see Diclofenac sodium						
Warfarin	T45.511	T45.512	T45.513	T45.514	T45.515	T45.516
rodenticide	T60.4X1-	T60.4X2-	T60.4X3-	T60.4X4-	—	—
sodium	T45.511	T45.512	T45.513	T45.514	T45.515	T45.516
Wasp (sting)	T63.461	T63.462	T63.463	T63.464	—	—
Water						
balance drug	T50.3X1	T50.3X2	T50.3X3	T50.3X4	T50.3X5	T50.3X6
distilled	T50.3X1	T50.3X2	T50.3X3	T50.3X4	T50.3X5	T50.3X6
gas — see Gas, water						
incomplete combustion of — see Carbon, monoxide, fuel, utility						
hemlock	T62.2X1	T62.2X2	T62.2X3	T62.2X4	—	—
moccasin (venom)	T63.061	T63.062	T63.063	T63.064	—	—
purified	T50.3X1	T50.3X2	T50.3X3	T50.3X4	T50.3X5	T50.3X6
Wax (paraffin) (petroleum)	T52.0X1	T52.0X2	T52.0X3	T52.0X4	—	—
automobile	T65.891	T65.892	T65.893	T65.894	—	—
floor	T52.0X1	T52.0X2	T52.0X3	T52.0X4	—	—
Weed killers NEC	T60.3X1	T60.3X2	T60.3X3	T60.3X4	—	—
Welldorm	T42.6X1	T42.6X2	T42.6X3	T42.6X4	T42.6X5	T42.6X6
White						
arsenic	T57.0X1	T57.0X2	T57.0X3	T57.0X4	—	—
hellebore	T62.2X1	T62.2X2	T62.2X3	T62.2X4	—	—
lotion (keratolytic)	T49.4X1	T49.4X2	T49.4X3	T49.4X4	T49.4X5	T49.4X6
spirit	T52.0X1	T52.0X2	T52.0X3	T52.0X4	—	—
Whitewash	T65.891	T65.892	T65.893	T65.894	—	—
Whole blood (human)	T45.8X1	T45.8X2	T45.8X3	T45.8X4	T45.8X5	T45.8X6
Wild						
black cherry	T62.2X1	T62.2X2	T62.2X3	T62.2X4	—	—
poisonous plants NEC	T62.2X1	T62.2X2	T62.2X3	T62.2X4	—	—
Window cleaning fluid	T65.891	T65.892	T65.893	T65.894	—	—
Wintergreen (oil)	T49.3X1	T49.3X2	T49.3X3	T49.3X4	T49.3X5	T49.3X6
Wisterine	T62.2X1	T62.2X2	T62.2X3	T62.2X4	—	—
Witch hazel	T49.2X1	T49.2X2	T49.2X3	T49.2X4	T49.2X5	T49.2X6
Wood alcohol or spirit	T51.1X1	T51.1X2	T51.1X3	T51.1X4	—	—
Wool fat (hydrous)	T49.3X1	T49.3X2	T49.3X3	T49.3X4	T49.3X5	T49.3X6
Woorali	T48.1X1	T48.1X2	T48.1X3	T48.1X4	T48.1X5	T48.1X6
Wormseed, American	T37.4X1	T37.4X2	T37.4X3	T37.4X4	T37.4X5	T37.4X6
Xamoterol	T44.5X1	T44.5X2	T44.5X3	T44.5X4	T44.5X5	T44.5X6
Xanthine diuretics	T50.2X1	T50.2X2	T50.2X3	T50.2X4	T50.2X5	T50.2X6
Xanthinol nicotinate	T46.7X1	T46.7X2	T46.7X3	T46.7X4	T46.7X5	T46.7X6
Xanthotoxin	T49.3X1	T49.3X2	T49.3X3	T49.3X4	T49.3X5	T49.3X6
Xantinol nicotinate	T46.7X1	T46.7X2	T46.7X3	T46.7X4	T46.7X5	T46.7X6
Xantocillin	T36.0X1	T36.0X2	T36.0X3	T36.0X4	T36.0X5	T36.0X6
Xenon (127Xe) (133Xe)	T50.8X1	T50.8X2	T50.8X3	T50.8X4	T50.8X5	T50.8X6
Xenysalate	T49.4X1	T49.4X2	T49.4X3	T49.4X4	T49.4X5	T49.4X6
Xibornol	T37.8X1	T37.8X2	T37.8X3	T37.8X4	T37.8X5	T37.8X6
Xigris	T45.511	T45.512	T45.513	T45.514	T45.515	T45.516
Xipamide	T50.2X1	T50.2X2	T50.2X3	T50.2X4	T50.2X5	T50.2X6
Xylene (vapor)	T52.2X1	T52.2X2	T52.2X3	T52.2X4	—	—
Xylocaine (infiltration) (topical)	T41.3X1	T41.3X2	T41.3X3	T41.3X4	T41.3X5	T41.3X6
nerve block (peripheral) (plexus)	T41.3X1	T41.3X2	T41.3X3	T41.3X4	T41.3X5	T41.3X6
spinal	T41.3X1	T41.3X2	T41.3X3	T41.3X4	T41.3X5	T41.3X6
Xylol (vapor)	T52.2X1	T52.2X2	T52.2X3	T52.2X4	—	—
Xylometazoline	T48.5X1	T48.5X2	T48.5X3	T48.5X4	T48.5X5	T48.5X6
Yeast	T45.2X1	T45.2X2	T45.2X3	T45.2X4	T45.2X5	T45.2X6
dried	T45.2X1	T45.2X2	T45.2X3	T45.2X4	T45.2X5	T45.2X6
Yellow						
fever vaccine	T50.B91	T50.B92	T50.B93	T50.B94	T50.B95	T50.B96
jasmine	T62.2X1	T62.2X2	T62.2X3	T62.2X4	—	—
phenolphthalein	T47.2X1	T47.2X2	T47.2X3	T47.2X4	T47.2X5	T47.2X6
Yew	T62.2X1	T62.2X2	T62.2X3	T62.2X4	—	—
Yohimbic acid	T40.991	T40.992	T40.993	T40.994	T40.995	T40.996
Zactane	T39.8X1	T39.8X2	T39.8X3	T39.8X4	T39.8X5	T39.8X6
Zalcitabine	T37.5X1	T37.5X2	T37.5X3	T37.5X4	T37.5X5	T37.5X6
Zaroxolyn	T50.2X1	T50.2X2	T50.2X3	T50.2X4	T50.2X5	T50.2X6
Zephiran (topical)	T49.0X1	T49.0X2	T49.0X3	T49.0X4	T49.0X5	T49.0X6
ophthalmic preparation	T49.5X1	T49.5X2	T49.5X3	T49.5X4	T49.5X5	T49.5X6
Zeranol	T38.7X1	T38.7X2	T38.7X3	T38.7X4	T38.7X5	T38.7X6
Zerone	T51.1X1	T51.1X2	T51.1X3	T51.1X4	—	—
Zidovudine	T37.5X1	T37.5X2	T37.5X3	T37.5X4	T37.5X5	T37.5X6
Zimeldine	T43.221	T43.222	T43.223	T43.224	T43.225	T43.226
Zinc (compounds) (fumes) (vapor) NEC	T56.5X1	T56.5X2	T56.5X3	T56.5X4	—	—
anti-infectives	T49.0X1	T49.0X2	T49.0X3	T49.0X4	T49.0X5	T49.0X6
antivaricose	T46.8X1	T46.8X2	T46.8X3	T46.8X4	T46.8X5	T46.8X6

Table of Drugs and Chemicals

Substance	Poisoning, Accidental (unintentional)	Poisoning, Intentional Self-harm	Poisoning, Assault	Poisoning, Undetermined	Adverse Effect	Under-dosing
Zinc (compounds) (fumes) (vapor)						
NEC — *continued*						
bacitracin	T49.0X1	T49.0X2	T49.0X3	T49.0X4	T49.0X5	T49.0X6
chloride (mouthwash)	T49.6X1	T49.6X2	T49.6X3	T49.6X4	T49.6X5	T49.6X6
chromate	T56.5X1	T56.5X2	T56.5X3	T56.5X4	—	—
gelatin	T49.3X1	T49.3X2	T49.3X3	T49.3X4	T49.3X5	T49.3X6
oxide	T49.3X1	T49.3X2	T49.3X3	T49.3X4	T49.3X5	T49.3X6
plaster	T49.3X1	T49.3X2	T49.3X3	T49.3X4	T49.3X5	T49.3X6
peroxide	T49.0X1	T49.0X2	T49.0X3	T49.0X4	T49.0X5	T49.0X6
pesticides	T56.5X1	T56.5X2	T56.5X3	T56.5X4	—	—
phosphide	T60.4X1	T60.4X2	T60.4X3	T60.4X4	—	—
pyrithionate	T49.4X1	T49.4X2	T49.4X3	T49.4X4	T49.4X5	T49.4X6
stearate	T49.3X1	T49.3X2	T49.3X3	T49.3X4	T49.3X5	T49.3X6
sulfate	T49.5X1	T49.5X2	T49.5X3	T49.5X4	T49.5X5	T49.5X6
ENT agent	T49.6X1	T49.6X2	T49.6X3	T49.6X4	T49.6X5	T49.6X6
ophthalmic solution	T49.5X1	T49.5X2	T49.5X3	T49.5X4	T49.5X5	T49.5X6
topical NEC	T49.0X1	T49.0X2	T49.0X3	T49.0X4	T49.0X5	T49.0X6
undecylenate	T49.0X1	T49.0X2	T49.0X3	T49.0X4	T49.0X5	T49.0X6
Zineb	T60.0X1	T60.0X2	T60.0X3	T60.0X4		
Zinostatin	T45.1X1	T45.1X2	T45.1X3	T45.1X4	T45.1X5	T45.1X6
Zipeprol	T48.3X1	T48.3X2	T48.3X3	T48.3X4	T48.3X5	T48.3X6
Zofenopril	T46.4X1	T46.4X2	T46.4X3	T46.4X4	T46.4X5	T46.4X6
Zolpidem	T42.6X1	T42.6X2	T42.6X3	T42.6X4	T42.6X5	T42.6X6
Zomepirac	T39.391	T39.392	T39.393	T39.394	T39.395	T39.396
Zopiclone	T42.6X1	T42.6X2	T42.6X3	T42.6X4	T42.6X5	T42.6X6
Zorubicin	T45.1X1	T45.1X2	T45.1X3	T45.1X4	T45.1X5	T45.1X6
Zotepine	T43.591	T43.592	T43.593	T43.594	T43.595	T43.596
Zovant	T45.511	T45.512	T45.513	T45.514	T45.515	T45.516
Zoxazolamine	T42.8X1	T42.8X2	T42.8X3	T42.8X4	T42.8X5	T42.8X6
Zuclopenthixol	T43.4X1	T43.4X2	T43.4X3	T43.4X4	T43.4X5	T43.4X6
Zygadenus (venenosus)	T62.2X1	T62.2X2	T62.2X3	T62.2X4	—	—
Zyprexa	T43.591	T43.592	T43.593	T43.594	T43.595	T43.596

A

Abandonment (causing exposure to weather conditions) (with intent to injure or kill) NEC X58 ☑

Abuse (adult) (child) (mental) (physical) (sexual) X58 ☑

Accident (to) X58 ☑
  aircraft (in transit) (powered) (*see also* Accident, transport, aircraft)
    due to, caused by cataclysm — *see* Forces of nature, by type
  animal-drawn vehicle — *see* Accident, transport, animal-drawn vehicle occupant
  animal-rider — *see* Accident, transport, animal-rider
  automobile — *see* Accident, transport, car occupant
  bare foot water skier V94.4 ☑
  boat, boating (*see also* Accident, watercraft)
    striking swimmer
      powered V94.11 ☑
      unpowered V94.12 ☑
  bus — *see* Accident, transport, bus occupant
  cable car, not on rails V98.0 ☑
    on rails — *see* Accident, transport, streetcar occupant
  car — *see* Accident, transport, car occupant
  caused by, due to
    animal NEC W64 ☑
    chain hoist W24.0 ☑
    cold (excessive) — *see* Exposure, cold
    corrosive liquid, substance — *see* Table of Drugs and Chemicals
    cutting or piercing instrument — *see* Contact, with, by type of instrument
    drive belt W24.0 ☑
    electric
      current — *see* Exposure, electric current
      motor (*see also* Contact, with, by type of machine) W31.3 ☑
        current (of) W86.8 ☑
    environmental factor NEC X58 ☑
    explosive material — *see* Explosion
    fire, flames — *see* Exposure, fire
    firearm missile — *see* Discharge, firearm by type
    heat (excessive) — *see* Heat
    hot — *see* Contact, with, hot
    ignition — *see* Ignition
    lifting device W24.0 ☑
    lightning — *see* subcategory T75.0 ☑
      causing fire — *see* Exposure, fire
    machine, machinery — *see* Contact, with, by type of machine
    natural factor NEC X58 ☑
    pulley (block) W24.0 ☑
    radiation — *see* Radiation
    steam X13.1 ☑
      inhalation X13.0 ☑
      pipe X16 ☑
    thunderbolt — *see* subcategory T75.0 ☑
      causing fire — *see* Exposure, fire
    transmission device W24.1 ☑
  coach — *see* Accident, transport, bus occupant
  coal car — *see* Accident, transport, industrial vehicle occupant
  diving (*see also* Fall, into, water)
    with
      drowning or submersion — *see* Drowning
  forklift — *see* Accident, transport, industrial vehicle occupant
  heavy transport vehicle NOS — *see* Accident, transport, truck occupant
  ice yacht V98.2 ☑
  in
    medical, surgical procedure
      as, or due to misadventure — *see* Misadventure
      causing an abnormal reaction or later complication without mention of misadventure (*see also* Complication of or following, by type of procedure) Y84.9
  land yacht V98.1 ☑
  late effect of — *see* W00-X58 with 7th character S
  logging car — *see* Accident, transport, industrial vehicle occupant
  machine, machinery (*see also* Contact, with, by type of machine)
    on board watercraft V93.69 ☑
      explosion — *see* Explosion, in, watercraft

Accident — *continued*
  machine, machinery (*see also* Contact, with, by type of machine) — *continued*
    on board watercraft — *continued*
      fire — *see* Burn, on board watercraft
      powered craft V93.63 ☑
        ferry boat V93.61 ☑
        fishing boat V93.62 ☑
        jetskis V93.63 ☑
        liner V93.61 ☑
        merchant ship V93.60 ☑
        passenger ship V93.61 ☑
        sailboat V93.64 ☑
  mine tram — *see* Accident, transport, industrial vehicle occupant
  mobility scooter (motorized) — *see* Accident, transport, pedestrian, conveyance, specified type NEC
  motor scooter — *see* Accident, transport, motorcyclist
  motor vehicle NOS (traffic) (*see also* Accident, transport) V89.2 ☑
    nontraffic V89.0 ☑
    three-wheeled NOS — *see* Accident, transport, three-wheeled motor vehicle occupant
  motorcycle NOS — *see* Accident, transport, motorcyclist
  nonmotor vehicle NOS (nontraffic) (*see also* Accident, transport) V89.1 ☑
    traffic NOS V89.3 ☑
  nontraffic (victim's mode of transport NOS) V88.9 ☑
    collision (between) V88.7 ☑
      bus and truck V88.5 ☑
      car and:
        bus V88.3 ☑
        pickup V88.2 ☑
        three-wheeled motor vehicle V88.0 ☑
        train V88.6 ☑
        truck V88.4 ☑
        two-wheeled motor vehicle V88.0 ☑
        van V88.2 ☑
      specified vehicle NEC and:
        three-wheeled motor vehicle V88.1 ☑
        two-wheeled motor vehicle V88.1 ☑
    known mode of transport — *see* Accident, transport, by type of vehicle
    noncollision V88.8 ☑
  on board watercraft V93.89 ☑
    powered craft V93.83 ☑
      ferry boat V93.81 ☑
      fishing boat V93.82 ☑
      jetskis V93.83 ☑
      liner V93.81 ☑
      merchant ship V93.80 ☑
      passenger ship V93.81 ☑
    unpowered craft V93.88 ☑
      canoe V93.85 ☑
      inflatable V93.86 ☑
        in tow
          recreational V94.31 ☑
          specified NEC V94.32 ☑
      kayak V93.85 ☑
      sailboat V93.84 ☑
      surf-board V93.88 ☑
      water skis V93.87 ☑
      windsurfer V93.88 ☑
  parachutist V97.29 ☑
    entangled in object V97.21 ☑
    injured on landing V97.22 ☑
  pedal cycle — *see* Accident, transport, pedal cyclist
  pedestrian (on foot)
    with
      another pedestrian W51 ☑
      on pedestrian conveyance NEC V00.09 ☑
      with fall W03 ☑
        due to ice or snow W00.0 ☑
      roller skater (in-line) V00.01 ☑
      skate boarder V00.02 ☑
      transport vehicle — *see* Accident, transport
    on pedestrian conveyance — *see* Accident, transport, pedestrian, conveyance
  pick-up truck or van — *see* Accident, transport, pickup truck occupant
  quarry truck — *see* Accident, transport, industrial vehicle occupant
  railway vehicle (any) (in motion) — *see* Accident, transport, railway vehicle occupant
    due to cataclysm — *see* Forces of nature, by type

Accident — *continued*
  scooter (non-motorized) — *see* Accident, transport, pedestrian, conveyance, scooter
  sequelae of — *see* categories W00-X58 with 7th character S
  skateboard — *see* Accident, transport, pedestrian, conveyance, skateboard
  ski(ing) — *see* Accident, transport, pedestrian, conveyance
    lift V98.3 ☑
  specified cause NEC X58 ☑
  streetcar — *see* Accident, transport, streetcar occupant
  traffic (victim's mode of transport NOS) V87.9 ☑
    collision (between) V87.7 ☑
      bus and truck V87.5 ☑
      car and:
        bus V87.3 ☑
        pickup V87.2 ☑
        three-wheeled motor vehicle V87.0 ☑
        train V87.6 ☑
        truck V87.4 ☑
        two-wheeled motor vehicle V87.0 ☑
        van V87.2 ☑
      specified vehicle NEC and:
        three-wheeled motor vehicle V87.1 ☑
        two-wheeled motor vehicle V87.1 ☑
    known mode of transport — *see* Accident, transport, by type of vehicle
    noncollision V87.8 ☑
  transport (involving injury to) V99 ☑
    18 wheeler — *see* Accident, transport, truck occupant
    agricultural vehicle occupant (nontraffic) V84.9 ☑
      driver V84.5 ☑
      hanger-on V84.7 ☑
      passenger V84.6 ☑
      traffic V84.3 ☑
        driver V84.0 ☑
        hanger-on V84.2 ☑
        passenger V84.1 ☑
      while boarding or alighting V84.4 ☑
    aircraft NEC V97.89 ☑
      military NEC V97.818 ☑
        civilian injured by V97.811 ☑
        with civilian aircraft V97.810 ☑
      occupant injured (in)
        nonpowered craft accident V96.9 ☑
          balloon V96.00 ☑
            collision V96.03 ☑
            crash V96.01 ☑
            explosion V96.05 ☑
            fire V96.04 ☑
            forced landing V96.02 ☑
            specified type NEC V96.09 ☑
          glider V96.20 ☑
            collision V96.23 ☑
            crash V96.21 ☑
            explosion V96.25 ☑
            fire V96.24 ☑
            forced landing V96.22 ☑
            specified type NEC V96.29 ☑
          hang glider V96.10 ☑
            collision V96.13 ☑
            crash V96.11 ☑
            explosion V96.15 ☑
            fire V96.14 ☑
            forced landing V96.12 ☑
            specified type NEC V96.19 ☑
          specified craft NEC V96.8 ☑
        powered craft accident V95.9 ☑
          fixed wing NEC
            commercial V95.30 ☑
              collision V95.33 ☑
              crash V95.31 ☑
              explosion V95.35 ☑
              fire V95.34 ☑
              forced landing V95.32 ☑
              specified type NEC V95.39 ☑
            private V95.20 ☑
              collision V95.23 ☑
              crash V95.21 ☑
              explosion V95.25 ☑
              fire V95.24 ☑
              forced landing V95.22 ☑
              specified type NEC V95.29 ☑
          glider V95.10 ☑

Accident — *continued*
  transport — *continued*
    aircraft — *continued*
      occupant injured — *continued*
        powered craft accident — *continued*
          glider — *continued*
            collision V95.13 ☑
            crash V95.11 ☑
            explosion V95.15 ☑
            fire V95.14 ☑
            forced landing V95.12 ☑
            specified type NEC V95.19 ☑
          helicopter V95.00 ☑
            collision V95.03 ☑
            crash V95.01 ☑
            explosion V95.05 ☑
            fire V95.04 ☑
            forced landing V95.02 ☑
            specified type NEC V95.09 ☑
          spacecraft V95.40 ☑
            collision V95.43 ☑
            crash V95.41 ☑
            explosion V95.45 ☑
            fire V95.44 ☑
            forced landing V95.42 ☑
            specified type NEC V95.49 ☑
          specified craft NEC V95.8 ☑
          ultralight V95.10 ☑
            collision V95.13 ☑
            crash V95.11 ☑
            explosion V95.15 ☑
            fire V95.14 ☑
            forced landing V95.12 ☑
            specified type NEC V95.19 ☑
        specified accident NEC V97.0 ☑
        while boarding or alighting V97.1 ☑
      person (injured by)
        falling from, in or on aircraft V97.0 ☑
        machinery on aircraft V97.89 ☑
        on ground with aircraft involvement V97.39 ☑
        rotating propeller V97.32 ☑
        struck by object falling from aircraft V97.31 ☑
        sucked into aircraft jet V97.33 ☑
        while boarding or alighting aircraft V97.1 ☑
    airport (battery-powered) passenger vehicle — *see* Accident, transport, industrial vehicle occupant
    all-terrain vehicle occupant (nontraffic) V86.95 ☑
      driver V86.55 ☑
      dune buggy — *see* Accident, transport, dune buggy occupant
      hanger-on V86.75 ☑
      passenger V86.65 ☑
      snowmobile — *see* Accident, transport, snowmobile occupant
      specified type NEC V86.99 ☑
      traffic V86.35 ☑
        driver V86.05 ☑
        hanger-on V86.25 ☑
        passenger V86.15 ☑
      while boarding or alighting V86.45 ☑
    ambulance occupant (traffic) V86.31 ☑
      driver V86.01 ☑
      hanger-on V86.21 ☑
      nontraffic V86.91 ☑
        driver V86.51 ☑
        hanger-on V86.71 ☑
        passenger V86.61 ☑
      passenger V86.11 ☑
      while boarding or alighting V86.41 ☑
    animal-drawn vehicle occupant (in) V80.929 ☑
      collision (with)
        animal V80.12 ☑
          being ridden V80.711 ☑
        animal-drawn vehicle V80.721 ☑
        bus V80.42 ☑
        car V80.42 ☑
        fixed or stationary object V80.82 ☑
        military vehicle V80.920 ☑
        nonmotor vehicle V80.791 ☑
        pedal cycle V80.22 ☑
        pedestrian V80.12 ☑
        pickup V80.42 ☑
        railway train or vehicle V80.62 ☑
        specified motor vehicle NEC V80.52 ☑

Accident — *continued*
  transport — *continued*
    animal-drawn vehicle occupant — *continued*
      collision — *continued*
        streetcar V80.731 ☑
        truck V80.42 ☑
        two- or three-wheeled motor vehicle V80.32 ☑
        van V80.42 ☑
      noncollision V80.02 ☑
      specified circumstance NEC V80.928 ☑
    animal-rider V80.919 ☑
      collision (with)
        animal V80.11 ☑
          being ridden V80.710 ☑
        animal-drawn vehicle V80.720 ☑
        bus V80.41 ☑
        car V80.41 ☑
        fixed or stationary object V80.81 ☑
        military vehicle V80.910 ☑
        nonmotor vehicle V80.790 ☑
        pedal cycle V80.21 ☑
        pedestrian V80.11 ☑
        pickup V80.41 ☑
        railway train or vehicle V80.61 ☑
        specified motor vehicle NEC V80.51 ☑
        streetcar V80.730 ☑
        truck V80.41 ☑
        two- or three-wheeled motor vehicle V80.31 ☑
        van V80.41 ☑
      noncollision V80.018 ☑
        specified as horse rider V80.010 ☑
      specified circumstance NEC V80.918 ☑
    armored car — *see* Accident, transport, truck occupant
    battery-powered truck (baggage) (mail) — *see* Accident, transport, industrial vehicle occupant
    bus occupant V79.9 ☑
      collision (with)
        animal (traffic) V70.9 ☑
          being ridden (traffic) V76.9 ☑
            nontraffic V76.3 ☑
            while boarding or alighting V76.4 ☑
          nontraffic V70.3 ☑
          while boarding or alighting V70.4 ☑
        animal-drawn vehicle (traffic) V76.9 ☑
          nontraffic V76.3 ☑
          while boarding or alighting V76.4 ☑
        bus (traffic) V74.9 ☑
          nontraffic V74.3 ☑
          while boarding or alighting V74.4 ☑
        car (traffic) V73.9 ☑
          nontraffic V73.3 ☑
          while boarding or alighting V73.4 ☑
        motor vehicle NOS (traffic) V79.60 ☑
          nontraffic V79.20 ☑
          specified type NEC (traffic) V79.69 ☑
            nontraffic V79.29 ☑
        pedal cycle (traffic) V71.9 ☑
          nontraffic V71.3 ☑
          while boarding or alighting V71.4 ☑
        pickup truck (traffic) V73.9 ☑
          nontraffic V73.3 ☑
          while boarding or alighting V73.4 ☑
        railway vehicle (traffic) V75.9 ☑
          nontraffic V75.3 ☑
          while boarding or alighting V75.4 ☑
        specified vehicle NEC (traffic) V76.9 ☑
          nontraffic V76.3 ☑
          while boarding or alighting V76.4 ☑
        stationary object (traffic) V77.9 ☑
          nontraffic V77.3 ☑
          while boarding or alighting V77.4 ☑
        streetcar (traffic) V76.9 ☑
          nontraffic V76.3 ☑
          while boarding or alighting V76.4 ☑
        three wheeled motor vehicle (traffic) V72.9 ☑
          nontraffic V72.3 ☑
          while boarding or alighting V72.4 ☑
        truck (traffic) V74.9 ☑
          nontraffic V74.3 ☑
          while boarding or alighting V74.4 ☑
        two wheeled motor vehicle (traffic) V72.9 ☑
          nontraffic V72.3 ☑
          while boarding or alighting V72.4 ☑

Accident — *continued*
  transport — *continued*
    bus occupant — *continued*
      collision — *continued*
        van (traffic) V73.9 ☑
          nontraffic V73.3 ☑
          while boarding or alighting V73.4 ☑
      driver
        collision (with)
          animal (traffic) V70.5 ☑
            being ridden (traffic) V76.5 ☑
              nontraffic V76.0 ☑
            nontraffic V70.0 ☑
          animal-drawn vehicle (traffic) V76.5 ☑
            nontraffic V76.0 ☑
          bus (traffic) V74.5 ☑
            nontraffic V74.0 ☑
          car (traffic) V73.5 ☑
            nontraffic V73.0 ☑
          motor vehicle NOS (traffic) V79.40 ☑
            nontraffic V79.00 ☑
            specified type NEC (traffic) V79.49 ☑
              nontraffic V79.09 ☑
          pedal cycle (traffic) V71.5 ☑
            nontraffic V71.0 ☑
          pickup truck (traffic) V73.5 ☑
            nontraffic V73.0 ☑
          railway vehicle (traffic) V75.5 ☑
            nontraffic V75.0 ☑
          specified vehicle NEC (traffic) V76.5 ☑
            nontraffic V76.0 ☑
          stationary object (traffic) V77.5 ☑
            nontraffic V77.0 ☑
          streetcar (traffic) V76.5 ☑
            nontraffic V76.0 ☑
          three wheeled motor vehicle (traffic) V72.5 ☑
            nontraffic V72.0 ☑
          truck (traffic) V74.5 ☑
            nontraffic V74.0 ☑
          two wheeled motor vehicle (traffic) V72.5 ☑
            nontraffic V72.0 ☑
          van (traffic) V73.5 ☑
            nontraffic V73.0 ☑
        noncollision accident (traffic) V78.5 ☑
          nontraffic V78.0 ☑
      hanger-on
        collision (with)
          animal (traffic) V70.7 ☑
            being ridden (traffic) V76.7 ☑
              nontraffic V76.2 ☑
            nontraffic V70.2 ☑
          animal-drawn vehicle (traffic) V76.7 ☑
            nontraffic V76.2 ☑
          bus (traffic) V74.7 ☑
            nontraffic V74.2 ☑
          car (traffic) V73.7 ☑
            nontraffic V73.2 ☑
          pedal cycle (traffic) V71.7 ☑
            nontraffic V71.2 ☑
          pickup truck (traffic) V73.7 ☑
            nontraffic V73.2 ☑
          railway vehicle (traffic) V75.7 ☑
            nontraffic V75.2 ☑
          specified vehicle NEC (traffic) V76.7 ☑
            nontraffic V76.2 ☑
          stationary object (traffic) V77.7 ☑
            nontraffic V77.2 ☑
          streetcar (traffic) V76.7 ☑
            nontraffic V76.2 ☑
          three wheeled motor vehicle (traffic) V72.7 ☑
            nontraffic V72.2 ☑
          truck (traffic) V74.7 ☑
            nontraffic V74.2 ☑
          two wheeled motor vehicle (traffic) V72.7 ☑
            nontraffic V72.2 ☑
          van (traffic) V73.7 ☑
            nontraffic V73.2 ☑
        noncollision accident (traffic) V78.7 ☑
          nontraffic V78.2 ☑
      noncollision accident (traffic) V78.9 ☑
        nontraffic V78.3 ☑
        while boarding or alighting V78.4 ☑

400   ☑ Additional Character Required — Refer to the Tabular List for Character Selection   ▽ Subterms under main terms may continue to next column or page

Accident — Accident

Accident — *continued*
  transport — *continued*
    bus occupant — *continued*
      nontraffic V79.3 ☑
      passenger
        collision (with)
          animal (traffic) V70.6 ☑
            being ridden (traffic) V76.6 ☑
              nontraffic V76.1 ☑
            nontraffic V70.1 ☑
          animal-drawn vehicle (traffic) V76.6 ☑
            nontraffic V76.1 ☑
          bus (traffic) V74.6 ☑
            nontraffic V74.1 ☑
          car (traffic) V73.6 ☑
            nontraffic V73.1 ☑
          motor vehicle NOS (traffic) V79.50 ☑
            nontraffic V79.10 ☑
            specified type NEC (traffic) V79.59 ☑
              nontraffic V79.19 ☑
          pedal cycle (traffic) V71.6 ☑
            nontraffic V71.1 ☑
          pickup truck (traffic) V73.6 ☑
            nontraffic V73.1 ☑
          railway vehicle (traffic) V75.6 ☑
            nontraffic V75.1 ☑
          specified vehicle NEC (traffic) V76.6 ☑
            nontraffic V76.1 ☑
          stationary object (traffic) V77.6 ☑
            nontraffic V77.1 ☑
          streetcar (traffic) V76.6 ☑
            nontraffic V76.1 ☑
          three wheeled motor vehicle (traffic) V72.6 ☑
            nontraffic V72.1 ☑
          truck (traffic) V74.6 ☑
            nontraffic V74.1 ☑
          two wheeled motor vehicle (traffic) V72.6 ☑
            nontraffic V72.1 ☑
          van (traffic) V73.6 ☑
            nontraffic V73.1 ☑
        noncollision accident (traffic) V78.6 ☑
          nontraffic V78.1 ☑
      specified type NEC V79.88 ☑
      military vehicle V79.81 ☑
    cable car, not on rails V98.0 ☑
      on rails — *see* Accident, transport, streetcar occupant
    car occupant V49.9 ☑
      ambulance occupant — *see* Accident, transport, ambulance occupant
      collision (with)
        animal (traffic) V40.9 ☑
          being ridden (traffic) V46.9 ☑
            nontraffic V46.3 ☑
            while boarding or alighting V46.4 ☑
          nontraffic V40.3 ☑
          while boarding or alighting V40.4 ☑
        animal-drawn vehicle (traffic) V46.9 ☑
          nontraffic V46.3 ☑
          while boarding or alighting V46.4 ☑
        bus (traffic) V44.9 ☑
          nontraffic V44.3 ☑
          while boarding or alighting V44.4 ☑
        car (traffic) V43.92 ☑
          nontraffic V43.32 ☑
          while boarding or alighting V43.42 ☑
        motor vehicle NOS (traffic) V49.60 ☑
          nontraffic V49.20 ☑
          specified type NEC (traffic) V49.69 ☑
            nontraffic V49.29 ☑
        pedal cycle (traffic) V41.9 ☑
          nontraffic V41.3 ☑
          while boarding or alighting V41.4 ☑
        pickup truck (traffic) V43.93 ☑
          nontraffic V43.33 ☑
          while boarding or alighting V43.43 ☑
        railway vehicle (traffic) V45.9 ☑
          nontraffic V45.3 ☑
          while boarding or alighting V45.4 ☑
        specified vehicle NEC (traffic) V46.9 ☑
          nontraffic V46.3 ☑
          while boarding or alighting V46.4 ☑
        sport utility vehicle (traffic) V43.91 ☑
          nontraffic V43.31 ☑

Accident — *continued*
  transport — *continued*
    car occupant — *continued*
      collision — *continued*
        sport utility vehicle — *continued*
          while boarding or alighting V43.41 ☑
        stationary object (traffic) V47.9 ☑
          nontraffic V47.3 ☑
          while boarding or alighting V47.4 ☑
        streetcar (traffic) V46.9 ☑
          nontraffic V46.3 ☑
          while boarding or alighting V46.4 ☑
        three wheeled motor vehicle (traffic) V42.9 ☑
          nontraffic V42.3 ☑
          while boarding or alighting V42.4 ☑
        truck (traffic) V44.9 ☑
          nontraffic V44.3 ☑
          while boarding or alighting V44.4 ☑
        two wheeled motor vehicle (traffic) V42.9 ☑
          nontraffic V42.3 ☑
          while boarding or alighting V42.4 ☑
        van (traffic) V43.94 ☑
          nontraffic V43.34 ☑
          while boarding or alighting V43.44 ☑
      driver
        collision (with)
          animal (traffic) V40.5 ☑
            being ridden (traffic) V46.5 ☑
              nontraffic V46.0 ☑
            nontraffic V40.0 ☑
          animal-drawn vehicle (traffic) V46.5 ☑
            nontraffic V46.0 ☑
          bus (traffic) V44.5 ☑
            nontraffic V44.0 ☑
          car (traffic) V43.52 ☑
            nontraffic V43.02 ☑
          motor vehicle NOS (traffic) V49.40 ☑
            nontraffic V49.00 ☑
            specified type NEC (traffic) V49.49 ☑
              nontraffic V49.09 ☑
          pedal cycle (traffic) V41.5 ☑
            nontraffic V41.0 ☑
          pickup truck (traffic) V43.53 ☑
            nontraffic V43.03 ☑
          railway vehicle (traffic) V45.5 ☑
            nontraffic V45.0 ☑
          specified vehicle NEC (traffic) V46.5 ☑
            nontraffic V46.0 ☑
          sport utility vehicle (traffic) V43.51 ☑
            nontraffic V43.01 ☑
          stationary object (traffic) V47.5 ☑
            nontraffic V47.0 ☑
          streetcar (traffic) V46.5 ☑
            nontraffic V46.0 ☑
          three wheeled motor vehicle (traffic) V42.5 ☑
            nontraffic V42.0 ☑
          truck (traffic) V44.5 ☑
            nontraffic V44.0 ☑
          two wheeled motor vehicle (traffic) V42.5 ☑
            nontraffic V42.0 ☑
          van (traffic) V43.54 ☑
            nontraffic V43.04 ☑
        noncollision accident (traffic) V48.5 ☑
          nontraffic V48.0 ☑
      hanger-on
        collision (with)
          animal (traffic) V40.7 ☑
            being ridden (traffic) V46.7 ☑
              nontraffic V46.2 ☑
            nontraffic V40.2 ☑
          animal-drawn vehicle (traffic) V46.7 ☑
            nontraffic V46.2 ☑
          bus (traffic) V44.7 ☑
            nontraffic V44.2 ☑
          car (traffic) V43.72 ☑
            nontraffic V43.22 ☑
          pedal cycle (traffic) V41.7 ☑
            nontraffic V41.2 ☑
          pickup truck (traffic) V43.73 ☑
            nontraffic V43.23 ☑
          railway vehicle (traffic) V45.7 ☑
            nontraffic V45.2 ☑
          specified vehicle NEC (traffic) V46.7 ☑
            nontraffic V46.2 ☑

Accident — *continued*
  transport — *continued*
    car occupant — *continued*
      hanger-on — *continued*
        collision — *continued*
          sport utility vehicle (traffic) V43.71 ☑
            nontraffic V43.21 ☑
          stationary object (traffic) V47.7 ☑
            nontraffic V47.2 ☑
          streetcar (traffic) V46.7 ☑
            nontraffic V46.2 ☑
          three wheeled motor vehicle (traffic) V42.7 ☑
            nontraffic V42.2 ☑
          truck (traffic) V44.7 ☑
            nontraffic V44.2 ☑
          two wheeled motor vehicle (traffic) V42.7 ☑
            nontraffic V42.2 ☑
          van (traffic) V43.74 ☑
            nontraffic V43.24 ☑
        noncollision accident (traffic) V48.7 ☑
          nontraffic V48.2 ☑
      noncollision accident (traffic) V48.9 ☑
        nontraffic V48.3 ☑
        while boarding or alighting V48.4 ☑
      nontraffic V49.3 ☑
      passenger
        collision (with)
          animal (traffic) V40.6 ☑
            being ridden (traffic) V46.6 ☑
              nontraffic V46.1 ☑
            nontraffic V40.1 ☑
          animal-drawn vehicle (traffic) V46.6 ☑
            nontraffic V46.1 ☑
          bus (traffic) V44.6 ☑
            nontraffic V44.1 ☑
          car (traffic) V43.62 ☑
            nontraffic V43.12 ☑
          motor vehicle NOS (traffic) V49.50 ☑
            nontraffic V49.10 ☑
            specified type NEC (traffic) V49.59 ☑
              nontraffic V49.19 ☑
          pedal cycle (traffic) V41.6 ☑
            nontraffic V41.1 ☑
          pickup truck (traffic) V43.63 ☑
            nontraffic V43.13 ☑
          railway vehicle (traffic) V45.6 ☑
            nontraffic V45.1 ☑
          specified vehicle NEC (traffic) V46.6 ☑
            nontraffic V46.1 ☑
          sport utility vehicle (traffic) V43.61 ☑
            nontraffic V43.11 ☑
          stationary object (traffic) V47.6 ☑
            nontraffic V47.1 ☑
          streetcar (traffic) V46.6 ☑
            nontraffic V46.1 ☑
          three wheeled motor vehicle (traffic) V42.6 ☑
            nontraffic V42.1 ☑
          truck (traffic) V44.6 ☑
            nontraffic V44.1 ☑
          two wheeled motor vehicle (traffic) V42.6 ☑
            nontraffic V42.1 ☑
          van (traffic) V43.64 ☑
            nontraffic V43.14 ☑
        noncollision accident (traffic) V48.6 ☑
          nontraffic V48.1 ☑
      specified type NEC V49.88 ☑
      military vehicle V49.81 ☑
    coal car — *see* Accident, transport, industrial vehicle occupant
    construction vehicle occupant (nontraffic) V85.9 ☑
      driver V85.5 ☑
      hanger-on V85.7 ☑
      passenger V85.6 ☑
      traffic V85.3 ☑
        driver V85.0 ☑
        hanger-on V85.2 ☑
        passenger V85.1 ☑
      while boarding or alighting V85.4 ☑
    dirt bike rider (nontraffic) V86.96 ☑
      driver V86.56 ☑
      hanger-on V86.76 ☑
      passenger V86.66 ☑

Accident — continued
  transport — continued
    dirt bike rider — continued
      traffic V86.36 ☑
        driver V86.06 ☑
        hanger-on V86.26 ☑
        passenger V86.16 ☑
      while boarding or alighting V86.46 ☑
    due to cataclysm — see Forces of nature, by type
    dune buggy occupant (nontraffic) V86.93 ☑
      driver V86.53 ☑
      hanger-on V86.73 ☑
      passenger V86.63 ☑
      traffic V86.33 ☑
        driver V86.03 ☑
        hanger-on V86.23 ☑
        passenger V86.13 ☑
      while boarding or alighting V86.43 ☑
    forklift — see Accident, transport, industrial vehicle occupant
    go cart — see Accident, transport, all-terrain vehicle occupant
    golf cart — see Accident, transport, all-terrain vehicle occupant
    heavy transport vehicle occupant — see Accident, transport, truck occupant
    ice yacht V98.2 ☑
    industrial vehicle occupant (nontraffic) V83.9 ☑
      driver V83.5 ☑
      hanger-on V83.7 ☑
      passenger V83.6 ☑
      traffic V83.3 ☑
        driver V83.0 ☑
        hanger-on V83.2 ☑
        passenger V83.1 ☑
      while boarding or alighting V83.4 ☑
    interurban electric car — see Accident, transport, streetcar
    land yacht V98.1 ☑
    logging car — see Accident, transport, industrial vehicle occupant
    military vehicle occupant (traffic) V86.34 ☑
      driver V86.04 ☑
      hanger-on V86.24 ☑
      nontraffic V86.94 ☑
        driver V86.54 ☑
        hanger-on V86.74 ☑
        passenger V86.64 ☑
      passenger V86.14 ☑
      while boarding or alighting V86.44 ☑
    mine tram — see Accident, transport, industrial vehicle occupant
    motor vehicle NEC occupant (traffic) V89.2 ☑
    motorcoach — see Accident, transport, bus occupant
    motor/cross bike rider (see also Accident, transport, dirt bike rider) V86.96 ☑
    motorcyclist V29.9 ☑
      collision (with)
        animal (traffic) V20.9 ☑
          being ridden (traffic) V26.9 ☑
            nontraffic V26.2 ☑
            while boarding or alighting V26.3 ☑
          nontraffic V20.2 ☑
          while boarding or alighting V20.3 ☑
        animal-drawn vehicle (traffic) V26.9 ☑
          nontraffic V26.2 ☑
          while boarding or alighting V26.3 ☑
        bus (traffic) V24.9 ☑
          nontraffic V24.2 ☑
          while boarding or alighting V24.3 ☑
        car (traffic) V23.9 ☑
          nontraffic V23.2 ☑
          while boarding or alighting V23.3 ☑
        motor vehicle NOS (traffic) V29.60 ☑
          nontraffic V29.20 ☑
          specified type NEC (traffic) V29.69 ☑
            nontraffic V29.29 ☑
        pedal cycle (traffic) V21.9 ☑
          nontraffic V21.2 ☑
          while boarding or alighting V21.3 ☑
        pickup truck (traffic) V23.9 ☑
          nontraffic V23.2 ☑
          while boarding or alighting V23.3 ☑
        railway vehicle (traffic) V25.9 ☑
          nontraffic V25.2 ☑

Accident — continued
  transport — continued
    motorcyclist — continued
      collision — continued
        railway vehicle — continued
          while boarding or alighting V25.3 ☑
        specified vehicle NEC (traffic) V26.9 ☑
          nontraffic V26.2 ☑
          while boarding or alighting V26.3 ☑
        stationary object (traffic) V27.9 ☑
          nontraffic V27.2 ☑
          while boarding or alighting V27.3 ☑
        streetcar (traffic) V26.9 ☑
          nontraffic V26.2 ☑
          while boarding or alighting V26.3 ☑
        three wheeled motor vehicle (traffic) V22.9 ☑
          nontraffic V22.2 ☑
          while boarding or alighting V22.3 ☑
        truck (traffic) V24.9 ☑
          nontraffic V24.2 ☑
          while boarding or alighting V24.3 ☑
        two wheeled motor vehicle (traffic) V22.9 ☑
          nontraffic V22.2 ☑
          while boarding or alighting V22.3 ☑
        van (traffic) V23.9 ☑
          nontraffic V23.2 ☑
          while boarding or alighting V23.3 ☑
      driver
        collision (with)
          animal (traffic) V20.4 ☑
            being ridden (traffic) V26.4 ☑
              nontraffic V26.0 ☑
            nontraffic V20.0 ☑
          animal-drawn vehicle (traffic) V26.4 ☑
            nontraffic V26.0 ☑
          bus (traffic) V24.4 ☑
            nontraffic V24.0 ☑
          car (traffic) V23.4 ☑
            nontraffic V23.0 ☑
          motor vehicle NOS (traffic) V29.40 ☑
            nontraffic V29.00 ☑
            specified type NEC (traffic) V29.49 ☑
              nontraffic V29.09 ☑
          pedal cycle (traffic) V21.4 ☑
            nontraffic V21.0 ☑
          pickup truck (traffic) V23.4 ☑
            nontraffic V23.0 ☑
          railway vehicle (traffic) V25.4 ☑
            nontraffic V25.0 ☑
          specified vehicle NEC (traffic) V26.4 ☑
            nontraffic V26.0 ☑
          stationary object (traffic) V27.4 ☑
            nontraffic V27.0 ☑
          streetcar (traffic) V26.4 ☑
            nontraffic V26.0 ☑
          three wheeled motor vehicle (traffic) V22.4 ☑
            nontraffic V22.0 ☑
          truck (traffic) V24.4 ☑
            nontraffic V24.0 ☑
          two wheeled motor vehicle (traffic) V22.4 ☑
            nontraffic V22.0 ☑
          van (traffic) V23.4 ☑
            nontraffic V23.0 ☑
        noncollision accident (traffic) V28.4 ☑
          nontraffic V28.0 ☑
      noncollision accident (traffic) V28.9 ☑
        nontraffic V28.2 ☑
        while boarding or alighting V28.3 ☑
      nontraffic V29.3 ☑
      passenger
        collision (with)
          animal (traffic) V20.5 ☑
            being ridden (traffic) V26.5 ☑
              nontraffic V26.1 ☑
            nontraffic V20.1 ☑
          animal-drawn vehicle (traffic) V26.5 ☑
            nontraffic V26.1 ☑
          bus (traffic) V24.5 ☑
            nontraffic V24.1 ☑
          car (traffic) V23.5 ☑
            nontraffic V23.1 ☑
          motor vehicle NOS (traffic) V29.50 ☑
            nontraffic V29.10 ☑
            specified type NEC (traffic) V29.59 ☑

Accident — continued
  transport — continued
    motorcyclist — continued
      passenger — continued
        collision — continued
          motor vehicle — continued
            specified type — continued
              nontraffic V29.19 ☑
          pedal cycle (traffic) V21.5 ☑
            nontraffic V21.1 ☑
          pickup truck (traffic) V23.5 ☑
            nontraffic V23.1 ☑
          railway vehicle (traffic) V25.5 ☑
            nontraffic V25.1 ☑
          specified vehicle NEC (traffic) V26.5 ☑
            nontraffic V26.1 ☑
          stationary object (traffic) V27.5 ☑
            nontraffic V27.1 ☑
          streetcar (traffic) V26.5 ☑
            nontraffic V26.1 ☑
          three wheeled motor vehicle (traffic) V22.5 ☑
            nontraffic V22.1 ☑
          truck (traffic) V24.5 ☑
            nontraffic V24.1 ☑
          two wheeled motor vehicle (traffic) V22.5 ☑
            nontraffic V22.1 ☑
          van (traffic) V23.5 ☑
            nontraffic V23.1 ☑
        noncollision accident (traffic) V28.5 ☑
          nontraffic V28.1 ☑
      specified type NEC V29.88 ☑
      military vehicle V29.81 ☑
    occupant (of)
      aircraft (powered) V95.9 ☑
        fixed wing
          commercial — see Accident, transport, aircraft, occupant, powered, fixed wing, commercial
          private — see Accident, transport, aircraft, occupant, powered, fixed wing, private
        nonpowered V96.9 ☑
        specified NEC V95.8 ☑
      airport battery-powered vehicle — see Accident, transport, industrial vehicle occupant
      all-terrain vehicle (ATV) — see Accident, transport, all-terrain vehicle occupant
      animal-drawn vehicle — see Accident, transport, animal-drawn vehicle occupant
      automobile — see Accident, transport, car occupant
      balloon V96.00 ☑
      battery-powered vehicle — see Accident, transport, industrial vehicle occupant
      bicycle — see Accident, transport, pedal cyclist
        motorized — see Accident, transport, motorcycle rider
      boat NEC — see Accident, watercraft
      bulldozer — see Accident, transport, construction vehicle occupant
      bus — see Accident, transport, bus occupant
      cable car (on rails) (see also Accident, transport, streetcar occupant)
        not on rails V98.0 ☑
      car (see also Accident, transport, car occupant)
        cable (on rails) (see also Accident, transport, streetcar occupant)
        not on rails V98.0 ☑
      coach — see Accident, transport, bus occupant
      coal-car — see Accident, transport, industrial vehicle occupant
      digger — see Accident, transport, construction vehicle occupant
      dump truck — see Accident, transport, construction vehicle occupant
      earth-leveler — see Accident, transport, construction vehicle occupant
      farm machinery (self-propelled) — see Accident, transport, agricultural vehicle occupant
      forklift — see Accident, transport, industrial vehicle occupant
      glider (unpowered) V96.20 ☑
        hang V96.10 ☑

☑ Additional Character Required — Refer to the Tabular List for Character Selection   Subterms under main terms may continue to next column or page

Accident — continued
　transport — continued
　　occupant — continued
　　　glider — continued
　　　　powered (microlight) (ultralight) — see Accident, transport, aircraft, occupant, powered, glider
　　　glider (unpowered) NEC V96.20 ☑
　　　hang-glider V96.10 ☑
　　　harvester — see Accident, transport, agricultural vehicle occupant
　　　heavy (transport) vehicle — see Accident, transport, truck occupant
　　　helicopter — see Accident, transport, aircraft, occupant, helicopter
　　　ice-yacht V98.2 ☑
　　　kite (carrying person) V96.8 ☑
　　　land-yacht V98.1 ☑
　　　logging car — see Accident, transport, industrial vehicle occupant
　　　mechanical shovel — see Accident, transport, construction vehicle occupant
　　　microlight — see Accident, transport, aircraft, occupant, powered, glider
　　　minibus — see Accident, transport, pickup truck occupant
　　　minivan — see Accident, transport, pickup truck occupant
　　　moped — see Accident, transport, motorcycle
　　　motor scooter — see Accident, transport, motorcycle
　　　motorcycle (with sidecar) — see Accident, transport, motorcycle
　　　off-road motor-vehicle (see also Accident, transport, all-terrain vehicle occupant) V86.99 ☑
　　　pedal cycle (see also Accident, transport, pedal cyclist)
　　　pick-up (truck) — see Accident, transport, pickup truck occupant
　　　railway (train) (vehicle) (subterranean) (elevated) — see Accident, transport, railway vehicle occupant
　　　rickshaw — see Accident, transport, pedal cycle
　　　　motorized — see Accident, transport, three-wheeled motor vehicle
　　　pedal driven — see Accident, transport, pedal cyclist
　　　road-roller — see Accident, transport, construction vehicle occupant
　　　ship NOS V94.9 ☑
　　　ski-lift (chair) (gondola) V98.3 ☑
　　　snowmobile — see Accident, transport, snowmobile occupant
　　　spacecraft, spaceship — see Accident, transport, aircraft, occupant, spacecraft
　　　sport utility vehicle — see Accident, transport, pickup truck occupant
　　　SUV — see Accident, transport, pickup truck occupant
　　　téléférique V98.0 ☑
　　　three-wheeled vehicle (motorized) (see also Accident, transport, three-wheeled motor vehicle occupant)
　　　　nonmotorized — see Accident, transport, pedal cycle
　　　tractor (farm) (and trailer) — see Accident, transport, agricultural vehicle occupant
　　　train — see Accident, transport, railway vehicle occupant
　　　tram — see Accident, transport, streetcar occupant
　　　　in mine or quarry — see Accident, transport, industrial vehicle occupant
　　　tricycle — see Accident, transport, pedal cycle
　　　　motorized — see Accident, transport, three-wheeled motor vehicle
　　　trolley — see Accident, transport, streetcar occupant
　　　　in mine or quarry — see Accident, transport, industrial vehicle occupant
　　　tub, in mine or quarry — see Accident, transport, industrial vehicle occupant

Accident — continued
　transport — continued
　　occupant — continued
　　　ultralight — see Accident, transport, aircraft, occupant, powered, glider
　　　van — see Accident, transport, van occupant
　　　vehicle NEC V89.9 ☑
　　　　heavy transport — see Accident, transport, truck occupant
　　　　motor (traffic) NEC V89.2 ☑
　　　　nontraffic NEC V89.0 ☑
　　　watercraft NOS V94.9 ☑
　　　　causing drowning — see Drowning, resulting from accident to boat
　　off-road motor-vehicle (see also Accident, transport, all-terrain vehicle occupant) V86.99 ☑
　　parachutist V97.29 ☑
　　　after accident to aircraft — see Accident, transport, aircraft
　　　entangled in object V97.21 ☑
　　　injured on landing V97.22 ☑
　　pedal cyclist V19.9 ☑
　　　collision (with)
　　　　animal (traffic) V10.9 ☑
　　　　　being ridden (traffic) V16.9 ☑
　　　　　　nontraffic V16.2 ☑
　　　　　　while boarding or alighting V16.3 ☑
　　　　　nontraffic V10.2 ☑
　　　　　while boarding or alighting V10.3 ☑
　　　　animal-drawn vehicle (traffic) V16.9 ☑
　　　　　nontraffic V16.2 ☑
　　　　　while boarding or alighting V16.3 ☑
　　　　bus (traffic) V14.9 ☑
　　　　　nontraffic V14.2 ☑
　　　　　while boarding or alighting V14.3 ☑
　　　　car (traffic) V13.9 ☑
　　　　　nontraffic V13.2 ☑
　　　　　while boarding or alighting V13.3 ☑
　　　　motor vehicle NOS (traffic) V19.60 ☑
　　　　　nontraffic V19.20 ☑
　　　　　specified type NEC (traffic) V19.69 ☑
　　　　　　nontraffic V19.29 ☑
　　　　pedal cycle (traffic) V11.9 ☑
　　　　　nontraffic V11.2 ☑
　　　　　while boarding or alighting V11.3 ☑
　　　　pickup truck (traffic) V13.9 ☑
　　　　　nontraffic V13.2 ☑
　　　　　while boarding or alighting V13.3 ☑
　　　　railway vehicle (traffic) V15.9 ☑
　　　　　nontraffic V15.2 ☑
　　　　　while boarding or alighting V15.3 ☑
　　　　specified vehicle NEC (traffic) V16.9 ☑
　　　　　nontraffic V16.2 ☑
　　　　　while boarding or alighting V16.3 ☑
　　　　stationary object (traffic) V17.9 ☑
　　　　　nontraffic V17.2 ☑
　　　　　while boarding or alighting V17.3 ☑
　　　　streetcar (traffic) V16.9 ☑
　　　　　nontraffic V16.2 ☑
　　　　　while boarding or alighting V16.3 ☑
　　　　three wheeled motor vehicle (traffic) V12.9 ☑
　　　　　nontraffic V12.2 ☑
　　　　　while boarding or alighting V12.3 ☑
　　　　truck (traffic) V14.9 ☑
　　　　　nontraffic V14.2 ☑
　　　　　while boarding or alighting V14.3 ☑
　　　　two wheeled motor vehicle (traffic) V12.9 ☑
　　　　　nontraffic V12.2 ☑
　　　　　while boarding or alighting V12.3 ☑
　　　　van (traffic) V13.9 ☑
　　　　　nontraffic V13.2 ☑
　　　　　while boarding or alighting V13.3 ☑
　　　driver
　　　　collision (with)
　　　　　animal (traffic) V10.4 ☑
　　　　　　being ridden (traffic) V16.4 ☑
　　　　　　　nontraffic V16.0 ☑
　　　　　　nontraffic V10.0 ☑
　　　　　animal-drawn vehicle (traffic) V16.4 ☑
　　　　　　nontraffic V16.0 ☑
　　　　　bus (traffic) V14.4 ☑
　　　　　　nontraffic V14.0 ☑
　　　　　car (traffic) V13.4 ☑
　　　　　　nontraffic V13.0 ☑
　　　　　motor vehicle NOS (traffic) V19.40 ☑
　　　　　　nontraffic V19.00 ☑

Accident — continued
　transport — continued
　　pedal cyclist — continued
　　　driver — continued
　　　　collision — continued
　　　　　motor vehicle — continued
　　　　　　specified type NEC (traffic) V19.49 ☑
　　　　　　　nontraffic V19.09 ☑
　　　　　pedal cycle (traffic) V11.4 ☑
　　　　　　nontraffic V11.0 ☑
　　　　　pickup truck (traffic) V13.4 ☑
　　　　　　nontraffic V13.0 ☑
　　　　　railway vehicle (traffic) V15.4 ☑
　　　　　　nontraffic V15.0 ☑
　　　　　specified vehicle NEC (traffic) V16.4 ☑
　　　　　　nontraffic V16.0 ☑
　　　　　stationary object (traffic) V17.4 ☑
　　　　　　nontraffic V17.0 ☑
　　　　　streetcar (traffic) V16.4 ☑
　　　　　　nontraffic V16.0 ☑
　　　　　three wheeled motor vehicle (traffic) V12.4 ☑
　　　　　　nontraffic V12.0 ☑
　　　　　truck (traffic) V14.4 ☑
　　　　　　nontraffic V14.0 ☑
　　　　　two wheeled motor vehicle (traffic) V12.4 ☑
　　　　　　nontraffic V12.0 ☑
　　　　　van (traffic) V13.4 ☑
　　　　　　nontraffic V13.0 ☑
　　　　noncollision accident (traffic) V18.4 ☑
　　　　　nontraffic V18.0 ☑
　　　noncollision accident (traffic) V18.9 ☑
　　　　nontraffic V18.2 ☑
　　　　while boarding or alighting V18.3 ☑
　　　nontraffic V19.3 ☑
　　　passenger
　　　　collision (with)
　　　　　animal (traffic) V10.5 ☑
　　　　　　being ridden (traffic) V16.5 ☑
　　　　　　　nontraffic V16.1 ☑
　　　　　　nontraffic V10.1 ☑
　　　　　animal-drawn vehicle (traffic) V16.5 ☑
　　　　　　nontraffic V16.1 ☑
　　　　　bus (traffic) V14.5 ☑
　　　　　　nontraffic V14.1 ☑
　　　　　car (traffic) V13.5 ☑
　　　　　　nontraffic V13.1 ☑
　　　　　motor vehicle NOS (traffic) V19.50 ☑
　　　　　　nontraffic V19.10 ☑
　　　　　specified type NEC (traffic) V19.59 ☑
　　　　　　nontraffic V19.19 ☑
　　　　　pedal cycle (traffic) V11.5 ☑
　　　　　　nontraffic V11.1 ☑
　　　　　pickup truck (traffic) V13.5 ☑
　　　　　　nontraffic V13.1 ☑
　　　　　railway vehicle (traffic) V15.5 ☑
　　　　　　nontraffic V15.1 ☑
　　　　　specified vehicle NEC (traffic) V16.5 ☑
　　　　　　nontraffic V16.1 ☑
　　　　　stationary object (traffic) V17.5 ☑
　　　　　　nontraffic V17.1 ☑
　　　　　streetcar (traffic) V16.5 ☑
　　　　　　nontraffic V16.1 ☑
　　　　　three wheeled motor vehicle (traffic) V12.5 ☑
　　　　　　nontraffic V12.1 ☑
　　　　　truck (traffic) V14.5 ☑
　　　　　　nontraffic V14.1 ☑
　　　　　two wheeled motor vehicle (traffic) V12.5 ☑
　　　　　　nontraffic V12.1 ☑
　　　　　van (traffic) V13.5 ☑
　　　　　　nontraffic V13.1 ☑
　　　　noncollision accident (traffic) V18.5 ☑
　　　　　nontraffic V18.1 ☑
　　　specified type NEC V19.88 ☑
　　　military vehicle V19.81 ☑
　　pedestrian
　　　conveyance (occupant) V09.9 ☑
　　　　baby stroller V00.828 ☑
　　　　collision (with) V09.9 ☑
　　　　　animal being ridden or animal drawn vehicle V06.99 ☑
　　　　　　nontraffic V06.09 ☑
　　　　　　traffic V06.19 ☑

◢ Subterms under main terms may continue to next column or page　　☑ Additional Character Required — Refer to the Tabular List for Character Selection　　**403**

Accident — Accident

Accident — *continued*
  transport — *continued*
    pedestrian — *continued*
      conveyance — *continued*
        baby stroller — *continued*
          collision — *continued*
            bus or heavy transport V04.99 ☑
              nontraffic V04.09 ☑
              traffic V04.19 ☑
            car V03.99 ☑
              nontraffic V03.09 ☑
              traffic V03.19 ☑
            pedal cycle V01.99 ☑
              nontraffic V01.09 ☑
              traffic V01.19 ☑
            pick-up truck or van V03.99 ☑
              nontraffic V03.09 ☑
              traffic V03.19 ☑
            railway (train) (vehicle) V05.99 ☑
              nontraffic V05.09 ☑
              traffic V05.19 ☑
            stationary object V00.822 ☑
            streetcar V06.99 ☑
              nontraffic V06.09 ☑
              traffic V06.19 ☑
            two- or three-wheeled motor vehicle V02.99 ☑
              nontraffic V02.09 ☑
              traffic V02.19 ☑
            vehicle V09.9 ☑
              animal-drawn V06.99 ☑
                nontraffic V06.09 ☑
                traffic V06.19 ☑
              motor
                nontraffic V09.00 ☑
                traffic V09.20 ☑
          fall V00.821 ☑
          nontraffic V09.1 ☑
            involving motor vehicle NEC V09.00 ☑
          traffic V09.3 ☑
            involving motor vehicle NEC V09.20 ☑
        flat-bottomed NEC V00.388 ☑
          collision (with) V09.9 ☑
            animal being ridden or animal drawn vehicle V06.99 ☑
              nontraffic V06.09 ☑
              traffic V06.19 ☑
            bus or heavy transport V04.99 ☑
              nontraffic V04.09 ☑
              traffic V04.19 ☑
            car V03.99 ☑
              nontraffic V03.09 ☑
              traffic V03.19 ☑
            pedal cycle V01.99 ☑
              nontraffic V01.09 ☑
              traffic V01.19 ☑
            pick-up truck or van V03.99 ☑
              nontraffic V03.09 ☑
              traffic V03.19 ☑
            railway (train) (vehicle) V05.99 ☑
              nontraffic V05.09 ☑
              traffic V05.19 ☑
            stationary object V00.382 ☑
            streetcar V06.99 ☑
              nontraffic V06.09 ☑
              traffic V06.19 ☑
            two- or three-wheeled motor vehicle V02.99 ☑
              nontraffic V02.09 ☑
              traffic V02.19 ☑
            vehicle V09.9 ☑
              animal-drawn V06.99 ☑
                nontraffic V06.09 ☑
                traffic V06.19 ☑
              motor
                nontraffic V09.00 ☑
                traffic V09.20 ☑
          fall V00.381 ☑
          nontraffic V09.1 ☑
            involving motor vehicle NEC V09.00 ☑
        snow
          board — *see* Accident, transport, pedestrian, conveyance, snow board
          ski — *see* Accident, transport, pedestrian, conveyance, skis (snow)

Accident — *continued*
  transport — *continued*
    pedestrian — *continued*
      conveyance — *continued*
        flat-bottomed — *continued*
          traffic V09.3 ☑
            involving motor vehicle NEC V09.20 ☑
        gliding type NEC V00.288 ☑
          collision (with) V09.9 ☑
            animal being ridden or animal drawn vehicle V06.99 ☑
              nontraffic V06.09 ☑
              traffic V06.19 ☑
            bus or heavy transport V04.99 ☑
              nontraffic V04.09 ☑
              traffic V04.19 ☑
            car V03.99 ☑
              nontraffic V03.09 ☑
              traffic V03.19 ☑
            pedal cycle V01.99 ☑
              nontraffic V01.09 ☑
              traffic V01.19 ☑
            pick-up truck or van V03.99 ☑
              nontraffic V03.09 ☑
              traffic V03.19 ☑
            railway (train) (vehicle) V05.99 ☑
              nontraffic V05.09 ☑
              traffic V05.19 ☑
            stationary object V00.282 ☑
            streetcar V06.99 ☑
              nontraffic V06.09 ☑
              traffic V02.19 ☑
            two- or three-wheeled motor vehicle V02.99 ☑
              nontraffic V02.09 ☑
              traffic V02.19 ☑
            vehicle V09.9 ☑
              animal-drawn V06.99 ☑
                nontraffic V06.09 ☑
                traffic V06.19 ☑
              motor
                nontraffic V09.00 ☑
                traffic V09.20 ☑
          fall V00.281 ☑
        heelies — *see* Accident, transport, pedestrian, conveyance, heelies
        ice skate — *see* Accident, transport, pedestrian, conveyance, ice skate
        nontraffic V09.1 ☑
          involving motor vehicle NEC V09.00 ☑
        sled — *see* Accident, transport, pedestrian, conveyance, sled
        traffic V09.3 ☑
          involving motor vehicle NEC V09.20 ☑
        wheelies — *see* Accident, transport, pedestrian, conveyance, heelies
      heelies V00.158 ☑
        colliding with stationary object V00.152 ☑
        fall V00.151 ☑
      ice skates V00.218 ☑
        collision (with) V09.9 ☑
          animal being ridden or animal drawn vehicle V06.99 ☑
            nontraffic V06.09 ☑
            traffic V06.19 ☑
          bus or heavy transport V04.99 ☑
            nontraffic V04.09 ☑
            traffic V04.19 ☑
          car V03.99 ☑
            nontraffic V03.09 ☑
            traffic V03.19 ☑
          pedal cycle V01.99 ☑
            nontraffic V01.09 ☑
            traffic V01.19 ☑
          pick-up truck or van V03.99 ☑
            nontraffic V03.09 ☑
            traffic V03.19 ☑
          railway (train) (vehicle) V05.99 ☑
            nontraffic V05.09 ☑
            traffic V05.19 ☑
          stationary object V00.212 ☑
          streetcar V06.99 ☑
            nontraffic V06.09 ☑
            traffic V06.19 ☑

Accident — *continued*
  transport — *continued*
    pedestrian — *continued*
      conveyance — *continued*
        ice skates — *continued*
          collision — *continued*
            two- or three-wheeled motor vehicle V02.99 ☑
              nontraffic V02.09 ☑
              traffic V02.19 ☑
            vehicle V09.9 ☑
              animal-drawn V06.99 ☑
                nontraffic V06.09 ☑
                traffic V06.19 ☑
              motor
                nontraffic V09.00 ☑
                traffic V09.20 ☑
          fall V00.211 ☑
          nontraffic V09.1 ☑
            involving motor vehicle NEC V09.00 ☑
          traffic V09.3 ☑
            involving motor vehicle NEC V09.20 ☑
      motorized mobility scooter V00.838 ☑
        collision with stationary object V00.832 ☑
        fall from V00.831 ☑
      nontraffic V09.1 ☑
        involving motor vehicle V09.00 ☑
          military V09.01 ☑
          specified type NEC V09.09 ☑
      roller skates (non in-line) V00.128 ☑
        collision (with) V09.9 ☑
          animal being ridden or animal drawn vehicle V06.91 ☑
            nontraffic V06.01 ☑
            traffic V06.11 ☑
          bus or heavy transport V04.91 ☑
            nontraffic V04.01 ☑
            traffic V04.11 ☑
          car V03.91 ☑
            nontraffic V03.01 ☑
            traffic V03.11 ☑
          pedal cycle V01.91 ☑
            nontraffic V01.01 ☑
            traffic V01.11 ☑
          pick-up truck or van V03.91 ☑
            nontraffic V03.01 ☑
            traffic V03.11 ☑
          railway (train) (vehicle) V05.91 ☑
            nontraffic V05.01 ☑
            traffic V05.11 ☑
          stationary object V00.122 ☑
          streetcar V06.91 ☑
            nontraffic V06.01 ☑
            traffic V06.11 ☑
          two- or three-wheeled motor vehicle V02.91 ☑
            nontraffic V02.01 ☑
            traffic V02.11 ☑
          vehicle V09.9 ☑
            animal-drawn V06.91 ☑
              nontraffic V06.01 ☑
              traffic V06.11 ☑
            motor
              nontraffic V09.00 ☑
              traffic V09.20 ☑
        fall V00.121 ☑
        in-line V00.118 ☑
          collision — *see also* Accident, transport, pedestrian, conveyance occupant, roller skates, collision with stationary object V00.112 ☑
          fall V00.111 ☑
        nontraffic V09.1 ☑
          involving motor vehicle NEC V09.00 ☑
        traffic V09.3 ☑
          involving motor vehicle NEC V09.20 ☑
      rolling shoes V00.158 ☑
        colliding with stationary object V00.152 ☑
        fall V00.151 ☑
      rolling type NEC V00.188 ☑
        collision (with) V09.9 ☑
          animal being ridden or animal drawn vehicle V06.99 ☑
            nontraffic V06.09 ☑

Accident — *continued*
  transport — *continued*
    pedestrian — *continued*
      conveyance — *continued*
        rolling type — *continued*
          collision — *continued*
            animal being ridden or animal drawn
              vehicle — *continued*
                traffic V06.19 ☑
            bus or heavy transport V04.99 ☑
              nontraffic V04.09 ☑
              traffic V04.19 ☑
            car V03.99 ☑
              nontraffic V03.09 ☑
              traffic V03.19 ☑
            pedal cycle V01.99 ☑
              nontraffic V01.09 ☑
              traffic V01.19 ☑
            pick-up truck or van V03.99 ☑
              nontraffic V03.09 ☑
              traffic V03.19 ☑
            railway (train) (vehicle) V05.99 ☑
              nontraffic V05.09 ☑
              traffic V05.19 ☑
            stationary object V00.182 ☑
            streetcar V06.99 ☑
              nontraffic V06.09 ☑
              traffic V06.19 ☑
            two- or three-wheeled motor vehicle
              V02.99 ☑
              nontraffic V02.09 ☑
              traffic V02.19 ☑
            vehicle V09.9 ☑
              animal-drawn V06.99 ☑
                nontraffic V06.09 ☑
                traffic V06.19 ☑
              motor
                nontraffic V09.00 ☑
                traffic V09.20 ☑
        fall V00.181 ☑
        in-line roller skate — *see* Accident,
          transport, pedestrian, conveyance,
          roller skate, in-line
        nontraffic V09.1 ☑
          involving motor vehicle NEC V09.00 ☑
        roller skate — *see* Accident, transport,
          pedestrian, conveyance, roller
          skate
        scooter (non-motorized) — *see* Accident,
          transport, pedestrian, conveyance,
          scooter
        skateboard — *see* Accident, transport,
          pedestrian, conveyance, skate-
          board
        traffic V09.3 ☑
          involving motor vehicle NEC V09.20 ☑
       scooter (non-motorized) V00.148 ☑
        collision (with) V09.9 ☑
          animal being ridden or animal drawn
            vehicle V06.99 ☑
            nontraffic V06.09 ☑
            traffic V06.19 ☑
          bus or heavy transport V04.99 ☑
            nontraffic V04.09 ☑
            traffic V04.19 ☑
          car V03.99 ☑
            nontraffic V03.09 ☑
            traffic V03.19 ☑
          pedal cycle V01.99 ☑
            nontraffic V01.09 ☑
            traffic V01.19 ☑
          pick-up truck or van V03.99 ☑
            nontraffic V03.09 ☑
            traffic V03.19 ☑
          railway (train) (vehicle) V05.99 ☑
            nontraffic V05.09 ☑
            traffic V05.19 ☑
          stationary object V00.142 ☑
          streetcar V06.99 ☑
            nontraffic V06.09 ☑
            traffic V06.19 ☑
          two- or three-wheeled motor vehicle
            V02.99 ☑
            nontraffic V02.09 ☑
            traffic V02.19 ☑
          vehicle V09.9 ☑

Accident — *continued*
  transport — *continued*
    pedestrian — *continued*
      conveyance — *continued*
        scooter — *continued*
          collision — *continued*
            vehicle — *continued*
              animal-drawn V06.99 ☑
                nontraffic V06.09 ☑
                traffic V06.19 ☑
              motor
                nontraffic V09.00 ☑
                traffic V09.20 ☑
        fall V00.141 ☑
        nontraffic V09.1 ☑
          involving motor vehicle NEC V09.00 ☑
        traffic V09.3 ☑
          involving motor vehicle NEC V09.20 ☑
       skate board V00.138 ☑
        collision (with) V09.9 ☑
          animal being ridden or animal drawn
            vehicle V06.92 ☑
            nontraffic V06.02 ☑
            traffic V06.12 ☑
          bus or heavy transport V04.92 ☑
            nontraffic V04.02 ☑
            traffic V04.12 ☑
          car V03.92 ☑
            nontraffic V03.02 ☑
            traffic V03.12 ☑
          pedal cycle V01.92 ☑
            nontraffic V01.02 ☑
            traffic V01.12 ☑
          pick-up truck or van V03.92 ☑
            nontraffic V03.02 ☑
            traffic V03.12 ☑
          railway (train) (vehicle) V05.92 ☑
            nontraffic V05.02 ☑
            traffic V05.12 ☑
          stationary object V00.132 ☑
          streetcar V06.92 ☑
            nontraffic V06.02 ☑
            traffic V06.12 ☑
          two- or three-wheeled motor vehicle
            V02.92 ☑
            nontraffic V02.02 ☑
            traffic V02.12 ☑
          vehicle V09.9 ☑
            animal-drawn V06.92 ☑
              nontraffic V06.02 ☑
              traffic V06.12 ☑
            motor
              nontraffic V09.00 ☑
              traffic V09.20 ☑
        fall V00.131 ☑
        nontraffic V09.1 ☑
          involving motor vehicle NEC V09.00 ☑
        traffic V09.3 ☑
          involving motor vehicle NEC V09.20 ☑
      skis (snow) V00.328 ☑
        collision (with) V09.9 ☑
          animal being ridden or animal drawn
            vehicle V06.99 ☑
            nontraffic V06.09 ☑
            traffic V06.19 ☑
          bus or heavy transport V04.99 ☑
            nontraffic V04.09 ☑
            traffic V04.19 ☑
          car V03.99 ☑
            nontraffic V03.09 ☑
            traffic V03.19 ☑
          pedal cycle V01.99 ☑
            nontraffic V01.09 ☑
            traffic V01.19 ☑
          pick-up truck or van V03.99 ☑
            nontraffic V03.09 ☑
            traffic V03.19 ☑
          railway (train) (vehicle) V05.99 ☑
            nontraffic V05.09 ☑
            traffic V05.19 ☑
          stationary object V00.322 ☑
          streetcar V06.99 ☑
            nontraffic V06.09 ☑
            traffic V06.19 ☑
          two- or three-wheeled motor vehicle
            V02.99 ☑

Accident — *continued*
  transport — *continued*
    pedestrian — *continued*
      conveyance — *continued*
        skis — *continued*
          collision — *continued*
            two- or three-wheeled motor vehicle
              — *continued*
              nontraffic V02.09 ☑
              traffic V02.19 ☑
            vehicle V09.9 ☑
              animal-drawn V06.99 ☑
                nontraffic V06.09 ☑
                traffic V06.19 ☑
              motor
                nontraffic V09.00 ☑
                traffic V09.20 ☑
        fall V00.321 ☑
        nontraffic V09.1 ☑
          involving motor vehicle NEC V09.00 ☑
        traffic V09.3 ☑
          involving motor vehicle NEC V09.20 ☑
      sled V00.228 ☑
        collision (with) V09.9 ☑
          animal being ridden or animal drawn
            vehicle V06.99 ☑
            nontraffic V06.09 ☑
            traffic V06.19 ☑
          bus or heavy transport V04.99 ☑
            nontraffic V04.09 ☑
            traffic V04.19 ☑
          car V03.99 ☑
            nontraffic V03.09 ☑
            traffic V03.19 ☑
          pedal cycle V01.99 ☑
            nontraffic V01.09 ☑
            traffic V01.19 ☑
          pick-up truck or van V03.99 ☑
            nontraffic V03.09 ☑
            traffic V03.19 ☑
          railway (train) (vehicle) V05.99 ☑
            nontraffic V05.09 ☑
            traffic V05.19 ☑
          stationary object V00.222 ☑
          streetcar V06.99 ☑
            nontraffic V06.09 ☑
            traffic V06.19 ☑
          two- or three-wheeled motor vehicle
            V02.99 ☑
            nontraffic V02.09 ☑
            traffic V02.19 ☑
          vehicle V09.9 ☑
            animal-drawn V06.99 ☑
              nontraffic V06.09 ☑
              traffic V06.19 ☑
            motor
              nontraffic V09.00 ☑
              traffic V09.20 ☑
        fall V00.221 ☑
        nontraffic V09.1 ☑
          involving motor vehicle NEC V09.00 ☑
        traffic V09.3 ☑
          involving motor vehicle NEC V09.20 ☑
      snow board V00.318 ☑
        collision (with) V09.9 ☑
          animal being ridden or animal drawn
            vehicle V06.99 ☑
            nontraffic V06.09 ☑
            traffic V06.19 ☑
          bus or heavy transport V04.99 ☑
            nontraffic V04.09 ☑
            traffic V04.19 ☑
          car V03.99 ☑
            nontraffic V03.09 ☑
            traffic V03.19 ☑
          pedal cycle V01.99 ☑
            nontraffic V01.09 ☑
            traffic V01.19 ☑
          pick-up truck or van V03.99 ☑
            nontraffic V03.09 ☑
            traffic V03.19 ☑
          railway (train) (vehicle) V05.99 ☑
            nontraffic V05.09 ☑
            traffic V05.19 ☑
          stationary object V00.312 ☑
          streetcar V06.99 ☑

Accident — *continued*
  transport — *continued*
    pedestrian — *continued*
      conveyance — *continued*
        snow board — *continued*
          collision — *continued*
            streetcar — *continued*
              nontraffic V06.09 ☑
              traffic V06.19 ☑
            two- or three-wheeled motor vehicle
              V02.99 ☑
              nontraffic V02.09 ☑
              traffic V02.19 ☑
            vehicle V09.9 ☑
              animal-drawn V06.99 ☑
                nontraffic V06.09 ☑
                traffic V06.19 ☑
              motor
                nontraffic V09.00 ☑
                traffic V09.20 ☑
           fall V00.311 ☑
          nontraffic V09.1 ☑
            involving motor vehicle NEC V09.00 ☑
          traffic V09.3 ☑
            involving motor vehicle NEC V09.20 ☑
         specified type NEC V00.898 ☑
         collision (with) V09.9 ☑
          animal being ridden or animal drawn
            vehicle V06.99 ☑
            nontraffic V06.09 ☑
            traffic V06.19 ☑
          bus or heavy transport V04.99 ☑
            nontraffic V04.09 ☑
            traffic V04.19 ☑
          car V03.99 ☑
            nontraffic V03.09 ☑
            traffic V03.19 ☑
          pedal cycle V01.99 ☑
            nontraffic V01.09 ☑
            traffic V01.19 ☑
          pick-up truck or van V03.99 ☑
            nontraffic V03.09 ☑
            traffic V03.19 ☑
          railway (train) (vehicle) V05.99 ☑
            nontraffic V05.09 ☑
            traffic V05.19 ☑
          stationary object V00.892 ☑
          streetcar V06.99 ☑
            nontraffic V06.09 ☑
            traffic V06.19 ☑
          two- or three-wheeled motor vehicle
            V02.99 ☑
            nontraffic V02.09 ☑
            traffic V02.19 ☑
          vehicle V09.9 ☑
            animal-drawn V06.99 ☑
              nontraffic V06.09 ☑
              traffic V06.19 ☑
            motor
              nontraffic V09.00 ☑
              traffic V09.20 ☑
         fall V00.891 ☑
        nontraffic V09.1 ☑
          involving motor vehicle NEC V09.00 ☑
        traffic V09.3 ☑
          involving motor vehicle NEC V09.20 ☑
      traffic V09.3 ☑
        involving motor vehicle V09.20 ☑
          military V09.21 ☑
          specified type NEC V09.29 ☑
      wheelchair (powered) V00.818 ☑
        collision (with) V09.9 ☑
          animal being ridden or animal drawn
            vehicle V06.99 ☑
            nontraffic V06.09 ☑
            traffic V06.19 ☑
          bus or heavy transport V04.99 ☑
            nontraffic V04.09 ☑
            traffic V04.19 ☑
          car V03.99 ☑
            nontraffic V03.09 ☑
            traffic V03.19 ☑
          pedal cycle V01.99 ☑
            nontraffic V01.09 ☑
            traffic V01.19 ☑
          pick-up truck or van V03.99 ☑

Accident — *continued*
  transport — *continued*
    pedestrian — *continued*
      conveyance — *continued*
        wheelchair — *continued*
          collision — *continued*
            pick-up truck or van — *continued*
              nontraffic V03.09 ☑
              traffic V03.19 ☑
            railway (train) (vehicle) V05.99 ☑
              nontraffic V05.09 ☑
              traffic V05.19 ☑
            stationary object V00.812 ☑
            streetcar V06.99 ☑
              nontraffic V06.09 ☑
              traffic V06.19 ☑
            two- or three-wheeled motor vehicle
              V02.99 ☑
              nontraffic V02.09 ☑
              traffic V02.19 ☑
            vehicle V09.9 ☑
              animal-drawn V06.99 ☑
                nontraffic V06.09 ☑
                traffic V06.19 ☑
              motor
                nontraffic V09.00 ☑
                traffic V09.20 ☑
         fall V00.811 ☑
        nontraffic V09.1 ☑
          involving motor vehicle NEC V09.00 ☑
        traffic V09.3 ☑
          involving motor vehicle NEC V09.20 ☑
      wheeled shoe V00.158 ☑
        colliding with stationary object
          V00.152 ☑
        fall V00.151 ☑
    on foot (*see also* Accident, pedestrian)
      collision (with)
        animal being ridden or animal drawn ve-
          hicle V06.90 ☑
          nontraffic V06.00 ☑
          traffic V06.10 ☑
        bus or heavy transport V04.90 ☑
          nontraffic V04.00 ☑
          traffic V04.10 ☑
        car V03.90 ☑
          nontraffic V03.00 ☑
          traffic V03.10 ☑
        pedal cycle V01.90 ☑
          nontraffic V01.00 ☑
          traffic V01.10 ☑
        pick-up truck or van V03.90 ☑
          nontraffic V03.00 ☑
          traffic V03.10 ☑
        railway (train) (vehicle) V05.90 ☑
          nontraffic V05.00 ☑
          traffic V05.10 ☑
        streetcar V06.90 ☑
          nontraffic V06.00 ☑
          traffic V06.10 ☑
        two- or three-wheeled motor vehicle
          V02.90 ☑
          nontraffic V02.00 ☑
          traffic V02.10 ☑
        vehicle V09.9 ☑
          animal-drawn V06.90 ☑
           nontraffic V06.00 ☑
           traffic V06.10 ☑
          motor
      nontraffic V09.1 ☑
        involving motor vehicle V09.00 ☑
          military V09.01 ☑
          specified type NEC V09.09 ☑
      traffic V09.3 ☑
        involving motor vehicle V09.20 ☑
          military V09.21 ☑
          specified type NEC V09.29 ☑
    person NEC (unknown way or transportation) V99 ☑
      collision (between)
        bus (with)
          heavy transport vehicle (traffic) V87.5 ☑
          nontraffic V88.5 ☑
        car (with)
          bus (traffic) V87.3 ☑
           nontraffic V88.3 ☑
          heavy transport vehicle (traffic) V87.4 ☑

Accident — *continued*
  transport — *continued*
    person — *continued*
      collision — *continued*
        car — *continued*
          heavy transport vehicle — *continued*
            nontraffic V88.4 ☑
            nontraffic V88.5 ☑
          pick-up truck or van (traffic) V87.2 ☑
            nontraffic V88.2 ☑
          train or railway vehicle (traffic) V87.6 ☑
            nontraffic V88.6 ☑
          two-or three-wheeled motor vehicle
            (traffic) V87.0 ☑
            nontraffic V88.0 ☑
         motor vehicle (traffic) NEC V87.7 ☑
          nontraffic V88.7 ☑
        two-or three-wheeled vehicle (with) (traffic)
          motor vehicle NEC V87.1 ☑
           nontraffic V88.1 ☑
        nonmotor vehicle (collision) (noncollision) (traf-
          fic) V87.9 ☑
        nontraffic V88.9 ☑
    pickup truck occupant V59.9 ☑
      collision (with)
        animal (traffic) V50.9 ☑
          being ridden (traffic) V56.9 ☑
           nontraffic V56.3 ☑
           while boarding or alighting V56.4 ☑
          nontraffic V50.3 ☑
          while boarding or alighting V50.4 ☑
        animal-drawn vehicle (traffic) V56.9 ☑
          nontraffic V56.3 ☑
          while boarding or alighting V56.4 ☑
        bus (traffic) V54.9 ☑
          nontraffic V54.3 ☑
          while boarding or alighting V54.4 ☑
        car (traffic) V53.9 ☑
          nontraffic V53.3 ☑
          while boarding or alighting V53.4 ☑
        motor vehicle NOS (traffic) V59.60 ☑
          nontraffic V59.20 ☑
          specified type NEC (traffic) V59.69 ☑
           nontraffic V59.29 ☑
        pedal cycle (traffic) V51.9 ☑
          nontraffic V51.3 ☑
          while boarding or alighting V51.4 ☑
        pickup truck (traffic) V53.9 ☑
          nontraffic V53.3 ☑
          while boarding or alighting V53.4 ☑
        railway vehicle (traffic) V55.9 ☑
          nontraffic V55.3 ☑
          while boarding or alighting V55.4 ☑
        specified vehicle NEC (traffic) V56.9 ☑
          nontraffic V56.3 ☑
          while boarding or alighting V56.4 ☑
        stationary object (traffic) V57.9 ☑
          nontraffic V57.3 ☑
          while boarding or alighting V57.4 ☑
        streetcar (traffic) V56.9 ☑
          nontraffic V56.3 ☑
          while boarding or alighting V56.4 ☑
        three wheeled motor vehicle (traffic) V52.9 ☑
          nontraffic V52.3 ☑
          while boarding or alighting V52.4 ☑
        truck (traffic) V54.9 ☑
          nontraffic V54.3 ☑
          while boarding or alighting V54.4 ☑
        two wheeled motor vehicle (traffic) V52.9 ☑
          nontraffic V52.3 ☑
          while boarding or alighting V52.4 ☑
        van (traffic) V53.9 ☑
          nontraffic V53.3 ☑
          while boarding or alighting V53.4 ☑
      driver
        collision (with)
          animal (traffic) V50.5 ☑
           being ridden (traffic) V56.5 ☑
            nontraffic V56.0 ☑
           nontraffic V50.0 ☑
          animal-drawn vehicle (traffic) V56.5 ☑
           nontraffic V56.0 ☑
          bus (traffic) V54.5 ☑
           nontraffic V54.0 ☑
          car (traffic) V53.5 ☑
           nontraffic V53.0 ☑

Accident — *continued*
 transport — *continued*
  pickup truck occupant — *continued*
   driver — *continued*
    collision — *continued*
     motor vehicle NOS (traffic) V59.40 ☑
      nontraffic V59.00 ☑
      specified type NEC (traffic) V59.49 ☑
       nontraffic V59.09 ☑
     pedal cycle (traffic) V51.5 ☑
      nontraffic V51.0 ☑
     pickup truck (traffic) V53.5 ☑
      nontraffic V53.0 ☑
     railway vehicle (traffic) V55.5 ☑
      nontraffic V55.0 ☑
     specified vehicle NEC (traffic) V56.5 ☑
      nontraffic V56.0 ☑
     stationary object (traffic) V57.5 ☑
      nontraffic V57.0 ☑
     streetcar (traffic) V56.5 ☑
      nontraffic V56.0 ☑
     three wheeled motor vehicle (traffic) V52.5 ☑
      nontraffic V52.0 ☑
     truck (traffic) V54.5 ☑
      nontraffic V54.0 ☑
     two wheeled motor vehicle (traffic) V52.5 ☑
      nontraffic V52.0 ☑
     van (traffic) V53.5 ☑
      nontraffic V53.0 ☑
    noncollision accident (traffic) V58.5 ☑
     nontraffic V58.0 ☑
   hanger-on
    collision (with)
     animal (traffic) V50.7 ☑
      being ridden (traffic) V56.7 ☑
       nontraffic V56.2 ☑
      nontraffic V50.2 ☑
     animal-drawn vehicle (traffic) V56.7 ☑
      nontraffic V56.2 ☑
     bus (traffic) V54.7 ☑
      nontraffic V54.2 ☑
     car (traffic) V53.7 ☑
      nontraffic V53.2 ☑
     pedal cycle (traffic) V51.7 ☑
      nontraffic V51.2 ☑
     pickup truck (traffic) V53.7 ☑
      nontraffic V53.2 ☑
     railway vehicle (traffic) V55.7 ☑
      nontraffic V55.2 ☑
     specified vehicle NEC (traffic) V56.7 ☑
      nontraffic V56.2 ☑
     stationary object (traffic) V57.7 ☑
      nontraffic V57.2 ☑
     streetcar (traffic) V56.7 ☑
      nontraffic V56.2 ☑
     three wheeled motor vehicle (traffic) V52.7 ☑
      nontraffic V52.2 ☑
     truck (traffic) V54.7 ☑
      nontraffic V54.2 ☑
     two wheeled motor vehicle (traffic) V52.7 ☑
      nontraffic V52.2 ☑
     van (traffic) V53.7 ☑
      nontraffic V53.2 ☑
    noncollision accident (traffic) V58.7 ☑
     nontraffic V58.2 ☑
   noncollision accident (traffic) V58.9 ☑
    nontraffic V58.3 ☑
    while boarding or alighting V58.4 ☑
   nontraffic V59.3 ☑
   passenger
    collision (with)
     animal (traffic) V50.6 ☑
      being ridden (traffic) V56.6 ☑
       nontraffic V56.1 ☑
      nontraffic V50.1 ☑
     animal-drawn vehicle (traffic) V56.6 ☑
      nontraffic V56.1 ☑
     bus (traffic) V54.6 ☑
      nontraffic V54.1 ☑
     car (traffic) V53.6 ☑
      nontraffic V53.1 ☑
     motor vehicle NOS (traffic) V59.50 ☑

Accident — *continued*
 transport — *continued*
  pickup truck occupant — *continued*
   passenger — *continued*
    collision — *continued*
     motor vehicle — *continued*
      nontraffic V59.10 ☑
      specified type NEC (traffic) V59.59 ☑
       nontraffic V59.19 ☑
     pedal cycle (traffic) V51.6 ☑
      nontraffic V51.1 ☑
     pickup truck (traffic) V53.6 ☑
      nontraffic V53.1 ☑
     railway vehicle (traffic) V55.6 ☑
      nontraffic V55.1 ☑
     specified vehicle NEC (traffic) V56.6 ☑
      nontraffic V56.1 ☑
     stationary object (traffic) V57.6 ☑
      nontraffic V57.1 ☑
     streetcar (traffic) V56.6 ☑
      nontraffic V56.1 ☑
     three wheeled motor vehicle (traffic) V52.6 ☑
      nontraffic V52.1 ☑
     truck (traffic) V54.6 ☑
      nontraffic V54.1 ☑
     two wheeled motor vehicle (traffic) V52.6 ☑
      nontraffic V52.1 ☑
     van (traffic) V53.6 ☑
      nontraffic V53.1 ☑
    noncollision accident (traffic) V58.6 ☑
     nontraffic V58.1 ☑
   specified type NEC V59.88 ☑
   military vehicle V59.81 ☑
  quarry truck — *see* Accident, transport, industrial vehicle occupant
  race car — *see* Accident, transport, motor vehicle NEC occupant
  railway vehicle occupant V81.9 ☑
   collision (with) V81.3 ☑
    motor vehicle (non-military) (traffic) V81.1 ☑
     military V81.83 ☑
     nontraffic V81.0 ☑
    rolling stock V81.2 ☑
    specified object NEC V81.3 ☑
   during derailment V81.7 ☑
    with antecedent collision — *see* Accident, transport, railway vehicle occupant, collision
   explosion V81.81 ☑
   fall (in railway vehicle) V81.5 ☑
    during derailment V81.7 ☑
     with antecedent collision — *see* Accident, transport, railway vehicle occupant, collision
    from railway vehicle V81.6 ☑
     during derailment V81.7 ☑
      with antecedent collision — *see* Accident, transport, railway vehicle occupant, collision
    while boarding or alighting V81.4 ☑
   fire V81.81 ☑
   object falling onto train V81.82 ☑
   specified type NEC V81.89 ☑
   while boarding or alighting V81.4 ☑
  ski lift V98.3 ☑
  snowmobile occupant (nontraffic) V86.92 ☑
   driver V86.52 ☑
   hanger-on V86.72 ☑
   passenger V86.62 ☑
   traffic V86.32 ☑
    driver V86.02 ☑
    hanger-on V86.22 ☑
    passenger V86.12 ☑
   while boarding or alighting V86.42 ☑
  specified NEC V98.8 ☑
  sport utility vehicle occupant (*see also* Accident, transport, pickup truck occupant)
  streetcar occupant V82.9 ☑
   collision (with) V82.3 ☑
    motor vehicle (traffic) V82.1 ☑
     nontraffic V82.0 ☑
    rolling stock V82.2 ☑
   during derailment V82.7 ☑

Accident — *continued*
 transport — *continued*
  streetcar occupant — *continued*
   during derailment — *continued*
    with antecedent collision — *see* Accident, transport, streetcar occupant, collision
   fall (in streetcar) V82.5 ☑
    during derailment V82.7 ☑
     with antecedent collision — *see* Accident, transport, streetcar occupant, collision
    from streetcar V82.6 ☑
     during derailment V82.7 ☑
      with antecedent collision — *see* Accident, transport, streetcar occupant, collision
    while boarding or alighting V82.4 ☑
   while boarding or alighting V82.4 ☑
   specified type NEC V82.8 ☑
   while boarding or alighting V82.4 ☑
  three-wheeled motor vehicle occupant V39.9 ☑
   collision (with)
    animal (traffic) V30.9 ☑
     being ridden (traffic) V36.9 ☑
      nontraffic V36.3 ☑
      while boarding or alighting V36.4 ☑
     nontraffic V30.3 ☑
     while boarding or alighting V30.4 ☑
    animal-drawn vehicle (traffic) V36.9 ☑
     nontraffic V36.3 ☑
     while boarding or alighting V36.4 ☑
    bus (traffic) V34.9 ☑
     nontraffic V34.3 ☑
     while boarding or alighting V34.4 ☑
    car (traffic) V33.9 ☑
     nontraffic V33.3 ☑
     while boarding or alighting V33.4 ☑
    motor vehicle NOS (traffic) V39.60 ☑
     nontraffic V39.20 ☑
     specified type NEC (traffic) V39.69 ☑
      nontraffic V39.29 ☑
    pedal cycle (traffic) V31.9 ☑
     nontraffic V31.3 ☑
     while boarding or alighting V31.4 ☑
    pickup truck (traffic) V33.9 ☑
     nontraffic V33.3 ☑
     while boarding or alighting V33.4 ☑
    railway vehicle (traffic) V35.9 ☑
     nontraffic V35.3 ☑
     while boarding or alighting V35.4 ☑
    specified vehicle NEC (traffic) V36.9 ☑
     nontraffic V36.3 ☑
     while boarding or alighting V36.4 ☑
    stationary object (traffic) V37.9 ☑
     nontraffic V37.3 ☑
     while boarding or alighting V37.4 ☑
    streetcar (traffic) V36.9 ☑
     nontraffic V36.3 ☑
     while boarding or alighting V36.4 ☑
    three wheeled motor vehicle (traffic) V32.9 ☑
     nontraffic V32.3 ☑
     while boarding or alighting V32.4 ☑
    truck (traffic) V34.9 ☑
     nontraffic V34.3 ☑
     while boarding or alighting V34.4 ☑
    two wheeled motor vehicle (traffic) V32.9 ☑
     nontraffic V32.3 ☑
     while boarding or alighting V32.4 ☑
    van (traffic) V33.9 ☑
     nontraffic V33.3 ☑
     while boarding or alighting V33.4 ☑
   driver
    collision (with)
     animal (traffic) V30.5 ☑
      being ridden (traffic) V36.5 ☑
       nontraffic V36.0 ☑
      nontraffic V30.0 ☑
     animal-drawn vehicle (traffic) V36.5 ☑
      nontraffic V36.0 ☑
     bus (traffic) V34.5 ☑
      nontraffic V34.0 ☑
     car (traffic) V33.5 ☑
      nontraffic V33.0 ☑
     motor vehicle NOS (traffic) V39.40 ☑
      nontraffic V39.00 ☑
      specified type NEC (traffic) V39.49 ☑

External Causes Index

Accident — *continued*
  transport — *continued*
    three-wheeled motor vehicle occupant — *continued*
      driver — *continued*
        collision — *continued*
          motor vehicle — *continued*
            specified type — *continued*
              nontraffic V39.09 ☑
          pedal cycle (traffic) V31.5 ☑
            nontraffic V31.0 ☑
          pickup truck (traffic) V33.5 ☑
            nontraffic V33.0 ☑
          railway vehicle (traffic) V35.5 ☑
            nontraffic V35.0 ☑
          specified vehicle NEC (traffic) V36.5 ☑
            nontraffic V36.0 ☑
          stationary object (traffic) V37.5 ☑
            nontraffic V37.0 ☑
          streetcar (traffic) V36.5 ☑
            nontraffic V36.0 ☑
          three wheeled motor vehicle (traffic) V32.5 ☑
            nontraffic V32.0 ☑
          truck (traffic) V34.5 ☑
            nontraffic V34.0 ☑
          two wheeled motor vehicle (traffic) V32.5 ☑
            nontraffic V32.0 ☑
          van (traffic) V33.5 ☑
            nontraffic V33.0 ☑
        noncollision accident (traffic) V38.5 ☑
          nontraffic V38.0 ☑
      hanger-on
        collision (with)
          animal (traffic) V30.7 ☑
            being ridden (traffic) V36.7 ☑
              nontraffic V36.2 ☑
            nontraffic V30.2 ☑
          animal-drawn vehicle (traffic) V36.7 ☑
            nontraffic V36.2 ☑
          bus (traffic) V34.7 ☑
            nontraffic V34.2 ☑
          car (traffic) V33.7 ☑
            nontraffic V33.2 ☑
          pedal cycle (traffic) V31.7 ☑
            nontraffic V31.2 ☑
          pickup truck (traffic) V33.7 ☑
            nontraffic V33.2 ☑
          railway vehicle (traffic) V35.7 ☑
            nontraffic V35.2 ☑
          specified vehicle NEC (traffic) V36.7 ☑
            nontraffic V36.2 ☑
          stationary object (traffic) V37.7 ☑
            nontraffic V37.2 ☑
          streetcar (traffic) V36.7 ☑
            nontraffic V36.2 ☑
          three wheeled motor vehicle (traffic) V32.7 ☑
            nontraffic V32.2 ☑
          truck (traffic) V34.7 ☑
            nontraffic V34.2 ☑
          two wheeled motor vehicle (traffic) V32.7 ☑
            nontraffic V32.2 ☑
          van (traffic) V33.7 ☑
            nontraffic V33.2 ☑
        noncollision accident (traffic) V38.7 ☑
          nontraffic V38.2 ☑
      noncollision accident (traffic) V38.9 ☑
        nontraffic V38.3 ☑
        while boarding or alighting V38.4 ☑
      nontraffic V39.3 ☑
      passenger
        collision (with)
          animal (traffic) V30.6 ☑
            being ridden (traffic) V36.6 ☑
              nontraffic V36.1 ☑
            nontraffic V30.1 ☑
          animal-drawn vehicle (traffic) V36.6 ☑
            nontraffic V36.1 ☑
          bus (traffic) V34.6 ☑
            nontraffic V34.1 ☑
          car (traffic) V33.6 ☑
            nontraffic V33.1 ☑
          motor vehicle NOS (traffic) V39.50 ☑

Accident — *continued*
  transport — *continued*
    three-wheeled motor vehicle occupant — *continued*
      passenger — *continued*
        collision — *continued*
          motor vehicle — *continued*
            nontraffic V39.10 ☑
            specified type NEC (traffic) V39.59 ☑
              nontraffic V39.19 ☑
          pedal cycle (traffic) V31.6 ☑
            nontraffic V31.1 ☑
          pickup truck (traffic) V33.6 ☑
            nontraffic V33.1 ☑
          railway vehicle (traffic) V35.6 ☑
            nontraffic V35.1 ☑
          specified vehicle NEC (traffic) V36.6 ☑
            nontraffic V36.1 ☑
          stationary object (traffic) V37.6 ☑
            nontraffic V37.1 ☑
          streetcar (traffic) V36.6 ☑
            nontraffic V36.1 ☑
          three wheeled motor vehicle (traffic) V32.6 ☑
            nontraffic V32.1 ☑
          truck (traffic) V34.6 ☑
            nontraffic V34.1 ☑
          two wheeled motor vehicle (traffic) V32.6 ☑
            nontraffic V32.1 ☑
          van (traffic) V33.6 ☑
            nontraffic V33.1 ☑
        noncollision accident (traffic) V38.6 ☑
          nontraffic V38.1 ☑
      specified type NEC V39.89 ☑
      military vehicle V39.81 ☑
    tractor (farm) (and trailer) — *see* Accident, transport, agricultural vehicle occupant
    tram — *see* Accident, transport, streetcar
      in mine or quarry — *see* Accident, transport, industrial vehicle occupant
    trolley — *see* Accident, transport, streetcar
      in mine or quarry — *see* Accident, transport, industrial vehicle occupant
    truck (heavy) occupant V69.9 ☑
      collision (with)
        animal (traffic) V60.9 ☑
          being ridden (traffic) V66.9 ☑
            nontraffic V66.3 ☑
            while boarding or alighting V66.4 ☑
          nontraffic V60.3 ☑
          while boarding or alighting V60.4 ☑
        animal-drawn vehicle (traffic) V66.9 ☑
          nontraffic V66.3 ☑
          while boarding or alighting V66.4 ☑
        bus (traffic) V64.9 ☑
          nontraffic V64.3 ☑
          while boarding or alighting V64.4 ☑
        car (traffic) V63.9 ☑
          nontraffic V63.3 ☑
          while boarding or alighting V63.4 ☑
        motor vehicle NOS (traffic) V69.60 ☑
          nontraffic V69.20 ☑
          specified type NEC (traffic) V69.69 ☑
            nontraffic V69.29 ☑
        pedal cycle (traffic) V61.9 ☑
          nontraffic V61.3 ☑
          while boarding or alighting V61.4 ☑
        pickup truck (traffic) V63.9 ☑
          nontraffic V63.3 ☑
          while boarding or alighting V63.4 ☑
        railway vehicle (traffic) V65.9 ☑
          nontraffic V65.3 ☑
          while boarding or alighting V65.4 ☑
        specified vehicle NEC (traffic) V66.9 ☑
          nontraffic V66.3 ☑
          while boarding or alighting V66.4 ☑
        stationary object (traffic) V67.9 ☑
          nontraffic V67.3 ☑
          while boarding or alighting V67.4 ☑
        streetcar (traffic) V66.9 ☑
          nontraffic V66.3 ☑
          while boarding or alighting V66.4 ☑
        three wheeled motor vehicle (traffic) V62.9 ☑
          nontraffic V62.3 ☑
          while boarding or alighting V62.4 ☑

Accident — *continued*
  transport — *continued*
    truck occupant — *continued*
      collision — *continued*
        truck (traffic) V64.9 ☑
          nontraffic V64.3 ☑
          while boarding or alighting V64.4 ☑
        two wheeled motor vehicle (traffic) V62.9 ☑
          nontraffic V62.3 ☑
          while boarding or alighting V62.4 ☑
        van (traffic) V63.9 ☑
          nontraffic V63.3 ☑
          while boarding or alighting V63.4 ☑
      driver
        collision (with)
          animal (traffic) V60.5 ☑
            being ridden (traffic) V66.5 ☑
              nontraffic V66.0 ☑
            nontraffic V60.0 ☑
          animal-drawn vehicle (traffic) V66.5 ☑
            nontraffic V66.0 ☑
          bus (traffic) V64.5 ☑
            nontraffic V64.0 ☑
          car (traffic) V63.5 ☑
            nontraffic V63.0 ☑
          motor vehicle NOS (traffic) V69.40 ☑
            nontraffic V69.00 ☑
            specified type NEC (traffic) V69.49 ☑
              nontraffic V69.09 ☑
          pedal cycle (traffic) V61.5 ☑
            nontraffic V61.0 ☑
          pickup truck (traffic) V63.5 ☑
            nontraffic V63.0 ☑
          railway vehicle (traffic) V65.5 ☑
            nontraffic V65.0 ☑
          specified vehicle NEC (traffic) V66.5 ☑
            nontraffic V66.0 ☑
          stationary object (traffic) V67.5 ☑
            nontraffic V67.0 ☑
          streetcar (traffic) V66.5 ☑
            nontraffic V66.0 ☑
          three wheeled motor vehicle (traffic) V62.5 ☑
            nontraffic V62.0 ☑
          truck (traffic) V64.5 ☑
            nontraffic V64.0 ☑
          two wheeled motor vehicle (traffic) V62.5 ☑
            nontraffic V62.0 ☑
          van (traffic) V63.5 ☑
            nontraffic V63.0 ☑
        noncollision accident (traffic) V68.5 ☑
          nontraffic V68.0 ☑
      dump — *see* Accident, transport, construction vehicle occupant
      hanger-on
        collision (with)
          animal (traffic) V60.7 ☑
            being ridden (traffic) V66.7 ☑
              nontraffic V66.2 ☑
            nontraffic V60.2 ☑
          animal-drawn vehicle (traffic) V66.7 ☑
            nontraffic V66.2 ☑
          bus (traffic) V64.7 ☑
            nontraffic V64.2 ☑
          car (traffic) V63.7 ☑
            nontraffic V63.2 ☑
          pedal cycle (traffic) V61.7 ☑
            nontraffic V61.2 ☑
          pickup truck (traffic) V63.7 ☑
            nontraffic V63.2 ☑
          railway vehicle (traffic) V65.7 ☑
            nontraffic V65.2 ☑
          specified vehicle NEC (traffic) V66.7 ☑
            nontraffic V66.2 ☑
          stationary object (traffic) V67.7 ☑
            nontraffic V67.2 ☑
          streetcar (traffic) V66.7 ☑
            nontraffic V66.2 ☑
          three wheeled motor vehicle (traffic) V62.7 ☑
            nontraffic V62.2 ☑
          truck (traffic) V64.7 ☑
            nontraffic V64.2 ☑
          two wheeled motor vehicle (traffic) V62.7 ☑

☑ Additional Character Required — Refer to the Tabular List for Character Selection   ▽ Subterms under main terms may continue to next column or page

Accident — Accident

Accident — *continued*
  transport — *continued*
    truck occupant — *continued*
      hanger-on — *continued*
        collision — *continued*
          two wheeled motor vehicle — *continued*
           nontraffic V62.2 ☑
           van (traffic) V63.7 ☑
           nontraffic V63.2 ☑
          noncollision accident (traffic) V68.7 ☑
           nontraffic V68.2 ☑
        noncollision accident (traffic) V68.9 ☑
          nontraffic V68.3 ☑
          while boarding or alighting V68.4 ☑
        nontraffic V69.3 ☑
      passenger
        collision (with)
          animal (traffic) V60.6 ☑
           being ridden (traffic) V66.6 ☑
            nontraffic V66.1-
           nontraffic V60.1
          animal-drawn vehicle (traffic) V66.6 ☑
           nontraffic V66.1 ☑
          bus (traffic) V64.6 ☑
           nontraffic V64.1 ☑
          car (traffic) V63.6 ☑
           nontraffic V63.1 ☑
          motor vehicle NOS (traffic) V69.50 ☑
           nontraffic V69.10 ☑
           specified type NEC (traffic) V69.59 ☑
            nontraffic V69.19 ☑
          pedal cycle (traffic) V61.6 ☑
           nontraffic V61.1 ☑
          pickup truck (traffic) V63.6 ☑
           nontraffic V63.1 ☑
          railway vehicle (traffic) V65.6 ☑
           nontraffic V65.1 ☑
          specified vehicle NEC (traffic) V66.6 ☑
           nontraffic V66.1 ☑
          stationary object (traffic) V67.6 ☑
           nontraffic V67.1 ☑
          streetcar (traffic) V66.6 ☑
           nontraffic V66.1 ☑
          three wheeled motor vehicle (traffic) V62.6 ☑
           nontraffic V62.1 ☑
          truck (traffic) V64.6 ☑
           nontraffic V64.1 ☑
          two wheeled motor vehicle (traffic) V62.6 ☑
           nontraffic V62.1 ☑
          van (traffic) V63.6 ☑
           nontraffic V63.1 ☑
        noncollision accident (traffic) V68.6 ☑
          nontraffic V68.1 ☑
      pickup — *see* Accident, transport, pickup truck occupant
      specified type NEC V69.88 ☑
      military vehicle V69.81 ☑
    van occupant V59.9 ☑
      collision (with)
        animal (traffic) V50.9 ☑
          being ridden (traffic) V56.9 ☑
           nontraffic V56.3 ☑
            while boarding or alighting V56.4 ☑
          nontraffic V50.3 ☑
          while boarding or alighting V50.4 ☑
         animal-drawn vehicle (traffic) V56.9 ☑
          nontraffic V56.3 ☑
          while boarding or alighting V56.4 ☑
         bus (traffic) V54.9 ☑
          nontraffic V54.3 ☑
          while boarding or alighting V54.4 ☑
         car (traffic) V53.9 ☑
          nontraffic V53.3 ☑
          while boarding or alighting V53.4 ☑
         motor vehicle NOS (traffic) V59.60 ☑
          nontraffic V59.20 ☑
          specified type NEC (traffic) V59.69 ☑
           nontraffic V59.29 ☑
         pedal cycle (traffic) V51.9 ☑
          nontraffic V51.3 ☑
          while boarding or alighting V51.4 ☑
         pickup truck (traffic) V53.9 ☑
          nontraffic V53.3 ☑

Accident — *continued*
  transport — *continued*
    van occupant — *continued*
      collision — *continued*
        pickup truck — *continued*
          while boarding or alighting V53.4 ☑
        railway vehicle (traffic) V55.9 ☑
          nontraffic V55.3 ☑
          while boarding or alighting V55.4 ☑
        specified vehicle NEC (traffic) V56.9 ☑
          nontraffic V56.3 ☑
          while boarding or alighting V56.4 ☑
        stationary object (traffic) V57.9 ☑
          nontraffic V57.3 ☑
          while boarding or alighting V57.4 ☑
        streetcar (traffic) V56.9 ☑
          nontraffic V56.3 ☑
          while boarding or alighting V56.4 ☑
        three wheeled motor vehicle (traffic) V52.9 ☑
          nontraffic V52.3 ☑
          while boarding or alighting V52.4 ☑
        truck (traffic) V54.9 ☑
          nontraffic V54.3 ☑
          while boarding or alighting V54.4 ☑
        two wheeled motor vehicle (traffic) V52.9 ☑
          nontraffic V52.3 ☑
          while boarding or alighting V52.4 ☑
        van (traffic) V53.9 ☑
          nontraffic V53.3 ☑
          while boarding or alighting V53.4 ☑
    driver
      collision (with)
        animal (traffic) V50.5 ☑
          being ridden (traffic) V56.5 ☑
           nontraffic V56.0 ☑
          nontraffic V50.0 ☑
        animal-drawn vehicle (traffic) V56.5 ☑
          nontraffic V56.0 ☑
        bus (traffic) V54.5 ☑
          nontraffic V54.0 ☑
        car (traffic) V53.5 ☑
          nontraffic V53.0 ☑
        motor vehicle NOS (traffic) V59.40 ☑
          nontraffic V59.00 ☑
          specified type NEC (traffic) V59.49 ☑
           nontraffic V59.09 ☑
        pedal cycle (traffic) V51.5 ☑
          nontraffic V51.0 ☑
        pickup truck (traffic) V53.5 ☑
          nontraffic V53.0 ☑
        railway vehicle (traffic) V55.5 ☑
          nontraffic V55.0 ☑
        specified vehicle NEC (traffic) V56.5 ☑
          nontraffic V56.0 ☑
        stationary object (traffic) V57.5 ☑
          nontraffic V57.0 ☑
        streetcar (traffic) V56.5 ☑
          nontraffic V56.0 ☑
        three wheeled motor vehicle (traffic) V52.5 ☑
          nontraffic V52.0 ☑
        truck (traffic) V54.5 ☑
          nontraffic V54.0 ☑
        two wheeled motor vehicle (traffic) V52.5 ☑
          nontraffic V52.0 ☑
        van (traffic) V53.5 ☑
          nontraffic V53.0 ☑
      noncollision accident (traffic) V58.5 ☑
        nontraffic V58.0 ☑
    hanger-on
      collision (with)
        animal (traffic) V50.7 ☑
          being ridden (traffic) V56.7 ☑
           nontraffic V56.2 ☑
          nontraffic V50.2 ☑
        animal-drawn vehicle (traffic) V56.7 ☑
          nontraffic V56.2 ☑
        bus (traffic) V54.7 ☑
          nontraffic V54.2 ☑
        car (traffic) V53.7 ☑
          nontraffic V53.2 ☑
        pedal cycle (traffic) V51.7 ☑
          nontraffic V51.2 ☑
        pickup truck (traffic) V53.7 ☑
          nontraffic V53.2 ☑

Accident — *continued*
  transport — *continued*
    van occupant — *continued*
      hanger-on — *continued*
        collision — *continued*
          railway vehicle (traffic) V55.7 ☑
           nontraffic V55.2 ☑
          specified vehicle NEC (traffic) V56.7 ☑
           nontraffic V56.2 ☑
          stationary object (traffic) V57.7 ☑
           nontraffic V57.2 ☑
          streetcar (traffic) V56.7 ☑
           nontraffic V56.2 ☑
          three wheeled motor vehicle (traffic) V52.7 ☑
           nontraffic V52.2 ☑
          truck (traffic) V54.7 ☑
           nontraffic V54.2 ☑
          two wheeled motor vehicle (traffic) V52.7 ☑
           nontraffic V52.2 ☑
          van (traffic) V53.7 ☑
           nontraffic V53.2 ☑
        noncollision accident (traffic) V58.7 ☑
          nontraffic V58.2 ☑
      noncollision accident (traffic) V58.9 ☑
        nontraffic V58.3 ☑
        while boarding or alighting V58.4 ☑
      nontraffic V59.3 ☑
      passenger
        collision (with)
          animal (traffic) V50.6 ☑
           being ridden (traffic) V56.6 ☑
            nontraffic V56.1 ☑
           nontraffic V50.1 ☑
          animal-drawn vehicle (traffic) V56.6 ☑
           nontraffic V56.1 ☑
          bus (traffic) V54.6 ☑
           nontraffic V54.1 ☑
          car (traffic) V53.6 ☑
           nontraffic V53.1 ☑
          motor vehicle NOS (traffic) V59.50 ☑
           nontraffic V59.10 ☑
           specified type NEC (traffic) V59.59 ☑
            nontraffic V59.19 ☑
          pedal cycle (traffic) V51.6 ☑
           nontraffic V51.1 ☑
          pickup truck (traffic) V53.6 ☑
           nontraffic V53.1 ☑
          railway vehicle (traffic) V55.6 ☑
           nontraffic V55.1 ☑
          specified vehicle NEC (traffic) V56.6 ☑
           nontraffic V56.1 ☑
          stationary object (traffic) V57.6 ☑
           nontraffic V57.1 ☑
          streetcar (traffic) V56.6 ☑
           nontraffic V56.1 ☑
          three wheeled motor vehicle (traffic) V52.6 ☑
           nontraffic V52.1 ☑
          truck (traffic) V54.6 ☑
           nontraffic V54.1 ☑
          two wheeled motor vehicle (traffic) V52.6 ☑
           nontraffic V52.1 ☑
          van (traffic) V53.6 ☑
           nontraffic V53.1 ☑
        noncollision accident (traffic) V58.6 ☑
          nontraffic V58.1 ☑
      specified type NEC V59.88 ☑
      military vehicle V59.81 ☑
    watercraft occupant — *see* Accident, watercraft
    vehicle NEC V89.9 ☑
    animal-drawn NEC — *see* Accident, transport, animal-drawn vehicle occupant
    special
      agricultural — *see* Accident, transport, agricultural vehicle occupant
      construction — *see* Accident, transport, construction vehicle occupant
      industrial — *see* Accident, transport, industrial vehicle occupant
      three-wheeled NEC (motorized) — *see* Accident, transport, three-wheeled motor vehicle occupant
  watercraft V94.9 ☑

▽ Subterms under main terms may continue to next column or page   ☑ Additional Character Required — Refer to the Tabular List for Character Selection   409

Accident — Accident

Accident — *continued*
  watercraft — *continued*
    causing
      drowning — *see* Drowning, due to, accident to, watercraft
      injury NEC V91.89 ☑
        crushed between craft and object V91.19 ☑
          powered craft V91.13 ☑
            ferry boat V91.11 ☑
            fishing boat V91.12 ☑
            jetskis V91.13 ☑
            liner V91.11 ☑
            merchant ship V91.10 ☑
            passenger ship V91.11 ☑
          unpowered craft V91.18 ☑
            canoe V91.15 ☑
            inflatable V91.16 ☑
            kayak V91.15 ☑
            sailboat V91.14 ☑
            surf-board V91.18 ☑
            windsurfer V91.18 ☑
      fall on board V91.29 ☑
        powered craft V91.23 ☑
          ferry boat V91.21 ☑
          fishing boat V91.22 ☑
          jetskis V91.23 ☑
          liner V91.21 ☑
          merchant ship V91.20 ☑
          passenger ship V91.21 ☑
        unpowered craft
          canoe V91.25 ☑
          inflatable V91.26 ☑
          kayak V91.25 ☑
          sailboat V91.24 ☑
      fire on board causing burn V91.09 ☑
        powered craft V91.03 ☑
          ferry boat V91.01 ☑
          fishing boat V91.02 ☑
          jetskis V91.03 ☑
          liner V91.01 ☑
          merchant ship V91.00 ☑
          passenger ship V91.01 ☑
        unpowered craft V91.08 ☑
          canoe V91.05 ☑
          inflatable V91.06 ☑
          kayak V91.05 ☑
          sailboat V91.04 ☑
          surf-board V91.08 ☑
          water skis V91.07 ☑
          windsurfer V91.08 ☑
      hit by falling object V91.39 ☑
        powered craft V91.33 ☑
          ferry boat V91.31 ☑
          fishing boat V91.32 ☑
          jetskis V91.33 ☑
          liner V91.31 ☑
          merchant ship V91.30 ☑
          passenger ship V91.31 ☑
        unpowered craft V91.38 ☑
          canoe V91.35 ☑
          inflatable V91.36 ☑
          kayak V91.35 ☑
          sailboat V91.34 ☑
          surf-board V91.38 ☑
          water skis V91.37 ☑
          windsurfer V91.38 ☑
      specified type NEC V91.89 ☑
        powered craft V91.83 ☑
          ferry boat V91.81 ☑
          fishing boat V91.82 ☑
          jetskis V91.83 ☑
          liner V91.81 ☑
          merchant ship V91.80 ☑
          passenger ship V91.81 ☑
        unpowered craft V91.88 ☑
          canoe V91.85 ☑
          inflatable V91.86 ☑
          kayak V91.85 ☑
          sailboat V91.84 ☑
          surf-board V91.88 ☑
          water skis V91.87 ☑
          windsurfer V91.88 ☑
    due to, caused by cataclysm — *see* Forces of nature, by type
    military NEC V94.818 ☑
      civilian in water injured by V94.811 ☑

Accident — *continued*
  watercraft — *continued*
    military — *continued*
      with civilian watercraft V94.810 ☑
    nonpowered, struck by
      nonpowered vessel V94.22 ☑
      powered vessel V94.21 ☑
    specified type NEC V94.89 ☑
    striking swimmer
      powered V94.11 ☑
      unpowered V94.12 ☑
Acid throwing (assault) Y08.89 ☑
Activity (involving) (of victim at time of event) Y93.9
  aerobic and step exercise (class) Y93.A3 (*following* Y93.7)
  alpine skiing Y93.23
  animal care NEC Y93.K9 (*following* Y93.7)
  arts and handcrafts NEC Y93.D9 (*following* Y93.7)
  athletics played as a team or group NEC Y93.69
  athletics played individually NEC Y93.59
  athletics NEC Y93.79
  baking Y93.G3 (*following* Y93.7)
  ballet Y93.41
  barbells Y93.B3 (*following* Y93.7)
  BASE (Building, Antenna, Span, Earth) jumping Y93.33
  baseball Y93.64
  basketball Y93.67
  bathing (personal) Y93.E1 (*following* Y93.7)
  beach volleyball Y93.68
  bike riding Y93.55
  blackout game Y93.85
  boogie boarding Y93.18
  bowling Y93.54
  boxing Y93.71
  brass instrument playing Y93.J4 (*following* Y93.7)
  building construction Y93.H3 (*following* Y93.7)
  bungee jumping Y93.34
  calisthenics Y93.A2 (*following* Y93.7)
  canoeing (in calm and turbulent water) Y93.16
  capture the flag Y93.6A
  cardiorespiratory exercise NEC Y93.A9 (*following* Y93.7)
  caregiving (providing) NEC Y93.F9 (*following* Y93.7)
    bathing Y93.F1 (*following* Y93.7)
    lifting Y93.F2 (*following* Y93.7)
  cellular
    communication device Y93.C2 (*following* Y93.7)
    telephone Y93.C2 (*following* Y93.7)
  challenge course Y93.A5 (*following* Y93.7)
  cheerleading Y93.45
  choking game Y93.85
  circuit training Y93.A4 (*following* Y93.7)
  cleaning
    floor Y93.E5 (*following* Y93.7)
  climbing NEC Y93.39
    mountain Y93.31
    rock Y93.31
    wall Y93.31
  clothing care and maintenance NEC Y93.E9 (*following* Y93.7)
  combatives Y93.75
  computer
    keyboarding Y93.C1 (*following* Y93.7)
    technology NEC Y93.C9 (*following* Y93.7)
  confidence course Y93.A5 (*following* Y93.7)
  construction (building) Y93.H3 (*following* Y93.7)
  cooking and baking Y93.G3 (*following* Y93.7)
  cool down exercises Y93.A2 (*following* Y93.7)
  cricket Y93.69
  crocheting Y93.D1 (*following* Y93.7)
  cross country skiing Y93.24
  dancing (all types) Y93.41
  digging
    dirt Y93.H1 (*following* Y93.7)
  dirt digging Y93.H1 (*following* Y93.7)
  dishwashing Y93.G1 (*following* Y93.7)
  diving (platform) (springboard) Y93.12
    underwater Y93.15
  dodge ball Y93.6A
  downhill skiing Y93.23
  drum playing Y93.J2 (*following* Y93.7)
  dumbbells Y93.B3 (*following* Y93.7)
  electronic
    devices NEC Y93.C9 (*following* Y93.7)
      hand held interactive Y93.C2 (*following* Y93.7)
    game playing (using) (with)
      interactive device Y93.C2 (*following* Y93.7)
      keyboard or other stationary device Y93.C1 (*following* Y93.7)

Activity — *continued*
  elliptical machine Y93.A1 (*following* Y93.7)
  exercise(s)
    machines ((primarily) for)
      cardiorespiratory conditioning Y93.A1 (*following* Y93.7)
      muscle strengthening Y93.B1 (*following* Y93.7)
    muscle strengthening (non-machine) NEC Y93.B9 (*following* Y93.7)
  external motion NEC Y93.I9 (*following* Y93.7)
    rollercoaster Y93.I1 (*following* Y93.7)
  fainting game Y93.85
  field hockey Y93.65
  figure skating (pairs) (singles) Y93.21
  flag football Y93.62
  floor mopping and cleaning Y93.E5 (*following* Y93.7)
  food preparation and clean up Y93.G1 (*following* Y93.7)
  football (American) NOS Y93.61
    flag Y93.62
    tackle Y93.61
    touch Y93.62
  four square Y93.6A
  free weights Y93.B3 (*following* Y93.7)
  frisbee (ultimate) Y93.74
  furniture
    building Y93.D3 (*following* Y93.7)
    finishing Y93.D3 (*following* Y93.7)
    repair Y93.D3 (*following* Y93.7)
  game playing (electronic)
    using interactive device Y93.C2 (*following* Y93.7)
    using keyboard or other stationary device Y93.C1 (*following* Y93.7)
  gardening Y93.H2 (*following* Y93.7)
  golf Y93.53
  grass drills Y93.A6 (*following* Y93.7)
  grilling and smoking food Y93.G2 (*following* Y93.7)
  grooming and shearing an animal Y93.K3 (*following* Y93.7)
  guerilla drills Y93.A6 (*following* Y93.7)
  gymnastics (rhythmic) Y93.43
  hand held interactive electronic device Y93.C2 (*following* Y93.7)
  handball Y93.73
  handcrafts NEC Y93.D9 (*following* Y93.7)
  hang gliding Y93.35
  hiking (on level or elevated terrain) Y93.01
  hockey (ice) Y93.22
    field Y93.65
  horseback riding Y93.52
  household (interior) maintenance NEC Y93.E9 (*following* Y93.7)
  ice NEC Y93.29
    dancing Y93.21
    hockey Y93.22
    skating Y93.21
  inline roller skating Y93.51
  ironing Y93.E4 (*following* Y93.7)
  judo Y93.75
  jumping jacks Y93.A2 (*following* Y93.7)
  jumping rope Y93.56
  jumping (off) NEC Y93.39
    BASE (Building, Antenna, Span, Earth) Y93.33
    bungee Y93.34
    jacks Y93.A2 (*following* Y93.7)
    rope Y93.56
  karate Y93.75
  kayaking (in calm and turbulent water) Y93.16
  keyboarding (computer) Y93.C1 (*following* Y93.7)
  kickball Y93.6A
  knitting Y93.D1 (*following* Y93.7)
  lacrosse Y93.65
  land maintenance NEC Y93.H9 (*following* Y93.7)
  landscaping Y93.H2 (*following* Y93.7)
  laundry Y93.E2 (*following* Y93.7)
  machines (exercise)
    primarily for cardiorespiratory conditioning Y93.A1 (*following* Y93.7)
    primarily for muscle strengthening Y93.B1 (*following* Y93.7)
  maintenance
    exterior building NEC Y93.H9 (*following* Y93.7)
    household (interior) NEC Y93.E9 (*following* Y93.7)
    land Y93.H9 (*following* Y93.7)
    property Y93.H9 (*following* Y93.7)
  marching (on level or elevated terrain) Y93.01
  martial arts Y93.75
  microwave oven Y93.G3 (*following* Y93.7)
  milking an animal Y93.K2 (*following* Y93.7)
  mopping (floor) Y93.E5 (*following* Y93.7)

Activity — *continued*
   mountain climbing Y93.31
   muscle strengthening
      exercises (non-machine) NEC Y93.B9 (*following* Y93.7)
      machines Y93.B1 (*following* Y93.7)
   musical keyboard (electronic) playing Y93.J1 (*following* Y93.7)
   nordic skiing Y93.24
   obstacle course Y93.A5 (*following* Y93.7)
   oven (microwave) Y93.G3 (*following* Y93.7)
   packing up and unpacking in moving to a new residence Y93.E6 (*following* Y93.7)
   parasailing Y93.19
   pass out game Y93.85
   percussion instrument playing NEC Y93.J2 (*following* Y93.7)
   personal
      bathing and showering Y93.E1 (*following* Y93.7)
      hygiene NEC Y93.E8 (*following* Y93.7)
      showering Y93.E1 (*following* Y93.7)
   physical games generally associated with school recess, summer camp and children Y93.6A
   physical training NEC Y93.A9 (*following* Y93.7)
   piano playing Y93.J1 (*following* Y93.7)
   pilates Y93.B4 (*following* Y93.7)
   platform diving Y93.12
   playing musical instrument
      brass instrument Y93.J4 (*following* Y93.7)
      drum Y93.J2 (*following* Y93.7)
      musical keyboard (electronic) Y93.J1 (*following* Y93.7)
      percussion instrument NEC Y93.J2 (*following* Y93.7)
      piano Y93.J1 (*following* Y93.7)
      string instrument Y93.J3 (*following* Y93.7)
      winds instrument Y93.J4 (*following* Y93.7)
   property maintenance
      exterior NEC Y93.H9 (*following* Y93.7)
      interior NEC Y93.E9 (*following* Y93.7)
   pruning (garden and lawn) Y93.H2 (*following* Y93.7)
   pull-ups Y93.B2 (*following* Y93.7)
   push-ups Y93.B2 (*following* Y93.7)
   racquetball Y93.73
   rafting (in calm and turbulent water) Y93.16
   raking (leaves) Y93.H1 (*following* Y93.7)
   rappelling Y93.32
   refereeing a sports activity Y93.81
   residential relocation Y93.E6 (*following* Y93.7)
   rhythmic gymnastics Y93.43
   rhythmic movement NEC Y93.49
   riding
      horseback Y93.52
      rollercoaster Y93.I1 (*following* Y93.7)
   rock climbing Y93.31
   roller skating (inline) Y93.51
   rollercoaster riding Y93.I1 (*following* Y93.7)
   rough housing and horseplay Y93.83
   rowing (in calm and turbulent water) Y93.16
   rugby Y93.63
   running Y93.02
   SCUBA diving Y93.15
   sewing Y93.D2 (*following* Y93.7)
   shoveling Y93.H1 (*following* Y93.7)
      dirt Y93.H1 (*following* Y93.7)
      snow Y93.H1 (*following* Y93.7)
   showering (personal) Y93.E1 (*following* Y93.7)
   sit-ups Y93.B2 (*following* Y93.7)
   skateboarding Y93.51
   skating (ice) Y93.21
      roller Y93.51
   skiing (alpine) (downhill) Y93.23
      cross country Y93.24
      nordic Y93.24
      water Y93.17
   sledding (snow) Y93.23
   sleeping (sleep) Y93.84
   smoking and grilling food Y93.G2 (*following* Y93.7)
   snorkeling Y93.15
   snow NEC Y93.29
      boarding Y93.23
      shoveling Y93.H1 (*following* Y93.7)
      sledding Y93.23
      tubing Y93.23
   soccer Y93.66
   softball Y93.64
   specified NEC Y93.89
   spectator at an event Y93.82
   sports NEC Y93.79
      sports played as a team or group NEC Y93.69

Activity — *continued*
   sports — *continued*
      sports played individually NEC Y93.59
   springboard diving Y93.12
   squash Y93.73
   stationary bike Y93.A1 (*following* Y93.7)
   step (stepping) exercise (class) Y93.A3 (*following* Y93.7)
   stepper machine Y93.A1 (*following* Y93.7)
   stove Y93.G3 (*following* Y93.7)
   string instrument playing Y93.J3 (*following* Y93.7)
   surfing Y93.18
      wind Y93.18
   swimming Y93.11
   tackle football Y93.61
   tap dancing Y93.41
   tennis Y93.73
   tobogganing Y93.23
   touch football Y93.62
   track and field events (non-running) Y93.57
      running Y93.02
   trampoline Y93.44
   treadmill Y93.A1 (*following* Y93.7)
   trimming shrubs Y93.H2 (*following* Y93.7)
   tubing (in calm and turbulent water) Y93.16
      snow Y93.23
   ultimate frisbee Y93.74
   underwater diving Y93.15
   unpacking in moving to a new residence Y93.E6 (*following* Y93.7)
   use of stove, oven and microwave oven Y93.G3 (*following* Y93.7)
   vacuuming Y93.E3 (*following* Y93.7)
   volleyball (beach) (court) Y93.68
   wake boarding Y93.17
   walking (on level or elevated terrain) Y93.01
      an animal Y93.K1 (*following* Y93.7)
   walking an animal Y93.K1 (*following* Y93.7)
   wall climbing Y93.31
   warm up and cool down exercises Y93.A2 (*following* Y93.7)
   water NEC Y93.19
      aerobics Y93.14
      craft NEC Y93.19
      exercise Y93.14
      polo Y93.13
      skiing Y93.17
      sliding Y93.18
      survival training and testing Y93.19
   weeding (garden and lawn) Y93.H2 (*following* Y93.7)
   wind instrument playing Y93.J4 (*following* Y93.7)
   windsurfing Y93.18
   wrestling Y93.72
   yoga Y93.42
Adverse effect of drugs — *see* Table of Drugs and Chemicals
Aerosinusitis — *see* Air, pressure
After-effect, late — *see* Sequelae
Air
   blast in war operations — *see* War operations, air blast
   pressure
      change, rapid
         during
            ascent W94.29 ☑
               while (in) (surfacing from)
                  aircraft W94.23 ☑
                  deep water diving W94.21 ☑
                  underground W94.22 ☑
            descent W94.39 ☑
               in
                  aircraft W94.31 ☑
                  water W94.32 ☑
      high, prolonged W94.0 ☑
      low, prolonged W94.12 ☑
         due to residence or long visit at high altitude W94.11 ☑
Alpine sickness W94.11 ☑
Altitude sickness W94.11 ☑
Anaphylactic shock, anaphylaxis — *see* Table of Drugs and Chemicals
Andes disease W94.11 ☑
Arachnidism, arachnoidism X58 ☑
Arson (with intent to injure or kill) X97 ☑
Asphyxia, asphyxiation
   by
      food (bone) (seed) — *see* categories T17 and T18
      gas (*see also* Table of Drugs and Chemicals)
         legal
            execution — *see* Legal, intervention, gas

Asphyxia, asphyxiation — *continued*
   by — *continued*
      gas (*see also* Table of Drugs and Chemicals) — *continued*
         legal — *continued*
            intervention — *see* Legal, intervention, gas
   from
      fire (*see also* Exposure, fire)
         in war operations — *see* War operations, fire
      ignition — *see* Ignition
      vomitus T17.81 ☑
   in war operations — *see* War operations, restriction of airway
Aspiration
   food (any type) (into respiratory tract) (with asphyxia, obstruction respiratory tract, suffocation) — *see* categories T17 and T18
   foreign body — *see* Foreign body, aspiration
   vomitus (with asphyxia, obstruction respiratory tract, suffocation) T17.81 ☑
Assassination (attempt) — *see* Assault
Assault (homicidal) (by) (in) Y09
   arson X97 ☑
   bite (of human being) Y04.1 ☑
   bodily force Y04.8 ☑
      bite Y04.1 ☑
      bumping into Y04.2 ☑
      sexual — *see* subcategories T74.0, T76.0 ☑
      unarmed fight Y04.0 ☑
   bomb X96.9 ☑
      antipersonnel X96.0 ☑
      fertilizer X96.3 ☑
      gasoline X96.1 ☑
      letter X96.2 ☑
      petrol X96.1 ☑
      pipe X96.3 ☑
      specified NEC X96.8 ☑
   brawl (hand) (fists) (foot) (unarmed) Y04.0 ☑
   burning, burns (by fire) NEC X97 ☑
      acid Y08.89 ☑
      caustic, corrosive substance Y08.89 ☑
      chemical from swallowing caustic, corrosive substance — *see* Table of Drugs and Chemicals
      cigarette(s) X97 ☑
      hot object X98.9 ☑
         fluid NEC X98.2 ☑
         household appliance X98.3 ☑
         specified NEC X98.8 ☑
         steam X98.0 ☑
         tap water X98.1 ☑
         vapors X98.0 ☑
      scalding — *see* Assault, burning
      steam X98.0 ☑
      vitriol Y08.89 ☑
   caustic, corrosive substance (gas) Y08.89 ☑
   crashing of
      aircraft Y08.81 ☑
      motor vehicle Y03.8 ☑
         pushed in front of Y02.0 ☑
         run over Y03.0 ☑
         specified NEC Y03.8 ☑
   cutting or piercing instrument X99.9 ☑
      dagger X99.2 ☑
      glass X99.0 ☑
      knife X99.1 ☑
      specified NEC X99.8 ☑
      sword X99.2 ☑
   dagger X99.2 ☑
   drowning (in) X92.9 ☑
      bathtub X92.0 ☑
      natural water X92.3 ☑
      specified NEC X92.8 ☑
      swimming pool X92.1 ☑
         following fall X92.2 ☑
   dynamite X96.8 ☑
   explosive(s) (material) X96.9 ☑
   fight (hand) (fists) (foot) (unarmed) Y04.0 ☑
      with weapon — *see* Assault, by type of weapon
   fire X97 ☑
   firearm X95.9 ☑
      airgun X95.01 ☑
      handgun X93 ☑
      hunting rifle X94.1 ☑
      larger X94.9 ☑
         specified NEC X94.8 ☑
      machine gun X94.2 ☑

Assault — *continued*
  firearm — *continued*
    shotgun X94.0 ☑
    specified NEC X95.8 ☑
  from high place Y01 ☑
  gunshot (wound) NEC — *see* Assault, firearm, by type
  incendiary device X97 ☑
  injury Y09
    to child due to criminal abortion attempt NEC
      Y08.89 ☑
  knife X99.1 ☑
  late effect of — *see* categories X92-Y08 with 7th character S
  placing before moving object NEC Y02.8 ☑
    motor vehicle Y02.0 ☑
  poisoning — *see* categories T36-T65 with 7th character S
  puncture, any part of body — *see* Assault, cutting or piercing instrument
  pushing
    before moving object NEC Y02.8 ☑
      motor vehicle Y02.0 ☑
      subway train Y02.1 ☑
      train Y02.1 ☑
    from high place Y01 ☑
  rape T74.2- ☑
  scalding — *see* Assault, burning
  sequelae of — *see* categories X92-Y08 with 7th character S
  sexual (by bodily force) T74.2- ☑
  shooting — *see* Assault, firearm
  specified means NEC Y08.89 ☑
  stab, any part of body — *see* Assault, cutting or piercing instrument
  steam X98.0 ☑
  striking against
    other person Y04.2 ☑
    sports equipment Y08.09 ☑
      baseball bat Y08.02 ☑
      hockey stick Y08.01 ☑
  struck by
    sports equipment Y08.09 ☑
      baseball bat Y08.02 ☑
      hockey stick Y08.01 ☑
  submersion — *see* Assault, drowning
  violence Y09
  weapon Y09
    blunt Y00 ☑
    cutting or piercing — *see* Assault, cutting or piercing instrument
    firearm — *see* Assault, firearm
  wound Y09
    cutting — *see* Assault, cutting or piercing instrument
    gunshot — *see* Assault, firearm
    knife X99.1 ☑
    piercing — *see* Assault, cutting or piercing instrument
    puncture — *see* Assault, cutting or piercing instrument
    stab — *see* Assault, cutting or piercing instrument
Attack by mammals NEC W55.89 ☑
Avalanche — *see* Landslide
Aviator's disease — *see* Air, pressure

B

Barotitis, barodontalgia, barosinusitis, barotrauma (otitic) (sinus) — *see* Air, pressure
Battered (baby) (child) (person) (syndrome) X58 ☑
Bayonet wound W26.1 ☑
  in
    legal intervention — *see* Legal, intervention, sharp object, bayonet
    war operations — *see* War operations, combat
  stated as undetermined whether accidental or intentional Y28.8 ☑
  suicide (attempt) X78.2 ☑
Bean in nose — *see* categories T17 and T18 ☑
Bed set on fire NEC — *see* Exposure, fire, uncontrolled, building, bed
Beheading (by guillotine)
  homicide X99.9 ☑
  legal execution — *see* Legal, intervention
Bending, injury in (prolonged) (static) X50.1 ☑
Bends — *see* Air, pressure, change

Bite, bitten by
  alligator W58.01 ☑
  arthropod (nonvenomous) NEC W57 ☑
  bull W55.21 ☑
  cat W55.01 ☑
  cow W55.21 ☑
  crocodile W58.11 ☑
  dog W54.0 ☑
  goat W55.31 ☑
  hoof stock NEC W55.31 ☑
  horse W55.11 ☑
  human being (accidentally) W50.3 ☑
    with intent to injure or kill Y04.1 ☑
    as, or caused by, a crowd or human stampede (with fall) W52 ☑
    assault Y04.1 ☑
    homicide (attempt) Y04.1 ☑
    in
      fight Y04.1 ☑
  insect (nonvenomous) W57 ☑
  lizard (nonvenomous) W59.01 ☑
  mammal NEC W55.81 ☑
    marine W56.31 ☑
  marine animal (nonvenomous) W56.81 ☑
  millipede W57 ☑
  moray eel W56.51 ☑
  mouse W53.01 ☑
  person(s) (accidentally) W50.3 ☑
    with intent to injure or kill Y04.1 ☑
    as, or caused by, a crowd or human stampede (with fall) W52 ☑
    assault Y04.1 ☑
    homicide (attempt) Y04.1 ☑
    in
      fight Y04.1 ☑
  pig W55.41 ☑
  raccoon W55.51 ☑
  rat W53.11 ☑
  reptile W59.81 ☑
    lizard W59.01 ☑
    snake W59.11 ☑
    turtle W59.21 ☑
      terrestrial W59.81 ☑
  rodent W53.81 ☑
    mouse W53.01 ☑
    rat W53.11 ☑
    specified NEC W53.81 ☑
    squirrel W53.21 ☑
  shark W56.41 ☑
  sheep W55.31 ☑
  snake (nonvenomous) W59.11 ☑
  spider (nonvenomous) W57 ☑
  squirrel W53.21 ☑
Blast (air) in war operations — *see* War operations, blast
Blizzard X37.2 ☑
Blood alcohol level Y90.9
  less than 20mg/100ml Y90.0
  presence in blood, level not specified Y90.9
  20-39mg/100ml Y90.1
  40-59mg/100ml Y90.2
  60-79mg/100ml Y90.3
  80-99mg/100ml Y90.4
  100-119mg/100ml Y90.5
  120-199mg/100ml Y90.6
  200-239mg/100ml Y90.7
Blow X58 ☑
  by law-enforcing agent, police (on duty) — *see* Legal, intervention, manhandling
  blunt object — *see* Legal, intervention, blunt object
Blowing up — *see* Explosion
Brawl (hand) (fists) (foot) Y04.0 ☑
Breakage (accidental) (part of)
  ladder (causing fall) W11 ☑
  scaffolding (causing fall) W12 ☑
Broken
  glass, contact with — *see* Contact, with, glass
  power line (causing electric shock) W85 ☑
Bumping against, into (accidentally)
  object W22.8 ☑
    caused by crowd or human stampede (with fall) W52 ☑
    sports equipment W21.9 ☑
    with fall — *see* Fall, due to, bumping against, object
  person(s) W51 ☑
    with fall W03 ☑
      due to ice or snow W00.0 ☑

Bumping against, into — *continued*
  person(s) — *continued*
    assault Y04.2 ☑
    caused by, a crowd or human stampede (with fall) W52 ☑
    homicide (attempt) Y04.2 ☑
  sports equipment W21.9 ☑
Burn, burned, burning (accidental) (by) (from) (on)
  acid NEC — *see* Table of Drugs and Chemicals
  bed linen — *see* Exposure, fire, uncontrolled, in building, bed
  blowtorch X08.8 ☑
    with ignition of clothing NEC X06.2 ☑
      nightwear X05 ☑
  bonfire, campfire (controlled) (*see also* Exposure, fire, controlled, not in building)
    uncontrolled — *see* Exposure, fire, uncontrolled, not in building
  candle X08.8 ☑
    with ignition of clothing NEC X06.2 ☑
      nightwear X05 ☑
  caustic liquid, substance (external) (internal) NEC — *see* Table of Drugs and Chemicals
  chemical (external) (internal) (*see also* Table of Drugs and Chemicals)
    in war operations — *see* War operations. fire
  cigar(s) or cigarette(s) X08.8 ☑
    with ignition of clothing NEC X06.2 ☑
      nightwear X05 ☑
  clothes, clothing NEC (from controlled fire) X06.2 ☑
    with conflagration — *see* Exposure, fire, uncontrolled, building
    not in building or structure — *see* Exposure, fire, uncontrolled, not in building
  cooker (hot) X15.8 ☑
    stated as undetermined whether accidental or intentional Y27.3 ☑
    suicide (attempt) X77.3 ☑
  electric blanket X16 ☑
  engine (hot) X17 ☑
  fire, flames — *see* Exposure, fire
  flare, Very pistol — *see* Discharge, firearm NEC
  heat
    from appliance (electrical) (household) X15.8 ☑
      cooker X15.8 ☑
      hotplate X15.2 ☑
      kettle X15.8 ☑
      light bulb X15.8 ☑
      saucepan X15.3 ☑
      skillet X15.3 ☑
      stated as undetermined whether accidental or intentional Y27.3 ☑
      stove X15.0 ☑
      suicide (attempt) X77.3 ☑
      toaster X15.1 ☑
    in local application or packing during medical or surgical procedure Y63.5
  heating
    appliance, radiator or pipe X16 ☑
  homicide (attempt) — *see* Assault, burning
  hot
    air X14.1 ☑
    cooker X15.8 ☑
    drink X10.0 ☑
    engine X17 ☑
    fat X10.2 ☑
    fluid NEC X12 ☑
    food X10.1 ☑
    gases X14.1 ☑
    heating appliance X16 ☑
    household appliance NEC X15.8 ☑
    kettle X15.8 ☑
    liquid NEC X12 ☑
    machinery X17 ☑
    metal (molten) (liquid) NEC X18 ☑
    object (not producing fire or flames) NEC X19 ☑
    oil (cooking) X10.2 ☑
    pipe(s) X16 ☑
    radiator X16 ☑
    saucepan (glass) (metal) X15.3 ☑
    stove (kitchen) X15.0 ☑
    substance NEC X19 ☑
      caustic or corrosive NEC — *see* Table of Drugs and Chemicals
    toaster X15.1 ☑
    tool X17 ☑

Burn, burned, burning — *continued*
- hot — *continued*
  - vapor X13.1 ☑
  - water (tap) — *see* Contact, with, hot, tap water
  - hotplate X15.2 ☑
    - suicide (attempt) X77.3 ☑
- ignition — *see* Ignition
- in war operations — *see* War operations, fire
- inflicted by other person X97 ☑
  - by hot objects, hot vapor, and steam — *see* Assault, burning, hot object
  - internal, from swallowed caustic, corrosive liquid, substance — *see* Table of Drugs and Chemicals
- iron (hot) X15.8 ☑
  - stated as undetermined whether accidental or intentional Y27.3 ☑
  - suicide (attempt) X77.3 ☑
- kettle (hot) X15.8 ☑
  - stated as undetermined whether accidental or intentional Y27.3 ☑
  - suicide (attempt) X77.3 ☑
- lamp (flame) X08.8 ☑
  - with ignition of clothing NEC X06.2 ☑
    - nightwear X05 ☑
- lighter (cigar) (cigarette) X08.8 ☑
  - with ignition of clothing NEC X06.2 ☑
    - nightwear X05 ☑
- lightning — *see* subcategory T75.0 ☑
  - causing fire — *see* Exposure, fire
- liquid (boiling) (hot) NEC X12 ☑
  - stated as undetermined whether accidental or intentional Y27.2 ☑
  - suicide (attempt) X77.2 ☑
- local application of externally applied substance in medical or surgical care Y63.5
- machinery (hot) X17 ☑
- matches X08.8 ☑
  - with ignition of clothing NEC X06.2 ☑
    - nightwear X05 ☑
- mattress — *see* Exposure, fire, uncontrolled, building, bed
- medicament, externally applied Y63.5
- metal (hot) (liquid) (molten) NEC X18 ☑
- nightwear (nightclothes, nightdress, gown, pajamas, robe) X05 ☑
- object (hot) NEC X19 ☑
- on board watercraft
  - due to
    - accident to watercraft V91.09 ☑
      - powered craft V91.03 ☑
        - ferry boat V91.01 ☑
        - fishing boat V91.02 ☑
        - jetskis V91.03 ☑
        - liner V91.01 ☑
        - merchant ship V91.00 ☑
        - passenger ship V91.01 ☑
      - unpowered craft V91.08 ☑
        - canoe V91.05 ☑
        - inflatable V91.06 ☑
        - kayak V91.05 ☑
        - sailboat V91.04 ☑
        - surf-board V91.08 ☑
        - water skis V91.07 ☑
        - windsurfer V91.08 ☑
    - fire on board V93.09 ☑
      - ferry boat V93.01 ☑
      - fishing boat V93.02 ☑
      - jetskis V93.03 ☑
      - liner V93.01 ☑
      - merchant ship V93.00 ☑
      - passenger ship V93.01 ☑
      - powered craft NEC V93.03 ☑
      - sailboat V93.04 ☑
    - specified heat source NEC on board V93.19 ☑
      - ferry boat V93.11 ☑
      - fishing boat V93.12 ☑
      - jetskis V93.13 ☑
      - liner V93.11 ☑
      - merchant ship V93.10 ☑
      - passenger ship V93.11 ☑
      - powered craft NEC V93.13 ☑
      - sailboat V93.14 ☑
- pipe (hot) X16 ☑
  - smoking X08.8 ☑
    - with ignition of clothing NEC X06.2 ☑
      - nightwear X05 ☑

Burn, burned, burning — *continued*
- powder — *see* Powder burn
- radiator (hot) X16 ☑
- saucepan (hot) (glass) (metal) X15.3 ☑
  - stated as undetermined whether accidental or intentional Y27.3 ☑
  - suicide (attempt) X77.3 ☑
- self-inflicted X76
  - stated as undetermined whether accidental or intentional Y26 ☑
- stated as undetermined whether accidental or intentional Y27.0 ☑
- steam X13.1 ☑
  - pipe X16 ☑
    - stated as undetermined whether accidental or intentional Y27.8 ☑
  - stated as undetermined whether accidental or intentional Y27.0 ☑
  - suicide (attempt) X77.0 ☑
- stove (hot) (kitchen) X15.0 ☑
  - stated as undetermined whether accidental or intentional Y27.3 ☑
  - suicide (attempt) X77.3 ☑
- substance (hot) NEC X19 ☑
  - boiling X12 ☑
    - stated as undetermined whether accidental or intentional Y27.2 ☑
    - suicide (attempt) X77.2 ☑
  - molten (metal) X18 ☑
- suicide (attempt) NEC X76 ☑
  - hot
    - household appliance X77.3 ☑
    - object X77.9 ☑
- therapeutic misadventure
  - heat in local application or packing during medical or surgical procedure Y63.5
  - overdose of radiation Y63.2
- toaster (hot) X15.1 ☑
  - stated as undetermined whether accidental or intentional Y27.3 ☑
  - suicide (attempt) X77.3 ☑
- tool (hot) X17 ☑
- torch, welding X08.8 ☑
  - with ignition of clothing NEC X06.2 ☑
    - nightwear X05 ☑
- trash fire (controlled) — *see* Exposure, fire, controlled, not in building
  - uncontrolled — *see* Exposure, fire, uncontrolled, not in building
- vapor (hot) X13.1 ☑
  - stated as undetermined whether accidental or intentional Y27.0 ☑
  - suicide (attempt) X77.0 ☑
- Very pistol — *see* Discharge, firearm NEC

Butted by animal W55.82 ☑
- bull W55.22 ☑
- cow W55.22 ☑
- goat W55.32 ☑
- horse W55.12 ☑
- pig W55.42 ☑
- sheep W55.32 ☑

C

Caisson disease — *see* Air, pressure, change
Campfire (exposure to) (controlled) (*see also* Exposure, fire, controlled, not in building)
- uncontrolled — *see* Exposure, fire, uncontrolled, not in building

Capital punishment (any means) — *see* Legal, intervention
Car sickness T75.3 ☑
Casualty (not due to war) NEC X58 ☑
- war — *see* War operations
Cat
- bite W55.01 ☑
- scratch W55.03 ☑
Cataclysm, cataclysmic (any injury) NEC — *see* Forces of nature
Catching fire — *see* Exposure, fire
Caught
- between
  - folding object W23.0 ☑
  - objects (moving) (stationary and moving) W23.0 ☑
    - and machinery — *see* Contact, with, by type of machine

Caught — *continued*
- between — *continued*
  - objects — *continued*
    - stationary W23.1 ☑
    - sliding door and door frame W23.0 ☑
  - by, in
    - machinery (moving parts of) — *see* Contact, with, by type of machine
    - washing-machine wringer W23.0 ☑
  - under packing crate (due to losing grip) W23.1 ☑
Cave-in caused by cataclysmic earth surface movement or eruption — *see* Landslide
Change(s) in air pressure — *see* Air, pressure, change
Choked, choking (on) (any object except food or vomitus)
- food (bone) (seed) — *see* categories T17 and T18 ☑
- vomitus T17.81-
Civil insurrection — *see* War operations
Cloudburst (any injury) X37.8 ☑
Cold, exposure to (accidental) (excessive) (extreme) (natural) (place) NEC — *see* Exposure, cold
Collapse
- building W20.1 ☑
  - burning (uncontrolled fire) X00.2 ☑
- dam or man-made structure (causing earth movement) X36.0 ☑
- machinery — *see* Contact, with, by type of machine
- structure W20.1 ☑
  - burning (uncontrolled fire) X00.2 ☑
Collision (accidental) NEC (*see also* Accident, transport) V89.9 ☑
- pedestrian W51 ☑
  - with fall W03 ☑
    - due to ice or snow W00.0 ☑
    - involving pedestrian conveyance — *see* Accident, transport, pedestrian, conveyance
  - and
    - crowd or human stampede (with fall) W52 ☑
    - object W22.8 ☑
      - with fall — *see* Fall, due to, bumping against, object
  - person(s) — *see* Collision, pedestrian
- transport vehicle NEC V89.9 ☑
  - and
    - avalanche, fallen or not moving — *see* Accident, transport
    - falling or moving — *see* Landslide
    - landslide, fallen or not moving — *see* Accident, transport
    - falling or moving — *see* Landslide
  - due to cataclysm — *see* Forces of nature, by type
  - intentional, purposeful suicide (attempt) — *see* Suicide, collision
Combustion, spontaneous — *see* Ignition
Complication (delayed) **of or following** (medical or surgical procedure) Y84.9
- with misadventure — *see* Misadventure
- amputation of limb(s) Y83.5
- anastomosis (arteriovenous) (blood vessel) (gastrojejunal) (tendon) (natural or artificial material) Y83.2
- aspiration (of fluid) Y84.4
  - tissue Y84.8
- biopsy Y84.8
- blood
  - sampling Y84.7
  - transfusion
    - procedure Y84.8
- bypass Y83.2
- catheterization (urinary) Y84.6
  - cardiac Y84.0
- colostomy Y83.3
- cystostomy Y83.3
- dialysis (kidney) Y84.1
- drug — *see* Table of Drugs and Chemicals
- due to misadventure — *see* Misadventure
- duodenostomy Y83.3
- electroshock therapy Y84.3
- external stoma, creation of Y83.3
- formation of external stoma Y83.3
- gastrostomy Y83.3
- graft Y83.2
- hypothermia (medically-induced) Y84.8
- implant, implantation (of)
  - artificial
    - internal device (cardiac pacemaker) (electrodes in brain) (heart valve prosthesis) (orthopedic) Y83.1

Complication (delayed) **of or following** — *continued*
  implant, implantation — *continued*
    artificial — *continued*
      material or tissue (for anastomosis or bypass) Y83.2
        with creation of external stoma Y83.3
      natural tissues (for anastomosis or bypass) Y83.2
        with creation of external stoma Y83.3
  infusion
    procedure Y84.8
  injection — *see* Table of Drugs and Chemicals
    procedure Y84.8
  insertion of gastric or duodenal sound Y84.5
  insulin-shock therapy Y84.3
  paracentesis (abdominal) (thoracic) (aspirative) Y84.4
  procedures other than surgical operation — *see* Complication of or following, by type of procedure
  radiological procedure or therapy Y84.2
  removal of organ (partial) (total) NEC Y83.6
  sampling
    blood Y84.7
    fluid NEC Y84.4
    tissue Y84.8
  shock therapy Y84.3
  surgical operation NEC (*see also* Complication of or following, by type of operation) Y83.9
    reconstructive NEC Y83.4
      with
        anastomosis, bypass or graft Y83.2
        formation of external stoma Y83.3
    specified NEC Y83.8
  transfusion (*see also* Table of Drugs and Chemicals)
    procedure Y84.8
  transplant, transplantation (heart) (kidney) (liver) (whole organ, any) Y83.0
    partial organ Y83.4
  ureterostomy Y83.3
  vaccination (*see also* Table of Drugs and Chemicals)
    procedure Y84.8

Compression
  divers' squeeze — *see* Air, pressure, change
  trachea by
    food (lodged in esophagus) — *see* categories T17 and T18 ☑
    vomitus (lodged in esophagus) T17.81- ☑

Conflagration — *see* Exposure, fire, uncontrolled

Constriction (external)
  hair W49.01 ☑
  jewelry W49.04 ☑
  ring W49.04 ☑
  rubber band W49.03 ☑
  specified item NEC W49.09 ☑
  string W49.02 ☑
  thread W49.02 ☑

Contact (accidental)
  with
    abrasive wheel (metalworking) W31.1 ☑
    alligator W58.09 ☑
      bite W58.01 ☑
      crushing W58.03 ☑
      strike W58.02 ☑
    amphibian W62.9 ☑
      frog W62.0 ☑
      toad W62.1 ☑
    animal (nonvenomous) NEC W64 ☑
      marine W56.89 ☑
        bite W56.81 ☑
        dolphin — *see* Contact, with, dolphin
        fish NEC — *see* Contact, with, fish
        mammal — *see* Contact, with, mammal, marine
        orca — *see* Contact, with, orca
        sea lion — *see* Contact, with, sea lion
        shark — *see* Contact, with, shark
        strike W56.82 ☑
    animate mechanical force NEC W64 ☑
    arrow W21.89 ☑
      not thrown, projected or falling W45.8 ☑
    arthropods (nonvenomous) W57 ☑
    axe W27.0 ☑
    band-saw (industrial) W31.2 ☑
    bayonet — *see* Bayonet wound
    bee(s) X58 ☑
    bench-saw (industrial) W31.2 ☑
    bird W61.99 ☑
      bite W61.91 ☑

Contact — *continued*
  with — *continued*
    bird — *continued*
      chicken — *see* Contact, with, chicken
      duck — *see* Contact, with, duck
      goose — *see* Contact, with, goose
      macaw — *see* Contact, with, macaw
      parrot — *see* Contact, with, parrot
      psittacine — *see* Contact, with, psittacine
      strike W61.92 ☑
      turkey — *see* Contact, with, turkey
    blender W29.0 ☑
    boiling water X12 ☑
      stated as undetermined whether accidental or intentional Y27.2 ☑
      suicide (attempt) X77.2 ☑
    bore, earth-drilling or mining (land) (seabed) W31.0 ☑
    buffalo — *see* Contact, with, hoof stock NEC
    bull W55.29 ☑
      bite W55.21 ☑
      gored W55.22 ☑
      strike W55.22 ☑
    bumper cars W31.81 ☑
    camel — *see* Contact, with, hoof stock NEC
    can
      lid W26.8 ☑
      opener W27.4 ☑
        powered W29.0 ☑
    cat W55.09 ☑
      bite W55.01 ☑
      scratch W55.03 ☑
    caterpillar (venomous) X58 ☑
    centipede (venomous) X58 ☑
    chain
      hoist W24.0 ☑
        agricultural operations W30.89 ☑
      saw W29.3 ☑
    chicken W61.39 ☑
      peck W61.33 ☑
      strike W61.32 ☑
    chisel W27.0 ☑
    circular saw W31.2 ☑
    cobra X58 ☑
    combine (harvester) W30.0 ☑
    conveyer belt W24.1 ☑
    cooker (hot) X15.8 ☑
      stated as undetermined whether accidental or intentional Y27.3 ☑
      suicide (attempt) X77.3 ☑
    coral X58 ☑
    cotton gin W31.82 ☑
    cow W55.29 ☑
      bite W55.21 ☑
      strike W55.22 ☑
    crane W24.0 ☑
      agricultural operations W30.89 ☑
    crocodile W58.19 ☑
      bite W58.11 ☑
      crushing W58.13 ☑
      strike W58.12 ☑
    dagger W26.1 ☑
      stated as undetermined whether accidental or intentional Y28.2 ☑
      suicide (attempt) X78.2 ☑
    dairy equipment W31.82 ☑
    dart W21.89 ☑
      not thrown, projected or falling W45.8 ☑
    deer — *see* Contact, with, hoof stock NEC
    derrick W24.0 ☑
      agricultural operations W30.89 ☑
      hay W30.2 ☑
    dog W54.8 ☑
      bite W54.0 ☑
      strike W54.1 ☑
    dolphin W56.09 ☑
      bite W56.01 ☑
      strike W56.02 ☑
    donkey — *see* Contact, with, hoof stock NEC
    drill (powered) W29.8 ☑
      earth (land) (seabed) W31.0 ☑
      nonpowered W27.8 ☑
    drive belt W24.0 ☑
      agricultural operations W30.89 ☑
    dry ice — *see* Exposure, cold, man-made
    dryer (clothes) (powered) (spin) W29.2 ☑

Contact — *continued*
  with — *continued*
    duck W61.69 ☑
      bite W61.61 ☑
      strike W61.62 ☑
    earth (-)
      drilling machine (industrial) W31.0 ☑
      scraping machine in stationary use W31.83 ☑
    edge of stiff paper W26.2 ☑
    electric
      beater W29.0 ☑
      blanket X16 ☑
      fan W29.2 ☑
        commercial W31.82 ☑
      knife W29.1 ☑
      mixer W29.0 ☑
    elevator (building) W24.0 ☑
      agricultural operations W30.89 ☑
        grain W30.3 ☑
    engine(s), hot NEC X17 ☑
    excavating machine W31.0 ☑
    farm machine W30.9 ☑
    feces — *see* Contact, with, by type of animal
    fer de lance X58 ☑
    fish W56.59 ☑
      bite W56.51 ☑
      shark — *see* Contact, with, shark
      strike W56.52 ☑
    flying horses W31.81 ☑
    forging (metalworking) machine W31.1 ☑
    fork W27.4 ☑
    forklift (truck) W24.0 ☑
      agricultural operations W30.89 ☑
    frog W62.0 ☑
    garden
      cultivator (powered) W29.3 ☑
        riding W30.89 ☑
      fork W27.1 ☑
    gas turbine W31.3 ☑
    Gila monster X58 ☑
    giraffe — *see* Contact, with, hoof stock NEC
    glass (sharp) (broken) W25 ☑
      assault X99.0 ☑
      due to fall — *see* Fall, by type
      stated as undetermined whether accidental or intentional Y28.0 ☑
      suicide (attempt) X78.0 ☑
      with subsequent fall W18.02 ☑
    goat W55.39 ☑
      bite W55.31 ☑
      strike W55.32 ☑
    goose W61.59 ☑
      bite W61.51 ☑
      strike W61.52 ☑
    hand
      saw W27.0 ☑
      tool (not powered) NEC W27.8 ☑
        powered W29.8 ☑
    harvester W30.0 ☑
    hay-derrick W30.2 ☑
    heating
      appliance (hot) X16 ☑
      pad (electric) X16 ☑
    heat NEC X19 ☑
      from appliance (electrical) (household) — *see* Contact, with, hot, household appliance
      heating appliance X16 ☑
    hedge-trimmer (powered) W29.3 ☑
    hoe W27.1 ☑
    hoist (chain) (shaft) NEC W24.0 ☑
      agricultural W30.89 ☑
    hoof stock NEC W55.39 ☑
      bite W55.31 ☑
      strike W55.32 ☑
    hornet(s) X58 ☑
    horse W55.19 ☑
      bite W55.11 ☑
      strike W55.12 ☑
    hot
      air X14.1 ☑
        inhalation X14.0 ☑
      cooker X15.8 ☑
      drinks X10.0 ☑
      engine X17 ☑
      fats X10.2 ☑
      fluids NEC X12 ☑

☑ **Additional Character Required** — Refer to the Tabular List for Character Selection ▽ᵘ **Subterms under main terms may continue to next column or page**

Contact — *continued*
  with — *continued*
    hot — *continued*
      fluids — *continued*
        assault X98.2 ☑
        suicide (attempt) X77.2 ☑
        undetermined whether accidental or intentional Y27.2 ☑
      food X10.1 ☑
      gases X14.1 ☑
        inhalation X14.0 ☑
      heating appliance X16 ☑
      household appliance X15.8 ☑
        assault X98.3 ☑
        cooker X15.8 ☑
        hotplate X15.2 ☑
        kettle X15.8 ☑
        light bulb X15.8 ☑
        object NEC X19 ☑
          assault X98.8 ☑
          stated as undetermined whether accidental or intentional Y27.9 ☑
          suicide (attempt) X77.8 ☑
        saucepan X15.3 ☑
        skillet X15.3 ☑
        stated as undetermined whether accidental or intentional Y27.3 ☑
        stove X15.0 ☑
        suicide (attempt) X77.3 ☑
        toaster X15.1 ☑
      kettle X15.8 ☑
      light bulb X15.8 ☑
      liquid NEC (*see also* Burn) X12 ☑
        drinks X10.0 ☑
        stated as undetermined whether accidental or intentional Y27.2 ☑
        suicide (attempt) X77.2 ☑
        tap water X11.8 ☑
          stated as undetermined whether accidental or intentional Y27.1 ☑
          suicide (attempt) X77.1 ☑
      machinery X17 ☑
      metal (molten) (liquid) NEC X18 ☑
      object (not producing fire or flames) NEC X19 ☑
      oil (cooking) X10.2 ☑
      pipe X16 ☑
      plate X15.2 ☑
      radiator X16 ☑
      saucepan (glass) (metal) X15.3 ☑
      skillet X15.3 ☑
      stove (kitchen) X15.0 ☑
      substance NEC X19 ☑
      tap-water X11.8 ☑
        assault X98.1 ☑
        heated on stove X12 ☑
          stated as undetermined whether accidental or intentional Y27.2 ☑
          suicide (attempt) X77.2 ☑
        in bathtub X11.0 ☑
        running X11.1 ☑
        stated as undetermined whether accidental or intentional Y27.1 ☑
        suicide (attempt) X77.1 ☑
      toaster X15.1 ☑
      tool X17 ☑
      vapors X13.1 ☑
        inhalation X13.0 ☑
      water (tap) X11.8 ☑
        boiling X12 ☑
          stated as undetermined whether accidental or intentional Y27.2 ☑
          suicide (attempt) X77.2 ☑
        heated on stove X12 ☑
          stated as undetermined whether accidental or intentional Y27.2 ☑
          suicide (attempt) X77.2 ☑
        in bathtub X11.0 ☑
        running X11.1 ☑
        stated as undetermined whether accidental or intentional Y27.1 ☑
        suicide (attempt) X77.1 ☑
    hotplate X15.2 ☑
    ice-pick W27.4 ☑
    insect (nonvenomous) NEC W57 ☑
    kettle (hot) X15.8 ☑
    knife W26.0 ☑

Contact — *continued*
  with — *continued*
    knife — *continued*
      assault X99.1 ☑
      electric W29.1 ☑
      stated as undetermined whether accidental or intentional Y28.1 ☑
      suicide (attempt) X78.1 ☑
    lathe (metalworking) W31.1 ☑
      turnings W45.8 ☑
      woodworking W31.2 ☑
    lawnmower (powered) (ridden) W28 ☑
      causing electrocution W86.8 ☑
        suicide (attempt) X83.1 ☑
      unpowered W27.1 ☑
    lift, lifting (devices) W24.0 ☑
      agricultural operations W30.89 ☑
      shaft W24.0 ☑
    liquefied gas — *see* Exposure, cold, man-made
    liquid air, hydrogen, nitrogen — *see* Exposure, cold, man-made
    lizard (nonvenomous) W59.09 ☑
      bite W59.01 ☑
      strike W59.02 ☑
    llama — *see* Contact, with, hoof stock NEC
    macaw W61.19 ☑
      bite W61.11 ☑
      strike W61.12 ☑
    machine, machinery W31.9 ☑
      abrasive wheel W31.1 ☑
      agricultural including animal-powered W30.9 ☑
        combine harvester W30.0 ☑
        grain storage elevator W30.3 ☑
        hay derrick W30.2 ☑
        power take-off device W30.1 ☑
        reaper W30.0 ☑
        specified NEC W30.89 ☑
        thresher W30.0 ☑
        transport vehicle, stationary W30.81 ☑
      band saw W31.2 ☑
      bench saw W31.2 ☑
      circular saw W31.2 ☑
      commercial NEC W31.82 ☑
      drilling, metal (industrial) W31.1 ☑
      earth-drilling W31.0 ☑
      earthmoving or scraping W31.89 ☑
      excavating W31.89 ☑
      forging machine W31.1 ☑
      gas turbine W31.3 ☑
      hot X17 ☑
      internal combustion engine W31.3 ☑
      land drill W31.0 ☑
      lathe W31.1 ☑
      lifting (devices) W24.0 ☑
      metal drill W31.1 ☑
      metalworking (industrial) W31.1 ☑
      milling, metal W31.1 ☑
      mining W31.0 ☑
      molding W31.2 ☑
      overhead plane W31.2 ☑
      power press, metal W31.1 ☑
      prime mover W31.3 ☑
      printing W31.89 ☑
      radial saw W31.2 ☑
      recreational W31.81 ☑
      roller-coaster W31.81 ☑
      rolling mill, metal W31.1 ☑
      sander W31.2 ☑
      seabed drill W31.0 ☑
      shaft
        hoist W31.0 ☑
        lift W31.0 ☑
      specified NEC W31.89 ☑
      spinning W31.89 ☑
      steam engine W31.3 ☑
      transmission W24.1 ☑
      undercutter W31.0 ☑
      water driven turbine W31.3 ☑
      weaving W31.89 ☑
      woodworking or forming (industrial) W31.2 ☑
    mammal (feces) (urine) W55.89 ☑
      bull — *see* Contact, with, bull
      cat — *see* Contact, with, cat
      cow — *see* Contact, with, cow
      goat — *see* Contact, with, goat
      hoof stock — *see* Contact, with, hoof stock

Contact — *continued*
  with — *continued*
    mammal — *continued*
      horse — *see* Contact, with, horse
      marine W56.39 ☑
        dolphin — *see* Contact, with, dolphin
        orca — *see* Contact, with, orca
        sea lion — *see* Contact, with, sea lion
        specified NEC W56.39 ☑
          bite W56.31 ☑
          strike W56.32 ☑
      pig — *see* Contact, with, pig
      raccoon — *see* Contact, with, raccoon
      rodent — *see* Contact, with, rodent
      sheep — *see* Contact, with, sheep
      specified NEC W55.89 ☑
        bite W55.81 ☑
        strike W55.82 ☑
    marine
      animal W56.89 ☑
        bite W56.81 ☑
        dolphin — *see* Contact, with, dolphin
        fish NEC — *see* Contact, with, fish
        mammal — *see* Contact, with, mammal, marine
        orca — *see* Contact, with, orca
        sea lion — *see* Contact, with, sea lion
        shark — *see* Contact, with, shark
        strike W56.82 ☑
    meat
      grinder (domestic) W29.0 ☑
        industrial W31.82 ☑
        nonpowered W27.4 ☑
      slicer (domestic) W29.0 ☑
        industrial W31.82 ☑
    merry go round W31.81 ☑
    metal, hot (liquid) (molten) NEC X18 ☑
    millipede W57 ☑
    nail W45.0 ☑
      gun W29.4 ☑
    needle (sewing) W27.3 ☑
      hypodermic W46.0 ☑
        contaminated W46.1 ☑
    object (blunt) NEC
      hot NEC X19 ☑
      legal intervention — *see* Legal, intervention, blunt object
      sharp NEC W45.8 ☑
        inflicted by other person NEC W45.8 ☑
          stated as
            intentional homicide (attempt) — *see* Assault, cutting or piercing instrument
        legal intervention — *see* Legal, intervention, sharp object
        self-inflicted X78.9 ☑
    orca W56.29 ☑
      bite W56.21 ☑
      strike W56.22 ☑
    overhead plane W31.2 ☑
    paper (as sharp object) W26.2 ☑
    paper-cutter W27.5 ☑
    parrot W61.09 ☑
      bite W61.01 ☑
      strike W61.02 ☑
    pig W55.49 ☑
      bite W55.41 ☑
      strike W55.42 ☑
    pipe, hot X16 ☑
    pitchfork W27.1 ☑
    plane (metal) (wood) W27.0 ☑
      overhead W31.2 ☑
    plant thorns, spines, sharp leaves or other mechanisms W60 ☑
    powered
      garden cultivator W29.3 ☑
      household appliance, implement, or machine W29.8 ☑
      saw (industrial) W31.2 ☑
        hand W29.8 ☑
    printing machine W31.89 ☑
    psittacine bird W61.29 ☑
      bite W61.21 ☑
      macaw — *see* Contact, with, macaw
      parrot — *see* Contact, with, parrot
      strike W61.22 ☑

Contact — *continued*
  with — *continued*
    pulley (block) (transmission) W24.0 ☑
      agricultural operations W30.89 ☑
    raccoon W55.59 ☑
      bite W55.51 ☑
      strike W55.52 ☑
    radial-saw (industrial) W31.2 ☑
    radiator (hot) X16 ☑
    rake W27.1 ☑
    rattlesnake X58 ☑
    reaper W30.0 ☑
    reptile W59.89 ☑
      lizard — *see* Contact, with, lizard
      snake — *see* Contact, with, snake
      specified NEC W59.89 ☑
        bite W59.81 ☑
        crushing W59.83 ☑
        strike W59.82 ☑
      turtle — *see* Contact, with, turtle
    rivet gun (powered) W29.4 ☑
    road scraper — *see* Accident, transport, construction
      vehicle
    rodent (feces) (urine) W53.89 ☑
      bite W53.81 ☑
      mouse W53.09 ☑
        bite W53.01 ☑
      rat W53.19 ☑
        bite W53.11 ☑
      specified NEC W53.89 ☑
        bite W53.81 ☑
      squirrel W53.29 ☑
        bite W53.21 ☑
    roller coaster W31.81 ☑
    rope NEC W24.0 ☑
      agricultural operations W30.89 ☑
    saliva — *see* Contact, with, by type of animal
    sander W29.8 ☑
      industrial W31.2 ☑
    saucepan (hot) (glass) (metal) X15.3 ☑
    saw W27.0 ☑
      band (industrial) W31.2 ☑
      bench (industrial) W31.2 ☑
      chain W29.3 ☑
      hand W27.0 ☑
    sawing machine, metal W31.1 ☑
    scissors W27.2 ☑
    scorpion X58 ☑
    screwdriver W27.0 ☑
      powered W29.8 ☑
    sea
      anemone, cucumber or urchin (spine) X58 ☑
      lion W56.19 ☑
        bite W56.11 ☑
        strike W56.12 ☑
    serpent — *see* Contact, with, snake, by type
    sewing-machine (electric) (powered) W29.2 ☑
      not powered W27.8 ☑
    shaft (hoist) (lift) (transmission) NEC W24.0 ☑
      agricultural W30.89 ☑
    shark W56.49 ☑
      bite W56.41 ☑
      strike W56.42 ☑
    sharp object(s) W26.9 ☑
      specified NEC W26.8 ☑
    shears (hand) W27.2 ☑
      powered (industrial) W31.1 ☑
        domestic W29.2 ☑
    sheep W55.39 ☑
      bite W55.31 ☑
      strike W55.32 ☑
    shovel W27.8 ☑
      steam — *see* Accident, transport, construction
        vehicle
    snake (nonvenomous) W59.19 ☑
      bite W59.11 ☑
      crushing W59.13 ☑
      strike W59.12 ☑
    spade W27.1 ☑
    spider (venomous) X58 ☑
    spin-drier W29.2 ☑
    spinning machine W31.89 ☑
    splinter W45.8 ☑
    sports equipment W21.9 ☑
    staple gun (powered) W29.8 ☑
    steam X13.1 ☑

Contact — *continued*
  with — *continued*
    steam — *continued*
      engine W31.3 ☑
      inhalation X13.0 ☑
      pipe X16 ☑
      shovel W31.89 ☑
    stove (hot) (kitchen) X15.0 ☑
    substance, hot NEC X19 ☑
      molten (metal) X18 ☑
    sword W26.1 ☑
      assault X99.2 ☑
      stated as undetermined whether accidental or
        intentional Y28.2 ☑
      suicide (attempt) X78.2 ☑
    tarantula X58 ☑
    thresher W30.0 ☑
    tin can lid W26.8 ☑
    toad W62.1 ☑
    toaster (hot) X15.1 ☑
    tool W27.8 ☑
      hand (not powered) W27.8 ☑
        auger W27.0 ☑
        axe W27.0 ☑
        can opener W27.4 ☑
        chisel W27.0 ☑
        fork W27.4 ☑
        garden W27.1 ☑
        handsaw W27.0 ☑
        hoe W27.1 ☑
        ice-pick W27.4 ☑
        kitchen utensil W27.4 ☑
        manual
          lawn mower W27.1 ☑
          sewing machine W27.8 ☑
        meat grinder W27.4 ☑
        needle (sewing) W27.3 ☑
          hypodermic W46.0 ☑
            contaminated W46.1 ☑
        paper cutter W27.5 ☑
        pitchfork W27.1 ☑
        rake W27.1 ☑
        scissors W27.2 ☑
        screwdriver W27.0 ☑
        specified NEC W27.8 ☑
        workbench W27.0 ☑
    hot X17 ☑
    powered W29.8 ☑
      blender W29.0 ☑
        commercial W31.82 ☑
      can opener W29.0 ☑
        commercial W31.82 ☑
      chainsaw W29.3 ☑
      clothes dryer W29.2 ☑
        commercial W31.82 ☑
      dishwasher W29.2 ☑
        commercial W31.82 ☑
      edger W29.3 ☑
      electric fan W29.2 ☑
        commercial W31.82 ☑
      electric knife W29.1 ☑
      food processor W29.0 ☑
        commercial W31.82 ☑
      garbage disposal W29.0 ☑
        commercial W31.82 ☑
      garden tool W29.3 ☑
      hedge trimmer W29.3 ☑
      ice maker W29.0 ☑
        commercial W31.82 ☑
      kitchen appliance W29.0 ☑
        commercial W31.82 ☑
      lawn mower W28 ☑
      meat grinder W29.0 ☑
        commercial W31.82 ☑
      mixer W29.0 ☑
        commercial W31.82 ☑
      rototiller W29.3 ☑
      sewing machine W29.2 ☑
        commercial W31.82 ☑
      washing machine W29.2 ☑
        commercial W31.82 ☑
    transmission device (belt, cable, chain, gear, pinion,
      shaft) W24.1 ☑
      agricultural operations W30.89 ☑
    turbine (gas) (water-driven) W31.3 ☑
    turkey W61.49 ☑

Contact — *continued*
  with — *continued*
    turkey — *continued*
      peck W61.43 ☑
      strike W61.42 ☑
    turtle (nonvenomous) W59.29 ☑
      bite W59.21 ☑
      strike W59.22 ☑
      terrestrial W59.89 ☑
        bite W59.81 ☑
        crushing W59.83 ☑
        strike W59.82 ☑
    under-cutter W31.0 ☑
    urine — *see* Contact, with, by type of animal
    vehicle
      agricultural use (transport) — *see* Accident,
        transport, agricultural vehicle
        not on public highway W30.81 ☑
      industrial use (transport) — *see* Accident, trans-
        port, industrial vehicle
        not on public highway W31.83 ☑
      off-road use (transport) — *see* Accident, trans-
        port, all-terrain or off-road vehicle
        not on public highway W31.83 ☑
      special construction use (transport) — *see* Acci-
        dent, transport, construction vehicle
        not on public highway W31.83 ☑
    venomous
      animal X58 ☑
      arthropods X58 ☑
      lizard X58 ☑
      marine animal NEC X58 ☑
      marine plant NEC X58 ☑
      millipedes (tropical) X58 ☑
      plant(s) X58 ☑
      snake X58 ☑
      spider X58 ☑
      viper X58 ☑
    washing-machine (powered) W29.2 ☑
    wasp X58 ☑
    weaving-machine W31.89 ☑
    winch W24.0 ☑
      agricultural operations W30.89 ☑
    wire NEC W24.0 ☑
      agricultural operations W30.89 ☑
    wood slivers W45.8 ☑
    yellow jacket X58 ☑
    zebra — *see* Contact, with, hoof stock NEC
  pressure X50.9 ☑
  stress X50.9 ☑
Coup de soleil X32 ☑
Crash
  aircraft (in transit) (powered) V95.9 ☑
    balloon V96.01 ☑
    fixed wing NEC (private) V95.21 ☑
      commercial V95.31 ☑
    glider V96.21 ☑
      hang V96.11 ☑
      powered V95.11 ☑
    helicopter V95.01 ☑
    in war operations — *see* War operations, destruction
      of aircraft
    microlight V95.11 ☑
    nonpowered V96.9 ☑
      specified NEC V96.8 ☑
    powered NEC V95.8 ☑
    stated as
      homicide (attempt) Y08.81 ☑
      suicide (attempt) X83.0 ☑
    ultralight V95.11 ☑
  spacecraft V95.41 ☑
  transport vehicle NEC (*see also* Accident, transport)
    V89.9 ☑
    homicide (attempt) Y03.8 ☑
    motor NEC (traffic) V89.2 ☑
      homicide (attempt) Y03.8 ☑
      suicide (attempt) — *see* Suicide, collision
Cruelty (mental) (physical) (sexual) X58 ☑
Crushed (accidentally) X58 ☑
  between objects (moving) (stationary and moving)
    W23.0 ☑
    stationary W23.1 ☑
  by
    alligator W58.03 ☑
    avalanche NEC — *see* Landslide
    cave-in W20.0 ☑

☑ Additional Character Required — Refer to the Tabular List for Character Selection ▽ Subterms under main terms may continue to next column or page

Crushed — *continued*
  by — *continued*
    cave-in — *continued*
      caused by cataclysmic earth surface movement
        — *see* Landslide
  crocodile W58.13 ☑
  crowd or human stampede W52 ☑
  falling
    aircraft V97.39 ☑
      in war operations — *see* War operations, destruction of aircraft
    earth, material W20.0 ☑
      caused by cataclysmic earth surface movement — *see* Landslide
    object NEC W20.8 ☑
  landslide NEC — *see* Landslide
  lizard (nonvenomous) W59.09 ☑
  machinery — *see* Contact, with, by type of machine
  reptile NEC W59.89 ☑
  snake (nonvenomous) W59.13 ☑
  in
    machinery — *see* Contact, with, by type of machine
Cut, cutting (any part of body) (accidental) (*see also* Contact, with, by object or machine)
  during medical or surgical treatment as misadventure — *see* Index to Diseases and Injuries, Complications
  homicide (attempt) — *see* Assault, cutting or piercing instrument
  inflicted by other person — *see* Assault, cutting or piercing instrument
  legal
    execution — *see* Legal, intervention
    intervention — *see* Legal, intervention, sharp object
  machine NEC (*see also* Contact, with, by type of machine) W31.9 ☑
  self-inflicted — *see* Suicide, cutting or piercing instrument
  suicide (attempt) — *see* Suicide, cutting or piercing instrument
Cyclone (any injury) X37.1 ☑

D

Decapitation (accidental circumstances) NEC X58 ☑
  homicide X99.9 ☑
  legal execution — *see* Legal, intervention
Dehydration from lack of water X58 ☑
Deprivation X58 ☑
Derailment (accidental)
  railway (rolling stock) (train) (vehicle) (without antecedent collision) V81.7 ☑
    with antecedent collision — *see* Accident, transport, railway vehicle occupant
  streetcar (without antecedent collision) V82.7 ☑
    with antecedent collision — *see* Accident, transport, streetcar occupant
Descent
  parachute (voluntary) (without accident to aircraft) V97.29 ☑
    due to accident to aircraft — *see* Accident, transport, aircraft
Desertion X58 ☑
Destitution X58 ☑
Disability, late effect or sequela of injury — *see* Sequelae
Discharge (accidental)
  airgun W34.010 ☑
    assault X95.01 ☑
    homicide (attempt) X95.01 ☑
    stated as undetermined whether accidental or intentional Y24.0 ☑
    suicide (attempt) X74.01 ☑
  BB gun — *see* Discharge, airgun
  firearm (accidental) W34.00 ☑
    assault X95.9 ☑
    handgun (pistol) (revolver) W32.0 ☑
      assault X93 ☑
      homicide (attempt) X93 ☑
      legal intervention — *see* Legal, intervention, firearm, handgun
      stated as undetermined whether accidental or intentional Y22 ☑
      suicide (attempt) X72 ☑
    homicide (attempt) X95.9 ☑
    hunting rifle W33.02 ☑

Discharge — *continued*
  firearm — *continued*
    hunting rifle — *continued*
      assault X94.1 ☑
      homicide (attempt) X94.1 ☑
      legal intervention
        injuring
          bystander Y35.032 ☑
          law enforcement personnel Y35.031 ☑
          suspect Y35.033 ☑
        stated as undetermined whether accidental or intentional Y23.1 ☑
        suicide (attempt) X73.1 ☑
    larger W33.00 ☑
      assault X94.9 ☑
      homicide (attempt) X94.9 ☑
      hunting rifle — *see* Discharge, firearm, hunting rifle
      legal intervention — *see* Legal, intervention, firearm by type of firearm
      machine gun — *see* Discharge, firearm, machine gun
      shotgun — *see* Discharge, firearm, shotgun
      specified NEC W33.09 ☑
        assault X94.8 ☑
        homicide (attempt) X94.8 ☑
        legal intervention
          injuring
            bystander Y35.092 ☑
            law enforcement personnel Y35.091 ☑
            suspect Y35.093 ☑
          stated as undetermined whether accidental or intentional Y23.8 ☑
          suicide (attempt) X73.8 ☑
      stated as undetermined whether accidental or intentional Y23.9 ☑
      suicide (attempt) X73.9 ☑
    legal intervention
      injuring
        bystander Y35.002 ☑
        law enforcement personnel Y35.001 ☑
        suspect Y35.03 ☑
      using rubber bullet
        injuring
          bystander Y35.042 ☑
          law enforcement personnel Y35.041 ☑
          suspect Y35.043 ☑
    machine gun W33.03 ☑
      assault X94.2 ☑
      homicide (attempt) X94.2 ☑
      legal intervention — *see* Legal, intervention, firearm, machine gun
      stated as undetermined whether accidental or intentional Y23.3 ☑
      suicide (attempt) X73.2 ☑
    pellet gun — *see* Discharge, airgun
    shotgun W33.01 ☑
      assault X94.0 ☑
      homicide (attempt) X94.0 ☑
      legal intervention — *see* Legal, intervention, firearm, specified NEC
      stated as undetermined whether accidental or intentional Y23.0 ☑
      suicide (attempt) X73.0 ☑
    specified NEC W34.09 ☑
      assault X95.8 ☑
      homicide (attempt) X95.8 ☑
      legal intervention — *see* Legal, intervention, firearm, specified NEC
      stated as undetermined whether accidental or intentional Y24.8 ☑
      suicide (attempt) X74.8 ☑
    stated as undetermined whether accidental or intentional Y24.9 ☑
    suicide (attempt) X74.9 ☑
    Very pistol W34.09 ☑
      assault X95.8 ☑
      homicide (attempt) X95.8 ☑
      stated as undetermined whether accidental or intentional Y24.8 ☑
      suicide (attempt) X74.8 ☑
  firework(s) W39 ☑
    stated as undetermined whether accidental or intentional Y25 ☑
  gas-operated gun NEC W34.018 ☑

Discharge — *continued*
  gas-operated gun — *continued*
    airgun — *see* Discharge, airgun
    assault X95.09 ☑
    homicide (attempt) X95.09 ☑
    paintball gun — *see* Discharge, paintball gun
    stated as undetermined whether accidental or intentional Y24.8 ☑
    suicide (attempt) X74.09 ☑
  gun NEC (*see also* Discharge, firearm NEC)
    air — *see* Discharge, airgun
    BB — *see* Discharge, airgun
    for single hand use — *see* Discharge, firearm, handgun
    hand — *see* Discharge, firearm, handgun
    machine — *see* Discharge, firearm, machine gun
    other specified — *see* Discharge, firearm NEC
    paintball — *see* Discharge, paintball gun
    pellet — *see* Discharge, airgun
  handgun — *see* Discharge, firearm, handgun
  machine gun — *see* Discharge, firearm, machine gun
  paintball gun W34.011 ☑
    assault X95.02 ☑
    homicide (attempt) X95.02 ☑
    stated as undetermined whether accidental or intentional Y24.8 ☑
    suicide (attempt) X74.02 ☑
  pistol — *see* Discharge, firearm, handgun
    flare — *see* Discharge, firearm, Very pistol
    pellet — *see* Discharge, airgun
    Very — *see* Discharge, firearm, Very pistol
  revolver — *see* Discharge, firearm, handgun
  rifle (hunting) — *see* Discharge, firearm, hunting rifle
  shotgun — *see* Discharge, firearm, shotgun
  spring-operated gun NEC W34.018 ☑
    assault X95.09 ☑
    homicide (attempt) X95.09 ☑
    stated as undetermined whether accidental or intentional Y24.8 ☑
    suicide (attempt) X74.09 ☑
Disease
  Andes W94.11 ☑
  aviator's — *see* Air, pressure
  range W94.11 ☑
Diver's disease, palsy, paralysis, squeeze — *see* Air, pressure
Diving (into water) — *see* Accident, diving
Dog bite W54.0 ☑
Dragged by transport vehicle NEC (*see also* Accident, transport) V09.9 ☑
Drinking poison (accidental) — *see* Table of Drugs and Chemicals
Dropped (accidentally) **while being carried or supported by other person** W04 ☑
Drowning (accidental) W74 ☑
  assault X92.9 ☑
  due to
    accident (to)
      machinery — *see* Contact, with, by type of machine
      watercraft V90.89 ☑
        burning V90.29 ☑
          powered V90.23 ☑
            fishing boat V90.22 ☑
            jetskis V90.23 ☑
            merchant ship V90.20 ☑
            passenger ship V90.21 ☑
          unpowered V90.28 ☑
            canoe V90.25 ☑
            inflatable V90.26 ☑
            kayak V90.25 ☑
            sailboat V90.24 ☑
            water skis V90.27 ☑
        crushed V90.39 ☑
          powered V90.33 ☑
            fishing boat V90.32 ☑
            jetskis V90.33 ☑
            merchant ship V90.30 ☑
            passenger ship V90.31 ☑
          unpowered V90.38 ☑
            canoe V90.35 ☑
            inflatable V90.36 ☑
            kayak V90.35 ☑
            sailboat V90.34 ☑
            water skis V90.37 ☑
        overturning V90.09 ☑

Drowning — *continued*
  due to — *continued*
    accident — *continued*
      watercraft — *continued*
        overturning — *continued*
          powered V90.03 ☑
            fishing boat V90.02 ☑
            jetskis V90.03 ☑
            merchant ship V90.00 ☑
            passenger ship V90.01 ☑
          unpowered V90.08 ☑
            canoe V90.05 ☑
            inflatable V90.06 ☑
            kayak V90.05 ☑
            sailboat V90.04 ☑
        sinking V90.19 ☑
          powered V90.13 ☑
            fishing boat V90.12 ☑
            jetskis V90.13 ☑
            merchant ship V90.10 ☑
            passenger ship V90.11 ☑
          unpowered V90.18 ☑
            canoe V90.15 ☑
            inflatable V90.16 ☑
            kayak V90.15 ☑
            sailboat V90.14 ☑
        specified type NEC V90.89 ☑
          powered V90.83 ☑
            fishing boat V90.82 ☑
            jetskis V90.83 ☑
            merchant ship V90.80 ☑
            passenger ship V90.81 ☑
          unpowered V90.88 ☑
            canoe V90.85 ☑
            inflatable V90.86 ☑
            kayak V90.85 ☑
            sailboat V90.84 ☑
            water skis V90.87 ☑
    avalanche — *see* Landslide
    cataclysmic
      earth surface movement NEC — *see* Forces of
        nature, earth movement
      storm — *see* Forces of nature, cataclysmic storm
    cloudburst X37.8 ☑
    cyclone X37.1 ☑
    fall overboard (from) V92.09 ☑
      powered craft V92.03 ☑
        ferry boat V92.01 ☑
        fishing boat V92.02 ☑
        jetskis V92.03 ☑
        liner V92.01 ☑
        merchant ship V92.00 ☑
        passenger ship V92.01 ☑
      resulting from
        accident to watercraft — *see* Drowning, due
          to, accident to, watercraft
        being washed overboard (from) V92.29 ☑
          powered craft V92.23 ☑
            ferry boat V92.21 ☑
            fishing boat V92.22 ☑
            jetskis V92.23 ☑
            liner V92.21 ☑
            merchant ship V92.20 ☑
            passenger ship V92.21 ☑
          unpowered craft V92.28 ☑
            canoe V92.25 ☑
            inflatable V92.26 ☑
            kayak V92.25 ☑
            sailboat V92.24 ☑
            surf-board V92.28 ☑
            water skis V92.27 ☑
            windsurfer V92.28 ☑
        motion of watercraft V92.19 ☑
          powered craft V92.13 ☑
            ferry boat V92.11 ☑
            fishing boat V92.12 ☑
            jetskis V92.13 ☑
            liner V92.11 ☑
            merchant ship V92.10 ☑
            passenger ship V92.11 ☑
          unpowered craft
            canoe V92.15 ☑
            inflatable V92.16 ☑
            kayak V92.15 ☑
            sailboat V92.14 ☑
      unpowered craft V92.08 ☑

Drowning — *continued*
  due to — *continued*
    fall overboard — *continued*
      unpowered craft — *continued*
        canoe V92.05 ☑
        inflatable V92.06 ☑
        kayak V92.05 ☑
        sailboat V92.04 ☑
        surf-board V92.08 ☑
        water skis V92.07 ☑
        windsurfer V92.08 ☑
    hurricane X37.0 ☑
    jumping into water from watercraft (involved in
      accident) (*see also* Drowning, due to, accident
      to, watercraft)
      without accident to or on watercraft W16.711 ☑
    tidal wave NEC — *see* Forces of nature, tidal wave
    torrential rain X37.8 ☑
  following
    fall
      into
        bathtub W16.211 ☑
        bucket W16.221 ☑
        fountain — *see* Drowning, following, fall, into,
          water, specified NEC
        quarry — *see* Drowning, following, fall, into,
          water, specified NEC
        reservoir — *see* Drowning, following, fall, into,
          water, specified NEC
        swimming-pool W16.011 ☑
          stated as undetermined whether acciden-
            tal or intentional Y21.3 ☑
          striking
            bottom W16.021 ☑
            wall W16.031 ☑
          suicide (attempt) X71.2 ☑
        water NOS W16.41 ☑
          natural (lake) (open sea) (river) (stream)
            (pond) W16.111 ☑
            striking
              bottom W16.121 ☑
              side W16.131 ☑
          specified NEC W16.311 ☑
            striking
              bottom W16.321 ☑
              wall W16.331 ☑
      overboard NEC — *see* Drowning, due to, fall
        overboard
    jump or dive
      from boat W16.711 ☑
        striking bottom W16.721 ☑
      into
        fountain — *see* Drowning, following, jump
          or dive, into, water, specified NEC
        quarry — *see* Drowning, following, jump or
          dive, into, water, specified NEC
        reservoir — *see* Drowning, following, jump
          or dive, into, water, specified NEC
        swimming-pool W16.511 ☑
          striking
            bottom W16.521 ☑
            wall W16.531 ☑
          suicide (attempt) X71.2 ☑
        water NOS W16.91 ☑
          natural (lake) (open sea) (river) (stream)
            (pond) W16.611 ☑
          specified NEC W16.811 ☑
            bottom W16.821 ☑
            striking
              bottom W16.821 ☑
              wall W16.831 ☑
          striking
            bottom W16.821 ☑
            wall W16.831 ☑
          striking bottom W16.621 ☑
  homicide (attempt) X92.9 ☑
  in
    bathtub (accidental) W65 ☑
      assault X92.0 ☑
      following fall W16.211 ☑
        stated as undetermined whether accidental
          or intentional Y21.1 ☑
      stated as undetermined whether accidental or
        intentional Y21.0 ☑
      suicide (attempt) X71.0 ☑
    lake — *see* Drowning, in, natural water

Drowning — *continued*
  in — *continued*
    natural water (lake) (open sea) (river) (stream)
      (pond) W69 ☑
      assault X92.3 ☑
      following
        dive or jump W16.611 ☑
          striking bottom W16.621 ☑
        fall W16.111 ☑
          striking
            bottom W16.121 ☑
            side W16.131 ☑
      stated as undetermined whether accidental or
        intentional Y21.4 ☑
      suicide (attempt) X71.3 ☑
    quarry — *see* Drowning, in, specified place NEC
    quenching tank — *see* Drowning, in, specified place
      NEC
    reservoir — *see* Drowning, in, specified place NEC
    river — *see* Drowning, in, natural water
    sea — *see* Drowning, in, natural water
    specified place NEC W73 ☑
      assault X92.8 ☑
      following
        dive or jump W16.811 ☑
          striking
            bottom W16.821 ☑
            wall W16.831 ☑
        fall W16.311 ☑
          striking
            bottom W16.321 ☑
            wall W16.331 ☑
      stated as undetermined whether accidental or
        intentional Y21.8 ☑
      suicide (attempt) X71.8 ☑
    stream — *see* Drowning, in, natural water
    swimming-pool W67 ☑
      assault X92.1 ☑
        following fall X92.2 ☑
      following
        dive or jump W16.511 ☑
          striking
            bottom W16.521 ☑
            wall W16.531 ☑
        fall W16.011 ☑
          striking
            bottom W16.021 ☑
            wall W16.031 ☑
      stated as undetermined whether accidental or
        intentional Y21.2 ☑
        following fall Y21.3 ☑
      suicide (attempt) X71.1 ☑
        following fall X71.2 ☑
    war operations — *see* War operations, restriction
      of airway
  resulting from accident to watercraft — *see* Drowning,
    due to, accident, watercraft
  self-inflicted X71.9 ☑
  stated as undetermined whether accidental or inten-
    tional Y21.9 ☑
  suicide (attempt) X71.9 ☑

E

Earth falling (on) W20.0 ☑
  caused by cataclysmic earth surface movement or
    eruption — *see* Landslide
Earth (surface) **movement NEC** — *see* Forces of nature,
  earth movement
Earthquake (any injury) X34 ☑
Effect(s) (adverse) **of**
  air pressure (any) — *see* Air, pressure
  cold, excessive (exposure to) — *see* Exposure, cold
  heat (excessive) — *see* Heat
  hot place (weather) — *see* Heat
  insolation X30 ☑
  late — *see* Sequelae
  motion — *see* Motion
  nuclear explosion or weapon in war operations — *se*
    War operations, nuclear weapon
  radiation — *see* Radiation
  travel — *see* Travel
Electric shock (accidental) (by) (in) — *see* Exposure,
  electric current
Electrocution (accidental) — *see* Exposure, electric cu
  rent

☑ **Additional Character Required — Refer to the Tabular List for Character Selection**   🔺 **Subterms under main terms may continue to next column or page**

Endotracheal tube wrongly placed during anesthetic procedure

Entanglement
- in
  - bed linen, causing suffocation T71 ☑
  - wheel of pedal cycle V19.88 ☑

Entry of foreign body or material — see Foreign body

Environmental pollution related condition — see category Z57

Execution, legal (any method) — see Legal, intervention

Exhaustion
- cold — see Exposure, cold
- due to excessive exertion (see also Overexertion) X50.9 ☑
- heat — see Heat

Explosion (accidental) (of) (with secondary fire) W40.9 ☑
- acetylene W40.1 ☑
- aerosol can W36.1 ☑
- air tank (compressed) (in machinery) W36.2 ☑
- aircraft (in transit) (powered) NEC V95.9 ☑
  - balloon V96.05 ☑
  - fixed wing NEC (private) V95.25 ☑
    - commercial V95.35 ☑
  - glider V96.25 ☑
    - hang V96.15 ☑
    - powered V95.15 ☑
  - helicopter V95.05 ☑
  - in war operations — see War operations, destruction of aircraft
  - microlight V95.15 ☑
  - nonpowered V96.9 ☑
    - specified NEC V96.8 ☑
  - powered NEC V95.8 ☑
  - stated as
    - homicide (attempt) Y03.8 ☑
    - suicide (attempt) X83.0 ☑
  - ultralight V95.15 ☑
- anesthetic gas in operating room W40.1 ☑
- antipersonnel bomb W40.8 ☑
  - assault X96.0 ☑
  - homicide (attempt) X96.0 ☑
  - suicide (attempt) X75 ☑
- assault X96.9 ☑
- bicycle tire W37.0 ☑
- blasting (cap) (materials) W40.0 ☑
- boiler (machinery), not on transport vehicle W35 ☑
  - on watercraft — see Explosion, in, watercraft
- butane W40.1 ☑
- caused by other person X96.9 ☑
- coal gas W40.1 ☑
- detonator W40.0 ☑
- dump (munitions) W40.8 ☑
- dynamite W40.0 ☑
  - in
    - assault X96.8 ☑
    - homicide (attempt) X96.8 ☑
    - legal intervention
      - injuring
        - bystander Y35.112 ☑
        - law enforcement personnel Y35.111 ☑
        - suspect Y35.113 ☑
    - suicide (attempt) X75 ☑
- explosive (material) W40.9 ☑
  - gas W40.1 ☑
  - in blasting operation W40.0 ☑
  - specified NEC W40.8 ☑
    - in
      - assault X96.8 ☑
      - homicide (attempt) X96.8 ☑
      - legal intervention
        - injuring
          - bystander Y35.192 ☑
          - law enforcement personnel Y35.191 ☑
          - suspect Y35.193 ☑
      - suicide (attempt) X75 ☑
- factory (munitions) W40.8 ☑
- fertilizer bomb W40.8 ☑
  - assault X96.3 ☑
  - homicide (attempt) X96.3 ☑
  - suicide (attempt) X75 ☑
- firearm (parts) NEC W34.19 ☑
  - airgun W34.110 ☑
  - BB gun W34.110 ☑
  - gas, air or spring-operated gun NEC W34.118 ☑
  - handgun W32.1 ☑

Explosion — continued
- firearm — continued
  - hunting rifle W33.12 ☑
  - larger firearm W33.10 ☑
    - specified NEC W33.19 ☑
  - machine gun W33.13 ☑
  - paintball gun W34.111 ☑
  - pellet gun W34.110 ☑
  - shotgun W33.11 ☑
  - Very pistol [flare] W34.19 ☑
- fire-damp W40.1 ☑
- fireworks W39 ☑
- gas (coal) (explosive) W40.1 ☑
  - cylinder W36.9 ☑
    - aerosol can W36.1 ☑
    - air tank W36.2 ☑
    - pressurized W36.3 ☑
    - specified NEC W36.8 ☑
- gasoline (fumes) (tank) not in moving motor vehicle W40.1 ☑
  - bomb W40.8 ☑
    - assault X96.1 ☑
    - homicide (attempt) X96.1 ☑
    - suicide (attempt) X75 ☑
  - in motor vehicle — see Accident, transport, by type of vehicle
- grain store W40.8 ☑
- grenade W40.8 ☑
  - in
    - assault X96.8 ☑
    - homicide (attempt) X96.8 ☑
    - legal intervention
      - injuring
        - bystander Y35.192 ☑
        - law enforcement personnel Y35.191 ☑
        - suspect Y35.193 ☑
    - suicide (attempt) X75 ☑
- handgun (parts) — see Explosion, firearm, hangun (parts)
- homicide (attempt) X96.9 ☑
  - antipersonnel bomb — see Explosion, antipersonnel bomb
  - fertilizer bomb — see Explosion, fertilizer bomb
  - gasoline bomb — see Explosion, gasoline bomb
  - letter bomb — see Explosion, letter bomb
  - pipe bomb — see Explosion, pipe bomb
  - specified NEC X96.8 ☑
- hose, pressurized W37.8 ☑
- hot water heater, tank (in machinery) W35 ☑
  - on watercraft — see Explosion, in, watercraft
- in, on
  - dump W40.8 ☑
  - factory W40.8 ☑
  - mine (of explosive gases) NEC W40.1 ☑
  - watercraft V93.59 ☑
    - powered craft V93.53 ☑
      - ferry boat V93.51 ☑
      - fishing boat V93.52 ☑
      - jetskis V93.53 ☑
      - liner V93.51 ☑
      - merchant ship V93.50 ☑
      - passenger ship V93.51 ☑
      - sailboat V93.54 ☑
- letter bomb W40.8 ☑
  - assault X96.2 ☑
  - homicide (attempt) X96.2 ☑
  - suicide (attempt) X75 ☑
- machinery (see also Contact, with, by type of machine)
  - on board watercraft — see Explosion, in, watercraft
  - pressure vessel — see Explosion, by type of vessel
- methane W40.1 ☑
- mine W40.1 ☑
- missile NEC W40.8 ☑
- mortar bomb W40.8 ☑
  - in
    - assault X96.8 ☑
    - homicide (attempt) X96.8 ☑
    - legal intervention
      - injuring
        - bystander Y35.192 ☑
        - law enforcement personnel Y35.191 ☑
        - suspect Y35.193 ☑
    - suicide (attempt) X75 ☑
- munitions (dump) (factory) W40.8 ☑
- pipe, pressurized W37.8 ☑
  - bomb W40.8 ☑

Explosion — continued
- pipe, pressurized — continued
  - bomb — continued
    - assault X96.4 ☑
    - homicide (attempt) X96.4 ☑
    - suicide (attempt) X75 ☑
- pressure, pressurized
  - cooker W38 ☑
  - gas tank (in machinery) W36.3 ☑
  - hose W37.8 ☑
  - pipe W37.8 ☑
  - specified device NEC W38 ☑
  - tire W37.8 ☑
    - bicycle W37.0 ☑
  - vessel (in machinery) W38 ☑
- propane W40.1 ☑
- self-inflicted X75 ☑
- shell (artillery) NEC W40.8 ☑
  - during war operations — see War operations, explosion
  - in
    - legal intervention
      - injuring
        - bystander Y35.122 ☑
        - law enforcement personnel Y35.121 ☑
        - suspect Y35.123 ☑
  - war — see War operations, explosion
- spacecraft V95.45 ☑
- stated as undetermined whether accidental or intentional Y25 ☑
- steam or water lines (in machinery) W37.8 ☑
- stove W40.9 ☑
- suicide (attempt) X75 ☑
- tire, pressurized W37.8 ☑
  - bicycle W37.0 ☑
- undetermined whether accidental or intentional Y25 ☑
- vehicle tire NEC W37.8 ☑
  - bicycle W37.0 ☑
- war operations — see War operations, explosion

Exposure (to) X58 ☑
- air pressure change — see Air, pressure
- cold (accidental) (excessive) (extreme) (natural) (place) X31 ☑
  - assault Y08.89 ☑
  - due to
    - man-made conditions W93.8 ☑
      - dry ice (contact) W93.01 ☑
        - inhalation W93.02 ☑
      - liquid air (contact) (hydrogen) (nitrogen) W93.11 ☑
        - inhalation W93.12 ☑
      - refrigeration unit (deep freeze) W93.2 ☑
      - suicide (attempt) X83.2 ☑
    - weather (conditions) X31 ☑
  - homicide (attempt) Y08.89 ☑
  - self-inflicted X83.2 ☑
- due to abandonment or neglect X58 ☑
- electric current W86.8 ☑
  - appliance (faulty) W86.8 ☑
    - domestic W86.0 ☑
  - caused by other person Y08.89 ☑
  - conductor (faulty) W86.1 ☑
  - control apparatus (faulty) W86.1 ☑
  - electric power generating plant, distribution station W86.1 ☑
  - electroshock gun — see Exposure, electric current, taser
  - high-voltage cable W85 ☑
  - homicide (attempt) Y08.89 ☑
  - legal execution — see Legal, intervention, specified means NEC
  - lightning — see subcategory T75.0 ☑
  - live rail W86.8 ☑
  - misadventure in medical or surgical procedure in electroshock therapy Y63.4
  - motor (electric) (faulty) W86.8 ☑
    - domestic W86.0 ☑
  - self-inflicted X83.1 ☑
  - specified NEC W86.8 ☑
    - domestic W86.0 ☑
  - stun gun — see Exposure, electric current, taser
  - suicide (attempt) X83.1 ☑
  - taser W86.8 ☑
    - assault Y08.89 ☑
    - legal intervention — see category Y35
    - self-harm (intentional) X83.8 ☑

Exposure — *continued*
electric current — *continued*
taser — *continued*
undetermined intent Y33 ☑
third rail W86.8 ☑
transformer (faulty) W86.1 ☑
transmission lines W85 ☑
environmental tobacco smoke X58 ☑
excessive
cold — *see* Exposure, cold
heat (natural) NEC X30 ☑
man-made W92 ☑
factor(s) NOS X58 ☑
environmental NEC X58 ☑
man-made NEC W99 ☑
natural NEC — *see* Forces of nature
specified NEC X58 ☑
fire, flames (accidental) X08.8 ☑
assault X97 ☑
campfire — *see* Exposure, fire, controlled, not in building
controlled (in)
with ignition (of) clothing (*see also* Ignition, clothes) X06.2 ☑
nightwear X05 ☑
bonfire — *see* Exposure, fire, controlled, not in building
brazier (in building or structure) (*see also* Exposure, fire, controlled, building)
not in building or structure — *see* Exposure, fire, controlled, not in building
building or structure X02.0 ☑
with
fall from building X02.3 ☑
from building X02.5 ☑
injury due to building collapse X02.2 ☑
smoke inhalation X02.1 ☑
hit by object from building X02.4 ☑
specified mode of injury NEC X02.8 ☑
fireplace, furnace or stove — *see* Exposure, fire, controlled, building
not in building or structure X03.0 ☑
with
fall X03.3 ☑
smoke inhalation X03.1 ☑
hit by object X03.4 ☑
specified mode of injury NEC X03.8 ☑
trash — *see* Exposure, fire, controlled, not in building
fireplace — *see* Exposure, fire, controlled, building
fittings or furniture (in building or structure) (uncontrolled) — *see* Exposure, fire, uncontrolled, building
forest (uncontrolled) — *see* Exposure, fire, uncontrolled, not in building
grass (uncontrolled) — *see* Exposure, fire, uncontrolled, not in building
hay (uncontrolled) — *see* Exposure, fire, uncontrolled, not in building
homicide (attempt) X97 ☑
ignition of highly flammable material X04 ☑
in, of, on, starting in
machinery — *see* Contact, with, by type of machine
motor vehicle (in motion) (*see also* Accident, transport, occupant by type of vehicle) V87.8 ☑
with collision — *see* Collision
railway rolling stock, train, vehicle V81.81 ☑
with collision — *see* Accident, transport, railway vehicle occupant
street car (in motion) V82.8 ☑
with collision — *see* Accident, transport, streetcar occupant
transport vehicle NEC (*see also* Accident, transport)
with collision — *see* Collision
war operations (*see also* War operations, fire)
from nuclear explosion — *see* War operations, nuclear weapons
watercraft (in transit) (not in transit) V91.09 ☑
localized — *see* Burn, on board watercraft, due to, fire on board
powered craft V91.03 ☑
ferry boat V91.01 ☑
fishing boat V91.02 ☑
jet skis V91.03 ☑

Exposure — *continued*
fire, flames — *continued*
in, of, on, starting in — *continued*
watercraft — *continued*
powered craft — *continued*
liner V91.01 ☑
merchant ship V91.00 ☑
passenger ship V91.01 ☑
unpowered craft V91.08 ☑
canoe V91.05 ☑
inflatable V91.06 ☑
kayak V91.05 ☑
sailboat V91.04 ☑
surf-board V91.08 ☑
waterskis V91.07 ☑
windsurfer V91.08 ☑
lumber (uncontrolled) — *see* Exposure, fire, uncontrolled, not in building
mine (uncontrolled) — *see* Exposure, fire, uncontrolled, not in building
prairie (uncontrolled) — *see* Exposure, fire, uncontrolled, not in building
resulting from
explosion — *see* Explosion
lightning X08.8 ☑
self-inflicted X76 ☑
specified NEC X08.8 ☑
started by other person X97 ☑
stated as undetermined whether accidental or intentional Y26 ☑
stove — *see* Exposure, fire, controlled, building
suicide (attempt) X76 ☑
tunnel (uncontrolled) — *see* Exposure, fire, uncontrolled, not in building
uncontrolled
in building or structure X00.0 ☑
with
fall from building X00.3 ☑
injury due to building collapse X00.2 ☑
jump from building X00.5 ☑
smoke inhalation X00.1 ☑
bed X08.00 ☑
due to
cigarette X08.01 ☑
specified material NEC X08.09 ☑
furniture NEC X08.20 ☑
due to
cigarette X08.21 ☑
specified material NEC X08.29 ☑
hit by object from building X00.4 ☑
sofa X08.10 ☑
due to
cigarette X08.11 ☑
specified material NEC X08.19 ☑
specified mode of injury NEC X08.8 ☑
not in building or structure (any) X01.0 ☑
with
fall X01.3 ☑
smoke inhalation X01.1 ☑
hit by object X01.4 ☑
specified mode of injury NEC X01.8 ☑
undetermined whether accidental or intentional Y26 ☑
forces of nature NEC — *see* Forces of nature
G-forces (abnormal) W49.9 ☑
gravitational forces (abnormal) W49.9 ☑
heat (natural) NEC — *see* Heat
high-pressure jet (hydraulic) (pneumatic) W49.9 ☑
hydraulic jet W49.9 ☑
inanimate mechanical force W49.9 ☑
jet, high-pressure (hydraulic) (pneumatic) W49.9 ☑
lightning — *see* subcategory T75.0 ☑
causing fire — *see* Exposure, fire
mechanical forces NEC W49.9 ☑
animate NEC W64 ☑
inanimate NEC W49.9 ☑
noise W42.9 ☑
supersonic W42.0 ☑
noxious substance — *see* Table of Drugs and Chemicals
pneumatic jet W49.9 ☑
prolonged in deep-freeze unit or refrigerator W93.2 ☑
radiation — *see* Radiation
smoke (*see also* Exposure, fire)
tobacco, second hand Z77.22
specified factors NEC X58 ☑
sunlight X32 ☑

Exposure — *continued*
sunlight — *continued*
man-made (sun lamp) W89.8 ☑
tanning bed W89.1 ☑
supersonic waves W42.0 ☑
transmission line(s), electric W85 ☑
vibration W49.9 ☑
waves
infrasound W49.9 ☑
sound W42.9 ☑
supersonic W42.0 ☑
weather NEC — *see* Forces of nature
External cause status Y99.9
child assisting in compensated work for family Y99.8
civilian activity done for financial or other compensation Y99.0
civilian activity done for income or pay Y99.0
family member assisting in compensated work for other family member Y99.8
hobby not done for income Y99.8
leisure activity Y99.8
military activity Y99.1
off-duty activity of military personnel Y99.8
recreation or sport not for income or while a student Y99.8
specified NEC Y99.8
student activity Y99.8
volunteer activity Y99.2

F

Factors, supplemental
alcohol
blood level
less than 20mg/100ml Y90.0
presence in blood, level not specified Y90.9
20-39mg/100ml Y90.1
40-59mg/100ml Y90.2
60-79mg/100ml Y90.3
80-99mg/100ml Y90.4
100-119mg/100ml Y90.5
120-199mg/100ml Y90.6
200-239mg/100ml Y90.7
240mg/100ml or more Y90.8
presence in blood, but level not specified Y90.9
environmental-pollution-related condition- *see* Z57 ☑
nosocomial condition Y95
work-related condition Y99.0
Failure
in suture or ligature during surgical procedure Y65.2
mechanical, of instrument or apparatus (any) (during any medical or surgical procedure) Y65.8
sterile precautions (during medical and surgical care) — *see* Misadventure, failure, sterile precautions, by type of procedure
to
introduce tube or instrument Y65.4
endotracheal tube during anesthesia Y65.3
make curve (transport vehicle) NEC — *see* Accident, transport
remove tube or instrument Y65.4
Fall, falling (accidental) W19 ☑
building W20.1 ☑
burning (uncontrolled fire) X00.3 ☑
down
embankment W17.81 ☑
escalator W10.0 ☑
hill W17.81 ☑
ladder W11 ☑
ramp W10.2 ☑
stairs, steps W10.9 ☑
due to
bumping against
object W18.00 ☑
sharp glass W18.02 ☑
specified NEC W18.09 ☑
sports equipment W18.01 ☑
person W03 ☑
due to ice or snow W00.0 ☑
on pedestrian conveyance — *see* Accident, transport, pedestrian, conveyance
collision with another person W03 ☑
due to ice or snow W00.0 ☑
involving pedestrian conveyance — *see* Accident, transport, pedestrian, conveyance
grocery cart tipping over W17.82 ☑
ice or snow W00.9 ☑

☑ Additional Character Required — Refer to the Tabular List for Character Selection   ⬚ Subterms under main terms may continue to next column or page

Fall, falling — continued
  due to — continued
    ice or snow — continued
      from one level to another W00.2 ☑
        on stairs or steps W00.1 ☑
      involving pedestrian conveyance — see Acci-
        dent, transport, pedestrian, conveyance
      on same level W00.0 ☑
    slipping (on moving sidewalk) W01.0 ☑
      with subsequent striking against object
        W01.10 ☑
        furniture W01.190 ☑
        sharp object W01.119 ☑
          glass W01.110 ☑
          power tool or machine W01.111 ☑
          specified NEC W01.118 ☑
        specified NEC W01.198 ☑
    striking against
      object W18.00 ☑
        sharp glass W18.02 ☑
        specified NEC W18.09 ☑
        sports equipment W18.01 ☑
      person W03 ☑
        due to ice or snow W00.0 ☑
        on pedestrian conveyance — see Accident,
          transport, pedestrian, conveyance
  earth (with asphyxia or suffocation (by pressure)) —
    see Earth, falling
  from, off, out of
    aircraft NEC (with accident to aircraft NEC) V97.0 ☑
      while boarding or alighting V97.1 ☑
    balcony W13.0 ☑
    bed W06 ☑
    boat, ship, watercraft NEC (with drowning or sub-
      mersion) — see Drowning, due to, fall over-
      board
      with hitting bottom or object V94.0 ☑
    bridge W13.1 ☑
    building W13.9 ☑
      burning (uncontrolled fire) X00.3 ☑
    cavity W17.2 ☑
    chair W07 ☑
    cherry picker W17.89 ☑
    cliff W15 ☑
    dock W17.4 ☑
    embankment W17.81 ☑
    escalator W10.0 ☑
    flagpole W13.8 ☑
    furniture NEC W08 ☑
    grocery cart W17.82 ☑
    haystack W17.89 ☑
    high place NEC W17.89 ☑
      stated as undetermined whether accidental or
        intentional Y30 ☑
    hole W17.2 ☑
    incline W10.2 ☑
    ladder W11 ☑
    lifting device W17.89 ☑
    machine, machinery (see also Contact, with, by type
      of machine)
      not in operation W17.89 ☑
    manhole W17.1 ☑
    mobile elevated work platform [MEWP] W17.89 ☑
    motorized mobility scooter W05.2 ☑
    one level to another NEC W17.89 ☑
      intentional, purposeful, suicide (attempt) X80 ☑
      stated as undetermined whether accidental or
        intentional Y30 ☑
    pit W17.2 ☑
    playground equipment W09.8 ☑
      jungle gym W09.2 ☑
      slide W09.0 ☑
      swing W09.1 ☑
    quarry W17.89 ☑
    railing W13.9 ☑
    ramp W10.2 ☑
    roof W13.2 ☑
    scaffolding W12 ☑
    scooter (nonmotorized) W05.1 ☑
      motorized mobility W05.2 ☑
    sky lift W17.89 ☑
    stairs, steps W10.9 ☑
      curb W10.1 ☑
      due to ice or snow W00.1 ☑
      escalator W10.0 ☑
      incline W10.2 ☑

Fall, falling — continued
  from, off, out of — continued
    stairs, steps — continued
      ramp W10.2 ☑
      sidewalk curb W10.1 ☑
      specified NEC W10.8 ☑
    stepladder W11 ☑
    storm drain W17.1 ☑
    streetcar NEC V82.6 ☑
      while boarding or alighting V82.4 ☑
      with antecedent collision — see Accident,
        transport, streetcar occupant
    structure NEC W13.8 ☑
      burning (uncontrolled fire) X00.3 ☑
    table W08 ☑
    toilet W18.11 ☑
      with subsequent striking against object
        W18.12 ☑
    train NEC V81.6 ☑
      during derailment (without antecedent collision)
        V81.7 ☑
        with antecedent collision — see Accident,
          transport, railway vehicle occupant
      while boarding or alighting V81.4 ☑
    transport vehicle after collision — see Accident,
      transport, by type of vehicle, collision
    tree W14 ☑
    vehicle (in motion) NEC (see also Accident, transport)
      V89.9 ☑
      motor NEC (see also Accident, transport, occu-
        pant, by type of vehicle) V87.8 ☑
      stationary W17.89 ☑
        while boarding or alighting — see Accident,
          transport, by type of vehicle, while
          boarding or alighting
    viaduct W13.8 ☑
    wall W13.8 ☑
    watercraft (see also Drowning, due to, fall over-
      board)
      with hitting bottom or object V94.0 ☑
    well W17.0 ☑
    wheelchair, non-moving W05.0 ☑
      powered — see Accident, transport, pedestrian,
        conveyance occupant, specified type NEC
    window W13.4 ☑
  in, on
    aircraft NEC V97.0 ☑
      while boarding or alighting V97.1 ☑
      with accident to aircraft V97.0 ☑
    bathtub (empty) W18.2 ☑
      filled W16.212 ☑
        causing drowning W16.211 ☑
    escalator W10.0 ☑
    incline W10.2 ☑
    ladder W11 ☑
    machine, machinery — see Contact, with, by type
      of machine
    object, edged, pointed or sharp (with cut) — see
      Fall, by type
    playground equipment W09.8 ☑
      jungle gym W09.2 ☑
      slide W09.0 ☑
      swing W09.1 ☑
    ramp W10.2 ☑
    scaffolding W12 ☑
    shower W18.2 ☑
      causing drowning W16.211 ☑
    staircase, stairs, steps W10.9 ☑
      curb W10.1 ☑
      due to ice or snow W00.1 ☑
      escalator W10.0 ☑
      incline W10.2 ☑
      specified NEC W10.8 ☑
    streetcar (without antecedent collision) V82.5 ☑
      with antecedent collision — see Accident,
        transport, streetcar occupant
      while boarding or alighting V82.4 ☑
    train (without antecedent collision) V81.5 ☑
      with antecedent collision — see Accident,
        transport, railway vehicle occupant
      during derailment (without antecedent collision)
        V81.7 ☑
        with antecedent collision — see Accident,
          transport, railway vehicle occupant
      while boarding or alighting V81.4 ☑

Fall, falling — continued
  in, on — continued
    transport vehicle after collision — see Accident,
      transport, by type of vehicle, collision
    watercraft V93.39 ☑
      due to
        accident to craft V91.29 ☑
          powered craft V91.23 ☑
            ferry boat V91.21 ☑
            fishing boat V91.22 ☑
            jetskis V91.23 ☑
            liner V91.21 ☑
            merchant ship V91.20 ☑
            passenger ship V91.21 ☑
          unpowered craft
            canoe V91.25 ☑
            inflatable V91.26 ☑
            kayak V91.25 ☑
            sailboat V91.24 ☑
        powered craft V93.33 ☑
          ferry boat V93.31 ☑
          fishing boat V93.32 ☑
          jetskis V93.33 ☑
          liner V93.31 ☑
          merchant ship V93.30 ☑
          passenger ship V93.31 ☑
        unpowered craft V93.38 ☑
          canoe V93.35 ☑
          inflatable V93.36 ☑
          kayak V93.35 ☑
          sailboat V93.34 ☑
          surf-board V93.38 ☑
          windsurfer V93.38 ☑
  into
    cavity W17.2 ☑
    dock W17.4 ☑
    fire — see Exposure, fire, by type
    haystack W17.89 ☑
    hole W17.2 ☑
    lake — see Fall, into, water
    manhole W17.1 ☑
    moving part of machinery — see Contact, with, by
      type of machine
    ocean — see Fall, into, water
    opening in surface NEC W17.89 ☑
    pit W17.2 ☑
    pond — see Fall, into, water
    quarry W17.89 ☑
    river — see Fall, into, water
    shaft W17.89 ☑
    storm drain W17.1 ☑
    stream — see Fall, into, water
    swimming pool (see also Fall, into, water, in, swim-
      ming pool)
      empty W17.3 ☑
    tank W17.89 ☑
    water W16.42 ☑
      causing drowning W16.41 ☑
      from watercraft — see Drowning, due to, fall
        overboard
      hitting diving board W21.4 ☑
      in
        bathtub W16.212 ☑
          causing drowning W16.211 ☑
        bucket W16.222 ☑
          causing drowning W16.221 ☑
        natural body of water W16.112 ☑
          causing drowning W16.111 ☑
          striking
            bottom W16.122 ☑
              causing drowning W16.121 ☑
            side W16.132 ☑
              causing drowning W16.131 ☑
        specified water NEC W16.312 ☑
          causing drowning W16.311 ☑
          striking
            bottom W16.322 ☑
              causing drowning W16.321 ☑
            wall W16.332 ☑
              causing drowning W16.331 ☑
        swimming pool W16.012 ☑
          causing drowning W16.011 ☑
          striking
            bottom W16.022 ☑
              causing drowning W16.031 ☑
            wall W16.032 ☑

Fall, falling — continued
  into — continued
    water — continued
      in — continued
        swimming pool — continued
          striking — continued
            wall — continued
              causing drowning W16.021 ☑
          utility bucket W16.222 ☑
            causing drowning W16.221 ☑
    well W17.0 ☑
  involving
    bed W06 ☑
    chair W07 ☑
    furniture NEC W08 ☑
    glass — see Fall, by type
    playground equipment W09.8 ☑
      jungle gym W09.2 ☑
      slide W09.0 ☑
      swing W09.1 ☑
    roller blades — see Accident, transport, pedestrian, conveyance
    skateboard(s) — see Accident, transport, pedestrian, conveyance
    skates (ice) (in line) (roller) — see Accident, transport, pedestrian, conveyance
    skis — see Accident, transport, pedestrian, conveyance
    table W08 ☑
    wheelchair, non-moving W05.0 ☑
      powered — see Accident, transport, pedestrian, conveyance, specified type NEC
  object — see Struck by, object, falling
  off
    toilet W18.11 ☑
      with subsequent striking against object W18.12 ☑
  on same level W18.30 ☑
    due to
      specified NEC W18.39 ☑
      stepping on an object W18.31 ☑
  out of
    bed W06 ☑
    building NEC W13.8 ☑
    chair W07 ☑
    furniture NEC W08 ☑
    wheelchair, non-moving W05.0 ☑
      powered — see Accident, transport, pedestrian, conveyance, specified type NEC
    window W13.4 ☑
  over
    animal W01.0 ☑
    cliff W15 ☑
    embankment W17.81 ☑
    small object W01.0 ☑
  rock W20.8 ☑
  same level W18.30 ☑
    from
      being crushed, pushed, or stepped on by a crowd or human stampede W52 ☑
      collision, pushing, shoving, by or with other person W03 ☑
      slipping, stumbling, tripping W01.0 ☑
    involving ice or snow W00.0 ☑
    involving skates (ice) (roller), skateboard, skis — see Accident, transport, pedestrian, conveyance
  snowslide (avalanche) — see Landslide
  stone W20.8 ☑
  structure W20.1 ☑
    burning (uncontrolled fire) X00.3 ☑
  through
    bridge W13.1 ☑
    floor W13.3 ☑
    roof W13.2 ☑
    wall W13.8 ☑
    window W13.4 ☑
  timber W20.8 ☑
  tree (caused by lightning) W20.8 ☑
  while being carried or supported by other person(s) W04 ☑

Fallen on by
  animal (not being ridden) NEC W55.89 ☑

Felo-de-se — see Suicide

Fight (hand) (fists) (foot) — see Assault, fight

Fire (accidental) — see Exposure, fire

Firearm discharge — see Discharge, firearm

Fireball effects from nuclear explosion in war operations — see War operations, nuclear weapons

Fireworks (explosion) W39 ☑

Flash burns from explosion — see Explosion

Flood (any injury) (caused by) X38 ☑
  collapse of man-made structure causing earth movement X36.0 ☑
  tidal wave — see Forces of nature, tidal wave

Food (any type) **in**
  air passages (with asphyxia, obstruction, or suffocation) — see categories T17 and T18 ☑
  alimentary tract causing asphyxia (due to compression of trachea) — see categories T17 and T18 ☑

Forces of nature X39.8 ☑
  avalanche X36.1 ☑
    causing transport accident — see Accident, transport, by type of vehicle
  blizzard X37.2 ☑
  cataclysmic storm X37.9 ☑
    with flood X38 ☑
    blizzard X37.2 ☑
    cloudburst X37.8 ☑
    cyclone X37.1 ☑
    dust storm X37.3 ☑
    hurricane X37.0 ☑
    specified storm NEC X37.8 ☑
    storm surge X37.0 ☑
    tornado X37.1 ☑
    twister X37.1 ☑
    typhoon X37.0 ☑
  cloudburst X37.8 ☑
  cold (natural) X31 ☑
  cyclone X37.1 ☑
  dam collapse causing earth movement X36.0 ☑
  dust storm X37.3 ☑
  earth movement X36.1 ☑
    caused by dam or structure collapse X36.0 ☑
    earthquake X34 ☑
  earthquake X34 ☑
  flood (caused by) X38 ☑
    dam collapse X36.0 ☑
    tidal wave — see Forces of nature, tidal wave
  heat (natural) X30 ☑
  hurricane X37.0 ☑
  landslide X36.1 ☑
    causing transport accident — see Accident, transport, by type of vehicle
  lightning — see subcategory T75.0 ☑
    causing fire — see Exposure, fire
  mudslide X36.1 ☑
    causing transport accident — see Accident, transport, by type of vehicle
  radiation (natural) X39.08 ☑
    radon X39.01 ☑
  radon X39.01 ☑
  specified force NEC X39.8 ☑
  storm surge X37.0 ☑
  structure collapse causing earth movement X36.0 ☑
  sunlight X32 ☑
  tidal wave X37.41 ☑
    due to
      earthquake X37.41 ☑
      landslide X37.43 ☑
      storm X37.42 ☑
      volcanic eruption X37.41 ☑
  tornado X37.1 ☑
  tsunami X37.41 ☑
  twister X37.1 ☑
  typhoon X37.0 ☑
  volcanic eruption X35 ☑

Foreign body
  aspiration — see Index to Diseases and Injuries, Foreign body, respiratory tract
  embedded in skin W45 ☑
  entering through skin W45.8 ☑
    can lid W26.8 ☑
    nail W45.0 ☑
    paper W26.2 ☑
    specified NEC W45.8 ☑
    splinter W45.8 ☑

Forest fire (exposure to) — see Exposure, fire, uncontrolled, not in building

Found injured X58 ☑
  from exposure (to) — see Exposure

Found injured — continued
  on
    highway, road(way), street V89.9 ☑
    railway right of way V81.9 ☑

Fracture (circumstances unknown or unspecified) X58 ☑
  due to specified cause NEC X58 ☑

Freezing — see Exposure, cold

Frostbite X31 ☑
  due to man-made conditions — see Exposure, cold, man-made

Frozen — see Exposure, cold

G

Gored by bull W55.22 ☑

Gunshot wound W34.00 ☑

H

Hailstones, injured by X39.8 ☑

Hanged herself or himself — see Hanging, self-inflicted

Hanging (accidental) (see also category) T71 ☑
  legal execution — see Legal, intervention, specified means NEC

Heat (effects of) (excessive) X30 ☑
  due to
    man-made conditions W92 ☑
      on board watercraft V93.29 ☑
        fishing boat V93.22 ☑
        merchant ship V93.20 ☑
        passenger ship V93.21 ☑
        sailboat V93.24 ☑
        specified powered craft NEC V93.23 ☑
      weather (conditions) X30 ☑
  from
    electric heating apparatus causing burning X16 ☑
    nuclear explosion in war operations — see War operations, nuclear weapons
  inappropriate in local application or packing in medical or surgical procedure Y63.5

Hemorrhage
  delayed following medical or surgical treatment without mention of misadventure — see Index to Diseases and Injuries, Complication(s)
  during medical or surgical treatment as misadventure — see Index to Diseases and Injuries, Complication(s)

High
  altitude (effects) — see Air, pressure, low
  level of radioactivity, effects — see Radiation
  pressure (effects) — see Air, pressure, high
  temperature, effects — see Heat

Hit, hitting (accidental) by — see Struck by

Hitting against — see Striking against

Homicide (attempt) (justifiable) — see Assault

Hot
  place, effects (see also Heat)
  weather, effects X30 ☑

House fire (uncontrolled) — see Exposure, fire, uncontrolled, building

Humidity, causing problem X39.8 ☑

Hunger X58 ☑

Hurricane (any injury) X37.0 ☑

Hypobarism, hypobaropathy — see Air, pressure, low

I

Ictus
  caloris (see also Heat)
  solaris X30 ☑

Ignition (accidental) (see also Exposure, fire) X08.8 ☑
  anesthetic gas in operating room W40.1 ☑
  apparel X06.2 ☑
    from highly flammable material X04 ☑
    nightwear X05 ☑
  bed linen (sheets) (spreads) (pillows) (mattress) — see Exposure, fire, uncontrolled, building, bed
  benzine X04 ☑
  clothes, clothing NEC (from controlled fire) X06.2 ☑
    from
      highly flammable material X04 ☑
  ether X04 ☑
    in operating room W40.1 ☑
  explosive material — see Explosion
  gasoline X04 ☑
  jewelry (plastic) (any) X06.0 ☑

Ignition — *continued*
  kerosene X04 ☑
  material
    explosive — *see* Explosion
    highly flammable with secondary explosion X04 ☑
  nightwear X05 ☑
  paraffin X04 ☑
  petrol X04 ☑
Immersion (accidental) (*see also* Drowning)
  hand or foot due to cold (excessive) X31 ☑
Implantation of quills of porcupine W55.89 ☑
Inanition (from) (hunger) X58 ☑
  thirst X58 ☑
Inappropriate operation performed
  correct operation on wrong side or body part (wrong side) (wrong site) Y65.53
  operation intended for another patient done on wrong patient Y65.52
  wrong operation performed on correct patient Y65.51
Inattention after, at birth (homicidal intent) (infanticidal intent) X58 ☑
Incident, adverse
  device
    anesthesiology Y70.8
      accessory Y70.2
      diagnostic Y70.0
      miscellaneous Y70.8
      monitoring Y70.0
      prosthetic Y70.2
      rehabilitative Y70.1
      surgical Y70.3
      therapeutic Y70.1
    cardiovascular Y71.8
      accessory Y71.2
      diagnostic Y71.0
      miscellaneous Y71.8
      monitoring Y71.0
      prosthetic Y71.2
      rehabilitative Y71.1
      surgical Y71.3
      therapeutic Y71.1
    gastroenterology Y73.8
      accessory Y73.2
      diagnostic Y73.0
      miscellaneous Y73.8
      monitoring Y73.0
      prosthetic Y73.2
      rehabilitative Y73.1
      surgical Y73.3
      therapeutic Y73.1
    general
      hospital Y74.8
        accessory Y74.2
        diagnostic Y74.0
        miscellaneous Y74.8
        monitoring Y74.0
        prosthetic Y74.2
        rehabilitative Y74.1
        surgical Y74.3
        therapeutic Y74.1
      surgical Y81.8
        accessory Y81.2
        diagnostic Y81.0
        miscellaneous Y81.8
        monitoring Y81.0
        prosthetic Y81.2
        rehabilitative Y81.1
        surgical Y81.3
        therapeutic Y81.1
    gynecological Y76.8
      accessory Y76.2
      diagnostic Y76.0
      miscellaneous Y76.8
      monitoring Y76.0
      prosthetic Y76.2
      rehabilitative Y76.1
      surgical Y76.3
      therapeutic Y76.1
    medical Y82.9
      specified type NEC Y82.8
    neurological Y75.8
      accessory Y75.2
      diagnostic Y75.0
      miscellaneous Y75.8
      monitoring Y75.0
      prosthetic Y75.2
      rehabilitative Y75.1
      surgical Y75.3

Incident, adverse — *continued*
  device — *continued*
    neurological — *continued*
      therapeutic Y75.1
    obstetrical Y76.8
      accessory Y76.2
      diagnostic Y76.0
      miscellaneous Y76.8
      monitoring Y76.0
      prosthetic Y76.2
      rehabilitative Y76.1
      surgical Y76.3
      therapeutic Y76.1
    ophthalmic Y77.8
      accessory Y77.2
      diagnostic Y77.0
      miscellaneous Y77.8
      monitoring Y77.0
      prosthetic Y77.2
      rehabilitative Y77.1
      surgical Y77.3
      therapeutic Y77.1
    orthopedic Y79.8
      accessory Y79.2
      diagnostic Y79.0
      miscellaneous Y79.8
      monitoring Y79.0
      prosthetic Y79.2
      rehabilitative Y79.1
      surgical Y79.3
      therapeutic Y79.1
    otorhinolaryngological Y72.8
      accessory Y72.2
      diagnostic Y72.0
      miscellaneous Y72.8
      monitoring Y72.0
      prosthetic Y72.2
      rehabilitative Y72.1
      surgical Y72.3
      therapeutic Y72.1
    personal use Y74.8
      accessory Y74.2
      diagnostic Y74.0
      miscellaneous Y74.8
      monitoring Y74.0
      prosthetic Y74.2
      rehabilitative Y74.1
      surgical Y74.3
      therapeutic Y74.1
    physical medicine Y80.8
      accessory Y80.2
      diagnostic Y80.0
      miscellaneous Y80.8
      monitoring Y80.0
      prosthetic Y80.2
      rehabilitative Y80.1
      surgical Y80.3
      therapeutic Y80.1
    plastic surgical Y81.8
      accessory Y81.2
      diagnostic Y81.0
      miscellaneous Y81.8
      monitoring Y81.0
      prosthetic Y81.2
      rehabilitative Y81.1
      surgical Y81.3
      therapeutic Y81.1
    radiological Y78.8
      accessory Y78.2
      diagnostic Y78.0
      miscellaneous Y78.8
      monitoring Y78.0
      prosthetic Y78.2
      rehabilitative Y78.1
      surgical Y78.3
      therapeutic Y78.1
    urology Y73.8
      accessory Y73.2
      diagnostic Y73.0
      miscellaneous Y73.8
      monitoring Y73.0
      prosthetic Y73.2
      rehabilitative Y73.1
      surgical Y73.3
      therapeutic Y73.1
Incineration (accidental) — *see* Exposure, fire
Infanticide — *see* Assault
Infrasound waves (causing injury) W49.9 ☑

Ingestion
  foreign body (causing injury) (with obstruction) — *see* Foreign body, alimentary canal
  poisonous
    plant(s) X58 ☑
    substance NEC — *see* Table of Drugs and Chemicals
Inhalation
  excessively cold substance, man-made — *see* Exposure, cold, man-made
  food (any type) (into respiratory tract) (with asphyxia, obstruction respiratory tract, suffocation) — *see* categories T17 and T18
  foreign body — *see* Foreign body, aspiration
  gastric contents (with asphyxia, obstruction respiratory passage, suffocation) T17.81- ☑
  hot air or gases X14.0 ☑
  liquid air, hydrogen, nitrogen W93.12 ☑
    suicide (attempt) X83.2 ☑
  steam X13.0 ☑
    assault X98.0 ☑
    stated as undetermined whether accidental or intentional Y27.0 ☑
    suicide (attempt) X77.0 ☑
  toxic gas — *see* Table of Drugs and Chemicals
  vomitus (with asphyxia, obstruction respiratory passage, suffocation) T17.81- ☑
Injury, injured (accidental(ly)) NOS X58 ☑
  by, caused by, from
    assault — *see* Assault
    law-enforcing agent, police, in course of legal intervention — *see* Legal intervention
    suicide (attempt) X83.8 ☑
  due to, in
    civil insurrection — *see* War operations
    fight (*see also* Assault, fight) Y04.0 ☑
    war operations — *see* War operations
  homicide (*see also* Assault) Y09
  inflicted (by)
    in course of arrest (attempted), suppression of disturbance, maintenance of order, by law-enforcing agents — *see* Legal intervention
    other person
      stated as
        accidental X58 ☑
        intentional, homicide (attempt) — *see* Assault
        undetermined whether accidental or intentional Y33 ☑
  purposely (inflicted) by other person(s) — *see* Assault
  self-inflicted X83.8 ☑
    stated as accidental X58 ☑
  specified cause NEC X58 ☑
  undetermined whether accidental or intentional Y33 ☑
Insolation, effects X30 ☑
Insufficient nourishment X58 ☑
Interruption of respiration (by)
  food (lodged in esophagus) — *see* categories T17 and T18 ☑
  vomitus (lodged in esophagus) T17.81- ☑
Intervention, legal — *see* Legal intervention
Intoxication
  drug — *see* Table of Drugs and Chemicals
  poison — *see* Table of Drugs and Chemicals

J

Jammed (accidentally)
  between objects (moving) (stationary and moving) W23.0 ☑
    stationary W23.1 ☑
Jumped, jumping
  before moving object NEC X81.8 ☑
    motor vehicle X81.0 ☑
    subway train X81.1 ☑
    train X81.1 ☑
    undetermined whether accidental or intentional Y31 ☑
  from
    boat (into water) voluntarily, without accident (to or on boat) W16.712 ☑
      striking bottom W16.722 ☑
        causing drowning W16.721 ☑
      with
        accident to or on boat — *see* Accident, watercraft
        drowning or submersion W16.711 ☑
          suicide (attempt) X71.3 ☑

Jumped, jumping — *continued*
  from — *continued*
    building (*see also* Jumped, from, high place)
        W13.9 ☑
      burning (uncontrolled fire) X00.5 ☑
    high place NEC W17.89 ☑
      suicide (attempt) X80 ☑
      undetermined whether accidental or intentional
          Y30 ☑
    structure (*see also* Jumped, from, high place)
        W13.9 ☑
      burning (uncontrolled fire) X00.5 ☑
  into water W16.92 ☑
    causing drowning W16.91 ☑
    from, off watercraft — *see* Jumped, from, boat
    in
      natural body W16.612 ☑
        causing drowning W16.611 ☑
        striking bottom W16.622 ☑
          causing drowning W16.621 ☑
      specified place NEC W16.812 ☑
        causing drowning W16.811 ☑
        striking
          bottom W16.822 ☑
            causing drowning W16.821 ☑
          wall W16.832 ☑
            causing drowning W16.831 ☑
      swimming pool W16.512 ☑
        causing drowning W16.511 ☑
        striking
          bottom W16.522 ☑
            causing drowning W16.521 ☑
          wall W16.532 ☑
            causing drowning W16.531 ☑
  suicide (attempt) X71.3 ☑

K

Kicked by
  animal NEC W55.82 ☑
  person(s) (accidentally) W50.1 ☑
    with intent to injure or kill Y04.0 ☑
    as, or caused by, a crowd or human stampede (with
        fall) W52 ☑
    assault Y04.0 ☑
    homicide (attempt) Y04.0 ☑
    in
      fight Y04.0 ☑
      legal intervention
        injuring
          bystander Y35.812 ☑
          law enforcement personnel Y35.811 ☑
          suspect Y35.813 ☑

Kicking
  against
    object W22.8 ☑
      sports equipment W21.9 ☑
      stationary W22.09 ☑
        sports equipment W21.89 ☑
    person — *see* Striking against, person
    sports equipment W21.9 ☑
  carpet stretcher with knee X50.3 ☑

Killed, killing (accidentally) NOS (*see also* Injury) X58 ☑
  in
    action — *see* War operations
    brawl, fight (hand) (fists) (foot) Y04.0 ☑
      by weapon (*see also* Assault)
        cutting, piercing — *see* Assault, cutting or
            piercing instrument
        firearm — *see* Discharge, firearm, by type,
            homicide
  self
    stated as
      accident NOS X58 ☑
      suicide — *see* Suicide
      undetermined whether accidental or intentional
          Y33 ☑

Kneeling (prolonged (static)) X50.1 ☑
Knocked down (accidentally) (by) NOS X58 ☑
  animal (not being ridden) NEC (*see also* Struck by, by
      type of animal)
  crowd or human stampede W52 ☑
  person W51 ☑
    in brawl, fight Y04.0 ☑
  transport vehicle NEC (*see also* Accident, transport)
      V09.9 ☑

L

Laceration NEC — *see* Injury
Lack of
  care (helpless person) (infant) (newborn) X58 ☑
  food except as result of abandonment or neglect
      X58 ☑
    due to abandonment or neglect X58 ☑
  water except as result of transport accident X58 ☑
    due to transport accident — *see* Accident, transport,
        by type
  helpless person, infant, newborn X58 ☑
Landslide (falling on transport vehicle) X36.1 ☑
  caused by collapse of man-made structure X36.0 ☑
Late effect — *see* Sequelae
Legal
  execution (any method) — *see* Legal, intervention
  intervention (by)
    baton — *see* Legal, intervention, blunt object, baton
    bayonet — *see* Legal, intervention, sharp object,
        bayonet
    blow — *see* Legal, intervention, manhandling
    blunt object
      baton
        injuring
          bystander Y35.312 ☑
          law enforcement personnel Y35.311 ☑
          suspect Y35.313 ☑
      injuring
        bystander Y35.302 ☑
        law enforcement personnel Y35.301 ☑
        suspect Y35.303 ☑
      specified NEC
        injuring
          bystander Y35.392 ☑
          law enforcement personnel Y35.391 ☑
          suspect Y35.393 ☑
      stave
        injuring
          bystander Y35.392 ☑
          law enforcement personnel Y35.391 ☑
          suspect Y35.393 ☑
    bomb — *see* Legal, intervention, explosive
    cutting or piercing instrument — *see* Legal, inter-
        vention, sharp object
    dynamite — *see* Legal, intervention, explosive, dy-
        namite
    explosive(s)
      dynamite
        injuring
          bystander Y35.112 ☑
          law enforcement personnel Y35.111 ☑
          suspect Y35.113 ☑
      grenade
        injuring
          bystander Y35.192 ☑
          law enforcement personnel Y35.191 ☑
          suspect Y35.193 ☑
      injuring
        bystander Y35.102 ☑
        law enforcement personnel Y35.101 ☑
        suspect Y35.103 ☑
      mortar bomb
        injuring
          bystander Y35.192 ☑
          law enforcement personnel Y35.191 ☑
          suspect Y35.193 ☑
      shell
        injuring
          bystander Y35.122 ☑
          law enforcement personnel Y35.121 ☑
          suspect Y35.123 ☑
      specified NEC
        injuring
          bystander Y35.192 ☑
          law enforcement personnel Y35.191 ☑
          suspect Y35.193 ☑
    firearm(s) (discharge)
      handgun
        injuring
          bystander Y35.022 ☑
          law enforcement personnel Y35.021 ☑
          suspect Y35.023 ☑
      injuring
        bystander Y35.002 ☑
        law enforcement personnel Y35.001 ☑

Legal — *continued*
  intervention — *continued*
    firearm(s) — *continued*
      injuring — *continued*
        suspect Y35.003 ☑
      machine gun
        injuring
          bystander Y35.012 ☑
          law enforcement personnel Y35.011 ☑
          suspect Y35.013 ☑
      rifle pellet
        injuring
          bystander Y35.032 ☑
          law enforcement personnel Y35.031 ☑
          suspect Y35.033 ☑
      rubber bullet
        injuring
          bystander Y35.042 ☑
          law enforcement personnel Y35.041 ☑
          suspect Y35.043 ☑
      shotgun — *see* Legal, intervention, firearm,
          specified NEC
      specified NEC
        injuring
          bystander Y35.092 ☑
          law enforcement personnel Y35.091 ☑
          suspect Y35.093 ☑
    gas (asphyxiation) (poisoning)
      injuring
        bystander Y35.202 ☑
        law enforcement personnel Y35.201 ☑
        suspect Y35.203 ☑
      specified NEC
        injuring
          bystander Y35.292 ☑
          law enforcement personnel Y35.291 ☑
          suspect Y35.293 ☑
      tear gas
        injuring
          bystander Y35.212 ☑
          law enforcement personnel Y35.211 ☑
          suspect Y35.213 ☑
    grenade — *see* Legal, intervention, explosive,
        grenade
    injuring
      bystander Y35.92 ☑
      law enforcement personnel Y35.91 ☑
      suspect Y35.93 ☑
    late effect (of) — *see* with 7th character S Y35 ☑
    manhandling
      injuring
        bystander Y35.812 ☑
        law enforcement personnel Y35.811 ☑
        suspect Y35.813 ☑
    sequelae (of) — *see* with 7th character S Y35 ☑
    sharp objects
      bayonet
        injuring
          bystander Y35.412 ☑
          law enforcement personnel Y35.411 ☑
          suspect Y35.413 ☑
      injuring
        bystander Y35.402 ☑
        law enforcement personnel Y35.401 ☑
        suspect Y35.403 ☑
      specified NEC
        injuring
          bystander Y35.492 ☑
          law enforcement personnel Y35.491 ☑
          suspect Y35.493 ☑
    specified means NEC
      injuring
        bystander Y35.892 ☑
        law enforcement personnel Y35.891 ☑
        suspect Y35.893 ☑
    stabbing — *see* Legal, intervention, sharp object
    stave — *see* Legal, intervention, blunt object, stave
    tear gas — *see* Legal, intervention, gas, tear gas
    truncheon — *see* Legal, intervention, blunt object,
        stave
Lifting — *see also* Overexertion
  heavy objects X50.0 ☑
  weights X50.0 ☑
Lightning (shock) (stroke) (struck by) — *see* subcategory
    T75.0 ☑
  causing fire — *see* Exposure, fire

☑ Additional Character Required — Refer to the Tabular List for Character Selection   ▽ Subterms under main terms may continue to next column or page

Loss of control (transport vehicle) NEC — *see* Accident, transport

Lost at sea NOS — *see* Drowning, due to, fall overboard

Low
 pressure (effects) — *see* Air, pressure, low
 temperature (effects) — *see* Exposure, cold

Lying before train, vehicle or other moving object X81.8 ✓
 subway train X81.1 ✓
 train X81.1 ✓
 undetermined whether accidental or intentional Y31 ✓

Lynching — *see* Assault

M

Malfunction (mechanism or component) (of)
 firearm W34.10 ✓
  airgun W34.110 ✓
  BB gun W34.110 ✓
  gas, air or spring-operated gun NEC W34.118 ✓
  handgun W32.1 ✓
  hunting rifle W33.12 ✓
  larger firearm W33.10 ✓
   specified NEC W33.19 ✓
  machine gun W33.13 ✓
  paintball gun W34.111 ✓
  pellet gun W34.110 ✓
  shotgun W33.11 ✓
  specified NEC W34.19 ✓
  Very pistol [flare] W34.19 ✓
  handgun — *see* Malfunction, firearm, handgun

Maltreatment — *see* Perpetrator

Mangled (accidentally) NOS X58 ✓

Manhandling (in brawl, fight) Y04.0 ✓
 legal intervention — *see* Legal, intervention, manhandling

Manslaughter (nonaccidental) — *see* Assault

Mauled by animal NEC W55.89 ✓

Medical procedure, complication of (delayed or as an abnormal reaction without mention of misadventure) — *see* Complication of or following, by specified type of procedure
 due to or as a result of misadventure — *see* Misadventure

Melting (due to fire) (*see also* Exposure, fire)
 apparel NEC X06.3 ✓
 clothes, clothing NEC X06.3 ✓
  nightwear X05 ✓
 fittings or furniture (burning building) (uncontrolled fire) X00.8 ✓
 nightwear X05 ✓
 plastic jewelry X06.1 ✓

Mental cruelty X58 ✓

Military operations (injuries to military and civilians occuring during peacetime on military property and during routine military exercises and operations) (by) (from) (involving) Y37.90- ✓
 air blast Y37.20- ✓
 aircraft
  destruction — *see* Military operations, destruction of aircraft
  airway restriction — *see* Military operations, restriction of airways
  asphyxiation — *see* Military operations, restriction of airways
 biological weapons Y37.6X- ✓
 blast Y37.20- ✓
 blast fragments Y37.20- ✓
 blast wave Y37.20- ✓
 blast wind Y37.20- ✓
 bomb Y37.20- ✓
  dirty Y37.50- ✓
  gasoline Y37.31- ✓
  incendiary Y37.31- ✓
  petrol Y37.31- ✓
 bullet Y37.43- ✓
  incendiary Y37.32- ✓
  rubber Y37.41- ✓
 chemical weapons Y37.7X- ✓
 combat
  hand to hand (unarmed) combat Y37.44- ✓
  using blunt or piercing object Y37.45- ✓
 conflagration — *see* Military operations, fire
 conventional warfare NEC Y37.49- ✓
 depth-charge Y37.01- ✓
 destruction of aircraft Y37.10- ✓

Military operations — *continued*
 destruction of aircraft — *continued*
  due to
   air to air missile Y37.11- ✓
   collision with other aircraft Y37.12- ✓
   detonation (accidental) of onboard munitions and explosives Y37.14- ✓
   enemy fire or explosives Y37.11- ✓
   explosive placed on aircraft Y37.11- ✓
   onboard fire Y37.13- ✓
   rocket propelled grenade [RPG] Y37.11- ✓
   small arms fire Y37.11- ✓
   surface to air missile Y37.11- ✓
   specified NEC Y37.19- ✓
 detonation (accidental) of
  onboard marine weapons Y37.05- ✓
  own munitions or munitions launch device Y37.24- ✓
 dirty bomb Y37.50- ✓
 explosion (of) Y37.20- ✓
  aerial bomb Y37.21- ✓
  bomb NOS (*see also* Military operations, bomb(s)) Y37.20- ✓
  fragments Y37.20- ✓
  grenade Y37.29- ✓
  guided missile Y37.22- ✓
  improvised explosive device [IED] (person-borne) (roadside) (vehicle-borne) Y37.23- ✓
  land mine Y37.29- ✓
  marine mine (at sea) (in harbor) Y37.02- ✓
  marine weapon Y37.00- ✓
   specified NEC Y37.09- ✓
  own munitions or munitions launch device (accidental) Y37.24- ✓
  sea-based artillery shell Y37.03- ✓
  specified NEC Y37.29- ✓
  torpedo Y37.04- ✓
 fire Y37.30- ✓
  specified NEC Y37.39- ✓
 firearms
  discharge Y37.43- ✓
  pellets Y37.42- ✓
 flamethrower Y37.33- ✓
 fragments (from) (of)
  improvised explosive device [IED] (person-borne) (roadside) (vehicle-borne) Y37.26- ✓
  munitions Y37.25- ✓
  specified NEC Y37.29- ✓
  weapons Y37.27- ✓
 friendly fire Y37.92- ✓
 hand to hand (unarmed) combat Y37.44- ✓
 hot substances — *see* Military operations, fire
 incendiary bullet Y37.32- ✓
 nuclear weapon (effects of) Y37.50- ✓
  acute radiation exposure Y37.54- ✓
  blast pressure Y37.51- ✓
  direct blast Y37.51- ✓
  direct heat Y37.53- ✓
  fallout exposure Y37.54- ✓
  fireball Y37.53- ✓
  indirect blast (struck or crushed by blast debris) (being thrown by blast) Y37.52- ✓
  ionizing radiation (immediate exposure) Y37.54- ✓
  nuclear radiation Y37.54- ✓
  radiation
   ionizing (immediate exposure) Y37.54- ✓
   nuclear Y37.54- ✓
   thermal Y37.53- ✓
  secondary effects Y37.54- ✓
  specified NEC Y37.59- ✓
  thermal radiation Y37.53- ✓
 restriction of air (airway)
  intentional Y37.46- ✓
  unintentional Y37.47- ✓
 rubber bullets Y37.41- ✓
 shrapnel NOS Y37.29- ✓
 suffocation — *see* Military operations, restriction of airways
 unconventional warfare NEC Y37.7X- ✓
 underwater blast NOS Y37.00- ✓
 warfare
  conventional NEC Y37.49- ✓
  unconventional NEC Y37.7X- ✓
 weapon of mass destruction [WMD] Y37.91- ✓
 weapons
  biological weapons Y37.6X- ✓

Military operations — *continued*
 weapons — *continued*
  chemical Y37.7X- ✓
  nuclear (effects of) Y37.50- ✓
   acute radiation exposure Y37.54- ✓
   blast pressure Y37.51- ✓
   direct blast Y37.51- ✓
   direct heat Y37.53- ✓
   fallout exposure Y37.54- ✓
   fireball Y37.53- ✓
   radiation
    ionizing (immediate exposure) Y37.54- ✓
    nuclear Y37.54- ✓
    thermal Y37.53- ✓
   secondary effects Y37.54- ✓
   specified NEC Y37.59- ✓
  of mass destruction [WMD] Y37.91- ✓

Misadventure(s) **to patient**(s) **during surgical or medical care** Y69
 contaminated medical or biological substance (blood, drug, fluid) Y64.9
  administered (by) NEC Y64.9
   immunization Y64.1
   infusion Y64.0
   injection Y64.1
   specified means NEC Y64.8
   transfusion Y64.0
   vaccination Y64.1
 excessive amount of blood or other fluid during transfusion or infusion Y63.0
 failure
  in dosage Y63.9
   electroshock therapy Y63.4
   inappropriate temperature (too hot or too cold) in local application and packing Y63.5
   infusion
    excessive amount of fluid Y63.0
    incorrect dilution of fluid Y63.1
   insulin-shock therapy Y63.4
   nonadministration of necessary drug or biological substance Y63.6
   overdose — *see* Table of Drugs and Chemicals
    radiation, in therapy Y63.2
   radiation
    overdose Y63.2
   specified procedure NEC Y63.8
   transfusion
    excessive amount of blood Y63.0
  mechanical, of instrument or apparatus (any) (during any procedure) Y65.8
  sterile precautions (during procedure) Y62.9
   aspiration of fluid or tissue (by puncture or catheterization, except heart) Y62.6
   biopsy (except needle aspiration) Y62.8
    needle (aspirating) Y62.6
   blood sampling Y62.6
   catheterization Y62.6
    heart Y62.5
   dialysis (kidney) Y62.2
   endoscopic examination Y62.4
   enema Y62.8
   immunization Y62.3
   infusion Y62.1
   injection Y62.3
   needle biopsy Y62.6
   paracentesis (abdominal) (thoracic) Y62.6
   perfusion Y62.2
   puncture (lumbar) Y62.6
   removal of catheter or packing Y62.8
   specified procedure NEC Y62.8
   surgical operation Y62.0
   transfusion Y62.1
   vaccination Y62.3
  suture or ligature during surgical procedure Y65.2
  to introduce or to remove tube or instrument — *see* Failure, to
 hemorrhage — *see* Index to Diseases and Injuries, Complication(s)
 inadvertent exposure of patient to radiation Y63.3
 inappropriate
  operation performed — *see* Inappropriate operation performed
  temperature (too hot or too cold) in local application or packing Y63.5
 infusion (*see also* Misadventure, by type, infusion) Y69
  excessive amount of fluid Y63.0
  incorrect dilution of fluid Y63.1
  wrong fluid Y65.1

Misadventure(s) **to patient**(s) **during surgical or medical care** — *continued*
  mismatched blood in transfusion Y65.0
  nonadministration of necessary drug or biological substance Y63.6
  overdose — *see* Table of Drugs and Chemicals
    radiation (in therapy) Y63.2
  perforation — *see* Index to Diseases and Injuries, Complication(s)
  performance of inappropriate operation — *see* Inappropriate operation performed
  puncture — *see* Index to Diseases and Injuries, Complication(s)
  specified type NEC Y65.8
    failure
      suture or ligature during surgical operation Y65.2
      to introduce or to remove tube or instrument — *see* Failure, to
    infusion of wrong fluid Y65.1
    performance of inappropriate operation — *see* Inappropriate operation performed
    transfusion of mismatched blood Y65.0
    wrong
      fluid in infusion Y65.1
      placement of endotracheal tube during anesthetic procedure Y65.3
  transfusion — *see* Misadventure, by type, transfusion
    excessive amount of blood Y63.0
    mismatched blood Y65.0
  wrong
    drug given in error — *see* Table of Drugs and Chemicals
    fluid in infusion Y65.1
    placement of endotracheal tube during anesthetic procedure Y65.3
Mismatched blood in transfusion Y65.0
Motion sickness T75.3 ☑
Mountain sickness W94.11 ☑
Mudslide (of cataclysmic nature) — *see* Landslide
Murder (attempt) — *see* Assault

N

Nail
  contact with W45.0 ☑
    gun W29.4 ☑
  embedded in skin W45.0 ☑
Neglect (criminal) (homicidal intent) X58 ☑
Noise (causing injury) (pollution) W42.9 ☑
  supersonic W42.0 ☑
Nonadministration (of)
  drug or biological substance (necessary) Y63.6
  surgical and medical care Y66
Nosocomial condition Y95

O

Object
  falling
    from, in, on, hitting
      machinery — *see* Contact, with, by type of machine
    set in motion by
      accidental explosion or rupture of pressure vessel W38 ☑
      firearm — *see* Discharge, firearm, by type
      machine(ry) — *see* Contact, with, by type of machine
Overdose (drug) — *see* Table of Drugs and Chemicals
  radiation Y63.2
Overexertion X50.9 ☑
  from
    prolonged static or awkward postures X50.1 ☑
    repetitive movements X50.3 ☑
    specified strenuous movements or postures NEC X50.9 ☑
    strenuous movement or load X50.0 ☑
Overexposure (accidental) (to)
  cold (*see also* Exposure, cold) X31 ☑
    due to man-made conditions — *see* Exposure, cold, man-made
  heat (*see also* Heat) X30 ☑
  radiation — *see* Radiation
  radioactivity W88.0 ☑
  sun (sunburn) X32 ☑
  weather NEC — *see* Forces of nature
  wind NEC — *see* Forces of nature

Overheated — *see* Heat
Overturning (accidental)
  machinery — *see* Contact, with, by type of machine
  transport vehicle NEC (*see also* Accident, transport) V89.9 ☑
  watercraft (causing drowning, submersion) (*see also* Drowning, due to, accident to, watercraft, overturning)
    causing injury except drowning or submersion — *see* Accident, watercraft, causing, injury NEC

P

Parachute descent (voluntary) (without accident to aircraft) V97.29 ☑
  due to accident to aircraft — *see* Accident, transport, aircraft
Pecked by bird W61.99 ☑
Perforation during medical or surgical treatment as misadventure — *see* Index to Diseases and Injuries, Complication(s)
Perpetrator, perpetration, of assault, maltreatment and neglect (by) Y07.9
  boyfriend Y07.03
  brother Y07.410
    stepbrother Y07.435
  coach Y07.53
  cousin
    female Y07.491
    male Y07.490
  daycare provider Y07.519
    at-home
      adult care Y07.512
      childcare Y07.510
    care center
      adult care Y07.513
      childcare Y07.511
  family member NEC Y07.499
  father Y07.11
    adoptive Y07.13
    foster Y07.420
    stepfather Y07.430
  foster father Y07.420
  foster mother Y07.421
  girl friend Y07.04
  healthcare provider Y07.529
    mental health Y07.521
    specified NEC Y07.528
  husband Y07.01
  instructor Y07.53
  mother Y07.12
    adoptive Y07.14
    foster Y07.421
    stepmother Y07.433
  multiple perpetrators Y07.6
  nonfamily member Y07.50
    specified NEC Y07.59
  nurse Y07.528
  occupational therapist Y07.528
  partner of parent
    female Y07.434
    male Y07.432
  physical therapist Y07.528
  sister Y07.411
  speech therapist Y07.528
  stepbrother Y07.435
  stepfather Y07.430
  stepmother Y07.433
  stepsister Y07.436
  teacher Y07.53
  wife Y07.02
Piercing — *see* Contact, with, by type of object or machine
Pinched
  between objects (moving) (stationary and moving) W23.0 ☑
    stationary W23.1 ☑
Pinned under machine(ry) — *see* Contact, with, by type of machine
Place of occurrence Y92.9
  abandoned house Y92.89
  airplane Y92.813
  airport Y92.520
  ambulatory health services establishment NEC Y92.538
  ambulatory surgery center Y92.530
  amusement park Y92.831
  apartment (co-op) — *see* Place of occurrence, residence, apartment

Place of occurrence — *continued*
  assembly hall Y92.29
  bank Y92.510
  barn Y92.71
  baseball field Y92.320
  basketball court Y92.310
  beach Y92.832
  boarding house — *see* Place of occurrence, residence, boarding house
  boat Y92.814
  bowling alley Y92.39
  bridge Y92.89
  building under construction Y92.61
  bus Y92.811
    station Y92.521
  cafe Y92.511
  campsite Y92.833
  campus — *see* Place of occurrence, school
  canal Y92.89
  car Y92.810
  casino Y92.59
  children's home — *see* Place of occurrence, residence, institutional, orphanage
  church Y92.22
  cinema Y92.26
  clubhouse Y92.29
  coal pit Y92.64
  college (community) Y92.214
  condominium — *see* Place of occurrence, residence, apartment
  construction area — *see* Place of occurrence, industrial and construction area
  convalescent home — *see* Place of occurrence, residence, institutional, nursing home
  court-house Y92.240
  cricket ground Y92.328
  cultural building Y92.258
    art gallery Y92.250
    museum Y92.251
    music hall Y92.252
    opera house Y92.253
    specified NEC Y92.258
    theater Y92.254
  dancehall Y92.252
  day nursery Y92.210
  dentist office Y92.531
  derelict house Y92.89
  desert Y92.820
  dockyard Y92.62
  dock NOS Y92.89
  doctor's office Y92.531
  dormitory — *see* Place of occurrence, residence, institutional, school dormitory
  dry dock Y92.62
  factory (building) (premises) Y92.63
  farm (land under cultivation) (outbuildings) Y92.79
    barn Y92.71
    chicken coop Y92.72
    field Y92.73
    hen house Y92.72
    house — *see* Place of occurrence, residence, house
    orchard Y92.74
    specified NEC Y92.79
  football field Y92.321
  forest Y92.821
  freeway Y92.411
  gallery Y92.250
  garage (commercial) Y92.59
    boarding house Y92.044
    military base Y92.135
    mobile home Y92.025
    nursing home Y92.124
    orphanage Y92.114
    private house Y92.015
    reform school Y92.155
  gas station Y92.524
  gasworks Y92.69
  golf course Y92.39
  gravel pit Y92.64
  grocery Y92.512
  gymnasium Y92.39
  handball court Y92.318
  harbor Y92.89
  harness racing course Y92.39
  healthcare provider office Y92.531
  highway (interstate) Y92.411
  hill Y92.828
  hockey rink Y92.330

☑ **Additional Character Required** — Refer to the Tabular List for Character Selection   ▽ **Subterms under main terms may continue to next column or page**

Place of occurrence — *continued*
  home — *see* Place of occurrence, residence
  hospice — *see* Place of occurrence, residence, institutional, nursing home
  hospital Y92.239
    cafeteria Y92.233
    corridor Y92.232
    operating room Y92.234
    patient
      bathroom Y92.231
      room Y92.230
    specified NEC Y92.238
  hotel Y92.59
  house (*see also* Place of occurrence, residence)
    abandoned Y92.89
    under construction Y92.61
  industrial and construction area (yard) Y92.69
    building under construction Y92.61
    dock Y92.62
    dry dock Y92.62
    factory Y92.63
    gasworks Y92.69
    mine Y92.64
    oil rig Y92.65
    pit Y92.64
    power station Y92.69
    shipyard Y92.62
    specified NEC Y92.69
    tunnel under construction Y92.69
    workshop Y92.69
  kindergarten Y92.211
  lacrosse field Y92.328
  lake Y92.828
  library Y92.241
  mall Y92.59
  market Y92.512
  marsh Y92.828
  military
    base — *see* Place of occurrence, residence, institutional, military base
    training ground Y92.84
  mine Y92.64
  mosque Y92.22
  motel Y92.59
  motorway (interstate) Y92.411
  mountain Y92.828
  movie-house Y92.26
  museum Y92.251
  music-hall Y92.252
  not applicable Y92.9
  nuclear power station Y92.69
  nursing home — *see* Place of occurrence, residence, institutional, nursing home
  office building Y92.59
  offshore installation Y92.65
  oil rig Y92.65
  old people's home — *see* Place of occurrence, residence, institutional, specified NEC
  opera-house Y92.253
  orphanage — *see* Place of occurrence, residence, institutional, orphanage
  outpatient surgery center Y92.530
  park (public) Y92.830
    amusement Y92.831
  parking garage Y92.89
    lot Y92.481
  pavement Y92.480
  physician office Y92.531
  polo field Y92.328
  pond Y92.828
  post office Y92.242
  power station Y92.69
  prairie Y92.828
  prison — *see* Place of occurrence, residence, institutional, prison
  public
    administration building Y92.248
      city hall Y92.243
      courthouse Y92.240
      library Y92.241
      post office Y92.242
      specified NEC Y92.248
    building NEC Y92.29
    hall Y92.29
    place NOS Y92.89
  race course Y92.39
  radio station Y92.59
  railway line (bridge) Y92.85

Place of occurrence — *continued*
  ranch (outbuildings) — *see* Place of occurrence, farm
  recreation area Y92.838
    amusement park Y92.831
    beach Y92.832
    campsite Y92.833
    park (public) Y92.830
    seashore Y92.832
    specified NEC Y92.838
  reform school - — *see* Place of occurrence, residence, institutional, reform school
  religious institution Y92.22
  residence (non-institutional) (private) Y92.009
    apartment Y92.039
      bathroom Y92.031
      bedroom Y92.032
      kitchen Y92.030
      specified NEC Y92.038
    bathroom Y92.002
    bedroom Y92.003
    boarding house Y92.049
      bathroom Y92.041
      bedroom Y92.042
      driveway Y92.043
      garage Y92.044
      garden Y92.046
      kitchen Y92.040
      specified NEC Y92.048
      swimming pool Y92.045
      yard Y92.046
    dining room Y92.001
    garden Y92.007
    home Y92.009
    house, single family Y92.019
      bathroom Y92.012
      bedroom Y92.013
      dining room Y92.011
      driveway Y92.014
      garage Y92.015
      garden Y92.017
      kitchen Y92.010
      specified NEC Y92.018
      swimming pool Y92.016
      yard Y92.017
    institutional Y92.10
      children's home — *see* Place of occurrence, residence, institutional, orphanage
      hospice — *see* Place of occurrence, residence, institutional, nursing home
      military base Y92.139
        barracks Y92.133
        garage Y92.135
        garden Y92.137
        kitchen Y92.130
        mess hall Y92.131
        specified NEC Y92.138
        swimming pool Y92.136
        yard Y92.137
      nursing home Y92.129
        bathroom Y92.121
        bedroom Y92.122
        driveway Y92.123
        garage Y92.124
        garden Y92.126
        kitchen Y92.120
        specified NEC Y92.128
        swimming pool Y92.125
        yard Y92.126
      orphanage Y92.119
        bathroom Y92.111
        bedroom Y92.112
        driveway Y92.113
        garage Y92.114
        garden Y92.116
        kitchen Y92.110
        specified NEC Y92.118
        swimming pool Y92.115
        yard Y92.116
      prison Y92.149
        bathroom Y92.142
        cell Y92.143
        courtyard Y92.147
        dining room Y92.141
        kitchen Y92.140
        specified NEC Y92.148
        swimming pool Y92.146
      reform school Y92.159
        bathroom Y92.152
        bedroom Y92.153

Place of occurrence — *continued*
  residence — *continued*
    institutional — *continued*
      reform school — *continued*
        dining room Y92.151
        driveway Y92.154
        garage Y92.155
        garden Y92.157
        kitchen Y92.150
        specified NEC Y92.158
        swimming pool Y92.156
        yard Y92.157
      school dormitory Y92.169
        bathroom Y92.162
        bedroom Y92.163
        dining room Y92.161
        kitchen Y92.160
        specified NEC Y92.168
      specified NEC Y92.199
        bathroom Y92.192
        bedroom Y92.193
        dining room Y92.191
        driveway Y92.194
        garage Y92.195
        garden Y92.197
        kitchen Y92.190
        specified NEC Y92.198
        swimming pool Y92.196
        yard Y92.197
    kitchen Y92.000
    mobile home Y92.029
      bathroom Y92.022
      bedroom Y92.023
      dining room Y92.021
      driveway Y92.024
      garage Y92.025
      garden Y92.027
      kitchen Y92.020
      specified NEC Y92.028
      swimming pool Y92.026
      yard Y92.027
    specified place in residence NEC Y92.008
    specified residence type NEC Y92.099
      bathroom Y92.091
      bedroom Y92.092
      driveway Y92.093
      garage Y92.094
      garden Y92.096
      kitchen Y92.090
      specified NEC Y92.098
      swimming pool Y92.095
      yard Y92.096
  restaurant Y92.511
  riding school Y92.39
  river Y92.828
  road Y92.410
  rodeo ring Y92.39
  rugby field Y92.328
  same day surgery center Y92.530
  sand pit Y92.64
  school (private) (public) (state) Y92.219
    college Y92.214
    daycare center Y92.210
    elementary school Y92.211
    high school Y92.213
    kindergarten Y92.211
    middle school Y92.212
    specified NEC Y92.218
    trace school Y92.215
    university Y92.214
    vocational school Y92.215
  sea (shore) Y92.832
  senior citizen center Y92.29
  service area
    airport Y92.520
    bus station Y92.521
    gas station Y92.524
    highway rest stop Y92.523
    railway station Y92.522
  shipyard Y92.62
  shop (commercial) Y92.513
  sidewalk Y92.480
  silo Y92.79
  skating rink (roller) Y92.331
    ice Y92.330
  slaughter house Y92.86
  soccer field Y92.322
  specified place NEC Y92.89
  sports area Y92.39

Place of occurrence — *continued*
  sports area — *continued*
    athletic
      court Y92.318
        basketball Y92.310
        specified NEC Y92.318
        squash Y92.311
        tennis Y92.312
      field Y92.328
        baseball Y92.320
        cricket ground Y92.328
        football Y92.321
        hockey Y92.328
        soccer Y92.322
        specified NEC Y92.328
    golf course Y92.39
    gymnasium Y92.39
    riding school Y92.39
    skating rink (roller) Y92.331
      ice Y92.330
    stadium Y92.39
    swimming pool Y92.34
  squash court Y92.311
  stadium Y92.39
  steeplechasing course Y92.39
  store Y92.512
  stream Y92.828
  street and highway Y92.410
    bike path Y92.482
    freeway Y92.411
    highway ramp Y92.415
    interstate highway Y92.411
    local residential or business street Y92.414
    motorway Y92.411
    parking lot Y92.481
    parkway Y92.412
    sidewalk Y92.480
    specified NEC Y92.488
    state road Y92.413
  subway car Y92.816
  supermarket Y92.512
  swamp Y92.828
  swimming pool (public) Y92.34
    private (at) Y92.095
      boarding house Y92.045
      military base Y92.136
      mobile home Y92.026
      nursing home Y92.125
      orphanage Y92.115
      prison Y92.146
      reform school Y92.156
      single family residence Y92.016
  synagogue Y92.22
  television station Y92.59
  tennis court Y92.312
  theater Y92.254
  trade area Y92.59
    bank Y92.510
    cafe Y92.511
    casino Y92.59
    garage Y92.59
    hotel Y92.59
    market Y92.512
    office building Y92.59
    radio station Y92.59
    restaurant Y92.511
    shop Y92.513
    shopping mall Y92.59
    store Y92.512
    supermarket Y92.512
    television station Y92.59
    warehouse Y92.59
  trailer park, residential — *see* Place of occurrence, residence, mobile home
  trailer site NOS Y92.89
  train Y92.815
    station Y92.522
  truck Y92.812
  tunnel under construction Y92.69
  university Y92.214
  urgent (health) care center Y92.532
  vehicle (transport) Y92.818
    airplane Y92.813
    boat Y92.814
    bus Y92.811
    car Y92.810
    specified NEC Y92.818
    subway car Y92.816
    train Y92.815

Place of occurrence — *continued*
  vehicle — *continued*
    truck Y92.812
    warehouse Y92.59
  water reservoir Y92.89
  wilderness area Y92.828
    desert Y92.820
    forest Y92.821
    marsh Y92.828
    mountain Y92.828
    prairie Y92.828
    specified NEC Y92.828
    swamp Y92.828
  workshop Y92.69
  yard, private Y92.096
    boarding house Y92.046
    mobile home Y92.027
    single family house Y92.017
  youth center Y92.29
  zoo (zoological garden) Y92.834
Plumbism — *see* Table of Drugs and Chemicals, lead
Poisoning (accidental) (by) (*see also* Table of Drugs and Chemicals)
  by plant, thorns, spines, sharp leaves or other mechanisms NEC X58 ☑
  carbon monoxide
    generated by
      motor vehicle — *see* Accident, transport
      watercraft (in transit) (not in transit) V93.89 ☑
        ferry boat V93.81 ☑
        fishing boat V93.82 ☑
        jet skis V93.83 ☑
        liner V93.81 ☑
        merchant ship V93.80 ☑
        passenger ship V93.81 ☑
        powered craft NEC V93.83 ☑
  caused by injection of poisons into skin by plant thorns, spines, sharp leaves X58 ☑
  marine or sea plants (venomous) X58 ☑
  execution — *see* Legal, intervention, gas
    intervention
      by gas — *see* Legal, intervention, gas
      other specified means — *see* Legal, intervention, specified means NEC
  exhaust gas
    generated by
      motor vehicle — *see* Accident, transport
      watercraft (in transit) (not in transit) V93.89 ☑
        ferry boat V93.81 ☑
        fishing boat V93.82 ☑
        jet skis V93.83 ☑
        liner V93.81 ☑
        merchant ship V93.80 ☑
        passenger ship V93.81 ☑
        powered craft NEC V93.83 ☑
  fumes or smoke due to
    explosion (*see also* Explosion) W40.9 ☑
    fire — *see* Exposure, fire
    ignition — *see* Ignition
  gas
    in legal intervention — *see* Legal, intervention, gas
    legal execution — *see* Legal, intervention, gas
  in war operations — *see* War operations
  legal
Powder burn (by) (from)
  airgun W34.110 ☑
  BB gun W34.110 ☑
  firearm NEC W34.19 ☑
  gas, air or spring-operated gun NEC W34.118 ☑
  handgun W32.1 ☑
  hunting rifle W33.12 ☑
  larger firearm W33.10 ☑
    specified NEC W33.19 ☑
  machine gun W33.13 ☑
  paintball gun W34.111 ☑
  pellet gun W34.110 ☑
  shotgun W33.11 ☑
  Very pistol [flare] W34.19 ☑
Premature cessation (of) **surgical and medical care** Y66
Privation (food) (water) X58 ☑
Procedure (operation)
  correct, on wrong side or body part (wrong side) (wrong site) Y65.53
  intended for another patient done on wrong patient Y65.52
  performed on patient not scheduled for surgery Y65.52

Procedure — *continued*
  performed on wrong patient Y65.52
  wrong, performed on correct patient Y65.51
Prolonged
  sitting in transport vehicle — *see* Travel, by type of vehicle
  stay in
    high altitude as cause of anoxia, barodontalgia, barotitis or hypoxia W94.11 ☑
    weightless environment X52 ☑
Pulling, excessive (*see also* Overexertion) X50.9- ☑
Puncture, puncturing (*see also* Contact, with, by type of object or machine)
  by
    plant thorns, spines, sharp leaves or other mechanisms NEC W60 ☑
  during medical or surgical treatment as misadventure — *see* Index to Diseases and Injuries, Complication(s)
Pushed, pushing (accidental) (injury in)
  by other person(s) (accidental) W51 ☑
  as, or caused by, a crowd or human stampede (with fall) W52 ☑
    before moving object NEC Y02.8 ☑
      motor vehicle Y02.0 ☑
      subway train Y02.1 ☑
      train Y02.1 ☑
    from
      high place NEC
        in accidental circumstances W17.89 ☑
        stated as
          intentional, homicide (attempt) Y01 ☑
          undetermined whether accidental or intentional Y30 ☑
      transport vehicle NEC (*see also* Accident, transport) V89.9 ☑
        stated as
          intentional, homicide (attempt) Y08.89 ☑
    with fall W03 ☑
      due to ice or snow W00.0 ☑
  overexertion X50.9 ☑

R

Radiation (exposure to)
  arc lamps W89.0 ☑
  atomic power plant (malfunction) NEC W88.1 ☑
  complication of or abnormal reaction to medical radiation therapy Y84.2
  electromagnetic, ionizing W88.0 ☑
  gamma rays W88.1 ☑
  in
    war operations (from or following nuclear explosion — *see* War operations
  inadvertent exposure of patient (receiving test or therapy) Y63.3
  infrared (heaters and lamps) W90.1 ☑
    excessive heat from W92 ☑
  ionized, ionizing (particles, artificially accelerated) W88.0 ☑
    radioisotopes W88.1 ☑
    specified NEC W88.8 ☑
    x-rays W88.0 ☑
  isotopes, radioactive — *see* Radiation, radioactive isotopes
  laser(s) W90.2 ☑
    in war operations — *see* War operations
    misadventure in medical care Y63.2
  light sources (man-made visible and ultraviolet) W89.9 ☑
    natural X32 ☑
    specified NEC W89.8 ☑
    tanning bed W89.1 ☑
    welding light W89.0 ☑
  man-made visible light W89.9 ☑
    specified NEC W89.8 ☑
    tanning bed W89.1 ☑
    welding light W89.0 ☑
  microwave W90.8 ☑
  misadventure in medical or surgical procedure Y63.
  natural NEC X39.08 ☑
    radon X39.01 ☑
  overdose (in medical or surgical procedure) Y63.2
  radar W90.0 ☑
  radioactive isotopes (any) W88.1 ☑
    atomic power plant malfunction W88.1 ☑
    misadventure in medical or surgical treatment Y6.

Radiation — *continued*
  radiofrequency W90.0 ☑
  radium NEC W88.1 ☑
  sun X32 ☑
  ultraviolet (light) (man-made) W89.9 ☑
    natural X32 ☑
    specified NEC W89.8 ☑
    tanning bed W89.1 ☑
    welding light W89.0 ☑
  welding arc, torch, or light W89.0 ☑
    excessive heat from W92 ☑
  x-rays (hard) (soft) W88.0 ☑
Range disease W94.11 ☑
Rape (attempted) T74.2- ☑
Rat bite W53.11 ☑
Reaching (prolonged) (static) X50.1 ☑
Reaction, abnormal to medical procedure (*see also* Complication of or following, by type of procedure) Y84.9
  biologicals — *see* Table of Drugs and Chemicals
  drugs — *see* Table of Drugs and Chemicals
  vaccine — *see* Table of Drugs and Chemicals
  with misadventure — *see* Misadventure
Recoil
  airgun W34.110 ☑
  BB gun W34.110 ☑
  firearm NEC W34.19 ☑
  gas, air or spring-operated gun NEC W34.118 ☑
  handgun W32.1 ☑
  hunting rifle W33.12 ☑
  larger firearm W33.10 ☑
    specified NEC W33.19 ☑
  machine gun W33.13 ☑
  paintball gun W34.111 ☑
  pellet W34.110 ☑
  shotgun W33.11 ☑
  Very pistol [flare] W34.19 ☑
Reduction in
  atmospheric pressure — *see* Air, pressure, change
Rock falling on or hitting (accidentally) (person) W20.8 ☑
  in cave-in W20.0 ☑
Run over (accidentally) (by)
  animal (not being ridden) NEC W55.89 ☑
  machinery — *see* Contact, with, by specified type of machine
  transport vehicle NEC (*see also* Accident, transport) V09.9 ☑
    intentional homicide (attempt) Y03.0 ☑
    motor NEC V09.20 ☑
      intentional homicide (attempt) Y03.0 ☑
Running
  before moving object X81.8 ☑
  motor vehicle X81.0 ☑
Running off, away
  animal (being ridden) (*see also* Accident, transport) V80.918 ☑
    not being ridden W55.89 ☑
  animal-drawn vehicle NEC (*see also* Accident, transport) V80.928 ☑
  highway, road(way), street
    transport vehicle NEC (*see also* Accident, transport) V89.9 ☑
Rupture pressurized devices — *see* Explosion, by type of device

S

Saturnism — *see* Table of Drugs and Chemicals, lead
Scald, scalding (accidental) (by) (from) (in) X19 ☑
  air (hot) X14.1 ☑
  gases (hot) X14.1 ☑
  homicide (attempt) — *see* Assault, burning, hot object
  inflicted by other person
    stated as intentional, homicide (attempt) — *see* Assault, burning, hot object
  liquid (boiling) (hot) NEC X12 ☑
    stated as undetermined whether accidental or intentional Y27.2 ☑
    suicide (attempt) X77.2 ☑
  local application of externally applied substance in medical or surgical care Y63.5
  metal (molten) (liquid) (hot) NEC X18 ☑
  self-inflicted X77.9 ☑
  stated as undetermined whether accidental or intentional Y27.8 ☑

Scald, scalding — *continued*
  steam X13.1 ☑
    assault X98.0 ☑
    stated as undetermined whether accidental or intentional Y27.0 ☑
    suicide (attempt) X77.0 ☑
  suicide (attempt) X77.9 ☑
  vapor (hot) X13.1 ☑
    assault X98.0 ☑
    stated as undetermined whether accidental or intentional Y27.0 ☑
    suicide (attempt) X77.0 ☑
Scratched by
  cat W55.03 ☑
  person(s) (accidentally) W50.4 ☑
    with intent to injure or kill Y04.0 ☑
    as, or caused by, a crowd or human stampede (with fall) W52
    assault Y04.0 ☑
    homicide (attempt) Y04.0 ☑
    in
      fight Y04.0 ☑
      legal intervention
        injuring
          bystander Y35.892 ☑
          law enforcement personnel Y35.891 ☑
          suspect Y35.893 ☑
Seasickness T75.3 ☑
Self-harm NEC (*see also* External cause by type, undetermined whether accidental or intentional)
  intentional — *see* Suicide
  poisoning NEC — *see* Table of Drugs and Chemicals, poisoning, accidental
Self-inflicted (injury) **NEC** (*see also* External cause by type, undetermined whether accidental or intentional)
  intentional — *see* Suicide
  poisoning NEC — *see* Table of Drugs and Chemicals, poisoning, accidental
Sequelae (of)
  accident NEC — *see* W00-X58 with 7th character S
  assault (homicidal) (any means) — *see* X92-Y08 with 7th character S
  homicide, attempt (any means) — *see* X92-Y08 with 7th character S
  injury undetermined whether accidentally or purposely inflicted — *see* Y21-Y33 with 7th character S
  intentional self-harm (classifiable to X71-X83) — *see* X71-X83 with 7th character S
  legal intervention — *see* with 7th character S Y35
  motor vehicle accident — *see* V00-V99 with 7th character S
  suicide, attempt (any means) — *see* X71-X83 with 7th character S
  transport accident — *see* V00-V99 with 7th character S
  war operations — *see* War operations
Shock
  electric — *see* Exposure, electric current
  from electric appliance (any) (faulty) W86.8 ☑
    domestic W86.0 ☑
    suicide (attempt) X83.1 ☑
Shooting, shot (accidental(ly)) (*see also* Discharge, firearm, by type)
  herself or himself — *see* Discharge, firearm by type, self-inflicted
  homicide (attempt) — *see* Discharge, firearm by type, homicide
  in war operations — *see* War operations
  inflicted by other person — *see* Discharge, firearm by type, homicide
    accidental — *see* Discharge, firearm, by type of firearm
  legal
    execution — *see* Legal, intervention, firearm
    intervention — *see* Legal, intervention, firearm
  self-inflicted — *see* Discharge, firearm by type, suicide
    accidental — *see* Discharge, firearm, by type of firearm
  suicide (attempt) — *see* Discharge, firearm by type, suicide
Shoving (accidentally) **by other person** — *see* Pushed, by other person
Sickness
  alpine W94.11 ☑
  motion — *see* Motion
  mountain W94.11 ☑

Sinking (accidental)
  watercraft (causing drowning, submersion) (*see also* Drowning, due to, accident to, watercraft, sinking)
  causing injury except drowning or submersion — *see* Accident, watercraft, causing, injury NEC
Siriasis X32 ☑
Sitting (prolonged) (static) X50.1 ☑
Slashed wrists — *see* Cut, self-inflicted
Slipping (accidental) (on same level) (with fall) W01.0 ☑
  on
    ice W00.0 ☑
      with skates — *see* Accident, transport, pedestrian, conveyance
    mud W01.0 ☑
    oil W01.0 ☑
    snow W00.0 ☑
      with skis — *see* Accident, transport, pedestrian, conveyance
    surface (slippery) (wet) NEC W01.0 ☑
  without fall W18.40 ☑
    due to
      specified NEC W18.49 ☑
      stepping from one level to another W18.43 ☑
      stepping into hole or opening W18.42 ☑
      stepping on object W18.41 ☑
Sliver, wood, contact with W45.8 ☑
Smoldering (due to fire) — *see* Exposure, fire
Sodomy (attempted) **by force** T74.2 ☑
Sound waves (causing injury) W42.9 ☑
  supersonic W42.0 ☑
Splinter, contact with W45.8 ☑
Stab, stabbing — *see* Cut
Standing (prolonged) (static) X50.1 ☑
Starvation X58 ☑
Status of external cause Y99.9
  child assisting in compensated work for family Y99.8
  civilian activity done for financial or other compensation Y99.0
  civilian activity done for income or pay Y99.0
  family member assisting in compensated work for other family member Y99.8
  hobby not done for income Y99.8
  leisure activity Y99.8
  military activity Y99.1
  off-duty activity of military personnel Y99.8
  recreation or sport not for income or while a student Y99.8
  specified NEC Y99.8
  student activity Y99.8
  volunteer activity Y99.2
Stepped on
  by
    animal (not being ridden) NEC W55.89 ☑
    crowd or human stampede W52
    person W50.0 ☑
Stepping on
  object W22.8 ☑
    sports equipment W21.9 ☑
    stationary W22.09 ☑
      sports equipment W21.89 ☑
    with fall W18.31 ☑
  person W51
    by crowd or human stampede W52 ☑
  sports equipment W21.9 ☑
Sting
  arthropod, nonvenomous W57 ☑
  insect, nonvenomous W57 ☑
Storm (cataclysmic) — *see* Forces of nature, cataclysmic storm
Straining, excessive (*see also* Overexertion) X50.9 ☑
Strangling — *see* Strangulation
Strangulation (accidental) T71 ☑
Strenuous movements (*see also* Overexertion) X50.9 ☑
Striking against
  airbag (automobile) W22.10 ☑
    driver side W22.11 ☑
    front passenger side W22.12 ☑
    specified NEC W22.19 ☑
  bottom when
    diving or jumping into water (in) W16.822 ☑
      causing drowning W16.821 ☑
      from boat W16.722 ☑
        causing drowning W16.721 ☑
      natural body W16.622 ☑
        causing drowning W16.821 ☑

Striking against — *continued*
  bottom when — *continued*
    diving or jumping into water — *continued*
      swimming pool W16.522 ☑
        causing drowning W16.521 ☑
    falling into water (in) W16.322 ☑
      causing drowning W16.321 ☑
      fountain — *see* Striking against, bottom when, falling into water, specified NEC
      natural body W16.122 ☑
        causing drowning W16.121 ☑
      reservoir — *see* Striking against, bottom when, falling into water, specified NEC
    specified NEC W16.322 ☑
      causing drowning W16.321 ☑
    swimming pool W16.022 ☑
      causing drowning W16.021 ☑
  diving board (swimming-pool) W21.4 ☑
  object W22.8 ☑
    caused by crowd or human stampede (with fall) W52 ☑
    furniture W22.03 ☑
    lamppost W22.02 ☑
    sports equipment W21.9 ☑
    stationary W22.09 ☑
      sports equipment W21.89 ☑
    wall W22.01 ☑
    with
      drowning or submersion — *see* Drowning
      fall — *see* Fall, due to, bumping against, object
  person(s) W51 ☑
    as, or caused by, a crowd or human stampede (with fall) W52 ☑
    assault Y04.2 ☑
    homicide (attempt) Y04.2 ☑
    with fall W03 ☑
      due to ice or snow W00.0 ☑
  sports equipment W21.9 ☑
  wall (when) W22.01 ☑
    diving or jumping into water (in) W16.832 ☑
      causing drowning W16.831 ☑
      swimming pool W16.532 ☑
        causing drowning W16.531 ☑
    falling into water (in) W16.332 ☑
      causing drowning W16.331 ☑
      fountain — *see* Striking against, wall when, falling into water, specified NEC
      natural body W16.132 ☑
        causing drowning W16.131 ☑
      reservoir — *see* Striking against, wall when, falling into water, specified NEC
    specified NEC W16.332 ☑
      causing drowning W16.331 ☑
    swimming pool W16.032 ☑
      causing drowning W16.031 ☑
    swimming pool (when) W22.042 ☑
      causing drowning W22.041 ☑
      diving or jumping into water W16.532 ☑
        causing drowning W16.531 ☑
      falling into water W16.032 ☑
        causing drowning W16.031 ☑

Struck (accidentally) **by**
  airbag (automobile) W22.10 ☑
    driver side W22.11 ☑
    front passenger side W22.12 ☑
    specified NEC W22.19 ☑
  alligator W58.02 ☑
  animal (not being ridden) NEC W55.89 ☑
  avalanche — *see* Landslide
  ball (hit) (thrown) W21.00 ☑
    assault Y08.09 ☑
    baseball W21.03 ☑
    basketball W21.05 ☑
    football W21.01 ☑
    golf ball W21.04 ☑
    soccer W21.02 ☑
    softball W21.07 ☑
    specified NEC W21.09 ☑
    volleyball W21.06 ☑
  bat or racquet
    baseball bat W21.11 ☑
      assault Y08.02 ☑
    golf club W21.13 ☑
      assault Y08.09 ☑
    specified NEC W21.19 ☑
      assault Y08.09 ☑

Struck (accidentally) **by** — *continued*
  bat or racquet — *continued*
    tennis racquet W21.12 ☑
      assault Y08.09 ☑
  bullet (*see also* Discharge, firearm by type)
    in war operations — *see* War operations
  crocodile W58.12 ☑
  dog W54.1 ☑
  flare, Very pistol — *see* Discharge, firearm NEC
  hailstones X39.8 ☑
  hockey (ice)
    field
      puck W21.221 ☑
      stick W21.211 ☑
    puck W21.220 ☑
    stick W21.210 ☑
      assault Y08.01 ☑
  landslide — *see* Landslide
  law-enforcement agent (on duty) — *see* Legal, intervention, manhandling
    with blunt object — *see* Legal, intervention, blunt object
  lightning T75.0 ☑
    causing fire — *see* Exposure, fire
  machine — *see* Contact, with, by type of machine
  mammal NEC W55.89 ☑
    marine W56.32 ☑
  marine animal W56.82 ☑
  missile
    firearm — *see* Discharge, firearm by type
    in war operations — *see* War operations, missile
  object W22.8 ☑
    blunt W22.8 ☑
      assault Y00 ☑
      suicide (attempt) X79 ☑
      undetermined whether accidental or intentional Y29 ☑
    falling W20.8 ☑
      from, in, on
        building W20.1 ☑
          burning (uncontrolled fire) X00.4 ☑
        cataclysmic
          earth surface movement NEC — *see* Landslide
          storm — *see* Forces of nature, cataclysmic storm
        cave-in W20.0 ☑
        earthquake X34 ☑
        machine (in operation) — *see* Contact, with, by type of machine
        structure W20.1 ☑
          burning X00.4 ☑
        transport vehicle (in motion) — *see* Accident, transport, by type of vehicle
        watercraft V93.49 ☑
          due to
            accident to craft V91.39 ☑
              powered craft V91.33 ☑
                ferry boat V91.31 ☑
                fishing boat V91.32 ☑
                jetskis V91.33 ☑
                liner V91.31 ☑
                merchant ship V91.30 ☑
                passenger ship V91.31 ☑
              unpowered craft V91.38 ☑
                canoe V91.35 ☑
                inflatable V91.36 ☑
                kayak V91.35 ☑
                sailboat V91.34 ☑
                surf-board V91.38 ☑
                windsurfer V91.38 ☑
            powered craft V93.43 ☑
              ferry boat V93.41 ☑
              fishing boat V93.42 ☑
              jetskis V93.43 ☑
              liner V93.41 ☑
              merchant ship V93.40 ☑
              passenger ship V93.41 ☑
            unpowered craft V93.48 ☑
              sailboat V93.44 ☑
              surf-board V93.48 ☑
              windsurfer V93.48 ☑
    moving NEC W20.8 ☑
    projected W20.8 ☑
      assault Y00 ☑
      in sports W21.9 ☑

Struck (accidentally) **by** — *continued*
  object — *continued*
    projected — *continued*
      in sports — *continued*
        assault Y08.09 ☑
        ball W21.00 ☑
          baseball W21.03 ☑
          basketball W21.05 ☑
          football W21.01 ☑
          golf ball W21.04 ☑
          soccer W21.02 ☑
          softball W21.07 ☑
          specified NEC W21.09 ☑
          volleyball W21.06 ☑
        bat or racquet
          baseball bat W21.11 ☑
            assault Y08.02 ☑
          golf club W21.13 ☑
            assault Y08.09 ☑
          specified NEC W21.19 ☑
            assault Y08.09 ☑
          tennis racquet W21.12 ☑
            assault Y08.09 ☑
        hockey (ice)
          field
            puck W21.221 ☑
            stick W21.211 ☑
          puck W21.220 ☑
          stick W21.210 ☑
            assault Y08.01 ☑
        specified NEC W21.89 ☑
    set in motion by explosion — *see* Explosion
    thrown W20.8 ☑
      assault Y00 ☑
      in sports W21.9 ☑
        assault Y08.09 ☑
        ball W21.00 ☑
          baseball W21.03 ☑
          basketball W21.05 ☑
          football W21.01 ☑
          golf ball W21.04 ☑
          soccer W21.02 ☑
          soft ball W21.07 ☑
          specified NEC W21.09 ☑
          volleyball W21.06 ☑
        bat or racquet
          baseball bat W21.11 ☑
            assault Y08.02 ☑
          golf club W21.13 ☑
            assault Y08.09 ☑
          specified NEC W21.19 ☑
            assault Y08.09 ☑
          tennis racquet W21.12 ☑
            assault Y08.09 ☑
        hockey (ice)
          field
            puck W21.221 ☑
            stick W21.211 ☑
          puck W21.220 ☑
          stick W21.210 ☑
            assault Y08.01 ☑
        specified NEC W21.89 ☑
  other person(s) W50.0 ☑
    with
      blunt object W22.8 ☑
        intentional, homicide (attempt) Y00 ☑
        sports equipment W21.9 ☑
        undetermined whether accidental or intentional Y29 ☑
      fall W03 ☑
        due to ice or snow W00.0 ☑
    as, or caused by, a crowd or human stampede (with fall) W52 ☑
    assault Y04.2 ☑
    homicide (attempt) Y04.2 ☑
    in legal intervention
      injuring
        bystander Y35.812 ☑
        law enforcement personnel Y35.811 ☑
        suspect Y35.813 ☑
    sports equipment W21.9 ☑
  police (on duty) — *see* Legal, intervention, manhandling
    with blunt object — *see* Legal, intervention, blunt object
  sports equipment W21.9 ☑

☑ **Additional Character Required — Refer to the Tabular List for Character Selection**   ▽ **Subterms under main terms may continue to next column or page**

Struck (accidentally) **by** — *continued*
  sports equipment — *continued*
    assault Y08.09 ☑
    ball W21.00 ☑
      baseball W21.03 ☑
      basketball W21.05 ☑
      football W21.01 ☑
      golf ball W21.04 ☑
      soccer W21.02 ☑
      soft ball W21.07 ☑
      specified NEC W21.09 ☑
      volleyball W21.06 ☑
    bat or racquet
      baseball bat W21.11 ☑
        assault Y08.02 ☑
      golf club W21.13 ☑
        assault Y08.09 ☑
      specified NEC W21.19 ☑
      tennis racquet W21.12 ☑
        assault Y08.09 ☑
    cleats (shoe) W21.31 ☑
    foot wear NEC W21.39 ☑
    football helmet W21.81 ☑
    hockey (ice)
      field
        puck W21.221 ☑
        stick W21.211 ☑
      puck W21.220 ☑
      stick W21.210 ☑
        assault Y08.01 ☑
    skate blades W21.32 ☑
    specified NEC W21.89 ☑
      assault Y08.09 ☑
  thunderbolt — *see* subcategory T75.0 ☑
    causing fire — *see* Exposure, fire
  transport vehicle NEC (*see also* Accident, transport)
      V09.9 ☑
    intentional, homicide (attempt) Y03.0 ☑
    motor NEC (*see also* Accident, transport) V09.20 ☑
      homicide Y03.0 ☑
  vehicle (transport) NEC — *see* Accident, transport, by
      type of vehicle
    stationary (falling from jack, hydraulic lift, ramp)
      W20.8 ☑
Stumbling
  over
    animal NEC W01.0 ☑
      with fall W18.09 ☑
    carpet, rug or (small) object W22.8 ☑
      with fall W18.09 ☑
    person W51 ☑
      with fall W03 ☑
        due to ice or snow W00.0 ☑
  without fall W18.40 ☑
    due to
      specified NEC W18.49 ☑
      stepping from one level to another W18.43 ☑
      stepping into hole or opening W18.42 ☑
      stepping on object W18.41 ☑
Submersion (accidental) — *see* Drowning
Suffocation (accidental) (by external means) (by pressure)
      (mechanical) (*see also* category) T71 ☑
  due to, by
    avalanche — *see* Landslide
    explosion — *see* Explosion
    fire — *see* Exposure, fire
    food, any type (aspiration) (ingestion) (inhalation)
        — *see* categories T17 and T18 ☑
    ignition — *see* Ignition
    landslide — *see* Landslide
    machine(ry) — *see* Contact, with, by type of ma-
        chine
    vomitus (aspiration) (inhalation) T17.81- ☑
  in
    burning building X00.8 ☑
Suicide, suicidal (attempted) (by) X83.8 ☑
  blunt object X79 ☑
  burning, burns X76 ☑
    hot object X77.9 ☑
      fluid NEC X77.2 ☑
      household appliance X77.3 ☑
      specified NEC X77.8 ☑
      steam X77.0 ☑
      tap water X77.1 ☑
      vapors X77.0 ☑
  caustic substance — *see* Table of Drugs and Chemicals

Suicide, suicidal — *continued*
  cold, extreme X83.2 ☑
  collision of motor vehicle with
    motor vehicle X82.0 ☑
    specified NEC X82.8 ☑
    train X82.1 ☑
    tree X82.2 ☑
  crashing of aircraft X83.0 ☑
  cut (any part of body) X78.9 ☑
  cutting or piercing instrument X78.9 ☑
    dagger X78.2 ☑
    glass X78.0 ☑
    knife X78.1 ☑
    specified NEC X78.8 ☑
    sword X78.2 ☑
  drowning (in) X71.9 ☑
    bathtub X71.0 ☑
    natural water X71.3 ☑
    specified NEC X71.8 ☑
    swimming pool X71.1 ☑
      following fall X71.2 ☑
  electrocution X83.1 ☑
  explosive(s) (material) X75 ☑
  fire, flames X76 ☑
  firearm X74.9 ☑
    airgun X74.01 ☑
    handgun X72 ☑
    hunting rifle X73.1 ☑
    larger X73.9 ☑
      specified NEC X73.8 ☑
    machine gun X73.2 ☑
    shotgun X73.0 ☑
    specified NEC X74.8 ☑
  hanging X83.8 ☑
  hot object — *see* Suicide, burning, hot object
  jumping
    before moving object X81.8 ☑
      motor vehicle X81.0 ☑
      subway train X81.1 ☑
      train X81.1 ☑
    from high place X80 ☑
  late effect of attempt — *see* X71-X83 with 7th character
      S
  lying before moving object, train, vehicle X81.8 ☑
  poisoning — *see* Table of Drugs and Chemicals
  puncture (any part of body) — *see* Suicide, cutting or
      piercing instrument
  scald — *see* Suicide, burning, hot object
  sequelae of attempt — *see* X71-X83 with 7th character
      S
  sharp object (any) — *see* Suicide, cutting or piercing
      instrument
  shooting — *see* Suicide, firearm
  specified means NEC X83.8 ☑
  stab (any part of body) — *see* Suicide, cutting or
      piercing instrument
  steam, hot vapors X77.0 ☑
  strangulation X83.8 ☑
  submersion — *see* Suicide, drowning
  suffocation X83.8 ☑
  wound NEC X83.8 ☑
Sunstroke X32 ☑
Supersonic waves (causing injury) W42.0 ☑
Surgical procedure, complication of (delayed or as an
      abnormal reaction without mention of misadven-
      ture) (*see also* Complication of or following, by type
      of procedure)
  due to or as a result of misadventure — *see* Misadven-
      ture
Swallowed, swallowing
  foreign body — *see* Foreign body, alimentary canal
  poison — *see* Table of Drugs and Chemicals
  substance
    caustic or corrosive — *see* Table of Drugs and
        Chemicals
    poisonous — *see* Table of Drugs and Chemicals

T

Tackle in sport W03 ☑
Terrorism (involving) Y38.80 ☑
  biological weapons Y38.6X- ☑
  chemical weapons Y38.7X- ☑
  conflagration Y38.3X- ☑
  drowning and submersion Y38.89- ☑
  explosion Y38.2X- ☑

Terrorism — *continued*
  explosion — *continued*
    destruction of aircraft Y38.1X- ☑
    marine weapons Y38.0X- ☑
    fire Y38.3X- ☑
    firearms Y38.4X- ☑
    hot substances Y38.3X- ☑
    lasers Y38.89- ☑
    nuclear weapons Y38.5X- ☑
    piercing or stabbing instruments Y38.89- ☑
    secondary effects Y38.9X- ☑
    specified method NEC Y38.89- ☑
    suicide bomber Y38.81- ☑
Thirst X58 ☑
Threat to breathing
  aspiration — *see* Aspiration
  due to cave-in, falling earth or substance NEC T71 ☑
Thrown (accidentally)
  against part (any) of or object in transport vehicle (in
        motion) NEC (*see also* Accident, transport)
  from
    high place, homicide (attempt) Y01 ☑
    machinery — *see* Contact, with, by type of machine
    transport vehicle NEC (*see also* Accident, transport)
        V89.9 ☑
  off — *see* Thrown, from
Thunderbolt — *see* subcategory T75.0 ☑
  causing fire — *see* Exposure, fire
Tidal wave (any injury) **NEC** — *see* Forces of nature, tidal
      wave
Took
  overdose (drug) — *see* Table of Drugs and Chemicals
  poison — *see* Table of Drugs and Chemicals
Tornado (any injury) X37.1 ☑
Torrential rain (any injury) X37.8 ☑
Torture X58 ☑
Trampled by animal NEC W55.89 ☑
Trapped (accidentally)
  between objects (moving) (stationary and moving) —
      see Caught
  by part (any) of
    motorcycle V29.88 ☑
    pedal cycle V19.88 ☑
    transport vehicle NEC (*see also* Accident, transport)
        V89.9 ☑
Travel (effects) (sickness) T75.3 ☑
Tree falling on or hitting (accidentally) (person)
      W20.8 ☑
Tripping
  over
    animal W01.0 ☑
      with fall W01.0 ☑
    carpet, rug or (small) object W22.8 ☑
      with fall W18.09 ☑
    person W51 ☑
      with fall W03 ☑
        due to ice or snow W00.0 ☑
  without fall W18.40 ☑
    due to
      specified NEC W18.49 ☑
      stepping from one level to another W18.43 ☑
      stepping into hole or opening W18.42 ☑
      stepping on object W18.41 ☑
Twisted by person(s) (accidentally) W50.2 ☑
  with intent to injure or kill Y04.0 ☑
  as, or caused by, a crowd or human stampede (with
      fall) W52 ☑
  assault Y04.0 ☑
  homicide (attempt) Y04.0 ☑
  in
    fight Y04.0 ☑
    legal intervention — *see* Legal, intervention, man-
        handling
Twisting (prolonged) (static) X50.1- ☑

U

**Underdosing of necessary drugs, medicaments or
      biological substances** Y63.6
Undetermined intent (contact) (exposure)
  automobile collision Y32 ☑
  blunt object Y29 ☑
  drowning (submersion) (in) Y21.9 ☑
    bathtub Y21.0 ☑
      after fall Y21.1 ☑

▽ Subterms under main terms may continue to next column or page   ☑ Additional Character Required — Refer to the Tabular List for Character Selection   431

Struck — Undetermined intent

Undetermined intent — *continued*
 drowning — *continued*
  natural water (lake) (ocean) (pond) (river) (stream) Y21.4 ☑
  specified place NEC Y21.8 ☑
  swimming pool Y21.2 ☑
   after fall Y21.3 ☑
 explosive material Y25 ☑
 fall, jump or push from high place Y30 ☑
 falling, lying or running before moving object Y31 ☑
 fire Y26 ☑
 firearm discharge Y24.9 ☑
  airgun (BB) (pellet) Y24.0 ☑
  handgun (pistol) (revolver) Y22 ☑
  hunting rifle Y23.1 ☑
  larger Y23.9 ☑
   hunting rifle Y23.1 ☑
   machine gun Y23.3 ☑
   military Y23.2 ☑
   shotgun Y23.0 ☑
   specified type NEC Y23.8 ☑
  machine gun Y23.3 ☑
  military Y23.2 ☑
  shotgun Y23.0 ☑
  specified type NEC Y24.8 ☑
  Very pistol Y24.8 ☑
 hot object Y27.9 ☑
  fluid NEC Y27.2 ☑
  household appliance Y27.3 ☑
  specified object NEC Y27.8 ☑
  steam Y27.0 ☑
  tap water Y27.1 ☑
  vapor Y27.0 ☑
 jump, fall or push from high place Y30 ☑
 lying, falling or running before moving object Y31 ☑
 motor vehicle crash Y32 ☑
 push, fall or jump from high place Y30 ☑
 running, falling or lying before moving object Y31 ☑
 sharp object Y28.9 ☑
  dagger Y28.2 ☑
  glass Y28.0 ☑
  knife Y28.1 ☑
  specified object NEC Y28.8 ☑
  sword Y28.2 ☑
 smoke Y26 ☑
 specified event NEC Y33 ☑
Use of hand as hammer X50.3 ☑

V

Vibration (causing injury) W49.9 ☑
Victim (of)
 avalanche — *see* Landslide
 earth movements NEC — *see* Forces of nature, earth movement
 earthquake X34 ☑
 flood — *see* Flood
 landslide — *see* Landslide
 lightning — *see* subcategory T75.0 ☑
  causing fire — *see* Exposure, fire
 storm (cataclysmic) NEC — *see* Forces of nature, cataclysmic storm
 volcanic eruption X35 ☑
Volcanic eruption (any injury) X35 ☑
Vomitus, gastric contents in air passages (with asphyxia, obstruction or suffocation) T17.81- ☑

W

Walked into stationary object (any) W22.09 ☑
 furniture W22.03 ☑
 lamppost W22.02 ☑
 wall W22.01 ☑
War operations (injuries to military personnel and civilians during war, civil insurrection and peacekeeping missions) (by) (from) (involving) Y36.90 ☑
 after cessation of hostilities Y36.89- ☑

War operations — *continued*
 after cessation of hostilities — *continued*
  explosion (of)
   bomb placed during war operations Y36.82- ☑
   mine placed during war operations Y36.81- ☑
  specified NEC Y36.88- ☑
 air blast Y36.20- ☑
 aircraft
  destruction — *see* War operations, destruction of aircraft
 airway restriction — *see* War operations, restriction of airways
 asphyxiation — *see* War operations, restriction of airways
 biological weapons Y36.6X- ☑
 blast Y36.20- ☑
 blast fragments Y36.20- ☑
 blast wave Y36.20- ☑
 blast wind Y36.20- ☑
 bomb Y36.20- ☑
  dirty Y36.50- ☑
  gasoline Y36.31- ☑
  incendiary Y36.31- ☑
  petrol Y36.31- ☑
 bullet Y36.43- ☑
  incendiary Y36.32- ☑
  rubber Y36.41- ☑
 chemical weapons Y36.7X- ☑
 combat
  hand to hand (unarmed) combat Y36.44- ☑
  using blunt or piercing object Y36.45- ☑
 conflagration — *see* War operations, fire
 conventional warfare NEC Y36.49- ☑
 depth-charge Y36.01- ☑
 destruction of aircraft Y36.10- ☑
  due to
   air to air missile Y36.11- ☑
   collision with other aircraft Y36.12- ☑
   detonation (accidental) of onboard munitions and explosives Y36.14- ☑
   enemy fire or explosives Y36.11- ☑
   explosive placed on aircraft Y36.11- ☑
   onboard fire Y36.13- ☑
   rocket propelled grenade [RPG] Y36.11- ☑
   small arms fire Y36.11- ☑
   surface to air missile Y36.11- ☑
  specified NEC Y36.19- ☑
 detonation (accidental) of
  onboard marine weapons Y36.05- ☑
  own munitions or munitions launch device Y36.24- ☑
 dirty bomb Y36.50- ☑
 explosion (of) Y36.20- ☑
  aerial bomb Y36.21- ☑
  after cessation of hostilities
   bomb placed during war operations Y36.82- ☑
   mine placed during war operations Y36.81- ☑
  bomb NOS (*see also* War operations, bomb(s)) Y36.20- ☑
  fragments Y36.20- ☑
  grenade Y36.29- ☑
  guided missile Y36.22- ☑
  improvised explosive device [IED] (person-borne) (roadside) (vehicle-borne) Y36.23- ☑
  land mine Y36.29- ☑
  marine mine (at sea) (in harbor) Y36.02- ☑
  marine weapon Y36.00- ☑
   specified NEC Y36.09- ☑
  own munitions or munitions launch device (accidental) Y36.24- ☑
  sea-based artillery shell Y36.03- ☑
  specified NEC Y36.29- ☑
  torpedo Y36.04- ☑
 fire Y36.30- ☑
  specified NEC Y36.39- ☑
 firearms
  discharge Y36.43- ☑
  pellets Y36.42- ☑

War operations — *continued*
 flamethrower Y36.33- ☑
 fragments (from) (of)
  improvised explosive device [IED] (person-borne) (roadside) (vehicle-borne) Y36.26- ☑
  munitions Y36.25- ☑
  specified NEC Y36.29- ☑
  weapons Y36.27- ☑
 friendly fire Y36.92 ☑
 hand to hand (unarmed) combat Y36.44- ☑
 hot substances — *see* War operations, fire
 incendiary bullet Y36.32- ☑
 nuclear weapon (effects of) Y36.50- ☑
  acute radiation exposure Y36.54- ☑
  blast pressure Y36.51- ☑
  direct blast Y36.51- ☑
  direct heat Y36.53- ☑
  fallout exposure Y36.54- ☑
  fireball Y36.53- ☑
  indirect blast (struck or crushed by blast debris) (being thrown by blast) Y36.52- ☑
  ionizing radiation (immediate exposure) Y36.54- ☑
  nuclear radiation Y36.54- ☑
  radiation
   ionizing (immediate exposure) Y36.54- ☑
   nuclear Y36.54- ☑
   thermal Y36.53- ☑
  secondary effects Y36.54- ☑
  specified NEC Y36.59- ☑
  thermal radiation Y36.53- ☑
 restriction of air (airway)
  intentional Y36.46- ☑
  unintentional Y36.47- ☑
 rubber bullets Y36.41- ☑
 shrapnel NOS Y36.29- ☑
 suffocation — *see* War operations, restriction of airways
 unconventional warfare NEC Y36.7X- ☑
 underwater blast NOS Y36.00- ☑
 warfare
  conventional NEC Y36.49- ☑
  unconventional NEC Y36.7X- ☑
 weapon of mass destruction [WMD] Y36.91 ☑
 weapons
  biological weapons Y36.6X- ☑
  chemical Y36.7X- ☑
  nuclear (effects of) Y36.50- ☑
   acute radiation exposure Y36.54- ☑
   blast pressure Y36.51- ☑
   direct blast Y36.51- ☑
   direct heat Y36.53- ☑
   fallout exposure Y36.54- ☑
   fireball Y36.53- ☑
   radiation
    ionizing (immediate exposure) Y36.54- ☑
    nuclear Y36.54- ☑
    thermal Y36.53- ☑
   secondary effects Y36.54- ☑
   specified NEC Y36.59- ☑
  of mass destruction [WMD] Y36.91 ☑
Washed
 away by flood — *see* Flood
 off road by storm (transport vehicle) — *see* Forces of nature, cataclysmic storm
Weather exposure NEC — *see* Forces of nature
Weightlessness (causing injury) (effects of) (in spacecraft, real or simulated) X52 ☑
Work related condition Y99.0
Wound (accidental) NEC (*see also* Injury) X58 ☑
 battle (*see also* War operations) Y36.90 ☑
 gunshot — *see* Discharge, firearm by type
Wreck transport vehicle NEC (*see also* Accident, transport) V89.9 ☑
Wrong
 device implanted into correct surgical site Y65.51
 fluid in infusion Y65.1
 patient, procedure performed on Y65.52
 procedure (operation) on correct patient Y65.51

☑ **Additional Character Required** — Refer to the Tabular List for Character Selection   ▽ **Subterms under main terms may continue to next column or page**

Chapter Specific Guidelines with Coding Examples

The chapter specific guidelines from the ICD-10-CM Official Guidelines for Coding and Reporting have been provided below. Along with these guidelines are coding examples, contained in the shaded boxes, that have been developed to help illustrate the coding and/or sequencing guidance found in these guidelines.

a. Human immunodeficiency virus (HIV) infections

1) Code only confirmed cases

Code only confirmed cases of HIV infection/illness. This is an exception to the hospital inpatient guideline Section II, H.

In this context, "confirmation" does not require documentation of positive serology or culture for HIV; the provider's diagnostic statement that the patient is HIV positive, or has an HIV-related illness is sufficient.

> Patient being seen for hypothyroidism with possible HIV infection
>
> **EØ3.9**   **Hypothyroidism, unspecified**
>
> *Explanation:* Only the hypothyroidism is coded in this scenario because it has not been confirmed that an HIV infection is present.

2) Selection and sequencing of HIV codes

(a) Patient admitted for HIV-related condition

If a patient is admitted for an HIV-related condition, the principal diagnosis should be B2Ø, Human immunodeficiency virus [HIV] disease followed by additional diagnosis codes for all reported HIV-related conditions.

> HIV with CMV
>
> **B2Ø**   **Human immunodeficiency virus [HIV] disease**
>
> **B25.9**   **Cytomegaloviral disease, unspecified**
>
> *Explanation:* Cytomegaloviral infection is an HIV related condition, so the HIV diagnosis code is reported first, followed by the code for the CMV.

(b) Patient with HIV disease admitted for unrelated condition

If a patient with HIV disease is admitted for an unrelated condition (such as a traumatic injury), the code for the unrelated condition (e.g., the nature of injury code) should be the principal diagnosis. Other diagnoses would be B2Ø followed by additional diagnosis codes for all reported HIV-related conditions.

> Sprain of the internal collateral ligament, right ankle; HIV
>
> **S93.491A**   **Sprain of other ligament of right ankle, initial encounter**
>
> **B2Ø**   **Human immunodeficiency virus [HIV] disease**
>
> *Explanation:* The ankle sprain is not related to HIV, so it is the first-listed diagnosis code, and HIV is reported secondarily.

(c) Whether the patient is newly diagnosed

Whether the patient is newly diagnosed or has had previous admissions/encounters for HIV conditions is irrelevant to the sequencing decision.

> Newly diagnosed multiple cutaneous Kaposi's sarcoma lesions in previously diagnosed HIV disease
>
> **B2Ø**   **Human immunodeficiency virus [HIV] disease**
>
> **C46.Ø**   **Kaposi's sarcoma of skin**
>
> *Explanation:* Even though the HIV was diagnosed on a previous encounter, it is still sequenced first when coded with an HIV related condition. Kaposi's sarcoma is an HIV-related condition.

(d) Asymptomatic human immunodeficiency virus

Z21, Asymptomatic human immunodeficiency virus [HIV] infection status, is to be applied when the patient without any documentation of symptoms is listed as being "HIV positive," "known HIV," "HIV test positive," or similar terminology. Do not use this code if the term "AIDS" is used or if the patient is treated for any HIV-related illness or is described as having any condition(s) resulting from his/her HIV positive status; use B2Ø in these cases.

> Patient is being seen for iron deficiency anemia. Status positive HIV test on Atripla, with no prior symptoms
>
> **D5Ø.9**   **Iron deficiency anemia, unspecified**
>
> **Z21**   **Asymptomatic human immunodeficiency virus [HIV] infection status**
>
> *Explanation:* Code Z21 is sequenced second since documentation indicates that the patient has had a positive HIV test but has been asymptomatic. Being on medication for HIV is not an indication that code B2Ø is used instead of Z21. Unless there has been documentation that the patient has had current or prior symptoms or HIV-related complications, code B2Ø is not used. The anemia is not an AIDS-related complication and is sequenced first.

(e) Patients with inconclusive HIV serology

Patients with inconclusive HIV serology, but no definitive diagnosis or manifestations of the illness, may be assigned code R75, Inconclusive laboratory evidence of human immunodeficiency virus [HIV].

(f) Previously diagnosed HIV-related illness

Patients with any known prior diagnosis of an HIV-related illness should be coded to B2Ø. Once a patient has developed an HIV-related illness, the patient should always be assigned code B2Ø on every subsequent admission/encounter. Patients previously diagnosed with any HIV illness (B2Ø) should never be assigned to R75 or Z21, Asymptomatic human immunodeficiency virus [HIV] infection status.

(g) HIV infection in pregnancy, childbirth and the puerperium

During pregnancy, childbirth or the puerperium, a patient admitted (or presenting for a health care encounter) because of an HIV-related illness should receive a principal diagnosis code of O98.7-, Human immunodeficiency [HIV] disease complicating pregnancy, childbirth and the puerperium, followed by B2Ø and the code(s) for the HIV-related illness(es). Codes from Chapter 15 always take sequencing priority.

Patients with asymptomatic HIV infection status admitted (or presenting for a health care encounter) during pregnancy, childbirth, or the puerperium should receive codes of O98.7- and Z21.

(h) Encounters for testing for HIV

If a patient is being seen to determine his/her HIV status, use code Z11.4, Encounter for screening for human immunodeficiency virus [HIV]. Use additional codes for any associated high risk behavior.

If a patient with signs or symptoms is being seen for HIV testing, code the signs and symptoms. An additional counseling code Z71.7, Human immunodeficiency virus [HIV] counseling, may be used if counseling is provided during the encounter for the test.

When a patient returns to be informed of his/her HIV test results and the test result is negative, use code Z71.7, Human immunodeficiency virus [HIV] counseling.

If the results are positive, see previous guidelines and assign codes as appropriate.

b. Infectious agents as the cause of diseases classified to other chapters

Certain infections are classified in chapters other than Chapter 1 and no organism is identified as part of the infection code. In these instances, it is necessary to use an additional code from Chapter 1 to identify the organism. A code from category B95, Streptococcus, Staphylococcus, and Enterococcus as the cause of diseases classified to other chapters, B96, Other bacterial agents as the cause of diseases classified to other chapters, or B97, Viral agents as the cause of diseases classified to other chapters, is to be used as an additional code to identify the organism. An instructional note will be found at the infection code advising that an additional organism code is required.

Acute *E. coli* cystitis

N30.00	**Acute cystitis without hematuria**
B96.20	**Unspecified Escherichia coli [E.coli] as the cause of diseases classified elsewhere**

Explanation: An instructional note under the category for the cystitis indicates to code also the specific organism.

c. Infections resistant to antibiotics

Many bacterial infections are resistant to current antibiotics. It is necessary to identify all infections documented as antibiotic resistant. Assign a code from category Z16, Resistance to antimicrobial drugs, following the infection code only if the infection code does not identify drug resistance.

Penicillin-resistant *Streptococcus pneumoniae* pneumonia

J13	**Pneumonia due to Streptococcus pneumoniae**
Z16.11	**Resistance to penicillins**

Explanation: Code Z16.11 is assigned as a secondary code to represent the penicillin resistance. This code includes resistance to amoxicillin and ampicillin.

d. Sepsis, severe sepsis, and septic shock

1) Coding of Sepsis and Severe Sepsis

(a) Sepsis

For a diagnosis of sepsis, assign the appropriate code for the underlying systemic infection. If the type of infection or causal organism is not further specified, assign code A41.9, Sepsis, unspecified organism.

A code from subcategory R65.2, Severe sepsis, should not be assigned unless severe sepsis or an associated acute organ dysfunction is documented.

Gram-negative sepsis

A41.50	**Gram-negative sepsis, unspecified**

Staphylococcal sepsis

A41.2	**Sepsis due to unspecified staphylococcus**

Explanation: In both examples above the organism causing the sepsis is identified, therefore A41.9 Sepsis, unspecified organism, would not be appropriate as this code would not capture the highest degree of specificity found in the documentation. Do not use an additional code for severe sepsis unless an acute organ dysfunction was also documented as "associated with" or "due to" the sepsis or the sepsis was documented as "severe."

(i) Negative or inconclusive blood cultures and sepsis

Negative or inconclusive blood cultures do not preclude a diagnosis of sepsis in patients with clinical evidence of the condition; however, the provider should be queried.

(ii) Urosepsis

The term urosepsis is a nonspecific term. It is not to be considered synonymous with sepsis. It has no default code in the Alphabetic Index. Should a provider use this term, he/she must be queried for clarification.

(iii) Sepsis with organ dysfunction

If a patient has sepsis and associated acute organ dysfunction or multiple organ dysfunction (MOD), follow the instructions for coding severe sepsis.

(iv) Acute organ dysfunction that is not clearly associated with the sepsis

If a patient has sepsis and an acute organ dysfunction, but the medical record documentation indicates that the acute organ dysfunction is related to a medical condition other than the sepsis, do not assign a code from subcategory R65.2, Severe sepsis. An acute organ dysfunction must be associated with the sepsis in order to assign the severe sepsis code. If the documentation is not clear as to whether an acute organ dysfunction is related to the sepsis or another medical condition, query the provider.

Sepsis and acute respiratory failure due to COPD exacerbation

A41.9	**Sepsis, unspecified organism**
J44.1	**Chronic obstructive pulmonary disease with (acute) exacerbation**
J96.00	**Acute respiratory failure, unspecified whether with hypoxia or hypercapnia**

Explanation: Although acute organ dysfunction is present in the form of acute respiratory failure, severe sepsis (R65.2) is not coded in this example, as the acute respiratory failure is attributed to the COPD exacerbation rather than the sepsis. Sequencing of these codes would be determined by the reason for the encounter.

(b) Severe sepsis

The coding of severe sepsis requires a minimum of 2 codes: first a code for the underlying systemic infection, followed by a code from subcategory R65.2, Severe sepsis. If the causal organism is not documented, assign code A41.9, Sepsis, unspecified organism, for the infection. Additional code(s) for the associated acute organ dysfunction are also required.

Due to the complex nature of severe sepsis, some cases may require querying the provider prior to assignment of the codes.

2) Septic shock

(a) Septic shock generally refers to circulatory failure associated with severe sepsis, and therefore, it represents a type of acute organ dysfunction.

For cases of septic shock, the code for the systemic infection should be sequenced first, followed by code R65.21, Severe sepsis with septic shock or code T81.12, Postprocedural septic shock. Any additional codes for the other acute organ dysfunctions should also be assigned. As noted in the sequencing instructions in the Tabular List, the code for septic shock cannot be assigned as a principal diagnosis.

Sepsis with septic shock

A41.9	**Sepsis, unspecified organism**
R65.21	**Severe sepsis with septic shock**

Explanation: Documentation of septic shock automatically implies severe sepsis as it is a form of acute organ dysfunction. Septic shock is not coded as the first-listed diagnosis; it is always preceded by the code for the systemic infection.

3) Sequencing of severe sepsis

If severe sepsis is present on admission, and meets the definition of principal diagnosis, the underlying systemic infection should be assigned as principal diagnosis followed by the appropriate code from subcategory R65.2 as required by the sequencing rules in the Tabular List. A code from subcategory R65.2 can never be assigned as a principal diagnosis.

When severe sepsis develops during an encounter (it was not present on admission), the underlying systemic infection and the appropriate code from subcategory R65.2 should be assigned as secondary diagnoses.

Severe sepsis may be present on admission, but the diagnosis may not be confirmed until sometime after admission. If the documentation is not clear whether severe sepsis was present on admission, the provider should be queried.

4) Sepsis and severe sepsis with a localized infection

If the reason for admission is both sepsis or severe sepsis and a localized infection, such as pneumonia or cellulitis, a code(s) for the underlying systemic infection should be assigned first and the code for the localized infection should be assigned as a secondary diagnosis. If the patient has severe sepsis, a code from subcategory R65.2 should also be assigned as a secondary diagnosis. If the patient is admitted with a localized infection, such as pneumonia, and sepsis/severe sepsis doesn't develop until after admission, the localized infection should be assigned first, followed by the appropriate sepsis/severe sepsis codes.

Patient presents with acute renal failure due to severe sepsis from *Pseudomonas pneumonia*

A41.52	Sepsis, due to Pseudomonas
J15.1	Pneumonia due to Pseudomonas
R65.20	Severe sepsis without septic shock
N17.9	Acute kidney failure, unspecified

Explanation: If all conditions are present, the systemic infection (sepsis) is sequenced first followed by the codes for the localized infection (pneumonia), severe sepsis and any organ dysfunction.

5) Sepsis due to a postprocedural infection

(a) Documentation of causal relationship

As with all postprocedural complications, code assignment is based on the provider's documentation of the relationship between the infection and the procedure.

(b) Sepsis due to a postprocedural infection

For **infections following a procedure, a code from** T81.**40, to T81.43** Infection following a procedure, or **a code from** O86.**00 to O86.03,** Infection of obstetric surgical wound, **that identifies the site of the infection** should be coded first, **if known. Assign an additional code for sepsis following a procedure (T81.44) or sepsis following an obstetrical procedure (O86.04). Use an additional code to identify the infectious agent.** If the patient has severe sepsis, the appropriate code from subcategory R65.2 should also be assigned with the additional code(s) for any acute organ dysfunction.

For **infections following infusion, transfusion, therapeutic injection, or immunization, a code from subcategory T80.2, Infections following infusion, transfusion, and therapeutic injection, or code T88.0-, Infection following immunization, should be coded first, followed by the code for the specific infection. If the patient has severe sepsis, the appropriate code from subcategory R65.2 should also be assigned, with the additional codes(s) for any acute organ dysfunction.**

(c) Postprocedural infection and postprocedural septic shock

If a postprocedural infection has resulted in postprocedural septic shock, **assign the codes indicated above for sepsis due to a postprocedural infection, followed by code T81.12-, Postprocedural septic shock. Do not assign code R65.21, Severe sepsis with septic shock. Additional code(s) should be assigned for any acute organ dysfunction.**

6) Sepsis and severe sepsis associated with a noninfectious process (condition)

In some cases a noninfectious process (condition), such as trauma, may lead to an infection which can result in sepsis or severe sepsis. If sepsis or severe sepsis is documented as associated with a noninfectious condition, such as a burn or serious injury, and this condition meets the definition for principal diagnosis, the code for the noninfectious condition should be sequenced first, followed by the code for the resulting infection. If severe sepsis is present, a code from subcategory R65.2 should also be assigned with any associated organ dysfunction(s) codes. It is not necessary to assign a code from subcategory R65.1, Systemic inflammatory response syndrome (SIRS) of non-infectious origin, for these cases.

If the infection meets the definition of principal diagnosis, it should be sequenced before the non-infectious condition. When both the associated non-infectious condition and the infection meet the definition of principal diagnosis, either may be assigned as principal diagnosis.

Only one code from category R65, Symptoms and signs specifically associated with systemic inflammation and infection, should be assigned. Therefore, when a non-infectious condition leads to an infection resulting in severe sepsis, assign the appropriate code from subcategory R65.2, Severe sepsis. Do not additionally assign a code from subcategory R65.1, Systemic inflammatory response syndrome (SIRS) of non-infectious origin.

See Section I.C.18. SIRS due to non-infectious process

7) Sepsis and septic shock complicating abortion, pregnancy, childbirth, and the puerperium

See Section I.C.15. Sepsis and septic shock complicating abortion, pregnancy, childbirth and the puerperium

8) Newborn sepsis

See Section I.C.16. f. Bacterial sepsis of Newborn

e. Methicillin resistant *Staphylococcus aureus* (MRSA) conditions

1) Selection and sequencing of MRSA codes

(a) Combination codes for MRSA infection

When a patient is diagnosed with an infection that is due to methicillin resistant *Staphylococcus aureus* (MRSA), and that infection has a combination code that includes the causal organism (e.g., sepsis, pneumonia) assign the appropriate combination code for the condition (e.g., code A41.02, Sepsis due to Methicillin resistant Staphylococcus aureus or code J15.212, Pneumonia due to Methicillin resistant Staphylococcus aureus). Do not assign code B95.62, Methicillin resistant Staphylococcus aureus infection as the cause of diseases classified elsewhere, as an additional code, because the combination code includes the type of infection and the MRSA organism. Do not assign a code from subcategory Z16.11, Resistance to penicillins, as an additional diagnosis.

See Section C.1. for instructions on coding and sequencing of sepsis and severe sepsis.

(b) Other codes for MRSA infection

When there is documentation of a current infection (e.g., wound infection, stitch abscess, urinary tract infection) due to MRSA, and that infection does not have a combination code that includes the causal organism, assign the appropriate code to identify the condition along with code B95.62, Methicillin resistant Staphylococcus aureus infection as the cause of diseases classified elsewhere for the MRSA infection. Do not assign a code from subcategory Z16.11, Resistance to penicillins.

(c) Methicillin susceptible Staphylococcus aureus (MSSA) and MRSA colonization

The condition or state of being colonized or carrying MSSA or MRSA is called colonization or carriage, while an individual person is described as being colonized or being a carrier. Colonization means that MSSA or MSRA is present on or in the body without necessarily causing illness. A positive MRSA colonization test might be documented by the provider as "MRSA screen positive" or "MRSA nasal swab positive".

Assign code Z22.322, Carrier or suspected carrier of Methicillin resistant Staphylococcus aureus, for patients documented as having MRSA colonization. Assign code Z22.321, Carrier or suspected carrier of Methicillin susceptible Staphylococcus aureus, for patient documented as having MSSA colonization. Colonization is not necessarily indicative of a disease process or as the cause of a specific condition the patient may have unless documented as such by the provider.

(d) MRSA colonization and infection

If a patient is documented as having both MRSA colonization and infection during a hospital admission, code Z22.322, Carrier or suspected carrier of Methicillin resistant Staphylococcus aureus, and a code for the MRSA infection may both be assigned.

f. Zika virus infections

1) Code only confirmed cases

Code only a confirmed diagnosis of Zika virus (A92.5, Zika virus disease) as documented by the provider. This is an exception to the hospital inpatient guideline Section II, H. In this context, "confirmation" does not require documentation of the type of test performed; the physician's diagnostic statement that the condition is confirmed is sufficient. This code should be assigned regardless of the stated mode of transmission.

If the provider documents "suspected", "possible" or "probable" Zika, do not assign code A92.5. Assign a code(s) explaining the reason for encounter (such as fever, rash, or joint pain) or Z20.**821**, Contact with and (suspected) exposure to **Zika virus.**

Chapter 1. Certain Infectious and Parasitic Diseases (A00–B99)

INCLUDES   diseases generally recognized as communicable or transmissible

Use additional code to identify resistance to antimicrobial drugs (Z16.-)

EXCLUDES 1   *certain localized infections - see body system-related chapters*

EXCLUDES 2   *carrier or suspected carrier of infectious disease (Z22.-)*

infectious and parasitic diseases complicating pregnancy, childbirth and the puerperium (O98.-)

infectious and parasitic diseases specific to the perinatal period (P35-P39)

influenza and other acute respiratory infections (J00-J22)

This chapter contains the following blocks:

A00-A09	Intestinal infectious diseases
A15-A19	Tuberculosis
A20-A28	Certain zoonotic bacterial diseases
A30-A49	Other bacterial diseases
A50-A64	Infections with a predominantly sexual mode of transmission
A65-A69	Other spirochetal diseases
A70-A74	Other diseases caused by chlamydiae
A75-A79	Rickettsioses
A80-A89	Viral and prion infections of the central nervous system
A90-A99	Arthropod-borne viral fevers and viral hemorrhagic fevers
B00-B09	Viral infections characterized by skin and mucous membrane lesions
B10	Other human herpesviruses
B15-B19	Viral hepatitis
B20	Human immunodeficiency virus [HIV] disease
B25-B34	Other viral diseases
B35-B49	Mycoses
B50-B64	Protozoal diseases
B65-B83	Helminthiases
B85-B89	Pediculosis, acariasis and other infestations
B90-B94	Sequelae of infectious and parasitic diseases
B95-B97	Bacterial and viral infectious agents
B99	Other infectious diseases

Intestinal infectious diseases (A00-A09)

✓4ᵗʰ **A00 Cholera**

DEF: Acute infection of the bowel due to vibrio cholerae that presents with profuse diarrhea, cramps, and vomiting, resulting in severe dehydration, electrolyte imbalance, and death. It is spread through ingestion of food or water contaminated with feces of infected persons.

     A00.0 Cholera due to Vibrio cholerae 01, biovar cholerae

         Classical cholera

     A00.1 Cholera due to Vibrio cholerae 01, biovar eltor

         Cholera eltor

     A00.9 Cholera, unspecified   ▽

✓4ᵗʰ **A01 Typhoid and paratyphoid fevers**

DEF: Typhoid fever: Acute generalized illness caused by *Salmonella typhi*. Clinical features include fever, headache, abdominal pain, cough, toxemia, leukopenia, abnormal pulse, rose spots on the skin, bacteremia, hyperplasia of intestinal lymph nodes, mesenteric lymphadenopathy, and Peyer's patches in the intestines.

DEF: Paratyphoid fever: Prolonged febrile illness, caused by *Salmonella* serotypes other than *S. typhi*, especially *S. enterica* serotypes paratyphi A, B, and C.

     ✓5ᵗʰ **A01.0 Typhoid fever**

         Infection due to Salmonella typhi

         A01.00 Typhoid fever, unspecified   ▽

         A01.01 Typhoid meningitis

         A01.02 Typhoid fever with heart involvement

             Typhoid endocarditis

             Typhoid myocarditis

         A01.03 Typhoid pneumonia   HCC

         A01.04 Typhoid arthritis   HCC

         A01.05 Typhoid osteomyelitis   HCC

         A01.09 Typhoid fever with other complications

     A01.1 Paratyphoid fever A

     A01.2 Paratyphoid fever B

     A01.3 Paratyphoid fever C

     A01.4 Paratyphoid fever, unspecified   ▽

         Infection due to Salmonella paratyphi NOS

✓4ᵗʰ **A02 Other salmonella infections**

     INCLUDES   infection or foodborne intoxication due to any Salmonella species other than S. typhi and S. paratyphi

     A02.0 Salmonella enteritis

         Salmonellosis

         TIP: Dehydration (E86.0) is a complication of salmonella enteritis and may be reported separately.

     A02.1 Salmonella sepsis   HCC

✓5ᵗʰ **A02.2 Localized salmonella infections**

     A02.20 Localized salmonella infection, unspecified   ▽

     A02.21 Salmonella meningitis

     A02.22 Salmonella pneumonia   HCC

     A02.23 Salmonella arthritis   HCC

     A02.24 Salmonella osteomyelitis   HCC

     A02.25 Salmonella pyelonephritis

         Salmonella tubulo-interstitial nephropathy

     A02.29 Salmonella with other localized infection

A02.8 Other specified salmonella infections

A02.9 Salmonella infection, unspecified   ▽

✓4ᵗʰ **A03 Shigellosis**

DEF: Infection caused by the genus the *Shigella*, of the family *Enterobacteriaceae* that is known to cause an acute dysenteric infection of the bowel with fever, drowsiness, anorexia, nausea, vomiting, bloody diarrhea, abdominal cramps, and distention.

     A03.0 Shigellosis due to Shigella dysenteriae

         Group A shigellosis [Shiga-Kruse dysentery]

     A03.1 Shigellosis due to Shigella flexneri

         Group B shigellosis

     A03.2 Shigellosis due to Shigella boydii

         Group C shigellosis

     A03.3 Shigellosis due to Shigella sonnei

         Group D shigellosis

     A03.8 Other shigellosis

     A03.9 Shigellosis, unspecified   ▽

         Bacillary dysentery NOS

✓4ᵗʰ **A04 Other bacterial intestinal infections**

     EXCLUDES 1   *bacterial foodborne intoxications, NEC (A05.-)*

            tuberculous enteritis (A18.32)

DEF: Escherichia coli: Gram negative, anaerobic of the family *Enterobacteriaceae* found in the large intestine of warm-blooded animals, generally as a nonpathologic entity aiding in digestion. They become pathogenic when an opportunity to grow somewhere outside this relationship presents itself, such as ingestion of fecal contaminated food or water.

     A04.0 Enteropathogenic Escherichia coli infection

     A04.1 Enterotoxigenic Escherichia coli infection

     A04.2 Enteroinvasive Escherichia coli infection

     A04.3 Enterohemorrhagic Escherichia coli infection

         DEF: *E. coli* infection penetrating the intestinal mucosa, producing microscopic ulceration and bleeding.

     A04.4 Other intestinal Escherichia coli infections

         Escherichia coli enteritis NOS

     A04.5 Campylobacter enteritis

         TIP: For Guillain-Barre syndrome occurring as a sequela of *Campylobacter enteritis*, assign code G61.0 as the first-listed diagnosis followed by B94.8 for the sequelae.

     A04.6 Enteritis due to Yersinia enterocolitica

         EXCLUDES 1   *extraintestinal yersiniosis (A28.2)*

     ✓5ᵗʰ **A04.7 Enterocolitis due to Clostridium difficile**

         Foodborne intoxication by Clostridium difficile

         Pseudomembraneous colitis

         AHA: 2017,4Q,4

         A04.71 Enterocolitis due to Clostridium difficile, recurrent

         A04.72 Enterocolitis due to Clostridium difficile, not specified as recurrent

     A04.8 Other specified bacterial intestinal infections

     A04.9 Bacterial intestinal infection, unspecified   ▽

         Bacterial enteritis NOS

✓4ᵗʰ **A05 Other bacterial foodborne intoxications, not elsewhere classified**

     EXCLUDES 1   *Clostridium difficile foodborne intoxication and infection (A04.7-)*

            Escherichia coli infection (A04.0-A04.4)

            listeriosis (A32.-)

            salmonella foodborne intoxication and infection (A02.-)

            toxic effect of noxious foodstuffs (T61-T62)

     A05.0 Foodborne staphylococcal intoxication

         TIP: Assign code A04.8 to report a staphylococcal infection when it is caused by the ingestion of contaminated food but not caused by *S. aureus* toxins.

A05.1 Botulism food poisoning
Botulism NOS
Classical foodborne intoxication due to Clostridium botulinum
> **EXCLUDES 1** infant botulism (A48.51)
> wound botulism (A48.52)

DEF: Muscle-paralyzing neurotoxic disease caused by ingesting pre-formed toxin from the bacterium *Clostridium botulinum*. It causes vomiting and diarrhea, vision problems, slurred speech, difficulty swallowing, paralysis, and death.

A05.2 Foodborne Clostridium perfringens [Clostridium welchii] intoxication
Enteritis necroticans
Pig-bel

A05.3 Foodborne Vibrio parahaemolyticus intoxication

A05.4 Foodborne Bacillus cereus intoxication

A05.5 Foodborne Vibrio vulnificus intoxication

A05.8 Other specified bacterial foodborne intoxications

A05.9 Bacterial foodborne intoxication, unspecified ▽

✓4ᵗʰ **A06 Amebiasis**
> **INCLUDES** infection due to Entamoeba histolytica
> **EXCLUDES 1** other protozoal intestinal diseases (A07.-)
> **EXCLUDES 2** acanthamebiasis (B60.1-)
> Naegleriasis (B60.2)

DEF: Infection with a single cell protozoan known as the amoeba. Transmission occurs through ingestion of feces, contaminated food or water, use of human feces as fertilizer, or person-to-person contact.

A06.0 Acute amebic dysentery
Acute amebiasis
Intestinal amebiasis NOS

A06.1 Chronic intestinal amebiasis

A06.2 Amebic nondysenteric colitis

A06.3 Ameboma of intestine
Ameboma NOS

A06.4 Amebic liver abscess
Hepatic amebiasis

A06.5 Amebic lung abscess   HCC
Amebic abscess of lung (and liver)

A06.6 Amebic brain abscess
Amebic abscess of brain (and liver) (and lung)

A06.7 Cutaneous amebiasis

✓5ᵗʰ **A06.8 Amebic infection of other sites**
A06.81 Amebic cystitis
A06.82 Other amebic genitourinary infections
Amebic balanitis
Amebic vesiculitis
Amebic vulvovaginitis
A06.89 Other amebic infections
Amebic appendicitis
Amebic splenic abscess

A06.9 Amebiasis, unspecified ▽

✓4ᵗʰ **A07 Other protozoal intestinal diseases**
DEF: Protozoa: Group comprised of the simplest, single celled organisms, ranging in size from micro to macroscopic. They can live alone or in colonies, and do not show any differentiation in tissues. Most are motile and can live free in nature, but some are parasitic, causing disease in the variety of hosts they inhabit.

A07.0 Balantidiasis
Balantidial dysentery

A07.1 Giardiasis [lambliasis]
DEF: Infection caused by the flagellate protozoan *Giardia lamblia* causing gastrointestinal problems such as vomiting, chronic diarrhea, and weight loss. The most common parasite in the US, this is usually transmitted by ingesting contaminated water while in the cyst state and latches onto the wall of the small intestine.

A07.2 Cryptosporidiosis   HCC
DEF: Microscopic parasite found in water and one of the most common causes of waterborne gastrointestinal infectious disease in the United States. It is usually transmitted by ingesting contaminated drinking water or recreational water and causes profuse watery diarrhea, flatulence, abdominal pain, and cramping.

A07.3 Isosporiasis
Infection due to Isospora belli and Isospora hominis
Intestinal coccidiosis
Isosporosis

A07.4 Cyclosporiasis

A07.8 Other specified protozoal intestinal diseases
Intestinal microsporidiosis
Intestinal trichomoniasis
Sarcocystosis
Sarcosporidiosis

A07.9 Protozoal intestinal disease, unspecified ▽
Flagellate diarrhea
Protozoal colitis
Protozoal diarrhea
Protozoal dysentery

✓4ᵗʰ **A08 Viral and other specified intestinal infections**
> **EXCLUDES 1** influenza with involvement of gastrointestinal tract (J09.X3, J10.2, J11.2)

A08.0 Rotaviral enteritis

✓5ᵗʰ **A08.1 Acute gastroenteropathy due to Norwalk agent and other small round viruses**
A08.11 Acute gastroenteropathy due to Norwalk agent
Acute gastroenteropathy due to Norovirus
Acute gastroenteropathy due to Norwalk-like agent
A08.19 Acute gastroenteropathy due to other small round viruses
Acute gastroenteropathy due to small round virus [SRV] NOS

A08.2 Adenoviral enteritis

✓5ᵗʰ **A08.3 Other viral enteritis**
A08.31 Calicivirus enteritis
A08.32 Astrovirus enteritis
A08.39 Other viral enteritis
Coxsackie virus enteritis
Echovirus enteritis
Enterovirus enteritis NEC
Torovirus enteritis

A08.4 Viral intestinal infection, unspecified ▽
Viral enteritis NOS
Viral gastroenteritis NOS
Viral gastroenteropathy NOS
AHA: 2016,3Q,12

A08.8 Other specified intestinal infections

A09 Infectious gastroenteritis and colitis, unspecified ▽
Infectious colitis NOS
Infectious enteritis NOS
Infectious gastroenteritis NOS
> **EXCLUDES 1** colitis NOS (K52.9)
> diarrhea NOS (R19.7)
> enteritis NOS (K52.9)
> gastroenteritis NOS (K52.9)
> noninfective gastroenteritis and colitis, unspecified (K52.9)

DEF: Colitis: Inflammation of mucous membranes of the colon.
DEF: Enteritis: Inflammation of mucous membranes of the small intestine.
DEF: Gastroenteritis: Inflammation of mucous membranes of the stomach and intestines.

| ✓ Additional Character Req | ✓x7ᵗʰ Placeholder Alert | **Manifestation** | ▽ Unspecified | ▶◀ Revised Text | ● New Code | ▲ Revised Code Title |

ICD-10-CM 2019   437

Tuberculosis (A15-A19)

INCLUDES infections due to Mycobacterium tuberculosis and Mycobacterium bovis

EXCLUDES 1 congenital tuberculosis (P37.0)
nonspecific reaction to test for tuberculosis without active tuberculosis (R76.1-)
pneumoconiosis associated with tuberculosis, any type in A15 (J65)
positive PPD (R76.11)
positive tuberculin skin test without active tuberculosis (R76.11)
sequelae of tuberculosis (B90.-)
silicotuberculosis (J65)

DEF: Bacterial infection that typically spreads by inhalation of an airborne agent that usually attacks the lungs, but may also affect other organs.

✓4ᵗʰ **A15 Respiratory tuberculosis**

A15.0 Tuberculosis of lung
Tuberculous bronchiectasis
Tuberculous fibrosis of lung
Tuberculous pneumonia
Tuberculous pneumothorax

Tuberculosis of Lung

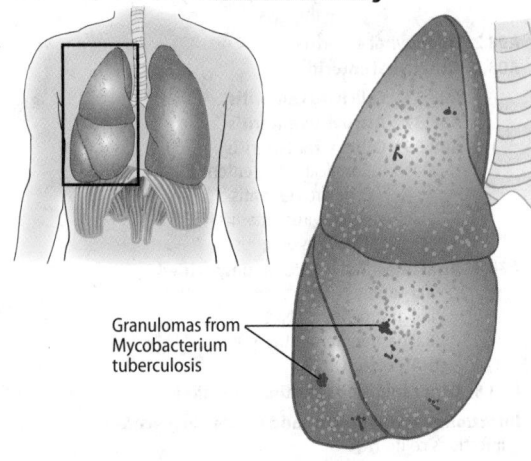

Granulomas from Mycobacterium tuberculosis

A15.4 Tuberculosis of intrathoracic lymph nodes
Tuberculosis of hilar lymph nodes
Tuberculosis of mediastinal lymph nodes
Tuberculosis of tracheobronchial lymph nodes
EXCLUDES 1 tuberculosis specified as primary (A15.7)

A15.5 Tuberculosis of larynx, trachea and bronchus
Tuberculosis of bronchus
Tuberculosis of glottis
Tuberculosis of larynx
Tuberculosis of trachea

A15.6 Tuberculous pleurisy
Tuberculosis of pleura Tuberculous empyema
EXCLUDES 1 primary respiratory tuberculosis (A15.7)

A15.7 Primary respiratory tuberculosis

A15.8 Other respiratory tuberculosis
Mediastinal tuberculosis
Nasopharyngeal tuberculosis
Tuberculosis of nose
Tuberculosis of sinus [any nasal]

A15.9 Respiratory tuberculosis unspecified   ▽

✓4ᵗʰ **A17 Tuberculosis of nervous system**

A17.0 Tuberculous meningitis
Tuberculosis of meninges (cerebral)(spinal)
Tuberculous leptomeningitis
EXCLUDES 1 tuberculous meningoencephalitis (A17.82)

A17.1 Meningeal tuberculoma
Tuberculoma of meninges (cerebral) (spinal)
EXCLUDES 2 tuberculoma of brain and spinal cord (A17.81)

✓5ᵗʰ **A17.8 Other tuberculosis of nervous system**

A17.81 Tuberculoma of brain and spinal cord
Tuberculous abscess of brain and spinal cord

A17.82 Tuberculous meningoencephalitis
Tuberculous myelitis

A17.83 Tuberculous neuritis
Tuberculous mononeuropathy

A17.89 Other tuberculosis of nervous system
Tuberculous polyneuropathy

A17.9 Tuberculosis of nervous system, unspecified   ▽

✓4ᵗʰ **A18 Tuberculosis of other organs**

✓5ᵗʰ **A18.0 Tuberculosis of bones and joints**

A18.01 Tuberculosis of spine
Pott's disease or curvature of spine
Tuberculous arthritis
Tuberculous osteomyelitis of spine
Tuberculous spondylitis

A18.02 Tuberculous arthritis of other joints
Tuberculosis of hip (joint)
Tuberculosis of knee (joint)

A18.03 Tuberculosis of other bones
Tuberculous mastoiditis
Tuberculous osteomyelitis

A18.09 Other musculoskeletal tuberculosis
Tuberculous myositis
Tuberculous synovitis
Tuberculous tenosynovitis

✓5ᵗʰ **A18.1 Tuberculosis of genitourinary system**

A18.10 Tuberculosis of genitourinary system, unspecified   ▽

A18.11 Tuberculosis of kidney and ureter

A18.12 Tuberculosis of bladder

A18.13 Tuberculosis of other urinary organs
Tuberculous urethritis

A18.14 Tuberculosis of prostate   A ♂

A18.15 Tuberculosis of other male genital organs   ♂

A18.16 Tuberculosis of cervix   ♀

A18.17 Tuberculous female pelvic inflammatory disease
Tuberculous endometritis
Tuberculous oophoritis and salpingitis   ♀

A18.18 Tuberculosis of other female genital organs   ♀
Tuberculous ulceration of vulva

A18.2 Tuberculous peripheral lymphadenopathy
Tuberculous adenitis
EXCLUDES 2 tuberculosis of bronchial and mediastinal lymph nodes (A15.4)
tuberculosis of mesenteric and retroperitoneal lymph nodes (A18.39)
tuberculous tracheobronchial adenopathy (A15.4)

✓5ᵗʰ **A18.3 Tuberculosis of intestines, peritoneum and mesenteric glands**

A18.31 Tuberculous peritonitis
Tuberculous ascites
DEF: Tuberculous inflammation of the membrane lining the abdomen.

A18.32 Tuberculous enteritis
Tuberculosis of anus and rectum
Tuberculosis of intestine (large) (small)

A18.39 Retroperitoneal tuberculosis
Tuberculosis of mesenteric glands
Tuberculosis of retroperitoneal (lymph glands)

A18.4 Tuberculosis of skin and subcutaneous tissue
Erythema induratum, tuberculous
Lupus excedens
Lupus vulgaris NOS
Lupus vulgaris of eyelid
Scrofuloderma
Tuberculosis of external ear
EXCLUDES 2 lupus erythematosus (L93.-)
lupus NOS (M32.9)
systemic (M32.-)

✓5ᵗʰ **A18.5 Tuberculosis of eye**
EXCLUDES 2 lupus vulgaris of eyelid (A18.4)

A18.50 Tuberculosis of eye, unspecified   ▽

A18.51 Tuberculous episcleritis

A18.52 Tuberculous keratitis
Tuberculous interstitial keratitis
Tuberculous keratoconjunctivitis (interstitial) (phlyctenular)

A18.53 Tuberculous chorioretinitis

A18.54 Tuberculous iridocyclitis

Chapter 1. Certain Infectious and Parasitic Diseases

    A18.59   **Other tuberculosis of eye**
       Tuberculous conjunctivitis
  A18.6   **Tuberculosis of (inner) (middle) ear**
      Tuberculous otitis media
      EXCLUDES 2   *tuberculosis of external ear (A18.4)*
             tuberculous mastoiditis (A18.03)
  A18.7   **Tuberculosis of adrenal glands**
      Tuberculous Addison's disease
 ✓5ᵗʰ **A18.8**   **Tuberculosis of other specified organs**
    A18.81   **Tuberculosis of thyroid gland**
    A18.82   **Tuberculosis of other endocrine glands**
       Tuberculosis of pituitary gland
       Tuberculosis of thymus gland
    A18.83   **Tuberculosis of digestive tract organs, not elsewhere classified**
       EXCLUDES 1   *tuberculosis of intestine (A18.32)*
    A18.84   **Tuberculosis of heart**
       Tuberculous cardiomyopathy
       Tuberculous endocarditis
       Tuberculous myocarditis
       Tuberculous pericarditis
    A18.85   **Tuberculosis of spleen**
    A18.89   **Tuberculosis of other sites**
       Tuberculosis of muscle
       Tuberculous cerebral arteritis

✓4ᵗʰ **A19**   **Miliary tuberculosis**
    INCLUDES   disseminated tuberculosis
         generalized tuberculosis
         tuberculous polyserositis
  A19.0   **Acute miliary tuberculosis of a single specified site**
  A19.1   **Acute miliary tuberculosis of multiple sites**
  A19.2   **Acute miliary tuberculosis, unspecified** ▽
  A19.8   **Other miliary tuberculosis**
  A19.9   **Miliary tuberculosis, unspecified** ▽

Certain zoonotic bacterial diseases (A20-A28)

✓4ᵗʰ **A20**   **Plague**
    INCLUDES   infection due to Yersinia pestis
  A20.0   **Bubonic plague**
  A20.1   **Cellulocutaneous plague**
  A20.2   **Pneumonic plague** HCC
  A20.3   **Plague meningitis**
  A20.7   **Septicemic plague** HCC
  A20.8   **Other forms of plague**
       Abortive plague
       Asymptomatic plague
       Pestis minor
  A20.9   **Plague, unspecified** ▽

✓4ᵗʰ **A21**   **Tularemia**
    INCLUDES   deer-fly fever
         infection due to Francisella tularensis
         rabbit fever
   DEF: Febrile disease transmitted to humans by the bites of deer flies, fleas, and ticks, by inhaling aerosolized *F. tularensis*, or by ingesting contaminated food or water. Patients quickly develop fever, chills, weakness, headache, backache, and malaise.
  A21.0   **Ulceroglandular tularemia**
  A21.1   **Oculoglandular tularemia**
       Ophthalmic tularemia
  A21.2   **Pulmonary tularemia** HCC
  A21.3   **Gastrointestinal tularemia**
       Abdominal tularemia
  A21.7   **Generalized tularemia**
  A21.8   **Other forms of tularemia**
  A21.9   **Tularemia, unspecified** ▽

✓4ᵗʰ **A22**   **Anthrax**
    INCLUDES   infection due to Bacillus anthracis
  A22.0   **Cutaneous anthrax**
       Malignant carbuncle
       Malignant pustule
  A22.1   **Pulmonary anthrax** HCC
       Inhalation anthrax
       Ragpicker's disease
       Woolsorter's disease
  A22.2   **Gastrointestinal anthrax**

  A22.7   **Anthrax sepsis** HCC
  A22.8   **Other forms of anthrax**
       Anthrax meningitis
  A22.9   **Anthrax, unspecified** ▽

✓4ᵗʰ **A23**   **Brucellosis**
    INCLUDES   Malta fever
         Mediterranean fever
         undulant fever
  A23.0   **Brucellosis due to Brucella melitensis**
  A23.1   **Brucellosis due to Brucella abortus**
  A23.2   **Brucellosis due to Brucella suis**
  A23.3   **Brucellosis due to Brucella canis**
  A23.8   **Other brucellosis**
  A23.9   **Brucellosis, unspecified** ▽

✓4ᵗʰ **A24**   **Glanders and melioidosis**
  A24.0   **Glanders**
       Infection due to Pseudomonas mallei
       Malleus
  A24.1   **Acute and fulminating melioidosis**
       Melioidosis pneumonia
       Melioidosis sepsis
  A24.2   **Subacute and chronic melioidosis**
  A24.3   **Other melioidosis**
  A24.9   **Melioidosis, unspecified** ▽
       Infection due to Pseudomonas pseudomallei NOS
       Whitmore's disease

✓4ᵗʰ **A25**   **Rat-bite fevers**
  A25.0   **Spirillosis**
       Sodoku
  A25.1   **Streptobacillosis**
       Epidemic arthritic erythema
       Haverhill fever
       Streptobacillary rat-bite fever
  A25.9   **Rat-bite fever, unspecified** ▽

✓4ᵗʰ **A26**   **Erysipeloid**
   DEF: Acute cutaneous infection typically caused by trauma to the skin. Presenting as cellulitis, it may become systemic affecting other organs. It is gram positive bacillus and mainly acquired by those who routinely handle meat.
  A26.0   **Cutaneous erysipeloid**
       Erythema migrans
  A26.7   **Erysipelothrix sepsis** HCC
  A26.8   **Other forms of erysipeloid**
  A26.9   **Erysipeloid, unspecified** ▽

✓4ᵗʰ **A27**   **Leptospirosis**
  A27.0   **Leptospirosis icterohemorrhagica**
       Leptospiral or spirochetal jaundice (hemorrhagic)
       Weil's disease
 ✓5ᵗʰ **A27.8**   **Other forms of leptospirosis**
    A27.81   **Aseptic meningitis in leptospirosis**
    A27.89   **Other forms of leptospirosis**
  A27.9   **Leptospirosis, unspecified** ▽

✓4ᵗʰ **A28**   **Other zoonotic bacterial diseases, not elsewhere classified**
  A28.0   **Pasteurellosis**
  A28.1   **Cat-scratch disease**
       Cat-scratch fever
  A28.2   **Extraintestinal yersiniosis**
       EXCLUDES 1   *enteritis due to Yersinia enterocolitica (A04.6)*
               plague (A20.-)
  A28.8   **Other specified zoonotic bacterial diseases, not elsewhere classified**
  A28.9   **Zoonotic bacterial disease, unspecified** ▽

Other bacterial diseases (A30-A49)

   AHA: 2016,3Q,8-14
✓4ᵗʰ **A30**   **Leprosy [Hansen's disease]**
    INCLUDES   infection due to Mycobacterium leprae
    EXCLUDES 1   *sequelae of leprosy (B92)*
  A30.0   **Indeterminate leprosy**
       I leprosy
  A30.1   **Tuberculoid leprosy**
       TT leprosy

A30.2 Borderline tuberculoid **leprosy**
BT leprosy

A30.3 Borderline **leprosy**
BB leprosy

A30.4 Borderline lepromatous **leprosy**
BL leprosy

A30.5 Lepromatous **leprosy**
LL leprosy

A30.8 Other forms of leprosy

A30.9 Leprosy, unspecified ▽

√4ᵗʰ **A31** Infection due to other mycobacteria

EXCLUDES 2 leprosy (A30.-)
tuberculosis (A15-A19)

A31.0 Pulmonary mycobacterial infection HCC
Infection due to Mycobacterium avium
Infection due to Mycobacterium intracellulare [Battey bacillus]
Infection due to Mycobacterium kansasii

A31.1 Cutaneous mycobacterial infection
Buruli ulcer
Infection due to Mycobacterium marinum
Infection due to Mycobacterium ulcerans

A31.2 Disseminated mycobacterium avium-intracellulare HCC
complex (DMAC)
MAC sepsis

A31.8 Other mycobacterial infections

A31.9 Mycobacterial infection, unspecified ▽
Atypical mycobacterial infection NOS
Mycobacteriosis NOS

√4ᵗʰ **A32** Listeriosis

INCLUDES listerial foodborne infection
EXCLUDES 1 neonatal (disseminated) listeriosis (P37.2)

A32.0 Cutaneous listeriosis

√5ᵗʰ **A32.1** Listerial meningitis and meningoencephalitis

A32.11 Listerial meningitis
A32.12 Listerial meningoencephalitis

A32.7 Listerial sepsis HCC

√5ᵗʰ **A32.8** Other forms of listeriosis

A32.81 Oculoglandular listeriosis
A32.82 Listerial endocarditis
A32.89 Other forms of listeriosis
Listerial cerebral arteritis

A32.9 Listeriosis, unspecified ▽

A33 Tetanus neonatorum N

A34 Obstetrical tetanus M ♀

A35 Other tetanus
Tetanus NOS
EXCLUDES 1 obstetrical tetanus (A34)
tetanus neonatorum (A33)

DEF: Tetanus: Acute, often fatal, infectious disease caused by the anaerobic, spore-forming bacillus *Clostridium tetani*. The bacillus enters the body through a contaminated wound, burns, surgical wounds, or cutaneous ulcers. Symptoms include lockjaw, spasms, seizures, and paralysis.

√4ᵗʰ **A36** Diphtheria

A36.0 Pharyngeal diphtheria
Diphtheritic membranous angina
Tonsillar diphtheria

A36.1 Nasopharyngeal diphtheria

A36.2 Laryngeal diphtheria
Diphtheritic laryngotracheitis

A36.3 Cutaneous diphtheria
EXCLUDES 2 erythrasma (L08.1)

√5ᵗʰ **A36.8** Other diphtheria

A36.81 Diphtheritic cardiomyopathy HCC
Diphtheritic myocarditis
A36.82 Diphtheritic radiculomyelitis
A36.83 Diphtheritic polyneuritis
A36.84 Diphtheritic tubulo-interstitial nephropathy
A36.85 Diphtheritic cystitis
A36.86 Diphtheritic conjunctivitis
A36.89 Other diphtheritic complications
Diphtheritic peritonitis

A36.9 Diphtheria, unspecified ▽

√4ᵗʰ **A37** Whooping cough
DEF: Acute, highly contagious respiratory tract infection caused by *Bordetella pertussis* and *B. bronchiseptica*. Whooping cough is known by its characteristic paroxysmal cough.

√5ᵗʰ **A37.0** Whooping cough due to Bordetella pertussis
A37.00 Whooping cough due to Bordetella pertussis without pneumonia
A37.01 Whooping cough due to Bordetella pertussis with pneumonia

√5ᵗʰ **A37.1** Whooping cough due to Bordetella parapertussis
A37.10 Whooping cough due to Bordetella parapertussis without pneumonia
A37.11 Whooping cough due to Bordetella parapertussis with pneumonia

√5ᵗʰ **A37.8** Whooping cough due to other Bordetella species
A37.80 Whooping cough due to other Bordetella species without pneumonia
A37.81 Whooping cough due to other Bordetella species with pneumonia

√5ᵗʰ **A37.9** Whooping cough, unspecified species
A37.90 Whooping cough, unspecified species without pneumonia ▽
A37.91 Whooping cough, unspecified species with pneumonia ▽

√4ᵗʰ **A38** Scarlet fever
INCLUDES scarlatina
EXCLUDES 2 streptococcal sore throat (J02.0)
DEF: Acute contagious disease caused by Group A bacteria, the same bacterium that causes strep throat. Individuals with strep throat can develop scarlet fever particularly if the infection is not treated with antibiotics. It is characterized by a red blush to the skin of the chest and abdomen and swelling of the nose, throat, and mouth.

A38.0 Scarlet fever with otitis media
A38.1 Scarlet fever with myocarditis
A38.8 Scarlet fever with other complications
A38.9 Scarlet fever, uncomplicated ▽
Scarlet fever, NOS

√4ᵗʰ **A39** Meningococcal infection
DEF: Condition caused by *Neisseria meningitidis*, a bacteria that may invade the spinal cord, brain, heart, joints, optic nerve, or bloodstream.

A39.0 Meningococcal meningitis
A39.1 Waterhouse-Friderichsen syndrome HCC
Meningococcal hemorrhagic adrenalitis
Meningococcic adrenal syndrome
A39.2 Acute meningococcemia HCC
A39.3 Chronic meningococcemia HCC
A39.4 Meningococcemia, unspecified HCC ▽

√5ᵗʰ **A39.5** Meningococcal heart disease
A39.50 Meningococcal carditis, unspecified ▽
A39.51 Meningococcal endocarditis
A39.52 Meningococcal myocarditis
A39.53 Meningococcal pericarditis

√5ᵗʰ **A39.8** Other meningococcal infections
A39.81 Meningococcal encephalitis
A39.82 Meningococcal retrobulbar neuritis
A39.83 Meningococcal arthritis HCC
A39.84 Postmeningococcal arthritis HCC
A39.89 Other meningococcal infections
Meningococcal conjunctivitis

A39.9 Meningococcal infection, unspecified ▽
Meningococcal disease NOS

√4ᵗʰ **A40** Streptococcal sepsis
Code first:
postprocedural streptococcal sepsis (T81.4-)
streptococcal sepsis during labor (O75.3)
streptococcal sepsis following abortion or ectopic or molar pregnancy (O03-O07, O08.0)
streptococcal sepsis following immunization (T88.0)
streptococcal sepsis following infusion, transfusion or therapeutic injection (T80.2-)
EXCLUDES 1 neonatal (P36.0-P36.1)
puerperal sepsis (O85)
sepsis due to Streptococcus, group D (A41.81)
AHA: 2018,1Q,16; 2016,1Q,32

A40.0 Sepsis due to streptococcus, group A HCC
A40.1 Sepsis due to streptococcus, group B HCC

A40.3 **Sepsis due to Streptococcus pneumoniae**   HCC
　　　 Pneumococcal sepsis

A40.8 **Other streptococcal sepsis**   HCC

A40.9 **Streptococcal sepsis, unspecified**   HCC ▽

√4ᵗʰ **A41 Other sepsis**
Code first:
postprocedural sepsis (T81.4-)
sepsis during labor (O75.3)
sepsis following abortion, ectopic or molar pregnancy (O03-O07, O08.0)
sepsis following immunization (T88.0)
sepsis following infusion, transfusion or therapeutic injection (T80.2-)

EXCLUDES 1   bacteremia NOS (R78.81)
neonatal (P36.-)
puerperal sepsis (O85)
streptococcal sepsis (A40.-)

EXCLUDES 2   sepsis (due to) (in) actinomycotic (A42.7)
sepsis (due to) (in) anthrax (A22.7)
sepsis (due to) (in) candidal (B37.7)
sepsis (due to) (in) Erysipelothrix (A26.7)
sepsis (due to) (in) extraintestinal yersiniosis (A28.2)
sepsis (due to) (in) gonococcal (A54.86)
sepsis (due to) (in) herpesviral (B00.7)
sepsis (due to) (in) listerial (A32.7)
sepsis (due to) (in) melioidosis (A24.1)
sepsis (due to) (in) meningococcal (A39.2-A39.4)
sepsis (due to) (in) plague (A20.7)
sepsis (due to) (in) tularemia (A21.7)
toxic shock syndrome (A48.3)

AHA: 2018,1Q,16; 2016,1Q,32; 2014,2Q,13

√5ᵗʰ **A41.0 Sepsis due to Staphylococcus aureus**

A41.01 **Sepsis due to Methicillin susceptible Staphylococcus aureus**   HCC Q
　　　 MSSA sepsis
　　　 Staphylococcus aureus sepsis NOS

A41.02 **Sepsis due to Methicillin resistant Staphylococcus aureus**   HCC

A41.1 **Sepsis due to other specified staphylococcus**   HCC
　　　 Coagulase negative staphylococcus sepsis

A41.2 **Sepsis due to unspecified staphylococcus**   HCC ▽

A41.3 **Sepsis due to Hemophilus influenzae**   HCC

A41.4 **Sepsis due to anaerobes**   HCC
　　　 EXCLUDES 1   gas gangrene (A48.0)

√5ᵗʰ **A41.5 Sepsis due to other Gram-negative organisms**

A41.50 **Gram-negative sepsis, unspecified**   HCC ▽
　　　 Gram-negative sepsis NOS

A41.51 **Sepsis due to Escherichia coli [E. coli]**   HCC

A41.52 **Sepsis due to Pseudomonas**   HCC
　　　 Pseudomonas aeroginosa

A41.53 **Sepsis due to Serratia**   HCC

A41.59 **Other Gram-negative sepsis**   HCC

√5ᵗʰ **A41.8 Other specified sepsis**

A41.81 **Sepsis due to Enterococcus**   HCC
　　　 TIP: E. faecium, is a species of Enterococcus that is highly resistant to multiple antibiotics. Assign a code from category Z16 when resistance to antimicrobial drugs is documented.

A41.89 **Other specified sepsis**   HCC
　　　 AHA: 2017,1Q,51; 2016,3Q,8-14

A41.9 **Sepsis, unspecified organism**   HCC ▽
　　　 Septicemia NOS

√4ᵗʰ **A42 Actinomycosis**
EXCLUDES 1   actinomycetoma (B47.1)

A42.0 **Pulmonary actinomycosis**   HCC

A42.1 **Abdominal actinomycosis**

A42.2 **Cervicofacial actinomycosis**

A42.7 **Actinomycotic sepsis**   HCC

√5ᵗʰ **A42.8 Other forms of actinomycosis**

A42.81 **Actinomycotic meningitis**

A42.82 **Actinomycotic encephalitis**

A42.89 **Other forms of actinomycosis**

A42.9 **Actinomycosis, unspecified**   ▽

√4ᵗʰ **A43 Nocardiosis**
DEF: Rare bacterial infection occurring most often in those with weakened immune systems. Can be acquired in soil, decaying plants, or standing water. It typically begins in the lungs and has a tendency to spread to other body systems.

A43.0 **Pulmonary nocardiosis**   HCC

A43.1 **Cutaneous nocardiosis**

A43.8 **Other forms of nocardiosis**

A43.9 **Nocardiosis, unspecified**   ▽

√4ᵗʰ **A44 Bartonellosis**

A44.0 **Systemic bartonellosis**
　　　 Oroya fever

A44.1 **Cutaneous and mucocutaneous bartonellosis**
　　　 Verruga peruana

A44.8 **Other forms of bartonellosis**

A44.9 **Bartonellosis, unspecified**   ▽

A46 Erysipelas
EXCLUDES 1   postpartum or puerperal erysipelas (O86.89)
DEF: Skin infection affecting the upper dermis and superficial dermal lymphatics. Lesion edges are well-demarcated with distinct raised borders. It is often caused by group A Streptococci.

√4ᵗʰ **A48 Other bacterial diseases, not elsewhere classified**
EXCLUDES 1   actinomycetoma (B47.1)

A48.0 **Gas gangrene**   HCC
　　　 Clostridial cellulitis
　　　 Clostridial myonecrosis
　　　 AHA: 2017,4Q,102

A48.1 **Legionnaires' disease**   HCC
　　　 DEF: Severe and often fatal infection by Legionella pneumophila. Symptoms include high fever, gastrointestinal pain, headache, myalgia, dry cough, and pneumonia and it is usually transmitted through airborne water droplets via air conditioning systems or hot tubs.

A48.2 **Nonpneumonic Legionnaires' disease [Pontiac fever]**

A48.3 **Toxic shock syndrome**   HCC
　　　 Use additional code to identify the organism (B95, B96)
　　　 EXCLUDES 1   endotoxic shock NOS (R57.8)
　　　　　　　　　　　 sepsis NOS (A41.9)
　　　 DEF: Bacteria producing an endotoxin, such as Staphylococci, flood the body with the toxins producing a high fever, vomiting and diarrhea, decreasing blood pressure, a skin rash, and shock. **Synonym(s):** TSS.

A48.4 **Brazilian purpuric fever**
　　　 Systemic Hemophilus aegyptius infection

√5ᵗʰ **A48.5 Other specified botulism**
　　　 Non-foodborne intoxication due to toxins of Clostridium botulinum [C. botulinum]
　　　 EXCLUDES 1   food poisoning due to toxins of Clostridium botulinum (A05.1)

A48.51 **Infant botulism**   P

A48.52 **Wound botulism**
　　　 Non-foodborne botulism NOS
　　　 Use additional code for associated wound

A48.8 **Other specified bacterial diseases**

√4ᵗʰ **A49 Bacterial infection of unspecified site**
EXCLUDES 1   bacterial agents as the cause of diseases classified elsewhere (B95-B96)
chlamydial infection NOS (A74.9)
meningococcal infection NOS (A39.9)
rickettsial infection NOS (A79.9)
spirochetal infection NOS (A69.9)

√5ᵗʰ **A49.0 Staphylococcal infection, unspecified site**

A49.01 **Methicillin susceptible Staphylococcus aureus infection, unspecified site**
　　　 Methicillin susceptible Staphylococcus aureus (MSSA) infection
　　　 Staphylococcus aureus infection NOS

A49.02 **Methicillin resistant Staphylococcus aureus infection, unspecified site**
　　　 Methicillin resistant Staphylococcus aureus (MRSA) infection

A49.1 **Streptococcal infection, unspecified site**

A49.2 **Hemophilus influenzae infection, unspecified site**

A49.3 **Mycoplasma infection, unspecified site**

A49.8 **Other bacterial infections of unspecified site**

☑ Additional Character Req   √x7ᵗʰ Placeholder Alert   Manifestation   ▽ Unspecified   ▶◀ Revised Text   ● New Code   ▲ Revised Code Title

ICD-10-CM 2019   441

Chapter 1. Certain Infectious and Parasitic Diseases

A40.3-A49.8

A49.9   **Bacterial infection, unspecified**   ▽
       EXCLUDES 1   *bacteremia NOS (R78.81)*

Infections with a predominantly sexual mode of transmission (A50-A64)

   EXCLUDES 1   *human immunodeficiency virus [HIV] disease (B20)*
                 nonspecific and nongonococcal urethritis (N34.1)
                 Reiter's disease (M02.3-)

✓4ᵗʰ **A50**   **Congenital syphilis**

✓5ᵗʰ   **A50.0**   **Early congenital syphilis, symptomatic**
          Any congenital syphilitic condition specified as early or manifest less than two years after birth.

       A50.01   **Early congenital syphilitic oculopathy**
       A50.02   **Early congenital syphilitic osteochondropathy**
       A50.03   **Early congenital syphilitic pharyngitis**
              Early congenital syphilitic laryngitis
       A50.04   **Early congenital syphilitic pneumonia**
       A50.05   **Early congenital syphilitic rhinitis**
       A50.06   **Early cutaneous congenital syphilis**
       A50.07   **Early mucocutaneous congenital syphilis**
       A50.08   **Early visceral congenital syphilis**
       A50.09   **Other early congenital syphilis, symptomatic**

   A50.1   **Early congenital syphilis, latent**
          Congenital syphilis without clinical manifestations, with positive serological reaction and negative spinal fluid test, less than two years after birth.

   A50.2   **Early congenital syphilis, unspecified**   ▽
          Congenital syphilis NOS less than two years after birth.

✓5ᵗʰ   **A50.3**   **Late congenital syphilitic oculopathy**
        EXCLUDES 1   *Hutchinson's triad (A50.53)*

       A50.30   **Late congenital syphilitic oculopathy, unspecified**   ▽
       A50.31   **Late congenital syphilitic interstitial keratitis**
       A50.32   **Late congenital syphilitic chorioretinitis**
       A50.39   **Other late congenital syphilitic oculopathy**

✓5ᵗʰ   **A50.4**   **Late congenital neurosyphilis [juvenile neurosyphilis]**
          Use additional code to identify any associated mental disorder
        EXCLUDES 1   *Hutchinson's triad (A50.53)*

       A50.40   **Late congenital neurosyphilis, unspecified**   ▽
              Juvenile neurosyphilis NOS
       A50.41   **Late congenital syphilitic meningitis**
       A50.42   **Late congenital syphilitic encephalitis**
       A50.43   **Late congenital syphilitic polyneuropathy**
       A50.44   **Late congenital syphilitic optic nerve atrophy**
       A50.45   **Juvenile general paresis**
              Dementia paralytica juvenilis
              Juvenile tabetoparetic neurosyphilis
       A50.49   **Other late congenital neurosyphilis**
              Juvenile tabes dorsalis

✓5ᵗʰ   **A50.5**   **Other late congenital syphilis, symptomatic**
          Any congenital syphilitic condition specified as late or manifest two years or more after birth.

       A50.51   **Clutton's joints**
       A50.52   **Hutchinson's teeth**
       A50.53   **Hutchinson's triad**
       A50.54   **Late congenital cardiovascular syphilis**
       A50.55   **Late congenital syphilitic arthropathy**   HCC
       A50.56   **Late congenital syphilitic osteochondropathy**
       A50.57   **Syphilitic saddle nose**
       A50.59   **Other late congenital syphilis, symptomatic**

   A50.6   **Late congenital syphilis, latent**
          Congenital syphilis without clinical manifestations, with positive serological reaction and negative spinal fluid test, two years or more after birth.

   A50.7   **Late congenital syphilis, unspecified**   ▽
          Congenital syphilis NOS two years or more after birth.

   A50.9   **Congenital syphilis, unspecified**   ▽

✓4ᵗʰ **A51**   **Early syphilis**
      DEF: Syphilis: Sexually transmitted disease caused by the treponema pallidum spirochete. Syphilis usually exhibits cutaneous manifestations and may exist for years without symptoms.

   A51.0   **Primary genital syphilis**
          Syphilitic chancre NOS
   A51.1   **Primary anal syphilis**
   A51.2   **Primary syphilis of other sites**

✓5ᵗʰ **A51.3**   **Secondary syphilis of skin and mucous membranes**
      DEF: Transitory or chronic cutaneous eruptions that present within two to 10 weeks following an initial syphilis infection that may include nontender lymphadenopathy along with alopecia and condylomata lata.

       A51.31   **Condyloma latum**
       A51.32   **Syphilitic alopecia**
       A51.39   **Other secondary syphilis of skin**
              Syphilitic leukoderma
              Syphilitic mucous patch
         EXCLUDES 1   *late syphilitic leukoderma (A52.79)*

✓5ᵗʰ **A51.4**   **Other secondary syphilis**

       A51.41   **Secondary syphilitic meningitis**
       A51.42   **Secondary syphilitic female pelvic disease**   ♀
       A51.43   **Secondary syphilitic oculopathy**
              Secondary syphilitic chorioretinitis
              Secondary syphilitic iridocyclitis, iritis
              Secondary syphilitic uveitis
       A51.44   **Secondary syphilitic nephritis**
       A51.45   **Secondary syphilitic hepatitis**
       A51.46   **Secondary syphilitic osteopathy**
       A51.49   **Other secondary syphilitic conditions**
              Secondary syphilitic lymphadenopathy
              Secondary syphilitic myositis

   A51.5   **Early syphilis, latent**
          Syphilis (acquired) without clinical manifestations, with positive serological reaction and negative spinal fluid test, less than two years after infection.

   A51.9   **Early syphilis, unspecified**   ▽

✓4ᵗʰ **A52**   **Late syphilis**

✓5ᵗʰ   **A52.0**   **Cardiovascular and cerebrovascular syphilis**

       A52.00   **Cardiovascular syphilis, unspecified**   ▽
       A52.01   **Syphilitic aneurysm of aorta**
       A52.02   **Syphilitic aortitis**
       A52.03   **Syphilitic endocarditis**
              Syphilitic aortic valve incompetence or stenosis
              Syphilitic mitral valve stenosis
              Syphilitic pulmonary valve regurgitation
       A52.04   **Syphilitic cerebral arteritis**
       A52.05   **Other cerebrovascular syphilis**
              Syphilitic cerebral aneurysm (ruptured) (non-ruptured)
              Syphilitic cerebral thrombosis
       A52.06   **Other syphilitic heart involvement**
              Syphilitic coronary artery disease
              Syphilitic myocarditis
              Syphilitic pericarditis
       A52.09   **Other cardiovascular syphilis**

✓5ᵗʰ   **A52.1**   **Symptomatic neurosyphilis**

       A52.10   **Symptomatic neurosyphilis, unspecified**   ▽
       A52.11   **Tabes dorsalis**
              Locomotor ataxia (progressive)
              Tabetic neurosyphilis
       A52.12   **Other cerebrospinal syphilis**
       A52.13   **Late syphilitic meningitis**
       A52.14   **Late syphilitic encephalitis**
       A52.15   **Late syphilitic neuropathy**
              Late syphilitic acoustic neuritis
              Late syphilitic optic (nerve) atrophy
              Late syphilitic polyneuropathy
              Late syphilitic retrobulbar neuritis
       A52.16   **Charcôt's arthropathy (tabetic)**
          DEF: Progressive neurologic arthropathy in which chronic degeneration of joints in the weight-bearing areas with peripheral hypertrophy occurs as a complication of a neuropathy disorder. Supporting structures relax from a loss of sensation resulting in chronic joint instability.
       A52.17   **General paresis**
              Dementia paralytica
       A52.19   **Other symptomatic neurosyphilis**
              Syphilitic parkinsonism

   A52.2   **Asymptomatic neurosyphilis**

A52.3 Neurosyphilis, unspecified ▽
- Gumma (syphilitic)
- Syphilis (late)
- Syphiloma

✓5ᵗʰ **A52.7 Other symptomatic late syphilis**

A52.71 Late syphilitic oculopathy
- Late syphilitic chorioretinitis
- Late syphilitic episcleritis

A52.72 Syphilis of lung and bronchus

A52.73 Symptomatic late syphilis of other respiratory organs

A52.74 Syphilis of liver and other viscera
- Late syphilitic peritonitis

A52.75 Syphilis of kidney and ureter
- Syphilitic glomerular disease

A52.76 Other genitourinary symptomatic late syphilis
- Late syphilitic female pelvic inflammatory disease

A52.77 Syphilis of bone and joint

A52.78 Syphilis of other musculoskeletal tissue
- Late syphilitic bursitis
- Syphilis [stage unspecified] of bursa
- Syphilis [stage unspecified] of muscle
- Syphilis [stage unspecified] of synovium
- Syphilis [stage unspecified] of tendon

A52.79 Other symptomatic late syphilis
- Late syphilitic leukoderma
- Syphilis of adrenal gland
- Syphilis of pituitary gland
- Syphilis of thyroid gland
- Syphilitic splenomegaly
- EXCLUDES 1   *syphilitic leukoderma (secondary) (A51.39)*

A52.8 Late syphilis, latent
- Syphilis (acquired) without clinical manifestations, with positive serological reaction and negative spinal fluid test, two years or more after infection

A52.9 Late syphilis, unspecified ▽

✓4ᵗʰ **A53 Other and unspecified syphilis**

A53.0 Latent syphilis, unspecified as early or late
- Latent syphilis NOS
- Positive serological reaction for syphilis

A53.9 Syphilis, unspecified ▽
- Infection due to Treponema pallidum NOS
- Syphilis (acquired) NOS
- EXCLUDES 1   *syphilis NOS under two years of age (A50.2)*

✓4ᵗʰ **A54 Gonococcal infection**
- **DEF:** Sexually transmitted bacterial infection caused by *Neisseria gonorrhoeae*. Women are often asymptomatic, while men tend to develop urinary symptoms quickly.

✓5ᵗʰ **A54.0 Gonococcal infection of lower genitourinary tract without periurethral or accessory gland abscess**
- EXCLUDES 1   *gonococcal infection with genitourinary gland abscess (A54.1)*
-       *gonococcal infection with periurethral abscess (A54.1)*

A54.00 Gonococcal infection of lower genitourinary tract, unspecified ▽

A54.01 Gonococcal cystitis and urethritis, unspecified ▽

A54.02 Gonococcal vulvovaginitis, unspecified ♀ ▽

A54.03 Gonococcal cervicitis, unspecified ♀ ▽

A54.09 Other gonococcal infection of lower genitourinary tract

A54.1 Gonococcal infection of lower genitourinary tract with periurethral and accessory gland abscess
- Gonococcal Bartholin's gland abscess

✓5ᵗʰ **A54.2 Gonococcal pelviperitonitis and other gonococcal genitourinary infection**

A54.21 Gonococcal infection of kidney and ureter

A54.22 Gonococcal prostatitis ♂

A54.23 Gonococcal infection of other male genital organs ♂
- Gonococcal epididymitis
- Gonococcal orchitis

A54.24 Gonococcal female pelvic inflammatory disease ♀
- Gonococcal pelviperitonitis
- EXCLUDES 1   *gonococcal peritonitis (A54.85)*

A54.29 Other gonococcal genitourinary infections

✓5ᵗʰ **A54.3 Gonococcal infection of eye**

A54.30 Gonococcal infection of eye, unspecified ▽

A54.31 Gonococcal conjunctivitis
- Ophthalmia neonatorum due to gonococcus

A54.32 Gonococcal iridocyclitis

A54.33 Gonococcal keratitis

A54.39 Other gonococcal eye infection
- Gonococcal endophthalmia

✓5ᵗʰ **A54.4 Gonococcal infection of musculoskeletal system**

A54.40 Gonococcal infection of musculoskeletal system, unspecified HCC ▽

A54.41 Gonococcal spondylopathy HCC

A54.42 Gonococcal arthritis HCC
- EXCLUDES 2   *gonococcal infection of spine (A54.41)*

A54.43 Gonococcal osteomyelitis HCC
- EXCLUDES 2   *gonococcal infection of spine (A54.41)*

A54.49 Gonococcal infection of other musculoskeletal tissue HCC
- Gonococcal bursitis
- Gonococcal myositis
- Gonococcal synovitis
- Gonococcal tenosynovitis

A54.5 Gonococcal pharyngitis

A54.6 Gonococcal infection of anus and rectum

✓5ᵗʰ **A54.8 Other gonococcal infections**

A54.81 Gonococcal meningitis

A54.82 Gonococcal brain abscess

A54.83 Gonococcal heart infection
- Gonococcal endocarditis
- Gonococcal myocarditis
- Gonococcal pericarditis

A54.84 Gonococcal pneumonia HCC

A54.85 Gonococcal peritonitis HCC
- EXCLUDES 1   *gonococcal pelviperitonitis (A54.24)*

A54.86 Gonococcal sepsis HCC

A54.89 Other gonococcal infections
- Gonococcal keratoderma
- Gonococcal lymphadenitis

A54.9 Gonococcal infection, unspecified ▽

A55 Chlamydial lymphogranuloma (venereum)
- Climatic or tropical bubo
- Durand-Nicolas-Favre disease
- Esthiomene
- Lymphogranuloma inguinale

✓4ᵗʰ **A56 Other sexually transmitted chlamydial diseases**
- INCLUDES   sexually transmitted diseases due to Chlamydia trachomatis
- EXCLUDES 1   *neonatal chlamydial conjunctivitis (P39.1)*
-       *neonatal chlamydial pneumonia (P23.1)*
- EXCLUDES 2   *chlamydial lymphogranuloma (A55)*
-       *conditions classified to A74.-*

✓5ᵗʰ **A56.0 Chlamydial infection of lower genitourinary tract**

A56.00 Chlamydial infection of lower genitourinary tract, unspecified ▽

A56.01 Chlamydial cystitis and urethritis

A56.02 Chlamydial vulvovaginitis ♀

A56.09 Other chlamydial infection of lower genitourinary tract
- Chlamydial cervicitis

✓5ᵗʰ **A56.1 Chlamydial infection of pelviperitoneum and other genitourinary organs**

A56.11 Chlamydial female pelvic inflammatory disease ♀

A56.19 Other chlamydial genitourinary infection
- Chlamydial epididymitis
- Chlamydial orchitis

A56.2 Chlamydial infection of genitourinary tract, unspecified ▽

A56.3 Chlamydial infection of anus and rectum

A56.4 Chlamydial infection of pharynx

A56.8 Sexually transmitted chlamydial infection of other sites

A57 Chancroid
Ulcus molle
DEF: Localized infection by *Haemophilus ducreyi,* causing genital ulcers and infecting the inguinal lymph nodes.

A58 Granuloma inguinale
Donovanosis

√4ᵗʰ **A59 Trichomoniasis**
EXCLUDES 2   *intestinal trichomoniasis (A07.8)*
DEF: Infection with the parasitic, flagellated protozoa of the genus *Trichomonas.* This protozoon is found in the intestinal and genitourinary tracts of humans and in the mouth around tartar, cavities, and areas of periodontal disease.

√5ᵗʰ **A59.0 Urogenital trichomoniasis**

A59.00 Urogenital trichomoniasis, unspecified ▽
Fluor (vaginalis) due to Trichomonas
Leukorrhea (vaginalis) due to Trichomonas

A59.01 Trichomonal vulvovaginitis ♀

A59.02 Trichomonal prostatitis ♂

A59.03 Trichomonal cystitis and urethritis

A59.09 Other urogenital trichomoniasis
Trichomonas cervicitis

A59.8 Trichomoniasis of other sites

A59.9 Trichomoniasis, unspecified ▽

√4ᵗʰ **A60 Anogenital herpesviral [herpes simplex] infections**

√5ᵗʰ **A60.0 Herpesviral infection of genitalia and urogenital tract**

A60.00 Herpesviral infection of urogenital system, unspecified ▽

A60.01 Herpesviral infection of penis ♂

A60.02 Herpesviral infection of other male genital organs ♂

A60.03 Herpesviral cervicitis ♀

A60.04 Herpesviral vulvovaginitis ♀
Herpesviral [herpes simplex] ulceration
Herpesviral [herpes simplex] vaginitis
Herpesviral [herpes simplex] vulvitis

A60.09 Herpesviral infection of other urogenital tract

A60.1 Herpesviral infection of perianal skin and rectum

A60.9 Anogenital herpesviral infection, unspecified ▽

√4ᵗʰ **A63 Other predominantly sexually transmitted diseases, not elsewhere classified**
EXCLUDES 2   *molluscum contagiosum (B08.1)*
papilloma of cervix (D26.0)

A63.0 Anogenital (venereal) warts
Anogenital warts due to (human) papillomavirus [HPV]
Condyloma acuminatum

A63.8 Other specified predominantly sexually transmitted diseases

A64 Unspecified sexually transmitted disease ▽

Other spirochetal diseases (A65-A69)

EXCLUDES 2   *leptospirosis (A27.-)*
syphilis (A50-A53)

A65 Nonvenereal syphilis
Bejel
Endemic syphilis
Njovera

√4ᵗʰ **A66 Yaws**
INCLUDES   bouba
frambesia (tropica)
pian

A66.0 Initial lesions of yaws
Chancre of yaws
Frambesia, initial or primary
Initial frambesial ulcer
Mother yaw

A66.1 Multiple papillomata and wet crab yaws
Frambesioma
Pianoma
Plantar or palmar papilloma of yaws

A66.2 Other early skin lesions of yaws
Cutaneous yaws, less than five years after infection
Early yaws (cutaneous) (macular) (maculopapular) (micropapular) (papular)
Frambeside of early yaws

A66.3 Hyperkeratosis of yaws
Ghoul hand
Hyperkeratosis, palmar or plantar (early) (late) due to yaws
Worm-eaten soles

A66.4 Gummata and ulcers of yaws
Gummatous frambeside
Nodular late yaws (ulcerated)

A66.5 Gangosa
Rhinopharyngitis mutilans

A66.6 Bone and joint lesions of yaws HCC
Yaws ganglion
Yaws goundou
Yaws gumma, bone
Yaws gummatous osteitis or periostitis
Yaws hydrarthrosis
Yaws osteitis
Yaws periostitis (hypertrophic)

A66.7 Other manifestations of yaws
Juxta-articular nodules of yaws
Mucosal yaws

A66.8 Latent yaws
Yaws without clinical manifestations, with positive serology

A66.9 Yaws, unspecified ▽

√4ᵗʰ **A67 Pinta [carate]**

A67.0 Primary lesions of pinta
Chancre (primary) of pinta
Papule (primary) of pinta

A67.1 Intermediate lesions of pinta
Erythematous plaques of pinta
Hyperchromic lesions of pinta
Hyperkeratosis of pinta
Pintids

A67.2 Late lesions of pinta
Achromic skin lesions of pinta
Cicatricial skin lesions of pinta
Dyschromic skin lesions of pinta

A67.3 Mixed lesions of pinta
Achromic with hyperchromic skin lesions of pinta [carate]

A67.9 Pinta, unspecified ▽

√4ᵗʰ **A68 Relapsing fevers**
INCLUDES   recurrent fever
EXCLUDES 2   *Lyme disease (A69.2-)*

A68.0 Louse-borne relapsing fever
Relapsing fever due to Borrelia recurrentis

A68.1 Tick-borne relapsing fever
Relapsing fever due to any Borrelia species other than Borrelia recurrentis

A68.9 Relapsing fever, unspecified ▽

√4ᵗʰ **A69 Other spirochetal infections**

A69.0 Necrotizing ulcerative stomatitis
Cancrum oris
Fusospirochetal gangrene
Noma
Stomatitis gangrenosa

A69.1 Other Vincent's infections
Fusospirochetal pharyngitis
Necrotizing ulcerative (acute) gingivitis
Necrotizing ulcerative (acute) gingivostomatitis
Spirochetal stomatitis
Trench mouth
Vincent's angina
Vincent's gingivitis

√5ᵗʰ **A69.2 Lyme disease**
Erythema chronicum migrans due to Borrelia burgdorferi
DEF: Recurrent multisystem disorder through tick bites that begins with lesions of erythema chronicum migrans and is followed by arthritis of the large joints, myalgia, malaise, and neurological and cardiac manifestations.

A69.20 Lyme disease, unspecified ▽

A69.21 Meningitis due to Lyme disease

A69.22 Other neurologic disorders in Lyme disease
Cranial neuritis
Meningoencephalitis
Polyneuropathy

A69.23 Arthritis due to Lyme disease HCC

A69.29   **Other conditions associated with Lyme disease**
Myopericarditis due to Lyme disease
AHA: 2016,3Q,12

A69.8   **Other specified spirochetal infections**

A69.9   **Spirochetal infection, unspecified** ▽

Other diseases caused by chlamydiae (A70-A74)

EXCLUDES 1   *sexually transmitted chlamydial diseases (A55-A56)*

A70 Chlamydia psittaci infections
Ornithosis
Parrot fever
Psittacosis

✓4th **A71 Trachoma**

     EXCLUDES 1   *sequelae of trachoma (B94.0)*

A71.0   **Initial stage of trachoma**
Trachoma dubium

A71.1   **Active stage of trachoma**
Granular conjunctivitis (trachomatous)
Trachomatous follicular conjunctivitis
Trachomatous pannus

A71.9   **Trachoma, unspecified** ▽

✓4th **A74 Other diseases caused by chlamydiae**

     EXCLUDES 1   *neonatal chlamydial conjunctivitis (P39.1)*
neonatal chlamydial pneumonia (P23.1)
Reiter's disease (M02.3-)
sexually transmitted chlamydial diseases (A55-A56)

     EXCLUDES 2   *chlamydial pneumonia (J16.0)*

A74.0   **Chlamydial conjunctivitis**
Paratrachoma

✓5th **A74.8**   **Other chlamydial diseases**

     A74.81   **Chlamydial peritonitis**
     A74.89   **Other chlamydial diseases**

A74.9   **Chlamydial infection, unspecified** ▽
Chlamydiosis NOS

Rickettsioses (A75-A79)

✓4th **A75 Typhus fever**

     EXCLUDES 1   *rickettsiosis due to Ehrlichia sennetsu (A79.81)*

A75.0   **Epidemic louse-borne typhus fever due to Rickettsia prowazekii**
Classical typhus (fever)
Epidemic (louse-borne) typhus

A75.1   **Recrudescent typhus [Brill's disease]**
Brill-Zinsser disease

A75.2   **Typhus fever due to Rickettsia typhi**
Murine (flea-borne) typhus

A75.3   **Typhus fever due to Rickettsia tsutsugamushi**
Scrub (mite-borne) typhus
Tsutsugamushi fever

A75.9   **Typhus fever, unspecified** ▽
Typhus (fever) NOS

✓4th **A77 Spotted fever [tick-borne rickettsioses]**

A77.0   **Spotted fever due to Rickettsia rickettsii**
Rocky Mountain spotted fever
Sao Paulo fever

A77.1   **Spotted fever due to Rickettsia conorii**
African tick typhus
Boutonneuse fever
India tick typhus
Kenya tick typhus
Marseilles fever
Mediterranean tick fever

A77.2   **Spotted fever due to Rickettsia siberica**
North Asian tick fever
Siberian tick typhus

A77.3   **Spotted fever due to Rickettsia australis**
Queensland tick typhus

✓5th **A77.4**   **Ehrlichiosis**

     EXCLUDES 1   *Rickettsiosis due to Ehrlichia sennetsu (A79.81)*

     A77.40   **Ehrlichiosis, unspecified** ▽
     A77.41   **Ehrlichiosis chafeensis [E. chafeensis]**
     A77.49   **Other ehrlichiosis**

A77.8   **Other spotted fevers**

A77.9   **Spotted fever, unspecified** ▽
Tick-borne typhus NOS

A78 Q fever
Infection due to Coxiella burnetii
Nine Mile fever
Quadrilateral fever

✓4th **A79 Other rickettsioses**

A79.0   **Trench fever**
Quintan fever
Wolhynian fever

A79.1   **Rickettsialpox due to Rickettsia akari**
Kew Garden fever
Vesicular rickettsiosis

✓5th **A79.8**   **Other specified rickettsioses**

     A79.81   **Rickettsiosis due to Ehrlichia sennetsu**
     A79.89   **Other specified rickettsioses**

A79.9   **Rickettsiosis, unspecified** ▽
Rickettsial infection NOS

Viral and prion infections of the central nervous system (A80-A89)

EXCLUDES 1   *postpolio syndrome (G14)*
sequelae of poliomyelitis (B91)
sequelae of viral encephalitis (B94.1)

✓4th **A80 Acute poliomyelitis**

A80.0   **Acute paralytic poliomyelitis, vaccine-associated**

A80.1   **Acute paralytic poliomyelitis, wild virus, imported**

A80.2   **Acute paralytic poliomyelitis, wild virus, indigenous**

✓5th **A80.3**   **Acute paralytic poliomyelitis, other and unspecified**

     A80.30   **Acute paralytic poliomyelitis, unspecified** ▽
     A80.39   **Other acute paralytic poliomyelitis**

A80.4   **Acute nonparalytic poliomyelitis**

A80.9   **Acute poliomyelitis, unspecified** ▽

✓4th **A81 Atypical virus infections of central nervous system**

     INCLUDES   diseases of the central nervous system caused by prions
Use additional code to identify:
dementia with behavioral disturbance (F02.81)
dementia without behavioral disturbance (F02.80)

✓5th **A81.0**   **Creutzfeldt-Jakob disease**

     DEF: Communicable, rare spongiform encephalopathy occurring later in life with progressive destruction of the pyramidal and extrapyramidal systems eventually leading to death. Progressive dementia, wasting of muscles, tremor, and other symptoms are present.

     A81.00   **Creutzfeldt-Jakob disease, unspecified** ▽
Jakob-Creutzfeldt disease, unspecified

     A81.01   **Variant Creutzfeldt-Jakob disease**
vCJD

     A81.09   **Other Creutzfeldt-Jakob disease**
CJD
Familial Creutzfeldt-Jakob disease
Iatrogenic Creutzfeldt-Jakob disease
Sporadic Creutzfeldt-Jakob disease
Subacute spongiform encephalopathy (with dementia)

A81.1   **Subacute sclerosing panencephalitis**
Dawson's inclusion body encephalitis
Van Bogaert's sclerosing leukoencephalopathy

A81.2   **Progressive multifocal leukoencephalopathy**
Multifocal leukoencephalopathy NOS

✓5th **A81.8**   **Other atypical virus infections of central nervous system**

     A81.81   **Kuru**
     A81.82   **Gerstmann-Sträussler-Scheinker syndrome**
GSS syndrome

     A81.83   **Fatal familial insomnia**
FFI

     A81.89   **Other atypical virus infections of central nervous system**

A81.9   **Atypical virus infection of central nervous system, unspecified** ▽
Prion diseases of the central nervous system NOS

✓4th **A82 Rabies**

A82.0   **Sylvatic rabies**

A82.1   **Urban rabies**

A82.9   **Rabies, unspecified** ▽

Chapter 1. Certain Infectious and Parasitic Diseases

✓4ᵗʰ **A83 Mosquito-borne viral encephalitis**

INCLUDES   mosquito-borne viral meningoencephalitis

EXCLUDES 2   *Venezuelan equine encephalitis (A92.2)*
West Nile fever (A92.3-)
West Nile virus (A92.3-)

A83.0 Japanese encephalitis

A83.1 Western equine encephalitis

A83.2 Eastern equine encephalitis

A83.3 St Louis encephalitis

A83.4 Australian encephalitis
Kunjin virus disease

A83.5 California encephalitis
California meningoencephalitis
La Crosse encephalitis

A83.6 Rocio virus disease

A83.8 Other mosquito-borne viral encephalitis

A83.9 Mosquito-borne viral encephalitis, unspecified ▽

✓4ᵗʰ **A84 Tick-borne viral encephalitis**

INCLUDES   tick-borne viral meningoencephalitis

A84.0 Far Eastern tick-borne encephalitis [Russian spring-summer encephalitis]

A84.1 Central European tick-borne encephalitis

A84.8 Other tick-borne viral encephalitis
Louping ill
Powassan virus disease

A84.9 Tick-borne viral encephalitis, unspecified ▽

✓4ᵗʰ **A85 Other viral encephalitis, not elsewhere classified**

INCLUDES   specified viral encephalomyelitis NEC
specified viral meningoencephalitis NEC

EXCLUDES 1   *benign myalgic encephalomyelitis (G93.3)*
encephalitis due to cytomegalovirus (B25.8)
encephalitis due to herpesvirus NEC (B10.0-)
encephalitis due to herpesvirus [herpes simplex] (B00.4)
encephalitis due to measles virus (B05.0)
encephalitis due to mumps virus (B26.2)
encephalitis due to poliomyelitis virus (A80.-)
encephalitis due to zoster (B02.0)
lymphocytic choriomeningitis (A87.2)

A85.0 Enteroviral encephalitis
Enteroviral encephalomyelitis

A85.1 Adenoviral encephalitis
Adenoviral meningoencephalitis

A85.2 Arthropod-borne viral encephalitis, unspecified ▽
EXCLUDES 1   *West nile virus with encephalitis (A92.31)*

A85.8 Other specified viral encephalitis
Encephalitis lethargica
Von Economo-Cruchet disease

A86 Unspecified viral encephalitis ▽
Viral encephalomyelitis NOS
Viral meningoencephalitis NOS

✓4ᵗʰ **A87 Viral meningitis**

EXCLUDES 1   *meningitis due to herpesvirus [herpes simplex] (B00.3)*
meningitis due to measles virus (B05.1)
meningitis due to mumps virus (B26.1)
meningitis due to poliomyelitis virus (A80.-)
meningitis due to zoster (B02.1)

DEF: Meningitis: Inflammation of the meningeal layers of the brain and spine.

A87.0 Enteroviral meningitis
Coxsackievirus meningitis
Echovirus meningitis

A87.1 Adenoviral meningitis

A87.2 Lymphocytic choriomeningitis
Lymphocytic meningoencephalitis

A87.8 Other viral meningitis

A87.9 Viral meningitis, unspecified ▽

✓4ᵗʰ **A88 Other viral infections of central nervous system, not elsewhere classified**

EXCLUDES 1   *viral encephalitis NOS (A86)*
viral meningitis NOS (A87.9)

A88.0 Enteroviral exanthematous fever [Boston exanthem]

A88.1 Epidemic vertigo

A88.8 Other specified viral infections of central nervous system

A89 Unspecified viral infection of central nervous system ▽

Arthropod-borne viral fevers and viral hemorrhagic fevers (A90-A99)

A90 Dengue fever [classical dengue]
EXCLUDES 1   *dengue hemorrhagic fever (A91)*
AHA: 2016,3Q,13

A91 Dengue hemorrhagic fever

✓4ᵗʰ **A92 Other mosquito-borne viral fevers**
EXCLUDES 1   *Ross River disease (B33.1)*

A92.0 Chikungunya virus disease
Chikungunya (hemorrhagic) fever

A92.1 O'nyong-nyong fever

A92.2 Venezuelan equine fever
Venezuelan equine encephalitis
Venezuelan equine encephalomyelitis virus disease

✓5ᵗʰ **A92.3 West Nile virus infection**
West Nile fever
AHA: 2016,3Q,12

A92.30 West Nile virus infection, unspecified ▽
West Nile fever NOS
West Nile fever without complications
West Nile virus NOS

A92.31 West Nile virus infection with encephalitis
West Nile encephalitis
West Nile encephalomyelitis

A92.32 West Nile virus infection with other neurologic manifestation
Use additional code to specify the neurologic manifestation

A92.39 West Nile virus infection with other complications
Use additional code to specify the other conditions

A92.4 Rift Valley fever

A92.5 Zika virus disease
Zika virus fever
Zika virus infection
Zika NOS
EXCLUDES 1   ▶*congenital Zika virus disease (P35.4)*◀
AHA: 2016,4Q,4-7
DEF: Virus transmitted via a bite from an infected Aedes species mosquito. Common symptoms of the virus include fever, rash, joint pain, and conjunctivitis; they are usually mild in nature and may last from several days to a week. Most people who have the Zika virus do not require medical attention; however, in pregnant women, the Zika virus can cause a serious birth defect called microcephaly, as well as other severe fetal brain defects.
TIP: Assign code Z71.1, when a patient requests testing for Zika virus but in the absence of symptoms or recent exposure to the virus.

A92.8 Other specified mosquito-borne viral fevers

A92.9 Mosquito-borne viral fever, unspecified ▽

✓4ᵗʰ **A93 Other arthropod-borne viral fevers, not elsewhere classified**

A93.0 Oropouche virus disease
Oropouche fever

A93.1 Sandfly fever
Pappataci fever
Phlebotomus fever

A93.2 Colorado tick fever

A93.8 Other specified arthropod-borne viral fevers
Piry virus disease
Vesicular stomatitis virus disease [Indiana fever]

A94 Unspecified arthropod-borne viral fever ▽
Arboviral fever NOS
Arbovirus infection NOS

✓4ᵗʰ **A95 Yellow fever**

A95.0 Sylvatic yellow fever
Jungle yellow fever

A95.1 Urban yellow fever

A95.9 Yellow fever, unspecified ▽

✓4ᵗʰ **A96 Arenaviral hemorrhagic fever**

A96.0 Junin hemorrhagic fever
Argentinian hemorrhagic fever

A96.1 Machupo hemorrhagic fever
Bolivian hemorrhagic fever

A96.2 Lassa fever

A96.8 Other arenaviral hemorrhagic fevers

A96.9   **Arenaviral hemorrhagic fever, unspecified**   ▽

☑4ᵗʰ **A98**   **Other viral hemorrhagic fevers, not elsewhere classified**
- EXCLUDES 1   *chikungunya hemorrhagic fever (A92.0)*
-      *dengue hemorrhagic fever (A91)*

A98.0   **Crimean-Congo hemorrhagic fever**
- Central Asian hemorrhagic fever

A98.1   **Omsk hemorrhagic fever**

A98.2   **Kyasanur Forest disease**

A98.3   **Marburg virus disease**

A98.4   **Ebola virus disease**

A98.5   **Hemorrhagic fever with renal syndrome**
- Epidemic hemorrhagic fever
- Korean hemorrhagic fever
- Russian hemorrhagic fever
- Hantaan virus disease
- Hantavirus disease with renal manifestations
- Nephropathia epidemica
- Songo fever
- EXCLUDES 1   *hantavirus (cardio)-pulmonary syndrome (B33.4)*

A98.8   **Other specified viral hemorrhagic fevers**

A99   **Unspecified viral hemorrhagic fever**   ▽

Viral infections characterized by skin and mucous membrane lesions (B00-B09)

☑4ᵗʰ **B00**   **Herpesviral [herpes simplex] infections**
- EXCLUDES 1   *congenital herpesviral infections (P35.2)*
- EXCLUDES 2   *anogenital herpesviral infection (A60.-)*
-      *gammaherpesviral mononucleosis (B27.0-)*
-      *herpangina (B08.5)*

B00.0   **Eczema herpeticum**
- Kaposi's varicelliform eruption

B00.1   **Herpesviral vesicular dermatitis**
- Herpes simplex facialis
- Herpes simplex labialis
- Herpes simplex otitis externa
- Vesicular dermatitis of ear
- Vesicular dermatitis of lip

B00.2   **Herpesviral gingivostomatitis and pharyngotonsillitis**
- Herpesviral pharyngitis

B00.3   **Herpesviral meningitis**

B00.4   **Herpesviral encephalitis**
- Herpesviral meningoencephalitis
- Simian B disease
- EXCLUDES 1   *herpesviral encephalitis due to herpesvirus 6 and 7 (B10.01, B10.09)*
-      *non-simplex herpesviral encephalitis (B10.0-)*

☑5ᵗʰ **B00.5**   **Herpesviral ocular disease**

    B00.50   **Herpesviral ocular disease, unspecified**   ▽

    B00.51   **Herpesviral iridocyclitis**
- Herpesviral iritis
- Herpesviral uveitis, anterior

    B00.52   **Herpesviral keratitis**
- Herpesviral keratoconjunctivitis

    B00.53   **Herpesviral conjunctivitis**

    B00.59   **Other herpesviral disease of eye**
- Herpesviral dermatitis of eyelid

B00.7   **Disseminated herpesviral disease**   HCC
- Herpesviral sepsis

☑5ᵗʰ **B00.8**   **Other forms of herpesviral infections**

    B00.81   **Herpesviral hepatitis**

    B00.82   **Herpes simplex myelitis**   HCC

    B00.89   **Other herpesviral infection**
- Herpesviral whitlow

B00.9   **Herpesviral infection, unspecified**   ▽
- Herpes simplex infection NOS

☑4ᵗʰ **B01**   **Varicella [chickenpox]**

B01.0   **Varicella meningitis**

☑5ᵗʰ **B01.1**   **Varicella encephalitis, myelitis and encephalomyelitis**
- Postchickenpox encephalitis, myelitis and encephalomyelitis

    B01.11   **Varicella encephalitis and encephalomyelitis**
- Postchickenpox encephalitis and encephalomyelitis

    B01.12   **Varicella myelitis**   HCC
- Postchickenpox myelitis

B01.2   **Varicella pneumonia**

☑5ᵗʰ **B01.8**   **Varicella with other complications**

    B01.81   **Varicella keratitis**

    B01.89   **Other varicella complications**

B01.9   **Varicella without complication**   ▽
- Varicella NOS

☑4ᵗʰ **B02**   **Zoster [herpes zoster]**
- INCLUDES   shingles
-      zona

B02.0   **Zoster encephalitis**
- Zoster meningoencephalitis

B02.1   **Zoster meningitis**

☑5ᵗʰ **B02.2**   **Zoster with other nervous system involvement**

    B02.21   **Postherpetic geniculate ganglionitis**

    B02.22   **Postherpetic trigeminal neuralgia**

    B02.23   **Postherpetic polyneuropathy**

    B02.24   **Postherpetic myelitis**   HCC
- Herpes zoster myelitis

    B02.29   **Other postherpetic nervous system involvement**
- Postherpetic radiculopathy

☑5ᵗʰ **B02.3**   **Zoster ocular disease**

    B02.30   **Zoster ocular disease, unspecified**   ▽

    B02.31   **Zoster conjunctivitis**

    B02.32   **Zoster iridocyclitis**

    B02.33   **Zoster keratitis**
- Herpes zoster keratoconjunctivitis

    B02.34   **Zoster scleritis**

    B02.39   **Other herpes zoster eye disease**
- Zoster blepharitis

B02.7   **Disseminated zoster**

B02.8   **Zoster with other complications**
- Herpes zoster otitis externa

B02.9   **Zoster without complications**   ▽
- Zoster NOS

B03   **Smallpox**
- NOTE   In 1980 the 33rd World Health Assembly declared that smallpox had been eradicated.
-      The classification is maintained for surveillance purposes.

B04   **Monkeypox**

☑4ᵗʰ **B05**   **Measles**
- INCLUDES   morbilli
- EXCLUDES 1   *subacute sclerosing panencephalitis (A81.1)*

B05.0   **Measles complicated by encephalitis**
- Postmeasles encephalitis

B05.1   **Measles complicated by meningitis**
- Postmeasles meningitis

B05.2   **Measles complicated by pneumonia**
- Postmeasles pneumonia

B05.3   **Measles complicated by otitis media**
- Postmeasles otitis media

B05.4   **Measles with intestinal complications**

☑5ᵗʰ **B05.8**   **Measles with other complications**

    B05.81   **Measles keratitis and keratoconjunctivitis**

    B05.89   **Other measles complications**

B05.9   **Measles without complication**   ▽
- Measles NOS

☑4ᵗʰ **B06**   **Rubella [German measles]**
- EXCLUDES 1   *congenital rubella (P35.0)*
- **DEF:** Highly contagious virus in which the symptoms are mild and short-lived in most people. Rubella during pregnancy, however, can result in abortion, stillbirth, or congenital defects.

☑5ᵗʰ **B06.0**   **Rubella with neurological complications**

    B06.00   **Rubella with neurological complication, unspecified**   ▽

    B06.01   **Rubella encephalitis**
- Rubella meningoencephalitis

    B06.02   **Rubella meningitis**

    B06.09   **Other neurological complications of rubella**

☑5ᵗʰ **B06.8**   **Rubella with other complications**

    B06.81   **Rubella pneumonia**

    B06.82   **Rubella arthritis**   HCC

    B06.89   **Other rubella complications**

☑ Additional Character Req   ☑ 7ᵗʰ Placeholder Alert   Manifestation   ▽ Unspecified   ►◄ Revised Text   ● New Code   ▲ Revised Code Title

ICD-10-CM 2019   447

B06.9 Rubella without complication ▽
Rubella NOS

✓4ᵗʰ **B07 Viral warts**
> INCLUDES   verruca simplex
> verruca vulgaris
> viral warts due to human papillomavirus
> EXCLUDES 2   *anogenital (venereal) warts (A63.0)*
> *papilloma of bladder (D41.4)*
> *papilloma of cervix (D26.0)*
> *papilloma larynx (D14.1)*

B07.0 Plantar wart
Verruca plantaris

B07.8 Other viral warts
Common wart
Flat wart
Verruca plana

B07.9 Viral wart, unspecified ▽

✓4ᵗʰ **B08 Other viral infections characterized by skin and mucous membrane lesions, not elsewhere classified**
> EXCLUDES 1   *vesicular stomatitis virus disease (A93.8)*

✓5ᵗʰ **B08.0 Other orthopoxvirus infections**
> EXCLUDES 2   *monkeypox (B04)*

✓6ᵗʰ **B08.01 Cowpox and vaccinia not from vaccine**

B08.010 Cowpox
> **DEF:** Disease contracted by milking infected cows. The vesicles usually appear on the fingers, hands, and adjacent areas and usually disappear without scarring. Other symptoms include local edema, lymphangitis, and regional lymphadenitis with or without fever.

B08.011 Vaccinia not from vaccine
> EXCLUDES 1   *vaccinia (from vaccination) (generalized) (T88.1)*

B08.02 Orf virus disease
Contagious pustular dermatitis
Ecthyma contagiosum

B08.03 Pseudocowpox [milker's node]

B08.04 Paravaccinia, unspecified ▽

B08.09 Other orthopoxvirus infections
Orthopoxvirus infection NOS

B08.1 Molluscum contagiosum
> **DEF:** Benign poxvirus infection causing small bumps on the skin or conjunctiva and is transmitted by close contact.

✓5ᵗʰ **B08.2 Exanthema subitum [sixth disease]**
Roseola infantum

B08.20 Exanthema subitum [sixth disease], unspecified P ▽
Roseola infantum, unspecified

B08.21 Exanthema subitum [sixth disease] due to human herpesvirus 6 P
Roseola infantum due to human herpesvirus 6

B08.22 Exanthema subitum [sixth disease] due to human herpesvirus 7 P
Roseola infantum due to human herpesvirus 7

B08.3 Erythema infectiosum [fifth disease]
> **DEF:** Infection with human parvovirus B19, mainly occurring in children. Symptoms include a low-grade fever, malaise, or a "cold" a few days before the appearance of a mild rash illness that presents as a "slapped-cheek" rash on the face and a lacy red rash on the trunk and limbs.

B08.4 Enteroviral vesicular stomatitis with exanthem
Hand, foot and mouth disease

B08.5 Enteroviral vesicular pharyngitis
Herpangina
> **DEF:** Acute infectious Coxsackie virus infection causing throat lesions, fever, and vomiting that generally affects children in the summer.

✓5ᵗʰ **B08.6 Parapoxvirus infections**

B08.60 Parapoxvirus infection, unspecified ▽
B08.61 Bovine stomatitis
B08.62 Sealpox
B08.69 Other parapoxvirus infections

✓5ᵗʰ **B08.7 Yatapoxvirus infections**

B08.70 Yatapoxvirus infection, unspecified ▽
B08.71 Tanapox virus disease

B08.72 Yaba pox virus disease
Yaba monkey tumor disease

B08.79 Other yatapoxvirus infections

B08.8 Other specified viral infections characterized by skin and mucous membrane lesions
Enteroviral lymphonodular pharyngitis
Foot-and-mouth disease
Poxvirus NEC

B09 Unspecified viral infection characterized by skin and mucous membrane lesions ▽
Viral enanthema NOS
Viral exanthema NOS

Other human herpesviruses (B10)

✓4ᵗʰ **B10 Other human herpesviruses**
> EXCLUDES 2   *cytomegalovirus (B25.9)*
> *Epstein-Barr virus (B27.0-)*
> *herpes NOS (B00.9)*
> *herpes simplex (B00.-)*
> *herpes zoster (B02.-)*
> *human herpesvirus NOS (B00.-)*
> *human herpesvirus 1 and 2 (B00.-)*
> *human herpesvirus 3 (B01.-, B02.-)*
> *human herpesvirus 4 (B27.0-)*
> *human herpesvirus 5 (B25.-)*
> *varicella (B01.-)*
> *zoster (B02.-)*

✓5ᵗʰ **B10.0 Other human herpesvirus encephalitis**
> EXCLUDES 2   *herpes encephalitis NOS (B00.4)*
> *herpes simplex encephalitis (B00.4)*
> *human herpesvirus encephalitis (B00.4)*
> *simian B herpes virus encephalitis (B00.4)*

B10.01 Human herpesvirus 6 encephalitis
B10.09 Other human herpesvirus encephalitis
Human herpesvirus 7 encephalitis

✓5ᵗʰ **B10.8 Other human herpesvirus infection**

B10.81 Human herpesvirus 6 infection
B10.82 Human herpesvirus 7 infection
B10.89 Other human herpesvirus infection
Human herpesvirus 8 infection
Kaposi's sarcoma-associated herpesvirus infection

Viral hepatitis (B15-B19)

> EXCLUDES 1   *sequelae of viral hepatitis (B94.2)*
> EXCLUDES 2   *cytomegaloviral hepatitis (B25.1)*
> *herpesviral [herpes simplex] hepatitis (B00.81)*

DEF: Hepatitis A: HAV infection that is self-limiting with flulike symptoms. Transmission is fecal-oral.
DEF: Hepatitis B: HBV infection that can be chronic and systemic. Transmission is bodily fluids.
DEF: Hepatitis C: HCV infection that can be chronic and systemic. Transmission is blood transfusion and unidentified agents.
DEF: Hepatitis D (delta): HDV that occurs only in the presence of hepatitis B virus. Transmission is contaminated blood in contact with mucous membranes.
DEF: Hepatitis E: HEV is an epidemic form. Transmission is fecal-oral, most often from contaminated water.

✓4ᵗʰ **B15 Acute hepatitis A**

B15.0 Hepatitis A with hepatic coma
B15.9 Hepatitis A without hepatic coma
Hepatitis A (acute)(viral) NOS

✓4ᵗʰ **B16 Acute hepatitis B**
> **AHA:** 2016,3Q,13

B16.0 Acute hepatitis B with delta-agent with hepatic coma
B16.1 Acute hepatitis B with delta-agent without hepatic coma
B16.2 Acute hepatitis B without delta-agent with hepatic coma
B16.9 Acute hepatitis B without delta-agent and without hepatic coma
Hepatitis B (acute) (viral) NOS

✓4ᵗʰ **B17 Other acute viral hepatitis**

B17.0 Acute delta-(super) infection of hepatitis B carrier

✓5ᵗʰ **B17.1 Acute hepatitis C**

B17.10 Acute hepatitis C without hepatic coma
Acute hepatitis C NOS

B17.11 Acute hepatitis C with hepatic coma

B17.2 Acute hepatitis E

B17.8   **Other specified acute viral hepatitis**
Hepatitis non-A non-B (acute) (viral) NEC

B17.9   **Acute viral hepatitis, unspecified** ▽
Acute hepatitis NOS
Acute infectious hepatitis NOS

✓4ᵗʰ **B18**   **Chronic viral hepatitis**
   INCLUDES   carrier of viral hepatitis
   AHA: 2017,1Q,41

B18.0   **Chronic viral hepatitis B with delta-agent**   HCC

B18.1   **Chronic viral hepatitis B without delta-agent**   HCC
Carrier of viral hepatitis B
Chronic (viral) hepatitis B

B18.2   **Chronic viral hepatitis C**   HCC
Carrier of viral hepatitis C
AHA: 2018,1Q,4

B18.8   **Other chronic viral hepatitis**   HCC
Carrier of other viral hepatitis

B18.9   **Chronic viral hepatitis, unspecified**   HCC ▽
Carrier of unspecified viral hepatitis

✓4ᵗʰ **B19**   **Unspecified viral hepatitis**

B19.0   **Unspecified viral hepatitis with hepatic coma** ▽

✓5ᵗʰ **B19.1**   **Unspecified viral hepatitis B**

B19.10   **Unspecified viral hepatitis B without hepatic coma** ▽
Unspecified viral hepatitis B NOS

B19.11   **Unspecified viral hepatitis B with hepatic coma** ▽

✓5ᵗʰ **B19.2**   **Unspecified viral hepatitis C**

B19.20   **Unspecified viral hepatitis C without hepatic coma** ▽
Viral hepatitis C NOS

B19.21   **Unspecified viral hepatitis C with hepatic coma** ▽

B19.9   **Unspecified viral hepatitis without hepatic coma** ▽
Viral hepatitis NOS

Human immunodeficiency virus [HIV] disease (B20)

B20   **Human immunodeficiency virus [HIV] disease**   HCC
   INCLUDES   acquired immune deficiency syndrome [AIDS]
     AIDS-related complex [ARC]
     HIV infection, symptomatic
Code first Human immunodeficiency virus [HIV] disease complicating pregnancy, childbirth and the puerperium, if applicable (O98.7-)
Use additional code(s) to identify all manifestations of HIV infection
   EXCLUDES 1   *asymptomatic human immunodeficiency virus [HIV] infection status (Z21)*
     exposure to HIV virus (Z20.6)
     inconclusive serologic evidence of HIV (R75)

Other viral diseases (B25-B34)

✓4ᵗʰ **B25**   **Cytomegaloviral disease**
   EXCLUDES 1   *congenital cytomegalovirus infection (P35.1)*
     cytomegaloviral mononucleosis (B27.1-)

B25.0   **Cytomegaloviral pneumonitis**   HCC
B25.1   **Cytomegaloviral hepatitis**   HCC
B25.2   **Cytomegaloviral pancreatitis**   HCC
B25.8   **Other cytomegaloviral diseases**   HCC
Cytomegaloviral encephalitis

B25.9   **Cytomegaloviral disease, unspecified**   HCC ▽

✓4ᵗʰ **B26**   **Mumps**
   INCLUDES   epidemic parotitis
     infectious parotitis

B26.0   **Mumps orchitis**   ♂
B26.1   **Mumps meningitis**
B26.2   **Mumps encephalitis**
B26.3   **Mumps pancreatitis**

✓5ᵗʰ **B26.8**   **Mumps with other complications**

B26.81   **Mumps hepatitis**
B26.82   **Mumps myocarditis**
B26.83   **Mumps nephritis**
B26.84   **Mumps polyneuropathy**
B26.85   **Mumps arthritis**   HCC
B26.89   **Other mumps complications**

B26.9   **Mumps without complication** ▽
Mumps NOS
Mumps parotitis NOS

✓4ᵗʰ **B27**   **Infectious mononucleosis**
   INCLUDES   glandular fever
     monocytic angina
     Pfeiffer's disease

✓5ᵗʰ **B27.0**   **Gammaherpesviral mononucleosis**
Mononucleosis due to Epstein-Barr virus

B27.00   **Gammaherpesviral mononucleosis without complication**
B27.01   **Gammaherpesviral mononucleosis with polyneuropathy**
B27.02   **Gammaherpesviral mononucleosis with meningitis**
B27.09   **Gammaherpesviral mononucleosis with other complications**
Hepatomegaly in gammaherpesviral mononucleosis

✓5ᵗʰ **B27.1**   **Cytomegaloviral mononucleosis**

B27.10   **Cytomegaloviral mononucleosis without complications**
B27.11   **Cytomegaloviral mononucleosis with polyneuropathy**
B27.12   **Cytomegaloviral mononucleosis with meningitis**
B27.19   **Cytomegaloviral mononucleosis with other complication**
Hepatomegaly in cytomegaloviral mononucleosis

✓5ᵗʰ **B27.8**   **Other infectious mononucleosis**

B27.80   **Other infectious mononucleosis without complication**
B27.81   **Other infectious mononucleosis with polyneuropathy**
B27.82   **Other infectious mononucleosis with meningitis**
B27.89   **Other infectious mononucleosis with other complication**
Hepatomegaly in other infectious mononucleosis

✓5ᵗʰ **B27.9**   **Infectious mononucleosis, unspecified**

B27.90   **Infectious mononucleosis, unspecified without complication** ▽
B27.91   **Infectious mononucleosis, unspecified with polyneuropathy** ▽
B27.92   **Infectious mononucleosis, unspecified with meningitis** ▽
B27.99   **Infectious mononucleosis, unspecified with other complication** ▽
Hepatomegaly in unspecified infectious mononucleosis

✓4ᵗʰ **B30**   **Viral conjunctivitis**
   EXCLUDES 1   *herpesviral [herpes simplex] ocular disease (B00.5)*
     ocular zoster (B02.3)

Viral Conjunctivitis

Normal conjunctiva

Inflamed conjunctiva

B30.0   **Keratoconjunctivitis due to adenovirus**
Epidemic keratoconjunctivitis
Shipyard eye

B30.1   **Conjunctivitis due to adenovirus**
     Acute adenoviral follicular conjunctivitis
     Swimming-pool conjunctivitis

B30.2   **Viral pharyngoconjunctivitis**

B30.3   **Acute epidemic hemorrhagic conjunctivitis (enteroviral)**
     Conjunctivitis due to coxsackievirus 24
     Conjunctivitis due to enterovirus 70
     Hemorrhagic conjunctivitis (acute)(epidemic)

B30.8   **Other viral conjunctivitis**
     Newcastle conjunctivitis

B30.9   **Viral conjunctivitis, unspecified**   ▽

✓4ᵗʰ **B33   Other viral diseases, not elsewhere classified**

B33.0   **Epidemic myalgia**
     Bornholm disease

B33.1   **Ross River disease**
     Epidemic polyarthritis and exanthema
     Ross River fever

✓5ᵗʰ **B33.2**   **Viral carditis**
     Coxsackie (virus) carditis

     B33.20   **Viral carditis, unspecified**   ▽
     B33.21   **Viral endocarditis**
     B33.22   **Viral myocarditis**
     B33.23   **Viral pericarditis**
     B33.24   **Viral cardiomyopathy**   HCC

B33.3   **Retrovirus infections, not elsewhere classified**
     Retrovirus infection NOS

B33.4   **Hantavirus (cardio)-pulmonary syndrome [HPS] [HCPS]**
     Hantavirus disease with pulmonary manifestations
     Sin nombre virus disease
     Use additional code to identify any associated acute kidney failure (N17.9)
     EXCLUDES 1   *hantavirus disease with renal manifestations (A98.5)*
               hemorrhagic fever with renal manifestations (A98.5)

B33.8   **Other specified viral diseases**
     EXCLUDES 1   *anogenital human papillomavirus infection (A63.0)*
               viral warts due to human papillomavirus infection (B07)

✓4ᵗʰ **B34   Viral infection of unspecified site**
     EXCLUDES 1   *anogenital human papillomavirus infection (A63.0)*
               cytomegaloviral disease NOS (B25.9)
               herpesvirus [herpes simplex] infection NOS (B00.9)
               retrovirus infection NOS (B33.3)
               viral agents as the cause of diseases classified elsewhere (B97.-)
               viral warts due to human papillomavirus infection (B07)

B34.0   **Adenovirus infection, unspecified**   ▽
B34.1   **Enterovirus infection, unspecified**   ▽
     Coxsackievirus infection NOS
     Echovirus infection NOS

B34.2   **Coronavirus infection, unspecified**   ▽
     EXCLUDES 1   *pneumonia due to SARS-associated coronavirus (J12.81)*

B34.3   **Parvovirus infection, unspecified**   ▽
B34.4   **Papovavirus infection, unspecified**   ▽
B34.8   **Other viral infections of unspecified site**   ▽
B34.9   **Viral infection, unspecified**   ▽
     Viremia NOS
     AHA: 2016,3Q,10

Mycoses (B35-B49)

EXCLUDES 2   *hypersensitivity pneumonitis due to organic dust (J67.-)*
               mycosis fungoides (C84.0-)

✓4ᵗʰ **B35   Dermatophytosis**
     INCLUDES   favus
              infections due to species of Epidermophyton, Micro-sporum and Trichophyton
              tinea, any type except those in B36.-
     DEF: Contagious superficial fungal infection of the skin that invades and grows in dead keratin.

B35.0   **Tinea barbae and tinea capitis**
     Beard ringworm
     Kerion
     Scalp ringworm
     Sycosis, mycotic

B35.1   **Tinea unguium**
     Dermatophytic onychia
     Dermatophytosis of nail
     Onychomycosis
     Ringworm of nails

B35.2   **Tinea manuum**
     Dermatophytosis of hand
     Hand ringworm

B35.3   **Tinea pedis**
     Athlete's foot
     Dermatophytosis of foot
     Foot ringworm

B35.4   **Tinea corporis**
     Ringworm of the body

B35.5   **Tinea imbricata**
     Tokelau

B35.6   **Tinea cruris**
     Dhobi itch
     Groin ringworm
     Jock itch

B35.8   **Other dermatophytoses**
     Disseminated dermatophytosis
     Granulomatous dermatophytosis

B35.9   **Dermatophytosis, unspecified**   ▽
     Ringworm NOS

✓4ᵗʰ **B36   Other superficial mycoses**

B36.0   **Pityriasis versicolor**
     Tinea flava
     Tinea versicolor

B36.1   **Tinea nigra**
     Keratomycosis nigricans palmaris
     Microsporosis nigra
     Pityriasis nigra

B36.2   **White piedra**
     Tinea blanca

B36.3   **Black piedra**

B36.8   **Other specified superficial mycoses**

B36.9   **Superficial mycosis, unspecified**   ▽

✓4ᵗʰ **B37   Candidiasis**
     INCLUDES   candidosis
              moniliasis
     EXCLUDES 1   *neonatal candidiasis (P37.5)*

B37.0   **Candidal stomatitis**
     Oral thrush

B37.1   **Pulmonary candidiasis**   HCC
     Candidal bronchitis
     Candidal pneumonia

B37.2   **Candidiasis of skin and nail**
     Candidal onychia
     Candidal paronychia
     EXCLUDES 2   *diaper dermatitis (L22)*

B37.3   **Candidiasis of vulva and vagina**   ♀
     Candidal vulvovaginitis
     Monilial vulvovaginitis
     Vaginal thrush

✓5ᵗʰ **B37.4**   **Candidiasis of other urogenital sites**

     B37.41   **Candidal cystitis and urethritis**
     B37.42   **Candidal balanitis**   ♂
     B37.49   **Other urogenital candidiasis**
             Candidal pyelonephritis

B37.5   **Candidal meningitis**
B37.6   **Candidal endocarditis**
B37.7   **Candidal sepsis**   HCC
     Disseminated candidiasis
     Systemic candidiasis
     AHA: 2014,4Q,46

✓5ᵗʰ **B37.8**   **Candidiasis of other sites**

     B37.81   **Candidal esophagitis**   HCC
     B37.82   **Candidal enteritis**
             Candidal proctitis
     B37.83   **Candidal cheilitis**
     B37.84   **Candidal otitis externa**
     B37.89   **Other sites of candidiasis**
             Candidal osteomyelitis

B37.9 Candidiasis, unspecified ▽
Thrush NOS

√4ᵗʰ **B38 Coccidioidomycosis**

B38.0 Acute pulmonary coccidioidomycosis HCC
B38.1 Chronic pulmonary coccidioidomycosis HCC
B38.2 Pulmonary coccidioidomycosis, unspecified HCC ▽
B38.3 Cutaneous coccidioidomycosis
B38.4 Coccidioidomycosis meningitis
DEF: *Coccidioides immitis* infection of the lining of the brain and/or spinal cord.
B38.7 Disseminated coccidioidomycosis
Generalized coccidioidomycosis
√5ᵗʰ **B38.8 Other forms of coccidioidomycosis**
B38.81 Prostatic coccidioidomycosis ♂
B38.89 Other forms of coccidioidomycosis
B38.9 Coccidioidomycosis, unspecified ▽

√4ᵗʰ **B39 Histoplasmosis**
Code first associated AIDS (B20)
Use additional code for any associated manifestations, such as:
endocarditis (I39)
meningitis (G02)
pericarditis (I32)
▶retinitis◀ (H32)
DEF: Type of lung infection caused by breathing in fungal spores often found in the droppings of bats and birds or soil contaminated by their droppings.

Histoplasmosis

Histoplasma capsulatum spores

Spores

B39.0 Acute pulmonary histoplasmosis capsulati HCC
B39.1 Chronic pulmonary histoplasmosis capsulati HCC
B39.2 Pulmonary histoplasmosis capsulati, unspecified HCC ▽
B39.3 Disseminated histoplasmosis capsulati
Generalized histoplasmosis capsulati
B39.4 Histoplasmosis capsulati, unspecified ▽
American histoplasmosis
B39.5 Histoplasmosis duboisii
African histoplasmosis
B39.9 Histoplasmosis, unspecified ▽

√4ᵗʰ **B40 Blastomycosis**
EXCLUDES 1 Brazilian blastomycosis (B41.-)
keloidal blastomycosis (B48.0)
B40.0 Acute pulmonary blastomycosis HCC
B40.1 Chronic pulmonary blastomycosis HCC
B40.2 Pulmonary blastomycosis, unspecified HCC ▽
B40.3 Cutaneous blastomycosis
B40.7 Disseminated blastomycosis
Generalized blastomycosis

√5ᵗʰ **B40.8 Other forms of blastomycosis**
B40.81 Blastomycotic meningoencephalitis
Meningomyelitis due to blastomycosis
B40.89 Other forms of blastomycosis
B40.9 Blastomycosis, unspecified ▽

√4ᵗʰ **B41 Paracoccidioidomycosis**
INCLUDES Brazilian blastomycosis
Lutz' disease
B41.0 Pulmonary paracoccidioidomycosis HCC
B41.7 Disseminated paracoccidioidomycosis
Generalized paracoccidioidomycosis
B41.8 Other forms of paracoccidioidomycosis
B41.9 Paracoccidioidomycosis, unspecified ▽

√4ᵗʰ **B42 Sporotrichosis**
B42.0 Pulmonary sporotrichosis
B42.1 Lymphocutaneous sporotrichosis
B42.7 Disseminated sporotrichosis
Generalized sporotrichosis
√5ᵗʰ **B42.8 Other forms of sporotrichosis**
B42.81 Cerebral sporotrichosis
Meningitis due to sporotrichosis
B42.82 Sporotrichosis arthritis HCC
B42.89 Other forms of sporotrichosis
B42.9 Sporotrichosis, unspecified ▽

√4ᵗʰ **B43 Chromomycosis and pheomycotic abscess**
B43.0 Cutaneous chromomycosis
Dermatitis verrucosa
B43.1 Pheomycotic brain abscess
Cerebral chromomycosis
B43.2 Subcutaneous pheomycotic abscess and cyst
B43.8 Other forms of chromomycosis
B43.9 Chromomycosis, unspecified ▽

√4ᵗʰ **B44 Aspergillosis**
INCLUDES aspergilloma
B44.0 Invasive pulmonary aspergillosis HCC
B44.1 Other pulmonary aspergillosis HCC
B44.2 Tonsillar aspergillosis HCC
B44.7 Disseminated aspergillosis HCC
Generalized aspergillosis
√5ᵗʰ **B44.8 Other forms of aspergillosis**
B44.81 Allergic bronchopulmonary aspergillosis HCC
B44.89 Other forms of aspergillosis HCC
B44.9 Aspergillosis, unspecified HCC ▽

√4ᵗʰ **B45 Cryptococcosis**
B45.0 Pulmonary cryptococcosis HCC
B45.1 Cerebral cryptococcosis HCC
Cryptococcal meningitis
Cryptococcosis meningocerebralis
B45.2 Cutaneous cryptococcosis HCC
B45.3 Osseous cryptococcosis HCC
B45.7 Disseminated cryptococcosis HCC
Generalized cryptococcosis
B45.8 Other forms of cryptococcosis HCC
B45.9 Cryptococcosis, unspecified HCC ▽

√4ᵗʰ **B46 Zygomycosis**
B46.0 Pulmonary mucormycosis HCC
B46.1 Rhinocerebral mucormycosis HCC
B46.2 Gastrointestinal mucormycosis HCC
B46.3 Cutaneous mucormycosis HCC
Subcutaneous mucormycosis
B46.4 Disseminated mucormycosis
Generalized mucormycosis
B46.5 Mucormycosis, unspecified HCC ▽
B46.8 Other zygomycoses HCC
Entomophthoromycosis
B46.9 Zygomycosis, unspecified HCC ▽
Phycomycosis NOS

√4ᵗʰ **B47 Mycetoma**
B47.0 Eumycetoma
Madura foot, mycotic
Maduromycosis
B47.1 Actinomycetoma

☑ Additional Character Req   √x7ᵗʰ Placeholder Alert   Manifestation   ▽ Unspecified   ▶◀ Revised Text   ● New Code   ▲ Revised Code Title

B47.9 **Mycetoma, unspecified**   ▽
Madura foot NOS

✓4ᵗʰ **B48 Other mycoses, not elsewhere classified**

     B48.0 **Lobomycosis**
Keloidal blastomycosis
Lobo's disease

     B48.1 **Rhinosporidiosis**

     B48.2 **Allescheriasis**
Infection due to Pseudallescheria boydii
    EXCLUDES 1   *eumycetoma (B47.0)*

     B48.3 **Geotrichosis**
Geotrichum stomatitis

     B48.4 **Penicillosis**   HCC

     B48.8 **Other specified mycoses**   HCC
Adiaspiromycosis
Infection of tissue and organs by Alternaria
Infection of tissue and organs by Drechslera
Infection of tissue and organs by Fusarium
Infection of tissue and organs by saprophytic fungi NEC
AHA: 2014,4Q,46; 2014,2Q,13

B49 Unspecified mycosis   ▽
Fungemia NOS

Protozoal diseases (B50-B64)

    EXCLUDES 1   *amebiasis (A06.-)*
other protozoal intestinal diseases (A07.-)

✓4ᵗʰ **B50 Plasmodium falciparum malaria**
    INCLUDES   mixed infections of Plasmodium falciparum with any other Plasmodium species

     B50.0 **Plasmodium falciparum malaria with cerebral complications**
Cerebral malaria NOS

     B50.8 **Other severe and complicated Plasmodium falciparum malaria**
Severe or complicated Plasmodium falciparum malaria NOS

     B50.9 **Plasmodium falciparum malaria, unspecified**   ▽

✓4ᵗʰ **B51 Plasmodium vivax malaria**
    INCLUDES   mixed infections of Plasmodium vivax with other Plasmodium species, except Plasmodium falciparum
    EXCLUDES 1   ►*Plasmodium vivax with Plasmodium falciparum*◄ *(B50.-)*

     B51.0 **Plasmodium vivax malaria with rupture of spleen**

     B51.8 **Plasmodium vivax malaria with other complications**

     B51.9 **Plasmodium vivax malaria without complication**   ▽
Plasmodium vivax malaria NOS

✓4ᵗʰ **B52 Plasmodium malariae malaria**
    INCLUDES   mixed infections of Plasmodium malariae with other Plasmodium species, except Plasmodium falciparum and Plasmodium vivax
    EXCLUDES 1   *Plasmodium falciparum (B50.-)*
Plasmodium vivax (B51.-)

     B52.0 **Plasmodium malariae malaria with nephropathy**

     B52.8 **Plasmodium malariae malaria with other complications**

     B52.9 **Plasmodium malariae malaria without complication**   ▽
Plasmodium malariae malaria NOS

✓4ᵗʰ **B53 Other specified malaria**

     B53.0 **Plasmodium ovale malaria**
    EXCLUDES 1   *Plasmodium ovale with Plasmodium falciparum (B50.-)*
Plasmodium ovale with Plasmodium malariae (B52.-)
Plasmodium ovale with Plasmodium vivax (B51.-)

     B53.1 **Malaria due to simian plasmodia**
    EXCLUDES 1   *malaria due to simian plasmodia with Plasmodium falciparum (B50.-)*
malaria due to simian plasmodia with Plasmodium malariae (B52.-)
malaria due to simian plasmodia with Plasmodium ovale (B53.0)
malaria due to simian plasmodia with Plasmodium vivax (B51.-)

     B53.8 **Other malaria, not elsewhere classified**

B54 Unspecified malaria   ▽

✓4ᵗʰ **B55 Leishmaniasis**

     B55.0 **Visceral leishmaniasis**
Kala-azar
Post-kala-azar dermal leishmaniasis

     B55.1 **Cutaneous leishmaniasis**

     B55.2 **Mucocutaneous leishmaniasis**

     B55.9 **Leishmaniasis, unspecified**   ▽

✓4ᵗʰ **B56 African trypanosomiasis**

     B56.0 **Gambiense trypanosomiasis**
Infection due to Trypanosoma brucei gambiense
West African sleeping sickness

     B56.1 **Rhodesiense trypanosomiasis**
East African sleeping sickness
Infection due to Trypanosoma brucei rhodesiense

     B56.9 **African trypanosomiasis, unspecified**   ▽
Sleeping sickness NOS

✓4ᵗʰ **B57 Chagas' disease**
    INCLUDES   American trypanosomiasis
infection due to Trypanosoma cruzi

     B57.0 **Acute Chagas' disease with heart involvement**
Acute Chagas' disease with myocarditis

     B57.1 **Acute Chagas' disease without heart involvement**
Acute Chagas' disease NOS

     B57.2 **Chagas' disease (chronic) with heart involvement**
American trypanosomiasis
Chagas' disease (chronic) NOS
Chagas' disease (chronic) with myocarditis
Trypanosomiasis NOS

✓5ᵗʰ   B57.3 **Chagas' disease (chronic) with digestive system involvement**

         B57.30 **Chagas' disease with digestive system involvement, unspecified**   ▽

         B57.31 **Megaesophagus in Chagas' disease**

         B57.32 **Megacolon in Chagas' disease**

         B57.39 **Other digestive system involvement in Chagas' disease**

✓5ᵗʰ   B57.4 **Chagas' disease (chronic) with nervous system involvement**

         B57.40 **Chagas' disease with nervous system involvement, unspecified**   ▽

         B57.41 **Meningitis in Chagas' disease**

         B57.42 **Meningoencephalitis in Chagas' disease**

         B57.49 **Other nervous system involvement in Chagas' disease**

     B57.5 **Chagas' disease (chronic) with other organ involvement**

✓4ᵗʰ **B58 Toxoplasmosis**
    INCLUDES   infection due to Toxoplasma gondii
    EXCLUDES 1   *congenital toxoplasmosis (P37.1)*

✓5ᵗʰ   B58.0 **Toxoplasma oculopathy**

         B58.00 **Toxoplasma oculopathy, unspecified**   ▽

         B58.01 **Toxoplasma chorioretinitis**

         B58.09 **Other toxoplasma oculopathy**
Toxoplasma uveitis

     B58.1 **Toxoplasma hepatitis**

     B58.2 **Toxoplasma meningoencephalitis**   HCC

     B58.3 **Pulmonary toxoplasmosis**   HCC

✓5ᵗʰ   B58.8 **Toxoplasmosis with other organ involvement**

         B58.81 **Toxoplasma myocarditis**

         B58.82 **Toxoplasma myositis**

         B58.83 **Toxoplasma tubulo-interstitial nephropathy**
Toxoplasma pyelonephritis

         B58.89 **Toxoplasmosis with other organ involvement**

     B58.9 **Toxoplasmosis, unspecified**   ▽

B59 Pneumocystosis   HCC
Pneumonia due to Pneumocystis carinii
Pneumonia due to Pneumocystis jiroveci

✓4ᵗʰ **B60 Other protozoal diseases, not elsewhere classified**
    EXCLUDES 1   *cryptosporidiosis (A07.2)*
intestinal microsporidiosis (A07.8)
isosporiasis (A07.3)

     B60.0 **Babesiosis**
Piroplasmosis

✓5ᵗʰ   B60.1 **Acanthamebiasis**

         B60.10 **Acanthamebiasis, unspecified**   ▽

         B60.11 **Meningoencephalitis due to Acanthamoeba (culbertsoni)**

B60.12 Conjunctivitis due to Acanthamoeba
B60.13 Keratoconjunctivitis due to Acanthamoeba
B60.19 Other acanthamebic disease
B60.2 Naegleriasis
Primary amebic meningoencephalitis
B60.8 Other specified protozoal diseases
Microsporidiosis

B64 Unspecified protozoal disease ▽

Helminthiases (B65-B83)

✓4ᵗʰ **B65 Schistosomiasis [bilharziasis]**
[INCLUDES] snail fever
B65.0 Schistosomiasis due to Schistosoma haematobium [urinary schistosomiasis]
B65.1 Schistosomiasis due to Schistosoma mansoni [intestinal schistosomiasis]
B65.2 Schistosomiasis due to Schistosoma japonicum
Asiatic schistosomiasis
B65.3 Cercarial dermatitis
Swimmer's itch
B65.8 Other schistosomiasis
Infection due to Schistosoma intercalatum
Infection due to Schistosoma mattheei
Infection due to Schistosoma mekongi
B65.9 Schistosomiasis, unspecified ▽

✓4ᵗʰ **B66 Other fluke infections**
B66.0 Opisthorchiasis
Infection due to cat liver fluke
Infection due to Opisthorchis (felineus)(viverrini)
B66.1 Clonorchiasis
Chinese liver fluke disease
Infection due to Clonorchis sinensis
Oriental liver fluke disease
B66.2 Dicroceliasis
Infection due to Dicrocoelium dendriticum
Lancet fluke infection
B66.3 Fascioliasis
Infection due to Fasciola gigantica
Infection due to Fasciola hepatica
Infection due to Fasciola indica
Sheep liver fluke disease
B66.4 Paragonimiasis HCC
Infection due to Paragonimus species
Lung fluke disease
Pulmonary distomiasis
B66.5 Fasciolopsiasis
Infection due to Fasciolopsis buski
Intestinal distomiasis
B66.8 Other specified fluke infections
Echinostomiasis
Heterophyiasis
Metagonimiasis
Nanophyetiasis
Watsoniasis
B66.9 Fluke infection, unspecified ▽

✓4ᵗʰ **B67 Echinococcosis**
[INCLUDES] hydatidosis
B67.0 Echinococcus granulosus infection of liver
B67.1 Echinococcus granulosus infection of lung HCC
B67.2 Echinococcus granulosus infection of bone
✓5ᵗʰ **B67.3 Echinococcus granulosus infection, other and multiple sites**
B67.31 Echinococcus granulosus infection, thyroid gland
B67.32 Echinococcus granulosus infection, multiple sites
B67.39 Echinococcus granulosus infection, other sites
B67.4 Echinococcus granulosus infection, unspecified ▽
Dog tapeworm (infection)
B67.5 Echinococcus multilocularis infection of liver
✓5ᵗʰ **B67.6 Echinococcus multilocularis infection, other and multiple sites**
B67.61 Echinococcus multilocularis infection, multiple sites
B67.69 Echinococcus multilocularis infection, other sites
B67.7 Echinococcus multilocularis infection, unspecified ▽
B67.8 Echinococcosis, unspecified, of liver ▽

✓5ᵗʰ **B67.9 Echinococcosis, other and unspecified**
B67.90 Echinococcosis, unspecified ▽
Echinococcosis NOS
B67.99 Other echinococcosis

✓4ᵗʰ **B68 Taeniasis**
[EXCLUDES 1] cysticercosis (B69.-)
B68.0 Taenia solium taeniasis
Pork tapeworm (infection)
B68.1 Taenia saginata taeniasis
Beef tapeworm (infection)
Infection due to adult tapeworm Taenia saginata
B68.9 Taeniasis, unspecified ▽

✓4ᵗʰ **B69 Cysticercosis**
[INCLUDES] cysticerciasis infection due to larval form of Taenia solium
DEF: Condition that is developed when larvae or eggs of the tapeworm *Taenia solium* are ingested, most commonly in fecally contaminated water or undercooked pork.
B69.0 Cysticercosis of central nervous system
B69.1 Cysticercosis of eye
✓5ᵗʰ **B69.8 Cysticercosis of other sites**
B69.81 Myositis in cysticercosis
B69.89 Cysticercosis of other sites
B69.9 Cysticercosis, unspecified ▽

✓4ᵗʰ **B70 Diphyllobothriasis and sparganosis**
B70.0 Diphyllobothriasis
Diphyllobothrium (adult) (latum) (pacificum) infection
Fish tapeworm (infection)
[EXCLUDES 2] larval diphyllobothriasis (B70.1)
B70.1 Sparganosis
Infection due to Sparganum (mansoni) (proliferum)
Infection due to Spirometra larva
Larval diphyllobothriasis
Spirometrosis

✓4ᵗʰ **B71 Other cestode infections**
B71.0 Hymenolepiasis
Dwarf tapeworm infection
Rat tapeworm (infection)
B71.1 Dipylidiasis
B71.8 Other specified cestode infections
Coenurosis
B71.9 Cestode infection, unspecified ▽
Tapeworm (infection) NOS

B72 Dracunculiasis
[INCLUDES] guinea worm infection
infection due to Dracunculus medinensis

✓4ᵗʰ **B73 Onchocerciasis**
[INCLUDES] onchocerca volvulus infection
onchocercosis
river blindness
✓5ᵗʰ **B73.0 Onchocerciasis with eye disease**
B73.00 Onchocerciasis with eye involvement, unspecified ▽
B73.01 Onchocerciasis with endophthalmitis
B73.02 Onchocerciasis with glaucoma
B73.09 Onchocerciasis with other eye involvement
Infestation of eyelid due to onchocerciasis
B73.1 Onchocerciasis without eye disease

✓4ᵗʰ **B74 Filariasis**
[EXCLUDES 2] onchocerciasis (B73)
tropical (pulmonary) eosinophilia NOS (J82)
B74.0 Filariasis due to Wuchereria bancrofti
Bancroftian elephantiasis
Bancroftian filariasis
B74.1 Filariasis due to Brugia malayi
B74.2 Filariasis due to Brugia timori
B74.3 Loiasis
Calabar swelling
Eyeworm disease of Africa
Loa loa infection

☑ Additional Character Req   ✓x7ᵗʰ Placeholder Alert   Manifestation   ▽ Unspecified   ▶◀ Revised Text   ● New Code   ▲ Revised Code Title

ICD-10-CM 2019   453

B74.4 Mansonelliasis
Infection due to Mansonella ozzardi
Infection due to Mansonella perstans
Infection due to Mansonella streptocerca

B74.8 Other filariases
Dirofilariasis

B74.9 Filariasis, unspecified ▽

B75 Trichinellosis
[INCLUDES] infection due to Trichinella species
trichiniasis
DEF: Infection by *Trichinella spiralis*, the smallest of the parasitic nematodes, that is transmitted by eating undercooked pork or bear meat. **Synonym(s):** Trichinosis.

✓4ᵗʰ B76 Hookworm diseases
[INCLUDES] uncinariasis

B76.0 Ancylostomiasis
Infection due to Ancylostoma species

B76.1 Necatoriasis
Infection due to Necator americanus

B76.8 Other hookworm diseases

B76.9 Hookworm disease, unspecified ▽
Cutaneous larva migrans NOS

✓4ᵗʰ B77 Ascariasis
[INCLUDES] ascaridiasis
roundworm infection

B77.0 Ascariasis with intestinal complications

✓5ᵗʰ B77.8 Ascariasis with other complications

B77.81 Ascariasis pneumonia

B77.89 Ascariasis with other complications

B77.9 Ascariasis, unspecified ▽

✓4ᵗʰ B78 Strongyloidiasis
[EXCLUDES 1] trichostrongyliasis (B81.2)

B78.0 Intestinal strongyloidiasis

B78.1 Cutaneous strongyloidiasis

B78.7 Disseminated strongyloidiasis

B78.9 Strongyloidiasis, unspecified ▽

B79 Trichuriasis
[INCLUDES] trichocephaliasis
whipworm (disease)(infection)

B80 Enterobiasis
[INCLUDES] oxyuriasis
pinworm infection
threadworm infection

✓4ᵗʰ B81 Other intestinal helminthiases, not elsewhere classified
[EXCLUDES 1] angiostrongyliasis due to:
angiostrongylus cantonensis (B83.2)
parastrongylus cantonensis (B83.2)

B81.0 Anisakiasis
Infection due to Anisakis larva

B81.1 Intestinal capillariasis
Capillariasis NOS
Infection due to Capillaria philippinensis
[EXCLUDES 2] hepatic capillariasis (B83.8)

B81.2 Trichostrongyliasis

B81.3 Intestinal angiostrongyliasis
Angiostrongyliasis due to:
angiostrongylus costaricensis
parastrongylus costaricensis

B81.4 Mixed intestinal helminthiases
Infection due to intestinal helminths classified to more than one of the categories B65.0-B81.3 and B81.8
Mixed helminthiasis NOS

B81.8 Other specified intestinal helminthiases
Infection due to Oesophagostomum species [esophagostomiasis]
Infection due to Ternidens diminutus [ternidensiasis]

✓4ᵗʰ B82 Unspecified intestinal parasitism

B82.0 Intestinal helminthiasis, unspecified ▽

B82.9 Intestinal parasitism, unspecified ▽

✓4ᵗʰ B83 Other helminthiases
[EXCLUDES 1] capillariasis NOS (B81.1)
[EXCLUDES 2] intestinal capillariasis (B81.1)

B83.0 Visceral larva migrans
Toxocariasis

B83.1 Gnathostomiasis
Wandering swelling

B83.2 Angiostrongyliasis due to Parastrongylus cantonensis
Eosinophilic meningoencephalitis due to Parastrongylus cantonensis
[EXCLUDES 2] intestinal angiostrongyliasis (B81.3)

B83.3 Syngamiasis
Syngamosis

B83.4 Internal hirudiniasis
[EXCLUDES 2] external hirudiniasis (B88.3)

B83.8 Other specified helminthiases
Acanthocephaliasis
Gongylonemiasis
Hepatic capillariasis
Metastrongyliasis
Thelaziasis

B83.9 Helminthiasis, unspecified ▽
Worms NOS
[EXCLUDES 1] intestinal helminthiasis NOS (B82.0)

Pediculosis, acariasis and other infestations (B85-B89)

✓4ᵗʰ B85 Pediculosis and phthiriasis

B85.0 Pediculosis due to Pediculus humanus capitis
Head-louse infestation

B85.1 Pediculosis due to Pediculus humanus corporis
Body-louse infestation

B85.2 Pediculosis, unspecified ▽

B85.3 Phthiriasis
Infestation by crab-louse
Infestation by Phthirus pubis

B85.4 Mixed pediculosis and phthiriasis
Infestation classifiable to more than one of the categories B85.0-B85.3

B86 Scabies
Sarcoptic itch
DEF: Mite infestation that is caused by *Sarcoptes scabiei*. Scabies causes intense itching and sometimes secondary infection.

✓4ᵗʰ B87 Myiasis
[INCLUDES] infestation by larva of flies

B87.0 Cutaneous myiasis
Creeping myiasis

B87.1 Wound myiasis
Traumatic myiasis

B87.2 Ocular myiasis

B87.3 Nasopharyngeal myiasis
Laryngeal myiasis

B87.4 Aural myiasis

✓5ᵗʰ B87.8 Myiasis of other sites

B87.81 Genitourinary myiasis

B87.82 Intestinal myiasis

B87.89 Myiasis of other sites

B87.9 Myiasis, unspecified ▽

✓4ᵗʰ B88 Other infestations

B88.0 Other acariasis
Acarine dermatitis
Dermatitis due to Demodex species
Dermatitis due to Dermanyssus gallinae
Dermatitis due to Liponyssoides sanguineus
Trombiculosis
[EXCLUDES 2] scabies (B86)

B88.1 Tungiasis [sandflea infestation]

B88.2 Other arthropod infestations
Scarabiasis

B88.3 External hirudiniasis
Leech infestation NOS
[EXCLUDES 2] internal hirudiniasis (B83.4)

B88.8 Other specified infestations
Ichthyoparasitism due to Vandellia cirrhosa
Linguatulosis
Porocephaliasis

B88.9 Infestation, unspecified ▽
Infestation (skin) NOS
Infestation by mites NOS
Skin parasites NOS

B89 Unspecified parasitic disease ▽

Sequelae of infectious and parasitic diseases (B90-B94)

NOTE   Categories B90-B94 are to be used to indicate conditions in categories A00-B89 as the cause of sequelae, which are themselves classified elsewhere. The "sequelae" include conditions specified as such; they also include residuals of diseases classifiable to the above categories if there is evidence that the disease itself is no longer present. Codes from these categories are not to be used for chronic infections. Code chronic current infections to active infectious disease as appropriate.

Code first condition resulting from (sequela) the infectious or parasitic disease

✓4ᵗʰ **B90 Sequelae of tuberculosis**

     B90.0 Sequelae of central nervous system tuberculosis
     B90.1 Sequelae of genitourinary tuberculosis
     B90.2 Sequelae of tuberculosis of bones and joints
     B90.8 Sequelae of tuberculosis of other organs
         EXCLUDES 2   sequelae of respiratory tuberculosis (B90.9)
     B90.9 Sequelae of respiratory and unspecified tuberculosis ▽
         Sequelae of tuberculosis NOS

B91 Sequelae of poliomyelitis
     EXCLUDES 1   postpolio syndrome (G14)

B92 Sequelae of leprosy

✓4ᵗʰ **B94 Sequelae of other and unspecified infectious and parasitic diseases**

     B94.0 Sequelae of trachoma
     B94.1 Sequelae of viral encephalitis
     B94.2 Sequelae of viral hepatitis
     B94.8 Sequelae of other specified infectious and parasitic diseases
         AHA: 2017,4Q,109
     B94.9 Sequelae of unspecified infectious and parasitic disease ▽

Bacterial and viral infectious agents (B95-B97)

NOTE   These categories are provided for use as supplementary or additional codes to identify the infectious agent(s) in diseases classified elsewhere.

AHA: 2018,1Q,16

✓4ᵗʰ **B95 Streptococcus, Staphylococcus, and Enterococcus as the cause of diseases classified elsewhere**

     B95.0 Streptococcus, group A, as the cause of diseases classified elsewhere
     B95.1 Streptococcus, group B, as the cause of diseases classified elsewhere
     B95.2 Enterococcus as the cause of diseases classified elsewhere
     B95.3 Streptococcus pneumoniae as the cause of diseases classified elsewhere
     B95.4 Other streptococcus as the cause of diseases classified elsewhere
     B95.5 Unspecified streptococcus as the cause of diseases classified elsewhere ▽

✓5ᵗʰ   **B95.6 Staphylococcus aureus as the cause of diseases classified elsewhere**
         B95.61 Methicillin susceptible Staphylococcus aureus infection as the cause of diseases classified elsewhere
             Methicillin susceptible Staphylococcus aureus (MSSA) infection as the cause of diseases classified elsewhere
             Staphylococcus aureus infection NOS as the cause of diseases classified elsewhere
         B95.62 Methicillin resistant Staphylococcus aureus infection as the cause of diseases classified elsewhere
             Methicillin resistant staphylococcus aureus (MRSA) infection as the cause of diseases classified elsewhere
             AHA: 2016,1Q,12

     B95.7 Other staphylococcus as the cause of diseases classified elsewhere

B95.8 Unspecified staphylococcus as the cause of diseases classified elsewhere ▽

✓4ᵗʰ **B96 Other bacterial agents as the cause of diseases classified elsewhere**

     B96.0 Mycoplasma pneumoniae [M. pneumoniae] as the cause of diseases classified elsewhere
         Pleuro-pneumonia-like-organism [PPLO]
     B96.1 Klebsiella pneumoniae [K. pneumoniae] as the cause of diseases classified elsewhere

✓5ᵗʰ   **B96.2 Escherichia coli [E. coli] as the cause of diseases classified elsewhere**
         B96.20 Unspecified Escherichia coli [E. coli] as the cause of diseases classified elsewhere ▽
             Escherichia coli [E. coli] NOS
         B96.21 Shiga toxin-producing Escherichia coli [E. coli] (STEC) O157 as the cause of diseases classified elsewhere
             E. coli O157:H- (nonmotile) with confirmation of Shiga toxin
             E. coli O157 with confirmation of Shiga toxin when H antigen is unknown, or is not H7
             O157:H7 Escherichia coli [E.coli] with or without confirmation of Shiga toxin-production
             Shiga toxin-producing Escherichia coli [E.coli] O157:H7 with or without confirmation of Shiga toxin-production
             STEC O157:H7 with or without confirmation of Shiga toxin-production
         B96.22 Other specified Shiga toxin-producing Escherichia coli [E. coli] (STEC) as the cause of diseases classified elsewhere
             Non-O157 Shiga toxin-producing Escherichia coli [E.coli]
             Non-O157 Shiga toxin-producing Escherichia coli [E.coli] with known O group
         B96.23 Unspecified Shiga toxin-producing Escherichia coli [E. coli] (STEC) as the cause of diseases classified elsewhere ▽
             Shiga toxin-producing Escherichia coli [E. coli] with unspecified O group
             STEC NOS
         B96.29 Other Escherichia coli [E. coli] as the cause of diseases classified elsewhere
             Non-Shiga toxin-producing E. coli

     B96.3 Hemophilus influenzae [H. influenzae] as the cause of diseases classified elsewhere
     B96.4 Proteus (mirabilis) (morganii) as the cause of diseases classified elsewhere
     B96.5 Pseudomonas (aeruginosa) (mallei) (pseudomallei) as the cause of diseases classified elsewhere
         AHA: 2015,1Q,18
     B96.6 Bacteroides fragilis [B. fragilis] as the cause of diseases classified elsewhere
     B96.7 Clostridium perfringens [C. perfringens] as the cause of diseases classified elsewhere

✓5ᵗʰ   **B96.8 Other specified bacterial agents as the cause of diseases classified elsewhere**
         B96.81 Helicobacter pylori [H. pylori] as the cause of diseases classified elsewhere
         B96.82 Vibrio vulnificus as the cause of diseases classified elsewhere
         B96.89 Other specified bacterial agents as the cause of diseases classified elsewhere

✓4ᵗʰ **B97 Viral agents as the cause of diseases classified elsewhere**
     AHA: 2016,3Q,8-10,14
     B97.0 Adenovirus as the cause of diseases classified elsewhere

✓5ᵗʰ   **B97.1 Enterovirus as the cause of diseases classified elsewhere**
         B97.10 Unspecified enterovirus as the cause of diseases classified elsewhere ▽
         B97.11 Coxsackievirus as the cause of diseases classified elsewhere
         B97.12 Echovirus as the cause of diseases classified elsewhere
         B97.19 Other enterovirus as the cause of diseases classified elsewhere

√5ᵗʰ **B97.2 Coronavirus as the cause of diseases classified elsewhere**

B97.21 SARS-associated coronavirus as the cause of diseases classified elsewhere

EXCLUDES 1   pneumonia due to SARS-associated coronavirus (J12.81)

B97.29 Other coronavirus as the cause of diseases classified elsewhere

√5ᵗʰ **B97.3 Retrovirus as the cause of diseases classified elsewhere**

EXCLUDES 1   human immunodeficiency virus [HIV] disease (B20)

B97.30 Unspecified retrovirus as the cause of diseases classified elsewhere   ▽

B97.31 Lentivirus as the cause of diseases classified elsewhere

B97.32 Oncovirus as the cause of diseases classified elsewhere

B97.33 Human T-cell lymphotrophic virus, type I [HTLV-I] as the cause of diseases classified elsewhere

B97.34 Human T-cell lymphotrophic virus, type II [HTLV-II] as the cause of diseases classified elsewhere

B97.35 Human immunodeficiency virus, type 2 [HIV 2] as the cause of diseases classified elsewhere   HCC

B97.39 Other retrovirus as the cause of diseases classified elsewhere

B97.4 Respiratory syncytial virus as the cause of diseases classified elsewhere

B97.5 Reovirus as the cause of diseases classified elsewhere

B97.6 Parvovirus as the cause of diseases classified elsewhere

B97.7 Papillomavirus as the cause of diseases classified elsewhere

√5ᵗʰ **B97.8 Other viral agents as the cause of diseases classified elsewhere**

B97.81 Human metapneumovirus as the cause of diseases classified elsewhere

B97.89 Other viral agents as the cause of diseases classified elsewhere

Other infectious diseases (B99)

√4ᵗʰ **B99 Other and unspecified infectious diseases**

B99.8 Other infectious disease

B99.9 Unspecified infectious disease   ▽

Chapter 2. Neoplasms (C00–D49)

Chapter Specific Guidelines with Coding Examples

The chapter specific guidelines from the ICD-10-CM Official Guidelines for Coding and Reporting have been provided below. Along with these guidelines are coding examples, contained in the shaded boxes, that have been developed to help illustrate the coding and/or sequencing guidance found in these guidelines.

General guidelines

Chapter 2 of the ICD-10-CM contains the codes for most benign and all malignant neoplasms. Certain benign neoplasms, such as prostatic adenomas, may be found in the specific body system chapters. To properly code a neoplasm it is necessary to determine from the record if the neoplasm is benign, in-situ, malignant, or of uncertain histologic behavior. If malignant, any secondary (metastatic) sites should also be determined.

Primary malignant neoplasms overlapping site boundaries

A primary malignant neoplasm that overlaps two or more contiguous (next to each other) sites should be classified to the subcategory/code .8 ('overlapping lesion'), unless the combination is specifically indexed elsewhere. For multiple neoplasms of the same site that are not contiguous such as tumors in different quadrants of the same breast, codes for each site should be assigned.

A 62-year-old female with a malignant lesion of the upper lip that extends from the lipstick area to the labial frenulum	
C00.8	**Malignant neoplasm of overlapping sites of lip**

Explanation: Because this is a single lesion that overlaps two contiguous sites, a single code for overlapping sites is assigned.

A 74-year-old male is treated for two distinct malignant lesions, one in the mucosa of the upper lip and a second in the mucosa of the lower lip.	
C00.3	**Malignant neoplasm of upper lip, inner aspect**
C00.4	**Malignant neoplasm of lower lip, inner aspect**

Explanation: This patient has two distinct malignant lesions of the upper and lower lips. Because the lesions are not contiguous, two codes are reported.

Malignant neoplasm of ectopic tissue

Malignant neoplasms of ectopic tissue are to be coded to the site of origin mentioned, e.g., ectopic pancreatic malignant neoplasms involving the stomach are coded to malignant neoplasm of pancreas, unspecified (C25.9).

The neoplasm table in the Alphabetic Index should be referenced first. However, if the histological term is documented, that term should be referenced first, rather than going immediately to the Neoplasm Table, in order to determine which column in the Neoplasm Table is appropriate. For example, if the documentation indicates "adenoma," refer to the term in the Alphabetic Index to review the entries under this term and the instructional note to "see also neoplasm, by site, benign." The table provides the proper code based on the type of neoplasm and the site. It is important to select the proper column in the table that corresponds to the type of neoplasm. The Tabular List should then be referenced to verify that the correct code has been selected from the table and that a more specific site code does not exist.

See Section I.C.21. Factors influencing health status and contact with health services, Status, for information regarding Z15.0, codes for genetic susceptibility to cancer.

a. Treatment directed at the malignancy

If the treatment is directed at the malignancy, designate the malignancy as the principal diagnosis.

The only exception to this guideline is if a patient admission/encounter is solely for the administration of chemotherapy, immunotherapy or external beam radiation therapy, assign the appropriate Z51.-- code as the first-listed or principal diagnosis, and the diagnosis or problem for which the service is being performed as a secondary diagnosis.

b. Treatment of secondary site

When a patient is admitted because of a primary neoplasm with metastasis and treatment is directed toward the secondary site only, the secondary neoplasm is designated as the principal diagnosis even though the primary malignancy is still present.

Patient with primary prostate cancer with metastasis to lungs presents for wedge resection of mass in right lung	
C78.01	**Secondary malignant neoplasm of right lung**
C61	**Malignant neoplasm of prostate**

Explanation: Since the encounter is for treatment of the lung metastasis, the secondary lung metastasis is sequenced before the primary prostate cancer.

c. Coding and sequencing of complications

Coding and sequencing of complications associated with the malignancies or with the therapy thereof are subject to the following guidelines:

1) Anemia associated with malignancy

When admission/encounter is for management of an anemia associated with the malignancy, and the treatment is only for anemia, the appropriate code for the malignancy is sequenced as the principal or first-listed diagnosis followed by the appropriate code for the anemia (such as code D63.0, Anemia in neoplastic disease).

Patient is seen for treatment of anemia in advanced primary liver cancer	
C22.8	**Malignant neoplasm of liver, primary, unspecified as to type**
D63.0	**Anemia in neoplastic disease**

Explanation: Even though the admission was solely to treat the anemia, this guideline indicates that the code for the malignancy is sequenced first.

2) Anemia associated with chemotherapy, immunotherapy and radiation therapy

When the admission/encounter is for management of an anemia associated with an adverse effect of the administration of chemotherapy or immunotherapy and the only treatment is for the anemia, the anemia code is sequenced first followed by the appropriate codes for the neoplasm and the adverse effect (T45.1X5, Adverse effect of antineoplastic and immunosuppressive drugs).

A 56-year-old Hispanic male with grade II follicular lymphoma involving multiple lymph node sites referred for blood transfusion to treat anemia due to chemotherapy	
D64.81	**Anemia due to antineoplastic chemotherapy**
C82.18	**Follicular lymphoma grade II, lymph nodes of multiple sites**
T45.1X5A	**Adverse effect of antineoplastic and immunosuppressive drugs, initial encounter**

Explanation: The code for the anemia is sequenced first followed by the code for the malignant neoplasm and lastly the code for the adverse effect.

When the admission/encounter is for management of an anemia associated with an adverse effect of radiotherapy, the anemia code should be sequenced first, followed by the appropriate neoplasm code and code Y84.2, Radiological procedure and radiotherapy as the cause of abnormal reaction of the patient, or of later complication, without mention of misadventure at the time of the procedure.

A 55-year-old male with a large malignant rectal tumor has been receiving external radiation therapy to shrink the tumor prior to planned surgery. He is referred today for a blood transfusion to treat anemia related to radiation therapy.

D64.89   **Other specified anemias**

C20   **Malignant neoplasm of rectum**

Y84.2   **Radiological procedure and radiotherapy as the cause of abnormal reaction of the patient, or of later complication, without mention of misadventure at the time of the procedure**

Explanation: The code for the anemia is sequenced first, followed by the code for the malignancy, and lastly the code for the abnormal reaction due to radiotherapy.

3) Management of dehydration due to the malignancy

When the admission/encounter is for management of dehydration due to the malignancy and only the dehydration is being treated (intravenous rehydration), the dehydration is sequenced first, followed by the code(s) for the malignancy.

4) Treatment of a complication resulting from a surgical procedure

When the admission/encounter is for treatment of a complication resulting from a surgical procedure, designate the complication as the principal or first-listed diagnosis if treatment is directed at resolving the complication.

d. Primary malignancy previously excised

When a primary malignancy has been previously excised or eradicated from its site and there is no further treatment directed to that site and there is no evidence of any existing primary malignancy **at that site**, a code from category Z85, Personal history of malignant neoplasm, should be used to indicate the former site of the malignancy. Any mention of extension, invasion, or metastasis to another site is coded as a secondary malignant neoplasm to that site. The secondary site may be the principal or first-listed with the Z85 code used as a secondary code.

History of lung cancer, left upper lobectomy 18 months ago with no current treatment; MRI of the brain shows metastatic disease in the brain

C79.31   **Secondary malignant neoplasm of brain**

Z85.118   **Personal history of other other malignant neoplasm of bronchifus and bronchfuls and lung**

Explanation: The patient has undergone a diagnostic procedure that revealed metastatic lung cancer in the brain. The code for the secondary (metastatic) site is sequenced first, followed by a personal history code to identify the former site of the primary malignancy.

e. Admissions/encounters involving chemotherapy, immunotherapy and radiation therapy

1) Episode of care involves surgical removal of neoplasm

When an episode of care involves the surgical removal of a neoplasm, primary or secondary site, followed by adjunct chemotherapy or radiation treatment during the same episode of care, the code for the neoplasm should be assigned as principal or first-listed diagnosis.

2) Patient admission/encounter solely for administration of chemotherapy, immunotherapy and radiation therapy

If a patient admission/encounter is solely for the administration of chemotherapy, immunotherapy or external beam radiation therapy assign code Z51.0, Encounter for antineoplastic radiation therapy, or Z51.11, Encounter for antineoplastic chemotherapy, or Z51.12, Encounter for antineoplastic immunotherapy as the first-listed or principal diagnosis. If a patient receives more than one of these therapies during the same admission more than one of these codes may be assigned, in any sequence.

The malignancy for which the therapy is being administered should be assigned as a secondary diagnosis.

If a patient admission/encounter is for the insertion or implantation of radioactive elements (e.g., brachytherapy) the appropriate code for the malignancy is sequenced as the principal or first-listed diagnosis. Code Z51.0 should not be assigned.

Patient presents for second round of rituximab and fludarabine for his chronic B cell lymphocytic leukemia

Z51.11   **Encounter for antineoplastic chemotherapy**

Z51.12   **Encounter for antineoplastic immunotherapy**

C91.10   **Chronic lymphocytic leukemia of B-cell type not having achieved remission**

Explanation: Rituximab is an antineoplastic immunotherapy while fludarabine is an antineoplastic chemotherapy. The two treatments are often used together. The encounter was solely for the purpose of administering this treatment and either can be sequenced first, before the neoplastic condition.

3) Patient admitted for radiation therapy, chemotherapy or immunotherapy and develops complications

When a patient is admitted for the purpose of external beam radiotherapy, immunotherapy or chemotherapy and develops complications such as uncontrolled nausea and vomiting or dehydration, the principal or first-listed diagnosis is Z51.0, Encounter for antineoplastic radiation therapy, or Z51.11, Encounter for antineoplastic chemotherapy, or Z51.12, Encounter for antineoplastic immunotherapy followed by any codes for the complications.

When a patient is admitted for the purpose of insertion or implantation of radioactive elements (e.g., brachytherapy) and develops complications such as uncontrolled nausea and vomiting or dehydration, the principal or first-listed diagnosis is the appropriate code for the malignancy followed by any codes for the complications.

f. Admission/encounter to determine extent of malignancy

When the reason for admission/encounter is to determine the extent of the malignancy, or for a procedure such as paracentesis or thoracentesis, the primary malignancy or appropriate metastatic site is designated as the principal or first-listed diagnosis, even though chemotherapy or radiotherapy is administered.

Patient with left lung cancer with malignant pleural effusion being seen for paracentesis and initiation/administration of chemotherapy

C34.92   **Malignant neoplasm of unspecified part of left bronchus or lung**

J91.0   **Malignant pleural effusion**

Z51.11   **Encounter for antineoplastic chemotherapy**

Explanation: The lung cancer is sequenced before the chemotherapy in this instance because the paracentesis for the malignant effusion is also being performed. An instructional note under the malignant effusion instructs that the lung cancer be sequenced first.

g. Symptoms, signs, and abnormal findings listed in Chapter 18 associated with neoplasms

Symptoms, signs, and ill-defined conditions listed in Chapter 18 characteristic of, or associated with, an existing primary or secondary site malignancy cannot be used to replace the malignancy as principal or first-listed diagnosis, regardless of the number of admissions or encounters for treatment and care of the neoplasm.

See Section I.C.21. Factors influencing health status and contact with health services, Encounter for prophylactic organ removal.

h. Admission/encounter for pain control/management

See Section I.C.6. for information on coding admission/encounter for pain control/management.

i. Malignancy in two or more noncontiguous sites

A patient may have more than one malignant tumor in the same organ. These tumors may represent different primaries or metastatic disease, depending on the site. Should the documentation be unclear, the provider should be queried as to the status of each tumor so that the correct codes can be assigned.

j. Disseminated malignant neoplasm, unspecified

Code C80.0, Disseminated malignant neoplasm, unspecified, is for use only in those cases where the patient has advanced metastatic disease and no known primary or secondary sites are specified. It should not be used in place of assigning codes for the primary site and all known secondary sites.

k. Malignant neoplasm without specification of site

Code C80.1, Malignant (primary) neoplasm, unspecified, equates to Cancer, unspecified. This code should only be used when no determination can be made as to the primary site of a malignancy. This code should rarely be used in the inpatient setting.

> Evaluation of painful hip leads to diagnosis of a metastatic bone lesion from an unknown primary neoplasm source
>
> **C79.51** **Secondary malignant neoplasm of bone**
>
> **C80.1** **Malignant (primary) neoplasm, unspecified**
>
> *Explanation*: If only the secondary site is known, use code C80.1 for the unknown primary site.

l. Sequencing of neoplasm codes

1) Encounter for treatment of primary malignancy

If the reason for the encounter is for treatment of a primary malignancy, assign the malignancy as the principal/first-listed diagnosis. The primary site is to be sequenced first, followed by any metastatic sites.

2) Encounter for treatment of secondary malignancy

When an encounter is for a primary malignancy with metastasis and treatment is directed toward the metastatic (secondary) site(s) only, the metastatic site(s) is designated as the principal/first-listed diagnosis. The primary malignancy is coded as an additional code.

> Patient has primary colon cancer with metastasis to rib and is evaluated for possible excision of portion of rib bone
>
> **C79.51** **Secondary malignant neoplasm of bone**
>
> **C18.9** **Malignant neoplasm of colon, unspecified**
>
> *Explanation*: The treatment for this encounter is focused on the metastasis to the rib bone rather than the primary colon cancer, thus indicating that the bone metastasis is sequenced as the first-listed code.

3) Malignant neoplasm in a pregnant patient

When a pregnant woman has a malignant neoplasm, a code from subcategory O9A.1-, Malignant neoplasm complicating pregnancy, childbirth, and the puerperium, should be sequenced first, followed by the appropriate code from Chapter 2 to indicate the type of neoplasm.

> A 30-year-old pregnant female in first trimester evaluated for pituitary gland malignancy
>
> **O9A.111** **Malignant neoplasm complicating pregnancy, first trimester**
>
> **C75.1** **Malignant neoplasm of pituitary gland**
>
> *Explanation*: Codes from chapter 15 describing complications of pregnancy are sequenced as first-listed codes, further specified by codes from other chapters such as neoplastic, unless the pregnancy is documented as incidental to the condition. See also guideline 1.C.15.a.1.

4) Encounter for complication associated with a neoplasm

When an encounter is for management of a complication associated with a neoplasm, such as dehydration, and the treatment is only for the complication, the complication is coded first, followed by the appropriate code(s) for the neoplasm.

The exception to this guideline is anemia. When the admission/encounter is for management of an anemia associated with the malignancy, and the treatment is only for anemia, the appropriate code for the malignancy is sequenced as the principal or first-listed diagnosis followed by code D63.0, Anemia in neoplastic disease.

> Patient with pancreatic cancer is seen for initiation of TPN for cancer-related moderate protein-calorie malnutrition
>
> **E44.0** **Moderate protein-calorie malnutrition**
>
> **C25.9** **Malignant neoplasm of pancreas, unspecified**
>
> *Explanation*: The encounter is to initiate treatment for malnutrition, a common complication of many types of neoplasms, and is sequenced first.

5) Complication from surgical procedure for treatment of a neoplasm

When an encounter is for treatment of a complication resulting from a surgical procedure performed for the treatment of the neoplasm, designate the complication as the principal/first-listed diagnosis. See guideline regarding the coding of a current malignancy versus personal history to determine if the code for the neoplasm should also be assigned.

6) Pathologic fracture due to a neoplasm

When an encounter is for a pathological fracture due to a neoplasm, and the focus of treatment is the fracture, a code from subcategory M84.5, Pathological fracture in neoplastic disease, should be sequenced first, followed by the code for the neoplasm.

If the focus of treatment is the neoplasm with an associated pathological fracture, the neoplasm code should be sequenced first, followed by a code from M84.5 for the pathological fracture.

m. Current malignancy versus personal history of malignancy

When a primary malignancy has been excised but further treatment, such as an additional surgery for the malignancy, radiation therapy or chemotherapy is directed to that site, the primary malignancy code should be used until treatment is completed.

When a primary malignancy has been previously excised or eradicated from its site, there is no further treatment (of the malignancy) directed to that site, and there is no evidence of any existing primary malignancy **at that site**, a code from category Z85, Personal history of malignant neoplasm, should be used to indicate the former site of the malignancy.

Subcategories Z85.0 – Z85.7 should only be assigned for the former site of a primary malignancy, not the site of a secondary malignancy. Codes from subcategory Z85.8-, may be assigned for the former site(s) of either a primary or secondary malignancy included in this subcategory.

See Section I.C.21. Factors influencing health status and contact with health services, History (of)

> Female patient with ongoing chemotherapy after right mastectomy for breast cancer
>
> **C50.911** **Malignant neoplasm of unspecified site of right female breast**
>
> **Z90.11** **Acquired absence of right breast and nipple**
>
> *Explanation*: Even though the breast has been removed, the breast cancer is still being treated with chemotherapy and therefore is still coded as a current condition rather than personal history.

n. Leukemia, multiple myeloma, and malignant plasma cell neoplasms in remission versus personal history

The categories for leukemia, and category C90, Multiple myeloma and malignant plasma cell neoplasms, have codes indicating whether or not the leukemia has achieved remission. There are also codes Z85.6, Personal history of leukemia, and Z85.79, Personal history of other malignant neoplasms of lymphoid, hematopoietic and related tissues. If the documentation is unclear as to whether the leukemia has achieved remission, the provider should be queried.

See Section I.C.21. Factors influencing health status and contact with health services, History (of)

o. Aftercare following surgery for neoplasm

See Section I.C.21. Factors influencing health status and contact with health services, Aftercare

p. Follow-up care for completed treatment of a malignancy

See Section I.C.21. Factors influencing health status and contact with health services, Follow-up

q. Prophylactic organ removal for prevention of malignancy

See Section I.C. 21, Factors influencing health status and contact with health services, Prophylactic organ removal

r. Malignant neoplasm associated with transplanted organ

A malignant neoplasm of a transplanted organ should be coded as a transplant complication. Assign first the appropriate code from category T86.-, Complications of transplanted organs and tissue, followed by code C80.2, Malignant neoplasm associated with transplanted organ. Use an additional code for the specific malignancy.

Chapter 2. Neoplasms (C00-D49)

NOTE

Functional activity

All neoplasms are classified in this chapter, whether they are functionally active or not. An additional code from Chapter 4 may be used, to identify functional activity associated with any neoplasm.

Morphology [Histology]

Chapter 2 classifies neoplasms primarily by site (topography), with broad groupings for behavior, malignant, in situ, benign, etc. The Table of Neoplasms should be used to identify the correct topography code. In a few cases, such as for malignant melanoma and certain neuroendocrine tumors, the morphology (histologic type) is included in the category and codes.

Primary malignant neoplasms overlapping site boundaries

A primary malignant neoplasm that overlaps two or more contiguous (next to each other) sites should be classified to the subcategory/code .8 ("overlapping lesion"), unless the combination is specifically indexed elsewhere. For multiple neoplasms of the same site that are not contiguous, such as tumors in different quadrants of the same breast, codes for each site should be assigned.

Malignant neoplasm of ectopic tissue

Malignant neoplasms of ectopic tissue are to be coded to the site mentioned, e.g., ectopic pancreatic malignant neoplasms are coded to pancreas, unspecified (C25.9).

AHA: 2017,4Q,103; 2017,1Q,4,5-6,8

This chapter contains the following blocks:

C00-C14	Malignant neoplasms of lip, oral cavity and pharynx
C15-C26	Malignant neoplasms of digestive organs
C30-C39	Malignant neoplasms of respiratory and intrathoracic organs
C40-C41	Malignant neoplasms of bone and articular cartilage
C43-C44	Melanoma and other malignant neoplasms of skin
C45-C49	Malignant neoplasms of mesothelial and soft tissue
C50	Malignant neoplasms of breast
C51-C58	Malignant neoplasms of female genital organs
C60-C63	Malignant neoplasms of male genital organs
C64-C68	Malignant neoplasms of urinary tract
C69-C72	Malignant neoplasms of eye, brain and other parts of central nervous system
C73-C75	Malignant neoplasms of thyroid and other endocrine glands
C7A	Malignant neuroendocrine tumors
C7B	Secondary neuroendocrine tumors
C76-C80	Malignant neoplasms of ill-defined, other secondary and unspecified sites
C81-C96	Malignant neoplasms of lymphoid, hematopoietic and related tissue
D00-D09	In situ neoplasms
D10-D36	Benign neoplasms, except benign neuroendocrine tumors
D3A	Benign neuroendocrine tumors
D37-D48	Neoplasms of uncertain behavior, polycythemia vera and myelodysplastic syndromes
D49	Neoplasms of unspecified behavior

Malignant Neoplasms (C00-C96)

Malignant neoplasms, stated or presumed to be primary (of specified sites), and certain specified histologies, except neuroendocrine, and of lymphoid, hematopoietic and related tissue (C00-C75)

TIP: Codes from this code block can be assigned based on the diagnosis listed in a pathology or cytology report when authenticated by a pathologist and available at the time of code assignment.

Malignant neoplasms of lip, oral cavity and pharynx (C00-C14)

√4th **C00 Malignant neoplasm of lip**

Use additional code to identify:
  alcohol abuse and dependence (F10.-)
  history of tobacco dependence (Z87.891)
  tobacco dependence (F17.-)
  tobacco use (Z72.0)

EXCLUDES 1   malignant melanoma of lip (C43.0)
      Merkel cell carcinoma of lip (C4A.0)
      other and unspecified malignant neoplasm of skin of lip (C44.0-)

C00.0 Malignant neoplasm of external upper lip
  Malignant neoplasm of lipstick area of upper lip
  Malignant neoplasm of upper lip NOS
  Malignant neoplasm of vermilion border of upper lip

C00.1 Malignant neoplasm of external lower lip
  Malignant neoplasm of lower lip NOS
  Malignant neoplasm of lipstick area of lower lip
  Malignant neoplasm of vermilion border of lower lip

C00.2 Malignant neoplasm of external lip, unspecified ▽
  Malignant neoplasm of vermilion border of lip NOS

C00.3 Malignant neoplasm of upper lip, inner aspect
  Malignant neoplasm of buccal aspect of upper lip
  Malignant neoplasm of frenulum of upper lip
  Malignant neoplasm of mucosa of upper lip
  Malignant neoplasm of oral aspect of upper lip

C00.4 Malignant neoplasm of lower lip, inner aspect
  Malignant neoplasm of buccal aspect of lower lip
  Malignant neoplasm of frenulum of lower lip
  Malignant neoplasm of mucosa of lower lip
  Malignant neoplasm of oral aspect of lower lip

C00.5 Malignant neoplasm of lip, unspecified, inner aspect ▽
  Malignant neoplasm of buccal aspect of lip, unspecified
  Malignant neoplasm of frenulum of lip, unspecified
  Malignant neoplasm of mucosa of lip, unspecified
  Malignant neoplasm of oral aspect of lip, unspecified

C00.6 Malignant neoplasm of commissure of lip, unspecified ▽

C00.8 Malignant neoplasm of overlapping sites of lip

C00.9 Malignant neoplasm of lip, unspecified ▽

C01 Malignant neoplasm of base of tongue HCC
  Malignant neoplasm of dorsal surface of base of tongue
  Malignant neoplasm of fixed part of tongue NOS
  Malignant neoplasm of posterior third of tongue
  Use additional code to identify:
    alcohol abuse and dependence (F10.-)
    history of tobacco dependence (Z87.891)
    tobacco dependence (F17.-)
    tobacco use (Z72.0)

Malignant Neoplasm of Tongue

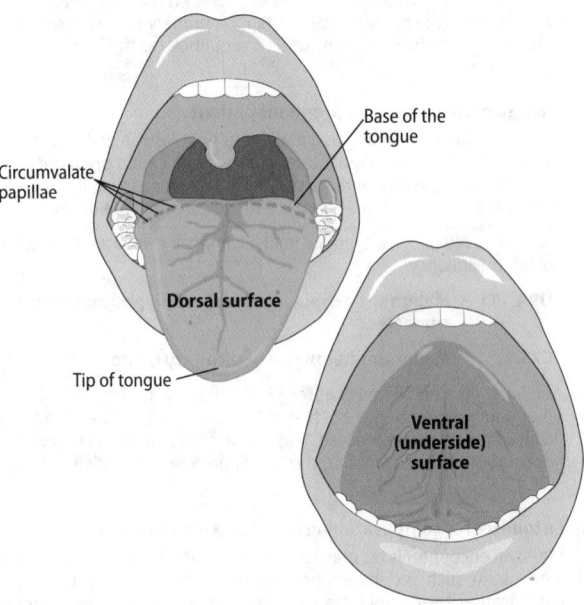

√4th C02 Malignant neoplasm of other and unspecified parts of tongue

Use additional code to identify:
  alcohol abuse and dependence (F10.-)
  history of tobacco dependence (Z87.891)
  tobacco dependence (F17.-)
  tobacco use (Z72.0)

C02.0 Malignant neoplasm of dorsal surface of tongue HCC
  Malignant neoplasm of anterior two-thirds of tongue, dorsal surface

EXCLUDES 2   malignant neoplasm of dorsal surface of base of tongue (C01)

C02.1 Malignant neoplasm of border of tongue HCC
  Malignant neoplasm of tip of tongue

C02.2 Malignant neoplasm of ventral surface of tongue HCC
  Malignant neoplasm of anterior two-thirds of tongue, ventral surface
  Malignant neoplasm of frenulum linguae

C02.3 Malignant neoplasm of anterior two-thirds of tongue, part unspecified HCC
  Malignant neoplasm of middle third of tongue NOS
  Malignant neoplasm of mobile part of tongue NOS

C02.4 Malignant neoplasm of lingual tonsil HCC
  EXCLUDES 2 malignant neoplasm of tonsil NOS (C09.9)

C02.8 Malignant neoplasm of overlapping sites of tongue HCC
  Malignant neoplasm of two or more contiguous sites of tongue

C02.9 Malignant neoplasm of tongue, unspecified HCC ▽

✓4th **C03 Malignant neoplasm of gum**
  INCLUDES malignant neoplasm of alveolar (ridge) mucosa
       malignant neoplasm of gingiva
  Use additional code to identify:
    alcohol abuse and dependence (F10.-)
    history of tobacco dependence (Z87.891)
    tobacco dependence (F17.-)
    tobacco use (Z72.0)
  EXCLUDES 2 malignant odontogenic neoplasms (C41.0-C41.1)

C03.0 Malignant neoplasm of upper gum HCC
C03.1 Malignant neoplasm of lower gum HCC
C03.9 Malignant neoplasm of gum, unspecified HCC ▽

✓4th **C04 Malignant neoplasm of floor of mouth**
  Use additional code to identify:
    alcohol abuse and dependence (F10.-)
    history of tobacco dependence (Z87.891)
    tobacco dependence (F17.-)
    tobacco use (Z72.0)

C04.0 Malignant neoplasm of anterior floor of mouth HCC
  Malignant neoplasm of anterior to the premolar-canine junction

C04.1 Malignant neoplasm of lateral floor of mouth HCC
C04.8 Malignant neoplasm of overlapping sites of floor of mouth HCC
C04.9 Malignant neoplasm of floor of mouth, unspecified HCC ▽

✓4th **C05 Malignant neoplasm of palate**
  Use additional code to identify:
    alcohol abuse and dependence (F10.-)
    history of tobacco dependence (Z87.891)
    tobacco dependence (F17.-)
    tobacco use (Z72.0)
  EXCLUDES 1 Kaposi's sarcoma of palate (C46.2)

C05.0 Malignant neoplasm of hard palate HCC
C05.1 Malignant neoplasm of soft palate HCC
  EXCLUDES 2 malignant neoplasm of nasopharyngeal surface of soft palate (C11.3)
C05.2 Malignant neoplasm of uvula HCC
C05.8 Malignant neoplasm of overlapping sites of palate HCC
C05.9 Malignant neoplasm of palate, unspecified HCC ▽
  Malignant neoplasm of roof of mouth

✓4th **C06 Malignant neoplasm of other and unspecified parts of mouth**
  Use additional code to identify:
    alcohol abuse and dependence (F10.-)
    history of tobacco dependence (Z87.891)
    tobacco dependence (F17.-)
    tobacco use (Z72.0)

C06.0 Malignant neoplasm of cheek mucosa HCC
  Malignant neoplasm of buccal mucosa NOS
  Malignant neoplasm of internal cheek

C06.1 Malignant neoplasm of vestibule of mouth HCC
  Malignant neoplasm of buccal sulcus (upper) (lower)
  Malignant neoplasm of labial sulcus (upper) (lower)

C06.2 Malignant neoplasm of retromolar area HCC

✓5th **C06.8 Malignant neoplasm of overlapping sites of other and unspecified parts of mouth**
  C06.80 Malignant neoplasm of overlapping sites of unspecified parts of mouth HCC ▽
  C06.89 Malignant neoplasm of overlapping sites of other parts of mouth HCC
    "book leaf" neoplasm [ventral surface of tongue and floor of mouth]

C06.9 Malignant neoplasm of mouth, unspecified HCC ▽
  Malignant neoplasm of minor salivary gland, unspecified site
  Malignant neoplasm of oral cavity NOS

C07 Malignant neoplasm of parotid gland HCC
  Use additional code to identify:
    alcohol abuse and dependence (F10.-)
    exposure to environmental tobacco smoke (Z77.22)
    exposure to tobacco smoke in the perinatal period (P96.81)
    history of tobacco dependence (Z87.891)
    occupational exposure to environmental tobacco smoke (Z57.31)
    tobacco dependence (F17.-)
    tobacco use (Z72.0)

✓4th **C08 Malignant neoplasm of other and unspecified major salivary glands**
  INCLUDES malignant neoplasm of salivary ducts
  Use additional code to identify:
    alcohol abuse and dependence (F10.-)
    exposure to environmental tobacco smoke (Z77.22)
    exposure to tobacco smoke in the perinatal period (P96.81)
    history of tobacco dependence (Z87.891)
    occupational exposure to environmental tobacco smoke (Z57.31)
    tobacco dependence (F17.-)
    tobacco use (Z72.0)
  EXCLUDES 1 malignant neoplasms of specified minor salivary glands which are classified according to their anatomical location
  EXCLUDES 2 malignant neoplasms of minor salivary glands NOS (C06.9)
         malignant neoplasm of parotid gland (C07)

C08.0 Malignant neoplasm of submandibular gland HCC
  Malignant neoplasm of submaxillary gland
C08.1 Malignant neoplasm of sublingual gland HCC
C08.9 Malignant neoplasm of major salivary gland, unspecified HCC ▽
  Malignant neoplasm of salivary gland (major) NOS

✓4th **C09 Malignant neoplasm of tonsil**
  Use additional code to identify:
    alcohol abuse and dependence (F10.-)
    exposure to environmental tobacco smoke (Z77.22)
    exposure to tobacco smoke in the perinatal period (P96.81)
    history of tobacco dependence (Z87.891)
    occupational exposure to environmental tobacco smoke (Z57.31)
    tobacco dependence (F17.-)
    tobacco use (Z72.0)
  EXCLUDES 2 malignant neoplasm of lingual tonsil (C02.4)
         malignant neoplasm of pharyngeal tonsil (C11.1)

C09.0 Malignant neoplasm of tonsillar fossa HCC
C09.1 Malignant neoplasm of tonsillar pillar (anterior) (posterior) HCC
C09.8 Malignant neoplasm of overlapping sites of tonsil HCC
C09.9 Malignant neoplasm of tonsil, unspecified HCC ▽
  Malignant neoplasm of tonsil NOS
  Malignant neoplasm of faucial tonsils
  Malignant neoplasm of palatine tonsils

✓4th **C10 Malignant neoplasm of oropharynx**
  Use additional code to identify:
    alcohol abuse and dependence (F10.-)
    exposure to environmental tobacco smoke (Z77.22)
    exposure to tobacco smoke in the perinatal period (P96.81)
    history of tobacco dependence (Z87.891)
    occupational exposure to environmental tobacco smoke (Z57.31)
    tobacco dependence (F17.-)
    tobacco use (Z72.0)
  EXCLUDES 2 malignant neoplasm of tonsil (C09.-)

C10.0 Malignant neoplasm of vallecula HCC
C10.1 Malignant neoplasm of anterior surface of epiglottis HCC
  Malignant neoplasm of epiglottis, free border [margin]
  Malignant neoplasm of glossoepiglottic fold(s)
  EXCLUDES 2 malignant neoplasm of epiglottis (suprahyoid portion) NOS (C32.1)
C10.2 Malignant neoplasm of lateral wall of oropharynx HCC
C10.3 Malignant neoplasm of posterior wall of oropharynx HCC
C10.4 Malignant neoplasm of branchial cleft HCC
  Malignant neoplasm of branchial cyst [site of neoplasm]
C10.8 Malignant neoplasm of overlapping sites of oropharynx HCC
  Malignant neoplasm of junctional region of oropharynx
C10.9 Malignant neoplasm of oropharynx, unspecified HCC ▽

✓4ᵗʰ **C11 Malignant neoplasm of nasopharynx**

Use additional code to identify:
exposure to environmental tobacco smoke (Z77.22)
exposure to tobacco smoke in the perinatal period (P96.81)
history of tobacco dependence (Z87.891)
occupational exposure to environmental tobacco smoke (Z57.31)
tobacco dependence (F17.-)
tobacco use (Z72.0)

C11.0 Malignant neoplasm of superior wall of   HCC
nasopharynx
Malignant neoplasm of roof of nasopharynx

C11.1 Malignant neoplasm of posterior wall of   HCC
nasopharynx
Malignant neoplasm of adenoid
Malignant neoplasm of pharyngeal tonsil

C11.2 Malignant neoplasm of lateral wall of nasopharynx   HCC
Malignant neoplasm of fossa of Rosenmüller
Malignant neoplasm of opening of auditory tube
Malignant neoplasm of pharyngeal recess

C11.3 Malignant neoplasm of anterior wall of   HCC
nasopharynx
Malignant neoplasm of floor of nasopharynx
Malignant neoplasm of nasopharyngeal (anterior) (posterior)
surface of soft palate
Malignant neoplasm of posterior margin of nasal choana
Malignant neoplasm of posterior margin of nasal septum

C11.8 Malignant neoplasm of overlapping sites of   HCC
nasopharynx

C11.9 Malignant neoplasm of nasopharynx, unspecified   HCC ▽
Malignant neoplasm of nasopharyngeal wall NOS

C12 Malignant neoplasm of pyriform sinus   HCC
Malignant neoplasm of pyriform fossa
Use additional code to identify:
exposure to environmental tobacco smoke (Z77.22)
exposure to tobacco smoke in the perinatal period (P96.81)
history of tobacco dependence (Z87.891)
occupational exposure to environmental tobacco smoke (Z57.31)
tobacco dependence (F17.-)
tobacco use (Z72.0)

✓4ᵗʰ **C13 Malignant neoplasm of hypopharynx**

Use additional code to identify:
exposure to environmental tobacco smoke (Z77.22)
exposure to tobacco smoke in the perinatal period (P96.81)
history of tobacco dependence (Z87.891)
occupational exposure to environmental tobacco smoke (Z57.31)
tobacco dependence (F17.-)
tobacco use (Z72.0)
EXCLUDES 2   malignant neoplasm of pyriform sinus (C12)

C13.0 Malignant neoplasm of postcricoid region   HCC
C13.1 Malignant neoplasm of aryepiglottic fold,   HCC
hypopharyngeal aspect
Malignant neoplasm of aryepiglottic fold, marginal zone
Malignant neoplasm of aryepiglottic fold NOS
Malignant neoplasm of interarytenoid fold, marginal zone
Malignant neoplasm of interarytenoid fold NOS
EXCLUDES 2   malignant neoplasm of aryepiglottic fold or
interarytenoid fold, laryngeal aspect (C32.1)

C13.2 Malignant neoplasm of posterior wall of   HCC
hypopharynx

C13.8 Malignant neoplasm of overlapping sites of   HCC
hypopharynx

C13.9 Malignant neoplasm of hypopharynx, unspecified   HCC ▽
Malignant neoplasm of hypopharyngeal wall NOS

✓4ᵗʰ **C14 Malignant neoplasm of other and ill-defined sites in the lip, oral cavity and pharynx**

Use additional code to identify:
alcohol abuse and dependence (F10.-)
exposure to environmental tobacco smoke (Z77.22)
exposure to tobacco smoke in the perinatal period (P96.81)
history of tobacco dependence (Z87.891)
occupational exposure to environmental tobacco smoke (Z57.31)
tobacco dependence (F17.-)
tobacco use (Z72.0)
EXCLUDES 1   malignant neoplasm of oral cavity NOS (C06.9)

C14.0 Malignant neoplasm of pharynx, unspecified   HCC ▽

C14.2 Malignant neoplasm of Waldeyer's ring   HCC
DEF: Waldeyer's ring: Ring of lymphoid tissue that is made up of
the two palatine tonsils, the pharyngeal tonsil (adenoid), and the
lingual tonsil. It functions as the defense against infection and
assists with the development of the immune system.

C14.8 Malignant neoplasm of overlapping sites of lip, oral   HCC
cavity and pharynx
Primary malignant neoplasm of two or more contiguous sites
of lip, oral cavity and pharynx
EXCLUDES 1   "book leaf" neoplasm [ventral surface of tongue and
floor of mouth] (C06.89)

Malignant neoplasms of digestive organs (C15-C26)

EXCLUDES 1   Kaposi's sarcoma of gastrointestinal sites (C46.4)
EXCLUDES 2   gastrointestinal stromal tumors (C49.A-)

✓4ᵗʰ **C15 Malignant neoplasm of esophagus**

Use additional code to identify:
alcohol abuse and dependence (F10.-)

C15.3 Malignant neoplasm of upper third of esophagus   HCC
C15.4 Malignant neoplasm of middle third of esophagus   HCC
C15.5 Malignant neoplasm of lower third of esophagus   HCC
EXCLUDES 1   malignant neoplasm of cardio-esophageal junction
(C16.0)

C15.8 Malignant neoplasm of overlapping sites of   HCC
esophagus

C15.9 Malignant neoplasm of esophagus, unspecified   HCC ▽

✓4ᵗʰ **C16 Malignant neoplasm of stomach**

Use additional code to identify:
alcohol abuse and dependence (F10.-)
EXCLUDES 2   malignant carcinoid tumor of the stomach (C7A.092)

C16.0 Malignant neoplasm of cardia   HCC
Malignant neoplasm of cardiac orifice
Malignant neoplasm of cardio-esophageal junction
Malignant neoplasm of esophagus and stomach
Malignant neoplasm of gastro-esophageal junction

C16.1 Malignant neoplasm of fundus of stomach   HCC
C16.2 Malignant neoplasm of body of stomach   HCC
C16.3 Malignant neoplasm of pyloric antrum   HCC
Malignant neoplasm of gastric antrum

C16.4 Malignant neoplasm of pylorus   HCC
Malignant neoplasm of prepylorus
Malignant neoplasm of pyloric canal

C16.5 Malignant neoplasm of lesser curvature of stomach,   HCC ▽
unspecified
Malignant neoplasm of lesser curvature of stomach, not
classifiable to C16.1-C16.4

C16.6 Malignant neoplasm of greater curvature of   HCC ▽
stomach, unspecified
Malignant neoplasm of greater curvature of stomach, not
classifiable to C16.0-C16.4

C16.8 Malignant neoplasm of overlapping sites of   HCC
stomach

C16.9 Malignant neoplasm of stomach, unspecified   HCC ▽
Gastric cancer NOS

✓4ᵗʰ **C17 Malignant neoplasm of small intestine**

EXCLUDES 1   malignant carcinoid tumors of the small intestine (C7A.01)
AHA: 2016,1Q,19

C17.0 Malignant neoplasm of duodenum   HCC
C17.1 Malignant neoplasm of jejunum   HCC
C17.2 Malignant neoplasm of ileum   HCC
EXCLUDES 1   malignant neoplasm of ileocecal valve (C18.0)

C17.3 Meckel's diverticulum, malignant   HCC
EXCLUDES 1   Meckel's diverticulum, congenital (Q43.0)
DEF: Congenital, abnormal remnant of embryonic digestive
system development that leaves a sacculation or outpouching
from the wall of the small intestine near the terminal part of the
ileum made of acid-secreting tissue as in the stomach.

C17.8 Malignant neoplasm of overlapping sites of small   HCC
intestine

C17.9 Malignant neoplasm of small intestine, unspecified   HCC ▽

✓4ᵗʰ C18 Malignant neoplasm of colon

     EXCLUDES 1   *malignant carcinoid tumors of the colon (C7A.02-)*

Colon

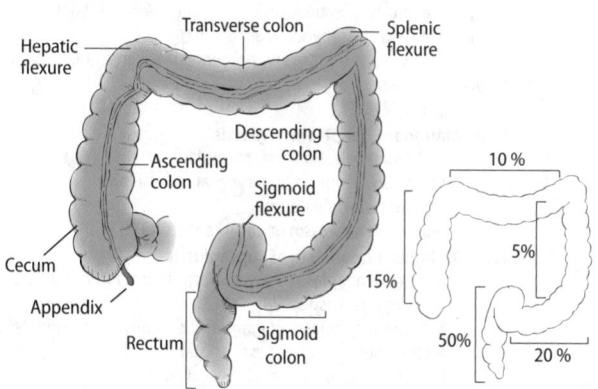

Anatomical distribution
of large bowel cancers

C18.0 Malignant neoplasm of cecum   HCC Q
     Malignant neoplasm of ileocecal valve

C18.1 Malignant neoplasm of appendix   HCC Q

C18.2 Malignant neoplasm of ascending colon   HCC Q

C18.3 Malignant neoplasm of hepatic flexure   HCC Q

C18.4 Malignant neoplasm of transverse colon   HCC Q

C18.5 Malignant neoplasm of splenic flexure   HCC Q

C18.6 Malignant neoplasm of descending colon   HCC Q

C18.7 Malignant neoplasm of sigmoid colon   HCC Q
     Malignant neoplasm of sigmoid (flexure)
     EXCLUDES 1   *malignant neoplasm of rectosigmoid junction (C19)*

C18.8 Malignant neoplasm of overlapping sites of colon   HCC Q

C18.9 Malignant neoplasm of colon, unspecified   HCC Q ▽
     Malignant neoplasm of large intestine NOS

C19 Malignant neoplasm of rectosigmoid junction   HCC Q
     Malignant neoplasm of colon with rectum
     Malignant neoplasm of rectosigmoid (colon)
     EXCLUDES 1   *malignant carcinoid tumors of the colon (C7A.02-)*

C20 Malignant neoplasm of rectum   HCC Q
     Malignant neoplasm of rectal ampulla
     EXCLUDES 1   *malignant carcinoid tumor of the rectum (C7A.026)*

✓4ᵗʰ C21 Malignant neoplasm of anus and anal canal

     EXCLUDES 2   *malignant carcinoid tumors of the colon (C7A.02-)*
             malignant melanoma of anal margin (C43.51)
             malignant melanoma of anal skin (C43.51)
             malignant melanoma of perianal skin (C43.51)
             other and unspecified malignant neoplasm of anal margin
                 (C44.500, C44.510, C44.520, C44.590)
             other and unspecified malignant neoplasm of anal skin
                 (C44.500, C44.510, C44.520, C44.590)
             other and unspecified malignant neoplasm of perianal skin
                 (C44.500, C44.510, C44.520, C44.590)

C21.0 Malignant neoplasm of anus, unspecified   HCC ▽

C21.1 Malignant neoplasm of anal canal   HCC
     Malignant neoplasm of anal sphincter

C21.2 Malignant neoplasm of cloacogenic zone   HCC Q

C21.8 Malignant neoplasm of overlapping sites of rectum, anus and anal canal   HCC Q
     Malignant neoplasm of anorectal junction
     Malignant neoplasm of anorectum
     Primary malignant neoplasm of two or more contiguous sites
        of rectum, anus and anal canal

✓4ᵗʰ C22 Malignant neoplasm of liver and intrahepatic bile ducts

     Use additional code to identify:
       alcohol abuse and dependence (F10.-)
       hepatitis B (B16.-, B18.0-B18.1)
       hepatitis C (B17.1-, B18.2)
     EXCLUDES 1   *malignant neoplasm of biliary tract NOS (C24.9)*
             secondary malignant neoplasm of liver and intrahepatic bile
               duct (C78.7)

C22.0 Liver cell carcinoma   HCC
     Hepatocellular carcinoma
     Hepatoma
     AHA: 2016,1Q,18

C22.1 Intrahepatic bile duct carcinoma   HCC
     Cholangiocarcinoma
     EXCLUDES 1   *malignant neoplasm of hepatic duct (C24.0)*

C22.2 Hepatoblastoma   HCC

C22.3 Angiosarcoma of liver   HCC
     Kupffer cell sarcoma

C22.4 Other sarcomas of liver   HCC

C22.7 Other specified carcinomas of liver   HCC

C22.8 Malignant neoplasm of liver, primary, unspecified as to type   HCC ▽

C22.9 Malignant neoplasm of liver, not specified as primary or secondary   HCC ▽

C23 Malignant neoplasm of gallbladder   HCC

✓4ᵗʰ C24 Malignant neoplasm of other and unspecified parts of biliary tract

     EXCLUDES 1   *malignant neoplasm of intrahepatic bile duct (C22.1)*

C24.0 Malignant neoplasm of extrahepatic bile duct   HCC
     Malignant neoplasm of biliary duct or passage NOS
     Malignant neoplasm of common bile duct
     Malignant neoplasm of cystic duct
     Malignant neoplasm of hepatic duct

C24.1 Malignant neoplasm of ampulla of Vater   HCC
     DEF: Malignant neoplasm in the area of dilation at the juncture
     of the common bile and pancreatic ducts near the opening into
     the lumen of the duodenum.

C24.8 Malignant neoplasm of overlapping sites of biliary tract   HCC
     Malignant neoplasm involving both intrahepatic and
       extrahepatic bile ducts
     Primary malignant neoplasm of two or more contiguous sites
       of biliary tract

C24.9 Malignant neoplasm of biliary tract, unspecified   HCC ▽

✓4ᵗʰ C25 Malignant neoplasm of pancreas

     Code also exocrine pancreatic insufficiency (K86.81)
     Use additional code to identify:
       alcohol abuse and dependence (F10.-)

Pancreas

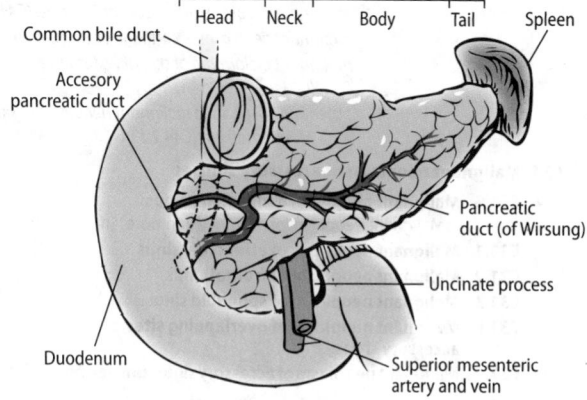

C25.0 Malignant neoplasm of head of pancreas   HCC Q

C25.1 Malignant neoplasm of body of pancreas   HCC Q

C25.2 Malignant neoplasm of tail of pancreas   HCC Q

C25.3 Malignant neoplasm of pancreatic duct   HCC Q

C25.4 Malignant neoplasm of endocrine pancreas   HCC Q
     Malignant neoplasm of islets of Langerhans
     Use additional code to identify any functional activity

☑ Additional Character Req   ✓x7ᵗʰ Placeholder Alert   Manifestation   ▽ Unspecified   ▶◀ Revised Text   ● New Code   ▲ Revised Code Title

ICD-10-CM 2019   463

C18–C25.4

Chapter 2. Neoplasms

C25.7–C34.31

C25.7 **Malignant neoplasm of other parts of pancreas** `HCC` `Q`
Malignant neoplasm of neck of pancreas

C25.8 **Malignant neoplasm of overlapping sites of pancreas** `HCC` `Q`

C25.9 **Malignant neoplasm of pancreas, unspecified** `HCC` `Q` ▽

✓4ᵗʰ **C26** **Malignant neoplasm of other and ill-defined digestive organs**
> **EXCLUDES 1** *malignant neoplasm of peritoneum and retroperitoneum (C48.-)*

C26.0 **Malignant neoplasm of intestinal tract, part unspecified** `HCC` ▽
Malignant neoplasm of intestine NOS

C26.1 **Malignant neoplasm of spleen** `HCC`
> **EXCLUDES 1** *Hodgkin lymphoma (C81.-)*
> *non-Hodgkin lymphoma (C82-C85)*

C26.9 **Malignant neoplasm of ill-defined sites within the digestive system** `HCC` ▽
Malignant neoplasm of alimentary canal or tract NOS
Malignant neoplasm of gastrointestinal tract NOS
> **EXCLUDES 1** *malignant neoplasm of abdominal NOS (C76.2)*
> *malignant neoplasm of intra-abdominal NOS (C76.2)*

Malignant neoplasms of respiratory and intrathoracic organs (C30-C39)

> **INCLUDES** malignant neoplasm of middle ear
> **EXCLUDES 1** mesothelioma (C45.-)

✓4ᵗʰ **C30** **Malignant neoplasm of nasal cavity and middle ear**

C30.0 **Malignant neoplasm of nasal cavity** `HCC`
Malignant neoplasm of cartilage of nose
Malignant neoplasm of nasal concha
Malignant neoplasm of internal nose
Malignant neoplasm of septum of nose
Malignant neoplasm of vestibule of nose
> **EXCLUDES 1** *malignant neoplasm of nasal bone (C41.0)*
> *malignant neoplasm of nose NOS (C76.0)*
> *malignant neoplasm of olfactory bulb (C72.2-)*
> *malignant neoplasm of posterior margin of nasal septum and choana (C11.3)*
> *malignant melanoma of skin of nose (C43.31)*
> *malignant neoplasm of turbinates (C41.0)*
> *other and unspecified malignant neoplasm of skin of nose (C44.301, C44.311, C44.321, C44.391)*

C30.1 **Malignant neoplasm of middle ear** `HCC`
Malignant neoplasm of antrum tympanicum
Malignant neoplasm of auditory tube
Malignant neoplasm of eustachian tube
Malignant neoplasm of inner ear
Malignant neoplasm of mastoid air cells
Malignant neoplasm of tympanic cavity
> **EXCLUDES 1** *malignant neoplasm of auricular canal (external) (C43.2-,C44.2-)*
> *malignant neoplasm of bone of ear (meatus) (C41.0)*
> *malignant neoplasm of cartilage of ear (C49.0)*
> *malignant melanoma of skin of (external) ear (C43.2-)*
> *other and unspecified malignant neoplasm of skin of (external) ear (C44.2-)*

✓4ᵗʰ **C31** **Malignant neoplasm of accessory sinuses**

C31.0 **Malignant neoplasm of maxillary sinus** `HCC`
Malignant neoplasm of antrum (Highmore) (maxillary)

C31.1 **Malignant neoplasm of ethmoidal sinus** `HCC`

C31.2 **Malignant neoplasm of frontal sinus** `HCC`

C31.3 **Malignant neoplasm of sphenoid sinus** `HCC`

C31.8 **Malignant neoplasm of overlapping sites of accessory sinuses** `HCC`

C31.9 **Malignant neoplasm of accessory sinus, unspecified** `HCC` ▽

✓4ᵗʰ **C32** **Malignant neoplasm of larynx**
Use additional code to identify:
  alcohol abuse and dependence (F10.-)
  exposure to environmental tobacco smoke (Z77.22)
  exposure to tobacco smoke in the perinatal period (P96.81)
  history of tobacco dependence (Z87.891)
  occupational exposure to environmental tobacco smoke (Z57.31)
  tobacco dependence (F17.-)
  tobacco use (Z72.0)

C32.0 **Malignant neoplasm of glottis** `HCC`
Malignant neoplasm of intrinsic larynx
Malignant neoplasm of laryngeal commissure (anterior)(posterior)
Malignant neoplasm of vocal cord (true) NOS

C32.1 **Malignant neoplasm of supraglottis** `HCC`
Malignant neoplasm of aryepiglottic fold or interarytenoid fold, laryngeal aspect
Malignant neoplasm of epiglottis (suprahyoid portion) NOS
Malignant neoplasm of extrinsic larynx
Malignant neoplasm of false vocal cord
Malignant neoplasm of posterior (laryngeal) surface of epiglottis
Malignant neoplasm of ventricular bands
> **EXCLUDES 2** *malignant neoplasm of anterior surface of epiglottis (C10.1)*
> *malignant neoplasm of aryepiglottic fold or interarytenoid fold, hypopharyngeal aspect (C13.1)*
> *malignant neoplasm of aryepiglottic fold or interarytenoid fold, marginal zone (C13.1)*
> *malignant neoplasm of aryepiglottic fold or interarytenoid fold NOS (C13.1)*

C32.2 **Malignant neoplasm of subglottis** `HCC`

C32.3 **Malignant neoplasm of laryngeal cartilage** `HCC`

C32.8 **Malignant neoplasm of overlapping sites of larynx** `HCC`

C32.9 **Malignant neoplasm of larynx, unspecified** `HCC` ▽

C33 **Malignant neoplasm of trachea** `HCC`
Use additional code to identify:
  exposure to environmental tobacco smoke (Z77.22)
  exposure to tobacco smoke in the perinatal period (P96.81)
  history of tobacco dependence (Z87.891)
  occupational exposure to environmental tobacco smoke (Z57.31)
  tobacco dependence (F17.-)
  tobacco use (Z72.0)

✓4ᵗʰ **C34** **Malignant neoplasm of bronchus and lung**
Use additional code to identify:
  exposure to environmental tobacco smoke (Z77.22)
  exposure to tobacco smoke in the perinatal period (P96.81)
  history of tobacco dependence (Z87.891)
  occupational exposure to environmental tobacco smoke (Z57.31)
  tobacco dependence (F17.-)
  tobacco use (Z72.0)
> **EXCLUDES 1** *Kaposi's sarcoma of lung (C46.5-)*
> *malignant carcinoid tumor of the bronchus and lung (C7A.090)*

✓5ᵗʰ **C34.0** **Malignant neoplasm of main bronchus**
Malignant neoplasm of carina
Malignant neoplasm of hilus (of lung)

C34.00 **Malignant neoplasm of unspecified main bronchus** `HCC` `Q` ▽

C34.01 **Malignant neoplasm of right main bronchus** `HCC` `Q`

C34.02 **Malignant neoplasm of left main bronchus** `HCC` `Q`

✓5ᵗʰ **C34.1** **Malignant neoplasm of upper lobe, bronchus or lung**

C34.10 **Malignant neoplasm of upper lobe, unspecified bronchus or lung** `HCC` `Q` ▽

C34.11 **Malignant neoplasm of upper lobe, right bronchus or lung** `HCC` `Q`

C34.12 **Malignant neoplasm of upper lobe, left bronchus or lung** `HCC` `Q`

C34.2 **Malignant neoplasm of middle lobe, bronchus or lung** `HCC` `Q`

✓5ᵗʰ **C34.3** **Malignant neoplasm of lower lobe, bronchus or lung**

C34.30 **Malignant neoplasm of lower lobe, unspecified bronchus or lung** `HCC` `Q` ▽

C34.31 **Malignant neoplasm of lower lobe, right bronchus or lung** `HCC` `Q`

C34.32   Malignant neoplasm of lower lobe, left bronchus or lung `HCC` `Q`

√5ᵗʰ **C34.8**   Malignant neoplasm of overlapping sites of bronchus and lung

C34.80   Malignant neoplasm of overlapping sites of unspecified bronchus and lung `HCC` `Q` ▽

C34.81   Malignant neoplasm of overlapping sites of right bronchus and lung `HCC` `Q`

C34.82   Malignant neoplasm of overlapping sites of left bronchus and lung `HCC` `Q`

√5ᵗʰ **C34.9**   Malignant neoplasm of unspecified part of bronchus or lung

C34.90   Malignant neoplasm of unspecified part of unspecified bronchus or lung `HCC` `Q` ▽
     Lung cancer NOS

C34.91   Malignant neoplasm of unspecified part of right bronchus or lung `HCC` `Q` ▽

C34.92   Malignant neoplasm of unspecified part of left bronchus or lung `HCC` `Q` ▽

C37   Malignant neoplasm of thymus `HCC`
   EXCLUDES 1   malignant carcinoid tumor of the thymus (C7A.Ø91)

√4ᵗʰ **C38**   Malignant neoplasm of heart, mediastinum and pleura
   EXCLUDES 1   mesothelioma (C45.-)

C38.Ø   Malignant neoplasm of heart `HCC`
     Malignant neoplasm of pericardium
     EXCLUDES 1   malignant neoplasm of great vessels (C49.3)

C38.1   Malignant neoplasm of anterior mediastinum `HCC`

C38.2   Malignant neoplasm of posterior mediastinum `HCC`

C38.3   Malignant neoplasm of mediastinum, part unspecified `HCC` ▽

C38.4   Malignant neoplasm of pleura `HCC`

C38.8   Malignant neoplasm of overlapping sites of heart, mediastinum and pleura `HCC`

√4ᵗʰ **C39**   Malignant neoplasm of other and ill-defined sites in the respiratory system and intrathoracic organs
     Use additional code to identify:
     exposure to environmental tobacco smoke (Z77.22)
     exposure to tobacco smoke in the perinatal period (P96.81)
     history of tobacco dependence (Z87.891)
     occupational exposure to environmental tobacco smoke (Z57.31)
     tobacco dependence (F17.-)
     tobacco use (Z72.Ø)
   EXCLUDES 1   intrathoracic malignant neoplasm NOS (C76.1)
          thoracic malignant neoplasm NOS (C76.1)

C39.Ø   Malignant neoplasm of upper respiratory tract, part unspecified `HCC` ▽

C39.9   Malignant neoplasm of lower respiratory tract, part unspecified `HCC` ▽
     Malignant neoplasm of respiratory tract NOS

Malignant neoplasms of bone and articular cartilage (C4Ø-C41)

INCLUDES   malignant neoplasm of cartilage (articular) (joint)
          malignant neoplasm of periosteum
EXCLUDES 1   malignant neoplasm of bone marrow NOS (C96.9)
          malignant neoplasm of synovia (C49.-)

√4ᵗʰ **C4Ø**   Malignant neoplasm of bone and articular cartilage of limbs
     Use additional code to identify major osseous defect, if applicable (M89.7-)

√5ᵗʰ **C4Ø.Ø**   Malignant neoplasm of scapula and long bones of upper limb

C4Ø.ØØ   Malignant neoplasm of scapula and long bones of unspecified upper limb `HCC` ▽

C4Ø.Ø1   Malignant neoplasm of scapula and long bones of right upper limb `HCC`

C4Ø.Ø2   Malignant neoplasm of scapula and long bones of left upper limb `HCC`

√5ᵗʰ **C4Ø.1**   Malignant neoplasm of short bones of upper limb

C4Ø.1Ø   Malignant neoplasm of short bones of unspecified upper limb `HCC` ▽

C4Ø.11   Malignant neoplasm of short bones of right upper limb `HCC`

C4Ø.12   Malignant neoplasm of short bones of left upper limb `HCC`

√5ᵗʰ **C4Ø.2**   Malignant neoplasm of long bones of lower limb

C4Ø.2Ø   Malignant neoplasm of long bones of unspecified lower limb `HCC` ▽

C4Ø.21   Malignant neoplasm of long bones of right lower limb `HCC`

C4Ø.22   Malignant neoplasm of long bones of left lower limb `HCC`

√5ᵗʰ **C4Ø.3**   Malignant neoplasm of short bones of lower limb

C4Ø.3Ø   Malignant neoplasm of short bones of unspecified lower limb `HCC` ▽

C4Ø.31   Malignant neoplasm of short bones of right lower limb `HCC`

C4Ø.32   Malignant neoplasm of short bones of left lower limb `HCC`

√5ᵗʰ **C4Ø.8**   Malignant neoplasm of overlapping sites of bone and articular cartilage of limb

C4Ø.8Ø   Malignant neoplasm of overlapping sites of bone and articular cartilage of unspecified limb `HCC` ▽

C4Ø.81   Malignant neoplasm of overlapping sites of bone and articular cartilage of right limb `HCC`

C4Ø.82   Malignant neoplasm of overlapping sites of bone and articular cartilage of left limb `HCC`

√5ᵗʰ **C4Ø.9**   Malignant neoplasm of unspecified bones and articular cartilage of limb

C4Ø.9Ø   Malignant neoplasm of unspecified bones and articular cartilage of unspecified limb `HCC` ▽

C4Ø.91   Malignant neoplasm of unspecified bones and articular cartilage of right limb `HCC` ▽

C4Ø.92   Malignant neoplasm of unspecified bones and articular cartilage of left limb `HCC` ▽

√4ᵗʰ **C41**   Malignant neoplasm of bone and articular cartilage of other and unspecified sites
   EXCLUDES 1   malignant neoplasm of bones of limbs (C4Ø.-)
          malignant neoplasm of cartilage of ear (C49.Ø)
          malignant neoplasm of cartilage of eyelid (C49.Ø)
          malignant neoplasm of cartilage of larynx (C32.3)
          malignant neoplasm of cartilage of limbs (C4Ø.-)
          malignant neoplasm of cartilage of nose (C3Ø.Ø)

C41.Ø   Malignant neoplasm of bones of skull and face `HCC`
     Malignant neoplasm of maxilla (superior)
     Malignant neoplasm of orbital bone
   EXCLUDES 2   carcinoma, any type except intraosseous or odontogenic of:
          maxillary sinus (C31.Ø)
          upper jaw (CØ3.Ø)
          malignant neoplasm of jaw bone (lower) (C41.1)

C41.1   Malignant neoplasm of mandible `HCC`
     Malignant neoplasm of inferior maxilla
     Malignant neoplasm of lower jaw bone
   EXCLUDES 2   carcinoma, any type except intraosseous or odontogenic of:
          jaw NOS (CØ3.9)
          lower (CØ3.1)
          malignant neoplasm of upper jaw bone (C41.Ø)

C41.2   Malignant neoplasm of vertebral column `HCC`
   EXCLUDES 1   malignant neoplasm of sacrum and coccyx (C41.4)

C41.3   Malignant neoplasm of ribs, sternum and clavicle `HCC`

C41.4   Malignant neoplasm of pelvic bones, sacrum and coccyx `HCC`

C41.9   Malignant neoplasm of bone and articular cartilage, unspecified `HCC` ▽

Melanoma and other malignant neoplasms of skin (C43-C44)

√4ᵗʰ **C43**   Malignant melanoma of skin
   EXCLUDES 1   melanoma in situ (DØ3.-)
   EXCLUDES 2   malignant melanoma of skin of genital organs (C51-C52, C6Ø.-, C63.-)
          Merkel cell carcinoma (C4A.-)
          sites other than skin - code to malignant neoplasm of the site

C43.Ø   Malignant melanoma of lip `HCC` `Q`
   EXCLUDES 1   malignant neoplasm of vermilion border of lip (CØØ.Ø-CØØ.2)

√5ᵗʰ **C43.1**   Malignant melanoma of eyelid, including canthus

C43.1Ø   Malignant melanoma of unspecified eyelid, including canthus `HCC` ▽

√6ᵗʰ **C43.11**   Malignant melanoma of right eyelid, including canthus

     ● **C43.111**   Malignant melanoma of right upper eyelid, including canthus

     ● **C43.112**   Malignant melanoma of right lower eyelid, including canthus

☑ Additional Character Req   √x7ᵗʰ Placeholder Alert   Manifestation   ▽ Unspecified   ►◄ Revised Text   ● New Code   ▲ Revised Code Title

ICD-10-CM 2019   465

✓6ᵗʰ **C43.12 Malignant melanoma of left eyelid, including canthus**
- **C43.121 Malignant melanoma of left upper eyelid, including canthus**
- **C43.122 Malignant melanoma of left lower eyelid, including canthus**

✓5ᵗʰ **C43.2 Malignant melanoma of ear and external auricular canal**
- **C43.2Ø Malignant melanoma of unspecified ear and external auricular canal** HCC Q ▽
- **C43.21 Malignant melanoma of right ear and external auricular canal** HCC Q
- **C43.22 Malignant melanoma of left ear and external auricular canal** HCC Q

✓5ᵗʰ **C43.3 Malignant melanoma of other and unspecified parts of face**
- **C43.3Ø Malignant melanoma of unspecified part of face** HCC Q ▽
- **C43.31 Malignant melanoma of nose** HCC Q
- **C43.39 Malignant melanoma of other parts of face** HCC Q

C43.4 Malignant melanoma of scalp and neck HCC Q

✓5ᵗʰ **C43.5 Malignant melanoma of trunk**
- EXCLUDES 2   *malignant neoplasm of anus NOS (C21.Ø)*
-     *malignant neoplasm of scrotum (C63.2)*
- **C43.51 Malignant melanoma of anal skin**
  - Malignant melanoma of anal margin
  - Malignant melanoma of perianal skin
- **C43.52 Malignant melanoma of skin of breast** HCC Q
- **C43.59 Malignant melanoma of other part of trunk** HCC Q

✓5ᵗʰ **C43.6 Malignant melanoma of upper limb, including shoulder**
- **C43.6Ø Malignant melanoma of unspecified upper limb, including shoulder** HCC Q ▽
- **C43.61 Malignant melanoma of right upper limb, including shoulder** HCC Q
- **C43.62 Malignant melanoma of left upper limb, including shoulder** HCC Q

✓5ᵗʰ **C43.7 Malignant melanoma of lower limb, including hip**
- **C43.7Ø Malignant melanoma of unspecified lower limb, including hip** HCC Q ▽
- **C43.71 Malignant melanoma of right lower limb, including hip** HCC Q
- **C43.72 Malignant melanoma of left lower limb, including hip** HCC Q

C43.8 Malignant melanoma of overlapping sites of skin HCC Q

C43.9 Malignant melanoma of skin, unspecified HCC Q ▽
- Malignant melanoma of unspecified site of skin
- Melanoma (malignant) NOS

✓4ᵗʰ **C4A Merkel cell carcinoma**

DEF: Malignant cutaneous cancer predominantly found in elderly patients with sun exposure that usually presents as a flesh-colored or bluish-red lump typically seen on the neck, head, and face.

C4A.Ø Merkel cell carcinoma of lip HCC
- EXCLUDES 1   *malignant neoplasm of vermilion border of lip (C00.0-C00.2)*

✓5ᵗʰ **C4A.1 Merkel cell carcinoma of eyelid, including canthus**
- **C4A.1Ø Merkel cell carcinoma of unspecified eyelid, including canthus** HCC ▽
- ✓6ᵗʰ **C4A.11 Merkel cell carcinoma of right eyelid, including canthus**
  - **C4A.111 Merkel cell carcinoma of right upper eyelid, including canthus**
  - **C4A.112 Merkel cell carcinoma of right lower eyelid, including canthus**
- ✓6ᵗʰ **C4A.12 Merkel cell carcinoma of left eyelid, including canthus**
  - **C4A.121 Merkel cell carcinoma of left upper eyelid, including canthus**
  - **C4A.122 Merkel cell carcinoma of left lower eyelid, including canthus**

✓5ᵗʰ **C4A.2 Merkel cell carcinoma of ear and external auricular canal**
- **C4A.2Ø Merkel cell carcinoma of unspecified ear and external auricular canal** HCC ▽
- **C4A.21 Merkel cell carcinoma of right ear and external auricular canal** HCC
- **C4A.22 Merkel cell carcinoma of left ear and external auricular canal** HCC

✓5ᵗʰ **C4A.3 Merkel cell carcinoma of other and unspecified parts of face**
- **C4A.3Ø Merkel cell carcinoma of unspecified part of face** HCC ▽

C4A.31 Merkel cell carcinoma of nose HCC

C4A.39 Merkel cell carcinoma of other parts of face HCC

C4A.4 Merkel cell carcinoma of scalp and neck HCC

✓5ᵗʰ **C4A.5 Merkel cell carcinoma of trunk**
- EXCLUDES 2   *malignant neoplasm of anus NOS (C21.Ø)*
-     *malignant neoplasm of scrotum (C63.2)*
- **C4A.51 Merkel cell carcinoma of anal skin** HCC
  - Merkel cell carcinoma of anal margin
  - Merkel cell carcinoma of perianal skin
- **C4A.52 Merkel cell carcinoma of skin of breast** HCC
- **C4A.59 Merkel cell carcinoma of other part of trunk** HCC

✓5ᵗʰ **C4A.6 Merkel cell carcinoma of upper limb, including shoulder**
- **C4A.6Ø Merkel cell carcinoma of unspecified upper limb, including shoulder** HCC ▽
- **C4A.61 Merkel cell carcinoma of right upper limb, including shoulder** HCC
- **C4A.62 Merkel cell carcinoma of left upper limb, including shoulder** HCC

✓5ᵗʰ **C4A.7 Merkel cell carcinoma of lower limb, including hip**
- **C4A.7Ø Merkel cell carcinoma of unspecified lower limb, including hip** HCC ▽
- **C4A.71 Merkel cell carcinoma of right lower limb, including hip** HCC
- **C4A.72 Merkel cell carcinoma of left lower limb, including hip** HCC

C4A.8 Merkel cell carcinoma of overlapping sites HCC

C4A.9 Merkel cell carcinoma, unspecified HCC ▽
- Merkel cell carcinoma of unspecified site
- Merkel cell carcinoma NOS

✓4ᵗʰ **C44 Other and unspecified malignant neoplasm of skin**

INCLUDES   malignant neoplasm of sebaceous glands
    malignant neoplasm of sweat glands

EXCLUDES 1   *Kaposi's sarcoma of skin (C46.Ø)*
    malignant melanoma of skin (C43.-)
    malignant neoplasm of skin of genital organs (C51-C52, C6Ø.-, C63.2)
    Merkel cell carcinoma (C4A.-)

DEF: Basal cell carcinoma: Abnormal growth of skin cells that arises from the deepest layer of the epidermis and may present as an open sore, red patches, pink growth, or scar. Typically caused by sun exposure, it is one of the most common forms of skin cancer.

DEF: Squamous cell carcinoma: Uncontrolled growth of abnormal skin cells that arises from the outer layers of the skin (epidermis) and may present as an open sore. It is characterized by a firm, red nodule, elevated growth with a central depression, or a flat sore with a scaly crust.

✓5ᵗʰ **C44.Ø Other and unspecified malignant neoplasm of skin of lip**
- EXCLUDES 1   *malignant neoplasm of lip (C00.-)*
- **C44.ØØ Unspecified malignant neoplasm of skin of lip** ▽
- **C44.Ø1 Basal cell carcinoma of skin of lip**
- **C44.Ø2 Squamous cell carcinoma of skin of lip**
- **C44.Ø9 Other specified malignant neoplasm of skin of lip**

✓5ᵗʰ **C44.1 Other and unspecified malignant neoplasm of skin of eyelid, including canthus**
- EXCLUDES 1   *connective tissue of eyelid (C49.Ø)*
- ✓6ᵗʰ **C44.1Ø Unspecified malignant neoplasm of skin of eyelid, including canthus**
  - **C44.1Ø1 Unspecified malignant neoplasm of skin of unspecified eyelid, including canthus** ▽
  - ✓7ᵗʰ **C44.1Ø2 Unspecified malignant neoplasm of skin of right eyelid, including canthus**
    - **C44.1Ø21 Unspecified malignant neoplasm of skin of right upper eyelid, including canthus** ▽
    - **C44.1Ø22 Unspecified malignant neoplasm of skin of right lower eyelid, including canthus** ▽
  - ✓7ᵗʰ **C44.1Ø9 Unspecified malignant neoplasm of skin of left eyelid, including canthus**

-    C44.1091   Unspecified malignant neoplasm of skin of left upper eyelid, including canthus   ▽
-    C44.1092   Unspecified malignant neoplasm of skin of left lower eyelid, including canthus   ▽

☑6ᵗʰ   **C44.11**   Basal cell carcinoma of skin of eyelid, including canthus

    C44.111   Basal cell carcinoma of skin of unspecified eyelid, including canthus   ▽

☑7ᵗʰ   C44.112   Basal cell carcinoma of skin of right eyelid, including canthus

-    C44.1121   Basal cell carcinoma of skin of right upper eyelid, including canthus
-    C44.1122   Basal cell carcinoma of skin of right lower eyelid, including canthus

☑7ᵗʰ   C44.119   Basal cell carcinoma of skin of left eyelid, including canthus

-    C44.1191   Basal cell carcinoma of skin of left upper eyelid, including canthus
-    C44.1192   Basal cell carcinoma of skin of left lower eyelid, including canthus

☑6ᵗʰ   **C44.12**   Squamous cell carcinoma of skin of eyelid, including canthus

    C44.121   Squamous cell carcinoma of skin of unspecified eyelid, including canthus   ▽

☑7ᵗʰ   C44.122   Squamous cell carcinoma of skin of right eyelid, including canthus

-    C44.1221   Squamous cell carcinoma of skin of right upper eyelid, including canthus
-    C44.1222   Squamous cell carcinoma of skin of right lower eyelid, including canthus

☑7ᵗʰ   C44.129   Squamous cell carcinoma of skin of left eyelid, including canthus

-    C44.1291   Squamous cell carcinoma of skin of left upper eyelid, including canthus
-    C44.1292   Squamous cell carcinoma of skin of left lower eyelid, including canthus

☑6ᵗʰ   **C44.13**   Sebaceous cell carcinoma of skin of eyelid, including canthus

    C44.131   Sebaceous cell carcinoma of skin of unspecified eyelid, including canthus   ▽

☑7ᵗʰ   C44.132   Sebaceous cell carcinoma of skin of right eyelid, including canthus

-    C44.1321   Sebaceous cell carcinoma of skin of right upper eyelid, including canthus
-    C44.1322   Sebaceous cell carcinoma of skin of right lower eyelid, including canthus

☑7ᵗʰ   C44.139   Sebaceous cell carcinoma of skin of left eyelid, including canthus

-    C44.1391   Sebaceous cell carcinoma of skin of left upper eyelid, including canthus
-    C44.1392   Sebaceous cell carcinoma of skin of left lower eyelid, including canthus

☑6ᵗʰ   **C44.19**   Other specified malignant neoplasm of skin of eyelid, including canthus

    C44.191   Other specified malignant neoplasm of skin of unspecified eyelid, including canthus   ▽

☑7ᵗʰ   C44.192   Other specified malignant neoplasm of skin of right eyelid, including canthus

-    C44.1921   Other specified malignant neoplasm of skin of right upper eyelid, including canthus

---

-    C44.1922   Other specified malignant neoplasm of skin of right lower eyelid, including canthus

☑7ᵗʰ   C44.199   Other specified malignant neoplasm of skin of left eyelid, including canthus

-    C44.1991   Other specified malignant neoplasm of skin of left upper eyelid, including canthus
-    C44.1992   Other specified malignant neoplasm of skin of left lower eyelid, including canthus

☑5ᵗʰ   **C44.2**   Other and unspecified malignant neoplasm of skin of ear and external auricular canal

    EXCLUDES 1   connective tissue of ear (C49.0)

☑6ᵗʰ   **C44.20**   Unspecified malignant neoplasm of skin of ear and external auricular canal

    C44.201   Unspecified malignant neoplasm of skin of unspecified ear and external auricular canal   ▽

    C44.202   Unspecified malignant neoplasm of skin of right ear and external auricular canal   ▽

    C44.209   Unspecified malignant neoplasm of skin of left ear and external auricular canal   ▽

☑6ᵗʰ   **C44.21**   Basal cell carcinoma of skin of ear and external auricular canal

    C44.211   Basal cell carcinoma of skin of unspecified ear and external auricular canal

    C44.212   Basal cell carcinoma of skin of right ear and external auricular canal

    C44.219   Basal cell carcinoma of skin of left ear and external auricular canal

☑6ᵗʰ   **C44.22**   Squamous cell carcinoma of skin of ear and external auricular canal

    C44.221   Squamous cell carcinoma of skin of unspecified ear and external auricular canal   ▽

    C44.222   Squamous cell carcinoma of skin of right ear and external auricular canal

    C44.229   Squamous cell carcinoma of skin of left ear and external auricular canal

☑6ᵗʰ   **C44.29**   Other specified malignant neoplasm of skin of ear and external auricular canal

    C44.291   Other specified malignant neoplasm of skin of unspecified ear and external auricular canal   ▽

    C44.292   Other specified malignant neoplasm of skin of right ear and external auricular canal

    C44.299   Other specified malignant neoplasm of skin of left ear and external auricular canal

☑5ᵗʰ   **C44.3**   Other and unspecified malignant neoplasm of skin of other and unspecified parts of face

☑6ᵗʰ   **C44.30**   Unspecified malignant neoplasm of skin of other and unspecified parts of face

    C44.300   Unspecified malignant neoplasm of skin of unspecified part of face   ▽

    C44.301   Unspecified malignant neoplasm of skin of nose   ▽

    C44.309   Unspecified malignant neoplasm of skin of other parts of face   ▽

☑6ᵗʰ   **C44.31**   Basal cell carcinoma of skin of other and unspecified parts of face

    C44.310   Basal cell carcinoma of skin of unspecified parts of face   ▽

    C44.311   Basal cell carcinoma of skin of nose

    C44.319   Basal cell carcinoma of skin of other parts of face

☑6ᵗʰ   **C44.32**   Squamous cell carcinoma of skin of other and unspecified parts of face

    C44.320   Squamous cell carcinoma of skin of unspecified parts of face   ▽

    C44.321   Squamous cell carcinoma of skin of nose

    C44.329   Squamous cell carcinoma of skin of other parts of face

---

☑ Additional Character Req   ✓x7ᵗʰ Placeholder Alert   Manifestation   ▽ Unspecified   ►◄ Revised Text   ● New Code   ▲ Revised Code Title

Chapter 2. Neoplasms

C44.39–C44.99

✓6ᵗʰ **C44.39** **Other specified malignant neoplasm of skin of other and unspecified parts of face**

C44.390 Other specified malignant neoplasm of skin of unspecified parts of face ▽

C44.391 Other specified malignant neoplasm of skin of nose

C44.399 Other specified malignant neoplasm of skin of other parts of face

✓5ᵗʰ **C44.4** **Other and unspecified malignant neoplasm of skin of scalp and neck**

C44.40 Unspecified malignant neoplasm of skin of scalp and neck ▽

C44.41 Basal cell carcinoma of skin of scalp and neck

C44.42 Squamous cell carcinoma of skin of scalp and neck

C44.49 Other specified malignant neoplasm of skin of scalp and neck

✓5ᵗʰ **C44.5** **Other and unspecified malignant neoplasm of skin of trunk**

     EXCLUDES 1   anus NOS (C21.0)
                    scrotum (C63.2)

✓6ᵗʰ **C44.50** Unspecified malignant neoplasm of skin of trunk

C44.500 Unspecified malignant neoplasm of anal skin ▽
       Unspecified malignant neoplasm of anal margin
       Unspecified malignant neoplasm of perianal skin

C44.501 Unspecified malignant neoplasm of skin of breast ▽

C44.509 Unspecified malignant neoplasm of skin of other part of trunk ▽

✓6ᵗʰ **C44.51** Basal cell carcinoma of skin of trunk

C44.510 Basal cell carcinoma of anal skin
       Basal cell carcinoma of anal margin
       Basal cell carcinoma of perianal skin

C44.511 Basal cell carcinoma of skin of breast

C44.519 Basal cell carcinoma of skin of other part of trunk

✓6ᵗʰ **C44.52** Squamous cell carcinoma of skin of trunk

C44.520 Squamous cell carcinoma of anal skin
       Squamous cell carcinoma of anal margin
       Squamous cell carcinoma of perianal skin

C44.521 Squamous cell carcinoma of skin of breast

C44.529 Squamous cell carcinoma of skin of other part of trunk

✓6ᵗʰ **C44.59** Other specified malignant neoplasm of skin of trunk

C44.590 Other specified malignant neoplasm of anal skin
       Other specified malignant neoplasm of anal margin
       Other specified malignant neoplasm of perianal skin

C44.591 Other specified malignant neoplasm of skin of breast

C44.599 Other specified malignant neoplasm of skin of other part of trunk

✓5ᵗʰ **C44.6** **Other and unspecified malignant neoplasm of skin of upper limb, including shoulder**

✓6ᵗʰ **C44.60** Unspecified malignant neoplasm of skin of upper limb, including shoulder

C44.601 Unspecified malignant neoplasm of skin of unspecified upper limb, including shoulder ▽

C44.602 Unspecified malignant neoplasm of skin of right upper limb, including shoulder ▽

C44.609 Unspecified malignant neoplasm of skin of left upper limb, including shoulder ▽

✓6ᵗʰ **C44.61** Basal cell carcinoma of skin of upper limb, including shoulder

C44.611 Basal cell carcinoma of skin of unspecified upper limb, including shoulder ▽

C44.612 Basal cell carcinoma of skin of right upper limb, including shoulder

C44.619 Basal cell carcinoma of skin of left upper limb, including shoulder

✓6ᵗʰ **C44.62** Squamous cell carcinoma of skin of upper limb, including shoulder

C44.621 Squamous cell carcinoma of skin of unspecified upper limb, including shoulder ▽

C44.622 Squamous cell carcinoma of skin of right upper limb, including shoulder

C44.629 Squamous cell carcinoma of skin of left upper limb, including shoulder

✓6ᵗʰ **C44.69** Other specified malignant neoplasm of skin of upper limb, including shoulder

C44.691 Other specified malignant neoplasm of skin of unspecified upper limb, including shoulder ▽

C44.692 Other specified malignant neoplasm of skin of right upper limb, including shoulder

C44.699 Other specified malignant neoplasm of skin of left upper limb, including shoulder

✓5ᵗʰ **C44.7** **Other and unspecified malignant neoplasm of skin of lower limb, including hip**

✓6ᵗʰ **C44.70** Unspecified malignant neoplasm of skin of lower limb, including hip

C44.701 Unspecified malignant neoplasm of skin of unspecified lower limb, including hip ▽

C44.702 Unspecified malignant neoplasm of skin of right lower limb, including hip ▽

C44.709 Unspecified malignant neoplasm of skin of left lower limb, including hip ▽

✓6ᵗʰ **C44.71** Basal cell carcinoma of skin of lower limb, including hip

C44.711 Basal cell carcinoma of skin of unspecified lower limb, including hip ▽

C44.712 Basal cell carcinoma of skin of right lower limb, including hip

C44.719 Basal cell carcinoma of skin of left lower limb, including hip

✓6ᵗʰ **C44.72** Squamous cell carcinoma of skin of lower limb, including hip

C44.721 Squamous cell carcinoma of skin of unspecified lower limb, including hip ▽

C44.722 Squamous cell carcinoma of skin of right lower limb, including hip

C44.729 Squamous cell carcinoma of skin of left lower limb, including hip

✓6ᵗʰ **C44.79** Other specified malignant neoplasm of skin of lower limb, including hip

C44.791 Other specified malignant neoplasm of skin of unspecified lower limb, including hip ▽

C44.792 Other specified malignant neoplasm of skin of right lower limb, including hip

C44.799 Other specified malignant neoplasm of skin of left lower limb, including hip

✓5ᵗʰ **C44.8** **Other and unspecified malignant neoplasm of overlapping sites of skin**

C44.80 Unspecified malignant neoplasm of overlapping sites of skin ▽

C44.81 Basal cell carcinoma of overlapping sites of skin

C44.82 Squamous cell carcinoma of overlapping sites of skin

C44.89 Other specified malignant neoplasm of overlapping sites of skin

✓5ᵗʰ **C44.9** **Other and unspecified malignant neoplasm of skin, unspecified**

C44.90 Unspecified malignant neoplasm of skin, unspecified ▽
       Malignant neoplasm of unspecified site of skin

C44.91 Basal cell carcinoma of skin, unspecified ▽

C44.92 Squamous cell carcinoma of skin, unspecified ▽

C44.99 Other specified malignant neoplasm of skin, unspecified ▽

Malignant neoplasms of mesothelial and soft tissue (C45-C49)

☑4ᵗʰ **C45 Mesothelioma**

DEF: Rare type of cancer that forms in the thin layer of protective tissue that covers the majority of internal organs (mesothelium).

C45.0 Mesothelioma of pleura   HCC
    EXCLUDES 1   *other malignant neoplasm of pleura (C38.4)*
    AHA: 2017,2Q,11

C45.1 Mesothelioma of peritoneum   HCC
    Mesothelioma of cul-de-sac
    Mesothelioma of mesentery
    Mesothelioma of mesocolon
    Mesothelioma of omentum
    Mesothelioma of peritoneum (parietal) (pelvic)
    EXCLUDES 1   *other malignant neoplasm of soft tissue of peritoneum (C48.-)*

C45.2 Mesothelioma of pericardium   HCC
    EXCLUDES 1   *other malignant neoplasm of pericardium (C38.0)*

C45.7 Mesothelioma of other sites   HCC

C45.9 Mesothelioma, unspecified   HCC ▽

☑4ᵗʰ **C46 Kaposi's sarcoma**

Code first any human immunodeficiency virus [HIV] disease (B20)
DEF: Malignant neoplasm that causes patches of abnormal tissue to grow under the skin, in the lining of the mouth, nose, and throat, in lymph nodes, or in other visceral organs. Kaposi's sarcoma is caused by human herpesvirus8 (HHV8).

C46.0 Kaposi's sarcoma of skin   HCC

C46.1 Kaposi's sarcoma of soft tissue   HCC
    Kaposi's sarcoma of blood vessel
    Kaposi's sarcoma of connective tissue
    Kaposi's sarcoma of fascia
    Kaposi's sarcoma of ligament
    Kaposi's sarcoma of lymphatic(s) NEC
    Kaposi's sarcoma of muscle
    EXCLUDES 2   *Kaposi's sarcoma of lymph glands and nodes (C46.3)*

C46.2 Kaposi's sarcoma of palate   HCC

C46.3 Kaposi's sarcoma of lymph nodes   HCC

C46.4 Kaposi's sarcoma of gastrointestinal sites   HCC

☑5ᵗʰ **C46.5 Kaposi's sarcoma of lung**

    C46.50 Kaposi's sarcoma of unspecified lung   HCC ▽
    C46.51 Kaposi's sarcoma of right lung   HCC
    C46.52 Kaposi's sarcoma of left lung   HCC

C46.7 Kaposi's sarcoma of other sites   HCC

C46.9 Kaposi's sarcoma, unspecified   HCC ▽
    Kaposi's sarcoma of unspecified site

☑4ᵗʰ **C47 Malignant neoplasm of peripheral nerves and autonomic nervous system**

    INCLUDES   malignant neoplasm of sympathetic and parasympathetic nerves and ganglia
    EXCLUDES 1   *Kaposi's sarcoma of soft tissue (C46.1)*

C47.0 Malignant neoplasm of peripheral nerves of head, face and neck   HCC
    EXCLUDES 1   *malignant neoplasm of peripheral nerves of orbit (C69.6-)*

☑5ᵗʰ **C47.1 Malignant neoplasm of peripheral nerves of upper limb, including shoulder**

    C47.10 Malignant neoplasm of peripheral nerves of unspecified upper limb, including shoulder   HCC ▽
    C47.11 Malignant neoplasm of peripheral nerves of right upper limb, including shoulder   HCC
    C47.12 Malignant neoplasm of peripheral nerves of left upper limb, including shoulder   HCC

☑5ᵗʰ **C47.2 Malignant neoplasm of peripheral nerves of lower limb, including hip**

    C47.20 Malignant neoplasm of peripheral nerves of unspecified lower limb, including hip   HCC ▽
    C47.21 Malignant neoplasm of peripheral nerves of right lower limb, including hip   HCC
    C47.22 Malignant neoplasm of peripheral nerves of left lower limb, including hip   HCC

C47.3 Malignant neoplasm of peripheral nerves of thorax   HCC

C47.4 Malignant neoplasm of peripheral nerves of abdomen   HCC

C47.5 Malignant neoplasm of peripheral nerves of pelvis   HCC

C47.6 Malignant neoplasm of peripheral nerves of trunk, unspecified   HCC ▽
    Malignant neoplasm of peripheral nerves of unspecified part of trunk

C47.8 Malignant neoplasm of overlapping sites of peripheral nerves and autonomic nervous system   HCC

C47.9 Malignant neoplasm of peripheral nerves and autonomic nervous system, unspecified   HCC ▽
    Malignant neoplasm of unspecified site of peripheral nerves and autonomic nervous system

☑4ᵗʰ **C48 Malignant neoplasm of retroperitoneum and peritoneum**

    EXCLUDES 1   *Kaposi's sarcoma of connective tissue (C46.1)*
              mesothelioma (C45.-)

C48.0 Malignant neoplasm of retroperitoneum   HCC

C48.1 Malignant neoplasm of specified parts of peritoneum   HCC
    Malignant neoplasm of cul-de-sac
    Malignant neoplasm of mesentery
    Malignant neoplasm of mesocolon
    Malignant neoplasm of omentum
    Malignant neoplasm of parietal peritoneum
    Malignant neoplasm of pelvic peritoneum

C48.2 Malignant neoplasm of peritoneum, unspecified   HCC ▽

C48.8 Malignant neoplasm of overlapping sites of retroperitoneum and peritoneum   HCC

☑4ᵗʰ **C49 Malignant neoplasm of other connective and soft tissue**

    INCLUDES   malignant neoplasm of blood vessel
             malignant neoplasm of bursa
             malignant neoplasm of cartilage
             malignant neoplasm of fascia
             malignant neoplasm of fat
             malignant neoplasm of ligament, except uterine
             malignant neoplasm of lymphatic vessel
             malignant neoplasm of muscle
             malignant neoplasm of synovia
             malignant neoplasm of tendon (sheath)
    EXCLUDES 1   *malignant neoplasm of cartilage (of):*
         articular (C40-C41)
         larynx (C32.3)
         nose (C30.0)
         malignant neoplasm of connective tissue of breast (C50.-)
    EXCLUDES 2   *Kaposi's sarcoma of soft tissue (C46.1)*
         malignant neoplasm of heart (C38.0)
         malignant neoplasm of peripheral nerves and autonomic nervous system (C47.-)
         malignant neoplasm of peritoneum (C48.2)
         malignant neoplasm of retroperitoneum (C48.0)
         malignant neoplasm of uterine ligament (C57.3)
         mesothelioma (C45.-)

C49.0 Malignant neoplasm of connective and soft tissue of head, face and neck   HCC
    Malignant neoplasm of connective tissue of ear
    Malignant neoplasm of connective tissue of eyelid
    EXCLUDES 1   *connective tissue of orbit (C69.6-)*

☑5ᵗʰ **C49.1 Malignant neoplasm of connective and soft tissue of upper limb, including shoulder**

    C49.10 Malignant neoplasm of connective and soft tissue of unspecified upper limb, including shoulder   HCC ▽
    C49.11 Malignant neoplasm of connective and soft tissue of right upper limb, including shoulder   HCC
    C49.12 Malignant neoplasm of connective and soft tissue of left upper limb, including shoulder   HCC

☑5ᵗʰ **C49.2 Malignant neoplasm of connective and soft tissue of lower limb, including hip**

    C49.20 Malignant neoplasm of connective and soft tissue of unspecified lower limb, including hip   HCC ▽
    C49.21 Malignant neoplasm of connective and soft tissue of right lower limb, including hip   HCC
    C49.22 Malignant neoplasm of connective and soft tissue of left lower limb, including hip   HCC

C49.3 Malignant neoplasm of connective and soft tissue `HCC`
of thorax
Malignant neoplasm of axilla
Malignant neoplasm of diaphragm
Malignant neoplasm of great vessels
EXCLUDES 1   *malignant neoplasm of breast (C50.-)*
malignant neoplasm of heart (C38.0)
malignant neoplasm of mediastinum (C38.1-C38.3)
malignant neoplasm of thymus (C37)
AHA: 2015,3Q,19

C49.4 Malignant neoplasm of connective and soft tissue `HCC`
of abdomen
Malignant neoplasm of abdominal wall
Malignant neoplasm of hypochondrium

C49.5 Malignant neoplasm of connective and soft tissue `HCC`
of pelvis
Malignant neoplasm of buttock
Malignant neoplasm of groin
Malignant neoplasm of perineum

C49.6 Malignant neoplasm of connective and soft tissue `HCC` ▽
of trunk, unspecified
Malignant neoplasm of back NOS

C49.8 Malignant neoplasm of overlapping sites of `HCC`
connective and soft tissue
Primary malignant neoplasm of two or more contiguous sites
of connective and soft tissue

C49.9 Malignant neoplasm of connective and soft tissue, `HCC` ▽
unspecified

√5ᵗʰ **C49.A Gastrointestinal stromal tumor**

AHA: 2016,4Q,8
DEF: Uncommon malignant tumor found in the GI tract that
originates from interstitial cells of the autonomic nervous system.
Most occur in the stomach or small intestine but can originate
anywhere in the GI tract.

C49.A0 Gastrointestinal stromal tumor, `HCC` ▽
unspecified site

C49.A1 Gastrointestinal stromal tumor of `HCC`
esophagus

C49.A2 Gastrointestinal stromal tumor of stomach `HCC`

C49.A3 Gastrointestinal stromal tumor of small `HCC`
intestine

C49.A4 Gastrointestinal stromal tumor of large `HCC`
intestine

C49.A5 Gastrointestinal stromal tumor of rectum `HCC`

C49.A9 Gastrointestinal stromal tumor of other `HCC`
sites

Malignant neoplasms of breast (C50)

√4ᵗʰ **C50 Malignant neoplasm of breast**
INCLUDES   connective tissue of breast
Paget's disease of breast
Paget's disease of nipple
Use additional code to identify estrogen receptor status (Z17.0, Z17.1)
EXCLUDES 1   *skin of breast (C44.501, C44.511, C44.521, C44.591)*
AHA: 2017,4Q,19

Female Breast

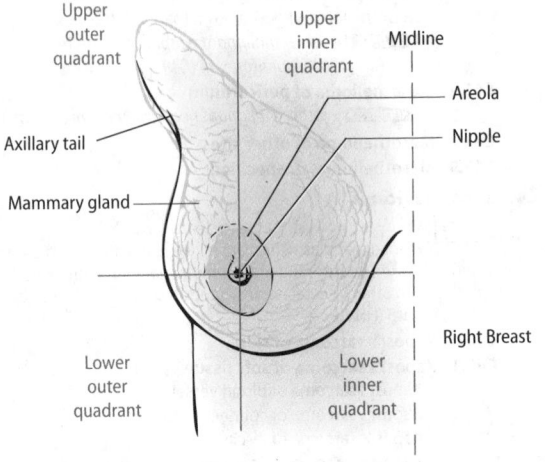

√5ᵗʰ **C50.0 Malignant neoplasm of nipple and areola**

√6ᵗʰ **C50.01 Malignant neoplasm of nipple and areola, female**

C50.011 Malignant neoplasm of nipple `HCC` 🄌 ♀
and areola, right female breast

C50.012 Malignant neoplasm of nipple `HCC` 🄌 ♀
and areola, left female breast

C50.019 Malignant neoplasm of nipple `HCC` 🄌♀▽
**and areola, unspecified female
breast**

√6ᵗʰ **C50.02 Malignant neoplasm of nipple and areola, male**

C50.021 Malignant neoplasm of nipple `HCC` 🄌 ♂
and areola, right male breast

C50.022 Malignant neoplasm of nipple `HCC` 🄌 ♂
and areola, left male breast

C50.029 Malignant neoplasm of nipple `HCC`🄌♂▽
**and areola, unspecified male
breast**

√5ᵗʰ **C50.1 Malignant neoplasm of central portion of breast**

√6ᵗʰ **C50.11 Malignant neoplasm of central portion of breast,
female**

C50.111 Malignant neoplasm of central `HCC` 🄌 ♀
portion of right female breast

C50.112 Malignant neoplasm of central `HCC` 🄌 ♀
portion of left female breast

C50.119 Malignant neoplasm of central `HCC`🄌♀▽
**portion of unspecified female
breast**

√6ᵗʰ **C50.12 Malignant neoplasm of central portion of breast,
male**

C50.121 Malignant neoplasm of central `HCC` 🄌 ♂
portion of right male breast

C50.122 Malignant neoplasm of central `HCC` 🄌 ♂
portion of left male breast

C50.129 Malignant neoplasm of central `HCC`🄌♂▽
**portion of unspecified male
breast**

√5ᵗʰ **C50.2 Malignant neoplasm of upper-inner quadrant of breast**

√6ᵗʰ **C50.21 Malignant neoplasm of upper-inner quadrant of
breast, female**

C50.211 Malignant neoplasm of `HCC` 🄌 ♀
**upper-inner quadrant of right
female breast**

C50.212 Malignant neoplasm of `HCC` 🄌 ♀
**upper-inner quadrant of left
female breast**

    C50.219 Malignant neoplasm of upper-inner quadrant of unspecified female breast   HCC ◨ ♀ ▽

   ✓6ᵗʰ **C50.22** Malignant neoplasm of upper-inner quadrant of breast, male

    C50.221 Malignant neoplasm of upper-inner quadrant of right male breast   HCC ◨ ♂

    C50.222 Malignant neoplasm of upper-inner quadrant of left male breast   HCC ◨ ♂

    C50.229 Malignant neoplasm of upper-inner quadrant of unspecified male breast   HCC ◨ ♂ ▽

✓5ᵗʰ **C50.3** Malignant neoplasm of lower-inner quadrant of breast

  ✓6ᵗʰ **C50.31** Malignant neoplasm of lower-inner quadrant of breast, female

    C50.311 Malignant neoplasm of lower-inner quadrant of right female breast   HCC ◨ ♀

    C50.312 Malignant neoplasm of lower-inner quadrant of left female breast   HCC ◨ ♀

    C50.319 Malignant neoplasm of lower-inner quadrant of unspecified female breast   HCC ◨ ♀ ▽

  ✓6ᵗʰ **C50.32** Malignant neoplasm of lower-inner quadrant of breast, male

    C50.321 Malignant neoplasm of lower-inner quadrant of right male breast   HCC ◨ ♂

    C50.322 Malignant neoplasm of lower-inner quadrant of left male breast   HCC ◨ ♂

    C50.329 Malignant neoplasm of lower-inner quadrant of unspecified male breast   HCC ◨ ♂ ▽

✓5ᵗʰ **C50.4** Malignant neoplasm of upper-outer quadrant of breast

  ✓6ᵗʰ **C50.41** Malignant neoplasm of upper-outer quadrant of breast, female

    C50.411 Malignant neoplasm of upper-outer quadrant of right female breast   HCC ◨ ♀

    C50.412 Malignant neoplasm of upper-outer quadrant of left female breast   HCC ◨ ♀

    C50.419 Malignant neoplasm of upper-outer quadrant of unspecified female breast   HCC ◨ ♀ ▽

  ✓6ᵗʰ **C50.42** Malignant neoplasm of upper-outer quadrant of breast, male

    C50.421 Malignant neoplasm of upper-outer quadrant of right male breast   HCC ◨ ♂

    C50.422 Malignant neoplasm of upper-outer quadrant of left male breast   HCC ◨ ♂

    C50.429 Malignant neoplasm of upper-outer quadrant of unspecified male breast   HCC ◨ ♂ ▽

✓5ᵗʰ **C50.5** Malignant neoplasm of lower-outer quadrant of breast

  ✓6ᵗʰ **C50.51** Malignant neoplasm of lower-outer quadrant of breast, female

    C50.511 Malignant neoplasm of lower-outer quadrant of right female breast   HCC ◨ ♀

    C50.512 Malignant neoplasm of lower-outer quadrant of left female breast   HCC ◨ ♀

    C50.519 Malignant neoplasm of lower-outer quadrant of unspecified female breast   HCC ◨ ♀ ▽

  ✓6ᵗʰ **C50.52** Malignant neoplasm of lower-outer quadrant of breast, male

    C50.521 Malignant neoplasm of lower-outer quadrant of right male breast   HCC ◨ ♂

    C50.522 Malignant neoplasm of lower-outer quadrant of left male breast   HCC ◨ ♂

    C50.529 Malignant neoplasm of lower-outer quadrant of unspecified male breast   HCC ◨ ♂ ▽

✓5ᵗʰ **C50.6** Malignant neoplasm of axillary tail of breast

  ✓6ᵗʰ **C50.61** Malignant neoplasm of axillary tail of breast, female

    C50.611 Malignant neoplasm of axillary tail of right female breast   HCC ◨ ♀

    C50.612 Malignant neoplasm of axillary tail of left female breast   HCC ◨ ♀

    C50.619 Malignant neoplasm of axillary tail of unspecified female breast   HCC ◨ ♀ ▽

  ✓6ᵗʰ **C50.62** Malignant neoplasm of axillary tail of breast, male

    C50.621 Malignant neoplasm of axillary tail of right male breast   HCC ◨ ♂

    C50.622 Malignant neoplasm of axillary tail of left male breast   HCC ◨ ♂

    C50.629 Malignant neoplasm of axillary tail of unspecified male breast   HCC ◨ ♂ ▽

✓5ᵗʰ **C50.8** Malignant neoplasm of overlapping sites of breast

  ✓6ᵗʰ **C50.81** Malignant neoplasm of overlapping sites of breast, female

    C50.811 Malignant neoplasm of overlapping sites of right female breast   HCC ◨ ♀

    C50.812 Malignant neoplasm of overlapping sites of left female breast   HCC ◨ ♀

    C50.819 Malignant neoplasm of overlapping sites of unspecified female breast   HCC ◨ ♀ ▽

  ✓6ᵗʰ **C50.82** Malignant neoplasm of overlapping sites of breast, male

    C50.821 Malignant neoplasm of overlapping sites of right male breast   HCC ◨ ♂

    C50.822 Malignant neoplasm of overlapping sites of left male breast   HCC ◨ ♂

    C50.829 Malignant neoplasm of overlapping sites of unspecified male breast   HCC ◨ ♂ ▽

✓5ᵗʰ **C50.9** Malignant neoplasm of breast of unspecified site

  ✓6ᵗʰ **C50.91** Malignant neoplasm of breast of unspecified site, female

    C50.911 Malignant neoplasm of unspecified site of right female breast   HCC ◨ ♀

    C50.912 Malignant neoplasm of unspecified site of left female breast   HCC ◨ ♀

    C50.919 Malignant neoplasm of unspecified site of unspecified female breast   HCC ◨ ♀ ▽

  ✓6ᵗʰ **C50.92** Malignant neoplasm of breast of unspecified site, male

    C50.921 Malignant neoplasm of unspecified site of right male breast   HCC ◨ ♂

    C50.922 Malignant neoplasm of unspecified site of left male breast   HCC ◨ ♂

    C50.929 Malignant neoplasm of unspecified site of unspecified male breast   HCC ◨ ♂ ▽

Malignant neoplasms of female genital organs (C51-C58)

INCLUDES   malignant neoplasm of skin of female genital organs

✓4ᵗʰ **C51 Malignant neoplasm of vulva**

   EXCLUDES 1   carcinoma in situ of vulva (D07.1)

  C51.0 Malignant neoplasm of labium majus   HCC ♀
      Malignant neoplasm of Bartholin's [greater vestibular] gland

  C51.1 Malignant neoplasm of labium minus   HCC ♀

  C51.2 Malignant neoplasm of clitoris   HCC ♀

  C51.8 Malignant neoplasm of overlapping sites of vulva   HCC ♀

  C51.9 Malignant neoplasm of vulva, unspecified   HCC ♀ ▽
      Malignant neoplasm of external female genitalia NOS
      Malignant neoplasm of pudendum

C52 Malignant neoplasm of vagina   HCC ♀
   EXCLUDES 1   carcinoma in situ of vagina (D07.2)

☑ Additional Character Req   ✓x7ᵗʰ Placeholder Alert   Manifestation   ▽ Unspecified   ►◄ Revised Text   ● New Code   ▲ Revised Code Title

Chapter 2. Neoplasms

C53–C63.9

√4ᵗʰ C53 Malignant neoplasm of cervix uteri
> **EXCLUDES 1**   carcinoma in situ of cervix uteri (D06.-)
> AHA: 2017,4Q,103

   C53.0 Malignant neoplasm of endocervix   HCC ♀
   C53.1 Malignant neoplasm of exocervix   HCC ♀
   C53.8 Malignant neoplasm of overlapping sites of cervix uteri   HCC ♀
   C53.9 Malignant neoplasm of cervix uteri, unspecified   HCC ♀ ▽

√4ᵗʰ C54 Malignant neoplasm of corpus uteri
   C54.0 Malignant neoplasm of isthmus uteri   HCC ♀
     Malignant neoplasm of lower uterine segment
   C54.1 Malignant neoplasm of endometrium   HCC ♀
   C54.2 Malignant neoplasm of myometrium   HCC ♀
   C54.3 Malignant neoplasm of fundus uteri   HCC ♀
   C54.8 Malignant neoplasm of overlapping sites of corpus uteri   HCC ♀
   C54.9 Malignant neoplasm of corpus uteri, unspecified   HCC ♀ ▽

C55 Malignant neoplasm of uterus, part unspecified   HCC ♀ ▽

√4ᵗʰ C56 Malignant neoplasm of ovary
> Use additional code to identify any functional activity

   C56.1 Malignant neoplasm of right ovary   HCC ♀
   C56.2 Malignant neoplasm of left ovary   HCC ♀
   C56.9 Malignant neoplasm of unspecified ovary   HCC ♀ ▽

√4ᵗʰ C57 Malignant neoplasm of other and unspecified female genital organs
   √5ᵗʰ C57.0 Malignant neoplasm of fallopian tube
     Malignant neoplasm of oviduct
     Malignant neoplasm of uterine tube
     C57.00 Malignant neoplasm of unspecified fallopian tube   HCC ♀ ▽
     C57.01 Malignant neoplasm of right fallopian tube   HCC ♀
     C57.02 Malignant neoplasm of left fallopian tube   HCC ♀
   √5ᵗʰ C57.1 Malignant neoplasm of broad ligament
     C57.10 Malignant neoplasm of unspecified broad ligament   HCC ♀ ▽
     C57.11 Malignant neoplasm of right broad ligament   HCC ♀
     C57.12 Malignant neoplasm of left broad ligament   HCC ♀
   √5ᵗʰ C57.2 Malignant neoplasm of round ligament
     C57.20 Malignant neoplasm of unspecified round ligament   HCC ♀ ▽
     C57.21 Malignant neoplasm of right round ligament   HCC ♀
     C57.22 Malignant neoplasm of left round ligament   HCC ♀
   C57.3 Malignant neoplasm of parametrium   HCC ♀
     Malignant neoplasm of uterine ligament NOS
   C57.4 Malignant neoplasm of uterine adnexa, unspecified   HCC ♀ ▽
   C57.7 Malignant neoplasm of other specified female genital organs
     Malignant neoplasm of wolffian body or duct
   C57.8 Malignant neoplasm of overlapping sites of female genital organs   HCC ♀
     Primary malignant neoplasm of two or more contiguous sites of the female genital organs whose point of origin cannot be determined
     Primary tubo-ovarian malignant neoplasm whose point of origin cannot be determined
     Primary utero-ovarian malignant neoplasm whose point of origin cannot be determined
   C57.9 Malignant neoplasm of female genital organ, unspecified   HCC ♀ ▽
     Malignant neoplasm of female genitourinary tract NOS

C58 Malignant neoplasm of placenta   HCC M ♀
> **INCLUDES**   choriocarcinoma NOS
>   chorionepithelioma NOS
> **EXCLUDES 1**   chorioadenoma (destruens) (D39.2)
>   hydatidiform mole NOS (O01.9)
>   invasive hydatidiform mole (D39.2)
>   male choriocarcinoma NOS (C62.9-)
>   malignant hydatidiform mole (D39.2)

Malignant neoplasms of male genital organs (C60-C63)

> **INCLUDES**   malignant neoplasm of skin of male genital organs

√4ᵗʰ C60 Malignant neoplasm of penis
   C60.0 Malignant neoplasm of prepuce   HCC ♂
     Malignant neoplasm of foreskin
   C60.1 Malignant neoplasm of glans penis   HCC ♂
   C60.2 Malignant neoplasm of body of penis   HCC ♂
     Malignant neoplasm of corpus cavernosum
   C60.8 Malignant neoplasm of overlapping sites of penis   HCC ♂
   C60.9 Malignant neoplasm of penis, unspecified   HCC ♂ ▽
     Malignant neoplasm of skin of penis NOS

C61 Malignant neoplasm of prostate   HCC Q ♂
> Use additional code to identify:
>   hormone sensitivity status (Z19.1-Z19.2)
>   rising PSA following treatment for malignant neoplasm of prostate (R97.21)
> **EXCLUDES 1**   malignant neoplasm of seminal vesicle (C63.7)
> AHA: 2017,1Q,17

√4ᵗʰ C62 Malignant neoplasm of testis
> Use additional code to identify any functional activity

   √5ᵗʰ C62.0 Malignant neoplasm of undescended testis
     Malignant neoplasm of ectopic testis
     Malignant neoplasm of retained testis
     C62.00 Malignant neoplasm of unspecified undescended testis   HCC ♂ ▽
     C62.01 Malignant neoplasm of undescended right testis   HCC ♂
     C62.02 Malignant neoplasm of undescended left testis   HCC ♂
   √5ᵗʰ C62.1 Malignant neoplasm of descended testis
     Malignant neoplasm of scrotal testis
     C62.10 Malignant neoplasm of unspecified descended testis   HCC ♂ ▽
     C62.11 Malignant neoplasm of descended right testis   HCC ♂
     C62.12 Malignant neoplasm of descended left testis   HCC ♂
   √5ᵗʰ C62.9 Malignant neoplasm of testis, unspecified whether descended or undescended
     C62.90 Malignant neoplasm of unspecified testis, unspecified whether descended or undescended   HCC ♂ ▽
      Malignant neoplasm of testis NOS
     C62.91 Malignant neoplasm of right testis, unspecified whether descended or undescended   HCC ♂ ▽
     C62.92 Malignant neoplasm of left testis, unspecified whether descended or undescended   HCC ♂ ▽

√4ᵗʰ C63 Malignant neoplasm of other and unspecified male genital organs
   √5ᵗʰ C63.0 Malignant neoplasm of epididymis
     C63.00 Malignant neoplasm of unspecified epididymis   HCC ♂ ▽
     C63.01 Malignant neoplasm of right epididymis   HCC ♂
     C63.02 Malignant neoplasm of left epididymis   HCC ♂
   √5ᵗʰ C63.1 Malignant neoplasm of spermatic cord
     C63.10 Malignant neoplasm of unspecified spermatic cord   HCC ♂ ▽
     C63.11 Malignant neoplasm of right spermatic cord   HCC ♂
     C63.12 Malignant neoplasm of left spermatic cord   HCC ♂
   C63.2 Malignant neoplasm of scrotum   HCC ♂
     Malignant neoplasm of skin of scrotum
   C63.7 Malignant neoplasm of other specified male genital organs   HCC ♂
     Malignant neoplasm of seminal vesicle
     Malignant neoplasm of tunica vaginalis
   C63.8 Malignant neoplasm of overlapping sites of male genital organs   HCC ♂
     Primary malignant neoplasm of two or more contiguous sites of male genital organs whose point of origin cannot be determined
   C63.9 Malignant neoplasm of male genital organ, unspecified   HCC ♂ ▽
     Malignant neoplasm of male genitourinary tract NOS

Malignant neoplasms of urinary tract (C64-C68)

✓4ᵗʰ C64 Malignant neoplasm of kidney, except renal pelvis

> **EXCLUDES 1**   *malignant carcinoid tumor of the kidney (C7A.093)*
> *malignant neoplasm of renal calyces (C65.-)*
> *malignant neoplasm of renal pelvis (C65.-)*

     C64.1 Malignant neoplasm of right kidney, except renal pelvis   HCC

     C64.2 Malignant neoplasm of left kidney, except renal pelvis   HCC

     C64.9 Malignant neoplasm of unspecified kidney, except renal pelvis   HCC ▽

✓4ᵗʰ C65 Malignant neoplasm of renal pelvis

> **INCLUDES**   malignant neoplasm of pelviureteric junction
> malignant neoplasm of renal calyces

     C65.1 Malignant neoplasm of right renal pelvis   HCC

     C65.2 Malignant neoplasm of left renal pelvis   HCC

     C65.9 Malignant neoplasm of unspecified renal pelvis   HCC ▽

✓4ᵗʰ C66 Malignant neoplasm of ureter

> **EXCLUDES 1**   *malignant neoplasm of ureteric orifice of bladder (C67.6)*

     C66.1 Malignant neoplasm of right ureter   HCC

     C66.2 Malignant neoplasm of left ureter   HCC

     C66.9 Malignant neoplasm of unspecified ureter   HCC ▽

✓4ᵗʰ C67 Malignant neoplasm of bladder

     C67.0 Malignant neoplasm of trigone of bladder   HCC

     C67.1 Malignant neoplasm of dome of bladder   HCC

     C67.2 Malignant neoplasm of lateral wall of bladder   HCC

     C67.3 Malignant neoplasm of anterior wall of bladder   HCC

     C67.4 Malignant neoplasm of posterior wall of bladder   HCC

     C67.5 Malignant neoplasm of bladder neck   HCC
         Malignant neoplasm of internal urethral orifice

     C67.6 Malignant neoplasm of ureteric orifice   HCC

     C67.7 Malignant neoplasm of urachus   HCC

     C67.8 Malignant neoplasm of overlapping sites of bladder   HCC

     C67.9 Malignant neoplasm of bladder, unspecified   HCC ▽
         AHA: 2016,1Q,19

✓4ᵗʰ C68 Malignant neoplasm of other and unspecified urinary organs

> **EXCLUDES 1**   *malignant neoplasm of female genitourinary tract NOS (C57.9)*
> *malignant neoplasm of male genitourinary tract NOS (C63.9)*

     C68.0 Malignant neoplasm of urethra   HCC
> **EXCLUDES 1**   *malignant neoplasm of urethral orifice of bladder (C67.5)*

     C68.1 Malignant neoplasm of paraurethral glands   HCC

     C68.8 Malignant neoplasm of overlapping sites of urinary organs   HCC
         Primary malignant neoplasm of two or more contiguous sites of urinary organs whose point of origin cannot be determined

     C68.9 Malignant neoplasm of urinary organ, unspecified   HCC ▽
         Malignant neoplasm of urinary system NOS

Malignant neoplasms of eye, brain and other parts of central nervous system (C69-C72)

✓4ᵗʰ C69 Malignant neoplasm of eye and adnexa

> **EXCLUDES 1**   *malignant neoplasm of connective tissue of eyelid (C49.0)*
> *malignant neoplasm of eyelid (skin) (C43.1-, C44.1-)*
> *malignant neoplasm of optic nerve (C72.3-)*

   ✓5ᵗʰ C69.0 Malignant neoplasm of conjunctiva

     C69.00 Malignant neoplasm of unspecified conjunctiva   HCC ▽

     C69.01 Malignant neoplasm of right conjunctiva   HCC

     C69.02 Malignant neoplasm of left conjunctiva   HCC

   ✓5ᵗʰ C69.1 Malignant neoplasm of cornea

     C69.10 Malignant neoplasm of unspecified cornea   HCC ▽

     C69.11 Malignant neoplasm of right cornea   HCC

     C69.12 Malignant neoplasm of left cornea   HCC

   ✓5ᵗʰ C69.2 Malignant neoplasm of retina

> **EXCLUDES 1**   *dark area on retina (D49.81)*
> *neoplasm of unspecified behavior of retina and choroid (D49.81)*
> *retinal freckle (D49.81)*

     C69.20 Malignant neoplasm of unspecified retina   HCC ▽

     C69.21 Malignant neoplasm of right retina   HCC

     C69.22 Malignant neoplasm of left retina   HCC

   ✓5ᵗʰ C69.3 Malignant neoplasm of choroid

     C69.30 Malignant neoplasm of unspecified choroid   HCC ▽

     C69.31 Malignant neoplasm of right choroid   HCC

     C69.32 Malignant neoplasm of left choroid   HCC

   ✓5ᵗʰ C69.4 Malignant neoplasm of ciliary body

     C69.40 Malignant neoplasm of unspecified ciliary body   HCC ▽

     C69.41 Malignant neoplasm of right ciliary body   HCC

     C69.42 Malignant neoplasm of left ciliary body   HCC

   ✓5ᵗʰ C69.5 Malignant neoplasm of lacrimal gland and duct

     Malignant neoplasm of lacrimal sac
     Malignant neoplasm of nasolacrimal duct

     C69.50 Malignant neoplasm of unspecified lacrimal gland and duct   HCC ▽

     C69.51 Malignant neoplasm of right lacrimal gland and duct   HCC

     C69.52 Malignant neoplasm of left lacrimal gland and duct   HCC

   ✓5ᵗʰ C69.6 Malignant neoplasm of orbit

     Malignant neoplasm of connective tissue of orbit
     Malignant neoplasm of extraocular muscle
     Malignant neoplasm of peripheral nerves of orbit
     Malignant neoplasm of retrobulbar tissue
     Malignant neoplasm of retro-ocular tissue
> **EXCLUDES 1**   *malignant neoplasm of orbital bone (C41.0)*

     C69.60 Malignant neoplasm of unspecified orbit   HCC ▽

     C69.61 Malignant neoplasm of right orbit   HCC

     C69.62 Malignant neoplasm of left orbit   HCC

   ✓5ᵗʰ C69.8 Malignant neoplasm of overlapping sites of eye and adnexa

     C69.80 Malignant neoplasm of overlapping sites of unspecified eye and adnexa   HCC ▽

     C69.81 Malignant neoplasm of overlapping sites of right eye and adnexa   HCC

     C69.82 Malignant neoplasm of overlapping sites of left eye and adnexa   HCC

   ✓5ᵗʰ C69.9 Malignant neoplasm of unspecified site of eye

     Malignant neoplasm of eyeball

     C69.90 Malignant neoplasm of unspecified site of unspecified eye   HCC ▽

     C69.91 Malignant neoplasm of unspecified site of right eye   HCC ▽

     C69.92 Malignant neoplasm of unspecified site of left eye   HCC ▽

✓4ᵗʰ C70 Malignant neoplasm of meninges

     C70.0 Malignant neoplasm of cerebral meninges   HCC

     C70.1 Malignant neoplasm of spinal meninges   HCC

     C70.9 Malignant neoplasm of meninges, unspecified   HCC ▽

✓4ᵗʰ **C71** **Malignant neoplasm of brain**

    EXCLUDES 1   malignant neoplasm of cranial nerves (C72.2-C72.5)

               retrobulbar malignant neoplasm (C69.6-)

Lobes of the Brain

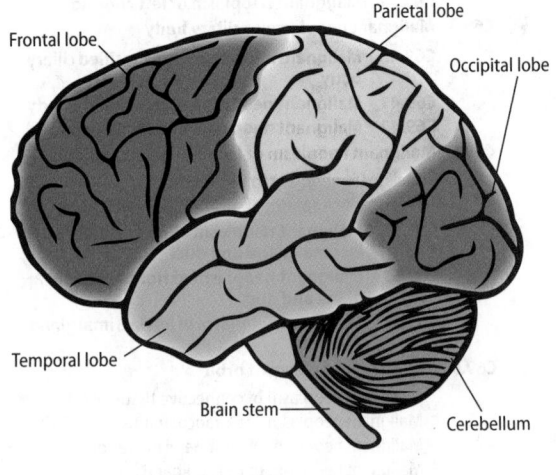

Frontal lobe — Parietal lobe — Occipital lobe — Temporal lobe — Brain stem — Cerebellum

  C71.Ø **Malignant neoplasm of cerebrum, except lobes and**   HCC
          ventricles
          Malignant neoplasm of supratentorial NOS

  C71.1 **Malignant neoplasm of frontal lobe**   HCC

  C71.2 **Malignant neoplasm of temporal lobe**   HCC

  C71.3 **Malignant neoplasm of parietal lobe**   HCC

  C71.4 **Malignant neoplasm of occipital lobe**   HCC

  C71.5 **Malignant neoplasm of cerebral ventricle**   HCC
         EXCLUDES 1   malignant neoplasm of fourth cerebral ventricle
                    (C71.7)

  C71.6 **Malignant neoplasm of cerebellum**   HCC

  C71.7 **Malignant neoplasm of brain stem**   HCC
          Malignant neoplasm of fourth cerebral ventricle
          Infratentorial malignant neoplasm NOS

  C71.8 **Malignant neoplasm of overlapping sites of brain**   HCC

  C71.9 **Malignant neoplasm of brain, unspecified**   HCC ▽
         AHA: 2014,3Q,3

✓4ᵗʰ **C72** **Malignant neoplasm of spinal cord, cranial nerves and other parts of central nervous system**

    EXCLUDES 1   malignant neoplasm of meninges (C70.-)

               malignant neoplasm of peripheral nerves and autonomic
               nervous system (C47.-)

  C72.Ø **Malignant neoplasm of spinal cord**   HCC

  C72.1 **Malignant neoplasm of cauda equina**   HCC

✓5ᵗʰ **C72.2** **Malignant neoplasm of olfactory nerve**
         Malignant neoplasm of olfactory bulb

    C72.2Ø **Malignant neoplasm of unspecified**   HCC ▽
              olfactory nerve

    C72.21 **Malignant neoplasm of right olfactory**   HCC
              nerve

    C72.22 **Malignant neoplasm of left olfactory**   HCC
              nerve

✓5ᵗʰ **C72.3** **Malignant neoplasm of optic nerve**

    C72.3Ø **Malignant neoplasm of unspecified optic**   HCC ▽
              nerve

    C72.31 **Malignant neoplasm of right optic nerve**   HCC

    C72.32 **Malignant neoplasm of left optic nerve**   HCC

✓5ᵗʰ **C72.4** **Malignant neoplasm of acoustic nerve**

    C72.4Ø **Malignant neoplasm of unspecified**   HCC ▽
              acoustic nerve

    C72.41 **Malignant neoplasm of right acoustic**   HCC
              nerve

    C72.42 **Malignant neoplasm of left acoustic nerve**   HCC

✓5ᵗʰ **C72.5** **Malignant neoplasm of other and unspecified cranial nerves**

    C72.5Ø **Malignant neoplasm of unspecified cranial**   HCC ▽
              nerve
              Malignant neoplasm of cranial nerve NOS

    C72.59 **Malignant neoplasm of other cranial**   HCC
              nerves

C72.9 **Malignant neoplasm of central nervous system,**   HCC ▽
     unspecified
        Malignant neoplasm of unspecified site of central nervous
        system
        Malignant neoplasm of nervous system NOS

Malignant neoplasms of thyroid and other endocrine glands (C73-C75)

C73 **Malignant neoplasm of thyroid gland**   HCC
      Use additional code to identify any functional activity

✓4ᵗʰ **C74** **Malignant neoplasm of adrenal gland**

     TIP: If an adrenal gland tumor is described as functional (producing too
     much of a hormone), additional codes should be assigned to report the
     functional activity.

✓5ᵗʰ **C74.Ø** **Malignant neoplasm of cortex of adrenal gland**

    C74.ØØ **Malignant neoplasm of cortex of**   HCC ▽
              unspecified adrenal gland

    C74.Ø1 **Malignant neoplasm of cortex of right**   HCC
              adrenal gland

    C74.Ø2 **Malignant neoplasm of cortex of left**   HCC
              adrenal gland

✓5ᵗʰ **C74.1** **Malignant neoplasm of medulla of adrenal gland**

    C74.1Ø **Malignant neoplasm of medulla of**   HCC ▽
              unspecified adrenal gland

    C74.11 **Malignant neoplasm of medulla of right**   HCC
              adrenal gland

    C74.12 **Malignant neoplasm of medulla of left**   HCC
              adrenal gland

✓5ᵗʰ **C74.9** **Malignant neoplasm of unspecified part of adrenal gland**

    C74.9Ø **Malignant neoplasm of unspecified part**   HCC ▽
              of unspecified adrenal gland

    C74.91 **Malignant neoplasm of unspecified part**   HCC ▽
              of right adrenal gland

    C74.92 **Malignant neoplasm of unspecified part**   HCC ▽
              of left adrenal gland

✓4ᵗʰ **C75** **Malignant neoplasm of other endocrine glands and related structures**

    EXCLUDES 1   malignant carcinoid tumors (C7A.Ø-)

             malignant neoplasm of adrenal gland (C74.-)

             malignant neoplasm of endocrine pancreas (C25.4)

             malignant neoplasm of islets of Langerhans (C25.4)

             malignant neoplasm of ovary (C56.-)

             malignant neoplasm of testis (C62.-)

             malignant neoplasm of thymus (C37)

             malignant neoplasm of thyroid gland (C73)

             malignant neuroendocrine tumors (C7A.-)

  C75.Ø **Malignant neoplasm of parathyroid gland**   HCC

  C75.1 **Malignant neoplasm of pituitary gland**   HCC

  C75.2 **Malignant neoplasm of craniopharyngeal duct**   HCC

  C75.3 **Malignant neoplasm of pineal gland**   HCC

  C75.4 **Malignant neoplasm of carotid body**   HCC

  C75.5 **Malignant neoplasm of aortic body and other**
         paraganglia

  C75.8 **Malignant neoplasm with pluriglandular**   HCC ▽
         involvement, unspecified

  C75.9 **Malignant neoplasm of endocrine gland,**   HCC ▽
         unspecified

Malignant neuroendocrine tumors (C7A)

✓4ᵗʰ **C7A** **Malignant neuroendocrine tumors**

     Code also any associated multiple endocrine neoplasia [MEN] syndromes
     (E31.2-)

     Use additional code to identify any associated endocrine syndrome,
     such as:

     carcinoid syndrome (E34.Ø)

    EXCLUDES 2   malignant pancreatic islet cell tumors (C25.4)

             Merkel cell carcinoma (C4A.-)

     DEF: Tumors comprised of cells that are capable of producing hormonal
     syndromes in which the normal hormonal balance required to support
     body system functions is adversely affected.

✓5ᵗʰ **C7A.Ø** **Malignant carcinoid tumors**

     DEF: Specific type of slow-growing benign or malignant
     neuroendocrine tumors. Carcinoid tumors occur most commonly
     in the hormone producing cells of the gastrointestinal tracts and
     can also occur in the pancreas, testes, ovaries, or lungs.

    C7A.ØØ **Malignant carcinoid tumor of unspecified**   HCC ▽
              site

✓6ᵗʰ **C7A.Ø1 Malignant carcinoid tumors of the** small intestine

     C7A.Ø1Ø Malignant carcinoid tumor of   HCC
         the duodenum

     C7A.Ø11 Malignant carcinoid tumor of   HCC
         the jejunum

     C7A.Ø12 Malignant carcinoid tumor of   HCC
         the ileum

     C7A.Ø19 Malignant carcinoid tumor of   HCC ▽
         the small intestine, unspecified
         portion

✓6ᵗʰ **C7A.Ø2 Malignant carcinoid tumors of the** appendix, large
     intestine, and rectum

     C7A.Ø2Ø Malignant carcinoid tumor of   HCC
         the appendix

     C7A.Ø21 Malignant carcinoid tumor of   HCC
         the cecum

     C7A.Ø22 Malignant carcinoid tumor of   HCC
         the ascending colon

     C7A.Ø23 Malignant carcinoid tumor of   HCC
         the transverse colon

     C7A.Ø24 Malignant carcinoid tumor of   HCC
         the descending colon

     C7A.Ø25 Malignant carcinoid tumor of   HCC
         the sigmoid colon

     C7A.Ø26 Malignant carcinoid tumor of   HCC
         the rectum

     C7A.Ø29 Malignant carcinoid tumor of   HCC ▽
         the large intestine, unspecified
         portion

            Malignant carcinoid tumor of the colon
              NOS

✓6ᵗʰ **C7A.Ø9 Malignant carcinoid tumors of other sites**

     C7A.Ø9Ø Malignant carcinoid tumor of   HCC
         the bronchus and lung

     C7A.Ø91 Malignant carcinoid tumor of   HCC
         the thymus

     C7A.Ø92 Malignant carcinoid tumor of   HCC
         the stomach

     C7A.Ø93 Malignant carcinoid tumor of   HCC
         the kidney

     C7A.Ø94 Malignant carcinoid tumor of   HCC ▽
         the foregut, unspecified

     C7A.Ø95 Malignant carcinoid tumor of   HCC ▽
         the midgut, unspecified

     C7A.Ø96 Malignant carcinoid tumor of   HCC ▽
         the hindgut, unspecified

     C7A.Ø98 Malignant carcinoid tumors of   HCC
         other sites

C7A.1 Malignant poorly differentiated neuroendocrine   HCC
tumors

    Malignant poorly differentiated neuroendocrine tumor NOS
    High grade neuroendocrine carcinoma, any site
    Malignant poorly differentiated neuroendocrine carcinoma,
    any site

C7A.8 Other malignant neuroendocrine tumors   HCC

Secondary neuroendocrine tumors (C7B)

✓4ᵗʰ **C7B Secondary** neuroendocrine tumors

    Use additional code to identify any functional activity

✓5ᵗʰ **C7B.Ø Secondary** carcinoid tumors

     C7B.ØØ Secondary carcinoid tumors, unspecified   HCC ▽
         site

     C7B.Ø1 Secondary carcinoid tumors of distant   HCC
         lymph nodes

     C7B.Ø2 Secondary carcinoid tumors of liver   HCC

     C7B.Ø3 Secondary carcinoid tumors of bone   HCC

     C7B.Ø4 Secondary carcinoid tumors of   HCC
         peritoneum

            Mesentary metastasis of carcinoid tumor

     C7B.Ø9 Secondary carcinoid tumors of other sites   HCC

C7B.1 Secondary Merkel cell carcinoma   HCC

    Merkel cell carcinoma nodal presentation
    Merkel cell carcinoma visceral metastatic presentation

C7B.8 Other secondary neuroendocrine tumors   HCC

Malignant neoplasms of ill-defined, other secondary and unspecified sites (C76-C8Ø)

✓4ᵗʰ **C76 Malignant neoplasm of other and ill-defined sites**

    EXCLUDES 1   *malignant neoplasm of female genitourinary tract NOS*
        (C57.9)
        malignant neoplasm of male genitourinary tract NOS (C63.9)
        malignant neoplasm of lymphoid, hematopoietic and related
          tissue (C81-C96)
        malignant neoplasm of skin (C44.-)
        malignant neoplasm of unspecified site NOS (C8Ø.1)

     C76.Ø Malignant neoplasm of head, face and neck   HCC
        Malignant neoplasm of cheek NOS
        Malignant neoplasm of nose NOS

     C76.1 Malignant neoplasm of thorax   HCC
        Intrathoracic malignant neoplasm NOS
        Malignant neoplasm of axilla NOS
        Thoracic malignant neoplasm NOS

     C76.2 Malignant neoplasm of abdomen   HCC

     C76.3 Malignant neoplasm of pelvis   HCC
        Malignant neoplasm of groin NOS
        Malignant neoplasm of sites overlapping systems within the
         pelvis
        Rectovaginal (septum) malignant neoplasm
        Rectovesical (septum) malignant neoplasm

✓5ᵗʰ   **C76.4 Malignant neoplasm of upper limb**

     C76.4Ø Malignant neoplasm of unspecified upper   HCC ▽
         limb

     C76.41 Malignant neoplasm of right upper limb   HCC

     C76.42 Malignant neoplasm of left upper limb   HCC

✓5ᵗʰ   **C76.5 Malignant neoplasm of lower limb**

     C76.5Ø Malignant neoplasm of unspecified lower   HCC ▽
         limb

     C76.51 Malignant neoplasm of right lower limb   HCC

     C76.52 Malignant neoplasm of left lower limb   HCC

     C76.8 Malignant neoplasm of other specified ill-defined   HCC
        sites
        Malignant neoplasm of overlapping ill-defined sites

✓4ᵗʰ **C77 Secondary and unspecified malignant neoplasm of lymph nodes**

    EXCLUDES 1   *malignant neoplasm of lymph nodes, specified as primary*
        (C81-C86, C88, C96.-)
        mesentary metastasis of carcinoid tumor (C7B.Ø4)
        secondary carcinoid tumors of distant lymph nodes (C7B.Ø1)

     C77.Ø Secondary and unspecified malignant neoplasm of   HCC 🄾
        lymph nodes of head, face and neck
        Secondary and unspecified malignant neoplasm of
         supraclavicular lymph nodes

     C77.1 Secondary and unspecified malignant neoplasm of   HCC 🄾
        intrathoracic lymph nodes

     C77.2 Secondary and unspecified malignant neoplasm of   HCC 🄾
        intra-abdominal lymph nodes

     C77.3 Secondary and unspecified malignant neoplasm of   HCC 🄾
        axilla and upper limb lymph nodes
        Secondary and unspecified malignant neoplasm of pectoral
         lymph nodes

     C77.4 Secondary and unspecified malignant neoplasm of   HCC 🄾
        inguinal and lower limb lymph nodes

     C77.5 Secondary and unspecified malignant neoplasm of   HCC 🄾
        intrapelvic lymph nodes

     C77.8 Secondary and unspecified malignant neoplasm of   HCC 🄾
        lymph nodes of multiple regions

     C77.9 Secondary and unspecified malignant neoplasm of   HCC 🄾 ▽
        lymph node, unspecified

✓4ᵗʰ **C78 Secondary malignant neoplasm of respiratory and digestive organs**

    EXCLUDES 1   *secondary carcinoid tumors of liver (C7B.Ø2)*
        secondary carcinoid tumors of peritoneum (C7B.Ø4)
    EXCLUDES 2   *lymph node metastases (C77.Ø)*

✓5ᵗʰ   **C78.Ø Secondary malignant neoplasm of lung**

     C78.ØØ Secondary malignant neoplasm of   HCC 🄾 ▽
         unspecified lung

     C78.Ø1 Secondary malignant neoplasm of right   HCC 🄾
         lung

     C78.Ø2 Secondary malignant neoplasm of left   HCC 🄾
         lung

     C78.1 Secondary malignant neoplasm of mediastinum   HCC 🄾

☑ Additional Character Req   ✓x7ᵗʰ Placeholder Alert   Manifestation   ▽ Unspecified   ►◄ Revised Text   ● New Code   ▲ Revised Code Title

ICD-10-CM 2019   475

C78.2 Secondary malignant neoplasm of pleura `HCC` `Q`

C78.3 Secondary malignant neoplasm of other and unspecified respiratory organs

  C78.30 Secondary malignant neoplasm of unspecified respiratory organ `HCC` `Q` ▽

  C78.39 Secondary malignant neoplasm of other respiratory organs `HCC` `Q`

C78.4 Secondary malignant neoplasm of small intestine `HCC` `Q`

C78.5 Secondary malignant neoplasm of large intestine and rectum `HCC` `Q`

C78.6 Secondary malignant neoplasm of retroperitoneum and peritoneum `HCC` `Q`
  AHA: 2017,2Q,12

C78.7 Secondary malignant neoplasm of liver and intrahepatic bile duct `HCC` `Q`

C78.8 Secondary malignant neoplasm of other and unspecified digestive organs

  C78.80 Secondary malignant neoplasm of unspecified digestive organ `HCC` `Q` ▽

  C78.89 Secondary malignant neoplasm of other digestive organs `HCC` `Q`
    Code also exocrine pancreatic insufficiency (K86.81)

C79 Secondary malignant neoplasm of other and unspecified sites
  EXCLUDES 1 secondary carcinoid tumors (C7B.-)
    secondary neuroendocrine tumors (C7B.-)

C79.0 Secondary malignant neoplasm of kidney and renal pelvis

  C79.00 Secondary malignant neoplasm of unspecified kidney and renal pelvis `HCC` `Q` ▽

  C79.01 Secondary malignant neoplasm of right kidney and renal pelvis `HCC` `Q`

  C79.02 Secondary malignant neoplasm of left kidney and renal pelvis `HCC` `Q`

C79.1 Secondary malignant neoplasm of bladder and other and unspecified urinary organs

  C79.10 Secondary malignant neoplasm of unspecified urinary organs `HCC` `Q` ▽

  C79.11 Secondary malignant neoplasm of bladder `HCC` `Q`
    EXCLUDES 2 lymph node metastases (C77.0)

  C79.19 Secondary malignant neoplasm of other urinary organs `HCC` `Q`

C79.2 Secondary malignant neoplasm of skin `HCC` `Q`
  EXCLUDES 1 secondary Merkel cell carcinoma (C7B.1)

C79.3 Secondary malignant neoplasm of brain and cerebral meninges

  C79.31 Secondary malignant neoplasm of brain `HCC` `Q`

  C79.32 Secondary malignant neoplasm of cerebral meninges `HCC` `Q`

C79.4 Secondary malignant neoplasm of other and unspecified parts of nervous system

  C79.40 Secondary malignant neoplasm of unspecified part of nervous system `HCC` `Q` ▽

  C79.49 Secondary malignant neoplasm of other parts of nervous system `HCC` `Q`

C79.5 Secondary malignant neoplasm of bone and bone marrow
  EXCLUDES 1 secondary carcinoid tumors of bone (C7B.03)

  C79.51 Secondary malignant neoplasm of bone `HCC` `Q`
    TIP: Do not assign in addition to a code from subcategory C90.0 when multiple myeloma is described as metastatic to the bone; bone involvement is integral to multiple myeloma.

  C79.52 Secondary malignant neoplasm of bone marrow `HCC` `Q`

C79.6 Secondary malignant neoplasm of ovary

  C79.60 Secondary malignant neoplasm of unspecified ovary `HCC` `Q` ♀ ▽

  C79.61 Secondary malignant neoplasm of right ovary `HCC` `Q` ♀

  C79.62 Secondary malignant neoplasm of left ovary `HCC` `Q` ♀

C79.7 Secondary malignant neoplasm of adrenal gland

  C79.70 Secondary malignant neoplasm of unspecified adrenal gland `HCC` `Q` ▽

  C79.71 Secondary malignant neoplasm of right adrenal gland `HCC` `Q`

  C79.72 Secondary malignant neoplasm of left adrenal gland `HCC` `Q`

C79.8 Secondary malignant neoplasm of other specified sites

  C79.81 Secondary malignant neoplasm of breast `HCC` `Q`

C79.82 Secondary malignant neoplasm of genital organs `HCC` `Q`

C79.89 Secondary malignant neoplasm of other specified sites `HCC` `Q`
  AHA: 2017,2Q,11

C79.9 Secondary malignant neoplasm of unspecified site `HCC` `Q` ▽
  Metastatic cancer NOS
  Metastatic disease NOS
  EXCLUDES 1 carcinomatosis NOS (C80.0)
    generalized cancer NOS (C80.0)
    malignant (primary) neoplasm of unspecified site (C80.1)

C80 Malignant neoplasm without specification of site
  EXCLUDES 1 malignant carcinoid tumor of unspecified site (C7A.00)
    malignant neoplasm of specified multiple sites - code to each site

C80.0 Disseminated malignant neoplasm, unspecified `HCC` ▽
  Carcinomatosis NOS
  Generalized cancer, unspecified site (primary) (secondary)
  Generalized malignancy, unspecified site (primary) (secondary)

C80.1 Malignant (primary) neoplasm, unspecified `HCC` ▽
  Cancer NOS
  Cancer unspecified site (primary)
  Carcinoma unspecified site (primary)
  Malignancy unspecified site (primary)
  EXCLUDES 1 secondary malignant neoplasm of unspecified site (C79.9)

C80.2 Malignant neoplasm associated with transplanted organ `HCC`
  Code first complication of transplanted organ (T86.-)
  Use additional code to identify the specific malignancy

Malignant neoplasms of lymphoid, hematopoietic and related tissue (C81-C96)

EXCLUDES 2 Kaposi's sarcoma of lymph nodes (C46.3)
  secondary and unspecified neoplasm of lymph nodes (C77.-)
  secondary neoplasm of bone marrow (C79.52)
  secondary neoplasm of spleen (C78.89)

C81 Hodgkin lymphoma
  EXCLUDES 1 personal history of Hodgkin lymphoma (Z85.71)
  DEF: Malignant disorder of lymphoid cells characterized by the presence of progressively swollen lymph nodes and spleen that may also involve the liver. A diagnosis of Hodgkin's lymphoma can be confirmed by the presence of Reed-Sternberg cells. Synonym(s): Hodgkin disease.

C81.0 Nodular lymphocyte predominant Hodgkin lymphoma

  C81.00 Nodular lymphocyte predominant Hodgkin lymphoma, unspecified site `HCC` ▽

  C81.01 Nodular lymphocyte predominant Hodgkin lymphoma, lymph nodes of head, face, and neck `HCC`

  C81.02 Nodular lymphocyte predominant Hodgkin lymphoma, intrathoracic lymph nodes `HCC`

  C81.03 Nodular lymphocyte predominant Hodgkin lymphoma, intra-abdominal lymph nodes `HCC`

  C81.04 Nodular lymphocyte predominant Hodgkin lymphoma, lymph nodes of axilla and upper limb `HCC`

  C81.05 Nodular lymphocyte predominant Hodgkin lymphoma, lymph nodes of inguinal region and lower limb `HCC`

  C81.06 Nodular lymphocyte predominant Hodgkin lymphoma, intrapelvic lymph nodes `HCC`

  C81.07 Nodular lymphocyte predominant Hodgkin lymphoma, spleen `HCC`

  C81.08 Nodular lymphocyte predominant Hodgkin lymphoma, lymph nodes of multiple sites `HCC`

  C81.09 Nodular lymphocyte predominant Hodgkin lymphoma, extranodal and solid organ sites `HCC`

C81.1 Nodular sclerosis Hodgkin lymphoma
  Nodular sclerosis classical Hodgkin lymphoma

  C81.10 Nodular sclerosis Hodgkin lymphoma, unspecified site `HCC` ▽

  C81.11 Nodular sclerosis Hodgkin lymphoma, lymph nodes of head, face, and neck `HCC`

C81.12   **Nodular sclerosis Hodgkin lymphoma, intrathoracic lymph nodes**   HCC

C81.13   **Nodular sclerosis Hodgkin lymphoma, intra-abdominal lymph nodes**   HCC

C81.14   **Nodular sclerosis Hodgkin lymphoma, lymph nodes of axilla and upper limb**   HCC

C81.15   **Nodular sclerosis Hodgkin lymphoma, lymph nodes of inguinal region and lower limb**   HCC

C81.16   **Nodular sclerosis Hodgkin lymphoma, intrapelvic lymph nodes**   HCC

C81.17   **Nodular sclerosis Hodgkin lymphoma, spleen**   HCC

C81.18   **Nodular sclerosis Hodgkin lymphoma, lymph nodes of multiple sites**   HCC

C81.19   **Nodular sclerosis Hodgkin lymphoma, extranodal and solid organ sites**   HCC

√5ᵗʰ **C81.2   Mixed cellularity Hodgkin lymphoma**

     Mixed cellularity classical Hodgkin lymphoma

C81.20   **Mixed cellularity Hodgkin lymphoma, unspecified site**   HCC ▽

C81.21   **Mixed cellularity Hodgkin lymphoma, lymph nodes of head, face, and neck**   HCC

C81.22   **Mixed cellularity Hodgkin lymphoma, intrathoracic lymph nodes**   HCC

C81.23   **Mixed cellularity Hodgkin lymphoma, intra-abdominal lymph nodes**   HCC

C81.24   **Mixed cellularity Hodgkin lymphoma, lymph nodes of axilla and upper limb**   HCC

C81.25   **Mixed cellularity Hodgkin lymphoma, lymph nodes of inguinal region and lower limb**   HCC

C81.26   **Mixed cellularity Hodgkin lymphoma, intrapelvic lymph nodes**   HCC

C81.27   **Mixed cellularity Hodgkin lymphoma, spleen**   HCC

C81.28   **Mixed cellularity Hodgkin lymphoma, lymph nodes of multiple sites**   HCC

C81.29   **Mixed cellularity Hodgkin lymphoma, extranodal and solid organ sites**   HCC

√5ᵗʰ **C81.3   Lymphocyte depleted Hodgkin lymphoma**

     Lymphocyte depleted classical Hodgkin lymphoma

C81.30   **Lymphocyte depleted Hodgkin lymphoma, unspecified site**   HCC ▽

C81.31   **Lymphocyte depleted Hodgkin lymphoma, lymph nodes of head, face, and neck**   HCC

C81.32   **Lymphocyte depleted Hodgkin lymphoma, intrathoracic lymph nodes**   HCC

C81.33   **Lymphocyte depleted Hodgkin lymphoma, intra-abdominal lymph nodes**   HCC

C81.34   **Lymphocyte depleted Hodgkin lymphoma, lymph nodes of axilla and upper limb**   HCC

C81.35   **Lymphocyte depleted Hodgkin lymphoma, lymph nodes of inguinal region and lower limb**   HCC

C81.36   **Lymphocyte depleted Hodgkin lymphoma, intrapelvic lymph nodes**   HCC

C81.37   **Lymphocyte depleted Hodgkin lymphoma, spleen**   HCC

C81.38   **Lymphocyte depleted Hodgkin lymphoma, lymph nodes of multiple sites**   HCC

C81.39   **Lymphocyte depleted Hodgkin lymphoma, extranodal and solid organ sites**   HCC

√5ᵗʰ **C81.4   Lymphocyte-rich Hodgkin lymphoma**

     Lymphocyte-rich classical Hodgkin lymphoma

     EXCLUDES 1   *nodular lymphocyte predominant Hodgkin lymphoma (C81.0-)*

C81.40   **Lymphocyte-rich Hodgkin lymphoma, unspecified site**   HCC ▽

C81.41   **Lymphocyte-rich Hodgkin lymphoma, lymph nodes of head, face, and neck**   HCC

C81.42   **Lymphocyte-rich Hodgkin lymphoma, intrathoracic lymph nodes**   HCC

C81.43   **Lymphocyte-rich Hodgkin lymphoma, intra-abdominal lymph nodes**   HCC

C81.44   **Lymphocyte-rich Hodgkin lymphoma, lymph nodes of axilla and upper limb**   HCC

C81.45   **Lymphocyte-rich Hodgkin lymphoma, lymph nodes of inguinal region and lower limb**   HCC

C81.46   **Lymphocyte-rich Hodgkin lymphoma, intrapelvic lymph nodes**   HCC

C81.47   **Lymphocyte-rich Hodgkin lymphoma, spleen**   HCC

C81.48   **Lymphocyte-rich Hodgkin lymphoma, lymph nodes of multiple sites**   HCC

C81.49   **Lymphocyte-rich Hodgkin lymphoma, extranodal and solid organ sites**   HCC

√5ᵗʰ **C81.7   Other Hodgkin lymphoma**

     Classical Hodgkin lymphoma NOS
     Other classical Hodgkin lymphoma

C81.70   **Other Hodgkin lymphoma, unspecified site**   HCC ▽

C81.71   **Other Hodgkin lymphoma, lymph nodes of head, face, and neck**   HCC

C81.72   **Other Hodgkin lymphoma, intrathoracic lymph nodes**   HCC

C81.73   **Other Hodgkin lymphoma, intra-abdominal lymph nodes**   HCC

C81.74   **Other Hodgkin lymphoma, lymph nodes of axilla and upper limb**   HCC

C81.75   **Other Hodgkin lymphoma, lymph nodes of inguinal region and lower limb**   HCC

C81.76   **Other Hodgkin lymphoma, intrapelvic lymph nodes**   HCC

C81.77   **Other Hodgkin lymphoma, spleen**   HCC

C81.78   **Other Hodgkin lymphoma, lymph nodes of multiple sites**   HCC

C81.79   **Other Hodgkin lymphoma, extranodal and solid organ sites**   HCC

√5ᵗʰ **C81.9   Hodgkin lymphoma, unspecified**

C81.90   **Hodgkin lymphoma, unspecified, unspecified site**   HCC ▽

C81.91   **Hodgkin lymphoma, unspecified, lymph nodes of head, face, and neck**   HCC ▽

C81.92   **Hodgkin lymphoma, unspecified, intrathoracic lymph nodes**   HCC ▽

C81.93   **Hodgkin lymphoma, unspecified, intra-abdominal lymph nodes**   HCC ▽

C81.94   **Hodgkin lymphoma, unspecified, lymph nodes of axilla and upper limb**   HCC ▽

C81.95   **Hodgkin lymphoma, unspecified, lymph nodes of inguinal region and lower limb**   HCC ▽

C81.96   **Hodgkin lymphoma, unspecified, intrapelvic lymph nodes**   HCC ▽

C81.97   **Hodgkin lymphoma, unspecified, spleen**   HCC ▽

C81.98   **Hodgkin lymphoma, unspecified, lymph nodes of multiple sites**   HCC ▽

C81.99   **Hodgkin lymphoma, unspecified, extranodal and solid organ sites**   HCC ▽

√4ᵗʰ **C82   Follicular lymphoma**

     INCLUDES   follicular lymphoma with or without diffuse areas

     EXCLUDES 1   *mature T/NK-cell lymphomas (C84.-)*

                personal history of non-Hodgkin lymphoma (Z85.72)

     DEF: Most common subgroup of non-Hodgkin lymphomas (NHL), accounting for 20 to 30 percent of all NHLs. NHL is a B-cell lymphoma that is slow growing and characterized by the circular pattern of malignant cell growth with the cells clustered into identifiable nodules or follicles.

√5ᵗʰ **C82.0   Follicular lymphoma grade I**

C82.00   **Follicular lymphoma grade I, unspecified site**   HCC ▽

C82.01   **Follicular lymphoma grade I, lymph nodes of head, face, and neck**   HCC

C82.02   **Follicular lymphoma grade I, intrathoracic lymph nodes**   HCC

C82.03   **Follicular lymphoma grade I, intra-abdominal lymph nodes**   HCC

C82.04   **Follicular lymphoma grade I, lymph nodes of axilla and upper limb**   HCC

C82.05   **Follicular lymphoma grade I, lymph nodes of inguinal region and lower limb**   HCC

C82.06   **Follicular lymphoma grade I, intrapelvic lymph nodes**   HCC

C82.07   **Follicular lymphoma grade I, spleen**   HCC

C82.08   **Follicular lymphoma grade I, lymph nodes of multiple sites**   HCC

☑ Additional Character Req   √x7ᵗʰ Placeholder Alert   **Manifestation**   ▽ Unspecified   ►◄ Revised Text   ● New Code   ▲ Revised Code Title

ICD-10-CM 2019   477

C82.Ø9   Follicular lymphoma grade I, extranodal and solid organ sites   HCC

✓5ᵗʰ **C82.1**   Follicular lymphoma grade II

C82.1Ø   Follicular lymphoma grade II, unspecified site   HCC ▽

C82.11   Follicular lymphoma grade II, lymph nodes of head, face, and neck   HCC

C82.12   Follicular lymphoma grade II, intrathoracic lymph nodes   HCC

C82.13   Follicular lymphoma grade II, intra-abdominal lymph nodes   HCC

C82.14   Follicular lymphoma grade II, lymph nodes of axilla and upper limb   HCC

C82.15   Follicular lymphoma grade II, lymph nodes of inguinal region and lower limb   HCC

C82.16   Follicular lymphoma grade II, intrapelvic lymph nodes   HCC

C82.17   Follicular lymphoma grade II, spleen   HCC

C82.18   Follicular lymphoma grade II, lymph nodes of multiple sites   HCC

C82.19   Follicular lymphoma grade II, extranodal and solid organ sites   HCC

✓5ᵗʰ **C82.2**   Follicular lymphoma grade III, unspecified

C82.2Ø   Follicular lymphoma grade III, unspecified, unspecified site   HCC ▽

C82.21   Follicular lymphoma grade III, unspecified, lymph nodes of head, face, and neck   HCC ▽

C82.22   Follicular lymphoma grade III, unspecified, intrathoracic lymph nodes   HCC ▽

C82.23   Follicular lymphoma grade III, unspecified, intra-abdominal lymph nodes   HCC ▽

C82.24   Follicular lymphoma grade III, unspecified, lymph nodes of axilla and upper limb   HCC ▽

C82.25   Follicular lymphoma grade III, unspecified, lymph nodes of inguinal region and lower limb   HCC ▽

C82.26   Follicular lymphoma grade III, unspecified, intrapelvic lymph nodes   HCC ▽

C82.27   Follicular lymphoma grade III, unspecified, spleen   HCC ▽

C82.28   Follicular lymphoma grade III, unspecified, lymph nodes of multiple sites   HCC ▽

C82.29   Follicular lymphoma grade III, unspecified, extranodal and solid organ sites   HCC ▽

✓5ᵗʰ **C82.3**   Follicular lymphoma grade IIIa

C82.3Ø   Follicular lymphoma grade IIIa, unspecified site   HCC ▽

C82.31   Follicular lymphoma grade IIIa, lymph nodes of head, face, and neck   HCC

C82.32   Follicular lymphoma grade IIIa, intrathoracic lymph nodes   HCC

C82.33   Follicular lymphoma grade IIIa, intra-abdominal lymph nodes   HCC

C82.34   Follicular lymphoma grade IIIa, lymph nodes of axilla and upper limb   HCC

C82.35   Follicular lymphoma grade IIIa, lymph nodes of inguinal region and lower limb   HCC

C82.36   Follicular lymphoma grade IIIa, intrapelvic lymph nodes   HCC

C82.37   Follicular lymphoma grade IIIa, spleen   HCC

C82.38   Follicular lymphoma grade IIIa, lymph nodes of multiple sites   HCC

C82.39   Follicular lymphoma grade IIIa, extranodal and solid organ sites   HCC

✓5ᵗʰ **C82.4**   Follicular lymphoma grade IIIb

C82.4Ø   Follicular lymphoma grade IIIb, unspecified site   HCC ▽

C82.41   Follicular lymphoma grade IIIb, lymph nodes of head, face, and neck   HCC

C82.42   Follicular lymphoma grade IIIb, intrathoracic lymph nodes   HCC

C82.43   Follicular lymphoma grade IIIb, intra-abdominal lymph nodes   HCC

C82.44   Follicular lymphoma grade IIIb, lymph nodes of axilla and upper limb   HCC

C82.45   Follicular lymphoma grade IIIb, lymph nodes of inguinal region and lower limb   HCC

C82.46   Follicular lymphoma grade IIIb, intrapelvic lymph nodes   HCC

C82.47   Follicular lymphoma grade IIIb, spleen   HCC

C82.48   Follicular lymphoma grade IIIb, lymph nodes of multiple sites   HCC

C82.49   Follicular lymphoma grade IIIb, extranodal and solid organ sites   HCC

✓5ᵗʰ **C82.5**   Diffuse follicle center lymphoma

C82.5Ø   Diffuse follicle center lymphoma, unspecified site   HCC ▽

C82.51   Diffuse follicle center lymphoma, lymph nodes of head, face, and neck   HCC

C82.52   Diffuse follicle center lymphoma, intrathoracic lymph nodes   HCC

C82.53   Diffuse follicle center lymphoma, intra-abdominal lymph nodes   HCC

C82.54   Diffuse follicle center lymphoma, lymph nodes of axilla and upper limb   HCC

C82.55   Diffuse follicle center lymphoma, lymph nodes of inguinal region and lower limb   HCC

C82.56   Diffuse follicle center lymphoma, intrapelvic lymph nodes   HCC

C82.57   Diffuse follicle center lymphoma, spleen   HCC

C82.58   Diffuse follicle center lymphoma, lymph nodes of multiple sites   HCC

C82.59   Diffuse follicle center lymphoma, extranodal and solid organ sites   HCC

✓5ᵗʰ **C82.6**   Cutaneous follicle center lymphoma

C82.6Ø   Cutaneous follicle center lymphoma, unspecified site   HCC ▽

C82.61   Cutaneous follicle center lymphoma, lymph nodes of head, face, and neck   HCC

C82.62   Cutaneous follicle center lymphoma, intrathoracic lymph nodes   HCC

C82.63   Cutaneous follicle center lymphoma, intra-abdominal lymph nodes   HCC

C82.64   Cutaneous follicle center lymphoma, lymph nodes of axilla and upper limb   HCC

C82.65   Cutaneous follicle center lymphoma, lymph nodes of inguinal region and lower limb   HCC

C82.66   Cutaneous follicle center lymphoma, intrapelvic lymph nodes   HCC

C82.67   Cutaneous follicle center lymphoma, spleen   HCC

C82.68   Cutaneous follicle center lymphoma, lymph nodes of multiple sites   HCC

C82.69   Cutaneous follicle center lymphoma, extranodal and solid organ sites   HCC

✓5ᵗʰ **C82.8**   Other types of follicular lymphoma

C82.8Ø   Other types of follicular lymphoma, unspecified site   HCC ▽

C82.81   Other types of follicular lymphoma, lymph nodes of head, face, and neck   HCC

C82.82   Other types of follicular lymphoma, intrathoracic lymph nodes   HCC

C82.83   Other types of follicular lymphoma, intra-abdominal lymph nodes   HCC

C82.84   Other types of follicular lymphoma, lymph nodes of axilla and upper limb   HCC

C82.85   Other types of follicular lymphoma, lymph nodes of inguinal region and lower limb   HCC

C82.86   Other types of follicular lymphoma, intrapelvic lymph nodes   HCC

C82.87   Other types of follicular lymphoma, spleen   HCC

C82.88   Other types of follicular lymphoma, lymph nodes of multiple sites   HCC

C82.89   Other types of follicular lymphoma, extranodal and solid organ sites   HCC

✓5ᵗʰ **C82.9**   Follicular lymphoma, unspecified

C82.9Ø   Follicular lymphoma, unspecified, unspecified site   HCC ▽

C82.91   Follicular lymphoma, unspecified, lymph nodes of head, face, and neck   HCC ▽

C82.92   Follicular lymphoma, unspecified, intrathoracic lymph nodes   HCC ▽

C82.93   Follicular lymphoma, unspecified, intra-abdominal lymph nodes   HCC ▽

C82.94   Follicular lymphoma, unspecified, lymph nodes of axilla and upper limb   HCC ▽

C82.95	Follicular lymphoma, unspecified, lymph nodes of **inguinal region and lower limb**	HCC ▽
C82.96	Follicular lymphoma, unspecified, **intrapelvic** lymph nodes	HCC ▽
C82.97	Follicular lymphoma, unspecified, **spleen**	HCC ▽
C82.98	Follicular lymphoma, unspecified, lymph nodes of **multiple sites**	HCC ▽
C82.99	Follicular lymphoma, unspecified, **extranodal and solid organ sites**	HCC ▽

√4ᵗʰ **C83** Non-follicular lymphoma

> EXCLUDES 1   *personal history of non-Hodgkin lymphoma (Z85.72)*

√5ᵗʰ **C83.0** Small cell B-cell lymphoma

> Lymphoplasmacytic lymphoma
> Nodal marginal zone lymphoma
> Non-leukemic variant of B-CLL
> Splenic marginal zone lymphoma
> EXCLUDES 1   *chronic lymphocytic leukemia (C91.1)*
>   *mature T/NK-cell lymphomas (C84.-)*
>   *Waldenström macroglobulinemia (C88.0)*
> **DEF:** Nonfollicular lymphoma that is rare, slow growing, and usually found in the older population.

C83.00	Small cell B-cell lymphoma, **unspecified site**	HCC ▽
C83.01	Small cell B-cell lymphoma, lymph nodes **of head, face, and neck**	HCC
C83.02	Small cell B-cell lymphoma, **intrathoracic lymph nodes**	HCC
C83.03	Small cell B-cell lymphoma, **intra-abdominal lymph nodes**	HCC
C83.04	Small cell B-cell lymphoma, lymph nodes **of axilla and upper limb**	HCC
C83.05	Small cell B-cell lymphoma, lymph nodes **of inguinal region and lower limb**	HCC
C83.06	Small cell B-cell lymphoma, **intrapelvic lymph nodes**	HCC
C83.07	Small cell B-cell lymphoma, **spleen**	HCC
C83.08	Small cell B-cell lymphoma, lymph nodes **of multiple sites**	HCC
C83.09	Small cell B-cell lymphoma, **extranodal and solid organ sites**	HCC

√5ᵗʰ **C83.1** Mantle cell lymphoma

> Centrocytic lymphoma
> Malignant lymphomatous polyposis
> **DEF:** Rare form of B-cell non-Hodgkin lymphoma named for the location of the tumor cell production, the mantle zone of the lymph nodes.

C83.10	Mantle cell lymphoma, **unspecified site**	HCC ▽
C83.11	Mantle cell lymphoma, lymph nodes of **head, face, and neck**	HCC
C83.12	Mantle cell lymphoma, **intrathoracic lymph nodes**	HCC
C83.13	Mantle cell lymphoma, **intra-abdominal lymph nodes**	HCC
C83.14	Mantle cell lymphoma, lymph nodes of **axilla and upper limb**	HCC
C83.15	Mantle cell lymphoma, lymph nodes of **inguinal region and lower limb**	HCC
C83.16	Mantle cell lymphoma, **intrapelvic** lymph nodes	HCC
C83.17	Mantle cell lymphoma, **spleen**	HCC
C83.18	Mantle cell lymphoma, lymph nodes of **multiple sites**	HCC
C83.19	Mantle cell lymphoma, **extranodal and solid organ sites**	HCC

√5ᵗʰ **C83.3** Diffuse large B-cell lymphoma

> Anaplastic diffuse large B-cell lymphoma
> CD30-positive diffuse large B-cell lymphoma
> Centroblastic diffuse large B-cell lymphoma
> Diffuse large B-cell lymphoma, subtype not specified
> Immunoblastic diffuse large B-cell lymphoma
> Plasmablastic diffuse large B-cell lymphoma
> T-cell rich diffuse large B-cell lymphoma
> EXCLUDES 1   *mediastinal (thymic) large B-cell lymphoma (C85.2-)*
>   *mature T/NK-cell lymphomas (C84.-)*
> **DEF:** Nonfollicular lymphoma that is one of the more common types of lymphoma. This cancer is fast growing and affects any age but is found mostly in the older population.

C83.30	Diffuse large B-cell lymphoma, **unspecified site**	HCC ▽

C83.31	Diffuse large B-cell lymphoma, lymph nodes of **head, face, and neck**	HCC
C83.32	Diffuse large B-cell lymphoma, **intrathoracic lymph nodes**	HCC
C83.33	Diffuse large B-cell lymphoma, **intra-abdominal lymph nodes**	HCC
C83.34	Diffuse large B-cell lymphoma, lymph nodes of **axilla and upper limb**	HCC
C83.35	Diffuse large B-cell lymphoma, lymph nodes of **inguinal region and lower limb**	HCC
C83.36	Diffuse large B-cell lymphoma, intrapelvic lymph nodes	HCC
C83.37	Diffuse large B-cell lymphoma, **spleen**	HCC
C83.38	Diffuse large B-cell lymphoma, lymph nodes of **multiple sites**	HCC
C83.39	Diffuse large B-cell lymphoma, **extranodal and solid organ sites**	HCC

√5ᵗʰ **C83.5** Lymphoblastic (diffuse) lymphoma

> B-precursor lymphoma
> Lymphoblastic B-cell lymphoma
> Lymphoblastic lymphoma NOS
> Lymphoblastic T-cell lymphoma
> T-precursor lymphoma
> **DEF:** Type of non-Hodgkin lymphoma considered lymphoma or leukemia—the determination is made based on the amount of bone marrow involvement. The cells are small to medium immature T-cells that often originate in the thymus where many of the T-cells are made.

C83.50	Lymphoblastic (diffuse) lymphoma, **unspecified site**	HCC ▽
C83.51	Lymphoblastic (diffuse) lymphoma, lymph nodes of **head, face, and neck**	HCC
C83.52	Lymphoblastic (diffuse) lymphoma, **intrathoracic lymph nodes**	HCC
C83.53	Lymphoblastic (diffuse) lymphoma, **intra-abdominal lymph nodes**	HCC
C83.54	Lymphoblastic (diffuse) lymphoma, lymph nodes of **axilla and upper limb**	HCC
C83.55	Lymphoblastic (diffuse) lymphoma, lymph nodes of **inguinal region and lower limb**	HCC
C83.56	Lymphoblastic (diffuse) lymphoma, **intrapelvic lymph nodes**	HCC
C83.57	Lymphoblastic (diffuse) lymphoma, **spleen**	HCC
C83.58	Lymphoblastic (diffuse) lymphoma, lymph nodes of **multiple sites**	HCC
C83.59	Lymphoblastic (diffuse) lymphoma, **extranodal and solid organ sites**	HCC

√5ᵗʰ **C83.7** Burkitt lymphoma

> Atypical Burkitt lymphoma
> Burkitt-like lymphoma
> EXCLUDES 1   *mature B-cell leukemia Burkitt type (C91.A-)*
> **DEF:** Malignancy of the lymphatic system, most often seen as a large bone-deteriorating lesion within the jaw or as an abdominal mass. It is a form of non-Hodgkin's lymphoma and is recognized as the fastest growing human tumor.

C83.70	Burkitt lymphoma, **unspecified site**	HCC ▽
C83.71	Burkitt lymphoma, lymph nodes of **head, face, and neck**	HCC
C83.72	Burkitt lymphoma, **intrathoracic lymph nodes**	HCC
C83.73	Burkitt lymphoma, **intra-abdominal lymph nodes**	HCC
C83.74	Burkitt lymphoma, lymph nodes of **axilla and upper limb**	HCC
C83.75	Burkitt lymphoma, lymph nodes of **inguinal region and lower limb**	HCC
C83.76	Burkitt lymphoma, **intrapelvic lymph nodes**	HCC
C83.77	Burkitt lymphoma, **spleen**	HCC
C83.78	Burkitt lymphoma, lymph nodes of **multiple sites**	HCC
C83.79	Burkitt lymphoma, **extranodal and solid organ sites**	HCC

√5ᵗʰ **C83.8** Other non-follicular lymphoma

> Intravascular large B-cell lymphoma
> Lymphoid granulomatosis
> Primary effusion B-cell lymphoma
> EXCLUDES 1   *mediastinal (thymic) large B-cell lymphoma (C85.2-)*
>   *T-cell rich B-cell lymphoma (C83.3-)*

C83.80	Other non-follicular lymphoma, **unspecified site**	HCC ▽

☑ Additional Character Req   √x7ᵗʰ Placeholder Alert   Manifestation   ▽ Unspecified   ►◄ Revised Text   ● New Code   ▲ Revised Code Title

ICD-10-CM 2019

479

C82.95–C83.80

Chapter 2. Neoplasms

C83.81   **Other non-follicular lymphoma, lymph nodes of head, face, and neck**   HCC

C83.82   **Other non-follicular lymphoma, intrathoracic lymph nodes**   HCC

C83.83   **Other non-follicular lymphoma, intra-abdominal lymph nodes**   HCC

C83.84   **Other non-follicular lymphoma, lymph nodes of axilla and upper limb**   HCC

C83.85   **Other non-follicular lymphoma, lymph nodes of inguinal region and lower limb**   HCC

C83.86   **Other non-follicular lymphoma, intrapelvic lymph nodes**   HCC

C83.87   **Other non-follicular lymphoma, spleen**   HCC

C83.88   **Other non-follicular lymphoma, lymph nodes of multiple sites**   HCC

C83.89   **Other non-follicular lymphoma, extranodal and solid organ sites**   HCC

√5ᵗʰ **C83.9**   **Non-follicular (diffuse) lymphoma, unspecified**

C83.90   **Non-follicular (diffuse) lymphoma, unspecified, unspecified site**   HCC ▽

C83.91   **Non-follicular (diffuse) lymphoma, unspecified, lymph nodes of head, face, and neck**   HCC ▽

C83.92   **Non-follicular (diffuse) lymphoma, unspecified, intrathoracic lymph nodes**   HCC ▽

C83.93   **Non-follicular (diffuse) lymphoma, unspecified, intra-abdominal lymph nodes**   HCC ▽

C83.94   **Non-follicular (diffuse) lymphoma, unspecified, lymph nodes of axilla and upper limb**   HCC ▽

C83.95   **Non-follicular (diffuse) lymphoma, unspecified, lymph nodes of inguinal region and lower limb**   HCC ▽

C83.96   **Non-follicular (diffuse) lymphoma, unspecified, intrapelvic lymph nodes**   HCC ▽

C83.97   **Non-follicular (diffuse) lymphoma, unspecified, spleen**   HCC ▽

C83.98   **Non-follicular (diffuse) lymphoma, unspecified, lymph nodes of multiple sites**   HCC ▽

C83.99   **Non-follicular (diffuse) lymphoma, unspecified, extranodal and solid organ sites**   HCC ▽

√4ᵗʰ **C84**   **Mature T/NK-cell lymphomas**

> **EXCLUDES 1**   *personal history of non-Hodgkin lymphoma (Z85.72)*

√5ᵗʰ **C84.0**   **Mycosis fungoides**

> **EXCLUDES 1**   *peripheral T-cell lymphoma, not classified (C84.4-)*
>
> **DEF:** Most common form of cutaneous T-cell lymphoma. A type of non-Hodgkin lymphoma in which white blood cells become cancerous and affect the skin and sometimes internal organs.
> **Synonym(s):** *Alibert-Bazin syndrome.*

C84.00   **Mycosis fungoides, unspecified site**   HCC ▽

C84.01   **Mycosis fungoides, lymph nodes of head, face, and neck**   HCC

C84.02   **Mycosis fungoides, intrathoracic lymph nodes**   HCC

C84.03   **Mycosis fungoides, intra-abdominal lymph nodes**   HCC

C84.04   **Mycosis fungoides, lymph nodes of axilla and upper limb**   HCC

C84.05   **Mycosis fungoides, lymph nodes of inguinal region and lower limb**   HCC

C84.06   **Mycosis fungoides, intrapelvic lymph nodes**   HCC

C84.07   **Mycosis fungoides, spleen**   HCC

C84.08   **Mycosis fungoides, lymph nodes of multiple sites**   HCC

C84.09   **Mycosis fungoides, extranodal and solid organ sites**   HCC

√5ᵗʰ **C84.1**   **Sézary disease**

> **DEF:** Extension of mycosis fungoides that affects the blood and all of the skin, appearing as sunburn, rather than patches. It spreads to the lymph nodes and is often linked to a weakened immune system.

C84.10   **Sézary disease, unspecified site**   HCC ▽

C84.11   **Sézary disease, lymph nodes of head, face, and neck**   HCC

C84.12   **Sézary disease, intrathoracic lymph nodes**   HCC

C84.13   **Sézary disease, intra-abdominal lymph nodes**   HCC

C84.14   **Sézary disease, lymph nodes of axilla and upper limb**   HCC

C84.15   **Sézary disease, lymph nodes of inguinal region and lower limb**   HCC

C84.16   **Sézary disease, intrapelvic lymph nodes**   HCC

C84.17   **Sézary disease, spleen**   HCC

C84.18   **Sézary disease, lymph nodes of multiple sites**   HCC

C84.19   **Sézary disease, extranodal and solid organ sites**   HCC

√5ᵗʰ **C84.4**   **Peripheral T-cell lymphoma, not classified**

> Lennert's lymphoma
> Lymphoepithelioid lymphoma
> Mature T-cell lymphoma, not elsewhere classified

C84.40   **Peripheral T-cell lymphoma, not classified, unspecified site**   HCC ▽

C84.41   **Peripheral T-cell lymphoma, not classified, lymph nodes of head, face, and neck**   HCC

C84.42   **Peripheral T-cell lymphoma, not classified, intrathoracic lymph nodes**   HCC

C84.43   **Peripheral T-cell lymphoma, not classified, intra-abdominal lymph nodes**   HCC

C84.44   **Peripheral T-cell lymphoma, not classified, lymph nodes of axilla and upper limb**   HCC

C84.45   **Peripheral T-cell lymphoma, not classified, lymph nodes of inguinal region and lower limb**   HCC

C84.46   **Peripheral T-cell lymphoma, not classified, intrapelvic lymph nodes**   HCC

C84.47   **Peripheral T-cell lymphoma, not classified, spleen**   HCC

C84.48   **Peripheral T-cell lymphoma, not classified, lymph nodes of multiple sites**   HCC

C84.49   **Peripheral T-cell lymphoma, not classified, extranodal and solid organ sites**   HCC

√5ᵗʰ **C84.6**   **Anaplastic large cell lymphoma, ALK-positive**

> Anaplastic large cell lymphoma, CD30-positive

C84.60   **Anaplastic large cell lymphoma, ALK-positive, unspecified site**   HCC ▽

C84.61   **Anaplastic large cell lymphoma, ALK-positive, lymph nodes of head, face, and neck**   HCC

C84.62   **Anaplastic large cell lymphoma, ALK-positive, intrathoracic lymph nodes**   HCC

C84.63   **Anaplastic large cell lymphoma, ALK-positive, intra-abdominal lymph nodes**   HCC

C84.64   **Anaplastic large cell lymphoma, ALK-positive, lymph nodes of axilla and upper limb**   HCC

C84.65   **Anaplastic large cell lymphoma, ALK-positive, lymph nodes of inguinal region and lower limb**   HCC

C84.66   **Anaplastic large cell lymphoma, ALK-positive, intrapelvic lymph nodes**   HCC

C84.67   **Anaplastic large cell lymphoma, ALK-positive, spleen**   HCC

C84.68   **Anaplastic large cell lymphoma, ALK-positive, lymph nodes of multiple sites**   HCC

C84.69   **Anaplastic large cell lymphoma, ALK-positive, extranodal and solid organ sites**   HCC

√5ᵗʰ **C84.7**   **Anaplastic large cell lymphoma, ALK-negative**

> **EXCLUDES 1**   *primary cutaneous CD30-positive T-cell proliferations (C86.6-)*

C84.70   **Anaplastic large cell lymphoma, ALK-negative, unspecified site**   HCC ▽

C84.71   **Anaplastic large cell lymphoma, ALK-negative, lymph nodes of head, face, and neck**   HCC

C84.72   **Anaplastic large cell lymphoma, ALK-negative, intrathoracic lymph nodes**   HCC

C84.73   **Anaplastic large cell lymphoma, ALK-negative, intra-abdominal lymph nodes**   HCC

C84.74   **Anaplastic large cell lymphoma, ALK-negative, lymph nodes of axilla and upper limb**   HCC

C84.75   **Anaplastic large cell lymphoma, ALK-negative, lymph nodes of inguinal region and lower limb**   HCC

C84.76   **Anaplastic large cell lymphoma, ALK-negative, intrapelvic lymph nodes**   HCC

C84.77 Anaplastic large cell lymphoma, ALK-negative, spleen   HCC

C84.78 Anaplastic large cell lymphoma, ALK-negative, lymph nodes of multiple sites   HCC

C84.79 Anaplastic large cell lymphoma, ALK-negative, extranodal and solid organ sites   HCC

√5ᵗʰ **C84.A** Cutaneous T-cell lymphoma, unspecified

C84.A0 Cutaneous T-cell lymphoma, unspecified, unspecified site   HCC ▽

C84.A1 Cutaneous T-cell lymphoma, unspecified, lymph nodes of head, face, and neck   HCC ▽

C84.A2 Cutaneous T-cell lymphoma, unspecified, intrathoracic lymph nodes   HCC ▽

C84.A3 Cutaneous T-cell lymphoma, unspecified, intra-abdominal lymph nodes   HCC ▽

C84.A4 Cutaneous T-cell lymphoma, unspecified, lymph nodes of axilla and upper limb   HCC ▽

C84.A5 Cutaneous T-cell lymphoma, unspecified, lymph nodes of inguinal region and lower limb   HCC ▽

C84.A6 Cutaneous T-cell lymphoma, unspecified, intrapelvic lymph nodes   HCC ▽

C84.A7 Cutaneous T-cell lymphoma, unspecified, spleen   HCC ▽

C84.A8 Cutaneous T-cell lymphoma, unspecified, lymph nodes of multiple sites   HCC ▽

C84.A9 Cutaneous T-cell lymphoma, unspecified, extranodal and solid organ sites   HCC ▽

√5ᵗʰ **C84.Z** Other mature T/NK-cell lymphomas

> **NOTE**   If T-cell lineage or involvement is mentioned in conjunction with a specific lymphoma, code to the more specific description.
>
> **EXCLUDES 1**   angioimmunoblastic T-cell lymphoma (C86.5)
> blastic NK-cell lymphoma (C86.4)
> enteropathy-type T-cell lymphoma (C86.2)
> extranodal NK-cell lymphoma, nasal type (C86.0)
> hepatosplenic T-cell lymphoma (C86.1)
> primary cutaneous CD30-positive T-cell proliferations (C86.6)
> subcutaneous panniculitis-like T-cell lymphoma (C86.3)
> T-cell leukemia (C91.1-)

C84.Z0 Other mature T/NK-cell lymphomas, unspecified site   HCC ▽

C84.Z1 Other mature T/NK-cell lymphomas, lymph nodes of head, face, and neck   HCC

C84.Z2 Other mature T/NK-cell lymphomas, intrathoracic lymph nodes   HCC

C84.Z3 Other mature T/NK-cell lymphomas, intra-abdominal lymph nodes   HCC

C84.Z4 Other mature T/NK-cell lymphomas, lymph nodes of axilla and upper limb   HCC

C84.Z5 Other mature T/NK-cell lymphomas, lymph nodes of inguinal region and lower limb   HCC

C84.Z6 Other mature T/NK-cell lymphomas, intrapelvic lymph nodes   HCC

C84.Z7 Other mature T/NK-cell lymphomas, spleen   HCC

C84.Z8 Other mature T/NK-cell lymphomas, lymph nodes of multiple sites   HCC

C84.Z9 Other mature T/NK-cell lymphomas, extranodal and solid organ sites   HCC

√5ᵗʰ **C84.9** Mature T/NK-cell lymphomas, unspecified

NK/T cell lymphoma NOS

> **EXCLUDES 1**   mature T-cell lymphoma, not elsewhere classified (C84.4-)

C84.90 Mature T/NK-cell lymphomas, unspecified, unspecified site   HCC ▽

C84.91 Mature T/NK-cell lymphomas, unspecified, lymph nodes of head, face, and neck   HCC ▽

C84.92 Mature T/NK-cell lymphomas, unspecified, intrathoracic lymph nodes   HCC ▽

C84.93 Mature T/NK-cell lymphomas, unspecified, intra-abdominal lymph nodes   HCC ▽

C84.94 Mature T/NK-cell lymphomas, unspecified, lymph nodes of axilla and upper limb   HCC ▽

C84.95 Mature T/NK-cell lymphomas, unspecified, lymph nodes of inguinal region and lower limb   HCC ▽

C84.96 Mature T/NK-cell lymphomas, unspecified, intrapelvic lymph nodes   HCC ▽

C84.97 Mature T/NK-cell lymphomas, unspecified, spleen   HCC ▽

C84.98 Mature T/NK-cell lymphomas, unspecified, lymph nodes of multiple sites   HCC ▽

C84.99 Mature T/NK-cell lymphomas, unspecified, extranodal and solid organ sites   HCC ▽

√4ᵗʰ **C85** Other specified and unspecified types of non-Hodgkin lymphoma

> **EXCLUDES 1**   other specified types of T/NK-cell lymphoma (C86.-)
> personal history of non-Hodgkin lymphoma (Z85.72)

√5ᵗʰ **C85.1** Unspecified B-cell lymphoma

> **NOTE**   If B-cell lineage or involvement is mentioned in conjunction with a specific lymphoma, code to the more specific description.

C85.10 Unspecified B-cell lymphoma, unspecified site   HCC ▽

C85.11 Unspecified B-cell lymphoma, lymph nodes of head, face, and neck   HCC ▽

C85.12 Unspecified B-cell lymphoma, intrathoracic lymph nodes   HCC ▽

C85.13 Unspecified B-cell lymphoma, intra-abdominal lymph nodes   HCC ▽

C85.14 Unspecified B-cell lymphoma, lymph nodes of axilla and upper limb   HCC ▽

C85.15 Unspecified B-cell lymphoma, lymph nodes of inguinal region and lower limb   HCC ▽

C85.16 Unspecified B-cell lymphoma, intrapelvic lymph nodes   HCC ▽

C85.17 Unspecified B-cell lymphoma, spleen   HCC ▽

C85.18 Unspecified B-cell lymphoma, lymph nodes of multiple sites   HCC ▽

C85.19 Unspecified B-cell lymphoma, extranodal and solid organ sites   HCC ▽

√5ᵗʰ **C85.2** Mediastinal (thymic) large B-cell lymphoma

C85.20 Mediastinal (thymic) large B-cell lymphoma, unspecified site   HCC ▽

C85.21 Mediastinal (thymic) large B-cell lymphoma, lymph nodes of head, face, and neck   HCC

C85.22 Mediastinal (thymic) large B-cell lymphoma, intrathoracic lymph nodes   HCC

C85.23 Mediastinal (thymic) large B-cell lymphoma, intra-abdominal lymph nodes   HCC

C85.24 Mediastinal (thymic) large B-cell lymphoma, lymph nodes of axilla and upper limb   HCC

C85.25 Mediastinal (thymic) large B-cell lymphoma, lymph nodes of inguinal region and lower limb   HCC

C85.26 Mediastinal (thymic) large B-cell lymphoma, intrapelvic lymph nodes   HCC

C85.27 Mediastinal (thymic) large B-cell lymphoma, spleen   HCC

C85.28 Mediastinal (thymic) large B-cell lymphoma, lymph nodes of multiple sites   HCC

C85.29 Mediastinal (thymic) large B-cell lymphoma, extranodal and solid organ sites   HCC

√5ᵗʰ **C85.8** Other specified types of non-Hodgkin lymphoma

C85.80 Other specified types of non-Hodgkin lymphoma, unspecified site   HCC ▽

C85.81 Other specified types of non-Hodgkin lymphoma, lymph nodes of head, face, and neck   HCC

C85.82 Other specified types of non-Hodgkin lymphoma, intrathoracic lymph nodes   HCC

C85.83 Other specified types of non-Hodgkin lymphoma, intra-abdominal lymph nodes   HCC

C85.84 Other specified types of non-Hodgkin lymphoma, lymph nodes of axilla and upper limb   HCC

C85.85 Other specified types of non-Hodgkin lymphoma, lymph nodes of inguinal region and lower limb   HCC

C85.86 Other specified types of non-Hodgkin lymphoma, intrapelvic lymph nodes   HCC

☑ Additional Character Req   √x7ᵗʰ Placeholder Alert   Manifestation   ▽ Unspecified   ►◄ Revised Text   ● New Code   ▲ Revised Code Title

ICD-10-CM 2019   481

Chapter 2. Neoplasms *(side tab)*

C85.87   **Other specified types of non-Hodgkin lymphoma, spleen**   `HCC`

C85.88   **Other specified types of non-Hodgkin lymphoma, lymph nodes of multiple sites**   `HCC`

C85.89   **Other specified types of non-Hodgkin lymphoma, extranodal and solid organ sites**   `HCC`

√5ᵗʰ **C85.9**   **Non-Hodgkin lymphoma, unspecified**

Lymphoma NOS
Malignant lymphoma NOS
Non-Hodgkin lymphoma NOS

C85.90   **Non-Hodgkin lymphoma, unspecified, unspecified site**   `HCC` ▽

C85.91   **Non-Hodgkin lymphoma, unspecified, lymph nodes of head, face, and neck**   `HCC` ▽

C85.92   **Non-Hodgkin lymphoma, unspecified, intrathoracic lymph nodes**   `HCC` ▽

C85.93   **Non-Hodgkin lymphoma, unspecified, intra-abdominal lymph nodes**   `HCC` ▽

C85.94   **Non-Hodgkin lymphoma, unspecified, lymph nodes of axilla and upper limb**   `HCC` ▽

C85.95   **Non-Hodgkin lymphoma, unspecified, lymph nodes of inguinal region and lower limb**   `HCC` ▽

C85.96   **Non-Hodgkin lymphoma, unspecified, intrapelvic lymph nodes**   `HCC` ▽

C85.97   **Non-Hodgkin lymphoma, unspecified, spleen**   `HCC` ▽

C85.98   **Non-Hodgkin lymphoma, unspecified, lymph nodes of multiple sites**   `HCC` ▽

C85.99   **Non-Hodgkin lymphoma, unspecified, extranodal and solid organ sites**   `HCC` ▽

√4ᵗʰ **C86**   **Other specified types of T/NK-cell lymphoma**

EXCLUDES 1   *anaplastic large cell lymphoma, ALK negative (C84.7-)*
anaplastic large cell lymphoma, ALK positive (C84.6-)
mature T/NK-cell lymphomas (C84.-)
other specified types of non-Hodgkin lymphoma (C85.8-)

C86.0   **Extranodal NK/T-cell lymphoma, nasal type**   `HCC`

C86.1   **Hepatosplenic T-cell lymphoma**   `HCC`
Alpha-beta and gamma delta types

C86.2   **Enteropathy-type (intestinal) T-cell lymphoma**   `HCC`
Enteropathy associated T-cell lymphoma

C86.3   **Subcutaneous panniculitis-like T-cell lymphoma**   `HCC`

C86.4   **Blastic NK-cell lymphoma**   `HCC`
Blastic plasmacytoid dendritic cell neoplasm (BPDCN)

C86.5   **Angioimmunoblastic T-cell lymphoma**   `HCC`
Angioimmunoblastic lymphadenopathy with dysproteinemia (AILD)

C86.6   **Primary cutaneous CD30-positive T-cell proliferations**   `HCC`
Lymphomatoid papulosis
Primary cutaneous anaplastic large cell lymphoma
Primary cutaneous CD30-positive large T-cell lymphoma

√4ᵗʰ **C88**   **Malignant immunoproliferative diseases and certain other B-cell lymphomas**

EXCLUDES 1   *B-cell lymphoma, unspecified (C85.1-)*
personal history of other malignant neoplasms of lymphoid, hematopoietic and related tissues (Z85.79)

C88.0   **Waldenström macroglobulinemia**   `HCC`
Lymphoplasmacytic lymphoma with IgM-production
Macroglobulinemia (idiopathic) (primary)
EXCLUDES 1   *small cell B-cell lymphoma (C83.0)*

C88.2   **Heavy chain disease**   `HCC`
Franklin disease
Gamma heavy chain disease
Mu heavy chain disease

C88.3   **Immunoproliferative small intestinal disease**   `HCC`
Alpha heavy chain disease
Mediterranean lymphoma

C88.4   **Extranodal marginal zone B-cell lymphoma of mucosa-associated lymphoid tissue [MALT-lymphoma]**   `HCC`
Lymphoma of skin-associated lymphoid tissue [SALT-lymphoma]
Lymphoma of bronchial-associated lymphoid tissue [BALT-lymphoma]
EXCLUDES 1   *high malignant (diffuse large B-cell) lymphoma (C83.3-)*

C88.8   **Other malignant immunoproliferative diseases**   `HCC`

C88.9   **Malignant immunoproliferative disease, unspecified**   `HCC` ▽
Immunoproliferative disease NOS

√4ᵗʰ **C90**   **Multiple myeloma and malignant plasma cell neoplasms**

EXCLUDES 1   *personal history of other malignant neoplasms of lymphoid, hematopoietic and related tissues (Z85.79)*

√5ᵗʰ **C90.0**   **Multiple myeloma**
Kahler's disease
Medullary plasmacytoma
Myelomatosis
Plasma cell myeloma
EXCLUDES 1   *solitary myeloma (C90.3-)*
solitary plasmactyoma (C90.3-)

TIP: Do not assign an additional code for bone metastasis (C79.51) when multiple myeloma is described as metastatic to the bone; bone involvement is integral to this disease process.

C90.00   **Multiple myeloma not having achieved remission**   `HCC`
Multiple myeloma with failed remission
Multiple myeloma NOS

C90.01   **Multiple myeloma in remission**   `HCC`

C90.02   **Multiple myeloma in relapse**   `HCC`

√5ᵗʰ **C90.1**   **Plasma cell leukemia**
Plasmacytic leukemia

C90.10   **Plasma cell leukemia not having achieved remission**   `HCC`
Plasma cell leukemia with failed remission
Plasma cell leukemia NOS

C90.11   **Plasma cell leukemia in remission**   `HCC`

C90.12   **Plasma cell leukemia in relapse**   `HCC`

√5ᵗʰ **C90.2**   **Extramedullary plasmacytoma**

C90.20   **Extramedullary plasmacytoma not having achieved remission**   `HCC`
Extramedullary plasmacytoma with failed remission
Extramedullary plasmacytoma NOS

C90.21   **Extramedullary plasmacytoma in remission**   `HCC`

C90.22   **Extramedullary plasmacytoma in relapse**   `HCC`

√5ᵗʰ **C90.3**   **Solitary plasmacytoma**
Localized malignant plasma cell tumor NOS
Plasmacytoma NOS
Solitary myeloma

C90.30   **Solitary plasmacytoma not having achieved remission**   `HCC`
Solitary plasmacytoma with failed remission
Solitary plasmacytoma NOS

C90.31   **Solitary plasmacytoma in remission**   `HCC`

C90.32   **Solitary plasmacytoma in relapse**   `HCC`

√4ᵗʰ **C91**   **Lymphoid leukemia**

EXCLUDES 1   *personal history of leukemia (Z85.6)*

DEF: Malignant proliferation of immature lymphocytes (white blood cells that make up lymphoid tissue), called lymphoblasts, that originate in the bone marrow. Can be acute (ALL) or chronic (CLL).

√5ᵗʰ **C91.0**   **Acute lymphoblastic leukemia [ALL]**

NOTE   Code C91.0 should only be used for T-cell and B-cell precursor leukemia

C91.00   **Acute lymphoblastic leukemia not having achieved remission**   `HCC`
Acute lymphoblastic leukemia with failed remission
Acute lymphoblastic leukemia NOS

C91.01   **Acute lymphoblastic leukemia, in remission**   `HCC`

C91.02   **Acute lymphoblastic leukemia, in relapse**   `HCC`

✓5th **C91.1 Chronic lymphocytic leukemia of B-cell type**

    Lymphoplasmacytic leukemia

    Richter syndrome

    EXCLUDES 1   *lymphoplasmacytic lymphoma (C83.0-)*

    C91.10 Chronic lymphocytic leukemia of B-cell   HCC

          type not having achieved remission

          Chronic lymphocytic leukemia of B-cell type with

            failed remission

          Chronic lymphocytic leukemia of B-cell type NOS

    C91.11 Chronic lymphocytic leukemia of B-cell   HCC

          type in remission

    C91.12 Chronic lymphocytic leukemia of B-cell   HCC

          type in relapse

✓5th **C91.3 Prolymphocytic leukemia of B-cell type**

    C91.30 Prolymphocytic leukemia of B-cell type   HCC

          not having achieved remission

          Prolymphocytic leukemia of B-cell type with failed

            remission

          Prolymphocytic leukemia of B-cell type NOS

    C91.31 Prolymphocytic leukemia of B-cell type,   HCC

          in remission

    C91.32 Prolymphocytic leukemia of B-cell type,   HCC

          in relapse

✓5th **C91.4 Hairy cell leukemia**

    Leukemic reticuloendotheliosis

    DEF: Rare type of leukemia that is slow growing and often also

    considered a type of lymphoma. The small B-cell lymphocytes

    appear with "hairy" projections under a microscope and are found

    mostly in the bone marrow, spleen, and blood.

    C91.40 Hairy cell leukemia not having achieved   HCC

          remission

          Hairy cell leukemia with failed remission

          Hairy cell leukemia NOS

    C91.41 Hairy cell leukemia, in remission   HCC

    C91.42 Hairy cell leukemia, in relapse   HCC

✓5th **C91.5 Adult T-cell lymphoma/leukemia (HTLV-1-associated)**

    Acute variant of adult T-cell lymphoma/leukemia

        (HTLV-1-associated)

    Chronic variant of adult T-cell lymphoma/leukemia

        (HTLV-1-associated)

    Lymphomatoid variant of adult T-cell lymphoma/leukemia

        (HTLV-1-associated)

    Smouldering variant of adult T-cell lymphoma/leukemia

        (HTLV-1-associated)

    C91.50 Adult T-cell lymphoma/leukemia   HCC A

          (HTLV-1-associated) not having achieved

          remission

          Adult T-cell lymphoma/leukemia (HTLV-1-associated)

            with failed remission

          Adult T-cell lymphoma/leukemia (HTLV-1-associated)

            NOS

    C91.51 Adult T-cell lymphoma/leukemia   HCC A

          (HTLV-1-associated), in remission

    C91.52 Adult T-cell lymphoma/leukemia   HCC A

          (HTLV-1-associated), in relapse

✓5th **C91.6 Prolymphocytic leukemia of T-cell type**

    C91.60 Prolymphocytic leukemia of T-cell type   HCC

          not having achieved remission

          Prolymphocytic leukemia of T-cell type with failed

            remission

          Prolymphocytic leukemia of T-cell type NOS

    C91.61 Prolymphocytic leukemia of T-cell type,   HCC

          in remission

    C91.62 Prolymphocytic leukemia of T-cell type,   HCC

          in relapse

✓5th **C91.A Mature B-cell leukemia Burkitt-type**

    EXCLUDES 1   *Burkitt lymphoma (C83.7-)*

    C91.A0 Mature B-cell leukemia Burkitt-type not   HCC

          having achieved remission

          Mature B-cell leukemia Burkitt-type with failed

            remission

          Mature B-cell leukemia Burkitt-type NOS

    C91.A1 Mature B-cell leukemia Burkitt-type, in   HCC

          remission

    C91.A2 Mature B-cell leukemia Burkitt-type, in   HCC

          relapse

✓5th **C91.Z Other lymphoid leukemia**

    T-cell large granular lymphocytic leukemia (associated with

        rheumatoid arthritis)

    C91.Z0 Other lymphoid leukemia not having   HCC

          achieved remission

          Other lymphoid leukemia with failed remission

          Other lymphoid leukemia NOS

    C91.Z1 Other lymphoid leukemia, in remission   HCC

    C91.Z2 Other lymphoid leukemia, in relapse   HCC

✓5th **C91.9 Lymphoid leukemia, unspecified**

    C91.90 Lymphoid leukemia, unspecified not   HCC ▽

          having achieved remission

          Lymphoid leukemia with failed remission

          Lymphoid leukemia NOS

    C91.91 Lymphoid leukemia, unspecified, in   HCC ▽

          remission

    C91.92 Lymphoid leukemia, unspecified, in   HCC ▽

          relapse

✓4th **C92 Myeloid leukemia**

    INCLUDES   granulocytic leukemia

             myelogenous leukemia

    EXCLUDES 1   *personal history of leukemia (Z85.6)*

    DEF: Cancer that develops in immature myelocytes called myeloblasts.

    These are the cells that become white blood cells (except lymphocytes),

    red blood cells, or platelet making cells. Can be acute (AML) or chronic

    (CML).

✓5th **C92.0 Acute myeloblastic leukemia**

    Acute myeloblastic leukemia, minimal differentiation

    Acute myeloblastic leukemia (with maturation)

    Acute myeloblastic leukemia 1/ETO

    Acute myeloblastic leukemia M0

    Acute myeloblastic leukemia M1

    Acute myeloblastic leukemia M2

    Acute myeloblastic leukemia with t(8;21)

    Acute myeloblastic leukemia (without a FAB classification) NOS

    Refractory anemia with excess blasts in transformation [RAEBT]

    EXCLUDES 1   *acute exacerbation of chronic myeloid leukemia*

             (C92.10)

             refractory anemia with excess of blasts not in

             transformation (D46.2-)

    C92.00 Acute myeloblastic leukemia, not having   HCC

          achieved remission

          Acute myeloblastic leukemia with failed remission

          Acute myeloblastic leukemia NOS

    C92.01 Acute myeloblastic leukemia, in remission   HCC

    C92.02 Acute myeloblastic leukemia, in relapse   HCC

✓5th **C92.1 Chronic myeloid leukemia, BCR/ABL-positive**

    Chronic myelogenous leukemia, Philadelphia chromosome

        (Ph1) positive

    Chronic myelogenous leukemia, t(9;22) (q34;q11)

    Chronic myelogenous leukemia with crisis of blast cells

    EXCLUDES 1   *atypical chronic myeloid leukemia BCR/ABL-negative*

             (C92.2-)

             chronic myelomonocytic leukemia (C93.1-)

             chronic myeloproliferative disease (D47.1)

    C92.10 Chronic myeloid leukemia,   HCC

          BCR/ABL-positive, not having achieved

          remission

          Chronic myeloid leukemia, BCR/ABL-positive with

            failed remission

          Chronic myeloid leukemia, BCR/ABL-positive NOS

    C92.11 Chronic myeloid leukemia,   HCC

          BCR/ABL-positive, in remission

    C92.12 Chronic myeloid leukemia,   HCC

          BCR/ABL-positive, in relapse

✓5th **C92.2 Atypical chronic myeloid leukemia, BCR/ABL-negative**

    C92.20 Atypical chronic myeloid leukemia,   HCC

          BCR/ABL-negative, not having achieved

          remission

          Atypical chronic myeloid leukemia, BCR/ABL-negative

            with failed remission

          Atypical chronic myeloid leukemia, BCR/ABL-negative

            NOS

    C92.21 Atypical chronic myeloid leukemia,   HCC

          BCR/ABL-negative, in remission

    C92.22 Atypical chronic myeloid leukemia,   HCC

          BCR/ABL-negative, in relapse

☑ Additional Character Req   ✓x7th Placeholder Alert   Manifestation   ▽ Unspecified   ►◄ Revised Text   ● New Code   ▲ Revised Code Title

Chapter 2. Neoplasms

C92.3–C94.02

√5ᵗʰ **C92.3** **Myeloid sarcoma**

A malignant tumor of immature myeloid cells

Chloroma

Granulocytic sarcoma

C92.30 **Myeloid sarcoma, not having achieved** HCC
remission

Myeloid sarcoma with failed remission

Myeloid sarcoma NOS

C92.31 **Myeloid sarcoma, in remission** HCC

C92.32 **Myeloid sarcoma, in relapse** HCC

√5ᵗʰ **C92.4** **Acute promyelocytic leukemia**

AML M3

AML Me with t(15;17) and variants

C92.40 **Acute promyelocytic leukemia, not having** HCC
achieved remission

Acute promyelocytic leukemia with failed remission

Acute promyelocytic leukemia NOS

C92.41 **Acute promyelocytic leukemia, in** HCC
remission

C92.42 **Acute promyelocytic leukemia, in relapse** HCC

√5ᵗʰ **C92.5** **Acute myelomonocytic leukemia**

AML M4

AML M4 Eo with inv(16) or t(16;16)

C92.50 **Acute myelomonocytic leukemia, not** HCC
having achieved remission

Acute myelomonocytic leukemia with failed remission

Acute myelomonocytic leukemia NOS

C92.51 **Acute myelomonocytic leukemia, in** HCC
remission

C92.52 **Acute myelomonocytic leukemia, in** HCC
relapse

√5ᵗʰ **C92.6** **Acute myeloid leukemia with 11q23-abnormality**

Acute myeloid leukemia with variation of MLL-gene

C92.60 **Acute myeloid leukemia with** HCC
11q23-abnormality not having achieved
remission

Acute myeloid leukemia with 11q23-abnormality with
failed remission

Acute myeloid leukemia with 11q23-abnormality NOS

C92.61 **Acute myeloid leukemia with** HCC
11q23-abnormality in remission

C92.62 **Acute myeloid leukemia with** HCC
11q23-abnormality in relapse

√5ᵗʰ **C92.A** **Acute myeloid leukemia with multilineage dysplasia**

Acute myeloid leukemia with dysplasia of remaining
hematopoesis and/or myelodysplastic disease in its history

C92.A0 **Acute myeloid leukemia with multilineage** HCC
dysplasia, not having achieved remission

Acute myeloid leukemia with multilineage dysplasia
with failed remission

Acute myeloid leukemia with multilineage dysplasia
NOS

C92.A1 **Acute myeloid leukemia with multilineage** HCC
dysplasia, in remission

C92.A2 **Acute myeloid leukemia with multilineage** HCC
dysplasia, in relapse

√5ᵗʰ **C92.Z** **Other myeloid leukemia**

C92.Z0 **Other myeloid leukemia not having** HCC
achieved remission

Myeloid leukemia NEC with failed remission

Myeloid leukemia NEC

C92.Z1 **Other myeloid leukemia, in remission** HCC

C92.Z2 **Other myeloid leukemia, in relapse** HCC

√5ᵗʰ **C92.9** **Myeloid leukemia, unspecified**

C92.90 **Myeloid leukemia, unspecified, not having** HCC ▽
achieved remission

Myeloid leukemia, unspecified with failed remission

Myeloid leukemia, unspecified NOS

C92.91 **Myeloid leukemia, unspecified in** HCC ▽
remission

C92.92 **Myeloid leukemia, unspecified in relapse** HCC ▽

√4ᵗʰ **C93** **Monocytic leukemia**

INCLUDES monocytoid leukemia

EXCLUDES 1 personal history of leukemia (Z85.6)

√5ᵗʰ **C93.0** **Acute monoblastic/monocytic leukemia**

AML M5

AML M5a

AML M5b

C93.00 **Acute monoblastic/monocytic leukemia,** HCC
not having achieved remission

Acute monoblastic/monocytic leukemia with failed
remission

Acute monoblastic/monocytic leukemia NOS

C93.01 **Acute monoblastic/monocytic leukemia,** HCC
in remission

C93.02 **Acute monoblastic/monocytic leukemia,** HCC
in relapse

√5ᵗʰ **C93.1** **Chronic myelomonocytic leukemia**

Chronic monocytic leukemia

CMML-1

CMML-2

CMML with eosinophilia

C93.10 **Chronic myelomonocytic leukemia not** HCC
having achieved remission

Chronic myelomonocytic leukemia with failed
remission

Chronic myelomonocytic leukemia NOS

C93.11 **Chronic myelomonocytic leukemia, in** HCC
remission

C93.12 **Chronic myelomonocytic leukemia, in** HCC
relapse

√5ᵗʰ **C93.3** **Juvenile myelomonocytic leukemia**

C93.30 **Juvenile myelomonocytic leukemia, not** HCC P
having achieved remission

Juvenile myelomonocytic leukemia with failed
remission

Juvenile myelomonocytic leukemia NOS

C93.31 **Juvenile myelomonocytic leukemia, in** HCC P
remission

C93.32 **Juvenile myelomonocytic leukemia, in** HCC P
relapse

√5ᵗʰ **C93.Z** **Other monocytic leukemia**

C93.Z0 **Other monocytic leukemia, not having** HCC
achieved remission

Other monocytic leukemia NOS

C93.Z1 **Other monocytic leukemia, in remission** HCC

C93.Z2 **Other monocytic leukemia, in relapse** HCC

√5ᵗʰ **C93.9** **Monocytic leukemia, unspecified**

C93.90 **Monocytic leukemia, unspecified, not** HCC ▽
having achieved remission

Monocytic leukemia, unspecified with failed remission

Monocytic leukemia, unspecified NOS

C93.91 **Monocytic leukemia, unspecified in** HCC ▽
remission

C93.92 **Monocytic leukemia, unspecified in** HCC ▽
relapse

√4ᵗʰ **C94** **Other leukemias of specified cell type**

EXCLUDES 1 leukemic reticuloendotheliosis (C91.4-)

myelodysplastic syndromes (D46.-)

personal history of leukemia (Z85.6)

plasma cell leukemia (C90.1-)

√5ᵗʰ **C94.0** **Acute erythroid leukemia**

Acute myeloid leukemia M6(a)(b)

Erythroleukemia

DEF: Erythroleukemia: Malignant blood dyscrasia (a
myeloproliferative disorder).

C94.00 **Acute erythroid leukemia, not having** HCC
achieved remission

Acute erythroid leukemia with failed remission

Acute erythroid leukemia NOS

C94.01 **Acute erythroid leukemia, in remission** HCC

C94.02 **Acute erythroid leukemia, in relapse** HCC

Chapter 2. Neoplasms

✓5ᵗʰ C94.2   Acute megakaryoblastic leukemia
Acute myeloid leukemia M7
Acute megakaryocytic leukemia

C94.20   Acute megakaryoblastic leukemia not having achieved remission   HCC
Acute megakaryoblastic leukemia with failed remission
Acute megakaryoblastic leukemia NOS

C94.21   Acute megakaryoblastic leukemia, in remission   HCC

C94.22   Acute megakaryoblastic leukemia, in relapse   HCC

✓5ᵗʰ C94.3   Mast cell leukemia
AHA: 2017,4Q,5

C94.30   Mast cell leukemia not having achieved remission   HCC
Mast cell leukemia with failed remission
Mast cell leukemia NOS

C94.31   Mast cell leukemia, in remission   HCC

C94.32   Mast cell leukemia, in relapse   HCC

✓5ᵗʰ C94.4   Acute panmyelosis with myelofibrosis
Acute myelofibrosis

EXCLUDES 1   *myelofibrosis NOS (D75.81)*
secondary myelofibrosis NOS (D75.81)

C94.40   Acute panmyelosis with myelofibrosis not having achieved remission   HCC
Acute myelofibrosis NOS
Acute panmyelosis with myelofibrosis with failed remission
Acute panmyelosis NOS

C94.41   Acute panmyelosis with myelofibrosis, in remission   HCC

C94.42   Acute panmyelosis with myelofibrosis, in relapse   HCC

C94.6   Myelodysplastic disease, not classified   HCC
Myeloproliferative disease, not classified

✓5ᵗʰ C94.8   Other specified leukemias
Aggressive NK-cell leukemia
Acute basophilic leukemia

C94.80   Other specified leukemias not having achieved remission   HCC
Other specified leukemia with failed remission
Other specified leukemias NOS

C94.81   Other specified leukemias, in remission   HCC

C94.82   Other specified leukemias, in relapse   HCC

✓4ᵗʰ C95   Leukemia of unspecified cell type
EXCLUDES 1   *personal history of leukemia (Z85.6)*

✓5ᵗʰ C95.0   Acute leukemia of unspecified cell type
Acute bilineal leukemia
Acute mixed lineage leukemia
Biphenotypic acute leukemia
Stem cell leukemia of unclear lineage

EXCLUDES 1   *acute exacerbation of unspecified chronic leukemia (C95.10)*

C95.00   Acute leukemia of unspecified cell type not having achieved remission   HCC
Acute leukemia of unspecified cell type with failed remission
Acute leukemia NOS

C95.01   Acute leukemia of unspecified cell type, in remission   HCC

C95.02   Acute leukemia of unspecified cell type, in relapse   HCC

✓5ᵗʰ C95.1   Chronic leukemia of unspecified cell type

C95.10   Chronic leukemia of unspecified cell type not having achieved remission   HCC
Chronic leukemia of unspecified cell type with failed remission
Chronic leukemia NOS

C95.11   Chronic leukemia of unspecified cell type, in remission   HCC

C95.12   Chronic leukemia of unspecified cell type, in relapse   HCC

✓5ᵗʰ C95.9   Leukemia, unspecified

C95.90   Leukemia, unspecified not having achieved remission   HCC ▽
Leukemia, unspecified with failed remission
Leukemia NOS

C95.91   Leukemia, unspecified, in remission   HCC ▽

C95.92   Leukemia, unspecified, in relapse   HCC ▽

✓4ᵗʰ C96   Other and unspecified malignant neoplasms of lymphoid, hematopoietic and related tissue
EXCLUDES 1   *personal history of other malignant neoplasms of lymphoid, hematopoietic and related tissues (Z85.79)*

C96.0   Multifocal and multisystemic (disseminated) Langerhans-cell histiocytosis   HCC
Histiocytosis X, multisystemic
Letterer-Siwe disease

EXCLUDES 1   *adult pulmonary Langerhans cell histiocytosis (J84.82)*
multifocal and unisystemic Langerhans-cell histiocytosis (C96.5)
unifocal Langerhans-cell histiocytosis (C96.6)

✓5ᵗʰ C96.2   Malignant mast cell neoplasm
EXCLUDES 1   *indolent mastocytosis (D47.02)*
mast cell leukemia (C94.30)
mastocytosis (congenital) (cutaneous) (Q82.2)

AHA: 2017,4Q,5
DEF: Mast cell: Type of white blood cell found in the loose connective tissue of blood vessels and bronchioles responsible for acute hypersensitivity reactions, including anaphylactic shock. The IgE receptors on these cells bind with allergens causing cell degranulation and diffuse, widespread histamine release that results in airway constriction and vasodilation with decreased systemic blood pressure.

C96.20   Malignant mast cell neoplasm, unspecified   HCC ▽

C96.21   Aggressive systemic mastocytosis   HCC

C96.22   Mast cell sarcoma   HCC

C96.29   Other malignant mast cell neoplasm   HCC

C96.4   Sarcoma of dendritic cells (accessory cells)   HCC
Follicular dendritic cell sarcoma
Interdigitating dendritic cell sarcoma
Langerhans cell sarcoma

C96.5   Multifocal and unisystemic Langerhans-cell histiocytosis   HCC
Hand-Schüller-Christian disease
Histiocytosis X, multifocal

EXCLUDES 1   *multifocal and multisystemic (disseminated) Langerhans-cell histiocytosis (C96.0)*
unifocal Langerhans-cell histiocytosis (C96.6)

C96.6   Unifocal Langerhans-cell histiocytosis   HCC
Eosinophilic granuloma
Histiocytosis X, unifocal
Histiocytosis X NOS
Langerhans-cell histiocytosis NOS

EXCLUDES 1   *multifocal and multisysemic (disseminated) Langerhans-cell histiocytosis (C96.0)*
multifocal and unisystemic Langerhans-cell histiocytosis (C96.5)

C96.A   Histiocytic sarcoma   HCC
Malignant histiocytosis

C96.Z   Other specified malignant neoplasms of lymphoid, hematopoietic and related tissue   HCC

C96.9   Malignant neoplasm of lymphoid, hematopoietic and related tissue, unspecified   HCC ▽

☑ Additional Character Req   ✓x7ᵗʰ Placeholder Alert   Manifestation   ▽ Unspecified   ▶◀ Revised Text   ● New Code   ▲ Revised Code Title

Chapter 2. Neoplasms

In situ neoplasms (D00-D09)

INCLUDES   Bowen's disease
erythroplasia
grade III intraepithelial neoplasia
Queyrat's erythroplasia

✓4ᵗʰ **D00   Carcinoma in situ of oral cavity, esophagus and stomach**
     EXCLUDES 1   *melanoma in situ (D03.-)*

✓5ᵗʰ **D00.0   Carcinoma in situ of lip, oral cavity and pharynx**
Use additional code to identify:
exposure to environmental tobacco smoke (Z77.22)
exposure to tobacco smoke in the perinatal period (P96.81)
history of tobacco dependence (Z87.891)
occupational exposure to environmental tobacco smoke (Z57.31)
tobacco dependence (F17.-)
tobacco use (Z72.0)
     EXCLUDES 1   *carcinoma in situ of aryepiglottic fold or interarytenoid fold, laryngeal aspect (D02.0)*
carcinoma in situ of epiglottis NOS (D02.0)
carcinoma in situ of epiglottis suprahyoid portion (D02.0)
carcinoma in situ of skin of lip (D03.0, D04.0)

     D00.00   Carcinoma in situ of oral cavity, unspecified site ▽
     D00.01   Carcinoma in situ of labial mucosa and vermilion border
     D00.02   Carcinoma in situ of buccal mucosa
     D00.03   Carcinoma in situ of gingiva and edentulous alveolar ridge
     D00.04   Carcinoma in situ of soft palate
     D00.05   Carcinoma in situ of hard palate
     D00.06   Carcinoma in situ of floor of mouth
     D00.07   Carcinoma in situ of tongue
     D00.08   Carcinoma in situ of pharynx
Carcinoma in situ of aryepiglottic fold NOS
Carcinoma in situ of hypopharyngeal aspect of aryepiglottic fold
Carcinoma in situ of marginal zone of aryepiglottic fold

     D00.1   Carcinoma in situ of esophagus
     D00.2   Carcinoma in situ of stomach

✓4ᵗʰ **D01   Carcinoma in situ of other and unspecified digestive organs**
     EXCLUDES 1   *melanoma in situ (D03.-)*

     D01.0   Carcinoma in situ of colon
     EXCLUDES 1   *carcinoma in situ of rectosigmoid junction (D01.1)*
     D01.1   Carcinoma in situ of rectosigmoid junction
     D01.2   Carcinoma in situ of rectum
     D01.3   Carcinoma in situ of anus and anal canal
Anal intraepithelial neoplasia III [AIN III]
Severe dysplasia of anus
     EXCLUDES 1   *anal intraepithelial neoplasia I and II [AIN I and AIN II] (K62.82)*
carcinoma in situ of anal margin (D04.5)
carcinoma in situ of anal skin (D04.5)
carcinoma in situ of perianal skin (D04.5)

✓5ᵗʰ **D01.4   Carcinoma in situ of other and unspecified parts of intestine**
     EXCLUDES 1   *carcinoma in situ of ampulla of Vater (D01.5)*
     D01.40   Carcinoma in situ of unspecified part of intestine ▽
     D01.49   Carcinoma in situ of other parts of intestine
     D01.5   Carcinoma in situ of liver, gallbladder and bile ducts
Carcinoma in situ of ampulla of Vater
     D01.7   Carcinoma in situ of other specified digestive organs
Carcinoma in situ of pancreas
     D01.9   Carcinoma in situ of digestive organ, unspecified ▽

✓4ᵗʰ **D02   Carcinoma in situ of middle ear and respiratory system**
Use additional code to identify:
exposure to environmental tobacco smoke (Z77.22)
exposure to tobacco smoke in the perinatal period (P96.81)
history of tobacco dependence (Z87.891)
occupational exposure to environmental tobacco smoke (Z57.31)
tobacco dependence (F17.-)
tobacco use (Z72.0)
     EXCLUDES 1   *melanoma in situ (D03.-)*

     D02.0   Carcinoma in situ of larynx
Carcinoma in situ of aryepiglottic fold or interarytenoid fold, laryngeal aspect
Carcinoma in situ of epiglottis (suprahyoid portion)
     EXCLUDES 1   *carcinoma in situ of aryepiglottic fold or interarytenoid fold NOS (D00.08)*
carcinoma in situ of hypopharyngeal aspect (D00.08)
carcinoma in situ of marginal zone (D00.08)

     D02.1   Carcinoma in situ of trachea
✓5ᵗʰ **D02.2   Carcinoma in situ of bronchus and lung**
     D02.20   Carcinoma in situ of unspecified bronchus and lung ▽
     D02.21   Carcinoma in situ of right bronchus and lung
     D02.22   Carcinoma in situ of left bronchus and lung
     D02.3   Carcinoma in situ of other parts of respiratory system
Carcinoma in situ of accessory sinuses
Carcinoma in situ of middle ear
Carcinoma in situ of nasal cavities
     EXCLUDES 1   *carcinoma in situ of ear (external) (skin) (D04.2-)*
carcinoma in situ of nose NOS (D09.8)
carcinoma in situ of skin of nose (D04.3)

     D02.4   Carcinoma in situ of respiratory system, unspecified ▽

✓4ᵗʰ **D03   Melanoma in situ**
     D03.0   Melanoma in situ of lip   HCC
✓5ᵗʰ **D03.1   Melanoma in situ of eyelid, including canthus**
     D03.10   Melanoma in situ of unspecified eyelid, including canthus   HCC ▽
     ✓6ᵗʰ **D03.11   Melanoma in situ of right eyelid, including canthus**
       D03.111   Melanoma in situ of right upper eyelid, including canthus
       D03.112   Melanoma in situ of right lower eyelid, including canthus
     ✓6ᵗʰ **D03.12   Melanoma in situ of left eyelid, including canthus**
       D03.121   Melanoma in situ of left upper eyelid, including canthus
       D03.122   Melanoma in situ of left lower eyelid, including canthus

✓5ᵗʰ **D03.2   Melanoma in situ of ear and external auricular canal**
     D03.20   Melanoma in situ of unspecified ear and external auricular canal   HCC ▽
     D03.21   Melanoma in situ of right ear and external auricular canal   HCC
     D03.22   Melanoma in situ of left ear and external auricular canal   HCC

✓5ᵗʰ **D03.3   Melanoma in situ of other and unspecified parts of face**
     D03.30   Melanoma in situ of unspecified part of face   HCC ▽
     D03.39   Melanoma in situ of other parts of face   HCC
     D03.4   Melanoma in situ of scalp and neck   HCC
✓5ᵗʰ **D03.5   Melanoma in situ of trunk**
     D03.51   Melanoma in situ of anal skin   HCC
Melanoma in situ of anal margin
Melanoma in situ of perianal skin
     D03.52   Melanoma in situ of breast (skin) (soft tissue)   HCC
     D03.59   Melanoma in situ of other part of trunk   HCC
✓5ᵗʰ **D03.6   Melanoma in situ of upper limb, including shoulder**
     D03.60   Melanoma in situ of unspecified upper limb, including shoulder   HCC ▽
     D03.61   Melanoma in situ of right upper limb, including shoulder   HCC
     D03.62   Melanoma in situ of left upper limb, including shoulder   HCC
✓5ᵗʰ **D03.7   Melanoma in situ of lower limb, including hip**
     D03.70   Melanoma in situ of unspecified lower limb, including hip   HCC

Chapter 2. Neoplasms

D03.71   Melanoma in situ of right lower limb, including hip   HCC

D03.72   Melanoma in situ of left lower limb, including hip   HCC

D03.8   **Melanoma in situ of other sites**   HCC
Melanoma in situ of scrotum
EXCLUDES 1   carcinoma in situ of scrotum (D07.61)

D03.9   **Melanoma in situ, unspecified**   HCC ▽

√4ᵗʰ **D04 Carcinoma in situ of skin**
EXCLUDES 1   erythroplasia of Queyrat (penis) NOS (D07.4)
melanoma in situ (D03.-)

D04.0   **Carcinoma in situ of skin of lip**
EXCLUDES 1   carcinoma in situ of vermilion border of lip (D00.01)

√5ᵗʰ D04.1   **Carcinoma in situ of skin of eyelid, including canthus**

D04.10   Carcinoma in situ of skin of unspecified eyelid, including canthus ▽

√6ᵗʰ D04.11   Carcinoma in situ of skin of right eyelid, including canthus

•   D04.111   Carcinoma in situ of skin of right upper eyelid, including canthus

•   D04.112   Carcinoma in situ of skin of right lower eyelid, including canthus

√6ᵗʰ D04.12   Carcinoma in situ of skin of left eyelid, including canthus

•   D04.121   Carcinoma in situ of skin of left upper eyelid, including canthus

•   D04.122   Carcinoma in situ of skin of left lower eyelid, including canthus

√5ᵗʰ D04.2   **Carcinoma in situ of skin of ear and external auricular canal**

D04.20   Carcinoma in situ of skin of unspecified ear and external auricular canal ▽

D04.21   Carcinoma in situ of skin of right ear and external auricular canal

D04.22   Carcinoma in situ of skin of left ear and external auricular canal

√5ᵗʰ D04.3   **Carcinoma in situ of skin of other and unspecified parts of face**

D04.30   Carcinoma in situ of skin of unspecified part of face ▽

D04.39   Carcinoma in situ of skin of other parts of face

D04.4   **Carcinoma in situ of skin of scalp and neck**

D04.5   **Carcinoma in situ of skin of trunk**
Carcinoma in situ of anal margin
Carcinoma in situ of anal skin
Carcinoma in situ of perianal skin
Carcinoma in situ of skin of breast
EXCLUDES 1   carcinoma in situ of anus NOS (D01.3)
carcinoma in situ of scrotum (D07.61)
carcinoma in situ of skin of genital organs (D07.-)

√5ᵗʰ D04.6   **Carcinoma in situ of skin of upper limb, including shoulder**

D04.60   Carcinoma in situ of skin of unspecified upper limb, including shoulder ▽

D04.61   Carcinoma in situ of skin of right upper limb, including shoulder

D04.62   Carcinoma in situ of skin of left upper limb, including shoulder

√5ᵗʰ D04.7   **Carcinoma in situ of skin of lower limb, including hip**

D04.70   Carcinoma in situ of skin of unspecified lower limb, including hip ▽

D04.71   Carcinoma in situ of skin of right lower limb, including hip

D04.72   Carcinoma in situ of skin of left lower limb, including hip

D04.8   **Carcinoma in situ of skin of other sites**

D04.9   **Carcinoma in situ of skin, unspecified** ▽

√4ᵗʰ **D05 Carcinoma in situ of breast**
EXCLUDES 1   carcinoma in situ of skin of breast (D04.5)
melanoma in situ of breast (skin) (D03.5)
Paget's disease of breast or nipple (C50.-)

√5ᵗʰ D05.0   **Lobular carcinoma in situ of breast**

D05.00   Lobular carcinoma in situ of unspecified breast ▽

D05.01   Lobular carcinoma in situ of right breast

D05.02   Lobular carcinoma in situ of left breast

√5ᵗʰ D05.1   **Intraductal carcinoma in situ of breast**

D05.10   Intraductal carcinoma in situ of unspecified breast ▽

D05.11   Intraductal carcinoma in situ of right breast

D05.12   Intraductal carcinoma in situ of left breast

√5ᵗʰ D05.8   **Other specified type of carcinoma in situ of breast**

D05.80   Other specified type of carcinoma in situ of unspecified breast ▽

D05.81   Other specified type of carcinoma in situ of right breast

D05.82   Other specified type of carcinoma in situ of left breast

√5ᵗʰ D05.9   **Unspecified type of carcinoma in situ of breast**

D05.90   Unspecified type of carcinoma in situ of unspecified breast ▽

D05.91   Unspecified type of carcinoma in situ of right breast ▽

D05.92   Unspecified type of carcinoma in situ of left breast ▽

√4ᵗʰ **D06 Carcinoma in situ of cervix uteri**
INCLUDES   cervical adenocarcinoma in situ
cervical intraepithelial glandular neoplasia
cervical intraepithelial neoplasia III [CIN III]
severe dysplasia of cervix uteri
EXCLUDES 1   cervical intraepithelial neoplasia II [CIN II] (N87.1)
cytologic evidence of malignancy of cervix without histologic confirmation (R87.614)
high grade squamous intraepithelial lesion (HGSIL) of cervix (R87.613)
melanoma in situ of cervix (D03.5)
moderate cervical dysplasia (N87.1)

D06.0   **Carcinoma in situ of endocervix**   ♀

D06.1   **Carcinoma in situ of exocervix**   ♀

D06.7   **Carcinoma in situ of other parts of cervix**   ♀

D06.9   **Carcinoma in situ of cervix, unspecified**   ♀ ▽

√4ᵗʰ **D07 Carcinoma in situ of other and unspecified genital organs**
EXCLUDES 1   melanoma in situ of trunk (D03.5)

D07.0   **Carcinoma in situ of endometrium**   ♀

D07.1   **Carcinoma in situ of vulva**   ♀
Severe dysplasia of vulva
Vulvar intraepithelial neoplasia III [VIN III]
EXCLUDES 1   moderate dysplasia of vulva (N90.1)
vulvar intraepithelial neoplasia II [VIN II] (N90.1)

D07.2   **Carcinoma in situ of vagina**   ♀
Severe dysplasia of vagina
Vaginal intraepithelial neoplasia III [VAIN III]
EXCLUDES 1   moderate dysplasia of vagina (N89.1)
vaginal intraepithelial neoplasia II [VIN II] (N89.1)

√5ᵗʰ D07.3   **Carcinoma in situ of other and unspecified female genital organs**

D07.30   Carcinoma in situ of unspecified female genital organs   ♀ ▽

D07.39   Carcinoma in situ of other female genital organs   ♀

D07.4   **Carcinoma in situ of penis**   ♂
Erythroplasia of Queyrat NOS

D07.5   **Carcinoma in situ of prostate**   ♂
Prostatic intraepithelial neoplasia III (PIN III)
Severe dysplasia of prostate
EXCLUDES 1   dysplasia (mild) (moderate) of prostate (N42.3-)
prostatic intraepithelial neoplasia II [PIN II] (N42.3-)

√5ᵗʰ D07.6   **Carcinoma in situ of other and unspecified male genital organs**

D07.60   Carcinoma in situ of unspecified male genital organs   ♂ ▽

D07.61   Carcinoma in situ of scrotum   ♂

D07.69   Carcinoma in situ of other male genital organs   ♂

√4ᵗʰ **D09 Carcinoma in situ of other and unspecified sites**
EXCLUDES 1   melanoma in situ (D03.-)

D09.0   **Carcinoma in situ of bladder**

√5ᵗʰ D09.1   **Carcinoma in situ of other and unspecified urinary organs**

D09.10   Carcinoma in situ of unspecified urinary organ ▽

D09.19   Carcinoma in situ of other urinary organs

√5ᵗʰ D09.2   **Carcinoma in situ of eye**
EXCLUDES 1   carcinoma in situ of skin of eyelid (D04.1-)

D09.20   Carcinoma in situ of unspecified eye ▽

D09.21   Carcinoma in situ of right eye

D09.22   Carcinoma in situ of left eye

D09.3   Carcinoma in situ of thyroid and other endocrine glands
> *EXCLUDES 1*   carcinoma in situ of endocrine pancreas (D01.7)
> carcinoma in situ of ovary (D07.39)
> carcinoma in situ of testis (D07.69)

D09.8   Carcinoma in situ of other specified sites

D09.9   Carcinoma in situ, unspecified   ▽

Benign neoplasms, except benign neuroendocrine tumors (D10-D36)

✓4ᵗʰ D10   **Benign neoplasm of mouth and pharynx**

D10.0   Benign neoplasm of lip
> Benign neoplasm of lip (frenulum) (inner aspect) (mucosa) (vermilion border)
> *EXCLUDES 1*   benign neoplasm of skin of lip (D22.0, D23.0)

D10.1   Benign neoplasm of tongue
> Benign neoplasm of lingual tonsil

D10.2   Benign neoplasm of floor of mouth

✓5ᵗʰ D10.3   Benign neoplasm of other and unspecified parts of mouth

     D10.30   Benign neoplasm of unspecified part of mouth   ▽

     D10.39   Benign neoplasm of other parts of mouth
> Benign neoplasm of minor salivary gland NOS
> *EXCLUDES 1*   benign odontogenic neoplasms (D16.4-D16.5)
> benign neoplasm of mucosa of lip (D10.0)
> benign neoplasm of nasopharyngeal surface of soft palate (D10.6)

D10.4   Benign neoplasm of tonsil
> Benign neoplasm of tonsil (faucial) (palatine)
> *EXCLUDES 1*   benign neoplasm of lingual tonsil (D10.1)
> benign neoplasm of pharyngeal tonsil (D10.6)
> benign neoplasm of tonsillar fossa (D10.5)
> benign neoplasm of tonsillar pillars (D10.5)

D10.5   Benign neoplasm of other parts of oropharynx
> Benign neoplasm of epiglottis, anterior aspect
> Benign neoplasm of tonsillar fossa
> Benign neoplasm of tonsillar pillars
> Benign neoplasm of vallecula
> *EXCLUDES 1*   benign neoplasm of epiglottis NOS (D14.1)
> benign neoplasm of epiglottis, suprahyoid portion (D14.1)

D10.6   Benign neoplasm of nasopharynx
> Benign neoplasm of pharyngeal tonsil
> Benign neoplasm of posterior margin of septum and choanae

D10.7   Benign neoplasm of hypopharynx

D10.9   Benign neoplasm of pharynx, unspecified   ▽

✓4ᵗʰ D11   **Benign neoplasm of major salivary glands**
> *EXCLUDES 1*   benign neoplasms of specified minor salivary glands which are classified according to their anatomical location
> benign neoplasms of minor salivary glands NOS (D10.39)

D11.0   Benign neoplasm of parotid gland

D11.7   Benign neoplasm of other major salivary glands
> Benign neoplasm of sublingual salivary gland
> Benign neoplasm of submandibular salivary gland

D11.9   Benign neoplasm of major salivary gland, unspecified   ▽

✓4ᵗʰ D12   **Benign neoplasm of colon, rectum, anus and anal canal**
> *EXCLUDES 1*   benign carcinoid tumors of the large intestine, and rectum (D3A.02-)
> AHA: 2018,2Q,14; 2017,1Q,15; 2015,2Q,14

D12.0   Benign neoplasm of cecum
> Benign neoplasm of ileocecal valve

D12.1   Benign neoplasm of appendix
> *EXCLUDES 1*   benign carcinoid tumor of the appendix (D3A.020)

D12.2   Benign neoplasm of ascending colon

D12.3   Benign neoplasm of transverse colon
> Benign neoplasm of hepatic flexure
> Benign neoplasm of splenic flexure
> AHA: 2017,1Q,16

D12.4   Benign neoplasm of descending colon

D12.5   Benign neoplasm of sigmoid colon

D12.6   Benign neoplasm of colon, unspecified   ▽
> Adenomatosis of colon
> Benign neoplasm of large intestine NOS
> Polyposis (hereditary) of colon
> *EXCLUDES 1*   inflammatory polyp of colon (K51.4-)
> polyp of colon NOS (K63.5)

D12.7   Benign neoplasm of rectosigmoid junction

D12.8   Benign neoplasm of rectum
> *EXCLUDES 1*   benign carcinoid tumor of the rectum (D3A.026)
> AHA: 2018,1Q,6

D12.9   Benign neoplasm of anus and anal canal
> Benign neoplasm of anus NOS
> *EXCLUDES 1*   benign neoplasm of anal margin (D22.5, D23.5)
> benign neoplasm of anal skin (D22.5, D23.5)
> benign neoplasm of perianal skin (D22.5, D23.5)

✓4ᵗʰ D13   **Benign neoplasm of other and ill-defined parts of digestive system**
> *EXCLUDES 1*   benign stromal tumors of digestive system (D21.4)

D13.0   Benign neoplasm of esophagus

D13.1   Benign neoplasm of stomach
> *EXCLUDES 1*   benign carcinoid tumor of the stomach (D3A.092)

D13.2   Benign neoplasm of duodenum
> *EXCLUDES 1*   benign carcinoid tumor of the duodenum (D3A.010)

✓5ᵗʰ D13.3   Benign neoplasm of other and unspecified parts of small intestine
> *EXCLUDES 1*   benign carcinoid tumors of the small intestine (D3A.01-)
> benign neoplasm of ileocecal valve (D12.0)

     D13.30   Benign neoplasm of unspecified part of small intestine   ▽

     D13.39   Benign neoplasm of other parts of small intestine

D13.4   Benign neoplasm of liver
> Benign neoplasm of intrahepatic bile ducts

D13.5   Benign neoplasm of extrahepatic bile ducts

D13.6   Benign neoplasm of pancreas
> *EXCLUDES 1*   benign neoplasm of endocrine pancreas (D13.7)

D13.7   Benign neoplasm of endocrine pancreas
> Benign neoplasm of islets of Langerhans
> Islet cell tumor
> Use additional code to identify any functional activity

D13.9   Benign neoplasm of ill-defined sites within the digestive system
> Benign neoplasm of digestive system NOS
> Benign neoplasm of intestine NOS
> Benign neoplasm of spleen

✓4ᵗʰ D14   **Benign neoplasm of middle ear and respiratory system**

D14.0   Benign neoplasm of middle ear, nasal cavity and accessory sinuses
> Benign neoplasm of cartilage of nose
> *EXCLUDES 1*   benign neoplasm of auricular canal (external) (D22.2-, D23.2-)
> benign neoplasm of bone of ear (D16.4)
> benign neoplasm of bone of nose (D16.4)
> benign neoplasm of cartilage of ear (D21.0)
> benign neoplasm of ear (external)(skin) (D22.2-, D23.2-)
> benign neoplasm of nose NOS (D36.7)
> benign neoplasm of skin of nose (D22.39, D23.39)
> benign neoplasm of olfactory bulb (D33.3)
> benign neoplasm of posterior margin of septum and choanae (D10.6)
> polyp of accessory sinus (J33.8)
> polyp of ear (middle) (H74.4)
> polyp of nasal (cavity) (J33.-)

D14.1   Benign neoplasm of larynx
> Adenomatous polyp of larynx
> Benign neoplasm of epiglottis (suprahyoid portion)
> *EXCLUDES 1*   benign neoplasm of epiglottis, anterior aspect (D10.5)
> polyp (nonadenomatous) of vocal cord or larynx (J38.1)

D14.2   Benign neoplasm of trachea

✓5ᵗʰ D14.3   Benign neoplasm of bronchus and lung
> *EXCLUDES 1*   benign carcinoid tumor of the bronchus and lung (D3A.090)

     D14.30   Benign neoplasm of unspecified bronchus and lung   ▽

D14.31   Benign neoplasm of **right** bronchus and lung

D14.32   Benign neoplasm of **left** bronchus and lung

D14.4   Benign neoplasm of **respiratory system, unspecified**   ▽

✓4ᵗʰ **D15**   Benign neoplasm of other and unspecified **intrathoracic organs**

     EXCLUDES 1   *benign neoplasm of mesothelial tissue (D19.-)*

D15.0   Benign neoplasm of **thymus**

     EXCLUDES 1   *benign carcinoid tumor of the thymus (D3A.091)*

D15.1   Benign neoplasm of **heart**

     EXCLUDES 1   *benign neoplasm of great vessels (D21.3)*

D15.2   Benign neoplasm of **mediastinum**

D15.7   Benign neoplasm of other specified intrathoracic organs

D15.9   Benign neoplasm of intrathoracic organ, unspecified   ▽

✓4ᵗʰ **D16**   Benign neoplasm of **bone and articular cartilage**

     EXCLUDES 1   *benign neoplasm of connective tissue of ear (D21.0)*
                     benign neoplasm of connective tissue of eyelid (D21.0)
                     benign neoplasm of connective tissue of larynx (D14.1)
                     benign neoplasm of connective tissue of nose (D14.0)
                     benign neoplasm of synovia (D21.-)

✓5ᵗʰ **D16.0**   Benign neoplasm of **scapula and long bones of upper limb**

     D16.00   Benign neoplasm of scapula and long bones of unspecified upper limb   ▽

     D16.01   Benign neoplasm of scapula and long bones of **right** upper limb

     D16.02   Benign neoplasm of scapula and long bones of **left** upper limb

✓5ᵗʰ **D16.1**   Benign neoplasm of **short bones of upper limb**

     D16.10   Benign neoplasm of short bones of unspecified upper limb   ▽

     D16.11   Benign neoplasm of short bones of **right** upper limb

     D16.12   Benign neoplasm of short bones of **left** upper limb

✓5ᵗʰ **D16.2**   Benign neoplasm of **long bones of lower limb**

     D16.20   Benign neoplasm of long bones of unspecified lower limb   ▽

     D16.21   Benign neoplasm of long bones of **right** lower limb

     D16.22   Benign neoplasm of long bones of **left** lower limb

✓5ᵗʰ **D16.3**   Benign neoplasm of **short bones of lower limb**

     D16.30   Benign neoplasm of short bones of unspecified lower limb   ▽

     D16.31   Benign neoplasm of short bones of **right** lower limb

     D16.32   Benign neoplasm of short bones of **left** lower limb

D16.4   Benign neoplasm of bones of **skull and face**

     Benign neoplasm of maxilla (superior)
     Benign neoplasm of orbital bone
     Keratocyst of maxilla
     Keratocystic odontogenic tumor of maxilla

     EXCLUDES 2   *benign neoplasm of lower jaw bone (D16.5)*

D16.5   Benign neoplasm of **lower jaw bone**

     Keratocyst of mandible
     Keratocystic odontogenic tumor of mandible

D16.6   Benign neoplasm of **vertebral column**

     EXCLUDES 1   *benign neoplasm of sacrum and coccyx (D16.8)*

D16.7   Benign neoplasm of **ribs, sternum and clavicle**

D16.8   Benign neoplasm of **pelvic bones, sacrum and coccyx**

D16.9   Benign neoplasm of bone and articular cartilage, unspecified   ▽

✓4ᵗʰ **D17**   Benign **lipomatous neoplasm**

D17.0   Benign lipomatous neoplasm of **skin and subcutaneous tissue of head, face and neck**

D17.1   Benign lipomatous neoplasm of **skin and subcutaneous tissue of trunk**

✓5ᵗʰ **D17.2**   Benign lipomatous neoplasm of **skin and subcutaneous tissue of limb**

     D17.20   Benign lipomatous neoplasm of skin and subcutaneous tissue of unspecified limb   ▽

     D17.21   Benign lipomatous neoplasm of skin and subcutaneous tissue of **right arm**

     D17.22   Benign lipomatous neoplasm of skin and subcutaneous tissue of **left arm**

     D17.23   Benign lipomatous neoplasm of skin and subcutaneous tissue of **right leg**

     D17.24   Benign lipomatous neoplasm of skin and subcutaneous tissue of **left leg**

✓5ᵗʰ **D17.3**   Benign lipomatous neoplasm of **skin and subcutaneous tissue** of other and unspecified sites

     D17.30   Benign lipomatous neoplasm of skin and subcutaneous tissue of unspecified sites   ▽

     D17.39   Benign lipomatous neoplasm of skin and subcutaneous tissue of other sites

D17.4   Benign lipomatous neoplasm of **intrathoracic organs**

D17.5   Benign lipomatous neoplasm of **intra-abdominal organs**

     EXCLUDES 1   *benign lipomatous neoplasm of peritoneum and retroperitoneum (D17.79)*

D17.6   Benign lipomatous neoplasm of **spermatic cord**   ♂

✓5ᵗʰ **D17.7**   Benign lipomatous neoplasm of **other sites**

     D17.71   Benign lipomatous neoplasm of **kidney**

     D17.72   Benign lipomatous neoplasm of other **genitourinary organ**

     D17.79   Benign lipomatous neoplasm of other sites
            Benign lipomatous neoplasm of peritoneum
            Benign lipomatous neoplasm of retroperitoneum

D17.9   Benign lipomatous neoplasm, unspecified   ▽
     Lipoma NOS

✓4ᵗʰ **D18**   **Hemangioma and lymphangioma, any site**

     EXCLUDES 1   *benign neoplasm of glomus jugulare (D35.6)*
                     blue or pigmented nevus (D22.-)
                     nevus NOS (D22.-)
                     vascular nevus (Q82.5)

✓5ᵗʰ **D18.0**   **Hemangioma**

     Angioma NOS
     Cavernous nevus
     DEF: Common benign tumor usually occurring in infancy that is composed of newly formed blood vessels due to malformation of the angioblastic tissue.

     D18.00   Hemangioma unspecified site   ▽

     D18.01   Hemangioma of **skin and subcutaneous tissue**

     D18.02   Hemangioma of **intracranial structures**   HCC

     D18.03   Hemangioma of **intra-abdominal structures**

     D18.09   Hemangioma of other sites

D18.1   Lymphangioma, any site
     AHA: 2018,2Q,13

✓4ᵗʰ **D19**   Benign neoplasm of **mesothelial tissue**

D19.0   Benign neoplasm of mesothelial tissue of **pleura**

D19.1   Benign neoplasm of mesothelial tissue of **peritoneum**

D19.7   Benign neoplasm of mesothelial tissue of other sites

D19.9   Benign neoplasm of mesothelial tissue, unspecified   ▽
     Benign mesothelioma NOS

✓4ᵗʰ **D20**   Benign neoplasm of soft tissue of **retroperitoneum and peritoneum**

     EXCLUDES 1   *benign lipomatous neoplasm of peritoneum and retroperitoneum (D17.79)*
                     benign neoplasm of mesothelial tissue (D19.-)

D20.0   Benign neoplasm of soft tissue of **retroperitoneum**

D20.1   Benign neoplasm of soft tissue of **peritoneum**

☑ Additional Character Req   ✓x7ᵗʰ Placeholder Alert   Manifestation   ▽ Unspecified   ▶◀ Revised Text   ● New Code   ▲ Revised Code Title

ICD-10-CM 2019   489

D14.31–D20.1

✓4ᵗʰ **D21 Other benign neoplasms of connective and other soft tissue**

INCLUDES   benign neoplasm of blood vessel
benign neoplasm of bursa
benign neoplasm of cartilage
benign neoplasm of fascia
benign neoplasm of fat
benign neoplasm of ligament, except uterine
benign neoplasm of lymphatic channel
benign neoplasm of muscle
benign neoplasm of synovia
benign neoplasm of tendon (sheath)
benign stromal tumors

EXCLUDES 1   benign neoplasm of articular cartilage (D16.-)
benign neoplasm of cartilage of larynx (D14.1)
benign neoplasm of cartilage of nose (D14.0)
benign neoplasm of connective tissue of breast (D24.-)
benign neoplasm of peripheral nerves and autonomic nervous
system (D36.1-)
benign neoplasm of peritoneum (D20.1)
benign neoplasm of retroperitoneum (D20.0)
benign neoplasm of uterine ligament, any (D28.2)
benign neoplasm of vascular tissue (D18.-)
hemangioma (D18.0-)
lipomatous neoplasm (D17.-)
lymphangioma (D18.1)
uterine leiomyoma (D25.-)

**D21.0 Benign neoplasm of connective and other soft tissue of head,
face and neck**
Benign neoplasm of connective tissue of ear
Benign neoplasm of connective tissue of eyelid
EXCLUDES 1   benign neoplasm of connective tissue of orbit
(D31.6-)

✓5ᵗʰ **D21.1 Benign neoplasm of connective and other soft tissue of upper
limb, including shoulder**
D21.10   Benign neoplasm of connective and other   ▽
soft tissue of unspecified upper limb,
including shoulder
D21.11   Benign neoplasm of connective and other soft
tissue of right upper limb, including shoulder
D21.12   Benign neoplasm of connective and other soft
tissue of left upper limb, including shoulder

✓5ᵗʰ **D21.2 Benign neoplasm of connective and other soft tissue of lower
limb, including hip**
D21.20   Benign neoplasm of connective and other   ▽
soft tissue of unspecified lower limb,
including hip
D21.21   Benign neoplasm of connective and other soft
tissue of right lower limb, including hip
D21.22   Benign neoplasm of connective and other soft
tissue of left lower limb, including hip

**D21.3 Benign neoplasm of connective and other soft tissue of
thorax**
Benign neoplasm of axilla
Benign neoplasm of diaphragm
Benign neoplasm of great vessels
EXCLUDES 1   benign neoplasm of heart (D15.1)
benign neoplasm of mediastinum (D15.2)
benign neoplasm of thymus (D15.0)

**D21.4 Benign neoplasm of connective and other soft tissue of
abdomen**
Benign stromal tumors of abdomen

D21.5 Benign neoplasm of connective and other soft tissue of pelvis
EXCLUDES 1   benign neoplasm of any uterine ligament (D28.2)
uterine leiomyoma (D25.-)

**D21.6 Benign neoplasm of connective and other soft   ▽
tissue of trunk, unspecified**
Benign neoplasm of back NOS

**D21.9 Benign neoplasm of connective and other soft   ▽
tissue, unspecified**

✓4ᵗʰ **D22 Melanocytic nevi**

INCLUDES   atypical nevus
blue hairy pigmented nevus
nevus NOS

D22.0 Melanocytic nevi of lip

✓5ᵗʰ **D22.1 Melanocytic nevi of eyelid, including canthus**
D22.10   Melanocytic nevi of unspecified eyelid,   ▽
including canthus

✓6ᵗʰ **D22.11 Melanocytic nevi of right eyelid, including canthus**
D22.111   Melanocytic nevi of right upper eyelid,
including canthus
D22.112   Melanocytic nevi of right lower eyelid,
including canthus

✓6ᵗʰ **D22.12 Melanocytic nevi of left eyelid, including canthus**
D22.121   Melanocytic nevi of left upper eyelid,
including canthus
D22.122   Melanocytic nevi of left lower eyelid,
including canthus

✓5ᵗʰ **D22.2 Melanocytic nevi of ear and external auricular canal**
D22.20   Melanocytic nevi of unspecified ear and   ▽
external auricular canal
D22.21   Melanocytic nevi of right ear and external auricular
canal
D22.22   Melanocytic nevi of left ear and external auricular
canal

✓5ᵗʰ **D22.3 Melanocytic nevi of other and unspecified parts of face**
D22.30   Melanocytic nevi of unspecified part of   ▽
face
D22.39   Melanocytic nevi of other parts of face

D22.4 Melanocytic nevi of scalp and neck

D22.5 Melanocytic nevi of trunk
Melanocytic nevi of anal margin
Melanocytic nevi of anal skin
Melanocytic nevi of perianal skin
Melanocytic nevi of skin of breast

✓5ᵗʰ **D22.6 Melanocytic nevi of upper limb, including shoulder**
D22.60   Melanocytic nevi of unspecified upper   ▽
limb, including shoulder
D22.61   Melanocytic nevi of right upper limb, including
shoulder
D22.62   Melanocytic nevi of left upper limb, including
shoulder

✓5ᵗʰ **D22.7 Melanocytic nevi of lower limb, including hip**
D22.70   Melanocytic nevi of unspecified lower   ▽
limb, including hip
D22.71   Melanocytic nevi of right lower limb, including hip
D22.72   Melanocytic nevi of left lower limb, including hip

D22.9 Melanocytic nevi, unspecified   ▽

✓4ᵗʰ **D23 Other benign neoplasms of skin**

INCLUDES   benign neoplasm of hair follicles
benign neoplasm of sebaceous glands
benign neoplasm of sweat glands
EXCLUDES 1   benign lipomatous neoplasms of skin (D17.0-D17.3)
melanocytic nevi (D22.-)

D23.0 Other benign neoplasm of skin of lip
EXCLUDES 1   benign neoplasm of vermilion border of lip (D10.0)

✓5ᵗʰ **D23.1 Other benign neoplasm of skin of eyelid, including canthus**
D23.10   Other benign neoplasm of skin of   ▽
unspecified eyelid, including canthus
✓6ᵗʰ D23.11   Other benign neoplasm of skin of right eyelid,
including canthus
D23.111   Other benign neoplasm of skin of right
upper eyelid, including canthus
D23.112   Other benign neoplasm of skin of right
lower eyelid, including canthus
✓6ᵗʰ D23.12   Other benign neoplasm of skin of left eyelid,
including canthus
D23.121   Other benign neoplasm of skin of left
upper eyelid, including canthus
D23.122   Other benign neoplasm of skin of left
lower eyelid, including canthus

✓5ᵗʰ **D23.2 Other benign neoplasm of skin of ear and external auricular
canal**
D23.20   Other benign neoplasm of skin of   ▽
unspecified ear and external auricular
canal
D23.21   Other benign neoplasm of skin of right ear and
external auricular canal
D23.22   Other benign neoplasm of skin of left ear and
external auricular canal

✓5ᵗʰ **D23.3 Other benign neoplasm of skin of other and unspecified parts
of face**
D23.30   Other benign neoplasm of skin of   ▽
unspecified part of face
D23.39   Other benign neoplasm of skin of other parts of
face

D23.4   **Other benign neoplasm of skin of** scalp and neck

D23.5   **Other benign neoplasm of skin of** trunk

     Other benign neoplasm of anal margin

     Other benign neoplasm of anal skin

     Other benign neoplasm of perianal skin

     Other benign neoplasm of skin of breast

     EXCLUDES 1   *benign neoplasm of anus NOS (D12.9)*

✓5ᵗʰ D23.6   **Other benign neoplasm of skin of** upper limb, including shoulder

     D23.60   **Other benign neoplasm of skin of** unspecified upper limb, including shoulder   ▽

     D23.61   **Other benign neoplasm of skin of** right upper limb, including shoulder

     D23.62   **Other benign neoplasm of skin of** left upper limb, including shoulder

✓5ᵗʰ D23.7   **Other benign neoplasm of skin of** lower limb, including hip

     D23.70   **Other benign neoplasm of skin of** unspecified lower limb, including hip   ▽

     D23.71   **Other benign neoplasm of skin of** right lower limb, including hip

     D23.72   **Other benign neoplasm of skin of** left lower limb, including hip

D23.9   **Other benign neoplasm of skin,** unspecified   ▽

✓4ᵗʰ **D24**   **Benign neoplasm of** breast

     INCLUDES   benign neoplasm of connective tissue of breast

           benign neoplasm of soft parts of breast

           fibroadenoma of breast

     EXCLUDES 2   *adenofibrosis of breast (N60.2)*

           benign cyst of breast (N60.-)

           benign mammary dysplasia (N60.-)

           benign neoplasm of skin of breast (D22.5, D23.5)

           fibrocystic disease of breast (N60.-)

D24.1   **Benign neoplasm of** right **breast**

D24.2   **Benign neoplasm of** left **breast**

D24.9   **Benign neoplasm of unspecified breast**   ▽

✓4ᵗʰ **D25**   **Leiomyoma of uterus**

     INCLUDES   uterine fibroid

           uterine fibromyoma

           uterine myoma

Uterine Leiomyomas (Fibroids)

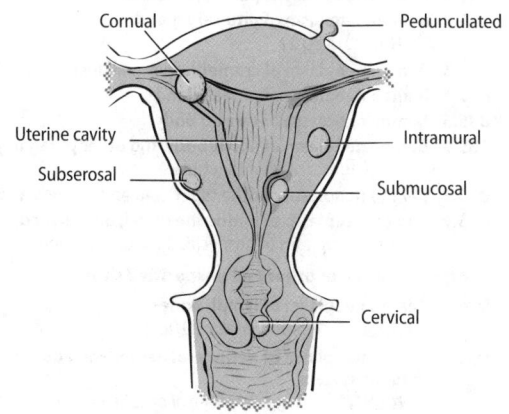

D25.0   **Submucous leiomyoma of uterus**   ♀

D25.1   **Intramural leiomyoma of uterus**   ♀

     Interstitial leiomyoma of uterus

D25.2   **Subserosal leiomyoma of uterus**   ♀

     Subperitoneal leiomyoma of uterus

D25.9   **Leiomyoma of uterus, unspecified**   ♀ ▽

✓4ᵗʰ **D26**   **Other benign neoplasms of** uterus

D26.0   **Other benign neoplasm of** cervix uteri   ♀

D26.1   **Other benign neoplasm of** corpus uteri   ♀

D26.7   **Other benign neoplasm of other** parts **of uterus**   ♀

D26.9   **Other benign neoplasm of uterus, unspecified**   ♀ ▽

✓4ᵗʰ **D27**   **Benign neoplasm of** ovary

     Use additional code to identify any functional activity

     EXCLUDES 2   *corpus albicans cyst (N83.2-)*

           corpus luteum cyst (N83.1-)

           endometrial cyst (N80.1)

           follicular (atretic) cyst (N83.0-)

           graafian follicle cyst (N83.0-)

           ovarian cyst NEC (N83.2-)

           ovarian retention cyst (N83.2-)

D27.0   **Benign neoplasm of** right **ovary**   ♀

D27.1   **Benign neoplasm of** left **ovary**   ♀

D27.9   **Benign neoplasm of unspecified ovary**   ♀ ▽

✓4ᵗʰ **D28**   **Benign neoplasm of other and unspecified** female genital organs

     INCLUDES   adenomatous polyp

           benign neoplasm of skin of female genital organs

           benign teratoma

     EXCLUDES 1   *epoophoron cyst (Q50.5)*

           fimbrial cyst (Q50.4)

           Gartner's duct cyst (Q52.4)

           parovarian cyst (Q50.5)

D28.0   **Benign neoplasm of** vulva   ♀

D28.1   **Benign neoplasm of** vagina   ♀

D28.2   **Benign neoplasm of** uterine tubes and ligaments   ♀

     Benign neoplasm of fallopian tube

     Benign neoplasm of uterine ligament (broad) (round)

D28.7   **Benign neoplasm of other specified female genital organs**   ♀

D28.9   **Benign neoplasm of female genital organ, unspecified**   ♀ ♀ ▽

✓4ᵗʰ **D29**   **Benign neoplasm of** male genital organs

     INCLUDES   benign neoplasm of skin of male genital organs

D29.0   **Benign neoplasm of** penis   ♂

D29.1   **Benign neoplasm of** prostate   ♂

     EXCLUDES 1   *enlarged prostate (N40.-)*

✓5ᵗʰ D29.2   **Benign neoplasm of** testis

     Use additional code to identify any functional activity

     D29.20   **Benign neoplasm of unspecified testis**   ♂ ▽

     D29.21   **Benign neoplasm of** right **testis**   ♂

     D29.22   **Benign neoplasm of** left **testis**   ♂

✓5ᵗʰ D29.3   **Benign neoplasm of** epididymis

     D29.30   **Benign neoplasm of unspecified epididymis**   ♂ ▽

     D29.31   **Benign neoplasm of** right **epididymis**   ♂

     D29.32   **Benign neoplasm of** left **epididymis**   ♂

D29.4   **Benign neoplasm of** scrotum   ♂

     Benign neoplasm of skin of scrotum

D29.8   **Benign neoplasm of other specified male genital organs**   ♂

     Benign neoplasm of seminal vesicle

     Benign neoplasm of spermatic cord

     Benign neoplasm of tunica vaginalis

D29.9   **Benign neoplasm of male genital organ, unspecified**   ♂ ▽

✓4ᵗʰ **D30**   **Benign neoplasm of** urinary organs

✓5ᵗʰ D30.0   **Benign neoplasm of** kidney

     EXCLUDES 1   *benign carcinoid tumor of the kidney (D3A.093)*

           benign neoplasm of renal calyces (D30.1-)

           benign neoplasm of renal pelvis (D30.1-)

     D30.00   **Benign neoplasm of unspecified kidney**   ▽

     D30.01   **Benign neoplasm of** right **kidney**

     D30.02   **Benign neoplasm of** left **kidney**

✓5ᵗʰ D30.1   **Benign neoplasm of** renal pelvis

     D30.10   **Benign neoplasm of unspecified renal pelvis**   ▽

     D30.11   **Benign neoplasm of** right **renal pelvis**

     D30.12   **Benign neoplasm of** left **renal pelvis**

✓5ᵗʰ D30.2   **Benign neoplasm of** ureter

     EXCLUDES 1   *benign neoplasm of ureteric orifice of bladder (D30.3)*

     D30.20   **Benign neoplasm of unspecified ureter**   ▽

     D30.21   **Benign neoplasm of** right **ureter**

     D30.22   **Benign neoplasm of** left **ureter**

D30.3   **Benign neoplasm of** bladder

     Benign neoplasm of ureteric orifice of bladder

     Benign neoplasm of urethral orifice of bladder

✔ Additional Character Req   ✔x7ᵗʰ Placeholder Alert   Manifestation   ▽ Unspecified   ►◄ Revised Text   ● New Code   ▲ Revised Code Title

ICD-10-CM 2019   491

D30.4   **Benign neoplasm of** urethra
   EXCLUDES 1   *benign neoplasm of urethral orifice of bladder (D30.3)*

D30.8   **Benign neoplasm of other specified urinary organs**
   Benign neoplasm of paraurethral glands

D30.9   **Benign neoplasm of urinary organ, unspecified** ▽
   Benign neoplasm of urinary system NOS

✓4ᵗʰ **D31**   **Benign neoplasm of** eye and adnexa
   EXCLUDES 1   *benign neoplasm of connective tissue of eyelid (D21.0)*
         benign neoplasm of optic nerve (D33.3)
         benign neoplasm of skin of eyelid (D22.1-, D23.1-)

✓5ᵗʰ **D31.0**   **Benign neoplasm of** conjunctiva

   D31.00   **Benign neoplasm of unspecified conjunctiva** ▽

   D31.01   **Benign neoplasm of** right **conjunctiva**

   D31.02   **Benign neoplasm of** left **conjunctiva**

✓5ᵗʰ **D31.1**   **Benign neoplasm of** cornea

   D31.10   **Benign neoplasm of unspecified cornea** ▽

   D31.11   **Benign neoplasm of** right **cornea**

   D31.12   **Benign neoplasm of** left **cornea**

✓5ᵗʰ **D31.2**   **Benign neoplasm of** retina
   EXCLUDES 1   *dark area on retina (D49.81)*
         hemangioma of retina (D49.81)
         neoplasm of unspecified behavior of retina and choroid (D49.81)
         retinal freckle (D49.81)

   D31.20   **Benign neoplasm of unspecified retina** ▽

   D31.21   **Benign neoplasm of** right **retina**

   D31.22   **Benign neoplasm of** left **retina**

✓5ᵗʰ **D31.3**   **Benign neoplasm of** choroid

   D31.30   **Benign neoplasm of unspecified choroid** ▽

   D31.31   **Benign neoplasm of** right **choroid**

   D31.32   **Benign neoplasm of** left **choroid**

✓5ᵗʰ **D31.4**   **Benign neoplasm of** ciliary body

   D31.40   **Benign neoplasm of unspecified ciliary body** ▽

   D31.41   **Benign neoplasm of** right **ciliary body**

   D31.42   **Benign neoplasm of** left **ciliary body**

✓5ᵗʰ **D31.5**   **Benign neoplasm of** lacrimal gland and duct
   Benign neoplasm of lacrimal sac
   Benign neoplasm of nasolacrimal duct

   D31.50   **Benign neoplasm of unspecified lacrimal gland and duct** ▽

   D31.51   **Benign neoplasm of** right **lacrimal gland and duct**

   D31.52   **Benign neoplasm of** left **lacrimal gland and duct**

✓5ᵗʰ **D31.6**   **Benign neoplasm of unspecified site of** orbit
   Benign neoplasm of connective tissue of orbit
   Benign neoplasm of extraocular muscle
   Benign neoplasm of peripheral nerves of orbit
   Benign neoplasm of retrobulbar tissue
   Benign neoplasm of retro-ocular tissue
   EXCLUDES 1   *benign neoplasm of orbital bone (D16.4)*

   D31.60   **Benign neoplasm of unspecified site of unspecified orbit** ▽

   D31.61   **Benign neoplasm of unspecified site of** right **orbit** ▽

   D31.62   **Benign neoplasm of unspecified site of** left **orbit** ▽

✓5ᵗʰ **D31.9**   **Benign neoplasm of unspecified** part of eye
   Benign neoplasm of eyeball

   D31.90   **Benign neoplasm of unspecified part of unspecified eye** ▽

   D31.91   **Benign neoplasm of unspecified part of** right **eye** ▽

   D31.92   **Benign neoplasm of unspecified part of** left **eye** ▽

✓4ᵗʰ **D32**   **Benign neoplasm of** meninges

   D32.0   **Benign neoplasm of** cerebral **meninges** ᴴᶜᶜ

   D32.1   **Benign neoplasm of** spinal **meninges** ᴴᶜᶜ

   D32.9   **Benign neoplasm of meninges, unspecified** ᴴᶜᶜ ▽
     Meningioma NOS

✓4ᵗʰ **D33**   **Benign neoplasm of** brain and other parts of central nervous system
   EXCLUDES 1   *angioma (D18.0-)*
         benign neoplasm of meninges (D32.-)
         benign neoplasm of peripheral nerves and autonomic nervous system (D36.1-)
         hemangioma (D18.0-)
         neurofibromatosis (Q85.0-)
         retro-ocular benign neoplasm (D31.6-)

   D33.0   **Benign neoplasm of** brain, supratentorial ᴴᶜᶜ
     Benign neoplasm of cerebral ventricle
     Benign neoplasm of cerebrum
     Benign neoplasm of frontal lobe
     Benign neoplasm of occipital lobe
     Benign neoplasm of parietal lobe
     Benign neoplasm of temporal lobe
     EXCLUDES 1   *benign neoplasm of fourth ventricle (D33.1)*

   D33.1   **Benign neoplasm of** brain, infratentorial ᴴᶜᶜ
     Benign neoplasm of brain stem
     Benign neoplasm of cerebellum
     Benign neoplasm of fourth ventricle

   D33.2   **Benign neoplasm of brain, unspecified** ᴴᶜᶜ ▽

   D33.3   **Benign neoplasm of** cranial nerves ᴴᶜᶜ
     Benign neoplasm of olfactory bulb

   D33.4   **Benign neoplasm of** spinal cord ᴴᶜᶜ

   D33.7   **Benign neoplasm of other specified parts of central nervous system** ᴴᶜᶜ

   D33.9   **Benign neoplasm of central nervous system, unspecified** ᴴᶜᶜ ▽
     Benign neoplasm of nervous system (central) NOS

D34   **Benign neoplasm of** thyroid gland
   Use additional code to identify any functional activity

✓4ᵗʰ **D35**   **Benign neoplasm of other and unspecified** endocrine glands
   Use additional code to identify any functional activity
   EXCLUDES 1   *benign neoplasm of endocrine pancreas (D13.7)*
         benign neoplasm of ovary (D27.-)
         benign neoplasm of testis (D29.2.-)
         benign neoplasm of thymus (D15.0)

✓5ᵗʰ **D35.0**   **Benign neoplasm of** adrenal gland

   D35.00   **Benign neoplasm of unspecified adrenal gland** ▽

   D35.01   **Benign neoplasm of** right **adrenal gland**

   D35.02   **Benign neoplasm of** left **adrenal gland**

   D35.1   **Benign neoplasm of** parathyroid gland

   D35.2   **Benign neoplasm of** pituitary gland ᴴᶜᶜ
     AHA: 2014,3Q,22

   D35.3   **Benign neoplasm of** craniopharyngeal duct ᴴᶜᶜ

   D35.4   **Benign neoplasm of** pineal gland ᴴᶜᶜ

   D35.5   **Benign neoplasm of** carotid body

   D35.6   **Benign neoplasm of** aortic body and other paraganglia
     Benign tumor of glomus jugulare

   D35.7   **Benign neoplasm of other specified endocrine glands**

   D35.9   **Benign neoplasm of endocrine gland, unspecified** ▽
     Benign neoplasm of unspecified endocrine gland

✓4ᵗʰ **D36**   **Benign neoplasm of other and unspecified sites**

   D36.0   **Benign neoplasm of** lymph nodes
     EXCLUDES 1   *lymphangioma (D18.1)*

✓5ᵗʰ **D36.1**   **Benign neoplasm of** peripheral nerves and autonomic nervous system
     EXCLUDES 1   *benign neoplasm of peripheral nerves of orbit (D31.6-)*
           neurofibromatosis (Q85.0-)

   D36.10   **Benign neoplasm of peripheral nerves and autonomic nervous system, unspecified** ▽

   D36.11   **Benign neoplasm of peripheral nerves and autonomic nervous system of** face, head, and neck

   D36.12   **Benign neoplasm of peripheral nerves and autonomic nervous system, upper limb, including shoulder**

   D36.13   **Benign neoplasm of peripheral nerves and autonomic nervous system of lower limb, including hip**

   D36.14   **Benign neoplasm of peripheral nerves and autonomic nervous system of** thorax

   D36.15   **Benign neoplasm of peripheral nerves and autonomic nervous system of** abdomen

D36.16	**Benign neoplasm of peripheral nerves and autonomic nervous system of** pelvis	
D36.17	**Benign neoplasm of peripheral nerves and autonomic nervous system of** trunk, unspecified	▽

D36.7 Benign neoplasm of other specified sites
    Benign neoplasm of nose NOS

D36.9 Benign neoplasm, unspecified site ▽

Benign neuroendocrine tumors (D3A)

✓4ᵗ **D3A Benign neuroendocrine tumors**

Code also any associated multiple endocrine neoplasia [MEN] syndromes (E31.2-)
Use additional code to identify any associated endocrine syndrome, such as:
carcinoid syndrome (E34.0)
EXCLUDES 2   *benign pancreatic islet cell tumors (D13.7)*

✓5ᵗ **D3A.0 Benign** carcinoid tumors

    D3A.00 Benign carcinoid tumor of unspecified site ▽
        Carcinoid tumor NOS

    ✓6ᵗ **D3A.01 Benign carcinoid tumors of the** small intestine

        D3A.010 Benign carcinoid tumor of the duodenum
        D3A.011 Benign carcinoid tumor of the jejunum
        D3A.012 Benign carcinoid tumor of the ileum
        D3A.019 Benign carcinoid tumor of the ▽
            small intestine, unspecified portion

    ✓6ᵗ **D3A.02 Benign carcinoid tumors of the** appendix, large intestine, and rectum

        D3A.020 Benign carcinoid tumor of the appendix
        D3A.021 Benign carcinoid tumor of the cecum
        D3A.022 Benign carcinoid tumor of the ascending colon
        D3A.023 Benign carcinoid tumor of the transverse colon
        D3A.024 Benign carcinoid tumor of the descending colon
        D3A.025 Benign carcinoid tumor of the sigmoid colon
        D3A.026 Benign carcinoid tumor of the rectum
        D3A.029 Benign carcinoid tumor of the ▽
            large intestine, unspecified portion
            Benign carcinoid tumor of the colon NOS

    ✓6ᵗ **D3A.09 Benign carcinoid tumors of other sites**

        D3A.090 Benign carcinoid tumor of the bronchus and lung
        D3A.091 Benign carcinoid tumor of the thymus
        D3A.092 Benign carcinoid tumor of the stomach
        D3A.093 Benign carcinoid tumor of the kidney
        D3A.094 Benign carcinoid tumor of the ▽
            foregut, unspecified
        D3A.095 Benign carcinoid tumor of the ▽
            midgut, unspecified
        D3A.096 Benign carcinoid tumor of the ▽
            hindgut, unspecified
        D3A.098 Benign carcinoid tumors of other sites

D3A.8 Other benign neuroendocrine tumors
    Neuroendocrine tumor NOS

Neoplasms of uncertain behavior, polycythemia vera and myelodysplastic syndromes (D37-D48)

NOTE   Categories D37-D44, and D48 classify by site neoplasms of uncertain behavior, i.e., histologic confirmation whether the neoplasm is malignant or benign cannot be made.

EXCLUDES 1   *neoplasms of unspecified behavior (D49.-)*

✓4ᵗ **D37 Neoplasm of uncertain behavior of** oral cavity and digestive organs

    EXCLUDES 1   *stromal tumors of uncertain behavior of digestive system (D48.1)*

✓5ᵗ **D37.0 Neoplasm of uncertain behavior of** lip, oral cavity and pharynx

    EXCLUDES 1   *neoplasm of uncertain behavior of aryepiglottic fold or interarytenoid fold, laryngeal aspect (D38.0)*
        neoplasm of uncertain behavior of epiglottis NOS (D38.0)
        neoplasm of uncertain behavior of skin of lip (D48.5)
        neoplasm of uncertain behavior of suprahyoid portion of epiglottis (D38.0)

    D37.01 Neoplasm of uncertain behavior of lip
        Neoplasm of uncertain behavior of vermilion border of lip

    D37.02 Neoplasm of uncertain behavior of tongue

    ✓6ᵗ **D37.03 Neoplasm of uncertain behavior of the** major salivary glands

        D37.030 Neoplasm of uncertain behavior of the parotid salivary glands
        D37.031 Neoplasm of uncertain behavior of the sublingual salivary glands
        D37.032 Neoplasm of uncertain behavior of the submandibular salivary glands
        D37.039 Neoplasm of uncertain behavior ▽
            of the major salivary glands, unspecified

    D37.04 Neoplasm of uncertain behavior of the minor salivary glands
        Neoplasm of uncertain behavior of submucosal salivary glands of lip
        Neoplasm of uncertain behavior of submucosal salivary glands of cheek
        Neoplasm of uncertain behavior of submucosal salivary glands of hard palate
        Neoplasm of uncertain behavior of submucosal salivary glands of soft palate

    D37.05 Neoplasm of uncertain behavior of pharynx
        Neoplasm of uncertain behavior of aryepiglottic fold of pharynx NOS
        Neoplasm of uncertain behavior of hypopharyngeal aspect of aryepiglottic fold of pharynx
        Neoplasm of uncertain behavior of marginal zone of aryepiglottic fold of pharynx

    D37.09 Neoplasm of uncertain behavior of other specified sites of the oral cavity

D37.1 Neoplasm of uncertain behavior of stomach

D37.2 Neoplasm of uncertain behavior of small intestine

D37.3 Neoplasm of uncertain behavior of appendix

D37.4 Neoplasm of uncertain behavior of colon

D37.5 Neoplasm of uncertain behavior of rectum
    Neoplasm of uncertain behavior of rectosigmoid junction

D37.6 Neoplasm of uncertain behavior of liver, gallbladder and bile ducts
    Neoplasm of uncertain behavior of ampulla of Vater

D37.8 Neoplasm of uncertain behavior of other specified digestive organs
    Neoplasm of uncertain behavior of anal canal
    Neoplasm of uncertain behavior of anal sphincter
    Neoplasm of uncertain behavior of anus NOS
    Neoplasm of uncertain behavior of esophagus
    Neoplasm of uncertain behavior of intestine NOS
    Neoplasm of uncertain behavior of pancreas
    EXCLUDES 1   *neoplasm of uncertain behavior of anal margin (D48.5)*
        neoplasm of uncertain behavior of anal skin (D48.5)
        neoplasm of uncertain behavior of perianal skin (D48.5)

D37.9 Neoplasm of uncertain behavior of digestive organ, unspecified ▽

Chapter 2. Neoplasms

✓4ᵗʰ **D38 Neoplasm of uncertain behavior of middle ear and respiratory and intrathoracic organs**
> EXCLUDES 1   *neoplasm of uncertain behavior of heart (D48.7)*

D38.0 Neoplasm of uncertain behavior of larynx
Neoplasm of uncertain behavior of aryepiglottic fold or interarytenoid fold, laryngeal aspect
Neoplasm of uncertain behavior of epiglottis (suprahyoid portion)
> EXCLUDES 1   *neoplasm of uncertain behavior of aryepiglottic fold or interarytenoid fold NOS (D37.05)*
> *neoplasm of uncertain behavior of hypopharyngeal aspect of aryepiglottic fold (D37.05)*
> *neoplasm of uncertain behavior of marginal zone of aryepiglottic fold (D37.05)*

D38.1 Neoplasm of uncertain behavior of trachea, bronchus and lung

D38.2 Neoplasm of uncertain behavior of pleura

D38.3 Neoplasm of uncertain behavior of mediastinum

D38.4 Neoplasm of uncertain behavior of thymus

D38.5 Neoplasm of uncertain behavior of other respiratory organs
Neoplasm of uncertain behavior of accessory sinuses
Neoplasm of uncertain behavior of cartilage of nose
Neoplasm of uncertain behavior of middle ear
Neoplasm of uncertain behavior of nasal cavities
> EXCLUDES 1   *neoplasm of uncertain behavior of ear (external) (skin) (D48.5)*
> *neoplasm of uncertain behavior of nose NOS (D48.7)*
> *neoplasm of uncertain behavior of skin of nose (D48.5)*

D38.6 Neoplasm of uncertain behavior of respiratory organ, unspecified ▽

✓4ᵗʰ **D39 Neoplasm of uncertain behavior of female genital organs**

D39.0 Neoplasm of uncertain behavior of uterus ♀

✓5ᵗʰ **D39.1 Neoplasm of uncertain behavior of ovary**
Use additional code to identify any functional activity

D39.10 Neoplasm of uncertain behavior of unspecified ovary ♀ ▽

D39.11 Neoplasm of uncertain behavior of right ovary ♀

D39.12 Neoplasm of uncertain behavior of left ovary ♀

D39.2 Neoplasm of uncertain behavior of placenta Ⓜ ♀
Chorioadenoma destruens
Invasive hydatidiform mole
Malignant hydatidiform mole
> EXCLUDES 1   *hydatidiform mole NOS (O01.9)*

D39.8 Neoplasm of uncertain behavior of other specified female genital organs ♀
Neoplasm of uncertain behavior of skin of female genital organs

D39.9 Neoplasm of uncertain behavior of female genital organ, unspecified ♀ ▽

✓4ᵗʰ **D40 Neoplasm of uncertain behavior of male genital organs**

D40.0 Neoplasm of uncertain behavior of prostate ♂

✓5ᵗʰ **D40.1 Neoplasm of uncertain behavior of testis**

D40.10 Neoplasm of uncertain behavior of unspecified testis ♂ ▽

D40.11 Neoplasm of uncertain behavior of right testis ♂

D40.12 Neoplasm of uncertain behavior of left testis ♂

D40.8 Neoplasm of uncertain behavior of other specified male genital organs ♂
Neoplasm of uncertain behavior of skin of male genital organs

D40.9 Neoplasm of uncertain behavior of male genital organ, unspecified ♂ ▽

✓4ᵗʰ **D41 Neoplasm of uncertain behavior of urinary organs**

✓5ᵗʰ **D41.0 Neoplasm of uncertain behavior of kidney**
> EXCLUDES 1   *neoplasm of uncertain behavior of renal pelvis (D41.1-)*

D41.00 Neoplasm of uncertain behavior of unspecified kidney ▽

D41.01 Neoplasm of uncertain behavior of right kidney

D41.02 Neoplasm of uncertain behavior of left kidney

✓5ᵗʰ **D41.1 Neoplasm of uncertain behavior of renal pelvis**

D41.10 Neoplasm of uncertain behavior of unspecified renal pelvis ▽

D41.11 Neoplasm of uncertain behavior of right renal pelvis

D41.12 Neoplasm of uncertain behavior of left renal pelvis

✓5ᵗʰ **D41.2 Neoplasm of uncertain behavior of ureter**

D41.20 Neoplasm of uncertain behavior of unspecified ureter ▽

D41.21 Neoplasm of uncertain behavior of right ureter

D41.22 Neoplasm of uncertain behavior of left ureter

D41.3 Neoplasm of uncertain behavior of urethra

D41.4 Neoplasm of uncertain behavior of bladder

D41.8 Neoplasm of uncertain behavior of other specified urinary organs

D41.9 Neoplasm of uncertain behavior of unspecified urinary organ ▽

✓4ᵗʰ **D42 Neoplasm of uncertain behavior of meninges**

D42.0 Neoplasm of uncertain behavior of cerebral meninges HCC

D42.1 Neoplasm of uncertain behavior of spinal meninges HCC

D42.9 Neoplasm of uncertain behavior of meninges, unspecified HCC ▽

✓4ᵗʰ **D43 Neoplasm of uncertain behavior of brain and central nervous system**
> EXCLUDES 1   *neoplasm of uncertain behavior of peripheral nerves and autonomic nervous system (D48.2)*

D43.0 Neoplasm of uncertain behavior of brain, supratentorial HCC
Neoplasm of uncertain behavior of cerebral ventricle
Neoplasm of uncertain behavior of cerebrum
Neoplasm of uncertain behavior of frontal lobe
Neoplasm of uncertain behavior of occipital lobe
Neoplasm of uncertain behavior of parietal lobe
Neoplasm of uncertain behavior of temporal lobe
> EXCLUDES 1   *neoplasm of uncertain behavior of fourth ventricle (D43.1)*

D43.1 Neoplasm of uncertain behavior of brain, infratentorial HCC
Neoplasm of uncertain behavior of brain stem
Neoplasm of uncertain behavior of cerebellum
Neoplasm of uncertain behavior of fourth ventricle

D43.2 Neoplasm of uncertain behavior of brain, unspecified HCC ▽

D43.3 Neoplasm of uncertain behavior of cranial nerves HCC

D43.4 Neoplasm of uncertain behavior of spinal cord HCC

D43.8 Neoplasm of uncertain behavior of other specified parts of central nervous system HCC

D43.9 Neoplasm of uncertain behavior of central nervous system, unspecified HCC ▽
Neoplasm of uncertain behavior of nervous system (central) NOS

✓4ᵗʰ **D44 Neoplasm of uncertain behavior of endocrine glands**
> EXCLUDES 1   *multiple endocrine adenomatosis (E31.2-)*
> *multiple endocrine neoplasia (E31.2-)*
> *neoplasm of uncertain behavior of endocrine pancreas (D37.8)*
> *neoplasm of uncertain behavior of ovary (D39.1-)*
> *neoplasm of uncertain behavior of testis (D40.1-)*
> *neoplasm of uncertain behavior of thymus (D38.4)*

D44.0 Neoplasm of uncertain behavior of thyroid gland

✓5ᵗʰ **D44.1 Neoplasm of uncertain behavior of adrenal gland**
Use additional code to identify any functional activity

D44.10 Neoplasm of uncertain behavior of unspecified adrenal gland ▽

D44.11 Neoplasm of uncertain behavior of right adrenal gland

D44.12 Neoplasm of uncertain behavior of left adrenal gland

D44.2 Neoplasm of uncertain behavior of parathyroid gland

D44.3 Neoplasm of uncertain behavior of pituitary gland HCC
Use additional code to identify any functional activity

D44.4 Neoplasm of uncertain behavior of craniopharyngeal duct HCC

D44.5 Neoplasm of uncertain behavior of pineal gland HCC

D44.6 Neoplasm of uncertain behavior of carotid body HCC

D44.7 Neoplasm of uncertain behavior of aortic body and other paraganglia HCC
AHA: 2016,4Q,26

D44.9 Neoplasm of uncertain behavior of unspecified endocrine gland ▽

D45 Polycythemia vera   `HCC`

     EXCLUDES 1   familial polycythemia (D75.0)

                 secondary polycythemia (D75.1)

   DEF: Abnormal proliferation of all bone marrow elements, increased red cell mass, and total blood volume. The etiology is unknown, but it is frequently associated with splenomegaly, leukocytosis, and thrombocythemia.

✓4ᵗʰ D46 Myelodysplastic syndromes

   Use additional code for adverse effect, if applicable, to identify drug (T36-T50 with fifth or sixth character 5)

     EXCLUDES 2   drug-induced aplastic anemia (D61.1)

   D46.0 Refractory anemia without ring sideroblasts, so stated   `HCC`

     Refractory anemia without sideroblasts, without excess of blasts

   D46.1 Refractory anemia with ring sideroblasts   `HCC`

     RARS

   ✓5ᵗʰ D46.2 Refractory anemia with excess of blasts [RAEB]

     D46.20 Refractory anemia with excess of blasts, unspecified   `HCC` ▽

         RAEB NOS

     D46.21 Refractory anemia with excess of blasts 1   `HCC`

         RAEB 1

     D46.22 Refractory anemia with excess of blasts 2   `HCC`

         RAEB 2

   D46.A Refractory cytopenia with multilineage dysplasia   `HCC`

   D46.B Refractory cytopenia with multilineage dysplasia and ring sideroblasts   `HCC`

     RCMD RS

   D46.C Myelodysplastic syndrome with isolated del(5q) chromosomal abnormality   `HCC`

     Myelodysplastic syndrome with 5q deletion

     5q minus syndrome NOS

   D46.4 Refractory anemia, unspecified   `HCC` ▽

   D46.Z Other myelodysplastic syndromes   `HCC`

     EXCLUDES 1   chronic myelomonocytic leukemia (C93.1-)

   D46.9 Myelodysplastic syndrome, unspecified   `HCC` ▽

     Myelodysplasia NOS

✓4ᵗʰ D47 Other neoplasms of uncertain behavior of lymphoid, hematopoietic and related tissue

   ✓5ᵗʰ D47.0 Mast cell neoplasms of uncertain behavior

     EXCLUDES 1   congenital cutaneous mastocytosis ▶(Q82.2)◀

                 histiocytic neoplasms of uncertain behavior (D47.Z9)

                 malignant mast cell neoplasm (C96.2-)

     AHA: 2017,4Q,5

     D47.01 Cutaneous mastocytosis

         Diffuse cutaneous mastocytosis

         Maculopapular cutaneous mastocytosis

         Solitary mastocytoma

         Telangiectasia macularis eruptiva perstans

         Urticaria pigmentosa

         EXCLUDES 1   congenital (diffuse) (maculopapular) cutaneous mastocytosis (Q82.2)

                 congenital urticaria pigmentosa (Q82.2)

                 extracutaneous mastocytoma (D47.09)

     D47.02 Systemic mastocytosis

         Indolent systemic mastocytosis

         Isolated bone marrow mastocytosis

         Smoldering systemic mastocytosis

         Systemic mastocytosis, with an associated hematological non-mast cell lineage disease (SM-AHNMD)

         Code also, if applicable, any associated hematological non-mast cell lineage disease, such as:

           acute myeloid leukemia (C92.6-, C92.A-)

           chronic myelomonocytic leukemia (C93.1-)

           essential thrombocytosis (D47.3)

           hypereosinophilic syndrome (D72.1)

           myelodysplastic syndrome (D46.9)

           myeloproliferative syndrome (D47.1)

           non-Hodgkin lymphoma (C82-C85)

           plasma cell myeloma (C90.0-)

           polycythemia vera (D45)

         EXCLUDES 1   aggressive systemic mastocytosis (C96.21)

                 mast cell leukemia (C94.3-)

     D47.09 Other mast cell neoplasms of uncertain behavior

         Extracutaneous mastocytoma

         Mast cell tumor NOS

         Mastocytoma NOS

         Mastocytosis NOS

   D47.1 Chronic myeloproliferative disease   `HCC`

     Chronic neutrophilic leukemia

     Myeloproliferative disease, unspecified

     EXCLUDES 1   atypical chronic myeloid leukemia BCR/ABL-negative (C92.2-)

                 chronic myeloid leukemia BCR/ABL-positive (C92.1-)

                 myelofibrosis NOS (D75.81)

                 myelophthisic anemia (D61.82)

                 myelophthisis (D61.82)

                 secondary myelofibrosis NOS (D75.81)

   D47.2 Monoclonal gammopathy

     Monoclonal gammopathy of undetermined significance [MGUS]

   D47.3 Essential (hemorrhagic) thrombocythemia   `HCC`

     Essential thrombocytosis

     Idiopathic hemorrhagic thrombocythemia

     DEF: Chronic myeloproliferative neoplasm involving production of excess blood platelets that may result in abnormal clotting or hemorrhaging.

   D47.4 Osteomyelofibrosis   `HCC`

     Chronic idiopathic myelofibrosis

     Myelofibrosis (idiopathic) (with myeloid metaplasia)

     Myelosclerosis (megakaryocytic) with myeloid metaplasia

     Secondary myelofibrosis in myeloproliferative disease

     EXCLUDES 1   acute myelofibrosis (C94.4-)

   ✓5ᵗʰ D47.Z Other specified neoplasms of uncertain behavior of lymphoid, hematopoietic and related tissue

     AHA: 2016,4Q,8

     D47.Z1 Post-transplant lymphoproliferative disorder (PTLD)   `HCC`

         Code first complications of transplanted organs and tissue (T86.-)

         DEF: Excessive proliferation of B-cell lymphocytes following Epstein-Barr virus infection in organ transplant patients. It may progress to non-Hodgkin lymphoma.

     D47.Z2 Castleman disease   `HCC`

         Code also if applicable human herpesvirus 8 infection (B10.89)

         EXCLUDES 2   Kaposi's sarcoma (C46-)

         DEF: Rare disease of the lymph nodes and lymphoid tissues that closely mimics lymphoma.

     D47.Z9 Other specified neoplasms of uncertain behavior of lymphoid, hematopoietic and related tissue   `HCC`

         Histiocytic tumors of uncertain behavior

   D47.9 Neoplasm of uncertain behavior of lymphoid, hematopoietic and related tissue, unspecified   `HCC` ▽

     Lymphoproliferative disease NOS

✓4ᵗʰ D48 Neoplasm of uncertain behavior of other and unspecified sites

     EXCLUDES 1   neurofibromatosis (nonmalignant) (Q85.0-)

   D48.0 Neoplasm of uncertain behavior of bone and articular cartilage

     EXCLUDES 1   neoplasm of uncertain behavior of cartilage of ear (D48.1)

                 neoplasm of uncertain behavior of cartilage of larynx (D38.0)

                 neoplasm of uncertain behavior of cartilage of nose (D38.5)

                 neoplasm of uncertain behavior of connective tissue of eyelid (D48.1)

                 neoplasm of uncertain behavior of synovia (D48.1)

☑ Additional Character Req   ✓x7ᵗʰ Placeholder Alert   Manifestation   ▽ Unspecified   ▶◀ Revised Text   ● New Code   ▲ Revised Code Title

ICD-10-CM 2019   495

D48.1 Neoplasm of uncertain behavior of connective and other soft tissue
    Neoplasm of uncertain behavior of connective tissue of ear
    Neoplasm of uncertain behavior of connective tissue of eyelid
    Stromal tumors of uncertain behavior of digestive system
    EXCLUDES 1   *neoplasm of uncertain behavior of articular cartilage (D48.0)*
            neoplasm of uncertain behavior of cartilage of larynx (D38.0)
            neoplasm of uncertain behavior of cartilage of nose (D38.5)
            neoplasm of uncertain behavior of connective tissue of breast (D48.6-)

D48.2 Neoplasm of uncertain behavior of peripheral nerves and autonomic nervous system
    EXCLUDES 1   *neoplasm of uncertain behavior of peripheral nerves of orbit (D48.7)*

D48.3 Neoplasm of uncertain behavior of retroperitoneum

D48.4 Neoplasm of uncertain behavior of peritoneum

D48.5 Neoplasm of uncertain behavior of skin
    Neoplasm of uncertain behavior of anal margin
    Neoplasm of uncertain behavior of anal skin
    Neoplasm of uncertain behavior of perianal skin
    Neoplasm of uncertain behavior of skin of breast
    EXCLUDES 1   *neoplasm of uncertain behavior of anus NOS (D37.8)*
            neoplasm of uncertain behavior of skin of genital organs (D39.8, D40.8)
            neoplasm of uncertain behavior of vermilion border of lip (D37.0)

√5ᵗʰ D48.6 Neoplasm of uncertain behavior of breast
    Neoplasm of uncertain behavior of connective tissue of breast
    Cystosarcoma phyllodes
    EXCLUDES 1   *neoplasm of uncertain behavior of skin of breast (D48.5)*

    D48.60 Neoplasm of uncertain behavior of unspecified breast ▽
    D48.61 Neoplasm of uncertain behavior of right breast
    D48.62 Neoplasm of uncertain behavior of left breast

D48.7 Neoplasm of uncertain behavior of other specified sites
    Neoplasm of uncertain behavior of eye
    Neoplasm of uncertain behavior of heart
    Neoplasm of uncertain behavior of peripheral nerves of orbit
    EXCLUDES 1   *neoplasm of uncertain behavior of connective tissue (D48.1)*
            neoplasm of uncertain behavior of skin of eyelid (D48.5)

D48.9 Neoplasm of uncertain behavior, unspecified ▽

Neoplasms of unspecified behavior (D49)

√4ᵗʰ D49 Neoplasms of unspecified behavior

    NOTE   Category D49 classifies by site neoplasms of unspecified morphology and behavior. The term "mass", unless otherwise stated, is not to be regarded as a neoplastic growth.

    INCLUDES   "growth" NOS
           neoplasm NOS
           new growth NOS
           tumor NOS
    EXCLUDES 1   *neoplasms of uncertain behavior (D37-D44, D48)*

D49.0 Neoplasm of unspecified behavior of digestive system
    EXCLUDES 1   *neoplasm of unspecified behavior of margin of anus (D49.2)*
            neoplasm of unspecified behavior of perianal skin (D49.2)
            neoplasm of unspecified behavior of skin of anus (D49.2)

D49.1 Neoplasm of unspecified behavior of respiratory system

D49.2 Neoplasm of unspecified behavior of bone, soft tissue, and skin
    EXCLUDES 1   *neoplasm of unspecified behavior of anal canal (D49.0)*
            neoplasm of unspecified behavior of anus NOS (D49.0)
            neoplasm of unspecified behavior of bone marrow (D49.89)
            neoplasm of unspecified behavior of cartilage of larynx (D49.1)
            neoplasm of unspecified behavior of cartilage of nose (D49.1)
            neoplasm of unspecified behavior of connective tissue of breast (D49.3)
            neoplasm of unspecified behavior of skin of genital organs (D49.59)
            neoplasm of unspecified behavior of vermilion border of lip (D49.0)

D49.3 Neoplasm of unspecified behavior of breast
    EXCLUDES 1   *neoplasm of unspecified behavior of skin of breast (D49.2)*

D49.4 Neoplasm of unspecified behavior of bladder

√5ᵗʰ D49.5 Neoplasm of unspecified behavior of other genitourinary organs
    AHA: 2016,4Q,9

    √6ᵗʰ D49.51 Neoplasm of unspecified behavior of kidney
        D49.511 Neoplasm of unspecified behavior of right kidney
        D49.512 Neoplasm of unspecified behavior of left kidney
        D49.519 Neoplasm of unspecified behavior of unspecified kidney ▽

    D49.59 Neoplasm of unspecified behavior of other genitourinary organ

D49.6 Neoplasm of unspecified behavior of brain HCC
    EXCLUDES 1   *neoplasm of unspecified behavior of cerebral meninges (D49.7)*
            neoplasm of unspecified behavior of cranial nerves (D49.7)

D49.7 Neoplasm of unspecified behavior of endocrine glands and other parts of nervous system
    EXCLUDES 1   *neoplasm of unspecified behavior of peripheral, sympathetic, and parasympathetic nerves and ganglia (D49.2)*

√5ᵗʰ D49.8 Neoplasm of unspecified behavior of other specified sites
    EXCLUDES 1   *neoplasm of unspecified behavior of eyelid (skin) (D49.2)*
            neoplasm of unspecified behavior of eyelid cartilage (D49.2)
            neoplasm of unspecified behavior of great vessels (D49.2)
            neoplasm of unspecified behavior of optic nerve (D49.7)

    D49.81 Neoplasm of unspecified behavior of retina and choroid
        Dark area on retina
        Retinal freckle

    D49.89 Neoplasm of unspecified behavior of other specified sites

D49.9 Neoplasm of unspecified behavior of unspecified site ▽

Chapter 3. Disease of the Blood and Blood-Forming Organs and Certain Disorders Involving the Immune Mechanism (D5Ø–D89)

Chapter Specific Coding Guidelines and Examples
Reserved for future guideline expansion.

Chapter 3. Diseases of the Blood and Blood-forming Organs and Certain Disorders Involving the Immune Mechanism (D50-D89)

EXCLUDES 2   autoimmune disease (systemic) NOS (M35.9)
certain conditions originating in the perinatal period (P00-P96)
complications of pregnancy, childbirth and the puerperium (O00-O9A)
congenital malformations, deformations and chromosomal abnormalities (Q00-Q99)
endocrine, nutritional and metabolic diseases (E00-E88)
human immunodeficiency virus [HIV] disease (B20)
injury, poisoning and certain other consequences of external causes (S00-T88)
neoplasms (C00-D49)
symptoms, signs and abnormal clinical and laboratory findings, not elsewhere classified (R00-R94)

This chapter contains the following blocks:
D50-D53   Nutritional anemias
D55-D59   Hemolytic anemias
D60-D64   Aplastic and other anemias and other bone marrow failure syndromes
D65-D69   Coagulation defects, purpura and other hemorrhagic conditions
D70-D77   Other disorders of blood and blood-forming organs
D78   Intraoperative and postprocedural complications of the spleen
D80-D89   Certain disorders involving the immune mechanism

Nutritional anemias (D50-D53)

DEF: Nutritional anemia: The result of inadequate intake or absorption of a vitamin or mineral that impacts the production of red blood cells or causes them to develop abnormally affecting the size and shape.
TIP: Documentation must identify a link between anemia and the nutritional deficiency; low levels of a particular nutrient may occur concurrently with anemia but not cause the anemia.

D50 Iron deficiency anemia
INCLUDES   asiderotic anemia
hypochromic anemia

D50.0 Iron deficiency anemia secondary to blood loss (chronic)
Posthemorrhagic anemia (chronic)
EXCLUDES 1   acute posthemorrhagic anemia (D62)
congenital anemia from fetal blood loss (P61.3)

D50.1 Sideropenic dysphagia
Kelly-Paterson syndrome
Plummer-Vinson syndrome

D50.8 Other iron deficiency anemias
Iron deficiency anemia due to inadequate dietary iron intake

D50.9 Iron deficiency anemia, unspecified

D51 Vitamin B12 deficiency anemia
EXCLUDES 1   vitamin B12 deficiency (E53.8)

D51.0 Vitamin B12 deficiency anemia due to intrinsic factor deficiency
Addison anemia
Biermer anemia
Pernicious (congenital) anemia
Congenital intrinsic factor deficiency
DEF: Chronic progressive anemia due to vitamin B12 malabsorption, caused by lack of secretion of intrinsic factor, which is produced by the gastric mucosa of the stomach.

D51.1 Vitamin B12 deficiency anemia due to selective vitamin B12 malabsorption with proteinuria
Imerslund (Gräsbeck) syndrome
Megaloblastic hereditary anemia

D51.2 Transcobalamin II deficiency

D51.3 Other dietary vitamin B12 deficiency anemia
Vegan anemia

D51.8 Other vitamin B12 deficiency anemias

D51.9 Vitamin B12 deficiency anemia, unspecified

D52 Folate deficiency anemia
EXCLUDES 1   folate deficiency without anemia (E53.8)
DEF: Deficiency in a B complex vitamin needed for the production of healthy red blood cells. Lack of folate, or folic acid, and other absorption conditions can cause anemia resulting in large, misshapen red blood cells called megaloblasts.

D52.0 Dietary folate deficiency anemia
Nutritional megaloblastic anemia
DEF: Result of a poor diet with inadequate intake of folate, which is needed to produce healthy red blood cells.

D52.1 Drug-induced folate deficiency anemia
Use additional code for adverse effect, if applicable, to identify drug (T36-T50 with fifth or sixth character 5)

D52.8 Other folate deficiency anemias
D52.9 Folate deficiency anemia, unspecified
Folic acid deficiency anemia NOS

D53 Other nutritional anemias
INCLUDES   megaloblastic anemia unresponsive to vitamin B12 or folate therapy

D53.0 Protein deficiency anemia
Amino-acid deficiency anemia
Orotaciduric anemia
EXCLUDES 1   Lesch-Nyhan syndrome (E79.1)

D53.1 Other megaloblastic anemias, not elsewhere classified
Megaloblastic anemia NOS
EXCLUDES 1   Di Guglielmo's disease (C94.0)

D53.2 Scorbutic anemia
EXCLUDES 1   scurvy (E54)

D53.8 Other specified nutritional anemias
Anemia associated with deficiency of copper
Anemia associated with deficiency of molybdenum
Anemia associated with deficiency of zinc
EXCLUDES 1   nutritional deficiencies without anemia, such as:
copper deficiency NOS (E61.0)
molybdenum deficiency NOS (E61.5)
zinc deficiency NOS (E60)

D53.9 Nutritional anemia, unspecified
Simple chronic anemia
EXCLUDES 1   anemia NOS (D64.9)

Hemolytic anemias (D55-D59)

D55 Anemia due to enzyme disorders
EXCLUDES 1   drug-induced enzyme deficiency anemia (D59.2)

D55.0 Anemia due to glucose-6-phosphate dehydrogenase [G6PD] deficiency HCC
Favism
G6PD deficiency anemia

D55.1 Anemia due to other disorders of glutathione metabolism HCC
Anemia (due to) enzyme deficiencies, except G6PD, related to the hexose monophosphate [HMP] shunt pathway
Anemia (due to) hemolytic nonspherocytic (hereditary), type I

D55.2 Anemia due to disorders of glycolytic enzymes HCC
Hemolytic nonspherocytic (hereditary) anemia, type II
Hexokinase deficiency anemia
Pyruvate kinase [PK] deficiency anemia
Triose-phosphate isomerase deficiency anemia
EXCLUDES 1   disorders of glycolysis not associated with anemia (E74.8)

D55.3 Anemia due to disorders of nucleotide metabolism HCC
D55.8 Other anemias due to enzyme disorders HCC
D55.9 Anemia due to enzyme disorder, unspecified HCC

☑️⁴ᵗʰ **D56 Thalassemia**

     EXCLUDES 1   *sickle-cell thalassemia (D57.4-)*

     DEF: Group of inherited disorders of hemoglobin metabolism causing mild to severe anemia. It is usually found in people of Mediterranean, African, Chinese, or Asian descent.

Thalassemia

Misshapen RBC

Misshapen RBC

Healthy RBC

   D56.Ø   **Alpha thalassemia**   HCC

      Alpha thalassemia major
      Hemoglobin H Constant Spring
      Hemoglobin H disease
      Hydrops fetalis due to alpha thalassemia
      Severe alpha thalassemia
      Triple gene defect alpha thalassemia
      Use additional code, if applicable, for hydrops fetalis due to alpha thalassemia (P56.99)

      EXCLUDES 1   *alpha thalassemia trait or minor (D56.3)*
                  asymptomatic alpha thalassemia (D56.3)
                  hydrops fetalis due to isoimmunization (P56.Ø)
                  hydrops fetalis not due to immune hemolysis (P83.2)

      DEF: HBA1 and HBA2 genetic variant of chromosome 16 prevalent among those of African and Southeast Asian descent. Alpha thalassemia is associated with a wide spectrum of anemic presentation and includes hemoglobin H disease subtypes.

   D56.1   **Beta thalassemia**   HCC

      Beta thalassemia major
      Cooley's anemia
      Homozygous beta thalassemia
      Severe beta thalassemia
      Thalassemia intermedia
      Thalassemia major

      EXCLUDES 1   *beta thalassemia minor (D56.3)*
                  beta thalassemia trait (D56.3)
                  delta-beta thalassemia (D56.2)
                  hemoglobin E-beta thalassemia (D56.5)
                  sickle-cell beta thalassemia (D57.4-)

   D56.2   **Delta-beta thalassemia**   HCC

      Homozygous delta-beta thalassemia

      EXCLUDES 1   *delta-beta thalassemia minor (D56.3)*
                  delta-beta thalassemia trait (D56.3)

   D56.3   **Thalassemia minor**

      Alpha thalassemia minor
      Alpha thalassemia silent carrier
      Alpha thalassemia trait
      Beta thalassemia minor
      Beta thalassemia trait
      Delta-beta thalassemia minor
      Delta-beta thalassemia trait
      Thalassemia trait NOS

      EXCLUDES 1   *alpha thalassemia (D56.Ø)*
                  beta thalassemia (D56.1)
                  delta-beta thalassemia (D56.2)
                  hemoglobin E-beta thalassemia (D56.5)
                  sickle-cell trait (D57.3)

      DEF: Solitary abnormal gene that identifies a carrier of the disease, yet with an absence of symptoms or a clinically mild anemic presentation.

   D56.4   **Hereditary persistence of fetal hemoglobin [HPFH]**   HCC

   D56.5   **Hemoglobin E-beta thalassemia**   HCC

      EXCLUDES 1   *beta thalassemia (D56.1)*
                  beta thalassemia minor (D56.3)
                  beta thalassemia trait (D56.3)
                  delta-beta thalassemia (D56.2)
                  delta-beta thalassemia trait (D56.3)
                  hemoglobin E disease (D58.2)
                  other hemoglobinopathies (D58.2)
                  sickle-cell beta thalassemia (D57.4-)

   D56.8   **Other thalassemias**   HCC

      Dominant thalassemia
      Hemoglobin C thalassemia
      Mixed thalassemia
      Thalassemia with other hemoglobinopathy

      EXCLUDES 1   *hemoglobin C disease (D58.2)*
                  hemoglobin E disease (D58.2)
                  other hemoglobinopathies (D58.2)
                  sickle-cell anemia (D57.-)
                  sickle-cell thalassemia (D57.4)

   D56.9   **Thalassemia, unspecified**   ▽

      Mediterranean anemia (with other hemoglobinopathy)

☑️⁴ᵗʰ **D57 Sickle-cell disorders**

     Use additional code for any associated fever (R5Ø.81)

     EXCLUDES 1   *other hemoglobinopathies (D58.-)*

     DEF: Severe, chronic inherited diseases caused by a genetic variation in hemoglobin protein of the red blood cell. The gene mutation causes the red blood cell to become hard, sticky, and crescent or sickle shaped making it harder for red blood cells to travel through the bloodstream disrupting blood flow and decreasing oxygen transport to tissues.

Sickle cell

Sickle cells

Normal RBCs

   ☑️⁵ᵗʰ **D57.Ø**   **Hb-SS disease with crisis**

        Sickle-cell disease NOS with crisis
        Hb-SS disease with vasoocclusive pain

        D57.ØØ   **Hb-SS disease with crisis, unspecified**   HCC ▽
        D57.Ø1   **Hb-SS disease with acute chest syndrome**   HCC
        D57.Ø2   **Hb-SS disease with splenic sequestration**   HCC

Chapter 3. Diseases of the Blood and Blood-forming Organs

D57.1 **Sickle-cell disease without crisis** HCC ▽
  Hb-SS disease without crisis
  Sickle-cell anemia NOS
  Sickle-cell disease NOS
  Sickle-cell disorder NOS

✓5ᵗʰ **D57.2** **Sickle-cell/Hb-C disease**
  Hb-SC disease
  Hb-S/Hb-C disease

   D57.20 **Sickle-cell/Hb-C disease without crisis** HCC ▽

✓6ᵗʰ **D57.21** **Sickle-cell/Hb-C disease with crisis**

     D57.211 **Sickle-cell/Hb-C disease with** HCC
        acute chest syndrome

     D57.212 **Sickle-cell/Hb-C disease with** HCC
        splenic sequestration

     D57.219 **Sickle-cell/Hb-C disease with** HCC ▽
        crisis, unspecified
         Sickle-cell/Hb-C disease with crisis NOS

D57.3 **Sickle-cell trait** HCC
  Hb-S trait
  Heterozygous hemoglobin S
  DEF: Heterozygous genetic makeup characterized by one gene for normal hemoglobin and one for sickle-cell hemoglobin. The clinical disease is rarely present.

✓5ᵗʰ **D57.4** **Sickle-cell thalassemia**
  Sickle-cell beta thalassemia
  Thalassemia Hb-S disease

   D57.40 **Sickle-cell thalassemia without crisis** HCC ▽
     Microdrepanocytosis
     Sickle-cell thalassemia NOS

✓6ᵗʰ **D57.41** **Sickle-cell thalassemia with crisis**
     Sickle-cell thalassemia with vasoocclusive pain

     D57.411 **Sickle-cell thalassemia with acute** HCC
        chest syndrome

     D57.412 **Sickle-cell thalassemia with** HCC
        splenic sequestration

     D57.419 **Sickle-cell thalassemia with crisis,** HCC ▽
        unspecified
         Sickle-cell thalassemia with crisis NOS

✓5ᵗʰ **D57.8** **Other sickle-cell disorders**
  Hb-SD disease
  Hb-SE disease

   D57.80 **Other sickle-cell disorders without crisis** HCC ▽

✓6ᵗʰ **D57.81** **Other sickle-cell disorders with crisis**

     D57.811 **Other sickle-cell disorders with** HCC
        acute chest syndrome

     D57.812 **Other sickle-cell disorders with** HCC
        splenic sequestration

     D57.819 **Other sickle-cell disorders with** HCC ▽
        crisis, unspecified
         Other sickle-cell disorders with crisis NOS

✓4ᵗʰ **D58** **Other hereditary hemolytic anemias**
  EXCLUDES 1   hemolytic anemia of the newborn (P55.-)

D58.0 **Hereditary spherocytosis** HCC
  Acholuric (familial) jaundice
  Congenital (spherocytic) hemolytic icterus
  Minkowski-Chauffard syndrome
  DEF: Inherited condition caused by mutations to genes responsible for the production of proteins that form the membranes of red blood cells. The shape and flexibility of the red blood cell membrane is altered diminishing the cells ability to traverse the spleen, therefore becoming trapped and destroyed before the red blood cell has reached maturity.

D58.1 **Hereditary elliptocytosis** HCC
  Elliptocytosis (congenital)
  Ovalocytosis (congenital) (hereditary)

D58.2 **Other hemoglobinopathies** HCC
  Abnormal hemoglobin NOS
  Congenital Heinz body anemia
  Hb-C disease
  Hb-D disease
  Hb-E disease
  Hemoglobinopathy NOS
  Unstable hemoglobin hemolytic disease
  EXCLUDES 1   *familial polycythemia (D75.0)*
       Hb-M disease (D74.0)
       hemoglobin E-beta thalassemia (D56.5)
       hereditary persistence of fetal hemoglobin [HPFH]
         (D56.4)
       high-altitude polycythemia (D75.1)
       methemoglobinemia (D74.-)
       other hemoglobinopathies with thalassemia (D56.8)

D58.8 **Other specified hereditary hemolytic anemias** HCC
  Stomatocytosis

D58.9 **Hereditary hemolytic anemia, unspecified** HCC ▽

✓4ᵗʰ **D59** **Acquired hemolytic anemia**
  DEF: Non-hereditary anemia characterized by premature destruction of red blood cells caused by infectious organisms, poisons, and physical agents.

D59.0 **Drug-induced autoimmune hemolytic anemia** HCC
  Use additional code for adverse effect, if applicable, to identify drug (T36-T50 with fifth or sixth character 5)

D59.1 **Other autoimmune hemolytic anemias** HCC
  Autoimmune hemolytic disease (cold type) (warm type)
  Chronic cold hemagglutinin disease
  Cold agglutinin disease
  Cold agglutinin hemoglobinuria
  Cold type (secondary) (symptomatic) hemolytic anemia
  Warm type (secondary) (symptomatic) hemolytic anemia
  EXCLUDES 1   *Evans syndrome (D69.41)*
       hemolytic disease of newborn (P55.-)
       paroxysmal cold hemoglobinuria (D59.6)

D59.2 **Drug-induced nonautoimmune hemolytic anemia** HCC
  Drug-induced enzyme deficiency anemia
  Use additional code for adverse effect, if applicable, to identify drug (T36-T50 with fifth or sixth character 5)

D59.3 **Hemolytic-uremic syndrome** HCC
  Use additional code to identify associated:
    E. coli infection (B96.2-)
    Pneumococcal pneumonia (J13)
    Shigella dysenteriae (A03.9)
  DEF: Condition typically precipitated by infection causing low platelets and destruction of red blood cells resulting in hemolytic anemia. This cell damage and blockage of renal capillaries lead to kidney failure. Mainly affects children.

D59.4 **Other nonautoimmune hemolytic anemias** HCC
  Mechanical hemolytic anemia
  Microangiopathic hemolytic anemia
  Toxic hemolytic anemia

D59.5 **Paroxysmal nocturnal hemoglobinuria** HCC
  [Marchiafava-Micheli]
  EXCLUDES 1   *hemoglobinuria NOS (R82.3)*

D59.6 **Hemoglobinuria due to hemolysis from other** HCC
  external causes
  Hemoglobinuria from exertion
  March hemoglobinuria
  Paroxysmal cold hemoglobinuria
  Use additional code (Chapter 20) to identify external cause
  EXCLUDES 1   *hemoglobinuria NOS (R82.3)*

D59.8 **Other acquired hemolytic anemias** HCC

D59.9 **Acquired hemolytic anemia, unspecified** HCC ▽
  Idiopathic hemolytic anemia, chronic

Aplastic and other anemias and other bone marrow failure syndromes (D60-D64)

✓4ᵗʰ **D60** **Acquired pure red cell aplasia [erythroblastopenia]**
  INCLUDES   red cell aplasia (acquired) (adult) (with thymoma)
  EXCLUDES 1   *congenital red cell aplasia (D61.01)*

D60.0 **Chronic acquired pure red cell aplasia** HCC

D60.1 **Transient acquired pure red cell aplasia** HCC

D60.8 **Other acquired pure red cell aplasias** HCC

D60.9 **Acquired pure red cell aplasia, unspecified** HCC ▽

√4th D61 Other aplastic anemias and other bone marrow failure syndromes

> EXCLUDES 1   neutropenia (D70.-)

> **AHA:** 2014,4Q,22

√5th D61.0 Constitutional aplastic anemia

D61.01 Constitutional (pure) red blood cell aplasia HCC

> Blackfan-Diamond syndrome
> Congenital (pure) red cell aplasia
> Familial hypoplastic anemia
> Primary (pure) red cell aplasia
> Red cell (pure) aplasia of infants
>
> > EXCLUDES 1   acquired red cell aplasia (D60.9)

D61.09 Other constitutional aplastic anemia HCC

> Fanconi's anemia
> Pancytopenia with malformations

D61.1 Drug-induced aplastic anemia HCC

> Use additional code for adverse effect, if applicable, to identify drug (T36-T50 with fifth or sixth character 5)

D61.2 Aplastic anemia due to other external agents HCC

> Code first, if applicable, toxic effects of substances chiefly nonmedicinal as to source (T51-T65)

D61.3 Idiopathic aplastic anemia HCC

√5th D61.8 Other specified aplastic anemias and other bone marrow failure syndromes

√6th D61.81 Pancytopenia

> > EXCLUDES 1   pancytopenia (due to) (with) aplastic anemia (D61.9)
> > pancytopenia (due to) (with) bone marrow infiltration (D61.82)
> > pancytopenia (due to) (with) congenital (pure) red cell aplasia (D61.01)
> > pancytopenia (due to) (with) hairy cell leukemia (C91.4-)
> > pancytopenia (due to) (with) human immunodeficiency virus disease (B20)
> > pancytopenia (due to) (with) leukoerythroblastic anemia (D61.82)
> > pancytopenia (due to) (with) myeloproliferative disease (D47.1)
> >
> > EXCLUDES 2   pancytopenia (due to) (with) myelodysplastic syndromes (D46.-)

> **DEF:** Shortage of all three blood cells: white, red, and platelets.

D61.810 Antineoplastic chemotherapy induced pancytopenia HCC

> > EXCLUDES 2   aplastic anemia due to antineoplastic chemotherapy (D61.1)

D61.811 Other drug-induced pancytopenia HCC

> > EXCLUDES 2   aplastic anemia due to drugs (D61.1)

D61.818 Other pancytopenia HCC

D61.82 Myelophthisis HCC

> Leukoerythroblastic anemia
> Myelophthisic anemia
> Panmyelophthisis
> Code also the underlying disorder, such as:
> > malignant neoplasm of breast (C50.-)
> > tuberculosis (A15.-)
>
> > EXCLUDES 1   idiopathic myelofibrosis (D47.1)
> > myelofibrosis NOS (D75.81)
> > myelofibrosis with myeloid metaplasia (D47.4)
> > primary myelofibrosis (D47.1)
> > secondary myelofibrosis (D75.81)

> **DEF:** Condition that occurs when normal hematopoietic tissue in the bone marrow is replaced with abnormal tissue, such as fibrous tissue or tumors. Most commonly seen during the advanced stages of cancer.

D61.89 Other specified aplastic anemias and other bone marrow failure syndromes HCC

D61.9 Aplastic anemia, unspecified HCC ▽

> Hypoplastic anemia NOS
> Medullary hypoplasia

D62 Acute posthemorrhagic anemia

> EXCLUDES 1   anemia due to chronic blood loss (D50.0)
> blood loss anemia NOS (D50.0)
> congenital anemia from fetal blood loss (P61.3)

√4th D63 Anemia in chronic diseases classified elsewhere

D63.0 Anemia in neoplastic disease

> Code first neoplasm (C00-D49)
>
> > EXCLUDES 1   aplastic anemia due to antineoplastic chemotherapy (D61.1)
> >
> > EXCLUDES 2   anemia due to antineoplastic chemotherapy (D64.81)

D63.1 Anemia in chronic kidney disease

> Erythropoietin resistant anemia (EPO resistant anemia)
> Code first underlying chronic kidney disease (CKD) (N18.-)

D63.8 Anemia in other chronic diseases classified elsewhere

> Code first underlying disease, such as:
> > diphyllobothriasis (B70.0)
> > hookworm disease (B76.0-B76.9)
> > hypothyroidism (E00.0-E03.9)
> > malaria (B50.0-B54)
> > symptomatic late syphilis (A52.79)
> > tuberculosis (A18.89)

√4th D64 Other anemias

> EXCLUDES 1   refractory anemia (D46.-)
> refractory anemia with excess blasts in transformation [RAEB T] (C92.0-)

> **DEF:** Sideroblastic anemia: Hereditary or secondary disorder in which the red blood cells cannot effectively use iron, a nutrient needed to make hemoglobin. Although the iron can enter the red blood cell it is not assimilated into the hemoglobin molecule and builds up ringed sideroblasts around the cell nucleus.

D64.0 Hereditary sideroblastic anemia HCC

> Sex-linked hypochromic sideroblastic anemia

D64.1 Secondary sideroblastic anemia due to disease HCC

> Code first underlying disease

D64.2 Secondary sideroblastic anemia due to drugs and toxins HCC

> Code first poisoning due to drug or toxin, if applicable (T36-T65 with fifth or sixth character 1-4 or 6)
> Use additional code for adverse effect, if applicable, to identify drug (T36-T50 with fifth or sixth character 5)

D64.3 Other sideroblastic anemias HCC

> Sideroblastic anemia NOS
> Pyridoxine-responsive sideroblastic anemia NEC

D64.4 Congenital dyserythropoietic anemia

> Dyshematopoietic anemia (congenital)
>
> > EXCLUDES 1   Blackfan-Diamond syndrome (D61.01)
> > Di Guglielmo's disease (C94.0)

√5th D64.8 Other specified anemias

D64.81 Anemia due to antineoplastic chemotherapy

> Antineoplastic chemotherapy induced anemia
>
> > EXCLUDES 1   aplastic anemia due to antineoplastic chemotherapy (D61.1)
> >
> > EXCLUDES 2   anemia in neoplastic disease (D63.0)

> **AHA:** 2014,4Q,22

> **DEF:** Reversible adverse effect of chemotherapy, causing inhibition of bone marrow production. A decrease in red blood cell production prevents adequate oxygenation of the tissues and organs causing fatigue, shortness of breath (SOB), and exacerbation of other medical conditions.

D64.89 Other specified anemias

> Infantile pseudoleukemia

D64.9 Anemia, unspecified ▽

> **AHA:** 2017,1Q,7

Coagulation defects, purpura and other hemorrhagic conditions (D65-D69)

D65 Disseminated intravascular coagulation [defibrination syndrome] `HCC`
Afibrinogenemia, acquired
Consumption coagulopathy
Diffuse or disseminated intravascular coagulation [DIC]
Fibrinolytic hemorrhage, acquired
Fibrinolytic purpura
Purpura fulminans
> **EXCLUDES 1** *disseminated intravascular coagulation (complicating):*
> *abortion or ectopic or molar pregnancy (O00-O07, O08.1)*
> *in newborn (P60)*
> *pregnancy, childbirth and the puerperium (O45.0, O46.0, O67.0, O72.3)*

Coagulation

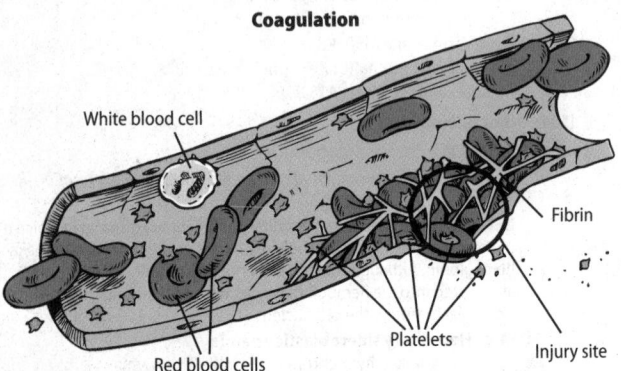

White blood cell
Fibrin
Platelets
Red blood cells
Injury site

D66 Hereditary factor VIII deficiency `HCC`
Classical hemophilia
Deficiency factor VIII (with functional defect)
Hemophilia A
Hemophilia NOS
> **EXCLUDES 1** *factor VIII deficiency with vascular defect (D68.0)*

DEF: Hereditary, sex-linked lack of antihemophilic globulin (AHG) (factor VIII) that causes abnormal coagulation characterized by increased bleeding; large bruises of skin; bleeding in the mouth, nose, and gastrointestinal tract; and hemorrhages into joints, resulting in swelling and impaired function.

D67 Hereditary factor IX deficiency `HCC`
Christmas disease
Factor IX deficiency (with functional defect)
Hemophilia B
Plasma thromboplastin component [PTC] deficiency

D68 Other coagulation defects ✓4ᵗʰ
> **EXCLUDES 1** *abnormal coagulation profile (R79.1)*
> *coagulation defects complicating abortion or ectopic or molar pregnancy (O00-O07, O08.1)*
> *coagulation defects complicating pregnancy, childbirth and the puerperium (O45.0, O46.0, O67.0, O72.3)*

AHA: 2016,1Q,14

D68.0 Von Willebrand's disease `HCC`
Angiohemophilia
Factor VIII deficiency with vascular defect
Vascular hemophilia
> **EXCLUDES 1** *capillary fragility (hereditary) (D69.8)*
> *factor VIII deficiency NOS (D66)*
> *factor VIII deficiency with functional defect (D66)*

DEF: Congenital, abnormal blood coagulation caused by deficient blood factor VII. Symptoms include excess or prolonged bleeding.

D68.1 Hereditary factor XI deficiency `HCC`
Hemophilia C
Plasma thromboplastin antecedent [PTA] deficiency
Rosenthal's disease

D68.2 Hereditary deficiency of other clotting factors `HCC`
AC globulin deficiency
Congenital afibrinogenemia
Deficiency of factor I [fibrinogen]
Deficiency of factor II [prothrombin]
Deficiency of factor V [labile]
Deficiency of factor VII [stable]
Deficiency of factor X [Stuart-Prower]
Deficiency of factor XII [Hageman]
Deficiency of factor XIII [fibrin stabilizing]
Dysfibrinogenemia (congenital)
Hypoproconvertinemia
Owren's disease
Proaccelerin deficiency

D68.3 Hemorrhagic disorder due to circulating anticoagulants ✓5ᵗʰ

D68.31 Hemorrhagic disorder due to intrinsic circulating anticoagulants, antibodies, or inhibitors ✓6ᵗʰ

D68.311 Acquired hemophilia `HCC`
Autoimmune hemophilia
Autoimmune inhibitors to clotting factors
Secondary hemophilia

D68.312 Antiphospholipid antibody with hemorrhagic disorder `HCC`
Lupus anticoagulant (LAC) with hemorrhagic disorder
Systemic lupus erythematosus [SLE] inhibitor with hemorrhagic disorder
> **EXCLUDES 1** *antiphospholipid antibody, finding without diagnosis (R76.0)*
> *antiphospholipid antibody syndrome (D68.61)*
> *antiphospholipid antibody with hypercoagulable state (D68.61)*
> *lupus anticoagulant (LAC) finding without diagnosis (R76.0)*
> *lupus anticoagulant (LAC) with hypercoagulable state (D68.62)*
> *systemic lupus erythematosus [SLE] inhibitor finding without diagnosis (R76.0)*
> *systemic lupus erythematosus [SLE] inhibitor with hypercoagulable state (D68.62)*

D68.318 Other hemorrhagic disorder due to intrinsic circulating anticoagulants, antibodies, or inhibitors `HCC`
Antithromboplastinemia
Antithromboplastinogenemia
Hemorrhagic disorder due to intrinsic increase in antithrombin
Hemorrhagic disorder due to intrinsic increase in anti-VIIIa
Hemorrhagic disorder due to intrinsic increase in anti-IXa
Hemorrhagic disorder due to intrinsic increase in anti-XIa

D68.32 Hemorrhagic disorder due to extrinsic circulating anticoagulants `HCC`
Drug-induced hemorrhagic disorder
Hemorrhagic disorder due to increase in anti-IIa
Hemorrhagic disorder due to increase in anti-Xa
Hyperheparinemia
Use additional code for adverse effect, if applicable, to identify drug (T45.515, T45.525)
AHA: 2016,1Q,14-15
TIP: Do not assign to identify routine therapeutic anticoagulation effects; assign only for documented adverse effects. An adverse effect code (T36–T50) identifying the specific therapeutic agent should also be assigned.

D68.4   Acquired coagulation factor deficiency   `HCC`
    Deficiency of coagulation factor due to liver disease
    Deficiency of coagulation factor due to vitamin K deficiency
     EXCLUDES 1   vitamin K deficiency of newborn (P53)

✓5th **D68.5   Primary thrombophilia**
    Primary hypercoagulable states
     EXCLUDES 1   antiphospholipid syndrome (D68.61)
             lupus anticoagulant (D68.62)
             secondary activated protein C resistance (D68.69)
             secondary antiphospholipid antibody syndrome
                 (D68.69)
             secondary lupus anticoagulant with hypercoagulable
                 state (D68.69)
             secondary systemic lupus erythematosus [SLE]
                 inhibitor with hypercoagulable state (D68.69)
             systemic lupus erythematosus [SLE] inhibitor finding
                 without diagnosis (R76.0)
             systemic lupus erythematosus [SLE] inhibitor with
                 hemorrhagic disorder (D68.312)
             thrombotic thrombocytopenic purpura (M31.1)
    DEF: Thrombophilia: Increased tendency of the blood to clot,
    which can lead to thrombus or embolus formation.

    D68.51   Activated protein C resistance   `HCC`
       Factor V Leiden mutation
    D68.52   Prothrombin gene mutation   `HCC`
    D68.59   Other primary thrombophilia   `HCC`
       Antithrombin III deficiency
       Hypercoagulable state NOS
       Primary hypercoagulable state NEC
       Primary thrombophilia NEC
       Protein C deficiency
       Protein S deficiency
       Thrombophilia NOS

✓5th **D68.6   Other thrombophilia**
    Other hypercoagulable states
     EXCLUDES 1   diffuse or disseminated intravascular coagulation
                [DIC] (D65)
             heparin induced thrombocytopenia (HIT) (D75.82)
             hyperhomocysteinemia (E72.11)

    D68.61   Antiphospholipid syndrome   `HCC`
       Anticardiolipin syndrome
       Antiphospholipid antibody syndrome
        EXCLUDES 1   anti-phospholipid antibody, finding
                   without diagnosis (R76.0)
                anti-phospholipid antibody with
                   hemorrhagic disorder (D68.312)
                lupus anticoagulant syndrome (D68.62)

    D68.62   Lupus anticoagulant syndrome   `HCC`
       Lupus anticoagulant
       Presence of systemic lupus erythematosus [SLE]
         inhibitor
        EXCLUDES 1   anticardiolipin syndrome (D68.61)
                antiphospholipid syndrome (D68.61)
                lupus anticoagulant (LAC) finding without
                   diagnosis (R76.0)
                lupus anticoagulant (LAC) with
                   hemorrhagic disorder (D68.312)

    D68.69   Other thrombophilia   `HCC`
       Hypercoagulable states NEC
       Secondary hypercoagulable state NOS

D68.8   Other specified coagulation defects   `HCC`
     EXCLUDES 1   hemorrhagic disease of newborn (P53)

D68.9   Coagulation defect, unspecified   `HCC` ▽

✓4th **D69   Purpura and other hemorrhagic conditions**
     EXCLUDES 1   benign hypergammaglobulinemic purpura (D89.0)
             cryoglobulinemic purpura (D89.1)
             essential (hemorrhagic) thrombocythemia (D47.3)
             hemorrhagic thrombocythemia (D47.3)
             purpura fulminans (D65)
             thrombotic thrombocytopenic purpura (M31.1)
             Waldenström hypergammaglobulinemic purpura (D89.0)

    D69.0   Allergic purpura   `HCC`
       Allergic vasculitis
       Nonthrombocytopenic hemorrhagic purpura
       Nonthrombocytopenic idiopathic purpura
       Purpura anaphylactoid
       Purpura Henoch(-Schönlein)
       Purpura rheumatica
       Vascular purpura
        EXCLUDES 1   thrombocytopenic hemorrhagic purpura (D69.3)
       DEF: Any hemorrhagic condition, thrombocytic or
       nonthrombocytopenic in origin, caused by a presumed allergic
       reaction.

    D69.1   Qualitative platelet defects   `HCC`
       Bernard-Soulier [giant platelet] syndrome
       Glanzmann's disease
       Grey platelet syndrome
       Thromboasthenia (hemorrhagic) (hereditary)
       Thrombocytopathy
        EXCLUDES 1   von Willebrand's disease (D68.0)

    D69.2   Other nonthrombocytopenic purpura   `HCC`
       Purpura NOS
       Purpura simplex
       Senile purpura

    D69.3   Immune thrombocytopenic purpura   `HCC`
       Hemorrhagic (thrombocytopenic) purpura
       Idiopathic thrombocytopenic purpura
       Tidal platelet dysgenesis
       DEF: Tidal platelet dysgenesis: Fluctuation of platelet counts
       from normal to very low within periods of 20 to 40 days and may
       involve autoimmune platelet destruction.

✓5th **D69.4   Other primary thrombocytopenia**
        EXCLUDES 1   transient neonatal thrombocytopenia (P61.0)
                 Wiskott-Aldrich syndrome (D82.0)

    D69.41   Evans syndrome   `HCC`
    D69.42   Congenital and hereditary   `HCC`
            thrombocytopenia purpura
       Congenital thrombocytopenia
       Hereditary thrombocytopenia
       Code first congenital or hereditary disorder, such as:
         thrombocytopenia with absent radius (TAR
         syndrome) (Q87.2)
    D69.49   Other primary thrombocytopenia   `HCC`
       Megakaryocytic hypoplasia
       Primary thrombocytopenia NOS

✓5th **D69.5   Secondary thrombocytopenia**
        EXCLUDES 1   heparin induced thrombocytopenia (HIT) (D75.82)
                 transient thrombocytopenia of newborn (P61.0)

    D69.51   Posttransfusion purpura
       Posttransfusion purpura from whole blood (fresh) or
         blood products
       PTP
    D69.59   Other secondary thrombocytopenia
       AHA: 2014,4Q,22

    D69.6   Thrombocytopenia, unspecified   `HCC` ▽
    D69.8   Other specified hemorrhagic conditions   `HCC`
       Capillary fragility (hereditary)
       Vascular pseudohemophilia

    D69.9   Hemorrhagic condition, unspecified   `HCC` ▽

☑ Additional Character Req   ✓x7th Placeholder Alert   Manifestation   ▽ Unspecified   ▶◀ Revised Text   ● New Code   ▲ Revised Code Title

ICD-10-CM 2019   **503**

Chapter 3. Diseases of the Blood and Blood-forming Organs

Other disorders of blood and blood-forming organs (D70-D77)

✓4ᵗʰ D70 Neutropenia

    INCLUDES   agranulocytosis
                decreased absolute neurophile count (ANC)

    Use additional code for any associated:
         fever (R50.81)
         mucositis (J34.81, K12.3-, K92.81, N76.81)

    EXCLUDES 1   *neutropenic splenomegaly (D73.81)*
                transient neonatal neutropenia (P61.5)

    DEF: Abnormally low number of neutrophils. Neutrophils are phagocytic, meaning they surround and consume harmful pathogens, primarily bacteria. When neutrophil counts decrease the risk of infection increases.

    D70.0 Congenital agranulocytosis   HCC
         Congenital neutropenia
         Infantile genetic agranulocytosis
         Kostmann's disease

    D70.1 Agranulocytosis secondary to cancer chemotherapy   HCC
         Use additional code for adverse effect, if applicable, to identify drug (T45.1X5)
         Code also underlying neoplasm
         AHA: 2014,4Q,22

    D70.2 Other drug-induced agranulocytosis   HCC
         Use additional code for adverse effect, if applicable, to identify drug (T36-T50 with fifth or sixth character 5)

    D70.3 Neutropenia due to infection   HCC

    D70.4 Cyclic neutropenia   HCC
         Cyclic hematopoiesis
         Periodic neutropenia

    D70.8 Other neutropenia   HCC

    D70.9 Neutropenia, unspecified   HCC ▽

D71 Functional disorders of polymorphonuclear neutrophils   HCC
     Cell membrane receptor complex [CR3] defect
     Chronic (childhood) granulomatous disease
     Congenital dysphagocytosis
     Progressive septic granulomatosis

✓4ᵗʰ D72 Other disorders of white blood cells

    EXCLUDES 1   *basophilia (D72.824)*
                immunity disorders (D80-D89)
                neutropenia (D70)
                preleukemia (syndrome) (D46.9)

    D72.0 Genetic anomalies of leukocytes   HCC
         Alder (granulation) (granulocyte) anomaly
         Alder syndrome
         Hereditary leukocytic hypersegmentation
         Hereditary leukocytic hyposegmentation
         Hereditary leukomelanopathy
         May-Hegglin (granulation) (granulocyte) anomaly
         May-Hegglin syndrome
         Pelger-Huët (granulation) (granulocyte) anomaly
         Pelger-Huët syndrome
         EXCLUDES 1   *Chédiak (-Steinbrinck)-Higashi syndrome (E70.330)*

    D72.1 Eosinophilia
         Allergic eosinophilia
         Hereditary eosinophilia
         EXCLUDES 1   *Löffler's syndrome (J82)*
                 pulmonary eosinophilia (J82)

    ✓5ᵗʰ D72.8 Other specified disorders of white blood cells
         EXCLUDES 1   *leukemia (C91-C95)*

        ✓6ᵗʰ D72.81 Decreased white blood cell count
             EXCLUDES 1   *neutropenia (D70.-)*

            D72.810 Lymphocytopenia
                 Decreased lymphocytes

            D72.818 Other decreased white blood cell count
                 Basophilic leukopenia
                 Eosinophilic leukopenia
                 Monocytopenia
                 Other decreased leukocytes
                 Plasmacytopenia

            D72.819 Decreased white blood cell count, unspecified   ▽
                 Decreased leukocytes, unspecified
                 Leukocytopenia, unspecified
                 Leukopenia
                 EXCLUDES 1   *malignant leukopenia (D70.9)*

        ✓6ᵗʰ D72.82 Elevated white blood cell count
             EXCLUDES 1   *eosinophilia (D72.1)*

            D72.820 Lymphocytosis (symptomatic)
                 Elevated lymphocytes

            D72.821 Monocytosis (symptomatic)
                 EXCLUDES 1   *infectious mononucleosis (B27.-)*

            D72.822 Plasmacytosis

            D72.823 Leukemoid reaction
                 Basophilic leukemoid reaction
                 Leukemoid reaction NOS
                 Lymphocytic leukemoid reaction
                 Monocytic leukemoid reaction
                 Myelocytic leukemoid reaction
                 Neutrophilic leukemoid reaction

            D72.824 Basophilia
                 DEF: Increase in the basophils of the blood, a type of white blood cell, often seen in conjunction with neoplastic disorders.

            D72.825 Bandemia
                 Bandemia without diagnosis of specific infection
                 EXCLUDES 1   *confirmed infection - code to infection*
                     leukemia (C91.-, C92.-, C93.-, C94.-, C95.-)
                 DEF: Increase in early neutrophil cells, called band cells that may indicate infection.

            D72.828 Other elevated white blood cell count

            D72.829 Elevated white blood cell count, unspecified   ▽
                 Elevated leukocytes, unspecified
                 Leukocytosis, unspecified

        D72.89 Other specified disorders of white blood cells
             Abnormality of white blood cells NEC

    D72.9 Disorder of white blood cells, unspecified   ▽
         Abnormal leukocyte differential NOS

✓4ᵗʰ D73 Diseases of spleen

    D73.0 Hyposplenism
         Atrophy of spleen
         EXCLUDES 1   *asplenia (congenital) (Q89.01)*
                 postsurgical absence of spleen (Z90.81)

    D73.1 Hypersplenism
         EXCLUDES 1   *neutropenic splenomegaly (D73.81)*
                 primary splenic neutropenia (D73.81)
                 splenitis, splenomegaly in late syphilis (A52.79)
                 splenitis, splenomegaly in tuberculosis (A18.85)
                 splenomegaly NOS (R16.1)
                 splenomegaly congenital (Q89.0)

    D73.2 Chronic congestive splenomegaly

    D73.3 Abscess of spleen

    D73.4 Cyst of spleen

    D73.5 Infarction of spleen
         Splenic rupture, nontraumatic
         Torsion of spleen
         EXCLUDES 1   *rupture of spleen due to Plasmodium vivax malaria (B51.0)*
                 traumatic rupture of spleen (S36.03-)

    ✓5ᵗʰ D73.8 Other diseases of spleen

        D73.81 Neutropenic splenomegaly
             Werner-Schultz disease

        D73.89 Other diseases of spleen
             Fibrosis of spleen NOS
             Perisplenitis
             Splenitis NOS

    D73.9 Disease of spleen, unspecified   ▽

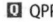

☑4ᵗʰ **D74 Methemoglobinemia**

    D74.0 Congenital methemoglobinemia
        Congenital NADH-methemoglobin reductase deficiency
        Hemoglobin-M [Hb-M] disease
        Methemoglobinemia, hereditary

    D74.8 Other methemoglobinemias
        Acquired methemoglobinemia (with sulfhemoglobinemia)
        Toxic methemoglobinemia

    D74.9 Methemoglobinemia, unspecified   ▽

☑4ᵗʰ **D75 Other and unspecified diseases of blood and blood-forming organs**

    EXCLUDES 2   acute lymphadenitis (L04.-)
                 chronic lymphadenitis (I88.1)
                 enlarged lymph nodes (R59.-)
                 hypergammaglobulinemia NOS (D89.2)
                 lymphadenitis NOS (I88.9)
                 mesenteric lymphadenitis (acute) (chronic) (I88.0)

    D75.0 Familial erythrocytosis
        Benign polycythemia
        Familial polycythemia
        EXCLUDES 1   hereditary ovalocytosis (D58.1)

    D75.1 Secondary polycythemia
        Acquired polycythemia
        Emotional polycythemia
        Erythrocytosis NOS
        Hypoxemic polycythemia
        Nephrogenous polycythemia
        Polycythemia due to erythropoietin
        Polycythemia due to fall in plasma volume
        Polycythemia due to high altitude
        Polycythemia due to stress
        Polycythemia NOS
        Relative polycythemia
        EXCLUDES 1   polycythemia neonatorum (P61.1)
                 polycythemia vera (D45)
        DEF: Elevated number of red blood cells in circulating blood as a result of reduced oxygen supply to the tissues.

☑5ᵗʰ **D75.8 Other specified diseases of blood and blood-forming organs**

        D75.81 Myelofibrosis   HCC
            Myelofibrosis NOS
            Secondary myelofibrosis NOS
            Code first the underlying disorder, such as:
                malignant neoplasm of breast (C50.-)
            Use additional code, if applicable, for associated therapy-related myelodysplastic syndrome (D46.-)
            Use additional code for adverse effect, if applicable, to identify drug (T45.1X5)
            EXCLUDES 1   acute myelofibrosis (C94.4-)
                   idiopathic myelofibrosis (D47.1)
                   leukoerythroblastic anemia (D61.82)
                   myelofibrosis with myeloid metaplasia (D47.4)
                   myelophthisic anemia (D61.82)
                   myelophthisis (D61.82)
                   primary myelofibrosis (D47.1)

        D75.82 Heparin induced thrombocytopenia (HIT)   HCC
            DEF: Immune-mediated reaction to heparin therapy causing an abrupt fall in platelet count and serious complications such as pulmonary embolism, stroke, AMI, or DVT.

        D75.89 Other specified diseases of blood and blood-forming organs

    D75.9 Disease of blood and blood-forming organs, unspecified   ▽

☑4ᵗʰ **D76 Other specified diseases with participation of lymphoreticular and reticulohistiocytic tissue**

    EXCLUDES 1   (Abt-) Letterer-Siwe disease (C96.0)
                 eosinophilic granuloma (C96.6)
                 Hand-Schüller-Christian disease (C96.5)
                 histiocytic medullary reticulosis (C96.9)
                 histiocytic sarcoma (C96.A)
                 histiocytosis X, multifocal (C96.5)
                 histiocytosis X, unifocal (C96.6)
                 Langerhans-cell histiocytosis, multifocal (C96.5)
                 Langerhans-cell histiocytosis NOS (C96.6)
                 Langerhans-cell histiocytosis, unifocal (C96.6)
                 leukemic reticuloendotheliosis (C91.4-)
                 lipomelanotic reticulosis (I89.8)
                 malignant histiocytosis (C96.A)
                 malignant reticulosis (C86.0)
                 nonlipid reticuloendotheliosis (C96.0)

    D76.1 Hemophagocytic lymphohistiocytosis   HCC
        Familial hemophagocytic reticulosis
        Histiocytoses of mononuclear phagocytes

    D76.2 Hemophagocytic syndrome, infection-associated   HCC
        Use additional code to identify infectious agent or disease

    D76.3 Other histiocytosis syndromes   HCC
        Reticulohistiocytoma (giant-cell)
        Sinus histiocytosis with massive lymphadenopathy
        Xanthogranuloma

D77 *Other disorders of blood and blood-forming organs in diseases classified elsewhere*

    Code first underlying disease, such as:
        amyloidosis (E85.-)
        congenital early syphilis (A50.0)
        echinococcosis (B67.0-B67.9)
        malaria (B50.0-B54)
        schistosomiasis [bilharziasis] (B65.0-B65.9)
        vitamin C deficiency (E54)
    EXCLUDES 1   rupture of spleen due to Plasmodium vivax malaria (B51.0)
                 splenitis, splenomegaly in late syphilis (A52.79)
                 splenitis, splenomegaly in tuberculosis (A18.85)

Intraoperative and postprocedural complications of the spleen (D78)

☑4ᵗʰ **D78 Intraoperative and postprocedural complications of the spleen**

    AHA: 2016,4Q,9-10

☑5ᵗʰ **D78.0 Intraoperative hemorrhage and hematoma of the spleen complicating a procedure**
        EXCLUDES 1   intraoperative hemorrhage and hematoma of the spleen due to accidental puncture or laceration during a procedure (D78.1-)

        D78.01 Intraoperative hemorrhage and hematoma of the spleen complicating a procedure on the spleen
        D78.02 Intraoperative hemorrhage and hematoma of the spleen complicating other procedure

☑5ᵗʰ **D78.1 Accidental puncture and laceration of the spleen during a procedure**
        D78.11 Accidental puncture and laceration of the spleen during a procedure on the spleen
        D78.12 Accidental puncture and laceration of the spleen during other procedure

☑5ᵗʰ **D78.2 Postprocedural hemorrhage of the spleen following a procedure**
        D78.21 Postprocedural hemorrhage of the spleen following a procedure on the spleen
        D78.22 Postprocedural hemorrhage of the spleen following other procedure

☑5ᵗʰ **D78.3 Postprocedural hematoma and seroma of the spleen following a procedure**
        D78.31 Postprocedural hematoma of the spleen following a procedure on the spleen
        D78.32 Postprocedural hematoma of the spleen following other procedure
        D78.33 Postprocedural seroma of the spleen following a procedure on the spleen
        D78.34 Postprocedural seroma of the spleen following other procedure

☑5ᵗʰ **D78.8 Other intraoperative and postprocedural complications of the spleen**
        Use additional code, if applicable, to further specify disorder
        D78.81 Other intraoperative complications of the spleen

---

☑ Additional Character Req   ✓x7ᵗʰ Placeholder Alert   Manifestation   ▽ Unspecified   ►◄ Revised Text   ● New Code   ▲ Revised Code Title

ICD-10-CM 2019   505

Chapter 3. Diseases of the Blood and Blood-forming Organs

D78.89   **Other postprocedural complications of the spleen**

Certain disorders involving the immune mechanism (D80-D89)

INCLUDES   defects in the complement system
immunodeficiency disorders, except human immunodeficiency
virus [HIV] disease
sarcoidosis

EXCLUDES 1   autoimmune disease (systemic) NOS (M35.9)
functional disorders of polymorphonuclear neutrophils (D71)
human immunodeficiency virus [HIV] disease (B20)

√4ᵗʰ **D80 Immunodeficiency with predominantly antibody defects**

D80.0   **Hereditary hypogammaglobulinemia**   HCC
Autosomal recessive agammaglobulinemia (Swiss type)
X-linked agammaglobulinemia [Bruton] (with growth hormone
deficiency)

D80.1   **Nonfamilial hypogammaglobulinemia**   HCC
Agammaglobulinemia with immunoglobulin-bearing
B-lymphocytes
Common variable agammaglobulinemia [CVAgamma]
Hypogammaglobulinemia NOS

D80.2   **Selective deficiency of immunoglobulin A [IgA]**   HCC

D80.3   **Selective deficiency of immunoglobulin G [IgG]
subclasses**   HCC

D80.4   **Selective deficiency of immunoglobulin M [IgM]**   HCC

D80.5   **Immunodeficiency with increased immunoglobulin
M [IgM]**   HCC

D80.6   **Antibody deficiency with near-normal
immunoglobulins or with hyperimmunoglobulinemia**   HCC

D80.7   **Transient hypogammaglobulinemia of infancy**   HCC

D80.8   **Other immunodeficiencies with predominantly
antibody defects**   HCC
Kappa light chain deficiency

D80.9   **Immunodeficiency with predominantly antibody
defects, unspecified**   HCC ▽

√4ᵗʰ **D81 Combined immunodeficiencies**

EXCLUDES 1   autosomal recessive agammaglobulinemia (Swiss type)
(D80.0)

D81.0   **Severe combined immunodeficiency [SCID] with
reticular dysgenesis**   HCC

D81.1   **Severe combined immunodeficiency [SCID] with low
T- and B-cell numbers**   HCC

D81.2   **Severe combined immunodeficiency [SCID] with low
or normal B-cell numbers**   HCC

D81.3   **Adenosine deaminase [ADA] deficiency**   HCC

D81.4   **Nezelof's syndrome**   HCC

D81.5   **Purine nucleoside phosphorylase [PNP] deficiency**   HCC

D81.6   **Major histocompatibility complex class I deficiency**   HCC
Bare lymphocyte syndrome

D81.7   **Major histocompatibility complex class II deficiency**   HCC

√5ᵗʰ D81.8   **Other combined immunodeficiencies**

√6ᵗʰ D81.81   **Biotin-dependent carboxylase deficiency**
Multiple carboxylase deficiency
EXCLUDES 1   biotin-dependent carboxylase deficiency
due to dietary deficiency of biotin
(E53.8)

D81.810   **Biotinidase deficiency**

D81.818   **Other biotin-dependent carboxylase
deficiency**
Holocarboxylase synthetase deficiency
Other multiple carboxylase deficiency

D81.819   **Biotin-dependent carboxylase
deficiency, unspecified** ▽
Multiple carboxylase deficiency,
unspecified

D81.89   **Other combined immunodeficiencies**   HCC

D81.9   **Combined immunodeficiency, unspecified**   HCC ▽
Severe combined immunodeficiency disorder [SCID] NOS

√4ᵗʰ **D82 Immunodeficiency associated with other major defects**

EXCLUDES 1   ataxia telangiectasia [Louis-Bar] (G11.3)

D82.0   **Wiskott-Aldrich syndrome**   HCC
Immunodeficiency with thrombocytopenia and eczema

D82.1   **Di George's syndrome**   HCC
Pharyngeal pouch syndrome
Thymic alymphoplasia
Thymic aplasia or hypoplasia with immunodeficiency

D82.2   **Immunodeficiency with short-limbed stature**   HCC

D82.3   **Immunodeficiency following hereditary defective
response to Epstein-Barr virus**   HCC
X-linked lymphoproliferative disease

D82.4   **Hyperimmunoglobulin E [IgE] syndrome**   HCC

D82.8   **Immunodeficiency associated with other specified
major defects**   HCC

D82.9   **Immunodeficiency associated with major defect,
unspecified**   HCC ▽

√4ᵗʰ **D83 Common variable immunodeficiency**

D83.0   **Common variable immunodeficiency with
predominant abnormalities of B-cell numbers and
function**   HCC

D83.1   **Common variable immunodeficiency with
predominant immunoregulatory T-cell disorders**   HCC

D83.2   **Common variable immunodeficiency with
autoantibodies to B- or T-cells**   HCC

D83.8   **Other common variable immunodeficiencies**   HCC

D83.9   **Common variable immunodeficiency, unspecified**   HCC ▽

√4ᵗʰ **D84 Other immunodeficiencies**

D84.0   **Lymphocyte function antigen-1 [LFA-1] defect**   HCC

D84.1   **Defects in the complement system**   HCC
C1 esterase inhibitor [C1-INH] deficiency

D84.8   **Other specified immunodeficiencies**   HCC

D84.9   **Immunodeficiency, unspecified**   HCC ▽

√4ᵗʰ **D86 Sarcoidosis**

D86.0   **Sarcoidosis of lung**   HCC

D86.1   **Sarcoidosis of lymph nodes**

D86.2   **Sarcoidosis of lung with sarcoidosis of lymph nodes**   HCC

D86.3   **Sarcoidosis of skin**

√5ᵗʰ D86.8   **Sarcoidosis of other sites**

D86.81   **Sarcoid meningitis**

D86.82   **Multiple cranial nerve palsies in sarcoidosis**   HCC

D86.83   **Sarcoid iridocyclitis**

D86.84   **Sarcoid pyelonephritis**
Tubulo-interstitial nephropathy in sarcoidosis

D86.85   **Sarcoid myocarditis**

D86.86   **Sarcoid arthropathy**
Polyarthritis in sarcoidosis

D86.87   **Sarcoid myositis**

D86.89   **Sarcoidosis of other sites**
Hepatic granuloma
Uveoparotid fever [Heerfordt]

D86.9   **Sarcoidosis, unspecified** ▽

√4ᵗʰ **D89 Other disorders involving the immune mechanism, not elsewhere
classified**

EXCLUDES 1   hyperglobulinemia NOS (R77.1)
monoclonal gammopathy (of undetermined significance)
(D47.2)

EXCLUDES 2   transplant failure and rejection (T86.-)

D89.0   **Polyclonal hypergammaglobulinemia**
Benign hypergammaglobulinemic purpura
Polyclonal gammopathy NOS

D89.1   **Cryoglobulinemia**   HCC
Cryoglobulinemic purpura
Cryoglobulinemic vasculitis
Essential cryoglobulinemia
Idiopathic cryoglobulinemia
Mixed cryoglobulinemia
Primary cryoglobulinemia
Secondary cryoglobulinemia

D89.2   **Hypergammaglobulinemia, unspecified** ▽

D89.3   **Immune reconstitution syndrome**   HCC
Immune reconstitution inflammatory syndrome [IRIS]
Use additional code for adverse effect, if applicable, to identify
drug (T36-T50 with fifth or sixth character 5)

HCC CMS-HCC   Q QPP   N Newborn : 0   P Pediatric : 0-17   M Maternity : 12-55   A Adult : 15-124

√5ᵗʰ **D89.4** **Mast cell activation syndrome and related disorders**

EXCLUDES 1   *aggressive systemic mastocytosis (C96.21)*
congenital cutaneous mastocytosis (Q82.2)
(non-congenital) cutaneous mastocytosis (D47.01)
(indolent) systemic mastocytosis (D47.02)
malignant mast cell neoplasm (C96.2-)
malignant mastocytoma (C96.29)
mastocytoma NOS (D47.09)
mast cell leukemia (C94.3-)
mast cell sarcoma (C96.22)
other mast cell neoplasms of uncertain behavior
    (D47.09)
systemic mastocytosis associated with a clonal
    hematologic non-mast cell lineage disease
    (SM-AHNMD) (D47.02)

AHA: 2016,4Q,11

D89.40 **Mast cell activation, unspecified**   HCC ▽
Mast cell activation disorder, unspecified
Mast cell activation syndrome, NOS

D89.41 **Monoclonal mast cell activation syndrome**   HCC

D89.42 **Idiopathic mast cell activation syndrome**   HCC

D89.43 **Secondary mast cell activation**   HCC
Secondary mast cell activation syndrome
Code also underlying etiology, if known

D89.49 **Other mast cell activation disorder**   HCC
Other mast cell activation syndrome

√5ᵗʰ **D89.8** **Other specified disorders involving the immune mechanism, not elsewhere classified**

√6ᵗʰ **D89.81** **Graft-versus-host disease**
Code first underlying cause, such as:
    complications of transplanted organs and tissue
      (T86.-)
    complications of blood transfusion (T80.89)
Use additional code to identify associated
    manifestations, such as:
    desquamative dermatitis (L30.8)
    diarrhea (R19.7)
    elevated bilirubin (R17)
    hair loss (L65.9)

D89.810 **Acute graft-versus-host disease**   HCC

D89.811 **Chronic graft-versus-host disease**   HCC

D89.812 **Acute on chronic**   HCC
graft-versus-host disease

D89.813 **Graft-versus-host disease,**   HCC ▽
unspecified

D89.82 **Autoimmune lymphoproliferative**   HCC
syndrome [ALPS]
DEF: Rare genetic alteration of the Fas protein that
impairs normal cellular apoptosis (normal cell death),
causing abnormal accumulation of lymphocytes in the
lymph glands, liver, and spleen. Symptoms include
neutropenia, anemia, and thrombocytopenia.

D89.89 **Other specified disorders involving the**   HCC
immune mechanism, not elsewhere
classified
EXCLUDES 1   *human immunodeficiency virus disease*
    (B20)
AHA: 2017,4Q,109

D89.9 **Disorder involving the immune mechanism,**   HCC ▽
unspecified
Immune disease NOS
AHA: 2015,3Q,22

Chapter 4. Endocrine, Nutritional, and Metabolic Diseases (E00–E89)

Chapter Specific Guidelines with Coding Examples

The chapter specific guidelines from the ICD-10-CM Official Guidelines for Coding and Reporting have been provided below. Along with these guidelines are coding examples, contained in the shaded boxes, that have been developed to help illustrate the coding and/or sequencing guidance found in these guidelines.

a. Diabetes mellitus

The diabetes mellitus codes are combination codes that include the type of diabetes mellitus, the body system affected, and the complications affecting that body system. As many codes within a particular category as are necessary to describe all of the complications of the disease may be used. They should be sequenced based on the reason for a particular encounter. Assign as many codes from categories E08–E13 as needed to identify all of the associated conditions that the patient has.

> Patient is seen for uncontrolled diabetes, type 2, with hyperglycemia diabetic nephropathy, and diabetic gastroparesis
>
> **E11.65**   **Type 2 diabetes mellitus with hyperglycemia**
>
> **E11.21**   **Type 2 diabetes mellitus with diabetic nephropathy**
>
> **E11.43**   **Type 2 diabetes mellitus with diabetic autonomic (poly)neuropathy**
>
> **K31.84**   **Gastroparesis**
>
> *Explanation*: Use as many codes to describe the diabetic complications as needed. Many are combination codes that describe more than one condition. Code first the reason for the encounter. The term "uncontrolled" can refer to either hyperglycemia or hypoglycemia. In this case, "uncontrolled" is described as "with hyperglycemia."

1) Type of diabetes

The age of a patient is not the sole determining factor, though most type 1 diabetics develop the condition before reaching puberty. For this reason type 1 diabetes mellitus is also referred to as juvenile diabetes.

> A 45-year-old patient is diagnosed with type 1 diabetes
>
> **E10.9**   **Type 1 diabetes mellitus without complications**
>
> *Explanation*: Although most type 1 diabetics are diagnosed in childhood or adolescence, it can also begin in adults.

2) Type of diabetes mellitus not documented

If the type of diabetes mellitus is not documented in the medical record the default is E11.-, Type 2 diabetes mellitus.

> Office visit lists diabetic retinopathy with macular edema and hypertension on patient problem list
>
> **E11.311**   **Type 2 diabetes mellitus with unspecified diabetic retinopathy with macular edema**
>
> **I10**   **Essential (primary) hypertension**
>
> *Explanation*: Since the type of diabetes was not documented, default to category E11.

3) Diabetes mellitus and the use of insulin and oral hypoglycemics

If the documentation in a medical record does not indicate the type of diabetes but does indicate that the patient uses insulin, code E11-, Type 2 diabetes mellitus, should be assigned. An additional code should be assigned from category Z79 to identify the long-term (current) use of insulin or oral hypoglycemic drugs. If the patient is treated with both oral medications and insulin, only the code for long-term (current) use of insulin should be assigned. Code Z79.4 should not be assigned if insulin is given temporarily to bring a type 2 patient's blood sugar under control during an encounter.

> Office visit lists chronic diabetes with daily insulin use on patient problem list
>
> **E11.9**   **Type 2 diabetes mellitus without complications**
>
> **Z79.4**   **Long term (current) use of insulin**
>
> *Explanation*: Do not assume that a patient on insulin must have type 1 diabetes. The default for diabetes without further specification defaults to type 2. Add the code for long term use of insulin.

4) Diabetes mellitus in pregnancy and gestational diabetes

See Section I.C.15. Diabetes mellitus in pregnancy.

See Section I.C.15. Gestational (pregnancy induced) diabetes

5) Complications due to insulin pump malfunction
(a) Underdose of insulin due to insulin pump failure

An underdose of insulin due to an insulin pump failure should be assigned to a code from subcategory T85.6, Mechanical complication of other specified internal and external prosthetic devices, implants and grafts, that specifies the type of pump malfunction, as the principal or first-listed code, followed by code T38.3X6-, Underdosing of insulin and oral hypoglycemic [antidiabetic] drugs. Additional codes for the type of diabetes mellitus and any associated complications due to the underdosing should also be assigned.

> A 24-year-old type 1 diabetic male treated in for hyperglycemia; insulin pump found to be malfunctioning and underdosing
>
> **T85.614A**   **Breakdown (mechanical) of insulin pump, initial encounter**
>
> **T38.3X6A**   **Underdosing of insulin and oral hypoglycemic [antidiabetic] drugs, initial encounter**
>
> **E10.65**   **Type 1 diabetes mellitus with hyperglycemia**
>
> *Explanation*: The complication code for the mechanical breakdown of the pump is sequenced first, followed by the underdosing code and type of diabetes with complication. Code all other diabetic complication codes necessary to describe the patient's condition.

(b) Overdose of insulin due to insulin pump failure

The principal or first-listed code for an encounter due to an insulin pump malfunction resulting in an overdose of insulin, should also be T85.6-, Mechanical complication of other specified internal and external prosthetic devices, implants and grafts, followed by code T38.3X1-, Poisoning by insulin and oral hypoglycemic [antidiabetic] drugs, accidental (unintentional).

> A 24-year-old type 1 diabetic male found down with diabetic coma, brought into ED and treated for hypoglycemia; insulin pump found to be malfunctioning and overdosing
>
> **T85.614A**   **Breakdown (mechanical) of insulin pump, initial encounter**
>
> **T38.3X1A**   **Poisoning by insulin and oral hypoglycemic [antidiabetic] drugs, accidental (unintentional), initial encounter**
>
> **E10.641**   **Type 1 diabetes mellitus with hypoglycemia with coma**
>
> *Explanation*: The complication code for the mechanical breakdown of the pump is sequenced first, followed by the poisoning code and type of diabetes with complication. All the characters in the combination code must be used to form a valid code and to fully describe the type of diabetes, the hypoglycemia, and the coma.

6) Secondary diabetes mellitus

Codes under categories E08, Diabetes mellitus due to underlying condition, E09, Drug or chemical induced diabetes mellitus, and E13, Other specified diabetes mellitus, identify complications/manifestations associated with secondary diabetes mellitus. Secondary diabetes is always caused by another condition or event (e.g., cystic fibrosis, malignant neoplasm of pancreas, pancreatectomy, adverse effect of drug, or poisoning).

(a) Secondary diabetes mellitus and the use of insulin or oral hypoglycemic drugs

For patients with secondary diabetes mellitus who routinely use insulin or oral hypoglycemic drugs, an additional code from category Z79 should be assigned to identify the long-term (current) use of insulin or oral hypoglycemic drugs. If the patient is treated with both oral medications and insulin, only the code for long-term (current) use of insulin should be assigned. Code Z79.4 should not be assigned if insulin is given temporarily to bring a secondary diabetic patient's blood sugar under control during an encounter.

> Type 2 diabetic with no complications, normally only on oral metformin, is given insulin for three days to maintain glucose control while in the hospital recovering from surgery
>
> **E11.9**   **Type 2 diabetes mellitus without complications**
>
> **Z79.84**   **Long term (current) use of oral hypoglycemic drugs**
>
> *Explanation*: Although the patient was given insulin for a short time during his hospital stay, the intent was only to maintain the patient's glucose levels while off his regular oral hypoglycemic medication, not for long term use. No code is needed for long term use of insulin, but a Z code for long term use of an oral hypoglycemic should be added to identify the chronic use of this drug.

> Type 2 diabetic with diabetic polyneuropathy on insulin
>
> **E11.42**   **Type 2 diabetes mellitus with diabetic polyneuropathy**
>
> **Z79.4**   **Long term (current) use of insulin**
>
> *Explanation*: Add the Z code for the long term use of insulin because the insulin is taken chronically.

(b) Assigning and sequencing secondary diabetes codes and its causes

The sequencing of the secondary diabetes codes in relationship to codes for the cause of the diabetes is based on the Tabular List instructions for categories E08, E09 and E13.

(i) Secondary diabetes mellitus due to pancreatectomy

For postpancreatectomy diabetes mellitus (lack of insulin due to the surgical removal of all or part of the pancreas), assign code E89.1, Postprocedural hypoinsulinemia. Assign a code from category E13 and a code from subcategory Z90.41-, Acquired absence of pancreas, as additional codes.

> Patient with newly diagnosed diabetes after surgical removal of part of pancreas
>
> **E89.1**   **Postprocedural hypoinsulinemia**
>
> **E13.9**   **Other specified diabetes mellitus without complications**
>
> **Z90.411**   **Acquired partial absence of pancreas**
>
> *Explanation*: Sequence the postprocedural complication of the hypoinsulinemia due to the partial removal of the pancreas as the first-listed code, followed by the other specified diabetes (NEC) with or without complications and the partial or total acquired absence of the pancreas.

(ii) Secondary diabetes due to drugs

Secondary diabetes may be caused by an adverse effect of correctly administered medications, poisoning or sequela of poisoning.

See section I.C.19.e for coding of adverse effects and poisoning, and section I.C.20 for external cause code reporting.

> Initial encounter for corticosteroid-induced diabetes mellitus
>
> **E09.9**   **Drug or chemical induced diabetes mellitus without complications**
>
> **T38.0X5A**   **Adverse effect of glucocorticoids and synthetic analogues, initial encounter**
>
> *Explanation*: If the diabetes is caused by an adverse effect of a drug, the diabetic condition is coded first. If it occurs from a poisoning or overdose, the poisoning code causing the diabetes is sequenced first.

Chapter 4. Endocrine, Nutritional and Metabolic Diseases (E00-E89)

> **NOTE** All neoplasms, whether functionally active or not, are classified in Chapter 2. Appropriate codes in this chapter (i.e.E05.8, E07.0, E16-E31, E34.-) may be used as additional codes to indicate either functional activity by neoplasms and ectopic endocrine tissue or hyperfunction and hypofunction of endocrine glands associated with neoplasms and other conditions classified elsewhere.

> **EXCLUDES 1** transitory endocrine and metabolic disorders specific to newborn (P70-P74)

AHA: 2018,2Q,6

This chapter contains the following blocks:

E00-E07   Disorders of thyroid gland
E08-E13   Diabetes mellitus
E15-E16   Other disorders of glucose regulation and pancreatic internal secretion
E20-E35   Disorders of other endocrine glands
E36   Intraoperative complications of endocrine system
E40-E46   Malnutrition
E50-E64   Other nutritional deficiencies
E65-E68   Overweight, obesity and other hyperalimentation
E70-E88   Metabolic disorders
E89   Postprocedural endocrine and metabolic complications and disorders, not elsewhere classified

Disorders of thyroid gland (E00-E07)

✓4ᵗʰ **E00 Congenital iodine-deficiency syndrome**

> Use additional code (F70-F79) to identify associated intellectual disabilities
> **EXCLUDES 1** subclinical iodine-deficiency hypothyroidism (E02)

E00.0 Congenital iodine-deficiency syndrome, neurological type
Endemic cretinism, neurological type

E00.1 Congenital iodine-deficiency syndrome, myxedematous type
Endemic hypothyroid cretinism
Endemic cretinism, myxedematous type

E00.2 Congenital iodine-deficiency syndrome, mixed type
Endemic cretinism, mixed type

E00.9 Congenital iodine-deficiency syndrome, unspecified   ▽
Congenital iodine-deficiency hypothyroidism NOS
Endemic cretinism NOS

✓4ᵗʰ **E01 Iodine-deficiency related thyroid disorders and allied conditions**

> **EXCLUDES 1** congenital iodine-deficiency syndrome (E00.-)
> subclinical iodine-deficiency hypothyroidism (E02)

E01.0 Iodine-deficiency related diffuse (endemic) goiter

E01.1 Iodine-deficiency related multinodular (endemic) goiter
Iodine-deficiency related nodular goiter

E01.2 Iodine-deficiency related (endemic) goiter, unspecified   ▽
Endemic goiter NOS

E01.8 Other iodine-deficiency related thyroid disorders and allied conditions
Acquired iodine-deficiency hypothyroidism NOS

E02 Subclinical iodine-deficiency hypothyroidism

✓4ᵗʰ **E03 Other hypothyroidism**

> **EXCLUDES 1** iodine-deficiency related hypothyroidism (E00-E02)
> postprocedural hypothyroidism (E89.0)

E03.0 Congenital hypothyroidism with diffuse goiter
Congenital parenchymatous goiter (nontoxic)
Congenital goiter (nontoxic) NOS
> **EXCLUDES 1** transitory congenital goiter with normal function (P72.0)

E03.1 Congenital hypothyroidism without goiter
Aplasia of thyroid (with myxedema)
Congenital atrophy of thyroid
Congenital hypothyroidism NOS

E03.2 Hypothyroidism due to medicaments and other exogenous substances
Code first poisoning due to drug or toxin, if applicable (T36-T65 with fifth or sixth character 1-4 or 6)
Use additional code for adverse effect, if applicable, to identify drug (T36-T50 with fifth or sixth character 5)

E03.3 Postinfectious hypothyroidism

E03.4 Atrophy of thyroid (acquired)
> **EXCLUDES 1** congenital atrophy of thyroid (E03.1)

E03.5 Myxedema coma   HCC

E03.8 Other specified hypothyroidism

E03.9 Hypothyroidism, unspecified   ▽
Myxedema NOS

✓4ᵗʰ **E04 Other nontoxic goiter**

> **EXCLUDES 1** congenital goiter (NOS) (diffuse) (parenchymatous) (E03.0)
> iodine-deficiency related goiter (E00-E02)

E04.0 Nontoxic diffuse goiter
Diffuse (colloid) nontoxic goiter
Simple nontoxic goiter

E04.1 Nontoxic single thyroid nodule
Colloid nodule (cystic) (thyroid)
Nontoxic uninodular goiter
Thyroid (cystic) nodule NOS
DEF: Enlarged thyroid, commonly due to decreased thyroid production, with a single nodule. No clinical hypothyroidism.

E04.2 Nontoxic multinodular goiter
Cystic goiter NOS
Multinodular (cystic) goiter NOS
DEF: Enlarged thyroid, commonly due to decreased thyroid production with multiple nodules. No clinical hypothyroidism.

E04.8 Other specified nontoxic goiter

E04.9 Nontoxic goiter, unspecified   ▽
Goiter NOS
Nodular goiter (nontoxic) NOS

✓4ᵗʰ **E05 Thyrotoxicosis [hyperthyroidism]**

> **EXCLUDES 1** chronic thyroiditis with transient thyrotoxicosis (E06.2)
> neonatal thyrotoxicosis (P72.1)

DEF: Excessive quantities of hormones from the thyroid gland caused by overproduction or loss of storage ability.

✓5ᵗʰ **E05.0 Thyrotoxicosis with diffuse goiter**
Exophthalmic or toxic goiter NOS
Graves' disease
Toxic diffuse goiter
DEF: Diffuse thyroid enlargement accompanied by hyperthyroidism, bulging eyes, and dermopathy.

E05.00 Thyrotoxicosis with diffuse goiter without thyrotoxic crisis or storm

E05.01 Thyrotoxicosis with diffuse goiter with thyrotoxic crisis or storm

Goiter

Pyramidal lobe
Thyroid cartilage
Healthy thyroid
Goiter (hyperfunctioning thyroid)

✓5ᵗʰ **E05.1 Thyrotoxicosis with toxic single thyroid nodule**
Thyrotoxicosis with toxic uninodular goiter
DEF: Symptomatic hyperthyroidism with a single nodule on the enlarged thyroid gland. Onset of symptoms can be abrupt and include extreme nervousness, insomnia, weight loss, tremors, and psychosis or coma.

E05.10 Thyrotoxicosis with toxic single thyroid nodule without thyrotoxic crisis or storm

E05.11 Thyrotoxicosis with toxic single thyroid nodule with thyrotoxic crisis or storm

✓5ᵗʰ **E05.2 Thyrotoxicosis with toxic multinodular goiter**
Toxic nodular goiter NOS

E05.20 Thyrotoxicosis with toxic multinodular goiter without thyrotoxic crisis or storm

E05.21 Thyrotoxicosis with toxic multinodular goiter with thyrotoxic crisis or storm

✓5ᵗʰ **E05.3 Thyrotoxicosis from ectopic thyroid tissue**

E05.30 Thyrotoxicosis from ectopic thyroid tissue without thyrotoxic crisis or storm

E05.31 Thyrotoxicosis from ectopic thyroid tissue with thyrotoxic crisis or storm

√5ᵗʰ **E05.4 Thyrotoxicosis factitia**

E05.40   **Thyrotoxicosis factitia** without thyrotoxic crisis or storm

E05.41   **Thyrotoxicosis factitia** with thyrotoxic crisis or storm

√5ᵗʰ **E05.8 Other thyrotoxicosis**

Overproduction of thyroid-stimulating hormone

E05.80   **Other thyrotoxicosis** without thyrotoxic crisis or storm

E05.81   **Other thyrotoxicosis** with thyrotoxic crisis or storm

√5ᵗʰ **E05.9 Thyrotoxicosis, unspecified**

Hyperthyroidism NOS

E05.90   **Thyrotoxicosis, unspecified** without thyrotoxic crisis or storm   ▽

E05.91   **Thyrotoxicosis, unspecified** with thyrotoxic crisis or storm   ▽

√4ᵗʰ **E06 Thyroiditis**

> **EXCLUDES 1**   *postpartum thyroiditis (O90.5)*
>
> **DEF:** Inflammation of the thyroid gland.

E06.0   **Acute thyroiditis**

Abscess of thyroid
Pyogenic thyroiditis
Suppurative thyroiditis
Use additional code (B95-B97) to identify infectious agent

E06.1   **Subacute thyroiditis**

de Quervain thyroiditis
Giant-cell thyroiditis
Granulomatous thyroiditis
Nonsuppurative thyroiditis
Viral thyroiditis

> **EXCLUDES 1**   *autoimmune thyroiditis (E06.3)*

E06.2   **Chronic thyroiditis with transient thyrotoxicosis**

> **EXCLUDES 1**   *autoimmune thyroiditis (E06.3)*

E06.3   **Autoimmune thyroiditis**

Hashimoto's thyroiditis
Hashitoxicosis (transient)
Lymphadenoid goiter
Lymphocytic thyroiditis
Struma lymphomatosa

E06.4   **Drug-induced thyroiditis**

Use additional code for adverse effect, if applicable, to identify drug (T36-T50 with fifth or sixth character 5)

E06.5   **Other chronic thyroiditis**

Chronic fibrous thyroiditis
Chronic thyroiditis NOS
Ligneous thyroiditis
Riedel thyroiditis

E06.9   **Thyroiditis, unspecified**   ▽

√4ᵗʰ **E07 Other disorders of thyroid**

E07.0   **Hypersecretion of calcitonin**

C-cell hyperplasia of thyroid
Hypersecretion of thyrocalcitonin

E07.1   **Dyshormogenetic goiter**

Familial dyshormogenetic goiter
Pendred's syndrome

> **EXCLUDES 1**   *transitory congenital goiter with normal function (P72.0)*

√5ᵗʰ **E07.8 Other specified disorders of thyroid**

E07.81   **Sick-euthyroid syndrome**

Euthyroid sick-syndrome

DEF: Thyroid dysfunction caused by abnormal levels of thyroid hormones T3 and/or T4. This syndrome is often associated with starvation or critical illness.

E07.89   **Other specified disorders of thyroid**

Abnormality of thyroid-binding globulin
Hemorrhage of thyroid
Infarction of thyroid

E07.9   **Disorder of thyroid, unspecified**   ▽

Diabetes mellitus (E08-E13)

AHA: 2018,2Q,6; 2017,4Q,6; 2017,1Q,42; 2016,4Q,11-13; 2016,2Q,36; 2016,1Q,11-13

TIP: There is no default code for diabetes mellitus documented only as uncontrolled. The provider must indicate whether the diabetic patient is hypoglycemic or hyperglycemic to determine the appropriate code.

√4ᵗʰ **E08 Diabetes mellitus due to underlying condition**

Code first the underlying condition, such as:
 congenital rubella (P35.0)
 Cushing's syndrome (E24.-)
 cystic fibrosis (E84.-)
 malignant neoplasm (C00-C96)
 malnutrition (E40-E46)
 pancreatitis and other diseases of the pancreas (K85-K86.-)
Use additional code to identify control using:
 insulin (Z79.4)
 oral antidiabetic drugs (Z79.84)
 oral hypoglycemic drugs (Z79.84)

> **EXCLUDES 1**   *drug or chemical induced diabetes mellitus (E09.-)*
> *gestational diabetes (O24.4-)*
> *neonatal diabetes mellitus (P70.2)*
> *postpancreatectomy diabetes mellitus (E13.-)*
> *postprocedural diabetes mellitus (E13.-)*
> *secondary diabetes mellitus NEC (E13.-)*
> *type 1 diabetes mellitus (E10.-)*
> *type 2 diabetes mellitus (E11.-)*

AHA: 2013,4Q,114; 2013,3Q,20

√5ᵗʰ **E08.0 Diabetes mellitus due to underlying condition with hyperosmolarity**

DEF: Diabetic hyperosmolarity: Extremely high levels of glucose in the blood without ketones.

E08.00   *Diabetes mellitus due to underlying condition with hyperosmolarity without nonketotic hyperglycemic-hyperosmolar coma (NKHHC)*   ʜᴄᴄ

E08.01   *Diabetes mellitus due to underlying condition with hyperosmolarity with coma*   ʜᴄᴄ

√5ᵗʰ **E08.1 Diabetes mellitus due to underlying condition with ketoacidosis**

DEF: Diabetic ketoacidosis: Potentially life-threatening complication due to a shortage of insulin in which the body switches to burning fatty acids and producing acidic ketone bodies.

E08.10   *Diabetes mellitus due to underlying condition with ketoacidosis without coma*   ʜᴄᴄ

E08.11   *Diabetes mellitus due to underlying condition with ketoacidosis with coma*   ʜᴄᴄ

√5ᵗʰ **E08.2 Diabetes mellitus due to underlying condition with kidney complications**

E08.21   *Diabetes mellitus due to underlying condition with diabetic nephropathy*   ʜᴄᴄ

Diabetes mellitus due to underlying condition with intercapillary glomerulosclerosis
Diabetes mellitus due to underlying condition with intracapillary glomerulonephrosis
Diabetes mellitus due to underlying condition with Kimmelstiel-Wilson disease

E08.22   *Diabetes mellitus due to underlying condition with diabetic chronic kidney disease*   ʜᴄᴄ

Use additional code to identify stage of chronic kidney disease (N18.1-N18.6)

E08.29   *Diabetes mellitus due to underlying condition with other diabetic kidney complication*   ʜᴄᴄ

Renal tubular degeneration in diabetes mellitus due to underlying condition

✓5th **E08.3** **Diabetes mellitus due to underlying condition with ophthalmic complications**

> One of the following 7th characters is to be assigned to codes in subcategories E08.32, E08.33, E08.34, E08.35, and E08.37 to designate laterality of the disease:
> 1   right eye
> 2   left eye
> 3   bilateral
> 9   unspecified eye

✓6th **E08.31** **Diabetes mellitus due to underlying condition with unspecified diabetic retinopathy**
> **DEF:** Diabetic retinopathy: Diabetic complication from damage to the retinal vessels resulting in vision problems that can progress to blindness.

     E08.311   *Diabetes mellitus due to underlying condition with unspecified diabetic retinopathy with macular edema*   HCC Q ▽

     E08.319   *Diabetes mellitus due to underlying condition with unspecified diabetic retinopathy without macular edema*   HCC Q ▽

✓6th **E08.32** **Diabetes mellitus due to underlying condition with mild nonproliferative diabetic retinopathy**
> Diabetes mellitus due to underlying condition with nonproliferative diabetic retinopathy NOS

     ✓7th *E08.321*   *Diabetes mellitus due to underlying condition with mild nonproliferative diabetic retinopathy with macular edema*   HCC Q

     ✓7th *E08.329*   *Diabetes mellitus due to underlying condition with mild nonproliferative diabetic retinopathy without macular edema*   HCC Q

✓6th **E08.33** **Diabetes mellitus due to underlying condition with moderate nonproliferative diabetic retinopathy**

     ✓7th *E08.331*   *Diabetes mellitus due to underlying condition with moderate nonproliferative diabetic retinopathy with macular edema*   HCC Q

     ✓7th *E08.339*   *Diabetes mellitus due to underlying condition with moderate nonproliferative diabetic retinopathy without macular edema*   HCC Q

✓6th **E08.34** **Diabetes mellitus due to underlying condition with severe nonproliferative diabetic retinopathy**

     ✓7th *E08.341*   *Diabetes mellitus due to underlying condition with severe nonproliferative diabetic retinopathy with macular edema*   HCC Q

     ✓7th *E08.349*   *Diabetes mellitus due to underlying condition with severe nonproliferative diabetic retinopathy without macular edema*   HCC Q

✓6th **E08.35** **Diabetes mellitus due to underlying condition with proliferative diabetic retinopathy**

     ✓7th *E08.351*   *Diabetes mellitus due to underlying condition with proliferative diabetic retinopathy with macular edema*   HCC Q

     ✓7th *E08.352*   *Diabetes mellitus due to underlying condition with proliferative diabetic retinopathy with traction retinal detachment involving the macula*   HCC Q

     ✓7th *E08.353*   *Diabetes mellitus due to underlying condition with proliferative diabetic retinopathy with traction retinal detachment not involving the macula*   HCC Q

     ✓7th *E08.354*   *Diabetes mellitus due to underlying condition with proliferative diabetic retinopathy with combined traction retinal detachment and rhegmatogenous retinal detachment*   HCC Q

     ✓7th *E08.355*   *Diabetes mellitus due to underlying condition with stable proliferative diabetic retinopathy*   HCC Q

     ✓7th *E08.359*   *Diabetes mellitus due to underlying condition with proliferative diabetic retinopathy without macular edema*   HCC Q

   E08.36   *Diabetes mellitus due to underlying condition with diabetic cataract*   HCC
> **AHA:** 2016,4Q,142

   ✓x7th *E08.37*   *Diabetes mellitus due to underlying condition with diabetic macular edema, resolved following treatment*   HCC

   E08.39   *Diabetes mellitus due to underlying condition with other diabetic ophthalmic complication*   HCC
> Use additional code to identify manifestation, such as:
>   diabetic glaucoma (H40-H42)

✓5th **E08.4** **Diabetes mellitus due to underlying condition with neurological complications**

   E08.40   *Diabetes mellitus due to underlying condition with diabetic neuropathy, unspecified*   HCC ▽

   E08.41   *Diabetes mellitus due to underlying condition with diabetic mononeuropathy*   HCC

   E08.42   *Diabetes mellitus due to underlying condition with diabetic polyneuropathy*   HCC
> Diabetes mellitus due to underlying condition with diabetic neuralgia

   E08.43   *Diabetes mellitus due to underlying condition with diabetic autonomic (poly)neuropathy*   HCC
> Diabetes mellitus due to underlying condition with diabetic gastroparesis
> **AHA:** 2013,4Q,114

   E08.44   *Diabetes mellitus due to underlying condition with diabetic amyotrophy*   HCC

   E08.49   *Diabetes mellitus due to underlying condition with other diabetic neurological complication*   HCC

✓5th **E08.5** **Diabetes mellitus due to underlying condition with circulatory complications**

   E08.51   *Diabetes mellitus due to underlying condition with diabetic peripheral angiopathy without gangrene*   HCC
> **AHA:** 2018,2Q,7

   E08.52   *Diabetes mellitus due to underlying condition with diabetic peripheral angiopathy with gangrene*   HCC
> Diabetes mellitus due to underlying condition with diabetic gangrene
> **AHA:** 2018,2Q,7; 2017,4Q,102

   E08.59   *Diabetes mellitus due to underlying condition with other circulatory complications*   HCC

✓5th **E08.6** **Diabetes mellitus due to underlying condition with other specified complications**

✓6th **E08.61** **Diabetes mellitus due to underlying condition with diabetic arthropathy**

     E08.610   *Diabetes mellitus due to underlying condition with diabetic neuropathic arthropathy*   HCC
> Diabetes mellitus due to underlying condition with Charcôt's joints
> **DEF:** Charcot's joint: Progressive neurologic arthropathy in which chronic degeneration of joints in the weight-bearing areas with peripheral hypertrophy occurs as a complication of a neuropathy disorder. Supporting structures relax from a loss of sensation resulting in chronic joint instability.

     E08.618   *Diabetes mellitus due to underlying condition with other diabetic arthropathy*   HCC
> **AHA:** 2018,2Q,6

✓6th **E08.62** **Diabetes mellitus due to underlying condition with skin complications**

     E08.620   *Diabetes mellitus due to underlying condition with diabetic dermatitis*   HCC
> Diabetes mellitus due to underlying condition with diabetic necrobiosis lipoidica

☑ Additional Character Req   ✓x7th Placeholder Alert   Manifestation   ▽ Unspecified   ►◄ Revised Text   ● New Code   ▲ Revised Code Title

ICD-10-CM 2019   513

Chapter 4. Endocrine, Nutritional and Metabolic Diseases

E08.621   *Diabetes mellitus due to underlying condition with foot ulcer*   HCC

Use additional code to identify site of ulcer (L97.4-, L97.5-)

TIP: Do not assign a code for diabetic ulcer when the ulcer is closed/resolved or to report history of diabetic ulcers; Z86.31 Personal history of diabetic foot ulcer, may be assigned.

E08.622   *Diabetes mellitus due to underlying condition with other skin ulcer*   HCC

Use additional code to identify site of ulcer (L97.1-L97.9, L98.41-L98.49)

AHA: 2017,4Q,17

E08.628   *Diabetes mellitus due to underlying condition with other skin complications*   HCC

AHA: 2017,4Q,100-101

√6ᵗʰ **E08.63**   **Diabetes mellitus due to underlying condition with oral complications**

E08.630   *Diabetes mellitus due to underlying condition with periodontal disease*   HCC

E08.638   *Diabetes mellitus due to underlying condition with other oral complications*   HCC

√6ᵗʰ **E08.64**   **Diabetes mellitus due to underlying condition with hypoglycemia**

E08.641   *Diabetes mellitus due to underlying condition with hypoglycemia with coma*   HCC

E08.649   *Diabetes mellitus due to underlying condition with hypoglycemia without coma*   HCC

AHA: 2016,3Q,42; 2015,3Q,21

E08.65   *Diabetes mellitus due to underlying condition with hyperglycemia*   HCC

E08.69   *Diabetes mellitus due to underlying condition with other specified complication*   HCC

Use additional code to identify complication

AHA: 2016,4Q,141; 2016,1Q,13

E08.8   *Diabetes mellitus due to underlying condition with unspecified complications*   HCC ▽

E08.9   *Diabetes mellitus due to underlying condition without complications*   HCC

√4ᵗʰ **E09**   **Drug or chemical induced diabetes mellitus**

Code first poisoning due to drug or toxin, if applicable (T36-T65 with fifth or sixth character 1-4 or 6)

Use additional code for adverse effect, if applicable, to identify drug (T36-T50 with fifth or sixth character 5)

Use additional code to identify control using:

insulin (Z79.4)

oral antidiabetic drugs (Z79.84)

oral hypoglycemic drugs (Z79.84)

EXCLUDES 1   *diabetes mellitus due to underlying condition (E08.-)*

gestational diabetes (O24.4-)

neonatal diabetes mellitus (P70.2)

postpancreatectomy diabetes mellitus (E13.-)

postprocedural diabetes mellitus (E13.-)

secondary diabetes mellitus NEC (E13.-)

type 1 diabetes mellitus (E10.-)

type 2 diabetes mellitus (E11.-)

AHA: 2013,4Q,114; 2013,3Q,20

√5ᵗʰ **E09.0**   **Drug or chemical induced diabetes mellitus with hyperosmolarity**

DEF: Diabetic hyperosmolarity: Extremely high levels of glucose in the blood without ketones.

E09.00   **Drug or chemical induced diabetes mellitus with hyperosmolarity without nonketotic hyperglycemic-hyperosmolar coma (NKHHC)**   HCC

E09.01   **Drug or chemical induced diabetes mellitus with hyperosmolarity with coma**   HCC

√5ᵗʰ **E09.1**   **Drug or chemical induced diabetes mellitus with ketoacidosis**

DEF: Diabetic ketoacidosis: Potentially life-threatening complication due to a shortage of insulin in which the body switches to burning fatty acids and producing acidic ketone bodies.

E09.10   **Drug or chemical induced diabetes mellitus with ketoacidosis without coma**   HCC

E09.11   **Drug or chemical induced diabetes mellitus with ketoacidosis with coma**   HCC

√5ᵗʰ **E09.2**   **Drug or chemical induced diabetes mellitus with kidney complications**

E09.21   **Drug or chemical induced diabetes mellitus with diabetic nephropathy**   HCC

Drug or chemical induced diabetes mellitus with intercapillary glomerulosclerosis

Drug or chemical induced diabetes mellitus with intracapillary glomerulonephrosis

Drug or chemical induced diabetes mellitus with Kimmelstiel-Wilson disease

E09.22   **Drug or chemical induced diabetes mellitus with diabetic chronic kidney disease**   HCC

Use additional code to identify stage of chronic kidney disease (N18.1-N18.6)

E09.29   **Drug or chemical induced diabetes mellitus with other diabetic kidney complication**   HCC

Drug or chemical induced diabetes mellitus with renal tubular degeneration

√5ᵗʰ **E09.3**   **Drug or chemical induced diabetes mellitus with ophthalmic complications**

One of the following 7th characters is to be assigned to codes in subcategories E09.32, E09.33, E09.34, E09.35, and E09.37 to designate laterality of the disease:

1   right eye

2   left eye

3   bilateral

9   unspecified eye

√6ᵗʰ **E09.31**   **Drug or chemical induced diabetes mellitus with unspecified diabetic retinopathy**

DEF: Diabetic retinopathy: Diabetic complication from damage to the retinal vessels resulting in vision problems that can progress to blindness.

E09.311   **Drug or chemical induced diabetes mellitus with unspecified diabetic retinopathy with macular edema**   HCC Q ▽

E09.319   **Drug or chemical induced diabetes mellitus with unspecified diabetic retinopathy without macular edema**   HCC Q ▽

√6ᵗʰ **E09.32**   **Drug or chemical induced diabetes mellitus with mild nonproliferative diabetic retinopathy**

Drug or chemical induced diabetes mellitus with nonproliferative diabetic retinopathy NOS

√7ᵗʰ **E09.321**   **Drug or chemical induced diabetes mellitus with mild nonproliferative diabetic retinopathy with macular edema**   HCC Q

√7ᵗʰ **E09.329**   **Drug or chemical induced diabetes mellitus with mild nonproliferative diabetic retinopathy without macular edema**   HCC Q

√6ᵗʰ **E09.33**   **Drug or chemical induced diabetes mellitus with moderate nonproliferative diabetic retinopathy**

√7ᵗʰ **E09.331**   **Drug or chemical induced diabetes mellitus with moderate nonproliferative diabetic retinopathy with macular edema**   HCC Q

√7ᵗʰ **E09.339**   **Drug or chemical induced diabetes mellitus with moderate nonproliferative diabetic retinopathy without macular edema**   HCC Q

√6ᵗʰ **E09.34**   **Drug or chemical induced diabetes mellitus with severe nonproliferative diabetic retinopathy**

√7ᵗʰ **E09.341**   **Drug or chemical induced diabetes mellitus with severe nonproliferative diabetic retinopathy with macular edema**   HCC Q

√7ᵗʰ **E09.349** **Drug or chemical induced diabetes mellitus with severe nonproliferative diabetic retinopathy** without macular edema HCC Q

√6ᵗʰ **E09.35** **Drug or chemical induced diabetes mellitus with** proliferative **diabetic** retinopathy

√7ᵗʰ **E09.351** **Drug or chemical induced diabetes mellitus with** proliferative diabetic retinopathy with macular edema HCC Q

√7ᵗʰ **E09.352** **Drug or chemical induced diabetes mellitus with** proliferative diabetic retinopathy with traction retinal detachment involving the macula HCC Q

√7ᵗʰ **E09.353** **Drug or chemical induced diabetes mellitus with** proliferative diabetic retinopathy with traction retinal detachment not involving the macula HCC Q

√7ᵗʰ **E09.354** **Drug or chemical induced diabetes mellitus with** proliferative diabetic retinopathy with combined traction retinal detachment and rhegmatogenous retinal detachment HCC Q

√7ᵗʰ **E09.355** **Drug or chemical induced diabetes mellitus with** stable proliferative diabetic retinopathy HCC Q

√7ᵗʰ **E09.359** **Drug or chemical induced diabetes mellitus with** proliferative diabetic retinopathy without macular edema HCC Q

E09.36 **Drug or chemical induced diabetes mellitus with diabetic** cataract HCC
    AHA: 2016,4Q,142

√x7ᵗʰ **E09.37** **Drug or chemical induced diabetes mellitus with diabetic** macular edema, resolved following treatment HCC

E09.39 **Drug or chemical induced diabetes mellitus with other diabetic ophthalmic complication** HCC
    Use additional code to identify manifestation, such as:
        diabetic glaucoma (H40-H42)

√5ᵗʰ **E09.4** **Drug or chemical induced diabetes mellitus with** neurological complications

E09.40 **Drug or chemical induced diabetes mellitus with neurological complications with diabetic** neuropathy, unspecified HCC ▽

E09.41 **Drug or chemical induced diabetes mellitus with neurological complications with diabetic** mononeuropathy HCC

E09.42 **Drug or chemical induced diabetes mellitus with neurological complications with diabetic** polyneuropathy HCC
    Drug or chemical induced diabetes mellitus with diabetic neuralgia

E09.43 **Drug or chemical induced diabetes mellitus with neurological complications with diabetic** autonomic (poly)neuropathy HCC
    Drug or chemical induced diabetes mellitus with diabetic gastroparesis
    AHA: 2013,4Q,114

E09.44 **Drug or chemical induced diabetes mellitus with neurological complications with diabetic** amyotrophy HCC

E09.49 **Drug or chemical induced diabetes mellitus with neurological complications with other diabetic neurological complication** HCC

√5ᵗʰ **E09.5** **Drug or chemical induced diabetes mellitus with** circulatory complications

E09.51 **Drug or chemical induced diabetes mellitus with diabetic** peripheral angiopathy without gangrene HCC
    AHA: 2018,2Q,7

E09.52 **Drug or chemical induced diabetes mellitus with diabetic** peripheral angiopathy with gangrene HCC
    Drug or chemical induced diabetes mellitus with diabetic gangrene
    AHA: 2018,2Q,7; 2017,4Q,102

E09.59 **Drug or chemical induced diabetes mellitus with other circulatory complications** HCC

√5ᵗʰ **E09.6** **Drug or chemical induced diabetes mellitus with other specified complications**

√6ᵗʰ **E09.61** **Drug or chemical induced diabetes mellitus with diabetic** arthropathy

E09.610 **Drug or chemical induced diabetes mellitus with diabetic neuropathic arthropathy** HCC
    Drug or chemical induced diabetes mellitus with Charcôt's joints
    DEF: Charcot's joint: Progressive neurologic arthropathy in which chronic degeneration of joints in the weight-bearing areas with peripheral hypertrophy occurs as a complication of a neuropathy disorder. Supporting structures relax from a loss of sensation resulting in chronic joint instability.

E09.618 **Drug or chemical induced diabetes mellitus with other diabetic arthropathy** HCC
    AHA: 2018,2Q,6

√6ᵗʰ **E09.62** **Drug or chemical induced diabetes mellitus with** skin complications

E09.620 **Drug or chemical induced diabetes mellitus with** diabetic dermatitis HCC
    Drug or chemical induced diabetes mellitus with diabetic necrobiosis lipoidica

E09.621 **Drug or chemical induced diabetes mellitus with foot ulcer** HCC
    Use additional code to identify site of ulcer (L97.4-, L97.5-)
    TIP: Do not assign a code for diabetic ulcer when the ulcer is closed/resolved or to report history of diabetic ulcers; Z86.31 Personal history of diabetic foot ulcer, may be assigned.

E09.622 **Drug or chemical induced diabetes mellitus with other skin ulcer** HCC
    Use additional code to identify site of ulcer (L97.1-L97.9, L98.41-L98.49)
    AHA: 2017,4Q,17

E09.628 **Drug or chemical induced diabetes mellitus with other skin complications** HCC
    AHA: 2017,4Q,100-101

√6ᵗʰ **E09.63** **Drug or chemical induced diabetes mellitus with** oral complications

E09.630 **Drug or chemical induced diabetes mellitus with** periodontal disease HCC

E09.638 **Drug or chemical induced diabetes mellitus with other oral complications** HCC

√6ᵗʰ **E09.64** **Drug or chemical induced diabetes mellitus with** hypoglycemia

E09.641 **Drug or chemical induced diabetes mellitus with hypoglycemia with coma** HCC

E09.649 **Drug or chemical induced diabetes mellitus with hypoglycemia** without coma HCC
    AHA: 2016,3Q,42; 2015,3Q,21

E09.65 **Drug or chemical induced diabetes mellitus with** hyperglycemia HCC

E09.69 **Drug or chemical induced diabetes mellitus with other specified complication** HCC
    Use additional code to identify complication
    AHA: 2016,4Q,141; 2016,1Q,13

E09.8 **Drug or chemical induced diabetes mellitus with unspecified complications** HCC ▽

E09.9 **Drug or chemical induced diabetes mellitus without complications** HCC

Chapter 4. Endocrine, Nutritional and Metabolic Diseases

E10–E10.59

✓4ᵗʰ **E10 Type 1 diabetes mellitus**

INCLUDES brittle diabetes (mellitus)
diabetes (mellitus) due to autoimmune process
diabetes (mellitus) due to immune mediated pancreatic
islet beta-cell destruction
idiopathic diabetes (mellitus)
juvenile onset diabetes (mellitus)
ketosis-prone diabetes (mellitus)

EXCLUDES 1 *diabetes mellitus due to underlying condition (E08.-)*
drug or chemical induced diabetes mellitus (E09.-)
gestational diabetes (O24.4-)
hyperglycemia NOS (R73.9)
neonatal diabetes mellitus (P70.2)
postpancreatectomy diabetes mellitus (E13.-)
postprocedural diabetes mellitus (E13.-)
secondary diabetes mellitus NEC (E13.-)
type 2 diabetes mellitus (E11.-)

AHA: 2013,4Q,114; 2013,3Q,20

✓5ᵗʰ **E10.1 Type 1 diabetes mellitus with** ketoacidosis

AHA: 2013,3Q,20
DEF: Diabetic ketoacidosis: Potentially life-threatening
complication due to a shortage of insulin in which the body
switches to burning fatty acids and producing acidic ketone
bodies.

E10.10 Type 1 diabetes mellitus with ketoacidosis HCC Q
without coma

E10.11 Type 1 diabetes mellitus with ketoacidosis HCC Q
with coma

✓5ᵗʰ **E10.2 Type 1 diabetes mellitus with** kidney complications

E10.21 Type 1 diabetes mellitus with diabetic HCC Q
nephropathy
Type 1 diabetes mellitus with intercapillary
glomerulosclerosis
Type 1 diabetes mellitus with intracapillary
glomerulonephrosis
Type 1 diabetes mellitus with Kimmelstiel-Wilson
disease

E10.22 Type 1 diabetes mellitus with diabetic HCC Q
chronic kidney disease
Use additional code to identify stage of chronic kidney
disease (N18.1-N18.6)

E10.29 Type 1 diabetes mellitus with other diabetic HCC Q
kidney complication
Type 1 diabetes mellitus with renal tubular
degeneration
AHA: 2016,1Q,13

✓5ᵗʰ **E10.3 Type 1 diabetes mellitus with** ophthalmic complications

One of the following 7th characters is to be assigned to codes
in subcategories E10.32, E10.33, E10.34, E10.35, and E10.37
to designate laterality of the disease:
1   right eye
2   left eye
3   bilateral
9   unspecified eye

✓6ᵗʰ **E10.31 Type 1 diabetes mellitus with unspecified diabetic**
retinopathy
DEF: Diabetic retinopathy: Diabetic complication from
damage to the retinal vessels resulting in vision
problems that can progress to blindness.

E10.311 Type 1 diabetes mellitus with HCC Q ▽
unspecified diabetic retinopathy
with macular edema

E10.319 Type 1 diabetes mellitus with HCC Q ▽
unspecified diabetic retinopathy
without macular edema

✓6ᵗʰ **E10.32 Type 1 diabetes mellitus with** mild nonproliferative
diabetic retinopathy
Type 1 diabetes mellitus with nonproliferative
diabetic retinopathy NOS

E10.321 Type 1 diabetes mellitus with HCC Q
mild nonproliferative diabetic
retinopathy with macular edema

E10.329 Type 1 diabetes mellitus with HCC Q
mild nonproliferative diabetic
retinopathy without macular
edema

✓6ᵗʰ **E10.33 Type 1 diabetes mellitus with** moderate
nonproliferative diabetic retinopathy

E10.331 Type 1 diabetes mellitus with HCC Q
moderate nonproliferative
diabetic retinopathy with
macular edema

E10.339 Type 1 diabetes mellitus with HCC Q
moderate nonproliferative
diabetic retinopathy without
macular edema

✓6ᵗʰ **E10.34 Type 1 diabetes mellitus with** severe
nonproliferative diabetic retinopathy

E10.341 Type 1 diabetes mellitus with HCC Q
severe nonproliferative diabetic
retinopathy with macular edema

E10.349 Type 1 diabetes mellitus with HCC Q
severe nonproliferative diabetic
retinopathy without macular
edema

✓6ᵗʰ **E10.35 Type 1 diabetes mellitus with** proliferative diabetic
retinopathy

E10.351 Type 1 diabetes mellitus with HCC Q
proliferative diabetic retinopathy
with macular edema

E10.352 Type 1 diabetes mellitus with HCC Q
proliferative diabetic retinopathy
with traction retinal detachment
involving the macula

E10.353 Type 1 diabetes mellitus with HCC Q
proliferative diabetic retinopathy
with traction retinal detachment
not involving the macula

E10.354 Type 1 diabetes mellitus with HCC Q
proliferative diabetic retinopathy
with combined traction retinal
detachment and
rhegmatogenous retinal
detachment

E10.355 Type 1 diabetes mellitus with HCC Q
stable proliferative diabetic
retinopathy

E10.359 Type 1 diabetes mellitus with HCC Q
proliferative diabetic retinopathy
without macular edema

E10.36 Type 1 diabetes mellitus with diabetic HCC Q
cataract
AHA: 2016,4Q,142

✓x7ᵗʰ **E10.37 Type 1 diabetes mellitus with diabetic** HCC Q
macular edema, resolved following
treatment

E10.39 Type 1 diabetes mellitus with other diabetic HCC Q
ophthalmic complication
Use additional code to identify manifestation, such
as:
diabetic glaucoma (H40-H42)

✓5ᵗʰ **E10.4 Type 1 diabetes mellitus with** neurological complications

E10.40 Type 1 diabetes mellitus with diabetic HCC Q ▽
neuropathy, unspecified

E10.41 Type 1 diabetes mellitus with diabetic HCC Q
mononeuropathy

E10.42 Type 1 diabetes mellitus with diabetic HCC Q
polyneuropathy
Type 1 diabetes mellitus with diabetic neuralgia

E10.43 Type 1 diabetes mellitus with diabetic HCC Q
autonomic (poly)neuropathy
Type 1 diabetes mellitus with diabetic gastroparesis
AHA: 2013,4Q,114

E10.44 Type 1 diabetes mellitus with diabetic HCC Q
amyotrophy

E10.49 Type 1 diabetes mellitus with other diabetic HCC Q
neurological complication

✓5ᵗʰ **E10.5 Type 1 diabetes mellitus with** circulatory complications

E10.51 Type 1 diabetes mellitus with diabetic HCC Q
peripheral angiopathy without gangrene
AHA: 2018,2Q,7

E10.52 Type 1 diabetes mellitus with diabetic HCC Q
peripheral angiopathy with gangrene
Type 1 diabetes mellitus with diabetic gangrene
AHA: 2018,2Q,7; 2017,4Q,102

E10.59 Type 1 diabetes mellitus with other HCC Q
circulatory complications

√5ᵗʰ **E10.6 Type 1 diabetes mellitus with other specified complications**

√6ᵗʰ **E10.61 Type 1 diabetes mellitus with diabetic arthropathy**

E10.610 Type 1 diabetes mellitus with diabetic neuropathic arthropathy `HCC` `Q`

Type 1 diabetes mellitus with Charcôt's joints

DEF: Charcot's joint: Progressive neurologic arthropathy in which chronic degeneration of joints in the weight-bearing areas with peripheral hypertrophy occurs as a complication of a neuropathy disorder. Supporting structures relax from a loss of sensation resulting in chronic joint instability.

E10.618 Type 1 diabetes mellitus with other diabetic arthropathy `HCC` `Q`

AHA: 2018,2Q,6

√6ᵗʰ **E10.62 Type 1 diabetes mellitus with skin complications**

E10.620 Type 1 diabetes mellitus with diabetic dermatitis `HCC` `Q`

Type 1 diabetes mellitus with diabetic necrobiosis lipoidica

E10.621 Type 1 diabetes mellitus with foot ulcer `HCC` `Q`

Use additional code to identify site of ulcer (L97.4-, L97.5-)

TIP: Do not assign a code for diabetic ulcer when the ulcer is closed/resolved or to report history of diabetic ulcers; Z86.31 Personal history of diabetic foot ulcer, may be assigned.

E10.622 Type 1 diabetes mellitus with other skin ulcer `HCC` `Q`

Use additional code to identify site of ulcer (L97.1-L97.9, L98.41-L98.49)

AHA: 2017,4Q,17

E10.628 Type 1 diabetes mellitus with other skin complications `HCC` `Q`

AHA: 2017,4Q,100-101

√6ᵗʰ **E10.63 Type 1 diabetes mellitus with oral complications**

E10.630 Type 1 diabetes mellitus with periodontal disease `HCC` `Q`

E10.638 Type 1 diabetes mellitus with other oral complications `HCC` `Q`

√6ᵗʰ **E10.64 Type 1 diabetes mellitus with hypoglycemia**

E10.641 Type 1 diabetes mellitus with hypoglycemia with coma `HCC` `Q`

E10.649 Type 1 diabetes mellitus with hypoglycemia without coma `HCC` `Q`

AHA: 2016,3Q,42; 2016,1Q,13; 2015,3Q,21

E10.65 Type 1 diabetes mellitus with hyperglycemia `HCC` `Q`

AHA: 2013,3Q,20

E10.69 Type 1 diabetes mellitus with other specified complication `HCC` `Q`

Use additional code to identify complication

AHA: 2016,4Q,141; 2016,1Q,13

E10.8 Type 1 diabetes mellitus with unspecified complications `HCC` `Q` ▽

E10.9 Type 1 diabetes mellitus without complications `HCC` `Q`

√4ᵗʰ **E11 Type 2 diabetes mellitus**

`INCLUDES` diabetes (mellitus) due to insulin secretory defect
diabetes NOS
insulin resistant diabetes (mellitus)

Use additional code to identify control using:
insulin (Z79.4)
oral antidiabetic drugs (Z79.84)
oral hypoglycemic drugs (Z79.84)

`EXCLUDES 1` diabetes mellitus due to underlying condition (E08.-)
drug or chemical induced diabetes mellitus (E09.-)
gestational diabetes (O24.4-)
neonatal diabetes mellitus (P70.2)
postpancreatectomy diabetes mellitus (E13.-)
postprocedural diabetes mellitus (E13.-)
secondary diabetes mellitus NEC (E13.-)
type 1 diabetes mellitus (E10.-)

AHA: 2016,2Q,10; 2013,4Q,114; 2013,3Q,20; 2013,1Q,26

√5ᵗʰ **E11.0 Type 2 diabetes mellitus with hyperosmolarity**

DEF: Diabetic hyperosmolarity: Extremely high levels of glucose in the blood without ketones.

E11.00 Type 2 diabetes mellitus with hyperosmolarity without nonketotic hyperglycemic-hyperosmolar coma (NKHHC) `HCC` `Q`

E11.01 Type 2 diabetes mellitus with hyperosmolarity with coma `HCC` `Q`

√5ᵗʰ **E11.1 Type 2 diabetes mellitus with ketoacidosis**

DEF: Diabetic ketoacidosis: Potentially life-threatening complication due to a shortage of insulin in which the body switches to burning fatty acids and producing acidic ketone bodies.

E11.10 Type 2 diabetes mellitus with ketoacidosis without coma `HCC`

E11.11 Type 2 diabetes mellitus with ketoacidosis with coma `HCC`

√5ᵗʰ **E11.2 Type 2 diabetes mellitus with kidney complications**

E11.21 Type 2 diabetes mellitus with diabetic nephropathy `HCC` `Q`

Type 2 diabetes mellitus with intercapillary glomerulosclerosis
Type 2 diabetes mellitus with intracapillary glomerulonephrosis
Type 2 diabetes mellitus with Kimmelstiel-Wilson disease

E11.22 Type 2 diabetes mellitus with diabetic chronic kidney disease `HCC` `Q`

Use additional code to identify stage of chronic kidney disease (N18.1-N18.6)

AHA: 2016,1Q,12

E11.29 Type 2 diabetes mellitus with other diabetic kidney complication `HCC` `Q`

Type 2 diabetes mellitus with renal tubular degeneration

√5ᵗʰ **E11.3 Type 2 diabetes mellitus with ophthalmic complications**

One of the following 7th characters is to be assigned to codes in subcategories E11.32, E11.33, E11.34, E11.35, and E11.37 to designate laterality of the disease:

1 right eye
2 left eye
3 bilateral
9 unspecified eye

√6ᵗʰ **E11.31 Type 2 diabetes mellitus with unspecified diabetic retinopathy**

DEF: Diabetic retinopathy: Diabetic complication from damage to the retinal vessels resulting in vision problems that can progress to blindness.

E11.311 Type 2 diabetes mellitus with unspecified diabetic retinopathy with macular edema `HCC` `Q` ▽

E11.319 Type 2 diabetes mellitus with unspecified diabetic retinopathy without macular edema `HCC` `Q` ▽

√6ᵗʰ **E11.32 Type 2 diabetes mellitus with mild nonproliferative diabetic retinopathy**

Type 2 diabetes mellitus with nonproliferative diabetic retinopathy NOS

√7ᵗʰ **E11.321 Type 2 diabetes mellitus with mild nonproliferative diabetic retinopathy with macular edema** `HCC` `Q`

| ☑ Additional Character Req | √ₓ7ᵗʰ Placeholder Alert | **Manifestation** | ▽ Unspecified | ▶◀ Revised Text | ● New Code | ▲ Revised Code Title |

ICD-10-CM 2019

517

E10.6–E11.321

Chapter 4. Endocrine, Nutritional and Metabolic Diseases

√7ᵗʰ **E11.329** **Type 2 diabetes mellitus with mild nonproliferative diabetic retinopathy** without macular edema ᴴᶜᶜ Q

√6ᵗʰ **E11.33** **Type 2 diabetes mellitus with moderate nonproliferative diabetic retinopathy**

 √7ᵗʰ **E11.331** **Type 2 diabetes mellitus with moderate nonproliferative diabetic retinopathy with** macular edema ᴴᶜᶜ Q

 √7ᵗʰ **E11.339** **Type 2 diabetes mellitus with moderate nonproliferative diabetic retinopathy without** macular edema ᴴᶜᶜ Q

√6ᵗʰ **E11.34** **Type 2 diabetes mellitus with severe nonproliferative diabetic retinopathy**

 √7ᵗʰ **E11.341** **Type 2 diabetes mellitus with severe nonproliferative diabetic retinopathy with macular edema** ᴴᶜᶜ Q

 √7ᵗʰ **E11.349** **Type 2 diabetes mellitus with severe nonproliferative diabetic retinopathy without macular edema** ᴴᶜᶜ Q

√6ᵗʰ **E11.35** **Type 2 diabetes mellitus with proliferative diabetic retinopathy**

 √7ᵗʰ **E11.351** **Type 2 diabetes mellitus with proliferative diabetic retinopathy with macular edema** ᴴᶜᶜ Q

 √7ᵗʰ **E11.352** **Type 2 diabetes mellitus with proliferative diabetic retinopathy with traction retinal detachment involving the macula** ᴴᶜᶜ Q

 √7ᵗʰ **E11.353** **Type 2 diabetes mellitus with proliferative diabetic retinopathy with traction retinal detachment not involving the macula** ᴴᶜᶜ Q

 √7ᵗʰ **E11.354** **Type 2 diabetes mellitus with proliferative diabetic retinopathy with combined traction retinal detachment and rhegmatogenous retinal detachment** ᴴᶜᶜ Q

 √7ᵗʰ **E11.355** **Type 2 diabetes mellitus with stable proliferative diabetic retinopathy** ᴴᶜᶜ Q

 √7ᵗʰ **E11.359** **Type 2 diabetes mellitus with proliferative diabetic retinopathy without macular edema** ᴴᶜᶜ Q

 E11.36 **Type 2 diabetes mellitus with diabetic cataract** ᴴᶜᶜ Q
  AHA: 2016,4Q,142

√x7ᵗʰ **E11.37** **Type 2 diabetes mellitus with diabetic macular edema, resolved following treatment** ᴴᶜᶜ Q

 E11.39 **Type 2 diabetes mellitus with other diabetic ophthalmic complication** ᴴᶜᶜ Q
  Use additional code to identify manifestation, such as:
  diabetic glaucoma (H40-H42)

√5ᵗʰ **E11.4** **Type 2 diabetes mellitus with neurological complications**

 E11.40 **Type 2 diabetes mellitus with diabetic neuropathy, unspecified** ᴴᶜᶜ Q ▽
  AHA: 2013,4Q,129

 E11.41 **Type 2 diabetes mellitus with diabetic mononeuropathy** ᴴᶜᶜ Q

 E11.42 **Type 2 diabetes mellitus with diabetic polyneuropathy** ᴴᶜᶜ Q
  Type 2 diabetes mellitus with diabetic neuralgia
  AHA: 2016,1Q,12

 E11.43 **Type 2 diabetes mellitus with diabetic autonomic (poly)neuropathy** ᴴᶜᶜ Q
  Type 2 diabetes mellitus with diabetic gastroparesis
  AHA: 2013,4Q,114

 E11.44 **Type 2 diabetes mellitus with diabetic amyotrophy** ᴴᶜᶜ Q

 E11.49 **Type 2 diabetes mellitus with other diabetic neurological complication** ᴴᶜᶜ Q

√5ᵗʰ **E11.5** **Type 2 diabetes mellitus with circulatory complications**

 E11.51 **Type 2 diabetes mellitus with diabetic peripheral angiopathy without gangrene** ᴴᶜᶜ Q
  AHA: 2018,2Q,7

 E11.52 **Type 2 diabetes mellitus with diabetic peripheral angiopathy with gangrene** ᴴᶜᶜ Q
  Type 2 diabetes mellitus with diabetic gangrene
  AHA: 2018,2Q,7; 2017,4Q,102

 E11.59 **Type 2 diabetes mellitus with other circulatory complications** ᴴᶜᶜ Q

√5ᵗʰ **E11.6** **Type 2 diabetes mellitus with other specified complications**

√6ᵗʰ **E11.61** **Type 2 diabetes mellitus with diabetic arthropathy**

 E11.610 **Type 2 diabetes mellitus with diabetic neuropathic arthropathy** ᴴᶜᶜ Q
  Type 2 diabetes mellitus with Charcôt's joints
  DEF: Charcot's joint: Progressive neurologic arthropathy in which chronic degeneration of joints in the weight-bearing areas with peripheral hypertrophy occurs as a complication of a neuropathy disorder. Supporting structures relax from a loss of sensation resulting in chronic joint instability.

 E11.618 **Type 2 diabetes mellitus with other diabetic arthropathy** ᴴᶜᶜ Q
  AHA: 2018,2Q,6

√6ᵗʰ **E11.62** **Type 2 diabetes mellitus with skin complications**

 E11.620 **Type 2 diabetes mellitus with diabetic dermatitis** ᴴᶜᶜ Q
  Type 2 diabetes mellitus with diabetic necrobiosis lipoidica

 E11.621 **Type 2 diabetes mellitus with foot ulcer** ᴴᶜᶜ Q
  Use additional code to identify site of ulcer (L97.4-, L97.5-)
  AHA: 2016,1Q,12
  TIP: Do not assign a code for diabetic ulcer when the ulcer is closed/resolved or to report history of diabetic ulcers; Z86.31 Personal history of diabetic foot ulcer, may be assigned.

 E11.622 **Type 2 diabetes mellitus with other skin ulcer** ᴴᶜᶜ Q
  Use additional code to identify site of ulcer (L97.1-L97.9, L98.41-L98.49)
  AHA: 2017,4Q,17

 E11.628 **Type 2 diabetes mellitus with other skin complications** ᴴᶜᶜ Q
  AHA: 2017,4Q,100-101

√6ᵗʰ **E11.63** **Type 2 diabetes mellitus with oral complications**

 E11.630 **Type 2 diabetes mellitus with periodontal disease** ᴴᶜᶜ Q

 E11.638 **Type 2 diabetes mellitus with other oral complications** ᴴᶜᶜ Q

√6ᵗʰ **E11.64** **Type 2 diabetes mellitus with hypoglycemia**

 E11.641 **Type 2 diabetes mellitus with hypoglycemia with coma** ᴴᶜᶜ Q

 E11.649 **Type 2 diabetes mellitus with hypoglycemia without coma** ᴴᶜᶜ Q
  AHA: 2016,3Q,42; 2015,3Q,21

 E11.65 **Type 2 diabetes mellitus with hyperglycemia** ᴴᶜᶜ Q
  AHA: 2013,3Q,20

 E11.69 **Type 2 diabetes mellitus with other specified complication** ᴴᶜᶜ Q
  Use additional code to identify complication
  AHA: 2016,4Q,141; 2016,1Q,13

E11.8 **Type 2 diabetes mellitus with unspecified complications** ᴴᶜᶜ Q ▽

E11.9 **Type 2 diabetes mellitus without complications** ᴴᶜᶜ Q

√4ᵗʰ E13 Other specified diabetes mellitus

  INCLUDES   diabetes mellitus due to genetic defects of beta-cell
                    function
            diabetes mellitus due to genetic defects in insulin action
            postpancreatectomy diabetes mellitus
            postprocedural diabetes mellitus
            secondary diabetes mellitus NEC
  Use additional code to identify control using:
  insulin (Z79.4)
  oral antidiabetic drugs (Z79.84)
  oral hypoglycemic drugs (Z79.84)
  EXCLUDES 1   diabetes (mellitus) due to autoimmune process (E10.-)
            diabetes (mellitus) due to immune mediated pancreatic islet
                    beta-cell destruction (E10.-)
            diabetes mellitus due to underlying condition (E08.-)
            drug or chemical induced diabetes mellitus (E09.-)
            gestational diabetes (O24.4-)
            neonatal diabetes mellitus (P70.2)
            type 1 diabetes mellitus (E10.-)
  AHA: 2013,4Q,114; 2013,3Q,20
  TIP: When postprocedural or postpancreatectomy hypoinsulinemia (E89.1)
  is documented with postprocedural or postpancreatectomy diabetes
  mellitus (E13.-), code E89.1 should be sequenced first.

√5ᵗʰ E13.0 Other specified diabetes mellitus with hyperosmolarity
            DEF: Diabetic hyperosmolarity: Extremely high levels of glucose
            in the blood without ketones.
      E13.00 Other specified diabetes mellitus with HCC Q
                hyperosmolarity without nonketotic
                hyperglycemic-hyperosmolar coma
                (NKHHC)
                EXCLUDES 2   type 2 diabetes mellitus (E11.-)
      E13.01 Other specified diabetes mellitus with HCC Q
                hyperosmolarity with coma

√5ᵗʰ E13.1 Other specified diabetes mellitus with ketoacidosis
            AHA: 2016,2Q,10; 2013,1Q,26
            DEF: Diabetic ketoacidosis: Potentially life-threatening
            complication due to a shortage of insulin in which the body
            switches to burning fatty acids and producing acidic ketone
            bodies.
      E13.10 Other specified diabetes mellitus with HCC Q
                ketoacidosis without coma
      E13.11 Other specified diabetes mellitus with HCC Q
                ketoacidosis with coma

√5ᵗʰ E13.2 Other specified diabetes mellitus with kidney complications
      E13.21 Other specified diabetes mellitus with HCC Q
                diabetic nephropathy
                Other specified diabetes mellitus with intercapillary
                    glomerulosclerosis
                Other specified diabetes mellitus with intracapillary
                    glomerulonephrosis
                Other specified diabetes mellitus with
                    Kimmelstiel-Wilson disease
      E13.22 Other specified diabetes mellitus with HCC Q
                diabetic chronic kidney disease
                Use additional code to identify stage of chronic kidney
                    disease (N18.1-N18.6)
      E13.29 Other specified diabetes mellitus with other HCC Q
                diabetic kidney complication
                Other specified diabetes mellitus with renal tubular
                    degeneration

**√5ᵗʰ E13.3 Other specified diabetes mellitus with ophthalmic
            complications**
            One of the following 7th characters is to be assigned to codes
            in subcategories E13.32, E13.33, E13.34, E13.35, and E13.37
            to designate laterality of the disease:
            1   right eye
            2   left eye
            3   bilateral
            9   unspecified eye
      **√6ᵗʰ E13.31 Other specified diabetes mellitus with unspecified
                diabetic retinopathy**
                DEF: Diabetic retinopathy: Diabetic complication from
                damage to the retinal vessels resulting in vision
                problems that can progress to blindness.
            E13.311 Other specified diabetes mellitus HCC Q ▽
                **with unspecified diabetic
                retinopathy with macular edema**

            E13.319 Other specified diabetes mellitus HCC Q ▽
                **with unspecified diabetic
                retinopathy without macular
                edema**
      **√6ᵗʰ E13.32 Other specified diabetes mellitus with mild
                nonproliferative diabetic retinopathy**
                Other specified diabetes mellitus with
                    nonproliferative diabetic retinopathy NOS
            √7ᵗʰ E13.321 Other specified diabetes mellitus HCC Q
                **with mild nonproliferative
                diabetic retinopathy with
                macular edema**
            √7ᵗʰ E13.329 Other specified diabetes mellitus HCC Q
                **with mild nonproliferative
                diabetic retinopathy without
                macular edema**
      **√6ᵗʰ E13.33 Other specified diabetes mellitus with moderate
                nonproliferative diabetic retinopathy**
            √7ᵗʰ E13.331 Other specified diabetes mellitus HCC Q
                **with moderate nonproliferative
                diabetic retinopathy with
                macular edema**
            √7ᵗʰ E13.339 Other specified diabetes mellitus HCC Q
                **with moderate nonproliferative
                diabetic retinopathy without
                macular edema**
      **√6ᵗʰ E13.34 Other specified diabetes mellitus with severe
                nonproliferative diabetic retinopathy**
            √7ᵗʰ E13.341 Other specified diabetes mellitus HCC Q
                **with severe nonproliferative
                diabetic retinopathy with
                macular edema**
            √7ᵗʰ E13.349 Other specified diabetes mellitus HCC Q
                **with severe nonproliferative
                diabetic retinopathy without
                macular edema**
      **√6ᵗʰ E13.35 Other specified diabetes mellitus with proliferative
                diabetic retinopathy**
            √7ᵗʰ E13.351 Other specified diabetes mellitus HCC Q
                **with proliferative diabetic
                retinopathy with macular edema**
            √7ᵗʰ E13.352 Other specified diabetes mellitus HCC Q
                **with proliferative diabetic
                retinopathy with traction retinal
                detachment involving the macula**
            √7ᵗʰ E13.353 Other specified diabetes mellitus HCC Q
                **with proliferative diabetic
                retinopathy with traction retinal
                detachment not involving the
                macula**
            √7ᵗʰ E13.354 Other specified diabetes mellitus HCC Q
                **with proliferative diabetic
                retinopathy with combined
                traction retinal detachment and
                rhegmatogenous retinal
                detachment**
            √7ᵗʰ E13.355 Other specified diabetes mellitus HCC Q
                **with stable proliferative diabetic
                retinopathy**
            √7ᵗʰ E13.359 Other specified diabetes mellitus HCC Q
                **with proliferative diabetic
                retinopathy without macular
                edema**
      E13.36 Other specified diabetes mellitus with HCC Q
                diabetic cataract
                AHA: 2016,4Q,142
      √x7ᵗʰ E13.37 Other specified diabetes mellitus with HCC Q
                **diabetic macular edema, resolved following
                treatment**
      E13.39 Other specified diabetes mellitus with other HCC Q
                diabetic ophthalmic complication
                Use additional code to identify manifestation, such
                    as:
                diabetic glaucoma (H40-H42)

**√5ᵗʰ E13.4 Other specified diabetes mellitus with neurological
            complications**
      E13.40 Other specified diabetes mellitus with HCC Q ▽
                diabetic neuropathy, unspecified
      E13.41 Other specified diabetes mellitus with HCC Q
                diabetic mononeuropathy

E13.42   **Other specified diabetes mellitus with** HCC Q
    diabetic polyneuropathy
    Other specified diabetes mellitus with diabetic
       neuralgia

E13.43   **Other specified diabetes mellitus with** HCC Q
    diabetic autonomic (poly)neuropathy
    Other specified diabetes mellitus with diabetic
       gastroparesis
    AHA: 2013,4Q,114

E13.44   **Other specified diabetes mellitus with** HCC Q
    diabetic amyotrophy

E13.49   **Other specified diabetes mellitus with other** HCC Q
    diabetic neurological complication

√5ᵗʰ **E13.5   Other specified diabetes mellitus with circulatory
    complications**

E13.51   **Other specified diabetes mellitus with** HCC Q
    **diabetic peripheral angiopathy without
    gangrene**
    AHA: 2018,2Q,7

E13.52   **Other specified diabetes mellitus with** HCC Q
    **diabetic peripheral angiopathy with
    gangrene**
    Other specified diabetes mellitus with diabetic
       gangrene
    AHA: 2018,2Q,7; 2017,4Q,102

E13.59   **Other specified diabetes mellitus with other** HCC Q
    circulatory complications

√5ᵗʰ **E13.6   Other specified diabetes mellitus with other specified
    complications**

√6ᵗʰ E13.61   **Other specified diabetes mellitus with diabetic
    arthropathy**

E13.610   **Other specified diabetes mellitus** HCC Q
    **with diabetic neuropathic
    arthropathy**
    Other specified diabetes mellitus with
       Charcôt's joints
    DEF: Charcôt's joint: Progressive neurologic
    arthropathy in which chronic degeneration
    of joints in the weight-bearing areas with
    peripheral hypertrophy occurs as a
    complication of a neuropathy disorder.
    Supporting structures relax from a loss of
    sensation resulting in chronic joint
    instability.

E13.618   **Other specified diabetes mellitus** HCC Q
    with other diabetic arthropathy
    AHA: 2018,2Q,6

√6ᵗʰ E13.62   **Other specified diabetes mellitus with skin
    complications**

E13.620   **Other specified diabetes mellitus** HCC Q
    with diabetic dermatitis
    Other specified diabetes mellitus with
       diabetic necrobiosis lipoidica

E13.621   **Other specified diabetes mellitus** HCC Q
    with foot ulcer
    Use additional code to identify site of ulcer
       (L97.4-, L97.5-)
    TIP: Do not assign a code for diabetic ulcer
    when the ulcer is closed/resolved or to
    report history of diabetic ulcers; Z86.31
    Personal history of diabetic foot ulcer, may
    be assigned.

E13.622   **Other specified diabetes mellitus** HCC Q
    with other skin ulcer
    Use additional code to identify site of ulcer
       (L97.1-L97.9, L98.41-L98.49)
    AHA: 2017,4Q,17

E13.628   **Other specified diabetes mellitus** HCC Q
    with other skin complications
    AHA: 2017,4Q,100-101

√6ᵗʰ E13.63   **Other specified diabetes mellitus with oral
    complications**

E13.630   **Other specified diabetes mellitus** HCC Q
    with periodontal disease

E13.638   **Other specified diabetes mellitus** HCC Q
    with other oral complications

√6ᵗʰ E13.64   **Other specified diabetes mellitus with
    hypoglycemia**

E13.641   **Other specified diabetes mellitus** HCC Q
    with hypoglycemia with coma

E13.649   **Other specified diabetes mellitus** HCC Q
    with hypoglycemia without coma
    AHA: 2016,3Q,42; 2015,3Q,21

E13.65   **Other specified diabetes mellitus with** HCC Q
    hyperglycemia

E13.69   **Other specified diabetes mellitus with other** HCC Q
    specified complication
    Use additional code to identify complication
    AHA: 2016,4Q,141; 2016,1Q,13

E13.8   **Other specified diabetes mellitus with unspecified** HCC Q ▽
    complications

E13.9   **Other specified diabetes mellitus without** HCC Q
    complications

Other disorders of glucose regulation and pancreatic internal secretion (E15-E16)

E15   **Nondiabetic hypoglycemic coma**   HCC
    [INCLUDES]   drug-induced insulin coma in nondiabetic
       hyperinsulinism with hypoglycemic coma
       hypoglycemic coma NOS

√4ᵗʰ **E16   Other disorders of pancreatic internal secretion**

E16.0   **Drug-induced hypoglycemia without coma**
    Use additional code for adverse effect, if applicable, to identify
       drug (T36-T50 with fifth or sixth character 5)
    EXCLUDES 1   *diabetes with hypoglycemia without coma (E09.649)*

E16.1   **Other hypoglycemia**
    Functional hyperinsulinism
    Functional nonhyperinsulinemic hypoglycemia
    Hyperinsulinism NOS
    Hyperplasia of pancreatic islet beta cells NOS
    EXCLUDES 1   *diabetes with hypoglycemia (E08.649, E10.649,*
       E11.649, E13.649)
       hypoglycemia in infant of diabetic mother (P70.1)
       neonatal hypoglycemia (P70.4)

E16.2   **Hypoglycemia, unspecified**   ▽
    EXCLUDES 1   *diabetes with hypoglycemia (E08.649, E10.649,*
       E11.649, E13.649)
    AHA: 2016,3Q,42
    TIP: Assign for nondiabetic hypoglycemic encephalopathy not
    further clarified in the documentation.

E16.3   **Increased secretion of glucagon**
    Hyperplasia of pancreatic endocrine cells with glucagon excess

E16.4   **Increased secretion of gastrin**
    Hypergastrinemia
    Hyperplasia of pancreatic endocrine cells with gastrin excess
    Zollinger-Ellison syndrome

E16.8   **Other specified disorders of pancreatic internal secretion**
    Increased secretion from endocrine pancreas of growth
       hormone-releasing hormone
    Increased secretion from endocrine pancreas of pancreatic
       polypeptide
    Increased secretion from endocrine pancreas of somatostatin
    Increased secretion from endocrine pancreas of
       vasoactive-intestinal polypeptide

E16.9   **Disorder of pancreatic internal secretion, unspecified**   ▽
    Islet-cell hyperplasia NOS
    Pancreatic endocrine cell hyperplasia NOS

Disorders of other endocrine glands (E20-E35)

    EXCLUDES 1   *galactorrhea (N64.3)*
       gynecomastia (N62)

√4ᵗʰ **E20   Hypoparathyroidism**
    EXCLUDES 1   *Di George's syndrome (D82.1)*
       postprocedural hypoparathyroidism (E89.2)
       tetany NOS (R29.0)
       transitory neonatal hypoparathyroidism (P71.4)

E20.0   **Idiopathic hypoparathyroidism**   HCC
    DEF: Abnormally low secretion of parathyroid hormones, with
    unknown cause, which causes decreased calcium and increased
    phosphorus in the blood, resulting in muscle cramps, tetany,
    tingling, or burning in the lips, fingers, and toes, and cataracts.

E20.1   **Pseudohypoparathyroidism**

E20.8   **Other hypoparathyroidism**   HCC

E20.9   **Hypoparathyroidism, unspecified**   HCC ▽
    Parathyroid tetany

√4ᵗʰ **E21 Hyperparathyroidism and other disorders of parathyroid gland**

    EXCLUDES 1   adult osteomalacia (M83.-)
                 ectopic hyperparathyroidism (E34.2)
                 familial hypocalciuric hypercalcemia (E83.52)
                 hungry bone syndrome (E83.81)
                 infantile and juvenile osteomalacia (E55.0)

E21.0   Primary hyperparathyroidism   HCC
     Hyperplasia of parathyroid
     Osteitis fibrosa cystica generalisata [von Recklinghausen's disease of bone]
     DEF: Parathyroid dysfunction commonly caused by hyperplasia of two or more glands. Symptoms include hypercalcemia and increased parathyroid hormone levels.

E21.1   Secondary hyperparathyroidism, not elsewhere classified   HCC
    EXCLUDES 1   secondary hyperparathyroidism of renal origin (N25.81)

E21.2   Other hyperparathyroidism   HCC
     Tertiary hyperparathyroidism
    EXCLUDES 1   familial hypocalciuric hypercalcemia (E83.52)

E21.3   Hyperparathyroidism, unspecified   HCC ▽

E21.4   Other specified disorders of parathyroid gland   HCC

E21.5   Disorder of parathyroid gland, unspecified   HCC ▽

√4ᵗʰ **E22 Hyperfunction of pituitary gland**

    EXCLUDES 1   Cushing's syndrome (E24.-)
                 Nelson's syndrome (E24.1)
                 overproduction of ACTH not associated with Cushing's disease (E27.0)
                 overproduction of pituitary ACTH (E24.0)
                 overproduction of thyroid-stimulating hormone (E05.8-)

E22.0   Acromegaly and pituitary gigantism   HCC
     Overproduction of growth hormone
    EXCLUDES 1   constitutional gigantism (E34.4)
                 constitutional tall stature (E34.4)
                 increased secretion from endocrine pancreas of growth hormone-releasing hormone (E16.8)
     DEF: Acromegaly: Chronic condition caused by overproduction of the pituitary growth hormone resulting in enlarged skeletal parts and facial features.

E22.1   Hyperprolactinemia   HCC
     Use additional code for adverse effect, if applicable, to identify drug (T36-T50 with fifth or sixth character 5)

E22.2   Syndrome of inappropriate secretion of antidiuretic hormone   HCC

E22.8   Other hyperfunction of pituitary gland   HCC
     Central precocious puberty

E22.9   Hyperfunction of pituitary gland, unspecified   HCC ▽

√4ᵗʰ **E23 Hypofunction and other disorders of the pituitary gland**

    INCLUDES   the listed conditions whether the disorder is in the pituitary or the hypothalamus
    EXCLUDES 1   postprocedural hypopituitarism (E89.3)

E23.0   Hypopituitarism   HCC
     Fertile eunuch syndrome
     Hypogonadotropic hypogonadism
     Idiopathic growth hormone deficiency
     Isolated deficiency of gonadotropin
     Isolated deficiency of growth hormone
     Isolated deficiency of pituitary hormone
     Kallmann's syndrome
     Lorain-Levi short stature
     Necrosis of pituitary gland (postpartum)
     Panhypopituitarism
     Pituitary cachexia
     Pituitary insufficiency NOS
     Pituitary short stature
     Sheehan's syndrome
     Simmonds' disease

E23.1   Drug-induced hypopituitarism   HCC
     Use additional code for adverse effect, if applicable, to identify drug (T36-T50 with fifth or sixth character 5)

E23.2   Diabetes insipidus   HCC
    EXCLUDES 1   nephrogenic diabetes insipidus (N25.1)

E23.3   Hypothalamic dysfunction, not elsewhere classified   HCC
    EXCLUDES 1   Prader-Willi syndrome (Q87.1)
                 Russell-Silver syndrome (Q87.1)

E23.6   Other disorders of pituitary gland   HCC
     Abscess of pituitary
     Adiposogenital dystrophy

E23.7   Disorder of pituitary gland, unspecified   HCC ▽

√4ᵗʰ **E24 Cushing's syndrome**

    EXCLUDES 1   congenital adrenal hyperplasia (E25.0)
     DEF: Abdominal striae, acne, hypertension, decreased carbohydrate tolerance, moon face, obesity, protein catabolism, and psychiatric disturbances resulting from increased adrenocortical secretion of cortisol caused by ACTH-dependent adrenocortical hyperplasia or tumor, or by steroid effects.

E24.0   Pituitary-dependent Cushing's disease   HCC
     Overproduction of pituitary ACTH
     Pituitary-dependent hypercorticalism

E24.1   Nelson's syndrome   HCC

E24.2   Drug-induced Cushing's syndrome   HCC
     Use additional code for adverse effect, if applicable, to identify drug (T36-T50 with fifth or sixth character 5)

E24.3   Ectopic ACTH syndrome   HCC

E24.4   Alcohol-induced pseudo-Cushing's syndrome   HCC

E24.8   Other Cushing's syndrome   HCC

E24.9   Cushing's syndrome, unspecified   HCC ▽

√4ᵗʰ **E25 Adrenogenital disorders**

    INCLUDES   adrenogenital syndromes, virilizing or feminizing, whether acquired or due to adrenal hyperplasia consequent on inborn enzyme defects in hormone synthesis
                 female adrenal pseudohermaphroditism
                 female heterosexual precocious pseudopuberty
                 male isosexual precocious pseudopuberty
                 male macrogenitosomia praecox
                 male sexual precocity with adrenal hyperplasia
                 male virilization (female)
    EXCLUDES 1   indeterminate sex and pseudohermaphroditism (Q56)
                 chromosomal abnormalities (Q90-Q99)

E25.0   Congenital adrenogenital disorders associated with enzyme deficiency   HCC
     Congenital adrenal hyperplasia
     21-Hydroxylase deficiency
     Salt-losing congenital adrenal hyperplasia

E25.8   Other adrenogenital disorders   HCC
     Idiopathic adrenogenital disorder
     Use additional code for adverse effect, if applicable, to identify drug (T36-T50 with fifth or sixth character 5)

E25.9   Adrenogenital disorder, unspecified   HCC ▽
     Adrenogenital syndrome NOS

√4ᵗʰ **E26 Hyperaldosteronism**

√5ᵗʰ **E26.0   Primary hyperaldosteronism**

    E26.01   Conn's syndrome   HCC
         Code also adrenal adenoma (D35.0-)

    E26.02   Glucocorticoid-remediable aldosteronism   HCC
         Familial aldosteronism type I
         DEF: Rare autosomal dominant familial form of primary aldosteronism in which the secretion of aldosterone is under the influence of adrenocorticotrophic hormone (ACTH) rather than the renin-angiotensin mechanism. Moderate hypersecretion of aldosterone and suppressed plasma renin activity that are rapidly reversed by administration of glucosteroids. Symptoms include hypertension and mild hypokalemia.

    E26.09   Other primary hyperaldosteronism   HCC
         Primary aldosteronism due to adrenal hyperplasia (bilateral)

E26.1   Secondary hyperaldosteronism   HCC

√5ᵗʰ **E26.8   Other hyperaldosteronism**

    E26.81   Bartter's syndrome   HCC

    E26.89   Other hyperaldosteronism   HCC

E26.9   Hyperaldosteronism, unspecified   HCC ▽
     Aldosteronism NOS
     Hyperaldosteronism NOS

√4ᵗʰ **E27 Other disorders of adrenal gland**

E27.0   Other adrenocortical overactivity   HCC
     Overproduction of ACTH, not associated with Cushing's disease
     Premature adrenarche
    EXCLUDES 1   Cushing's syndrome (E24.-)

☑ Additional Character Req   √x 7ᵗʰ Placeholder Alert   Manifestation   ▽ Unspecified   ►◄ Revised Text   ● New Code   ▲ Revised Code Title

Chapter 4. Endocrine, Nutritional and Metabolic Diseases

E27.1   Primary adrenocortical insufficiency `HCC`
Addison's disease
Autoimmune adrenalitis
> EXCLUDES 1   Addison only phenotype adrenoleukodystrophy
> (E71.528)
> amyloidosis (E85.-)
> tuberculous Addison's disease (A18.7)
> Waterhouse-Friderichsen syndrome (A39.1)

E27.2   Addisonian crisis `HCC`
Adrenal crisis
Adrenocortical crisis
DEF: Life-threatening condition that occurs when there is not enough cortisol excreted from the adrenal glands. This condition may be due to injury to the adrenal glands or to the pituitary gland, which controls adrenal hormone secretion, or when a patient stops hydrocortisone treatment too quickly or too early.

E27.3   Drug-induced adrenocortical insufficiency `HCC`
Use additional code for adverse effect, if applicable, to identify drug (T36-T50 with fifth or sixth character 5)

✓5ᵗʰ **E27.4   Other and unspecified adrenocortical insufficiency**
> EXCLUDES 1   adrenoleukodystrophy [Addison-Schilder] (E71.528)
> Waterhouse-Friderichsen syndrome (A39.1)

     E27.40   Unspecified adrenocortical insufficiency `HCC` ▽
Adrenocortical insufficiency NOS
Hypoaldosteronism

     E27.49   Other adrenocortical insufficiency `HCC`
Adrenal hemorrhage
Adrenal infarction

E27.5   Adrenomedullary hyperfunction `HCC`
Adrenomedullary hyperplasia
Catecholamine hypersecretion

E27.8   Other specified disorders of adrenal gland `HCC`
Abnormality of cortisol-binding globulin

E27.9   Disorder of adrenal gland, unspecified `HCC` ▽

✓4ᵗʰ **E28   Ovarian dysfunction**
> EXCLUDES 1   isolated gonadotropin deficiency (E23.0)
> postprocedural ovarian failure (E89.4-)

E28.0   Estrogen excess ♀
Use additional code for adverse effect, if applicable, to identify drug (T36-T50 with fifth or sixth character 5)

E28.1   Androgen excess ♀
Hypersecretion of ovarian androgens
Use additional code for adverse effect, if applicable, to identify drug (T36-T50 with fifth or sixth character 5)

E28.2   Polycystic ovarian syndrome ♀
Sclerocystic ovary syndrome
Stein-Leventhal syndrome
DEF: Common hormonal disorder among women of reproductive age that involves enlarged ovaries with numerous small cysts located along the outer ovarian edge.

✓5ᵗʰ **E28.3   Primary ovarian failure**
> EXCLUDES 1   pure gonadal dysgenesis (Q99.1)
> Turner's syndrome (Q96.-)

     ✓6ᵗʰ **E28.31   Premature menopause**
         E28.310   Symptomatic premature menopause Ⓐ ♀
Symptoms such as flushing, sleeplessness, headache, lack of concentration, associated with premature menopause

         E28.319   Asymptomatic premature menopause Ⓐ ♀
Premature menopause NOS

     E28.39   Other primary ovarian failure ♀
Decreased estrogen
Resistant ovary syndrome

E28.8   Other ovarian dysfunction ♀
Ovarian hyperfunction NOS
> EXCLUDES 1   postprocedural ovarian failure (E89.4-)

E28.9   Ovarian dysfunction, unspecified ♀ ▽

✓4ᵗʰ **E29   Testicular dysfunction**
> EXCLUDES 1   androgen insensitivity syndrome (E34.5-)
> azoospermia or oligospermia NOS (N46.0-N46.1)
> isolated gonadotropin deficiency (E23.0)
> Klinefelter's syndrome (Q98.0-Q98.1, Q98.4)

E29.0   Testicular hyperfunction ♂
Hypersecretion of testicular hormones

E29.1   Testicular hypofunction ♂
Defective biosynthesis of testicular androgen NOS
5-delta-Reductase deficiency (with male pseudohermaphroditism)
Testicular hypogonadism NOS
Use additional code for adverse effect, if applicable, to identify drug (T36-T50 with fifth or sixth character 5)
> EXCLUDES 1   postprocedural testicular hypofunction (E89.5)

E29.8   Other testicular dysfunction ♂
E29.9   Testicular dysfunction, unspecified ♂ ▽

✓4ᵗʰ **E30   Disorders of puberty, not elsewhere classified**

E30.0   Delayed puberty
Constitutional delay of puberty
Delayed sexual development

E30.1   Precocious puberty Ⓟ
Precocious menstruation
> EXCLUDES 1   Albright (-McCune) (-Sternberg) syndrome (Q78.1)
> central precocious puberty (E22.8)
> congenital adrenal hyperplasia (E25.0)
> female heterosexual precocious pseudopuberty (E25.-)
> male isosexual precocious pseudopuberty (E25.-)

E30.8   Other disorders of puberty Ⓟ
Premature thelarche

E30.9   Disorder of puberty, unspecified ▽

✓4ᵗʰ **E31   Polyglandular dysfunction**
> EXCLUDES 1   ataxia telangiectasia [Louis-Bar] (G11.3)
> dystrophia myotonica [Steinert] (G71.11)
> pseudohypoparathyroidism (E20.1)

E31.0   Autoimmune polyglandular failure `HCC`
Schmidt's syndrome

E31.1   Polyglandular hyperfunction `HCC`
> EXCLUDES 1   multiple endocrine adenomatosis (E31.2-)
> multiple endocrine neoplasia (E31.2-)

✓5ᵗʰ **E31.2   Multiple endocrine neoplasia [MEN] syndromes**
Multiple endocrine adenomatosis
Code also any associated malignancies and other conditions associated with the syndromes

     E31.20   Multiple endocrine neoplasia [MEN] syndrome, unspecified `HCC` ▽
Multiple endocrine adenomatosis NOS
Multiple endocrine neoplasia [MEN] syndrome NOS

     E31.21   Multiple endocrine neoplasia [MEN] type I `HCC`
Wermer's syndrome

     E31.22   Multiple endocrine neoplasia [MEN] type IIA `HCC`
Sipple's syndrome

     E31.23   Multiple endocrine neoplasia [MEN] type IIB `HCC`

E31.8   Other polyglandular dysfunction `HCC`
E31.9   Polyglandular dysfunction, unspecified `HCC` ▽

✓4ᵗʰ **E32   Diseases of thymus**
> EXCLUDES 1   aplasia or hypoplasia of thymus with immunodeficiency (D82.1)
> myasthenia gravis (G70.0)

E32.0   Persistent hyperplasia of thymus `HCC`
Hypertrophy of thymus

E32.1   Abscess of thymus `HCC`
E32.8   Other diseases of thymus `HCC`
> EXCLUDES 1   aplasia or hypoplasia with immunodeficiency (D82.1)
> thymoma (D15.0)

E32.9   Disease of thymus, unspecified `HCC` ▽

Chapter 4. Endocrine, Nutritional and Metabolic Diseases

E34 Other endocrine disorders
EXCLUDES 1 pseudohypoparathyroidism (E20.1)

E34.0 Carcinoid syndrome [HCC]
NOTE May be used as an additional code to identify functional activity associated with a carcinoid tumor.

E34.1 Other hypersecretion of intestinal hormones

E34.2 Ectopic hormone secretion, not elsewhere classified
EXCLUDES 1 ectopic ACTH syndrome (E24.3)

E34.3 Short stature due to endocrine disorder
Constitutional short stature
Laron-type short stature
EXCLUDES 1 achondroplastic short stature (Q77.4)
hypochondroplastic short stature (Q77.4)
nutritional short stature (E45)
pituitary short stature (E23.0)
progeria (E34.8)
renal short stature (N25.0)
Russell-Silver syndrome (Q87.1)
short-limbed stature with immunodeficiency (D82.2)
short stature in specific dysmorphic syndromes - code to syndrome - see Alphabetical Index
short stature NOS (R62.52)

E34.4 Constitutional tall stature [HCC]
Constitutional gigantism

E34.5 Androgen insensitivity syndrome
DEF: X-linked recessive condition in which individuals that are chromosomally male fail to develop normal male external genitalia due to an abnormality on the X chromosome that prohibits the body, completely or in part, from recognizing the androgens produced. *Synonym(s): AIS*

E34.50 Androgen insensitivity syndrome, unspecified ▽
Androgen insensitivity NOS

E34.51 Complete androgen insensitivity syndrome
Complete androgen insensitivity
de Quervain syndrome
Goldberg-Maxwell syndrome

E34.52 Partial androgen insensitivity syndrome
Partial androgen insensitivity
Reifenstein syndrome

E34.8 Other specified endocrine disorders
Pineal gland dysfunction
Progeria
EXCLUDES 2 pseudohypoparathyroidism (E20.1)

E34.9 Endocrine disorder, unspecified ▽
Endocrine disturbance NOS
Hormone disturbance NOS

E35 Disorders of endocrine glands in diseases classified elsewhere
Code first underlying disease, such as:
late congenital syphilis of thymus gland [Dubois disease] (A50.5)
Use additional code, if applicable, to identify:
sequelae of tuberculosis of other organs (B90.8)
EXCLUDES 1 Echinococcus granulosus infection of thyroid gland (B67.3)
meningococcal hemorrhagic adrenalitis (A39.1)
syphilis of endocrine gland (A52.79)
tuberculosis of adrenal gland, except calcification (A18.7)
tuberculosis of endocrine gland NEC (A18.82)
tuberculosis of thyroid gland (A18.81)
Waterhouse-Friderichsen syndrome (A39.1)

Intraoperative complications of endocrine system (E36)

E36 Intraoperative complications of endocrine system
EXCLUDES 2 postprocedural endocrine and metabolic complications and disorders, not elsewhere classified (E89.-)

E36.0 Intraoperative hemorrhage and hematoma of an endocrine system organ or structure complicating a procedure
EXCLUDES 1 intraoperative hemorrhage and hematoma of an endocrine system organ or structure due to accidental puncture or laceration during a procedure (E36.1-)

E36.01 Intraoperative hemorrhage and hematoma of an endocrine system organ or structure complicating an endocrine system procedure

E36.02 Intraoperative hemorrhage and hematoma of an endocrine system organ or structure complicating other procedure

E36.1 Accidental puncture and laceration of an endocrine system organ or structure during a procedure

E36.11 Accidental puncture and laceration of an endocrine system organ or structure during an endocrine system procedure

E36.12 Accidental puncture and laceration of an endocrine system organ or structure during other procedure

E36.8 Other intraoperative complications of endocrine system
Use additional code, if applicable, to further specify disorder

Malnutrition (E40-E46)
EXCLUDES 1 intestinal malabsorption (K90.-)
sequelae of protein-calorie malnutrition (E64.0)
EXCLUDES 2 nutritional anemias (D50-D53)
starvation (T73.0)
AHA: 2017,4Q,108; 2017,3Q,25
TIP: Assign additional code for BMI from category Z68, when documented. BMI can be based on documentation from clinicians who are not the patient's provider.

E40 Kwashiorkor [HCC]
Severe malnutrition with nutritional edema with dyspigmentation of skin and hair
EXCLUDES 1 marasmic kwashiorkor (E42)

E41 Nutritional marasmus [HCC]
Severe malnutrition with marasmus
EXCLUDES 1 marasmic kwashiorkor (E42)
AHA: 2017,3Q,24
DEF: Protein-calorie malabsorption or malnutrition in children characterized by tissue wasting, dehydration, and subcutaneous fat depletion. It may occur with infectious disease.
TIP: Assign code R64 when emaciated or emaciation is documented without documentation of malnutrition.

E42 Marasmic kwashiorkor [HCC]
Intermediate form severe protein-calorie malnutrition
Severe protein-calorie malnutrition with signs of both kwashiorkor and marasmus

E43 Unspecified severe protein-calorie malnutrition [HCC] ▽
Starvation edema
AHA: 2017,4Q,108

E44 Protein-calorie malnutrition of moderate and mild degree
E44.0 Moderate protein-calorie malnutrition [HCC]
E44.1 Mild protein-calorie malnutrition [HCC]

E45 Retarded development following protein-calorie malnutrition [HCC]
Nutritional short stature
Nutritional stunting
Physical retardation due to malnutrition

E46 Unspecified protein-calorie malnutrition [HCC] ▽
Malnutrition NOS
Protein-calorie imbalance NOS
EXCLUDES 1 nutritional deficiency NOS (E63.9)

Other nutritional deficiencies (E50-E64)
EXCLUDES 2 nutritional anemias (D50-D53)

E50 Vitamin A deficiency
EXCLUDES 1 sequelae of vitamin A deficiency (E64.1)

E50.0 Vitamin A deficiency with conjunctival xerosis
E50.1 Vitamin A deficiency with Bitot's spot and conjunctival xerosis
Bitot's spot in the young child
DEF: Vitamin A deficiency with conjunctival dryness and superficial spots of keratinized epithelium.

E50.2 Vitamin A deficiency with corneal xerosis
E50.3 Vitamin A deficiency with corneal ulceration and xerosis
E50.4 Vitamin A deficiency with keratomalacia
DEF: Vitamin A deficiency creating corneal dryness that progresses to corneal insensitivity, softness, and necrosis. It is usually bilateral.

E50.5 Vitamin A deficiency with night blindness
E50.6 Vitamin A deficiency with xerophthalmic scars of cornea
E50.7 Other ocular manifestations of vitamin A deficiency
Xerophthalmia NOS

Chapter 4. Endocrine, Nutritional and Metabolic Diseases

E50.8   Other manifestations of vitamin A deficiency
Follicular keratosis
Xeroderma

E50.9   Vitamin A deficiency, unspecified ▽
Hypovitaminosis A NOS

√4ᵗʰ **E51   Thiamine deficiency**
     EXCLUDES 1   sequelae of thiamine deficiency (E64.8)

√5ᵗʰ **E51.1   Beriberi**

E51.11   Dry beriberi
Beriberi NOS
Beriberi with polyneuropathy

E51.12   Wet beriberi
Beriberi with cardiovascular manifestations
Cardiovascular beriberi
Shoshin disease

E51.2   Wernicke's encephalopathy
     DEF: Deficiency of vitamin B1 resulting in a triad of acute mental confusion, ataxia, and ophthalmoplegia. The vast majority of affected patients are alcoholics.

E51.8   Other manifestations of thiamine deficiency

E51.9   Thiamine deficiency, unspecified ▽

E52   Niacin deficiency [pellagra]
Niacin (-tryptophan) deficiency
Nicotinamide deficiency
Pellagra (alcoholic)
     EXCLUDES 1   sequelae of niacin deficiency (E64.8)

√4ᵗʰ **E53   Deficiency of other B group vitamins**
     EXCLUDES 1   sequelae of vitamin B deficiency (E64.8)

E53.0   Riboflavin deficiency
Ariboflavinosis
Vitamin B2 deficiency

E53.1   Pyridoxine deficiency
Vitamin B6 deficiency
     EXCLUDES 1   pyridoxine-responsive sideroblastic anemia (D64.3)

E53.8   Deficiency of other specified B group vitamins
Biotin deficiency
Cyanocobalamin deficiency
Folate deficiency
Folic acid deficiency
Pantothenic acid deficiency
Vitamin B12 deficiency
     EXCLUDES 1   folate deficiency anemia (D52.-)
                  vitamin B12 deficiency anemia (D51.-)

E53.9   Vitamin B deficiency, unspecified ▽

E54   Ascorbic acid deficiency
Deficiency of vitamin C
Scurvy
     EXCLUDES 1   scorbutic anemia (D53.2)
                  sequelae of vitamin C deficiency (E64.2)
     DEF: Vitamin C deficiency causing swollen gums, myalgia, weight loss, and weakness.

√4ᵗʰ **E55   Vitamin D deficiency**
     EXCLUDES 1   adult osteomalacia (M83.-)
                  osteoporosis (M80.-)
                  sequelae of rickets (E64.3)

E55.0   Rickets, active
Infantile osteomalacia
Juvenile osteomalacia
     EXCLUDES 1   celiac rickets (K90.0)
                  Crohn's rickets (K50.-)
                  hereditary vitamin D-dependent rickets (E83.32)
                  inactive rickets (E64.3)
                  renal rickets (N25.0)
                  sequelae of rickets (E64.3)
                  vitamin D-resistant rickets (E83.31)
     DEF: Rickets: Softening or weakening of the bones due to a lack of vitamin D, calcium, and phosphate.

E55.9   Vitamin D deficiency, unspecified ▽
Avitaminosis D

√4ᵗʰ **E56   Other vitamin deficiencies**
     EXCLUDES 1   sequelae of other vitamin deficiencies (E64.8)

E56.0   Deficiency of vitamin E

E56.1   Deficiency of vitamin K
     EXCLUDES 1   deficiency of coagulation factor due to vitamin K deficiency (D68.4)
                  vitamin K deficiency of newborn (P53)

E56.8   Deficiency of other vitamins

E56.9   Vitamin deficiency, unspecified ▽

E58   Dietary calcium deficiency
     EXCLUDES 1   disorders of calcium metabolism (E83.5-)
                  sequelae of calcium deficiency (E64.8)

E59   Dietary selenium deficiency
Keshan disease
     EXCLUDES 1   sequelae of selenium deficiency (E64.8)

E60   Dietary zinc deficiency

√4ᵗʰ **E61   Deficiency of other nutrient elements**
Use additional code for adverse effect, if applicable, to identify drug (T36-T50 with fifth or sixth character 5)
     EXCLUDES 1   disorders of mineral metabolism (E83.-)
                  iodine deficiency related thyroid disorders (E00-E02)
                  sequelae of malnutrition and other nutritional deficiencies (E64.-)

E61.0   Copper deficiency

E61.1   Iron deficiency
     EXCLUDES 1   iron deficiency anemia (D50.-)

E61.2   Magnesium deficiency

E61.3   Manganese deficiency

E61.4   Chromium deficiency

E61.5   Molybdenum deficiency

E61.6   Vanadium deficiency

E61.7   Deficiency of multiple nutrient elements

E61.8   Deficiency of other specified nutrient elements

E61.9   Deficiency of nutrient element, unspecified ▽

√4ᵗʰ **E63   Other nutritional deficiencies**
     EXCLUDES 1   dehydration (E86.0)
                  failure to thrive, adult (R62.7)
                  failure to thrive, child (R62.51)
                  feeding problems in newborn (P92.-)
                  sequelae of malnutrition and other nutritional deficiencies (E64.-)

E63.0   Essential fatty acid [EFA] deficiency

E63.1   Imbalance of constituents of food intake

E63.8   Other specified nutritional deficiencies

E63.9   Nutritional deficiency, unspecified ▽

√4ᵗʰ **E64   Sequelae of malnutrition and other nutritional deficiencies**
     NOTE   This category is to be used to indicate conditions in categories E43, E44, E46, E50-E63 as the cause of sequelae, which are themselves classified elsewhere. The 'sequelae' include conditions specified as such; they also include the late effects of diseases classifiable to the above categories if the disease itself is no longer present
Code first condition resulting from (sequela) of malnutrition and other nutritional deficiencies

E64.0   Sequelae of protein-calorie malnutrition   HCC
     EXCLUDES 2   retarded development following protein-calorie malnutrition (E45)

E64.1   Sequelae of vitamin A deficiency

E64.2   Sequelae of vitamin C deficiency

E64.3   Sequelae of rickets

E64.8   Sequelae of other nutritional deficiencies

E64.9   Sequelae of unspecified nutritional deficiency ▽

Overweight, obesity and other hyperalimentation (E65-E68)

E65   Localized adiposity
Fat pad

☑4ᵗʰ **E66 Overweight and obesity**

Code first obesity complicating pregnancy, childbirth and the puerperium, if applicable (O99.21-)

Use additional code to identify body mass index (BMI), if known (Z68.-)

EXCLUDES 1   *adiposogenital dystrophy (E23.6)*

lipomatosis NOS (E88.2)

lipomatosis dolorosa [Dercum] (E88.2)

Prader-Willi syndrome (Q87.1)

☑5ᵗʰ **E66.0 Obesity** due to excess calories

E66.01 Morbid (severe) obesity due to excess calories   HCC

EXCLUDES 1   *morbid (severe) obesity with alveolar hypoventilation (E66.2)*

E66.09 Other obesity due to excess calories

E66.1 Drug-induced obesity

Use additional code for adverse effect, if applicable, to identify drug (T36-T50 with fifth or sixth character 5)

E66.2 Morbid (severe) obesity with alveolar hypoventilation   HCC

Obesity hypoventilation syndrome (OHS)

Pickwickian syndrome

E66.3 Overweight

E66.8 Other obesity

E66.9 Obesity, unspecified   ▽

Obesity NOS

☑4ᵗʰ **E67 Other hyperalimentation**

EXCLUDES 1   *hyperalimentation NOS (R63.2)*

sequelae of hyperalimentation (E68)

E67.0 Hypervitaminosis A

▲ **E67.1 Hypercarotenemia**

DEF: Elevated blood carotene level as a result of excessive carotenoid ingestion or an inability to convert carotenoids to vitamin A. Characteristics often include yellow discoloration of the skin, which may follow overeating of carotenoid-rich foods such as carrots, sweet potatoes, or squash.

E67.2 Megavitamin-B6 syndrome

E67.3 Hypervitaminosis D

E67.8 Other specified hyperalimentation

E68 Sequelae of hyperalimentation

Code first condition resulting from (sequela) of hyperalimentation

Metabolic disorders (E70-E88)

EXCLUDES 1   *androgen insensitivity syndrome (E34.5-)*

congenital adrenal hyperplasia (E25.0)

Ehlers-Danlos syndrome (Q79.6)

hemolytic anemias attributable to enzyme disorders (D55.-)

Marfan's syndrome (Q87.4)

5-alpha-reductase deficiency (E29.1)

AHA: 2018,2Q,6

☑4ᵗʰ **E70 Disorders of aromatic amino-acid metabolism**

E70.0 Classical phenylketonuria   HCC

E70.1 Other hyperphenylalaninemias   HCC

☑5ᵗʰ **E70.2 Disorders of tyrosine metabolism**

EXCLUDES 1   *transitory tyrosinemia of newborn (P74.5)*

E70.20 Disorder of tyrosine metabolism, unspecified   HCC ▽

E70.21 Tyrosinemia   HCC

Hypertyrosinemia

E70.29 Other disorders of tyrosine metabolism   HCC

Alkaptonuria

Ochronosis

☑5ᵗʰ **E70.3 Albinism**

DEF: Absence of pigment in skin, hair, and eyes. This genetic condition is often accompanied by astigmatism, photophobia, and nystagmus.

E70.30 Albinism, unspecified   HCC ▽

☑6ᵗʰ **E70.31 Ocular albinism**

E70.310 X-linked ocular albinism   HCC

E70.311 Autosomal recessive ocular albinism   HCC

E70.318 Other ocular albinism   HCC

E70.319 Ocular albinism, unspecified   HCC ▽

☑6ᵗʰ **E70.32 Oculocutaneous albinism**

EXCLUDES 1   *Chediak-Higashi syndrome (E70.330)*

Hermansky-Pudlak syndrome (E70.331)

E70.320 Tyrosinase negative oculocutaneous albinism   HCC

Albinism I

Oculocutaneous albinism ty-neg

E70.321 Tyrosinase positive oculocutaneous albinism   HCC

Albinism II

Oculocutaneous albinism ty-pos

E70.328 Other oculocutaneous albinism   HCC

Cross syndrome

E70.329 Oculocutaneous albinism, unspecified   HCC ▽

☑6ᵗʰ **E70.33 Albinism with hematologic abnormality**

E70.330 Chediak-Higashi syndrome   HCC

E70.331 Hermansky-Pudlak syndrome   HCC

E70.338 Other albinism with hematologic abnormality   HCC

E70.339 Albinism with hematologic abnormality, unspecified   HCC ▽

E70.39 Other specified albinism   HCC

Piebaldism

☑5ᵗʰ **E70.4 Disorders of histidine metabolism**

E70.40 Disorders of histidine metabolism, unspecified   HCC ▽

E70.41 Histidinemia   HCC

E70.49 Other disorders of histidine metabolism   HCC

E70.5 Disorders of tryptophan metabolism   HCC

E70.8 Other disorders of aromatic amino-acid metabolism   HCC

E70.9 Disorder of aromatic amino-acid metabolism, unspecified   HCC ▽

☑4ᵗʰ **E71 Disorders of branched-chain amino-acid metabolism and fatty-acid metabolism**

E71.0 Maple-syrup-urine disease   HCC

☑5ᵗʰ **E71.1 Other disorders of branched-chain amino-acid metabolism**

☑6ᵗʰ **E71.11 Branched-chain organic acidurias**

E71.110 Isovaleric acidemia   HCC

E71.111 3-methylglutaconic aciduria   HCC

E71.118 Other branched-chain organic acidurias   HCC

☑6ᵗʰ **E71.12 Disorders of propionate metabolism**

E71.120 Methylmalonic acidemia   HCC

E71.121 Propionic acidemia   HCC

E71.128 Other disorders of propionate metabolism   HCC

E71.19 Other disorders of branched-chain amino-acid metabolism   HCC

Hyperleucine-isoleucinemia

Hypervalinemia

E71.2 Disorder of branched-chain amino-acid metabolism, unspecified   HCC ▽

☑5ᵗʰ **E71.3 Disorders of fatty-acid metabolism**

EXCLUDES 1   *peroxisomal disorders (E71.5)*

Refsum's disease (G60.1)

Schilder's disease (G37.0)

EXCLUDES 2   *carnitine deficiency due to inborn error of metabolism (E71.42)*

E71.30 Disorder of fatty-acid metabolism, unspecified   ▽

☑6ᵗʰ **E71.31 Disorders of fatty-acid oxidation**

E71.310 Long chain/very long chain acyl CoA dehydrogenase deficiency   HCC

LCAD

VLCAD

E71.311 Medium chain acyl CoA dehydrogenase deficiency   HCC

MCAD

E71.312 Short chain acyl CoA dehydrogenase deficiency   HCC

SCAD

☑ Additional Character Req   ✓x7ᵗʰ Placeholder Alert   Manifestation   ▽ Unspecified   ▶◀ Revised Text   ● New Code   ▲ Revised Code Title

Chapter 4. Endocrine, Nutritional and Metabolic Diseases

E71.313   **Glutaric aciduria type II**   HCC
       Glutaric aciduria type II A
       Glutaric aciduria type II B
       Glutaric aciduria type II C
       EXCLUDES 1   *glutaric aciduria (type 1) NOS (E72.3)*

E71.314   **Muscle carnitine palmitoyltransferase deficiency**   HCC

E71.318   **Other disorders of fatty-acid oxidation**   HCC

E71.32   **Disorders of ketone metabolism**   HCC

E71.39   **Other disorders of fatty-acid metabolism**   HCC

√5ᵗʰ   **E71.4**   **Disorders of carnitine metabolism**
     EXCLUDES 1   *muscle carnitine palmitoyltransferase deficiency (E71.314)*

E71.40   **Disorder of carnitine metabolism, unspecified**   HCC ▽

E71.41   **Primary carnitine deficiency**   HCC

E71.42   **Carnitine deficiency due to inborn errors of metabolism**   HCC
       Code also associated inborn error or metabolism

E71.43   **Iatrogenic carnitine deficiency**   HCC
       Carnitine deficiency due to hemodialysis
       Carnitine deficiency due to Valproic acid therapy

√6ᵗʰ   **E71.44**   **Other secondary carnitine deficiency**

     E71.440   **Ruvalcaba-Myhre-Smith syndrome**   HCC

     E71.448   **Other secondary carnitine deficiency**   HCC

√5ᵗʰ   **E71.5**   **Peroxisomal disorders**
     EXCLUDES 1   *Schilder's disease (G37.0)*

E71.50   **Peroxisomal disorder, unspecified**   HCC ▽

√6ᵗʰ   **E71.51**   **Disorders of peroxisome biogenesis**
     Group 1 peroxisomal disorders
     EXCLUDES 1   *Refsum's disease (G60.1)*

     E71.510   **Zellweger syndrome**   HCC

     E71.511   **Neonatal adrenoleukodystrophy**   HCC
       EXCLUDES 1   *X-linked adrenoleukodystrophy (E71.42-)*

     E71.518   **Other disorders of peroxisome biogenesis**   HCC

√6ᵗʰ   **E71.52**   **X-linked adrenoleukodystrophy**

     E71.520   **Childhood cerebral X-linked adrenoleukodystrophy**   HCC

     E71.521   **Adolescent X-linked adrenoleukodystrophy**   HCC

     E71.522   **Adrenomyeloneuropathy**   HCC

     E71.528   **Other X-linked adrenoleukodystrophy**   HCC
       Addison only phenotype adrenoleukodystrophy
       Addison-Schilder adrenoleukodystrophy

     E71.529   **X-linked adrenoleukodystrophy, unspecified type**   HCC ▽

E71.53   **Other group 2 peroxisomal disorders**   HCC

√6ᵗʰ   **E71.54**   **Other peroxisomal disorders**

     E71.540   **Rhizomelic chondrodysplasia punctata**   HCC
       EXCLUDES 1   *chondrodysplasia punctata NOS (Q77.3)*

     E71.541   **Zellweger-like syndrome**   HCC

     E71.542   **Other group 3 peroxisomal disorders**   HCC

     E71.548   **Other peroxisomal disorders**   HCC

√4ᵗʰ   **E72**   **Other disorders of amino-acid metabolism**
     EXCLUDES 1   *disorders of:*
       aromatic amino-acid metabolism (E70.-)
       branched-chain amino-acid metabolism (E71.0-E71.2)
       fatty-acid metabolism (E71.3)
       purine and pyrimidine metabolism (E79.-)
       gout (M1A.-, M10.-)

√5ᵗʰ   **E72.0**   **Disorders of amino-acid transport**
     EXCLUDES 1   *disorders of tryptophan metabolism (E70.5)*

     E72.00   **Disorders of amino-acid transport, unspecified**   HCC ▽

     E72.01   **Cystinuria**   HCC

     E72.02   **Hartnup's disease**   HCC

E72.03   **Lowe's syndrome**   HCC
       Use additional code for associated glaucoma (H42)

E72.04   **Cystinosis**   HCC
       Fanconi (-de Toni) (-Debré) syndrome with cystinosis
       EXCLUDES 1   *Fanconi (-de Toni) (-Debré) syndrome without cystinosis (E72.09)*

E72.09   **Other disorders of amino-acid transport**   HCC
       Fanconi (-de Toni) (-Debré) syndrome, unspecified

√5ᵗʰ   **E72.1**   **Disorders of sulfur-bearing amino-acid metabolism**
     EXCLUDES 1   *cystinosis (E72.04)*
       cystinuria (E72.01)
       transcobalamin II deficiency (D51.2)

E72.10   **Disorders of sulfur-bearing amino-acid metabolism, unspecified**   HCC ▽

E72.11   **Homocystinuria**   HCC
       Cystathionine synthase deficiency

E72.12   **Methylenetetrahydrofolate reductase deficiency**   HCC

E72.19   **Other disorders of sulfur-bearing amino-acid metabolism**   HCC
       Cystathioninuria
       Methioninemia
       Sulfite oxidase deficiency

√5ᵗʰ   **E72.2**   **Disorders of urea cycle metabolism**
     EXCLUDES 1   *disorders of ornithine metabolism (E72.4)*

E72.20   **Disorder of urea cycle metabolism, unspecified**   HCC ▽
       Hyperammonemia
       EXCLUDES 1   *hyperammonemia- hyperornithinemia-homocitrullinemia syndrome E72.4*
       transient hyperammonemia of newborn (P74.6)

E72.21   **Argininemia**   HCC

E72.22   **Arginosuccinic aciduria**   HCC

E72.23   **Citrullinemia**   HCC

E72.29   **Other disorders of urea cycle metabolism**   HCC

E72.3   **Disorders of lysine and hydroxylysine metabolism**   HCC
       Glutaric aciduria NOS
       Glutaric aciduria (type I)
       Hydroxylysinemia
       Hyperlysinemia
     EXCLUDES 1   *glutaric aciduria type II (E71.313)*
       Refsum's disease (G60.1)
       Zellweger syndrome (E71.510)

E72.4   **Disorders of ornithine metabolism**   HCC
       Hyperammonemia-Hyperornithinemia-Homocitrullinemia syndrome
       Ornithinemia (types I, II)
       Ornithine transcarbamylase deficiency
     EXCLUDES 1   *hereditary choroidal dystrophy (H31.2-)*

√5ᵗʰ   **E72.5**   **Disorders of glycine metabolism**

E72.50   **Disorder of glycine metabolism, unspecified**   HCC ▽

E72.51   **Non-ketotic hyperglycinemia**   HCC

E72.52   **Trimethylaminuria**   HCC

E72.53   **Primary hyperoxaluria**   HCC
       Oxalosis
       Oxaluria

E72.59   **Other disorders of glycine metabolism**   HCC
       D-glycericacidemia
       Hyperhydroxyprolinemia
       Hyperprolinemia (types I, II)
       Sarcosinemia

√5ᵗʰ   **E72.8**   **Other specified disorders of amino-acid metabolism**
       ~~Disorders of beta-amino-acid metabolism~~
       ~~Disorders of gamma-glutamyl cycle~~

     E72.81   **Disorders of gamma aminobutyric acid metabolism**
       4-hydroxybutyric aciduria
       Disorders of GABA metabolism
       GABA metabolic defect
       GABA transaminase deficiency
       GABA-T deficiency
       Gamma-hydroxybutyric aciduria
       SSADHD
       Succinic semialdehyde dehydrogenase deficiency

E72.89   **Other specified disorders of amino-acid metabolism**
    Disorders of beta-amino-acid metabolism
    Disorders of gamma-glutamyl cycle

E72.9   **Disorder of amino-acid metabolism, unspecified**   HCC ▽

✓4ᵗʰ **E73   Lactose intolerance**
    DEF: Inability to break down sugar in dairy products due to a deficiency in the enzyme lactase.

E73.0   **Congenital lactase deficiency**

E73.1   **Secondary lactase deficiency**

E73.8   **Other lactose intolerance**

E73.9   **Lactose intolerance, unspecified**   ▽

✓4ᵗʰ **E74   Other disorders of carbohydrate metabolism**
    EXCLUDES 1   diabetes mellitus (E08-E13)
           hypoglycemia NOS (E16.2)
           increased secretion of glucagon (E16.3)
           mucopolysaccharidosis (E76.0-E76.3)

✓5ᵗʰ E74.0   **Glycogen storage disease**

E74.00   **Glycogen storage disease, unspecified**   HCC ▽

E74.01   **von Gierke disease**   HCC
    Type I glycogen storage disease

E74.02   **Pompe disease**   HCC
    Cardiac glycogenosis
    Type II glycogen storage disease

E74.03   **Cori disease**   HCC
    Forbes disease
    Type III glycogen storage disease

E74.04   **McArdle disease**   HCC
    Type V glycogen storage disease

E74.09   **Other glycogen storage disease**   HCC
    Andersen disease
    Hers disease
    Tauri disease
    Glycogen storage disease, types 0, IV, VI-XI
    Liver phosphorylase deficiency
    Muscle phosphofructokinase deficiency

✓5ᵗʰ E74.1   **Disorders of fructose metabolism**
    EXCLUDES 1   muscle phosphofructokinase deficiency (E74.09)

E74.10   **Disorder of fructose metabolism, unspecified**   ▽

E74.11   **Essential fructosuria**
    Fructokinase deficiency

E74.12   **Hereditary fructose intolerance**
    Fructosemia

E74.19   **Other disorders of fructose metabolism**
    Fructose-1, 6-diphosphatase deficiency

✓5ᵗʰ E74.2   **Disorders of galactose metabolism**

E74.20   **Disorders of galactose metabolism, unspecified**   HCC ▽

E74.21   **Galactosemia**   HCC
    DEF: Any of three genetic disorders caused by a defective galactose metabolism. Symptoms include failure to thrive in infancy, jaundice, liver and spleen damage, cataracts, and mental retardation.

E74.29   **Other disorders of galactose metabolism**   HCC
    Galactokinase deficiency

✓5ᵗʰ E74.3   **Other disorders of intestinal carbohydrate absorption**
    EXCLUDES 2   lactose intolerance (E73.-)

E74.31   **Sucrase-isomaltase deficiency**

E74.39   **Other disorders of intestinal carbohydrate absorption**
    Disorder of intestinal carbohydrate absorption NOS
    Glucose-galactose malabsorption
    Sucrase deficiency

E74.4   **Disorders of pyruvate metabolism and gluconeogenesis**   HCC
    Deficiency of phosphoenolpyruvate carboxykinase
    Deficiency of pyruvate carboxylase
    Deficiency of pyruvate dehydrogenase
    EXCLUDES 1   disorders of pyruvate metabolism and gluconeogenesis with anemia (D55.-)
           Leigh's syndrome (G31.82)

E74.8   **Other specified disorders of carbohydrate metabolism**   HCC
    Essential pentosuria
    Renal glycosuria

E74.9   **Disorder of carbohydrate metabolism, unspecified**   HCC ▽

✓4ᵗʰ **E75   Disorders of sphingolipid metabolism and other lipid storage disorders**
    EXCLUDES 1   mucolipidosis, types I-III (E77.0-E77.1)
           Refsum's disease (G60.1)

✓5ᵗʰ E75.0   **GM2 gangliosidosis**

E75.00   **GM2 gangliosidosis, unspecified**   ▽

E75.01   **Sandhoff disease**

E75.02   **Tay-Sachs disease**
    DEF: Genetic mutation of the HEXA gene that inhibits the breakdown of a toxic substance called ganglioside. The accumulation of ganglioside results in destruction of the neurons in the brain and spinal cord.

Tay-Sachs Disease

Healthy neuron

Lysosome

Neuron affected by Tay-Sachs

Bulging lysosome

E75.09   **Other GM2 gangliosidosis**
    Adult GM2 gangliosidosis
    Juvenile GM2 gangliosidosis

✓5ᵗʰ E75.1   **Other and unspecified gangliosidosis**

E75.10   **Unspecified gangliosidosis**   ▽
    Gangliosidosis NOS

E75.11   **Mucolipidosis IV**

E75.19   **Other gangliosidosis**
    GM1 gangliosidosis
    GM3 gangliosidosis

✓5ᵗʰ E75.2   **Other sphingolipidosis**
    EXCLUDES 1   adrenoleukodystrophy [Addison-Schilder] (E71.528)

E75.21   **Fabry (-Anderson) disease**   HCC

E75.22   **Gaucher disease**   HCC

E75.23   **Krabbe disease**

✓6ᵗʰ E75.24   **Niemann-Pick disease**

E75.240   **Niemann-Pick disease type A**   HCC

E75.241   **Niemann-Pick disease type B**   HCC

E75.242   **Niemann-Pick disease type C**   HCC

E75.243   **Niemann-Pick disease type D**   HCC

E75.248   **Other Niemann-Pick disease**   HCC

E75.249   **Niemann-Pick disease, unspecified**   HCC ▽

E75.25   **Metachromatic leukodystrophy**

E75.26   **Sulfatase deficiency**
    Multiple sulfatase deficiency (MSD)

E75.29   **Other sphingolipidosis**
    Farber's syndrome
    ~~Sulfatase deficiency~~
    Sulfatide lipidosis

E75.3   **Sphingolipidosis, unspecified**   HCC ▽

E75.4   **Neuronal ceroid lipofuscinosis**
    Batten disease
    Bielschowsky-Jansky disease
    Kufs disease
    Spielmeyer-Vogt disease

☑ Additional Character Req   ✓x7ᵗʰ Placeholder Alert   Manifestation   ▽ Unspecified   ▶◀ Revised Text   ● New Code   ▲ Revised Code Title

E75.5　Other lipid storage disorders
　Cerebrotendinous cholesterosis [van Bogaert-Scherer-Epstein]
　Wolman's disease

E75.6　Lipid storage disorder, unspecified ▽

✓4ᵗʰ **E76　Disorders of glycosaminoglycan metabolism**

　✓5ᵗʰ **E76.0　Mucopolysaccharidosis, type I**

　　E76.01　Hurler's syndrome HCC
　　E76.02　Hurler-Scheie syndrome HCC
　　E76.03　Scheie's syndrome HCC

　E76.1　Mucopolysaccharidosis, type II HCC
　　Hunter's syndrome

　✓5ᵗʰ **E76.2　Other mucopolysaccharidoses**

　　✓6ᵗʰ **E76.21　Morquio mucopolysaccharidoses**

　　　E76.210　Morquio A HCC
　　　　mucopolysaccharidoses
　　　　Classic Morquio syndrome
　　　　Morquio syndrome A
　　　　Mucopolysaccharidosis, type IVA

　　　E76.211　Morquio B HCC
　　　　mucopolysaccharidoses
　　　　Morquio-like mucopolysaccharidoses
　　　　Morquio-like syndrome
　　　　Morquio syndrome B
　　　　Mucopolysaccharidosis, type IVB

　　　E76.219　Morquio mucopolysaccharidoses, HCC ▽
　　　　unspecified
　　　　Morquio syndrome
　　　　Mucopolysaccharidosis, type IV

　　E76.22　Sanfilippo mucopolysaccharidoses HCC
　　　Mucopolysaccharidosis, type III (A) (B) (C) (D)
　　　Sanfilippo A syndrome
　　　Sanfilippo B syndrome
　　　Sanfilippo C syndrome
　　　Sanfilippo D syndrome

　　E76.29　Other mucopolysaccharidoses HCC
　　　beta-Glucuronidase deficiency
　　　Maroteaux-Lamy (mild) (severe) syndrome
　　　Mucopolysaccharidosis, types VI, VII

　E76.3　Mucopolysaccharidosis, unspecified HCC ▽
　E76.8　Other disorders of glucosaminoglycan metabolism HCC
　E76.9　Glucosaminoglycan metabolism disorder, unspecified HCC ▽

✓4ᵗʰ **E77　Disorders of glycoprotein metabolism**

　E77.0　Defects in post-translational modification of HCC
　　lysosomal enzymes
　　Mucolipidosis II [I-cell disease]
　　Mucolipidosis III [pseudo-Hurler polydystrophy]

　E77.1　Defects in glycoprotein degradation HCC
　　Aspartylglucosaminuria
　　Fucosidosis
　　Mannosidosis
　　Sialidosis [mucolipidosis I]

　E77.8　Other disorders of glycoprotein metabolism HCC
　E77.9　Disorder of glycoprotein metabolism, unspecified HCC ▽

✓4ᵗʰ **E78　Disorders of lipoprotein metabolism and other lipidemias**

　　EXCLUDES 1　sphingolipidosis (E75.0-E75.3)

　✓5ᵗʰ **E78.0　Pure hypercholesterolemia**

　　AHA: 2016,4Q,13-14

　　E78.00　Pure hypercholesterolemia, unspecified ▽
　　　Fredrickson's hyperlipoproteinemia, type IIa
　　　Hyperbetalipoproteinemia
　　　Low-density-lipoprotein-type [LDL]
　　　　hyperlipoproteinemia
　　　(Pure) hypercholesterolemia NOS

　　E78.01　Familial hypercholesterolemia

　E78.1　Pure hyperglyceridemia
　　Elevated fasting triglycerides
　　Endogenous hyperglyceridemia
　　Fredrickson's hyperlipoproteinemia, type IV
　　Hyperlipidemia, group B
　　Hyperprebetalipoproteinemia
　　Very-low-density-lipoprotein-type [VLDL] hyperlipoproteinemia

E78.2　Mixed hyperlipidemia
　Broad- or floating-betalipoproteinemia
　Combined hyperlipidemia NOS
　Elevated cholesterol with elevated triglycerides NEC
　Fredrickson's hyperlipoproteinemia, type IIb or III
　Hyperbetalipoproteinemia with prebetalipoproteinemia
　Hypercholesteremia with endogenous hyperglyceridemia
　Hyperlipidemia, group C
　Tubo-eruptive xanthoma
　Xanthoma tuberosum
　EXCLUDES 1　cerebrotendinous cholesterosis [van Bogaert-Scherer-Epstein] (E75.5)
　　　　　　familial combined hyperlipidemia ▶(E78.49)◀

E78.3　Hyperchylomicronemia
　Chylomicron retention disease
　Fredrickson's hyperlipoproteinemia, type I or V
　Hyperlipidemia, group D
　Mixed hyperglyceridemia

✓5ᵗʰ **E78.4　Other hyperlipidemia**
　Familial combined hyperlipidemia

　● **E78.41　Elevated Lipoprotein(a)**
　　　Elevated Lp(a)

　● **E78.49　Other hyperlipidemia**
　　　Familial combined hyperlipidemia

E78.5　Hyperlipidemia, unspecified ▽

E78.6　Lipoprotein deficiency
　Abetalipoproteinemia
　Depressed HDL cholesterol
　High-density lipoprotein deficiency
　Hypoalphalipoproteinemia
　Hypobetalipoproteinemia (familial)
　Lecithin cholesterol acyltransferase deficiency
　Tangier disease

✓5ᵗʰ **E78.7　Disorders of bile acid and cholesterol metabolism**
　　EXCLUDES 1　Niemann-Pick disease type C (E75.242)

　E78.70　Disorder of bile acid and cholesterol ▽
　　metabolism, unspecified
　E78.71　Barth syndrome
　E78.72　Smith-Lemli-Opitz syndrome
　E78.79　Other disorders of bile acid and cholesterol
　　metabolism

✓5ᵗʰ **E78.8　Other disorders of lipoprotein metabolism**

　E78.81　Lipoid dermatoarthritis
　E78.89　Other lipoprotein metabolism disorders

E78.9　Disorder of lipoprotein metabolism, unspecified ▽

✓4ᵗʰ **E79　Disorders of purine and pyrimidine metabolism**

　　EXCLUDES 1　Ataxia-telangiectasia (G11.3)
　　　　　　Bloom's syndrome (Q82.8)
　　　　　　Cockayne's syndrome (Q87.1)
　　　　　　calculus of kidney (N20.0)
　　　　　　combined immunodeficiency disorders (D81.-)
　　　　　　Fanconi's anemia (D61.09)
　　　　　　gout (M1A.-, M10.-)
　　　　　　orotaciduric anemia (D53.0)
　　　　　　progeria (E34.8)
　　　　　　Werner's syndrome (E34.8)
　　　　　　xeroderma pigmentosum (Q82.1)

　E79.0　Hyperuricemia without signs of inflammatory arthritis and
　　tophaceous disease
　　Asymptomatic hyperuricemia

　E79.1　Lesch-Nyhan syndrome HCC
　　HGPRT deficiency

　E79.2　Myoadenylate deaminase deficiency HCC
　E79.8　Other disorders of purine and pyrimidine metabolism HCC
　　Hereditary xanthinuria
　E79.9　Disorder of purine and pyrimidine metabolism, HCC ▽
　　unspecified

✓4ᵗʰ **E80　Disorders of porphyrin and bilirubin metabolism**
　　INCLUDES　defects of catalase and peroxidase

　E80.0　Hereditary erythropoietic porphyria HCC
　　Congenital erythropoietic porphyria
　　Erythropoietic protoporphyria

　E80.1　Porphyria cutanea tarda HCC

√5ᵗʰ E80.2 Other and unspecified porphyria

    E80.20 Unspecified porphyria   HCC ▽
         Porphyria NOS

    E80.21 Acute intermittent (hepatic) porphyria   HCC

    E80.29 Other porphyria   HCC
         Hereditary coproporphyria

E80.3 Defects of catalase and peroxidase   HCC
     Acatalasia [Takahara]

E80.4 Gilbert syndrome

E80.5 Crigler-Najjar syndrome

E80.6 Other disorders of bilirubin metabolism
     Dubin-Johnson syndrome
     Rotor's syndrome

E80.7 Disorder of bilirubin metabolism, unspecified   ▽

√4ᵗʰ E83 Disorders of mineral metabolism

     EXCLUDES 1   dietary mineral deficiency (E58-E61)
                 parathyroid disorders (E20-E21)
                 vitamin D deficiency (E55.-)

√5ᵗʰ E83.0 Disorders of copper metabolism

    E83.00 Disorder of copper metabolism, unspecified   ▽

    E83.01 Wilson's disease
         Code also associated Kayser Fleischer ring (H18.04-)

    E83.09 Other disorders of copper metabolism
         Menkes' (kinky hair) (steely hair) disease

√5ᵗʰ E83.1 Disorders of iron metabolism

     EXCLUDES 1   iron deficiency anemia (D50.-)
                 sideroblastic anemia (D64.0-D64.3)

    E83.10 Disorder of iron metabolism, unspecified   ▽

    √6ᵗʰ E83.11 Hemochromatosis

         EXCLUDES 1   GALD (P78.84)
                     Gestational alloimmune liver disease
                           (P78.84)
                     Neonatal hemochromatosis (P78.84)

        E83.110 Hereditary hemochromatosis   HCC
              Bronzed diabetes
              Pigmentary cirrhosis (of liver)
              Primary (hereditary) hemochromatosis

        E83.111 Hemochromatosis due to repeated red blood cell transfusions
              Iron overload due to repeated red blood cell transfusions
              Transfusion (red blood cell) associated hemochromatosis

        E83.118 Other hemochromatosis

        E83.119 Hemochromatosis, unspecified   ▽

    E83.19 Other disorders of iron metabolism
         Use additional code, if applicable, for idiopathic pulmonary hemosiderosis (J84.03)

E83.2 Disorders of zinc metabolism
     Acrodermatitis enteropathica

√5ᵗʰ E83.3 Disorders of phosphorus metabolism and phosphatases

     EXCLUDES 1   adult osteomalacia (M83.-)
                 osteoporosis (M80.-)

    E83.30 Disorder of phosphorus metabolism, unspecified   ▽

    E83.31 Familial hypophosphatemia
         Vitamin D-resistant osteomalacia
         Vitamin D-resistant rickets
         EXCLUDES 1   vitamin D-deficiency rickets (E55.0)

    E83.32 Hereditary vitamin D-dependent rickets (type 1) (type 2)
         25-hydroxyvitamin D 1-alpha-hydroxylase deficiency
         Pseudovitamin D deficiency
         Vitamin D receptor defect

    E83.39 Other disorders of phosphorus metabolism
         Acid phosphatase deficiency
         Hypophosphatasia

√5ᵗʰ E83.4 Disorders of magnesium metabolism

    E83.40 Disorders of magnesium metabolism, unspecified   ▽

    E83.41 Hypermagnesemia
         AHA: 2016,4Q,54

    E83.42 Hypomagnesemia

    E83.49 Other disorders of magnesium metabolism

√5ᵗʰ E83.5 Disorders of calcium metabolism

     EXCLUDES 1   chondrocalcinosis (M11.1-M11.2)
                 hungry bone syndrome (E83.81)
                 hyperparathyroidism (E21.0-E21.3)

    E83.50 Unspecified disorder of calcium metabolism   ▽

    E83.51 Hypocalcemia

    E83.52 Hypercalcemia
         Familial hypocalciuric hypercalcemia

    E83.59 Other disorders of calcium metabolism
         ~~Idiopathic hypercalciuria~~

√5ᵗʰ E83.8 Other disorders of mineral metabolism

    E83.81 Hungry bone syndrome

    E83.89 Other disorders of mineral metabolism

E83.9 Disorder of mineral metabolism, unspecified   ▽

√4ᵗʰ E84 Cystic fibrosis

     INCLUDES   mucoviscidosis

     Code also exocrine pancreatic insufficiency (K86.81)

     DEF: Genetic disorder affecting the respiratory, digestive, and reproductive systems in infants to young adults by disturbing exocrine gland function and causing chronic pulmonary disease with excess mucus production and pancreatic deficiency.

E84.0 Cystic fibrosis with pulmonary manifestations   HCC
     Use additional code to identify any infectious organism present, such as:
         Pseudomonas (B96.5)

√5ᵗʰ E84.1 Cystic fibrosis with intestinal manifestations

    E84.11 Meconium ileus in cystic fibrosis   HCC N
         EXCLUDES 1   meconium ileus not due to cystic fibrosis (P76.0)

    E84.19 Cystic fibrosis with other intestinal manifestations   HCC
         Distal intestinal obstruction syndrome

E84.8 Cystic fibrosis with other manifestations   HCC

E84.9 Cystic fibrosis, unspecified   HCC ▽

√4ᵗʰ E85 Amyloidosis

     EXCLUDES 2   Alzheimer's disease (G30.0-)

     DEF: Conditions of diverse etiologies characterized by the accumulation of insoluble fibrillar proteins (amyloid) in various organs and tissues of the body, compromising vital functions.

E85.0 Non-neuropathic heredofamilial amyloidosis   HCC
     Hereditary amyloid nephropathy
     Code also associated disorders, such as:
         autoinflammatory syndromes (M04.-)
     EXCLUDES 2   Transthyretin-related (ATTR) familial amyloid cardiomyopathy (E85.4)

E85.1 Neuropathic heredofamilial amyloidosis   HCC
     Amyloid polyneuropathy (Portuguese)
     Transthyretin-related (ATTR) familial amyloid polyneuropathy
     AHA: 2012,4Q,99

E85.2 Heredofamilial amyloidosis, unspecified   HCC ▽

E85.3 Secondary systemic amyloidosis   HCC
     Hemodialysis-associated amyloidosis

E85.4 Organ-limited amyloidosis   HCC
     Localized amyloidosis
     Transthyretin-related (ATTR) familial amyloid cardiomyopathy

√5ᵗʰ E85.8 Other amyloidosis

     AHA: 2017,4Q,7

    E85.81 Light chain (AL) amyloidosis   HCC

    E85.82 Wild-type transthyretin-related (ATTR) amyloidosis   HCC
         Senile systemic amyloidosis (SSA)

    E85.89 Other amyloidosis   HCC

E85.9 Amyloidosis, unspecified   HCC ▽

√4ᵗʰ E86 Volume depletion

     Use additional code(s) for any associated disorders of electrolyte and acid-base balance (E87.-)

     EXCLUDES 1   dehydration of newborn (P74.1)
                 hypovolemic shock NOS (R57.1)
                 postprocedural hypovolemic shock (T81.19)
                 traumatic hypovolemic shock (T79.4)

     AHA: 2018,2Q,6

E86.0 Dehydration
     AHA: 2014,1Q,7
     TIP: Can be assigned in addition to hypernatremia (E87.0) or hyponatremia (E87.1), when documented.

✔ Additional Character Req   √x7ᵗʰ Placeholder Alert   Manifestation   ▽ Unspecified   ▶◀ Revised Text   ● New Code   ▲ Revised Code Title

E86.1 Hypovolemia
Depletion of volume of plasma

E86.9 Volume depletion, unspecified ▽
DEF: Depletion of total body water (dehydration) and/or contraction of total intravascular plasma (hypovolemia).

✓4ᵗʰ **E87 Other disorders of fluid, electrolyte and acid-base balance**
EXCLUDES 1   *diabetes insipidus (E23.2)*
electrolyte imbalance associated with hyperemesis gravidarum (O21.1)
electrolyte imbalance following ectopic or molar pregnancy (O08.5)
familial periodic paralysis (G72.3)
AHA: 2018,2Q,6

E87.0 Hyperosmolality and hypernatremia
Sodium [Na] excess
Sodium [Na] overload
AHA: 2014,1Q,7
TIP: Assign an additional code for dehydration (E86.0), when documented.

E87.1 Hypo-osmolality and hyponatremia
Sodium [Na] deficiency
EXCLUDES 1   *syndrome of inappropriate secretion of antidiuretic hormone (E22.2)*
AHA: 2014,1Q,7
TIP: Assign an additional code for dehydration (E86.0), when documented.

E87.2 Acidosis
Acidosis NOS
Lactic acidosis
Metabolic acidosis
Respiratory acidosis
EXCLUDES 1   *diabetic acidosis - see categories E08-E10, E13 with ketoacidosis*
DEF: Reduction of alkaline in the blood and tissues caused by an increase in acid and decrease in bicarbonate.

E87.3 Alkalosis
Alkalosis NOS
Metabolic alkalosis
Respiratory alkalosis

E87.4 Mixed disorder of acid-base balance

E87.5 Hyperkalemia
Potassium [K] excess
Potassium [K] overload

E87.6 Hypokalemia
Potassium [K] deficiency

✓5ᵗʰ **E87.7 Fluid overload**
EXCLUDES 1   *edema NOS (R60.9)*
fluid retention (R60.9)

E87.70 Fluid overload, unspecified ▽

E87.71 Transfusion associated circulatory overload
Fluid overload due to transfusion (blood) (blood components)
TACO

E87.79 Other fluid overload

E87.8 Other disorders of electrolyte and fluid balance, not elsewhere classified
Electrolyte imbalance NOS
Hyperchloremia
Hypochloremia

✓4ᵗʰ **E88 Other and unspecified metabolic disorders**
Use additional codes for associated conditions
EXCLUDES 1   *histiocytosis X (chronic) (C96.6)*

✓5ᵗʰ **E88.0 Disorders of plasma-protein metabolism, not elsewhere classified**
EXCLUDES 1   *disorder of lipoprotein metabolism (E78.-)*
monoclonal gammopathy (of undetermined significance) (D47.2)
polyclonal hypergammaglobulinemia (D89.0)
Waldenström macroglobulinemia (C88.0)

E88.01 Alpha-1-antitrypsin deficiency HCC
AAT deficiency

● **E88.02 Plasminogen deficiency**
Dysplasminogenemia
Hypoplasminogenemia
Type 1 plasminogen deficiency
Type 2 plasminogen deficiency
Code also, if applicable, ligneous conjunctivitis (H10.51)
Use additional code for associated findings, such as:
hydrocephalus (G91.4)
ligneous conjunctivitis (H10.51)
otitis media (H67.-)
respiratory disorder related to plasminogen deficiency (J99)

E88.09 Other disorders of plasma-protein metabolism, not elsewhere classified
Bisalbuminemia

E88.1 Lipodystrophy, not elsewhere classified
Lipodystrophy NOS
EXCLUDES 1   *Whipple's disease (K90.81)*

E88.2 Lipomatosis, not elsewhere classified
Lipomatosis NOS
Lipomatosis (Check) dolorosa [Dercum]

E88.3 Tumor lysis syndrome
Tumor lysis syndrome (spontaneous)
Tumor lysis syndrome following antineoplastic drug chemotherapy
Use additional code for adverse effect, if applicable, to identify drug (T45.1X5)
DEF: Potentially fatal metabolic complication of tumor necrosis caused by spontaneous or treatment-related accumulation of byproducts from dying cancer cells. Symptoms include hyperkalemia, hyperphosphatemia, hypocalcemia, hyperuricemia, and hyperuricosuria.

✓5ᵗʰ **E88.4 Mitochondrial metabolism disorders**
EXCLUDES 1   *disorders of pyruvate metabolism (E74.4)*
Kearns-Sayre syndrome (H49.81)
Leber's disease (H47.22)
Leigh's encephalopathy (G31.82)
Mitochondrial myopathy, NEC (G71.3)
Reye's syndrome (G93.7)

E88.40 Mitochondrial metabolism disorder, unspecified HCC ▽

E88.41 MELAS syndrome HCC
Mitochondrial myopathy, encephalopathy, lactic acidosis and stroke-like episodes

E88.42 MERRF syndrome HCC
Myoclonic epilepsy associated with ragged-red fibers
Code also progressive myoclonic epilepsy (G40.3-)

E88.49 Other mitochondrial metabolism disorders HCC

✓5ᵗʰ **E88.8 Other specified metabolic disorders**

E88.81 Metabolic syndrome
Dysmetabolic syndrome X
Use additional codes for associated manifestations, such as:
obesity (E66.-)
DEF: Group of health risks that increase the likelihood of developing heart disease, stroke, and diabetes. These risks include certain parameters for blood pressure, cholesterol, and glucose levels.

E88.89 Other specified metabolic disorders HCC
Launois-Bensaude adenolipomatosis
EXCLUDES 1   *adult pulmonary Langerhans cell histiocytosis (J84.82)*

E88.9 Metabolic disorder, unspecified ▽

Postprocedural endocrine and metabolic complications and disorders, not elsewhere classified (E89)

✓4ᵗʰ **E89 Postprocedural endocrine and metabolic complications and disorders, not elsewhere classified**
EXCLUDES 2   *intraoperative complications of endocrine system organ or structure (E36.0-, E36.1-, E36.8)*

E89.0 Postprocedural hypothyroidism
Postirradiation hypothyroidism
Postsurgical hypothyroidism

E89.1　**Postprocedural hypoinsulinemia**
　　　Postpancreatectomy hyperglycemia
　　　Postsurgical hypoinsulinemia
　　　Use additional code, if applicable, to identify:
　　　　acquired absence of pancreas (Z90.41-)
　　　　diabetes mellitus (postpancreatectomy) (postprocedural)
　　　　　(E13.-)
　　　　insulin use (Z79.4)
　　　　　EXCLUDES 1　transient postprocedural hyperglycemia (R73.9)
　　　　　　　　　　 transient postprocedural hypoglycemia (E16.2)

E89.2　**Postprocedural hypoparathyroidism**　　HCC
　　　Parathyroprival tetany

E89.3　**Postprocedural hypopituitarism**　　HCC
　　　Postirradiation hypopituitarism

✓5ᵗʰ **E89.4**　**Postprocedural ovarian failure**

　　E89.40　**Asymptomatic postprocedural ovarian**　♀
　　　　　　failure
　　　　　　Postprocedural ovarian failure NOS

　　E89.41　**Symptomatic postprocedural ovarian**　♀
　　　　　　failure
　　　　　　Symptoms such as flushing, sleeplessness, headache,
　　　　　　　lack of concentration, associated with
　　　　　　　postprocedural menopause

E89.5　**Postprocedural testicular hypofunction**　　♂

E89.6　**Postprocedural adrenocortical (-medullary)**　HCC
　　　hypofunction

✓5ᵗʰ **E89.8**　**Other postprocedural endocrine and metabolic complications**
　　　and disorders
　　　AHA: 2016,4Q,9-10

　　✓6ᵗʰ **E89.81**　**Postprocedural hemorrhage of an endocrine system**
　　　　　　organ or structure following a procedure
　　　　　E89.810　**Postprocedural hemorrhage of an**
　　　　　　　　　endocrine system organ or structure
　　　　　　　　　following an endocrine system procedure
　　　　　E89.811　**Postprocedural hemorrhage of an**
　　　　　　　　　endocrine system organ or structure
　　　　　　　　　following other procedure

　　✓6ᵗʰ **E89.82**　**Postprocedural hematoma and seroma of an**
　　　　　　endocrine system organ or structure
　　　　　E89.820　**Postprocedural hematoma of an**
　　　　　　　　　endocrine system organ or structure
　　　　　　　　　following an endocrine system procedure
　　　　　E89.821　**Postprocedural hematoma of an**
　　　　　　　　　endocrine system organ or structure
　　　　　　　　　following other procedure
　　　　　E89.822　**Postprocedural seroma of an endocrine**
　　　　　　　　　system organ or structure following an
　　　　　　　　　endocrine system procedure
　　　　　E89.823　**Postprocedural seroma of an endocrine**
　　　　　　　　　system organ or structure following other
　　　　　　　　　procedure

　　E89.89　**Other postprocedural endocrine and metabolic**
　　　　　　complications and disorders
　　　　　　Use additional code, if applicable, to further specify
　　　　　　　disorder

Chapter 5. Mental, Behavioral and Neurodevelopmental Disorders (FØ1–F99)

Chapter Specific Guidelines with Coding Examples

The chapter specific guidelines from the ICD-10-CM Official Guidelines for Coding and Reporting have been provided below. Along with these guidelines are coding examples, contained in the shaded boxes, that have been developed to help illustrate the coding and/or sequencing guidance found in these guidelines.

a. Pain disorders related to psychological factors

Assign code F45.41, for pain that is exclusively related to psychological disorders. As indicated by the Excludes 1 note under category G89, a code from category G89 should not be assigned with code F45.41.

> Chest pain determined to be persistent somatoform pain disorder
>
> **F45.41   Pain disorder exclusively related to psychological factors**
>
> *Explanation*: This pain was diagnosed as being exclusively psychological; therefore, no code from category G89 is added.

Code F45.42, Pain disorders with related psychological factors, should be used with a code from category G89, Pain, not elsewhere classified, if there is documentation of a psychological component for a patient with acute or chronic pain.

See Section I.C.6. Pain

b. Mental and behavioral disorders due to psychoactive substance use

1) In remission

Selection of codes for "in remission" for categories F10-F19, Mental and behavioral disorders due to psychoactive substance use (categories F10-F19 with -.11, -.21) requires the provider's clinical judgment. The appropriate codes for "in remission" are assigned only on the basis of provider documentation (as defined in the Official Guidelines for Coding and Reporting), unless otherwise instructed by the classification.

Mild substance use disorders in early or sustained remission are classified to the appropriate codes for substance abuse in remission, and moderate or severe substance use disorders in early or sustained remission are classified to the appropriate codes for substance dependence in remission.

> Physician documentation indicates the patient is seen to monitor progress on quitting cigarette smoking. The problem list indicates mild tobacco use disorder that is currently in remission.
>
> **F17.211   Nicotine dependence, cigarettes, in remission**
>
> *Explanation*: According to the index, Disorder, tobacco use, cigarettes (mild) (moderate) (severe), in remission (early) (sustained) is categorized to dependence (F17.211). Since the physician clearly documents mild cigarette use "disorder" and that the disorder is in remission, a code for nicotine dependence "in remission" is appropriate.

2) Psychoactive substance use, abuse and dependence

When the provider documentation refers to use, abuse and dependence of the same substance (e.g. alcohol, opioid, cannabis, etc.), only one code should be assigned to identify the pattern of use based on the following hierarchy:

- If both use and abuse are documented, assign only the code for abuse
- If both abuse and dependence are documented, assign only the code for dependence
- If use, abuse and dependence are all documented, assign only the code for dependence
- If both use and dependence are documented, assign only the code for dependence.

> History and physical notes cannabis dependence and ongoing cannabis abuse
>
> **F12.20   Cannabis dependence, uncomplicated**
>
> *Explanation*: In the hierarchy, the dependence code is used if both abuse and dependence are documented.

> Current problem list indicates daily opioid use with opioid abuse.
>
> **F11.10   Opioid abuse, uncomplicated**
>
> *Explanation*: In the hierarchy, the abuse code is used if both abuse and use are documented.

3) Psychoactive substance use, *unspecified*

As with all other **unspecified** diagnoses, the codes for **unspecified** psychoactive substance use disorders (F10.9-, F11.9-, F12.9-, F13.9-, F14.9-, F15.9-, F16.9-, **F18.9-, F19.9-**) should only be assigned based on provider documentation and when they meet the definition of a reportable diagnosis (see Section III, Reporting Additional Diagnoses). The**se** codes are to be used only when the psychoactive substance use is associated with a physical, mental or behavioral disorder, and such a relationship is documented by the provider.

c. Factitious disorder

Factitious disorder imposed on self or Munchausen's syndrome is a disorder in which a person falsely reports or causes his or her own physical or psychological signs or symptoms. For patients with documented factitious disorder on self or Munchausen's syndrome, assign the appropriate code from subcategory F68.1-, Factitious disorder imposed on self.

Munchausen's syndrome by proxy (MSBP) is a disorder in which a caregiver (perpetrator) falsely reports or causes an illness or injury in another person (victim) under his or her care, such as a child, an elderly adult, or a person who has a disability. The condition is also referred to as "factitious disorder imposed on another" or "factitious disorder by proxy." The perpetrator, not the victim, receives this diagnosis. Assign code F68.A, Factitious disorder imposed on another, to the perpetrator's record. For the victim of a patient suffering from MSBP, assign the appropriate code from categories T74, Adult and child abuse, neglect and other maltreatment, confirmed, or T76, Adult and child abuse, neglect and other maltreatment, suspected.

See Section I.C.19.f. Adult and child abuse, neglect and other maltreatment

Chapter 5. Mental, Behavioral and Neurodevelopmental Disorders (F01-F99)

INCLUDES disorders of psychological development

EXCLUDES 2 *symptoms, signs and abnormal clinical laboratory findings, not elsewhere classified (R00-R99)*

This chapter contains the following blocks:

F01-F09 Mental disorders due to known physiological conditions
F10-F19 Mental and behavioral disorders due to psychoactive substance use
F20-F29 Schizophrenia, schizotypal, delusional, and other non-mood psychotic disorders
F30-F39 Mood [affective] disorders
F40-F48 Anxiety, dissociative, stress-related, somatoform and other nonpsychotic mental disorders
F50-F59 Behavioral syndromes associated with physiological disturbances and physical factors
F60-F69 Disorders of adult personality and behavior
F70-F79 Intellectual disabilities
F80-F89 Pervasive and specific developmental disorders
F90-F98 Behavioral and emotional disorders with onset usually occurring in childhood and adolescence
F99 Unspecified mental disorder

Mental disorders due to known physiological conditions (F01-F09)

NOTE This block comprises a range of mental disorders grouped together on the basis of their having in common a demonstrable etiology in cerebral disease, brain injury, or other insult leading to cerebral dysfunction. The dysfunction may be primary, as in diseases, injuries, and insults that affect the brain directly and selectively; or secondary, as in systemic diseases and disorders that attack the brain only as one of the multiple organs or systems of the body that are involved.

✓4ᵗʰ F01 Vascular dementia

Vascular dementia as a result of infarction of the brain due to vascular disease, including hypertensive cerebrovascular disease.

INCLUDES arteriosclerotic dementia

Code first the underlying physiological condition or sequelae of cerebrovascular disease.

✓5ᵗʰ F01.5 Vascular dementia

F01.50 Vascular dementia without behavioral disturbance 🅐

Major neurocognitive disorder without behavioral disturbance

F01.51 Vascular dementia with behavioral disturbance 🆀 🅐

Major neurocognitive disorder due to vascular disease, with behavioral disturbance
Major neurocognitive disorder with aggressive behavior
Major neurocognitive disorder with combative behavior
Major neurocognitive disorder with violent behavior
Vascular dementia with aggressive behavior
Vascular dementia with combative behavior
Vascular dementia with violent behavior
Use additional code, if applicable, to identify wandering in vascular dementia (Z91.83)

✓4ᵗʰ F02 Dementia in other diseases classified elsewhere

INCLUDES major neurocognitive disorder in other diseases classified elsewhere

Code first the underlying physiological condition, such as:
Alzheimer's (G30.-)
cerebral lipidosis (E75.4)
Creutzfeldt-Jakob disease (A81.0-)
dementia with Lewy bodies (G31.83)
dementia with Parkinsonism (G31.83)
epilepsy and recurrent seizures (G40.-)
frontotemporal dementia (G31.09)
hepatolenticular degeneration (E83.0)
human immunodeficiency virus [HIV] disease (B20)
Huntington's disease (G10)
hypercalcemia (E83.52)
hypothyroidism, acquired (E00-E03.-)
intoxications (T36-T65)
Jakob-Creutzfeldt disease (A81.0-)
multiple sclerosis (G35)
neurosyphilis (A52.17)
niacin deficiency [pellagra] (E52)
Parkinson's disease (G20)
Pick's disease (G31.01)
polyarteritis nodosa (M30.0)
prion disease (A81.9)
systemic lupus erythematosus (M32.-)
traumatic brain injury (S06.-)
trypanosomiasis (B56.-, B57.-)
vitamin B deficiency (E53.8)

EXCLUDES 2 *dementia in alcohol and psychoactive substance disorders (F10-F19, with .17, .27, .97)*
vascular dementia (F01.5-)

✓5ᵗʰ F02.8 Dementia in other diseases classified elsewhere

AHA: 2017,2Q,7; 2016,4Q,141; 2016,2Q,6
TIP: A code from this subcategory should always be assigned with a code from category G30 when Alzheimer's disease is documented, even in the absence of documented dementia.

F02.80 Dementia in other diseases classified elsewhere without behavioral disturbance
Dementia in other diseases classified elsewhere NOS
Major neurocognitive disorder in other diseases classified elsewhere

F02.81 Dementia in other diseases classified elsewhere with behavioral disturbance
Dementia in other diseases classified elsewhere with aggressive behavior
Dementia in other diseases classified elsewhere with combative behavior
Dementia in other diseases classified elsewhere with violent behavior
Major neurocognitive disorder in other diseases classified elsewhere with aggressive behavior
Major neurocognitive disorder in other diseases classified elsewhere with combative behavior
Major neurocognitive disorder in other diseases classified elsewhere with violent behavior
Use additional code, if applicable, to identify wandering in dementia in conditions classified elsewhere (Z91.83)

✓4ᵗʰ F03 Unspecified dementia

Presenile dementia NOS
Presenile psychosis NOS
Primary degenerative dementia NOS
Senile dementia NOS
Senile dementia depressed or paranoid type
Senile psychosis NOS

EXCLUDES 1 *senility NOS (R41.81)*

EXCLUDES 2 *mild memory disturbance due to known physiological condition (F06.8)*
senile dementia with delirium or acute confusional state (F05)

✓5ᵗʰ F03.9 Unspecified dementia

F03.90 Unspecified dementia without behavioral disturbance 🅐 ▽
Dementia NOS
AHA: 2012,4Q,92

F03.91 Unspecified dementia with behavioral disturbance △ ▽

Unspecified dementia with aggressive behavior

Unspecified dementia with combative behavior

Unspecified dementia with violent behavior

Use additional code, if applicable, to identify wandering in unspecified dementia (Z91.83)

F04 Amnestic disorder due to known physiological condition

Korsakov's psychosis or syndrome, nonalcoholic

Code first the underlying physiological condition

EXCLUDES 1   amnesia NOS (R41.3)

anterograde amnesia (R41.1)

dissociative amnesia (F44.0)

retrograde amnesia (R41.2)

EXCLUDES 2   alcohol-induced or unspecified Korsakov's syndrome (F10.26, F10.96)

Korsakov's syndrome induced by other psychoactive substances (F13.26, F13.96, F19.16, F19.26, F19.96)

F05 Delirium due to known physiological condition

Acute or subacute brain syndrome

Acute or subacute confusional state (nonalcoholic)

Acute or subacute infective psychosis

Acute or subacute organic reaction

Acute or subacute psycho-organic syndrome

Delirium of mixed etiology

Delirium superimposed on dementia

Sundowning

Code first the underlying physiological condition

EXCLUDES 1   delirium NOS (R41.0)

EXCLUDES 2   delirium tremens alcohol-induced or unspecified (F10.231, F10.921)

✓4ᵗʰ F06 Other mental disorders due to known physiological condition

INCLUDES   mental disorders due to endocrine disorder

mental disorders due to exogenous hormone

mental disorders due to exogenous toxic substance

mental disorders due to primary cerebral disease

mental disorders due to somatic illness

mental disorders due to systemic disease affecting the brain

Code first the underlying physiological condition

EXCLUDES 1   unspecified dementia (F03)

EXCLUDES 2   delirium due to known physiological condition (F05)

dementia as classified in F01-F02

other mental disorders associated with alcohol and other psychoactive substances (F10-F19)

F06.0 Psychotic disorder with hallucinations due to known physiological condition

Organic hallucinatory state (nonalcoholic)

EXCLUDES 2   hallucinations and perceptual disturbance induced by alcohol and other psychoactive substances (F10-F19 with .151, .251, .951)

schizophrenia (F20.-)

F06.1 Catatonic disorder due to known physiological condition

Catatonia associated with another mental disorder

Catatonia NOS

EXCLUDES 1   catatonic stupor (R40.1)

stupor NOS (R40.1)

EXCLUDES 2   catatonic schizophrenia (F20.2)

dissociative stupor (F44.2)

DEF: Catatonic: Abnormal neuropsychiatric state characterized by stupor, immobility or purposeless movements, or unresponsiveness in a person who otherwise appears awake.

F06.2 Psychotic disorder with delusions due to known physiological condition

Paranoid and paranoid-hallucinatory organic states

Schizophrenia-like psychosis in epilepsy

EXCLUDES 2   alcohol and drug-induced psychotic disorder (F10-F19 with .150, .250, .950)

brief psychotic disorder (F23)

delusional disorder (F22)

schizophrenia (F20.-)

✓5ᵗʰ F06.3 Mood disorder due to known physiological condition

EXCLUDES 2   mood disorders due to alcohol and other psychoactive substances (F10-F19 with .14, .24, .94)

mood disorders, not due to known physiological condition or unspecified (F30-F39)

F06.30 Mood disorder due to known physiological condition, unspecified ▽

F06.31 Mood disorder due to known physiological condition with depressive features

Depressive disorder due to known physiological condition, with depressive features

F06.32 Mood disorder due to known physiological condition with major depressive-like episode

Depressive disorder due to known physiological condition, with major depressive-like episode

F06.33 Mood disorder due to known physiological condition with manic features

Bipolar and related disorder due to a known physiological condition, with manic features

Bipolar and related disorder due to known physiological condition, with manic- or hypomanic-like episodes

F06.34 Mood disorder due to known physiological condition with mixed features

Bipolar and related disorder due to known physiological condition, with mixed features

Depressive disorder due to known physiological condition, with mixed features

F06.4 Anxiety disorder due to known physiological condition

EXCLUDES 2   anxiety disorders due to alcohol and other psychoactive substances (F10-F19 with .180, .280, .980)

anxiety disorders, not due to known physiological condition or unspecified (F40.-, F41.-)

F06.8 Other specified mental disorders due to known physiological condition

Epileptic psychosis NOS

Obsessive-compulsive and related disorder due to a known physiological condition

Organic dissociative disorder

Organic emotionally labile [asthenic] disorder

✓4ᵗʰ F07 Personality and behavioral disorders due to known physiological condition

Code first the underlying physiological condition

F07.0 Personality change due to known physiological condition

Frontal lobe syndrome

Limbic epilepsy personality syndrome

Lobotomy syndrome

Organic personality disorder

Organic pseudopsychopathic personality

Organic pseudoretarded personality

Postleucotomy syndrome

Code first underlying physiological condition

EXCLUDES 1   mild cognitive impairment (G31.84)

postconcussional syndrome (F07.81)

postencephalitic syndrome (F07.89)

signs and symptoms involving emotional state (R45.-)

EXCLUDES 2   specific personality disorder (F60.-)

✓5ᵗʰ F07.8 Other personality and behavioral disorders due to known physiological condition

F07.81 Postconcussional syndrome

Postcontusional syndrome (encephalopathy)

Post-traumatic brain syndrome, nonpsychotic

Use additional code to identify associated post-traumatic headache, if applicable (G44.3-)

EXCLUDES 1   current concussion (brain) (S06.0-)

postencephalitic syndrome (F07.89)

DEF: Concussion symptoms that persist for weeks or months after a head injury. These symptoms may include headache, giddiness, fatigue, insomnia, mood fluctuation, and a subjective feeling of impaired intellectual function with extreme reaction to normal stressors.

F07.89 Other personality and behavioral disorders due to known physiological condition

Postencephalitic syndrome

Right hemispheric organic affective disorder

✓ Additional Character Req   ✓x7ᵗʰ Placeholder Alert   **Manifestation**   ▽ Unspecified   ►◄ Revised Text   ● New Code   ▲ Revised Code Title

ICD-10-CM 2019   535

Chapter 5. Mental, Behavioral and Neurodevelopmental Disorders

F07.9–F10.26

F07.9 Unspecified personality and behavioral disorder due to known physiological condition ▽
Organic psychosyndrome

F09 Unspecified mental disorder due to known physiological condition ▽
Mental disorder NOS due to known physiological condition
Organic brain syndrome NOS
Organic mental disorder NOS
Organic psychosis NOS
Symptomatic psychosis NOS
Code first the underlying physiological condition
EXCLUDES 1   psychosis NOS (F29)

Mental and behavioral disorders due to psychoactive substance use (F10-F19)

AHA: 2017,4Q,8; 2017,2Q,27

✓4ᵗʰ **F10 Alcohol related disorders**
Use additional code for blood alcohol level, if applicable (Y90.-)

✓5ᵗʰ **F10.1 Alcohol abuse**
EXCLUDES 1   alcohol dependence (F10.2-)
alcohol use, unspecified (F10.9-)
AHA: 2018,1Q,16; 2015,2Q,15
TIP: Alcohol withdrawal is classified to dependence only (F10.23-); there is no combination code for alcohol abuse with withdrawal. When alcohol abuse and alcohol withdrawal are documented for the same encounter, query the provider for clarification.
TIP: Assign when documentation indicates alcohol withdrawal without dependence; do not assign an additional code for withdrawal.

F10.10 Alcohol abuse, uncomplicated
Alcohol use disorder, mild

F10.11 Alcohol abuse, in remission
Alcohol use disorder, mild, in early remission
Alcohol use disorder, mild, in sustained remission

✓6ᵗʰ **F10.12 Alcohol abuse with intoxication**
F10.120 Alcohol abuse with intoxication, uncomplicated HCC
F10.121 Alcohol abuse with intoxication delirium HCC
F10.129 Alcohol abuse with intoxication, unspecified HCC ▽

F10.14 Alcohol abuse with alcohol-induced mood disorder HCC
Alcohol use disorder, mild, with alcohol-induced bipolar or related disorder
Alcohol use disorder, mild, with alcohol-induced depressive disorder

✓6ᵗʰ **F10.15 Alcohol abuse with alcohol-induced psychotic disorder**
F10.150 Alcohol abuse with alcohol-induced psychotic disorder with delusions HCC
F10.151 Alcohol abuse with alcohol-induced psychotic disorder with hallucinations HCC
DEF: Psychosis lasting less than six months with slight or no clouding of consciousness in which auditory hallucinations predominate.
F10.159 Alcohol abuse with alcohol-induced psychotic disorder, unspecified HCC ▽

✓6ᵗʰ **F10.18 Alcohol abuse with other alcohol-induced disorders**
F10.180 Alcohol abuse with alcohol-induced anxiety disorder HCC
F10.181 Alcohol abuse with alcohol-induced sexual dysfunction HCC
F10.182 Alcohol abuse with alcohol-induced sleep disorder HCC
F10.188 Alcohol abuse with other alcohol-induced disorder HCC

F10.19 Alcohol abuse with unspecified alcohol-induced disorder HCC ▽

✓5ᵗʰ **F10.2 Alcohol dependence**
EXCLUDES 1   alcohol abuse (F10.1-)
alcohol use, unspecified (F10.9-)
EXCLUDES 2   toxic effect of alcohol (T51.0-)

F10.20 Alcohol dependence, uncomplicated HCC
Alcohol use disorder, moderate
Alcohol use disorder, severe

F10.21 Alcohol dependence, in remission HCC
Alcohol use disorder, moderate, in early remission
Alcohol use disorder, moderate, in sustained remission
Alcohol use disorder, severe, in early remission
Alcohol use disorder, severe, in sustained remission

✓6ᵗʰ **F10.22 Alcohol dependence with intoxication**
Acute drunkenness (in alcoholism)
EXCLUDES 2   alcohol dependence with withdrawal (F10.23-)
F10.220 Alcohol dependence with intoxication, uncomplicated HCC
F10.221 Alcohol dependence with intoxication delirium HCC
F10.229 Alcohol dependence with intoxication, unspecified HCC ▽

✓6ᵗʰ **F10.23 Alcohol dependence with withdrawal**
EXCLUDES 2   alcohol dependence with intoxication (F10.22-)
AHA: 2018,1Q,16; 2015,2Q,15
TIP: Do not assign a code from this subcategory when documentation indicates alcohol withdrawal without dependence.
F10.230 Alcohol dependence with withdrawal, uncomplicated HCC
F10.231 Alcohol dependence with withdrawal delirium HCC
F10.232 Alcohol dependence with withdrawal with perceptual disturbance HCC
F10.239 Alcohol dependence with withdrawal, unspecified HCC ▽

F10.24 Alcohol dependence with alcohol-induced mood disorder HCC
Alcohol use disorder, moderate, with alcohol-induced bipolar or related disorder
Alcohol use disorder, moderate, with alcohol-induced depressive disorder
Alcohol use disorder, severe, with alcohol-induced bipolar or related disorder
Alcohol use disorder, severe, with alcohol-induced depressive disorder

✓6ᵗʰ **F10.25 Alcohol dependence with alcohol-induced psychotic disorder**
F10.250 Alcohol dependence with alcohol-induced psychotic disorder with delusions HCC
F10.251 Alcohol dependence with alcohol-induced psychotic disorder with hallucinations HCC
F10.259 Alcohol dependence with alcohol-induced psychotic disorder, unspecified HCC ▽

F10.26 Alcohol dependence with alcohol-induced persisting amnestic disorder HCC
Alcohol use disorder, moderate, with alcohol-induced major neurocognitive disorder, amnestic-confabulatory type
Alcohol use disorder, severe, with alcohol-induced major neurocognitive disorder, amnestic-confabulatory type
DEF: Prominent and lasting reduced memory span and disordered time appreciation and confabulation that occurs in alcoholics as sequel to acute alcoholic psychosis.

F10.27 Alcohol dependence with alcohol-induced persisting dementia `HCC`
> Alcohol use disorder, moderate, with alcohol-induced major neurocognitive disorder, nonamnestic-confabulatory type
> Alcohol use disorder, severe, with alcohol-induced major neurocognitive disorder, nonamnestic-confabulatory type

√6th **F10.28 Alcohol dependence with other alcohol-induced disorders**
     F10.280 Alcohol dependence with alcohol-induced anxiety disorder `HCC`
     F10.281 Alcohol dependence with alcohol-induced sexual dysfunction `HCC`
     F10.282 Alcohol dependence with alcohol-induced sleep disorder `HCC`
     F10.288 Alcohol dependence with other alcohol-induced disorder `HCC`
> > Alcohol use disorder, moderate, with alcohol-induced mild neurocognitive disorder
> > Alcohol use disorder, severe, with alcohol-induced mild neurocognitive disorder

     F10.29 Alcohol dependence with unspecified alcohol-induced disorder `HCC` ▽

√5th **F10.9 Alcohol use, unspecified**
> *EXCLUDES 1*   alcohol abuse (F10.1-)
>   alcohol dependence (F10.2-)
> **AHA:** 2018,2Q,10-11

√6th **F10.92 Alcohol use, unspecified with intoxication**
     F10.920 Alcohol use, unspecified with intoxication, uncomplicated `HCC`
> > **AHA:** 2018,2Q,10-11
     F10.921 Alcohol use, unspecified with intoxication delirium `HCC`
     F10.929 Alcohol use, unspecified with intoxication, unspecified `HCC` ▽

     F10.94 Alcohol use, unspecified with alcohol-induced mood disorder `HCC`
> Alcohol induced bipolar or related disorder, without use disorder
> Alcohol induced depressive disorder, without use disorder

√6th **F10.95 Alcohol use, unspecified with alcohol-induced psychotic disorder**
     F10.950 Alcohol use, unspecified with alcohol-induced psychotic disorder with delusions `HCC`
     F10.951 Alcohol use, unspecified with alcohol-induced psychotic disorder with hallucinations `HCC`
     F10.959 Alcohol use, unspecified with alcohol-induced psychotic disorder, unspecified `HCC` ▽
> > Alcohol-induced psychotic disorder without use disorder

     F10.96 Alcohol use, unspecified with alcohol-induced persisting amnestic disorder `HCC`
> Alcohol-induced major neurocognitive disorder, amnestic-confabulatory type, without use disorder

     F10.97 Alcohol use, unspecified with alcohol-induced persisting dementia `HCC`
> Alcohol-induced major neurocognitive disorder, nonamnestic-confabulatory type, without use disorder

√6th **F10.98 Alcohol use, unspecified with other alcohol-induced disorders**
     F10.980 Alcohol use, unspecified with alcohol-induced anxiety disorder `HCC`
> > Alcohol induced anxiety disorder, without use disorder
     F10.981 Alcohol use, unspecified with alcohol-induced sexual dysfunction `HCC`
> > Alcohol induced sexual dysfunction, without use disorder

     F10.982 Alcohol use, unspecified with alcohol-induced sleep disorder `HCC`
> > Alcohol induced sleep disorder, without use disorder
     F10.988 Alcohol use, unspecified with other alcohol-induced disorder `HCC`
> > Alcohol induced mild neurocognitive disorder, without use disorder

     F10.99 Alcohol use, unspecified with unspecified alcohol-induced disorder `HCC` ▽

√4th **F11 Opioid related disorders**
√5th **F11.1 Opioid abuse**
> *EXCLUDES 1*   opioid dependence (F11.2-)
>   opioid use, unspecified (F11.9-)

     F11.10 Opioid abuse, uncomplicated
> Opioid use disorder, mild
     F11.11 Opioid abuse, in remission
> Opioid use disorder, mild, in early remission
> Opioid use disorder, mild, in sustained remission

√6th **F11.12 Opioid abuse with intoxication**
     F11.120 Opioid abuse with intoxication, uncomplicated `HCC`
     F11.121 Opioid abuse with intoxication delirium `HCC`
     F11.122 Opioid abuse with intoxication with perceptual disturbance `HCC`
     F11.129 Opioid abuse with intoxication, unspecified `HCC` ▽

     F11.14 Opioid abuse with opioid-induced mood disorder `HCC`
> Opioid use disorder, mild, with opioid-induced depressive disorder

√6th **F11.15 Opioid abuse with opioid-induced psychotic disorder**
     F11.150 Opioid abuse with opioid-induced psychotic disorder with delusions `HCC`
     F11.151 Opioid abuse with opioid-induced psychotic disorder with hallucinations `HCC`
     F11.159 Opioid abuse with opioid-induced psychotic disorder, unspecified `HCC` ▽

√6th **F11.18 Opioid abuse with other opioid-induced disorder**
     F11.181 Opioid abuse with opioid-induced sexual dysfunction `HCC`
     F11.182 Opioid abuse with opioid-induced sleep disorder `HCC`
     F11.188 Opioid abuse with other opioid-induced disorder `HCC`

     F11.19 Opioid abuse with unspecified opioid-induced disorder `HCC` ▽

√5th **F11.2 Opioid dependence**
> *EXCLUDES 1*   opioid abuse (F11.1-)
>   opioid use, unspecified (F11.9-)
> *EXCLUDES 2*   opioid poisoning (T40.0-T40.2-)

     F11.20 Opioid dependence, uncomplicated `HCC`
> Opioid use disorder, moderate
> Opioid use disorder, severe
     F11.21 Opioid dependence, in remission `HCC`
> Opioid use disorder, moderate, in early remission
> Opioid use disorder, moderate, in sustained remission
> Opioid use disorder, severe, in early remission
> Opioid use disorder, severe, in sustained remission

√6th **F11.22 Opioid dependence with intoxication**
> *EXCLUDES 1*   opioid dependence with withdrawal (F11.23)
     F11.220 Opioid dependence with intoxication, uncomplicated `HCC`
     F11.221 Opioid dependence with intoxication delirium `HCC`
     F11.222 Opioid dependence with intoxication with perceptual disturbance `HCC`
     F11.229 Opioid dependence with intoxication, unspecified `HCC` ▽

     F11.23 Opioid dependence with withdrawal `HCC`
> *EXCLUDES 1*   opioid dependence with intoxication (F11.22-)

✓ Additional Character Req   √x7th Placeholder Alert   Manifestation   ▽ Unspecified   ►◄ Revised Text   ● New Code   ▲ Revised Code Title

ICD-10-CM 2019   537

Chapter 5. Mental, Behavioral and Neurodevelopmental Disorders

F11.24 **Opioid dependence with opioid-induced mood disorder** `HCC`
Opioid use disorder, moderate, with opioid induced depressive disorder

√6th F11.25 **Opioid dependence with opioid-induced psychotic disorder**
     F11.250 **Opioid dependence with opioid-induced psychotic disorder with delusions** `HCC`
     F11.251 **Opioid dependence with opioid-induced psychotic disorder with hallucinations** `HCC`
     F11.259 **Opioid dependence with opioid-induced psychotic disorder, unspecified** `HCC` ▽

√6th F11.28 **Opioid dependence with other opioid-induced disorder**
     F11.281 **Opioid dependence with opioid-induced sexual dysfunction** `HCC`
     F11.282 **Opioid dependence with opioid-induced sleep disorder** `HCC`
     F11.288 **Opioid dependence with other opioid-induced disorder** `HCC`

F11.29 **Opioid dependence with unspecified opioid-induced disorder** `HCC` ▽

√5th F11.9 **Opioid use, unspecified**
     EXCLUDES 1   *opioid abuse (F11.1-)*
                 opioid dependence (F11.2-)

F11.90 **Opioid use, unspecified, uncomplicated**
     AHA: 2018,2Q,10-11

√6th F11.92 **Opioid use, unspecified with intoxication**
     EXCLUDES 1   *opioid use, unspecified with withdrawal (F11.93)*
     F11.920 **Opioid use, unspecified with intoxication, uncomplicated** `HCC`
     F11.921 **Opioid use, unspecified with intoxication delirium** `HCC`
               Opioid-induced delirium
     F11.922 **Opioid use, unspecified with intoxication with perceptual disturbance** `HCC`
     F11.929 **Opioid use, unspecified with intoxication, unspecified** `HCC` ▽

F11.93 **Opioid use, unspecified with withdrawal** `HCC`
     EXCLUDES 1   *opioid use, unspecified with intoxication (F11.92-)*

F11.94 **Opioid use, unspecified with opioid-induced mood disorder** `HCC`
     Opioid induced depressive disorder, without use disorder

√6th F11.95 **Opioid use, unspecified with opioid-induced psychotic disorder**
     F11.950 **Opioid use, unspecified with opioid-induced psychotic disorder with delusions** `HCC`
     F11.951 **Opioid use, unspecified with opioid-induced psychotic disorder with hallucinations** `HCC`
     F11.959 **Opioid use, unspecified with opioid-induced psychotic disorder, unspecified** `HCC` ▽

√6th F11.98 **Opioid use, unspecified with other specified opioid-induced disorder**
     F11.981 **Opioid use, unspecified with opioid-induced sexual dysfunction** `HCC`
               Opioid induced sexual dysfunction, without use disorder
     F11.982 **Opioid use, unspecified with opioid-induced sleep disorder** `HCC`
               Opioid induced sleep disorder, without use disorder
     F11.988 **Opioid use, unspecified with other opioid-induced disorder** `HCC`
               Opioid induced anxiety disorder, without use disorder

F11.99 **Opioid use, unspecified with unspecified opioid-induced disorder** `HCC` ▽

√4th F12 **Cannabis related disorders**
     INCLUDES   marijuana

√5th F12.1 **Cannabis abuse**
     EXCLUDES 1   *cannabis dependence (F12.2-)*
                 cannabis use, unspecified (F12.9-)

F12.10 **Cannabis abuse, uncomplicated**
     Cannabis use disorder, mild

F12.11 **Cannabis abuse, in remission**
     Cannabis use disorder, mild, in early remission
     Cannabis use disorder, mild, in sustained remission

√6th F12.12 **Cannabis abuse with intoxication**
     F12.120 **Cannabis abuse with intoxication, uncomplicated** `HCC`
     F12.121 **Cannabis abuse with intoxication delirium** `HCC`
     F12.122 **Cannabis abuse with intoxication with perceptual disturbance** `HCC`
     F12.129 **Cannabis abuse with intoxication, unspecified** `HCC` ▽

√6th F12.15 **Cannabis abuse with psychotic disorder**
     F12.150 **Cannabis abuse with psychotic disorder with delusions** `HCC`
     F12.151 **Cannabis abuse with psychotic disorder with hallucinations** `HCC`
     F12.159 **Cannabis abuse with psychotic disorder, unspecified** `HCC` ▽

√6th F12.18 **Cannabis abuse with other cannabis-induced disorder**
     F12.180 **Cannabis abuse with cannabis-induced anxiety disorder** `HCC`
     F12.188 **Cannabis abuse with other cannabis-induced disorder** `HCC`
               Cannabis use disorder, mild, with cannabis-induced sleep disorder

F12.19 **Cannabis abuse with unspecified cannabis-induced disorder** `HCC` ▽

√5th F12.2 **Cannabis dependence**
     EXCLUDES 1   *cannabis abuse (F12.1-)*
                 cannabis use, unspecified (F12.9-)
     EXCLUDES 2   *cannabis poisoning (T40.7-)*

F12.20 **Cannabis dependence, uncomplicated** `HCC`
     Cannabis use disorder, moderate
     Cannabis use disorder, severe

F12.21 **Cannabis dependence, in remission** `HCC`
     Cannabis use disorder, moderate, in early remission
     Cannabis use disorder, moderate, in sustained remission
     Cannabis use disorder, severe, in early remission
     Cannabis use disorder, severe, in sustained remission

√6th F12.22 **Cannabis dependence with intoxication**
     F12.220 **Cannabis dependence with intoxication, uncomplicated** `HCC`
     F12.221 **Cannabis dependence with intoxication delirium** `HCC`
     F12.222 **Cannabis dependence with intoxication with perceptual disturbance** `HCC`
     F12.229 **Cannabis dependence with intoxication, unspecified** `HCC` ▽

F12.23 **Cannabis dependence with withdrawal**

√6th F12.25 **Cannabis dependence with psychotic disorder**
     F12.250 **Cannabis dependence with psychotic disorder with delusions** `HCC`
     F12.251 **Cannabis dependence with psychotic disorder with hallucinations** `HCC`
     F12.259 **Cannabis dependence with psychotic disorder, unspecified** `HCC` ▽

√6th F12.28 **Cannabis dependence with other cannabis-induced disorder**
     F12.280 **Cannabis dependence with cannabis-induced anxiety disorder** `HCC`

F12.288 Cannabis dependence with other `HCC`
cannabis-induced disorder
Cannabis use disorder, moderate, with
cannabis-induced sleep disorder
Cannabis use disorder, severe, with
cannabis-induced sleep disorder
~~Cannabis withdrawal~~

F12.29 Cannabis dependence with unspecified `HCC` ▽
cannabis-induced disorder

√5ᵗʰ **F12.9 Cannabis use, unspecified**
EXCLUDES 1 *cannabis abuse (F12.1-)*
cannabis dependence (F12.2-)

F12.90 Cannabis use, unspecified, uncomplicated
AHA: 2018,2Q,10-11

√6ᵗʰ **F12.92 Cannabis use, unspecified with intoxication**
F12.920 Cannabis use, unspecified with `HCC`
intoxication, uncomplicated
F12.921 Cannabis use, unspecified with `HCC`
intoxication delirium
F12.922 Cannabis use, unspecified with `HCC`
intoxication with perceptual
disturbance
F12.929 Cannabis use, unspecified with `HCC` ▽
intoxication, unspecified

● **F12.93 Cannabis use, unspecified with withdrawal**

√6ᵗʰ **F12.95 Cannabis use, unspecified with psychotic disorder**
F12.950 Cannabis use, unspecified with `HCC`
psychotic disorder with delusions
F12.951 Cannabis use, unspecified with `HCC`
psychotic disorder with
hallucinations
F12.959 Cannabis use, unspecified with `HCC` ▽
psychotic disorder, unspecified
Cannabis induced psychotic disorder,
without use disorder

√6ᵗʰ **F12.98 Cannabis use, unspecified with other**
cannabis-induced disorder
F12.980 Cannabis use, unspecified with `HCC`
anxiety disorder
Cannabis induced anxiety disorder,
without use disorder
F12.988 Cannabis use, unspecified with `HCC`
other cannabis-induced disorder
Cannabis induced sleep disorder, without
use disorder

F12.99 Cannabis use, unspecified with unspecified `HCC` ▽
cannabis-induced disorder

√4ᵗʰ **F13 Sedative, hypnotic, or anxiolytic related disorders**

√5ᵗʰ **F13.1 Sedative, hypnotic or anxiolytic-related abuse**
EXCLUDES 1 *sedative, hypnotic or anxiolytic-related dependence*
(F13.2-)
sedative, hypnotic, or anxiolytic use, unspecified
(F13.9-)

F13.10 Sedative, hypnotic or anxiolytic abuse,
uncomplicated
Sedative, hypnotic, or anxiolytic use disorder, mild

F13.11 Sedative, hypnotic or anxiolytic abuse, in remission
Sedative, hypnotic or anxiolytic use disorder, mild, in
early remission
Sedative, hypnotic or anxiolytic use disorder, mild, in
sustained remission

√6ᵗʰ **F13.12 Sedative, hypnotic or anxiolytic abuse with**
intoxication
F13.120 Sedative, hypnotic or anxiolytic `HCC`
abuse with intoxication,
uncomplicated
F13.121 Sedative, hypnotic or anxiolytic `HCC`
abuse with intoxication delirium
F13.129 Sedative, hypnotic or anxiolytic `HCC` ▽
abuse with intoxication,
unspecified

F13.14 Sedative, hypnotic or anxiolytic abuse with `HCC`
sedative, hypnotic or anxiolytic-induced
mood disorder
Sedative, hypnotic, or anxiolytic use disorder, mild,
with sedative, hypnotic, or anxiolytic-induced
bipolar or related disorder
Sedative, hypnotic, or anxiolytic use disorder, mild,
with sedative, hypnotic, or anxiolytic-induced
depressive disorder

√6ᵗʰ **F13.15 Sedative, hypnotic or anxiolytic abuse with**
sedative, hypnotic or anxiolytic-induced psychotic
disorder
F13.150 Sedative, hypnotic or anxiolytic `HCC`
abuse with sedative, hypnotic or
anxiolytic-induced psychotic
disorder with delusions
F13.151 Sedative, hypnotic or anxiolytic `HCC`
abuse with sedative, hypnotic or
anxiolytic-induced psychotic
disorder with hallucinations
F13.159 Sedative, hypnotic or anxiolytic `HCC` ▽
abuse with sedative, hypnotic or
anxiolytic-induced psychotic
disorder, unspecified

√6ᵗʰ **F13.18 Sedative, hypnotic or anxiolytic abuse with other**
sedative, hypnotic or anxiolytic-induced disorders
F13.180 Sedative, hypnotic or anxiolytic `HCC`
abuse with sedative, hypnotic or
anxiolytic-induced anxiety
disorder
F13.181 Sedative, hypnotic or anxiolytic `HCC`
abuse with sedative, hypnotic or
anxiolytic-induced sexual
dysfunction
F13.182 Sedative, hypnotic or anxiolytic `HCC`
abuse with sedative, hypnotic or
anxiolytic-induced sleep disorder
F13.188 Sedative, hypnotic or anxiolytic `HCC`
abuse with other sedative,
hypnotic or anxiolytic-induced
disorder

F13.19 Sedative, hypnotic or anxiolytic abuse with `HCC` ▽
unspecified sedative, hypnotic or
anxiolytic-induced disorder

√5ᵗʰ **F13.2 Sedative, hypnotic or anxiolytic-related dependence**
EXCLUDES 1 *sedative, hypnotic or anxiolytic-related abuse (F13.1-)*
sedative, hypnotic, or anxiolytic use, unspecified
(F13.9-)
EXCLUDES 2 *sedative, hypnotic, or anxiolytic poisoning (T42.-)*

F13.20 Sedative, hypnotic or anxiolytic `HCC`
dependence, uncomplicated
F13.21 Sedative, hypnotic or anxiolytic `HCC`
dependence, in remission
Sedative, hypnotic or anxiolytic use disorder,
moderate, in early remission
Sedative, hypnotic or anxiolytic use disorder,
moderate, in sustained remission
Sedative, hypnotic or anxiolytic use disorder, severe,
in early remission
Sedative, hypnotic or anxiolytic use disorder, severe,
in sustained remission

√6ᵗʰ **F13.22 Sedative, hypnotic or anxiolytic dependence with**
intoxication
EXCLUDES 1 *sedative, hypnotic or anxiolytic*
dependence with withdrawal
(F13.23-)
F13.220 Sedative, hypnotic or anxiolytic `HCC`
dependence with intoxication,
uncomplicated
F13.221 Sedative, hypnotic or anxiolytic `HCC`
dependence with intoxication
delirium
F13.229 Sedative, hypnotic or anxiolytic `HCC` ▽
dependence with intoxication,
unspecified

| ☑ Additional Character Req | √x7ᵗʰ Placeholder Alert | Manifestation | ▽ Unspecified | ►◄ Revised Text | ● New Code | ▲ Revised Code Title |

ICD-10-CM 2019   539

✓6ᵗʰ F13.23 Sedative, hypnotic or anxiolytic dependence with withdrawal
Sedative, hypnotic, or anxiolytic use disorder, moderate
Sedative, hypnotic, or anxiolytic use disorder, severe
EXCLUDES 1 *sedative, hypnotic or anxiolytic dependence with intoxication (F13.22-)*

    F13.230 Sedative, hypnotic or anxiolytic dependence with withdrawal, uncomplicated HCC

    F13.231 Sedative, hypnotic or anxiolytic dependence with withdrawal delirium HCC

    F13.232 Sedative, hypnotic or anxiolytic dependence with withdrawal with perceptual disturbance HCC
Sedative, hypnotic, or anxiolytic withdrawal with perceptual disturbances

    F13.239 Sedative, hypnotic or anxiolytic dependence with withdrawal, unspecified HCC ▽
Sedative, hypnotic, or anxiolytic withdrawal without perceptual disturbances

F13.24 Sedative, hypnotic or anxiolytic dependence with sedative, hypnotic or anxiolytic-induced mood disorder HCC
Sedative, hypnotic, or anxiolytic use disorder, moderate, with sedative, hypnotic, or anxiolytic-induced bipolar or related disorder
Sedative, hypnotic, or anxiolytic use disorder, moderate, with sedative, hypnotic, or anxiolytic-induced depressive disorder
Sedative, hypnotic, or anxiolytic use disorder, severe, with sedative, hypnotic, or anxiolytic-induced bipolar or related disorder
Sedative, hypnotic, or anxiolytic use disorder, severe, with sedative, hypnotic, or anxiolytic-induced depressive disorder

✓6ᵗʰ F13.25 Sedative, hypnotic or anxiolytic dependence with sedative, hypnotic or anxiolytic-induced psychotic disorder

    F13.250 Sedative, hypnotic or anxiolytic dependence with sedative, hypnotic or anxiolytic-induced psychotic disorder with delusions HCC

    F13.251 Sedative, hypnotic or anxiolytic dependence with sedative, hypnotic or anxiolytic-induced psychotic disorder with hallucinations HCC

    F13.259 Sedative, hypnotic or anxiolytic dependence with sedative, hypnotic or anxiolytic-induced psychotic disorder, unspecified HCC ▽

F13.26 Sedative, hypnotic or anxiolytic dependence with sedative, hypnotic or anxiolytic-induced persisting amnestic disorder HCC

F13.27 Sedative, hypnotic or anxiolytic dependence with sedative, hypnotic or anxiolytic-induced persisting dementia HCC
Sedative, hypnotic, or anxiolytic use disorder, moderate, with sedative, hypnotic, or anxiolytic induced major neurocognitive disorder
Sedative, hypnotic, or anxiolytic use disorder, severe, with sedative, hypnotic, or anxiolytic-induced major neurocognitive disorder

✓6ᵗʰ F13.28 Sedative, hypnotic or anxiolytic dependence with other sedative, hypnotic or anxiolytic-induced disorders

    F13.280 Sedative, hypnotic or anxiolytic dependence with sedative, hypnotic or anxiolytic-induced anxiety disorder HCC

    F13.281 Sedative, hypnotic or anxiolytic dependence with sedative, hypnotic or anxiolytic-induced sexual dysfunction HCC

    F13.282 Sedative, hypnotic or anxiolytic dependence with sedative, hypnotic or anxiolytic-induced sleep disorder HCC

    F13.288 Sedative, hypnotic or anxiolytic dependence with other sedative, hypnotic or anxiolytic-induced disorder HCC
Sedative, hypnotic, or anxiolytic use disorder, moderate, with sedative, hypnotic, or anxiolytic-induced mild neurocognitive disorder
Sedative, hypnotic, or anxiolytic use disorder, severe, with sedative, hypnotic, or anxiolytic-induced mild neurocognitive disorder

F13.29 Sedative, hypnotic or anxiolytic dependence with unspecified sedative, hypnotic or anxiolytic-induced disorder HCC ▽

✓5ᵗʰ F13.9 Sedative, hypnotic or anxiolytic-related use, unspecified
EXCLUDES 1 *sedative, hypnotic or anxiolytic-related abuse (F13.1-)*
sedative, hypnotic or anxiolytic-related dependence (F13.2-)

F13.90 Sedative, hypnotic, or anxiolytic use, unspecified, uncomplicated
AHA: 2018,2Q,10-11

✓6ᵗʰ F13.92 Sedative, hypnotic or anxiolytic use, unspecified with intoxication
EXCLUDES 1 *sedative, hypnotic or anxiolytic use, unspecified with withdrawal (F13.93-)*

    F13.920 Sedative, hypnotic or anxiolytic use, unspecified with intoxication, uncomplicated HCC

    F13.921 Sedative, hypnotic or anxiolytic use, unspecified with intoxication delirium HCC
Sedative, hypnotic, or anxiolytic-induced delirium

    F13.929 Sedative, hypnotic or anxiolytic use, unspecified with intoxication, unspecified HCC ▽

✓6ᵗʰ F13.93 Sedative, hypnotic or anxiolytic use, unspecified with withdrawal
EXCLUDES 1 *sedative, hypnotic or anxiolytic use, unspecified with intoxication (F13.92-)*

    F13.930 Sedative, hypnotic or anxiolytic use, unspecified with withdrawal, uncomplicated HCC

    F13.931 Sedative, hypnotic or anxiolytic use, unspecified with withdrawal delirium HCC

    F13.932 Sedative, hypnotic or anxiolytic use, unspecified with withdrawal with perceptual disturbances HCC

    F13.939 Sedative, hypnotic or anxiolytic use, unspecified with withdrawal, unspecified HCC ▽

F13.94 Sedative, hypnotic or anxiolytic use, unspecified with sedative, hypnotic or anxiolytic-induced mood disorder HCC
Sedative, hypnotic, or anxiolytic-induced bipolar or related disorder, without use disorder
Sedative, hypnotic, or anxiolytic-induced depressive disorder, without use disorder

✓6ᵗʰ F13.95 Sedative, hypnotic or anxiolytic use, unspecified with sedative, hypnotic or anxiolytic-induced psychotic disorder

    F13.950 Sedative, hypnotic or anxiolytic use, unspecified with sedative, hypnotic or anxiolytic-induced psychotic disorder with delusions HCC

    F13.951 Sedative, hypnotic or anxiolytic use, unspecified with sedative, hypnotic or anxiolytic-induced psychotic disorder with hallucinations HCC

F13.959   Sedative, hypnotic or anxiolytic use, unspecified with sedative, hypnotic or anxiolytic-induced psychotic disorder, unspecified   HCC ▽
     Sedative, hypnotic, or anxiolytic-induced psychotic disorder, without use disorder

F13.96   Sedative, hypnotic or anxiolytic use, unspecified with sedative, hypnotic or anxiolytic-induced persisting amnestic disorder   HCC

F13.97   Sedative, hypnotic or anxiolytic use, unspecified with sedative, hypnotic or anxiolytic-induced persisting dementia   HCC
     Sedative, hypnotic, or anxiolytic-induced major neurocognitive disorder, without use disorder

√6ᵗʰ **F13.98**   Sedative, hypnotic or anxiolytic use, unspecified with other sedative, hypnotic or anxiolytic-induced disorders

     F13.980   Sedative, hypnotic or anxiolytic use, unspecified with sedative, hypnotic or anxiolytic-induced anxiety disorder   HCC
         Sedative, hypnotic, or anxiolytic-induced anxiety disorder, without use disorder

     F13.981   Sedative, hypnotic or anxiolytic use, unspecified with sedative, hypnotic or anxiolytic-induced sexual dysfunction   HCC
         Sedative, hypnotic, or anxiolytic-induced sexual dysfunction disorder, without use disorder

     F13.982   Sedative, hypnotic or anxiolytic use, unspecified with sedative, hypnotic or anxiolytic-induced sleep disorder   HCC
         Sedative, hypnotic, or anxiolytic-induced sleep disorder, without use disorder

     F13.988   Sedative, hypnotic or anxiolytic use, unspecified with other sedative, hypnotic or anxiolytic-induced disorder   HCC
         Sedative, hypnotic, or anxiolytic-induced mild neurocognitive disorder

F13.99   Sedative, hypnotic or anxiolytic use, unspecified with unspecified sedative, hypnotic or anxiolytic-induced disorder   HCC ▽

√4ᵗʰ **F14**   **Cocaine related disorders**
     EXCLUDES 2   other stimulant-related disorders (F15.-)

√5ᵗʰ **F14.1**   **Cocaine abuse**
     EXCLUDES 1   cocaine dependence (F14.2-)
              cocaine use, unspecified (F14.9-)

     F14.10   Cocaine abuse, uncomplicated
         Cocaine use disorder, mild

     F14.11   Cocaine abuse, in remission
         Cocaine use disorder, mild, in early remission
         Cocaine use disorder, mild, in sustained remission

√6ᵗʰ **F14.12**   Cocaine abuse with intoxication

     F14.120   Cocaine abuse with intoxication, uncomplicated   HCC

     F14.121   Cocaine abuse with intoxication with delirium   HCC

     F14.122   Cocaine abuse with intoxication with perceptual disturbance   HCC

     F14.129   Cocaine abuse with intoxication, unspecified   HCC ▽

     F14.14   Cocaine abuse with cocaine-induced mood disorder   HCC
         Cocaine use disorder, mild, with cocaine-induced bipolar or related disorder
         Cocaine use disorder, mild, with cocaine-induced depressive disorder

√6ᵗʰ **F14.15**   Cocaine abuse with cocaine-induced psychotic disorder

     F14.150   Cocaine abuse with cocaine-induced psychotic disorder with delusions   HCC

     F14.151   Cocaine abuse with cocaine-induced psychotic disorder with hallucinations   HCC

     F14.159   Cocaine abuse with cocaine-induced psychotic disorder, unspecified   HCC ▽

√6ᵗʰ **F14.18**   Cocaine abuse with other cocaine-induced disorder

     F14.180   Cocaine abuse with cocaine-induced anxiety disorder   HCC

     F14.181   Cocaine abuse with cocaine-induced sexual dysfunction   HCC

     F14.182   Cocaine abuse with cocaine-induced sleep disorder   HCC

     F14.188   Cocaine abuse with other cocaine-induced disorder   HCC
         Cocaine use disorder, mild, with cocaine-induced obsessive compulsive or related disorder

     F14.19   Cocaine abuse with unspecified cocaine-induced disorder   HCC

√5ᵗʰ **F14.2**   **Cocaine dependence**
     EXCLUDES 1   cocaine abuse (F14.1-)
              cocaine use, unspecified (F14.9-)
     EXCLUDES 2   cocaine poisoning (T40.5-)

     F14.20   Cocaine dependence, uncomplicated   HCC
         Cocaine use disorder, moderate
         Cocaine use disorder, severe

     F14.21   Cocaine dependence, in remission   HCC
         Cocaine use disorder, moderate, in early remission
         Cocaine use disorder, moderate, in sustained remission
         Cocaine use disorder, severe, in early remission
         Cocaine use disorder, severe, in sustained remission

√6ᵗʰ **F14.22**   Cocaine dependence with intoxication
     EXCLUDES 1   cocaine dependence with withdrawal (F14.23)

     F14.220   Cocaine dependence with intoxication, uncomplicated   HCC

     F14.221   Cocaine dependence with intoxication delirium   HCC

     F14.222   Cocaine dependence with intoxication with perceptual disturbance   HCC

     F14.229   Cocaine dependence with intoxication, unspecified   HCC ▽

     F14.23   Cocaine dependence with withdrawal   HCC
     EXCLUDES 1   cocaine dependence with intoxication (F14.22-)

     F14.24   Cocaine dependence with cocaine-induced mood disorder   HCC
         Cocaine use disorder, moderate, with cocaine-induced bipolar or related disorder
         Cocaine use disorder, moderate, with cocaine-induced depressive disorder
         Cocaine use disorder, severe, with cocaine-induced bipolar or related disorder
         Cocaine use disorder, severe, with cocaine-induced depressive disorder

√6ᵗʰ **F14.25**   Cocaine dependence with cocaine-induced psychotic disorder

     F14.250   Cocaine dependence with cocaine-induced psychotic disorder with delusions   HCC

     F14.251   Cocaine dependence with cocaine-induced psychotic disorder with hallucinations   HCC

     F14.259   Cocaine dependence with cocaine-induced psychotic disorder, unspecified   HCC ▽

√6ᵗʰ **F14.28**   Cocaine dependence with other cocaine-induced disorder

     F14.280   Cocaine dependence with cocaine-induced anxiety disorder   HCC

     F14.281   Cocaine dependence with cocaine-induced sexual dysfunction   HCC

     F14.282   Cocaine dependence with cocaine-induced sleep disorder   HCC

☑ Additional Character Req   √x7ᵗʰ Placeholder Alert   Manifestation   ▽ Unspecified   ►◄ Revised Text   ● New Code   ▲ Revised Code Title

Chapter 5. Mental, Behavioral and Neurodevelopmental Disorders

F14.288   **Cocaine dependence with other cocaine-induced disorder**   HCC
     Cocaine use disorder, moderate, with cocaine-induced obsessive compulsive or related disorder
     Cocaine use disorder, severe, with cocaine-induced obsessive compulsive or related disorder

F14.29   **Cocaine dependence with unspecified cocaine-induced disorder**   HCC ▽

√5ᵗʰ **F14.9**   **Cocaine use, unspecified**
     EXCLUDES 1   *cocaine abuse (F14.1-)*
              cocaine dependence (F14.2-)

    F14.90   **Cocaine use, unspecified, uncomplicated**
       AHA: 2018,2Q,10-11

√6ᵗʰ   **F14.92**   **Cocaine use, unspecified with intoxication**
     F14.920   **Cocaine use, unspecified with intoxication, uncomplicated**   HCC
     F14.921   **Cocaine use, unspecified with intoxication delirium**   HCC
     F14.922   **Cocaine use, unspecified with intoxication with perceptual disturbance**   HCC
     F14.929   **Cocaine use, unspecified with intoxication, unspecified**   HCC ▽

    F14.94   **Cocaine use, unspecified with cocaine-induced mood disorder**   HCC
     Cocaine induced bipolar or related disorder, without use disorder
     Cocaine induced depressive disorder, without use disorder

√6ᵗʰ   **F14.95**   **Cocaine use, unspecified with cocaine-induced psychotic disorder**
     F14.950   **Cocaine use, unspecified with cocaine-induced psychotic disorder with delusions**   HCC
     F14.951   **Cocaine use, unspecified with cocaine-induced psychotic disorder with hallucinations**   HCC
     F14.959   **Cocaine use, unspecified with cocaine-induced psychotic disorder, unspecified**   HCC ▽
       Cocaine induced psychotic disorder, without use disorder

√6ᵗʰ   **F14.98**   **Cocaine use, unspecified with other specified cocaine-induced disorder**
     F14.980   **Cocaine use, unspecified with cocaine-induced anxiety disorder**   HCC
       Cocaine induced anxiety disorder, without use disorder
     F14.981   **Cocaine use, unspecified with cocaine-induced sexual dysfunction**   HCC
       Cocaine induced sexual dysfunction, without use disorder
     F14.982   **Cocaine use, unspecified with cocaine-induced sleep disorder**   HCC
       Cocaine induced sleep disorder, without use disorder
     F14.988   **Cocaine use, unspecified with other cocaine-induced disorder**   HCC
       Cocaine induced obsessive compulsive or related disorder

    F14.99   **Cocaine use, unspecified with unspecified cocaine-induced disorder**   HCC ▽

√4ᵗʰ **F15**   **Other stimulant related disorders**
     INCLUDES   amphetamine-related disorders
                caffeine
     EXCLUDES 2   *cocaine-related disorders (F14.-)*

√5ᵗʰ   **F15.1**   **Other stimulant abuse**
     EXCLUDES 1   *other stimulant dependence (F15.2-)*
              other stimulant use, unspecified (F15.9-)

    F15.10   **Other stimulant abuse, uncomplicated**
     Amphetamine type substance use disorder, mild
     Other or unspecified stimulant use disorder, mild

F15.11   **Other stimulant abuse, in remission**
     Amphetamine type substance use disorder, mild, in early remission
     Amphetamine type substance use disorder, mild, in sustained remission
     Other or unspecified stimulant use disorder, mild, in early remission
     Other or unspecified stimulant use disorder, mild, in sustained remission

√6ᵗʰ   **F15.12**   **Other stimulant abuse with intoxication**
     F15.120   **Other stimulant abuse with intoxication, uncomplicated**   HCC
     F15.121   **Other stimulant abuse with intoxication delirium**   HCC
     F15.122   **Other stimulant abuse with intoxication with perceptual disturbance**   HCC
       Amphetamine or other stimulant use disorder, mild, with amphetamine or other stimulant intoxication, with perceptual disturbances
     F15.129   **Other stimulant abuse with intoxication, unspecified**   HCC ▽
       Amphetamine or other stimulant use disorder, mild, with amphetamine or other stimulant intoxication, without perceptual disturbances

    F15.14   **Other stimulant abuse with stimulant-induced mood disorder**   HCC
     Amphetamine or other stimulant use disorder, mild, with amphetamine or other stimulant induced bipolar or related disorder
     Amphetamine or other stimulant use disorder, mild, with amphetamine or other stimulant induced depressive disorder

√6ᵗʰ   **F15.15**   **Other stimulant abuse with stimulant-induced psychotic disorder**
     F15.150   **Other stimulant abuse with stimulant-induced psychotic disorder with delusions**   HCC
     F15.151   **Other stimulant abuse with stimulant-induced psychotic disorder with hallucinations**   HCC
     F15.159   **Other stimulant abuse with stimulant-induced psychotic disorder, unspecified**   HCC ▽

√6ᵗʰ   **F15.18**   **Other stimulant abuse with other stimulant-induced disorder**
     F15.180   **Other stimulant abuse with stimulant-induced anxiety disorder**   HCC
     F15.181   **Other stimulant abuse with stimulant-induced sexual dysfunction**   HCC
     F15.182   **Other stimulant abuse with stimulant-induced sleep disorder**   HCC
     F15.188   **Other stimulant abuse with other stimulant-induced disorder**   HCC
       Amphetamine or other stimulant use disorder, mild, with amphetamine or other stimulant induced obsessive-compulsive or related disorder

    F15.19   **Other stimulant abuse with unspecified stimulant-induced disorder**   HCC ▽

√5ᵗʰ   **F15.2**   **Other stimulant dependence**
     EXCLUDES 1   *other stimulant abuse (F15.1-)*
              other stimulant use, unspecified (F15.9-)

    F15.20   **Other stimulant dependence, uncomplicated**   HCC
     Amphetamine type substance use disorder, moderate
     Amphetamine type substance use disorder, severe
     Other or unspecified stimulant use disorder, moderate
     Other or unspecified stimulant use disorder, severe

F15.21 **Other stimulant dependence, in remission** `HCC`
Amphetamine type substance use disorder, moderate, in early remission
Amphetamine type substance use disorder, moderate, in sustained remission
Amphetamine type substance use disorder, severe, in early remission
Amphetamine type substance use disorder, severe, in sustained remission
Other or unspecified stimulant use disorder, moderate, in early remission
Other or unspecified stimulant use disorder, moderate, in sustained remission
Other or unspecified stimulant use disorder, severe, in early remission
Other or unspecified stimulant use disorder, severe, in sustained remission

√6ᵗʰ **F15.22** **Other stimulant dependence with intoxication**
EXCLUDES 1 *other stimulant dependence with withdrawal (F15.23)*

F15.220 **Other stimulant dependence with intoxication, uncomplicated** `HCC`
F15.221 **Other stimulant dependence with intoxication delirium** `HCC`
F15.222 **Other stimulant dependence with intoxication with perceptual disturbance** `HCC`
Amphetamine or other stimulant use disorder, moderate, with amphetamine or other stimulant intoxication, with perceptual disturbances
Amphetamine or other stimulant use disorder, severe, with amphetamine or other stimulant intoxication, with perceptual disturbances
F15.229 **Other stimulant dependence with intoxication, unspecified** `HCC` ▽
Amphetamine or other stimulant use disorder, moderate, with amphetamine or other stimulant intoxication, without perceptual disturbances
Amphetamine or other stimulant use disorder, severe, with amphetamine or other stimulant intoxication, without perceptual disturbances

F15.23 **Other stimulant dependence with withdrawal** `HCC`
Amphetamine or other stimulant withdrawal
EXCLUDES 1 *other stimulant dependence with intoxication (F15.22-)*

F15.24 **Other stimulant dependence with stimulant-induced mood disorder** `HCC`
Amphetamine or other stimulant use disorder, moderate, with amphetamine or other stimulant-induced bipolar or related disorder
Amphetamine or other stimulant use disorder, moderate, with amphetamine or other stimulant induced depressive disorder
Amphetamine or other stimulant use disorder, severe, with amphetamine or other stimulant-induced bipolar or related disorder
Amphetamine or other stimulant use disorder, severe, with amphetamine or other stimulant-induced depressive disorder

√6ᵗʰ **F15.25** **Other stimulant dependence with stimulant-induced psychotic disorder**
F15.250 **Other stimulant dependence with stimulant-induced psychotic disorder with delusions** `HCC`
F15.251 **Other stimulant dependence with stimulant-induced psychotic disorder with hallucinations** `HCC`
F15.259 **Other stimulant dependence with stimulant-induced psychotic disorder, unspecified** `HCC` ▽

√6ᵗʰ **F15.28** **Other stimulant dependence with other stimulant-induced disorder**
F15.280 **Other stimulant dependence with stimulant-induced anxiety disorder** `HCC`
F15.281 **Other stimulant dependence with stimulant-induced sexual dysfunction** `HCC`
F15.282 **Other stimulant dependence with stimulant-induced sleep disorder** `HCC`
F15.288 **Other stimulant dependence with other stimulant-induced disorder** `HCC`
Amphetamine or other stimulant use disorder, moderate, with amphetamine or other stimulant induced obsessive compulsive or related disorder
Amphetamine or other stimulant use disorder, severe, with amphetamine or other stimulant induced obsessive compulsive or related disorder

F15.29 **Other stimulant dependence with unspecified stimulant-induced disorder** `HCC` ▽

√5ᵗʰ **F15.9** **Other stimulant use, unspecified**
EXCLUDES 1 *other stimulant abuse (F15.1-)*
other stimulant dependence (F15.2-)

F15.90 **Other stimulant use, unspecified, uncomplicated**
AHA: 2018,2Q,10-11

√6ᵗʰ **F15.92** **Other stimulant use, unspecified with intoxication**
EXCLUDES 1 *other stimulant use, unspecified with withdrawal (F15.93)*

F15.920 **Other stimulant use, unspecified with intoxication, uncomplicated** `HCC`
F15.921 **Other stimulant use, unspecified with intoxication delirium** `HCC`
Amphetamine or other stimulant-induced delirium
F15.922 **Other stimulant use, unspecified with intoxication with perceptual disturbance** `HCC`
F15.929 **Other stimulant use, unspecified with intoxication, unspecified** `HCC` ▽
Caffeine intoxication

F15.93 **Other stimulant use, unspecified with withdrawal** `HCC`
Caffeine withdrawal
EXCLUDES 1 *other stimulant use, unspecified with intoxication (F15.92-)*

F15.94 **Other stimulant use, unspecified with stimulant-induced mood disorder** `HCC`
Amphetamine or other stimulant-induced bipolar or related disorder, without use disorder
Amphetamine or other stimulant-induced depressive disorder, without use disorder

√6ᵗʰ **F15.95** **Other stimulant use, unspecified with stimulant-induced psychotic disorder**
F15.950 **Other stimulant use, unspecified with stimulant-induced psychotic disorder with delusions** `HCC`
F15.951 **Other stimulant use, unspecified with stimulant-induced psychotic disorder with hallucinations** `HCC`
F15.959 **Other stimulant use, unspecified with stimulant-induced psychotic disorder, unspecified** `HCC` ▽
Amphetamine or other stimulant-induced psychotic disorder, without use disorder

√6ᵗʰ **F15.98** **Other stimulant use, unspecified with other stimulant-induced disorder**
F15.980 **Other stimulant use, unspecified with stimulant-induced anxiety disorder** `HCC`
Amphetamine or other stimulant-induced anxiety disorder, without use disorder
Caffeine induced anxiety disorder, without use disorder

Chapter 5. Mental, Behavioral and Neurodevelopmental Disorders

F15.981 **Other stimulant use, unspecified with stimulant-induced sexual dysfunction** HCC
Amphetamine or other stimulant-induced sexual dysfunction, without use disorder

F15.982 **Other stimulant use, unspecified with stimulant-induced sleep disorder** HCC
Amphetamine or other stimulant-induced sleep disorder, without use disorder
Caffeine induced sleep disorder, without use disorder

F15.988 **Other stimulant use, unspecified with other stimulant-induced disorder** HCC
Amphetamine or other stimulant-induced obsessive compulsive or related disorder, without use disorder

F15.99 **Other stimulant use, unspecified with unspecified stimulant-induced disorder** HCC ▽

✓4ᵗʰ **F16** **Hallucinogen related disorders**
INCLUDES   ecstasy
PCP
phencyclidine

✓5ᵗʰ **F16.1** **Hallucinogen abuse**
EXCLUDES 1   *hallucinogen dependence (F16.2-)*
hallucinogen use, unspecified (F16.9-)

F16.10 **Hallucinogen abuse, uncomplicated**
Other hallucinogen use disorder, mild
Phencyclidine use disorder, mild

F16.11 **Hallucinogen abuse, in remission**
Other hallucinogen use disorder, mild, in early remission
Other hallucinogen use disorder, mild, in sustained remission
Phencyclidine use disorder, mild, in early remission
Phencyclidine use disorder, mild, in sustained remission

✓6ᵗʰ **F16.12** **Hallucinogen abuse with intoxication**

F16.120 **Hallucinogen abuse with intoxication, uncomplicated** HCC

F16.121 **Hallucinogen abuse with intoxication with delirium** HCC

F16.122 **Hallucinogen abuse with intoxication with perceptual disturbance** HCC

F16.129 **Hallucinogen abuse with intoxication, unspecified** HCC ▽

F16.14 **Hallucinogen abuse with hallucinogen-induced mood disorder** HCC
Other hallucinogen use disorder, mild, with other hallucinogen induced bipolar or related disorder
Other hallucinogen use disorder, mild, with other hallucinogen induced depressive disorder
Phencyclidine use disorder, mild, with phencyclidine induced bipolar or related disorder
Phencyclidine use disorder, mild, with phencyclidine induced depressive disorder

✓6ᵗʰ **F16.15** **Hallucinogen abuse with hallucinogen-induced psychotic disorder**

F16.150 **Hallucinogen abuse with hallucinogen-induced psychotic disorder with delusions** HCC

F16.151 **Hallucinogen abuse with hallucinogen-induced psychotic disorder with hallucinations** HCC

F16.159 **Hallucinogen abuse with hallucinogen-induced psychotic disorder, unspecified** HCC ▽

✓6ᵗʰ **F16.18** **Hallucinogen abuse with other hallucinogen-induced disorder**

F16.180 **Hallucinogen abuse with hallucinogen-induced anxiety disorder** HCC

F16.183 **Hallucinogen abuse with hallucinogen persisting perception disorder (flashbacks)** HCC

F16.188 **Hallucinogen abuse with other hallucinogen-induced disorder** HCC

F16.19 **Hallucinogen abuse with unspecified hallucinogen-induced disorder** HCC ▽

✓5ᵗʰ **F16.2** **Hallucinogen dependence**
EXCLUDES 1   *hallucinogen abuse (F16.1-)*
hallucinogen use, unspecified (F16.9-)

F16.20 **Hallucinogen dependence, uncomplicated** HCC
Other hallucinogen use disorder, moderate
Other hallucinogen use disorder, severe
Phencyclidine use disorder, moderate
Phencyclidine use disorder, severe

F16.21 **Hallucinogen dependence, in remission** HCC
Other hallucinogen use disorder, moderate, in early remission
Other hallucinogen use disorder, moderate, in sustained remission
Other hallucinogen use disorder, severe, in early remission
Other hallucinogen use disorder, severe, in sustained remission
Phencyclidine use disorder, moderate, in early remission
Phencyclidine use disorder, moderate, in sustained remission
Phencyclidine use disorder, severe, in early remission
Phencyclidine use disorder, severe, in sustained remission

✓6ᵗʰ **F16.22** **Hallucinogen dependence with intoxication**

F16.220 **Hallucinogen dependence with intoxication, uncomplicated** HCC

F16.221 **Hallucinogen dependence with intoxication with delirium** HCC

F16.229 **Hallucinogen dependence with intoxication, unspecified** HCC ▽

F16.24 **Hallucinogen dependence with hallucinogen-induced mood disorder** HCC
Other hallucinogen use disorder, moderate, with other hallucinogen induced bipolar or related disorder
Other hallucinogen use disorder, moderate, with other hallucinogen induced depressive disorder
Other hallucinogen use disorder, severe, with other hallucinogen-induced bipolar or related disorder
Other hallucinogen use disorder, severe, with other hallucinogen-induced depressive disorder
Phencyclidine use disorder, moderate, with phencyclidine induced bipolar or related disorder
Phencyclidine use disorder, moderate, with phencyclidine induced depressive disorder
Phencyclidine use disorder, severe, with phencyclidine induced bipolar or related disorder
Phencyclidine use disorder, severe, with phencyclidine-induced depressive disorder

✓6ᵗʰ **F16.25** **Hallucinogen dependence with hallucinogen-induced psychotic disorder**

F16.250 **Hallucinogen dependence with hallucinogen-induced psychotic disorder with delusions** HCC

F16.251 **Hallucinogen dependence with hallucinogen-induced psychotic disorder with hallucinations** HCC

F16.259 **Hallucinogen dependence with hallucinogen-induced psychotic disorder, unspecified** HCC ▽

✓6ᵗʰ **F16.28** **Hallucinogen dependence with other hallucinogen-induced disorder**

F16.280 **Hallucinogen dependence with hallucinogen-induced anxiety disorder** HCC

F16.283 **Hallucinogen dependence with hallucinogen persisting perception disorder (flashbacks)** HCC

F16.288 **Hallucinogen dependence with other hallucinogen-induced disorder** HCC

F16.29 **Hallucinogen dependence with unspecified hallucinogen-induced disorder** HCC ▽

√5ᵗʰ **F16.9 Hallucinogen use, unspecified**

      EXCLUDES 1   *hallucinogen abuse (F16.1-)*
                 hallucinogen dependence (F16.2-)

    F16.90 Hallucinogen use, unspecified, uncomplicated
        AHA: 2018,2Q,10-11

√6ᵗʰ **F16.92 Hallucinogen use, unspecified with intoxication**

      F16.920 Hallucinogen use, unspecified HCC
             with intoxication, uncomplicated

      F16.921 Hallucinogen use, unspecified HCC
             with intoxication with delirium
                 Other hallucinogen intoxication delirium

      F16.929 Hallucinogen use, unspecified HCC ▽
             with intoxication, unspecified

    F16.94 Hallucinogen use, unspecified with HCC
        hallucinogen-induced mood disorder
           Other hallucinogen induced bipolar or related
               disorder, without use disorder
           Other hallucinogen induced depressive disorder,
               without use disorder
           Phencyclidine induced bipolar or related disorder,
               without use disorder
           Phencyclidine induced depressive disorder, without
               use disorder

√6ᵗʰ **F16.95 Hallucinogen use, unspecified with**
        hallucinogen-induced psychotic disorder

      F16.950 Hallucinogen use, unspecified HCC
             with hallucinogen-induced
             psychotic disorder with delusions

      F16.951 Hallucinogen use, unspecified HCC
             with hallucinogen-induced
             psychotic disorder with
             hallucinations

      F16.959 Hallucinogen use, unspecified HCC ▽
             with hallucinogen-induced
             psychotic disorder, unspecified
                 Other hallucinogen induced psychotic
                    disorder, without use disorder
                 Phencyclidine induced psychotic disorder,
                    without use disorder

√6ᵗʰ **F16.98 Hallucinogen use, unspecified with other specified**
        hallucinogen-induced disorder

      F16.980 Hallucinogen use, unspecified HCC
             with hallucinogen-induced
             anxiety disorder
                 Other hallucinogen-induced anxiety
                    disorder, without use disorder
                 Phencyclidine induced anxiety disorder,
                    without use disorder

      F16.983 Hallucinogen use, unspecified HCC
             with hallucinogen persisting
             perception disorder (flashbacks)

      F16.988 Hallucinogen use, unspecified HCC
             with other hallucinogen-induced
             disorder

    F16.99 Hallucinogen use, unspecified with HCC ▽
        unspecified hallucinogen-induced disorder

√4ᵗʰ **F17 Nicotine dependence**

    EXCLUDES 1   *history of tobacco dependence (Z87.891)*
                 tobacco use NOS (Z72.0)

    EXCLUDES 2   *tobacco use (smoking) during pregnancy, childbirth and the*
                    puerperium (O99.33-)
                 toxic effect of nicotine (T65.2-)

  AHA: 2013,4Q,108-109

√5ᵗʰ **F17.2 Nicotine dependence**

√6ᵗʰ **F17.20 Nicotine dependence, unspecified**

      F17.200 Nicotine dependence,   ▽
             unspecified, uncomplicated
                 Tobacco use disorder, mild
                 Tobacco use disorder, moderate
                 Tobacco use disorder, severe
             AHA: 2016,1Q,36
             TIP: Assign when provider documentation
             indicates "smoker" without further
             specification.

      F17.201 Nicotine dependence,   ▽
             unspecified, in remission
                 Tobacco use disorder, mild, in early
                    remission
                 Tobacco use disorder, mild, in sustained
                    remission
                 Tobacco use disorder, moderate, in early
                    remission
                 Tobacco use disorder, moderate, in
                    sustained remission
                 Tobacco use disorder, severe, in early
                    remission
                 Tobacco use disorder, severe, in sustained
                    remission

      F17.203 Nicotine dependence unspecified, ▽
             with withdrawal
                 Tobacco withdrawal

      F17.208 Nicotine dependence,   ▽
             unspecified, with other
             nicotine-induced disorders

      F17.209 Nicotine dependence,   ▽
             unspecified, with unspecified
             nicotine-induced disorders

√6ᵗʰ **F17.21 Nicotine dependence, cigarettes**

      F17.210 Nicotine dependence, cigarettes,
             uncomplicated
             AHA: 2017,2Q,28-29

      F17.211 Nicotine dependence, cigarettes, in
             remission
                 Tobacco use disorder, cigarettes, mild, in
                    early remission
                 Tobacco use disorder, cigarettes, mild, in
                    sustained remission
                 Tobacco use disorder, cigarettes,
                    moderate, in early remission
                 Tobacco use disorder, cigarettes,
                    moderate, in sustained remission
                 Tobacco use disorder, cigarettes, severe,
                    in early remission
                 Tobacco use disorder, cigarettes, severe,
                    in sustained remission

      F17.213 Nicotine dependence, cigarettes, with
             withdrawal

      F17.218 Nicotine dependence, cigarettes, with
             other nicotine-induced disorders

      F17.219 Nicotine dependence, cigarettes, ▽
             with unspecified
             nicotine-induced disorders

√6ᵗʰ **F17.22 Nicotine dependence, chewing tobacco**

      F17.220 Nicotine dependence, chewing tobacco,
             uncomplicated

      F17.221 Nicotine dependence, chewing tobacco,
             in remission
                 Tobacco use disorder, chewing tobacco,
                    mild, in early remission
                 Tobacco use disorder, chewing tobacco,
                    mild, in sustained remission
                 Tobacco use disorder, chewing tobacco,
                    moderate, in early remission
                 Tobacco use disorder, chewing tobacco,
                    moderate, in sustained remission
                 Tobacco use disorder, chewing tobacco,
                    severe, in early remission
                 Tobacco use disorder, chewing tobacco,
                    severe, in sustained remission

      F17.223 Nicotine dependence, chewing tobacco,
             with withdrawal

      F17.228 Nicotine dependence, chewing tobacco,
             with other nicotine-induced disorders

      F17.229 Nicotine dependence, chewing ▽
             tobacco, with unspecified
             nicotine-induced disorders

√6ᵗʰ **F17.29 Nicotine dependence, other tobacco product**

      F17.290 Nicotine dependence, other tobacco
             product, uncomplicated
             AHA: 2017,2Q,28-29

✔ Additional Character Req	✔x7ᵗʰ Placeholder Alert	Manifestation	▽ Unspecified	►◄ Revised Text	● New Code	▲ Revised Code Title

F17.291   **Nicotine dependence, other tobacco product, in remission**
Tobacco use disorder, other tobacco product, mild, in early remission
Tobacco use disorder, other tobacco product, mild, in sustained remission
Tobacco use disorder, other tobacco product, moderate, in early remission
Tobacco use disorder, other tobacco product, moderate, in sustained remission
Tobacco use disorder, other tobacco product, severe, in early remission
Tobacco use disorder, other tobacco product, severe, in sustained remission

F17.293   **Nicotine dependence, other tobacco product, with withdrawal**

F17.298   **Nicotine dependence, other tobacco product, with other nicotine-induced disorders**

F17.299   **Nicotine dependence, other tobacco product, with unspecified nicotine-induced disorders** ▽

✓4th **F18**   **Inhalant related disorders**
   INCLUDES   volatile solvents

✓5th **F18.1**   **Inhalant abuse**
   EXCLUDES 1   *inhalant dependence (F18.2-)*
            inhalant use, unspecified (F18.9-)

F18.10   **Inhalant abuse, uncomplicated**
Inhalant use disorder, mild

F18.11   **Inhalant abuse, in remission**
Inhalant use disorder, mild, in early remission
Inhalant use disorder, mild, in sustained remission

✓6th **F18.12**   **Inhalant abuse with intoxication**
   F18.120   **Inhalant abuse with intoxication, uncomplicated** HCC
   F18.121   **Inhalant abuse with intoxication delirium** HCC
   F18.129   **Inhalant abuse with intoxication, unspecified** HCC ▽

F18.14   **Inhalant abuse with inhalant-induced mood disorder** HCC
Inhalant use disorder, mild, with inhalant induced depressive disorder

✓6th **F18.15**   **Inhalant abuse with inhalant-induced psychotic disorder**
   F18.150   **Inhalant abuse with inhalant-induced psychotic disorder with delusions** HCC
   F18.151   **Inhalant abuse with inhalant-induced psychotic disorder with hallucinations** HCC
   F18.159   **Inhalant abuse with inhalant-induced psychotic disorder, unspecified** HCC ▽

F18.17   **Inhalant abuse with inhalant-induced dementia** HCC
Inhalant use disorder, mild, with inhalant induced major neurocognitive disorder

✓6th **F18.18**   **Inhalant abuse with other inhalant-induced disorders**
   F18.180   **Inhalant abuse with inhalant-induced anxiety disorder** HCC
   F18.188   **Inhalant abuse with other inhalant-induced disorder** HCC
Inhalant use disorder, mild, with inhalant induced mild neurocognitive disorder

F18.19   **Inhalant abuse with unspecified inhalant-induced disorder** HCC ▽

✓5th **F18.2**   **Inhalant dependence**
   EXCLUDES 1   *inhalant abuse (F18.1-)*
            inhalant use, unspecified (F18.9-)

F18.20   **Inhalant dependence, uncomplicated** HCC
Inhalant use disorder, moderate
Inhalant use disorder, severe

F18.21   **Inhalant dependence, in remission** HCC
Inhalant use disorder, moderate, in early remission
Inhalant use disorder, moderate, in sustained remission
Inhalant use disorder, severe, in early remission
Inhalant use disorder, severe, in sustained remission

✓6th **F18.22**   **Inhalant dependence with intoxication**
   F18.220   **Inhalant dependence with intoxication, uncomplicated** HCC
   F18.221   **Inhalant dependence with intoxication delirium** HCC
   F18.229   **Inhalant dependence with intoxication, unspecified** HCC ▽

F18.24   **Inhalant dependence with inhalant-induced mood disorder** HCC
Inhalant use disorder, moderate, with inhalant induced depressive disorder
Inhalant use disorder, severe, with inhalant induced depressive disorder

✓6th **F18.25**   **Inhalant dependence with inhalant-induced psychotic disorder**
   F18.250   **Inhalant dependence with inhalant-induced psychotic disorder with delusions** HCC
   F18.251   **Inhalant dependence with inhalant-induced psychotic disorder with hallucinations** HCC
   F18.259   **Inhalant dependence with inhalant-induced psychotic disorder, unspecified** HCC ▽

F18.27   **Inhalant dependence with inhalant-induced dementia** HCC
Inhalant use disorder, moderate, with inhalant induced major neurocognitive disorder
Inhalant use disorder, severe, with inhalant induced major neurocognitive disorder

✓6th **F18.28**   **Inhalant dependence with other inhalant-induced disorders**
   F18.280   **Inhalant dependence with inhalant-induced anxiety disorder** HCC
   F18.288   **Inhalant dependence with other inhalant-induced disorder** HCC
Inhalant use disorder, moderate, with inhalant-induced mild neurocognitive disorder
Inhalant use disorder, severe, with inhalant-induced mild neurocognitive disorder

F18.29   **Inhalant dependence with unspecified inhalant-induced disorder** HCC ▽

✓5th **F18.9**   **Inhalant use, unspecified**
   EXCLUDES 1   *inhalant abuse (F18.1-)*
            inhalant dependence (F18.2-)

F18.90   **Inhalant use, unspecified, uncomplicated**
   AHA: 2018,2Q,10-11

✓6th **F18.92**   **Inhalant use, unspecified with intoxication**
   F18.920   **Inhalant use, unspecified with intoxication, uncomplicated** HCC
   F18.921   **Inhalant use, unspecified with intoxication with delirium** HCC
   F18.929   **Inhalant use, unspecified with intoxication, unspecified** HCC ▽

F18.94   **Inhalant use, unspecified with inhalant-induced mood disorder** HCC
Inhalant induced depressive disorder

✓6th **F18.95**   **Inhalant use, unspecified with inhalant-induced psychotic disorder**
   F18.950   **Inhalant use, unspecified with inhalant-induced psychotic disorder with delusions** HCC
   F18.951   **Inhalant use, unspecified with inhalant-induced psychotic disorder with hallucinations** HCC
   F18.959   **Inhalant use, unspecified with inhalant-induced psychotic disorder, unspecified** HCC ▽

F18.97   **Inhalant use, unspecified with inhalant-induced persisting dementia** HCC
Inhalant-induced major neurocognitive disorder

√6ᵗʰ **F18.98** **Inhalant use, unspecified with other inhalant-induced disorders**

    F18.980 **Inhalant use, unspecified with inhalant-induced** anxiety **disorder** `HCC`

    F18.988 **Inhalant use, unspecified with other inhalant-induced disorder** `HCC`
        Inhalant-induced mild neurocognitive disorder

  F18.99 **Inhalant use, unspecified with unspecified inhalant-induced disorder** `HCC` ▽

√4ᵗʰ **F19** **Other** psychoactive **substance related disorders**
    INCLUDES   polysubstance drug use (indiscriminate drug use)

√5ᵗʰ **F19.1** **Other psychoactive substance** abuse
    EXCLUDES 1   *other psychoactive substance dependence (F19.2-)*
               other psychoactive substance use, unspecified (F19.9-)

  F19.10 **Other psychoactive substance abuse, uncomplicated**
    Other (or unknown) substance use disorder, mild

  F19.11 **Other psychoactive substance abuse, in remission**
    Other (or unknown) substance use disorder, mild, in early remission
    Other (or unknown) substance use disorder, mild, in sustained remission

√6ᵗʰ **F19.12** **Other psychoactive substance abuse with intoxication**

    F19.120 **Other psychoactive substance abuse with intoxication, uncomplicated** `HCC`

    F19.121 **Other psychoactive substance abuse with intoxication** delirium `HCC`

    F19.122 **Other psychoactive substance abuse with intoxication with** perceptual disturbances `HCC`

    F19.129 **Other psychoactive substance abuse with intoxication, unspecified** `HCC` ▽

  F19.14 **Other psychoactive substance abuse with psychoactive substance-induced** mood **disorder** `HCC`
    Other (or unknown) substance use disorder, mild, with other (or unknown) substance-induced bipolar or related disorder
    Other (or unknown) substance use disorder, mild, with other (or unknown) substance-induced depressive disorder

√6ᵗʰ **F19.15** **Other psychoactive substance abuse with psychoactive substance-induced** psychotic **disorder**

    F19.150 **Other psychoactive substance abuse with psychoactive substance-induced psychotic disorder with** delusions `HCC`

    F19.151 **Other psychoactive substance abuse with psychoactive substance-induced psychotic disorder with** hallucinations `HCC`

    F19.159 **Other psychoactive substance abuse with psychoactive substance-induced psychotic disorder, unspecified** `HCC` ▽

  F19.16 **Other psychoactive substance abuse with psychoactive substance-induced** persisting **amnestic disorder** `HCC`

  F19.17 **Other psychoactive substance abuse with psychoactive substance-induced** persisting **dementia** `HCC`
    Other (or unknown) substance use disorder, mild, with other (or unknown) substance-induced major neurocognitive disorder

√6ᵗʰ **F19.18** **Other psychoactive substance abuse with other psychoactive substance-induced disorders**

    F19.180 **Other psychoactive substance abuse with psychoactive substance-induced** anxiety **disorder** `HCC`

    F19.181 **Other psychoactive substance abuse with psychoactive substance-induced** sexual **dysfunction** `HCC`

    F19.182 **Other psychoactive substance abuse with psychoactive substance-induced** sleep **disorder** `HCC`

    F19.188 **Other psychoactive substance abuse with other psychoactive substance-induced disorder** `HCC`
        Other (or unknown) substance use disorder, mild, with other (or unknown) substance induced mild neurocognitive disorder
        Other (or unknown) substance use disorder, mild, with other (or unknown) substance induced obsessive-compulsive or related disorder

  F19.19 **Other psychoactive substance abuse with unspecified psychoactive substance-induced disorder** `HCC` ▽

√5ᵗʰ **F19.2** **Other psychoactive substance** dependence
    EXCLUDES 1   *other psychoactive substance abuse (F19.1-)*
               other psychoactive substance use, unspecified (F19.9-)

  F19.20 **Other psychoactive substance dependence, uncomplicated** `HCC`
    Other (or unknown) substance use disorder, moderate
    Other (or unknown) substance use disorder, severe

  F19.21 **Other psychoactive substance dependence, in remission** `HCC`
    Other (or unknown) substance use disorder, moderate, in early remission
    Other (or unknown) substance use disorder, moderate, in sustained remission
    Other (or unknown) substance use disorder, severe, in early remission
    ▶Other (or unknown) substance use disorder, severe, in sustained remission◀

√6ᵗʰ **F19.22** **Other psychoactive substance dependence with intoxication**
    EXCLUDES 1   *other psychoactive substance dependence with withdrawal (F19.23-)*

    F19.220 **Other psychoactive substance dependence with intoxication, uncomplicated** `HCC`

    F19.221 **Other psychoactive substance dependence with intoxication** delirium `HCC`

    F19.222 **Other psychoactive substance dependence with intoxication with** perceptual disturbance `HCC`

    F19.229 **Other psychoactive substance dependence with intoxication, unspecified** `HCC` ▽

√6ᵗʰ **F19.23** **Other psychoactive substance dependence with withdrawal**
    EXCLUDES 1   *other psychoactive substance dependence with intoxication (F19.22-)*

    F19.230 **Other psychoactive substance dependence with withdrawal, uncomplicated** `HCC`

    F19.231 **Other psychoactive substance dependence with withdrawal** delirium `HCC`

    F19.232 **Other psychoactive substance dependence with withdrawal with** perceptual disturbance `HCC`

    F19.239 **Other psychoactive substance dependence with withdrawal, unspecified** `HCC` ▽

☑ Additional Character Req   √x7ᵗʰ Placeholder Alert   ~~Manifestation~~   ▽ Unspecified   ▶◀ Revised Text   ● New Code   ▲ Revised Code Title

Chapter 5. Mental, Behavioral and Neurodevelopmental Disorders

F19.24   **Other psychoactive substance dependence with psychoactive substance-induced mood disorder**   HCC
Other (or unknown) substance use disorder, moderate, with other (or unknown) substance induced bipolar or related disorder
Other (or unknown) substance use disorder, moderate, with other (or unknown) substance induced depressive disorder
Other (or unknown) substance use disorder, severe, with other (or unknown) substance induced bipolar or related disorder
Other (or unknown) substance use disorder, severe, with other (or unknown) substance induced depressive disorder

√6ᵗʰ **F19.25**   **Other psychoactive substance dependence with psychoactive substance-induced psychotic disorder**

     F19.250   Other psychoactive substance dependence with psychoactive substance-induced psychotic disorder with delusions   HCC

     F19.251   Other psychoactive substance dependence with psychoactive substance-induced psychotic disorder with hallucinations   HCC

     F19.259   Other psychoactive substance dependence with psychoactive substance-induced psychotic disorder, unspecified   HCC ▽

F19.26   **Other psychoactive substance dependence with psychoactive substance-induced persisting amnestic disorder**   HCC

F19.27   **Other psychoactive substance dependence with psychoactive substance-induced persisting dementia**   HCC
Other (or unknown) substance use disorder, moderate, with other (or unknown) substance induced major neurocognitive disorder
Other (or unknown) substance use disorder, severe, with other (or unknown) substance induced major neurocognitive disorder

√6ᵗʰ **F19.28**   **Other psychoactive substance dependence with other psychoactive substance-induced disorders**

     F19.280   Other psychoactive substance dependence with psychoactive substance-induced anxiety disorder   HCC

     F19.281   Other psychoactive substance dependence with psychoactive substance-induced sexual dysfunction   HCC

     F19.282   Other psychoactive substance dependence with psychoactive substance-induced sleep disorder   HCC

     F19.288   Other psychoactive substance dependence with other psychoactive substance-induced disorder   HCC
Other (or unknown) substance use disorder, moderate, with other (or unknown) substance induced mild neurocognitive disorder
Other (or unknown) substance use disorder, severe, with other (or unknown) substance induced mild neurocognitive disorder
Other (or unknown) substance use disorder, moderate, with other (or unknown) substance induced obsessive compulsive or related disorder
Other (or unknown) substance use disorder, severe, with other (or unknown) substance induced obsessive-compulsive or related disorder

F19.29   **Other psychoactive substance dependence with unspecified psychoactive substance-induced disorder**   HCC ▽

√5ᵗʰ **F19.9**   **Other psychoactive substance use, unspecified**
     EXCLUDES 1   *other psychoactive substance abuse (F19.1-)*
         other psychoactive substance dependence (F19.2-)

     F19.90   **Other psychoactive substance use, unspecified, uncomplicated**
         AHA: 2018,2Q,10-11

√6ᵗʰ **F19.92**   **Other psychoactive substance use, unspecified with intoxication**
     EXCLUDES 1   *other psychoactive substance use, unspecified with withdrawal (F19.93)*

     F19.920   Other psychoactive substance use, unspecified with intoxication, uncomplicated   HCC

     F19.921   Other psychoactive substance use, unspecified with intoxication with delirium   HCC
Other (or unknown) substance-induced delirium

     F19.922   Other psychoactive substance use, unspecified with intoxication with perceptual disturbance   HCC

     F19.929   Other psychoactive substance use, unspecified with intoxication, unspecified   HCC ▽

√6ᵗʰ **F19.93**   **Other psychoactive substance use, unspecified with withdrawal**
     EXCLUDES 1   *other psychoactive substance use, unspecified with intoxication (F19.92-)*

     F19.930   Other psychoactive substance use, unspecified with withdrawal, uncomplicated   HCC

     F19.931   Other psychoactive substance use, unspecified with withdrawal delirium   HCC

     F19.932   Other psychoactive substance use, unspecified with withdrawal with perceptual disturbance   HCC

     F19.939   Other psychoactive substance use, unspecified with withdrawal, unspecified   HCC ▽

     F19.94   **Other psychoactive substance use, unspecified with psychoactive substance-induced mood disorder**   HCC
Other (or unknown) substance-induced bipolar or related disorder, without use disorder
Other (or unknown) substance-induced depressive disorder, without use disorder

√6ᵗʰ **F19.95**   **Other psychoactive substance use, unspecified with psychoactive substance-induced psychotic disorder**

     F19.950   Other psychoactive substance use, unspecified with psychoactive substance-induced psychotic disorder with delusions   HCC

     F19.951   Other psychoactive substance use, unspecified with psychoactive substance-induced psychotic disorder with hallucinations   HCC

     F19.959   Other psychoactive substance use, unspecified with psychoactive substance-induced psychotic disorder, unspecified   HCC ▽
Other or unknown substance-induced psychotic disorder, without use disorder

     F19.96   **Other psychoactive substance use, unspecified with psychoactive substance-induced persisting amnestic disorder**   HCC

     F19.97   **Other psychoactive substance use, unspecified with psychoactive substance-induced persisting dementia**   HCC
Other (or unknown) substance-induced major neurocognitive disorder, without use disorder

√6th **F19.98** **Other psychoactive substance use, unspecified with other psychoactive substance-induced disorders**

    F19.980 **Other psychoactive substance use, unspecified with psychoactive substance-induced anxiety disorder** `HCC`

        Other (or unknown) substance-induced anxiety disorder, without use disorder

    F19.981 **Other psychoactive substance use, unspecified with psychoactive substance-induced sexual dysfunction** `HCC`

        Other (or unknown) substance-induced sexual dysfunction, without use disorder

    F19.982 **Other psychoactive substance use, unspecified with psychoactive substance-induced sleep disorder** `HCC`

        Other (or unknown) substance-induced sleep disorder, without use disorder

    F19.988 **Other psychoactive substance use, unspecified with other psychoactive substance-induced disorder** `HCC`

        Other (or unknown) substance-induced mild neurocognitive disorder, without use disorder

        Other (or unknown) substance-induced obsessive-compulsive or related disorder, without use disorder

    F19.99 **Other psychoactive substance use, unspecified with unspecified psychoactive substance-induced disorder** `HCC` ▽

Schizophrenia, schizotypal, delusional, and other non-mood psychotic disorders (F20-F29)

√4th **F20** **Schizophrenia**

    `EXCLUDES 1`   *brief psychotic disorder (F23)*
              cyclic schizophrenia (F25.0)
              mood [affective] disorders with psychotic symptoms (F30.2, F31.2, F31.5, F31.64, F32.3, F33.3)
              schizoaffective disorder (F25.-)
              schizophrenic reaction NOS (F23)
    `EXCLUDES 2`   *schizophrenic reaction in:*
              alcoholism (F10.15-, F10.25-, F10.95-)
              brain disease (F06.2)
              epilepsy (F06.2)
              psychoactive drug use (F11-F19 with .15, .25, .95)
              schizotypal disorder (F21)

    DEF: Group of disorders with disturbances in thought (delusions, hallucinations), mood (blunted, flattened, inappropriate affect), and sense of self. Schizophrenia also includes bizarre, purposeless behavior, repetitious activity, or inactivity.

    F20.0 **Paranoid schizophrenia** `HCC`
        Paraphrenic schizophrenia
        `EXCLUDES 1` *involutional paranoid state (F22)*
                paranoia (F22)
        DEF: Preoccupied with delusional suspicions and auditory hallucinations related to a single theme. This type of schizophrenia is usually hostile, grandiose, threatening, persecutory, and occasionally hypochondriacal.

    F20.1 **Disorganized schizophrenia** `HCC`
        Hebephrenic schizophrenia
        Hebephrenia

    F20.2 **Catatonic schizophrenia** `HCC`
        Schizophrenic catalepsy
        Schizophrenic catatonia
        Schizophrenic flexibilitas cerea
        `EXCLUDES 1` *catatonic stupor (R40.1)*
        DEF: Extreme changes in motor activity. One extreme is a decreased response or reaction to the environment and the other is spontaneous activity.

    F20.3 **Undifferentiated schizophrenia** `HCC`
        Atypical schizophrenia
        `EXCLUDES 1` *acute schizophrenia-like psychotic disorder (F23)*
        `EXCLUDES 2` *post-schizophrenic depression(F32.89)*

    F20.5 **Residual schizophrenia** `HCC`
        Restzustand (schizophrenic)
        Schizophrenic residual state

√5th **F20.8** **Other schizophrenia**

    F20.81 **Schizophreniform disorder** `HCC`
        Schizophreniform psychosis NOS

    F20.89 **Other schizophrenia** `HCC`
        Cenesthopathic schizophrenia
        Simple schizophrenia

    F20.9 **Schizophrenia, unspecified** `HCC` ▽

F21 **Schizotypal disorder**
    Borderline schizophrenia
    Latent schizophrenia
    Latent schizophrenic reaction
    Prepsychotic schizophrenia
    Prodromal schizophrenia
    Pseudoneurotic schizophrenia
    Pseudopsychopathic schizophrenia
    Schizotypal personality disorder
    `EXCLUDES 2` *Asperger's syndrome (F84.5)*
              schizoid personality disorder (F60.1)
    DEF: Disorder characterized by various oddities of thinking, perception, communication, and behavior that may be manifested as magical thinking, ideas of reference, paranoid ideation, recurrent illusions and derealization (depersonalization), or social isolation.

F22 **Delusional disorders** `HCC`
    Delusional dysmorphophobia
    Involutional paranoid state
    Paranoia
    Paranoia querulans
    Paranoid psychosis
    Paranoid state
    Paraphrenia (late)
    Sensitiver Beziehungswahn
    `EXCLUDES 1` *mood [affective] disorders with psychotic symptoms (F30.2, F31.2, F31.5, F31.64, F32.3, F33.3)*
              paranoid schizophrenia (F20.0)
    `EXCLUDES 2` *paranoid personality disorder (F60.0)*
              paranoid psychosis, psychogenic (F23)
              paranoid reaction (F23)

F23 **Brief psychotic disorder**
    Paranoid reaction
    Psychogenic paranoid psychosis
    `EXCLUDES 2` *mood [affective] disorders with psychotic symptoms (F30.2, F31.2, F31.5, F31.64, F32.3, F33.3)*

F24 **Shared psychotic disorder** `HCC`
    Folie à deux
    Induced paranoid disorder
    Induced psychotic disorder

√4th **F25** **Schizoaffective disorders**
    `EXCLUDES 1` *mood [affective] disorders with psychotic symptoms (F30.2, F31.2, F31.5, F31.64, F32.3, F33.3)*
              schizophrenia (F20.-)

    F25.0 **Schizoaffective disorder, bipolar type** `HCC`
        Cyclic schizophrenia
        Schizoaffective disorder, manic type
        Schizoaffective disorder, mixed type
        Schizoaffective psychosis, bipolar type

    F25.1 **Schizoaffective disorder, depressive type** `HCC`
        Schizoaffective psychosis, depressive type

    F25.8 **Other schizoaffective disorders** `HCC`

    F25.9 **Schizoaffective disorder, unspecified** `HCC` ▽
        Schizoaffective psychosis NOS

F28 **Other psychotic disorder not due to a substance or known physiological condition**
    Chronic hallucinatory psychosis
    Other specified schizophrenia spectrum and other psychotic disorder

F29 **Unspecified psychosis not due to a substance or known physiological condition** ▽
    Psychosis NOS
    Unspecified schizophrenia spectrum and other psychotic disorder
    `EXCLUDES 1` *mental disorder NOS (F99)*
              unspecified mental disorder due to known physiological condition (F09)

Chapter 5. Mental, Behavioral and Neurodevelopmental Disorders

F30–F32.4

Mood [affective] disorders (F30-F39)

✓4th F30 Manic episode

INCLUDES   bipolar disorder, single manic episode
       mixed affective episode

EXCLUDES 1   *bipolar disorder (F31.-)*
       major depressive disorder, recurrent (F33.-)
       major depressive disorder, single episode (F32.-)

DEF: Mania: Characterized by abnormal states of elation or excitement out of keeping with the individual's circumstances and varying from enhanced liveliness (hypomania) to violent, almost uncontrollable, excitement. Aggression and anger, flight of ideas, distractibility, impaired judgment, and grandiose ideas are common.

✓5th F30.1 Manic episode without psychotic symptoms

- **F30.10** Manic episode without psychotic symptoms, unspecified   HCC ▽
- **F30.11** Manic episode without psychotic symptoms, mild   HCC
- **F30.12** Manic episode without psychotic symptoms, moderate   HCC
- **F30.13** Manic episode, severe, without psychotic symptoms   HCC

F30.2 Manic episode, severe with psychotic symptoms   HCC
     Manic stupor
     Mania with mood-congruent psychotic symptoms
     Mania with mood-incongruent psychotic symptoms

F30.3 Manic episode in partial remission   HCC
F30.4 Manic episode in full remission   HCC
F30.8 Other manic episodes   HCC
     Hypomania

F30.9 Manic episode, unspecified   HCC ▽
     Mania NOS

✓4th F31 Bipolar disorder

INCLUDES   bipolar I disorder
       bipolar type I disorder
       manic-depressive illness
       manic-depressive psychosis
       manic-depressive reaction

EXCLUDES 1   *bipolar disorder, single manic episode (F30.-)*
       major depressive disorder, recurrent (F33.-)
       major depressive disorder, single episode (F32.-)

EXCLUDES 2   *cyclothymia (F34.0)*

F31.0 Bipolar disorder, current episode hypomanic   HCC

✓5th F31.1 Bipolar disorder, current episode manic without psychotic features

- **F31.10** Bipolar disorder, current episode manic without psychotic features, unspecified   HCC Q ▽
- **F31.11** Bipolar disorder, current episode manic without psychotic features, mild   HCC Q
- **F31.12** Bipolar disorder, current episode manic without psychotic features, moderate   HCC Q
- **F31.13** Bipolar disorder, current episode manic without psychotic features, severe   HCC Q

F31.2 Bipolar disorder, current episode manic severe with psychotic features   HCC Q
     Bipolar disorder, current episode manic with mood-congruent psychotic symptoms
     Bipolar disorder, current episode manic with mood-incongruent psychotic symptoms
     Bipolar I disorder, current or most recent episode manic with psychotic features

✓5th F31.3 Bipolar disorder, current episode depressed, mild or moderate severity

- **F31.30** Bipolar disorder, current episode depressed, mild or moderate severity, unspecified   HCC Q ▽
- **F31.31** Bipolar disorder, current episode depressed, mild   HCC Q
- **F31.32** Bipolar disorder, current episode depressed, moderate   HCC Q

F31.4 Bipolar disorder, current episode depressed, severe, without psychotic features   HCC Q

F31.5 Bipolar disorder, current episode depressed, severe, with psychotic features   HCC Q
     Bipolar disorder, current episode depressed with mood-congruent psychotic symptoms
     Bipolar disorder, current episode depressed with mood-incongruent psychotic symptoms
     Bipolar I disorder, current or most recent episode depressed, with psychotic features

✓5th F31.6 Bipolar disorder, current episode mixed

- **F31.60** Bipolar disorder, current episode mixed, unspecified   HCC Q ▽
- **F31.61** Bipolar disorder, current episode mixed, mild   HCC Q
- **F31.62** Bipolar disorder, current episode mixed, moderate   HCC Q
- **F31.63** Bipolar disorder, current episode mixed, severe, without psychotic features   HCC Q
- **F31.64** Bipolar disorder, current episode mixed, severe, with psychotic features   HCC Q
     Bipolar disorder, current episode mixed with mood-congruent psychotic symptoms
     Bipolar disorder, current episode mixed with mood-incongruent psychotic symptoms

✓5th F31.7 Bipolar disorder, currently in remission

- **F31.70** Bipolar disorder, currently in remission, most recent episode unspecified   HCC Q ▽
- **F31.71** Bipolar disorder, in partial remission, most recent episode hypomanic   HCC Q
- **F31.72** Bipolar disorder, in full remission, most recent episode hypomanic   HCC Q
- **F31.73** Bipolar disorder, in partial remission, most recent episode manic   HCC Q
- **F31.74** Bipolar disorder, in full remission, most recent episode manic   HCC Q
- **F31.75** Bipolar disorder, in partial remission, most recent episode depressed   HCC Q
- **F31.76** Bipolar disorder, in full remission, most recent episode depressed   HCC Q
- **F31.77** Bipolar disorder, in partial remission, most recent episode mixed   HCC Q
- **F31.78** Bipolar disorder, in full remission, most recent episode mixed   HCC Q

✓5th F31.8 Other bipolar disorders

- **F31.81** Bipolar II disorder   HCC Q
     Bipolar disorder, type 2
- **F31.89** Other bipolar disorder   HCC Q
     Recurrent manic episodes NOS

F31.9 Bipolar disorder, unspecified   HCC Q ▽
     Manic depression

✓4th F32 Major depressive disorder, single episode

INCLUDES   single episode of agitated depression
       single episode of depressive reaction
       single episode of major depression
       single episode of psychogenic depression
       single episode of reactive depression
       single episode of vital depression

EXCLUDES 1   *bipolar disorder (F31.-)*
       manic episode (F30.-)
       recurrent depressive disorder (F33.-)

EXCLUDES 2   *adjustment disorder (F43.2)*

DEF: Mood disorder that produces depression that may exhibit as sadness, low self-esteem, or guilt feelings. Other manifestations may be withdrawal from friends and family and interrupted sleep.

F32.0 Major depressive disorder, single episode, mild   HCC Q
F32.1 Major depressive disorder, single episode, moderate   HCC Q
F32.2 Major depressive disorder, single episode, severe without psychotic features   HCC Q
F32.3 Major depressive disorder, single episode, severe with psychotic features   HCC Q
     Single episode of major depression with mood-congruent psychotic symptoms
     Single episode of major depression with mood-incongruent psychotic symptoms
     Single episode of major depression with psychotic symptoms
     Single episode of psychogenic depressive psychosis
     Single episode of psychotic depression
     Single episode of reactive depressive psychosis

F32.4 Major depressive disorder, single episode, in partial remission   HCC Q

F32.5   **Major depressive disorder, single episode, in full remission**   HCC 0

✓5ᵗʰ **F32.8**   **Other depressive episodes**

    AHA: 2016,4Q,14

    F32.81   **Premenstrual dysphoric disorder**   ♀

       EXCLUDES 1   *premenstrual tension syndrome (N94.3)*

       DEF: Severe manifestation of premenstrual syndrome (PMS) that can be disabling and destructive to day-to-day activities. It can exacerbate pre-existing emotional disorders, like depression and anxiety, and cause feelings of loss of control, fatigue, and irritability.

    F32.89   **Other specified depressive episodes**

       Atypical depression

       Post-schizophrenic depression

       Single episode of 'masked' depression NOS

F32.9   **Major depressive disorder, single episode, unspecified**   0 ▽

    Depression NOS

    Depressive disorder NOS

    Major depression NOS

    AHA: 2013,4Q,107

✓4ᵗʰ **F33**   **Major depressive disorder, recurrent**

    INCLUDES   recurrent episodes of depressive reaction

       recurrent episodes of endogenous depression

       recurrent episodes of major depression

       recurrent episodes of psychogenic depression

       recurrent episodes of reactive depression

       recurrent episodes of seasonal depressive disorder

       recurrent episodes of vital depression

    EXCLUDES 1   *bipolar disorder (F31.-)*

       manic episode (F30.-)

    F33.0   **Major depressive disorder, recurrent, mild**   HCC 0

    F33.1   **Major depressive disorder, recurrent, moderate**   HCC 0

    F33.2   **Major depressive disorder, recurrent, severe without psychotic features**   HCC 0

    F33.3   **Major depressive disorder, recurrent, severe with psychotic symptoms**   HCC 0

       Endogenous depression with psychotic symptoms

       Major depressive disorder, recurrent, with psychotic features

       Recurrent severe episodes of major depression with mood-congruent psychotic symptoms

       Recurrent severe episodes of major depression with mood-incongruent psychotic symptoms

       Recurrent severe episodes of major depression with psychotic symptoms

       Recurrent severe episodes of psychogenic depressive psychosis

       Recurrent severe episodes of psychotic depression

       Recurrent severe episodes of reactive depressive psychosis

✓5ᵗʰ **F33.4**   **Major depressive disorder, recurrent, in remission**

    F33.40   **Major depressive disorder, recurrent, in remission, unspecified**   HCC 0 ▽

    F33.41   **Major depressive disorder, recurrent, in partial remission**   HCC 0

    F33.42   **Major depressive disorder, recurrent, in full remission**   HCC 0

    F33.8   **Other recurrent depressive disorders**   HCC 0

       Recurrent brief depressive episodes

    F33.9   **Major depressive disorder, recurrent, unspecified**   HCC 0 ▽

       Monopolar depression NOS

✓4ᵗʰ **F34**   **Persistent mood [affective] disorders**

    F34.0   **Cyclothymic disorder**

       Affective personality disorder

       Cycloid personality

       Cyclothymia

       Cyclothymic personality

       DEF: Mood disorder characterized by fast and repeated alterations between hypomanic and depressed moods.

F34.1   **Dysthymic disorder**   0

    Depressive neurosis

    Depressive personality disorder

    Dysthymia

    Neurotic depression

    Persistent anxiety depression

    Persistent depressive disorder

    EXCLUDES 2   *anxiety depression (mild or not persistent) (F41.8)*

    DEF: Depression without psychosis. It is a less severe but persistent depression and is considered a mild to moderate chronic form of depression.

✓5ᵗʰ **F34.8**   **Other persistent mood [affective] disorders**   HCC

    AHA: 2016,4Q,14

    F34.81   **Disruptive mood dysregulation disorder**   HCC 0

    F34.89   **Other specified persistent mood disorders**   HCC 0

    F34.9   **Persistent mood [affective] disorder, unspecified**   HCC ▽

F39   **Unspecified mood [affective] disorder**   HCC ▽

    Affective psychosis NOS

Anxiety, dissociative, stress-related, somatoform and other nonpsychotic mental disorders (F40-F48)

✓4ᵗʰ **F40**   **Phobic anxiety disorders**

✓5ᵗʰ **F40.0**   **Agoraphobia**

    DEF: Profound anxiety or fear of leaving familiar settings like home, or being in unfamiliar locations or with strangers or crowds. Agoraphobia may or may not be preceded by recurrent panic attacks.

    F40.00   **Agoraphobia, unspecified**   ▽

    F40.01   **Agoraphobia with panic disorder**

       Panic disorder with agoraphobia

       EXCLUDES 1   *panic disorder without agoraphobia (F41.0)*

    F40.02   **Agoraphobia without panic disorder**

✓5ᵗʰ **F40.1**   **Social phobias**

    Anthropophobia

    Social anxiety disorder

    Social anxiety disorder of childhood

    Social neurosis

    F40.10   **Social phobia, unspecified**   ▽

    F40.11   **Social phobia, generalized**

✓5ᵗʰ **F40.2**   **Specific (isolated) phobias**

    EXCLUDES 2   *dysmorphophobia (nondelusional) (F45.22)*

       nosophobia (F45.22)

    ✓6ᵗʰ **F40.21**   **Animal type phobia**

       F40.210   **Arachnophobia**

          Fear of spiders

       F40.218   **Other animal type phobia**

    ✓6ᵗʰ **F40.22**   **Natural environment type phobia**

       F40.220   **Fear of thunderstorms**

       F40.228   **Other natural environment type phobia**

    ✓6ᵗʰ **F40.23**   **Blood, injection, injury type phobia**

       F40.230   **Fear of blood**

       F40.231   **Fear of injections and transfusions**

       F40.232   **Fear of other medical care**

       F40.233   **Fear of injury**

    ✓6ᵗʰ **F40.24**   **Situational type phobia**

       F40.240   **Claustrophobia**

       F40.241   **Acrophobia**

       F40.242   **Fear of bridges**

       F40.243   **Fear of flying**

       F40.248   **Other situational type phobia**

    ✓6ᵗʰ **F40.29**   **Other specified phobia**

       F40.290   **Androphobia**

          Fear of men

       F40.291   **Gynephobia**

          Fear of women

       F40.298   **Other specified phobia**

    F40.8   **Other phobic anxiety disorders**

       Phobic anxiety disorder of childhood

    F40.9   **Phobic anxiety disorder, unspecified**   ▽

       Phobia NOS

       Phobic state NOS

| ✓ Additional Character Req | ✓x7ᵗʰ Placeholder Alert | Manifestation | ▽ Unspecified | ▶◀ Revised Text | ● New Code | ▲ Revised Code Title |

Chapter 5. Mental, Behavioral and Neurodevelopmental Disorders

F41–F44.9

✓4ᵗʰ **F41 Other anxiety disorders**

EXCLUDES 2　*anxiety in:*
- *acute stress reaction (F43.0)*
- *neurasthenia (F48.8)*
- *psychophysiologic disorders (F45.-)*
- *transient adjustment reaction (F43.2)*
- *separation anxiety (F93.0)*

F41.0 Panic disorder [episodic paroxysmal anxiety]
- Panic attack
- Panic state

EXCLUDES 1　*panic disorder with agoraphobia (F40.01)*

DEF: Neurotic disorder characterized by recurrent panic or anxiety, apprehension, fear, or terror. Symptoms include shortness of breath, palpitations, dizziness, and shakiness; fear of dying may persist.

F41.1 Generalized anxiety disorder
- Anxiety neurosis
- Anxiety reaction
- Anxiety state
- Overanxious disorder

EXCLUDES 2　*neurasthenia (F48.8)*

F41.3 Other mixed anxiety disorders

F41.8 Other specified anxiety disorders
- Anxiety depression (mild or not persistent)
- Anxiety hysteria
- Mixed anxiety and depressive disorder

F41.9 Anxiety disorder, unspecified　　▽
- Anxiety NOS

✓4ᵗʰ **F42 Obsessive-compulsive disorder**

EXCLUDES 2　*obsessive-compulsive personality (disorder) (F60.5)*
- *obsessive-compulsive symptoms occurring in depression (F32-F33)*
- *obsessive-compulsive symptoms occurring in schizophrenia (F20.-)*

AHA: 2016,4Q,14-15

F42.2 Mixed obsessional thoughts and acts

F42.3 Hoarding disorder

F42.4 Excoriation (skin-picking) disorder

EXCLUDES 1　*factitial dermatitis (L98.1)*
- *other specified behavioral and emotional disorders with onset usually occurring in early childhood and adolescence (F98.8)*

F42.8 Other obsessive-compulsive disorder
- Anancastic neurosis
- Obsessive-compulsive neurosis

F42.9 Obsessive-compulsive disorder, unspecified　　▽

✓4ᵗʰ **F43 Reaction to severe stress, and adjustment disorders**

F43.0 Acute stress reaction
- Acute crisis reaction
- Acute reaction to stress
- Combat and operational stress reaction
- Combat fatigue
- Crisis state
- Psychic shock

✓5ᵗʰ **F43.1 Post-traumatic stress disorder (PTSD)**
- Traumatic neurosis

DEF: Preoccupation with traumatic events beyond normal experience (i.e., rape, personal assault, etc.) that may also include recurring flashbacks of the trauma. Symptoms include difficulty remembering, sleeping, or concentrating, and guilt feelings for surviving.

F43.10 Post-traumatic stress disorder, unspecified　　▽

F43.11 Post-traumatic stress disorder, acute

F43.12 Post-traumatic stress disorder, chronic

✓5ᵗʰ **F43.2 Adjustment disorders**
- Culture shock
- Grief reaction
- Hospitalism in children

EXCLUDES 2　*separation anxiety disorder of childhood (F93.0)*

F43.20 Adjustment disorder, unspecified　　▽

F43.21 Adjustment disorder with depressed mood　　Q

AHA: 2014,1Q,25

F43.22 Adjustment disorder with anxiety

F43.23 Adjustment disorder with mixed anxiety and depressed mood　　Q

F43.24 Adjustment disorder with disturbance of conduct

F43.25 Adjustment disorder with mixed disturbance of emotions and conduct

F43.29 Adjustment disorder with other symptoms

F43.8 Other reactions to severe stress
- Other specified trauma and stressor-related disorder

F43.9 Reaction to severe stress, unspecified　　▽
- Trauma and stressor-related disorder, NOS

✓4ᵗʰ **F44 Dissociative and conversion disorders**

INCLUDES　conversion hysteria
- conversion reaction
- hysteria
- hysterical psychosis

EXCLUDES 2　*malingering [conscious simulation] (Z76.5)*

F44.0 Dissociative amnesia

EXCLUDES 1　*amnesia NOS (R41.3)*
- *anterograde amnesia (R41.1)*
- *dissociative amnesia with dissociative fugue (F44.1)*
- *retrograde amnesia (R41.2)*

EXCLUDES 2　*alcohol-or other psychoactive substance-induced amnestic disorder (F10, F13, F19 with .26, .96)*
- *amnestic disorder due to known physiological condition (F04)*
- *postictal amnesia in epilepsy (G40.-)*

F44.1 Dissociative fugue
- Dissociative amnesia with dissociative fugue

EXCLUDES 2　*postictal fugue in epilepsy (G40.-)*

DEF: Dissociative hysteria identified by memory loss and flight from familiar surroundings to a completely separate environment. Episodes may last hours or days. Conscious activity is not associated with perception of surroundings and there is no later memory of the episode.

F44.2 Dissociative stupor

EXCLUDES 1　*catatonic stupor (R40.1)*
- *stupor NOS (R40.1)*

EXCLUDES 2　*catatonic disorder due to known physiological condition (F06.1)*
- *depressive stupor (F32, F33)*
- *manic stupor (F30, F31)*

F44.4 Conversion disorder with motor symptom or deficit
- Conversion disorder with abnormal movement
- Conversion disorder with speech symptoms
- Conversion disorder with swallowing symptoms
- Conversion disorder with weakness/paralysis
- Dissociative motor disorders
- Psychogenic aphonia
- Psychogenic dysphonia

F44.5 Conversion disorder with seizures or convulsions
- Conversion disorder with attacks or seizures
- Dissociative convulsions

F44.6 Conversion disorder with sensory symptom or deficit
- Conversion disorder with anesthesia or sensory loss
- Conversion disorder with special sensory symptoms
- Dissociative anesthesia and sensory loss
- Psychogenic deafness

F44.7 Conversion disorder with mixed symptom presentation

✓5ᵗʰ **F44.8 Other dissociative and conversion disorders**

F44.81 Dissociative identity disorder
- Multiple personality disorder

F44.89 Other dissociative and conversion disorders
- Ganser's syndrome
- Psychogenic confusion
- Psychogenic twilight state
- Trance and possession disorders

F44.9 Dissociative and conversion disorder, unspecified　　▽
- Dissociative disorder NOS

✓4ᵗʰ F45 Somatoform disorders

> EXCLUDES 2   dissociative and conversion disorders (F44.-)
>
> factitious disorders ▶(F68.1-, F68.A)◀
>
> hair-plucking (F63.3)
>
> lalling (F80.0)
>
> lisping (F80.0)
>
> malingering [conscious simulation] (Z76.5)
>
> nail-biting (F98.8)
>
> psychological or behavioral factors associated with disorders or diseases classified elsewhere (F54)
>
> sexual dysfunction, not due to a substance or known physiological condition (F52.-)
>
> thumb-sucking (F98.8)
>
> tic disorders (in childhood and adolescence) (F95.-)
>
> Tourette's syndrome (F95.2)
>
> trichotillomania (F63.3)

DEF: Types of disorders causing inconsistent physical symptoms that cannot be explained.

F45.0 Somatization disorder
Briquet's disorder
Multiple psychosomatic disorder

F45.1 Undifferentiated somatoform disorder
Somatic symptom disorder
Undifferentiated psychosomatic disorder

✓5ᵗʰ F45.2 Hypochondriacal disorders

> EXCLUDES 2   delusional dysmorphophobia (F22)
>
> fixed delusions about bodily functions or shape (F22)

    F45.20 Hypochondriacal disorder, unspecified ▽

    F45.21 Hypochondriasis
        Hypochondriacal neurosis
        Illness anxiety disorder

    F45.22 Body dysmorphic disorder
        Dysmorphophobia (nondelusional)
        Nosophobia

    F45.29 Other hypochondriacal disorders

✓5ᵗʰ F45.4 Pain disorders related to psychological factors

> EXCLUDES 1   pain NOS (R52)

    F45.41 Pain disorder exclusively related to psychological factors
        Somatoform pain disorder (persistent)

    F45.42 Pain disorder with related psychological factors
        Code also associated acute or chronic pain (G89.-)

F45.8 Other somatoform disorders
Psychogenic dysmenorrhea
Psychogenic dysphagia, including 'globus hystericus'
Psychogenic pruritus
Psychogenic torticollis
Somatoform autonomic dysfunction
Teeth grinding

> EXCLUDES 1   sleep related teeth grinding (G47.63)

F45.9 Somatoform disorder, unspecified ▽
Psychosomatic disorder NOS

✓4ᵗʰ F48 Other nonpsychotic mental disorders

F48.1 Depersonalization-derealization syndrome

F48.2 Pseudobulbar affect
Involuntary emotional expression disorder
Code first underlying cause, if known, such as:
   amyotrophic lateral sclerosis (G12.21)
   multiple sclerosis (G35)
   sequelae of cerebrovascular disease (I69.-)
   sequelae of traumatic intracranial injury (S06.-)

F48.8 Other specified nonpsychotic mental disorders
Dhat syndrome
Neurasthenia
Occupational neurosis, including writer's cramp
Psychasthenia
Psychasthenic neurosis
Psychogenic syncope

F48.9 Nonpsychotic mental disorder, unspecified ▽
Neurosis NOS

Behavioral syndromes associated with physiological disturbances and physical factors (F50-F59)

✓4ᵗʰ F50 Eating disorders

> EXCLUDES 1   anorexia NOS (R63.0)
>
> feeding difficulties (R63.3)
>
> feeding problems of newborn (P92.-)
>
> polyphagia (R63.2)
>
> EXCLUDES 2   feeding disorder in infancy or childhood (F98.2-)

TIP: Assign additional code for BMI from category Z68, when documented. BMI can be based on documentation from clinicians who are not the patient's provider.

✓5ᵗʰ F50.0 Anorexia nervosa

> EXCLUDES 1   loss of appetite (R63.0)
>
> psychogenic loss of appetite (F50.89)

DEF: Psychological eating disorder characterized by an intense fear of gaining weight and an unrealistic perception of body image that perpetuates the feeling of being fat or having too much fat. Avoidance of food and restrictive or unhealthy eating are common.

    F50.00 Anorexia nervosa, unspecified ▽

    F50.01 Anorexia nervosa, restricting type

    F50.02 Anorexia nervosa, binge eating/purging type

> EXCLUDES 1   bulimia nervosa (F50.2)

F50.2 Bulimia nervosa
Bulimia NOS
Hyperorexia nervosa

> EXCLUDES 1   anorexia nervosa, binge eating/purging type (F50.02)

DEF: Episodic pattern of overeating (binge eating) followed by purging or extreme exercise accompanied by an awareness of the abnormal eating pattern with a fear of not being able to stop eating.

✓5ᵗʰ F50.8 Other eating disorders

> EXCLUDES 2   pica of infancy and childhood (F98.3)

AHA: 2017,4Q,9; 2016,4Q,15-16

    F50.81 Binge eating disorder

    F50.82 Avoidant/restrictive food intake disorder

    F50.89 Other specified eating disorder
        Pica in adults
        Psychogenic loss of appetite

F50.9 Eating disorder, unspecified ▽
Atypical anorexia nervosa
Atypical bulimia nervosa
Feeding or eating disorder, unspecified
Other specified feeding disorder

✓4ᵗʰ F51 Sleep disorders not due to a substance or known physiological condition

> EXCLUDES 2   organic sleep disorders (G47.-)

✓5ᵗʰ F51.0 Insomnia not due to a substance or known physiological condition

> EXCLUDES 2   alcohol related insomnia (F10.182, F10.282, F10.982)
>
> drug-related insomnia (F11.182, F11.282, F11.982, F13.182, F13.282, F13.982, F14.182, F14.282, F14.982, F15.182, F15.282, F15.982, F19.182, F19.282, F19.982)
>
> insomnia NOS (G47.0-)
>
> insomnia due to known physiological condition (G47.0-)
>
> organic insomnia (G47.0-)
>
> sleep deprivation (Z72.820)

    F51.01 Primary insomnia
        Idiopathic insomnia

    F51.02 Adjustment insomnia

    F51.03 Paradoxical insomnia

    F51.04 Psychophysiologic insomnia

    F51.05 Insomnia due to other mental disorder
        Code also associated mental disorder

    F51.09 Other insomnia not due to a substance or known physiological condition

---

✓ Additional Character Req   ✓x7ᵗʰ Placeholder Alert   Manifestation   ▽ Unspecified   ▶◀ Revised Text   ● New Code   ▲ Revised Code Title

Chapter 5. Mental, Behavioral and Neurodevelopmental Disorders

√5ᵗʰ **F51.1 Hypersomnia not due to a substance or known physiological condition**
    EXCLUDES 2   *alcohol related hypersomnia (F10.182, F10.282, F10.982)*
        drug-related hypersomnia (F11.182, F11.282, F11.982, F13.182, F13.282, F13.982, F14.182, F14.282, F14.982, F15.182, F15.282, F15.982, F19.182, F19.282, F19.982)
        hypersomnia NOS (G47.10)
        hypersomnia due to known physiological condition (G47.10)
        idiopathic hypersomnia (G47.11, G47.12)
        narcolepsy (G47.4-)

    F51.11 Primary hypersomnia
    F51.12 Insufficient sleep syndrome
        EXCLUDES 1   *sleep deprivation (Z72.820)*
    F51.13 Hypersomnia due to other mental disorder
        Code also associated mental disorder
    F51.19 Other hypersomnia not due to a substance or known physiological condition

F51.3 Sleepwalking [somnambulism]
    Non-rapid eye movement sleep arousal disorders, sleepwalking type

F51.4 Sleep terrors [night terrors]
    Non-rapid eye movement sleep arousal disorders, sleep terror type

F51.5 Nightmare disorder
    Dream anxiety disorder

F51.8 Other sleep disorders not due to a substance or known physiological condition

F51.9 Sleep disorder not due to a substance or known ▽ **physiological condition, unspecified**
    Emotional sleep disorder NOS

√4ᵗʰ **F52 Sexual dysfunction not due to a substance or known physiological condition**
    EXCLUDES 2   *Dhat syndrome (F48.8)*

F52.0 Hypoactive sexual desire disorder
    Lack or loss of sexual desire
    Male hypoactive sexual desire disorder
    Sexual anhedonia
    EXCLUDES 1   *decreased libido (R68.82)*

F52.1 Sexual aversion disorder
    Sexual aversion and lack of sexual enjoyment

√5ᵗʰ **F52.2 Sexual arousal disorders**
    Failure of genital response
    F52.21 Male erectile disorder ♂
        Erectile disorder
        Psychogenic impotence
        EXCLUDES 1   *impotence of organic origin (N52.-)*
                impotence NOS (N52.-)
    F52.22 Female sexual arousal disorder ♀
        Female sexual interest/arousal disorder

√5ᵗʰ **F52.3 Orgasmic disorder**
    Inhibited orgasm
    Psychogenic anorgasmy
    F52.31 Female orgasmic disorder ♀
    F52.32 Male orgasmic disorder ♂
        Delayed ejaculation

F52.4 Premature ejaculation ♂

F52.5 Vaginismus not due to a substance or known ♀ **physiological condition**
    Psychogenic vaginismus
    EXCLUDES 2   *vaginismus (due to a known physiological condition) (N94.2)*
    DEF: Psychogenic response resulting in painful contractions of the vaginal canal muscles. This condition can be severe enough to prevent sexual intercourse.

F52.6 Dyspareunia not due to a substance or known physiological condition
    Genito-pelvic pain penetration disorder
    Psychogenic dyspareunia
    EXCLUDES 2   *dyspareunia (due to a known physiological condition) (N94.1-)*

F52.8 Other sexual dysfunction not due to a substance or known physiological condition
    Excessive sexual drive
    Nymphomania
    Satyriasis

F52.9 Unspecified sexual dysfunction not due to a ▽ **substance or known physiological condition**
    Sexual dysfunction NOS

▲ √4ᵗʰ **F53 Mental and behavioral disorders associated with the puerperium, not elsewhere classified**
    ~~Postpartum depression~~
    EXCLUDES 1   *mood disorders with psychotic features (F30.2, F31.2, F31.5, F31.64, F32.3, F33.3)*
        postpartum dysphoria (O90.6)
        psychosis in schizophrenia, schizotypal, delusional, and other psychotic disorders (F20-F29)

● **F53.0 Postpartum depression**
    Postnatal depression, NOS
    Postpartum depression, NOS

● **F53.1 Puerperal psychosis**
    Postpartum psychosis
    Puerperal psychosis, NOS

F54 Psychological and behavioral factors associated with disorders or diseases classified elsewhere
    Psychological factors affecting physical conditions
    Code first the associated physical disorder, such as:
    asthma (J45.-)
    dermatitis (L23-L25)
    gastric ulcer (K25.-)
    mucous colitis (K58.-)
    ulcerative colitis (K51.-)
    urticaria (L50.-)
    EXCLUDES 2   *tension-type headache (G44.2)*

√4ᵗʰ **F55 Abuse of non-psychoactive substances**
    EXCLUDES 2   *abuse of psychoactive substances (F10-F19)*

    F55.0 Abuse of antacids
    F55.1 Abuse of herbal or folk remedies
    F55.2 Abuse of laxatives
    F55.3 Abuse of steroids or hormones
    F55.4 Abuse of vitamins
    F55.8 Abuse of other non-psychoactive substances

F59 Unspecified behavioral syndromes associated with ▽ **physiological disturbances and physical factors**
    Psychogenic physiological dysfunction NOS

Disorders of adult personality and behavior (F60-F69)

√4ᵗʰ **F60 Specific personality disorders**

    F60.0 Paranoid personality disorder
    Expansive paranoid personality (disorder)
    Fanatic personality (disorder)
    Paranoid personality (disorder)
    Querulant personality (disorder)
    Sensitive paranoid personality (disorder)
    EXCLUDES 2   *paranoia (F22)*
        paranoia querulans (F22)
        paranoid psychosis (F22)
        paranoid schizophrenia (F20.0)
        paranoid state (F22)

    F60.1 Schizoid personality disorder
    EXCLUDES 2   *Asperger's syndrome (F84.5)*
        delusional disorder (F22)
        schizoid disorder of childhood (F84.5)
        schizophrenia (F20.-)
        schizotypal disorder (F21)

    F60.2 Antisocial personality disorder
    Amoral personality (disorder)
    Asocial personality (disorder)
    Dissocial personality disorder
    Psychopathic personality (disorder)
    Sociopathic personality (disorder)
    EXCLUDES 1   *conduct disorders (F91.-)*
    EXCLUDES 2   *borderline personality disorder (F60.3)*

F60.3 Borderline personality disorder
Aggressive personality (disorder)
Emotionally unstable personality disorder
Explosive personality (disorder)
EXCLUDES 2   *antisocial personality disorder (F60.2)*

F60.4 Histrionic personality disorder
Hysterical personality (disorder)
Psychoinfantile personality (disorder)

F60.5 Obsessive-compulsive personality disorder
Anankastic personality (disorder)
Compulsive personality (disorder)
Obsessional personality (disorder)
EXCLUDES 2   *obsessive-compulsive disorder (F42-)*

F60.6 Avoidant personality disorder
Anxious personality disorder

F60.7 Dependent personality disorder
Asthenic personality (disorder)
Inadequate personality (disorder)
Passive personality (disorder)
DEF: Lack of self-confidence, fear of abandonment, and an obsessive need to be taken care of.

✓5ᵗʰ **F60.8 Other specific personality disorders**

     F60.81 Narcissistic personality disorder

     F60.89 Other specific personality disorders
         Eccentric personality disorder
         "Haltlose" type personality disorder
         Immature personality disorder
         Passive-aggressive personality disorder
         Psychoneurotic personality disorder
         Self-defeating personality disorder

F60.9 Personality disorder, unspecified ▽
Character disorder NOS
Character neurosis NOS
Pathological personality NOS

✓4ᵗʰ **F63 Impulse disorders**
EXCLUDES 2   *habitual excessive use of alcohol or psychoactive substances (F10-F19)*
          impulse disorders involving sexual behavior (F65.-)

F63.0 Pathological gambling
Compulsive gambling
Gambling disorder
EXCLUDES 1   *gambling and betting NOS (Z72.6)*
EXCLUDES 2   *excessive gambling by manic patients (F30, F31)*
          gambling in antisocial personality disorder (F60.2)

F63.1 Pyromania
Pathological fire-setting
EXCLUDES 2   *fire-setting (by) (in):*
          adult with antisocial personality disorder (F60.2)
          alcohol or psychoactive substance intoxication (F10-F19)
          conduct disorders (F91.-)
          mental disorders due to known physiological condition (F01-F09)
          schizophrenia (F20.-)

F63.2 Kleptomania
Pathological stealing
EXCLUDES 1   *shoplifting as the reason for observation for suspected mental disorder (Z03.8)*
EXCLUDES 2   *depressive disorder with stealing (F31-F33)*
          stealing due to underlying mental condition - code to mental condition
          stealing in mental disorders due to known physiological condition (F01-F09)

F63.3 Trichotillomania
Hair plucking
EXCLUDES 2   *other stereotyped movement disorder (F98.4)*

✓5ᵗʰ **F63.8 Other impulse disorders**

     F63.81 Intermittent explosive disorder

     F63.89 Other impulse disorders

F63.9 Impulse disorder, unspecified ▽
Impulse control disorder NOS

✓4ᵗʰ **F64 Gender identity disorders**
AHA: 2016,4Q,16

F64.0 Transsexualism
Gender identity disorder in adolescence and adulthood
Gender dysphoria in adolescents and adults

F64.1 Dual role transvestism
Use additional code to identify sex reassignment status (Z87.890)
EXCLUDES 1   *gender identity disorder in childhood (F64.2)*
EXCLUDES 2   *fetishistic transvestism (F65.1)*

F64.2 Gender identity disorder of childhood ℗
Gender dysphoria in children
EXCLUDES 1   *gender identity disorder in adolescence and adulthood (F64.0)*
EXCLUDES 2   *sexual maturation disorder (F66)*

F64.8 Other gender identity disorders
Other specified gender dysphoria

F64.9 Gender identity disorder, unspecified ▽
Gender dysphoria, unspecified
Gender-role disorder NOS

✓4ᵗʰ **F65 Paraphilias**

F65.0 Fetishism
Fetishistic disorder

F65.1 Transvestic fetishism
Fetishistic transvestism
Transvestic disorder

F65.2 Exhibitionism
Exhibitionistic disorder

F65.3 Voyeurism
Voyeuristic disorder

F65.4 Pedophilia
Pedophilic disorder

✓5ᵗʰ **F65.5 Sadomasochism**

     F65.50 Sadomasochism, unspecified ▽

     F65.51 Sexual masochism
         Sexual masochism disorder

     F65.52 Sexual sadism
         Sexual sadism disorder

✓5ᵗʰ **F65.8 Other paraphilias**

     F65.81 Frotteurism
         Frotteuristic disorder

     F65.89 Other paraphilias
         Necrophilia
         Other specified paraphilic disorder

F65.9 Paraphilia, unspecified ▽
Paraphilic disorder, unspecified
Sexual deviation NOS

F66 Other sexual disorders
Sexual maturation disorder
Sexual relationship disorder

✓4ᵗʰ **F68 Other disorders of adult personality and behavior**

▲   ✓5ᵗʰ **F68.1 Factitious disorder imposed on self**
Compensation neurosis
Elaboration of physical symptoms for psychological reasons
Hospital hopper syndrome
Münchausen's syndrome
Peregrinating patient
EXCLUDES 2   *factitial dermatitis (L98.1)*
          person feigning illness (with obvious motivation) (Z76.5)

▲   **F68.10 Factitious disorder imposed on self, unspecified** ▽

▲   **F68.11 Factitious disorder imposed on self, with predominantly psychological signs and symptoms**

▲   **F68.12 Factitious disorder imposed on self, with predominantly physical signs and symptoms**

▲   **F68.13 Factitious disorder imposed on self, with combined psychological and physical signs and symptoms**

●   **F68.A Factitious disorder imposed on another**
         Factitious disorder by proxy
         Münchausen's by proxy

     F68.8 Other specified disorders of adult personality and behavior

F69 Unspecified disorder of adult personality and behavior Ⓐ ▽

Chapter 5. Mental, Behavioral and Neurodevelopmental Disorders

F70–F84.0

Intellectual disabilities (F70-F79)

Code first any associated physical or developmental disorders

EXCLUDES 1   *borderline intellectual functioning, IQ above 70 to 84 (R41.83)*

F70   **Mild intellectual disabilities**
     IQ level 50-55 to approximately 70
     Mild mental subnormality

F71   **Moderate intellectual disabilities**
     IQ level 35-40 to 50-55
     Moderate mental subnormality

F72   **Severe intellectual disabilities**
     IQ 20-25 to 35-40
     Severe mental subnormality

F73   **Profound intellectual disabilities**
     IQ level below 20-25
     Profound mental subnormality

F78   **Other intellectual disabilities**

F79   **Unspecified intellectual disabilities**   ▽
     Mental deficiency NOS
     Mental subnormality NOS

Pervasive and specific developmental disorders (F80-F89)

✓4ᵗʰ   **F80**   **Specific developmental disorders of speech and language**

   F80.0   **Phonological disorder**
       Dyslalia
       Functional speech articulation disorder
       Lalling
       Lisping
       Phonological developmental disorder
       Speech articulation developmental disorder
       Speech-sound disorder
       EXCLUDES 1   *speech articulation impairment due to aphasia NOS (R47.01)*
              speech articulation impairment due to apraxia (R48.2)
       EXCLUDES 2   *speech articulation impairment due to hearing loss (F80.4)*
              speech articulation impairment due to intellectual disabilities (F70-F79)
              speech articulation impairment with expressive language developmental disorder (F80.1)
              speech articulation impairment with mixed receptive expressive language developmental disorder (F80.2)

   F80.1   **Expressive language disorder**
       Developmental dysphasia or aphasia, expressive type
       EXCLUDES 1   *mixed receptive-expressive language disorder (F80.2)*
              dysphasia and aphasia NOS (R47.-)
       EXCLUDES 2   *acquired aphasia with epilepsy [Landau-Kleffner] (G40.80-)*
              selective mutism (F94.0)
              intellectual disabilities (F70-F79)
              pervasive developmental disorders (F84.-)

   F80.2   **Mixed receptive-expressive language disorder**
       Developmental dysphasia or aphasia, receptive type
       Developmental Wernicke's aphasia
       EXCLUDES 1   *central auditory processing disorder (H93.25)*
              dysphasia or aphasia NOS (R47.-)
              expressive language disorder (F80.1)
              expressive type dysphasia or aphasia (F80.1)
              word deafness (H93.25)
       EXCLUDES 2   *acquired aphasia with epilepsy [Landau-Kleffner] (G40.80-)*
              pervasive developmental disorders (F84.-)
              selective mutism (F94.0)
              intellectual disabilities (F70-F79)

   F80.4   **Speech and language development delay due to hearing loss**
       Code also type of hearing loss (H90.-, H91.-)

✓5ᵗʰ   **F80.8**   **Other developmental disorders of speech and language**
       AHA: 2017,1Q,27

   F80.81   **Childhood onset fluency disorder**
       Cluttering NOS
       Stuttering NOS
       EXCLUDES 1   *adult onset fluency disorder (F98.5)*
              fluency disorder in conditions classified elsewhere (R47.82)
              fluency disorder (stuttering) following cerebrovascular disease (I69. with final characters -23)

   F80.82   **Social pragmatic communication disorder**
       EXCLUDES 1   *Asperger's syndrome (F84.5)*
              autistic disorder (F84.0)
       AHA: 2016,4Q,16

   F80.89   **Other developmental disorders of speech and language**

   F80.9   **Developmental disorder of speech and language, unspecified**   ▽
       Communication disorder NOS
       Language disorder NOS

✓4ᵗʰ   **F81**   **Specific developmental disorders of scholastic skills**

   F81.0   **Specific reading disorder**
       "Backward reading"
       Developmental dyslexia
       Specific learning disorder, with impairment in reading
       Specific reading retardation
       EXCLUDES 1   *alexia NOS (R48.0)*
              dyslexia NOS (R48.0)
       DEF: Serious impairment of reading skills unexplained in relation to general intelligence and teaching processes.

   F81.2   **Mathematics disorder**
       Developmental acalculia
       Developmental arithmetical disorder
       Developmental Gerstmann's syndrome
       Specific learning disorder, with impairment in mathematics
       EXCLUDES 1   *acalculia NOS (R48.8)*
       EXCLUDES 2   *arithmetical difficulties associated with a reading disorder (F81.0)*
              arithmetical difficulties associated with a spelling disorder (F81.81)
              arithmetical difficulties due to inadequate teaching (Z55.8)

✓5ᵗʰ   **F81.8**   **Other developmental disorders of scholastic skills**

   F81.81   **Disorder of written expression**
       Specific learning disorder, with impairment in written expression
       Specific spelling disorder

   F81.89   **Other developmental disorders of scholastic skills**

   F81.9   **Developmental disorder of scholastic skills, unspecified**   ▽
       Knowledge acquisition disability NOS
       Learning disability NOS
       Learning disorder NOS

F82   **Specific developmental disorder of motor function**
     Clumsy child syndrome
     Developmental coordination disorder
     Developmental dyspraxia
     EXCLUDES 1   *abnormalities of gait and mobility (R26.-)*
            lack of coordination (R27.-)
     EXCLUDES 2   *lack of coordination secondary to intellectual disabilities (F70-F79)*

✓4ᵗʰ   **F84**   **Pervasive developmental disorders**
     Use additional code to identify any associated medical condition and intellectual disabilities.

   F84.0   **Autistic disorder**
       Autism spectrum disorder
       Infantile autism
       Infantile psychosis
       Kanner's syndrome
       EXCLUDES 1   *Asperger's syndrome (F84.5)*
       AHA: 2017,1Q,27
       TIP: When the encounter is focused on treatment of conditions related to autism spectrum disorder, first assign codes to identify the problem or manifestation receiving therapeutic services.

F84.2 Rett's syndrome
> EXCLUDES 1   *Asperger's syndrome (F84.5)*
>   *autistic disorder (F84.0)*
>   *other childhood disintegrative disorder (F84.3)*

F84.3 Other childhood disintegrative disorder   P
> Dementia infantilis
> Disintegrative psychosis
> Heller's syndrome
> Symbiotic psychosis
> Use additional code to identify any associated neurological condition
> EXCLUDES 1   *Asperger's syndrome (F84.5)*
>   *autistic disorder (F84.0)*
>   *Rett's syndrome (F84.2)*

F84.5 Asperger's syndrome
> Asperger's disorder
> Autistic psychopathy
> Schizoid disorder of childhood
> **DEF:** High-functioning form of autism. Children with this syndrome usually develop speech on schedule, are generally very intelligent, and communicate well, but have considerable social shortcomings. *Synonym(s):* AS.

F84.8 Other pervasive developmental disorders
> Overactive disorder associated with intellectual disabilities and stereotyped movements

F84.9 Pervasive developmental disorder, unspecified   ▽
> Atypical autism

F88 Other disorders of psychological development
> Developmental agnosia
> Global developmental delay
> Other specified neurodevelopmental disorder

F89 Unspecified disorder of psychological development   ▽
> Developmental disorder NOS
> Neurodevelopmental disorder NOS

Behavioral and emotional disorders with onset usually occurring in childhood and adolescence (F90-F98)

> NOTE   Codes within categories F90-F98 may be used regardless of the age of a patient. These disorders generally have onset within the childhood or adolescent years, but may continue throughout life or not be diagnosed until adulthood

✓4th F90 Attention-deficit hyperactivity disorders
> INCLUDES   attention deficit disorder with hyperactivity
>   attention deficit syndrome with hyperactivity
> EXCLUDES 2   *anxiety disorders (F40.-, F41.-)*
>   *mood [affective] disorders (F30-F39)*
>   *pervasive developmental disorders (F84.-)*
>   *schizophrenia (F20.-)*

F90.0 Attention-deficit hyperactivity disorder, predominantly inattentive type
> Attention-deficit/hyperactivity disorder, predominantly inattentive presentation

F90.1 Attention-deficit hyperactivity disorder, predominantly hyperactive type
> Attention-deficit/hyperactivity disorder, predominantly hyperactive impulsive presentation

F90.2 Attention-deficit hyperactivity disorder, combined type
> Attention-deficit/hyperactivity disorder, combined presentation

F90.8 Attention-deficit hyperactivity disorder, other type

F90.9 Attention-deficit hyperactivity disorder, unspecified type   ▽
> Attention-deficit hyperactivity disorder of childhood or adolescence NOS
> Attention-deficit hyperactivity disorder NOS

✓4th F91 Conduct disorders
> EXCLUDES 1   *antisocial behavior (Z72.81-)*
>   *antisocial personality disorder (F60.2)*
> EXCLUDES 2   *conduct problems associated with attention-deficit hyperactivity disorder (F90.-)*
>   *mood [affective] disorders (F30-F39)*
>   *pervasive developmental disorders (F84.-)*
>   *schizophrenia (F20.-)*

F91.0 Conduct disorder confined to family context

F91.1 Conduct disorder, childhood-onset type
> Unsocialized conduct disorder
> Conduct disorder, solitary aggressive type
> Unsocialized aggressive disorder

F91.2 Conduct disorder, adolescent-onset type
> Socialized conduct disorder
> Conduct disorder, group type

F91.3 Oppositional defiant disorder

F91.8 Other conduct disorders
> Other specified conduct disorder
> Other specified disruptive disorder

F91.9 Conduct disorder, unspecified   ▽
> Behavioral disorder NOS
> Conduct disorder NOS
> Disruptive behavior disorder NOS
> Disruptive disorder NOS

✓4th F93 Emotional disorders with onset specific to childhood
F93.0 Separation anxiety disorder of childhood
> EXCLUDES 2   *mood [affective] disorders (F30-F39)*
>   *nonpsychotic mental disorders (F40-F48)*
>   *phobic anxiety disorder of childhood (F40.8)*
>   *social phobia (F40.1)*

F93.8 Other childhood emotional disorders
> Identity disorder
> EXCLUDES 2   *gender identity disorder of childhood (F64.2)*

F93.9 Childhood emotional disorder, unspecified   ▽

✓4th F94 Disorders of social functioning with onset specific to childhood and adolescence
F94.0 Selective mutism
> Elective mutism
> EXCLUDES 2   *pervasive developmental disorders (F84.-)*
>   *schizophrenia (F20.-)*
>   *specific developmental disorders of speech and language (F80.-)*
>   *transient mutism as part of separation anxiety in young children (F93.0)*

F94.1 Reactive attachment disorder of childhood
> Use additional code to identify any associated failure to thrive or growth retardation
> EXCLUDES 1   *disinhibited attachment disorder of childhood (F94.2)*
>   *normal variation in pattern of selective attachment*
> EXCLUDES 2   *Asperger's syndrome (F84.5)*
>   *maltreatment syndromes (T74.-)*
>   *sexual or physical abuse in childhood, resulting in psychosocial problems (Z62.81-)*

F94.2 Disinhibited attachment disorder of childhood
> Affectionless psychopathy
> Institutional syndrome
> EXCLUDES 1   *reactive attachment disorder of childhood (F94.1)*
> EXCLUDES 2   *Asperger's syndrome (F84.5)*
>   *attention-deficit hyperactivity disorders (F90.-)*
>   *hospitalism in children (F43.2-)*

F94.8 Other childhood disorders of social functioning

F94.9 Childhood disorder of social functioning, unspecified   ▽

✓4th F95 Tic disorder
F95.0 Transient tic disorder
> Provisional tic disorder

F95.1 Chronic motor or vocal tic disorder

F95.2 Tourette's disorder
> Combined vocal and multiple motor tic disorder [de la Tourette]
> Tourette's syndrome

F95.8 Other tic disorders

F95.9 Tic disorder, unspecified   ▽
> Tic NOS

☑ Additional Character Req   ✓x7th Placeholder Alert   Manifestation   ▽ Unspecified   ►◄ Revised Text   ● New Code   ▲ Revised Code Title

Chapter 5. Mental, Behavioral and Neurodevelopmental Disorders

✓4ᵗʰ **F98 Other behavioral and emotional disorders with onset usually occurring in childhood and adolescence**

> EXCLUDES 2   breath-holding spells (R06.89)
> gender identity disorder of childhood (F64.2)
> Kleine-Levin syndrome (G47.13)
> obsessive-compulsive disorder (F42-)
> sleep disorders not due to a substance or known physiological condition (F51.-)

F98.0 Enuresis not due to a substance or known physiological condition   🄌

> Enuresis (primary) (secondary) of nonorganic origin
> Functional enuresis
> Psychogenic enuresis
> Urinary incontinence of nonorganic origin
> > EXCLUDES 1   enuresis NOS (R32)

F98.1 Encopresis not due to a substance or known physiological condition

> Functional encopresis
> Incontinence of feces of nonorganic origin
> Psychogenic encopresis
> Use additional code to identify the cause of any coexisting constipation
> > EXCLUDES 1   encopresis NOS (R15.-)

✓5ᵗʰ **F98.2 Other feeding disorders of infancy and childhood**

> EXCLUDES 1   feeding difficulties (R63.3)
> EXCLUDES 2   anorexia nervosa and other eating disorders (F50.-)
> feeding problems of newborn (P92.-)
> pica of infancy or childhood (F98.3)

     F98.21 Rumination disorder of infancy
     F98.29 Other feeding disorders of infancy and early childhood

F98.3 Pica of infancy and childhood

F98.4 Stereotyped movement disorders

> Stereotype/habit disorder
> > EXCLUDES 1   abnormal involuntary movements (R25.-)
> > EXCLUDES 2   compulsions in obsessive-compulsive disorder (F42-)
> > hair plucking (F63.3)
> > movement disorders of organic origin (G20-G25)
> > nail-biting (F98.8)
> > nose-picking (F98.8)
> > stereotypies that are part of a broader psychiatric condition (F01-F95)
> > thumb-sucking (F98.8)
> > tic disorders (F95.-)
> > trichotillomania (F63.3)

F98.5 Adult onset fluency disorder

> EXCLUDES 1   childhood onset fluency disorder (F80.81)
> dysphasia (R47.02)
> fluency disorder in conditions classified elsewhere (R47.82)
> fluency disorder (stuttering) following cerebrovascular disease (I69. with final characters -23)
> tic disorders (F95.-)

F98.8 Other specified behavioral and emotional disorders with onset usually occurring in childhood and adolescence

> Excessive masturbation
> Nail-biting
> Nose-picking
> Thumb-sucking

F98.9 Unspecified behavioral and emotional disorders with onset usually occurring in childhood and adolescence   ▽

Unspecified mental disorder (F99)

F99 Mental disorder, not otherwise specified

> Mental illness NOS
> > EXCLUDES 1   unspecified mental disorder due to known physiological condition (F09)

Chapter 6. Diseases of the Nervous System (G00-G99)

Chapter Specific Guidelines with Coding Examples

The chapter specific guidelines from the ICD-10-CM Official Guidelines for Coding and Reporting have been provided below. Along with these guidelines are coding examples, contained in the shaded boxes, that have been developed to help illustrate the coding and/or sequencing guidance found in these guidelines.

a. Dominant/nondominant side

Codes from category G81, Hemiplegia and hemiparesis, and subcategories G83.1, Monoplegia of lower limb, G83.2, Monoplegia of upper limb, and G83.3, Monoplegia, unspecified, identify whether the dominant or nondominant side is affected. Should the affected side be documented, but not specified as dominant or nondominant, and the classification system does not indicate a default, code selection is as follows:

- For ambidextrous patients, the default should be dominant.
- If the left side is affected, the default is non-dominant.
- If the right side is affected, the default is dominant.

> Hemiplegia affecting left side of ambidextrous patient
>
> **G81.92   Hemiplegia, unspecified affecting left dominant side**
>
> *Explanation*: Documentation states that the left side is affected and dominant is used for ambidextrous persons.

> Right spastic hemiplegia, unknown whether patient is right- or left-handed
>
> **G81.11   Spastic hemiplegia affecting right dominant side**
>
> *Explanation*: Since it is unknown whether the patient is right- or left-handed, if the right side is affected, the default is dominant.

b. Pain—Category G89

1) General coding information

Codes in category G89, Pain, not elsewhere classified, may be used in conjunction with codes from other categories and chapters to provide more detail about acute or chronic pain and neoplasm-related pain, unless otherwise indicated below.

If the pain is not specified as acute or chronic, post-thoracotomy, postprocedural, or neoplasm-related, do not assign codes from category G89.

A code from category G89 should not be assigned if the underlying (definitive) diagnosis is known, unless the reason for the encounter is pain control/ management and not management of the underlying condition.

When an admission or encounter is for a procedure aimed at treating the underlying condition (e.g., spinal fusion, kyphoplasty), a code for the underlying condition (e.g., vertebral fracture, spinal stenosis) should be assigned as the principal diagnosis. No code from category G89 should be assigned.

> Elderly patient with back pain is admitted for outpatient kyphoplasty for age-related osteopathic compression fracture at vertebra T3
>
> **M80.08XA   Age-related osteoporosis with current pathological fracture, vertebra(e), initial encounter for fracture**
>
> *Explanation*: No code is assigned for the pain as it is inherent in the underlying condition being treated.

(a) Category G89 codes as principal or first-listed diagnosis

Category G89 codes are acceptable as principal diagnosis or the first-listed code:

- When pain control or pain management is the reason for the admission/encounter (e.g., a patient with displaced intervertebral disc, nerve impingement and severe back pain presents for injection of steroid into the spinal canal). The underlying cause of the pain should be reported as an additional diagnosis, if known.

> Patient presents for steroid injection in the right elbow due to chronic pain associated with primary degenerative joint disease.
>
> **G89.29   Other chronic pain**
>
> **M19.021   Primary osteoarthritis, right elbow**
>
> *Explanation*: Since the encounter is for control of pain, not treating the underlying condition, the pain code is sequenced first followed by the underlying condition. The M25 pain code is not necessary as the underlying condition code represents the specific site.

- When a patient is admitted for the insertion of a neurostimulator for pain control, assign the appropriate pain code as the principal or first-listed diagnosis. When an admission or encounter is for a procedure aimed at treating the underlying condition and a neurostimulator is inserted for pain control during the same admission/encounter, a code for the underlying condition should be assigned as the principal diagnosis and the appropriate pain code should be assigned as a secondary diagnosis.

(b) Use of category G89 codes in conjunction with site specific pain codes

(i) Assigning category G89 and site-specific pain codes

Codes from category G89 may be used in conjunction with codes that identify the site of pain (including codes from chapter 18) if the category G89 code provides additional information. For example, if the code describes the site of the pain, but does not fully describe whether the pain is acute or chronic, then both codes should be assigned.

> Patient is seen to evaluate chronic right knee pain
>
> **M25.561   Pain in right knee**
>
> **G89.29   Other chronic pain**
>
> *Explanation*: No underlying condition has been determined yet so the pain would be the reason for the visit. The M25 pain code in this instance does not fully describe the condition as it does not represent that the pain is chronic. The G89 chronic pain code is assigned to provide specificity.

(ii) Sequencing of category G89 codes with site-specific pain codes

The sequencing of category G89 codes with site-specific pain codes (including chapter 18 codes), is dependent on the circumstances of the encounter/admission as follows:

- If the encounter is for pain control or pain management, assign the code from category G89 followed by the code identifying the specific site of pain (e.g., encounter for pain management for acute neck pain from trauma is assigned code G89.11, Acute pain due to trauma, followed by code M54.2, Cervicalgia, to identify the site of pain).

> Management of acute, traumatic left shoulder pain
>
> **G89.11   Acute pain due to trauma**
>
> **M25.512   Pain in left shoulder**
>
> *Explanation*: The reason for the encounter is to manage or control the pain, not to treat or evaluate an underlying condition. The G89 pain code is assigned as the first-listed diagnosis but in this instance does not fully describe the condition as it does not include the site and laterality. The M25 pain code is added to provide this information.

- If the encounter is for any other reason except pain control or pain management, and a related definitive diagnosis has not been established (confirmed) by the provider, assign the code for the specific site of pain first, followed by the appropriate code from category G89.

> Tests are performed to investigate the source of the patient's chronic epigastric abdominal pain
>
> **R10.13   Epigastric pain**
>
> **G89.29   Other chronic pain**
>
> *Explanation*: In this instance the patient's epigastric pain is not being treated; rather the source of the pain is being investigated. A code from chapter 18 for epigastric pain is sequenced before the additional specificity of the G89 code for the chronic pain.

2) Pain due to devices, implants and grafts

See Section I.C.19. Pain due to medical devices

3) Postoperative Pain

The provider's documentation should be used to guide the coding of postoperative pain, as well as *Section III. Reporting Additional Diagnoses* and *Section IV. Diagnostic Coding and Reporting in the Outpatient Setting.*

The default for post-thoracotomy and other postoperative pain not specified as acute or chronic is the code for the acute form.

Routine or expected postoperative pain immediately after surgery should not be coded.

> Pain pump dose is increased for the patient's unexpected, extreme pain post-thoracotomy
>
> **G89.12   Acute post-thoracotomy pain**
>
> *Explanation*: When acute or chronic is not documented, default to acute. The use of "unexpected, extreme" and the increase of medication dosage indicate that the pain was more than routine or expected.

(a) Postoperative pain not associated with specific postoperative complication

Postoperative pain not associated with a specific postoperative complication is assigned to the appropriate postoperative pain code in category G89.

(b) Postoperative pain associated with specific postoperative complication

Postoperative pain associated with a specific postoperative complication (such as painful wire sutures) is assigned to the appropriate code(s) found in Chapter 19, Injury, poisoning, and certain other consequences of external causes. If appropriate, use additional code(s) from category G89 to identify acute or chronic pain (G89.18 or G89.28).

4) Chronic pain

Chronic pain is classified to subcategory G89.2. There is no time frame defining when pain becomes chronic pain. The provider's documentation should be used to guide use of these codes.

5) Neoplasm related pain

Code G89.3 is assigned to pain documented as being related, associated or due to cancer, primary or secondary malignancy, or tumor. This code is assigned regardless of whether the pain is acute or chronic.

This code may be assigned as the principal or first-listed code when the stated reason for the admission/encounter is documented as pain control/pain management. The underlying neoplasm should be reported as an additional diagnosis.

> Patient referred today for pain management due to acute pain related to malignancy of the right breast.
>
> **G89.3   Neoplasm related pain (acute)(chronic)**
>
> **C50.911   Malignant neoplasm of unspecified site of right female breast**
>
> *Explanation*: Since the encounter was for pain medication management, the pain, rather than the neoplasm, was the reason for the encounter and is sequenced first. This "neoplasm-related pain" code includes both acute and chronic pain.

When the reason for the admission/encounter is management of the neoplasm and the pain associated with the neoplasm is also documented, code G89.3 may be assigned as an additional diagnosis. It is not necessary to assign an additional code for the site of the pain.

See Section I.C.2 for instructions on the sequencing of neoplasms for all other stated reasons for the admission/encounter (except for pain control/pain management).

> Patient with lung cancer presents with acute hip pain and is evaluated and found to have iliac bone metastasis
>
> **C79.51   Secondary malignant neoplasm of bone**
>
> **C34.90   Malignant neoplasm of unspecified part of unspecified bronchus or lung**
>
> **G89.3   Neoplasm related pain (acute)(chronic)**
>
> *Explanation*: The reason for the encounter was the evaluation and diagnosis of the bone metastasis, whose code would be assigned as first-listed, followed by codes for the primary neoplasm and the pain due to the iliac bone metastasis.

6) Chronic pain syndrome

Central pain syndrome (G89.0) and chronic pain syndrome (G89.4) are different than the term "chronic pain," and therefore codes should only be used when the provider has specifically documented this condition.

See Section I.C.5. Pain disorders related to psychological factors

Chapter 6. Diseases of the Nervous System (G00-G99)

EXCLUDES 2   certain conditions originating in the perinatal period (P04-P96)

certain infectious and parasitic diseases (A00-B99)

complications of pregnancy, childbirth and the puerperium (O00-O9A)

congenital malformations, deformations, and chromosomal abnormalities (Q00-Q99)

endocrine, nutritional and metabolic diseases (E00-E88)

injury, poisoning and certain other consequences of external causes (S00-T88)

neoplasms (C00-D49)

symptoms, signs and abnormal clinical and laboratory findings, not elsewhere classified (R00-R94)

This chapter contains the following blocks:

G00-G09   Inflammatory diseases of the central nervous system
G10-G14   Systemic atrophies primarily affecting the central nervous system
G20-G26   Extrapyramidal and movement disorders
G30-G32   Other degenerative diseases of the nervous system
G35-G37   Demyelinating diseases of the central nervous system
G40-G47   Episodic and paroxysmal disorders
G50-G59   Nerve, nerve root and plexus disorders
G60-G65   Polyneuropathies and other disorders of the peripheral nervous system
G70-G73   Diseases of myoneural junction and muscle
G80-G83   Cerebral palsy and other paralytic syndromes
G89-G99   Other disorders of the nervous system

Inflammatory diseases of the central nervous system (G00-G09)

☑4ᵗʰ **G00**   **Bacterial meningitis, not elsewhere classified**

INCLUDES   bacterial arachnoiditis
bacterial leptomeningitis
bacterial meningitis
bacterial pachymeningitis

EXCLUDES 1   *bacterial meningoencephalitis (G04.2)*
bacterial meningomyelitis (G04.2)

DEF: Inflammation of meningeal layers of the brain and spinal cord due to a bacterial infection.

G00.0   **Hemophilus meningitis**
Meningitis due to Hemophilus influenzae

G00.1   **Pneumococcal meningitis**
Meningtitis due to Streptococcal pneumoniae

G00.2   **Streptococcal meningitis**
Use additional code to further identify organism (B95.0-B95.5)

G00.3   **Staphylococcal meningitis**
Use additional code to further identify organism (B95.61-B95.8)

G00.8   **Other bacterial meningitis**
Meningitis due to Escherichia coli
Meningitis due to Friedländer's bacillus
Meningitis due to Klebsiella
Use additional code to further identify organism (B96.-)

G00.9   **Bacterial meningitis, unspecified**   ▽
Meningitis due to gram-negative bacteria, unspecified
Purulent meningitis NOS
Pyogenic meningitis NOS
Suppurative meningitis NOS

G01   *Meningitis in bacterial diseases classified elsewhere*
Code first underlying disease

EXCLUDES 1   meningitis (in):
gonococcal (A54.81)
leptospirosis (A27.81)
listeriosis (A32.11)
Lyme disease (A69.21)
meningococcal (A39.0)
neurosyphilis (A52.13)
tuberculosis (A17.0)
meningoencephalitis and meningomyelitis in bacterial diseases classified elsewhere (G05)

G02   *Meningitis in other infectious and parasitic diseases classified elsewhere*
Code first underlying disease, such as:
African trypanosomiasis (B56.-)
poliovirus infection (A80.-)

EXCLUDES 1   *candidal meningitis (B37.5)*
coccidioidomycosis meningitis (B38.4)
cryptococcal meningitis (B45.1)
herpesviral [herpes simplex] meningitis (B00.3)
infectious mononucleosis complicated by meningitis (B27.- with fourth character 2)
measles complicated by meningitis (B05.1)
meningoencephalitis and meningomyelitis in other infectious and parasitic diseases classified elsewhere (G05)
mumps meningitis (B26.1)
rubella meningitis (B06.02)
varicella [chickenpox] meningitis (B01.0)
zoster meningitis (B02.1)

☑4ᵗʰ **G03**   **Meningitis due to other and unspecified causes**

INCLUDES   arachnoiditis NOS
leptomeningitis NOS
meningitis NOS
pachymeningitis NOS

EXCLUDES 1   *meningoencephalitis (G04.-)*
meningomyelitis (G04.-)

G03.0   **Nonpyogenic meningitis**
Aseptic meningitis
Nonbacterial meningitis
DEF: Type of meningitis where no bacterial, viral, or other infectious source exists that explains the meningitis symptomology.

G03.1   **Chronic meningitis**

G03.2   **Benign recurrent meningitis [Mollaret]**
DEF: Aseptic or noninfectious inflammation of the meninges with the presence of Mollaret cells in the spinal fluid. The patient experiences recurrent bouts of inflammation, lasting anywhere from two to five days.

G03.8   **Meningitis due to other specified causes**

G03.9   **Meningitis, unspecified**   ▽
Arachnoiditis (spinal) NOS

☑4ᵗʰ **G04**   **Encephalitis, myelitis and encephalomyelitis**

INCLUDES   acute ascending myelitis
meningoencephalitis
meningomyelitis

EXCLUDES 1   *encephalopathy NOS (G93.40)*
EXCLUDES 2   *acute transverse myelitis (G37.3-)*
alcoholic encephalopathy (G31.2)
benign myalgic encephalomyelitis (G93.3)
multiple sclerosis (G35)
subacute necrotizing myelitis (G37.4)
toxic encephalitis (G92)
toxic encephalopathy (G92)

DEF: Encephalitis: Inflammation of the brain, often caused by viral or bacterial infection.
DEF: Encephalomyelitis: Inflammatory disease, often viral in nature, that affects the brain and spinal cord.
DEF: Myelitis: Inflammation of the spinal cord.

☑5ᵗʰ **G04.0**   **Acute disseminated encephalitis and encephalomyelitis (ADEM)**

EXCLUDES 1   *acute necrotizing hemorrhagic encephalopathy (G04.3-)*
other noninfectious acute disseminated encephalomyelitis (noninfectious ADEM) (G04.81)

G04.00   **Acute disseminated encephalitis and**   ▽
encephalomyelitis, unspecified

G04.01   **Postinfectious acute disseminated encephalitis and encephalomyelitis (postinfectious ADEM)**

EXCLUDES 1   *post chickenpox encephalitis (B01.1)*
post measles encephalitis (B05.0)
post measles myelitis (B05.1)

☑ Additional Character Req   ☑x7ᵗʰ Placeholder Alert   Manifestation   ▽ Unspecified   ►◄ Revised Text   ● New Code   ▲ Revised Code Title

ICD-10-CM 2019   561

Chapter 6. Diseases of the Nervous System

G04.02   Postimmunization acute disseminated encephalitis, myelitis and encephalomyelitis
Encephalitis, post immunization
Encephalomyelitis, post immunization
Use additional code to identify the vaccine (T50.A-, T50.B-, T50.Z-)

G04.1   Tropical spastic paraplegia   HCC

G04.2   Bacterial meningoencephalitis and meningomyelitis, not elsewhere classified

✓5ᵗʰ **G04.3**   Acute necrotizing hemorrhagic encephalopathy
EXCLUDES 1   acute disseminated encephalitis and encephalomyelitis (G04.0-)

G04.30   Acute necrotizing hemorrhagic encephalopathy, unspecified   ▽

G04.31   Postinfectious acute necrotizing hemorrhagic encephalopathy

G04.32   Postimmunization acute necrotizing hemorrhagic encephalopathy
Use additional code to identify the vaccine (T50.A-, T50.B-, T50.Z-)

G04.39   Other acute necrotizing hemorrhagic encephalopathy
Code also underlying etiology, if applicable

✓5ᵗʰ **G04.8**   Other encephalitis, myelitis and encephalomyelitis
Code also any associated seizure (G40.-, R56.9)

G04.81   Other encephalitis and encephalomyelitis
Noninfectious acute disseminated encephalomyelitis (noninfectious ADEM)

G04.89   Other myelitis   HCC

✓5ᵗʰ **G04.9**   Encephalitis, myelitis and encephalomyelitis, unspecified

G04.90   Encephalitis and encephalomyelitis, unspecified   ▽
Ventriculitis (cerebral) NOS

G04.91   Myelitis, unspecified   HCC   ▽

✓4ᵗʰ **G05**   Encephalitis, myelitis and encephalomyelitis in diseases classified elsewhere
Code first underlying disease, such as:
human immunodeficiency virus [HIV] disease (B20)
poliovirus (A80.-)
suppurative otitis media (H66.01-H66.4)
trichinellosis (B75)
EXCLUDES 1   adenoviral encephalitis, myelitis and encephalomyelitis (A85.1)
congenital toxoplasmosis encephalitis, myelitis and encephalomyelitis (P37.1)
cytomegaloviral encephalitis, myelitis and encephalomyelitis (B25.8)
encephalitis, myelitis and encephalomyelitis (in) measles (B05.0)
encephalitis, myelitis and encephalomyelitis (in) systemic lupus erythematosus (M32.19)
enteroviral encephalitis, myelitis and encephalomyelitis (A85.0)
eosinophilic meningoencephalitis (B83.2)
herpesviral [herpes simplex] encephalitis, myelitis and encephalomyelitis (B00.4)
listerial encephalitis, myelitis and encephalomyelitis (A32.12)
meningococcal encephalitis, myelitis and encephalomyelitis (A39.81)
mumps encephalitis, myelitis and encephalomyelitis (B26.2)
postchickenpox encephalitis, myelitis and encephalomyelitis (B01.1-)
rubella encephalitis, myelitis and encephalomyelitis (B06.01)
toxoplasmosis encephalitis, myelitis and encephalomyelitis (B58.2)
zoster encephalitis, myelitis and encephalomyelitis (B02.0)

G05.3   Encephalitis and encephalomyelitis in diseases classified elsewhere
Meningoencephalitis in diseases classified elsewhere

G05.4   Myelitis in diseases classified elsewhere   HCC
Meningomyelitis in diseases classified elsewhere

✓4ᵗʰ **G06**   Intracranial and intraspinal abscess and granuloma
Use additional code (B95-B97) to identify infectious agent
DEF: Abscess: Circumscribed collection of pus resulting from bacteria, frequently associated with swelling and other signs of inflammation.
DEF: Granuloma: Abnormal, dense collections or cells forming a mass or nodule of chronically inflamed tissue with granulations that is usually associated with an infective process.

G06.0   Intracranial abscess and granuloma
Brain [any part] abscess (embolic)
Cerebellar abscess (embolic)
Cerebral abscess (embolic)
Intracranial epidural abscess or granuloma
Intracranial extradural abscess or granuloma
Intracranial subdural abscess or granuloma
Otogenic abscess (embolic)
EXCLUDES 1   tuberculous intracranial abscess and granuloma (A17.81)

G06.1   Intraspinal abscess and granuloma
Abscess (embolic) of spinal cord [any part]
Intraspinal epidural abscess or granuloma
Intraspinal extradural abscess or granuloma
Intraspinal subdural abscess or granuloma
EXCLUDES 1   tuberculous intraspinal abscess and granuloma (A17.81)

G06.2   Extradural and subdural abscess, unspecified   ▽

G07   Intracranial and intraspinal abscess and granuloma in diseases classified elsewhere
Code first underlying disease, such as:
schistosomiasis granuloma of brain (B65.-)
EXCLUDES 1   abscess of brain:
amebic (A06.6)
chromomycotic (B43.1)
gonococcal (A54.82)
tuberculous (A17.81)
tuberculoma of meninges (A17.1)

G08   Intracranial and intraspinal phlebitis and thrombophlebitis
Septic embolism of intracranial or intraspinal venous sinuses and veins
Septic endophlebitis of intracranial or intraspinal venous sinuses and veins
Septic phlebitis of intracranial or intraspinal venous sinuses and veins
Septic thrombophlebitis of intracranial or intraspinal venous sinuses and veins
Septic thrombosis of intracranial or intraspinal venous sinuses and veins
EXCLUDES 1   intracranial phlebitis and thrombophlebitis complicating:
abortion, ectopic or molar pregnancy (O00-O07, O08.7)
pregnancy, childbirth and the puerperium (O22.5, O87.3)
nonpyogenic intracranial phlebitis and thrombophlebitis (I67.6)
EXCLUDES 2   intracranial phlebitis and thrombophlebitis complicating nonpyogenic intraspinal phlebitis and thrombophlebitis (G95.1)
DEF: Inflammation and formation of a blood clot in a vein within the brain or spine, or their linings.

G09   Sequelae of inflammatory diseases of central nervous system
NOTE   Category G09 is to be used to indicate conditions whose primary classification is to G00-G08 as the cause of sequelae, themselves classifiable elsewhere. The "sequelae" include conditions specified as residuals.
Code first condition resulting from (sequela) of inflammatory diseases of central nervous system

Systemic atrophies primarily affecting the central nervous system (G10-G14)

G10   Huntington's disease   HCC
Huntington's chorea
Huntington's dementia
Code also dementia in other diseases classified elsewhere without behavioral disturbance (F02.80)
DEF: Genetic disease caused by degeneration of nerve cells in the brain, characterized by chronic progressive mental deterioration. Dementia and death occur within 15 to 20 years of onset.

√4ᵗʰ **G11 Hereditary ataxia**

     EXCLUDES 2   cerebral palsy (G80.-)

                 hereditary and idiopathic neuropathy (G60.-)

                 metabolic disorders (E70-E88)

     DEF: Ataxia: Defect in muscular control or coordination due to a central nervous system disorder, particularly when voluntary muscular movements are attempted.

     G11.0 Congenital nonprogressive ataxia   HCC

     G11.1 Early-onset cerebellar ataxia   HCC

           Early-onset cerebellar ataxia with essential tremor

           Early-onset cerebellar ataxia with myoclonus [Hunt's ataxia]

           Early-onset cerebellar ataxia with retained tendon reflexes

           Friedreich's ataxia (autosomal recessive)

           X-linked recessive spinocerebellar ataxia

     G11.2 Late-onset cerebellar ataxia   HCC A

     G11.3 Cerebellar ataxia with defective DNA repair   HCC

           Ataxia telangiectasia [Louis-Bar]

           EXCLUDES 2   Cockayne's syndrome (Q87.1)

                   other disorders of purine and pyrimidine metabolism (E79.-)

                   xeroderma pigmentosum (Q82.1)

     G11.4 Hereditary spastic paraplegia   HCC

     G11.8 Other hereditary ataxias   HCC

     G11.9 Hereditary ataxia, unspecified   HCC ▽

           Hereditary cerebellar ataxia NOS

           Hereditary cerebellar degeneration

           Hereditary cerebellar disease

           Hereditary cerebellar syndrome

√4ᵗʰ **G12 Spinal muscular atrophy and related syndromes**

     G12.0 Infantile spinal muscular atrophy, type I [Werdnig-Hoffman]   HCC

     G12.1 Other inherited spinal muscular atrophy   HCC

           Adult form spinal muscular atrophy

           Childhood form, type II spinal muscular atrophy

           Distal spinal muscular atrophy

           Juvenile form, type III spinal muscular atrophy [Kugelberg-Welander]

           Progressive bulbar palsy of childhood [Fazio-Londe]

           Scapuloperoneal form spinal muscular atrophy

     √5ᵗʰ **G12.2 Motor neuron disease**

         AHA: 2017,4Q,9-10

         G12.20 Motor neuron disease, unspecified   HCC ▽

         G12.21 Amyotrophic lateral sclerosis   HCC A

         G12.22 Progressive bulbar palsy   HCC

         G12.23 Primary lateral sclerosis   HCC

         G12.24 Familial motor neuron disease   HCC

         G12.25 Progressive spinal muscle atrophy   HCC

         G12.29 Other motor neuron disease   HCC

     G12.8 Other spinal muscular atrophies and related syndromes   HCC

     G12.9 Spinal muscular atrophy, unspecified   HCC ▽

√4ᵗʰ **G13 Systemic atrophies primarily affecting central nervous system in diseases classified elsewhere**

     G13.0 Paraneoplastic neuromyopathy and neuropathy   HCC

           Carcinomatous neuromyopathy

           Sensorial paraneoplastic neuropathy [Denny Brown]

           Code first underlying neoplasm (C00-D49)

     G13.1 Other systemic atrophy primarily affecting central nervous system in neoplastic disease   HCC

           Paraneoplastic limbic encephalopathy

           Code first underlying neoplasm (C00-D49)

     G13.2 Systemic atrophy primarily affecting the central nervous system in myxedema

           Code first underlying disease, such as:

              hypothyroidism (E03.-)

              myxedematous congenital iodine deficiency (E00.1)

     G13.8 Systemic atrophy primarily affecting central nervous system in other diseases classified elsewhere

           Code first underlying disease

     G14 Postpolio syndrome

       INCLUDES   postpolio myelitic syndrome

       EXCLUDES 1   sequelae of poliomyelitis (B91)

Extrapyramidal and movement disorders (G20-G26)

     G20 Parkinson's disease   HCC

           Hemiparkinsonism

           Idiopathic Parkinsonism or Parkinson's disease

           Paralysis agitans

           Parkinsonism or Parkinson's disease NOS

           Primary Parkinsonism or Parkinson's disease

       EXCLUDES 1   dementia with Parkinsonism (G31.83)

       AHA: 2017,2Q,7; 2016,2Q,6

       TIP: Repeated falls (R29.6) are not integral to Parkinson's disease and can be separately coded.

     √4ᵗʰ **G21 Secondary parkinsonism**

       EXCLUDES 1   dementia with Parkinsonism (G31.83)

                 Huntington's disease (G10)

                 Shy-Drager syndrome (G90.3)

                 syphilitic Parkinsonism (A52.19)

       G21.0 Malignant neuroleptic syndrome

           Use additional code for adverse effect, if applicable, to identify drug (T43.3X5, T43.4X5, T43.5X5, T43.595)

           EXCLUDES 1   neuroleptic induced parkinsonism (G21.11)

     √5ᵗʰ **G21.1 Other drug-induced secondary parkinsonism**

         G21.11 Neuroleptic induced parkinsonism   HCC

              Use additional code for adverse effect, if applicable, to identify drug (T43.3X5, T43.4X5, T43.5X5, T43.595)

              EXCLUDES 1   malignant neuroleptic syndrome (G21.0)

         G21.19 Other drug induced secondary parkinsonism

              Other medication-induced parkinsonism

              Use additional code for adverse effect, if applicable, to identify drug (T36-T50 with fifth or sixth character 5)

       G21.2 Secondary parkinsonism due to other external agents   HCC

           Code first (T51-T65) to identify external agent

       G21.3 Postencephalitic parkinsonism   HCC

       G21.4 Vascular parkinsonism   HCC

       G21.8 Other secondary parkinsonism   HCC

       G21.9 Secondary parkinsonism, unspecified   HCC ▽

     √4ᵗʰ **G23 Other degenerative diseases of basal ganglia**

       EXCLUDES 2   multi-system degeneration of the autonomic nervous system (G90.3)

       G23.0 Hallervorden-Spatz disease   HCC

           Pigmentary pallidal degeneration

       G23.1 Progressive supranuclear ophthalmoplegia [Steele-Richardson-Olszewski]   HCC

           Progressive supranuclear palsy

       G23.2 Striatonigral degeneration   HCC

       G23.8 Other specified degenerative diseases of basal ganglia   HCC

           Calcification of basal ganglia

       G23.9 Degenerative disease of basal ganglia, unspecified   HCC ▽

     √4ᵗʰ **G24 Dystonia**

       INCLUDES   dyskinesia

       EXCLUDES 2   athetoid cerebral palsy (G80.3)

       DEF: Disorder of abnormal muscle tone, excessive or inadequate. Involuntary movements and prolonged muscle contractions result in tremors, abnormalities in posture, and twisting body motions that affect an isolated area or the whole body.

     √5ᵗʰ **G24.0 Drug induced dystonia**

           Use additional code for adverse effect, if applicable, to identify drug (T36-T50 with fifth or sixth character 5)

         G24.01 Drug induced subacute dyskinesia

              Drug induced blepharospasm

              Drug induced orofacial dyskinesia

              Neuroleptic induced tardive dyskinesia

              Tardive dyskinesia

         G24.02 Drug induced acute dystonia

              Acute dystonic reaction to drugs

              Neuroleptic induced acute dystonia

         G24.09 Other drug induced dystonia

✓ Additional Character Req   √x7ᵗʰ Placeholder Alert   Manifestation   ▽ Unspecified   ►◄ Revised Text   ● New Code   ▲ Revised Code Title

ICD-10-CM 2019   **563**

G24.1 **Genetic torsion dystonia**
Dystonia deformans progressiva
Dystonia musculorum deformans
Familial torsion dystonia
Idiopathic familial dystonia
Idiopathic (torsion) dystonia NOS
(Schwalbe-) Ziehen-Oppenheim disease

G24.2 **Idiopathic nonfamilial dystonia**

G24.3 **Spasmodic torticollis**
EXCLUDES 1   *congenital torticollis (Q68.0)*
hysterical torticollis (F44.4)
ocular torticollis (R29.891)
psychogenic torticollis (F45.8)
torticollis NOS (M43.6)
traumatic recurrent torticollis (S13.4)
DEF: Twisted, unnatural position of the neck due to contracted cervical muscles that pull the head to one side or cause involuntary shaking of the head.

G24.4 **Idiopathic orofacial dystonia**
Orofacial dyskinesia
EXCLUDES 1   *drug induced orofacial dyskinesia (G24.01)*

G24.5 **Blepharospasm**
EXCLUDES 1   *drug induced blepharospasm (G24.01)*
DEF: Involuntary contraction of the orbicularis oculi muscle, resulting in the eyelids being completely closed.

G24.8 **Other dystonia**
Acquired torsion dystonia NOS

G24.9 **Dystonia, unspecified**   ▽
Dyskinesia NOS

√4th **G25** **Other extrapyramidal and movement disorders**
EXCLUDES 2   *sleep related movement disorders (G47.6-)*

G25.0 **Essential tremor**
Familial tremor
EXCLUDES 1   *tremor NOS (R25.1)*

G25.1 **Drug-induced tremor**
Use additional code for adverse effect, if applicable, to identify drug (T36-T50 with fifth or sixth character 5)

G25.2 **Other specified forms of tremor**
Intention tremor

G25.3 **Myoclonus**
Drug-induced myoclonus
Palatal myoclonus
Use additional code for adverse effect, if applicable, to identify drug (T36-T50 with fifth or sixth character 5)
EXCLUDES 1   *facial myokymia (G51.4)*
myoclonic epilepsy (G40.-)
DEF: Spasmodic, brief, involuntary muscle contractions that can be due to an undetermined etiology, drug-induced, or caused by a disease process.

G25.4 **Drug-induced chorea**
Use additional code for adverse effect, if applicable, to identify drug (T36-T50 with fifth or sixth character 5)

G25.5 **Other chorea**
Chorea NOS
EXCLUDES 1   *chorea NOS with heart involvement (I02.0)*
Huntington's chorea (G10)
rheumatic chorea (I02.-)
Sydenham's chorea (I02.-)

√5th **G25.6** **Drug induced tics and other tics of organic origin**

G25.61 **Drug induced tics**
Use additional code for adverse effect, if applicable, to identify drug (T36-T50 with fifth or sixth character 5)

G25.69 **Other tics of organic origin**
EXCLUDES 1   *habit spasm (F95.9)*
tic NOS (F95.9)
Tourette's syndrome (F95.2)

√5th **G25.7** **Other and unspecified drug induced movement disorders**
Use additional code for adverse effect, if applicable, to identify drug (T36-T50 with fifth or sixth character 5)

G25.70 **Drug induced movement disorder, unspecified**   ▽

G25.71 **Drug induced akathisia**
Drug induced acathisia
Neuroleptic induced acute akathisia
Tardive akathisia

G25.79 **Other drug induced movement disorders**

√5th **G25.8** **Other specified extrapyramidal and movement disorders**

G25.81 **Restless legs syndrome**
DEF: Neurological disorder of unknown etiology creating an irresistible urge to move the legs, which may temporarily relieve the symptoms. This syndrome is accompanied by motor restlessness and sensations of pain, burning, prickling, or tingling.

G25.82 **Stiff-man syndrome**

G25.83 **Benign shuddering attacks**

G25.89 **Other specified extrapyramidal and movement disorders**

G25.9 **Extrapyramidal and movement disorder, unspecified**   ▽

G26 *Extrapyramidal and movement disorders in diseases classified elsewhere*
Code first underlying disease

Other degenerative diseases of the nervous system (G30-G32)

√4th **G30** **Alzheimer's disease**
INCLUDES   Alzheimer's dementia senile and presenile forms
Use additional code to identify:
delirium, if applicable (F05)
dementia with behavioral disturbance (F02.81)
dementia without behavioral disturbance (F02.80)
EXCLUDES 1   *senile degeneration of brain NEC (G31.1)*
senile dementia NOS (F03)
senility NOS (R41.81)
AHA: 2017,1Q,43
TIP: A code from subcategory F02.8 should always be assigned with a code from this category, even in the absence of documented dementia.
TIP: Functional quadriplegia (R53.2) is not integral to Alzheimer's disease and can be coded in addition to codes from category G30.

G30.0 **Alzheimer's disease with early onset**

G30.1 **Alzheimer's disease with late onset**   A

G30.8 **Other Alzheimer's disease**

G30.9 **Alzheimer's disease, unspecified**   ▽
AHA: 2016,2Q,6; 2012,4Q,95

√4th **G31** **Other degenerative diseases of nervous system, not elsewhere classified**
Use additional code to identify:
dementia with behavioral disturbance (F02.81)
dementia without behavioral disturbance (F02.80)
EXCLUDES 2   *Reye's syndrome (G93.7)*

√5th **G31.0** **Frontotemporal dementia**

G31.01 **Pick's disease**
Primary progressive aphasia
Progressive isolated aphasia
DEF: Progressive frontotemporal dementia with asymmetrical atrophy of the frontal and temporal regions of the cerebral cortex and abnormal rounded brain cells called Pick cells with the presence of abnormal staining of protein (called tau). Symptoms include prominent apathy, behavioral changes such as disinhibition and restlessness, echolalia, impairment of language, memory, and intellect, increased carelessness, poor personal hygiene, and decreased attention span.

G31.09 **Other frontotemporal dementia**
Frontal dementia

G31.1 **Senile degeneration of brain, not elsewhere classified**
EXCLUDES 1   *Alzheimer's disease (G30.-)*
senility NOS (R41.81)

G31.2 **Degeneration of nervous system due to alcohol**
Alcoholic cerebellar ataxia
Alcoholic cerebellar degeneration
Alcoholic cerebral degeneration
Alcoholic encephalopathy
Dysfunction of the autonomic nervous system due to alcohol
Code also associated alcoholism (F10.-)

√5th **G31.8** **Other specified degenerative diseases of nervous system**

G31.81 **Alpers disease**
Grey-matter degeneration

G31.82   **Leigh's disease**
       Subacute necrotizing encephalopathy

G31.83   **Dementia with Lewy bodies**
       Dementia with Parkinsonism
       Lewy body dementia
       Lewy body disease
       AHA: 2017,2Q,7; 2016,4Q,141
       DEF: Cerebral dementia with neurophysiologic changes, increased hippocampal volume, hypoperfusion in the occipital lobes, beta amyloid deposits with neurofibrillary tangles, and atrophy of the cortex and brainstem. Hallmark neuropsychological characteristics include fluctuating cognition with pronounced variation in attention and alertness, recurrent hallucinations, and Parkinsonism.

G31.84   **Mild cognitive impairment, so stated**
       Mild neurocognitive disorder
       EXCLUDES 1   *age related cognitive decline (R41.81)*
                  altered mental status (R41.82)
                  cerebral degeneration (G31.9)
                  change in mental status (R41.82)
                  cognitive deficits following (sequelae of) cerebral hemorrhage or infarction (I69.01-, I69.11-, I69.21-, I69.31-, I69.81-, I69.91-)
                  cognitive impairment due to intracranial or head injury (S06.-)
                  dementia (F01.-, F02.-, F03)
                  mild memory disturbance (F06.8)
                  neurologic neglect syndrome (R41.4)
                  personality change, nonpsychotic (F68.8)

G31.85   **Corticobasal degeneration**

G31.89   **Other specified degenerative diseases of nervous system**

G31.9   **Degenerative disease of nervous system, unspecified**   ▽

✓4ᵗʰ **G32**   **Other degenerative disorders of nervous system in diseases classified elsewhere**

     G32.0   *Subacute combined degeneration of spinal cord in diseases classified elsewhere*   HCC
           Dana-Putnam syndrome
           Sclerosis of spinal cord (combined) (dorsolateral) (posterolateral)
           Code first underlying disease, such as:
              anemia (D51.9)
              dietary (D51.3)
              pernicious (D51.0)
              vitamin B12 deficiency (E53.8)
           EXCLUDES 1   *syphilitic combined degeneration of spinal cord (A52.11)*

     ✓5ᵗʰ **G32.8**   **Other specified degenerative disorders of nervous system in diseases classified elsewhere**
           Code first underlying disease, such as:
              amyloidosis cerebral degeneration (E85.-)
              cerebral degeneration (due to) hypothyroidism (E00.0-E03.9)
              cerebral degeneration (due to) neoplasm (C00-D49)
              cerebral degeneration (due to) vitamin B deficiency, except thiamine (E52-E53.-)
           EXCLUDES 1   *superior hemorrhagic polioencephalitis [Wernicke's encephalopathy] (E51.2)*

         G32.81   *Cerebellar ataxia in diseases classified elsewhere*   HCC
              Code first underlying disease, such as:
                celiac disease (with gluten ataxia) (K90.0)
                cerebellar ataxia (in) neoplastic disease (paraneoplastic cerebellar degeneration) (C00-D49)
                non-celiac gluten ataxia (M35.9)
             EXCLUDES 1   *systemic atrophy primarily affecting the central nervous system in alcoholic cerebellar ataxia (G31.2)*
                       systemic atrophy primarily affecting the central nervous system in myxedema (G13.2)

         G32.89   *Other specified degenerative disorders of nervous system in diseases classified elsewhere*
              Degenerative encephalopathy in diseases classified elsewhere

Demyelinating diseases of the central nervous system (G35-G37)

G35   **Multiple sclerosis**   HCC
       Disseminated multiple sclerosis
       Generalized multiple sclerosis
       Multiple sclerosis NOS
       Multiple sclerosis of brain stem
       Multiple sclerosis of cord

✓4ᵗʰ **G36**   **Other acute disseminated demyelination**
       EXCLUDES 1   *postinfectious encephalitis and encephalomyelitis NOS (G04.01)*
       DEF: Demyelination: Abnormal loss of myelin, the protective white matter that insulates nerve endings and facilitates neuroreception and neurotransmission. When this substance is damaged, the nerve is short-circuited, resulting in impaired or loss of function.

     G36.0   **Neuromyelitis optica [Devic]**   HCC
           Demyelination in optic neuritis
         EXCLUDES 1   *optic neuritis NOS (H46)*

     G36.1   **Acute and subacute hemorrhagic leukoencephalitis [Hurst]**   HCC

     G36.8   **Other specified acute disseminated demyelination**   HCC

     G36.9   **Acute disseminated demyelination, unspecified**   HCC ▽

✓4ᵗʰ **G37**   **Other demyelinating diseases of central nervous system**

     G37.0   **Diffuse sclerosis of central nervous system**   HCC
           Periaxial encephalitis
           Schilder's disease
         EXCLUDES 1   *X linked adrenoleukodystrophy (E71.52-)*

     G37.1   **Central demyelination of corpus callosum**   HCC

     G37.2   **Central pontine myelinolysis**   HCC

     G37.3   **Acute transverse myelitis in demyelinating disease of central nervous system**   HCC
           Acute transverse myelitis NOS
           Acute transverse myelopathy
         EXCLUDES 1   *multiple sclerosis (G35)*
                       neuromyelitis optica [Devic] (G36.0)

     G37.4   **Subacute necrotizing myelitis of central nervous system**   HCC

     G37.5   **Concentric sclerosis [Balo] of central nervous system**   HCC

     G37.8   **Other specified demyelinating diseases of central nervous system**   HCC

     G37.9   **Demyelinating disease of central nervous system, unspecified**   HCC ▽

☑ Additional Character Req   ✓x7ᵗʰ Placeholder Alert   Manifestation   ▽ Unspecified   ►◄ Revised Text   ● New Code   ▲ Revised Code Title

Chapter 6. Diseases of the Nervous System

Episodic and paroxysmal disorders (G40-G47)

✓4ᵗʰ **G40 Epilepsy and recurrent seizures**

> **NOTE** The following terms are to be considered equivalent to intractable: pharmacoresistant (pharmacologically resistant), treatment resistant, refractory (medically) and poorly controlled

> **EXCLUDES 1** conversion disorder with seizures (F44.5)
> convulsions NOS (R56.9)
> post traumatic seizures (R56.1)
> seizure (convulsive) NOS (R56.9)
> seizure of newborn (P90)

> **EXCLUDES 2** hippocampal sclerosis (G93.81)
> mesial temporal sclerosis (G93.81)
> temporal sclerosis (G93.81)
> Todd's paralysis (G83.84)

✓5ᵗʰ **G40.0 Localization-related (focal) (partial) idiopathic epilepsy and epileptic syndromes with seizures of localized onset**
Benign childhood epilepsy with centrotemporal EEG spikes
Childhood epilepsy with occipital EEG paroxysms
> **EXCLUDES 1** adult onset localization-related epilepsy (G40.1-, G40.2-)

✓6ᵗʰ **G40.00 Localization-related (focal) (partial) idiopathic epilepsy and epileptic syndromes with seizures of localized onset, not intractable**
Localization-related (focal) (partial) idiopathic epilepsy and epileptic syndromes with seizures of localized onset without intractability

G40.001 Localization-related (focal) HCC **(partial) idiopathic epilepsy and epileptic syndromes with seizures of localized onset, not intractable, with status epilepticus**

G40.009 Localization-related (focal) HCC **(partial) idiopathic epilepsy and epileptic syndromes with seizures of localized onset, not intractable, without status epilepticus**
Localization-related (focal) (partial) idiopathic epilepsy and epileptic syndromes with seizures of localized onset NOS

✓6ᵗʰ **G40.01 Localization-related (focal) (partial) idiopathic epilepsy and epileptic syndromes with seizures of localized onset, intractable**

G40.011 Localization-related (focal) HCC **(partial) idiopathic epilepsy and epileptic syndromes with seizures of localized onset, intractable, with status epilepticus**

G40.019 Localization-related (focal) HCC **(partial) idiopathic epilepsy and epileptic syndromes with seizures of localized onset, intractable, without status epilepticus**

✓5ᵗʰ **G40.1 Localization-related (focal) (partial) symptomatic epilepsy and epileptic syndromes with simple partial seizures**
Attacks without alteration of consciousness
Epilepsia partialis continua [Kozhevnikof]
Simple partial seizures developing into secondarily generalized seizures

✓6ᵗʰ **G40.10 Localization-related (focal) (partial) symptomatic epilepsy and epileptic syndromes with simple partial seizures, not intractable**
Localization-related (focal) (partial) symptomatic epilepsy and epileptic syndromes with simple partial seizures without intractability

G40.101 Localization-related (focal) HCC **(partial) symptomatic epilepsy and epileptic syndromes with simple partial seizures, not intractable, with status epilepticus**

G40.109 Localization-related (focal) HCC ◻ **(partial) symptomatic epilepsy and epileptic syndromes with simple partial seizures, not intractable, without status epilepticus**
Localization-related (focal) (partial) symptomatic epilepsy and epileptic syndromes with simple partial seizures NOS

✓6ᵗʰ **G40.11 Localization-related (focal) (partial) symptomatic epilepsy and epileptic syndromes with simple partial seizures, intractable**

G40.111 Localization-related (focal) HCC **(partial) symptomatic epilepsy and epileptic syndromes with simple partial seizures, intractable, with status epilepticus**

G40.119 Localization-related (focal) HCC ◻ **(partial) symptomatic epilepsy and epileptic syndromes with simple partial seizures, intractable, without status epilepticus**

✓5ᵗʰ **G40.2 Localization-related (focal) (partial) symptomatic epilepsy and epileptic syndromes with complex partial seizures**
Attacks with alteration of consciousness, often with automatisms
Complex partial seizures developing into secondarily generalized seizures

✓6ᵗʰ **G40.20 Localization-related (focal) (partial) symptomatic epilepsy and epileptic syndromes with complex partial seizures, not intractable**
Localization-related (focal) (partial) symptomatic epilepsy and epileptic syndromes with complex partial seizures without intractability

G40.201 Localization-related (focal) HCC **(partial) symptomatic epilepsy and epileptic syndromes with complex partial seizures, not intractable, with status epilepticus**

G40.209 Localization-related (focal) HCC ◻ **(partial) symptomatic epilepsy and epileptic syndromes with complex partial seizures, not intractable, without status epilepticus**
Localization-related (focal) (partial) symptomatic epilepsy and epileptic syndromes with complex partial seizures NOS

✓6ᵗʰ **G40.21 Localization-related (focal) (partial) symptomatic epilepsy and epileptic syndromes with complex partial seizures, intractable**

G40.211 Localization-related (focal) HCC **(partial) symptomatic epilepsy and epileptic syndromes with complex partial seizures, intractable, with status epilepticus**

G40.219 Localization-related (focal) HCC ◻ **(partial) symptomatic epilepsy and epileptic syndromes with complex partial seizures, intractable, without status epilepticus**

✓5ᵗʰ **G40.3 Generalized idiopathic epilepsy and epileptic syndromes**
Code also MERRF syndrome, if applicable (E88.42)

✓6ᵗʰ **G40.30 Generalized idiopathic epilepsy and epileptic syndromes, not intractable**
Generalized idiopathic epilepsy and epileptic syndromes without intractability

G40.301 Generalized idiopathic epilepsy HCC **and epileptic syndromes, not intractable, with status epilepticus**

G40.309   **Generalized idiopathic epilepsy** `HCC` `Q`
    and epileptic syndromes, not
    intractable, without status
    epilepticus
        Generalized idiopathic epilepsy and
        epileptic syndromes NOS

√6ᵗʰ **G40.31**   **Generalized idiopathic epilepsy and epileptic**
    syndromes, intractable

    G40.311   **Generalized idiopathic epilepsy** `HCC`
        and epileptic syndromes,
        intractable, with status
        epilepticus

    G40.319   **Generalized idiopathic epilepsy** `HCC`
        and epileptic syndromes,
        intractable, without status
        epilepticus

√5ᵗʰ **G40.A**   **Absence epileptic syndrome**

    Childhood absence epilepsy [pyknolepsy]
    Juvenile absence epilepsy
    Absence epileptic syndrome, NOS

√6ᵗʰ **G40.A0**   **Absence epileptic syndrome, not intractable**

    G40.A01   **Absence epileptic syndrome, not** `HCC`
        intractable, with status
        epilepticus

    G40.A09   **Absence epileptic syndrome, not** `HCC` `Q`
        intractable, without status
        epilepticus

√6ᵗʰ **G40.A1**   **Absence epileptic syndrome, intractable**

    G40.A11   **Absence epileptic syndrome,** `HCC`
        intractable, with status
        epilepticus

    G40.A19   **Absence epileptic syndrome,** `HCC` `Q`
        intractable, without status
        epilepticus

√5ᵗʰ **G40.B**   **Juvenile myoclonic epilepsy [impulsive petit mal]**

√6ᵗʰ **G40.B0**   **Juvenile myoclonic epilepsy, not intractable**

    G40.B01   **Juvenile myoclonic epilepsy, not** `HCC`
        intractable, with status
        epilepticus

    G40.B09   **Juvenile myoclonic epilepsy, not** `HCC`
        intractable, without status
        epilepticus

√6ᵗʰ **G40.B1**   **Juvenile myoclonic epilepsy, intractable**

    G40.B11   **Juvenile myoclonic epilepsy,** `HCC`
        intractable, with status
        epilepticus

    G40.B19   **Juvenile myoclonic epilepsy,** `HCC`
        intractable, without status
        epilepticus

√5ᵗʰ **G40.4**   **Other generalized epilepsy and epileptic syndromes**

    Epilepsy with grand mal seizures on awakening
    Epilepsy with myoclonic absences
    Epilepsy with myoclonic-astatic seizures
    Grand mal seizure NOS
    Nonspecific atonic epileptic seizures
    Nonspecific clonic epileptic seizures
    Nonspecific myoclonic epileptic seizures
    Nonspecific tonic epileptic seizures
    Nonspecific tonic-clonic epileptic seizures
    Symptomatic early myoclonic encephalopathy

√6ᵗʰ **G40.40**   **Other generalized epilepsy and epileptic**
    syndromes, not intractable
        Other generalized epilepsy and epileptic syndromes
           without intractability
        Other generalized epilepsy and epileptic syndromes
           NOS

    G40.401   **Other generalized epilepsy and** `HCC`
        epileptic syndromes, not
        intractable, with status
        epilepticus

    G40.409   **Other generalized epilepsy and** `HCC` `Q`
        epileptic syndromes, not
        intractable, without status
        epilepticus

√6ᵗʰ **G40.41**   **Other generalized epilepsy and epileptic**
    syndromes, intractable

    G40.411   **Other generalized epilepsy and** `HCC` `Q`
        epileptic syndromes, intractable,
        with status epilepticus

    G40.419   **Other generalized epilepsy and** `HCC`
        epileptic syndromes, intractable,
        without status epilepticus

√5ᵗʰ **G40.5**   **Epileptic seizures related to external causes**

    Epileptic seizures related to alcohol
    Epileptic seizures related to drugs
    Epileptic seizures related to hormonal changes
    Epileptic seizures related to sleep deprivation
    Epileptic seizures related to stress
    Code also, if applicable, associated epilepsy and recurrent
        seizures (G40.-)
    Use additional code for adverse effect, if applicable, to identify
        drug (T36-T50 with fifth or sixth character 5)

√6ᵗʰ **G40.50**   **Epileptic seizures related to external causes, not**
    intractable

    G40.501   **Epileptic seizures related to** `HCC`
        external causes, not intractable,
        with status epilepticus

    G40.509   **Epileptic seizures related to** `HCC`
        external causes, not intractable,
        without status epilepticus
           Epileptic seizures related to external
           causes, NOS

√5ᵗʰ **G40.8**   **Other epilepsy and recurrent seizures**

    Epilepsies and epileptic syndromes undetermined as to whether
        they are focal or generalized
    Landau-Kleffner syndrome

√6ᵗʰ **G40.80**   **Other epilepsy**

    G40.801   **Other epilepsy, not intractable,** `HCC`
        with status epilepticus
           Other epilepsy without intractability with
           status epilepticus

    G40.802   **Other epilepsy, not intractable,** `HCC`
        without status epilepticus
           Other epilepsy NOS
           Other epilepsy without intractability
           without status epilepticus

    G40.803   **Other epilepsy, intractable, with** `HCC`
        status epilepticus

    G40.804   **Other epilepsy, intractable,** `HCC`
        without status epilepticus

√6ᵗʰ **G40.81**   **Lennox-Gastaut syndrome**

    DEF: Severe form of epilepsy with usual onset in early
        childhood. Seizures are frequent and difficult to treat,
        causing falls and intellectual impairment.

    G40.811   **Lennox-Gastaut syndrome, not** `HCC`
        intractable, with status
        epilepticus

    G40.812   **Lennox-Gastaut syndrome, not** `HCC`
        intractable, without status
        epilepticus

    G40.813   **Lennox-Gastaut syndrome,** `HCC`
        intractable, with status
        epilepticus

    G40.814   **Lennox-Gastaut syndrome,** `HCC`
        intractable, without status
        epilepticus

√6ᵗʰ **G40.82**   **Epileptic spasms**

    Infantile spasms
    Salaam attacks
    West's syndrome

    G40.821   **Epileptic spasms, not intractable,** `HCC`
        with status epilepticus

    G40.822   **Epileptic spasms, not intractable,** `HCC` `Q`
        without status epilepticus

    G40.823   **Epileptic spasms, intractable,** `HCC`
        with status epilepticus

    G40.824   **Epileptic spasms, intractable,** `HCC` `Q`
        without status epilepticus

    G40.89   **Other seizures** `HCC`
        EXCLUDES 1   post traumatic seizures (R56.1)
                recurrent seizures NOS (G40.909)
                seizure NOS (R56.9)

√5ᵗʰ **G40.9**   **Epilepsy, unspecified**

√6ᵗʰ **G40.90**   **Epilepsy, unspecified, not intractable**
        Epilepsy, unspecified, without intractability

    G40.901   **Epilepsy, unspecified, not** `HCC` ▽
        intractable, with status
        epilepticus

☑ Additional Character Req   √x7ᵗʰ Placeholder Alert   Manifestation   ▽ Unspecified   ►◄ Revised Text   ● New Code   ▲ Revised Code Title

G40.909   **Epilepsy, unspecified, not intractable, without status epilepticus**   HCC Q ▽
Epilepsy NOS
Epileptic convulsions NOS
Epileptic fits NOS
Epileptic seizures NOS
Recurrent seizures NOS
Seizure disorder NOS

√6ᵗʰ **G40.91**   **Epilepsy, unspecified, intractable**
Intractable seizure disorder NOS

G40.911   **Epilepsy, unspecified, intractable, with status epilepticus**   HCC ▽

G40.919   **Epilepsy, unspecified, intractable, without status epilepticus**   HCC ▽

√4ᵗʰ **G43**   **Migraine**

> NOTE   The following terms are to be considered equivalent to intractable: pharmacoresistant (pharmacologically resistant), treatment resistant, refractory (medically) and poorly controlled

Use additional code for adverse effect, if applicable, to identify drug (T36-T50 with fifth or sixth character 5)

EXCLUDES 1   headache NOS (R51)
           lower half migraine (G44.00)
EXCLUDES 2   headache syndromes (G44.-)

DEF: Headaches that occur periodically on one or both sides of the head that may be associated with nausea and vomiting, sensitivity to light and sound, dizziness, distorted vision, and cognitive disturbances.

√5ᵗʰ **G43.0**   **Migraine without aura**
Common migraine
EXCLUDES 1   chronic migraine without aura (G43.7-)

√6ᵗʰ **G43.00**   **Migraine without aura, not intractable**
Migraine without aura without mention of refractory migraine

G43.001   **Migraine without aura, not intractable, with status migrainosus**   Q

G43.009   **Migraine without aura, not intractable, without status migrainosus**   Q
Migraine without aura NOS

√6ᵗʰ **G43.01**   **Migraine without aura, intractable**
Migraine without aura with refractory migraine

G43.011   **Migraine without aura, intractable, with status migrainosus**   Q

G43.019   **Migraine without aura, intractable, without status migrainosus**   Q

√5ᵗʰ **G43.1**   **Migraine with aura**
Basilar migraine
Classical migraine
Migraine equivalents
Migraine preceded or accompanied by transient focal neurological phenomena
Migraine triggered seizures
Migraine with acute-onset aura
Migraine with aura without headache (migraine equivalents)
Migraine with prolonged aura
Migraine with typical aura
Retinal migraine
Code also any associated seizure (G40.-, R56.9)
EXCLUDES 1   persistent migraine aura (G43.5-, G43.6-)

√6ᵗʰ **G43.10**   **Migraine with aura, not intractable**
Migraine with aura without mention of refractory migraine

G43.101   **Migraine with aura, not intractable, with status migrainosus**   Q

G43.109   **Migraine with aura, not intractable, without status migrainosus**   Q
Migraine with aura NOS

√6ᵗʰ **G43.11**   **Migraine with aura, intractable**
Migraine with aura with refractory migraine

G43.111   **Migraine with aura, intractable, with status migrainosus**   Q

G43.119   **Migraine with aura, intractable, without status migrainosus**   Q

√5ᵗʰ **G43.4**   **Hemiplegic migraine**
Familial migraine
Sporadic migraine

√6ᵗʰ **G43.40**   **Hemiplegic migraine, not intractable**
Hemiplegic migraine without refractory migraine

G43.401   **Hemiplegic migraine, not intractable, with status migrainosus**   Q

G43.409   **Hemiplegic migraine, not intractable, without status migrainosus**   Q
Hemiplegic migraine NOS

√6ᵗʰ **G43.41**   **Hemiplegic migraine, intractable**
Hemiplegic migraine with refractory migraine

G43.411   **Hemiplegic migraine, intractable, with status migrainosus**   Q

G43.419   **Hemiplegic migraine, intractable, without status migrainosus**   Q

√5ᵗʰ **G43.5**   **Persistent migraine aura without cerebral infarction**

√6ᵗʰ **G43.50**   **Persistent migraine aura without cerebral infarction, not intractable**
Persistent migraine aura without cerebral infarction, without refractory migraine

G43.501   **Persistent migraine aura without cerebral infarction, not intractable, with status migrainosus**   Q

G43.509   **Persistent migraine aura without cerebral infarction, not intractable, without status migrainosus**   Q
Persistent migraine aura NOS

√6ᵗʰ **G43.51**   **Persistent migraine aura without cerebral infarction, intractable**
Persistent migraine aura without cerebral infarction, with refractory migraine

G43.511   **Persistent migraine aura without cerebral infarction, intractable, with status migrainosus**   Q

G43.519   **Persistent migraine aura without cerebral infarction, intractable, without status migrainosus**   Q

√5ᵗʰ **G43.6**   **Persistent migraine aura with cerebral infarction**
Code also the type of cerebral infarction (I63.-)

√6ᵗʰ **G43.60**   **Persistent migraine aura with cerebral infarction, not intractable**
Persistent migraine aura with cerebral infarction, without refractory migraine

G43.601   **Persistent migraine aura with cerebral infarction, not intractable, with status migrainosus**   Q

G43.609   **Persistent migraine aura with cerebral infarction, not intractable, without status migrainosus**   Q

√6ᵗʰ **G43.61**   **Persistent migraine aura with cerebral infarction, intractable**
Persistent migraine aura with cerebral infarction, with refractory migraine

G43.611   **Persistent migraine aura with cerebral infarction, intractable, with status migrainosus**   Q

G43.619   **Persistent migraine aura with cerebral infarction, intractable, without status migrainosus**   Q

√5ᵗʰ **G43.7**   **Chronic migraine without aura**
Transformed migraine
EXCLUDES 1   migraine without aura (G43.0-)

√6ᵗʰ **G43.70**   **Chronic migraine without aura, not intractable**
Chronic migraine without aura, without refractory migraine

G43.701   **Chronic migraine without aura, not intractable, with status migrainosus**   Q

G43.709   **Chronic migraine without aura, not intractable, without status migrainosus**   Q
Chronic migraine without aura NOS

√6ᵗʰ **G43.71　Chronic migraine without aura, intractable**
Chronic migraine without aura, with refractory migraine

G43.711　Chronic migraine without aura, intractable, with status migrainosus Q

G43.719　Chronic migraine without aura, intractable, without status migrainosus

√5ᵗʰ **G43.A　Cyclical vomiting**
TIP: Assign K31.89 Other diseases of stomach and duodenum, along with the appropriate code from category R11 Nausea and vomiting, to identify cyclical vomiting not related to migraine.

G43.AØ　Cyclical vomiting, not intractable
Cyclical vomiting, without refractory migraine

G43.A1　Cyclical vomiting, intractable
Cyclical vomiting, with refractory migraine

√5ᵗʰ **G43.B　Ophthalmoplegic migraine**

G43.BØ　Ophthalmoplegic migraine, not intractable Q
Ophthalmoplegic migraine, without refractory migraine

G43.B1　Ophthalmoplegic migraine, intractable Q
Ophthalmoplegic migraine, with refractory migraine

√5ᵗʰ **G43.C　Periodic headache syndromes in child or adult**

G43.CØ　Periodic headache syndromes in child or adult, not intractable Q
Periodic headache syndromes in child or adult, without refractory migraine

G43.C1　Periodic headache syndromes in child or adult, intractable Q
Periodic headache syndromes in child or adult, with refractory migraine

√5ᵗʰ **G43.D　Abdominal migraine**

G43.DØ　Abdominal migraine, not intractable
Abdominal migraine, without refractory migraine

G43.D1　Abdominal migraine, intractable
Abdominal migraine, with refractory migraine

√5ᵗʰ **G43.8　Other migraine**

√6ᵗʰ **G43.8Ø　Other migraine, not intractable**
Other migraine, without refractory migraine

G43.8Ø1　Other migraine, not intractable, with status migrainosus Q

G43.8Ø9　Other migraine, not intractable, without status migrainosus Q

√6ᵗʰ **G43.81　Other migraine, intractable**
Other migraine, with refractory migraine

G43.811　Other migraine, intractable, with status migrainosus Q

G43.819　Other migraine, intractable, without status migrainosus Q

√6ᵗʰ **G43.82　Menstrual migraine, not intractable**
Menstrual headache, not intractable
Menstrual migraine, without refractory migraine
Menstrually related migraine, not intractable
Pre-menstrual headache, not intractable
Pre-menstrual migraine, not intractable
Pure menstrual migraine, not intractable
Code also associated premenstrual tension syndrome (N94.3)

G43.821　Menstrual migraine, not intractable, with status migrainosus ♀

G43.829　Menstrual migraine, not intractable, without status migrainosus ♀
Menstrual migraine NOS

√6ᵗʰ **G43.83　Menstrual migraine, intractable**
Menstrual headache, intractable
Menstrual migraine, with refractory migraine
Menstrually related migraine, intractable
Pre-menstrual headache, intractable
Pre-menstrual migraine, intractable
Pure menstrual migraine, intractable
Code also associated premenstrual tension syndrome (N94.3)

G43.831　Menstrual migraine, intractable, with status migrainosus ♀

G43.839　Menstrual migraine, intractable, without status migrainosus ♀

√5ᵗʰ **G43.9　Migraine, unspecified**

√6ᵗʰ **G43.9Ø　Migraine, unspecified, not intractable**
Migraine, unspecified, without refractory migraine

G43.9Ø1　Migraine, unspecified, not intractable, with status migrainosus Q ▽
Status migrainosus NOS

G43.9Ø9　Migraine, unspecified, not intractable, without status migrainosus Q ▽
Migraine NOS

√6ᵗʰ **G43.91　Migraine, unspecified, intractable**
Migraine, unspecified, with refractory migraine

G43.911　Migraine, unspecified, intractable, with status migrainosus Q ▽

G43.919　Migraine, unspecified, intractable, without status migrainosus Q ▽

√4ᵗʰ **G44　Other headache syndromes**

EXCLUDES 1　headache NOS (R51)

EXCLUDES 2　atypical facial pain (G50.1)
headache due to lumbar puncture (G97.1)
migraines (G43.-)
trigeminal neuralgia (G50.Ø)

√5ᵗʰ **G44.Ø　Cluster headaches and other trigeminal autonomic cephalgias (TAC)**
DEF: Cluster headache: Characteristic grouping or clustering of headaches that can last for a number of weeks or months and then completely disappear for months or years. They are typically not associated with gastrointestinal upset or light sensitivity as experienced in migraines.

√6ᵗʰ **G44.ØØ　Cluster headache syndrome, unspecified**
Ciliary neuralgia
Cluster headache NOS
Histamine cephalgia
Lower half migraine
Migrainous neuralgia

G44.ØØ1　Cluster headache syndrome, unspecified, intractable Q ▽

G44.ØØ9　Cluster headache syndrome, unspecified, not intractable Q ▽
Cluster headache syndrome NOS

√6ᵗʰ **G44.Ø1　Episodic cluster headache**

G44.Ø11　Episodic cluster headache, intractable Q

G44.Ø19　Episodic cluster headache, not intractable Q
Episodic cluster headache NOS

√6ᵗʰ **G44.Ø2　Chronic cluster headache**

G44.Ø21　Chronic cluster headache, intractable Q

G44.Ø29　Chronic cluster headache, not intractable Q
Chronic cluster headache NOS

√6ᵗʰ **G44.Ø3　Episodic paroxysmal hemicrania**
Paroxysmal hemicrania NOS

G44.Ø31　Episodic paroxysmal hemicrania, intractable Q

G44.Ø39　Episodic paroxysmal hemicrania, not intractable Q
Episodic paroxysmal hemicrania NOS

√6ᵗʰ **G44.Ø4　Chronic paroxysmal hemicrania**

G44.Ø41　Chronic paroxysmal hemicrania, intractable Q

G44.Ø49　Chronic paroxysmal hemicrania, not intractable Q
Chronic paroxysmal hemicrania NOS

√6ᵗʰ **G44.Ø5　Short lasting unilateral neuralgiform headache with conjunctival injection and tearing (SUNCT)**

G44.Ø51　Short lasting unilateral neuralgiform headache with conjunctival injection and tearing (SUNCT), intractable Q

| ☑ Additional Character Req | √x7ᵗʰ Placeholder Alert | Manifestation | ▽ Unspecified | ►◄ Revised Text | ● New Code | ▲ Revised Code Title |

ICD-10-CM 2019　　569

G44.059 **Short lasting unilateral neuralgiform headache with conjunctival injection and tearing (SUNCT), not intractable**   ◘

Short lasting unilateral neuralgiform headache with conjunctival injection and tearing (SUNCT) NOS

√6ᵗʰ **G44.09** **Other trigeminal autonomic cephalgias (TAC)**

G44.091 **Other trigeminal autonomic cephalgias (TAC), intractable**   ◘

G44.099 **Other trigeminal autonomic cephalgias (TAC), not intractable**   ◘

G44.1 **Vascular headache, not elsewhere classified**   ◘

EXCLUDES 2   cluster headache (G44.0)

complicated headache syndromes (G44.5-)

drug-induced headache (G44.4-)

migraine (G43.-)

other specified headache syndromes (G44.8-)

post-traumatic headache (G44.3-)

tension-type headache (G44.2-)

√5ᵗʰ **G44.2** **Tension-type headache**

√6ᵗʰ **G44.20** **Tension-type headache, unspecified**

G44.201 **Tension-type headache, unspecified, intractable**   ◘ ▽

G44.209 **Tension-type headache, unspecified, not intractable**   ◘ ▽

Tension headache NOS

√6ᵗʰ **G44.21** **Episodic tension-type headache**

G44.211 **Episodic tension-type headache, intractable**   ◘

G44.219 **Episodic tension-type headache, not intractable**   ◘

Episodic tension-type headache NOS

√6ᵗʰ **G44.22** **Chronic tension-type headache**

G44.221 **Chronic tension-type headache, intractable**   ◘

G44.229 **Chronic tension-type headache, not intractable**   ◘

Chronic tension-type headache NOS

√5ᵗʰ **G44.3** **Post-traumatic headache**

√6ᵗʰ **G44.30** **Post-traumatic headache, unspecified**

G44.301 **Post-traumatic headache, unspecified, intractable**   ▽

G44.309 **Post-traumatic headache, unspecified, not intractable**   ▽

Post-traumatic headache NOS

√6ᵗʰ **G44.31** **Acute post-traumatic headache**

G44.311 **Acute post-traumatic headache, intractable**

G44.319 **Acute post-traumatic headache, not intractable**

Acute post-traumatic headache NOS

√6ᵗʰ **G44.32** **Chronic post-traumatic headache**

G44.321 **Chronic post-traumatic headache, intractable**

G44.329 **Chronic post-traumatic headache, not intractable**

Chronic post-traumatic headache NOS

√5ᵗʰ **G44.4** **Drug-induced headache, not elsewhere classified**

Medication overuse headache

Use additional code for adverse effect, if applicable, to identify drug (T36-T50 with fifth or sixth character 5)

G44.40 **Drug-induced headache, not elsewhere classified, not intractable**

G44.41 **Drug-induced headache, not elsewhere classified, intractable**

√5ᵗʰ **G44.5** **Complicated headache syndromes**

G44.51 **Hemicrania continua**   ◘

DEF: Persistent primary headache of unknown causation occurring on one side of the face and head. May last for more than three months, with daily and continuous pain of moderate intensity with severe exacerbations.

G44.52 **New daily persistent headache (NDPH)**   ◘

G44.53 **Primary thunderclap headache**   ◘

G44.59 **Other complicated headache syndrome**   ◘

√5ᵗʰ **G44.8** **Other specified headache syndromes**

G44.81 **Hypnic headache**   ◘

G44.82 **Headache associated with sexual activity**

Orgasmic headache

Preorgasmic headache

G44.83 **Primary cough headache**   ◘

G44.84 **Primary exertional headache**   ◘

G44.85 **Primary stabbing headache**   ◘

G44.89 **Other headache syndrome**   ◘

√4ᵗʰ **G45** **Transient cerebral ischemic attacks and related syndromes**

EXCLUDES 1   neonatal cerebral ischemia (P91.0)

transient retinal artery occlusion (H34.0-)

AHA: 2018,2Q,9

DEF: Transient cerebral ischemic attack: Intermittent or brief cerebral dysfunction from lack of oxygenation with no persistent neurological deficits associated with occlusive vascular disease. TIA may denote an impending cerebrovascular accident.

G45.0 **Vertebro-basilar artery syndrome**

G45.1 **Carotid artery syndrome (hemispheric)**

G45.2 **Multiple and bilateral precerebral artery syndromes**

G45.3 **Amaurosis fugax**

G45.4 **Transient global amnesia**

EXCLUDES 1   amnesia NOS (R41.3)

G45.8 **Other transient cerebral ischemic attacks and related syndromes**

G45.9 **Transient cerebral ischemic attack, unspecified**   ▽

Spasm of cerebral artery

TIA

Transient cerebral ischemia NOS

√4ᵗʰ **G46** **Vascular syndromes of brain in cerebrovascular diseases**

Code first underlying cerebrovascular disease (I60-I69)

G46.0 **Middle cerebral artery syndrome**

G46.1 **Anterior cerebral artery syndrome**

G46.2 **Posterior cerebral artery syndrome**

G46.3 **Brain stem stroke syndrome**

Benedikt syndrome

Claude syndrome

Foville syndrome

Millard-Gubler syndrome

Wallenberg syndrome

Weber syndrome

G46.4 **Cerebellar stroke syndrome**

G46.5 **Pure motor lacunar syndrome**

G46.6 **Pure sensory lacunar syndrome**

G46.7 **Other lacunar syndromes**

G46.8 **Other vascular syndromes of brain in cerebrovascular diseases**

√4ᵗʰ **G47** **Sleep disorders**

EXCLUDES 2   nightmares (F51.5)

nonorganic sleep disorders (F51.-)

sleep terrors (F51.4)

sleepwalking (F51.3)

√5ᵗʰ **G47.0** **Insomnia**

EXCLUDES 2   alcohol related insomnia (F10.182, F10.282, F10.982)

drug-related insomnia (F11.182, F11.282, F11.982, F13.182, F13.282, F13.982, F14.182, F14.282, F14.982, F15.182, F15.282, F15.982, F19.182, F19.282, F19.982)

idiopathic insomnia (F51.01)

insomnia due to a mental disorder (F51.05)

insomnia not due to a substance or known physiological condition (F51.0-)

nonorganic insomnia (F51.0-)

primary insomnia (F51.01)

sleep apnea (G47.3-)

G47.00 **Insomnia, unspecified**   ▽

Insomnia NOS

G47.01 **Insomnia due to medical condition**

Code also associated medical condition

G47.09 **Other insomnia**

√5ᵗʰ **G47.1 Hypersomnia**

> EXCLUDES 2   alcohol-related hypersomnia (F10.182, F10.282, F10.982)
>
> drug-related hypersomnia (F11.182, F11.282, F11.982, F13.182, F13.282, F13.982, F14.182, F14.282, F14.982, F15.182, F15.282, F15.982, F19.182, F19.282, F19.982)
>
> hypersomnia due to a mental disorder (F51.13)
>
> hypersomnia not due to a substance or known physiological condition (F51.1-)
>
> primary hypersomnia (F51.11)
>
> sleep apnea (G47.3-)

G47.10 Hypersomnia, unspecified ▽
Hypersomnia NOS

G47.11 Idiopathic hypersomnia with long sleep time
Idiopathic hypersomnia NOS

G47.12 Idiopathic hypersomnia without long sleep time

G47.13 Recurrent hypersomnia
Kleine-Levin syndrome
Menstrual related hypersomnia

G47.14 Hypersomnia due to medical condition
Code also associated medical condition

G47.19 Other hypersomnia

√5ᵗʰ **G47.2 Circadian rhythm sleep disorders**

Disorders of the sleep wake schedule
Inversion of nyctohemeral rhythm
Inversion of sleep rhythm

G47.20 Circadian rhythm sleep disorder, unspecified type ▽
Sleep wake schedule disorder NOS

G47.21 Circadian rhythm sleep disorder, delayed sleep phase type
Delayed sleep phase syndrome

G47.22 Circadian rhythm sleep disorder, advanced sleep phase type

G47.23 Circadian rhythm sleep disorder, irregular sleep wake type
Irregular sleep-wake pattern

G47.24 Circadian rhythm sleep disorder, free running type
Circadian rhythm sleep disorder, non-24-hour sleep-wake type

G47.25 Circadian rhythm sleep disorder, jet lag type

G47.26 Circadian rhythm sleep disorder, shift work type

G47.27 Circadian rhythm sleep disorder in conditions classified elsewhere
Code first underlying condition

G47.29 Other circadian rhythm sleep disorder

√5ᵗʰ **G47.3 Sleep apnea**

Code also any associated underlying condition

> EXCLUDES 1   apnea NOS (R06.81)
>
> Cheyne-Stokes breathing (R06.3)
>
> pickwickian syndrome (E66.2)
>
> sleep apnea of newborn (P28.3)

G47.30 Sleep apnea, unspecified ▽
Sleep apnea NOS

G47.31 Primary central sleep apnea
Idiopathic central sleep apnea

G47.32 High altitude periodic breathing

G47.33 Obstructive sleep apnea (adult) (pediatric)
Obstructive sleep apnea hypopnea

> EXCLUDES 1   obstructive sleep apnea of newborn (P28.3)

G47.34 Idiopathic sleep related nonobstructive alveolar hypoventilation
Sleep related hypoxia

G47.35 Congenital central alveolar hypoventilation syndrome

G47.36 Sleep related hypoventilation in conditions classified elsewhere
Sleep related hypoxemia in conditions classified elsewhere
Code first underlying condition

G47.37 Central sleep apnea in conditions classified elsewhere
Code first underlying condition

G47.39 Other sleep apnea

√5ᵗʰ **G47.4 Narcolepsy and cataplexy**

√6ᵗʰ **G47.41 Narcolepsy**

G47.411 Narcolepsy with cataplexy

G47.419 Narcolepsy without cataplexy
Narcolepsy NOS

√6ᵗʰ **G47.42 Narcolepsy in conditions classified elsewhere**
Code first underlying condition

G47.421 Narcolepsy in conditions classified elsewhere with cataplexy

G47.429 Narcolepsy in conditions classified elsewhere without cataplexy

√5ᵗʰ **G47.5 Parasomnia**

> EXCLUDES 1   alcohol induced parasomnia (F10.182, F10.282, F10.982)
>
> drug induced parasomnia (F11.182, F11.282, F11.982, F13.182, F13.282, F13.982, F14.182, F14.282, F14.982, F15.182, F15.282, F15.982, F19.182, F19.282, F19.982)
>
> parasomnia not due to a substance or known physiological condition (F51.8)

G47.50 Parasomnia, unspecified ▽
Parasomnia NOS

G47.51 Confusional arousals

G47.52 REM sleep behavior disorder

G47.53 Recurrent isolated sleep paralysis

G47.54 Parasomnia in conditions classified elsewhere
Code first underlying condition

G47.59 Other parasomnia

√5ᵗʰ **G47.6 Sleep related movement disorders**

> EXCLUDES 2   restless legs syndrome (G25.81)

G47.61 Periodic limb movement disorder

G47.62 Sleep related leg cramps

G47.63 Sleep related bruxism

> EXCLUDES 1   psychogenic bruxism (F45.8)

G47.69 Other sleep related movement disorders

G47.8 Other sleep disorders
Other specified sleep-wake disorder

G47.9 Sleep disorder, unspecified ▽
Sleep disorder NOS
Unspecified sleep-wake disorder

☑ Additional Character Req   √7ᵗʰ Placeholder Alert   Manifestation   ▽ Unspecified   ▶◀ Revised Text   ● New Code   ▲ Revised Code Title

Chapter 6. Diseases of the Nervous System

Nerve, nerve root and plexus disorders (G50-G59)

> **EXCLUDES 1**   current traumatic nerve, nerve root and plexus disorders - see Injury, nerve by body region
> neuralgia NOS (M79.2)
> neuritis NOS (M79.2)
> peripheral neuritis in pregnancy (O26.82-)
> radiculitis NOS (M54.1-)

✓4ᵗʰ G50   Disorders of trigeminal nerve

> **INCLUDES**   disorders of 5th cranial nerve

Trigeminal and Facial Nerve Branches

Supratrochlear nerve
Supraorbital nerve
V2 branch
Infraorbital nerve
V1 branch
Trigeminal nerve (CN V) branches in infratemporal fossa
V3 branch
Mental nerve
Mental foramen

G50.0   **Trigeminal neuralgia**
Syndrome of paroxysmal facial pain
Tic douloureux

G50.1   **Atypical facial pain**

G50.8   **Other disorders of trigeminal nerve**

G50.9   **Disorder of trigeminal nerve, unspecified**   ▽

✓4ᵗʰ G51   Facial nerve disorders

> **INCLUDES**   disorders of 7th cranial nerve

G51.0   **Bell's palsy**
Facial palsy

G51.1   **Geniculate ganglionitis**
> **EXCLUDES 1**   postherpetic geniculate ganglionitis (B02.21)

G51.2   **Melkersson's syndrome**
Melkersson-Rosenthal syndrome

✓5ᵗʰ G51.3   **Clonic hemifacial spasm**

-   **G51.31**   **Clonic hemifacial spasm, right**
-   **G51.32**   **Clonic hemifacial spasm, left**
-   **G51.33**   **Clonic hemifacial spasm, bilateral**
-   **G51.39**   **Clonic hemifacial spasm, unspecified**   ▽

G51.4   **Facial myokymia**

G51.8   **Other disorders of facial nerve**

G51.9   **Disorder of facial nerve, unspecified**   ▽

✓4ᵗʰ G52   Disorders of other cranial nerves

> **EXCLUDES 2**   disorders of acoustic [8th] nerve (H93.3)
> disorders of optic [2nd] nerve (H46, H47.0)
> paralytic strabismus due to nerve palsy (H49.0-H49.2)

G52.0   **Disorders of olfactory nerve**
Disorders of 1st cranial nerve

G52.1   **Disorders of glossopharyngeal nerve**
Disorder of 9th cranial nerve
Glossopharyngeal neuralgia

G52.2   **Disorders of vagus nerve**
Disorders of pneumogastric [10th] nerve

G52.3   **Disorders of hypoglossal nerve**
Disorders of 12th cranial nerve

G52.7   **Disorders of multiple cranial nerves**
Polyneuritis cranialis

G52.8   **Disorders of other specified cranial nerves**

G52.9   **Cranial nerve disorder, unspecified**   ▽

G53   *Cranial nerve disorders in diseases classified elsewhere*

Code first underlying disease, such as:
neoplasm (C00-D49)

> **EXCLUDES 1**   multiple cranial nerve palsy in sarcoidosis (D86.82)
> multiple cranial nerve palsy in syphilis (A52.15)
> postherpetic geniculate ganglionitis (B02.21)
> postherpetic trigeminal neuralgia (B02.22)

✓4ᵗʰ G54   Nerve root and plexus disorders

> **EXCLUDES 1**   current traumatic nerve root and plexus disorders - see nerve injury by body region
> intervertebral disc disorders (M50-M51)
> neuralgia or neuritis NOS (M79.2)
> neuritis or radiculitis brachial NOS (M54.13)
> neuritis or radiculitis lumbar NOS (M54.16)
> neuritis or radiculitis lumbosacral NOS (M54.17)
> neuritis or radiculitis thoracic NOS (M54.14)
> radiculitis NOS (M54.10)
> radiculopathy NOS (M54.10)
> spondylosis (M47.-)

G54.0   **Brachial plexus disorders**
Thoracic outlet syndrome
DEF: Acquired disorder affecting the spinal nerves that send signals to the shoulder, arm, and hand, causing corresponding motor and sensory dysfunction. This disorder is characterized by regional paresthesia, pain, muscle weakness, and in severe cases paralysis.

G54.1   **Lumbosacral plexus disorders**

G54.2   **Cervical root disorders, not elsewhere classified**

G54.3   **Thoracic root disorders, not elsewhere classified**

G54.4   **Lumbosacral root disorders, not elsewhere classified**

G54.5   **Neuralgic amyotrophy**
Parsonage-Aldren-Turner syndrome
Shoulder-girdle neuritis
> **EXCLUDES 1**   neuralgic amyotrophy in diabetes mellitus (E08-E13 with .44)

G54.6   **Phantom limb syndrome with pain**   ᴴᶜᶜ

G54.7   **Phantom limb syndrome without pain**   ᴴᶜᶜ
Phantom limb syndrome NOS

G54.8   **Other nerve root and plexus disorders**

G54.9   **Nerve root and plexus disorder, unspecified**   ▽

G55   *Nerve root and plexus compressions in diseases classified elsewhere*

Code first underlying disease, such as:
neoplasm (C00-D49)

> **EXCLUDES 1**   nerve root compression (due to) (in) ankylosing spondylitis (M45.-)
> nerve root compression (due to) (in) dorsopathies (M53.-, M54.-)
> nerve root compression (due to) (in) intervertebral disc disorders (M50.1.-, M51.1.-)
> nerve root compression (due to) (in) spondylopathies (M46.-, M48.-)
> nerve root compression (due to) (in) spondylosis (M47.0-M47.2-)

√4ᵗʰ G56 Mononeuropathies of upper limb

    EXCLUDES 1   *current traumatic nerve disorder - see nerve injury by body region*

    AHA: 2016,4Q,17-18

Nerves of Upper Limb

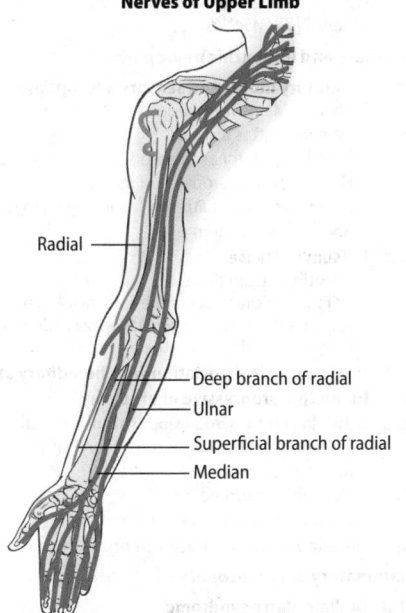

Radial

Deep branch of radial
Ulnar
Superficial branch of radial
Median

√5ᵗʰ G56.0   Carpal tunnel syndrome

  G56.00   Carpal tunnel syndrome, unspecified upper limb   ▽

  G56.01   Carpal tunnel syndrome, right upper limb

  G56.02   Carpal tunnel syndrome, left upper limb

  G56.03   Carpal tunnel syndrome, bilateral upper limbs

√5ᵗʰ G56.1   Other lesions of median nerve

  G56.10   Other lesions of median nerve, unspecified upper limb   ▽

  G56.11   Other lesions of median nerve, right upper limb

  G56.12   Other lesions of median nerve, left upper limb

  G56.13   Other lesions of median nerve, bilateral upper limbs

√5ᵗʰ G56.2   Lesion of ulnar nerve

    Tardy ulnar nerve palsy

  G56.20   Lesion of ulnar nerve, unspecified upper limb   ▽

  G56.21   Lesion of ulnar nerve, right upper limb

  G56.22   Lesion of ulnar nerve, left upper limb

  G56.23   Lesion of ulnar nerve, bilateral upper limbs

√5ᵗʰ G56.3   Lesion of radial nerve

  G56.30   Lesion of radial nerve, unspecified upper limb   ▽

  G56.31   Lesion of radial nerve, right upper limb

  G56.32   Lesion of radial nerve, left upper limb

  G56.33   Lesion of radial nerve, bilateral upper limbs

√5ᵗʰ G56.4   Causalgia of upper limb

    Complex regional pain syndrome II of upper limb

    EXCLUDES 1   *complex regional pain syndrome I of lower limb (G90.52-)*

           complex regional pain syndrome I of upper limb (G90.51-)

           complex regional pain syndrome II of lower limb (G57.7-)

           reflex sympathetic dystrophy of lower limb (G90.52-)

           reflex sympathetic dystrophy of upper limb (G90.51-)

  G56.40   Causalgia of unspecified upper limb   ▽

  G56.41   Causalgia of right upper limb

  G56.42   Causalgia of left upper limb

  G56.43   Causalgia of bilateral upper limbs

√5ᵗʰ G56.8   Other specified mononeuropathies of upper limb

    Interdigital neuroma of upper limb

  G56.80   Other specified mononeuropathies of unspecified upper limb   ▽

  G56.81   Other specified mononeuropathies of right upper limb

---

  G56.82   Other specified mononeuropathies of left upper limb

  G56.83   Other specified mononeuropathies of bilateral upper limbs

√5ᵗʰ G56.9   Unspecified mononeuropathy of upper limb

  G56.90   Unspecified mononeuropathy of unspecified upper limb   ▽

  G56.91   Unspecified mononeuropathy of right upper limb   ▽

  G56.92   Unspecified mononeuropathy of left upper limb   ▽

  G56.93   Unspecified mononeuropathy of bilateral upper limbs   ▽

√4ᵗʰ G57 Mononeuropathies of lower limb

    EXCLUDES 1   *current traumatic nerve disorder - see nerve injury by body region*

    AHA: 2016,4Q,17-18

Nerves of Lower Limb

Obturator nerve

Sciatic nerve

Femoral nerve

Saphenous nerve

Common fibular (peroneal) nerve

Deep fibular (peroneal) nerve

Tibial nerve

Superficial fibular (peroneal) nerve

√5ᵗʰ G57.0   Lesion of sciatic nerve

    EXCLUDES 1   *sciatica NOS (M54.3-)*

    EXCLUDES 2   *sciatica attributed to intervertebral disc disorder (M51.1.-)*

  G57.00   Lesion of sciatic nerve, unspecified lower limb   ▽

  G57.01   Lesion of sciatic nerve, right lower limb

  G57.02   Lesion of sciatic nerve, left lower limb

  G57.03   Lesion of sciatic nerve, bilateral lower limbs

√5ᵗʰ G57.1   Meralgia paresthetica

    Lateral cutaneous nerve of thigh syndrome

  G57.10   Meralgia paresthetica, unspecified lower limb   ▽

  G57.11   Meralgia paresthetica, right lower limb

  G57.12   Meralgia paresthetica, left lower limb

  G57.13   Meralgia paresthetica, bilateral lower limbs

√5ᵗʰ G57.2   Lesion of femoral nerve

  G57.20   Lesion of femoral nerve, unspecified lower limb   ▽

  G57.21   Lesion of femoral nerve, right lower limb

  G57.22   Lesion of femoral nerve, left lower limb

  G57.23   Lesion of femoral nerve, bilateral lower limbs

√5ᵗʰ G57.3   Lesion of lateral popliteal nerve

    Peroneal nerve palsy

  G57.30   Lesion of lateral popliteal nerve, unspecified lower limb   ▽

  G57.31   Lesion of lateral popliteal nerve, right lower limb

  G57.32   Lesion of lateral popliteal nerve, left lower limb

  G57.33   Lesion of lateral popliteal nerve, bilateral lower limbs

---

✓ Additional Character Req   ✓x7ᵗʰ Placeholder Alert   Manifestation   ▽ Unspecified   ▶◀ Revised Text   ● New Code   ▲ Revised Code Title

✓5ᵗʰ **G57.4 Lesion of** medial popliteal nerve

G57.40   **Lesion of medial popliteal nerve,** ▽
unspecified lower limb

G57.41   **Lesion of medial popliteal nerve, right lower limb**

G57.42   **Lesion of medial popliteal nerve, left lower limb**

G57.43   **Lesion of medial popliteal nerve, bilateral lower
limbs**

✓5ᵗʰ **G57.5 Tarsal tunnel syndrome**

G57.50   **Tarsal tunnel syndrome, unspecified lower** ▽
limb

G57.51   **Tarsal tunnel syndrome, right lower limb**

G57.52   **Tarsal tunnel syndrome, left lower limb**

G57.53   **Tarsal tunnel syndrome, bilateral lower limbs**

✓5ᵗʰ **G57.6 Lesion of** plantar nerve

Morton's metatarsalgia

G57.60   **Lesion of plantar nerve, unspecified lower** ▽
limb

G57.61   **Lesion of plantar nerve, right lower limb**

G57.62   **Lesion of plantar nerve, left lower limb**

G57.63   **Lesion of plantar nerve, bilateral lower limbs**

✓5ᵗʰ **G57.7 Causalgia of lower limb**

Complex regional pain syndrome II of lower limb

EXCLUDES 1   *complex regional pain syndrome I of lower limb
(G90.52-)*

*complex regional pain syndrome I of upper limb
(G90.51-)*

*complex regional pain syndrome II of upper limb
(G56.4-)*

reflex sympathetic dystrophy of lower limb (G90.52-)

reflex sympathetic dystrophy of upper limb (G90.51-)

G57.70   **Causalgia of unspecified lower limb** ▽

G57.71   **Causalgia of right lower limb**

G57.72   **Causalgia of left lower limb**

G57.73   **Causalgia of bilateral lower limbs**

✓5ᵗʰ **G57.8 Other specified mononeuropathies of lower limb**

Interdigital neuroma of lower limb

G57.80   **Other specified mononeuropathies of** ▽
unspecified lower limb

G57.81   **Other specified mononeuropathies of right lower
limb**

G57.82   **Other specified mononeuropathies of left lower
limb**

G57.83   **Other specified mononeuropathies of bilateral
lower limbs**

✓5ᵗʰ **G57.9 Unspecified mononeuropathy of lower limb**

G57.90   **Unspecified mononeuropathy of** ▽
unspecified lower limb

G57.91   **Unspecified mononeuropathy of right lower** ▽
limb

G57.92   **Unspecified mononeuropathy of left lower** ▽
limb

G57.93   **Unspecified mononeuropathy of bilateral** ▽
lower limbs

✓4ᵗʰ **G58 Other mononeuropathies**

G58.0 Intercostal neuropathy

G58.7 Mononeuritis multiplex

G58.8 Other specified mononeuropathies

G58.9 Mononeuropathy, unspecified ▽

G59 *Mononeuropathy in diseases classified elsewhere*

Code first underlying disease

EXCLUDES 1   *diabetic mononeuropathy (E08-E13 with .41)*

syphilitic nerve paralysis (A52.19)

syphilitic neuritis (A52.15)

tuberculous mononeuropathy (A17.83)

Polyneuropathies and other disorders of the peripheral nervous system (G60-G65)

EXCLUDES 1   *neuralgia NOS (M79.2)*
neuritis NOS (M79.2)
peripheral neuritis in pregnancy (O26.82-)
radiculitis NOS (M54.10)

✓4ᵗʰ **G60 Hereditary and idiopathic neuropathy**

G60.0 Hereditary motor and sensory neuropathy

Charcôt-Marie-Tooth disease

Déjérine-Sottas disease

Hereditary motor and sensory neuropathy, types I-IV

Hypertrophic neuropathy of infancy

Peroneal muscular atrophy (axonal type) (hypertrophic type)

Roussy-Levy syndrome

G60.1 Refsum's disease

Infantile Refsum disease

DEF: Genetic disorder of the lipid metabolism characterized by
retinitis pigmentosa, degenerative nerve disease, ataxia, and dry,
rough, scaly skin.

G60.2 Neuropathy in association with hereditary ataxia

G60.3 Idiopathic progressive neuropathy

G60.8 Other hereditary and idiopathic neuropathies

Dominantly inherited sensory neuropathy

Morvan's disease

Nelaton's syndrome

Recessively inherited sensory neuropathy

G60.9 Hereditary and idiopathic neuropathy, unspecified ▽

✓4ᵗʰ **G61 Inflammatory polyneuropathy**

G61.0 Guillain-Barre syndrome   HCC

Acute (post-)infective polyneuritis

Miller Fisher syndrome

AHA: 2014,2Q,4

DEF: Autoimmune disorder due to an immune response to foreign
antigens with paraplegia of limbs, flaccid paralysis,
ophthalmoplegia, ataxia, and areflexia. In most cases, this disorder
is triggered by a mild viral infection, surgery, or following an
immunization.

TIP: Guillain-Barre syndrome can occur as a sequela of
Campylobacter enteritis. Assign code B94.8 for the sequelae as an
additional diagnosis.

G61.1 Serum neuropathy   HCC

Use additional code for adverse effect, if applicable, to identify
serum (T50.-)

✓5ᵗʰ **G61.8 Other inflammatory polyneuropathies**

G61.81   **Chronic inflammatory demyelinating**   HCC
polyneuritis

G61.82   **Multifocal motor neuropathy**   HCC

MMN

AHA: 2016,4Q,18

G61.89   **Other inflammatory polyneuropathies**   HCC

G61.9 Inflammatory polyneuropathy, unspecified   HCC ▽

✓4ᵗʰ **G62 Other and unspecified polyneuropathies**

G62.0 Drug-induced polyneuropathy   HCC

Use additional code for adverse effect, if applicable, to identify
drug (T36-T50 with fifth or sixth character 5)

G62.1 Alcoholic polyneuropathy   HCC

G62.2 Polyneuropathy due to other toxic agents   HCC

Code first (T51-T65) to identify toxic agent

✓5ᵗʰ **G62.8 Other specified polyneuropathies**

G62.81   **Critical illness polyneuropathy**   HCC

Acute motor neuropathy

G62.82   **Radiation-induced polyneuropathy**   HCC

Use additional external cause code (W88-W90, X39.0-)
to identify cause

G62.89   **Other specified polyneuropathies**

AHA: 2016,2Q,11

G62.9 Polyneuropathy, unspecified ▽

Neuropathy NOS

G63   *Polyneuropathy in diseases classified elsewhere*   HCC

     Code first underlying disease, such as:
       amyloidosis (E85.-)
       endocrine disease, except diabetes (E00-E07, E15-E16, E20-E34)
       metabolic diseases (E70-E88)
       neoplasm (C00-D49)
       nutritional deficiency (E40-E64)

     EXCLUDES 1   *polyneuropathy (in):*
         diabetes mellitus (E08-E13 with .42)
         diphtheria (A36.83)
         infectious mononucleosis (B27.0-B27.9 with 1)
         Lyme disease (A69.22)
         mumps (B26.84)
         postherpetic (B02.23)
         rheumatoid arthritis (M05.33)
         scleroderma (M34.83)
         systemic lupus erythematosus (M32.19)

     AHA: 2012,4Q,99

G64   **Other disorders of peripheral nervous system**
     Disorder of peripheral nervous system NOS

✓4th **G65**   **Sequelae of inflammatory and toxic polyneuropathies**
     Code first condition resulting from (sequela) of inflammatory and toxic polyneuropathies

     G65.0   **Sequelae of Guillain-Barré syndrome**   HCC
     G65.1   **Sequelae of other inflammatory polyneuropathy**   HCC
     G65.2   **Sequelae of toxic polyneuropathy**   HCC

Diseases of myoneural junction and muscle (G70-G73)

✓4th **G70**   **Myasthenia gravis and other myoneural disorders**
     EXCLUDES 1   *botulism (A05.1, A48.51-A48.52)*
         transient neonatal myasthenia gravis (P94.0)

     ✓5th **G70.0**   **Myasthenia gravis**
         DEF: Autoimmune neuromuscular disorder caused by antibodies to the acetylcholine receptors at the neuromuscular junction, interfering with proper binding of the neurotransmitter from the neuron to the target muscle, causing muscle weakness, fatigue, and exhaustion, without pain or atrophy.

         G70.00   **Myasthenia gravis without (acute) exacerbation**   HCC
           Myasthenia gravis NOS
         G70.01   **Myasthenia gravis with (acute) exacerbation**   HCC
           Myasthenia gravis in crisis

     G70.1   **Toxic myoneural disorders**   HCC
       Code first (T51-T65) to identify toxic agent
     G70.2   **Congenital and developmental myasthenia**   HCC
     ✓5th **G70.8**   **Other specified myoneural disorders**
         G70.80   **Lambert-Eaton syndrome, unspecified**   HCC ▽
           Lambert-Eaton syndrome NOS
         G70.81   *Lambert-Eaton syndrome in disease classified elsewhere*   HCC
           Code first underlying disease
           EXCLUDES 1   *Lambert-Eaton syndrome in neoplastic disease (G73.1)*
         G70.89   **Other specified myoneural disorders**   HCC
     G70.9   **Myoneural disorder, unspecified**   HCC ▽

✓4th **G71**   **Primary disorders of muscles**
     EXCLUDES 2   *arthrogryposis multiplex congenita (Q74.3)*
         metabolic disorders (E70-E88)
         myositis (M60.-)

     ✓5th **G71.0**   **Muscular dystrophy**
       ~~Autosomal recessive, childhood type, muscular dystrophy resembling Duchenne or Becker muscular dystrophy~~
       ~~Benign [Becker] muscular dystrophy~~
       ~~Benign scapuloperoneal muscular dystrophy with early contractures [Emery-Dreifuss]~~
       ~~Congenital muscular dystrophy NOS~~
       ~~Congenital muscular dystrophy with specific morphological abnormalities of the muscle fiber~~
       ~~Distal muscular dystrophy~~
       ~~Facioscapulohumeral muscular dystrophy~~
       ~~Limb-girdle muscular dystrophy~~
       ~~Ocular muscular dystrophy~~
       ~~Oculopharyngeal muscular dystrophy~~
       ~~Scapuloperoneal muscular dystrophy~~
       ~~Severe [Duchenne] muscular dystrophy~~

         ● **G71.00**   **Muscular dystrophy, unspecified**   ▽
         ● **G71.01**   **Duchenne or Becker muscular dystrophy**
           Autosomal recessive, childhood type, muscular dystrophy resembling Duchenne or Becker muscular dystrophy
           Benign [Becker] muscular dystrophy
           Severe [Duchenne] muscular dystrophy
         ● **G71.02**   **Facioscapulohumeral muscular dystrophy**
           Scapulohumeral muscular dystrophy
         ● **G71.09**   **Other specified muscular dystrophies**
           Benign scapuloperoneal muscular dystrophy with early contractures [Emery-Dreifuss]
           Congenital muscular dystrophy NOS
           Congenital muscular dystrophy with specific morphological abnormalities of the muscle fiber
           Distal muscular dystrophy
           Limb-girdle muscular dystrophy
           Ocular muscular dystrophy
           Oculopharyngeal muscular dystrophy
           Scapuloperoneal muscular dystrophy

     ✓5th **G71.1**   **Myotonic disorders**
         G71.11   **Myotonic muscular dystrophy**   HCC
           Dystrophia myotonica [Steinert]
           Myotonia atrophica
           Myotonic dystrophy
           Proximal myotonic myopathy (PROMM)
           Steinert disease
         G71.12   **Myotonia congenita**
           Acetazolamide responsive myotonia congenita
           Dominant myotonia congenita [Thomsen disease]
           Myotonia levior
           Recessive myotonia congenita [Becker disease]
         G71.13   **Myotonic chondrodystrophy**
           Chondrodystrophic myotonia
           Congenital myotonic chondrodystrophy
           Schwartz-Jampel disease
         G71.14   **Drug induced myotonia**
           Use additional code for adverse effect, if applicable, to identify drug (T36-T50 with fifth or sixth character 5)
         G71.19   **Other specified myotonic disorders**
           Myotonia fluctuans
           Myotonia permanens
           Neuromyotonia [Isaacs]
           Paramyotonia congenita (of von Eulenburg)
           Pseudomyotonia
           Symptomatic myotonia

     G71.2   **Congenital myopathies**   HCC
       Central core disease
       Fiber-type disproportion
       Minicore disease
       Multicore disease
       Myotubular (centronuclear) myopathy
       Nemaline myopathy
       EXCLUDES 1   *arthrogryposis multiplex congenita (Q74.3)*

✓ Additional Character Req   ✓x7th Placeholder Alert   Manifestation   ▽ Unspecified   ►◄ Revised Text   ● New Code   ▲ Revised Code Title

Chapter 6. Diseases of the Nervous System

G71.3 Mitochondrial myopathy, not elsewhere classified
> EXCLUDES 1   Kearns-Sayre syndrome (H49.81)
> Leber's disease (H47.21)
> Leigh's encephalopathy (G31.82)
> mitochondrial metabolism disorders (E88.4.-)
> Reye's syndrome (G93.7)

G71.8 Other primary disorders of muscles

G71.9 Primary disorder of muscle, unspecified ▽
> Hereditary myopathy NOS

✓4ᵗʰ G72 Other and unspecified myopathies
> EXCLUDES 1   arthrogryposis multiplex congenita (Q74.3)
> dermatopolymyositis (M33.-)
> ischemic infarction of muscle (M62.2-)
> myositis (M6Ø.-)
> polymyositis (M33.2.-)

G72.Ø Drug-induced myopathy
> Use additional code for adverse effect, if applicable, to identify drug (T36-T5Ø with fifth or sixth character 5)

G72.1 Alcoholic myopathy
> Use additional code to identify alcoholism (F1Ø.-)

G72.2 Myopathy due to other toxic agents
> Code first (T51-T65) to identify toxic agent

G72.3 Periodic paralysis
> Familial periodic paralysis
> Hyperkalemic periodic paralysis (familial)
> Hypokalemic periodic paralysis (familial)
> Myotonic periodic paralysis (familial)
> Normokalemic paralysis (familial)
> Potassium sensitive periodic paralysis
> EXCLUDES 1   paramyotonia congenita (of von Eulenburg) (G71.19)

✓5ᵗʰ G72.4 Inflammatory and immune myopathies, not elsewhere classified
> **G72.41 Inclusion body myositis [IBM]**
> **G72.49 Other inflammatory and immune myopathies, not elsewhere classified**
> Inflammatory myopathy NOS

✓5ᵗʰ G72.8 Other specified myopathies
> **G72.81 Critical illness myopathy**
> Acute necrotizing myopathy
> Acute quadriplegic myopathy
> Intensive care (ICU) myopathy
> Myopathy of critical illness
> **G72.89 Other specified myopathies**

G72.9 Myopathy, unspecified ▽

✓4ᵗʰ G73 Disorders of myoneural junction and muscle in diseases classified elsewhere
> *G73.1 Lambert-Eaton syndrome in neoplastic disease*   HCC
> Code first underlying neoplasm (CØØ-D49)
> EXCLUDES 1   Lambert-Eaton syndrome not associated with neoplasm (G7Ø.8Ø-G7Ø.81)
>
> *G73.3 Myasthenic syndromes in other diseases classified elsewhere*   HCC
> Code first underlying disease, such as:
> neoplasm (CØØ-D49)
> thyrotoxicosis (EØ5.-)
>
> *G73.7 Myopathy in diseases classified elsewhere*
> Code first underlying disease, such as:
> hyperparathyroidism (E21.Ø, E21.3)
> hypoparathyroidism (E2Ø.-)
> glycogen storage disease (E74.Ø)
> lipid storage disorders (E75.-)
> EXCLUDES 1   myopathy in:
> rheumatoid arthritis (MØ5.32)
> sarcoidosis (D86.87)
> scleroderma (M34.82)
> sicca syndrome [Sjögren] (M35.Ø3)
> systemic lupus erythematosus (M32.19)

Cerebral palsy and other paralytic syndromes (G8Ø-G83)

✓4ᵗʰ G8Ø Cerebral palsy
> EXCLUDES 1   hereditary spastic paraplegia (G11.4)

G8Ø.Ø Spastic quadriplegic cerebral palsy   HCC
> Congenital spastic paralysis (cerebral)

G8Ø.1 Spastic diplegic cerebral palsy   HCC
> Spastic cerebral palsy NOS

G8Ø.2 Spastic hemiplegic cerebral palsy   HCC

G8Ø.3 Athetoid cerebral palsy   HCC
> Double athetosis (syndrome)
> Dyskinetic cerebral palsy
> Dystonic cerebral palsy
> Vogt disease

G8Ø.4 Ataxic cerebral palsy   HCC

G8Ø.8 Other cerebral palsy   HCC
> Mixed cerebral palsy syndromes

G8Ø.9 Cerebral palsy, unspecified   HCC ▽
> Cerebral palsy NOS

✓4ᵗʰ G81 Hemiplegia and hemiparesis
> NOTE   This category is to be used only when hemiplegia (complete)(incomplete) is reported without further specification, or is stated to be old or longstanding but of unspecified cause. The category is also for use in multiple coding to identify these types of hemiplegia resulting from any cause.
>
> EXCLUDES 1   congenital cerebral palsy (G8Ø.-)
> hemiplegia and hemiparesis due to sequela of cerebrovascular disease (I69.Ø5-, I69.15-, I69.25-, I69.35-, I69.85-, I69.95-)
>
> **AHA:** 2015,1Q,25
> **TIP:** If the documentation specifies the affected side but not whether it is the dominant or nondominant side, the default is as follows: for ambidextrous patients, the default is dominant; when the left side is affected, the default is nondominant; and when the right side is affected, the default is dominant.

✓5ᵗʰ G81.Ø Flaccid hemiplegia
> **G81.ØØ Flaccid hemiplegia affecting unspecified side**   HCC ▽
> **G81.Ø1 Flaccid hemiplegia affecting right dominant side**   HCC
> **G81.Ø2 Flaccid hemiplegia affecting left dominant side**   HCC
> **G81.Ø3 Flaccid hemiplegia affecting right nondominant side**   HCC
> **G81.Ø4 Flaccid hemiplegia affecting left nondominant side**   HCC

✓5ᵗʰ G81.1 Spastic hemiplegia
> **G81.1Ø Spastic hemiplegia affecting unspecified side**   HCC ▽
> **G81.11 Spastic hemiplegia affecting right dominant side**   HCC
> **G81.12 Spastic hemiplegia affecting left dominant side**   HCC
> **G81.13 Spastic hemiplegia affecting right nondominant side**   HCC
> **G81.14 Spastic hemiplegia affecting left nondominant side**   HCC

✓5ᵗʰ G81.9 Hemiplegia, unspecified
> **AHA:** 2014,1Q,23
> **G81.9Ø Hemiplegia, unspecified affecting unspecified side**   HCC ▽
> **G81.91 Hemiplegia, unspecified affecting right dominant side**   HCC ▽
> **G81.92 Hemiplegia, unspecified affecting left dominant side**   HCC ▽
> **G81.93 Hemiplegia, unspecified affecting right nondominant side**   HCC ▽
> **G81.94 Hemiplegia, unspecified affecting left nondominant side**   HCC ▽

✓4ᵗʰ **G82 Paraplegia (paraparesis) and quadriplegia (quadriparesis)**

> **NOTE**   This category is to be used only when the listed conditions are reported without further specification, or are stated to be old or longstanding but of unspecified cause. The category is also for use in multiple coding to identify these conditions resulting from any cause
>
> **EXCLUDES 1**   congenital cerebral palsy (G80.-)
>   functional quadriplegia (R53.2)
>   hysterical paralysis (F44.4)

   ✓5ᵗʰ **G82.2 Paraplegia**

       Paralysis of both lower limbs NOS
       Paraparesis (lower) NOS
       Paraplegia (lower) NOS
       AHA: 2017,3Q,3

       G82.20 Paraplegia, unspecified   HCC ▽
       G82.21 Paraplegia, complete   HCC
       G82.22 Paraplegia, incomplete   HCC

   ✓5ᵗʰ **G82.5 Quadriplegia**

       G82.50 Quadriplegia, unspecified   HCC ▽
       G82.51 Quadriplegia, C1-C4 complete   HCC
       G82.52 Quadriplegia, C1-C4 incomplete   HCC
       G82.53 Quadriplegia, C5-C7 complete   HCC
       G82.54 Quadriplegia, C5-C7 incomplete   HCC

✓4ᵗʰ **G83 Other paralytic syndromes**

> **NOTE**   This category is to be used only when the listed conditions are reported without further specification, or are stated to be old or longstanding but of unspecified cause. The category is also for use in multiple coding to identify these conditions resulting from any cause.
>
> **INCLUDES**   paralysis (complete) (incomplete), except as in G80-G82

   G83.0 Diplegia of upper limbs   HCC
       Diplegia (upper)
       Paralysis of both upper limbs

   ✓5ᵗʰ **G83.1 Monoplegia of lower limb**

       Paralysis of lower limb
       EXCLUDES 1   monoplegia of lower limbs due to sequela of cerebrovascular disease (I69.04-, I69.14-, I69.24-, I69.34-, I69.84-, I69.94-)

       TIP: If the documentation specifies the affected side but not whether it is the dominant or nondominant side, the default is as follows: for ambidextrous patients, the default is dominant; when the left side is affected, the default is nondominant; and when the right side is affected, the default is dominant.

       G83.10 Monoplegia of lower limb affecting unspecified side   HCC ▽
       G83.11 Monoplegia of lower limb affecting right dominant side   HCC
       G83.12 Monoplegia of lower limb affecting left dominant side   HCC
       G83.13 Monoplegia of lower limb affecting right nondominant side   HCC
       G83.14 Monoplegia of lower limb affecting left nondominant side   HCC

   ✓5ᵗʰ **G83.2 Monoplegia of upper limb**

       Paralysis of upper limb
       EXCLUDES 1   monoplegia of upper limbs due to sequela of cerebrovascular disease (I69.03-, I69.13-, I69.23-, I69.33-, I69.83-, I69.93-)

       TIP: If the documentation specifies the affected side but not whether it is the dominant or nondominant side, the default is as follows: for ambidextrous patients, the default is dominant; when the left side is affected, the default is nondominant; and when the right side is affected, the default is dominant.

       G83.20 Monoplegia of upper limb affecting unspecified side   HCC ▽
       G83.21 Monoplegia of upper limb affecting right dominant side   HCC
       G83.22 Monoplegia of upper limb affecting left dominant side   HCC
       G83.23 Monoplegia of upper limb affecting right nondominant side   HCC
       G83.24 Monoplegia of upper limb affecting left nondominant side   HCC

   ✓5ᵗʰ **G83.3 Monoplegia, unspecified**

       TIP: If the documentation specifies the affected side but not whether it is the dominant or nondominant side, the default is as follows: for ambidextrous patients, the default is dominant; when the left side is affected, the default is nondominant; and when the right side is affected, the default is dominant.

       G83.30 Monoplegia, unspecified affecting unspecified side   HCC ▽
       G83.31 Monoplegia, unspecified affecting right dominant side   HCC ▽
       G83.32 Monoplegia, unspecified affecting left dominant side   HCC ▽
       G83.33 Monoplegia, unspecified affecting right nondominant side   HCC ▽
       G83.34 Monoplegia, unspecified affecting left nondominant side   HCC ▽

   G83.4 Cauda equina syndrome   HCC
       Neurogenic bladder due to cauda equina syndrome
       EXCLUDES 1   cord bladder NOS (G95.89)
                   neurogenic bladder NOS (N31.9)

       DEF: Compression of the spinal nerve roots presenting with pain and tingling radiating down the buttocks, back of the thigh and calf, and into the foot in a sciatic manner with aching in the bladder, perineum, and sacrum. Loss of bowel and bladder control may also occur.

   G83.5 Locked-in state   HCC

   ✓5ᵗʰ **G83.8 Other specified paralytic syndromes**

       EXCLUDES 1   paralytic syndromes due to current spinal cord injury - code to spinal cord injury (S14, S24, S34)

       G83.81 Brown-Séquard syndrome   HCC
       G83.82 Anterior cord syndrome   HCC
       G83.83 Posterior cord syndrome   HCC
       G83.84 Todd's paralysis (postepileptic)   HCC
       G83.89 Other specified paralytic syndromes   HCC

   G83.9 Paralytic syndrome, unspecified   HCC ▽

✔ Additional Character Req   ✓x7ᵗʰ Placeholder Alert   **Manifestation**   ▽ Unspecified   ▶◀ Revised Text   ● New Code   ▲ Revised Code Title

Other disorders of the nervous system (G89-G99)

✓4ᵗʰ G89   Pain, not elsewhere classified

Code also related psychological factors associated with pain (F45.42)

EXCLUDES 1   generalized pain NOS (R52)

pain disorders exclusively related to psychological factors (F45.41)

pain NOS (R52)

EXCLUDES 2   atypical face pain (G50.1)

headache syndromes (G44.-)

localized pain, unspecified type - code to pain by site, such as:

abdomen pain (R10.-)

back pain (M54.9)

breast pain (N64.4)

chest pain (R07.1-R07.9)

ear pain (H92.0-)

eye pain (H57.1)

headache (R51)

joint pain (M25.5-)

limb pain (M79.6-)

lumbar region pain (M54.5)

painful urination (R30.9)

pelvic and perineal pain (R10.2)

renal colic (N23)

shoulder pain (M25.51-)

spine pain (M54.-)

throat pain (R07.0)

tongue pain (K14.6)

tooth pain (K08.8)

migraines (G43.-)

myalgia ▶(M79.1-)◀

pain from prosthetic devices, implants, and grafts (T82.84, T83.84, T84.84, T85.84-)

phantom limb syndrome with pain (G54.6)

vulvar vestibulitis (N94.810)

vulvodynia (N94.81-)

G89.0   Central pain syndrome

Déjérine-Roussy syndrome

Myelopathic pain syndrome

Thalamic pain syndrome (hyperesthetic)

✓5ᵗʰ G89.1   Acute pain, not elsewhere classified

G89.11   Acute pain due to trauma

G89.12   Acute post-thoracotomy pain

Post-thoracotomy pain NOS

G89.18   Other acute postprocedural pain

Postoperative pain NOS

Postprocedural pain NOS

✓5ᵗʰ G89.2   Chronic pain, not elsewhere classified

EXCLUDES 1   causalgia, lower limb (G57.7-)

causalgia, upper limb (G56.4-)

central pain syndrome (G89.0)

chronic pain syndrome (G89.4)

complex regional pain syndrome II, lower limb (G57.7-)

complex regional pain syndrome II, upper limb (G56.4-)

neoplasm related chronic pain (G89.3)

reflex sympathetic dystrophy (G90.5-)

G89.21   Chronic pain due to trauma

G89.22   Chronic post-thoracotomy pain

G89.28   Other chronic postprocedural pain

Other chronic postoperative pain

G89.29   Other chronic pain

G89.3   Neoplasm related pain (acute) (chronic)

Cancer associated pain

Pain due to malignancy (primary) (secondary)

Tumor associated pain

G89.4   Chronic pain syndrome

Chronic pain associated with significant psychosocial dysfunction

✓4ᵗʰ G90   Disorders of autonomic nervous system

EXCLUDES 1   dysfunction of the autonomic nervous system due to alcohol (G31.2)

✓5ᵗʰ G90.0   Idiopathic peripheral autonomic neuropathy

G90.01   Carotid sinus syncope

Carotid sinus syndrome

DEF: Vagal activation caused by pressure on the carotid sinus baroreceptors. Sympathetic nerve impulses may cause sinus arrest or AV block.

G90.09   Other idiopathic peripheral autonomic neuropathy

Idiopathic peripheral autonomic neuropathy NOS

G90.1   Familial dysautonomia [Riley-Day]   HCC

G90.2   Horner's syndrome

Bernard(-Horner) syndrome

Cervical sympathetic dystrophy or paralysis

G90.3   Multi-system degeneration of the autonomic nervous system   HCC

Neurogenic orthostatic hypotension [Shy-Drager]

EXCLUDES 1   orthostatic hypotension NOS (I95.1)

G90.4   Autonomic dysreflexia

Use additional code to identify the cause, such as:

fecal impaction (K56.41)

pressure ulcer (pressure area) (L89.-)

urinary tract infection (N39.0)

✓5ᵗʰ G90.5   Complex regional pain syndrome I (CRPS I)

Reflex sympathetic dystrophy

EXCLUDES 1   causalgia of lower limb (G57.7-)

causalgia of upper limb (G56.4-)

complex regional pain syndrome II of lower limb (G57.7-)

complex regional pain syndrome II of upper limb (G56.4-)

G90.50   Complex regional pain syndrome I, unspecified   ▽

✓6ᵗʰ G90.51   Complex regional pain syndrome I of upper limb

G90.511   Complex regional pain syndrome I of right upper limb

G90.512   Complex regional pain syndrome I of left upper limb

G90.513   Complex regional pain syndrome I of upper limb, bilateral

G90.519   Complex regional pain syndrome I of unspecified upper limb   ▽

✓6ᵗʰ G90.52   Complex regional pain syndrome I of lower limb

G90.521   Complex regional pain syndrome I of right lower limb

G90.522   Complex regional pain syndrome I of left lower limb

G90.523   Complex regional pain syndrome I of lower limb, bilateral

G90.529   Complex regional pain syndrome I of unspecified lower limb   ▽

G90.59   Complex regional pain syndrome I of other specified site

G90.8   Other disorders of autonomic nervous system

G90.9   Disorder of the autonomic nervous system, unspecified   ▽

√4ᵗʰ G91 Hercephalus

> INCLUDES   acquired hydrocephalus
> EXCLUDES 1   *Arnold-Chiari syndrome with hydrocephalus (Q07.-)*
> *congenital hydrocephalus (Q03.-)*
> *spina bifida with hydrocephalus (Q05.-)*

Hydrocephalus (Acquired)

Normal ventricles   Hydrocephalic ventricles

G91.0 Communicating hydrocephalus
> Secondary normal pressure hydrocephalus

G91.1 Obstructive hydrocephalus
> **DEF:** Obstruction of the cerebrospinal fluid passage from the brain into the spinal canal characterized by headaches, drowsiness, poor coordination, urinary incontinence, nausea, vomiting, and papilledema.

G91.2 (Idiopathic) normal pressure hydrocephalus
> Normal pressure hydrocephalus NOS

G91.3 Post-traumatic hydrocephalus, unspecified   ▽

G91.4 *Hydrocephalus in diseases classified elsewhere*
> Code first underlying condition, such as:
> congenital syphilis (A50.4-)
> neoplasm (C00-D49)
> ▶plasminogen deficiency (E88.02)◀
> EXCLUDES 1   *hydrocephalus due to congenital toxoplasmosis (P37.1)*
> **AHA:** 2014,3Q,3

G91.8 Other hydrocephalus
G91.9 Hydrocephalus, unspecified   ▽

G92 Toxic encephalopathy
> Toxic encephalitis
> Toxic metabolic encephalopathy
> Code first, if applicable, drug induced (T36-T50)
> Code first (T51-T65) to identify toxic agent
> **AHA:** 2017,1Q,39-40
> **DEF:** Brain tissue degeneration due to a toxic substance.

√4ᵗʰ G93 Other disorders of brain

G93.0 Cerebral cysts
> Arachnoid cyst
> Porencephalic cyst, acquired
> EXCLUDES 1   *acquired periventricular cysts of newborn (P91.1)*
> *congenital cerebral cysts (Q04.6)*

G93.1 Anoxic brain damage, not elsewhere classified   HCC
> EXCLUDES 1   *cerebral anoxia due to anesthesia during labor and delivery (O74.3)*
> *cerebral anoxia due to anesthesia during the puerperium (O89.2)*
> *neonatal anoxia (P84)*
> **DEF:** Brain injury not resulting from birth trauma that is due to lack of oxygen. Brain cells, when deprived of oxygen; begin to expire after 4 minutes.

G93.2 Benign intracranial hypertension
> EXCLUDES 1   *hypertensive encephalopathy (I67.4)*

G93.3 Postviral fatigue syndrome
> Benign myalgic encephalomyelitis
> EXCLUDES 1   *chronic fatigue syndrome NOS (R53.82)*

√5ᵗʰ G93.4 Other and unspecified encephalopathy
> EXCLUDES 1   *alcoholic encephalopathy (G31.2)*
> *encephalopathy in diseases classified elsewhere (G94)*
> *hypertensive encephalopathy (I67.4)*
> *toxic (metabolic) encephalopathy (G92)*

G93.40 Encephalopathy, unspecified   ▽
> **AHA:** 2017,2Q,8

G93.41 Metabolic encephalopathy
> Septic encephalopathy
> **AHA:** 2017,2Q,8; 2016,3Q,42; 2015,3Q,21
> **TIP:** Assign separately when documented with diabetic hypoglycemia (E08.649, E09.649, E10.649, E11.649, E13.649).

G93.49 Other encephalopathy
> Encephalopathy NEC
> **AHA:** 2018,2Q,22,24; 2017,2Q,9

G93.5 Compression of brain   HCC
> Arnold-Chiari type 1 compression of brain
> Compression of brain (stem)
> Herniation of brain (stem)
> EXCLUDES 1   *diffuse traumatic compression of brain (S06.2-)*
> *focal traumatic compression of brain (S06.3-)*

G93.6 Cerebral edema   HCC
> EXCLUDES 1   *cerebral edema due to birth injury (P11.0)*
> *traumatic cerebral edema (S06.1-)*

G93.7 Reye's syndrome   P
> Code first poisoning due to salicylates, if applicable (T39.0-, with sixth character 1-4)
> Use additional code for adverse effect due to salicylates, if applicable (T39.0-, with sixth character 5)
> **DEF:** Rare childhood illness often developed after a viral upper respiratory infection. Symptoms include vomiting, elevated serum transaminase, brain swelling, disturbances of consciousness, seizures, and changes in liver and other viscera and it can be fatal.

√5ᵗʰ G93.8 Other specified disorders of brain

G93.81 Temporal sclerosis
> Hippocampal sclerosis
> Mesial temporal sclerosis

G93.82 Brain death
G93.89 Other specified disorders of brain
> Postradiation encephalopathy

G93.9 Disorder of brain, unspecified   ▽

G94 *Other disorders of brain in diseases classified elsewhere*
> Code first underlying disease
> EXCLUDES 1   *encephalopathy in congenital syphilis (A50.49)*
> *encephalopathy in influenza (J09.X9, J10.81, J11.81)*
> *encephalopathy in syphilis (A52.19)*
> *hydrocephalus in diseases classified elsewhere (G91.4)*
> **AHA:** 2018,2Q,22; 2017,2Q,8-9

√4ᵗʰ G95 Other and unspecified diseases of spinal cord
> EXCLUDES 2   *myelitis (G04.-)*

G95.0 Syringomyelia and syringobulbia   HCC

√5ᵗʰ G95.1 Vascular myelopathies
> EXCLUDES 2   *intraspinal phlebitis and thrombophlebitis, except non-pyogenic (G08)*

G95.11 Acute infarction of spinal cord (embolic) (nonembolic)   HCC
> Anoxia of spinal cord
> Arterial thrombosis of spinal cord

G95.19 Other vascular myelopathies   HCC
> Edema of spinal cord
> Hematomyelia
> Nonpyogenic intraspinal phlebitis and thrombophlebitis
> Subacute necrotic myelopathy

√5ᵗʰ G95.2 Other and unspecified cord compression

G95.20 Unspecified cord compression   HCC ▽
G95.29 Other cord compression   HCC

√5ᵗʰ G95.8 Other specified diseases of spinal cord
> EXCLUDES 1   *neurogenic bladder NOS (N31.9)*
> *neurogenic bladder due to cauda equina syndrome (G83.4)*
> *neuromuscular dysfunction of bladder without spinal cord lesion (N31.-)*

G95.81 Conus medullaris syndrome   HCC

☑ Additional Character Req   √x7ᵗʰ Placeholder Alert   Manifestation   ▽ Unspecified   ▶◀ Revised Text   ● New Code   ▲ Revised Code Title

G95.89   **Other specified diseases of spinal cord**   HCC
Cord bladder NOS
Drug-induced myelopathy
Radiation-induced myelopathy
EXCLUDES 1   *myelopathy NOS (G95.9)*

G95.9   **Disease of spinal cord, unspecified**   HCC ▽
Myelopathy NOS

✓4ᵗʰ **G96**   **Other disorders of central nervous system**

G96.0   **Cerebrospinal fluid leak**
EXCLUDES 1   *cerebrospinal fluid leak from spinal puncture (G97.0)*
AHA: 2018,2Q,13
DEF: Cerebrospinal fluid discharging from the nose or the ear caused by a fracture of the frontal bone with tearing of dura mater and arachnoid. It is characterized by watery drainage usually from only one side of the nose or one ear, headache, vision changes, and hearing loss.

✓5ᵗʰ **G96.1**   **Disorders of meninges, not elsewhere classified**

G96.11   **Dural tear**
EXCLUDES 1   *accidental puncture or laceration of dura during a procedure (G97.41)*
AHA: 2014,4Q,24

G96.12   **Meningeal adhesions (cerebral) (spinal)**

G96.19   **Other disorders of meninges, not elsewhere classified**

G96.8   **Other specified disorders of central nervous system**

G96.9   **Disorder of central nervous system, unspecified**   ▽

✓4ᵗʰ **G97**   **Intraoperative and postprocedural complications and disorders of nervous system, not elsewhere classified**
EXCLUDES 2   *intraoperative and postprocedural cerebrovascular infarction (I97.81-, I97.82-)*
AHA: 2016,4Q,9-10

G97.0   **Cerebrospinal fluid leak from spinal puncture**

Spinal Puncture

Spinal cord
Epidural space
Subarachnoid space
Vertebra
Spinal needle

Lumbar area

G97.1   **Other reaction to spinal and lumbar puncture**
Headache due to lumbar puncture

G97.2   **Intracranial hypotension following ventricular shunting**

✓5ᵗʰ **G97.3**   **Intraoperative hemorrhage and hematoma of a nervous system organ or structure complicating a procedure**
EXCLUDES 1   *intraoperative hemorrhage and hematoma of a nervous system organ or structure due to accidental puncture and laceration during a procedure (G97.4-)*

G97.31   **Intraoperative hemorrhage and hematoma of a nervous system organ or structure complicating a nervous system procedure**

G97.32   **Intraoperative hemorrhage and hematoma of a nervous system organ or structure complicating other procedure**

✓5ᵗʰ **G97.4**   **Accidental puncture and laceration of a nervous system organ or structure during a procedure**

G97.41   **Accidental puncture or laceration of dura during a procedure**
Incidental (inadvertent) durotomy
AHA: 2014,4Q,24

G97.48   **Accidental puncture and laceration of other nervous system organ or structure during a nervous system procedure**

G97.49   **Accidental puncture and laceration of other nervous system organ or structure during other procedure**

✓5ᵗʰ **G97.5**   **Postprocedural hemorrhage of a nervous system organ or structure following a procedure**

G97.51   **Postprocedural hemorrhage of a nervous system organ or structure following a nervous system procedure**

G97.52   **Postprocedural hemorrhage of a nervous system organ or structure following other procedure**

✓5ᵗʰ **G97.6**   **Postprocedural hematoma and seroma of a nervous system organ or structure following a procedure**

G97.61   **Postprocedural hematoma of a nervous system organ or structure following a nervous system procedure**

G97.62   **Postprocedural hematoma of a nervous system organ or structure following other procedure**

G97.63   **Postprocedural seroma of a nervous system organ or structure following a nervous system procedure**

G97.64   **Postprocedural seroma of a nervous system organ or structure following other procedure**

✓5ᵗʰ **G97.8**   **Other intraoperative and postprocedural complications and disorders of nervous system**
Use additional code to further specify disorder

G97.81   **Other intraoperative complications of nervous system**

G97.82   **Other postprocedural complications and disorders of nervous system**

✓4ᵗʰ **G98**   **Other disorders of nervous system not elsewhere classified**
INCLUDES   nervous system disorder NOS

G98.0   **Neurogenic arthritis, not elsewhere classified**
Nonsyphilitic neurogenic arthropathy NEC
Nonsyphilitic neurogenic spondylopathy NEC
EXCLUDES 1   *spondylopathy (in):*
     syringomyelia and syringobulbia (G95.0)
     tabes dorsalis (A52.11)

G98.8   **Other disorders of nervous system**
Nervous system disorder NOS

✓4ᵗʰ **G99**   **Other disorders of nervous system in diseases classified elsewhere**

G99.0   *Autonomic neuropathy in diseases classified elsewhere*
Code first underlying disease, such as:
amyloidosis (E85.-)
gout (M1A.-, M10.-)
hyperthyroidism (E05.-)
EXCLUDES 1   *diabetic autonomic neuropathy (E08-E13 with .43)*

G99.2   *Myelopathy in diseases classified elsewhere*   HCC
Code first underlying disease, such as:
neoplasm (C00-D49)
EXCLUDES 1   *myelopathy in:*
     intervertebral disease (M50.0-, M51.0-)
     spondylosis (M47.0-, M47.1-)

G99.8   *Other specified disorders of nervous system in diseases classified elsewhere*
Code first underlying disorder, such as:
amyloidosis (E85.-)
avitaminosis (E56.9)
EXCLUDES 1   *nervous system involvement in:*
     cysticercosis (B69.0)
     rubella (B06.0-)
     syphilis (A52.1-)

Chapter 7. Diseases of the Eye and Adnexa (H00–H59)

Chapter Specific Guidelines with Coding Examples

The chapter specific guidelines from the ICD-10-CM Official Guidelines for Coding and Reporting have been provided below. Along with these guidelines are coding examples, contained in the shaded boxes, that have been developed to help illustrate the coding and/or sequencing guidance found in these guidelines.

a. Glaucoma

1) Assigning glaucoma codes

Assign as many codes from category H40, Glaucoma, as needed to identify the type of glaucoma, the affected eye, and the glaucoma stage.

2) Bilateral glaucoma with same type and stage

When a patient has bilateral glaucoma and both eyes are documented as being the same type and stage, and there is a code for bilateral glaucoma, report only the code for the type of glaucoma, bilateral, with the seventh character for the stage.

> Bilateral mild stage primary open-angle glaucoma
>
> **H40.1131   Primary open-angle glaucoma, bilateral, mild stage**
>
> *Explanation*: In this scenario, the patient has the same type and stage of glaucoma in both eyes. As this type of glaucoma has a code for bilateral, assign only the code for the bilateral glaucoma with the seventh character for the stage.

When a patient has bilateral glaucoma and both eyes are documented as being the same type and stage, and the classification does not provide a code for bilateral glaucoma (i.e. subcategories H40.10 and H40.20) report only one code for the type of glaucoma with the appropriate seventh character for the stage.

> Bilateral open-angle glaucoma, severe stage; not specified as to type
>
> **H40.10X3   Unspecified open-angle glaucoma, severe stage**
>
> *Explanation*: In this scenario, the patient has glaucoma of the same type and stage of both eyes, but there is no code specifically for bilateral glaucoma. Only one code is assigned with the appropriate seventh character for the stage.

3) Bilateral glaucoma stage with different types or stages

When a patient has bilateral glaucoma and each eye is documented as having a different type or stage, and the classification distinguishes laterality, assign the appropriate code for each eye rather than the code for bilateral glaucoma.

> Bilateral chronic angle-closure glaucoma; right eye is documented as mild stage and left eye as moderate stage
>
> **H40.2211   Chronic angle-closure glaucoma, right eye, mild stage**
>
> **H40.2222   Chronic angle-closure glaucoma, left eye, moderate stage**
>
> *Explanation*: In this scenario the patient has the same type of glaucoma in both eyes, but each eye is at a different stage. Because the subcategory for this condition identifies laterality, one code is assigned for the right eye and one code is assigned for the left eye, each with the appropriate seventh character for the stage appended.

When a patient has bilateral glaucoma and each eye is documented as having a different type, and the classification does not distinguish laterality (i.e. subcategories H40.10 and H40.20), assign one code for each type of glaucoma with the appropriate seventh character for the stage.

> Documentation relates mild, unspecified primary angle-closure glaucoma of the left eye with mild unspecified open-angle glaucoma of the right eye
>
> **H40.20X1   Unspecified primary angle-closure glaucoma, mild stage**
>
> **H40.10X1   Unspecified open-angle glaucoma, mild stage**
>
> *Explanation*: In this scenario the patient has a different type of glaucoma in each eye and the classification does not distinguish laterality. A code for each type of glaucoma is assigned, each with the appropriate seventh character for the stage.

When a patient has bilateral glaucoma and each eye is documented as having the same type, but different stage, and the classification does not distinguish laterality (i.e. subcategories H40.10 and H40.20), assign a code for the type of glaucoma for each eye with the seventh character for the specific glaucoma stage documented for each eye.

> Bilateral open-angle glaucoma, not specified as to type; the right eye is documented to be in mild stage and the left eye as being in moderate stage
>
> **H40.10X1   Unspecified open-angle glaucoma, mild stage**
>
> **H40.10X2   Unspecified open-angle glaucoma, moderate stage**
>
> *Explanation*: In this scenario the patient has the same type of glaucoma in each eye but each eye is at a different stage, and the classification does not distinguish laterality at this subcategory level. Two codes are assigned; both codes represent the same type of glaucoma but each has a different seventh character identifying the appropriate stage for each eye.

4) Patient admitted with glaucoma and stage evolves during the admission

If a patient is admitted with glaucoma and the stage progresses during the admission, assign the code for highest stage documented.

5) Indeterminate stage glaucoma

Assignment of the seventh character "4" for "indeterminate stage" should be based on the clinical documentation. The seventh character "4" is used for glaucomas whose stage cannot be clinically determined. This seventh character should not be confused with the seventh character "0", unspecified, which should be assigned when there is no documentation regarding the stage of the glaucoma.

b. Blindness

If "blindness" or "low vision" of both eyes is documented but the visual impairment category is not documented, assign code H54.3, Unqualified visual loss, both eyes. If "blindness" or "low vision" in one eye is documented but the visual impairment category is not documented, assign a code from H54.6-, Unqualified visual loss, one eye. If "blindness" or "visual loss" is documented without any information about whether one or both eyes are affected, assign code H54.7, Unspecified visual loss.

> Patient assessment indicates moderately impaired/low vision in the left eye with no visual impairments in the right eye
>
> **H54.62   Unqualified visual loss, left eye, normal vision right eye**
>
> Report unqualified visual loss when the visual impairment category is not specified. In this case, only the left eye is impacted by visual loss with normal vision of the right eye documented.

Chapter 7. Diseases of the Eye and Adnexa

Chapter 7. Diseases of the Eye and Adnexa (H00-H59)

NOTE   Use an external cause code following the code for the eye condition, if applicable, to identify the cause of the eye condition.

EXCLUDES 2   certain conditions originating in the perinatal period (P04-P96)
certain infectious and parasitic diseases (A00-B99)
complications of pregnancy, childbirth and the puerperium (O00-O9A)
congenital malformations, deformations, and chromosomal abnormalities (Q00-Q99)
diabetes mellitus related eye conditions (E09.3-, E10.3-, E11.3-, E13.3-)
endocrine, nutritional and metabolic diseases (E00-E88)
injury (trauma) of eye and orbit (S05.-)
injury, poisoning and certain other consequences of external causes (S00-T88)
neoplasms (C00-D49)
symptoms, signs and abnormal clinical and laboratory findings, not elsewhere classified (R00-R94)
syphilis related eye disorders (A50.01, A50.3-, A51.43, A52.71)

This chapter contains the following blocks:
H00-H05   Disorders of eyelid, lacrimal system and orbit
H10-H11   Disorders of conjunctiva
H15-H22   Disorders of sclera, cornea, iris and ciliary body
H25-H28   Disorders of lens
H30-H36   Disorders of choroid and retina
H40-H42   Glaucoma
H43-H44   Disorders of vitreous body and globe
H46-H47   Disorders of optic nerve and visual pathways
H49-H52   Disorders of ocular muscles, binocular movement, accommodation and refraction
H53-H54   Visual disturbances and blindness
H55-H57   Other disorders of eye and adnexa
H59   Intraoperative and postprocedural complications and disorders of eye and adnexa, not elsewhere classified

Disorders of eyelid, lacrimal system and orbit (H00-H05)

EXCLUDES 2   open wound of eyelid (S01.1-)
superficial injury of eyelid (S00.1-, S00.2-)

✓4ᵗʰ **H00   Hordeolum and chalazion**

   ✓5ᵗʰ **H00.0   Hordeolum (externum) (internum) of eyelid**

      DEF: Acute localized infection of the gland of Zeis (external hordeolum) or Molt or of the meibomian glands (internal hordeolum) of the orbit.

     ✓6ᵗʰ **H00.01   Hordeolum externum**

       Hordeolum NOS
       Stye

       H00.011   Hordeolum externum right upper eyelid
       H00.012   Hordeolum externum right lower eyelid
       H00.013   Hordeolum externum right eye, unspecified eyelid ▽
       H00.014   Hordeolum externum left upper eyelid
       H00.015   Hordeolum externum left lower eyelid
       H00.016   Hordeolum externum left eye, unspecified eyelid ▽
       H00.019   Hordeolum externum unspecified eye, unspecified eyelid ▽

     ✓6ᵗʰ **H00.02   Hordeolum internum**

       Infection of meibomian gland

       H00.021   Hordeolum internum right upper eyelid
       H00.022   Hordeolum internum right lower eyelid
       H00.023   Hordeolum internum right eye, unspecified eyelid ▽
       H00.024   Hordeolum internum left upper eyelid
       H00.025   Hordeolum internum left lower eyelid
       H00.026   Hordeolum internum left eye, unspecified eyelid ▽
       H00.029   Hordeolum internum unspecified eye, unspecified eyelid ▽

     ✓6ᵗʰ **H00.03   Abscess of eyelid**

       Furuncle of eyelid

       H00.031   Abscess of right upper eyelid
       H00.032   Abscess of right lower eyelid
       H00.033   Abscess of eyelid right eye, unspecified eyelid ▽
       H00.034   Abscess of left upper eyelid
       H00.035   Abscess of left lower eyelid
       H00.036   Abscess of eyelid left eye, unspecified eyelid ▽
       H00.039   Abscess of eyelid unspecified eye, unspecified eyelid ▽

✓5ᵗʰ **H00.1   Chalazion**

   Meibomian (gland) cyst

   EXCLUDES 2   infected meibomian gland (H00.02-)

   DEF: Noninfectious, obstructive mass in the oil gland of the eyelid that results in a small chronic lump or inflammation.

   H00.11   Chalazion right upper eyelid
   H00.12   Chalazion right lower eyelid
   H00.13   Chalazion right eye, unspecified eyelid ▽
   H00.14   Chalazion left upper eyelid
   H00.15   Chalazion left lower eyelid
   H00.16   Chalazion left eye, unspecified eyelid ▽
   H00.19   Chalazion unspecified eye, unspecified eyelid ▽

✓4ᵗʰ **H01   Other inflammation of eyelid**

   ✓5ᵗʰ **H01.0   Blepharitis**

     EXCLUDES 1   blepharoconjunctivitis (H10.5-)

     ✓6ᵗʰ **H01.00   Unspecified blepharitis**

       H01.001   Unspecified blepharitis right upper eyelid ▽
       H01.002   Unspecified blepharitis right lower eyelid ▽
       H01.003   Unspecified blepharitis right eye, unspecified eyelid ▽
       H01.004   Unspecified blepharitis left upper eyelid ▽
       H01.005   Unspecified blepharitis left lower eyelid ▽
       H01.006   Unspecified blepharitis left eye, unspecified eyelid ▽
       H01.009   Unspecified blepharitis unspecified eye, unspecified eyelid ▽
●   H01.00A   Unspecified blepharitis right eye, upper and lower eyelids ▽
●   H01.00B   Unspecified blepharitis left eye, upper and lower eyelids ▽

     ✓6ᵗʰ **H01.01   Ulcerative blepharitis**

       H01.011   Ulcerative blepharitis right upper eyelid
       H01.012   Ulcerative blepharitis right lower eyelid
       H01.013   Ulcerative blepharitis right eye, unspecified eyelid ▽
       H01.014   Ulcerative blepharitis left upper eyelid
       H01.015   Ulcerative blepharitis left lower eyelid
       H01.016   Ulcerative blepharitis left eye, unspecified eyelid ▽
       H01.019   Ulcerative blepharitis unspecified eye, unspecified eyelid ▽
●   H01.01A   Ulcerative blepharitis right eye, upper and lower eyelids
●   H01.01B   Ulcerative blepharitis left eye, upper and lower eyelids

     ✓6ᵗʰ **H01.02   Squamous blepharitis**

       H01.021   Squamous blepharitis right upper eyelid
       H01.022   Squamous blepharitis right lower eyelid
       H01.023   Squamous blepharitis right eye, unspecified eyelid
       H01.024   Squamous blepharitis left upper eyelid
       H01.025   Squamous blepharitis left lower eyelid
       H01.026   Squamous blepharitis left eye, unspecified eyelid ▽
       H01.029   Squamous blepharitis unspecified eye, unspecified eyelid ▽
●   H01.02A   Squamous blepharitis right eye, upper and lower eyelids
●   H01.02B   Squamous blepharitis left eye, upper and lower eyelids

   ✓5ᵗʰ **H01.1   Noninfectious dermatoses of eyelid**

     ✓6ᵗʰ **H01.11   Allergic dermatitis of eyelid**

       Contact dermatitis of eyelid

       H01.111   Allergic dermatitis of right upper eyelid
       H01.112   Allergic dermatitis of right lower eyelid
       H01.113   Allergic dermatitis of right eye, unspecified eyelid ▽
       H01.114   Allergic dermatitis of left upper eyelid
       H01.115   Allergic dermatitis of left lower eyelid
       H01.116   Allergic dermatitis of left eye, unspecified eyelid ▽
       H01.119   Allergic dermatitis of unspecified eye, unspecified eyelid ▽

√6ᵗʰ **H01.12** **Discoid lupus erythematosus of eyelid**

    H01.121 **Discoid lupus erythematosus of** right upper **eyelid**

    H01.122 **Discoid lupus erythematosus of** right lower **eyelid**

    H01.123 **Discoid lupus erythematosus of** right eye, unspecified eyelid ▽

    H01.124 **Discoid lupus erythematosus of** left upper eyelid

    H01.125 **Discoid lupus erythematosus of** left lower eyelid

    H01.126 **Discoid lupus erythematosus of** left eye, unspecified eyelid ▽

    H01.129 **Discoid lupus erythematosus of unspecified eye, unspecified eyelid** ▽

√6ᵗʰ **H01.13** **Eczematous dermatitis of eyelid**

    H01.131 **Eczematous dermatitis of** right upper eyelid

    H01.132 **Eczematous dermatitis of** right lower eyelid

    H01.133 **Eczematous dermatitis of** right eye, unspecified eyelid ▽

    H01.134 **Eczematous dermatitis of** left upper eyelid

    H01.135 **Eczematous dermatitis of** left lower eyelid

    H01.136 **Eczematous dermatitis of** left eye, unspecified eyelid ▽

    H01.139 **Eczematous dermatitis of unspecified eye, unspecified eyelid** ▽

√6ᵗʰ **H01.14** **Xeroderma of eyelid**

    H01.141 **Xeroderma of** right upper **eyelid**

    H01.142 **Xeroderma of** right lower **eyelid**

    H01.143 **Xeroderma of** right eye, unspecified eyelid ▽

    H01.144 **Xeroderma of** left upper **eyelid**

    H01.145 **Xeroderma of** left lower **eyelid**

    H01.146 **Xeroderma of** left eye, unspecified eyelid ▽

    H01.149 **Xeroderma of unspecified eye, unspecified eyelid** ▽

H01.8 **Other specified inflammations of eyelid**

H01.9 **Unspecified inflammation of eyelid** ▽

    Inflammation of eyelid NOS

√4ᵗʰ **H02** **Other disorders of eyelid**

    EXCLUDES 1   congenital malformations of eyelid (Q10.0-Q10.3)

Entropion and Ectropion

Normal eyelid   Entropion   Ectropion

√5ᵗʰ **H02.0** **Entropion and trichiasis of eyelid**

    DEF: Entropion: Inversion of the eyelid, turning the edge in toward the eyeball and causing irritation from contact of the lashes with the surface of the eye.

    DEF: Trichiasis: Condition wherein the eyelid is in a normal position but lashes are ingrown or misdirected in their growth so that they irritate the tissues of the eye.

√6ᵗʰ **H02.00** **Unspecified entropion of eyelid**

    H02.001 **Unspecified entropion of** right upper **eyelid** ▽

    H02.002 **Unspecified entropion of** right lower **eyelid** ▽

    H02.003 **Unspecified entropion of** right eye, unspecified eyelid ▽

    H02.004 **Unspecified entropion of** left upper **eyelid**

    H02.005 **Unspecified entropion of** left lower eyelid ▽

    H02.006 **Unspecified entropion of** left eye, unspecified eyelid ▽

    H02.009 **Unspecified entropion of unspecified eye, unspecified eyelid** ▽

√6ᵗʰ **H02.01** **Cicatricial entropion of eyelid**

    H02.011 **Cicatricial entropion of** right upper **eyelid**

    H02.012 **Cicatricial entropion of** right lower **eyelid**

    H02.013 **Cicatricial entropion of** right eye, unspecified eyelid ▽

    H02.014 **Cicatricial entropion of** left upper **eyelid**

    H02.015 **Cicatricial entropion of** left lower **eyelid**

    H02.016 **Cicatricial entropion of** left eye, unspecified eyelid ▽

    H02.019 **Cicatricial entropion of unspecified eye, unspecified eyelid** ▽

√6ᵗʰ **H02.02** **Mechanical entropion of eyelid**

    H02.021 **Mechanical entropion of** right upper **eyelid**

    H02.022 **Mechanical entropion of** right lower **eyelid**

    H02.023 **Mechanical entropion of** right eye, unspecified eyelid ▽

    H02.024 **Mechanical entropion of** left upper **eyelid**

    H02.025 **Mechanical entropion of** left lower **eyelid**

    H02.026 **Mechanical entropion of** left eye, unspecified eyelid ▽

    H02.029 **Mechanical entropion of unspecified eye, unspecified eyelid** ▽

√6ᵗʰ **H02.03** **Senile entropion of eyelid**

    H02.031 **Senile entropion of** right upper **eyelid** 🅐

    H02.032 **Senile entropion of** right lower **eyelid** 🅐

    H02.033 **Senile entropion of** right eye, unspecified eyelid 🅐 ▽

    H02.034 **Senile entropion of** left upper **eyelid** 🅐

    H02.035 **Senile entropion of** left lower **eyelid** 🅐

    H02.036 **Senile entropion of** left eye, unspecified eyelid 🅐 ▽

    H02.039 **Senile entropion of unspecified eye, unspecified eyelid** 🅐 ▽

√6ᵗʰ **H02.04** **Spastic entropion of eyelid**

    H02.041 **Spastic entropion of** right upper **eyelid**

    H02.042 **Spastic entropion of** right lower **eyelid**

    H02.043 **Spastic entropion of** right eye, unspecified eyelid ▽

    H02.044 **Spastic entropion of** left upper **eyelid**

    H02.045 **Spastic entropion of** left lower **eyelid**

    H02.046 **Spastic entropion of** left eye, unspecified eyelid ▽

    H02.049 **Spastic entropion of unspecified eye, unspecified eyelid** ▽

√6ᵗʰ **H02.05** **Trichiasis without entropion**

    H02.051 **Trichiasis without entropion** right upper eyelid

    H02.052 **Trichiasis without entropion** right lower eyelid

    H02.053 **Trichiasis without entropion** right eye, unspecified eyelid ▽

    H02.054 **Trichiasis without entropion** left upper eyelid

    H02.055 **Trichiasis without entropion** left lower eyelid

    H02.056 **Trichiasis without entropion** left eye, unspecified eyelid ▽

    H02.059 **Trichiasis without entropion unspecified eye, unspecified eyelid** ▽

✔ Additional Character Req   √x7ᵗʰ Placeholder Alert   Manifestation   ▽ Unspecified   ►◄ Revised Text   ● New Code   🔺 Revised Code Title

ICD-10-CM 2019   583

Chapter 7. Diseases of the Eye and Adnexa

✓5ᵗʰ **H02.1 Ectropion of eyelid**

> **DEF:** Drooping of the lower eyelid away from the eye or outward turning or eversion of the edge of the eyelid, exposing the palpebral conjunctiva and causing irritation.

✓6ᵗʰ **H02.10 Unspecified ectropion of eyelid**

- H02.101 Unspecified ectropion of right upper eyelid ▽
- H02.102 Unspecified ectropion of right lower eyelid ▽
- H02.103 Unspecified ectropion of right eye, unspecified eyelid ▽
- H02.104 Unspecified ectropion of left upper eyelid ▽
- H02.105 Unspecified ectropion of left lower eyelid ▽
- H02.106 Unspecified ectropion of left eye, unspecified eyelid ▽
- H02.109 Unspecified ectropion of unspecified eye, unspecified eyelid ▽

✓6ᵗʰ **H02.11 Cicatricial ectropion of eyelid**

- H02.111 Cicatricial ectropion of right upper eyelid
- H02.112 Cicatricial ectropion of right lower eyelid
- H02.113 Cicatricial ectropion of right eye, unspecified eyelid ▽
- H02.114 Cicatricial ectropion of left upper eyelid
- H02.115 Cicatricial ectropion of left lower eyelid
- H02.116 Cicatricial ectropion of left eye, unspecified eyelid ▽
- H02.119 Cicatricial ectropion of unspecified eye, unspecified eyelid ▽

✓6ᵗʰ **H02.12 Mechanical ectropion of eyelid**

- H02.121 Mechanical ectropion of right upper eyelid
- H02.122 Mechanical ectropion of right lower eyelid
- H02.123 Mechanical ectropion of right eye, unspecified eyelid ▽
- H02.124 Mechanical ectropion of left upper eyelid
- H02.125 Mechanical ectropion of left lower eyelid
- H02.126 Mechanical ectropion of left eye, unspecified eyelid ▽
- H02.129 Mechanical ectropion of unspecified eye, unspecified eyelid ▽

✓6ᵗʰ **H02.13 Senile ectropion of eyelid**

- H02.131 Senile ectropion of right upper eyelid 🅐
- H02.132 Senile ectropion of right lower eyelid 🅐
- H02.133 Senile ectropion of right eye, unspecified eyelid 🅐 ▽
- H02.134 Senile ectropion of left upper eyelid 🅐
- H02.135 Senile ectropion of left lower eyelid 🅐
- H02.136 Senile ectropion of left eye, unspecified eyelid 🅐 ▽
- H02.139 Senile ectropion of unspecified eye, unspecified eyelid 🅐 ▽

✓6ᵗʰ **H02.14 Spastic ectropion of eyelid**

- H02.141 Spastic ectropion of right upper eyelid
- H02.142 Spastic ectropion of right lower eyelid
- H02.143 Spastic ectropion of right eye, unspecified eyelid ▽
- H02.144 Spastic ectropion of left upper eyelid
- H02.145 Spastic ectropion of left lower eyelid
- H02.146 Spastic ectropion of left eye, unspecified eyelid ▽
- H02.149 Spastic ectropion of unspecified eye, unspecified eyelid ▽

• ✓6ᵗʰ **H02.15 Paralytic ectropion of eyelid**

- • H02.151 Paralytic ectropion of right upper eyelid
- • H02.152 Paralytic ectropion of right lower eyelid
- • H02.153 Paralytic ectropion of right eye, unspecified eyelid ▽
- • H02.154 Paralytic ectropion of left upper eyelid
- • H02.155 Paralytic ectropion of left lower eyelid

- • H02.156 Paralytic ectropion of left eye, unspecified eyelid ▽
- • H02.159 Paralytic ectropion of unspecified eye, unspecified eyelid ▽

✓5ᵗʰ **H02.2 Lagophthalmos**

> **DEF:** Condition of the eye that prevents it from closing completely.

✓6ᵗʰ **H02.20 Unspecified lagophthalmos**

- H02.201 Unspecified lagophthalmos right upper eyelid ▽
- H02.202 Unspecified lagophthalmos right lower eyelid ▽
- H02.203 Unspecified lagophthalmos right eye, unspecified eyelid ▽
- H02.204 Unspecified lagophthalmos left upper eyelid ▽
- H02.205 Unspecified lagophthalmos left lower eyelid ▽
- H02.206 Unspecified lagophthalmos left eye, unspecified eyelid ▽
- H02.209 Unspecified lagophthalmos unspecified eye, unspecified eyelid ▽
- • H02.20A Unspecified lagophthalmos right eye, upper and lower eyelids ▽
- • H02.20B Unspecified lagophthalmos left eye, upper and lower eyelids ▽
- • H02.20C Unspecified lagophthalmos, bilateral, upper and lower eyelids ▽

✓6ᵗʰ **H02.21 Cicatricial lagophthalmos**

- H02.211 Cicatricial lagophthalmos right upper eyelid
- H02.212 Cicatricial lagophthalmos right lower eyelid
- H02.213 Cicatricial lagophthalmos right eye, unspecified eyelid ▽
- H02.214 Cicatricial lagophthalmos left upper eyelid
- H02.215 Cicatricial lagophthalmos left lower eyelid
- H02.216 Cicatricial lagophthalmos left eye, unspecified eyelid ▽
- H02.219 Cicatricial lagophthalmos unspecified eye, unspecified eyelid ▽
- • H02.21A Cicatricial lagophthalmos right eye, upper and lower eyelids
- • H02.21B Cicatricial lagophthalmos left eye, upper and lower eyelids
- • H02.21C Cicatricial lagophthalmos, bilateral, upper and lower eyelids

✓6ᵗʰ **H02.22 Mechanical lagophthalmos**

- H02.221 Mechanical lagophthalmos right upper eyelid
- H02.222 Mechanical lagophthalmos right lower eyelid
- H02.223 Mechanical lagophthalmos right eye, unspecified eyelid ▽
- H02.224 Mechanical lagophthalmos left upper eyelid
- H02.225 Mechanical lagophthalmos left lower eyelid
- H02.226 Mechanical lagophthalmos left eye, unspecified eyelid ▽
- H02.229 Mechanical lagophthalmos unspecified eye, unspecified eyelid ▽
- • H02.22A Mechanical lagophthalmos right eye, upper and lower eyelids
- • H02.22B Mechanical lagophthalmos left eye, upper and lower eyelids
- • H02.22C Mechanical lagophthalmos, bilateral, upper and lower eyelids

✓6ᵗʰ **H02.23 Paralytic lagophthalmos**

- H02.231 Paralytic lagophthalmos right upper eyelid
- H02.232 Paralytic lagophthalmos right lower eyelid
- H02.233 Paralytic lagophthalmos right eye, unspecified eyelid ▽
- H02.234 Paralytic lagophthalmos left upper eyelid
- H02.235 Paralytic lagophthalmos left lower eyelid

H02.236 **Paralytic lagophthalmos** left eye, unspecified eyelid ▽

H02.239 **Paralytic lagophthalmos** unspecified eye, unspecified eyelid ▽

● H02.23A **Paralytic lagophthalmos** right eye, upper and lower eyelids

● H02.23B **Paralytic lagophthalmos** left eye, upper and lower eyelids

● H02.23C **Paralytic lagophthalmos,** bilateral, upper and lower eyelids

√5ᵗʰ **H02.3 Blepharochalasis**

Pseudoptosis

DEF: Loss of elasticity and relaxation of skin of the eyelid, thickened or indurated skin on the eyelid associated with recurrent episodes of edema, and intracellular atrophy.

H02.30 **Blepharochalasis** unspecified eye, unspecified eyelid ▽

H02.31 **Blepharochalasis** right upper eyelid

H02.32 **Blepharochalasis** right lower eyelid

H02.33 **Blepharochalasis** right eye, unspecified eyelid ▽

H02.34 **Blepharochalasis** left upper eyelid

H02.35 **Blepharochalasis** left lower eyelid

H02.36 **Blepharochalasis** left eye, unspecified eyelid ▽

√5ᵗʰ **H02.4 Ptosis of eyelid**

√6ᵗʰ H02.40 **Unspecified ptosis of eyelid**

H02.401 **Unspecified ptosis of** right eyelid ▽

H02.402 **Unspecified ptosis of** left eyelid ▽

H02.403 **Unspecified ptosis of** bilateral eyelids ▽

H02.409 **Unspecified ptosis of** unspecified eyelid ▽

√6ᵗʰ H02.41 **Mechanical ptosis of eyelid**

H02.411 **Mechanical ptosis of** right eyelid

H02.412 **Mechanical ptosis of** left eyelid

H02.413 **Mechanical ptosis of** bilateral eyelids

H02.419 **Mechanical ptosis of** unspecified eyelid ▽

√6ᵗʰ H02.42 **Myogenic ptosis of eyelid**

H02.421 **Myogenic ptosis of** right eyelid

H02.422 **Myogenic ptosis of** left eyelid

H02.423 **Myogenic ptosis of** bilateral eyelids

H02.429 **Myogenic ptosis of** unspecified eyelid ▽

√6ᵗʰ H02.43 **Paralytic ptosis of eyelid**

Neurogenic ptosis of eyelid

H02.431 **Paralytic ptosis of** right eyelid

H02.432 **Paralytic ptosis of** left eyelid

H02.433 **Paralytic ptosis of** bilateral eyelids

H02.439 **Paralytic ptosis** unspecified eyelid ▽

√5ᵗʰ **H02.5 Other disorders affecting eyelid function**

EXCLUDES 2 blepharospasm (G24.5)
organic tic (G25.69)
psychogenic tic (F95.-)

√6ᵗʰ H02.51 **Abnormal innervation syndrome**

H02.511 **Abnormal innervation syndrome** right upper eyelid

H02.512 **Abnormal innervation syndrome** right lower eyelid

H02.513 **Abnormal innervation syndrome** right eye, unspecified eyelid ▽

H02.514 **Abnormal innervation syndrome** left upper eyelid

H02.515 **Abnormal innervation syndrome** left lower eyelid

H02.516 **Abnormal innervation syndrome** left eye, unspecified eyelid ▽

H02.519 **Abnormal innervation syndrome** unspecified eye, unspecified eyelid ▽

√6ᵗʰ H02.52 **Blepharophimosis**

Ankyloblepharon

H02.521 **Blepharophimosis** right upper eyelid

H02.522 **Blepharophimosis** right lower eyelid

H02.523 **Blepharophimosis** right eye, unspecified eyelid ▽

H02.524 **Blepharophimosis** left upper eyelid

H02.525 **Blepharophimosis** left lower eyelid

H02.526 **Blepharophimosis** left eye, unspecified eyelid ▽

H02.529 **Blepharophimosis** unspecified eye, unspecified lid ▽

√6ᵗʰ H02.53 **Eyelid retraction**

Eyelid lag

H02.531 **Eyelid retraction** right upper eyelid

H02.532 **Eyelid retraction** right lower eyelid

H02.533 **Eyelid retraction** right eye, unspecified eyelid ▽

H02.534 **Eyelid retraction** left upper eyelid

H02.535 **Eyelid retraction** left lower eyelid

H02.536 **Eyelid retraction** left eye, unspecified eyelid ▽

H02.539 **Eyelid retraction** unspecified eye, unspecified lid ▽

H02.59 **Other disorders affecting eyelid function**

Deficient blink reflex

Sensory disorders

√5ᵗʰ **H02.6 Xanthelasma of eyelid**

DEF: Condition in which there are small yellow tumors that occur on the eyelid, usually appearing near the nose.

H02.60 **Xanthelasma of** unspecified eye, unspecified eyelid ▽

H02.61 **Xanthelasma of** right upper eyelid

H02.62 **Xanthelasma of** right lower eyelid

H02.63 **Xanthelasma of** right eye, unspecified eyelid ▽

H02.64 **Xanthelasma of** left upper eyelid

H02.65 **Xanthelasma of** left lower eyelid

H02.66 **Xanthelasma of** left eye, unspecified eyelid ▽

√5ᵗʰ **H02.7 Other and unspecified degenerative disorders of eyelid and periocular area**

H02.70 **Unspecified degenerative disorders of eyelid and periocular area** ▽

√6ᵗʰ H02.71 **Chloasma of eyelid and periocular area**

Dyspigmentation of eyelid

Hyperpigmentation of eyelid

H02.711 **Chloasma of** right upper eyelid and periocular area

H02.712 **Chloasma of** right lower eyelid and periocular area

H02.713 **Chloasma of** right eye, unspecified eyelid and periocular area ▽

H02.714 **Chloasma of** left upper eyelid and periocular area

H02.715 **Chloasma of** left lower eyelid and periocular area

H02.716 **Chloasma of** left eye, unspecified eyelid and periocular area ▽

H02.719 **Chloasma of** unspecified eye, unspecified eyelid and periocular area ▽

√6ᵗʰ H02.72 **Madarosis of eyelid and periocular area**

Hypotrichosis of eyelid

H02.721 **Madarosis of** right upper eyelid and periocular area

H02.722 **Madarosis of** right lower eyelid and periocular area

H02.723 **Madarosis of** right eye, unspecified eyelid and periocular area ▽

H02.724 **Madarosis of** left upper eyelid and periocular area

H02.725 **Madarosis of** left lower eyelid and periocular area

H02.726 **Madarosis of** left eye, unspecified eyelid and periocular area ▽

H02.729 **Madarosis of** unspecified eye, unspecified eyelid and periocular area ▽

√6ᵗʰ H02.73 **Vitiligo of eyelid and periocular area**

Hypopigmentation of eyelid

H02.731 **Vitiligo of** right upper eyelid and periocular area

H02.732 **Vitiligo of** right lower eyelid and periocular area

H02.733 **Vitiligo of** right eye, unspecified eyelid and periocular area ▽

☑ Additional Character Req   √x7ᵗʰ Placeholder Alert   **Manifestation**   ▽ Unspecified   ►◄ Revised Text   ● New Code   ▲ Revised Code Title

Chapter 7. Diseases of the Eye and Adnexa

H02.734 Vitiligo of left upper eyelid and periocular area

H02.735 Vitiligo of left lower eyelid and periocular area

H02.736 Vitiligo of left eye, unspecified eyelid and periocular area ▽

H02.739 Vitiligo of unspecified eye, unspecified eyelid and periocular area ▽

H02.79 Other degenerative disorders of eyelid and periocular area

✓5ᵗʰ **H02.8** Other specified disorders of eyelid

✓6ᵗʰ **H02.81** Retained foreign body in eyelid

Use additional code to identify the type of retained foreign body (Z18.-)

EXCLUDES 1   laceration of eyelid with foreign body (S01.12-)

retained intraocular foreign body (H44.6-, H44.7-)

superficial foreign body of eyelid and periocular area (S00.25-)

H02.811 Retained foreign body in right upper eyelid

H02.812 Retained foreign body in right lower eyelid

H02.813 Retained foreign body in right eye, unspecified eyelid ▽

H02.814 Retained foreign body in left upper eyelid

H02.815 Retained foreign body in left lower eyelid

H02.816 Retained foreign body in left eye, unspecified eyelid ▽

H02.819 Retained foreign body in unspecified eye, unspecified eyelid ▽

✓6ᵗʰ **H02.82** Cysts of eyelid

Sebaceous cyst of eyelid

H02.821 Cysts of right upper eyelid

H02.822 Cysts of right lower eyelid

H02.823 Cysts of right eye, unspecified eyelid ▽

H02.824 Cysts of left upper eyelid

H02.825 Cysts of left lower eyelid

H02.826 Cysts of left eye, unspecified eyelid ▽

H02.829 Cysts of unspecified eye, unspecified eyelid ▽

✓6ᵗʰ **H02.83** Dermatochalasis of eyelid

DEF: Acquired form of connective tissue disorder associated with decreased elastic tissue and abnormal elastin formation, resulting in loss of elasticity of the skin of the eyelid. It is generally associated with aging.

H02.831 Dermatochalasis of right upper eyelid

H02.832 Dermatochalasis of right lower eyelid

H02.833 Dermatochalasis of right eye, unspecified eyelid ▽

H02.834 Dermatochalasis of left upper eyelid

H02.835 Dermatochalasis of left lower eyelid

H02.836 Dermatochalasis of left eye, unspecified eyelid ▽

H02.839 Dermatochalasis of unspecified eye, unspecified eyelid ▽

✓6ᵗʰ **H02.84** Edema of eyelid

Hyperemia of eyelid

H02.841 Edema of right upper eyelid

H02.842 Edema of right lower eyelid

H02.843 Edema of right eye, unspecified eyelid ▽

H02.844 Edema of left upper eyelid

H02.845 Edema of left lower eyelid

H02.846 Edema of left eye, unspecified eyelid ▽

H02.849 Edema of unspecified eye, unspecified eyelid ▽

✓6ᵗʰ **H02.85** Elephantiasis of eyelid

H02.851 Elephantiasis of right upper eyelid

H02.852 Elephantiasis of right lower eyelid

H02.853 Elephantiasis of right eye, unspecified eyelid ▽

H02.854 Elephantiasis of left upper eyelid

H02.855 Elephantiasis of left lower eyelid

H02.856 Elephantiasis of left eye, unspecified eyelid ▽

H02.859 Elephantiasis of unspecified eye, unspecified eyelid ▽

✓6ᵗʰ **H02.86** Hypertrichosis of eyelid

H02.861 Hypertrichosis of right upper eyelid

H02.862 Hypertrichosis of right lower eyelid

H02.863 Hypertrichosis of right eye, unspecified eyelid

H02.864 Hypertrichosis of left upper eyelid

H02.865 Hypertrichosis of left lower eyelid

H02.866 Hypertrichosis of left eye, unspecified eyelid ▽

H02.869 Hypertrichosis of unspecified eye, unspecified eyelid ▽

✓6ᵗʰ **H02.87** Vascular anomalies of eyelid

H02.871 Vascular anomalies of right upper eyelid

H02.872 Vascular anomalies of right lower eyelid

H02.873 Vascular anomalies of right eye, unspecified eyelid ▽

H02.874 Vascular anomalies of left upper eyelid

H02.875 Vascular anomalies of left lower eyelid

H02.876 Vascular anomalies of left eye, unspecified eyelid ▽

H02.879 Vascular anomalies of unspecified eye, unspecified eyelid ▽

✓6ᵗʰ **H02.88** Meibomian gland dysfunction of eyelid

H02.881 Meibomian gland dysfunction right upper eyelid

H02.882 Meibomian gland dysfunction right lower eyelid

H02.883 Meibomian gland dysfunction of right eye, unspecified eyelid ▽

H02.884 Meibomian gland dysfunction left upper eyelid

H02.885 Meibomian gland dysfunction left lower eyelid

H02.886 Meibomian gland dysfunction of left eye, unspecified eyelid ▽

H02.889 Meibomian gland dysfunction of unspecified eye, unspecified eyelid ▽

H02.88A Meibomian gland dysfunction right eye, upper and lower eyelids

H02.88B Meibomian gland dysfunction left eye, upper and lower eyelids

H02.89 Other specified disorders of eyelid

Hemorrhage of eyelid

H02.9 Unspecified disorder of eyelid ▽

Disorder of eyelid NOS

✓4ᵗʰ **H04** Disorders of lacrimal system

EXCLUDES 1   congenital malformations of lacrimal system (Q10.4-Q10.6)

✓5ᵗʰ **H04.0** Dacryoadenitis

DEF: Inflammation of the lacrimal gland.

✓6ᵗʰ **H04.00** Unspecified dacryoadenitis

H04.001 Unspecified dacryoadenitis, right lacrimal gland ▽

H04.002 Unspecified dacryoadenitis, left lacrimal gland ▽

H04.003 Unspecified dacryoadenitis, bilateral lacrimal glands ▽

H04.009 Unspecified dacryoadenitis, unspecified lacrimal gland ▽

✓6ᵗʰ **H04.01** Acute dacryoadenitis

H04.011 Acute dacryoadenitis, right lacrimal gland

H04.012 Acute dacryoadenitis, left lacrimal gland

H04.013 Acute dacryoadenitis, bilateral lacrimal glands

H04.019 Acute dacryoadenitis, unspecified lacrimal gland ▽

✓6ᵗʰ **H04.02** Chronic dacryoadenitis

H04.021 Chronic dacryoadenitis, right lacrimal gland

H04.022 Chronic dacryoadenitis, left lacrimal gland

H04.023 Chronic dacryoadenitis, bilateral lacrimal gland

H04.029 Chronic dacryoadenitis, unspecified lacrimal gland ▽

✓6ᵗʰ H04.03 Chronic enlargement of lacrimal gland

    H04.031 Chronic enlargement of right lacrimal gland

    H04.032 Chronic enlargement of left lacrimal gland

    H04.033 Chronic enlargement of bilateral lacrimal glands

    H04.039 Chronic enlargement of unspecified lacrimal gland ▽

✓5ᵗʰ H04.1 Other disorders of lacrimal gland

  ✓6ᵗʰ H04.11 Dacryops

    H04.111 Dacryops of right lacrimal gland

    H04.112 Dacryops of left lacrimal gland

    H04.113 Dacryops of bilateral lacrimal glands

    H04.119 Dacryops of unspecified lacrimal gland ▽

  ✓6ᵗʰ H04.12 Dry eye syndrome

    Tear film insufficiency, NOS

    H04.121 Dry eye syndrome of right lacrimal gland

    H04.122 Dry eye syndrome of left lacrimal gland

    H04.123 Dry eye syndrome of bilateral lacrimal glands

    H04.129 Dry eye syndrome of unspecified lacrimal gland ▽

  ✓6ᵗʰ H04.13 Lacrimal cyst

    Lacrimal cystic degeneration

    H04.131 Lacrimal cyst, right lacrimal gland

    H04.132 Lacrimal cyst, left lacrimal gland

    H04.133 Lacrimal cyst, bilateral lacrimal glands

    H04.139 Lacrimal cyst, unspecified lacrimal gland ▽

  ✓6ᵗʰ H04.14 Primary lacrimal gland atrophy

    H04.141 Primary lacrimal gland atrophy, right lacrimal gland

    H04.142 Primary lacrimal gland atrophy, left lacrimal gland

    H04.143 Primary lacrimal gland atrophy, bilateral lacrimal glands

    H04.149 Primary lacrimal gland atrophy, unspecified lacrimal gland ▽

  ✓6ᵗʰ H04.15 Secondary lacrimal gland atrophy

    H04.151 Secondary lacrimal gland atrophy, right lacrimal gland

    H04.152 Secondary lacrimal gland atrophy, left lacrimal gland

    H04.153 Secondary lacrimal gland atrophy, bilateral lacrimal glands

    H04.159 Secondary lacrimal gland atrophy, unspecified lacrimal gland ▽

  ✓6ᵗʰ H04.16 Lacrimal gland dislocation

    H04.161 Lacrimal gland dislocation, right lacrimal gland

    H04.162 Lacrimal gland dislocation, left lacrimal gland

    H04.163 Lacrimal gland dislocation, bilateral lacrimal glands

    H04.169 Lacrimal gland dislocation, unspecified lacrimal gland ▽

  H04.19 Other specified disorders of lacrimal gland

✓5ᵗʰ H04.2 Epiphora

  DEF: Excessive tearing or overflow of tears down the cheeks often due to a stricture in the lacrimal passages but can be caused by other conditions.

  ✓6ᵗʰ H04.20 Unspecified epiphora

▲   H04.201 Unspecified epiphora, right side ▽

▲   H04.202 Unspecified epiphora, left side ▽

▲   H04.203 Unspecified epiphora, bilateral ▽

▲   H04.209 Unspecified epiphora, unspecified side

  ✓6ᵗʰ H04.21 Epiphora due to excess lacrimation

    H04.211 Epiphora due to excess lacrimation, right lacrimal gland

    H04.212 Epiphora due to excess lacrimation, left lacrimal gland

    H04.213 Epiphora due to excess lacrimation, bilateral lacrimal glands

    H04.219 Epiphora due to excess lacrimation, unspecified lacrimal gland ▽

  ✓6ᵗʰ H04.22 Epiphora due to insufficient drainage

▲   H04.221 Epiphora due to insufficient drainage, right side

▲   H04.222 Epiphora due to insufficient drainage, left side

▲   H04.223 Epiphora due to insufficient drainage, bilateral

▲   H04.229 Epiphora due to insufficient drainage, unspecified side ▽

✓5ᵗʰ H04.3 Acute and unspecified inflammation of lacrimal passages

  EXCLUDES 1 *neonatal dacryocystitis (P39.1)*

  ✓6ᵗʰ H04.30 Unspecified dacryocystitis

    H04.301 Unspecified dacryocystitis of right lacrimal passage ▽

    H04.302 Unspecified dacryocystitis of left lacrimal passage ▽

    H04.303 Unspecified dacryocystitis of bilateral lacrimal passages ▽

    H04.309 Unspecified dacryocystitis of unspecified lacrimal passage ▽

  ✓6ᵗʰ H04.31 Phlegmonous dacryocystitis

    H04.311 Phlegmonous dacryocystitis of right lacrimal passage

    H04.312 Phlegmonous dacryocystitis of left lacrimal passage

    H04.313 Phlegmonous dacryocystitis of bilateral lacrimal passages

    H04.319 Phlegmonous dacryocystitis of unspecified lacrimal passage ▽

  ✓6ᵗʰ H04.32 Acute dacryocystitis

    Acute dacryopericystitis

    H04.321 Acute dacryocystitis of right lacrimal passage

    H04.322 Acute dacryocystitis of left lacrimal passage

    H04.323 Acute dacryocystitis of bilateral lacrimal passages

    H04.329 Acute dacryocystitis of unspecified lacrimal passage ▽

  ✓6ᵗʰ H04.33 Acute lacrimal canaliculitis

    H04.331 Acute lacrimal canaliculitis of right lacrimal passage

    H04.332 Acute lacrimal canaliculitis of left lacrimal passage

    H04.333 Acute lacrimal canaliculitis of bilateral lacrimal passages

    H04.339 Acute lacrimal canaliculitis of unspecified lacrimal passage ▽

✓5ᵗʰ H04.4 Chronic inflammation of lacrimal passages

  ✓6ᵗʰ H04.41 Chronic dacryocystitis

    H04.411 Chronic dacryocystitis of right lacrimal passage

    H04.412 Chronic dacryocystitis of left lacrimal passage

    H04.413 Chronic dacryocystitis of bilateral lacrimal passages

    H04.419 Chronic dacryocystitis of unspecified lacrimal passage ▽

  ✓6ᵗʰ H04.42 Chronic lacrimal canaliculitis

    H04.421 Chronic lacrimal canaliculitis of right lacrimal passage

    H04.422 Chronic lacrimal canaliculitis of left lacrimal passage

    H04.423 Chronic lacrimal canaliculitis of bilateral lacrimal passages

    H04.429 Chronic lacrimal canaliculitis of unspecified lacrimal passage ▽

  ✓6ᵗʰ H04.43 Chronic lacrimal mucocele

    H04.431 Chronic lacrimal mucocele of right lacrimal passage

    H04.432 Chronic lacrimal mucocele of left lacrimal passage

    H04.433 Chronic lacrimal mucocele of bilateral lacrimal passages

    H04.439 Chronic lacrimal mucocele of unspecified lacrimal passage ▽

✓ Additional Character Req   ✓x7ᵗʰ Placeholder Alert   Manifestation   ▽ Unspecified   ►◄ Revised Text   ● New Code   ▲ Revised Code Title

✓5th **H04.5** **Stenosis and insufficiency of lacrimal passages**

  ✓6th **H04.51** **Dacryolith**

    H04.511 **Dacryolith of** right **lacrimal passage**

    H04.512 **Dacryolith of** left **lacrimal passage**

    H04.513 **Dacryolith of** bilateral **lacrimal passages**

    H04.519 **Dacryolith of unspecified lacrimal** ▽
       passage

  ✓6th **H04.52** **Eversion of lacrimal** punctum

    H04.521 **Eversion of** right **lacrimal punctum**

    H04.522 **Eversion of** left **lacrimal punctum**

    H04.523 **Eversion of** bilateral **lacrimal punctum**

    H04.529 **Eversion of unspecified lacrimal** ▽
       punctum

  ✓6th **H04.53** **Neonatal obstruction of nasolacrimal duct**

      EXCLUDES 1 *congenital stenosis and stricture of*
      lacrimal duct (Q10.5)

    H04.531 **Neonatal obstruction of** right 　Ⓝ
       nasolacrimal duct

    H04.532 **Neonatal obstruction of** left 　Ⓝ
       nasolacrimal duct

    H04.533 **Neonatal obstruction of** bilateral 　Ⓝ
       nasolacrimal duct

    H04.539 **Neonatal obstruction of** 　　Ⓝ ▽
       unspecified nasolacrimal duct

  ✓6th **H04.54** **Stenosis of lacrimal** canaliculi

    H04.541 **Stenosis of** right **lacrimal canaliculi**

    H04.542 **Stenosis of** left **lacrimal canaliculi**

    H04.543 **Stenosis of** bilateral **lacrimal canaliculi**

    H04.549 **Stenosis of unspecified lacrimal** ▽
       canaliculi

  ✓6th **H04.55** **Acquired stenosis of nasolacrimal** duct

    H04.551 **Acquired stenosis of** right **nasolacrimal**
       duct

    H04.552 **Acquired stenosis of** left **nasolacrimal**
       duct

    H04.553 **Acquired stenosis of** bilateral
       nasolacrimal duct

    H04.559 **Acquired stenosis of unspecified** ▽
       nasolacrimal duct

  ✓6th **H04.56** **Stenosis of lacrimal** punctum

    H04.561 **Stenosis of** right **lacrimal punctum**

    H04.562 **Stenosis of** left **lacrimal punctum**

    H04.563 **Stenosis of** bilateral **lacrimal punctum**

    H04.569 **Stenosis of unspecified lacrimal** ▽
       punctum

  ✓6th **H04.57** **Stenosis of lacrimal** sac

    H04.571 **Stenosis of** right **lacrimal sac**

    H04.572 **Stenosis of** left **lacrimal sac**

    H04.573 **Stenosis of** bilateral **lacrimal sac**

    H04.579 **Stenosis of unspecified lacrimal** ▽
       sac

✓5th **H04.6** **Other changes of lacrimal passages**

  ✓6th **H04.61** **Lacrimal** fistula

    H04.611 **Lacrimal fistula** right **lacrimal passage**

    H04.612 **Lacrimal fistula** left **lacrimal passage**

    H04.613 **Lacrimal fistula** bilateral **lacrimal**
       passages

    H04.619 **Lacrimal fistula unspecified** ▽
       lacrimal passage

    H04.69 **Other changes of lacrimal passages**

✓5th **H04.8** **Other disorders of lacrimal system**

  ✓6th **H04.81** **Granuloma of lacrimal passages**

    H04.811 **Granuloma of** right **lacrimal passage**

    H04.812 **Granuloma of** left **lacrimal passage**

    H04.813 **Granuloma of** bilateral **lacrimal passages**

    H04.819 **Granuloma of unspecified** ▽
       lacrimal passage

    H04.89 **Other disorders of lacrimal system**

  H04.9 **Disorder of lacrimal system, unspecified** ▽

✓4th **H05** **Disorders of orbit**

    EXCLUDES 1 *congenital malformation of orbit (Q10.7)*

  ✓5th **H05.0** **Acute inflammation of orbit**

    H05.00 **Unspecified acute inflammation of orbit** ▽

  ✓6th **H05.01** **Cellulitis of orbit**

      Abscess of orbit

    H05.011 **Cellulitis of** right **orbit**

    H05.012 **Cellulitis of** left **orbit**

    H05.013 **Cellulitis of** bilateral **orbits**

    H05.019 **Cellulitis of unspecified orbit** ▽

  ✓6th **H05.02** **Osteomyelitis of orbit**

    H05.021 **Osteomyelitis of** right **orbit**

    H05.022 **Osteomyelitis of** left **orbit**

    H05.023 **Osteomyelitis of** bilateral **orbits**

    H05.029 **Osteomyelitis of unspecified orbit** ▽

  ✓6th **H05.03** **Periostitis of orbit**

    H05.031 **Periostitis of** right **orbit**

    H05.032 **Periostitis of** left **orbit**

    H05.033 **Periostitis of** bilateral **orbits**

    H05.039 **Periostitis of unspecified orbit** ▽

  ✓6th **H05.04** **Tenonitis of orbit**

    H05.041 **Tenonitis of** right **orbit**

    H05.042 **Tenonitis of** left **orbit**

    H05.043 **Tenonitis of** bilateral **orbits**

    H05.049 **Tenonitis of unspecified orbit** ▽

✓5th **H05.1** **Chronic inflammatory disorders of orbit**

  H05.10 **Unspecified chronic inflammatory disorders** ▽
    of orbit

  ✓6th **H05.11** **Granuloma of orbit**

      Pseudotumor (inflammatory) of orbit

    H05.111 **Granuloma of** right **orbit**

    H05.112 **Granuloma of** left **orbit**

    H05.113 **Granuloma of** bilateral **orbits**

    H05.119 **Granuloma of unspecified orbit** ▽

  ✓6th **H05.12** **Orbital** myositis

    H05.121 **Orbital myositis,** right **orbit**

    H05.122 **Orbital myositis,** left **orbit**

    H05.123 **Orbital myositis,** bilateral

    H05.129 **Orbital myositis, unspecified orbit** ▽

✓5th **H05.2** **Exophthalmic conditions**

  H05.20 **Unspecified exophthalmos** ▽

  ✓6th **H05.21** **Displacement (lateral) of globe**

    H05.211 **Displacement (lateral) of globe,** right **eye**

    H05.212 **Displacement (lateral) of globe,** left **eye**

    H05.213 **Displacement (lateral) of globe,** bilateral

    H05.219 **Displacement (lateral) of globe,** ▽
       unspecified eye

  ✓6th **H05.22** **Edema of orbit**

      Orbital congestion

    H05.221 **Edema of** right **orbit**

    H05.222 **Edema of** left **orbit**

    H05.223 **Edema of** bilateral **orbit**

    H05.229 **Edema of unspecified orbit** ▽

  ✓6th **H05.23** **Hemorrhage of orbit**

    H05.231 **Hemorrhage of** right **orbit**

    H05.232 **Hemorrhage of** left **orbit**

    H05.233 **Hemorrhage of** bilateral **orbit**

    H05.239 **Hemorrhage of unspecified orbit** ▽

  ✓6th **H05.24** **Constant** exophthalmos

    H05.241 **Constant exophthalmos,** right **eye**

    H05.242 **Constant exophthalmos,** left **eye**

    H05.243 **Constant exophthalmos,** bilateral

    H05.249 **Constant exophthalmos,** ▽
       unspecified eye

  ✓6th **H05.25** **Intermittent** exophthalmos

    H05.251 **Intermittent exophthalmos,** right **eye**

    H05.252 **Intermittent exophthalmos,** left **eye**

    H05.253 **Intermittent exophthalmos,** bilateral

    H05.259 **Intermittent exophthalmos,** ▽
       unspecified eye

  ✓6th **H05.26** **Pulsating** exophthalmos

    H05.261 **Pulsating exophthalmos,** right **eye**

    H05.262 **Pulsating exophthalmos,** left **eye**

    H05.263 **Pulsating exophthalmos,** bilateral

    H05.269 **Pulsating exophthalmos,** ▽
       unspecified eye

✓5th **H05.3** **Deformity of orbit**

    EXCLUDES 1 *congenital deformity of orbit (Q10.7)*
       hypertelorism (Q75.2)

  H05.30 **Unspecified deformity of orbit** ▽

  ✓6th **H05.31** **Atrophy of orbit**

    H05.311 **Atrophy of** right **orbit**

    H05.312 **Atrophy of** left **orbit**

    H05.313 **Atrophy of** bilateral **orbit**

H05.319   **Atrophy of unspecified orbit** ▽

√6ᵗʰ **H05.32 Deformity of orbit** due to bone disease

Code also associated bone disease

H05.321   **Deformity of** right **orbit due to bone disease**

H05.322   **Deformity of** left **orbit due to bone disease**

H05.323   **Deformity of** bilateral **orbits due to bone disease**

H05.329   **Deformity of unspecified orbit due to bone disease** ▽

√6ᵗʰ **H05.33 Deformity of orbit** due to trauma or surgery

H05.331   **Deformity of** right **orbit due to trauma or surgery**

H05.332   **Deformity of** left **orbit due to trauma or surgery**

H05.333   **Deformity of** bilateral **orbits due to trauma or surgery**

H05.339   **Deformity of unspecified orbit due to trauma or surgery** ▽

√6ᵗʰ **H05.34 Enlargement of orbit**

H05.341   **Enlargement of** right **orbit**

H05.342   **Enlargement of** left **orbit**

H05.343   **Enlargement of** bilateral **orbits**

H05.349   **Enlargement of unspecified orbit** ▽

√6ᵗʰ **H05.35 Exostosis of orbit**

H05.351   **Exostosis of** right **orbit**

H05.352   **Exostosis of** left **orbit**

H05.353   **Exostosis of** bilateral **orbits**

H05.359   **Exostosis of unspecified orbit** ▽

√5ᵗʰ **H05.4 Enophthalmos**

√6ᵗʰ **H05.40 Unspecified enophthalmos**

H05.401   **Unspecified enophthalmos,** right **eye** ▽

H05.402   **Unspecified enophthalmos,** left **eye** ▽

H05.403   **Unspecified enophthalmos,** bilateral ▽

H05.409   **Unspecified enophthalmos, unspecified eye** ▽

√6ᵗʰ **H05.41 Enophthalmos** due to atrophy of orbital tissue

H05.411   **Enophthalmos due to atrophy of orbital tissue,** right **eye**

H05.412   **Enophthalmos due to atrophy of orbital tissue,** left **eye**

H05.413   **Enophthalmos due to atrophy of orbital tissue,** bilateral

H05.419   **Enophthalmos due to atrophy of orbital tissue, unspecified eye** ▽

√6ᵗʰ **H05.42 Enophthalmos** due to trauma or surgery

H05.421   **Enophthalmos due to trauma or surgery,** right **eye**

H05.422   **Enophthalmos due to trauma or surgery,** left **eye**

H05.423   **Enophthalmos due to trauma or surgery,** bilateral

H05.429   **Enophthalmos due to trauma or surgery, unspecified eye** ▽

√5ᵗʰ **H05.5 Retained (old) foreign body following penetrating wound of orbit**

Retrobulbar foreign body

Use additional code to identify the type of retained foreign body (Z18.-)

EXCLUDES 1   current penetrating wound of orbit (S05.4-)

EXCLUDES 2   retained foreign body of eyelid (H02.81-)

retained intraocular foreign body (H44.6-, H44.7-)

H05.50   **Retained (old) foreign body following penetrating wound of unspecified orbit** ▽

H05.51   **Retained (old) foreign body following penetrating wound of** right **orbit**

H05.52   **Retained (old) foreign body following penetrating wound of** left **orbit**

H05.53   **Retained (old) foreign body following penetrating wound of** bilateral **orbits**

√5ᵗʰ **H05.8 Other disorders of orbit**

√6ᵗʰ **H05.81 Cyst of orbit**

Encephalocele of orbit

H05.811   **Cyst of** right **orbit**

H05.812   **Cyst of** left **orbit**

H05.813   **Cyst of** bilateral **orbits**

H05.819   **Cyst of unspecified orbit** ▽

√6ᵗʰ **H05.82 Myopathy of extraocular muscles**

H05.821   **Myopathy of extraocular muscles,** right **orbit**

H05.822   **Myopathy of extraocular muscles,** left **orbit**

H05.823   **Myopathy of extraocular muscles,** bilateral

H05.829   **Myopathy of extraocular muscles, unspecified orbit** ▽

H05.89   **Other disorders of orbit**

H05.9 Unspecified disorder of orbit ▽

Disorders of conjunctiva (H10-H11)

√4ᵗʰ **H10 Conjunctivitis**

EXCLUDES 1   keratoconjunctivitis (H16.2-)

√5ᵗʰ **H10.0 Mucopurulent conjunctivitis**

√6ᵗʰ **H10.01 Acute follicular conjunctivitis**

H10.011   **Acute follicular conjunctivitis,** right **eye**

H10.012   **Acute follicular conjunctivitis,** left **eye**

H10.013   **Acute follicular conjunctivitis,** bilateral

H10.019   **Acute follicular conjunctivitis, unspecified eye** ▽

√6ᵗʰ **H10.02 Other mucopurulent conjunctivitis**

H10.021   **Other mucopurulent conjunctivitis,** right **eye**

H10.022   **Other mucopurulent conjunctivitis,** left **eye**

H10.023   **Other mucopurulent conjunctivitis,** bilateral

H10.029   **Other mucopurulent conjunctivitis, unspecified eye** ▽

√5ᵗʰ **H10.1 Acute atopic conjunctivitis**

Acute papillary conjunctivitis

H10.10   **Acute atopic conjunctivitis, unspecified eye** ▽

H10.11   **Acute atopic conjunctivitis,** right **eye**

H10.12   **Acute atopic conjunctivitis,** left **eye**

H10.13   **Acute atopic conjunctivitis,** bilateral

√5ᵗʰ **H10.2 Other acute conjunctivitis**

√6ᵗʰ **H10.21 Acute toxic conjunctivitis**

Acute chemical conjunctivitis

Code first (T51-T65) to identify chemical and intent

EXCLUDES 1   burn and corrosion of eye and adnexa (T26.-)

H10.211   **Acute toxic conjunctivitis,** right **eye**

H10.212   **Acute toxic conjunctivitis,** left **eye**

H10.213   **Acute toxic conjunctivitis,** bilateral

H10.219   **Acute toxic conjunctivitis, unspecified eye** ▽

√6ᵗʰ **H10.22 Pseudomembranous conjunctivitis**

H10.221   **Pseudomembranous conjunctivitis,** right **eye**

H10.222   **Pseudomembranous conjunctivitis,** left **eye**

H10.223   **Pseudomembranous conjunctivitis,** bilateral

H10.229   **Pseudomembranous conjunctivitis, unspecified eye** ▽

√6ᵗʰ **H10.23 Serous conjunctivitis, except viral**

EXCLUDES 1   viral conjunctivitis (B30.-)

H10.231   **Serous conjunctivitis, except viral,** right **eye**

H10.232   **Serous conjunctivitis, except viral,** left **eye**

H10.233   **Serous conjunctivitis, except viral,** bilateral

H10.239   **Serous conjunctivitis, except viral, unspecified eye** ▽

√5ᵗʰ **H10.3 Unspecified acute conjunctivitis**

EXCLUDES 1   ophthalmia neonatorum NOS (P39.1)

H10.30   **Unspecified acute conjunctivitis, unspecified eye** ▽

H10.31   **Unspecified acute conjunctivitis,** right **eye** ▽

H10.32   **Unspecified acute conjunctivitis,** left **eye** ▽

H10.33   **Unspecified acute conjunctivitis,** bilateral ▽

☑ Additional Character Req   √x7ᵗʰ Placeholder Alert   <u>Manifestation</u>   ▽ Unspecified   ►◄ Revised Text   ● New Code   ▲ Revised Code Title

Chapter 7. Diseases of the Eye and Adnexa

H10.4–H11.069

√5th **H10.4 Chronic conjunctivitis**

√6th **H10.40 Unspecified chronic conjunctivitis**

H10.401 Unspecified chronic conjunctivitis, **right** eye ▽

H10.402 Unspecified chronic conjunctivitis, **left** eye ▽

H10.403 Unspecified chronic conjunctivitis, **bilateral** ▽

H10.409 Unspecified chronic conjunctivitis, unspecified eye ▽

√6th **H10.41 Chronic giant papillary conjunctivitis**

H10.411 Chronic giant papillary conjunctivitis, **right** eye

H10.412 Chronic giant papillary conjunctivitis, **left** eye

H10.413 Chronic giant papillary conjunctivitis, **bilateral**

H10.419 Chronic giant papillary conjunctivitis, unspecified eye ▽

√6th **H10.42 Simple chronic conjunctivitis**

H10.421 Simple chronic conjunctivitis, **right** eye

H10.422 Simple chronic conjunctivitis, **left** eye

H10.423 Simple chronic conjunctivitis, **bilateral**

H10.429 Simple chronic conjunctivitis, unspecified eye ▽

√6th **H10.43 Chronic follicular conjunctivitis**

H10.431 Chronic follicular conjunctivitis, **right** eye

H10.432 Chronic follicular conjunctivitis, **left** eye

H10.433 Chronic follicular conjunctivitis, **bilateral**

H10.439 Chronic follicular conjunctivitis, unspecified eye ▽

H10.44 Vernal conjunctivitis

EXCLUDES 1   *vernal keratoconjunctivitis with limbar and corneal involvement (H16.26-)*

H10.45 Other chronic allergic conjunctivitis

√5th **H10.5 Blepharoconjunctivitis**

√6th **H10.50 Unspecified blepharoconjunctivitis**

H10.501 Unspecified blepharoconjunctivitis, **right** eye ▽

H10.502 Unspecified blepharoconjunctivitis, **left** eye ▽

H10.503 Unspecified blepharoconjunctivitis, **bilateral** ▽

H10.509 Unspecified blepharoconjunctivitis, unspecified eye ▽

√6th **H10.51 Ligneous conjunctivitis**

▶Code also underlying condition if known, such as:◀
▶plasminogen deficiency (E88.02)◀

H10.511 Ligneous conjunctivitis, **right** eye

H10.512 Ligneous conjunctivitis, **left** eye

H10.513 Ligneous conjunctivitis, **bilateral**

H10.519 Ligneous conjunctivitis, unspecified eye ▽

√6th **H10.52 Angular blepharoconjunctivitis**

H10.521 Angular blepharoconjunctivitis, **right** eye

H10.522 Angular blepharoconjunctivitis, **left** eye

H10.523 Angular blepharoconjunctivitis, **bilateral**

H10.529 Angular blepharoconjunctivitis, unspecified eye ▽

√6th **H10.53 Contact blepharoconjunctivitis**

H10.531 Contact blepharoconjunctivitis, **right** eye

H10.532 Contact blepharoconjunctivitis, **left** eye

H10.533 Contact blepharoconjunctivitis, **bilateral**

H10.539 Contact blepharoconjunctivitis, unspecified eye ▽

√5th **H10.8 Other conjunctivitis**

√6th **H10.81 Pingueculitis**

EXCLUDES 1   *pinguecula (H11.15-)*

H10.811 Pingueculitis, **right** eye

H10.812 Pingueculitis, **left** eye

H10.813 Pingueculitis, **bilateral**

H10.819 Pingueculitis, unspecified eye ▽

● √6th **H10.82 Rosacea conjunctivitis**

Code first underlying rosacea dermatitis (L71.-)

● H10.821 Rosacea conjunctivitis, **right** eye

● H10.822 Rosacea conjunctivitis, **left** eye

● H10.823 Rosacea conjunctivitis, **bilateral**

● H10.829 Rosacea conjunctivitis, unspecified eye ▽

H10.89 **Other conjunctivitis**

H10.9 **Unspecified conjunctivitis** ▽

√4th **H11 Other disorders of conjunctiva**

EXCLUDES 1   *keratoconjunctivitis (H16.2-)*

√5th **H11.0 Pterygium of eye**

EXCLUDES 1   *pseudopterygium (H11.81-)*

Pterygium

Pterygium

√6th **H11.00 Unspecified pterygium of eye**

H11.001 Unspecified pterygium of **right** eye ▽

H11.002 Unspecified pterygium of **left** eye ▽

H11.003 Unspecified pterygium of eye, **bilateral** ▽

H11.009 Unspecified pterygium of unspecified eye ▽

√6th **H11.01 Amyloid pterygium**

H11.011 Amyloid pterygium of **right** eye

H11.012 Amyloid pterygium of **left** eye

H11.013 Amyloid pterygium of eye, **bilateral**

H11.019 Amyloid pterygium of unspecified eye ▽

√6th **H11.02 Central pterygium of eye**

H11.021 Central pterygium of **right** eye

H11.022 Central pterygium of **left** eye

H11.023 Central pterygium of eye, **bilateral**

H11.029 Central pterygium of unspecified eye ▽

√6th **H11.03 Double pterygium of eye**

H11.031 Double pterygium of **right** eye

H11.032 Double pterygium of **left** eye

H11.033 Double pterygium of eye, **bilateral**

H11.039 Double pterygium of unspecified eye ▽

√6th **H11.04 Peripheral pterygium of eye, stationary**

H11.041 Peripheral pterygium, stationary, **right** eye

H11.042 Peripheral pterygium, stationary, **left** eye

H11.043 Peripheral pterygium, stationary, **bilateral**

H11.049 Peripheral pterygium, stationary, unspecified eye ▽

√6th **H11.05 Peripheral pterygium of eye, progressive**

H11.051 Peripheral pterygium, progressive, **right** eye

H11.052 Peripheral pterygium, progressive, **left** eye

H11.053 Peripheral pterygium, progressive, **bilateral**

H11.059 Peripheral pterygium, progressive, unspecified eye ▽

√6th **H11.06 Recurrent pterygium of eye**

H11.061 Recurrent pterygium of **right** eye

H11.062 Recurrent pterygium of **left** eye

H11.063 Recurrent pterygium of eye, **bilateral**

H11.069 Recurrent pterygium of unspecified eye

√5ᵗʰ **H11.1** **Conjunctival degenerations and deposits**
     EXCLUDES 2   *pseudopterygium (H11.81)*
   H11.10 **Unspecified conjunctival degenerations** ▽
√6ᵗʰ **H11.11** **Conjunctival deposits**
     H11.111 **Conjunctival deposits, right eye**
     H11.112 **Conjunctival deposits, left eye**
     H11.113 **Conjunctival deposits, bilateral**
     H11.119 **Conjunctival deposits, unspecified eye** ▽
√6ᵗʰ **H11.12** **Conjunctival concretions**
     H11.121 **Conjunctival concretions, right eye**
     H11.122 **Conjunctival concretions, left eye**
     H11.123 **Conjunctival concretions, bilateral**
     H11.129 **Conjunctival concretions, unspecified eye** ▽
√6ᵗʰ **H11.13** **Conjunctival pigmentations**
     Conjunctival argyrosis [argyria]
     H11.131 **Conjunctival pigmentations, right eye**
     H11.132 **Conjunctival pigmentations, left eye**
     H11.133 **Conjunctival pigmentations, bilateral**
     H11.139 **Conjunctival pigmentations, unspecified eye** ▽
√6ᵗʰ **H11.14** **Conjunctival xerosis, unspecified**
     EXCLUDES 1   *xerosis of conjunctiva due to vitamin A deficiency (E50.0, E50.1)*
     DEF: Abnormal dryness of the conjunctiva due to lack of insufficient tears or conjunctival secretions.
     H11.141 **Conjunctival xerosis, unspecified, right eye** ▽
     H11.142 **Conjunctival xerosis, unspecified, left eye** ▽
     H11.143 **Conjunctival xerosis, unspecified, bilateral** ▽
     H11.149 **Conjunctival xerosis, unspecified, unspecified eye** ▽
√6ᵗʰ **H11.15** **Pinguecula**
     EXCLUDES 1   *pingueculitis (H10.81-)*

Pinguecula

Pinguecula

     H11.151 **Pinguecula, right eye**
     H11.152 **Pinguecula, left eye**
     H11.153 **Pinguecula, bilateral**
     H11.159 **Pinguecula, unspecified eye** ▽
√5ᵗʰ **H11.2** **Conjunctival scars**
√6ᵗʰ **H11.21** **Conjunctival adhesions and strands (localized)**
     H11.211 **Conjunctival adhesions and strands (localized), right eye**
     H11.212 **Conjunctival adhesions and strands (localized), left eye**
     H11.213 **Conjunctival adhesions and strands (localized), bilateral**
     H11.219 **Conjunctival adhesions and strands (localized), unspecified eye** ▽
√6ᵗʰ **H11.22** **Conjunctival granuloma**
     H11.221 **Conjunctival granuloma, right eye**
     H11.222 **Conjunctival granuloma, left eye**
     H11.223 **Conjunctival granuloma, bilateral**
     H11.229 **Conjunctival granuloma, unspecified** ▽

√6ᵗʰ **H11.23** **Symblepharon**
     H11.231 **Symblepharon, right eye**
     H11.232 **Symblepharon, left eye**
     H11.233 **Symblepharon, bilateral**
     H11.239 **Symblepharon, unspecified eye** ▽
√6ᵗʰ **H11.24** **Scarring of conjunctiva**
     H11.241 **Scarring of conjunctiva, right eye**
     H11.242 **Scarring of conjunctiva, left eye**
     H11.243 **Scarring of conjunctiva, bilateral**
     H11.249 **Scarring of conjunctiva, unspecified eye** ▽
√5ᵗʰ **H11.3** **Conjunctival hemorrhage**
     Subconjunctival hemorrhage
   H11.30 **Conjunctival hemorrhage, unspecified eye** ▽
   H11.31 **Conjunctival hemorrhage, right eye**
   H11.32 **Conjunctival hemorrhage, left eye**
   H11.33 **Conjunctival hemorrhage, bilateral**
√5ᵗʰ **H11.4** **Other conjunctival vascular disorders and cysts**
√6ᵗʰ **H11.41** **Vascular abnormalities of conjunctiva**
     Conjunctival aneurysm
     H11.411 **Vascular abnormalities of conjunctiva, right eye**
     H11.412 **Vascular abnormalities of conjunctiva, left eye**
     H11.413 **Vascular abnormalities of conjunctiva, bilateral**
     H11.419 **Vascular abnormalities of conjunctiva, unspecified eye** ▽
√6ᵗʰ **H11.42** **Conjunctival edema**
     H11.421 **Conjunctival edema, right eye**
     H11.422 **Conjunctival edema, left eye**
     H11.423 **Conjunctival edema, bilateral**
     H11.429 **Conjunctival edema, unspecified eye** ▽
√6ᵗʰ **H11.43** **Conjunctival hyperemia**
     H11.431 **Conjunctival hyperemia, right eye**
     H11.432 **Conjunctival hyperemia, left eye**
     H11.433 **Conjunctival hyperemia, bilateral**
     H11.439 **Conjunctival hyperemia, unspecified eye** ▽
√6ᵗʰ **H11.44** **Conjunctival cysts**
     H11.441 **Conjunctival cysts, right eye**
     H11.442 **Conjunctival cysts, left eye**
     H11.443 **Conjunctival cysts, bilateral**
     H11.449 **Conjunctival cysts, unspecified eye** ▽
√5ᵗʰ **H11.8** **Other specified disorders of conjunctiva**
√6ᵗʰ **H11.81** **Pseudopterygium of conjunctiva**
     H11.811 **Pseudopterygium of conjunctiva, right eye**
     H11.812 **Pseudopterygium of conjunctiva, left eye**
     H11.813 **Pseudopterygium of conjunctiva, bilateral**
     H11.819 **Pseudopterygium of conjunctiva, unspecified eye** ▽
√6ᵗʰ **H11.82** **Conjunctivochalasis**
     H11.821 **Conjunctivochalasis, right eye**
     H11.822 **Conjunctivochalasis, left eye**
     H11.823 **Conjunctivochalasis, bilateral**
     H11.829 **Conjunctivochalasis, unspecified eye** ▽
   H11.89 **Other specified disorders of conjunctiva**
   H11.9 **Unspecified disorder of conjunctiva** ▽

Disorders of sclera, cornea, iris and ciliary body (H15-H22)

√4ᵗʰ **H15** **Disorders of sclera**
√5ᵗʰ **H15.0** **Scleritis**
√6ᵗʰ **H15.00** **Unspecified scleritis**
     H15.001 **Unspecified scleritis, right eye** ▽
     H15.002 **Unspecified scleritis, left eye** ▽
     H15.003 **Unspecified scleritis, bilateral** ▽
     H15.009 **Unspecified scleritis, unspecified eye** ▽
√6ᵗʰ **H15.01** **Anterior scleritis**
     H15.011 **Anterior scleritis, right eye** ▽
     H15.012 **Anterior scleritis, left eye** ▽

        H15.013 Anterior scleritis, bilateral
        H15.019 Anterior scleritis, unspecified eye ▽

√6ᵗʰ **H15.02** Brawny scleritis
        H15.021 Brawny scleritis, right eye
        H15.022 Brawny scleritis, left eye
        H15.023 Brawny scleritis, bilateral
        H15.029 Brawny scleritis, unspecified eye ▽

√6ᵗʰ **H15.03** Posterior scleritis
      Sclerotenonitis
        H15.031 Posterior scleritis, right eye
        H15.032 Posterior scleritis, left eye
        H15.033 Posterior scleritis, bilateral
        H15.039 Posterior scleritis, unspecified eye ▽

√6ᵗʰ **H15.04** Scleritis with corneal involvement
        H15.041 Scleritis with corneal involvement, right eye
        H15.042 Scleritis with corneal involvement, left eye
        H15.043 Scleritis with corneal involvement, bilateral
        H15.049 Scleritis with corneal involvement, unspecified eye ▽

√6ᵗʰ **H15.05** Scleromalacia perforans
        H15.051 Scleromalacia perforans, right eye
        H15.052 Scleromalacia perforans, left eye
        H15.053 Scleromalacia perforans, bilateral
        H15.059 Scleromalacia perforans, unspecified eye ▽

√6ᵗʰ **H15.09** Other scleritis
      Scleral abscess
        H15.091 Other scleritis, right eye
        H15.092 Other scleritis, left eye
        H15.093 Other scleritis, bilateral
        H15.099 Other scleritis, unspecified eye ▽

√5ᵗʰ **H15.1** Episcleritis
√6ᵗʰ **H15.10** Unspecified episcleritis
        H15.101 Unspecified episcleritis, right eye ▽
        H15.102 Unspecified episcleritis, left eye ▽
        H15.103 Unspecified episcleritis, bilateral ▽
        H15.109 Unspecified episcleritis, unspecified eye ▽

√6ᵗʰ **H15.11** Episcleritis periodica fugax
        H15.111 Episcleritis periodica fugax, right eye
        H15.112 Episcleritis periodica fugax, left eye
        H15.113 Episcleritis periodica fugax, bilateral
        H15.119 Episcleritis periodica fugax, unspecified eye ▽

√6ᵗʰ **H15.12** Nodular episcleritis
        H15.121 Nodular episcleritis, right eye
        H15.122 Nodular episcleritis, left eye
        H15.123 Nodular episcleritis, bilateral
        H15.129 Nodular episcleritis, unspecified eye ▽

√5ᵗʰ **H15.8** Other disorders of sclera
      EXCLUDES 2 blue sclera (Q13.5)
                degenerative myopia (H44.2-)

√6ᵗʰ **H15.81** Equatorial staphyloma
        H15.811 Equatorial staphyloma, right eye
        H15.812 Equatorial staphyloma, left eye
        H15.813 Equatorial staphyloma, bilateral
        H15.819 Equatorial staphyloma, unspecified eye ▽

√6ᵗʰ **H15.82** Localized anterior staphyloma
        H15.821 Localized anterior staphyloma, right eye
        H15.822 Localized anterior staphyloma, left eye
        H15.823 Localized anterior staphyloma, bilateral
        H15.829 Localized anterior staphyloma, unspecified eye ▽

√6ᵗʰ **H15.83** Staphyloma posticum
        H15.831 Staphyloma posticum, right eye
        H15.832 Staphyloma posticum, left eye
        H15.833 Staphyloma posticum, bilateral
        H15.839 Staphyloma posticum, unspecified eye ▽

√6ᵗʰ **H15.84** Scleral ectasia
        H15.841 Scleral ectasia, right eye

        H15.842 Scleral ectasia, left eye
        H15.843 Scleral ectasia, bilateral
        H15.849 Scleral ectasia, unspecified eye ▽

√6ᵗʰ **H15.85** Ring staphyloma
        H15.851 Ring staphyloma, right eye
        H15.852 Ring staphyloma, left eye
        H15.853 Ring staphyloma, bilateral
        H15.859 Ring staphyloma, unspecified eye ▽

      H15.89 Other disorders of sclera
H15.9 Unspecified disorder of sclera ▽

√4ᵗʰ **H16** **Keratitis**
      DEF: Condition in which the cornea becomes inflamed and irritated.

√5ᵗʰ **H16.0** Corneal ulcer
√6ᵗʰ **H16.00** Unspecified corneal ulcer
        H16.001 Unspecified corneal ulcer, right eye ▽
        H16.002 Unspecified corneal ulcer, left eye ▽
        H16.003 Unspecified corneal ulcer, bilateral ▽
        H16.009 Unspecified corneal ulcer, unspecified eye ▽

√6ᵗʰ **H16.01** Central corneal ulcer
        H16.011 Central corneal ulcer, right eye
        H16.012 Central corneal ulcer, left eye
        H16.013 Central corneal ulcer, bilateral
        H16.019 Central corneal ulcer, unspecified eye ▽

√6ᵗʰ **H16.02** Ring corneal ulcer
        H16.021 Ring corneal ulcer, right eye
        H16.022 Ring corneal ulcer, left eye
        H16.023 Ring corneal ulcer, bilateral
        H16.029 Ring corneal ulcer, unspecified eye ▽

√6ᵗʰ **H16.03** Corneal ulcer with hypopyon
        H16.031 Corneal ulcer with hypopyon, right eye
        H16.032 Corneal ulcer with hypopyon, left eye
        H16.033 Corneal ulcer with hypopyon, bilateral
        H16.039 Corneal ulcer with hypopyon, unspecified eye ▽

√6ᵗʰ **H16.04** Marginal corneal ulcer
        H16.041 Marginal corneal ulcer, right eye
        H16.042 Marginal corneal ulcer, left eye
        H16.043 Marginal corneal ulcer, bilateral
        H16.049 Marginal corneal ulcer, unspecified eye ▽

√6ᵗʰ **H16.05** Mooren's corneal ulcer
        H16.051 Mooren's corneal ulcer, right eye
        H16.052 Mooren's corneal ulcer, left eye
        H16.053 Mooren's corneal ulcer, bilateral
        H16.059 Mooren's corneal ulcer, unspecified eye ▽

√6ᵗʰ **H16.06** Mycotic corneal ulcer
        H16.061 Mycotic corneal ulcer, right eye
        H16.062 Mycotic corneal ulcer, left eye
        H16.063 Mycotic corneal ulcer, bilateral
        H16.069 Mycotic corneal ulcer, unspecified eye ▽

√6ᵗʰ **H16.07** Perforated corneal ulcer
        H16.071 Perforated corneal ulcer, right eye
        H16.072 Perforated corneal ulcer, left eye
        H16.073 Perforated corneal ulcer, bilateral
        H16.079 Perforated corneal ulcer, unspecified eye ▽

√5ᵗʰ **H16.1** Other and unspecified superficial keratitis without conjunctivitis
√6ᵗʰ **H16.10** Unspecified superficial keratitis
        H16.101 Unspecified superficial keratitis, right eye ▽
        H16.102 Unspecified superficial keratitis, left eye ▽
        H16.103 Unspecified superficial keratitis, bilateral ▽
        H16.109 Unspecified superficial keratitis, unspecified eye ▽

✓6ᵗʰ **H16.11** **Macular keratitis**

    Areolar keratitis
    Nummular keratitis
    Stellate keratitis
    Striate keratitis

    H16.111 **Macular keratitis, right eye**
    H16.112 **Macular keratitis, left eye**
    H16.113 **Macular keratitis, bilateral**
    H16.119 **Macular keratitis, unspecified eye** ▽

✓6ᵗʰ **H16.12** **Filamentary keratitis**

    H16.121 **Filamentary keratitis, right eye**
    H16.122 **Filamentary keratitis, left eye**
    H16.123 **Filamentary keratitis, bilateral**
    H16.129 **Filamentary keratitis, unspecified eye** ▽

✓6ᵗʰ **H16.13** **Photokeratitis**

    Snow blindness
    Welders keratitis

    H16.131 **Photokeratitis, right eye**
    H16.132 **Photokeratitis, left eye**
    H16.133 **Photokeratitis, bilateral**
    H16.139 **Photokeratitis, unspecified eye** ▽

✓6ᵗʰ **H16.14** **Punctate keratitis**

    H16.141 **Punctate keratitis, right eye**
    H16.142 **Punctate keratitis, left eye**
    H16.143 **Punctate keratitis, bilateral**
    H16.149 **Punctate keratitis, unspecified eye** ▽

✓5ᵗʰ **H16.2** **Keratoconjunctivitis**

✓6ᵗʰ **H16.20** **Unspecified keratoconjunctivitis**

    Superficial keratitis with conjunctivitis NOS

    H16.201 **Unspecified keratoconjunctivitis, right eye** ▽
    H16.202 **Unspecified keratoconjunctivitis, left eye** ▽
    H16.203 **Unspecified keratoconjunctivitis, bilateral** ▽
    H16.209 **Unspecified keratoconjunctivitis, unspecified eye** ▽

✓6ᵗʰ **H16.21** **Exposure keratoconjunctivitis**

    H16.211 **Exposure keratoconjunctivitis, right eye**
    H16.212 **Exposure keratoconjunctivitis, left eye**
    H16.213 **Exposure keratoconjunctivitis, bilateral**
    H16.219 **Exposure keratoconjunctivitis, unspecified eye** ▽

✓6ᵗʰ **H16.22** **Keratoconjunctivitis sicca, not specified as Sjögren's**

    EXCLUDES 1   *Sjögren's syndrome (M35.01)*

    H16.221 **Keratoconjunctivitis sicca, not specified as Sjögren's, right eye**
    H16.222 **Keratoconjunctivitis sicca, not specified as Sjögren's, left eye**
    H16.223 **Keratoconjunctivitis sicca, not specified as Sjögren's, bilateral**
    H16.229 **Keratoconjunctivitis sicca, not specified as Sjögren's, unspecified eye** ▽

✓6ᵗʰ **H16.23** **Neurotrophic keratoconjunctivitis**

    H16.231 **Neurotrophic keratoconjunctivitis, right eye**
    H16.232 **Neurotrophic keratoconjunctivitis, left eye**
    H16.233 **Neurotrophic keratoconjunctivitis, bilateral**
    H16.239 **Neurotrophic keratoconjunctivitis, unspecified eye** ▽

✓6ᵗʰ **H16.24** **Ophthalmia nodosa**

    H16.241 **Ophthalmia nodosa, right eye**
    H16.242 **Ophthalmia nodosa, left eye**
    H16.243 **Ophthalmia nodosa, bilateral**
    H16.249 **Ophthalmia nodosa, unspecified eye** ▽

✓6ᵗʰ **H16.25** **Phlyctenular keratoconjunctivitis**

    H16.251 **Phlyctenular keratoconjunctivitis, right eye**
    H16.252 **Phlyctenular keratoconjunctivitis, left eye**
    H16.253 **Phlyctenular keratoconjunctivitis, bilateral**

    H16.259 **Phlyctenular keratoconjunctivitis, unspecified eye** ▽

✓6ᵗʰ **H16.26** **Vernal keratoconjunctivitis, with limbar and corneal involvement**

    EXCLUDES 1   *vernal conjunctivitis without limbar and corneal involvement (H10.44)*

    H16.261 **Vernal keratoconjunctivitis, with limbar and corneal involvement, right eye**
    H16.262 **Vernal keratoconjunctivitis, with limbar and corneal involvement, left eye**
    H16.263 **Vernal keratoconjunctivitis, with limbar and corneal involvement, bilateral**
    H16.269 **Vernal keratoconjunctivitis, with limbar and corneal involvement, unspecified eye** ▽

✓6ᵗʰ **H16.29** **Other keratoconjunctivitis**

    H16.291 **Other keratoconjunctivitis, right eye**
    H16.292 **Other keratoconjunctivitis, left eye**
    H16.293 **Other keratoconjunctivitis, bilateral**
    H16.299 **Other keratoconjunctivitis, unspecified eye** ▽

✓5ᵗʰ **H16.3** **Interstitial and deep keratitis**

✓6ᵗʰ **H16.30** **Unspecified interstitial keratitis**

    H16.301 **Unspecified interstitial keratitis, right eye** ▽
    H16.302 **Unspecified interstitial keratitis, left eye** ▽
    H16.303 **Unspecified interstitial keratitis, bilateral** ▽
    H16.309 **Unspecified interstitial keratitis, unspecified eye** ▽

✓6ᵗʰ **H16.31** **Corneal abscess**

    H16.311 **Corneal abscess, right eye**
    H16.312 **Corneal abscess, left eye**
    H16.313 **Corneal abscess, bilateral**
    H16.319 **Corneal abscess, unspecified eye** ▽

✓6ᵗʰ **H16.32** **Diffuse interstitial keratitis**

    Cogan's syndrome

    H16.321 **Diffuse interstitial keratitis, right eye**
    H16.322 **Diffuse interstitial keratitis, left eye**
    H16.323 **Diffuse interstitial keratitis, bilateral**
    H16.329 **Diffuse interstitial keratitis, unspecified eye** ▽

✓6ᵗʰ **H16.33** **Sclerosing keratitis**

    H16.331 **Sclerosing keratitis, right eye**
    H16.332 **Sclerosing keratitis, left eye**
    H16.333 **Sclerosing keratitis, bilateral**
    H16.339 **Sclerosing keratitis, unspecified eye** ▽

✓6ᵗʰ **H16.39** **Other interstitial and deep keratitis**

    H16.391 **Other interstitial and deep keratitis, right eye**
    H16.392 **Other interstitial and deep keratitis, left eye**
    H16.393 **Other interstitial and deep keratitis, bilateral**
    H16.399 **Other interstitial and deep keratitis, unspecified eye** ▽

✓5ᵗʰ **H16.4** **Corneal neovascularization**

✓6ᵗʰ **H16.40** **Unspecified corneal neovascularization**

    H16.401 **Unspecified corneal neovascularization, right eye** ▽
    H16.402 **Unspecified corneal neovascularization, left eye** ▽
    H16.403 **Unspecified corneal neovascularization, bilateral** ▽
    H16.409 **Unspecified corneal neovascularization, unspecified eye** ▽

✓6ᵗʰ **H16.41** **Ghost vessels (corneal)**

    H16.411 **Ghost vessels (corneal), right eye**
    H16.412 **Ghost vessels (corneal), left eye**
    H16.413 **Ghost vessels (corneal), bilateral**
    H16.419 **Ghost vessels (corneal), unspecified eye** ▽

✓6ᵗʰ **H16.42** **Pannus (corneal)**

    H16.421 **Pannus (corneal), right eye**
    H16.422 **Pannus (corneal), left eye**
    H16.423 **Pannus (corneal), bilateral**

☑ Additional Character Req   ✓x7ᵗʰ Placeholder Alert   Manifestation   ▽ Unspecified   ►◄ Revised Text   ● New Code   ▲ Revised Code Title

H16.429   Pannus (corneal), unspecified eye ▽

√6ᵗʰ H16.43   Localized vascularization of cornea

H16.431   Localized vascularization of cornea, right eye

H16.432   Localized vascularization of cornea, left eye

H16.433   Localized vascularization of cornea, bilateral

H16.439   Localized vascularization of cornea, unspecified eye ▽

√6ᵗʰ H16.44   Deep vascularization of cornea

H16.441   Deep vascularization of cornea, right eye

H16.442   Deep vascularization of cornea, left eye

H16.443   Deep vascularization of cornea, bilateral

H16.449   Deep vascularization of cornea, unspecified eye ▽

H16.8   Other keratitis

H16.9   Unspecified keratitis ▽

√4ᵗʰ **H17   Corneal scars and opacities**

√5ᵗʰ H17.0   Adherent leukoma

H17.00   Adherent leukoma, unspecified eye ▽

H17.01   Adherent leukoma, right eye

H17.02   Adherent leukoma, left eye

H17.03   Adherent leukoma, bilateral

√5ᵗʰ H17.1   Central corneal opacity

H17.10   Central corneal opacity, unspecified eye ▽

H17.11   Central corneal opacity, right eye

H17.12   Central corneal opacity, left eye

H17.13   Central corneal opacity, bilateral

√5ᵗʰ H17.8   Other corneal scars and opacities

√6ᵗʰ H17.81   Minor opacity of cornea

Corneal nebula

H17.811   Minor opacity of cornea, right eye

H17.812   Minor opacity of cornea, left eye

H17.813   Minor opacity of cornea, bilateral

H17.819   Minor opacity of cornea, unspecified eye ▽

√6ᵗʰ H17.82   Peripheral opacity of cornea

H17.821   Peripheral opacity of cornea, right eye

H17.822   Peripheral opacity of cornea, left eye

H17.823   Peripheral opacity of cornea, bilateral

H17.829   Peripheral opacity of cornea, unspecified eye ▽

H17.89   Other corneal scars and opacities

H17.9   Unspecified corneal scar and opacity ▽

√4ᵗʰ **H18   Other disorders of cornea**

√5ᵗʰ H18.0   Corneal pigmentations and deposits

√6ᵗʰ H18.00   Unspecified corneal deposit

H18.001   Unspecified corneal deposit, right eye ▽

H18.002   Unspecified corneal deposit, left eye ▽

H18.003   Unspecified corneal deposit, bilateral ▽

H18.009   Unspecified corneal deposit, unspecified eye ▽

√6ᵗʰ H18.01   Anterior corneal pigmentations

Staehli's line

H18.011   Anterior corneal pigmentations, right eye

H18.012   Anterior corneal pigmentations, left eye

H18.013   Anterior corneal pigmentations, bilateral

H18.019   Anterior corneal pigmentations, unspecified eye ▽

√6ᵗʰ H18.02   Argentous corneal deposits

H18.021   Argentous corneal deposits, right eye

H18.022   Argentous corneal deposits, left eye

H18.023   Argentous corneal deposits, bilateral

H18.029   Argentous corneal deposits, unspecified eye ▽

√6ᵗʰ H18.03   Corneal deposits in metabolic disorders

Code also associated metabolic disorder

H18.031   Corneal deposits in metabolic disorders, right eye

H18.032   Corneal deposits in metabolic disorders, left eye

H18.033   Corneal deposits in metabolic disorders, bilateral

H18.039   Corneal deposits in metabolic disorders, unspecified eye ▽

√6ᵗʰ H18.04   Kayser-Fleischer ring

Code also associated Wilson's disease (E83.01)

H18.041   Kayser-Fleischer ring, right eye

H18.042   Kayser-Fleischer ring, left eye

H18.043   Kayser-Fleischer ring, bilateral

H18.049   Kayser-Fleischer ring, unspecified eye ▽

√6ᵗʰ H18.05   Posterior corneal pigmentations

Krukenberg's spindle

H18.051   Posterior corneal pigmentations, right eye

H18.052   Posterior corneal pigmentations, left eye

H18.053   Posterior corneal pigmentations, bilateral

H18.059   Posterior corneal pigmentations, unspecified eye ▽

√6ᵗʰ H18.06   Stromal corneal pigmentations

Hematocornea

H18.061   Stromal corneal pigmentations, right eye

H18.062   Stromal corneal pigmentations, left eye

H18.063   Stromal corneal pigmentations, bilateral

H18.069   Stromal corneal pigmentations, unspecified eye ▽

√5ᵗʰ H18.1   Bullous keratopathy

DEF: Corneal swelling due to a damaged corneal endothelium. Bullous keratopathy is characterized by recurring, rupturing epithelial blisters causing glaucoma, iridocyclitis, and Fuchs dystrophy.

H18.10   Bullous keratopathy, unspecified eye ▽

H18.11   Bullous keratopathy, right eye

H18.12   Bullous keratopathy, left eye

H18.13   Bullous keratopathy, bilateral

√5ᵗʰ H18.2   Other and unspecified corneal edema

H18.20   Unspecified corneal edema ▽

√6ᵗʰ H18.21   Corneal edema secondary to contact lens

EXCLUDES 2   other corneal disorders due to contact lens (H18.82-)

H18.211   Corneal edema secondary to contact lens, right eye

H18.212   Corneal edema secondary to contact lens, left eye

H18.213   Corneal edema secondary to contact lens, bilateral

H18.219   Corneal edema secondary to contact lens, unspecified eye

√6ᵗʰ H18.22   Idiopathic corneal edema

H18.221   Idiopathic corneal edema, right eye

H18.222   Idiopathic corneal edema, left eye

H18.223   Idiopathic corneal edema, bilateral

H18.229   Idiopathic corneal edema, unspecified eye ▽

√6ᵗʰ H18.23   Secondary corneal edema

H18.231   Secondary corneal edema, right eye

H18.232   Secondary corneal edema, left eye

H18.233   Secondary corneal edema, bilateral

H18.239   Secondary corneal edema, unspecified eye ▽

√5ᵗʰ H18.3   Changes of corneal membranes

H18.30   Unspecified corneal membrane change ▽

√6ᵗʰ H18.31   Folds and rupture in Bowman's membrane

H18.311   Folds and rupture in Bowman's membrane, right eye

H18.312   Folds and rupture in Bowman's membrane, left eye

H18.313   Folds and rupture in Bowman's membrane, bilateral

H18.319   Folds and rupture in Bowman's membrane, unspecified eye ▽

√6ᵗʰ H18.32   Folds in Descemet's membrane

H18.321   Folds in Descemet's membrane, right eye

H18.322   Folds in Descemet's membrane, left eye

H18.323   Folds in Descemet's membrane, bilateral

H18.329   Folds in Descemet's membrane, unspecified eye ▽

√6ᵗʰ **H18.33** Rupture in Descemet's membrane

   H18.331 Rupture in Descemet's membrane, **right eye**

   H18.332 Rupture in Descemet's membrane, **left eye**

   H18.333 Rupture in Descemet's membrane, **bilateral**

   H18.339 Rupture in Descemet's membrane, unspecified eye ▽

√5ᵗʰ **H18.4** Corneal degeneration

   EXCLUDES 1 Mooren's ulcer (H16.Ø-)
                recurrent erosion of cornea (H18.83-)

   H18.40 Unspecified corneal degeneration ▽

√6ᵗʰ **H18.41** Arcus senilis

      Senile corneal changes

      H18.411 Arcus senilis, **right eye**

      H18.412 Arcus senilis, **left eye**

      H18.413 Arcus senilis, **bilateral**

      H18.419 Arcus senilis, unspecified eye ▽

√6ᵗʰ **H18.42** Band keratopathy

      H18.421 Band keratopathy, **right eye**

      H18.422 Band keratopathy, **left eye**

      H18.423 Band keratopathy, **bilateral**

      H18.429 Band keratopathy, unspecified eye ▽

   H18.43 Other calcerous corneal degeneration

√6ᵗʰ **H18.44** Keratomalacia

         EXCLUDES 1 keratomalacia due to vitamin A deficiency (E5Ø.4)

      H18.441 Keratomalacia, **right eye**

      H18.442 Keratomalacia, **left eye**

      H18.443 Keratomalacia, **bilateral**

      H18.449 Keratomalacia, unspecified eye ▽

√6ᵗʰ **H18.45** Nodular corneal degeneration

      H18.451 Nodular corneal degeneration, **right eye**

      H18.452 Nodular corneal degeneration, **left eye**

      H18.453 Nodular corneal degeneration, **bilateral**

      H18.459 Nodular corneal degeneration, unspecified eye ▽

√6ᵗʰ **H18.46** Peripheral corneal degeneration

      H18.461 Peripheral corneal degeneration, **right eye**

      H18.462 Peripheral corneal degeneration, **left eye**

      H18.463 Peripheral corneal degeneration, **bilateral**

      H18.469 Peripheral corneal degeneration, unspecified eye ▽

   H18.49 Other corneal degeneration

√5ᵗʰ **H18.5** Hereditary corneal dystrophies

   H18.50 Unspecified hereditary corneal dystrophies ▽

   H18.51 Endothelial corneal dystrophy

      Fuchs' dystrophy

   H18.52 Epithelial (juvenile) corneal dystrophy

   H18.53 Granular corneal dystrophy

   H18.54 Lattice corneal dystrophy

   H18.55 Macular corneal dystrophy

   H18.59 Other hereditary corneal dystrophies

√5ᵗʰ **H18.6** Keratoconus

√6ᵗʰ **H18.60** Keratoconus, unspecified

      H18.6Ø1 Keratoconus, unspecified, **right eye** ▽

      H18.6Ø2 Keratoconus, unspecified, **left eye** ▽

      H18.6Ø3 Keratoconus, unspecified, **bilateral** ▽

      H18.6Ø9 Keratoconus, unspecified, unspecified eye ▽

√6ᵗʰ **H18.61** Keratoconus, stable

      H18.611 Keratoconus, stable, **right eye**

      H18.612 Keratoconus, stable, **left eye**

      H18.613 Keratoconus, stable, **bilateral**

      H18.619 Keratoconus, stable, unspecified eye ▽

√6ᵗʰ **H18.62** Keratoconus, unstable

      Acute hydrops

      H18.621 Keratoconus, unstable, **right eye**

      H18.622 Keratoconus, unstable, **left eye**

      H18.623 Keratoconus, unstable, **bilateral**

      H18.629 Keratoconus, unstable, unspecified eye ▽

√5ᵗʰ **H18.7** Other and unspecified corneal deformities

      EXCLUDES 1 congenital malformations of cornea (Q13.3-Q13.4)

   H18.70 Unspecified corneal deformity ▽

√6ᵗʰ **H18.71** Corneal ectasia

      H18.711 Corneal ectasia, **right eye**

      H18.712 Corneal ectasia, **left eye**

      H18.713 Corneal ectasia, **bilateral**

      H18.719 Corneal ectasia, unspecified eye ▽

√6ᵗʰ **H18.72** Corneal staphyloma

      H18.721 Corneal staphyloma, **right eye**

      H18.722 Corneal staphyloma, **left eye**

      H18.723 Corneal staphyloma, **bilateral**

      H18.729 Corneal staphyloma, unspecified eye ▽

√6ᵗʰ **H18.73** Descemetocele

      H18.731 Descemetocele, **right eye**

      H18.732 Descemetocele, **left eye**

      H18.733 Descemetocele, **bilateral**

      H18.739 Descemetocele, unspecified eye ▽

√6ᵗʰ **H18.79** Other corneal deformities

      H18.791 Other corneal deformities, **right eye**

      H18.792 Other corneal deformities, **left eye**

      H18.793 Other corneal deformities, **bilateral**

      H18.799 Other corneal deformities, unspecified eye ▽

√5ᵗʰ **H18.8** Other specified disorders of cornea

√6ᵗʰ **H18.81** Anesthesia and hypoesthesia of cornea

      H18.811 Anesthesia and hypoesthesia of cornea, **right eye**

      H18.812 Anesthesia and hypoesthesia of cornea, **left eye**

      H18.813 Anesthesia and hypoesthesia of cornea, **bilateral**

      H18.819 Anesthesia and hypoesthesia of cornea, unspecified eye ▽

√6ᵗʰ **H18.82** Corneal disorder due to contact lens

         EXCLUDES 2 corneal edema due to contact lens (H18.21-)

      H18.821 Corneal disorder due to contact lens, **right eye**

      H18.822 Corneal disorder due to contact lens, **left eye**

      H18.823 Corneal disorder due to contact lens, **bilateral**

      H18.829 Corneal disorder due to contact lens, unspecified eye ▽

√6ᵗʰ **H18.83** Recurrent erosion of cornea

      H18.831 Recurrent erosion of cornea, **right eye**

      H18.832 Recurrent erosion of cornea, **left eye**

      H18.833 Recurrent erosion of cornea, **bilateral**

      H18.839 Recurrent erosion of cornea, unspecified eye ▽

√6ᵗʰ **H18.89** Other specified disorders of cornea

      H18.891 Other specified disorders of cornea, **right eye**

      H18.892 Other specified disorders of cornea, **left eye**

      H18.893 Other specified disorders of cornea, **bilateral**

      H18.899 Other specified disorders of cornea, unspecified eye ▽

   H18.9 Unspecified disorder of cornea ▽

☑ Additional Character Req   √x7ᵗʰ Placeholder Alert   Manifestation   ▽ Unspecified   ►◄ Revised Text   ● New Code   ▲ Revised Code Title

Chapter 7. Diseases of the Eye and Adnexa

H20–H21.232

√4th **H20 Iridocyclitis**

√5th **H20.0 Acute and subacute iridocyclitis**

Acute anterior uveitis
Acute cyclitis
Acute iritis
Subacute anterior uveitis
Subacute cyclitis
Subacute iritis

EXCLUDES 1   iridocyclitis, iritis, uveitis (due to) (in) diabetes mellitus (E08-E13 with .39)
iridocyclitis, iritis, uveitis (due to) (in) diphtheria (A36.89)
iridocyclitis, iritis, uveitis (due to) (in) gonococcal (A54.32)
iridocyclitis, iritis, uveitis (due to) (in) herpes (simplex) (B00.51)
iridocyclitis, iritis, uveitis (due to) (in) herpes zoster (B02.32)
iridocyclitis, iritis, uveitis (due to) (in) late congenital syphilis (A50.39)
iridocyclitis, iritis, uveitis (due to) (in) late syphilis (A52.71)
iridocyclitis, iritis, uveitis (due to) (in) sarcoidosis (D86.83)
iridocyclitis, iritis, uveitis (due to) (in) syphilis (A51.43)
iridocyclitis, iritis, uveitis (due to) (in) toxoplasmosis (B58.09)
iridocyclitis, iritis, uveitis (due to) (in) tuberculosis (A18.54)

     H20.00 Unspecified acute and subacute iridocyclitis ▽

√6th **H20.01 Primary iridocyclitis**

     H20.011 Primary iridocyclitis, right eye
     H20.012 Primary iridocyclitis, left eye
     H20.013 Primary iridocyclitis, bilateral
     H20.019 Primary iridocyclitis, unspecified eye ▽

√6th **H20.02 Recurrent acute iridocyclitis**

     H20.021 Recurrent acute iridocyclitis, right eye
     H20.022 Recurrent acute iridocyclitis, left eye
     H20.023 Recurrent acute iridocyclitis, bilateral
     H20.029 Recurrent acute iridocyclitis, unspecified eye ▽

√6th **H20.03 Secondary infectious iridocyclitis**

     H20.031 Secondary infectious iridocyclitis, right eye
     H20.032 Secondary infectious iridocyclitis, left eye
     H20.033 Secondary infectious iridocyclitis, bilateral
     H20.039 Secondary infectious iridocyclitis, unspecified eye ▽

√6th **H20.04 Secondary noninfectious iridocyclitis**

     H20.041 Secondary noninfectious iridocyclitis, right eye
     H20.042 Secondary noninfectious iridocyclitis, left eye
     H20.043 Secondary noninfectious iridocyclitis, bilateral
     H20.049 Secondary noninfectious iridocyclitis, unspecified eye ▽

√6th **H20.05 Hypopyon**

     H20.051 Hypopyon, right eye
     H20.052 Hypopyon, left eye
     H20.053 Hypopyon, bilateral
     H20.059 Hypopyon, unspecified eye ▽

√5th **H20.1 Chronic iridocyclitis**

Use additional code for any associated cataract (H26.21-)
EXCLUDES 2   posterior cyclitis (H30.2-)

     H20.10 Chronic iridocyclitis, unspecified eye ▽
     H20.11 Chronic iridocyclitis, right eye
     H20.12 Chronic iridocyclitis, left eye
     H20.13 Chronic iridocyclitis, bilateral

√5th **H20.2 Lens-induced iridocyclitis**

     H20.20 Lens-induced iridocyclitis, unspecified eye ▽
     H20.21 Lens-induced iridocyclitis, right eye
     H20.22 Lens-induced iridocyclitis, left eye
     H20.23 Lens-induced iridocyclitis, bilateral

√5th **H20.8 Other iridocyclitis**

EXCLUDES 2   glaucomatocyclitis crises (H40.4-)
posterior cyclitis (H30.2-)
sympathetic uveitis (H44.13-)

√6th **H20.81 Fuchs' heterochromic cyclitis**

     H20.811 Fuchs' heterochromic cyclitis, right eye
     H20.812 Fuchs' heterochromic cyclitis, left eye
     H20.813 Fuchs' heterochromic cyclitis, bilateral
     H20.819 Fuchs' heterochromic cyclitis, unspecified eye ▽

√6th **H20.82 Vogt-Koyanagi syndrome**

     H20.821 Vogt-Koyanagi syndrome, right eye
     H20.822 Vogt-Koyanagi syndrome, left eye
     H20.823 Vogt-Koyanagi syndrome, bilateral
     H20.829 Vogt-Koyanagi syndrome, unspecified eye ▽

H20.9 Unspecified iridocyclitis ▽
Uveitis NOS

√4th **H21 Other disorders of iris and ciliary body**

EXCLUDES 2   sympathetic uveitis (H44.1-)

√5th **H21.0 Hyphema**

EXCLUDES 1   traumatic hyphema (S05.1-)

Hyphema

Iris
Cornea
Hyphema

     H21.00 Hyphema, unspecified eye ▽
     H21.01 Hyphema, right eye
     H21.02 Hyphema, left eye
     H21.03 Hyphema, bilateral

√5th **H21.1 Other vascular disorders of iris and ciliary body**

Neovascularization of iris or ciliary body
Rubeosis iridis
Rubeosis of iris

√6th **H21.1X Other vascular disorders of iris and ciliary body**

     H21.1X1 Other vascular disorders of iris and ciliary body, right eye
     H21.1X2 Other vascular disorders of iris and ciliary body, left eye
     H21.1X3 Other vascular disorders of iris and ciliary body, bilateral
     H21.1X9 Other vascular disorders of iris and ciliary body, unspecified eye ▽

√5th **H21.2 Degeneration of iris and ciliary body**

√6th **H21.21 Degeneration of chamber angle**

     H21.211 Degeneration of chamber angle, right eye
     H21.212 Degeneration of chamber angle, left eye
     H21.213 Degeneration of chamber angle, bilateral
     H21.219 Degeneration of chamber angle, unspecified eye ▽

√6th **H21.22 Degeneration of ciliary body**

     H21.221 Degeneration of ciliary body, right eye
     H21.222 Degeneration of ciliary body, left eye
     H21.223 Degeneration of ciliary body, bilateral
     H21.229 Degeneration of ciliary body, unspecified eye ▽

√6th **H21.23 Degeneration of iris (pigmentary)**

Translucency of iris

     H21.231 Degeneration of iris (pigmentary), right eye
     H21.232 Degeneration of iris (pigmentary), left eye

H21.233   **Degeneration of iris (pigmentary), bilateral**

H21.239   **Degeneration of iris (pigmentary), unspecified eye** ▽

√6ᵗʰ **H21.24**   **Degeneration of** pupillary margin

H21.241   **Degeneration of pupillary margin,** right eye

H21.242   **Degeneration of pupillary margin,** left eye

H21.243   **Degeneration of pupillary margin,** bilateral

H21.249   **Degeneration of pupillary margin, unspecified eye** ▽

√6ᵗʰ **H21.25**   **Iridoschisis**

H21.251   **Iridoschisis,** right eye

H21.252   **Iridoschisis,** left eye

H21.253   **Iridoschisis,** bilateral

H21.259   **Iridoschisis, unspecified eye** ▽

√6ᵗʰ **H21.26**   **Iris** atrophy **(essential) (progressive)**

H21.261   **Iris atrophy (essential) (progressive),** right eye

H21.262   **Iris atrophy (essential) (progressive),** left eye

H21.263   **Iris atrophy (essential) (progressive),** bilateral

H21.269   **Iris atrophy (essential) (progressive), unspecified eye** ▽

√6ᵗʰ **H21.27**   **Miotic pupillary cyst**

H21.271   **Miotic pupillary cyst,** right eye

H21.272   **Miotic pupillary cyst,** left eye

H21.273   **Miotic pupillary cyst,** bilateral

H21.279   **Miotic pupillary cyst, unspecified eye** ▽

H21.29   **Other iris atrophy**

√5ᵗʰ **H21.3**   **Cyst of iris, ciliary body and anterior chamber**

EXCLUDES 2   *miotic pupillary cyst (H21.27-)*

√6ᵗʰ **H21.30**   **Idiopathic** cysts of iris, ciliary body or anterior chamber

Cyst of iris, ciliary body or anterior chamber NOS

H21.301   **Idiopathic cysts of iris, ciliary body or anterior chamber,** right eye

H21.302   **Idiopathic cysts of iris, ciliary body or anterior chamber,** left eye

H21.303   **Idiopathic cysts of iris, ciliary body or anterior chamber,** bilateral

H21.309   **Idiopathic cysts of iris, ciliary body or anterior chamber, unspecified eye** ▽

√6ᵗʰ **H21.31**   **Exudative** cysts of iris or anterior chamber

H21.311   **Exudative cysts of iris or anterior chamber,** right eye

H21.312   **Exudative cysts of iris or anterior chamber,** left eye

H21.313   **Exudative cysts of iris or anterior chamber,** bilateral

H21.319   **Exudative cysts of iris or anterior chamber, unspecified eye** ▽

√6ᵗʰ **H21.32**   **Implantation** cysts of iris, ciliary body or anterior chamber

H21.321   **Implantation cysts of iris, ciliary body or anterior chamber,** right eye

H21.322   **Implantation cysts of iris, ciliary body or anterior chamber,** left eye

H21.323   **Implantation cysts of iris, ciliary body or anterior chamber,** bilateral

H21.329   **Implantation cysts of iris, ciliary body or anterior chamber, unspecified eye** ▽

√6ᵗʰ **H21.33**   **Parasitic** cyst of iris, ciliary body or anterior chamber

H21.331   **Parasitic cyst of iris, ciliary body or anterior chamber,** right eye

H21.332   **Parasitic cyst of iris, ciliary body or anterior chamber,** left eye

H21.333   **Parasitic cyst of iris, ciliary body or anterior chamber,** bilateral

H21.339   **Parasitic cyst of iris, ciliary body or anterior chamber, unspecified eye** ▽

√6ᵗʰ **H21.34**   **Primary** cyst of pars plana

H21.341   **Primary cyst of pars plana,** right eye

H21.342   **Primary cyst of pars plana,** left eye

H21.343   **Primary cyst of pars plana,** bilateral

H21.349   **Primary cyst of pars plana, unspecified eye** ▽

√6ᵗʰ **H21.35**   **Exudative cyst of** pars plana

DEF: Protein, fatty-filled bullous elevation of the nonpigmented outermost ciliary epithelium of pars plana, due to fluid leak from blood vessels.

H21.351   **Exudative cyst of pars plana,** right eye

H21.352   **Exudative cyst of pars plana,** left eye

H21.353   **Exudative cyst of pars plana,** bilateral

H21.359   **Exudative cyst of pars plana, unspecified eye** ▽

√5ᵗʰ **H21.4**   **Pupillary membranes**

Iris bombé

Pupillary occlusion

Pupillary seclusion

EXCLUDES 1   *congenital pupillary membranes (Q13.8)*

H21.40   **Pupillary membranes, unspecified eye** ▽

H21.41   **Pupillary membranes,** right eye

H21.42   **Pupillary membranes,** left eye

H21.43   **Pupillary membranes,** bilateral

√5ᵗʰ **H21.5**   **Other and unspecified adhesions and disruptions of iris and ciliary body**

EXCLUDES 1   *corectopia (Q13.2)*

√6ᵗʰ **H21.50**   **Unspecified adhesions of iris**

Synechia (iris) NOS

H21.501   **Unspecified adhesions of iris,** right eye ▽

H21.502   **Unspecified adhesions of iris,** left eye ▽

H21.503   **Unspecified adhesions of iris,** bilateral ▽

H21.509   **Unspecified adhesions of iris and ciliary body, unspecified eye** ▽

√6ᵗʰ **H21.51**   **Anterior synechiae (iris)**

H21.511   **Anterior synechiae (iris),** right eye

H21.512   **Anterior synechiae (iris),** left eye

H21.513   **Anterior synechiae (iris),** bilateral

H21.519   **Anterior synechiae (iris), unspecified eye** ▽

√6ᵗʰ **H21.52**   **Goniosynechiae**

H21.521   **Goniosynechiae,** right eye

H21.522   **Goniosynechiae,** left eye

H21.523   **Goniosynechiae,** bilateral

H21.529   **Goniosynechiae, unspecified eye** ▽

√6ᵗʰ **H21.53**   **Iridodialysis**

H21.531   **Iridodialysis,** right eye

H21.532   **Iridodialysis,** left eye

H21.533   **Iridodialysis,** bilateral

H21.539   **Iridodialysis, unspecified eye** ▽

√6ᵗʰ **H21.54**   **Posterior synechiae (iris)**

H21.541   **Posterior synechiae (iris),** right eye

H21.542   **Posterior synechiae (iris),** left eye

H21.543   **Posterior synechiae (iris),** bilateral

H21.549   **Posterior synechiae (iris), unspecified eye** ▽

√6ᵗʰ **H21.55**   **Recession of chamber angle**

H21.551   **Recession of chamber angle,** right eye

H21.552   **Recession of chamber angle,** left eye

H21.553   **Recession of chamber angle,** bilateral

H21.559   **Recession of chamber angle, unspecified eye** ▽

√6ᵗʰ **H21.56**   **Pupillary abnormalities**

Deformed pupil

Ectopic pupil

Rupture of sphincter, pupil

EXCLUDES 1   *congenital deformity of pupil (Q13.2-)*

H21.561   **Pupillary abnormality,** right eye

H21.562   **Pupillary abnormality,** left eye

H21.563   **Pupillary abnormality,** bilateral

H21.569   **Pupillary abnormality, unspecified eye** ▽

✓ Additional Character Req   ✓x 7ᵗʰ Placeholder Alert   Manifestation   ▽ Unspecified   ▶◀ Revised Text   ● New Code   ▲ Revised Code Title

Chapter 7. Diseases of the Eye and Adnexa *(left margin)*

H21.8–H26.042 *(left margin)*

√5ᵗʰ **H21.8 Other specified disorders of iris and ciliary body**

   H21.81 Floppy iris syndrome
Intraoperative floppy iris syndrome (IFIS)
Use additional code for adverse effect, if applicable, to identify drug (T36-T50 with fifth or sixth character 5)

   H21.82 Plateau iris syndrome (post-iridectomy) (postprocedural)

   H21.89 Other specified disorders of iris and ciliary body

H21.9 Unspecified disorder of iris and ciliary body ▽

H22 Disorders of iris and ciliary body in diseases classified elsewhere
Code first underlying disease, such as:
gout (M1A.-, M10.-)
leprosy (A30.-)
parasitic disease (B89)

Disorders of lens (H25-H28)

√4ᵗʰ **H25 Age-related cataract**
Senile cataract
EXCLUDES 2 *capsular glaucoma with pseudoexfoliation of lens (H40.1-)*

Cataracts

Normal lens

Clouded lens

Lens affected by cataracts

√5ᵗʰ **H25.0 Age-related incipient cataract**

√6ᵗʰ **H25.01 Cortical age-related cataract**

   H25.011 Cortical age-related cataract, right eye Ⓐ

   H25.012 Cortical age-related cataract, left eye Ⓐ

   H25.013 Cortical age-related cataract, bilateral Ⓐ

   H25.019 Cortical age-related cataract, unspecified eye Ⓐ ▽

√6ᵗʰ **H25.03 Anterior subcapsular polar age-related cataract**

   H25.031 Anterior subcapsular polar age-related cataract, right eye Ⓐ

   H25.032 Anterior subcapsular polar age-related cataract, left eye Ⓐ

   H25.033 Anterior subcapsular polar age-related cataract, bilateral Ⓐ

   H25.039 Anterior subcapsular polar age-related cataract, unspecified eye Ⓐ ▽

√6ᵗʰ **H25.04 Posterior subcapsular polar age-related cataract**

   H25.041 Posterior subcapsular polar age-related cataract, right eye Ⓐ

   H25.042 Posterior subcapsular polar age-related cataract, left eye Ⓐ

   H25.043 Posterior subcapsular polar age-related cataract, bilateral Ⓐ

   H25.049 Posterior subcapsular polar age-related cataract, unspecified eye Ⓐ ▽

√6ᵗʰ **H25.09 Other age-related incipient cataract**
Coronary age-related cataract
Punctate age-related cataract
Water clefts

   H25.091 Other age-related incipient cataract, right eye Ⓐ

   H25.092 Other age-related incipient cataract, left eye Ⓐ

   H25.093 Other age-related incipient cataract, bilateral Ⓐ

   H25.099 Other age-related incipient cataract, unspecified eye Ⓐ ▽

√5ᵗʰ **H25.1 Age-related nuclear cataract**
Cataracta brunescens
Nuclear sclerosis cataract
AHA: 2016,1Q,32

   H25.10 Age-related nuclear cataract, unspecified eye Ⓐ ▽

   H25.11 Age-related nuclear cataract, right eye Ⓐ

   H25.12 Age-related nuclear cataract, left eye Ⓐ

   H25.13 Age-related nuclear cataract, bilateral Ⓐ

√5ᵗʰ **H25.2 Age-related cataract, morgagnian type**
Age-related hypermature cataract

   H25.20 Age-related cataract, morgagnian type, unspecified eye Ⓐ ▽

   H25.21 Age-related cataract, morgagnian type, right eye Ⓐ

   H25.22 Age-related cataract, morgagnian type, left eye Ⓐ

   H25.23 Age-related cataract, morgagnian type, bilateral Ⓐ

√5ᵗʰ **H25.8 Other age-related cataract**

√6ᵗʰ **H25.81 Combined forms of age-related cataract**

   H25.811 Combined forms of age-related cataract, right eye Ⓐ

   H25.812 Combined forms of age-related cataract, left eye Ⓐ

   H25.813 Combined forms of age-related cataract, bilateral Ⓐ

   H25.819 Combined forms of age-related cataract, unspecified eye Ⓐ ▽

   H25.89 Other age-related cataract Ⓐ

H25.9 Unspecified age-related cataract Ⓐ ▽

√4ᵗʰ **H26 Other cataract**
EXCLUDES 1 *congenital cataract (Q12.0)*

√5ᵗʰ **H26.0 Infantile and juvenile cataract**

√6ᵗʰ **H26.00 Unspecified infantile and juvenile cataract**

   H26.001 Unspecified infantile and juvenile cataract, right eye ℙ ▽

   H26.002 Unspecified infantile and juvenile cataract, left eye ℙ ▽

   H26.003 Unspecified infantile and juvenile cataract, bilateral ℙ ▽

   H26.009 Unspecified infantile and juvenile cataract, unspecified eye ℙ ▽

√6ᵗʰ **H26.01 Infantile and juvenile cortical, lamellar, or zonular cataract**

   H26.011 Infantile and juvenile cortical, lamellar, or zonular cataract, right eye ℙ

   H26.012 Infantile and juvenile cortical, lamellar, or zonular cataract, left eye ℙ

   H26.013 Infantile and juvenile cortical, lamellar, or zonular cataract, bilateral ℙ

   H26.019 Infantile and juvenile cortical, lamellar, or zonular cataract, unspecified eye ℙ ▽

√6ᵗʰ **H26.03 Infantile and juvenile nuclear cataract**

   H26.031 Infantile and juvenile nuclear cataract, right eye ℙ

   H26.032 Infantile and juvenile nuclear cataract, left eye ℙ

   H26.033 Infantile and juvenile nuclear cataract, bilateral ℙ

   H26.039 Infantile and juvenile nuclear cataract, unspecified eye ℙ ▽

√6ᵗʰ **H26.04 Anterior subcapsular polar infantile and juvenile cataract**

   H26.041 Anterior subcapsular polar infantile and juvenile cataract, right eye ℙ

   H26.042 Anterior subcapsular polar infantile and juvenile cataract, left eye ℙ

H26.043 **Anterior subcapsular polar infantile and juvenile cataract, bilateral** P

H26.049 **Anterior subcapsular polar infantile and juvenile cataract, unspecified eye** P ▽

√6ᵗʰ H26.05 **Posterior subcapsular polar infantile and juvenile cataract**

H26.051 **Posterior subcapsular polar infantile and juvenile cataract, right eye** P

H26.052 **Posterior subcapsular polar infantile and juvenile cataract, left eye** P

H26.053 **Posterior subcapsular polar infantile and juvenile cataract, bilateral** P

H26.059 **Posterior subcapsular polar infantile and juvenile cataract, unspecified eye** P ▽

√6ᵗʰ H26.06 **Combined forms of infantile and juvenile cataract**

H26.061 **Combined forms of infantile and juvenile cataract, right eye** P

H26.062 **Combined forms of infantile and juvenile cataract, left eye** P

H26.063 **Combined forms of infantile and juvenile cataract, bilateral** P

H26.069 **Combined forms of infantile and juvenile cataract, unspecified eye** P ▽

H26.09 **Other infantile and juvenile cataract** P

√5ᵗʰ H26.1 **Traumatic cataract**

Use additional code (Chapter 20) to identify external cause

√6ᵗʰ H26.10 **Unspecified traumatic cataract**

H26.101 **Unspecified traumatic cataract, right eye** ▽

H26.102 **Unspecified traumatic cataract, left eye** ▽

H26.103 **Unspecified traumatic cataract, bilateral** ▽

H26.109 **Unspecified traumatic cataract, unspecified eye** ▽

√6ᵗʰ H26.11 **Localized traumatic opacities**

H26.111 **Localized traumatic opacities, right eye**

H26.112 **Localized traumatic opacities, left eye**

H26.113 **Localized traumatic opacities, bilateral**

H26.119 **Localized traumatic opacities, unspecified eye** ▽

√6ᵗʰ H26.12 **Partially resolved traumatic cataract**

H26.121 **Partially resolved traumatic cataract, right eye**

H26.122 **Partially resolved traumatic cataract, left eye**

H26.123 **Partially resolved traumatic cataract, bilateral**

H26.129 **Partially resolved traumatic cataract, unspecified eye** ▽

√6ᵗʰ H26.13 **Total traumatic cataract**

H26.131 **Total traumatic cataract, right eye**

H26.132 **Total traumatic cataract, left eye**

H26.133 **Total traumatic cataract, bilateral**

H26.139 **Total traumatic cataract, unspecified eye** ▽

√5ᵗʰ H26.2 **Complicated cataract**

H26.20 **Unspecified complicated cataract** ▽
Cataracta complicata NOS

√6ᵗʰ H26.21 **Cataract with neovascularization**

Code also associated condition, such as:
chronic iridocyclitis (H20.1-)

H26.211 **Cataract with neovascularization, right eye**

H26.212 **Cataract with neovascularization, left eye**

H26.213 **Cataract with neovascularization, bilateral**

H26.219 **Cataract with neovascularization, unspecified eye** ▽

√6ᵗʰ H26.22 **Cataract secondary to ocular disorders (degenerative) (inflammatory)**
Code also associated ocular disorder

H26.221 **Cataract secondary to ocular disorders (degenerative) (inflammatory), right eye**

H26.222 **Cataract secondary to ocular disorders (degenerative) (inflammatory), left eye**

H26.223 **Cataract secondary to ocular disorders (degenerative) (inflammatory), bilateral**

H26.229 **Cataract secondary to ocular disorders (degenerative) (inflammatory), unspecified eye** ▽

√6ᵗʰ H26.23 **Glaucomatous flecks (subcapsular)**
Code first underlying glaucoma (H40-H42)

H26.231 **Glaucomatous flecks (subcapsular), right eye**

H26.232 **Glaucomatous flecks (subcapsular), left eye**

H26.233 **Glaucomatous flecks (subcapsular), bilateral**

H26.239 **Glaucomatous flecks (subcapsular), unspecified eye** ▽

√5ᵗʰ H26.3 **Drug-induced cataract**
Toxic cataract
Use additional code for adverse effect, if applicable, to identify drug (T36-T50 with fifth or sixth character 5)

H26.30 **Drug-induced cataract, unspecified eye** ▽

H26.31 **Drug-induced cataract, right eye**

H26.32 **Drug-induced cataract, left eye**

H26.33 **Drug-induced cataract, bilateral**

√5ᵗʰ H26.4 **Secondary cataract**

H26.40 **Unspecified secondary cataract** ▽

√6ᵗʰ H26.41 **Soemmering's ring**

H26.411 **Soemmering's ring, right eye**

H26.412 **Soemmering's ring, left eye**

H26.413 **Soemmering's ring, bilateral**

H26.419 **Soemmering's ring, unspecified eye** ▽

√6ᵗʰ H26.49 **Other secondary cataract**
AHA: 2018,2Q,14

H26.491 **Other secondary cataract, right eye**

H26.492 **Other secondary cataract, left eye**

H26.493 **Other secondary cataract, bilateral**

H26.499 **Other secondary cataract, unspecified eye** ▽

H26.8 **Other specified cataract**

H26.9 **Unspecified cataract** ▽

√4ᵗʰ H27 **Other disorders of lens**

EXCLUDES 1 *congenital lens malformations (Q12.-)*
mechanical complications of intraocular lens implant (T85.2)
pseudophakia (Z96.1)

√5ᵗʰ H27.0 **Aphakia**
Acquired absence of lens
Acquired aphakia
Aphakia due to trauma
EXCLUDES 1 *cataract extraction status (Z98.4-)*
congenital absence of lens (Q12.3)
congenital aphakia (Q12.3)

H27.00 **Aphakia, unspecified eye** ▽

H27.01 **Aphakia, right eye**

H27.02 **Aphakia, left eye**

H27.03 **Aphakia, bilateral**

√5ᵗʰ H27.1 **Dislocation of lens**

H27.10 **Unspecified dislocation of lens** ▽

√6ᵗʰ H27.11 **Subluxation of lens**

H27.111 **Subluxation of lens, right eye**

H27.112 **Subluxation of lens, left eye**

H27.113 **Subluxation of lens, bilateral**

H27.119 **Subluxation of lens, unspecified eye** ▽

√6ᵗʰ H27.12 **Anterior dislocation of lens**

H27.121 **Anterior dislocation of lens, right eye**

H27.122 **Anterior dislocation of lens, left eye**

H27.123 **Anterior dislocation of lens, bilateral**

H27.129 **Anterior dislocation of lens, unspecified eye** ▽

√6ᵗʰ H27.13 **Posterior dislocation of lens**

H27.131 **Posterior dislocation of lens, right eye**

H27.132 **Posterior dislocation of lens, left eye**

H27.133 **Posterior dislocation of lens, bilateral**

H27.139 **Posterior dislocation of lens, unspecified eye** ▽

Chapter 7. Diseases of the Eye and Adnexa

H27.8   Other specified disorders of lens

H27.9   Unspecified disorder of lens   ▽

H28   *Cataract in diseases classified elsewhere*

Code first underlying disease, such as:
- hypoparathyroidism (E20.-)
- myotonia (G71.1-)
- myxedema (E03.-)
- protein-calorie malnutrition (E40-E46)

EXCLUDES 1   cataract in diabetes mellitus (E08.36, E09.36, E10.36, E11.36, E13.36)

Disorders of choroid and retina (H30-H36)

H30   Chorioretinal inflammation

H30.0   Focal chorioretinal inflammation

- Focal chorioretinitis
- Focal choroiditis
- Focal retinitis
- Focal retinochoroiditis

H30.00   Unspecified focal chorioretinal inflammation
- Focal chorioretinitis NOS
- Focal choroiditis NOS
- Focal retinitis NOS
- Focal retinochoroiditis NOS

H30.001   Unspecified focal chorioretinal inflammation, right eye ▽

H30.002   Unspecified focal chorioretinal inflammation, left eye ▽

H30.003   Unspecified focal chorioretinal inflammation, bilateral ▽

H30.009   Unspecified focal chorioretinal inflammation, unspecified eye ▽

H30.01   Focal chorioretinal inflammation, juxtapapillary

H30.011   Focal chorioretinal inflammation, juxtapapillary, right eye

H30.012   Focal chorioretinal inflammation, juxtapapillary, left eye

H30.013   Focal chorioretinal inflammation, juxtapapillary, bilateral

H30.019   Focal chorioretinal inflammation, juxtapapillary, unspecified eye ▽

H30.02   Focal chorioretinal inflammation of posterior pole

H30.021   Focal chorioretinal inflammation of posterior pole, right eye

H30.022   Focal chorioretinal inflammation of posterior pole, left eye

H30.023   Focal chorioretinal inflammation of posterior pole, bilateral

H30.029   Focal chorioretinal inflammation of posterior pole, unspecified eye ▽

H30.03   Focal chorioretinal inflammation, peripheral

H30.031   Focal chorioretinal inflammation, peripheral, right eye

H30.032   Focal chorioretinal inflammation, peripheral, left eye

H30.033   Focal chorioretinal inflammation, peripheral, bilateral

H30.039   Focal chorioretinal inflammation, peripheral, unspecified eye ▽

H30.04   Focal chorioretinal inflammation, macular or paramacular

H30.041   Focal chorioretinal inflammation, macular or paramacular, right eye

H30.042   Focal chorioretinal inflammation, macular or paramacular, left eye

H30.043   Focal chorioretinal inflammation, macular or paramacular, bilateral

H30.049   Focal chorioretinal inflammation, macular or paramacular, unspecified eye ▽

H30.1   Disseminated chorioretinal inflammation
- Disseminated chorioretinitis
- Disseminated choroiditis
- Disseminated retinitis
- Disseminated retinochoroiditis

EXCLUDES 2   exudative retinopathy (H35.02-)

H30.10   Unspecified disseminated chorioretinal inflammation
- Disseminated chorioretinitis NOS
- Disseminated choroiditis NOS
- Disseminated retinitis NOS
- Disseminated retinochoroiditis NOS

H30.101   Unspecified disseminated chorioretinal inflammation, right eye ▽

H30.102   Unspecified disseminated chorioretinal inflammation, left eye ▽

H30.103   Unspecified disseminated chorioretinal inflammation, bilateral ▽

H30.109   Unspecified disseminated chorioretinal inflammation, unspecified eye ▽

H30.11   Disseminated chorioretinal inflammation of posterior pole

H30.111   Disseminated chorioretinal inflammation of posterior pole, right eye

H30.112   Disseminated chorioretinal inflammation of posterior pole, left eye

H30.113   Disseminated chorioretinal inflammation of posterior pole, bilateral

H30.119   Disseminated chorioretinal inflammation of posterior pole, unspecified eye ▽

H30.12   Disseminated chorioretinal inflammation, peripheral

H30.121   Disseminated chorioretinal inflammation, peripheral right eye

H30.122   Disseminated chorioretinal inflammation, peripheral, left eye

H30.123   Disseminated chorioretinal inflammation, peripheral, bilateral

H30.129   Disseminated chorioretinal inflammation, peripheral, unspecified eye ▽

H30.13   Disseminated chorioretinal inflammation, generalized

H30.131   Disseminated chorioretinal inflammation, generalized, right eye

H30.132   Disseminated chorioretinal inflammation, generalized, left eye

H30.133   Disseminated chorioretinal inflammation, generalized, bilateral

H30.139   Disseminated chorioretinal inflammation, generalized, unspecified eye ▽

H30.14   Acute posterior multifocal placoid pigment epitheliopathy

H30.141   Acute posterior multifocal placoid pigment epitheliopathy, right eye

H30.142   Acute posterior multifocal placoid pigment epitheliopathy, left eye

H30.143   Acute posterior multifocal placoid pigment epitheliopathy, bilateral

H30.149   Acute posterior multifocal placoid pigment epitheliopathy, unspecified eye ▽

H30.2   Posterior cyclitis
- Pars planitis

H30.20   Posterior cyclitis, unspecified eye ▽

H30.21   Posterior cyclitis, right eye

H30.22   Posterior cyclitis, left eye

H30.23   Posterior cyclitis, bilateral

H30.8   Other chorioretinal inflammations

H30.81   Harada's disease

H30.811   Harada's disease, right eye

H30.812   Harada's disease, left eye

H30.813   Harada's disease, bilateral

H30.819   Harada's disease, unspecified eye ▽

✓6ᵗʰ **H30.89** **Other chorioretinal inflammations**

    H30.891 **Other chorioretinal inflammations, right eye**

    H30.892 **Other chorioretinal inflammations, left eye**

    H30.893 **Other chorioretinal inflammations, bilateral**

    H30.899 **Other chorioretinal inflammations, unspecified eye** ▽

✓5ᵗʰ **H30.9** **Unspecified chorioretinal inflammation**

    Chorioretinitis NOS
    Choroiditis NOS
    Neuroretinitis NOS
    Retinitis NOS
    Retinochoroiditis NOS

    H30.90 **Unspecified chorioretinal inflammation, unspecified eye** ▽

    H30.91 **Unspecified chorioretinal inflammation, right eye** ▽

    H30.92 **Unspecified chorioretinal inflammation, left eye** ▽

    H30.93 **Unspecified chorioretinal inflammation, bilateral** ▽

✓4ᵗʰ **H31** **Other disorders of choroid**

✓5ᵗʰ **H31.0** **Chorioretinal scars**

    EXCLUDES 2 *postsurgical chorioretinal scars (H59.81-)*

✓6ᵗʰ **H31.00** **Unspecified chorioretinal scars**

    H31.001 **Unspecified chorioretinal scars, right eye** ▽

    H31.002 **Unspecified chorioretinal scars, left eye** ▽

    H31.003 **Unspecified chorioretinal scars, bilateral** ▽

    H31.009 **Unspecified chorioretinal scars, unspecified eye** ▽

✓6ᵗʰ **H31.01** **Macula scars of posterior pole (postinflammatory) (post-traumatic)**

    EXCLUDES 1 *postprocedural chorioretinal scar (H59.81-)*

    H31.011 **Macula scars of posterior pole (postinflammatory) (post-traumatic), right eye**

    H31.012 **Macula scars of posterior pole (postinflammatory) (post-traumatic), left eye**

    H31.013 **Macula scars of posterior pole (postinflammatory) (post-traumatic), bilateral**

    H31.019 **Macula scars of posterior pole (postinflammatory) (post-traumatic), unspecified eye** ▽

✓6ᵗʰ **H31.02** **Solar retinopathy**

    H31.021 **Solar retinopathy, right eye**

    H31.022 **Solar retinopathy, left eye**

    H31.023 **Solar retinopathy, bilateral**

    H31.029 **Solar retinopathy, unspecified eye** ▽

✓6ᵗʰ **H31.09** **Other chorioretinal scars**

    H31.091 **Other chorioretinal scars, right eye**

    H31.092 **Other chorioretinal scars, left eye**

    H31.093 **Other chorioretinal scars, bilateral**

    H31.099 **Other chorioretinal scars, unspecified eye** ▽

✓5ᵗʰ **H31.1** **Choroidal degeneration**

    EXCLUDES 2 *angioid streaks of macula (H35.33)*

✓6ᵗʰ **H31.10** **Unspecified choroidal degeneration**

    Choroidal sclerosis NOS

    H31.101 **Choroidal degeneration, unspecified, right eye** ▽

    H31.102 **Choroidal degeneration, unspecified, left eye** ▽

    H31.103 **Choroidal degeneration, unspecified, bilateral** ▽

    H31.109 **Choroidal degeneration, unspecified, unspecified eye** ▽

✓6ᵗʰ **H31.11** **Age-related choroidal atrophy**

    H31.111 **Age-related choroidal atrophy, right eye** Ⓐ

    H31.112 **Age-related choroidal atrophy, left eye** Ⓐ

    H31.113 **Age-related choroidal atrophy, bilateral** Ⓐ

    H31.119 **Age-related choroidal atrophy, unspecified eye** Ⓐ ▽

✓6ᵗʰ **H31.12** **Diffuse secondary atrophy of choroid**

    H31.121 **Diffuse secondary atrophy of choroid, right eye**

    H31.122 **Diffuse secondary atrophy of choroid, left eye**

    H31.123 **Diffuse secondary atrophy of choroid, bilateral**

    H31.129 **Diffuse secondary atrophy of choroid, unspecified eye** ▽

✓5ᵗʰ **H31.2** **Hereditary choroidal dystrophy**

    EXCLUDES 2 *hyperornithinemia (E72.4)*
                    ornithinemia (E72.4)

    H31.20 **Hereditary choroidal dystrophy, unspecified** ▽

    H31.21 **Choroideremia**

    H31.22 **Choroidal dystrophy (central areolar) (generalized) (peripapillary)**

    H31.23 **Gyrate atrophy, choroid**

    H31.29 **Other hereditary choroidal dystrophy**

✓5ᵗʰ **H31.3** **Choroidal hemorrhage and rupture**

✓6ᵗʰ **H31.30** **Unspecified choroidal hemorrhage**

    H31.301 **Unspecified choroidal hemorrhage, right eye** ▽

    H31.302 **Unspecified choroidal hemorrhage, left eye** ▽

    H31.303 **Unspecified choroidal hemorrhage, bilateral** ▽

    H31.309 **Unspecified choroidal hemorrhage, unspecified eye** ▽

✓6ᵗʰ **H31.31** **Expulsive choroidal hemorrhage**

    H31.311 **Expulsive choroidal hemorrhage, right eye**

    H31.312 **Expulsive choroidal hemorrhage, left eye**

    H31.313 **Expulsive choroidal hemorrhage, bilateral**

    H31.319 **Expulsive choroidal hemorrhage, unspecified eye** ▽

✓6ᵗʰ **H31.32** **Choroidal rupture**

    H31.321 **Choroidal rupture, right eye**

    H31.322 **Choroidal rupture, left eye**

    H31.323 **Choroidal rupture, bilateral**

    H31.329 **Choroidal rupture, unspecified eye** ▽

✓5ᵗʰ **H31.4** **Choroidal detachment**

✓6ᵗʰ **H31.40** **Unspecified choroidal detachment**

    H31.401 **Unspecified choroidal detachment, right eye** ▽

    H31.402 **Unspecified choroidal detachment, left eye** ▽

    H31.403 **Unspecified choroidal detachment, bilateral** ▽

    H31.409 **Unspecified choroidal detachment, unspecified eye** ▽

✓6ᵗʰ **H31.41** **Hemorrhagic choroidal detachment**

    H31.411 **Hemorrhagic choroidal detachment, right eye**

    H31.412 **Hemorrhagic choroidal detachment, left eye**

    H31.413 **Hemorrhagic choroidal detachment, bilateral**

    H31.419 **Hemorrhagic choroidal detachment, unspecified eye** ▽

✓6ᵗʰ **H31.42** **Serous choroidal detachment**

    H31.421 **Serous choroidal detachment, right eye**

    H31.422 **Serous choroidal detachment, left eye**

    H31.423 **Serous choroidal detachment, bilateral**

    H31.429 **Serous choroidal detachment, unspecified eye** ▽

H31.8 **Other specified disorders of choroid**

H31.9 **Unspecified disorder of choroid** ▽

✓ Additional Character Req	✓x7ᵗʰ Placeholder Alert	Manifestation	▽ Unspecified	►◄ Revised Text	● New Code	▲ Revised Code Title

ICD-10-CM 2019   **601**

H32 Chorioretinal disorders in diseases classified elsewhere

Code first underlying disease, such as:
congenital toxoplasmosis (P37.1)
histoplasmosis (B39.-)
leprosy (A30.-)

EXCLUDES 1   chorioretinitis (in):
     toxoplasmosis (acquired) (B58.01)
     tuberculosis (A18.53)

✓4ᵗʰ **H33 Retinal detachments and breaks**

EXCLUDES 1   detachment of retinal pigment epithelium (H35.72-, H35.73-)

Retinal Detachment

Lens, Vitreous, Choroid, Area of detachment, Iris, Retina, Cornea, Sclera

✓5ᵗʰ **H33.0 Retinal detachment with retinal break**

Rhegmatogenous retinal detachment

EXCLUDES 1   serous retinal detachment (without retinal break) (H33.2-)

✓6ᵗʰ **H33.00 Unspecified retinal detachment with retinal break**

     H33.001   Unspecified retinal detachment with retinal break, right eye ▽

     H33.002   Unspecified retinal detachment with retinal break, left eye ▽

     H33.003   Unspecified retinal detachment with retinal break, bilateral ▽

     H33.009   Unspecified retinal detachment with retinal break, unspecified eye ▽

✓6ᵗʰ **H33.01 Retinal detachment with single break**

     H33.011   Retinal detachment with single break, right eye

     H33.012   Retinal detachment with single break, left eye

     H33.013   Retinal detachment with single break, bilateral

     H33.019   Retinal detachment with single break, unspecified eye ▽

✓6ᵗʰ **H33.02 Retinal detachment with multiple breaks**

     H33.021   Retinal detachment with multiple breaks, right eye

     H33.022   Retinal detachment with multiple breaks, left eye

     H33.023   Retinal detachment with multiple breaks, bilateral

     H33.029   Retinal detachment with multiple breaks, unspecified eye ▽

✓6ᵗʰ **H33.03 Retinal detachment with giant retinal tear**

     H33.031   Retinal detachment with giant retinal tear, right eye

     H33.032   Retinal detachment with giant retinal tear, left eye

     H33.033   Retinal detachment with giant retinal tear, bilateral

     H33.039   Retinal detachment with giant retinal tear, unspecified eye ▽

✓6ᵗʰ **H33.04 Retinal detachment with retinal dialysis**

     H33.041   Retinal detachment with retinal dialysis, right eye

     H33.042   Retinal detachment with retinal dialysis, left eye

     H33.043   Retinal detachment with retinal dialysis, bilateral

     H33.049   Retinal detachment with retinal dialysis, unspecified eye ▽

✓6ᵗʰ **H33.05 Total retinal detachment**

     H33.051   Total retinal detachment, right eye

     H33.052   Total retinal detachment, left eye

     H33.053   Total retinal detachment, bilateral

     H33.059   Total retinal detachment, unspecified eye ▽

✓5ᵗʰ **H33.1 Retinoschisis and retinal cysts**

EXCLUDES 1   congenital retinoschisis (Q14.1)
     microcystoid degeneration of retina (H35.42-)

✓6ᵗʰ **H33.10 Unspecified retinoschisis**

     H33.101   Unspecified retinoschisis, right eye ▽

     H33.102   Unspecified retinoschisis, left eye ▽

     H33.103   Unspecified retinoschisis, bilateral ▽

     H33.109   Unspecified retinoschisis, unspecified eye ▽

✓6ᵗʰ **H33.11 Cyst of ora serrata**

     H33.111   Cyst of ora serrata, right eye

     H33.112   Cyst of ora serrata, left eye

     H33.113   Cyst of ora serrata, bilateral

     H33.119   Cyst of ora serrata, unspecified eye ▽

✓6ᵗʰ **H33.12 Parasitic cyst of retina**

     H33.121   Parasitic cyst of retina, right eye

     H33.122   Parasitic cyst of retina, left eye

     H33.123   Parasitic cyst of retina, bilateral

     H33.129   Parasitic cyst of retina, unspecified eye ▽

✓6ᵗʰ **H33.19 Other retinoschisis and retinal cysts**

Pseudocyst of retina

     H33.191   Other retinoschisis and retinal cysts, right eye

     H33.192   Other retinoschisis and retinal cysts, left eye

     H33.193   Other retinoschisis and retinal cysts, bilateral

     H33.199   Other retinoschisis and retinal cysts, unspecified eye ▽

✓5ᵗʰ **H33.2 Serous retinal detachment**

Retinal detachment NOS
Retinal detachment without retinal break

EXCLUDES 1   central serous chorioretinopathy (H35.71-)

     H33.20   Serous retinal detachment, unspecified eye ▽

     H33.21   Serous retinal detachment, right eye

     H33.22   Serous retinal detachment, left eye

     H33.23   Serous retinal detachment, bilateral

✓5ᵗʰ **H33.3 Retinal breaks without detachment**

EXCLUDES 1   chorioretinal scars after surgery for detachment (H59.81-)
     peripheral retinal degeneration without break (H35.4-)

✓6ᵗʰ **H33.30 Unspecified retinal break**

     H33.301   Unspecified retinal break, right eye ▽

     H33.302   Unspecified retinal break, left eye ▽

     H33.303   Unspecified retinal break, bilateral ▽

     H33.309   Unspecified retinal break, unspecified eye ▽

✓6ᵗʰ **H33.31 Horseshoe tear of retina without detachment**

Operculum of retina without detachment

     H33.311   Horseshoe tear of retina without detachment, right eye

     H33.312   Horseshoe tear of retina without detachment, left eye

     H33.313   Horseshoe tear of retina without detachment, bilateral

     H33.319   Horseshoe tear of retina without detachment, unspecified eye ▽

✓6ᵗʰ **H33.32 Round hole of retina without detachment**

     H33.321   Round hole, right eye

     H33.322   Round hole, left eye

     H33.323   Round hole, bilateral

     H33.329   Round hole, unspecified eye ▽

√6ʰ H33.33 Multiple defects of retina without detachment
- **H33.331** Multiple defects of retina without detachment, **right** eye
- **H33.332** Multiple defects of retina without detachment, **left** eye
- **H33.333** Multiple defects of retina without detachment, **bilateral**
- **H33.339** Multiple defects of retina without detachment, **unspecified eye** ▽

√5ʰ H33.4 Traction detachment of retina
Proliferative vitreo-retinopathy with retinal detachment
- **H33.40** Traction detachment of retina, unspecified eye ▽
- **H33.41** Traction detachment of retina, **right** eye
- **H33.42** Traction detachment of retina, **left** eye
- **H33.43** Traction detachment of retina, **bilateral**

H33.8 Other retinal detachments

√4ʰ H34 Retinal vascular occlusions
EXCLUDES 1   amaurosis fugax (G45.3)

√5ʰ H34.0 Transient retinal artery occlusion
- **H34.00** Transient retinal artery occlusion, unspecified eye ▽
- **H34.01** Transient retinal artery occlusion, **right** eye
- **H34.02** Transient retinal artery occlusion, **left** eye
- **H34.03** Transient retinal artery occlusion, **bilateral**

√5ʰ H34.1 Central retinal artery occlusion
- **H34.10** Central retinal artery occlusion, unspecified eye ▽
- **H34.11** Central retinal artery occlusion, **right** eye
- **H34.12** Central retinal artery occlusion, **left** eye
- **H34.13** Central retinal artery occlusion, **bilateral**

√5ʰ H34.2 Other retinal artery occlusions

√6ʰ H34.21 Partial retinal artery occlusion
Hollenhorst's plaque
Retinal microembolism
- **H34.211** Partial retinal artery occlusion, **right** eye
- **H34.212** Partial retinal artery occlusion, **left** eye
- **H34.213** Partial retinal artery occlusion, **bilateral**
- **H34.219** Partial retinal artery occlusion, **unspecified eye** ▽

√6ʰ H34.23 Retinal artery branch occlusion
- **H34.231** Retinal artery branch occlusion, **right** eye
- **H34.232** Retinal artery branch occlusion, **left** eye
- **H34.233** Retinal artery branch occlusion, **bilateral**
- **H34.239** Retinal artery branch occlusion, **unspecified eye** ▽

√5ʰ H34.8 Other retinal vascular occlusions
AHA: 2016,4Q,19

√6ʰ H34.81 Central retinal vein occlusion
One of the following 7th characters is to be assigned to codes in subcategory H34.81 to designate the severity of the occlusion:
- Ø with macular edema
- 1 with retinal neovascularization
- 2 stable
- old central retinal vein occlusion
- **√7ʰ H34.811** Central retinal vein occlusion, **right** eye
- **√7ʰ H34.812** Central retinal vein occlusion, **left** eye
- **√7ʰ H34.813** Central retinal vein occlusion, **bilateral**
- **√7ʰ H34.819** Central retinal vein occlusion, **unspecified eye** ▽

√6ʰ H34.82 Venous engorgement
Incipient retinal vein occlusion
Partial retinal vein occlusion
- **H34.821** Venous engorgement, **right** eye
- **H34.822** Venous engorgement, **left** eye
- **H34.823** Venous engorgement, **bilateral**
- **H34.829** Venous engorgement, **unspecified eye** ▽

√6ʰ H34.83 Tributary (branch) retinal vein occlusion
One of the following 7th characters is to be assigned to codes in subcategory H34.83 to designate the severity of the occlusion:
- Ø with macular edema
- 1 with retinal neovascularization
- 2 stable
- old tributary (branch) retinal vein occlusion
- **√7ʰ H34.831** Tributary (branch) retinal vein occlusion, **right** eye
- **√7ʰ H34.832** Tributary (branch) retinal vein occlusion, **left** eye
- **√7ʰ H34.833** Tributary (branch) retinal vein occlusion, **bilateral**
- **√7ʰ H34.839** Tributary (branch) retinal vein occlusion, unspecified eye ▽

H34.9 Unspecified retinal vascular occlusion ▽

√4ʰ H35 Other retinal disorders
EXCLUDES 2   diabetic retinal disorders (E08.311-E08.359, E09.311-E09.359, E10.311-E10.359, E11.311-E11.359, E13.311-E13.359)

√5ʰ H35.0 Background retinopathy and retinal vascular changes
Code also any associated hypertension (I10.-)
- **H35.00** Unspecified background retinopathy ▽

√6ʰ H35.01 Changes in retinal vascular appearance
Retinal vascular sheathing
- **H35.011** Changes in retinal vascular appearance, **right** eye
- **H35.012** Changes in retinal vascular appearance, **left** eye
- **H35.013** Changes in retinal vascular appearance, **bilateral**
- **H35.019** Changes in retinal vascular appearance, **unspecified eye** ▽

√6ʰ H35.02 Exudative retinopathy
Coats retinopathy
- **H35.021** Exudative retinopathy, **right** eye
- **H35.022** Exudative retinopathy, **left** eye
- **H35.023** Exudative retinopathy, **bilateral**
- **H35.029** Exudative retinopathy, **unspecified eye** ▽

√6ʰ H35.03 Hypertensive retinopathy
- **H35.031** Hypertensive retinopathy, **right** eye
- **H35.032** Hypertensive retinopathy, **left** eye
- **H35.033** Hypertensive retinopathy, **bilateral**
- **H35.039** Hypertensive retinopathy, **unspecified eye** ▽

√6ʰ H35.04 Retinal micro-aneurysms, unspecified
- **H35.041** Retinal micro-aneurysms, unspecified, **right** eye ▽
- **H35.042** Retinal micro-aneurysms, unspecified, **left** eye ▽
- **H35.043** Retinal micro-aneurysms, unspecified, **bilateral** ▽
- **H35.049** Retinal micro-aneurysms, unspecified, **unspecified eye** ▽

√6ʰ H35.05 Retinal neovascularization, unspecified
- **H35.051** Retinal neovascularization, unspecified, **right** eye ▽
- **H35.052** Retinal neovascularization, unspecified, **left** eye ▽
- **H35.053** Retinal neovascularization, unspecified, **bilateral** ▽
- **H35.059** Retinal neovascularization, unspecified, **unspecified eye** ▽

√6ʰ H35.06 Retinal vasculitis
Eales disease
Retinal perivasculitis
DEF: Sight-threatening intraocular inflammation of the retinal blood vessels that causes minimal, partial, or even complete blindness.
- **H35.061** Retinal vasculitis, **right** eye
- **H35.062** Retinal vasculitis, **left** eye
- **H35.063** Retinal vasculitis, **bilateral**
- **H35.069** Retinal vasculitis, unspecified eye ▽

√6ʰ H35.07 Retinal telangiectasis
- **H35.071** Retinal telangiectasis, **right** eye
- **H35.072** Retinal telangiectasis, **left** eye
- **H35.073** Retinal telangiectasis, **bilateral**

H35.Ø79   **Retinal telangiectasis, unspecified eye** ▽

H35.Ø9   **Other intraretinal microvascular abnormalities**
Retinal varices

✓5ᵗʰ **H35.1   Retinopathy of prematurity**

✓6ᵗʰ H35.1Ø   **Retinopathy of prematurity, unspecified**
Retinopathy of prematurity NOS

H35.1Ø1   **Retinopathy of prematurity, unspecified, right eye** ▽

H35.1Ø2   **Retinopathy of prematurity, unspecified, left eye** ▽

H35.1Ø3   **Retinopathy of prematurity, unspecified, bilateral** ▽

H35.1Ø9   **Retinopathy of prematurity, unspecified, unspecified eye** ▽

✓6ᵗʰ H35.11   **Retinopathy of prematurity, stage Ø**

H35.111   **Retinopathy of prematurity, stage Ø, right eye**

H35.112   **Retinopathy of prematurity, stage Ø, left eye**

H35.113   **Retinopathy of prematurity, stage Ø, bilateral**

H35.119   **Retinopathy of prematurity, stage Ø, unspecified eye** ▽

✓6ᵗʰ H35.12   **Retinopathy of prematurity, stage 1**

H35.121   **Retinopathy of prematurity, stage 1, right eye**

H35.122   **Retinopathy of prematurity, stage 1, left eye**

H35.123   **Retinopathy of prematurity, stage 1, bilateral**

H35.129   **Retinopathy of prematurity, stage 1, unspecified eye** ▽

✓6ᵗʰ H35.13   **Retinopathy of prematurity, stage 2**

H35.131   **Retinopathy of prematurity, stage 2, right eye**

H35.132   **Retinopathy of prematurity, stage 2, left eye**

H35.133   **Retinopathy of prematurity, stage 2, bilateral**

H35.139   **Retinopathy of prematurity, stage 2, unspecified eye** ▽

✓6ᵗʰ H35.14   **Retinopathy of prematurity, stage 3**

H35.141   **Retinopathy of prematurity, stage 3, right eye**

H35.142   **Retinopathy of prematurity, stage 3, left eye**

H35.143   **Retinopathy of prematurity, stage 3, bilateral**

H35.149   **Retinopathy of prematurity, stage 3, unspecified eye** ▽

✓6ᵗʰ H35.15   **Retinopathy of prematurity, stage 4**

H35.151   **Retinopathy of prematurity, stage 4, right eye**

H35.152   **Retinopathy of prematurity, stage 4, left eye**

H35.153   **Retinopathy of prematurity, stage 4, bilateral**

H35.159   **Retinopathy of prematurity, stage 4, unspecified eye** ▽

✓6ᵗʰ H35.16   **Retinopathy of prematurity, stage 5**

H35.161   **Retinopathy of prematurity, stage 5, right eye**

H35.162   **Retinopathy of prematurity, stage 5, left eye**

H35.163   **Retinopathy of prematurity, stage 5, bilateral**

H35.169   **Retinopathy of prematurity, stage 5, unspecified eye** ▽

✓6ᵗʰ H35.17   **Retrolental fibroplasia**

H35.171   **Retrolental fibroplasia, right eye**

H35.172   **Retrolental fibroplasia, left eye**

H35.173   **Retrolental fibroplasia, bilateral**

H35.179   **Retrolental fibroplasia, unspecified eye** ▽

✓5ᵗʰ **H35.2   Other non-diabetic proliferative retinopathy**
Proliferative vitreo-retinopathy

EXCLUDES 1   *proliferative vitreo-retinopathy with retinal detachment (H33.4-)*

H35.2Ø   **Other non-diabetic proliferative retinopathy, unspecified eye** ▽

H35.21   **Other non-diabetic proliferative retinopathy, right eye**

H35.22   **Other non-diabetic proliferative retinopathy, left eye**

H35.23   **Other non-diabetic proliferative retinopathy, bilateral**

✓5ᵗʰ **H35.3   Degeneration of macula and posterior pole**

H35.3Ø   **Unspecified macular degeneration** ⓠ Ⓐ ▽
Age-related macular degeneration

✓6ᵗʰ H35.31   **Nonexudative age-related macular degeneration**
Atrophic age-related macular degeneration
Dry age-related macular degeneration
AHA: 2016,4Q,20-21

One of the following 7th characters is to be assigned to each code in subcategory H35.31 to designate the stage of the disease:
Ø   stage unspecified
1   early dry stage
2   intermediate dry stage
3   advanced atrophic without subfoveal involvement
advanced dry stage
4   advanced atrophic with subfoveal involvement

✓7ᵗʰ H35.311   **Nonexudative age-related macular degeneration, right eye** ⓠ Ⓐ

✓7ᵗʰ H35.312   **Nonexudative age-related macular degeneration, left eye** ⓠ Ⓐ

✓7ᵗʰ H35.313   **Nonexudative age-related macular degeneration, bilateral** ⓠ Ⓐ

✓7ᵗʰ H35.319   **Nonexudative age-related macular degeneration, unspecified eye** Ⓐ ▽

✓6ᵗʰ H35.32   **Exudative age-related macular degeneration**
Wet age-related macular degeneration
AHA: 2016,4Q,20-21

One of the following 7th characters is to be assigned to each code in subcategory H35.32 to designate the stage of the disease:
Ø   stage unspecified
1   with active choroidal neovascularization
2   with inactive choroidal neovascularization
with involuted or regressed neovascularization
3   with inactive scar

✓7ᵗʰ H35.321   **Exudative age-related macular degeneration, right eye** HCC ⓠ Ⓐ

✓7ᵗʰ H35.322   **Exudative age-related macular degeneration, left eye** HCC ⓠ Ⓐ

✓7ᵗʰ H35.323   **Exudative age-related macular degeneration, bilateral** HCC ⓠ Ⓐ

✓7ᵗʰ H35.329   **Exudative age-related macular degeneration, unspecified eye** HCC Ⓐ ▽

H35.33   **Angioid streaks of macula**
DEF: Degeneration of the choroid; characterized by broad, irregular, dark brown streaks radiating from optic disc; occurs with pseudoxanthoma elasticum or Paget's disease.

✓6ᵗʰ H35.34   **Macular cyst, hole, or pseudohole**

H35.341   **Macular cyst, hole, or pseudohole, right eye**

H35.342   **Macular cyst, hole, or pseudohole, left eye**

H35.343   **Macular cyst, hole, or pseudohole, bilateral**

H35.349   **Macular cyst, hole, or pseudohole, unspecified eye** ▽

✓6ᵗʰ H35.35   **Cystoid macular degeneration**

EXCLUDES 1   *cystoid macular edema following cataract surgery (H59.Ø3-)*

H35.351   **Cystoid macular degeneration, right eye**

H35.352   **Cystoid macular degeneration, left eye**

H35.353   **Cystoid macular degeneration, bilateral**

H35.359   **Cystoid macular degeneration, unspecified eye** ▽

√6ᵗʰ **H35.36** **Drusen (degenerative) of macula**
     AHA: 2017,1Q,51; 2016,4Q,21
     H35.361 **Drusen (degenerative) of macula, right eye**
     H35.362 **Drusen (degenerative) of macula, left eye**
     H35.363 **Drusen (degenerative) of macula, bilateral**
     H35.369 **Drusen (degenerative) of macula, unspecified eye** ▽

√6ᵗʰ **H35.37** **Puckering of macula**
     H35.371 **Puckering of macula, right eye**
     H35.372 **Puckering of macula, left eye**
     H35.373 **Puckering of macula, bilateral**
     H35.379 **Puckering of macula, unspecified eye** ▽

√6ᵗʰ **H35.38** **Toxic maculopathy**
     Code first poisoning due to drug or toxin, if applicable (T36-T65 with fifth or sixth character 1-4 or 6)
     Use additional code for adverse effect, if applicable, to identify drug (T36-T50 with fifth or sixth character 5)
     H35.381 **Toxic maculopathy, right eye**
     H35.382 **Toxic maculopathy, left eye**
     H35.383 **Toxic maculopathy, bilateral**
     H35.389 **Toxic maculopathy, unspecified eye** ▽

√5ᵗʰ **H35.4** **Peripheral retinal degeneration**
     EXCLUDES 1   hereditary retinal degeneration (dystrophy) (H35.5-)
                 peripheral retinal degeneration with retinal break (H33.3-)
     H35.40 **Unspecified peripheral retinal degeneration** ▽
√6ᵗʰ **H35.41** **Lattice degeneration of retina**
     Palisade degeneration of retina
     DEF: Degeneration of the retina, often bilateral, that is usually benign. It is characterized by lines intersecting at irregular intervals in the peripheral retina. Retinal thinning and retinal holes may occur.
     H35.411 **Lattice degeneration of retina, right eye**
     H35.412 **Lattice degeneration of retina, left eye**
     H35.413 **Lattice degeneration of retina, bilateral**
     H35.419 **Lattice degeneration of retina, unspecified eye** ▽
√6ᵗʰ **H35.42** **Microcystoid degeneration of retina**
     H35.421 **Microcystoid degeneration of retina, right eye**
     H35.422 **Microcystoid degeneration of retina, left eye**
     H35.423 **Microcystoid degeneration of retina, bilateral**
     H35.429 **Microcystoid degeneration of retina, unspecified eye** ▽
√6ᵗʰ **H35.43** **Paving stone degeneration of retina**
     H35.431 **Paving stone degeneration of retina, right eye**
     H35.432 **Paving stone degeneration of retina, left eye**
     H35.433 **Paving stone degeneration of retina, bilateral**
     H35.439 **Paving stone degeneration of retina, unspecified eye** ▽
√6ᵗʰ **H35.44** **Age-related reticular degeneration of retina**
     H35.441 **Age-related reticular degeneration of retina, right eye** A
     H35.442 **Age-related reticular degeneration of retina, left eye** A
     H35.443 **Age-related reticular degeneration of retina, bilateral** A
     H35.449 **Age-related reticular degeneration of retina, unspecified eye** A ▽
√6ᵗʰ **H35.45** **Secondary pigmentary degeneration**
     H35.451 **Secondary pigmentary degeneration, right eye**
     H35.452 **Secondary pigmentary degeneration, left eye**
     H35.453 **Secondary pigmentary degeneration, bilateral**
     H35.459 **Secondary pigmentary degeneration, unspecified eye** ▽

√6ᵗʰ **H35.46** **Secondary vitreoretinal degeneration**
     H35.461 **Secondary vitreoretinal degeneration, right eye**
     H35.462 **Secondary vitreoretinal degeneration, left eye**
     H35.463 **Secondary vitreoretinal degeneration, bilateral**
     H35.469 **Secondary vitreoretinal degeneration, unspecified eye** ▽

√5ᵗʰ **H35.5** **Hereditary retinal dystrophy**
     EXCLUDES 1   dystrophies primarily involving Bruch's membrane (H31.1-)
     H35.50 **Unspecified hereditary retinal dystrophy** ▽
     H35.51 **Vitreoretinal dystrophy**
     H35.52 **Pigmentary retinal dystrophy**
         Albipunctate retinal dystrophy
         Retinitis pigmentosa
         Tapetoretinal dystrophy
     H35.53 **Other dystrophies primarily involving the sensory retina**
         Stargardt's disease
     H35.54 **Dystrophies primarily involving the retinal pigment epithelium**
         Vitelliform retinal dystrophy

√5ᵗʰ **H35.6** **Retinal hemorrhage**
     H35.60 **Retinal hemorrhage, unspecified eye** ▽
     H35.61 **Retinal hemorrhage, right eye**
     H35.62 **Retinal hemorrhage, left eye**
     H35.63 **Retinal hemorrhage, bilateral**

√5ᵗʰ **H35.7** **Separation of retinal layers**
     EXCLUDES 1   retinal detachment (serous) (H33.2-)
                 rhegmatogenous retinal detachment (H33.0-)
     H35.70 **Unspecified separation of retinal layers** ▽
√6ᵗʰ **H35.71** **Central serous chorioretinopathy**
     H35.711 **Central serous chorioretinopathy, right eye**
     H35.712 **Central serous chorioretinopathy, left eye**
     H35.713 **Central serous chorioretinopathy, bilateral**
     H35.719 **Central serous chorioretinopathy, unspecified eye** ▽
√6ᵗʰ **H35.72** **Serous detachment of retinal pigment epithelium**
     H35.721 **Serous detachment of retinal pigment epithelium, right eye**
     H35.722 **Serous detachment of retinal pigment epithelium, left eye**
     H35.723 **Serous detachment of retinal pigment epithelium, bilateral**
     H35.729 **Serous detachment of retinal pigment epithelium, unspecified eye** ▽
√6ᵗʰ **H35.73** **Hemorrhagic detachment of retinal pigment epithelium**
     H35.731 **Hemorrhagic detachment of retinal pigment epithelium, right eye**
     H35.732 **Hemorrhagic detachment of retinal pigment epithelium, left eye**
     H35.733 **Hemorrhagic detachment of retinal pigment epithelium, bilateral**
     H35.739 **Hemorrhagic detachment of retinal pigment epithelium, unspecified eye** ▽

√5ᵗʰ **H35.8** **Other specified retinal disorders**
     EXCLUDES 2   retinal hemorrhage (H35.6-)
     H35.81 **Retinal edema**
         Retinal cotton wool spots
     H35.82 **Retinal ischemia**
     H35.89 **Other specified retinal disorders**
H35.9 **Unspecified retinal disorder** ▽

H36 *Retinal disorders in diseases classified elsewhere*
     Code first underlying disease, such as:
         lipid storage disorders (E75.-)
         sickle-cell disorders (D57.-)
     EXCLUDES 1   arteriosclerotic retinopathy (H35.0-)
                 diabetic retinopathy (E08.3-, E09.3-, E10.3-, E11.3-, E13.3-)

☑ Additional Character Req   √x7ᵗʰ Placeholder Alert   Manifestation   ▽ Unspecified   ▶◀ Revised Text   ● New Code   ▲ Revised Code Title

Chapter 7. Diseases of the Eye and Adnexa

Glaucoma (H40–H42)

✓4ᵗʰ H40 Glaucoma

EXCLUDES 1   absolute glaucoma (H44.51-)
congenital glaucoma (Q15.0)
traumatic glaucoma due to birth injury (P15.3)

Open Angle/Angle Closure Glaucoma

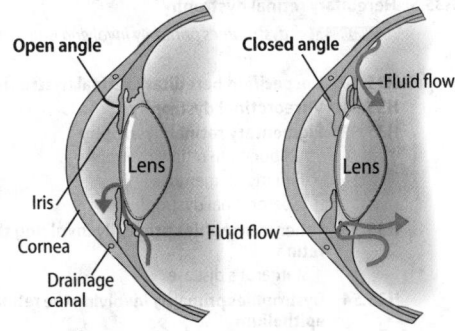

✓5ᵗʰ H40.0 Glaucoma suspect

✓6ᵗʰ H40.00 Preglaucoma, unspecified
- H40.001 Preglaucoma, unspecified, right eye ▽
- H40.002 Preglaucoma, unspecified, left eye ▽
- H40.003 Preglaucoma, unspecified, bilateral ▽
- H40.009 Preglaucoma, unspecified, unspecified eye ▽

✓6ᵗʰ H40.01 Open angle with borderline findings, low risk
Open angle, low risk
- H40.011 Open angle with borderline findings, low risk, right eye
- H40.012 Open angle with borderline findings, low risk, left eye
- H40.013 Open angle with borderline findings, low risk, bilateral
- H40.019 Open angle with borderline findings, low risk, unspecified eye ▽

✓6ᵗʰ H40.02 Open angle with borderline findings, high risk
Open angle, high risk
- H40.021 Open angle with borderline findings, high risk, right eye
- H40.022 Open angle with borderline findings, high risk, left eye
- H40.023 Open angle with borderline findings, high risk, bilateral
- H40.029 Open angle with borderline findings, high risk, unspecified eye ▽

✓6ᵗʰ H40.03 Anatomical narrow angle
Primary angle closure suspect
- H40.031 Anatomical narrow angle, right eye
- H40.032 Anatomical narrow angle, left eye
- H40.033 Anatomical narrow angle, bilateral
- H40.039 Anatomical narrow angle, unspecified eye ▽

✓6ᵗʰ H40.04 Steroid responder
- H40.041 Steroid responder, right eye
- H40.042 Steroid responder, left eye
- H40.043 Steroid responder, bilateral
- H40.049 Steroid responder, unspecified eye ▽

✓6ᵗʰ H40.05 Ocular hypertension
- H40.051 Ocular hypertension, right eye
- H40.052 Ocular hypertension, left eye
- H40.053 Ocular hypertension, bilateral
- H40.059 Ocular hypertension, unspecified eye ▽

✓6ᵗʰ H40.06 Primary angle closure without glaucoma damage
- H40.061 Primary angle closure without glaucoma damage, right eye
- H40.062 Primary angle closure without glaucoma damage, left eye
- H40.063 Primary angle closure without glaucoma damage, bilateral
- H40.069 Primary angle closure without glaucoma damage, unspecified eye ▽

✓5ᵗʰ H40.1 Open-angle glaucoma

> One of the following 7th characters is to be assigned to each code in subcategories H40.10, H40.11, H40.12, H40.13, and H40.14 to designate the stage of glaucoma.
> 0 stage unspecified
> 1 mild stage
> 2 moderate stage
> 3 severe stage
> 4 indeterminate stage

✓x7ᵗʰ H40.10 Unspecified open-angle glaucoma 🄠 ▽
> TIP: Only one code from this subcategory should be assigned when both left and right eyes are the same stage.

✓6ᵗʰ H40.11 Primary open-angle glaucoma
Chronic simple glaucoma
AHA: 2016,4Q,22
- ✓7ᵗʰ H40.111 Primary open-angle glaucoma, right eye 🄠
- ✓7ᵗʰ H40.112 Primary open-angle glaucoma, left eye 🄠
- ✓7ᵗʰ H40.113 Primary open-angle glaucoma, bilateral 🄠
- ✓7ᵗʰ H40.119 Primary open-angle glaucoma, unspecified eye 🄠 ▽

✓6ᵗʰ H40.12 Low-tension glaucoma
- ✓7ᵗʰ H40.121 Low-tension glaucoma, right eye 🄠
- ✓7ᵗʰ H40.122 Low-tension glaucoma, left eye 🄠
- ✓7ᵗʰ H40.123 Low-tension glaucoma, bilateral 🄠
- ✓7ᵗʰ H40.129 Low-tension glaucoma, unspecified eye 🄠 ▽

✓6ᵗʰ H40.13 Pigmentary glaucoma
- ✓7ᵗʰ H40.131 Pigmentary glaucoma, right eye
- ✓7ᵗʰ H40.132 Pigmentary glaucoma, left eye
- ✓7ᵗʰ H40.133 Pigmentary glaucoma, bilateral
- ✓7ᵗʰ H40.139 Pigmentary glaucoma, unspecified ▽

✓6ᵗʰ H40.14 Capsular glaucoma with pseudoexfoliation of lens
- ✓7ᵗʰ H40.141 Capsular glaucoma with pseudoexfoliation of lens, right eye
- ✓7ᵗʰ H40.142 Capsular glaucoma with pseudoexfoliation of lens, left eye
- ✓7ᵗʰ H40.143 Capsular glaucoma with pseudoexfoliation of lens, bilateral
- ✓7ᵗʰ H40.149 Capsular glaucoma with pseudoexfoliation of lens, unspecified eye ▽

✓6ᵗʰ H40.15 Residual stage of open-angle glaucoma
- H40.151 Residual stage of open-angle glaucoma, right eye 🄠
- H40.152 Residual stage of open-angle glaucoma, left eye 🄠
- H40.153 Residual stage of open-angle glaucoma, bilateral 🄠
- H40.159 Residual stage of open-angle glaucoma, unspecified eye 🄠 ▽

✓5ᵗʰ H40.2 Primary angle-closure glaucoma

EXCLUDES 1   aqueous misdirection (H40.83-)
malignant glaucoma (H40.83-)

> One of the following 7th characters is to be assigned to code H40.20 and H40.22- to designate the stage of glaucoma.
> 0 stage unspecified
> 1 mild stage
> 2 moderate stage
> 3 severe stage
> 4 indeterminate stage

✓x7ᵗʰ H40.20 Unspecified primary angle-closure glaucoma ▽
> TIP: Only one code from this subcategory should be assigned when both left and right eyes are the same stage.

√6ᵗʰ **H40.21** Acute angle-closure glaucoma

Acute angle-closure glaucoma attack
Acute angle-closure glaucoma crisis

H40.211 Acute angle-closure glaucoma, right eye
H40.212 Acute angle-closure glaucoma, left eye
H40.213 Acute angle-closure glaucoma, bilateral
H40.219 Acute angle-closure glaucoma, unspecified eye   ▽

√6ᵗʰ **H40.22** Chronic angle-closure glaucoma

Chronic primary angle closure glaucoma

√7ᵗʰ **H40.221** Chronic angle-closure glaucoma, right eye
√7ᵗʰ **H40.222** Chronic angle-closure glaucoma, left eye
√7ᵗʰ **H40.223** Chronic angle-closure glaucoma, bilateral
√7ᵗʰ **H40.229** Chronic angle-closure glaucoma, unspecified eye   ▽

√6ᵗʰ **H40.23** Intermittent angle-closure glaucoma

H40.231 Intermittent angle-closure glaucoma, right eye
H40.232 Intermittent angle-closure glaucoma, left eye
H40.233 Intermittent angle-closure glaucoma, bilateral
H40.239 Intermittent angle-closure glaucoma, unspecified eye   ▽

√6ᵗʰ **H40.24** Residual stage of angle-closure glaucoma

H40.241 Residual stage of angle-closure glaucoma, right eye
H40.242 Residual stage of angle-closure glaucoma, left eye
H40.243 Residual stage of angle-closure glaucoma, bilateral
H40.249 Residual stage of angle-closure glaucoma, unspecified eye   ▽

√5ᵗʰ **H40.3** Glaucoma secondary to eye trauma

Code also underlying condition

> One of the following 7th characters is to be assigned to each code in subcategory H40.3- to designate the stage of glaucoma.
> 0   stage unspecified
> 1   mild stage
> 2   moderate stage
> 3   severe stage
> 4   indeterminate stage

√x7ᵗʰ **H40.30** Glaucoma secondary to eye trauma, unspecified eye   ▽
√x7ᵗʰ **H40.31** Glaucoma secondary to eye trauma, right eye
√x7ᵗʰ **H40.32** Glaucoma secondary to eye trauma, left eye
√x7ᵗʰ **H40.33** Glaucoma secondary to eye trauma, bilateral

√5ᵗʰ **H40.4** Glaucoma secondary to eye inflammation

Code also underlying condition

> One of the following 7th characters is to be assigned to each code in subcategory H40.4- to designate the stage of glaucoma.
> 0   stage unspecified
> 1   mild stage
> 2   moderate stage
> 3   severe stage
> 4   indeterminate stage

√x7ᵗʰ **H40.40** Glaucoma secondary to eye inflammation, unspecified eye   ▽
√x7ᵗʰ **H40.41** Glaucoma secondary to eye inflammation, right eye
√x7ᵗʰ **H40.42** Glaucoma secondary to eye inflammation, left eye
√x7ᵗʰ **H40.43** Glaucoma secondary to eye inflammation, bilateral

√5ᵗʰ **H40.5** Glaucoma secondary to other eye disorders

Code also underlying eye disorder

> One of the following 7th characters is to be assigned to each code in subcategory H40.5- to designate the stage of glaucoma.
> 0   stage unspecified
> 1   mild stage
> 2   moderate stage
> 3   severe stage
> 4   indeterminate stage

√x7ᵗʰ **H40.50** Glaucoma secondary to other eye disorders, unspecified eye   ▽
√x7ᵗʰ **H40.51** Glaucoma secondary to other eye disorders, right eye
√x7ᵗʰ **H40.52** Glaucoma secondary to other eye disorders, left eye
√x7ᵗʰ **H40.53** Glaucoma secondary to other eye disorders, bilateral

√5ᵗʰ **H40.6** Glaucoma secondary to drugs

Use additional code for adverse effect, if applicable, to identify drug (T36-T50 with fifth or sixth character 5)

> One of the following 7th characters is to be assigned to each code in subcategory H40.6- to designate the stage of glaucoma
> 0   stage unspecified
> 1   mild stage
> 2   moderate stage
> 3   severe stage
> 4   indeterminate stage

√x7ᵗʰ **H40.60** Glaucoma secondary to drugs, unspecified eye   ▽
√x7ᵗʰ **H40.61** Glaucoma secondary to drugs, right eye
√x7ᵗʰ **H40.62** Glaucoma secondary to drugs, left eye
√x7ᵗʰ **H40.63** Glaucoma secondary to drugs, bilateral

√5ᵗʰ **H40.8** Other glaucoma

√6ᵗʰ **H40.81** Glaucoma with increased episcleral venous pressure

H40.811 Glaucoma with increased episcleral venous pressure, right eye
H40.812 Glaucoma with increased episcleral venous pressure, left eye
H40.813 Glaucoma with increased episcleral venous pressure, bilateral
H40.819 Glaucoma with increased episcleral venous pressure, unspecified eye   ▽

√6ᵗʰ **H40.82** Hypersecretion glaucoma

H40.821 Hypersecretion glaucoma, right eye
H40.822 Hypersecretion glaucoma, left eye
H40.823 Hypersecretion glaucoma, bilateral
H40.829 Hypersecretion glaucoma, unspecified eye   ▽

√6ᵗʰ **H40.83** Aqueous misdirection

Malignant glaucoma

H40.831 Aqueous misdirection, right eye
H40.832 Aqueous misdirection, left eye
H40.833 Aqueous misdirection, bilateral
H40.839 Aqueous misdirection, unspecified eye   ▽

H40.89 Other specified glaucoma

H40.9 Unspecified glaucoma   ▽

H42 *Glaucoma in diseases classified elsewhere*

Code first underlying condition, such as:
amyloidosis (E85.-)
aniridia (Q13.1)
glaucoma (in) diabetes mellitus (E08.39, E09.39, E10.39, E11.39, E13.39)
Lowe's syndrome (E72.03)
Reiger's anomaly (Q13.81)
specified metabolic disorder (E70-E88)

EXCLUDES 1   *glaucoma (in) onchocerciasis (B73.02)*
          glaucoma (in) syphilis (A52.71)
          glaucoma (in) tuberculous (A18.59)

☑ Additional Character Req   √x7ᵗʰ Placeholder Alert   Manifestation   ▽ Unspecified   ►◄ Revised Text   ● New Code   ▲ Revised Code Title

Disorders of vitreous body and globe (H43-H44)

✓4ᵗʰ **H43 Disorders of vitreous body**

  ✓5ᵗʰ **H43.0 Vitreous prolapse**

    EXCLUDES 1   traumatic vitreous prolapse (S05.2-)

       vitreous syndrome following cataract surgery (H59.0-)

     H43.00   Vitreous prolapse, unspecified eye ▽

     H43.01   Vitreous prolapse, right eye

     H43.02   Vitreous prolapse, left eye

     H43.03   Vitreous prolapse, bilateral

  ✓5ᵗʰ **H43.1 Vitreous hemorrhage**

     H43.10   Vitreous hemorrhage, unspecified eye HCC ▽

     H43.11   Vitreous hemorrhage, right eye HCC

     H43.12   Vitreous hemorrhage, left eye HCC

     H43.13   Vitreous hemorrhage, bilateral HCC

  ✓5ᵗʰ **H43.2 Crystalline deposits in vitreous body**

     H43.20   Crystalline deposits in vitreous body, unspecified eye ▽

     H43.21   Crystalline deposits in vitreous body, right eye

     H43.22   Crystalline deposits in vitreous body, left eye

     H43.23   Crystalline deposits in vitreous body, bilateral

  ✓5ᵗʰ **H43.3 Other vitreous opacities**

    ✓6ᵗʰ **H43.31   Vitreous membranes and strands**

       H43.311   Vitreous membranes and strands, right eye

       H43.312   Vitreous membranes and strands, left eye

       H43.313   Vitreous membranes and strands, bilateral

       H43.319   Vitreous membranes and strands, unspecified eye ▽

    ✓6ᵗʰ **H43.39   Other vitreous opacities**

       Vitreous floaters

       H43.391   Other vitreous opacities, right eye

       H43.392   Other vitreous opacities, left eye

       H43.393   Other vitreous opacities, bilateral

       H43.399   Other vitreous opacities, unspecified eye ▽

  ✓5ᵗʰ **H43.8 Other disorders of vitreous body**

    EXCLUDES 1   proliferative vitreo-retinopathy with retinal detachment (H33.4-)

    EXCLUDES 2   vitreous abscess (H44.02-)

    ✓6ᵗʰ **H43.81   Vitreous degeneration**

       Vitreous detachment

       H43.811   Vitreous degeneration, right eye

       H43.812   Vitreous degeneration, left eye

       H43.813   Vitreous degeneration, bilateral

       H43.819   Vitreous degeneration, unspecified eye ▽

    ✓6ᵗʰ **H43.82   Vitreomacular adhesion**

       Vitreomacular traction

       H43.821   Vitreomacular adhesion, right eye A

       H43.822   Vitreomacular adhesion, left eye A

       H43.823   Vitreomacular adhesion, bilateral A

       H43.829   Vitreomacular adhesion, unspecified eye A ▽

     H43.89   Other disorders of vitreous body

   H43.9   Unspecified disorder of vitreous body ▽

✓4ᵗʰ **H44 Disorders of globe**

  INCLUDES   disorders affecting multiple structures of eye

  ✓5ᵗʰ **H44.0 Purulent endophthalmitis**

     Use additional code to identify organism

    EXCLUDES 1   bleb associated endophthalmitis (H59.4-)

    ✓6ᵗʰ **H44.00   Unspecified purulent endophthalmitis**

       H44.001   Unspecified purulent endophthalmitis, right eye ▽

       H44.002   Unspecified purulent endophthalmitis, left eye ▽

       H44.003   Unspecified purulent endophthalmitis, bilateral ▽

       H44.009   Unspecified purulent endophthalmitis, unspecified eye ▽

    ✓6ᵗʰ **H44.01   Panophthalmitis (acute)**

       H44.011   Panophthalmitis (acute), right eye

       H44.012   Panophthalmitis (acute), left eye

       H44.013   Panophthalmitis (acute), bilateral

       H44.019   Panophthalmitis (acute), unspecified eye ▽

    ✓6ᵗʰ **H44.02   Vitreous abscess (chronic)**

       H44.021   Vitreous abscess (chronic), right eye

       H44.022   Vitreous abscess (chronic), left eye

       H44.023   Vitreous abscess (chronic), bilateral

       H44.029   Vitreous abscess (chronic), unspecified eye ▽

  ✓5ᵗʰ **H44.1 Other endophthalmitis**

    EXCLUDES 1   bleb associated endophthalmitis (H59.4-)

    EXCLUDES 2   ophthalmia nodosa (H16.2-)

    ✓6ᵗʰ **H44.11   Panuveitis**

       DEF: Inflammation of all layers of the uvea of the eye, including the choroid, iris, and ciliary body. It also typically involves the lens, retina, optic nerve, and vitreous and causes reduced vision or blindness.

       H44.111   Panuveitis, right eye

       H44.112   Panuveitis, left eye

       H44.113   Panuveitis, bilateral

       H44.119   Panuveitis, unspecified eye ▽

    ✓6ᵗʰ **H44.12   Parasitic endophthalmitis, unspecified** ▽

       H44.121   Parasitic endophthalmitis, unspecified, right eye ▽

       H44.122   Parasitic endophthalmitis, unspecified, left eye ▽

       H44.123   Parasitic endophthalmitis, unspecified, bilateral ▽

       H44.129   Parasitic endophthalmitis, unspecified, unspecified eye ▽

    ✓6ᵗʰ **H44.13   Sympathetic uveitis**

       H44.131   Sympathetic uveitis, right eye

       H44.132   Sympathetic uveitis, left eye

       H44.133   Sympathetic uveitis, bilateral

       H44.139   Sympathetic uveitis, unspecified eye ▽

     H44.19   Other endophthalmitis

  ✓5ᵗʰ **H44.2 Degenerative myopia**

     Malignant myopia

     AHA: 2017,4Q,10-11

     H44.20   Degenerative myopia, unspecified eye ▽

     H44.21   Degenerative myopia, right eye

     H44.22   Degenerative myopia, left eye

     H44.23   Degenerative myopia, bilateral

    ✓6ᵗʰ **H44.2A   Degenerative myopia with choroidal neovascularization**

       Use additional code for any associated choroid disorders (H31.-)

       H44.2A1   Degenerative myopia with choroidal neovascularization, right eye

       H44.2A2   Degenerative myopia with choroidal neovascularization, left eye

       H44.2A3   Degenerative myopia with choroidal neovascularization, bilateral eye

       H44.2A9   Degenerative myopia with choroidal neovascularization, unspecified eye ▽

    ✓6ᵗʰ **H44.2B   Degenerative myopia with macular hole**

       H44.2B1   Degenerative myopia with macular hole, right eye

       H44.2B2   Degenerative myopia with macular hole, left eye

       H44.2B3   Degenerative myopia with macular hole, bilateral, eye

       H44.2B9   Degenerative myopia with macular hole, unspecified eye ▽

    ✓6ᵗʰ **H44.2C   Degenerative myopia with retinal detachment**

       Use additional code to identify the retinal detachment (H33.-)

       H44.2C1   Degenerative myopia with retinal detachment, right eye

       H44.2C2   Degenerative myopia with retinal detachment, left eye

       H44.2C3   Degenerative myopia with retinal detachment, bilateral eye

       H44.2C9   Degenerative myopia with retinal detachment, unspecified eye ▽

✓6ᵗʰ H44.2D Degenerative myopia with foveoschisis

    H44.2D1 Degenerative myopia with foveoschisis, **right eye**

    H44.2D2 Degenerative myopia with foveoschisis, **left eye**

    H44.2D3 Degenerative myopia with foveoschisis, **bilateral eye**

    H44.2D9 Degenerative myopia with foveoschisis, unspecified eye ▽

✓6ᵗʰ H44.2E Degenerative myopia with other maculopathy

    H44.2E1 Degenerative myopia with other maculopathy, **right eye**

    H44.2E2 Degenerative myopia with other maculopathy, **left eye**

    H44.2E3 Degenerative myopia with other maculopathy, **bilateral eye**

    H44.2E9 Degenerative myopia with other maculopathy, unspecified eye ▽

✓5ᵗʰ H44.3 Other and unspecified degenerative disorders of globe

    H44.30 Unspecified degenerative disorder of globe ▽

✓6ᵗʰ H44.31 Chalcosis

    H44.311 Chalcosis, **right eye**

    H44.312 Chalcosis, **left eye**

    H44.313 Chalcosis, **bilateral**

    H44.319 Chalcosis, unspecified eye ▽

✓6ᵗʰ H44.32 Siderosis of eye

    DEF: Iron pigment deposits within tissue of the eyeball caused by high iron content of the blood. Symptoms include cataracts, rust-colored anterior subcapsular deposits, iris heterochromia, pupillary mydriasis, and depressed electroretinogram amplitudes.

    H44.321 Siderosis of eye, **right eye**

    H44.322 Siderosis of eye, **left eye**

    H44.323 Siderosis of eye, **bilateral**

    H44.329 Siderosis of eye, unspecified eye ▽

✓6ᵗʰ H44.39 Other degenerative disorders of globe

    H44.391 Other degenerative disorders of globe, **right eye**

    H44.392 Other degenerative disorders of globe, **left eye**

    H44.393 Other degenerative disorders of globe, **bilateral**

    H44.399 Other degenerative disorders of globe, unspecified eye ▽

✓5ᵗʰ H44.4 Hypotony of eye

    H44.40 Unspecified hypotony of eye ▽

✓6ᵗʰ H44.41 Flat anterior chamber hypotony of eye

    H44.411 Flat anterior chamber hypotony of **right eye**

    H44.412 Flat anterior chamber hypotony of **left eye**

    H44.413 Flat anterior chamber hypotony of eye, **bilateral**

    H44.419 Flat anterior chamber hypotony of unspecified eye ▽

✓6ᵗʰ H44.42 Hypotony of eye due to ocular fistula

    H44.421 Hypotony of **right eye** due to ocular fistula

    H44.422 Hypotony of **left eye** due to ocular fistula

    H44.423 Hypotony of eye due to ocular fistula, **bilateral**

    H44.429 Hypotony of unspecified eye due to ocular fistula ▽

✓6ᵗʰ H44.43 Hypotony of eye due to other ocular disorders

    H44.431 Hypotony of eye due to other ocular disorders, **right eye**

    H44.432 Hypotony of eye due to other ocular disorders, **left eye**

    H44.433 Hypotony of eye due to other ocular disorders, **bilateral**

    H44.439 Hypotony of eye due to other ocular disorders, unspecified eye ▽

✓6ᵗʰ H44.44 Primary hypotony of eye

    H44.441 Primary hypotony of **right eye**

    H44.442 Primary hypotony of **left eye**

    H44.443 Primary hypotony of eye, **bilateral**

    H44.449 Primary hypotony of unspecified eye ▽

✓5ᵗʰ H44.5 Degenerated conditions of globe

    H44.50 Unspecified degenerated conditions of globe ▽

✓6ᵗʰ H44.51 Absolute glaucoma

    H44.511 Absolute glaucoma, **right eye**

    H44.512 Absolute glaucoma, **left eye**

    H44.513 Absolute glaucoma, **bilateral**

    H44.519 Absolute glaucoma, unspecified eye ▽

✓6ᵗʰ H44.52 Atrophy of globe

    Phthisis bulbi

    H44.521 Atrophy of globe, **right eye**

    H44.522 Atrophy of globe, **left eye**

    H44.523 Atrophy of globe, **bilateral**

    H44.529 Atrophy of globe, unspecified eye ▽

✓6ᵗʰ H44.53 Leucocoria

    H44.531 Leucocoria, **right eye**

    H44.532 Leucocoria, **left eye**

    H44.533 Leucocoria, **bilateral**

    H44.539 Leucocoria, unspecified eye ▽

✓5ᵗʰ H44.6 Retained (old) intraocular foreign body, magnetic

    Use additional code to identify magnetic foreign body (Z18.11)

    EXCLUDES 1   current intraocular foreign body (S05.-)

    EXCLUDES 2   retained foreign body in eyelid (H02.81-)

                 retained (old) foreign body following penetrating wound of orbit (H05.5-)

                  retained (old) intraocular foreign body, nonmagnetic (H44.7-)

✓6ᵗʰ H44.60 Unspecified retained (old) intraocular foreign body, magnetic

    H44.601 Unspecified retained (old) intraocular foreign body, magnetic, **right eye** ▽

    H44.602 Unspecified retained (old) intraocular foreign body, magnetic, **left eye** ▽

    H44.603 Unspecified retained (old) intraocular foreign body, magnetic, **bilateral** ▽

    H44.609 Unspecified retained (old) intraocular foreign body, magnetic, unspecified eye ▽

✓6ᵗʰ H44.61 Retained (old) magnetic foreign body in anterior chamber

    H44.611 Retained (old) magnetic foreign body in anterior chamber, **right eye**

    H44.612 Retained (old) magnetic foreign body in anterior chamber, **left eye**

    H44.613 Retained (old) magnetic foreign body in anterior chamber, **bilateral**

    H44.619 Retained (old) magnetic foreign body in anterior chamber, unspecified eye ▽

✓6ᵗʰ H44.62 Retained (old) magnetic foreign body in iris or ciliary body

    H44.621 Retained (old) magnetic foreign body in iris or ciliary body, **right eye**

    H44.622 Retained (old) magnetic foreign body in iris or ciliary body, **left eye**

    H44.623 Retained (old) magnetic foreign body in iris or ciliary body, **bilateral**

    H44.629 Retained (old) magnetic foreign body in iris or ciliary body, unspecified eye ▽

✓6ᵗʰ H44.63 Retained (old) magnetic foreign body in lens

    H44.631 Retained (old) magnetic foreign body in lens, **right eye**

    H44.632 Retained (old) magnetic foreign body in lens, **left eye**

    H44.633 Retained (old) magnetic foreign body in lens, **bilateral**

    H44.639 Retained (old) magnetic foreign body in lens, unspecified eye ▽

✓6ᵗʰ H44.64 Retained (old) magnetic foreign body in posterior wall of globe

    H44.641 Retained (old) magnetic foreign body in posterior wall of globe, **right eye**

    H44.642 Retained (old) magnetic foreign body in posterior wall of globe, **left eye**

    H44.643 Retained (old) magnetic foreign body in posterior wall of globe, **bilateral**

☑ Additional Character Req   ✓ˣ7ᵗʰ Placeholder Alert   Manifestation   ▽ Unspecified   ►◄ Revised Text   ● New Code   ▲ Revised Code Title

H44.649 Retained (old) magnetic foreign body in posterior wall of globe, unspecified eye ▽

√6ᵗʰ **H44.65** Retained (old) magnetic foreign body in vitreous body

H44.651 Retained (old) magnetic foreign body in vitreous body, right eye

H44.652 Retained (old) magnetic foreign body in vitreous body, left eye

H44.653 Retained (old) magnetic foreign body in vitreous body, bilateral

H44.659 Retained (old) magnetic foreign body in vitreous body, unspecified eye

√6ᵗʰ **H44.69** Retained (old) intraocular foreign body, magnetic, in other or multiple sites

H44.691 Retained (old) intraocular foreign body, magnetic, in other or multiple sites, right eye

H44.692 Retained (old) intraocular foreign body, magnetic, in other or multiple sites, left eye

H44.693 Retained (old) intraocular foreign body, magnetic, in other or multiple sites, bilateral

H44.699 Retained (old) intraocular foreign body, magnetic, in other or multiple sites, unspecified eye ▽

√5ᵗʰ **H44.7** Retained (old) intraocular foreign body, nonmagnetic

Use additional code to identify nonmagnetic foreign body (Z18.01-Z18.10, Z18.12, Z18.2-Z18.9)

EXCLUDES 1   *current intraocular foreign body (S05.-)*

EXCLUDES 2   *retained foreign body in eyelid (H02.81-)*
             retained (old) foreign body following penetrating wound of orbit (H05.5-)
             retained (old) intraocular foreign body, magnetic (H44.6-)

√6ᵗʰ **H44.70** Unspecified retained (old) intraocular foreign body, nonmagnetic

H44.701 Unspecified retained (old) intraocular foreign body, nonmagnetic, right eye ▽

H44.702 Unspecified retained (old) intraocular foreign body, nonmagnetic, left eye ▽

H44.703 Unspecified retained (old) intraocular foreign body, nonmagnetic, bilateral ▽

H44.709 Unspecified retained (old) intraocular foreign body, nonmagnetic, unspecified eye ▽

Retained (old) intraocular foreign body NOS

√6ᵗʰ **H44.71** Retained (nonmagnetic) (old) foreign body in anterior chamber

H44.711 Retained (nonmagnetic) (old) foreign body in anterior chamber, right eye

H44.712 Retained (nonmagnetic) (old) foreign body in anterior chamber, left eye

H44.713 Retained (nonmagnetic) (old) foreign body in anterior chamber, bilateral

H44.719 Retained (nonmagnetic) (old) foreign body in anterior chamber, unspecified eye ▽

√6ᵗʰ **H44.72** Retained (nonmagnetic) (old) foreign body in iris or ciliary body

H44.721 Retained (nonmagnetic) (old) foreign body in iris or ciliary body, right eye

H44.722 Retained (nonmagnetic) (old) foreign body in iris or ciliary body, left eye

H44.723 Retained (nonmagnetic) (old) foreign body in iris or ciliary body, bilateral

H44.729 Retained (nonmagnetic) (old) foreign body in iris or ciliary body, unspecified eye ▽

√6ᵗʰ **H44.73** Retained (nonmagnetic) (old) foreign body in lens

H44.731 Retained (nonmagnetic) (old) foreign body in lens, right eye

H44.732 Retained (nonmagnetic) (old) foreign body in lens, left eye

H44.733 Retained (nonmagnetic) (old) foreign body in lens, bilateral

H44.739 Retained (nonmagnetic) (old) foreign body in lens, unspecified eye ▽

√6ᵗʰ **H44.74** Retained (nonmagnetic) (old) foreign body in posterior wall of globe

H44.741 Retained (nonmagnetic) (old) foreign body in posterior wall of globe, right eye

H44.742 Retained (nonmagnetic) (old) foreign body in posterior wall of globe, left eye

H44.743 Retained (nonmagnetic) (old) foreign body in posterior wall of globe, bilateral

H44.749 Retained (nonmagnetic) (old) foreign body in posterior wall of globe, unspecified eye ▽

√6ᵗʰ **H44.75** Retained (nonmagnetic) (old) foreign body in vitreous body

H44.751 Retained (nonmagnetic) (old) foreign body in vitreous body, right eye

H44.752 Retained (nonmagnetic) (old) foreign body in vitreous body, left eye

H44.753 Retained (nonmagnetic) (old) foreign body in vitreous body, bilateral

H44.759 Retained (nonmagnetic) (old) foreign body in vitreous body, unspecified eye ▽

√6ᵗʰ **H44.79** Retained (old) intraocular foreign body, nonmagnetic, in other or multiple sites

H44.791 Retained (old) intraocular foreign body, nonmagnetic, in other or multiple sites, right eye

H44.792 Retained (old) intraocular foreign body, nonmagnetic, in other or multiple sites, left eye

H44.793 Retained (old) intraocular foreign body, nonmagnetic, in other or multiple sites, bilateral

H44.799 Retained (old) intraocular foreign body, nonmagnetic, in other or multiple sites, unspecified eye ▽

√5ᵗʰ **H44.8** Other disorders of globe

√6ᵗʰ **H44.81** Hemophthalmos

DEF: Pool of blood within the eyeball, not from a current injury.

H44.811 Hemophthalmos, right eye

H44.812 Hemophthalmos, left eye

H44.813 Hemophthalmos, bilateral

H44.819 Hemophthalmos, unspecified eye ▽

√6ᵗʰ **H44.82** Luxation of globe

H44.821 Luxation of globe, right eye

H44.822 Luxation of globe, left eye

H44.823 Luxation of globe, bilateral

H44.829 Luxation of globe, unspecified eye ▽

H44.89 Other disorders of globe

H44.9 Unspecified disorder of globe ▽

Disorders of optic nerve and visual pathways (H46-H47)

√4ᵗʰ **H46** Optic neuritis

EXCLUDES 2   *ischemic optic neuropathy (H47.01-)*
             neuromyelitis optica [Devic] (G36.0)

√5ᵗʰ **H46.0** Optic papillitis

H46.00 Optic papillitis, unspecified eye ▽

H46.01 Optic papillitis, right eye

H46.02 Optic papillitis, left eye

H46.03 Optic papillitis, bilateral

√5ᵗʰ **H46.1** Retrobulbar neuritis

Retrobulbar neuritis NOS

EXCLUDES 1   *syphilitic retrobulbar neuritis (A52.15)*

H46.10 Retrobulbar neuritis, unspecified eye ▽

H46.11 Retrobulbar neuritis, right eye

H46.12 Retrobulbar neuritis, left eye

H46.13 Retrobulbar neuritis, bilateral

H46.2 Nutritional optic neuropathy

H46.3 Toxic optic neuropathy

Code first (T51-T65) to identify cause

H46.8 Other optic neuritis

H46.9 Unspecified optic neuritis ▽

☑4ᵗʰ **H47**   **Other disorders of optic [2nd] nerve and visual pathways**

    ☑5ᵗʰ **H47.0**   **Disorders of optic nerve, not elsewhere classified**

       ☑6ᵗʰ **H47.01**   **Ischemic** optic neuropathy

          H47.011   Ischemic optic neuropathy, right eye
          H47.012   Ischemic optic neuropathy, left eye
          H47.013   Ischemic optic neuropathy, bilateral
          H47.019   Ischemic optic neuropathy,   ▽
                unspecified eye

       ☑6ᵗʰ **H47.02**   **Hemorrhage** in optic nerve sheath

          H47.021   Hemorrhage in optic nerve sheath, right eye
          H47.022   Hemorrhage in optic nerve sheath, left eye
          H47.023   Hemorrhage in optic nerve sheath, bilateral
          H47.029   Hemorrhage in optic nerve   ▽
                sheath, unspecified eye

       ☑6ᵗʰ **H47.03**   **Optic nerve** hypoplasia

          H47.031   Optic nerve hypoplasia, right eye
          H47.032   Optic nerve hypoplasia, left eye
          H47.033   Optic nerve hypoplasia, bilateral
          H47.039   Optic nerve hypoplasia,   ▽
                unspecified eye

       ☑6ᵗʰ **H47.09**   **Other disorders of optic nerve, not elsewhere classified**

          Compression of optic nerve

          H47.091   Other disorders of optic nerve, not elsewhere classified, right eye
          H47.092   Other disorders of optic nerve, not elsewhere classified, left eye
          H47.093   Other disorders of optic nerve, not elsewhere classified, bilateral
          H47.099   Other disorders of optic nerve,   ▽
                not elsewhere classified, unspecified eye

    ☑5ᵗʰ **H47.1**   **Papilledema**

       DEF: Swelling of the optic papilla, the raised area connected to the optic disk made up of nerves that enter the eyeball. It may be caused by increased intracranial pressure, decreased ocular pressure, or a retinal disorder.

       H47.10   **Unspecified papilledema**   ▽
       H47.11   **Papilledema associated with** increased intracranial pressure
       H47.12   **Papilledema associated with** decreased ocular pressure
       H47.13   **Papilledema associated with** retinal disorder
       ☑6ᵗʰ **H47.14**   **Foster-Kennedy syndrome**

          H47.141   Foster-Kennedy syndrome, right eye
          H47.142   Foster-Kennedy syndrome, left eye
          H47.143   Foster-Kennedy syndrome, bilateral
          H47.149   Foster-Kennedy syndrome,   ▽
                unspecified eye

    ☑5ᵗʰ **H47.2**   **Optic atrophy**

       H47.20   **Unspecified optic atrophy**   ▽
       ☑6ᵗʰ **H47.21**   **Primary** optic atrophy

          H47.211   Primary optic atrophy, right eye
          H47.212   Primary optic atrophy, left eye
          H47.213   Primary optic atrophy, bilateral
          H47.219   Primary optic atrophy,   ▽
                unspecified eye

       H47.22   **Hereditary** optic atrophy

          Leber's optic atrophy

       ☑6ᵗʰ **H47.23**   **Glaucomatous** optic atrophy

          H47.231   Glaucomatous optic atrophy, right eye
          H47.232   Glaucomatous optic atrophy, left eye
          H47.233   Glaucomatous optic atrophy, bilateral
          H47.239   Glaucomatous optic atrophy,   ▽
                unspecified eye

       ☑6ᵗʰ **H47.29**   **Other optic atrophy**

          Temporal pallor of optic disc

          H47.291   Other optic atrophy, right eye
          H47.292   Other optic atrophy, left eye
          H47.293   Other optic atrophy, bilateral
          H47.299   Other optic atrophy, unspecified   ▽
                eye

    ☑5ᵗʰ **H47.3**   **Other disorders of optic disc**

       ☑6ᵗʰ **H47.31**   **Coloboma** of optic disc

          H47.311   Coloboma of optic disc, right eye

          H47.312   Coloboma of optic disc, left eye
          H47.313   Coloboma of optic disc, bilateral
          H47.319   Coloboma of optic disc,   ▽
                unspecified eye

       ☑6ᵗʰ **H47.32**   **Drusen** of optic disc

          H47.321   Drusen of optic disc, right eye
          H47.322   Drusen of optic disc, left eye
          H47.323   Drusen of optic disc, bilateral
          H47.329   Drusen of optic disc, unspecified   ▽
                eye

       ☑6ᵗʰ **H47.33**   **Pseudopapilledema** of optic disc

          H47.331   Pseudopapilledema of optic disc, right eye
          H47.332   Pseudopapilledema of optic disc, left eye
          H47.333   Pseudopapilledema of optic disc, bilateral
          H47.339   Pseudopapilledema of optic disc,   ▽
                unspecified eye

       ☑6ᵗʰ **H47.39**   **Other disorders of optic disc**

          H47.391   Other disorders of optic disc, right eye
          H47.392   Other disorders of optic disc, left eye
          H47.393   Other disorders of optic disc, bilateral
          H47.399   Other disorders of optic disc,   ▽
                unspecified eye

    ☑5ᵗʰ **H47.4**   **Disorders of optic chiasm**

       Code also underlying condition

       H47.41   **Disorders of optic chiasm in (due to)** inflammatory disorders
       H47.42   **Disorders of optic chiasm in (due to)** neoplasm
       H47.43   **Disorders of optic chiasm in (due to)** vascular disorders
       H47.49   **Disorders of optic chiasm in (due to) other disorders**

    ☑5ᵗʰ **H47.5**   **Disorders of other visual pathways**

       Disorders of optic tracts, geniculate nuclei and optic radiations
       Code also underlying condition

       ☑6ᵗʰ **H47.51**   **Disorders of visual pathways in (due to) inflammatory disorders**

          H47.511   Disorders of visual pathways in (due to) inflammatory disorders, right side
          H47.512   Disorders of visual pathways in (due to) inflammatory disorders, left side
          H47.519   Disorders of visual pathways in   ▽
                (due to) inflammatory disorders, unspecified side

       ☑6ᵗʰ **H47.52**   **Disorders of visual pathways in (due to)** neoplasm

          H47.521   Disorders of visual pathways in (due to) neoplasm, right side
          H47.522   Disorders of visual pathways in (due to) neoplasm, left side
          H47.529   Disorders of visual pathways in   ▽
                (due to) neoplasm, unspecified side

       ☑6ᵗʰ **H47.53**   **Disorders of visual pathways in (due to) vascular disorders**

          H47.531   Disorders of visual pathways in (due to) vascular disorders, right side
          H47.532   Disorders of visual pathways in (due to) vascular disorders, left side
          H47.539   Disorders of visual pathways in   ▽
                (due to) vascular disorders, unspecified side

    ☑5ᵗʰ **H47.6**   **Disorders of visual cortex**

       Code also underlying condition

       EXCLUDES 1   injury to visual cortex S04.04

       ☑6ᵗʰ **H47.61**   **Cortical blindness**

          H47.611   Cortical blindness, right side of brain
          H47.612   Cortical blindness, left side of brain
          H47.619   Cortical blindness, unspecified   ▽
                side of brain

       ☑6ᵗʰ **H47.62**   **Disorders of visual cortex in (due to)** inflammatory disorders

          H47.621   Disorders of visual cortex in (due to) inflammatory disorders, right side of brain
          H47.622   Disorders of visual cortex in (due to) inflammatory disorders, left side of brain
          H47.629   Disorders of visual cortex in (due   ▽
                to) inflammatory disorders, unspecified side of brain

---

☑ Additional Character Req   ⁷ˣ⁷ᵗʰ Placeholder Alert   Manifestation   ▽ Unspecified   ▶◀ Revised Text   ● New Code   ▲ Revised Code Title

ICD-10-CM 2019   **611**

Chapter 7. Diseases of the Eye and Adnexa

H47.63–H50.132

√6ᵗʰ **H47.63** **Disorders of visual cortex in (due to)** neoplasm

     H47.631 **Disorders of visual cortex in (due to) neoplasm,** right **side of brain**

     H47.632 **Disorders of visual cortex in (due to) neoplasm,** left **side of brain**

     H47.639 **Disorders of visual cortex in (due to) neoplasm, unspecified side of brain** ▽

√6ᵗʰ **H47.64** **Disorders of visual cortex in (due to)** vascular **disorders**

     H47.641 **Disorders of visual cortex in (due to) vascular disorders,** right **side of brain**

     H47.642 **Disorders of visual cortex in (due to) vascular disorders,** left **side of brain**

     H47.649 **Disorders of visual cortex in (due to) vascular disorders, unspecified side of brain** ▽

H47.9 **Unspecified disorder of visual pathways** ▽

Disorders of ocular muscles, binocular movement, accommodation and refraction (H49-H52)

EXCLUDES 2   *nystagmus and other irregular eye movements (H55)*

√4ᵗʰ **H49** **Paralytic strabismus**

EXCLUDES 2   *internal ophthalmoplegia (H52.51-)*
                 internuclear ophthalmoplegia (H51.2-)
                 progressive supranuclear ophthalmoplegia (G23.1)

DEF: Strabismus: Misalignment of the eyes with the inability to move and focus in the same direction due to conditions affecting the muscles controlling them.

√5ᵗʰ **H49.0** **Third [oculomotor] nerve palsy**

     H49.00 **Third [oculomotor] nerve palsy, unspecified eye** ▽

     H49.01 **Third [oculomotor] nerve palsy,** right **eye**

     H49.02 **Third [oculomotor] nerve palsy,** left **eye**

     H49.03 **Third [oculomotor] nerve palsy,** bilateral

√5ᵗʰ **H49.1** **Fourth [trochlear] nerve palsy**

     H49.10 **Fourth [trochlear] nerve palsy, unspecified eye** ▽

     H49.11 **Fourth [trochlear] nerve palsy,** right **eye**

     H49.12 **Fourth [trochlear] nerve palsy,** left **eye**

     H49.13 **Fourth [trochlear] nerve palsy,** bilateral

√5ᵗʰ **H49.2** **Sixth [abducent] nerve palsy**

     H49.20 **Sixth [abducent] nerve palsy, unspecified eye** ▽

     H49.21 **Sixth [abducent] nerve palsy,** right **eye**

     H49.22 **Sixth [abducent] nerve palsy,** left **eye**

     H49.23 **Sixth [abducent] nerve palsy,** bilateral

√5ᵗʰ **H49.3** **Total (external) ophthalmoplegia**

     H49.30 **Total (external) ophthalmoplegia, unspecified eye** ▽

     H49.31 **Total (external) ophthalmoplegia,** right **eye**

     H49.32 **Total (external) ophthalmoplegia,** left **eye**

     H49.33 **Total (external) ophthalmoplegia,** bilateral

√5ᵗʰ **H49.4** **Progressive external ophthalmoplegia**

EXCLUDES 1   *Kearns-Sayre syndrome (H49.81-)*

     H49.40 **Progressive external ophthalmoplegia, unspecified eye** ▽

     H49.41 **Progressive external ophthalmoplegia,** right **eye**

     H49.42 **Progressive external ophthalmoplegia,** left **eye**

     H49.43 **Progressive external ophthalmoplegia,** bilateral

√5ᵗʰ **H49.8** **Other paralytic strabismus**

√6ᵗʰ **H49.81** **Kearns-Sayre syndrome**

     Progressive external ophthalmoplegia with pigmentary retinopathy
     Use additional code for other manifestation, such as: heart block (I45.9)

     H49.811 **Kearns-Sayre syndrome,** right **eye** HCC

     H49.812 **Kearns-Sayre syndrome,** left **eye** HCC

     H49.813 **Kearns-Sayre syndrome,** bilateral HCC

     H49.819 **Kearns-Sayre syndrome, unspecified eye** HCC ▽

√6ᵗʰ **H49.88** **Other paralytic strabismus**

     External ophthalmoplegia NOS

     H49.881 **Other paralytic strabismus,** right **eye**

     H49.882 **Other paralytic strabismus,** left **eye**

     H49.883 **Other paralytic strabismus,** bilateral

     H49.889 **Other paralytic strabismus, unspecified eye** ▽

H49.9 **Unspecified paralytic strabismus** ▽

√4ᵗʰ **H50** **Other strabismus**

DEF: Strabismus: Misalignment of the eyes with the inability to move and focus in the same direction due to conditions affecting the muscles controlling them.

√5ᵗʰ **H50.0** **Esotropia**

     Convergent concomitant strabismus

EXCLUDES 1   *intermittent esotropia (H50.31-, H50.32)*

     H50.00 **Unspecified esotropia** ▽

√6ᵗʰ **H50.01** **Monocular esotropia**

     H50.011 **Monocular esotropia,** right **eye**

     H50.012 **Monocular esotropia,** left **eye**

√6ᵗʰ **H50.02** **Monocular esotropia with** A **pattern**

     H50.021 **Monocular esotropia with A pattern,** right **eye**

     H50.022 **Monocular esotropia with A pattern,** left **eye**

√6ᵗʰ **H50.03** **Monocular esotropia with** V **pattern**

     H50.031 **Monocular esotropia with V pattern,** right **eye**

     H50.032 **Monocular esotropia with V pattern,** left **eye**

√6ᵗʰ **H50.04** **Monocular esotropia with** other noncomitancies

     H50.041 **Monocular esotropia with other noncomitancies,** right **eye**

     H50.042 **Monocular esotropia with other noncomitancies,** left **eye**

     H50.05 **Alternating esotropia**

     H50.06 **Alternating esotropia with** A **pattern**

     H50.07 **Alternating esotropia with** V **pattern**

     H50.08 **Alternating esotropia with other noncomitancies**

Eye Muscle Diseases

R.   L.
Monocular (one eye only) esotropia (inward)

Monocular exotropia (outward)

Monocular hypertropia (upward)

√5ᵗʰ **H50.1** **Exotropia**

     Divergent concomitant strabismus

EXCLUDES 1   *intermittent exotropia (H50.33-, H50.34)*

     H50.10 **Unspecified exotropia** ▽

√6ᵗʰ **H50.11** **Monocular exotropia**

     H50.111 **Monocular exotropia,** right **eye**

     H50.112 **Monocular exotropia,** left **eye**

√6ᵗʰ **H50.12** **Monocular exotropia with** A **pattern**

     H50.121 **Monocular exotropia with A pattern,** right **eye**

     H50.122 **Monocular exotropia with A pattern,** left **eye**

√6ᵗʰ **H50.13** **Monocular exotropia with** V **pattern**

     H50.131 **Monocular exotropia with V pattern,** right **eye**

     H50.132 **Monocular exotropia with V pattern,** left **eye**

√6ᵗʰ **H50.14** Monocular exotropia with other noncomitancies

    H50.141 Monocular exotropia with other noncomitancies, right eye

    H50.142 Monocular exotropia with other noncomitancies, left eye

H50.15 Alternating exotropia

H50.16 Alternating exotropia with A pattern

H50.17 Alternating exotropia with V pattern

H50.18 Alternating exotropia with other noncomitancies

√5ᵗʰ **H50.2** Vertical strabismus

    Hypertropia

H50.21 Vertical strabismus, right eye

H50.22 Vertical strabismus, left eye

√5ᵗʰ **H50.3** Intermittent heterotropia

H50.30 Unspecified intermittent heterotropia ▽

√6ᵗʰ **H50.31** Intermittent monocular esotropia

    H50.311 Intermittent monocular esotropia, right eye

    H50.312 Intermittent monocular esotropia, left eye

H50.32 Intermittent alternating esotropia

√6ᵗʰ **H50.33** Intermittent monocular exotropia

    H50.331 Intermittent monocular exotropia, right eye

    H50.332 Intermittent monocular exotropia, left eye

H50.34 Intermittent alternating exotropia

√5ᵗʰ **H50.4** Other and unspecified heterotropia

H50.40 Unspecified heterotropia ▽

√6ᵗʰ **H50.41** Cyclotropia

    H50.411 Cyclotropia, right eye

    H50.412 Cyclotropia, left eye

H50.42 Monofixation syndrome

H50.43 Accommodative component in esotropia

√5ᵗʰ **H50.5** Heterophoria

H50.50 Unspecified heterophoria ▽

H50.51 Esophoria

H50.52 Exophoria

H50.53 Vertical heterophoria

H50.54 Cyclophoria

H50.55 Alternating heterophoria

√5ᵗʰ **H50.6** Mechanical strabismus

H50.60 Mechanical strabismus, unspecified ▽

√6ᵗʰ **H50.61** Brown's sheath syndrome

    H50.611 Brown's sheath syndrome, right eye

    H50.612 Brown's sheath syndrome, left eye

H50.69 Other mechanical strabismus

    Strabismus due to adhesions

    Traumatic limitation of duction of eye muscle

√5ᵗʰ **H50.8** Other specified strabismus

√6ᵗʰ **H50.81** Duane's syndrome

    H50.811 Duane's syndrome, right eye

    H50.812 Duane's syndrome, left eye

H50.89 Other specified strabismus

H50.9 Unspecified strabismus ▽

√4ᵗʰ **H51** Other disorders of binocular movement

H51.0 Palsy (spasm) of conjugate gaze

√5ᵗʰ **H51.1** Convergence insufficiency and excess

H51.11 Convergence insufficiency

H51.12 Convergence excess

√5ᵗʰ **H51.2** Internuclear ophthalmoplegia

H51.20 Internuclear ophthalmoplegia, unspecified eye ▽

H51.21 Internuclear ophthalmoplegia, right eye

H51.22 Internuclear ophthalmoplegia, left eye

H51.23 Internuclear ophthalmoplegia, bilateral

H51.8 Other specified disorders of binocular movement

H51.9 Unspecified disorder of binocular movement ▽

√4ᵗʰ **H52** Disorders of refraction and accommodation

√5ᵗʰ **H52.0** Hypermetropia

H52.00 Hypermetropia, unspecified eye ▽

H52.01 Hypermetropia, right eye

H52.02 Hypermetropia, left eye

H52.03 Hypermetropia, bilateral

√5ᵗʰ **H52.1** Myopia

    EXCLUDES 1   degenerative myopia (H44.2-)

H52.10 Myopia, unspecified eye ▽

H52.11 Myopia, right eye

H52.12 Myopia, left eye

H52.13 Myopia, bilateral

√5ᵗʰ **H52.2** Astigmatism

√6ᵗʰ **H52.20** Unspecified astigmatism

    H52.201 Unspecified astigmatism, right eye ▽

    H52.202 Unspecified astigmatism, left eye ▽

    H52.203 Unspecified astigmatism, bilateral

    H52.209 Unspecified astigmatism, unspecified eye ▽

√6ᵗʰ **H52.21** Irregular astigmatism

    H52.211 Irregular astigmatism, right eye

    H52.212 Irregular astigmatism, left eye

    H52.213 Irregular astigmatism, bilateral

    H52.219 Irregular astigmatism, unspecified eye ▽

√6ᵗʰ **H52.22** Regular astigmatism

    H52.221 Regular astigmatism, right eye

    H52.222 Regular astigmatism, left eye

    H52.223 Regular astigmatism, bilateral

    H52.229 Regular astigmatism, unspecified eye ▽

√5ᵗʰ **H52.3** Anisometropia and aniseikonia

H52.31 Anisometropia

H52.32 Aniseikonia

H52.4 Presbyopia

√5ᵗʰ **H52.5** Disorders of accommodation

√6ᵗʰ **H52.51** Internal ophthalmoplegia (complete) (total)

    H52.511 Internal ophthalmoplegia (complete) (total), right eye

    H52.512 Internal ophthalmoplegia (complete) (total), left eye

    H52.513 Internal ophthalmoplegia (complete) (total), bilateral

    H52.519 Internal ophthalmoplegia (complete) (total), unspecified eye ▽

√6ᵗʰ **H52.52** Paresis of accommodation

    H52.521 Paresis of accommodation, right eye

    H52.522 Paresis of accommodation, left eye

    H52.523 Paresis of accommodation, bilateral

    H52.529 Paresis of accommodation, unspecified eye ▽

√6ᵗʰ **H52.53** Spasm of accommodation

    H52.531 Spasm of accommodation, right eye

    H52.532 Spasm of accommodation, left eye

    H52.533 Spasm of accommodation, bilateral

    H52.539 Spasm of accommodation, unspecified eye ▽

H52.6 Other disorders of refraction

H52.7 Unspecified disorder of refraction ▽

Visual disturbances and blindness (H53-H54)

√4ᵗʰ **H53** Visual disturbances

√5ᵗʰ **H53.0** Amblyopia ex anopsia

    EXCLUDES 1   amblyopia due to vitamin A deficiency (E50.5)

√6ᵗʰ **H53.00** Unspecified amblyopia

    H53.001 Unspecified amblyopia, right eye ▽

    H53.002 Unspecified amblyopia, left eye ▽

    H53.003 Unspecified amblyopia, bilateral ▽

    H53.009 Unspecified amblyopia, unspecified eye ▽

√6ᵗʰ **H53.01** Deprivation amblyopia

    H53.011 Deprivation amblyopia, right eye

    H53.012 Deprivation amblyopia, left eye

    H53.013 Deprivation amblyopia, bilateral

    H53.019 Deprivation amblyopia, unspecified eye ▽

√6ᵗʰ **H53.02** Refractive amblyopia

    H53.021 Refractive amblyopia, right eye

    H53.022 Refractive amblyopia, left eye

☑ Additional Character Req   √x7ᵗʰ Placeholder Alert   Manifestation   ▽ Unspecified   ►◄ Revised Text   ● New Code   ▲ Revised Code Title

ICD-10-CM 2019   613

     H53.Ø23 **Refractive amblyopia, bilateral**

     H53.Ø29 **Refractive amblyopia, unspecified eye** ▽

  ✓6ᵗʰ H53.Ø3 **Strabismic amblyopia**

     EXCLUDES 1   *strabismus (H5Ø.-)*

     H53.Ø31 **Strabismic amblyopia, right eye**

     H53.Ø32 **Strabismic amblyopia, left eye**

     H53.Ø33 **Strabismic amblyopia, bilateral**

     H53.Ø39 **Strabismic amblyopia, unspecified eye** ▽

  ✓6ᵗʰ H53.Ø4 **Amblyopia suspect**

     AHA: 2016,4Q,22-23

     H53.Ø41 **Amblyopia suspect, right eye**

     H53.Ø42 **Amblyopia suspect, left eye**

     H53.Ø43 **Amblyopia suspect, bilateral**

     H53.Ø49 **Amblyopia suspect, unspecified eye** ▽

✓5ᵗʰ **H53.1 Subjective visual disturbances**

   EXCLUDES 1   *subjective visual disturbances due to vitamin A deficiency (E5Ø.5)*

       visual hallucinations (R44.1)

  H53.10 **Unspecified subjective visual disturbances** ▽

  H53.11 **Day blindness**

     Hemeralopia

  ✓6ᵗʰ H53.12 **Transient visual loss**

     Scintillating scotoma

     EXCLUDES 1   *amaurosis fugax (G45.3-)*

       transient retinal artery occlusion (H34.Ø-)

     H53.121 **Transient visual loss, right eye**

     H53.122 **Transient visual loss, left eye**

     H53.123 **Transient visual loss, bilateral**

     H53.129 **Transient visual loss, unspecified eye** ▽

  ✓6ᵗʰ H53.13 **Sudden visual loss**

     H53.131 **Sudden visual loss, right eye**

     H53.132 **Sudden visual loss, left eye**

     H53.133 **Sudden visual loss, bilateral**

     H53.139 **Sudden visual loss, unspecified eye** ▽

  ✓6ᵗʰ H53.14 **Visual discomfort**

     Asthenopia

     Photophobia

     H53.141 **Visual discomfort, right eye**

     H53.142 **Visual discomfort, left eye**

     H53.143 **Visual discomfort, bilateral**

     H53.149 **Visual discomfort, unspecified** ▽

  H53.15 **Visual distortions of shape and size**

     Metamorphopsia

  H53.16 **Psychophysical visual disturbances**

  H53.19 **Other subjective visual disturbances**

     Visual halos

H53.2 Diplopia

  Double vision

✓5ᵗʰ **H53.3 Other and unspecified disorders of binocular vision**

  H53.30 **Unspecified disorder of binocular vision** ▽

  H53.31 **Abnormal retinal correspondence**

  H53.32 **Fusion with defective stereopsis**

  H53.33 **Simultaneous visual perception without fusion**

  H53.34 **Suppression of binocular vision**

✓5ᵗʰ **H53.4 Visual field defects**

  H53.40 **Unspecified visual field defects** ▽

  ✓6ᵗʰ H53.41 **Scotoma involving central area**

     Central scotoma

     H53.411 **Scotoma involving central area, right eye**

     H53.412 **Scotoma involving central area, left eye**

     H53.413 **Scotoma involving central area, bilateral**

     H53.419 **Scotoma involving central area, unspecified eye** ▽

  ✓6ᵗʰ H53.42 **Scotoma of blind spot area**

     Enlarged blind spot

     H53.421 **Scotoma of blind spot area, right eye**

     H53.422 **Scotoma of blind spot area, left eye**

     H53.423 **Scotoma of blind spot area, bilateral**

     H53.429 **Scotoma of blind spot area, unspecified eye** ▽

  ✓6ᵗʰ H53.43 **Sector or arcuate defects**

     Arcuate scotoma

     Bjerrum scotoma

     H53.431 **Sector or arcuate defects, right eye**

     H53.432 **Sector or arcuate defects, left eye**

     H53.433 **Sector or arcuate defects, bilateral**

     H53.439 **Sector or arcuate defects, unspecified eye** ▽

  ✓6ᵗʰ H53.45 **Other localized visual field defect**

     Peripheral visual field defect

     Ring scotoma NOS

     Scotoma NOS

     H53.451 **Other localized visual field defect, right eye**

     H53.452 **Other localized visual field defect, left eye**

     H53.453 **Other localized visual field defect, bilateral**

     H53.459 **Other localized visual field defect, unspecified eye** ▽

  ✓6ᵗʰ H53.46 **Homonymous bilateral field defects**

     Homonymous hemianopia

     Homonymous hemianopsia

     Quadrant anopia

     Quadrant anopsia

     H53.461 **Homonymous bilateral field defects, right side**

     H53.462 **Homonymous bilateral field defects, left side**

     H53.469 **Homonymous bilateral field defects, unspecified side** ▽

       Homonymous bilateral field defects NOS

  H53.47 **Heteronymous bilateral field defects**

     Heteronymous hemianop(s)ia

  ✓6ᵗʰ H53.48 **Generalized contraction of visual field**

     H53.481 **Generalized contraction of visual field, right eye**

     H53.482 **Generalized contraction of visual field, left eye**

     H53.483 **Generalized contraction of visual field, bilateral**

     H53.489 **Generalized contraction of visual field, unspecified eye** ▽

✓5ᵗʰ **H53.5 Color vision deficiencies**

  Color blindness

  EXCLUDES 2   *day blindness (H53.11)*

  H53.50 **Unspecified color vision deficiencies** ▽

     Color blindness NOS

  H53.51 **Achromatopsia**

     DEF: Nonprogressive genetic visual disorder characterized by complete color blindness, decreased vision, and light sensitivity.

  H53.52 **Acquired color vision deficiency**

  H53.53 **Deuteranomaly**

     Deuteranopia

     DEF: Male-only genetic disorder causing difficulty in distinguishing green and red; no shortened spectrum.

  H53.54 **Protanomaly**

     Protanopia

  H53.55 **Tritanomaly**

     Tritanopia

  H53.59 **Other color vision deficiencies**

✓5ᵗʰ **H53.6 Night blindness**

  EXCLUDES 1   *night blindness due to vitamin A deficiency (E5Ø.5)*

  H53.60 **Unspecified night blindness** ▽

  H53.61 **Abnormal dark adaptation curve**

  H53.62 **Acquired night blindness**

  H53.63 **Congenital night blindness**

  H53.69 **Other night blindness**

✓5ᵗʰ **H53.7 Vision sensitivity deficiencies**

  H53.71 **Glare sensitivity**

  H53.72 **Impaired contrast sensitivity**

H53.8 Other visual disturbances

H53.9 Unspecified visual disturbance ▽

✓4th **H54   Blindness and low vision**

> NOTE   For definition of visual impairment categories see table below
>
> Code first any associated underlying cause of the blindness
>
> EXCLUDES 1   *amaurosis fugax (G45.3)*
>
> AHA: 2017,4Q,11-12

✓5th **H54.0   Blindness, both eyes**

> Visual impairment categories 3, 4, 5 in both eyes.

> ✓6th **H54.0X   Blindness, both eyes, different category levels**

>> ✓7th **H54.0X3   Blindness right eye, category 3**

>>> **H54.0X33   Blindness right eye category 3, blindness left eye category 3**
>>>
>>> **H54.0X34   Blindness right eye category 3, blindness left eye category 4**
>>>
>>> **H54.0X35   Blindness right eye category 3, blindness left eye category 5**

>> ✓7th **H54.0X4   Blindness right eye, category 4**

>>> **H54.0X43   Blindness right eye category 4, blindness left eye category 3**
>>>
>>> **H54.0X44   Blindness right eye category 4, blindness left eye category 4**
>>>
>>> **H54.0X45   Blindness right eye category 4, blindness left eye category 5**

>> ✓7th **H54.0X5   Blindness right eye, category 5**

>>> **H54.0X53   Blindness right eye category 5, blindness left eye category 3**
>>>
>>> **H54.0X54   Blindness right eye category 5, blindness left eye category 4**
>>>
>>> **H54.0X55   Blindness right eye category 5, blindness left eye category 5**

✓5th **H54.1   Blindness, one eye, low vision other eye**

> Visual impairment categories 3, 4, 5 in one eye, with categories 1 or 2 in the other eye.

> **H54.10   Blindness, one eye, low vision other eye, unspecified eyes** ▽

> ✓6th **H54.11   Blindness, right eye, low vision left eye**

>> ✓7th **H54.113   Blindness right eye category 3, low vision left eye**

>>> **H54.1131   Blindness right eye category 3, low vision left eye category 1**
>>>
>>> **H54.1132   Blindness right eye category 3, low vision left eye category 2**

>> ✓7th **H54.114   Blindness right eye category 4, low vision left eye**

>>> **H54.1141   Blindness right eye category 4, low vision left eye category 1**
>>>
>>> **H54.1142   Blindness right eye category 4, low vision left eye category 2**

>> ✓7th **H54.115   Blindness right eye category 5, low vision left eye**

>>> **H54.1151   Blindness right eye category 5, low vision left eye category 1**
>>>
>>> **H54.1152   Blindness right eye category 5, low vision left eye category 2**

> ✓6th **H54.12   Blindness, left eye, low vision right eye**

>> ✓7th **H54.121   Low vision right eye category 1, blindness left eye**

>>> **H54.1213   Low vision right eye category 1, blindness left eye category 3**
>>>
>>> **H54.1214   Low vision right eye category 1, blindness left eye category 4**
>>>
>>> **H54.1215   Low vision right eye category 1, blindness left eye category 5**

>> ✓7th **H54.122   Low vision right eye category 2, blindness left eye**

>>> **H54.1223   Low vision right eye category 2, blindness left eye category 3**
>>>
>>> **H54.1224   Low vision right eye category 2, blindness left eye category 4**
>>>
>>> **H54.1225   Low vision right eye category 2, blindness left eye category 5**

✓5th **H54.2   Low vision, both eyes**

> Visual impairment categories 1 or 2 in both eyes.

> ✓6th **H54.2X   Low vision, both eyes, different category levels**

>> ✓7th **H54.2X1   Low vision, right eye, category 1**

>>> **H54.2X11   Low vision right eye category 1, low vision left eye category 1**
>>>
>>> **H54.2X12   Low vision right eye category 1, low vision left eye category 2**

>> ✓7th **H54.2X2   Low vision, right eye, category 2**

>>> **H54.2X21   Low vision right eye category 2, low vision left eye category 1**
>>>
>>> **H54.2X22   Low vision right eye category 2, low vision left eye category 2**

H54.3   Unqualified visual loss, both eyes

> Visual impairment category 9 in both eyes.
>
> TIP: Assign only when both eyes are documented as affected by blindness or low vision but the visual impairment category is not documented.

✓5th **H54.4   Blindness, one eye**

> Visual impairment categories 3, 4, 5 in one eye [normal vision in other eye]

> **H54.40   Blindness, one eye, unspecified eye** ▽

> ✓6th **H54.41   Blindness, right eye, normal vision left eye**

>> ✓7th **H54.413   Blindness, right eye, category 3**

>>> **H54.413A   Blindness right eye category 3, normal vision left eye**

>> ✓7th **H54.414   Blindness, right eye, category 4**

>>> **H54.414A   Blindness right eye category 4, normal vision left eye**

>> ✓7th **H54.415   Blindness, right eye, category 5**

>>> **H54.415A   Blindness right eye category 5, normal vision left eye**

> ✓6th **H54.42   Blindness, left eye, normal vision right eye**

>> ✓7th **H54.42A   Blindness, left eye, category 3-5**

>>> **H54.42A3   Blindness left eye category 3, normal vision right eye**
>>>
>>> **H54.42A4   Blindness left eye category 4, normal vision right eye**
>>>
>>> **H54.42A5   Blindness left eye category 5, normal vision right eye**

✓5th **H54.5   Low vision, one eye**

> Visual impairment categories 1 or 2 in one eye [normal vision in other eye].

> **H54.50   Low vision, one eye, unspecified eye** ▽

> ✓6th **H54.51   Low vision, right eye, normal vision left eye**

>> ✓7th **H54.511   Low vision, right eye, category 1-2**

>>> **H54.511A   Low vision right eye category 1, normal vision left eye**
>>>
>>> **H54.512A   Low vision right eye category 2, normal vision left eye**

> ✓7th **H54.52   Low vision, left eye, normal vision right eye**

>> ✓7th **H54.52A   Low vision, left eye, category 1-2**

>>> **H54.52A1   Low vision left eye category 1, normal vision right eye**
>>>
>>> **H54.52A2   Low vision left eye category 2, normal vision right eye**

✓5th **H54.6   Unqualified visual loss, one eye**

> Visual impairment category 9 in one eye [normal vision in other eye].
>
> TIP: Assign a code from this category only when one eye is documented as affected by blindness or low vision but the visual impairment category is not documented.

> **H54.60   Unqualified visual loss, one eye, unspecified** ▽
>
> **H54.61   Unqualified visual loss, right eye, normal vision left eye**
>
> **H54.62   Unqualified visual loss, left eye, normal vision right eye**

H54.7   Unspecified visual loss ▽

> Visual impairment category 9 NOS
>
> TIP: Assign only when documentation specifies blindness, visual loss, or low vision but not whether one or both eyes are affected or the visual impairment category.

✓ Additional Character Req   ✓x7th Placeholder Alert   Manifestation   ▽ Unspecified   ►◄ Revised Text   ● New Code   ▲ Revised Code Title

Chapter 7. Diseases of the Eye and Adnexa

H54.8   Legal blindness, as defined in USA
Blindness NOS according to USA definition
EXCLUDES 1   *legal blindness with specification of impairment level (H54.0-H54.7)*

NOTE   The table below gives a classification of severity of visual impairment recommended by a WHO Study Group on the Prevention of Blindness, Geneva, 6-10 November 1972.

The term "low vision" in category H54 comprises categories 1 and 2 of the table, the term "blindness" categories 3, 4 and 5, and the term "unqualified visual loss" category 9.

If the extent of the visual field is taken into account, patients with a field no greater than 10 but greater than 5 around central fixation should be placed in category 3 and patients with a field no greater than 5 around central fixation should be placed in category 4, even if the central acuity is not impaired.

Category of visual impairment	Visual acuity with best possible correction	
	Maximum less than:	**Minimum equal to or better than:**
1	6/18 3/10 (0.3) 20/70	6/60 1/10 (0.1) 20/200
2	6/60 1/10 (0.1) 20/200	3/60 1/20 (0.05) 20/400
3	3/60 1/200 (0.05) 20/400	1/60 (finger counting at one meter) 1/50 (0.02) 5/300 (20/1200)
4	1/60 (finger counting at one meter) 1/50 (0.02) 5/300	Light perception
5	No light perception	
9	Undetermined or unspecified	

Other disorders of eye and adnexa (H55-H57)

√4ᵗʰ **H55   Nystagmus and other irregular eye movements**

    √5ᵗʰ **H55.0   Nystagmus**
       DEF: Rapid, rhythmic, involuntary movements of the eyeball in vertical, horizontal, rotational, or mixed directions.

       H55.00   Unspecified nystagmus   ▽
       H55.01   Congenital nystagmus
       H55.02   Latent nystagmus
       H55.03   Visual deprivation nystagmus
       H55.04   Dissociated nystagmus
       H55.09   Other forms of nystagmus

    √5ᵗʰ **H55.8   Other irregular eye movements**
       H55.81   Saccadic eye movements
       H55.89   Other irregular eye movements

√4ᵗʰ **H57   Other disorders of eye and adnexa**

    √5ᵗʰ **H57.0   Anomalies of pupillary function**
       H57.00   Unspecified anomaly of pupillary function   ▽
       H57.01   Argyll Robertson pupil, atypical
          EXCLUDES 1   *syphilitic Argyll Robertson pupil (A52.19)*
       H57.02   Anisocoria
       H57.03   Miosis
       H57.04   Mydriasis
     √6ᵗʰ **H57.05   Tonic pupil**
       H57.051   Tonic pupil, right eye
       H57.052   Tonic pupil, left eye
       H57.053   Tonic pupil, bilateral
       H57.059   Tonic pupil, unspecified eye   ▽
       H57.09   Other anomalies of pupillary function

    √5ᵗʰ **H57.1   Ocular pain**
       H57.10   Ocular pain, unspecified eye   ▽
       H57.11   Ocular pain, right eye

       H57.12   Ocular pain, left eye
       H57.13   Ocular pain, bilateral

    √5ᵗʰ **H57.8   Other specified disorders of eye and adnexa**
     √6ᵗʰ **H57.81   Brow ptosis**
       H57.811   Brow ptosis, right
       H57.812   Brow ptosis, left
       H57.813   Brow ptosis, bilateral
       H57.819   Brow ptosis, unspecified   ▽
       H57.89   Other specified disorders of eye and adnexa

    H57.9   Unspecified disorder of eye and adnexa   ▽

Intraoperative and postprocedural complications and disorders of eye and adnexa, not elsewhere classified (H59)

√4ᵗʰ **H59   Intraoperative and postprocedural complications and disorders of eye and adnexa, not elsewhere classified**
    EXCLUDES 1   *mechanical complication of intraocular lens (T85.2)*
              mechanical complication of other ocular prosthetic devices, implants and grafts (T85.3)
              pseudophakia (Z96.1)
              secondary cataracts (H26.4-)

    √5ᵗʰ **H59.0   Disorders of the eye following cataract surgery**
     √6ᵗʰ **H59.01   Keratopathy (bullous aphakic) following cataract surgery**
       Vitreal corneal syndrome
       Vitreous (touch) syndrome
       H59.011   Keratopathy (bullous aphakic) following cataract surgery, right eye
       H59.012   Keratopathy (bullous aphakic) following cataract surgery, left eye
       H59.013   Keratopathy (bullous aphakic) following cataract surgery, bilateral
       H59.019   Keratopathy (bullous aphakic) following cataract surgery, unspecified eye   ▽
     √6ᵗʰ **H59.02   Cataract (lens) fragments in eye following cataract surgery**
       H59.021   Cataract (lens) fragments in eye following cataract surgery, right eye
       H59.022   Cataract (lens) fragments in eye following cataract surgery, left eye
       H59.023   Cataract (lens) fragments in eye following cataract surgery, bilateral
       H59.029   Cataract (lens) fragments in eye following cataract surgery, unspecified eye   ▽
     √6ᵗʰ **H59.03   Cystoid macular edema following cataract surgery**
       H59.031   Cystoid macular edema following cataract surgery, right eye
       H59.032   Cystoid macular edema following cataract surgery, left eye
       H59.033   Cystoid macular edema following cataract surgery, bilateral
       H59.039   Cystoid macular edema following cataract surgery, unspecified eye   ▽
     √6ᵗʰ **H59.09   Other disorders of the eye following cataract surgery**
       H59.091   Other disorders of the right eye following cataract surgery
       H59.092   Other disorders of the left eye following cataract surgery
       H59.093   Other disorders of the eye following cataract surgery, bilateral
       H59.099   Other disorders of unspecified eye following cataract surgery   ▽

    √5ᵗʰ **H59.1   Intraoperative hemorrhage and hematoma of eye and adnexa complicating a procedure**
       EXCLUDES 1   *intraoperative hemorrhage and hematoma of eye and adnexa due to accidental puncture or laceration during a procedure (H59.2-)*
     √6ᵗʰ **H59.11   Intraoperative hemorrhage and hematoma of eye and adnexa complicating an ophthalmic procedure**
       H59.111   Intraoperative hemorrhage and hematoma of right eye and adnexa complicating an ophthalmic procedure
       H59.112   Intraoperative hemorrhage and hematoma of left eye and adnexa complicating an ophthalmic procedure

H59.113 Intraoperative hemorrhage and hematoma of eye and adnexa complicating an ophthalmic procedure, bilateral

H59.119 Intraoperative hemorrhage and hematoma of unspecified eye and adnexa complicating an ophthalmic procedure ▽

√6th H59.12 Intraoperative hemorrhage and hematoma of eye and adnexa complicating other procedure

H59.121 Intraoperative hemorrhage and hematoma of right eye and adnexa complicating other procedure

H59.122 Intraoperative hemorrhage and hematoma of left eye and adnexa complicating other procedure

H59.123 Intraoperative hemorrhage and hematoma of eye and adnexa complicating other procedure, bilateral

H59.129 Intraoperative hemorrhage and hematoma of unspecified eye and adnexa complicating other procedure ▽

√5th H59.2 Accidental puncture and laceration of eye and adnexa during a procedure

√6th H59.21 Accidental puncture and laceration of eye and adnexa during an ophthalmic procedure

H59.211 Accidental puncture and laceration of right eye and adnexa during an ophthalmic procedure

H59.212 Accidental puncture and laceration of left eye and adnexa during an ophthalmic procedure

H59.213 Accidental puncture and laceration of eye and adnexa during an ophthalmic procedure, bilateral

H59.219 Accidental puncture and laceration of unspecified eye and adnexa during an ophthalmic procedure ▽

√6th H59.22 Accidental puncture and laceration of eye and adnexa during other procedure

H59.221 Accidental puncture and laceration of right eye and adnexa during other procedure

H59.222 Accidental puncture and laceration of left eye and adnexa during other procedure

H59.223 Accidental puncture and laceration of eye and adnexa during other procedure, bilateral

H59.229 Accidental puncture and laceration of unspecified eye and adnexa during other procedure ▽

√5th H59.3 Postprocedural hemorrhage, hematoma, and seroma of eye and adnexa following a procedure

AHA: 2016,4Q,9-10

√6th H59.31 Postprocedural hemorrhage of eye and adnexa following an ophthalmic procedure

H59.311 Postprocedural hemorrhage of right eye and adnexa following an ophthalmic procedure

H59.312 Postprocedural hemorrhage of left eye and adnexa following an ophthalmic procedure

H59.313 Postprocedural hemorrhage of eye and adnexa following an ophthalmic procedure, bilateral

H59.319 Postprocedural hemorrhage of unspecified eye and adnexa following an ophthalmic procedure ▽

√6th H59.32 Postprocedural hemorrhage of eye and adnexa following other procedure

H59.321 Postprocedural hemorrhage of right eye and adnexa following other procedure

H59.322 Postprocedural hemorrhage of left eye and adnexa following other procedure

H59.323 Postprocedural hemorrhage of eye and adnexa following other procedure, bilateral

H59.329 Postprocedural hemorrhage of unspecified eye and adnexa following other procedure ▽

√6th H59.33 Postprocedural hematoma of eye and adnexa following an ophthalmic procedure

H59.331 Postprocedural hematoma of right eye and adnexa following an ophthalmic procedure

H59.332 Postprocedural hematoma of left eye and adnexa following an ophthalmic procedure

H59.333 Postprocedural hematoma of eye and adnexa following an ophthalmic procedure, bilateral

H59.339 Postprocedural hematoma of unspecified eye and adnexa following an ophthalmic procedure ▽

√6th H59.34 Postprocedural hematoma of eye and adnexa following other procedure

H59.341 Postprocedural hematoma of right eye and adnexa following other procedure

H59.342 Postprocedural hematoma of left eye and adnexa following other procedure

H59.343 Postprocedural hematoma of eye and adnexa following other procedure, bilateral

H59.349 Postprocedural hematoma of unspecified eye and adnexa following other procedure ▽

√6th H59.35 Postprocedural seroma of eye and adnexa following an ophthalmic procedure

H59.351 Postprocedural seroma of right eye and adnexa following an ophthalmic procedure

H59.352 Postprocedural seroma of left eye and adnexa following an ophthalmic procedure

H59.353 Postprocedural seroma of eye and adnexa following an ophthalmic procedure, bilateral

H59.359 Postprocedural seroma of unspecified eye and adnexa following an ophthalmic procedure ▽

√6th H59.36 Postprocedural seroma of eye and adnexa following other procedure

H59.361 Postprocedural seroma of right eye and adnexa following other procedure

H59.362 Postprocedural seroma of left eye and adnexa following other procedure

H59.363 Postprocedural seroma of eye and adnexa following other procedure, bilateral

H59.369 Postprocedural seroma of unspecified eye and adnexa following other procedure ▽

√5th H59.4 Inflammation (infection) of postprocedural bleb

Postprocedural blebitis

EXCLUDES 1 filtering (vitreous) bleb after glaucoma surgery status (Z98.83)

H59.40 Inflammation (infection) of postprocedural bleb, unspecified ▽

H59.41 Inflammation (infection) of postprocedural bleb, stage 1

H59.42 Inflammation (infection) of postprocedural bleb, stage 2

H59.43 Inflammation (infection) of postprocedural bleb, stage 3

Bleb endophthalmitis

√5th H59.8 Other intraoperative and postprocedural complications and disorders of eye and adnexa, not elsewhere classified

√6th H59.81 Chorioretinal scars after surgery for detachment

H59.811 Chorioretinal scars after surgery for detachment, right eye

H59.812 Chorioretinal scars after surgery for detachment, left eye

H59.813 Chorioretinal scars after surgery for detachment, bilateral

H59.819 Chorioretinal scars after surgery for detachment, unspecified eye ▽

H59.88 Other intraoperative complications of eye and adnexa, not elsewhere classified

H59.89 Other postprocedural complications and disorders of eye and adnexa, not elsewhere classified

---

☑ Additional Character Req   √x7th Placeholder Alert   Manifestation   ▽ Unspecified   ▶◀ Revised Text   ● New Code   ▲ Revised Code Title

Chapter 8. Diseases of the Ear and Mastoid Process (H6Ø–H95)

Chapter Specific Coding Guidelines and Examples
Reserved for future guideline expansion.

Chapter 8. Diseases of the Ear and Mastoid Process (H60-H95)

NOTE   Use an external cause code following the code for the ear condition, if applicable, to identify the cause of the ear condition

EXCLUDES 2   certain conditions originating in the perinatal period (P04-P96)
certain infectious and parasitic diseases (A00-B99)
complications of pregnancy, childbirth and the puerperium (O00-O9A)
congenital malformations, deformations and chromosomal abnormalities (Q00-Q99)
endocrine, nutritional and metabolic diseases (E00-E88)
injury, poisoning and certain other consequences of external causes (S00-T88)
neoplasms (C00-D49)
symptoms, signs and abnormal clinical and laboratory findings, not elsewhere classified (R00-R94)

This chapter contains the following blocks:

H60-H62   Diseases of external ear
H65-H75   Diseases of middle ear and mastoid
H80-H83   Diseases of inner ear
H90-H94   Other disorders of ear
H95   Intraoperative and postprocedural complications and disorders of ear and mastoid process, not elsewhere classified

Diseases of external ear (H60-H62)

✓4ᵗʰ **H60 Otitis externa**

TIP: When the specific infectious agent is identified, a code from Chapter 1 is assigned instead of a code from this category.

✓5ᵗʰ **H60.0 Abscess of external ear**

Boil of external ear
Carbuncle of auricle or external auditory canal
Furuncle of external ear

H60.00   Abscess of external ear, unspecified ear ▽
H60.01   Abscess of **right** external ear
H60.02   Abscess of **left** external ear
H60.03   Abscess of external ear, **bilateral**

✓5ᵗʰ **H60.1 Cellulitis of external ear**

Cellulitis of auricle
Cellulitis of external auditory canal

H60.10   Cellulitis of external ear, unspecified ear ▽
H60.11   Cellulitis of **right** external ear
H60.12   Cellulitis of **left** external ear
H60.13   Cellulitis of external ear, **bilateral**

✓5ᵗʰ **H60.2 Malignant otitis externa**

H60.20   Malignant otitis externa, unspecified ear ▽
H60.21   Malignant otitis externa, **right** ear
H60.22   Malignant otitis externa, **left** ear
H60.23   Malignant otitis externa, **bilateral**

✓5ᵗʰ **H60.3 Other infective otitis externa**

✓6ᵗʰ **H60.31 Diffuse otitis externa**

H60.311   Diffuse otitis externa, **right** ear Q
H60.312   Diffuse otitis externa, **left** ear Q
H60.313   Diffuse otitis externa, **bilateral** Q
H60.319   Diffuse otitis externa, unspecified ear Q ▽

✓6ᵗʰ **H60.32 Hemorrhagic otitis externa**

H60.321   Hemorrhagic otitis externa, **right** ear Q
H60.322   Hemorrhagic otitis externa, **left** ear Q
H60.323   Hemorrhagic otitis externa, **bilateral** Q
H60.329   Hemorrhagic otitis externa, unspecified ear Q ▽

✓6ᵗʰ **H60.33 Swimmer's ear**

DEF: Commonly occurs when water gets trapped in the ear after swimming.

H60.331   Swimmer's ear, **right** ear Q
H60.332   Swimmer's ear, **left** ear Q
H60.333   Swimmer's ear, **bilateral** Q
H60.339   Swimmer's ear, unspecified ear Q ▽

✓6ᵗʰ **H60.39 Other infective otitis externa**

H60.391   Other infective otitis externa, **right** ear Q
H60.392   Other infective otitis externa, **left** ear Q
H60.393   Other infective otitis externa, **bilateral** Q

H60.399   Other infective otitis externa, unspecified ear Q ▽

✓5ᵗʰ **H60.4 Cholesteatoma of external ear**

Keratosis obturans of external ear (canal)

EXCLUDES 2   cholesteatoma of middle ear (H71.-)
recurrent cholesteatoma of postmastoidectomy cavity (H95.0-)

DEF: Cholesteatoma: Noncancerous cyst-like mass of cell debris, including cholesterol and epithelial cells resulting from trauma, repeated or improperly healed infections, and congenital enclosure of epidermal cells.

H60.40   Cholesteatoma of external ear, unspecified ear ▽
H60.41   Cholesteatoma of **right** external ear
H60.42   Cholesteatoma of **left** external ear
H60.43   Cholesteatoma of external ear, **bilateral**

✓5ᵗʰ **H60.5 Acute noninfective otitis externa**

✓6ᵗʰ **H60.50 Unspecified acute noninfective otitis externa**

Acute otitis externa NOS

H60.501   Unspecified acute noninfective otitis externa, **right** ear Q ▽
H60.502   Unspecified acute noninfective otitis externa, **left** ear Q ▽
H60.503   Unspecified acute noninfective otitis externa, **bilateral** Q ▽
H60.509   Unspecified acute noninfective otitis externa, unspecified ear Q ▽

✓6ᵗʰ **H60.51 Acute actinic otitis externa**

H60.511   Acute actinic otitis externa, **right** ear Q
H60.512   Acute actinic otitis externa, **left** ear Q
H60.513   Acute actinic otitis externa, **bilateral** Q
H60.519   Acute actinic otitis externa, unspecified ear Q ▽

✓6ᵗʰ **H60.52 Acute chemical otitis externa**

H60.521   Acute chemical otitis externa, **right** ear Q
H60.522   Acute chemical otitis externa, **left** ear Q
H60.523   Acute chemical otitis externa, **bilateral** Q
H60.529   Acute chemical otitis externa, unspecified ear Q ▽

✓6ᵗʰ **H60.53 Acute contact otitis externa**

H60.531   Acute contact otitis externa, **right** ear Q
H60.532   Acute contact otitis externa, **left** ear Q
H60.533   Acute contact otitis externa, **bilateral** Q
H60.539   Acute contact otitis externa, unspecified ear Q ▽

✓6ᵗʰ **H60.54 Acute eczematoid otitis externa**

H60.541   Acute eczematoid otitis externa, **right** ear Q
H60.542   Acute eczematoid otitis externa, **left** ear Q
H60.543   Acute eczematoid otitis externa, **bilateral** Q
H60.549   Acute eczematoid otitis externa, unspecified ear Q ▽

✓6ᵗʰ **H60.55 Acute reactive otitis externa**

H60.551   Acute reactive otitis externa, **right** ear Q
H60.552   Acute reactive otitis externa, **left** ear Q
H60.553   Acute reactive otitis externa, **bilateral** Q
H60.559   Acute reactive otitis externa, unspecified ear Q ▽

✓6ᵗʰ **H60.59 Other noninfective acute otitis externa**

H60.591   Other noninfective acute otitis externa, **right** ear Q
H60.592   Other noninfective acute otitis externa, **left** ear Q
H60.593   Other noninfective acute otitis externa, **bilateral** Q

H60.599   Other noninfective acute otitis externa, unspecified ear   🔟 ▽

√5ᵗʰ **H60.6**   Unspecified chronic otitis externa

    H60.60   Unspecified chronic otitis externa, unspecified ear   ▽

    H60.61   Unspecified chronic otitis externa, right ear   ▽

    H60.62   Unspecified chronic otitis externa, left ear   ▽

    H60.63   Unspecified chronic otitis externa, bilateral   ▽

√5ᵗʰ **H60.8**   Other otitis externa

   √6ᵗʰ **H60.8X**   Other otitis externa

     H60.8X1   Other otitis externa, right ear

     H60.8X2   Other otitis externa, left ear

     H60.8X3   Other otitis externa, bilateral   🔟

     H60.8X9   Other otitis externa, unspecified ear   ▽

√5ᵗʰ **H60.9**   Unspecified otitis externa

    H60.90   Unspecified otitis externa, unspecified ear   ▽

    H60.91   Unspecified otitis externa, right ear   ▽

    H60.92   Unspecified otitis externa, left ear   ▽

    H60.93   Unspecified otitis externa, bilateral   ▽

√4ᵗʰ **H61**   **Other disorders of external ear**

  √5ᵗʰ **H61.0**   Chondritis and perichondritis of external ear

    Chondrodermatitis nodularis chronica helicis

    Perichondritis of auricle

    Perichondritis of pinna

   √6ᵗʰ **H61.00**   Unspecified perichondritis of external ear

     H61.001   Unspecified perichondritis of right external ear   ▽

     H61.002   Unspecified perichondritis of left external ear   ▽

     H61.003   Unspecified perichondritis of external ear, bilateral   ▽

     H61.009   Unspecified perichondritis of external ear, unspecified ear   ▽

   √6ᵗʰ **H61.01**   Acute perichondritis of external ear

     H61.011   Acute perichondritis of right external ear

     H61.012   Acute perichondritis of left external ear

     H61.013   Acute perichondritis of external ear, bilateral

     H61.019   Acute perichondritis of external ear, unspecified ear   ▽

   √6ᵗʰ **H61.02**   Chronic perichondritis of external ear

     H61.021   Chronic perichondritis of right external ear

     H61.022   Chronic perichondritis of left external ear

     H61.023   Chronic perichondritis of external ear, bilateral

     H61.029   Chronic perichondritis of external ear, unspecified ear   ▽

   √6ᵗʰ **H61.03**   Chondritis of external ear

    Chondritis of auricle

    Chondritis of pinna

    AHA: 2015,1Q,18

    DEF: Infection that has progressed into the cartilage and presents as indurated and edematous skin over the pinna. Vascular compromise occurs with tissue necrosis and deformity.

     H61.031   Chondritis of right external ear

     H61.032   Chondritis of left external ear

     H61.033   Chondritis of external ear, bilateral

     H61.039   Chondritis of external ear, unspecified ear   ▽

  √5ᵗʰ **H61.1**   Noninfective disorders of pinna

    EXCLUDES 2   cauliflower ear (M95.1-)

              gouty tophi of ear (M1A.-)

   √6ᵗʰ **H61.10**   Unspecified noninfective disorders of pinna

    Disorder of pinna NOS

     H61.101   Unspecified noninfective disorders of pinna, right ear   ▽

     H61.102   Unspecified noninfective disorders of pinna, left ear   ▽

     H61.103   Unspecified noninfective disorders of pinna, bilateral   ▽

     H61.109   Unspecified noninfective disorders of pinna, unspecified ear   ▽

   √6ᵗʰ **H61.11**   Acquired deformity of pinna

    Acquired deformity of auricle

    EXCLUDES 2   cauliflower ear (M95.1-)

     H61.111   Acquired deformity of pinna, right ear

     H61.112   Acquired deformity of pinna, left ear

     H61.113   Acquired deformity of pinna, bilateral

     H61.119   Acquired deformity of pinna, unspecified ear   ▽

   √6ᵗʰ **H61.12**   Hematoma of pinna

    Hematoma of auricle

     H61.121   Hematoma of pinna, right ear

     H61.122   Hematoma of pinna, left ear

     H61.123   Hematoma of pinna, bilateral

     H61.129   Hematoma of pinna, unspecified ear   ▽

   √6ᵗʰ **H61.19**   Other noninfective disorders of pinna

     H61.191   Noninfective disorders of pinna, right ear

     H61.192   Noninfective disorders of pinna, left ear

     H61.193   Noninfective disorders of pinna, bilateral

     H61.199   Noninfective disorders of pinna, unspecified ear   ▽

  √5ᵗʰ **H61.2**   Impacted cerumen

    Wax in ear

    H61.20   Impacted cerumen, unspecified ear   ▽

    H61.21   Impacted cerumen, right ear

    H61.22   Impacted cerumen, left ear

    H61.23   Impacted cerumen, bilateral

  √5ᵗʰ **H61.3**   Acquired stenosis of external ear canal

    Collapse of external ear canal

    EXCLUDES 1   postprocedural stenosis of external ear canal (H95.81-)

   √6ᵗʰ **H61.30**   Acquired stenosis of external ear canal, unspecified

     H61.301   Acquired stenosis of right external ear canal, unspecified   ▽

     H61.302   Acquired stenosis of left external ear canal, unspecified   ▽

     H61.303   Acquired stenosis of external ear canal, unspecified, bilateral   ▽

     H61.309   Acquired stenosis of external ear canal, unspecified, unspecified ear   ▽

   √6ᵗʰ **H61.31**   Acquired stenosis of external ear canal secondary to trauma

     H61.311   Acquired stenosis of right external ear canal secondary to trauma

     H61.312   Acquired stenosis of left external ear canal secondary to trauma

     H61.313   Acquired stenosis of external ear canal secondary to trauma, bilateral

     H61.319   Acquired stenosis of external ear canal secondary to trauma, unspecified ear   ▽

   √6ᵗʰ **H61.32**   Acquired stenosis of external ear canal secondary to inflammation and infection

    DEF: Narrowing of the external ear canal due to chronic inflammation or infection.

     H61.321   Acquired stenosis of right external ear canal secondary to inflammation and infection

     H61.322   Acquired stenosis of left external ear canal secondary to inflammation and infection

     H61.323   Acquired stenosis of external ear canal secondary to inflammation and infection, bilateral

     H61.329   Acquired stenosis of external ear canal secondary to inflammation and infection, unspecified ear   ▽

   √6ᵗʰ **H61.39**   Other acquired stenosis of external ear canal

     H61.391   Other acquired stenosis of right external ear canal

     H61.392   Other acquired stenosis of left external ear canal

     H61.393   Other acquired stenosis of external ear canal, bilateral

     H61.399   Other acquired stenosis of external ear canal, unspecified ear   ▽

☑ Additional Character Req   ▽×7ᵗʰ Placeholder Alert   Manifestation   ▽ Unspecified   ▶◀ Revised Text   ● New Code   ▲ Revised Code Title

ICD-10-CM 2019   621

√5ᵗʰ **H61.8** **Other specified disorders of external ear**

√6ᵗʰ **H61.81** **Exostosis of external canal**

H61.811 **Exostosis of right external canal**

H61.812 **Exostosis of left external canal**

H61.813 **Exostosis of external canal, bilateral**

H61.819 **Exostosis of external canal, unspecified ear** ▽

√6ᵗʰ **H61.89** **Other specified disorders of external ear**

H61.891 **Other specified disorders of right external ear**

H61.892 **Other specified disorders of left external ear**

H61.893 **Other specified disorders of external ear, bilateral**

H61.899 **Other specified disorders of external ear, unspecified ear** ▽

√5ᵗʰ **H61.9** **Disorder of external ear, unspecified**

H61.90 **Disorder of external ear, unspecified, unspecified ear** ▽

H61.91 **Disorder of right external ear, unspecified** ▽

H61.92 **Disorder of left external ear, unspecified** ▽

H61.93 **Disorder of external ear, unspecified, bilateral** ▽

√4ᵗʰ **H62** **Disorders of external ear in diseases classified elsewhere**

√5ᵗʰ **H62.4** **Otitis externa in other diseases classified elsewhere**

Code first underlying disease, such as:
erysipelas (A46)
impetigo (L01.0)

EXCLUDES 1   otitis externa (in):
candidiasis (B37.84)
herpes viral [herpes simplex] (B00.1)
herpes zoster (B02.8)

H62.40 *Otitis externa in other diseases classified elsewhere, unspecified ear* 0 ▽

H62.41 *Otitis externa in other diseases classified elsewhere, right ear* 0

H62.42 *Otitis externa in other diseases classified elsewhere, left ear* 0

H62.43 *Otitis externa in other diseases classified elsewhere, bilateral* 0

√5ᵗʰ **H62.8** **Other disorders of external ear in diseases classified elsewhere**

Code first underlying disease, such as:
gout (M1A.-, M10.-)

√6ᵗʰ **H62.8X** **Other disorders of external ear in diseases classified elsewhere**

H62.8X1 *Other disorders of right external ear in diseases classified elsewhere*

H62.8X2 *Other disorders of left external ear in diseases classified elsewhere*

H62.8X3 *Other disorders of external ear in diseases classified elsewhere, bilateral*

H62.8X9 *Other disorders of external ear in diseases classified elsewhere, unspecified ear* ▽

Diseases of middle ear and mastoid (H65-H75)

√4ᵗʰ **H65** **Nonsuppurative otitis media**

INCLUDES   nonsuppurative otitis media with myringitis

Use additional code for any associated perforated tympanic membrane (H72.-)

Use additional code to identify:
exposure to environmental tobacco smoke (Z77.22)
exposure to tobacco smoke in the perinatal period (P96.81)
history of tobacco dependence (Z87.891)
occupational exposure to environmental tobacco smoke (Z57.31)
tobacco dependence (F17.-)
tobacco use (Z72.0)

√5ᵗʰ **H65.0** **Acute serous otitis media**

Acute and subacute secretory otitis

H65.00 **Acute serous otitis media, unspecified ear** ▽

H65.01 **Acute serous otitis media, right ear**

H65.02 **Acute serous otitis media, left ear**

H65.03 **Acute serous otitis media, bilateral**

H65.04 **Acute serous otitis media, recurrent, right ear**

H65.05 **Acute serous otitis media, recurrent, left ear**

H65.06 **Acute serous otitis media, recurrent, bilateral**

H65.07 **Acute serous otitis media, recurrent, unspecified ear** ▽

√5ᵗʰ **H65.1** **Other acute nonsuppurative otitis media**

EXCLUDES 1   otitic barotrauma (T70.0)
otitis media (acute) NOS (H66.9)

√6ᵗʰ **H65.11** **Acute and subacute allergic otitis media (mucoid) (sanguinous) (serous)**

H65.111 **Acute and subacute allergic otitis media (mucoid) (sanguinous) (serous), right ear**

H65.112 **Acute and subacute allergic otitis media (mucoid) (sanguinous) (serous), left ear**

H65.113 **Acute and subacute allergic otitis media (mucoid) (sanguinous) (serous), bilateral**

H65.114 **Acute and subacute allergic otitis media (mucoid) (sanguinous) (serous), recurrent, right ear**

H65.115 **Acute and subacute allergic otitis media (mucoid) (sanguinous) (serous), recurrent, left ear**

H65.116 **Acute and subacute allergic otitis media (mucoid) (sanguinous) (serous), recurrent, bilateral**

H65.117 **Acute and subacute allergic otitis media (mucoid) (sanguinous) (serous), recurrent, unspecified ear** ▽

H65.119 **Acute and subacute allergic otitis media (mucoid) (sanguinous) (serous), unspecified ear** ▽

√6ᵗʰ **H65.19** **Other acute nonsuppurative otitis media**

Acute and subacute mucoid otitis media
Acute and subacute nonsuppurative otitis media NOS
Acute and subacute sanguinous otitis media
Acute and subacute seromucinous otitis media

H65.191 **Other acute nonsuppurative otitis media, right ear**

H65.192 **Other acute nonsuppurative otitis media, left ear**

H65.193 **Other acute nonsuppurative otitis media, bilateral**

H65.194 **Other acute nonsuppurative otitis media, recurrent, right ear**

H65.195 **Other acute nonsuppurative otitis media, recurrent, left ear**

H65.196 **Other acute nonsuppurative otitis media, recurrent, bilateral**

H65.197 **Other acute nonsuppurative otitis media recurrent, unspecified ear** ▽

H65.199 **Other acute nonsuppurative otitis media, unspecified ear** ▽

√5ᵗʰ **H65.2** **Chronic serous otitis media**

Chronic tubotympanal catarrh

H65.20 **Chronic serous otitis media, unspecified ear** ▽

H65.21 **Chronic serous otitis media, right ear**

H65.22 **Chronic serous otitis media, left ear**

H65.23 **Chronic serous otitis media, bilateral**

√5ᵗʰ **H65.3** **Chronic mucoid otitis media**

Chronic mucinous otitis media
Chronic secretory otitis media
Chronic transudative otitis media
Glue ear

EXCLUDES 1   adhesive middle ear disease (H74.1)

H65.30 **Chronic mucoid otitis media, unspecified ear** ▽

H65.31 **Chronic mucoid otitis media, right ear**

H65.32 **Chronic mucoid otitis media, left ear**

H65.33 **Chronic mucoid otitis media, bilateral**

√5ᵗʰ **H65.4** **Other chronic nonsuppurative otitis media**

√6ᵗʰ **H65.41** **Chronic allergic otitis media**

H65.411 **Chronic allergic otitis media, right ear**

H65.412 **Chronic allergic otitis media, left ear**

H65.413 **Chronic allergic otitis media, bilateral**

H65.419 **Chronic allergic otitis media, unspecified ear** ▽

✓6ᵗʰ **H65.49 Other chronic nonsuppurative otitis media**
>Chronic exudative otitis media
>Chronic nonsuppurative otitis media NOS
>Chronic otitis media with effusion (nonpurulent)
>Chronic seromucinous otitis media

> **H65.491 Other chronic nonsuppurative otitis media, right ear**

> **H65.492 Other chronic nonsuppurative otitis media, left ear**

> **H65.493 Other chronic nonsuppurative otitis media, bilateral**

> **H65.499 Other chronic nonsuppurative otitis media, unspecified ear** ▽

✓5ᵗʰ **H65.9 Unspecified nonsuppurative otitis media**
>Allergic otitis media NOS
>Catarrhal otitis media NOS
>Exudative otitis media NOS
>Mucoid otitis media NOS
>Otitis media with effusion (nonpurulent) NOS
>Secretory otitis media NOS
>Seromucinous otitis media NOS
>Serous otitis media NOS
>Transudative otitis media NOS

> **H65.90 Unspecified nonsuppurative otitis media, unspecified ear** ▽

> **H65.91 Unspecified nonsuppurative otitis media, right ear** ▽

> **H65.92 Unspecified nonsuppurative otitis media, left ear** ▽

> **H65.93 Unspecified nonsuppurative otitis media, bilateral** ▽

✓4ᵗʰ **H66 Suppurative and unspecified otitis media**

> **INCLUDES** suppurative and unspecified otitis media with myringitis
> Use additional code to identify:
> exposure to environmental tobacco smoke (Z77.22)
> exposure to tobacco smoke in the perinatal period (P96.81)
> history of tobacco dependence (Z87.891)
> occupational exposure to environmental tobacco smoke (Z57.31)
> tobacco dependence (F17.-)
> tobacco use (Z72.0)
> **AHA:** 2016,1Q,34

✓5ᵗʰ **H66.0 Acute suppurative otitis media**

> ✓6ᵗʰ **H66.00 Acute suppurative otitis media without spontaneous rupture of ear drum**

>> **H66.001 Acute suppurative otitis media without spontaneous rupture of ear drum, right ear**

>> **H66.002 Acute suppurative otitis media without spontaneous rupture of ear drum, left ear**

>> **H66.003 Acute suppurative otitis media without spontaneous rupture of ear drum, bilateral**

>> **H66.004 Acute suppurative otitis media without spontaneous rupture of ear drum, recurrent, right ear**

>> **H66.005 Acute suppurative otitis media without spontaneous rupture of ear drum, recurrent, left ear**

>> **H66.006 Acute suppurative otitis media without spontaneous rupture of ear drum, recurrent, bilateral**

>> **H66.007 Acute suppurative otitis media without spontaneous rupture of ear drum, recurrent, unspecified ear** ▽

>> **H66.009 Acute suppurative otitis media without spontaneous rupture of ear drum, unspecified ear** ▽

> ✓6ᵗʰ **H66.01 Acute suppurative otitis media with spontaneous rupture of ear drum**
>> **DEF:** Sudden, severe inflammation of the middle ear, causing pressure that perforates the ear drum tissue.

>> **H66.011 Acute suppurative otitis media with spontaneous rupture of ear drum, right ear**

>> **H66.012 Acute suppurative otitis media with spontaneous rupture of ear drum, left ear**

>> **H66.013 Acute suppurative otitis media with spontaneous rupture of ear drum, bilateral**

>> **H66.014 Acute suppurative otitis media with spontaneous rupture of ear drum, recurrent, right ear**

>> **H66.015 Acute suppurative otitis media with spontaneous rupture of ear drum, recurrent, left ear**

>> **H66.016 Acute suppurative otitis media with spontaneous rupture of ear drum, recurrent, bilateral**

>> **H66.017 Acute suppurative otitis media with spontaneous rupture of ear drum, recurrent, unspecified ear** ▽

>> **H66.019 Acute suppurative otitis media with spontaneous rupture of ear drum, unspecified ear** ▽

✓5ᵗʰ **H66.1 Chronic tubotympanic suppurative otitis media**
>Benign chronic suppurative otitis media
>Chronic tubotympanic disease
>Use additional code for any associated perforated tympanic membrane (H72.-)

> **H66.10 Chronic tubotympanic suppurative otitis media, unspecified** ▽

> **H66.11 Chronic tubotympanic suppurative otitis media, right ear**

> **H66.12 Chronic tubotympanic suppurative otitis media, left ear**

> **H66.13 Chronic tubotympanic suppurative otitis media, bilateral**

✓5ᵗʰ **H66.2 Chronic atticoantral suppurative otitis media**
>Chronic atticoantral disease
>Use additional code for any associated perforated tympanic membrane (H72.-)

> **H66.20 Chronic atticoantral suppurative otitis media, unspecified ear** ▽

> **H66.21 Chronic atticoantral suppurative otitis media, right ear**

> **H66.22 Chronic atticoantral suppurative otitis media, left ear**

> **H66.23 Chronic atticoantral suppurative otitis media, bilateral**

✓5ᵗʰ **H66.3 Other chronic suppurative otitis media**
>Chronic suppurative otitis media NOS
>Use additional code for any associated perforated tympanic membrane (H72.-)
> **EXCLUDES 1** tuberculous otitis media (A18.6)

> ✓6ᵗʰ **H66.3X Other chronic suppurative otitis media**

>> **H66.3X1 Other chronic suppurative otitis media, right ear**

>> **H66.3X2 Other chronic suppurative otitis media, left ear**

>> **H66.3X3 Other chronic suppurative otitis media, bilateral**

>> **H66.3X9 Other chronic suppurative otitis media, unspecified ear** ▽

✓5ᵗʰ **H66.4 Suppurative otitis media, unspecified**
>Purulent otitis media NOS
>Use additional code for any associated perforated tympanic membrane (H72.-)

> **H66.40 Suppurative otitis media, unspecified, unspecified ear** ▽

> **H66.41 Suppurative otitis media, unspecified, right ear**

> **H66.42 Suppurative otitis media, unspecified, left ear**

> **H66.43 Suppurative otitis media, unspecified, bilateral**

✓5ᵗʰ **H66.9 Otitis media, unspecified**
>Otitis media NOS
>Acute otitis media NOS
>Chronic otitis media NOS
>Use additional code for any associated perforated tympanic membrane (H72.-)

> **H66.90 Otitis media, unspecified, unspecified ear** ▽

> **H66.91 Otitis media, unspecified, right ear** ▽

> **H66.92 Otitis media, unspecified, left ear** ▽

> **H66.93 Otitis media, unspecified, bilateral** ▽

✓4ᵗʰ **H67** **Otitis media in diseases classified elsewhere**

Code first underlying disease, such as:
▶plasminogen deficiency (E88.02)◀
viral disease NEC (B00-B34)
Use additional code for any associated perforated tympanic membrane (H72.-)

EXCLUDES 1   otitis media in:
influenza (J09.X9, J10.83, J11.83)
measles (B05.3)
scarlet fever (A38.0)
tuberculosis (A18.6)

H67.1 *Otitis media in diseases classified elsewhere, right ear*
H67.2 *Otitis media in diseases classified elsewhere, left ear*
H67.3 *Otitis media in diseases classified elsewhere, bilateral*
H67.9 *Otitis media in diseases classified elsewhere, unspecified ear* ▽

✓4ᵗʰ **H68** **Eustachian salpingitis and obstruction**

✓5ᵗʰ **H68.0** **Eustachian salpingitis**

✓6ᵗʰ **H68.00** **Unspecified Eustachian salpingitis**

H68.001 **Unspecified Eustachian salpingitis, right ear** ▽
H68.002 **Unspecified Eustachian salpingitis, left ear** ▽
H68.003 **Unspecified Eustachian salpingitis, bilateral** ▽
H68.009 **Unspecified Eustachian salpingitis, unspecified ear** ▽

✓6ᵗʰ **H68.01** **Acute Eustachian salpingitis**

H68.011 **Acute Eustachian salpingitis, right ear**
H68.012 **Acute Eustachian salpingitis, left ear**
H68.013 **Acute Eustachian salpingitis, bilateral**
H68.019 **Acute Eustachian salpingitis, unspecified ear** ▽

✓6ᵗʰ **H68.02** **Chronic Eustachian salpingitis**

H68.021 **Chronic Eustachian salpingitis, right ear**
H68.022 **Chronic Eustachian salpingitis, left ear**
H68.023 **Chronic Eustachian salpingitis, bilateral**
H68.029 **Chronic Eustachian salpingitis, unspecified ear** ▽

✓5ᵗʰ **H68.1** **Obstruction of Eustachian tube**

Stenosis of Eustachian tube
Stricture of Eustachian tube

✓6ᵗʰ **H68.10** **Unspecified obstruction of Eustachian tube**

H68.101 **Unspecified obstruction of Eustachian tube, right ear** ▽
H68.102 **Unspecified obstruction of Eustachian tube, left ear** ▽
H68.103 **Unspecified obstruction of Eustachian tube, bilateral** ▽
H68.109 **Unspecified obstruction of Eustachian tube, unspecified ear** ▽

✓6ᵗʰ **H68.11** **Osseous obstruction of Eustachian tube**

H68.111 **Osseous obstruction of Eustachian tube, right ear**
H68.112 **Osseous obstruction of Eustachian tube, left ear**
H68.113 **Osseous obstruction of Eustachian tube, bilateral**
H68.119 **Osseous obstruction of Eustachian tube, unspecified ear** ▽

✓6ᵗʰ **H68.12** **Intrinsic cartilagenous obstruction of Eustachian tube**

H68.121 **Intrinsic cartilagenous obstruction of Eustachian tube, right ear**
H68.122 **Intrinsic cartilagenous obstruction of Eustachian tube, left ear**
H68.123 **Intrinsic cartilagenous obstruction of Eustachian tube, bilateral**
H68.129 **Intrinsic cartilagenous obstruction of Eustachian tube, unspecified ear** ▽

✓6ᵗʰ **H68.13** **Extrinsic cartilagenous obstruction of Eustachian tube**

Compression of Eustachian tube

H68.131 **Extrinsic cartilagenous obstruction of Eustachian tube, right ear**
H68.132 **Extrinsic cartilagenous obstruction of Eustachian tube, left ear**

H68.133 **Extrinsic cartilagenous obstruction of Eustachian tube, bilateral**
H68.139 **Extrinsic cartilagenous obstruction of Eustachian tube, unspecified ear** ▽

✓4ᵗʰ **H69** **Other and unspecified disorders of Eustachian tube**

✓5ᵗʰ **H69.0** **Patulous Eustachian tube**

H69.00 **Patulous Eustachian tube, unspecified ear** ▽
H69.01 **Patulous Eustachian tube, right ear**
H69.02 **Patulous Eustachian tube, left ear**
H69.03 **Patulous Eustachian tube, bilateral**

✓5ᵗʰ **H69.8** **Other specified disorders of Eustachian tube**

H69.80 **Other specified disorders of Eustachian tube, unspecified ear** ▽
H69.81 **Other specified disorders of Eustachian tube, right ear**
H69.82 **Other specified disorders of Eustachian tube, left ear**
H69.83 **Other specified disorders of Eustachian tube, bilateral**

✓5ᵗʰ **H69.9** **Unspecified Eustachian tube disorder**

H69.90 **Unspecified Eustachian tube disorder, unspecified ear** ▽
H69.91 **Unspecified Eustachian tube disorder, right ear** ▽
H69.92 **Unspecified Eustachian tube disorder, left ear** ▽
H69.93 **Unspecified Eustachian tube disorder, bilateral** ▽

✓4ᵗʰ **H70** **Mastoiditis and related conditions**

✓5ᵗʰ **H70.0** **Acute mastoiditis**

Abscess of mastoid
Empyema of mastoid

✓6ᵗʰ **H70.00** **Acute mastoiditis without complications**

H70.001 **Acute mastoiditis without complications, right ear**
H70.002 **Acute mastoiditis without complications, left ear**
H70.003 **Acute mastoiditis without complications, bilateral**
H70.009 **Acute mastoiditis without complications, unspecified ear** ▽

✓6ᵗʰ **H70.01** **Subperiosteal abscess of mastoid**

H70.011 **Subperiosteal abscess of mastoid, right ear**
H70.012 **Subperiosteal abscess of mastoid, left ear**
H70.013 **Subperiosteal abscess of mastoid, bilateral**
H70.019 **Subperiosteal abscess of mastoid, unspecified ear** ▽

✓6ᵗʰ **H70.09** **Acute mastoiditis with other complications**

H70.091 **Acute mastoiditis with other complications, right ear**
H70.092 **Acute mastoiditis with other complications, left ear**
H70.093 **Acute mastoiditis with other complications, bilateral**
H70.099 **Acute mastoiditis with other complications, unspecified ear** ▽

✓5ᵗʰ **H70.1** **Chronic mastoiditis**

Caries of mastoid
Fistula of mastoid

EXCLUDES 1   tuberculous mastoiditis (A18.03)

H70.10 **Chronic mastoiditis, unspecified ear** ▽
H70.11 **Chronic mastoiditis, right ear**
H70.12 **Chronic mastoiditis, left ear**
H70.13 **Chronic mastoiditis, bilateral**

✓5ᵗʰ **H70.2** **Petrositis**

Inflammation of petrous bone

✓6ᵗʰ **H70.20** **Unspecified petrositis**

H70.201 **Unspecified petrositis, right ear** ▽
H70.202 **Unspecified petrositis, left ear** ▽
H70.203 **Unspecified petrositis, bilateral** ▽
H70.209 **Unspecified petrositis, unspecified ear** ▽

√6ᵗʰ **H70.21** Acute **petrositis**

DEF: Sudden, severe inflammation of the petrous temporal bone behind the ear, associated with a middle ear infection.

H70.211 Acute petrositis, right ear
H70.212 Acute petrositis, left ear
H70.213 Acute petrositis, bilateral
H70.219 Acute petrositis, unspecified ear ▽

√6ᵗʰ **H70.22** Chronic **petrositis**

H70.221 Chronic petrositis, right ear
H70.222 Chronic petrositis, left ear
H70.223 Chronic petrositis, bilateral
H70.229 Chronic petrositis, unspecified ear ▽

√5ᵗʰ **H70.8** Other mastoiditis and related conditions

EXCLUDES 1   preauricular sinus and cyst (Q18.1)
sinus, fistula, and cyst of branchial cleft (Q18.0)

√6ᵗʰ **H70.81** Postauricular fistula

H70.811 Postauricular fistula, right ear
H70.812 Postauricular fistula, left ear
H70.813 Postauricular fistula, bilateral
H70.819 Postauricular fistula, unspecified ear ▽

√6ᵗʰ **H70.89** Other mastoiditis and related conditions

H70.891 Other mastoiditis and related conditions, right ear
H70.892 Other mastoiditis and related conditions, left ear
H70.893 Other mastoiditis and related conditions, bilateral
H70.899 Other mastoiditis and related conditions, unspecified ear ▽

√5ᵗʰ **H70.9** Unspecified mastoiditis

H70.90 Unspecified mastoiditis, unspecified ear ▽
H70.91 Unspecified mastoiditis, right ear ▽
H70.92 Unspecified mastoiditis, left ear ▽
H70.93 Unspecified mastoiditis, bilateral ▽

√4ᵗʰ **H71** Cholesteatoma of middle ear

EXCLUDES 2   cholesteatoma of external ear (H60.4-)
recurrent cholesteatoma of postmastoidectomy cavity (H95.0-)

DEF: Cholesteatoma: Noncancerous cyst-like mass of cell debris, including cholesterol and epithelial cells resulting from trauma, repeated or improperly healed infections, and congenital enclosure of epidermal cells.

Cholesteatoma of Middle Ear

Middle ear chamber

Ear drum

Cholesteatoma sac

√5ᵗʰ **H71.0** Cholesteatoma of attic

H71.00 Cholesteatoma of attic, unspecified ear ▽
H71.01 Cholesteatoma of attic, right ear
H71.02 Cholesteatoma of attic, left ear
H71.03 Cholesteatoma of attic, bilateral

√5ᵗʰ **H71.1** Cholesteatoma of tympanum

H71.10 Cholesteatoma of tympanum, unspecified ear ▽
H71.11 Cholesteatoma of tympanum, right ear
H71.12 Cholesteatoma of tympanum, left ear
H71.13 Cholesteatoma of tympanum, bilateral

√5ᵗʰ **H71.2** Cholesteatoma of mastoid

H71.20 Cholesteatoma of mastoid, unspecified ear ▽
H71.21 Cholesteatoma of mastoid, right ear
H71.22 Cholesteatoma of mastoid, left ear
H71.23 Cholesteatoma of mastoid, bilateral

√5ᵗʰ **H71.3** Diffuse cholesteatosis

H71.30 Diffuse cholesteatosis, unspecified ear ▽
H71.31 Diffuse cholesteatosis, right ear
H71.32 Diffuse cholesteatosis, left ear
H71.33 Diffuse cholesteatosis, bilateral

√5ᵗʰ **H71.9** Unspecified cholesteatoma

H71.90 Unspecified cholesteatoma, unspecified ear ▽
H71.91 Unspecified cholesteatoma, right ear ▽
H71.92 Unspecified cholesteatoma, left ear ▽
H71.93 Unspecified cholesteatoma, bilateral ▽

√4ᵗʰ **H72** Perforation of tympanic membrane

INCLUDES   persistent post-traumatic perforation of ear drum
postinflammatory perforation of ear drum

Code first any associated otitis media (H65.-, H66.1-, H66.2-, H66.3-, H66.4-, H66.9-, H67.-)

EXCLUDES 1   acute suppurative otitis media with rupture of the tympanic membrane (H66.01-)
traumatic rupture of ear drum (S09.2-)

√5ᵗʰ **H72.0** Central perforation of tympanic membrane

H72.00 Central perforation of tympanic membrane, unspecified ear ▽
H72.01 Central perforation of tympanic membrane, right ear
H72.02 Central perforation of tympanic membrane, left ear
H72.03 Central perforation of tympanic membrane, bilateral

√5ᵗʰ **H72.1** Attic perforation of tympanic membrane

Perforation of pars flaccida

H72.10 Attic perforation of tympanic membrane, unspecified ear ▽
H72.11 Attic perforation of tympanic membrane, right ear
H72.12 Attic perforation of tympanic membrane, left ear
H72.13 Attic perforation of tympanic membrane, bilateral

√5ᵗʰ **H72.2** Other marginal perforations of tympanic membrane

√6ᵗʰ **H72.2X** Other marginal perforations of tympanic membrane

H72.2X1 Other marginal perforations of tympanic membrane, right ear
H72.2X2 Other marginal perforations of tympanic membrane, left ear
H72.2X3 Other marginal perforations of tympanic membrane, bilateral
H72.2X9 Other marginal perforations of tympanic membrane, unspecified ear ▽

√5ᵗʰ **H72.8** Other perforations of tympanic membrane

√6ᵗʰ **H72.81** Multiple perforations of tympanic membrane

H72.811 Multiple perforations of tympanic membrane, right ear
H72.812 Multiple perforations of tympanic membrane, left ear
H72.813 Multiple perforations of tympanic membrane, bilateral
H72.819 Multiple perforations of tympanic membrane, unspecified ear ▽

√6ᵗʰ **H72.82** Total perforations of tympanic membrane

H72.821 Total perforations of tympanic membrane, right ear
H72.822 Total perforations of tympanic membrane, left ear
H72.823 Total perforations of tympanic membrane, bilateral
H72.829 Total perforations of tympanic membrane, unspecified ear ▽

√5ᵗʰ **H72.9** Unspecified perforation of tympanic membrane

H72.90 Unspecified perforation of tympanic membrane, unspecified ear ▽
H72.91 Unspecified perforation of tympanic membrane, right ear ▽
H72.92 Unspecified perforation of tympanic membrane, left ear ▽

Chapter 8. Diseases of the Ear and Mastoid Process

H70.21–H72.92

H72.93   Unspecified perforation of tympanic membrane, **bilateral**   ▽

✓4ᵗʰ **H73   Other disorders of tympanic membrane**

✓5ᵗʰ **H73.0   Acute myringitis**

EXCLUDES 1   *acute myringitis with otitis media (H65, H66)*

✓6ᵗʰ **H73.00   Unspecified acute myringitis**

Acute tympanitis NOS

H73.001   Acute myringitis, **right ear**
H73.002   Acute myringitis, **left ear**
H73.003   Acute myringitis, **bilateral**
H73.009   Acute myringitis, **unspecified ear**   ▽

✓6ᵗʰ **H73.01   Bullous myringitis**

DEF: Bacterial or viral otitis media that is characterized by the appearance of serous or hemorrhagic blebs on the ear drum and sudden onset of severe pain in ear.

H73.011   Bullous myringitis, **right ear**
H73.012   Bullous myringitis, **left ear**
H73.013   Bullous myringitis, **bilateral**
H73.019   Bullous myringitis, **unspecified ear**   ▽

✓6ᵗʰ **H73.09   Other acute myringitis**

H73.091   Other acute myringitis, **right ear**
H73.092   Other acute myringitis, **left ear**
H73.093   Other acute myringitis, **bilateral**
H73.099   Other acute myringitis, **unspecified ear**   ▽

✓5ᵗʰ **H73.1   Chronic myringitis**

Chronic tympanitis

EXCLUDES 1   *chronic myringitis with otitis media (H65, H66)*

H73.10   Chronic myringitis, **unspecified ear**   ▽
H73.11   Chronic myringitis, **right ear**
H73.12   Chronic myringitis, **left ear**
H73.13   Chronic myringitis, **bilateral**

✓5ᵗʰ **H73.2   Unspecified myringitis**

H73.20   Unspecified myringitis, **unspecified ear**   ▽
H73.21   Unspecified myringitis, **right ear**   ▽
H73.22   Unspecified myringitis, **left ear**   ▽
H73.23   Unspecified myringitis, **bilateral**   ▽

✓5ᵗʰ **H73.8   Other specified disorders of tympanic membrane**

✓6ᵗʰ **H73.81   Atrophic flaccid tympanic membrane**

H73.811   Atrophic flaccid tympanic membrane, **right ear**
H73.812   Atrophic flaccid tympanic membrane, **left ear**
H73.813   Atrophic flaccid tympanic membrane, **bilateral**
H73.819   Atrophic flaccid tympanic membrane, **unspecified ear**   ▽

✓6ᵗʰ **H73.82   Atrophic nonflaccid tympanic membrane**

H73.821   Atrophic nonflaccid tympanic membrane, **right ear**
H73.822   Atrophic nonflaccid tympanic membrane, **left ear**
H73.823   Atrophic nonflaccid tympanic membrane, **bilateral**
H73.829   Atrophic nonflaccid tympanic membrane, **unspecified ear**   ▽

✓6ᵗʰ **H73.89   Other specified disorders of tympanic membrane**

H73.891   Other specified disorders of tympanic membrane, **right ear**
H73.892   Other specified disorders of tympanic membrane, **left ear**
H73.893   Other specified disorders of tympanic membrane, **bilateral**
H73.899   Other specified disorders of tympanic membrane, **unspecified ear**   ▽

✓5ᵗʰ **H73.9   Unspecified disorder of tympanic membrane**

H73.90   Unspecified disorder of tympanic membrane, **unspecified ear**   ▽
H73.91   Unspecified disorder of tympanic membrane, **right ear**   ▽
H73.92   Unspecified disorder of tympanic membrane, **left ear**   ▽
H73.93   Unspecified disorder of tympanic membrane, **bilateral**   ▽

✓4ᵗʰ **H74   Other disorders of middle ear mastoid**

EXCLUDES 2   *mastoiditis (H70.-)*

✓5ᵗʰ **H74.0   Tympanosclerosis**

DEF: Calcification of tissue in the ear drum, middle ear bones, and middle ear canal.

H74.01   Tympanosclerosis, **right ear**
H74.02   Tympanosclerosis, **left ear**
H74.03   Tympanosclerosis, **bilateral**
H74.09   Tympanosclerosis, **unspecified ear**   ▽

✓5ᵗʰ **H74.1   Adhesive middle ear disease**

Adhesive otitis

EXCLUDES 1   *glue ear (H65.3-)*

H74.11   Adhesive **right** middle ear disease
H74.12   Adhesive **left** middle ear disease
H74.13   Adhesive middle ear disease, **bilateral**
H74.19   Adhesive middle ear disease, **unspecified ear**   ▽

✓5ᵗʰ **H74.2   Discontinuity and dislocation of ear ossicles**

H74.20   Discontinuity and dislocation of ear ossicles, **unspecified ear**   ▽
H74.21   Discontinuity and dislocation of **right** ear ossicles
H74.22   Discontinuity and dislocation of **left** ear ossicles
H74.23   Discontinuity and dislocation of ear ossicles, **bilateral**

✓5ᵗʰ **H74.3   Other acquired abnormalities of ear ossicles**

✓6ᵗʰ **H74.31   Ankylosis of ear ossicles**

H74.311   Ankylosis of ear ossicles, **right ear**
H74.312   Ankylosis of ear ossicles, **left ear**
H74.313   Ankylosis of ear ossicles, **bilateral**
H74.319   Ankylosis of ear ossicles, **unspecified ear**   ▽

✓6ᵗʰ **H74.32   Partial loss of ear ossicles**

H74.321   Partial loss of ear ossicles, **right ear**
H74.322   Partial loss of ear ossicles, **left ear**
H74.323   Partial loss of ear ossicles, **bilateral**
H74.329   Partial loss of ear ossicles, **unspecified ear**   ▽

✓6ᵗʰ **H74.39   Other acquired abnormalities of ear ossicles**

H74.391   Other acquired abnormalities of **right** ear ossicles
H74.392   Other acquired abnormalities of **left** ear ossicles
H74.393   Other acquired abnormalities of ear ossicles, **bilateral**
H74.399   Other acquired abnormalities of ear ossicles, **unspecified ear**   ▽

✓5ᵗʰ **H74.4   Polyp of middle ear**

H74.40   Polyp of middle ear, **unspecified ear**   ▽
H74.41   Polyp of **right** middle ear
H74.42   Polyp of **left** middle ear
H74.43   Polyp of middle ear, **bilateral**

✓5ᵗʰ **H74.8   Other specified disorders of middle ear and mastoid**

✓6ᵗʰ **H74.8X   Other specified disorders of middle ear and mastoid**

H74.8X1   Other specified disorders of **right** middle ear and mastoid
H74.8X2   Other specified disorders of **left** middle ear and mastoid
H74.8X3   Other specified disorders of middle ear and mastoid, **bilateral**
H74.8X9   Other specified disorders of middle ear and mastoid, **unspecified ear**   ▽

✓5ᵗʰ **H74.9   Unspecified disorder of middle ear and mastoid**

H74.90   Unspecified disorder of middle ear and mastoid, **unspecified ear**   ▽
H74.91   Unspecified disorder of **right** middle ear and mastoid   ▽
H74.92   Unspecified disorder of **left** middle ear and mastoid   ▽
H74.93   Unspecified disorder of middle ear and mastoid, **bilateral**   ▽

√4ᵗʰ **H75 Other disorders of middle ear and mastoid in diseases classified elsewhere**

Code first underlying disease

√5ᵗʰ **H75.0 Mastoiditis in infectious and parasitic diseases classified elsewhere**

EXCLUDES 1   mastoiditis (in):
     syphilis (A52.77)
     tuberculosis (A18.03)

H75.00   *Mastoiditis in infectious and parasitic diseases classified elsewhere, unspecified ear* ▽

H75.01   *Mastoiditis in infectious and parasitic diseases classified elsewhere, right ear*

H75.02   *Mastoiditis in infectious and parasitic diseases classified elsewhere, left ear*

H75.03   *Mastoiditis in infectious and parasitic diseases classified elsewhere, bilateral*

√5ᵗʰ **H75.8 Other specified disorders of middle ear and mastoid in diseases classified elsewhere**

H75.80   *Other specified disorders of middle ear and mastoid in diseases classified elsewhere, unspecified ear* ▽

H75.81   *Other specified disorders of right middle ear and mastoid in diseases classified elsewhere*

H75.82   *Other specified disorders of left middle ear and mastoid in diseases classified elsewhere*

H75.83   *Other specified disorders of middle ear and mastoid in diseases classified elsewhere, bilateral*

Diseases of inner ear (H80-H83)

√4ᵗʰ **H80 Otosclerosis**

INCLUDES   otospongiosis

√5ᵗʰ **H80.0 Otosclerosis involving oval window, nonobliterative**

H80.00   Otosclerosis involving oval window, nonobliterative, unspecified ear ▽

H80.01   Otosclerosis involving oval window, nonobliterative, right ear

H80.02   Otosclerosis involving oval window, nonobliterative, left ear

H80.03   Otosclerosis involving oval window, nonobliterative, bilateral

√5ᵗʰ **H80.1 Otosclerosis involving oval window, obliterative**

H80.10   Otosclerosis involving oval window, obliterative, unspecified ear ▽

H80.11   Otosclerosis involving oval window, obliterative, right ear

H80.12   Otosclerosis involving oval window, obliterative, left ear

H80.13   Otosclerosis involving oval window, obliterative, bilateral

√5ᵗʰ **H80.2 Cochlear otosclerosis**

Otosclerosis involving otic capsule
Otosclerosis involving round window

H80.20   Cochlear otosclerosis, unspecified ear ▽

H80.21   Cochlear otosclerosis, right ear

H80.22   Cochlear otosclerosis, left ear

H80.23   Cochlear otosclerosis, bilateral

√5ᵗʰ **H80.8 Other otosclerosis**

H80.80   Other otosclerosis, unspecified ear ▽

H80.81   Other otosclerosis, right ear

H80.82   Other otosclerosis, left ear

H80.83   Other otosclerosis, bilateral

√5ᵗʰ **H80.9 Unspecified otosclerosis**

H80.90   Unspecified otosclerosis, unspecified ear ▽

H80.91   Unspecified otosclerosis, right ear ▽

H80.92   Unspecified otosclerosis, left ear ▽

H80.93   Unspecified otosclerosis, bilateral ▽

√4ᵗʰ **H81 Disorders of vestibular function**

EXCLUDES 1   epidemic vertigo (A88.1)
     vertigo NOS (R42)

√5ᵗʰ **H81.0 Ménière's disease**

Labyrinthine hydrops
Ménière's syndrome or vertigo

DEF: Distended membranous labyrinth of the middle ear from fluctuating pressure of fluid (hydrops) that causes vertigo, tinnitus, pressure, and hearing loss that may last on and off for several hours. Episodes may occur in clusters or may subside for weeks, months, or even years.

H81.01   Ménière's disease, right ear

H81.02   Ménière's disease, left ear

H81.03   Ménière's disease, bilateral

H81.09   Ménière's disease, unspecified ear ▽

√5ᵗʰ **H81.1 Benign paroxysmal vertigo**

H81.10   Benign paroxysmal vertigo, unspecified ear 🄾 ▽

H81.11   Benign paroxysmal vertigo, right ear 🄾

H81.12   Benign paroxysmal vertigo, left ear 🄾

H81.13   Benign paroxysmal vertigo, bilateral 🄾

√5ᵗʰ **H81.2 Vestibular neuronitis**

DEF: Transient benign vertigo caused by inflammation of the vestibular nerve. It is characterized by response to caloric stimulation on one side and nystagmus with rhythmic movement of the eyes. Normal auditory function is present.

H81.20   Vestibular neuronitis, unspecified ear ▽

H81.21   Vestibular neuronitis, right ear

H81.22   Vestibular neuronitis, left ear

H81.23   Vestibular neuronitis, bilateral

√5ᵗʰ **H81.3 Other peripheral vertigo**

√6ᵗʰ **H81.31 Aural vertigo**

H81.311   Aural vertigo, right ear

H81.312   Aural vertigo, left ear

H81.313   Aural vertigo, bilateral

H81.319   Aural vertigo, unspecified ear ▽

√6ᵗʰ **H81.39 Other peripheral vertigo**

Lermoyez' syndrome
Otogenic vertigo
Peripheral vertigo NOS

H81.391   Other peripheral vertigo, right ear

H81.392   Other peripheral vertigo, left ear

H81.393   Other peripheral vertigo, bilateral

H81.399   Other peripheral vertigo, unspecified ear ▽

√5ᵗʰ **H81.4 Vertigo of central origin**

Central positional nystagmus

H81.41   Vertigo of central origin, right ear

H81.42   Vertigo of central origin, left ear

H81.43   Vertigo of central origin, bilateral

H81.49   Vertigo of central origin, unspecified ear ▽

√5ᵗʰ **H81.8 Other disorders of vestibular function**

√6ᵗʰ **H81.8X Other disorders of vestibular function**

H81.8X1   Other disorders of vestibular function, right ear

H81.8X2   Other disorders of vestibular function, left ear

H81.8X3   Other disorders of vestibular function, bilateral

H81.8X9   Other disorders of vestibular function, unspecified ear ▽

√5ᵗʰ **H81.9 Unspecified disorder of vestibular function**

Vertiginous syndrome NOS

H81.90   Unspecified disorder of vestibular function, unspecified ear ▽

H81.91   Unspecified disorder of vestibular function, right ear ▽

H81.92   Unspecified disorder of vestibular function, left ear ▽

H81.93   Unspecified disorder of vestibular function, bilateral ▽

√4ᵗʰ **H82 Vertiginous syndromes in diseases classified elsewhere**

Code first underlying disease

EXCLUDES 1   epidemic vertigo (A88.1)

H82.1   *Vertiginous syndromes in diseases classified elsewhere, right ear*

H82.2   *Vertiginous syndromes in diseases classified elsewhere, left ear*

✓ Additional Character Req   √x7ᵗʰ Placeholder Alert   Manifestation   ▽ Unspecified   ▶◀ Revised Text   ● New Code   ▲ Revised Code Title

Chapter 8. Diseases of the Ear and Mastoid Process *(side margin)*

*H82.3–H91.13 (side margin)*

H82.3 *Vertiginous syndromes in diseases classified elsewhere, bilateral*

H82.9 *Vertiginous syndromes in diseases classified elsewhere, unspecified ear* ▽

✓4ᵗʰ **H83 Other diseases of inner ear**

  ✓5ᵗʰ **H83.0 Labyrinthitis**

    DEF: Inflammation of the inner ear, or labyrinth, characterized by pus, vertigo, dizziness, nausea, and hearing loss.

    H83.01 Labyrinthitis, right ear
    H83.02 Labyrinthitis, left ear
    H83.03 Labyrinthitis, bilateral
    H83.09 Labyrinthitis, unspecified ear ▽

  ✓5ᵗʰ **H83.1 Labyrinthine fistula**

    H83.11 Labyrinthine fistula, right ear
    H83.12 Labyrinthine fistula, left ear
    H83.13 Labyrinthine fistula, bilateral
    H83.19 Labyrinthine fistula, unspecified ear ▽

  ✓5ᵗʰ **H83.2 Labyrinthine dysfunction**

    Labyrinthine hypersensitivity
    Labyrinthine hypofunction
    Labyrinthine loss of function
    DEF: Decreased function of the labyrinth sensors.

    ✓6ᵗʰ **H83.2X Labyrinthine dysfunction**

      H83.2X1 Labyrinthine dysfunction, right ear
      H83.2X2 Labyrinthine dysfunction, left ear
      H83.2X3 Labyrinthine dysfunction, bilateral
      H83.2X9 Labyrinthine dysfunction, unspecified ear ▽

  ✓5ᵗʰ **H83.3 Noise effects on inner ear**

    Acoustic trauma of inner ear
    Noise-induced hearing loss of inner ear

    ✓6ᵗʰ **H83.3X Noise effects on inner ear**

      H83.3X1 Noise effects on right inner ear
      H83.3X2 Noise effects on left inner ear
      H83.3X3 Noise effects on inner ear, bilateral
      H83.3X9 Noise effects on inner ear, unspecified ear ▽

  ✓5ᵗʰ **H83.8 Other specified diseases of inner ear**

    ✓6ᵗʰ **H83.8X Other specified diseases of inner ear**

      H83.8X1 Other specified diseases of right inner ear
      H83.8X2 Other specified diseases of left inner ear
      H83.8X3 Other specified diseases of inner ear, bilateral
      H83.8X9 Other specified diseases of inner ear, unspecified ear ▽

  ✓5ᵗʰ **H83.9 Unspecified disease of inner ear**

    H83.90 Unspecified disease of inner ear, unspecified ear ▽
    H83.91 Unspecified disease of right inner ear ▽
    H83.92 Unspecified disease of left inner ear ▽
    H83.93 Unspecified disease of inner ear, bilateral ▽

Other disorders of ear (H90-H94)

✓4ᵗʰ **H90 Conductive and sensorineural hearing loss**

  EXCLUDES 1   deaf nonspeaking NEC (H91.3) (~H91.3)
         deafness NOS (H91.9-)
         hearing loss NOS (H91.9-)
         noise-induced hearing loss (H83.3-)
         ototoxic hearing loss (H91.0-)
         sudden (idiopathic) hearing loss (H91.2-)

  AHA: 2015,2Q,7
  DEF: Conductive hearing loss: Hearing Loss due to the inability of sound waves to move from the outer (external ear) to the inner ear.
  DEF: Sensorineural hearing loss: Hearing loss that occurs from damage to the hair cells of the inner ear or problems with the nerve pathways from the inner ear to the brain.

  H90.0 Conductive hearing loss, bilateral

  ✓5ᵗʰ **H90.1 Conductive hearing loss, unilateral with unrestricted hearing on the contralateral side**

    H90.11 Conductive hearing loss, unilateral, right ear, with unrestricted hearing on the contralateral side
    H90.12 Conductive hearing loss, unilateral, left ear, with unrestricted hearing on the contralateral side

  H90.2 Conductive hearing loss, unspecified ▽
    Conductive deafness NOS

  H90.3 Sensorineural hearing loss, bilateral

✓5ᵗʰ **H90.4 Sensorineural hearing loss, unilateral with unrestricted hearing on the contralateral side**

  H90.41 Sensorineural hearing loss, unilateral, right ear, with unrestricted hearing on the contralateral side
  H90.42 Sensorineural hearing loss, unilateral, left ear, with unrestricted hearing on the contralateral side

H90.5 Unspecified sensorineural hearing loss ▽
  Central hearing loss NOS
  Congenital deafness NOS
  Neural hearing loss NOS
  Perceptive hearing loss NOS
  Sensorineural deafness NOS
  Sensory hearing loss NOS
  EXCLUDES 1   abnormal auditory perception (H93.2-)
          psychogenic deafness (F44.6)

H90.6 Mixed conductive and sensorineural hearing loss, bilateral
  AHA: 2015,2Q,7

✓5ᵗʰ **H90.7 Mixed conductive and sensorineural hearing loss, unilateral with unrestricted hearing on the contralateral side**

  H90.71 Mixed conductive and sensorineural hearing loss, unilateral, right ear, with unrestricted hearing on the contralateral side
  H90.72 Mixed conductive and sensorineural hearing loss, unilateral, left ear, with unrestricted hearing on the contralateral side

H90.8 Mixed conductive and sensorineural hearing loss, unspecified ▽

✓5ᵗʰ **H90.A Conductive and sensorineural hearing loss with restricted hearing on the contralateral side**
  AHA: 2016,4Q,23-25

  ✓6ᵗʰ **H90.A1 Conductive hearing loss, unilateral, with restricted hearing on the contralateral side**

    H90.A11 Conductive hearing loss, unilateral, right ear with restricted hearing on the contralateral side
    H90.A12 Conductive hearing loss, unilateral, left ear with restricted hearing on the contralateral side

  ✓6ᵗʰ **H90.A2 Sensorineural hearing loss, unilateral, with restricted hearing on the contralateral side**

    H90.A21 Sensorineural hearing loss, unilateral, right ear, with restricted hearing on the contralateral side
    H90.A22 Sensorineural hearing loss, unilateral, left ear, with restricted hearing on the contralateral side

  ✓6ᵗʰ **H90.A3 Mixed conductive and sensorineural hearing loss, unilateral with restricted hearing on the contralateral side**

    H90.A31 Mixed conductive and sensorineural hearing loss, unilateral, right ear with restricted hearing on the contralateral side
    H90.A32 Mixed conductive and sensorineural hearing loss, unilateral, left ear with restricted hearing on the contralateral side

✓4ᵗʰ **H91 Other and unspecified hearing loss**

  EXCLUDES 1   abnormal auditory perception (H93.2-)
         hearing loss as classified in H90.-
         impacted cerumen (H61.2-)
         noise-induced hearing loss (H83.3-)
         psychogenic deafness (F44.6)
         transient ischemic deafness (H93.01-)

  ✓5ᵗʰ **H91.0 Ototoxic hearing loss**

    Code first poisoning due to drug or toxin, if applicable (T36-T65 with fifth or sixth character 1-4 or 6)
    Use additional code for adverse effect, if applicable, to identify drug (T36-T50 with fifth or sixth character 5)

    H91.01 Ototoxic hearing loss, right ear
    H91.02 Ototoxic hearing loss, left ear
    H91.03 Ototoxic hearing loss, bilateral
    H91.09 Ototoxic hearing loss, unspecified ear ▽

  ✓5ᵗʰ **H91.1 Presbycusis**

    Presbyacusia

    H91.10 Presbycusis, unspecified ear ▽
    H91.11 Presbycusis, right ear
    H91.12 Presbycusis, left ear
    H91.13 Presbycusis, bilateral

√5ᵗʰ **H91.2**   **Sudden idiopathic hearing loss**
     Sudden hearing loss NOS

     H91.20   **Sudden idiopathic hearing loss, unspecified** ▽
                 ear
     H91.21   **Sudden idiopathic hearing loss, right ear**
     H91.22   **Sudden idiopathic hearing loss, left ear**
     H91.23   **Sudden idiopathic hearing loss, bilateral**

H91.3   **Deaf nonspeaking, not elsewhere classified**

√5ᵗʰ **H91.8**   **Other specified hearing loss**

   √6ᵗʰ **H91.8X**   **Other specified hearing loss**

       H91.8X1   **Other specified hearing loss, right ear**
       H91.8X2   **Other specified hearing loss, left ear**
       H91.8X3   **Other specified hearing loss, bilateral**
       H91.8X9   **Other specified hearing loss,** ▽
                   unspecified ear

√5ᵗʰ **H91.9**   **Unspecified hearing loss**
     Deafness NOS
     High frequency deafness
     Low frequency deafness

     H91.90   **Unspecified hearing loss, unspecified ear** ▽
     H91.91   **Unspecified hearing loss, right ear** ▽
     H91.92   **Unspecified hearing loss, left ear** ▽
     H91.93   **Unspecified hearing loss, bilateral** ▽

√4ᵗʰ **H92**   **Otalgia and effusion of ear**

√5ᵗʰ **H92.0**   **Otalgia**

     H92.01   **Otalgia, right ear**
     H92.02   **Otalgia, left ear**
     H92.03   **Otalgia, bilateral**
     H92.09   **Otalgia, unspecified ear** ▽

√5ᵗʰ **H92.1**   **Otorrhea**

     EXCLUDES 1   *leakage of cerebrospinal fluid through ear (G96.0)*

     H92.10   **Otorrhea, unspecified ear** ▽
     H92.11   **Otorrhea, right ear**
     H92.12   **Otorrhea, left ear**
     H92.13   **Otorrhea, bilateral**

√5ᵗʰ **H92.2**   **Otorrhagia**

     EXCLUDES 1   *traumatic otorrhagia - code to injury*

     H92.20   **Otorrhagia, unspecified ear** ▽
     H92.21   **Otorrhagia, right ear**
     H92.22   **Otorrhagia, left ear**
     H92.23   **Otorrhagia, bilateral**

√4ᵗʰ **H93**   **Other disorders of ear, not elsewhere classified**

√5ᵗʰ **H93.0**   **Degenerative and vascular disorders of ear**

     EXCLUDES 1   *presbycusis (H91.1)*

   √6ᵗʰ **H93.01**   **Transient ischemic deafness**

       H93.011   **Transient ischemic deafness, right ear**
       H93.012   **Transient ischemic deafness, left ear**
       H93.013   **Transient ischemic deafness, bilateral**
       H93.019   **Transient ischemic deafness,** ▽
                 unspecified ear

   √6ᵗʰ **H93.09**   **Unspecified degenerative and vascular disorders of ear**

       H93.091   **Unspecified degenerative and** ▽
                 vascular disorders of right ear
       H93.092   **Unspecified degenerative and** ▽
                 vascular disorders of left ear
       H93.093   **Unspecified degenerative and** ▽
                 vascular disorders of ear, bilateral
       H93.099   **Unspecified degenerative and** ▽
                 vascular disorders of unspecified
                 ear

√5ᵗʰ **H93.1**   **Tinnitus**

     H93.11   **Tinnitus, right ear**
     H93.12   **Tinnitus, left ear**
     H93.13   **Tinnitus, bilateral**
     H93.19   **Tinnitus, unspecified ear** ▽

√5ᵗʰ **H93.A**   **Pulsatile tinnitus**

     AHA: 2016,4Q,25-26

     H93.A1   **Pulsatile tinnitus, right ear**
     H93.A2   **Pulsatile tinnitus, left ear**
     H93.A3   **Pulsatile tinnitus, bilateral**
     H93.A9   **Pulsatile tinnitus, unspecified ear** ▽

√5ᵗʰ **H93.2**   **Other abnormal auditory perceptions**

     EXCLUDES 2   *auditory hallucinations (R44.0)*

   √6ᵗʰ **H93.21**   **Auditory recruitment**

       H93.211   **Auditory recruitment, right ear**
       H93.212   **Auditory recruitment, left ear**
       H93.213   **Auditory recruitment, bilateral**
       H93.219   **Auditory recruitment, unspecified** ▽
                 ear

   √6ᵗʰ **H93.22**   **Diplacusis**

       H93.221   **Diplacusis, right ear**
       H93.222   **Diplacusis, left ear**
       H93.223   **Diplacusis, bilateral**
       H93.229   **Diplacusis, unspecified ear** ▽

   √6ᵗʰ **H93.23**   **Hyperacusis**

       DEF: Exceptionally acute sense of hearing caused by such conditions as Bell's palsy. This term may also refer to painful sensitivity to sounds.

       H93.231   **Hyperacusis, right ear**
       H93.232   **Hyperacusis, left ear**
       H93.233   **Hyperacusis, bilateral**
       H93.239   **Hyperacusis, unspecified ear** ▽

   √6ᵗʰ **H93.24**   **Temporary auditory threshold shift**

       H93.241   **Temporary auditory threshold shift, right ear**
       H93.242   **Temporary auditory threshold shift, left ear**
       H93.243   **Temporary auditory threshold shift, bilateral**
       H93.249   **Temporary auditory threshold** ▽
                 shift, unspecified ear

     H93.25   **Central auditory processing disorder**
       Congenital auditory imperception
       Word deafness
       EXCLUDES 1   *mixed receptive-expressive language disorder (F80.2)*

   √6ᵗʰ **H93.29**   **Other abnormal auditory perceptions**

       H93.291   **Other abnormal auditory perceptions, right ear**
       H93.292   **Other abnormal auditory perceptions, left ear**
       H93.293   **Other abnormal auditory perceptions, bilateral**
       H93.299   **Other abnormal auditory** ▽
                 perceptions, unspecified ear

√5ᵗʰ **H93.3**   **Disorders of acoustic nerve**
     Disorder of 8th cranial nerve
     EXCLUDES 1   *acoustic neuroma (D33.3)*
                 syphilitic acoustic neuritis (A52.15)

   √6ᵗʰ **H93.3X**   **Disorders of acoustic nerve**

       H93.3X1   **Disorders of right acoustic nerve**
       H93.3X2   **Disorders of left acoustic nerve**
       H93.3X3   **Disorders of bilateral acoustic nerves**
       H93.3X9   **Disorders of unspecified acoustic** ▽
                 nerve

√5ᵗʰ **H93.8**   **Other specified disorders of ear**

   √6ᵗʰ **H93.8X**   **Other specified disorders of ear**

       H93.8X1   **Other specified disorders of right ear**
       H93.8X2   **Other specified disorders of left ear**
       H93.8X3   **Other specified disorders of ear, bilateral**
       H93.8X9   **Other specified disorders of ear,** ▽
                 unspecified ear

√5ᵗʰ **H93.9**   **Unspecified disorder of ear**

     H93.90   **Unspecified disorder of ear, unspecified ear** ▽
     H93.91   **Unspecified disorder of right ear** ▽
     H93.92   **Unspecified disorder of left ear** ▽
     H93.93   **Unspecified disorder of ear, bilateral** ▽

√4ᵗʰ **H94**   **Other disorders of ear in diseases classified elsewhere**

√5ᵗʰ **H94.0**   **Acoustic neuritis in infectious and parasitic diseases classified elsewhere**
     Code first underlying disease, such as:
     parasitic disease (B65-B89)
     EXCLUDES 1   *acoustic neuritis (in):*
                 herpes zoster (B02.29)
                 syphilis (A52.15)

     H94.00   *Acoustic neuritis in infectious and parasitic* ▽
                 diseases classified elsewhere, unspecified ear

☑ Additional Character Req   √x7ᵗʰ Placeholder Alert   Manifestation   ▽ Unspecified   ►◄ Revised Text   ● New Code   ▲ Revised Code Title

ICD-10-CM 2019   629

H94.Ø1   **Acoustic neuritis in infectious and parasitic diseases classified elsewhere,** *right ear*

H94.Ø2   **Acoustic neuritis in infectious and parasitic diseases classified elsewhere,** *left ear*

H94.Ø3   **Acoustic neuritis in infectious and parasitic diseases classified elsewhere,** *bilateral*

√5ᵗʰ   **H94.8**   **Other specified disorders of ear in diseases classified elsewhere**

     Code first underlying disease, such as:
       congenital syphilis (A5Ø.Ø)

     EXCLUDES 1   aural myiasis (B87.4)
              syphilitic labyrinthitis (A52.79)

H94.8Ø   **Other specified disorders of ear in diseases classified elsewhere, unspecified ear** ▽

H94.81   **Other specified disorders of** *right* **ear in diseases classified elsewhere**

H94.82   **Other specified disorders of** *left* **ear in diseases classified elsewhere**

H94.83   **Other specified disorders of ear in diseases classified elsewhere,** *bilateral*

Intraoperative and postprocedural complications and disorders of ear and mastoid process, not elsewhere classified (H95)

√4ᵗʰ   **H95**   **Intraoperative and postprocedural complications and disorders of ear and mastoid process, not elsewhere classified**

     AHA: 2016,4Q,9-10

√5ᵗʰ   **H95.Ø**   **Recurrent cholesteatoma of postmastoidectomy cavity**

     H95.ØØ   **Recurrent cholesteatoma of** ▽
              postmastoidectomy cavity, unspecified ear

     H95.Ø1   **Recurrent cholesteatoma of postmastoidectomy cavity, right ear**

     H95.Ø2   **Recurrent cholesteatoma of postmastoidectomy cavity, left ear**

     H95.Ø3   **Recurrent cholesteatoma of postmastoidectomy cavity, bilateral ears**

√5ᵗʰ   **H95.1**   **Other disorders of ear and mastoid process following mastoidectomy**

   √6ᵗʰ   **H95.11**   **Chronic inflammation of postmastoidectomy cavity**

       H95.111   **Chronic inflammation of postmastoidectomy cavity, right ear**

       H95.112   **Chronic inflammation of postmastoidectomy cavity, left ear**

       H95.113   **Chronic inflammation of postmastoidectomy cavity, bilateral ears**

       H95.119   **Chronic inflammation of** ▽
               postmastoidectomy cavity, unspecified ear

   √6ᵗʰ   **H95.12**   **Granulation of postmastoidectomy cavity**

       H95.121   **Granulation of postmastoidectomy cavity, right ear**

       H95.122   **Granulation of postmastoidectomy cavity, left ear**

       H95.123   **Granulation of postmastoidectomy cavity, bilateral ears**

       H95.129   **Granulation of** ▽
               postmastoidectomy cavity, unspecified ear

   √6ᵗʰ   **H95.13**   **Mucosal cyst of postmastoidectomy cavity**

       H95.131   **Mucosal cyst of postmastoidectomy cavity, right ear**

       H95.132   **Mucosal cyst of postmastoidectomy cavity, left ear**

       H95.133   **Mucosal cyst of postmastoidectomy cavity, bilateral ears**

       H95.139   **Mucosal cyst of** ▽
               postmastoidectomy cavity, unspecified ear

   √6ᵗʰ   **H95.19**   **Other disorders following mastoidectomy**

       H95.191   **Other disorders following mastoidectomy, right ear**

       H95.192   **Other disorders following mastoidectomy, left ear**

       H95.193   **Other disorders following mastoidectomy, bilateral ears**

       H95.199   **Other disorders following** ▽
               mastoidectomy, unspecified ear

√5ᵗʰ   **H95.2**   **Intraoperative hemorrhage and hematoma of ear and mastoid process complicating a procedure**

     EXCLUDES 1   *intraoperative hemorrhage and hematoma of ear and mastoid process due to accidental puncture or laceration during a procedure (H95.3-)*

     H95.21   **Intraoperative hemorrhage and hematoma of ear and mastoid process complicating a procedure on the ear and mastoid process**

     H95.22   **Intraoperative hemorrhage and hematoma of ear and mastoid process complicating other procedure**

√5ᵗʰ   **H95.3**   **Accidental puncture and laceration of ear and mastoid process during a procedure**

     H95.31   **Accidental puncture and laceration of the ear and mastoid process during a procedure on the ear and mastoid process**

     H95.32   **Accidental puncture and laceration of the ear and mastoid process during other procedure**

√5ᵗʰ   **H95.4**   **Postprocedural hemorrhage of ear and mastoid process following a procedure**

     H95.41   **Postprocedural hemorrhage of ear and mastoid process following a procedure on the ear and mastoid process**

     H95.42   **Postprocedural hemorrhage of ear and mastoid process following other procedure**

√5ᵗʰ   **H95.5**   **Postprocedural hematoma and seroma of ear and mastoid process following a procedure**

     H95.51   **Postprocedural hematoma of ear and mastoid process following a procedure on the ear and mastoid process**

     H95.52   **Postprocedural hematoma of ear and mastoid process following other procedure**

     H95.53   **Postprocedural seroma of ear and mastoid process following a procedure on the ear and mastoid process**

     H95.54   **Postprocedural seroma of ear and mastoid process following other procedure**

√5ᵗʰ   **H95.8**   **Other intraoperative and postprocedural complications and disorders of the ear and mastoid process, not elsewhere classified**

     EXCLUDES 2   *postprocedural complications and disorders following mastoidectomy (H95.Ø-, H95.1-)*

   √6ᵗʰ   **H95.81**   **Postprocedural stenosis of external ear canal**

       H95.811   **Postprocedural stenosis of right external ear canal**

       H95.812   **Postprocedural stenosis of left external ear canal**

       H95.813   **Postprocedural stenosis of external ear canal, bilateral**

       H95.819   **Postprocedural stenosis of** ▽
               unspecified external ear canal

     H95.88   **Other intraoperative complications and disorders of the ear and mastoid process, not elsewhere classified**

       Use additional code, if applicable, to further specify disorder

     H95.89   **Other postprocedural complications and disorders of the ear and mastoid process, not elsewhere classified**

       Use additional code, if applicable, to further specify disorder

Chapter 9. Diseases of the Circulatory System (I00–I99)

Chapter Specific Guidelines with Coding Examples

The chapter specific guidelines from the ICD-10-CM Official Guidelines for Coding and Reporting have been provided below. Along with these guidelines are coding examples, contained in the shaded boxes, that have been developed to help illustrate the coding and/or sequencing guidance found in these guidelines.

a. Hypertension

The classification presumes a causal relationship between hypertension and heart involvement and between hypertension and kidney involvement, as the two conditions are linked by the term "with" in the Alphabetic Index. These conditions should be coded as related even in the absence of provider documentation explicitly linking them, unless the documentation clearly states the conditions are unrelated.

For hypertension and conditions not specifically linked by relational terms such as "with," "associated with" or "due to" in the classification, provider documentation must link the conditions in order to code them as related.

1) Hypertension with heart disease

Hypertension with heart conditions classified to I50.- or **I51.4-I51.7, I51.89, I51.9**, are assigned to a code from category I11, Hypertensive heart disease. Use additional code(s) from category I50, Heart failure, to identify the type(s) of heart failure in those patients with heart failure.

The same heart conditions (I50.-, **I51.4-I51.7, I51.89, I51.9**) with hypertension are coded separately if the provider has **documented they are unrelated to the hypertension.** Sequence according to the circumstances of the admission/encounter.

> Patient is treated for left heart failure. Patient also has a history of hypertension managed by medication.
>
> **I11.0**   **Hypertensive heart disease with heart failure**
>
> **I50.1**   **Left ventricular failure, unspecified**
>
> *Explanation*: Without a diagnostic statement to the contrary, hypertension and heart failure have an assumed causal relationship, and a combination code should be used. An additional code to identify the type of heart failure (I50.-) should also be provided.

2) Hypertensive chronic kidney disease

Assign codes from category I12, Hypertensive chronic kidney disease, when both hypertension and a condition classifiable to category N18, Chronic kidney disease (CKD), are present. CKD should not be coded as hypertensive if the **provider indicates the CKD is not related to the hypertension.**

The appropriate code from category N18 should be used as a secondary code with a code from category I12 to identify the stage of chronic kidney disease.

See Section I.C.14. Chronic kidney disease.

If a patient has hypertensive chronic kidney disease and acute renal failure, an additional code for the acute renal failure is required.

> Patient presents with stage IV chronic kidney disease (CKD). The patient also has documented hypertension secondary to primary hyperparathyroidism.
>
> **N18.4**   **Chronic kidney disease, stage 4 (severe)**
>
> **I10**   **Essential (primary) hypertension**
>
> **E21.0**   **Primary hyperparathyroidism**
>
> *Explanation*: A combination code describing a relationship between hypertension and CKD is not used due to the physician documentation identifying the primary hyperparathyroidism as the cause for the hypertension.

3) Hypertensive heart and chronic kidney disease

Assign codes from combination category I13, Hypertensive heart and chronic kidney disease, when there is hypertension with both heart and kidney involvement. If heart failure is present, assign an additional code from category I50 to identify the type of heart failure.

The appropriate code from category N18, Chronic kidney disease, should be used as a secondary code with a code from category I13 to identify the stage of chronic kidney disease.

See Section I.C.14. Chronic kidney disease.

The codes in category I13, Hypertensive heart and chronic kidney disease, are combination codes that include hypertension, heart disease and chronic kidney disease. The Includes note at I13 specifies that the conditions included at I11 and I12 are included together in I13. If a patient has hypertension, heart disease and chronic kidney disease, then a code

from I13 should be used, not individual codes for hypertension, heart disease and chronic kidney disease, or codes from I11 or I12.

For patients with both acute renal failure and chronic kidney disease, an additional code for acute renal failure is required.

> Hypertensive heart and kidney disease with congestive heart failure and stage 2 chronic kidney disease
>
> **I13.0**   **Hypertensive heart and chronic kidney disease with heart failure and stage 1 through stage 4 chronic kidney disease, or unspecified chronic kidney disease**
>
> **I50.9**   **Heart failure, unspecified**
>
> **N18.2**   **Chronic kidney disease, stage 2 (mild)**
>
> *Explanation*: Combination codes in category I13 are used to report conditions classifiable to *both* categories I11 and I12. Do not report conditions classifiable to I11 and I12 separately. Use additional codes to report type of heart failure and stage of CKD.

4) Hypertensive cerebrovascular disease

For hypertensive cerebrovascular disease, first assign the appropriate code from categories I60-I69, followed by the appropriate hypertension code.

> Rupture of cerebral aneurysm caused by malignant hypertension
>
> **I60.7**   **Nontraumatic subarachnoid hemorrhage from unspecified introcranial artery**
>
> **I10**   **Essential (primary) hypertension**
>
> *Explanation*: Hypertensive cerebrovascular disease requires two codes: the appropriate I60–I69 code followed by the appropriate hypertension code.

5) Hypertensive retinopathy

Subcategory H35.0, Background retinopathy and retinal vascular changes, should be used with a code from category I10 – I15, Hypertensive disease to include the systemic hypertension. The sequencing is based on the reason for the encounter.

6) Hypertension, secondary

Secondary hypertension is due to an underlying condition. Two codes are required: one to identify the underlying etiology and one from category I15 to identify the hypertension. Sequencing of codes is determined by the reason for admission/encounter.

> Renovascular hypertension due to renal artery atherosclerosis
>
> **I15.0**   **Renovascular hypertension**
>
> **I70.1**   **Atherosclerosis of renal artery**
>
> *Explanation*: Secondary hypertension requires two codes: a code to identify the etiology and the appropriate I15 code.

7) Hypertension, transient

Assign code R03.0, Elevated blood pressure reading without diagnosis of hypertension, unless patient has an established diagnosis of hypertension. Assign code O13.-, Gestational [pregnancy-induced] hypertension without significant proteinuria, or O14.-, Pre-eclampsia, for transient hypertension of pregnancy.

8) Hypertension, controlled

This diagnostic statement usually refers to an existing state of hypertension under control by therapy. Assign the appropriate code from categories I10-I15, Hypertensive diseases.

9) Hypertension, uncontrolled

Uncontrolled hypertension may refer to untreated hypertension or hypertension not responding to current therapeutic regimen. In either case, assign the appropriate code from categories I10-I15, Hypertensive diseases.

10) Hypertensive crisis

Assign a code from category I16, Hypertensive crisis, for documented hypertensive urgency, hypertensive emergency or unspecified hypertensive crisis. Code also any identified hypertensive disease (I10-I15). The sequencing is based on the reason for the encounter.

11) Pulmonary hypertension

Pulmonary hypertension is classified to category I27, Other pulmonary heart diseases. For secondary pulmonary hypertension (I27.1, I27.2-), code also any associated conditions or adverse effects of drugs or toxins. The sequencing is based on the reason for the encounter, **except for adverse effects of drugs (See Section I.C.19.e.).**

b. Atherosclerotic coronary artery disease and angina

ICD-10-CM has combination codes for atherosclerotic heart disease with angina pectoris. The subcategories for these codes are I25.11, Atherosclerotic heart disease of native coronary artery with angina pectoris and I25.7, Atherosclerosis of coronary artery bypass graft(s) and coronary artery of transplanted heart with angina pectoris.

When using one of these combination codes it is not necessary to use an additional code for angina pectoris. A causal relationship can be assumed in a patient with both atherosclerosis and angina pectoris, unless the documentation indicates the angina is due to something other than the atherosclerosis.

If a patient with coronary artery disease is admitted due to an acute myocardial infarction (AMI), the AMI should be sequenced before the coronary artery disease.

See Section I.C.9. Acute myocardial infarction (AMI)

> Patient is being seen for spastic angina pectoris. She also has a documented history of progressive coronary artery disease of the native vessels.
>
> **I25.111   Atherosclerotic heart disease of native coronary artery with angina pectoris with documented spasm**
>
> *Explanation*: Report the combination code for atherosclerotic heart disease (coronary artery disease) with angina pectoris. A causal relationship is assumed in a patient with both atherosclerosis and angina pectoris, unless the documentation indicates the angina is due to something other than the atherosclerosis. When using one of these combination codes, it is not necessary to use an additional code for angina pectoris.

c. Intraoperative and postprocedural cerebrovascular accident

Medical record documentation should clearly specify the cause- and- effect relationship between the medical intervention and the cerebrovascular accident in order to assign a code for intraoperative or postprocedural cerebrovascular accident.

Proper code assignment depends on whether it was an infarction or hemorrhage and whether it occurred intraoperatively or postoperatively. If it was a cerebral hemorrhage, code assignment depends on the type of procedure performed.

> Embolic cerebral infarction of the right middle cerebral artery that occurred during hip replacement surgery. The surgeon documented as due to the surgery.
>
> **I97.811   Intraoperative cerebrovascular infarction during other surgery**
>
> **I63.411   Cerebral infarction due to embolism of right middle cerebral artery**
>
> *Explanation*: Code assignment for intraoperative or postprocedural cerebrovascular accident is based on the provider's documentation of a cause-and-effect relationship between the condition and the procedure. Proper code assignment also depends on whether the cerebrovascular accident was an infarction or hemorrhage, occurred intraoperatively or postoperatively, and the type of procedure performed.

d. Sequelae of cerebrovascular disease

1) Category I69, Sequelae of cerebrovascular disease

Category I69 is used to indicate conditions classifiable to categories I60-I67 as the causes of sequela (neurologic deficits), themselves classified elsewhere. These "late effects" include neurologic deficits that persist after initial onset of conditions classifiable to categories I60-I67. The neurologic deficits caused by cerebrovascular disease may be present from the onset or may arise at any time after the onset of the condition classifiable to categories I60-I67.

Codes from category I69, Sequelae of cerebrovascular disease, that specify hemiplegia, hemiparesis and monoplegia identify whether the dominant or nondominant side is affected. Should the affected side be documented, but not specified as dominant or nondominant, and the classification system does not indicate a default, code selection is as follows:

- For ambidextrous patients, the default should be dominant.
- If the left side is affected, the default is non-dominant.
- If the right side is affected, the default is dominant.

2) Codes from category I69 with codes from I60–I67

Codes from category I69 may be assigned on a health care record with codes from I60-I67, if the patient has a current cerebrovascular disease and deficits from an old cerebrovascular disease.

3) Codes from category I69 and personal history of transient ischemic attack (TIA) and cerebral infarction (Z86.73)

Codes from category I69 should not be assigned if the patient does not have neurologic deficits.

See Section I.C.21. 4. History (of) for use of personal history codes

e. Acute myocardial infarction (AMI)

1) Type 1 ST elevation myocardial infarction (STEMI) and non-ST elevation myocardial infarction (NSTEMI)

The ICD-10-CM codes for type 1 acute myocardial infarction (AMI) identify the site, such as anterolateral wall or true posterior wall. Subcategories I21.0-I21.2 and code I21.3 are used for type 1 ST elevation myocardial infarction (STEMI). Code I21.4, Non-ST elevation (NSTEMI) myocardial infarction, is used for type 1 non ST elevation myocardial infarction (NSTEMI) and nontransmural MIs.

If a type 1 NSTEMI evolves to STEMI, assign the STEMI code. If a type 1 STEMI converts to NSTEMI due to thrombolytic therapy, it is still coded as STEMI.

For encounters occurring while the myocardial infarction is equal to, or less than, four weeks old, including transfers to another acute setting or a postacute setting, and the myocardial infarction meets the definition for "other diagnoses" (see Section III, Reporting Additional Diagnoses), codes from category I21 may continue to be reported. For encounters after the 4 week time frame and the patient is still receiving care related to the myocardial infarction, the appropriate aftercare code should be assigned, rather than a code from category I21. For old or healed myocardial infarctions not requiring further care, code I25.2, Old myocardial infarction, may be assigned.

2) Acute myocardial infarction, unspecified

Code I21.9, Acute myocardial infarction, unspecified, is the default for unspecified acute myocardial infarction or unspecified type. If only type 1 STEMI or transmural MI without the site is documented, assign code I21.3, ST elevation (STEMI) myocardial infarction of unspecified site.

3) AMI documented as nontransmural or subendocardial but site provided

If an AMI is documented as nontransmural or subendocardial, but the site is provided, it is still coded as a subendocardial AMI.

See Section I.C.21.3 for information on coding status post administration of tPA in a different facility within the last 24 hours.

> Acute inferior subendocardial myocardial infarction (NSTEMI)
>
> **I21.4   Non-ST elevation (NSTEMI) myocardial infarction**
>
> *Explanation*: An AMI documented as subendocardial or nontransmural is coded as such (I21.4, I22.2), even if the site of infarction is specified.

4) Subsequent acute myocardial infarction

A code from category I22, Subsequent ST elevation (STEMI) and non-ST elevation (NSTEMI) myocardial infarction, is to be used when a patient who has suffered a type 1 or unspecified AMI has a new AMI within the 4 week time frame of the initial AMI. A code from category I22 must be used in conjunction with a code from category I21. The sequencing of the I22 and I21 codes depends on the circumstances of the encounter.

Do not assign code I22 for subsequent myocardial infarctions other than type 1 or unspecified. For subsequent type 2 AMI assign only code I21.A1. For subsequent type 4 or type 5 AMI, assign only code I21.A9.

If a subsequent myocardial infarction of one type occurs within 4 weeks of a myocardial infarction of a different type, assign the appropriate codes from category I21 to identify each type. Do not assign a code from I22. Codes from category I22 should only be assigned if both the initial and subsequent myocardial infarctions are type 1 or unspecified.

5) Other Types of Myocardial Infarction

The ICD-10-CM provides codes for different types of myocardial infarction. Type 1 myocardial infarctions are assigned to codes I21.0-I21.4 **and I21.9.**

Type 2 myocardial infarction (myocardial infarction due to demand ischemia or secondary to ischemic balance) is assigned to code I21.A1, Myocardial infarction type 2 with a code for the underlying cause. Do not assign code I24.8, Other forms of acute ischemic heart disease for the demand ischemia. Sequencing of type 2 AMI or the underlying cause is dependent on the circumstances of admission. When a type 2 AMI code is described as NSTEMI or STEMI, only assign code I21.A1. Codes I21.01-I21.4 should only be assigned for type 1 AMIs.

Acute myocardial infarctions type 3, 4a, 4b, 4c and 5 are assigned to code I21.A9, Other myocardial infarction type.

The "Code also" and "Code first" notes should be followed related to complications, and for coding of postprocedural myocardial infarctions during or following cardiac surgery.

Chapter 9. Diseases of the Circulatory System (I00-I99)

EXCLUDES 2
certain conditions originating in the perinatal period (P04-P96)
certain infectious and parasitic diseases (A00-B99)
complications of pregnancy, childbirth and the puerperium (O00-O9A)
congenital malformations, deformations, and chromosomal abnormalities (Q00-Q99)
endocrine, nutritional and metabolic diseases (E00-E88)
injury, poisoning and certain other consequences of external causes (S00-T88)
neoplasms (C00-D49)
symptoms, signs and abnormal clinical and laboratory findings, not elsewhere classified (R00-R94)
systemic connective tissue disorders (M30-M36)
transient cerebral ischemic attacks and related syndromes (G45.-)

This chapter contains the following blocks:

I00-I02	Acute rheumatic fever
I05-I09	Chronic rheumatic heart diseases
I10-I16	Hypertensive diseases
I20-I25	Ischemic heart diseases
I26-I28	Pulmonary heart disease and diseases of pulmonary circulation
I30-I52	Other forms of heart disease
I60-I69	Cerebrovascular diseases
I70-I79	Diseases of arteries, arterioles and capillaries
I80-I89	Diseases of veins, lymphatic vessels and lymph nodes, not elsewhere classified
I95-I99	Other and unspecified disorders of the circulatory system

Acute rheumatic fever (I00-I02)

DEF: Inflammatory disease that can follow a throat infection by group A streptococci. Complications can involve the joints (arthritis), subcutaneous tissue (nodules), skin (erythema marginatum), heart (carditis), or brain (chorea).

I00 Rheumatic fever without heart involvement
    INCLUDES   arthritis, rheumatic, acute or subacute
    EXCLUDES 1   rheumatic fever with heart involvement (I01.0-I01.9)

✓4ᵗʰ I01 Rheumatic fever with heart involvement
    EXCLUDES 1   chronic diseases of rheumatic origin (I05-I09) unless rheumatic fever is also present or there is evidence of reactivation or activity of the rheumatic process

   I01.0 Acute rheumatic pericarditis
      Any condition in I00 with pericarditis
      Rheumatic pericarditis (acute)
      EXCLUDES 1   acute pericarditis not specified as rheumatic (I30.-)

   I01.1 Acute rheumatic endocarditis
      Any condition in I00 with endocarditis or valvulitis
      Acute rheumatic valvulitis

   I01.2 Acute rheumatic myocarditis
      Any condition in I00 with myocarditis

   I01.8 Other acute rheumatic heart disease
      Any condition in I00 with other or multiple types of heart involvement
      Acute rheumatic pancarditis

   I01.9 Acute rheumatic heart disease, unspecified   ▽
      Any condition in I00 with unspecified type of heart involvement
      Rheumatic carditis, acute
      Rheumatic heart disease, active or acute

✓4ᵗʰ I02 Rheumatic chorea
    INCLUDES   Sydenham's chorea
    EXCLUDES 1   chorea NOS (G25.5)
           Huntington's chorea (G10)

   I02.0 Rheumatic chorea with heart involvement
      Chorea NOS with heart involvement
      Rheumatic chorea with heart involvement of any type classifiable under I01.-

   I02.9 Rheumatic chorea without heart involvement
      Rheumatic chorea NOS

Chronic rheumatic heart diseases (I05-I09)

✓4ᵗʰ I05 Rheumatic mitral valve diseases
    INCLUDES   conditions classifiable to both I05.0 and I05.2-I05.9, whether specified as rheumatic or not
    EXCLUDES 1   mitral valve disease specified as nonrheumatic (I34.-)
           mitral valve disease with aortic and/or tricuspid valve involvement (I08.-)

   I05.0 Rheumatic mitral stenosis
      Mitral (valve) obstruction (rheumatic)
      DEF: Narrowing of the mitral valve between the left atrium and left ventricle due to rheumatic fever. Symptoms include shortness of breath during or after exercise, fatigue, palpitations, chest discomfort, and swelling of feet or legs.

   I05.1 Rheumatic mitral insufficiency
      Rheumatic mitral incompetence
      Rheumatic mitral regurgitation
      EXCLUDES 1   mitral insufficiency not specified as rheumatic (I34.0)

   I05.2 Rheumatic mitral stenosis with insufficiency
      Rheumatic mitral stenosis with incompetence or regurgitation

   I05.8 Other rheumatic mitral valve diseases
      Rheumatic mitral (valve) failure

   I05.9 Rheumatic mitral valve disease, unspecified   ▽
      Rheumatic mitral (valve) disorder (chronic) NOS

✓4ᵗʰ I06 Rheumatic aortic valve diseases
    EXCLUDES 1   aortic valve disease not specified as rheumatic (I35.-)
           aortic valve disease with mitral and/or tricuspid valve involvement (I08.-)

   I06.0 Rheumatic aortic stenosis
      Rheumatic aortic (valve) obstruction

   I06.1 Rheumatic aortic insufficiency
      Rheumatic aortic incompetence
      Rheumatic aortic regurgitation

   I06.2 Rheumatic aortic stenosis with insufficiency
      Rheumatic aortic stenosis with incompetence or regurgitation

   I06.8 Other rheumatic aortic valve diseases

   I06.9 Rheumatic aortic valve disease, unspecified   ▽
      Rheumatic aortic (valve) disease NOS

✓4ᵗʰ I07 Rheumatic tricuspid valve diseases
    INCLUDES   rheumatic tricuspid valve diseases specified as rheumatic or unspecified
    EXCLUDES 1   tricuspid valve disease specified as nonrheumatic (I36.-)
           tricuspid valve disease with aortic and/or mitral valve involvement (I08.-)

   I07.0 Rheumatic tricuspid stenosis
      Tricuspid (valve) stenosis (rheumatic)

   I07.1 Rheumatic tricuspid insufficiency
      Tricuspid (valve) insufficiency (rheumatic)

   I07.2 Rheumatic tricuspid stenosis and insufficiency

   I07.8 Other rheumatic tricuspid valve diseases

   I07.9 Rheumatic tricuspid valve disease, unspecified   ▽
      Rheumatic tricuspid valve disorder NOS

✓4ᵗʰ I08 Multiple valve diseases
    INCLUDES   multiple valve diseases specified as rheumatic or unspecified
    EXCLUDES 1   endocarditis, valve unspecified (I38)
           multiple valve disease specified a nonrheumatic (I34.-, I35.-, I36.-, I37.-, I38.-, Q22.-, Q23.-, Q24.8-)
           rheumatic valve disease NOS (I09.1)

   I08.0 Rheumatic disorders of both mitral and aortic valves
      Involvement of both mitral and aortic valves specified as rheumatic or unspecified

   I08.1 Rheumatic disorders of both mitral and tricuspid valves

   I08.2 Rheumatic disorders of both aortic and tricuspid valves

   I08.3 Combined rheumatic disorders of mitral, aortic and tricuspid valves

   I08.8 Other rheumatic multiple valve diseases

   I08.9 Rheumatic multiple valve disease, unspecified   ▽

✓4ᵗʰ I09 Other rheumatic heart diseases

   I09.0 Rheumatic myocarditis
      EXCLUDES 1   myocarditis not specified as rheumatic (I51.4)

☑ Additional Character Req   ✓x7ᵗʰ Placeholder Alert   Manifestation   ▽ Unspecified   ►◄ Revised Text   ● New Code   ▲ Revised Code Title

I09.1 Rheumatic diseases of endocardium, valve unspecified ▽
Rheumatic endocarditis (chronic)
Rheumatic valvulitis (chronic)
EXCLUDES 1 endocarditis, valve unspecified (I38)

I09.2 Chronic rheumatic pericarditis
Adherent pericardium, rheumatic
Chronic rheumatic mediastinopericarditis
Chronic rheumatic myopericarditis
EXCLUDES 1 chronic pericarditis not specified as rheumatic (I31.-)

✓5ᵗʰ **I09.8 Other specified rheumatic heart diseases**
I09.81 Rheumatic heart failure HCC
Use additional code to identify type of heart failure (I50.-)
DEF: Decreased cardiac output, edema, and hypertension due to rheumatic heart disease.
I09.89 Other specified rheumatic heart diseases
Rheumatic disease of pulmonary valve

I09.9 Rheumatic heart disease, unspecified ▽
Rheumatic carditis
EXCLUDES 1 rheumatoid carditis (M05.31)

Hypertensive diseases (I10-I16)

Use additional code to identify:
exposure to environmental tobacco smoke (Z77.22)
history of tobacco dependence (Z87.891)
occupational exposure to environmental tobacco smoke (Z57.31)
tobacco dependence (F17.-)
tobacco use (Z72.0)
EXCLUDES 1 neonatal hypertension (P29.2)
primary pulmonary hypertension (I27.0)
EXCLUDES 2 hypertensive disease complicating pregnancy, childbirth and the puerperium (O10-O11, O13-O16)

I10 Essential (primary) hypertension Q
INCLUDES high blood pressure
hypertension (arterial) (benign) (essential) (malignant) (primary) (systemic)
EXCLUDES 1 hypertensive disease complicating pregnancy, childbirth and the puerperium (O10-O11, O13-O16)
EXCLUDES 2 essential (primary) hypertension involving vessels of brain (I60-I69)
essential (primary) hypertension involving vessels of eye (H35.0-)
AHA: 2018,2Q,9; 2016,4Q,27

✓4ᵗʰ **I11 Hypertensive heart disease**
INCLUDES any condition in I50.-, I51.4-I51.9 due to hypertension
AHA: 2018,2Q,9
TIP: Do not assign a code from this category when provider documentation indicates the heart disease is attributable to another cause.
I11.0 Hypertensive heart disease with heart failure HCC
Hypertensive heart failure
Use additional code to identify type of heart failure (I50.-)
AHA: 2017,1Q,47
I11.9 Hypertensive heart disease without heart failure ▽
Hypertensive heart disease NOS

✓4ᵗʰ **I12 Hypertensive chronic kidney disease**
INCLUDES any condition in N18 and N26 - due to hypertension
arteriosclerosis of kidney
arteriosclerotic nephritis (chronic) (interstitial)
hypertensive nephropathy
nephrosclerosis
EXCLUDES 1 hypertension due to kidney disease (I15.0, I15.1)
renovascular hypertension (I15.0)
secondary hypertension (I15.-)
EXCLUDES 2 acute kidney failure (N17.-)
AHA: 2016,3Q,22
TIP: Do not assign a code from this category when provider documentation indicates the chronic kidney disease (CKD) is attributable to another cause.
I12.0 Hypertensive chronic kidney disease with stage 5 HCC **chronic kidney disease or end stage renal disease**
Use additional code to identify the stage of chronic kidney disease (N18.5, N18.6)

I12.9 Hypertensive chronic kidney disease with stage 1 ▽ **through stage 4 chronic kidney disease, or unspecified chronic kidney disease**
Hypertensive chronic kidney disease NOS
Hypertensive renal disease NOS
Use additional code to identify the stage of chronic kidney disease (N18.1-N18.4, N18.9)

✓4ᵗʰ **I13 Hypertensive heart and chronic kidney disease**
INCLUDES any condition in I11.- with any condition in I12.-
cardiorenal disease
cardiovascular renal disease
TIP: Do not assign a code from this category when provider documentation indicates the heart and/or chronic kidney disease is attributable to another cause.
I13.0 Hypertensive heart and chronic kidney disease with HCC **heart failure and stage 1 through stage 4 chronic kidney disease, or unspecified chronic kidney disease**
Use additional code to identify type of heart failure (I50.-)
Use additional code to identify stage of chronic kidney disease (N18.1-N18.4, N18.9)

✓5ᵗʰ **I13.1 Hypertensive heart and chronic kidney disease without heart failure**
I13.10 Hypertensive heart and chronic kidney ▽ **disease without heart failure, with stage 1 through stage 4 chronic kidney disease, or unspecified chronic kidney disease**
Hypertensive heart disease and hypertensive chronic kidney disease NOS
Use additional code to identify the stage of chronic kidney disease (N18.1-N18.4, N18.9)
I13.11 Hypertensive heart and chronic kidney HCC **disease without heart failure, with stage 5 chronic kidney disease, or end stage renal disease**
Use additional code to identify the stage of chronic kidney disease (N18.5, N18.6)
I13.2 Hypertensive heart and chronic kidney disease with HCC **heart failure and with stage 5 chronic kidney disease, or end stage renal disease**
Use additional code to identify type of heart failure (I50.-)
Use additional code to identify the stage of chronic kidney disease (N18.5, N18.6)

✓4ᵗʰ **I15 Secondary hypertension**
Code also underlying condition
EXCLUDES 1 postprocedural hypertension (I97.3)
EXCLUDES 2 secondary hypertension involving vessels of brain (I60-I69)
secondary hypertension involving vessels of eye (H35.0-)
I15.0 Renovascular hypertension
I15.1 Hypertension secondary to other renal disorders
AHA: 2016,3Q,22
I15.2 Hypertension secondary to endocrine disorders
I15.8 Other secondary hypertension
I15.9 Secondary hypertension, unspecified ▽

✓4ᵗʰ **I16 Hypertensive crisis**
Code also any identified hypertensive disease (I10-I15)
AHA: 2016,4Q,26-28
I16.0 Hypertensive urgency
I16.1 Hypertensive emergency
I16.9 Hypertensive crisis, unspecified ▽

Ischemic heart diseases (I20-I25)

Use additional code to identify presence of hypertension (I10-I16)

✓4ᵗʰ I20 Angina pectoris

Use additional code to identify:
exposure to environmental tobacco smoke (Z77.22)
history of tobacco dependence (Z87.891)
occupational exposure to environmental tobacco smoke (Z57.31)
tobacco dependence (F17.-)
tobacco use (Z72.0)

EXCLUDES 1   angina pectoris with atherosclerotic heart disease of native coronary arteries (I25.1-)
atherosclerosis of coronary artery bypass graft(s) and coronary artery of transplanted heart with angina pectoris (I25.7-)
postinfarction angina (I23.7)

DEF: Chest pain due to reduced blood flow resulting in a lack of oxygen to the heart muscles.

I20.0   Unstable angina   HCC Q
Accelerated angina
Crescendo angina
De novo effort angina
Intermediate coronary syndrome
Preinfarction syndrome
Worsening effort angina
DEF: Condition representing an intermediate stage between angina of effort and acute myocardial infarction.

I20.1   Angina pectoris with documented spasm   HCC
Angiospastic angina
Prinzmetal angina
Spasm-induced angina
Variant angina

I20.8   Other forms of angina pectoris   HCC Q
Angina equivalent
Angina of effort
Coronary slow flow syndrome
Stable angina
Stenocardia
Use additional code(s) for symptoms associated with angina equivalent

I20.9   Angina pectoris, unspecified   HCC Q ▽
Angina NOS
Anginal syndrome
Cardiac angina
Ischemic chest pain

✓4ᵗʰ I21 Acute myocardial infarction

INCLUDES   cardiac infarction
coronary (artery) embolism
coronary (artery) occlusion
coronary (artery) rupture
coronary (artery) thrombosis
infarction of heart, myocardium, or ventricle
myocardial infarction specified as acute or with a stated duration of 4 weeks (28 days) or less from onset

Use additional code, if applicable, to identify:
exposure to environmental tobacco smoke (Z77.22)
history of tobacco dependence (Z87.891)
occupational exposure to environmental tobacco smoke (Z57.31)
status post administration of tPA (rtPA) in a different facility within the last 24 hours prior to admission to current facility (Z92.82)
tobacco dependence (F17.-)
tobacco use (Z72.0)

EXCLUDES 2   old myocardial infarction (I25.2)
postmyocardial infarction syndrome (I24.1)
subsequent type 1 myocardial infarction (I22.-)

AHA: 2017,4Q,12-14; 2017,1Q,44-45; 2016,4Q,140; 2015,2Q,16; 2013,1Q,25; 2012,4Q,96,102-103

✓5ᵗʰ I21.0   ST elevation (STEMI) myocardial infarction of anterior wall
Type 1 ST elevation myocardial infarction of anterior wall
DEF: ST elevation myocardial infarction: Complete obstruction of one or more coronary arteries causing decreased blood flow (ischemia) and necrosis of myocardial muscle cells.

I21.01   ST elevation (STEMI) myocardial infarction   HCC Q
involving left main coronary artery

I21.02   ST elevation (STEMI) myocardial infarction   HCC Q
involving left anterior descending coronary artery
ST elevation (STEMI) myocardial infarction involving diagonal coronary artery
AHA: 2013,1Q,25

I21.09   ST elevation (STEMI) myocardial infarction   HCC Q
involving other coronary artery of anterior wall
Acute transmural myocardial infarction of anterior wall
Anteroapical transmural (Q wave) infarction (acute)
Anterolateral transmural (Q wave) infarction (acute)
Anteroseptal transmural (Q wave) infarction (acute)
Transmural (Q wave) infarction (acute) (of) anterior (wall) NOS
AHA: 2012,4Q,102-103

✓5ᵗʰ I21.1   ST elevation (STEMI) myocardial infarction of inferior wall
Type 1 ST elevation myocardial infarction of inferior wall
DEF: ST elevation myocardial infarction: Complete obstruction of one or more coronary arteries causing decreased blood flow (ischemia) and necrosis of myocardial muscle cells.

I21.11   ST elevation (STEMI) myocardial infarction   HCC Q
involving right coronary artery
Inferoposterior transmural (Q wave) infarction (acute)

I21.19   ST elevation (STEMI) myocardial infarction   HCC Q
involving other coronary artery of inferior wall
Acute transmural myocardial infarction of inferior wall
Inferolateral transmural (Q wave) infarction (acute)
Transmural (Q wave) infarction (acute) (of) diaphragmatic wall
Transmural (Q wave) infarction (acute) (of) inferior (wall) NOS
EXCLUDES 2   ST elevation (STEMI) myocardial infarction involving left circumflex coronary artery (I21.21)
AHA: 2012,4Q,96

✓5ᵗʰ I21.2   ST elevation (STEMI) myocardial infarction of other sites
Type 1 ST elevation myocardial infarction of other sites
DEF: ST elevation myocardial infarction: Complete obstruction of one or more coronary arteries causing decreased blood flow (ischemia) and necrosis of myocardial muscle cells.

I21.21   ST elevation (STEMI) myocardial infarction   HCC Q
involving left circumflex coronary artery
ST elevation (STEMI) myocardial infarction involving oblique marginal coronary artery

I21.29   ST elevation (STEMI) myocardial infarction   HCC Q
involving other sites
Acute transmural myocardial infarction of other sites
Apical-lateral transmural (Q wave) infarction (acute)
Basal-lateral transmural (Q wave) infarction (acute)
High lateral transmural (Q wave) infarction (acute)
Lateral (wall) NOS transmural (Q wave) infarction (acute)
Posterior (true) transmural (Q wave) infarction (acute)
Posterobasal transmural (Q wave) infarction (acute)
Posterolateral transmural (Q wave) infarction (acute)
Posteroseptal transmural (Q wave) infarction (acute)
Septal transmural (Q wave) infarction (acute) NOS

I21.3   ST elevation (STEMI) myocardial infarction of unspecified site   HCC Q ▽
Acute transmural myocardial infarction of unspecified site
Transmural (Q wave) myocardial infarction NOS
Type 1 ST elevation myocardial infarction of unspecified site
DEF: ST elevation myocardial infarction: Complete obstruction of one or more coronary arteries causing decreased blood flow (ischemia) and necrosis of myocardial muscle cells.

I21.4   Non-ST elevation (NSTEMI) myocardial infarction   HCC Q
Acute subendocardial myocardial infarction
Non-Q wave myocardial infarction NOS
Nontransmural myocardial infarction NOS
Type 1 non-ST elevation myocardial infarction
AHA: 2017,1Q,44-45
DEF: Partial obstruction of one or more coronary arteries that causes decreased blood flow (ischemia) and may cause partial thickness necrosis of myocardial muscle cells.

✔ Additional Character Req   ✓x7ᵗʰ Placeholder Alert   Manifestation   ▽ Unspecified   ►◄ Revised Text   ● New Code   ▲ Revised Code Title

ICD-10-CM 2019   635

I21.9   **Acute myocardial infarction, unspecified**   HCC ▽
Myocardial infarction (acute) NOS

✓5ᵗʰ **I21.A**   **Other type of myocardial infarction**

I21.A1   **Myocardial infarction type 2**   HCC
Myocardial infarction due to demand ischemia
Myocardial infarction secondary to ischemic
imbalance
Code also the underlying cause, if known and
applicable, such as:
anemia (D50.0-D64.9)
chronic obstructive pulmonary disease (J44.-)
heart failure (I50.-)
paroxysmal tachycardia (I47.0-I47.9)
renal failure (N17.0-N19)
shock (R57.0-R57.9)
AHA: 2017,4Q,13-14
DEF: Often referred to as due to demand ischemia,
myocardial infarction (MI) type 2 refers to an MI due to
ischemia and necrosis resulting from an oxygen
imbalance to the heart. This mismatch between oxygen
decreased supply and increased demand is caused by
conditions other than coronary artery disease such as
vasospasm, embolism, anemia, hypertension,
hypotension, or arrhythmias.

I21.A9   **Other myocardial infarction type**   HCC
Myocardial infarction associated with
revascularization procedure
Myocardial infarction type 3
Myocardial infarction type 4a
Myocardial infarction type 4b
Myocardial infarction type 4c
Myocardial infarction type 5
Code first, if applicable, postprocedural myocardial
infarction following cardiac surgery (I97.190), or
postprocedural myocardial infarction during
cardiac surgery (I97.790)
Code also complication, if known and applicable, such
as:
(acute) stent occlusion (T82.897-)
(acute) stent stenosis (T82.857-)
(acute) stent thrombosis (T82.867-)
cardiac arrest due to underlying cardiac condition
(I46.2)
complication of percutaneous coronary intervention
(PCI) (I97.89)
occlusion of coronary artery bypass graft (T82.218-)

✓4ᵗʰ **I22**   **Subsequent ST elevation (STEMI) and non-ST elevation (NSTEMI) myocardial infarction**

INCLUDES   acute myocardial infarction occurring within four weeks
(28 days) of a previous acute myocardial infarction,
regardless of site
cardiac infarction
coronary (artery) embolism
coronary (artery) occlusion
coronary (artery) rupture
coronary (artery) thrombosis
infarction of heart, myocardium, or ventricle
recurrent myocardial infarction
reinfarction of myocardium
rupture of heart, myocardium, or ventricle
subsequent type 1 myocardial infarction
Use additional code, if applicable, to identify:
exposure to environmental tobacco smoke (Z77.22)
history of tobacco dependence (Z87.891)
occupational exposure to environmental tobacco smoke (Z57.31)
status post administration of tPA (rtPA) in a different facility within
the last 24 hours prior to admission to current facility (Z92.82)
tobacco dependence (F17.-)
tobacco use (Z72.0)
EXCLUDES 1   subsequent myocardial infarction, type 2 (I21.A1)
subsequent myocardial infarction of other type (type 3) (type
4) (type 5) (I21.A9)
AHA: 2017,4Q,12-13; 2017,2Q,11; 2013,1Q,25; 2012,4Q,97,102-103
DEF: ST elevation myocardial infarction: Complete obstruction of one or
more coronary arteries causing decreased blood flow (ischemia) and
necrosis of myocardial muscle cells.
DEF: Non-ST elevation myocardial infarction: Partial obstruction of one
or more coronary arteries that causes decreased blood flow (ischemia)
and may cause partial thickness necrosis of myocardial muscle cells.

I22.0   **Subsequent ST elevation (STEMI) myocardial**   HCC
infarction of anterior wall
Subsequent acute transmural myocardial infarction of anterior
wall
Subsequent transmural (Q wave) infarction (acute)(of) anterior
(wall) NOS
Subsequent anteroapical transmural (Q wave) infarction (acute)
Subsequent anterolateral transmural (Q wave) infarction (acute)
Subsequent anteroseptal transmural (Q wave) infarction (acute)

I22.1   **Subsequent ST elevation (STEMI) myocardial**   HCC
infarction of inferior wall
Subsequent acute transmural myocardial infarction of inferior
wall
Subsequent transmural (Q wave) infarction (acute)(of)
diaphragmatic wall
Subsequent transmural (Q wave) infarction (acute)(of) inferior
(wall) NOS
Subsequent inferolateral transmural (Q wave) infarction (acute)
Subsequent inferoposterior transmural (Q wave) infarction
(acute)
AHA: 2012,4Q,102

I22.2   **Subsequent non-ST elevation (NSTEMI) myocardial**   HCC
infarction
Subsequent acute subendocardial myocardial infarction
Subsequent non-Q wave myocardial infarction NOS
Subsequent nontransmural myocardial infarction NOS

I22.8 **Subsequent ST elevation (STEMI) myocardial infarction of other sites** `HCC`

Subsequent acute transmural myocardial infarction of other sites

Subsequent apical-lateral transmural (Q wave) myocardial infarction (acute)

Subsequent basal-lateral transmural (Q wave) myocardial infarction (acute)

Subsequent high lateral transmural (Q wave) myocardial infarction (acute)

Subsequent transmural (Q wave) myocardial infarction (acute)(of) lateral (wall) NOS

Subsequent posterior (true) transmural (Q wave) myocardial infarction (acute)

Subsequent posterobasal transmural (Q wave) myocardial infarction (acute)

Subsequent posterolateral transmural (Q wave) myocardial infarction (acute)

Subsequent posteroseptal transmural (Q wave) myocardial infarction (acute)

Subsequent septal NOS transmural (Q wave) myocardial infarction (acute)

I22.9 **Subsequent ST elevation (STEMI) myocardial infarction of unspecified site** `HCC` ▽

Subsequent acute myocardial infarction of unspecified site

Subsequent myocardial infarction (acute) NOS

✓4th **I23** **Certain current complications following ST elevation (STEMI) and non-ST elevation (NSTEMI) myocardial infarction (within the 28 day period)**

AHA: 2017,2Q,11

DEF: ST elevation myocardial infarction: Complete obstruction of one or more coronary arteries causing decreased blood flow (ischemia) and necrosis of myocardial muscle cells.

DEF: Non-ST elevation myocardial infarction: Partial obstruction of one or more coronary arteries that causes decreased blood flow (ischemia) and may cause partial thickness necrosis of myocardial muscle cells.

I23.0 **Hemopericardium as current complication following acute myocardial infarction** `HCC` `A`

EXCLUDES 1   *hemopericardium not specified as current complication following acute myocardial infarction (I31.2)*

I23.1 **Atrial septal defect as current complication following acute myocardial infarction** `HCC` `A`

EXCLUDES 1   *acquired atrial septal defect not specified as current complication following acute myocardial infarction (I51.0)*

I23.2 **Ventricular septal defect as current complication following acute myocardial infarction** `HCC` `A`

EXCLUDES 1   *acquired ventricular septal defect not specified as current complication following acute myocardial infarction (I51.0)*

I23.3 **Rupture of cardiac wall without hemopericardium as current complication following acute myocardial infarction** `HCC` `A`

I23.4 **Rupture of chordae tendineae as current complication following acute myocardial infarction** `HCC`

EXCLUDES 1   *rupture of chordae tendineae not specified as current complication following acute myocardial infarction (I51.1)*

I23.5 **Rupture of papillary muscle as current complication following acute myocardial infarction** `HCC`

EXCLUDES 1   *rupture of papillary muscle not specified as current complication following acute myocardial infarction (I51.2)*

I23.6 **Thrombosis of atrium, auricular appendage, and ventricle as current complications following acute myocardial infarction** `HCC` `A`

EXCLUDES 1   *thrombosis of atrium, auricular appendage, and ventricle not specified as current complication following acute myocardial infarction (I51.3)*

I23.7 **Postinfarction angina** `HCC` `A`

AHA: 2015,2Q,16

I23.8 **Other current complications following acute myocardial infarction** `HCC` `A`

✓4th **I24** **Other acute ischemic heart diseases**

EXCLUDES 1   *angina pectoris (I20.-)*

transient myocardial ischemia in newborn (P29.4)

I24.0 **Acute coronary thrombosis not resulting in myocardial infarction** `HCC` `0`

Acute coronary (artery) (vein) embolism not resulting in myocardial infarction

Acute coronary (artery) (vein) occlusion not resulting in myocardial infarction

Acute coronary (artery) (vein) thromboembolism not resulting in myocardial infarction

EXCLUDES 1   *atherosclerotic heart disease (I25.1-)*

AHA: 2013,1Q,24

I24.1 **Dressler's syndrome** `HCC`

Postmyocardial infarction syndrome

EXCLUDES 1   *postinfarction angina (I23.7)*

DEF: Fever, leukocytosis, chest pain, evidence of pericarditis, pleurisy, and pneumonia occurring days or weeks after a myocardial infarction.

I24.8 **Other forms of acute ischemic heart disease** `HCC` `0`

EXCLUDES 1   *myocardial infarction due to demand ischemia (I21.A1)*

AHA: 2017,4Q,13

I24.9 **Acute ischemic heart disease, unspecified** `HCC` `0` ▽

EXCLUDES 1   *ischemic heart disease (chronic) NOS (I25.9)*

✓4th **I25** **Chronic ischemic heart disease**

Use additional code to identify:

chronic total occlusion of coronary artery (I25.82)

exposure to environmental tobacco smoke (Z77.22)

history of tobacco dependence (Z87.891)

occupational exposure to environmental tobacco smoke (Z57.31)

tobacco dependence (F17.-)

tobacco use (Z72.0)

✓5th **I25.1** **Atherosclerotic heart disease of native coronary artery**

Atherosclerotic cardiovascular disease

Coronary (artery) atheroma

Coronary (artery) atherosclerosis

Coronary (artery) disease

Coronary (artery) sclerosis

Use additional code, if applicable, to identify:

coronary atherosclerosis due to calcified coronary lesion (I25.84)

coronary atherosclerosis due to lipid rich plaque (I25.83)

EXCLUDES 2   *atheroembolism (I75.-)*

atherosclerosis of coronary artery bypass graft(s) and transplanted heart (I25.7-)

Atheromas

Atheromas (fatty tissue and/or plaque)   Lumen

I25.10 **Atherosclerotic heart disease of native coronary artery without angina pectoris** `0` `A` ▽

Atherosclerotic heart disease NOS

AHA: 2015,2Q,16; 2012,4Q,92

✓6th **I25.11** **Atherosclerotic heart disease of native coronary artery with angina pectoris**

I25.110 **Atherosclerotic heart disease of native coronary artery with unstable angina pectoris** `HCC` `0` `A`

EXCLUDES 1   *unstable angina without atherosclerotic heart disease (I20.0)*

☑ Additional Character Req   ✓×7th Placeholder Alert   Manifestation   ▽ Unspecified   ▶◀ Revised Text   ● New Code   ▲ Revised Code Title

ICD-10-CM 2019   637

Chapter 9. Diseases of the Circulatory System

I25.111   **Atherosclerotic heart disease of** HCC Q A **native coronary artery with angina pectoris with documented spasm**
> *EXCLUDES 1*   *angina pectoris with documented spasm without atherosclerotic heart disease (I20.1)*

I25.118   **Atherosclerotic heart disease of** HCC Q A **native coronary artery with other forms of angina pectoris**
> *EXCLUDES 1*   *other forms of angina pectoris without atherosclerotic heart disease (I20.8)*

> **AHA:** 2015,2Q,16

I25.119   **Atherosclerotic heart disease of** HCC Q A ▽ **native coronary artery with unspecified angina pectoris**
> Atherosclerotic heart disease with angina NOS
> Atherosclerotic heart disease with ischemic chest pain
> *EXCLUDES 1*   *unspecified angina pectoris without atherosclerotic heart disease (I20.9)*

I25.2   Old myocardial infarction
> Healed myocardial infarction
> Past myocardial infarction diagnosed by ECG or other investigation, but currently presenting no symptoms

I25.3   Aneurysm of heart
> Mural aneurysm
> Ventricular aneurysm

√5ᵗʰ **I25.4   Coronary artery aneurysm and dissection**

I25.41   **Coronary artery aneurysm**
> Coronary arteriovenous fistula, acquired
> *EXCLUDES 1*   *congenital coronary (artery) aneurysm (Q24.5)*

I25.42   **Coronary artery dissection**
> **DEF:** Tear in the intimal arterial wall of a coronary artery resulting in the sudden intrusion of blood within the layers of the wall.

I25.5   Ischemic cardiomyopathy   Q
> *EXCLUDES 2*   *coronary atherosclerosis (I25.1-, I25.7-)*

I25.6   Silent myocardial ischemia   Q

√5ᵗʰ **I25.7   Atherosclerosis of coronary artery bypass graft(s) and coronary artery of transplanted heart with angina pectoris**
> Use additional code, if applicable, to identify:
> coronary atherosclerosis due to calcified coronary lesion (I25.84)
> coronary atherosclerosis due to lipid rich plaque (I25.83)
> *EXCLUDES 1*   *atherosclerosis of bypass graft(s) of transplanted heart without angina pectoris (I25.812)*
> *atherosclerosis of coronary artery bypass graft(s) without angina pectoris (I25.810)*
> *atherosclerosis of native coronary artery of transplanted heart without angina pectoris (I25.811)*

√6ᵗʰ I25.70   **Atherosclerosis of coronary artery bypass graft(s), unspecified, with angina pectoris**

I25.700   **Atherosclerosis of coronary** HCC Q A ▽ **artery bypass graft(s), unspecified, with unstable angina pectoris**
> *EXCLUDES 1*   *unstable angina pectoris without atherosclerosis of coronary artery bypass graft (I20.0)*

I25.701   **Atherosclerosis of coronary** HCC Q A ▽ **artery bypass graft(s), unspecified, with angina pectoris with documented spasm**
> *EXCLUDES 1*   *angina pectoris with documented spasm without atherosclerosis of coronary artery bypass graft (I20.1)*

I25.708   **Atherosclerosis of coronary** HCC Q A ▽ **artery bypass graft(s), unspecified, with other forms of angina pectoris**
> *EXCLUDES 1*   *other forms of angina pectoris without atherosclerosis of coronary artery bypass graft (I20.8)*

I25.709   **Atherosclerosis of coronary** HCC Q A ▽ **artery bypass graft(s), unspecified, with unspecified angina pectoris**
> *EXCLUDES 1*   *unspecified angina pectoris without atherosclerosis of coronary artery bypass graft (I20.9)*

√6ᵗʰ I25.71   **Atherosclerosis of autologous vein coronary artery bypass graft(s) with angina pectoris**

I25.710   **Atherosclerosis of autologous** HCC Q A **vein coronary artery bypass graft(s) with unstable angina pectoris**
> *EXCLUDES 1*   *unstable angina without atherosclerosis of autologous vein coronary artery bypass graft(s) (I20.0)*
> *EXCLUDES 2*   *embolism or thrombus of coronary artery bypass graft(s) (T82.8-)*

I25.711   **Atherosclerosis of autologous** HCC Q A **vein coronary artery bypass graft(s) with angina pectoris with documented spasm**
> *EXCLUDES 1*   *angina pectoris with documented spasm without atherosclerosis of autologous vein coronary artery bypass graft(s) (I20.1)*

I25.718   **Atherosclerosis of autologous** HCC Q A **vein coronary artery bypass graft(s) with other forms of angina pectoris**
> *EXCLUDES 1*   *other forms of angina pectoris without atherosclerosis of autologous vein coronary artery bypass graft(s) (I20.8)*

I25.719   **Atherosclerosis of autologous** HCC Q A ▽ **vein coronary artery bypass graft(s) with unspecified angina pectoris**
> *EXCLUDES 1*   *unspecified angina pectoris without atherosclerosis of autologous vein coronary artery bypass graft(s) (I20.9)*

√6ᵗʰ I25.72   **Atherosclerosis of autologous artery coronary artery bypass graft(s) with angina pectoris**
> Atherosclerosis of internal mammary artery graft with angina pectoris

I25.720   **Atherosclerosis of autologous** HCC Q A **artery coronary artery bypass graft(s) with unstable angina pectoris**
> *EXCLUDES 1*   *unstable angina without atherosclerosis of autologous artery coronary artery bypass graft(s) (I20.0)*

I25.721 **Atherosclerosis of autologous** `HCC` `Q` `A`
**artery coronary artery bypass
graft(s) with documented spasm**
> *EXCLUDES 1*   *angina pectoris with
> documented spasm
> without atherosclerosis of
> autologous artery
> coronary artery bypass
> graft(s) (I20.1)*

I25.728 **Atherosclerosis of autologous** `HCC` `Q` `A`
**artery coronary artery bypass
graft(s) with other forms of
angina pectoris**
> *EXCLUDES 1*   *other forms of angina pectoris
> without atherosclerosis of
> autologous artery
> coronary artery bypass
> graft(s) (I20.8)*

I25.729 **Atherosclerosis of autologous** `HCC` `Q` `A` `▽`
**artery coronary artery bypass
graft(s) with unspecified angina
pectoris**
> *EXCLUDES 1*   *unspecified angina pectoris
> without atherosclerosis of
> autologous artery
> coronary artery bypass
> graft(s) (I20.9)*

`√6ᵗʰ` **I25.73 Atherosclerosis of nonautologous biological
coronary artery bypass graft(s) with angina pectoris**

I25.730 **Atherosclerosis of** `HCC` `Q` `A`
**nonautologous biological
coronary artery bypass graft(s)
with unstable angina pectoris**
> *EXCLUDES 1*   *unstable angina without
> atherosclerosis of
> nonautologous biological
> coronary artery bypass
> graft(s) (I20.0)*

I25.731 **Atherosclerosis of** `HCC` `Q` `A`
**nonautologous biological
coronary artery bypass graft(s)
with angina pectoris with
documented spasm**
> *EXCLUDES 1*   *angina pectoris with
> documented spasm
> without atherosclerosis of
> nonautologous biological
> coronary artery bypass
> graft(s) (I20.1)*

I25.738 **Atherosclerosis of** `HCC` `Q` `A`
**nonautologous biological
coronary artery bypass graft(s)
with other forms of angina
pectoris**
> *EXCLUDES 1*   *other forms of angina pectoris
> without atherosclerosis of
> nonautologous biological
> coronary artery bypass
> graft(s) (I20.8)*

I25.739 **Atherosclerosis of** `HCC` `Q` `A` `▽`
**nonautologous biological
coronary artery bypass graft(s)
with unspecified angina
pectoris**
> *EXCLUDES 1*   *unspecified angina pectoris
> without atherosclerosis of
> nonautologous biological
> coronary artery bypass
> graft(s) (I20.9)*

`√6ᵗʰ` **I25.75 Atherosclerosis of native coronary artery of
transplanted heart with angina pectoris**
> *EXCLUDES 1*   *atherosclerosis of native coronary artery
> of transplanted heart without angina
> pectoris (I25.811)*

I25.750 **Atherosclerosis of native** `HCC` `Q`
**coronary artery of transplanted
heart with unstable angina**

I25.751 **Atherosclerosis of native** `HCC` `Q`
**coronary artery of transplanted
heart with angina pectoris with
documented spasm**

I25.758 **Atherosclerosis of native** `HCC` `Q`
**coronary artery of transplanted
heart with other forms of
angina pectoris**

I25.759 **Atherosclerosis of native** `HCC` `Q` `▽`
**coronary artery of transplanted
heart with unspecified angina
pectoris**

`√6ᵗʰ` **I25.76 Atherosclerosis of bypass graft of coronary artery
of transplanted heart with angina pectoris**
> *EXCLUDES 1*   *atherosclerosis of bypass graft of coronary
> artery of transplanted heart without
> angina pectoris (I25.812)*

I25.760 **Atherosclerosis of bypass graft** `HCC` `Q` `A`
**of coronary artery of
transplanted heart with
unstable angina**

I25.761 **Atherosclerosis of bypass graft** `HCC` `Q` `A`
**of coronary artery of
transplanted heart with angina
pectoris with documented
spasm**

I25.768 **Atherosclerosis of bypass graft** `HCC` `Q` `A`
**of coronary artery of
transplanted heart with other
forms of angina pectoris**

I25.769 **Atherosclerosis of bypass graft** `HCC` `Q` `A` `▽`
**of coronary artery of
transplanted heart with
unspecified angina pectoris**

`√6ᵗʰ` **I25.79 Atherosclerosis of other coronary artery bypass
graft(s) with angina pectoris**

I25.790 **Atherosclerosis of other** `HCC` `Q` `A`
**coronary artery bypass graft(s)
with unstable angina pectoris**
> *EXCLUDES 1*   *unstable angina without
> atherosclerosis of other
> coronary artery bypass
> graft(s) (I20.0)*

I25.791 **Atherosclerosis of other** `HCC` `Q` `A`
**coronary artery bypass graft(s)
with angina pectoris with
documented spasm**
> *EXCLUDES 1*   *angina pectoris with
> documented spasm
> without atherosclerosis of
> other coronary artery
> bypass graft(s) (I20.1)*

I25.798 **Atherosclerosis of other** `HCC` `Q` `A`
**coronary artery bypass graft(s)
with other forms of angina
pectoris**
> *EXCLUDES 1*   *other forms of angina pectoris
> without atherosclerosis of
> other coronary artery
> bypass graft(s) (I20.8)*

I25.799 **Atherosclerosis of other** `HCC` `Q` `A` `▽`
**coronary artery bypass graft(s)
with unspecified angina
pectoris**
> *EXCLUDES 1*   *unspecified angina pectoris
> without atherosclerosis of
> other coronary artery
> bypass graft(s) (I20.9)*

☑ Additional Character Req   `√x7ᵗʰ` Placeholder Alert   Manifestation   ▽ Unspecified   ►◄ Revised Text   ● New Code   ▲ Revised Code Title

ICD-10-CM 2019   **639**

✓5ᵗʰ **I25.8   Other forms of chronic ischemic heart disease**

    ✓6ᵗʰ **I25.81   Atherosclerosis of other coronary vessels** without angina pectoris

        Use additional code, if applicable, to identify:
            coronary atherosclerosis due to calcified coronary lesion (I25.84)
            coronary atherosclerosis due to lipid rich plaque (I25.83)

        EXCLUDES 1   atherosclerotic heart disease of native coronary artery without angina pectoris (I25.10)

        I25.810   Atherosclerosis of coronary artery bypass graft(s) without angina pectoris Q A

            Atherosclerosis of coronary artery bypass graft NOS

            EXCLUDES 1 atherosclerosis of coronary bypass graft(s) with angina pectoris (I25.70-I25.73-, I25.79-)

        I25.811   Atherosclerosis of native **coronary artery of** transplanted **heart without angina pectoris** Q

            Atherosclerosis of native coronary artery of transplanted heart NOS

            EXCLUDES 1 atherosclerosis of native coronary artery of transplanted heart with angina pectoris (I25.75-)

        I25.812   Atherosclerosis of bypass graft of coronary artery of transplanted heart without **angina pectoris** Q A

            Atherosclerosis of bypass graft of transplanted heart NOS

            EXCLUDES 1 atherosclerosis of bypass graft of transplanted heart with angina pectoris (I25.76)

    I25.82   Chronic total occlusion of coronary artery Q

        Complete occlusion of coronary artery
        Total occlusion of coronary artery
        Code first coronary atherosclerosis (I25.1-, I25.7-, I25.81-)

        EXCLUDES 1 acute coronary occlusion with myocardial infarction (I21.0-I21.9, I22.-)
                acute coronary occlusion without myocardial infarction (I24.0)

        DEF: Complete blockage of the coronary artery due to plaque accumulation over an extended period of time, resulting in substantial reduction of blood flow. Symptoms include angina or chest pain.

    I25.83   Coronary atherosclerosis due to lipid rich plaque Q A

        Code first coronary atherosclerosis (I25.1-, I25.7-, I25.81-)

    I25.84   Coronary atherosclerosis due to calcified coronary lesion Q

        Coronary atherosclerosis due to severely calcified coronary lesion
        Code first coronary atherosclerosis (I25.1-, I25.7-, I25.81-)

    I25.89   Other forms of chronic ischemic heart disease Q

I25.9   Chronic ischemic heart disease, unspecified Q ▽

    Ischemic heart disease (chronic) NOS

Pulmonary heart disease and diseases of pulmonary circulation (I26-I28)

✓4ᵗʰ **I26   Pulmonary embolism**

  INCLUDES pulmonary (acute)(artery)(vein) infarction
          pulmonary (acute) (artery)(vein) thromboembolism
          pulmonary (acute)(artery)(vein) thrombosis

  EXCLUDES 2 chronic pulmonary embolism (I27.82)
          personal history of pulmonary embolism (Z86.711)
          pulmonary embolism complicating abortion, ectopic or molar pregnancy (O00-O07, O08.2)
          pulmonary embolism complicating pregnancy, childbirth and the puerperium (O88.-)
          pulmonary embolism due to trauma (T79.0, T79.1)
          pulmonary embolism due to complications of surgical and medical care (T80.0, T81.7-, T82.8-)
          septic (non-pulmonary) arterial embolism (I76)

  ✓5ᵗʰ **I26.0   Pulmonary embolism** with acute cor pulmonale

        I26.01   Septic pulmonary embolism with acute cor pulmonale HCC

            Code first underlying infection

        I26.02   Saddle embolus of pulmonary artery with acute cor pulmonale HCC

        I26.09   Other pulmonary embolism with acute cor pulmonale HCC

            Acute cor pulmonale NOS
            AHA: 2014,4Q,21

  ✓5ᵗʰ **I26.9   Pulmonary embolism** without acute cor pulmonale

        I26.90   Septic pulmonary embolism without acute cor pulmonale HCC

            Code first underlying infection

        I26.92   Saddle embolus of pulmonary artery without acute cor pulmonale HCC

        I26.99   Other pulmonary embolism without acute cor pulmonale HCC

            Acute pulmonary embolism NOS
            Pulmonary embolism NOS

✓4ᵗʰ **I27   Other pulmonary heart diseases**

  I27.0   Primary pulmonary hypertension HCC

      Heritable pulmonary arterial hypertension
      Idiopathic pulmonary arterial hypertension
      Primary group 1 pulmonary hypertension
      Primary pulmonary arterial hypertension

      EXCLUDES 1 persistent pulmonary hypertension of newborn (P29.30)
             pulmonary hypertension NOS (I27.20)
             secondary pulmonary arterial hypertension (I27.21)
             secondary pulmonary hypertension (I27.29)

      DEF: Condition that occurs when pressure within the pulmonary artery is elevated and vascular resistance is observed in the lungs.

  I27.1   Kyphoscoliotic heart disease HCC

  ✓5ᵗʰ **I27.2   Other secondary pulmonary hypertension**

      Code also associated underlying condition

      EXCLUDES 1 Eisenmenger's syndrome (I27.83)

      AHA: 2017,4Q,14-15; 2014,4Q,21

      DEF: Condition that occurs when pressure within the pulmonary artery is elevated and vascular resistance is observed in the lungs.

      I27.20   Pulmonary hypertension, unspecified HCC ▽

          Pulmonary hypertension NOS

I27.21   **Secondary pulmonary arterial hypertension**   `HCC`
(Associated) (drug-induced) (toxin-induced) pulmonary arterial hypertension NOS
(Associated) (drug-induced) (toxin-induced) (secondary) group 1 pulmonary hypertension
Code also associated conditions if applicable, or adverse effects of drugs or toxins, such as:
adverse effect of appetite depressants (T50.5X5)
congenital heart disease (Q20-Q28)
human immunodeficiency virus [HIV] disease (B20)
polymyositis (M33.2-)
portal hypertension (K76.6)
rheumatoid arthritis (M05.-)
schistosomiasis (B65.-)
Sjögren syndrome (M35.0-)
systemic sclerosis (M34.-)

I27.22   **Pulmonary hypertension due to left heart disease**   `HCC`
Group 2 pulmonary hypertension
Code also associated left heart disease, if known, such as:
multiple valve disease (I08.-)
rheumatic aortic valve diseases (I06.-)
rheumatic mitral valve diseases (I05.-)

I27.23   **Pulmonary hypertension due to lung diseases and hypoxia**   `HCC`
Group 3 pulmonary hypertension
Code also associated lung disease, if known, such as:
bronchiectasis (J47.-)
cystic fibrosis with pulmonary manifestations (E84.0)
interstitial lung disease (J84.-)
pleural effusion (J90)
sleep apnea (G47.3-)

I27.24   **Chronic thromboembolic pulmonary hypertension**   `HCC`
Group 4 pulmonary hypertension
Code also associated pulmonary embolism, if applicable (I26.-, I27.82)

I27.29   **Other secondary pulmonary hypertension**   `HCC`
Group 5 pulmonary hypertension
Pulmonary hypertension with unclear multifactorial mechanisms
Pulmonary hypertension due to hematologic disorders
Pulmonary hypertension due to metabolic disorders
Pulmonary hypertension due to other systemic disorders
Code also other associated disorders, if known, such as:
chronic myeloid leukemia (C92.10- C92.22)
essential thrombocythemia (D47.3)
Gaucher disease (E75.22)
hypertensive chronic kidney disease with end stage renal disease ►(I12.0, I13.11, I13.2)◄
hyperthyroidism (E05.-)
hypothyroidism (E00-E03)
polycythemia vera (D45)
sarcoidosis (D86.-)
AHA: 2016,2Q,8

`√5ᵗʰ` **I27.8**   **Other specified pulmonary heart diseases**

I27.81   **Cor pulmonale (chronic)**   `HCC`
Cor pulmonale NOS
`EXCLUDES 1`   *acute cor pulmonale (I26.0-)*
AHA: 2014,4Q,21

I27.82   **Chronic pulmonary embolism**   `HCC`
Use additional code, if applicable, for associated long-term (current) use of anticoagulants (Z79.01)
`EXCLUDES 1`   *personal history of pulmonary embolism (Z86.711)*
DEF: Long-standing condition commonly associated with pulmonary hypertension in which small blood clots travel to the lungs repeatedly over many weeks, months, or years, requiring continuation of established anticoagulant or thrombolytic therapy.

I27.83   **Eisenmenger's syndrome**   `HCC`
Eisenmenger's complex
(Irreversible) Eisenmenger's disease
Pulmonary hypertension with right to left shunt related to congenital heart disease
Code also underlying heart defect, if known, such as:
atrial septal defect (Q21.1)
Eisenmenger's defect (Q21.8)
patent ductus arteriosus (Q25.0)
ventricular septal defect (Q21.0)
DEF: Pulmonary hypertension with congenital communication between two circulations resulting in a right to left shunt. This causes reduced oxygen saturation in the arterial blood, leading to cyanosis and organ damage. Once it develops, this life-threating condition is irreversible.

I27.89   **Other specified pulmonary heart diseases**   `HCC`

I27.9   **Pulmonary heart disease, unspecified**   `HCC` ▽
Chronic cardiopulmonary disease

`√4ᵗʰ` **I28**   **Other diseases of pulmonary vessels**

I28.0   **Arteriovenous fistula of pulmonary vessels**   `HCC`
`EXCLUDES 1`   *congenital arteriovenous fistula (Q25.72)*

I28.1   **Aneurysm of pulmonary artery**   `HCC`
`EXCLUDES 1`   *congenital aneurysm (Q25.79)*
congenital arteriovenous aneurysm (Q25.72)

I28.8   **Other diseases of pulmonary vessels**   `HCC`
Pulmonary arteritis
Pulmonary endarteritis
Rupture of pulmonary vessels
Stenosis of pulmonary vessels
Stricture of pulmonary vessels

I28.9   **Disease of pulmonary vessels, unspecified**   `HCC` ▽

Other forms of heart disease (I30-I52)

`√4ᵗʰ` **I30**   **Acute pericarditis**
`INCLUDES`   acute mediastinopericarditis
acute myopericarditis
acute pericardial effusion
acute pleuropericarditis
acute pneumopericarditis
`EXCLUDES 1`   *Dressler's syndrome (I24.1)*
rheumatic pericarditis (acute) (I01.0)
viral pericarditis due to Coxsakie virus (B33.23)
DEF: Pericarditis: Inflammation affecting the pericardium, the fibroserous membrane that surrounds the heart.

I30.0   **Acute nonspecific idiopathic pericarditis**

I30.1   **Infective pericarditis**
Pneumococcal pericarditis
Pneumopyopericardium
Purulent pericarditis
Pyopericarditis
Pyopericardium
Pyopneumopericardium
Staphylococcal pericarditis
Streptococcal pericarditis
Suppurative pericarditis
Viral pericarditis
Use additional code (B95-B97) to identify infectious agent

I30.8   **Other forms of acute pericarditis**

I30.9   **Acute pericarditis, unspecified**   ▽

`√4ᵗʰ` **I31**   **Other diseases of pericardium**
`EXCLUDES 1`   *diseases of pericardium specified as rheumatic (I09.2)*
postcardiotomy syndrome (I97.0)
traumatic injury to pericardium (S26.-)

I31.0   **Chronic adhesive pericarditis**
Accretio cordis
Adherent pericardium
Adhesive mediastinopericarditis

I31.1   **Chronic constrictive pericarditis**
Concretio cordis
Pericardial calcification

I31.2 Hemopericardium, not elsewhere classified

EXCLUDES 1   *hemopericardium as current complication following acute myocardial infarction (I23.0)*

DEF: Presence of blood in the pericardial sac (pericardium). It can lead to potentially fatal cardiac tamponade if enough blood enters the pericardial cavity.

I31.3 Pericardial effusion (noninflammatory)

Chylopericardium

EXCLUDES 1   *acute pericardial effusion (I30.9)*

I31.4 Cardiac tamponade

Code first underlying cause

DEF: Life-threatening condition in which fluid or blood accumulates in the space between the muscle of the heart (myocardium) and the outer sac that covers the heart (pericardium), resulting in compression of the heart.

Cardiac Tamponade

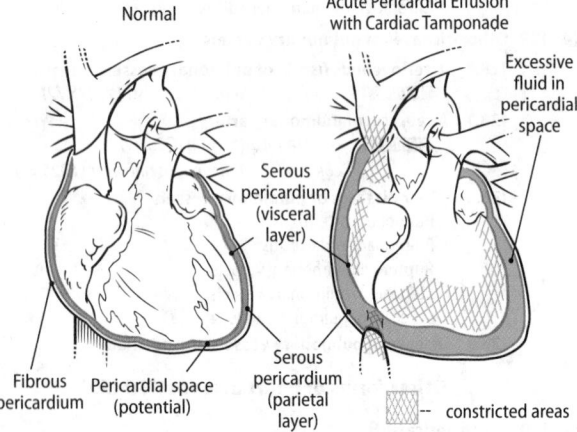

Normal

Acute Pericardial Effusion with Cardiac Tamponade

Excessive fluid in pericardial space

Serous pericardium (visceral layer)

Fibrous pericardium

Pericardial space (potential)

Serous pericardium (parietal layer)

constricted areas

I31.8 Other specified diseases of pericardium

Epicardial plaques

Focal pericardial adhesions

I31.9 Disease of pericardium, unspecified ▽

Pericarditis (chronic) NOS

I32 Pericarditis in diseases classified elsewhere

Code first underlying disease

EXCLUDES 1   *pericarditis (in):*

coxsackie (virus) (B33.23)

gonococcal (A54.83)

meningococcal (A39.53)

rheumatoid (arthritis) (M05.31)

syphilitic (A52.06)

systemic lupus erythematosus (M32.12)

tuberculosis (A18.84)

DEF: Pericarditis: Inflammation affecting the pericardium, the fibroserous membrane that surrounds the heart.

☑4ᵗʰ I33 Acute and subacute endocarditis

EXCLUDES 1   *acute rheumatic endocarditis (I01.1)*

endocarditis NOS (I38)

DEF: Endocarditis: Inflammatory disease of the interior lining of the heart chamber and heart valves.

I33.0 Acute and subacute infective endocarditis

Bacterial endocarditis (acute) (subacute)

Infective endocarditis (acute) (subacute) NOS

Endocarditis lenta (acute) (subacute)

Malignant endocarditis (acute) (subacute)

Purulent endocarditis (acute) (subacute)

Septic endocarditis (acute) (subacute)

Ulcerative endocarditis (acute) (subacute)

Vegetative endocarditis (acute) (subacute)

Use additional code (B95-B97) to identify infectious agent

I33.9 Acute and subacute endocarditis, unspecified ▽

Acute endocarditis NOS

Acute myoendocarditis NOS

Acute periendocarditis NOS

Subacute endocarditis NOS

Subacute myoendocarditis NOS

Subacute periendocarditis NOS

☑4ᵗʰ I34 Nonrheumatic mitral valve disorders

EXCLUDES 1   *mitral valve disease (I05.9)*

mitral valve failure (I05.8)

mitral valve stenosis (I05.0)

mitral valve disorder of unspecified cause with diseases of aortic and/or tricuspid valve(s) (I08.-)

mitral valve disorder of unspecified cause with mitral stenosis or obstruction (I05.0)

mitral valve disorder specified as congenital (Q23.2, Q23.9)

mitral valve disorder specified as rheumatic (I05.-)

I34.0 Nonrheumatic mitral (valve) insufficiency

Nonrheumatic mitral (valve) incompetence NOS

Nonrheumatic mitral (valve) regurgitation NOS

I34.1 Nonrheumatic mitral (valve) prolapse

Floppy nonrheumatic mitral valve syndrome

EXCLUDES 1   *Marfan's syndrome (Q87.4-)*

I34.2 Nonrheumatic mitral (valve) stenosis

I34.8 Other nonrheumatic mitral valve disorders

I34.9 Nonrheumatic mitral valve disorder, unspecified ▽

☑4ᵗʰ I35 Nonrheumatic aortic valve disorders

EXCLUDES 1   *aortic valve disorder of unspecified cause but with diseases of mitral and/or tricuspid valve(s) (I08.-)*

aortic valve disorder specified as congenital (Q23.0, Q23.1)

aortic valve disorder specified as rheumatic (I06.-)

hypertrophic subaortic stenosis (I42.1)

I35.0 Nonrheumatic aortic (valve) stenosis

I35.1 Nonrheumatic aortic (valve) insufficiency

Nonrheumatic aortic (valve) incompetence NOS

Nonrheumatic aortic (valve) regurgitation NOS

I35.2 Nonrheumatic aortic (valve) stenosis with insufficiency

I35.8 Other nonrheumatic aortic valve disorders

I35.9 Nonrheumatic aortic valve disorder, unspecified ▽

☑4ᵗʰ I36 Nonrheumatic tricuspid valve disorders

EXCLUDES 1   *tricuspid valve disorders of unspecified cause (I07.-)*

tricuspid valve disorders specified as congenital (Q22.4, Q22.8, Q22.9)

tricuspid valve disorders specified as rheumatic (I07.-)

tricuspid valve disorders with aortic and/or mitral valve involvement (I08.-)

I36.0 Nonrheumatic tricuspid (valve) stenosis

I36.1 Nonrheumatic tricuspid (valve) insufficiency

Nonrheumatic tricuspid (valve) incompetence

Nonrheumatic tricuspid (valve) regurgitation

I36.2 Nonrheumatic tricuspid (valve) stenosis with insufficiency

I36.8 Other nonrheumatic tricuspid valve disorders

I36.9 Nonrheumatic tricuspid valve disorder, unspecified ▽

☑4ᵗʰ I37 Nonrheumatic pulmonary valve disorders

EXCLUDES 1   *pulmonary valve disorder specified as congenital (Q22.1, Q22.2, Q22.3)*

pulmonary valve disorder specified as rheumatic (I09.89)

I37.0 Nonrheumatic pulmonary valve stenosis

I37.1 Nonrheumatic pulmonary valve insufficiency

Nonrheumatic pulmonary valve incompetence

Nonrheumatic pulmonary valve regurgitation

I37.2 Nonrheumatic pulmonary valve stenosis with insufficiency

I37.8 Other nonrheumatic pulmonary valve disorders

I37.9 Nonrheumatic pulmonary valve disorder, unspecified ▽

I38 Endocarditis, valve unspecified ▽

INCLUDES   endocarditis (chronic) NOS

valvular incompetence NOS

valvular insufficiency NOS

valvular regurgitation NOS

valvular stenosis NOS

valvulitis (chronic) NOS

EXCLUDES 1   *congenital insufficiency of cardiac valve NOS (Q24.8)*

congenital stenosis of cardiac valve NOS (Q24.8)

endocardial fibroelastosis (I42.4)

endocarditis specified as rheumatic (I09.1)

DEF: Endocarditis: Inflammatory disease of the interior lining of the heart chamber and heart valves.

I39 Endocarditis and heart valve disorders in diseases classified elsewhere
Code first underlying disease, such as:
Q fever (A78)
EXCLUDES 1   endocardial involvement in:
candidiasis (B37.6)
gonococcal infection (A54.83)
Libman-Sacks disease (M32.11)
listerosis (A32.82)
meningococcal infection (A39.51)
rheumatoid arthritis (MØ5.31)
syphilis (A52.Ø3)
tuberculosis (A18.84)
typhoid fever (AØ1.Ø2)
DEF: Endocarditis: Inflammatory disease of the interior lining of the heart chamber and heart valves.

✓4ᵗʰ **I4Ø Acute myocarditis**
INCLUDES   subacute myocarditis
EXCLUDES 1   acute rheumatic myocarditis (IØ1.2)
DEF: Myocarditis: Inflammation of the middle layer of the heart, which is composed of muscle tissue.

I4Ø.Ø Infective myocarditis
Septic myocarditis
Use additional code (B95-B97) to identify infectious agent

I4Ø.1 Isolated myocarditis
Fiedler's myocarditis
Giant cell myocarditis
Idiopathic myocarditis

I4Ø.8 Other acute myocarditis
I4Ø.9 Acute myocarditis, unspecified   ▽

I41 Myocarditis in diseases classified elsewhere
Code first underlying disease, such as:
typhus (A75.Ø-A75.9)
EXCLUDES 1   myocarditis (in):
Chagas' disease (chronic) (B57.2)
acute (B57.Ø)
coxsackie (virus) infection (B33.22)
diphtheritic (A36.81)
gonococcal (A54.83)
influenzal (JØ9.X9, J1Ø.82, J11.82)
meningococcal (A39.52)
mumps (B26.82)
rheumatoid arthritis (MØ5.31)
sarcoid (D86.85)
syphilis (A52.Ø6)
toxoplasmosis (B58.81)
tuberculous (A18.84)
DEF: Myocarditis: Inflammation of the middle layer of the heart, which is composed of muscle tissue.

✓4ᵗʰ **I42 Cardiomyopathy**
INCLUDES   myocardiopathy
Code first pre-existing cardiomyopathy complicating pregnancy and puerperium (O99.4)
EXCLUDES 2   ischemic cardiomyopathy (I25.5)
peripartum cardiomyopathy (O9Ø.3)
ventricular hypertrophy (I51.7)

I42.Ø Dilated cardiomyopathy   HCC
Congestive cardiomyopathy

I42.1 Obstructive hypertrophic cardiomyopathy   HCC
Hypertrophic subaortic stenosis (idiopathic)
DEF: Cardiomyopathy marked by left ventricle hypertrophy and an enlarged septum that result in obstructed blood flow, arrhythmias, mitral regurgitation, and sudden cardiac death.
TIP: When this condition is described as inherited, assign code Q24.8.

I42.2 Other hypertrophic cardiomyopathy   HCC
Nonobstructive hypertrophic cardiomyopathy

I42.3 Endomyocardial (eosinophilic) disease   HCC
Endomyocardial (tropical) fibrosis
Löffler's endocarditis

I42.4 Endocardial fibroelastosis   HCC
Congenital cardiomyopathy
Elastomyofibrosis

I42.5 Other restrictive cardiomyopathy   HCC
Constrictive cardiomyopathy NOS

I42.6 Alcoholic cardiomyopathy   HCC
Code also presence of alcoholism (F1Ø.-)

I42.7 Cardiomyopathy due to drug and external agent   HCC
Code first poisoning due to drug or toxin, if applicable (T36-T65 with fifth or sixth character 1-4 or 6)
Use additional code for adverse effect, if applicable, to identify drug (T36-T5Ø with fifth or sixth character 5)

I42.8 Other cardiomyopathies   HCC
I42.9 Cardiomyopathy, unspecified   HCC ▽
Cardiomyopathy (primary) (secondary) NOS

I43 Cardiomyopathy in diseases classified elsewhere   HCC
Code first underlying disease, such as:
amyloidosis (E85.-)
glycogen storage disease (E74.Ø)
gout (M1Ø.Ø-)
thyrotoxicosis (EØ5.Ø-EØ5.9-)
EXCLUDES 1   cardiomyopathy (in):
coxsackie (virus) (B33.24)
diphtheria (A36.81)
sarcoidosis (D86.85)
tuberculosis (A18.84)

✓4ᵗʰ **I44 Atrioventricular and left bundle-branch block**

I44.Ø Atrioventricular block, first degree
I44.1 Atrioventricular block, second degree
Atrioventricular block, type I and II
Möbitz block, type I and II
Second degree block, type I and II
Wenckebach's block

I44.2 Atrioventricular block, complete   HCC
Complete heart block NOS
Third degree block

✓5ᵗʰ **I44.3 Other and unspecified atrioventricular block**
Atrioventricular block NOS
I44.3Ø Unspecified atrioventricular block   ▽
I44.39 Other atrioventricular block

I44.4 Left anterior fascicular block
I44.5 Left posterior fascicular block

✓5ᵗʰ **I44.6 Other and unspecified fascicular block**
I44.6Ø Unspecified fascicular block   ▽
Left bundle-branch hemiblock NOS
I44.69 Other fascicular block

I44.7 Left bundle-branch block, unspecified   ▽

Conduction Disorders

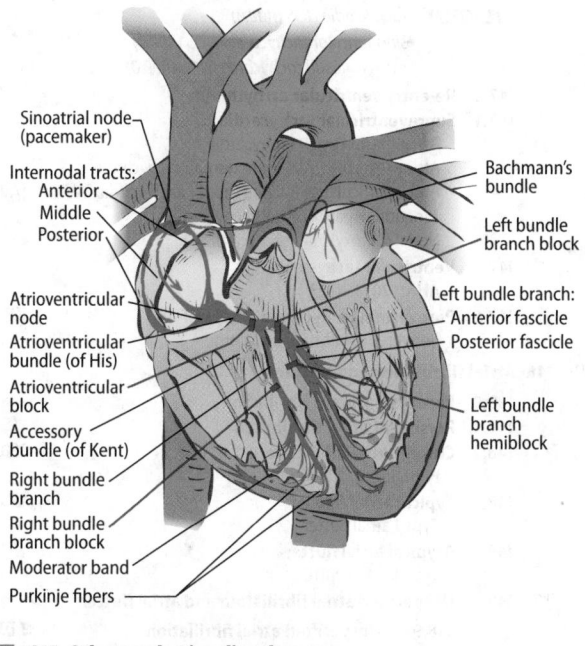

Sinoatrial node (pacemaker)
Internodal tracts:
Anterior
Middle
Posterior
Atrioventricular node
Atrioventricular bundle (of His)
Atrioventricular block
Accessory bundle (of Kent)
Right bundle branch
Right bundle branch block
Moderator band
Purkinje fibers
Bachmann's bundle
Left bundle branch block
Left bundle branch:
Anterior fascicle
Posterior fascicle
Left bundle branch hemiblock

✓4ᵗʰ **I45 Other conduction disorders**

I45.Ø Right fascicular block

I45.1 Other and unspecified right bundle-branch block
- **I45.10 Unspecified right bundle-branch block** ▽
  - Right bundle-branch block NOS
- **I45.19 Other right bundle-branch block**

I45.2 Bifascicular block

I45.3 Trifascicular block

I45.4 Nonspecific intraventricular block
- Bundle-branch block NOS

I45.5 Other specified heart block
- Sinoatrial block
- Sinoauricular block
  - EXCLUDES 1   heart block NOS (I45.9)

I45.6 Pre-excitation syndrome
- Accelerated atrioventricular conduction
- Accessory atrioventricular conduction
- Anomalous atrioventricular excitation
- Lown-Ganong-Levine syndrome
- Pre-excitation atrioventricular conduction
- Wolff-Parkinson-White syndrome

I45.8 Other specified conduction disorders
- **I45.81 Long QT syndrome**
  - DEF: Condition characterized by recurrent syncope, malignant arrhythmias, and sudden death. This syndrome has a characteristic prolonged Q-T interval on an electrocardiogram.
- **I45.89 Other specified conduction disorders**
  - Atrioventricular [AV] dissociation
  - Interference dissociation
  - Isorhythmic dissociation
  - Nonparoxysmal AV nodal tachycardia
  - AHA: 2013,2Q,31

I45.9 Conduction disorder, unspecified ▽
- Heart block NOS
- Stokes-Adams syndrome

I46 Cardiac arrest
- EXCLUDES 1   cardiogenic shock (R57.0)

I46.2 Cardiac arrest due to underlying cardiac condition HCC
- Code first underlying cardiac condition

I46.8 Cardiac arrest due to other underlying condition HCC
- Code first underlying condition

I46.9 Cardiac arrest, cause unspecified HCC ▽

I47 Paroxysmal tachycardia
- Code first tachycardia complicating:
  - abortion or ectopic or molar pregnancy (O00-O07, O08.8)
  - obstetric surgery and procedures (O75.4)
  - EXCLUDES 1   tachycardia NOS (R00.0)
  - sinoauricular tachycardia NOS (R00.0)
  - sinus [sinusal] tachycardia NOS (R00.0)

I47.0 Re-entry ventricular arrhythmia HCC

I47.1 Supraventricular tachycardia HCC
- Atrial (paroxysmal) tachycardia
- Atrioventricular [AV] (paroxysmal) tachycardia
- Atrioventricular re-entrant (nodal) tachycardia [AVNRT] [AVRT]
- Junctional (paroxysmal) tachycardia
- Nodal (paroxysmal) tachycardia

I47.2 Ventricular tachycardia HCC
- AHA: 2013,3Q,23

I47.9 Paroxysmal tachycardia, unspecified HCC ▽
- Bouveret (-Hoffman) syndrome

I48 Atrial fibrillation and flutter

I48.0 Paroxysmal atrial fibrillation HCC Q

I48.1 Persistent atrial fibrillation HCC Q

I48.2 Chronic atrial fibrillation HCC Q
- Permanent atrial fibrillation

I48.3 Typical atrial flutter HCC Q
- Type I atrial flutter

I48.4 Atypical atrial flutter HCC Q
- Type II atrial flutter

I48.9 Unspecified atrial fibrillation and atrial flutter
- **I48.91 Unspecified atrial fibrillation** HCC Q ▽
- **I48.92 Unspecified atrial flutter** HCC Q ▽

I49 Other cardiac arrhythmias
- Code first cardiac arrhythmia complicating:
  - abortion or ectopic or molar pregnancy (O00-O07, O08.8)
  - obstetric surgery and procedures (O75.4)
  - EXCLUDES 1   neonatal dysrhythmia (P29.1-)
  - sinoatrial bradycardia (R00.1)
  - sinus bradycardia (R00.1)
  - vagal bradycardia (R00.1)
  - EXCLUDES 2   bradycardia NOS (R00.1)

I49.0 Ventricular fibrillation and flutter
- **I49.01 Ventricular fibrillation** HCC
- **I49.02 Ventricular flutter** HCC

I49.1 Atrial premature depolarization
- Atrial premature beats

I49.2 Junctional premature depolarization HCC

I49.3 Ventricular premature depolarization

I49.4 Other and unspecified premature depolarization
- **I49.40 Unspecified premature depolarization** ▽
  - Premature beats NOS
- **I49.49 Other premature depolarization**
  - Ectopic beats
  - Extrasystoles
  - Extrasystolic arrhythmias
  - Premature contractions

I49.5 Sick sinus syndrome HCC
- Tachycardia-bradycardia syndrome
- TIP: Do not assign when sick sinus syndrome (SSS) is controlled by a pacemaker and no management of the condition is required during the encounter; assign only code Z95.0 Presence of cardiac pacemaker.
- TIP: When the purpose of the encounter is to interrogate the pacemaker, sick sinus syndrome (SSS) should be coded only when the interrogation identifies problems with this condition.

I49.8 Other specified cardiac arrhythmias
- Brugada syndrome
- Coronary sinus rhythm disorder
- Ectopic rhythm disorder
- Nodal rhythm disorder

I49.9 Cardiac arrhythmia, unspecified ▽
- Arrhythmia (cardiac) NOS

I50 Heart failure
- Code first:
  - heart failure complicating abortion or ectopic or molar pregnancy (O00-O07, O08.8)
  - heart failure due to hypertension (I11.0)
  - heart failure due to hypertension with chronic kidney disease (I13.-)
  - heart failure following surgery (I97.13-)
  - obstetric surgery and procedures (O75.4)
  - rheumatic heart failure (I09.81)
  - EXCLUDES 1   neonatal cardiac failure (P29.0)
  - EXCLUDES 2   cardiac arrest (I46.-)
  - AHA: 2018,2Q,9; 2017,1Q,47; 2014,1Q,25; 2013,2Q,33

I50.1 Left ventricular failure, unspecified HCC ▽
- Cardiac asthma
- Edema of lung with heart disease NOS
- Edema of lung with heart failure
- Left heart failure
- Pulmonary edema with heart disease NOS
- Pulmonary edema with heart failure
  - EXCLUDES 1   edema of lung without heart disease or heart failure (J81.-)
  - pulmonary edema without heart disease or failure (J81.-)

I50.2 Systolic (congestive) heart failure
- Heart failure with reduced ejection fraction [HFrEF]
- Systolic left ventricular heart failure
- Code also end stage heart failure, if applicable (I50.84)
  - EXCLUDES 1   combined systolic (congestive) and diastolic (congestive) heart failure (I50.4-)
  - AHA: 2017,1Q,46; 2016,1Q,10
- **I50.20 Unspecified systolic (congestive) heart failure** HCC ▽
- **I50.21 Acute systolic (congestive) heart failure** HCC
- **I50.22 Chronic systolic (congestive) heart failure** HCC
- **I50.23 Acute on chronic systolic (congestive) heart failure** HCC

✓5ᵗʰ **I50.3** **Diastolic (congestive) heart failure**
Diastolic left ventricular heart failure
Heart failure with normal ejection fraction
Heart failure with preserved ejection fraction [HFpEF]
Code also end stage heart failure, if applicable (I50.84)
> EXCLUDES 1   combined systolic (congestive) and diastolic (congestive) heart failure (I50.4-)

AHA: 2017,1Q,46; 2016,1Q,10

I50.30   **Unspecified diastolic (congestive) heart failure**   HCC ▽

I50.31   **Acute diastolic (congestive) heart failure**   HCC

I50.32   **Chronic diastolic (congestive) heart failure**   HCC

I50.33   **Acute on chronic diastolic (congestive) heart failure**   HCC

✓5ᵗʰ **I50.4** **Combined systolic (congestive) and diastolic (congestive) heart failure**
Combined systolic and diastolic left ventricular heart failure
Heart failure with reduced ejection fraction and diastolic dysfunction
Code also end stage heart failure, if applicable (I50.84)
AHA: 2017,1Q,46; 2016,1Q,10

I50.40   **Unspecified combined systolic (congestive) and diastolic (congestive) heart failure**   HCC ▽

I50.41   **Acute combined systolic (congestive) and diastolic (congestive) heart failure**   HCC

I50.42   **Chronic combined systolic (congestive) and diastolic (congestive) heart failure**   HCC

I50.43   **Acute on chronic combined systolic (congestive) and diastolic (congestive) heart failure**   HCC

✓5ᵗʰ **I50.8** **Other heart failure**
AHA: 2017,4Q,15-16

✓6ᵗʰ **I50.81**   **Right heart failure**
Right ventricular failure

I50.810   **Right heart failure, unspecified**   HCC ▽
Right heart failure without mention of left heart failure
Right ventricular failure NOS

I50.811   **Acute right heart failure**   HCC
Acute isolated right heart failure
Acute (isolated) right ventricular failure

I50.812   **Chronic right heart failure**   HCC
Chronic isolated right heart failure
Chronic (isolated) right ventricular failure

I50.813   **Acute on chronic right heart failure**   HCC
Acute on chronic isolated right heart failure
Acute on chronic (isolated) right ventricular failure
Acute decompensation of chronic (isolated) right ventricular failure
Acute exacerbation of chronic (isolated) right ventricular failure

I50.814   **Right heart failure due to left heart failure**   HCC
Right ventricular failure secondary to left ventricular failure
Code also the type of left ventricular failure, if known (I50.2-I50.43)
> EXCLUDES 1   right heart failure with but not due to left heart failure (I50.82)

I50.82   **Biventricular heart failure**   HCC
Code also the type of left ventricular failure as systolic, diastolic, or combined, if known (I50.2-I50.43)

I50.83   **High output heart failure**   HCC
DEF: Occurs when the high demand for blood exceeds the capacity of a normally functioning heart to meet the demand.

I50.84   **End stage heart failure**   HCC
Stage D heart failure
Code also the type of heart failure as systolic, diastolic, or combined, if known (I50.2-I50.43)

I50.89   **Other heart failure**   HCC

I50.9 **Heart failure, unspecified**   HCC ▽
Cardiac, heart or myocardial failure NOS
Congestive heart disease
Congestive heart failure NOS
> EXCLUDES 2   fluid overload (E87.70)

AHA: 2017,4Q,15-16; 2017,1Q,45-46; 2014,4Q,21; 2012,4Q,92

✓4ᵗʰ **I51** **Complications and ill-defined descriptions of heart disease**
> EXCLUDES 1   any condition in I51.4-I51.9 due to hypertension (I11.-)
> any condition in I51.4-I51.9 due to hypertension and chronic kidney disease (I13.-)
> heart disease specified as rheumatic (I00-I09)

I51.0 **Cardiac septal defect, acquired**   A
Acquired septal atrial defect (old)
Acquired septal auricular defect (old)
Acquired septal ventricular defect (old)
> EXCLUDES 1   cardiac septal defect as current complication following acute myocardial infarction (I23.1, I23.2)

DEF: Abnormal communication between opposite heart chambers due to a defect of the septum. It is not present at birth.

I51.1 **Rupture of chordae tendineae, not elsewhere classified**   HCC
> EXCLUDES 1   rupture of chordae tendineae as current complication following acute myocardial infarction (I23.4)

I51.2 **Rupture of papillary muscle, not elsewhere classified**   HCC
> EXCLUDES 1   rupture of papillary muscle as current complication following acute myocardial infarction (I23.5)

I51.3 **Intracardiac thrombosis, not elsewhere classified**
Apical thrombosis (old)
Atrial thrombosis (old)
Auricular thrombosis (old)
Mural thrombosis (old)
Ventricular thrombosis (old)
> EXCLUDES 1   intracardiac thrombosis as current complication following acute myocardial infarction (I23.6)

AHA: 2013,1Q,24

I51.4 **Myocarditis, unspecified**   HCC ▽
Chronic (interstitial) myocarditis
Myocardial fibrosis
Myocarditis NOS
> EXCLUDES 1   acute or subacute myocarditis (I40.-)

AHA: 2018,2Q,9

I51.5 **Myocardial degeneration**   HCC
Fatty degeneration of heart or myocardium
Myocardial disease
Senile degeneration of heart or myocardium
AHA: 2018,2Q,9

I51.7 **Cardiomegaly**
Cardiac dilatation
Cardiac hypertrophy
Ventricular dilatation
AHA: 2018,2Q,9

✓5ᵗʰ **I51.8** **Other ill-defined heart diseases**
AHA: 2018,2Q,9

I51.81   **Takotsubo syndrome**
Reversible left ventricular dysfunction following sudden emotional stress
Stress induced cardiomyopathy
Takotsubo cardiomyopathy
Transient left ventricular apical ballooning syndrome
DEF: Complex of symptoms mimicking myocardial infarct in absence of heart disease, with the majority of cases occurring in postmenopausal women. Heart muscles are temporarily weakened, and a sudden, massive surge of adrenalin stuns the heart, greatly reducing the ability to pump blood.

I51.89   **Other ill-defined heart diseases**
Carditis (acute)(chronic)
Pancarditis (acute)(chronic)

I51.9 **Heart disease, unspecified**   ▽
AHA: 2018,2Q,9

Chapter 9. Diseases of the Circulatory System

152 **Other heart disorders in diseases classified elsewhere**

Code first underlying disease, such as:
congenital syphilis (A5Ø.5)
mucopolysaccharidosis (E76.3)
schistosomiasis (B65.Ø-B65.9)

EXCLUDES 1   heart disease (in):
gonococcal infection (A54.83)
meningococcal infection (A39.5Ø)
rheumatoid arthritis (MØ5.31)
syphilis (A52.Ø6)

Cerebrovascular diseases (I6Ø-I69)

Use additional code to identify presence of:
alcohol abuse and dependence (F1Ø.-)
exposure to environmental tobacco smoke (Z77.22)
history of tobacco dependence (Z87.891)
hypertension ▶(I1Ø-I16)◀
occupational exposure to environmental tobacco smoke (Z57.31)
tobacco dependence (F17.-)
tobacco use (Z72.Ø)

EXCLUDES 1   traumatic intracranial hemorrhage (SØ6.-)

AHA: 2014,3Q,5; 2012,4Q,91-92

√4ᵗʰ **I6Ø** **Nontraumatic subarachnoid hemorrhage**

EXCLUDES 1   syphilitic ruptured cerebral aneurysm (A52.Ø5)
EXCLUDES 2   sequelae of subarachnoid hemorrhage (I69.Ø-)

√5ᵗʰ **I6Ø.Ø** **Nontraumatic subarachnoid hemorrhage from carotid siphon and bifurcation**

     I6Ø.ØØ **Nontraumatic subarachnoid hemorrhage from unspecified carotid siphon and bifurcation** HCC ▽

     I6Ø.Ø1 **Nontraumatic subarachnoid hemorrhage from right carotid siphon and bifurcation** . HCC

     I6Ø.Ø2 **Nontraumatic subarachnoid hemorrhage from left carotid siphon and bifurcation** HCC

√5ᵗʰ **I6Ø.1** **Nontraumatic subarachnoid hemorrhage from middle cerebral artery**

     I6Ø.1Ø **Nontraumatic subarachnoid hemorrhage from unspecified middle cerebral artery** HCC ▽

     I6Ø.11 **Nontraumatic subarachnoid hemorrhage from right middle cerebral artery** HCC

     I6Ø.12 **Nontraumatic subarachnoid hemorrhage from left middle cerebral artery** HCC

I6Ø.2 **Nontraumatic subarachnoid hemorrhage from anterior communicating artery** HCC

√5ᵗʰ **I6Ø.3** **Nontraumatic subarachnoid hemorrhage from posterior communicating artery**

     I6Ø.3Ø **Nontraumatic subarachnoid hemorrhage from unspecified posterior communicating artery** HCC ▽

     I6Ø.31 **Nontraumatic subarachnoid hemorrhage from right posterior communicating artery** HCC

     I6Ø.32 **Nontraumatic subarachnoid hemorrhage from left posterior communicating artery** HCC

I6Ø.4 **Nontraumatic subarachnoid hemorrhage from basilar artery** HCC

√5ᵗʰ **I6Ø.5** **Nontraumatic subarachnoid hemorrhage from vertebral artery**

     I6Ø.5Ø **Nontraumatic subarachnoid hemorrhage from unspecified vertebral artery** HCC ▽

     I6Ø.51 **Nontraumatic subarachnoid hemorrhage from right vertebral artery** HCC

     I6Ø.52 **Nontraumatic subarachnoid hemorrhage from left vertebral artery** HCC

I6Ø.6 **Nontraumatic subarachnoid hemorrhage from other intracranial arteries** HCC

I6Ø.7 **Nontraumatic subarachnoid hemorrhage from unspecified intracranial artery** HCC ▽

Ruptured (congenital) berry aneurysm
Ruptured (congenital) cerebral aneurysm
Subarachnoid hemorrhage (nontraumatic) from cerebral artery NOS
Subarachnoid hemorrhage (nontraumatic) from communicating artery NOS

EXCLUDES 1   berry aneurysm, nonruptured (I67.1)

I6Ø.8 **Other nontraumatic subarachnoid hemorrhage** HCC

Meningeal hemorrhage
Rupture of cerebral arteriovenous malformation

I6Ø.9 **Nontraumatic subarachnoid hemorrhage, unspecified** HCC ▽

√4ᵗʰ **I61** **Nontraumatic intracerebral hemorrhage**

EXCLUDES 2   sequelae of intracerebral hemorrhage (I69.1-)

AHA: 2017,2Q,9-10

I61.Ø **Nontraumatic intracerebral hemorrhage in hemisphere, subcortical** HCC

Deep intracerebral hemorrhage (nontraumatic)
AHA: 2016,4Q,27

I61.1 **Nontraumatic intracerebral hemorrhage in hemisphere, cortical** HCC

Cerebral lobe hemorrhage (nontraumatic)
Superficial intracerebral hemorrhage (nontraumatic)

I61.2 **Nontraumatic intracerebral hemorrhage in hemisphere, unspecified** HCC ▽

I61.3 **Nontraumatic intracerebral hemorrhage in brain stem** HCC

I61.4 **Nontraumatic intracerebral hemorrhage in cerebellum** HCC

I61.5 **Nontraumatic intracerebral hemorrhage, intraventricular** HCC

I61.6 **Nontraumatic intracerebral hemorrhage, multiple localized** HCC

I61.8 **Other nontraumatic intracerebral hemorrhage** HCC

I61.9 **Nontraumatic intracerebral hemorrhage, unspecified** HCC ▽

√4ᵗʰ **I62** **Other and unspecified nontraumatic intracranial hemorrhage**

EXCLUDES 2   sequelae of intracranial hemorrhage (I69.2)

√5ᵗʰ **I62.Ø** **Nontraumatic subdural hemorrhage**

     I62.ØØ **Nontraumatic subdural hemorrhage, unspecified** HCC ▽

     I62.Ø1 **Nontraumatic acute subdural hemorrhage** HCC

     I62.Ø2 **Nontraumatic subacute subdural hemorrhage** HCC

     I62.Ø3 **Nontraumatic chronic subdural hemorrhage** HCC

I62.1 **Nontraumatic extradural hemorrhage** HCC

Nontraumatic epidural hemorrhage

I62.9 **Nontraumatic intracranial hemorrhage, unspecified** HCC ▽

√4ᵗʰ **I63** **Cerebral infarction**

INCLUDES   occlusion and stenosis of cerebral and precerebral arteries, resulting in cerebral infarction

Use additional code, if applicable, to identify status post administration of tPA (rtPA) in a different facility within the last 24 hours prior to admission to current facility (Z92.82)

Use additional code, if known, to indicate National Institutes of Health Stroke Scale (NIHSS) score (R29.7-)

EXCLUDES 2   sequelae of cerebral infarction (I69.3-)

AHA: 2017,2Q,9-10; 2016,4Q,28,61-62; 2014,1Q,23

TIP: Weakness on one side of the body documented as secondary to stroke is synonymous with hemiparesis/hemiplegia (G81.-). Weakness of one limb documented as secondary to stroke is synonymous with monoplegia (G83.1-, G83.2-, G83.3-).

√5ᵗʰ **I63.Ø** **Cerebral infarction due to thrombosis of precerebral arteries**

     I63.ØØ **Cerebral infarction due to thrombosis of unspecified precerebral artery** HCC ▽

     √6ᵗʰ **I63.Ø1** **Cerebral infarction due to thrombosis of vertebral artery**

         I63.Ø11 **Cerebral infarction due to thrombosis of right vertebral artery** HCC

         I63.Ø12 **Cerebral infarction due to thrombosis of left vertebral artery** HCC

         I63.Ø13 **Cerebral infarction due to thrombosis of bilateral vertebral arteries** HCC Q

         I63.Ø19 **Cerebral infarction due to thrombosis of unspecified vertebral artery** HCC ▽

     I63.Ø2 **Cerebral infarction due to thrombosis of basilar artery** HCC

     √6ᵗʰ **I63.Ø3** **Cerebral infarction due to thrombosis of carotid artery**

         I63.Ø31 **Cerebral infarction due to thrombosis of right carotid artery** HCC

         I63.Ø32 **Cerebral infarction due to thrombosis of left carotid artery** HCC

I63.033   Cerebral infarction due to thrombosis of bilateral carotid arteries   HCC Q

I63.039   Cerebral infarction due to thrombosis of unspecified carotid artery   HCC ▽

I63.09   Cerebral infarction due to thrombosis of other precerebral artery   HCC

√5ᵗʰ **I63.1**   Cerebral infarction due to embolism of precerebral arteries

I63.10   Cerebral infarction due to embolism of unspecified precerebral artery   HCC ▽

√6ᵗʰ I63.11   Cerebral infarction due to embolism of vertebral artery

I63.111   Cerebral infarction due to embolism of right vertebral artery   HCC

I63.112   Cerebral infarction due to embolism of left vertebral artery   HCC

I63.113   Cerebral infarction due to embolism of bilateral vertebral arteries   HCC Q

I63.119   Cerebral infarction due to embolism of unspecified vertebral artery   HCC ▽

I63.12   Cerebral infarction due to embolism of basilar artery   HCC

√6ᵗʰ I63.13   Cerebral infarction due to embolism of carotid artery

I63.131   Cerebral infarction due to embolism of right carotid artery   HCC

I63.132   Cerebral infarction due to embolism of left carotid artery   HCC

I63.133   Cerebral infarction due to embolism of bilateral carotid arteries   HCC

I63.139   Cerebral infarction due to embolism of unspecified carotid artery   HCC ▽

I63.19   Cerebral infarction due to embolism of other precerebral artery   HCC

√5ᵗʰ **I63.2**   Cerebral infarction due to unspecified occlusion or stenosis of precerebral arteries

I63.20   Cerebral infarction due to unspecified occlusion or stenosis of unspecified precerebral arteries   HCC Q ▽

√6ᵗʰ I63.21   Cerebral infarction due to unspecified occlusion or stenosis of vertebral arteries

I63.211   Cerebral infarction due to unspecified occlusion or stenosis of right vertebral artery   HCC Q

I63.212   Cerebral infarction due to unspecified occlusion or stenosis of left vertebral artery   HCC Q

I63.213   Cerebral infarction due to unspecified occlusion or stenosis of bilateral vertebral arteries   HCC Q

▲   I63.219   Cerebral infarction due to unspecified occlusion or stenosis of unspecified vertebral artery   HCC Q ▽

I63.22   Cerebral infarction due to unspecified occlusion or stenosis of basilar artery   HCC Q

√6ᵗʰ I63.23   Cerebral infarction due to unspecified occlusion or stenosis of carotid arteries

I63.231   Cerebral infarction due to unspecified occlusion or stenosis of right carotid arteries   HCC Q

I63.232   Cerebral infarction due to unspecified occlusion or stenosis of left carotid arteries   HCC Q

I63.233   Cerebral infarction due to unspecified occlusion or stenosis of bilateral carotid arteries   HCC Q

▲   I63.239   Cerebral infarction due to unspecified occlusion or stenosis of unspecified carotid artery   HCC Q ▽

I63.29   Cerebral infarction due to unspecified occlusion or stenosis of other precerebral arteries   HCC

√5ᵗʰ **I63.3**   Cerebral infarction due to thrombosis of cerebral arteries

I63.30   Cerebral infarction due to thrombosis of unspecified cerebral artery   HCC ▽

√6ᵗʰ I63.31   Cerebral infarction due to thrombosis of middle cerebral artery

I63.311   Cerebral infarction due to thrombosis of right middle cerebral artery   HCC

I63.312   Cerebral infarction due to thrombosis of left middle cerebral artery   HCC

I63.313   Cerebral infarction due to thrombosis of bilateral middle cerebral arteries   HCC Q

I63.319   Cerebral infarction due to thrombosis of unspecified middle cerebral artery   HCC ▽

√6ᵗʰ I63.32   Cerebral infarction due to thrombosis of anterior cerebral artery

I63.321   Cerebral infarction due to thrombosis of right anterior cerebral artery   HCC

I63.322   Cerebral infarction due to thrombosis of left anterior cerebral artery   HCC

I63.323   Cerebral infarction due to thrombosis of bilateral anterior cerebral arteries   HCC Q

I63.329   Cerebral infarction due to thrombosis of unspecified anterior cerebral artery   HCC ▽

√6ᵗʰ I63.33   Cerebral infarction due to thrombosis of posterior cerebral artery

I63.331   Cerebral infarction due to thrombosis of right posterior cerebral artery   HCC

I63.332   Cerebral infarction due to thrombosis of left posterior cerebral artery   HCC

I63.333   Cerebral infarction due to thrombosis of bilateral posterior cerebral arteries   HCC Q

I63.339   Cerebral infarction due to thrombosis of unspecified posterior cerebral artery   HCC ▽

√6ᵗʰ I63.34   Cerebral infarction due to thrombosis of cerebellar artery

I63.341   Cerebral infarction due to thrombosis of right cerebellar artery   HCC

I63.342   Cerebral infarction due to thrombosis of left cerebellar artery   HCC

▲   I63.343   Cerebral infarction due to thrombosis of bilateral cerebellar arteries   HCC

I63.349   Cerebral infarction due to thrombosis of unspecified cerebellar artery   HCC ▽

I63.39   Cerebral infarction due to thrombosis of other cerebral artery   HCC

√5ᵗʰ **I63.4**   Cerebral infarction due to embolism of cerebral arteries

I63.40   Cerebral infarction due to embolism of unspecified cerebral artery   HCC ▽

√6ᵗʰ I63.41   Cerebral infarction due to embolism of middle cerebral artery

I63.411   Cerebral infarction due to embolism of right middle cerebral artery   HCC

I63.412   Cerebral infarction due to embolism of left middle cerebral artery   HCC

I63.413   Cerebral infarction due to embolism of bilateral middle cerebral arteries   HCC Q

I63.419   Cerebral infarction due to embolism of unspecified middle cerebral artery   HCC ▽

√6ᵗʰ I63.42   Cerebral infarction due to embolism of anterior cerebral artery

I63.421   Cerebral infarction due to embolism of right anterior cerebral artery   HCC

✔ Additional Character Req   ✔x 7ᵗʰ Placeholder Alert   Manifestation   ▽ Unspecified   ►◄ Revised Text   ● New Code   ▲ Revised Code Title

ICD-10-CM 2019   **647**

Chapter 9. Diseases of the Circulatory System

I63.422 Cerebral infarction due to embolism of left anterior cerebral artery — HCC

I63.423 Cerebral infarction due to embolism of bilateral anterior cerebral arteries — HCC Q

I63.429 Cerebral infarction due to embolism of unspecified anterior cerebral artery — HCC Q ▽

I63.43 Cerebral infarction due to embolism of posterior cerebral artery
- I63.431 Cerebral infarction due to embolism of right posterior cerebral artery — HCC Q
- I63.432 Cerebral infarction due to embolism of left posterior cerebral artery — HCC Q
- I63.433 Cerebral infarction due to embolism of bilateral posterior cerebral arteries — HCC Q
- I63.439 Cerebral infarction due to embolism of unspecified posterior cerebral artery — HCC Q ▽

I63.44 Cerebral infarction due to embolism of cerebellar artery
- I63.441 Cerebral infarction due to embolism of right cerebellar artery — HCC Q
- I63.442 Cerebral infarction due to embolism of left cerebellar artery — HCC Q
- I63.443 Cerebral infarction due to embolism of bilateral cerebellar arteries — HCC
- I63.449 Cerebral infarction due to embolism of unspecified cerebellar artery — HCC Q ▽

I63.49 Cerebral infarction due to embolism of other cerebral artery — HCC Q

I63.5 Cerebral infarction due to unspecified occlusion or stenosis of cerebral arteries
- I63.50 Cerebral infarction due to unspecified occlusion or stenosis of unspecified cerebral artery — HCC Q ▽
- I63.51 Cerebral infarction due to unspecified occlusion or stenosis of middle cerebral artery
  - I63.511 Cerebral infarction due to unspecified occlusion or stenosis of right middle cerebral artery — HCC Q
  - I63.512 Cerebral infarction due to unspecified occlusion or stenosis of left middle cerebral artery — HCC Q
  - I63.513 Cerebral infarction due to unspecified occlusion or stenosis of bilateral middle cerebral arteries — HCC Q
  - I63.519 Cerebral infarction due to unspecified occlusion or stenosis of unspecified middle cerebral artery — HCC Q ▽
- I63.52 Cerebral infarction due to unspecified occlusion or stenosis of anterior cerebral artery
  - I63.521 Cerebral infarction due to unspecified occlusion or stenosis of right anterior cerebral artery — HCC Q
  - I63.522 Cerebral infarction due to unspecified occlusion or stenosis of left anterior cerebral artery — HCC Q
  - I63.523 Cerebral infarction due to unspecified occlusion or stenosis of bilateral anterior cerebral arteries — HCC Q
  - I63.529 Cerebral infarction due to unspecified occlusion or stenosis of unspecified anterior cerebral artery — HCC Q ▽

I63.53 Cerebral infarction due to unspecified occlusion or stenosis of posterior cerebral artery
- I63.531 Cerebral infarction due to unspecified occlusion or stenosis of right posterior cerebral artery — HCC Q
- I63.532 Cerebral infarction due to unspecified occlusion or stenosis of left posterior cerebral artery — HCC Q
- I63.533 Cerebral infarction due to unspecified occlusion or stenosis of bilateral posterior cerebral arteries — HCC Q
- I63.539 Cerebral infarction due to unspecified occlusion or stenosis of unspecified posterior cerebral artery — HCC Q ▽

I63.54 Cerebral infarction due to unspecified occlusion or stenosis of cerebellar artery
- I63.541 Cerebral infarction due to unspecified occlusion or stenosis of right cerebellar artery — HCC Q
- I63.542 Cerebral infarction due to unspecified occlusion or stenosis of left cerebellar artery — HCC Q
- I63.543 Cerebral infarction due to unspecified occlusion or stenosis of bilateral cerebellar arteries — HCC Q
- I63.549 Cerebral infarction due to unspecified occlusion or stenosis of unspecified cerebellar artery — HCC Q ▽

I63.59 Cerebral infarction due to unspecified occlusion or stenosis of other cerebral artery — HCC Q

I63.6 Cerebral infarction due to cerebral venous thrombosis, nonpyogenic — HCC Q

I63.8 Other cerebral infarction
- I63.81 Other cerebral infarction due to occlusion or stenosis of small artery
  Lacunar infarction
- I63.89 Other cerebral infarction

I63.9 Cerebral infarction, unspecified — HCC Q ▽
Stroke NOS
EXCLUDES 2 transient cerebral ischemic attacks and related syndromes (G45.-)
AHA: 2015,1Q,25
TIP: When provider documentation does not identify the location of an infarction, imaging reports can be used to pinpoint the location and lead to a more specific infarction code.

I65 Occlusion and stenosis of precerebral arteries, not resulting in cerebral infarction
INCLUDES embolism of precerebral artery
narrowing of precerebral artery
obstruction (complete) (partial) of precerebral artery
thrombosis of precerebral artery
EXCLUDES 1 insufficiency, NOS, of precerebral artery (G45.-)
insufficiency of precerebral arteries causing cerebral infarction (I63.0-I63.2)
AHA: 2018,2Q,9

I65.0 Occlusion and stenosis of vertebral artery
- I65.01 Occlusion and stenosis of right vertebral artery — Q
- I65.02 Occlusion and stenosis of left vertebral artery — Q
- I65.03 Occlusion and stenosis of bilateral vertebral arteries — Q
- I65.09 Occlusion and stenosis of unspecified vertebral artery — Q ▽

I65.1 Occlusion and stenosis of basilar artery — Q

I65.2 Occlusion and stenosis of carotid artery
- I65.21 Occlusion and stenosis of right carotid artery — Q
- I65.22 Occlusion and stenosis of left carotid artery — Q
- I65.23 Occlusion and stenosis of bilateral carotid arteries — Q

I65.29   **Occlusion and stenosis of unspecified carotid artery**   ▣ ▽

I65.8   **Occlusion and stenosis of other precerebral arteries**   ▣

I65.9   **Occlusion and stenosis of unspecified precerebral artery**   ▣ ▽
     Occlusion and stenosis of precerebral artery NOS

✓4th **I66**   **Occlusion and stenosis of** cerebral **arteries, not resulting in cerebral infarction**

     INCLUDES   embolism of cerebral artery
                narrowing of cerebral artery
                obstruction (complete) (partial) of cerebral artery
                thrombosis of cerebral artery

     EXCLUDES 1   *occlusion and stenosis of cerebral artery causing cerebral infarction (I63.3-I63.5)*

✓5th **I66.0**   **Occlusion and stenosis of** middle **cerebral artery**

     I66.01   **Occlusion and stenosis of** right **middle cerebral artery**   ▣

     I66.02   **Occlusion and stenosis of** left **middle cerebral artery**   ▣

     I66.03   **Occlusion and stenosis of** bilateral **middle cerebral arteries**   ▣

     I66.09   **Occlusion and stenosis of unspecified middle cerebral artery**   ▣ ▽

✓5th **I66.1**   **Occlusion and stenosis of** anterior **cerebral artery**

     I66.11   **Occlusion and stenosis of** right **anterior cerebral artery**   ▣

     I66.12   **Occlusion and stenosis of** left **anterior cerebral artery**   ▣

     I66.13   **Occlusion and stenosis of** bilateral **anterior cerebral arteries**   ▣

     I66.19   **Occlusion and stenosis of unspecified anterior cerebral artery**   ▣ ▽

✓5th **I66.2**   **Occlusion and stenosis of** posterior **cerebral artery**

     I66.21   **Occlusion and stenosis of** right **posterior cerebral artery**   ▣

     I66.22   **Occlusion and stenosis of** left **posterior cerebral artery**   ▣

     I66.23   **Occlusion and stenosis of** bilateral **posterior cerebral arteries**   ▣

     I66.29   **Occlusion and stenosis of unspecified posterior cerebral artery**   ▣ ▽

I66.3   **Occlusion and stenosis of** cerebellar **arteries**   ▣

I66.8   **Occlusion and stenosis of other cerebral arteries**   ▣
     Occlusion and stenosis of perforating arteries

I66.9   **Occlusion and stenosis of unspecified cerebral artery**   ▣ ▽

✓4th **I67**   **Other cerebrovascular diseases**

     EXCLUDES 2   *sequelae of the listed conditions (I69.8)*

     I67.0   **Dissection of cerebral arteries, nonruptured**   HCC
         EXCLUDES 1   *ruptured cerebral arteries (I60.7)*

I67.1   **Cerebral aneurysm, nonruptured**
     Cerebral aneurysm NOS
     Cerebral arteriovenous fistula, acquired
     Internal carotid artery aneurysm, intracranial portion
     Internal carotid artery aneurysm, NOS
     EXCLUDES 1   *congenital cerebral aneurysm, nonruptured (Q28.-)*
                     ruptured cerebral aneurysm (I60.7)

Berry Aneurysm

Berry aneurysms form at the site of a weakness in an arterial wall, often at a junction

Common sites of berry aneurysms in the circle of Willis arteries

I67.2   **Cerebral atherosclerosis**   ▣ Ⓐ
     Atheroma of cerebral and precerebral arteries

I67.3   **Progressive vascular leukoencephalopathy**
     Binswanger's disease

I67.4   **Hypertensive encephalopathy**
     EXCLUDES 2   *insufficiency, NOS, of precerebral arteries (G45.2)*

I67.5   **Moyamoya disease**
     DEF: Cerebrovascular ischemia. Vessels occlude and rupture, causing tiny hemorrhages at the base of brain. It affects predominantly Japanese people.

I67.6   **Nonpyogenic thrombosis of intracranial venous system**
     Nonpyogenic thrombosis of cerebral vein
     Nonpyogenic thrombosis of intracranial venous sinus
     EXCLUDES 1   *nonpyogenic thrombosis of intracranial venous system causing infarction (I63.6)*

I67.7   **Cerebral arteritis, not elsewhere classified**
     Granulomatous angiitis of the nervous system
     EXCLUDES 1   *allergic granulomatous angiitis (M30.1)*

✓5th **I67.8**   **Other specified cerebrovascular diseases**

     I67.81   **Acute cerebrovascular insufficiency**
         Acute cerebrovascular insufficiency unspecified as to location or reversibility

     I67.82   **Cerebral ischemia**
         Chronic cerebral ischemia

     I67.83   **Posterior reversible encephalopathy syndrome**
         PRES

     ✓6th I67.84   **Cerebral vasospasm and vasoconstriction**

         I67.841   **Reversible cerebrovascular vasoconstriction syndrome**
             Call-Fleming syndrome
             Code first underlying condition, if applicable, such as eclampsia (O15.00-O15.9)

         I67.848   **Other cerebrovascular vasospasm and vasoconstriction**

✓ Additional Character Req   √x7th Placeholder Alert   Manifestation   ▽ Unspecified   ▶◀ Revised Text   ● New Code   ▲ Revised Code Title

ICD-10-CM 2019   **649**

Chapter 9. Diseases of the Circulatory System

● ✓6ᵗʰ **I67.85 Hereditary cerebrovascular diseases**

I67.850 Cerebral autosomal dominant arteriopathy with subcortical infarcts and leukoencephalopathy
CADASIL
Code also any associated diagnoses, such as:
epilepsy (G40.-)
stroke (I63.-)
vascular dementia (F01.-)

● **I67.858 Other hereditary cerebrovascular disease**

I67.89 Other cerebrovascular disease

I67.9 Cerebrovascular disease, unspecified ▽

✓4ᵗʰ **I68 Cerebrovascular disorders in diseases classified elsewhere**

I68.0 Cerebral amyloid angiopathy
Code first underlying amyloidosis (E85.-)

I68.2 Cerebral arteritis in other diseases classified elsewhere
Code first underlying disease
EXCLUDES 1   cerebral arteritis (in):
listerosis (A32.89)
syphilis (A52.04)
systemic lupus erythematosus (M32.19)
tuberculosis (A18.89)

I68.8 Other cerebrovascular disorders in diseases classified elsewhere
Code first underlying disease
EXCLUDES 1   syphilitic cerebral aneurysm (A52.05)

✓4ᵗʰ **I69 Sequelae of cerebrovascular disease**

NOTE   Category I69 is to be used to indicate conditions in I60-I67 as the cause of sequelae. The "sequelae" include conditions specified as such or as residuals which may occur at any time after the onset of the causal condition

EXCLUDES 1   personal history of cerebral infarction without residual deficit (Z86.73)
personal history of prolonged reversible ischemic neurologic deficit (PRIND) (Z86.73)
personal history of reversible ischemic neurologcial deficit (RIND) (Z86.73)
sequelae of traumatic intracranial injury (S06.-)

AHA: 2017,1Q,47; 2016,4Q,28; 2015,1Q,25; 2012,4Q,106
TIP: Weakness on one side of the body (unilateral weakness) documented as secondary to old cerebrovascular disease is synonymous with hemiparesis/hemiplegia. Weakness of one limb documented as secondary to old cerebrovascular disease is synonymous with monoplegia.
TIP: For codes describing hemiplegia, hemiparesis, and monoplegia; if the documentation identifies the affected side but not whether it is the dominant or nondominant side, the default is as follows: for ambidextrous patients, the default is dominant; when the left side is affected, the default is nondominant; and when the right side is affected, the default is dominant.

✓5ᵗʰ **I69.0 Sequelae of nontraumatic subarachnoid hemorrhage**

I69.00 Unspecified sequelae of nontraumatic subarachnoid hemorrhage ▽

✓6ᵗʰ **I69.01 Cognitive deficits following nontraumatic subarachnoid hemorrhage**

I69.010 Attention and concentration deficit following nontraumatic subarachnoid hemorrhage

I69.011 Memory deficit following nontraumatic subarachnoid hemorrhage

I69.012 Visuospatial deficit and spatial neglect following nontraumatic subarachnoid hemorrhage

I69.013 Psychomotor deficit following nontraumatic subarachnoid hemorrhage

I69.014 Frontal lobe and executive function deficit following nontraumatic subarachnoid hemorrhage

I69.015 Cognitive social or emotional deficit following nontraumatic subarachnoid hemorrhage

I69.018 Other symptoms and signs involving cognitive functions following nontraumatic subarachnoid hemorrhage

I69.019 Unspecified symptoms and signs involving cognitive functions following nontraumatic subarachnoid hemorrhage ▽

✓6ᵗʰ **I69.02 Speech and language deficits following nontraumatic subarachnoid hemorrhage**

I69.020 Aphasia following nontraumatic subarachnoid hemorrhage

I69.021 Dysphasia following nontraumatic subarachnoid hemorrhage

I69.022 Dysarthria following nontraumatic subarachnoid hemorrhage

I69.023 Fluency disorder following nontraumatic subarachnoid hemorrhage
Stuttering following nontraumatic subarachnoid hemorrhage

I69.028 Other speech and language deficits following nontraumatic subarachnoid hemorrhage

✓6ᵗʰ **I69.03 Monoplegia of upper limb following nontraumatic subarachnoid hemorrhage**
AHA: 2017,1Q,47

I69.031 Monoplegia of upper limb following nontraumatic subarachnoid hemorrhage affecting right dominant side HCC

I69.032 Monoplegia of upper limb following nontraumatic subarachnoid hemorrhage affecting left dominant side HCC

I69.033 Monoplegia of upper limb following nontraumatic subarachnoid hemorrhage affecting right non-dominant side HCC

I69.034 Monoplegia of upper limb following nontraumatic subarachnoid hemorrhage affecting left non-dominant side HCC

I69.039 Monoplegia of upper limb following nontraumatic subarachnoid hemorrhage affecting unspecified side HCC ▽

✓6ᵗʰ **I69.04 Monoplegia of lower limb following nontraumatic subarachnoid hemorrhage**
AHA: 2017,1Q,47

I69.041 Monoplegia of lower limb following nontraumatic subarachnoid hemorrhage affecting right dominant side HCC

I69.042 Monoplegia of lower limb following nontraumatic subarachnoid hemorrhage affecting left dominant side HCC

I69.043 Monoplegia of lower limb following nontraumatic subarachnoid hemorrhage affecting right non-dominant side HCC

I69.044 Monoplegia of lower limb following nontraumatic subarachnoid hemorrhage affecting left non-dominant side HCC

I69.049 Monoplegia of lower limb following nontraumatic subarachnoid hemorrhage affecting unspecified side HCC ▽

✓6ᵗʰ **I69.05 Hemiplegia and hemiparesis following nontraumatic subarachnoid hemorrhage**
AHA: 2015,1Q,25

I69.051 Hemiplegia and hemiparesis following nontraumatic subarachnoid hemorrhage affecting right dominant side HCC

I69.052 Hemiplegia and hemiparesis following nontraumatic subarachnoid hemorrhage affecting left dominant side HCC

I69.053 Hemiplegia and hemiparesis following nontraumatic subarachnoid hemorrhage affecting right non-dominant side HCC

I69.054 Hemiplegia and hemiparesis following nontraumatic subarachnoid hemorrhage affecting left non-dominant side HCC

I69.059   **Hemiplegia and hemiparesis following nontraumatic subarachnoid hemorrhage affecting unspecified side** `HCC` ▽

✓6ᵗʰ   I69.06   **Other paralytic syndrome following nontraumatic subarachnoid hemorrhage**

Use additional code to identify type of paralytic syndrome, such as:
locked-in state (G83.5)
quadriplegia (G82.5-)

EXCLUDES 1   *hemiplegia/hemiparesis following nontraumatic subarachnoid hemorrhage (I69.05-)*
monoplegia of lower limb following nontraumatic subarachnoid hemorrhage (I69.04-)
monoplegia of upper limb following nontraumatic subarachnoid hemorrhage (I69.03-)

I69.061   **Other paralytic syndrome following nontraumatic subarachnoid hemorrhage affecting right dominant side** `HCC`

I69.062   **Other paralytic syndrome following nontraumatic subarachnoid hemorrhage affecting left dominant side** `HCC`

I69.063   **Other paralytic syndrome following nontraumatic subarachnoid hemorrhage affecting right non-dominant side** `HCC`

I69.064   **Other paralytic syndrome following nontraumatic subarachnoid hemorrhage affecting left non-dominant side** `HCC`

I69.065   **Other paralytic syndrome following nontraumatic subarachnoid hemorrhage, bilateral** `HCC`

I69.069   **Other paralytic syndrome following nontraumatic subarachnoid hemorrhage affecting unspecified side** `HCC` ▽

✓6ᵗʰ   I69.09   **Other sequelae of nontraumatic subarachnoid hemorrhage**

I69.090   **Apraxia following nontraumatic subarachnoid hemorrhage**

I69.091   **Dysphagia following nontraumatic subarachnoid hemorrhage**

Use additional code to identify the type of dysphagia, if known (R13.1-)

I69.092   **Facial weakness following nontraumatic subarachnoid hemorrhage**

Facial droop following nontraumatic subarachnoid hemorrhage

I69.093   **Ataxia following nontraumatic subarachnoid hemorrhage**

I69.098   **Other sequelae following nontraumatic subarachnoid hemorrhage**

Alterations of sensation following nontraumatic subarachnoid hemorrhage
Disturbance of vision following nontraumatic subarachnoid hemorrhage
Use additional code to identify the sequelae

✓5ᵗʰ   **I69.1   Sequelae of nontraumatic intracerebral hemorrhage**

I69.10   **Unspecified sequelae of nontraumatic intracerebral hemorrhage** ▽

✓6ᵗʰ   I69.11   **Cognitive deficits following nontraumatic intracerebral hemorrhage**

I69.110   **Attention and concentration deficit following nontraumatic intracerebral hemorrhage**

I69.111   **Memory deficit following nontraumatic intracerebral hemorrhage**

I69.112   **Visuospatial deficit and spatial neglect following nontraumatic intracerebral hemorrhage**

I69.113   **Psychomotor deficit following nontraumatic intracerebral hemorrhage**

I69.114   **Frontal lobe and executive function deficit following nontraumatic intracerebral hemorrhage**

I69.115   **Cognitive social or emotional deficit following nontraumatic intracerebral hemorrhage**

I69.118   **Other symptoms and signs involving cognitive functions following nontraumatic intracerebral hemorrhage**

I69.119   **Unspecified symptoms and signs involving cognitive functions following nontraumatic intracerebral hemorrhage** ▽

✓6ᵗʰ   I69.12   **Speech and language deficits following nontraumatic intracerebral hemorrhage**

I69.120   **Aphasia following nontraumatic intracerebral hemorrhage**

I69.121   **Dysphasia following nontraumatic intracerebral hemorrhage**

I69.122   **Dysarthria following nontraumatic intracerebral hemorrhage**

I69.123   **Fluency disorder following nontraumatic intracerebral hemorrhage**

Stuttering following nontraumatic intracerebral hemorrhage

I69.128   **Other speech and language deficits following nontraumatic intracerebral hemorrhage**

✓6ᵗʰ   I69.13   **Monoplegia of upper limb following nontraumatic intracerebral hemorrhage**

AHA: 2017,1Q,47

I69.131   **Monoplegia of upper limb following nontraumatic intracerebral hemorrhage affecting right dominant side** `HCC`

I69.132   **Monoplegia of upper limb following nontraumatic intracerebral hemorrhage affecting left dominant side** `HCC`

I69.133   **Monoplegia of upper limb following nontraumatic intracerebral hemorrhage affecting right non-dominant side** `HCC`

I69.134   **Monoplegia of upper limb following nontraumatic intracerebral hemorrhage affecting left non-dominant side** `HCC`

I69.139   **Monoplegia of upper limb following nontraumatic intracerebral hemorrhage affecting unspecified side** `HCC` ▽

✓6ᵗʰ   I69.14   **Monoplegia of lower limb following nontraumatic intracerebral hemorrhage**

AHA: 2017,1Q,47

I69.141   **Monoplegia of lower limb following nontraumatic intracerebral hemorrhage affecting right dominant side** `HCC`

I69.142   **Monoplegia of lower limb following nontraumatic intracerebral hemorrhage affecting left dominant side** `HCC`

I69.143   **Monoplegia of lower limb following nontraumatic intracerebral hemorrhage affecting right non-dominant side** `HCC`

I69.144   **Monoplegia of lower limb following nontraumatic intracerebral hemorrhage affecting left non-dominant side** `HCC`

I69.149   **Monoplegia of lower limb following nontraumatic intracerebral hemorrhage affecting unspecified side** `HCC`

☑ Additional Character Req   ✓x7ᵗʰ Placeholder Alert   Manifestation   ▽ Unspecified   ►◄ Revised Text   ● New Code   ▲ Revised Code Title

√6ᵗʰ **I69.15** Hemiplegia and hemiparesis following nontraumatic intracerebral hemorrhage

AHA: 2015,1Q,25

I69.151 Hemiplegia and hemiparesis following nontraumatic intracerebral hemorrhage affecting right dominant side   HCC

I69.152 Hemiplegia and hemiparesis following nontraumatic intracerebral hemorrhage affecting left dominant side   HCC

I69.153 Hemiplegia and hemiparesis following nontraumatic intracerebral hemorrhage affecting right non-dominant side   HCC

I69.154 Hemiplegia and hemiparesis following nontraumatic intracerebral hemorrhage affecting left non-dominant side   HCC

I69.159 Hemiplegia and hemiparesis following nontraumatic intracerebral hemorrhage affecting unspecified side   HCC ▽

√6ᵗʰ **I69.16** Other paralytic syndrome following nontraumatic intracerebral hemorrhage

Use additional code to identify type of paralytic syndrome, such as:
locked-in state (G83.5)
quadriplegia (G82.5-)

EXCLUDES 1   *hemiplegia/hemiparesis following nontraumatic intracerebral hemorrhage (I69.15-)*
monoplegia of lower limb following nontraumatic intracerebral hemorrhage (I69.14-)
monoplegia of upper limb following nontraumatic intracerebral hemorrhage (I69.13-)

I69.161 Other paralytic syndrome following nontraumatic intracerebral hemorrhage affecting right dominant side   HCC

I69.162 Other paralytic syndrome following nontraumatic intracerebral hemorrhage affecting left dominant side   HCC

I69.163 Other paralytic syndrome following nontraumatic intracerebral hemorrhage affecting right non-dominant side   HCC

I69.164 Other paralytic syndrome following nontraumatic intracerebral hemorrhage affecting left non-dominant side   HCC

I69.165 Other paralytic syndrome following nontraumatic intracerebral hemorrhage, bilateral   HCC

I69.169 Other paralytic syndrome following nontraumatic intracerebral hemorrhage affecting unspecified side   HCC ▽

√6ᵗʰ **I69.19** Other sequelae of nontraumatic intracerebral hemorrhage

I69.190 Apraxia following nontraumatic intracerebral hemorrhage

I69.191 Dysphagia following nontraumatic intracerebral hemorrhage

Use additional code to identify the type of dysphagia, if known (R13.1-)

I69.192 Facial weakness following nontraumatic intracerebral hemorrhage

Facial droop following nontraumatic intracerebral hemorrhage

I69.193 Ataxia following nontraumatic intracerebral hemorrhage

I69.198 Other sequelae of nontraumatic intracerebral hemorrhage

Alteration of sensations following nontraumatic intracerebral hemorrhage

Disturbance of vision following nontraumatic intracerebral hemorrhage

Use additional code to identify the sequelae

√5ᵗʰ **I69.2** Sequelae of other nontraumatic intracranial hemorrhage

I69.20 Unspecified sequelae of other nontraumatic intracranial hemorrhage   ▽

√6ᵗʰ **I69.21** Cognitive deficits following other nontraumatic intracranial hemorrhage

I69.210 Attention and concentration deficit following other nontraumatic intracranial hemorrhage

I69.211 Memory deficit following other nontraumatic intracranial hemorrhage

I69.212 Visuospatial deficit and spatial neglect following other nontraumatic intracranial hemorrhage

I69.213 Psychomotor deficit following other nontraumatic intracranial hemorrhage

I69.214 Frontal lobe and executive function deficit following other nontraumatic intracranial hemorrhage

I69.215 Cognitive social or emotional deficit following other nontraumatic intracranial hemorrhage

I69.218 Other symptoms and signs involving cognitive functions following other nontraumatic intracranial hemorrhage

I69.219 Unspecified symptoms and signs involving cognitive functions following other nontraumatic intracranial hemorrhage   ▽

√6ᵗʰ **I69.22** Speech and language deficits following other nontraumatic intracranial hemorrhage

I69.220 Aphasia following other nontraumatic intracranial hemorrhage

I69.221 Dysphasia following other nontraumatic intracranial hemorrhage

I69.222 Dysarthria following other nontraumatic intracranial hemorrhage

I69.223 Fluency disorder following other nontraumatic intracranial hemorrhage

Stuttering following other nontraumatic intracranial hemorrhage

I69.228 Other speech and language deficits following other nontraumatic intracranial hemorrhage

√6ᵗʰ **I69.23** Monoplegia of upper limb following other nontraumatic intracranial hemorrhage

AHA: 2017,1Q,47

I69.231 Monoplegia of upper limb following other nontraumatic intracranial hemorrhage affecting right dominant side   HCC

I69.232 Monoplegia of upper limb following other nontraumatic intracranial hemorrhage affecting left dominant side   HCC

I69.233 Monoplegia of upper limb following other nontraumatic intracranial hemorrhage affecting right non-dominant side   HCC

I69.234 Monoplegia of upper limb following other nontraumatic intracranial hemorrhage affecting left non-dominant side   HCC

I69.239 Monoplegia of upper limb following other nontraumatic intracranial hemorrhage affecting unspecified side   HCC ▽

✓6ᵗʰ **I69.24** **Monoplegia of lower limb** following other nontraumatic intracranial hemorrhage
    AHA: 2017,1Q,47

    I69.241 **Monoplegia of lower limb** following other nontraumatic intracranial hemorrhage affecting **right dominant** side   HCC

    I69.242 **Monoplegia of lower limb** following other nontraumatic intracranial hemorrhage affecting **left dominant** side   HCC

    I69.243 **Monoplegia of lower limb** following other nontraumatic intracranial hemorrhage affecting **right non-dominant** side   HCC

    I69.244 **Monoplegia of lower limb** following other nontraumatic intracranial hemorrhage affecting **left non-dominant** side   HCC

    I69.249 **Monoplegia of lower limb** following other nontraumatic intracranial hemorrhage affecting **unspecified side**   HCC ▽

✓6ᵗʰ **I69.25** **Hemiplegia and hemiparesis** following other nontraumatic intracranial hemorrhage
    AHA: 2015,1Q,25

    I69.251 **Hemiplegia and hemiparesis** following other nontraumatic intracranial hemorrhage affecting **right dominant** side   HCC

    I69.252 **Hemiplegia and hemiparesis** following other nontraumatic intracranial hemorrhage affecting **left dominant** side   HCC

    I69.253 **Hemiplegia and hemiparesis** following other nontraumatic intracranial hemorrhage affecting **right non-dominant** side   HCC

    I69.254 **Hemiplegia and hemiparesis** following other nontraumatic intracranial hemorrhage affecting **left non-dominant** side   HCC

    I69.259 **Hemiplegia and hemiparesis** following other nontraumatic intracranial hemorrhage affecting **unspecified side**   HCC ▽

✓6ᵗʰ **I69.26** **Other paralytic syndrome** following other nontraumatic intracranial hemorrhage
    Use additional code to identify type of paralytic syndrome, such as:
    locked-in state (G83.5)
    quadriplegia (G82.5-)

    EXCLUDES 1   hemiplegia/hemiparesis following other nontraumatic intracranial hemorrhage (I69.25-)
        monoplegia of lower limb following other nontraumatic intracranial hemorrhage (I69.24-)
        monoplegia of upper limb following other nontraumatic intracranial hemorrhage (I69.23-)

    I69.261 **Other paralytic syndrome** following other nontraumatic intracranial hemorrhage affecting **right dominant** side   HCC

    I69.262 **Other paralytic syndrome** following other nontraumatic intracranial hemorrhage affecting **left dominant** side   HCC

    I69.263 **Other paralytic syndrome** following other nontraumatic intracranial hemorrhage affecting **right non-dominant** side   HCC

    I69.264 **Other paralytic syndrome** following other nontraumatic intracranial hemorrhage affecting **left non-dominant** side   HCC

    I69.265 **Other paralytic syndrome** following other nontraumatic intracranial hemorrhage, **bilateral**   HCC

    I69.269 **Other paralytic syndrome** following other nontraumatic intracranial hemorrhage **affecting unspecified side**   HCC ▽

✓6ᵗʰ **I69.29** **Other sequelae of other nontraumatic intracranial hemorrhage**

    I69.290 **Apraxia** following other nontraumatic intracranial hemorrhage

    I69.291 **Dysphagia** following other nontraumatic intracranial hemorrhage
      Use additional code to identify the type of dysphagia, if known (R13.1-)

    I69.292 **Facial weakness** following other nontraumatic intracranial hemorrhage
      Facial droop following other nontraumatic intracranial hemorrhage

    I69.293 **Ataxia** following other nontraumatic intracranial hemorrhage

    I69.298 **Other sequelae** of other nontraumatic intracranial hemorrhage
      Alteration of sensation following other nontraumatic intracranial hemorrhage
      Disturbance of vision following other nontraumatic intracranial hemorrhage
      Use additional code to identify the sequelae

✓5ᵗʰ **I69.3** **Sequelae of** cerebral infarction
    Sequelae of stroke NOS
    AHA: 2013,4Q,127-128; 2012,4Q,92,94

    I69.30 **Unspecified sequelae of cerebral infarction**   ▽

✓6ᵗʰ **I69.31** **Cognitive** deficits following cerebral infarction

    I69.310 **Attention and concentration** deficit following cerebral infarction

    I69.311 **Memory** deficit following cerebral infarction

    I69.312 **Visuospatial** deficit and spatial neglect following cerebral infarction

    I69.313 **Psychomotor** deficit following cerebral infarction

    I69.314 **Frontal lobe and executive function** deficit following cerebral infarction

    I69.315 **Cognitive social or emotional** deficit following cerebral infarction

    I69.318 **Other symptoms and signs involving cognitive functions** following cerebral infarction

    I69.319 **Unspecified symptoms and signs involving cognitive functions** following cerebral infarction   ▽

✓6ᵗʰ **I69.32** **Speech and language deficits** following cerebral infarction

    I69.320 **Aphasia** following cerebral infarction

    I69.321 **Dysphasia** following cerebral infarction
      AHA: 2012,4Q,91

    I69.322 **Dysarthria** following cerebral infarction
      EXCLUDES 2   transient ischemic attack (TIA) (G45.9)

    I69.323 **Fluency disorder** following cerebral infarction
      Stuttering following cerebral infarction

    I69.328 **Other speech and language deficits** following cerebral infarction

✓6ᵗʰ **I69.33** **Monoplegia of upper limb** following cerebral infarction
    AHA: 2017,1Q,47

    I69.331 **Monoplegia of upper limb** following cerebral infarction affecting **right dominant** side   HCC

    I69.332 **Monoplegia of upper limb** following cerebral infarction affecting **left dominant** side   HCC

    I69.333 **Monoplegia of upper limb** following cerebral infarction affecting **right non-dominant** side   HCC

    I69.334 **Monoplegia of upper limb** following cerebral infarction affecting **left non-dominant** side   HCC

✅ Additional Character Req   ✓x7ᵗʰ Placeholder Alert   Manifestation   ▽ Unspecified   ▶◀ Revised Text   ● New Code   ▲ Revised Code Title

ICD-10-CM 2019   653

I69.339 Monoplegia of upper limb following cerebral infarction affecting unspecified side   HCC ▽

√6ᵗʰ **I69.34** Monoplegia of lower limb following cerebral infarction

AHA: 2017,1Q,47

I69.341 Monoplegia of lower limb following cerebral infarction affecting right dominant side   HCC

I69.342 Monoplegia of lower limb following cerebral infarction affecting left dominant side   HCC

I69.343 Monoplegia of lower limb following cerebral infarction affecting right non-dominant side   HCC

I69.344 Monoplegia of lower limb following cerebral infarction affecting left non-dominant side   HCC

I69.349 Monoplegia of lower limb following cerebral infarction affecting unspecified side   HCC ▽

√6ᵗʰ **I69.35** Hemiplegia and hemiparesis following cerebral infarction

AHA: 2015,1Q,25

I69.351 Hemiplegia and hemiparesis following cerebral infarction affecting right dominant side   HCC

> EXCLUDES 2   transient ischemic attack (TIA) (G45.9)

I69.352 Hemiplegia and hemiparesis following cerebral infarction affecting left dominant side   HCC

I69.353 Hemiplegia and hemiparesis following cerebral infarction affecting right non-dominant side   HCC

I69.354 Hemiplegia and hemiparesis following cerebral infarction affecting left non-dominant side   HCC

AHA: 2012,4Q,91

I69.359 Hemiplegia and hemiparesis following cerebral infarction affecting unspecified side   HCC ▽

√6ᵗʰ **I69.36** Other paralytic syndrome following cerebral infarction

Use additional code to identify type of paralytic syndrome, such as:

locked-in state (G83.5)
quadriplegia (G82.5-)

> EXCLUDES 1   hemiplegia/hemiparesis following cerebral infarction (I69.35-)
> monoplegia of lower limb following cerebral infarction (I69.34-)
> monoplegia of upper limb following cerebral infarction (I69.33-)

I69.361 Other paralytic syndrome following cerebral infarction affecting right dominant side   HCC

I69.362 Other paralytic syndrome following cerebral infarction affecting left dominant side   HCC

I69.363 Other paralytic syndrome following cerebral infarction affecting right non-dominant side   HCC

I69.364 Other paralytic syndrome following cerebral infarction affecting left non-dominant side   HCC

I69.365 Other paralytic syndrome following cerebral infarction, bilateral   HCC

I69.369 Other paralytic syndrome following cerebral infarction affecting unspecified side   HCC ▽

√6ᵗʰ **I69.39** Other sequelae of cerebral infarction

I69.390 Apraxia following cerebral infarction

I69.391 Dysphagia following cerebral infarction

Use additional code to identify the type of dysphagia, if known (R13.1-)

I69.392 Facial weakness following cerebral infarction

Facial droop following cerebral infarction

I69.393 Ataxia following cerebral infarction

I69.398 Other sequelae of cerebral infarction

Alteration of sensation following cerebral infarction

Disturbance of vision following cerebral infarction

Use additional code to identify the sequelae

√5ᵗʰ **I69.8** Sequelae of other cerebrovascular diseases

> EXCLUDES 1   sequelae of traumatic intracranial injury (S06.-)

I69.80 Unspecified sequelae of other cerebrovascular disease   ▽

√6ᵗʰ **I69.81** Cognitive deficits following other cerebrovascular disease

I69.810 Attention and concentration deficit following other cerebrovascular disease

I69.811 Memory deficit following other cerebrovascular disease

I69.812 Visuospatial deficit and spatial neglect following other cerebrovascular disease

I69.813 Psychomotor deficit following other cerebrovascular disease

I69.814 Frontal lobe and executive function deficit following other cerebrovascular disease

I69.815 Cognitive social or emotional deficit following other cerebrovascular disease

I69.818 Other symptoms and signs involving cognitive functions following other cerebrovascular disease

I69.819 Unspecified symptoms and signs involving cognitive functions following other cerebrovascular disease   ▽

√6ᵗʰ **I69.82** Speech and language deficits following other cerebrovascular disease

I69.820 Aphasia following other cerebrovascular disease

I69.821 Dysphasia following other cerebrovascular disease

I69.822 Dysarthria following other cerebrovascular disease

I69.823 Fluency disorder following other cerebrovascular disease

Stuttering following other cerebrovascular disease

I69.828 Other speech and language deficits following other cerebrovascular disease

√6ᵗʰ **I69.83** Monoplegia of upper limb following other cerebrovascular disease

AHA: 2017,1Q,47

I69.831 Monoplegia of upper limb following other cerebrovascular disease affecting right dominant side   HCC

I69.832 Monoplegia of upper limb following other cerebrovascular disease affecting left dominant side   HCC

I69.833 Monoplegia of upper limb following other cerebrovascular disease affecting right non-dominant side   HCC

I69.834 Monoplegia of upper limb following other cerebrovascular disease affecting left non-dominant side   HCC

I69.839 Monoplegia of upper limb following other cerebrovascular disease affecting unspecified side   HCC ▽

√6ᵗʰ **I69.84** Monoplegia of lower limb following other cerebrovascular disease

AHA: 2017,1Q,47

I69.841 Monoplegia of lower limb following other cerebrovascular disease affecting right dominant side   HCC

I69.842 Monoplegia of lower limb following other cerebrovascular disease affecting left dominant side `HCC`

I69.843 Monoplegia of lower limb following other cerebrovascular disease affecting right non-dominant side `HCC`

I69.844 Monoplegia of lower limb following other cerebrovascular disease affecting left non-dominant side `HCC`

I69.849 Monoplegia of lower limb following other cerebrovascular disease affecting unspecified side `HCC` ▽

√6ᵗʰ **I69.85** Hemiplegia and hemiparesis following other cerebrovascular disease
     AHA: 2015,1Q,25

I69.851 Hemiplegia and hemiparesis following other cerebrovascular disease affecting right dominant side `HCC`

I69.852 Hemiplegia and hemiparesis following other cerebrovascular disease affecting left dominant side `HCC`

I69.853 Hemiplegia and hemiparesis following other cerebrovascular disease affecting right non-dominant side `HCC`

I69.854 Hemiplegia and hemiparesis following other cerebrovascular disease affecting left non-dominant side `HCC`

I69.859 Hemiplegia and hemiparesis following other cerebrovascular disease affecting unspecified side `HCC` ▽

√6ᵗʰ **I69.86** Other paralytic syndrome following other cerebrovascular disease
     Use additional code to identify type of paralytic syndrome, such as:
     locked-in state (G83.5)
     quadriplegia (G82.5-)
     EXCLUDES 1   hemiplegia/hemiparesis following other cerebrovascular disease (I69.85-)
            monoplegia of lower limb following other cerebrovascular disease (I69.84-)
            monoplegia of upper limb following other cerebrovascular disease (I69.83-)

I69.861 Other paralytic syndrome following other cerebrovascular disease affecting right dominant side `HCC`

I69.862 Other paralytic syndrome following other cerebrovascular disease affecting left dominant side `HCC`

I69.863 Other paralytic syndrome following other cerebrovascular disease affecting right non-dominant side `HCC`

I69.864 Other paralytic syndrome following other cerebrovascular disease affecting left non-dominant side `HCC`

I69.865 Other paralytic syndrome following other cerebrovascular disease, bilateral `HCC`

I69.869 Other paralytic syndrome following other cerebrovascular disease affecting unspecified side `HCC` ▽

√6ᵗʰ **I69.89** Other sequelae of other cerebrovascular disease

I69.890 Apraxia following other cerebrovascular disease

I69.891 Dysphagia following other cerebrovascular disease
     Use additional code to identify the type of dysphagia, if known (R13.1-)

I69.892 Facial weakness following other cerebrovascular disease
     Facial droop following other cerebrovascular disease

I69.893 Ataxia following other cerebrovascular disease

I69.898 Other sequelae of other cerebrovascular disease
     Alteration of sensation following other cerebrovascular disease
     Disturbance of vision following other cerebrovascular disease
     Use additional code to identify the sequelae

√5ᵗʰ **I69.9** Sequelae of unspecified cerebrovascular diseases
     EXCLUDES 1   sequelae of stroke (I69.3)
            sequelae of traumatic intracranial injury (S06.-)

I69.90 Unspecified sequelae of unspecified cerebrovascular disease ▽

√6ᵗʰ **I69.91** Cognitive deficits following unspecified cerebrovascular disease

I69.910 Attention and concentration deficit following unspecified cerebrovascular disease ▽

I69.911 Memory deficit following unspecified cerebrovascular disease ▽

I69.912 Visuospatial deficit and spatial neglect following unspecified cerebrovascular disease ▽

I69.913 Psychomotor deficit following unspecified cerebrovascular disease ▽

I69.914 Frontal lobe and executive function deficit following unspecified cerebrovascular disease ▽

I69.915 Cognitive social or emotional deficit following unspecified cerebrovascular disease ▽

I69.918 Other symptoms and signs involving cognitive functions following unspecified cerebrovascular disease ▽

I69.919 Unspecified symptoms and signs involving cognitive functions following unspecified cerebrovascular disease ▽

√6ᵗʰ **I69.92** Speech and language deficits following unspecified cerebrovascular disease

I69.920 Aphasia following unspecified cerebrovascular disease ▽

I69.921 Dysphasia following unspecified cerebrovascular disease ▽

I69.922 Dysarthria following unspecified cerebrovascular disease ▽

I69.923 Fluency disorder following unspecified cerebrovascular disease ▽
     Stuttering following unspecified cerebrovascular disease

I69.928 Other speech and language deficits following unspecified cerebrovascular disease ▽

√6ᵗʰ **I69.93** Monoplegia of upper limb following unspecified cerebrovascular disease
     AHA: 2017,1Q,47

I69.931 Monoplegia of upper limb following unspecified cerebrovascular disease affecting right dominant side `HCC` ▽

I69.932 Monoplegia of upper limb following unspecified cerebrovascular disease affecting left dominant side `HCC` ▽

I69.933 Monoplegia of upper limb following unspecified cerebrovascular disease affecting right non-dominant side `HCC` ▽

     I69.934   **Monoplegia of upper limb following unspecified cerebrovascular disease affecting** left non-dominant **side** `HCC` ▽

     I69.939   **Monoplegia of upper limb following unspecified cerebrovascular disease affecting unspecified side** `HCC` ▽

✓6ᵗʰ **I69.94**   **Monoplegia of lower limb** following unspecified cerebrovascular disease

      AHA: 2017,1Q,47

     I69.941   **Monoplegia of lower limb following unspecified cerebrovascular disease affecting** right dominant **side** `HCC` ▽

     I69.942   **Monoplegia of lower limb following unspecified cerebrovascular disease affecting** left dominant **side** `HCC` ▽

     I69.943   **Monoplegia of lower limb following unspecified cerebrovascular disease affecting** right non-dominant **side** `HCC` ▽

     I69.944   **Monoplegia of lower limb following unspecified cerebrovascular disease affecting** left non-dominant **side** `HCC` ▽

     I69.949   **Monoplegia of lower limb following unspecified cerebrovascular disease affecting unspecified side** `HCC` ▽

✓6ᵗʰ **I69.95**   **Hemiplegia and hemiparesis following unspecified cerebrovascular disease**

      AHA: 2015,1Q,25

     I69.951   **Hemiplegia and hemiparesis following unspecified cerebrovascular disease affecting** right dominant **side** `HCC` ▽

     I69.952   **Hemiplegia and hemiparesis following unspecified cerebrovascular disease affecting** left dominant **side** `HCC` ▽

     I69.953   **Hemiplegia and hemiparesis following unspecified cerebrovascular disease affecting** right non-dominant **side** `HCC` ▽

     I69.954   **Hemiplegia and hemiparesis following unspecified cerebrovascular disease affecting** left non-dominant **side** `HCC` ▽

     I69.959   **Hemiplegia and hemiparesis following unspecified cerebrovascular disease affecting unspecified side** `HCC` ▽

✓6ᵗʰ **I69.96**   **Other** paralytic syndrome **following unspecified cerebrovascular disease**

      Use additional code to identify type of paralytic syndrome, such as:
      locked-in state (G83.5)
      quadriplegia (G82.5-)

     EXCLUDES 1   *hemiplegia/hemiparesis following unspecified cerebrovascular disease (I69.95-)*
      monoplegia of lower limb following unspecified cerebrovascular disease (I69.94-)
      monoplegia of upper limb following unspecified cerebrovascular disease (I69.93-)

     I69.961   **Other paralytic syndrome following unspecified cerebrovascular disease affecting** right dominant **side** `HCC` ▽

     I69.962   **Other paralytic syndrome following unspecified cerebrovascular disease affecting** left dominant **side** `HCC` ▽

     I69.963   **Other paralytic syndrome following unspecified cerebrovascular disease affecting** right non-dominant **side** `HCC` ▽

     I69.964   **Other paralytic syndrome following unspecified cerebrovascular disease affecting** left non-dominant **side** `HCC` ▽

     I69.965   **Other paralytic syndrome following unspecified cerebrovascular disease, bilateral** `HCC` ▽

     I69.969   **Other paralytic syndrome following unspecified cerebrovascular disease affecting unspecified side** `HCC` ▽

✓6ᵗʰ **I69.99**   **Other sequelae of unspecified cerebrovascular disease**

     I69.990   **Apraxia following unspecified cerebrovascular disease** ▽

     I69.991   **Dysphagia following unspecified cerebrovascular disease** ▽
      Use additional code to identify the type of dysphagia, if known (R13.1-)

     I69.992   **Facial weakness following unspecified cerebrovascular disease** ▽
      Facial droop following unspecified cerebrovascular disease

     I69.993   **Ataxia following unspecified cerebrovascular disease** ▽

     I69.998   **Other sequelae following unspecified cerebrovascular disease** ▽
      Alteration in sensation following unspecified cerebrovascular disease
      Disturbance of vision following unspecified cerebrovascular disease
      Use additional code to identify the sequelae

Diseases of arteries, arterioles and capillaries (I70-I79)

✓4ᵗʰ **I70**   **Atherosclerosis**

      `INCLUDES`   arterial degeneration
      arteriolosclerosis
      arteriosclerosis
      arteriosclerotic vascular disease
      arteriovascular degeneration
      atheroma
      endarteritis deformans or obliterans
      senile arteritis
      senile endarteritis
      vascular degeneration

      Use additional code to identify:
      exposure to environmental tobacco smoke (Z77.22)
      history of tobacco dependence (Z87.891)
      occupational exposure to environmental tobacco smoke (Z57.31)
      tobacco dependence (F17.-)
      tobacco use (Z72.0)

      EXCLUDES 2   *arteriosclerotic cardiovascular disease (I25.1-)*
      arteriosclerotic heart disease (I25.1-)
      atheroembolism (I75.-)
      cerebral atherosclerosis (I67.2)
      coronary atherosclerosis (I25.1-)
      mesenteric atherosclerosis (K55.1)
      precerebral atherosclerosis (I67.2)
      primary pulmonary atherosclerosis (I27.0)

I70.0   **Atherosclerosis of aorta** `HCC` `Q` `A`

I70.1   **Atherosclerosis of renal artery** `HCC` `Q` `A`
      Goldblatt's kidney
      EXCLUDES 2   *atherosclerosis of renal arterioles (I12.-)*

✓5ᵗʰ I70.2 Atherosclerosis of native arteries of the extremities
     Mönckeberg's (medial) sclerosis
     Use additional code, if applicable, to identify chronic total
       occlusion of artery of extremity (I70.92)
     EXCLUDES 2   atherosclerosis of bypass graft of extremities
         (I70.30–I70.79)
     AHA: 2018,2Q,7

   ✓6ᵗʰ **I70.20 Unspecified atherosclerosis of native arteries of extremities**

     I70.201 Unspecified atherosclerosis of HCC Q A ▽
         native arteries of extremities, right leg

     I70.202 Unspecified atherosclerosis of HCC Q A ▽
         native arteries of extremities, left leg

     I70.203 Unspecified atherosclerosis of HCC Q A ▽
         native arteries of extremities, bilateral legs

     I70.208 Unspecified atherosclerosis of HCC Q A ▽
         native arteries of extremities, other extremity

     I70.209 Unspecified atherosclerosis of HCC Q A ▽
         native arteries of extremities, unspecified extremity

   ✓6ᵗʰ **I70.21 Atherosclerosis of native arteries of extremities with intermittent claudication**

     I70.211 Atherosclerosis of native HCC Q A
         arteries of extremities with intermittent claudication, right leg

     I70.212 Atherosclerosis of native HCC Q A
         arteries of extremities with intermittent claudication, left leg

     I70.213 Atherosclerosis of native HCC Q A
         arteries of extremities with intermittent claudication, bilateral legs

     I70.218 Atherosclerosis of native HCC Q A
         arteries of extremities with intermittent claudication, other extremity

     I70.219 Atherosclerosis of native HCC Q A ▽
         arteries of extremities with intermittent claudication, unspecified extremity

   ✓6ᵗʰ **I70.22 Atherosclerosis of native arteries of extremities with rest pain**
     INCLUDES   any condition classifiable to I70.21-

     I70.221 Atherosclerosis of native HCC Q A
         arteries of extremities with rest pain, right leg

     I70.222 Atherosclerosis of native HCC Q A
         arteries of extremities with rest pain, left leg

     I70.223 Atherosclerosis of native HCC Q A
         arteries of extremities with rest pain, bilateral legs

     I70.228 Atherosclerosis of native HCC Q A
         arteries of extremities with rest pain, other extremity

     I70.229 Atherosclerosis of native HCC Q A ▽
         arteries of extremities with rest pain, unspecified extremity

   ✓6ᵗʰ **I70.23 Atherosclerosis of native arteries of right leg with ulceration**
     INCLUDES   any condition classifiable to I70.211 and
         I70.221
     Use additional code to identify severity of ulcer (L97.-)

     I70.231 Atherosclerosis of native HCC Q A
         arteries of right leg with ulceration of thigh

     I70.232 Atherosclerosis of native HCC Q A
         arteries of right leg with ulceration of calf

     I70.233 Atherosclerosis of native HCC Q A
         arteries of right leg with ulceration of ankle

     I70.234 Atherosclerosis of native HCC Q A
         arteries of right leg with ulceration of heel and midfoot
         Atherosclerosis of native arteries of right
           leg with ulceration of plantar surface
           of midfoot

     I70.235 Atherosclerosis of native HCC Q A
         arteries of right leg with ulceration of other part of foot
         Atherosclerosis of native arteries of right
           leg extremities with ulceration of toe

     I70.238 Atherosclerosis of native HCC Q A
         arteries of right leg with ulceration of other part of lower right leg

     I70.239 Atherosclerosis of native HCC Q A ▽
         arteries of right leg with ulceration of unspecified site

   ✓6ᵗʰ **I70.24 Atherosclerosis of native arteries of left leg with ulceration**
     INCLUDES   any condition classifiable to I70.212 and
         I70.222
     Use additional code to identify severity of ulcer (L97.-)

     I70.241 Atherosclerosis of native HCC Q A
         arteries of left leg with ulceration of thigh

     I70.242 Atherosclerosis of native HCC Q A
         arteries of left leg with ulceration of calf

     I70.243 Atherosclerosis of native HCC Q A
         arteries of left leg with ulceration of ankle

     I70.244 Atherosclerosis of native HCC Q A
         arteries of left leg with ulceration of heel and midfoot
         Atherosclerosis of native arteries of left leg
           with ulceration of plantar surface of
           midfoot

     I70.245 Atherosclerosis of native HCC Q A
         arteries of left leg with ulceration of other part of foot
         Atherosclerosis of native arteries of left leg
           extremities with ulceration of toe

     I70.248 Atherosclerosis of native HCC Q A
         arteries of left leg with ulceration of other part of lower left leg

     I70.249 Atherosclerosis of native HCC Q A ▽
         arteries of left leg with ulceration of unspecified site

   I70.25 Atherosclerosis of native arteries of other HCC Q A
     extremities with ulceration
     INCLUDES   any condition classifiable to I70.218 and
         I70.228
     Use additional code to identify the severity of the
       ulcer (L98.49-)

   ✓6ᵗʰ **I70.26 Atherosclerosis of native arteries of extremities with gangrene**
     INCLUDES   any condition classifiable to I70.21-,
         I70.22-, I70.23-, I70.24-, and I70.25-
     Use additional code to identify the severity of any
       ulcer (L97.-, L98.49-), if applicable

     I70.261 Atherosclerosis of native HCC Q A
         arteries of extremities with gangrene, right leg

     I70.262 Atherosclerosis of native HCC Q A
         arteries of extremities with gangrene, left leg

     I70.263 Atherosclerosis of native HCC Q A
         arteries of extremities with gangrene, bilateral legs

     I70.268 Atherosclerosis of native HCC Q A
         arteries of extremities with gangrene, other extremity

     I70.269 Atherosclerosis of native HCC Q A ▽
         arteries of extremities with gangrene, unspecified extremity

   ✓6ᵗʰ **I70.29 Other atherosclerosis of native arteries of extremities**

     I70.291 Other atherosclerosis of native HCC Q A
         arteries of extremities, right leg

✓ Additional Character Req   ✓x7ᵗʰ Placeholder Alert   Manifestation   ▽ Unspecified   ►◄ Revised Text   ● New Code   ▲ Revised Code Title

ICD-10-CM 2019   657

I70.292 Other atherosclerosis of native HCC Q A arteries of extremities, left leg

I70.293 Other atherosclerosis of native HCC Q A arteries of extremities, bilateral legs

I70.298 Other atherosclerosis of native HCC Q A arteries of extremities, other extremity

I70.299 Other atherosclerosis of native HCC Q A ▽ arteries of extremities, unspecified extremity

√5ᵗʰ **I70.3** Atherosclerosis of unspecified type of bypass graft(s) of the extremities

Use additional code, if applicable, to identify chronic total occlusion of artery of extremity (I70.92)

EXCLUDES 1   embolism or thrombus of bypass graft(s) of extremities (T82.8-)

√6ᵗʰ **I70.30** Unspecified atherosclerosis of unspecified type of bypass graft(s) of the extremities

I70.301 Unspecified atherosclerosis of HCC Q A ▽ unspecified type of bypass graft(s) of the extremities, right leg

I70.302 Unspecified atherosclerosis of HCC Q A ▽ unspecified type of bypass graft(s) of the extremities, left leg

I70.303 Unspecified atherosclerosis of HCC Q A ▽ unspecified type of bypass graft(s) of the extremities, bilateral legs

I70.308 Unspecified atherosclerosis of HCC Q A ▽ unspecified type of bypass graft(s) of the extremities, other extremity

I70.309 Unspecified atherosclerosis of HCC Q A ▽ unspecified type of bypass graft(s) of the extremities, unspecified extremity

√6ᵗʰ **I70.31** Atherosclerosis of unspecified type of bypass graft(s) of the extremities with intermittent claudication

I70.311 Atherosclerosis of unspecified HCC Q A type of bypass graft(s) of the extremities with intermittent claudication, right leg

I70.312 Atherosclerosis of unspecified HCC Q A type of bypass graft(s) of the extremities with intermittent claudication, left leg

I70.313 Atherosclerosis of unspecified HCC Q A type of bypass graft(s) of the extremities with intermittent claudication, bilateral legs

I70.318 Atherosclerosis of unspecified HCC Q A type of bypass graft(s) of the extremities with intermittent claudication, other extremity

I70.319 Atherosclerosis of unspecified HCC Q A ▽ type of bypass graft(s) of the extremities with intermittent claudication, unspecified extremity

√6ᵗʰ **I70.32** Atherosclerosis of unspecified type of bypass graft(s) of the extremities with rest pain

INCLUDES   any condition classifiable to I70.31-

I70.321 Atherosclerosis of unspecified HCC Q A type of bypass graft(s) of the extremities with rest pain, right leg

I70.322 Atherosclerosis of unspecified HCC Q A type of bypass graft(s) of the extremities with rest pain, left leg

I70.323 Atherosclerosis of unspecified HCC Q A type of bypass graft(s) of the extremities with rest pain, bilateral legs

I70.328 Atherosclerosis of unspecified HCC Q A type of bypass graft(s) of the extremities with rest pain, other extremity

I70.329 Atherosclerosis of unspecified HCC Q A ▽ type of bypass graft(s) of the extremities with rest pain, unspecified extremity

√6ᵗʰ **I70.33** Atherosclerosis of unspecified type of bypass graft(s) of the right leg with ulceration

INCLUDES   any condition classifiable to I70.311 and I70.321

Use additional code to identify severity of ulcer (L97.-)

I70.331 Atherosclerosis of unspecified HCC Q A type of bypass graft(s) of the right leg with ulceration of thigh

I70.332 Atherosclerosis of unspecified HCC Q A type of bypass graft(s) of the right leg with ulceration of calf

I70.333 Atherosclerosis of unspecified HCC Q A type of bypass graft(s) of the right leg with ulceration of ankle

I70.334 Atherosclerosis of unspecified HCC Q A type of bypass graft(s) of the right leg with ulceration of heel and midfoot

Atherosclerosis of unspecified type of bypass graft(s) of right leg with ulceration of plantar surface of midfoot

I70.335 Atherosclerosis of unspecified HCC Q A type of bypass graft(s) of the right leg with ulceration of other part of foot

Atherosclerosis of unspecified type of bypass graft(s) of the right leg with ulceration of toe

I70.338 Atherosclerosis of unspecified HCC Q A type of bypass graft(s) of the right leg with ulceration of other part of lower leg

I70.339 Atherosclerosis of unspecified HCC Q A ▽ type of bypass graft(s) of the right leg with ulceration of unspecified site

√6ᵗʰ **I70.34** Atherosclerosis of unspecified type of bypass graft(s) of the left leg with ulceration

INCLUDES   any condition classifiable to I70.312 and I70.322

Use additional code to identify severity of ulcer (L97.-)

I70.341 Atherosclerosis of unspecified HCC Q A type of bypass graft(s) of the left leg with ulceration of thigh

I70.342 Atherosclerosis of unspecified HCC Q A type of bypass graft(s) of the left leg with ulceration of calf

I70.343 Atherosclerosis of unspecified HCC Q A type of bypass graft(s) of the left leg with ulceration of ankle

I70.344 Atherosclerosis of unspecified HCC Q A type of bypass graft(s) of the left leg with ulceration of heel and midfoot

Atherosclerosis of unspecified type of bypass graft(s) of left leg with ulceration of plantar surface of midfoot

I70.345 Atherosclerosis of unspecified HCC Q A type of bypass graft(s) of the left leg with ulceration of other part of foot

Atherosclerosis of unspecified type of bypass graft(s) of the left leg with ulceration of toe

I70.348 Atherosclerosis of unspecified HCC Q A type of bypass graft(s) of the left leg with ulceration of other part of lower leg

I70.349 Atherosclerosis of unspecified HCC Q A ▽ type of bypass graft(s) of the left leg with ulceration of unspecified site

I70.35 Atherosclerosis of unspecified type of bypass graft(s) of other extremity with ulceration ᴴᶜᶜ Q A
  INCLUDES any condition classifiable to I70.318 and I70.328
  Use additional code to identify severity of ulcer (L98.49-)

√6ᵗʰ **I70.36** Atherosclerosis of unspecified type of bypass graft(s) of the extremities with gangrene
  INCLUDES any condition classifiable to I70.31-, I70.32-, I70.33-, I70.34-, I70.35
  Use additional code to identify the severity of any ulcer (L97.-, L98.49-), if applicable

  I70.361 Atherosclerosis of unspecified ᴴᶜᶜ Q A type of bypass graft(s) of the extremities with gangrene, right leg
  I70.362 Atherosclerosis of unspecified ᴴᶜᶜ Q A type of bypass graft(s) of the extremities with gangrene, left leg
  I70.363 Atherosclerosis of unspecified ᴴᶜᶜ Q A type of bypass graft(s) of the extremities with gangrene, bilateral legs
  I70.368 Atherosclerosis of unspecified ᴴᶜᶜ Q A type of bypass graft(s) of the extremities with gangrene, other extremity
  I70.369 Atherosclerosis of unspecified ᴴᶜᶜ Q A ▽ type of bypass graft(s) of the extremities with gangrene, unspecified extremity

√6ᵗʰ **I70.39** Other atherosclerosis of unspecified type of bypass graft(s) of the extremities

  I70.391 Other atherosclerosis of ᴴᶜᶜ Q A unspecified type of bypass graft(s) of the extremities, right leg
  I70.392 Other atherosclerosis of ᴴᶜᶜ Q A unspecified type of bypass graft(s) of the extremities, left leg
  I70.393 Other atherosclerosis of ᴴᶜᶜ Q A unspecified type of bypass graft(s) of the extremities, bilateral legs
  I70.398 Other atherosclerosis of ᴴᶜᶜ Q A unspecified type of bypass graft(s) of the extremities, other extremity
  I70.399 Other atherosclerosis of ᴴᶜᶜ Q A ▽ unspecified type of bypass graft(s) of the extremities, unspecified extremity

√5ᵗʰ **I70.4** Atherosclerosis of autologous vein bypass graft(s) of the extremities
  Use additional code, if applicable, to identify chronic total occlusion of artery of extremity (I70.92)

√6ᵗʰ **I70.40** Unspecified atherosclerosis of autologous vein bypass graft(s) of the extremities

  I70.401 Unspecified atherosclerosis of ᴴᶜᶜ Q A ▽ autologous vein bypass graft(s) of the extremities, right leg
  I70.402 Unspecified atherosclerosis of ᴴᶜᶜ Q A ▽ autologous vein bypass graft(s) of the extremities, left leg
  I70.403 Unspecified atherosclerosis of ᴴᶜᶜ Q A ▽ autologous vein bypass graft(s) of the extremities, bilateral legs
  I70.408 Unspecified atherosclerosis of ᴴᶜᶜ Q A ▽ autologous vein bypass graft(s) of the extremities, other extremity
  I70.409 Unspecified atherosclerosis of ᴴᶜᶜ Q A ▽ autologous vein bypass graft(s) of the extremities, unspecified extremity

√6ᵗʰ **I70.41** Atherosclerosis of autologous vein bypass graft(s) of the extremities with intermittent claudication

  I70.411 Atherosclerosis of autologous ᴴᶜᶜ Q A vein bypass graft(s) of the extremities with intermittent claudication, right leg

  I70.412 Atherosclerosis of autologous ᴴᶜᶜ Q A vein bypass graft(s) of the extremities with intermittent claudication, left leg
  I70.413 Atherosclerosis of autologous ᴴᶜᶜ Q A vein bypass graft(s) of the extremities with intermittent claudication, bilateral legs
  I70.418 Atherosclerosis of autologous ᴴᶜᶜ Q A vein bypass graft(s) of the extremities with intermittent claudication, other extremity
  I70.419 Atherosclerosis of autologous ᴴᶜᶜ Q A ▽ vein bypass graft(s) of the extremities with intermittent claudication, unspecified extremity

√6ᵗʰ **I70.42** Atherosclerosis of autologous vein bypass graft(s) of the extremities with rest pain
  INCLUDES any condition classifiable to I70.41-

  I70.421 Atherosclerosis of autologous ᴴᶜᶜ Q A vein bypass graft(s) of the extremities with rest pain, right leg
  I70.422 Atherosclerosis of autologous ᴴᶜᶜ Q A vein bypass graft(s) of the extremities with rest pain, left leg
  I70.423 Atherosclerosis of autologous ᴴᶜᶜ Q A vein bypass graft(s) of the extremities with rest pain, bilateral legs
  I70.428 Atherosclerosis of autologous ᴴᶜᶜ Q A vein bypass graft(s) of the extremities with rest pain, other extremity
  I70.429 Atherosclerosis of autologous ᴴᶜᶜ Q A ▽ vein bypass graft(s) of the extremities with rest pain, unspecified extremity

√6ᵗʰ **I70.43** Atherosclerosis of autologous vein bypass graft(s) of the right leg with ulceration
  INCLUDES any condition classifiable to I70.411 and I70.421
  Use additional code to identify severity of ulcer (L97.-)

  I70.431 Atherosclerosis of autologous ᴴᶜᶜ Q A vein bypass graft(s) of the right leg with ulceration of thigh
  I70.432 Atherosclerosis of autologous ᴴᶜᶜ Q A vein bypass graft(s) of the right leg with ulceration of calf
  I70.433 Atherosclerosis of autologous ᴴᶜᶜ Q A vein bypass graft(s) of the right leg with ulceration of ankle
  I70.434 Atherosclerosis of autologous ᴴᶜᶜ Q A vein bypass graft(s) of the right leg with ulceration of heel and midfoot
    Atherosclerosis of autologous vein bypass graft(s) of right leg with ulceration of plantar surface of midfoot
  I70.435 Atherosclerosis of autologous ᴴᶜᶜ Q A vein bypass graft(s) of the right leg with ulceration of other part of foot
    Atherosclerosis of autologous vein bypass graft(s) of right leg with ulceration of toe
  I70.438 Atherosclerosis of autologous ᴴᶜᶜ Q A vein bypass graft(s) of the right leg with ulceration of other part of lower leg
  I70.439 Atherosclerosis of autologous ᴴᶜᶜ Q A ▽ vein bypass graft(s) of the right leg with ulceration of unspecified site

√6ᵗʰ **I70.44** Atherosclerosis of autologous vein bypass graft(s) of the left leg with ulceration
  INCLUDES any condition classifiable to I70.412 and I70.422
  Use additional code to identify severity of ulcer (L97.-)

  I70.441 Atherosclerosis of autologous ᴴᶜᶜ Q A vein bypass graft(s) of the left leg with ulceration of thigh

✓ Additional Character Req   √x7ᵗʰ Placeholder Alert   Manifestation   ▽ Unspecified   ►◄ Revised Text   ● New Code   ▲ Revised Code Title

ICD-10-CM 2019
659
Chapter 9. Diseases of the Circulatory System
I70.35–I70.441

I70.442   **Atherosclerosis of autologous** HCC Q A **vein bypass graft(s) of the left leg with ulceration of** calf

I70.443   **Atherosclerosis of autologous** HCC Q A **vein bypass graft(s) of the left leg with ulceration of** ankle

I70.444   **Atherosclerosis of autologous** HCC Q A **vein bypass graft(s) of the left leg with ulceration of** heel and midfoot
    Atherosclerosis of autologous vein bypass graft(s) of left leg with ulceration of plantar surface of midfoot

I70.445   **Atherosclerosis of autologous** HCC Q A **vein bypass graft(s) of the left leg with ulceration of other part of foot**
    Atherosclerosis of autologous vein bypass graft(s) of left leg with ulceration of toe

I70.448   **Atherosclerosis of autologous** HCC Q A **vein bypass graft(s) of the left leg with ulceration of other part of lower leg**

I70.449   **Atherosclerosis of autologous** HCC Q A ▽ **vein bypass graft(s) of the left leg with ulceration of unspecified site**

I70.45   **Atherosclerosis of autologous vein bypass** HCC Q A **graft(s) of other extremity with** ulceration
   INCLUDES   any condition classifiable to I70.418, I70.428, and I70.438
   Use additional code to identify severity of ulcer (L98.49)

√6ᵗʰ I70.46   **Atherosclerosis of autologous vein bypass graft(s) of the extremities with** gangrene
   INCLUDES   any condition classifiable to I70.41-, I70.42-, and I70.43-, I70.44-, I70.45
   Use additional code to identify the severity of any ulcer (L97.-, L98.49-), if applicable

I70.461   **Atherosclerosis of autologous** HCC Q A **vein bypass graft(s) of the extremities with gangrene,** right leg

I70.462   **Atherosclerosis of autologous** HCC Q A **vein bypass graft(s) of the extremities with gangrene,** left leg

I70.463   **Atherosclerosis of autologous** HCC Q A **vein bypass graft(s) of the extremities with gangrene,** bilateral legs

I70.468   **Atherosclerosis of autologous** HCC Q A **vein bypass graft(s) of the extremities with gangrene, other extremity**

I70.469   **Atherosclerosis of autologous** HCC Q A ▽ **vein bypass graft(s) of the extremities with gangrene, unspecified extremity**

√6ᵗʰ I70.49   **Other atherosclerosis of autologous vein bypass graft(s) of the extremities**

I70.491   **Other atherosclerosis of** HCC Q A **autologous vein bypass graft(s) of the extremities,** right leg

I70.492   **Other atherosclerosis of** HCC Q A **autologous vein bypass graft(s) of the extremities,** left leg

I70.493   **Other atherosclerosis of** HCC Q A **autologous vein bypass graft(s) of the extremities,** bilateral legs

I70.498   **Other atherosclerosis of** HCC Q A **autologous vein bypass graft(s) of the extremities, other extremity**

I70.499   **Other atherosclerosis of** HCC Q A ▽ **autologous vein bypass graft(s) of the extremities, unspecified extremity**

√5ᵗʰ I70.5   **Atherosclerosis of** nonautologous biological bypass graft(s) **of the** extremities
   Use additional code, if applicable, to identify chronic total occlusion of artery of extremity (I70.92)

√6ᵗʰ I70.50   **Unspecified atherosclerosis of nonautologous biological bypass graft(s) of the extremities**

I70.501   **Unspecified atherosclerosis of** HCC Q A ▽ **nonautologous biological bypass graft(s) of the extremities,** right leg

I70.502   **Unspecified atherosclerosis of** HCC Q A ▽ **nonautologous biological bypass graft(s) of the extremities,** left leg

I70.503   **Unspecified atherosclerosis of** HCC Q A ▽ **nonautologous biological bypass graft(s) of the extremities,** bilateral legs

I70.508   **Unspecified atherosclerosis of** HCC Q A ▽ **nonautologous biological bypass graft(s) of the extremities, other extremity**

I70.509   **Unspecified atherosclerosis of** HCC Q A ▽ **nonautologous biological bypass graft(s) of the extremities, unspecified extremity**

√6ᵗʰ I70.51   **Atherosclerosis of nonautologous biological bypass graft(s) of the extremities** intermittent claudication

I70.511   **Atherosclerosis of** HCC Q A **nonautologous biological bypass graft(s) of the extremities with intermittent claudication,** right leg

I70.512   **Atherosclerosis of** HCC Q A **nonautologous biological bypass graft(s) of the extremities with intermittent claudication,** left leg

I70.513   **Atherosclerosis of** HCC Q A **nonautologous biological bypass graft(s) of the extremities with intermittent claudication,** bilateral legs

I70.518   **Atherosclerosis of** HCC Q A **nonautologous biological bypass graft(s) of the extremities with intermittent claudication, other extremity**

I70.519   **Atherosclerosis of** HCC Q A ▽ **nonautologous biological bypass graft(s) of the extremities with intermittent claudication, unspecified extremity**

√6ᵗʰ I70.52   **Atherosclerosis of nonautologous biological bypass graft(s) of the extremities with** rest pain
   INCLUDES   any condition classifiable to I70.51-

I70.521   **Atherosclerosis of** HCC Q A **nonautologous biological bypass graft(s) of the extremities with rest pain,** right leg

I70.522   **Atherosclerosis of** HCC Q A **nonautologous biological bypass graft(s) of the extremities with rest pain,** left leg

I70.523   **Atherosclerosis of** HCC Q A **nonautologous biological bypass graft(s) of the extremities with rest pain,** bilateral legs

I70.528   **Atherosclerosis of** HCC Q A **nonautologous biological bypass graft(s) of the extremities with rest pain, other extremity**

I70.529   **Atherosclerosis of** HCC Q A ▽ **nonautologous biological bypass graft(s) of the extremities with rest pain, unspecified extremity**

√6ᵗʰ **I70.53** **Atherosclerosis of nonautologous biological bypass graft(s) of the right leg with ulceration**
      INCLUDES any condition classifiable to I70.511 and I70.521
      Use additional code to identify severity of ulcer (L97.-)

    I70.531 Atherosclerosis of nonautologous biological bypass graft(s) of the right leg with ulceration of thigh HCC Q A

    I70.532 Atherosclerosis of nonautologous biological bypass graft(s) of the right leg with ulceration of calf HCC Q A

    I70.533 Atherosclerosis of nonautologous biological bypass graft(s) of the right leg with ulceration of ankle HCC Q A

    I70.534 Atherosclerosis of nonautologous biological bypass graft(s) of the right leg with ulceration of heel and midfoot HCC Q A
        Atherosclerosis of nonautologous biological bypass graft(s) of right leg with ulceration of plantar surface of midfoot

    I70.535 Atherosclerosis of nonautologous biological bypass graft(s) of the right leg with ulceration of other part of foot HCC Q A
        Atherosclerosis of nonautologous biological bypass graft(s) of the right leg with ulceration of toe

    I70.538 Atherosclerosis of nonautologous biological bypass graft(s) of the right leg with ulceration of other part of lower leg HCC Q A

    I70.539 Atherosclerosis of nonautologous biological bypass graft(s) of the right leg with ulceration of unspecified site HCC Q A ▽

√6ᵗʰ **I70.54** **Atherosclerosis of nonautologous biological bypass graft(s) of the left leg with ulceration**
      INCLUDES any condition classifiable to I70.512 and I70.522
      Use additional code to identify severity of ulcer (L97.-)

    I70.541 Atherosclerosis of nonautologous biological bypass graft(s) of the left leg with ulceration of thigh HCC Q A

    I70.542 Atherosclerosis of nonautologous biological bypass graft(s) of the left leg with ulceration of calf HCC Q A

    I70.543 Atherosclerosis of nonautologous biological bypass graft(s) of the left leg with ulceration of ankle HCC Q A

    I70.544 Atherosclerosis of nonautologous biological bypass graft(s) of the left leg with ulceration of heel and midfoot HCC Q A
        Atherosclerosis of nonautologous biological bypass graft(s) of left leg with ulceration of plantar surface of midfoot

    I70.545 Atherosclerosis of nonautologous biological bypass graft(s) of the left leg with ulceration of other part of foot HCC Q A
        Atherosclerosis of nonautologous biological bypass graft(s) of the left leg with ulceration of toe

    I70.548 Atherosclerosis of nonautologous biological bypass graft(s) of the left leg with ulceration of other part of lower leg HCC Q A

    I70.549 Atherosclerosis of nonautologous biological bypass graft(s) of the left leg with ulceration of unspecified site HCC Q A ▽

I70.55 **Atherosclerosis of nonautologous biological bypass graft(s) of other extremity with ulceration** HCC Q A
      INCLUDES any condition classifiable to I70.518, I70.528, and I70.538
      Use additional code to identify severity of ulcer (L98.49)

√6ᵗʰ **I70.56** **Atherosclerosis of nonautologous biological bypass graft(s) of the extremities with gangrene**
      INCLUDES any condition classifiable to I70.51-, I70.52-, and I70.53-, I70.54-, I70.55
      Use additional code to identify the severity of any ulcer (L97.-, L98.49-), if applicable

    I70.561 Atherosclerosis of nonautologous biological bypass graft(s) of the extremities with gangrene, right leg HCC Q A

    I70.562 Atherosclerosis of nonautologous biological bypass graft(s) of the extremities with gangrene, left leg HCC Q A

    I70.563 Atherosclerosis of nonautologous biological bypass graft(s) of the extremities with gangrene, bilateral legs HCC Q A

    I70.568 Atherosclerosis of nonautologous biological bypass graft(s) of the extremities with gangrene, other extremity HCC Q A

    I70.569 Atherosclerosis of nonautologous biological bypass graft(s) of the extremities with gangrene, unspecified extremity HCC Q A ▽

√6ᵗʰ **I70.59** **Other atherosclerosis of nonautologous biological bypass graft(s) of the extremities**

    I70.591 Other atherosclerosis of nonautologous biological bypass graft(s) of the extremities, right leg HCC Q A

    I70.592 Other atherosclerosis of nonautologous biological bypass graft(s) of the extremities, left leg HCC Q A

    I70.593 Other atherosclerosis of nonautologous biological bypass graft(s) of the extremities, bilateral legs HCC Q A

    I70.598 Other atherosclerosis of nonautologous biological bypass graft(s) of the extremities, other extremity HCC Q A

    I70.599 Other atherosclerosis of nonautologous biological bypass graft(s) of the extremities, unspecified extremity HCC Q A ▽

√5ᵗʰ **I70.6** **Atherosclerosis of nonbiological bypass graft(s) of the extremities**
      Use additional code, if applicable, to identify chronic total occlusion of artery of extremity (I70.92)

√6ᵗʰ **I70.60** **Unspecified atherosclerosis of nonbiological bypass graft(s) of the extremities**

    I70.601 Unspecified atherosclerosis of nonbiological bypass graft(s) of the extremities, right leg HCC Q A ▽

    I70.602 Unspecified atherosclerosis of nonbiological bypass graft(s) of the extremities, left leg HCC Q A ▽

    I70.603 Unspecified atherosclerosis of nonbiological bypass graft(s) of the extremities, bilateral legs HCC Q A ▽

    I70.608 Unspecified atherosclerosis of nonbiological bypass graft(s) of the extremities, other extremity HCC Q A ▽

✓ Additional Character Req   √x7ᵗʰ Placeholder Alert   Manifestation   ▽ Unspecified   ►◄ Revised Text   ● New Code   ▲ Revised Code Title

I70.609   Unspecified atherosclerosis of `HCC` `Q` `A` ▽ nonbiological bypass graft(s) of the extremities, unspecified extremity

✓6ᵗʰ   I70.61   Atherosclerosis of nonbiological bypass graft(s) of the extremities with intermittent claudication

I70.611   Atherosclerosis of nonbiological `HCC` `Q` `A` bypass graft(s) of the extremities with intermittent claudication, right leg

I70.612   Atherosclerosis of nonbiological `HCC` `Q` `A` bypass graft(s) of the extremities with intermittent claudication, left leg

I70.613   Atherosclerosis of nonbiological `HCC` `Q` `A` bypass graft(s) of the extremities with intermittent claudication, bilateral legs

I70.618   Atherosclerosis of nonbiological `HCC` `Q` `A` bypass graft(s) of the extremities with intermittent claudication, other extremity

I70.619   Atherosclerosis of nonbiological `HCC` `Q` `A` ▽ bypass graft(s) of the extremities with intermittent claudication, unspecified extremity

✓6ᵗʰ   I70.62   Atherosclerosis of nonbiological bypass graft(s) of the extremities with rest pain

INCLUDES   any condition classifiable to I70.61-

I70.621   Atherosclerosis of nonbiological `HCC` `Q` `A` bypass graft(s) of the extremities with rest pain, right leg

I70.622   Atherosclerosis of nonbiological `HCC` `Q` `A` bypass graft(s) of the extremities with rest pain, left leg

I70.623   Atherosclerosis of nonbiological `HCC` `Q` `A` bypass graft(s) of the extremities with rest pain, bilateral legs

I70.628   Atherosclerosis of nonbiological `HCC` `Q` `A` bypass graft(s) of the extremities with rest pain, other extremity

I70.629   Atherosclerosis of nonbiological `HCC` `Q` `A` ▽ bypass graft(s) of the extremities with rest pain, unspecified extremity

✓6ᵗʰ   I70.63   Atherosclerosis of nonbiological bypass graft(s) of the right leg with ulceration

INCLUDES   any condition classifiable to I70.611 and I70.621

Use additional code to identify severity of ulcer (L97.-)

I70.631   Atherosclerosis of nonbiological `HCC` `Q` `A` bypass graft(s) of the right leg with ulceration of thigh

I70.632   Atherosclerosis of nonbiological `HCC` `Q` `A` bypass graft(s) of the right leg with ulceration of calf

I70.633   Atherosclerosis of nonbiological `HCC` `Q` `A` bypass graft(s) of the right leg with ulceration of ankle

I70.634   Atherosclerosis of nonbiological `HCC` `Q` `A` bypass graft(s) of the right leg with ulceration of heel and midfoot

Atherosclerosis of nonbiological bypass graft(s) of right leg with ulceration of plantar surface of midfoot

I70.635   Atherosclerosis of nonbiological `HCC` `Q` `A` bypass graft(s) of the right leg with ulceration of other part of foot

Atherosclerosis of nonbiological bypass graft(s) of the right leg with ulceration of toe

I70.638   Atherosclerosis of nonbiological `HCC` `Q` `A` bypass graft(s) of the right leg with ulceration of other part of lower leg

I70.639   Atherosclerosis of nonbiological `HCC` `Q` `A` ▽ bypass graft(s) of the right leg with ulceration of unspecified site

✓6ᵗʰ   I70.64   Atherosclerosis of nonbiological bypass graft(s) of the left leg with ulceration

INCLUDES   any condition classifiable to I70.612 and I70.622

Use additional code to identify severity of ulcer (L97.-)

I70.641   Atherosclerosis of nonbiological `HCC` `Q` `A` bypass graft(s) of the left leg with ulceration of thigh

I70.642   Atherosclerosis of nonbiological `HCC` `Q` `A` bypass graft(s) of the left leg with ulceration of calf

I70.643   Atherosclerosis of nonbiological `HCC` `Q` `A` bypass graft(s) of the left leg with ulceration of ankle

I70.644   Atherosclerosis of nonbiological `HCC` `Q` `A` bypass graft(s) of the left leg with ulceration of heel and midfoot

Atherosclerosis of nonbiological bypass graft(s) of left leg with ulceration of plantar surface of midfoot

I70.645   Atherosclerosis of nonbiological `HCC` `Q` `A` bypass graft(s) of the left leg with ulceration of other part of foot

Atherosclerosis of nonbiological bypass graft(s) of the left leg with ulceration of toe

I70.648   Atherosclerosis of nonbiological `HCC` `Q` `A` bypass graft(s) of the left leg with ulceration of other part of lower leg

I70.649   Atherosclerosis of nonbiological `HCC` `Q` `A` ▽ bypass graft(s) of the left leg with ulceration of unspecified site

I70.65   Atherosclerosis of nonbiological bypass `HCC` `Q` `A` graft(s) of other extremity with ulceration

INCLUDES   any condition classifiable to I70.618 and I70.628

Use additional code to identify severity of ulcer (L98.49)

✓6ᵗʰ   I70.66   Atherosclerosis of nonbiological bypass graft(s) of the extremities with gangrene

INCLUDES   any condition classifiable to I70.61-, I70.62-, I70.63-, I70.64-, I70.65

Use additional code to identify the severity of any ulcer (L97.-, L98.49-), if applicable

I70.661   Atherosclerosis of nonbiological `HCC` `Q` `A` bypass graft(s) of the extremities with gangrene, right leg

I70.662   Atherosclerosis of nonbiological `HCC` `Q` `A` bypass graft(s) of the extremities with gangrene, left leg

I70.663   Atherosclerosis of nonbiological `HCC` `Q` `A` bypass graft(s) of the extremities with gangrene, bilateral legs

I70.668   Atherosclerosis of nonbiological `HCC` `Q` `A` bypass graft(s) of the extremities with gangrene, other extremity

I70.669   Atherosclerosis of nonbiological `HCC` `Q` `A` ▽ bypass graft(s) of the extremities with gangrene, unspecified extremity

✓6ᵗʰ   I70.69   Other atherosclerosis of nonbiological bypass graft(s) of the extremities

I70.691   Other atherosclerosis of `HCC` `Q` `A` nonbiological bypass graft(s) of the extremities, right leg

I70.692   Other atherosclerosis of `HCC` `Q` `A` nonbiological bypass graft(s) of the extremities, left leg

I70.693   Other atherosclerosis of `HCC` `Q` `A` nonbiological bypass graft(s) of the extremities, bilateral legs

I70.698   **Other atherosclerosis of** HCC Q A **nonbiological bypass graft(s) of the extremities, other extremity**

I70.699   **Other atherosclerosis of** HCC Q A ▽ **nonbiological bypass graft(s) of the extremities, unspecified extremity**

✓5ᵗʰ   I70.7   **Atherosclerosis of** other type of bypass graft(s) of the extremities

Use additional code, if applicable, to identify chronic total occlusion of artery of extremity (I70.92)

✓6ᵗʰ   I70.70   **Unspecified atherosclerosis of other type of bypass graft(s) of the extremities**

I70.701   **Unspecified atherosclerosis of** HCC Q A ▽ **other type of bypass graft(s) of the extremities,** right leg

I70.702   **Unspecified atherosclerosis of** HCC Q A ▽ **other type of bypass graft(s) of the extremities,** left leg

I70.703   **Unspecified atherosclerosis of** HCC Q A ▽ **other type of bypass graft(s) of the extremities,** bilateral legs

I70.708   **Unspecified atherosclerosis of** HCC Q A ▽ **other type of bypass graft(s) of the extremities, other extremity**

I70.709   **Unspecified atherosclerosis of** HCC Q A ▽ **other type of bypass graft(s) of the extremities, unspecified extremity**

✓6ᵗʰ   I70.71   **Atherosclerosis of other type of bypass graft(s) of the extremities with** intermittent claudication

I70.711   **Atherosclerosis of other type of** HCC Q A **bypass graft(s) of the extremities with intermittent claudication,** right leg

I70.712   **Atherosclerosis of other type of** HCC Q A **bypass graft(s) of the extremities with intermittent claudication,** left leg

I70.713   **Atherosclerosis of other type of** HCC Q A **bypass graft(s) of the extremities with intermittent claudication,** bilateral legs

I70.718   **Atherosclerosis of other type of** HCC Q A **bypass graft(s) of the extremities with intermittent claudication, other extremity**

I70.719   **Atherosclerosis of other type of** HCC Q A ▽ **bypass graft(s) of the extremities with intermittent claudication, unspecified extremity**

✓6ᵗʰ   I70.72   **Atherosclerosis of other type of bypass graft(s) of the extremities with** rest pain

INCLUDES   any condition classifiable to I70.71-

I70.721   **Atherosclerosis of other type of** HCC Q A **bypass graft(s) of the extremities with rest pain,** right leg

I70.722   **Atherosclerosis of other type of** HCC Q A **bypass graft(s) of the extremities with rest pain,** left leg

I70.723   **Atherosclerosis of other type of** HCC Q A **bypass graft(s) of the extremities with rest pain,** bilateral legs

I70.728   **Atherosclerosis of other type of** HCC Q A **bypass graft(s) of the extremities with rest pain, other extremity**

I70.729   **Atherosclerosis of other type of** HCC Q A ▽ **bypass graft(s) of the extremities with rest pain, unspecified extremity**

✓6ᵗʰ   I70.73   **Atherosclerosis of other type of bypass graft(s) of the** right leg with ulceration

INCLUDES   any condition classifiable to I70.711 and I70.721

Use additional code to identify severity of ulcer (L97.-)

I70.731   **Atherosclerosis of other type of** HCC Q A **bypass graft(s) of the right leg with ulceration of** thigh

I70.732   **Atherosclerosis of other type of** HCC Q A **bypass graft(s) of the right leg with ulceration of** calf

I70.733   **Atherosclerosis of other type of** HCC Q A **bypass graft(s) of the right leg with ulceration of** ankle

I70.734   **Atherosclerosis of other type of** HCC Q A **bypass graft(s) of the right leg with ulceration of** heel and midfoot

Atherosclerosis of other type of bypass graft(s) of right leg with ulceration of plantar surface of midfoot

I70.735   **Atherosclerosis of other type of** HCC Q A **bypass graft(s) of the right leg with ulceration of other part of foot**

Atherosclerosis of other type of bypass graft(s) of right leg with ulceration of toe

I70.738   **Atherosclerosis of other type of** HCC Q A **bypass graft(s) of the right leg with ulceration of other part of lower leg**

I70.739   **Atherosclerosis of other type of** HCC Q A ▽ **bypass graft(s) of the right leg with ulceration of unspecified site**

✓6ᵗʰ   I70.74   **Atherosclerosis of other type of bypass graft(s) of the** left leg with ulceration

INCLUDES   any condition classifiable to I70.712 and I70.722

Use additional code to identify severity of ulcer (L97.-)

I70.741   **Atherosclerosis of other type of** HCC Q A **bypass graft(s) of the left leg with ulceration of** thigh

I70.742   **Atherosclerosis of other type of** HCC Q A **bypass graft(s) of the left leg with ulceration of** calf

I70.743   **Atherosclerosis of other type of** HCC Q A **bypass graft(s) of the left leg with ulceration of** ankle

I70.744   **Atherosclerosis of other type of** HCC Q A **bypass graft(s) of the left leg with ulceration of** heel and midfoot

Atherosclerosis of other type of bypass graft(s) of left leg with ulceration of plantar surface of midfoot

I70.745   **Atherosclerosis of other type of** HCC Q A **bypass graft(s) of the left leg with ulceration of other part of foot**

Atherosclerosis of other type of bypass graft(s) of left leg with ulceration of toe

I70.748   **Atherosclerosis of other type of** HCC Q A **bypass graft(s) of the left leg with ulceration of other part of lower leg**

I70.749   **Atherosclerosis of other type of** HCC Q A ▽ **bypass graft(s) of the left leg with ulceration of unspecified site**

I70.75   **Atherosclerosis of other type of bypass** HCC Q A **graft(s) of other extremity with** ulceration

INCLUDES   any condition classifiable to I70.718 and I70.728

Use additional code to identify severity of ulcer (L98.49)

✓6ᵗʰ   I70.76   **Atherosclerosis of other type of bypass graft(s) of the extremities with** gangrene

INCLUDES   any condition classifiable to I70.71-, I70.72-, I70.73-, I70.74-, I70.75

Use additional code to identify the severity of any ulcer (L97.-, L98.49-), if applicable

I70.761   **Atherosclerosis of other type of** HCC Q A **bypass graft(s) of the extremities with gangrene,** right leg

✓ Additional Character Req   ✓x7ᵗʰ Placeholder Alert   Manifestation   ▽ Unspecified   ►◄ Revised Text   ● New Code   ▲ Revised Code Title

ICD-10-CM 2019   663

I70.762 Atherosclerosis of other type of HCC Q A bypass graft(s) of the extremities with gangrene, left leg

I70.763 Atherosclerosis of other type of HCC Q A bypass graft(s) of the extremities with gangrene, bilateral legs

I70.768 Atherosclerosis of other type of HCC Q A bypass graft(s) of the extremities with gangrene, other extremity

I70.769 Atherosclerosis of other type of HCC Q A ▽ bypass graft(s) of the extremities with gangrene, unspecified extremity

✓6ᵗʰ **I70.79** Other atherosclerosis of other type of bypass graft(s) of the extremities

I70.791 Other atherosclerosis of other HCC Q A type of bypass graft(s) of the extremities, right leg

I70.792 Other atherosclerosis of other HCC Q A type of bypass graft(s) of the extremities, left leg

I70.793 Other atherosclerosis of other HCC Q A type of bypass graft(s) of the extremities, bilateral legs

I70.798 Other atherosclerosis of other HCC Q A type of bypass graft(s) of the extremities, other extremity

I70.799 Other atherosclerosis of other HCC Q A ▽ type of bypass graft(s) of the extremities, unspecified extremity

I70.8 Atherosclerosis of other arteries   Q A

   TIP: Arteriosclerosis of the iliac arteries is coded here.

✓5ᵗʰ **I70.9** Other and unspecified atherosclerosis

I70.90 Unspecified atherosclerosis   Q A ▽

I70.91 Generalized atherosclerosis   Q A

I70.92 Chronic total occlusion of artery of the HCC Q A extremities

   Complete occlusion of artery of the extremities

   Total occlusion of artery of the extremities

   Code first atherosclerosis of arteries of the extremities (I70.2-, I70.3-, I70.4-, I70.5-, I70.6-, I70.7-)

✓4ᵗʰ **I71 Aortic aneurysm and dissection**

  EXCLUDES 1   aortic ectasia (I77.81-)

        syphilitic aortic aneurysm (A52.01)

        traumatic aortic aneurysm (S25.09, S35.09)

✓5ᵗʰ **I71.0** Dissection of aorta

I71.00 Dissection of unspecified site of aorta   HCC ▽

I71.01 Dissection of thoracic aorta   HCC

I71.02 Dissection of abdominal aorta   HCC

I71.03 Dissection of thoracoabdominal aorta   HCC

I71.1 Thoracic aortic aneurysm, ruptured   HCC

I71.2 Thoracic aortic aneurysm, without rupture   HCC

I71.3 Abdominal aortic aneurysm, ruptured   HCC

I71.4 Abdominal aortic aneurysm, without rupture   HCC

I71.5 Thoracoabdominal aortic aneurysm, ruptured   HCC

I71.6 Thoracoabdominal aortic aneurysm, without rupture   HCC

I71.8 Aortic aneurysm of unspecified site, ruptured   HCC ▽

   Rupture of aorta NOS

I71.9 Aortic aneurysm of unspecified site, without   HCC ▽ rupture

   Aneurysm of aorta

   Dilatation of aorta

   Hyaline necrosis of aorta

✓4ᵗʰ **I72 Other aneurysm**

  INCLUDES   aneurysm (cirsoid) (false) (ruptured)

  EXCLUDES 2   acquired aneurysm (I77.0)

        aneurysm (of) aorta (I71.-)

        aneurysm (of) arteriovenous NOS (Q27.3-)

        carotid artery dissection (I77.71)

        cerebral (nonruptured) aneurysm (I67.1)

        coronary aneurysm (I25.4)

        coronary artery dissection (I25.42)

        dissection of artery NEC (I77.79)

        dissection of precerebral artery, congenital (nonruptured) (Q28.1)

        heart aneurysm (I25.3)

        iliac artery dissection (I77.72)

        precerebral artery, congential (nonruptured) (Q28.1)

        pulmonary artery aneurysm (I28.1)

        renal artery dissection (I77.73)

        retinal aneurysm (H35.0)

        ruptured cerebral aneurysm (I60.7)

        varicose aneurysm (I77.0)

        vertebral artery dissection (I77.74)

  AHA: 2016,4Q,28-29

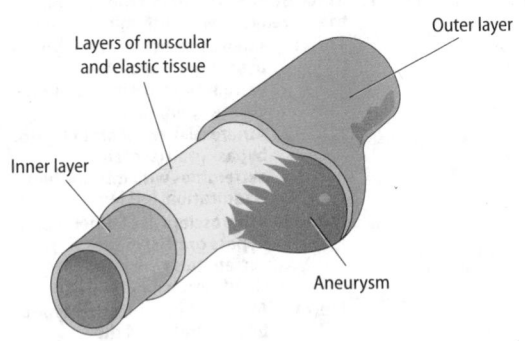

Aneurysm

Outer layer

Layers of muscular and elastic tissue

Inner layer

Aneurysm

I72.0 Aneurysm of carotid artery   HCC

   Aneurysm of common carotid artery

   Aneurysm of external carotid artery

   Aneurysm of internal carotid artery, extracranial portion

  EXCLUDES 1   aneurysm of internal carotid artery, intracranial portion (I67.1)

        aneurysm of internal carotid artery NOS (I67.1)

I72.1 Aneurysm of artery of upper extremity   HCC

I72.2 Aneurysm of renal artery   HCC

I72.3 Aneurysm of iliac artery   HCC

I72.4 Aneurysm of artery of lower extremity   HCC

I72.5 Aneurysm of other precerebral arteries   HCC

   Aneurysm of basilar artery (trunk)

  EXCLUDES 2   aneurysm of carotid artery (I72.0)

        aneurysm of vertebral artery (I72.6)

        dissection of carotid artery (I77.71)

        dissection of other precerebral arteries (I77.75)

        dissection of vertebral artery (I77.74)

I72.6 Aneurysm of vertebral artery   HCC

  EXCLUDES 2   dissection of vertebral artery (I77.74)

I72.8 Aneurysm of other specified arteries   HCC

I72.9 Aneurysm of unspecified site   HCC ▽

✓4ᵗʰ I73 Other peripheral vascular diseases

     EXCLUDES 2   chilblains (T69.1)

                   frostbite (T33-T34)

                   immersion hand or foot (T69.0-)

                   spasm of cerebral artery (G45.9)

✓5ᵗʰ I73.0 Raynaud's syndrome

Raynaud's disease

Raynaud's phenomenon (secondary)

DEF: Constriction of the arteries of the digits caused by cold or by nerve or arterial damage and can be prompted by stress or emotion. Blood cannot reach the skin and soft tissues and the skin turns white with blue mottling.

    I73.00   **Raynaud's syndrome without gangrene**

    I73.01   **Raynaud's syndrome with gangrene**   HCC

I73.1 Thromboangiitis obliterans [Buerger's disease]   HCC

DEF: Inflammatory disease of the extremity blood vessels, mainly the lower blood vessels. This disease is associated with heavy tobacco use. The arteries are more affected than veins. It occurs primarily in young men and leads to tissue ischemia and gangrene.

✓5ᵗʰ I73.8 Other specified peripheral vascular diseases

     EXCLUDES 1   diabetic (peripheral) angiopathy (E08-E13 with .51-.52)

    I73.81   **Erythromelalgia**   HCC

    I73.89   **Other specified peripheral vascular diseases**   HCC

Acrocyanosis

Erythrocyanosis

Simple acroparesthesia [Schultze's type]

Vasomotor acroparesthesia [Nothnagel's type]

I73.9 Peripheral vascular disease, unspecified   HCC ▽

Intermittent claudication

Peripheral angiopathy NOS

Spasm of artery

     EXCLUDES 1   atherosclerosis of the extremities (I70.2-I70.7-)

     AHA: 2018,2Q,7

✓4ᵗʰ I74 Arterial embolism and thrombosis

     INCLUDES   embolic infarction

                   embolic occlusion

                   thrombotic infarction

                   thrombotic occlusion

Code first:

     embolism and thrombosis complicating abortion or ectopic or molar pregnancy (O00-O07, O08.2)

     embolism and thrombosis complicating pregnancy, childbirth and the puerperium (O88.-)

     EXCLUDES 2   atheroembolism (I75.-)

                   basilar embolism and thrombosis (I63.0-I63.2, I65.1)

                   carotid embolism and thrombosis (I63.0-I63.2, I65.2)

                   cerebral embolism and thrombosis (I63.3-I63.5, I66.-)

                   coronary embolism and thrombosis (I21-I25)

                   mesenteric embolism and thrombosis (K55.0-)

                   ophthalmic embolism and thrombosis (H34.-)

                   precerebral embolism and thrombosis NOS (I63.0-I63.2, I65.9)

                   pulmonary embolism and thrombosis (I26.-)

                   renal embolism and thrombosis (N28.0)

                   retinal embolism and thrombosis (H34.-)

                   septic embolism and thrombosis (I76)

                   vertebral embolism and thrombosis (I63.0-I63.2, I65.0)

✓5ᵗʰ I74.0 Embolism and thrombosis of abdominal aorta

    I74.01   **Saddle embolus of abdominal aorta**   HCC Q

    I74.09   **Other arterial embolism and thrombosis of abdominal aorta**   HCC Q

Aortic bifurcation syndrome

Aortoiliac obstruction

Leriche's syndrome

✓5ᵗʰ I74.1 Embolism and thrombosis of other and unspecified parts of aorta

    I74.10   **Embolism and thrombosis of unspecified parts of aorta**   HCC Q ▽

    I74.11   **Embolism and thrombosis of thoracic aorta**   HCC Q

    I74.19   **Embolism and thrombosis of other parts of aorta**   HCC Q

I74.2 Embolism and thrombosis of arteries of the upper extremities   HCC Q

I74.3 Embolism and thrombosis of arteries of the lower extremities   HCC Q

I74.4 Embolism and thrombosis of arteries of extremities, unspecified   HCC Q ▽

Peripheral arterial embolism NOS

I74.5 Embolism and thrombosis of iliac artery   HCC Q

I74.8 Embolism and thrombosis of other arteries   HCC Q

I74.9 Embolism and thrombosis of unspecified artery   HCC Q ▽

✓4ᵗʰ I75 Atheroembolism

     INCLUDES   atherothrombotic microembolism

                   cholesterol embolism

✓5ᵗʰ I75.0 Atheroembolism of extremities

✓6ᵗʰ I75.01 Atheroembolism of upper extremity

       I75.011   **Atheroembolism of right upper extremity**   HCC Q

       I75.012   **Atheroembolism of left upper extremity**   HCC Q

       I75.013   **Atheroembolism of bilateral upper extremities**   HCC Q

       I75.019   **Atheroembolism of unspecified upper extremity**   HCC Q ▽

✓6ᵗʰ I75.02 Atheroembolism of lower extremity

       I75.021   **Atheroembolism of right lower extremity**   HCC Q

       I75.022   **Atheroembolism of left lower extremity**   HCC Q

       I75.023   **Atheroembolism of bilateral lower extremities**   HCC Q

       I75.029   **Atheroembolism of unspecified lower extremity**   HCC Q ▽

✓5ᵗʰ I75.8 Atheroembolism of other sites

    I75.81   **Atheroembolism of kidney**   HCC Q

Use additional code for any associated acute kidney failure and chronic kidney disease (N17.-, N18.-)

    I75.89   **Atheroembolism of other site**   HCC Q

I76 Septic arterial embolism   HCC

Code first underlying infection, such as:

     infective endocarditis (I33.0)

     lung abscess (J85.-)

Use additional code to identify the site of the embolism (I74.-)

     EXCLUDES 2   septic pulmonary embolism (I26.01, I26.90)

✓4ᵗʰ I77 Other disorders of arteries and arterioles

     EXCLUDES 2   collagen (vascular) diseases (M30-M36)

                   hypersensitivity angiitis (M31.0)

                   pulmonary artery (I28.-)

I77.0 Arteriovenous fistula, acquired   HCC

Aneurysmal varix

Arteriovenous aneurysm, acquired

     EXCLUDES 1   arteriovenous aneurysm NOS (Q27.3-)

                   presence of arteriovenous shunt (fistula) for dialysis (Z99.2)

                   traumatic - see injury of blood vessel by body region

     EXCLUDES 2   cerebral (I67.1)

                   coronary (I25.4)

DEF: Communication between an artery and vein caused by trauma or invasive procedures.

I77.1 Stricture of artery   HCC

Narrowing of artery

I77.2 Rupture of artery   HCC

Erosion of artery

Fistula of artery

Ulcer of artery

     EXCLUDES 1   traumatic rupture of artery - see injury of blood vessel by body region

I77.3 Arterial fibromuscular dysplasia   HCC

Fibromuscular hyperplasia (of) carotid artery

Fibromuscular hyperplasia (of) renal artery

I77.4 Celiac artery compression syndrome   HCC

I77.5 Necrosis of artery   HCC

I77.6 Arteritis, unspecified ▽

Aortitis NOS

Endarteritis NOS

EXCLUDES 1   arteritis or endarteritis:

aortic arch (M31.4)

cerebral NEC (I67.7)

coronary (I25.89)

deformans (I70.-)

giant cell ▶(M31.5, M31.6)◀

obliterans (I70.-)

senile (I70.-)

√5ᵗʰ I77.7 Other arterial dissection

EXCLUDES 2   dissection of aorta (I71.0-)

dissection of coronary artery (I25.42)

AHA: 2016,4Q,28-29

I77.70   **Dissection of unspecified artery** HCC ▽

I77.71   **Dissection of carotid artery** HCC

I77.72   **Dissection of iliac artery** HCC

I77.73   **Dissection of renal artery** HCC

I77.74   **Dissection of vertebral artery** HCC

    EXCLUDES 2   aneurysm of vertebral artery (I72.6)

I77.75   **Dissection of other precerebral arteries** HCC

Dissection of basilar artery (trunk)

    EXCLUDES 2   aneurysm of carotid artery (I72.0)

aneurysm of other precerebral arteries (I72.5)

aneurysm of vertebral artery (I72.6)

dissection of carotid artery (I77.71)

dissection of vertebral artery (I77.74)

I77.76   **Dissection of artery of upper extremity** HCC

I77.77   **Dissection of artery of lower extremity** HCC

I77.79   **Dissection of other specified artery** HCC

√5ᵗʰ I77.8 Other specified disorders of arteries and arterioles

√6ᵗʰ I77.81 Aortic ectasia

Ectasis aorta

    EXCLUDES 1   aortic aneurysm and dissection (I71.0-)

I77.810   **Thoracic aortic ectasia** HCC

I77.811   **Abdominal aortic ectasia** HCC

I77.812   **Thoracoabdominal aortic ectasia** HCC

I77.819   **Aortic ectasia, unspecified site** HCC ▽

I77.89 Other specified disorders of arteries and arterioles HCC

I77.9 Disorder of arteries and arterioles, unspecified HCC ▽

AHA: 2018,2Q,7

√4ᵗʰ I78 Diseases of capillaries

I78.0 Hereditary hemorrhagic telangiectasia HCC

Rendu-Osler-Weber disease

I78.1 Nevus, non-neoplastic

Araneus nevus

Senile nevus

Spider nevus

Stellar nevus

EXCLUDES 1   nevus NOS (D22.-)

vascular NOS (Q82.5)

EXCLUDES 2   blue nevus (D22.-)

flammeus nevus (Q82.5)

hairy nevus (D22.-)

melanocytic nevus (D22.-)

pigmented nevus (D22.-)

portwine nevus (Q82.5)

sanguineous nevus (Q82.5)

strawberry nevus (Q82.5)

verrucous nevus (Q82.5)

I78.8 Other diseases of capillaries

I78.9 Disease of capillaries, unspecified ▽

√4ᵗʰ I79 Disorders of arteries, arterioles and capillaries in diseases classified elsewhere

I79.0 Aneurysm of aorta in diseases classified elsewhere HCC

Code first underlying disease

    EXCLUDES 1   syphilitic aneurysm (A52.01)

I79.1 Aortitis in diseases classified elsewhere HCC

Code first underlying disease

    EXCLUDES 1   syphilitic aortitis (A52.02)

I79.8 Other disorders of arteries, arterioles and capillaries in diseases classified elsewhere HCC

Code first underlying disease, such as:

amyloidosis (E85.-)

    EXCLUDES 1   diabetic (peripheral) angiopathy (E08-E13 with .51-.52)

syphilitic endarteritis (A52.09)

tuberculous endarteritis (A18.89)

Diseases of veins, lymphatic vessels and lymph nodes, not elsewhere classified (I80-I89)

√4ᵗʰ I80 Phlebitis and thrombophlebitis

INCLUDES   endophlebitis

inflammation, vein

periphlebitis

suppurative phlebitis

Code first:

phlebitis and thrombophlebitis complicating abortion, ectopic or molar pregnancy (O00-O07, O08.7)

phlebitis and thrombophlebitis complicating pregnancy, childbirth and the puerperium (O22.-, O87.-)

    EXCLUDES 1   venous embolism and thrombosis of lower extremities (I82.4-, I82.5-, I82.81-)

√5ᵗʰ I80.0 Phlebitis and thrombophlebitis of superficial vessels of lower extremities

Phlebitis and thrombophlebitis of femoropopliteal vein

I80.00   **Phlebitis and thrombophlebitis of superficial vessels of unspecified lower extremity** ▽

I80.01   **Phlebitis and thrombophlebitis of superficial vessels of right lower extremity**

I80.02   **Phlebitis and thrombophlebitis of superficial vessels of left lower extremity**

I80.03   **Phlebitis and thrombophlebitis of superficial vessels of lower extremities, bilateral**

√5ᵗʰ I80.1 Phlebitis and thrombophlebitis of femoral vein

I80.10   **Phlebitis and thrombophlebitis of unspecified femoral vein** HCC ▽

I80.11   **Phlebitis and thrombophlebitis of right femoral vein** HCC

I80.12   **Phlebitis and thrombophlebitis of left femoral vein** HCC

I80.13   **Phlebitis and thrombophlebitis of femoral vein, bilateral** HCC

√5ᵗʰ I80.2 Phlebitis and thrombophlebitis of other and unspecified deep vessels of lower extremities

√6ᵗʰ I80.20 Phlebitis and thrombophlebitis of unspecified deep vessels of lower extremities

I80.201   **Phlebitis and thrombophlebitis of unspecified deep vessels of right lower extremity** HCC

I80.202   **Phlebitis and thrombophlebitis of unspecified deep vessels of left lower extremity** HCC

I80.203   **Phlebitis and thrombophlebitis of unspecified deep vessels of lower extremities, bilateral** HCC

I80.209   **Phlebitis and thrombophlebitis of unspecified deep vessels of unspecified lower extremity** HCC ▽

√6ᵗʰ I80.21 Phlebitis and thrombophlebitis of iliac vein

I80.211   **Phlebitis and thrombophlebitis of right iliac vein** HCC

I80.212   **Phlebitis and thrombophlebitis of left iliac vein** HCC

I80.213   **Phlebitis and thrombophlebitis of iliac vein, bilateral** HCC

I80.219   **Phlebitis and thrombophlebitis of unspecified iliac vein** HCC ▽

√6ᵗʰ I80.22 Phlebitis and thrombophlebitis of popliteal vein

I80.221   **Phlebitis and thrombophlebitis of right popliteal vein** HCC

I80.222   **Phlebitis and thrombophlebitis of left popliteal vein** HCC

I80.223   **Phlebitis and thrombophlebitis of popliteal vein, bilateral** HCC

I80.229   **Phlebitis and thrombophlebitis of unspecified popliteal vein** HCC ▽

√6ᵗʰ **I80.23** **Phlebitis and thrombophlebitis of tibial vein**

     I80.231 **Phlebitis and thrombophlebitis of right tibial vein** `HCC`

     I80.232 **Phlebitis and thrombophlebitis of left tibial vein** `HCC`

     I80.233 **Phlebitis and thrombophlebitis of tibial vein, bilateral** `HCC`

     I80.239 **Phlebitis and thrombophlebitis of unspecified tibial vein** `HCC` ▽

√6ᵗʰ **I80.29** **Phlebitis and thrombophlebitis of other deep vessels of lower extremities**

     I80.291 **Phlebitis and thrombophlebitis of other deep vessels of right lower extremity** `HCC`

     I80.292 **Phlebitis and thrombophlebitis of other deep vessels of left lower extremity** `HCC`

     I80.293 **Phlebitis and thrombophlebitis of other deep vessels of lower extremity, bilateral** `HCC`

     I80.299 **Phlebitis and thrombophlebitis of other deep vessels of unspecified lower extremity** `HCC` ▽

I80.3 **Phlebitis and thrombophlebitis of lower extremities, unspecified** ▽

I80.8 **Phlebitis and thrombophlebitis of other sites**

I80.9 **Phlebitis and thrombophlebitis of unspecified site** ▽

I81 **Portal vein thrombosis**
Portal (vein) obstruction
> *EXCLUDES 2*   hepatic vein thrombosis (I82.0)
>   phlebitis of portal vein (K75.1)

√4ᵗʰ **I82** **Other venous embolism and thrombosis**
Code first venous embolism and thrombosis complicating:
   abortion, ectopic or molar pregnancy (O00–O07, O08.7)
   pregnancy, childbirth and the puerperium (O22.-, O87.-)
> *EXCLUDES 2*   venous embolism and thrombosis (of):
>   cerebral (I63.6, I67.6)
>   coronary (I21–I25)
>   intracranial and intraspinal, septic or NOS (G08)
>   intracranial, nonpyogenic (I67.6)
>   intraspinal, nonpyogenic (G95.1)
>   mesenteric (K55.0-)
>   portal (I81)
>   pulmonary (I26.-)

I82.0 **Budd-Chiari syndrome** `HCC`
Hepatic vein thrombosis
DEF: Thrombosis or other obstruction of the hepatic veins. Symptoms include an enlarged liver, extensive collateral vessels, intractable ascites, and severe portal hypertension.

I82.1 **Thrombophlebitis migrans**

√5ᵗʰ **I82.2** **Embolism and thrombosis of vena cava and other thoracic veins**

   √6ᵗʰ **I82.21** **Embolism and thrombosis of superior vena cava**

     I82.210 **Acute embolism and thrombosis of superior vena cava** `HCC`
Embolism and thrombosis of superior vena cava NOS

     I82.211 **Chronic embolism and thrombosis of superior vena cava** `HCC`

   √6ᵗʰ **I82.22** **Embolism and thrombosis of inferior vena cava**

     I82.220 **Acute embolism and thrombosis of inferior vena cava** `HCC`
Embolism and thrombosis of inferior vena cava NOS

     I82.221 **Chronic embolism and thrombosis of inferior vena cava** `HCC`

   √6ᵗʰ **I82.29** **Embolism and thrombosis of other thoracic veins**
Embolism and thrombosis of brachiocephalic (innominate) vein

     I82.290 **Acute embolism and thrombosis of other thoracic veins** `HCC`

     I82.291 **Chronic embolism and thrombosis of other thoracic veins** `HCC`

I82.3 **Embolism and thrombosis of renal vein** `HCC`

√5ᵗʰ **I82.4** **Acute embolism and thrombosis of deep veins of lower extremity**

   √6ᵗʰ **I82.40** **Acute embolism and thrombosis of unspecified deep veins of lower extremity**
Deep vein thrombosis NOS
DVT NOS
> *EXCLUDES 1*   acute embolism and thrombosis of unspecified deep veins of distal lower extremity (I82.4Z-)
>   acute embolism and thrombosis of unspecified deep veins of proximal lower extremity (I82.4Y-)

     I82.401 **Acute embolism and thrombosis of unspecified deep veins of right lower extremity** `HCC` ▽

     I82.402 **Acute embolism and thrombosis of unspecified deep veins of left lower extremity** `HCC` ▽

     I82.403 **Acute embolism and thrombosis of unspecified deep veins of lower extremity, bilateral** `HCC` ▽

     I82.409 **Acute embolism and thrombosis of unspecified deep veins of unspecified lower extremity** `HCC` ▽

   √6ᵗʰ **I82.41** **Acute embolism and thrombosis of femoral vein**

     I82.411 **Acute embolism and thrombosis of right femoral vein** `HCC`

     I82.412 **Acute embolism and thrombosis of left femoral vein** `HCC`

     I82.413 **Acute embolism and thrombosis of femoral vein, bilateral** `HCC`

     I82.419 **Acute embolism and thrombosis of unspecified femoral vein** `HCC` ▽

   √6ᵗʰ **I82.42** **Acute embolism and thrombosis of iliac vein**

     I82.421 **Acute embolism and thrombosis of right iliac vein** `HCC`

     I82.422 **Acute embolism and thrombosis of left iliac vein** `HCC`

     I82.423 **Acute embolism and thrombosis of iliac vein, bilateral** `HCC`

     I82.429 **Acute embolism and thrombosis of unspecified iliac vein** `HCC` ▽

   √6ᵗʰ **I82.43** **Acute embolism and thrombosis of popliteal vein**

     I82.431 **Acute embolism and thrombosis of right popliteal vein** `HCC`

     I82.432 **Acute embolism and thrombosis of left popliteal vein** `HCC`

     I82.433 **Acute embolism and thrombosis of popliteal vein, bilateral** `HCC`

     I82.439 **Acute embolism and thrombosis of unspecified popliteal vein** `HCC` ▽

   √6ᵗʰ **I82.44** **Acute embolism and thrombosis of tibial vein**

     I82.441 **Acute embolism and thrombosis of right tibial vein** `HCC`

     I82.442 **Acute embolism and thrombosis of left tibial vein** `HCC`

     I82.443 **Acute embolism and thrombosis of tibial vein, bilateral** `HCC`

     I82.449 **Acute embolism and thrombosis of unspecified tibial vein** `HCC` ▽

   √6ᵗʰ **I82.49** **Acute embolism and thrombosis of other specified deep vein of lower extremity**

     I82.491 **Acute embolism and thrombosis of other specified deep vein of right lower extremity** `HCC`

     I82.492 **Acute embolism and thrombosis of other specified deep vein of left lower extremity** `HCC`

     I82.493 **Acute embolism and thrombosis of other specified deep vein of lower extremity, bilateral** `HCC`

     I82.499 **Acute embolism and thrombosis of other specified deep vein of unspecified lower extremity** `HCC` ▽

| ☑ Additional Character Req | ✓x7ᵗʰ Placeholder Alert | Manifestation | ▽ Unspecified | ►◄ Revised Text | ● New Code | ▲ Revised Code Title |

✓6ᵗʰ **I82.4Y** **Acute embolism and thrombosis of unspecified deep veins of proximal lower extremity**
Acute embolism and thrombosis of deep vein of thigh NOS
Acute embolism and thrombosis of deep vein of upper leg NOS

I82.4Y1 **Acute embolism and thrombosis of unspecified deep veins of right proximal lower extremity** HCC ▽

I82.4Y2 **Acute embolism and thrombosis of unspecified deep veins of left proximal lower extremity** HCC ▽

I82.4Y3 **Acute embolism and thrombosis of unspecified deep veins of proximal lower extremity, bilateral** HCC ▽

I82.4Y9 **Acute embolism and thrombosis of unspecified deep veins of unspecified proximal lower extremity** HCC ▽

✓6ᵗʰ **I82.4Z** **Acute embolism and thrombosis of unspecified deep veins of distal lower extremity**
Acute embolism and thrombosis of deep vein of calf NOS
Acute embolism and thrombosis of deep vein of lower leg NOS

I82.4Z1 **Acute embolism and thrombosis of unspecified deep veins of right distal lower extremity** HCC ▽

I82.4Z2 **Acute embolism and thrombosis of unspecified deep veins of left distal lower extremity** HCC ▽

I82.4Z3 **Acute embolism and thrombosis of unspecified deep veins of distal lower extremity, bilateral** HCC ▽

I82.4Z9 **Acute embolism and thrombosis of unspecified deep veins of unspecified distal lower extremity** HCC ▽

✓5ᵗʰ **I82.5** **Chronic embolism and thrombosis of deep veins of lower extremity**
Use additional code, if applicable, for associated long-term (current) use of anticoagulants (Z79.01)
EXCLUDES 1 *personal history of venous embolism and thrombosis (Z86.718)*

✓6ᵗʰ **I82.50** **Chronic embolism and thrombosis of unspecified deep veins of lower extremity**
EXCLUDES 1 *chronic embolism and thrombosis of unspecified deep veins of distal lower extremity (I82.5Z-)*
chronic embolism and thrombosis of unspecified deep veins of proximal lower extremity (I82.5Y-)

I82.501 **Chronic embolism and thrombosis of unspecified deep veins of right lower extremity** HCC ▽

I82.502 **Chronic embolism and thrombosis of unspecified deep veins of left lower extremity** HCC ▽

I82.503 **Chronic embolism and thrombosis of unspecified deep veins of lower extremity, bilateral** HCC ▽

I82.509 **Chronic embolism and thrombosis of unspecified deep veins of unspecified lower extremity** HCC ▽

✓6ᵗʰ **I82.51** **Chronic embolism and thrombosis of femoral vein**

I82.511 **Chronic embolism and thrombosis of right femoral vein** HCC

I82.512 **Chronic embolism and thrombosis of left femoral vein** HCC

I82.513 **Chronic embolism and thrombosis of femoral vein, bilateral** HCC

I82.519 **Chronic embolism and thrombosis of unspecified femoral vein** HCC ▽

✓6ᵗʰ **I82.52** **Chronic embolism and thrombosis of iliac vein**

I82.521 **Chronic embolism and thrombosis of right iliac vein** HCC

I82.522 **Chronic embolism and thrombosis of left iliac vein** HCC

I82.523 **Chronic embolism and thrombosis of iliac vein, bilateral** HCC

I82.529 **Chronic embolism and thrombosis of unspecified iliac vein** HCC ▽

✓6ᵗʰ **I82.53** **Chronic embolism and thrombosis of popliteal vein**

I82.531 **Chronic embolism and thrombosis of right popliteal vein** HCC

I82.532 **Chronic embolism and thrombosis of left popliteal vein** HCC

I82.533 **Chronic embolism and thrombosis of popliteal vein, bilateral** HCC

I82.539 **Chronic embolism and thrombosis of unspecified popliteal vein** HCC ▽

✓6ᵗʰ **I82.54** **Chronic embolism and thrombosis of tibial vein**

I82.541 **Chronic embolism and thrombosis of right tibial vein** HCC

I82.542 **Chronic embolism and thrombosis of left tibial vein** HCC

I82.543 **Chronic embolism and thrombosis of tibial vein, bilateral** HCC

I82.549 **Chronic embolism and thrombosis of unspecified tibial vein** HCC ▽

✓6ᵗʰ **I82.59** **Chronic embolism and thrombosis of other specified deep vein of lower extremity**

I82.591 **Chronic embolism and thrombosis of other specified deep vein of right lower extremity** HCC

I82.592 **Chronic embolism and thrombosis of other specified deep vein of left lower extremity** HCC

I82.593 **Chronic embolism and thrombosis of other specified deep vein of lower extremity, bilateral** HCC

I82.599 **Chronic embolism and thrombosis of other specified deep vein of unspecified lower extremity** HCC ▽

✓6ᵗʰ **I82.5Y** **Chronic embolism and thrombosis of unspecified deep veins of proximal lower extremity**
Chronic embolism and thrombosis of deep veins of thigh NOS
Chronic embolism and thrombosis of deep veins of upper leg NOS

I82.5Y1 **Chronic embolism and thrombosis of unspecified deep veins of right proximal lower extremity** HCC ▽

I82.5Y2 **Chronic embolism and thrombosis of unspecified deep veins of left proximal lower extremity** HCC ▽

I82.5Y3 **Chronic embolism and thrombosis of unspecified deep veins of proximal lower extremity, bilateral** HCC ▽

I82.5Y9 **Chronic embolism and thrombosis of unspecified deep veins of unspecified proximal lower extremity** HCC ▽

✓6ᵗʰ **I82.5Z** **Chronic embolism and thrombosis of unspecified deep veins of distal lower extremity**
Chronic embolism and thrombosis of deep veins of calf NOS
Chronic embolism and thrombosis of deep veins of lower leg NOS

I82.5Z1 **Chronic embolism and thrombosis of unspecified deep veins of right distal lower extremity** HCC ▽

I82.5Z2 **Chronic embolism and thrombosis of unspecified deep veins of left distal lower extremity** HCC ▽

I82.5Z3   Chronic embolism and thrombosis of unspecified deep veins of distal lower extremity, bilateral   HCC ▽

I82.5Z9   Chronic embolism and thrombosis of unspecified deep veins of unspecified distal lower extremity   HCC ▽

√5ᵗʰ   **I82.6**   Acute embolism and thrombosis of veins of upper extremity

√6ᵗʰ   **I82.60**   **Acute embolism and thrombosis of unspecified veins of upper extremity**

I82.601   Acute embolism and thrombosis of unspecified veins of right upper extremity ▽

I82.602   Acute embolism and thrombosis of unspecified veins of left upper extremity ▽

I82.603   Acute embolism and thrombosis of unspecified veins of upper extremity, bilateral ▽

I82.609   Acute embolism and thrombosis of unspecified veins of unspecified upper extremity ▽

√6ᵗʰ   **I82.61**   **Acute embolism and thrombosis of superficial veins of upper extremity**
     Acute embolism and thrombosis of antecubital vein
     Acute embolism and thrombosis of basilic vein
     Acute embolism and thrombosis of cephalic vein

I82.611   Acute embolism and thrombosis of superficial veins of right upper extremity

I82.612   Acute embolism and thrombosis of superficial veins of left upper extremity

I82.613   Acute embolism and thrombosis of superficial veins of upper extremity, bilateral

I82.619   Acute embolism and thrombosis of superficial veins of unspecified upper extremity ▽

√6ᵗʰ   **I82.62**   **Acute embolism and thrombosis of deep veins of upper extremity**
     Acute embolism and thrombosis of brachial vein
     Acute embolism and thrombosis of radial vein
     Acute embolism and thrombosis of ulnar vein

I82.621   Acute embolism and thrombosis of deep veins of right upper extremity   HCC

I82.622   Acute embolism and thrombosis of deep veins of left upper extremity   HCC

I82.623   Acute embolism and thrombosis of deep veins of upper extremity, bilateral   HCC

I82.629   Acute embolism and thrombosis of deep veins of unspecified upper extremity   HCC ▽

√5ᵗʰ   **I82.7**   Chronic embolism and thrombosis of veins of upper extremity
     Use additional code, if applicable, for associated long-term (current) use of anticoagulants (Z79.01)
     EXCLUDES 1   *personal history of venous embolism and thrombosis (Z86.718)*

√6ᵗʰ   **I82.70**   **Chronic embolism and thrombosis of unspecified veins of upper extremity**

I82.701   Chronic embolism and thrombosis of unspecified veins of right upper extremity ▽

I82.702   Chronic embolism and thrombosis of unspecified veins of left upper extremity ▽

I82.703   Chronic embolism and thrombosis of unspecified veins of upper extremity, bilateral ▽

I82.709   Chronic embolism and thrombosis of unspecified veins of unspecified upper extremity ▽

√6ᵗʰ   **I82.71**   **Chronic embolism and thrombosis of superficial veins of upper extremity**
     Chronic embolism and thrombosis of antecubital vein
     Chronic embolism and thrombosis of basilic vein
     Chronic embolism and thrombosis of cephalic vein

I82.711   Chronic embolism and thrombosis of superficial veins of right upper extremity

I82.712   Chronic embolism and thrombosis of superficial veins of left upper extremity

I82.713   Chronic embolism and thrombosis of superficial veins of upper extremity, bilateral

I82.719   Chronic embolism and thrombosis of superficial veins of unspecified upper extremity ▽

√6ᵗʰ   **I82.72**   **Chronic embolism and thrombosis of deep veins of upper extremity**
     Chronic embolism and thrombosis of brachial vein
     Chronic embolism and thrombosis of radial vein
     Chronic embolism and thrombosis of ulnar vein

I82.721   Chronic embolism and thrombosis of deep veins of right upper extremity   HCC

I82.722   Chronic embolism and thrombosis of deep veins of left upper extremity   HCC

I82.723   Chronic embolism and thrombosis of deep veins of upper extremity, bilateral   HCC

I82.729   Chronic embolism and thrombosis of deep veins of unspecified upper extremity   HCC ▽

√5ᵗʰ   **I82.A**   Embolism and thrombosis of axillary vein

√6ᵗʰ   **I82.A1**   Acute embolism and thrombosis of axillary vein

I82.A11   Acute embolism and thrombosis of right axillary vein   HCC

I82.A12   Acute embolism and thrombosis of left axillary vein   HCC

I82.A13   Acute embolism and thrombosis of axillary vein, bilateral   HCC

I82.A19   Acute embolism and thrombosis of unspecified axillary vein   HCC ▽

√6ᵗʰ   **I82.A2**   Chronic embolism and thrombosis of axillary vein

I82.A21   Chronic embolism and thrombosis of right axillary vein   HCC

I82.A22   Chronic embolism and thrombosis of left axillary vein   HCC

I82.A23   Chronic embolism and thrombosis of axillary vein, bilateral   HCC

I82.A29   Chronic embolism and thrombosis of unspecified axillary vein   HCC ▽

√5ᵗʰ   **I82.B**   Embolism and thrombosis of subclavian vein

√6ᵗʰ   **I82.B1**   Acute embolism and thrombosis of subclavian vein

I82.B11   Acute embolism and thrombosis of right subclavian vein   HCC

I82.B12   Acute embolism and thrombosis of left subclavian vein   HCC

I82.B13   Acute embolism and thrombosis of subclavian vein, bilateral   HCC

I82.B19   Acute embolism and thrombosis of unspecified subclavian vein   HCC ▽

√6ᵗʰ   **I82.B2**   Chronic embolism and thrombosis of subclavian vein

I82.B21   Chronic embolism and thrombosis of right subclavian vein   HCC

I82.B22   Chronic embolism and thrombosis of left subclavian vein   HCC

I82.B23   Chronic embolism and thrombosis of subclavian vein, bilateral   HCC

I82.B29   Chronic embolism and thrombosis of unspecified subclavian vein   HCC ▽

√5ᵗʰ   **I82.C**   Embolism and thrombosis of internal jugular vein

√6ᵗʰ   **I82.C1**   Acute embolism and thrombosis of internal jugular vein

I82.C11   Acute embolism and thrombosis of right internal jugular vein   HCC

I82.C12   Acute embolism and thrombosis of left internal jugular vein   HCC

I82.C13   Acute embolism and thrombosis of internal jugular vein, bilateral   HCC

☑ Additional Character Req   √x7ᵗʰ Placeholder Alert   Manifestation   ▽ Unspecified   ►◄ Revised Text   ● New Code   ▲ Revised Code Title

    I82.C19   **Acute embolism and thrombosis** HCC ▽
of unspecified internal jugular
vein

  √6ᵗʰ   **I82.C2**   **Chronic embolism and thrombosis of internal**
jugular vein

    I82.C21   **Chronic embolism and** HCC
thrombosis of right internal
jugular vein

    I82.C22   **Chronic embolism and** HCC
thrombosis of left internal
jugular vein

    I82.C23   **Chronic embolism and** HCC
thrombosis of internal jugular
vein, bilateral

    I82.C29   **Chronic embolism and** HCC ▽
thrombosis of unspecified
internal jugular vein

√5ᵗʰ   **I82.8**   **Embolism and thrombosis of other specified veins**

    Use additional code, if applicable, for associated long-term
(current) use of anticoagulants (Z79.Ø1)

  √6ᵗʰ   **I82.81**   **Embolism and thrombosis of superficial veins of**
lower extremities

    Embolism and thrombosis of saphenous vein (greater)
(lesser)

    I82.811   **Embolism and thrombosis of superficial**
veins of right lower extremity

    I82.812   **Embolism and thrombosis of superficial**
veins of left lower extremity

    I82.813   **Embolism and thrombosis of superficial**
veins of lower extremities, bilateral

    I82.819   **Embolism and thrombosis of** ▽
superficial veins of unspecified
lower extremity

  √6ᵗʰ   **I82.89**   **Embolism and thrombosis of other specified veins**

    I82.89Ø   **Acute embolism and thrombosis of other**
specified veins

    I82.891   **Chronic embolism and thrombosis of**
other specified veins

√5ᵗʰ   **I82.9**   **Embolism and thrombosis of unspecified vein**

    I82.9Ø   **Acute embolism and thrombosis of** ▽
unspecified vein

    Embolism of vein NOS
Thrombosis (vein) NOS

    I82.91   **Chronic embolism and thrombosis of** ▽
unspecified vein

√4ᵗʰ   **I83**   **Varicose veins of lower extremities**

    EXCLUDES 1   *varicose veins complicating pregnancy (O22.Ø-)*
varicose veins complicating the puerperium (O87.4)

√5ᵗʰ   **I83.Ø**   **Varicose veins of lower extremities with ulcer**

    Use additional code to identify severity of ulcer (L97.-)

  √6ᵗʰ   **I83.ØØ**   **Varicose veins of unspecified lower extremity with**
ulcer

    I83.ØØ1   **Varicose veins of unspecified** HCC A ▽
lower extremity with ulcer of
thigh

    I83.ØØ2   **Varicose veins of unspecified** HCC A ▽
lower extremity with ulcer of
calf

    I83.ØØ3   **Varicose veins of unspecified** HCC A ▽
lower extremity with ulcer of
ankle

    I83.ØØ4   **Varicose veins of unspecified** HCC A ▽
lower extremity with ulcer of
heel and midfoot

    Varicose veins of unspecified lower
extremity with ulcer of plantar surface
of midfoot

    I83.ØØ5   **Varicose veins of unspecified** HCC A ▽
lower extremity with ulcer other
part of foot

    Varicose veins of unspecified lower
extremity with ulcer of toe

    I83.ØØ8   **Varicose veins of unspecified** HCC A ▽
lower extremity with ulcer other
part of lower leg

    I83.ØØ9   **Varicose veins of unspecified** HCC A ▽
lower extremity with ulcer of
unspecified site

  √6ᵗʰ   **I83.Ø1**   **Varicose veins of right lower extremity with ulcer**

    I83.Ø11   **Varicose veins of right lower** HCC A
extremity with ulcer of thigh

    I83.Ø12   **Varicose veins of right lower** HCC A
extremity with ulcer of calf

    I83.Ø13   **Varicose veins of right lower** HCC A
extremity with ulcer of ankle

    I83.Ø14   **Varicose veins of right lower** HCC A
extremity with ulcer of heel and
midfoot

    Varicose veins of right lower extremity with
ulcer of plantar surface of midfoot

    I83.Ø15   **Varicose veins of right lower** HCC A
extremity with ulcer other part
of foot

    Varicose veins of right lower extremity with
ulcer of toe

    I83.Ø18   **Varicose veins of right lower** HCC A
extremity with ulcer other part
of lower leg

    I83.Ø19   **Varicose veins of right lower** HCC A ▽
extremity with ulcer of
unspecified site

  √6ᵗʰ   **I83.Ø2**   **Varicose veins of left lower extremity with ulcer**

    I83.Ø21   **Varicose veins of left lower** HCC A
extremity with ulcer of thigh

    I83.Ø22   **Varicose veins of left lower** HCC A
extremity with ulcer of calf

    I83.Ø23   **Varicose veins of left lower** HCC A
extremity with ulcer of ankle

    I83.Ø24   **Varicose veins of left lower** HCC A
extremity with ulcer of heel and
midfoot

    Varicose veins of left lower extremity with
ulcer of plantar surface of midfoot

    I83.Ø25   **Varicose veins of left lower** HCC A
extremity with ulcer other part
of foot

    Varicose veins of left lower extremity with
ulcer of toe

    I83.Ø28   **Varicose veins of left lower** HCC A
extremity with ulcer other part
of lower leg

    I83.Ø29   **Varicose veins of left lower** HCC A ▽
extremity with ulcer of
unspecified site

√5ᵗʰ   **I83.1**   **Varicose veins of lower extremities with inflammation**

    I83.1Ø   **Varicose veins of unspecified lower** A ▽
extremity with inflammation

    I83.11   **Varicose veins of right lower extremity** A
with inflammation

    I83.12   **Varicose veins of left lower extremity with** A
inflammation

√5ᵗʰ   **I83.2**   **Varicose veins of lower extremities with both ulcer and**
inflammation

    Use additional code to identify severity of ulcer (L97.-)

  √6ᵗʰ   **I83.2Ø**   **Varicose veins of unspecified lower extremity with**
both ulcer and inflammation

    I83.2Ø1   **Varicose veins of unspecified** HCC A ▽
lower extremity with both ulcer
of thigh and inflammation

    I83.2Ø2   **Varicose veins of unspecified** HCC A ▽
lower extremity with both ulcer
of calf and inflammation

    I83.2Ø3   **Varicose veins of unspecified** HCC A ▽
lower extremity with both ulcer
of ankle and inflammation

    I83.2Ø4   **Varicose veins of unspecified** HCC A ▽
lower extremity with both ulcer
of heel and midfoot and
inflammation

    Varicose veins of unspecified lower
extremity with both ulcer of plantar
surface of midfoot and inflammation

    I83.2Ø5   **Varicose veins of unspecified** HCC A ▽
lower extremity with both ulcer
of other part of foot and
inflammation

    Varicose veins of unspecified lower
extremity with both ulcer of toe and
inflammation

    I83.2Ø8   **Varicose veins of unspecified** HCC A ▽
lower extremity with both ulcer
of other part of lower extremity
and inflammation

I83.209   **Varicose veins of unspecified lower extremity with both ulcer of unspecified site and inflammation** HCC A ▽

√6ᵗʰ   I83.21   **Varicose veins of right lower extremity with both ulcer and inflammation**

    I83.211   **Varicose veins of right lower extremity with both ulcer of thigh and inflammation** HCC A

    I83.212   **Varicose veins of right lower extremity with both ulcer of calf and inflammation** HCC A

    I83.213   **Varicose veins of right lower extremity with both ulcer of ankle and inflammation** HCC A

    I83.214   **Varicose veins of right lower extremity with both ulcer of heel and midfoot and inflammation** HCC A

       Varicose veins of right lower extremity with both ulcer of plantar surface of midfoot and inflammation

    I83.215   **Varicose veins of right lower extremity with both ulcer other part of foot and inflammation** HCC A

       Varicose veins of right lower extremity with both ulcer of toe and inflammation

    I83.218   **Varicose veins of right lower extremity with both ulcer of other part of lower extremity and inflammation** HCC A

    I83.219   **Varicose veins of right lower extremity with both ulcer of unspecified site and inflammation** HCC A ▽

√6ᵗʰ   I83.22   **Varicose veins of left lower extremity with both ulcer and inflammation**

    I83.221   **Varicose veins of left lower extremity with both ulcer of thigh and inflammation** HCC A

    I83.222   **Varicose veins of left lower extremity with both ulcer of calf and inflammation** HCC A

    I83.223   **Varicose veins of left lower extremity with both ulcer of ankle and inflammation** HCC A

    I83.224   **Varicose veins of left lower extremity with both ulcer of heel and midfoot and inflammation** HCC A

       Varicose veins of left lower extremity with both ulcer of plantar surface of midfoot and inflammation

    I83.225   **Varicose veins of left lower extremity with both ulcer other part of foot and inflammation** HCC A

       Varicose veins of left lower extremity with both ulcer of toe and inflammation

    I83.228   **Varicose veins of left lower extremity with both ulcer of other part of lower extremity and inflammation** HCC A

    I83.229   **Varicose veins of left lower extremity with both ulcer of unspecified site and inflammation** HCC A ▽

√5ᵗʰ   I83.8   **Varicose veins of lower extremities with other complications**

√6ᵗʰ   I83.81   **Varicose veins of lower extremities with pain**

    I83.811   **Varicose veins of right lower extremity with pain** A

    I83.812   **Varicose veins of left lower extremity with pain** A

    I83.813   **Varicose veins of bilateral lower extremities with pain** A

    I83.819   **Varicose veins of unspecified lower extremity with pain** A ▽

√6ᵗʰ   I83.89   **Varicose veins of lower extremities with other complications**

       Varicose veins of lower extremities with edema

       Varicose veins of lower extremities with swelling

    I83.891   **Varicose veins of right lower extremity with other complications** A

    I83.892   **Varicose veins of left lower extremity with other complications** A

    I83.893   **Varicose veins of bilateral lower extremities with other complications** A

    I83.899   **Varicose veins of unspecified lower extremity with other complications** A ▽

√5ᵗʰ   I83.9   **Asymptomatic varicose veins of lower extremities**

       Phlebectasia of lower extremities

       Varicose veins of lower extremities

       Varix of lower extremities

    I83.90   **Asymptomatic varicose veins of unspecified lower extremity** A ▽

       Varicose veins NOS

    I83.91   **Asymptomatic varicose veins of right lower extremity** A

    I83.92   **Asymptomatic varicose veins of left lower extremity** A

    I83.93   **Asymptomatic varicose veins of bilateral lower extremities** A

√4ᵗʰ   **I85   Esophageal varices**

    Use additional code to identify:

    alcohol abuse and dependence (F10.-)

√5ᵗʰ   I85.0   **Esophageal varices**

       Idiopathic esophageal varices

       Primary esophageal varices

    I85.00   **Esophageal varices without bleeding** HCC

       Esophageal varices NOS

    I85.01   **Esophageal varices with bleeding** HCC

√5ᵗʰ   I85.1   **Secondary esophageal varices**

       Esophageal varices secondary to alcoholic liver disease

       Esophageal varices secondary to cirrhosis of liver

       Esophageal varices secondary to schistosomiasis

       Esophageal varices secondary to toxic liver disease

       Code first underlying disease

    I85.10   **Secondary esophageal varices without bleeding** HCC

    I85.11   **Secondary esophageal varices with bleeding** HCC

√4ᵗʰ   **I86   Varicose veins of other sites**

    EXCLUDES 1   *varicose veins of unspecified site (I83.9-)*

    EXCLUDES 2   *retinal varices (H35.0-)*

    I86.0   **Sublingual varices**

       DEF: Distended, tortuous veins beneath the tongue.

    I86.1   **Scrotal varices** ♂

       Varicocele

    I86.2   **Pelvic varices**

    I86.3   **Vulval varices** ♀

       EXCLUDES 1   *vulval varices complicating childbirth and the puerperium (O87.8)*

           vulval varices complicating pregnancy (O22.1-)

    I86.4   **Gastric varices**

    I86.8   **Varicose veins of other specified sites** A

       Varicose ulcer of nasal septum

√4ᵗʰ   **I87   Other disorders of veins**

√5ᵗʰ   I87.0   **Postthrombotic syndrome**

       Chronic venous hypertension due to deep vein thrombosis

       Postphlebitic syndrome

       EXCLUDES 1   *chronic venous hypertension without deep vein thrombosis (I87.3-)*

√6ᵗʰ   I87.00   **Postthrombotic syndrome without complications**

       Asymptomatic postthrombotic syndrome

    I87.001   **Postthrombotic syndrome without complications of right lower extremity**

    I87.002   **Postthrombotic syndrome without complications of left lower extremity**

    I87.003   **Postthrombotic syndrome without complications of bilateral lower extremity**

    I87.009   **Postthrombotic syndrome without complications of unspecified extremity** ▽

       Postthrombotic syndrome NOS

☑ Additional Character Req   ✓x7ᵗʰ Placeholder Alert   Manifestation   ▽ Unspecified   ►◄ Revised Text   ● New Code   ▲ Revised Code Title

ICD-10-CM 2019   671

Chapter 9. Diseases of the Circulatory System

√6ᵗʰ **187.01** **Postthrombotic syndrome with** ulcer

    Use additional code to specify site and severity of ulcer (L97.-)

187.011 **Postthrombotic syndrome with ulcer of** right lower **extremity**   HCC

187.012 **Postthrombotic syndrome with ulcer of** left lower **extremity**   HCC

187.013 **Postthrombotic syndrome with ulcer of** bilateral lower **extremity**   HCC

187.019 **Postthrombotic syndrome with ulcer of unspecified lower extremity**   HCC ▽

√6ᵗʰ **187.02** **Postthrombotic syndrome with** inflammation

187.021 **Postthrombotic syndrome with inflammation of** right lower **extremity**

187.022 **Postthrombotic syndrome with inflammation of** left lower **extremity**

187.023 **Postthrombotic syndrome with inflammation of** bilateral lower **extremity**

187.029 **Postthrombotic syndrome with inflammation of unspecified lower extremity**   ▽

√6ᵗʰ **187.03** **Postthrombotic syndrome with** ulcer and inflammation

    Use additional code to specify site and severity of ulcer (L97.-)

187.031 **Postthrombotic syndrome with ulcer and inflammation of** right lower **extremity**   HCC

187.032 **Postthrombotic syndrome with ulcer and inflammation of** left lower **extremity**   HCC

187.033 **Postthrombotic syndrome with ulcer and inflammation of** bilateral lower **extremity**   HCC

187.039 **Postthrombotic syndrome with ulcer and inflammation of unspecified lower extremity**   HCC ▽

√6ᵗʰ **187.09** **Postthrombotic syndrome with other complications**

187.091 **Postthrombotic syndrome with other complications of** right lower **extremity**

187.092 **Postthrombotic syndrome with other complications of** left lower **extremity**

187.093 **Postthrombotic syndrome with other complications of** bilateral lower **extremity**

187.099 **Postthrombotic syndrome with other complications of unspecified lower extremity**   ▽

187.1 **Compression of vein**

    Stricture of vein

    Vena cava syndrome (inferior) (superior)

    EXCLUDES 2   *compression of pulmonary vein (I28.8)*

187.2 **Venous insufficiency (chronic) (peripheral)**

    Stasis dermatitis

    EXCLUDES 1   *stasis dermatitis with varicose veins of lower extremities (I83.1-, I83.2-)*

    DEF: Insufficient drainage of venous blood in any part of the body that results in edema or dermatosis.

√5ᵗʰ **187.3** **Chronic venous hypertension (idiopathic)**

    Stasis edema

    EXCLUDES 1   *chronic venous hypertension due to deep vein thrombosis (I87.0-)*

        varicose veins of lower extremities (I83.-)

√6ᵗʰ **187.30** **Chronic venous hypertension (idiopathic) without complications**

    Asymptomatic chronic venous hypertension (idiopathic)

187.301 **Chronic venous hypertension (idiopathic) without complications of** right lower **extremity**

187.302 **Chronic venous hypertension (idiopathic) without complications of** left lower **extremity**

187.303 **Chronic venous hypertension (idiopathic) without complications of** bilateral lower **extremity**

187.309 **Chronic venous hypertension (idiopathic) without complications of unspecified lower extremity**   ▽

    Chronic venous hypertension NOS

√6ᵗʰ **187.31** **Chronic venous hypertension (idiopathic) with** ulcer

    Use additional code to specify site and severity of ulcer (L97.-)

187.311 **Chronic venous hypertension (idiopathic) with ulcer of** right lower **extremity**   HCC

187.312 **Chronic venous hypertension (idiopathic) with ulcer of** left lower **extremity**   HCC

187.313 **Chronic venous hypertension (idiopathic) with ulcer of** bilateral lower **extremity**   HCC

187.319 **Chronic venous hypertension (idiopathic) with ulcer of unspecified lower extremity**   HCC ▽

√6ᵗʰ **187.32** **Chronic venous hypertension (idiopathic) with** inflammation

187.321 **Chronic venous hypertension (idiopathic) with inflammation of** right lower **extremity**

187.322 **Chronic venous hypertension (idiopathic) with inflammation of** left lower **extremity**

187.323 **Chronic venous hypertension (idiopathic) with inflammation of** bilateral lower **extremity**

187.329 **Chronic venous hypertension (idiopathic) with inflammation of unspecified lower extremity**   ▽

√6ᵗʰ **187.33** **Chronic venous hypertension (idiopathic) with** ulcer and inflammation

    Use additional code to specify site and severity of ulcer (L97.-)

187.331 **Chronic venous hypertension (idiopathic) with ulcer and inflammation of** right lower **extremity**   HCC

187.332 **Chronic venous hypertension (idiopathic) with ulcer and inflammation of** left lower **extremity**   HCC

187.333 **Chronic venous hypertension (idiopathic) with ulcer and inflammation of** bilateral lower **extremity**   HCC

187.339 **Chronic venous hypertension (idiopathic) with ulcer and inflammation of unspecified lower extremity**   HCC ▽

√6ᵗʰ **187.39** **Chronic venous hypertension (idiopathic) with other complications**

187.391 **Chronic venous hypertension (idiopathic) with other complications of** right lower **extremity**

187.392 **Chronic venous hypertension (idiopathic) with other complications of** left lower **extremity**

187.393 **Chronic venous hypertension (idiopathic) with other complications of** bilateral lower **extremity**

187.399 **Chronic venous hypertension (idiopathic) with other complications of unspecified lower extremity**   ▽

187.8 **Other specified disorders of veins**

    Phlebosclerosis

    Venofibrosis

187.9 **Disorder of vein, unspecified**   ▽

√4ᵗʰ **188** **Nonspecific lymphadenitis**

    EXCLUDES 1   *acute lymphadenitis, except mesenteric (L04.-)*

        enlarged lymph nodes NOS (R59.-)

        human immunodeficiency virus [HIV] disease resulting in generalized lymphadenopathy (B20)

188.0 **Nonspecific mesenteric lymphadenitis**

    Mesenteric lymphadenitis (acute)(chronic)

I88.1 **Chronic lymphadenitis, except mesenteric**
Adenitis
Lymphadenitis

I88.8 **Other nonspecific lymphadenitis**

I88.9 **Nonspecific lymphadenitis, unspecified** ▽
Lymphadenitis NOS

✓4ᵗʰ **I89** **Other noninfective disorders of lymphatic vessels and lymph nodes**

　　EXCLUDES 1　chylocele, tunica vaginalis (nonfilarial) NOS (N50.89)
　　　　　　　enlarged lymph nodes NOS (R59.-)
　　　　　　　filarial chylocele (B74.-)
　　　　　　　hereditary lymphedema (Q82.0)

I89.0 **Lymphedema, not elsewhere classified**
Elephantiasis (nonfilarial) NOS
Lymphangiectasis
Obliteration, lymphatic vessel
Praecox lymphedema
Secondary lymphedema
　　EXCLUDES 1　postmastectomy lymphedema (I97.2)

I89.1 **Lymphangitis**
Chronic lymphangitis
Lymphangitis NOS
Subacute lymphangitis
　　EXCLUDES 1　acute lymphangitis (L03.-)

I89.8 **Other specified noninfective disorders of lymphatic vessels and lymph nodes**
Chylocele (nonfilarial)
Chylous ascites
Chylous cyst
Lipomelanotic reticulosis
Lymph node or vessel fistula
Lymph node or vessel infarction
Lymph node or vessel rupture

I89.9 **Noninfective disorder of lymphatic vessels and lymph nodes, unspecified** ▽
Disease of lymphatic vessels NOS

Other and unspecified disorders of the circulatory system (I95-I99)

✓4ᵗʰ **I95** **Hypotension**
　　EXCLUDES 1　cardiovascular collapse (R57.9) (~R57.9)
　　　　　　　maternal hypotension syndrome (O26.5-)
　　　　　　　nonspecific low blood pressure reading NOS (R03.1)

I95.0 **Idiopathic hypotension**

I95.1 **Orthostatic hypotension**
Hypotension, postural
　　EXCLUDES 1　neurogenic orthostatic hypotension [Shy-Drager] (G90.3)
　　　　　　　orthostatic hypotension due to drugs (I95.2)

I95.2 **Hypotension due to drugs**
Orthostatic hypotension due to drugs
Use additional code for adverse effect, if applicable, to identify drug (T36-T50 with fifth or sixth character 5)

I95.3 **Hypotension of hemodialysis**
Intra-dialytic hypotension

✓5ᵗʰ **I95.8** **Other hypotension**

I95.81 **Postprocedural hypotension**

I95.89 **Other hypotension**
Chronic hypotension

I95.9 **Hypotension, unspecified** ▽

I96 **Gangrene, not elsewhere classified**　　HCC
Gangrenous cellulitis
　　EXCLUDES 1　gangrene in atherosclerosis of native arteries of the extremities (I70.26)
　　　　　　　gangrene in hernia (K40.1, K40.4, K41.1, K41.4, K42.1, K43.1-, K44.1, K45.1, K46.1)
　　　　　　　gangrene in other peripheral vascular diseases (I73.-)
　　　　　　　gangrene of certain specified sites - see Alphabetical Index
　　　　　　　gas gangrene (A48.0)
　　　　　　　pyoderma gangrenosum (L88)
　　EXCLUDES 2　gangrene in diabetes mellitus (E08-E13 with .52)
　　AHA: 2017,3Q,6; 2013,2Q,34

✓4ᵗʰ **I97** **Intraoperative and postprocedural complications and disorders of circulatory system, not elsewhere classified**
　　EXCLUDES 2　postprocedural shock (T81.1-)

I97.0 **Postcardiotomy syndrome**

✓5ᵗʰ **I97.1** **Other postprocedural cardiac functional disturbances**
　　EXCLUDES 2　acute pulmonary insufficiency following thoracic surgery (J95.1)
　　　　　　　intraoperative cardiac functional disturbances (I97.7-)

✓6ᵗʰ **I97.11** **Postprocedural cardiac insufficiency**

I97.110 **Postprocedural cardiac insufficiency following cardiac surgery**

I97.111 **Postprocedural cardiac insufficiency following other surgery**

✓6ᵗʰ **I97.12** **Postprocedural cardiac arrest**

I97.120 **Postprocedural cardiac arrest following cardiac surgery**

I97.121 **Postprocedural cardiac arrest following other surgery**

✓6ᵗʰ **I97.13** **Postprocedural heart failure**
Use additional code to identify the heart failure (I50.-)

I97.130 **Postprocedural heart failure following cardiac surgery**

I97.131 **Postprocedural heart failure following other surgery**

✓6ᵗʰ **I97.19** **Other postprocedural cardiac functional disturbances**
Use additional code, if applicable, to further specify disorder

I97.190 **Other postprocedural cardiac functional disturbances following cardiac surgery**
Use additional code, if applicable, for type 4 or type 5 myocardial infarction, to further specify disorder

I97.191 **Other postprocedural cardiac functional disturbances following other surgery**

I97.2 **Postmastectomy lymphedema syndrome** ▲
Elephantiasis due to mastectomy
Obliteration of lymphatic vessels

I97.3 **Postprocedural hypertension**

✓5ᵗʰ **I97.4** **Intraoperative hemorrhage and hematoma of a circulatory system organ or structure complicating a procedure**
　　EXCLUDES 1　intraoperative hemorrhage and hematoma of a circulatory system organ or structure due to accidental puncture and laceration during a procedure (I97.5-)
　　EXCLUDES 2　intraoperative cerebrovascular hemorrhage complicating a procedure (G97.3-)

✓6ᵗʰ **I97.41** **Intraoperative hemorrhage and hematoma of a circulatory system organ or structure complicating a circulatory system procedure**

I97.410 **Intraoperative hemorrhage and hematoma of a circulatory system organ or structure complicating a cardiac catheterization**

I97.411 **Intraoperative hemorrhage and hematoma of a circulatory system organ or structure complicating a cardiac bypass**

I97.418 **Intraoperative hemorrhage and hematoma of a circulatory system organ or structure complicating other circulatory system procedure**

I97.42 **Intraoperative hemorrhage and hematoma of a circulatory system organ or structure complicating other procedure**

✓5ᵗʰ **I97.5** **Accidental puncture and laceration of a circulatory system organ or structure during a procedure**
　　EXCLUDES 2　accidental puncture and laceration of brain during a procedure (G97.4-)

I97.51 **Accidental puncture and laceration of a circulatory system organ or structure during a circulatory system procedure**

I97.52 **Accidental puncture and laceration of a circulatory system organ or structure during other procedure**

☑ Additional Character Req　　✓ₓ7ᵗʰ Placeholder Alert　　Manifestation　　▽ Unspecified　　▶◀ Revised Text　　● New Code　　▲ Revised Code Title

Chapter 9. Diseases of the Circulatory System

✓5ᵗʰ **I97.6 Postprocedural hemorrhage, hematoma and seroma** of a circulatory system organ or structure following a procedure

    EXCLUDES 2   *postprocedural cerebrovascular hemorrhage complicating a procedure (G97.5-)*

    AHA: 2016,4Q,9-10

✓6ᵗʰ **I97.61 Postprocedural hemorrhage** of a circulatory system organ or structure following a **circulatory system procedure**

    I97.610 Postprocedural hemorrhage of a circulatory system organ or structure following a **cardiac catheterization**

    I97.611 Postprocedural hemorrhage of a circulatory system organ or structure following **cardiac bypass**

    I97.618 Postprocedural hemorrhage of a circulatory system organ or structure following **other circulatory system procedure**

✓6ᵗʰ **I97.62 Postprocedural hemorrhage, hematoma and seroma** of a circulatory system organ or structure following **other procedure**

    I97.620 Postprocedural **hemorrhage** of a circulatory system organ or structure following other procedure

    I97.621 Postprocedural **hematoma** of a circulatory system organ or structure following other procedure

    I97.622 Postprocedural **seroma** of a circulatory system organ or structure following other procedure

✓6ᵗʰ **I97.63 Postprocedural hematoma** of a circulatory system organ or structure following a **circulatory system procedure**

    I97.630 Postprocedural hematoma of a circulatory system organ or structure following a **cardiac catheterization**

    I97.631 Postprocedural hematoma of a circulatory system organ or structure following **cardiac bypass**

    I97.638 Postprocedural hematoma of a circulatory system organ or structure following **other circulatory system procedure**

✓6ᵗʰ **I97.64 Postprocedural seroma** of a circulatory system organ or structure following a circulatory system procedure

    I97.640 Postprocedural seroma of a circulatory system organ or structure following a **cardiac catheterization**

    I97.641 Postprocedural seroma of a circulatory system organ or structure following **cardiac bypass**

    I97.648 Postprocedural seroma of a circulatory system organ or structure following other circulatory system procedure

✓5ᵗʰ **I97.7 Intraoperative cardiac functional disturbances**

    EXCLUDES 2   *acute pulmonary insufficiency following thoracic surgery (J95.1)*

              postprocedural cardiac functional disturbances (I97.1-)

✓6ᵗʰ **I97.71 Intraoperative cardiac arrest**

    I97.710 Intraoperative cardiac arrest during **cardiac surgery**

    I97.711 Intraoperative cardiac arrest during **other surgery**

✓6ᵗʰ **I97.79 Other intraoperative cardiac functional disturbances**

    Use additional code, if applicable, to further specify disorder

    I97.790 Other intraoperative cardiac functional disturbances during **cardiac surgery**

    I97.791 Other intraoperative cardiac functional disturbances during **other surgery**

✓5ᵗʰ **I97.8 Other intraoperative and postprocedural complications and disorders of the circulatory system, not elsewhere classified**

    Use additional code, if applicable, to further specify disorder

✓6ᵗʰ **I97.81 Intraoperative cerebrovascular infarction**

    I97.810 Intraoperative cerebrovascular infarction during **cardiac surgery**   HCC

    I97.811 Intraoperative cerebrovascular infarction during **other surgery**   HCC

✓6ᵗʰ **I97.82 Postprocedural cerebrovascular infarction**

    I97.820 Postprocedural cerebrovascular infarction following **cardiac surgery**   HCC

    I97.821 Postprocedural cerebrovascular infarction following **other surgery**   HCC

    I97.88 Other intraoperative complications of the circulatory system, not elsewhere classified

    I97.89 Other postprocedural complications and disorders of the circulatory system, not elsewhere classified

✓4ᵗʰ **I99 Other and unspecified disorders of circulatory system**

    I99.8 Other disorder of circulatory system

    I99.9 Unspecified disorder of circulatory system   ▽

Chapter 10. Diseases of the Respiratory System (JØØ–J99)

Chapter Specific Guidelines with Coding Examples

The chapter specific guidelines from the ICD-10-CM Official Guidelines for Coding and Reporting have been provided below. Along with these guidelines are coding examples, contained in the shaded boxes, that have been developed to help illustrate the coding and/or sequencing guidance found in these guidelines.

a. Chronic obstructive pulmonary disease [COPD] and asthma

1) Acute exacerbation of chronic obstructive bronchitis and asthma

The codes in categories J44 and J45 distinguish between uncomplicated cases and those in acute exacerbation. An acute exacerbation is a worsening or a decompensation of a chronic condition. An acute exacerbation is not equivalent to an infection superimposed on a chronic condition, though an exacerbation may be triggered by an infection.

Acute streptococcal bronchitis with acute exacerbation of COPD

J20.2   **Acute bronchitis due to streptococcus**

J44.0   **Chronic obstructive pulmonary disease with acute lower respiratory infection**

J44.1   **Chronic obstructive pulmonary disease with (acute) exacerbation**

Explanation: ICD-10-CM uses combination codes to create organism-specific classifications for acute bronchitis. Category J44 codes include combination codes with severity components, which differentiate between COPD with acute lower respiratory infection (acute bronchitis), COPD with acute exacerbation, and COPD without mention of a complication (unspecified).

An acute exacerbation is a worsening or a decompensation of a chronic condition. An acute exacerbation is not equivalent to an infection superimposed on a chronic condition, though an exacerbation may be triggered by an infection, as in this example.

Exacerbation of moderate persistent asthma with status asthmaticus

J45.42   **Moderate persistent asthma with status asthmaticus**

Explanation: Category J45 Asthma includes severity-specific subcategories and fifth-character codes to distinguish between uncomplicated cases, those in acute exacerbation, and those with status asthmaticus.

---

b. Acute respiratory failure

1) Acute respiratory failure as principal diagnosis

A code from subcategory J96.0, Acute respiratory failure, or subcategory J96.2, Acute and chronic respiratory failure, may be assigned as a principal diagnosis when it is the condition established after study to be chiefly responsible for occasioning the admission to the hospital, and the selection is supported by the Alphabetic Index and Tabular List. However, chapter-specific coding guidelines (such as obstetrics, poisoning, HIV, newborn) that provide sequencing direction take precedence.

Acute hypoxic respiratory failure due to exacerbation of chronic obstructive bronchitis

J96.01   **Acute respiratory failure with hypoxia**

J44.1   **Chronic obstructive pulmonary disease with (acute) exacerbation**

Explanation: Category J96 classifies respiratory failure with combination codes that designate the severity and the presence of hypoxia and hypercapnia. Code J96.01 is sequenced as the first-listed diagnosis, as the reason for the encounter. Respiratory failure may be assigned as a principal diagnosis when it is the condition established after study to be chiefly responsible for occasioning the encounter and the selection is supported by the Alphabetic Index and Tabular List.

---

2) Acute respiratory failure as secondary diagnosis

Respiratory failure may be listed as a secondary diagnosis if it occurs after admission, or if it is present on admission, but does not meet the definition of principal diagnosis.

Acute respiratory failure due to accidental oxycodone overdose

T40.2X1A   **Poisoning by other opioids, accidental (unintentional), initial encounter**

J96.00   **Acute respiratory failure, unspecified whether with hypoxia or hypercapnia**

Explanation: Respiratory failure may be assigned as a principal diagnosis when it is the condition established after study to be chiefly responsible for occasioning the encounter, and the selection is supported by the Alphabetic Index and Tabular List. However, chapter-specific coding guidelines, such as poisoning, that provide sequencing direction take precedence. When coding a poisoning or reaction to the improper use of a medication (e.g. overdose, wrong substance given or taken in error, wrong route of administration), first assign the appropriate code from categories T36–T50. Use additional code(s) for all manifestations of the poisoning. In this instance, the respiratory failure is a manifestation of the poisoning and is sequenced as a secondary diagnosis.

---

3) Sequencing of acute respiratory failure and another acute condition

When a patient is admitted with respiratory failure and another acute condition, (e.g., myocardial infarction, cerebrovascular accident, aspiration pneumonia), the principal diagnosis will not be the same in every situation. This applies whether the other acute condition is a respiratory or nonrespiratory condition. Selection of the principal diagnosis will be dependent on the circumstances of admission. If both the respiratory failure and the other acute condition are equally responsible for occasioning the admission to the hospital, and there are no chapter-specific sequencing rules, the guideline regarding two or more diagnoses that equally meet the definition for principal diagnosis (*Section II, C.*) may be applied in these situations.

If the documentation is not clear as to whether acute respiratory failure and another condition are equally responsible for occasioning the admission, query the provider for clarification.

Patient presents with acute pneumococcal pneumonia and acute respiratory failure

J96.00   **Acute respiratory failure, unspecified whether with hypoxia or hypercapnia**

J13   **Pneumonia due to Streptococcus pneumoniae**

Explanation: When a patient is seen for respiratory failure and another acute condition, such as a bacterial pneumonia, the principal or first-listed diagnosis is not the same in every situation. This applies whether the other acute condition is a respiratory or nonrespiratory condition. The principal diagnosis depends on the problem chiefly responsible for the encounter.

---

c. Influenza due to certain identified influenza viruses

Code only confirmed cases of influenza due to certain identified influenza viruses (category J09), and due to other identified influenza virus (category J10). This is an exception to the hospital inpatient guideline Section II, H. (Uncertain Diagnosis).

In this context, "confirmation" does not require documentation of positive laboratory testing specific for avian or other novel influenza A or other identified influenza virus. However, coding should be based on the provider's diagnostic statement that the patient has avian influenza, or other novel influenza A, for category J09, or has another particular identified strain of influenza, such as H1N1 or H3N2, but not identified as novel or variant, for category J10.

If the provider records "suspected" or "possible" or "probable" avian influenza, or novel influenza, or other identified influenza, then the appropriate influenza code from category J11, Influenza due to unidentified influenza virus, should be assigned. A code from category J09, Influenza due to certain identified influenza viruses, should not be assigned nor should a code from category J10, Influenza due to other identified influenza virus.

Influenza due to avian influenza virus with pneumonia

J09.X1   Influenza due to identified novel influenza A virus with pneumonia

Explanation: Codes in category J09 Influenza due to certain identified influenza viruses should be assigned only for confirmed cases. "Confirmation" does not require positive laboratory testing of a specific influenza virus but does need to be based on the provider's diagnostic statement, which should not include terms such as "possible," "probable," or "suspected."

d. Ventilator associated pneumonia

1) Documentation of ventilator associated pneumonia

As with all procedural or postprocedural complications, code assignment is based on the provider's documentation of the relationship between the condition and the procedure.

Code J95.851, Ventilator associated pneumonia, should be assigned only when the provider has documented ventilator associated pneumonia (VAP). An additional code to identify the organism (e.g., Pseudomonas aeruginosa, code B96.5) should also be assigned. Do not assign an additional code from categories J12-J18 to identify the type of pneumonia.

Code J95.851 should not be assigned for cases where the patient has pneumonia and is on a mechanical ventilator and the provider has not specifically stated that the pneumonia is ventilator-associated pneumonia. If the documentation is unclear as to whether the patient has a pneumonia that is a complication attributable to the mechanical ventilator, query the provider.

2) Ventilator associated pneumonia develops after admission

A patient may be admitted with one type of pneumonia (e.g., code J13, Pneumonia due to Streptococcus pneumonia) and subsequently develop VAP. In this instance, the principal diagnosis would be the appropriate code from categories J12-J18 for the pneumonia diagnosed at the time of admission. Code J95.851, Ventilator associated pneumonia, would be assigned as an additional diagnosis when the provider has also documented the presence of ventilator associated pneumonia.

Chapter 10. Diseases of the Respiratory System (J00-J99)

NOTE   When a respiratory condition is described as occurring in more than one site and is not specifically indexed, it should be classified to the lower anatomic site (e.g., tracheobronchitis to bronchitis in J40).

Use additional code, where applicable, to identify:
exposure to environmental tobacco smoke (Z77.22)
exposure to tobacco smoke in the perinatal period (P96.81)
history of tobacco dependence (Z87.891)
occupational exposure to environmental tobacco smoke (Z57.31)
tobacco dependence (F17.-)
tobacco use (Z72.0)

EXCLUDES 2   certain conditions originating in the perinatal period (P04-P96)
certain infectious and parasitic diseases (A00-B99)
complications of pregnancy, childbirth and the puerperium (O00-O9A)
congenital malformations, deformations and chromosomal abnormalities (Q00-Q99)
endocrine, nutritional and metabolic diseases (E00-E88)
injury, poisoning and certain other consequences of external causes (S00-T88)
neoplasms (C00-D49)
smoke inhalation (T59.81-)
symptoms, signs and abnormal clinical and laboratory findings, not elsewhere classified (R00-R94)

This chapter contains the following blocks:
J00-J06   Acute upper respiratory infections
J09-J18   Influenza and pneumonia
J20-J22   Other acute lower respiratory infections
J30-J39   Other diseases of upper respiratory tract
J40-J47   Chronic lower respiratory diseases
J60-J70   Lung diseases due to external agents
J80-J84   Other respiratory diseases principally affecting the interstitium
J85-J86   Suppurative and necrotic conditions of the lower respiratory tract
J90-J94   Other diseases of the pleura
J95   Intraoperative and postprocedural complications and disorders of respiratory system, not elsewhere classified
J96-J99   Other diseases of the respiratory system

Acute upper respiratory infections (J00-J06)

EXCLUDES 1   chronic obstructive pulmonary disease with acute lower respiratory infection (J44.0)
influenza virus with other respiratory manifestations (J09.X2, J10.1, J11.1)

J00   Acute nasopharyngitis [common cold]
Acute rhinitis
Coryza (acute)
Infective nasopharyngitis NOS
Infective rhinitis
Nasal catarrh, acute
Nasopharyngitis NOS

EXCLUDES 1   acute pharyngitis (J02.-)
acute sore throat NOS (J02.9)
pharyngitis NOS (J02.9)
rhinitis NOS (J31.0)
sore throat NOS (J02.9)

EXCLUDES 2   allergic rhinitis (J30.1-J30.9)
chronic pharyngitis (J31.2)
chronic rhinitis (J31.0)
chronic sore throat (J31.2)
nasopharyngitis, chronic (J31.1)
vasomotor rhinitis (J30.0)

DEF: Acute inflammation of the mucous membranes that extends from the nares to the pharynx. It is characterized by nasal obstruction, sneezing, runny nose, and sore throat.

☑4ᵗʰ J01   Acute sinusitis
INCLUDES   acute abscess of sinus
acute empyema of sinus
acute infection of sinus
acute inflammation of sinus
acute suppuration of sinus
Use additional code (B95-B97) to identify infectious agent
EXCLUDES 1   sinusitis NOS (J32.9)
EXCLUDES 2   chronic sinusitis (J32.0-J32.8)

☑5ᵗʰ J01.0   Acute maxillary sinusitis
Acute antritis
J01.00   Acute maxillary sinusitis, unspecified   ▽
J01.01   Acute recurrent maxillary sinusitis

☑5ᵗʰ J01.1   Acute frontal sinusitis
J01.10   Acute frontal sinusitis, unspecified   ▽
J01.11   Acute recurrent frontal sinusitis
☑5ᵗʰ J01.2   Acute ethmoidal sinusitis
J01.20   Acute ethmoidal sinusitis, unspecified   ▽
J01.21   Acute recurrent ethmoidal sinusitis
☑5ᵗʰ J01.3   Acute sphenoidal sinusitis
J01.30   Acute sphenoidal sinusitis, unspecified   ▽
J01.31   Acute recurrent sphenoidal sinusitis
☑5ᵗʰ J01.4   Acute pansinusitis
J01.40   Acute pansinusitis, unspecified   ▽
J01.41   Acute recurrent pansinusitis
☑5ᵗʰ J01.8   Other acute sinusitis
J01.80   Other acute sinusitis
Acute sinusitis involving more than one sinus but not pansinusitis
J01.81   Other acute recurrent sinusitis
Acute recurrent sinusitis involving more than one sinus but not pansinusitis
☑5ᵗʰ J01.9   Acute sinusitis, unspecified
J01.90   Acute sinusitis, unspecified   ▽
J01.91   Acute recurrent sinusitis, unspecified   ▽

☑4ᵗʰ J02   Acute pharyngitis
INCLUDES   acute sore throat
EXCLUDES 1   acute laryngopharyngitis (J06.0)
peritonsillar abscess (J36)
pharyngeal abscess (J39.1)
retropharyngeal abscess (J39.0)
EXCLUDES 2   chronic pharyngitis (J31.2)

J02.0   Streptococcal pharyngitis
Septic pharyngitis
Streptococcal sore throat
EXCLUDES 2   scarlet fever (A38.-)

J02.8   Acute pharyngitis due to other specified organisms
Use additional code (B95-B97) to identify infectious agent
EXCLUDES 1   acute pharyngitis due to coxsackie virus (B08.5)
acute pharyngitis due to gonococcus (A54.5)
acute pharyngitis due to herpes [simplex] virus (B00.2)
acute pharyngitis due to infectious mononucleosis (B27.-)
enteroviral vesicular pharyngitis (B08.5)

J02.9   Acute pharyngitis, unspecified   ▽
Gangrenous pharyngitis (acute)
Infective pharyngitis (acute) NOS
Pharyngitis (acute) NOS
Sore throat (acute) NOS
Suppurative pharyngitis (acute)
Ulcerative pharyngitis (acute)

☑4ᵗʰ J03   Acute tonsillitis
EXCLUDES 1   acute sore throat (J02.-)
hypertrophy of tonsils (J35.1)
peritonsillar abscess (J36)
sore throat NOS (J02.9)
streptococcal sore throat (J02.0)
EXCLUDES 2   chronic tonsillitis (J35.0)

☑5ᵗʰ J03.0   Streptococcal tonsillitis
J03.00   Acute streptococcal tonsillitis, unspecified   ▽
J03.01   Acute recurrent streptococcal tonsillitis
☑5ᵗʰ J03.8   Acute tonsillitis due to other specified organisms
Use additional code (B95-B97) to identify infectious agent
EXCLUDES 1   diphtheritic tonsillitis (A36.0)
herpesviral pharyngotonsillitis (B00.2)
streptococcal tonsillitis (J03.0)
tuberculous tonsillitis (A15.8)
Vincent's tonsillitis (A69.1)
J03.80   Acute tonsillitis due to other specified organisms
J03.81   Acute recurrent tonsillitis due to other specified organisms

| ☑ Additional Character Req | ✓x7ᵗʰ Placeholder Alert | Manifestation | ▽ Unspecified | ►◄ Revised Text | ● New Code | ▲ Revised Code Title |

ICD-10-CM 2019   **677**

√5ᵗʰ **J03.9** **Acute tonsillitis, unspecified**
Follicular tonsillitis (acute)
Gangrenous tonsillitis (acute)
Infective tonsillitis (acute)
Tonsillitis (acute) NOS
Ulcerative tonsillitis (acute)

     J03.90 **Acute tonsillitis, unspecified** ▽

     J03.91 **Acute recurrent tonsillitis, unspecified** ▽

√4ᵗʰ **J04** **Acute laryngitis and tracheitis**
Use additional code (B95-B97) to identify infectious agent
   EXCLUDES 1   *acute obstructive laryngitis [croup] and epiglottitis (J05.-)*
   EXCLUDES 2   *laryngismus (stridulus) (J38.5)*

   J04.0 **Acute laryngitis**
Edematous laryngitis (acute)
Laryngitis (acute) NOS
Subglottic laryngitis (acute)
Suppurative laryngitis (acute)
Ulcerative laryngitis (acute)
     EXCLUDES 1   *acute obstructive laryngitis (J05.0)*
     EXCLUDES 2   *chronic laryngitis (J37.0)*

√5ᵗʰ **J04.1** **Acute tracheitis**
Acute viral tracheitis
Catarrhal tracheitis (acute)
Tracheitis (acute) NOS
     EXCLUDES 2   *chronic tracheitis (J42)*

     J04.10 **Acute tracheitis without obstruction**

     J04.11 **Acute tracheitis with obstruction**

   J04.2 **Acute laryngotracheitis**
Laryngotracheitis NOS
Tracheitis (acute) with laryngitis (acute)
     EXCLUDES 1   *acute obstructive laryngotracheitis (J05.0)*
     EXCLUDES 2   *chronic laryngotracheitis (J37.1)*

√5ᵗʰ **J04.3** **Supraglottitis, unspecified**

     J04.30 **Supraglottitis, unspecified, without obstruction** ▽

     J04.31 **Supraglottitis, unspecified, with obstruction** ▽

√4ᵗʰ **J05** **Acute obstructive laryngitis [croup] and epiglottitis**
Use additional code (B95-B97) to identify infectious agent

   J05.0 **Acute obstructive laryngitis [croup]**
Obstructive laryngitis (acute) NOS
Obstructive laryngotracheitis NOS
DEF: Acute laryngeal obstruction due to allergies, foreign bodies, or in the majority of cases a viral infection. Symptoms include a harsh, barking cough, hoarseness, and a persistent, high-pitched respiratory sound (stridor).

√5ᵗʰ **J05.1** **Acute epiglottitis**
     EXCLUDES 2   *epiglottitis, chronic (J37.0)*

     J05.10 **Acute epiglottitis without obstruction**
Epiglottitis NOS

     J05.11 **Acute epiglottitis with obstruction**

√4ᵗʰ **J06** **Acute upper respiratory infections of multiple and unspecified sites**
   EXCLUDES 1   *acute respiratory infection NOS (J22)*
                streptococcal pharyngitis (J02.0)

   J06.0 **Acute laryngopharyngitis**

   J06.9 **Acute upper respiratory infection, unspecified** ▽
Upper respiratory disease, acute
Upper respiratory infection NOS

Influenza and pneumonia (J09-J18)

   EXCLUDES 2   *allergic or eosinophilic pneumonia (J82)*
                aspiration pneumonia NOS (J69.0)
                meconium pneumonia (P24.01)
                neonatal aspiration pneumonia (P24.-)
                pneumonia due to solids and liquids (J69.-)
                congenital pneumonia (P23.9)
                lipid pneumonia (J69.1)
                rheumatic pneumonia (I00)
                ventilator associated pneumonia (J95.851)
AHA: 2017,4Q,96
TIP: Hemoptysis (R04.2) is not customarily associated with pneumonia and may be reported separately.

√4ᵗʰ **J09** **Influenza due to certain identified influenza viruses**
     EXCLUDES 1   *influenza A/H1N1 (J10.-)*
                  influenza due to other identified influenza virus (J10.-)
                  influenza due to unidentified influenza virus (J11.-)
                  seasonal influenza due to other identified influenza virus (J10.-)
                  seasonal influenza due to unidentified influenza virus (J11.-)

√5ᵗʰ **J09.X** **Influenza due to identified novel influenza A virus**
Avian influenza
Bird influenza
Influenza A/H5N1
Influenza of other animal origin, not bird or swine
Swine influenza virus (viruses that normally cause infections in pigs)
AHA: 2016,3Q,10

     J09.X1 **Influenza due to identified novel influenza A virus with pneumonia**
Code also, if applicable, associated:
lung abscess (J85.1)
other specified type of pneumonia

     J09.X2 **Influenza due to identified novel influenza A virus with other respiratory manifestations**
Influenza due to identified novel influenza A virus NOS
Influenza due to identified novel influenza A virus with laryngitis
Influenza due to identified novel influenza A virus with pharyngitis
Influenza due to identified novel influenza A virus with upper respiratory symptoms
Use additional code, if applicable, for associated:
pleural effusion (J91.8)
sinusitis (J01.-)

     J09.X3 **Influenza due to identified novel influenza A virus with gastrointestinal manifestations**
Influenza due to identified novel influenza A virus gastroenteritis
     EXCLUDES 1   *'intestinal flu' [viral gastroenteritis] (A08.-)*

     J09.X9 **Influenza due to identified novel influenza A virus with other manifestations**
Influenza due to identified novel influenza A virus with encephalopathy
Influenza due to identified novel influenza A virus with myocarditis
Influenza due to identified novel influenza A virus with otitis media
Use additional code to identify manifestation

√4ᵗʰ **J10** **Influenza due to other identified influenza virus**
     EXCLUDES 1   *influenza due to avian influenza virus (J09.X-)*
                  influenza due to swine flu (J09.X-)
                  influenza due to unidentifed influenza virus (J11.-)

√5ᵗʰ **J10.0** **Influenza due to other identified influenza virus with pneumonia**
Code also associated lung abscess, if applicable (J85.1)

     J10.00 **Influenza due to other identified influenza virus with unspecified type of pneumonia** ▽

     J10.01 **Influenza due to other identified influenza virus with the same other identified influenza virus pneumonia**

     J10.08 **Influenza due to other identified influenza virus with other specified pneumonia**
Code also other specified type of pneumonia

J10.1   **Influenza due to other identified influenza virus with other respiratory manifestations**

    Influenza due to other identified influenza virus NOS

    Influenza due to other identified influenza virus with laryngitis

    Influenza due to other identified influenza virus with pharyngitis

    Influenza due to other identified influenza virus with upper respiratory symptoms

    Use additional code for associated pleural effusion, if applicable (J91.8)

    Use additional code for associated sinusitis, if applicable (J01.-)

    AHA: 2016,3Q,10-11

J10.2   **Influenza due to other identified influenza virus with gastrointestinal manifestations**

    Influenza due to other identified influenza virus gastroenteritis

    EXCLUDES 1   "intestinal flu" [viral gastroenteritis] (A08.-)

√5ᵗʰ **J10.8**   **Influenza due to other identified influenza virus with other manifestations**

   J10.81   **Influenza due to other identified influenza virus with encephalopathy**

   J10.82   **Influenza due to other identified influenza virus with myocarditis**

   J10.83   **Influenza due to other identified influenza virus with otitis media**

     Use additional code for any associated perforated tympanic membrane (H72.-)

   J10.89   **Influenza due to other identified influenza virus with other manifestations**

     Use additional codes to identify the manifestations

√4ᵗʰ **J11**   **Influenza due to unidentified influenza virus**

√5ᵗʰ **J11.0**   **Influenza due to unidentified influenza virus with pneumonia**

    Code also associated lung abscess, if applicable (J85.1)

    AHA: 2016,3Q,11

   J11.00   **Influenza due to unidentified influenza virus with unspecified type of pneumonia**   ▽

     Influenza with pneumonia NOS

   J11.08   **Influenza due to unidentified influenza virus with specified pneumonia**

     Code also other specified type of pneumonia

J11.1   **Influenza due to unidentified influenza virus with other respiratory manifestations**

    Influenza NOS

    Influenzal laryngitis NOS

    Influenzal pharyngitis NOS

    Influenza with upper respiratory symptoms NOS

    Use additional code for associated pleural effusion, if applicable (J91.8)

    Use additional code for associated sinusitis, if applicable (J01.-)

J11.2   **Influenza due to unidentified influenza virus with gastrointestinal manifestations**

    Influenza gastroenteritis NOS

    EXCLUDES 1   "intestinal flu" [viral gastroenteritis] (A08.-)

√5ᵗʰ **J11.8**   **Influenza due to unidentified influenza virus with other manifestations**

   J11.81   **Influenza due to unidentified influenza virus with encephalopathy**

     Influenzal encephalopathy NOS

   J11.82   **Influenza due to unidentified influenza virus with myocarditis**

     Influenzal myocarditis NOS

   J11.83   **Influenza due to unidentified influenza virus with otitis media**

     Influenzal otitis media NOS

     Use additional code for any associated perforated tympanic membrane (H72.-)

   J11.89   **Influenza due to unidentified influenza virus with other manifestations**

     Use additional codes to identify the manifestations

√4ᵗʰ **J12**   **Viral pneumonia, not elsewhere classified**

   INCLUDES   bronchopneumonia due to viruses other than influenza viruses

   Code first associated influenza, if applicable (J09.X1, J10.0-, J11.0-)

   Code also associated abscess, if applicable (J85.1)

   EXCLUDES 1   aspiration pneumonia due to anesthesia during labor and delivery (O74.0)

     aspiration pneumonia due to anesthesia during pregnancy (O29)

     aspiration pneumonia due to anesthesia during puerperium (O89.0)

     aspiration pneumonia due to solids and liquids (J69.-)

     aspiration pneumonia NOS (J69.0)

     congenital pneumonia (P23.0)

     congenital rubella pneumonitis (P35.0)

     interstitial pneumonia NOS (J84.9)

     lipid pneumonia (J69.1)

     neonatal aspiration pneumonia (P24.-)

   AHA: 2016,3Q,15; 2013,4Q,118

  J12.0   **Adenoviral pneumonia**

  J12.1   **Respiratory syncytial virus pneumonia**

  J12.2   **Parainfluenza virus pneumonia**

  J12.3   **Human metapneumovirus pneumonia**

√5ᵗʰ **J12.8**   **Other viral pneumonia**

   J12.81   **Pneumonia due to SARS-associated coronavirus**

     Severe acute respiratory syndrome NOS

     DEF: Severe adult respiratory syndrome caused by the coronavirus, specified as inflammation of the lungs with consolidation.

   J12.89   **Other viral pneumonia**

  J12.9   **Viral pneumonia, unspecified**   ▽

J13   **Pneumonia due to Streptococcus pneumoniae**   HCC

   Bronchopneumonia due to S. pneumoniae

   Code first associated influenza, if applicable (J09.X1, J10.0-, J11.0-)

   Code also associated abscess, if applicable (J85.1)

   EXCLUDES 1   congenital pneumonia due to S. pneumoniae (P23.6)

     lobar pneumonia, unspecified organism (J18.1)

     pneumonia due to other streptococci (J15.3-J15.4)

   AHA: 2016,3Q,15; 2013,4Q,118

J14   **Pneumonia due to Hemophilus influenzae**   HCC

   Bronchopneumonia due to H. influenzae

   Code first associated influenza, if applicable (J09.X1, J10.0-, J11.0-)

   Code also associated abscess, if applicable (J85.1)

   EXCLUDES 1   congenital pneumonia due to H. influenzae (P23.6)

   AHA: 2016,3Q,15; 2013,4Q,118

√4ᵗʰ **J15**   **Bacterial pneumonia, not elsewhere classified**

   INCLUDES   Bronchopneumonia due to bacteria other than S. pneumoniae and H. influenzae

   Code first associated influenza, if applicable (J09.X1, J10.0-, -J11.0-)

   Code also associated abscess, if applicable (J85.1)

   EXCLUDES 1   chlamydial pneumonia (J16.0)

     congenital pneumonia (P23.-)

     Legionnaires' disease (A48.1)

     spirochetal pneumonia (A69.8)

   AHA: 2016,3Q,15; 2013,4Q,118

  J15.0   **Pneumonia due to Klebsiella pneumoniae**   HCC

  J15.1   **Pneumonia due to Pseudomonas**   HCC

√5ᵗʰ **J15.2**   **Pneumonia due to staphylococcus**

   J15.20   **Pneumonia due to staphylococcus, unspecified**   HCC ▽

√6ᵗʰ **J15.21**   **Pneumonia due to Staphylococcus aureus**

    J15.211   **Pneumonia due to methicillin susceptible Staphylococcus aureus**   HCC

     MSSA pneumonia

     Pneumonia due to Staphylococcus aureus NOS

    J15.212   **Pneumonia due to methicillin resistant Staphylococcus aureus**   HCC

   J15.29   **Pneumonia due to other staphylococcus**   HCC

  J15.3   **Pneumonia due to streptococcus, group B**   HCC

  J15.4   **Pneumonia due to other streptococci**   HCC

   EXCLUDES 1   pneumonia due to streptococcus, group B (J15.3)

     pneumonia due to Streptococcus pneumoniae (J13)

  J15.5   **Pneumonia due to Escherichia coli**   HCC

☑ Additional Character Req   ✓ˣ⁷ᵗʰ Placeholder Alert   Manifestation   ▽ Unspecified   ►◄ Revised Text   ● New Code   ▲ Revised Code Title

ICD-10-CM 2019   679

J10.1–J15.5

Chapter 10. Diseases of the Respiratory System

J15.6   **Pneumonia due to other Gram-negative bacteria**   HCC
Pneumonia due to other aerobic Gram-negative bacteria
Pneumonia due to Serratia marcescens

J15.7   **Pneumonia due to Mycoplasma pneumoniae**

J15.8   **Pneumonia due to other specified bacteria**   HCC

J15.9   **Unspecified bacterial pneumonia**   ▽
Pneumonia due to gram-positive bacteria

✓4ᵗʰ **J16**   **Pneumonia due to other infectious organisms, not elsewhere classified**
Code first associated influenza, if applicable (J09.X1, J10.0-, J11.0-)
Code also associated abscess, if applicable (J85.1)

> EXCLUDES 1   *congenital pneumonia (P23.-)*
> *ornithosis (A70)*
> *pneumocystosis (B59)*
> *pneumonia NOS (J18.9)*

AHA: 2016,3Q,15; 2013,4Q,118

J16.0   **Chlamydial pneumonia**

J16.8   **Pneumonia due to other specified infectious organisms**

J17   *Pneumonia in diseases classified elsewhere*
Code first underlying disease, such as:
Q fever (A78)
rheumatic fever (I00)
schistosomiasis (B65.0-B65.9)

> EXCLUDES 1   *candidial pneumonia (B37.1)*
> *chlamydial pneumonia (J16.0)*
> *gonorrheal pneumonia (A54.84)*
> *histoplasmosis pneumonia (B39.0-B39.2)*
> *measles pneumonia (B05.2)*
> *nocardiosis pneumonia (A43.0)*
> *pneumocystosis (B59)*
> *pneumonia due to Pneumocystis carinii (B59)*
> *pneumonia due to Pneumocystis jiroveci (B59)*
> *pneumonia in actinomycosis (A42.0)*
> *pneumonia in anthrax (A22.1)*
> *pneumonia in ascariasis (B77.81)*
> *pneumonia in aspergillosis (B44.0-B44.1)*
> *pneumonia in coccidioidomycosis (B38.0-B38.2)*
> *pneumonia in cytomegalovirus disease (B25.0)*
> *pneumonia in toxoplasmosis (B58.3)*
> *rubella pneumonia (B06.81)*
> *salmonella pneumonia (A02.22)*
> *spirochetal infection NEC with pneumonia (A69.8)*
> *tularemia pneumonia (A21.2)*
> *typhoid fever with pneumonia (A01.03)*
> *varicella pneumonia (B01.2)*
> *whooping cough with pneumonia (A37 with fifth character 1)*

AHA: 2016,3Q,15; 2013,4Q,118

✓4ᵗʰ **J18**   **Pneumonia, unspecified organism**
Code first associated influenza, if applicable (J09.X1, J10.0-, J11.0-)

> EXCLUDES 1   *abscess of lung with pneumonia (J85.1)*
> *aspiration pneumonia due to anesthesia during labor and delivery (O74.0)*
> *aspiration pneumonia due to anesthesia during pregnancy (O29)*
> *aspiration pneumonia due to anesthesia during puerperium (O89.0)*
> *aspiration pneumonia due to solids and liquids (J69.-)*
> *aspiration pneumonia NOS (J69.0)*
> *congenital pneumonia (P23.0)*
> *drug-induced interstitial lung disorder (J70.2-J70.4)*
> *interstitial pneumonia NOS (J84.9)*
> *lipid pneumonia (J69.1)*
> *neonatal aspiration pneumonia (P24.-)*
> *pneumonitis due to external agents (J67-J70)*
> *pneumonitis due to fumes and vapors (J68.0)*
> *usual interstitial pneumonia (J84.17)*

AHA: 2016,3Q,15; 2013,4Q,118

J18.0   **Bronchopneumonia, unspecified organism**   ▽
> EXCLUDES 1   *hypostatic bronchopneumonia (J18.2)*
> *lipid pneumonia (J69.1)*
> EXCLUDES 2   *acute bronchiolitis (J21.-)*
> *chronic bronchiolitis (J44.9)*

J18.1   **Lobar pneumonia, unspecified organism**   HCC ▽

J18.2   **Hypostatic pneumonia, unspecified organism**   ▽
Hypostatic bronchopneumonia
Passive pneumonia

J18.8   **Other pneumonia, unspecified organism**   ▽

J18.9   **Pneumonia, unspecified organism**   ▽
AHA: 2014,3Q,4; 2013,4Q,119; 2012,4Q,94

Other acute lower respiratory infections (J20-J22)

> EXCLUDES 2   *chronic obstructive pulmonary disease with acute lower respiratory infection (J44.0)*

✓4ᵗʰ **J20**   **Acute bronchitis**
> INCLUDES   acute and subacute bronchitis (with) bronchospasm
> acute and subacute bronchitis (with) tracheitis
> acute and subacute bronchitis (with) tracheobronchitis, acute
> acute and subacute fibrinous bronchitis
> acute and subacute membranous bronchitis
> acute and subacute purulent bronchitis
> acute and subacute septic bronchitis
> EXCLUDES 1   *bronchitis NOS (J40)*
> *tracheobronchitis NOS (J40)*
> EXCLUDES 2   *acute bronchitis with bronchiectasis (J47.0)*
> *acute bronchitis with chronic obstructive asthma (J44.0)*
> *acute bronchitis with chronic obstructive pulmonary disease (J44.0)*
> *allergic bronchitis NOS (J45.909-)*
> *bronchitis due to chemicals, fumes and vapors (J68.0)*
> *chronic bronchitis NOS (J42)*
> *chronic mucopurulent bronchitis (J41.1)*
> *chronic obstructive bronchitis (J44.-)*
> *chronic obstructive tracheobronchitis (J44.-)*
> *chronic simple bronchitis (J41.0)*
> *chronic tracheobronchitis (J42)*

AHA: 2016,3Q,10,16
DEF: Acute inflammation of the main branches of the bronchial tree due to infectious or irritant agents. Symptoms include cough with a varied production of sputum, fever, substernal soreness, and lung rales. Bronchitis usually lasts three to 10 days.

J20.0   **Acute bronchitis due to Mycoplasma pneumoniae**

J20.1   **Acute bronchitis due to Hemophilus influenzae**

J20.2   **Acute bronchitis due to streptococcus**

J20.3   **Acute bronchitis due to coxsackievirus**

J20.4   **Acute bronchitis due to parainfluenza virus**

J20.5   **Acute bronchitis due to respiratory syncytial virus**

J20.6   **Acute bronchitis due to rhinovirus**

J20.7   **Acute bronchitis due to echovirus**

J20.8   **Acute bronchitis due to other specified organisms**

J20.9   **Acute bronchitis, unspecified**   ▽

✓4ᵗʰ **J21**   **Acute bronchiolitis**
> INCLUDES   acute bronchiolitis with bronchospasm
> EXCLUDES 2   *respiratory bronchiolitis interstitial lung disease (J84.115)*

J21.0   **Acute bronchiolitis due to respiratory syncytial virus**

J21.1   **Acute bronchiolitis due to human metapneumovirus**

J21.8   **Acute bronchiolitis due to other specified organisms**

J21.9   **Acute bronchiolitis, unspecified**   ▽
Bronchiolitis (acute)
> EXCLUDES 1   *chronic bronchiolitis (J44.-)*

J22   **Unspecified acute lower respiratory infection**   ▽
Acute (lower) respiratory (tract) infection NOS
> EXCLUDES 1   *upper respiratory infection (acute) (J06.9)*

Other diseases of upper respiratory tract (J30-J39)

✓4ᵗʰ **J30**   **Vasomotor and allergic rhinitis**
> INCLUDES   spasmodic rhinorrhea
> EXCLUDES 1   *allergic rhinitis with asthma (bronchial) (J45.909)*
> *rhinitis NOS (J31.0)*

J30.0   **Vasomotor rhinitis**
DEF: Noninfectious and nonallergic type of rhinitis for which the cause is often unknown. Symptoms often mimic those of allergic rhinitis with a diagnosis of vasomotor rhinitis typically made after ruling out allergens as the cause.

J30.1   Allergic rhinitis due to pollen
   Allergy NOS due to pollen
   Hay fever
   Pollinosis

J30.2   Other seasonal allergic rhinitis

J30.5   Allergic rhinitis due to food

√5ᵗʰ **J30.8   Other allergic rhinitis**

   J30.81   Allergic rhinitis due to animal (cat) (dog) hair and dander

   J30.89   Other allergic rhinitis
      Perennial allergic rhinitis

J30.9   Allergic rhinitis, unspecified   ▽

√4ᵗʰ **J31   Chronic rhinitis, nasopharyngitis and pharyngitis**
   Use additional code to identify:
      exposure to environmental tobacco smoke (Z77.22)
      exposure to tobacco smoke in the perinatal period (P96.81)
      history of tobacco dependence (Z87.891)
      occupational exposure to environmental tobacco smoke (Z57.31)
      tobacco dependence (F17.-)
      tobacco use (Z72.0)

   J31.0   Chronic rhinitis
      Atrophic rhinitis (chronic)
      Granulomatous rhinitis (chronic)
      Hypertrophic rhinitis (chronic)
      Obstructive rhinitis (chronic)
      Ozena
      Purulent rhinitis (chronic)
      Rhinitis (chronic) NOS
      Ulcerative rhinitis (chronic)
      EXCLUDES 1   *allergic rhinitis (J30.1-J30.9)*
                     vasomotor rhinitis (J30.0)
      DEF: Persistent inflammation of the mucous membranes of the nose, characterized by a postnasal drip.

   J31.1   Chronic nasopharyngitis
      EXCLUDES 2   *acute nasopharyngitis (J00)*
      DEF: Persistent inflammation of the mucous membranes extending from the nares to the pharynx. It is characterized by constant irritation in the nasopharynx and postnasal drip.

   J31.2   Chronic pharyngitis
      Atrophic pharyngitis (chronic)
      Chronic sore throat
      Granular pharyngitis (chronic)
      Hypertrophic pharyngitis (chronic)
      EXCLUDES 2   *acute pharyngitis (J02.9)*

√4ᵗʰ **J32   Chronic sinusitis**
   INCLUDES   sinus abscess
               sinus empyema
               sinus infection
               sinus suppuration
   Use additional code to identify:
      exposure to environmental tobacco smoke (Z77.22)
      exposure to tobacco smoke in the perinatal period (P96.81)
      history of tobacco dependence (Z87.891)
      infectious agent (B95-B97)
      occupational exposure to environmental tobacco smoke (Z57.31)
      tobacco dependence (F17.-)
      tobacco use (Z72.0)
   EXCLUDES 2   *acute sinusitis (J01.-)*

   J32.0   Chronic maxillary sinusitis
      Antritis (chronic)
      Maxillary sinusitis NOS

   J32.1   Chronic frontal sinusitis
      Frontal sinusitis NOS

   J32.2   Chronic ethmoidal sinusitis
      Ethmoidal sinusitis NOS
      EXCLUDES 1   *Woakes' ethmoiditis (J33.1)*

   J32.3   Chronic sphenoidal sinusitis
      Sphenoidal sinusitis NOS

   J32.4   Chronic pansinusitis
      Pansinusitis NOS

   J32.8   Other chronic sinusitis
      Sinusitis (chronic) involving more than one sinus but not pansinusitis

   J32.9   Chronic sinusitis, unspecified   ▽
      Sinusitis (chronic) NOS

√4ᵗʰ **J33   Nasal polyp**
   Use additional code to identify:
      exposure to environmental tobacco smoke (Z77.22)
      exposure to tobacco smoke in the perinatal period (P96.81)
      history of tobacco dependence (Z87.891)
      occupational exposure to environmental tobacco smoke (Z57.31)
      tobacco dependence (F17.-)
      tobacco use (Z72.0)
   EXCLUDES 1   *adenomatous polyps (D14.0)*

   J33.0   Polyp of nasal cavity
      Choanal polyp
      Nasopharyngeal polyp

   J33.1   Polypoid sinus degeneration
      Woakes' syndrome or ethmoiditis

   J33.8   Other polyp of sinus
      Accessory polyp of sinus
      Ethmoidal polyp of sinus
      Maxillary polyp of sinus
      Sphenoidal polyp of sinus

   J33.9   Nasal polyp, unspecified   ▽

√4ᵗʰ **J34   Other and unspecified disorders of nose and nasal sinuses**
   EXCLUDES 2   *varicose ulcer of nasal septum (I86.8)*

   J34.0   Abscess, furuncle and carbuncle of nose
      Cellulitis of nose
      Necrosis of nose
      Ulceration of nose

   J34.1   Cyst and mucocele of nose and nasal sinus

   J34.2   Deviated nasal septum
      Deflection or deviation of septum (nasal) (acquired)
      EXCLUDES 1   *congenital deviated nasal septum (Q67.4)*
      DEF: Condition in which the nasal septum, a thin wall composed of cartilage and bone that separates the two nostrils, is crooked or displaced from the midline.

   J34.3   Hypertrophy of nasal turbinates
      DEF: Overgrowth of bones within the nasal turbinate, which are ridges of bone and soft tissue that project from the sidewalls of the nasal passages. Hypertrophy can cause obstruction of the nasal passages.

   √5ᵗʰ **J34.8   Other specified disorders of nose and nasal sinuses**

      J34.81   Nasal mucositis (ulcerative)
         Code also type of associated therapy, such as:
            antineoplastic and immunosuppressive drugs (T45.1X-)
            radiological procedure and radiotherapy (Y84.2)
         EXCLUDES 2   *gastrointestinal mucositis (ulcerative) (K92.81)*
                        mucositis (ulcerative) of vagina and vulva (N76.81)
                        oral mucositis (ulcerative) (K12.3-)

      J34.89   Other specified disorders of nose and nasal sinuses
         Perforation of nasal septum NOS
         Rhinolith

   J34.9   Unspecified disorder of nose and nasal sinuses   ▽

√4ᵗʰ **J35   Chronic diseases of tonsils and adenoids**
   Use additional code to identify:
      exposure to environmental tobacco smoke (Z77.22)
      exposure to tobacco smoke in the perinatal period (P96.81)
      history of tobacco dependence (Z87.891)
      occupational exposure to environmental tobacco smoke (Z57.31)
      tobacco dependence (F17.-)
      tobacco use (Z72.0)

   √5ᵗʰ **J35.0   Chronic tonsillitis and adenoiditis**
      EXCLUDES 2   *acute tonsillitis (J03.-)*

      J35.01   Chronic tonsillitis
      J35.02   Chronic adenoiditis
      J35.03   Chronic tonsillitis and adenoiditis

   J35.1   Hypertrophy of tonsils
      Enlargement of tonsils
      EXCLUDES 1   *hypertrophy of tonsils with tonsillitis (J35.0-)*

   J35.2   Hypertrophy of adenoids
      Enlargement of adenoids
      EXCLUDES 1   *hypertrophy of adenoids with adenoiditis (J35.0-)*

   J35.3   Hypertrophy of tonsils with hypertrophy of adenoids
      EXCLUDES 1   *hypertrophy of tonsils and adenoids with tonsillitis and adenoiditis (J35.03)*

Chapter 10. Diseases of the Respiratory System

J35.8   **Other chronic diseases of tonsils and adenoids**
Adenoid vegetations
Amygdalolith
Calculus, tonsil
Cicatrix of tonsil (and adenoid)
Tonsillar tag
Ulcer of tonsil

J35.9   **Chronic disease of tonsils and adenoids, unspecified** ▽
Disease (chronic) of tonsils and adenoids NOS

J36   **Peritonsillar abscess**
INCLUDES   abscess of tonsil
peritonsillar cellulitis
quinsy
Use additional code (B95-B97) to identify infectious agent
EXCLUDES 1   *acute tonsillitis (J03.-)*
chronic tonsillitis (J35.0)
retropharyngeal abscess (J39.0)
tonsillitis NOS (J03.9-)

✓4ᵗʰ J37   **Chronic laryngitis and laryngotracheitis**
Use additional code to identify:
exposure to environmental tobacco smoke (Z77.22)
exposure to tobacco smoke in the perinatal period (P96.81)
history of tobacco dependence (Z87.891)
infectious agent (B95-B97)
occupational exposure to environmental tobacco smoke (Z57.31)
tobacco dependence (F17.-)
tobacco use (Z72.0)

J37.0   **Chronic laryngitis**
Catarrhal laryngitis
Hypertrophic laryngitis
Sicca laryngitis
EXCLUDES 2   *acute laryngitis (J04.0)*
obstructive (acute) laryngitis (J05.0)

J37.1   **Chronic laryngotracheitis**
Laryngitis, chronic, with tracheitis (chronic)
Tracheitis, chronic, with laryngitis
EXCLUDES 1   *chronic tracheitis (J42)*
EXCLUDES 2   *acute laryngotracheitis (J04.2)*
acute tracheitis (J04.1)

✓4ᵗʰ J38   **Diseases of vocal cords and larynx, not elsewhere classified**
Use additional code to identify:
exposure to environmental tobacco smoke (Z77.22)
exposure to tobacco smoke in the perinatal period (P96.81)
history of tobacco dependence (Z87.891)
occupational exposure to environmental tobacco smoke (Z57.31)
tobacco dependence (F17.-)
tobacco use (Z72.0)
EXCLUDES 1   *congenital laryngeal stridor (P28.89)*
obstructive laryngitis (acute) (J05.0)
postprocedural subglottic stenosis (J95.5)
stridor (R06.1)
ulcerative laryngitis (J04.0)

✓5ᵗʰ J38.0   **Paralysis of vocal cords and larynx**
Laryngoplegia
Paralysis of glottis

J38.00   **Paralysis of vocal cords and larynx, unspecified** ▽

J38.01   **Paralysis of vocal cords and larynx, unilateral**

J38.02   **Paralysis of vocal cords and larynx, bilateral**

J38.1   **Polyp of vocal cord and larynx**
EXCLUDES 1   *adenomatous polyps (D14.1)*

J38.2   **Nodules of vocal cords**
Chorditis (fibrinous)(nodosa)(tuberosa)
Singer's nodes
Teacher's nodes

J38.3   **Other diseases of vocal cords**
Abscess of vocal cords
Cellulitis of vocal cords
Granuloma of vocal cords
Leukokeratosis of vocal cords
Leukoplakia of vocal cords

J38.4   **Edema of larynx**
Edema (of) glottis
Subglottic edema
Supraglottic edema
EXCLUDES 1   *acute obstructive laryngitis [croup] (J05.0)*
edematous laryngitis (J04.0)

J38.5   **Laryngeal spasm**
Laryngismus (stridulus)

J38.6   **Stenosis of larynx**

J38.7   **Other diseases of larynx**
Abscess of larynx
Cellulitis of larynx
Disease of larynx NOS
Necrosis of larynx
Pachyderma of larynx
Perichondritis of larynx
Ulcer of larynx

✓4ᵗʰ J39   **Other diseases of upper respiratory tract**
EXCLUDES 1   *acute respiratory infection NOS (J22)*
acute upper respiratory infection (J06.9)
upper respiratory inflammation due to chemicals, gases, fumes or vapors (J68.2)

J39.0   **Retropharyngeal and parapharyngeal abscess**
Peripharyngeal abscess
EXCLUDES 1   *peritonsillar abscess (J36)*
DEF: Purulent infection behind the pharynx and the front of the precerebral fascia, characterized by neck stiffness, cervical lymphadenopathy, sore throat, fever, and stridor.

J39.1   **Other abscess of pharynx**
Cellulitis of pharynx
Nasopharyngeal abscess

J39.2   **Other diseases of pharynx**
Cyst of pharynx
Edema of pharynx
EXCLUDES 2   *chronic pharyngitis (J31.2)*
ulcerative pharyngitis (J02.9)

J39.3   **Upper respiratory tract hypersensitivity reaction, site unspecified** ▽
EXCLUDES 1   *hypersensitivity reaction of upper respiratory tract, such as:*
extrinsic allergic alveolitis (J67.9)
pneumoconiosis (J60-J67.9)

J39.8   **Other specified diseases of upper respiratory tract**

J39.9   **Disease of upper respiratory tract, unspecified** ▽

Chronic lower respiratory diseases (J40-J47)

EXCLUDES 1   *bronchitis due to chemicals, gases, fumes and vapors (J68.0)*
EXCLUDES 2   *cystic fibrosis (E84.-)*

J40   **Bronchitis, not specified as acute or chronic** ▽
Bronchitis NOS
Bronchitis with tracheitis NOS
Catarrhal bronchitis
Tracheobronchitis NOS
Use additional code to identify:
exposure to environmental tobacco smoke (Z77.22)
exposure to tobacco smoke in the perinatal period (P96.81)
history of tobacco dependence (Z87.891)
occupational exposure to environmental tobacco smoke (Z57.31)
tobacco dependence (F17.-)
tobacco use (Z72.0)
EXCLUDES 1   *acute bronchitis (J20.-)*
allergic bronchitis NOS (J45.909-)
asthmatic bronchitis NOS (J45.9-)
bronchitis due to chemicals, gases, fumes and vapors (J68.0)

✓4ᵗʰ J41   **Simple and mucopurulent chronic bronchitis**
Use additional code to identify:
exposure to environmental tobacco smoke (Z77.22)
exposure to tobacco smoke in the perinatal period (P96.81)
history of tobacco dependence (Z87.891)
occupational exposure to environmental tobacco smoke (Z57.31)
tobacco dependence (F17.-)
tobacco use (Z72.0)
EXCLUDES 1   *chronic bronchitis NOS (J42)*
chronic obstructive bronchitis (J44.-)

J41.0   **Simple chronic bronchitis**   HCC 0

J41.1   **Mucopurulent chronic bronchitis**   HCC 0

J41.8 Mixed simple and mucopurulent chronic bronchitis HCC ☐

J42 Unspecified chronic bronchitis HCC ☐ ▽

Chronic bronchitis NOS
Chronic tracheitis
Chronic tracheobronchitis

Use additional code to identify:
exposure to environmental tobacco smoke (Z77.22)
exposure to tobacco smoke in the perinatal period (P96.81)
history of tobacco dependence (Z87.891)
occupational exposure to environmental tobacco smoke (Z57.31)
tobacco dependence (F17.-)
tobacco use (Z72.0)

EXCLUDES 1   *chronic asthmatic bronchitis (J44.-)*
chronic bronchitis with airways obstruction (J44.-)
chronic emphysematous bronchitis (J44.-)
chronic obstructive pulmonary disease NOS (J44.9)
simple and mucopurulent chronic bronchitis (J41.-)

✓4th **J43 Emphysema**

Use additional code to identify:
exposure to environmental tobacco smoke (Z77.22)
history of tobacco dependence (Z87.891)
occupational exposure to environmental tobacco smoke (Z57.31)
tobacco dependence (F17.-)
tobacco use (Z72.0)

EXCLUDES 1   *compensatory emphysema (J98.3)*
emphysema due to inhalation of chemicals, gases, fumes or vapors (J68.4)
emphysema with chronic (obstructive) bronchitis (J44.-)
emphysematous (obstructive) bronchitis (J44.-)
interstitial emphysema (J98.2)
mediastinal emphysema (J98.2)
neonatal interstitial emphysema (P25.0)
surgical (subcutaneous) emphysema (T81.82)
traumatic subcutaneous emphysema (T79.7)

DEF: Pathological condition in which there is destructive enlargement of the air sacs in the lungs resulting in damage and lack of elasticity to the alveolar walls, commonly seen in long-term smokers.

Emphysema

Healthy alveoli   Alveoli w/ Emphysema

Patent bronchiole
Collapsed bronchiole
Well-vascularized
Enlarged alveoli
Broken/fewer capillaries
Dilated alveoli
Alveolar membranes break down
Excess mucus

J43.0 Unilateral pulmonary emphysema [MacLeod's syndrome] HCC ☐

Swyer-James syndrome
Unilateral emphysema
Unilateral hyperlucent lung
Unilateral pulmonary artery functional hypoplasia
Unilateral transparency of lung

J43.1 Panlobular emphysema HCC ☐
Panacinar emphysema

J43.2 Centrilobular emphysema HCC ☐

J43.8 Other emphysema HCC ☐

J43.9 Emphysema, unspecified HCC ☐ ▽
Bullous emphysema (lung)(pulmonary)
Emphysema (lung)(pulmonary) NOS
Emphysematous bleb
Vesicular emphysema (lung)(pulmonary)
AHA: 2017,4Q,97-98

✓4th **J44 Other chronic obstructive pulmonary disease**

INCLUDES   asthma with chronic obstructive pulmonary disease
chronic asthmatic (obstructive) bronchitis
chronic bronchitis with airways obstruction
chronic bronchitis with emphysema
chronic emphysematous bronchitis
chronic obstructive asthma
chronic obstructive bronchitis
chronic obstructive tracheobronchitis

Code also type of asthma, if applicable (J45.-)
Use additional code to identify:
exposure to environmental tobacco smoke (Z77.22)
history of tobacco dependence (Z87.891)
occupational exposure to environmental tobacco smoke (Z57.31)
tobacco dependence (F17.-)
tobacco use (Z72.0)

EXCLUDES 1   *bronchiectasis (J47.-)*
chronic bronchitis NOS (J42)
chronic simple and mucopurulent bronchitis (J41.-)
chronic tracheitis (J42)
chronic tracheobronchitis (J42)
emphysema without chronic bronchitis (J43.-)

AHA: 2017,4Q,97-98; 2017,1Q,25-26; 2016,3Q,15-16; 2013,4Q,109

J44.0 Chronic obstructive pulmonary disease with acute lower respiratory infection HCC ☐
Code also to identify the infection
AHA: 2017,4Q,96; 2017,1Q,24-25
TIP: Do not assign when only aspiration pneumonia is present. Aspiration pneumonia is not classified as a respiratory infection.

J44.1 Chronic obstructive pulmonary disease with (acute) exacerbation HCC ☐
Decompensated COPD
Decompensated COPD with (acute) exacerbation
EXCLUDES 2   *chronic obstructive pulmonary disease [COPD] with acute bronchitis (J44.0)*
lung diseases due to external agents (J60-J70)
AHA: 2017,4Q,96; 2017,1Q,26; 2016,1Q,36
TIP: Exacerbation of COPD should not be assumed based upon worsening of a concomitant respiratory disease or when COPD is described as end-stage.
TIP: Assign J43.9 when COPD exacerbation with emphysema is documented.

J44.9 Chronic obstructive pulmonary disease, unspecified HCC ☐ ▽
Chronic obstructive airway disease NOS
Chronic obstructive lung disease NOS
EXCLUDES 2   *lung diseases due to external agents (J60-J70)*
AHA: 2017,4Q,96-97; 2016,1Q,36; 2014,4Q,21; 2013,4Q,109

Chapter 10. Diseases of the Respiratory System

J45–J63.6

✓4ᵗʰ J45 Asthma

INCLUDES   allergic (predominantly) asthma
allergic bronchitis NOS
allergic rhinitis with asthma
atopic asthma
extrinsic allergic asthma
hay fever with asthma
idiosyncratic asthma
intrinsic nonallergic asthma
nonallergic asthma

Use additional code to identify:
exposure to environmental tobacco smoke (Z77.22)
exposure to tobacco smoke in the perinatal period (P96.81)
history of tobacco dependence (Z87.891)
occupational exposure to environmental tobacco smoke (Z57.31)
tobacco dependence (F17.-)
tobacco use (Z72.0)

EXCLUDES 1   detergent asthma (J69.8)
eosinophilic asthma (J82)
miner's asthma (J60)
wheezing NOS (R06.2)
wood asthma (J67.8)

EXCLUDES 2   asthma with chronic obstructive pulmonary disease (J44.9)
chronic asthmatic (obstructive) bronchitis (J44.9)
chronic obstructive asthma (J44.9)

AHA: 2017,1Q,25-26; 2012,4Q,99
DEF: Status asthmaticus: Severe, intractable episode of asthma that is unresponsive to normal therapeutic measures.

Asthma

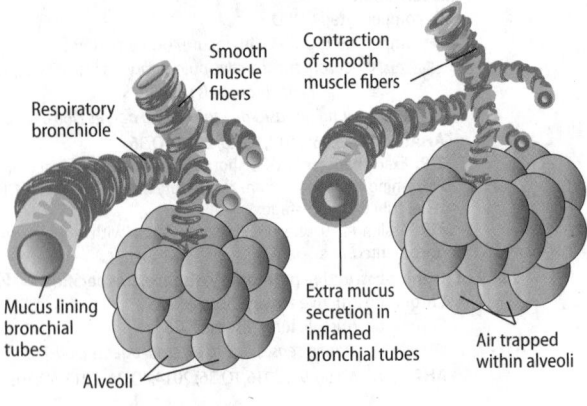

Smooth muscle fibers
Contraction of smooth muscle fibers
Respiratory bronchiole
Mucus lining bronchial tubes
Extra mucus secretion in inflamed bronchial tubes
Air trapped within alveoli
Alveoli

Normal alveoli   Asthmatic alveoli

✓5ᵗʰ J45.2 Mild intermittent asthma

J45.20 Mild intermittent asthma, uncomplicated
Mild intermittent asthma NOS
J45.21 Mild intermittent asthma with (acute) exacerbation
J45.22 Mild intermittent asthma with status asthmaticus

✓5ᵗʰ J45.3 Mild persistent asthma

J45.30 Mild persistent asthma, uncomplicated
Mild persistent asthma NOS
J45.31 Mild persistent asthma with (acute) exacerbation
AHA: 2016,1Q,35
J45.32 Mild persistent asthma with status asthmaticus

✓5ᵗʰ J45.4 Moderate persistent asthma

J45.40 Moderate persistent asthma, uncomplicated
Moderate persistent asthma NOS
J45.41 Moderate persistent asthma with (acute) exacerbation
AHA: 2017,1Q,26
J45.42 Moderate persistent asthma with status asthmaticus

✓5ᵗʰ J45.5 Severe persistent asthma

J45.50 Severe persistent asthma, uncomplicated
Severe persistent asthma NOS
J45.51 Severe persistent asthma with (acute) exacerbation
J45.52 Severe persistent asthma with status asthmaticus

✓5ᵗʰ J45.9 Other and unspecified asthma

✓6ᵗʰ **J45.90 Unspecified asthma**
Asthmatic bronchitis NOS
Childhood asthma NOS
Late onset asthma
AHA: 2017,4Q,96; 2017,1Q,25

J45.901 Unspecified asthma with (acute) exacerbation ▽
J45.902 Unspecified asthma with status asthmaticus ▽
J45.909 Unspecified asthma, uncomplicated ▽
Asthma NOS
EXCLUDES 2   lung diseases due to external agents (J60-J70)
AHA: 2017,1Q,25

✓6ᵗʰ **J45.99 Other asthma**
J45.990 Exercise induced bronchospasm
J45.991 Cough variant asthma
J45.998 Other asthma

✓4ᵗʰ J47 Bronchiectasis

INCLUDES   bronchiolectasis

Use additional code to identify:
exposure to environmental tobacco smoke (Z77.22)
exposure to tobacco smoke in the perinatal period (P96.81)
history of tobacco dependence (Z87.891)
occupational exposure to environmental tobacco smoke (Z57.31)
tobacco dependence (F17.-)
tobacco use (Z72.0)

EXCLUDES 1   congenital bronchiectasis (Q33.4)
tuberculous bronchiectasis (current disease) (A15.0)

DEF: Dilation of the bronchi with mucus production and persistent cough due to infection or chronic conditions that causes diminished lung capacity and frequent infections of the lung.

J47.0 Bronchiectasis with acute lower respiratory infection HCC
Bronchiectasis with acute bronchitis
Use additional code to identify the infection
J47.1 Bronchiectasis with (acute) exacerbation HCC
J47.9 Bronchiectasis, uncomplicated HCC ▽
Bronchiectasis NOS

Lung diseases due to external agents (J60-J70)

EXCLUDES 2   asthma (J45.-)
malignant neoplasm of bronchus and lung (C34.-)

DEF: Pneumoconiosis: Condition caused by inhaling inorganic dust particles, typically associated with occupations that require regular exposure to mineral dusts. A form of interstitial lung disease that contributes to the inflammation of the air sacs, causing the lung tissue to harden.

J60 Coalworker's pneumoconiosis HCC A
Anthracosilicosis
Anthracosis
Black lung disease
Coalworker's lung
EXCLUDES 1   coalworker pneumoconiosis with tuberculosis, any type in A15 (J65)

J61 Pneumoconiosis due to asbestos and other mineral fibers HCC A
Asbestosis
EXCLUDES 1   pleural plaque with asbestosis (J92.0)
pneumoconiosis with tuberculosis, any type in A15 (J65)

✓4ᵗʰ J62 Pneumoconiosis due to dust containing silica

INCLUDES   silicotic fibrosis (massive) of lung
EXCLUDES 1   pneumoconiosis with tuberculosis, any type in A15 (J65)

J62.0 Pneumoconiosis due to talc dust HCC
J62.8 Pneumoconiosis due to other dust containing silica HCC
Silicosis NOS

✓4ᵗʰ J63 Pneumoconiosis due to other inorganic dusts

EXCLUDES 1   pneumoconiosis with tuberculosis, any type in A15 (J65)

J63.0 Aluminosis (of lung) HCC
J63.1 Bauxite fibrosis (of lung) HCC
J63.2 Berylliosis HCC
J63.3 Graphite fibrosis (of lung) HCC
J63.4 Siderosis HCC
J63.5 Stannosis HCC
J63.6 Pneumoconiosis due to other specified inorganic dusts

J64 Unspecified pneumoconiosis HCC ▽
     EXCLUDES 1   pneumonoconiosis with tuberculosis, any type in A15 (J65)

J65 Pneumoconiosis associated with tuberculosis HCC
     Any condition in J60-J64 with tuberculosis, any type in A15
     Silicotuberculosis

√4ᵗʰ **J66 Airway disease due to specific organic dust**
     EXCLUDES 2   allergic alveolitis (J67.-)
              asbestosis (J61)
              bagassosis (J67.1)
              farmer's lung (J67.0)
              hypersensitivity pneumonitis due to organic dust (J67.-)
              reactive airways dysfunction syndrome (J68.3)

J66.0 Byssinosis HCC
     Airway disease due to cotton dust

J66.1 Flax-dressers' disease HCC

J66.2 Cannabinosis HCC

J66.8 Airway disease due to other specific organic dusts HCC

√4ᵗʰ **J67 Hypersensitivity pneumonitis due to organic dust**
     INCLUDES   allergic alveolitis and pneumonitis due to inhaled organic dust and particles of fungal, actinomycetic or other origin
     EXCLUDES 1   pneumonitis due to inhalation of chemicals, gases, fumes or vapors (J68.0)

J67.0 Farmer's lung HCC
     Harvester's lung
     Haymaker's lung
     Moldy hay disease

J67.1 Bagassosis HCC
     Bagasse disease
     Bagasse pneumonitis

J67.2 Bird fancier's lung HCC
     Budgerigar fancier's disease or lung
     Pigeon fancier's disease or lung

J67.3 Suberosis HCC
     Corkhandler's disease or lung
     Corkworker's disease or lung

J67.4 Maltworker's lung HCC
     Alveolitis due to Aspergillus clavatus

J67.5 Mushroom-worker's lung HCC

J67.6 Maple-bark-stripper's lung HCC
     Alveolitis due to Cryptostroma corticale
     Cryptostromosis

J67.7 Air conditioner and humidifier lung HCC
     Allergic alveolitis due to fungal, thermophilic actinomycetes and other organisms growing in ventilation [air conditioning] systems

J67.8 Hypersensitivity pneumonitis due to other organic dusts HCC
     Cheese-washer's lung
     Coffee-worker's lung
     Fish-meal worker's lung
     Furrier's lung
     Sequoiosis

J67.9 Hypersensitivity pneumonitis due to unspecified organic dust HCC ▽
     Allergic alveolitis (extrinsic) NOS
     Hypersensitivity pneumonitis NOS

√4ᵗʰ **J68 Respiratory conditions due to inhalation of chemicals, gases, fumes and vapors**
     Code first (T51-T65) to identify cause
     Use additional code to identify associated respiratory conditions, such as:
     acute respiratory failure (J96.0-)

J68.0 Bronchitis and pneumonitis due to chemicals, gases, fumes and vapors HCC
     Chemical bronchitis (acute)

J68.1 Pulmonary edema due to chemicals, gases, fumes and vapors HCC
     Chemical pulmonary edema (acute) (chronic)
     EXCLUDES 1   pulmonary edema (acute) (chronic) NOS (J81.-)

J68.2 Upper respiratory inflammation due to chemicals, gases, fumes and vapors, not elsewhere classified HCC

J68.3 Other acute and subacute respiratory conditions due to chemicals, gases, fumes and vapors HCC
     Reactive airways dysfunction syndrome

J68.4 Chronic respiratory conditions due to chemicals, gases, fumes and vapors HCC
     Emphysema (diffuse) (chronic) due to inhalation of chemicals, gases, fumes and vapors
     Obliterative bronchiolitis (chronic) (subacute) due to inhalation of chemicals, gases, fumes and vapors
     Pulmonary fibrosis (chronic) due to inhalation of chemicals, gases, fumes and vapors
     EXCLUDES 1   chronic pulmonary edema due to chemicals, gases, fumes and vapors (J68.1)

J68.8 Other respiratory conditions due to chemicals, gases, fumes and vapors HCC

J68.9 Unspecified respiratory condition due to chemicals, gases, fumes and vapors HCC ▽

√4ᵗʰ **J69 Pneumonitis due to solids and liquids**
     EXCLUDES 1   neonatal aspiration syndromes (P24.-)
              postprocedural pneumonitis (J95.4)
     AHA: 2017,1Q,24
     DEF: Pneumonitis: Noninfectious inflammation of the walls of the alveoli in the lung tissue due to inhalation of food, vomit, oils, essences, or other solids or liquids.

J69.0 Pneumonitis due to inhalation of food and vomit HCC
     Aspiration pneumonia NOS
     Aspiration pneumonia (due to) food (regurgitated)
     Aspiration pneumonia (due to) gastric secretions
     Aspiration pneumonia (due to) milk
     Aspiration pneumonia (due to) vomit
     Code also any associated foreign body in respiratory tract (T17.-)
     EXCLUDES 1   chemical pneumonitis due to anesthesia (J95.4)
              obstetric aspiration pneumonitis (O74.0)

J69.1 Pneumonitis due to inhalation of oils and essences HCC
     Exogenous lipoid pneumonia
     Lipid pneumonia NOS
     Code first (T51-T65) to identify substance
     EXCLUDES 1   endogenous lipoid pneumonia (J84.89)

J69.8 Pneumonitis due to inhalation of other solids and liquids HCC
     Pneumonitis due to aspiration of blood
     Pneumonitis due to aspiration of detergent
     Code first (T51-T65) to identify substance

√4ᵗʰ **J70 Respiratory conditions due to other external agents**

J70.0 Acute pulmonary manifestations due to radiation HCC
     Radiation pneumonitis
     Use additional code (W88-W90, X39.0-) to identify the external cause

J70.1 Chronic and other pulmonary manifestations due to radiation HCC
     Fibrosis of lung following radiation
     Use additional code (W88-W90, X39.0-) to identify the external cause

J70.2 Acute drug-induced interstitial lung disorders HCC
     Use additional code for adverse effect, if applicable, to identify drug (T36-T50 with fifth or sixth character 5)
     EXCLUDES 1   interstitial pneumonia NOS (J84.9)
              lymphoid interstitial pneumonia (J84.2)

J70.3 Chronic drug-induced interstitial lung disorders HCC
     Use additional code for adverse effect, if applicable, to identify drug (T36-T50 with fifth or sixth character 5)
     EXCLUDES 1   interstitial pneumonia NOS (J84.9)
              lymphoid interstitial pneumonia (J84.2)

J70.4 Drug-induced interstitial lung disorders, unspecified HCC ▽
     Use additional code for adverse effect, if applicable, to identify drug (T36-T50 with fifth or sixth character 5)
     EXCLUDES 1   interstitial pneumonia NOS (J84.9)
              lymphoid interstitial pneumonia (J84.2)

J70.5 Respiratory conditions due to smoke inhalation HCC
     Smoke inhalation NOS
     EXCLUDES 1   smoke inhalation due to chemicals, gases, fumes and vapors (J68.9)
     AHA: 2013,4Q,121

J70.8 Respiratory conditions due to other specified external agents HCC
     Code first (T51-T65) to identify the external agent

J70.9 Respiratory conditions due to unspecified external agent HCC ▽
     Code first (T51-T65) to identify the external agent

✓ Additional Character Req   ✓x7ᵗʰ Placeholder Alert   Manifestation   ▽ Unspecified   ▶◀ Revised Text   ● New Code   ▲ Revised Code Title

Chapter 10. Diseases of the Respiratory System

Other respiratory diseases principally affecting the interstitium (J80-J84)

J80 Acute respiratory distress syndrome
Acute respiratory distress syndrome in adult or child
Adult hyaline membrane disease
EXCLUDES 1   *respiratory distress syndrome in newborn (perinatal) (P22.0)*
AHA: 2017,1Q,26

✓4ᵗʰ J81 Pulmonary edema
Use additional code to identify:
   exposure to environmental tobacco smoke (Z77.22)
   history of tobacco dependence (Z87.891)
   occupational exposure to environmental tobacco smoke (Z57.31)
   tobacco dependence (F17.-)
   tobacco use (Z72.0)
EXCLUDES 1   *chemical (acute) pulmonary edema (J68.1)*
     hypostatic pneumonia (J18.2)
     passive pneumonia (J18.2)
     pulmonary edema due to external agents (J60-J70)
     pulmonary edema with heart disease NOS (I50.1)
     pulmonary edema with heart failure (I50.1)
DEF: Accumulation of fluid in the air sacs of the lungs, making it difficult to breath.

J81.0 Acute pulmonary edema   HCC
   Acute edema of lung

J81.1 Chronic pulmonary edema
   Pulmonary congestion (chronic) (passive)
   Pulmonary edema NOS

J82 Pulmonary eosinophilia, not elsewhere classified   HCC
Allergic pneumonia
Eosinophilic asthma
Eosinophilic pneumonia
Löffler's pneumonia
Tropical (pulmonary) eosinophilia NOS
EXCLUDES 1   *pulmonary eosinophilia due to aspergillosis (B44.-)*
     pulmonary eosinophilia due to drugs (J70.2-J70.4)
     pulmonary eosinophilia due to specified parasitic infection (B50-B83)
     pulmonary eosinophilia due to systemic connective tissue disorders (M30-M36)
     pulmonary infiltrate NOS (R91.8)
DEF: Infiltration of eosinophils (white blood cells of the immune system) into the parenchyma of the lungs, resulting in cough, fever, and dyspnea.

✓4ᵗʰ J84 Other interstitial pulmonary diseases
EXCLUDES 1   *drug-induced interstitial lung disorders (J70.2-J70.4)*
     interstitial emphysema (J98.2)
EXCLUDES 2   *lung diseases due to external agents (J60-J70)*

✓5ᵗʰ J84.0 Alveolar and parieto-alveolar conditions

J84.01 Alveolar proteinosis   HCC
   DEF: Reduced ventilation due to proteinaceous deposits on alveoli. Symptoms include dyspnea, cough, chest pain, weakness, weight loss, and hemoptysis.

J84.02 Pulmonary alveolar microlithiasis   HCC

J84.03 Idiopathic pulmonary hemosiderosis   HCC
   Essential brown induration of lung
   Code first underlying disease, such as:
     disorders of iron metabolism (E83.1-)
   EXCLUDES 1   *acute idiopathic pulmonary hemorrhage in infants [AIPHI] (R04.81)*
   DEF: Fibrosis of the alveolar walls marked by abnormal accumulation of iron as hemosiderin in the lungs. It primarily affects children and symptoms include anemia, fluid in the lungs, and blood in the sputum. Etiology is unknown.

J84.09 Other alveolar and parieto-alveolar conditions   HCC

✓5ᵗʰ J84.1 Other interstitial pulmonary diseases with fibrosis
EXCLUDES 1   *pulmonary fibrosis (chronic) due to inhalation of chemicals, gases, fumes or vapors (J68.4)*
     pulmonary fibrosis (chronic) following radiation (J70.1)

J84.10 Pulmonary fibrosis, unspecified   HCC ▽
   Capillary fibrosis of lung
   Cirrhosis of lung (chronic) NOS
   Fibrosis of lung (atrophic) (chronic) (confluent) (massive) (perialveolar) (peribronchial) NOS
   Induration of lung (chronic) NOS
   Postinflammatory pulmonary fibrosis

✓6ᵗʰ J84.11 Idiopathic interstitial pneumonia
EXCLUDES 1   *lymphoid interstitial pneumonia (J84.2)*
     pneumocystis pneumonia (B59)

J84.111 Idiopathic interstitial pneumonia, not otherwise specified   HCC ▽

J84.112 Idiopathic pulmonary fibrosis   HCC
   Cryptogenic fibrosing alveolitis
   Idiopathic fibrosing alveolitis

J84.113 Idiopathic non-specific interstitial pneumonitis   HCC
   EXCLUDES 1   *non-specific interstitial pneumonia NOS, or due to known underlying cause (J84.89)*

J84.114 Acute interstitial pneumonitis   HCC
   Hamman-Rich syndrome
   EXCLUDES 1   *pneumocystis pneumonia (B59)*

J84.115 Respiratory bronchiolitis interstitial lung disease   HCC

J84.116 Cryptogenic organizing pneumonia   HCC
   EXCLUDES 1   *organizing pneumonia NOS, or due to known underlying cause (J84.89)*

J84.117 Desquamative interstitial pneumonia   HCC

J84.17 Other interstitial pulmonary diseases with fibrosis in diseases classified elsewhere   HCC
   Interstitial pneumonia (nonspecific) (usual) due to collagen vascular disease
   Interstitial pneumonia (nonspecific) (usual) in diseases classified elsewhere
   Organizing pneumonia due to collagen vascular disease
   Organizing pneumonia in diseases classified elsewhere
   Code first underlying disease, such as:
     progressive systemic sclerosis (M34.0)
     rheumatoid arthritis (M05.00-M06.9)
     systemic lupus erythematosis (M32.0-M32.9)

J84.2 Lymphoid interstitial pneumonia   HCC
Lymphoid interstitial pneumonitis

✓5ᵗʰ J84.8 Other specified interstitial pulmonary diseases
EXCLUDES 1   *exogenous lipoid pneumonia (J69.1)*
     unspecified lipoid pneumonia (J69.1)

J84.81 Lymphangioleiomyomatosis   HCC
   Lymphangiomyomatosis

J84.82 Adult pulmonary Langerhans cell histiocytosis   HCC A
   Adult PLCH

J84.83 Surfactant mutations of the lung   HCC
   DEF: Genetic disorder resulting in insufficient secretion of a complex mixture of phospholipids and proteins that reduce surface tension in the alveoli following the onset of breathing to facilitate lung expansion in the newborn. It is the leading indication for pediatric lung transplantation.

✓6ᵗʰ J84.84 Other interstitial lung diseases of childhood

J84.841 Neuroendocrine cell hyperplasia of infancy   HCC

J84.842 Pulmonary interstitial glycogenosis   HCC

J84.843 Alveolar capillary dysplasia with vein misalignment   HCC

J84.848 Other interstitial lung diseases of childhood   HCC

J84.89 **Other specified interstitial pulmonary diseases** HCC
    Endogenous lipoid pneumonia
    Interstitial pneumonitis
    Non-specific interstitial pneumonitis NOS
    Organizing pneumonia NOS
    Code first, if applicable:
      poisoning due to drug or toxin (T51-T65 with fifth or sixth character to indicate intent), for toxic pneumonopathy
      underlying cause of pneumonopathy, if known
    Use additional code, for adverse effect, to identify drug (T36-T50 with fifth or sixth character 5), if drug-induced
      EXCLUDES 1   *cryptogenic organizing pneumonia (J84.116)*
            idiopathic non-specific interstitial pneumonitis (J84.113)
            lipoid pneumonia, exogenous or unspecified (J69.1)
            lymphoid interstitial pneumonia (J84.2)

J84.9 **Interstitial pulmonary disease, unspecified** HCC ▽
    Interstitial pneumonia NOS

Suppurative and necrotic conditions of the lower respiratory tract (J85-J86)

√4ᵗʰ **J85** **Abscess of lung and mediastinum**
    Use additional code (B95-B97) to identify infectious agent

J85.0 **Gangrene and necrosis of lung** HCC

J85.1 **Abscess of lung with pneumonia** HCC
    Code also the type of pneumonia

J85.2 **Abscess of lung without pneumonia** HCC
    Abscess of lung NOS

J85.3 **Abscess of mediastinum** HCC

√4ᵗʰ **J86** **Pyothorax**
    Use additional code (B95-B97) to identify infectious agent
    EXCLUDES 1   *abscess of lung (J85.-)*
            pyothorax due to tuberculosis (A15.6)
    DEF: Collection of pus in the pleural space that is commonly caused by an infection that spreads from the lung, such as bacterial pneumonia or a lung abscess.

J86.0 **Pyothorax with fistula** HCC
    Bronchocutaneous fistula
    Bronchopleural fistula
    Hepatopleural fistula
    Mediastinal fistula
    Pleural fistula
    Thoracic fistula
    Any condition classifiable to J86.9 with fistula
    DEF: Purulent infection of the respiratory cavity, with communication from a cavity to another structure.

J86.9 **Pyothorax without fistula** HCC
    Abscess of pleura
    Abscess of thorax
    Empyema (chest) (lung) (pleura)
    Fibrinopurulent pleurisy
    Purulent pleurisy
    Pyopneumothorax
    Septic pleurisy
    Seropurulent pleurisy
    Suppurative pleurisy

Other diseases of the pleura (J90-J94)

J90 **Pleural effusion, not elsewhere classified**
    Encysted pleurisy
    Pleural effusion NOS
    Pleurisy with effusion (exudative) (serous)
    EXCLUDES 1   *chylous (pleural) effusion (J94.0)*
            malignant pleural effusion (J91.0))
            pleurisy NOS (R09.1)
            tuberculous pleural effusion (A15.6)
    DEF: Collection of lymph and other fluid within the pleural space.

Pleural Effusion

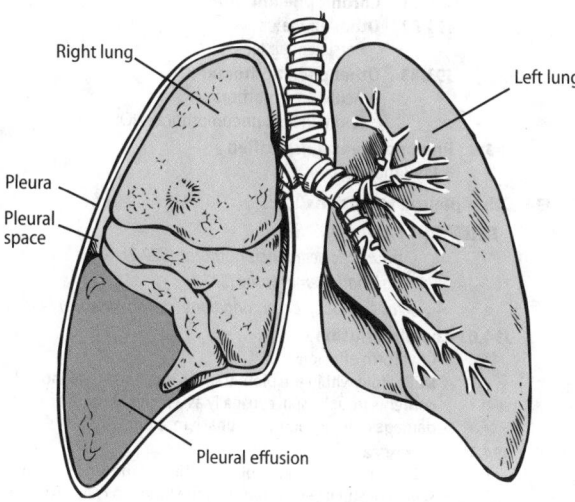

Right lung — Left lung — Pleura — Pleural space — Pleural effusion

√4ᵗʰ **J91** **Pleural effusion in conditions classified elsewhere**
    EXCLUDES 2   *pleural effusion in heart failure (I50.-)*
            pleural effusion in systemic lupus erythematosus (M32.13)
    DEF: Collection of lymph and other fluid within the pleural space.

J91.0 ***Malignant pleural effusion***
    Code first underlying neoplasm

J91.8 ***Pleural effusion in other conditions classified elsewhere***
    Code first underlying disease, such as:
      filariasis (B74.0-B74.9)
      influenza (J09.X2, J10.1, J11.1)
    AHA: 2015,2Q,15

√4ᵗʰ **J92** **Pleural plaque**
    INCLUDES   pleural thickening
    DEF: Areas of fibrous thickening that form on the parietal or visceral pleura, the membranes that line the ribs and lungs.

J92.0 **Pleural plaque with presence of asbestos**

J92.9 **Pleural plaque without asbestos**
    Pleural plaque NOS

√4ᵗʰ **J93** **Pneumothorax and air leak**
    EXCLUDES 1   *congenital or perinatal pneumothorax (P25.1)*
            postprocedural air leak (J95.812)
            postprocedural pneumothorax (J95.811)
            pyopneumothorax (J86.-)
            traumatic pneumothorax (S27.0)
            tuberculous (current disease) pneumothorax (A15.-)
    DEF: Pneumothorax: Lung displacement due to abnormal leakage of air or gas that is trapped in the pleural space formed by the membrane that encloses the lungs and lines the thoracic cavity.

J93.0 **Spontaneous tension pneumothorax**
    DEF: Leaking air from the lung into the lining, causing collapse.

√5ᵗʰ **J93.1** **Other spontaneous pneumothorax**

J93.11 **Primary spontaneous pneumothorax**

J93.12 Secondary spontaneous pneumothorax
Code first underlying condition, such as:
catamenial pneumothorax due to endometriosis (N80.8)
cystic fibrosis (E84.-)
eosinophilic pneumonia (J82)
lymphangioleiomyomatosis (J84.81)
malignant neoplasm of bronchus and lung (C34.-)
Marfan's syndrome (Q87.4)
pneumonia due to Pneumocystis carinii (B59)
secondary malignant neoplasm of lung (C78.0-)
spontaneous rupture of the esophagus (K22.3)

√5ᵗʰ **J93.8 Other pneumothorax and air leak**

J93.81 Chronic pneumothorax
J93.82 Other air leak
Persistent air leak

J93.83 Other pneumothorax
Acute pneumothorax
Spontaneous pneumothorax NOS

J93.9 Pneumothorax, unspecified ▽
Pneumothorax NOS

√4ᵗʰ **J94 Other pleural conditions**
EXCLUDES 1   pleurisy NOS (R09.1)
traumatic hemopneumothorax (S27.2)
traumatic hemothorax (S27.1)
tuberculous pleural conditions (current disease) (A15.-)

J94.0 Chylous effusion
Chyliform effusion
DEF: Fluid within the pleural space due to the leaking of lymph contents into the space, usually as a result of thoracic duct damage or injury or mediastinal lymphoma.

J94.1 Fibrothorax
DEF: Fibrosis within the pleural lining of the lungs commonly seen as a stiff layer surrounding the lung typically attributed to traumatic hemothorax or pleural effusion.

J94.2 Hemothorax
Hemopneumothorax

J94.8 Other specified pleural conditions
Hydropneumothorax
Hydrothorax

J94.9 Pleural condition, unspecified ▽

Intraoperative and postprocedural complications and disorders of respiratory system, not elsewhere classified (J95)

√4ᵗʰ **J95 Intraoperative and postprocedural complications and disorders of respiratory system, not elsewhere classified**
EXCLUDES 2   aspiration pneumonia (J69.-)
emphysema (subcutaneous) resulting from a procedure (T81.82)
hypostatic pneumonia (J18.2)
pulmonary manifestations due to radiation (J70.0-J70.1)

√5ᵗʰ **J95.0 Tracheostomy complications**

Tracheostomy

Tracheostomy in place

Incision in trachea
Tracheostomy tube
Trachea

J95.00 Unspecified tracheostomy complication HCC ▽
J95.01 Hemorrhage from tracheostomy stoma HCC
J95.02 Infection of tracheostomy stoma HCC
Use additional code to identify type of infection, such as:
cellulitis of neck (L03.221)
sepsis (A40, A41.-)

J95.03 Malfunction of tracheostomy stoma HCC
Mechanical complication of tracheostomy stoma
Obstruction of tracheostomy airway
Tracheal stenosis due to tracheostomy

J95.04 Tracheo-esophageal fistula following tracheostomy HCC

J95.09 Other tracheostomy complication HCC

J95.1 Acute pulmonary insufficiency following thoracic surgery HCC
EXCLUDES 2   functional disturbances following cardiac surgery (I97.0, I97.1-)

J95.2 Acute pulmonary insufficiency following nonthoracic surgery HCC
EXCLUDES 2   functional disturbances following cardiac surgery (I97.0, I97.1-)

J95.3 Chronic pulmonary insufficiency following surgery HCC
EXCLUDES 2   functional disturbances following cardiac surgery (I97.0, I97.1-)

J95.4 Chemical pneumonitis due to anesthesia
Mendelson's syndrome
Postprocedural aspiration pneumonia
Use additional code for adverse effect, if applicable, to identify drug (T41.- with fifth or sixth character 5)
EXCLUDES 1   aspiration pneumonitis due to anesthesia complicating labor and delivery (O74.0)
aspiration pneumonitis due to anesthesia complicating pregnancy (O29)
aspiration pneumonitis due to anesthesia complicating the puerperium (O89.01)

J95.5 Postprocedural subglottic stenosis

☑5ᵗʰ **J95.6 Intraoperative hemorrhage and hematoma of a respiratory system organ or structure complicating a procedure**

> EXCLUDES 1   intraoperative hemorrhage and hematoma of a respiratory system organ or structure due to accidental puncture and laceration during procedure (J95.7-)

J95.61 Intraoperative hemorrhage and hematoma of a respiratory system organ or structure complicating a respiratory system procedure

J95.62 Intraoperative hemorrhage and hematoma of a respiratory system organ or structure complicating other procedure

☑5ᵗʰ **J95.7 Accidental puncture and laceration of a respiratory system organ or structure during a procedure**

> EXCLUDES 2   postprocedural pneumothorax (J95.811)

J95.71 Accidental puncture and laceration of a respiratory system organ or structure during a respiratory system procedure

J95.72 Accidental puncture and laceration of a respiratory system organ or structure during other procedure

☑5ᵗʰ **J95.8 Other intraoperative and postprocedural complications and disorders of respiratory system, not elsewhere classified**

AHA: 2016,4Q,9-10

☑6ᵗʰ **J95.81 Postprocedural pneumothorax and air leak**

J95.811 Postprocedural pneumothorax

J95.812 Postprocedural air leak

☑6ᵗʰ **J95.82 Postprocedural respiratory failure**

> EXCLUDES 1   respiratory failure in other conditions (J96.-)

J95.821 Acute postprocedural respiratory failure HCC

> Postprocedural respiratory failure NOS

J95.822 Acute and chronic postprocedural respiratory failure HCC

☑6ᵗʰ **J95.83 Postprocedural hemorrhage of a respiratory system organ or structure following a procedure**

J95.830 Postprocedural hemorrhage of a respiratory system organ or structure following a respiratory system procedure

J95.831 Postprocedural hemorrhage of a respiratory system organ or structure following other procedure

J95.84 Transfusion-related acute lung injury (TRALI)

> DEF: Relatively rare, but serious, pulmonary complication of blood transfusion, with acute respiratory distress, noncardiogenic pulmonary edema, cyanosis, hypoxemia, hypotension, fever, and chills.

☑6ᵗʰ **J95.85 Complication of respirator [ventilator]**

J95.850 Mechanical complication of respirator HCC

> EXCLUDES 1   encounter for respirator [ventilator] dependence during power failure (Z99.12)

J95.851 Ventilator associated pneumonia HCC

> Ventilator associated pneumonitis
> Use additional code to identify the organism, if known (B95.-, B96.-, B97.-)
> EXCLUDES 1   ventilator lung in newborn (P27.8)
> AHA: 2017,1Q,25

J95.859 Other complication of respirator [ventilator] HCC

☑6ᵗʰ **J95.86 Postprocedural hematoma and seroma of a respiratory system organ or structure following a procedure**

J95.860 Postprocedural hematoma of a respiratory system organ or structure following a respiratory system procedure

J95.861 Postprocedural hematoma of a respiratory system organ or structure following other procedure

J95.862 Postprocedural seroma of a respiratory system organ or structure following a respiratory system procedure

J95.863 Postprocedural seroma of a respiratory system organ or structure following other procedure

J95.88 Other intraoperative complications of respiratory system, not elsewhere classified

J95.89 Other postprocedural complications and disorders of respiratory system, not elsewhere classified

> Use additional code to identify disorder, such as:
> aspiration pneumonia (J69.-)
> bacterial or viral pneumonia (J12-J18)
> EXCLUDES 2   acute pulmonary insufficiency following thoracic surgery (J95.1)
> postprocedural subglottic stenosis (J95.5)

Other diseases of the respiratory system (J96-J99)

☑4ᵗʰ **J96 Respiratory failure, not elsewhere classified**

> EXCLUDES 1   acute respiratory distress syndrome (J80)
> cardiorespiratory failure (R09.2)
> newborn respiratory distress syndrome (P22.0)
> postprocedural respiratory failure (J95.82-)
> respiratory arrest (R09.2)
> respiratory arrest of newborn (P28.81)
> respiratory failure of newborn (P28.5)

☑5ᵗʰ **J96.0 Acute respiratory failure**

J96.00 Acute respiratory failure, unspecified whether with hypoxia or hypercapnia HCC ▽

> AHA: 2016,3Q,14; 2013,4Q,121

J96.01 Acute respiratory failure with hypoxia HCC

J96.02 Acute respiratory failure with hypercapnia HCC

☑5ᵗʰ **J96.1 Chronic respiratory failure**

J96.10 Chronic respiratory failure, unspecified whether with hypoxia or hypercapnia HCC ▽

> AHA: 2016,1Q,38; 2015,1Q,21

J96.11 Chronic respiratory failure with hypoxia HCC

> AHA: 2013,4Q,129

J96.12 Chronic respiratory failure with hypercapnia HCC

☑5ᵗʰ **J96.2 Acute and chronic respiratory failure**

> Acute on chronic respiratory failure

J96.20 Acute and chronic respiratory failure, unspecified whether with hypoxia or hypercapnia HCC ▽

J96.21 Acute and chronic respiratory failure with hypoxia HCC

J96.22 Acute and chronic respiratory failure with hypercapnia HCC

☑5ᵗʰ **J96.9 Respiratory failure, unspecified**

J96.90 Respiratory failure, unspecified, unspecified whether with hypoxia or hypercapnia HCC ▽

J96.91 Respiratory failure, unspecified with hypoxia HCC ▽

J96.92 Respiratory failure, unspecified with hypercapnia HCC ▽

☑4ᵗʰ **J98 Other respiratory disorders**

> Use additional code to identify:
> exposure to environmental tobacco smoke (Z77.22)
> exposure to tobacco smoke in the perinatal period (P96.81)
> history of tobacco dependence (Z87.891)
> occupational exposure to environmental tobacco smoke (Z57.31)
> tobacco dependence (F17.-)
> tobacco use (Z72.0)
> EXCLUDES 1   newborn apnea (P28.4)
> newborn sleep apnea (P28.3)
> EXCLUDES 2   apnea NOS (R06.81)
> sleep apnea (G47.3-)

☑5ᵗʰ **J98.0 Diseases of bronchus, not elsewhere classified**

J98.01 Acute bronchospasm

> EXCLUDES 1   acute bronchiolitis with bronchospasm (J21.-)
> acute bronchitis with bronchospasm (J20.-)
> asthma (J45.-)
> exercise induced bronchospasm (J45.990)

J98.09 Other diseases of bronchus, not elsewhere classified

> Broncholithiasis
> Calcification of bronchus
> Stenosis of bronchus
> Tracheobronchial collapse
> Tracheobronchial dyskinesia
> Ulcer of bronchus

☑ Additional Character Req   ✓x7ᵗʰ Placeholder Alert   Manifestation   ▽ Unspecified   ▶◀ Revised Text   ● New Code   ▲ Revised Code Title

ICD-10-CM 2019   689

Chapter 10. Diseases of the Respiratory System

✓5ᵗʰ **J98.1 Pulmonary collapse**

     EXCLUDES 1   therapeutic collapse of lung status (Z98.3)

     J98.11 Atelectasis

         EXCLUDES 1   newborn atelectasis

                     tuberculous atelectasis (current disease) (A15)

         DEF: Collapse of lung tissue affecting part or all of one lung, preventing normal oxygen absorption to healthy tissues.

     J98.19 Other pulmonary collapse

J98.2 Interstitial emphysema   HCC

     Mediastinal emphysema

     EXCLUDES 1   emphysema NOS (J43.9)

                 emphysema in newborn (P25.0)

                 surgical emphysema (subcutaneous) (T81.82)

                 traumatic subcutaneous emphysema (T79.7)

J98.3 Compensatory emphysema   HCC

     DEF: Distention of all or part of the lung caused by disease processes or surgical intervention that decreased volume in another part of the lung, causing an overcompensation reaction. Compensatory emphysema occurs in association with pneumonias, pleural effusions, atelectasis, empyema, and pneumothorax.

J98.4 Other disorders of lung

     Calcification of lung

     Cystic lung disease (acquired)

     Lung disease NOS

     Pulmolithiasis

     EXCLUDES 1   acute interstitial pneumonitis (J84.114)

                 pulmonary insufficiency following surgery (J95.1-J95.2)

✓5ᵗʰ **J98.5 Diseases of mediastinum, not elsewhere classified**

     EXCLUDES 2   abscess of mediastinum (J85.3)

     AHA: 2016,4Q,29

     J98.51 Mediastinitis

         Code first underlying condition, if applicable, such as postoperative mediastinitis (T81.-)

     J98.59 Other diseases of mediastinum, not elsewhere classified

         Fibrosis of mediastinum

         Hernia of mediastinum

         Retraction of mediastinum

J98.6 Disorders of diaphragm

     Diaphragmatitis

     Paralysis of diaphragm

     Relaxation of diaphragm

     EXCLUDES 1   congenital malformation of diaphragm NEC (Q79.1)

                 congenital diaphragmatic hernia (Q79.0)

     EXCLUDES 2   diaphragmatic hernia (K44.-)

J98.8 Other specified respiratory disorders

J98.9 Respiratory disorder, unspecified   ▽

     Respiratory disease (chronic) NOS

J99 Respiratory disorders in diseases classified elsewhere   HCC

     Code first underlying disease, such as:

     amyloidosis (E85.-)

     ankylosing spondylitis (M45)

     congenital syphilis (A50.5)

     cryoglobulinemia (D89.1)

     early congenital syphilis (A50.0)

     ▶plasminogen deficiency (E88.02)◀

     schistosomiasis (B65.0-B65.9)

     EXCLUDES 1   respiratory disorders in:

                 amebiasis (A06.5)

                 blastomycosis (B40.0-B40.2)

                 candidiasis (B37.1)

                 coccidioidomycosis (B38.0-B38.2)

                 cystic fibrosis with pulmonary manifestations (E84.0)

                 dermatomyositis (M33.01, M33.11)

                 histoplasmosis (B39.0-B39.2)

                 late syphilis (A52.72, A52.73)

                 polymyositis (M33.21)

                 sicca syndrome (M35.02)

                 systemic lupus erythematosus (M32.13)

                 systemic sclerosis (M34.81)

                 Wegener's granulomatosis (M31.30-M31.31)

Chapter 11. Diseases of the Digestive System (K00–K95)

Chapter Specific Coding Guidelines and Examples
Reserved for future guideline expansion.

Chapter 11. Diseases of the Digestive System

Chapter 11. Diseases of the Digestive System (K00-K95)

EXCLUDES 2   certain conditions originating in the perinatal period (P04-P96)
certain infectious and parasitic diseases (A00-B99)
complications of pregnancy, childbirth and the puerperium (O00-O9A)
congenital malformations, deformations and chromosomal abnormalities (Q00-Q99)
endocrine, nutritional and metabolic diseases (E00-E88)
injury, poisoning and certain other consequences of external causes (S00-T88)
neoplasms (C00-D49)
symptoms, signs and abnormal clinical and laboratory findings, not elsewhere classified (R00-R94)

This chapter contains the following blocks:

K00-K14   Diseases of oral cavity and salivary glands
K20-K31   Diseases of esophagus, stomach and duodenum
K35-K38   Diseases of appendix
K40-K46   Hernia
K50-K52   Noninfective enteritis and colitis
K55-K64   Other diseases of intestines
K65-K68   Diseases of peritoneum and retroperitoneum
K70-K77   Diseases of liver
K80-K87   Disorders of gallbladder, biliary tract and pancreas
K90-K95   Other diseases of the digestive system

Diseases of oral cavity and salivary glands (K00-K14)

✓4ᵗʰ K00   Disorders of tooth development and eruption

EXCLUDES 2   embedded and impacted teeth (K01.-)

K00.0   Anodontia
Hypodontia
Oligodontia
EXCLUDES 1   acquired absence of teeth (K08.1-)
DEF: Partial or complete absence of teeth due to a congenital defect involving the tooth bud.

K00.1   Supernumerary teeth
Distomolar
Fourth molar
Mesiodens
Paramolar
Supplementary teeth
EXCLUDES 2   supernumerary roots (K00.2)

K00.2   Abnormalities of size and form of teeth
Concrescence of teeth
Dens evaginatus
Dens in dente
Dens invaginatus
Enamel pearls
Fusion of teeth
Gemination of teeth
Macrodontia
Microdontia
Peg-shaped [conical] teeth
Supernumerary roots
Taurodontism
Tuberculum paramolare
EXCLUDES 1   abnormalities of teeth due to congenital syphilis (A50.5)
tuberculum Carabelli, which is regarded as a normal variation and should not be coded

K00.3   Mottled teeth
Dental fluorosis
Mottling of enamel
Nonfluoride enamel opacities
EXCLUDES 2   deposits [accretions] on teeth (K03.6)

K00.4   Disturbances in tooth formation
Aplasia and hypoplasia of cementum
Dilaceration of tooth
Enamel hypoplasia (neonatal) (postnatal) (prenatal)
Regional odontodysplasia
Turner's tooth
EXCLUDES 1   Hutchinson's teeth and mulberry molars in congenital syphilis (A50.5)
EXCLUDES 2   mottled teeth (K00.3)

K00.5   Hereditary disturbances in tooth structure, not elsewhere classified
Amelogenesis imperfecta
Dentinogenesis imperfecta
Odontogenesis imperfecta
Dentinal dysplasia
Shell teeth

K00.6   Disturbances in tooth eruption
Dentia praecox
Natal tooth
Neonatal tooth
Premature eruption of tooth
Premature shedding of primary [deciduous] tooth
Prenatal teeth
Retained [persistent] primary tooth
EXCLUDES 2   embedded and impacted teeth (K01.-)

K00.7   Teething syndrome

K00.8   Other disorders of tooth development
Color changes during tooth formation
Intrinsic staining of teeth NOS
EXCLUDES 2   posteruptive color changes (K03.7)

K00.9   Disorder of tooth development, unspecified   ▽
Disorder of odontogenesis NOS

✓4ᵗʰ K01   Embedded and impacted teeth
EXCLUDES 1   abnormal position of fully erupted teeth (M26.3-)

K01.0   Embedded teeth
K01.1   Impacted teeth

✓4ᵗʰ K02   Dental caries
INCLUDES   caries of dentine
dental cavities
early childhood caries
pre-eruptive caries
recurrent caries (dentino enamel junction) (enamel) (to the pulp)
tooth decay

Tooth Anatomy

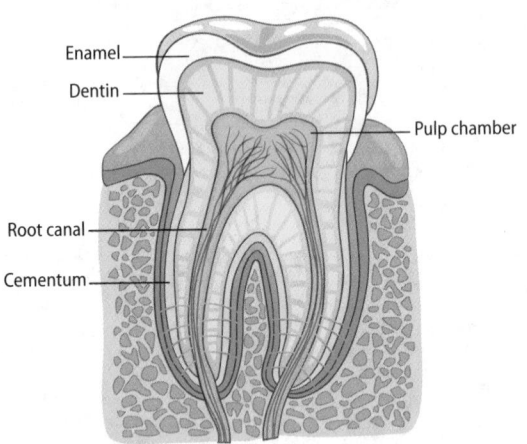

Enamel
Dentin
Pulp chamber
Root canal
Cementum

K02.3   Arrested dental caries
Arrested coronal and root caries

✓5ᵗʰ K02.5   Dental caries on pit and fissure surface
Dental caries on chewing surface of tooth

K02.51   Dental caries on pit and fissure surface limited to enamel
White spot lesions [initial caries] on pit and fissure surface of tooth

K02.52   Dental caries on pit and fissure surface penetrating into dentin
Primary dental caries, cervical origin

K02.53   Dental caries on pit and fissure surface penetrating into pulp

✓5ᵗʰ K02.6   Dental caries on smooth surface

K02.61   Dental caries on smooth surface limited to enamel
White spot lesions [initial caries] on smooth surface of tooth

K02.62   Dental caries on smooth surface penetrating into dentin

K02.63   Dental caries on smooth surface penetrating into pulp

K02.7   Dental root caries

K02.9   Dental caries, unspecified   ▽

✓4ᵗʰ **K03**   Other diseases of hard tissues of teeth

> EXCLUDES 2   *bruxism (F45.8)*
> *dental caries (K02.-)*
> *teeth-grinding NOS (F45.8)*

K03.0   Excessive attrition of teeth
Approximal wear of teeth
Occlusal wear of teeth
DEF: Attrition: In dentistry, wearing away or erosion of tooth surface from abrasive food or grinding teeth.

K03.1   Abrasion of teeth
Dentifrice abrasion of teeth
Habitual abrasion of teeth
Occupational abrasion of teeth
Ritual abrasion of teeth
Traditional abrasion of teeth
Wedge defect NOS

K03.2   Erosion of teeth
Erosion of teeth due to diet
Erosion of teeth due to drugs and medicaments
Erosion of teeth due to persistent vomiting
Erosion of teeth NOS
Idiopathic erosion of teeth
Occupational erosion of teeth

K03.3   Pathological resorption of teeth
Internal granuloma of pulp
Resorption of teeth (external)

K03.4   Hypercementosis
Cementation hyperplasia

K03.5   Ankylosis of teeth

K03.6   Deposits [accretions] on teeth
Betel deposits [accretions] on teeth
Black deposits [accretions] on teeth
Extrinsic staining of teeth NOS
Green deposits [accretions] on teeth
Materia alba deposits [accretions] on teeth
Orange deposits [accretions] on teeth
Staining of teeth NOS
Subgingival dental calculus
Supragingival dental calculus
Tobacco deposits [accretions] on teeth

K03.7   Posteruptive color changes of dental hard tissues
> EXCLUDES 2   *deposits [accretions] on teeth (K03.6)*

✓5ᵗʰ **K03.8**   Other specified diseases of hard tissues of teeth

> **K03.81**   Cracked tooth
> > EXCLUDES 1   *asymptomatic craze lines in enamel - omit code*
> > *broken or fractured tooth due to trauma (S02.5)*
>
> **K03.89**   Other specified diseases of hard tissues of teeth

K03.9   Disease of hard tissues of teeth, unspecified   ▽

✓4ᵗʰ **K04**   Diseases of pulp and periapical tissues
AHA: 2016,4Q,29-30

✓5ᵗʰ **K04.0**   Pulpitis
Acute pulpitis
Chronic (hyperplastic) (ulcerative) pulpitis

> **K04.01**   Reversible pulpitis
> **K04.02**   Irreversible pulpitis

K04.1   Necrosis of pulp
Pulpal gangrene

K04.2   Pulp degeneration
Denticles
Pulpal calcifications
Pulpal stones

K04.3   Abnormal hard tissue formation in pulp
Secondary or irregular dentine

K04.4   Acute apical periodontitis of pulpal origin
Acute apical periodontitis NOS
> EXCLUDES 1   *acute periodontitis (K05.2-)*
DEF: Severe inflammation of the area surrounding the tip of a tooth's root that is often secondary to infection or trauma.

K04.5   Chronic apical periodontitis
Apical or periapical granuloma
Apical periodontitis NOS
> EXCLUDES 1   *chronic periodontitis (K05.3-)*

K04.6   Periapical abscess with sinus
Dental abscess with sinus
Dentoalveolar abscess with sinus

K04.7   Periapical abscess without sinus
Dental abscess without sinus
Dentoalveolar abscess without sinus

K04.8   Radicular cyst
Apical (periodontal) cyst
Periapical cyst
Residual radicular cyst
> EXCLUDES 2   *lateral periodontal cyst (K09.0)*
DEF: Most common odontogenic cyst in tissue around the tooth apex due to chronic inflammation of dental pulp.

✓5ᵗʰ **K04.9**   Other and unspecified diseases of pulp and periapical tissues

> **K04.90**   Unspecified diseases of pulp and periapical tissues   ▽
> **K04.99**   Other diseases of pulp and periapical tissues

✓4ᵗʰ **K05**   Gingivitis and periodontal diseases
Use additional code to identify:
alcohol abuse and dependence (F10.-)
exposure to environmental tobacco smoke (Z77.22)
exposure to tobacco smoke in the perinatal period (P96.81)
history of tobacco dependence (Z87.891)
occupational exposure to environmental tobacco smoke (Z57.31)
tobacco dependence (F17.-)
tobacco use (Z72.0)
AHA: 2016,4Q,29-30

✓5ᵗʰ **K05.0**   Acute gingivitis
> EXCLUDES 1   *acute necrotizing ulcerative gingivitis (A69.1)*
> *herpesviral [herpes simplex] gingivostomatitis (B00.2)*

> **K05.00**   Acute gingivitis, plaque induced
> Acute gingivitis NOS
> Plaque induced gingival disease
>
> **K05.01**   Acute gingivitis, non-plaque induced

✓5ᵗʰ **K05.1**   Chronic gingivitis
Desquamative gingivitis (chronic)
Gingivitis (chronic) NOS
Hyperplastic gingivitis (chronic)
Pregnancy associated gingivitis
Simple marginal gingivitis (chronic)
Ulcerative gingivitis (chronic)
Code first, if applicable, diseases of the digestive system complicating pregnacy (O99.61-)

> **K05.10**   Chronic gingivitis, plaque induced
> Chronic gingivitis NOS
> Gingivitis NOS
>
> **K05.11**   Chronic gingivitis, non-plaque induced

✓5ᵗʰ **K05.2**   Aggressive periodontitis
Acute pericoronitis
> EXCLUDES 1   *acute apical periodontitis (K04.4)*
> *periapical abscess (K04.7)*
> *periapical abscess with sinus (K04.6)*

> **K05.20**   Aggressive periodontitis, unspecified   ▽
>
> ✓6ᵗʰ **K05.21**   Aggressive periodontitis, localized
> Periodontal abscess
> > **K05.211** Aggressive periodontitis, localized, slight
> > **K05.212** Aggressive periodontitis, localized, moderate
> > **K05.213** Aggressive periodontitis, localized, severe
> > **K05.219** Aggressive periodontitis, localized, unspecified severity   ▽
>
> ✓6ᵗʰ **K05.22**   Aggressive periodontitis, generalized
> > **K05.221** Aggressive periodontitis, generalized, slight
> > **K05.222** Aggressive periodontitis, generalized, moderate
> > **K05.223** Aggressive periodontitis, generalized, severe
> > **K05.229** Aggressive periodontitis, generalized, unspecified severity   ▽

☑ Additional Character Req   ✓x7ᵗʰ Placeholder Alert   Manifestation   ▽ Unspecified   ▶◀ Revised Text   ● New Code   ▲ Revised Code Title
ICD-10-CM 2019

693

✓5ᵗʰ **K05.3 Chronic periodontitis**
Chronic pericoronitis
Complex periodontitis
Periodontitis NOS
Simplex periodontitis
     EXCLUDES 1   *chronic apical periodontitis (K04.5)*

     K05.30 Chronic periodontitis, unspecified ▽
     ✓6ᵗʰ **K05.31 Chronic periodontitis, localized**
       K05.311 Chronic periodontitis, localized, slight
       K05.312 Chronic periodontitis, localized, moderate
       K05.313 Chronic periodontitis, localized, severe
       K05.319 Chronic periodontitis, localized, unspecified severity ▽

     ✓6ᵗʰ **K05.32 Chronic periodontitis, generalized**
       K05.321 Chronic periodontitis, generalized, slight
       K05.322 Chronic periodontitis, generalized, moderate
       K05.323 Chronic periodontitis, generalized, severe
       K05.329 Chronic periodontitis, generalized, unspecified ▽

K05.4 Periodontosis
Juvenile periodontosis
K05.5 Other periodontal diseases
Combined periodontic-endodontic lesion
Narrow gingival width (of periodontal soft tissue)
     EXCLUDES 2   *leukoplakia of gingiva (K13.21)*
K05.6 Periodontal disease, unspecified ▽

✓4ᵗʰ **K06 Other disorders of gingiva and edentulous alveolar ridge**
     EXCLUDES 2   *acute gingivitis (K05.0)*
          atrophy of edentulous alveolar ridge (K08.2)
          chronic gingivitis (K05.1)
          gingivitis NOS (K05.1)

     AHA: 2016,4Q,29-30
✓5ᵗʰ **K06.0 Gingival recession**
Gingival recession (postinfective) (postprocedural)
     AHA: 2017,4Q,16
     ✓6ᵗʰ **K06.01 Gingival recession, localized**
       K06.010 Localized gingival recession, unspecified ▽
         Localized gingival recession, NOS
       K06.011 Localized gingival recession, minimal
       K06.012 Localized gingival recession, moderate
       K06.013 Localized gingival recession, severe
     ✓6ᵗʰ **K06.02 Gingival recession, generalized**
       K06.020 Generalized gingival recession, unspecified ▽
         Generalized gingival recession, NOS
       K06.021 Generalized gingival recession, minimal
       K06.022 Generalized gingival recession, moderate
       K06.023 Generalized gingival recession, severe

K06.1 Gingival enlargement
Gingival fibromatosis
K06.2 Gingival and edentulous alveolar ridge lesions associated with trauma
Irritative hyperplasia of edentulous ridge [denture hyperplasia]
Use additional code (Chapter 20) to identify external cause or denture status (Z97.2)
K06.3 Horizontal alveolar bone loss
K06.8 Other specified disorders of gingiva and edentulous alveolar ridge
Fibrous epulis
Flabby alveolar ridge
Giant cell epulis
Peripheral giant cell granuloma of gingiva
Pyogenic granuloma of gingiva
Vertical ridge deficiency
     EXCLUDES 2   *gingival cyst (K09.0)*
K06.9 Disorder of gingiva and edentulous alveolar ridge, unspecified ▽

✓4ᵗʰ **K08 Other disorders of teeth and supporting structures**
     EXCLUDES 2   *dentofacial anomalies [including malocclusion] (M26.-)*
          disorders of jaw (M27.-)
     AHA: 2016,4Q,29-30
K08.0 Exfoliation of teeth due to systemic causes
Code also underlying systemic condition
✓5ᵗʰ **K08.1 Complete loss of teeth**
Acquired loss of teeth, complete
     EXCLUDES 1   *congenital absence of teeth (K00.0)*
          exfoliation of teeth due to systemic causes (K08.0)
          partial loss of teeth (K08.4-)
     DEF: Loss of all teeth as a result of caries, trauma, extraction, periodontal disease, or other specified or unspecified causes.
     Synonym(s): complete edentulism
     ✓6ᵗʰ **K08.10 Complete loss of teeth, unspecified cause**
       K08.101 Complete loss of teeth, unspecified cause, class I ▽
       K08.102 Complete loss of teeth, unspecified cause, class II ▽
       K08.103 Complete loss of teeth, unspecified cause, class III ▽
       K08.104 Complete loss of teeth, unspecified cause, class IV ▽
       K08.109 Complete loss of teeth, unspecified cause, unspecified class ▽
         Edentulism NOS
     ✓6ᵗʰ **K08.11 Complete loss of teeth due to trauma**
       K08.111 Complete loss of teeth due to trauma, class I
       K08.112 Complete loss of teeth due to trauma, class II
       K08.113 Complete loss of teeth due to trauma, class III
       K08.114 Complete loss of teeth due to trauma, class IV
       K08.119 Complete loss of teeth due to trauma, unspecified class ▽
     ✓6ᵗʰ **K08.12 Complete loss of teeth due to periodontal diseases**
       K08.121 Complete loss of teeth due to periodontal diseases, class I
       K08.122 Complete loss of teeth due to periodontal diseases, class II
       K08.123 Complete loss of teeth due to periodontal diseases, class III
       K08.124 Complete loss of teeth due to periodontal diseases, class IV
       K08.129 Complete loss of teeth due to periodontal diseases, unspecified class ▽
     ✓6ᵗʰ **K08.13 Complete loss of teeth due to caries**
       K08.131 Complete loss of teeth due to caries, class I
       K08.132 Complete loss of teeth due to caries, class II
       K08.133 Complete loss of teeth due to caries, class III
       K08.134 Complete loss of teeth due to caries, class IV
       K08.139 Complete loss of teeth due to caries, unspecified class ▽
     ✓6ᵗʰ **K08.19 Complete loss of teeth due to other specified cause**
       K08.191 Complete loss of teeth due to other specified cause, class I
       K08.192 Complete loss of teeth due to other specified cause, class II
       K08.193 Complete loss of teeth due to other specified cause, class III
       K08.194 Complete loss of teeth due to other specified cause, class IV
       K08.199 Complete loss of teeth due to other specified cause, unspecified class ▽
     ✓5ᵗʰ **K08.2 Atrophy of edentulous alveolar ridge**
       K08.20 Unspecified atrophy of edentulous alveolar ridge ▽
         Atrophy of the mandible NOS
         Atrophy of the maxilla NOS

KØ8.21   **Minimal atrophy of the mandible**
     Minimal atrophy of the edentulous mandible

KØ8.22   **Moderate atrophy of the mandible**
     Moderate atrophy of the edentulous mandible

KØ8.23   **Severe atrophy of the mandible**
     Severe atrophy of the edentulous mandible

KØ8.24   **Minimal atrophy of maxilla**
     Minimal atrophy of the edentulous maxilla

KØ8.25   **Moderate atrophy of maxilla**
     Moderate atrophy of the edentulous maxilla

KØ8.26   **Severe atrophy of maxilla**
     Severe atrophy of the edentulous maxilla

KØ8.3   **Retained dental root**

✓5ᵗʰ KØ8.4   **Partial loss of teeth**
     Acquired loss of teeth, partial
     EXCLUDES 1   complete loss of teeth (KØ8.1-)
         congenital absence of teeth (KØØ.Ø)
     EXCLUDES 2   exfoliation of teeth due to systemic causes (KØ8.Ø)

   ✓6ᵗʰ KØ8.40   **Partial loss of teeth, unspecified cause**

     KØ8.401   **Partial loss of teeth, unspecified cause, class I** ▽

     KØ8.402   **Partial loss of teeth, unspecified cause, class II** ▽

     KØ8.403   **Partial loss of teeth, unspecified cause, class III** ▽

     KØ8.404   **Partial loss of teeth, unspecified cause, class IV** ▽

     KØ8.409   **Partial loss of teeth, unspecified cause, unspecified class** ▽
         Tooth extraction status NOS

   ✓6ᵗʰ KØ8.41   **Partial loss of teeth due to trauma**

     KØ8.411   **Partial loss of teeth due to trauma, class I**

     KØ8.412   **Partial loss of teeth due to trauma, class II**

     KØ8.413   **Partial loss of teeth due to trauma, class III**

     KØ8.414   **Partial loss of teeth due to trauma, class IV**

     KØ8.419   **Partial loss of teeth due to trauma, unspecified class** ▽

   ✓6ᵗʰ KØ8.42   **Partial loss of teeth due to periodontal diseases**

     KØ8.421   **Partial loss of teeth due to periodontal diseases, class I**

     KØ8.422   **Partial loss of teeth due to periodontal diseases, class II**

     KØ8.423   **Partial loss of teeth due to periodontal diseases, class III**

     KØ8.424   **Partial loss of teeth due to periodontal diseases, class IV**

     KØ8.429   **Partial loss of teeth due to periodontal diseases, unspecified class** ▽

   ✓6ᵗʰ KØ8.43   **Partial loss of teeth due to caries**

     KØ8.431   **Partial loss of teeth due to caries, class I**

     KØ8.432   **Partial loss of teeth due to caries, class II**

     KØ8.433   **Partial loss of teeth due to caries, class III**

     KØ8.434   **Partial loss of teeth due to caries, class IV**

     KØ8.439   **Partial loss of teeth due to caries, unspecified class** ▽

   ✓6ᵗʰ KØ8.49   **Partial loss of teeth due to other specified cause**

     KØ8.491   **Partial loss of teeth due to other specified cause, class I**

     KØ8.492   **Partial loss of teeth due to other specified cause, class II**

     KØ8.493   **Partial loss of teeth due to other specified cause, class III**

     KØ8.494   **Partial loss of teeth due to other specified cause, class IV**

     KØ8.499   **Partial loss of teeth due to other specified cause, unspecified class** ▽

✓5ᵗʰ KØ8.5   **Unsatisfactory restoration of tooth**
     Defective bridge, crown, filling
     Defective dental restoration
     EXCLUDES 1   dental restoration status (Z98.811)
     EXCLUDES 2   endosseous dental implant failure (M27.6-)
         unsatisfactory endodontic treatment (M27.5-)

   KØ8.50   **Unsatisfactory restoration of tooth, unspecified** ▽
     Defective dental restoration NOS

   KØ8.51   **Open restoration margins of tooth**
     Dental restoration failure of marginal integrity
     Open margin on tooth restoration
     Poor gingival margin to tooth restoration

   KØ8.52   **Unrepairable overhanging of dental restorative materials**
     Overhanging of tooth restoration

   ✓6ᵗʰ KØ8.53   **Fractured dental restorative material**
     EXCLUDES 1   cracked tooth (KØ3.81)
         traumatic fracture of tooth (SØ2.5)

     KØ8.530   **Fractured dental restorative material without loss of material**

     KØ8.531   **Fractured dental restorative material with loss of material**

     KØ8.539   **Fractured dental restorative material, unspecified** ▽

   KØ8.54   **Contour of existing restoration of tooth biologically incompatible with oral health**
     Dental restoration failure of periodontal anatomical integrity
     Unacceptable contours of existing restoration of tooth
     Unacceptable morphology of existing restoration of tooth

   KØ8.55   **Allergy to existing dental restorative material**
     Use additional code to identify the specific type of allergy

   KØ8.56   **Poor aesthetic of existing restoration of tooth**
     Dental restoration aesthetically inadequate or displeasing

   KØ8.59   **Other unsatisfactory restoration of tooth**
     Other defective dental restoration

✓5ᵗʰ KØ8.8   **Other specified disorders of teeth and supporting structures**

   KØ8.81   **Primary occlusal trauma**

   KØ8.82   **Secondary occlusal trauma**

   KØ8.89   **Other specified disorders of teeth and supporting structures**
     Enlargement of alveolar ridge NOS
     Insufficient anatomic crown height
     Insufficient clinical crown length
     Irregular alveolar process
     Toothache NOS

KØ8.9   **Disorder of teeth and supporting structures, unspecified** ▽

✓4ᵗʰ **KØ9**   **Cysts of oral region, not elsewhere classified**
     INCLUDES   lesions showing histological features both of aneurysmal cyst and of another fibro-osseous lesion
     EXCLUDES 2   cysts of jaw (M27.Ø-, M27.4-)
         radicular cyst (KØ4.8)

KØ9.Ø   **Developmental odontogenic cysts**
     Dentigerous cyst
     Eruption cyst
     Follicular cyst
     Gingival cyst
     Lateral periodontal cyst
     Primordial cyst
     EXCLUDES 2   keratocysts (D16.4, D16.5)
         odontogenic keratocystic tumors (D16.4, D16.5)

KØ9.1   **Developmental (nonodontogenic) cysts of oral region**
     Cyst (of) incisive canal
     Cyst (of) palatine of papilla
     Globulomaxillary cyst
     Median palatal cyst
     Nasoalveolar cyst
     Nasolabial cyst
     Nasopalatine duct cyst

K09.8 **Other cysts of oral region, not elsewhere classified**
Dermoid cyst
Epidermoid cyst
Lymphoepithelial cyst
Epstein's pearl

K09.9 **Cyst of oral region, unspecified** ▽

✓4ᵗʰ **K11** **Diseases of salivary glands**
Use additional code to identify:
alcohol abuse and dependence (F10.-)
exposure to environmental tobacco smoke (Z77.22)
exposure to tobacco smoke in the perinatal period (P96.81)
history of tobacco dependence (Z87.891)
occupational exposure to environmental tobacco smoke (Z57.31)
tobacco dependence (F17.-)
tobacco use (Z72.0)

K11.0 **Atrophy of salivary gland**

K11.1 **Hypertrophy of salivary gland**
DEF: Overgrowth of or enlarged salivary gland tissue caused by infection, salivary duct blockage, autoimmune diseases, and benign and malignant tumors.

✓5ᵗʰ **K11.2** **Sialoadenitis**
Parotitis
EXCLUDES 1 *epidemic parotitis (B26.-)*
mumps (B26.-)
uveoparotid fever [Heerfordt] (D86.89)
DEF: Inflammation of the salivary gland.
K11.20 **Sialoadenitis, unspecified** ▽
K11.21 **Acute sialoadenitis**
EXCLUDES 1 *acute recurrent sialoadenitis (K11.22)*
K11.22 **Acute recurrent sialoadenitis**
K11.23 **Chronic sialoadenitis**

K11.3 **Abscess of salivary gland**

K11.4 **Fistula of salivary gland**
EXCLUDES 1 *congenital fistula of salivary gland (Q38.4)*

K11.5 **Sialolithiasis**
Calculus of salivary gland or duct
Stone of salivary gland or duct

K11.6 **Mucocele of salivary gland**
Mucous extravasation cyst of salivary gland
Mucous retention cyst of salivary gland
Ranula

K11.7 **Disturbances of salivary secretion**
Hypoptyalism
Ptyalism
Xerostomia
EXCLUDES 2 *dry mouth NOS (R68.2)*

K11.8 **Other diseases of salivary glands**
Benign lymphoepithelial lesion of salivary gland
Mikulicz' disease
Necrotizing sialometaplasia
Sialectasia
Stenosis of salivary duct
Stricture of salivary duct
EXCLUDES 1 *sicca syndrome [Sjögren] (M35.0-)*

K11.9 **Disease of salivary gland, unspecified** ▽
Sialoadenopathy NOS

✓4ᵗʰ **K12** **Stomatitis and related lesions**
Use additional code to identify:
alcohol abuse and dependence (F10.-)
exposure to environmental tobacco smoke (Z77.22)
exposure to tobacco smoke in the perinatal period (P96.81)
history of tobacco dependence (Z87.891)
occupational exposure to environmental tobacco smoke (Z57.31)
tobacco dependence (F17.-)
tobacco use (Z72.0)
EXCLUDES 1 *cancrum oris (A69.0)*
cheilitis (K13.0)
gangrenous stomatitis (A69.0)
herpesviral [herpes simplex] gingivostomatitis (B00.2)
noma (A69.0)

K12.0 **Recurrent oral aphthae**
Aphthous stomatitis (major) (minor)
Bednar's aphthae
Periadenitis mucosa necrotica recurrens
Recurrent aphthous ulcer
Stomatitis herpetiformis
DEF: Disorder of unknown etiology with small oval or round painful ulcers of the mouth marked by a grayish exudate and a red halo effect.

K12.1 **Other forms of stomatitis**
Stomatitis NOS
Denture stomatitis
Ulcerative stomatitis
Vesicular stomatitis
EXCLUDES 1 *acute necrotizing ulcerative stomatitis (A69.1)*
Vincent's stomatitis (A69.1)

K12.2 **Cellulitis and abscess of mouth**
Cellulitis of mouth (floor)
Submandibular abscess
EXCLUDES 2 *abscess of salivary gland (K11.3)*
abscess of tongue (K14.0)
periapical abscess (K04.6-K04.7)
periodontal abscess (K05.21)
peritonsillar abscess (J36)

✓5ᵗʰ **K12.3** **Oral mucositis (ulcerative)**
Mucositis (oral) (oropharyneal)
EXCLUDES 2 *gastrointestinal mucositis (ulcerative) (K92.81)*
mucositis (ulcerative) of vagina and vulva (N76.81)
nasal mucositis (ulcerative) (J34.81)
K12.30 **Oral mucositis (ulcerative), unspecified** ▽
K12.31 **Oral mucositis (ulcerative) due to antineoplastic therapy**
Use additional code for adverse effect, if applicable, to identify antineoplastic and immunosuppressive drugs (T45.1X5)
Use additional code for other antineoplastic therapy, such as:
radiological procedure and radiotherapy (Y84.2)
K12.32 **Oral mucositis (ulcerative) due to other drugs**
Use additional code for adverse effect, if applicable, to identify drug (T36-T50 with fifth or sixth character 5)
K12.33 **Oral mucositis (ulcerative) due to radiation**
Use additional external cause code (W88-W90, X39.0-) to identify cause
K12.39 **Other oral mucositis (ulcerative)**
Viral oral mucositis (ulcerative)

☑4ᵗʰ **K13** **Other diseases of lip and oral mucosa**

    INCLUDES   epithelial disturbances of tongue

    Use additional code to identify:
      alcohol abuse and dependence (F10.-)
      exposure to environmental tobacco smoke (Z77.22)
      exposure to tobacco smoke in the perinatal period (P96.81)
      history of tobacco dependence (Z87.891)
      occupational exposure to environmental tobacco smoke (Z57.31)
      tobacco dependence (F17.-)
      tobacco use (Z72.0)

    EXCLUDES 2   certain disorders of gingiva and edentulous alveolar ridge
            (K05-K06)
           cysts of oral region (K09.-)
           diseases of tongue (K14.-)
           stomatitis and related lesions (K12.-)

   K13.0 **Diseases of lips**
      Abscess of lips
      Angular cheilitis
      Cellulitis of lips
      Cheilitis NOS
      Cheilodynia
      Cheilosis
      Exfoliative cheilitis
      Fistula of lips
      Glandular cheilitis
      Hypertrophy of lips
      Perlèche NEC

      EXCLUDES 1   ariboflavinosis (E53.0)
             cheilitis due to radiation-related disorders (L55-L59)
             congenital fistula of lips (Q38.0)
             congenital hypertrophy of lips (Q18.6)
             perlèche due to candidiasis (B37.83)
             perlèche due to riboflavin deficiency (E53.0)

   K13.1 **Cheek and lip biting**

☑5ᵗʰ **K13.2** **Leukoplakia and other disturbances of oral epithelium, including tongue**

      EXCLUDES 1   carcinoma in situ of oral epithelium (D00.0-)
             hairy leukoplakia (K13.3)

     DEF: Leukoplakia: Thickened white patches or lesions appearing
     on a mucous membrane, such as oral mucosa or tongue.

     K13.21 **Leukoplakia of oral mucosa, including tongue**
         Leukokeratosis of oral mucosa
         Leukoplakia of gingiva, lips, tongue
         EXCLUDES 1   hairy leukoplakia (K13.3)
                leukokeratosis nicotina palati (K13.24)

     K13.22 **Minimal keratinized residual ridge mucosa**
         Minimal keratinization of alveolar ridge mucosa

     K13.23 **Excessive keratinized residual ridge mucosa**
         Excessive keratinization of alveolar ridge mucosa

     K13.24 **Leukokeratosis nicotina palati**
         Smoker's palate

     K13.29 **Other disturbances of oral epithelium, including tongue**
         Erythroplakia of mouth or tongue
         Focal epithelial hyperplasia of mouth or tongue
         Leukoedema of mouth or tongue
         Other oral epithelium disturbances

   K13.3 **Hairy leukoplakia**

   K13.4 **Granuloma and granuloma-like lesions of oral mucosa**
      Eosinophilic granuloma
      Granuloma pyogenicum
      Verrucous xanthoma

   K13.5 **Oral submucous fibrosis**
      Submucous fibrosis of tongue

   K13.6 **Irritative hyperplasia of oral mucosa**
      EXCLUDES 2   irritative hyperplasia of edentulous ridge [denture
             hyperplasia] (K06.2)

☑5ᵗʰ **K13.7** **Other and unspecified lesions of oral mucosa**
     K13.70 **Unspecified lesions of oral mucosa**   ▽
     K13.79 **Other lesions of oral mucosa**
         Focal oral mucinosis

☑4ᵗʰ **K14** **Diseases of tongue**

    Use additional code to identify:
      alcohol abuse and dependence (F10.-)
      exposure to environmental tobacco smoke (Z77.22)
      history of tobacco dependence (Z87.891)
      occupational exposure to environmental tobacco smoke (Z57.31)
      tobacco dependence (F17.-)
      tobacco use (Z72.0)

    EXCLUDES 2   erythroplakia (K13.29)
           focal epithelial hyperplasia (K13.29)
           leukedema of tongue (K13.29)
           leukoplakia of tongue (K13.21)
           hairy leukoplakia (K13.3)
           macroglossia (congenital) (Q38.2)
           submucous fibrosis of tongue (K13.5)

   K14.0 **Glossitis**
      Abscess of tongue
      Ulceration (traumatic) of tongue
      EXCLUDES 1   atrophic glossitis (K14.4)
     DEF: Inflammation and swelling of the tongue that may be
     associated with infection, adverse drug reactions, smoking, or
     injury.

   K14.1 **Geographic tongue**
      Benign migratory glossitis
      Glossitis areata exfoliativa

   K14.2 **Median rhomboid glossitis**

   K14.3 **Hypertrophy of tongue papillae**
      Black hairy tongue
      Coated tongue
      Hypertrophy of foliate papillae
      Lingua villosa nigra

   K14.4 **Atrophy of tongue papillae**
      Atrophic glossitis

   K14.5 **Plicated tongue**
      Fissured tongue
      Furrowed tongue
      Scrotal tongue
      EXCLUDES 1   fissured tongue, congenital (Q38.3)

   K14.6 **Glossodynia**
      Glossopyrosis
      Painful tongue

   K14.8 **Other diseases of tongue**
      Atrophy of tongue
      Crenated tongue
      Enlargement of tongue
      Glossocele
      Glossoptosis
      Hypertrophy of tongue

   K14.9 **Disease of tongue, unspecified**   ▽
      Glossopathy NOS

Diseases of esophagus, stomach and duodenum (K20-K31)

    EXCLUDES 2   hiatus hernia (K44.-)

☑4ᵗʰ **K20** **Esophagitis**

    Use additional code to identify:
      alcohol abuse and dependence (F10.-)
    EXCLUDES 1   erosion of esophagus (K22.1-)
           esophagitis with gastro-esophageal reflux disease (K21.0)
           reflux esophagitis (K21.0)
           ulcerative esophagitis (K22.1-)
    EXCLUDES 2   eosinophilic gastritis or gastroenteritis (K52.81)

   K20.0 **Eosinophilic esophagitis**
   K20.8 **Other esophagitis**
      Abscess of esophagus
   K20.9 **Esophagitis, unspecified**   ▽
      Esophagitis NOS

☑4ᵗʰ **K21** **Gastro-esophageal reflux disease**
    EXCLUDES 1   newborn esophageal reflux (P78.83)

   K21.0 **Gastro-esophageal reflux disease with esophagitis**
      Reflux esophagitis

   K21.9 **Gastro-esophageal reflux disease without esophagitis**
      Esophageal reflux NOS
      AHA: 2016,1Q,18

☑ Additional Character Req   ✓x7ᵗʰ Placeholder Alert   Manifestation   ▽ Unspecified   ►◄ Revised Text   ● New Code   ▲ Revised Code Title

Chapter 11. Diseases of the Digestive System   K22–K26.9

✓4ᵗʰ K22 Other diseases of esophagus

EXCLUDES 2   esophageal varices (I85.-)

K22.0 Achalasia of cardia
Achalasia NOS
Cardiospasm
EXCLUDES 1   congenital cardiospasm (Q39.5)
DEF: Esophageal motility disorder that is caused by absence of the esophageal peristalsis and impaired relaxation of the lower esophageal sphincter. It is characterized by dysphagia, regurgitation, and heartburn.

✓5ᵗʰ K22.1 Ulcer of esophagus
Barrett's ulcer
Erosion of esophagus
Fungal ulcer of esophagus
Peptic ulcer of esophagus
Ulcer of esophagus due to ingestion of chemicals
Ulcer of esophagus due to ingestion of drugs and medicaments
Ulcerative esophagitis
Code first poisoning due to drug or toxin, if applicable (T36-T65 with fifth or sixth character 1-4 or 6)
Use additional code for adverse effect, if applicable, to identify drug (T36-T50 with fifth or sixth character 5)
EXCLUDES 1   Barrett's esophagus (K22.7-)
AHA: 2017,3Q,27
TIP: For bleeding ulcers resulting from anticoagulant therapy, code D68.32 Hemorrhagic disorder due to extrinsic circulating anticoagulant, and an adverse-effect code from subcategory T45.5- should also be assigned.

K22.10 Ulcer of esophagus without bleeding
Ulcer of esophagus NOS

K22.11 Ulcer of esophagus with bleeding
EXCLUDES 2   bleeding esophageal varices (I85.01, I85.11)

K22.2 Esophageal obstruction
Compression of esophagus
Constriction of esophagus
Stenosis of esophagus
Stricture of esophagus
EXCLUDES 1   congenital stenosis or stricture of esophagus (Q39.3)

K22.3 Perforation of esophagus
Rupture of esophagus
EXCLUDES 1   traumatic perforation of (thoracic) esophagus (S27.8-)

K22.4 Dyskinesia of esophagus
Corkscrew esophagus
Diffuse esophageal spasm
Spasm of esophagus
EXCLUDES 1   cardiospasm (K22.0)

K22.5 Diverticulum of esophagus, acquired
Esophageal pouch, acquired
EXCLUDES 1   diverticulum of esophagus (congenital) (Q39.6)

K22.6 Gastro-esophageal laceration-hemorrhage syndrome
Mallory-Weiss syndrome

✓5ᵗʰ K22.7 Barrett's esophagus
Barrett's disease
Barrett's syndrome
EXCLUDES 1   Barrett's ulcer (K22.1)
     malignant neoplasm of esophagus (C15.-)
DEF: Metaplastic disorder in which specialized columnar epithelial cells replace the normal squamous epithelial cells. Secondary to chronic gastroesophageal reflux damage to the mucosa, this disorder increases the risk of developing adenocarcinoma.

K22.70 Barrett's esophagus without dysplasia 🆀
Barrett's esophagus NOS

✓6ᵗʰ K22.71 Barrett's esophagus with dysplasia

    K22.710 Barrett's esophagus with low grade dysplasia 🆀

    K22.711 Barrett's esophagus with high grade dysplasia 🆀

    K22.719 Barrett's esophagus with dysplasia, unspecified 🆀 ▽

K22.8 Other specified diseases of esophagus
Hemorrhage of esophagus NOS
EXCLUDES 2   esophageal varices (I85.-)
     Paterson-Kelly syndrome (D50.1)

K22.9 Disease of esophagus, unspecified   ▽

K23 Disorders of esophagus in diseases classified elsewhere
Code first underlying disease, such as:
congenital syphilis (A50.5)
EXCLUDES 1   late syphilis (A52.79)
     megaesophagus due to Chagas' disease (B57.31)
     tuberculosis (A18.83)

✓4ᵗʰ K25 Gastric ulcer
INCLUDES   erosion (acute) of stomach
     pylorus ulcer (peptic)
     stomach ulcer (peptic)
Use additional code to identify:
alcohol abuse and dependence (F10.-)
EXCLUDES 1   acute gastritis (K29.0-)
     peptic ulcer NOS (K27.-)
AHA: 2017,3Q,27
TIP: For bleeding ulcers resulting from anticoagulant therapy, code D68.32 Hemorrhagic disorder due to extrinsic circulating anticoagulant, and an adverse-effect code from subcategory T45.5- should also be assigned.

Gastrointestinal Ulcers

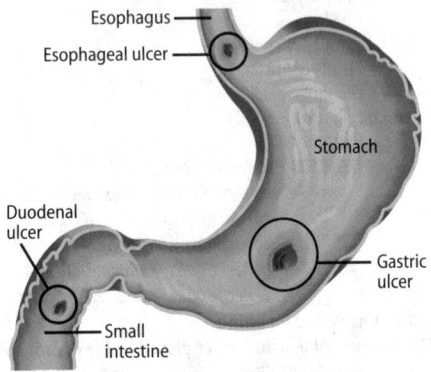

K25.0 Acute gastric ulcer with hemorrhage
K25.1 Acute gastric ulcer with perforation   HCC
K25.2 Acute gastric ulcer with both hemorrhage and perforation   HCC
K25.3 Acute gastric ulcer without hemorrhage or perforation
K25.4 Chronic or unspecified gastric ulcer with hemorrhage
K25.5 Chronic or unspecified gastric ulcer with perforation   HCC
K25.6 Chronic or unspecified gastric ulcer with both hemorrhage and perforation   HCC
K25.7 Chronic gastric ulcer without hemorrhage or perforation
K25.9 Gastric ulcer, unspecified as acute or chronic, without hemorrhage or perforation   ▽

✓4ᵗʰ K26 Duodenal ulcer
INCLUDES   erosion (acute) of duodenum
     duodenum ulcer (peptic)
     postpyloric ulcer (peptic)
Use additional code to identify:
alcohol abuse and dependence (F10.-)
EXCLUDES 1   peptic ulcer NOS (K27.-)
AHA: 2017,3Q,27
TIP: For bleeding ulcers resulting from anticoagulant therapy, code D68.32 Hemorrhagic disorder due to extrinsic circulating anticoagulant, and an adverse-effect code from subcategory T45.5- should also be assigned.

K26.0 Acute duodenal ulcer with hemorrhage
K26.1 Acute duodenal ulcer with perforation   HCC
K26.2 Acute duodenal ulcer with both hemorrhage and perforation   HCC
K26.3 Acute duodenal ulcer without hemorrhage or perforation
K26.4 Chronic or unspecified duodenal ulcer with hemorrhage
AHA: 2016,1Q,14
K26.5 Chronic or unspecified duodenal ulcer with perforation   HCC
K26.6 Chronic or unspecified duodenal ulcer with both hemorrhage and perforation   HCC
K26.7 Chronic duodenal ulcer without hemorrhage or perforation
K26.9 Duodenal ulcer, unspecified as acute or chronic, without hemorrhage or perforation   ▽

Chapter 11. Diseases of the Digestive System

☑4ᵗʰ **K27 Peptic ulcer, site unspecified**

INCLUDES gastroduodenal ulcer NOS
peptic ulcer NOS

Use additional code to identify:
alcohol abuse and dependence (F10.-)

EXCLUDES 1 *peptic ulcer of newborn (P78.82)*

AHA: 2017,3Q,27

TIP: For bleeding ulcers resulting from anticoagulant therapy, code D68.32 Hemorrhagic disorder due to extrinsic circulating anticoagulant, and an adverse-effect code from subcategory T45.5- should also be assigned.

K27.0 **Acute peptic ulcer, site unspecified, with hemorrhage**

K27.1 **Acute peptic ulcer, site unspecified, with perforation**   HCC

K27.2 **Acute peptic ulcer, site unspecified, with both hemorrhage and perforation**   HCC

K27.3 **Acute peptic ulcer, site unspecified, without hemorrhage or perforation**

K27.4 **Chronic or unspecified peptic ulcer, site unspecified, with hemorrhage**

K27.5 **Chronic or unspecified peptic ulcer, site unspecified, with perforation**   HCC

K27.6 **Chronic or unspecified peptic ulcer, site unspecified, with both hemorrhage and perforation**   HCC

K27.7 **Chronic peptic ulcer, site unspecified, without hemorrhage or perforation**

K27.9 **Peptic ulcer, site unspecified, unspecified as acute or chronic, without hemorrhage or perforation**   ▽

☑4ᵗʰ **K28 Gastrojejunal ulcer**

INCLUDES anastomotic ulcer (peptic) or erosion
gastrocolic ulcer (peptic) or erosion
gastrointestinal ulcer (peptic) or erosion
gastrojejunal ulcer (peptic) or erosion
jejunal ulcer (peptic) or erosion
marginal ulcer (peptic) or erosion
stomal ulcer (peptic) or erosion

Use additional code to identify:
alcohol abuse and dependence (F10.-)

EXCLUDES 1 *primary ulcer of small intestine (K63.3)*

AHA: 2017,3Q,27

TIP: For bleeding ulcers resulting from anticoagulant therapy, code D68.32 Hemorrhagic disorder due to extrinsic circulating anticoagulant, and an adverse-effect code from subcategory T45.5- should also be assigned.

K28.0 **Acute gastrojejunal ulcer with hemorrhage**

K28.1 **Acute gastrojejunal ulcer with perforation**   HCC

K28.2 **Acute gastrojejunal ulcer with both hemorrhage and perforation**   HCC

K28.3 **Acute gastrojejunal ulcer without hemorrhage or perforation**

K28.4 **Chronic or unspecified gastrojejunal ulcer with hemorrhage**

K28.5 **Chronic or unspecified gastrojejunal ulcer with perforation**   HCC

K28.6 **Chronic or unspecified gastrojejunal ulcer with both hemorrhage and perforation**   HCC

K28.7 **Chronic gastrojejunal ulcer without hemorrhage or perforation**

K28.9 **Gastrojejunal ulcer, unspecified as acute or chronic, without hemorrhage or perforation**   ▽

☑4ᵗʰ **K29 Gastritis and duodenitis**

EXCLUDES 1 *eosinophilic gastritis or gastroenteritis (K52.81)*
Zollinger-Ellison syndrome (E16.4)

TIP: For bleeding resulting from anticoagulant therapy, code D68.32 Hemorrhagic disorder due to extrinsic circulating anticoagulant, and an adverse-effect code from subcategory T45.5- should also be assigned.

☑5ᵗʰ **K29.0 Acute gastritis**

Use additional code to identify:
alcohol abuse and dependence (F10.-)

EXCLUDES 1 *erosion (acute) of stomach (K25.-)*

K29.00 **Acute gastritis without bleeding**

K29.01 **Acute gastritis with bleeding**

☑5ᵗʰ **K29.2 Alcoholic gastritis**

Use additional code to identify:
alcohol abuse and dependence (F10.-)

K29.20 **Alcoholic gastritis without bleeding**

K29.21 **Alcoholic gastritis with bleeding**

☑5ᵗʰ **K29.3 Chronic superficial gastritis**

K29.30 **Chronic superficial gastritis without bleeding**

K29.31 **Chronic superficial gastritis with bleeding**

☑5ᵗʰ **K29.4 Chronic atrophic gastritis**

Gastric atrophy

K29.40 **Chronic atrophic gastritis without bleeding**

K29.41 **Chronic atrophic gastritis with bleeding**

☑5ᵗʰ **K29.5 Unspecified chronic gastritis**

Chronic antral gastritis
Chronic fundal gastritis

K29.50 **Unspecified chronic gastritis without bleeding**   ▽

K29.51 **Unspecified chronic gastritis with bleeding**   ▽

☑5ᵗʰ **K29.6 Other gastritis**

Giant hypertrophic gastritis
Granulomatous gastritis
Ménétrier's disease

K29.60 **Other gastritis without bleeding**

K29.61 **Other gastritis with bleeding**

☑5ᵗʰ **K29.7 Gastritis, unspecified**

K29.70 **Gastritis, unspecified, without bleeding**   ▽

K29.71 **Gastritis, unspecified, with bleeding**   ▽

☑5ᵗʰ **K29.8 Duodenitis**

K29.80 **Duodenitis without bleeding**

K29.81 **Duodenitis with bleeding**

☑5ᵗʰ **K29.9 Gastroduodenitis, unspecified**

K29.90 **Gastroduodenitis, unspecified, without bleeding**   ▽

K29.91 **Gastroduodenitis, unspecified, with bleeding**   ▽

K30 Functional dyspepsia

Indigestion

EXCLUDES 1 *dyspepsia NOS (R10.13)*
heartburn (R12)
nervous dyspepsia (F45.8)
neurotic dyspepsia (F45.8)
psychogenic dyspepsia (F45.8)

☑4ᵗʰ **K31 Other diseases of stomach and duodenum**

INCLUDES functional disorders of stomach

EXCLUDES 2 *diabetic gastroparesis (E08.43, E09.43, E10.43, E11.43, E13.43)*
diverticulum of duodenum (K57.00-K57.13)

K31.0 **Acute dilatation of stomach**

Acute distention of stomach

K31.1 **Adult hypertrophic pyloric stenosis**   Ⓐ

Pyloric stenosis NOS

EXCLUDES 1 *congenital or infantile pyloric stenosis (Q40.0)*

K31.2 **Hourglass stricture and stenosis of stomach**

EXCLUDES 1 *congenital hourglass stomach (Q40.2)*
hourglass contraction of stomach (K31.89)

K31.3 **Pylorospasm, not elsewhere classified**

EXCLUDES 1 *congenital or infantile pylorospasm (Q40.0)*
neurotic pylorospasm (F45.8)
psychogenic pylorospasm (F45.8)

K31.4 **Gastric diverticulum**

EXCLUDES 1 *congenital diverticulum of stomach (Q40.2)*

K31.5 **Obstruction of duodenum**

Constriction of duodenum
Duodenal ileus (chronic)
Stenosis of duodenum
Stricture of duodenum
Volvulus of duodenum

EXCLUDES 1 *congenital stenosis of duodenum (Q41.0)*

K31.6 **Fistula of stomach and duodenum**

Gastrocolic fistula
Gastrojejunocolic fistula

K31.7 **Polyp of stomach and duodenum**

EXCLUDES 1 *adenomatous polyp of stomach (D13.1)*

☑5ᵗʰ **K31.8 Other specified diseases of stomach and duodenum**

☑6ᵗʰ **K31.81 Angiodysplasia of stomach and duodenum**

K31.811 **Angiodysplasia of stomach and duodenum with bleeding**

K31.819 **Angiodysplasia of stomach and duodenum without bleeding**

Angiodysplasia of stomach and duodenum NOS

☑ Additional Character Req   ✓x7ᵗʰ Placeholder Alert   Manifestation   ▽ Unspecified   ►◄ Revised Text   ● New Code   ▲ Revised Code Title

ICD-10-CM 2019   **699**

K31.82 Dieulafoy lesion (hemorrhagic) of stomach and duodenum
> **EXCLUDES 2** *Dieulafoy lesion of intestine (K63.81)*
> **DEF:** Abnormally large submucosal artery protruding through a defect in the stomach mucosa or intestines that can cause massive and life-threatening hemorrhaging.

K31.83 Achlorhydria
> **DEF:** Absence of hydrochloric acid in gastric secretions due to gastric mucosa atrophy. Achlorhydria is unresponsive to histamines.

K31.84 Gastroparesis
> Gastroparalysis
> Code first underlying disease, if known, such as:
>   anorexia nervosa (F50.0-)
>   diabetes mellitus (E08.43, E09.43, E10.43, E11.43, E13.43)
>   scleroderma (M34.-)
> **AHA:** 2013,4Q,114

K31.89 Other diseases of stomach and duodenum
> **AHA:** 2017,1Q,28
> **TIP:** Assign for cyclical vomiting not related to migraine, along with a code from category R11 Nausea and vomiting.

K31.9 Disease of stomach and duodenum, unspecified   ▽

Diseases of appendix (K35-K38)

√4ᵗʰ **K35 Acute appendicitis**

√5ᵗʰ **K35.2 Acute appendicitis with generalized peritonitis**
> Appendicitis (acute) with generalized (diffuse) peritonitis following rupture or perforation of appendix
> ~~Perforated appendix NOS~~
> ~~Ruptured appendix NOS~~

● **K35.20 Acute appendicitis with generalized peritonitis, without abscess**
> (Acute) appendicitis with generalized peritonitis NOS

● **K35.21 Acute appendicitis with generalized peritonitis, with abscess**

√5ᵗʰ **K35.3 Acute appendicitis with localized peritonitis**
> ~~Acute appendicitis with or without perforation or rupture with peritonitis NOS~~
> ~~Acute appendicitis with or without perforation or rupture with localized peritonitis~~
> ~~Acute appendicitis with peritoneal abscess~~

● **K35.30 Acute appendicitis with localized peritonitis, without perforation or gangrene**
> Acute appendicitis with localized peritonitis NOS

● **K35.31 Acute appendicitis with localized peritonitis and gangrene, without perforation**

● **K35.32 Acute appendicitis with perforation and localized peritonitis, without abscess**
> (Acute) appendicitis with perforation NOS
> Perforated appendix NOS
> Ruptured appendix (with localized peritonitis) NOS

● **K35.33 Acute appendicitis with perforation and localized peritonitis, with abscess**
> (Acute) appendicitis with (peritoneal) abscess NOS
> Ruptured appendix with localized peritonitis and abscess

√5ᵗʰ **K35.8 Other and unspecified acute appendicitis**

K35.80 Unspecified acute appendicitis   ▽
> Acute appendicitis NOS
> Acute appendicitis without (localized) (generalized) peritonitis

√6ᵗʰ **K35.89 Other acute appendicitis**

● **K35.890 Other acute appendicitis without perforation or gangrene**

● **K35.891 Other acute appendicitis without perforation, with gangrene**
> (Acute) appendicitis with gangrene NOS

K36 Other appendicitis
> Chronic appendicitis
> Recurrent appendicitis

K37 Unspecified appendicitis   ▽
> **EXCLUDES 1** *unspecified appendicitis with peritonitis ▶(K35.2-, K35.3-)◀*

√4ᵗʰ **K38 Other diseases of appendix**

K38.0 Hyperplasia of appendix

K38.1 Appendicular concretions
> Fecalith of appendix
> Stercolith of appendix

K38.2 Diverticulum of appendix

K38.3 Fistula of appendix

K38.8 Other specified diseases of appendix
> Intussusception of appendix

K38.9 Disease of appendix, unspecified   ▽

Hernia (K40-K46)

> **NOTE** Hernia with both gangrene and obstruction is classified to hernia with gangrene.
> **INCLUDES** acquired hernia
> congenital [except diaphragmatic or hiatus] hernia
> recurrent hernia

√4ᵗʰ **K40 Inguinal hernia**
> **INCLUDES** bubonocele
> direct inguinal hernia
> double inguinal hernia
> indirect inguinal hernia
> inguinal hernia NOS
> oblique inguinal hernia
> scrotal hernia

√5ᵗʰ **K40.0 Bilateral inguinal hernia, with obstruction, without gangrene**
> Inguinal hernia (bilateral) causing obstruction without gangrene
> Incarcerated inguinal hernia (bilateral) without gangrene
> Irreducible inguinal hernia (bilateral) without gangrene
> Strangulated inguinal hernia (bilateral) without gangrene

K40.00 Bilateral inguinal hernia, with obstruction, without gangrene, not specified as recurrent
> Bilateral inguinal hernia, with obstruction, without gangrene NOS

K40.01 Bilateral inguinal hernia, with obstruction, without gangrene, recurrent

√5ᵗʰ **K40.1 Bilateral inguinal hernia, with gangrene**

K40.10 Bilateral inguinal hernia, with gangrene, not specified as recurrent
> Bilateral inguinal hernia, with gangrene NOS

K40.11 Bilateral inguinal hernia, with gangrene, recurrent

√5ᵗʰ **K40.2 Bilateral inguinal hernia, without obstruction or gangrene**

K40.20 Bilateral inguinal hernia, without obstruction or gangrene, not specified as recurrent
> Bilateral inguinal hernia NOS

K40.21 Bilateral inguinal hernia, without obstruction or gangrene, recurrent

√5ᵗʰ **K40.3 Unilateral inguinal hernia, with obstruction, without gangrene**
> Inguinal hernia (unilateral) causing obstruction without gangrene
> Incarcerated inguinal hernia (unilateral) without gangrene
> Irreducible inguinal hernia (unilateral) without gangrene
> Strangulated inguinal hernia (unilateral) without gangrene

K40.30 Unilateral inguinal hernia, with obstruction, without gangrene, not specified as recurrent
> Inguinal hernia, with obstruction NOS
> Unilateral inguinal hernia, with obstruction, without gangrene NOS

K40.31 Unilateral inguinal hernia, with obstruction, without gangrene, recurrent

√5ᵗʰ **K40.4 Unilateral inguinal hernia, with gangrene**

K40.40 Unilateral inguinal hernia, with gangrene, not specified as recurrent
> Inguinal hernia with gangrene NOS
> Unilateral inguinal hernia with gangrene NOS

K40.41 Unilateral inguinal hernia, with gangrene, recurrent

√5ᵗʰ **K40.9 Unilateral inguinal hernia, without obstruction or gangrene**

K40.90 Unilateral inguinal hernia, without obstruction or gangrene, not specified as recurrent
> Inguinal hernia NOS
> Unilateral inguinal hernia NOS

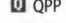

K40.91   Unilateral inguinal hernia, without obstruction or gangrene, **recurrent**

Hernia Sites

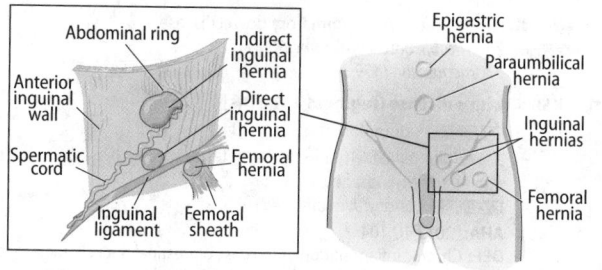

Labels: Abdominal ring, Indirect inguinal hernia, Direct inguinal hernia, Anterior inguinal wall, Spermatic cord, Femoral hernia, Inguinal ligament, Femoral sheath, Epigastric hernia, Paraumbilical hernia, Inguinal hernias, Femoral hernia

☑4ᵗʰ **K41   Femoral hernia**

☑5ᵗʰ **K41.0   Bilateral femoral hernia, with obstruction, without gangrene**
Femoral hernia (bilateral) causing obstruction, without gangrene
Incarcerated femoral hernia (bilateral), without gangrene
Irreducible femoral hernia (bilateral), without gangrene
Strangulated femoral hernia (bilateral), without gangrene

   K41.00   Bilateral femoral hernia, with obstruction, without gangrene, not specified as recurrent ▲
Bilateral femoral hernia, with obstruction, without gangrene NOS

   K41.01   Bilateral femoral hernia, with obstruction, without gangrene, recurrent

☑5ᵗʰ **K41.1   Bilateral femoral hernia, with gangrene**

   K41.10   Bilateral femoral hernia, with gangrene, not specified as recurrent
Bilateral femoral hernia, with gangrene NOS

   K41.11   Bilateral femoral hernia, with gangrene, recurrent

☑5ᵗʰ **K41.2   Bilateral femoral hernia, without obstruction or gangrene**

   K41.20   Bilateral femoral hernia, without obstruction or gangrene, not specified as recurrent
Bilateral femoral hernia NOS

   K41.21   Bilateral femoral hernia, without obstruction or gangrene, recurrent

☑5ᵗʰ **K41.3   Unilateral femoral hernia, with obstruction, without gangrene**
Femoral hernia (unilateral) causing obstruction, without gangrene
Incarcerated femoral hernia (unilateral), without gangrene
Irreducible femoral hernia (unilateral), without gangrene
Strangulated femoral hernia (unilateral), without gangrene

   K41.30   Unilateral femoral hernia, with obstruction, without gangrene, not specified as recurrent
Femoral hernia, with obstruction NOS
Unilateral femoral hernia, with obstruction NOS

   K41.31   Unilateral femoral hernia, with obstruction, without gangrene, recurrent

☑5ᵗʰ **K41.4   Unilateral femoral hernia, with gangrene**

   K41.40   Unilateral femoral hernia, with gangrene, not specified as recurrent
Femoral hernia, with gangrene NOS
Unilateral femoral hernia, with gangrene NOS

   K41.41   Unilateral femoral hernia, with gangrene, recurrent

☑5ᵗʰ **K41.9   Unilateral femoral hernia, without obstruction or gangrene**

   K41.90   Unilateral femoral hernia, without obstruction or gangrene, not specified as recurrent
Femoral hernia NOS
Unilateral femoral hernia NOS

   K41.91   Unilateral femoral hernia, without obstruction or gangrene, recurrent

☑4ᵗʰ **K42   Umbilical hernia**
   INCLUDES   paraumbilical hernia
   EXCLUDES 1   *omphalocele (Q79.2)*

   K42.0   Umbilical hernia with obstruction, without gangrene
Umbilical hernia causing obstruction, without gangrene
Incarcerated umbilical hernia, without gangrene
Irreducible umbilical hernia, without gangrene
Strangulated umbilical hernia, without gangrene

K42.1   Umbilical hernia with gangrene
Gangrenous umbilical hernia

K42.9   Umbilical hernia without obstruction or gangrene
Umbilical hernia NOS

☑4ᵗʰ **K43   Ventral hernia**
   DEF: Condition in which a loop of bowel protrudes through a weakness in the abdominal wall muscles that may occur as a birth defect, past surgical site (incisional), or form at a stomal site (parastomal).

   K43.0   Incisional hernia with obstruction, without gangrene
Incisional hernia causing obstruction, without gangrene
Incarcerated incisional hernia, without gangrene
Irreducible incisional hernia, without gangrene
Strangulated incisional hernia, without gangrene

   K43.1   Incisional hernia with gangrene
Gangrenous incisional hernia

   K43.2   Incisional hernia without obstruction or gangrene
Incisional hernia NOS

   K43.3   Parastomal hernia with obstruction, without gangrene
Incarcerated parastomal hernia, without gangrene
Irreducible parastomal hernia, without gangrene
Parastomal hernia causing obstruction, without gangrene
Strangulated parastomal hernia, without gangrene

   K43.4   Parastomal hernia with gangrene
Gangrenous parastomal hernia

   K43.5   Parastomal hernia without obstruction or gangrene
Parastomal hernia NOS

   K43.6   Other and unspecified ventral hernia with obstruction, without gangrene ▽
Epigastric hernia causing obstruction, without gangrene
Hypogastric hernia causing obstruction, without gangrene
Incarcerated epigastric hernia without gangrene
Incarcerated hypogastric hernia without gangrene
Incarcerated midline hernia without gangrene
Incarcerated spigelian hernia without gangrene
Incarcerated subxiphoid hernia without gangrene
Irreducible epigastric hernia without gangrene
Irreducible hypogastric hernia without gangrene
Irreducible midline hernia without gangrene
Irreducible spigelian hernia without gangrene
Irreducible subxiphoid hernia without gangrene
Midline hernia causing obstruction, without gangrene
Spigelian hernia causing obstruction, without gangrene
Strangulated epigastric hernia without gangrene
Strangulated hypogastric hernia without gangrene
Strangulated midline hernia without gangrene
Strangulated spigelian hernia without gangrene
Strangulated subxiphoid hernia without gangrene
Subxiphoid hernia causing obstruction, without gangrene

   K43.7   Other and unspecified ventral hernia with gangrene ▽
Any condition listed under K43.6 specified as gangrenous

   K43.9   Ventral hernia without obstruction or gangrene
Epigastric hernia
Ventral hernia NOS

✓4ᵗʰ **K44 Diaphragmatic hernia**

INCLUDES hiatus hernia (esophageal) (sliding)
paraesophageal hernia

EXCLUDES 1 *congenital diaphragmatic hernia (Q79.0)*
congenital hiatus hernia (Q40.1)

DEF: Protrusion of an abdominal organ, usually the stomach, through the esophageal opening within the diaphragm and occurring in two types: the sliding hiatal hernia and the paraesophageal hernia.

Hiatal Hernia

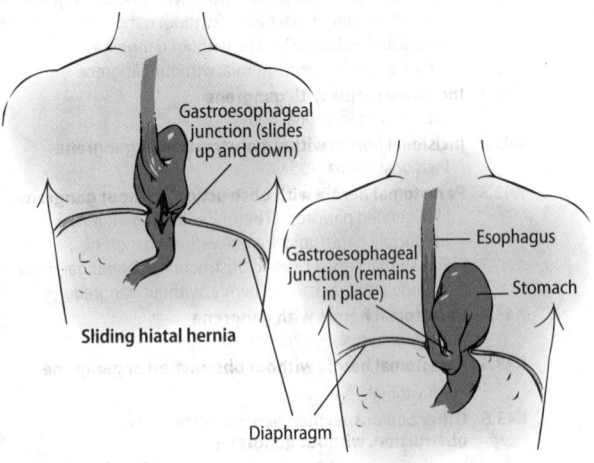

Gastroesophageal junction (slides up and down)

Sliding hiatal hernia

Gastroesophageal junction (remains in place)

Esophagus

Stomach

Diaphragm

Paraesophageal hiatal hernia

K44.0 Diaphragmatic hernia with obstruction, without gangrene
Diaphragmatic hernia causing obstruction
Incarcerated diaphragmatic hernia
Irreducible diaphragmatic hernia
Strangulated diaphragmatic hernia

K44.1 Diaphragmatic hernia with gangrene
Gangrenous diaphragmatic hernia

K44.9 Diaphragmatic hernia without obstruction or gangrene
Diaphragmatic hernia NOS

✓4ᵗʰ **K45 Other abdominal hernia**

INCLUDES abdominal hernia, specified site NEC
lumbar hernia
obturator hernia
pudendal hernia
retroperitoneal hernia
sciatic hernia

K45.0 Other specified abdominal hernia with obstruction, without gangrene
Other specified abdominal hernia causing obstruction
Other specified incarcerated abdominal hernia
Other specified irreducible abdominal hernia
Other specified strangulated abdominal hernia

K45.1 Other specified abdominal hernia with gangrene
Any condition listed under K45 specified as gangrenous

K45.8 Other specified abdominal hernia without obstruction or gangrene

✓4ᵗʰ **K46 Unspecified abdominal hernia**

INCLUDES enterocele
epiplocele
hernia NOS
interstitial hernia
intestinal hernia
intra-abdominal hernia

EXCLUDES 1 *vaginal enterocele (N81.5)*

K46.0 Unspecified abdominal hernia with obstruction, without gangrene ▽
Unspecified abdominal hernia causing obstruction
Unspecified incarcerated abdominal hernia
Unspecified irreducible abdominal hernia
Unspecified strangulated abdominal hernia

K46.1 Unspecified abdominal hernia with gangrene ▽
Any condition listed under K46 specified as gangrenous

K46.9 Unspecified abdominal hernia without obstruction or gangrene ▽
Abdominal hernia NOS

Noninfective enteritis and colitis (K50-K52)

INCLUDES noninfective inflammatory bowel disease
EXCLUDES 1 *irritable bowel syndrome (K58.-)*
megacolon (K59.3-)

✓4ᵗʰ **K50 Crohn's disease [regional enteritis]**

INCLUDES granulomatous enteritis
Use additional code to identify manifestations, such as:
pyoderma gangrenosum (L88)

EXCLUDES 1 *ulcerative colitis (K51.-)*

AHA: 2012,4Q,104

DEF: Chronic inflammation of the gastrointestinal tract characterized by chronic granulomatous disease, most commonly affecting the intestines and the terminal ileum.

✓5ᵗʰ **K50.0 Crohn's disease of small intestine**
Crohn's disease [regional enteritis] of duodenum
Crohn's disease [regional enteritis] of ileum
Crohn's disease [regional enteritis] of jejunum
Regional ileitis
Terminal ileitis

EXCLUDES 1 *Crohn's disease of both small and large intestine (K50.8-)*

K50.00 Crohn's disease of small intestine without complications ᴴᶜᶜ

✓6ᵗʰ **K50.01 Crohn's disease of small intestine with complications**

K50.011 Crohn's disease of small intestine with rectal bleeding ᴴᶜᶜ

K50.012 Crohn's disease of small intestine with intestinal obstruction ᴴᶜᶜ

K50.013 Crohn's disease of small intestine with fistula ᴴᶜᶜ

K50.014 Crohn's disease of small intestine with abscess ᴴᶜᶜ
AHA: 2012,4Q,104

K50.018 Crohn's disease of small intestine with other complication ᴴᶜᶜ

K50.019 Crohn's disease of small intestine with unspecified complications ᴴᶜᶜ ▽

✓5ᵗʰ **K50.1 Crohn's disease of large intestine**
Crohn's disease [regional enteritis] of colon
Crohn's disease [regional enteritis] of large bowel
Crohn's disease [regional enteritis] of rectum
Granulomatous colitis
Regional colitis

EXCLUDES 1 *Crohn's disease of both small and large intestine (K50.8)*

K50.10 Crohn's disease of large intestine without complications ᴴᶜᶜ

✓6ᵗʰ **K50.11 Crohn's disease of large intestine with complications**

K50.111 Crohn's disease of large intestine with rectal bleeding ᴴᶜᶜ

K50.112 Crohn's disease of large intestine with intestinal obstruction ᴴᶜᶜ

K50.113 Crohn's disease of large intestine with fistula ᴴᶜᶜ

K50.114 Crohn's disease of large intestine with abscess ᴴᶜᶜ

K50.118 Crohn's disease of large intestine with other complication ᴴᶜᶜ

K50.119 Crohn's disease of large intestine with unspecified complications ᴴᶜᶜ ▽

✓5ᵗʰ **K50.8 Crohn's disease of both small and large intestine**

K50.80 Crohn's disease of both small and large intestine without complications ᴴᶜᶜ

✓6ᵗʰ **K50.81 Crohn's disease of both small and large intestine with complications**

K50.811 Crohn's disease of both small and large intestine with rectal bleeding ᴴᶜᶜ

K50.812 Crohn's disease of both small and large intestine with intestinal obstruction ᴴᶜᶜ

K50.813 Crohn's disease of both small and large intestine with fistula ᴴᶜᶜ

K50.814 Crohn's disease of both small and large intestine with abscess `HCC`

K50.818 Crohn's disease of both small and large intestine with other complication `HCC`

K50.819 Crohn's disease of both small and large intestine with unspecified complications `HCC` ▽

√5ᵗʰ **K50.9** Crohn's disease, unspecified

K50.90 Crohn's disease, unspecified, without complications `HCC` ▽

Crohn's disease NOS

Regional enteritis NOS

√6ᵗʰ **K50.91** Crohn's disease, unspecified, with complications

K50.911 Crohn's disease, unspecified, with rectal bleeding `HCC` ▽

K50.912 Crohn's disease, unspecified, with intestinal obstruction `HCC` ▽

K50.913 Crohn's disease, unspecified, with fistula `HCC` ▽

K50.914 Crohn's disease, unspecified, with abscess `HCC` ▽

K50.918 Crohn's disease, unspecified, with other complication `HCC` ▽

K50.919 Crohn's disease, unspecified, with unspecified complications `HCC` ▽

√4ᵗʰ **K51** Ulcerative colitis

Use additional code to identify manifestations, such as:

pyoderma gangrenosum (L88)

EXCLUDES 1 Crohn's disease [regional enteritis] (K50.-)

√5ᵗʰ **K51.0** Ulcerative (chronic) pancolitis

Backwash ileitis

K51.00 Ulcerative (chronic) pancolitis without complications `HCC`

Ulcerative (chronic) pancolitis NOS

√6ᵗʰ **K51.01** Ulcerative (chronic) pancolitis with complications

K51.011 Ulcerative (chronic) pancolitis with rectal bleeding `HCC`

K51.012 Ulcerative (chronic) pancolitis with intestinal obstruction `HCC`

K51.013 Ulcerative (chronic) pancolitis with fistula `HCC`

K51.014 Ulcerative (chronic) pancolitis with abscess `HCC`

K51.018 Ulcerative (chronic) pancolitis with other complication `HCC`

K51.019 Ulcerative (chronic) pancolitis with unspecified complications `HCC` ▽

√5ᵗʰ **K51.2** Ulcerative (chronic) proctitis

K51.20 Ulcerative (chronic) proctitis without complications `HCC`

Ulcerative (chronic) proctitis NOS

√6ᵗʰ **K51.21** Ulcerative (chronic) proctitis with complications

K51.211 Ulcerative (chronic) proctitis with rectal bleeding `HCC`

K51.212 Ulcerative (chronic) proctitis with intestinal obstruction `HCC`

K51.213 Ulcerative (chronic) proctitis with fistula `HCC`

K51.214 Ulcerative (chronic) proctitis with abscess `HCC`

K51.218 Ulcerative (chronic) proctitis with other complication `HCC`

K51.219 Ulcerative (chronic) proctitis with unspecified complications `HCC` ▽

√5ᵗʰ **K51.3** Ulcerative (chronic) rectosigmoiditis

K51.30 Ulcerative (chronic) rectosigmoiditis without complications `HCC`

Ulcerative (chronic) rectosigmoiditis NOS

√6ᵗʰ **K51.31** Ulcerative (chronic) rectosigmoiditis with complications

K51.311 Ulcerative (chronic) rectosigmoiditis with rectal bleeding `HCC`

K51.312 Ulcerative (chronic) rectosigmoiditis with intestinal obstruction `HCC`

K51.313 Ulcerative (chronic) rectosigmoiditis with fistula `HCC`

K51.314 Ulcerative (chronic) rectosigmoiditis with abscess `HCC`

K51.318 Ulcerative (chronic) rectosigmoiditis with other complication `HCC`

K51.319 Ulcerative (chronic) rectosigmoiditis with unspecified complications `HCC` ▽

√5ᵗʰ **K51.4** Inflammatory polyps of colon

EXCLUDES 1 adenomatous polyp of colon (D12.6)

polyposis of colon (D12.6)

polyps of colon NOS (K63.5)

K51.40 Inflammatory polyps of colon without complications `HCC`

Inflammatory polyps of colon NOS

√6ᵗʰ **K51.41** Inflammatory polyps of colon with complications

K51.411 Inflammatory polyps of colon with rectal bleeding `HCC`

K51.412 Inflammatory polyps of colon with intestinal obstruction `HCC`

K51.413 Inflammatory polyps of colon with fistula `HCC`

K51.414 Inflammatory polyps of colon with abscess `HCC`

K51.418 Inflammatory polyps of colon with other complication `HCC`

K51.419 Inflammatory polyps of colon with unspecified complications `HCC` ▽

√5ᵗʰ **K51.5** Left sided colitis

Left hemicolitis

K51.50 Left sided colitis without complications `HCC`

Left sided colitis NOS

√6ᵗʰ **K51.51** Left sided colitis with complications

K51.511 Left sided colitis with rectal bleeding `HCC`

K51.512 Left sided colitis with intestinal obstruction `HCC`

K51.513 Left sided colitis with fistula `HCC`

K51.514 Left sided colitis with abscess `HCC`

K51.518 Left sided colitis with other complication `HCC`

K51.519 Left sided colitis with unspecified complications `HCC` ▽

√5ᵗʰ **K51.8** Other ulcerative colitis

K51.80 Other ulcerative colitis without complications `HCC`

√6ᵗʰ **K51.81** Other ulcerative colitis with complications

K51.811 Other ulcerative colitis with rectal bleeding `HCC`

K51.812 Other ulcerative colitis with intestinal obstruction `HCC`

K51.813 Other ulcerative colitis with fistula `HCC`

K51.814 Other ulcerative colitis with abscess `HCC`

K51.818 Other ulcerative colitis with other complication `HCC`

K51.819 Other ulcerative colitis with unspecified complications `HCC` ▽

√5ᵗʰ **K51.9** Ulcerative colitis, unspecified

K51.90 Ulcerative colitis, unspecified, without complications `HCC` ▽

√6ᵗʰ **K51.91** Ulcerative colitis, unspecified, with complications

K51.911 Ulcerative colitis, unspecified with rectal bleeding `HCC` ▽

K51.912 Ulcerative colitis, unspecified with intestinal obstruction `HCC` ▽

K51.913 Ulcerative colitis, unspecified with fistula `HCC` ▽

K51.914 Ulcerative colitis, unspecified with abscess `HCC` ▽

K51.918 Ulcerative colitis, unspecified with other complication `HCC` ▽

K51.919 Ulcerative colitis, unspecified with unspecified complications `HCC` ▽

√4ᵗʰ **K52** Other and unspecified noninfective gastroenteritis and colitis

AHA: 2016,4Q,30-31

K52.0 Gastroenteritis and colitis due to radiation

☑ Additional Character Req | √x7ᵗʰ Placeholder Alert | Manifestation | ▽ Unspecified | ►◄ Revised Text | ● New Code | ▲ Revised Code Title

ICD-10-CM 2019

703

Chapter 11. Diseases of the Digestive System

K50.814–K52.0

K52.1 **Toxic** gastroenteritis and colitis

Drug-induced gastroenteritis and colitis

Code first (T51-T65) to identify toxic agent

Use additional code for adverse effect, if applicable, to identify drug (T36-T50 with fifth or sixth character 5)

√5th **K52.2** **Allergic and dietetic gastroenteritis and colitis**

Food hypersensitivity gastroenteritis or colitis

Use additional code to identify type of food allergy (Z91.01-, Z91.02-)

EXCLUDES 2   allergic eosinophilic colitis (K52.82)

allergic eosinophilic esophagitis (K20.0)

allergic eosinophilic gastritis (K52.81)

allergic eosinophilic gastroenteritis (K52.81)

food protein-induced proctocolitis (K52.82)

DEF: True immunoglobulin E (IgE)-mediated allergic reaction of the lining of the stomach, intestines, or colon to food proteins. It causes nausea, vomiting, diarrhea, and abdominal cramping.

K52.21 **Food protein-induced enterocolitis syndrome**

▶FPIES◀

Use additional code for hypovolemic shock, if present (R57.1)

K52.22 **Food protein-induced enteropathy**

K52.29 **Other allergic and dietetic gastroenteritis and colitis**

Food hypersensitivity gastroenteritis or colitis

Immediate gastrointestinal hypersensitivity

K52.3 **Indeterminate colitis**

Colonic inflammatory bowel disease unclassified (IBDU)

EXCLUDES 1   unspecified colitis (K52.9)

√5th **K52.8** **Other specified noninfective gastroenteritis and colitis**

K52.81 **Eosinophilic gastritis or gastroenteritis**

Eosinophilic enteritis

EXCLUDES 2   eosinophilic esophagitis (K20.0)

DEF: Disorder involving the accumulation of eosinophil in the lining of the stomach or multiple levels of the gastrointestinal tract, but without a known cause such as connective tissue disease, drug reaction, malignancy, or parasitic infection.

K52.82 **Eosinophilic colitis**

Allergic proctocolitis

Food-induced eosinophilic proctocolitis

Food protein-induced proctocolitis

Milk protein-induced proctocolitis

DEF: Disorder involving the accumulation of eosinophil in the tissues lining the colon, but without a known cause such as connective tissue disease, drug reaction, malignancy, or parasitic infection. The resultant inflammation may cause extreme abdominal pain, diarrhea, or bloody stool.

√6th **K52.83** **Microscopic colitis**

K52.831 **Collagenous colitis**

K52.832 **Lymphocytic colitis**

K52.838 **Other microscopic colitis**

K52.839 **Microscopic colitis, unspecified** ▽

K52.89 **Other specified noninfective gastroenteritis and colitis**

K52.9 **Noninfective gastroenteritis and colitis, unspecified** ▽

Colitis NOS

Enteritis NOS

Gastroenteritis NOS

Ileitis NOS

Jejunitis NOS

Sigmoiditis NOS

EXCLUDES 1   diarrhea NOS (R19.7)

functional diarrhea (K59.1)

infectious gastroenteritis and colitis NOS (A09)

neonatal diarrhea (noninfective) (P78.3)

psychogenic diarrhea (F45.8)

Other diseases of intestines (K55-K64)

√4th **K55** **Vascular disorders of intestine**

EXCLUDES 1   necrotizing enterocolitis of newborn (P77.-)

AHA: 2016,4Q,32

√5th **K55.0** **Acute vascular disorders of intestine**   HCC

Infarction of appendices epiploicae

Mesenteric (artery) (vein) embolism

Mesenteric (artery) (vein) infarction

Mesenteric (artery) (vein) thrombosis

√6th **K55.01** **Acute (reversible) ischemia of small intestine**

K55.011 **Focal (segmental) acute (reversible) ischemia of small intestine**   HCC

K55.012 **Diffuse acute (reversible) ischemia of small intestine**   HCC

K55.019 **Acute (reversible) ischemia of small intestine, extent unspecified**   HCC ▽

√6th **K55.02** **Acute infarction of small intestine**

Gangrene of small intestine

Necrosis of small intestine

K55.021 **Focal (segmental) acute infarction of small intestine**   HCC

K55.022 **Diffuse acute infarction of small intestine**   HCC

K55.029 **Acute infarction of small intestine, extent unspecified**   HCC ▽

√6th **K55.03** **Acute (reversible) ischemia of large intestine**

Acute fulminant ischemic colitis

Subacute ischemic colitis

K55.031 **Focal (segmental) acute (reversible) ischemia of large intestine**   HCC

K55.032 **Diffuse acute (reversible) ischemia of large intestine**   HCC

K55.039 **Acute (reversible) ischemia of large intestine, extent unspecified**   HCC ▽

√6th **K55.04** **Acute infarction of large intestine**

Gangrene of large intestine

Necrosis of large intestine

K55.041 **Focal (segmental) acute infarction of large intestine**   HCC

K55.042 **Diffuse acute infarction of large intestine**   HCC

K55.049 **Acute infarction of large intestine, extent unspecified**   HCC ▽

√6th **K55.05** **Acute (reversible) ischemia of intestine, part unspecified**

K55.051 **Focal (segmental) acute (reversible) ischemia of intestine, part unspecified**   HCC ▽

K55.052 **Diffuse acute (reversible) ischemia of intestine, part unspecified**   HCC ▽

K55.059 **Acute (reversible) ischemia of intestine, part and extent unspecified**   HCC ▽

√6th **K55.06** **Acute infarction of intestine, part unspecified**

Acute intestinal infarction

Gangrene of intestine

Necrosis of intestine

K55.061 **Focal (segmental) acute infarction of intestine, part unspecified**   HCC ▽

K55.062 **Diffuse acute infarction of intestine, part unspecified**   HCC ▽

K55.069 **Acute infarction of intestine, part and extent unspecified**   HCC ▽

K55.1 **Chronic vascular disorders of intestine**   HCC

Chronic ischemic colitis

Chronic ischemic enteritis

Chronic ischemic enterocolitis

Ischemic stricture of intestine

Mesenteric atherosclerosis

Mesenteric vascular insufficiency

√5th **K55.2** **Angiodysplasia of colon**

K55.20 **Angiodysplasia of colon without hemorrhage**

K55.21 **Angiodysplasia of colon with hemorrhage**
> **DEF:** Small vascular abnormalities due to fragile blood vessels in the colon, resulting in blood loss from the gastrointestinal (GI) tract.

√5ᵗʰ **K55.3** **Necrotizing enterocolitis**
> *EXCLUDES 1*   necrotizing enterocolitis of newborn (P77.-)
> *EXCLUDES 2*   necrotizing enterocolitis due to Clostridium difficile (A04.7-)

K55.30 **Necrotizing enterocolitis, unspecified** HCC ▽
> Necrotizing enterocolitis, NOS

K55.31 **Stage 1 necrotizing enterocolitis** HCC
> Necrotizing enterocolitis without pneumatosis, without perforation

K55.32 **Stage 2 necrotizing enterocolitis** HCC
> Necrotizing enterocolitis with pneumatosis, without perforation

K55.33 **Stage 3 necrotizing enterocolitis** HCC
> Necrotizing enterocolitis with perforation
> Necrotizing enterocolitis with pneumatosis and perforation

K55.8 **Other vascular disorders of intestine** HCC

K55.9 **Vascular disorder of intestine, unspecified** HCC ▽
> Ischemic colitis
> Ischemic enteritis
> Ischemic enterocolitis

√4ᵗʰ **K56** **Paralytic ileus and intestinal obstruction without hernia**
> *EXCLUDES 1*   congenital stricture or stenosis of intestine (Q41-Q42)
> cystic fibrosis with meconium ileus (E84.11)
> ischemic stricture of intestine (K55.1)
> meconium ileus NOS (P76.0)
> neonatal intestinal obstructions classifiable to P76.-
> obstruction of duodenum (K31.5)
> postprocedural intestinal obstruction (K91.3-)
> stenosis of anus or rectum (K62.4)

K56.0 **Paralytic ileus** HCC
> Paralysis of bowel
> Paralysis of colon
> Paralysis of intestine
> *EXCLUDES 1*   gallstone ileus (K56.3)
> ileus NOS (K56.7)
> obstructive ileus NOS (K56.69-)
> **DEF:** Intestinal obstruction due to paralysis of bowel motility or peristalsis.

K56.1 **Intussusception** HCC
> Intussusception or invagination of bowel
> Intussusception or invagination of colon
> Intussusception or invagination of intestine
> Intussusception or invagination of rectum
> *EXCLUDES 2*   intussusception of appendix (K38.8)
> **DEF:** Intestinal obstruction due to prolapse of a bowel section into an adjacent section. It occurs primarily in children and symptoms include acute abdominal pain, vomiting, and passage of blood and mucus from the rectum.

K56.2 **Volvulus** HCC
> Strangulation of colon or intestine
> Torsion of colon or intestine
> Twist of colon or intestine
> *EXCLUDES 2*   volvulus of duodenum (K31.5)
> **DEF:** Twisting, knotting, or entanglement of the bowel on itself that may quickly compromise oxygen supply to the intestinal tissues. A volvulus usually occurs at the sigmoid and ileocecal areas of the intestines.

Volvulus

Knotted intestine (volvulus)

K56.3 **Gallstone ileus** HCC
> Obstruction of intestine by gallstone

√5ᵗʰ **K56.4** **Other impaction of intestine**

K56.41 **Fecal impaction** HCC
> *EXCLUDES 1*   constipation (K59.0-)
> incomplete defecation (R15.0)

K56.49 **Other impaction of intestine** HCC

√5ᵗʰ **K56.5** **Intestinal adhesions [bands] with obstruction (postinfection)**
> Abdominal hernia due to adhesions with obstruction
> Peritoneal adhesions [bands] with intestinal obstruction (postinfection)
> **AHA:** 2017,4Q,16-17

K56.50 **Intestinal adhesions [bands], unspecified as to partial versus complete obstruction** HCC ▽
> Intestinal adhesions with obstruction NOS

K56.51 **Intestinal adhesions [bands], with partial obstruction** HCC
> Intestinal adhesions with incomplete obstruction

K56.52 **Intestinal adhesions [bands] with complete obstruction** HCC

√5ᵗʰ **K56.6** **Other and unspecified intestinal obstruction**
> **AHA:** 2017,4Q,16-17; 2017,2Q,12

√6ᵗʰ **K56.60** **Unspecified intestinal obstruction**
> *EXCLUDES 1*   intestinal obstruction due to specified condition - code to condition

K56.600 **Partial intestinal obstruction, unspecified as to cause** HCC ▽
> Incomplete intestinal obstruction, NOS

K56.601 **Complete intestinal obstruction, unspecified as to cause** HCC ▽

K56.609 **Unspecified intestinal obstruction, unspecified as to partial versus complete obstruction** HCC ▽
> Intestinal obstruction NOS

☑ Additional Character Req   √x7ᵗʰ Placeholder Alert   Manifestation   ▽ Unspecified   ▶◀ Revised Text   ● New Code   ▲ Revised Code Title

ICD-10-CM 2019

705

K55.21–K56.609

Chapter 11. Diseases of the Digestive System

✓6ᵗʰ **K56.69 Other intestinal obstruction**
Enterostenosis NOS
Obstructive ileus NOS
Occlusion of colon or intestine NOS
Stenosis of colon or intestine NOS
Stricture of colon or intestine NOS
EXCLUDES 1   *intestinal obstruction due to specified condition - code to condition*

     K56.690 Other partial intestinal   HCC
          obstruction
          Other incomplete intestinal obstruction

     K56.691 Other complete intestinal   HCC
          obstruction

     K56.699 Other intestinal obstruction   HCC ▽
          unspecified as to partial versus
          complete obstruction
          Other intestinal obstruction, NEC

K56.7 Ileus, unspecified   HCC ▽
   EXCLUDES 1   *obstructive ileus (K56.69-)*
   EXCLUDES 2   *intestinal obstruction with hernia (K40-K46)*
   AHA: 2017,1Q,40

✓4ᵗʰ **K57 Diverticular disease of intestine**
▶Code also if applicable peritonitis K65.-◀
   EXCLUDES 1   *congenital diverticulum of intestine (Q43.8)*
               Meckel's diverticulum (Q43.0)
   EXCLUDES 2   *diverticulum of appendix (K38.2)*

✓5ᵗʰ **K57.0 Diverticulitis of small intestine with perforation and abscess**
Diverticulitis of small intestine with peritonitis
   EXCLUDES 1   *diverticulitis of both small and large intestine with perforation and abscess (K57.4-)*

     K57.00 Diverticulitis of small intestine with perforation and abscess without bleeding

     K57.01 Diverticulitis of small intestine with perforation and abscess with bleeding

✓5ᵗʰ **K57.1 Diverticular disease of small intestine without perforation or abscess**
   EXCLUDES 1   *diverticular disease of both small and large intestine without perforation or abscess (K57.5-)*

     K57.10 Diverticulosis of small intestine without perforation or abscess without bleeding
          Diverticular disease of small intestine NOS

     K57.11 Diverticulosis of small intestine without perforation or abscess with bleeding

     K57.12 Diverticulitis of small intestine without perforation or abscess without bleeding

     K57.13 Diverticulitis of small intestine without perforation or abscess with bleeding

✓5ᵗʰ **K57.2 Diverticulitis of large intestine with perforation and abscess**
Diverticulitis of colon with peritonitis
   EXCLUDES 1   *diverticulitis of both small and large intestine with perforation and abscess (K57.4-)*

     K57.20 Diverticulitis of large intestine with perforation and abscess without bleeding

     K57.21 Diverticulitis of large intestine with perforation and abscess with bleeding

✓5ᵗʰ **K57.3 Diverticular disease of large intestine without perforation or abscess**
   EXCLUDES 1   *diverticular disease of both small and large intestine without perforation or abscess (K57.5-)*

     K57.30 Diverticulosis of large intestine without perforation or abscess without bleeding
          Diverticular disease of colon NOS

     K57.31 Diverticulosis of large intestine without perforation or abscess with bleeding

     K57.32 Diverticulitis of large intestine without perforation or abscess without bleeding

     K57.33 Diverticulitis of large intestine without perforation or abscess with bleeding

✓5ᵗʰ **K57.4 Diverticulitis of both small and large intestine with perforation and abscess**
Diverticulitis of both small and large intestine with peritonitis

     K57.40 Diverticulitis of both small and large intestine with perforation and abscess without bleeding

     K57.41 Diverticulitis of both small and large intestine with perforation and abscess with bleeding

✓5ᵗʰ **K57.5 Diverticular disease of both small and large intestine without perforation or abscess**

     K57.50 Diverticulosis of both small and large intestine without perforation or abscess without bleeding
          Diverticular disease of both small and large intestine NOS

     K57.51 Diverticulosis of both small and large intestine without perforation or abscess with bleeding

     K57.52 Diverticulitis of both small and large intestine without perforation or abscess without bleeding

     K57.53 Diverticulitis of both small and large intestine without perforation or abscess with bleeding

✓5ᵗʰ **K57.8 Diverticulitis of intestine, part unspecified, with perforation and abscess**
Diverticulitis of intestine NOS with peritonitis

     K57.80 Diverticulitis of intestine, part unspecified, with perforation and abscess without bleeding   ▽

     K57.81 Diverticulitis of intestine, part unspecified, with perforation and abscess with bleeding   ▽

✓5ᵗʰ **K57.9 Diverticular disease of intestine, part unspecified, without perforation or abscess**

     K57.90 Diverticulosis of intestine, part unspecified, without perforation or abscess without bleeding   ▽
          Diverticular disease of intestine NOS

     K57.91 Diverticulosis of intestine, part unspecified, without perforation or abscess with bleeding   ▽

     K57.92 Diverticulitis of intestine, part unspecified, without perforation or abscess without bleeding   ▽

     K57.93 Diverticulitis of intestine, part unspecified, without perforation or abscess with bleeding   ▽

✓4ᵗʰ **K58 Irritable bowel syndrome**
   INCLUDES   irritable colon
              spastic colon
   AHA: 2016,4Q,32-33

   K58.0 Irritable bowel syndrome with diarrhea
   K58.1 Irritable bowel syndrome with constipation
   K58.2 Mixed irritable bowel syndrome
   K58.8 Other irritable bowel syndrome
   K58.9 Irritable bowel syndrome without diarrhea
     Irritable bowel syndrome NOS

✓4ᵗʰ **K59 Other functional intestinal disorders**
   EXCLUDES 1   *change in bowel habit NOS (R19.4)*
               intestinal malabsorption (K90.-)
               psychogenic intestinal disorders (F45.8)
   EXCLUDES 2   *functional disorders of stomach (K31.-)*

✓5ᵗʰ **K59.0 Constipation**
Use additional code for adverse effect, if applicable, to identify drug (T36-T50 with fifth or sixth character 5)
   EXCLUDES 1   *fecal impaction (K56.41)*
               incomplete defecation (R15.0)
   AHA: 2016,4Q,33

     K59.00 Constipation, unspecified   ▽
     K59.01 Slow transit constipation
          DEF: Delay in the transit of fecal material through the colon secondary to smooth muscle dysfunction or decreased peristaltic contractions along the colon.

     K59.02 Outlet dysfunction constipation
     K59.03 Drug induced constipation
          Use additional code for adverse effect, if applicable, to identify drug (T36-T50 with fifth or sixth character 5)

     K59.04 Chronic idiopathic constipation
          Functional constipation

     K59.09 Other constipation
          Chronic constipation

   K59.1 Functional diarrhea
     EXCLUDES 1   *diarrhea NOS (R19.7)*
               irritable bowel syndrome with diarrhea (K58.0)

K59.2 Neurogenic bowel, not elsewhere classified
> **DEF:** Disorder of bowel due to a spinal cord lesion due to injury or as a complication of conditions such as multiple sclerosis (MS) or spina bifida. Loss of bowel control is the primary symptom, manifested as constipation or bowel incontinence.

√5ᵗʰ **K59.3 Megacolon, not elsewhere classified**
> Dilatation of colon
> Code first, if applicable (T51-T65) to identify toxic agent
> **EXCLUDES 1**   congenital megacolon (aganglionic) (Q43.1)
>   megacolon (due to) (in) Chagas' disease (B57.32)
>   megacolon (due to) (in) Clostridium difficile (A04.7-)
>   megacolon (due to) (in) Hirschsprung's disease (Q43.1)
> **AHA:** 2016,4Q,33-34

     K59.31 Toxic megacolon   HCC

     K59.39 Other megacolon
> Megacolon NOS

K59.4 Anal spasm
> Proctalgia fugax

K59.8 Other specified functional intestinal disorders
> Atony of colon
> Pseudo-obstruction (acute) (chronic) of intestine

K59.9 Functional intestinal disorder, unspecified ▽

√4ᵗʰ **K60 Fissure and fistula of anal and rectal regions**
> **EXCLUDES 1**   fissure and fistula of anal and rectal regions with abscess or cellulitis (K61.-)
> **EXCLUDES 2**   anal sphincter tear (healed) (nontraumatic) (old) (K62.81)

K60.0 Acute anal fissure

K60.1 Chronic anal fissure

K60.2 Anal fissure, unspecified ▽

K60.3 Anal fistula

K60.4 Rectal fistula
> Fistula of rectum to skin
> **EXCLUDES 1**   rectovaginal fistula (N82.3)
>   vesicorectal fistual (N32.1)

K60.5 Anorectal fistula

√4ᵗʰ **K61 Abscess of anal and rectal regions**
> **INCLUDES**   abscess of anal and rectal regions
>   cellulitis of anal and rectal regions

K61.0 Anal abscess
> Perianal abscess
> **EXCLUDES 1**   intrasphincteric abscess (K61.4)
> **EXCLUDES 2**   ▶intrasphincteric abscess (K61.4)◀

K61.1 Rectal abscess
> Perirectal abscess
> **EXCLUDES 1**   ischiorectal abscess ▶(K61.39)◀
> **AHA:** 2012,4Q,104

K61.2 Anorectal abscess

√5ᵗʰ **K61.3 Ischiorectal abscess**
> Abscess of ischiorectal fossa

    ●   **K61.31 Horseshoe abscess**

    ●   **K61.39 Other ischiorectal abscess**
> Abscess of ischiorectal fossa
> Ischiorectal abscess, NOS

K61.4 Intrasphincteric abscess
> ▶Intersphincteric abscess◀

    ● **K61.5 Supralevator abscess**

√4ᵗʰ **K62 Other diseases of anus and rectum**
> **INCLUDES**   anal canal
> **EXCLUDES 2**   colostomy and enterostomy malfunction (K94.0-, K94.1-)
>   fecal incontinence (R15.-)
>   hemorrhoids (K64.-)

K62.0 Anal polyp

K62.1 Rectal polyp
> **EXCLUDES 1**   adenomatous polyp (D12.8)
> **AHA:** 2018,1Q,6

K62.2 Anal prolapse
> Prolapse of anal canal

K62.3 Rectal prolapse
> Prolapse of rectal mucosa

K62.4 Stenosis of anus and rectum
> Stricture of anus (sphincter)

K62.5 Hemorrhage of anus and rectum
> **EXCLUDES 1**   gastrointestinal bleeding NOS (K92.2)
>   melena (K92.1)
>   neonatal rectal hemorrhage (P54.2)

K62.6 Ulcer of anus and rectum
> Solitary ulcer of anus and rectum
> Stercoral ulcer of anus and rectum
> **EXCLUDES 1**   fissure and fistula of anus and rectum (K60.-)
>   ulcerative colitis (K51.-)

K62.7 Radiation proctitis
> Use additional code to identify the type of radiation (W90.-)

√5ᵗʰ **K62.8 Other specified diseases of anus and rectum**
> **EXCLUDES 2**   ulcerative proctitis (K51.2)

     K62.81 Anal sphincter tear (healed) (nontraumatic) (old)
> Tear of anus, nontraumatic
> Use additional code for any associated fecal incontinence (R15.-)
> **EXCLUDES 2**   anal fissure (K60.-)
>   anal sphincter tear (healed) (old) complicating delivery (O34.7-)
>   traumatic tear of anal sphincter (S31.831)

     K62.82 Dysplasia of anus
> Anal intraepithelial neoplasia I and II (AIN I and II) (histologically confirmed)
> Dysplasia of anus NOS
> Mild and moderate dysplasia of anus (histologically confirmed)
> **EXCLUDES 1**   abnormal results from anal cytologic examination without histologic confirmation (R85.61-)
>   anal intraepithelial neoplasia III (D01.3)
>   carcinoma in situ of anus (D01.3)
>   HGSIL of anus (R85.613)
>   severe dysplasia of anus (D01.3)

     K62.89 Other specified diseases of anus and rectum
> Proctitis NOS
> Use additional code for any associated fecal incontinence (R15.-)

K62.9 Disease of anus and rectum, unspecified ▽

√4ᵗʰ **K63 Other diseases of intestine**

K63.0 Abscess of intestine
> **EXCLUDES 1**   abscess of intestine with Crohn's disease (K50.014, K50.114, K50.814, K50.914)
>   abscess of intestine with diverticular disease (K57.0, K57.2, K57.4, K57.8)
>   abscess of intestine with ulcerative colitis (K51.014, K51.214, K51.314, K51.414, K51.514, K51.814, K51.914)
> **EXCLUDES 2**   abscess of anal and rectal regions (K61.-)
>   abscess of appendix ▶(K35.3-)◀

K63.1 Perforation of intestine (nontraumatic)   HCC
> Perforation (nontraumatic) of rectum
> **EXCLUDES 1**   perforation (nontraumatic) of duodenum (K26.-)
>   perforation (nontraumatic) of intestine with diverticular disease (K57.0, K57.2, K57.4, K57.8)
> **EXCLUDES 2**   perforation (nontraumatic) of appendix ▶(K35.2-, K35.3-)◀

K63.2 Fistula of intestine
> **EXCLUDES 1**   fistula of duodenum (K31.6)
>   fistula of intestine with Crohn's disease (K50.013, K50.113, K50.813, K50.913)
>   fistula of intestine with ulcerative colitis (K51.013, K51.213, K51.313, K51.413, K51.513, K51.813, K51.913)
> **EXCLUDES 2**   fistula of anal and rectal regions (K60.-)
>   fistula of appendix (K38.3)
>   intestinal-genital fistula, female (N82.2-N82.4)
>   vesicointestinal fistula (N32.1)
> **AHA:** 2017,3Q,4

☑ Additional Character Req   √x7ᵗʰ Placeholder Alert   Manifestation   ▽ Unspecified   ▶◀ Revised Text   ● New Code   ▲ Revised Code Title

K63.3   Ulcer of intestine
Primary ulcer of small intestine
- **EXCLUDES 1**   *duodenal ulcer (K26.-)*
  gastrointestinal ulcer (K28.-)
  gastrojejunal ulcer (K28.-)
  jejunal ulcer (K28.-)
  peptic ulcer, site unspecified (K27.-)
  ulcer of intestine with perforation (K63.1)
  ulcer of anus or rectum (K62.6)
  ulcerative colitis (K51.-)

K63.4   Enteroptosis

K63.5   Polyp of colon
- **EXCLUDES 1**   *adenomatous polyp of colon (D12.6)*
  inflammatory polyp of colon (K51.4-)
  polyposis of colon (D12.6)

     AHA: 2018,2Q,14; 2017,1Q,15; 2015,2Q,14

✓5th   K63.8   Other specified diseases of intestine

K63.81   Dieulafoy lesion of intestine
- **EXCLUDES 2**   *Dieulafoy lesion of stomach and duodenum (K31.82)*

DEF: Abnormally large submucosal artery protruding through a defect in the stomach mucosa or intestines that can cause massive and life-threatening hemorrhaging.

K63.89   Other specified diseases of intestine
     AHA: 2013,2Q,31

K63.9   Disease of intestine, unspecified   ▽

✓4th   K64   Hemorrhoids and perianal venous thrombosis
- **INCLUDES**   piles
- **EXCLUDES 1**   *hemorrhoids complicating childbirth and the puerperium (O87.2)*
  hemorrhoids complicating pregnancy (O22.4)

Hemorrhoids

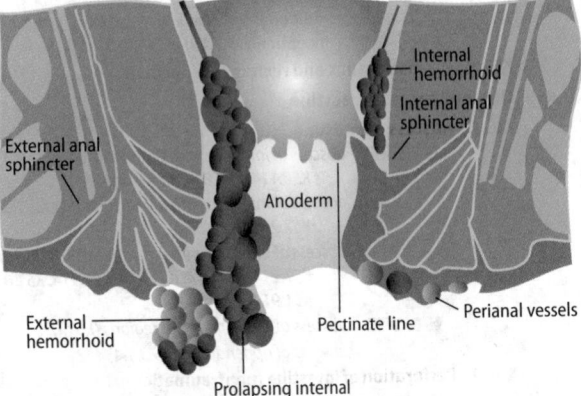

External anal sphincter
Internal hemorrhoid
Internal anal sphincter
Anoderm
External hemorrhoid
Pectinate line
Perianal vessels
Prolapsing internal hemorrhoid

K64.0   First degree hemorrhoids
Grade/stage I hemorrhoids
Hemorrhoids (bleeding) without prolapse outside of anal canal

K64.1   Second degree hemorrhoids
Grade/stage II hemorrhoids
Hemorrhoids (bleeding) that prolapse with straining, but retract spontaneously

K64.2   Third degree hemorrhoids
Grade/stage III hemorrhoids
Hemorrhoids (bleeding) that prolapse with straining and require manual replacement back inside anal canal

K64.3   Fourth degree hemorrhoids
Grade/stage IV hemorrhoids
Hemorrhoids (bleeding) with prolapsed tissue that cannot be manually replaced

K64.4   Residual hemorrhoidal skin tags
External hemorrhoids, NOS
Skin tags of anus

K64.5   Perianal venous thrombosis
External hemorrhoids with thrombosis
Perianal hematoma
Thrombosed hemorrhoids NOS

K64.8   Other hemorrhoids
Internal hemorrhoids, without mention of degree
Prolapsed hemorrhoids, degree not specified

K64.9   Unspecified hemorrhoids   ▽
Hemorrhoids (bleeding) NOS
Hemorrhoids (bleeding) without mention of degree

Diseases of peritoneum and retroperitoneum (K65-K68)

✓4th   K65   Peritonitis
▶ Use additional code (B95-B97), to identify infectious agent, if known ◀
▶ Code also if applicable diverticular disease of intestine (K57.-) ◀
- **EXCLUDES 1**   *acute appendicitis with generalized peritonitis ▶(K35.2-)◀*
  aseptic peritonitis (T81.6)
  benign paroxysmal peritonitis (E85.0)
  chemical peritonitis (T81.6)
  ~~*diverticulitis of both small and large intestine with peritonitis (K57.4-)*~~
  ~~*diverticulitis of colon with peritonitis (K57.2-)*~~
  ~~*diverticulitis of intestine, NOS, with peritonitis (K57.8-)*~~
  ~~*diverticulitis of small intestine with peritonitis (K57.0-)*~~
  gonococcal peritonitis (A54.85)
  neonatal peritonitis (P78.0-P78.1)
  pelvic peritonitis, female (N73.3-N73.5)
  periodic familial peritonitis (E85.0)
  peritonitis due to talc or other foreign substance (T81.6)
  peritonitis in chlamydia (A74.81)
  peritonitis in diphtheria (A36.89)
  peritonitis in syphilis (late) (A52.74)
  peritonitis in tuberculosis (A18.31)
  peritonitis with or following abortion or ectopic or molar pregnancy (O00-O07, O08.0)
  peritonitis with or following appendicitis (K35.-)
  ~~*peritonitis with or following diverticular disease of intestine (K57.-)*~~
  puerperal peritonitis (O85)
  retroperitoneal infections (K68.-)

K65.0   Generalized (acute) peritonitis   HCC
Pelvic peritonitis (acute), male
Subphrenic peritonitis (acute)
Suppurative peritonitis (acute)

K65.1   Peritoneal abscess   HCC
Abdominopelvic abscess
Abscess (of) omentum
Abscess (of) peritoneum
Mesenteric abscess
Retrocecal abscess
Subdiaphragmatic abscess
Subhepatic abscess
Subphrenic abscess

K65.2   Spontaneous bacterial peritonitis   HCC
- **EXCLUDES 1**   *bacterial peritonitis NOS (K65.9)*

K65.3   Choleperitonitis   HCC
Peritonitis due to bile
DEF: Inflammation of the peritoneum due to leakage of bile into the peritoneal cavity resulting from rupture of the bile passages or gallbladder.

K65.4   Sclerosing mesenteritis   HCC
Fat necrosis of peritoneum
(Idiopathic) sclerosing mesenteric fibrosis
Mesenteric lipodystrophy
Mesenteric panniculitis
Retractile mesenteritis

K65.8   Other peritonitis   HCC
Chronic proliferative peritonitis
Peritonitis due to urine

K65.9   Peritonitis, unspecified   HCC ▽
Bacterial peritonitis NOS
AHA: 2013,2Q,31

√4ᵗʰ **K66 Other disorders of peritoneum**

    EXCLUDES 2   *ascites (R18.-)*
                   peritoneal effusion (chronic) (R18.8)

    K66.0 Peritoneal adhesions (postprocedural) (postinfection)
         Adhesions (of) abdominal (wall)
         Adhesions (of) diaphragm
         Adhesions (of) intestine
         Adhesions (of) male pelvis
         Adhesions (of) omentum
         Adhesions (of) stomach
         Adhesive bands
         Mesenteric adhesions
         EXCLUDES 1   *female pelvic adhesions [bands] (N73.6)*
                       peritoneal adhesions with intestinal obstruction (K56.5-)

    K66.1 Hemoperitoneum
         EXCLUDES 1   *traumatic hemoperitoneum (S36.8-)*

    K66.8 Other specified disorders of peritoneum
    K66.9 Disorder of peritoneum, unspecified ▽

K67 Disorders of peritoneum in infectious diseases classified elsewhere   HCC

     Code first underlying disease, such as:
         congenital syphilis (A50.0)
         helminthiasis (B65.0-B83.9)
         EXCLUDES 1   *peritonitis in chlamydia (A74.81)*
                       peritonitis in diphtheria (A36.89)
                       peritonitis in gonococcal (A54.85)
                       peritonitis in syphilis (late) (A52.74)
                       peritonitis in tuberculosis (A18.31)

√4ᵗʰ **K68 Disorders of retroperitoneum**

√5ᵗʰ   **K68.1 Retroperitoneal abscess**

         K68.11 Postprocedural retroperitoneal abscess
               EXCLUDES 2   ▶*infection following procedure (T81.4-)*◀
         K68.12 Psoas muscle abscess   HCC
         K68.19 Other retroperitoneal abscess   HCC
    K68.9 Other disorders of retroperitoneum

Diseases of liver (K70-K77)

     EXCLUDES 1   *jaundice NOS (R17)*
     EXCLUDES 2   *hemochromatosis (E83.11-)*
                   Reye's syndrome (G93.7)
                   viral hepatitis (B15-B19)
                   Wilson's disease (E83.0)

√4ᵗʰ **K70 Alcoholic liver disease**

     Use additional code to identify:
         alcohol abuse and dependence (F10.-)

    K70.0 Alcoholic fatty liver   A

√5ᵗʰ   **K70.1 Alcoholic hepatitis**
         K70.10 Alcoholic hepatitis without ascites   A
         K70.11 Alcoholic hepatitis with ascites   A
    K70.2 Alcoholic fibrosis and sclerosis of liver   A

√5ᵗʰ   **K70.3 Alcoholic cirrhosis of liver**
         Alcoholic cirrhosis NOS
         K70.30 Alcoholic cirrhosis of liver without ascites   HCC A
         K70.31 Alcoholic cirrhosis of liver with ascites   HCC A
               AHA: 2018,1Q,4

√5ᵗʰ   **K70.4 Alcoholic hepatic failure**
         Acute alcoholic hepatic failure
         Alcoholic hepatic failure NOS
         Chronic alcoholic hepatic failure
         Subacute alcoholic hepatic failure
         K70.40 Alcoholic hepatic failure without coma   HCC A
         K70.41 Alcoholic hepatic failure with coma   HCC A
    K70.9 Alcoholic liver disease, unspecified   HCC A ▽

√4ᵗʰ **K71 Toxic liver disease**

     INCLUDES   drug-induced idiosyncratic (unpredictable) liver disease
                   drug-induced toxic (predictable) liver disease
     Code first poisoning due to drug or toxin, if applicable (T36-T65 with fifth or sixth character 1-4 or 6)
     Use additional code for adverse effect, if applicable, to identify drug (T36-T50 with fifth or sixth character 5)
     EXCLUDES 2   *alcoholic liver disease (K70.-)*
                   Budd-Chiari syndrome (I82.0)

    K71.0 Toxic liver disease with cholestasis
         Cholestasis with hepatocyte injury
         "Pure" cholestasis

√5ᵗʰ   **K71.1 Toxic liver disease with hepatic necrosis**
         Hepatic failure (acute) (chronic) due to drugs
         K71.10 Toxic liver disease with hepatic necrosis, without coma
         K71.11 Toxic liver disease with hepatic necrosis, with coma   HCC

    K71.2 Toxic liver disease with acute hepatitis
    K71.3 Toxic liver disease with chronic persistent hepatitis
    K71.4 Toxic liver disease with chronic lobular hepatitis

√5ᵗʰ   **K71.5 Toxic liver disease with chronic active hepatitis**
         Toxic liver disease with lupoid hepatitis
         K71.50 Toxic liver disease with chronic active hepatitis without ascites
         K71.51 Toxic liver disease with chronic active hepatitis with ascites
               AHA: 2018,1Q,4

    K71.6 Toxic liver disease with hepatitis, not elsewhere classified
    K71.7 Toxic liver disease with fibrosis and cirrhosis of liver
    K71.8 Toxic liver disease with other disorders of liver
         Toxic liver disease with focal nodular hyperplasia
         Toxic liver disease with hepatic granulomas
         Toxic liver disease with peliosis hepatis
         Toxic liver disease with veno-occlusive disease of liver
    K71.9 Toxic liver disease, unspecified ▽

√4ᵗʰ **K72 Hepatic failure, not elsewhere classified**

     INCLUDES   fulminant hepatitis NEC, with hepatic failure
                   hepatic encephalopathy NOS
                   liver (cell) necrosis with hepatic failure
                   malignant hepatitis NEC, with hepatic failure
                   yellow liver atrophy or dystrophy
     EXCLUDES 1   *alcoholic hepatic failure (K70.4)*
                   hepatic failure with toxic liver disease (K71.1-)
                   icterus of newborn (P55-P59)
                   postprocedural hepatic failure (K91.82)
     EXCLUDES 2   *hepatic failure complicating abortion or ectopic or molar pregnancy (O00-O07, O08.8)*
                   hepatic failure complicating pregnancy, childbirth and the puerperium (O26.6-)
                   viral hepatitis with hepatic coma (B15-B19)
     AHA: 2017,1Q,41

√5ᵗʰ   **K72.0 Acute and subacute hepatic failure**
         Acute non-viral hepatitis NOS
         AHA: 2015,2Q,17; 2014,2Q,13
         K72.00 Acute and subacute hepatic failure without coma
         K72.01 Acute and subacute hepatic failure with coma   HCC

√5ᵗʰ   **K72.1 Chronic hepatic failure**
         K72.10 Chronic hepatic failure without coma   HCC
         K72.11 Chronic hepatic failure with coma   HCC

√5ᵗʰ   **K72.9 Hepatic failure, unspecified**
         K72.90 Hepatic failure, unspecified without coma   HCC ▽
               AHA: 2016,2Q,35
         K72.91 Hepatic failure, unspecified with coma   HCC ▽
               Hepatic coma NOS

√4ᵗʰ **K73 Chronic hepatitis, not elsewhere classified**

     EXCLUDES 1   *alcoholic hepatitis (chronic) (K70.1-)*
                   drug-induced hepatitis (chronic) (K71.-)
                   granulomatous hepatitis (chronic) NEC (K75.3)
                   reactive, nonspecific hepatitis (chronic) (K75.2)
                   viral hepatitis (chronic) (B15-B19)

    K73.0 Chronic persistent hepatitis, not elsewhere classified   HCC
    K73.1 Chronic lobular hepatitis, not elsewhere classified   HCC
    K73.2 Chronic active hepatitis, not elsewhere classified   HCC

☑ Additional Character Req   ✓x7ᵗʰ Placeholder Alert   **Manifestation**   ▽ Unspecified   ▶◀ Revised Text   ● New Code   ▲ Revised Code Title

ICD-10-CM 2019   709

Chapter 11. Diseases of the Digestive System

K73.8   **Other chronic hepatitis, not elsewhere classified**   HCC

K73.9   **Chronic hepatitis, unspecified**   HCC ▽

√4ᵗʰ **K74**   **Fibrosis and cirrhosis of liver**

Code also, if applicable, viral hepatitis (acute) (chronic) (B15-B19)

EXCLUDES 1   *alcoholic cirrhosis (of liver) (K70.3)*
alcoholic fibrosis of liver (K70.2)
cardiac sclerosis of liver (K76.1)
cirrhosis (of liver) with toxic liver disease (K71.7)
congenital cirrhosis (of liver) (P78.81)
pigmentary cirrhosis (of liver) (E83.110)

K74.0   **Hepatic fibrosis**

K74.1   **Hepatic sclerosis**

K74.2   **Hepatic fibrosis with hepatic sclerosis**

K74.3   **Primary biliary cirrhosis**   HCC
Chronic nonsuppurative destructive cholangitis
▶Primary biliary cholangitis◀
EXCLUDES 2   ▶*primary sclerosing cholangitis (K83.01)*◀

K74.4   **Secondary biliary cirrhosis**   HCC

K74.5   **Biliary cirrhosis, unspecified**   HCC ▽

√5ᵗʰ **K74.6**   **Other and unspecified cirrhosis of liver**   HCC ▽

     K74.60   **Unspecified cirrhosis of liver**
Cirrhosis (of liver) NOS
AHA: 2018,1Q,4

     K74.69   **Other cirrhosis of liver**   HCC
Cryptogenic cirrhosis (of liver)
Macronodular cirrhosis (of liver)
Micronodular cirrhosis (of liver)
Mixed type cirrhosis (of liver)
Portal cirrhosis (of liver)
Postnecrotic cirrhosis (of liver)

√4ᵗʰ **K75**   **Other inflammatory liver diseases**

EXCLUDES 2   *toxic liver disease (K71.-)*

K75.0   **Abscess of liver**
Cholangitic hepatic abscess
Hematogenic hepatic abscess
Hepatic abscess NOS
Lymphogenic hepatic abscess
Pylephlebitic hepatic abscess
EXCLUDES 1   *amebic liver abscess (A06.4)*
cholangitis without liver abscess ▶(K83.09)◀
pylephlebitis without liver abscess (K75.1)
EXCLUDES 2   *acute or subacute hepatitis NOS (B17.9)*
acute or subacute non-viral hepatitis (K72.0)
chronic hepatitis NEC (K73.8)

K75.1   **Phlebitis of portal vein**
Pylephlebitis
EXCLUDES 1   *pylephlebitic liver abscess (K75.0)*
DEF: Inflammation of the portal vein or branches due to diverticulitis, perforated appendicitis, or peritonitis. Symptoms include fever, chills, jaundice, sweating, and abscess in various body parts.

K75.2   **Nonspecific reactive hepatitis**
EXCLUDES 1   *acute or subacute hepatitis (K72.0-)*
chronic hepatitis NEC (K73.-)
viral hepatitis (B15-B19)

K75.3   **Granulomatous hepatitis, not elsewhere classified**
EXCLUDES 1   *acute or subacute hepatitis (K72.0-)*
chronic hepatitis NEC (K73.-)
viral hepatitis (B15-B19)

K75.4   **Autoimmune hepatitis**   HCC
Lupoid hepatitis NEC

√5ᵗʰ **K75.8**   **Other specified inflammatory liver diseases**

     K75.81   **Nonalcoholic steatohepatitis (NASH)**

     K75.89   **Other specified inflammatory liver diseases**

K75.9   **Inflammatory liver disease, unspecified**   ▽
Hepatitis NOS
EXCLUDES 1   *acute or subacute hepatitis (K72.0-)*
chronic hepatitis NEC (K73.-)
viral hepatitis (B15-B19)
AHA: 2015,2Q,17

√4ᵗʰ **K76**   **Other diseases of liver**

EXCLUDES 2   *alcoholic liver disease (K70.-)*
amyloid degeneration of liver (E85.-)
cystic disease of liver (congenital) (Q44.6)
hepatic vein thrombosis (I82.0)
hepatomegaly NOS (R16.0)
pigmentary cirrhosis (of liver) (E83.110)
portal vein thrombosis (I81)
toxic liver disease (K71.-)

K76.0   **Fatty (change of) liver, not elsewhere classified**
Nonalcoholic fatty liver disease (NAFLD)
EXCLUDES 1   *nonalcoholic steatohepatitis (NASH) (K75.81)*

K76.1   **Chronic passive congestion of liver**
Cardiac cirrhosis
Cardiac sclerosis

K76.2   **Central hemorrhagic necrosis of liver**
EXCLUDES 1   *liver necrosis with hepatic failure (K72.-)*

K76.3   **Infarction of liver**

K76.4   **Peliosis hepatis**
Hepatic angiomatosis

K76.5   **Hepatic veno-occlusive disease**
EXCLUDES 1   *Budd-Chiari syndrome (I82.0)*

K76.6   **Portal hypertension**   HCC
Use additional code for any associated complications, such as:
portal hypertensive gastropathy (K31.89)

K76.7   **Hepatorenal syndrome**   HCC
EXCLUDES 1   *hepatorenal syndrome following labor and delivery (O90.4)*
postprocedural hepatorenal syndrome (K91.83)

√5ᵗʰ **K76.8**   **Other specified diseases of liver**

     K76.81   **Hepatopulmonary syndrome**   HCC
Code first underlying liver disease, such as:
alcoholic cirrhosis of liver (K70.3-)
cirrhosis of liver without mention of alcohol (K74.6-)

     K76.89   **Other specified diseases of liver**
Cyst (simple) of liver
Focal nodular hyperplasia of liver
Hepatoptosis

K76.9   **Liver disease, unspecified**   ▽

K77   ***Liver disorders in diseases classified elsewhere***
Code first underlying disease, such as:
amyloidosis (E85.-)
congenital syphilis (A50.0, A50.5)
congenital toxoplasmosis (P37.1)
schistosomiasis (B65.0-B65.9)
EXCLUDES 1   *alcoholic hepatitis (K70.1-)*
alcoholic liver disease (K70.-)
cytomegaloviral hepatitis (B25.1)
herpesviral [herpes simplex] hepatitis (B00.81)
infectious mononucleosis with liver disease (B27.0-B27.9 with .9)
mumps hepatitis (B26.81)
sarcoidosis with liver disease (D86.89)
secondary syphilis with liver disease (A51.45)
syphilis (late) with liver disease (A52.74)
toxoplasmosis (acquired) hepatitis (B58.1)
tuberculosis with liver disease (A18.83)

Disorders of gallbladder, biliary tract and pancreas (K80-K87)

√4ᵗʰ **K80   Cholelithiasis**

> **EXCLUDES 1**   *retained cholelithiasis following cholecystectomy (K91.86)*
> **DEF:** Presence or formation of concretions (calculi or "gallstones") in the gallbladder. The stones contain cholesterol, calcium carbonate, or calcium bilirubinate in pure forms or in various combinations.

Cholelithiasis

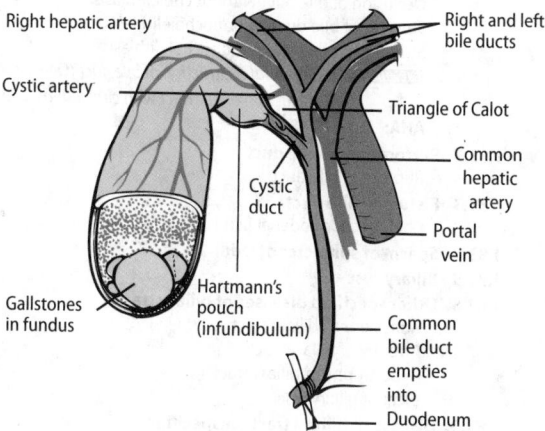

Right hepatic artery
Right and left bile ducts
Cystic artery
Triangle of Calot
Cystic duct
Common hepatic artery
Portal vein
Gallstones in fundus
Hartmann's pouch (infundibulum)
Common bile duct empties into Duodenum

√5ᵗʰ **K80.0   Calculus of gallbladder with acute cholecystitis**

> Any condition listed in K80.2 with acute cholecystitis
> ►Use additional code if applicable for associated gangrene of gallbladder (K82.A1), or perforation of gallbladder (K82.A2)◄

    K80.00   Calculus of gallbladder with acute cholecystitis without obstruction

    K80.01   Calculus of gallbladder with acute cholecystitis with obstruction

√5ᵗʰ **K80.1   Calculus of gallbladder with other cholecystitis**

> ►Use additional code if applicable for associated gangrene of gallbladder (K82.A1), or perforation of gallbladder (K82.A2)◄

    K80.10   Calculus of gallbladder with chronic cholecystitis without obstruction
        Cholelithiasis with cholecystitis NOS

    K80.11   Calculus of gallbladder with chronic cholecystitis with obstruction

    K80.12   Calculus of gallbladder with acute and chronic cholecystitis without obstruction

    K80.13   Calculus of gallbladder with acute and chronic cholecystitis with obstruction

    K80.18   Calculus of gallbladder with other cholecystitis without obstruction

    K80.19   Calculus of gallbladder with other cholecystitis with obstruction

√5ᵗʰ **K80.2   Calculus of gallbladder without cholecystitis**

> Cholecystolithiasis without cholecystitis
> Cholelithiasis (without cholecystitis)
> Colic (recurrent) of gallbladder (without cholecystitis)
> Gallstone (impacted) of cystic duct (without cholecystitis)
> Gallstone (impacted) of gallbladder (without cholecystitis)

    K80.20   Calculus of gallbladder without cholecystitis without obstruction

    K80.21   Calculus of gallbladder without cholecystitis with obstruction

√5ᵗʰ **K80.3   Calculus of bile duct with cholangitis**

> Any condition listed in K80.5 with cholangitis
> **DEF:** Cholangitis: Inflammation of the bile ducts.

    K80.30   Calculus of bile duct with cholangitis, unspecified, without obstruction   ▽

    K80.31   Calculus of bile duct with cholangitis, unspecified, with obstruction   ▽

    K80.32   Calculus of bile duct with acute cholangitis without obstruction

    K80.33   Calculus of bile duct with acute cholangitis with obstruction

    K80.34   Calculus of bile duct with chronic cholangitis without obstruction

    K80.35   Calculus of bile duct with chronic cholangitis with obstruction

    K80.36   Calculus of bile duct with acute and chronic cholangitis without obstruction

    K80.37   Calculus of bile duct with acute and chronic cholangitis with obstruction

√5ᵗʰ **K80.4   Calculus of bile duct with cholecystitis**

> Any condition listed in K80.5 with cholecystitis (with cholangitis)
> ►Use additional code if applicable for associated gangrene of gallbladder (K82.A1), or perforation of gallbladder (K82.A2)◄

    K80.40   Calculus of bile duct with cholecystitis, unspecified, without obstruction   ▽

    K80.41   Calculus of bile duct with cholecystitis, unspecified, with obstruction   ▽

    K80.42   Calculus of bile duct with acute cholecystitis without obstruction

    K80.43   Calculus of bile duct with acute cholecystitis with obstruction

    K80.44   Calculus of bile duct with chronic cholecystitis without obstruction

    K80.45   Calculus of bile duct with chronic cholecystitis with obstruction

    K80.46   Calculus of bile duct with acute and chronic cholecystitis without obstruction

    K80.47   Calculus of bile duct with acute and chronic cholecystitis with obstruction

√5ᵗʰ **K80.5   Calculus of bile duct without cholangitis or cholecystitis**

> Choledocholithiasis (without cholangitis or cholecystitis)
> Gallstone (impacted) of bile duct NOS (without cholangitis or cholecystitis)
> Gallstone (impacted) of common duct (without cholangitis or cholecystitis)
> Gallstone (impacted) of hepatic duct (without cholangitis or cholecystitis)
> Hepatic cholelithiasis (without cholangitis or cholecystitis)
> Hepatic colic (recurrent) (without cholangitis or cholecystitis)
> **DEF:** Cholangitis: Inflammation of the bile ducts.

    K80.50   Calculus of bile duct without cholangitis or cholecystitis without obstruction

    K80.51   Calculus of bile duct without cholangitis or cholecystitis with obstruction

√5ᵗʰ **K80.6   Calculus of gallbladder and bile duct with cholecystitis**

> ►Use additional code if applicable for associated gangrene of gallbladder (K82.A1), or perforation of gallbladder (K82.A2)◄

    K80.60   Calculus of gallbladder and bile duct with cholecystitis, unspecified, without obstruction   ▽

    K80.61   Calculus of gallbladder and bile duct with cholecystitis, unspecified, with obstruction   ▽

    K80.62   Calculus of gallbladder and bile duct with acute cholecystitis without obstruction

    K80.63   Calculus of gallbladder and bile duct with acute cholecystitis with obstruction

    K80.64   Calculus of gallbladder and bile duct with chronic cholecystitis without obstruction

    K80.65   Calculus of gallbladder and bile duct with chronic cholecystitis with obstruction

    K80.66   Calculus of gallbladder and bile duct with acute and chronic cholecystitis without obstruction

    K80.67   Calculus of gallbladder and bile duct with acute and chronic cholecystitis with obstruction

√5ᵗʰ **K80.7   Calculus of gallbladder and bile duct without cholecystitis**

    K80.70   Calculus of gallbladder and bile duct without cholecystitis without obstruction

    K80.71   Calculus of gallbladder and bile duct without cholecystitis with obstruction

√5ᵗʰ **K80.8   Other cholelithiasis**

    K80.80   Other cholelithiasis without obstruction
    K80.81   Other cholelithiasis with obstruction

☑ Additional Character Req   √x7ᵗʰ Placeholder Alert   <u>Manifestation</u>   ▽ Unspecified   ►◄ Revised Text   ● New Code   ▲ Revised Code Title

ICD-10-CM 2019

711

Chapter 11. Diseases of the Digestive System

K81–K85.92

✓4ᵗʰ **K81 Cholecystitis**
▶Use additional code if applicable for associated gangrene of gallbladder (K82.A1), or perforation of gallbladder (K82.A2)◀
EXCLUDES 1   cholecystitis with cholelithiasis (K80.-)

K81.0 Acute cholecystitis
Abscess of gallbladder
Angiocholecystitis
Emphysematous (acute) cholecystitis
Empyema of gallbladder
Gangrene of gallbladder
Gangrenous cholecystitis
Suppurative cholecystitis

K81.1 Chronic cholecystitis
K81.2 Acute cholecystitis with chronic cholecystitis
K81.9 Cholecystitis, unspecified   ▽

✓4ᵗʰ **K82 Other diseases of gallbladder**
EXCLUDES 1   nonvisualization of gallbladder (R93.2)
postcholecystectomy syndrome (K91.5)

K82.0 Obstruction of gallbladder
Occlusion of cystic duct or gallbladder without cholelithiasis
Stenosis of cystic duct or gallbladder without cholelithiasis
Stricture of cystic duct or gallbladder without cholelithiasis
EXCLUDES 1   obstruction of gallbladder with cholelithiasis (K80.-)

K82.1 Hydrops of gallbladder
Mucocele of gallbladder

K82.2 Perforation of gallbladder
Rupture of cystic duct or gallbladder
EXCLUDES 1   ▶perforation of gallbladder in cholecystitis (K82.A2)◀

K82.3 Fistula of gallbladder
Cholecystocolic fistula
Cholecystoduodenal fistula

K82.4 Cholesterolosis of gallbladder
Strawberry gallbladder
EXCLUDES 1   cholesterolosis of gallbladder with cholecystitis (K81.-)
cholesterolosis of gallbladder with cholelithiasis (K80.-)

K82.8 Other specified diseases of gallbladder
Adhesions of cystic duct or gallbladder
Atrophy of cystic duct or gallbladder
Cyst of cystic duct or gallbladder
Dyskinesia of cystic duct or gallbladder
Hypertrophy of cystic duct or gallbladder
Nonfunctioning of cystic duct or gallbladder
Ulcer of cystic duct or gallbladder

K82.9 Disease of gallbladder, unspecified   ▽

● ✓5ᵗʰ **K82.A Disorders of gallbladder in diseases classified elsewhere**
Code first the type of cholecystitis (K81.-), or cholelithiasis with cholecystitis (K80.00-K80.19, K80.40-K80.47, K80.60-K80.67)

● **K82.A1 Gangrene of gallbladder in cholecystitis**

● **K82.A2 Perforation of gallbladder in cholecystitis**

✓4ᵗʰ **K83 Other diseases of biliary tract**
EXCLUDES 1   postcholecystectomy syndrome (K91.5)
EXCLUDES 2   conditions involving the gallbladder (K81-K82)
conditions involving the cystic duct (K81-K82)

✓5ᵗʰ **K83.0 Cholangitis**
~~Ascending cholangitis~~
~~Cholangitis NOS~~
~~Primary cholangitis~~
~~Recurrent cholangitis~~
~~Sclerosing cholangitis~~
~~Secondary cholangitis~~
~~Stenosing cholangitis~~
~~Suppurative cholangitis~~
EXCLUDES 1   cholangitic liver abscess (K75.0)
cholangitis with choledocholithiasis (K80.3-, K80.4-)
~~chronic nonsuppurative destructive cholangitis (K74.3)~~
EXCLUDES 2   ▶chronic nonsuppurative destructive cholangitis (K74.3)◀
▶primary biliary cholangitis (K74.3)◀
▶primary biliary cirrhosis (K74.3)◀

● **K83.01 Primary sclerosing cholangitis**

K83.09 Other cholangitis
Ascending cholangitis
Cholangitis NOS
Primary cholangitis
Recurrent cholangitis
Sclerosing cholangitis
Secondary cholangitis
Stenosing cholangitis
Suppurative cholangitis

K83.1 Obstruction of bile duct
Occlusion of bile duct without cholelithiasis
Stenosis of bile duct without cholelithiasis
Stricture of bile duct without cholelithiasis
EXCLUDES 1   congenital obstruction of bile duct (Q44.3)
obstruction of bile duct with cholelithiasis (K80.-)
AHA: 2016,1Q,18

K83.2 Perforation of bile duct
Rupture of bile duct

K83.3 Fistula of bile duct
Choledochoduodenal fistula

K83.4 Spasm of sphincter of Oddi

K83.5 Biliary cyst

K83.8 Other specified diseases of biliary tract
Adhesions of biliary tract
Atrophy of biliary tract
Hypertrophy of biliary tract
Ulcer of biliary tract

K83.9 Disease of biliary tract, unspecified   ▽

✓4ᵗʰ **K85 Acute pancreatitis**
INCLUDES   acute (recurrent) pancreatitis
subacute pancreatitis
AHA: 2016,4Q,34

✓5ᵗʰ **K85.0 Idiopathic acute pancreatitis**
K85.00 Idiopathic acute pancreatitis without necrosis or infection
K85.01 Idiopathic acute pancreatitis with uninfected necrosis
K85.02 Idiopathic acute pancreatitis with infected necrosis

✓5ᵗʰ **K85.1 Biliary acute pancreatitis**
Gallstone pancreatitis
K85.10 Biliary acute pancreatitis without necrosis or infection
K85.11 Biliary acute pancreatitis with uninfected necrosis
K85.12 Biliary acute pancreatitis with infected necrosis

✓5ᵗʰ **K85.2 Alcohol induced acute pancreatitis**
EXCLUDES 2   alcohol induced chronic pancreatitis (K86.0)
K85.20 Alcohol induced acute pancreatitis without necrosis or infection
K85.21 Alcohol induced acute pancreatitis with uninfected necrosis
K85.22 Alcohol induced acute pancreatitis with infected necrosis

✓5ᵗʰ **K85.3 Drug induced acute pancreatitis**
Use additional code for adverse effect, if applicable, to identify drug (T36-T50 with fifth or sixth character 5)
Use additional code to identify drug abuse and dependence (F11.- F17.-)
K85.30 Drug induced acute pancreatitis without necrosis or infection
K85.31 Drug induced acute pancreatitis with uninfected necrosis
K85.32 Drug induced acute pancreatitis with infected necrosis

✓5ᵗʰ **K85.8 Other acute pancreatitis**
K85.80 Other acute pancreatitis without necrosis or infection
K85.81 Other acute pancreatitis with uninfected necrosis
K85.82 Other acute pancreatitis with infected necrosis

✓5ᵗʰ **K85.9 Acute pancreatitis, unspecified**
Pancreatitis NOS
K85.90 Acute pancreatitis without necrosis or infection, unspecified   ▽
K85.91 Acute pancreatitis with uninfected necrosis, unspecified   ▽
K85.92 Acute pancreatitis with infected necrosis, unspecified   ▽

✓4ᵗʰ K86 Other diseases of pancreas

> *EXCLUDES 2*   fibrocystic disease of pancreas (E84.-)
> islet cell tumor (of pancreas) (D13.7)
> pancreatic steatorrhea (K90.3)

K86.0 Alcohol-induced chronic pancreatitis   ⬛HCC

     Use additional code to identify:
       alcohol abuse and dependence (F10.-)
     Code also exocrine pancreatic insufficiency (K86.81)
> *EXCLUDES 2*   alcohol induced acute pancreatitis (K85.2-)

K86.1 Other chronic pancreatitis   ⬛HCC

     Chronic pancreatitis NOS
     Infectious chronic pancreatitis
     Recurrent chronic pancreatitis
     Relapsing chronic pancreatitis
     Code also exocrine pancreatic insufficiency (K86.81)

K86.2 Cyst of pancreas

K86.3 Pseudocyst of pancreas

✓5ᵗʰ K86.8 Other specified diseases of pancreas

     AHA: 2016,4Q,34-35

K86.81 Exocrine pancreatic insufficiency

K86.89 Other specified diseases of pancreas

     Aseptic pancreatic necrosis, unrelated to acute
       pancreatitis
     Atrophy of pancreas
     Calculus of pancreas
     Cirrhosis of pancreas
     Fibrosis of pancreas
     Pancreatic fat necrosis, unrelated to acute pancreatitis
     Pancreatic infantilism
     Pancreatic necrosis NOS, unrelated to acute
       pancreatitis

K86.9 Disease of pancreas, unspecified   ▽

K87 *Disorders of gallbladder, biliary tract and pancreas in diseases classified elsewhere*

     Code first underlying disease
> *EXCLUDES 1*   cytomegaloviral pancreatitis (B25.2)
> mumps pancreatitis (B26.3)
> syphilitic gallbladder (A52.74)
> syphilitic pancreas (A52.74)
> tuberculosis of gallbladder (A18.83)
> tuberculosis of pancreas (A18.83)

Other diseases of the digestive system (K90-K95)

✓4ᵗʰ K90 Intestinal malabsorption

> *EXCLUDES 1*   intestinal malabsorption following gastrointestinal surgery
> (K91.2)

     AHA: 2017,4Q,108

K90.0 Celiac disease

     Celiac disease with steatorrhea
     Celiac gluten-sensitive enteropathy
     Nontropical sprue
     Use additional code for associated disorders including:
       dermatitis herpetiformis (L13.0)
       gluten ataxia (G32.81)
     Code also exocrine pancreatic insufficiency (K86.81)
     DEF: Malabsorption syndrome due to gluten consumption.
     Symptoms include fetid, bulky, frothy, oily stools; a distended
     abdomen; gas; asthenia; electrolyte depletion; and vitamin B, D,
     and K deficiency.

K90.1 Tropical sprue

     Sprue NOS
     Tropical steatorrhea

K90.2 Blind loop syndrome, not elsewhere classified

     Blind loop syndrome NOS
> *EXCLUDES 1*   congenital blind loop syndrome (Q43.8)
> postsurgical blind loop syndrome (K91.2)

K90.3 Pancreatic steatorrhea

✓5ᵗʰ K90.4 Other malabsorption due to intolerance

> *EXCLUDES 2*   celiac gluten-sensitive enteropathy (K90.0)
> lactose intolerance (E73.-)

     AHA: 2016,4Q,35-36

K90.41 Non-celiac gluten sensitivity

     Gluten sensitivity NOS
     Non-celiac gluten sensitive enteropathy

K90.49 Malabsorption due to intolerance, not elsewhere classified

     Malabsorption due to intolerance to carbohydrate
     Malabsorption due to intolerance to fat
     Malabsorption due to intolerance to protein
     Malabsorption due to intolerance to starch

✓5ᵗʰ K90.8 Other intestinal malabsorption

K90.81 Whipple's disease

K90.89 Other intestinal malabsorption

K90.9 Intestinal malabsorption, unspecified   ▽

✓4ᵗʰ K91 Intraoperative and postprocedural complications and disorders of digestive system, not elsewhere classified

> *EXCLUDES 2*   complications of artificial opening of digestive system (K94.-)
> complications of bariatric procedures (K95.-)
> gastrojejunal ulcer (K28.-)
> postprocedural (radiation) retroperitoneal abscess (K68.11)
> radiation colitis (K52.0)
> radiation gastroenteritis (K52.0)
> radiation proctitis (K62.7)

     AHA: 2016,4Q,9-10

K91.0 Vomiting following gastrointestinal surgery

K91.1 Postgastric surgery syndromes

     Dumping syndrome
     Postgastrectomy syndrome
     Postvagotomy syndrome

K91.2 Postsurgical malabsorption, not elsewhere classified

     Postsurgical blind loop syndrome
> *EXCLUDES 1*   malabsorption osteomalacia in adults (M83.2)
> malabsorption osteoporosis, postsurgical (M80.8-,
> M81.8)

✓5ᵗʰ K91.3 Postprocedural intestinal obstruction

     AHA: 2017,4Q,16-17; 2017,1Q,40

K91.30 Postprocedural intestinal obstruction, unspecified as to partial versus complete   ▽

     Postprocedural intestinal obstruction NOS

K91.31 Postprocedural partial intestinal obstruction

     Postprocedural incomplete intestinal obstruction

K91.32 Postprocedural complete intestinal obstruction

K91.5 Postcholecystectomy syndrome

✓5ᵗʰ K91.6 Intraoperative hemorrhage and hematoma of a digestive system organ or structure complicating a procedure

> *EXCLUDES 1*   intraoperative hemorrhage and hematoma of a
> digestive system organ or structure due to
> accidental puncture and laceration during a
> procedure (K91.7-)

K91.61 Intraoperative hemorrhage and hematoma of a digestive system organ or structure complicating a digestive system procedure

K91.62 Intraoperative hemorrhage and hematoma of a digestive system organ or structure complicating other procedure

✓5ᵗʰ K91.7 Accidental puncture and laceration of a digestive system organ or structure during a procedure

K91.71 Accidental puncture and laceration of a digestive system organ or structure during a digestive system procedure

K91.72 Accidental puncture and laceration of a digestive system organ or structure during other procedure

✓5ᵗʰ K91.8 Other intraoperative and postprocedural complications and disorders of digestive system

K91.81 Other intraoperative complications of digestive system

K91.82 Postprocedural hepatic failure

K91.83 Postprocedural hepatorenal syndrome

✓6ᵗʰ K91.84 Postprocedural hemorrhage of a digestive system organ or structure following a procedure

K91.840 Postprocedural hemorrhage of a digestive system organ or structure following a digestive system procedure

     AHA: 2016,1Q,15

K91.841 Postprocedural hemorrhage of a digestive system organ or structure following other procedure

☑ Additional Character Req   ✓x7ᵗʰ Placeholder Alert   Manifestation   ▽ Unspecified   ►◄ Revised Text   ● New Code   ▲ Revised Code Title

ICD-10-CM 2019   **713**

✓6ᵗʰ **K91.85** **Complications of intestinal pouch**

    K91.85Ø **Pouchitis** HCC
        Inflammation of internal ileoanal pouch
        DEF: Inflammatory complication of an
        existing surgically created ileoanal pouch,
        resulting in multiple GI complaints,
        including diarrhea, abdominal pain, rectal
        bleeding, fecal urgency, or incontinence.

    K91.858 **Other complications of intestinal** HCC
        pouch

K91.86 **Retained cholelithiasis following cholecystectomy**

✓6ᵗʰ **K91.87** **Postprocedural hematoma and seroma of a**
digestive system organ or structure following a
procedure

    K91.87Ø **Postprocedural hematoma of a digestive**
        system organ or structure following a
        digestive system procedure

    K91.871 **Postprocedural hematoma of a digestive**
        system organ or structure following other
        procedure

    K91.872 **Postprocedural seroma of a digestive**
        system organ or structure following a
        digestive system procedure

    K91.873 **Postprocedural seroma of a digestive**
        system organ or structure following other
        procedure

K91.89 **Other postprocedural complications and disorders**
of digestive system
    Use additional code, if applicable, to further specify
    disorder
    EXCLUDES 2   postprocedural retroperitoneal abscess
        (K68.11)

    AHA: 2017,1Q,40

✓4ᵗʰ **K92** **Other diseases of digestive system**
    EXCLUDES 1   neonatal gastrointestinal hemorrhage (P54.Ø-P54.3)

K92.Ø **Hematemesis**

K92.1 **Melena**
    EXCLUDES 1   occult blood in feces (R19.5)

K92.2 **Gastrointestinal hemorrhage, unspecified** ▽
    Gastric hemorrhage NOS
    Intestinal hemorrhage NOS
    EXCLUDES 1   acute hemorrhagic gastritis (K29.Ø1)
        hemorrhage of anus and rectum (K62.5)
        angiodysplasia of stomach with hemorrhage
        (K31.811)
        diverticular disease with hemorrhage (K57.-)
        gastritis and duodenitis with hemorrhage (K29.-)
        peptic ulcer with hemorrhage (K25-K28)

✓5ᵗʰ **K92.8** **Other specified diseases of the digestive system**

    K92.81 **Gastrointestinal mucositis (ulcerative)**
        Code also type of associated therapy, such as:
        antineoplastic and immunosuppressive drugs
        (T45.1X-)
        radiological procedure and radiotherapy (Y84.2)
        EXCLUDES 2   mucositis (ulcerative) of vagina and vulva
            (N76.81)
            nasal mucositis (ulcerative) (J34.81)
            oral mucositis (ulcerative) (K12.3-)

    K92.89 **Other specified diseases of the digestive system**

K92.9 **Disease of digestive system, unspecified** ▽

✓4ᵗʰ **K94** **Complications of artificial openings of the digestive system**

✓5ᵗʰ **K94.Ø** **Colostomy complications**

    K94.ØØ **Colostomy complication, unspecified** HCC ▽
    K94.Ø1 **Colostomy hemorrhage** HCC
    K94.Ø2 **Colostomy infection** HCC
        Use additional code to specify type of infection, such
        as:
        cellulitis of abdominal wall (LØ3.311)
        sepsis (A4Ø.-, A41.-)
    K94.Ø3 **Colostomy malfunction** HCC
        Mechanical complication of colostomy
    K94.Ø9 **Other complications of colostomy** HCC

✓5ᵗʰ **K94.1** **Enterostomy complications**

    K94.1Ø **Enterostomy complication, unspecified** HCC ▽
    K94.11 **Enterostomy hemorrhage** HCC

    K94.12 **Enterostomy infection** HCC
        Use additional code to specify type of infection, such
        as:
        cellulitis of abdominal wall (LØ3.311)
        sepsis (A4Ø.-, A41.-)
    K94.13 **Enterostomy malfunction** HCC
        Mechanical complication of enterostomy
    K94.19 **Other complications of enterostomy** HCC

✓5ᵗʰ **K94.2** **Gastrostomy complications**

    K94.2Ø **Gastrostomy complication, unspecified** HCC ▽
    K94.21 **Gastrostomy hemorrhage** HCC
    K94.22 **Gastrostomy infection** HCC
        Use additional code to specify type of infection, such
        as:
        cellulitis of abdominal wall (LØ3.311)
        sepsis (A4Ø.-, A41.-)
    K94.23 **Gastrostomy malfunction** HCC
        Mechanical complication of gastrostomy
    K94.29 **Other complications of gastrostomy** HCC

✓5ᵗʰ **K94.3** **Esophagostomy complications**

    K94.3Ø **Esophagostomy complications, unspecified** HCC ▽
    K94.31 **Esophagostomy hemorrhage** HCC
    K94.32 **Esophagostomy infection** HCC
        Use additional code to identify the infection
    K94.33 **Esophagostomy malfunction** HCC
        Mechanical complication of esophagostomy
    K94.39 **Other complications of esophagostomy** HCC

✓4ᵗʰ **K95** **Complications of bariatric procedures**

✓5ᵗʰ **K95.Ø** **Complications of gastric band procedure**

    K95.Ø1 **Infection due to gastric band procedure**
        Use additional code to specify type of infection or
        organism, such as:
        bacterial and viral infectious agents (B95.-, B96.-)
        cellulitis of abdominal wall (LØ3.311)
        sepsis (A4Ø.-, A41.-)
    K95.Ø9 **Other complications of gastric band procedure**
        Use additional code, if applicable, to further specify
        complication

✓5ᵗʰ **K95.8** **Complications of other bariatric procedure**
    EXCLUDES 1   complications of gastric band surgery (K95.Ø-)

    K95.81 **Infection due to other bariatric procedure**
        Use additional code to specify type of infection or
        organism, such as:
        bacterial and viral infectious agents (B95.-, B96.-)
        cellulitis of abdominal wall (LØ3.311)
        sepsis (A4Ø.-, A41.-)
    K95.89 **Other complications of other bariatric procedure**
        Use additional code, if applicable, to further specify
        complication

Chapter 12. Diseases of the Skin and Subcutaneous Tissue (L00–L99)

Chapter Specific Guidelines with Coding Examples

The chapter specific guidelines from the ICD-10-CM Official Guidelines for Coding and Reporting have been provided below. Along with these guidelines are coding examples, contained in the shaded boxes, that have been developed to help illustrate the coding and/or sequencing guidance found in these guidelines.

a. Pressure ulcer stage codes

1) Pressure ulcer stages

Codes from category L89, Pressure ulcer, identify the site of the pressure ulcer as well as the stage of the ulcer.

The ICD-10-CM classifies pressure ulcer stages based on severity, which is designated by stages 1-4, unspecified stage and unstageable.

Assign as many codes from category L89 as needed to identify all the pressure ulcers the patient has, if applicable.

See Section I.B.14 for pressure ulcer stage documentation by clinicians other than patient's provider

> Stage 3 pressure ulcer left ankle, 6 x 7 cm that invades the fascia; stage 2 pressure ulcer of left hip
>
> **L89.523**   **Pressure ulcer of left ankle, stage 3**
>
> **L89.222**   **Pressure ulcer of left hip, stage 2**
>
> *Explanation:* Patient has a left ankle pressure ulcer documented as stage 3 and a left hip pressure ulcer documented as stage 2. Combination codes from category L89 Pressure ulcer, identify the site of the pressure ulcer as well as the stage. Assign as many codes from category L89 as needed to identify all the pressure ulcers the patient has.

2) Unstageable pressure ulcers

Assignment of the code for unstageable pressure ulcer (L89.--0) should be based on the clinical documentation. These codes are used for pressure ulcers whose stage cannot be clinically determined (e.g., the ulcer is covered by eschar or has been treated with a skin or muscle graft) and pressure ulcers that are documented as deep tissue injury but not documented as due to trauma. This code should not be confused with the codes for unspecified stage (L89.--9). When there is no documentation regarding the stage of the pressure ulcer, assign the appropriate code for unspecified stage (L89.--9).

> Pressure ulcer of the right lower back documented as unstageable due to the presence of thick eschar covering the ulcer
>
> **L89.130**   **Pressure ulcer of right lower back, unstageable**
>
> *Explanation:* Codes for unstageable pressure ulcers are assigned when the stage cannot be clinically determined (e.g., the ulcer is covered by eschar or has been treated with a skin or muscle graft).

3) Documented pressure ulcer stage

Assignment of the pressure ulcer stage code should be guided by clinical documentation of the stage or documentation of the terms found in the Alphabetic Index. For clinical terms describing the stage that are not found in the Alphabetic Index, and there is no documentation of the stage, the provider should be queried.

> Left heel pressure ulcer with partial thickness skin loss involving the dermis
>
> **L89.622**   **Pressure ulcer of left heel, stage 2**
>
> *Explanation:* Code assignment for the pressure ulcer stage should be guided by either the clinical documentation of the stage or the documentation of terms found in the Alphabetic Index. The clinical documentation describing the left heel pressure ulcer "partial thickness skin loss involving the dermis" matches the ICD-10-CM index parenthetical description for stage 2 "(abrasion, blister, partial thickness skin loss involving epidermis and/or dermis)."

4) Patients admitted with pressure ulcers documented as healed

No code is assigned if the documentation states that the pressure ulcer is completely healed.

> Patient receiving follow-up examination of a completely healed pressure ulcer of the foot
>
> **Z09**   **Encounter for follow-up examination after completed treatment for conditions other than malignant neoplasm**
>
> **Z87.2**   **Personal history of diseases of the skin and subcutaneous tissue**
>
> *Explanation:* Assign only codes for the reason for the encounter and the personal history of the pressure ulcer. Personal history code Z87.2 includes conditions classifiable to L00–L99 such as pressure ulcer. No code is assigned for a pressure ulcer documented as completely healed.

5) Patients admitted with pressure ulcers documented as healing

Pressure ulcers described as healing should be assigned the appropriate pressure ulcer stage code based on the documentation in the medical record. If the documentation does not provide information about the stage of the healing pressure ulcer, assign the appropriate code for unspecified stage.

If the documentation is unclear as to whether the patient has a current (new) pressure ulcer or if the patient is being treated for a healing pressure ulcer, query the provider.

For ulcers that were present on admission but healed at the time of discharge, assign the code for the site and stage of the pressure ulcer at the time of admission.

6) Patient admitted with pressure ulcer evolving into another stage during the admission

If a patient is admitted to an inpatient hospital with a pressure ulcer at one stage and it progresses to a higher stage, two separate codes should be assigned: one code for the site and stage of the ulcer on admission and a second code for the same ulcer site and the highest stage reported during the stay.

b. Non-pressure chronic ulcers

1) Patients admitted with non-pressure ulcers documented as healed

No code is assigned if the documentation states that the non-pressure ulcer is completely healed.

2) Patients admitted with non-pressure ulcers documented as healing

Non-pressure ulcers described as healing should be assigned the appropriate non-pressure ulcer code based on the documentation in the medical record. If the documentation does not provide information about the severity of the healing non-pressure ulcer, assign the appropriate code for unspecified severity.

If the documentation is unclear as to whether the patient has a current (new) non-pressure ulcer or if the patient is being treated for a healing non-pressure ulcer, query the provider.

For ulcers that were present on admission but healed at the time of discharge, assign the code for the site and severity of the non-pressure ulcer at the time of admission.

3) Patient admitted with non-pressure ulcer that progresses to another severity level during the admission

If a patient is admitted to an inpatient hospital with a non-pressure ulcer at one severity level and it progresses to a higher severity level, two separate codes should be assigned: one code for the site and severity level of the ulcer on admission and a second code for the same ulcer site and the highest severity level reported during the stay.

See Section I.B.14 for pressure ulcer stage documentation by clinicians other than patient's provider

Chapter 12. Diseases of the Skin and Subcutaneous Tissue (L00-L99)

EXCLUDES 2   *certain conditions originating in the perinatal period (P04-P96)*
certain infectious and parasitic diseases (A00-B99)
complications of pregnancy, childbirth and the puerperium (O00-O9A)
congenital malformations, deformations, and chromosomal abnormalities (Q00-Q99)
endocrine, nutritional and metabolic diseases (E00-E88)
lipomelanotic reticulosis (I89.8)
neoplasms (C00-D49)
symptoms, signs and abnormal clinical and laboratory findings, not elsewhere classified (R00-R94)
systemic connective tissue disorders (M30-M36)
viral warts (B07.-)

This chapter contains the following blocks:
L00-L08   Infections of the skin and subcutaneous tissue
L10-L14   Bullous disorders
L20-L30   Dermatitis and eczema
L40-L45   Papulosquamous disorders
L49-L54   Urticaria and erythema
L55-L59   Radiation-related disorders of the skin and subcutaneous tissue
L60-L75   Disorders of skin appendages
L76   Intraoperative and postprocedural complications of skin and subcutaneous tissue
L80-L99   Other disorders of the skin and subcutaneous tissue

Infections of the skin and subcutaneous tissue (L00-L08)

Use additional code (B95-B97) to identify infectious agent
EXCLUDES 2   *hordeolum (H00.0)*
infective dermatitis (L30.3)
local infections of skin classified in Chapter 1
lupus panniculitis (L93.2)
panniculitis NOS (M79.3)
panniculitis of neck and back (M54.0-)
perlèche NOS (K13.0)
perlèche due to candidiasis (B37.0)
perlèche due to riboflavin deficiency (E53.0)
pyogenic granuloma (L98.0)
relapsing panniculitis [Weber-Christian] (M35.6)
viral warts (B07.-)
zoster (B02.-)

L00   Staphylococcal scalded skin syndrome
Ritter's disease
Use additional code to identify percentage of skin exfoliation (L49.-)
EXCLUDES 1   *bullous impetigo (L01.03)*
pemphigus neonatorum (L01.03)
toxic epidermal necrolysis [Lyell] (L51.2)
DEF: Infectious skin disease of children younger than 5 years marked by eruptions ranging from a few localized blisters to widespread, easily ruptured, fine vesicles and bullae affecting almost the entire body. It results in exfoliation of large planes of skin and leaves raw areas.

✓4ᵗʰ L01   Impetigo
EXCLUDES 1   *impetigo herpetiformis (L40.1)*
DEF: Acute, superficial, highly contagious skin infection commonly occurring in children. Skin lesions usually appear on the face and consist of vesicles and bullae that burst and form yellow crusts.

   ✓5ᵗʰ L01.0   Impetigo
     Impetigo contagiosa
     Impetigo vulgaris
     L01.00   Impetigo, unspecified   ▽
       Impetigo NOS
     L01.01   Non-bullous impetigo
     L01.02   Bockhart's impetigo
       Impetigo follicularis
       Perifolliculitis NOS
       Superficial pustular perifolliculitis
       DEF: Superficial inflammation of the hair follicles most commonly caused by staph aureus that manifests as rounded, sphere-shaped, pustular eruptions in the areas of the scalp, beard, underarms, extremities, and buttocks.
     L01.03   Bullous impetigo
       Impetigo neonatorum
       Pemphigus neonatorum
     L01.09   Other impetigo
       Ulcerative impetigo
   L01.1   Impetiginization of other dermatoses

✓4ᵗʰ L02   Cutaneous abscess, furuncle and carbuncle
Use additional code to identify organism (B95-B96)
EXCLUDES 2   *abscess of anus and rectal regions (K61.-)*
abscess of female genital organs (external) (N76.4)
abscess of male genital organs (external) (N48.2, N49.-)
DEF: Carbuncle: Infection of the skin that arises from a collection of interconnected infected boils or furuncles, usually from hair follicles infected by *Staphylococcus*. This condition can produce pus and form drainage cavities.
DEF: Furuncle: Inflamed, painful abscess, cyst, or nodule on the skin caused by bacteria, often *Staphylococcus*, entering along the hair follicle.

  ✓5ᵗʰ L02.0   Cutaneous abscess, furuncle and carbuncle of face
     EXCLUDES 2   *abscess of ear, external (H60.0)*
      abscess of eyelid (H00.0)
      abscess of head [any part, except face] (L02.8)
      abscess of lacrimal gland (H04.0)
      abscess of lacrimal passages (H04.3)
      abscess of mouth (K12.2)
      abscess of nose (J34.0)
      abscess of orbit (H05.0)
      submandibular abscess (K12.2)
     L02.01   Cutaneous abscess of face
     L02.02   Furuncle of face
       Boil of face
       Folliculitis of face
     L02.03   Carbuncle of face
  ✓5ᵗʰ L02.1   Cutaneous abscess, furuncle and carbuncle of neck
     L02.11   Cutaneous abscess of neck
     L02.12   Furuncle of neck
       Boil of neck
       Folliculitis of neck
     L02.13   Carbuncle of neck
  ✓5ᵗʰ L02.2   Cutaneous abscess, furuncle and carbuncle of trunk
     EXCLUDES 1   *non-newborn omphalitis (L08.82)*
      omphalitis of newborn (P38.-)
     EXCLUDES 2   *abscess of breast (N61.1)*
      abscess of buttocks (L02.3)
      abscess of female external genital organs (N76.4)
      abscess of hip (L02.4)
      abscess of male external genital organs (N48.2, N49.-)
   ✓6ᵗʰ L02.21   Cutaneous abscess of trunk
     L02.211   Cutaneous abscess of abdominal wall
     L02.212   Cutaneous abscess of back [any part, except buttock]
     L02.213   Cutaneous abscess of chest wall
     L02.214   Cutaneous abscess of groin
     L02.215   Cutaneous abscess of perineum
     L02.216   Cutaneous abscess of umbilicus
     L02.219   Cutaneous abscess of trunk, unspecified   ▽
   ✓6ᵗʰ L02.22   Furuncle of trunk
     Boil of trunk
     Folliculitis of trunk
     L02.221   Furuncle of abdominal wall
     L02.222   Furuncle of back [any part, except buttock]
     L02.223   Furuncle of chest wall
     L02.224   Furuncle of groin
     L02.225   Furuncle of perineum
     L02.226   Furuncle of umbilicus
     L02.229   Furuncle of trunk, unspecified   ▽
   ✓6ᵗʰ L02.23   Carbuncle of trunk
     L02.231   Carbuncle of abdominal wall
     L02.232   Carbuncle of back [any part, except buttock]
     L02.233   Carbuncle of chest wall
     L02.234   Carbuncle of groin
     L02.235   Carbuncle of perineum
     L02.236   Carbuncle of umbilicus
     L02.239   Carbuncle of trunk, unspecified   ▽
  ✓5ᵗʰ L02.3   Cutaneous abscess, furuncle and carbuncle of buttock
     EXCLUDES 1   *pilonidal cyst with abscess (L05.01)*
     L02.31   Cutaneous abscess of buttock
       Cutaneous abscess of gluteal region

L02.32   **Furuncle of buttock**
     Boil of buttock
     Folliculitis of buttock
     Furuncle of gluteal region

L02.33   **Carbuncle of buttock**
     Carbuncle of gluteal region

✓5ᵗʰ **L02.4**   **Cutaneous abscess, furuncle and carbuncle of limb**

     EXCLUDES 2   *cutaneous abscess, furuncle and carbuncle of groin (L02.214, L02.224, L02.234)*
         cutaneous abscess, furuncle and carbuncle of hand (L02.5-)
         cutaneous abscess, furuncle and carbuncle of foot (L02.6-)

   ✓6ᵗʰ **L02.41**   **Cutaneous abscess of limb**

     L02.411   **Cutaneous abscess of right axilla**
     L02.412   **Cutaneous abscess of left axilla**
     L02.413   **Cutaneous abscess of right upper limb**
     L02.414   **Cutaneous abscess of left upper limb**
     L02.415   **Cutaneous abscess of right lower limb**
     L02.416   **Cutaneous abscess of left lower limb**
     L02.419   **Cutaneous abscess of limb, unspecified**   ▽

   ✓6ᵗʰ **L02.42**   **Furuncle of limb**
     Boil of limb
     Folliculitis of limb

     L02.421   **Furuncle of right axilla**
     L02.422   **Furuncle of left axilla**
     L02.423   **Furuncle of right upper limb**
     L02.424   **Furuncle of left upper limb**
     L02.425   **Furuncle of right lower limb**
     L02.426   **Furuncle of left lower limb**
     L02.429   **Furuncle of limb, unspecified**   ▽

   ✓6ᵗʰ **L02.43**   **Carbuncle of limb**

     L02.431   **Carbuncle of right axilla**
     L02.432   **Carbuncle of left axilla**
     L02.433   **Carbuncle of right upper limb**
     L02.434   **Carbuncle of left upper limb**
     L02.435   **Carbuncle of right lower limb**
     L02.436   **Carbuncle of left lower limb**
     L02.439   **Carbuncle of limb, unspecified**   ▽

✓5ᵗʰ **L02.5**   **Cutaneous abscess, furuncle and carbuncle of hand**

   ✓6ᵗʰ **L02.51**   **Cutaneous abscess of hand**

     L02.511   **Cutaneous abscess of right hand**
     L02.512   **Cutaneous abscess of left hand**
     L02.519   **Cutaneous abscess of unspecified hand**   ▽

   ✓6ᵗʰ **L02.52**   **Furuncle hand**
     Boil of hand
     Folliculitis of hand

     L02.521   **Furuncle right hand**
     L02.522   **Furuncle left hand**
     L02.529   **Furuncle unspecified hand**   ▽

   ✓6ᵗʰ **L02.53**   **Carbuncle of hand**

     L02.531   **Carbuncle of right hand**
     L02.532   **Carbuncle of left hand**
     L02.539   **Carbuncle of unspecified hand**   ▽

✓5ᵗʰ **L02.6**   **Cutaneous abscess, furuncle and carbuncle of foot**

   ✓6ᵗʰ **L02.61**   **Cutaneous abscess of foot**

     L02.611   **Cutaneous abscess of right foot**
     L02.612   **Cutaneous abscess of left foot**
     L02.619   **Cutaneous abscess of unspecified foot**   ▽

   ✓6ᵗʰ **L02.62**   **Furuncle of foot**
     Boil of foot
     Folliculitis of foot

     L02.621   **Furuncle of right foot**
     L02.622   **Furuncle of left foot**
     L02.629   **Furuncle of unspecified foot**   ▽

   ✓6ᵗʰ **L02.63**   **Carbuncle of foot**

     L02.631   **Carbuncle of right foot**
     L02.632   **Carbuncle of left foot**
     L02.639   **Carbuncle of unspecified foot**   ▽

✓5ᵗʰ **L02.8**   **Cutaneous abscess, furuncle and carbuncle of other sites**

   ✓6ᵗʰ **L02.81**   **Cutaneous abscess of other sites**

     L02.811   **Cutaneous abscess of head [any part, except face]**

     L02.818   **Cutaneous abscess of other sites**

   ✓6ᵗʰ **L02.82**   **Furuncle of other sites**

     Boil of other sites
     Folliculitis of other sites

     L02.821   **Furuncle of head [any part, except face]**
     L02.828   **Furuncle of other sites**

   ✓6ᵗʰ **L02.83**   **Carbuncle of other sites**

     L02.831   **Carbuncle of head [any part, except face]**
     L02.838   **Carbuncle of other sites**

✓5ᵗʰ **L02.9**   **Cutaneous abscess, furuncle and carbuncle, unspecified**

     L02.91   **Cutaneous abscess, unspecified**   ▽
     L02.92   **Furuncle, unspecified**   ▽
         Boil NOS
         Furunculosis NOS
     L02.93   **Carbuncle, unspecified**   ▽

✓4ᵗʰ **L03**   **Cellulitis and acute lymphangitis**

     EXCLUDES 2   *cellulitis of anal and rectal region (K61.-)*
         cellulitis of external auditory canal (H60.1)
         cellulitis of eyelid (H00.0)
         cellulitis of female external genital organs (N76.4)
         cellulitis of lacrimal apparatus (H04.3)
         cellulitis of male external genital organs (N48.2, N49.-)
         cellulitis of mouth (K12.2)
         cellulitis of nose (J34.0)
         eosinophilic cellulitis [Wells] (L98.3)
         febrile neutrophilic dermatosis [Sweet] (L98.2)
         lymphangitis (chronic) (subacute) (I89.1)

     AHA: 2017,4Q,100
     DEF: Cellulitis: Infection of the skin and subcutaneous tissues, most often caused by *Staphylococcus* or *Streptococcus* bacteria secondary to a cutaneous lesion. Progression of the inflammation may lead to abscess and tissue death, or even systemic infection-like bacteremia.
     DEF: Lymphangitis: Inflammation of the lymph channels most often caused by *Streptococcus*.

   ✓5ᵗʰ **L03.0**   **Cellulitis and acute lymphangitis of finger and toe**
     Infection of nail
     Onychia
     Paronychia
     Perionychia

     ✓6ᵗʰ **L03.01**   **Cellulitis of finger**
         Felon
         Whitlow
         EXCLUDES 1   *herpetic whitlow (B00.89)*
         DEF: Felon: Superficial bacterial skin infection at the tip of the finger.
         L03.011   **Cellulitis of right finger**
         L03.012   **Cellulitis of left finger**
         L03.019   **Cellulitis of unspecified finger**   ▽

     ✓6ᵗʰ **L03.02**   **Acute lymphangitis of finger**
         Hangnail with lymphangitis of finger
         L03.021   **Acute lymphangitis of right finger**
         L03.022   **Acute lymphangitis of left finger**
         L03.029   **Acute lymphangitis of unspecified finger**   ▽

     ✓6ᵗʰ **L03.03**   **Cellulitis of toe**
         L03.031   **Cellulitis of right toe**
         L03.032   **Cellulitis of left toe**
         L03.039   **Cellulitis of unspecified toe**   ▽

     ✓6ᵗʰ **L03.04**   **Acute lymphangitis of toe**
         Hangnail with lymphangitis of toe
         L03.041   **Acute lymphangitis of right toe**
         L03.042   **Acute lymphangitis of left toe**
         L03.049   **Acute lymphangitis of unspecified toe**   ▽

   ✓5ᵗʰ **L03.1**   **Cellulitis and acute lymphangitis of other parts of limb**

     ✓6ᵗʰ **L03.11**   **Cellulitis of other parts of limb**
         EXCLUDES 2   *cellulitis of fingers (L03.01-)*
           cellulitis of toes (L03.03-)
           groin (L03.314)
         L03.111   **Cellulitis of right axilla**
         L03.112   **Cellulitis of left axilla**
         L03.113   **Cellulitis of right upper limb**
         L03.114   **Cellulitis of left upper limb**
         L03.115   **Cellulitis of right lower limb**
         L03.116   **Cellulitis of left lower limb**

L03.119 Cellulitis of unspecified part of limb ▽

✓6ᵗʰ **L03.12 Acute lymphangitis of other parts of limb**
  EXCLUDES 2 acute lymphangitis of fingers (L03.2-)
  acute lymphangitis of groin (L03.324)
  acute lymphangitis of toes (L03.04-)

L03.121 Acute lymphangitis of right axilla
L03.122 Acute lymphangitis of left axilla
L03.123 Acute lymphangitis of right upper limb
L03.124 Acute lymphangitis of left upper limb
L03.125 Acute lymphangitis of right lower limb
L03.126 Acute lymphangitis of left lower limb
L03.129 Acute lymphangitis of unspecified part of limb ▽

✓5ᵗʰ **L03.2 Cellulitis and acute lymphangitis of face and neck**

✓6ᵗʰ **L03.21 Cellulitis and acute lymphangitis of face**

L03.211 Cellulitis of face
  EXCLUDES 2 abscess of orbit (H05.01-)
  cellulitis of ear (H60.1-)
  cellulitis of eyelid (H00.0-)
  cellulitis of head (L03.81)
  cellulitis of lacrimal apparatus (H04.3)
  cellulitis of lip (K13.0)
  cellulitis of mouth (K12.2)
  cellulitis of nose (internal) (J34.0)
  cellulitis of orbit (H05.01-)
  cellulitis of scalp (L03.81)
  AHA: 2013,4Q,123

L03.212 Acute lymphangitis of face
L03.213 Periorbital cellulitis
  Preseptal cellulitis
  AHA: 2016,4Q,36

✓6ᵗʰ **L03.22 Cellulitis and acute lymphangitis of neck**

L03.221 Cellulitis of neck
L03.222 Acute lymphangitis of neck

✓5ᵗʰ **L03.3 Cellulitis and acute lymphangitis of trunk**

✓6ᵗʰ **L03.31 Cellulitis of trunk**
  EXCLUDES 2 cellulitis of anal and rectal regions (K61.-)
  cellulitis of breast NOS (N61.0)
  cellulitis of female external genital organs (N76.4)
  cellulitis of male external genital organs (N48.2, N49.-)
  omphalitis of newborn (P38.-)
  puerperal cellulitis of breast (O91.2)

L03.311 Cellulitis of abdominal wall
  EXCLUDES 2 cellulitis of umbilicus (L03.316)
  cellulitis of groin (L03.314)

L03.312 Cellulitis of back [any part except buttock]
L03.313 Cellulitis of chest wall
L03.314 Cellulitis of groin
L03.315 Cellulitis of perineum
L03.316 Cellulitis of umbilicus
L03.317 Cellulitis of buttock
L03.319 Cellulitis of trunk, unspecified ▽

✓6ᵗʰ **L03.32 Acute lymphangitis of trunk**

L03.321 Acute lymphangitis of abdominal wall
L03.322 Acute lymphangitis of back [any part except buttock]
L03.323 Acute lymphangitis of chest wall
L03.324 Acute lymphangitis of groin
L03.325 Acute lymphangitis of perineum
L03.326 Acute lymphangitis of umbilicus
L03.327 Acute lymphangitis of buttock
L03.329 Acute lymphangitis of trunk, unspecified ▽

✓5ᵗʰ **L03.8 Cellulitis and acute lymphangitis of other sites**

✓6ᵗʰ **L03.81 Cellulitis of other sites**

L03.811 Cellulitis of head [any part, except face]
  Cellulitis of scalp
  EXCLUDES 2 cellulitis of face (L03.211)

L03.818 Cellulitis of other sites

✓6ᵗʰ **L03.89 Acute lymphangitis of other sites**

L03.891 Acute lymphangitis of head [any part, except face]
L03.898 Acute lymphangitis of other sites

✓5ᵗʰ **L03.9 Cellulitis and acute lymphangitis, unspecified**

L03.90 Cellulitis, unspecified ▽
L03.91 Acute lymphangitis, unspecified ▽
  EXCLUDES 1 lymphangitis NOS (I89.1)

✓4ᵗʰ **L04 Acute lymphadenitis**

  INCLUDES abscess (acute) of lymph nodes, except mesenteric
  acute lymphadenitis, except mesenteric

  EXCLUDES 1 chronic or subacute lymphadenitis, except mesenteric (I88.1)
  enlarged lymph nodes (R59.-)
  human immunodeficiency virus [HIV] disease resulting in generalized lymphadenopathy (B20)
  lymphadenitis NOS (I88.9)
  nonspecific mesenteric lymphadenitis (I88.0)

  DEF: Inflammation or enlargement of the lymph nodes.

L04.0 Acute lymphadenitis of face, head and neck
L04.1 Acute lymphadenitis of trunk
L04.2 Acute lymphadenitis of upper limb
  Acute lymphadenitis of axilla
  Acute lymphadenitis of shoulder
L04.3 Acute lymphadenitis of lower limb
  Acute lymphadenitis of hip
  EXCLUDES 2 acute lymphadenitis of groin (L04.1)
L04.8 Acute lymphadenitis of other sites
L04.9 Acute lymphadenitis, unspecified ▽

✓4ᵗʰ **L05 Pilonidal cyst and sinus**

Pilonidal Cyst

- Skin
- Fistula
- Pilonidal cyst
- Fat
- Bone

✓5ᵗʰ **L05.0 Pilonidal cyst and sinus with abscess**

L05.01 Pilonidal cyst with abscess
  Pilonidal abscess
  Pilonidal dimple with abscess
  Postanal dimple with abscess
  EXCLUDES 2 congenital sacral dimple (Q82.6)
  parasacral dimple (Q82.6)

L05.02 Pilonidal sinus with abscess
  Coccygeal fistula with abscess
  Coccygeal sinus with abscess
  Pilonidal fistula with abscess

✓5ᵗʰ **L05.9 Pilonidal cyst and sinus without abscess**

L05.91 Pilonidal cyst without abscess
  Pilonidal dimple
  Postanal dimple
  Pilonidal cyst NOS
  EXCLUDES 2 congenital sacral dimple (Q82.6)
  parasacral dimple (Q82.6)

L05.92 Pilonidal sinus without abscess
  Coccygeal fistula
  Coccygeal sinus without abscess
  Pilonidal fistula

✓4ᵗʰ L08 Other local infections of skin and subcutaneous tissue

     L08.0 Pyoderma
         Dermatitis gangrenosa
         Purulent dermatitis
         Septic dermatitis
         Suppurative dermatitis
         EXCLUDES 1   *pyoderma gangrenosum (L88)*
                      pyoderma vegetans (L08.81)
         DEF: Any superficial skin disease commonly characterized by the discharging of pus not attributed to another condition.

     L08.1 Erythrasma
         DEF: Chronic, superficial skin infection of brown scaly patches, commonly found in skin folds most prevalent in the overweight or diabetic population.

     ✓5ᵗʰ L08.8 Other specified local infections of the skin and subcutaneous tissue
         L08.81 Pyoderma vegetans
             EXCLUDES 1   *pyoderma gangrenosum (L88)*
                      pyoderma NOS (L08.0)
         L08.82 Omphalitis not of newborn
             EXCLUDES 1   *omphalitis of newborn (P38.-)*
         L08.89 Other specified local infections of the skin and subcutaneous tissue

     L08.9 Local infection of the skin and subcutaneous tissue, unspecified ▽

Bullous disorders (L10-L14)

     EXCLUDES 1   *benign familial pemphigus [Hailey-Hailey] (Q82.8)*
                    staphylococcal scalded skin syndrome (L00)
                    toxic epidermal necrolysis [Lyell] (L51.2)

✓4ᵗʰ L10 Pemphigus
     EXCLUDES 1   *pemphigus neonatorum (L01.03)*

     L10.0 Pemphigus vulgaris
     L10.1 Pemphigus vegetans
     L10.2 Pemphigus foliaceous
     L10.3 Brazilian pemphigus [fogo selvagem]
     L10.4 Pemphigus erythematosus
         Senear-Usher syndrome
     L10.5 Drug-induced pemphigus
         Use additional code for adverse effect, if applicable, to identify drug (T36-T50 with fifth or sixth character 5)
     ✓5ᵗʰ L10.8 Other pemphigus
         L10.81 Paraneoplastic pemphigus
         L10.89 Other pemphigus
     L10.9 Pemphigus, unspecified ▽

✓4ᵗʰ L11 Other acantholytic disorders
     L11.0 Acquired keratosis follicularis
         EXCLUDES 1   *keratosis follicularis (congenital) [Darier-White] (Q82.8)*
     L11.1 Transient acantholytic dermatosis [Grover]
     L11.8 Other specified acantholytic disorders
     L11.9 Acantholytic disorder, unspecified ▽

✓4ᵗʰ L12 Pemphigoid
     EXCLUDES 1   *herpes gestationis (O26.4-)*
                 impetigo herpetiformis (L40.1)

     L12.0 Bullous pemphigoid
     L12.1 Cicatricial pemphigoid
         Benign mucous membrane pemphigoid
         DEF: Chronic autoimmune disease characterized by subepidermal blistering lesions of the mucosa, including the conjunctiva. It is seen predominantly in the elderly and produces adhesions and scarring.
     L12.2 Chronic bullous disease of childhood P
         Juvenile dermatitis herpetiformis
     ✓5ᵗʰ L12.3 Acquired epidermolysis bullosa
         EXCLUDES 1   *epidermolysis bullosa (congenital) (Q81.-)*
         L12.30 Acquired epidermolysis bullosa, unspecified HCC ▽
         L12.31 Epidermolysis bullosa due to drug HCC
             Use additional code for adverse effect, if applicable, to identify drug (T36-T50 with fifth or sixth character 5)
         L12.35 Other acquired epidermolysis bullosa HCC
     L12.8 Other pemphigoid
     L12.9 Pemphigoid, unspecified ▽

✓4ᵗʰ L13 Other bullous disorders
     L13.0 Dermatitis herpetiformis
         Duhring's disease
         Hydroa herpetiformis
         EXCLUDES 1   *juvenile dermatitis herpetiformis (L12.2)*
                      senile dermatitis herpetiformis (L12.0)
         DEF: Skin disease to which people are genetically predisposed resulting from an immunological response to gluten. Dermatitis herpetiformis is an extremely pruritic eruption of various lesions that frequently heal, leaving hyperpigmentation or hypopigmentation and occasionally scarring. It is usually associated with asymptomatic gluten-sensitive enteropathy.
     L13.1 Subcorneal pustular dermatitis
         Sneddon-Wilkinson disease
     L13.8 Other specified bullous disorders
     L13.9 Bullous disorder, unspecified ▽

*L14 **Bullous disorders in diseases classified elsewhere***
     Code first underlying disease

Dermatitis and eczema (L20-L30)

   NOTE   In this block the terms dermatitis and eczema are used synonymously and interchangeably.

   EXCLUDES 2   *chronic (childhood) granulomatous disease (D71)*
                 dermatitis gangrenosa (L08.0)
                 dermatitis herpetiformis (L13.0)
                 dry skin dermatitis (L85.3)
                 factitial dermatitis (L98.1)
                 perioral dermatitis (L71.0)
                 radiation-related disorders of the skin and subcutaneous tissue (L55-L59)
                 stasis dermatitis (I87.2)

✓4ᵗʰ L20 Atopic dermatitis
     L20.0 Besnier's prurigo
     ✓5ᵗʰ L20.8 Other atopic dermatitis
         EXCLUDES 2   *circumscribed neurodermatitis (L28.0)*
         L20.81 Atopic neurodermatitis
             Diffuse neurodermatitis
         L20.82 Flexural eczema
         L20.83 Infantile (acute) (chronic) eczema P
         L20.84 Intrinsic (allergic) eczema
         L20.89 Other atopic dermatitis
     L20.9 Atopic dermatitis, unspecified ▽

✓4ᵗʰ L21 Seborrheic dermatitis
     EXCLUDES 2   *infective dermatitis (L30.3)*
                 seborrheic keratosis (L82.-)
     L21.0 Seborrhea capitis
         Cradle cap
         AHA: 2018,1Q,6
         TIP: Assign for dandruff in an adult patient.
     L21.1 Seborrheic infantile dermatitis P
     L21.8 Other seborrheic dermatitis
     L21.9 Seborrheic dermatitis, unspecified ▽
         Seborrhea NOS

L22 Diaper dermatitis
     Diaper erythema
     Diaper rash
     Psoriasiform diaper rash

✓4ᵗʰ L23 Allergic contact dermatitis
     EXCLUDES 1   *allergy NOS (T78.40)*
                 contact dermatitis NOS (L25.9)
                 dermatitis NOS (L30.9)
     EXCLUDES 2   *dermatitis due to substances taken internally (L27.-)*
                 dermatitis of eyelid (H01.1-)
                 diaper dermatitis (L22)
                 eczema of external ear (H60.5-)
                 irritant contact dermatitis (L24.-)
                 perioral dermatitis (L71.0)
                 radiation-related disorders of the skin and subcutaneous tissue (L55-L59)
     L23.0 Allergic contact dermatitis due to metals
         Allergic contact dermatitis due to chromium
         Allergic contact dermatitis due to nickel
     L23.1 Allergic contact dermatitis due to adhesives
     L23.2 Allergic contact dermatitis due to cosmetics

✓ Additional Character Req   ✓x7ᵗʰ Placeholder Alert   Manifestation   ▽ Unspecified   ►◄ Revised Text   ● New Code   ▲ Revised Code Title

ICD-10-CM 2019   719

Chapter 12. Diseases of the Skin and Subcutaneous Tissue

L23.3   **Allergic contact dermatitis due to drugs in contact with skin**
Use additional code for adverse effect, if applicable, to identify drug (T36-T50 with fifth or sixth character 5)
EXCLUDES 2   dermatitis due to ingested drugs and medicaments (L27.0-L27.1)

L23.4   **Allergic contact dermatitis due to dyes**

L23.5   **Allergic contact dermatitis due to other chemical products**
Allergic contact dermatitis due to cement
Allergic contact dermatitis due to insecticide
Allergic contact dermatitis due to plastic
Allergic contact dermatitis due to rubber

L23.6   **Allergic contact dermatitis due to food in contact with the skin**
EXCLUDES 2   dermatitis due to ingested food (L27.2)

L23.7   **Allergic contact dermatitis due to plants, except food**
EXCLUDES 2   allergy NOS due to pollen (J30.1)

√5th **L23.8**   **Allergic contact dermatitis due to other agents**

     L23.81   **Allergic contact dermatitis due to animal (cat) (dog) dander**
Allergic contact dermatitis due to animal (cat) (dog) hair

     L23.89   **Allergic contact dermatitis due to other agents**

L23.9   **Allergic contact dermatitis, unspecified cause** ▽
Allergic contact eczema NOS

√4th **L24**   **Irritant contact dermatitis**
EXCLUDES 1   allergy NOS (T78.40)
contact dermatitis NOS (L25.9)
dermatitis NOS (L30.9)
EXCLUDES 2   allergic contact dermatitis (L23.-)
dermatitis due to substances taken internally (L27.-)
dermatitis of eyelid (H01.1-)
diaper dermatitis (L22)
eczema of external ear (H60.5-)
perioral dermatitis (L71.0)
radiation-related disorders of the skin and subcutaneous tissue (L55-L59)

L24.0   **Irritant contact dermatitis due to detergents**

L24.1   **Irritant contact dermatitis due to oils and greases**

L24.2   **Irritant contact dermatitis due to solvents**
Irritant contact dermatitis due to chlorocompound
Irritant contact dermatitis due to cyclohexane
Irritant contact dermatitis due to ester
Irritant contact dermatitis due to glycol
Irritant contact dermatitis due to hydrocarbon
Irritant contact dermatitis due to ketone

L24.3   **Irritant contact dermatitis due to cosmetics**

L24.4   **Irritant contact dermatitis due to drugs in contact with skin**
Use additional code for adverse effect, if applicable, to identify drug (T36-T50 with fifth or sixth character 5)

L24.5   **Irritant contact dermatitis due to other chemical products**
Irritant contact dermatitis due to cement
Irritant contact dermatitis due to insecticide
Irritant contact dermatitis due to plastic
Irritant contact dermatitis due to rubber

L24.6   **Irritant contact dermatitis due to food in contact with skin**
EXCLUDES 2   dermatitis due to ingested food (L27.2)

L24.7   **Irritant contact dermatitis due to plants, except food**
EXCLUDES 2   allergy NOS to pollen (J30.1)

√5th **L24.8**   **Irritant contact dermatitis due to other agents**

     L24.81   **Irritant contact dermatitis due to metals**
Irritant contact dermatitis due to chromium
Irritant contact dermatitis due to nickel

     L24.89   **Irritant contact dermatitis due to other agents**
Irritant contact dermatitis due to dyes

L24.9   **Irritant contact dermatitis, unspecified cause** ▽
Irritant contact eczema NOS

√4th **L25**   **Unspecified contact dermatitis**
EXCLUDES 1   allergic contact dermatitis (L23.-)
allergy NOS (T78.40)
dermatitis NOS (L30.9)
irritant contact dermatitis (L24.-)
EXCLUDES 2   dermatitis due to ingested substances (L27.-)
dermatitis of eyelid (H01.1-)
eczema of external ear (H60.5-)
perioral dermatitis (L71.0)
radiation-related disorders of the skin and subcutaneous tissue (L55-L59)

L25.0   **Unspecified contact dermatitis due to cosmetics** ▽

L25.1   **Unspecified contact dermatitis due to drugs in contact with skin** ▽
Use additional code for adverse effect, if applicable, to identify drug (T36-T50 with fifth or sixth character 5)
EXCLUDES 2   dermatitis due to ingested drugs and medicaments (L27.0-L27.1)

L25.2   **Unspecified contact dermatitis due to dyes** ▽

L25.3   **Unspecified contact dermatitis due to other chemical products** ▽
Unspecified contact dermatitis due to cement
Unspecified contact dermatitis due to insecticide

L25.4   **Unspecified contact dermatitis due to food in contact with skin** ▽
EXCLUDES 2   dermatitis due to ingested food (L27.2)

L25.5   **Unspecified contact dermatitis due to plants, except food** ▽
EXCLUDES 1   nettle rash (L50.9)
EXCLUDES 2   allergy NOS due to pollen (J30.1)

L25.8   **Unspecified contact dermatitis due to other agents** ▽

L25.9   **Unspecified contact dermatitis, unspecified cause** ▽
Contact dermatitis (occupational) NOS
Contact eczema (occupational) NOS

L26   **Exfoliative dermatitis**
Hebra's pityriasis
EXCLUDES 1   Ritter's disease (L00)

√4th **L27**   **Dermatitis due to substances taken internally**
EXCLUDES 1   allergy NOS (T78.40)
EXCLUDES 2   adverse food reaction, except dermatitis (T78.0-T78.1)
contact dermatitis (L23-L25)
drug photoallergic response (L56.1)
drug phototoxic response (L56.0)
urticaria (L50.-)

L27.0   **Generalized skin eruption due to drugs and medicaments taken internally**
Use additional code for adverse effect, if applicable, to identify drug (T36-T50 with fifth or sixth character 5)

L27.1   **Localized skin eruption due to drugs and medicaments taken internally**
Use additional code for adverse effect, if applicable, to identify drug (T36-T50 with fifth or sixth character 5)

L27.2   **Dermatitis due to ingested food**
EXCLUDES 2   dermatitis due to food in contact with skin (L23.6, L24.6, L25.4)

L27.8   **Dermatitis due to other substances taken internally**

L27.9   **Dermatitis due to unspecified substance taken internally** ▽

√4th **L28**   **Lichen simplex chronicus and prurigo**

L28.0   **Lichen simplex chronicus**
Circumscribed neurodermatitis
Lichen NOS

L28.1   **Prurigo nodularis**

L28.2   **Other prurigo**
Prurigo NOS
Prurigo Hebra
Prurigo mitis
Urticaria papulosa

√4th **L29**   **Pruritus**
EXCLUDES 1   neurotic excoriation (L98.1)
psychogenic pruritus (F45.8)

L29.0   **Pruritus ani**
L29.1   **Pruritus scroti** ♂
L29.2   **Pruritus vulvae** ♀
L29.3   **Anogenital pruritus, unspecified** ▽

L29.8   **Other pruritus**

L29.9   **Pruritus, unspecified**   ▽
      Itch NOS

✓4ᵗʰ **L30   Other and unspecified dermatitis**
      EXCLUDES 2   *contact dermatitis (L23-L25)*
                       dry skin dermatitis (L85.3)
                       small plaque parapsoriasis (L41.3)
                       stasis dermatitis (I87.2)

L30.0   **Nummular dermatitis**

L30.1   **Dyshidrosis [pompholyx]**

L30.2   **Cutaneous autosensitization**
      Candidid [levurid]
      Dermatophytid
      Eczematid

L30.3   **Infective dermatitis**
      Infectious eczematoid dermatitis

L30.4   **Erythema intertrigo**

L30.5   **Pityriasis alba**
      AHA: 2018,1Q,6

L30.8   **Other specified dermatitis**

L30.9   **Dermatitis, unspecified**   ▽
      Eczema NOS

Papulosquamous disorders (L40-L45)

✓4ᵗʰ **L40   Psoriasis**
      DEF: Chronic autoimmune condition that speeds up skin cell growth, causing excessive immature skin cells to form raised, rounded erythematous lesions covered by dry, silvery scaling patches. Most commonly found on the scalp, elbows, knees, hands, feet, and genitals, it can also affect the joints with stiffness and swelling.

L40.0   **Psoriasis vulgaris**
      Nummular psoriasis
      Plaque psoriasis

L40.1   **Generalized pustular psoriasis**
      Impetigo herpetiformis
      Von Zumbusch's disease

L40.2   **Acrodermatitis continua**

L40.3   **Pustulosis palmaris et plantaris**

L40.4   **Guttate psoriasis**

✓5ᵗʰ L40.5   **Arthropathic psoriasis**

      L40.50   **Arthropathic psoriasis, unspecified**   HCC ▽

      L40.51   **Distal interphalangeal psoriatic arthropathy**   HCC

      L40.52   **Psoriatic arthritis mutilans**   HCC

      L40.53   **Psoriatic spondylitis**   HCC

      L40.54   **Psoriatic juvenile arthropathy**   HCC

      L40.59   **Other psoriatic arthropathy**   HCC

L40.8   **Other psoriasis**
      Flexural psoriasis

L40.9   **Psoriasis, unspecified**   ▽

✓4ᵗʰ **L41   Parapsoriasis**
      EXCLUDES 1   *poikiloderma vasculare atrophicans (L94.5)*

L41.0   **Pityriasis lichenoides et varioliformis acuta**
      Mucha-Habermann disease

L41.1   **Pityriasis lichenoides chronica**

L41.3   **Small plaque parapsoriasis**

L41.4   **Large plaque parapsoriasis**

L41.5   **Retiform parapsoriasis**

L41.8   **Other parapsoriasis**

L41.9   **Parapsoriasis, unspecified**   ▽

L42   **Pityriasis rosea**

✓4ᵗʰ **L43   Lichen planus**
      EXCLUDES 1   *lichen planopilaris (L66.1)*

L43.0   **Hypertrophic lichen planus**

L43.1   **Bullous lichen planus**

L43.2   **Lichenoid drug reaction**
      Use additional code for adverse effect, if applicable, to identify drug (T36-T50 with fifth or sixth character 5)

L43.3   **Subacute (active) lichen planus**
      Lichen planus tropicus

L43.8   **Other lichen planus**

L43.9   **Lichen planus, unspecified**   ▽

✓4ᵗʰ **L44   Other papulosquamous disorders**

L44.0   **Pityriasis rubra pilaris**

L44.1   **Lichen nitidus**
      DEF: Chronic, inflammatory, asymptomatic skin disorder, characterized by numerous glistening, flat-topped, discrete, skin-colored micropapules, most often on the penis, lower abdomen, inner thighs, wrists, forearms, breasts, and buttocks.

L44.2   **Lichen striatus**

L44.3   **Lichen ruber moniliformis**

L44.4   **Infantile papular acrodermatitis [Gianotti-Crosti]**   P

L44.8   **Other specified papulosquamous disorders**

L44.9   **Papulosquamous disorder, unspecified**   ▽

*L45   **Papulosquamous disorders in diseases classified elsewhere***
      Code first underlying disease

Urticaria and erythema (L49-L54)

      EXCLUDES 1   *Lyme disease (A69.2-)*
                       rosacea (L71.-)

✓4ᵗʰ **L49   Exfoliation due to erythematous conditions according to extent of body surface involved**
      Code first erythematous condition causing exfoliation, such as:
      Ritter's disease (L00)
      (Staphylococcal) scalded skin syndrom (L00)
      Stevens-Johnson syndrome (L51.1)
      Stevens-Johnson syndrome-toxic epidermal necrolysis overlap syndrome (L51.3)
      toxic epidermal necrolysis (L51.2)
      DEF: Exfoliation: Falling or sloughing off skin in layers.

L49.0   **Exfoliation due to erythematous condition involving less than 10 percent of body surface**
      Exfoliation due to erythematous condition NOS

L49.1   **Exfoliation due to erythematous condition involving 10-19 percent of body surface**

L49.2   **Exfoliation due to erythematous condition involving 20-29 percent of body surface**

L49.3   **Exfoliation due to erythematous condition involving 30-39 percent of body surface**

L49.4   **Exfoliation due to erythematous condition involving 40-49 percent of body surface**

L49.5   **Exfoliation due to erythematous condition involving 50-59 percent of body surface**

L49.6   **Exfoliation due to erythematous condition involving 60-69 percent of body surface**

L49.7   **Exfoliation due to erythematous condition involving 70-79 percent of body surface**

L49.8   **Exfoliation due to erythematous condition involving 80-89 percent of body surface**

L49.9   **Exfoliation due to erythematous condition involving 90 or more percent of body surface**

✓4ᵗʰ **L50   Urticaria**
      EXCLUDES 1   *allergic contact dermatitis (L23.-)*
                       angioneurotic edema (T78.3)
                       giant urticaria (T78.3)
                       hereditary angio-edema (D84.1)
                       Quincke's edema (T78.3)
                       serum urticaria (T80.6-)
                       solar urticaria (L56.3)
                       urticaria neonatorum (P83.8)
                       urticaria papulosa (L28.2)
                       urticaria pigmentosa (Q82.2)
      DEF: Eruption of itching edema of the skin. **Synonym(s):** *hives.*

L50.0   **Allergic urticaria**

L50.1   **Idiopathic urticaria**

L50.2   **Urticaria due to cold and heat**
      EXCLUDES 2   *familial cold urticaria (M04.2)*

L50.3   **Dermatographic urticaria**

L50.4   **Vibratory urticaria**

L50.5   **Cholinergic urticaria**

L50.6   **Contact urticaria**

L50.8   **Other urticaria**
      Chronic urticaria
      Recurrent periodic urticaria

L50.9   **Urticaria, unspecified**   ▽

✓ Additional Character Req   ✓7ᵗʰ Placeholder Alert   Manifestation   ▽ Unspecified   ►◄ Revised Text   ● New Code   ▲ Revised Code Title

Chapter 12. Diseases of the Skin and Subcutaneous Tissue *(left margin)*

L51–L59.9 *(left margin)*

√4ᵗʰ **L51 Erythema multiforme**

Use additional code for adverse effect, if applicable, to identify drug (T36-T50 with fifth or sixth character 5)

Use additional code to identify associated manifestations, such as:
arthropathy associated with dermatological disorders (M14.8-)
conjunctival edema (H11.42)
conjunctivitis (H10.22-)
corneal scars and opacities (H17.-)
corneal ulcer (H16.0-)
edema of eyelid ▶(H02.84-)◀
inflammation of eyelid (H01.8)
keratoconjunctivitis sicca (H16.22-)
mechanical lagophthalmos (H02.22-)
stomatitis (K12.-)
symblepharon (H11.23-)

Use additional code to identify percentage of skin exfoliation (L49.-)

EXCLUDES 1   *staphylococcal scalded skin syndrome (L00)*
Ritter's disease (L00)

DEF: Acute complex of symptoms with a varied pattern of skin eruptions, such as macular, bullous, popular, nodose, or vesicular lesions on the neck, face, and legs. Erythema (redness of skin and mucous membranes) multiforme (multiple forms) is a hypersensitivity (allergic) reaction that can occur at any age but primarily affects children or young adults.

L51.0 Nonbullous erythema multiforme

L51.1 Stevens-Johnson syndrome   HCC

L51.2 Toxic epidermal necrolysis [Lyell]   HCC

L51.3 Stevens-Johnson syndrome-toxic epidermal necrolysis overlap syndrome   HCC
SJS-TEN overlap syndrome

L51.8 Other erythema multiforme

L51.9 Erythema multiforme, unspecified   ▽
Erythema iris
Erythema multiforme major NOS
Erythema multiforme minor NOS
Herpes iris

L52 Erythema nodosum

EXCLUDES 1   *tuberculous erythema nodosum (A18.4)*

DEF: Form of panniculitis (inflammation of the fat layer beneath the skin) most often occurring in women. Commonly seen as a hypersensitivity reaction to infections, drugs, sarcoidosis, and specific enteropathies. The acute stage is associated with fever, malaise, and arthralgia. The lesions are pink to blue in color as tender nodules and are found on the front of the legs below the knees.

√4ᵗʰ **L53 Other erythematous conditions**

EXCLUDES 1   *erythema ab igne (L59.0)*
erythema due to external agents in contact with skin (L23-L25)
erythema intertrigo (L30.4)

L53.0 Toxic erythema
Code first poisoning due to drug or toxin, if applicable (T36-T65 with fifth or sixth character 1-4 or 6)
Use additional code for adverse effect, if applicable, to identify drug (T36-T50 with fifth or sixth character 5)

EXCLUDES 1   *neonatal erythema toxicum (P83.1)*

L53.1 Erythema annulare centrifugum

L53.2 Erythema marginatum

L53.3 Other chronic figurate erythema

L53.8 Other specified erythematous conditions

L53.9 Erythematous condition, unspecified   ▽
Erythema NOS
Erythroderma NOS

L54 Erythema in diseases classified elsewhere
Code first underlying disease

Radiation-related disorders of the skin and subcutaneous tissue (L55-L59)

√4ᵗʰ **L55 Sunburn**

L55.0 Sunburn of first degree

L55.1 Sunburn of second degree

L55.2 Sunburn of third degree

L55.9 Sunburn, unspecified   ▽

√4ᵗʰ **L56 Other acute skin changes due to ultraviolet radiation**

Use additional code to identify the source of the ultraviolet radiation (W89, X32)

L56.0 Drug phototoxic response
Use additional code for adverse effect, if applicable, to identify drug (T36-T50 with fifth or sixth character 5)

L56.1 Drug photoallergic response
Use additional code for adverse effect, if applicable, to identify drug (T36-T50 with fifth or sixth character 5)

L56.2 Photocontact dermatitis [berloque dermatitis]

L56.3 Solar urticaria

L56.4 Polymorphous light eruption

L56.5 Disseminated superficial actinic porokeratosis (DSAP)
DEF: Autosomal dominant skin condition occurring in sun-exposed areas of the skin (particularly the arms and legs), characterized by superficial annular, keratotic, brownish-red spots or thickenings with depressed centers and sharp, ridged borders. It may evolve into squamous cell carcinoma.

L56.8 Other specified acute skin changes due to ultraviolet radiation

L56.9 Acute skin change due to ultraviolet radiation, unspecified   ▽

√4ᵗʰ **L57 Skin changes due to chronic exposure to nonionizing radiation**

Use additional code to identify the source of the ultraviolet radiation (W89)

L57.0 Actinic keratosis
Keratosis NOS
Senile keratosis
Solar keratosis

L57.1 Actinic reticuloid

L57.2 Cutis rhomboidalis nuchae

L57.3 Poikiloderma of Civatte

L57.4 Cutis laxa senilis
Elastosis senilis

L57.5 Actinic granuloma

L57.8 Other skin changes due to chronic exposure to nonionizing radiation
Farmer's skin
Sailor's skin
Solar dermatitis

L57.9 Skin changes due to chronic exposure to nonionizing radiation, unspecified   ▽

√4ᵗʰ **L58 Radiodermatitis**

Use additional code to identify the source of the radiation (W88, W90)

L58.0 Acute radiodermatitis

L58.1 Chronic radiodermatitis

L58.9 Radiodermatitis, unspecified   ▽

√4ᵗʰ **L59 Other disorders of skin and subcutaneous tissue related to radiation**

L59.0 Erythema ab igne [dermatitis ab igne]

L59.8 Other specified disorders of the skin and subcutaneous tissue related to radiation
AHA: 2017,1Q,33

L59.9 Disorder of the skin and subcutaneous tissue related to radiation, unspecified   ▽

Disorders of skin appendages (L60-L75)

EXCLUDES1   *congenital malformations of integument (Q84.-)*

✓4ᵗʰ **L60 Nail disorders**

   EXCLUDES2   *clubbing of nails (R68.3)*
                    onychia and paronychia (L03.0-)

Nail Disorders

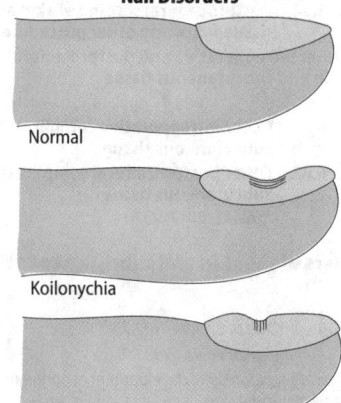

Normal

Koilonychia

Beau's Lines

   L60.0 Ingrowing nail
   L60.1 Onycholysis
   L60.2 Onychogryphosis
   L60.3 Nail dystrophy
   L60.4 Beau's lines
   L60.5 Yellow nail syndrome
   L60.8 Other nail disorders
   L60.9 Nail disorder, unspecified ▽

L62 *Nail disorders in diseases classified elsewhere*
   Code first underlying disease, such as:
     pachydermoperiostosis (M89.4-)

✓4ᵗʰ **L63 Alopecia areata**

   L63.0 Alopecia (capitis) totalis
   L63.1 Alopecia universalis
   L63.2 Ophiasis
   L63.8 Other alopecia areata
   L63.9 Alopecia areata, unspecified ▽

✓4ᵗʰ **L64 Androgenic alopecia**

   INCLUDES   male-pattern baldness

   L64.0 Drug-induced androgenic alopecia
     Use additional code for adverse effect, if applicable, to identify
       drug (T36-T50 with fifth or sixth character 5)

   L64.8 Other androgenic alopecia
   L64.9 Androgenic alopecia, unspecified ▽

✓4ᵗʰ **L65 Other nonscarring hair loss**

   Use additional code for adverse effect, if applicable, to identify drug
     (T36-T50 with fifth or sixth character 5)

   EXCLUDES1   *trichotillomania (F63.3)*

   L65.0 Telogen effluvium
     DEF: Form of nonscarring alopecia characterized by shedding of
     hair from premature telogen development in follicles due to
     stress, including shock, childbirth, surgery, drugs, or weight loss.

   L65.1 Anagen effluvium
   L65.2 Alopecia mucinosa
   L65.8 Other specified nonscarring hair loss
   L65.9 Nonscarring hair loss, unspecified ▽
     Alopecia NOS

✓4ᵗʰ **L66 Cicatricial alopecia [scarring hair loss]**

   L66.0 Pseudopelade
   L66.1 Lichen planopilaris
     Follicular lichen planus
   L66.2 Folliculitis decalvans
   L66.3 Perifolliculitis capitis abscedens
   L66.4 Folliculitis ulerythematosa reticulata

   L66.8 Other cicatricial alopecia
     AHA: 2015,1Q,19
   L66.9 Cicatricial alopecia, unspecified ▽

✓4ᵗʰ **L67 Hair color and hair shaft abnormalities**

   EXCLUDES1   *monilethrix (Q84.1)*
                pili annulati (Q84.1)
                telogen effluvium (L65.0)

   L67.0 Trichorrhexis nodosa
   L67.1 Variations in hair color
     Canities
     Greyness, hair (premature)
     Heterochromia of hair
     Poliosis circumscripta, acquired
     Poliosis NOS
   L67.8 Other hair color and hair shaft abnormalities
     Fragilitas crinium
   L67.9 Hair color and hair shaft abnormality, unspecified ▽

✓4ᵗʰ **L68 Hypertrichosis**

   INCLUDES   excess hair
   EXCLUDES1   *congenital hypertrichosis (Q84.2)*
                persistent lanugo (Q84.2)

   L68.0 Hirsutism
   L68.1 Acquired hypertrichosis lanuginosa
   L68.2 Localized hypertrichosis
   L68.3 Polytrichia
   L68.8 Other hypertrichosis
   L68.9 Hypertrichosis, unspecified ▽

✓4ᵗʰ **L70 Acne**

   EXCLUDES2   *acne keloid (L73.0)*

   L70.0 Acne vulgaris
   L70.1 Acne conglobata
   L70.2 Acne varioliformis
     Acne necrotica miliaris
     DEF: Rare form of acne characterized by development of
     persistent brown papulopustules followed by scar formation. This
     type of acne usually presents on the brow and temporoparietal
     part of the scalp.
   L70.3 Acne tropica
   L70.4 Infantile acne ℙ
   L70.5 Acné excoriée
     Acné excoriée des jeunes filles
     Picker's acne
   L70.8 Other acne
   L70.9 Acne, unspecified ▽

✓4ᵗʰ **L71 Rosacea**

   Use additional code for adverse effect, if applicable, to identify drug
     (T36-T50 with fifth or sixth character 5)

   L71.0 Perioral dermatitis
   L71.1 Rhinophyma
   L71.8 Other rosacea
   L71.9 Rosacea, unspecified ▽

✓4ᵗʰ **L72 Follicular cysts of skin and subcutaneous tissue**

   L72.0 Epidermal cyst
   ✓5ᵗʰ **L72.1 Pilar and trichodermal cyst**
     L72.11 Pilar cyst
     L72.12 Trichodermal cyst
       Trichilemmal (proliferating) cyst
   L72.2 Steatocystoma multiplex
   L72.3 Sebaceous cyst
     EXCLUDES2   *pilar cyst (L72.11)*
                trichilemmal (proliferating) cyst (L72.12)
   L72.8 Other follicular cysts of the skin and subcutaneous tissue
   L72.9 Follicular cyst of the skin and subcutaneous tissue, unspecified ▽

✓4ᵗʰ **L73 Other follicular disorders**

   L73.0 Acne keloid
   L73.1 Pseudofolliculitis barbae
   L73.2 Hidradenitis suppurativa
   L73.8 Other specified follicular disorders
     Sycosis barbae
   L73.9 Follicular disorder, unspecified ▽

☑ Additional Character Req   ✓x7ᵗʰ Placeholder Alert   Manifestation   ▽ Unspecified   ▶◀ Revised Text   ● New Code   ▲ Revised Code Title

Chapter 12. Diseases of the Skin and Subcutaneous Tissue

L74–L85.9

√4ᵗʰ L74 Eccrine sweat disorders

EXCLUDES 2   generalized hyperhidrosis (R61)

DEF: Eccrine sweat glands: Glands found in the dermal and hypodermal layer of the skin throughout the body, particularly on the forehead, scalp, axillae, palms, and soles. These glands produce watery and neutral or slightly acidic sweat.

L74.0 Miliaria rubra

L74.1 Miliaria crystallina

L74.2 Miliaria profunda
Miliaria tropicalis

L74.3 Miliaria, unspecified ▽

L74.4 Anhidrosis
Hypohidrosis
DEF: Inability to sweat normally. When the body can't cool itself through perspiration it can lead to heatstroke, a life-threatening condition.

√5ᵗʰ L74.5 Focal hyperhidrosis

   √6ᵗʰ L74.51 Primary focal hyperhidrosis

      L74.510 Primary focal hyperhidrosis, axilla

      L74.511 Primary focal hyperhidrosis, face

      L74.512 Primary focal hyperhidrosis, palms

      L74.513 Primary focal hyperhidrosis, soles

      L74.519 Primary focal hyperhidrosis, unspecified ▽

   L74.52 Secondary focal hyperhidrosis
      Frey's syndrome

L74.8 Other eccrine sweat disorders

L74.9 Eccrine sweat disorder, unspecified ▽
Sweat gland disorder NOS

√4ᵗʰ L75 Apocrine sweat disorders

EXCLUDES 1   dyshidrosis (L30.1)
           hidradenitis suppurativa (L73.2)

DEF: Apocrine sweat glands: Found in the axilla, areola, and circumanal region, these glands begin to function in puberty and produce viscid milky secretions in response to external stimuli.

L75.0 Bromhidrosis

L75.1 Chromhidrosis

L75.2 Apocrine miliaria
Fox-Fordyce disease
DEF: Chronic, usually pruritic disease evidenced by small follicular papular eruptions, especially in the axillary and pubic areas. Apocrine miliaria develops from the closure and rupture of the affected apocrine glands' intraepidermal portion of the ducts.

L75.8 Other apocrine sweat disorders

L75.9 Apocrine sweat disorder, unspecified ▽

Intraoperative and postprocedural complications of skin and subcutaneous tissue (L76)

√4ᵗʰ L76 Intraoperative and postprocedural complications of skin and subcutaneous tissue
AHA: 2016,4Q,9-10

√5ᵗʰ L76.0 Intraoperative hemorrhage and hematoma of skin and subcutaneous tissue complicating a procedure

EXCLUDES 1   intraoperative hemorrhage and hematoma of skin and subcutaneous tissue due to accidental puncture and laceration during a procedure (L76.1-)

   L76.01 Intraoperative hemorrhage and hematoma of skin and subcutaneous tissue complicating a dermatologic procedure

   L76.02 Intraoperative hemorrhage and hematoma of skin and subcutaneous tissue complicating other procedure

√5ᵗʰ L76.1 Accidental puncture and laceration of skin and subcutaneous tissue during a procedure

   L76.11 Accidental puncture and laceration of skin and subcutaneous tissue during a dermatologic procedure

   L76.12 Accidental puncture and laceration of skin and subcutaneous tissue during other procedure

√5ᵗʰ L76.2 Postprocedural hemorrhage of skin and subcutaneous tissue following a procedure

   L76.21 Postprocedural hemorrhage of skin and subcutaneous tissue following a dermatologic procedure

   L76.22 Postprocedural hemorrhage of skin and subcutaneous tissue following other procedure

√5ᵗʰ L76.3 Postprocedural hematoma and seroma of skin and subcutaneous tissue following a procedure

   L76.31 Postprocedural hematoma of skin and subcutaneous tissue following a dermatologic procedure

   L76.32 Postprocedural hematoma of skin and subcutaneous tissue following other procedure

   L76.33 Postprocedural seroma of skin and subcutaneous tissue following a dermatologic procedure

   L76.34 Postprocedural seroma of skin and subcutaneous tissue following other procedure

√5ᵗʰ L76.8 Other intraoperative and postprocedural complications of skin and subcutaneous tissue
Use additional code, if applicable, to further specify disorder

   L76.81 Other intraoperative complications of skin and subcutaneous tissue

   L76.82 Other postprocedural complications of skin and subcutaneous tissue
AHA: 2017,3Q,6

Other disorders of the skin and subcutaneous tissue (L80-L99)

L80 Vitiligo

EXCLUDES 2   vitiligo of eyelids (H02.73-)
           vitiligo of vulva (N90.89)

DEF: Persistent, progressive development of nonpigmented white patches on otherwise normal skin.

√4ᵗʰ L81 Other disorders of pigmentation

EXCLUDES 1   birthmark NOS (Q82.5)
           Peutz-Jeghers syndrome (Q85.8)

EXCLUDES 2   nevus - see Alphabetical Index

L81.0 Postinflammatory hyperpigmentation

L81.1 Chloasma

L81.2 Freckles

L81.3 Café au lait spots

L81.4 Other melanin hyperpigmentation
Lentigo

L81.5 Leukoderma, not elsewhere classified

L81.6 Other disorders of diminished melanin formation

L81.7 Pigmented purpuric dermatosis
Angioma serpiginosum

L81.8 Other specified disorders of pigmentation
Iron pigmentation
Tattoo pigmentation

L81.9 Disorder of pigmentation, unspecified ▽

√4ᵗʰ L82 Seborrheic keratosis

INCLUDES   basal cell papilloma
        dermatosis papulosa nigra
        Leser-Trélat disease

EXCLUDES 2   seborrheic dermatitis (L21.-)

DEF: Common, benign, noninvasive, lightly pigmented, warty growth composed of basaloid cells that usually appear at middle age as soft, easily crumbling plaques on the face, trunk, and extremities.

L82.0 Inflamed seborrheic keratosis

L82.1 Other seborrheic keratosis
Seborrheic keratosis NOS

L83 Acanthosis nigricans
Confluent and reticulated papillomatosis
DEF: Diffuse, velvety hyperplasia of the spinous skin layer of the axilla and other body folds marked by gray, brown, or black pigmentation. In adult form, it is often associated with malignant acanthosis nigricans in a benign, nevoid form relatively generalized.

L84 Corns and callosities
Callus
Clavus

√4ᵗʰ L85 Other epidermal thickening

EXCLUDES 2   hypertrophic disorders of the skin (L91.-)

L85.0 Acquired ichthyosis
EXCLUDES 1   congenital ichthyosis (Q80.-)

L85.1 Acquired keratosis [keratoderma] palmaris et plantaris
EXCLUDES 1   inherited keratosis palmaris et plantaris (Q82.8)

L85.2 Keratosis punctata (palmaris et plantaris)

L85.3 Xerosis cutis
Dry skin dermatitis

L85.8 Other specified epidermal thickening
Cutaneous horn

L85.9 Epidermal thickening, unspecified ▽

L86 *Keratoderma in diseases classified elsewhere*

Code first underlying disease, such as:

Reiter's disease (M02.3-)

EXCLUDES 1   gonococcal keratoderma (A54.89)

gonococcal keratosis (A54.89)

keratoderma due to vitamin A deficiency (E50.8)

keratosis due to vitamin A deficiency (E50.8)

xeroderma due to vitamin A deficiency (E50.8)

✓4ᵗʰ L87 Transepidermal elimination disorders

EXCLUDES 1   granuloma annulare (perforating) (L92.0)

L87.0 Keratosis follicularis et parafollicularis in cutem penetrans

Hyperkeratosis follicularis penetrans

Kyrle disease

L87.1 Reactive perforating collagenosis

L87.2 Elastosis perforans serpiginosa

L87.8 Other transepidermal elimination disorders

L87.9 Transepidermal elimination disorder, unspecified ▽

L88 Pyoderma gangrenosum

Phagedenic pyoderma

EXCLUDES 1   dermatitis gangrenosa (L08.0)

DEF: Persistent debilitating skin disease characterized by irregular, boggy, blue-red ulcerations, with central healing and undermined edges.

✓4ᵗʰ L89 Pressure ulcer

INCLUDES   bed sore

decubitus ulcer

plaster ulcer

pressure area

pressure sore

Code first any associated gangrene (I96)

EXCLUDES 2   decubitus (trophic) ulcer of cervix (uteri) (N86)

diabetic ulcers (E08.621, E08.622, E09.621, E09.622, E10.621, E10.622, E11.621, E11.622, E13.621, E13.622)

non-pressure chronic ulcer of skin (L97.-)

skin infections (L00-L08)

varicose ulcer (I83.0, I83.2)

AHA: 2018,2Q,21; 2017,4Q,109; 2017,1Q,49; 2016,4Q,143

TIP: The stage of a diagnosed pressure ulcer can be based on documentation from clinicians who are not the patient's provider.

Four Stages of Pressure Ulcer

Stage 1
Persistent focal edema

Stage 2
Abrasion, blister, partial thickness skin loss involving epidermis and/or dermis

Stage 3
Full thickness skin loss involving damage or necrosis of subcutaneous tissue

Stage 4
Necrosis of soft tissues through to underlying muscle, tendon, or bone

✓5ᵗʰ L89.0 Pressure ulcer of elbow

✓6ᵗʰ L89.00 Pressure ulcer of unspecified elbow

L89.000 Pressure ulcer of unspecified elbow, unstageable HCC ▽

L89.001 Pressure ulcer of unspecified elbow, stage 1 ▽

Healing pressure ulcer of unspecified elbow, stage 1

Pressure pre-ulcer skin changes limited to persistent focal edema, unspecified elbow

L89.002 Pressure ulcer of unspecified elbow, stage 2 ▽

Healing pressure ulcer of unspecified elbow, stage 2

Pressure ulcer with abrasion, blister, partial thickness skin loss involving epidermis and/or dermis, unspecified elbow

L89.003 Pressure ulcer of unspecified elbow, stage 3 HCC ▽

Healing pressure ulcer of unspecified elbow, stage 3

Pressure ulcer with full thickness skin loss involving damage or necrosis of subcutaneous tissue, unspecified elbow

L89.004 Pressure ulcer of unspecified elbow, stage 4 HCC ▽

Healing pressure ulcer of unspecified elbow, stage 4

Pressure ulcer with necrosis of soft tissues through to underlying muscle, tendon, or bone, unspecified elbow

L89.009 Pressure ulcer of unspecified elbow, unspecified stage ▽

Healing pressure ulcer of elbow NOS

Healing pressure ulcer of unspecified elbow, unspecified stage

✓6ᵗʰ L89.01 Pressure ulcer of right elbow

L89.010 Pressure ulcer of right elbow, unstageable HCC

L89.011 Pressure ulcer of right elbow, stage 1

Healing pressure ulcer of right elbow, stage 1

Pressure pre-ulcer skin changes limited to persistent focal edema, right elbow

L89.012 Pressure ulcer of right elbow, stage 2

Healing pressure ulcer of right elbow, stage 2

Pressure ulcer with abrasion, blister, partial thickness skin loss involving epidermis and/or dermis, right elbow

L89.013 Pressure ulcer of right elbow, stage 3 HCC

Healing pressure ulcer of right elbow, stage 3

Pressure ulcer with full thickness skin loss involving damage or necrosis of subcutaneous tissue, right elbow

L89.014 Pressure ulcer of right elbow, stage 4 HCC

Healing pressure ulcer of right elbow, stage 4

Pressure ulcer with necrosis of soft tissues through to underlying muscle, tendon, or bone, right elbow

L89.019 Pressure ulcer of right elbow, unspecified stage ▽

Healing pressure right of elbow NOS

Healing pressure ulcer of right elbow, unspecified stage

✓6ᵗʰ L89.02 Pressure ulcer of left elbow

L89.020 Pressure ulcer of left elbow, unstageable HCC

L89.021 Pressure ulcer of left elbow, stage 1

Healing pressure ulcer of left elbow, stage 1

Pressure pre-ulcer skin changes limited to persistent focal edema, left elbow

L89.022 Pressure ulcer of left elbow, stage 2

Healing pressure ulcer of left elbow, stage 2

Pressure ulcer with abrasion, blister, partial thickness skin loss involving epidermis and/or dermis, left elbow

✓ Additional Character Req   ✓x7ᵗʰ Placeholder Alert   Manifestation   ▽ Unspecified   ▶◀ Revised Text   ● New Code   ▲ Revised Code Title

ICD-10-CM 2019   725

L89.023 **Pressure ulcer of left elbow,** HCC
     stage 3
     Healing pressure ulcer of left elbow,
       stage 3
     Pressure ulcer with full thickness skin loss
       involving damage or necrosis of
       subcutaneous tissue, left elbow

L89.024 **Pressure ulcer of left elbow,** HCC
     stage 4
     Healing pressure ulcer of left elbow,
       stage 4
     Pressure ulcer with necrosis of soft tissues
       through to underlying muscle,
       tendon, or bone, left elbow

L89.029 **Pressure ulcer of left elbow,** ▽
     unspecified stage
     Healing pressure ulcer of left of elbow NOS
     Healing pressure ulcer of left elbow,
       unspecified stage

✓5ᵗʰ **L89.1**   **Pressure ulcer of back**

  ✓6ᵗʰ **L89.10**   **Pressure ulcer of unspecified part of back**

L89.100 **Pressure ulcer of unspecified part** HCC ▽
     of back, unstageable

L89.101 **Pressure ulcer of unspecified part** ▽
     of back, stage 1
     Healing pressure ulcer of unspecified part
       of back, stage 1
     Pressure pre-ulcer skin changes limited to
       persistent focal edema, unspecified
       part of back

L89.102 **Pressure ulcer of unspecified part** ▽
     of back, stage 2
     Healing pressure ulcer of unspecified part
       of back, stage 2
     Pressure ulcer with abrasion, blister, partial
       thickness skin loss involving
       epidermis and/or dermis, unspecified
       part of back

L89.103 **Pressure ulcer of unspecified part** HCC ▽
     of back, stage 3
     Healing pressure ulcer of unspecified part
       of back, stage 3
     Pressure ulcer with full thickness skin loss
       involving damage or necrosis of
       subcutaneous tissue, unspecified part
       of back

L89.104 **Pressure ulcer of unspecified part** HCC ▽
     of back, stage 4
     Healing pressure ulcer of unspecified part
       of back, stage 4
     Pressure ulcer with necrosis of soft tissues
       through to underlying muscle,
       tendon, or bone, unspecified part of
       back

L89.109 **Pressure ulcer of unspecified part** ▽
     of back, unspecified stage
     Healing pressure ulcer of unspecified part
       of back NOS
     Healing pressure ulcer of unspecified part
       of back, unspecified stage

  ✓6ᵗʰ **L89.11**   **Pressure ulcer of right upper back**
     Pressure ulcer of right shoulder blade

L89.110 **Pressure ulcer of right upper** HCC
     back, unstageable

L89.111 **Pressure ulcer of right upper back, stage 1**
     Healing pressure ulcer of right upper back,
       stage 1
     Pressure pre-ulcer skin changes limited to
       persistent focal edema, right upper
       back

L89.112 **Pressure ulcer of right upper back, stage 2**
     Healing pressure ulcer of right upper back,
       stage 2
     Pressure ulcer with abrasion, blister, partial
       thickness skin loss involving
       epidermis and/or dermis, right upper
       back

L89.113 **Pressure ulcer of right upper** HCC
     back, stage 3
     Healing pressure ulcer of right upper back,
       stage 3
     Pressure ulcer with full thickness skin loss
       involving damage or necrosis of
       subcutaneous tissue, right upper back

L89.114 **Pressure ulcer of right upper** HCC
     back, stage 4
     Healing pressure ulcer of right upper back,
       stage 4
     Pressure ulcer with necrosis of soft tissues
       through to underlying muscle,
       tendon, or bone, right upper back

L89.119 **Pressure ulcer of right upper** ▽
     back, unspecified stage
     Healing pressure ulcer of right upper back
       NOS
     Healing pressure ulcer of right upper back,
       unspecified stage

  ✓6ᵗʰ **L89.12**   **Pressure ulcer of left upper back**
     Pressure ulcer of left shoulder blade

L89.120 **Pressure ulcer of left upper back,** HCC
     unstageable

L89.121 **Pressure ulcer of left upper back, stage 1**
     Healing pressure ulcer of left upper back,
       stage 1
     Pressure pre-ulcer skin changes limited to
       persistent focal edema, left upper
       back

L89.122 **Pressure ulcer of left upper back, stage 2**
     Healing pressure ulcer of left upper back,
       stage 2
     Pressure ulcer with abrasion, blister, partial
       thickness skin loss involving
       epidermis and/or dermis, left upper
       back

L89.123 **Pressure ulcer of left upper back,** HCC
     stage 3
     Healing pressure ulcer of left upper back,
       stage 3
     Pressure ulcer with full thickness skin loss
       involving damage or necrosis of
       subcutaneous tissue, left upper back

L89.124 **Pressure ulcer of left upper back,** HCC
     stage 4
     Healing pressure ulcer of left upper back,
       stage 4
     Pressure ulcer with necrosis of soft tissues
       through to underlying muscle,
       tendon, or bone, left upper back

L89.129 **Pressure ulcer of left upper back,** ▽
     unspecified stage
     Healing pressure ulcer of left upper back
       NOS
     Healing pressure ulcer of left upper back,
       unspecified stage

  ✓6ᵗʰ **L89.13**   **Pressure ulcer of right lower back**

L89.130 **Pressure ulcer of right lower back,** HCC
     unstageable

L89.131 **Pressure ulcer of right lower back, stage 1**
     Healing pressure ulcer of right lower back,
       stage 1
     Pressure pre-ulcer skin changes limited to
       persistent focal edema, right lower
       back

L89.132 **Pressure ulcer of right lower back, stage 2**
     Healing pressure ulcer of right lower back,
       stage 2
     Pressure ulcer with abrasion, blister, partial
       thickness skin loss involving
       epidermis and/or dermis, right lower
       back

L89.133 **Pressure ulcer of right lower back,** HCC
    stage 3
    Healing pressure ulcer of right lower back,
      stage 3
    Pressure ulcer with full thickness skin loss
      involving damage or necrosis of
      subcutaneous tissue, right lower back

L89.134 **Pressure ulcer of right lower back,** HCC
    stage 4
    Healing pressure ulcer of right lower back,
      stage 4
    Pressure ulcer with necrosis of soft tissues
      through to underlying muscle,
      tendon, or bone, right lower back

L89.139 **Pressure ulcer of right lower back,** ▽
    unspecified stage
    Healing pressure ulcer of right lower back
      NOS
    Healing pressure ulcer of right lower back,
      unspecified stage

✓6ᵗʰ **L89.14** **Pressure ulcer of left lower back**

L89.140 **Pressure ulcer of left lower back,** HCC
    unstageable

L89.141 **Pressure ulcer of left lower back, stage 1**
    Healing pressure ulcer of left lower back,
      stage 1
    Pressure pre-ulcer skin changes limited to
      persistent focal edema, left lower
      back

L89.142 **Pressure ulcer of left lower back, stage 2**
    Healing pressure ulcer of left lower back,
      stage 2
    Pressure ulcer with abrasion, blister, partial
      thickness skin loss involving
      epidermis and/or dermis, left lower
      back

L89.143 **Pressure ulcer of left lower back,** HCC
    stage 3
    Healing pressure ulcer of left lower back,
      stage 3
    Pressure ulcer with full thickness skin loss
      involving damage or necrosis of
      subcutaneous tissue, left lower back

L89.144 **Pressure ulcer of left lower back,** HCC
    stage 4
    Healing pressure ulcer of left lower back,
      stage 4
    Pressure ulcer with necrosis of soft tissues
      through to underlying muscle,
      tendon, or bone, left lower back

L89.149 **Pressure ulcer of left lower back,** ▽
    unspecified stage
    Healing pressure ulcer of left lower back
      NOS
    Healing pressure ulcer of left lower back,
      unspecified stage

✓6ᵗʰ **L89.15** **Pressure ulcer of sacral region**
    Pressure ulcer of coccyx
    Pressure ulcer of tailbone

L89.150 **Pressure ulcer of sacral region,** HCC
    unstageable

L89.151 **Pressure ulcer of sacral region, stage 1**
    Healing pressure ulcer of sacral region,
      stage 1
    Pressure pre-ulcer skin changes limited to
      persistent focal edema, sacral region

L89.152 **Pressure ulcer of sacral region, stage 2**
    Healing pressure ulcer of sacral region,
      stage 2
    Pressure ulcer with abrasion, blister, partial
      thickness skin loss involving
      epidermis and/or dermis, sacral
      region

L89.153 **Pressure ulcer of sacral region,** HCC
    stage 3
    Healing pressure ulcer of sacral region,
      stage 3
    Pressure ulcer with full thickness skin loss
      involving damage or necrosis of
      subcutaneous tissue, sacral region

L89.154 **Pressure ulcer of sacral region,** HCC
    stage 4
    Healing pressure ulcer of sacral region,
      stage 4
    Pressure ulcer with necrosis of soft tissues
      through to underlying muscle,
      tendon, or bone, sacral region

L89.159 **Pressure ulcer of sacral region,** ▽
    unspecified stage
    Healing pressure ulcer of sacral region NOS
    Healing pressure ulcer of sacral region,
      unspecified stage

✓5ᵗʰ **L89.2** **Pressure ulcer of hip**

✓6ᵗʰ **L89.20** **Pressure ulcer of unspecified hip**

L89.200 **Pressure ulcer of unspecified hip,** HCC ▽
    unstageable

L89.201 **Pressure ulcer of unspecified hip,** ▽
    stage 1
    Healing pressure ulcer of unspecified hip
      back, stage 1
    Pressure pre-ulcer skin changes limited to
      persistent focal edema, unspecified
      hip

L89.202 **Pressure ulcer of unspecified hip,** ▽
    stage 2
    Healing pressure ulcer of unspecified hip,
      stage 2
    Pressure ulcer with abrasion, blister, partial
      thickness skin loss involving
      epidermis and/or dermis, unspecified
      hip

L89.203 **Pressure ulcer of unspecified hip,** HCC ▽
    stage 3
    Healing pressure ulcer of unspecified hip,
      stage 3
    Pressure ulcer with full thickness skin loss
      involving damage or necrosis of
      subcutaneous tissue, unspecified hip

L89.204 **Pressure ulcer of unspecified hip,** HCC ▽
    stage 4
    Healing pressure ulcer of unspecified hip,
      stage 4
    Pressure ulcer with necrosis of soft tissues
      through to underlying muscle,
      tendon, or bone, unspecified hip

L89.209 **Pressure ulcer of unspecified hip,** ▽
    unspecified stage
    Healing pressure ulcer of unspecified hip
      NOS
    Healing pressure ulcer of unspecified hip,
      unspecified stage

✓6ᵗʰ **L89.21** **Pressure ulcer of right hip**

L89.210 **Pressure ulcer of right hip,** HCC
    unstageable

L89.211 **Pressure ulcer of right hip, stage 1**
    Healing pressure ulcer of right hip back,
      stage 1
    Pressure pre-ulcer skin changes limited to
      persistent focal edema, right hip

L89.212 **Pressure ulcer of right hip, stage 2**
    Healing pressure ulcer of right hip, stage 2
    Pressure ulcer with abrasion, blister, partial
      thickness skin loss involving
      epidermis and/or dermis, right hip

L89.213 **Pressure ulcer of right hip, stage 3** HCC
    Healing pressure ulcer of right hip, stage 3
    Pressure ulcer with full thickness skin loss
      involving damage or necrosis of
      subcutaneous tissue, right hip

✓ Additional Character Req   ✓x7ᵗʰ Placeholder Alert   Manifestation   ▽ Unspecified   ▶◀ Revised Text   ● New Code   ▲ Revised Code Title

L89.214 Pressure ulcer of right hip, stage 4 HCC
Healing pressure ulcer of right hip, stage 4
Pressure ulcer with necrosis of soft tissues through to underlying muscle, tendon, or bone, right hip

L89.219 Pressure ulcer of right hip, unspecified stage ▽
Healing pressure ulcer of right hip NOS
Healing pressure ulcer of right hip, unspecified stage

√6ᵗʰ **L89.22 Pressure ulcer of left hip**

L89.220 Pressure ulcer of left hip, unstageable HCC

L89.221 Pressure ulcer of left hip, stage 1
Healing pressure ulcer of left hip back, stage 1
Pressure pre-ulcer skin changes limited to persistent focal edema, left hip

L89.222 Pressure ulcer of left hip, stage 2
Healing pressure ulcer of left hip, stage 2
Pressure ulcer with abrasion, blister, partial thickness skin loss involving epidermis and/or dermis, left hip

L89.223 Pressure ulcer of left hip, stage 3 HCC
Healing pressure ulcer of left hip, stage 3
Pressure ulcer with full thickness skin loss involving damage or necrosis of subcutaneous tissue, left hip

L89.224 Pressure ulcer of left hip, stage 4 HCC
Healing pressure ulcer of left hip, stage 4
Pressure ulcer with necrosis of soft tissues through to underlying muscle, tendon, or bone, left hip

L89.229 Pressure ulcer of left hip, unspecified stage ▽
Healing pressure ulcer of left hip NOS
Healing pressure ulcer of left hip, unspecified stage

√5ᵗʰ **L89.3 Pressure ulcer of buttock**

√6ᵗʰ **L89.30 Pressure ulcer of unspecified buttock**

L89.300 Pressure ulcer of unspecified buttock, unstageable HCC ▽

L89.301 Pressure ulcer of unspecified buttock, stage 1 ▽
Healing pressure ulcer of unspecified buttock, stage 1
Pressure pre-ulcer skin changes limited to persistent focal edema, unspecified buttock

L89.302 Pressure ulcer of unspecified buttock, stage 2 ▽
Healing pressure ulcer of unspecified buttock, stage 2
Pressure ulcer with abrasion, blister, partial thickness skin loss involving epidermis and/or dermis, unspecified buttock

L89.303 Pressure ulcer of unspecified buttock, stage 3 HCC ▽
Healing pressure ulcer of unspecified buttock, stage 3
Pressure ulcer with full thickness skin loss involving damage or necrosis of subcutaneous tissue, unspecified buttock

L89.304 Pressure ulcer of unspecified buttock, stage 4 HCC ▽
Healing pressure ulcer of unspecified buttock, stage 4
Pressure ulcer with necrosis of soft tissues through to underlying muscle, tendon, or bone, unspecified buttock

L89.309 Pressure ulcer of unspecified buttock, unspecified stage ▽
Healing pressure ulcer of unspecified buttock NOS
Healing pressure ulcer of unspecified buttock, unspecified stage

√6ᵗʰ **L89.31 Pressure ulcer of right buttock**

L89.310 Pressure ulcer of right buttock, unstageable HCC

L89.311 Pressure ulcer of right buttock, stage 1
Healing pressure ulcer of right buttock, stage 1
Pressure pre-ulcer skin changes limited to persistent focal edema, right buttock

L89.312 Pressure ulcer of right buttock, stage 2
Healing pressure ulcer of right buttock, stage 2
Pressure ulcer with abrasion, blister, partial thickness skin loss involving epidermis and/or dermis, right buttock

L89.313 Pressure ulcer of right buttock, stage 3 HCC
Healing pressure ulcer of right buttock, stage 3
Pressure ulcer with full thickness skin loss involving damage or necrosis of subcutaneous tissue, right buttock

L89.314 Pressure ulcer of right buttock, stage 4 HCC
Healing pressure ulcer of right buttock, stage 4
Pressure ulcer with necrosis of soft tissues through to underlying muscle, tendon, or bone, right buttock

L89.319 Pressure ulcer of right buttock, unspecified stage ▽
Healing pressure ulcer of right buttock NOS
Healing pressure ulcer of right buttock, unspecified stage

√6ᵗʰ **L89.32 Pressure ulcer of left buttock**

L89.320 Pressure ulcer of left buttock, unstageable HCC

L89.321 Pressure ulcer of left buttock, stage 1
Healing pressure ulcer of left buttock, stage 1
Pressure pre-ulcer skin changes limited to persistent focal edema, left buttock

L89.322 Pressure ulcer of left buttock, stage 2
Healing pressure ulcer of left buttock, stage 2
Pressure ulcer with abrasion, blister, partial thickness skin loss involving epidermis and/or dermis, left buttock

L89.323 Pressure ulcer of left buttock, stage 3 HCC
Healing pressure ulcer of left buttock, stage 3
Pressure ulcer with full thickness skin loss involving damage or necrosis of subcutaneous tissue, left buttock

L89.324 Pressure ulcer of left buttock, stage 4 HCC
Healing pressure ulcer of left buttock, stage 4
Pressure ulcer with necrosis of soft tissues through to underlying muscle, tendon, or bone, left buttock

L89.329 Pressure ulcer of left buttock, unspecified stage ▽
Healing pressure ulcer of left buttock NOS
Healing pressure ulcer of left buttock, unspecified stage

√5ᵗʰ **L89.4 Pressure ulcer of contiguous site of back, buttock and hip**

L89.40 Pressure ulcer of contiguous site of back, buttock and hip, unspecified stage ▽
Healing pressure ulcer of contiguous site of back, buttock and hip NOS
Healing pressure ulcer of contiguous site of back, buttock and hip, unspecified stage

L89.41 Pressure ulcer of contiguous site of back, buttock and hip, stage 1
Healing pressure ulcer of contiguous site of back, buttock and hip, stage 1
Pressure pre-ulcer skin changes limited to persistent focal edema, contiguous site of back, buttock and hip

L89.42 Pressure ulcer of contiguous site of back, buttock and hip, stage 2
Healing pressure ulcer of contiguous site of back, buttock and hip, stage 2
Pressure ulcer with abrasion, blister, partial thickness skin loss involving epidermis and/or dermis, contiguous site of back, buttock and hip

L89.43 Pressure ulcer of contiguous site of back, buttock and hip, stage 3 HCC
Healing pressure ulcer of contiguous site of back, buttock and hip, stage 3
Pressure ulcer with full thickness skin loss involving damage or necrosis of subcutaneous tissue, contiguous site of back, buttock and hip

L89.44 Pressure ulcer of contiguous site of back, buttock and hip, stage 4 HCC
Healing pressure ulcer of contiguous site of back, buttock and hip, stage 4
Pressure ulcer with necrosis of soft tissues through to underlying muscle, tendon, or bone, contiguous site of back, buttock and hip

L89.45 Pressure ulcer of contiguous site of back, buttock and hip, unstageable HCC

√5th **L89.5 Pressure ulcer of ankle**

√6th **L89.50 Pressure ulcer of unspecified ankle**

L89.500 Pressure ulcer of unspecified ankle, unstageable HCC ▽

L89.501 Pressure ulcer of unspecified ankle, stage 1 ▽
Healing pressure ulcer of unspecified ankle, stage 1
Pressure pre-ulcer skin changes limited to persistent focal edema, unspecified ankle

L89.502 Pressure ulcer of unspecified ankle, stage 2 ▽
Healing pressure ulcer of unspecified ankle, stage 2
Pressure ulcer with abrasion, blister, partial thickness skin loss involving epidermis and/or dermis, unspecified ankle

L89.503 Pressure ulcer of unspecified ankle, stage 3 HCC ▽
Healing pressure ulcer of unspecified ankle, stage 3
Pressure ulcer with full thickness skin loss involving damage or necrosis of subcutaneous tissue, unspecified ankle

L89.504 Pressure ulcer of unspecified ankle, stage 4 HCC ▽
Healing pressure ulcer of unspecified ankle, stage 4
Pressure ulcer with necrosis of soft tissues through to underlying muscle, tendon, or bone, unspecified ankle

L89.509 Pressure ulcer of unspecified ankle, unspecified stage ▽
Healing pressure ulcer of unspecified ankle NOS
Healing pressure ulcer of unspecified ankle, unspecified stage

√6th **L89.51 Pressure ulcer of right ankle**

L89.510 Pressure ulcer of right ankle, unstageable HCC

L89.511 Pressure ulcer of right ankle, stage 1
Healing pressure ulcer of right ankle, stage 1
Pressure pre-ulcer skin changes limited to persistent focal edema, right ankle

L89.512 Pressure ulcer of right ankle, stage 2
Healing pressure ulcer of right ankle, stage 2
Pressure ulcer with abrasion, blister, partial thickness skin loss involving epidermis and/or dermis, right ankle

L89.513 Pressure ulcer of right ankle, stage 3 HCC
Healing pressure ulcer of right ankle, stage 3
Pressure ulcer with full thickness skin loss involving damage or necrosis of subcutaneous tissue, right ankle

L89.514 Pressure ulcer of right ankle, stage 4 HCC
Healing pressure ulcer of right ankle, stage 4
Pressure ulcer with necrosis of soft tissues through to underlying muscle, tendon, or bone, right ankle

L89.519 Pressure ulcer of right ankle, unspecified stage ▽
Healing pressure ulcer of right ankle NOS
Healing pressure ulcer of right ankle, unspecified stage

√6th **L89.52 Pressure ulcer of left ankle**

L89.520 Pressure ulcer of left ankle, unstageable HCC

L89.521 Pressure ulcer of left ankle, stage 1
Healing pressure ulcer of left ankle, stage 1
Pressure pre-ulcer skin changes limited to persistent focal edema, left ankle

L89.522 Pressure ulcer of left ankle, stage 2
Healing pressure ulcer of left ankle, stage 2
Pressure ulcer with abrasion, blister, partial thickness skin loss involving epidermis and/or dermis, left ankle

L89.523 Pressure ulcer of left ankle, stage 3 HCC
Healing pressure ulcer of left ankle, stage 3
Pressure ulcer with full thickness skin loss involving damage or necrosis of subcutaneous tissue, left ankle

L89.524 Pressure ulcer of left ankle, stage 4 HCC
Healing pressure ulcer of left ankle, stage 4
Pressure ulcer with necrosis of soft tissues through to underlying muscle, tendon, or bone, left ankle

L89.529 Pressure ulcer of left ankle, unspecified stage ▽
Healing pressure ulcer of left ankle NOS
Healing pressure ulcer of left ankle, unspecified stage

√5th **L89.6 Pressure ulcer of heel**

√6th **L89.60 Pressure ulcer of unspecified heel**

L89.600 Pressure ulcer of unspecified heel, unstageable HCC ▽

L89.601 Pressure ulcer of unspecified heel, stage 1 ▽
Healing pressure ulcer of unspecified heel, stage 1
Pressure pre-ulcer skin changes limited to persistent focal edema, unspecified heel

L89.602 Pressure ulcer of unspecified heel, stage 2 ▽
Healing pressure ulcer of unspecified heel, stage 2
Pressure ulcer with abrasion, blister, partial thickness skin loss involving epidermis and/or dermis, unspecified heel

Chapter 12. Diseases of the Skin and Subcutaneous Tissue

L89.6Ø3–L89.92

L89.6Ø3   **Pressure ulcer of unspecified heel, stage 3**   HCC ▽
Healing pressure ulcer of unspecified heel, stage 3
Pressure ulcer with full thickness skin loss involving damage or necrosis of subcutaneous tissue, unspecified heel

L89.6Ø4   **Pressure ulcer of unspecified heel, stage 4**   HCC ▽
Healing pressure ulcer of unspecified heel, stage 4
Pressure ulcer with necrosis of soft tissues through to underlying muscle, tendon, or bone, unspecified heel

L89.6Ø9   **Pressure ulcer of unspecified heel, unspecified stage**   ▽
Healing pressure ulcer of unspecified heel NOS
Healing pressure ulcer of unspecified heel, unspecified stage

✓6ᵗʰ **L89.61**   **Pressure ulcer of right heel**

L89.61Ø   **Pressure ulcer of right heel, unstageable**   HCC

L89.611   **Pressure ulcer of right heel, stage 1**
Healing pressure ulcer of right heel, stage 1
Pressure pre-ulcer skin changes limited to persistent focal edema, right heel

L89.612   **Pressure ulcer of right heel, stage 2**
Healing pressure ulcer of right heel, stage 2
Pressure ulcer with abrasion, blister, partial thickness skin loss involving epidermis and/or dermis, right heel

L89.613   **Pressure ulcer of right heel, stage 3**   HCC
Healing pressure ulcer of right heel, stage 3
Pressure ulcer with full thickness skin loss involving damage or necrosis of subcutaneous tissue, right heel

L89.614   **Pressure ulcer of right heel, stage 4**   HCC
Healing pressure ulcer of right heel, stage 4
Pressure ulcer with necrosis of soft tissues through to underlying muscle, tendon, or bone, right heel

L89.619   **Pressure ulcer of right heel, unspecified stage**   ▽
Healing pressure ulcer of right heel NOS
Healing pressure ulcer of right heel, unspecified stage

✓6ᵗʰ **L89.62**   **Pressure ulcer of left heel**

L89.62Ø   **Pressure ulcer of left heel, unstageable**   HCC

L89.621   **Pressure ulcer of left heel, stage 1**
Healing pressure ulcer of left heel, stage 1
Pressure pre-ulcer skin changes limited to persistent focal edema, left heel

L89.622   **Pressure ulcer of left heel, stage 2**
Healing pressure ulcer of left heel, stage 2
Pressure ulcer with abrasion, blister, partial thickness skin loss involving epidermis and/or dermis, left heel

L89.623   **Pressure ulcer of left heel, stage 3**   HCC
Healing pressure ulcer of left heel, stage 3
Pressure ulcer with full thickness skin loss involving damage or necrosis of subcutaneous tissue, left heel

L89.624   **Pressure ulcer of left heel, stage 4**   HCC
Healing pressure ulcer of left heel, stage 4
Pressure ulcer with necrosis of soft tissues through to underlying muscle, tendon, or bone, left heel

L89.629   **Pressure ulcer of left heel, unspecified stage**   ▽
Healing pressure ulcer of left heel NOS
Healing pressure ulcer of left heel, unspecified stage

✓5ᵗʰ **L89.8**   **Pressure ulcer of other site**

✓6ᵗʰ **L89.81**   **Pressure ulcer of head**
Pressure ulcer of face

L89.81Ø   **Pressure ulcer of head, unstageable**   HCC

L89.811   **Pressure ulcer of head, stage 1**
Healing pressure ulcer of head, stage 1
Pressure pre-ulcer skin changes limited to persistent focal edema, head

L89.812   **Pressure ulcer of head, stage 2**
Healing pressure ulcer of head, stage 2
Pressure ulcer with abrasion, blister, partial thickness skin loss involving epidermis and/or dermis, head

L89.813   **Pressure ulcer of head, stage 3**   HCC
Healing pressure ulcer of head, stage 3
Pressure ulcer with full thickness skin loss involving damage or necrosis of subcutaneous tissue, head

L89.814   **Pressure ulcer of head, stage 4**   HCC
Healing pressure ulcer of head, stage 4
Pressure ulcer with necrosis of soft tissues through to underlying muscle, tendon, or bone, head

L89.819   **Pressure ulcer of head, unspecified stage**   ▽
Healing pressure ulcer of head NOS
Healing pressure ulcer of head, unspecified stage

✓6ᵗʰ **L89.89**   **Pressure ulcer of other site**

L89.89Ø   **Pressure ulcer of other site, unstageable**   HCC

L89.891   **Pressure ulcer of other site, stage 1**
Healing pressure ulcer of other site, stage 1
Pressure pre-ulcer skin changes limited to persistent focal edema, other site

L89.892   **Pressure ulcer of other site, stage 2**
Healing pressure ulcer of other site, stage 2
Pressure ulcer with abrasion, blister, partial thickness skin loss involving epidermis and/or dermis, other site

L89.893   **Pressure ulcer of other site, stage 3**   HCC
Healing pressure ulcer of other site, stage 3
Pressure ulcer with full thickness skin loss involving damage or necrosis of subcutaneous tissue, other site

L89.894   **Pressure ulcer of other site, stage 4**   HCC
Healing pressure ulcer of other site, stage 4
Pressure ulcer with necrosis of soft tissues through to underlying muscle, tendon, or bone, other site

L89.899   **Pressure ulcer of other site, unspecified stage**   ▽
Healing pressure ulcer of other site NOS
Healing pressure ulcer of other site, unspecified stage

✓5ᵗʰ **L89.9**   **Pressure ulcer of unspecified site**

L89.9Ø   **Pressure ulcer of unspecified site, unspecified stage**   ▽
Healing pressure ulcer of unspecified site NOS
Healing pressure ulcer of unspecified site, unspecified stage

L89.91   **Pressure ulcer of unspecified site, stage 1**   ▽
Healing pressure ulcer of unspecified site, stage 1
Pressure pre-ulcer skin changes limited to persistent focal edema, unspecified site

L89.92   **Pressure ulcer of unspecified site, stage 2**   ▽
Healing pressure ulcer of unspecified site, stage 2
Pressure ulcer with abrasion, blister, partial thickness skin loss involving epidermis and/or dermis, unspecified site

L89.93 Pressure ulcer of unspecified site, stage 3 HCC ▽
Healing pressure ulcer of unspecified site, stage 3
Pressure ulcer with full thickness skin loss involving damage or necrosis of subcutaneous tissue, unspecified site

L89.94 Pressure ulcer of unspecified site, stage 4 HCC ▽
Healing pressure ulcer of unspecified site, stage 4
Pressure ulcer with necrosis of soft tissues through to underlying muscle, tendon, or bone, unspecified site

L89.95 Pressure ulcer of unspecified site, unstageable HCC ▽

✓4th **L90 Atrophic disorders of skin**

L90.0 Lichen sclerosus et atrophicus
> EXCLUDES 2   *lichen sclerosus of external female genital organs (N90.4)*
> *lichen sclerosus of external male genital organs (N48.0)*

L90.1 Anetoderma of Schweninger-Buzzi

L90.2 Anetoderma of Jadassohn-Pellizzari

L90.3 Atrophoderma of Pasini and Pierini

L90.4 Acrodermatitis chronica atrophicans

L90.5 Scar conditions and fibrosis of skin
Adherent scar (skin)
Cicatrix
Disfigurement of skin due to scar
Fibrosis of skin NOS
Scar NOS
> EXCLUDES 2   *hypertrophic scar (L91.0)*
> *keloid scar (L91.0)*
> **AHA:** 2016,2Q,5; 2015,1Q,19

L90.6 Striae atrophicae

L90.8 Other atrophic disorders of skin

L90.9 Atrophic disorder of skin, unspecified ▽

✓4th **L91 Hypertrophic disorders of skin**

L91.0 Hypertrophic scar
Keloid
Keloid scar
> EXCLUDES 2   *acne keloid (L73.0)*
> *scar NOS (L90.5)*
> **DEF:** Overgrowth of scar tissue due to excess amounts of collagen during connective tissue repair, occurring mainly on the upper trunk and face.

L91.8 Other hypertrophic disorders of the skin

L91.9 Hypertrophic disorder of the skin, unspecified ▽

✓4th **L92 Granulomatous disorders of skin and subcutaneous tissue**
> EXCLUDES 2   *actinic granuloma (L57.5)*

L92.0 Granuloma annulare
Perforating granuloma annulare

L92.1 Necrobiosis lipoidica, not elsewhere classified
> EXCLUDES 1   *necrobiosis lipoidica associated with diabetes mellitus (E08-E13 with .620)*

L92.2 Granuloma faciale [eosinophilic granuloma of skin]

L92.3 Foreign body granuloma of the skin and subcutaneous tissue
Use additional code to identify the type of retained foreign body (Z18.-)

L92.8 Other granulomatous disorders of the skin and subcutaneous tissue

L92.9 Granulomatous disorder of the skin and subcutaneous tissue, unspecified ▽
> EXCLUDES 2   *umbilical granuloma (P83.81)*
> **AHA:** 2017,4Q,21-22

✓4th **L93 Lupus erythematosus**
Use additional code for adverse effect, if applicable, to identify drug (T36-T50 with fifth or sixth character 5)
> EXCLUDES 1   *lupus exedens (A18.4)*
> *lupus vulgaris (A18.4)*
> *scleroderma (M34.-)*
> *systemic lupus erythematosus (M32.-)*
> **DEF:** Inflammatory, autoimmune skin condition in which the body's autoimmune system attacks healthy tissue of the integumentary system.

L93.0 Discoid lupus erythematosus
Lupus erythematosus NOS

L93.1 Subacute cutaneous lupus erythematosus

L93.2 Other local lupus erythematosus
Lupus erythematosus profundus
Lupus panniculitis

✓4th **L94 Other localized connective tissue disorders**
> EXCLUDES 1   *systemic connective tissue disorders (M30-M36)*

L94.0 Localized scleroderma [morphea]
Circumscribed scleroderma

L94.1 Linear scleroderma
En coup de sabre lesion

L94.2 Calcinosis cutis

L94.3 Sclerodactyly

L94.4 Gottron's papules

L94.5 Poikiloderma vasculare atrophicans

L94.6 Ainhum

L94.8 Other specified localized connective tissue disorders

L94.9 Localized connective tissue disorder, unspecified ▽

✓4th **L95 Vasculitis limited to skin, not elsewhere classified**
> EXCLUDES 1   *angioma serpiginosum (L81.7)*
> *Henoch(-Schönlein) purpura (D69.0)*
> *hypersensitivity angiitis (M31.0)*
> *lupus panniculitis (L93.2)*
> *panniculitis NOS (M79.3)*
> *panniculitis of neck and back (M54.0-)*
> *polyarteritis nodosa (M30.0)*
> *relapsing panniculitis (M35.6)*
> *rheumatoid vasculitis (M05.2)*
> *serum sickness (T80.6-)*
> *urticaria (L50.-)*
> *Wegener's granulomatosis (M31.3-)*

L95.0 Livedoid vasculitis
Atrophie blanche (en plaque)

L95.1 Erythema elevatum diutinum

L95.8 Other vasculitis limited to the skin

L95.9 Vasculitis limited to the skin, unspecified ▽

✓4th **L97 Non-pressure chronic ulcer of lower limb, not elsewhere classified**
> INCLUDES   chronic ulcer of skin of lower limb NOS
> non-healing ulcer of skin
> non-infected sinus of skin
> trophic ulcer NOS
> tropical ulcer NOS
> ulcer of skin of lower limb NOS

Code first any associated underlying condition, such as:
any associated gangrene (I96)
atherosclerosis of the lower extremities (I70.23-, I70.24-, I70.33-, I70.34-, I70.43-, I70.44-, I70.53-, I70.54-, I70.63-, I70.64-, I70.73-, I70.74-)
chronic venous hypertension (I87.31-, I87.33-)
diabetic ulcers (E08.621, E08.622, E09.621, E09.622, E10.621, E10.622, E11.621, E11.622, E13.621, E13.622)
postphlebitic syndrome (I87.01-, I87.03-)
postthrombotic syndrome (I87.01-, I87.03-)
varicose ulcer (I83.0-, I83.2-)
> EXCLUDES 2   *pressure ulcer (pressure area) (L89.-)*
> *skin infections (L00-L08)*
> *specific infections classified to A00-B99*

AHA: 2017,4Q,17
TIP: The depth and/or severity of a diagnosed nonpressure ulcer can be determined based on medical record documentation from clinicians who are not the patient's provider.
TIP: Assign a code from this category/subcategory for nonpressure ulcers documented as acute.

✓5th **L97.1 Non-pressure chronic ulcer of thigh**

✓6th **L97.10 Non-pressure chronic ulcer of unspecified thigh**

L97.101 Non-pressure chronic ulcer of unspecified thigh limited to breakdown of skin HCC ▽

L97.102 Non-pressure chronic ulcer of unspecified thigh with fat layer exposed HCC ▽

L97.103 Non-pressure chronic ulcer of unspecified thigh with necrosis of muscle HCC ▽

L97.104 Non-pressure chronic ulcer of unspecified thigh with necrosis of bone HCC ▽

L97.105   Non-pressure chronic ulcer of unspecified thigh with muscle involvement without evidence of necrosis   HCC ▽

L97.106   Non-pressure chronic ulcer of unspecified thigh with bone involvement without evidence of necrosis   HCC ▽

L97.108   Non-pressure chronic ulcer of unspecified thigh with other specified severity   HCC ▽

L97.109   Non-pressure chronic ulcer of unspecified thigh with unspecified severity   HCC ▽

√6th **L97.11**   Non-pressure chronic ulcer of right thigh

L97.111   Non-pressure chronic ulcer of right thigh limited to breakdown of skin   HCC

L97.112   Non-pressure chronic ulcer of right thigh with fat layer exposed   HCC

L97.113   Non-pressure chronic ulcer of right thigh with necrosis of muscle   HCC

L97.114   Non-pressure chronic ulcer of right thigh with necrosis of bone   HCC

L97.115   Non-pressure chronic ulcer of right thigh with muscle involvement without evidence of necrosis   HCC

L97.116   Non-pressure chronic ulcer of right thigh with bone involvement without evidence of necrosis   HCC

L97.118   Non-pressure chronic ulcer of right thigh with other specified severity   HCC

L97.119   Non-pressure chronic ulcer of right thigh with unspecified severity   HCC ▽

√6th **L97.12**   Non-pressure chronic ulcer of left thigh

L97.121   Non-pressure chronic ulcer of left thigh limited to breakdown of skin   HCC

L97.122   Non-pressure chronic ulcer of left thigh with fat layer exposed   HCC

L97.123   Non-pressure chronic ulcer of left thigh with necrosis of muscle   HCC

L97.124   Non-pressure chronic ulcer of left thigh with necrosis of bone   HCC

L97.125   Non-pressure chronic ulcer of left thigh with muscle involvement without evidence of necrosis   HCC

L97.126   Non-pressure chronic ulcer of left thigh with bone involvement without evidence of necrosis   HCC

L97.128   Non-pressure chronic ulcer of left thigh with other specified severity   HCC

L97.129   Non-pressure chronic ulcer of left thigh with unspecified severity   HCC ▽

√5th **L97.2**   Non-pressure chronic ulcer of calf

√6th **L97.20**   Non-pressure chronic ulcer of unspecified calf

L97.201   Non-pressure chronic ulcer of unspecified calf limited to breakdown of skin   HCC ▽

L97.202   Non-pressure chronic ulcer of unspecified calf with fat layer exposed   HCC ▽

L97.203   Non-pressure chronic ulcer of unspecified calf with necrosis of muscle   HCC ▽

L97.204   Non-pressure chronic ulcer of unspecified calf with necrosis of bone   HCC ▽

L97.205   Non-pressure chronic ulcer of unspecified calf with muscle involvement without evidence of necrosis   HCC ▽

L97.206   Non-pressure chronic ulcer of unspecified calf with bone involvement without evidence of necrosis   HCC ▽

L97.208   Non-pressure chronic ulcer of unspecified calf with other specified severity   HCC ▽

L97.209   Non-pressure chronic ulcer of unspecified calf with unspecified severity   HCC ▽

√6th **L97.21**   Non-pressure chronic ulcer of right calf

L97.211   Non-pressure chronic ulcer of right calf limited to breakdown of skin   HCC

L97.212   Non-pressure chronic ulcer of right calf with fat layer exposed   HCC

L97.213   Non-pressure chronic ulcer of right calf with necrosis of muscle   HCC

L97.214   Non-pressure chronic ulcer of right calf with necrosis of bone   HCC

L97.215   Non-pressure chronic ulcer of right calf with muscle involvement without evidence of necrosis   HCC

L97.216   Non-pressure chronic ulcer of right calf with bone involvement without evidence of necrosis   HCC

L97.218   Non-pressure chronic ulcer of right calf with other specified severity   HCC

L97.219   Non-pressure chronic ulcer of right calf with unspecified severity   HCC ▽

√6th **L97.22**   Non-pressure chronic ulcer of left calf

L97.221   Non-pressure chronic ulcer of left calf limited to breakdown of skin   HCC

L97.222   Non-pressure chronic ulcer of left calf with fat layer exposed   HCC

L97.223   Non-pressure chronic ulcer of left calf with necrosis of muscle   HCC

L97.224   Non-pressure chronic ulcer of left calf with necrosis of bone   HCC

L97.225   Non-pressure chronic ulcer of left calf with muscle involvement without evidence of necrosis   HCC

L97.226   Non-pressure chronic ulcer of left calf with bone involvement without evidence of necrosis   HCC

L97.228   Non-pressure chronic ulcer of left calf with other specified severity   HCC

L97.229   Non-pressure chronic ulcer of left calf with unspecified severity   HCC ▽

√5th **L97.3**   Non-pressure chronic ulcer of ankle

√6th **L97.30**   Non-pressure chronic ulcer of unspecified ankle

L97.301   Non-pressure chronic ulcer of unspecified ankle limited to breakdown of skin   HCC ▽

L97.302   Non-pressure chronic ulcer of unspecified ankle with fat layer exposed   HCC ▽

L97.303   Non-pressure chronic ulcer of unspecified ankle with necrosis of muscle   HCC ▽

L97.304   Non-pressure chronic ulcer of unspecified ankle with necrosis of bone   HCC ▽

L97.305   Non-pressure chronic ulcer of unspecified ankle with muscle involvement without evidence of necrosis   HCC ▽

L97.306   Non-pressure chronic ulcer of unspecified ankle with bone involvement without evidence of necrosis   HCC ▽

L97.308   Non-pressure chronic ulcer of unspecified ankle with other specified severity   HCC ▽

L97.309   Non-pressure chronic ulcer of unspecified ankle with unspecified severity   HCC ▽

√6th **L97.31**   Non-pressure chronic ulcer of right ankle

L97.311   Non-pressure chronic ulcer of right ankle limited to breakdown of skin   HCC

L97.312   Non-pressure chronic ulcer of right ankle with fat layer exposed   HCC

L97.313   Non-pressure chronic ulcer of right ankle with necrosis of muscle   `HCC`

L97.314   Non-pressure chronic ulcer of right ankle with necrosis of bone   `HCC`

L97.315   Non-pressure chronic ulcer of right ankle with muscle involvement without evidence of necrosis   `HCC`

L97.316   Non-pressure chronic ulcer of right ankle with bone involvement without evidence of necrosis   `HCC`

L97.318   Non-pressure chronic ulcer of right ankle with other specified severity   `HCC`

L97.319   Non-pressure chronic ulcer of right ankle with unspecified severity   `HCC` ▽

✓6ᵗʰ **L97.32**   Non-pressure chronic ulcer of left ankle

L97.321   Non-pressure chronic ulcer of left ankle limited to breakdown of skin   `HCC`

L97.322   Non-pressure chronic ulcer of left ankle with fat layer exposed   `HCC`

L97.323   Non-pressure chronic ulcer of left ankle with necrosis of muscle   `HCC`

L97.324   Non-pressure chronic ulcer of left ankle with necrosis of bone   `HCC`

L97.325   Non-pressure chronic ulcer of left ankle with muscle involvement without evidence of necrosis   `HCC`

L97.326   Non-pressure chronic ulcer of left ankle with bone involvement without evidence of necrosis   `HCC`

L97.328   Non-pressure chronic ulcer of left ankle with other specified severity   `HCC`

L97.329   Non-pressure chronic ulcer of left ankle with unspecified severity   `HCC` ▽

✓5ᵗʰ **L97.4**   Non-pressure chronic ulcer of heel and midfoot

Non-pressure chronic ulcer of plantar surface of midfoot

✓6ᵗʰ **L97.40**   Non-pressure chronic ulcer of unspecified heel and midfoot

L97.401   Non-pressure chronic ulcer of unspecified heel and midfoot limited to breakdown of skin   `HCC` ▽

L97.402   Non-pressure chronic ulcer of unspecified heel and midfoot with fat layer exposed   `HCC` ▽

L97.403   Non-pressure chronic ulcer of unspecified heel and midfoot with necrosis of muscle   `HCC` ▽

L97.404   Non-pressure chronic ulcer of unspecified heel and midfoot with necrosis of bone   `HCC` ▽

L97.405   Non-pressure chronic ulcer of unspecified heel and midfoot with muscle involvement without evidence of necrosis   `HCC` ▽

L97.406   Non-pressure chronic ulcer of unspecified heel and midfoot with bone involvement without evidence of necrosis   `HCC` ▽

L97.408   Non-pressure chronic ulcer of unspecified heel and midfoot with other specified severity   `HCC` ▽

L97.409   Non-pressure chronic ulcer of unspecified heel and midfoot with unspecified severity   `HCC` ▽

✓6ᵗʰ **L97.41**   Non-pressure chronic ulcer of right heel and midfoot

L97.411   Non-pressure chronic ulcer of right heel and midfoot limited to breakdown of skin   `HCC`

L97.412   Non-pressure chronic ulcer of right heel and midfoot with fat layer exposed   `HCC`

L97.413   Non-pressure chronic ulcer of right heel and midfoot with necrosis of muscle   `HCC`

L97.414   Non-pressure chronic ulcer of right heel and midfoot with necrosis of bone   `HCC`

L97.415   Non-pressure chronic ulcer of right heel and midfoot with muscle involvement without evidence of necrosis   `HCC`

L97.416   Non-pressure chronic ulcer of right heel and midfoot with bone involvement without evidence of necrosis   `HCC`

L97.418   Non-pressure chronic ulcer of right heel and midfoot with other specified severity   `HCC`

L97.419   Non-pressure chronic ulcer of right heel and midfoot with unspecified severity   `HCC` ▽

✓6ᵗʰ **L97.42**   Non-pressure chronic ulcer of left heel and midfoot

L97.421   Non-pressure chronic ulcer of left heel and midfoot limited to breakdown of skin   `HCC`

     AHA: 2016,1Q,12

L97.422   Non-pressure chronic ulcer of left heel and midfoot with fat layer exposed   `HCC`

L97.423   Non-pressure chronic ulcer of left heel and midfoot with necrosis of muscle   `HCC`

L97.424   Non-pressure chronic ulcer of left heel and midfoot with necrosis of bone   `HCC`

L97.425   Non-pressure chronic ulcer of left heel and midfoot with muscle involvement without evidence of necrosis   `HCC`

L97.426   Non-pressure chronic ulcer of left heel and midfoot with bone involvement without evidence of necrosis   `HCC`

L97.428   Non-pressure chronic ulcer of left heel and midfoot with other specified severity   `HCC`

L97.429   Non-pressure chronic ulcer of left heel and midfoot with unspecified severity   `HCC` ▽

✓5ᵗʰ **L97.5**   Non-pressure chronic ulcer of other part of foot

Non-pressure chronic ulcer of toe

✓6ᵗʰ **L97.50**   Non-pressure chronic ulcer of other part of unspecified foot

L97.501   Non-pressure chronic ulcer of other part of unspecified foot limited to breakdown of skin   `HCC` ▽

L97.502   Non-pressure chronic ulcer of other part of unspecified foot with fat layer exposed   `HCC` ▽

L97.503   Non-pressure chronic ulcer of other part of unspecified foot with necrosis of muscle   `HCC` ▽

L97.504   Non-pressure chronic ulcer of other part of unspecified foot with necrosis of bone   `HCC` ▽

L97.505   Non-pressure chronic ulcer of other part of unspecified foot with muscle involvement without evidence of necrosis   `HCC` ▽

L97.506   Non-pressure chronic ulcer of other part of unspecified foot with bone involvement without evidence of necrosis   `HCC` ▽

L97.508   Non-pressure chronic ulcer of other part of unspecified foot with other specified severity   `HCC` ▽

L97.509   Non-pressure chronic ulcer of other part of unspecified foot with unspecified severity   `HCC` ▽

✓6ᵗʰ **L97.51**   Non-pressure chronic ulcer of other part of right foot

L97.511   Non-pressure chronic ulcer of other part of right foot limited to breakdown of skin   `HCC`

L97.512   Non-pressure chronic ulcer of other part of right foot with fat layer exposed   `HCC`

L97.513   Non-pressure chronic ulcer of other part of right foot with necrosis of muscle   `HCC`

☑ Additional Character Req   ✓x7ᵗʰ Placeholder Alert   Manifestation   ▽ Unspecified   ►◄ Revised Text   ● New Code   ▲ Revised Code Title

L97.514 Non-pressure chronic ulcer of other part of right foot with necrosis of bone `HCC`

L97.515 Non-pressure chronic ulcer of other part of right foot with muscle involvement without evidence of necrosis `HCC`

L97.516 Non-pressure chronic ulcer of other part of right foot with bone involvement without evidence of necrosis `HCC`

L97.518 Non-pressure chronic ulcer of other part of right foot with other specified severity `HCC`

L97.519 Non-pressure chronic ulcer of other part of right foot with unspecified severity `HCC` ▽

√6ᵗʰ L97.52 Non-pressure chronic ulcer of other part of left foot

L97.521 Non-pressure chronic ulcer of other part of left foot limited to breakdown of skin `HCC`

L97.522 Non-pressure chronic ulcer of other part of left foot with fat layer exposed `HCC`

L97.523 Non-pressure chronic ulcer of other part of left foot with necrosis of muscle `HCC`

L97.524 Non-pressure chronic ulcer of other part of left foot with necrosis of bone `HCC`

L97.525 Non-pressure chronic ulcer of other part of left foot with muscle involvement without evidence of necrosis `HCC`

L97.526 Non-pressure chronic ulcer of other part of left foot with bone involvement without evidence of necrosis `HCC`

L97.528 Non-pressure chronic ulcer of other part of left foot with other specified severity `HCC`

L97.529 Non-pressure chronic ulcer of other part of left foot with unspecified severity `HCC` ▽

√5ᵗʰ L97.8 Non-pressure chronic ulcer of other part of lower leg

√6ᵗʰ L97.80 Non-pressure chronic ulcer of other part of unspecified lower leg

L97.801 Non-pressure chronic ulcer of other part of unspecified lower leg limited to breakdown of skin `HCC` ▽

L97.802 Non-pressure chronic ulcer of other part of unspecified lower leg with fat layer exposed `HCC` ▽

L97.803 Non-pressure chronic ulcer of other part of unspecified lower leg with necrosis of muscle `HCC` ▽

L97.804 Non-pressure chronic ulcer of other part of unspecified lower leg with necrosis of bone `HCC` ▽

L97.805 Non-pressure chronic ulcer of other part of unspecified lower leg with muscle involvement without evidence of necrosis `HCC` ▽

L97.806 Non-pressure chronic ulcer of other part of unspecified lower leg with bone involvement without evidence of necrosis `HCC` ▽

L97.808 Non-pressure chronic ulcer of other part of unspecified lower leg with other specified severity `HCC` ▽

L97.809 Non-pressure chronic ulcer of other part of unspecified lower leg with unspecified severity `HCC` ▽

√6ᵗʰ L97.81 Non-pressure chronic ulcer of other part of right lower leg

L97.811 Non-pressure chronic ulcer of other part of right lower leg limited to breakdown of skin `HCC`

L97.812 Non-pressure chronic ulcer of other part of right lower leg with fat layer exposed `HCC`

L97.813 Non-pressure chronic ulcer of other part of right lower leg with necrosis of muscle `HCC`

L97.814 Non-pressure chronic ulcer of other part of right lower leg with necrosis of bone `HCC`

L97.815 Non-pressure chronic ulcer of other part of right lower leg with muscle involvement without evidence of necrosis `HCC`

L97.816 Non-pressure chronic ulcer of other part of right lower leg with bone involvement without evidence of necrosis `HCC`

L97.818 Non-pressure chronic ulcer of other part of right lower leg with other specified severity `HCC`

L97.819 Non-pressure chronic ulcer of other part of right lower leg with unspecified severity `HCC` ▽

√6ᵗʰ L97.82 Non-pressure chronic ulcer of other part of left lower leg

L97.821 Non-pressure chronic ulcer of other part of left lower leg limited to breakdown of skin `HCC`

L97.822 Non-pressure chronic ulcer of other part of left lower leg with fat layer exposed `HCC`

L97.823 Non-pressure chronic ulcer of other part of left lower leg with necrosis of muscle `HCC`

L97.824 Non-pressure chronic ulcer of other part of left lower leg with necrosis of bone `HCC`

L97.825 Non-pressure chronic ulcer of other part of left lower leg with muscle involvement without evidence of necrosis `HCC`

L97.826 Non-pressure chronic ulcer of other part of left lower leg with bone involvement without evidence of necrosis `HCC`

L97.828 Non-pressure chronic ulcer of other part of left lower leg with other specified severity `HCC`

L97.829 Non-pressure chronic ulcer of other part of left lower leg with unspecified severity `HCC` ▽

√5ᵗʰ L97.9 Non-pressure chronic ulcer of unspecified part of lower leg

√6ᵗʰ L97.90 Non-pressure chronic ulcer of unspecified part of unspecified lower leg

L97.901 Non-pressure chronic ulcer of unspecified part of unspecified lower leg limited to breakdown of skin `HCC` ▽

L97.902 Non-pressure chronic ulcer of unspecified part of unspecified lower leg with fat layer exposed `HCC` ▽

L97.903 Non-pressure chronic ulcer of unspecified part of unspecified lower leg with necrosis of muscle `HCC` ▽

L97.904 Non-pressure chronic ulcer of unspecified part of unspecified lower leg with necrosis of bone `HCC` ▽

L97.905 Non-pressure chronic ulcer of unspecified part of unspecified lower leg with muscle involvement without evidence of necrosis `HCC` ▽

L97.906 Non-pressure chronic ulcer of unspecified part of unspecified lower leg with bone involvement without evidence of necrosis `HCC` ▽

L97.908 Non-pressure chronic ulcer of unspecified part of unspecified lower leg with other specified severity `HCC` ▽

L97.909 Non-pressure chronic ulcer of unspecified part of unspecified lower leg with unspecified severity `HCC` ▽

√6ᵗʰ L97.91 Non-pressure chronic ulcer of unspecified part of right lower leg

L97.911 Non-pressure chronic ulcer of unspecified part of right lower leg limited to breakdown of skin `HCC` ▽

L97.912 **Non-pressure chronic ulcer of unspecified part of right lower leg with fat layer exposed** HCC ▽

L97.913 **Non-pressure chronic ulcer of unspecified part of right lower leg with necrosis of muscle** HCC ▽

L97.914 **Non-pressure chronic ulcer of unspecified part of right lower leg with necrosis of bone** HCC ▽

L97.915 **Non-pressure chronic ulcer of unspecified part of right lower leg with muscle involvement without evidence of necrosis** HCC ▽

L97.916 **Non-pressure chronic ulcer of unspecified part of right lower leg with bone involvement without evidence of necrosis** HCC ▽

L97.918 **Non-pressure chronic ulcer of unspecified part of right lower leg with other specified severity** HCC ▽

L97.919 **Non-pressure chronic ulcer of unspecified part of right lower leg with unspecified severity** HCC ▽

√6ᵗʰ **L97.92 Non-pressure chronic ulcer of unspecified part of left lower leg**

L97.921 **Non-pressure chronic ulcer of unspecified part of left lower leg limited to breakdown of skin** HCC ▽

L97.922 **Non-pressure chronic ulcer of unspecified part of left lower leg with fat layer exposed** HCC ▽

L97.923 **Non-pressure chronic ulcer of unspecified part of left lower leg with necrosis of muscle** HCC ▽

L97.924 **Non-pressure chronic ulcer of unspecified part of left lower leg with necrosis of bone** HCC ▽

L97.925 **Non-pressure chronic ulcer of unspecified part of left lower leg with muscle involvement without evidence of necrosis** HCC ▽

L97.926 **Non-pressure chronic ulcer of unspecified part of left lower leg with bone involvement without evidence of necrosis** HCC ▽

L97.928 **Non-pressure chronic ulcer of unspecified part of left lower leg with other specified severity** HCC ▽

L97.929 **Non-pressure chronic ulcer of unspecified part of left lower leg with unspecified severity** HCC ▽

√4ᵗʰ **L98 Other disorders of skin and subcutaneous tissue, not elsewhere classified**

L98.0 Pyogenic granuloma

EXCLUDES 2   pyogenic granuloma of gingiva (K06.8)

pyogenic granuloma of maxillary alveolar ridge (K04.5)

pyogenic granuloma of oral mucosa (K13.4)

DEF: Solitary polypoid capillary hemangioma often associated with local irritation, trauma, and superimposed inflammation. Located on the skin and gingival or oral mucosa, they bleed easily and may ulcerate and form crusted sores.

L98.1 Factitial dermatitis

Neurotic excoriation

EXCLUDES 1   excoriation (skin-picking) disorder (F42.4)

AHA: 2016,4Q,15

DEF: Self-inflicted skin lesions to satisfy an unconscious psychological or emotional need. Methods used to injure the skin include deep excoriations with a sharp instrument, scarification with a knife, or the application of caustic chemicals and burning, sometimes with a cigarette.

L98.2 Febrile neutrophilic dermatosis [Sweet]

L98.3 Eosinophilic cellulitis [Wells]

√5ᵗʰ **L98.4 Non-pressure chronic ulcer of skin, not elsewhere classified**

Chronic ulcer of skin NOS

Tropical ulcer NOS

Ulcer of skin NOS

EXCLUDES 2   gangrene (I96)

pressure ulcer (pressure area) (L89.-)

skin infections (L00-L08)

specific infections classified to A00-B99

ulcer of lower limb NEC (L97.-)

varicose ulcer (I83.0-I82.2)

AHA: 2017,4Q,17

TIP: The depth and/or severity of a diagnosed nonpressure ulcer can be determined based on medical record documentation from clinicians who are not the patient's provider.

TIP: Assign a code from this category/subcategory for nonpressure ulcers documented as acute.

√6ᵗʰ **L98.41 Non-pressure chronic ulcer of buttock**

L98.411 **Non-pressure chronic ulcer of buttock limited to breakdown of skin** HCC

L98.412 **Non-pressure chronic ulcer of buttock with fat layer exposed** HCC

L98.413 **Non-pressure chronic ulcer of buttock with necrosis of muscle** HCC

L98.414 **Non-pressure chronic ulcer of buttock with necrosis of bone** HCC

L98.415 **Non-pressure chronic ulcer of buttock with muscle involvement without evidence of necrosis** HCC

L98.416 **Non-pressure chronic ulcer of buttock with bone involvement without evidence of necrosis** HCC

L98.418 **Non-pressure chronic ulcer of buttock with other specified severity** HCC

L98.419 **Non-pressure chronic ulcer of buttock with unspecified severity** HCC ▽

√6ᵗʰ **L98.42 Non-pressure chronic ulcer of back**

L98.421 **Non-pressure chronic ulcer of back limited to breakdown of skin** HCC

L98.422 **Non-pressure chronic ulcer of back with fat layer exposed** HCC

L98.423 **Non-pressure chronic ulcer of back with necrosis of muscle** HCC

L98.424 **Non-pressure chronic ulcer of back with necrosis of bone** HCC

L98.425 **Non-pressure chronic ulcer of back with muscle involvement without evidence of necrosis** HCC

L98.426 **Non-pressure chronic ulcer of back with bone involvement without evidence of necrosis** HCC

L98.428 **Non-pressure chronic ulcer of back with other specified severity** HCC

L98.429 **Non-pressure chronic ulcer of back with unspecified severity** HCC ▽

√6ᵗʰ **L98.49 Non-pressure chronic ulcer of skin of other sites**

Non-pressure chronic ulcer of skin NOS

L98.491 **Non-pressure chronic ulcer of skin of other sites limited to breakdown of skin** HCC

L98.492 **Non-pressure chronic ulcer of skin of other sites with fat layer exposed** HCC

L98.493 **Non-pressure chronic ulcer of skin of other sites with necrosis of muscle** HCC

L98.494 **Non-pressure chronic ulcer of skin of other sites with necrosis of bone** HCC

L98.495 **Non-pressure chronic ulcer of skin of other sites with muscle involvement without evidence of necrosis** HCC

▲ L98.496 **Non-pressure chronic ulcer of skin of other sites with bone involvement without evidence of necrosis** HCC

▲ L98.498 **Non-pressure chronic ulcer of skin of other sites with other specified severity** HCC

☑ Additional Character Req   √x7ᵗʰ Placeholder Alert   Manifestation   ▽ Unspecified   ▶◀ Revised Text   ● New Code   ▲ Revised Code Title

      L98.499   **Non-pressure chronic ulcer of skin** HCC ▽
              of other sites with unspecified
              severity

L98.5   **Mucinosis of the skin**
     Focal mucinosis
     Lichen myxedematosus
     Reticular erythematous mucinosis
     EXCLUDES 1   *focal oral mucinosis (K13.79)*
                myxedema (E03.9)

L98.6   **Other infiltrative disorders of the skin and subcutaneous**
     tissue
     EXCLUDES 1   *hyalinosis cutis et mucosae (E78.89)*

L98.7   **Excessive and redundant skin and subcutaneous tissue**
     Loose or sagging skin, following bariatric surgery weight loss
     Loose or sagging skin following dietary weight loss
     Loose or sagging skin, NOS
     EXCLUDES 2   *acquired excess or redundant skin of eyelid (H02.3-)*
                congenital excess or redundant skin of eyelid (Q10.3)
                skin changes due to chronic exposure to nonionizing
                    radiation (L57.-)

     AHA: 2016,4Q,36

L98.8   **Other specified disorders of the skin and subcutaneous tissue**
     AHA: 2013,2Q,32

L98.9   **Disorder of the skin and subcutaneous tissue,**   ▽
     unspecified

L99   *Other disorders of skin and subcutaneous tissue in diseases classified elsewhere*

     Code first underlying disease, such as:
     amyloidosis (E85.-)
     EXCLUDES 1   *skin disorders in diabetes (E08-E13 with .62)*
                skin disorders in gonorrhea (A54.89)
                skin disorders in syphilis (A51.31, A52.79)

Chapter 13. Diseases of the Musculoskeletal System and Connective Tissue (M00–M99)

Chapter Specific Guidelines with Coding Examples

The chapter specific guidelines from the ICD-10-CM Official Guidelines for Coding and Reporting have been provided below. Along with these guidelines are coding examples, contained in the shaded boxes, that have been developed to help illustrate the coding and/or sequencing guidance found in these guidelines.

a. Site and laterality

Most of the codes within Chapter 13 have site and laterality designations. The site represents the bone, joint or the muscle involved. For some conditions where more than one bone, joint or muscle is usually involved, such as osteoarthritis, there is a "multiple sites" code available. For categories where no multiple site code is provided and more than one bone, joint or muscle is involved, multiple codes should be used to indicate the different sites involved.

> Olecranon bursitis of the left elbow
>
> **M70.22   Olecranon bursitis, left elbow**
>
> *Explanation:* Most of the codes within chapter 13 have site and laterality designations. The site represents the bone, joint, or the muscle involved.

> Rheumatoid arthritis of multiple sites without rheumatoid factor
>
> **M06.09   Rheumatoid arthritis without rheumatoid factor, multiple sites**
>
> *Explanation:* For some conditions where more than one bone, joint or muscle is usually involved, such as osteoarthritis, there is a "multiple sites" code available.

> Adolescent scoliosis in the upper thoracic region and the lumbar vertebrae
>
> **M41.124   Adolescent idiopathic scoliosis, thoracic region**
>
> **M41.126   Adolescent idiopathic scoliosis, lumbar region**
>
> *Explanation:* For categories without a multiple site code and more than one bone, joint, or muscle is involved, multiple codes should be used to indicate the different sites involved.

1) Bone versus joint

For certain conditions, the bone may be affected at the upper or lower end, (e.g., avascular necrosis of bone, M87, Osteoporosis, M80, M81). Though the portion of the bone affected may be at the joint, the site designation will be the bone, not the joint.

> Idiopathic avascular necrosis of the femoral head of the left hip joint
>
> **M87.052   Idiopathic aseptic necrosis of left femur**
>
> *Explanation:* For certain conditions such as avascular necrosis, the bone may be affected at the joint, but the site designation is the bone, not the joint.

b. Acute traumatic versus chronic or recurrent musculoskeletal conditions

Many musculoskeletal conditions are a result of previous injury or trauma to a site, or are recurrent conditions. Bone, joint or muscle conditions that are the result of a healed injury are usually found in chapter 13. Recurrent bone, joint or muscle conditions are also usually found in chapter 13. Any current, acute injury should be coded to the appropriate injury code from chapter 19. Chronic or recurrent conditions should generally be coded with a code from chapter 13. If it is difficult to determine from the documentation in the record which code is best to describe a condition, query the provider.

> Acute traumatic bucket handle tear of right medial meniscus
>
> **S83.211A   Bucket-handle tear of medial meniscus, current injury, right knee, initial encounter**
>
> *Explanation:* Any current, acute injury is not coded in chapter 13. It should instead be coded to the appropriate injury code from chapter 19.

> Old bucket handle tear of right medial meniscus
>
> **M23.203   Derangement of unspecified medial meniscus due to old tear or injury, right knee**
>
> *Explanation:* Chronic or recurrent conditions should generally be coded with a code from chapter 13.

c. Coding of Pathologic Fractures

7th character A is for use as long as the patient is receiving active treatment for the fracture. Examples of active treatment are: surgical treatment, emergency department encounter, evaluation and continuing treatment by the same or a different physician. While the patient may be seen by a new or different provider over the course of treatment for a pathological fracture, assignment of the 7th character is based on whether the patient is undergoing active treatment and not whether the provider is seeing the patient for the first time.

> Pathologic fracture of left foot, unknown cause, currently under active treatment by a follow-up provider
>
> **M84.475A   Pathological fracture, left foot, initial encounter for fracture**
>
> *Explanation:* Seventh character A is for use as long as the patient is receiving active treatment for a pathologic fracture. Examples of active treatment are surgical treatment, emergency department encounter, evaluation, and continuing treatment by the same or a different physician.
>
> The seventh character is based on whether the patient is undergoing active treatment and not whether the provider is seeing the patient for the first time.

7th character D is to be used for encounters after the patient has completed active treatment for the fracture and is receiving routine care for the fracture during the healing or recovery phase. The other 7th characters, listed under each subcategory in the Tabular List, are to be used for subsequent encounters for treatment of problems associated with the healing, such as malunions, nonunions, and sequelae.

Care for complications of surgical treatment for fracture repairs during the healing or recovery phase should be coded with the appropriate complication codes.

See Section I.C.19. Coding of traumatic fractures.

d. Osteoporosis

Osteoporosis is a systemic condition, meaning that all bones of the musculoskeletal system are affected. Therefore, site is not a component of the codes under category M81, Osteoporosis without current pathological fracture. The site codes under category M80, Osteoporosis with current pathological fracture, identify the site of the fracture, not the osteoporosis.

1) Osteoporosis without pathological fracture

Category M81, Osteoporosis without current pathological fracture, is for use for patients with osteoporosis who do not currently have a pathologic fracture due to the osteoporosis, even if they have had a fracture in the past. For patients with a history of osteoporosis fractures, status code Z87.310, Personal history of (healed) osteoporosis fracture, should follow the code from M81.

> Age-related osteoporosis with healed osteoporotic fracture of the lumbar vertebra
>
> **M81.0   Age-related osteoporosis without current pathological fracture**
>
> **Z87.310   Personal history of (healed) osteoporosis fracture**
>
> *Explanation:* Category M81 is used for patients with osteoporosis who do not currently have a pathologic fracture due to the osteoporosis. To report a previous (healed) fracture, status code Z87.310 Personal history of (healed) osteoporosis fracture, should follow the code from M81.

2) Osteoporosis with current pathological fracture

Category M80, Osteoporosis with current pathological fracture, is for patients who have a current pathologic fracture at the time of an encounter. The codes under M80 identify the site of the fracture. A code from category M80, not a traumatic fracture code, should be used for any patient with known osteoporosis who suffers a fracture, even if the patient had a minor fall or trauma, if that fall or trauma would not usually break a normal, healthy bone.

> Disuse osteoporosis with current fracture of right shoulder sustained lifting a grocery bag, initial encounter
>
> **M80.811A   Other osteoporosis with current pathological fracture, right shoulder, initial encounter for fracture**
>
> *Explanation:* A code from category M80, not a traumatic fracture code, should be used for any patient with known osteoporosis who suffers a fracture, even if the patient had a minor fall or trauma, if that fall or trauma would not usually break a normal, healthy bone.

Muscle/Tendon Table

ICD-10-CM categorizes certain muscles and tendons in the upper and lower extremities by their action (e.g., extension, flexion), their anatomical location (e.g., posterior, anterior), and/or whether they are intrinsic or extrinsic to a certain anatomical area. The Muscle/Tendon Table is provided at the beginning of chapters 13 and 19 as a resource to help users when code selection depends on one or more of these characteristics. A **TIP** has been placed at those categories and/or subcategories that relate to this table. Please note that this table is not all-inclusive, and proper code assignment should be based on the provider's documentation.

Body Region	Muscle	Extensor Tendon	Flexor Tendon	Other Tendon
Shoulder				
	Deltoid	Posterior deltoid	Anterior deltoid	
	Rotator cuff			
	Infraspinatus			Infraspinatus
	Subscapularis			Subscapularis
	Supraspinatus			Supraspinatus
	Teres minor			Teres minor
	Teres major	Teres major		
Upper arm				
	Anterior muscles			
	Biceps brachii — long head		Biceps brachii — long head	
	Biceps brachii — short head		Biceps brachii — short head	
	Brachialis		Brachialis	
	Coracobrachialis		Coracobrachialis	
	Posterior muscles			
	Triceps brachii	Triceps brachii		
Forearm				
	Anterior muscles			
	Flexors			
	Deep			
	Flexor digitorum profundus		Flexor digitorum profundus	
	Flexor pollicis longus		Flexor pollicis longus	
	Intermediate			
	Flexor digitorum superficialis		Flexor digitorum superficialis	
	Superficial			
	Flexor carpi radialis		Flexor carpi radialis	
	Flexor carpi ulnaris		Flexor carpi ulnaris	
	Palmaris longus		Palmaris longus	
	Pronators			
	Pronator quadratus			Pronator quadratus
	Pronator teres			Pronator teres
	Posterior muscles			
	Extensors			
	Deep			
	Abductor pollicis longus			Abductor pollicis longus
	Extensor indicis	Extensor indicis		
	Extensor pollicis brevis	Extensor pollicis brevis		
	Extensor pollicis longus	Extensor pollicis longus		
	Superficial			
	Brachioradialis			Brachioradialis
	Extensor carpi radialis brevis	Extensor carpi radialis brevis		
	Extensor carpi radialis longus	Extensor carpi radialis longus		
	Extensor carpi ulnaris	Extensor carpi ulnaris		
	Extensor digiti minimi	Extensor digiti minimi		
	Extensor digitorum	Extensor digitorum		
	Anconeus	Anconeus		
	Supinator			Supinator

Body Region	Muscle	Extensor Tendon	Flexor Tendon	Other Tendon
Hand				
Extrinsic — attach to a site in the forearm as well as a site in the hand with action related to hand movement at the wrist				
	Extensor carpi radialis brevis	Extensor carpi radialis brevis		
	Extensor carpi radialis longus	Extensor carpie radialis longus		
	Extensor carpi ulnaris	Extensor carpi ulnaris		
	Flexor carpi radialis		Flexor carpi radialis	
	Flexor carpi ulnaris		Flexor carpi ulnaris	
	Flexor digitorum superficialis		Flexor digitorum superficialis	
	Palmaris longus		Palmaris longus	
Extrinsic — attach to a site in the forearm as well as a site in the hand with action in the hand related to finger movement				
	Adductor pollicis longus			Adductor pollicis longus
	Extensor digiti minimi	Extensor digiti minimi		
	Extensor digitorum	Extensor digitorum		
	Extensor indicis	Extensor indicis		
	Flexor digitorum profundus		Flexor digitorum profundus	
	Flexor digitorum superficialis		Flexor digitorum superficialis	
Extrinsic — attach to a site in the forearm as well as a site in the hand with action in the hand related to thumb movement				
	Extensor pollicis brevis	Extensor pollicis brevis		
	Extensor pollicis longus	Extensor pollicis longus		
	Flexor pollicis longus		Flexor pollicis longus	
Intrinsic — found within the hand only				
	Adductor pollicis			Adductor pollicis
	Dorsal interossei	Dorsal interossei	Dorsal interossei	
	Lumbricals	Lumbricals	Lumbricals	
	Palmaris brevis			Palmaris brevis
	Palmar interossei	Palmar interossei	Palmar interossei	
	Hypothenar muscles			
	Abductor digiti minimi			Abductor digiti minimi
	Flexor digiti minimi brevis		Flexor digiti minimi brevis	
	Oppenens digiti minimi		Oppenens digiti minimi	
	Thenar muscles			
	Abductor pollicis brevis			Abductor pollicis brevis
	Flexor pollicis brevis		Flexor pollicis brevis	
	Oppenens pollicis		Oppenens pollicis	
Thigh				
	Anterior muscles			
	Iliopsoas		Iliopsoas	
	Pectineus		Pectineus	
	Quadriceps	Quadriceps		
	Rectus femoris	Rectus femoris — Extends knee	Rectus femoris — Flexes hip	
	Vastus intermedius	Vastus intermedius		
	Vastus lateralis	Vastus lateralis		
	Vastus medialis	Vastus medialis		
	Sartorius		Sartorius	
	Medial muscles			
	Adductor brevis			Adductor brevis
	Adductor longus			Adductor longus
	Adductor magnus			Adductor magnus
	Gracilis			Gracilis
	Obturator externus			Obturator externus
	Posterior muscles			
	Hamstring	Hamstring — Extends hip	Hamstring — Flexes knee	
	Biceps femoris	Biceps femoris	Biceps femoris	
	Semimembranosus	Semimembranosus	Semimembranosus	
	Semitendinosus	Semitendinosus	Semitendinosus	

Body Region	Muscle	Extensor Tendon	Flexor Tendon	Other Tendon
Lower leg				
	Anterior muscles			
	Extensor digitorum longus	Extensor digitorum longus		
	Extensor hallucis longus	Extensor hallucis longus		
	Fibularis (peroneus) tertius	Fibularis (peroneus) tertius		
	Tibialis anterior	Tibialis anterior		Tibialis anterior
	Lateral muscles			
	Fibularis (peroneus) brevis		Fibularis (peroneus) brevis	
	Fibularis (peroneus) longus		Fibularis (peroneus) longus	
	Posterior muscles			
	Deep			
	Flexor digitorum longus		Flexor digitorum longus	
	Flexor hallucis longus		Flexor hallucis longus	
	Popliteus		Popliteus	
	Tibialis posterior		Tibialis posterior	
	Superficial			
	Gastrocnemius		Gastrocnemius	
	Plantaris		Plantaris	
	Soleus		Soleus	
				Calcaneal (Achilles)
Ankle/Foot				
Extrinsic — attach to a site in the lower leg as well as a site in the foot with action related to foot movement at the ankle				
	Plantaris		Plantaris	
	Soleus		Soleus	
	Tibialis anterior	Tibialis anterior		
	Tibialis posterior		Tibialis posterior	
Extrinsic — attach to a site in the lower leg as well as a site in the foot with action in the foot related to toe movement				
	Extensor digitorum longus	Extensor digitorum longus		
	Extensor hallicus longus	Extensor hallicus longus		
	Flexor digitorum longus		Flexor digitorum longus	
	Flexor hallucis longus		Flexor hallucis longus	
Intrinsic — found within the ankle/foot only				
	Dorsal muscles			
	Extensor digitorum brevis	Extensor digitorum brevis		
	Extensor hallucis brevis	Extensor hallucis brevis		
	Plantar muscles			
	Abductor digiti minimi		Abductor digiti minimi	
	Abductor hallucis		Abductor hallucis	
	Dorsal interossei	Dorsal interossei	Dorsal interossei	
	Flexor digiti minimi brevis		Flexor digiti minimi brevis	
	Flexor digitorum brevis		Flexor digitorum brevis	
	Flexor hallucis brevis		Flexor hallucis brevis	
	Lumbricals	Lumbricals	Lumbricals	
	Quadratus plantae		Quadratus plantae	
	Plantar interossei	Plantar interossei	Plantar interossei	

Chapter 13. Diseases of the Musculoskeletal System and Connective Tissue (M00-M99)

NOTE   Use an external cause code following the code for the musculoskeletal condition, if applicable, to identify the cause of the musculoskeletal condition

EXCLUDES 2   arthropathic psoriasis (L40.5-)
certain conditions originating in the perinatal period (P04-P96)
certain infectious and parasitic diseases (A00-B99)
compartment syndrome (traumatic) (T79.A-)
complications of pregnancy, childbirth and the puerperium (O00-O9A)
congenital malformations, deformations, and chromosomal abnormalities (Q00-Q99)
endocrine, nutritional and metabolic diseases (E00-E88)
injury, poisoning and certain other consequences of external causes (S00-T88)
neoplasms (C00-D49)
symptoms, signs and abnormal clinical and laboratory findings, not elsewhere classified (R00-R94)

This chapter contains the following blocks:

M00-M02   Infectious arthropathies
►M04◄   ►Autoinflammatory syndromes◄
M05-M14   Inflammatory polyarthropathies
M15-M19   Osteoarthritis
M20-M25   Other joint disorders
M26-M27   Dentofacial anomalies [including malocclusion] and other disorders of jaw
M30-M36   Systemic connective tissue disorders
M40-M43   Deforming dorsopathies
M45-M49   Spondylopathies
M50-M54   Other dorsopathies
M60-M63   Disorders of muscles
M65-M67   Disorders of synovium and tendon
M70-M79   Other soft tissue disorders
M80-M85   Disorders of bone density and structure
M86-M90   Other osteopathies
M91-M94   Chondropathies
M95   Other disorders of the musculoskeletal system and connective tissue
M96   Intraoperative and postprocedural complications and disorders of musculoskeletal system, not elsewhere classified
►M97◄   ►Periprosthetic fracture around internal prosthetic joint◄
M99   Biomechanical lesions, not elsewhere classified

Arthropathies (M00-M25)

INCLUDES   disorders affecting predominantly peripheral (limb) joints

Infectious arthropathies (M00-M02)

NOTE   This block comprises arthropathies due to microbiological agents. Distinction is made between the following types of etiological relationship:

a) direct infection of joint, where organisms invade synovial tissue and microbial antigen is present in the joint;

b) indirect infection, which may be of two types: a reactive arthropathy, where microbial infection of the body is established but neither organisms nor antigens can be identified in the joint, and a postinfective arthropathy, where microbial antigen is present but recovery of an organism is inconstant and evidence of local multiplication is lacking.

✓4ᵗʰ **M00**   **Pyogenic arthritis**

   DEF: Pyogenic: Relating to or involving pus production, often referred to as suppurative or purulent.

✓5ᵗʰ **M00.0**   **Staphylococcal arthritis and polyarthritis**

   Use additional code (B95.61-B95.8) to identify bacterial agent
   EXCLUDES 2   infection and inflammatory reaction due to internal joint prosthesis (T84.5-)

   M00.00   Staphylococcal arthritis, unspecified joint   HCC ▽
✓6ᵗʰ   **M00.01**   Staphylococcal arthritis, shoulder
    M00.011   Staphylococcal arthritis, right shoulder   HCC
    M00.012   Staphylococcal arthritis, left shoulder   HCC
    M00.019   Staphylococcal arthritis, unspecified shoulder   HCC ▽
✓6ᵗʰ   **M00.02**   Staphylococcal arthritis, elbow
    M00.021   Staphylococcal arthritis, right elbow   HCC
    M00.022   Staphylococcal arthritis, left elbow   HCC
    M00.029   Staphylococcal arthritis, unspecified elbow   HCC ▽

✓6ᵗʰ **M00.03**   **Staphylococcal arthritis, wrist**
   Staphylococcal arthritis of carpal bones
    M00.031   Staphylococcal arthritis, right wrist   HCC
    M00.032   Staphylococcal arthritis, left wrist   HCC
    M00.039   Staphylococcal arthritis, unspecified wrist   HCC ▽
✓6ᵗʰ **M00.04**   **Staphylococcal arthritis, hand**
   Staphylococcal arthritis of metacarpus and phalanges
    M00.041   Staphylococcal arthritis, right hand   HCC
    M00.042   Staphylococcal arthritis, left hand   HCC
    M00.049   Staphylococcal arthritis, unspecified hand   HCC ▽
✓6ᵗʰ **M00.05**   **Staphylococcal arthritis, hip**
    M00.051   Staphylococcal arthritis, right hip   HCC
    M00.052   Staphylococcal arthritis, left hip   HCC
    M00.059   Staphylococcal arthritis, unspecified hip   HCC ▽
✓6ᵗʰ **M00.06**   **Staphylococcal arthritis, knee**
    M00.061   Staphylococcal arthritis, right knee   HCC
    M00.062   Staphylococcal arthritis, left knee   HCC
    M00.069   Staphylococcal arthritis, unspecified knee   HCC ▽
✓6ᵗʰ **M00.07**   **Staphylococcal arthritis, ankle and foot**
   Staphylococcal arthritis, tarsus, metatarsus and phalanges
    M00.071   Staphylococcal arthritis, right ankle and foot   HCC
    M00.072   Staphylococcal arthritis, left ankle and foot   HCC
    M00.079   Staphylococcal arthritis, unspecified ankle and foot   HCC ▽
   M00.08   Staphylococcal arthritis, vertebrae   HCC
   M00.09   Staphylococcal polyarthritis   HCC
✓5ᵗʰ **M00.1**   **Pneumococcal arthritis and polyarthritis**
   M00.10   Pneumococcal arthritis, unspecified joint   HCC ▽
✓6ᵗʰ **M00.11**   **Pneumococcal arthritis, shoulder**
    M00.111   Pneumococcal arthritis, right shoulder   HCC
    M00.112   Pneumococcal arthritis, left shoulder   HCC
    M00.119   Pneumococcal arthritis, unspecified shoulder   HCC ▽
✓6ᵗʰ **M00.12**   **Pneumococcal arthritis, elbow**
    M00.121   Pneumococcal arthritis, right elbow   HCC
    M00.122   Pneumococcal arthritis, left elbow   HCC
    M00.129   Pneumococcal arthritis, unspecified elbow   HCC ▽
✓6ᵗʰ **M00.13**   **Pneumococcal arthritis, wrist**
   Pneumococcal arthritis of carpal bones
    M00.131   Pneumococcal arthritis, right wrist   HCC
    M00.132   Pneumococcal arthritis, left wrist   HCC
    M00.139   Pneumococcal arthritis, unspecified wrist   HCC ▽
✓6ᵗʰ **M00.14**   **Pneumococcal arthritis, hand**
   Pneumococcal arthritis of metacarpus and phalanges
    M00.141   Pneumococcal arthritis, right hand   HCC
    M00.142   Pneumococcal arthritis, left hand   HCC
    M00.149   Pneumococcal arthritis, unspecified hand   HCC ▽
✓6ᵗʰ **M00.15**   **Pneumococcal arthritis, hip**
    M00.151   Pneumococcal arthritis, right hip   HCC
    M00.152   Pneumococcal arthritis, left hip   HCC
    M00.159   Pneumococcal arthritis, unspecified hip   HCC ▽
✓6ᵗʰ **M00.16**   **Pneumococcal arthritis, knee**
    M00.161   Pneumococcal arthritis, right knee   HCC
    M00.162   Pneumococcal arthritis, left knee   HCC
    M00.169   Pneumococcal arthritis, unspecified knee   HCC ▽

✓ Additional Character Req   ✓x7ᵗʰ Placeholder Alert   **Manifestation**   ▽ Unspecified   ►◄ Revised Text   ● New Code   ▲ Revised Code Title

√6ᵗʰ **M00.17** **Pneumococcal arthritis,** ankle and foot

Pneumococcal arthritis, tarsus, metatarsus and phalanges

    M00.171 **Pneumococcal arthritis,** right ankle and foot `HCC`

    M00.172 **Pneumococcal arthritis,** left ankle and foot `HCC`

    M00.179 **Pneumococcal arthritis,** unspecified ankle and foot `HCC` ▽

M00.18 **Pneumococcal arthritis,** vertebrae `HCC`

M00.19 **Pneumococcal** polyarthritis `HCC`

√5ᵗʰ **M00.2** **Other streptococcal arthritis and polyarthritis**

Use additional code (B95.0-B95.2, B95.4-B95.5) to identify bacterial agent

M00.20 **Other streptococcal arthritis, unspecified joint** `HCC` ▽

√6ᵗʰ **M00.21** **Other streptococcal arthritis,** shoulder

    M00.211 **Other streptococcal arthritis,** right shoulder `HCC`

    M00.212 **Other streptococcal arthritis,** left shoulder `HCC`

    M00.219 **Other streptococcal arthritis,** unspecified shoulder `HCC` ▽

√6ᵗʰ **M00.22** **Other streptococcal arthritis,** elbow

    M00.221 **Other streptococcal arthritis,** right elbow `HCC`

    M00.222 **Other streptococcal arthritis,** left elbow `HCC`

    M00.229 **Other streptococcal arthritis,** unspecified elbow `HCC` ▽

√6ᵗʰ **M00.23** **Other streptococcal arthritis,** wrist

Other streptococcal arthritis of carpal bones

    M00.231 **Other streptococcal arthritis,** right wrist `HCC`

    M00.232 **Other streptococcal arthritis,** left wrist `HCC`

    M00.239 **Other streptococcal arthritis,** unspecified wrist `HCC` ▽

√6ᵗʰ **M00.24** **Other streptococcal arthritis,** hand

Other streptococcal arthritis metacarpus and phalanges

    M00.241 **Other streptococcal arthritis,** right hand `HCC`

    M00.242 **Other streptococcal arthritis,** left hand `HCC`

    M00.249 **Other streptococcal arthritis,** unspecified hand `HCC` ▽

√6ᵗʰ **M00.25** **Other streptococcal arthritis,** hip

    M00.251 **Other streptococcal arthritis,** right hip `HCC`

    M00.252 **Other streptococcal arthritis,** left hip `HCC`

    M00.259 **Other streptococcal arthritis,** unspecified hip `HCC` ▽

√6ᵗʰ **M00.26** **Other streptococcal arthritis,** knee

    M00.261 **Other streptococcal arthritis,** right knee `HCC`

    M00.262 **Other streptococcal arthritis,** left knee `HCC`

    M00.269 **Other streptococcal arthritis,** unspecified knee `HCC` ▽

√6ᵗʰ **M00.27** **Other streptococcal arthritis,** ankle and foot

Other streptococcal arthritis, tarsus, metatarsus and phalanges

    M00.271 **Other streptococcal arthritis,** right ankle and foot `HCC`

    M00.272 **Other streptococcal arthritis,** left ankle and foot `HCC`

    M00.279 **Other streptococcal arthritis,** unspecified ankle and foot `HCC` ▽

M00.28 **Other streptococcal arthritis,** vertebrae `HCC`

M00.29 **Other streptococcal** polyarthritis `HCC`

√5ᵗʰ **M00.8** **Arthritis and polyarthritis due to other bacteria**

Use additional code (B96) to identify bacteria

M00.80 **Arthritis due to other bacteria, unspecified joint** `HCC` ▽

√6ᵗʰ **M00.81** **Arthritis due to other bacteria,** shoulder

    M00.811 **Arthritis due to other bacteria,** right shoulder `HCC`

    M00.812 **Arthritis due to other bacteria,** left shoulder `HCC`

    M00.819 **Arthritis due to other bacteria,** unspecified shoulder `HCC` ▽

√6ᵗʰ **M00.82** **Arthritis due to other bacteria,** elbow

    M00.821 **Arthritis due to other bacteria,** right elbow `HCC`

    M00.822 **Arthritis due to other bacteria,** left elbow `HCC`

    M00.829 **Arthritis due to other bacteria,** unspecified elbow `HCC` ▽

√6ᵗʰ **M00.83** **Arthritis due to other bacteria,** wrist

Arthritis due to other bacteria, carpal bones

    M00.831 **Arthritis due to other bacteria,** right wrist `HCC`

    M00.832 **Arthritis due to other bacteria,** left wrist `HCC`

    M00.839 **Arthritis due to other bacteria,** unspecified wrist `HCC` ▽

√6ᵗʰ **M00.84** **Arthritis due to other bacteria,** hand

Arthritis due to other bacteria, metacarpus and phalanges

    M00.841 **Arthritis due to other bacteria,** right hand `HCC`

    M00.842 **Arthritis due to other bacteria,** left hand `HCC`

    M00.849 **Arthritis due to other bacteria,** unspecified hand `HCC` ▽

√6ᵗʰ **M00.85** **Arthritis due to other bacteria,** hip

    M00.851 **Arthritis due to other bacteria,** right hip `HCC`

    M00.852 **Arthritis due to other bacteria,** left hip `HCC`

    M00.859 **Arthritis due to other bacteria,** unspecified hip `HCC` ▽

√6ᵗʰ **M00.86** **Arthritis due to other bacteria,** knee

    M00.861 **Arthritis due to other bacteria,** right knee `HCC`

    M00.862 **Arthritis due to other bacteria,** left knee `HCC`

    M00.869 **Arthritis due to other bacteria,** unspecified knee `HCC` ▽

√6ᵗʰ **M00.87** **Arthritis due to other bacteria,** ankle and foot

Arthritis due to other bacteria, tarsus, metatarsus, and phalanges

    M00.871 **Arthritis due to other bacteria,** right ankle and foot `HCC`

    M00.872 **Arthritis due to other bacteria,** left ankle and foot `HCC`

    M00.879 **Arthritis due to other bacteria,** unspecified ankle and foot `HCC` ▽

M00.88 **Arthritis due to other bacteria,** vertebrae `HCC`

M00.89 **Polyarthritis** due to other bacteria `HCC`

M00.9 **Pyogenic arthritis, unspecified** `HCC` ▽

Infective arthritis NOS

√4ᵗʰ **M01** **Direct infections of joint in infectious and parasitic diseases classified elsewhere**

Code first underlying disease, such as:

leprosy [Hansen's disease] (A30.-)

mycoses (B35-B49)

O'nyong-nyong fever (A92.1)

paratyphoid fever (A01.1-A01.4)

EXCLUDES 1   arthropathy in Lyme disease (A69.23)

gonococcal arthritis (A54.42)

meningococcal arthritis (A39.83)

mumps arthritis (B26.85)

postinfective arthropathy (M02.-)

postmeningococcal arthritis (A39.84)

reactive arthritis (M02.3)

rubella arthritis (B06.82)

sarcoidosis arthritis (D86.86)

typhoid fever arthritis (A01.04)

tuberculosis arthritis (A18.01-A18.02)

√5ᵗʰ **M01.X** **Direct infection of joint in infectious and parasitic diseases classified elsewhere**

    M01.X0 *Direct infection of unspecified joint in infectious and parasitic diseases classified elsewhere* `HCC` ▽

√6ᵗʰ **M01.X1** **Direct infection of** shoulder **joint in infectious and parasitic diseases classified elsewhere**

     M01.X11   *Direct infection of* right *shoulder in infectious and parasitic diseases classified elsewhere*   HCC

     M01.X12   *Direct infection of* left *shoulder in infectious and parasitic diseases classified elsewhere*   HCC

     M01.X19   *Direct infection of unspecified shoulder in infectious and parasitic diseases classified elsewhere*   HCC ▽

√6ᵗʰ **M01.X2** **Direct infection of** elbow **in infectious and parasitic diseases classified elsewhere**

     M01.X21   *Direct infection of* right *elbow in infectious and parasitic diseases classified elsewhere*   HCC

     M01.X22   *Direct infection of* left *elbow in infectious and parasitic diseases classified elsewhere*   HCC

     M01.X29   *Direct infection of unspecified elbow in infectious and parasitic diseases classified elsewhere*   HCC ▽

√6ᵗʰ **M01.X3** **Direct infection of** wrist **in infectious and parasitic diseases classified elsewhere**

     Direct infection of carpal bones in infectious and parasitic diseases classified elsewhere

     M01.X31   *Direct infection of* right *wrist in infectious and parasitic diseases classified elsewhere*   HCC

     M01.X32   *Direct infection of* left *wrist in infectious and parasitic diseases classified elsewhere*   HCC

     M01.X39   *Direct infection of unspecified wrist in infectious and parasitic diseases classified elsewhere*   HCC ▽

√6ᵗʰ **M01.X4** **Direct infection of** hand **in infectious and parasitic diseases classified elsewhere**

     Direct infection of metacarpus and phalanges in infectious and parasitic diseases classified elsewhere

     M01.X41   *Direct infection of* right *hand in infectious and parasitic diseases classified elsewhere*   HCC

     M01.X42   *Direct infection of* left *hand in infectious and parasitic diseases classified elsewhere*   HCC

     M01.X49   *Direct infection of unspecified hand in infectious and parasitic diseases classified elsewhere*   HCC ▽

√6ᵗʰ **M01.X5** **Direct infection of** hip **in infectious and parasitic diseases classified elsewhere**

     M01.X51   *Direct infection of* right *hip in infectious and parasitic diseases classified elsewhere*   HCC

     M01.X52   *Direct infection of* left *hip in infectious and parasitic diseases classified elsewhere*   HCC

     M01.X59   *Direct infection of unspecified hip in infectious and parasitic diseases classified elsewhere*   HCC ▽

√6ᵗʰ **M01.X6** **Direct infection of** knee **in infectious and parasitic diseases classified elsewhere**

     M01.X61   *Direct infection of* right *knee in infectious and parasitic diseases classified elsewhere*   HCC

     M01.X62   *Direct infection of* left *knee in infectious and parasitic diseases classified elsewhere*   HCC

     M01.X69   *Direct infection of unspecified knee in infectious and parasitic diseases classified elsewhere*   HCC ▽

√6ᵗʰ **M01.X7** **Direct infection of** ankle and foot **in infectious and parasitic diseases classified elsewhere**

     Direct infection of tarsus, metatarsus and phalanges in infectious and parasitic diseases classified elsewhere

     M01.X71   *Direct infection of* right *ankle and foot in infectious and parasitic diseases classified elsewhere*   HCC

     M01.X72   *Direct infection of* left *ankle and foot in infectious and parasitic diseases classified elsewhere*   HCC

     M01.X79   *Direct infection of unspecified ankle and foot in infectious and parasitic diseases classified elsewhere*   HCC ▽

     M01.X8   **Direct infection of** vertebrae **in infectious and parasitic diseases classified elsewhere**   HCC

     M01.X9   **Direct infection of** multiple joints **in infectious and parasitic diseases classified elsewhere**   HCC

√4ᵗʰ **M02** **Postinfective and reactive arthropathies**

Code first underlying disease, such as:
congenital syphilis [Clutton's joints] (A50.5)
enteritis due to Yersinia enterocolitica (A04.6)
infective endocarditis (I33.0)
viral hepatitis (B15-B19)

> EXCLUDES 1   Behçet's disease (M35.2)
> direct infections of joint in infectious and parasitic diseases classified elsewhere (M01.-)
> mumps arthritis (B26.85)
> postmeningococcal arthritis (A39.84)
> rheumatic fever (I00)
> rubella arthritis (B06.82)
> syphilis arthritis (late) (A52.77)
> tabetic arthropathy [Charcôt's] (A52.16)

√5ᵗʰ **M02.0** **Arthropathy** following intestinal bypass

     M02.00   **Arthropathy following intestinal bypass, unspecified site**   ▽

√6ᵗʰ   **M02.01**   **Arthropathy following intestinal bypass,** shoulder

     M02.011   **Arthropathy following intestinal bypass,** right **shoulder**

     M02.012   **Arthropathy following intestinal bypass,** left **shoulder**

     M02.019   **Arthropathy following intestinal bypass, unspecified shoulder**   ▽

√6ᵗʰ   **M02.02**   **Arthropathy following intestinal bypass,** elbow

     M02.021   **Arthropathy following intestinal bypass,** right **elbow**

     M02.022   **Arthropathy following intestinal bypass,** left **elbow**

     M02.029   **Arthropathy following intestinal bypass, unspecified elbow**   ▽

√6ᵗʰ   **M02.03**   **Arthropathy following intestinal bypass,** wrist

     Arthropathy following intestinal bypass, carpal bones

     M02.031   **Arthropathy following intestinal bypass,** right **wrist**

     M02.032   **Arthropathy following intestinal bypass,** left **wrist**

     M02.039   **Arthropathy following intestinal bypass, unspecified wrist**   ▽

√6ᵗʰ   **M02.04**   **Arthropathy following intestinal bypass,** hand

     Arthropathy following intestinal bypass, metacarpals and phalanges

     M02.041   **Arthropathy following intestinal bypass,** right **hand**

     M02.042   **Arthropathy following intestinal bypass,** left **hand**

     M02.049   **Arthropathy following intestinal bypass, unspecified hand**   ▽

√6ᵗʰ   **M02.05**   **Arthropathy following intestinal bypass,** hip

     M02.051   **Arthropathy following intestinal bypass,** right **hip**

     M02.052   **Arthropathy following intestinal bypass,** left **hip**

     M02.059   **Arthropathy following intestinal bypass, unspecified hip**   ▽

√6ᵗʰ   **M02.06**   **Arthropathy following intestinal bypass,** knee

     M02.061   **Arthropathy following intestinal bypass,** right **knee**

     M02.062   **Arthropathy following intestinal bypass,** left **knee**

     M02.069   **Arthropathy following intestinal bypass, unspecified knee**   ▽

√6ᵗʰ   **M02.07**   **Arthropathy following intestinal bypass,** ankle and foot

     Arthropathy following intestinal bypass, tarsus, metatarsus and phalanges

     M02.071   **Arthropathy following intestinal bypass,** right **ankle and foot**

     M02.072   **Arthropathy following intestinal bypass,** left **ankle and foot**

✓ Additional Character Req   ✓x7ᵗʰ Placeholder Alert   Manifestation   ▽ Unspecified   ►◄ Revised Text   ● New Code   ▲ Revised Code Title

ICD-10-CM 2019   743

M02.079 Arthropathy following intestinal bypass, unspecified ankle and foot ▽

M02.08 Arthropathy following intestinal bypass, vertebrae

M02.09 Arthropathy following intestinal bypass, multiple sites

✓5ᵗʰ **M02.1** Postdysenteric arthropathy

    M02.10 Postdysenteric arthropathy, unspecified site HCC ▽

    ✓6ᵗʰ **M02.11** Postdysenteric arthropathy, shoulder

        M02.111 Postdysenteric arthropathy, right shoulder HCC

        M02.112 Postdysenteric arthropathy, left shoulder HCC

        M02.119 Postdysenteric arthropathy, unspecified shoulder HCC ▽

    ✓6ᵗʰ **M02.12** Postdysenteric arthropathy, elbow

        M02.121 Postdysenteric arthropathy, right elbow HCC

        M02.122 Postdysenteric arthropathy, left elbow HCC

        M02.129 Postdysenteric arthropathy, unspecified elbow HCC ▽

    ✓6ᵗʰ **M02.13** Postdysenteric arthropathy, wrist

        Postdysenteric arthropathy, carpal bones

        M02.131 Postdysenteric arthropathy, right wrist HCC

        M02.132 Postdysenteric arthropathy, left wrist HCC

        M02.139 Postdysenteric arthropathy, unspecified wrist HCC ▽

    ✓6ᵗʰ **M02.14** Postdysenteric arthropathy, hand

        Postdysenteric arthropathy, metacarpus and phalanges

        M02.141 Postdysenteric arthropathy, right hand HCC

        M02.142 Postdysenteric arthropathy, left hand HCC

        M02.149 Postdysenteric arthropathy, unspecified hand HCC ▽

    ✓6ᵗʰ **M02.15** Postdysenteric arthropathy, hip

        M02.151 Postdysenteric arthropathy, right hip HCC

        M02.152 Postdysenteric arthropathy, left hip HCC

        M02.159 Postdysenteric arthropathy, unspecified hip HCC ▽

    ✓6ᵗʰ **M02.16** Postdysenteric arthropathy, knee

        M02.161 Postdysenteric arthropathy, right knee HCC

        M02.162 Postdysenteric arthropathy, left knee HCC

        M02.169 Postdysenteric arthropathy, unspecified knee HCC ▽

    ✓6ᵗʰ **M02.17** Postdysenteric arthropathy, ankle and foot

        Postdysenteric arthropathy, tarsus, metatarsus and phalanges

        M02.171 Postdysenteric arthropathy, right ankle and foot HCC

        M02.172 Postdysenteric arthropathy, left ankle and foot HCC

        M02.179 Postdysenteric arthropathy, unspecified ankle and foot HCC ▽

    M02.18 Postdysenteric arthropathy, vertebrae HCC

    M02.19 Postdysenteric arthropathy, multiple sites HCC

✓5ᵗʰ **M02.2** Postimmunization arthropathy

    M02.20 Postimmunization arthropathy, unspecified site ▽

    ✓6ᵗʰ **M02.21** Postimmunization arthropathy, shoulder

        M02.211 Postimmunization arthropathy, right shoulder

        M02.212 Postimmunization arthropathy, left shoulder

        M02.219 Postimmunization arthropathy, unspecified shoulder ▽

    ✓6ᵗʰ **M02.22** Postimmunization arthropathy, elbow

        M02.221 Postimmunization arthropathy, right elbow

        M02.222 Postimmunization arthropathy, left elbow

M02.229 Postimmunization arthropathy, unspecified elbow ▽

✓6ᵗʰ **M02.23** Postimmunization arthropathy, wrist

    Postimmunization arthropathy, carpal bones

    M02.231 Postimmunization arthropathy, right wrist

    M02.232 Postimmunization arthropathy, left wrist

    M02.239 Postimmunization arthropathy, unspecified wrist ▽

✓6ᵗʰ **M02.24** Postimmunization arthropathy, hand

    Postimmunization arthropathy, metacarpus and phalanges

    M02.241 Postimmunization arthropathy, right hand

    M02.242 Postimmunization arthropathy, left hand

    M02.249 Postimmunization arthropathy, unspecified hand ▽

✓6ᵗʰ **M02.25** Postimmunization arthropathy, hip

    M02.251 Postimmunization arthropathy, right hip

    M02.252 Postimmunization arthropathy, left hip

    M02.259 Postimmunization arthropathy, unspecified hip ▽

✓6ᵗʰ **M02.26** Postimmunization arthropathy, knee

    M02.261 Postimmunization arthropathy, right knee

    M02.262 Postimmunization arthropathy, left knee

    M02.269 Postimmunization arthropathy, unspecified knee ▽

✓6ᵗʰ **M02.27** Postimmunization arthropathy, ankle and foot

    Postimmunization arthropathy, tarsus, metatarsus and phalanges

    M02.271 Postimmunization arthropathy, right ankle and foot

    M02.272 Postimmunization arthropathy, left ankle and foot

    M02.279 Postimmunization arthropathy, unspecified ankle and foot ▽

M02.28 Postimmunization arthropathy, vertebrae

M02.29 Postimmunization arthropathy, multiple sites

✓5ᵗʰ **M02.3** Reiter's disease

    Reactive arthritis

    DEF: Arthritis, iridocyclitis, and urethritis, sometimes with diarrhea. While symptoms may recur, arthritis is constant.

    M02.30 Reiter's disease, unspecified site HCC ▽

    ✓6ᵗʰ **M02.31** Reiter's disease, shoulder

        M02.311 Reiter's disease, right shoulder HCC

        M02.312 Reiter's disease, left shoulder HCC

        M02.319 Reiter's disease, unspecified shoulder HCC ▽

    ✓6ᵗʰ **M02.32** Reiter's disease, elbow

        M02.321 Reiter's disease, right elbow HCC

        M02.322 Reiter's disease, left elbow HCC

        M02.329 Reiter's disease, unspecified elbow HCC ▽

    ✓6ᵗʰ **M02.33** Reiter's disease, wrist

        Reiter's disease, carpal bones

        M02.331 Reiter's disease, right wrist HCC

        M02.332 Reiter's disease, left wrist HCC

        M02.339 Reiter's disease, unspecified wrist HCC ▽

    ✓6ᵗʰ **M02.34** Reiter's disease, hand

        Reiter's disease, metacarpus and phalanges

        M02.341 Reiter's disease, right hand HCC

        M02.342 Reiter's disease, left hand HCC

        M02.349 Reiter's disease, unspecified hand HCC ▽

    ✓6ᵗʰ **M02.35** Reiter's disease, hip

        M02.351 Reiter's disease, right hip HCC

        M02.352 Reiter's disease, left hip HCC

        M02.359 Reiter's disease, unspecified hip HCC ▽

    ✓6ᵗʰ **M02.36** Reiter's disease, knee

        M02.361 Reiter's disease, right knee HCC

        M02.362 Reiter's disease, left knee HCC

        M02.369 Reiter's disease, unspecified knee HCC ▽

    ✓6ᵗʰ **M02.37** Reiter's disease, ankle and foot

        Reiter's disease, tarsus, metatarsus and phalanges

        M02.371 Reiter's disease, right ankle and foot HCC

        M02.372 Reiter's disease, left ankle and foot HCC

M02.379 Reiter's disease, unspecified ankle and foot `HCC` ▽

M02.38 Reiter's disease, vertebrae `HCC`

M02.39 Reiter's disease, multiple sites `HCC`

✓5ᵗʰ **M02.8 Other reactive arthropathies**

M02.80 *Other reactive arthropathies, unspecified site* `HCC` ▽

✓6ᵗʰ **M02.81 Other reactive arthropathies, shoulder**

M02.811 *Other reactive arthropathies, right shoulder* `HCC`

M02.812 *Other reactive arthropathies, left shoulder* `HCC`

M02.819 *Other reactive arthropathies, unspecified shoulder* `HCC` ▽

✓6ᵗʰ **M02.82 Other reactive arthropathies, elbow**

M02.821 *Other reactive arthropathies, right elbow* `HCC`

M02.822 *Other reactive arthropathies, left elbow* `HCC`

M02.829 *Other reactive arthropathies, unspecified elbow* `HCC` ▽

✓6ᵗʰ **M02.83 Other reactive arthropathies, wrist**

Other reactive arthropathies, carpal bones

M02.831 *Other reactive arthropathies, right wrist* `HCC`

M02.832 *Other reactive arthropathies, left wrist* `HCC`

M02.839 *Other reactive arthropathies, unspecified wrist* `HCC` ▽

✓6ᵗʰ **M02.84 Other reactive arthropathies, hand**

Other reactive arthropathies, metacarpus and phalanges

M02.841 *Other reactive arthropathies, right hand* `HCC`

M02.842 *Other reactive arthropathies, left hand* `HCC`

M02.849 *Other reactive arthropathies, unspecified hand* `HCC` ▽

✓6ᵗʰ **M02.85 Other reactive arthropathies, hip**

M02.851 *Other reactive arthropathies, right hip* `HCC`

M02.852 *Other reactive arthropathies, left hip* `HCC`

M02.859 *Other reactive arthropathies, unspecified hip* `HCC` ▽

✓6ᵗʰ **M02.86 Other reactive arthropathies, knee**

M02.861 *Other reactive arthropathies, right knee* `HCC`

M02.862 *Other reactive arthropathies, left knee* `HCC`

M02.869 *Other reactive arthropathies, unspecified knee* `HCC` ▽

✓6ᵗʰ **M02.87 Other reactive arthropathies, ankle and foot**

Other reactive arthropathies, tarsus, metatarsus and phalanges

M02.871 *Other reactive arthropathies, right ankle and foot* `HCC`

M02.872 *Other reactive arthropathies, left ankle and foot* `HCC`

M02.879 *Other reactive arthropathies, unspecified ankle and foot* `HCC` ▽

M02.88 *Other reactive arthropathies, vertebrae* `HCC`

M02.89 *Other reactive arthropathies, multiple sites* `HCC`

M02.9 *Reactive arthropathy, unspecified* `HCC` ▽

Autoinflammatory syndromes (M04)

AHA: 2016,4Q,37

✓4ᵗʰ **M04 Autoinflammatory syndromes**

EXCLUDES 2 *Crohn's disease (K50.-)*

M04.1 Periodic fever syndromes `HCC`

Familial Mediterranean fever

Hyperimmunoglobin D syndrome

Mevalonate kinase deficiency

Tumor necrosis factor receptor associated periodic syndrome [TRAPS]

M04.2 Cryopyrin-associated periodic syndromes `HCC`

Chronic infantile neurological, cutaneous and articular syndrome [CINCA]

Familial cold autoinflammatory syndrome

Familial cold urticaria

Muckle-Wells syndrome

Neonatal onset multisystemic inflammatory disorder [NOMID]

M04.8 Other autoinflammatory syndromes `HCC`

Blau syndrome

Deficiency of interleukin 1 receptor antagonist [DIRA]

Majeed syndrome

Periodic fever, aphthous stomatitis, pharyngitis, and adenopathy syndrome [PFAPA]

Pyogenic arthritis, pyoderma gangrenosum, and acne syndrome [PAPA]

M04.9 Autoinflammatory syndrome, unspecified `HCC` ▽

Inflammatory polyarthropathies (M05-M14)

✓4ᵗʰ **M05 Rheumatoid arthritis with rheumatoid factor**

EXCLUDES 1 *rheumatic fever (I00)*

juvenile rheumatoid arthritis (M08.-)

rheumatoid arthritis of spine (M45.-)

DEF: Rheumatoid arthritis: Autoimmune systemic disease that causes chronic inflammation of the joints and other areas of the body, manifested by inflammatory changes in articular structures and synovial membranes, atrophy, and loss in bone density.

✓5ᵗʰ **M05.0 Felty's syndrome**

Rheumatoid arthritis with splenoadenomegaly and leukopenia

M05.00 Felty's syndrome, unspecified site `HCC` ▽

✓6ᵗʰ **M05.01 Felty's syndrome, shoulder**

M05.011 Felty's syndrome, right shoulder `HCC`

M05.012 Felty's syndrome, left shoulder `HCC`

M05.019 Felty's syndrome, unspecified shoulder `HCC` ▽

✓6ᵗʰ **M05.02 Felty's syndrome, elbow**

M05.021 Felty's syndrome, right elbow `HCC`

M05.022 Felty's syndrome, left elbow `HCC`

M05.029 Felty's syndrome, unspecified elbow `HCC` ▽

✓6ᵗʰ **M05.03 Felty's syndrome, wrist**

Felty's syndrome, carpal bones

M05.031 Felty's syndrome, right wrist `HCC`

M05.032 Felty's syndrome, left wrist `HCC`

M05.039 Felty's syndrome, unspecified wrist `HCC` ▽

✓6ᵗʰ **M05.04 Felty's syndrome, hand**

Felty's syndrome, metacarpus and phalanges

M05.041 Felty's syndrome, right hand `HCC`

M05.042 Felty's syndrome, left hand `HCC`

M05.049 Felty's syndrome, unspecified hand `HCC` ▽

✓6ᵗʰ **M05.05 Felty's syndrome, hip**

M05.051 Felty's syndrome, right hip `HCC`

M05.052 Felty's syndrome, left hip `HCC`

M05.059 Felty's syndrome, unspecified hip `HCC` ▽

✓6ᵗʰ **M05.06 Felty's syndrome, knee**

M05.061 Felty's syndrome, right knee `HCC`

M05.062 Felty's syndrome, left knee `HCC`

M05.069 Felty's syndrome, unspecified knee `HCC` ▽

✓6ᵗʰ **M05.07 Felty's syndrome, ankle and foot**

Felty's syndrome, tarsus, metatarsus and phalanges

M05.071 Felty's syndrome, right ankle and foot `HCC`

M05.072 Felty's syndrome, left ankle and foot `HCC`

M05.079 Felty's syndrome, unspecified ankle and foot `HCC` ▽

M05.09 Felty's syndrome, multiple sites `HCC`

✓5ᵗʰ **M05.1 Rheumatoid lung disease with rheumatoid arthritis**

DEF: Lung disorders associated with rheumatoid arthritis.

M05.10 Rheumatoid lung disease with rheumatoid arthritis of unspecified site `HCC` ▽

☑ Additional Character Req ✓x7ᵗʰ Placeholder Alert Manifestation ▽ Unspecified ►◄ Revised Text ● New Code ▲ Revised Code Title

Chapter 13. Diseases of the Musculoskeletal System and Connective Tissue

M05.11–M05.30

√6ᵗʰ **M05.11** **Rheumatoid lung disease with rheumatoid arthritis of shoulder**

    M05.111 **Rheumatoid lung disease with rheumatoid arthritis of right shoulder**   HCC

    M05.112 **Rheumatoid lung disease with rheumatoid arthritis of left shoulder**   HCC

    M05.119 **Rheumatoid lung disease with rheumatoid arthritis of unspecified shoulder**   HCC ▽

√6ᵗʰ **M05.12** **Rheumatoid lung disease with rheumatoid arthritis of elbow**

    M05.121 **Rheumatoid lung disease with rheumatoid arthritis of right elbow**   HCC

    M05.122 **Rheumatoid lung disease with rheumatoid arthritis of left elbow**   HCC

    M05.129 **Rheumatoid lung disease with rheumatoid arthritis of unspecified elbow**   HCC ▽

√6ᵗʰ **M05.13** **Rheumatoid lung disease with rheumatoid arthritis of wrist**

    Rheumatoid lung disease with rheumatoid arthritis, carpal bones

    M05.131 **Rheumatoid lung disease with rheumatoid arthritis of right wrist**   HCC

    M05.132 **Rheumatoid lung disease with rheumatoid arthritis of left wrist**   HCC

    M05.139 **Rheumatoid lung disease with rheumatoid arthritis of unspecified wrist**   HCC ▽

√6ᵗʰ **M05.14** **Rheumatoid lung disease with rheumatoid arthritis of hand**

    Rheumatoid lung disease with rheumatoid arthritis, metacarpus and phalanges

    M05.141 **Rheumatoid lung disease with rheumatoid arthritis of right hand**   HCC

    M05.142 **Rheumatoid lung disease with rheumatoid arthritis of left hand**   HCC

    M05.149 **Rheumatoid lung disease with rheumatoid arthritis of unspecified hand**   HCC ▽

√6ᵗʰ **M05.15** **Rheumatoid lung disease with rheumatoid arthritis of hip**

    M05.151 **Rheumatoid lung disease with rheumatoid arthritis of right hip**   HCC

    M05.152 **Rheumatoid lung disease with rheumatoid arthritis of left hip**   HCC

    M05.159 **Rheumatoid lung disease with rheumatoid arthritis of unspecified hip**   HCC ▽

√6ᵗʰ **M05.16** **Rheumatoid lung disease with rheumatoid arthritis of knee**

    M05.161 **Rheumatoid lung disease with rheumatoid arthritis of right knee**   HCC

    M05.162 **Rheumatoid lung disease with rheumatoid arthritis of left knee**   HCC

    M05.169 **Rheumatoid lung disease with rheumatoid arthritis of unspecified knee**   HCC ▽

√6ᵗʰ **M05.17** **Rheumatoid lung disease with rheumatoid arthritis of ankle and foot**

    Rheumatoid lung disease with rheumatoid arthritis, tarsus, metatarsus and phalanges

    M05.171 **Rheumatoid lung disease with rheumatoid arthritis of right ankle and foot**   HCC

    M05.172 **Rheumatoid lung disease with rheumatoid arthritis of left ankle and foot**   HCC

    M05.179 **Rheumatoid lung disease with rheumatoid arthritis of unspecified ankle and foot**   HCC ▽

    M05.19 **Rheumatoid lung disease with rheumatoid arthritis of multiple sites**   HCC

√5ᵗʰ **M05.2** **Rheumatoid vasculitis with rheumatoid arthritis**

    M05.20 **Rheumatoid vasculitis with rheumatoid arthritis of unspecified site**   HCC ▽

√6ᵗʰ **M05.21** **Rheumatoid vasculitis with rheumatoid arthritis of shoulder**

    M05.211 **Rheumatoid vasculitis with rheumatoid arthritis of right shoulder**   HCC

    M05.212 **Rheumatoid vasculitis with rheumatoid arthritis of left shoulder**   HCC

    M05.219 **Rheumatoid vasculitis with rheumatoid arthritis of unspecified shoulder**   HCC ▽

√6ᵗʰ **M05.22** **Rheumatoid vasculitis with rheumatoid arthritis of elbow**

    M05.221 **Rheumatoid vasculitis with rheumatoid arthritis of right elbow**   HCC

    M05.222 **Rheumatoid vasculitis with rheumatoid arthritis of left elbow**   HCC

    M05.229 **Rheumatoid vasculitis with rheumatoid arthritis of unspecified elbow**   HCC ▽

√6ᵗʰ **M05.23** **Rheumatoid vasculitis with rheumatoid arthritis of wrist**

    Rheumatoid vasculitis with rheumatoid arthritis, carpal bones

    M05.231 **Rheumatoid vasculitis with rheumatoid arthritis of right wrist**   HCC

    M05.232 **Rheumatoid vasculitis with rheumatoid arthritis of left wrist**   HCC

    M05.239 **Rheumatoid vasculitis with rheumatoid arthritis of unspecified wrist**   HCC ▽

√6ᵗʰ **M05.24** **Rheumatoid vasculitis with rheumatoid arthritis of hand**

    Rheumatoid vasculitis with rheumatoid arthritis, metacarpus and phalanges

    M05.241 **Rheumatoid vasculitis with rheumatoid arthritis of right hand**   HCC

    M05.242 **Rheumatoid vasculitis with rheumatoid arthritis of left hand**   HCC

    M05.249 **Rheumatoid vasculitis with rheumatoid arthritis of unspecified hand**   HCC ▽

√6ᵗʰ **M05.25** **Rheumatoid vasculitis with rheumatoid arthritis of hip**

    M05.251 **Rheumatoid vasculitis with rheumatoid arthritis of right hip**   HCC

    M05.252 **Rheumatoid vasculitis with rheumatoid arthritis of left hip**   HCC

    M05.259 **Rheumatoid vasculitis with rheumatoid arthritis of unspecified hip**   HCC ▽

√6ᵗʰ **M05.26** **Rheumatoid vasculitis with rheumatoid arthritis of knee**

    M05.261 **Rheumatoid vasculitis with rheumatoid arthritis of right knee**   HCC

    M05.262 **Rheumatoid vasculitis with rheumatoid arthritis of left knee**   HCC

    M05.269 **Rheumatoid vasculitis with rheumatoid arthritis of unspecified knee**   HCC ▽

√6ᵗʰ **M05.27** **Rheumatoid vasculitis with rheumatoid arthritis of ankle and foot**

    Rheumatoid vasculitis with rheumatoid arthritis, tarsus, metatarsus and phalanges

    M05.271 **Rheumatoid vasculitis with rheumatoid arthritis of right ankle and foot**   HCC

    M05.272 **Rheumatoid vasculitis with rheumatoid arthritis of left ankle and foot**   HCC

    M05.279 **Rheumatoid vasculitis with rheumatoid arthritis of unspecified ankle and foot**   HCC ▽

    M05.29 **Rheumatoid vasculitis with rheumatoid arthritis of multiple sites**   HCC

√5ᵗʰ **M05.3** **Rheumatoid heart disease with rheumatoid arthritis**

    Rheumatoid carditis
    Rheumatoid endocarditis
    Rheumatoid myocarditis
    Rheumatoid pericarditis

    M05.30 **Rheumatoid heart disease with rheumatoid arthritis of unspecified site**   HCC ▽

√6ᵗʰ **M05.31 Rheumatoid heart disease with rheumatoid arthritis of shoulder**

M05.311 Rheumatoid heart disease with rheumatoid arthritis of right shoulder HCC

M05.312 Rheumatoid heart disease with rheumatoid arthritis of left shoulder HCC

M05.319 Rheumatoid heart disease with rheumatoid arthritis of unspecified shoulder HCC ▽

√6ᵗʰ **M05.32 Rheumatoid heart disease with rheumatoid arthritis of elbow**

M05.321 Rheumatoid heart disease with rheumatoid arthritis of right elbow HCC

M05.322 Rheumatoid heart disease with rheumatoid arthritis of left elbow HCC

M05.329 Rheumatoid heart disease with rheumatoid arthritis of unspecified elbow HCC ▽

√6ᵗʰ **M05.33 Rheumatoid heart disease with rheumatoid arthritis of wrist**
Rheumatoid heart disease with rheumatoid arthritis, carpal bones

M05.331 Rheumatoid heart disease with rheumatoid arthritis of right wrist HCC

M05.332 Rheumatoid heart disease with rheumatoid arthritis of left wrist HCC

M05.339 Rheumatoid heart disease with rheumatoid arthritis of unspecified wrist HCC ▽

√6ᵗʰ **M05.34 Rheumatoid heart disease with rheumatoid arthritis of hand**
Rheumatoid heart disease with rheumatoid arthritis, metacarpus and phalanges

M05.341 Rheumatoid heart disease with rheumatoid arthritis of right hand HCC

M05.342 Rheumatoid heart disease with rheumatoid arthritis of left hand HCC

M05.349 Rheumatoid heart disease with rheumatoid arthritis of unspecified hand HCC ▽

√6ᵗʰ **M05.35 Rheumatoid heart disease with rheumatoid arthritis of hip**

M05.351 Rheumatoid heart disease with rheumatoid arthritis of right hip HCC

M05.352 Rheumatoid heart disease with rheumatoid arthritis of left hip HCC

M05.359 Rheumatoid heart disease with rheumatoid arthritis of unspecified hip HCC ▽

√6ᵗʰ **M05.36 Rheumatoid heart disease with rheumatoid arthritis of knee**

M05.361 Rheumatoid heart disease with rheumatoid arthritis of right knee HCC

M05.362 Rheumatoid heart disease with rheumatoid arthritis of left knee HCC

M05.369 Rheumatoid heart disease with rheumatoid arthritis of unspecified knee HCC ▽

√6ᵗʰ **M05.37 Rheumatoid heart disease with rheumatoid arthritis of ankle and foot**
Rheumatoid heart disease with rheumatoid arthritis, tarsus, metatarsus and phalanges

M05.371 Rheumatoid heart disease with rheumatoid arthritis of right ankle and foot HCC

M05.372 Rheumatoid heart disease with rheumatoid arthritis of left ankle and foot HCC

M05.379 Rheumatoid heart disease with rheumatoid arthritis of unspecified ankle and foot HCC ▽

M05.39 Rheumatoid heart disease with rheumatoid arthritis of multiple sites HCC

√5ᵗʰ **M05.4 Rheumatoid myopathy with rheumatoid arthritis**

M05.40 Rheumatoid myopathy with rheumatoid arthritis of unspecified site HCC ▽

√6ᵗʰ **M05.41 Rheumatoid myopathy with rheumatoid arthritis of shoulder**

M05.411 Rheumatoid myopathy with rheumatoid arthritis of right shoulder HCC

M05.412 Rheumatoid myopathy with rheumatoid arthritis of left shoulder HCC

M05.419 Rheumatoid myopathy with rheumatoid arthritis of unspecified shoulder HCC ▽

√6ᵗʰ **M05.42 Rheumatoid myopathy with rheumatoid arthritis of elbow**

M05.421 Rheumatoid myopathy with rheumatoid arthritis of right elbow HCC

M05.422 Rheumatoid myopathy with rheumatoid arthritis of left elbow HCC

M05.429 Rheumatoid myopathy with rheumatoid arthritis of unspecified elbow HCC ▽

√6ᵗʰ **M05.43 Rheumatoid myopathy with rheumatoid arthritis of wrist**
Rheumatoid myopathy with rheumatoid arthritis, carpal bones

M05.431 Rheumatoid myopathy with rheumatoid arthritis of right wrist HCC

M05.432 Rheumatoid myopathy with rheumatoid arthritis of left wrist HCC

M05.439 Rheumatoid myopathy with rheumatoid arthritis of unspecified wrist HCC ▽

√6ᵗʰ **M05.44 Rheumatoid myopathy with rheumatoid arthritis of hand**
Rheumatoid myopathy with rheumatoid arthritis, metacarpus and phalanges

M05.441 Rheumatoid myopathy with rheumatoid arthritis of right hand HCC

M05.442 Rheumatoid myopathy with rheumatoid arthritis of left hand HCC

M05.449 Rheumatoid myopathy with rheumatoid arthritis of unspecified hand HCC ▽

√6ᵗʰ **M05.45 Rheumatoid myopathy with rheumatoid arthritis of hip**

M05.451 Rheumatoid myopathy with rheumatoid arthritis of right hip HCC

M05.452 Rheumatoid myopathy with rheumatoid arthritis of left hip HCC

M05.459 Rheumatoid myopathy with rheumatoid arthritis of unspecified hip HCC ▽

√6ᵗʰ **M05.46 Rheumatoid myopathy with rheumatoid arthritis of knee**

M05.461 Rheumatoid myopathy with rheumatoid arthritis of right knee HCC

M05.462 Rheumatoid myopathy with rheumatoid arthritis of left knee HCC

M05.469 Rheumatoid myopathy with rheumatoid arthritis of unspecified knee HCC ▽

√6ᵗʰ **M05.47 Rheumatoid myopathy with rheumatoid arthritis of ankle and foot**
Rheumatoid myopathy with rheumatoid arthritis, tarsus, metatarsus and phalanges

M05.471 Rheumatoid myopathy with rheumatoid arthritis of right ankle and foot HCC

M05.472 Rheumatoid myopathy with rheumatoid arthritis of left ankle and foot HCC

M05.479 Rheumatoid myopathy with rheumatoid arthritis of unspecified ankle and foot HCC ▽

M05.49 Rheumatoid myopathy with rheumatoid arthritis of multiple sites HCC

√5ᵗʰ **M05.5 Rheumatoid polyneuropathy with rheumatoid arthritis**

M05.50 Rheumatoid polyneuropathy with rheumatoid arthritis of unspecified site HCC ▽

✓ Additional Character Req | √x7ᵗʰ Placeholder Alert | Manifestation | ▽ Unspecified | ►◄ Revised Text | ● New Code | ▲ Revised Code Title

ICD-10-CM 2019 | 747

Chapter 13. Diseases of the Musculoskeletal System and Connective Tissue

√6ᵗʰ **M05.51 Rheumatoid polyneuropathy with rheumatoid arthritis of shoulder**

     M05.511 Rheumatoid polyneuropathy with rheumatoid arthritis of right shoulder   HCC

     M05.512 Rheumatoid polyneuropathy with rheumatoid arthritis of left shoulder   HCC

     M05.519 Rheumatoid polyneuropathy with rheumatoid arthritis of unspecified shoulder   HCC ▽

√6ᵗʰ **M05.52 Rheumatoid polyneuropathy with rheumatoid arthritis of elbow**

     M05.521 Rheumatoid polyneuropathy with rheumatoid arthritis of right elbow   HCC

     M05.522 Rheumatoid polyneuropathy with rheumatoid arthritis of left elbow   HCC

     M05.529 Rheumatoid polyneuropathy with rheumatoid arthritis of unspecified elbow   HCC ▽

√6ᵗʰ **M05.53 Rheumatoid polyneuropathy with rheumatoid arthritis of wrist**

     Rheumatoid polyneuropathy with rheumatoid arthritis, carpal bones

     M05.531 Rheumatoid polyneuropathy with rheumatoid arthritis of right wrist   HCC

     M05.532 Rheumatoid polyneuropathy with rheumatoid arthritis of left wrist   HCC

     M05.539 Rheumatoid polyneuropathy with rheumatoid arthritis of unspecified wrist   HCC ▽

√6ᵗʰ **M05.54 Rheumatoid polyneuropathy with rheumatoid arthritis of hand**

     Rheumatoid polyneuropathy with rheumatoid arthritis, metacarpus and phalanges

     M05.541 Rheumatoid polyneuropathy with rheumatoid arthritis of right hand   HCC

     M05.542 Rheumatoid polyneuropathy with rheumatoid arthritis of left hand   HCC

     M05.549 Rheumatoid polyneuropathy with rheumatoid arthritis of unspecified hand   HCC ▽

√6ᵗʰ **M05.55 Rheumatoid polyneuropathy with rheumatoid arthritis of hip**

     M05.551 Rheumatoid polyneuropathy with rheumatoid arthritis of right hip   HCC

     M05.552 Rheumatoid polyneuropathy with rheumatoid arthritis of left hip   HCC

     M05.559 Rheumatoid polyneuropathy with rheumatoid arthritis of unspecified hip   HCC ▽

√6ᵗʰ **M05.56 Rheumatoid polyneuropathy with rheumatoid arthritis of knee**

     M05.561 Rheumatoid polyneuropathy with rheumatoid arthritis of right knee   HCC

     M05.562 Rheumatoid polyneuropathy with rheumatoid arthritis of left knee   HCC

     M05.569 Rheumatoid polyneuropathy with rheumatoid arthritis of unspecified knee   HCC ▽

√6ᵗʰ **M05.57 Rheumatoid polyneuropathy with rheumatoid arthritis of ankle and foot**

     Rheumatoid polyneuropathy with rheumatoid arthritis, tarsus, metatarsus and phalanges

     M05.571 Rheumatoid polyneuropathy with rheumatoid arthritis of right ankle and foot   HCC

     M05.572 Rheumatoid polyneuropathy with rheumatoid arthritis of left ankle and foot   HCC

     M05.579 Rheumatoid polyneuropathy with rheumatoid arthritis of unspecified ankle and foot   HCC ▽

     M05.59 Rheumatoid polyneuropathy with rheumatoid arthritis of multiple sites   HCC

√5ᵗʰ **M05.6 Rheumatoid arthritis with involvement of other organs and systems**

     M05.60 Rheumatoid arthritis of unspecified site with involvement of other organs and systems   HCC ▽

√6ᵗʰ **M05.61 Rheumatoid arthritis of shoulder with involvement of other organs and systems**

     M05.611 Rheumatoid arthritis of right shoulder with involvement of other organs and systems   HCC

     M05.612 Rheumatoid arthritis of left shoulder with involvement of other organs and systems   HCC

     M05.619 Rheumatoid arthritis of unspecified shoulder with involvement of other organs and systems   HCC ▽

√6ᵗʰ **M05.62 Rheumatoid arthritis of elbow with involvement of other organs and systems**

     M05.621 Rheumatoid arthritis of right elbow with involvement of other organs and systems   HCC

     M05.622 Rheumatoid arthritis of left elbow with involvement of other organs and systems   HCC

     M05.629 Rheumatoid arthritis of unspecified elbow with involvement of other organs and systems   HCC ▽

√6ᵗʰ **M05.63 Rheumatoid arthritis of wrist with involvement of other organs and systems**

     Rheumatoid arthritis of carpal bones with involvement of other organs and systems

     M05.631 Rheumatoid arthritis of right wrist with involvement of other organs and systems   HCC

     M05.632 Rheumatoid arthritis of left wrist with involvement of other organs and systems   HCC

     M05.639 Rheumatoid arthritis of unspecified wrist with involvement of other organs and systems   HCC ▽

√6ᵗʰ **M05.64 Rheumatoid arthritis of hand with involvement of other organs and systems**

     Rheumatoid arthritis of metacarpus and phalanges with involvement of other organs and systems

     M05.641 Rheumatoid arthritis of right hand with involvement of other organs and systems   HCC

     M05.642 Rheumatoid arthritis of left hand with involvement of other organs and systems   HCC

     M05.649 Rheumatoid arthritis of unspecified hand with involvement of other organs and systems   HCC ▽

√6ᵗʰ **M05.65 Rheumatoid arthritis of hip with involvement of other organs and systems**

     M05.651 Rheumatoid arthritis of right hip with involvement of other organs and systems   HCC

     M05.652 Rheumatoid arthritis of left hip with involvement of other organs and systems   HCC

     M05.659 Rheumatoid arthritis of unspecified hip with involvement of other organs and systems   HCC ▽

√6ᵗʰ **M05.66 Rheumatoid arthritis of knee with involvement of other organs and systems**

     M05.661 Rheumatoid arthritis of right knee with involvement of other organs and systems   HCC

     M05.662 Rheumatoid arthritis of left knee with involvement of other organs and systems   HCC

     M05.669 Rheumatoid arthritis of unspecified knee with involvement of other organs and systems   HCC ▽

√6ᵗʰ **M05.67 Rheumatoid arthritis of ankle and foot with involvement of other organs and systems**

     Rheumatoid arthritis of tarsus, metatarsus and phalanges with involvement of other organs and systems

     M05.671 Rheumatoid arthritis of right ankle and foot with involvement of other organs and systems   HCC

        M05.672 Rheumatoid arthritis of left ankle and foot with involvement of other organs and systems `HCC`

        M05.679 Rheumatoid arthritis of unspecified ankle and foot with involvement of other organs and systems `HCC` ▽

    M05.69 Rheumatoid arthritis of multiple sites with involvement of other organs and systems `HCC`

✓5ᵗʰ **M05.7** Rheumatoid arthritis with rheumatoid factor without organ or systems involvement

    M05.70 Rheumatoid arthritis with rheumatoid factor of unspecified site without organ or systems involvement `HCC` ▽

✓6ᵗʰ **M05.71** Rheumatoid arthritis with rheumatoid factor of shoulder without organ or systems involvement

        M05.711 Rheumatoid arthritis with rheumatoid factor of right shoulder without organ or systems involvement `HCC`

        M05.712 Rheumatoid arthritis with rheumatoid factor of left shoulder without organ or systems involvement `HCC`

        M05.719 Rheumatoid arthritis with rheumatoid factor of unspecified shoulder without organ or systems involvement `HCC` ▽

✓6ᵗʰ **M05.72** Rheumatoid arthritis with rheumatoid factor of elbow without organ or systems involvement

        M05.721 Rheumatoid arthritis with rheumatoid factor of right elbow without organ or systems involvement `HCC`

        M05.722 Rheumatoid arthritis with rheumatoid factor of left elbow without organ or systems involvement `HCC`

        M05.729 Rheumatoid arthritis with rheumatoid factor of unspecified elbow without organ or systems involvement `HCC` ▽

✓6ᵗʰ **M05.73** Rheumatoid arthritis with rheumatoid factor of wrist without organ or systems involvement

        M05.731 Rheumatoid arthritis with rheumatoid factor of right wrist without organ or systems involvement `HCC`

        M05.732 Rheumatoid arthritis with rheumatoid factor of left wrist without organ or systems involvement `HCC`

        M05.739 Rheumatoid arthritis with rheumatoid factor of unspecified wrist without organ or systems involvement `HCC` ▽

✓6ᵗʰ **M05.74** Rheumatoid arthritis with rheumatoid factor of hand without organ or systems involvement

        M05.741 Rheumatoid arthritis with rheumatoid factor of right hand without organ or systems involvement `HCC`

        M05.742 Rheumatoid arthritis with rheumatoid factor of left hand without organ or systems involvement `HCC`

        M05.749 Rheumatoid arthritis with rheumatoid factor of unspecified hand without organ or systems involvement `HCC` ▽

✓6ᵗʰ **M05.75** Rheumatoid arthritis with rheumatoid factor of hip without organ or systems involvement

        M05.751 Rheumatoid arthritis with rheumatoid factor of right hip without organ or systems involvement `HCC`

        M05.752 Rheumatoid arthritis with rheumatoid factor of left hip without organ or systems involvement `HCC`

        M05.759 Rheumatoid arthritis with rheumatoid factor of unspecified hip without organ or systems involvement `HCC` ▽

✓6ᵗʰ **M05.76** Rheumatoid arthritis with rheumatoid factor of knee without organ or systems involvement

        M05.761 Rheumatoid arthritis with rheumatoid factor of right knee without organ or systems involvement `HCC`

        M05.762 Rheumatoid arthritis with rheumatoid factor of left knee without organ or systems involvement `HCC`

        M05.769 Rheumatoid arthritis with rheumatoid factor of unspecified knee without organ or systems involvement `HCC` ▽

✓6ᵗʰ **M05.77** Rheumatoid arthritis with rheumatoid factor of ankle and foot without organ or systems involvement

        M05.771 Rheumatoid arthritis with rheumatoid factor of right ankle and foot without organ or systems involvement `HCC`

        M05.772 Rheumatoid arthritis with rheumatoid factor of left ankle and foot without organ or systems involvement `HCC`

        M05.779 Rheumatoid arthritis with rheumatoid factor of unspecified ankle and foot without organ or systems involvement `HCC` ▽

    M05.79 Rheumatoid arthritis with rheumatoid factor of multiple sites without organ or systems involvement `HCC`

✓5ᵗʰ **M05.8** Other rheumatoid arthritis with rheumatoid factor

    M05.80 Other rheumatoid arthritis with rheumatoid factor of unspecified site `HCC` ▽

✓6ᵗʰ **M05.81** Other rheumatoid arthritis with rheumatoid factor of shoulder

        M05.811 Other rheumatoid arthritis with rheumatoid factor of right shoulder `HCC`

        M05.812 Other rheumatoid arthritis with rheumatoid factor of left shoulder `HCC`

        M05.819 Other rheumatoid arthritis with rheumatoid factor of unspecified shoulder `HCC` ▽

✓6ᵗʰ **M05.82** Other rheumatoid arthritis with rheumatoid factor of elbow

        M05.821 Other rheumatoid arthritis with rheumatoid factor of right elbow `HCC`

        M05.822 Other rheumatoid arthritis with rheumatoid factor of left elbow `HCC`

        M05.829 Other rheumatoid arthritis with rheumatoid factor of unspecified elbow `HCC` ▽

✓6ᵗʰ **M05.83** Other rheumatoid arthritis with rheumatoid factor of wrist

        M05.831 Other rheumatoid arthritis with rheumatoid factor of right wrist `HCC`

        M05.832 Other rheumatoid arthritis with rheumatoid factor of left wrist `HCC`

        M05.839 Other rheumatoid arthritis with rheumatoid factor of unspecified wrist `HCC` ▽

✓6ᵗʰ **M05.84** Other rheumatoid arthritis with rheumatoid factor of hand

        M05.841 Other rheumatoid arthritis with rheumatoid factor of right hand `HCC`

        M05.842 Other rheumatoid arthritis with rheumatoid factor of left hand `HCC`

        M05.849 Other rheumatoid arthritis with rheumatoid factor of unspecified hand `HCC` ▽

✓6ᵗʰ **M05.85** Other rheumatoid arthritis with rheumatoid factor of hip

        M05.851 Other rheumatoid arthritis with rheumatoid factor of right hip `HCC`

        M05.852 Other rheumatoid arthritis with rheumatoid factor of left hip `HCC`

        M05.859 Other rheumatoid arthritis with rheumatoid factor of unspecified hip `HCC` ▽

Chapter 13. Diseases of the Musculoskeletal System and Connective Tissue

√6ᵗʰ **M05.86** Other rheumatoid arthritis with rheumatoid factor of knee

     M05.861 Other rheumatoid arthritis with rheumatoid factor of right knee   HCC

     M05.862 Other rheumatoid arthritis with rheumatoid factor of left knee   HCC

     M05.869 Other rheumatoid arthritis with rheumatoid factor of unspecified knee   HCC ▽

√6ᵗʰ **M05.87** Other rheumatoid arthritis with rheumatoid factor of ankle and foot

     M05.871 Other rheumatoid arthritis with rheumatoid factor of right ankle and foot   HCC

     M05.872 Other rheumatoid arthritis with rheumatoid factor of left ankle and foot   HCC

     M05.879 Other rheumatoid arthritis with rheumatoid factor of unspecified ankle and foot   HCC ▽

     M05.89 Other rheumatoid arthritis with rheumatoid factor of multiple sites   HCC

     M05.9 Rheumatoid arthritis with rheumatoid factor, unspecified   HCC ▽

√4ᵗʰ **M06** Other rheumatoid arthritis

DEF: Rheumatoid arthritis: Autoimmune systemic disease that causes chronic inflammation of the joints and other areas of the body, manifested by inflammatory changes in articular structures and synovial membranes, atrophy, and loss in bone density.

√5ᵗʰ **M06.0** Rheumatoid arthritis without rheumatoid factor

     M06.00 Rheumatoid arthritis without rheumatoid factor, unspecified site   HCC ▽

√6ᵗʰ **M06.01** Rheumatoid arthritis without rheumatoid factor, shoulder

     M06.011 Rheumatoid arthritis without rheumatoid factor, right shoulder   HCC

     M06.012 Rheumatoid arthritis without rheumatoid factor, left shoulder   HCC

     M06.019 Rheumatoid arthritis without rheumatoid factor, unspecified shoulder   HCC ▽

√6ᵗʰ **M06.02** Rheumatoid arthritis without rheumatoid factor, elbow

     M06.021 Rheumatoid arthritis without rheumatoid factor, right elbow   HCC

     M06.022 Rheumatoid arthritis without rheumatoid factor, left elbow   HCC

     M06.029 Rheumatoid arthritis without rheumatoid factor, unspecified elbow   HCC ▽

√6ᵗʰ **M06.03** Rheumatoid arthritis without rheumatoid factor, wrist

     M06.031 Rheumatoid arthritis without rheumatoid factor, right wrist   HCC

     M06.032 Rheumatoid arthritis without rheumatoid factor, left wrist   HCC

     M06.039 Rheumatoid arthritis without rheumatoid factor, unspecified wrist   HCC ▽

√6ᵗʰ **M06.04** Rheumatoid arthritis without rheumatoid factor, hand

     M06.041 Rheumatoid arthritis without rheumatoid factor, right hand   HCC

     M06.042 Rheumatoid arthritis without rheumatoid factor, left hand   HCC

     M06.049 Rheumatoid arthritis without rheumatoid factor, unspecified hand   HCC ▽

√6ᵗʰ **M06.05** Rheumatoid arthritis without rheumatoid factor, hip

     M06.051 Rheumatoid arthritis without rheumatoid factor, right hip   HCC

     M06.052 Rheumatoid arthritis without rheumatoid factor, left hip   HCC

     M06.059 Rheumatoid arthritis without rheumatoid factor, unspecified hip   HCC ▽

√6ᵗʰ **M06.06** Rheumatoid arthritis without rheumatoid factor, knee

     M06.061 Rheumatoid arthritis without rheumatoid factor, right knee   HCC

     M06.062 Rheumatoid arthritis without rheumatoid factor, left knee   HCC

     M06.069 Rheumatoid arthritis without rheumatoid factor, unspecified knee   HCC ▽

√6ᵗʰ **M06.07** Rheumatoid arthritis without rheumatoid factor, ankle and foot

     M06.071 Rheumatoid arthritis without rheumatoid factor, right ankle and foot   HCC

     M06.072 Rheumatoid arthritis without rheumatoid factor, left ankle and foot   HCC

     M06.079 Rheumatoid arthritis without rheumatoid factor, unspecified ankle and foot   HCC ▽

     M06.08 Rheumatoid arthritis without rheumatoid factor, vertebrae   HCC

     M06.09 Rheumatoid arthritis without rheumatoid factor, multiple sites   HCC

M06.1 Adult-onset Still's disease   HCC A

     EXCLUDES 1   Still's disease NOS (M08.2-)

     DEF: Type of systemic arthritis characterized by a transient rash and spiking fevers. This condition may resolve or develop into a chronic condition and may affect internal organs, as well as joints. **Synonym(s):** AOSD

√5ᵗʰ **M06.2** Rheumatoid bursitis

     M06.20 Rheumatoid bursitis, unspecified site   HCC ▽

√6ᵗʰ **M06.21** Rheumatoid bursitis, shoulder

     M06.211 Rheumatoid bursitis, right shoulder   HCC

     M06.212 Rheumatoid bursitis, left shoulder   HCC

     M06.219 Rheumatoid bursitis, unspecified shoulder   HCC ▽

√6ᵗʰ **M06.22** Rheumatoid bursitis, elbow

     M06.221 Rheumatoid bursitis, right elbow   HCC

     M06.222 Rheumatoid bursitis, left elbow   HCC

     M06.229 Rheumatoid bursitis, unspecified elbow   HCC ▽

√6ᵗʰ **M06.23** Rheumatoid bursitis, wrist

     M06.231 Rheumatoid bursitis, right wrist   HCC

     M06.232 Rheumatoid bursitis, left wrist   HCC

     M06.239 Rheumatoid bursitis, unspecified wrist   HCC ▽

√6ᵗʰ **M06.24** Rheumatoid bursitis, hand

     M06.241 Rheumatoid bursitis, right hand   HCC

     M06.242 Rheumatoid bursitis, left hand   HCC

     M06.249 Rheumatoid bursitis, unspecified hand   HCC ▽

√6ᵗʰ **M06.25** Rheumatoid bursitis, hip

     M06.251 Rheumatoid bursitis, right hip   HCC

     M06.252 Rheumatoid bursitis, left hip   HCC

     M06.259 Rheumatoid bursitis, unspecified hip   HCC ▽

√6ᵗʰ **M06.26** Rheumatoid bursitis, knee

     M06.261 Rheumatoid bursitis, right knee   HCC

     M06.262 Rheumatoid bursitis, left knee   HCC

     M06.269 Rheumatoid bursitis, unspecified knee   HCC ▽

√6ᵗʰ **M06.27** Rheumatoid bursitis, ankle and foot

     M06.271 Rheumatoid bursitis, right ankle and foot   HCC

     M06.272 Rheumatoid bursitis, left ankle and foot   HCC

     M06.279 Rheumatoid bursitis, unspecified ankle and foot   HCC ▽

     M06.28 Rheumatoid bursitis, vertebrae   HCC

     M06.29 Rheumatoid bursitis, multiple sites   HCC

√5ᵗʰ **M06.3** Rheumatoid nodule

     M06.30 Rheumatoid nodule, unspecified site   HCC ▽

√6ᵗʰ **M06.31** Rheumatoid nodule, shoulder

     M06.311 Rheumatoid nodule, right shoulder   HCC

     M06.312 Rheumatoid nodule, left shoulder   HCC

     M06.319 Rheumatoid nodule, unspecified shoulder   HCC ▽

√6ᵗʰ **M06.32** Rheumatoid nodule, elbow

     M06.321 Rheumatoid nodule, right elbow   HCC

     M06.322 Rheumatoid nodule, left elbow   HCC

M06.329 Rheumatoid nodule, unspecified elbow HCC ▽

√6ᵗʰ M06.33 Rheumatoid nodule, wrist
   M06.331 Rheumatoid nodule, right wrist HCC
   M06.332 Rheumatoid nodule, left wrist HCC
   M06.339 Rheumatoid nodule, unspecified wrist HCC ▽

√6ᵗʰ M06.34 Rheumatoid nodule, hand
   M06.341 Rheumatoid nodule, right hand HCC
   M06.342 Rheumatoid nodule, left hand HCC
   M06.349 Rheumatoid nodule, unspecified hand HCC ▽

√6ᵗʰ M06.35 Rheumatoid nodule, hip
   M06.351 Rheumatoid nodule, right hip HCC
   M06.352 Rheumatoid nodule, left hip HCC
   M06.359 Rheumatoid nodule, unspecified hip HCC ▽

√6ᵗʰ M06.36 Rheumatoid nodule, knee
   M06.361 Rheumatoid nodule, right knee HCC
   M06.362 Rheumatoid nodule, left knee HCC
   M06.369 Rheumatoid nodule, unspecified knee HCC ▽

√6ᵗʰ M06.37 Rheumatoid nodule, ankle and foot
   M06.371 Rheumatoid nodule, right ankle and foot HCC
   M06.372 Rheumatoid nodule, left ankle and foot HCC
   M06.379 Rheumatoid nodule, unspecified ankle and foot HCC ▽

M06.38 Rheumatoid nodule, vertebrae HCC
M06.39 Rheumatoid nodule, multiple sites HCC

M06.4 Inflammatory polyarthropathy HCC
   EXCLUDES 1 polyarthritis NOS (M13.0)

√5ᵗʰ M06.8 Other specified rheumatoid arthritis
   M06.80 Other specified rheumatoid arthritis, unspecified site HCC ▽

√6ᵗʰ M06.81 Other specified rheumatoid arthritis, shoulder
   M06.811 Other specified rheumatoid arthritis, right shoulder HCC
   M06.812 Other specified rheumatoid arthritis, left shoulder HCC
   M06.819 Other specified rheumatoid arthritis, unspecified shoulder HCC ▽

√6ᵗʰ M06.82 Other specified rheumatoid arthritis, elbow
   M06.821 Other specified rheumatoid arthritis, right elbow HCC
   M06.822 Other specified rheumatoid arthritis, left elbow HCC
   M06.829 Other specified rheumatoid arthritis, unspecified elbow HCC ▽

√6ᵗʰ M06.83 Other specified rheumatoid arthritis, wrist
   M06.831 Other specified rheumatoid arthritis, right wrist HCC
   M06.832 Other specified rheumatoid arthritis, left wrist HCC
   M06.839 Other specified rheumatoid arthritis, unspecified wrist HCC ▽

√6ᵗʰ M06.84 Other specified rheumatoid arthritis, hand
   M06.841 Other specified rheumatoid arthritis, right hand HCC
   M06.842 Other specified rheumatoid arthritis, left hand HCC
   M06.849 Other specified rheumatoid arthritis, unspecified hand HCC ▽

√6ᵗʰ M06.85 Other specified rheumatoid arthritis, hip
   M06.851 Other specified rheumatoid arthritis, right hip HCC
   M06.852 Other specified rheumatoid arthritis, left hip HCC
   M06.859 Other specified rheumatoid arthritis, unspecified hip HCC ▽

√6ᵗʰ M06.86 Other specified rheumatoid arthritis, knee
   M06.861 Other specified rheumatoid arthritis, right knee HCC
   M06.862 Other specified rheumatoid arthritis, left knee HCC
   M06.869 Other specified rheumatoid arthritis, unspecified knee HCC ▽

√6ᵗʰ M06.87 Other specified rheumatoid arthritis, ankle and foot
   M06.871 Other specified rheumatoid arthritis, right ankle and foot HCC
   M06.872 Other specified rheumatoid arthritis, left ankle and foot HCC
   M06.879 Other specified rheumatoid arthritis, unspecified ankle and foot HCC ▽

M06.88 Other specified rheumatoid arthritis, vertebrae HCC
M06.89 Other specified rheumatoid arthritis, multiple sites HCC

M06.9 Rheumatoid arthritis, unspecified HCC ▽

√4ᵗʰ M07 Enteropathic arthropathies
Code also associated enteropathy, such as:
   regional enteritis [Crohn's disease] (K50.-)
   ulcerative colitis (K51.-)
   EXCLUDES 1 psoriatic arthropathies (L40.5-)

√5ᵗʰ M07.6 Enteropathic arthropathies
   M07.60 Enteropathic arthropathies, unspecified site ▽

√6ᵗʰ M07.61 Enteropathic arthropathies, shoulder
   M07.611 Enteropathic arthropathies, right shoulder
   M07.612 Enteropathic arthropathies, left shoulder
   M07.619 Enteropathic arthropathies, unspecified shoulder ▽

√6ᵗʰ M07.62 Enteropathic arthropathies, elbow
   M07.621 Enteropathic arthropathies, right elbow
   M07.622 Enteropathic arthropathies, left elbow
   M07.629 Enteropathic arthropathies, unspecified elbow ▽

√6ᵗʰ M07.63 Enteropathic arthropathies, wrist
   M07.631 Enteropathic arthropathies, right wrist
   M07.632 Enteropathic arthropathies, left wrist
   M07.639 Enteropathic arthropathies, unspecified wrist ▽

√6ᵗʰ M07.64 Enteropathic arthropathies, hand
   M07.641 Enteropathic arthropathies, right hand
   M07.642 Enteropathic arthropathies, left hand
   M07.649 Enteropathic arthropathies, unspecified hand ▽

√6ᵗʰ M07.65 Enteropathic arthropathies, hip
   M07.651 Enteropathic arthropathies, right hip
   M07.652 Enteropathic arthropathies, left hip
   M07.659 Enteropathic arthropathies, unspecified hip ▽

√6ᵗʰ M07.66 Enteropathic arthropathies, knee
   M07.661 Enteropathic arthropathies, right knee
   M07.662 Enteropathic arthropathies, left knee
   M07.669 Enteropathic arthropathies, unspecified knee ▽

√6ᵗʰ M07.67 Enteropathic arthropathies, ankle and foot
   M07.671 Enteropathic arthropathies, right ankle and foot
   M07.672 Enteropathic arthropathies, left ankle and foot
   M07.679 Enteropathic arthropathies, unspecified ankle and foot ▽

M07.68 Enteropathic arthropathies, vertebrae
M07.69 Enteropathic arthropathies, multiple sites

√4ᵗʰ M08 Juvenile arthritis
Code also any associated underlying condition, such as:
   regional enteritis [Crohn's disease] (K50.-)
   ulcerative colitis (K51.-)
   EXCLUDES 1 arthropathy in Whipple's disease (M14.8)
   Felty's syndrome (M05.0)
   juvenile dermatomyositis (M33.0-)
   psoriatic juvenile arthropathy (L40.54)

√5ᵗʰ M08.0 Unspecified juvenile rheumatoid arthritis
Juvenile rheumatoid arthritis with or without rheumatoid factor
   M08.00 Unspecified juvenile rheumatoid arthritis of unspecified site HCC ▽

√6ᵗʰ M08.01 Unspecified juvenile rheumatoid arthritis, shoulder
   M08.011 Unspecified juvenile rheumatoid arthritis, right shoulder HCC ▽

M08.012 Unspecified juvenile rheumatoid HCC ▽
arthritis, **left shoulder**

M08.019 Unspecified juvenile rheumatoid HCC ▽
arthritis, **unspecified shoulder**

√6ᵗʰ **M08.02** Unspecified juvenile rheumatoid arthritis of **elbow**

M08.021 Unspecified juvenile rheumatoid HCC ▽
arthritis, **right elbow**

M08.022 Unspecified juvenile rheumatoid HCC ▽
arthritis, **left elbow**

M08.029 Unspecified juvenile rheumatoid HCC ▽
arthritis, **unspecified elbow**

√6ᵗʰ **M08.03** Unspecified juvenile rheumatoid arthritis, **wrist**

M08.031 Unspecified juvenile rheumatoid HCC ▽
arthritis, **right wrist**

M08.032 Unspecified juvenile rheumatoid HCC ▽
arthritis, **left wrist**

M08.039 Unspecified juvenile rheumatoid HCC ▽
arthritis, **unspecified wrist**

√6ᵗʰ **M08.04** Unspecified juvenile rheumatoid arthritis, **hand**

M08.041 Unspecified juvenile rheumatoid HCC ▽
arthritis, **right hand**

M08.042 Unspecified juvenile rheumatoid HCC ▽
arthritis, **left hand**

M08.049 Unspecified juvenile rheumatoid HCC ▽
arthritis, **unspecified hand**

√6ᵗʰ **M08.05** Unspecified juvenile rheumatoid arthritis, **hip**

M08.051 Unspecified juvenile rheumatoid HCC ▽
arthritis, **right hip**

M08.052 Unspecified juvenile rheumatoid HCC ▽
arthritis, **left hip**

M08.059 Unspecified juvenile rheumatoid HCC ▽
arthritis, **unspecified hip**

√6ᵗʰ **M08.06** Unspecified juvenile rheumatoid arthritis, **knee**

M08.061 Unspecified juvenile rheumatoid HCC ▽
arthritis, **right knee**

M08.062 Unspecified juvenile rheumatoid HCC ▽
arthritis, **left knee**

M08.069 Unspecified juvenile rheumatoid HCC ▽
arthritis, **unspecified knee**

√6ᵗʰ **M08.07** Unspecified juvenile rheumatoid arthritis, **ankle
and foot**

M08.071 Unspecified juvenile rheumatoid HCC ▽
arthritis, **right ankle and foot**

M08.072 Unspecified juvenile rheumatoid HCC ▽
arthritis, **left ankle and foot**

M08.079 Unspecified juvenile rheumatoid HCC ▽
arthritis, **unspecified ankle and
foot**

M08.08 Unspecified juvenile rheumatoid arthritis, HCC ▽
vertebrae

M08.09 Unspecified juvenile rheumatoid arthritis, HCC ▽
multiple sites

M08.1 Juvenile **ankylosing spondylitis** HCC

> *EXCLUDES 1* ankylosing spondylitis in adults (M45.0-)

√5ᵗʰ **M08.2** Juvenile rheumatoid arthritis **with systemic onset**

Still's disease NOS

> *EXCLUDES 1* adult-onset Still's disease (M06.1-)

DEF: Systemic juvenile rheumatoid arthritis characterized by a
transient rash and spiking fevers that may affect internal organs,
as well as joints.

M08.20 Juvenile rheumatoid arthritis with systemic HCC ▽
onset, **unspecified site**

√6ᵗʰ **M08.21** Juvenile rheumatoid arthritis with systemic onset,
shoulder

M08.211 Juvenile rheumatoid arthritis HCC
with systemic onset, **right
shoulder**

M08.212 Juvenile rheumatoid arthritis HCC
with systemic onset, **left shoulder**

M08.219 Juvenile rheumatoid arthritis HCC ▽
with systemic onset, **unspecified
shoulder**

√6ᵗʰ **M08.22** Juvenile rheumatoid arthritis with systemic onset,
elbow

M08.221 Juvenile rheumatoid arthritis HCC
with systemic onset, **right elbow**

M08.222 Juvenile rheumatoid arthritis HCC
with systemic onset, **left elbow**

M08.229 Juvenile rheumatoid arthritis HCC ▽
with systemic onset, **unspecified
elbow**

√6ᵗʰ **M08.23** Juvenile rheumatoid arthritis with systemic onset,
wrist

M08.231 Juvenile rheumatoid arthritis HCC
with systemic onset, **right wrist**

M08.232 Juvenile rheumatoid arthritis HCC
with systemic onset, **left wrist**

M08.239 Juvenile rheumatoid arthritis HCC ▽
with systemic onset, **unspecified
wrist**

√6ᵗʰ **M08.24** Juvenile rheumatoid arthritis with systemic onset,
hand

M08.241 Juvenile rheumatoid arthritis HCC
with systemic onset, **right hand**

M08.242 Juvenile rheumatoid arthritis HCC
with systemic onset, **left hand**

M08.249 Juvenile rheumatoid arthritis HCC ▽
with systemic onset, **unspecified
hand**

√6ᵗʰ **M08.25** Juvenile rheumatoid arthritis with systemic onset,
hip

M08.251 Juvenile rheumatoid arthritis HCC
with systemic onset, **right hip**

M08.252 Juvenile rheumatoid arthritis HCC
with systemic onset, **left hip**

M08.259 Juvenile rheumatoid arthritis HCC ▽
with systemic onset, **unspecified
hip**

√6ᵗʰ **M08.26** Juvenile rheumatoid arthritis with systemic onset,
knee

M08.261 Juvenile rheumatoid arthritis HCC
with systemic onset, **right knee**

M08.262 Juvenile rheumatoid arthritis HCC
with systemic onset, **left knee**

M08.269 Juvenile rheumatoid arthritis HCC ▽
with systemic onset, **unspecified
knee**

√6ᵗʰ **M08.27** Juvenile rheumatoid arthritis with systemic onset,
ankle and foot

M08.271 Juvenile rheumatoid arthritis HCC
with systemic onset, **right ankle
and foot**

M08.272 Juvenile rheumatoid arthritis HCC
with systemic onset, **left ankle
and foot**

M08.279 Juvenile rheumatoid arthritis HCC ▽
with systemic onset, **unspecified
ankle and foot**

M08.28 Juvenile rheumatoid arthritis with systemic HCC
onset, **vertebrae**

M08.29 Juvenile rheumatoid arthritis with systemic HCC
onset, **multiple sites**

M08.3 Juvenile rheumatoid **polyarthritis (seronegative)** HCC

√5ᵗʰ **M08.4** **Pauciarticular** juvenile rheumatoid arthritis

M08.40 Pauciarticular juvenile rheumatoid arthritis, HCC ▽
unspecified site

√6ᵗʰ **M08.41** Pauciarticular juvenile rheumatoid arthritis,
shoulder

M08.411 Pauciarticular juvenile HCC
rheumatoid arthritis, **right
shoulder**

M08.412 Pauciarticular juvenile HCC
rheumatoid arthritis, **left
shoulder**

M08.419 Pauciarticular juvenile HCC ▽
rheumatoid arthritis, **unspecified
shoulder**

√6ᵗʰ **M08.42** Pauciarticular juvenile rheumatoid arthritis, **elbow**

M08.421 Pauciarticular juvenile HCC
rheumatoid arthritis, **right elbow**

M08.422 Pauciarticular juvenile HCC
rheumatoid arthritis, **left elbow**

M08.429 Pauciarticular juvenile HCC ▽
rheumatoid arthritis, **unspecified
elbow**

√6ᵗʰ **M08.43** Pauciarticular juvenile rheumatoid arthritis, **wrist**

M08.431 Pauciarticular juvenile HCC
rheumatoid arthritis, **right wrist**

M08.432 Pauciarticular juvenile HCC
rheumatoid arthritis, **left wrist**

M08.439 Pauciarticular juvenile HCC ▽
rheumatoid arthritis, **unspecified
wrist**

√6ᵗʰ **MØ8.44** Pauciarticular juvenile rheumatoid arthritis, hand

    MØ8.441 Pauciarticular juvenile rheumatoid arthritis, right hand   HCC

    MØ8.442 Pauciarticular juvenile rheumatoid arthritis, left hand   HCC

    MØ8.449 Pauciarticular juvenile rheumatoid arthritis, unspecified hand   HCC ▽

√6ᵗʰ **MØ8.45** Pauciarticular juvenile rheumatoid arthritis, hip

    MØ8.451 Pauciarticular juvenile rheumatoid arthritis, right hip   HCC

    MØ8.452 Pauciarticular juvenile rheumatoid arthritis, left hip   HCC

    MØ8.459 Pauciarticular juvenile rheumatoid arthritis, unspecified hip   HCC ▽

√6ᵗʰ **MØ8.46** Pauciarticular juvenile rheumatoid arthritis, knee

    MØ8.461 Pauciarticular juvenile rheumatoid arthritis, right knee   HCC

    MØ8.462 Pauciarticular juvenile rheumatoid arthritis, left knee   HCC

    MØ8.469 Pauciarticular juvenile rheumatoid arthritis, unspecified knee   HCC ▽

√6ᵗʰ **MØ8.47** Pauciarticular juvenile rheumatoid arthritis, ankle and foot

    MØ8.471 Pauciarticular juvenile rheumatoid arthritis, right ankle and foot   HCC

    MØ8.472 Pauciarticular juvenile rheumatoid arthritis, left ankle and foot   HCC

    MØ8.479 Pauciarticular juvenile rheumatoid arthritis, unspecified ankle and foot   HCC ▽

MØ8.48 Pauciarticular juvenile rheumatoid arthritis, vertebrae   HCC

√5ᵗʰ **MØ8.8** Other juvenile arthritis

    MØ8.80 Other juvenile arthritis, unspecified site   HCC ▽

√6ᵗʰ **MØ8.81** Other juvenile arthritis, shoulder

    MØ8.811 Other juvenile arthritis, right shoulder   HCC

    MØ8.812 Other juvenile arthritis, left shoulder   HCC

    MØ8.819 Other juvenile arthritis, unspecified shoulder   HCC ▽

√6ᵗʰ **MØ8.82** Other juvenile arthritis, elbow

    MØ8.821 Other juvenile arthritis, right elbow   HCC

    MØ8.822 Other juvenile arthritis, left elbow   HCC

    MØ8.829 Other juvenile arthritis, unspecified elbow   HCC ▽

√6ᵗʰ **MØ8.83** Other juvenile arthritis, wrist

    MØ8.831 Other juvenile arthritis, right wrist   HCC

    MØ8.832 Other juvenile arthritis, left wrist   HCC

    MØ8.839 Other juvenile arthritis, unspecified wrist   HCC ▽

√6ᵗʰ **MØ8.84** Other juvenile arthritis, hand

    MØ8.841 Other juvenile arthritis, right hand   HCC

    MØ8.842 Other juvenile arthritis, left hand   HCC

    MØ8.849 Other juvenile arthritis, unspecified hand   HCC ▽

√6ᵗʰ **MØ8.85** Other juvenile arthritis, hip

    MØ8.851 Other juvenile arthritis, right hip   HCC

    MØ8.852 Other juvenile arthritis, left hip   HCC

    MØ8.859 Other juvenile arthritis, unspecified hip   HCC ▽

√6ᵗʰ **MØ8.86** Other juvenile arthritis, knee

    MØ8.861 Other juvenile arthritis, right knee   HCC

    MØ8.862 Other juvenile arthritis, left knee   HCC

    MØ8.869 Other juvenile arthritis, unspecified knee   HCC ▽

√6ᵗʰ **MØ8.87** Other juvenile arthritis, ankle and foot

    MØ8.871 Other juvenile arthritis, right ankle and foot   HCC

    MØ8.872 Other juvenile arthritis, left ankle and foot   HCC

    MØ8.879 Other juvenile arthritis, unspecified ankle and foot   HCC ▽

    MØ8.88 Other juvenile arthritis, other specified site   HCC

        Other juvenile arthritis, vertebrae

    MØ8.89 Other juvenile arthritis, multiple sites   HCC

√5ᵗʰ **MØ8.9** Juvenile arthritis, unspecified

    EXCLUDES 1   *juvenile rheumatoid arthritis, unspecified (MØ8.Ø-)*

    MØ8.90 Juvenile arthritis, unspecified, unspecified site   HCC ▽

√6ᵗʰ **MØ8.91** Juvenile arthritis, unspecified, shoulder

    MØ8.911 Juvenile arthritis, unspecified, right shoulder   HCC ▽

    MØ8.912 Juvenile arthritis, unspecified, left shoulder   HCC ▽

    MØ8.919 Juvenile arthritis, unspecified, unspecified shoulder   HCC ▽

√6ᵗʰ **MØ8.92** Juvenile arthritis, unspecified, elbow

    MØ8.921 Juvenile arthritis, unspecified, right elbow   HCC ▽

    MØ8.922 Juvenile arthritis, unspecified, left elbow   HCC ▽

    MØ8.929 Juvenile arthritis, unspecified, unspecified elbow   HCC ▽

√6ᵗʰ **MØ8.93** Juvenile arthritis, unspecified, wrist

    MØ8.931 Juvenile arthritis, unspecified, right wrist   HCC ▽

    MØ8.932 Juvenile arthritis, unspecified, left wrist   HCC ▽

    MØ8.939 Juvenile arthritis, unspecified, unspecified wrist   HCC ▽

√6ᵗʰ **MØ8.94** Juvenile arthritis, unspecified, hand

    MØ8.941 Juvenile arthritis, unspecified, right hand   HCC ▽

    MØ8.942 Juvenile arthritis, unspecified, left hand   HCC ▽

    MØ8.949 Juvenile arthritis, unspecified, unspecified hand   HCC ▽

√6ᵗʰ **MØ8.95** Juvenile arthritis, unspecified, hip

    MØ8.951 Juvenile arthritis, unspecified, right hip   HCC ▽

    MØ8.952 Juvenile arthritis, unspecified, left hip   HCC ▽

    MØ8.959 Juvenile arthritis, unspecified, unspecified hip   HCC ▽

√6ᵗʰ **MØ8.96** Juvenile arthritis, unspecified, knee

    MØ8.961 Juvenile arthritis, unspecified, right knee   HCC ▽

    MØ8.962 Juvenile arthritis, unspecified, left knee   HCC ▽

    MØ8.969 Juvenile arthritis, unspecified, unspecified knee   HCC ▽

√6ᵗʰ **MØ8.97** Juvenile arthritis, unspecified, ankle and foot

    MØ8.971 Juvenile arthritis, unspecified, right ankle and foot   HCC ▽

    MØ8.972 Juvenile arthritis, unspecified, left ankle and foot   HCC ▽

    MØ8.979 Juvenile arthritis, unspecified, unspecified ankle and foot   HCC ▽

    MØ8.98 Juvenile arthritis, unspecified, vertebrae   HCC ▽

    MØ8.99 Juvenile arthritis, unspecified, multiple sites   HCC ▽

✓ Additional Character Req   √x7ᵗʰ Placeholder Alert   Manifestation   ▽ Unspecified   ►◄ Revised Text   ● New Code   ▲ Revised Code Title

ICD-10-CM 2019   753

Chapter 13. Diseases of the Musculoskeletal System and Connective Tissue

M1A–M1A.29

√4ᵗʰ **M1A   Chronic gout**

Use additional code to identify:
autonomic neuropathy in diseases classified elsewhere (G99.0)
calculus of urinary tract in diseases classified elsewhere (N22)
cardiomyopathy in diseases classified elsewhere (I43)
disorders of external ear in diseases classified elsewhere (H61.1-,
   H62.8-)
disorders of iris and ciliary body in diseases classified elsewhere (H22)
glomerular disorders in diseases classified elsewhere (N08)

EXCLUDES 1   gout NOS (M10.-)
EXCLUDES 2   acute gout (M10.-)

> The appropriate 7th character is to be added to each code from
> category M1A.
> Ø   without tophus (tophi)
> 1   with tophus (tophi)

√5ᵗʰ **M1A.Ø   Idiopathic chronic gout**

Chronic gouty bursitis
Primary chronic gout

√x7ᵗʰ **M1A.ØØ   Idiopathic chronic gout, unspecified site**   ▽

√6ᵗʰ **M1A.Ø1   Idiopathic chronic gout, shoulder**

√7ᵗʰ **M1A.Ø11   Idiopathic chronic gout, right shoulder**

√7ᵗʰ **M1A.Ø12   Idiopathic chronic gout, left shoulder**

√7ᵗʰ **M1A.Ø19   Idiopathic chronic gout,
unspecified shoulder**   ▽

√6ᵗʰ **M1A.Ø2   Idiopathic chronic gout, elbow**

√7ᵗʰ **M1A.Ø21   Idiopathic chronic gout, right elbow**

√7ᵗʰ **M1A.Ø22   Idiopathic chronic gout, left elbow**

√7ᵗʰ **M1A.Ø29   Idiopathic chronic gout,
unspecified elbow**   ▽

√6ᵗʰ **M1A.Ø3   Idiopathic chronic gout, wrist**

√7ᵗʰ **M1A.Ø31   Idiopathic chronic gout, right wrist**

√7ᵗʰ **M1A.Ø32   Idiopathic chronic gout, left wrist**

√7ᵗʰ **M1A.Ø39   Idiopathic chronic gout,
unspecified wrist**   ▽

√6ᵗʰ **M1A.Ø4   Idiopathic chronic gout, hand**

√7ᵗʰ **M1A.Ø41   Idiopathic chronic gout, right hand**

√7ᵗʰ **M1A.Ø42   Idiopathic chronic gout, left hand**

√7ᵗʰ **M1A.Ø49   Idiopathic chronic gout,
unspecified hand**   ▽

√6ᵗʰ **M1A.Ø5   Idiopathic chronic gout, hip**

√7ᵗʰ **M1A.Ø51   Idiopathic chronic gout, right hip**

√7ᵗʰ **M1A.Ø52   Idiopathic chronic gout, left hip**

√7ᵗʰ **M1A.Ø59   Idiopathic chronic gout,
unspecified hip**   ▽

√6ᵗʰ **M1A.Ø6   Idiopathic chronic gout, knee**

√7ᵗʰ **M1A.Ø61   Idiopathic chronic gout, right knee**

√7ᵗʰ **M1A.Ø62   Idiopathic chronic gout, left knee**

√7ᵗʰ **M1A.Ø69   Idiopathic chronic gout,
unspecified knee**   ▽

√6ᵗʰ **M1A.Ø7   Idiopathic chronic gout, ankle and foot**

√7ᵗʰ **M1A.Ø71   Idiopathic chronic gout, right ankle and
foot**

√7ᵗʰ **M1A.Ø72   Idiopathic chronic gout, left ankle and
foot**

√7ᵗʰ **M1A.Ø79   Idiopathic chronic gout,
unspecified ankle and foot**   ▽

√x7ᵗʰ **M1A.Ø8   Idiopathic chronic gout, vertebrae**

√x7ᵗʰ **M1A.Ø9   Idiopathic chronic gout, multiple sites**

√5ᵗʰ **M1A.1   Lead-induced chronic gout**

Code first toxic effects of lead and its compounds (T56.Ø-)

√x7ᵗʰ **M1A.1Ø   Lead-induced chronic gout, unspecified site**   ▽

√6ᵗʰ **M1A.11   Lead-induced chronic gout, shoulder**

√7ᵗʰ **M1A.111   Lead-induced chronic gout, right
shoulder**

√7ᵗʰ **M1A.112   Lead-induced chronic gout, left shoulder**

√7ᵗʰ **M1A.119   Lead-induced chronic gout,
unspecified shoulder**   ▽

√6ᵗʰ **M1A.12   Lead-induced chronic gout, elbow**

√7ᵗʰ **M1A.121   Lead-induced chronic gout, right elbow**

√7ᵗʰ **M1A.122   Lead-induced chronic gout, left elbow**

√7ᵗʰ **M1A.129   Lead-induced chronic gout,
unspecified elbow**   ▽

√6ᵗʰ **M1A.13   Lead-induced chronic gout, wrist**

√7ᵗʰ **M1A.131   Lead-induced chronic gout, right wrist**

√7ᵗʰ **M1A.132   Lead-induced chronic gout, left wrist**

√7ᵗʰ **M1A.139   Lead-induced chronic gout,
unspecified wrist**   ▽

√6ᵗʰ **M1A.14   Lead-induced chronic gout, hand**

√7ᵗʰ **M1A.141   Lead-induced chronic gout, right hand**

√7ᵗʰ **M1A.142   Lead-induced chronic gout, left hand**

√7ᵗʰ **M1A.149   Lead-induced chronic gout,
unspecified hand**   ▽

√6ᵗʰ **M1A.15   Lead-induced chronic gout, hip**

√7ᵗʰ **M1A.151   Lead-induced chronic gout, right hip**

√7ᵗʰ **M1A.152   Lead-induced chronic gout, left hip**

√7ᵗʰ **M1A.159   Lead-induced chronic gout,
unspecified hip**   ▽

√6ᵗʰ **M1A.16   Lead-induced chronic gout, knee**

√7ᵗʰ **M1A.161   Lead-induced chronic gout, right knee**

√7ᵗʰ **M1A.162   Lead-induced chronic gout, left knee**

√7ᵗʰ **M1A.169   Lead-induced chronic gout,
unspecified knee**   ▽

√6ᵗʰ **M1A.17   Lead-induced chronic gout, ankle and foot**

√7ᵗʰ **M1A.171   Lead-induced chronic gout, right ankle
and foot**

√7ᵗʰ **M1A.172   Lead-induced chronic gout, left ankle and
foot**

√7ᵗʰ **M1A.179   Lead-induced chronic gout,
unspecified ankle and foot**   ▽

√x7ᵗʰ **M1A.18   Lead-induced chronic gout, vertebrae**

√x7ᵗʰ **M1A.19   Lead-induced chronic gout, multiple sites**

√5ᵗʰ **M1A.2   Drug-induced chronic gout**

Use additional code for adverse effect, if applicable, to identify
drug (T36-T50 with fifth or sixth character 5)

√x7ᵗʰ **M1A.2Ø   Drug-induced chronic gout, unspecified site**   ▽

√6ᵗʰ **M1A.21   Drug-induced chronic gout, shoulder**

√7ᵗʰ **M1A.211   Drug-induced chronic gout, right
shoulder**

√7ᵗʰ **M1A.212   Drug-induced chronic gout, left shoulder**

√7ᵗʰ **M1A.219   Drug-induced chronic gout,
unspecified shoulder**   ▽

√6ᵗʰ **M1A.22   Drug-induced chronic gout, elbow**

√7ᵗʰ **M1A.221   Drug-induced chronic gout, right elbow**

√7ᵗʰ **M1A.222   Drug-induced chronic gout, left elbow**

√7ᵗʰ **M1A.229   Drug-induced chronic gout,
unspecified elbow**   ▽

√6ᵗʰ **M1A.23   Drug-induced chronic gout, wrist**

√7ᵗʰ **M1A.231   Drug-induced chronic gout, right wrist**

√7ᵗʰ **M1A.232   Drug-induced chronic gout, left wrist**

√7ᵗʰ **M1A.239   Drug-induced chronic gout,
unspecified wrist**   ▽

√6ᵗʰ **M1A.24   Drug-induced chronic gout, hand**

√7ᵗʰ **M1A.241   Drug-induced chronic gout, right hand**

√7ᵗʰ **M1A.242   Drug-induced chronic gout, left hand**

√7ᵗʰ **M1A.249   Drug-induced chronic gout,
unspecified hand**   ▽

√6ᵗʰ **M1A.25   Drug-induced chronic gout, hip**

√7ᵗʰ **M1A.251   Drug-induced chronic gout, right hip**

√7ᵗʰ **M1A.252   Drug-induced chronic gout, left hip**

√7ᵗʰ **M1A.259   Drug-induced chronic gout,
unspecified hip**   ▽

√6ᵗʰ **M1A.26   Drug-induced chronic gout, knee**

√7ᵗʰ **M1A.261   Drug-induced chronic gout, right knee**

√7ᵗʰ **M1A.262   Drug-induced chronic gout, left knee**

√7ᵗʰ **M1A.269   Drug-induced chronic gout,
unspecified knee**   ▽

√6ᵗʰ **M1A.27   Drug-induced chronic gout, ankle and foot**

√7ᵗʰ **M1A.271   Drug-induced chronic gout, right ankle
and foot**

√7ᵗʰ **M1A.272   Drug-induced chronic gout, left ankle and
foot**

√7ᵗʰ **M1A.279   Drug-induced chronic gout,
unspecified ankle and foot**   ▽

√x7ᵗʰ **M1A.28   Drug-induced chronic gout, vertebrae**

√x7ᵗʰ **M1A.29   Drug-induced chronic gout, multiple sites**

√5ᵗʰ **M1A.3** Chronic gout due to renal impairment

Code first associated renal disease

√x7ᵗʰ **M1A.30** Chronic gout due to renal impairment, unspecified site ▽

√6ᵗʰ **M1A.31** Chronic gout due to renal impairment, shoulder

√7ᵗʰ **M1A.311** Chronic gout due to renal impairment, right shoulder

√7ᵗʰ **M1A.312** Chronic gout due to renal impairment, left shoulder

√7ᵗʰ **M1A.319** Chronic gout due to renal impairment, unspecified shoulder ▽

√6ᵗʰ **M1A.32** Chronic gout due to renal impairment, elbow

√7ᵗʰ **M1A.321** Chronic gout due to renal impairment, right elbow

√7ᵗʰ **M1A.322** Chronic gout due to renal impairment, left elbow

√7ᵗʰ **M1A.329** Chronic gout due to renal impairment, unspecified elbow ▽

√6ᵗʰ **M1A.33** Chronic gout due to renal impairment, wrist

√7ᵗʰ **M1A.331** Chronic gout due to renal impairment, right wrist

√7ᵗʰ **M1A.332** Chronic gout due to renal impairment, left wrist

√7ᵗʰ **M1A.339** Chronic gout due to renal impairment, unspecified wrist ▽

√6ᵗʰ **M1A.34** Chronic gout due to renal impairment, hand

√7ᵗʰ **M1A.341** Chronic gout due to renal impairment, right hand

√7ᵗʰ **M1A.342** Chronic gout due to renal impairment, left hand

√7ᵗʰ **M1A.349** Chronic gout due to renal impairment, unspecified hand ▽

√6ᵗʰ **M1A.35** Chronic gout due to renal impairment, hip

√7ᵗʰ **M1A.351** Chronic gout due to renal impairment, right hip

√7ᵗʰ **M1A.352** Chronic gout due to renal impairment, left hip

√7ᵗʰ **M1A.359** Chronic gout due to renal impairment, unspecified hip ▽

√6ᵗʰ **M1A.36** Chronic gout due to renal impairment, knee

√7ᵗʰ **M1A.361** Chronic gout due to renal impairment, right knee

√7ᵗʰ **M1A.362** Chronic gout due to renal impairment, left knee

√7ᵗʰ **M1A.369** Chronic gout due to renal impairment, unspecified knee ▽

√6ᵗʰ **M1A.37** Chronic gout due to renal impairment, ankle and foot

√7ᵗʰ **M1A.371** Chronic gout due to renal impairment, right ankle and foot

√7ᵗʰ **M1A.372** Chronic gout due to renal impairment, left ankle and foot

√7ᵗʰ **M1A.379** Chronic gout due to renal impairment, unspecified ankle and foot ▽

√x7ᵗʰ **M1A.38** Chronic gout due to renal impairment, vertebrae

√x7ᵗʰ **M1A.39** Chronic gout due to renal impairment, multiple sites

√5ᵗʰ **M1A.4** Other secondary chronic gout

Code first associated condition

√x7ᵗʰ **M1A.40** Other secondary chronic gout, unspecified site ▽

√6ᵗʰ **M1A.41** Other secondary chronic gout, shoulder

√7ᵗʰ **M1A.411** Other secondary chronic gout, right shoulder

√7ᵗʰ **M1A.412** Other secondary chronic gout, left shoulder

√7ᵗʰ **M1A.419** Other secondary chronic gout, unspecified shoulder ▽

√6ᵗʰ **M1A.42** Other secondary chronic gout, elbow

√7ᵗʰ **M1A.421** Other secondary chronic gout, right elbow

√7ᵗʰ **M1A.422** Other secondary chronic gout, left elbow

√7ᵗʰ **M1A.429** Other secondary chronic gout, unspecified elbow ▽

√6ᵗʰ **M1A.43** Other secondary chronic gout, wrist

√7ᵗʰ **M1A.431** Other secondary chronic gout, right wrist

√7ᵗʰ **M1A.432** Other secondary chronic gout, left wrist

√7ᵗʰ **M1A.439** Other secondary chronic gout, unspecified wrist ▽

√6ᵗʰ **M1A.44** Other secondary chronic gout, hand

√7ᵗʰ **M1A.441** Other secondary chronic gout, right hand

√7ᵗʰ **M1A.442** Other secondary chronic gout, left hand

√7ᵗʰ **M1A.449** Other secondary chronic gout, unspecified hand ▽

√6ᵗʰ **M1A.45** Other secondary chronic gout, hip

√7ᵗʰ **M1A.451** Other secondary chronic gout, right hip

√7ᵗʰ **M1A.452** Other secondary chronic gout, left hip

√7ᵗʰ **M1A.459** Other secondary chronic gout, unspecified hip ▽

√6ᵗʰ **M1A.46** Other secondary chronic gout, knee

√7ᵗʰ **M1A.461** Other secondary chronic gout, right knee

√7ᵗʰ **M1A.462** Other secondary chronic gout, left knee

√7ᵗʰ **M1A.469** Other secondary chronic gout, unspecified knee ▽

√6ᵗʰ **M1A.47** Other secondary chronic gout, ankle and foot

√7ᵗʰ **M1A.471** Other secondary chronic gout, right ankle and foot

√7ᵗʰ **M1A.472** Other secondary chronic gout, left ankle and foot

√7ᵗʰ **M1A.479** Other secondary chronic gout, unspecified ankle and foot ▽

√x7ᵗʰ **M1A.48** Other secondary chronic gout, vertebrae

√x7ᵗʰ **M1A.49** Other secondary chronic gout, multiple sites

√x7ᵗʰ **M1A.9** Chronic gout, unspecified ▽

√4ᵗʰ **M10** Gout

Acute gout

Gout attack

Gout flare

Podagra

Use additional code to identify:

autonomic neuropathy in diseases classified elsewhere (G99.0)

calculus of urinary tract in diseases classified elsewhere (N22)

cardiomyopathy in diseases classified elsewhere (I43)

disorders of external ear in diseases classified elsewhere (H61.1-, H62.8-)

disorders of iris and ciliary body in diseases classified elsewhere (H22)

glomerular disorders in diseases classified elsewhere (N08)

EXCLUDES 2   *chronic gout (M1A.-)*

DEF: Purine and pyrimidine metabolic disorders, manifested by hyperuricemia and recurrent acute inflammatory arthritis. Monosodium urate or monohydrate crystals may be deposited in and around the joints, leading to joint destruction and severe crippling.

√5ᵗʰ **M10.0** Idiopathic gout

Gouty bursitis

Primary gout

M10.00 Idiopathic gout, unspecified site ▽

√6ᵗʰ **M10.01** Idiopathic gout, shoulder

M10.011 Idiopathic gout, right shoulder

M10.012 Idiopathic gout, left shoulder

M10.019 Idiopathic gout, unspecified shoulder ▽

√6ᵗʰ **M10.02** Idiopathic gout, elbow

M10.021 Idiopathic gout, right elbow

M10.022 Idiopathic gout, left elbow

M10.029 Idiopathic gout, unspecified elbow ▽

√6ᵗʰ **M10.03** Idiopathic gout, wrist

M10.031 Idiopathic gout, right wrist

M10.032 Idiopathic gout, left wrist

M10.039 Idiopathic gout, unspecified wrist ▽

√6ᵗʰ **M10.04** Idiopathic gout, hand

M10.041 Idiopathic gout, right hand

M10.042 Idiopathic gout, left hand

M10.049 Idiopathic gout, unspecified hand ▽

√6ᵗʰ **M10.05** Idiopathic gout, hip

M10.051 Idiopathic gout, right hip

M10.052 Idiopathic gout, left hip

M10.059 Idiopathic gout, unspecified hip ▽

√6ᵗʰ **M10.06** Idiopathic gout, knee

M10.061 Idiopathic gout, right knee

M10.062 Idiopathic gout, left knee

M10.069 Idiopathic gout, unspecified knee ▽

☑ Additional Character Req   √x7ᵗʰ Placeholder Alert   Manifestation   ▽ Unspecified   ▶◀ Revised Text   ● New Code   ▲ Revised Code Title

ICD-10-CM 2019   755

√6ᵗʰ **M10.07 Idiopathic gout,** ankle and foot
- M10.071 Idiopathic gout, right ankle and foot
- M10.072 Idiopathic gout, left ankle and foot
- M10.079 Idiopathic gout, unspecified ankle and foot ▽

M10.08 Idiopathic gout, vertebrae
M10.09 Idiopathic gout, multiple sites

√5ᵗʰ **M10.1 Lead-induced gout**
  Code first toxic effects of lead and its compounds (T56.0-)
- M10.10 Lead-induced gout, unspecified site ▽

√6ᵗʰ **M10.11 Lead-induced gout,** shoulder
- M10.111 Lead-induced gout, right shoulder
- M10.112 Lead-induced gout, left shoulder
- M10.119 Lead-induced gout, unspecified shoulder ▽

√6ᵗʰ **M10.12 Lead-induced gout,** elbow
- M10.121 Lead-induced gout, right elbow
- M10.122 Lead-induced gout, left elbow
- M10.129 Lead-induced gout, unspecified elbow ▽

√6ᵗʰ **M10.13 Lead-induced gout,** wrist
- M10.131 Lead-induced gout, right wrist
- M10.132 Lead-induced gout, left wrist
- M10.139 Lead-induced gout, unspecified wrist ▽

√6ᵗʰ **M10.14 Lead-induced gout,** hand
- M10.141 Lead-induced gout, right hand
- M10.142 Lead-induced gout, left hand
- M10.149 Lead-induced gout, unspecified hand ▽

√6ᵗʰ **M10.15 Lead-induced gout,** hip
- M10.151 Lead-induced gout, right hip
- M10.152 Lead-induced gout, left hip
- M10.159 Lead-induced gout, unspecified hip ▽

√6ᵗʰ **M10.16 Lead-induced gout,** knee
- M10.161 Lead-induced gout, right knee
- M10.162 Lead-induced gout, left knee
- M10.169 Lead-induced gout, unspecified knee ▽

√6ᵗʰ **M10.17 Lead-induced gout,** ankle and foot
- M10.171 Lead-induced gout, right ankle and foot
- M10.172 Lead-induced gout, left ankle and foot
- M10.179 Lead-induced gout, unspecified ankle and foot ▽

M10.18 Lead-induced gout, vertebrae
M10.19 Lead-induced gout, multiple sites

√5ᵗʰ **M10.2 Drug-induced gout**
  Use additional code for adverse effect, if applicable, to identify drug (T36-T50 with fifth or sixth character 5)
- M10.20 Drug-induced gout, unspecified site ▽

√6ᵗʰ **M10.21 Drug-induced gout,** shoulder
- M10.211 Drug-induced gout, right shoulder
- M10.212 Drug-induced gout, left shoulder
- M10.219 Drug-induced gout, unspecified shoulder ▽

√6ᵗʰ **M10.22 Drug-induced gout,** elbow
- M10.221 Drug-induced gout, right elbow
- M10.222 Drug-induced gout, left elbow
- M10.229 Drug-induced gout, unspecified elbow ▽

√6ᵗʰ **M10.23 Drug-induced gout,** wrist
- M10.231 Drug-induced gout, right wrist
- M10.232 Drug-induced gout, left wrist
- M10.239 Drug-induced gout, unspecified wrist ▽

√6ᵗʰ **M10.24 Drug-induced gout,** hand
- M10.241 Drug-induced gout, right hand
- M10.242 Drug-induced gout, left hand
- M10.249 Drug-induced gout, unspecified hand ▽

√6ᵗʰ **M10.25 Drug-induced gout,** hip
- M10.251 Drug-induced gout, right hip
- M10.252 Drug-induced gout, left hip
- M10.259 Drug-induced gout, unspecified hip ▽

√6ᵗʰ **M10.26 Drug-induced gout,** knee
- M10.261 Drug-induced gout, right knee
- M10.262 Drug-induced gout, left knee
- M10.269 Drug-induced gout, unspecified knee ▽

√6ᵗʰ **M10.27 Drug-induced gout,** ankle and foot
- M10.271 Drug-induced gout, right ankle and foot
- M10.272 Drug-induced gout, left ankle and foot
- M10.279 Drug-induced gout, unspecified ankle and foot ▽

M10.28 Drug-induced gout, vertebrae
M10.29 Drug-induced gout, multiple sites

√5ᵗʰ **M10.3 Gout due to renal impairment**
  Code first associated renal disease
- M10.30 Gout due to renal impairment, unspecified site ▽

√6ᵗʰ **M10.31 Gout due to renal impairment,** shoulder
- M10.311 Gout due to renal impairment, right shoulder
- M10.312 Gout due to renal impairment, left shoulder
- M10.319 Gout due to renal impairment, unspecified shoulder ▽

√6ᵗʰ **M10.32 Gout due to renal impairment,** elbow
- M10.321 Gout due to renal impairment, right elbow
- M10.322 Gout due to renal impairment, left elbow
- M10.329 Gout due to renal impairment, unspecified elbow ▽

√6ᵗʰ **M10.33 Gout due to renal impairment,** wrist
- M10.331 Gout due to renal impairment, right wrist
- M10.332 Gout due to renal impairment, left wrist
- M10.339 Gout due to renal impairment, unspecified wrist ▽

√6ᵗʰ **M10.34 Gout due to renal impairment,** hand
- M10.341 Gout due to renal impairment, right hand
- M10.342 Gout due to renal impairment, left hand
- M10.349 Gout due to renal impairment, unspecified hand ▽

√6ᵗʰ **M10.35 Gout due to renal impairment,** hip
- M10.351 Gout due to renal impairment, right hip
- M10.352 Gout due to renal impairment, left hip
- M10.359 Gout due to renal impairment, unspecified hip ▽

√6ᵗʰ **M10.36 Gout due to renal impairment,** knee
- M10.361 Gout due to renal impairment, right knee
- M10.362 Gout due to renal impairment, left knee
- M10.369 Gout due to renal impairment, unspecified knee ▽

√6ᵗʰ **M10.37 Gout due to renal impairment,** ankle and foot
- M10.371 Gout due to renal impairment, right ankle and foot
- M10.372 Gout due to renal impairment, left ankle and foot
- M10.379 Gout due to renal impairment, unspecified ankle and foot ▽

M10.38 Gout due to renal impairment, vertebrae
M10.39 Gout due to renal impairment, multiple sites

√5ᵗʰ **M10.4 Other secondary gout**
  Code first associated condition
- M10.40 Other secondary gout, unspecified site ▽

√6ᵗʰ **M10.41 Other secondary gout,** shoulder
- M10.411 Other secondary gout, right shoulder
- M10.412 Other secondary gout, left shoulder
- M10.419 Other secondary gout, unspecified shoulder ▽

√6ᵗʰ **M10.42 Other secondary gout,** elbow
- M10.421 Other secondary gout, right elbow
- M10.422 Other secondary gout, left elbow
- M10.429 Other secondary gout, unspecified elbow ▽

√6ᵗʰ **M10.43 Other secondary gout,** wrist
- M10.431 Other secondary gout, right wrist
- M10.432 Other secondary gout, left wrist
- M10.439 Other secondary gout, unspecified wrist ▽

√6ᵗʰ **M10.44** Other secondary gout, hand

    M10.441 Other secondary gout, right hand
    M10.442 Other secondary gout, left hand
    M10.449 Other secondary gout,   ▽
             unspecified hand

√6ᵗʰ **M10.45** Other secondary gout, hip

    M10.451 Other secondary gout, right hip
    M10.452 Other secondary gout, left hip
    M10.459 Other secondary gout,   ▽
             unspecified hip

√6ᵗʰ **M10.46** Other secondary gout, knee

    M10.461 Other secondary gout, right knee
    M10.462 Other secondary gout, left knee
    M10.469 Other secondary gout,   ▽
             unspecified knee

√6ᵗʰ **M10.47** Other secondary gout, ankle and foot

    M10.471 Other secondary gout, right ankle and foot
    M10.472 Other secondary gout, left ankle and foot
    M10.479 Other secondary gout,   ▽
             unspecified ankle and foot

  M10.48 Other secondary gout, vertebrae
  M10.49 Other secondary gout, multiple sites

M10.9 Gout, unspecified   ▽
     Gout NOS

√4ᵗʰ **M11** Other crystal arthropathies

√5ᵗʰ **M11.0** Hydroxyapatite deposition disease

    DEF: Disease caused by deposits of calcium phosphate crystals in the soft tissues close to the joint (especially tendons) or in the joints. These calcifications can be mono or polyarticular and can cause destruction of the joint involved.

    M11.00 Hydroxyapatite deposition disease,   ▽
           unspecified site

√6ᵗʰ   **M11.01** Hydroxyapatite deposition disease, shoulder

    M11.011 Hydroxyapatite deposition disease, right shoulder
    M11.012 Hydroxyapatite deposition disease, left shoulder
    M11.019 Hydroxyapatite deposition   ▽
            disease, unspecified shoulder

√6ᵗʰ   **M11.02** Hydroxyapatite deposition disease, elbow

    M11.021 Hydroxyapatite deposition disease, right elbow
    M11.022 Hydroxyapatite deposition disease, left elbow
    M11.029 Hydroxyapatite deposition   ▽
            disease, unspecified elbow

√6ᵗʰ   **M11.03** Hydroxyapatite deposition disease, wrist

    M11.031 Hydroxyapatite deposition disease, right wrist
    M11.032 Hydroxyapatite deposition disease, left wrist
    M11.039 Hydroxyapatite deposition   ▽
            disease, unspecified wrist

√6ᵗʰ   **M11.04** Hydroxyapatite deposition disease, hand

    M11.041 Hydroxyapatite deposition disease, right hand
    M11.042 Hydroxyapatite deposition disease, left hand
    M11.049 Hydroxyapatite deposition   ▽
            disease, unspecified hand

√6ᵗʰ   **M11.05** Hydroxyapatite deposition disease, hip

    M11.051 Hydroxyapatite deposition disease, right hip
    M11.052 Hydroxyapatite deposition disease, left hip
    M11.059 Hydroxyapatite deposition   ▽
            disease, unspecified hip

√6ᵗʰ   **M11.06** Hydroxyapatite deposition disease, knee

    M11.061 Hydroxyapatite deposition disease, right knee
    M11.062 Hydroxyapatite deposition disease, left knee
    M11.069 Hydroxyapatite deposition   ▽
            disease, unspecified knee

√6ᵗʰ   **M11.07** Hydroxyapatite deposition disease, ankle and foot

    M11.071 Hydroxyapatite deposition disease, right ankle and foot

    M11.072 Hydroxyapatite deposition disease, left ankle and foot
    M11.079 Hydroxyapatite deposition   ▽
            disease, unspecified ankle and foot

  M11.08 Hydroxyapatite deposition disease, vertebrae
  M11.09 Hydroxyapatite deposition disease, multiple sites

√5ᵗʰ **M11.1** Familial chondrocalcinosis

  M11.10 Familial chondrocalcinosis, unspecified site   ▽

√6ᵗʰ   **M11.11** Familial chondrocalcinosis, shoulder

    M11.111 Familial chondrocalcinosis, right shoulder
    M11.112 Familial chondrocalcinosis, left shoulder
    M11.119 Familial chondrocalcinosis,   ▽
            unspecified shoulder

√6ᵗʰ   **M11.12** Familial chondrocalcinosis, elbow

    M11.121 Familial chondrocalcinosis, right elbow
    M11.122 Familial chondrocalcinosis, left elbow
    M11.129 Familial chondrocalcinosis,   ▽
            unspecified elbow

√6ᵗʰ   **M11.13** Familial chondrocalcinosis, wrist

    M11.131 Familial chondrocalcinosis, right wrist
    M11.132 Familial chondrocalcinosis, left wrist
    M11.139 Familial chondrocalcinosis,   ▽
            unspecified wrist

√6ᵗʰ   **M11.14** Familial chondrocalcinosis, hand

    M11.141 Familial chondrocalcinosis, right hand
    M11.142 Familial chondrocalcinosis, left hand
    M11.149 Familial chondrocalcinosis,   ▽
            unspecified hand

√6ᵗʰ   **M11.15** Familial chondrocalcinosis, hip

    M11.151 Familial chondrocalcinosis, right hip
    M11.152 Familial chondrocalcinosis, left hip
    M11.159 Familial chondrocalcinosis,   ▽
            unspecified hip

√6ᵗʰ   **M11.16** Familial chondrocalcinosis, knee

    M11.161 Familial chondrocalcinosis, right knee
    M11.162 Familial chondrocalcinosis, left knee
    M11.169 Familial chondrocalcinosis,   ▽
            unspecified knee

√6ᵗʰ   **M11.17** Familial chondrocalcinosis, ankle and foot

    M11.171 Familial chondrocalcinosis, right ankle and foot
    M11.172 Familial chondrocalcinosis, left ankle and foot
    M11.179 Familial chondrocalcinosis,   ▽
            unspecified ankle and foot

  M11.18 Familial chondrocalcinosis, vertebrae
  M11.19 Familial chondrocalcinosis, multiple sites

√5ᵗʰ **M11.2** Other chondrocalcinosis

     Chondrocalcinosis NOS

  M11.20 Other chondrocalcinosis, unspecified site   ▽

√6ᵗʰ   **M11.21** Other chondrocalcinosis, shoulder

    M11.211 Other chondrocalcinosis, right shoulder
    M11.212 Other chondrocalcinosis, left shoulder
    M11.219 Other chondrocalcinosis,   ▽
            unspecified shoulder

√6ᵗʰ   **M11.22** Other chondrocalcinosis, elbow

    M11.221 Other chondrocalcinosis, right elbow
    M11.222 Other chondrocalcinosis, left elbow
    M11.229 Other chondrocalcinosis,   ▽
            unspecified elbow

√6ᵗʰ   **M11.23** Other chondrocalcinosis, wrist

    M11.231 Other chondrocalcinosis, right wrist
    M11.232 Other chondrocalcinosis, left wrist
    M11.239 Other chondrocalcinosis,   ▽
            unspecified wrist

√6ᵗʰ   **M11.24** Other chondrocalcinosis, hand

    M11.241 Other chondrocalcinosis, right hand
    M11.242 Other chondrocalcinosis, left hand
    M11.249 Other chondrocalcinosis,   ▽
            unspecified hand

√6ᵗʰ   **M11.25** Other chondrocalcinosis, hip

    M11.251 Other chondrocalcinosis, right hip
    M11.252 Other chondrocalcinosis, left hip
    M11.259 Other chondrocalcinosis,   ▽
            unspecified hip

☑ Additional Character Req   √x7ᵗʰ Placeholder Alert   Manifestation   ▽ Unspecified   ▶◀ Revised Text   ● New Code   ▲ Revised Code Title

ICD-10-CM 2019   757

Chapter 13. Diseases of the Musculoskeletal System and Connective Tissue

M11.26–M12.122

√6ᵗʰ M11.26 Other chondrocalcinosis, knee
- M11.261 Other chondrocalcinosis, right knee
- M11.262 Other chondrocalcinosis, left knee
- M11.269 Other chondrocalcinosis, unspecified knee ▽

√6ᵗʰ M11.27 Other chondrocalcinosis, ankle and foot
- M11.271 Other chondrocalcinosis, right ankle and foot
- M11.272 Other chondrocalcinosis, left ankle and foot
- M11.279 Other chondrocalcinosis, unspecified ankle and foot ▽

- M11.28 Other chondrocalcinosis, vertebrae
- M11.29 Other chondrocalcinosis, multiple sites

√5ᵗʰ M11.8 Other specified crystal arthropathies
- M11.80 Other specified crystal arthropathies, unspecified site ▽

√6ᵗʰ M11.81 Other specified crystal arthropathies, shoulder
- M11.811 Other specified crystal arthropathies, right shoulder
- M11.812 Other specified crystal arthropathies, left shoulder
- M11.819 Other specified crystal arthropathies, unspecified shoulder ▽

√6ᵗʰ M11.82 Other specified crystal arthropathies, elbow
- M11.821 Other specified crystal arthropathies, right elbow
- M11.822 Other specified crystal arthropathies, left elbow
- M11.829 Other specified crystal arthropathies, unspecified elbow ▽

√6ᵗʰ M11.83 Other specified crystal arthropathies, wrist
- M11.831 Other specified crystal arthropathies, right wrist
- M11.832 Other specified crystal arthropathies, left wrist
- M11.839 Other specified crystal arthropathies, unspecified wrist ▽

√6ᵗʰ M11.84 Other specified crystal arthropathies, hand
- M11.841 Other specified crystal arthropathies, right hand
- M11.842 Other specified crystal arthropathies, left hand
- M11.849 Other specified crystal arthropathies, unspecified hand ▽

√6ᵗʰ M11.85 Other specified crystal arthropathies, hip
- M11.851 Other specified crystal arthropathies, right hip
- M11.852 Other specified crystal arthropathies, left hip
- M11.859 Other specified crystal arthropathies, unspecified hip ▽

√6ᵗʰ M11.86 Other specified crystal arthropathies, knee
- M11.861 Other specified crystal arthropathies, right knee
- M11.862 Other specified crystal arthropathies, left knee
- M11.869 Other specified crystal arthropathies, unspecified knee ▽

√6ᵗʰ M11.87 Other specified crystal arthropathies, ankle and foot
- M11.871 Other specified crystal arthropathies, right ankle and foot
- M11.872 Other specified crystal arthropathies, left ankle and foot
- M11.879 Other specified crystal arthropathies, unspecified ankle and foot ▽

- M11.88 Other specified crystal arthropathies, vertebrae
- M11.89 Other specified crystal arthropathies, multiple sites
- M11.9 Crystal arthropathy, unspecified ▽

√4ᵗʰ M12 Other and unspecified arthropathy

EXCLUDES 1   arthrosis (M15-M19)
   cricoarytenoid arthropathy (J38.7)

√5ᵗʰ M12.0 Chronic postrheumatic arthropathy [Jaccoud]
- M12.00 Chronic postrheumatic arthropathy [Jaccoud], unspecified site   HCC ▽

√6ᵗʰ M12.01 Chronic postrheumatic arthropathy [Jaccoud], shoulder
- M12.011 Chronic postrheumatic arthropathy [Jaccoud], right shoulder   HCC
- M12.012 Chronic postrheumatic arthropathy [Jaccoud], left shoulder   HCC
- M12.019 Chronic postrheumatic arthropathy [Jaccoud], unspecified shoulder   HCC ▽

√6ᵗʰ M12.02 Chronic postrheumatic arthropathy [Jaccoud], elbow
- M12.021 Chronic postrheumatic arthropathy [Jaccoud], right elbow   HCC
- M12.022 Chronic postrheumatic arthropathy [Jaccoud], left elbow   HCC
- M12.029 Chronic postrheumatic arthropathy [Jaccoud], unspecified elbow   HCC ▽

√6ᵗʰ M12.03 Chronic postrheumatic arthropathy [Jaccoud], wrist
- M12.031 Chronic postrheumatic arthropathy [Jaccoud], right wrist   HCC
- M12.032 Chronic postrheumatic arthropathy [Jaccoud], left wrist   HCC
- M12.039 Chronic postrheumatic arthropathy [Jaccoud], unspecified wrist   HCC ▽

√6ᵗʰ M12.04 Chronic postrheumatic arthropathy [Jaccoud], hand
- M12.041 Chronic postrheumatic arthropathy [Jaccoud], right hand   HCC
- M12.042 Chronic postrheumatic arthropathy [Jaccoud], left hand   HCC
- M12.049 Chronic postrheumatic arthropathy [Jaccoud], unspecified hand   HCC ▽

√6ᵗʰ M12.05 Chronic postrheumatic arthropathy [Jaccoud], hip
- M12.051 Chronic postrheumatic arthropathy [Jaccoud], right hip   HCC
- M12.052 Chronic postrheumatic arthropathy [Jaccoud], left hip   HCC
- M12.059 Chronic postrheumatic arthropathy [Jaccoud], unspecified hip   HCC ▽

√6ᵗʰ M12.06 Chronic postrheumatic arthropathy [Jaccoud], knee
- M12.061 Chronic postrheumatic arthropathy [Jaccoud], right knee   HCC
- M12.062 Chronic postrheumatic arthropathy [Jaccoud], left knee   HCC
- M12.069 Chronic postrheumatic arthropathy [Jaccoud], unspecified knee   HCC ▽

√6ᵗʰ M12.07 Chronic postrheumatic arthropathy [Jaccoud], ankle and foot
- M12.071 Chronic postrheumatic arthropathy [Jaccoud], right ankle and foot   HCC
- M12.072 Chronic postrheumatic arthropathy [Jaccoud], left ankle and foot   HCC
- M12.079 Chronic postrheumatic arthropathy [Jaccoud], unspecified ankle and foot   HCC ▽

- M12.08 Chronic postrheumatic arthropathy [Jaccoud], other specified site   HCC
  Chronic postrheumatic arthropathy [Jaccoud], vertebrae
- M12.09 Chronic postrheumatic arthropathy [Jaccoud], multiple sites   HCC

√5ᵗʰ M12.1 Kaschin-Beck disease
  Osteochondroarthrosis deformans endemica
- M12.10 Kaschin-Beck disease, unspecified site ▽

√6ᵗʰ M12.11 Kaschin-Beck disease, shoulder
- M12.111 Kaschin-Beck disease, right shoulder
- M12.112 Kaschin-Beck disease, left shoulder
- M12.119 Kaschin-Beck disease, unspecified shoulder ▽

√6ᵗʰ M12.12 Kaschin-Beck disease, elbow
- M12.121 Kaschin-Beck disease, right elbow
- M12.122 Kaschin-Beck disease, left elbow

M12.129   Kaschin-Beck disease, unspecified elbow ▽

√6ᵗʰ   **M12.13**   Kaschin-Beck disease, wrist

    M12.131   Kaschin-Beck disease, right wrist
    M12.132   Kaschin-Beck disease, left wrist
    M12.139   Kaschin-Beck disease, unspecified wrist ▽

√6ᵗʰ   **M12.14**   Kaschin-Beck disease, hand

    M12.141   Kaschin-Beck disease, right hand
    M12.142   Kaschin-Beck disease, left hand
    M12.149   Kaschin-Beck disease, unspecified hand ▽

√6ᵗʰ   **M12.15**   Kaschin-Beck disease, hip

    M12.151   Kaschin-Beck disease, right hip
    M12.152   Kaschin-Beck disease, left hip
    M12.159   Kaschin-Beck disease, unspecified hip ▽

√6ᵗʰ   **M12.16**   Kaschin-Beck disease, knee

    M12.161   Kaschin-Beck disease, right knee
    M12.162   Kaschin-Beck disease, left knee
    M12.169   Kaschin-Beck disease, unspecified knee ▽

√6ᵗʰ   **M12.17**   Kaschin-Beck disease, ankle and foot

    M12.171   Kaschin-Beck disease, right ankle and foot
    M12.172   Kaschin-Beck disease, left ankle and foot
    M12.179   Kaschin-Beck disease, unspecified ankle and foot ▽

    M12.18   Kaschin-Beck disease, vertebrae
    M12.19   Kaschin-Beck disease, multiple sites

√5ᵗʰ   **M12.2**   Villonodular synovitis (pigmented)

    M12.20   Villonodular synovitis (pigmented), unspecified site ▽

√6ᵗʰ   **M12.21**   Villonodular synovitis (pigmented), shoulder

    M12.211   Villonodular synovitis (pigmented), right shoulder
    M12.212   Villonodular synovitis (pigmented), left shoulder
    M12.219   Villonodular synovitis (pigmented), unspecified shoulder ▽

√6ᵗʰ   **M12.22**   Villonodular synovitis (pigmented), elbow

    M12.221   Villonodular synovitis (pigmented), right elbow
    M12.222   Villonodular synovitis (pigmented), left elbow
    M12.229   Villonodular synovitis (pigmented), unspecified elbow ▽

√6ᵗʰ   **M12.23**   Villonodular synovitis (pigmented), wrist

    M12.231   Villonodular synovitis (pigmented), right wrist
    M12.232   Villonodular synovitis (pigmented), left wrist
    M12.239   Villonodular synovitis (pigmented), unspecified wrist ▽

√6ᵗʰ   **M12.24**   Villonodular synovitis (pigmented), hand

    M12.241   Villonodular synovitis (pigmented), right hand
    M12.242   Villonodular synovitis (pigmented), left hand
    M12.249   Villonodular synovitis (pigmented), unspecified hand ▽

√6ᵗʰ   **M12.25**   Villonodular synovitis (pigmented), hip

    M12.251   Villonodular synovitis (pigmented), right hip
    M12.252   Villonodular synovitis (pigmented), left hip
    M12.259   Villonodular synovitis (pigmented), unspecified hip ▽

√6ᵗʰ   **M12.26**   Villonodular synovitis (pigmented), knee

    M12.261   Villonodular synovitis (pigmented), right knee
    M12.262   Villonodular synovitis (pigmented), left knee
    M12.269   Villonodular synovitis (pigmented), unspecified knee ▽

√6ᵗʰ   **M12.27**   Villonodular synovitis (pigmented), ankle and foot

    M12.271   Villonodular synovitis (pigmented), right ankle and foot

M12.272   Villonodular synovitis (pigmented), left ankle and foot

M12.279   Villonodular synovitis (pigmented), unspecified ankle and foot ▽

    M12.28   Villonodular synovitis (pigmented), other specified site
       Villonodular synovitis (pigmented), vertebrae

    M12.29   Villonodular synovitis (pigmented), multiple sites

√5ᵗʰ   **M12.3**   Palindromic rheumatism

    DEF: Sudden and recurring attacks of moderate to severe joint pain and swelling generally occurring in the hands or feet of unknown etiology. After the attack subsides, the joints appear normal again.

    M12.30   Palindromic rheumatism, unspecified site ▽

√6ᵗʰ   **M12.31**   Palindromic rheumatism, shoulder

    M12.311   Palindromic rheumatism, right shoulder
    M12.312   Palindromic rheumatism, left shoulder
    M12.319   Palindromic rheumatism, unspecified shoulder ▽

√6ᵗʰ   **M12.32**   Palindromic rheumatism, elbow

    M12.321   Palindromic rheumatism, right elbow
    M12.322   Palindromic rheumatism, left elbow
    M12.329   Palindromic rheumatism, unspecified elbow ▽

√6ᵗʰ   **M12.33**   Palindromic rheumatism, wrist

    M12.331   Palindromic rheumatism, right wrist
    M12.332   Palindromic rheumatism, left wrist
    M12.339   Palindromic rheumatism, unspecified wrist ▽

√6ᵗʰ   **M12.34**   Palindromic rheumatism, hand

    M12.341   Palindromic rheumatism, right hand
    M12.342   Palindromic rheumatism, left hand
    M12.349   Palindromic rheumatism, unspecified hand ▽

√6ᵗʰ   **M12.35**   Palindromic rheumatism, hip

    M12.351   Palindromic rheumatism, right hip
    M12.352   Palindromic rheumatism, left hip
    M12.359   Palindromic rheumatism, unspecified hip ▽

√6ᵗʰ   **M12.36**   Palindromic rheumatism, knee

    M12.361   Palindromic rheumatism, right knee
    M12.362   Palindromic rheumatism, left knee
    M12.369   Palindromic rheumatism, unspecified knee ▽

√6ᵗʰ   **M12.37**   Palindromic rheumatism, ankle and foot

    M12.371   Palindromic rheumatism, right ankle and foot
    M12.372   Palindromic rheumatism, left ankle and foot
    M12.379   Palindromic rheumatism, unspecified ankle and foot ▽

    M12.38   Palindromic rheumatism, other specified site
       Palindromic rheumatism, vertebrae

    M12.39   Palindromic rheumatism, multiple sites

√5ᵗʰ   **M12.4**   Intermittent hydrarthrosis

    M12.40   Intermittent hydrarthrosis, unspecified site ▽

√6ᵗʰ   **M12.41**   Intermittent hydrarthrosis, shoulder

    M12.411   Intermittent hydrarthrosis, right shoulder
    M12.412   Intermittent hydrarthrosis, left shoulder
    M12.419   Intermittent hydrarthrosis, unspecified shoulder ▽

√6ᵗʰ   **M12.42**   Intermittent hydrarthrosis, elbow

    M12.421   Intermittent hydrarthrosis, right elbow
    M12.422   Intermittent hydrarthrosis, left elbow
    M12.429   Intermittent hydrarthrosis, unspecified elbow ▽

√6ᵗʰ   **M12.43**   Intermittent hydrarthrosis, wrist

    M12.431   Intermittent hydrarthrosis, right wrist
    M12.432   Intermittent hydrarthrosis, left wrist
    M12.439   Intermittent hydrarthrosis, unspecified wrist ▽

√6ᵗʰ   **M12.44**   Intermittent hydrarthrosis, hand

    M12.441   Intermittent hydrarthrosis, right hand
    M12.442   Intermittent hydrarthrosis, left hand
    M12.449   Intermittent hydrarthrosis, unspecified hand ▽

✓ Additional Character Req   √x7ᵗʰ Placeholder Alert   Manifestation   ▽ Unspecified   ►◄ Revised Text   ● New Code   ▲ Revised Code Title

√6ᵗʰ **M12.45 Intermittent hydrarthrosis, hip**
- **M12.451 Intermittent hydrarthrosis, right hip**
- **M12.452 Intermittent hydrarthrosis, left hip**
- **M12.459 Intermittent hydrarthrosis, unspecified hip** ▽

√6ᵗʰ **M12.46 Intermittent hydrarthrosis, knee**
- **M12.461 Intermittent hydrarthrosis, right knee**
- **M12.462 Intermittent hydrarthrosis, left knee**
- **M12.469 Intermittent hydrarthrosis, unspecified knee** ▽

√6ᵗʰ **M12.47 Intermittent hydrarthrosis, ankle and foot**
- **M12.471 Intermittent hydrarthrosis, right ankle and foot**
- **M12.472 Intermittent hydrarthrosis, left ankle and foot**
- **M12.479 Intermittent hydrarthrosis, unspecified ankle and foot** ▽

M12.48 Intermittent hydrarthrosis, other site
M12.49 Intermittent hydrarthrosis, multiple sites

√5ᵗʰ **M12.5 Traumatic arthropathy**

EXCLUDES 1   current injury–see Alphabetic Index
post-traumatic osteoarthritis of first carpometacarpal joint (M18.2-M18.3)
post-traumatic osteoarthritis of hip (M16.4-M16.5)
post-traumatic osteoarthritis of knee (M17.2-M17.3)
post-traumatic osteoarthritis NOS (M19.1-)
post-traumatic osteoarthritis of other single joints (M19.1-)

AHA: 2015,1Q,17

M12.50 Traumatic arthropathy, unspecified site ▽

√6ᵗʰ **M12.51 Traumatic arthropathy, shoulder**
- **M12.511 Traumatic arthropathy, right shoulder**
- **M12.512 Traumatic arthropathy, left shoulder**
- **M12.519 Traumatic arthropathy, unspecified shoulder** ▽

√6ᵗʰ **M12.52 Traumatic arthropathy, elbow**
- **M12.521 Traumatic arthropathy, right elbow**
- **M12.522 Traumatic arthropathy, left elbow**
- **M12.529 Traumatic arthropathy, unspecified elbow** ▽

√6ᵗʰ **M12.53 Traumatic arthropathy, wrist**
- **M12.531 Traumatic arthropathy, right wrist**
- **M12.532 Traumatic arthropathy, left wrist**
- **M12.539 Traumatic arthropathy, unspecified wrist** ▽

√6ᵗʰ **M12.54 Traumatic arthropathy, hand**
- **M12.541 Traumatic arthropathy, right hand**
- **M12.542 Traumatic arthropathy, left hand**
- **M12.549 Traumatic arthropathy, unspecified hand** ▽

√6ᵗʰ **M12.55 Traumatic arthropathy, hip**
- **M12.551 Traumatic arthropathy, right hip**
- **M12.552 Traumatic arthropathy, left hip**
- **M12.559 Traumatic arthropathy, unspecified hip** ▽

√6ᵗʰ **M12.56 Traumatic arthropathy, knee**
- **M12.561 Traumatic arthropathy, right knee**
- **M12.562 Traumatic arthropathy, left knee**
- **M12.569 Traumatic arthropathy, unspecified knee** ▽

√6ᵗʰ **M12.57 Traumatic arthropathy, ankle and foot**
- **M12.571 Traumatic arthropathy, right ankle and foot**
- **M12.572 Traumatic arthropathy, left ankle and foot**
- **M12.579 Traumatic arthropathy, unspecified ankle and foot** ▽

M12.58 Traumatic arthropathy, other specified site
Traumatic arthropathy, vertebrae

M12.59 Traumatic arthropathy, multiple sites

√5ᵗʰ **M12.8 Other specific arthropathies, not elsewhere classified**
Transient arthropathy

M12.80 Other specific arthropathies, not elsewhere classified, unspecified site ▽

√6ᵗʰ **M12.81 Other specific arthropathies, not elsewhere classified, shoulder**
- **M12.811 Other specific arthropathies, not elsewhere classified, right shoulder**
- **M12.812 Other specific arthropathies, not elsewhere classified, left shoulder**
- **M12.819 Other specific arthropathies, not elsewhere classified, unspecified shoulder** ▽

√6ᵗʰ **M12.82 Other specific arthropathies, not elsewhere classified, elbow**
- **M12.821 Other specific arthropathies, not elsewhere classified, right elbow**
- **M12.822 Other specific arthropathies, not elsewhere classified, left elbow**
- **M12.829 Other specific arthropathies, not elsewhere classified, unspecified elbow** ▽

√6ᵗʰ **M12.83 Other specific arthropathies, not elsewhere classified, wrist**
- **M12.831 Other specific arthropathies, not elsewhere classified, right wrist**
- **M12.832 Other specific arthropathies, not elsewhere classified, left wrist**
- **M12.839 Other specific arthropathies, not elsewhere classified, unspecified wrist** ▽

√6ᵗʰ **M12.84 Other specific arthropathies, not elsewhere classified, hand**
- **M12.841 Other specific arthropathies, not elsewhere classified, right hand**
- **M12.842 Other specific arthropathies, not elsewhere classified, left hand**
- **M12.849 Other specific arthropathies, not elsewhere classified, unspecified hand** ▽

√6ᵗʰ **M12.85 Other specific arthropathies, not elsewhere classified, hip**
- **M12.851 Other specific arthropathies, not elsewhere classified, right hip**
- **M12.852 Other specific arthropathies, not elsewhere classified, left hip**
- **M12.859 Other specific arthropathies, not elsewhere classified, unspecified hip** ▽

√6ᵗʰ **M12.86 Other specific arthropathies, not elsewhere classified, knee**
- **M12.861 Other specific arthropathies, not elsewhere classified, right knee**
- **M12.862 Other specific arthropathies, not elsewhere classified, left knee**
- **M12.869 Other specific arthropathies, not elsewhere classified, unspecified knee** ▽

√6ᵗʰ **M12.87 Other specific arthropathies, not elsewhere classified, ankle and foot**
- **M12.871 Other specific arthropathies, not elsewhere classified, right ankle and foot**
- **M12.872 Other specific arthropathies, not elsewhere classified, left ankle and foot**
- **M12.879 Other specific arthropathies, not elsewhere classified, unspecified ankle and foot** ▽

M12.88 Other specific arthropathies, not elsewhere classified, other specified site
Other specific arthropathies, not elsewhere classified, vertebrae

M12.89 Other specific arthropathies, not elsewhere classified, multiple sites

M12.9 Arthropathy, unspecified ▽

√4ᵗʰ **M13 Other arthritis**

EXCLUDES 1   arthrosis (M15-M19)
osteoarthritis (M15-M19)

M13.0 Polyarthritis, unspecified ▽

√5ᵗʰ **M13.1 Monoarthritis, not elsewhere classified**

M13.10 Monoarthritis, not elsewhere classified, unspecified site ▽

√6ᵗʰ **M13.11 Monoarthritis, not elsewhere classified, shoulder**
- **M13.111 Monoarthritis, not elsewhere classified, right shoulder**
- **M13.112 Monoarthritis, not elsewhere classified, left shoulder**

M13.119   Monoarthritis, not elsewhere classified, unspecified shoulder ▽

√6ᵗʰ M13.12   Monoarthritis, not elsewhere classified, elbow

M13.121   Monoarthritis, not elsewhere classified, right elbow

M13.122   Monoarthritis, not elsewhere classified, left elbow

M13.129   Monoarthritis, not elsewhere classified, unspecified elbow ▽

√6ᵗʰ M13.13   Monoarthritis, not elsewhere classified, wrist

M13.131   Monoarthritis, not elsewhere classified, right wrist

M13.132   Monoarthritis, not elsewhere classified, left wrist

M13.139   Monoarthritis, not elsewhere classified, unspecified wrist ▽

√6ᵗʰ M13.14   Monoarthritis, not elsewhere classified, hand

M13.141   Monoarthritis, not elsewhere classified, right hand

M13.142   Monoarthritis, not elsewhere classified, left hand

M13.149   Monoarthritis, not elsewhere classified, unspecified hand ▽

√6ᵗʰ M13.15   Monoarthritis, not elsewhere classified, hip

M13.151   Monoarthritis, not elsewhere classified, right hip

M13.152   Monoarthritis, not elsewhere classified, left hip

M13.159   Monoarthritis, not elsewhere classified, unspecified hip ▽

√6ᵗʰ M13.16   Monoarthritis, not elsewhere classified, knee

M13.161   Monoarthritis, not elsewhere classified, right knee

M13.162   Monoarthritis, not elsewhere classified, left knee

M13.169   Monoarthritis, not elsewhere classified, unspecified knee ▽

√6ᵗʰ M13.17   Monoarthritis, not elsewhere classified, ankle and foot

M13.171   Monoarthritis, not elsewhere classified, right ankle and foot

M13.172   Monoarthritis, not elsewhere classified, left ankle and foot

M13.179   Monoarthritis, not elsewhere classified, unspecified ankle and foot ▽

√5ᵗʰ M13.8   Other specified arthritis

Allergic arthritis

EXCLUDES 1   osteoarthritis (M15-M19)

M13.80   Other specified arthritis, unspecified site ▽

√6ᵗʰ M13.81   Other specified arthritis, shoulder

M13.811   Other specified arthritis, right shoulder

M13.812   Other specified arthritis, left shoulder

M13.819   Other specified arthritis, unspecified shoulder ▽

√6ᵗʰ M13.82   Other specified arthritis, elbow

M13.821   Other specified arthritis, right elbow

M13.822   Other specified arthritis, left elbow

M13.829   Other specified arthritis, unspecified elbow ▽

√6ᵗʰ M13.83   Other specified arthritis, wrist

M13.831   Other specified arthritis, right wrist

M13.832   Other specified arthritis, left wrist

M13.839   Other specified arthritis, unspecified wrist ▽

√6ᵗʰ M13.84   Other specified arthritis, hand

M13.841   Other specified arthritis, right hand

M13.842   Other specified arthritis, left hand

M13.849   Other specified arthritis, unspecified hand ▽

√6ᵗʰ M13.85   Other specified arthritis, hip

M13.851   Other specified arthritis, right hip

M13.852   Other specified arthritis, left hip

M13.859   Other specified arthritis, unspecified hip ▽

√6ᵗʰ M13.86   Other specified arthritis, knee

M13.861   Other specified arthritis, right knee

M13.862   Other specified arthritis, left knee

M13.869   Other specified arthritis, unspecified knee ▽

√6ᵗʰ M13.87   Other specified arthritis, ankle and foot

M13.871   Other specified arthritis, right ankle and foot

M13.872   Other specified arthritis, left ankle and foot

M13.879   Other specified arthritis, unspecified ankle and foot ▽

M13.88   Other specified arthritis, other site

M13.89   Other specified arthritis, multiple sites

√4ᵗʰ M14   Arthropathies in other diseases classified elsewhere

EXCLUDES 1   arthropathy in:

diabetes mellitus (E08-E13 with .61-)

hematological disorders (M36.2-M36.3)

hypersensitivity reactions (M36.4)

neoplastic disease (M36.1)

neurosyphillis (A52.16)

sarcoidosis (D86.86)

enteropathic arthropathies (M07.-)

juvenile psoriatic arthropathy (L40.54)

lipoid dermatoarthritis (E78.81)

√5ᵗʰ M14.6   Charcôt's joint

Neuropathic arthropathy

EXCLUDES 1   Charcôt's joint in diabetes mellitus (E08-E13 with .610)

Charcôt's joint in tabes dorsalis (A52.16)

DEF: Progressive neurologic arthropathy in which chronic degeneration of joints in the weight-bearing areas with peripheral hypertrophy occurs as a complication of a neuropathy disorder. Supporting structures relax from a loss of sensation resulting in chronic joint instability.

M14.60   Charcôt's joint, unspecified site ▽

√6ᵗʰ M14.61   Charcôt's joint, shoulder

M14.611   Charcôt's joint, right shoulder

M14.612   Charcôt's joint, left shoulder

M14.619   Charcôt's joint, unspecified shoulder ▽

√6ᵗʰ M14.62   Charcôt's joint, elbow

M14.621   Charcôt's joint, right elbow

M14.622   Charcôt's joint, left elbow

M14.629   Charcôt's joint, unspecified elbow ▽

√6ᵗʰ M14.63   Charcôt's joint, wrist

M14.631   Charcôt's joint, right wrist

M14.632   Charcôt's joint, left wrist

M14.639   Charcôt's joint, unspecified wrist ▽

√6ᵗʰ M14.64   Charcôt's joint, hand

M14.641   Charcôt's joint, right hand

M14.642   Charcôt's joint, left hand

M14.649   Charcôt's joint, unspecified hand ▽

√6ᵗʰ M14.65   Charcôt's joint, hip

M14.651   Charcôt's joint, right hip

M14.652   Charcôt's joint, left hip

M14.659   Charcôt's joint, unspecified hip ▽

√6ᵗʰ M14.66   Charcôt's joint, knee

M14.661   Charcôt's joint, right knee

M14.662   Charcôt's joint, left knee

M14.669   Charcôt's joint, unspecified knee ▽

√6ᵗʰ M14.67   Charcôt's joint, ankle and foot

M14.671   Charcôt's joint, right ankle and foot

M14.672   Charcôt's joint, left ankle and foot

M14.679   Charcôt's joint, unspecified ankle and foot ▽

M14.68   Charcôt's joint, vertebrae

M14.69   Charcôt's joint, multiple sites

✓ Additional Character Req   ✓x7ᵗʰ Placeholder Alert   Manifestation   ▽ Unspecified   ►◄ Revised Text   ● New Code   ▲ Revised Code Title

ICD-10-CM 2019   761

Chapter 13. Diseases of the Musculoskeletal System and Connective Tissue

M14.8–M17.4

√5ᵗʰ **M14.8 Arthropathies in other specified diseases classified elsewhere**

Code first underlying disease, such as:
amyloidosis (E85.-)
erythema multiforme (L51.-)
erythema nodosum (L52)
hemochromatosis (E83.11-)
hyperparathyroidism (E21.-)
hypothyroidism (E00-E03)
sickle-cell disorders (D57.-)
thyrotoxicosis [hyperthyroidism] (E05.-)
Whipple's disease (K90.81)

M14.80 **Arthropathies in other specified diseases** ▽
classified elsewhere, unspecified site

√6ᵗʰ **M14.81 Arthropathies in other specified diseases classified elsewhere, shoulder**

M14.811 *Arthropathies in other specified diseases classified elsewhere, right shoulder*

M14.812 *Arthropathies in other specified diseases classified elsewhere, left shoulder*

M14.819 *Arthropathies in other specified* ▽ *diseases classified elsewhere, unspecified shoulder*

√6ᵗʰ **M14.82 Arthropathies in other specified diseases classified elsewhere, elbow**

M14.821 *Arthropathies in other specified diseases classified elsewhere, right elbow*

M14.822 *Arthropathies in other specified diseases classified elsewhere, left elbow*

M14.829 *Arthropathies in other specified* ▽ *diseases classified elsewhere, unspecified elbow*

√6ᵗʰ **M14.83 Arthropathies in other specified diseases classified elsewhere, wrist**

M14.831 *Arthropathies in other specified diseases classified elsewhere, right wrist*

M14.832 *Arthropathies in other specified diseases classified elsewhere, left wrist*

M14.839 *Arthropathies in other specified* ▽ *diseases classified elsewhere, unspecified wrist*

√6ᵗʰ **M14.84 Arthropathies in other specified diseases classified elsewhere, hand**

M14.841 *Arthropathies in other specified diseases classified elsewhere, right hand*

M14.842 *Arthropathies in other specified diseases classified elsewhere, left hand*

M14.849 *Arthropathies in other specified* ▽ *diseases classified elsewhere, unspecified hand*

√6ᵗʰ **M14.85 Arthropathies in other specified diseases classified elsewhere, hip**

M14.851 *Arthropathies in other specified diseases classified elsewhere, right hip*

M14.852 *Arthropathies in other specified diseases classified elsewhere, left hip*

M14.859 *Arthropathies in other specified* ▽ *diseases classified elsewhere, unspecified hip*

√6ᵗʰ **M14.86 Arthropathies in other specified diseases classified elsewhere, knee**

M14.861 *Arthropathies in other specified diseases classified elsewhere, right knee*

M14.862 *Arthropathies in other specified diseases classified elsewhere, left knee*

M14.869 *Arthropathies in other specified* ▽ *diseases classified elsewhere, unspecified knee*

√6ᵗʰ **M14.87 Arthropathies in other specified diseases classified elsewhere, ankle and foot**

M14.871 *Arthropathies in other specified diseases classified elsewhere, right ankle and foot*

M14.872 *Arthropathies in other specified diseases classified elsewhere, left ankle and foot*

M14.879 *Arthropathies in other specified* ▽ *diseases classified elsewhere, unspecified ankle and foot*

M14.88 **Arthropathies in other specified diseases classified elsewhere, vertebrae**

M14.89 **Arthropathies in other specified diseases classified elsewhere, multiple sites**

Osteoarthritis (M15-M19)

EXCLUDES 2   osteoarthritis of spine (M47.-)

TIP: Assign a primary osteoarthritis code when the type of osteoarthritis—primary, secondary, or generalized—is not specified in the documentation. Primary is considered the default.

√4ᵗʰ **M15 Polyosteoarthritis**

INCLUDES   arthritis of multiple sites

EXCLUDES 1   *bilateral involvement of single joint (M16-M19)*

M15.0 Primary generalized (osteo)arthritis   Q

M15.1 Heberden's nodes (with arthropathy)   Q
Interphalangeal distal osteoarthritis

M15.2 Bouchard's nodes (with arthropathy)   Q
Juxtaphalangeal distal osteoarthritis

M15.3 Secondary multiple arthritis   Q
Post-traumatic polyosteoarthritis

M15.4 Erosive (osteo)arthritis   Q

M15.8 Other polyosteoarthritis   Q

M15.9 Polyosteoarthritis, unspecified   Q ▽
Generalized osteoarthritis NOS

√4ᵗʰ **M16 Osteoarthritis of hip**

AHA: 2016,4Q,146

M16.0 Bilateral primary osteoarthritis of hip   Q
AHA: 2018,2Q,15

√5ᵗʰ **M16.1 Unilateral primary osteoarthritis of hip**

Primary osteoarthritis of hip NOS
AHA: 2018,2Q,15

M16.10 Unilateral primary osteoarthritis,   Q ▽
unspecified hip

M16.11 Unilateral primary osteoarthritis, right hip   Q

M16.12 Unilateral primary osteoarthritis, left hip   Q

M16.2 Bilateral osteoarthritis resulting from hip dysplasia   Q

√5ᵗʰ **M16.3 Unilateral osteoarthritis resulting from hip dysplasia**

Dysplastic osteoarthritis of hip NOS

M16.30 Unilateral osteoarthritis resulting from hip   Q ▽
dysplasia, unspecified hip

M16.31 Unilateral osteoarthritis resulting from hip   Q
dysplasia, right hip

M16.32 Unilateral osteoarthritis resulting from hip   Q
dysplasia, left hip

M16.4 Bilateral post-traumatic osteoarthritis of hip   Q

√5ᵗʰ **M16.5 Unilateral post-traumatic osteoarthritis of hip**

Post-traumatic osteoarthritis of hip NOS

M16.50 Unilateral post-traumatic osteoarthritis,   Q ▽
unspecified hip

M16.51 Unilateral post-traumatic osteoarthritis,   Q
right hip

M16.52 Unilateral post-traumatic osteoarthritis,   Q
left hip

M16.6 Other bilateral secondary osteoarthritis of hip   Q

M16.7 Other unilateral secondary osteoarthritis of hip   Q
Secondary osteoarthritis of hip NOS

M16.9 Osteoarthritis of hip, unspecified   Q ▽

√4ᵗʰ **M17 Osteoarthritis of knee**

AHA: 2016,4Q,146-147

M17.0 Bilateral primary osteoarthritis of knee   Q
AHA: 2018,2Q,15

√5ᵗʰ **M17.1 Unilateral primary osteoarthritis of knee**

Primary osteoarthritis of knee NOS
AHA: 2018,2Q,15

M17.10 Unilateral primary osteoarthritis,   Q ▽
unspecified knee

M17.11 Unilateral primary osteoarthritis, right knee   Q

M17.12 Unilateral primary osteoarthritis, left knee   Q

M17.2 Bilateral post-traumatic osteoarthritis of knee   Q

√5ᵗʰ **M17.3 Unilateral post-traumatic osteoarthritis of knee**

Post-traumatic osteoarthritis of knee NOS

M17.30 Unilateral post-traumatic osteoarthritis,   Q ▽
unspecified knee

M17.31 Unilateral post-traumatic osteoarthritis,   Q
right knee

M17.32 Unilateral post-traumatic osteoarthritis,   Q
left knee

M17.4 Other bilateral secondary osteoarthritis of knee   Q

M17.5 **Other unilateral secondary osteoarthritis of knee** ▢
  Secondary osteoarthritis of knee NOS
M17.9 **Osteoarthritis of knee, unspecified** ▢ ▽

✓4ᵗʰ **M18 Osteoarthritis of first carpometacarpal joint**

M18.0 **Bilateral primary osteoarthritis of first carpometacarpal joints** ▢
✓5ᵗʰ M18.1 **Unilateral primary osteoarthritis of first carpometacarpal joint**
  Primary osteoarthritis of first carpometacarpal joint NOS
  M18.10 **Unilateral primary osteoarthritis of first carpometacarpal joint, unspecified hand** ▢ ▽
  M18.11 **Unilateral primary osteoarthritis of first carpometacarpal joint, right hand** ▢
  M18.12 **Unilateral primary osteoarthritis of first carpometacarpal joint, left hand** ▢
M18.2 **Bilateral post-traumatic osteoarthritis of first carpometacarpal joints** ▢
✓5ᵗʰ M18.3 **Unilateral post-traumatic osteoarthritis of first carpometacarpal joint**
  Post-traumatic osteoarthritis of first carpometacarpal joint NOS
  M18.30 **Unilateral post-traumatic osteoarthritis of first carpometacarpal joint, unspecified hand** ▢ ▽
  M18.31 **Unilateral post-traumatic osteoarthritis of first carpometacarpal joint, right hand** ▢
  M18.32 **Unilateral post-traumatic osteoarthritis of first carpometacarpal joint, left hand** ▢
M18.4 **Other bilateral secondary osteoarthritis of first carpometacarpal joints** ▢
✓5ᵗʰ M18.5 **Other unilateral secondary osteoarthritis of first carpometacarpal joint**
  Secondary osteoarthritis of first carpometacarpal joint NOS
  M18.50 **Other unilateral secondary osteoarthritis of first carpometacarpal joint, unspecified hand** ▢ ▽
  M18.51 **Other unilateral secondary osteoarthritis of first carpometacarpal joint, right hand** ▢
  M18.52 **Other unilateral secondary osteoarthritis of first carpometacarpal joint, left hand** ▢
M18.9 **Osteoarthritis of first carpometacarpal joint, unspecified** ▢ ▽

✓4ᵗʰ **M19 Other and unspecified osteoarthritis**
  EXCLUDES 1 polyarthritis (M15.-)
  EXCLUDES 2 arthrosis of spine (M47.-)
    hallux rigidus (M20.2)
    osteoarthritis of spine (M47.-)

✓5ᵗʰ M19.0 **Primary osteoarthritis of other joints**
  AHA: 2018,2Q,15; 2016,4Q,145
  ✓6ᵗʰ M19.01 **Primary osteoarthritis, shoulder**
    M19.011 **Primary osteoarthritis, right shoulder** ▢
    M19.012 **Primary osteoarthritis, left shoulder** ▢
    M19.019 **Primary osteoarthritis, unspecified shoulder** ▢ ▽
  ✓6ᵗʰ M19.02 **Primary osteoarthritis, elbow**
    M19.021 **Primary osteoarthritis, right elbow** ▢
    M19.022 **Primary osteoarthritis, left elbow** ▢
    M19.029 **Primary osteoarthritis, unspecified elbow** ▢ ▽
  ✓6ᵗʰ M19.03 **Primary osteoarthritis, wrist**
    M19.031 **Primary osteoarthritis, right wrist** ▢
    M19.032 **Primary osteoarthritis, left wrist** ▢
    M19.039 **Primary osteoarthritis, unspecified wrist** ▢ ▽
  ✓6ᵗʰ M19.04 **Primary osteoarthritis, hand**
    EXCLUDES 2 primary osteoarthritis of first carpometacarpal joint (M18.0-, M18.1-)
    M19.041 **Primary osteoarthritis, right hand** ▢
    M19.042 **Primary osteoarthritis, left hand** ▢
    M19.049 **Primary osteoarthritis, unspecified hand** ▢ ▽
  ✓6ᵗʰ M19.07 **Primary osteoarthritis ankle and foot**
    M19.071 **Primary osteoarthritis, right ankle and foot** ▢
    M19.072 **Primary osteoarthritis, left ankle and foot** ▢

M19.079 **Primary osteoarthritis, unspecified ankle and foot** ▢ ▽
✓5ᵗʰ M19.1 **Post-traumatic osteoarthritis of other joints**
  ✓6ᵗʰ M19.11 **Post-traumatic osteoarthritis, shoulder**
    M19.111 **Post-traumatic osteoarthritis, right shoulder** ▢
    M19.112 **Post-traumatic osteoarthritis, left shoulder** ▢
    M19.119 **Post-traumatic osteoarthritis, unspecified shoulder** ▢ ▽
  ✓6ᵗʰ M19.12 **Post-traumatic osteoarthritis, elbow**
    M19.121 **Post-traumatic osteoarthritis, right elbow** ▢
    M19.122 **Post-traumatic osteoarthritis, left elbow** ▢
    M19.129 **Post-traumatic osteoarthritis, unspecified elbow** ▢ ▽
  ✓6ᵗʰ M19.13 **Post-traumatic osteoarthritis, wrist**
    M19.131 **Post-traumatic osteoarthritis, right wrist** ▢
    M19.132 **Post-traumatic osteoarthritis, left wrist** ▢
    M19.139 **Post-traumatic osteoarthritis, unspecified wrist** ▢ ▽
  ✓6ᵗʰ M19.14 **Post-traumatic osteoarthritis, hand**
    EXCLUDES 2 post-traumatic osteoarthritis of first carpometacarpal joint (M18.2-, M18.3-)
    M19.141 **Post-traumatic osteoarthritis, right hand** ▢
    M19.142 **Post-traumatic osteoarthritis, left hand** ▢
    M19.149 **Post-traumatic osteoarthritis, unspecified hand** ▢ ▽
  ✓6ᵗʰ M19.17 **Post-traumatic osteoarthritis, ankle and foot**
    M19.171 **Post-traumatic osteoarthritis, right ankle and foot** ▢
    M19.172 **Post-traumatic osteoarthritis, left ankle and foot** ▢
    M19.179 **Post-traumatic osteoarthritis, unspecified ankle and foot** ▢ ▽
✓5ᵗʰ M19.2 **Secondary osteoarthritis of other joints**
  ✓6ᵗʰ M19.21 **Secondary osteoarthritis, shoulder**
    M19.211 **Secondary osteoarthritis, right shoulder** ▢
    M19.212 **Secondary osteoarthritis, left shoulder** ▢
    M19.219 **Secondary osteoarthritis, unspecified shoulder** ▢ ▽
  ✓6ᵗʰ M19.22 **Secondary osteoarthritis, elbow**
    M19.221 **Secondary osteoarthritis, right elbow** ▢
    M19.222 **Secondary osteoarthritis, left elbow** ▢
    M19.229 **Secondary osteoarthritis, unspecified elbow** ▢ ▽
  ✓6ᵗʰ M19.23 **Secondary osteoarthritis, wrist**
    M19.231 **Secondary osteoarthritis, right wrist** ▢
    M19.232 **Secondary osteoarthritis, left wrist** ▢
    M19.239 **Secondary osteoarthritis, unspecified wrist** ▢ ▽
  ✓6ᵗʰ M19.24 **Secondary osteoarthritis, hand**
    M19.241 **Secondary osteoarthritis, right hand** ▢
    M19.242 **Secondary osteoarthritis, left hand** ▢
    M19.249 **Secondary osteoarthritis, unspecified hand** ▢ ▽
  ✓6ᵗʰ M19.27 **Secondary osteoarthritis, ankle and foot**
    M19.271 **Secondary osteoarthritis, right ankle and foot** ▢
    M19.272 **Secondary osteoarthritis, left ankle and foot** ▢
    M19.279 **Secondary osteoarthritis, unspecified ankle and foot** ▢ ▽

☑ Additional Character Req   ✓x7ᵗʰ Placeholder Alert   Manifestation   ▽ Unspecified   ▶◀ Revised Text   ● New Code   ▲ Revised Code Title

√5ᵗʰ **M19.9 Osteoarthritis, unspecified site**

M19.90 Unspecified osteoarthritis, unspecified site ◘ ▽
Arthrosis NOS
Arthritis NOS
Osteoarthritis NOS
AHA: 2016,4Q,147

M19.91 Primary osteoarthritis, unspecified site ◘ ▽
Primary osteoarthritis NOS

M19.92 Post-traumatic osteoarthritis, unspecified site ◘ ▽
Post-traumatic osteoarthritis NOS

M19.93 Secondary osteoarthritis, unspecified site ◘ ▽
Secondary osteoarthritis NOS

Other joint disorders (M20-M25)

EXCLUDES 2   *joints of the spine (M40-M54)*

√4ᵗʰ **M20 Acquired deformities of fingers and toes**
EXCLUDES 1   *acquired absence of fingers and toes (Z89.-)*
congenital absence of fingers and toes (Q71.3-, Q72.3-)
congenital deformities and malformations of fingers and toes (Q66.-, Q68-Q70, Q74.-)

√5ᵗʰ **M20.0 Deformity of finger(s)**
EXCLUDES 1   *clubbing of fingers (R68.3)*
palmar fascial fibromatosis [Dupuytren] (M72.0)
trigger finger (M65.3)

√6ᵗʰ **M20.00 Unspecified deformity of finger(s)**
M20.001 Unspecified deformity of right finger(s) ▽
M20.002 Unspecified deformity of left finger(s) ▽
M20.009 Unspecified deformity of unspecified finger(s) ▽

√6ᵗʰ **M20.01 Mallet finger**
M20.011 Mallet finger of right finger(s)
M20.012 Mallet finger of left finger(s)
M20.019 Mallet finger of unspecified finger(s) ▽

√6ᵗʰ **M20.02 Boutonnière deformity**
DEF: Deformity of the finger caused by flexion of the proximal interphalangeal joint and hyperextension of the distal joint. The deformity results from rheumatoid arthritis, osteoarthritis, or injury.
M20.021 Boutonnière deformity of right finger(s)
M20.022 Boutonnière deformity of left finger(s)
M20.029 Boutonnière deformity of unspecified finger(s) ▽

√6ᵗʰ **M20.03 Swan-neck deformity**
DEF: Flexed distal and hyperextended proximal interphalangeal joint most commonly caused by rheumatoid arthritis.
M20.031 Swan-neck deformity of right finger(s)
M20.032 Swan-neck deformity of left finger(s)
M20.039 Swan-neck deformity of unspecified finger(s) ▽

√6ᵗʰ **M20.09 Other deformity of finger(s)**
M20.091 Other deformity of right finger(s)
M20.092 Other deformity of left finger(s)
M20.099 Other deformity of finger(s), unspecified finger(s) ▽

√5ᵗʰ **M20.1 Hallux valgus (acquired)**
EXCLUDES 2   *bunion (M21.6-)*
AHA: 2016,4Q,38
DEF: Deformity in which the great toe deviates toward the other toes and may even be positioned over or under the second toe.

Hallux Valgus

Hallux valgus

Medial eminence of metatarsal bone

Right foot

M20.10 Hallux valgus (acquired), unspecified foot ▽
M20.11 Hallux valgus (acquired), right foot
M20.12 Hallux valgus (acquired), left foot

√5ᵗʰ **M20.2 Hallux rigidus**
M20.20 Hallux rigidus, unspecified foot ▽
M20.21 Hallux rigidus, right foot
M20.22 Hallux rigidus, left foot

√5ᵗʰ **M20.3 Hallux varus (acquired)**
DEF: Deformity in which the great toe deviates away from the other toes.
M20.30 Hallux varus (acquired), unspecified foot ▽
M20.31 Hallux varus (acquired), right foot
M20.32 Hallux varus (acquired), left foot

√5ᵗʰ **M20.4 Other hammer toe(s) (acquired)**
M20.40 Other hammer toe(s) (acquired), unspecified foot ▽
M20.41 Other hammer toe(s) (acquired), right foot
M20.42 Other hammer toe(s) (acquired), left foot

√5ᵗʰ **M20.5 Other deformities of toe(s) (acquired)**
√6ᵗʰ **M20.5X Other deformities of toe(s) (acquired)**
M20.5X1 Other deformities of toe(s) (acquired), right foot
M20.5X2 Other deformities of toe(s) (acquired), left foot
M20.5X9 Other deformities of toe(s) (acquired), unspecified foot ▽

√5ᵗʰ **M20.6 Acquired deformities of toe(s), unspecified**
M20.60 Acquired deformities of toe(s), unspecified, unspecified foot ▽
M20.61 Acquired deformities of toe(s), unspecified, right foot ▽
M20.62 Acquired deformities of toe(s), unspecified, left foot ▽

√4ᵗʰ **M21 Other acquired deformities of limbs**
EXCLUDES 1   *acquired absence of limb (Z89.-)*
congenital absence of limbs (Q71-Q73)
congenital deformities and malformations of limbs (Q65-Q66, Q68-Q74)
EXCLUDES 2   *acquired deformities of fingers or toes (M20.-)*
coxa plana (M91.2)

√5ᵗʰ **M21.0 Valgus deformity, not elsewhere classified**
EXCLUDES 1   *metatarsus valgus (Q66.6)*
talipes calcaneovalgus (Q66.4)

M21.00 Valgus deformity, not elsewhere classified, unspecified site ▽

√6ᵗʰ **M21.02** **Valgus deformity, not elsewhere classified, elbow**
   Cubitus valgus
   M21.021 **Valgus deformity, not elsewhere classified, right elbow**
   M21.022 **Valgus deformity, not elsewhere classified, left elbow**
   M21.029 **Valgus deformity, not elsewhere classified, unspecified elbow** ▽

√6ᵗʰ **M21.05** **Valgus deformity, not elsewhere classified, hip**
   M21.051 **Valgus deformity, not elsewhere classified, right hip**
   M21.052 **Valgus deformity, not elsewhere classified, left hip**
   M21.059 **Valgus deformity, not elsewhere classified, unspecified hip** ▽

√6ᵗʰ **M21.06** **Valgus deformity, not elsewhere classified, knee**
   Genu valgum
   Knock knee
   DEF: Genu valga/valgum: Condition in which the thighs slant inward, causing the knees to be angled abnormally close together, leaving the space between the ankles wider than normal.

Genu Valga (knock-knee)

   M21.061 **Valgus deformity, not elsewhere classified, right knee**
   M21.062 **Valgus deformity, not elsewhere classified, left knee**
   M21.069 **Valgus deformity, not elsewhere classified, unspecified knee** ▽

√6ᵗʰ **M21.07** **Valgus deformity, not elsewhere classified, ankle**
   M21.071 **Valgus deformity, not elsewhere classified, right ankle**
   M21.072 **Valgus deformity, not elsewhere classified, left ankle**
   M21.079 **Valgus deformity, not elsewhere classified, unspecified ankle** ▽

√5ᵗʰ **M21.1** **Varus deformity, not elsewhere classified**
   EXCLUDES 1   metatarsus varus (Q66.22)
                tibia vara (M92.5)
   M21.10 **Varus deformity, not elsewhere classified, unspecified site** ▽

√6ᵗʰ **M21.12** **Varus deformity, not elsewhere classified, elbow**
   Cubitus varus, elbow
   M21.121 **Varus deformity, not elsewhere classified, right elbow**
   M21.122 **Varus deformity, not elsewhere classified, left elbow**
   M21.129 **Varus deformity, not elsewhere classified, unspecified elbow** ▽

√6ᵗʰ **M21.15** **Varus deformity, not elsewhere classified, hip**
   M21.151 **Varus deformity, not elsewhere classified, right hip**
   M21.152 **Varus deformity, not elsewhere classified, left hip**

M21.159 **Varus deformity, not elsewhere classified, unspecified** ▽

√6ᵗʰ **M21.16** **Varus deformity, not elsewhere classified, knee**
   Bow leg
   Genu varum
   DEF: Genu varus/varum: Condition in which the thighs and/or legs are bowed in an outward curve with an abnormally increased space between the knees.

Genu Varus (bowleg)

   M21.161 **Varus deformity, not elsewhere classified, right knee**
   M21.162 **Varus deformity, not elsewhere classified, left knee**
   M21.169 **Varus deformity, not elsewhere classified, unspecified knee** ▽

√6ᵗʰ **M21.17** **Varus deformity, not elsewhere classified, ankle**
   M21.171 **Varus deformity, not elsewhere classified, right ankle**
   M21.172 **Varus deformity, not elsewhere classified, left ankle**
   M21.179 **Varus deformity, not elsewhere classified, unspecified ankle** ▽

√5ᵗʰ **M21.2** **Flexion deformity**
   M21.20 **Flexion deformity, unspecified site** ▽

√6ᵗʰ **M21.21** **Flexion deformity, shoulder**
   M21.211 **Flexion deformity, right shoulder**
   M21.212 **Flexion deformity, left shoulder**
   M21.219 **Flexion deformity, unspecified shoulder** ▽

√6ᵗʰ **M21.22** **Flexion deformity, elbow**
   M21.221 **Flexion deformity, right elbow**
   M21.222 **Flexion deformity, left elbow**
   M21.229 **Flexion deformity, unspecified elbow** ▽

√6ᵗʰ **M21.23** **Flexion deformity, wrist**
   M21.231 **Flexion deformity, right wrist**
   M21.232 **Flexion deformity, left wrist**
   M21.239 **Flexion deformity, unspecified wrist** ▽

√6ᵗʰ **M21.24** **Flexion deformity, finger joints**
   M21.241 **Flexion deformity, right finger joints**
   M21.242 **Flexion deformity, left finger joints**
   M21.249 **Flexion deformity, unspecified finger joints** ▽

√6ᵗʰ **M21.25** **Flexion deformity, hip**
   M21.251 **Flexion deformity, right hip**
   M21.252 **Flexion deformity, left hip**
   M21.259 **Flexion deformity, unspecified hip** ▽

√6ᵗʰ **M21.26** **Flexion deformity, knee**
   M21.261 **Flexion deformity, right knee**
   M21.262 **Flexion deformity, left knee**

M21.269 Flexion deformity, unspecified knee ▽

√6ᵗʰ M21.27 **Flexion deformity, ankle and toes**

M21.271 Flexion deformity, right ankle and toes
M21.272 Flexion deformity, left ankle and toes
M21.279 Flexion deformity, unspecified ankle and toes ▽

√5ᵗʰ M21.3 **Wrist or foot drop (acquired)**

√6ᵗʰ M21.33 **Wrist drop (acquired)**

M21.331 Wrist drop, right wrist
M21.332 Wrist drop, left wrist
M21.339 Wrist drop, unspecified wrist ▽

√6ᵗʰ M21.37 **Foot drop (acquired)**

M21.371 Foot drop, right foot
M21.372 Foot drop, left foot
M21.379 Foot drop, unspecified foot ▽

√5ᵗʰ M21.4 **Flat foot [pes planus] (acquired)**

EXCLUDES 1   congenital pes planus (Q66.5-)

M21.40 Flat foot [pes planus] (acquired), unspecified foot ▽
M21.41 Flat foot [pes planus] (acquired), right foot
M21.42 Flat foot [pes planus] (acquired), left foot

√5ᵗʰ M21.5 **Acquired clawhand, clubhand, clawfoot and clubfoot**

EXCLUDES 1   clubfoot, not specified as acquired (Q66.89)

√6ᵗʰ M21.51 **Acquired clawhand**

M21.511 Acquired clawhand, right hand
M21.512 Acquired clawhand, left hand
M21.519 Acquired clawhand, unspecified hand ▽

√6ᵗʰ M21.52 **Acquired clubhand**

M21.521 Acquired clubhand, right hand
M21.522 Acquired clubhand, left hand
M21.529 Acquired clubhand, unspecified hand ▽

√6ᵗʰ M21.53 **Acquired clawfoot**

DEF: High foot arch with hyperextended toes at the metatarsophalangeal joint and flexed toes at the distal joints.

M21.531 Acquired clawfoot, right foot
M21.532 Acquired clawfoot, left foot
M21.539 Acquired clawfoot, unspecified foot ▽

√6ᵗʰ M21.54 **Acquired clubfoot**

DEF: Acquired anomaly of the foot with the heel elevated and rotated outward and the toes pointing inward.

M21.541 Acquired clubfoot, right foot
M21.542 Acquired clubfoot, left foot
M21.549 Acquired clubfoot, unspecified foot ▽

√5ᵗʰ M21.6 **Other acquired deformities of foot**

EXCLUDES 2   deformities of toe (acquired) (M20.1-M20.6-)
AHA: 2016,4Q,38

√6ᵗʰ M21.61 **Bunion**

M21.611 Bunion of right foot
M21.612 Bunion of left foot
M21.619 Bunion of unspecified foot ▽

√6ᵗʰ M21.62 **Bunionette**

M21.621 Bunionette of right foot
M21.622 Bunionette of left foot
M21.629 Bunionette of unspecified foot ▽

√6ᵗʰ M21.6X **Other acquired deformities of foot**

M21.6X1 Other acquired deformities of right foot
M21.6X2 Other acquired deformities of left foot
M21.6X9 Other acquired deformities of unspecified foot ▽

√5ᵗʰ M21.7 **Unequal limb length (acquired)**

NOTE   The site used should correspond to the shorter limb

M21.70 Unequal limb length (acquired), unspecified site ▽

√6ᵗʰ M21.72 **Unequal limb length (acquired), humerus**

M21.721 Unequal limb length (acquired), right humerus
M21.722 Unequal limb length (acquired), left humerus

M21.729 Unequal limb length (acquired), unspecified humerus ▽

√6ᵗʰ M21.73 **Unequal limb length (acquired), ulna and radius**

M21.731 Unequal limb length (acquired), right ulna
M21.732 Unequal limb length (acquired), left ulna
M21.733 Unequal limb length (acquired), right radius
M21.734 Unequal limb length (acquired), left radius
M21.739 Unequal limb length (acquired), unspecified ulna and radius ▽

√6ᵗʰ M21.75 **Unequal limb length (acquired), femur**

M21.751 Unequal limb length (acquired), right femur
M21.752 Unequal limb length (acquired), left femur
M21.759 Unequal limb length (acquired), unspecified femur ▽

√6ᵗʰ M21.76 **Unequal limb length (acquired), tibia and fibula**

M21.761 Unequal limb length (acquired), right tibia
M21.762 Unequal limb length (acquired), left tibia
M21.763 Unequal limb length (acquired), right fibula
M21.764 Unequal limb length (acquired), left fibula
M21.769 Unequal limb length (acquired), unspecified tibia and fibula ▽

√5ᵗʰ M21.8 **Other specified acquired deformities of limbs**

EXCLUDES 2   coxa plana (M91.2)

M21.80 Other specified acquired deformities of unspecified limb ▽

√6ᵗʰ M21.82 **Other specified acquired deformities of upper arm**

M21.821 Other specified acquired deformities of right upper arm
M21.822 Other specified acquired deformities of left upper arm
M21.829 Other specified acquired deformities of unspecified upper arm ▽

√6ᵗʰ M21.83 **Other specified acquired deformities of forearm**

M21.831 Other specified acquired deformities of right forearm
M21.832 Other specified acquired deformities of left forearm
M21.839 Other specified acquired deformities of unspecified forearm ▽

√6ᵗʰ M21.85 **Other specified acquired deformities of thigh**

M21.851 Other specified acquired deformities of right thigh
M21.852 Other specified acquired deformities of left thigh
M21.859 Other specified acquired deformities of unspecified thigh ▽

√6ᵗʰ M21.86 **Other specified acquired deformities of lower leg**

M21.861 Other specified acquired deformities of right lower leg
M21.862 Other specified acquired deformities of left lower leg
M21.869 Other specified acquired deformities of unspecified lower leg ▽

√5ᵗʰ M21.9 **Unspecified acquired deformity of limb and hand**

M21.90 Unspecified acquired deformity of unspecified limb ▽

√6ᵗʰ M21.92 **Unspecified acquired deformity of upper arm**

M21.921 Unspecified acquired deformity of right upper arm ▽
M21.922 Unspecified acquired deformity of left upper arm ▽
M21.929 Unspecified acquired deformity of unspecified upper arm ▽

√6ᵗʰ M21.93 **Unspecified acquired deformity of forearm**

M21.931 Unspecified acquired deformity of right forearm ▽
M21.932 Unspecified acquired deformity of left forearm ▽

M21.939   Unspecified acquired deformity of unspecified forearm ▽

√6ᵗʰ   **M21.94**   Unspecified acquired deformity of hand

M21.941   Unspecified acquired deformity of hand, right hand ▽

M21.942   Unspecified acquired deformity of hand, left hand ▽

M21.949   Unspecified acquired deformity of hand, unspecified hand ▽

√6ᵗʰ   **M21.95**   Unspecified acquired deformity of thigh

M21.951   Unspecified acquired deformity of right thigh ▽

M21.952   Unspecified acquired deformity of left thigh ▽

M21.959   Unspecified acquired deformity of unspecified thigh ▽

√6ᵗʰ   **M21.96**   Unspecified acquired deformity of lower leg

M21.961   Unspecified acquired deformity of right lower leg ▽

M21.962   Unspecified acquired deformity of left lower leg ▽

M21.969   Unspecified acquired deformity of unspecified lower leg ▽

√4ᵗʰ   **M22**   **Disorder of patella**

EXCLUDES 1   traumatic dislocation of patella (S83.0-)

√5ᵗʰ   **M22.0**   Recurrent dislocation of patella

M22.00   Recurrent dislocation of patella, unspecified knee ▽

M22.01   Recurrent dislocation of patella, right knee

M22.02   Recurrent dislocation of patella, left knee

√5ᵗʰ   **M22.1**   Recurrent subluxation of patella

Incomplete dislocation of patella

M22.10   Recurrent subluxation of patella, unspecified knee ▽

M22.11   Recurrent subluxation of patella, right knee

M22.12   Recurrent subluxation of patella, left knee

√5ᵗʰ   **M22.2**   Patellofemoral disorders

√6ᵗʰ   **M22.2X**   Patellofemoral disorders

M22.2X1   Patellofemoral disorders, right knee

M22.2X2   Patellofemoral disorders, left knee

M22.2X9   Patellofemoral disorders, unspecified knee ▽

√5ᵗʰ   **M22.3**   Other derangements of patella

√6ᵗʰ   **M22.3X**   Other derangements of patella

M22.3X1   Other derangements of patella, right knee

M22.3X2   Other derangements of patella, left knee

M22.3X9   Other derangements of patella, unspecified knee ▽

√5ᵗʰ   **M22.4**   Chondromalacia patellae

M22.40   Chondromalacia patellae, unspecified knee ▽

M22.41   Chondromalacia patellae, right knee

M22.42   Chondromalacia patellae, left knee

√5ᵗʰ   **M22.8**   Other disorders of patella

√6ᵗʰ   **M22.8X**   Other disorders of patella

M22.8X1   Other disorders of patella, right knee

M22.8X2   Other disorders of patella, left knee

M22.8X9   Other disorders of patella, unspecified knee ▽

√5ᵗʰ   **M22.9**   Unspecified disorder of patella

M22.90   Unspecified disorder of patella, unspecified knee ▽

M22.91   Unspecified disorder of patella, right knee ▽

M22.92   Unspecified disorder of patella, left knee ▽

√4ᵗʰ   **M23**   **Internal derangement of knee**

EXCLUDES 1   ankylosis (M24.66)

current injury - see injury of knee and lower leg (S80-S89)

deformity of knee (M21.-)

osteochondritis dissecans (M93.2)

recurrent dislocation or subluxation of joints (M24.4)

recurrent dislocation or subluxation of patella (M22.0-M22.1)

√5ᵗʰ   **M23.0**   Cystic meniscus

√6ᵗʰ   **M23.00**   Cystic meniscus, unspecified meniscus

Cystic meniscus, unspecified lateral meniscus

Cystic meniscus, unspecified medial meniscus

M23.000   Cystic meniscus, unspecified lateral meniscus, right knee

M23.001   Cystic meniscus, unspecified lateral meniscus, left knee

M23.002   Cystic meniscus, unspecified lateral meniscus, unspecified knee ▽

M23.003   Cystic meniscus, unspecified medial meniscus, right knee

M23.004   Cystic meniscus, unspecified medial meniscus, left knee

M23.005   Cystic meniscus, unspecified medial meniscus, unspecified knee ▽

M23.006   Cystic meniscus, unspecified meniscus, right knee

M23.007   Cystic meniscus, unspecified meniscus, left knee

M23.009   Cystic meniscus, unspecified meniscus, unspecified knee ▽

√6ᵗʰ   **M23.01**   Cystic meniscus, anterior horn of medial meniscus

M23.011   Cystic meniscus, anterior horn of medial meniscus, right knee

M23.012   Cystic meniscus, anterior horn of medial meniscus, left knee

M23.019   Cystic meniscus, anterior horn of medial meniscus, unspecified knee ▽

√6ᵗʰ   **M23.02**   Cystic meniscus, posterior horn of medial meniscus

M23.021   Cystic meniscus, posterior horn of medial meniscus, right knee

M23.022   Cystic meniscus, posterior horn of medial meniscus, left knee

M23.029   Cystic meniscus, posterior horn of medial meniscus, unspecified knee ▽

√6ᵗʰ   **M23.03**   Cystic meniscus, other medial meniscus

M23.031   Cystic meniscus, other medial meniscus, right knee

M23.032   Cystic meniscus, other medial meniscus, left knee

M23.039   Cystic meniscus, other medial meniscus, unspecified knee ▽

√6ᵗʰ   **M23.04**   Cystic meniscus, anterior horn of lateral meniscus

M23.041   Cystic meniscus, anterior horn of lateral meniscus, right knee

M23.042   Cystic meniscus, anterior horn of lateral meniscus, left knee

M23.049   Cystic meniscus, anterior horn of lateral meniscus, unspecified knee ▽

√6ᵗʰ   **M23.05**   Cystic meniscus, posterior horn of lateral meniscus

M23.051   Cystic meniscus, posterior horn of lateral meniscus, right knee

M23.052   Cystic meniscus, posterior horn of lateral meniscus, left knee

M23.059   Cystic meniscus, posterior horn of lateral meniscus, unspecified knee ▽

√6ᵗʰ   **M23.06**   Cystic meniscus, other lateral meniscus

M23.061   Cystic meniscus, other lateral meniscus, right knee

M23.062   Cystic meniscus, other lateral meniscus, left knee

M23.069   Cystic meniscus, other lateral meniscus, unspecified knee ▽

✓ Additional Character Req   ✓x7ᵗʰ Placeholder Alert   Manifestation   ▽ Unspecified   ▶◀ Revised Text   ● New Code   ▲ Revised Code Title

ICD-10-CM 2019

767

✓5ᵗʰ **M23.2** **Derangement of meniscus due to old tear or injury**
Old bucket-handle tear

Derangement of Meniscus

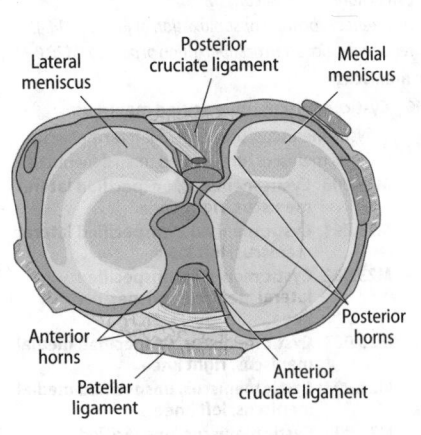

Lateral meniscus
Posterior cruciate ligament
Medial meniscus
Anterior horns
Patellar ligament
Posterior horns
Anterior cruciate ligament

Overhead view of right knee

Bucket handle tear

Radial tear

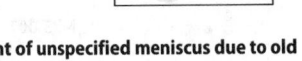
Meniscus

✓6ᵗʰ **M23.20** **Derangement of unspecified meniscus due to old tear or injury**
Derangement of unspecified lateral meniscus due to old tear or injury
Derangement of unspecified medial meniscus due to old tear or injury

M23.200 Derangement of unspecified lateral meniscus due to old tear or injury, right knee ▽

M23.201 Derangement of unspecified lateral meniscus due to old tear or injury, left knee ▽

M23.202 Derangement of unspecified lateral meniscus due to old tear or injury, unspecified knee ▽

M23.203 Derangement of unspecified medial meniscus due to old tear or injury, right knee ▽

M23.204 Derangement of unspecified medial meniscus due to old tear or injury, left knee ▽

M23.205 Derangement of unspecified medial meniscus due to old tear or injury, unspecified knee ▽

M23.206 Derangement of unspecified meniscus due to old tear or injury, right knee ▽

M23.207 Derangement of unspecified meniscus due to old tear or injury, left knee ▽

M23.209 Derangement of unspecified meniscus due to old tear or injury, unspecified knee ▽

✓6ᵗʰ **M23.21** **Derangement of anterior horn of medial meniscus due to old tear or injury**

M23.211 Derangement of anterior horn of medial meniscus due to old tear or injury, right knee

M23.212 Derangement of anterior horn of medial meniscus due to old tear or injury, left knee

M23.219 Derangement of anterior horn of medial meniscus due to old tear or injury, unspecified knee ▽

✓6ᵗʰ **M23.22** **Derangement of posterior horn of medial meniscus due to old tear or injury**

M23.221 Derangement of posterior horn of medial meniscus due to old tear or injury, right knee

M23.222 Derangement of posterior horn of medial meniscus due to old tear or injury, left knee

M23.229 Derangement of posterior horn of medial meniscus due to old tear or injury, unspecified knee ▽

✓6ᵗʰ **M23.23** **Derangement of other medial meniscus due to old tear or injury**

M23.231 Derangement of other medial meniscus due to old tear or injury, right knee

M23.232 Derangement of other medial meniscus due to old tear or injury, left knee

M23.239 Derangement of other medial meniscus due to old tear or injury, unspecified knee ▽

✓6ᵗʰ **M23.24** **Derangement of anterior horn of lateral meniscus due to old tear or injury**

M23.241 Derangement of anterior horn of lateral meniscus due to old tear or injury, right knee

M23.242 Derangement of anterior horn of lateral meniscus due to old tear or injury, left knee

M23.249 Derangement of anterior horn of lateral meniscus due to old tear or injury, unspecified knee ▽

✓6ᵗʰ **M23.25** **Derangement of posterior horn of lateral meniscus due to old tear or injury**

M23.251 Derangement of posterior horn of lateral meniscus due to old tear or injury, right knee

M23.252 Derangement of posterior horn of lateral meniscus due to old tear or injury, left knee

M23.259 Derangement of posterior horn of lateral meniscus due to old tear or injury, unspecified knee ▽

✓6ᵗʰ **M23.26** **Derangement of other lateral meniscus due to old tear or injury**

M23.261 Derangement of other lateral meniscus due to old tear or injury, right knee

M23.262 Derangement of other lateral meniscus due to old tear or injury, left knee

M23.269 Derangement of other lateral meniscus due to old tear or injury, unspecified knee ▽

✓5ᵗʰ **M23.3** **Other meniscus derangements**
Degenerate meniscus
Detached meniscus
Retained meniscus

✓6ᵗʰ **M23.30** **Other meniscus derangements, unspecified meniscus**
Other meniscus derangements, unspecified lateral meniscus
Other meniscus derangements, unspecified medial meniscus

M23.300 Other meniscus derangements, unspecified lateral meniscus, right knee ▽

M23.301 Other meniscus derangements, unspecified lateral meniscus, left knee ▽

M23.302 Other meniscus derangements, unspecified lateral meniscus, unspecified knee ▽

M23.303 Other meniscus derangements, unspecified medial meniscus, right knee ▽

M23.304 Other meniscus derangements, unspecified medial meniscus, left knee ▽

M23.305 Other meniscus derangements, unspecified medial meniscus, unspecified knee ▽

M23.306 Other meniscus derangements, unspecified meniscus, right knee ▽

M23.307 Other meniscus derangements, unspecified meniscus, left knee ▽

M23.309 Other meniscus derangements, unspecified meniscus, unspecified knee ▽

✓6ᵗʰ **M23.31** **Other meniscus derangements, anterior horn of medial meniscus**

M23.311 Other meniscus derangements, anterior horn of medial meniscus, right knee

M23.312 Other meniscus derangements, anterior horn of medial meniscus, left knee

M23.319 Other meniscus derangements, anterior horn of medial meniscus, unspecified knee ▽

√6ᵗʰ M23.32 Other meniscus derangements, posterior horn of medial meniscus

M23.321 Other meniscus derangements, posterior horn of medial meniscus, right knee

M23.322 Other meniscus derangements, posterior horn of medial meniscus, left knee

M23.329 Other meniscus derangements, posterior horn of medial meniscus, unspecified knee ▽

√6ᵗʰ M23.33 Other meniscus derangements, other medial meniscus

M23.331 Other meniscus derangements, other medial meniscus, right knee

M23.332 Other meniscus derangements, other medial meniscus, left knee

M23.339 Other meniscus derangements, other medial meniscus, unspecified knee ▽

√6ᵗʰ M23.34 Other meniscus derangements, anterior horn of lateral meniscus

M23.341 Other meniscus derangements, anterior horn of lateral meniscus, right knee

M23.342 Other meniscus derangements, anterior horn of lateral meniscus, left knee

M23.349 Other meniscus derangements, anterior horn of lateral meniscus, unspecified knee ▽

√6ᵗʰ M23.35 Other meniscus derangements, posterior horn of lateral meniscus

M23.351 Other meniscus derangements, posterior horn of lateral meniscus, right knee

M23.352 Other meniscus derangements, posterior horn of lateral meniscus, left knee

M23.359 Other meniscus derangements, posterior horn of lateral meniscus, unspecified knee ▽

√6ᵗʰ M23.36 Other meniscus derangements, other lateral meniscus

M23.361 Other meniscus derangements, other lateral meniscus, right knee

M23.362 Other meniscus derangements, other lateral meniscus, left knee

M23.369 Other meniscus derangements, other lateral meniscus, unspecified knee ▽

√5ᵗʰ M23.4 Loose body in knee

M23.40 Loose body in knee, unspecified knee ▽
M23.41 Loose body in knee, right knee
M23.42 Loose body in knee, left knee

√5ᵗʰ M23.5 Chronic instability of knee

M23.50 Chronic instability of knee, unspecified knee ▽
M23.51 Chronic instability of knee, right knee
M23.52 Chronic instability of knee, left knee

√5ᵗʰ M23.6 Other spontaneous disruption of ligament(s) of knee

√6ᵗʰ M23.60 Other spontaneous disruption of unspecified ligament of knee

M23.601 Other spontaneous disruption of unspecified ligament of right knee ▽

M23.602 Other spontaneous disruption of unspecified ligament of left knee ▽

M23.609 Other spontaneous disruption of unspecified ligament of unspecified knee ▽

√6ᵗʰ M23.61 Other spontaneous disruption of anterior cruciate ligament of knee

M23.611 Other spontaneous disruption of anterior cruciate ligament of right knee

M23.612 Other spontaneous disruption of anterior cruciate ligament of left knee

M23.619 Other spontaneous disruption of anterior cruciate ligament of unspecified knee ▽

√6ᵗʰ M23.62 Other spontaneous disruption of posterior cruciate ligament of knee

M23.621 Other spontaneous disruption of posterior cruciate ligament of right knee

M23.622 Other spontaneous disruption of posterior cruciate ligament of left knee

M23.629 Other spontaneous disruption of posterior cruciate ligament of unspecified knee ▽

√6ᵗʰ M23.63 Other spontaneous disruption of medial collateral ligament of knee

M23.631 Other spontaneous disruption of medial collateral ligament of right knee

M23.632 Other spontaneous disruption of medial collateral ligament of left knee

M23.639 Other spontaneous disruption of medial collateral ligament of unspecified knee ▽

√6ᵗʰ M23.64 Other spontaneous disruption of lateral collateral ligament of knee

M23.641 Other spontaneous disruption of lateral collateral ligament of right knee

M23.642 Other spontaneous disruption of lateral collateral ligament of left knee

M23.649 Other spontaneous disruption of lateral collateral ligament of unspecified knee ▽

√6ᵗʰ M23.67 Other spontaneous disruption of capsular ligament of knee

M23.671 Other spontaneous disruption of capsular ligament of right knee

M23.672 Other spontaneous disruption of capsular ligament of left knee

M23.679 Other spontaneous disruption of capsular ligament of unspecified knee ▽

√5ᵗʰ M23.8 Other internal derangements of knee

Laxity of ligament of knee
Snapping knee

√6ᵗʰ M23.8X Other internal derangements of knee

M23.8X1 Other internal derangements of right knee

M23.8X2 Other internal derangements of left knee

M23.8X9 Other internal derangements of unspecified knee ▽

√5ᵗʰ M23.9 Unspecified internal derangement of knee

M23.90 Unspecified internal derangement of unspecified knee ▽

M23.91 Unspecified internal derangement of right knee ▽

M23.92 Unspecified internal derangement of left knee ▽

√4ᵗʰ **M24 Other specific joint derangements**

EXCLUDES 1 current injury - see injury of joint by body region
EXCLUDES 2 ganglion (M67.4)
snapping knee (M23.8-)
temporomandibular joint disorders (M26.6-)

√5ᵗʰ M24.0 Loose body in joint

EXCLUDES 2 loose body in knee (M23.4)

M24.00 Loose body in unspecified joint ▽

√6ᵗʰ M24.01 Loose body in shoulder

M24.011 Loose body in right shoulder
M24.012 Loose body in left shoulder
M24.019 Loose body in unspecified shoulder ▽

√6ᵗʰ M24.02 Loose body in elbow

M24.021 Loose body in right elbow
M24.022 Loose body in left elbow
M24.029 Loose body in unspecified elbow ▽

√6ᵗʰ M24.03 Loose body in wrist

M24.031 Loose body in right wrist
M24.032 Loose body in left wrist
M24.039 Loose body in unspecified wrist ▽

√6ᵗʰ M24.04 Loose body in finger joints

M24.041 Loose body in right finger joint(s)
M24.042 Loose body in left finger joint(s)
M24.049 Loose body in unspecified finger joint(s) ▽

√6ᵗʰ M24.05 Loose body in hip

M24.051 Loose body in right hip
M24.052 Loose body in left hip
M24.059 Loose body in unspecified hip ▽

√6ᵗʰ **M24.07** **Loose body in** ankle and toe joints

     M24.071 **Loose body in** right ankle

     M24.072 **Loose body in** left ankle

     M24.073 **Loose body in unspecified ankle** ▽

     M24.074 **Loose body in** right toe joint(s)

     M24.075 **Loose body in** left toe joint(s)

     M24.076 **Loose body in unspecified toe** ▽
               joints

     M24.08 **Loose body, other site**

√5ᵗʰ **M24.1** **Other articular cartilage disorders**

     EXCLUDES 2   chondrocalcinosis (M11.1, M11.2-)

                 internal derangement of knee (M23.-)

                 metastatic calcification (E83.5)

                 ochronosis (E70.2)

     M24.10 **Other articular cartilage disorders,** ▽
               unspecified site

√6ᵗʰ **M24.11** **Other articular cartilage disorders,** shoulder

     M24.111 **Other articular cartilage disorders,** right
               shoulder

     M24.112 **Other articular cartilage disorders,** left
               shoulder

     M24.119 **Other articular cartilage** ▽
               disorders, unspecified shoulder

√6ᵗʰ **M24.12** **Other articular cartilage disorders,** elbow

     M24.121 **Other articular cartilage disorders,** right
               elbow

     M24.122 **Other articular cartilage disorders,** left
               elbow

     M24.129 **Other articular cartilage** ▽
               disorders, unspecified elbow

√6ᵗʰ **M24.13** **Other articular cartilage disorders,** wrist

     M24.131 **Other articular cartilage disorders,** right
               wrist

     M24.132 **Other articular cartilage disorders,** left
               wrist

     M24.139 **Other articular cartilage** ▽
               disorders, unspecified wrist

√6ᵗʰ **M24.14** **Other articular cartilage disorders,** hand

     M24.141 **Other articular cartilage disorders,** right
               hand

     M24.142 **Other articular cartilage disorders,** left
               hand

     M24.149 **Other articular cartilage** ▽
               disorders, unspecified hand

√6ᵗʰ **M24.15** **Other articular cartilage disorders,** hip

     M24.151 **Other articular cartilage disorders,** right
               hip

     M24.152 **Other articular cartilage disorders,** left
               hip

     M24.159 **Other articular cartilage** ▽
               disorders, unspecified hip

√6ᵗʰ **M24.17** **Other articular cartilage disorders,** ankle and foot

     M24.171 **Other articular cartilage disorders,** right
               ankle

     M24.172 **Other articular cartilage disorders,** left
               ankle

     M24.173 **Other articular cartilage** ▽
               disorders, unspecified ankle

     M24.174 **Other articular cartilage disorders,** right
               foot

     M24.175 **Other articular cartilage disorders,** left
               foot

     M24.176 **Other articular cartilage** ▽
               disorders, unspecified foot

√5ᵗʰ **M24.2** **Disorder of ligament**

     Instability secondary to old ligament injury

     Ligamentous laxity NOS

     EXCLUDES 1   familial ligamentous laxity (M35.7)

     EXCLUDES 2   internal derangement of knee (M23.5-M23.89)

     M24.20 **Disorder of ligament, unspecified site** ▽

√6ᵗʰ **M24.21** **Disorder of ligament,** shoulder

     M24.211 **Disorder of ligament,** right shoulder

     M24.212 **Disorder of ligament,** left shoulder

     M24.219 **Disorder of ligament, unspecified** ▽
               shoulder

√6ᵗʰ **M24.22** **Disorder of ligament,** elbow

     M24.221 **Disorder of ligament,** right elbow

     M24.222 **Disorder of ligament,** left elbow

     M24.229 **Disorder of ligament, unspecified** ▽
               elbow

√6ᵗʰ **M24.23** **Disorder of ligament,** wrist

     M24.231 **Disorder of ligament,** right wrist

     M24.232 **Disorder of ligament,** left wrist

     M24.239 **Disorder of ligament, unspecified** ▽
               wrist

√6ᵗʰ **M24.24** **Disorder of ligament,** hand

     M24.241 **Disorder of ligament,** right hand

     M24.242 **Disorder of ligament,** left hand

     M24.249 **Disorder of ligament, unspecified** ▽
               hand

√6ᵗʰ **M24.25** **Disorder of ligament,** hip

     M24.251 **Disorder of ligament,** right hip

     M24.252 **Disorder of ligament,** left hip

     M24.259 **Disorder of ligament, unspecified** ▽
               hip

√6ᵗʰ **M24.27** **Disorder of ligament,** ankle and foot

     M24.271 **Disorder of ligament,** right ankle

     M24.272 **Disorder of ligament,** left ankle

     M24.273 **Disorder of ligament, unspecified** ▽
               ankle

     M24.274 **Disorder of ligament,** right foot

     M24.275 **Disorder of ligament,** left foot

     M24.276 **Disorder of ligament, unspecified** ▽
               foot

     M24.28 **Disorder of ligament,** vertebrae

√5ᵗʰ **M24.3** **Pathological dislocation of joint, not elsewhere classified**

     EXCLUDES 1   congenital dislocation or displacement of joint - see
                     congenital malformations and deformations of
                     the musculoskeletal system (Q65-Q79)

                 current injury - see injury of joints and ligaments by
                     body region

                 recurrent dislocation of joint (M24.4-)

     M24.30 **Pathological dislocation of unspecified** ▽
               joint, not elsewhere classified

√6ᵗʰ **M24.31** **Pathological dislocation of shoulder, not elsewhere classified**

     M24.311 **Pathological dislocation of** right
               shoulder, not elsewhere classified

     M24.312 **Pathological dislocation of** left shoulder,
               not elsewhere classified

     M24.319 **Pathological dislocation of** ▽
               unspecified shoulder, not
               elsewhere classified

√6ᵗʰ **M24.32** **Pathological dislocation of elbow, not elsewhere classified**

     M24.321 **Pathological dislocation of right elbow,**
               not elsewhere classified

     M24.322 **Pathological dislocation of left elbow, not**
               elsewhere classified

     M24.329 **Pathological dislocation of** ▽
               unspecified elbow, not elsewhere
               classified

√6ᵗʰ **M24.33** **Pathological dislocation of wrist, not elsewhere classified**

     M24.331 **Pathological dislocation of right wrist,**
               not elsewhere classified

     M24.332 **Pathological dislocation of left wrist, not**
               elsewhere classified

     M24.339 **Pathological dislocation of** ▽
               unspecified wrist, not elsewhere
               classified

√6ᵗʰ **M24.34** **Pathological dislocation of hand, not elsewhere classified**

     M24.341 **Pathological dislocation of right hand,**
               not elsewhere classified

     M24.342 **Pathological dislocation of left hand, not**
               elsewhere classified

     M24.349 **Pathological dislocation of** ▽
               unspecified hand, not elsewhere
               classified

√6ᵗʰ **M24.35** **Pathological dislocation of hip, not elsewhere classified**

     M24.351 **Pathological dislocation of right hip, not**
               elsewhere classified

     M24.352 **Pathological dislocation of left hip, not**
               elsewhere classified

     M24.359 **Pathological dislocation of** ▽
               unspecified hip, not elsewhere
               classified

√6th **M24.36 Pathological dislocation of knee, not elsewhere classified**

    M24.361 Pathological dislocation of right knee, not elsewhere classified

    M24.362 Pathological dislocation of left knee, not elsewhere classified

    M24.369 Pathological dislocation of unspecified knee, not elsewhere classified ▽

√6th **M24.37 Pathological dislocation of ankle and foot, not elsewhere classified**

    M24.371 Pathological dislocation of right ankle, not elsewhere classified

    M24.372 Pathological dislocation of left ankle, not elsewhere classified

    M24.373 Pathological dislocation of unspecified ankle, not elsewhere classified ▽

    M24.374 Pathological dislocation of right foot, not elsewhere classified

    M24.375 Pathological dislocation of left foot, not elsewhere classified

    M24.376 Pathological dislocation of unspecified foot, not elsewhere classified ▽

√5th **M24.4 Recurrent dislocation of joint**

Recurrent subluxation of joint

EXCLUDES 2   recurrent dislocation of patella (M22.0-M22.1)

           recurrent vertebral dislocation (M43.3-, M43.4, M43.5-)

    M24.40 Recurrent dislocation, unspecified joint ▽

√6th **M24.41** Recurrent dislocation, shoulder

    M24.411 Recurrent dislocation, right shoulder

    M24.412 Recurrent dislocation, left shoulder

    M24.419 Recurrent dislocation, unspecified shoulder ▽

√6th **M24.42** Recurrent dislocation, elbow

    M24.421 Recurrent dislocation, right elbow

    M24.422 Recurrent dislocation, left elbow

    M24.429 Recurrent dislocation, unspecified elbow ▽

√6th **M24.43** Recurrent dislocation, wrist

    M24.431 Recurrent dislocation, right wrist

    M24.432 Recurrent dislocation, left wrist

    M24.439 Recurrent dislocation, unspecified wrist ▽

√6th **M24.44** Recurrent dislocation, hand and finger(s)

    M24.441 Recurrent dislocation, right hand

    M24.442 Recurrent dislocation, left hand

    M24.443 Recurrent dislocation, unspecified hand ▽

    M24.444 Recurrent dislocation, right finger

    M24.445 Recurrent dislocation, left finger

    M24.446 Recurrent dislocation, unspecified finger ▽

√6th **M24.45** Recurrent dislocation, hip

    M24.451 Recurrent dislocation, right hip

    M24.452 Recurrent dislocation, left hip

    M24.459 Recurrent dislocation, unspecified hip ▽

√6th **M24.46** Recurrent dislocation, knee

    M24.461 Recurrent dislocation, right knee

    M24.462 Recurrent dislocation, left knee

    M24.469 Recurrent dislocation, unspecified knee ▽

√6th **M24.47** Recurrent dislocation, ankle, foot and toes

    M24.471 Recurrent dislocation, right ankle

    M24.472 Recurrent dislocation, left ankle

    M24.473 Recurrent dislocation, unspecified ankle ▽

    M24.474 Recurrent dislocation, right foot

    M24.475 Recurrent dislocation, left foot

    M24.476 Recurrent dislocation, unspecified foot ▽

    M24.477 Recurrent dislocation, right toe(s)

    M24.478 Recurrent dislocation, left toe(s)

    M24.479 Recurrent dislocation, unspecified toe(s) ▽

√5th **M24.5 Contracture of joint**

EXCLUDES 1   contracture of muscle without contracture of joint (M62.4-)

           contracture of tendon (sheath) without contracture of joint (M62.4-)

           Dupuytren's contracture (M72.0)

EXCLUDES 2   acquired deformities of limbs (M20-M21)

AHA: 2016,2Q,6

    M24.50 Contracture, unspecified joint ▽

√6th **M24.51** Contracture, shoulder

    M24.511 Contracture, right shoulder

    M24.512 Contracture, left shoulder

    M24.519 Contracture, unspecified shoulder ▽

√6th **M24.52** Contracture, elbow

    M24.521 Contracture, right elbow

    M24.522 Contracture, left elbow

    M24.529 Contracture, unspecified elbow ▽

√6th **M24.53** Contracture, wrist

    M24.531 Contracture, right wrist

    M24.532 Contracture, left wrist

    M24.539 Contracture, unspecified wrist ▽

√6th **M24.54** Contracture, hand

    M24.541 Contracture, right hand

    M24.542 Contracture, left hand

    M24.549 Contracture, unspecified hand ▽

√6th **M24.55** Contracture, hip

    M24.551 Contracture, right hip

    M24.552 Contracture, left hip

    M24.559 Contracture, unspecified hip ▽

√6th **M24.56** Contracture, knee

    M24.561 Contracture, right knee

    M24.562 Contracture, left knee

    M24.569 Contracture, unspecified knee ▽

√6th **M24.57** Contracture, ankle and foot

    M24.571 Contracture, right ankle

    M24.572 Contracture, left ankle

    M24.573 Contracture, unspecified ankle ▽

    M24.574 Contracture, right foot

    M24.575 Contracture, left foot

    M24.576 Contracture, unspecified foot ▽

√5th **M24.6 Ankylosis of joint**

EXCLUDES 1   stiffness of joint without ankylosis (M25.6-)

EXCLUDES 2   spine (M43.2-)

DEF: Ankylosis: Abnormal union or fusion of bones in a joint, which is normally moveable.

    M24.60 Ankylosis, unspecified joint ▽

√6th **M24.61** Ankylosis, shoulder

    M24.611 Ankylosis, right shoulder

    M24.612 Ankylosis, left shoulder

    M24.619 Ankylosis, unspecified shoulder ▽

√6th **M24.62** Ankylosis, elbow

    M24.621 Ankylosis, right elbow

    M24.622 Ankylosis, left elbow

    M24.629 Ankylosis, unspecified elbow ▽

√6th **M24.63** Ankylosis, wrist

    M24.631 Ankylosis, right wrist

    M24.632 Ankylosis, left wrist

    M24.639 Ankylosis, unspecified wrist ▽

√6th **M24.64** Ankylosis, hand

    M24.641 Ankylosis, right hand

    M24.642 Ankylosis, left hand

    M24.649 Ankylosis, unspecified hand ▽

√6th **M24.65** Ankylosis, hip

    M24.651 Ankylosis, right hip

    M24.652 Ankylosis, left hip

    M24.659 Ankylosis, unspecified hip ▽

√6th **M24.66** Ankylosis, knee

    M24.661 Ankylosis, right knee

    M24.662 Ankylosis, left knee

    M24.669 Ankylosis, unspecified knee ▽

√6th **M24.67** Ankylosis, ankle and foot

    M24.671 Ankylosis, right ankle

    M24.672 Ankylosis, left ankle

    M24.673 Ankylosis, unspecified ankle ▽

    M24.674 Ankylosis, right foot

☑ Additional Character Req   √x7th Placeholder Alert   Manifestation   ▽ Unspecified   ►◄ Revised Text   ● New Code   ▲ Revised Code Title

M24.675   Ankylosis, left foot
M24.676   Ankylosis, unspecified foot ▽

M24.7   Protrusio acetabuli
     DEF: Intrapelvic protrusion of the acetabulum characterized by the sinking of the floor of the acetabulum, causing the femoral head to protrude. It limits hip movement and is of unknown etiology. *Synonym(s): Otto's pelvis.*

√5ᵗʰ **M24.8   Other specific joint derangements, not elsewhere classified**
     EXCLUDES 2   iliotibial band syndrome (M76.3)

     M24.80   Other specific joint derangements of unspecified joint, not elsewhere classified ▽

√6ᵗʰ   **M24.81   Other specific joint derangements of shoulder, not elsewhere classified**
     M24.811   Other specific joint derangements of right shoulder, not elsewhere classified
     M24.812   Other specific joint derangements of left shoulder, not elsewhere classified
     M24.819   Other specific joint derangements of unspecified shoulder, not elsewhere classified ▽

√6ᵗʰ   **M24.82   Other specific joint derangements of elbow, not elsewhere classified**
     M24.821   Other specific joint derangements of right elbow, not elsewhere classified
     M24.822   Other specific joint derangements of left elbow, not elsewhere classified
     M24.829   Other specific joint derangements of unspecified elbow, not elsewhere classified ▽

√6ᵗʰ   **M24.83   Other specific joint derangements of wrist, not elsewhere classified**
     M24.831   Other specific joint derangements of right wrist, not elsewhere classified
     M24.832   Other specific joint derangements of left wrist, not elsewhere classified
     M24.839   Other specific joint derangements of unspecified wrist, not elsewhere classified ▽

√6ᵗʰ   **M24.84   Other specific joint derangements of hand, not elsewhere classified**
     M24.841   Other specific joint derangements of right hand, not elsewhere classified
     M24.842   Other specific joint derangements of left hand, not elsewhere classified
     M24.849   Other specific joint derangements of unspecified hand, not elsewhere classified ▽

√6ᵗʰ   **M24.85   Other specific joint derangements of hip, not elsewhere classified**
     Irritable hip
     M24.851   Other specific joint derangements of right hip, not elsewhere classified
     M24.852   Other specific joint derangements of left hip, not elsewhere classified
     M24.859   Other specific joint derangements of unspecified hip, not elsewhere classified ▽

√6ᵗʰ   **M24.87   Other specific joint derangements of ankle and foot, not elsewhere classified**
     M24.871   Other specific joint derangements of right ankle, not elsewhere classified
     M24.872   Other specific joint derangements of left ankle, not elsewhere classified
     M24.873   Other specific joint derangements of unspecified ankle, not elsewhere classified ▽
     M24.874   Other specific joint derangements of right foot, not elsewhere classified
     M24.875   Other specific joint derangements of left foot, not elsewhere classified
     M24.876   Other specific joint derangements of unspecified foot, not elsewhere classified ▽

M24.9   Joint derangement, unspecified ▽

√4ᵗʰ **M25   Other joint disorder, not elsewhere classified**
     EXCLUDES 2   abnormality of gait and mobility (R26.-)
          acquired deformities of limb (M20-M21)
          calcification of bursa (M71.4-)
          calcification of shoulder (joint) (M75.3)
          calcification of tendon (M65.2-)
          difficulty in walking (R26.2)
          temporomandibular joint disorder (M26.6-)

√5ᵗʰ **M25.0   Hemarthrosis**
     EXCLUDES 1   current injury - see injury of joint by body region
          hemophilic arthropathy (M36.2)

     M25.00   Hemarthrosis, unspecified joint ▽

√6ᵗʰ   **M25.01   Hemarthrosis, shoulder**
     M25.011   Hemarthrosis, right shoulder
     M25.012   Hemarthrosis, left shoulder
     M25.019   Hemarthrosis, unspecified shoulder ▽

√6ᵗʰ   **M25.02   Hemarthrosis, elbow**
     M25.021   Hemarthrosis, right elbow
     M25.022   Hemarthrosis, left elbow
     M25.029   Hemarthrosis, unspecified elbow ▽

√6ᵗʰ   **M25.03   Hemarthrosis, wrist**
     M25.031   Hemarthrosis, right wrist
     M25.032   Hemarthrosis, left wrist
     M25.039   Hemarthrosis, unspecified wrist ▽

√6ᵗʰ   **M25.04   Hemarthrosis, hand**
     M25.041   Hemarthrosis, right hand
     M25.042   Hemarthrosis, left hand
     M25.049   Hemarthrosis, unspecified hand ▽

√6ᵗʰ   **M25.05   Hemarthrosis, hip**
     M25.051   Hemarthrosis, right hip
     M25.052   Hemarthrosis, left hip
     M25.059   Hemarthrosis, unspecified hip ▽

√6ᵗʰ   **M25.06   Hemarthrosis, knee**
     M25.061   Hemarthrosis, right knee
     M25.062   Hemarthrosis, left knee
     M25.069   Hemarthrosis, unspecified knee ▽

√6ᵗʰ   **M25.07   Hemarthrosis, ankle and foot**
     M25.071   Hemarthrosis, right ankle
     M25.072   Hemarthrosis, left ankle
     M25.073   Hemarthrosis, unspecified ankle ▽
     M25.074   Hemarthrosis, right foot
     M25.075   Hemarthrosis, left foot
     M25.076   Hemarthrosis, unspecified foot ▽

     M25.08   Hemarthrosis, other specified site
     Hemarthrosis, vertebrae

√5ᵗʰ **M25.1   Fistula of joint**
     M25.10   Fistula, unspecified joint ▽

√6ᵗʰ   **M25.11   Fistula, shoulder**
     M25.111   Fistula, right shoulder
     M25.112   Fistula, left shoulder
     M25.119   Fistula, unspecified shoulder ▽

√6ᵗʰ   **M25.12   Fistula, elbow**
     M25.121   Fistula, right elbow
     M25.122   Fistula, left elbow
     M25.129   Fistula, unspecified elbow ▽

√6ᵗʰ   **M25.13   Fistula, wrist**
     M25.131   Fistula, right wrist
     M25.132   Fistula, left wrist
     M25.139   Fistula, unspecified wrist ▽

√6ᵗʰ   **M25.14   Fistula, hand**
     M25.141   Fistula, right hand
     M25.142   Fistula, left hand
     M25.149   Fistula, unspecified hand ▽

√6ᵗʰ   **M25.15   Fistula, hip**
     M25.151   Fistula, right hip
     M25.152   Fistula, left hip
     M25.159   Fistula, unspecified hip ▽

√6ᵗʰ   **M25.16   Fistula, knee**
     M25.161   Fistula, right knee
     M25.162   Fistula, left knee
     M25.169   Fistula, unspecified knee ▽

√6ᵗʰ   **M25.17   Fistula, ankle and foot**
     M25.171   Fistula, right ankle

M25.172 Fistula, left ankle
M25.173 Fistula, unspecified ankle ▽
M25.174 Fistula, right foot
M25.175 Fistula, left foot
M25.176 Fistula, unspecified foot ▽
M25.18 Fistula, other specified site
Fistula, vertebrae

√5ᵗʰ M25.2 Flail joint
DEF: Hinged joint that exhibits an abnormal or excessive degree of range and mobility.
M25.20 Flail joint, unspecified joint ▽
√6ᵗʰ M25.21 Flail joint, shoulder
M25.211 Flail joint, right shoulder
M25.212 Flail joint, left shoulder
M25.219 Flail joint, unspecified shoulder ▽
√6ᵗʰ M25.22 Flail joint, elbow
M25.221 Flail joint, right elbow
M25.222 Flail joint, left elbow
M25.229 Flail joint, unspecified elbow ▽
√6ᵗʰ M25.23 Flail joint, wrist
M25.231 Flail joint, right wrist
M25.232 Flail joint, left wrist
M25.239 Flail joint, unspecified wrist ▽
√6ᵗʰ M25.24 Flail joint, hand
M25.241 Flail joint, right hand
M25.242 Flail joint, left hand
M25.249 Flail joint, unspecified hand ▽
√6ᵗʰ M25.25 Flail joint, hip
M25.251 Flail joint, right hip
M25.252 Flail joint, left hip
M25.259 Flail joint, unspecified hip ▽
√6ᵗʰ M25.26 Flail joint, knee
M25.261 Flail joint, right knee
M25.262 Flail joint, left knee
M25.269 Flail joint, unspecified knee ▽
√6ᵗʰ M25.27 Flail joint, ankle and foot
M25.271 Flail joint, right ankle and foot
M25.272 Flail joint, left ankle and foot
M25.279 Flail joint, unspecified ankle and foot ▽
M25.28 Flail joint, other site

√5ᵗʰ M25.3 Other instability of joint
EXCLUDES 1 instability of joint secondary to old ligament injury (M24.2-)
instability of joint secondary to removal of joint prosthesis (M96.8-)
EXCLUDES 2 spinal instabilities (M53.2-)
M25.30 Other instability, unspecified joint ▽
√6ᵗʰ M25.31 Other instability, shoulder
M25.311 Other instability, right shoulder
M25.312 Other instability, left shoulder
M25.319 Other instability, unspecified shoulder ▽
√6ᵗʰ M25.32 Other instability, elbow
M25.321 Other instability, right elbow
M25.322 Other instability, left elbow
M25.329 Other instability, unspecified elbow ▽
√6ᵗʰ M25.33 Other instability, wrist
M25.331 Other instability, right wrist
M25.332 Other instability, left wrist
M25.339 Other instability, unspecified wrist ▽
√6ᵗʰ M25.34 Other instability, hand
M25.341 Other instability, right hand
M25.342 Other instability, left hand
M25.349 Other instability, unspecified hand ▽
√6ᵗʰ M25.35 Other instability, hip
M25.351 Other instability, right hip
M25.352 Other instability, left hip
M25.359 Other instability, unspecified hip ▽
√6ᵗʰ M25.36 Other instability, knee
M25.361 Other instability, right knee
M25.362 Other instability, left knee

M25.369 Other instability, unspecified knee ▽
√6ᵗʰ M25.37 Other instability, ankle and foot
M25.371 Other instability, right ankle
M25.372 Other instability, left ankle
M25.373 Other instability, unspecified ankle ▽
M25.374 Other instability, right foot
M25.375 Other instability, left foot
M25.376 Other instability, unspecified foot ▽

√5ᵗʰ M25.4 Effusion of joint
EXCLUDES 1 hydrarthrosis in yaws (A66.6)
intermittent hydrarthrosis (M12.4-)
other infective (teno)synovitis (M65.1-)
M25.40 Effusion, unspecified joint ▽
√6ᵗʰ M25.41 Effusion, shoulder
M25.411 Effusion, right shoulder
M25.412 Effusion, left shoulder
M25.419 Effusion, unspecified shoulder ▽
√6ᵗʰ M25.42 Effusion, elbow
M25.421 Effusion, right elbow
M25.422 Effusion, left elbow
M25.429 Effusion, unspecified elbow ▽
√6ᵗʰ M25.43 Effusion, wrist
M25.431 Effusion, right wrist
M25.432 Effusion, left wrist
M25.439 Effusion, unspecified wrist ▽
√6ᵗʰ M25.44 Effusion, hand
M25.441 Effusion, right hand
M25.442 Effusion, left hand
M25.449 Effusion, unspecified hand ▽
√6ᵗʰ M25.45 Effusion, hip
M25.451 Effusion, right hip
M25.452 Effusion, left hip
M25.459 Effusion, unspecified hip ▽
√6ᵗʰ M25.46 Effusion, knee
M25.461 Effusion, right knee
M25.462 Effusion, left knee
M25.469 Effusion, unspecified knee ▽
√6ᵗʰ M25.47 Effusion, ankle and foot
M25.471 Effusion, right ankle
M25.472 Effusion, left ankle
M25.473 Effusion, unspecified ankle ▽
M25.474 Effusion, right foot
M25.475 Effusion, left foot
M25.476 Effusion, unspecified foot ▽
M25.48 Effusion, other site

√5ᵗʰ M25.5 Pain in joint
EXCLUDES 2 pain in hand (M79.64-)
pain in fingers (M79.64-)
pain in foot (M79.67-)
pain in limb (M79.6-)
pain in toes (M79.67-)
M25.50 Pain in unspecified joint ▽
√6ᵗʰ M25.51 Pain in shoulder
M25.511 Pain in right shoulder
M25.512 Pain in left shoulder
M25.519 Pain in unspecified shoulder ▽
√6ᵗʰ M25.52 Pain in elbow
M25.521 Pain in right elbow
M25.522 Pain in left elbow
M25.529 Pain in unspecified elbow ▽
√6ᵗʰ M25.53 Pain in wrist
M25.531 Pain in right wrist
M25.532 Pain in left wrist
M25.539 Pain in unspecified wrist ▽
√6ᵗʰ M25.54 Pain in joints of hand
AHA: 2016,4Q,38
M25.541 Pain in joints of right hand
M25.542 Pain in joints of left hand
M25.549 Pain in joints of unspecified hand ▽
Pain in joints of hand NOS
√6ᵗʰ M25.55 Pain in hip
M25.551 Pain in right hip
M25.552 Pain in left hip

M25.559 Pain in unspecified hip ▽

✓6ᵗʰ M25.56 Pain in knee
    M25.561 Pain in right knee
    M25.562 Pain in left knee
    M25.569 Pain in unspecified knee ▽

✓6ᵗʰ M25.57 Pain in ankle and joints of foot
    M25.571 Pain in right ankle and joints of right foot
    M25.572 Pain in left ankle and joints of left foot
    M25.579 Pain in unspecified ankle and ▽
        joints of unspecified foot

✓5ᵗʰ M25.6 Stiffness of joint, not elsewhere classified
    EXCLUDES 1   ankylosis of joint (M24.6-)
            contracture of joint (M24.5-)

    M25.60 Stiffness of unspecified joint, not elsewhere ▽
        classified

✓6ᵗʰ M25.61 Stiffness of shoulder, not elsewhere classified
    M25.611 Stiffness of right shoulder, not elsewhere
        classified
    M25.612 Stiffness of left shoulder, not elsewhere
        classified
    M25.619 Stiffness of unspecified shoulder, ▽
        not elsewhere classified

✓6ᵗʰ M25.62 Stiffness of elbow, not elsewhere classified
    M25.621 Stiffness of right elbow, not elsewhere
        classified
    M25.622 Stiffness of left elbow, not elsewhere
        classified
    M25.629 Stiffness of unspecified elbow, ▽
        not elsewhere classified

✓6ᵗʰ M25.63 Stiffness of wrist, not elsewhere classified
    M25.631 Stiffness of right wrist, not elsewhere
        classified
    M25.632 Stiffness of left wrist, not elsewhere
        classified
    M25.639 Stiffness of unspecified wrist, not ▽
        elsewhere classified

✓6ᵗʰ M25.64 Stiffness of hand, not elsewhere classified
    M25.641 Stiffness of right hand, not elsewhere
        classified
    M25.642 Stiffness of left hand, not elsewhere
        classified
    M25.649 Stiffness of unspecified hand, not ▽
        elsewhere classified

✓6ᵗʰ M25.65 Stiffness of hip, not elsewhere classified
    M25.651 Stiffness of right hip, not elsewhere
        classified
    M25.652 Stiffness of left hip, not elsewhere
        classified
    M25.659 Stiffness of unspecified hip, not ▽
        elsewhere classified

✓6ᵗʰ M25.66 Stiffness of knee, not elsewhere classified
    M25.661 Stiffness of right knee, not elsewhere
        classified
    M25.662 Stiffness of left knee, not elsewhere
        classified
    M25.669 Stiffness of unspecified knee, not ▽
        elsewhere classified

✓6ᵗʰ M25.67 Stiffness of ankle and foot, not elsewhere classified
    M25.671 Stiffness of right ankle, not elsewhere
        classified
    M25.672 Stiffness of left ankle, not elsewhere
        classified
    M25.673 Stiffness of unspecified ankle, not ▽
        elsewhere classified
    M25.674 Stiffness of right foot, not elsewhere
        classified
    M25.675 Stiffness of left foot, not elsewhere
        classified
    M25.676 Stiffness of unspecified foot, not ▽
        elsewhere classified

✓5ᵗʰ M25.7 Osteophyte
    M25.70 Osteophyte, unspecified joint ▽
✓6ᵗʰ M25.71 Osteophyte, shoulder
    M25.711 Osteophyte, right shoulder
    M25.712 Osteophyte, left shoulder
    M25.719 Osteophyte, unspecified shoulder ▽
✓6ᵗʰ M25.72 Osteophyte, elbow
    M25.721 Osteophyte, right elbow
    M25.722 Osteophyte, left elbow

    M25.729 Osteophyte, unspecified elbow ▽
✓6ᵗʰ M25.73 Osteophyte, wrist
    M25.731 Osteophyte, right wrist
    M25.732 Osteophyte, left wrist
    M25.739 Osteophyte, unspecified wrist ▽
✓6ᵗʰ M25.74 Osteophyte, hand
    M25.741 Osteophyte, right hand
    M25.742 Osteophyte, left hand
    M25.749 Osteophyte, unspecified hand ▽
✓6ᵗʰ M25.75 Osteophyte, hip
    M25.751 Osteophyte, right hip
    M25.752 Osteophyte, left hip
    M25.759 Osteophyte, unspecified hip ▽
✓6ᵗʰ M25.76 Osteophyte, knee
    M25.761 Osteophyte, right knee
    M25.762 Osteophyte, left knee
    M25.769 Osteophyte, unspecified knee ▽
✓6ᵗʰ M25.77 Osteophyte, ankle and foot
    M25.771 Osteophyte, right ankle
    M25.772 Osteophyte, left ankle
    M25.773 Osteophyte, unspecified ankle ▽
    M25.774 Osteophyte, right foot
    M25.775 Osteophyte, left foot
    M25.776 Osteophyte, unspecified foot ▽
    M25.78 Osteophyte, vertebrae

✓5ᵗʰ M25.8 Other specified joint disorders
    M25.80 Other specified joint disorders, unspecified ▽
        joint
✓6ᵗʰ M25.81 Other specified joint disorders, shoulder
    M25.811 Other specified joint disorders, right
        shoulder
    M25.812 Other specified joint disorders, left
        shoulder
    M25.819 Other specified joint disorders, ▽
        unspecified shoulder
✓6ᵗʰ M25.82 Other specified joint disorders, elbow
    M25.821 Other specified joint disorders, right
        elbow
    M25.822 Other specified joint disorders, left elbow
    M25.829 Other specified joint disorders, ▽
        unspecified elbow
✓6ᵗʰ M25.83 Other specified joint disorders, wrist
    M25.831 Other specified joint disorders, right wrist
    M25.832 Other specified joint disorders, left wrist
    M25.839 Other specified joint disorders, ▽
        unspecified wrist
✓6ᵗʰ M25.84 Other specified joint disorders, hand
    M25.841 Other specified joint disorders, right hand
    M25.842 Other specified joint disorders, left hand
    M25.849 Other specified joint disorders, ▽
        unspecified hand
✓6ᵗʰ M25.85 Other specified joint disorders, hip
    AHA: 2014,4Q,25
    M25.851 Other specified joint disorders, right hip
    M25.852 Other specified joint disorders, left hip
    M25.859 Other specified joint disorders, ▽
        unspecified hip
✓6ᵗʰ M25.86 Other specified joint disorders, knee
    M25.861 Other specified joint disorders, right knee
    M25.862 Other specified joint disorders, left knee
    M25.869 Other specified joint disorders, ▽
        unspecified knee
✓6ᵗʰ M25.87 Other specified joint disorders, ankle and foot
    M25.871 Other specified joint disorders, right
        ankle and foot
    M25.872 Other specified joint disorders, left ankle
        and foot
    M25.879 Other specified joint disorders, ▽
        unspecified ankle and foot

M25.9 Joint disorder, unspecified ▽

Dentofacial anomalies [including malocclusion] and other disorders of jaw (M26-M27)

EXCLUDES 1　hemifacial atrophy or hypertrophy (Q67.4)
unilateral condylar hyperplasia or hypoplasia (M27.8)

✓4ᵗʰ **M26　Dentofacial anomalies [including malocclusion]**

✓5ᵗʰ **M26.0　Major anomalies of jaw size**

EXCLUDES 1　acromegaly (E22.0)
Robin's syndrome (Q87.0)

M26.00　Unspecified anomaly of jaw size　▽
M26.01　Maxillary hyperplasia
M26.02　Maxillary hypoplasia
　　　　AHA: 2014,3Q,23
M26.03　Mandibular hyperplasia
M26.04　Mandibular hypoplasia
M26.05　Macrogenia
M26.06　Microgenia
M26.07　Excessive tuberosity of jaw
　　　　Entire maxillary tuberosity
M26.09　Other specified anomalies of jaw size

✓5ᵗʰ **M26.1　Anomalies of jaw-cranial base relationship**

M26.10　Unspecified anomaly of jaw-cranial base relationship　▽
M26.11　Maxillary asymmetry
M26.12　Other jaw asymmetry
M26.19　Other specified anomalies of jaw-cranial base relationship

✓5ᵗʰ **M26.2　Anomalies of dental arch relationship**

M26.20　Unspecified anomaly of dental arch relationship　▽

✓6ᵗʰ M26.21　Malocclusion, Angle's class
　　M26.211　Malocclusion, Angle's class I
　　　　　　Neutro-occlusion
　　M26.212　Malocclusion, Angle's class II
　　　　　　Disto-occlusion Division I
　　　　　　Disto-occlusion Division II
　　M26.213　Malocclusion, Angle's class III
　　　　　　Mesio-occlusion
　　M26.219　Malocclusion, Angle's class, unspecified　▽

✓6ᵗʰ M26.22　Open occlusal relationship
　　M26.220　Open anterior occlusal relationship
　　　　　　▶Anterior open bite◀
　　M26.221　Open posterior occlusal relationship
　　　　　　▶Posterior open bite◀

M26.23　Excessive horizontal overlap
　　　　Excessive horizontal overjet
M26.24　Reverse articulation
　　　　Crossbite (anterior) (posterior)
M26.25　Anomalies of interarch distance
M26.29　Other anomalies of dental arch relationship
　　　　Midline deviation of dental arch
　　　　Overbite (excessive) deep
　　　　Overbite (excessive) horizontal
　　　　Overbite (excessive) vertical
　　　　Posterior lingual occlusion of mandibular teeth

✓5ᵗʰ **M26.3　Anomalies of tooth position of fully erupted tooth or teeth**

EXCLUDES 2　embedded and impacted teeth (K01.-)

M26.30　Unspecified anomaly of tooth position of fully erupted tooth or teeth　▽
　　　　Abnormal spacing of fully erupted tooth or teeth NOS
　　　　Displacement of fully erupted tooth or teeth NOS
　　　　Transposition of fully erupted tooth or teeth NOS
M26.31　Crowding of fully erupted teeth
M26.32　Excessive spacing of fully erupted teeth
　　　　Diastema of fully erupted tooth or teeth NOS
M26.33　Horizontal displacement of fully erupted tooth or teeth
　　　　Tipped tooth or teeth
　　　　Tipping of fully erupted tooth
M26.34　Vertical displacement of fully erupted tooth or teeth
　　　　Extruded tooth
　　　　Infraeruption of tooth or teeth
　　　　Supraeruption of tooth or teeth
M26.35　Rotation of fully erupted tooth or teeth

M26.36　Insufficient interocclusal distance of fully erupted teeth (ridge)
　　　　Lack of adequate intermaxillary vertical dimension of fully erupted teeth
M26.37　Excessive interocclusal distance of fully erupted teeth
　　　　Excessive intermaxillary vertical dimension of fully erupted teeth
　　　　Loss of occlusal vertical dimension of fully erupted teeth
M26.39　Other anomalies of tooth position of fully erupted tooth or teeth

M26.4　Malocclusion, unspecified　▽

✓5ᵗʰ **M26.5　Dentofacial functional abnormalities**

EXCLUDES 1　bruxism (F45.8)
teeth-grinding NOS (F45.8)

M26.50　Dentofacial functional abnormalities, unspecified　▽
M26.51　Abnormal jaw closure
M26.52　Limited mandibular range of motion
M26.53　Deviation in opening and closing of the mandible
M26.54　Insufficient anterior guidance
　　　　Insufficient anterior occlusal guidance
M26.55　Centric occlusion maximum intercuspation discrepancy
　　　　EXCLUDES 1　centric occlusion NOS (M26.59)
M26.56　Non-working side interference
　　　　Balancing side interference
M26.57　Lack of posterior occlusal support
M26.59　Other dentofacial functional abnormalities
　　　　Centric occlusion (of teeth) NOS
　　　　Malocclusion due to abnormal swallowing
　　　　Malocclusion due to mouth breathing
　　　　Malocclusion due to tongue, lip or finger habits

✓5ᵗʰ **M26.6　Temporomandibular joint disorders**

EXCLUDES 2　current temporomandibular joint dislocation (S03.0)
current temporomandibular joint sprain (S03.4)

AHA: 2016,4Q,38-39

Temporomandibular Joint

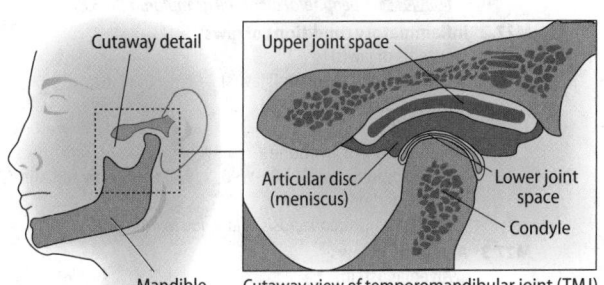

Cutaway detail　Upper joint space
Articular disc (meniscus)　Lower joint space
Condyle
Mandible　Cutaway view of temporomandibular joint (TMJ)

✓6ᵗʰ M26.60　Temporomandibular joint disorder, unspecified
　　M26.601　Right temporomandibular joint disorder, unspecified　▽
　　M26.602　Left temporomandibular joint disorder, unspecified　▽
　　M26.603　Bilateral temporomandibular joint disorder, unspecified　▽
　　M26.609　Unspecified temporomandibular joint disorder, unspecified side　▽
　　　　　　Temporomandibular joint disorder NOS

✓6ᵗʰ M26.61　Adhesions and ankylosis of temporomandibular joint
　　M26.611　Adhesions and ankylosis of right temporomandibular joint
　　M26.612　Adhesions and ankylosis of left temporomandibular joint
　　M26.613　Adhesions and ankylosis of bilateral temporomandibular joint
　　M26.619　Adhesions and ankylosis of temporomandibular joint, unspecified side　▽

✓6ᵗʰ M26.62　Arthralgia of temporomandibular joint
▲　　M26.621　Arthralgia of right temporomandibular joint

✓ Additional Character Req　　✓x7ᵗʰ Placeholder Alert　　Manifestation　　▽ Unspecified　　▶◀ Revised Text　　● New Code　　▲ Revised Code Title

ICD-10-CM 2019　　　　　　　　　　　　　　　　　　　　　　　　　　　　　　　　　　　　　775

M26.622 **Arthralgia of** left **temporomandibular joint**

M26.623 **Arthralgia of** bilateral **temporomandibular joint**

M26.629 **Arthralgia of temporomandibular joint, unspecified side** ▽

✓6ᵗʰ M26.63 Articular disc disorder of temporomandibular joint

M26.631 **Articular disc disorder of** right **temporomandibular joint**

M26.632 **Articular disc disorder of** left **temporomandibular joint**

M26.633 **Articular disc disorder of** bilateral **temporomandibular joint**

M26.639 **Articular disc disorder of** ▽ **temporomandibular joint, unspecified side**

M26.69 **Other specified disorders of temporomandibular joint**

✓5ᵗʰ M26.7 **Dental alveolar anomalies**

M26.70 **Unspecified alveolar anomaly** ▽

M26.71 **Alveolar** maxillary hyperplasia

M26.72 **Alveolar** mandibular hyperplasia

M26.73 **Alveolar** maxillary hypoplasia

M26.74 **Alveolar** mandibular hypoplasia

M26.79 **Other specified alveolar anomalies**

✓5ᵗʰ M26.8 **Other dentofacial anomalies**

M26.81 **Anterior soft tissue impingement**
Anterior soft tissue impingement on teeth

M26.82 **Posterior soft tissue impingement**
Posterior soft tissue impingement on teeth

M26.89 **Other dentofacial anomalies**

M26.9 **Dentofacial anomaly, unspecified** ▽

✓4ᵗʰ **M27 Other diseases of jaws**

M27.0 **Developmental disorders of jaws**
Latent bone cyst of jaw
Stafne's cyst
Torus mandibularis
Torus palatinus

M27.1 **Giant cell granuloma, central**
Giant cell granuloma NOS
EXCLUDES 1 *peripheral giant cell granuloma (K06.8)*

M27.2 **Inflammatory conditions of jaws**
Osteitis of jaw(s)
Osteomyelitis (neonatal) jaw(s)
Osteoradionecrosis jaw(s)
Periostitis jaw(s)
Sequestrum of jaw bone
Use additional code (W88-W90, X39.0) to identify radiation, if radiation-induced
EXCLUDES 2 *osteonecrosis of jaw due to drug (M87.180)*

M27.3 **Alveolitis of jaws**
Alveolar osteitis
Dry socket

✓5ᵗʰ M27.4 **Other and unspecified cysts of jaw**
EXCLUDES 1 *cysts of oral region (K09.-)*
latent bone cyst of jaw (M27.0)
Stafne's cyst (M27.0)

M27.40 **Unspecified cyst of jaw** ▽
Cyst of jaw NOS

M27.49 **Other cysts of jaw**
Aneurysmal cyst of jaw
Hemorrhagic cyst of jaw
Traumatic cyst of jaw

✓5ᵗʰ M27.5 **Periradicular pathology associated with previous endodontic treatment**

M27.51 **Perforation of root canal space due to endodontic treatment**

M27.52 **Endodontic overfill**

M27.53 **Endodontic underfill**

M27.59 **Other periradicular pathology associated with previous endodontic treatment**

✓5ᵗʰ M27.6 **Endosseous dental implant failure**

M27.61 **Osseointegration failure of dental implant**
Hemorrhagic complications of dental implant placement
Iatrogenic osseointegration failure of dental implant
Osseointegration failure of dental implant due to complications of systemic disease
Osseointegration failure of dental implant due to poor bone quality
Pre-integration failure of dental implant NOS
Pre-osseointegration failure of dental implant

M27.62 **Post-osseointegration biological failure of dental implant**
Failure of dental implant due to lack of attached gingiva
Failure of dental implant due to occlusal trauma (caused by poor prosthetic design)
Failure of dental implant due to parafunctional habits
Failure of dental implant due to periodontal infection (peri-implantitis)
Failure of dental implant due to poor oral hygiene
Iatrogenic post-osseointegration failure of dental implant
Post-osseointegration failure of dental implant due to complications of systemic disease

M27.63 **Post-osseointegration mechanical failure of dental implant**
Failure of dental prosthesis causing loss of dental implant
Fracture of dental implant
EXCLUDES 2 *cracked tooth (K03.81)*
fractured dental restorative material with loss of material (K08.531)
fractured dental restorative material without loss of material (K08.530)
fractured tooth (S02.5)

M27.69 **Other endosseous dental implant failure**
Dental implant failure NOS

M27.8 **Other specified diseases of jaws**
Cherubism
Exostosis
Fibrous dysplasia
Unilateral condylar hyperplasia
Unilateral condylar hypoplasia
EXCLUDES 1 *jaw pain (R68.84)*

M27.9 **Disease of jaws, unspecified** ▽

Systemic connective tissue disorders (M30-M36)

INCLUDES autoimmune disease NOS
collagen (vascular) disease NOS
systemic autoimmune disease
systemic collagen (vascular) disease
EXCLUDES 1 *autoimmune disease, single organ or single cell-type-code to relevant condition category*

✓4ᵗʰ **M30 Polyarteritis nodosa and related conditions**
EXCLUDES 1 *microscopic polyarteritis (M31.7)*

M30.0 **Polyarteritis nodosa** HCC

M30.1 **Polyarteritis with lung involvement [Churg-Strauss]** HCC
Allergic granulomatous angiitis

M30.2 **Juvenile polyarteritis** HCC

M30.3 **Mucocutaneous lymph node syndrome [Kawasaki]** HCC

M30.8 **Other conditions related to polyarteritis nodosa** HCC
Polyangiitis overlap syndrome

✓4ᵗʰ **M31 Other necrotizing vasculopathies**

M31.0 **Hypersensitivity angiitis** HCC
Goodpasture's syndrome

M31.1 **Thrombotic microangiopathy** HCC
Thrombotic thrombocytopenic purpura

M31.2 **Lethal midline granuloma** HCC

✓5ᵗʰ M31.3 **Wegener's granulomatosis**
Necrotizing respiratory granulomatosis

M31.30 **Wegener's granulomatosis without renal involvement** HCC
Wegener's granulomatosis NOS

M31.31 **Wegener's granulomatosis with renal involvement** HCC

M31.4 **Aortic arch syndrome [Takayasu]** HCC

M31.5 **Giant cell arteritis with polymyalgia rheumatica** HCC
M31.6 **Other giant cell arteritis** HCC
M31.7 **Microscopic polyangiitis** HCC
    Microscopic polyarteritis
    EXCLUDES 1   polyarteritis nodosa (M30.0)
M31.8 **Other specified necrotizing vasculopathies** HCC
    Hypocomplementemic vasculitis
    Septic vasculitis
M31.9 **Necrotizing vasculopathy, unspecified** HCC ▽

✓4ᵗʰ **M32 Systemic lupus erythematosus (SLE)**
    EXCLUDES 1   lupus erythematosus (discoid) (NOS) (L93.0)
M32.0 **Drug-induced systemic lupus erythematosus** HCC
    Use additional code for adverse effect, if applicable, to identify drug (T36-T50 with fifth or sixth character 5)
✓5ᵗʰ M32.1 **Systemic lupus erythematosus with organ or system involvement**
    M32.10 **Systemic lupus erythematosus, organ or system involvement unspecified** HCC ▽
    M32.11 **Endocarditis in systemic lupus erythematosus** HCC
       Libman-Sacks disease
    M32.12 **Pericarditis in systemic lupus erythematosus** HCC
       Lupus pericarditis
    M32.13 **Lung involvement in systemic lupus erythematosus** HCC
       Pleural effusion due to systemic lupus erythematosus
    M32.14 **Glomerular disease in systemic lupus erythematosus** HCC
       Lupus renal disease NOS
       AHA: 2013,4Q,125
    M32.15 **Tubulo-interstitial nephropathy in systemic lupus erythematosus** HCC
    M32.19 **Other organ or system involvement in systemic lupus erythematosus**
M32.8 **Other forms of systemic lupus erythematosus** HCC
M32.9 **Systemic lupus erythematosus, unspecified** HCC ▽
    SLE NOS
    Systemic lupus erythematosus NOS
    Systemic lupus erythematosus without organ involvement

✓4ᵗʰ **M33 Dermatopolymyositis**
    AHA: 2017,4Q,18
✓5ᵗʰ M33.0 **Juvenile dermatomyositis**
    M33.00 **Juvenile dermatomyositis, organ involvement unspecified** HCC ▽
    M33.01 **Juvenile dermatomyositis with respiratory involvement** HCC
    M33.02 **Juvenile dermatomyositis with myopathy** HCC
    M33.03 **Juvenile dermatomyositis without myopathy** HCC
    M33.09 **Juvenile dermatomyositis with other organ involvement** HCC
✓5ᵗʰ M33.1 **Other dermatomyositis**
    Adult dermatomyositis
    M33.10 **Other dermatomyositis, organ involvement unspecified** HCC ▽
    M33.11 **Other dermatomyositis with respiratory involvement** HCC
    M33.12 **Other dermatomyositis with myopathy** HCC
    M33.13 **Other dermatomyositis without myopathy** HCC
       Dermatomyositis NOS
    M33.19 **Other dermatomyositis with other organ involvement** HCC
✓5ᵗʰ M33.2 **Polymyositis**
    M33.20 **Polymyositis, organ involvement unspecified** HCC ▽
    M33.21 **Polymyositis with respiratory involvement** HCC
    M33.22 **Polymyositis with myopathy** HCC
    M33.29 **Polymyositis with other organ involvement** HCC
✓5ᵗʰ M33.9 **Dermatopolymyositis, unspecified**
    M33.90 **Dermatopolymyositis, unspecified, organ involvement unspecified** HCC ▽
    M33.91 **Dermatopolymyositis, unspecified with respiratory involvement** HCC ▽
    M33.92 **Dermatopolymyositis, unspecified with myopathy** HCC ▽
    M33.93 **Dermatopolymyositis, unspecified without myopathy** HCC ▽

M33.99 **Dermatopolymyositis, unspecified with other organ involvement** HCC ▽
✓4ᵗʰ **M34 Systemic sclerosis [scleroderma]**
    EXCLUDES 1   circumscribed scleroderma (L94.0)
       neonatal scleroderma (P83.8)
M34.0 **Progressive systemic sclerosis** HCC
M34.1 **CR(E)ST syndrome** HCC
    Combination of calcinosis, Raynaud's phenomenon, esophageal dysfunction, sclerodactyly, telangiectasia
M34.2 **Systemic sclerosis induced by drug and chemical** HCC
    Code first poisoning due to drug or toxin, if applicable (T36-T65 with fifth or sixth character 1-4 or 6)
    Use additional code for adverse effect, if applicable, to identify drug (T36-T50 with fifth or sixth character 5)
✓5ᵗʰ M34.8 **Other forms of systemic sclerosis**
    M34.81 **Systemic sclerosis with lung involvement** HCC
    M34.82 **Systemic sclerosis with myopathy** HCC
    M34.83 **Systemic sclerosis with polyneuropathy** HCC
    M34.89 **Other systemic sclerosis** HCC
M34.9 **Systemic sclerosis, unspecified** HCC ▽
✓4ᵗʰ **M35 Other systemic involvement of connective tissue**
    EXCLUDES 1   reactive perforating collagenosis (L87.1)
✓5ᵗʰ M35.0 **Sicca syndrome [Sjögren]**
    DEF: Autoimmune disease associated with keratoconjunctivitis, laryngopharyngitis, rhinitis, dry mouth, enlarged parotid gland, and chronic polyarthritis.
    M35.00 **Sicca syndrome, unspecified** HCC ▽
    M35.01 **Sicca syndrome with keratoconjunctivitis** HCC
    M35.02 **Sicca syndrome with lung involvement** HCC
    M35.03 **Sicca syndrome with myopathy** HCC
    M35.04 **Sicca syndrome with tubulo-interstitial nephropathy** HCC
       Renal tubular acidosis in sicca syndrome
    M35.09 **Sicca syndrome with other organ involvement** HCC
M35.1 **Other overlap syndromes** HCC
    Mixed connective tissue disease
    EXCLUDES 1   polyangiitis overlap syndrome (M30.8)
M35.2 **Behçet's disease** HCC
M35.3 **Polymyalgia rheumatica** HCC
    EXCLUDES 1   polymyalgia rheumatica with giant cell arteritis (M31.5)
M35.4 **Diffuse (eosinophilic) fasciitis**
M35.5 **Multifocal fibrosclerosis** HCC
M35.6 **Relapsing panniculitis [Weber-Christian]**
    EXCLUDES 1   lupus panniculitis (L93.2)
       panniculitis NOS (M79.3-)
M35.7 **Hypermobility syndrome**
    Familial ligamentous laxity
    EXCLUDES 1   Ehlers-Danlos syndrome (Q79.6)
       ligamentous laxity, NOS (M24.2-)
M35.8 **Other specified systemic involvement of connective tissue** HCC
M35.9 **Systemic involvement of connective tissue, unspecified** HCC ▽
    Autoimmune disease (systemic) NOS
    Collagen (vascular) disease NOS
✓4ᵗʰ **M36 Systemic disorders of connective tissue in diseases classified elsewhere**
    EXCLUDES 2   arthropathies in diseases classified elsewhere (M14.-)
M36.0 *Dermato(poly)myositis in neoplastic disease* HCC
    Code first underlying neoplasm (C00-D49)
M36.1 *Arthropathy in neoplastic disease*
    Code first underlying neoplasm, such as:
       leukemia (C91-C95)
       malignant histiocytosis (C96.A)
       multiple myeloma (C90.0)

M36.2   *Hemophilic arthropathy*
    Hemarthrosis in hemophilic arthropathy
    Code first underlying disease, such as:
       factor VIII deficiency (D66)
         with vascular defect (D68.0)
       factor IX deficiency (D67)
       hemophilia (classical) (D66)
       hemophilia B (D67)
       hemophilia C (D68.1)

M36.3   *Arthropathy in other blood disorders*

M36.4   *Arthropathy in hypersensitivity reactions classified elsewhere*
    Code first underlying disease, such as:
       Henoch (-Schönlein) purpura (D69.0)
       serum sickness (T80.6-)

M36.8   *Systemic disorders of connective tissue in other*   HCC
    diseases classified elsewhere
    Code first underlying disease, such as:
       alkaptonuria (E70.2)
       hypogammaglobulinemia (D80.-)
       ochronosis (E70.2)

Dorsopathies (M40-M54)

Deforming dorsopathies (M40-M43)

✓4ᵗʰ **M40**   **Kyphosis and lordosis**
    EXCLUDES 1   *congenital kyphosis and lordosis (Q76.4)*
               kyphoscoliosis (M41.-)
               postprocedural kyphosis and lordosis (M96.-)

Kyphosis and Lordosis

Kyphosis: Excessive convexity in the thoracic region

Lordosis: Excessive concavity in the lumbar region

✓5ᵗʰ **M40.0**   **Postural kyphosis**
    EXCLUDES 1   *osteochondrosis of spine (M42.-)*
    M40.00   **Postural kyphosis, site unspecified**   ▽
    M40.03   **Postural kyphosis, cervicothoracic region**
    M40.04   **Postural kyphosis, thoracic region**
    M40.05   **Postural kyphosis, thoracolumbar region**

✓5ᵗʰ **M40.1**   **Other secondary kyphosis**
    M40.10   **Other secondary kyphosis, site unspecified**   ▽
    M40.12   **Other secondary kyphosis, cervical region**
    M40.13   **Other secondary kyphosis, cervicothoracic region**
    M40.14   **Other secondary kyphosis, thoracic region**
    M40.15   **Other secondary kyphosis, thoracolumbar region**

✓5ᵗʰ **M40.2**   **Other and unspecified kyphosis**
    ✓6ᵗʰ **M40.20**   **Unspecified kyphosis**
       M40.202   **Unspecified kyphosis, cervical**   ▽
               region
       M40.203   **Unspecified kyphosis,**   ▽
               cervicothoracic region
       M40.204   **Unspecified kyphosis, thoracic**   ▽
               region
       M40.205   **Unspecified kyphosis,**   ▽
               thoracolumbar region
       M40.209   **Unspecified kyphosis, site**   ▽
               unspecified
    ✓6ᵗʰ **M40.29**   **Other kyphosis**
       M40.292   **Other kyphosis, cervical region**

       M40.293   **Other kyphosis, cervicothoracic region**
       M40.294   **Other kyphosis, thoracic region**
       M40.295   **Other kyphosis, thoracolumbar region**
       M40.299   **Other kyphosis, site unspecified**   ▽

✓5ᵗʰ **M40.3**   **Flatback syndrome**
    M40.30   **Flatback syndrome, site unspecified**   ▽
    M40.35   **Flatback syndrome, thoracolumbar region**
    M40.36   **Flatback syndrome, lumbar region**
    M40.37   **Flatback syndrome, lumbosacral region**

✓5ᵗʰ **M40.4**   **Postural lordosis**
    Acquired lordosis
    M40.40   **Postural lordosis, site unspecified**   ▽
    M40.45   **Postural lordosis, thoracolumbar region**
    M40.46   **Postural lordosis, lumbar region**
    M40.47   **Postural lordosis, lumbosacral region**

✓5ᵗʰ **M40.5**   **Lordosis, unspecified**
    M40.50   **Lordosis, unspecified, site unspecified**   ▽
    M40.55   **Lordosis, unspecified, thoracolumbar region**
    M40.56   **Lordosis, unspecified, lumbar region**
    M40.57   **Lordosis, unspecified, lumbosacral region**

✓4ᵗʰ **M41**   **Scoliosis**
    INCLUDES   kyphoscoliosis
    EXCLUDES 1   *congenital scoliosis due to bony malformation (Q76.3)*
               congenital scoliosis NOS (Q67.5)
               kyphoscoliotic heart disease (I27.1)
               postprocedural scoliosis (M96.-)
               postural congenital scoliosis (Q67.5)

Scoliosis

Lateral curvature of spine

✓5ᵗʰ **M41.0**   **Infantile idiopathic scoliosis**
    AHA: 2014,4Q,26
    M41.00   **Infantile idiopathic scoliosis, site**   ▽
               unspecified
    M41.02   **Infantile idiopathic scoliosis, cervical region**
    M41.03   **Infantile idiopathic scoliosis, cervicothoracic region**
    M41.04   **Infantile idiopathic scoliosis, thoracic region**
    M41.05   **Infantile idiopathic scoliosis, thoracolumbar region**
    M41.06   **Infantile idiopathic scoliosis, lumbar region**
    M41.07   **Infantile idiopathic scoliosis, lumbosacral region**
    M41.08   **Infantile idiopathic scoliosis, sacral and sacrococcygeal region**

✓5ᵗʰ **M41.1**   **Juvenile and adolescent idiopathic scoliosis**
    ✓6ᵗʰ **M41.11**   **Juvenile idiopathic scoliosis**
       AHA: 2014,4Q,28
       M41.112   **Juvenile idiopathic scoliosis, cervical region**
       M41.113   **Juvenile idiopathic scoliosis, cervicothoracic region**
       M41.114   **Juvenile idiopathic scoliosis, thoracic region**
       M41.115   **Juvenile idiopathic scoliosis, thoracolumbar region**
       M41.116   **Juvenile idiopathic scoliosis, lumbar region**

M41.117 Juvenile idiopathic scoliosis, **lumbosacral region**

M41.119 Juvenile idiopathic scoliosis, site unspecified ▽

✓6ᵗʰ **M41.12 Adolescent scoliosis**

M41.122 Adolescent idiopathic scoliosis, **cervical region**

M41.123 Adolescent idiopathic scoliosis, **cervicothoracic region**

M41.124 Adolescent idiopathic scoliosis, **thoracic region**

M41.125 Adolescent idiopathic scoliosis, **thoracolumbar region**

M41.126 Adolescent idiopathic scoliosis, **lumbar region**

M41.127 Adolescent idiopathic scoliosis, **lumbosacral region**

M41.129 Adolescent idiopathic scoliosis, site unspecified ▽

✓5ᵗʰ **M41.2 Other** idiopathic scoliosis

M41.20 Other idiopathic scoliosis, site unspecified ▽
M41.22 Other idiopathic scoliosis, **cervical region**
M41.23 Other idiopathic scoliosis, **cervicothoracic region**
M41.24 Other idiopathic scoliosis, **thoracic region**
M41.25 Other idiopathic scoliosis, **thoracolumbar region**
M41.26 Other idiopathic scoliosis, **lumbar region**
M41.27 Other idiopathic scoliosis, **lumbosacral region**

✓5ᵗʰ **M41.3** Thoracogenic scoliosis

M41.30 Thoracogenic scoliosis, site unspecified ▽
M41.34 Thoracogenic scoliosis, **thoracic region**
M41.35 Thoracogenic scoliosis, **thoracolumbar region**

✓5ᵗʰ **M41.4 Neuromuscular scoliosis**

Scoliosis secondary to cerebral palsy, Friedreich's ataxia, poliomyelitis and other neuromuscular disorders
Code also underlying condition
AHA: 2014,4Q,27

M41.40 Neuromuscular scoliosis, site unspecified ▽
M41.41 Neuromuscular scoliosis, **occipito-atlanto-axial region**
M41.42 Neuromuscular scoliosis, **cervical region**
M41.43 Neuromuscular scoliosis, **cervicothoracic region**
M41.44 Neuromuscular scoliosis, **thoracic region**
M41.45 Neuromuscular scoliosis, **thoracolumbar region**
M41.46 Neuromuscular scoliosis, **lumbar region**
M41.47 Neuromuscular scoliosis, **lumbosacral region**

✓5ᵗʰ **M41.5 Other** secondary scoliosis

M41.50 Other secondary scoliosis, site unspecified ▽
M41.52 Other secondary scoliosis, **cervical region**
M41.53 Other secondary scoliosis, **cervicothoracic region**
M41.54 Other secondary scoliosis, **thoracic region**
M41.55 Other secondary scoliosis, **thoracolumbar region**
M41.56 Other secondary scoliosis, **lumbar region**
M41.57 Other secondary scoliosis, **lumbosacral region**

✓5ᵗʰ **M41.8 Other forms of scoliosis**

M41.80 Other forms of scoliosis, site unspecified ▽
M41.82 Other forms of scoliosis, **cervical region**
M41.83 Other forms of scoliosis, **cervicothoracic region**
M41.84 Other forms of scoliosis, **thoracic region**
M41.85 Other forms of scoliosis, **thoracolumbar region**
M41.86 Other forms of scoliosis, **lumbar region**
M41.87 Other forms of scoliosis, **lumbosacral region**

M41.9 Scoliosis, unspecified ▽

✓4ᵗʰ **M42 Spinal osteochondrosis**

✓5ᵗʰ **M42.0 Juvenile** osteochondrosis of spine

Calvé's disease
Scheuermann's disease
EXCLUDES 1 postural kyphosis (M40.0)

M42.00 Juvenile osteochondrosis of spine, site unspecified ▽
M42.01 Juvenile osteochondrosis of spine, **occipito-atlanto-axial region**
M42.02 Juvenile osteochondrosis of spine, **cervical region**
M42.03 Juvenile osteochondrosis of spine, **cervicothoracic region**
M42.04 Juvenile osteochondrosis of spine, **thoracic region**
M42.05 Juvenile osteochondrosis of spine, **thoracolumbar region**

M42.06 Juvenile osteochondrosis of spine, **lumbar region**
M42.07 Juvenile osteochondrosis of spine, **lumbosacral region**
M42.08 Juvenile osteochondrosis of spine, **sacral and sacrococcygeal region**
M42.09 Juvenile osteochondrosis of spine, **multiple sites in spine**

✓5ᵗʰ **M42.1 Adult** osteochondrosis of spine

M42.10 Adult osteochondrosis of spine, site unspecified 🄰 ▽
M42.11 Adult osteochondrosis of spine, **occipito-atlanto-axial region** 🄰
M42.12 Adult osteochondrosis of spine, **cervical region** 🄰
M42.13 Adult osteochondrosis of spine, **cervicothoracic region** 🄰
M42.14 Adult osteochondrosis of spine, **thoracic region** 🄰
M42.15 Adult osteochondrosis of spine, **thoracolumbar region** 🄰
M42.16 Adult osteochondrosis of spine, **lumbar region** 🄰
M42.17 Adult osteochondrosis of spine, **lumbosacral region** 🄰
M42.18 Adult osteochondrosis of spine, sacral and sacrococcygeal region 🄰
M42.19 Adult osteochondrosis of spine, multiple sites in spine 🄰

M42.9 Spinal osteochondrosis, unspecified ▽

✓4ᵗʰ **M43 Other deforming dorsopathies**

EXCLUDES 1 congenital spondylolysis and spondylolisthesis (Q76.2)
hemivertebra (Q76.3-Q76.4)
Klippel-Feil syndrome (Q76.1)
lumbarization and sacralization (Q76.4)
platyspondylisis (Q76.4)
spina bifida occulta (Q76.0)
spinal curvature in osteoporosis (M80.-)
spinal curvature in Paget's disease of bone [osteitis deformans] (M88.-)

✓5ᵗʰ **M43.0 Spondylolysis**

EXCLUDES 1 congenital spondylolysis (Q76.2)
spondylolisthesis (M43.1)

M43.00 Spondylolysis, site unspecified ▽
M43.01 Spondylolysis, **occipito-atlanto-axial region**
M43.02 Spondylolysis, **cervical region**
M43.03 Spondylolysis, **cervicothoracic region**
M43.04 Spondylolysis, **thoracic region**
M43.05 Spondylolysis, **thoracolumbar region**
M43.06 Spondylolysis, **lumbar region**
M43.07 Spondylolysis, **lumbosacral region**
M43.08 Spondylolysis, **sacral and sacrococcygeal region**
M43.09 Spondylolysis, **multiple sites in spine**

✓5ᵗʰ **M43.1 Spondylolisthesis**

EXCLUDES 1 acute traumatic of lumbosacral region (S33.1)
acute traumatic of sites other than lumbosacral- code to Fracture, vertebra, by region
congenital spondylolisthesis (Q76.2)

M43.10 Spondylolisthesis, site unspecified ▽
M43.11 Spondylolisthesis, **occipito-atlanto-axial region**
M43.12 Spondylolisthesis, **cervical region**
M43.13 Spondylolisthesis, **cervicothoracic region**
M43.14 Spondylolisthesis, **thoracic region**
M43.15 Spondylolisthesis, **thoracolumbar region**
M43.16 Spondylolisthesis, **lumbar region**
M43.17 Spondylolisthesis, **lumbosacral region**
M43.18 Spondylolisthesis, **sacral and sacrococcygeal region**
M43.19 Spondylolisthesis, **multiple sites in spine**

✓5ᵗʰ **M43.2 Fusion of spine**

Ankylosis of spinal joint
EXCLUDES 1 ankylosing spondylitis (M45.0-)
congenital fusion of spine (Q76.4)
EXCLUDES 2 arthrodesis status (Z98.1)
pseudoarthrosis after fusion or arthrodesis (M96.0)

M43.20 Fusion of spine, site unspecified ▽
M43.21 Fusion of spine, **occipito-atlanto-axial region**
M43.22 Fusion of spine, **cervical region**
M43.23 Fusion of spine, **cervicothoracic region**

☑ Additional Character Req   ✓x7ᵗʰ Placeholder Alert   Manifestation   ▽ Unspecified   ►◄ Revised Text   ● New Code   ▲ Revised Code Title

ICD-10-CM 2019   779

M43.24   **Fusion of spine, thoracic region**
M43.25   **Fusion of spine, thoracolumbar region**
M43.26   **Fusion of spine, lumbar region**
M43.27   **Fusion of spine, lumbosacral region**
M43.28   **Fusion of spine, sacral and sacrococcygeal region**

M43.3   **Recurrent atlantoaxial dislocation with myelopathy**
M43.4   **Other recurrent atlantoaxial dislocation**

√5ᵗʰ   M43.5   **Other recurrent vertebral dislocation**

> EXCLUDES 1   biomechanical lesions NEC (M99.-)

√6ᵗʰ   M43.5X   **Other recurrent vertebral dislocation**

M43.5X2   **Other recurrent vertebral dislocation, cervical region**
M43.5X3   **Other recurrent vertebral dislocation, cervicothoracic region**
M43.5X4   **Other recurrent vertebral dislocation, thoracic region**
M43.5X5   **Other recurrent vertebral dislocation, thoracolumbar region**
M43.5X6   **Other recurrent vertebral dislocation, lumbar region**
M43.5X7   **Other recurrent vertebral dislocation, lumbosacral region**
M43.5X8   **Other recurrent vertebral dislocation, sacral and sacrococcygeal region**
M43.5X9   **Other recurrent vertebral dislocation, site unspecified** ▽

M43.6   **Torticollis**

> EXCLUDES 1   congenital (sternomastoid) torticollis (Q68.0)
> current injury - see Injury, of spine, by body region
> ocular torticollis (R29.891)
> psychogenic torticollis (F45.8)
> spasmodic torticollis (G24.3)
> torticollis due to birth injury (P15.2)

> **DEF:** Twisted, unnatural position of the neck due to contracted cervical muscles that pull the head to one side.

√5ᵗʰ   M43.8   **Other specified deforming dorsopathies**

> EXCLUDES 2   kyphosis and lordosis (M40.-)
> scoliosis (M41.-)

√6ᵗʰ   M43.8X   **Other specified deforming dorsopathies**

M43.8X1   **Other specified deforming dorsopathies, occipito-atlanto-axial region**
M43.8X2   **Other specified deforming dorsopathies, cervical region**
M43.8X3   **Other specified deforming dorsopathies, cervicothoracic region**
M43.8X4   **Other specified deforming dorsopathies, thoracic region**
M43.8X5   **Other specified deforming dorsopathies, thoracolumbar region**
M43.8X6   **Other specified deforming dorsopathies, lumbar region**
M43.8X7   **Other specified deforming dorsopathies, lumbosacral region**
M43.8X8   **Other specified deforming dorsopathies, sacral and sacrococcygeal region**
M43.8X9   **Other specified deforming dorsopathies, site unspecified** ▽

M43.9   **Deforming dorsopathy, unspecified** ▽
Curvature of spine NOS

Spondylopathies (M45-M49)

√4ᵗʰ   **M45   Ankylosing spondylitis**

Rheumatoid arthritis of spine

> EXCLUDES 1   arthropathy in Reiter's disease (M02.3-)
> juvenile (ankylosing) spondylitis (M08.1)

> EXCLUDES 2   Behçet's disease (M35.2)

M45.0   **Ankylosing spondylitis of multiple sites in spine** HCC
M45.1   **Ankylosing spondylitis of occipito-atlanto-axial region** HCC
M45.2   **Ankylosing spondylitis of cervical region** HCC
M45.3   **Ankylosing spondylitis of cervicothoracic region** HCC
M45.4   **Ankylosing spondylitis of thoracic region** HCC
M45.5   **Ankylosing spondylitis of thoracolumbar region** HCC
M45.6   **Ankylosing spondylitis lumbar region** HCC
M45.7   **Ankylosing spondylitis of lumbosacral region** HCC
M45.8   **Ankylosing spondylitis sacral and sacrococcygeal region** HCC
M45.9   **Ankylosing spondylitis of unspecified sites in spine** HCC ▽

√4ᵗʰ   **M46   Other inflammatory spondylopathies**

√5ᵗʰ   M46.0   **Spinal enthesopathy**

Disorder of ligamentous or muscular attachments of spine

M46.00   **Spinal enthesopathy, site unspecified** HCC ▽
M46.01   **Spinal enthesopathy, occipito-atlanto-axial region** HCC
M46.02   **Spinal enthesopathy, cervical region** HCC
M46.03   **Spinal enthesopathy, cervicothoracic region** HCC
M46.04   **Spinal enthesopathy, thoracic region** HCC
M46.05   **Spinal enthesopathy, thoracolumbar region** HCC
M46.06   **Spinal enthesopathy, lumbar region** HCC
M46.07   **Spinal enthesopathy, lumbosacral region** HCC
M46.08   **Spinal enthesopathy, sacral and sacrococcygeal region** HCC
M46.09   **Spinal enthesopathy, multiple sites in spine** HCC

M46.1   **Sacroiliitis, not elsewhere classified** HCC

> **DEF:** Inflammation of the sacroiliac joint (situated at the juncture of the sacrum and hip). Symptoms include pain in the buttocks or lower back that can extend down one or both legs.

√5ᵗʰ   M46.2   **Osteomyelitis of vertebra**

M46.20   **Osteomyelitis of vertebra, site unspecified** HCC ▽
M46.21   **Osteomyelitis of vertebra, occipito-atlanto-axial region** HCC
M46.22   **Osteomyelitis of vertebra, cervical region** HCC
M46.23   **Osteomyelitis of vertebra, cervicothoracic region** HCC
M46.24   **Osteomyelitis of vertebra, thoracic region** HCC
M46.25   **Osteomyelitis of vertebra, thoracolumbar region** HCC
M46.26   **Osteomyelitis of vertebra, lumbar region** HCC
M46.27   **Osteomyelitis of vertebra, lumbosacral region** HCC
M46.28   **Osteomyelitis of vertebra, sacral and sacrococcygeal region** HCC

√5ᵗʰ   M46.3   **Infection of intervertebral disc (pyogenic)**

Use additional code (B95-B97) to identify infectious agent

M46.30   **Infection of intervertebral disc (pyogenic), site unspecified** HCC ▽
M46.31   **Infection of intervertebral disc (pyogenic), occipito-atlanto-axial region** HCC
M46.32   **Infection of intervertebral disc (pyogenic), cervical region** HCC
M46.33   **Infection of intervertebral disc (pyogenic), cervicothoracic region** HCC
M46.34   **Infection of intervertebral disc (pyogenic), thoracic region** HCC
M46.35   **Infection of intervertebral disc (pyogenic), thoracolumbar region** HCC
M46.36   **Infection of intervertebral disc (pyogenic), lumbar region** HCC
M46.37   **Infection of intervertebral disc (pyogenic), lumbosacral region** HCC
M46.38   **Infection of intervertebral disc (pyogenic), sacral and sacrococcygeal region** HCC
M46.39   **Infection of intervertebral disc (pyogenic), multiple sites in spine** HCC

√5ᵗʰ   M46.4   **Discitis, unspecified**

M46.40   **Discitis, unspecified, site unspecified** ▽
M46.41   **Discitis, unspecified, occipito-atlanto-axial region** ▽
M46.42   **Discitis, unspecified, cervical region** ▽
M46.43   **Discitis, unspecified, cervicothoracic region** ▽
M46.44   **Discitis, unspecified, thoracic region** ▽
M46.45   **Discitis, unspecified, thoracolumbar region** ▽
M46.46   **Discitis, unspecified, lumbar region** ▽
M46.47   **Discitis, unspecified, lumbosacral region** ▽
M46.48   **Discitis, unspecified, sacral and sacrococcygeal region** ▽
M46.49   **Discitis, unspecified, multiple sites in spine** ▽

√5ᵗʰ   M46.5   **Other infective spondylopathies**

M46.50   **Other infective spondylopathies, site unspecified** HCC ▽
M46.51   **Other infective spondylopathies, occipito-atlanto-axial region** HCC
M46.52   **Other infective spondylopathies, cervical region** HCC
M46.53   **Other infective spondylopathies, cervicothoracic region** HCC

M46.54   Other infective spondylopathies, thoracic region   `HCC`

M46.55   Other infective spondylopathies, thoracolumbar region   `HCC`

M46.56   Other infective spondylopathies, lumbar region   `HCC`

M46.57   Other infective spondylopathies, lumbosacral region   `HCC`

M46.58   Other infective spondylopathies, sacral and sacrococcygeal region   `HCC`

M46.59   Other infective spondylopathies, multiple sites in spine   `HCC`

√5ᵗʰ **M46.8 Other specified inflammatory spondylopathies**

M46.80   Other specified inflammatory spondylopathies, site unspecified   `HCC` ▽

M46.81   Other specified inflammatory spondylopathies, occipito-atlanto-axial region   `HCC`

M46.82   Other specified inflammatory spondylopathies, cervical region   `HCC`

M46.83   Other specified inflammatory spondylopathies, cervicothoracic region   `HCC`

M46.84   Other specified inflammatory spondylopathies, thoracic region   `HCC`

M46.85   Other specified inflammatory spondylopathies, thoracolumbar region   `HCC`

M46.86   Other specified inflammatory spondylopathies, lumbar region   `HCC`

M46.87   Other specified inflammatory spondylopathies, lumbosacral region   `HCC`

M46.88   Other specified inflammatory spondylopathies, sacral and sacrococcygeal region   `HCC`

M46.89   Other specified inflammatory spondylopathies, multiple sites in spine   `HCC`

√5ᵗʰ **M46.9 Unspecified inflammatory spondylopathy**

M46.90   Unspecified inflammatory spondylopathy, site unspecified   `HCC` ▽

M46.91   Unspecified inflammatory spondylopathy, occipito-atlanto-axial region   `HCC` ▽

M46.92   Unspecified inflammatory spondylopathy, cervical region   `HCC` ▽

M46.93   Unspecified inflammatory spondylopathy, cervicothoracic region   `HCC` ▽

M46.94   Unspecified inflammatory spondylopathy, thoracic region   `HCC` ▽

M46.95   Unspecified inflammatory spondylopathy, thoracolumbar region   `HCC` ▽

M46.96   Unspecified inflammatory spondylopathy, lumbar region   `HCC` ▽

M46.97   Unspecified inflammatory spondylopathy, lumbosacral region   `HCC` ▽

M46.98   Unspecified inflammatory spondylopathy, sacral and sacrococcygeal region   `HCC` ▽

M46.99   Unspecified inflammatory spondylopathy, multiple sites in spine   `HCC` ▽

√4ᵗʰ **M47 Spondylosis**

   `INCLUDES`   arthrosis or osteoarthritis of spine

        degeneration of facet joints

√5ᵗʰ **M47.0 Anterior spinal and vertebral artery compression syndromes**

√6ᵗʰ **M47.01 Anterior spinal artery compression syndromes**

M47.011   Anterior spinal artery compression syndromes, occipito-atlanto-axial region

M47.012   Anterior spinal artery compression syndromes, cervical region

M47.013   Anterior spinal artery compression syndromes, cervicothoracic region

M47.014   Anterior spinal artery compression syndromes, thoracic region

M47.015   Anterior spinal artery compression syndromes, thoracolumbar region

M47.016   Anterior spinal artery compression syndromes, lumbar region

M47.019   Anterior spinal artery compression syndromes, site unspecified   ▽

√6ᵗʰ **M47.02 Vertebral artery compression syndromes**

M47.021   Vertebral artery compression syndromes, occipito-atlanto-axial region

M47.022   Vertebral artery compression syndromes, cervical region

M47.029   Vertebral artery compression syndromes, site unspecified   ▽

√5ᵗʰ **M47.1 Other spondylosis with myelopathy**

   Spondylogenic compression of spinal cord

   `EXCLUDES 1`   vertebral subluxation (M43.3-M43.59)

M47.10   Other spondylosis with myelopathy, site unspecified   ▽

M47.11   Other spondylosis with myelopathy, occipito-atlanto-axial region

M47.12   Other spondylosis with myelopathy, cervical region

M47.13   Other spondylosis with myelopathy, cervicothoracic region

M47.14   Other spondylosis with myelopathy, thoracic region

M47.15   Other spondylosis with myelopathy, thoracolumbar region

M47.16   Other spondylosis with myelopathy, lumbar region

√5ᵗʰ **M47.2 Other spondylosis with radiculopathy**

M47.20   Other spondylosis with radiculopathy, site unspecified   ▽

M47.21   Other spondylosis with radiculopathy, occipito-atlanto-axial region

M47.22   Other spondylosis with radiculopathy, cervical region

M47.23   Other spondylosis with radiculopathy, cervicothoracic region

M47.24   Other spondylosis with radiculopathy, thoracic region

M47.25   Other spondylosis with radiculopathy, thoracolumbar region

M47.26   Other spondylosis with radiculopathy, lumbar region

M47.27   Other spondylosis with radiculopathy, lumbosacral region

M47.28   Other spondylosis with radiculopathy, sacral and sacrococcygeal region

√5ᵗʰ **M47.8 Other spondylosis**

√6ᵗʰ **M47.81 Spondylosis without myelopathy or radiculopathy**

    AHA: 2018,2Q,14

M47.811   Spondylosis without myelopathy or radiculopathy, occipito-atlanto-axial region

M47.812   Spondylosis without myelopathy or radiculopathy, cervical region

M47.813   Spondylosis without myelopathy or radiculopathy, cervicothoracic region

M47.814   Spondylosis without myelopathy or radiculopathy, thoracic region

M47.815   Spondylosis without myelopathy or radiculopathy, thoracolumbar region

M47.816   Spondylosis without myelopathy or radiculopathy, lumbar region

M47.817   Spondylosis without myelopathy or radiculopathy, lumbosacral region

M47.818   Spondylosis without myelopathy or radiculopathy, sacral and sacrococcygeal region

M47.819   Spondylosis without myelopathy or radiculopathy, site unspecified   ▽

√6ᵗʰ **M47.89 Other spondylosis**

M47.891   Other spondylosis, occipito-atlanto-axial region

M47.892   Other spondylosis, cervical region

M47.893   Other spondylosis, cervicothoracic region

M47.894   Other spondylosis, thoracic region

M47.895   Other spondylosis, thoracolumbar region

M47.896   Other spondylosis, lumbar region

M47.897   Other spondylosis, lumbosacral region

M47.898   Other spondylosis, sacral and sacrococcygeal region

M47.899   Other spondylosis, site unspecified   ▽

M47.9   Spondylosis, unspecified   ▽

√4ᵗʰ **M48 Other spondylopathies**

√5ᵗʰ **M48.0 Spinal stenosis**

   Caudal stenosis

M48.00   Spinal stenosis, site unspecified   ▽

M48.01   Spinal stenosis, occipito-atlanto-axial region

M48.02   Spinal stenosis, cervical region

M48.03   Spinal stenosis, cervicothoracic region

☑ Additional Character Req   √x7ᵗʰ Placeholder Alert   Manifestation   ▽ Unspecified   ▶◀ Revised Text   ● New Code   ▲ Revised Code Title

ICD-10-CM 2019   781

    M48.04   **Spinal stenosis, thoracic region**

    M48.05   **Spinal stenosis, thoracolumbar region**

✓6th   **M48.06**   **Spinal stenosis, lumbar region**

         AHA: 2017,4Q,18-19

         DEF: Spinal canal narrowing in the lumbar area with nerve root compression, causing muscle pain, fatigue, and weakness during extension of the lumbar spine. Pain is relieved by sitting or bending.

         M48.061   **Spinal stenosis, lumbar region** without neurogenic claudication

             Spinal stenosis, lumbar region NOS

         M48.062   **Spinal stenosis, lumbar region** with neurogenic claudication

    M48.07   **Spinal stenosis, lumbosacral region**

    M48.08   **Spinal stenosis, sacral and sacrococcygeal region**

✓5th   **M48.1**   **Ankylosing hyperostosis [Forestier]**

     Diffuse idiopathic skeletal hyperostosis [DISH]

    M48.10   **Ankylosing hyperostosis [Forestier], site unspecified** ▽

    M48.11   **Ankylosing hyperostosis [Forestier], occipito-atlanto-axial region**

    M48.12   **Ankylosing hyperostosis [Forestier], cervical region**

    M48.13   **Ankylosing hyperostosis [Forestier], cervicothoracic region**

    M48.14   **Ankylosing hyperostosis [Forestier], thoracic region**

    M48.15   **Ankylosing hyperostosis [Forestier], thoracolumbar region**

    M48.16   **Ankylosing hyperostosis [Forestier], lumbar region**

    M48.17   **Ankylosing hyperostosis [Forestier], lumbosacral region**

    M48.18   **Ankylosing hyperostosis [Forestier], sacral and sacrococcygeal region**

    M48.19   **Ankylosing hyperostosis [Forestier], multiple sites in spine**

✓5th   **M48.2**   **Kissing spine**

    M48.20   **Kissing spine, site unspecified** ▽

    M48.21   **Kissing spine, occipito-atlanto-axial region**

    M48.22   **Kissing spine, cervical region**

    M48.23   **Kissing spine, cervicothoracic region**

    M48.24   **Kissing spine, thoracic region**

    M48.25   **Kissing spine, thoracolumbar region**

    M48.26   **Kissing spine, lumbar region**

    M48.27   **Kissing spine, lumbosacral region**

✓5th   **M48.3**   **Traumatic spondylopathy**

    M48.30   **Traumatic spondylopathy, site unspecified** ▽

    M48.31   **Traumatic spondylopathy, occipito-atlanto-axial region**

    M48.32   **Traumatic spondylopathy, cervical region**

    M48.33   **Traumatic spondylopathy, cervicothoracic region**

    M48.34   **Traumatic spondylopathy, thoracic region**

    M48.35   **Traumatic spondylopathy, thoracolumbar region**

    M48.36   **Traumatic spondylopathy, lumbar region**

    M48.37   **Traumatic spondylopathy, lumbosacral region**

    M48.38   **Traumatic spondylopathy, sacral and sacrococcygeal region**

✓5th   **M48.4**   **Fatigue fracture of vertebra**

     Stress fracture of vertebra

     EXCLUDES 1   *pathological fracture NOS (M84.4-)*

         pathological fracture of vertebra due to neoplasm (M84.58)

         pathological fracture of vertebra due to osteoporosis (M80.-)

         pathological fracture of vertebra due to other diagnosis (M84.68)

         traumatic fracture of vertebrae (S12.0-S12.3-, S22.0-, S32.0-)

     The appropriate 7th character is to be added to each code from subcategory M48.4.

     A   initial encounter for fracture
     D   subsequent encounter for fracture with routine healing
     G   subsequent encounter for fracture with delayed healing
     S   sequela of fracture

✓x7th   **M48.40**   **Fatigue fracture of vertebra, site unspecified** Q ▽

✓x7th   **M48.41**   **Fatigue fracture of vertebra, occipito-atlanto-axial region** Q

✓x7th   **M48.42**   **Fatigue fracture of vertebra, cervical region** Q

✓x7th   **M48.43**   **Fatigue fracture of vertebra, cervicothoracic region** Q

✓x7th   **M48.44**   **Fatigue fracture of vertebra, thoracic region** Q

✓x7th   **M48.45**   **Fatigue fracture of vertebra, thoracolumbar region** Q

✓x7th   **M48.46**   **Fatigue fracture of vertebra, lumbar region** Q

✓x7th   **M48.47**   **Fatigue fracture of vertebra, lumbosacral region** Q

✓x7th   **M48.48**   **Fatigue fracture of vertebra, sacral and sacrococcygeal region** Q

✓5th   **M48.5**   **Collapsed vertebra, not elsewhere classified**

     Collapsed vertebra NOS

     Compression fracture of vertebra NOS

     Wedging of vertebra NOS

     EXCLUDES 1   *current injury - see Injury of spine, by body region*

         fatigue fracture of vertebra (M48.4)

         pathological fracture NOS (M84.4-)

         pathological fracture of vertebra due to neoplasm (M84.58)

         pathological fracture of vertebra due to osteoporosis (M80.-)

         pathological fracture of vertebra due to other diagnosis (M84.68)

         stress fracture of vertebra (M48.4-)

         traumatic fracture of vertebra (S12.-, S22.-, S32.-)

     The appropriate 7th character is to be added to each code from subcategory M48.5.

     A   initial encounter for fracture
     D   subsequent encounter for fracture with routine healing
     G   subsequent encounter for fracture with delayed healing
     S   sequela of fracture

[1] ✓x7th   **M48.50**   **Collapsed vertebra, not elsewhere classified, site unspecified** HCC ▽

[1] ✓x7th   **M48.51**   **Collapsed vertebra, not elsewhere classified, occipito-atlanto-axial region** HCC

[1] ✓x7th   **M48.52**   **Collapsed vertebra, not elsewhere classified, cervical region** HCC

[1] ✓x7th   **M48.53**   **Collapsed vertebra, not elsewhere classified, cervicothoracic region** HCC

[1] ✓x7th   **M48.54**   **Collapsed vertebra, not elsewhere classified, thoracic region** HCC

[1] ✓x7th   **M48.55**   **Collapsed vertebra, not elsewhere classified, thoracolumbar region** HCC

[1] ✓x7th   **M48.56**   **Collapsed vertebra, not elsewhere classified, lumbar region** HCC

[1] ✓x7th   **M48.57**   **Collapsed vertebra, not elsewhere classified, lumbosacral region** HCC

[1] ✓x7th   **M48.58**   **Collapsed vertebra, not elsewhere classified, sacral and sacrococcygeal region** HCC

✓5th   **M48.8**   **Other specified spondylopathies**

     Ossification of posterior longitudinal ligament

✓6th   **M48.8X**   **Other specified spondylopathies**

    M48.8X1   **Other specified spondylopathies, occipito-atlanto-axial region** HCC

    M48.8X2   **Other specified spondylopathies, cervical region** HCC

    M48.8X3   **Other specified spondylopathies, cervicothoracic region** HCC

    M48.8X4   **Other specified spondylopathies, thoracic region** HCC

    M48.8X5   **Other specified spondylopathies, thoracolumbar region** HCC

    M48.8X6   **Other specified spondylopathies, lumbar region** HCC

    M48.8X7   **Other specified spondylopathies, lumbosacral region** HCC

    M48.8X8   **Other specified spondylopathies, sacral and sacrococcygeal region** HCC

    M48.8X9   **Other specified spondylopathies, site unspecified** HCC ▽

    M48.9   **Spondylopathy, unspecified** ▽

√4ᵗʰ **M49 Spondylopathies in diseases classified elsewhere**

INCLUDES   curvature of spine in diseases classified elsewhere
deformity of spine in diseases classified elsewhere
kyphosis in diseases classified elsewhere
scoliosis in diseases classified elsewhere
spondylopathy in diseases classified elsewhere

Code first underlying disease, such as:
brucellosis (A23.-)
Charcôt-Marie-Tooth disease (G60.0)
enterobacterial infections (A01-A04)
osteitis fibrosa cystica (E21.0)

EXCLUDES 1   curvature of spine in tuberculosis [Pott's] (A18.01)
enteropathic arthropathies (M07.-)
gonococcal spondylitis (A54.41)
neuropathic spondylopathy in syringomyelia (G95.0)
neuropathic spondylopathy in tabes dorsalis (A52.11)
neuropathic [tabes dorsalis] spondylitis (A52.11)
nonsyphilitic neuropathic spondylopathy NEC (G98.0)
spondylitis in syphilis (acquired) (A52.77)
tuberculous spondylitis (A18.01)
typhoid fever spondylitis (A01.05)

√5ᵗʰ **M49.8 Spondylopathy in diseases classified elsewhere**

M49.80   *Spondylopathy in diseases classified*   HCC ▽
elsewhere, site unspecified

M49.81   *Spondylopathy in diseases classified*   HCC
elsewhere, occipito-atlanto-axial region

M49.82   *Spondylopathy in diseases classified*   HCC
elsewhere, cervical region

M49.83   *Spondylopathy in diseases classified*   HCC
elsewhere, cervicothoracic region

M49.84   *Spondylopathy in diseases classified*   HCC
elsewhere, thoracic region

M49.85   *Spondylopathy in diseases classified*   HCC
elsewhere, thoracolumbar region

M49.86   *Spondylopathy in diseases classified*   HCC
elsewhere, lumbar region

M49.87   *Spondylopathy in diseases classified*   HCC
elsewhere, lumbosacral region

M49.88   *Spondylopathy in diseases classified*   HCC
elsewhere, sacral and sacrococcygeal region

M49.89   *Spondylopathy in diseases classified*   HCC
elsewhere, multiple sites in spine

Other dorsopathies (M50-M54)

EXCLUDES 1   current injury - see injury of spine by body region
discitis NOS (M46.4-)

√4ᵗʰ **M50 Cervical disc disorders**

NOTE   Code to the most superior level of disorder

INCLUDES   cervicothoracic disc disorders
cervicothoracic disc disorders with cervicalgia

AHA: 2016,4Q,39-40; 2016,1Q,17

√5ᵗʰ **M50.0 Cervical disc disorder with myelopathy**

M50.00   **Cervical disc disorder with myelopathy,**   ▽
unspecified cervical region

▲   M50.01   **Cervical disc disorder with myelopathy, high**
cervical region
C2-C3 disc disorder with myelopathy
C3-C4 disc disorder with myelopathy

√6ᵗʰ   M50.02   **Cervical disc disorder with myelopathy, mid-cervical**
region

M50.020   **Cervical disc disorder with**   ▽
myelopathy, mid-cervical region,
unspecified level

M50.021   **Cervical disc disorder at C4-C5 level with**
myelopathy
C4-C5 disc disorder with myelopathy

M50.022   **Cervical disc disorder at C5-C6 level with**
myelopathy
C5-C6 disc disorder with myelopathy

M50.023   **Cervical disc disorder at C6-C7 level with**
myelopathy
C6-C7 disc disorder with myelopathy

M50.03   **Cervical disc disorder with myelopathy,**
cervicothoracic region
C7-T1 disc disorder with myelopathy

√5ᵗʰ **M50.1 Cervical disc disorder with radiculopathy**

EXCLUDES 2   brachial radiculitis NOS (M54.13)

M50.10   **Cervical disc disorder with radiculopathy,**   ▽
unspecified cervical region

▲   M50.11   **Cervical disc disorder with radiculopathy, high**
cervical region
C2-C3 disc disorder with radiculopathy
C3 radiculopathy due to disc disorder
C3-C4 disc disorder with radiculopathy
C4 radiculopathy due to disc disorder

√6ᵗʰ   M50.12   **Cervical disc disorder with radiculopathy,**
mid-cervical region

M50.120   **Mid-cervical disc disorder,**   ▽
unspecified

M50.121   **Cervical disc disorder at C4-C5 level with**
radiculopathy
C4-C5 disc disorder with radiculopathy
C5 radiculopathy due to disc disorder

M50.122   **Cervical disc disorder at C5-C6 level with**
radiculopathy
C5-C6 disc disorder with radiculopathy
C6 radiculopathy due to disc disorder

M50.123   **Cervical disc disorder at C6-C7 level with**
radiculopathy
C6-C7 disc disorder with radiculopathy
C7 radiculopathy due to disc disorder

M50.13   **Cervical disc disorder with radiculopathy,**
cervicothoracic region
C7-T1 disc disorder with radiculopathy
C8 radiculopathy due to disc disorder

√5ᵗʰ **M50.2 Other cervical disc displacement**

M50.20   **Other cervical disc displacement,**   ▽
unspecified cervical region

▲   M50.21   **Other cervical disc displacement, high cervical**
region
Other C2-C3 cervical disc displacement
Other C3-C4 cervical disc displacement

√6ᵗʰ   M50.22   **Other cervical disc displacement, mid-cervical**
region

M50.220   **Other cervical disc displacement,**   ▽
mid-cervical region, unspecified
level

M50.221   **Other cervical disc displacement at C4-C5**
level
Other C4-C5 cervical disc displacement

M50.222   **Other cervical disc displacement at C5-C6**
level
Other C5-C6 cervical disc displacement

M50.223   **Other cervical disc displacement at C6-C7**
level
Other C6-C7 cervical disc displacement

M50.23   **Other cervical disc displacement, cervicothoracic**
region
Other C7-T1 cervical disc displacement

√5ᵗʰ **M50.3 Other cervical disc degeneration**

M50.30   **Other cervical disc degeneration,**   ▽
unspecified cervical region

▲   M50.31   **Other cervical disc degeneration, high cervical**
region
Other C2-C3 cervical disc degeneration
Other C3-C4 cervical disc degeneration

√6ᵗʰ   M50.32   **Other cervical disc degeneration, mid-cervical**
region

M50.320   **Other cervical disc degeneration,**   ▽
mid-cervical region, unspecified
level

M50.321   **Other cervical disc degeneration at C4-C5**
level
Other C4-C5 cervical disc degeneration

M50.322   **Other cervical disc degeneration at C5-C6**
level
Other C5-C6 cervical disc degeneration

M50.323   **Other cervical disc degeneration at C6-C7**
level
Other C6-C7 cervical disc degeneration

M50.33   **Other cervical disc degeneration, cervicothoracic**
region
Other C7-T1 cervical disc degeneration

☑ Additional Character Req   √x7ᵗʰ Placeholder Alert   **Manifestation**   ▽ Unspecified   ►◄ Revised Text   ● New Code   ▲ Revised Code Title

Chapter 13. Diseases of the Musculoskeletal System and Connective Tissue

M50.8–M53.2X9

✓5ᵗʰ **M50.8 Other cervical disc disorders**

M50.80 Other cervical disc disorders, unspecified cervical region ▽

▲ **M50.81 Other cervical disc disorders, high cervical region**
Other C2-C3 cervical disc disorders
Other C3-C4 cervical disc disorders

✓6ᵗʰ **M50.82 Other cervical disc disorders, mid-cervical region**

M50.820 Other cervical disc disorders, mid-cervical region, unspecified level ▽

M50.821 Other cervical disc disorders at C4-C5 level
Other C4-C5 cervical disc disorders

M50.822 Other cervical disc disorders at C5-C6 level
Other C5-C6 cervical disc disorders

M50.823 Other cervical disc disorders at C6-C7 level
Other C6-C7 cervical disc disorders

M50.83 Other cervical disc disorders, cervicothoracic region
Other C7-T1 cervical disc disorders

✓5ᵗʰ **M50.9 Cervical disc disorder, unspecified**

M50.90 Cervical disc disorder, unspecified, unspecified cervical region ▽

▲ **M50.91 Cervical disc disorder, unspecified, high cervical region** ▽
C2-C3 cervical disc disorder, unspecified
C3-C4 cervical disc disorder, unspecified

✓6ᵗʰ **M50.92 Cervical disc disorder, unspecified, mid-cervical region**

M50.920 Unspecified cervical disc disorder, mid-cervical region, unspecified level ▽

M50.921 Unspecified cervical disc disorder at C4-C5 level ▽
Unspecified C4-C5 cervical disc disorder

M50.922 Unspecified cervical disc disorder at C5-C6 level ▽
Unspecified C5-C6 cervical disc disorder

M50.923 Unspecified cervical disc disorder at C6-C7 level ▽
Unspecified C6-C7 cervical disc disorder

M50.93 Cervical disc disorder, unspecified, cervicothoracic region ▽
C7-T1 cervical disc disorder, unspecified

✓4ᵗʰ **M51 Thoracic, thoracolumbar, and lumbosacral intervertebral disc disorders**

EXCLUDES 2 cervical and cervicothoracic disc disorders (M50.-)
sacral and sacrococcygeal disorders (M53.3)

✓5ᵗʰ **M51.0 Thoracic, thoracolumbar and lumbosacral intervertebral disc disorders with myelopathy**

M51.04 Intervertebral disc disorders with myelopathy, thoracic region

M51.05 Intervertebral disc disorders with myelopathy, thoracolumbar region

M51.06 Intervertebral disc disorders with myelopathy, lumbar region

✓5ᵗʰ **M51.1 Thoracic, thoracolumbar and lumbosacral intervertebral disc disorders with radiculopathy**
Sciatica due to intervertebral disc disorder
EXCLUDES 1 lumbar radiculitis NOS (M54.16)
sciatica NOS (M54.3)

M51.14 Intervertebral disc disorders with radiculopathy, thoracic region

M51.15 Intervertebral disc disorders with radiculopathy, thoracolumbar region

M51.16 Intervertebral disc disorders with radiculopathy, lumbar region

M51.17 Intervertebral disc disorders with radiculopathy, lumbosacral region

✓5ᵗʰ **M51.2 Other thoracic, thoracolumbar and lumbosacral intervertebral disc displacement**
Lumbago due to displacement of intervertebral disc

Displacement Intervertebral Disc

Normal Top View   Herniated Top View

Lamina
Ligamentum flavum
Disc annulus
Nucleus pulposus
Nucleus pulposus
Spinal cord
Herniates through annulus
Spinal nerve

M51.24 Other intervertebral disc displacement, thoracic region

M51.25 Other intervertebral disc displacement, thoracolumbar region

M51.26 Other intervertebral disc displacement, lumbar region

M51.27 Other intervertebral disc displacement, lumbosacral region

✓5ᵗʰ **M51.3 Other thoracic, thoracolumbar and lumbosacral intervertebral disc degeneration**
AHA: 2018,2Q,15; 2013,3Q,22

M51.34 Other intervertebral disc degeneration, thoracic region

M51.35 Other intervertebral disc degeneration, thoracolumbar region

M51.36 Other intervertebral disc degeneration, lumbar region

M51.37 Other intervertebral disc degeneration, lumbosacral region

✓5ᵗʰ **M51.4 Schmorl's nodes**
DEF: Irregular bone defect in the margin of the vertebral body that causes herniation into the end plate of the vertebral body.

M51.44 Schmorl's nodes, thoracic region

M51.45 Schmorl's nodes, thoracolumbar region

M51.46 Schmorl's nodes, lumbar region

M51.47 Schmorl's nodes, lumbosacral region

✓5ᵗʰ **M51.8 Other thoracic, thoracolumbar and lumbosacral intervertebral disc disorders**

M51.84 Other intervertebral disc disorders, thoracic region

M51.85 Other intervertebral disc disorders, thoracolumbar region

M51.86 Other intervertebral disc disorders, lumbar region

M51.87 Other intervertebral disc disorders, lumbosacral region

M51.9 Unspecified thoracic, thoracolumbar and lumbosacral intervertebral disc disorder ▽

✓4ᵗʰ **M53 Other and unspecified dorsopathies, not elsewhere classified**

M53.0 Cervicocranial syndrome
Posterior cervical sympathetic syndrome

M53.1 Cervicobrachial syndrome
EXCLUDES 2 cervical disc disorder (M50.-)
thoracic outlet syndrome (G54.0)

✓5ᵗʰ **M53.2 Spinal instabilities**

✓6ᵗʰ **M53.2X Spinal instabilities**

M53.2X1 Spinal instabilities, occipito-atlanto-axial region

M53.2X2 Spinal instabilities, cervical region

M53.2X3 Spinal instabilities, cervicothoracic region

M53.2X4 Spinal instabilities, thoracic region

M53.2X5 Spinal instabilities, thoracolumbar region

M53.2X6 Spinal instabilities, lumbar region

M53.2X7 Spinal instabilities, lumbosacral region

M53.2X8 Spinal instabilities, sacral and sacrococcygeal region

M53.2X9 Spinal instabilities, site unspecified ▽

M53.3 **Sacrococcygeal disorders, not elsewhere classified**
    Coccygodynia

√5ᵗʰ M53.8 **Other specified dorsopathies**

    M53.80 **Other specified dorsopathies, site unspecified** ▽

    M53.81 **Other specified dorsopathies, occipito-atlanto-axial region**

    M53.82 **Other specified dorsopathies, cervical region**

    M53.83 **Other specified dorsopathies, cervicothoracic region**

    M53.84 **Other specified dorsopathies, thoracic region**

    M53.85 **Other specified dorsopathies, thoracolumbar region**

    M53.86 **Other specified dorsopathies, lumbar region**

    M53.87 **Other specified dorsopathies, lumbosacral region**

    M53.88 **Other specified dorsopathies, sacral and sacrococcygeal region**

M53.9 **Dorsopathy, unspecified** ▽

√4ᵗʰ **M54 Dorsalgia**

    EXCLUDES 1   psychogenic dorsalgia (F45.41)

√5ᵗʰ M54.0 **Panniculitis affecting regions of neck and back**

    EXCLUDES 1   lupus panniculitis (L93.2)
               panniculitis NOS (M79.3)
               relapsing [Weber-Christian] panniculitis (M35.6)

    M54.00 **Panniculitis affecting regions of neck and back, site unspecified** ▽

    M54.01 **Panniculitis affecting regions of neck and back, occipito-atlanto-axial region**

    M54.02 **Panniculitis affecting regions of neck and back, cervical region**

    M54.03 **Panniculitis affecting regions of neck and back, cervicothoracic region**

    M54.04 **Panniculitis affecting regions of neck and back, thoracic region**

    M54.05 **Panniculitis affecting regions of neck and back, thoracolumbar region**

    M54.06 **Panniculitis affecting regions of neck and back, lumbar region**

    M54.07 **Panniculitis affecting regions of neck and back, lumbosacral region**

    M54.08 **Panniculitis affecting regions of neck and back, sacral and sacrococcygeal region**

    M54.09 **Panniculitis affecting regions, neck and back, multiple sites in spine**

√5ᵗʰ M54.1 **Radiculopathy**

    Brachial neuritis or radiculitis NOS
    Lumbar neuritis or radiculitis NOS
    Lumbosacral neuritis or radiculitis NOS
    Thoracic neuritis or radiculitis NOS
    Radiculitis NOS

    EXCLUDES 1   neuralgia and neuritis NOS (M79.2)
               radiculopathy with cervical disc disorder (M50.1)
               radiculopathy with lumbar and other intervertebral disc disorder (M51.1-)
               radiculopathy with spondylosis (M47.2-)

    M54.10 **Radiculopathy, site unspecified** ▽

    M54.11 **Radiculopathy, occipito-atlanto-axial region**

    M54.12 **Radiculopathy, cervical region**

    M54.13 **Radiculopathy, cervicothoracic region**

    M54.14 **Radiculopathy, thoracic region**

    M54.15 **Radiculopathy, thoracolumbar region**

    M54.16 **Radiculopathy, lumbar region**

    M54.17 **Radiculopathy, lumbosacral region**

    M54.18 **Radiculopathy, sacral and sacrococcygeal region**

M54.2 **Cervicalgia**

    EXCLUDES 1   cervicalgia due to intervertebral cervical disc disorder (M50.-)

√5ᵗʰ M54.3 **Sciatica**

    EXCLUDES 1   lesion of sciatic nerve (G57.0)
               sciatica due to intervertebral disc disorder (M51.1-)
               sciatica with lumbago (M54.4-)

    M54.30 **Sciatica, unspecified side** ▽

    M54.31 **Sciatica, right side**

    M54.32 **Sciatica, left side**

√5ᵗʰ M54.4 **Lumbago with sciatica**

    EXCLUDES 1   lumbago with sciatica due to intervertebral disc disorder (M51.1-)

    AHA: 2016,2Q,7

    M54.40 **Lumbago with sciatica, unspecified side** ▽

    M54.41 **Lumbago with sciatica, right side**

    M54.42 **Lumbago with sciatica, left side**

M54.5 **Low back pain**

    Loin pain
    Lumbago NOS

    EXCLUDES 1   low back strain (S39.012)
               lumbago due to intervertebral disc displacement (M51.2-)
               lumbago with sciatica (M54.4-)

M54.6 **Pain in thoracic spine**

    EXCLUDES 1   pain in thoracic spine due to intervertebral disc disorder (M51.-)

√5ᵗʰ M54.8 **Other dorsalgia**

    EXCLUDES 1   dorsalgia in thoracic region (M54.6)
               low back pain (M54.5)

    M54.81 **Occipital neuralgia**

    M54.89 **Other dorsalgia**

M54.9 **Dorsalgia, unspecified** ▽

    Backache NOS
    Back pain NOS

Soft Tissue Disorders (M60-M79)

Disorders of muscles (M60-M63)

EXCLUDES 1   dermatopolymyositis (M33.-)
               muscular dystrophies and myopathies (G71-G72)
               myopathy in amyloidosis (E85.-)
               myopathy in polyarteritis nodosa (M30.0)
               myopathy in rheumatoid arthritis (M05.32)
               myopathy in scleroderma (M34.-)
               myopathy in Sjögren's syndrome (M35.03)
               myopathy in systemic lupus erythematosus (M32.-)

√4ᵗʰ **M60 Myositis**

    EXCLUDES 2   inclusion body myositis [IBM] (G72.41)

√5ᵗʰ M60.0 **Infective myositis**

    Tropical pyomyositis
    Use additional code (B95-B97) to identify infectious agent

    √6ᵗʰ M60.00 **Infective myositis, unspecified site**

       M60.000 **Infective myositis, unspecified right arm**
          Infective myositis, right upper limb NOS

       M60.001 **Infective myositis, unspecified left arm**
          Infective myositis, left upper limb NOS

       M60.002 **Infective myositis, unspecified arm** ▽
          Infective myositis, upper limb NOS

       M60.003 **Infective myositis, unspecified right leg**
          Infective myositis, right lower limb NOS

       M60.004 **Infective myositis, unspecified left leg**
          Infective myositis, left lower limb NOS

       M60.005 **Infective myositis, unspecified leg**
          Infective myositis, lower limb NOS

       M60.009 **Infective myositis, unspecified site** ▽

    √6ᵗʰ M60.01 **Infective myositis, shoulder**

       M60.011 **Infective myositis, right shoulder**

       M60.012 **Infective myositis, left shoulder**

       M60.019 **Infective myositis, unspecified shoulder** ▽

    √6ᵗʰ M60.02 **Infective myositis, upper arm**

       M60.021 **Infective myositis, right upper arm**

       M60.022 **Infective myositis, left upper arm**

       M60.029 **Infective myositis, unspecified upper arm** ▽

    √6ᵗʰ M60.03 **Infective myositis, forearm**

       M60.031 **Infective myositis, right forearm**

       M60.032 **Infective myositis, left forearm**

       M60.039 **Infective myositis, unspecified forearm** ▽

    √6ᵗʰ M60.04 **Infective myositis, hand and fingers**

       M60.041 **Infective myositis, right hand**

       M60.042 **Infective myositis, left hand**

☑ Additional Character Req   ✓x7ᵗʰ Placeholder Alert   Manifestation   ▽ Unspecified   ▶◀ Revised Text   ● New Code   ▲ Revised Code Title

ICD-10-CM 2019   **785**

M60.043 Infective myositis, unspecified hand ▽
M60.044 Infective myositis, right finger(s)
M60.045 Infective myositis, left finger(s)
M60.046 Infective myositis, unspecified finger(s) ▽

√6ᵗʰ M60.05 Infective myositis, thigh
M60.051 Infective myositis, right thigh
M60.052 Infective myositis, left thigh
M60.059 Infective myositis, unspecified thigh ▽

√6ᵗʰ M60.06 Infective myositis, lower leg
M60.061 Infective myositis, right lower leg
M60.062 Infective myositis, left lower leg
M60.069 Infective myositis, unspecified lower leg ▽

√6ᵗʰ M60.07 Infective myositis, ankle, foot and toes
M60.070 Infective myositis, right ankle
M60.071 Infective myositis, left ankle
M60.072 Infective myositis, unspecified ankle ▽
M60.073 Infective myositis, right foot
M60.074 Infective myositis, left foot
M60.075 Infective myositis, unspecified foot ▽
M60.076 Infective myositis, right toe(s)
M60.077 Infective myositis, left toe(s)
M60.078 Infective myositis, unspecified toe(s) ▽

M60.08 Infective myositis, other site
M60.09 Infective myositis, multiple sites

√5ᵗʰ M60.1 Interstitial myositis
M60.10 Interstitial myositis of unspecified site ▽

√6ᵗʰ M60.11 Interstitial myositis, shoulder
M60.111 Interstitial myositis, right shoulder
M60.112 Interstitial myositis, left shoulder
M60.119 Interstitial myositis, unspecified shoulder ▽

√6ᵗʰ M60.12 Interstitial myositis, upper arm
M60.121 Interstitial myositis, right upper arm
M60.122 Interstitial myositis, left upper arm
M60.129 Interstitial myositis, unspecified upper arm ▽

√6ᵗʰ M60.13 Interstitial myositis, forearm
M60.131 Interstitial myositis, right forearm
M60.132 Interstitial myositis, left forearm
M60.139 Interstitial myositis, unspecified forearm ▽

√6ᵗʰ M60.14 Interstitial myositis, hand
M60.141 Interstitial myositis, right hand
M60.142 Interstitial myositis, left hand
M60.149 Interstitial myositis, unspecified hand ▽

√6ᵗʰ M60.15 Interstitial myositis, thigh
M60.151 Interstitial myositis, right thigh
M60.152 Interstitial myositis, left thigh
M60.159 Interstitial myositis, unspecified thigh ▽

√6ᵗʰ M60.16 Interstitial myositis, lower leg
M60.161 Interstitial myositis, right lower leg
M60.162 Interstitial myositis, left lower leg
M60.169 Interstitial myositis, unspecified lower leg ▽

√6ᵗʰ M60.17 Interstitial myositis, ankle and foot
M60.171 Interstitial myositis, right ankle and foot
M60.172 Interstitial myositis, left ankle and foot
M60.179 Interstitial myositis, unspecified ankle and foot ▽

M60.18 Interstitial myositis, other site
M60.19 Interstitial myositis, multiple sites

√5ᵗʰ M60.2 Foreign body granuloma of soft tissue, not elsewhere classified
Use additional code to identify the type of retained foreign body (Z18.-)
EXCLUDES 1 foreign body granuloma of skin and subcutaneous tissue (L92.3)

M60.20 Foreign body granuloma of soft tissue, not elsewhere classified, unspecified site ▽

√6ᵗʰ M60.21 Foreign body granuloma of soft tissue, not elsewhere classified, shoulder
M60.211 Foreign body granuloma of soft tissue, not elsewhere classified, right shoulder
M60.212 Foreign body granuloma of soft tissue, not elsewhere classified, left shoulder
M60.219 Foreign body granuloma of soft tissue, not elsewhere classified, unspecified shoulder ▽

√6ᵗʰ M60.22 Foreign body granuloma of soft tissue, not elsewhere classified, upper arm
M60.221 Foreign body granuloma of soft tissue, not elsewhere classified, right upper arm
M60.222 Foreign body granuloma of soft tissue, not elsewhere classified, left upper arm
M60.229 Foreign body granuloma of soft tissue, not elsewhere classified, unspecified upper arm ▽

√6ᵗʰ M60.23 Foreign body granuloma of soft tissue, not elsewhere classified, forearm
M60.231 Foreign body granuloma of soft tissue, not elsewhere classified, right forearm
M60.232 Foreign body granuloma of soft tissue, not elsewhere classified, left forearm
M60.239 Foreign body granuloma of soft tissue, not elsewhere classified, unspecified forearm ▽

√6ᵗʰ M60.24 Foreign body granuloma of soft tissue, not elsewhere classified, hand
M60.241 Foreign body granuloma of soft tissue, not elsewhere classified, right hand
M60.242 Foreign body granuloma of soft tissue, not elsewhere classified, left hand
M60.249 Foreign body granuloma of soft tissue, not elsewhere classified, unspecified hand ▽

√6ᵗʰ M60.25 Foreign body granuloma of soft tissue, not elsewhere classified, thigh
M60.251 Foreign body granuloma of soft tissue, not elsewhere classified, right thigh
M60.252 Foreign body granuloma of soft tissue, not elsewhere classified, left thigh
M60.259 Foreign body granuloma of soft tissue, not elsewhere classified, unspecified thigh ▽

√6ᵗʰ M60.26 Foreign body granuloma of soft tissue, not elsewhere classified, lower leg
M60.261 Foreign body granuloma of soft tissue, not elsewhere classified, right lower leg
M60.262 Foreign body granuloma of soft tissue, not elsewhere classified, left lower leg
M60.269 Foreign body granuloma of soft tissue, not elsewhere classified, unspecified lower leg ▽

√6ᵗʰ M60.27 Foreign body granuloma of soft tissue, not elsewhere classified, ankle and foot
M60.271 Foreign body granuloma of soft tissue, not elsewhere classified, right ankle and foot
M60.272 Foreign body granuloma of soft tissue, not elsewhere classified, left ankle and foot
M60.279 Foreign body granuloma of soft tissue, not elsewhere classified, unspecified ankle and foot ▽

M60.28 Foreign body granuloma of soft tissue, not elsewhere classified, other site

√5ᵗʰ M60.8 Other myositis
M60.80 Other myositis, unspecified site ▽

√6ᵗʰ M60.81 Other myositis shoulder
M60.811 Other myositis, right shoulder
M60.812 Other myositis, left shoulder
M60.819 Other myositis, unspecified shoulder ▽

√6ᵗʰ M60.82 Other myositis, upper arm
M60.821 Other myositis, right upper arm
M60.822 Other myositis, left upper arm
M60.829 Other myositis, unspecified upper arm ▽

√6ᵗʰ M60.83 Other myositis, forearm
M60.831 Other myositis, right forearm
M60.832 Other myositis, left forearm

M60.839   Other myositis, unspecified forearm   ▽

✓6ᵗʰ   **M60.84**   **Other myositis, hand**

    M60.841   Other myositis, right hand
    M60.842   Other myositis, left hand
    M60.849   Other myositis, unspecified hand   ▽

✓6ᵗʰ   **M60.85**   **Other myositis, thigh**

    M60.851   Other myositis, right thigh
    M60.852   Other myositis, left thigh
    M60.859   Other myositis, unspecified thigh   ▽

✓6ᵗʰ   **M60.86**   **Other myositis, lower leg**

    M60.861   Other myositis, right lower leg
    M60.862   Other myositis, left lower leg
    M60.869   Other myositis, unspecified lower leg   ▽

✓6ᵗʰ   **M60.87**   **Other myositis, ankle and foot**

    M60.871   Other myositis, right ankle and foot
    M60.872   Other myositis, left ankle and foot
    M60.879   Other myositis, unspecified ankle and foot   ▽

    M60.88   **Other myositis, other site**
    M60.89   **Other myositis, multiple sites**

   M60.9   **Myositis, unspecified**   ▽

✓4ᵗʰ   **M61**   **Calcification and ossification of muscle**

✓5ᵗʰ   **M61.0**   **Myositis ossificans traumatica**

    M61.00   **Myositis ossificans traumatica, unspecified site**   ▽

✓6ᵗʰ   **M61.01**   **Myositis ossificans traumatica, shoulder**

    M61.011   Myositis ossificans traumatica, right shoulder
    M61.012   Myositis ossificans traumatica, left shoulder
    M61.019   Myositis ossificans traumatica, unspecified shoulder   ▽

✓6ᵗʰ   **M61.02**   **Myositis ossificans traumatica, upper arm**

    M61.021   Myositis ossificans traumatica, right upper arm
    M61.022   Myositis ossificans traumatica, left upper arm
    M61.029   Myositis ossificans traumatica, unspecified upper arm   ▽

✓6ᵗʰ   **M61.03**   **Myositis ossificans traumatica, forearm**

    M61.031   Myositis ossificans traumatica, right forearm
    M61.032   Myositis ossificans traumatica, left forearm
    M61.039   Myositis ossificans traumatica, unspecified forearm   ▽

✓6ᵗʰ   **M61.04**   **Myositis ossificans traumatica, hand**

    M61.041   Myositis ossificans traumatica, right hand
    M61.042   Myositis ossificans traumatica, left hand
    M61.049   Myositis ossificans traumatica, unspecified hand   ▽

✓6ᵗʰ   **M61.05**   **Myositis ossificans traumatica, thigh**

    M61.051   Myositis ossificans traumatica, right thigh
    M61.052   Myositis ossificans traumatica, left thigh
    M61.059   Myositis ossificans traumatica, unspecified thigh   ▽

✓6ᵗʰ   **M61.06**   **Myositis ossificans traumatica, lower leg**

    M61.061   Myositis ossificans traumatica, right lower leg
    M61.062   Myositis ossificans traumatica, left lower leg
    M61.069   Myositis ossificans traumatica, unspecified lower leg   ▽

✓6ᵗʰ   **M61.07**   **Myositis ossificans traumatica, ankle and foot**

    M61.071   Myositis ossificans traumatica, right ankle and foot
    M61.072   Myositis ossificans traumatica, left ankle and foot
    M61.079   Myositis ossificans traumatica, unspecified ankle and foot   ▽

    M61.08   **Myositis ossificans traumatica, other site**
    M61.09   **Myositis ossificans traumatica, multiple sites**

✓5ᵗʰ   **M61.1**   **Myositis ossificans progressiva**

    Fibrodysplasia ossificans progressiva

    M61.10   **Myositis ossificans progressiva, unspecified site**   ▽

✓6ᵗʰ   **M61.11**   **Myositis ossificans progressiva, shoulder**

    M61.111   Myositis ossificans progressiva, right shoulder
    M61.112   Myositis ossificans progressiva, left shoulder
    M61.119   Myositis ossificans progressiva, unspecified shoulder   ▽

✓6ᵗʰ   **M61.12**   **Myositis ossificans progressiva, upper arm**

    M61.121   Myositis ossificans progressiva, right upper arm
    M61.122   Myositis ossificans progressiva, left upper arm
    M61.129   Myositis ossificans progressiva, unspecified arm   ▽

✓6ᵗʰ   **M61.13**   **Myositis ossificans progressiva, forearm**

    M61.131   Myositis ossificans progressiva, right forearm
    M61.132   Myositis ossificans progressiva, left forearm
    M61.139   Myositis ossificans progressiva, unspecified forearm   ▽

✓6ᵗʰ   **M61.14**   **Myositis ossificans progressiva, hand and finger(s)**

    M61.141   Myositis ossificans progressiva, right hand
    M61.142   Myositis ossificans progressiva, left hand
    M61.143   Myositis ossificans progressiva, unspecified hand
    M61.144   Myositis ossificans progressiva, right finger(s)
    M61.145   Myositis ossificans progressiva, left finger(s)
    M61.146   Myositis ossificans progressiva, unspecified finger(s)   ▽

✓6ᵗʰ   **M61.15**   **Myositis ossificans progressiva, thigh**

    M61.151   Myositis ossificans progressiva, right thigh
    M61.152   Myositis ossificans progressiva, left thigh
    M61.159   Myositis ossificans progressiva, unspecified thigh   ▽

✓6ᵗʰ   **M61.16**   **Myositis ossificans progressiva, lower leg**

    M61.161   Myositis ossificans progressiva, right lower leg
    M61.162   Myositis ossificans progressiva, left lower leg
    M61.169   Myositis ossificans progressiva, unspecified lower leg   ▽

✓6ᵗʰ   **M61.17**   **Myositis ossificans progressiva, ankle, foot and toe(s)**

    M61.171   Myositis ossificans progressiva, right ankle
    M61.172   Myositis ossificans progressiva, left ankle
    M61.173   Myositis ossificans progressiva, unspecified ankle   ▽
    M61.174   Myositis ossificans progressiva, right foot
    M61.175   Myositis ossificans progressiva, left foot
    M61.176   Myositis ossificans progressiva, unspecified foot   ▽
    M61.177   Myositis ossificans progressiva, right toe(s)
    M61.178   Myositis ossificans progressiva, left toe(s)
    M61.179   Myositis ossificans progressiva, unspecified toe(s)   ▽

    M61.18   **Myositis ossificans progressiva, other site**
    M61.19   **Myositis ossificans progressiva, multiple sites**

✓5ᵗʰ   **M61.2**   **Paralytic calcification and ossification of muscle**

    Myositis ossificans associated with quadriplegia or paraplegia

    M61.20   **Paralytic calcification and ossification of muscle, unspecified site**   ▽

✓6ᵗʰ   **M61.21**   **Paralytic calcification and ossification of muscle, shoulder**

    M61.211   Paralytic calcification and ossification of muscle, right shoulder
    M61.212   Paralytic calcification and ossification of muscle, left shoulder
    M61.219   Paralytic calcification and ossification of muscle, unspecified shoulder   ▽

✓6ᵗʰ   **M61.22**   **Paralytic calcification and ossification of muscle, upper arm**

    M61.221   Paralytic calcification and ossification of muscle, right upper arm

| ✓ Additional Character Req | ✓x7ᵗʰ Placeholder Alert | **Manifestation** | ▽ Unspecified | ►◄ Revised Text | ● New Code | ▲ Revised Code Title |

ICD-10-CM 2019   787

M61.222 Paralytic calcification and ossification of muscle, left upper arm
M61.229 Paralytic calcification and ossification of muscle, unspecified upper arm ▽

M61.23 Paralytic calcification and ossification of muscle, forearm
M61.231 Paralytic calcification and ossification of muscle, right forearm
M61.232 Paralytic calcification and ossification of muscle, left forearm
M61.239 Paralytic calcification and ossification of muscle, unspecified forearm ▽

M61.24 Paralytic calcification and ossification of muscle, hand
M61.241 Paralytic calcification and ossification of muscle, right hand
M61.242 Paralytic calcification and ossification of muscle, left hand
M61.249 Paralytic calcification and ossification of muscle, unspecified hand ▽

M61.25 Paralytic calcification and ossification of muscle, thigh
M61.251 Paralytic calcification and ossification of muscle, right thigh
M61.252 Paralytic calcification and ossification of muscle, left thigh
M61.259 Paralytic calcification and ossification of muscle, unspecified thigh ▽

M61.26 Paralytic calcification and ossification of muscle, lower leg
M61.261 Paralytic calcification and ossification of muscle, right lower leg
M61.262 Paralytic calcification and ossification of muscle, left lower leg
M61.269 Paralytic calcification and ossification of muscle, unspecified lower leg ▽

M61.27 Paralytic calcification and ossification of muscle, ankle and foot
M61.271 Paralytic calcification and ossification of muscle, right ankle and foot
M61.272 Paralytic calcification and ossification of muscle, left ankle and foot
M61.279 Paralytic calcification and ossification of muscle, unspecified ankle and foot ▽

M61.28 Paralytic calcification and ossification of muscle, other site
M61.29 Paralytic calcification and ossification of muscle, multiple sites

M61.3 Calcification and ossification of muscles associated with burns
Myositis ossificans associated with burns
M61.30 Calcification and ossification of muscles associated with burns, unspecified site ▽
M61.31 Calcification and ossification of muscles associated with burns, shoulder
M61.311 Calcification and ossification of muscles associated with burns, right shoulder
M61.312 Calcification and ossification of muscles associated with burns, left shoulder
M61.319 Calcification and ossification of muscles associated with burns, unspecified shoulder ▽
M61.32 Calcification and ossification of muscles associated with burns, upper arm
M61.321 Calcification and ossification of muscles associated with burns, right upper arm
M61.322 Calcification and ossification of muscles associated with burns, left upper arm
M61.329 Calcification and ossification of muscles associated with burns, unspecified upper arm ▽
M61.33 Calcification and ossification of muscles associated with burns, forearm
M61.331 Calcification and ossification of muscles associated with burns, right forearm
M61.332 Calcification and ossification of muscles associated with burns, left forearm

M61.339 Calcification and ossification of muscles associated with burns, unspecified forearm ▽
M61.34 Calcification and ossification of muscles associated with burns, hand
M61.341 Calcification and ossification of muscles associated with burns, right hand
M61.342 Calcification and ossification of muscles associated with burns, left hand
M61.349 Calcification and ossification of muscles associated with burns, unspecified hand ▽
M61.35 Calcification and ossification of muscles associated with burns, thigh
M61.351 Calcification and ossification of muscles associated with burns, right thigh
M61.352 Calcification and ossification of muscles associated with burns, left thigh
M61.359 Calcification and ossification of muscles associated with burns, unspecified thigh ▽
M61.36 Calcification and ossification of muscles associated with burns, lower leg
M61.361 Calcification and ossification of muscles associated with burns, right lower leg
M61.362 Calcification and ossification of muscles associated with burns, left lower leg
M61.369 Calcification and ossification of muscles associated with burns, unspecified lower leg ▽
M61.37 Calcification and ossification of muscles associated with burns, ankle and foot
M61.371 Calcification and ossification of muscles associated with burns, right ankle and foot
M61.372 Calcification and ossification of muscles associated with burns, left ankle and foot
M61.379 Calcification and ossification of muscles associated with burns, unspecified ankle and foot ▽
M61.38 Calcification and ossification of muscles associated with burns, other site
M61.39 Calcification and ossification of muscles associated with burns, multiple sites

M61.4 Other calcification of muscle
EXCLUDES 1 calcific tendinitis NOS (M65.2-)
calcific tendinitis of shoulder (M75.3)
M61.40 Other calcification of muscle, unspecified site ▽
M61.41 Other calcification of muscle, shoulder
M61.411 Other calcification of muscle, right shoulder
M61.412 Other calcification of muscle, left shoulder
M61.419 Other calcification of muscle, unspecified shoulder ▽
M61.42 Other calcification of muscle, upper arm
M61.421 Other calcification of muscle, right upper arm
M61.422 Other calcification of muscle, left upper arm
M61.429 Other calcification of muscle, unspecified upper arm ▽
M61.43 Other calcification of muscle, forearm
M61.431 Other calcification of muscle, right forearm
M61.432 Other calcification of muscle, left forearm
M61.439 Other calcification of muscle, unspecified forearm ▽
M61.44 Other calcification of muscle, hand
M61.441 Other calcification of muscle, right hand
M61.442 Other calcification of muscle, left hand
M61.449 Other calcification of muscle, unspecified hand ▽
M61.45 Other calcification of muscle, thigh
M61.451 Other calcification of muscle, right thigh
M61.452 Other calcification of muscle, left thigh
M61.459 Other calcification of muscle, unspecified thigh ▽

√6ᵗʰ **M61.46** Other calcification of muscle, lower leg

     M61.461 Other calcification of muscle, right lower leg

     M61.462 Other calcification of muscle, left lower leg

     M61.469 Other calcification of muscle, unspecified lower leg ▽

√6ᵗʰ **M61.47** Other calcification of muscle, ankle and foot

     M61.471 Other calcification of muscle, right ankle and foot

     M61.472 Other calcification of muscle, left ankle and foot

     M61.479 Other calcification of muscle, unspecified ankle and foot ▽

     M61.48 Other calcification of muscle, other site

     M61.49 Other calcification of muscle, multiple sites

√5ᵗʰ **M61.5** Other ossification of muscle

     M61.50 Other ossification of muscle, unspecified site ▽

√6ᵗʰ **M61.51** Other ossification of muscle, shoulder

     M61.511 Other ossification of muscle, right shoulder

     M61.512 Other ossification of muscle, left shoulder

     M61.519 Other ossification of muscle, unspecified shoulder ▽

√6ᵗʰ **M61.52** Other ossification of muscle, upper arm

     M61.521 Other ossification of muscle, right upper arm

     M61.522 Other ossification of muscle, left upper arm

     M61.529 Other ossification of muscle, unspecified upper arm ▽

√6ᵗʰ **M61.53** Other ossification of muscle, forearm

     M61.531 Other ossification of muscle, right forearm

     M61.532 Other ossification of muscle, left forearm

     M61.539 Other ossification of muscle, unspecified forearm ▽

√6ᵗʰ **M61.54** Other ossification of muscle, hand

     M61.541 Other ossification of muscle, right hand

     M61.542 Other ossification of muscle, left hand

     M61.549 Other ossification of muscle, unspecified hand ▽

√6ᵗʰ **M61.55** Other ossification of muscle, thigh

     M61.551 Other ossification of muscle, right thigh

     M61.552 Other ossification of muscle, left thigh

     M61.559 Other ossification of muscle, unspecified thigh ▽

√6ᵗʰ **M61.56** Other ossification of muscle, lower leg

     M61.561 Other ossification of muscle, right lower leg

     M61.562 Other ossification of muscle, left lower leg

     M61.569 Other ossification of muscle, unspecified lower leg ▽

√6ᵗʰ **M61.57** Other ossification of muscle, ankle and foot

     M61.571 Other ossification of muscle, right ankle and foot

     M61.572 Other ossification of muscle, left ankle and foot

     M61.579 Other ossification of muscle, unspecified ankle and foot ▽

     M61.58 Other ossification of muscle, other site

     M61.59 Other ossification of muscle, multiple sites

M61.9 Calcification and ossification of muscle, unspecified ▽

√4ᵗʰ **M62** Other disorders of muscle

     EXCLUDES 1   alcoholic myopathy (G72.1)
                cramp and spasm (R25.2)
                drug-induced myopathy (G72.0)
                myalgia ▶(M79.1-)◀
                stiff-man syndrome (G25.82)

     EXCLUDES 2   nontraumatic hematoma of muscle (M79.81)

√5ᵗʰ **M62.0** Separation of muscle (nontraumatic)

     Diastasis of muscle

     EXCLUDES 1   diastasis recti complicating pregnancy, labor and delivery (O71.8)
                traumatic separation of muscle - see strain of muscle by body region

     M62.00 Separation of muscle (nontraumatic), unspecified site ▽

√6ᵗʰ **M62.01** Separation of muscle (nontraumatic), shoulder

     M62.011 Separation of muscle (nontraumatic), right shoulder

     M62.012 Separation of muscle (nontraumatic), left shoulder

     M62.019 Separation of muscle (nontraumatic), unspecified shoulder ▽

√6ᵗʰ **M62.02** Separation of muscle (nontraumatic), upper arm

     M62.021 Separation of muscle (nontraumatic), right upper arm

     M62.022 Separation of muscle (nontraumatic), left upper arm

     M62.029 Separation of muscle (nontraumatic), unspecified upper arm ▽

√6ᵗʰ **M62.03** Separation of muscle (nontraumatic), forearm

     M62.031 Separation of muscle (nontraumatic), right forearm

     M62.032 Separation of muscle (nontraumatic), left forearm

     M62.039 Separation of muscle (nontraumatic), unspecified forearm ▽

√6ᵗʰ **M62.04** Separation of muscle (nontraumatic), hand

     M62.041 Separation of muscle (nontraumatic), right hand

     M62.042 Separation of muscle (nontraumatic), left hand

     M62.049 Separation of muscle (nontraumatic), unspecified hand ▽

√6ᵗʰ **M62.05** Separation of muscle (nontraumatic), thigh

     M62.051 Separation of muscle (nontraumatic), right thigh

     M62.052 Separation of muscle (nontraumatic), left thigh

     M62.059 Separation of muscle (nontraumatic), unspecified thigh ▽

√6ᵗʰ **M62.06** Separation of muscle (nontraumatic), lower leg

     M62.061 Separation of muscle (nontraumatic), right lower leg

     M62.062 Separation of muscle (nontraumatic), left lower leg

     M62.069 Separation of muscle (nontraumatic), unspecified lower leg ▽

√6ᵗʰ **M62.07** Separation of muscle (nontraumatic), ankle and foot

     M62.071 Separation of muscle (nontraumatic), right ankle and foot

     M62.072 Separation of muscle (nontraumatic), left ankle and foot

     M62.079 Separation of muscle (nontraumatic), unspecified ankle and foot ▽

     M62.08 Separation of muscle (nontraumatic), other site

√5ᵗʰ **M62.1** Other rupture of muscle (nontraumatic)

     EXCLUDES 1   traumatic rupture of muscle - see strain of muscle by body region

     EXCLUDES 2   rupture of tendon (M66.-)

     M62.10 Other rupture of muscle (nontraumatic), unspecified site ▽

☑ Additional Character Req   √x7ᵗʰ Placeholder Alert   Manifestation   ▽ Unspecified   ▶◀ Revised Text   ● New Code   ▲ Revised Code Title

ICD-10-CM 2019   789

Chapter 13. Diseases of the Musculoskeletal System and Connective Tissue

√6ᵗ **M62.11** Other rupture of muscle (nontraumatic), shoulder

    M62.111 Other rupture of muscle (nontraumatic), right shoulder

    M62.112 Other rupture of muscle (nontraumatic), left shoulder

    M62.119 Other rupture of muscle (nontraumatic), unspecified shoulder ▽

√6ᵗ **M62.12** Other rupture of muscle (nontraumatic), upper arm

    M62.121 Other rupture of muscle (nontraumatic), right upper arm

    M62.122 Other rupture of muscle (nontraumatic), left upper arm

    M62.129 Other rupture of muscle (nontraumatic), unspecified upper arm ▽

√6ᵗ **M62.13** Other rupture of muscle (nontraumatic), forearm

    M62.131 Other rupture of muscle (nontraumatic), right forearm

    M62.132 Other rupture of muscle (nontraumatic), left forearm

    M62.139 Other rupture of muscle (nontraumatic), unspecified forearm ▽

√6ᵗ **M62.14** Other rupture of muscle (nontraumatic), hand

    M62.141 Other rupture of muscle (nontraumatic), right hand

    M62.142 Other rupture of muscle (nontraumatic), left hand

    M62.149 Other rupture of muscle (nontraumatic), unspecified hand ▽

√6ᵗ **M62.15** Other rupture of muscle (nontraumatic), thigh

    M62.151 Other rupture of muscle (nontraumatic), right thigh

    M62.152 Other rupture of muscle (nontraumatic), left thigh

    M62.159 Other rupture of muscle (nontraumatic), unspecified thigh ▽

√6ᵗ **M62.16** Other rupture of muscle (nontraumatic), lower leg

    M62.161 Other rupture of muscle (nontraumatic), right lower leg

    M62.162 Other rupture of muscle (nontraumatic), left lower leg

    M62.169 Other rupture of muscle (nontraumatic), unspecified lower leg ▽

√6ᵗ **M62.17** Other rupture of muscle (nontraumatic), ankle and foot

    M62.171 Other rupture of muscle (nontraumatic), right ankle and foot

    M62.172 Other rupture of muscle (nontraumatic), left ankle and foot

    M62.179 Other rupture of muscle (nontraumatic), unspecified ankle and foot ▽

    M62.18 Other rupture of muscle (nontraumatic), other site

√5ᵗ **M62.2 Nontraumatic ischemic infarction of muscle**

    EXCLUDES 1   compartment syndrome (traumatic) (T79.A-)
            nontraumatic compartment syndrome (M79.A-)
            rhabdomyolysis (M62.82)
            traumatic ischemia of muscle (T79.6)
            Volkmann's ischemic contracture (T79.6)

    M62.20 Nontraumatic ischemic infarction of muscle, unspecified site ▽

√6ᵗ **M62.21** Nontraumatic ischemic infarction of muscle, shoulder

    M62.211 Nontraumatic ischemic infarction of muscle, right shoulder

    M62.212 Nontraumatic ischemic infarction of muscle, left shoulder

    M62.219 Nontraumatic ischemic infarction of muscle, unspecified shoulder ▽

√6ᵗ **M62.22** Nontraumatic ischemic infarction of muscle, upper arm

    M62.221 Nontraumatic ischemic infarction of muscle, right upper arm

    M62.222 Nontraumatic ischemic infarction of muscle, left upper arm

    M62.229 Nontraumatic ischemic infarction of muscle, unspecified upper arm ▽

√6ᵗ **M62.23** Nontraumatic ischemic infarction of muscle, forearm

    M62.231 Nontraumatic ischemic infarction of muscle, right forearm

    M62.232 Nontraumatic ischemic infarction of muscle, left forearm

    M62.239 Nontraumatic ischemic infarction of muscle, unspecified forearm ▽

√6ᵗ **M62.24** Nontraumatic ischemic infarction of muscle, hand

    M62.241 Nontraumatic ischemic infarction of muscle, right hand

    M62.242 Nontraumatic ischemic infarction of muscle, left hand

    M62.249 Nontraumatic ischemic infarction of muscle, unspecified hand ▽

√6ᵗ **M62.25** Nontraumatic ischemic infarction of muscle, thigh

    M62.251 Nontraumatic ischemic infarction of muscle, right thigh

    M62.252 Nontraumatic ischemic infarction of muscle, left thigh

    M62.259 Nontraumatic ischemic infarction of muscle, unspecified thigh ▽

√6ᵗ **M62.26** Nontraumatic ischemic infarction of muscle, lower leg

    M62.261 Nontraumatic ischemic infarction of muscle, right lower leg

    M62.262 Nontraumatic ischemic infarction of muscle, left lower leg

    M62.269 Nontraumatic ischemic infarction of muscle, unspecified lower leg ▽

√6ᵗ **M62.27** Nontraumatic ischemic infarction of muscle, ankle and foot

    M62.271 Nontraumatic ischemic infarction of muscle, right ankle and foot

    M62.272 Nontraumatic ischemic infarction of muscle, left ankle and foot

    M62.279 Nontraumatic ischemic infarction of muscle, unspecified ankle and foot ▽

    M62.28 Nontraumatic ischemic infarction of muscle, other site

M62.3 Immobility syndrome (paraplegic)

√5ᵗ **M62.4 Contracture of muscle**

    Contracture of tendon (sheath)
    EXCLUDES 1   contracture of joint (M24.5-)

    M62.40 Contracture of muscle, unspecified site ▽

√6ᵗ **M62.41** Contracture of muscle, shoulder

    M62.411 Contracture of muscle, right shoulder
    M62.412 Contracture of muscle, left shoulder
    M62.419 Contracture of muscle, unspecified shoulder ▽

√6ᵗ **M62.42** Contracture of muscle, upper arm

    M62.421 Contracture of muscle, right upper arm
    M62.422 Contracture of muscle, left upper arm
    M62.429 Contracture of muscle, unspecified upper arm ▽

√6ᵗ **M62.43** Contracture of muscle, forearm

    M62.431 Contracture of muscle, right forearm
    M62.432 Contracture of muscle, left forearm
    M62.439 Contracture of muscle, unspecified forearm ▽

√6ᵗ **M62.44** Contracture of muscle, hand

    M62.441 Contracture of muscle, right hand
    M62.442 Contracture of muscle, left hand
    M62.449 Contracture of muscle, unspecified hand ▽

√6ᵗ **M62.45** Contracture of muscle, thigh

    M62.451 Contracture of muscle, right thigh
    M62.452 Contracture of muscle, left thigh
    M62.459 Contracture of muscle, unspecified thigh ▽

√6ᵗ **M62.46** Contracture of muscle, lower leg

    M62.461 Contracture of muscle, right lower leg
    M62.462 Contracture of muscle, left lower leg
    M62.469 Contracture of muscle, unspecified lower leg ▽

√6ᵗ **M62.47** Contracture of muscle, ankle and foot

    M62.471 Contracture of muscle, right ankle and foot

M62.472　Contracture of muscle, left ankle and foot
M62.479　Contracture of muscle, unspecified ankle and foot ▽
M62.48　Contracture of muscle, other site
M62.49　Contracture of muscle, multiple sites

☑5ᵗʰ　M62.5　Muscle wasting and atrophy, not elsewhere classified
Disuse atrophy NEC
EXCLUDES 1　neuralgic amyotrophy (G54.5)
　　　　　　progressive muscular atrophy (G12.21)
　　　　　　sarcopenia (M62.84)
EXCLUDES 2　pelvic muscle wasting (N81.84)

M62.50　Muscle wasting and atrophy, not elsewhere classified, unspecified site ▽

☑6ᵗʰ　M62.51　Muscle wasting and atrophy, not elsewhere classified, shoulder
M62.511　Muscle wasting and atrophy, not elsewhere classified, right shoulder
M62.512　Muscle wasting and atrophy, not elsewhere classified, left shoulder
M62.519　Muscle wasting and atrophy, not elsewhere classified, unspecified shoulder ▽

☑6ᵗʰ　M62.52　Muscle wasting and atrophy, not elsewhere classified, upper arm
M62.521　Muscle wasting and atrophy, not elsewhere classified, right upper arm
M62.522　Muscle wasting and atrophy, not elsewhere classified, left upper arm
M62.529　Muscle wasting and atrophy, not elsewhere classified, unspecified upper arm ▽

☑6ᵗʰ　M62.53　Muscle wasting and atrophy, not elsewhere classified, forearm
M62.531　Muscle wasting and atrophy, not elsewhere classified, right forearm
M62.532　Muscle wasting and atrophy, not elsewhere classified, left forearm
M62.539　Muscle wasting and atrophy, not elsewhere classified, unspecified forearm ▽

☑6ᵗʰ　M62.54　Muscle wasting and atrophy, not elsewhere classified, hand
M62.541　Muscle wasting and atrophy, not elsewhere classified, right hand
M62.542　Muscle wasting and atrophy, not elsewhere classified, left hand
M62.549　Muscle wasting and atrophy, not elsewhere classified, unspecified hand ▽

☑6ᵗʰ　M62.55　Muscle wasting and atrophy, not elsewhere classified, thigh
M62.551　Muscle wasting and atrophy, not elsewhere classified, right thigh
M62.552　Muscle wasting and atrophy, not elsewhere classified, left thigh
M62.559　Muscle wasting and atrophy, not elsewhere classified, unspecified thigh ▽

☑6ᵗʰ　M62.56　Muscle wasting and atrophy, not elsewhere classified, lower leg
M62.561　Muscle wasting and atrophy, not elsewhere classified, right lower leg
M62.562　Muscle wasting and atrophy, not elsewhere classified, left lower leg
M62.569　Muscle wasting and atrophy, not elsewhere classified, unspecified lower leg ▽

☑6ᵗʰ　M62.57　Muscle wasting and atrophy, not elsewhere classified, ankle and foot
M62.571　Muscle wasting and atrophy, not elsewhere classified, right ankle and foot
M62.572　Muscle wasting and atrophy, not elsewhere classified, left ankle and foot
M62.579　Muscle wasting and atrophy, not elsewhere classified, unspecified ankle and foot ▽
M62.58　Muscle wasting and atrophy, not elsewhere classified, other site
M62.59　Muscle wasting and atrophy, not elsewhere classified, multiple sites

☑5ᵗʰ　M62.8　Other specified disorders of muscle
EXCLUDES 2　nontraumatic hematoma of muscle (M79.81)

M62.81　Muscle weakness (generalized)
EXCLUDES 1　muscle weakness in sarcopenia (M62.84)

M62.82　Rhabdomyolysis
EXCLUDES 1　traumatic rhabdomyolysis (T79.6)
DEF: Rapid disintegration or destruction of skeletal muscle caused by direct or indirect injury, resulting in the excretion of muscle protein myoglobin into the urine.

☑6ᵗʰ　M62.83　Muscle spasm
M62.830　Muscle spasm of back
M62.831　Muscle spasm of calf
Charley-horse
M62.838　Other muscle spasm

M62.84　Sarcopenia
Age-related sarcopenia
Code first underlying disease, if applicable, such as:
　disorders of myoneural junction and muscle disease in diseases classified elsewhere (G73.-)
　other and unspecified myopathies (G72.-)
　primary disorders of muscles (G71.-)
AHA: 2016,4Q,41

M62.89　Other specified disorders of muscle
Muscle (sheath) hernia

M62.9　Disorder of muscle, unspecified ▽

☑4ᵗʰ　M63　Disorders of muscle in diseases classified elsewhere
Code first underlying disease, such as:
　leprosy (A30.-)
　neoplasm (C49.-, C79.89, D21.-, D48.1)
　schistosomiasis (B65.-)
　trichinellosis (B75)
EXCLUDES 1　myopathy in cysticercosis (B69.81)
　　　　　　myopathy in endocrine diseases (G73.7)
　　　　　　myopathy in metabolic diseases (G73.7)
　　　　　　myopathy in sarcoidosis (D86.87)
　　　　　　myopathy in secondary syphilis (A51.49)
　　　　　　myopathy in syphilis (late) (A52.78)
　　　　　　myopathy in toxoplasmosis (B58.82)
　　　　　　myopathy in tuberculosis (A18.09)

☑5ᵗʰ　M63.8　Disorders of muscle in diseases classified elsewhere

M63.80　*Disorders of muscle in diseases classified elsewhere, unspecified site* ▽

☑6ᵗʰ　M63.81　Disorders of muscle in diseases classified elsewhere, shoulder
M63.811　*Disorders of muscle in diseases classified elsewhere, right shoulder*
M63.812　*Disorders of muscle in diseases classified elsewhere, left shoulder*
M63.819　*Disorders of muscle in diseases classified elsewhere, unspecified shoulder* ▽

☑6ᵗʰ　M63.82　Disorders of muscle in diseases classified elsewhere, upper arm
M63.821　*Disorders of muscle in diseases classified elsewhere, right upper arm*
M63.822　*Disorders of muscle in diseases classified elsewhere, left upper arm*
M63.829　*Disorders of muscle in diseases classified elsewhere, unspecified upper arm* ▽

☑6ᵗʰ　M63.83　Disorders of muscle in diseases classified elsewhere, forearm
M63.831　*Disorders of muscle in diseases classified elsewhere, right forearm*
M63.832　*Disorders of muscle in diseases classified elsewhere, left forearm*
M63.839　*Disorders of muscle in diseases classified elsewhere, unspecified forearm* ▽

☑6ᵗʰ　M63.84　Disorders of muscle in diseases classified elsewhere, hand
M63.841　*Disorders of muscle in diseases classified elsewhere, right hand*
M63.842　*Disorders of muscle in diseases classified elsewhere, left hand*
M63.849　*Disorders of muscle in diseases classified elsewhere, unspecified hand* ▽

☑ Additional Character Req　　✓x7ᵗʰ Placeholder Alert　　Manifestation　　▽ Unspecified　　►◄ Revised Text　　● New Code　　▲ Revised Code Title

ICD-10-CM 2019　　　**791**

Chapter 13. Diseases of the Musculoskeletal System and Connective Tissue

M63.85–M65.269

√6ᵗʰ **M63.85** **Disorders of muscle in diseases classified elsewhere, thigh**

    M63.851 *Disorders of muscle in diseases classified elsewhere, right thigh*

    M63.852 *Disorders of muscle in diseases classified elsewhere, left thigh*

    M63.859 *Disorders of muscle in diseases classified elsewhere, unspecified thigh* ▽

√6ᵗʰ **M63.86** **Disorders of muscle in diseases classified elsewhere, lower leg**

    M63.861 *Disorders of muscle in diseases classified elsewhere, right lower leg*

    M63.862 *Disorders of muscle in diseases classified elsewhere, left lower leg*

    M63.869 *Disorders of muscle in diseases classified elsewhere, unspecified lower leg* ▽

√6ᵗʰ **M63.87** **Disorders of muscle in diseases classified elsewhere, ankle and foot**

    M63.871 *Disorders of muscle in diseases classified elsewhere, right ankle and foot*

    M63.872 *Disorders of muscle in diseases classified elsewhere, left ankle and foot*

    M63.879 *Disorders of muscle in diseases classified elsewhere, unspecified ankle and foot* ▽

   M63.88 *Disorders of muscle in diseases classified elsewhere, other site*

   M63.89 *Disorders of muscle in diseases classified elsewhere, multiple sites*

Disorders of synovium and tendon (M65-M67)

√4ᵗʰ **M65** **Synovitis and tenosynovitis**

   EXCLUDES 1   *chronic crepitant synovitis of hand and wrist (M70.0-)*
              current injury - see injury of ligament or tendon by body region
              soft tissue disorders related to use, overuse and pressure (M70.-)

√5ᵗʰ **M65.0** **Abscess of tendon sheath**

   Use additional code (B95-B96) to identify bacterial agent.

   M65.00 **Abscess of tendon sheath, unspecified site** ▽

  √6ᵗʰ **M65.01** **Abscess of tendon sheath, shoulder**

    M65.011 **Abscess of tendon sheath, right shoulder**

    M65.012 **Abscess of tendon sheath, left shoulder**

    M65.019 **Abscess of tendon sheath, unspecified shoulder** ▽

  √6ᵗʰ **M65.02** **Abscess of tendon sheath, upper arm**

    M65.021 **Abscess of tendon sheath, right upper arm**

    M65.022 **Abscess of tendon sheath, left upper arm**

    M65.029 **Abscess of tendon sheath, unspecified upper arm** ▽

  √6ᵗʰ **M65.03** **Abscess of tendon sheath, forearm**

    M65.031 **Abscess of tendon sheath, right forearm**

    M65.032 **Abscess of tendon sheath, left forearm**

    M65.039 **Abscess of tendon sheath, unspecified forearm** ▽

  √6ᵗʰ **M65.04** **Abscess of tendon sheath, hand**

    M65.041 **Abscess of tendon sheath, right hand**

    M65.042 **Abscess of tendon sheath, left hand**

    M65.049 **Abscess of tendon sheath, unspecified hand** ▽

  √6ᵗʰ **M65.05** **Abscess of tendon sheath, thigh**

    M65.051 **Abscess of tendon sheath, right thigh**

    M65.052 **Abscess of tendon sheath, left thigh**

    M65.059 **Abscess of tendon sheath, unspecified thigh** ▽

  √6ᵗʰ **M65.06** **Abscess of tendon sheath, lower leg**

    M65.061 **Abscess of tendon sheath, right lower leg**

    M65.062 **Abscess of tendon sheath, left lower leg**

    M65.069 **Abscess of tendon sheath, unspecified lower leg** ▽

  √6ᵗʰ **M65.07** **Abscess of tendon sheath, ankle and foot**

    M65.071 **Abscess of tendon sheath, right ankle and foot**

    M65.072 **Abscess of tendon sheath, left ankle and foot**

    M65.079 **Abscess of tendon sheath, unspecified ankle and foot** ▽

   M65.08 **Abscess of tendon sheath, other site**

√5ᵗʰ **M65.1** **Other infective (teno)synovitis**

   M65.10 **Other infective (teno)synovitis, unspecified site** ▽

  √6ᵗʰ **M65.11** **Other infective (teno)synovitis, shoulder**

    M65.111 **Other infective (teno)synovitis, right shoulder**

    M65.112 **Other infective (teno)synovitis, left shoulder**

    M65.119 **Other infective (teno)synovitis, unspecified shoulder** ▽

  √6ᵗʰ **M65.12** **Other infective (teno)synovitis, elbow**

    M65.121 **Other infective (teno)synovitis, right elbow**

    M65.122 **Other infective (teno)synovitis, left elbow**

    M65.129 **Other infective (teno)synovitis, unspecified elbow** ▽

  √6ᵗʰ **M65.13** **Other infective (teno)synovitis, wrist**

    M65.131 **Other infective (teno)synovitis, right wrist**

    M65.132 **Other infective (teno)synovitis, left wrist**

    M65.139 **Other infective (teno)synovitis, unspecified wrist** ▽

  √6ᵗʰ **M65.14** **Other infective (teno)synovitis, hand**

    M65.141 **Other infective (teno)synovitis, right hand**

    M65.142 **Other infective (teno)synovitis, left hand**

    M65.149 **Other infective (teno)synovitis, unspecified hand** ▽

  √6ᵗʰ **M65.15** **Other infective (teno)synovitis, hip**

    M65.151 **Other infective (teno)synovitis, right hip**

    M65.152 **Other infective (teno)synovitis, left hip**

    M65.159 **Other infective (teno)synovitis, unspecified hip** ▽

  √6ᵗʰ **M65.16** **Other infective (teno)synovitis, knee**

    M65.161 **Other infective (teno)synovitis, right knee**

    M65.162 **Other infective (teno)synovitis, left knee**

    M65.169 **Other infective (teno)synovitis, unspecified knee** ▽

  √6ᵗʰ **M65.17** **Other infective (teno)synovitis, ankle and foot**

    M65.171 **Other infective (teno)synovitis, right ankle and foot**

    M65.172 **Other infective (teno)synovitis, left ankle and foot**

    M65.179 **Other infective (teno)synovitis, unspecified ankle and foot** ▽

   M65.18 **Other infective (teno)synovitis, other site**

   M65.19 **Other infective (teno)synovitis, multiple sites**

√5ᵗʰ **M65.2** **Calcific tendinitis**

   EXCLUDES 1   *tendinitis as classified in M75-M77*
              calcified tendinitis of shoulder (M75.3)

   M65.20 **Calcific tendinitis, unspecified site** ▽

  √6ᵗʰ **M65.22** **Calcific tendinitis, upper arm**

    M65.221 **Calcific tendinitis, right upper arm**

    M65.222 **Calcific tendinitis, left upper arm**

    M65.229 **Calcific tendinitis, unspecified upper arm** ▽

  √6ᵗʰ **M65.23** **Calcific tendinitis, forearm**

    M65.231 **Calcific tendinitis, right forearm**

    M65.232 **Calcific tendinitis, left forearm**

    M65.239 **Calcific tendinitis, unspecified forearm** ▽

  √6ᵗʰ **M65.24** **Calcific tendinitis, hand**

    M65.241 **Calcific tendinitis, right hand**

    M65.242 **Calcific tendinitis, left hand**

    M65.249 **Calcific tendinitis, unspecified hand** ▽

  √6ᵗʰ **M65.25** **Calcific tendinitis, thigh**

    M65.251 **Calcific tendinitis, right thigh**

    M65.252 **Calcific tendinitis, left thigh**

    M65.259 **Calcific tendinitis, unspecified thigh** ▽

  √6ᵗʰ **M65.26** **Calcific tendinitis, lower leg**

    M65.261 **Calcific tendinitis, right lower leg**

    M65.262 **Calcific tendinitis, left lower leg**

    M65.269 **Calcific tendinitis, unspecified lower leg** ▽

√6ᵗʰ **M65.27 Calcific tendinitis, ankle and foot**

     M65.271 Calcific tendinitis, right ankle and foot
     M65.272 Calcific tendinitis, left ankle and foot
     M65.279 Calcific tendinitis, unspecified ankle and foot ▽

M65.28 Calcific tendinitis, other site
M65.29 Calcific tendinitis, multiple sites

√5ᵗʰ **M65.3 Trigger finger**

     Nodular tendinous disease

M65.30 Trigger finger, unspecified finger ▽

√6ᵗʰ **M65.31 Trigger thumb**

     M65.311 Trigger thumb, right thumb
     M65.312 Trigger thumb, left thumb
     M65.319 Trigger thumb, unspecified thumb ▽

√6ᵗʰ **M65.32 Trigger finger, index finger**

     M65.321 Trigger finger, right index finger
     M65.322 Trigger finger, left index finger
     M65.329 Trigger finger, unspecified index finger ▽

√6ᵗʰ **M65.33 Trigger finger, middle finger**

     M65.331 Trigger finger, right middle finger
     M65.332 Trigger finger, left middle finger
     M65.339 Trigger finger, unspecified middle finger ▽

√6ᵗʰ **M65.34 Trigger finger, ring finger**

     M65.341 Trigger finger, right ring finger
     M65.342 Trigger finger, left ring finger
     M65.349 Trigger finger, unspecified ring finger ▽

√6ᵗʰ **M65.35 Trigger finger, little finger**

     M65.351 Trigger finger, right little finger
     M65.352 Trigger finger, left little finger
     M65.359 Trigger finger, unspecified little finger ▽

M65.4 Radial styloid tenosynovitis [de Quervain]

√5ᵗʰ **M65.8 Other synovitis and tenosynovitis**

M65.80 Other synovitis and tenosynovitis, unspecified site ▽

√6ᵗʰ **M65.81 Other synovitis and tenosynovitis, shoulder**

     M65.811 Other synovitis and tenosynovitis, right shoulder
     M65.812 Other synovitis and tenosynovitis, left shoulder
     M65.819 Other synovitis and tenosynovitis, unspecified shoulder ▽

√6ᵗʰ **M65.82 Other synovitis and tenosynovitis, upper arm**

     M65.821 Other synovitis and tenosynovitis, right upper arm
     M65.822 Other synovitis and tenosynovitis, left upper arm
     M65.829 Other synovitis and tenosynovitis, unspecified upper arm ▽

√6ᵗʰ **M65.83 Other synovitis and tenosynovitis, forearm**

     M65.831 Other synovitis and tenosynovitis, right forearm
     M65.832 Other synovitis and tenosynovitis, left forearm
     M65.839 Other synovitis and tenosynovitis, unspecified forearm ▽

√6ᵗʰ **M65.84 Other synovitis and tenosynovitis, hand**

     M65.841 Other synovitis and tenosynovitis, right hand
     M65.842 Other synovitis and tenosynovitis, left hand
     M65.849 Other synovitis and tenosynovitis, unspecified hand ▽

√6ᵗʰ **M65.85 Other synovitis and tenosynovitis, thigh**

     M65.851 Other synovitis and tenosynovitis, right thigh
     M65.852 Other synovitis and tenosynovitis, left thigh
     M65.859 Other synovitis and tenosynovitis, unspecified thigh ▽

√6ᵗʰ **M65.86 Other synovitis and tenosynovitis, lower leg**

     M65.861 Other synovitis and tenosynovitis, right lower leg
     M65.862 Other synovitis and tenosynovitis, left lower leg
     M65.869 Other synovitis and tenosynovitis, unspecified lower leg ▽

√6ᵗʰ **M65.87 Other synovitis and tenosynovitis, ankle and foot**

     M65.871 Other synovitis and tenosynovitis, right ankle and foot
     M65.872 Other synovitis and tenosynovitis, left ankle and foot
     M65.879 Other synovitis and tenosynovitis, unspecified ankle and foot ▽

M65.88 Other synovitis and tenosynovitis, other site
M65.89 Other synovitis and tenosynovitis, multiple sites

M65.9 Synovitis and tenosynovitis, unspecified ▽

√4ᵗʰ **M66 Spontaneous rupture of synovium and tendon**

     INCLUDES   rupture that occurs when a normal force is applied to tissues that are inferred to have less than normal strength

     EXCLUDES 2   *rotator cuff syndrome (M75.1-)*
         rupture where an abnormal force is applied to normal tissue - see injury of tendon by body region

M66.0 Rupture of popliteal cyst

√5ᵗʰ **M66.1 Rupture of synovium**

     Rupture of synovial cyst
     EXCLUDES 2   *rupture of popliteal cyst (M66.0)*

M66.10 Rupture of synovium, unspecified joint ▽

√6ᵗʰ **M66.11 Rupture of synovium, shoulder**

     M66.111 Rupture of synovium, right shoulder
     M66.112 Rupture of synovium, left shoulder
     M66.119 Rupture of synovium, unspecified shoulder ▽

√6ᵗʰ **M66.12 Rupture of synovium, elbow**

     M66.121 Rupture of synovium, right elbow
     M66.122 Rupture of synovium, left elbow
     M66.129 Rupture of synovium, unspecified elbow ▽

√6ᵗʰ **M66.13 Rupture of synovium, wrist**

     M66.131 Rupture of synovium, right wrist
     M66.132 Rupture of synovium, left wrist
     M66.139 Rupture of synovium, unspecified wrist ▽

√6ᵗʰ **M66.14 Rupture of synovium, hand and fingers**

     M66.141 Rupture of synovium, right hand
     M66.142 Rupture of synovium, left hand
     M66.143 Rupture of synovium, unspecified hand ▽
     M66.144 Rupture of synovium, right finger(s)
     M66.145 Rupture of synovium, left finger(s)
     M66.146 Rupture of synovium, unspecified finger(s) ▽

√6ᵗʰ **M66.15 Rupture of synovium, hip**

     M66.151 Rupture of synovium, right hip
     M66.152 Rupture of synovium, left hip
     M66.159 Rupture of synovium, unspecified hip ▽

√6ᵗʰ **M66.17 Rupture of synovium, ankle, foot and toes**

     M66.171 Rupture of synovium, right ankle
     M66.172 Rupture of synovium, left ankle
     M66.173 Rupture of synovium, unspecified ankle ▽
     M66.174 Rupture of synovium, right foot
     M66.175 Rupture of synovium, left foot
     M66.176 Rupture of synovium, unspecified foot ▽
     M66.177 Rupture of synovium, right toe(s)
     M66.178 Rupture of synovium, left toe(s)
     M66.179 Rupture of synovium, unspecified toe(s) ▽

M66.18 Rupture of synovium, other site

☑ Additional Character Req   √ˣ⁷ᵗʰ Placeholder Alert   Manifestation   ▽ Unspecified   ▶◀ Revised Text   ● New Code   ▲ Revised Code Title

ICD-10-CM 2019   793

✓5ᵗʰ **M66.2 Spontaneous rupture of extensor tendons**

> **TIP:** Refer to the Muscle/Tendon table at the beginning of this chapter.

M66.20 Spontaneous rupture of extensor tendons, unspecified site ▽

✓6ᵗʰ **M66.21 Spontaneous rupture of extensor tendons, shoulder**

M66.211 Spontaneous rupture of extensor tendons, right shoulder

M66.212 Spontaneous rupture of extensor tendons, left shoulder

M66.219 Spontaneous rupture of extensor tendons, unspecified shoulder ▽

✓6ᵗʰ **M66.22 Spontaneous rupture of extensor tendons, upper arm**

M66.221 Spontaneous rupture of extensor tendons, right upper arm

M66.222 Spontaneous rupture of extensor tendons, left upper arm

M66.229 Spontaneous rupture of extensor tendons, unspecified upper arm ▽

✓6ᵗʰ **M66.23 Spontaneous rupture of extensor tendons, forearm**

M66.231 Spontaneous rupture of extensor tendons, right forearm

M66.232 Spontaneous rupture of extensor tendons, left forearm

M66.239 Spontaneous rupture of extensor tendons, unspecified forearm ▽

✓6ᵗʰ **M66.24 Spontaneous rupture of extensor tendons, hand**

M66.241 Spontaneous rupture of extensor tendons, right hand

M66.242 Spontaneous rupture of extensor tendons, left hand

M66.249 Spontaneous rupture of extensor tendons, unspecified hand ▽

✓6ᵗʰ **M66.25 Spontaneous rupture of extensor tendons, thigh**

M66.251 Spontaneous rupture of extensor tendons, right thigh

M66.252 Spontaneous rupture of extensor tendons, left thigh

M66.259 Spontaneous rupture of extensor tendons, unspecified thigh ▽

✓6ᵗʰ **M66.26 Spontaneous rupture of extensor tendons, lower leg**

M66.261 Spontaneous rupture of extensor tendons, right lower leg

M66.262 Spontaneous rupture of extensor tendons, left lower leg

M66.269 Spontaneous rupture of extensor tendons, unspecified lower leg ▽

✓6ᵗʰ **M66.27 Spontaneous rupture of extensor tendons, ankle and foot**

M66.271 Spontaneous rupture of extensor tendons, right ankle and foot

M66.272 Spontaneous rupture of extensor tendons, left ankle and foot

M66.279 Spontaneous rupture of extensor tendons, unspecified ankle and foot ▽

M66.28 Spontaneous rupture of extensor tendons, other site

M66.29 Spontaneous rupture of extensor tendons, multiple sites

✓5ᵗʰ **M66.3 Spontaneous rupture of flexor tendons**

> **TIP:** Refer to the Muscle/Tendon table at the beginning of this chapter.

M66.30 Spontaneous rupture of flexor tendons, unspecified site ▽

✓6ᵗʰ **M66.31 Spontaneous rupture of flexor tendons, shoulder**

M66.311 Spontaneous rupture of flexor tendons, right shoulder

M66.312 Spontaneous rupture of flexor tendons, left shoulder

M66.319 Spontaneous rupture of flexor tendons, unspecified shoulder ▽

✓6ᵗʰ **M66.32 Spontaneous rupture of flexor tendons, upper arm**

M66.321 Spontaneous rupture of flexor tendons, right upper arm

M66.322 Spontaneous rupture of flexor tendons, left upper arm

M66.329 Spontaneous rupture of flexor tendons, unspecified upper arm ▽

✓6ᵗʰ **M66.33 Spontaneous rupture of flexor tendons, forearm**

M66.331 Spontaneous rupture of flexor tendons, right forearm

M66.332 Spontaneous rupture of flexor tendons, left forearm

M66.339 Spontaneous rupture of flexor tendons, unspecified forearm ▽

✓6ᵗʰ **M66.34 Spontaneous rupture of flexor tendons, hand**

M66.341 Spontaneous rupture of flexor tendons, right hand

M66.342 Spontaneous rupture of flexor tendons, left hand

M66.349 Spontaneous rupture of flexor tendons, unspecified hand ▽

✓6ᵗʰ **M66.35 Spontaneous rupture of flexor tendons, thigh**

M66.351 Spontaneous rupture of flexor tendons, right thigh

M66.352 Spontaneous rupture of flexor tendons, left thigh

M66.359 Spontaneous rupture of flexor tendons, unspecified thigh ▽

✓6ᵗʰ **M66.36 Spontaneous rupture of flexor tendons, lower leg**

M66.361 Spontaneous rupture of flexor tendons, right lower leg

M66.362 Spontaneous rupture of flexor tendons, left lower leg

M66.369 Spontaneous rupture of flexor tendons, unspecified lower leg ▽

✓6ᵗʰ **M66.37 Spontaneous rupture of flexor tendons, ankle and foot**

M66.371 Spontaneous rupture of flexor tendons, right ankle and foot

M66.372 Spontaneous rupture of flexor tendons, left ankle and foot

M66.379 Spontaneous rupture of flexor tendons, unspecified ankle and foot ▽

M66.38 Spontaneous rupture of flexor tendons, other site

M66.39 Spontaneous rupture of flexor tendons, multiple sites

✓5ᵗʰ **M66.8 Spontaneous rupture of other tendons**

> **TIP:** Refer to the Muscle/Tendon table at the beginning of this chapter.

M66.80 Spontaneous rupture of other tendons, unspecified site ▽

✓6ᵗʰ **M66.81 Spontaneous rupture of other tendons, shoulder**

M66.811 Spontaneous rupture of other tendons, right shoulder

M66.812 Spontaneous rupture of other tendons, left shoulder

M66.819 Spontaneous rupture of other tendons, unspecified shoulder ▽

✓6ᵗʰ **M66.82 Spontaneous rupture of other tendons, upper arm**

M66.821 Spontaneous rupture of other tendons, right upper arm

M66.822 Spontaneous rupture of other tendons, left upper arm

M66.829 Spontaneous rupture of other tendons, unspecified upper arm ▽

✓6ᵗʰ **M66.83 Spontaneous rupture of other tendons, forearm**

M66.831 Spontaneous rupture of other tendons, right forearm

M66.832 Spontaneous rupture of other tendons, left forearm

M66.839 Spontaneous rupture of other tendons, unspecified forearm ▽

✓6ᵗʰ **M66.84 Spontaneous rupture of other tendons, hand**

M66.841 Spontaneous rupture of other tendons, right hand

M66.842 Spontaneous rupture of other tendons, left hand

M66.849 Spontaneous rupture of other tendons, unspecified hand ▽

✓6ᵗʰ **M66.85 Spontaneous rupture of other tendons, thigh**

M66.851 Spontaneous rupture of other tendons, right thigh

M66.852 Spontaneous rupture of other tendons, left thigh

M66.859 Spontaneous rupture of other tendons, unspecified thigh ▽

✓6ᵗʰ **M66.86** Spontaneous rupture of other tendons, lower leg

    M66.861 Spontaneous rupture of other tendons, right lower leg

    M66.862 Spontaneous rupture of other tendons, left lower leg

    M66.869 Spontaneous rupture of other tendons, unspecified lower leg ▽

✓6ᵗʰ **M66.87** Spontaneous rupture of other tendons, ankle and foot

    M66.871 Spontaneous rupture of other tendons, right ankle and foot

    M66.872 Spontaneous rupture of other tendons, left ankle and foot

    M66.879 Spontaneous rupture of other tendons, unspecified ankle and foot ▽

  M66.88 Spontaneous rupture of other tendons, other

  M66.89 Spontaneous rupture of other tendons, multiple sites

 M66.9 Spontaneous rupture of unspecified tendon ▽
    Rupture at musculotendinous junction, nontraumatic

✓4ᵗʰ **M67** **Other disorders of synovium and tendon**

  EXCLUDES 1 *palmar fascial fibromatosis [Dupuytren] (M72.0)*
    tendinitis NOS (M77.9-)
    xanthomatosis localized to tendons (E78.2)

✓5ᵗʰ **M67.0** Short Achilles tendon (acquired)

  M67.00 Short Achilles tendon (acquired), unspecified ankle ▽

  M67.01 Short Achilles tendon (acquired), right ankle

  M67.02 Short Achilles tendon (acquired), left ankle

✓5ᵗʰ **M67.2** Synovial hypertrophy, not elsewhere classified

  EXCLUDES 1 *villonodular synovitis (pigmented) (M12.2-)*

  M67.20 Synovial hypertrophy, not elsewhere classified, unspecified site ▽

✓6ᵗʰ **M67.21** Synovial hypertrophy, not elsewhere classified, shoulder

    M67.211 Synovial hypertrophy, not elsewhere classified, right shoulder

    M67.212 Synovial hypertrophy, not elsewhere classified, left shoulder

    M67.219 Synovial hypertrophy, not elsewhere classified, unspecified shoulder ▽

✓6ᵗʰ **M67.22** Synovial hypertrophy, not elsewhere classified, upper arm

    M67.221 Synovial hypertrophy, not elsewhere classified, right upper arm

    M67.222 Synovial hypertrophy, not elsewhere classified, left upper arm

    M67.229 Synovial hypertrophy, not elsewhere classified, unspecified upper arm ▽

✓6ᵗʰ **M67.23** Synovial hypertrophy, not elsewhere classified, forearm

    M67.231 Synovial hypertrophy, not elsewhere classified, right forearm

    M67.232 Synovial hypertrophy, not elsewhere classified, left forearm

    M67.239 Synovial hypertrophy, not elsewhere classified, unspecified forearm ▽

✓6ᵗʰ **M67.24** Synovial hypertrophy, not elsewhere classified, hand

    M67.241 Synovial hypertrophy, not elsewhere classified, right hand

    M67.242 Synovial hypertrophy, not elsewhere classified, left hand

    M67.249 Synovial hypertrophy, not elsewhere classified, unspecified hand ▽

✓6ᵗʰ **M67.25** Synovial hypertrophy, not elsewhere classified, thigh

    M67.251 Synovial hypertrophy, not elsewhere classified, right thigh

    M67.252 Synovial hypertrophy, not elsewhere classified, left thigh

    M67.259 Synovial hypertrophy, not elsewhere classified, unspecified thigh ▽

✓6ᵗʰ **M67.26** Synovial hypertrophy, not elsewhere classified, lower leg

    M67.261 Synovial hypertrophy, not elsewhere classified, right lower leg

    M67.262 Synovial hypertrophy, not elsewhere classified, left lower leg

    M67.269 Synovial hypertrophy, not elsewhere classified, unspecified lower leg ▽

✓6ᵗʰ **M67.27** Synovial hypertrophy, not elsewhere classified, ankle and foot

    M67.271 Synovial hypertrophy, not elsewhere classified, right ankle and foot

    M67.272 Synovial hypertrophy, not elsewhere classified, left ankle and foot

    M67.279 Synovial hypertrophy, not elsewhere classified, unspecified ankle and foot ▽

  M67.28 Synovial hypertrophy, not elsewhere classified, other site

  M67.29 Synovial hypertrophy, not elsewhere classified, multiple sites

✓5ᵗʰ **M67.3** Transient synovitis

  Toxic synovitis
  EXCLUDES 1 *palindromic rheumatism (M12.3-)*

  M67.30 Transient synovitis, unspecified site ▽

✓6ᵗʰ **M67.31** Transient synovitis, shoulder

    M67.311 Transient synovitis, right shoulder

    M67.312 Transient synovitis, left shoulder

    M67.319 Transient synovitis, unspecified shoulder ▽

✓6ᵗʰ **M67.32** Transient synovitis, elbow

    M67.321 Transient synovitis, right elbow

    M67.322 Transient synovitis, left elbow

    M67.329 Transient synovitis, unspecified elbow ▽

✓6ᵗʰ **M67.33** Transient synovitis, wrist

    M67.331 Transient synovitis, right wrist

    M67.332 Transient synovitis, left wrist

    M67.339 Transient synovitis, unspecified wrist ▽

✓6ᵗʰ **M67.34** Transient synovitis, hand

    M67.341 Transient synovitis, right hand

    M67.342 Transient synovitis, left hand

    M67.349 Transient synovitis, unspecified hand ▽

✓6ᵗʰ **M67.35** Transient synovitis, hip

    M67.351 Transient synovitis, right hip

    M67.352 Transient synovitis, left hip

    M67.359 Transient synovitis, unspecified hip ▽

✓6ᵗʰ **M67.36** Transient synovitis, knee

    M67.361 Transient synovitis, right knee

    M67.362 Transient synovitis, left knee

    M67.369 Transient synovitis, unspecified knee ▽

✓6ᵗʰ **M67.37** Transient synovitis, ankle and foot

    M67.371 Transient synovitis, right ankle and foot

    M67.372 Transient synovitis, left ankle and foot

    M67.379 Transient synovitis, unspecified ankle and foot ▽

  M67.38 Transient synovitis, other site

  M67.39 Transient synovitis, multiple sites

✓5ᵗʰ **M67.4** Ganglion

  Ganglion of joint or tendon (sheath)
  EXCLUDES 1 *ganglion in yaws (A66.6)*
  EXCLUDES 2 *cyst of bursa (M71.2-M71.3)*
    cyst of synovium (M71.2-M71.3)

  DEF: Fluid-filled, benign cyst appearing on a tendon sheath or aponeurosis, frequently connecting to an underlying joint.

  M67.40 Ganglion, unspecified site ▽

✓6ᵗʰ **M67.41** Ganglion, shoulder

    M67.411 Ganglion, right shoulder

    M67.412 Ganglion, left shoulder

    M67.419 Ganglion, unspecified shoulder ▽

✓6ᵗʰ **M67.42** Ganglion, elbow

    M67.421 Ganglion, right elbow

    M67.422 Ganglion, left elbow

✓ Additional Character Req   ✓x7ᵗʰ Placeholder Alert   **Manifestation**   ▽ Unspecified   ▶◀ Revised Text   ● New Code   ▲ Revised Code Title

        M67.429   Ganglion, unspecified elbow   ▽
√6ᵗʰ M67.43   Ganglion, wrist

Ganglion of Wrist

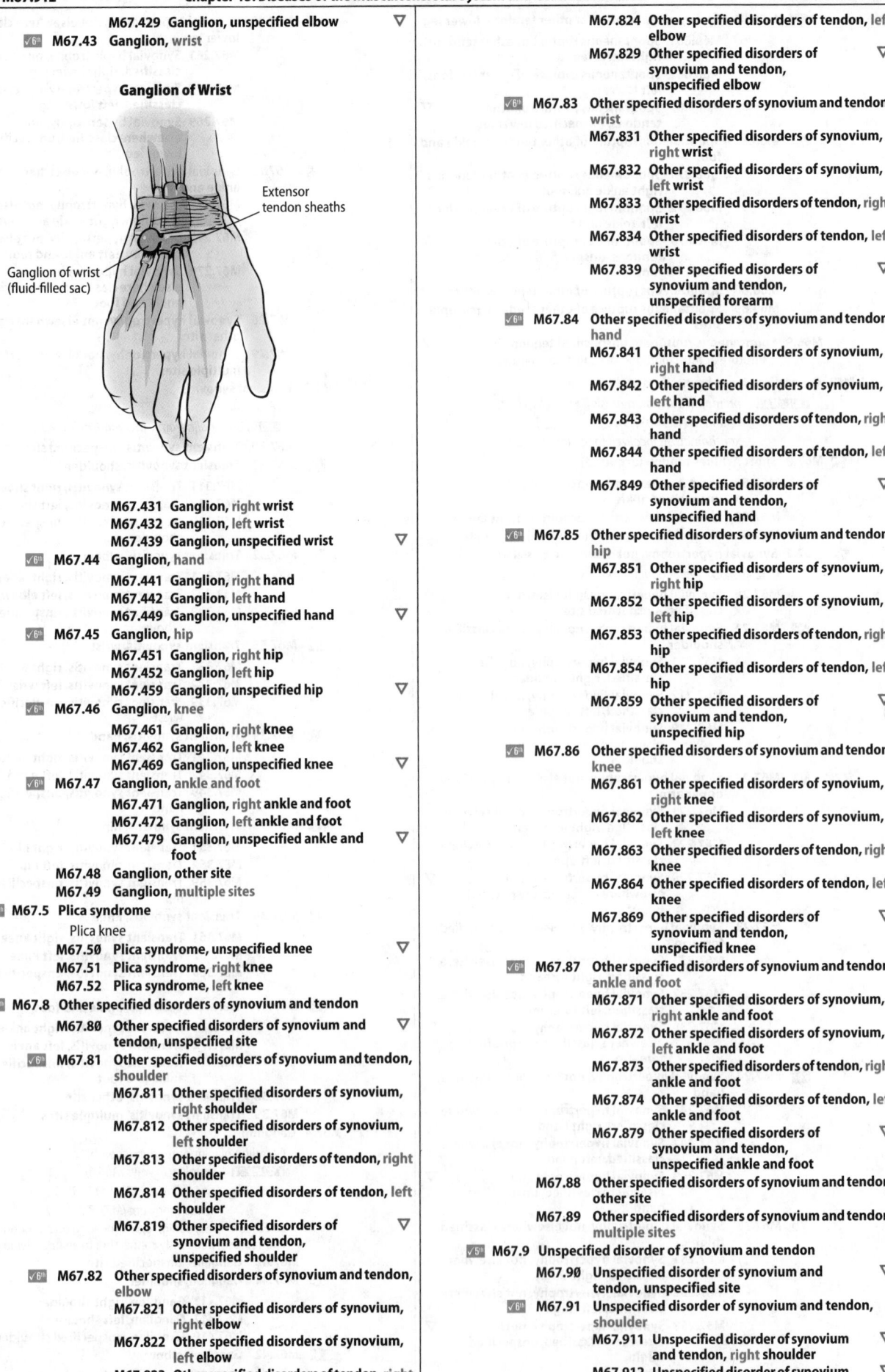

Extensor tendon sheaths

Ganglion of wrist (fluid-filled sac)

        M67.431   Ganglion, right wrist
        M67.432   Ganglion, left wrist
        M67.439   Ganglion, unspecified wrist   ▽
√6ᵗʰ M67.44   Ganglion, hand
        M67.441   Ganglion, right hand
        M67.442   Ganglion, left hand
        M67.449   Ganglion, unspecified hand   ▽
√6ᵗʰ M67.45   Ganglion, hip
        M67.451   Ganglion, right hip
        M67.452   Ganglion, left hip
        M67.459   Ganglion, unspecified hip   ▽
√6ᵗʰ M67.46   Ganglion, knee
        M67.461   Ganglion, right knee
        M67.462   Ganglion, left knee
        M67.469   Ganglion, unspecified knee   ▽
√6ᵗʰ M67.47   Ganglion, ankle and foot
        M67.471   Ganglion, right ankle and foot
        M67.472   Ganglion, left ankle and foot
        M67.479   Ganglion, unspecified ankle and foot   ▽
    M67.48   Ganglion, other site
    M67.49   Ganglion, multiple sites
√5ᵗʰ M67.5   Plica syndrome
    Plica knee
    M67.50   Plica syndrome, unspecified knee   ▽
    M67.51   Plica syndrome, right knee
    M67.52   Plica syndrome, left knee
√5ᵗʰ M67.8   Other specified disorders of synovium and tendon
    M67.80   Other specified disorders of synovium and tendon, unspecified site   ▽
√6ᵗʰ M67.81   Other specified disorders of synovium and tendon, shoulder
        M67.811   Other specified disorders of synovium, right shoulder
        M67.812   Other specified disorders of synovium, left shoulder
        M67.813   Other specified disorders of tendon, right shoulder
        M67.814   Other specified disorders of tendon, left shoulder
        M67.819   Other specified disorders of synovium and tendon, unspecified shoulder   ▽
√6ᵗʰ M67.82   Other specified disorders of synovium and tendon, elbow
        M67.821   Other specified disorders of synovium, right elbow
        M67.822   Other specified disorders of synovium, left elbow
        M67.823   Other specified disorders of tendon, right elbow

        M67.824   Other specified disorders of tendon, left elbow
        M67.829   Other specified disorders of synovium and tendon, unspecified elbow   ▽
√6ᵗʰ M67.83   Other specified disorders of synovium and tendon, wrist
        M67.831   Other specified disorders of synovium, right wrist
        M67.832   Other specified disorders of synovium, left wrist
        M67.833   Other specified disorders of tendon, right wrist
        M67.834   Other specified disorders of tendon, left wrist
        M67.839   Other specified disorders of synovium and tendon, unspecified forearm   ▽
√6ᵗʰ M67.84   Other specified disorders of synovium and tendon, hand
        M67.841   Other specified disorders of synovium, right hand
        M67.842   Other specified disorders of synovium, left hand
        M67.843   Other specified disorders of tendon, right hand
        M67.844   Other specified disorders of tendon, left hand
        M67.849   Other specified disorders of synovium and tendon, unspecified hand   ▽
√6ᵗʰ M67.85   Other specified disorders of synovium and tendon, hip
        M67.851   Other specified disorders of synovium, right hip
        M67.852   Other specified disorders of synovium, left hip
        M67.853   Other specified disorders of tendon, right hip
        M67.854   Other specified disorders of tendon, left hip
        M67.859   Other specified disorders of synovium and tendon, unspecified hip   ▽
√6ᵗʰ M67.86   Other specified disorders of synovium and tendon, knee
        M67.861   Other specified disorders of synovium, right knee
        M67.862   Other specified disorders of synovium, left knee
        M67.863   Other specified disorders of tendon, right knee
        M67.864   Other specified disorders of tendon, left knee
        M67.869   Other specified disorders of synovium and tendon, unspecified knee   ▽
√6ᵗʰ M67.87   Other specified disorders of synovium and tendon, ankle and foot
        M67.871   Other specified disorders of synovium, right ankle and foot
        M67.872   Other specified disorders of synovium, left ankle and foot
        M67.873   Other specified disorders of tendon, right ankle and foot
        M67.874   Other specified disorders of tendon, left ankle and foot
        M67.879   Other specified disorders of synovium and tendon, unspecified ankle and foot   ▽
    M67.88   Other specified disorders of synovium and tendon, other site
    M67.89   Other specified disorders of synovium and tendon, multiple sites
√5ᵗʰ M67.9   Unspecified disorder of synovium and tendon
    M67.90   Unspecified disorder of synovium and tendon, unspecified site   ▽
√6ᵗʰ M67.91   Unspecified disorder of synovium and tendon, shoulder
        M67.911   Unspecified disorder of synovium and tendon, right shoulder   ▽
        M67.912   Unspecified disorder of synovium and tendon, left shoulder   ▽

M67.919   Unspecified disorder of synovium and tendon, unspecified shoulder ▽

✓6ᵗʰ M67.92   Unspecified disorder of synovium and tendon, upper arm

     M67.921   Unspecified disorder of synovium and tendon, right upper arm ▽

     M67.922   Unspecified disorder of synovium and tendon, left upper arm ▽

     M67.929   Unspecified disorder of synovium and tendon, unspecified upper arm ▽

✓6ᵗʰ M67.93   Unspecified disorder of synovium and tendon, forearm

     M67.931   Unspecified disorder of synovium and tendon, right forearm ▽

     M67.932   Unspecified disorder of synovium and tendon, left forearm ▽

     M67.939   Unspecified disorder of synovium and tendon, unspecified forearm ▽

✓6ᵗʰ M67.94   Unspecified disorder of synovium and tendon, hand

     M67.941   Unspecified disorder of synovium and tendon, right hand ▽

     M67.942   Unspecified disorder of synovium and tendon, left hand ▽

     M67.949   Unspecified disorder of synovium and tendon, unspecified hand ▽

✓6ᵗʰ M67.95   Unspecified disorder of synovium and tendon, thigh

     M67.951   Unspecified disorder of synovium and tendon, right thigh ▽

     M67.952   Unspecified disorder of synovium and tendon, left thigh ▽

     M67.959   Unspecified disorder of synovium and tendon, unspecified thigh ▽

✓6ᵗʰ M67.96   Unspecified disorder of synovium and tendon, lower leg

     M67.961   Unspecified disorder of synovium and tendon, right lower leg ▽

     M67.962   Unspecified disorder of synovium and tendon, left lower leg ▽

     M67.969   Unspecified disorder of synovium and tendon, unspecified lower leg ▽

✓6ᵗʰ M67.97   Unspecified disorder of synovium and tendon, ankle and foot

     M67.971   Unspecified disorder of synovium and tendon, right ankle and foot ▽

     M67.972   Unspecified disorder of synovium and tendon, left ankle and foot ▽

     M67.979   Unspecified disorder of synovium and tendon, unspecified ankle and foot ▽

M67.98   Unspecified disorder of synovium and tendon, other site ▽

M67.99   Unspecified disorder of synovium and tendon, multiple sites ▽

Other soft tissue disorders (M70-M79)

✓4ᵗʰ **M70**   **Soft tissue disorders related to use, overuse and pressure**

   INCLUDES   soft tissue disorders of occupational origin

   Use additional external cause code to identify activity causing disorder (Y93.-)

   EXCLUDES 1   bursitis NOS (M71.9-)

   EXCLUDES 2   bursitis of shoulder (M75.5)

            enthesopathies (M76-M77)

            pressure ulcer (pressure area) (L89.-)

✓5ᵗʰ M70.0   Crepitant synovitis (acute) (chronic) of hand and wrist

✓6ᵗʰ M70.03   Crepitant synovitis (acute) (chronic), wrist

     M70.031   Crepitant synovitis (acute) (chronic), right wrist

     M70.032   Crepitant synovitis (acute) (chronic), left wrist

     M70.039   Crepitant synovitis (acute) (chronic), unspecified wrist ▽

✓6ᵗʰ M70.04   Crepitant synovitis (acute) (chronic), hand

     M70.041   Crepitant synovitis (acute) (chronic), right hand

     M70.042   Crepitant synovitis (acute) (chronic), left hand

     M70.049   Crepitant synovitis (acute) (chronic), unspecified hand ▽

✓5ᵗʰ M70.1   Bursitis of hand

     M70.10   Bursitis, unspecified hand ▽

     M70.11   Bursitis, right hand

     M70.12   Bursitis, left hand

✓5ᵗʰ M70.2   Olecranon bursitis

     M70.20   Olecranon bursitis, unspecified elbow ▽

     M70.21   Olecranon bursitis, right elbow

     M70.22   Olecranon bursitis, left elbow

✓5ᵗʰ M70.3   Other bursitis of elbow

     M70.30   Other bursitis of elbow, unspecified elbow ▽

     M70.31   Other bursitis of elbow, right elbow

     M70.32   Other bursitis of elbow, left elbow

✓5ᵗʰ M70.4   Prepatellar bursitis

     M70.40   Prepatellar bursitis, unspecified knee ▽

     M70.41   Prepatellar bursitis, right knee

     M70.42   Prepatellar bursitis, left knee

✓5ᵗʰ M70.5   Other bursitis of knee

     M70.50   Other bursitis of knee, unspecified knee ▽

     M70.51   Other bursitis of knee, right knee

     M70.52   Other bursitis of knee, left knee

✓5ᵗʰ M70.6   Trochanteric bursitis

     Trochanteric tendinitis

     M70.60   Trochanteric bursitis, unspecified hip ▽

     M70.61   Trochanteric bursitis, right hip

     M70.62   Trochanteric bursitis, left hip

✓5ᵗʰ M70.7   Other bursitis of hip

     Ischial bursitis

     M70.70   Other bursitis of hip, unspecified hip ▽

     M70.71   Other bursitis of hip, right hip

     M70.72   Other bursitis of hip, left hip

✓5ᵗʰ M70.8   Other soft tissue disorders related to use, overuse and pressure

     M70.80   Other soft tissue disorders related to use, overuse and pressure of unspecified site ▽

   ✓6ᵗʰ M70.81   Other soft tissue disorders related to use, overuse and pressure of shoulder

     M70.811   Other soft tissue disorders related to use, overuse and pressure, right shoulder

     M70.812   Other soft tissue disorders related to use, overuse and pressure, left shoulder

     M70.819   Other soft tissue disorders related to use, overuse and pressure, unspecified shoulder ▽

   ✓6ᵗʰ M70.82   Other soft tissue disorders related to use, overuse and pressure of upper arm

     M70.821   Other soft tissue disorders related to use, overuse and pressure, right upper arm

     M70.822   Other soft tissue disorders related to use, overuse and pressure, left upper arm

     M70.829   Other soft tissue disorders related to use, overuse and pressure, unspecified upper arms ▽

   ✓6ᵗʰ M70.83   Other soft tissue disorders related to use, overuse and pressure of forearm

     M70.831   Other soft tissue disorders related to use, overuse and pressure, right forearm

     M70.832   Other soft tissue disorders related to use, overuse and pressure, left forearm

     M70.839   Other soft tissue disorders related to use, overuse and pressure, unspecified forearm ▽

   ✓6ᵗʰ M70.84   Other soft tissue disorders related to use, overuse and pressure of hand

     M70.841   Other soft tissue disorders related to use, overuse and pressure, right hand

     M70.842   Other soft tissue disorders related to use, overuse and pressure, left hand

     M70.849   Other soft tissue disorders related to use, overuse and pressure, unspecified hand ▽

   ✓6ᵗʰ M70.85   Other soft tissue disorders related to use, overuse and pressure of thigh

     M70.851   Other soft tissue disorders related to use, overuse and pressure, right thigh

     M70.852   Other soft tissue disorders related to use, overuse and pressure, left thigh

     M70.859   Other soft tissue disorders related to use, overuse and pressure, unspecified thigh ▽

✓ Additional Character Req   ✓x7ᵗʰ Placeholder Alert   Manifestation   ▽ Unspecified   ▶◀ Revised Text   ● New Code   ▲ Revised Code Title

ICD-10-CM 2019   797

Chapter 13. Diseases of the Musculoskeletal System and Connective Tissue

M70.86–M71.119

√6ᵗʰ **M70.86** Other soft tissue disorders related to use, overuse and pressure lower leg

    M70.861 Other soft tissue disorders related to use, overuse and pressure, right lower leg

    M70.862 Other soft tissue disorders related to use, overuse and pressure, left lower leg

    M70.869 Other soft tissue disorders related to use, overuse and pressure, unspecified leg ▽

√6ᵗʰ **M70.87** Other soft tissue disorders related to use, overuse and pressure of ankle and foot

    M70.871 Other soft tissue disorders related to use, overuse and pressure, right ankle and foot

    M70.872 Other soft tissue disorders related to use, overuse and pressure, left ankle and foot

    M70.879 Other soft tissue disorders related to use, overuse and pressure, unspecified ankle and foot ▽

M70.88 Other soft tissue disorders related to use, overuse and pressure other site

M70.89 Other soft tissue disorders related to use, overuse and pressure multiple sites

√5ᵗʰ **M70.9** Unspecified soft tissue disorder related to use, overuse and pressure

    M70.90 Unspecified soft tissue disorder related to use, overuse and pressure of unspecified site ▽

√6ᵗʰ **M70.91** Unspecified soft tissue disorder related to use, overuse and pressure of shoulder

    M70.911 Unspecified soft tissue disorder related to use, overuse and pressure, right shoulder ▽

    M70.912 Unspecified soft tissue disorder related to use, overuse and pressure, left shoulder ▽

    M70.919 Unspecified soft tissue disorder related to use, overuse and pressure, unspecified shoulder ▽

√6ᵗʰ **M70.92** Unspecified soft tissue disorder related to use, overuse and pressure of upper arm

    M70.921 Unspecified soft tissue disorder related to use, overuse and pressure, right upper arm ▽

    M70.922 Unspecified soft tissue disorder related to use, overuse and pressure, left upper arm ▽

    M70.929 Unspecified soft tissue disorder related to use, overuse and pressure, unspecified upper arm ▽

√6ᵗʰ **M70.93** Unspecified soft tissue disorder related to use, overuse and pressure of forearm

    M70.931 Unspecified soft tissue disorder related to use, overuse and pressure, right forearm ▽

    M70.932 Unspecified soft tissue disorder related to use, overuse and pressure, left forearm ▽

    M70.939 Unspecified soft tissue disorder related to use, overuse and pressure, unspecified forearm ▽

√6ᵗʰ **M70.94** Unspecified soft tissue disorder related to use, overuse and pressure of hand

    M70.941 Unspecified soft tissue disorder related to use, overuse and pressure, right hand ▽

    M70.942 Unspecified soft tissue disorder related to use, overuse and pressure, left hand ▽

    M70.949 Unspecified soft tissue disorder related to use, overuse and pressure, unspecified hand ▽

√6ᵗʰ **M70.95** Unspecified soft tissue disorder related to use, overuse and pressure of thigh

    M70.951 Unspecified soft tissue disorder related to use, overuse and pressure, right thigh ▽

    M70.952 Unspecified soft tissue disorder related to use, overuse and pressure, left thigh ▽

    M70.959 Unspecified soft tissue disorder related to use, overuse and pressure, unspecified thigh ▽

√6ᵗʰ **M70.96** Unspecified soft tissue disorder related to use, overuse and pressure lower leg

    M70.961 Unspecified soft tissue disorder related to use, overuse and pressure, right lower leg ▽

    M70.962 Unspecified soft tissue disorder related to use, overuse and pressure, left lower leg ▽

    M70.969 Unspecified soft tissue disorder related to use, overuse and pressure, unspecified lower leg ▽

√6ᵗʰ **M70.97** Unspecified soft tissue disorder related to use, overuse and pressure of ankle and foot

    M70.971 Unspecified soft tissue disorder related to use, overuse and pressure, right ankle and foot ▽

    M70.972 Unspecified soft tissue disorder related to use, overuse and pressure, left ankle and foot ▽

    M70.979 Unspecified soft tissue disorder related to use, overuse and pressure, unspecified ankle and foot ▽

M70.98 Unspecified soft tissue disorder related to use, overuse and pressure other ▽

M70.99 Unspecified soft tissue disorder related to use, overuse and pressure multiple sites ▽

√4ᵗʰ **M71** Other bursopathies

    EXCLUDES 1 bunion (M20.1)
         bursitis related to use, overuse or pressure (M70.-)
         enthesopathies (M76-M77)

√5ᵗʰ **M71.0** Abscess of bursa

    Use additional code (B95.-, B96.-) to identify causative organism

    M71.00 Abscess of bursa, unspecified site ▽

√6ᵗʰ   **M71.01** Abscess of bursa, shoulder

    M71.011 Abscess of bursa, right shoulder
    M71.012 Abscess of bursa, left shoulder
    M71.019 Abscess of bursa, unspecified shoulder ▽

√6ᵗʰ   **M71.02** Abscess of bursa, elbow

    M71.021 Abscess of bursa, right elbow
    M71.022 Abscess of bursa, left elbow
    M71.029 Abscess of bursa, unspecified elbow ▽

√6ᵗʰ   **M71.03** Abscess of bursa, wrist

    M71.031 Abscess of bursa, right wrist
    M71.032 Abscess of bursa, left wrist
    M71.039 Abscess of bursa, unspecified wrist ▽

√6ᵗʰ   **M71.04** Abscess of bursa, hand

    M71.041 Abscess of bursa, right hand
    M71.042 Abscess of bursa, left hand
    M71.049 Abscess of bursa, unspecified hand ▽

√6ᵗʰ   **M71.05** Abscess of bursa, hip

    M71.051 Abscess of bursa, right hip
    M71.052 Abscess of bursa, left hip
    M71.059 Abscess of bursa, unspecified hip ▽

√6ᵗʰ   **M71.06** Abscess of bursa, knee

    M71.061 Abscess of bursa, right knee
    M71.062 Abscess of bursa, left knee
    M71.069 Abscess of bursa, unspecified knee ▽

√6ᵗʰ   **M71.07** Abscess of bursa, ankle and foot

    M71.071 Abscess of bursa, right ankle and foot
    M71.072 Abscess of bursa, left ankle and foot
    M71.079 Abscess of bursa, unspecified ankle and foot ▽

    M71.08 Abscess of bursa, other site
    M71.09 Abscess of bursa, multiple sites

√5ᵗʰ **M71.1** Other infective bursitis

    Use additional code (B95.-, B96.-) to identify causative organism

    M71.10 Other infective bursitis, unspecified site ▽

√6ᵗʰ   **M71.11** Other infective bursitis, shoulder

    M71.111 Other infective bursitis, right shoulder
    M71.112 Other infective bursitis, left shoulder
    M71.119 Other infective bursitis, unspecified shoulder ▽

✓6ᵗʰ **M71.12 Other infective bursitis,** elbow

    M71.121 Other infective bursitis, right elbow
    M71.122 Other infective bursitis, left elbow
    M71.129 Other infective bursitis, ▽
        unspecified elbow

✓6ᵗʰ **M71.13 Other infective bursitis,** wrist

    M71.131 Other infective bursitis, right wrist
    M71.132 Other infective bursitis, left wrist
    M71.139 Other infective bursitis, ▽
        unspecified wrist

✓6ᵗʰ **M71.14 Other infective bursitis,** hand

    M71.141 Other infective bursitis, right hand
    M71.142 Other infective bursitis, left hand
    M71.149 Other infective bursitis, ▽
        unspecified hand

✓6ᵗʰ **M71.15 Other infective bursitis,** hip

    M71.151 Other infective bursitis, right hip
    M71.152 Other infective bursitis, left hip
    M71.159 Other infective bursitis, ▽
        unspecified hip

✓6ᵗʰ **M71.16 Other infective bursitis,** knee

    M71.161 Other infective bursitis, right knee
    M71.162 Other infective bursitis, left knee
    M71.169 Other infective bursitis, ▽
        unspecified knee

✓6ᵗʰ **M71.17 Other infective bursitis,** ankle and foot

    M71.171 Other infective bursitis, right ankle and
        foot
    M71.172 Other infective bursitis, left ankle and
        foot
    M71.179 Other infective bursitis, ▽
        unspecified ankle and foot

   M71.18 Other infective bursitis, other site
   M71.19 Other infective bursitis, multiple sites

✓5ᵗʰ **M71.2 Synovial cyst of popliteal space [Baker]**

    EXCLUDES 1   *synovial cyst of popliteal space with rupture (M66.0)*

Baker's Cyst

Baker's cyst
connected to
knee joint
synovial cavity

   M71.20 Synovial cyst of popliteal space [Baker], ▽
       unspecified knee
   M71.21 Synovial cyst of popliteal space [Baker], right knee
   M71.22 Synovial cyst of popliteal space [Baker], left knee

✓5ᵗʰ **M71.3 Other bursal cyst**

   Synovial cyst NOS
    EXCLUDES 1   *synovial cyst with rupture (M66.1-)*

   M71.30 Other bursal cyst, unspecified site ▽

✓6ᵗʰ **M71.31 Other bursal cyst,** shoulder

    M71.311 Other bursal cyst, right shoulder
    M71.312 Other bursal cyst, left shoulder
    M71.319 Other bursal cyst, unspecified ▽
        shoulder

✓6ᵗʰ **M71.32 Other bursal cyst,** elbow

    M71.321 Other bursal cyst, right elbow
    M71.322 Other bursal cyst, left elbow

    M71.329 Other bursal cyst, unspecified ▽
        elbow

✓6ᵗʰ **M71.33 Other bursal cyst,** wrist

    M71.331 Other bursal cyst, right wrist
    M71.332 Other bursal cyst, left wrist
    M71.339 Other bursal cyst, unspecified ▽
        wrist

✓6ᵗʰ **M71.34 Other bursal cyst,** hand

    M71.341 Other bursal cyst, right hand
    M71.342 Other bursal cyst, left hand
    M71.349 Other bursal cyst, unspecified ▽
        hand

✓6ᵗʰ **M71.35 Other bursal cyst,** hip

    M71.351 Other bursal cyst, right hip
    M71.352 Other bursal cyst, left hip
    M71.359 Other bursal cyst, unspecified hip ▽

✓6ᵗʰ **M71.37 Other bursal cyst,** ankle and foot

    M71.371 Other bursal cyst, right ankle and foot
    M71.372 Other bursal cyst, left ankle and foot
    M71.379 Other bursal cyst, unspecified ▽
        ankle and foot

   M71.38 Other bursal cyst, other site
   M71.39 Other bursal cyst, multiple sites

✓5ᵗʰ **M71.4 Calcium deposit in bursa**

    EXCLUDES 2   *calcium deposit in bursa of shoulder (M75.3)*

   M71.40 Calcium deposit in bursa, unspecified site ▽

✓6ᵗʰ **M71.42 Calcium deposit in bursa,** elbow

    M71.421 Calcium deposit in bursa, right elbow
    M71.422 Calcium deposit in bursa, left elbow
    M71.429 Calcium deposit in bursa, ▽
        unspecified elbow

✓6ᵗʰ **M71.43 Calcium deposit in bursa,** wrist

    M71.431 Calcium deposit in bursa, right wrist
    M71.432 Calcium deposit in bursa, left wrist
    M71.439 Calcium deposit in bursa, ▽
        unspecified wrist

✓6ᵗʰ **M71.44 Calcium deposit in bursa,** hand

    M71.441 Calcium deposit in bursa, right hand
    M71.442 Calcium deposit in bursa, left hand
    M71.449 Calcium deposit in bursa, ▽
        unspecified hand

✓6ᵗʰ **M71.45 Calcium deposit in bursa,** hip

    M71.451 Calcium deposit in bursa, right hip
    M71.452 Calcium deposit in bursa, left hip
    M71.459 Calcium deposit in bursa, ▽
        unspecified hip

✓6ᵗʰ **M71.46 Calcium deposit in bursa,** knee

    M71.461 Calcium deposit in bursa, right knee
    M71.462 Calcium deposit in bursa, left knee
    M71.469 Calcium deposit in bursa, ▽
        unspecified knee

✓6ᵗʰ **M71.47 Calcium deposit in bursa,** ankle and foot

    M71.471 Calcium deposit in bursa, right ankle and
        foot
    M71.472 Calcium deposit in bursa, left ankle and
        foot
    M71.479 Calcium deposit in bursa, ▽
        unspecified ankle and foot

   M71.48 Calcium deposit in bursa, other site
   M71.49 Calcium deposit in bursa, multiple sites

✓5ᵗʰ **M71.5 Other bursitis, not elsewhere classified**

    EXCLUDES 1   *bursitis NOS (M71.9-)*
    EXCLUDES 2   *bursitis of shoulder (M75.5)*
            bursitis of tibial collateral [Pellegrini-Stieda] (M76.4-)

   M71.50 Other bursitis, not elsewhere classified, ▽
       unspecified site

✓6ᵗʰ **M71.52 Other bursitis, not elsewhere classified,** elbow

    M71.521 Other bursitis, not elsewhere classified,
        right elbow
    M71.522 Other bursitis, not elsewhere classified,
        left elbow
    M71.529 Other bursitis, not elsewhere ▽
        classified, unspecified elbow

✓6ᵗʰ **M71.53 Other bursitis, not elsewhere classified,** wrist

    M71.531 Other bursitis, not elsewhere classified,
        right wrist

✓ Additional Character Req   ✓x7ᵗʰ Placeholder Alert   **Manifestation**   ▽ Unspecified   ▶◀ Revised Text   ● New Code   ▲ Revised Code Title

ICD-10-CM 2019   799

M71.532 Other bursitis, not elsewhere classified, **left** wrist

M71.539 Other bursitis, not elsewhere classified, unspecified wrist ▽

✓6ᵗʰ **M71.54** Other bursitis, not elsewhere classified, **hand**

M71.541 Other bursitis, not elsewhere classified, **right** hand

M71.542 Other bursitis, not elsewhere classified, **left** hand

M71.549 Other bursitis, not elsewhere classified, unspecified hand ▽

✓6ᵗʰ **M71.55** Other bursitis, not elsewhere classified, **hip**

M71.551 Other bursitis, not elsewhere classified, **right** hip

M71.552 Other bursitis, not elsewhere classified, **left** hip

M71.559 Other bursitis, not elsewhere classified, unspecified hip ▽

✓6ᵗʰ **M71.56** Other bursitis, not elsewhere classified, **knee**

M71.561 Other bursitis, not elsewhere classified, **right** knee

M71.562 Other bursitis, not elsewhere classified, **left** knee

M71.569 Other bursitis, not elsewhere classified, unspecified knee ▽

✓6ᵗʰ **M71.57** Other bursitis, not elsewhere classified, **ankle and foot**

M71.571 Other bursitis, not elsewhere classified, **right** ankle and foot

M71.572 Other bursitis, not elsewhere classified, **left** ankle and foot

M71.579 Other bursitis, not elsewhere classified, unspecified ankle and foot ▽

M71.58 Other bursitis, not elsewhere classified, other site

✓5ᵗʰ **M71.8** Other specified bursopathies

M71.80 Other specified bursopathies, unspecified site ▽

✓6ᵗʰ **M71.81** Other specified bursopathies, **shoulder**

M71.811 Other specified bursopathies, **right** shoulder

M71.812 Other specified bursopathies, **left** shoulder

M71.819 Other specified bursopathies, unspecified shoulder ▽

✓6ᵗʰ **M71.82** Other specified bursopathies, **elbow**

M71.821 Other specified bursopathies, **right** elbow

M71.822 Other specified bursopathies, **left** elbow

M71.829 Other specified bursopathies, unspecified elbow ▽

✓6ᵗʰ **M71.83** Other specified bursopathies, **wrist**

M71.831 Other specified bursopathies, **right** wrist

M71.832 Other specified bursopathies, **left** wrist

M71.839 Other specified bursopathies, unspecified wrist ▽

✓6ᵗʰ **M71.84** Other specified bursopathies, **hand**

M71.841 Other specified bursopathies, **right** hand

M71.842 Other specified bursopathies, **left** hand

M71.849 Other specified bursopathies, unspecified hand ▽

✓6ᵗʰ **M71.85** Other specified bursopathies, **hip**

M71.851 Other specified bursopathies, **right** hip

M71.852 Other specified bursopathies, **left** hip

M71.859 Other specified bursopathies, unspecified hip ▽

✓6ᵗʰ **M71.86** Other specified bursopathies, **knee**

M71.861 Other specified bursopathies, **right** knee

M71.862 Other specified bursopathies, **left** knee

M71.869 Other specified bursopathies, unspecified knee ▽

✓6ᵗʰ **M71.87** Other specified bursopathies, **ankle and foot**

M71.871 Other specified bursopathies, **right** ankle and foot

M71.872 Other specified bursopathies, **left** ankle and foot

M71.879 Other specified bursopathies, unspecified ankle and foot ▽

M71.88 Other specified bursopathies, other site

M71.89 Other specified bursopathies, **multiple sites**

M71.9 Bursopathy, unspecified ▽
Bursitis NOS

✓4ᵗʰ **M72** Fibroblastic disorders
EXCLUDES 2   retroperitoneal fibromatosis (D48.3)

M72.0 Palmar fascial fibromatosis [Dupuytren] Ⓐ
DEF: Dupuytren's contracture: Flexion deformity of a finger, due to shortened, thickened fibrosing of palmar fascia. The cause is unknown, but it is associated with long-standing epilepsy.

M72.1 Knuckle pads

M72.2 Plantar fascial fibromatosis
Plantar fasciitis
DEF: Rapid-growing and multiplanar nodular swellings and pain in the foot that is not associated with contractures.

M72.4 Pseudosarcomatous fibromatosis
Nodular fasciitis

M72.6 Necrotizing fasciitis Ⓗᴄᴄ
Use additional code (B95.-, B96.-) to identify causative organism

M72.8 Other fibroblastic disorders
Abscess of fascia
Fasciitis NEC
Other infective fasciitis
Use additional code to (B95.-, B96.-) identify causative organism
EXCLUDES 1   diffuse (eosinophilic) fasciitis (M35.4)
necrotizing fasciitis (M72.6)
nodular fasciitis (M72.4)
perirenal fasciitis NOS (N13.5)
perirenal fasciitis with infection (N13.6)
plantar fasciitis (M72.2)

M72.9 Fibroblastic disorder, unspecified ▽
Fasciitis NOS
Fibromatosis NOS

✓4ᵗʰ **M75** Shoulder lesions
EXCLUDES 2   shoulder-hand syndrome (M89.0-)

✓5ᵗʰ **M75.0** Adhesive capsulitis of shoulder
Frozen shoulder
Periarthritis of shoulder
AHA: 2015,2Q,23

M75.00 Adhesive capsulitis of unspecified shoulder ▽

M75.01 Adhesive capsulitis of **right** shoulder

M75.02 Adhesive capsulitis of **left** shoulder

✓5ᵗʰ **M75.1** Rotator cuff tear or rupture, not specified as traumatic
Rotator cuff syndrome
Supraspinatus syndrome
Supraspinatus tear or rupture, not specified as traumatic
EXCLUDES 1   tear of rotator cuff, traumatic (S46.01-)

✓6ᵗʰ **M75.10** Unspecified rotator cuff tear or rupture, not specified as traumatic

M75.100 Unspecified rotator cuff tear or rupture of unspecified shoulder, not specified as traumatic ▽

M75.101 Unspecified rotator cuff tear or rupture of **right** shoulder, not specified as traumatic ▽

M75.102 Unspecified rotator cuff tear or rupture of **left** shoulder, not specified as traumatic ▽

✓6ᵗʰ **M75.11** Incomplete rotator cuff tear or rupture not specified as traumatic

M75.110 Incomplete rotator cuff tear or rupture of unspecified shoulder, not specified as traumatic ▽

M75.111 Incomplete rotator cuff tear or rupture of **right** shoulder, not specified as traumatic

M75.112 Incomplete rotator cuff tear or rupture of **left** shoulder, not specified as traumatic

✓6ᵗʰ **M75.12** Complete rotator cuff tear or rupture not specified as traumatic

M75.120 Complete rotator cuff tear or rupture of unspecified shoulder, not specified as traumatic ▽

M75.121 Complete rotator cuff tear or rupture of **right** shoulder, not specified as traumatic

M75.122 Complete rotator cuff tear or rupture of **left** shoulder, not specified as traumatic

✓5ᵗʰ **M75.2** Bicipital tendinitis

M75.20 Bicipital tendinitis, unspecified shoulder ▽

M75.21   **Bicipital tendinitis**, right shoulder
M75.22   **Bicipital tendinitis**, left shoulder

√5ᵗʰ **M75.3**   **Calcific tendinitis of shoulder**
     Calcified bursa of shoulder
M75.30   **Calcific tendinitis of unspecified shoulder** ▽
M75.31   **Calcific tendinitis of** right **shoulder**
M75.32   **Calcific tendinitis of** left **shoulder**

√5ᵗʰ **M75.4**   **Impingement syndrome of shoulder**
M75.40   **Impingement syndrome of unspecified shoulder** ▽
M75.41   **Impingement syndrome of** right **shoulder**
M75.42   **Impingement syndrome of** left **shoulder**

√5ᵗʰ **M75.5**   **Bursitis of shoulder**
M75.50   **Bursitis of unspecified shoulder** ▽
M75.51   **Bursitis of** right **shoulder**
M75.52   **Bursitis of** left **shoulder**

√5ᵗʰ **M75.8**   **Other shoulder lesions**
M75.80   **Other shoulder lesions, unspecified shoulder** ▽
M75.81   **Other shoulder lesions,** right **shoulder**
M75.82   **Other shoulder lesions,** left **shoulder**

√5ᵗʰ **M75.9**   **Shoulder lesion, unspecified**
M75.90   **Shoulder lesion, unspecified, unspecified shoulder** ▽
M75.91   **Shoulder lesion, unspecified,** right **shoulder** ▽
M75.92   **Shoulder lesion, unspecified,** left **shoulder** ▽

√4ᵗʰ **M76**   **Enthesopathies, lower limb, excluding foot**
   EXCLUDES 2   bursitis due to use, overuse and pressure (M70.-)
           enthesopathies of ankle and foot (M77.5-)

√5ᵗʰ **M76.0**   **Gluteal tendinitis**
M76.00   **Gluteal tendinitis, unspecified hip** ▽
M76.01   **Gluteal tendinitis,** right **hip**
M76.02   **Gluteal tendinitis,** left **hip**

√5ᵗʰ **M76.1**   **Psoas tendinitis**
M76.10   **Psoas tendinitis, unspecified hip** ▽
M76.11   **Psoas tendinitis,** right **hip**
M76.12   **Psoas tendinitis,** left **hip**

√5ᵗʰ **M76.2**   **Iliac crest spur**
M76.20   **Iliac crest spur, unspecified hip** ▽
M76.21   **Iliac crest spur,** right **hip**
M76.22   **Iliac crest spur,** left **hip**

√5ᵗʰ **M76.3**   **Iliotibial band syndrome**
M76.30   **Iliotibial band syndrome, unspecified leg** ▽
M76.31   **Iliotibial band syndrome,** right **leg**
M76.32   **Iliotibial band syndrome,** left **leg**

√5ᵗʰ **M76.4**   **Tibial collateral bursitis [Pellegrini-Stieda]**
M76.40   **Tibial collateral bursitis [Pellegrini-Stieda], unspecified leg** ▽
M76.41   **Tibial collateral bursitis [Pellegrini-Stieda],** right **leg**
M76.42   **Tibial collateral bursitis [Pellegrini-Stieda],** left **leg**

√5ᵗʰ **M76.5**   **Patellar tendinitis**
M76.50   **Patellar tendinitis, unspecified knee** ▽
M76.51   **Patellar tendinitis,** right **knee**
M76.52   **Patellar tendinitis,** left **knee**

√5ᵗʰ **M76.6**   **Achilles tendinitis**
     Achilles bursitis
M76.60   **Achilles tendinitis, unspecified leg** ▽
M76.61   **Achilles tendinitis,** right **leg**
M76.62   **Achilles tendinitis,** left **leg**

√5ᵗʰ **M76.7**   **Peroneal tendinitis**
M76.70   **Peroneal tendinitis, unspecified leg** ▽
M76.71   **Peroneal tendinitis,** right **leg**
M76.72   **Peroneal tendinitis,** left **leg**

√5ᵗʰ **M76.8**   **Other specified enthesopathies of lower limb, excluding foot**
   √6ᵗʰ **M76.81**   **Anterior tibial syndrome**
     M76.811   **Anterior tibial syndrome,** right **leg**
     M76.812   **Anterior tibial syndrome,** left **leg**
     M76.819   **Anterior tibial syndrome, unspecified leg** ▽
   √6ᵗʰ **M76.82**   **Posterior tibial tendinitis**
     M76.821   **Posterior tibial tendinitis,** right **leg**
     M76.822   **Posterior tibial tendinitis,** left **leg**

M76.829   **Posterior tibial tendinitis, unspecified leg** ▽

√6ᵗʰ **M76.89**   **Other specified enthesopathies of** lower limb, excluding foot
M76.891   **Other specified enthesopathies of** right **lower limb, excluding foot**
M76.892   **Other specified enthesopathies of** left **lower limb, excluding foot**
M76.899   **Other specified enthesopathies of unspecified lower limb, excluding foot**

M76.9   **Unspecified enthesopathy, lower limb, excluding foot** ▽

√4ᵗʰ **M77**   **Other enthesopathies**
   EXCLUDES 1   bursitis NOS (M71.9-)
   EXCLUDES 2   bursitis due to use, overuse and pressure (M70.-)
           osteophyte (M25.7)
           spinal enthesopathy (M46.0-)

√5ᵗʰ **M77.0**   **Medial epicondylitis**
M77.00   **Medial epicondylitis, unspecified elbow** ▽
M77.01   **Medial epicondylitis,** right **elbow**
M77.02   **Medial epicondylitis,** left **elbow**

√5ᵗʰ **M77.1**   **Lateral epicondylitis**
     Tennis elbow
M77.10   **Lateral epicondylitis, unspecified elbow** ▽
M77.11   **Lateral epicondylitis,** right **elbow**
M77.12   **Lateral epicondylitis,** left **elbow**

√5ᵗʰ **M77.2**   **Periarthritis of wrist**
M77.20   **Periarthritis, unspecified wrist** ▽
M77.21   **Periarthritis,** right **wrist**
M77.22   **Periarthritis,** left **wrist**

√5ᵗʰ **M77.3**   **Calcaneal spur**
   DEF: Overgrowth of calcaneus bone on the underside of the heel that causes pain on walking. Calcaneal spur is due to a chronic avulsion injury of the plantar fascia from the calcaneus.
M77.30   **Calcaneal spur, unspecified foot** ▽
M77.31   **Calcaneal spur,** right **foot**
M77.32   **Calcaneal spur,** left **foot**

√5ᵗʰ **M77.4**   **Metatarsalgia**
   EXCLUDES 1   Morton's metatarsalgia (G57.6)
M77.40   **Metatarsalgia, unspecified foot** ▽
M77.41   **Metatarsalgia,** right **foot**
M77.42   **Metatarsalgia,** left **foot**

√5ᵗʰ **M77.5**   **Other enthesopathy of** foot
M77.50   **Other enthesopathy of unspecified foot** ▽
M77.51   **Other enthesopathy of** right **foot**
M77.52   **Other enthesopathy of** left **foot**

M77.8   **Other enthesopathies, not elsewhere classified**
M77.9   **Enthesopathy, unspecified** ▽
     Bone spur NOS
     Capsulitis NOS
     Periarthritis NOS
     Tendinitis NOS

√4ᵗʰ **M79**   **Other and unspecified soft tissue disorders, not elsewhere classified**
   EXCLUDES 1   psychogenic rheumatism (F45.8)
           soft tissue pain, psychogenic (F45.41)

M79.0   **Rheumatism, unspecified** ▽
   EXCLUDES 1   fibromyalgia (M79.7)
           palindromic rheumatism (M12.3-)

√5ᵗʰ **M79.1**   **Myalgia**
     Myofascial pain syndrome
   EXCLUDES 1   fibromyalgia (M79.7)
           myositis (M60.-)
●   M79.10   **Myalgia, unspecified site** ▽
●   M79.11   **Myalgia of** mastication muscle
●   M79.12   **Myalgia of** auxiliary muscles, **head and neck**
●   M79.18   **Myalgia, other site**

✓ Additional Character Req   ✓x7ᵗʰ Placeholder Alert   **Manifestation**   ▽ Unspecified   ►◄ Revised Text   ● New Code   ▲ Revised Code Title

ICD-10-CM 2019   **801**

Chapter 13. Diseases of the Musculoskeletal System and Connective Tissue

M75.21–M79.18

M79.2 Neuralgia and neuritis, unspecified ▽
　EXCLUDES 1　brachial radiculitis NOS (M54.1)
　　　　lumbosacral radiculitis NOS (M54.1)
　　　　mononeuropathies (G56-G58)
　　　　radiculitis NOS (M54.1)
　　　　sciatica (M54.3-M54.4)
　TIP: Assign for documented neuropathic pain.

M79.3 Panniculitis, unspecified ▽
　EXCLUDES 1　lupus panniculitis (L93.2)
　　　　neck and back panniculitis (M54.0-)
　　　　relapsing [Weber-Christian] panniculitis (M35.6)

M79.4 Hypertrophy of (infrapatellar) fat pad

M79.5 Residual foreign body in soft tissue
　EXCLUDES 1　foreign body granuloma of skin and subcutaneous tissue (L92.3)
　　　　foreign body granuloma of soft tissue (M60.2-)

√5ᵗʰ **M79.6 Pain in limb, hand, foot, fingers and toes**
　EXCLUDES 2　pain in joint (M25.5-)
　√6ᵗʰ **M79.60 Pain in limb, unspecified**
　　M79.601 Pain in right arm
　　　Pain in right upper limb NOS
　　M79.602 Pain in left arm
　　　Pain in left upper limb NOS
　　M79.603 Pain in arm, unspecified ▽
　　　Pain in upper limb NOS
　　M79.604 Pain in right leg
　　　Pain in right lower limb NOS
　　M79.605 Pain in left leg
　　　Pain in left lower limb NOS
　　M79.606 Pain in leg, unspecified ▽
　　　Pain in lower limb NOS
　　M79.609 Pain in unspecified limb ▽
　　　Pain in limb NOS
　√6ᵗʰ **M79.62 Pain in upper arm**
　　　Pain in axillary region
　　M79.621 Pain in right upper arm
　　M79.622 Pain in left upper arm
　　M79.629 Pain in unspecified upper arm ▽
　√6ᵗʰ **M79.63 Pain in forearm**
　　M79.631 Pain in right forearm
　　M79.632 Pain in left forearm
　　M79.639 Pain in unspecified forearm ▽
　√6ᵗʰ **M79.64 Pain in hand and fingers**
　　M79.641 Pain in right hand
　　M79.642 Pain in left hand
　　M79.643 Pain in unspecified hand ▽
　　M79.644 Pain in right finger(s)
　　M79.645 Pain in left finger(s)
　　M79.646 Pain in unspecified finger(s) ▽
　√6ᵗʰ **M79.65 Pain in thigh**
　　M79.651 Pain in right thigh
　　M79.652 Pain in left thigh
　　M79.659 Pain in unspecified thigh ▽
　√6ᵗʰ **M79.66 Pain in lower leg**
　　M79.661 Pain in right lower leg
　　M79.662 Pain in left lower leg
　　M79.669 Pain in unspecified lower leg ▽
　√6ᵗʰ **M79.67 Pain in foot and toes**
　　M79.671 Pain in right foot
　　M79.672 Pain in left foot
　　M79.673 Pain in unspecified foot ▽
　　M79.674 Pain in right toe(s)
　　M79.675 Pain in left toe(s)
　　M79.676 Pain in unspecified toe(s) ▽

M79.7 Fibromyalgia
　Fibromyositis
　Fibrositis
　Myofibrositis

√5ᵗʰ **M79.A Nontraumatic compartment syndrome**
　Code first, if applicable, associated postprocedural complication
　EXCLUDES 1　compartment syndrome NOS (T79.A-)
　　　　fibromyalgia (M79.7)
　　　　nontraumatic ischemic infarction of muscle (M62.2-)
　　　　traumatic compartment syndrome (T79.A-)
　√6ᵗʰ **M79.A1 Nontraumatic compartment syndrome of upper extremity**
　　Nontraumatic compartment syndrome of shoulder, arm, forearm, wrist, hand, and fingers
　　M79.A11 Nontraumatic compartment syndrome of right upper extremity
　　M79.A12 Nontraumatic compartment syndrome of left upper extremity
　　M79.A19 Nontraumatic compartment syndrome of unspecified upper extremity ▽
　√6ᵗʰ **M79.A2 Nontraumatic compartment syndrome of lower extremity**
　　Nontraumatic compartment syndrome of hip, buttock, thigh, leg, foot, and toes
　　M79.A21 Nontraumatic compartment syndrome of right lower extremity
　　M79.A22 Nontraumatic compartment syndrome of left lower extremity
　　M79.A29 Nontraumatic compartment syndrome of unspecified lower extremity ▽
　　M79.A3 Nontraumatic compartment syndrome of abdomen
　　M79.A9 Nontraumatic compartment syndrome of other sites

√5ᵗʰ **M79.8 Other specified soft tissue disorders**
　M79.81 Nontraumatic hematoma of soft tissue
　　Nontraumatic hematoma of muscle
　　Nontraumatic seroma of muscle and soft tissue
　M79.89 Other specified soft tissue disorders
　　Polyalgia

M79.9 Soft tissue disorder, unspecified ▽

Osteopathies And Chondropathies (M80-M94)

Disorders of bone density and structure (M80-M85)

√4ᵗʰ **M80 Osteoporosis with current pathological fracture**
　INCLUDES　osteoporosis with current fragility fracture
　Use additional code to identify major osseous defect, if applicable (M89.7-)
　EXCLUDES 1　collapsed vertebra NOS (M48.5)
　　　　pathological fracture NOS (M84.4)
　　　　wedging of vertebra NOS (M48.5)
　EXCLUDES 2　personal history of (healed) osteoporosis fracture (Z87.310)
　AHA: 2018,2Q,12
　TIP: The site codes in this category identify the site of the fracture, not the site of the osteoporosis.

　The appropriate 7th character is to be added to each code from category M80:
　A　initial encounter for fracture
　D　subsequent encounter for fracture with routine healing
　G　subsequent encounter for fracture with delayed healing
　K　subsequent encounter for fracture with nonunion
　P　subsequent encounter for fracture with malunion
　S　sequela

√5ᵗʰ **M80.0 Age-related osteoporosis with current pathological fracture**
　Involutional osteoporosis with current pathological fracture
　Osteoporosis NOS with current pathological fracture
　Postmenopausal osteoporosis with current pathological fracture
　Senile osteoporosis with current pathological fracture
　√x7ᵗʰ **M80.00 Age-related osteoporosis with current pathological fracture, unspecified site** Q A ▽
　√6ᵗʰ **M80.01 Age-related osteoporosis with current pathological fracture, shoulder**
　　√7ᵗʰ **M80.011 Age-related osteoporosis with current pathological fracture, right shoulder** Q A
　　√7ᵗʰ **M80.012 Age-related osteoporosis with current pathological fracture, left shoulder** Q A

✓7ᵗʰ **M80.019** Age-related osteoporosis with current pathological fracture, unspecified shoulder   Q A ▽

✓6ᵗʰ **M80.02** Age-related osteoporosis with current pathological fracture, humerus

✓7ᵗʰ **M80.021** Age-related osteoporosis with current pathological fracture, right humerus   Q A

✓7ᵗʰ **M80.022** Age-related osteoporosis with current pathological fracture, left humerus   Q A

✓7ᵗʰ **M80.029** Age-related osteoporosis with current pathological fracture, unspecified humerus   Q A ▽

✓6ᵗʰ **M80.03** Age-related osteoporosis with current pathological fracture, forearm

Age-related osteoporosis with current pathological fracture of wrist

✓7ᵗʰ **M80.031** Age-related osteoporosis with current pathological fracture, right forearm   Q A

✓7ᵗʰ **M80.032** Age-related osteoporosis with current pathological fracture, left forearm   Q A

✓7ᵗʰ **M80.039** Age-related osteoporosis with current pathological fracture, unspecified forearm   Q A ▽

✓6ᵗʰ **M80.04** Age-related osteoporosis with current pathological fracture, hand

✓7ᵗʰ **M80.041** Age-related osteoporosis with current pathological fracture, right hand   Q A

✓7ᵗʰ **M80.042** Age-related osteoporosis with current pathological fracture, left hand   Q A

✓7ᵗʰ **M80.049** Age-related osteoporosis with current pathological fracture, unspecified hand   Q A ▽

✓6ᵗʰ **M80.05** Age-related osteoporosis with current pathological fracture, femur

Age-related osteoporosis with current pathological fracture of hip

¹ ✓7ᵗʰ **M80.051** Age-related osteoporosis with current pathological fracture, right femur   HCC Q A

¹ ✓7ᵗʰ **M80.052** Age-related osteoporosis with current pathological fracture, left femur   HCC Q A

¹ ✓7ᵗʰ **M80.059** Age-related osteoporosis with current pathological fracture, unspecified femur   HCC Q A ▽

✓6ᵗʰ **M80.06** Age-related osteoporosis with current pathological fracture, lower leg

✓7ᵗʰ **M80.061** Age-related osteoporosis with current pathological fracture, right lower leg   Q A

✓7ᵗʰ **M80.062** Age-related osteoporosis with current pathological fracture, left lower leg   Q A

✓7ᵗʰ **M80.069** Age-related osteoporosis with current pathological fracture, unspecified lower leg   Q A ▽

✓6ᵗʰ **M80.07** Age-related osteoporosis with current pathological fracture, ankle and foot

✓7ᵗʰ **M80.071** Age-related osteoporosis with current pathological fracture, right ankle and foot   Q A

✓7ᵗʰ **M80.072** Age-related osteoporosis with current pathological fracture, left ankle and foot   Q A

✓7ᵗʰ **M80.079** Age-related osteoporosis with current pathological fracture, unspecified ankle and foot   Q A ▽

¹ ✓x7ᵗʰ **M80.08** Age-related osteoporosis with current pathological fracture, vertebra(e)   HCC Q A

✓5ᵗʰ **M80.8** Other osteoporosis with current pathological fracture

Drug-induced osteoporosis with current pathological fracture
Idiopathic osteoporosis with current pathological fracture
Osteoporosis of disuse with current pathological fracture
Postoophorectomy osteoporosis with current pathological fracture
Postsurgical malabsorption osteoporosis with current pathological fracture
Post-traumatic osteoporosis with current pathological fracture
Use additional code for adverse effect, if applicable, to identify drug (T36-T50 with fifth or sixth character 5)

✓x7ᵗʰ **M80.80** Other osteoporosis with current pathological fracture, unspecified site   Q ▽

✓6ᵗʰ **M80.81** Other osteoporosis with pathological fracture, shoulder

✓7ᵗʰ **M80.811** Other osteoporosis with current pathological fracture, right shoulder   Q

✓7ᵗʰ **M80.812** Other osteoporosis with current pathological fracture, left shoulder   Q

✓7ᵗʰ **M80.819** Other osteoporosis with current pathological fracture, unspecified shoulder   Q ▽

✓6ᵗʰ **M80.82** Other osteoporosis with current pathological fracture, humerus

✓7ᵗʰ **M80.821** Other osteoporosis with current pathological fracture, right humerus   Q

✓7ᵗʰ **M80.822** Other osteoporosis with current pathological fracture, left humerus   Q

✓7ᵗʰ **M80.829** Other osteoporosis with current pathological fracture, unspecified humerus   Q ▽

✓6ᵗʰ **M80.83** Other osteoporosis with current pathological fracture, forearm

Other osteoporosis with current pathological fracture of wrist

✓7ᵗʰ **M80.831** Other osteoporosis with current pathological fracture, right forearm   Q

✓7ᵗʰ **M80.832** Other osteoporosis with current pathological fracture, left forearm   Q

✓7ᵗʰ **M80.839** Other osteoporosis with current pathological fracture, unspecified forearm   Q ▽

✓6ᵗʰ **M80.84** Other osteoporosis with current pathological fracture, hand

✓7ᵗʰ **M80.841** Other osteoporosis with current pathological fracture, right hand   Q

✓7ᵗʰ **M80.842** Other osteoporosis with current pathological fracture, left hand   Q

✓7ᵗʰ **M80.849** Other osteoporosis with current pathological fracture, unspecified hand   Q ▽

✓6ᵗʰ **M80.85** Other osteoporosis with current pathological fracture, femur

Other osteoporosis with current pathological fracture of hip

¹ ✓7ᵗʰ **M80.851** Other osteoporosis with current pathological fracture, right femur   HCC Q

¹ ✓7ᵗʰ **M80.852** Other osteoporosis with current pathological fracture, left femur   HCC Q

¹ ✓7ᵗʰ **M80.859** Other osteoporosis with current pathological fracture, unspecified femur   HCC Q ▽

✓6ᵗʰ **M80.86** Other osteoporosis with current pathological fracture, lower leg

✓7ᵗʰ **M80.861** Other osteoporosis with current pathological fracture, right lower leg   Q

✓7ᵗʰ **M80.862** Other osteoporosis with current pathological fracture, left lower leg   Q

✓7ᵗʰ **M80.869** Other osteoporosis with current pathological fracture, unspecified lower leg   Q ▽

☑ Additional Character Req   ✓x7ᵗʰ Placeholder Alert   Manifestation   ▽ Unspecified   ►◄ Revised Text   ● New Code   ▲ Revised Code Title

ICD-10-CM 2019

803

Chapter 13. Diseases of the Musculoskeletal System and Connective Tissue

M80.019–M80.869

✓6ᵗʰ **M80.87** **Other osteoporosis with current pathological fracture,** ankle and foot

    ✓7ᵗʰ **M80.871** **Other osteoporosis with current pathological fracture,** right **ankle and foot**   🔲

    ✓7ᵗʰ **M80.872** **Other osteoporosis with current pathological fracture,** left **ankle and foot**   🔲

    ✓7ᵗʰ **M80.879** **Other osteoporosis with current pathological fracture, unspecified ankle and foot**   🔲 ▽

1 ✓x7ᵗʰ **M80.88** **Other osteoporosis with current pathological fracture,** vertebra(e)   HCC 🔲

✓4ᵗʰ **M81 Osteoporosis** without current pathological fracture

Use additional code to identify:

major osseous defect, if applicable (M89.7-)

personal history of (healed) osteoporosis fracture, if applicable (Z87.310)

    EXCLUDES 1   *osteoporosis with current pathological fracture (M80.-)*

         Sudeck's atrophy (M89.0)

M81.0 **Age-related osteoporosis without current pathological fracture**   🔲 Ⓐ

    Involutional osteoporosis without current pathological fracture

    Osteoporosis NOS

    Postmenopausal osteoporosis without current pathological fracture

    Senile osteoporosis without current pathological fracture

M81.6 **Localized osteoporosis [Lequesne]**   🔲

    EXCLUDES 1   *Sudeck's atrophy (M89.0)*

M81.8 **Other osteoporosis without current pathological fracture**   🔲

    Drug-induced osteoporosis without current pathological fracture

    Idiopathic osteoporosis without current pathological fracture

    Osteoporosis of disuse without current pathological fracture

    Postoophorectomy osteoporosis without current pathological fracture

    Postsurgical malabsorption osteoporosis without current pathological fracture

    Post-traumatic osteoporosis without current pathological fracture

    Use additional code for adverse effect, if applicable, to identify drug (T36-T50 with fifth or sixth character 5)

✓4ᵗʰ **M83 Adult osteomalacia**

    EXCLUDES 1   *infantile and juvenile osteomalacia (E55.0)*

         renal osteodystrophy (N25.0)

         rickets (active) (E55.0)

         rickets (active) sequelae (E64.3)

         vitamin D-resistant osteomalacia (E83.3)

         vitamin D-resistant rickets (active) (E83.3)

M83.0 **Puerperal osteomalacia**   Ⓜ ♀

M83.1 **Senile osteomalacia**   Ⓐ

M83.2 **Adult osteomalacia due to malabsorption**   Ⓐ

    Postsurgical malabsorption osteomalacia in adults

M83.3 **Adult osteomalacia due to malnutrition**   Ⓐ

M83.4 **Aluminum bone disease**

M83.5 **Other drug-induced osteomalacia in adults**   Ⓐ

    Use additional code for adverse effect, if applicable, to identify drug (T36-T50 with fifth or sixth character 5)

M83.8 **Other adult osteomalacia**   Ⓐ

M83.9 **Adult osteomalacia, unspecified**   Ⓐ ▽

✓4ᵗʰ **M84 Disorder of continuity of bone**

    EXCLUDES 2   *traumatic fracture of bone-see fracture, by site*

✓5ᵗʰ **M84.3 Stress fracture**

    Fatigue fracture

    March fracture

    Stress fracture NOS

    Stress reaction

    Use additional external cause code(s) to identify the cause of the stress fracture

    EXCLUDES 1   *pathological fracture due to osteoporosis (M80.-)*

         pathological fracture NOS (M84.4.-)

         traumatic fracture (S12.-, S22.-, S32.-, S42.-, S52.-, S62.-, S72.-, S82.-, S92.-)

    EXCLUDES 2   *personal history of (healed) stress (fatigue) fracture (Z87.312)*

         stress fracture of vertebra (M48.4-)

The appropriate 7th character is to be added to each code from subcategory M84.3.

A   initial encounter for fracture

D   subsequent encounter for fracture with routine healing

G   subsequent encounter for fracture with delayed healing

K   subsequent encounter for fracture with nonunion

P   subsequent encounter for fracture with malunion

S   sequela

✓x7ᵗʰ **M84.30** **Stress fracture, unspecified site**   ▽

✓6ᵗʰ **M84.31** **Stress fracture,** shoulder

    ✓7ᵗʰ **M84.311** **Stress fracture,** right **shoulder**   🔲

    ✓7ᵗʰ **M84.312** **Stress fracture,** left **shoulder**   🔲

    ✓7ᵗʰ **M84.319** **Stress fracture, unspecified shoulder**   🔲 ▽

✓6ᵗʰ **M84.32** **Stress fracture,** humerus

    ✓7ᵗʰ **M84.321** **Stress fracture,** right **humerus**   🔲

    ✓7ᵗʰ **M84.322** **Stress fracture,** left **humerus**   🔲

    ✓7ᵗʰ **M84.329** **Stress fracture, unspecified humerus**   🔲 ▽

✓6ᵗʰ **M84.33** **Stress fracture,** ulna and radius

    ✓7ᵗʰ **M84.331** **Stress fracture,** right **ulna**   🔲

    ✓7ᵗʰ **M84.332** **Stress fracture,** left **ulna**   🔲

    ✓7ᵗʰ **M84.333** **Stress fracture,** right **radius**   🔲

    ✓7ᵗʰ **M84.334** **Stress fracture,** left **radius**   🔲

    ✓7ᵗʰ **M84.339** **Stress fracture, unspecified ulna and radius**   🔲 ▽

✓6ᵗʰ **M84.34** **Stress fracture,** hand and fingers

    ✓7ᵗʰ **M84.341** **Stress fracture,** right **hand**   🔲

    ✓7ᵗʰ **M84.342** **Stress fracture,** left **hand**   🔲

    ✓7ᵗʰ **M84.343** **Stress fracture, unspecified hand**   🔲 ▽

    ✓7ᵗʰ **M84.344** **Stress fracture,** right **finger(s)**

    ✓7ᵗʰ **M84.345** **Stress fracture,** left **finger(s)**

    ✓7ᵗʰ **M84.346** **Stress fracture, unspecified finger(s)**   ▽

✓6ᵗʰ **M84.35** **Stress fracture,** pelvis and femur

    Stress fracture, hip

    ✓7ᵗʰ **M84.350** **Stress fracture,** pelvis   🔲

    ✓7ᵗʰ **M84.351** **Stress fracture,** right **femur**   🔲

    ✓7ᵗʰ **M84.352** **Stress fracture,** left **femur**   🔲

    ✓7ᵗʰ **M84.353** **Stress fracture, unspecified femur**   🔲 ▽

    ✓7ᵗʰ **M84.359** **Stress fracture, hip, unspecified**   🔲 ▽

✓6ᵗʰ **M84.36** **Stress fracture,** tibia and fibula

    ✓7ᵗʰ **M84.361** **Stress fracture,** right **tibia**   🔲

    ✓7ᵗʰ **M84.362** **Stress fracture,** left **tibia**   🔲

    ✓7ᵗʰ **M84.363** **Stress fracture,** right **fibula**   🔲

    ✓7ᵗʰ **M84.364** **Stress fracture,** left **fibula**   🔲

    ✓7ᵗʰ **M84.369** **Stress fracture, unspecified tibia and fibula**   🔲 ▽

✓6ᵗʰ **M84.37** **Stress fracture,** ankle, foot and toes

    ✓7ᵗʰ **M84.371** **Stress fracture,** right **ankle**   🔲

    ✓7ᵗʰ **M84.372** **Stress fracture,** left **ankle**   🔲

    ✓7ᵗʰ **M84.373** **Stress fracture, unspecified ankle**   🔲 ▽

    ✓7ᵗʰ **M84.374** **Stress fracture,** right **foot**   🔲

    ✓7ᵗʰ **M84.375** **Stress fracture,** left **foot**   🔲

    ✓7ᵗʰ **M84.376** **Stress fracture, unspecified foot**   🔲 ▽

√7ᵗʰ **M84.377** Stress fracture, right toe(s)

√7ᵗʰ **M84.378** Stress fracture, left toe(s)

√7ᵗʰ **M84.379** Stress fracture, unspecified toe(s) ▽

√x7ᵗʰ **M84.38** Stress fracture, other site   0

     EXCLUDES 2   stress fracture of vertebra (M48.4-)

√5ᵗʰ **M84.4** Pathological fracture, not elsewhere classified

     Chronic fracture

     Pathological fracture NOS

     EXCLUDES 1   collapsed vertebra NEC (M48.5)

            pathological fracture in neoplastic disease (M84.5-)

            pathological fracture in osteoporosis (M80.-)

            pathological fracture in other disease (M84.6-)

            stress fracture (M84.3-)

            traumatic fracture (S12.-, S22.-, S32.-, S42.-, S52.-, S62.-, S72.-, S82.-, S92.-)

     EXCLUDES 2   personal history of (healed) pathological fracture (Z87.311)

The appropriate 7th character is to be added to each code from subcategory M84.4.
A   initial encounter for fracture
D   subsequent encounter for fracture with routine healing
G   subsequent encounter for fracture with delayed healing
K   subsequent encounter for fracture with nonunion
P   subsequent encounter for fracture with malunion
S   sequela

√x7ᵗʰ **M84.40** Pathological fracture, unspecified site ▽

√6ᵗʰ **M84.41** Pathological fracture, shoulder

√7ᵗʰ **M84.411** Pathological fracture, right shoulder

√7ᵗʰ **M84.412** Pathological fracture, left shoulder

√7ᵗʰ **M84.419** Pathological fracture, unspecified shoulder ▽

√6ᵗʰ **M84.42** Pathological fracture, humerus

√7ᵗʰ **M84.421** Pathological fracture, right humerus

√7ᵗʰ **M84.422** Pathological fracture, left humerus

√7ᵗʰ **M84.429** Pathological fracture, unspecified humerus ▽

√6ᵗʰ **M84.43** Pathological fracture, ulna and radius

√7ᵗʰ **M84.431** Pathological fracture, right ulna

√7ᵗʰ **M84.432** Pathological fracture, left ulna

√7ᵗʰ **M84.433** Pathological fracture, right radius

√7ᵗʰ **M84.434** Pathological fracture, left radius

√7ᵗʰ **M84.439** Pathological fracture, unspecified ulna and radius ▽

√6ᵗʰ **M84.44** Pathological fracture, hand and fingers

√7ᵗʰ **M84.441** Pathological fracture, right hand

√7ᵗʰ **M84.442** Pathological fracture, left hand

√7ᵗʰ **M84.443** Pathological fracture, unspecified hand ▽

√7ᵗʰ **M84.444** Pathological fracture, right finger(s)

√7ᵗʰ **M84.445** Pathological fracture, left finger(s)

√7ᵗʰ **M84.446** Pathological fracture, unspecified finger(s) ▽

√6ᵗʰ **M84.45** Pathological fracture, femur and pelvis

     AHA: 2016,4Q,43

1 √7ᵗʰ **M84.451** Pathological fracture, right femur   HCC

1 √7ᵗʰ **M84.452** Pathological fracture, left femur   HCC

1 √7ᵗʰ **M84.453** Pathological fracture, unspecified femur   HCC ▽

√7ᵗʰ **M84.454** Pathological fracture, pelvis

1 √7ᵗʰ **M84.459** Pathological fracture, hip, unspecified   HCC ▽

√6ᵗʰ **M84.46** Pathological fracture, tibia and fibula

√7ᵗʰ **M84.461** Pathological fracture, right tibia

√7ᵗʰ **M84.462** Pathological fracture, left tibia

√7ᵗʰ **M84.463** Pathological fracture, right fibula

√7ᵗʰ **M84.464** Pathological fracture, left fibula

√7ᵗʰ **M84.469** Pathological fracture, unspecified tibia and fibula ▽

√6ᵗʰ **M84.47** Pathological fracture, ankle, foot and toes

√7ᵗʰ **M84.471** Pathological fracture, right ankle

√7ᵗʰ **M84.472** Pathological fracture, left ankle

√7ᵗʰ **M84.473** Pathological fracture, unspecified ankle ▽

√7ᵗʰ **M84.474** Pathological fracture, right foot

√7ᵗʰ **M84.475** Pathological fracture, left foot

√7ᵗʰ **M84.476** Pathological fracture, unspecified foot ▽

√7ᵗʰ **M84.477** Pathological fracture, right toe(s)

√7ᵗʰ **M84.478** Pathological fracture, left toe(s)

√7ᵗʰ **M84.479** Pathological fracture, unspecified toe(s) ▽

√x7ᵗʰ **M84.48** Pathological fracture, other site

√5ᵗʰ **M84.5** Pathological fracture in neoplastic disease

     Code also underlying neoplasm

The appropriate 7th character is to be added to each code from subcategory M84.5.
A   initial encounter for fracture
D   subsequent encounter for fracture with routine healing
G   subsequent encounter for fracture with delayed healing
K   subsequent encounter for fracture with nonunion
P   subsequent encounter for fracture with malunion
S   sequela

√x7ᵗʰ **M84.50** Pathological fracture in neoplastic disease, unspecified site ▽

√6ᵗʰ **M84.51** Pathological fracture in neoplastic disease, shoulder

√7ᵗʰ **M84.511** Pathological fracture in neoplastic disease, right shoulder

√7ᵗʰ **M84.512** Pathological fracture in neoplastic disease, left shoulder

√7ᵗʰ **M84.519** Pathological fracture in neoplastic disease, unspecified shoulder ▽

√6ᵗʰ **M84.52** Pathological fracture in neoplastic disease, humerus

√7ᵗʰ **M84.521** Pathological fracture in neoplastic disease, right humerus

√7ᵗʰ **M84.522** Pathological fracture in neoplastic disease, left humerus

√7ᵗʰ **M84.529** Pathological fracture in neoplastic disease, unspecified humerus ▽

√6ᵗʰ **M84.53** Pathological fracture in neoplastic disease, ulna and radius

√7ᵗʰ **M84.531** Pathological fracture in neoplastic disease, right ulna

√7ᵗʰ **M84.532** Pathological fracture in neoplastic disease, left ulna

√7ᵗʰ **M84.533** Pathological fracture in neoplastic disease, right radius

√7ᵗʰ **M84.534** Pathological fracture in neoplastic disease, left radius

√7ᵗʰ **M84.539** Pathological fracture in neoplastic disease, unspecified ulna and radius ▽

√6ᵗʰ **M84.54** Pathological fracture in neoplastic disease, hand

√7ᵗʰ **M84.541** Pathological fracture in neoplastic disease, right hand

√7ᵗʰ **M84.542** Pathological fracture in neoplastic disease, left hand

√7ᵗʰ **M84.549** Pathological fracture in neoplastic disease, unspecified hand ▽

√6ᵗʰ **M84.55** Pathological fracture in neoplastic disease, pelvis and femur

√7ᵗʰ **M84.550** Pathological fracture in neoplastic disease, pelvis

1 √7ᵗʰ **M84.551** Pathological fracture in neoplastic disease, right femur   HCC

1 √7ᵗʰ **M84.552** Pathological fracture in neoplastic disease, left femur   HCC

1 √7ᵗʰ **M84.553** Pathological fracture in neoplastic disease, unspecified femur   HCC ▽

1 √7ᵗʰ **M84.559** Pathological fracture in neoplastic disease, hip, unspecified   HCC ▽

√6ᵗʰ **M84.56** Pathological fracture in neoplastic disease, tibia and fibula

√7ᵗʰ **M84.561** Pathological fracture in neoplastic disease, right tibia

✓ Additional Character Req   √x7ᵗʰ Placeholder Alert   Manifestation   ▽ Unspecified   ►◄ Revised Text   ● New Code   ▲ Revised Code Title

ICD-10-CM 2019   805

✓7ᵗʰ **M84.562** Pathological fracture in neoplastic disease, **left tibia**

✓7ᵗʰ **M84.563** Pathological fracture in neoplastic disease, **right fibula**

✓7ᵗʰ **M84.564** Pathological fracture in neoplastic disease, **left fibula**

✓7ᵗʰ **M84.569** Pathological fracture in neoplastic disease, unspecified tibia and fibula ▽

✓6ᵗʰ **M84.57** Pathological fracture in neoplastic disease, **ankle and foot**

✓7ᵗʰ **M84.571** Pathological fracture in neoplastic disease, **right ankle**

✓7ᵗʰ **M84.572** Pathological fracture in neoplastic disease, **left ankle**

✓7ᵗʰ **M84.573** Pathological fracture in neoplastic disease, unspecified ankle ▽

✓7ᵗʰ **M84.574** Pathological fracture in neoplastic disease, **right foot**

✓7ᵗʰ **M84.575** Pathological fracture in neoplastic disease, **left foot**

✓7ᵗʰ **M84.576** Pathological fracture in neoplastic disease, unspecified foot ▽

✓x7ᵗʰ **M84.58** Pathological fracture in neoplastic disease, other specified site

Pathological fracture in neoplastic disease, vertebrae

✓5ᵗʰ **M84.6** Pathological fracture in other disease

Code also underlying condition

EXCLUDES 1   *pathological fracture in osteoporosis (M80.-)*

The appropriate 7th character is to be added to each code from subcategory M84.6.
A   initial encounter for fracture
D   subsequent encounter for fracture with routine healing
G   subsequent encounter for fracture with delayed healing
K   subsequent encounter for fracture with nonunion
P   subsequent encounter for fracture with malunion
S   sequela

✓x7ᵗʰ **M84.60** Pathological fracture in other disease, unspecified site ▽

✓6ᵗʰ **M84.61** Pathological fracture in other disease, **shoulder**

✓7ᵗʰ **M84.611** Pathological fracture in other disease, **right shoulder**

✓7ᵗʰ **M84.612** Pathological fracture in other disease, **left shoulder**

✓7ᵗʰ **M84.619** Pathological fracture in other disease, unspecified shoulder ▽

✓6ᵗʰ **M84.62** Pathological fracture in other disease, **humerus**

✓7ᵗʰ **M84.621** Pathological fracture in other disease, **right humerus**

✓7ᵗʰ **M84.622** Pathological fracture in other disease, **left humerus**

✓7ᵗʰ **M84.629** Pathological fracture in other disease, unspecified humerus ▽

✓6ᵗʰ **M84.63** Pathological fracture in other disease, **ulna and radius**

✓7ᵗʰ **M84.631** Pathological fracture in other disease, **right ulna**

✓7ᵗʰ **M84.632** Pathological fracture in other disease, **left ulna**

✓7ᵗʰ **M84.633** Pathological fracture in other disease, **right radius**

✓7ᵗʰ **M84.634** Pathological fracture in other disease, **left radius**

✓7ᵗʰ **M84.639** Pathological fracture in other disease, unspecified ulna and radius ▽

✓6ᵗʰ **M84.64** Pathological fracture in other disease, **hand**

✓7ᵗʰ **M84.641** Pathological fracture in other disease, **right hand**

✓7ᵗʰ **M84.642** Pathological fracture in other disease, **left hand**

✓7ᵗʰ **M84.649** Pathological fracture in other disease, unspecified hand ▽

✓6ᵗʰ **M84.65** Pathological fracture in other disease, **pelvis and femur**

✓7ᵗʰ **M84.650** Pathological fracture in other disease, **pelvis**

¹ ✓7ᵗʰ **M84.651** Pathological fracture in other disease, **right femur** HCC

¹ ✓7ᵗʰ **M84.652** Pathological fracture in other disease, **left femur** HCC

¹ ✓7ᵗʰ **M84.653** Pathological fracture in other disease, **unspecified femur** HCC ▽

¹ ✓7ᵗʰ **M84.659** Pathological fracture in other disease, **hip, unspecified** HCC ▽

✓6ᵗʰ **M84.66** Pathological fracture in other disease, **tibia and fibula**

✓7ᵗʰ **M84.661** Pathological fracture in other disease, **right tibia**

✓7ᵗʰ **M84.662** Pathological fracture in other disease, **left tibia**

✓7ᵗʰ **M84.663** Pathological fracture in other disease, **right fibula**

✓7ᵗʰ **M84.664** Pathological fracture in other disease, **left fibula**

✓7ᵗʰ **M84.669** Pathological fracture in other disease, unspecified tibia and fibula ▽

✓6ᵗʰ **M84.67** Pathological fracture in other disease, **ankle and foot**

✓7ᵗʰ **M84.671** Pathological fracture in other disease, **right ankle**

✓7ᵗʰ **M84.672** Pathological fracture in other disease, **left ankle**

✓7ᵗʰ **M84.673** Pathological fracture in other disease, unspecified ankle ▽

✓7ᵗʰ **M84.674** Pathological fracture in other disease, **right foot**

✓7ᵗʰ **M84.675** Pathological fracture in other disease, **left foot**

✓7ᵗʰ **M84.676** Pathological fracture in other disease, unspecified foot ▽

✓x7ᵗʰ **M84.68** Pathological fracture in other disease, other site

✓5ᵗʰ **M84.7** Nontraumatic fracture, not elsewhere classified

✓6ᵗʰ **M84.75** **Atypical** femoral fracture

AHA: 2016,4Q,41-42

The appropriate 7th character is to be added to each code from M84.75.
A   initial encounter for fracture
D   subsequent encounter for fracture with routine healing
G   subsequent encounter for fracture with delayed healing
K   subsequent encounter for fracture with nonunion
P   subsequent encounter for fracture with malunion
S   sequela

✓7ᵗʰ **M84.750** **Atypical** femoral fracture, unspecified Q ▽

✓7ᵗʰ **M84.751** **Incomplete atypical** femoral fracture, **right leg** Q

✓7ᵗʰ **M84.752** **Incomplete atypical** femoral fracture, **left leg** Q

✓7ᵗʰ **M84.753** **Incomplete atypical** femoral fracture, **unspecified leg** Q ▽

¹ ✓7ᵗʰ **M84.754** **Complete transverse atypical** femoral fracture, **right leg** HCC Q

¹ ✓7ᵗʰ **M84.755** **Complete transverse atypical** femoral fracture, **left leg** HCC Q

¹ ✓7ᵗʰ **M84.756** **Complete transverse atypical** femoral fracture, **unspecified leg** HCC Q ▽

¹ ✓7ᵗʰ **M84.757** **Complete oblique atypical** femoral fracture, **right leg** HCC Q

¹ ✓7ᵗʰ **M84.758** **Complete oblique atypical** femoral fracture, **left leg** HCC

¹ ✓7ᵗʰ **M84.759** **Complete oblique atypical** femoral fracture, **unspecified leg** HCC Q ▽

✓5ᵗʰ **M84.8** Other disorders of continuity of bone

M84.80 Other disorders of continuity of bone, unspecified site ▽

✓6ᵗʰ **M84.81** Other disorders of continuity of bone, **shoulder**

M84.811 Other disorders of continuity of bone, **right shoulder**

M84.812 Other disorders of continuity of bone, **left shoulder**

M84.819 Other disorders of continuity of bone, unspecified shoulder ▽

√6ᵗʰ **M84.82 Other disorders of continuity of bone,** humerus

     M84.821 Other disorders of continuity of bone, right **humerus**

     M84.822 Other disorders of continuity of bone, left **humerus**

     M84.829 Other disorders of continuity of bone, unspecified humerus ▽

√6ᵗʰ **M84.83 Other disorders of continuity of bone,** ulna and radius

     M84.831 Other disorders of continuity of bone, right **ulna**

     M84.832 Other disorders of continuity of bone, left **ulna**

     M84.833 Other disorders of continuity of bone, right **radius**

     M84.834 Other disorders of continuity of bone, left **radius**

     M84.839 Other disorders of continuity of bone, unspecified ulna and radius ▽

√6ᵗʰ **M84.84 Other disorders of continuity of bone,** hand

     M84.841 Other disorders of continuity of bone, right **hand**

     M84.842 Other disorders of continuity of bone, left **hand**

     M84.849 Other disorders of continuity of bone, unspecified hand ▽

√6ᵗʰ **M84.85 Other disorders of continuity of bone,** pelvic region and thigh

     M84.851 Other disorders of continuity of bone, right **pelvic region and thigh**

     M84.852 Other disorders of continuity of bone, left **pelvic region and thigh**

     M84.859 Other disorders of continuity of bone, unspecified pelvic region and thigh ▽

√6ᵗʰ **M84.86 Other disorders of continuity of bone,** tibia and fibula

     M84.861 Other disorders of continuity of bone, right **tibia**

     M84.862 Other disorders of continuity of bone, left **tibia**

     M84.863 Other disorders of continuity of bone, right **fibula**

     M84.864 Other disorders of continuity of bone, left **fibula**

     M84.869 Other disorders of continuity of bone, unspecified tibia and fibula ▽

√6ᵗʰ **M84.87 Other disorders of continuity of bone,** ankle and foot

     M84.871 Other disorders of continuity of bone, right **ankle and foot**

     M84.872 Other disorders of continuity of bone, left **ankle and foot**

     M84.879 Other disorders of continuity of bone, unspecified ankle and foot ▽

     M84.88 Other disorders of continuity of bone, other site

     M84.9 Disorder of continuity of bone, unspecified ▽

√4ᵗʰ **M85 Other disorders of bone density and structure**

     EXCLUDES 1   osteogenesis imperfecta (Q78.0)

              osteopetrosis (Q78.2)

              osteopoikilosis (Q78.8)

              polyostotic fibrous dysplasia (Q78.1)

√5ᵗʰ **M85.0 Fibrous dysplasia (monostotic)**

     EXCLUDES 2   fibrous dysplasia of jaw (M27.8)

     M85.00 Fibrous dysplasia (monostotic), unspecified site ▽

√6ᵗʰ **M85.01 Fibrous dysplasia (monostotic),** shoulder

     M85.011 Fibrous dysplasia (monostotic), right **shoulder**

     M85.012 Fibrous dysplasia (monostotic), left **shoulder**

     M85.019 Fibrous dysplasia (monostotic), unspecified shoulder ▽

√6ᵗʰ **M85.02 Fibrous dysplasia (monostotic),** upper arm

     M85.021 Fibrous dysplasia (monostotic), right **upper arm**

     M85.022 Fibrous dysplasia (monostotic), left **upper arm**

     M85.029 Fibrous dysplasia (monostotic), unspecified upper arm ▽

√6ᵗʰ **M85.03 Fibrous dysplasia (monostotic),** forearm

     M85.031 Fibrous dysplasia (monostotic), right **forearm**

     M85.032 Fibrous dysplasia (monostotic), left **forearm**

     M85.039 Fibrous dysplasia (monostotic), unspecified forearm ▽

√6ᵗʰ **M85.04 Fibrous dysplasia (monostotic),** hand

     M85.041 Fibrous dysplasia (monostotic), right **hand**

     M85.042 Fibrous dysplasia (monostotic), left **hand**

     M85.049 Fibrous dysplasia (monostotic), unspecified hand ▽

√6ᵗʰ **M85.05 Fibrous dysplasia (monostotic),** thigh

     M85.051 Fibrous dysplasia (monostotic), right **thigh**

     M85.052 Fibrous dysplasia (monostotic), left **thigh**

     M85.059 Fibrous dysplasia (monostotic), unspecified thigh ▽

√6ᵗʰ **M85.06 Fibrous dysplasia (monostotic),** lower leg

     M85.061 Fibrous dysplasia (monostotic), right **lower leg**

     M85.062 Fibrous dysplasia (monostotic), left **lower leg**

     M85.069 Fibrous dysplasia (monostotic), unspecified lower leg ▽

√6ᵗʰ **M85.07 Fibrous dysplasia (monostotic),** ankle and foot

     M85.071 Fibrous dysplasia (monostotic), right **ankle and foot**

     M85.072 Fibrous dysplasia (monostotic), left **ankle and foot**

     M85.079 Fibrous dysplasia (monostotic), unspecified ankle and foot ▽

     M85.08 Fibrous dysplasia (monostotic), other site

     M85.09 Fibrous dysplasia (monostotic), multiple sites

√5ᵗʰ **M85.1 Skeletal fluorosis**

     M85.10 Skeletal fluorosis, unspecified site ▽

√6ᵗʰ **M85.11 Skeletal fluorosis,** shoulder

     M85.111 Skeletal fluorosis, right **shoulder**

     M85.112 Skeletal fluorosis, left **shoulder**

     M85.119 Skeletal fluorosis, unspecified shoulder ▽

√6ᵗʰ **M85.12 Skeletal fluorosis,** upper arm

     M85.121 Skeletal fluorosis, right **upper arm**

     M85.122 Skeletal fluorosis, left **upper arm**

     M85.129 Skeletal fluorosis, unspecified upper arm ▽

√6ᵗʰ **M85.13 Skeletal fluorosis,** forearm

     M85.131 Skeletal fluorosis, right **forearm**

     M85.132 Skeletal fluorosis, left **forearm**

     M85.139 Skeletal fluorosis, unspecified forearm ▽

√6ᵗʰ **M85.14 Skeletal fluorosis,** hand

     M85.141 Skeletal fluorosis, right **hand**

     M85.142 Skeletal fluorosis, left **hand**

     M85.149 Skeletal fluorosis, unspecified hand ▽

√6ᵗʰ **M85.15 Skeletal fluorosis,** thigh

     M85.151 Skeletal fluorosis, right **thigh**

     M85.152 Skeletal fluorosis, left **thigh**

     M85.159 Skeletal fluorosis, unspecified thigh ▽

√6ᵗʰ **M85.16 Skeletal fluorosis,** lower leg

     M85.161 Skeletal fluorosis, right **lower leg**

     M85.162 Skeletal fluorosis, left **lower leg**

     M85.169 Skeletal fluorosis, unspecified lower leg ▽

√6ᵗʰ **M85.17 Skeletal fluorosis,** ankle and foot

     M85.171 Skeletal fluorosis, right **ankle and foot**

     M85.172 Skeletal fluorosis, left **ankle and foot**

     M85.179 Skeletal fluorosis, unspecified ankle and foot ▽

     M85.18 Skeletal fluorosis, other site

     M85.19 Skeletal fluorosis, multiple sites

M85.2 Hyperostosis of skull

     DEF: Abnormal bone growth on the inner aspect of the cranial bones.

☑ Additional Character Req   √x 7ᵗʰ Placeholder Alert   Manifestation   ▽ Unspecified   ►◄ Revised Text   ● New Code   ▲ Revised Code Title

√5ᵗʰ **M85.3 Osteitis condensans**

    M85.30 Osteitis condensans, unspecified site ▽

  √6ᵗʰ **M85.31** Osteitis condensans, shoulder

      M85.311 Osteitis condensans, right shoulder
      M85.312 Osteitis condensans, left shoulder
      M85.319 Osteitis condensans, unspecified shoulder ▽

  √6ᵗʰ **M85.32** Osteitis condensans, upper arm

      M85.321 Osteitis condensans, right upper arm
      M85.322 Osteitis condensans, left upper arm
      M85.329 Osteitis condensans, unspecified upper arm ▽

  √6ᵗʰ **M85.33** Osteitis condensans, forearm

      M85.331 Osteitis condensans, right forearm
      M85.332 Osteitis condensans, left forearm
      M85.339 Osteitis condensans, unspecified forearm ▽

  √6ᵗʰ **M85.34** Osteitis condensans, hand

      M85.341 Osteitis condensans, right hand
      M85.342 Osteitis condensans, left hand
      M85.349 Osteitis condensans, unspecified hand ▽

  √6ᵗʰ **M85.35** Osteitis condensans, thigh

      M85.351 Osteitis condensans, right thigh
      M85.352 Osteitis condensans, left thigh
      M85.359 Osteitis condensans, unspecified thigh ▽

  √6ᵗʰ **M85.36** Osteitis condensans, lower leg

      M85.361 Osteitis condensans, right lower leg
      M85.362 Osteitis condensans, left lower leg
      M85.369 Osteitis condensans, unspecified lower leg ▽

  √6ᵗʰ **M85.37** Osteitis condensans, ankle and foot

      M85.371 Osteitis condensans, right ankle and foot
      M85.372 Osteitis condensans, left ankle and foot
      M85.379 Osteitis condensans, unspecified ankle and foot ▽

    M85.38 Osteitis condensans, other site

    M85.39 Osteitis condensans, multiple sites

√5ᵗʰ **M85.4 Solitary bone cyst**

    EXCLUDES 2   *solitary cyst of jaw (M27.4)*

    M85.40 Solitary bone cyst, unspecified site ▽

  √6ᵗʰ **M85.41** Solitary bone cyst, shoulder

      M85.411 Solitary bone cyst, right shoulder
      M85.412 Solitary bone cyst, left shoulder
      M85.419 Solitary bone cyst, unspecified shoulder ▽

  √6ᵗʰ **M85.42** Solitary bone cyst, humerus

      M85.421 Solitary bone cyst, right humerus
      M85.422 Solitary bone cyst, left humerus
      M85.429 Solitary bone cyst, unspecified humerus ▽

  √6ᵗʰ **M85.43** Solitary bone cyst, ulna and radius

      M85.431 Solitary bone cyst, right ulna and radius
      M85.432 Solitary bone cyst, left ulna and radius
      M85.439 Solitary bone cyst, unspecified ulna and radius ▽

  √6ᵗʰ **M85.44** Solitary bone cyst, hand

      M85.441 Solitary bone cyst, right hand
      M85.442 Solitary bone cyst, left hand
      M85.449 Solitary bone cyst, unspecified hand ▽

  √6ᵗʰ **M85.45** Solitary bone cyst, pelvis

      M85.451 Solitary bone cyst, right pelvis
      M85.452 Solitary bone cyst, left pelvis
      M85.459 Solitary bone cyst, unspecified pelvis ▽

  √6ᵗʰ **M85.46** Solitary bone cyst, tibia and fibula

      M85.461 Solitary bone cyst, right tibia and fibula
      M85.462 Solitary bone cyst, left tibia and fibula
      M85.469 Solitary bone cyst, unspecified tibia and fibula ▽

  √6ᵗʰ **M85.47** Solitary bone cyst, ankle and foot

      M85.471 Solitary bone cyst, right ankle and foot
      M85.472 Solitary bone cyst, left ankle and foot
      M85.479 Solitary bone cyst, unspecified ankle and foot ▽

    M85.48 Solitary bone cyst, other site

√5ᵗʰ **M85.5 Aneurysmal bone cyst**

    EXCLUDES 2   *aneurysmal cyst of jaw (M27.4)*

    DEF: Solitary bone lesion that bulges into the periosteum and is marked by a calcified rim.

    M85.50 Aneurysmal bone cyst, unspecified site ▽

  √6ᵗʰ **M85.51** Aneurysmal bone cyst, shoulder

      M85.511 Aneurysmal bone cyst, right shoulder
      M85.512 Aneurysmal bone cyst, left shoulder
      M85.519 Aneurysmal bone cyst, unspecified shoulder ▽

  √6ᵗʰ **M85.52** Aneurysmal bone cyst, upper arm

      M85.521 Aneurysmal bone cyst, right upper arm
      M85.522 Aneurysmal bone cyst, left upper arm
      M85.529 Aneurysmal bone cyst, unspecified upper arm

  √6ᵗʰ **M85.53** Aneurysmal bone cyst, forearm

      M85.531 Aneurysmal bone cyst, right forearm
      M85.532 Aneurysmal bone cyst, left forearm
      M85.539 Aneurysmal bone cyst, unspecified forearm ▽

  √6ᵗʰ **M85.54** Aneurysmal bone cyst, hand

      M85.541 Aneurysmal bone cyst, right hand
      M85.542 Aneurysmal bone cyst, left hand
      M85.549 Aneurysmal bone cyst, unspecified hand ▽

  √6ᵗʰ **M85.55** Aneurysmal bone cyst, thigh

      M85.551 Aneurysmal bone cyst, right thigh
      M85.552 Aneurysmal bone cyst, left thigh
      M85.559 Aneurysmal bone cyst, unspecified thigh ▽

  √6ᵗʰ **M85.56** Aneurysmal bone cyst, lower leg

      M85.561 Aneurysmal bone cyst, right lower leg
      M85.562 Aneurysmal bone cyst, left lower leg
      M85.569 Aneurysmal bone cyst, unspecified lower leg ▽

  √6ᵗʰ **M85.57** Aneurysmal bone cyst, ankle and foot

      M85.571 Aneurysmal bone cyst, right ankle and foot
      M85.572 Aneurysmal bone cyst, left ankle and foot
      M85.579 Aneurysmal bone cyst, unspecified ankle and foot ▽

    M85.58 Aneurysmal bone cyst, other site

    M85.59 Aneurysmal bone cyst, multiple sites

√5ᵗʰ **M85.6 Other cyst of bone**

    EXCLUDES 1   *cyst of jaw NEC (M27.4)*

                osteitis fibrosa cystica generalisata [von Recklinghausen's disease of bone] (E21.0)

    M85.60 Other cyst of bone, unspecified site ▽

  √6ᵗʰ **M85.61** Other cyst of bone, shoulder

      M85.611 Other cyst of bone, right shoulder
      M85.612 Other cyst of bone, left shoulder
      M85.619 Other cyst of bone, unspecified shoulder ▽

  √6ᵗʰ **M85.62** Other cyst of bone, upper arm

      M85.621 Other cyst of bone, right upper arm
      M85.622 Other cyst of bone, left upper arm
      M85.629 Other cyst of bone, unspecified upper arm ▽

  √6ᵗʰ **M85.63** Other cyst of bone, forearm

      M85.631 Other cyst of bone, right forearm
      M85.632 Other cyst of bone, left forearm
      M85.639 Other cyst of bone, unspecified forearm ▽

  √6ᵗʰ **M85.64** Other cyst of bone, hand

      M85.641 Other cyst of bone, right hand
      M85.642 Other cyst of bone, left hand
      M85.649 Other cyst of bone, unspecified hand ▽

  √6ᵗʰ **M85.65** Other cyst of bone, thigh

      M85.651 Other cyst of bone, right thigh
      M85.652 Other cyst of bone, left thigh
      M85.659 Other cyst of bone, unspecified thigh ▽

  √6ᵗʰ **M85.66** Other cyst of bone, lower leg

      M85.661 Other cyst of bone, right lower leg
      M85.662 Other cyst of bone, left lower leg

M85.669 Other cyst of bone, unspecified ▽
lower leg

√6ᵗʰ M85.67 Other cyst of bone, ankle and foot

M85.671 Other cyst of bone, right ankle and foot
M85.672 Other cyst of bone, left ankle and foot
M85.679 Other cyst of bone, unspecified ▽
ankle and foot

M85.68 Other cyst of bone, other site
M85.69 Other cyst of bone, multiple sites

√5ᵗʰ M85.8 Other specified disorders of bone density and structure

Hyperostosis of bones, except skull
Osteosclerosis, acquired

EXCLUDES 1 diffuse idiopathic skeletal hyperostosis [DISH] (M48.1)
osteosclerosis congenita (Q77.4)
osteosclerosis fragilitas (generalista) (Q78.2)
osteosclerosis myelofibrosis (D75.81)

M85.80 Other specified disorders of bone density ▽
and structure, unspecified site

√6ᵗʰ M85.81 Other specified disorders of bone density and structure, shoulder

M85.811 Other specified disorders of bone density and structure, right shoulder
M85.812 Other specified disorders of bone density and structure, left shoulder
M85.819 Other specified disorders of bone ▽
density and structure,
unspecified shoulder

√6ᵗʰ M85.82 Other specified disorders of bone density and structure, upper arm

M85.821 Other specified disorders of bone density and structure, right upper arm
M85.822 Other specified disorders of bone density and structure, left upper arm
M85.829 Other specified disorders of bone ▽
density and structure,
unspecified upper arm

√6ᵗʰ M85.83 Other specified disorders of bone density and structure, forearm

M85.831 Other specified disorders of bone density and structure, right forearm
M85.832 Other specified disorders of bone density and structure, left forearm
M85.839 Other specified disorders of bone ▽
density and structure,
unspecified forearm

√6ᵗʰ M85.84 Other specified disorders of bone density and structure, hand

M85.841 Other specified disorders of bone density and structure, right hand
M85.842 Other specified disorders of bone density and structure, left hand
M85.849 Other specified disorders of bone ▽
density and structure,
unspecified hand

√6ᵗʰ M85.85 Other specified disorders of bone density and structure, thigh

M85.851 Other specified disorders of bone density and structure, right thigh
M85.852 Other specified disorders of bone density and structure, left thigh
M85.859 Other specified disorders of bone ▽
density and structure,
unspecified thigh

√6ᵗʰ M85.86 Other specified disorders of bone density and structure, lower leg

M85.861 Other specified disorders of bone density and structure, right lower leg
M85.862 Other specified disorders of bone density and structure, left lower leg
M85.869 Other specified disorders of bone ▽
density and structure,
unspecified lower leg

√6ᵗʰ M85.87 Other specified disorders of bone density and structure, ankle and foot

M85.871 Other specified disorders of bone density and structure, right ankle and foot
M85.872 Other specified disorders of bone density and structure, left ankle and foot
M85.879 Other specified disorders of bone ▽
density and structure,
unspecified ankle and foot

M85.88 Other specified disorders of bone density and structure, other site

M85.89 Other specified disorders of bone density and structure, multiple sites

M85.9 Disorder of bone density and structure, unspecified ▽

Other osteopathies (M86-M90)

EXCLUDES 1 postprocedural osteopathies (M96.-)

√4ᵗʰ M86 Osteomyelitis

Use additional code (B95-B97) to identify infectious agent
Use additional code to identify major osseous defect, if applicable (M89.7-)

EXCLUDES 1 osteomyelitis due to:
echinococcus (B67.2)
gonococcus (A54.43)
salmonella (A02.24)

EXCLUDES 2 ostemyelitis of:
orbit (H05.0-)
petrous bone (H70.2-)
vertebra (M46.2-)

√5ᵗʰ M86.0 Acute hematogenous osteomyelitis

M86.00 Acute hematogenous osteomyelitis, HCC ▽
unspecified site

√6ᵗʰ M86.01 Acute hematogenous osteomyelitis, shoulder

M86.011 Acute hematogenous HCC
osteomyelitis, right shoulder
M86.012 Acute hematogenous HCC
osteomyelitis, left shoulder
M86.019 Acute hematogenous HCC ▽
osteomyelitis, unspecified
shoulder

√6ᵗʰ M86.02 Acute hematogenous osteomyelitis, humerus

M86.021 Acute hematogenous HCC
osteomyelitis, right humerus
M86.022 Acute hematogenous HCC
osteomyelitis, left humerus
M86.029 Acute hematogenous HCC ▽
osteomyelitis, unspecified
humerus

√6ᵗʰ M86.03 Acute hematogenous osteomyelitis, radius and ulna

M86.031 Acute hematogenous HCC
osteomyelitis, right radius and
ulna
M86.032 Acute hematogenous HCC
osteomyelitis, left radius and ulna
M86.039 Acute hematogenous HCC ▽
osteomyelitis, unspecified radius
and ulna

√6ᵗʰ M86.04 Acute hematogenous osteomyelitis, hand

M86.041 Acute hematogenous HCC
osteomyelitis, right hand
M86.042 Acute hematogenous HCC
osteomyelitis, left hand
M86.049 Acute hematogenous HCC ▽
osteomyelitis, unspecified hand

√6ᵗʰ M86.05 Acute hematogenous osteomyelitis, femur

M86.051 Acute hematogenous HCC
osteomyelitis, right femur
M86.052 Acute hematogenous HCC
osteomyelitis, left femur
M86.059 Acute hematogenous HCC ▽
osteomyelitis, unspecified femur

√6ᵗʰ M86.06 Acute hematogenous osteomyelitis, tibia and fibula

M86.061 Acute hematogenous HCC
osteomyelitis, right tibia and
fibula
M86.062 Acute hematogenous HCC
osteomyelitis, left tibia and fibula
M86.069 Acute hematogenous HCC ▽
osteomyelitis, unspecified tibia
and fibula

√6ᵗʰ M86.07 Acute hematogenous osteomyelitis, ankle and foot

M86.071 Acute hematogenous HCC
osteomyelitis, right ankle and
foot
M86.072 Acute hematogenous HCC
osteomyelitis, left ankle and foot

M86.079   Acute hematogenous osteomyelitis, unspecified ankle and foot   HCC ▽

M86.08   Acute hematogenous osteomyelitis, other sites   HCC

M86.09   Acute hematogenous osteomyelitis, multiple sites   HCC

✓5th M86.1   **Other acute osteomyelitis**

M86.10   Other acute osteomyelitis, unspecified site   HCC ▽

✓6th M86.11   Other acute osteomyelitis, shoulder

M86.111   Other acute osteomyelitis, right shoulder   HCC

M86.112   Other acute osteomyelitis, left shoulder   HCC

M86.119   Other acute osteomyelitis, unspecified shoulder   HCC ▽

✓6th M86.12   Other acute osteomyelitis, humerus

M86.121   Other acute osteomyelitis, right humerus   HCC

M86.122   Other acute osteomyelitis, left humerus   HCC

M86.129   Other acute osteomyelitis, unspecified humerus   HCC ▽

✓6th M86.13   Other acute osteomyelitis, radius and ulna

M86.131   Other acute osteomyelitis, right radius and ulna   HCC

M86.132   Other acute osteomyelitis, left radius and ulna   HCC

M86.139   Other acute osteomyelitis, unspecified radius and ulna   HCC ▽

✓6th M86.14   Other acute osteomyelitis, hand

M86.141   Other acute osteomyelitis, right hand   HCC

M86.142   Other acute osteomyelitis, left hand   HCC

M86.149   Other acute osteomyelitis, unspecified hand   HCC ▽

✓6th M86.15   Other acute osteomyelitis, femur

M86.151   Other acute osteomyelitis, right femur   HCC

M86.152   Other acute osteomyelitis, left femur   HCC

M86.159   Other acute osteomyelitis, unspecified femur   HCC ▽

✓6th M86.16   Other acute osteomyelitis, tibia and fibula

M86.161   Other acute osteomyelitis, right tibia and fibula   HCC

M86.162   Other acute osteomyelitis, left tibia and fibula   HCC

M86.169   Other acute osteomyelitis, unspecified tibia and fibula   HCC ▽

✓6th M86.17   Other acute osteomyelitis, ankle and foot

M86.171   Other acute osteomyelitis, right ankle and foot   HCC

M86.172   Other acute osteomyelitis, left ankle and foot   HCC

M86.179   Other acute osteomyelitis, unspecified ankle and foot   HCC ▽

M86.18   Other acute osteomyelitis, other site   HCC

M86.19   Other acute osteomyelitis, multiple sites   HCC

✓5th M86.2   **Subacute osteomyelitis**

M86.20   Subacute osteomyelitis, unspecified site   HCC ▽

✓6th M86.21   Subacute osteomyelitis, shoulder

M86.211   Subacute osteomyelitis, right shoulder   HCC

M86.212   Subacute osteomyelitis, left shoulder   HCC

M86.219   Subacute osteomyelitis, unspecified shoulder   HCC ▽

✓6th M86.22   Subacute osteomyelitis, humerus

M86.221   Subacute osteomyelitis, right humerus   HCC

M86.222   Subacute osteomyelitis, left humerus   HCC

M86.229   Subacute osteomyelitis, unspecified humerus   HCC ▽

✓6th M86.23   Subacute osteomyelitis, radius and ulna

M86.231   Subacute osteomyelitis, right radius and ulna   HCC

M86.232   Subacute osteomyelitis, left radius and ulna   HCC

M86.239   Subacute osteomyelitis, unspecified radius and ulna   HCC ▽

✓6th M86.24   Subacute osteomyelitis, hand

M86.241   Subacute osteomyelitis, right hand   HCC

M86.242   Subacute osteomyelitis, left hand   HCC

M86.249   Subacute osteomyelitis, unspecified hand   HCC ▽

✓6th M86.25   Subacute osteomyelitis, femur

M86.251   Subacute osteomyelitis, right femur   HCC

M86.252   Subacute osteomyelitis, left femur   HCC

M86.259   Subacute osteomyelitis, unspecified femur   HCC ▽

✓6th M86.26   Subacute osteomyelitis, tibia and fibula

M86.261   Subacute osteomyelitis, right tibia and fibula   HCC

M86.262   Subacute osteomyelitis, left tibia and fibula   HCC

M86.269   Subacute osteomyelitis, unspecified tibia and fibula   HCC ▽

✓6th M86.27   Subacute osteomyelitis, ankle and foot

M86.271   Subacute osteomyelitis, right ankle and foot   HCC

M86.272   Subacute osteomyelitis, left ankle and foot   HCC

M86.279   Subacute osteomyelitis, unspecified ankle and foot   HCC ▽

M86.28   Subacute osteomyelitis, other site   HCC

M86.29   Subacute osteomyelitis, multiple sites   HCC

✓5th M86.3   **Chronic multifocal osteomyelitis**

M86.30   Chronic multifocal osteomyelitis, unspecified site   HCC ▽

✓6th M86.31   Chronic multifocal osteomyelitis, shoulder

M86.311   Chronic multifocal osteomyelitis, right shoulder   HCC

M86.312   Chronic multifocal osteomyelitis, left shoulder   HCC

M86.319   Chronic multifocal osteomyelitis, unspecified shoulder   HCC ▽

✓6th M86.32   Chronic multifocal osteomyelitis, humerus

M86.321   Chronic multifocal osteomyelitis, right humerus   HCC

M86.322   Chronic multifocal osteomyelitis, left humerus   HCC

M86.329   Chronic multifocal osteomyelitis, unspecified humerus   HCC ▽

✓6th M86.33   Chronic multifocal osteomyelitis, radius and ulna

M86.331   Chronic multifocal osteomyelitis, right radius and ulna   HCC

M86.332   Chronic multifocal osteomyelitis, left radius and ulna   HCC

M86.339   Chronic multifocal osteomyelitis, unspecified radius and ulna   HCC ▽

✓6th M86.34   Chronic multifocal osteomyelitis, hand

M86.341   Chronic multifocal osteomyelitis, right hand   HCC

M86.342   Chronic multifocal osteomyelitis, left hand   HCC

M86.349   Chronic multifocal osteomyelitis, unspecified hand   HCC ▽

✓6th M86.35   Chronic multifocal osteomyelitis, femur

M86.351   Chronic multifocal osteomyelitis, right femur   HCC

M86.352   Chronic multifocal osteomyelitis, left femur   HCC

M86.359   Chronic multifocal osteomyelitis, unspecified femur   HCC ▽

✓6th M86.36   Chronic multifocal osteomyelitis, tibia and fibula

M86.361   Chronic multifocal osteomyelitis, right tibia and fibula   HCC

M86.362   Chronic multifocal osteomyelitis, left tibia and fibula   HCC

M86.369   Chronic multifocal osteomyelitis, unspecified tibia and fibula   HCC ▽

√6ᵗʰ **M86.37** Chronic multifocal osteomyelitis, ankle and foot

     M86.371 Chronic multifocal osteomyelitis, right ankle and foot   HCC

     M86.372 Chronic multifocal osteomyelitis, left ankle and foot   HCC

     M86.379 Chronic multifocal osteomyelitis, unspecified ankle and foot   HCC ▽

   M86.38 Chronic multifocal osteomyelitis, other site   HCC

   M86.39 Chronic multifocal osteomyelitis, multiple sites   HCC

√5ᵗʰ **M86.4** Chronic osteomyelitis with draining sinus

   M86.40 Chronic osteomyelitis with draining sinus, unspecified site   HCC ▽

√6ᵗʰ **M86.41** Chronic osteomyelitis with draining sinus, shoulder

     M86.411 Chronic osteomyelitis with draining sinus, right shoulder   HCC

     M86.412 Chronic osteomyelitis with draining sinus, left shoulder   HCC

     M86.419 Chronic osteomyelitis with draining sinus, unspecified shoulder   HCC ▽

√6ᵗʰ **M86.42** Chronic osteomyelitis with draining sinus, humerus

     M86.421 Chronic osteomyelitis with draining sinus, right humerus   HCC

     M86.422 Chronic osteomyelitis with draining sinus, left humerus   HCC

     M86.429 Chronic osteomyelitis with draining sinus, unspecified humerus   HCC ▽

√6ᵗʰ **M86.43** Chronic osteomyelitis with draining sinus, radius and ulna

     M86.431 Chronic osteomyelitis with draining sinus, right radius and ulna   HCC

     M86.432 Chronic osteomyelitis with draining sinus, left radius and ulna   HCC

     M86.439 Chronic osteomyelitis with draining sinus, unspecified radius and ulna   HCC ▽

√6ᵗʰ **M86.44** Chronic osteomyelitis with draining sinus, hand

     M86.441 Chronic osteomyelitis with draining sinus, right hand   HCC

     M86.442 Chronic osteomyelitis with draining sinus, left hand   HCC

     M86.449 Chronic osteomyelitis with draining sinus, unspecified hand   HCC ▽

√6ᵗʰ **M86.45** Chronic osteomyelitis with draining sinus, femur

     M86.451 Chronic osteomyelitis with draining sinus, right femur   HCC

     M86.452 Chronic osteomyelitis with draining sinus, left femur   HCC

     M86.459 Chronic osteomyelitis with draining sinus, unspecified femur   HCC ▽

√6ᵗʰ **M86.46** Chronic osteomyelitis with draining sinus, tibia and fibula

     M86.461 Chronic osteomyelitis with draining sinus, right tibia and fibula   HCC

     M86.462 Chronic osteomyelitis with draining sinus, left tibia and fibula   HCC

     M86.469 Chronic osteomyelitis with draining sinus, unspecified tibia and fibula   HCC ▽

√6ᵗʰ **M86.47** Chronic osteomyelitis with draining sinus, ankle and foot

     M86.471 Chronic osteomyelitis with draining sinus, right ankle and foot   HCC

     M86.472 Chronic osteomyelitis with draining sinus, left ankle and foot   HCC

     M86.479 Chronic osteomyelitis with draining sinus, unspecified ankle and foot   HCC ▽

   M86.48 Chronic osteomyelitis with draining sinus, other site   HCC

   M86.49 Chronic osteomyelitis with draining sinus, multiple sites   HCC

√5ᵗʰ **M86.5** Other chronic hematogenous osteomyelitis

   M86.50 Other chronic hematogenous osteomyelitis, unspecified site   HCC ▽

√6ᵗʰ **M86.51** Other chronic hematogenous osteomyelitis, shoulder

     M86.511 Other chronic hematogenous osteomyelitis, right shoulder   HCC

     M86.512 Other chronic hematogenous osteomyelitis, left shoulder   HCC

     M86.519 Other chronic hematogenous osteomyelitis, unspecified shoulder   HCC ▽

√6ᵗʰ **M86.52** Other chronic hematogenous osteomyelitis, humerus

     M86.521 Other chronic hematogenous osteomyelitis, right humerus   HCC

     M86.522 Other chronic hematogenous osteomyelitis, left humerus   HCC

     M86.529 Other chronic hematogenous osteomyelitis, unspecified humerus   HCC ▽

√6ᵗʰ **M86.53** Other chronic hematogenous osteomyelitis, radius and ulna

     M86.531 Other chronic hematogenous osteomyelitis, right radius and ulna   HCC

     M86.532 Other chronic hematogenous osteomyelitis, left radius and ulna   HCC

     M86.539 Other chronic hematogenous osteomyelitis, unspecified radius and ulna   HCC ▽

√6ᵗʰ **M86.54** Other chronic hematogenous osteomyelitis, hand

     M86.541 Other chronic hematogenous osteomyelitis, right hand   HCC

     M86.542 Other chronic hematogenous osteomyelitis, left hand   HCC

     M86.549 Other chronic hematogenous osteomyelitis, unspecified hand   HCC ▽

√6ᵗʰ **M86.55** Other chronic hematogenous osteomyelitis, femur

     M86.551 Other chronic hematogenous osteomyelitis, right femur   HCC

     M86.552 Other chronic hematogenous osteomyelitis, left femur   HCC

     M86.559 Other chronic hematogenous osteomyelitis, unspecified femur   HCC ▽

√6ᵗʰ **M86.56** Other chronic hematogenous osteomyelitis, tibia and fibula

     M86.561 Other chronic hematogenous osteomyelitis, right tibia and fibula   HCC

     M86.562 Other chronic hematogenous osteomyelitis, left tibia and fibula   HCC

     M86.569 Other chronic hematogenous osteomyelitis, unspecified tibia and fibula   HCC ▽

√6ᵗʰ **M86.57** Other chronic hematogenous osteomyelitis, ankle and foot

     M86.571 Other chronic hematogenous osteomyelitis, right ankle and foot   HCC

     M86.572 Other chronic hematogenous osteomyelitis, left ankle and foot   HCC

     M86.579 Other chronic hematogenous osteomyelitis, unspecified ankle and foot   HCC ▽

   M86.58 Other chronic hematogenous osteomyelitis, other site   HCC

   M86.59 Other chronic hematogenous osteomyelitis, multiple sites   HCC

√5ᵗʰ **M86.6** Other chronic osteomyelitis

   M86.60 Other chronic osteomyelitis, unspecified site   HCC ▽

√6ᵗʰ **M86.61** Other chronic osteomyelitis, shoulder

     M86.611 Other chronic osteomyelitis, right shoulder   HCC

     M86.612 Other chronic osteomyelitis, left shoulder   HCC

     M86.619 Other chronic osteomyelitis, unspecified shoulder   HCC ▽

√6ᵗʰ **M86.62** Other chronic osteomyelitis, humerus

▲   **M86.621** Other chronic osteomyelitis, right humerus   HCC

▲   **M86.622** Other chronic osteomyelitis, left humerus   HCC

✓ Additional Character Req   ✓x7ᵗʰ Placeholder Alert   Manifestation   ▽ Unspecified   ▶◀ Revised Text   ● New Code   ▲ Revised Code Title

Chapter 13. Diseases of the Musculoskeletal System and Connective Tissue

M86.629 Other chronic osteomyelitis, unspecified humerus `HCC` ▽

√6ᵗʰ M86.63 Other chronic osteomyelitis, radius and ulna
  M86.631 Other chronic osteomyelitis, right radius and ulna `HCC`
  M86.632 Other chronic osteomyelitis, left radius and ulna `HCC`
  M86.639 Other chronic osteomyelitis, unspecified radius and ulna `HCC` ▽

√6ᵗʰ M86.64 Other chronic osteomyelitis, hand
  M86.641 Other chronic osteomyelitis, right hand `HCC`
  M86.642 Other chronic osteomyelitis, left hand `HCC`
  M86.649 Other chronic osteomyelitis, unspecified hand `HCC` ▽

√6ᵗʰ M86.65 Other chronic osteomyelitis, thigh
  M86.651 Other chronic osteomyelitis, right thigh `HCC`
  M86.652 Other chronic osteomyelitis, left thigh `HCC`
  M86.659 Other chronic osteomyelitis, unspecified thigh `HCC` ▽

√6ᵗʰ M86.66 Other chronic osteomyelitis, tibia and fibula
  M86.661 Other chronic osteomyelitis, right tibia and fibula `HCC`
  M86.662 Other chronic osteomyelitis, left tibia and fibula `HCC`
  M86.669 Other chronic osteomyelitis, unspecified tibia and fibula `HCC` ▽

√6ᵗʰ M86.67 Other chronic osteomyelitis, ankle and foot
  M86.671 Other chronic osteomyelitis, right ankle and foot `HCC`
    AHA: 2016,1Q,13
  M86.672 Other chronic osteomyelitis, left ankle and foot `HCC`
  M86.679 Other chronic osteomyelitis, unspecified ankle and foot `HCC` ▽

M86.68 Other chronic osteomyelitis, other site `HCC`
M86.69 Other chronic osteomyelitis, multiple sites `HCC`

√5ᵗʰ M86.8 Other osteomyelitis
  Brodie's abscess
  √6ᵗʰ M86.8X Other osteomyelitis
    M86.8X0 Other osteomyelitis, multiple sites `HCC`
    M86.8X1 Other osteomyelitis, shoulder `HCC`
    M86.8X2 Other osteomyelitis, upper arm `HCC`
    M86.8X3 Other osteomyelitis, forearm `HCC`
    M86.8X4 Other osteomyelitis, hand `HCC`
    M86.8X5 Other osteomyelitis, thigh `HCC`
    M86.8X6 Other osteomyelitis, lower leg `HCC`
    M86.8X7 Other osteomyelitis, ankle and foot `HCC`
    M86.8X8 Other osteomyelitis, other site `HCC`
    M86.8X9 Other osteomyelitis, unspecified sites `HCC` ▽

M86.9 Osteomyelitis, unspecified `HCC` ▽
  Infection of bone NOS
  Periostitis without osteomyelitis

√4ᵗʰ **M87 Osteonecrosis**
  INCLUDES avascular necrosis of bone
  Use additional code to identify major osseous defect, if applicable (M89.7-)
  EXCLUDES 1 juvenile osteonecrosis (M91-M92)
    osteochondropathies (M90-M93)

√5ᵗʰ M87.0 Idiopathic aseptic necrosis of bone
  M87.00 Idiopathic aseptic necrosis of unspecified bone `HCC` ▽
  √6ᵗʰ M87.01 Idiopathic aseptic necrosis of shoulder
    Idiopathic aseptic necrosis of clavicle and scapula
    M87.011 Idiopathic aseptic necrosis of right shoulder `HCC`
    M87.012 Idiopathic aseptic necrosis of left shoulder `HCC`
    M87.019 Idiopathic aseptic necrosis of unspecified shoulder `HCC` ▽

√6ᵗʰ M87.02 Idiopathic aseptic necrosis of humerus
  M87.021 Idiopathic aseptic necrosis of right humerus `HCC`
  M87.022 Idiopathic aseptic necrosis of left humerus `HCC`
  M87.029 Idiopathic aseptic necrosis of unspecified humerus `HCC` ▽

√6ᵗʰ M87.03 Idiopathic aseptic necrosis of radius, ulna and carpus
  M87.031 Idiopathic aseptic necrosis of right radius `HCC`
  M87.032 Idiopathic aseptic necrosis of left radius `HCC`
  M87.033 Idiopathic aseptic necrosis of unspecified radius `HCC` ▽
  M87.034 Idiopathic aseptic necrosis of right ulna `HCC`
  M87.035 Idiopathic aseptic necrosis of left ulna `HCC`
  M87.036 Idiopathic aseptic necrosis of unspecified ulna `HCC` ▽
  M87.037 Idiopathic aseptic necrosis of right carpus `HCC`
  M87.038 Idiopathic aseptic necrosis of left carpus `HCC`
  M87.039 Idiopathic aseptic necrosis of unspecified carpus `HCC` ▽

√6ᵗʰ M87.04 Idiopathic aseptic necrosis of hand and fingers
  Idiopathic aseptic necrosis of metacarpals and phalanges of hands
  M87.041 Idiopathic aseptic necrosis of right hand `HCC`
  M87.042 Idiopathic aseptic necrosis of left hand `HCC`
  M87.043 Idiopathic aseptic necrosis of unspecified hand `HCC` ▽
  M87.044 Idiopathic aseptic necrosis of right finger(s) `HCC`
  M87.045 Idiopathic aseptic necrosis of left finger(s) `HCC`
  M87.046 Idiopathic aseptic necrosis of unspecified finger(s) `HCC` ▽

√6ᵗʰ M87.05 Idiopathic aseptic necrosis of pelvis and femur
  M87.050 Idiopathic aseptic necrosis of pelvis `HCC`
  M87.051 Idiopathic aseptic necrosis of right femur `HCC`
  M87.052 Idiopathic aseptic necrosis of left femur `HCC`
  M87.059 Idiopathic aseptic necrosis of unspecified femur `HCC` ▽
    Idiopathic aseptic necrosis of hip NOS

√6ᵗʰ M87.06 Idiopathic aseptic necrosis of tibia and fibula
  M87.061 Idiopathic aseptic necrosis of right tibia `HCC`
  M87.062 Idiopathic aseptic necrosis of left tibia `HCC`
  M87.063 Idiopathic aseptic necrosis of unspecified tibia `HCC` ▽
  M87.064 Idiopathic aseptic necrosis of right fibula `HCC`
  M87.065 Idiopathic aseptic necrosis of left fibula `HCC`
  M87.066 Idiopathic aseptic necrosis of unspecified fibula `HCC` ▽

√6ᵗʰ M87.07 Idiopathic aseptic necrosis of ankle, foot and toes
  Idiopathic aseptic necrosis of metatarsus, tarsus, and phalanges of toes
  M87.071 Idiopathic aseptic necrosis of right ankle `HCC`
  M87.072 Idiopathic aseptic necrosis of left ankle `HCC`
  M87.073 Idiopathic aseptic necrosis of unspecified ankle `HCC` ▽
  M87.074 Idiopathic aseptic necrosis of right foot `HCC`
  M87.075 Idiopathic aseptic necrosis of left foot `HCC`
  M87.076 Idiopathic aseptic necrosis of unspecified foot `HCC` ▽
  M87.077 Idiopathic aseptic necrosis of right toe(s) `HCC`

M87.Ø78	Idiopathic aseptic necrosis of left toe(s)	HCC
M87.Ø79	Idiopathic aseptic necrosis of unspecified toe(s)	HCC ▽
M87.Ø8	**Idiopathic aseptic necrosis of bone, other site**	HCC
M87.Ø9	**Idiopathic aseptic necrosis of bone, multiple sites**	HCC

✓5ᵗʰ **M87.1 Osteonecrosis due to drugs**

Use additional code for adverse effect, if applicable, to identify drug (T36-T5Ø with fifth or sixth character 5)

M87.1Ø	**Osteonecrosis due to drugs, unspecified bone**	HCC ▽

✓6ᵗʰ **M87.11 Osteonecrosis due to drugs, shoulder**

M87.111	Osteonecrosis due to drugs, right shoulder	HCC
M87.112	Osteonecrosis due to drugs, left shoulder	HCC
M87.119	Osteonecrosis due to drugs, unspecified shoulder	HCC ▽

✓6ᵗʰ **M87.12 Osteonecrosis due to drugs, humerus**

M87.121	Osteonecrosis due to drugs, right humerus	HCC
M87.122	Osteonecrosis due to drugs, left humerus	HCC
M87.129	Osteonecrosis due to drugs, unspecified humerus	HCC ▽

✓6ᵗʰ **M87.13 Osteonecrosis due to drugs of radius, ulna and carpus**

M87.131	Osteonecrosis due to drugs of right radius	HCC
M87.132	Osteonecrosis due to drugs of left radius	HCC
M87.133	Osteonecrosis due to drugs of unspecified radius	HCC ▽
M87.134	Osteonecrosis due to drugs of right ulna	HCC
M87.135	Osteonecrosis due to drugs of left ulna	HCC
M87.136	Osteonecrosis due to drugs of unspecified ulna	HCC ▽
M87.137	Osteonecrosis due to drugs of right carpus	HCC
M87.138	Osteonecrosis due to drugs of left carpus	HCC
M87.139	Osteonecrosis due to drugs of unspecified carpus	HCC ▽

✓6ᵗʰ **M87.14 Osteonecrosis due to drugs, hand and fingers**

M87.141	Osteonecrosis due to drugs, right hand	HCC
M87.142	Osteonecrosis due to drugs, left hand	HCC
M87.143	Osteonecrosis due to drugs, unspecified hand	HCC ▽
M87.144	Osteonecrosis due to drugs, right finger(s)	HCC
M87.145	Osteonecrosis due to drugs, left finger(s)	HCC
M87.146	Osteonecrosis due to drugs, unspecified finger(s)	HCC ▽

✓6ᵗʰ **M87.15 Osteonecrosis due to drugs, pelvis and femur**

M87.15Ø	Osteonecrosis due to drugs, pelvis	HCC
M87.151	Osteonecrosis due to drugs, right femur	HCC
M87.152	Osteonecrosis due to drugs, left femur	HCC
M87.159	Osteonecrosis due to drugs, unspecified femur	HCC ▽

✓6ᵗʰ **M87.16 Osteonecrosis due to drugs, tibia and fibula**

M87.161	Osteonecrosis due to drugs, right tibia	HCC
M87.162	Osteonecrosis due to drugs, left tibia	HCC
M87.163	Osteonecrosis due to drugs, unspecified tibia	HCC ▽
M87.164	Osteonecrosis due to drugs, right fibula	HCC
M87.165	Osteonecrosis due to drugs, left fibula	HCC
M87.166	Osteonecrosis due to drugs, unspecified fibula	HCC ▽

✓6ᵗʰ **M87.17 Osteonecrosis due to drugs, ankle, foot and toes**

M87.171	Osteonecrosis due to drugs, right ankle	HCC
M87.172	Osteonecrosis due to drugs, left ankle	HCC
M87.173	Osteonecrosis due to drugs, unspecified ankle	HCC ▽
M87.174	Osteonecrosis due to drugs, right foot	HCC
M87.175	Osteonecrosis due to drugs, left foot	HCC
M87.176	Osteonecrosis due to drugs, unspecified foot	HCC ▽
M87.177	Osteonecrosis due to drugs, right toe(s)	HCC
M87.178	Osteonecrosis due to drugs, left toe(s)	HCC
M87.179	Osteonecrosis due to drugs, unspecified toe(s)	HCC ▽

✓6ᵗʰ **M87.18 Osteonecrosis due to drugs, other site**

M87.18Ø	Osteonecrosis due to drugs, jaw	HCC
M87.188	Osteonecrosis due to drugs, other site	HCC
M87.19	**Osteonecrosis due to drugs, multiple sites**	HCC

✓5ᵗʰ **M87.2 Osteonecrosis due to previous trauma**

M87.2Ø	**Osteonecrosis due to previous trauma, unspecified bone**	HCC ▽

✓6ᵗʰ **M87.21 Osteonecrosis due to previous trauma, shoulder**

M87.211	Osteonecrosis due to previous trauma, right shoulder	HCC
M87.212	Osteonecrosis due to previous trauma, left shoulder	HCC
M87.219	Osteonecrosis due to previous trauma, unspecified shoulder	HCC ▽

✓6ᵗʰ **M87.22 Osteonecrosis due to previous trauma, humerus**

M87.221	Osteonecrosis due to previous trauma, right humerus	HCC
M87.222	Osteonecrosis due to previous trauma, left humerus	HCC
M87.229	Osteonecrosis due to previous trauma, unspecified humerus	HCC ▽

✓6ᵗʰ **M87.23 Osteonecrosis due to previous trauma of radius, ulna and carpus**

M87.231	Osteonecrosis due to previous trauma of right radius	HCC
M87.232	Osteonecrosis due to previous trauma of left radius	HCC
M87.233	Osteonecrosis due to previous trauma of unspecified radius	HCC ▽
M87.234	Osteonecrosis due to previous trauma of right ulna	HCC
M87.235	Osteonecrosis due to previous trauma of left ulna	HCC
M87.236	Osteonecrosis due to previous trauma of unspecified ulna	HCC ▽
M87.237	Osteonecrosis due to previous trauma of right carpus	HCC
M87.238	Osteonecrosis due to previous trauma of left carpus	HCC
M87.239	Osteonecrosis due to previous trauma of unspecified carpus	HCC ▽

✓6ᵗʰ **M87.24 Osteonecrosis due to previous trauma, hand and fingers**

M87.241	Osteonecrosis due to previous trauma, right hand	HCC
M87.242	Osteonecrosis due to previous trauma, left hand	HCC
M87.243	Osteonecrosis due to previous trauma, unspecified hand	HCC ▽
M87.244	Osteonecrosis due to previous trauma, right finger(s)	HCC
M87.245	Osteonecrosis due to previous trauma, left finger(s)	HCC
M87.246	Osteonecrosis due to previous trauma, unspecified finger(s)	HCC ▽

✓6ᵗʰ **M87.25 Osteonecrosis due to previous trauma, pelvis and femur**

M87.25Ø	Osteonecrosis due to previous trauma, pelvis	HCC
M87.251	Osteonecrosis due to previous trauma, right femur	HCC

☑ Additional Character Req	✓x7ᵗʰ Placeholder Alert	Manifestation	▽ Unspecified	▶◀ Revised Text	● New Code	▲ Revised Code Title

M87.252   Osteonecrosis due to previous trauma, left femur   HCC

M87.256   Osteonecrosis due to previous trauma, unspecified femur   HCC ▽

√6ᵗʰ   **M87.26**   Osteonecrosis due to previous trauma, tibia and fibula

    M87.261   Osteonecrosis due to previous trauma, right tibia   HCC

    M87.262   Osteonecrosis due to previous trauma, left tibia   HCC

    M87.263   Osteonecrosis due to previous trauma, unspecified tibia   HCC ▽

    M87.264   Osteonecrosis due to previous trauma, right fibula   HCC

    M87.265   Osteonecrosis due to previous trauma, left fibula   HCC

    M87.266   Osteonecrosis due to previous trauma, unspecified fibula   HCC ▽

√6ᵗʰ   **M87.27**   Osteonecrosis due to previous trauma, ankle, foot and toes

    M87.271   Osteonecrosis due to previous trauma, right ankle   HCC

    M87.272   Osteonecrosis due to previous trauma, left ankle   HCC

    M87.273   Osteonecrosis due to previous trauma, unspecified ankle   HCC ▽

    M87.274   Osteonecrosis due to previous trauma, right foot   HCC

    M87.275   Osteonecrosis due to previous trauma, left foot   HCC

    M87.276   Osteonecrosis due to previous trauma, unspecified foot   HCC ▽

    M87.277   Osteonecrosis due to previous trauma, right toe(s)   HCC

    M87.278   Osteonecrosis due to previous trauma, left toe(s)   HCC

    M87.279   Osteonecrosis due to previous trauma, unspecified toe(s)   HCC ▽

M87.28   Osteonecrosis due to previous trauma, other site   HCC

M87.29   Osteonecrosis due to previous trauma, multiple sites   HCC

√5ᵗʰ   **M87.3**   Other secondary osteonecrosis

M87.30   Other secondary osteonecrosis, unspecified bone   HCC ▽

√6ᵗʰ   **M87.31**   Other secondary osteonecrosis, shoulder

    M87.311   Other secondary osteonecrosis, right shoulder   HCC

    M87.312   Other secondary osteonecrosis, left shoulder   HCC

    M87.319   Other secondary osteonecrosis, unspecified shoulder   HCC ▽

√6ᵗʰ   **M87.32**   Other secondary osteonecrosis, humerus

    M87.321   Other secondary osteonecrosis, right humerus   HCC

    M87.322   Other secondary osteonecrosis, left humerus   HCC

    M87.329   Other secondary osteonecrosis, unspecified humerus   HCC ▽

√6ᵗʰ   **M87.33**   Other secondary osteonecrosis of radius, ulna and carpus

    M87.331   Other secondary osteonecrosis of right radius   HCC

    M87.332   Other secondary osteonecrosis of left radius   HCC

    M87.333   Other secondary osteonecrosis of unspecified radius   HCC ▽

    M87.334   Other secondary osteonecrosis of right ulna   HCC

    M87.335   Other secondary osteonecrosis of left ulna   HCC

    M87.336   Other secondary osteonecrosis of unspecified ulna   HCC ▽

    M87.337   Other secondary osteonecrosis of right carpus   HCC

    M87.338   Other secondary osteonecrosis of left carpus   HCC

    M87.339   Other secondary osteonecrosis of unspecified carpus   HCC ▽

√6ᵗʰ   **M87.34**   Other secondary osteonecrosis, hand and fingers

    M87.341   Other secondary osteonecrosis, right hand   HCC

    M87.342   Other secondary osteonecrosis, left hand   HCC

    M87.343   Other secondary osteonecrosis, unspecified hand   HCC ▽

    M87.344   Other secondary osteonecrosis, right finger(s)   HCC

    M87.345   Other secondary osteonecrosis, left finger(s)   HCC

    M87.346   Other secondary osteonecrosis, unspecified finger(s)   HCC ▽

√6ᵗʰ   **M87.35**   Other secondary osteonecrosis, pelvis and femur

    M87.350   Other secondary osteonecrosis, pelvis   HCC

    M87.351   Other secondary osteonecrosis, right femur   HCC

    M87.352   Other secondary osteonecrosis, left femur   HCC

    M87.353   Other secondary osteonecrosis, unspecified femur   HCC ▽

√6ᵗʰ   **M87.36**   Other secondary osteonecrosis, tibia and fibula

    M87.361   Other secondary osteonecrosis, right tibia   HCC

    M87.362   Other secondary osteonecrosis, left tibia   HCC

    M87.363   Other secondary osteonecrosis, unspecified tibia   HCC ▽

    M87.364   Other secondary osteonecrosis, right fibula   HCC

    M87.365   Other secondary osteonecrosis, left fibula   HCC

    M87.366   Other secondary osteonecrosis, unspecified fibula   HCC ▽

√6ᵗʰ   **M87.37**   Other secondary osteonecrosis, ankle and foot

    M87.371   Other secondary osteonecrosis, right ankle   HCC

    M87.372   Other secondary osteonecrosis, left ankle   HCC

    M87.373   Other secondary osteonecrosis, unspecified ankle   HCC ▽

    M87.374   Other secondary osteonecrosis, right foot   HCC

    M87.375   Other secondary osteonecrosis, left foot   HCC

    M87.376   Other secondary osteonecrosis, unspecified foot   HCC ▽

    M87.377   Other secondary osteonecrosis, right toe(s)   HCC

    M87.378   Other secondary osteonecrosis, left toe(s)   HCC

    M87.379   Other secondary osteonecrosis, unspecified toe(s)   HCC ▽

M87.38   Other secondary osteonecrosis, other site   HCC

M87.39   Other secondary osteonecrosis, multiple sites   HCC

√5ᵗʰ   **M87.8**   Other osteonecrosis

M87.80   Other osteonecrosis, unspecified bone   HCC ▽

√6ᵗʰ   **M87.81**   Other osteonecrosis, shoulder

    M87.811   Other osteonecrosis, right shoulder   HCC

    M87.812   Other osteonecrosis, left shoulder   HCC

    M87.819   Other osteonecrosis, unspecified shoulder   HCC ▽

√6ᵗʰ   **M87.82**   Other osteonecrosis, humerus

    M87.821   Other osteonecrosis, right humerus   HCC

    M87.822   Other osteonecrosis, left humerus   HCC

    M87.829   Other osteonecrosis, unspecified humerus   HCC ▽

√6ᵗʰ   **M87.83**   Other osteonecrosis of radius, ulna and carpus

    M87.831   Other osteonecrosis of right radius   HCC

    M87.832   Other osteonecrosis of left radius   HCC

    M87.833   Other osteonecrosis of unspecified radius   HCC ▽

    M87.834   Other osteonecrosis of right ulna   HCC

    M87.835   Other osteonecrosis of left ulna   HCC

    M87.836   Other osteonecrosis of unspecified ulna   HCC ▽

    M87.837   Other osteonecrosis of right carpus   HCC

    M87.838   Other osteonecrosis of left carpus   HCC

M87.839 Other osteonecrosis of unspecified carpus   HCC ▽

√6th **M87.84** Other osteonecrosis, hand and fingers

     M87.841 Other osteonecrosis, right hand   HCC

     M87.842 Other osteonecrosis, left hand   HCC

     M87.843 Other osteonecrosis, unspecified hand   HCC ▽

     M87.844 Other osteonecrosis, right finger(s)   HCC

     M87.845 Other osteonecrosis, left finger(s)   HCC

     M87.849 Other osteonecrosis, unspecified finger(s)   HCC ▽

√6th **M87.85** Other osteonecrosis, pelvis and femur

     M87.850 Other osteonecrosis, pelvis   HCC

     M87.851 Other osteonecrosis, right femur   HCC

     M87.852 Other osteonecrosis, left femur   HCC

     M87.859 Other osteonecrosis, unspecified femur   HCC ▽

√6th **M87.86** Other osteonecrosis, tibia and fibula

     M87.861 Other osteonecrosis, right tibia   HCC

     M87.862 Other osteonecrosis, left tibia   HCC

     M87.863 Other osteonecrosis, unspecified tibia   HCC ▽

     M87.864 Other osteonecrosis, right fibula   HCC

     M87.865 Other osteonecrosis, left fibula   HCC

     M87.869 Other osteonecrosis, unspecified fibula   HCC ▽

√6th **M87.87** Other osteonecrosis, ankle, foot and toes

     M87.871 Other osteonecrosis, right ankle   HCC

     M87.872 Other osteonecrosis, left ankle   HCC

     M87.873 Other osteonecrosis, unspecified ankle   HCC ▽

     M87.874 Other osteonecrosis, right foot   HCC

     M87.875 Other osteonecrosis, left foot   HCC

     M87.876 Other osteonecrosis, unspecified foot   HCC ▽

     M87.877 Other osteonecrosis, right toe(s)   HCC

     M87.878 Other osteonecrosis, left toe(s)   HCC

     M87.879 Other osteonecrosis, unspecified toe(s)   HCC ▽

M87.88 Other osteonecrosis, other site   HCC

M87.89 Other osteonecrosis, multiple sites   HCC

M87.9 Osteonecrosis, unspecified   HCC ▽
     Necrosis of bone NOS

√4th **M88** Osteitis deformans [Paget's disease of bone]

     EXCLUDES 1   *osteitis deformans in neoplastic disease (M90.6)*

     DEF: Bone disease characterized by numerous cycles of bone resorption by the body. Resorption is followed by accelerated repair attempts, causing bone deformities and bowing, with associated fractures and pain.

M88.0 Osteitis deformans of skull

M88.1 Osteitis deformans of vertebrae

√5th **M88.8** Osteitis deformans of other bones

     √6th **M88.81** Osteitis deformans of shoulder

         M88.811 Osteitis deformans of right shoulder

         M88.812 Osteitis deformans of left shoulder

         M88.819 Osteitis deformans of unspecified shoulder   ▽

     √6th **M88.82** Osteitis deformans of upper arm

         M88.821 Osteitis deformans of right upper arm

         M88.822 Osteitis deformans of left upper arm

         M88.829 Osteitis deformans of unspecified upper arm   ▽

     √6th **M88.83** Osteitis deformans of forearm

         M88.831 Osteitis deformans of right forearm

         M88.832 Osteitis deformans of left forearm

         M88.839 Osteitis deformans of unspecified forearm   ▽

     √6th **M88.84** Osteitis deformans of hand

         M88.841 Osteitis deformans of right hand

         M88.842 Osteitis deformans of left hand

         M88.849 Osteitis deformans of unspecified hand   ▽

     √6th **M88.85** Osteitis deformans of thigh

         M88.851 Osteitis deformans of right thigh

         M88.852 Osteitis deformans of left thigh

         M88.859 Osteitis deformans of unspecified thigh   ▽

√6th **M88.86** Osteitis deformans of lower leg

     M88.861 Osteitis deformans of right lower leg

     M88.862 Osteitis deformans of left lower leg

     M88.869 Osteitis deformans of unspecified lower leg   ▽

√6th **M88.87** Osteitis deformans of ankle and foot

     M88.871 Osteitis deformans of right ankle and foot

     M88.872 Osteitis deformans of left ankle and foot

     M88.879 Osteitis deformans of unspecified ankle and foot   ▽

M88.88 Osteitis deformans of other bones

     EXCLUDES 2   *osteitis deformans of skull (M88.0)*

                 osteitis deformans of vertebrae (M88.1)

M88.89 Osteitis deformans of multiple sites

M88.9 Osteitis deformans of unspecified bone   ▽

√4th **M89** Other disorders of bone

     √5th **M89.0** Algoneurodystrophy

         Shoulder-hand syndrome

         Sudeck's atrophy

         EXCLUDES 1   *causalgia, lower limb (G57.7-)*

                 causalgia, upper limb (G56.4-)

                 complex regional pain syndrome II, lower limb (G57.7-)

                 complex regional pain syndrome II, upper limb (G56.4-)

                 reflex sympathetic dystrophy (G90.5-)

         M89.00 Algoneurodystrophy, unspecified site   ▽

     √6th **M89.01** Algoneurodystrophy, shoulder

         M89.011 Algoneurodystrophy, right shoulder

         M89.012 Algoneurodystrophy, left shoulder

         M89.019 Algoneurodystrophy, unspecified shoulder   ▽

     √6th **M89.02** Algoneurodystrophy, upper arm

         M89.021 Algoneurodystrophy, right upper arm

         M89.022 Algoneurodystrophy, left upper arm

         M89.029 Algoneurodystrophy, unspecified upper arm   ▽

     √6th **M89.03** Algoneurodystrophy, forearm

         M89.031 Algoneurodystrophy, right forearm

         M89.032 Algoneurodystrophy, left forearm

         M89.039 Algoneurodystrophy, unspecified forearm   ▽

     √6th **M89.04** Algoneurodystrophy, hand

         M89.041 Algoneurodystrophy, right hand

         M89.042 Algoneurodystrophy, left hand

         M89.049 Algoneurodystrophy, unspecified hand   ▽

     √6th **M89.05** Algoneurodystrophy, thigh

         M89.051 Algoneurodystrophy, right thigh

         M89.052 Algoneurodystrophy, left thigh

         M89.059 Algoneurodystrophy, unspecified thigh   ▽

     √6th **M89.06** Algoneurodystrophy, lower leg

         M89.061 Algoneurodystrophy, right lower leg

         M89.062 Algoneurodystrophy, left lower leg

         M89.069 Algoneurodystrophy, unspecified lower leg   ▽

     √6th **M89.07** Algoneurodystrophy, ankle and foot

         M89.071 Algoneurodystrophy, right ankle and foot

         M89.072 Algoneurodystrophy, left ankle and foot

         M89.079 Algoneurodystrophy, unspecified ankle and foot   ▽

         M89.08 Algoneurodystrophy, other site

         M89.09 Algoneurodystrophy, multiple sites

     √5th **M89.1** Physeal arrest

         Arrest of growth plate

         Epiphyseal arrest

         Growth plate arrest

     √6th **M89.12** Physeal arrest, humerus

         M89.121 Complete physeal arrest, right proximal humerus

         M89.122 Complete physeal arrest, left proximal humerus

         M89.123 Partial physeal arrest, right proximal humerus

✓ Additional Character Req   ✓x7th Placeholder Alert   Manifestation   ▽ Unspecified   ►◄ Revised Text   ● New Code   ▲ Revised Code Title

ICD-10-CM 2019   815

M89.124 **Partial** physeal arrest, **left proximal humerus**
M89.125 **Complete** physeal arrest, **right distal humerus**
M89.126 **Complete** physeal arrest, **left distal humerus**
M89.127 **Partial** physeal arrest, **right distal humerus**
M89.128 **Partial** physeal arrest, **left distal humerus**
M89.129 Physeal arrest, humerus, unspecified ▽

√6ᵗʰ **M89.13** Physeal arrest, **forearm**
M89.131 **Complete** physeal arrest, **right distal radius**
M89.132 **Complete** physeal arrest, **left distal radius**
M89.133 **Partial** physeal arrest, **right distal radius**
M89.134 **Partial** physeal arrest, **left distal radius**
M89.138 Other physeal arrest of forearm
M89.139 Physeal arrest, forearm, unspecified ▽

√6ᵗʰ **M89.15** Physeal arrest, **femur**
M89.151 **Complete** physeal arrest, **right proximal femur**
M89.152 **Complete** physeal arrest, **left proximal femur**
M89.153 **Partial** physeal arrest, **right proximal femur**
M89.154 **Partial** physeal arrest, **left proximal femur**
M89.155 **Complete** physeal arrest, **right distal femur**
M89.156 **Complete** physeal arrest, **left distal femur**
M89.157 **Partial** physeal arrest, **right distal femur**
M89.158 **Partial** physeal arrest, **left distal femur**
M89.159 Physeal arrest, femur, unspecified ▽

√6ᵗʰ **M89.16** Physeal arrest, **lower leg**
M89.160 **Complete** physeal arrest, **right proximal tibia**
M89.161 **Complete** physeal arrest, **left proximal tibia**
M89.162 **Partial** physeal arrest, **right proximal tibia**
M89.163 **Partial** physeal arrest, **left proximal tibia**
M89.164 **Complete** physeal arrest, **right distal tibia**
M89.165 **Complete** physeal arrest, **left distal tibia**
M89.166 **Partial** physeal arrest, **right distal tibia**
M89.167 **Partial** physeal arrest, **left distal tibia**
M89.168 Other physeal arrest of lower leg
M89.169 Physeal arrest, lower leg, unspecified ▽

M89.18 Physeal arrest, other site

√5ᵗʰ **M89.2** Other disorders of bone development and growth
M89.20 Other disorders of bone development and growth, unspecified site ▽

√6ᵗʰ **M89.21** Other disorders of bone development and growth, **shoulder**
M89.211 Other disorders of bone development and growth, **right shoulder**
M89.212 Other disorders of bone development and growth, **left shoulder**
M89.219 Other disorders of bone development and growth, unspecified shoulder ▽

√6ᵗʰ **M89.22** Other disorders of bone development and growth, **humerus**
M89.221 Other disorders of bone development and growth, **right humerus**
M89.222 Other disorders of bone development and growth, **left humerus**
M89.229 Other disorders of bone development and growth, unspecified humerus ▽

√6ᵗʰ **M89.23** Other disorders of bone development and growth, **ulna and radius**
M89.231 Other disorders of bone development and growth, **right ulna**
M89.232 Other disorders of bone development and growth, **left ulna**
M89.233 Other disorders of bone development and growth, **right radius**
M89.234 Other disorders of bone development and growth, **left radius**

M89.239 Other disorders of bone development and growth, unspecified ulna and radius ▽

√6ᵗʰ **M89.24** Other disorders of bone development and growth, **hand**
M89.241 Other disorders of bone development and growth, **right hand**
M89.242 Other disorders of bone development and growth, **left hand**
M89.249 Other disorders of bone development and growth, unspecified hand ▽

√6ᵗʰ **M89.25** Other disorders of bone development and growth, **femur**
M89.251 Other disorders of bone development and growth, **right femur**
M89.252 Other disorders of bone development and growth, **left femur**
M89.259 Other disorders of bone development and growth, unspecified femur ▽

√6ᵗʰ **M89.26** Other disorders of bone development and growth, **tibia and fibula**
M89.261 Other disorders of bone development and growth, **right tibia**
M89.262 Other disorders of bone development and growth, **left tibia**
M89.263 Other disorders of bone development and growth, **right fibula**
M89.264 Other disorders of bone development and growth, **left fibula**
M89.269 Other disorders of bone development and growth, unspecified lower leg ▽

√6ᵗʰ **M89.27** Other disorders of bone development and growth, **ankle and foot**
M89.271 Other disorders of bone development and growth, **right ankle and foot**
M89.272 Other disorders of bone development and growth, **left ankle and foot**
M89.279 Other disorders of bone development and growth, unspecified ankle and foot ▽

M89.28 Other disorders of bone development and growth, other site
M89.29 Other disorders of bone development and growth, **multiple sites**

√5ᵗʰ **M89.3** Hypertrophy of bone
M89.30 Hypertrophy of bone, unspecified site ▽

√6ᵗʰ **M89.31** Hypertrophy of bone, **shoulder**
M89.311 Hypertrophy of bone, **right shoulder**
M89.312 Hypertrophy of bone, **left shoulder**
M89.319 Hypertrophy of bone, unspecified shoulder ▽

√6ᵗʰ **M89.32** Hypertrophy of bone, **humerus**
M89.321 Hypertrophy of bone, **right humerus**
M89.322 Hypertrophy of bone, **left humerus**
M89.329 Hypertrophy of bone, unspecified humerus ▽

√6ᵗʰ **M89.33** Hypertrophy of bone, **ulna and radius**
M89.331 Hypertrophy of bone, **right ulna**
M89.332 Hypertrophy of bone, **left ulna**
M89.333 Hypertrophy of bone, **right radius**
M89.334 Hypertrophy of bone, **left radius**
M89.339 Hypertrophy of bone, unspecified ulna and radius ▽

√6ᵗʰ **M89.34** Hypertrophy of bone, **hand**
M89.341 Hypertrophy of bone, **right hand**
M89.342 Hypertrophy of bone, **left hand**
M89.349 Hypertrophy of bone, unspecified hand ▽

√6ᵗʰ **M89.35** Hypertrophy of bone, **femur**
M89.351 Hypertrophy of bone, **right femur**
M89.352 Hypertrophy of bone, **left femur**
M89.359 Hypertrophy of bone, unspecified femur ▽

√6ᵗʰ **M89.36** Hypertrophy of bone, **tibia and fibula**
M89.361 Hypertrophy of bone, **right tibia**
M89.362 Hypertrophy of bone, **left tibia**
M89.363 Hypertrophy of bone, **right fibula**
M89.364 Hypertrophy of bone, **left fibula**

M89.369   Hypertrophy of bone, unspecified tibia and fibula   ▽

✓6ᵗʰ M89.37   **Hypertrophy of bone, ankle and foot**

     M89.371   Hypertrophy of bone, right ankle and foot

     M89.372   Hypertrophy of bone, left ankle and foot

     M89.379   Hypertrophy of bone, unspecified ankle and foot

M89.38   **Hypertrophy of bone, other site**

M89.39   **Hypertrophy of bone, multiple sites**

✓5ᵗʰ **M89.4   Other hypertrophic osteoarthropathy**

     Marie-Bamberger disease

     Pachydermoperiostosis

M89.40   **Other hypertrophic osteoarthropathy, unspecified site**   ▽

✓6ᵗʰ M89.41   **Other hypertrophic osteoarthropathy, shoulder**

     M89.411   Other hypertrophic osteoarthropathy, right shoulder

     M89.412   Other hypertrophic osteoarthropathy, left shoulder

     M89.419   Other hypertrophic osteoarthropathy, unspecified shoulder   ▽

✓6ᵗʰ M89.42   **Other hypertrophic osteoarthropathy, upper arm**

     M89.421   Other hypertrophic osteoarthropathy, right upper arm

     M89.422   Other hypertrophic osteoarthropathy, left upper arm

     M89.429   Other hypertrophic osteoarthropathy, unspecified upper arm   ▽

✓6ᵗʰ M89.43   **Other hypertrophic osteoarthropathy, forearm**

     M89.431   Other hypertrophic osteoarthropathy, right forearm

     M89.432   Other hypertrophic osteoarthropathy, left forearm

     M89.439   Other hypertrophic osteoarthropathy, unspecified forearm   ▽

✓6ᵗʰ M89.44   **Other hypertrophic osteoarthropathy, hand**

     M89.441   Other hypertrophic osteoarthropathy, right hand

     M89.442   Other hypertrophic osteoarthropathy, left hand

     M89.449   Other hypertrophic osteoarthropathy, unspecified hand   ▽

✓6ᵗʰ M89.45   **Other hypertrophic osteoarthropathy, thigh**

     M89.451   Other hypertrophic osteoarthropathy, right thigh

     M89.452   Other hypertrophic osteoarthropathy, left thigh

     M89.459   Other hypertrophic osteoarthropathy, unspecified thigh   ▽

✓6ᵗʰ M89.46   **Other hypertrophic osteoarthropathy, lower leg**

     M89.461   Other hypertrophic osteoarthropathy, right lower leg

     M89.462   Other hypertrophic osteoarthropathy, left lower leg

     M89.469   Other hypertrophic osteoarthropathy, unspecified lower leg   ▽

✓6ᵗʰ M89.47   **Other hypertrophic osteoarthropathy, ankle and foot**

     M89.471   Other hypertrophic osteoarthropathy, right ankle and foot

     M89.472   Other hypertrophic osteoarthropathy, left ankle and foot

     M89.479   Other hypertrophic osteoarthropathy, unspecified ankle and foot   ▽

M89.48   **Other hypertrophic osteoarthropathy, other site**

M89.49   **Other hypertrophic osteoarthropathy, multiple sites**

✓5ᵗʰ **M89.5   Osteolysis**

     Use additional code to identify major osseous defect, if applicable (M89.7-)

     EXCLUDES 2   *periprosthetic osteolysis of internal prosthetic joint (T84.05-)*

M89.50   **Osteolysis, unspecified site**   ▽

✓6ᵗʰ M89.51   **Osteolysis, shoulder**

     M89.511   Osteolysis, right shoulder

     M89.512   Osteolysis, left shoulder

     M89.519   Osteolysis, unspecified shoulder   ▽

✓6ᵗʰ M89.52   **Osteolysis, upper arm**

     M89.521   Osteolysis, right upper arm

     M89.522   Osteolysis, left upper arm

     M89.529   Osteolysis, unspecified upper arm   ▽

✓6ᵗʰ M89.53   **Osteolysis, forearm**

     M89.531   Osteolysis, right forearm

     M89.532   Osteolysis, left forearm

     M89.539   Osteolysis, unspecified forearm   ▽

✓6ᵗʰ M89.54   **Osteolysis, hand**

     M89.541   Osteolysis, right hand

     M89.542   Osteolysis, left hand

     M89.549   Osteolysis, unspecified hand   ▽

✓6ᵗʰ M89.55   **Osteolysis, thigh**

     M89.551   Osteolysis, right thigh

     M89.552   Osteolysis, left thigh

     M89.559   Osteolysis, unspecified thigh   ▽

✓6ᵗʰ M89.56   **Osteolysis, lower leg**

     M89.561   Osteolysis, right lower leg

     M89.562   Osteolysis, left lower leg

     M89.569   Osteolysis, unspecified lower leg   ▽

✓6ᵗʰ M89.57   **Osteolysis, ankle and foot**

     M89.571   Osteolysis, right ankle and foot

     M89.572   Osteolysis, left ankle and foot

     M89.579   Osteolysis, unspecified ankle and foot   ▽

M89.58   **Osteolysis, other site**

M89.59   **Osteolysis, multiple sites**

✓5ᵗʰ **M89.6   Osteopathy after poliomyelitis**

     Use additional code (B91) to identify previous poliomyelitis

     EXCLUDES 1   *postpolio syndrome (G14)*

M89.60   **Osteopathy after poliomyelitis, unspecified site**   HCC ▽

✓6ᵗʰ M89.61   **Osteopathy after poliomyelitis, shoulder**

     M89.611   Osteopathy after poliomyelitis, right shoulder   HCC

     M89.612   Osteopathy after poliomyelitis, left shoulder   HCC

     M89.619   Osteopathy after poliomyelitis, unspecified shoulder   HCC ▽

✓6ᵗʰ M89.62   **Osteopathy after poliomyelitis, upper arm**

     M89.621   Osteopathy after poliomyelitis, right upper arm   HCC

     M89.622   Osteopathy after poliomyelitis, left upper arm   HCC

     M89.629   Osteopathy after poliomyelitis, unspecified upper arm   HCC ▽

✓6ᵗʰ M89.63   **Osteopathy after poliomyelitis, forearm**

     M89.631   Osteopathy after poliomyelitis, right forearm   HCC

     M89.632   Osteopathy after poliomyelitis, left forearm   HCC

     M89.639   Osteopathy after poliomyelitis, unspecified forearm   HCC ▽

✓6ᵗʰ M89.64   **Osteopathy after poliomyelitis, hand**

     M89.641   Osteopathy after poliomyelitis, right hand   HCC

     M89.642   Osteopathy after poliomyelitis, left hand   HCC

     M89.649   Osteopathy after poliomyelitis, unspecified hand   HCC ▽

✓6ᵗʰ M89.65   **Osteopathy after poliomyelitis, thigh**

     M89.651   Osteopathy after poliomyelitis, right thigh   HCC

     M89.652   Osteopathy after poliomyelitis, left thigh   HCC

     M89.659   Osteopathy after poliomyelitis, unspecified thigh   HCC ▽

✓6ᵗʰ M89.66   **Osteopathy after poliomyelitis, lower leg**

     M89.661   Osteopathy after poliomyelitis, right lower leg   HCC

     M89.662   Osteopathy after poliomyelitis, left lower leg   HCC

     M89.669   Osteopathy after poliomyelitis, unspecified lower leg   HCC ▽

✓ Additional Character Req   ✓x7ᵗʰ Placeholder Alert   Manifestation   ▽ Unspecified   ▶◀ Revised Text   ● New Code   ▲ Revised Code Title

ICD-10-CM 2019   817

√6ᵗʰ **M89.67 Osteopathy after poliomyelitis, ankle and foot**

M89.671 Osteopathy after poliomyelitis, HCC
right ankle and foot

M89.672 Osteopathy after poliomyelitis, HCC
left ankle and foot

M89.679 Osteopathy after poliomyelitis, HCC ▽
unspecified ankle and foot

M89.68 Osteopathy after poliomyelitis, other site HCC

M89.69 Osteopathy after poliomyelitis, multiple HCC
sites

√5ᵗʰ **M89.7 Major osseous defect**

Code first underlying disease, if known, such as:
aseptic necrosis of bone (M87.-)
malignant neoplasm of bone (C40.-)
osteolysis (M89.5)
osteomyelitis (M86.-)
osteonecrosis (M87.-)
osteoporosis (M80.-, M81.-)
periprosthetic osteolysis (T84.05-)

M89.70 Major osseous defect, unspecified site ▽

√6ᵗʰ **M89.71 Major osseous defect, shoulder region**

Major osseous defect clavicle or scapula

M89.711 Major osseous defect, right shoulder
region

M89.712 Major osseous defect, left shoulder region

M89.719 Major osseous defect, unspecified ▽
shoulder region

√6ᵗʰ **M89.72 Major osseous defect, humerus**

M89.721 Major osseous defect, right humerus

M89.722 Major osseous defect, left humerus

M89.729 Major osseous defect, unspecified ▽
humerus

√6ᵗʰ **M89.73 Major osseous defect, forearm**

Major osseous defect of radius and ulna

M89.731 Major osseous defect, right forearm

M89.732 Major osseous defect, left forearm

M89.739 Major osseous defect, unspecified ▽
forearm

√6ᵗʰ **M89.74 Major osseous defect, hand**

Major osseous defect of carpus, fingers, metacarpus

M89.741 Major osseous defect, right hand

M89.742 Major osseous defect, left hand

M89.749 Major osseous defect, unspecified ▽
hand

√5ᵗʰ **M89.75 Major osseous defect, pelvic region and thigh**

Major osseous defect of femur and pelvis

M89.751 Major osseous defect, right pelvic region
and thigh

M89.752 Major osseous defect, left pelvic region
and thigh

M89.759 Major osseous defect, unspecified ▽
pelvic region and thigh

√6ᵗʰ **M89.76 Major osseous defect, lower leg**

Major osseous defect of fibula and tibia

M89.761 Major osseous defect, right lower leg

M89.762 Major osseous defect, left lower leg

M89.769 Major osseous defect, unspecified ▽
lower leg

√6ᵗʰ **M89.77 Major osseous defect, ankle and foot**

Major osseous defect of metatarsus, tarsus, toes

M89.771 Major osseous defect, right ankle and
foot

M89.772 Major osseous defect, left ankle and foot

M89.779 Major osseous defect, unspecified ▽
ankle and foot

M89.78 Major osseous defect, other site

M89.79 Major osseous defect, multiple sites

√5ᵗʰ **M89.8 Other specified disorders of bone**

Infantile cortical hyperostoses
Post-traumatic subperiosteal ossification

√6ᵗʰ **M89.8X Other specified disorders of bone**

M89.8X0 Other specified disorders of bone,
multiple sites

M89.8X1 Other specified disorders of bone,
shoulder

M89.8X2 Other specified disorders of bone, upper
arm

M89.8X3 Other specified disorders of bone,
forearm

M89.8X4 Other specified disorders of bone, hand

M89.8X5 Other specified disorders of bone, thigh

M89.8X6 Other specified disorders of bone, lower
leg

M89.8X7 Other specified disorders of bone, ankle
and foot

M89.8X8 Other specified disorders of bone, other
site

M89.8X9 Other specified disorders of bone, ▽
unspecified site

M89.9 Disorder of bone, unspecified ▽

√4ᵗʰ **M90 Osteopathies in diseases classified elsewhere**

EXCLUDES 1 osteochondritis, osteomyelitis, and osteopathy (in):
cryptococcosis (B45.3)
diabetes mellitus (E08-E13 with .69-)
gonococcal (A54.43)
neurogenic syphilis (A52.11)
renal osteodystrophy (N25.0)
salmonellosis (A02.24)
secondary syphilis (A51.46)
syphilis (late) (A52.77)

√5ᵗʰ **M90.5 Osteonecrosis in diseases classified elsewhere**

Code first underlying disease, such as:
caisson disease (T70.3)
hemoglobinopathy (D50-D64)

M90.50 Osteonecrosis in diseases classified HCC ▽
elsewhere, unspecified site

√6ᵗʰ **M90.51 Osteonecrosis in diseases classified elsewhere,**
shoulder

M90.511 Osteonecrosis in diseases classified HCC
elsewhere, right shoulder

M90.512 Osteonecrosis in diseases classified HCC
elsewhere, left shoulder

M90.519 Osteonecrosis in diseases classified HCC ▽
elsewhere, unspecified shoulder

√6ᵗʰ **M90.52 Osteonecrosis in diseases classified elsewhere,**
upper arm

M90.521 Osteonecrosis in diseases classified HCC
elsewhere, right upper arm

M90.522 Osteonecrosis in diseases classified HCC
elsewhere, left upper arm

M90.529 Osteonecrosis in diseases classified HCC ▽
elsewhere, unspecified upper arm

√6ᵗʰ **M90.53 Osteonecrosis in diseases classified elsewhere,**
forearm

M90.531 Osteonecrosis in diseases classified HCC
elsewhere, right forearm

M90.532 Osteonecrosis in diseases classified HCC
elsewhere, left forearm

M90.539 Osteonecrosis in diseases classified HCC ▽
elsewhere, unspecified forearm

√6ᵗʰ **M90.54 Osteonecrosis in diseases classified elsewhere, hand**

M90.541 Osteonecrosis in diseases classified HCC
elsewhere, right hand

M90.542 Osteonecrosis in diseases classified HCC
elsewhere, left hand

M90.549 Osteonecrosis in diseases classified HCC ▽
elsewhere, unspecified hand

√6ᵗʰ **M90.55 Osteonecrosis in diseases classified elsewhere,**
thigh

M90.551 Osteonecrosis in diseases classified HCC
elsewhere, right thigh

M90.552 Osteonecrosis in diseases classified HCC
elsewhere, left thigh

M90.559 Osteonecrosis in diseases classified HCC ▽
elsewhere, unspecified thigh

√6ᵗʰ **M90.56 Osteonecrosis in diseases classified elsewhere,**
lower leg

M90.561 Osteonecrosis in diseases classified HCC
elsewhere, right lower leg

M90.562 Osteonecrosis in diseases classified HCC
elsewhere, left lower leg

M90.569 Osteonecrosis in diseases classified HCC ▽
elsewhere, unspecified lower leg

√6ᵗʰ **M90.57 Osteonecrosis in diseases classified elsewhere,**
ankle and foot

M90.571 Osteonecrosis in diseases classified HCC
elsewhere, right ankle and foot

M90.572   Osteonecrosis in diseases classified elsewhere, *left ankle and foot*   HCC

M90.579   Osteonecrosis in diseases classified elsewhere, *unspecified ankle and foot*   HCC ▽

M90.58   Osteonecrosis in diseases classified elsewhere, other site   HCC

M90.59   Osteonecrosis in diseases classified elsewhere, *multiple sites*   HCC

√5th **M90.6**   **Osteitis deformans in neoplastic diseases**

Osteitis deformans in malignant neoplasm of bone

Code first the neoplasm (C40.-, C41.-)

EXCLUDES 1   osteitis deformans [Paget's disease of bone] (M88.-)

M90.60   Osteitis deformans in neoplastic diseases, unspecified site ▽

√6th M90.61   Osteitis deformans in neoplastic diseases, shoulder

M90.611   Osteitis deformans in neoplastic diseases, *right shoulder*

M90.612   Osteitis deformans in neoplastic diseases, *left shoulder*

M90.619   Osteitis deformans in neoplastic diseases, unspecified shoulder ▽

√6th M90.62   Osteitis deformans in neoplastic diseases, upper arm

M90.621   Osteitis deformans in neoplastic diseases, *right upper arm*

M90.622   Osteitis deformans in neoplastic diseases, *left upper arm*

M90.629   Osteitis deformans in neoplastic diseases, unspecified upper arm ▽

√6th M90.63   Osteitis deformans in neoplastic diseases, forearm

M90.631   Osteitis deformans in neoplastic diseases, *right forearm*

M90.632   Osteitis deformans in neoplastic diseases, *left forearm*

M90.639   Osteitis deformans in neoplastic diseases, unspecified forearm ▽

√6th M90.64   Osteitis deformans in neoplastic diseases, hand

M90.641   Osteitis deformans in neoplastic diseases, *right hand*

M90.642   Osteitis deformans in neoplastic diseases, *left hand*

M90.649   Osteitis deformans in neoplastic diseases, unspecified hand ▽

√6th M90.65   Osteitis deformans in neoplastic diseases, thigh

M90.651   Osteitis deformans in neoplastic diseases, *right thigh*

M90.652   Osteitis deformans in neoplastic diseases, *left thigh*

M90.659   Osteitis deformans in neoplastic diseases, unspecified thigh ▽

√6th M90.66   Osteitis deformans in neoplastic diseases, lower leg

M90.661   Osteitis deformans in neoplastic diseases, *right lower leg*

M90.662   Osteitis deformans in neoplastic diseases, *left lower leg*

M90.669   Osteitis deformans in neoplastic diseases, unspecified lower leg ▽

√6th M90.67   Osteitis deformans in neoplastic diseases, ankle and foot

M90.671   Osteitis deformans in neoplastic diseases, *right ankle and foot*

M90.672   Osteitis deformans in neoplastic diseases, *left ankle and foot*

M90.679   Osteitis deformans in neoplastic diseases, unspecified ankle and foot ▽

M90.68   Osteitis deformans in neoplastic diseases, other site

M90.69   Osteitis deformans in neoplastic diseases, *multiple sites*

√5th **M90.8**   **Osteopathy in diseases classified elsewhere**

Code first underlying disease, such as:

rickets (E55.0)

vitamin-D-resistant rickets (E83.3)

M90.80   Osteopathy in diseases classified elsewhere, unspecified site ▽

√6th M90.81   Osteopathy in diseases classified elsewhere, shoulder

M90.811   Osteopathy in diseases classified elsewhere, *right shoulder*

M90.812   Osteopathy in diseases classified elsewhere, *left shoulder*

M90.819   Osteopathy in diseases classified elsewhere, *unspecified shoulder* ▽

√6th M90.82   Osteopathy in diseases classified elsewhere, upper arm

M90.821   Osteopathy in diseases classified elsewhere, *right upper arm*

M90.822   Osteopathy in diseases classified elsewhere, *left upper arm*

M90.829   Osteopathy in diseases classified elsewhere, *unspecified upper arm* ▽

√6th M90.83   Osteopathy in diseases classified elsewhere, forearm

M90.831   Osteopathy in diseases classified elsewhere, *right forearm*

M90.832   Osteopathy in diseases classified elsewhere, *left forearm*

M90.839   Osteopathy in diseases classified elsewhere, *unspecified forearm* ▽

√6th M90.84   Osteopathy in diseases classified elsewhere, hand

M90.841   Osteopathy in diseases classified elsewhere, *right hand*

M90.842   Osteopathy in diseases classified elsewhere, *left hand*

M90.849   Osteopathy in diseases classified elsewhere, *unspecified hand* ▽

√6th M90.85   Osteopathy in diseases classified elsewhere, thigh

M90.851   Osteopathy in diseases classified elsewhere, *right thigh*

M90.852   Osteopathy in diseases classified elsewhere, *left thigh*

M90.859   Osteopathy in diseases classified elsewhere, *unspecified thigh* ▽

√6th M90.86   Osteopathy in diseases classified elsewhere, lower leg

M90.861   Osteopathy in diseases classified elsewhere, *right lower leg*

M90.862   Osteopathy in diseases classified elsewhere, *left lower leg*

M90.869   Osteopathy in diseases classified elsewhere, *unspecified lower leg* ▽

√6th M90.87   Osteopathy in diseases classified elsewhere, ankle and foot

M90.871   Osteopathy in diseases classified elsewhere, *right ankle and foot*

M90.872   Osteopathy in diseases classified elsewhere, *left ankle and foot*

M90.879   Osteopathy in diseases classified elsewhere, *unspecified ankle and foot* ▽

M90.88   Osteopathy in diseases classified elsewhere, other site

M90.89   Osteopathy in diseases classified elsewhere, *multiple sites*

Chondropathies (M91-M94)

EXCLUDES 1   postprocedural chondropathies (M96.-)

√4th **M91**   **Juvenile osteochondrosis of hip and pelvis**

EXCLUDES 1   slipped upper femoral epiphysis (nontraumatic) (M93.0)

M91.0   **Juvenile osteochondrosis of pelvis**

Osteochondrosis (juvenile) of acetabulum

Osteochondrosis (juvenile) of iliac crest [Buchanan]

Osteochondrosis (juvenile) of ischiopubic synchondrosis [van Neck]

Osteochondrosis (juvenile) of symphysis pubis [Pierson]

√5th **M91.1**   **Juvenile osteochondrosis of head of femur [Legg-Calvé-Perthes]**

M91.10   Juvenile osteochondrosis of head of femur [Legg-Calvé-Perthes], unspecified leg ▽

M91.11   Juvenile osteochondrosis of head of femur [Legg-Calvé-Perthes], right leg

M91.12   Juvenile osteochondrosis of head of femur [Legg-Calvé-Perthes], left leg

√5th **M91.2**   **Coxa plana**

Hip deformity due to previous juvenile osteochondrosis

M91.20   Coxa plana, unspecified hip ▽

M91.21   Coxa plana, right hip

M91.22   Coxa plana, left hip

☑ Additional Character Req   √x7th Placeholder Alert   Manifestation   ▽ Unspecified   ►◄ Revised Text   ● New Code   ▲ Revised Code Title

ICD-10-CM 2019   819

✓5ᵗʰ **M91.3** Pseudocoxalgia

     M91.30 Pseudocoxalgia, unspecified hip ▽

     M91.31 Pseudocoxalgia, right hip

     M91.32 Pseudocoxalgia, left hip

✓5ᵗʰ **M91.4** Coxa magna

     M91.40 Coxa magna, unspecified hip ▽

     M91.41 Coxa magna, right hip

     M91.42 Coxa magna, left hip

✓5ᵗʰ **M91.8** Other juvenile osteochondrosis of hip and pelvis

     Juvenile osteochondrosis after reduction of congenital dislocation of hip

     M91.80 Other juvenile osteochondrosis of hip and pelvis, unspecified leg ▽

     M91.81 Other juvenile osteochondrosis of hip and pelvis, right leg

     M91.82 Other juvenile osteochondrosis of hip and pelvis, left leg

✓5ᵗʰ **M91.9** Juvenile osteochondrosis of hip and pelvis, unspecified

     M91.90 Juvenile osteochondrosis of hip and pelvis, unspecified, unspecified leg ▽

     M91.91 Juvenile osteochondrosis of hip and pelvis, unspecified, right leg ▽

     M91.92 Juvenile osteochondrosis of hip and pelvis, unspecified, left leg ▽

✓4ᵗʰ **M92** Other juvenile osteochondrosis

  ✓5ᵗʰ **M92.0** Juvenile osteochondrosis of humerus

     Osteochondrosis (juvenile) of capitulum of humerus [Panner]

     Osteochondrosis (juvenile) of head of humerus [Haas]

     M92.00 Juvenile osteochondrosis of humerus, unspecified arm ▽

     M92.01 Juvenile osteochondrosis of humerus, right arm

     M92.02 Juvenile osteochondrosis of humerus, left arm

  ✓5ᵗʰ **M92.1** Juvenile osteochondrosis of radius and ulna

     Osteochondrosis (juvenile) of lower ulna [Burns]

     Osteochondrosis (juvenile) of radial head [Brailsford]

     M92.10 Juvenile osteochondrosis of radius and ulna, unspecified arm ▽

     M92.11 Juvenile osteochondrosis of radius and ulna, right arm

     M92.12 Juvenile osteochondrosis of radius and ulna, left arm

  ✓5ᵗʰ **M92.2** Juvenile osteochondrosis, hand

    ✓6ᵗʰ **M92.20** Unspecified juvenile osteochondrosis, hand

       M92.201 Unspecified juvenile osteochondrosis, right hand ▽

       M92.202 Unspecified juvenile osteochondrosis, left hand ▽

       M92.209 Unspecified juvenile osteochondrosis, unspecified hand ▽

    ✓6ᵗʰ **M92.21** Osteochondrosis (juvenile) of carpal lunate [Kienböck]

       M92.211 Osteochondrosis (juvenile) of carpal lunate [Kienböck], right hand

       M92.212 Osteochondrosis (juvenile) of carpal lunate [Kienböck], left hand

       M92.219 Osteochondrosis (juvenile) of carpal lunate [Kienböck], unspecified hand ▽

    ✓6ᵗʰ **M92.22** Osteochondrosis (juvenile) of metacarpal heads [Mauclaire]

       M92.221 Osteochondrosis (juvenile) of metacarpal heads [Mauclaire], right hand

       M92.222 Osteochondrosis (juvenile) of metacarpal heads [Mauclaire], left hand

       M92.229 Osteochondrosis (juvenile) of metacarpal heads [Mauclaire], unspecified hand ▽

    ✓6ᵗʰ **M92.29** Other juvenile osteochondrosis, hand

       M92.291 Other juvenile osteochondrosis, right hand

       M92.292 Other juvenile osteochondrosis, left hand

       M92.299 Other juvenile osteochondrosis, unspecified hand ▽

  ✓5ᵗʰ **M92.3** Other juvenile osteochondrosis, upper limb

     M92.30 Other juvenile osteochondrosis, unspecified upper limb ▽

     M92.31 Other juvenile osteochondrosis, right upper limb

M92.32 Other juvenile osteochondrosis, left upper limb

✓5ᵗʰ **M92.4** Juvenile osteochondrosis of patella

     Osteochondrosis (juvenile) of primary patellar center [Köhler]

     Osteochondrosis (juvenile) of secondary patellar centre [Sinding Larsen]

     M92.40 Juvenile osteochondrosis of patella, unspecified knee ▽

     M92.41 Juvenile osteochondrosis of patella, right knee

     M92.42 Juvenile osteochondrosis of patella, left knee

✓5ᵗʰ **M92.5** Juvenile osteochondrosis of tibia and fibula

     Osteochondrosis (juvenile) of proximal tibia [Blount]

     Osteochondrosis (juvenile) of tibial tubercle [Osgood-Schlatter]

     Tibia vara

     M92.50 Juvenile osteochondrosis of tibia and fibula, unspecified leg ▽

     M92.51 Juvenile osteochondrosis of tibia and fibula, right leg

     M92.52 Juvenile osteochondrosis of tibia and fibula, left leg

✓5ᵗʰ **M92.6** Juvenile osteochondrosis of tarsus

     Osteochondrosis (juvenile) of calcaneum [Sever]

     Osteochondrosis (juvenile) of os tibiale externum [Haglund]

     Osteochondrosis (juvenile) of talus [Diaz]

     Osteochondrosis (juvenile) of tarsal navicular [Köhler]

     M92.60 Juvenile osteochondrosis of tarsus, unspecified ankle ▽

     M92.61 Juvenile osteochondrosis of tarsus, right ankle

     M92.62 Juvenile osteochondrosis of tarsus, left ankle

✓5ᵗʰ **M92.7** Juvenile osteochondrosis of metatarsus

     Osteochondrosis (juvenile) of fifth metatarsus [Iselin]

     Osteochondrosis (juvenile) of second metatarsus [Freiberg]

     M92.70 Juvenile osteochondrosis of metatarsus, unspecified foot ▽

     M92.71 Juvenile osteochondrosis of metatarsus, right foot

     M92.72 Juvenile osteochondrosis of metatarsus, left foot

M92.8 Other specified juvenile osteochondrosis

     Calcaneal apophysitis

M92.9 Juvenile osteochondrosis, unspecified ▽

     Juvenile apophysitis NOS

     Juvenile epiphysitis NOS

     Juvenile osteochondritis NOS

     Juvenile osteochondrosis NOS

✓4ᵗʰ **M93** Other osteochondropathies

     EXCLUDES 2   osteochondrosis of spine (M42.-)

  ✓5ᵗʰ **M93.0** Slipped upper femoral epiphysis (nontraumatic)

     Use additional code for associated chondrolysis (M94.3)

    ✓6ᵗʰ **M93.00** Unspecified slipped upper femoral epiphysis (nontraumatic)

       M93.001 Unspecified slipped upper femoral epiphysis (nontraumatic), right hip ▽

       M93.002 Unspecified slipped upper femoral epiphysis (nontraumatic), left hip ▽

       M93.003 Unspecified slipped upper femoral epiphysis (nontraumatic), unspecified hip ▽

    ✓6ᵗʰ **M93.01** Acute slipped upper femoral epiphysis (nontraumatic)

       M93.011 Acute slipped upper femoral epiphysis (nontraumatic), right hip

       M93.012 Acute slipped upper femoral epiphysis (nontraumatic), left hip

       M93.013 Acute slipped upper femoral epiphysis (nontraumatic), unspecified hip ▽

    ✓6ᵗʰ **M93.02** Chronic slipped upper femoral epiphysis (nontraumatic)

       M93.021 Chronic slipped upper femoral epiphysis (nontraumatic), right hip

       M93.022 Chronic slipped upper femoral epiphysis (nontraumatic), left hip

       M93.023 Chronic slipped upper femoral epiphysis (nontraumatic), unspecified hip ▽

    ✓6ᵗʰ **M93.03** Acute on chronic slipped upper femoral epiphysis (nontraumatic)

       M93.031 Acute on chronic slipped upper femoral epiphysis (nontraumatic), right hip

      M93.032 Acute on chronic slipped upper femoral epiphysis (nontraumatic), left hip

      M93.033 Acute on chronic slipped upper femoral epiphysis (nontraumatic), unspecified hip

M93.1 Kienböck's disease of adults   Ⓐ
    Adult osteochondrosis of carpal lunates

√5ᵗʰ **M93.2** Osteochondritis dissecans

    DEF: Avascular necrosis caused by lack of blood flow to the bone and cartilage of a joint causing the bone to die. This can result in splinters or pieces of cartilage breaking off in the joint.

    M93.20 Osteochondritis dissecans of unspecified site   ▽

    √6ᵗʰ **M93.21** Osteochondritis dissecans of shoulder

      M93.211 Osteochondritis dissecans, right shoulder
      M93.212 Osteochondritis dissecans, left shoulder
      M93.219 Osteochondritis dissecans, unspecified shoulder   ▽

    √6ᵗʰ **M93.22** Osteochondritis dissecans of elbow

      M93.221 Osteochondritis dissecans, right elbow
      M93.222 Osteochondritis dissecans, left elbow
      M93.229 Osteochondritis dissecans, unspecified elbow   ▽

    √6ᵗʰ **M93.23** Osteochondritis dissecans of wrist

      M93.231 Osteochondritis dissecans, right wrist
      M93.232 Osteochondritis dissecans, left wrist
      M93.239 Osteochondritis dissecans, unspecified wrist   ▽

    √6ᵗʰ **M93.24** Osteochondritis dissecans of joints of hand

      M93.241 Osteochondritis dissecans, joints of right hand
      M93.242 Osteochondritis dissecans, joints of left hand
      M93.249 Osteochondritis dissecans, joints of unspecified hand   ▽

    √6ᵗʰ **M93.25** Osteochondritis dissecans of hip

      M93.251 Osteochondritis dissecans, right hip
      M93.252 Osteochondritis dissecans, left hip
      M93.259 Osteochondritis dissecans, unspecified hip   ▽

    √6ᵗʰ **M93.26** Osteochondritis dissecans knee

      M93.261 Osteochondritis dissecans, right knee
      M93.262 Osteochondritis dissecans, left knee
      M93.269 Osteochondritis dissecans, unspecified knee   ▽

    √6ᵗʰ **M93.27** Osteochondritis dissecans of ankle and joints of foot

      M93.271 Osteochondritis dissecans, right ankle and joints of right foot
      M93.272 Osteochondritis dissecans, left ankle and joints of left foot
      M93.279 Osteochondritis dissecans, unspecified ankle and joints of foot   ▽

    M93.28 Osteochondritis dissecans other site

    M93.29 Osteochondritis dissecans multiple sites

√5ᵗʰ **M93.8** Other specified osteochondropathies

    M93.80 Other specified osteochondropathies of unspecified site   ▽

    √6ᵗʰ **M93.81** Other specified osteochondropathies of shoulder

      M93.811 Other specified osteochondropathies, right shoulder
      M93.812 Other specified osteochondropathies, left shoulder
      M93.819 Other specified osteochondropathies, unspecified shoulder   ▽

    √6ᵗʰ **M93.82** Other specified osteochondropathies of upper arm

      M93.821 Other specified osteochondropathies, right upper arm
      M93.822 Other specified osteochondropathies, left upper arm
      M93.829 Other specified osteochondropathies, unspecified upper arm   ▽

    √6ᵗʰ **M93.83** Other specified osteochondropathies of forearm

      M93.831 Other specified osteochondropathies, right forearm
      M93.832 Other specified osteochondropathies, left forearm

      M93.839 Other specified osteochondropathies, unspecified forearm   ▽

    √6ᵗʰ **M93.84** Other specified osteochondropathies of hand

      M93.841 Other specified osteochondropathies, right hand
      M93.842 Other specified osteochondropathies, left hand
      M93.849 Other specified osteochondropathies, unspecified hand   ▽

    √6ᵗʰ **M93.85** Other specified osteochondropathies of thigh

      M93.851 Other specified osteochondropathies, right thigh
      M93.852 Other specified osteochondropathies, left thigh
      M93.859 Other specified osteochondropathies, unspecified thigh   ▽

    √6ᵗʰ **M93.86** Other specified osteochondropathies lower leg

      M93.861 Other specified osteochondropathies, right lower leg
      M93.862 Other specified osteochondropathies, left lower leg
      M93.869 Other specified osteochondropathies, unspecified lower leg   ▽

    √6ᵗʰ **M93.87** Other specified osteochondropathies of ankle and foot

      M93.871 Other specified osteochondropathies, right ankle and foot
      M93.872 Other specified osteochondropathies, left ankle and foot
      M93.879 Other specified osteochondropathies, unspecified ankle and foot   ▽

    M93.88 Other specified osteochondropathies other site

    M93.89 Other specified osteochondropathies multiple sites

√5ᵗʰ **M93.9** Osteochondropathy, unspecified

    Apophysitis NOS
    Epiphysitis NOS
    Osteochondritis NOS
    Osteochondrosis NOS

    M93.90 Osteochondropathy, unspecified of unspecified site   ▽

    √6ᵗʰ **M93.91** Osteochondropathy, unspecified of shoulder

      M93.911 Osteochondropathy, unspecified, right shoulder   ▽
      M93.912 Osteochondropathy, unspecified, left shoulder   ▽
      M93.919 Osteochondropathy, unspecified, unspecified shoulder   ▽

    √6ᵗʰ **M93.92** Osteochondropathy, unspecified of upper arm

      M93.921 Osteochondropathy, unspecified, right upper arm   ▽
      M93.922 Osteochondropathy, unspecified, left upper arm   ▽
      M93.929 Osteochondropathy, unspecified, unspecified upper arm   ▽

    √6ᵗʰ **M93.93** Osteochondropathy, unspecified of forearm

      M93.931 Osteochondropathy, unspecified, right forearm   ▽
      M93.932 Osteochondropathy, unspecified, left forearm   ▽
      M93.939 Osteochondropathy, unspecified, unspecified forearm   ▽

    √6ᵗʰ **M93.94** Osteochondropathy, unspecified of hand

      M93.941 Osteochondropathy, unspecified, right hand   ▽
      M93.942 Osteochondropathy, unspecified, left hand   ▽
      M93.949 Osteochondropathy, unspecified, unspecified hand   ▽

    √6ᵗʰ **M93.95** Osteochondropathy, unspecified of thigh

      M93.951 Osteochondropathy, unspecified, right thigh   ▽
      M93.952 Osteochondropathy, unspecified, left thigh   ▽
      M93.959 Osteochondropathy, unspecified, unspecified thigh   ▽

☑ Additional Character Req   √x7ᵗʰ Placeholder Alert   <u>Manifestation</u>   ▽ Unspecified   ▶◀ Revised Text   ● New Code   ▲ Revised Code Title

✓6ᵗʰ **M93.96 Osteochondropathy, unspecified** lower leg

  M93.961 Osteochondropathy, unspecified, right lower leg ▽

  M93.962 Osteochondropathy, unspecified, left lower leg ▽

  M93.969 Osteochondropathy, unspecified, unspecified lower leg ▽

✓6ᵗʰ **M93.97 Osteochondropathy, unspecified of** ankle and foot

  M93.971 Osteochondropathy, unspecified, right ankle and foot ▽

  M93.972 Osteochondropathy, unspecified, left ankle and foot ▽

  M93.979 Osteochondropathy, unspecified, unspecified ankle and foot ▽

M93.98 Osteochondropathy, unspecified other site ▽

M93.99 Osteochondropathy, unspecified multiple sites ▽

✓4ᵗʰ **M94 Other disorders of cartilage**

  M94.0 Chondrocostal junction syndrome [Tietze]

    Costochondritis

  M94.1 Relapsing polychondritis

✓5ᵗʰ **M94.2 Chondromalacia**

    EXCLUDES 1   chondromalacia patellae (M22.4)

  M94.20 Chondromalacia, unspecified site ▽

✓6ᵗʰ **M94.21 Chondromalacia, shoulder**

  M94.211 Chondromalacia, right shoulder

  M94.212 Chondromalacia, left shoulder

  M94.219 Chondromalacia, unspecified shoulder ▽

✓6ᵗʰ **M94.22 Chondromalacia, elbow**

  M94.221 Chondromalacia, right elbow

  M94.222 Chondromalacia, left elbow

  M94.229 Chondromalacia, unspecified elbow ▽

✓6ᵗʰ **M94.23 Chondromalacia, wrist**

  M94.231 Chondromalacia, right wrist

  M94.232 Chondromalacia, left wrist

  M94.239 Chondromalacia, unspecified wrist ▽

✓6ᵗʰ **M94.24 Chondromalacia, joints of hand**

  M94.241 Chondromalacia, joints of right hand

  M94.242 Chondromalacia, joints of left hand

  M94.249 Chondromalacia, joints of unspecified hand ▽

✓6ᵗʰ **M94.25 Chondromalacia, hip**

  M94.251 Chondromalacia, right hip

  M94.252 Chondromalacia, left hip

  M94.259 Chondromalacia, unspecified hip ▽

✓6ᵗʰ **M94.26 Chondromalacia, knee**

  M94.261 Chondromalacia, right knee

  M94.262 Chondromalacia, left knee

  M94.269 Chondromalacia, unspecified knee ▽

✓6ᵗʰ **M94.27 Chondromalacia, ankle and joints of foot**

  M94.271 Chondromalacia, right ankle and joints of right foot

  M94.272 Chondromalacia, left ankle and joints of left foot

  M94.279 Chondromalacia, unspecified ankle and joints of foot ▽

M94.28 Chondromalacia, other site

M94.29 Chondromalacia, multiple sites

✓5ᵗʰ **M94.3 Chondrolysis**

  Code first any associated slipped upper femoral epiphysis (nontraumatic) (M93.0-)

✓6ᵗʰ **M94.35 Chondrolysis, hip**

  M94.351 Chondrolysis, right hip

  M94.352 Chondrolysis, left hip

  M94.359 Chondrolysis, unspecified hip ▽

✓5ᵗʰ **M94.8 Other specified disorders of cartilage**

✓6ᵗʰ **M94.8X Other specified disorders of cartilage**

  M94.8X0 Other specified disorders of cartilage, multiple sites

  M94.8X1 Other specified disorders of cartilage, shoulder

  M94.8X2 Other specified disorders of cartilage, upper arm

  M94.8X3 Other specified disorders of cartilage, forearm

  M94.8X4 Other specified disorders of cartilage, hand

  M94.8X5 Other specified disorders of cartilage, thigh

  M94.8X6 Other specified disorders of cartilage, lower leg

  M94.8X7 Other specified disorders of cartilage, ankle and foot

  M94.8X8 Other specified disorders of cartilage, other site

  M94.8X9 Other specified disorders of cartilage, unspecified sites ▽

M94.9 Disorder of cartilage, unspecified ▽

Other disorders of the musculoskeletal system and connective tissue (M95)

✓4ᵗʰ **M95 Other acquired deformities of musculoskeletal system and connective tissue**

  EXCLUDES 2   acquired absence of limbs and organs (Z89-Z90)

    acquired deformities of limbs (M20-M21)

    congenital malformations and deformations of the musculoskeletal system (Q65-Q79)

    deforming dorsopathies (M40-M43)

    dentofacial anomalies [including malocclusion] (M26.-)

    postprocedural musculoskeletal disorders (M96.-)

  M95.0 Acquired deformity of nose

    EXCLUDES 2   deviated nasal septum (J34.2)

✓5ᵗʰ **M95.1 Cauliflower ear**

    EXCLUDES 2   other acquired deformities of ear (H61.1)

    DEF: Acquired deformity of the external ear due to injury or subsequent perichondritis.

  M95.10 Cauliflower ear, unspecified ear ▽

  M95.11 Cauliflower ear, right ear

  M95.12 Cauliflower ear, left ear

  M95.2 Other acquired deformity of head

  M95.3 Acquired deformity of neck

  M95.4 Acquired deformity of chest and rib

    AHA: 2014,4Q,26-27

  M95.5 Acquired deformity of pelvis

    EXCLUDES 1   maternal care for known or suspected disproportion (O33.-)

  M95.8 Other specified acquired deformities of musculoskeletal system

  M95.9 Acquired deformity of musculoskeletal system, unspecified ▽

Intraoperative and postprocedural complications and disorders of musculoskeletal system, not elsewhere classified (M96)

✓4ᵗʰ **M96 Intraoperative and postprocedural complications and disorders of musculoskeletal system, not elsewhere classified**

  EXCLUDES 2   arthropathy following intestinal bypass (M02.0-)

    complications of internal orthopedic prosthetic devices, implants and grafts (T84.-)

    disorders associated with osteoporosis (M80)

    periprosthetic fracture around internal prosthetic joint (M97.-)

    presence of functional implants and other devices (Z96-Z97)

  M96.0 Pseudarthrosis after fusion or arthrodesis

  M96.1 Postlaminectomy syndrome, not elsewhere classified

  M96.2 Postradiation kyphosis

  M96.3 Postlaminectomy kyphosis

  M96.4 Postsurgical lordosis

  M96.5 Postradiation scoliosis

✓5ᵗʰ **M96.6 Fracture of bone following insertion of orthopedic implant, joint prosthesis, or bone plate**

  Intraoperative fracture of bone during insertion of orthopedic implant, joint prosthesis, or bone plate

    EXCLUDES 2   complication of internal orthopedic devices, implants or grafts (T84.-)

✓6ᵗʰ **M96.62 Fracture of** humerus **following insertion of orthopedic implant, joint prosthesis, or bone plate**

  M96.621 Fracture of humerus following insertion of orthopedic implant, joint prosthesis, or bone plate, right arm HCC

√6ᵗʰ **M96.622** Fracture of humerus following insertion of orthopedic implant, joint prosthesis, or bone plate, left arm `HCC`

M96.629 Fracture of humerus following insertion of orthopedic implant, joint prosthesis, or bone plate, unspecified arm `HCC` ▽

√6ᵗʰ **M96.63** Fracture of radius or ulna following insertion of orthopedic implant, joint prosthesis, or bone plate

M96.631 Fracture of radius or ulna following insertion of orthopedic implant, joint prosthesis, or bone plate, right arm `HCC`

M96.632 Fracture of radius or ulna following insertion of orthopedic implant, joint prosthesis, or bone plate, left arm `HCC`

M96.639 Fracture of radius or ulna following insertion of orthopedic implant, joint prosthesis, or bone plate, unspecified arm `HCC` ▽

M96.65 Fracture of pelvis following insertion of orthopedic implant, joint prosthesis, or bone plate `HCC`

√6ᵗʰ **M96.66** Fracture of femur following insertion of orthopedic implant, joint prosthesis, or bone plate

M96.661 Fracture of femur following insertion of orthopedic implant, joint prosthesis, or bone plate, right leg `HCC`

M96.662 Fracture of femur following insertion of orthopedic implant, joint prosthesis, or bone plate, left leg `HCC`

M96.669 Fracture of femur following insertion of orthopedic implant, joint prosthesis, or bone plate, unspecified leg `HCC` ▽

√6ᵗʰ **M96.67** Fracture of tibia or fibula following insertion of orthopedic implant, joint prosthesis, or bone plate

M96.671 Fracture of tibia or fibula following insertion of orthopedic implant, joint prosthesis, or bone plate, right leg `HCC`

M96.672 Fracture of tibia or fibula following insertion of orthopedic implant, joint prosthesis, or bone plate, left leg `HCC`

M96.679 Fracture of tibia or fibula following insertion of orthopedic implant, joint prosthesis, or bone plate, unspecified leg `HCC` ▽

M96.69 Fracture of other bone following insertion of orthopedic implant, joint prosthesis, or bone plate `HCC`

√5ᵗʰ **M96.8** Other intraoperative and postprocedural complications and disorders of musculoskeletal system, not elsewhere classified

AHA: 2016,4Q,9-10

√6ᵗʰ **M96.81** Intraoperative hemorrhage and hematoma of a musculoskeletal structure complicating a procedure

`EXCLUDES 1`   intraoperative hemorrhage and hematoma of a musculoskeletal structure due to accidental puncture and laceration during a procedure (M96.82-)

M96.810 Intraoperative hemorrhage and hematoma of a musculoskeletal structure complicating a musculoskeletal system procedure

M96.811 Intraoperative hemorrhage and hematoma of a musculoskeletal structure complicating other procedure

√6ᵗʰ **M96.82** Accidental puncture and laceration of a musculoskeletal structure during a procedure

M96.820 Accidental puncture and laceration of a musculoskeletal structure during a musculoskeletal system procedure

M96.821 Accidental puncture and laceration of a musculoskeletal structure during other procedure

√6ᵗʰ **M96.83** Postprocedural hemorrhage of a musculoskeletal structure following a procedure

M96.830 Postprocedural hemorrhage of a musculoskeletal structure following a musculoskeletal system procedure

M96.831 Postprocedural hemorrhage of a musculoskeletal structure following other procedure

√6ᵗʰ **M96.84** Postprocedural hematoma and seroma of a musculoskeletal structure following a procedure

M96.840 Postprocedural hematoma of a musculoskeletal structure following a musculoskeletal system procedure

M96.841 Postprocedural hematoma of a musculoskeletal structure following other procedure

AHA: 2016,4Q,10

M96.842 Postprocedural seroma of a musculoskeletal structure following a musculoskeletal system procedure

M96.843 Postprocedural seroma of a musculoskeletal structure following other procedure

M96.89 Other intraoperative and postprocedural complications and disorders of the musculoskeletal system

Instability of joint secondary to removal of joint prosthesis

Use additional code, if applicable, to further specify disorder

Periprosthetic fractures around internal prosthetic joint (M97)

√4ᵗʰ **M97** **Periprosthetic fracture around internal prosthetic joint**

`EXCLUDES 2`   breakage (fracture) of prosthetic joint (T84.01-)
fracture of bone following insertion of orthopedic implant, joint prosthesis or bone plate (M96.6-)

AHA: 2016,4Q,42-43

> The appropriate 7th character is to be added to each code from category M97.
> A   initial encounter
> D   subsequent encounter
> S   sequela

√5ᵗʰ **M97.0** Periprosthetic fracture around internal prosthetic hip joint

AHA: 2018,1Q,21; 2016,4Q,42

¹ √x7ᵗʰ **M97.01** Periprosthetic fracture around internal prosthetic right hip joint `HCC`

¹ √x7ᵗʰ **M97.02** Periprosthetic fracture around internal prosthetic left hip joint `HCC`

√5ᵗʰ **M97.1** Periprosthetic fracture around internal prosthetic knee joint

√x7ᵗʰ **M97.11** Periprosthetic fracture around internal prosthetic right knee joint

√x7ᵗʰ **M97.12** Periprosthetic fracture around internal prosthetic left knee joint

√5ᵗʰ **M97.2** Periprosthetic fracture around internal prosthetic ankle joint

√x7ᵗʰ **M97.21** Periprosthetic fracture around internal prosthetic right ankle joint

√x7ᵗʰ **M97.22** Periprosthetic fracture around internal prosthetic left ankle joint

√5ᵗʰ **M97.3** Periprosthetic fracture around internal prosthetic shoulder joint

√x7ᵗʰ **M97.31** Periprosthetic fracture around internal prosthetic right shoulder joint

√x7ᵗʰ **M97.32** Periprosthetic fracture around internal prosthetic left shoulder joint

√5ᵗʰ **M97.4** Periprosthetic fracture around internal prosthetic elbow joint

√x7ᵗʰ **M97.41** Periprosthetic fracture around internal prosthetic right elbow joint

√x7ᵗʰ **M97.42** Periprosthetic fracture around internal prosthetic left elbow joint

√x7ᵗʰ **M97.8** Periprosthetic fracture around other internal prosthetic joint

Periprosthetic fracture around internal prosthetic finger joint
Periprosthetic fracture around internal prosthetic spinal joint
Periprosthetic fracture around internal prosthetic toe joint
Periprosthetic fracture around internal prosthetic wrist joint
Use additional code to identify the joint (Z96.6-)

√x7ᵗʰ **M97.9** Periprosthetic fracture around unspecified internal prosthetic joint   ▽

☑ Additional Character Req   √x7ᵗʰ Placeholder Alert   Manifestation   ▽ Unspecified   ▶◀ Revised Text   ● New Code   ▲ Revised Code Title

Biomechanical lesions, not elsewhere classified (M99)

√4ᵗʰ M99 Biomechanical lesions, not elsewhere classified

> **NOTE**   This category should not be used if the condition can be classified elsewhere.

> **DEF:** Biomechanical lesion: Term used by osteopathic and chiropractic physicians to describe musculoskeletal conditions treated that are not more appropriately classified elsewhere.

√5ᵗʰ M99.0 Segmental and somatic dysfunction

- M99.00 Segmental and somatic dysfunction of head region
- M99.01 Segmental and somatic dysfunction of cervical region
- M99.02 Segmental and somatic dysfunction of thoracic region
- M99.03 Segmental and somatic dysfunction of lumbar region
- M99.04 Segmental and somatic dysfunction of sacral region
- M99.05 Segmental and somatic dysfunction of pelvic region
- M99.06 Segmental and somatic dysfunction of lower extremity
- M99.07 Segmental and somatic dysfunction of upper extremity
- M99.08 Segmental and somatic dysfunction of rib cage
- M99.09 Segmental and somatic dysfunction of abdomen and other regions

√5ᵗʰ M99.1 Subluxation complex (vertebral)

- M99.10 Subluxation complex (vertebral) of head region
- M99.11 Subluxation complex (vertebral) of cervical region
- M99.12 Subluxation complex (vertebral) of thoracic region
- M99.13 Subluxation complex (vertebral) of lumbar region
- M99.14 Subluxation complex (vertebral) of sacral region
- M99.15 Subluxation complex (vertebral) of pelvic region
- M99.16 Subluxation complex (vertebral) of lower extremity
- M99.17 Subluxation complex (vertebral) of upper extremity
- M99.18 Subluxation complex (vertebral) of rib cage
- M99.19 Subluxation complex (vertebral) of abdomen and other regions

√5ᵗʰ M99.2 Subluxation stenosis of neural canal

- M99.20 Subluxation stenosis of neural canal of head region
- M99.21 Subluxation stenosis of neural canal of cervical region
- M99.22 Subluxation stenosis of neural canal of thoracic region
- M99.23 Subluxation stenosis of neural canal of lumbar region
- M99.24 Subluxation stenosis of neural canal of sacral region
- M99.25 Subluxation stenosis of neural canal of pelvic region
- M99.26 Subluxation stenosis of neural canal of lower extremity
- M99.27 Subluxation stenosis of neural canal of upper extremity
- M99.28 Subluxation stenosis of neural canal of rib cage
- M99.29 Subluxation stenosis of neural canal of abdomen and other regions

√5ᵗʰ M99.3 Osseous stenosis of neural canal

- M99.30 Osseous stenosis of neural canal of head region
- M99.31 Osseous stenosis of neural canal of cervical region
- M99.32 Osseous stenosis of neural canal of thoracic region
- M99.33 Osseous stenosis of neural canal of lumbar region
- M99.34 Osseous stenosis of neural canal of sacral region
- M99.35 Osseous stenosis of neural canal of pelvic region
- M99.36 Osseous stenosis of neural canal of lower extremity
- M99.37 Osseous stenosis of neural canal of upper extremity
- M99.38 Osseous stenosis of neural canal of rib cage
- M99.39 Osseous stenosis of neural canal of abdomen and other regions

√5ᵗʰ M99.4 Connective tissue stenosis of neural canal

- M99.40 Connective tissue stenosis of neural canal of head region
- M99.41 Connective tissue stenosis of neural canal of cervical region
- M99.42 Connective tissue stenosis of neural canal of thoracic region
- M99.43 Connective tissue stenosis of neural canal of lumbar region
- M99.44 Connective tissue stenosis of neural canal of sacral region
- M99.45 Connective tissue stenosis of neural canal of pelvic region
- M99.46 Connective tissue stenosis of neural canal of lower extremity
- M99.47 Connective tissue stenosis of neural canal of upper extremity
- M99.48 Connective tissue stenosis of neural canal of rib cage
- M99.49 Connective tissue stenosis of neural canal of abdomen and other regions

√5ᵗʰ M99.5 Intervertebral disc stenosis of neural canal

- M99.50 Intervertebral disc stenosis of neural canal of head region
- M99.51 Intervertebral disc stenosis of neural canal of cervical region
- M99.52 Intervertebral disc stenosis of neural canal of thoracic region
- M99.53 Intervertebral disc stenosis of neural canal of lumbar region
- M99.54 Intervertebral disc stenosis of neural canal of sacral region
- M99.55 Intervertebral disc stenosis of neural canal of pelvic region
- M99.56 Intervertebral disc stenosis of neural canal of lower extremity
- M99.57 Intervertebral disc stenosis of neural canal of upper extremity
- M99.58 Intervertebral disc stenosis of neural canal of rib cage
- M99.59 Intervertebral disc stenosis of neural canal of abdomen and other regions

√5ᵗʰ M99.6 Osseous and subluxation stenosis of intervertebral foramina

- M99.60 Osseous and subluxation stenosis of intervertebral foramina of head region
- M99.61 Osseous and subluxation stenosis of intervertebral foramina of cervical region
- M99.62 Osseous and subluxation stenosis of intervertebral foramina of thoracic region
- M99.63 Osseous and subluxation stenosis of intervertebral foramina of lumbar region
- M99.64 Osseous and subluxation stenosis of intervertebral foramina of sacral region
- M99.65 Osseous and subluxation stenosis of intervertebral foramina of pelvic region
- M99.66 Osseous and subluxation stenosis of intervertebral foramina of lower extremity
- M99.67 Osseous and subluxation stenosis of intervertebral foramina of upper extremity
- M99.68 Osseous and subluxation stenosis of intervertebral foramina of rib cage
- M99.69 Osseous and subluxation stenosis of intervertebral foramina of abdomen and other regions

√5ᵗʰ M99.7 Connective tissue and disc stenosis of intervertebral foramina

- M99.70 Connective tissue and disc stenosis of intervertebral foramina of head region
- M99.71 Connective tissue and disc stenosis of intervertebral foramina of cervical region
- M99.72 Connective tissue and disc stenosis of intervertebral foramina of thoracic region
- M99.73 Connective tissue and disc stenosis of intervertebral foramina of lumbar region
- M99.74 Connective tissue and disc stenosis of intervertebral foramina of sacral region
- M99.75 Connective tissue and disc stenosis of intervertebral foramina of pelvic region
- M99.76 Connective tissue and disc stenosis of intervertebral foramina of lower extremity
- M99.77 Connective tissue and disc stenosis of intervertebral foramina of upper extremity
- M99.78 Connective tissue and disc stenosis of intervertebral foramina of rib cage
- M99.79 Connective tissue and disc stenosis of intervertebral foramina of abdomen and other regions

√5ᵗʰ M99.8 Other biomechanical lesions

- M99.80 Other biomechanical lesions of head region
- M99.81 Other biomechanical lesions of cervical region
- M99.82 Other biomechanical lesions of thoracic region
- M99.83 Other biomechanical lesions of lumbar region
- M99.84 Other biomechanical lesions of sacral region
- M99.85 Other biomechanical lesions of pelvic region
- M99.86 Other biomechanical lesions of lower extremity

    M99.87   **Other biomechanical lesions of** upper extremity

    M99.88   **Other biomechanical lesions of** rib cage

    M99.89   **Other biomechanical lesions of** abdomen and other regions

  M99.9   **Biomechanical lesion, unspecified**   ▽

☑ Additional Character Req	ᴠₓ⁷ᵗʰ Placeholder Alert	Manifestation	▽ Unspecified	►◄ Revised Text	● New Code	▲ Revised Code Title

Chapter 14. Diseases of Genitourinary System (NØØ–N99)

Chapter Specific Guidelines with Coding Examples

The chapter specific guidelines from the ICD-10-CM Official Guidelines for Coding and Reporting have been provided below. Along with these guidelines are coding examples, contained in the shaded boxes, that have been developed to help illustrate the coding and/or sequencing guidance found in these guidelines.

a. Chronic kidney disease

1) Stages of chronic kidney disease (CKD)

The ICD-10-CM classifies CKD based on severity. The severity of CKD is designated by stages 1-5. Stage 2, code N18.2, equates to mild CKD; stage 3, code N18.3, equates to moderate CKD; and stage 4, code N18.4, equates to severe CKD. Code N18.6, End stage renal disease (ESRD), is assigned when the provider has documented end-stage-renal disease (ESRD).

If both a stage of CKD and ESRD are documented, assign code N18.6 only.

> Stage 5 chronic kidney disease with ESRD requiring chronic dialysis
>
> **N18.6**   **End stage renal disease**
>
> **Z99.2**   **Dependence on renal dialysis**
>
> *Explanation:* The diagnostic statement indicates the patient has chronic kidney disease, documented both as stage 5 and as ESRD requiring chronic dialysis. Code N18.6 End stage renal disease (ESRD), is assigned when the provider has documented end-stage-renal disease (ESRD). If both a stage of CKD and ESRD are documented, assign code N18.6 only.

2) Chronic kidney disease and kidney transplant status

Patients who have undergone kidney transplant may still have some form of chronic kidney disease (CKD) because the kidney transplant may not fully restore kidney function. Therefore, the presence of CKD alone does not constitute a transplant complication. Assign the appropriate N18 code for the patient's stage of CKD and code Z94.Ø, Kidney transplant status. If a transplant complication such as failure or rejection or other transplant complication is documented, see section I.C.19.g for information on coding complications of a kidney transplant. If the documentation is unclear as to whether the patient has a complication of the transplant, query the provider.

> Patient with residual chronic kidney disease stage 1 after kidney transplant
>
> **N18.1**   **Chronic kidney disease, stage 1**
>
> **Z94.Ø**   **Kidney transplant status**
>
> *Explanation:* Patients who have undergone kidney transplant may still have some form of chronic kidney disease (CKD) because the kidney transplant may not fully restore kidney function. The presence of CKD alone does not constitute a transplant complication. Assign the appropriate N18 code for the patient's stage of CKD and code Z94.Ø Kidney transplant status.

3) Chronic kidney disease with other conditions

Patients with CKD may also suffer from other serious conditions, most commonly diabetes mellitus and hypertension. The sequencing of the CKD code in relationship to codes for other contributing conditions is based on the conventions in the Tabular List.

See I.C.9. Hypertensive chronic kidney disease.

See I.C.19. Chronic kidney disease and kidney transplant complications.

> Type 1 diabetic chronic kidney disease, stage 2
>
> **E10.22**   **Type 1 diabetes mellitus with diabetic chronic kidney disease**
>
> **N18.2**   **Chronic kidney disease, stage 2 (mild)**
>
> *Explanation:* Patients with CKD may also suffer from other serious conditions such as diabetes mellitus. The sequencing of the CKD code in relationship to codes for other contributing conditions is based on the conventions in the Tabular List. Diabetic CKD code E10.22 includes an instructional note to "Use additional code to identify stage of chronic kidney disease (N18.1–N18.6)," thus providing sequencing direction.

Chapter 14. Diseases of the Genitourinary System (N00–N99)

EXCLUDES 2
    certain conditions originating in the perinatal period (P04-P96)
    certain infectious and parasitic diseases (A00-B99)
    complications of pregnancy, childbirth and the puerperium (O00-O9A)
    congenital malformations, deformations and chromosomal abnormalities (Q00-Q99)
    endocrine, nutritional and metabolic diseases (E00-E88)
    injury, poisoning and certain other consequences of external causes (S00-T88)
    neoplasms (C00-D49)
    symptoms, signs and abnormal clinical and laboratory findings, not elsewhere classified (R00-R94)

This chapter contains the following blocks:

N00-N08   Glomerular diseases
N10-N16   Renal tubulo-interstitial diseases
N17-N19   Acute kidney failure and chronic kidney disease
N20-N23   Urolithiasis
N25-N29   Other disorders of kidney and ureter
N30-N39   Other diseases of the urinary system
N40-N53   Diseases of male genital organs
N60-N65   Disorders of breast
N70-N77   Inflammatory diseases of female pelvic organs
N80-N98   Noninflammatory disorders of female genital tract
N99   Intraoperative and postprocedural complications and disorders of genitourinary system, not elsewhere classified

Glomerular diseases (N00-N08)

Code also any associated kidney failure (N17-N19).
EXCLUDES 1   hypertensive chronic kidney disease (I12.-)
DEF: Glomeruli: Clusters of microscopic blood vessels located within the kidneys containing small pores through which waste products are filtered from the blood and urine is formed.
DEF: Glomerulonephritis: Disease of the kidney with diffuse inflammation of the capillary loops of the glomeruli.

✓4ᵗʰ **N00 Acute nephritic syndrome**

    INCLUDES   acute glomerular disease
                    acute glomerulonephritis
                    acute nephritis
    EXCLUDES 1   acute tubulo-interstitial nephritis (N10)
                    nephritic syndrome NOS (N05.-)

    N00.0 Acute nephritic syndrome with minor glomerular abnormality
        Acute nephritic syndrome with minimal change lesion

    N00.1 Acute nephritic syndrome with focal and segmental glomerular lesions
        Acute nephritic syndrome with focal and segmental hyalinosis
        Acute nephritic syndrome with focal and segmental sclerosis
        Acute nephritic syndrome with focal glomerulonephritis

    N00.2 Acute nephritic syndrome with diffuse membranous glomerulonephritis

    N00.3 Acute nephritic syndrome with diffuse mesangial proliferative glomerulonephritis

    N00.4 Acute nephritic syndrome with diffuse endocapillary proliferative glomerulonephritis

    N00.5 Acute nephritic syndrome with diffuse mesangiocapillary glomerulonephritis
        Acute nephritic syndrome with membranoproliferative glomerulonephritis, types 1 and 3, or NOS

    N00.6 Acute nephritic syndrome with dense deposit disease
        Acute nephritic syndrome with membranoproliferative glomerulonephritis, type 2

    N00.7 Acute nephritic syndrome with diffuse crescentic glomerulonephritis
        Acute nephritic syndrome with extracapillary glomerulonephritis

    N00.8 Acute nephritic syndrome with other morphologic changes
        Acute nephritic syndrome with proliferative glomerulonephritis NOS

    N00.9 Acute nephritic syndrome with unspecified morphologic changes ▽

✓4ᵗʰ **N01 Rapidly progressive nephritic syndrome**

    INCLUDES   rapidly progressive glomerular disease
                    rapidly progressive glomerulonephritis
                    rapidly progressive nephritis
    EXCLUDES 1   nephritic syndrome NOS (N05.-)

    N01.0 Rapidly progressive nephritic syndrome with minor glomerular abnormality
        Rapidly progressive nephritic syndrome with minimal change lesion

    N01.1 Rapidly progressive nephritic syndrome with focal and segmental glomerular lesions
        Rapidly progressive nephritic syndrome with focal and segmental hyalinosis
        Rapidly progressive nephritic syndrome with focal and segmental sclerosis
        Rapidly progressive nephritic syndrome with focal glomerulonephritis

    N01.2 Rapidly progressive nephritic syndrome with diffuse membranous glomerulonephritis

    N01.3 Rapidly progressive nephritic syndrome with diffuse mesangial proliferative glomerulonephritis

    N01.4 Rapidly progressive nephritic syndrome with diffuse endocapillary proliferative glomerulonephritis

    N01.5 Rapidly progressive nephritic syndrome with diffuse mesangiocapillary glomerulonephritis
        Rapidly progressive nephritic syndrome with membranoproliferative glomerulonephritis, types 1 and 3, or NOS

    N01.6 Rapidly progressive nephritic syndrome with dense deposit disease
        Rapidly progressive nephritic syndrome with membranoproliferative glomerulonephritis, type 2

    N01.7 Rapidly progressive nephritic syndrome with diffuse crescentic glomerulonephritis
        Rapidly progressive nephritic syndrome with extracapillary glomerulonephritis

    N01.8 Rapidly progressive nephritic syndrome with other morphologic changes
        Rapidly progressive nephritic syndrome with proliferative glomerulonephritis NOS

    N01.9 Rapidly progressive nephritic syndrome with unspecified morphologic changes ▽

✓4ᵗʰ **N02 Recurrent and persistent hematuria**

    EXCLUDES 1   acute cystitis with hematuria (N30.01)
                    hematuria NOS (R31.9)
                    hematuria not associated with specified morphologic lesions (R31.-)

    N02.0 Recurrent and persistent hematuria with minor glomerular abnormality
        Recurrent and persistent hematuria with minimal change lesion

    N02.1 Recurrent and persistent hematuria with focal and segmental glomerular lesions
        Recurrent and persistent hematuria with focal and segmental hyalinosis
        Recurrent and persistent hematuria with focal and segmental sclerosis
        Recurrent and persistent hematuria with focal glomerulonephritis

    N02.2 Recurrent and persistent hematuria with diffuse membranous glomerulonephritis

    N02.3 Recurrent and persistent hematuria with diffuse mesangial proliferative glomerulonephritis

    N02.4 Recurrent and persistent hematuria with diffuse endocapillary proliferative glomerulonephritis

    N02.5 Recurrent and persistent hematuria with diffuse mesangiocapillary glomerulonephritis
        Recurrent and persistent hematuria with membranoproliferative glomerulonephritis, types 1 and 3, or NOS

    N02.6 Recurrent and persistent hematuria with dense deposit disease
        Recurrent and persistent hematuria with membranoproliferative glomerulonephritis, type 2

    N02.7 Recurrent and persistent hematuria with diffuse crescentic glomerulonephritis
        Recurrent and persistent hematuria with extracapillary glomerulonephritis

N02.8   **Recurrent and persistent hematuria with other morphologic changes**
     Recurrent and persistent hematuria with proliferative glomerulonephritis NOS

N02.9   **Recurrent and persistent hematuria with unspecified morphologic changes** ▽
     AHA: 2017,2Q,5

☑4ᵗʰ **N03**   **Chronic nephritic syndrome**
     INCLUDES   chronic glomerular disease
              chronic glomerulonephritis
              chronic nephritis
     EXCLUDES 1   *chronic tubulo-interstitial nephritis (N11.-)*
              diffuse sclerosing glomerulonephritis (N05.8-)
              nephritic syndrome NOS (N05.-)
     DEF: Slow, progressive type of nephritis characterized by inflammation of the capillary loops in the glomeruli of the kidney, which leads to renal failure.

N03.0   **Chronic nephritic syndrome with minor glomerular abnormality**
     Chronic nephritic syndrome with minimal change lesion

N03.1   **Chronic nephritic syndrome with focal and segmental glomerular lesions**
     Chronic nephritic syndrome with focal and segmental hyalinosis
     Chronic nephritic syndrome with focal and segmental sclerosis
     Chronic nephritic syndrome with focal glomerulonephritis

N03.2   **Chronic nephritic syndrome with diffuse membranous glomerulonephritis**

N03.3   **Chronic nephritic syndrome with diffuse mesangial proliferative glomerulonephritis**

N03.4   **Chronic nephritic syndrome with diffuse endocapillary proliferative glomerulonephritis**

N03.5   **Chronic nephritic syndrome with diffuse mesangiocapillary glomerulonephritis**
     Chronic nephritic syndrome with membranoproliferative glomerulonephritis, types 1 and 3, or NOS

N03.6   **Chronic nephritic syndrome with dense deposit disease**
     Chronic nephritic syndrome with membranoproliferative glomerulonephritis, type 2

N03.7   **Chronic nephritic syndrome with diffuse crescentic glomerulonephritis**
     Chronic nephritic syndrome with extracapillary glomerulonephritis

N03.8   **Chronic nephritic syndrome with other morphologic changes**
     Chronic nephritic syndrome with proliferative glomerulonephritis NOS

N03.9   **Chronic nephritic syndrome with unspecified morphologic changes** ▽

N04   **Nephrotic syndrome**
☑4ᵗʰ
     INCLUDES   congenital nephrotic syndrome
              lipoid nephrosis

N04.0   **Nephrotic syndrome with minor glomerular abnormality**
     Nephrotic syndrome with minimal change lesion

N04.1   **Nephrotic syndrome with focal and segmental glomerular lesions**
     Nephrotic syndrome with focal and segmental hyalinosis
     Nephrotic syndrome with focal and segmental sclerosis
     Nephrotic syndrome with focal glomerulonephritis

N04.2   **Nephrotic syndrome with diffuse membranous glomerulonephritis**

N04.3   **Nephrotic syndrome with diffuse mesangial proliferative glomerulonephritis**

N04.4   **Nephrotic syndrome with diffuse endocapillary proliferative glomerulonephritis**

N04.5   **Nephrotic syndrome with diffuse mesangiocapillary glomerulonephritis**
     Nephrotic syndrome with membranoproliferative glomerulonephritis, types 1 and 3, or NOS

N04.6   **Nephrotic syndrome with dense deposit disease**
     Nephrotic syndrome with membranoproliferative glomerulonephritis, type 2

N04.7   **Nephrotic syndrome with diffuse crescentic glomerulonephritis**
     Nephrotic syndrome with extracapillary glomerulonephritis

N04.8   **Nephrotic syndrome with other morphologic changes**
     Nephrotic syndrome with proliferative glomerulonephritis NOS

N04.9   **Nephrotic syndrome with unspecified morphologic changes** ▽

☑4ᵗʰ **N05**   **Unspecified nephritic syndrome**
     INCLUDES   glomerular disease NOS
              glomerulonephritis NOS
              nephritis NOS
              nephropathy NOS and renal disease NOS with morphological lesion specified in .0-.8
     EXCLUDES 1   *nephropathy NOS with no stated morphological lesion (N28.9)*
              renal disease NOS with no stated morphological lesion (N28.9)
              tubulo-interstitial nephritis NOS (N12)

N05.0   **Unspecified nephritic syndrome with minor glomerular abnormality** ▽
     Unspecified nephritic syndrome with minimal change lesion

N05.1   **Unspecified nephritic syndrome with focal and segmental glomerular lesions** ▽
     Unspecified nephritic syndrome with focal and segmental hyalinosis
     Unspecified nephritic syndrome with focal and segmental sclerosis
     Unspecified nephritic syndrome with focal glomerulonephritis

N05.2   **Unspecified nephritic syndrome with diffuse membranous glomerulonephritis** ▽

N05.3   **Unspecified nephritic syndrome with diffuse mesangial proliferative glomerulonephritis** ▽

N05.4   **Unspecified nephritic syndrome with diffuse endocapillary proliferative glomerulonephritis** ▽

N05.5   **Unspecified nephritic syndrome with diffuse mesangiocapillary glomerulonephritis** ▽
     Unspecified nephritic syndrome with membranoproliferative glomerulonephritis, types 1 and 3, or NOS

N05.6   **Unspecified nephritic syndrome with dense deposit disease** ▽
     Unspecified nephritic syndrome with membranoproliferative glomerulonephritis, type 2

N05.7   **Unspecified nephritic syndrome with diffuse crescentic glomerulonephritis** ▽
     Unspecified nephritic syndrome with extracapillary glomerulonephritis

N05.8   **Unspecified nephritic syndrome with other morphologic changes** ▽
     Unspecified nephritic syndrome with proliferative glomerulonephritis NOS

N05.9   **Unspecified nephritic syndrome with unspecified morphologic changes** ▽

☑4ᵗʰ **N06**   **Isolated proteinuria with specified morphological lesion**
     EXCLUDES 1   *proteinuria not associated with specific morphologic lesions (R80.0)*

N06.0   **Isolated proteinuria with minor glomerular abnormality**
     Isolated proteinuria with minimal change lesion

N06.1   **Isolated proteinuria with focal and segmental glomerular lesions**
     Isolated proteinuria with focal and segmental hyalinosis
     Isolated proteinuria with focal and segmental sclerosis
     Isolated proteinuria with focal glomerulonephritis

N06.2   **Isolated proteinuria with diffuse membranous glomerulonephritis**

N06.3   **Isolated proteinuria with diffuse mesangial proliferative glomerulonephritis**

N06.4   **Isolated proteinuria with diffuse endocapillary proliferative glomerulonephritis**

N06.5   **Isolated proteinuria with diffuse mesangiocapillary glomerulonephritis**
     Isolated proteinuria with membranoproliferative glomerulonephritis, types 1 and 3, or NOS

N06.6   **Isolated proteinuria with dense deposit disease**
     Isolated proteinuria with membranoproliferative glomerulonephritis, type 2

N06.7   **Isolated proteinuria with diffuse crescentic glomerulonephritis**
     Isolated proteinuria with extracapillary glomerulonephritis

N06.8   **Isolated proteinuria with other morphologic lesion**
     Isolated proteinuria with proliferative glomerulonephritis NOS

N06.9   **Isolated proteinuria with unspecified morphologic lesion** ▽

☑ Additional Character Req   6ˣ7ᵗʰ Placeholder Alert   **Manifestation**   ▽ Unspecified   ▶◀ Revised Text   ● New Code   ▲ Revised Code Title

✓4ᵗʰ **N07 Hereditary nephropathy, not elsewhere classified**

     EXCLUDES 2   *Alport's syndrome (Q87.81-)*
               hereditary amyloid nephropathy (E85.-)
               nail patella syndrome (Q87.2)
               non-neuropathic heredofamilial amyloidosis (E85.-)

N07.0 Hereditary nephropathy, not elsewhere classified with minor glomerular abnormality
     Hereditary nephropathy, not elsewhere classified with minimal change lesion

N07.1 Hereditary nephropathy, not elsewhere classified with focal and segmental glomerular lesions
     Hereditary nephropathy, not elsewhere classified with focal and segmental hyalinosis
     Hereditary nephropathy, not elsewhere classified with focal and segmental sclerosis
     Hereditary nephropathy, not elsewhere classified with focal glomerulonephritis

N07.2 Hereditary nephropathy, not elsewhere classified with diffuse membranous glomerulonephritis

N07.3 Hereditary nephropathy, not elsewhere classified with diffuse mesangial proliferative glomerulonephritis

N07.4 Hereditary nephropathy, not elsewhere classified with diffuse endocapillary proliferative glomerulonephritis

N07.5 Hereditary nephropathy, not elsewhere classified with diffuse mesangiocapillary glomerulonephritis
     Hereditary nephropathy, not elsewhere classified with membranoproliferative glomerulonephritis, types 1 and 3, or NOS

N07.6 Hereditary nephropathy, not elsewhere classified with dense deposit disease
     Hereditary nephropathy, not elsewhere classified with membranoproliferative glomerulonephritis, type 2

N07.7 Hereditary nephropathy, not elsewhere classified with diffuse crescentic glomerulonephritis
     Hereditary nephropathy, not elsewhere classified with extracapillary glomerulonephritis

N07.8 Hereditary nephropathy, not elsewhere classified with other morphologic lesions
     Hereditary nephropathy, not elsewhere classified with proliferative glomerulonephritis NOS

N07.9 Hereditary nephropathy, not elsewhere classified with unspecified morphologic lesions ▽

N08 *Glomerular disorders in diseases classified elsewhere*
     Glomerulonephritis
     Nephritis
     Nephropathy
     Code first underlying disease, such as:
         amyloidosis (E85.-)
         congenital syphilis (A50.5)
         cryoglobulinemia (D89.1)
         disseminated intravascular coagulation (D65)
         gout (M1A.-, M10.-)
         microscopic polyangiitis (M31.7)
         multiple myeloma (C90.0-)
         sepsis (A40.0-A41.9)
         sickle-cell disease (D57.0-D57.8)

       EXCLUDES 1   *glomerulonephritis, nephritis and nephropathy (in):*
               antiglomerular basement membrane disease (M31.0)
               diabetes (E08-E13 with .21)
               gonococcal (A54.21)
               Goodpasture's syndrome (M31.0)
               hemolytic-uremic syndrome (D59.3)
               lupus (M32.14)
               mumps (B26.83)
               syphilis (A52.75)
               systemic lupus erythematosus (M32.14)
               Wegener's granulomatosis (M31.31)
           pyelonephritis in diseases classified elsewhere (N16)
           renal tubulo-interstitial disorders classified elsewhere (N16)

Renal tubulo-interstitial diseases (N10-N16)

     INCLUDES   pyelonephritis
     EXCLUDES 1   *pyeloureteritis cystica (N28.85)*

N10 Acute pyelonephritis
     Acute infectious interstitial nephritis
     Acute pyelitis
     Acute tubulo-interstitial nephritis
     Hemoglobin nephrosis
     Myoglobin nephrosis
     Use additional code (B95-B97), to identify infectious agent

✓4ᵗʰ **N11 Chronic tubulo-interstitial nephritis**

     INCLUDES   chronic infectious interstitial nephritis
               chronic pyelitis
               chronic pyelonephritis
     Use additional code (B95-B97), to identify infectious agent

N11.0 Nonobstructive reflux-associated chronic pyelonephritis
     Pyelonephritis (chronic) associated with (vesicoureteral) reflux
       EXCLUDES 1   *vesicoureteral reflux NOS (N13.70)*

N11.1 Chronic obstructive pyelonephritis
     Pyelonephritis (chronic) associated with anomaly of pelviureteric junction
     Pyelonephritis (chronic) associated with anomaly of pyeloureteric junction
     Pyelonephritis (chronic) associated with crossing of vessel
     Pyelonephritis (chronic) associated with kinking of ureter
     Pyelonephritis (chronic) associated with obstruction of ureter
     Pyelonephritis (chronic) associated with stricture of pelviureteric junction
     Pyelonephritis (chronic) associated with stricture of ureter
       EXCLUDES 1   *calculous pyelonephritis (N20.9)*
               obstructive uropathy (N13.-)

N11.8 Other chronic tubulo-interstitial nephritis
     Nonobstructive chronic pyelonephritis NOS

N11.9 Chronic tubulo-interstitial nephritis, unspecified ▽
     Chronic interstitial nephritis NOS
     Chronic pyelitis NOS
     Chronic pyelonephritis NOS

N12 Tubulo-interstitial nephritis, not specified as acute or chronic
     Interstitial nephritis NOS
     Pyelitis NOS
     Pyelonephritis NOS
       EXCLUDES 1   *calculous pyelonephritis (N20.9)*

✓4ᵗʰ N13   Obstructive and reflux uropathy

> **EXCLUDES 2**   calculus of kidney and ureter without hydronephrosis (N20.-)
> congenital obstructive defects of renal pelvis and ureter (Q62.0-Q62.3)
> hydronephrosis with ureteropelvic junction obstruction (Q62.11)
> obstructive pyelonephritis (N11.1)

DEF: Hydronephrosis: Distension of the kidney caused by an accumulation of urine that cannot flow out due to an obstruction that may be caused by conditions such as kidney stones or vesicoureteral reflux.

N13.0   Hydronephrosis with ureteropelvic junction obstruction
Hydronephrosis due to acquired occlusion of ureteropelvic junction

> **EXCLUDES 2**   hydronephrosis with ureteropelvic junction obstruction due to calculus (N13.2)

AHA: 2016,4Q,43

Hydronephrosis/UPJ Obstruction

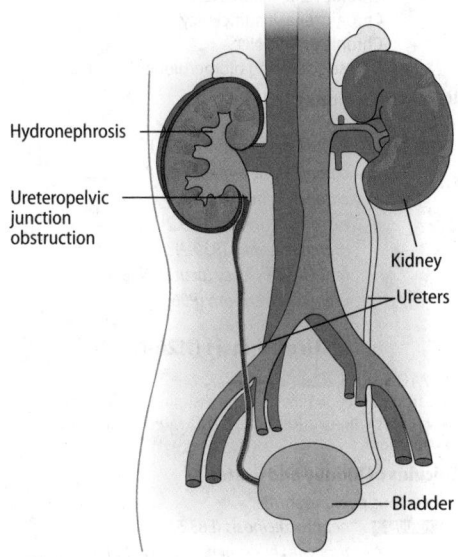

Hydronephrosis

Ureteropelvic junction obstruction

Kidney

Ureters

Bladder

N13.1   Hydronephrosis with ureteral stricture, not elsewhere classified
> **EXCLUDES 1**   hydronephrosis with ureteral stricture with infection (N13.6)

N13.2   Hydronephrosis with renal and ureteral calculous obstruction
> **EXCLUDES 1**   hydronephrosis with renal and ureteral calculous obstruction with infection (N13.6)

✓5ᵗʰ N13.3   Other and unspecified hydronephrosis
> **EXCLUDES 1**   hydronephrosis with infection (N13.6)

N13.30   Unspecified hydronephrosis   ▽
N13.39   Other hydronephrosis

N13.4   Hydroureter
> **EXCLUDES 1**   congenital hydroureter (Q62.3-)
> hydroureter with infection (N13.6)
> vesicoureteral-reflux with hydroureter (N13.73-)

DEF: Abnormal enlargement or distension of the ureter with water or urine caused by an obstruction.

N13.5   Crossing vessel and stricture of ureter without hydronephrosis
Kinking and stricture of ureter without hydronephrosis
> **EXCLUDES 1**   crossing vessel and stricture of ureter without hydronephrosis with infection (N13.6)

N13.6   Pyonephrosis
Conditions in N13.0-N13.5 with infection
Obstructive uropathy with infection
Use additional code (B95-B97), to identify infectious agent
AHA: 2018,2Q,21

✓5ᵗʰ N13.7   Vesicoureteral-reflux

> **EXCLUDES 1**   reflux-associated pyelonephritis (N11.0)

DEF: Urine passage from the bladder flows backward up into the ureter and kidneys that can lead to bacterial infection and an increase in hydrostatic pressure, causing kidney damage.

Vesicoureteral Reflux

Kidneys

Ureters

Bladder

Normal flow of urine   Urine flowing the wrong way (VUR)

N13.70   Vesicoureteral-reflux, unspecified   ▽
Vesicoureteral-reflux NOS
N13.71   Vesicoureteral-reflux without reflux nephropathy
✓6ᵗʰ N13.72   Vesicoureteral-reflux with reflux nephropathy without hydroureter
N13.721   Vesicoureteral-reflux with reflux nephropathy without hydroureter, unilateral
N13.722   Vesicoureteral-reflux with reflux nephropathy without hydroureter, bilateral
N13.729   Vesicoureteral-reflux with reflux nephropathy without hydroureter, unspecified   ▽
✓6ᵗʰ N13.73   Vesicoureteral-reflux with reflux nephropathy with hydroureter
N13.731   Vesicoureteral-reflux with reflux nephropathy with hydroureter, unilateral
N13.732   Vesicoureteral-reflux with reflux nephropathy with hydroureter, bilateral
N13.739   Vesicoureteral-reflux with reflux nephropathy with hydroureter, unspecified   ▽

N13.8   Other obstructive and reflux uropathy
Urinary tract obstruction due to specified cause
Code first, if applicable, any causal condition, such as:
   enlarged prostate (N40.1)

N13.9   Obstructive and reflux uropathy, unspecified   ▽
Urinary tract obstruction NOS

✓4ᵗʰ N14   Drug- and heavy-metal-induced tubulo-interstitial and tubular conditions
Code first poisoning due to drug or toxin, if applicable (T36-T65 with fifth or sixth character 1-4 or 6)
Use additional code for adverse effect, if applicable, to identify drug (T36-T50 with fifth or sixth character 5)

N14.0   Analgesic nephropathy
N14.1   Nephropathy induced by other drugs, medicaments and biological substances
N14.2   Nephropathy induced by unspecified drug, medicament or biological substance   ▽
N14.3   Nephropathy induced by heavy metals
N14.4   Toxic nephropathy, not elsewhere classified

✓4ᵗʰ N15   Other renal tubulo-interstitial diseases

N15.0   Balkan nephropathy
Balkan endemic nephropathy

N15.1   Renal and perinephric abscess
N15.8   Other specified renal tubulo-interstitial diseases
N15.9   Renal tubulo-interstitial disease, unspecified   ▽
Infection of kidney NOS
> **EXCLUDES 1**   urinary tract infection NOS (N39.0)

☑ Additional Character Req   ✓x7ᵗʰ Placeholder Alert   **Manifestation**   ▽ Unspecified   ▶◀ Revised Text   ● New Code   ▲ Revised Code Title

ICD-10-CM 2019   831

N16   *Renal tubulo-interstitial disorders in diseases classified elsewhere*
Pyelonephritis
Tubulo-interstitial nephritis
Code first underlying disease, such as:
    brucellosis (A23.0-A23.9)
    cryoglobulinemia (D89.1)
    glycogen storage disease (E74.0)
    leukemia (C91-C95)
    lymphoma (C81.0-C85.9, C96.0-C96.9)
    multiple myeloma (C90.0-)
    sepsis (A40.0-A41.9)
    Wilson's disease (E83.0)

    EXCLUDES 1   *diphtheritic pyelonephritis and tubulo-interstitial nephritis (A36.84)*
        pyelonephritis and tubulo-interstitial nephritis in candidiasis (B37.49)
        pyelonephritis and tubulo-interstitial nephritis in cystinosis (E72.04)
        pyelonephritis and tubulo-interstitial nephritis in salmonella infection (A02.25)
        pyelonephritis and tubulo-interstitial nephritis in sarcoidosis (D86.84)
        pyelonephritis and tubulo-interstitial nephritis in sicca syndrome [Sjogren's] (M35.04)
        pyelonephritis and tubulo-interstitial nephritis in systemic lupus erythematosus (M32.15)
        pyelonephritis and tubulo-interstitial nephritis in toxoplasmosis (B58.83)
        renal tubular degeneration in diabetes (E08-E13 with .29)
        syphilitic pyelonephritis and tubulo-interstitial nephritis (A52.75)

Acute kidney failure and chronic kidney disease (N17-N19)

    EXCLUDES 2   *congenital renal failure (P96.0)*
        drug- and heavy-metal-induced tubulo-interstitial and tubular conditions (N14.-)
        extrarenal uremia (R39.2)
        hemolytic-uremic syndrome (D59.3)
        hepatorenal syndrome (K76.7)
        postpartum hepatorenal syndrome (O90.4)
        posttraumatic renal failure (T79.5)
        prerenal uremia (R39.2)
        renal failure complicating abortion or ectopic or molar pregnancy (O00-O07, O08.4)
        renal failure following labor and delivery (O90.4)
        renal failure postprocedural (N99.0)

✓4ᵗʰ N17   **Acute kidney failure**
Code also associated underlying condition
    EXCLUDES 1   *posttraumatic renal failure (T79.5)*
AHA: 2013,4Q,124

  N17.0   **Acute kidney failure with tubular necrosis**   HCC
    Acute tubular necrosis
    Renal tubular necrosis
    Tubular necrosis NOS

  N17.1   **Acute kidney failure with acute cortical necrosis**   HCC
    Acute cortical necrosis
    Cortical necrosis NOS
    Renal cortical necrosis

  N17.2   **Acute kidney failure with medullary necrosis**   HCC
    Medullary [papillary] necrosis NOS
    Acute medullary [papillary] necrosis
    Renal medullary [papillary] necrosis

  N17.8   **Other acute kidney failure**   HCC

  N17.9   **Acute kidney failure, unspecified**   HCC ▽
    Acute kidney injury (nontraumatic)
    EXCLUDES 2   *traumatic kidney injury (S37.0-)*

✓4ᵗʰ N18   **Chronic kidney disease (CKD)**
Code first any associated:
    diabetic chronic kidney disease (E08.22, E09.22, E10.22, E11.22, E13.22)
    hypertensive chronic kidney disease (I12.-, I13.-)
Use additional code to identify kidney transplant status, if applicable, (Z94.0)
AHA: 2013,1Q,24
TIP: CKD/ESRD occurring in an individual with a history of kidney transplant should not be assumed to be a transplant complication unless specifically indicated as such by provider documentation.

  N18.1   **Chronic kidney disease, stage 1**

  N18.2   **Chronic kidney disease, stage 2 (mild)**

  N18.3   **Chronic kidney disease, stage 3 (moderate)**

  N18.4   **Chronic kidney disease, stage 4 (severe)**   HCC

  N18.5   **Chronic kidney disease, stage 5**   HCC
    EXCLUDES 1   *chronic kidney disease, stage 5 requiring chronic dialysis (N18.6)*
    DEF: End-stage renal disease (ESRD) with a GFR value of 15 ml/min or less not yet requiring chronic dialysis.
    TIP: When both ESRD and CKD 5 are documented, code only for ESRD.

  N18.6   **End stage renal disease**   HCC
    Chronic kidney disease requiring chronic dialysis
    Use additional code to identify dialysis status (Z99.2)
    AHA: 2016,3Q,22; 2016,1Q,12; 2013,4Q,124-125
    TIP: When both ESRD and CKD 5 are documented, code only for ESRD.

  N18.9   **Chronic kidney disease, unspecified**   ▽
    Chronic renal disease
    Chronic renal failure NOS
    Chronic renal insufficiency
    Chronic uremia NOS
    Diffuse sclerosing glomerulonephritis NOS

N19   **Unspecified kidney failure**   ▽
Uremia NOS
    EXCLUDES 1   *acute kidney failure (N17.-)*
        chronic kidney disease (N18.-)
        chronic uremia (N18.9)
        extrarenal uremia (R39.2)
        prerenal uremia (R39.2)
        renal insufficiency (acute) (N28.9)
        uremia of newborn (P96.0)

Urolithiasis (N20-N23)

AHA: 2017,1Q,5; 2015,2Q,8
TIP: Codes from this code block can be assigned based on the diagnosis listed in a radiology report when authenticated by a radiologist and available at the time of code assignment.

✓4ᵗʰ N20   **Calculus of kidney and ureter**
Calculous pyelonephritis
    EXCLUDES 1   *nephrocalcinosis (E83.5)*
        that with hydronephrosis (N13.2)

  N20.0   **Calculus of kidney**
    Nephrolithiasis NOS
    Renal calculus
    Renal stone
    Staghorn calculus
    Stone in kidney

  N20.1   **Calculus of ureter**
    Ureteric stone
    AHA: 2016,3Q,22

  N20.2   **Calculus of kidney with calculus of ureter**

  N20.9   **Urinary calculus, unspecified**   ▽

✓4ᵗʰ N21   **Calculus of lower urinary tract**
Calculus of lower urinary tract with cystitis and urethritis

  N21.0   **Calculus in bladder**
    Calculus in diverticulum of bladder
    Urinary bladder stone
    EXCLUDES 2   *staghorn calculus (N20.0)*

  N21.1   **Calculus in urethra**
    EXCLUDES 2   *calculus of prostate (N42.0)*

  N21.8   **Other lower urinary tract calculus**

  N21.9   **Calculus of lower urinary tract, unspecified**   ▽
    EXCLUDES 1   *calculus of urinary tract NOS (N20.9)*

N22   *Calculus of urinary tract in diseases classified elsewhere*
Code first underlying disease, such as:
    gout (M1A.-, M10.-)
    schistosomiasis (B65.0-B65.9)

N23   **Unspecified renal colic**   ▽

Other disorders of kidney and ureter (N25-N29)

EXCLUDES 2   *disorders of kidney and ureter with urolithiasis (N20-N23)*

√4ᵗʰ **N25 Disorders resulting from impaired renal tubular function**

N25.0 Renal osteodystrophy
Azotemic osteodystrophy
Phosphate-losing tubular disorders
Renal rickets
Renal short stature
EXCLUDES 2   *metabolic disorders classifiable to E70-E88*
DEF: Various bone diseases occurring when kidney function is impaired or fails. Abnormal levels of phosphorous and calcium can lead to osteomalacia, osteoporosis, or osteosclerosis.

N25.1 Nephrogenic diabetes insipidus   HCC
EXCLUDES 1   *diabetes insipidus NOS (E23.2)*
DEF: Type of diabetes due to the inability of renal tubules to reabsorb water back into the body. It is not responsive to vasopressin (antidiuretic hormone) and it is characterized by excessive thirst and excessive urine production. It may develop into chronic renal insufficiency.

√5ᵗʰ **N25.8 Other disorders resulting from impaired renal tubular function**

N25.81 Secondary hyperparathyroidism of renal origin   HCC
EXCLUDES 1   *secondary hyperparathyroidism, non-renal (E21.1)*
EXCLUDES 2   *metabolic disorders classifiable to E70-E88*
DEF: Parathyroid dysfunction caused by chronic renal failure. Phosphate clearance and vitamin D production is impaired resulting in lowered calcium blood levels and an excessive production of parathyroid hormone.

N25.89 Other disorders resulting from impaired renal tubular function
Hypokalemic nephropathy
Lightwood-Albright syndrome
Renal tubular acidosis NOS

N25.9 Disorder resulting from impaired renal tubular function, unspecified   ▽

√4ᵗʰ **N26 Unspecified contracted kidney**
EXCLUDES 1   *contracted kidney due to hypertension (I12.-)*
diffuse sclerosing glomerulonephritis (N05.8.-)
hypertensive nephrosclerosis (arteriolar) (arteriosclerotic) (I12.-)
small kidney of unknown cause (N27.-)

N26.1 Atrophy of kidney (terminal)
N26.2 Page kidney
N26.9 Renal sclerosis, unspecified   ▽

√4ᵗʰ **N27 Small kidney of unknown cause**
INCLUDES   oligonephronia
N27.0 Small kidney, unilateral
N27.1 Small kidney, bilateral
N27.9 Small kidney, unspecified   ▽

√4ᵗʰ **N28 Other disorders of kidney and ureter, not elsewhere classified**

N28.0 Ischemia and infarction of kidney   HCC
Renal artery embolism
Renal artery obstruction
Renal artery occlusion
Renal artery thrombosis
Renal infarct
EXCLUDES 1   *atherosclerosis of renal artery (extrarenal part) (I70.1)*
congenital stenosis of renal artery (Q27.1)
Goldblatt's kidney (I70.1)

N28.1 Cyst of kidney, acquired
Cyst (multiple) (solitary) of kidney (acquired)
EXCLUDES 1   *cystic kidney disease (congenital) (Q61.-)*

√5ᵗʰ **N28.8 Other specified disorders of kidney and ureter**
EXCLUDES 1   *hydroureter (N13.4)*
ureteric stricture with hydronephrosis (N13.1)
ureteric stricture without hydronephrosis (N13.5)

N28.81 Hypertrophy of kidney
N28.82 Megaloureter
N28.83 Nephroptosis
N28.84 Pyelitis cystica
N28.85 Pyeloureteritis cystica
N28.86 Ureteritis cystica
N28.89 Other specified disorders of kidney and ureter

N28.9 Disorder of kidney and ureter, unspecified   ▽
Nephropathy NOS
Renal disease (acute) NOS
Renal insufficiency (acute)
EXCLUDES 1   *chronic renal insufficiency (N18.9)*
unspecified nephritic syndrome (N05.-)
AHA: 2016,1Q,13

N29 Other disorders of kidney and ureter in diseases classified elsewhere
Code first underlying disease, such as:
amyloidosis (E85.-)
nephrocalcinosis (E83.5)
schistosomiasis (B65.0-B65.9)
EXCLUDES 1   *disorders of kidney and ureter in:*
cystinosis (E72.0)
gonorrhea (A54.21)
syphilis (A52.75)
tuberculosis (A18.11)

Other diseases of the urinary system (N30-N39)

EXCLUDES 1   *urinary infection (complicating):*
abortion or ectopic or molar pregnancy (O00-O07, O08.8)
pregnancy, childbirth and the puerperium (O23.-, O75.3, O86.2-)

√4ᵗʰ **N30 Cystitis**
Use additional code to identify infectious agent (B95-B97)
EXCLUDES 1   *prostatocystitis (N41.3)*
AHA: 2017,1Q,6
DEF: Inflammation of the urinary bladder. Symptoms include dysuria, frequency of urination, urgency, and hematuria.

√5ᵗʰ **N30.0 Acute cystitis**
EXCLUDES 1   *irradiation cystitis (N30.4-)*
trigonitis (N30.3-)
N30.00 Acute cystitis without hematuria
N30.01 Acute cystitis with hematuria

√5ᵗʰ **N30.1 Interstitial cystitis (chronic)**
N30.10 Interstitial cystitis (chronic) without hematuria
N30.11 Interstitial cystitis (chronic) with hematuria

√5ᵗʰ **N30.2 Other chronic cystitis**
N30.20 Other chronic cystitis without hematuria
N30.21 Other chronic cystitis with hematuria

√5ᵗʰ **N30.3 Trigonitis**
Urethrotrigonitis
N30.30 Trigonitis without hematuria
N30.31 Trigonitis with hematuria

√5ᵗʰ **N30.4 Irradiation cystitis**
N30.40 Irradiation cystitis without hematuria
N30.41 Irradiation cystitis with hematuria

√5ᵗʰ **N30.8 Other cystitis**
Abscess of bladder
N30.80 Other cystitis without hematuria
N30.81 Other cystitis with hematuria

√5ᵗʰ **N30.9 Cystitis, unspecified**
N30.90 Cystitis, unspecified without hematuria   ▽
N30.91 Cystitis, unspecified with hematuria   ▽

√4ᵗʰ **N31 Neuromuscular dysfunction of bladder, not elsewhere classified**
Use additional code to identify any associated urinary incontinence (N39.3-N39.4-)
EXCLUDES 1   *cord bladder NOS (G95.89)*
neurogenic bladder due to cauda equina syndrome (G83.4)
neuromuscular dysfunction due to spinal cord lesion (G95.89)

N31.0 Uninhibited neuropathic bladder, not elsewhere classified
N31.1 Reflex neuropathic bladder, not elsewhere classified
N31.2 Flaccid neuropathic bladder, not elsewhere classified
Atonic (motor) (sensory) neuropathic bladder
Autonomous neuropathic bladder
Nonreflex neuropathic bladder
N31.8 Other neuromuscular dysfunction of bladder
N31.9 Neuromuscular dysfunction of bladder, unspecified   ▽
Neurogenic bladder dysfunction NOS

☑ Additional Character Req   √x7ᵗʰ Placeholder Alert   Manifestation   ▽ Unspecified   ▶◀ Revised Text   ● New Code   ▲ Revised Code Title

☑4ᵗʰ **N32 Other disorders of bladder**

     EXCLUDES 2   calculus of bladder (N21.0)

           cystocele (N81.1-)

           hernia or prolapse of bladder, female (N81.1-)

N32.0 Bladder-neck obstruction

     Bladder-neck stenosis (acquired)

     EXCLUDES 1   congenital bladder-neck obstruction (Q64.3-)

     DEF: Bladder outlet and vesicourethral obstruction that occurs as a consequence of benign prostatic hypertrophy or prostatic cancer. It may also occur in either sex due to strictures, radiation, cystoscopy, catheterization, injury, infection, blood clots, bladder cancer, impaction, or other disease that compresses the bladder neck.

N32.1 Vesicointestinal fistula

     Vesicorectal fistula

N32.2 Vesical fistula, not elsewhere classified

     EXCLUDES 1   fistula between bladder and female genital tract (N82.0-N82.1)

N32.3 Diverticulum of bladder

     EXCLUDES 1   congenital diverticulum of bladder (Q64.6)

           diverticulitis of bladder (N30.8-)

☑5ᵗʰ **N32.8 Other specified disorders of bladder**

     N32.81 Overactive bladder

         Detrusor muscle hyperactivity

         EXCLUDES 1   frequent urination due to specified bladder condition — code to condition

         DEF: Sudden involuntary contractions of the muscular wall of the bladder that results in a sudden, strong urge to urinate.

     N32.89 Other specified disorders of bladder

         Bladder hemorrhage

         Bladder hypertrophy

         Calcified bladder

         Contracted bladder

N32.9 Bladder disorder, unspecified   ▽

N33 *Bladder disorders in diseases classified elsewhere*

     Code first underlying disease, such as:

         schistosomiasis (B65.0-B65.9)

     EXCLUDES 1   bladder disorder in syphilis (A52.76)

           bladder disorder in tuberculosis (A18.12)

           candidal cystitis (B37.41)

           chlamydial cystitis (A56.01)

           cystitis in gonorrhea (A54.01)

           cystitis in neurogenic bladder (N31.-)

           diphtheritic cystitis (A36.85)

           neurogenic bladder (N31.-)

           syphilitic cystitis (A52.76)

           trichomonal cystitis (A59.03)

☑4ᵗʰ **N34 Urethritis and urethral syndrome**

     Use additional code (B95-B97), to identify infectious agent

     EXCLUDES 2   Reiter's disease (M02.3-)

           urethritis in diseases with a predominantly sexual mode of transmission (A50-A64)

           urethrotrigonitis (N30.3-)

     AHA: 2017,1Q,6

N34.0 Urethral abscess

     Abscess (of) Cowper's gland

     Abscess (of) Littré's gland

     Abscess (of) urethral (gland)

     Periurethral abscess

     EXCLUDES 1   urethral caruncle (N36.2)

N34.1 Nonspecific urethritis

     Nongonococcal urethritis

     Nonvenereal urethritis

N34.2 Other urethritis

     Meatitis, urethral

     Postmenopausal urethritis

     Ulcer of urethra (meatus)

     Urethritis NOS

N34.3 Urethral syndrome, unspecified   ▽

☑4ᵗʰ **N35 Urethral stricture**

     EXCLUDES 1   congenital urethral stricture (Q64.3-)

           postprocedural urethral stricture (N99.1-)

☑5ᵗʰ **N35.0 Post-traumatic urethral stricture**

     Urethral stricture due to injury

     EXCLUDES 1   postprocedural urethral stricture (N99.1-)

     ☑6ᵗʰ **N35.01 Post-traumatic urethral stricture, male**

         N35.010 Post-traumatic urethral stricture, male, meatal   ♂

         N35.011 Post-traumatic bulbous urethral stricture   ♂

         N35.012 Post-traumatic membranous urethral stricture   ♂

         N35.013 Post-traumatic anterior urethral stricture   ♂

         N35.014 Post-traumatic urethral stricture, male, unspecified   ♂ ▽

         ● **N35.016 Post-traumatic urethral stricture, male, overlapping sites**

     ☑6ᵗʰ **N35.02 Post-traumatic urethral stricture, female**

         N35.021 Urethral stricture due to childbirth   ♀

         N35.028 Other post-traumatic urethral stricture, female   ♀

☑5ᵗʰ **N35.1 Postinfective urethral stricture, not elsewhere classified**

     EXCLUDES 1   gonococcal urethral stricture (A54.01)

           syphilitic urethral stricture (A52.76)

           urethral stricture associated with schistosomiasis (B65.-, N29)

     ☑6ᵗʰ **N35.11 Postinfective urethral stricture, not elsewhere classified, male**

         N35.111 Postinfective urethral stricture, not elsewhere classified, male, meatal   ♂

         N35.112 Postinfective bulbous urethral stricture, not elsewhere classified, male   ♂

         N35.113 Postinfective membranous urethral stricture, not elsewhere classified, male   ♂

         N35.114 Postinfective anterior urethral stricture, not elsewhere classified, male   ♂

         ● **N35.116 Postinfective urethral stricture, not elsewhere classified, male, overlapping sites**

         N35.119 Postinfective urethral stricture, not elsewhere classified, male, unspecified   ♂ ▽

     N35.12 Postinfective urethral stricture, not elsewhere classified, female   ♀

☑5ᵗʰ **N35.8 Other urethral stricture**

     EXCLUDES 1   postprocedural urethral stricture (N99.1-)

     ● ☑6ᵗʰ **N35.81 Other urethral stricture, male**

         ● **N35.811 Other urethral stricture, male, meatal**

         ● **N35.812 Other urethral bulbous stricture, male**

         ● **N35.813 Other membranous urethral stricture, male**

         ● **N35.814 Other anterior urethral stricture, male, anterior**

         ● **N35.816 Other urethral stricture, male, overlapping sites**

         N35.819 Other urethral stricture, male, unspecified site   ▽

     ● **N35.82 Other urethral stricture, female**

☑5ᵗʰ **N35.9 Urethral stricture, unspecified**

     ● ☑6ᵗʰ **N35.91 Urethral stricture, unspecified, male**

         ● **N35.911 Unspecified urethral stricture, male, meatal**   ▽

         ● **N35.912 Unspecified bulbous urethral stricture, male**   ▽

         ● **N35.913 Unspecified membranous urethral stricture, male**   ▽

         ● **N35.914 Unspecified anterior urethral stricture, male**   ▽

         ● **N35.916 Unspecified urethral stricture, male, overlapping sites**   ▽

HCC CMS-HCC   Q QPP   N Newborn : 0   P Pediatric : 0-17   M Maternity : 12-55   A Adult : 15-124

●   **N35.919** **Unspecified urethral stricture,** ▽
                male, unspecified site
                Pinhole meatus NOS
                Urethral stricture NOS

●   **N35.92** **Unspecified urethral stricture, female** ▽

✓4ᵗʰ **N36** **Other disorders of urethra**

    N36.0 **Urethral** *fistula*
        Urethroperineal fistula
        Urethrorectal fistula
        Urinary fistula NOS
        EXCLUDES 1   urethroscrotal fistula (N50.89)
                urethrovaginal fistula (N82.1)
                urethrovesicovaginal fistula (N82.1)

    N36.1 **Urethral** *diverticulum*

    N36.2 **Urethral** *caruncle*

✓5ᵗʰ **N36.4** **Urethral** *functional and muscular disorders*
        Use additional code to identify associated urinary stress
          incontinence (N39.3)
        N36.41 **Hypermobility of urethra**
        N36.42 **Intrinsic sphincter deficiency (ISD)**
        N36.43 **Combined hypermobility of urethra and intrinsic
                 sphincter deficiency**
        N36.44 **Muscular disorders of urethra**
             Bladder sphincter dyssynergy

    N36.5 **Urethral** *false passage*

    N36.8 **Other specified disorders of urethra**
        EXCLUDES 1   congenital urethrocele (Q64.7)
                female urethrocele (N81.0)

    N36.9 **Urethral disorder, unspecified** ▽

N37 *Urethral disorders in diseases classified elsewhere*
    Code first underlying disease
    EXCLUDES 1   urethritis (in):
             candidal infection (B37.41)
             chlamydial (A56.01)
             gonorrhea (A54.01)
             syphilis (A52.76)
             trichomonal infection (A59.03)
             tuberculosis (A18.13)

✓4ᵗʰ **N39** **Other disorders of urinary system**
    EXCLUDES 2   hematuria NOS (R31.-)
             recurrent or persistent hematuria (N02.-)
             recurrent or persistent hematuria with specified
                morphological lesion (N02.-)
             proteinuria NOS (R80.-)

    N39.0 **Urinary tract infection, site not specified** ▽
        Use additional code (B95-B97), to identify infectious agent
        EXCLUDES 1   candidiasis of urinary tract (B37.4-)
              neonatal urinary tract infection (P39.3)
              urinary tract infection of specified site, such as:
                cystitis (N30.-)
                urethritis (N34.-)
        AHA: 2018,2Q,21,22; 2018,1Q,16; 2017,1Q,6; 2012,4Q,94

    N39.3 **Stress incontinence (female) (male)** ⓪
        Code also any associated overactive bladder (N32.81)
        EXCLUDES 1   mixed incontinence (N39.46)

✓5ᵗʰ **N39.4** **Other specified urinary incontinence**
        Code also any associated overactive bladder (N32.81)
        EXCLUDES 1   enuresis NOS (R32)
              functional urinary incontinence (R39.81)
              urinary incontinence associated with cognitive
                impairment (R39.81)
              urinary incontinence NOS (R32)
              urinary incontinence of nonorganic origin (F98.0)
        N39.41 **Urge incontinence** ⓪
            EXCLUDES 1   mixed incontinence (N39.46)
        N39.42 **Incontinence without sensory awareness** ⓪
            Insensible (urinary) incontinence
        N39.43 **Post-void dribbling** ⓪
        N39.44 **Nocturnal enuresis** ⓪
        N39.45 **Continuous leakage** ⓪
        N39.46 **Mixed incontinence** ⓪
            Urge and stress incontinence

✓6ᵗʰ **N39.49** **Other specified urinary incontinence**
        AHA: 2016,4Q,44
        N39.490 **Overflow incontinence** ⓪
        N39.491 **Coital incontinence** ⓪
        N39.492 **Postural (urinary) incontinence** ⓪
        N39.498 **Other specified urinary
              incontinence**
            Reflex incontinence
            Total incontinence

    N39.8 **Other specified disorders of urinary system**

    N39.9 **Disorder of urinary system, unspecified** ▽

Diseases of male genital organs (N40-N53)

✓4ᵗʰ **N40** **Benign prostatic hyperplasia**
    INCLUDES   adenofibromatous hypertrophy of prostate
             benign hypertrophy of the prostate
             benign prostatic hypertrophy
             BPH
             enlarged prostate
             nodular prostate
             polyp of prostate
    EXCLUDES 1   *benign neoplasms of prostate (adenoma, benign)
             (fibroadenoma) (fibroma) (myoma) (D29.1)*
    EXCLUDES 2   *malignant neoplasm of prostate (C61)*
    DEF: Enlargement of the prostate gland due to an abnormal proliferation
    of fibrostromal tissue in the paraurethral glands. This condition causes
    impingement of the urethra resulting in obstructed urinary flow.

    N40.0 **Benign prostatic hyperplasia without lower urinary** 🅰 ♂
        tract symptoms
        Enlarged prostate NOS
        Enlarged prostate without LUTS

    N40.1 **Benign prostatic hyperplasia with lower urinary tract** 🅰 ♂
        symptoms
        Enlarged prostate with LUTS
        Use additional code for associated symptoms, when specified:
          incomplete bladder emptying (R39.14)
          nocturia (R35.1)
          straining on urination (R39.16)
          urinary frequency (R35.0)
          urinary hesitancy (R39.11)
          urinary incontinence (N39.4-)
          urinary obstruction (N13.8)
          urinary retention (R33.8)
          urinary urgency (R39.15)
          weak urinary stream (R39.12)

    N40.2 **Nodular prostate without lower urinary tract** 🅰 ♂
        symptoms
        Nodular prostate without LUTS

    N40.3 **Nodular prostate with lower urinary tract symptoms** 🅰 ♂
        Use additional code for associated symptoms, when specified:
          incomplete bladder emptying (R39.14)
          nocturia (R35.1)
          straining on urination (R39.16)
          urinary frequency (R35.0)
          urinary hesitancy (R39.11)
          urinary incontinence (N39.4-)
          urinary obstruction (N13.8)
          urinary retention (R33.8)
          urinary urgency (R39.15)
          weak urinary stream (R39.12)

✓4ᵗʰ **N41** **Inflammatory diseases of prostate**
    Use additional code (B95-B97), to identify infectious agent
    N41.0 **Acute prostatitis** 🅰 ♂
    N41.1 **Chronic prostatitis** 🅰 ♂
    N41.2 **Abscess of prostate** 🅰 ♂
    N41.3 **Prostatocystitis** 🅰 ♂
    N41.4 **Granulomatous prostatitis** 🅰 ♂
    N41.8 **Other inflammatory diseases of prostate** 🅰 ♂
    N41.9 **Inflammatory disease of prostate, unspecified** 🅰 ♂ ▽
        Prostatitis NOS

✓4ᵗʰ **N42** **Other and unspecified disorders of prostate**
    N42.0 **Calculus of prostate** 🅰 ♂
        Prostatic stone
        DEF: Formation of a small, solid stone often composed of calcium
        carbonate or calcium phosphate in the prostate gland.

☑ Additional Character Req   ✓7ᵗʰ Placeholder Alert   Manifestation   ▽ Unspecified   ►◄ Revised Text   ● New Code   ▲ Revised Code Title

ICD-10-CM 2019   **835**

Chapter 14. Diseases of the Genitourinary System

N42.1   **Congestion and hemorrhage of prostate**   A ♂
> EXCLUDES 1   enlarged prostate (N40.-)
> hematuria (R31.-)
> hyperplasia of prostate (N40.-)
> inflammatory diseases of prostate (N41.-)

✓5ᵗʰ **N42.3**   **Dysplasia of prostate**
> **AHA:** 2016,4Q,44

   N42.30   **Unspecified dysplasia of prostate**   ♂ ▽
   N42.31   **Prostatic intraepithelial neoplasia**   ♂
> PIN
> Prostatic intraepithelial neoplasia I (PIN I)
> Prostatic intraepithelial neoplasia II (PIN II)
> EXCLUDES 1   prostatic intraepithelial neoplasia III (PIN III) (D07.5)
> **DEF:** Abnormality of shape and size of the intraepithelial tissues of the prostate. It is a premalignant condition characterized by stalks and absence of a basilar cell layer.

   N42.32   **Atypical small acinar proliferation of prostate**   ♂
   N42.39   **Other dysplasia of prostate**   ♂

✓5ᵗʰ **N42.8**   **Other specified disorders of prostate**
   N42.81   **Prostatodynia syndrome**   A ♂
> Painful prostate syndrome

   N42.82   **Prostatosis syndrome**   A ♂
   N42.83   **Cyst of prostate**   A ♂
   N42.89   **Other specified disorders of prostate**   A ♂
N42.9   **Disorder of prostate, unspecified**   A ♂ ▽

✓4ᵗʰ **N43**   **Hydrocele and spermatocele**
> INCLUDES   hydrocele of spermatic cord, testis or tunica vaginalis
> EXCLUDES 1   congenital hydrocele (P83.5)
> **DEF:** Hydrocele: Serous fluid that collects in the tunica vaginalis of the scrotum along the spermatic cord in males.

N43.0   **Encysted hydrocele**   ♂
N43.1   **Infected hydrocele**   ♂
> Use additional code (B95-B97), to identify infectious agent

N43.2   **Other hydrocele**   ♂

Hydrocele

Normal   Noncommunicating hydrocele   Communicating hydrocele   Hydrocele of the cord

N43.3   **Hydrocele, unspecified**   ♂ ▽
✓5ᵗʰ **N43.4**   **Spermatocele of epididymis**
> Spermatic cyst
> **DEF:** Spermatocele: Noncancerous accumulation of fluid and dead sperm cells normally located at the head of the epididymis that exhibits itself as a hard, smooth scrotal mass and do not normally require treatment unless they become enlarged or cause pain.

   N43.40   **Spermatocele of epididymis, unspecified**   ♂ ▽
   N43.41   **Spermatocele of epididymis, single**   ♂
   N43.42   **Spermatocele of epididymis, multiple**   ♂

✓4ᵗʰ **N44**   **Noninflammatory disorders of testis**
✓5ᵗʰ **N44.0**   **Torsion of testis**
   N44.00   **Torsion of testis, unspecified**   ♂ ▽
   N44.01   **Extravaginal torsion of spermatic cord**   ♂
> **DEF:** Torsion of the spermatic cord just below the tunica vaginalis attachments.

   N44.02   **Intravaginal torsion of spermatic cord**   ♂
> Torsion of spermatic cord NOS

   N44.03   **Torsion of appendix testis**   ♂
   N44.04   **Torsion of appendix epididymis**   ♂
N44.1   **Cyst of tunica albuginea testis**   ♂

N44.2   **Benign cyst of testis**   ♂
N44.8   **Other noninflammatory disorders of the testis**   ♂

✓4ᵗʰ **N45**   **Orchitis and epididymitis**
> Use additional code (B95-B97), to identify infectious agent

N45.1   **Epididymitis**   ♂
N45.2   **Orchitis**   ♂
N45.3   **Epididymo-orchitis**   ♂
N45.4   **Abscess of epididymis or testis**   ♂

✓4ᵗʰ **N46**   **Male infertility**
> EXCLUDES 1   vasectomy status (Z98.52)

✓5ᵗʰ **N46.0**   **Azoospermia**
> Absolute male infertility
> Male infertility due to germinal (cell) aplasia
> Male infertility due to spermatogenic arrest (complete)

   N46.01   **Organic azoospermia**   A ♂
> Azoospermia NOS

✓6ᵗʰ   **N46.02**   **Azoospermia due to extratesticular causes**
> Code also associated cause

    N46.021   **Azoospermia due to drug therapy**   A ♂
    N46.022   **Azoospermia due to infection**   A ♂
    N46.023   **Azoospermia due to obstruction of efferent ducts**   A ♂
    N46.024   **Azoospermia due to radiation**   A ♂
    N46.025   **Azoospermia due to systemic disease**   A ♂
    N46.029   **Azoospermia due to other extratesticular causes**   A ♂

✓5ᵗʰ **N46.1**   **Oligospermia**
> Male infertility due to germinal cell desquamation
> Male infertility due to hypospermatogenesis
> Male infertility due to incomplete spermatogenic arrest

   N46.11   **Organic oligospermia**   A ♂
> Oligospermia NOS

✓6ᵗʰ   **N46.12**   **Oligospermia due to extratesticular causes**
> Code also associated cause

    N46.121   **Oligospermia due to drug therapy**   A ♂
    N46.122   **Oligospermia due to infection**   A ♂
    N46.123   **Oligospermia due to obstruction of efferent ducts**   A ♂
    N46.124   **Oligospermia due to radiation**   A ♂
    N46.125   **Oligospermia due to systemic disease**   A ♂
    N46.129   **Oligospermia due to other extratesticular causes**   A ♂

N46.8   **Other male infertility**   A ♂
N46.9   **Male infertility, unspecified**   A ♂ ▽

✓4ᵗʰ **N47**   **Disorders of prepuce**
N47.0   **Adherent prepuce, newborn**   N ♂
N47.1   **Phimosis**   ♂
> **DEF:** Condition in which the foreskin is contracted and cannot be drawn back behind the glans penis.

N47.2   **Paraphimosis**   ♂
N47.3   **Deficient foreskin**   ♂
N47.4   **Benign cyst of prepuce**   ♂
N47.5   **Adhesions of prepuce and glans penis**   ♂
N47.6   **Balanoposthitis**   ♂
> Use additional code (B95-B97), to identify infectious agent
> EXCLUDES 1   balanitis (N48.1)

N47.7   **Other inflammatory diseases of prepuce**   ♂
> Use additional code (B95-B97), to identify infectious agent

N47.8   **Other disorders of prepuce**   ♂

✓4ᵗʰ **N48**   **Other disorders of penis**
N48.0   **Leukoplakia of penis**   ♂
> Balanitis xerotica obliterans
> Kraurosis of penis
> Lichen sclerosus of external male genital organs
> EXCLUDES 1   carcinoma in situ of penis (D07.4)

N48.1 **Balanitis** ♂
Use additional code (B95-B97), to identify infectious agent
> **EXCLUDES 1**   amebic balanitis (A06.8)
> balanitis xerotica obliterans (N48.0)
> candidal balanitis (B37.42)
> gonococcal balanitis (A54.23)
> herpesviral [herpes simplex] balanitis (A60.01)

DEF: Inflammation of the glans penis, most often affecting uncircumcised males.

√5ᵗʰ **N48.2** **Other inflammatory disorders of penis**
Use additional code (B95-B97), to identify infectious agent
> **EXCLUDES 1**   balanitis (N48.1)
> balanitis xerotica obliterans (N48.0)
> balanoposthitis (N47.6)

    N48.21 **Abscess of corpus cavernosum and penis** ♂
    N48.22 **Cellulitis of corpus cavernosum and penis** ♂
    N48.29 **Other inflammatory disorders of penis** ♂

√5ᵗʰ **N48.3** **Priapism**
Painful erection
Code first underlying cause

    N48.30 **Priapism, unspecified** ♂ ▽
    N48.31 **Priapism** due to trauma ♂
    N48.32 *Priapism due to disease classified elsewhere* ♂
    N48.33 **Priapism,** drug-induced ♂
    N48.39 **Other priapism** ♂

N48.5 **Ulcer of penis** ♂
N48.6 **Induration penis plastica** ♂
Peyronie's disease
Plastic induration of penis

√5ᵗʰ **N48.8** **Other specified disorders of penis**
    N48.81 **Thrombosis of superficial vein of penis** ♂
    N48.82 **Acquired torsion of penis** ♂
Acquired torsion of penis NOS
> **EXCLUDES 1**   congenital torsion of penis (Q55.63)

    N48.83 **Acquired buried penis** ♂
> **EXCLUDES 1**   congenital hidden penis (Q55.64)

    N48.89 **Other specified disorders of penis** ♂
N48.9 **Disorder of penis, unspecified** ♂ ▽

√4ᵗʰ **N49** **Inflammatory disorders of male genital organs, not elsewhere classified**
Use additional code (B95-B97), to identify infectious agent
> **EXCLUDES 1**   inflammation of penis (N48.1, N48.2-)
> orchitis and epididymitis (N45.-)

N49.0 **Inflammatory disorders of** seminal vesicle ♂
Vesiculitis NOS
N49.1 **Inflammatory disorders of** spermatic cord, tunica ♂
vaginalis and vas deferens
Vasitis
N49.2 **Inflammatory disorders of** scrotum ♂
N49.3 **Fournier gangrene** ♂
N49.8 **Inflammatory disorders of other specified male** ♂
genital organs
Inflammation of multiple sites in male genital organs
N49.9 **Inflammatory disorder of unspecified male genital** ♂ ▽
organ
Abscess of unspecified male genital organ
Boil of unspecified male genital organ
Carbuncle of unspecified male genital organ
Cellulitis of unspecified male genital organ

√4ᵗʰ **N50** **Other and unspecified disorders of male genital organs**
> **EXCLUDES 2**   torsion of testis (N44.0-)

N50.0 **Atrophy of testis** ♂
N50.1 **Vascular disorders of male genital organs** ♂
Hematocele, NOS, of male genital organs
Hemorrhage of male genital organs
Thrombosis of male genital organs
N50.3 **Cyst of epididymis** ♂
√5ᵗʰ **N50.8** **Other specified disorders of male genital organs**
AHA: 2016,4Q,45
√6ᵗʰ **N50.81** **Testicular pain**
    N50.811 **Right testicular pain** ♂
    N50.812 **Left testicular pain** ♂
    N50.819 **Testicular pain, unspecified** ♂ ▽
    N50.82 **Scrotal pain** ♂

N50.89 **Other specified disorders of the male** ♂
genital organs
Atrophy of scrotum, seminal vesicle, spermatic cord, tunica vaginalis and vas deferens
Chylocele, tunica vaginalis (nonfilarial) NOS
Edema of scrotum, seminal vesicle, spermatic cord, tunica vaginalis and vas deferens
Hypertrophy of scrotum, seminal vesicle, spermatic cord, tunica vaginalis and vas deferens
Stricture of spermatic cord, tunica vaginalis, and vas deferens
Ulcer of scrotum, seminal vesicle, spermatic cord, testis, tunica vaginalis and vas deferens
Urethroscrotal fistula

N50.9 **Disorder of male genital organs, unspecified** ♂ ▽

√ *N51* *Disorders of male genital organs in diseases classified* ♂
elsewhere
Code first underlying disease, such as:
filariasis (B74.0-B74.9)
> **EXCLUDES 1**   amebic balanitis (A06.8)
> candidal balanitis (B37.42)
> gonococcal balanitis (A54.23)
> gonococcal prostatitis (A54.22)
> herpesviral [herpes simplex] balanitis (A60.01)
> trichomonal prostatitis (A59.02)
> tuberculous prostatitis (A18.14)

√4ᵗʰ **N52** **Male erectile dysfunction**
> **EXCLUDES 1**   psychogenic impotence (F52.21)

√5ᵗʰ **N52.0** **Vasculogenic** erectile dysfunction
    N52.01 **Erectile dysfunction due to** arterial 🅐 ♂
insufficiency
    N52.02 **Corporo-venous occlusive** erectile 🅐 ♂
dysfunction
    N52.03 **Combined arterial insufficiency and** 🅐 ♂
corporo-venous occlusive **erectile**
dysfunction

√ *N52.1* *Erectile dysfunction due to diseases classified* 🅐 ♂
elsewhere
Code first underlying disease
N52.2 **Drug-induced** erectile dysfunction 🅐 ♂
√5ᵗʰ **N52.3** **Postprocedural** erectile dysfunction
AHA: 2016,4Q,45
    N52.31 **Erectile dysfunction following** radical 🅐 ♂
prostatectomy
    N52.32 **Erectile dysfunction following** radical 🅐 ♂
cystectomy
    N52.33 **Erectile dysfunction following** urethral 🅐 ♂
surgery
    N52.34 **Erectile dysfunction following** simple 🅐 ♂
prostatectomy
    N52.35 **Erectile dysfunction following** radiation 🅐 ♂
therapy
    N52.36 **Erectile dysfunction following** interstitial 🅐 ♂
seed therapy
    N52.37 **Erectile dysfunction following** prostate 🅐 ♂
ablative therapy
Erectile dysfunction following cryotherapy
Erectile dysfunction following other prostate ablative therapies
Erectile dysfunction following ultrasound ablative therapies
    N52.39 **Other and unspecified postprocedural** 🅐 ♂ ▽
erectile dysfunction
N52.8 **Other male erectile dysfunction** 🅐 ♂
N52.9 **Male erectile dysfunction, unspecified** 🅐 ♂ ▽
Impotence NOS

√4ᵗʰ **N53** **Other male sexual dysfunction**
> **EXCLUDES 1**   psychogenic sexual dysfunction (F52.-)

√5ᵗʰ **N53.1** **Ejaculatory dysfunction**
> **EXCLUDES 1**   premature ejaculation (F52.4)

    N53.11 **Retarded ejaculation** ♂
    N53.12 **Painful ejaculation** ♂
    N53.13 **Anejaculatory orgasm** ♂

☑ Additional Character Req   √x7ᵗʰ Placeholder Alert   Manifestation   ▽ Unspecified   ▶◀ Revised Text   ● New Code   ▲ Revised Code Title

Chapter 14. Diseases of the Genitourinary System

N53.14   **Retrograde ejaculation**   ♂
     DEF: Form of male sexual dysfunction in which the semen enters the bladder instead of going out through the urethra during ejaculation.

N53.19   **Other ejaculatory dysfunction**   ♂
     Ejaculatory dysfunction NOS

N53.8   **Other male sexual dysfunction**   ♂

N53.9   **Unspecified male sexual dysfunction**   ♂ ▽

Disorders of breast (N60-N65)

   EXCLUDES 1   disorders of breast associated with childbirth (O91-O92)

√4ᵗ **N60**   **Benign mammary dysplasia**
     INCLUDES   fibrocystic mastopathy

√5ᵗ **N60.0**   **Solitary cyst of breast**
     Cyst of breast
     N60.01   **Solitary cyst of right breast**
     N60.02   **Solitary cyst of left breast**
     N60.09   **Solitary cyst of unspecified breast**   ▽

√5ᵗ **N60.1**   **Diffuse cystic mastopathy**
     Cystic breast
     Fibrocystic disease of breast
     EXCLUDES 1   diffuse cystic mastopathy with epithelial proliferation (N60.3-)
     N60.11   **Diffuse cystic mastopathy of right breast**   A
     N60.12   **Diffuse cystic mastopathy of left breast**   A
     N60.19   **Diffuse cystic mastopathy of unspecified breast**   A ▽

√5ᵗ **N60.2**   **Fibroadenosis of breast**
     Adenofibrosis of breast
     EXCLUDES 2   fibroadenoma of breast (D24.-)
     N60.21   **Fibroadenosis of right breast**
     N60.22   **Fibroadenosis of left breast**
     N60.29   **Fibroadenosis of unspecified breast**   ▽

√5ᵗ **N60.3**   **Fibrosclerosis of breast**
     Cystic mastopathy with epithelial proliferation
     N60.31   **Fibrosclerosis of right breast**
     N60.32   **Fibrosclerosis of left breast**
     N60.39   **Fibrosclerosis of unspecified breast**   ▽

√5ᵗ **N60.4**   **Mammary duct ectasia**
     N60.41   **Mammary duct ectasia of right breast**
     N60.42   **Mammary duct ectasia of left breast**
     N60.49   **Mammary duct ectasia of unspecified breast**   ▽

√5ᵗ **N60.8**   **Other benign mammary dysplasias**
     N60.81   **Other benign mammary dysplasias of right breast**
     N60.82   **Other benign mammary dysplasias of left breast**
     N60.89   **Other benign mammary dysplasias of unspecified breast**   ▽

√5ᵗ **N60.9**   **Unspecified benign mammary dysplasia**
     N60.91   **Unspecified benign mammary dysplasia of right breast**   ▽
     N60.92   **Unspecified benign mammary dysplasia of left breast**   ▽
     N60.99   **Unspecified benign mammary dysplasia of unspecified breast**   ▽

√4ᵗ **N61**   **Inflammatory disorders of breast**
     EXCLUDES 1   inflammatory carcinoma of breast (C50.9)
        inflammatory disorder of breast associated with childbirth (O91.-)
        neonatal infective mastitis (P39.0)
        thrombophlebitis of breast [Mondor's disease] (I80.8)

   N61.0   **Mastitis without abscess**
     Infective mastitis (acute) (nonpuerperal) (subacute)
     Mastitis (acute) (nonpuerperal) (subacute) NOS
     Cellulitis (acute) (nonpuerperal) (subacute) of breast NOS
     Cellulitis (acute) (nonpuerperal) (subacute) of nipple NOS

   N61.1   **Abscess of the breast and nipple**
     Abscess (acute) (chronic) (nonpuerperal) of areola
     Abscess (acute) (chronic) (nonpuerperal) of breast
     Carbuncle of breast
     Mastitis with abscess

N62   **Hypertrophy of breast**
     Gynecomastia
     Hypertrophy of breast NOS
     Massive pubertal hypertrophy of breast
     EXCLUDES 1   breast engorgement of newborn (P83.4)
        disproportion of reconstructed breast (N65.1)

√4ᵗ **N63**   **Unspecified lump in breast**
     Nodule(s) NOS in breast
     AHA: 2017,4Q,19

▲   **N63.0**   **Unspecified lump in unspecified breast**   ▽

√5ᵗ **N63.1**   **Unspecified lump in the right breast**
     N63.10   **Unspecified lump in the right breast, unspecified quadrant**   ▽
     N63.11   **Unspecified lump in the right breast, upper outer quadrant**   ▽
     N63.12   **Unspecified lump in the right breast, upper inner quadrant**   ▽
     N63.13   **Unspecified lump in the right breast, lower outer quadrant**   ▽
     N63.14   **Unspecified lump in the right breast, lower inner quadrant**   ▽

√5ᵗ **N63.2**   **Unspecified lump in the left breast**
     N63.20   **Unspecified lump in the left breast, unspecified quadrant**   ▽
     N63.21   **Unspecified lump in the left breast, upper outer quadrant**   ▽
     N63.22   **Unspecified lump in the left breast, upper inner quadrant**   ▽
     N63.23   **Unspecified lump in the left breast, lower outer quadrant**   ▽
     N63.24   **Unspecified lump in the left breast, lower inner quadrant**   ▽

√5ᵗ **N63.3**   **Unspecified lump in axillary tail**
     N63.31   **Unspecified lump in axillary tail of the right breast**   ▽
     N63.32   **Unspecified lump in axillary tail of the left breast**   ▽

√5ᵗ **N63.4**   **Unspecified lump in breast, subareolar**
     N63.41   **Unspecified lump in right breast, subareolar**   ▽
     N63.42   **Unspecified lump in left breast, subareolar**   ▽

√4ᵗ **N64**   **Other disorders of breast**
     EXCLUDES 2   mechanical complication of breast prosthesis and implant (T85.4-)

   N64.0   **Fissure and fistula of nipple**

   N64.1   **Fat necrosis of breast**
     Fat necrosis (segmental) of breast
     Code first breast necrosis due to breast graft (T85.898)

   N64.2   **Atrophy of breast**

   N64.3   **Galactorrhea not associated with childbirth**

   N64.4   **Mastodynia**

√5ᵗ **N64.5**   **Other signs and symptoms in breast**
     EXCLUDES 2   abnormal findings on diagnostic imaging of breast (R92.-)
     N64.51   **Induration of breast**
     N64.52   **Nipple discharge**
        EXCLUDES 1   abnormal findings in nipple discharge (R89.-)
     N64.53   **Retraction of nipple**
     N64.59   **Other signs and symptoms in breast**

√5ᵗ **N64.8**   **Other specified disorders of breast**
     N64.81   **Ptosis of breast**   A
        EXCLUDES 1   ptosis of native breast in relation to reconstructed breast (N65.1)
     N64.82   **Hypoplasia of breast**   A
        Micromastia
        EXCLUDES 1   congenital absence of breast (Q83.0)
          hypoplasia of native breast in relation to reconstructed breast (N65.1)
     N64.89   **Other specified disorders of breast**
        Galactocele
        Subinvolution of breast (postlactational)
        AHA: 2018,1Q,3

   N64.9   **Disorder of breast, unspecified**   ▽

✓4ᵗʰ **N65**   **Deformity and disproportion of reconstructed breast**

     N65.0   **Deformity of reconstructed breast**   ▲

         Contour irregularity in reconstructed breast

         Excess tissue in reconstructed breast

         Misshapen reconstructed breast

     N65.1   **Disproportion of reconstructed breast**   ▲

         Breast asymmetry between native breast and reconstructed breast

         Disproportion between native breast and reconstructed breast

Inflammatory diseases of female pelvic organs (N70-N77)

EXCLUDES 1   inflammatory diseases of female pelvic organs complicating:

     abortion or ectopic or molar pregnancy (O00-O07, O08.0)

     pregnancy, childbirth and the puerperium (O23.-, O75.3, O85, O86.-)

✓4ᵗʰ **N70**   **Salpingitis and oophoritis**

     INCLUDES   abscess (of) fallopian tube

         abscess (of) ovary

         pyosalpinx

         salpingo-oophoritis

         tubo-ovarian abscess

         tubo-ovarian inflammatory disease

     Use additional code (B95-B97), to identify infectious agent

     EXCLUDES 1   gonococcal infection (A54.24)

         tuberculous infection (A18.17)

     ✓5ᵗʰ **N70.0**   **Acute salpingitis and oophoritis**

         N70.01   **Acute salpingitis**   ♀

         N70.02   **Acute oophoritis**   ♀

         N70.03   **Acute salpingitis and oophoritis**   ♀

     ✓5ᵗʰ **N70.1**   **Chronic salpingitis and oophoritis**

         Hydrosalpinx

         N70.11   **Chronic salpingitis**   ♀

         N70.12   **Chronic oophoritis**   ♀

         N70.13   **Chronic salpingitis and oophoritis**   ♀

     ✓5ᵗʰ **N70.9**   **Salpingitis and oophoritis, unspecified**

         N70.91   **Salpingitis, unspecified**   ♀ ▽

         N70.92   **Oophoritis, unspecified**   ♀ ▽

         N70.93   **Salpingitis and oophoritis, unspecified**   ♀ ▽

✓4ᵗʰ **N71**   **Inflammatory disease of uterus, except cervix**

     INCLUDES   endo (myo) metritis

         metritis

         myometritis

         pyometra

         uterine abscess

     Use additional code (B95-B97), to identify infectious agent

     EXCLUDES 1   hyperplastic endometritis (N85.0-)

         infection of uterus following delivery (O85, O86.-)

     N71.0   **Acute inflammatory disease of uterus**   ♀

     N71.1   **Chronic inflammatory disease of uterus**   ♀

     N71.9   **Inflammatory disease of uterus, unspecified**   ♀ ▽

N72   **Inflammatory disease of cervix uteri**   ♀

     INCLUDES   cervicitis (with or without erosion or ectropion)

         endocervicitis (with or without erosion or ectropion)

         exocervicitis (with or without erosion or ectropion)

     Use additional code (B95-B97), to identify infectious agent

     EXCLUDES 1   erosion and ectropion of cervix without cervicitis (N86)

✓4ᵗʰ **N73**   **Other female pelvic inflammatory diseases**

     Use additional code (B95-B97), to identify infectious agent

     N73.0   **Acute parametritis and pelvic cellulitis**   ♀

         Abscess of broad ligament

         Abscess of parametrium

         Pelvic cellulitis, female

         DEF: Parametritis: Inflammation of the parametrium.

     N73.1   **Chronic parametritis and pelvic cellulitis**   ♀

         Any condition in N73.0 specified as chronic

         EXCLUDES 1   tuberculous parametritis and pelvic cellultis (A18.17)

     N73.2   **Unspecified parametritis and pelvic cellulitis**   ♀ ▽

         Any condition in N73.0 unspecified whether acute or chronic

     N73.3   **Female acute pelvic peritonitis**   ♀

     N73.4   **Female chronic pelvic peritonitis**   ♀

         EXCLUDES 1   tuberculous pelvic (female) peritonitis (A18.17)

     N73.5   **Female pelvic peritonitis, unspecified**   ♀ ▽

     N73.6   **Female pelvic peritoneal adhesions (postinfective)**   ♀

         EXCLUDES 2   postprocedural pelvic peritoneal adhesions (N99.4)

         AHA: 2014,1Q,6

     N73.8   **Other specified female pelvic inflammatory diseases**   ♀

     N73.9   **Female pelvic inflammatory disease, unspecified**   ♀ ▽

         Female pelvic infection or inflammation NOS

N74   *Female pelvic inflammatory disorders in diseases classified elsewhere*   ♀

     Code first underlying disease

     EXCLUDES 1   chlamydial cervicitis (A56.02)

         chlamydial pelvic inflammatory disease (A56.11)

         gonococcal cervicitis (A54.03)

         gonococcal pelvic inflammatory disease (A54.24)

         herpesviral [herpes simplex] cervicitis (A60.03)

         herpesviral [herpes simplex] pelvic inflammatory disease (A60.09)

         syphilitic cervicitis (A52.76)

         syphilitic pelvic inflammatory disease (A52.76)

         trichomonal cervicitis (A59.09)

         tuberculous cervicitis (A18.16)

         tuberculous pelvic inflammatory disease (A18.17)

✓4ᵗʰ **N75**   **Diseases of Bartholin's gland**

     DEF: Bartholin's gland: Mucous-producing gland found in the vestibular bulbs on either side of the vaginal orifice and connected to the mucosal membrane at the opening by a duct.

     N75.0   **Cyst of Bartholin's gland**   ♀

     N75.1   **Abscess of Bartholin's gland**   ♀

     N75.8   **Other diseases of Bartholin's gland**   ♀

         Bartholinitis

     N75.9   **Disease of Bartholin's gland, unspecified**   ♀ ▽

✓4ᵗʰ **N76**   **Other inflammation of vagina and vulva**

     Use additional code (B95-B97), to identify infectious agent

     EXCLUDES 2   senile (atrophic) vaginitis (N95.2)

         vulvar vestibulitis (N94.810)

     N76.0   **Acute vaginitis**   ♀

         Acute vulvovaginitis

         Vaginitis NOS

         Vulvovaginitis NOS

     N76.1   **Subacute and chronic vaginitis**   ♀

         Chronic vulvovaginitis

         Subacute vulvovaginitis

     N76.2   **Acute vulvitis**   ♀

         Vulvitis NOS

     N76.3   **Subacute and chronic vulvitis**   ♀

     N76.4   **Abscess of vulva**   ♀

         Furuncle of vulva

     N76.5   **Ulceration of vagina**   ♀

     N76.6   **Ulceration of vulva**   ♀

     ✓5ᵗʰ **N76.8**   **Other specified inflammation of vagina and vulva**

         N76.81   **Mucositis (ulcerative) of vagina and vulva**   ♀

             Code also type of associated therapy, such as:

             antineoplastic and immunosuppressive drugs (T45.1X-)

             radiological procedure and radiotherapy (Y84.2)

             EXCLUDES 2   gastrointestinal mucositis (ulcerative) (K92.81)

                 nasal mucositis (ulcerative) (J34.81)

                 oral mucositis (ulcerative) (K12.3-)

         N76.89   **Other specified inflammation of vagina and vulva**   ♀

✓4ᵗʰ **N77**   **Vulvovaginal ulceration and inflammation in diseases classified elsewhere**

     N77.0   *Ulceration of vulva in diseases classified elsewhere*   ♀

         Code first underlying disease, such as:

         Behçet's disease (M35.2)

         EXCLUDES 1   ulceration of vulva in gonococcal infection (A54.02)

             ulceration of vulva in herpesviral [herpes simplex] infection (A60.04)

             ulceration of vulva in syphilis (A51.0)

             ulceration of vulva in tuberculosis (A18.18)

☑ Additional Character Req   ✓×7ᵗʰ Placeholder Alert   Manifestation   ▽ Unspecified   ►◄ Revised Text   ● New Code   ▲ Revised Code Title

ICD-10-CM 2019   839

Chapter 14. Diseases of the Genitourinary System

N77.1   **Vaginitis, vulvitis and vulvovaginitis in diseases classified elsewhere**   ♀

Code first underlying disease, such as:
pinworm (B80)

EXCLUDES 1   candidal vulvovaginitis (B37.3)
chlamydial vulvovaginitis (A56.02)
gonococcal vulvovaginitis (A54.02)
herpesviral [herpes simplex] vulvovaginitis (A60.04)
trichomonal vulvovaginitis (A59.01)
tuberculous vulvovaginitis (A18.18)
vulvovaginitis in early syphilis (A51.0)
vulvovaginitis in late syphilis (A52.76)

Noninflammatory disorders of female genital tract (N80-N98)

√4ᵗʰ **N80**   **Endometriosis**

DEF: Aberrant uterine mucosal tissue appearing in areas of the pelvic cavity outside of its normal location, lining the uterus, and inflaming surrounding tissues often resulting in infertility or spontaneous abortion.

N80.0   **Endometriosis of uterus**   ♀
Adenomyosis
EXCLUDES 1   stromal endometriosis (D39.0)

N80.1   **Endometriosis of ovary**   ♀

N80.2   **Endometriosis of fallopian tube**   ♀

N80.3   **Endometriosis of pelvic peritoneum**   ♀

N80.4   **Endometriosis of rectovaginal septum and vagina**   ♀

N80.5   **Endometriosis of intestine**   ♀

N80.6   **Endometriosis in cutaneous scar**   ♀

N80.8   **Other endometriosis**   ♀
Endometriosis of thorax

N80.9   **Endometriosis, unspecified**   ♀ ▽

√4ᵗʰ **N81**   **Female genital prolapse**

EXCLUDES 1   genital prolapse complicating pregnancy, labor or delivery (O34.5-)
prolapse and hernia of ovary and fallopian tube (N83.4-)
prolapse of vaginal vault after hysterectomy (N99.3)

Types of Pelvic Organ Prolapse

Urethrocele — Bladder, Uterus, Rectum, Urethra, Vaginal canal, Urethrocele

Cystocele — Bladder, Uterus, Rectum, Urethra, Vaginal canal, Cystocele

Rectocele — Bladder, Uterus, Rectum, Urethra, Vaginal canal, Rectocele

Enterocele — Bladder, Uterus, Enterocele, Urethra, Terminal ileum, Vaginal canal

N81.0   **Urethrocele**   ♀
EXCLUDES 1   urethrocele with cystocele (N81.1-)
urethrocele with prolapse of uterus (N81.2-N81.4)

√5ᵗʰ **N81.1**   **Cystocele**
Cystocele with urethrocele
Cystourethrocele
EXCLUDES 1   cystocele with prolapse of uterus (N81.2-N81.4)

N81.10   **Cystocele, unspecified**   ◘ ♀ ▽
Prolapse of (anterior) vaginal wall NOS

N81.11   **Cystocele, midline**   ◘ ♀

N81.12   **Cystocele, lateral**   ◘ ♀
Paravaginal cystocele
DEF: Detachment of the lateral support connections of the vagina at the arcus tendineus fasciae pelvis (ATFP) that results in bladder drop. The bladder herniates into the vagina laterally.

N81.2   **Incomplete uterovaginal prolapse**   ◘ ♀
First degree uterine prolapse
Prolapse of cervix NOS
Second degree uterine prolapse
EXCLUDES 1   cervical stump prolapse (N81.85)

N81.3   **Complete uterovaginal prolapse**   ◘ ♀
Procidentia (uteri) NOS
Third degree uterine prolapse

N81.4   **Uterovaginal prolapse, unspecified**   ◘ ♀ ▽
Prolapse of uterus NOS

N81.5   **Vaginal enterocele**   ♀
EXCLUDES 1   enterocele with prolapse of uterus (N81.2-N81.4)

N81.6   **Rectocele**   ♀
Prolapse of posterior vaginal wall
Use additional code for any associated fecal incontinence, if applicable (R15.-)
EXCLUDES 2   perineocele (N81.81)
rectal prolapse (K62.3)
rectocele with prolapse of uterus (N81.2-N81.4)

√5ᵗʰ **N81.8**   **Other female genital prolapse**

N81.81   **Perineocele**   ♀

N81.82   **Incompetence or weakening of pubocervical tissue**   ♀

N81.83   **Incompetence or weakening of rectovaginal tissue**   ♀

N81.84   **Pelvic muscle wasting**   ♀
Disuse atrophy of pelvic muscles and anal sphincter

N81.85   **Cervical stump prolapse**   ♀

N81.89   **Other female genital prolapse**   ◘ ♀
Deficient perineum
Old laceration of muscles of pelvic floor

N81.9   **Female genital prolapse, unspecified**   ◘ ♀ ▽

√4ᵗʰ **N82**   **Fistulae involving female genital tract**
EXCLUDES 1   vesicointestinal fistulae (N32.1)

N82.0   **Vesicovaginal fistula**   ♀

N82.1   **Other female urinary-genital tract fistulae**   ♀
Cervicovesical fistula
Ureterovaginal fistula
Urethrovaginal fistula
Uteroureteric fistula
Uterovesical fistula
AHA: 2017,3Q,3

N82.2   **Fistula of vagina to small intestine**   ♀

N82.3   **Fistula of vagina to large intestine**   ♀
Rectovaginal fistula

N82.4   **Other female intestinal-genital tract fistulae**   ♀
Intestinouterine fistula

N82.5   **Female genital tract-skin fistulae**   ♀
Uterus to abdominal wall fistula
Vaginoperineal fistula

N82.8   **Other female genital tract fistulae**   ♀

N82.9   **Female genital tract fistula, unspecified**   ♀ ▽

√4ᵗʰ **N83**   **Noninflammatory disorders of ovary, fallopian tube and broad ligament**
EXCLUDES 2   hydrosalpinx (N70.1-)
AHA: 2016,4Q,46

√5ᵗʰ **N83.0**   **Follicular cyst of ovary**
Cyst of graafian follicle
Hemorrhagic follicular cyst (of ovary)

N83.00   **Follicular cyst of ovary, unspecified side**   ♀ ▽

N83.01   **Follicular cyst of right ovary**   ♀

N83.02   **Follicular cyst of left ovary**   ♀

√5ᵗʰ **N83.1**   **Corpus luteum cyst**
Hemorrhagic corpus luteum cyst

N83.10   **Corpus luteum cyst of ovary, unspecified side**   ♀ ▽

N83.11   **Corpus luteum cyst of right ovary**   ♀

N83.12   **Corpus luteum cyst of left ovary**   ♀

✓5ᵗʰ **N83.2** **Other and unspecified ovarian cysts**

> EXCLUDES 1   *developmental ovarian cyst (Q50.1)*
> *neoplastic ovarian cyst (D27.-)*
> *polycystic ovarian syndrome (E28.2)*
> *Stein-Leventhal syndrome (E28.2)*

     ✓6ᵗʰ **N83.20** **Unspecified ovarian cysts**

         N83.201 **Unspecified ovarian cyst, right side** ♀ ▽

         N83.202 **Unspecified ovarian cyst, left side** ♀ ▽

         N83.209 **Unspecified ovarian cyst, unspecified side** ♀ ▽
            Ovarian cyst, NOS

     ✓6ᵗʰ **N83.29** **Other ovarian cysts**
         Retention cyst of ovary
         Simple cyst of ovary

         N83.291 **Other ovarian cyst, right side** ♀

         N83.292 **Other ovarian cyst, left side** ♀

         N83.299 **Other ovarian cyst, unspecified side** ♀ ▽

✓5ᵗʰ **N83.3** **Acquired atrophy of ovary and fallopian tube**

     ✓6ᵗʰ **N83.31** **Acquired atrophy of ovary**

         N83.311 **Acquired atrophy of right ovary** ♀

         N83.312 **Acquired atrophy of left ovary** ♀

         N83.319 **Acquired atrophy of ovary, unspecified side** ♀ ▽
            Acquired atrophy of ovary, NOS

     ✓6ᵗʰ **N83.32** **Acquired atrophy of fallopian tube**

         N83.321 **Acquired atrophy of right fallopian tube** ♀

         N83.322 **Acquired atrophy of left fallopian tube** ♀

         N83.329 **Acquired atrophy of fallopian tube, unspecified side** ♀ ▽
            Acquired atrophy of fallopian tube, NOS

     ✓6ᵗʰ **N83.33** **Acquired atrophy of ovary and fallopian tube**

         N83.331 **Acquired atrophy of right ovary and fallopian tube** ♀

         N83.332 **Acquired atrophy of left ovary and fallopian tube** ♀

         N83.339 **Acquired atrophy of ovary and fallopian tube, unspecified side** ♀ ▽
            Acquired atrophy of ovary and fallopian tube, NOS

✓5ᵗʰ **N83.4** **Prolapse and hernia of ovary and fallopian tube**

     N83.40 **Prolapse and hernia of ovary and fallopian tube, unspecified side** ♀ ▽
         Prolapse and hernia of ovary and fallopian tube, NOS

     N83.41 **Prolapse and hernia of right ovary and fallopian tube** ♀

     N83.42 **Prolapse and hernia of left ovary and fallopian tube** ♀

✓5ᵗʰ **N83.5** **Torsion of ovary, ovarian pedicle and fallopian tube**
     Torsion of accessory tube

     ✓6ᵗʰ **N83.51** **Torsion of ovary and ovarian pedicle**

         N83.511 **Torsion of right ovary and ovarian pedicle** ♀

         N83.512 **Torsion of left ovary and ovarian pedicle** ♀

         N83.519 **Torsion of ovary and ovarian pedicle, unspecified side** ♀ ▽
            Torsion of ovary and ovarian pedicle, NOS

     ✓6ᵗʰ **N83.52** **Torsion of fallopian tube**
         Torsion of hydatid of Morgagni

         N83.521 **Torsion of right fallopian tube** ♀

         N83.522 **Torsion of left fallopian tube** ♀

         N83.529 **Torsion of fallopian tube, unspecified side** ♀ ▽
            Torsion of fallopian tube, NOS

     N83.53 **Torsion of ovary, ovarian pedicle and fallopian tube** ♀

N83.6 **Hematosalpinx**

> EXCLUDES 1   *hematosalpinx (with) (in):*
> *hematocolpos (N89.7)*
> *hematometra (N85.7)*
> *tubal pregnancy (O00.1-)*

N83.7 **Hematoma of broad ligament** ♀

N83.8 **Other noninflammatory disorders of ovary, fallopian tube and broad ligament** ♀
     Broad ligament laceration syndrome [Allen-Masters]

N83.9 **Noninflammatory disorder of ovary, fallopian tube and broad ligament, unspecified** ♀ ▽

✓4ᵗʰ **N84** **Polyp of female genital tract**

> EXCLUDES 1   *adenomatous polyp (D28.-)*
> *placental polyp (O90.89)*

N84.0 **Polyp of corpus uteri** ♀
     Polyp of endometrium
     Polyp of uterus NOS
> EXCLUDES 1   *polypoid endometrial hyperplasia (N85.0-)*

N84.1 **Polyp of cervix uteri** ♀
     Mucous polyp of cervix

N84.2 **Polyp of vagina** ♀

N84.3 **Polyp of vulva** ♀
     Polyp of labia

N84.8 **Polyp of other parts of female genital tract** ♀

N84.9 **Polyp of female genital tract, unspecified** ♀ ▽

✓4ᵗʰ **N85** **Other noninflammatory disorders of uterus, except cervix**

> EXCLUDES 1   *endometriosis (N80.-)*
> *inflammatory diseases of uterus (N71.-)*
> *noninflammatory disorders of cervix, except malposition (N86-N88)*
> *polyp of corpus uteri (N84.0)*
> *uterine prolapse (N81.-)*

     ✓5ᵗʰ **N85.0** **Endometrial hyperplasia**

         N85.00 **Endometrial hyperplasia, unspecified** ♀ ▽
            Hyperplasia (adenomatous) (cystic) (glandular) of endometrium
            Hyperplastic endometritis

         N85.01 **Benign endometrial hyperplasia** ♀
            Endometrial hyperplasia (complex) (simple) without atypia

         N85.02 **Endometrial intraepithelial neoplasia [EIN]** ♀
            Endometrial hyperplasia with atypia
> EXCLUDES 1   *malignant neoplasm of endometrium (with endometrial intraepithelial neoplasia [EIN]) (C54.1)*

     N85.2 **Hypertrophy of uterus** ♀
         Bulky or enlarged uterus
> EXCLUDES 1   *puerperal hypertrophy of uterus (O90.89)*

     N85.3 **Subinvolution of uterus** ♀
> EXCLUDES 1   *puerperal subinvolution of uterus (O90.89)*

     N85.4 **Malposition of uterus** ♀
         Anteversion of uterus
         Retroflexion of uterus
         Retroversion of uterus
> EXCLUDES 1   *malposition of uterus complicating pregnancy, labor or delivery (O34.5-, O65.5)*

     N85.5 **Inversion of uterus** ♀
> EXCLUDES 1   *current obstetric trauma (O71.2)*
> *postpartum inversion of uterus (O71.2)*

     DEF: Abnormality in which the uterus turns inside out.

Inversion of Uterus

Uterus

     N85.6 **Intrauterine synechiae** ♀

☑ Additional Character Req   ✓x7ᵗʰ Placeholder Alert   Manifestation   ▽ Unspecified   ▶◀ Revised Text   ● New Code   ▲ Revised Code Title

ICD-10-CM 2019   **841**

Chapter 14. Diseases of the Genitourinary System

N85.7-N91.2

N85.7 Hematometra ♀
Hematosalpinx with hematometra
EXCLUDES 1 hematometra with hematocolpos (N89.7)
DEF: Accumulation of blood within the uterus.

N85.8 Other specified noninflammatory disorders of uterus ♀
Atrophy of uterus, acquired
Fibrosis of uterus NOS

N85.9 Noninflammatory disorder of uterus, unspecified ♀ ▽
Disorder of uterus NOS

N86 Erosion and ectropion of cervix uteri ♀
Decubitus (trophic) ulcer of cervix
Eversion of cervix
EXCLUDES 1 erosion and ectropion of cervix with cervicitis (N72)

✓4ᵗʰ **N87 Dysplasia of cervix uteri**
EXCLUDES 1 abnormal results from cervical cytologic examination without histologic confirmation (R87.61-)
carcinoma in situ of cervix uteri (D06.-)
cervical intraepithelial neoplasia III [CIN III] (D06.-)
HGSIL of cervix (R87.613)
severe dysplasia of cervix uteri (D06.-)

N87.0 Mild cervical dysplasia ♀
Cervical intraepithelial neoplasia I [CIN I]

N87.1 Moderate cervical dysplasia ♀
Cervical intraepithelial neoplasia II [CIN II]

N87.9 Dysplasia of cervix uteri, unspecified ♀ ▽
Anaplasia of cervix
Cervical atypism
Cervical dysplasia NOS

✓4ᵗʰ **N88 Other noninflammatory disorders of cervix uteri**
EXCLUDES 2 inflammatory disease of cervix (N72)
polyp of cervix (N84.1)

N88.0 Leukoplakia of cervix uteri ♀

N88.1 Old laceration of cervix uteri ♀
Adhesions of cervix
EXCLUDES 1 current obstetric trauma (O71.3)

N88.2 Stricture and stenosis of cervix uteri ♀
EXCLUDES 1 stricture and stenosis of cervix uteri complicating labor (O65.5)

N88.3 Incompetence of cervix uteri ♀
Investigation and management of (suspected) cervical incompetence in a nonpregnant woman
EXCLUDES 1 cervical incompetence complicating pregnancy (O34.3-)

N88.4 Hypertrophic elongation of cervix uteri ♀

N88.8 Other specified noninflammatory disorders of cervix uteri ♀
EXCLUDES 1 current obstetric trauma (O71.3)

N88.9 Noninflammatory disorder of cervix uteri, unspecified ♀ ▽

✓4ᵗʰ **N89 Other noninflammatory disorders of vagina**
EXCLUDES 1 abnormal results from vaginal cytologic examination without histologic confirmation (R87.62-)
carcinoma in situ of vagina (D07.2)
HGSIL of vagina (R87.623)
inflammation of vagina (N76.-)
senile (atrophic) vaginitis (N95.2)
severe dysplasia of vagina (D07.2)
trichomonal leukorrhea (A59.00)
vaginal intraepithelial neoplasia [VAIN], grade III (D07.2)

N89.0 Mild vaginal dysplasia ♀
Vaginal intraepithelial neoplasia [VAIN], grade I

N89.1 Moderate vaginal dysplasia ♀
Vaginal intraepithelial neoplasia [VAIN], grade II

N89.3 Dysplasia of vagina, unspecified ♀ ▽

N89.4 Leukoplakia of vagina ♀

N89.5 Stricture and atresia of vagina ♀
Vaginal adhesions
Vaginal stenosis
EXCLUDES 1 congenital atresia or stricture (Q52.4)
postprocedural adhesions of vagina (N99.2)

N89.6 Tight hymenal ring ♀
Rigid hymen
Tight introitus
EXCLUDES 1 imperforate hymen (Q52.3)

N89.7 Hematocolpos ♀
Hematocolpos with hematometra or hematosalpinx
AHA: 2016,4Q,58

N89.8 Other specified noninflammatory disorders of vagina ♀
Leukorrhea NOS
Old vaginal laceration
Pessary ulcer of vagina
EXCLUDES 1 current obstetric trauma (O70.-, O71.4, O71.7-O71.8)
old laceration involving muscles of pelvic floor (N81.8)

N89.9 Noninflammatory disorder of vagina, unspecified ♀ ▽

✓4ᵗʰ **N90 Other noninflammatory disorders of vulva and perineum**
EXCLUDES 1 anogenital (venereal) warts (A63.0)
carcinoma in situ of vulva (D07.1)
condyloma acuminatum (A63.0)
current obstetric trauma (O70.-, O71.7-O71.8)
inflammation of vulva (N76.-)
severe dysplasia of vulva (D07.1)
vulvar intraepithelial neoplasm III [VIN III] (D07.1)

N90.0 Mild vulvar dysplasia ♀
Vulvar intraepithelial neoplasia [VIN], grade I

N90.1 Moderate vulvar dysplasia ♀
Vulvar intraepithelial neoplasia [VIN], grade II

N90.3 Dysplasia of vulva, unspecified ♀ ▽

N90.4 Leukoplakia of vulva ♀
Dystrophy of vulva
Kraurosis of vulva
Lichen sclerosus of external female genital organs

N90.5 Atrophy of vulva ♀
Stenosis of vulva

✓5ᵗʰ **N90.6 Hypertrophy of vulva**
AHA: 2016,4Q,46

N90.60 Unspecified hypertrophy of vulva ♀ ▽
Unspecified hypertrophy of labia

N90.61 Childhood asymmetric labium majus enlargement ♀
CALME

N90.69 Other specified hypertrophy of vulva ♀
Other specified hypertrophy of labia

N90.7 Vulvar cyst ♀

✓5ᵗʰ **N90.8 Other specified noninflammatory disorders of vulva and perineum**

✓6ᵗʰ **N90.81 Female genital mutilation status**
Female genital cutting status

N90.810 Female genital mutilation status, unspecified ♀ ▽
Female genital cutting status, unspecified
Female genital mutilation status NOS

N90.811 Female genital mutilation Type I status ♀
Clitorectomy status
Female genital cutting Type I status

N90.812 Female genital mutilation Type II status ♀
Clitorectomy with excision of labia minora status
Female genital cutting Type II status

N90.813 Female genital mutilation Type III status ♀
Female genital cutting Type III status
Infibulation status

N90.818 Other female genital mutilation status ♀
Female genital cutting Type IV status
Female genital mutilation Type IV status
Other female genital cutting status

N90.89 Other specified noninflammatory disorders of vulva and perineum ♀
Adhesions of vulva
Hypertrophy of clitoris

N90.9 Noninflammatory disorder of vulva and perineum, unspecified ♀ ▽

✓4ᵗʰ **N91 Absent, scanty and rare menstruation**
EXCLUDES 1 ovarian dysfunction (E28.-)

N91.0 Primary amenorrhea ♀

N91.1 Secondary amenorrhea ♀

N91.2 Amenorrhea, unspecified ♀ ▽

N91.3   **Primary oligomenorrhea**   ♀

N91.4   **Secondary oligomenorrhea**   ♀

N91.5   **Oligomenorrhea, unspecified**   ♀ ▽
       Hypomenorrhea NOS

√4ᵗʰ **N92**   **Excessive, frequent and irregular menstruation**
     EXCLUDES 1   postmenopausal bleeding (N95.0)
             precocious puberty (menstruation) (E30.1)

N92.0   **Excessive and frequent menstruation with regular cycle**   ♀
       Heavy periods NOS
       Menorrhagia NOS
       Polymenorrhea

N92.1   **Excessive and frequent menstruation with irregular cycle**   ♀
       Irregular intermenstrual bleeding
       Irregular, shortened intervals between menstrual bleeding
       Menometrorrhagia
       Metrorrhagia

N92.2   **Excessive menstruation at puberty**   P ♀
       Excessive bleeding associated with onset of menstrual periods
       Pubertal menorrhagia
       Puberty bleeding

N92.3   **Ovulation bleeding**   ♀
       Regular intermenstrual bleeding

N92.4   **Excessive bleeding in the premenopausal period**   ♀
       Climacteric menorrhagia or metrorrhagia
       Menopausal menorrhagia or metrorrhagia
       Preclimacteric menorrhagia or metrorrhagia
       Premenopausal menorrhagia or metrorrhagia

N92.5   **Other specified irregular menstruation**   ♀

N92.6   **Irregular menstruation, unspecified**   ♀ ▽
       Irregular bleeding NOS
       Irregular periods NOS
     EXCLUDES 1   irregular menstruation with:
             lengthened intervals or scanty bleeding (N91.3-N91.5)
             shortened intervals or excessive bleeding (N92.1)

√4ᵗʰ **N93**   **Other abnormal uterine and vaginal bleeding**
     EXCLUDES 1   neonatal vaginal hemorrhage (P54.6)
             precocious puberty (menstruation) (E30.1)
             pseudomenses (P54.6)

N93.0   **Postcoital and contact bleeding**   ♀

N93.1   **Pre-pubertal vaginal bleeding**   ♀
       AHA: 2016,4Q,47

N93.8   **Other specified abnormal uterine and vaginal bleeding**   ♀
       Dysfunctional or functional uterine or vaginal bleeding NOS

N93.9   **Abnormal uterine and vaginal bleeding, unspecified**   ♀ ▽

√4ᵗʰ **N94**   **Pain and other conditions associated with female genital organs and menstrual cycle**

N94.0   **Mittelschmerz**   ♀
       DEF: One-sided, lower abdominal pain occurring between menstrual periods that is associated with ovulation.

√5ᵗʰ **N94.1**   **Dyspareunia**
     EXCLUDES 1   psychogenic dyspareunia (F52.6)
       AHA: 2016,4Q,47

       N94.10   **Unspecified dyspareunia**   ♀ ▽

       N94.11   **Superficial (introital) dyspareunia**   ♀

       N94.12   **Deep dyspareunia**   ♀

       N94.19   **Other specified dyspareunia**   ♀

N94.2   **Vaginismus**
     EXCLUDES 1   psychogenic vaginismus (F52.5)
       DEF: Spontaneous contractions of the muscles surrounding the vagina, causing it to constrict or close.

N94.3   **Premenstrual tension syndrome**
       Code also associated menstrual migraine (G43.82-, G43.83-)
     EXCLUDES 1   premenstrual dysphoric disorder (F32.81)

N94.4   **Primary dysmenorrhea**   ♀

N94.5   **Secondary dysmenorrhea**   ♀

N94.6   **Dysmenorrhea, unspecified**   ♀ ▽
     EXCLUDES 1   psychogenic dysmenorrhea (F45.8)

√5ᵗʰ **N94.8**   **Other specified conditions associated with female genital organs and menstrual cycle**

     √6ᵗʰ **N94.81**   **Vulvodynia**

          N94.810   **Vulvar vestibulitis**   ♀

          N94.818   **Other vulvodynia**   ♀

          N94.819   **Vulvodynia, unspecified**   ♀ ▽
             Vulvodynia NOS

       N94.89   **Other specified conditions associated with female genital organs and menstrual cycle**
          DEF: Hydrocele: Serous fluid that collects in the canal of Nuck in females.

N94.9   **Unspecified condition associated with female genital organs and menstrual cycle**   ♀ ▽

√4ᵗʰ **N95**   **Menopausal and other perimenopausal disorders**
     Menopausal and other perimenopausal disorders due to naturally occurring (age-related) menopause and perimenopause
     EXCLUDES 1   excessive bleeding in the premenopausal period (N92.4)
             menopausal and perimenopausal disorders due to artificial or premature menopause (E89.4-, E28.31-)
             premature menopause (E28.31-)
     EXCLUDES 2   postmenopausal osteoporosis (M81.0-)
             postmenopausal osteoporosis with current pathological fracture (M80.0-)
             postmenopausal urethritis (N34.2)

N95.0   **Postmenopausal bleeding**   ♀

N95.1   **Menopausal and female climacteric states**   ♀
       Symptoms such as flushing, sleeplessness, headache, lack of concentration, associated with natural (age-related) menopause
       Use additional code for associated symptoms
     EXCLUDES 1   asymptomatic menopausal state (Z78.0)
             symptoms associated with artificial menopause (E89.41)
             symptoms associated with premature menopause (E28.310)

N95.2   **Postmenopausal atrophic vaginitis**   ♀
       Senile (atrophic) vaginitis

N95.8   **Other specified menopausal and perimenopausal disorders**   ♀

N95.9   **Unspecified menopausal and perimenopausal disorder**   ♀ ▽

N96   **Recurrent pregnancy loss**   ♀
     Investigation or care in a nonpregnant woman with history of recurrent pregnancy loss
     EXCLUDES 1   recurrent pregnancy loss with current pregnancy (O26.2-)

√4ᵗʰ **N97**   **Female infertility**
     INCLUDES   inability to achieve a pregnancy
             sterility, female NOS
     EXCLUDES 1   female infertility associated with:
             hypopituitarism (E23.0)
             Stein-Leventhal syndrome (E28.2)
     EXCLUDES 2   incompetence of cervix uteri (N88.3)
     DEF: Infertility: Inability to conceive for at least one year with regular intercourse.
     DEF: Primary infertility: Infertility occurring in patients who have never conceived.
     DEF: Secondary infertility: Infertility occurring in patients who have previously conceived.

N97.0   **Female infertility associated with anovulation**   ♀

N97.1   **Female infertility of tubal origin**   ♀
       Female infertility associated with congenital anomaly of tube
       Female infertility due to tubal block
       Female infertility due to tubal occlusion
       Female infertility due to tubal stenosis

N97.2   **Female infertility of uterine origin**   ♀
       Female infertility associated with congenital anomaly of uterus
       Female infertility due to nonimplantation of ovum

N97.8   **Female infertility of other origin**   ♀

N97.9   **Female infertility, unspecified**   ♀ ▽

√4ᵗʰ **N98**   **Complications associated with artificial fertilization**

N98.0   **Infection associated with artificial insemination**   ♀

N98.1   **Hyperstimulation of ovaries**   ♀
       Hyperstimulation of ovaries NOS
       Hyperstimulation of ovaries associated with induced ovulation

N98.2   **Complications of attempted introduction of fertilized ovum following in vitro fertilization**   ♀

N98.3   **Complications of attempted introduction of embryo in embryo transfer**   ♀

N98.8   **Other complications associated with artificial fertilization**   ♀

N98.9   **Complication associated with artificial fertilization, unspecified**   ♀ ▽

✔ Additional Character Req   √x7ᵗʰ Placeholder Alert   Manifestation   ▽ Unspecified   ▶◀ Revised Text   ● New Code   ▲ Revised Code Title

Intraoperative and postprocedural complications and disorders of genitourinary system, not elsewhere classified (N99)

✓4ᵗʰ N99 Intraoperative and postprocedural complications and disorders of genitourinary system, not elsewhere classified

EXCLUDES 2   *irradiation cystitis (N30.4-)*

postoophorectomy osteoporosis with current pathological fracture (M80.8-)

postoophorectomy osteoporosis without current pathological fracture (M81.8)

N99.0 Postprocedural (acute) (chronic) kidney failure

Use additional code to type of kidney disease

✓5ᵗʰ N99.1 Postprocedural urethral stricture

Postcatheterization urethral stricture

✓6ᵗʰ N99.11 Postprocedural urethral stricture, male

AHA: 2016,4Q,47-48

N99.110 Postprocedural urethral stricture, male, meatal ♂

N99.111 Postprocedural bulbous urethral stricture, male ♂

N99.112 Postprocedural membranous urethral stricture, male ♂

N99.113 Postprocedural anterior bulbous urethral stricture, male ♂

N99.114 Postprocedural urethral stricture, male, unspecified ♂ ▽

N99.115 Postprocedural fossa navicularis urethral stricture ♂

N99.116 Postprocedural urethral stricture, male, overlapping sites

N99.12 Postprocedural urethral stricture, female ♀

N99.2 Postprocedural adhesions of vagina ♀

N99.3 Prolapse of vaginal vault after hysterectomy ♀

N99.4 Postprocedural pelvic peritoneal adhesions

EXCLUDES 2   *pelvic peritoneal adhesions NOS (N73.6)*

postinfective pelvic peritoneal adhesions (N73.6)

✓5ᵗʰ N99.5 Complications of stoma of urinary tract

EXCLUDES 2   *mechanical complication of urinary catheter (T83.0-)*

AHA: 2016,4Q,48

✓6ᵗʰ N99.51 Complication of cystostomy

N99.510 Cystostomy hemorrhage HCC

N99.511 Cystostomy infection HCC

N99.512 Cystostomy malfunction HCC

N99.518 Other cystostomy complication HCC

✓6ᵗʰ N99.52 Complication of incontinent external stoma of urinary tract

N99.520 Hemorrhage of incontinent external stoma of urinary tract HCC

N99.521 Infection of incontinent external stoma of urinary tract HCC

N99.522 Malfunction of incontinent external stoma of urinary tract HCC

N99.523 Herniation of incontinent stoma of urinary tract HCC

N99.524 Stenosis of incontinent stoma of urinary tract HCC

N99.528 Other complication of incontinent external stoma of urinary tract HCC

✓6ᵗʰ N99.53 Complication of continent stoma of urinary tract

N99.530 Hemorrhage of continent stoma of urinary tract HCC

N99.531 Infection of continent stoma of urinary tract HCC

N99.532 Malfunction of continent stoma of urinary tract HCC

N99.533 Herniation of continent stoma of urinary tract HCC

N99.534 Stenosis of continent stoma of urinary tract HCC

N99.538 Other complication of continent stoma of urinary tract HCC

✓5ᵗʰ N99.6 Intraoperative hemorrhage and hematoma of a genitourinary system organ or structure complicating a procedure

EXCLUDES 1   *intraoperative hemorrhage and hematoma of a genitourinary system organ or structure due to accidental puncture or laceration during a procedure (N99.7-)*

N99.61 Intraoperative hemorrhage and hematoma of a genitourinary system organ or structure complicating a genitourinary system procedure

N99.62 Intraoperative hemorrhage and hematoma of a genitourinary system organ or structure complicating other procedure

✓5ᵗʰ N99.7 Accidental puncture and laceration of a genitourinary system organ or structure during a procedure

N99.71 Accidental puncture and laceration of a genitourinary system organ or structure during a genitourinary system procedure

N99.72 Accidental puncture and laceration of a genitourinary system organ or structure during other procedure

✓5ᵗʰ N99.8 Other intraoperative and postprocedural complications and disorders of genitourinary system

AHA: 2016,4Q,9-10

N99.81 Other intraoperative complications of genitourinary system

✓6ᵗʰ N99.82 Postprocedural hemorrhage of a genitourinary system organ or structure following a procedure

N99.820 Postprocedural hemorrhage of a genitourinary system organ or structure following a genitourinary system procedure

N99.821 Postprocedural hemorrhage of a genitourinary system organ or structure following other procedure

N99.83 Residual ovary syndrome ♀

✓6ᵗʰ N99.84 Postprocedural hematoma and seroma of a genitourinary system organ or structure following a procedure

N99.840 Postprocedural hematoma of a genitourinary system organ or structure following a genitourinary system procedure

N99.841 Postprocedural hematoma of a genitourinary system organ or structure following other procedure

N99.842 Postprocedural seroma of a genitourinary system organ or structure following a genitourinary system procedure

N99.843 Postprocedural seroma of a genitourinary system organ or structure following other procedure

N99.89 Other postprocedural complications and disorders of genitourinary system

Chapter 15. Pregnancy, Childbirth, and the Puerperium (O00–O9A)

Chapter Specific Guidelines with Coding Examples
The chapter specific guidelines from the ICD-10-CM Official Guidelines for Coding and Reporting have been provided below. Along with these guidelines are coding examples, contained in the shaded boxes, that have been developed to help illustrate the coding and/or sequencing guidance found in these guidelines.

a. General rules for obstetric cases

1) Codes from Chapter 15 and sequencing priority
Obstetric cases require codes from chapter 15, codes in the range O00-O9A, Pregnancy, Childbirth, and the Puerperium. Chapter 15 codes have sequencing priority over codes from other chapters. Additional codes from other chapters may be used in conjunction with chapter 15 codes to further specify conditions. Should the provider document that the pregnancy is incidental to the encounter, then code Z33.1, Pregnant state, incidental, should be used in place of any chapter 15 codes. It is the provider's responsibility to state that the condition being treated is not affecting the pregnancy.

> Bladder abscess in pregnant patient at 25 weeks' gestation
>
> **O23.12   Infections of bladder in pregnancy, second trimester**
>
> **N30.80   Other cystitis without hematuria**
>
> **Z3A.25   25 weeks gestation of pregnancy**
>
> *Explanation:* The documentation does not indicate that the pregnancy is incidental or in any way unaffected by the bladder abscess; therefore, an obstetrics code should be sequenced first. An additional code was provided to identify the specific bladder condition as this information is not called out specifically in the obstetrics code.

2) Chapter 15 codes used only on the maternal record
Chapter 15 codes are to be used only on the maternal record, never on the record of the newborn.

3) Final character for trimester
The majority of codes in Chapter 15 have a final character indicating the trimester of pregnancy. The timeframes for the trimesters are indicated at the beginning of the chapter. If trimester is not a component of a code, it is because the condition always occurs in a specific trimester, or the concept of trimester of pregnancy is not applicable. Certain codes have characters for only certain trimesters because the condition does not occur in all trimesters, but it may occur in more than just one. Assignment of the final character for trimester should be based on the provider's documentation of the trimester (or number of weeks) for the current admission/encounter. This applies to the assignment of trimester for pre-existing conditions as well as those that develop during or are due to the pregnancy. The provider's documentation of the number of weeks may be used to assign the appropriate code identifying the trimester.

Whenever delivery occurs during the current admission, and there is an "in childbirth" option for the obstetric complication being coded, the "in childbirth" code should be assigned.

> Pregnant patient at 21 weeks' gestation admitted with excessive vomiting
>
> **O21.2   Late vomiting of pregnancy**
>
> **Z3A.21   21 weeks gestation of pregnancy**
>
> *Explanation:* Category O21 classifies vomiting in pregnancy. Although code selection is based on whether the vomiting is before or after 20 completed weeks, these codes are not further classified by trimester. If vomiting only in the second trimester was documented, the provider should be queried for the specific week of gestation, as this will affect code selection.

4) Selection of trimester for inpatient admissions that encompass more than one trimester
In instances when a patient is admitted to a hospital for complications of pregnancy during one trimester and remains in the hospital into a subsequent trimester, the trimester character for the antepartum complication code should be assigned on the basis of the trimester when the complication developed, not the trimester of the discharge. If the condition developed prior to the current admission/encounter or represents a pre-existing condition, the trimester character for the trimester at the time of the admission/encounter should be assigned.

5) Unspecified trimester
Each category that includes codes for trimester has a code for "unspecified trimester." The "unspecified trimester" code should rarely be used, such as when the documentation in the record is insufficient to determine the trimester and it is not possible to obtain clarification.

6) 7th character for fetus identification
Where applicable, a 7th character is to be assigned for certain categories (O31, O32, O33.3 - O33.6, O35, O36, O40, O41, O60.1, O60.2, O64, and O69) to identify the fetus for which the complication code applies.

Assign 7th character "0":
- For single gestations
- When the documentation in the record is insufficient to determine the fetus affected and it is not possible to obtain clarification.
- When it is not possible to clinically determine which fetus is affected.

> Maternal patient with twin gestations is seen after ultrasound identifies fetus B to be in breech presentation
>
> **O32.1XX2   Maternal care for breech presentation, fetus 2**
>
> *Explanation:* The documentation indicates that although there are two fetuses, only one fetus is determined to be in breech presentation. Whether fetus 2 or fetus B is used, the coder can assign the seventh character of 2 to identify the second fetus as the one in breech.

b. Selection of OB principal or first-listed diagnosis

1) Routine outpatient prenatal visits
For routine outpatient prenatal visits when no complications are present, a code from category Z34, Encounter for supervision of normal pregnancy, should be used as the first-listed diagnosis. These codes should not be used in conjunction with chapter 15 codes.

2) Supervision of high-risk pregnancy
Codes from category O09, Supervision of high-risk pregnancy, are intended for use only during the prenatal period. For complications during the labor or delivery episode as a result of a high-risk pregnancy, assign the applicable complication codes from Chapter 15. If there are no complications during the labor or delivery episode, assign code O80, Encounter for full-term uncomplicated delivery.

For routine prenatal outpatient visits for patients with high-risk pregnancies, a code from category O09, Supervision of high-risk pregnancy, should be used as the first-listed diagnosis. Secondary chapter 15 codes may be used in conjunction with these codes if appropriate.

> 36-year-old seen in labor with second child at 39 weeks' gestation, delivered a healthy baby, delivery complicated by tear of fourchette that was repaired
>
> **O70.0   First degree perineal laceration during delivery**
>
> **Z3A.39   39 weeks gestation of pregnancy**
>
> **Z37.0   Single live birth**
>
> Explanation: Although this patient is over 35 and having her second child (elderly multigravida), do not append a code from subcategory O09.52-. A code describing the tear of the fourchette, which complicated the delivery, should be used in addition to the applicable Z codes.

3) Episodes when no delivery occurs
In episodes when no delivery occurs, the principal diagnosis should correspond to the principal complication of the pregnancy which necessitated the encounter. Should more than one complication exist, all of which are treated or monitored, any of the complications codes may be sequenced first.

4) When a delivery occurs
When an obstetric patient is admitted and delivers during that admission, the condition that prompted the admission should be sequenced as the principal diagnosis. If multiple conditions prompted the admission, sequence the one most related to the delivery as the principal diagnosis. A code for any complication of the delivery should be assigned as an additional diagnosis. In cases of cesarean delivery, if the patient was admitted with a condition that resulted in the performance of a cesarean procedure, that condition should be selected as the principal diagnosis. If the reason for the admission was unrelated to the condition resulting in

the cesarean delivery, the condition related to the reason for the admission should be selected as the principal diagnosis.

> Maternal patient with diet-controlled gestational diabetes was seen at 38 weeks' gestation in obstructed labor due to footling presentation; cesarean performed for the malpresentation
>
> **O64.8XX0** **Obstructed labor due to other malposition and malpresentation, not applicable or unspecified**
>
> **O24.420** **Gestational diabetes mellitus in childbirth, diet controlled**
>
> **Z3A.38** **38 weeks gestation of pregnancy**
>
> **Z37.0** **Single live birth**
>
> *Explanation:* The obstructed labor necessitated the cesarean procedure.

5) Outcome of delivery

A code from category Z37, Outcome of delivery, should be included on every maternal record when a delivery has occurred. These codes are not to be used on subsequent records or on the newborn record.

c. Pre-existing conditions versus conditions due to the pregnancy

Certain categories in Chapter 15 distinguish between conditions of the mother that existed prior to pregnancy (pre-existing) and those that are a direct result of pregnancy. When assigning codes from Chapter 15, it is important to assess if a condition was pre-existing prior to pregnancy or developed during or due to the pregnancy in order to assign the correct code.

Categories that do not distinguish between pre-existing and pregnancy-related conditions may be used for either. It is acceptable to use codes specifically for the puerperium with codes complicating pregnancy and childbirth if a condition arises postpartum during the delivery encounter.

> Type 2 diabetic patient presents at 19 weeks gestation for glucose check. Patient has been taking oral metformin for several years and currently is experiencing no diabetic complications.
>
> **O24.112** **Pre-existing type 2 diabetes mellitus, in pregnancy, second trimester**
>
> **E11.9** **Type 2 diabetes mellitus without complications**
>
> **Z79.84** **Long term (current) use of oral hypoglycemic drugs**
>
> *Explanation:* The documentation states that the patient has been on a diabetic medication (oral metformin) for several years, indicating the patient was diabetic prior to becoming pregnant. Reporting pre-existing Type 2 diabetes in a pregnant patient requires two codes to capture the condition, a code from category O24 and a code from category E11. A note at E11 indicates that the code for long-term use of oral hypoglycemic drugs should also be reported.

d. Pre-existing hypertension in pregnancy

Category O10, Pre-existing hypertension complicating pregnancy, childbirth and the puerperium, includes codes for hypertensive heart and hypertensive chronic kidney disease. When assigning one of the O10 codes that includes hypertensive heart disease or hypertensive chronic kidney disease, it is necessary to add a secondary code from the appropriate hypertension category to specify the type of heart failure or chronic kidney disease. *See Section I.C.9. Hypertension.*

e. Fetal conditions affecting the management of the mother

1) Codes from categories O35 and O36

Codes from categories O35, Maternal care for known or suspected fetal abnormality and damage, and O36, Maternal care for other fetal problems, are assigned only when the fetal condition is actually responsible for modifying the management of the mother, i.e., by requiring diagnostic studies, additional observation, special care, or termination of pregnancy. The fact that the fetal condition exists does not justify assigning a code from this series to the mother's record.

> A patient with twin gestation is seen for spotting 15 weeks into her pregnancy; the doctors also suspect fetal hydrocephalus. Patient is instructed to return in one week for additional diagnostic testing, sooner if the problem worsens.
>
> **O35.0XX0** **Maternal care for (suspected) central nervous system malformation in fetus, not applicable or unspecified**
>
> **O26.852** **Spotting complicating pregnancy, second trimester**
>
> **Z3A.15** **15 weeks gestation of pregnancy**
>
> *Explanation:* Whether the fetal hydrocephalus was suspected or confirmed, an additional code is warranted for this condition since documentation indicates the patient is to return sooner than her routine visit for further testing.

2) In utero surgery

In cases when surgery is performed on the fetus, a diagnosis code from category O35, Maternal care for known or suspected fetal abnormality and damage, should be assigned identifying the fetal condition. Assign the appropriate procedure code for the procedure performed.

No code from Chapter 16, the perinatal codes, should be used on the mother's record to identify fetal conditions. Surgery performed in utero on a fetus is still to be coded as an obstetric encounter.

f. HIV infection in pregnancy, childbirth and the puerperium

During pregnancy, childbirth or the puerperium, a patient admitted because of an HIV-related illness should receive a principal diagnosis from subcategory O98.7-, Human immunodeficiency [HIV] disease complicating pregnancy, childbirth and the puerperium, followed by the code(s) for the HIV-related illness(es).

Patients with asymptomatic HIV infection status admitted during pregnancy, childbirth, or the puerperium should receive codes of O98.7- and Z21, Asymptomatic human immunodeficiency virus [HIV] infection status.

> A previously asymptomatic HIV patient who is 13 weeks pregnant is evaluated for HIV-related candidal bronchitis
>
> **O98.711** **Human immunodeficiency virus [HIV] disease complicating pregnancy, first trimester**
>
> **B20** **Human immunodeficiency virus [HIV] disease**
>
> **B37.1** **Candidal bronchitis**
>
> **Z3A.13** **13 weeks gestation of pregnancy**
>
> *Explanation:* Because candidal bronchitis is an AIDS-related condition, this patient is now considered to have HIV disease. An obstetrics code indicating that HIV is complicating the pregnancy is coded first, followed by B20 for HIV disease as well as a code for the candidal bronchitis.

g. Diabetes mellitus in pregnancy

Diabetes mellitus is a significant complicating factor in pregnancy. Pregnant women who are diabetic should be assigned a code from category O24, Diabetes mellitus in pregnancy, childbirth, and the puerperium, first, followed by the appropriate diabetes code(s) (E08-E13) from Chapter 4.

h. Long term use of insulin and oral hypoglycemics

See section I.C.4.a.3 for information on the long term use of insulin and oral hypoglycemic.

i. Gestational (pregnancy induced) diabetes

Gestational (pregnancy induced) diabetes can occur during the second and third trimester of pregnancy in women who were not diabetic prior to pregnancy. Gestational diabetes can cause complications in the pregnancy similar to those of pre-existing diabetes mellitus. It also puts the woman at greater risk of developing diabetes after the pregnancy. Codes for gestational diabetes are in subcategory O24.4, Gestational diabetes mellitus. No other code from category O24, Diabetes mellitus in pregnancy, childbirth, and the puerperium, should be used with a code from O24.4.

The codes under subcategory O24.4 include diet controlled, insulin controlled, and controlled by oral hypoglycemic drugs. If a patient with gestational diabetes is treated with both diet and insulin, only the code for insulin-controlled is required. If a patient with gestational diabetes is treated with both diet and oral hypoglycemic medications, only the code for "controlled by oral hypoglycemic drugs" is required. Code Z79.4, Long-term (current) use of insulin or code Z79.84, Long-term (current) use of oral hypoglycemic drugs, should not be assigned with codes from subcategory O24.4.

An abnormal glucose tolerance in pregnancy is assigned a code from subcategory O99.81, Abnormal glucose complicating pregnancy, childbirth, and the puerperium.

j. Sepsis and septic shock complicating abortion, pregnancy, childbirth and the puerperium

When assigning a chapter 15 code for sepsis complicating abortion, pregnancy, childbirth, and the puerperium, a code for the specific type of infection should be assigned as an additional diagnosis. If severe sepsis is present, a code from subcategory R65.2, Severe sepsis, and code(s) for associated organ dysfunction(s) should also be assigned as additional diagnoses.

Patient is seen several days after a miscarriage with sepsis; cultures return MSSA

| O03.87 | Sepsis following complete or unspecified spontaneous abortion |
| B95.61 | Methicillin susceptible Staphylococcus aureus infection as the cause of diseases classified elsewhere |

Explanation: The type of infection that caused this patient to become septic was methicillin susceptible *Staphylococcus aureus* (MSSA), which as a secondary code helps capture all aspects related to this patient's septic condition.

---

k. Puerperal sepsis

Code O85, Puerperal sepsis, should be assigned with a secondary code to identify the causal organism (e.g., for a bacterial infection, assign a code from category B95-B96, Bacterial infections in conditions classified elsewhere). A code from category A40, Streptococcal sepsis, or A41, Other sepsis, should not be used for puerperal sepsis. If applicable, use additional codes to identify severe sepsis (R65.2-) and any associated acute organ dysfunction.

l. Alcohol, tobacco *and drug* use during pregnancy, childbirth and the puerperium

1) Alcohol use during pregnancy, childbirth and the puerperium

Codes under subcategory O99.31, Alcohol use complicating pregnancy, childbirth, and the puerperium, should be assigned for any pregnancy case when a mother uses alcohol during the pregnancy or postpartum. A secondary code from category F10, Alcohol related disorders, should also be assigned to identify manifestations of the alcohol use.

2) Tobacco use during pregnancy, childbirth and the puerperium

Codes under subcategory O99.33, Smoking (tobacco) complicating pregnancy, childbirth, and the puerperium, should be assigned for any pregnancy case when a mother uses any type of tobacco product during the pregnancy or postpartum. A secondary code from category F17, Nicotine dependence, should also be assigned to identify the type of nicotine dependence.

3) Drug use during pregnancy, childbirth and the puerperium

Codes under subcategory O99.32, Drug use complicating pregnancy, childbirth, and the puerperium, should be assigned for any pregnancy case when a mother uses drugs during the pregnancy or postpartum. This can involve illegal drugs, or inappropriate use or abuse of prescription drugs. Secondary code(s) from categories F11-F16 and F18-F19 should also be assigned to identify manifestations of the drug use.

m. Poisoning, toxic effects, adverse effects and underdosing in a pregnant patient

A code from subcategory O9A.2, Injury, poisoning and certain other consequences of external causes complicating pregnancy, childbirth, and the puerperium, should be sequenced first, followed by the appropriate injury, poisoning, toxic effect, adverse effect or underdosing code, and then the additional code(s) that specifies the condition caused by the poisoning, toxic effect, adverse effect or underdosing.

See Section I.C.19. Adverse effects, poisoning, underdosing and toxic effects.

Patient treated for accidental carbon monoxide poisoning from a gas heating implement; the patient is 18 weeks' pregnant

O9A.212	Injury, poisoning and certain other consequences of external causes complicating pregnancy, second trimester
T58.11XA	Toxic effect of carbon monoxide from utility gas, accidental (unintentional), initial encounter
Z3A.18	18 weeks gestation of pregnancy

Explanation: Although the carbon monoxide poisoning is the reason for the encounter, a code from the obstetrics chapter must be sequenced first. Chapter 15 codes have sequencing priority over codes from other chapters.

---

n. Normal delivery, code O80

1) Encounter for full term uncomplicated delivery

Code O80 should be assigned when a woman is admitted for a full-term normal delivery and delivers a single, healthy infant without any complications antepartum, during the delivery, or postpartum during the delivery episode. Code O80 is always a principal diagnosis. It is not to be used if any other code from chapter 15 is needed to describe a current complication of the antenatal, delivery, or perinatal period. Additional codes from other chapters may be used with code O80 if they are not related to or are in any way complicating the pregnancy.

2) Uncomplicated delivery with resolved antepartum complication

Code O80 may be used if the patient had a complication at some point during the pregnancy, but the complication is not present at the time of the admission for delivery.

Patient presents in labor at 39 weeks' gestation and delivers a healthy newborn; patient had abnormal glucose levels in her first trimester, which have since resolved

| O80 | Encounter for full-term uncomplicated delivery |
| Z37.0 | Single live birth |

Explanation: The abnormal glucose levels during the first trimester cannot be coded if they are not affecting the patient's current trimester. Without additional complications associated with the pregnancy, fetus, or mother, code O80 is appropriate.

---

3) Outcome of delivery for O80

Z37.0, Single live birth, is the only outcome of delivery code appropriate for use with O80.

o. The peripartum and postpartum periods

1) Peripartum and postpartum periods

The postpartum period begins immediately after delivery and continues for six weeks following delivery. The peripartum period is defined as the last month of pregnancy to five months postpartum.

2) Peripartum and postpartum complication

A postpartum complication is any complication occurring within the six-week period.

3) Pregnancy-related complications after 6 week period

Chapter 15 codes may also be used to describe pregnancy-related complications after the peripartum or postpartum period if the provider documents that a condition is pregnancy related.

Patient referred for varicose veins. She had a baby boy three months ago; the varicose veins started to appear one month ago. The doctor attributes the patient's pregnancy as the cause of the varicose veins, which continue to be painful and bother the patient. She is seeking surgical relief.

| O87.4 | Varicose veins of the lower extremity in the puerperium |

Explanation: Although the varicose veins occurred several months after the delivery of the newborn, the doctor attributed the varicose veins to pregnancy and therefore a code from chapter 15 is appropriate.

---

4) Admission for routine postpartum care following delivery outside hospital

When the mother delivers outside the hospital prior to admission and is admitted for routine postpartum care and no complications are noted, code Z39.0, Encounter for care and examination of mother immediately after delivery, should be assigned as the principal diagnosis.

5) Pregnancy associated cardiomyopathy

Pregnancy associated cardiomyopathy, code O90.3, is unique in that it may be diagnosed in the third trimester of pregnancy but may continue to progress months after delivery. For this reason, it is referred to as peripartum cardiomyopathy. Code O90.3 is only for use when the cardiomyopathy develops as a result of pregnancy in a woman who did not have pre-existing heart disease.

p. Code O94, Sequelae of complication of pregnancy, childbirth, and the puerperium

1) Code O94

Code O94, Sequelae of complication of pregnancy, childbirth, and the puerperium, is for use in those cases when an initial complication of a pregnancy develops a sequelae requiring care or treatment at a future date.

2) After the initial postpartum period

This code may be used at any time after the initial postpartum period.

3) Sequencing of code O94

This code, like all sequela codes, is to be sequenced following the code describing the sequelae of the complication.

q. Termination of pregnancy and spontaneous abortions

1) Abortion with Liveborn Fetus

When an attempted termination of pregnancy results in a liveborn fetus, assign code Z33.2, Encounter for elective termination of pregnancy and a code from category Z37, Outcome of Delivery.

2) Retained Products of Conception following an abortion

Subsequent encounters for retained products of conception following a spontaneous abortion or elective termination of pregnancy, without complications are assigned O03.4, Incomplete spontaneous abortion without complication, or code O07.4, Failed attempted termination of pregnancy without complication. This advice is appropriate even when the patient was discharged previously with a discharge diagnosis of complete abortion. If the patient has a specific complication associated with the spontaneous abortion or elective termination of pregnancy in addition to retained products of conception, assign the appropriate complication in category O03 or O07 instead of code O03.4 or O07.4

> Patient was seen two days ago for complete spontaneous abortion but returns today for urinary tract infection (UTI) with ultrasound showing retained products of conception
>
> **O03.38   Urinary tract infection following incomplete spontaneous abortion**
>
> *Explanation:* Although the diagnosis from the patient's previous stay indicated that the patient had a complete abortion, it is now determined that there were actually retained products of conception (POC). An abortion with retained POC is considered incomplete and in this case resulted in the patient developing a UTI.

3) Complications leading to abortion

Codes from Chapter 15 may be used as additional codes to identify any documented complications of the pregnancy in conjunction with codes in categories in O04, O07 and O08.

r. Abuse in a pregnant patient

For suspected or confirmed cases of abuse of a pregnant patient, a code(s) from subcategories O9A.3, Physical abuse complicating pregnancy, childbirth, and the puerperium, O9A.4, Sexual abuse complicating pregnancy, childbirth, and the puerperium, and O9A.5, Psychological abuse complicating pregnancy, childbirth, and the puerperium, should be sequenced first, followed by the appropriate codes (if applicable) to identify any associated current injury due to physical abuse, sexual abuse, and the perpetrator of abuse.

See Section I.C.19. Adult and child abuse, neglect and other maltreatment.

Chapter 15. Pregnancy, Childbirth and the Puerperium (O00-O9A)

NOTE   CODES FROM THIS CHAPTER ARE FOR USE ONLY ON MATERNAL RECORDS, NEVER ON NEWBORN RECORDS

Codes from this chapter are for use for conditions related to or aggravated by the pregnancy, childbirth, or by the puerperium (maternal causes or obstetric causes)

NOTE   Trimesters are counted from the first day of the last menstrual period. They are defined as follows:

1st trimester- less than 14 weeks Ø days

2nd trimester- 14 weeks Ø days to less than 28 weeks Ø days

3rd trimester- 28 weeks Ø days until delivery

Use additional code from category Z3A, Weeks of gestation, to identify the specific week of the pregnancy, if known.

EXCLUDES 1   supervision of normal pregnancy (Z34.-)

EXCLUDES 2   mental and behavioral disorders associated with the puerperium ▶(F53.-)◀

obstetrical tetanus (A34)

postpartum necrosis of pituitary gland (E23.Ø)

puerperal osteomalacia (M83.Ø)

AHA: 2016,1Q,3-5; 2014,3Q,17

This chapter contains the following blocks:

O00-O08   Pregnancy with abortive outcome
O09   Supervision of high risk pregnancy
O10-O16   Edema, proteinuria and hypertensive disorders in pregnancy, childbirth and the puerperium
O20-O29   Other maternal disorders predominantly related to pregnancy
O30-O48   Maternal care related to the fetus and amniotic cavity and possible delivery problems
O60-O77   Complications of labor and delivery
O80-O82   Encounter for delivery
O85-O92   Complications predominantly related to the puerperium
O94-O9A   Other obstetric conditions, not elsewhere classified

Pregnancy with abortive outcome (O00-O08)

EXCLUDES 1   continuing pregnancy in multiple gestation after abortion of one fetus or more (O31.1-, O31.3-)

TIP: Do not assign a code from category Z3A with codes in this code block.

✓4th O00 Ectopic pregnancy

INCLUDES   ruptured ectopic pregnancy

Use additional code from category O08 to identify any associated complication

AHA: 2016,4Q,48-50; 2014,3Q,17

DEF: Implantation of a fertilized egg outside the uterus, usually in the fallopian tube or abdomen that requires emergency treatment.

Ectopic Pregnancy

Cornual/interstitial
Isthmic
Ampullar
Tubal (fallopian)
Infundibular
Ovarian
Intraligamentous
Abdominal
Cervical
Intramural/mural

✓5th O00.Ø Abdominal pregnancy

EXCLUDES 1   maternal care for viable fetus in abdominal pregnancy (O36.7-)

O00.00   **Abdominal pregnancy** without intrauterine pregnancy   Ⓜ ♀
Abdominal pregnancy NOS

O00.01   **Abdominal pregnancy** with intrauterine pregnancy   Ⓜ ♀

✓5th O00.1 Tubal pregnancy

Fallopian pregnancy
Rupture of (fallopian) tube due to pregnancy
Tubal abortion

AHA: 2017,4Q,20

✓6th O00.10   **Tubal pregnancy** without intrauterine pregnancy
Tubal pregnancy NOS

O00.101   **Right tubal pregnancy without intrauterine pregnancy**   Ⓜ ♀

O00.102   **Left tubal pregnancy without intrauterine pregnancy**   Ⓜ ♀

O00.109   **Unspecified tubal pregnancy without intrauterine pregnancy**   Ⓜ ♀ ▽

✓6th O00.11   **Tubal pregnancy** with intrauterine pregnancy

O00.111   **Right tubal pregnancy with intrauterine pregnancy**   Ⓜ ♀

O00.112   **Left tubal pregnancy with intrauterine pregnancy**   Ⓜ ♀

O00.119   **Unspecified tubal pregnancy with intrauterine pregnancy**   Ⓜ ♀ ▽

✓5th O00.2 Ovarian pregnancy

AHA: 2017,4Q,20

✓6th O00.20   **Ovarian pregnancy** without intrauterine pregnancy
Ovarian pregnancy NOS

O00.201   **Right ovarian pregnancy** without intrauterine pregnancy   Ⓜ ♀

O00.202   **Left ovarian pregnancy without intrauterine pregnancy**   Ⓜ ♀

O00.209   **Unspecified ovarian pregnancy without intrauterine pregnancy**   Ⓜ ♀ ▽

✓6th O00.21   **Ovarian pregnancy** with intrauterine pregnancy

O00.211   **Right ovarian pregnancy with intrauterine pregnancy**   Ⓜ ♀

O00.212   **Left ovarian pregnancy with intrauterine pregnancy**   Ⓜ ♀

O00.219   **Unspecified ovarian pregnancy with intrauterine pregnancy**   Ⓜ ♀ ▽

✓5th O00.8 Other ectopic pregnancy

Cervical pregnancy
Cornual pregnancy
Intraligamentous pregnancy
Mural pregnancy

O00.80   **Other ectopic pregnancy** without intrauterine pregnancy   ⓞ Ⓜ ♀
Other ectopic pregnancy NOS

O00.81   **Other ectopic pregnancy** with intrauterine pregnancy   ⓞ Ⓜ ♀

✓5th O00.9 Ectopic pregnancy, unspecified

O00.90   **Unspecified ectopic pregnancy** without intrauterine pregnancy   ⓞ Ⓜ ♀ ▽
Ectopic pregnancy NOS

O00.91   **Unspecified ectopic pregnancy** with intrauterine pregnancy   ⓞ Ⓜ ♀ ▽

✓4th O01 Hydatidiform mole

Use additional code from category O08 to identify any associated complication

EXCLUDES 1   chorioadenoma (destruens) (D39.2)
malignant hydatidiform mole (D39.2)

AHA: 2014,3Q,17

DEF: Abnormal product of pregnancy, marked by a mass of cysts resembling a bunch of grapes due to chorionic villi proliferation and dissolution. It must be surgically removed.

O01.Ø   **Classical hydatidiform mole**   Ⓜ ♀
Complete hydatidiform mole

O01.1   **Incomplete and partial hydatidiform mole**   Ⓜ ♀

O01.9   **Hydatidiform mole, unspecified**   Ⓜ ♀ ▽
Trophoblastic disease NOS
Vesicular mole NOS

☑ Additional Character Req   ✓x7th Placeholder Alert   Manifestation   ▽ Unspecified   ▶◀ Revised Text   ● New Code   ▲ Revised Code Title

Chapter 15. Pregnancy, Childbirth and the Puerperium

✓4ᵗʰ **O02 Other abnormal products of conception**

Use additional code from category O08 to identify any associated complication

EXCLUDES 1   *papyraceous fetus (O31.0-)*

AHA: 2014,3Q,17

O02.0 Blighted ovum and nonhydatidiform mole   Ⓜ ♀

Carneous mole
Fleshy mole
Intrauterine mole NOS
Molar pregnancy NEC
Pathological ovum

O02.1 Missed abortion   Ⓠ Ⓜ ♀

Early fetal death, before completion of 20 weeks of gestation, with retention of dead fetus

EXCLUDES 1   *failed induced abortion (O07.-)*
fetal death (intrauterine) (late) (O36.4)
missed abortion with blighted ovum (O02.0)
missed abortion with hydatidiform mole (O01.-)
missed abortion with nonhydatidiform (O02.0)
missed abortion with other abnormal products of conception (O02.8-)
missed delivery (O36.4)
stillbirth (P95)

✓5ᵗʰ **O02.8 Other specified abnormal products of conception**

EXCLUDES 1   *abnormal products of conception with blighted ovum (O02.0)*
abnormal products of conception with hydatidiform mole (O01.-)
abnormal products of conception with nonhydatidiform mole (O02.0)

O02.81 Inappropriate change in quantitative human chorionic gonadotropin (hCG) in early pregnancy   Ⓜ ♀

Biochemical pregnancy
Chemical pregnancy
Inappropriate level of quantitative human chorionic gonadotropin (hCG) for gestational age in early pregnancy

O02.89 Other abnormal products of conception   Ⓜ ♀

O02.9 Abnormal product of conception, unspecified   Ⓜ ♀ ▽

✓4ᵗʰ **O03 Spontaneous abortion**

NOTE   Incomplete abortion includes retained products of conception following spontaneous abortion

INCLUDES   miscarriage

O03.0 Genital tract and pelvic infection following incomplete spontaneous abortion   Ⓜ ♀

Endometritis following incomplete spontaneous abortion
Oophoritis following incomplete spontaneous abortion
Parametritis following incomplete spontaneous abortion
Pelvic peritonitis following incomplete spontaneous abortion
Salpingitis following incomplete spontaneous abortion
Salpingo-oophoritis following incomplete spontaneous abortion

EXCLUDES 1   *sepsis following incomplete spontaneous abortion (O03.37)*
urinary tract infection following incomplete spontaneous abortion (O03.38)

O03.1 Delayed or excessive hemorrhage following incomplete spontaneous abortion   Ⓠ Ⓜ ♀

Afibrinogenemia following incomplete spontaneous abortion
Defibrination syndrome following incomplete spontaneous abortion
Hemolysis following incomplete spontaneous abortion
Intravascular coagulation following incomplete spontaneous abortion

O03.2 Embolism following incomplete spontaneous abortion   Ⓜ ♀

Air embolism following incomplete spontaneous abortion
Amniotic fluid embolism following incomplete spontaneous abortion
Blood-clot embolism following incomplete spontaneous abortion
Embolism NOS following incomplete spontaneous abortion
Fat embolism following incomplete spontaneous abortion
Pulmonary embolism following incomplete spontaneous abortion
Pyemic embolism following incomplete spontaneous abortion
Septic or septicopyemic embolism following incomplete spontaneous abortion
Soap embolism following incomplete spontaneous abortion

✓5ᵗʰ **O03.3 Other and unspecified complications following incomplete spontaneous abortion**

O03.30 Unspecified complication following incomplete spontaneous abortion   Ⓜ ♀ ▽

O03.31 Shock following incomplete spontaneous abortion   Ⓜ ♀

Circulatory collapse following incomplete spontaneous abortion
Shock (postprocedural) following incomplete spontaneous abortion

EXCLUDES 1   *shock due to infection following incomplete spontaneous abortion (O03.37)*

O03.32 Renal failure following incomplete spontaneous abortion   Ⓜ ♀

Kidney failure (acute) following incomplete spontaneous abortion
Oliguria following incomplete spontaneous abortion
Renal shutdown following incomplete spontaneous abortion
Renal tubular necrosis following incomplete spontaneous abortion
Uremia following incomplete spontaneous abortion

O03.33 Metabolic disorder following incomplete spontaneous abortion   Ⓜ ♀

O03.34 Damage to pelvic organs following incomplete spontaneous abortion   Ⓜ ♀

Laceration, perforation, tear or chemical damage of bladder following incomplete spontaneous abortion.
Laceration, perforation, tear or chemical damage of bowel following incomplete spontaneous abortion
Laceration, perforation, tear or chemical damage of broad ligament following incomplete spontaneous abortion
Laceration, perforation, tear or chemical damage of cervix following incomplete spontaneous abortion
Laceration, perforation, tear or chemical damage of periurethral tissue following incomplete spontaneous abortion
Laceration, perforation, tear or chemical damage of uterus following incomplete spontaneous abortion
Laceration, perforation, tear or chemical damage of vagina following incomplete spontaneous abortion

O03.35 Other venous complications following incomplete spontaneous abortion   Ⓜ ♀

O03.36 Cardiac arrest following incomplete spontaneous abortion   Ⓜ ♀

O03.37 Sepsis following incomplete spontaneous abortion   Ⓜ ♀

Use additional code to identify infectious agent (B95-B97)
Use additional code to identify severe sepsis, if applicable (R65.2-)

EXCLUDES 1   *septic or septicopyemic embolism following incomplete spontaneous abortion (O03.2)*

O03.38   **Urinary tract infection following**   M ♀
incomplete spontaneous abortion
     Cystitis following incomplete spontaneous abortion

O03.39   **Incomplete spontaneous abortion with**   M ♀
other complications

O03.4   **Incomplete spontaneous abortion without**   M ♀
complication

O03.5   **Genital tract and pelvic infection following**   M ♀
complete or unspecified spontaneous abortion
     Endometritis following complete or unspecified spontaneous abortion
     Oophoritis following complete or unspecified abortion
     Parametritis following complete or unspecified spontaneous abortion
     Pelvic peritonitis following complete or unspecified spontaneous abortion
     Salpingitis following complete or unspecified spontaneous abortion
     Salpingo-oophoritis following complete or unspecified spontaneous abortion
     EXCLUDES 1   *sepsis following complete or unspecified spontaneous abortion (O03.87)*
            urinary tract infection following complete or unspecified spontaneous abortion (O03.88)

O03.6   **Delayed or excessive hemorrhage following**   ◖ M ♀
complete or unspecified spontaneous abortion
     Afibrinogenemia following complete or unspecified spontaneous abortion
     Defibrination syndrome following complete or unspecified spontaneous abortion
     Hemolysis following complete or unspecified spontaneous abortion
     Intravascular coagulation following complete or unspecified spontaneous abortion

O03.7   **Embolism following complete or unspecified**   M ♀
spontaneous abortion
     Air embolism following complete or unspecified spontaneous abortion
     Amniotic fluid embolism following complete or unspecified spontaneous abortion
     Blood-clot embolism following complete or unspecified spontaneous abortion
     Embolism NOS following complete or unspecified spontaneous abortion
     Fat embolism following complete or unspecified spontaneous abortion
     Pulmonary embolism following complete or unspecified spontaneous abortion
     Pyemic embolism following complete or unspecified spontaneous abortion
     Septic or septicopyemic embolism following complete or unspecified spontaneous abortion
     Soap embolism following complete or unspecified spontaneous abortion

✓5ᵗʰ **O03.8**   **Other and unspecified complications following complete or unspecified spontaneous abortion**

O03.80   **Unspecified complication following**   M ♀ ▽
complete or unspecified spontaneous abortion

O03.81   **Shock following complete or unspecified**   M ♀
spontaneous abortion
     Circulatory collapse following complete or unspecified spontaneous abortion
     Shock (postprocedural) following complete or unspecified spontaneous abortion
     EXCLUDES 1   *shock due to infection following complete or unspecified spontaneous abortion (O03.87)*

O03.82   **Renal failure following complete or**   M ♀
unspecified spontaneous abortion
     Kidney failure (acute) following complete or unspecified spontaneous abortion
     Oliguria following complete or unspecified spontaneous abortion
     Renal shutdown following complete or unspecified spontaneous abortion
     Renal tubular necrosis following complete or unspecified spontaneous abortion
     Uremia following complete or unspecified spontaneous abortion

O03.83   **Metabolic disorder following complete or**   M ♀
unspecified spontaneous abortion

O03.84   **Damage to pelvic organs following**   M ♀
complete or unspecified spontaneous abortion
     Laceration, perforation, tear or chemical damage of bladder following complete or unspecified spontaneous abortion
     Laceration, perforation, tear or chemical damage of bowel following complete or unspecified spontaneous abortion
     Laceration, perforation, tear or chemical damage of broad ligament following complete or unspecified spontaneous abortion
     Laceration, perforation, tear or chemical damage of cervix following complete or unspecified spontaneous abortion
     Laceration, perforation, tear or chemical damage of periurethral tissue following complete or unspecified spontaneous abortion
     Laceration, perforation, tear or chemical damage of uterus following complete or unspecified spontaneous abortion
     Laceration, perforation, tear or chemical damage of vagina following complete or unspecified spontaneous abortion

O03.85   **Other venous complications following**   M ♀
complete or unspecified spontaneous abortion

O03.86   **Cardiac arrest following complete or**   M ♀
unspecified spontaneous abortion

O03.87   **Sepsis following complete or unspecified**   M ♀
spontaneous abortion
     Use additional code to identify infectious agent (B95-B97)
     Use additional code to identify severe sepsis, if applicable (R65.2-)
     EXCLUDES 1   *septic or septicopyemic embolism following complete or unspecified spontaneous abortion (O03.7)*

O03.88   **Urinary tract infection following complete**   M ♀
or unspecified spontaneous abortion
     Cystitis following complete or unspecified spontaneous abortion

O03.89   **Complete or unspecified spontaneous**   M ♀
abortion with other complications

O03.9   **Complete or unspecified spontaneous abortion**   M ♀ ▽
without complication
     Miscarriage NOS
     Spontaneous abortion NOS

Chapter 15. Pregnancy, Childbirth and the Puerperium

☑4ᵗʰ **O04 Complications following (induced) termination of pregnancy**

INCLUDES   complications following (induced) termination of pregnancy

EXCLUDES 1   *encounter for elective termination of pregnancy, uncomplicated (Z33.2)*

failed attempted termination of pregnancy (O07.-)

O04.5 Genital tract and pelvic infection following Ⓜ ♀
(induced) termination of pregnancy

Endometritis following (induced) termination of pregnancy
Oophoritis following (induced) termination of pregnancy
Parametritis following (induced) termination of pregnancy
Pelvic peritonitis following (induced) termination of pregnancy
Salpingitis following (induced) termination of pregnancy
Salpingo-oophoritis following (induced) termination of pregnancy

EXCLUDES 1   *sepsis following (induced) termination of pregnancy (O04.87)*

urinary tract infection following (induced) termination of pregnancy (O04.88)

O04.6 Delayed or excessive hemorrhage following Ⓠ Ⓜ ♀
(induced) termination of pregnancy

Afibrinogenemia following (induced) termination of pregnancy
Defibrination syndrome following (induced) termination of pregnancy
Hemolysis following (induced) termination of pregnancy
Intravascular coagulation following (induced) termination of pregnancy

O04.7 Embolism following (induced) termination of Ⓜ ♀
pregnancy

Air embolism following (induced) termination of pregnancy
Amniotic fluid embolism following (induced) termination of pregnancy
Blood-clot embolism following (induced) termination of pregnancy
Embolism NOS following (induced) termination of pregnancy
Fat embolism following (induced) termination of pregnancy
Pulmonary embolism following (induced) termination of pregnancy
Pyemic embolism following (induced) termination of pregnancy
Septic or septicopyemic embolism following (induced) termination of pregnancy
Soap embolism following (induced) termination of pregnancy

☑5ᵗʰ **O04.8 (Induced) termination of pregnancy with other and unspecified complications**

O04.80 (Induced) termination of pregnancy with Ⓜ ♀ ▽
unspecified complications

O04.81 Shock following (induced) termination of Ⓜ ♀
pregnancy

Circulatory collapse following (induced) termination of pregnancy
Shock (postprocedural) following (induced) termination of pregnancy

EXCLUDES 1   *shock due to infection following (induced) termination of pregnancy (O04.87)*

O04.82 Renal failure following (induced) Ⓜ ♀
termination of pregnancy

Kidney failure (acute) following (induced) termination of pregnancy
Oliguria following (induced) termination of pregnancy
Renal shutdown following (induced) termination of pregnancy
Renal tubular necrosis following (induced) termination of pregnancy
Uremia following (induced) termination of pregnancy

O04.83 Metabolic disorder following (induced) Ⓜ ♀
termination of pregnancy

O04.84 Damage to pelvic organs following Ⓜ ♀
(induced) termination of pregnancy

Laceration, perforation, tear or chemical damage of bladder following (induced) termination of pregnancy
Laceration, perforation, tear or chemical damage of bowel following (induced) termination of pregnancy
Laceration, perforation, tear or chemical damage of broad ligament following (induced) termination of pregnancy
Laceration, perforation, tear or chemical damage of cervix following (induced) termination of pregnancy
Laceration, perforation, tear or chemical damage of periurethral tissue following (induced) termination of pregnancy
Laceration, perforation, tear or chemical damage of uterus following (induced) termination of pregnancy
Laceration, perforation, tear or chemical damage of vagina following (induced) termination of pregnancy

O04.85 Other venous complications following Ⓜ ♀
(induced) termination of pregnancy

O04.86 Cardiac arrest following (induced) Ⓜ ♀
termination of pregnancy

O04.87 Sepsis following (induced) termination of Ⓜ ♀
pregnancy

Use additional code to identify infectious agent (B95-B97)

Use additional code to identify severe sepsis, if applicable (R65.2-)

EXCLUDES 1   *septic or septicopyemic embolism following (induced) termination of pregnancy (O04.7)*

O04.88 Urinary tract infection following (induced) Ⓜ ♀
termination of pregnancy

Cystitis following (induced) termination of pregnancy

O04.89 (Induced) termination of pregnancy with Ⓜ ♀
other complications

☑4ᵗʰ **O07 Failed attempted termination of pregnancy**

INCLUDES   failure of attempted induction of termination of pregnancy
incomplete elective abortion

EXCLUDES 1   *incomplete spontaneous abortion (O03.0-)*

O07.0 Genital tract and pelvic infection following failed Ⓜ ♀
attempted termination of pregnancy

Endometritis following failed attempted termination of pregnancy
Oophoritis following failed attempted termination of pregnancy
Parametritis following failed attempted termination of pregnancy
Pelvic peritonitis following failed attempted termination of pregnancy
Salpingitis following failed attempted termination of pregnancy
Salpingo-oophoritis following failed attempted termination of pregnancy

EXCLUDES 1   *sepsis following failed attempted termination of pregnancy (O07.37)*

urinary tract infection following failed attempted termination of pregnancy (O07.38)

O07.1 Delayed or excessive hemorrhage following failed Ⓠ Ⓜ ♀
attempted termination of pregnancy

Afibrinogenemia following failed attempted termination of pregnancy
Defibrination syndrome following failed attempted termination of pregnancy
Hemolysis following failed attempted termination of pregnancy
Intravascular coagulation following failed attempted termination of pregnancy

O07.2 Embolism following failed attempted termination of pregnancy   Ⓜ ♀

Air embolism following failed attempted termination of pregnancy

Amniotic fluid embolism following failed attempted termination of pregnancy

Blood-clot embolism following failed attempted termination of pregnancy

Embolism NOS following failed attempted termination of pregnancy

Fat embolism following failed attempted termination of pregnancy

Pulmonary embolism following failed attempted termination of pregnancy

Pyemic embolism following failed attempted termination of pregnancy

Septic or septicopyemic embolism following failed attempted termination of pregnancy

Soap embolism following failed attempted termination of pregnancy

✓5ᵗʰ O07.3 Failed attempted termination of pregnancy with other and unspecified complications

O07.30 Failed attempted termination of pregnancy with unspecified complications   Ⓜ ♀ ▽

O07.31 Shock following failed attempted termination of pregnancy   Ⓜ ♀

Circulatory collapse following failed attempted termination of pregnancy

Shock (postprocedural) following failed attempted termination of pregnancy

EXCLUDES 1   shock due to infection following failed attempted termination of pregnancy (O07.37)

O07.32 Renal failure following failed attempted termination of pregnancy   Ⓜ ♀

Kidney failure (acute) following failed attempted termination of pregnancy

Oliguria following failed attempted termination of pregnancy

Renal shutdown following failed attempted termination of pregnancy

Renal tubular necrosis following failed attempted termination of pregnancy

Uremia following failed attempted termination of pregnancy

O07.33 Metabolic disorder following failed attempted termination of pregnancy   Ⓜ ♀

O07.34 Damage to pelvic organs following failed attempted termination of pregnancy   Ⓜ ♀

Laceration, perforation, tear or chemical damage of bladder following failed attempted termination of pregnancy

Laceration, perforation, tear or chemical damage of bowel following failed attempted termination of pregnancy

Laceration, perforation, tear or chemical damage of broad ligament following failed attempted termination of pregnancy

Laceration, perforation, tear or chemical damage of cervix following failed attempted termination of pregnancy

Laceration, perforation, tear or chemical damage of periurethral tissue following failed attempted termination of pregnancy

Laceration, perforation, tear or chemical damage of uterus following failed attempted termination of pregnancy

Laceration, perforation, tear or chemical damage of vagina following failed attempted termination of pregnancy

O07.35 Other venous complications following failed attempted termination of pregnancy   Ⓜ ♀

O07.36 Cardiac arrest following failed attempted termination of pregnancy   Ⓜ ♀

O07.37 Sepsis following failed attempted termination of pregnancy   Ⓜ ♀

Use additional code (B95-B97), to identify infectious agent

Use additional code (R65.2-) to identify severe sepsis, if applicable

EXCLUDES 1   septic or septicopyemic embolism following failed attempted termination of pregnancy (O07.2)

O07.38 Urinary tract infection following failed attempted termination of pregnancy   Ⓜ ♀

Cystitis following failed attempted termination of pregnancy

O07.39 Failed attempted termination of pregnancy with other complications   Ⓜ ♀

O07.4 Failed attempted termination of pregnancy without complication   Ⓜ ♀

✓4ᵗʰ O08 Complications following ectopic and molar pregnancy

This category is for use with categories O00-O02 to identify any associated complications

O08.0 Genital tract and pelvic infection following ectopic and molar pregnancy   Ⓜ ♀

Endometritis following ectopic and molar pregnancy

Oophoritis following ectopic and molar pregnancy

Parametritis following ectopic and molar pregnancy

Pelvic peritonitis following ectopic and molar pregnancy

Salpingitis following ectopic and molar pregnancy

Salpingo-oophoritis following ectopic and molar pregnancy

EXCLUDES 1   sepsis following ectopic and molar pregnancy (O08.82)

urinary tract infection (O08.83)

O08.1 Delayed or excessive hemorrhage following ectopic and molar pregnancy   ⓪ Ⓜ ♀

Afibrinogenemia following ectopic and molar pregnancy

Defibrination syndrome following ectopic and molar pregnancy

Hemolysis following ectopic and molar pregnancy

Intravascular coagulation following ectopic and molar pregnancy

EXCLUDES 1   delayed or excessive hemorrhage due to incomplete abortion (O03.1)

O08.2 Embolism following ectopic and molar pregnancy   Ⓜ ♀

Air embolism following ectopic and molar pregnancy

Amniotic fluid embolism following ectopic and molar pregnancy

Blood-clot embolism following ectopic and molar pregnancy

Embolism NOS following ectopic and molar pregnancy

Fat embolism following ectopic and molar pregnancy

Pulmonary embolism following ectopic and molar pregnancy

Pyemic embolism following ectopic and molar pregnancy

Septic or septicopyemic embolism following ectopic and molar pregnancy

Soap embolism following ectopic and molar pregnancy

O08.3 Shock following ectopic and molar pregnancy   Ⓜ ♀

Circulatory collapse following ectopic and molar pregnancy

Shock (postprocedural) following ectopic and molar pregnancy

EXCLUDES 1   shock due to infection following ectopic and molar pregnancy (O08.82)

O08.4 Renal failure following ectopic and molar pregnancy   Ⓜ ♀

Kidney failure (acute) following ectopic and molar pregnancy

Oliguria following ectopic and molar pregnancy

Renal shutdown following ectopic and molar pregnancy

Renal tubular necrosis following ectopic and molar pregnancy

Uremia following ectopic and molar pregnancy

O08.5 Metabolic disorders following an ectopic and molar pregnancy   Ⓜ ♀

✓ Additional Character Req   ✓x7ᵗʰ Placeholder Alert   Manifestation   ▽ Unspecified   ►◄ Revised Text   ● New Code   ▲ Revised Code Title

ICD-10-CM 2019   853

O08.6 **Damage to pelvic organs and tissues following an ectopic and molar pregnancy**   M ♀
  Laceration, perforation, tear or chemical damage of bladder following an ectopic and molar pregnancy
  Laceration, perforation, tear or chemical damage of bowel following an ectopic and molar pregnancy
  Laceration, perforation, tear or chemical damage of broad ligament following an ectopic and molar pregnancy
  Laceration, perforation, tear or chemical damage of cervix following an ectopic and molar pregnancy
  Laceration, perforation, tear or chemical damage of periurethral tissue following an ectopic and molar pregnancy
  Laceration, perforation, tear or chemical damage of uterus following an ectopic and molar pregnancy
  Laceration, perforation, tear or chemical damage of vagina following an ectopic and molar pregnancy

O08.7 **Other venous complications following an ectopic and molar pregnancy**   M ♀

✓5ᵗʰ **O08.8** **Other complications following an ectopic and molar pregnancy**

    O08.81 **Cardiac arrest following an ectopic and molar pregnancy**   M ♀

    O08.82 **Sepsis following ectopic and molar pregnancy**   M ♀
      Use additional code (B95-B97), to identify infectious agent
      Use additional code (R65.2-) to identify severe sepsis, if applicable
      EXCLUDES 1   septic or septicopyemic embolism following ectopic and molar pregnancy (O08.2)

    O08.83 **Urinary tract infection following an ectopic and molar pregnancy**   M ♀
      Cystitis following an ectopic and molar pregnancy

    O08.89 **Other complications following an ectopic and molar pregnancy**   M ♀

O08.9 **Unspecified complication following an ectopic and molar pregnancy**   M ♀ ▽

Supervision of high risk pregnancy (O09)

✓4ᵗʰ **O09** **Supervision of high risk pregnancy**
    AHA: 2016,4Q,48-50,150

✓5ᵗʰ **O09.0** **Supervision of pregnancy with history of infertility**
    DEF: Infertility: Inability to conceive for at least one year with regular intercourse.

    O09.00 **Supervision of pregnancy with history of infertility, unspecified trimester**   M ♀ ▽

    O09.01 **Supervision of pregnancy with history of infertility, first trimester**   M ♀

    O09.02 **Supervision of pregnancy with history of infertility, second trimester**   M ♀

    O09.03 **Supervision of pregnancy with history of infertility, third trimester**   M ♀

✓5ᵗʰ **O09.1** **Supervision of pregnancy with history of ectopic pregnancy**
    DEF: Ectopic pregnancy: Implantation of a fertilized egg outside the uterus, usually in the fallopian tube or abdomen that requires emergency treatment.

    O09.10 **Supervision of pregnancy with history of ectopic pregnancy, unspecified trimester**   M ♀ ▽

    O09.11 **Supervision of pregnancy with history of ectopic pregnancy, first trimester**   M ♀

    O09.12 **Supervision of pregnancy with history of ectopic pregnancy, second trimester**   M ♀

    O09.13 **Supervision of pregnancy with history of ectopic pregnancy, third trimester**   M ♀

✓5ᵗʰ **O09.A** **Supervision of pregnancy with history of molar pregnancy**
    DEF: Molar pregnancy: Trophoblastic neoplasm that mimics pregnancy by proliferating from a pathologic ovum and resulting only in a mass of cysts resembling grapes, 80 percent of which are benign, but require surgical removal.

    O09.A0 **Supervision of pregnancy with history of molar pregnancy, unspecified trimester**   M ♀ ▽

    O09.A1 **Supervision of pregnancy with history of molar pregnancy, first trimester**   M ♀

    O09.A2 **Supervision of pregnancy with history of molar pregnancy, second trimester**   M ♀

    O09.A3 **Supervision of pregnancy with history of molar pregnancy, third trimester**   M ♀

✓5ᵗʰ **O09.2** **Supervision of pregnancy with other poor reproductive or obstetric history**
    EXCLUDES 2   pregnancy care for patient with history of recurrent pregnancy loss (O26.2-)

✓6ᵗʰ **O09.21** **Supervision of pregnancy with history of pre-term labor**

    O09.211 **Supervision of pregnancy with history of pre-term labor, first trimester**   M ♀

    O09.212 **Supervision of pregnancy with history of pre-term labor, second trimester**   M ♀

    O09.213 **Supervision of pregnancy with history of pre-term labor, third trimester**   M ♀

    O09.219 **Supervision of pregnancy with history of pre-term labor, unspecified trimester**   M ♀ ▽

✓6ᵗʰ **O09.29** **Supervision of pregnancy with other poor reproductive or obstetric history**
    Supervision of pregnancy with history of neonatal death
    Supervision of pregnancy with history of stillbirth

    O09.291 **Supervision of pregnancy with other poor reproductive or obstetric history, first trimester**   M ♀

    O09.292 **Supervision of pregnancy with other poor reproductive or obstetric history, second trimester**   M ♀

    O09.293 **Supervision of pregnancy with other poor reproductive or obstetric history, third trimester**   M ♀

    O09.299 **Supervision of pregnancy with other poor reproductive or obstetric history, unspecified trimester**   M ♀ ▽

✓5ᵗʰ **O09.3** **Supervision of pregnancy with insufficient antenatal care**
    Supervision of concealed pregnancy
    Supervision of hidden pregnancy

    O09.30 **Supervision of pregnancy with insufficient antenatal care, unspecified trimester**   M ♀ ▽

    O09.31 **Supervision of pregnancy with insufficient antenatal care, first trimester**   M ♀

    O09.32 **Supervision of pregnancy with insufficient antenatal care, second trimester**   M ♀

    O09.33 **Supervision of pregnancy with insufficient antenatal care, third trimester**   M ♀

✓5ᵗʰ **O09.4** **Supervision of pregnancy with grand multiparity**

    O09.40 **Supervision of pregnancy with grand multiparity, unspecified trimester**   M ♀ ▽

    O09.41 **Supervision of pregnancy with grand multiparity, first trimester**   M ♀

    O09.42 **Supervision of pregnancy with grand multiparity, second trimester**   M ♀

    O09.43 **Supervision of pregnancy with grand multiparity, third trimester**   M ♀

✓5ᵗʰ **O09.5** **Supervision of elderly primigravida and multigravida**
    Pregnancy for a female 35 years and older at expected date of delivery

✓6ᵗʰ **O09.51** **Supervision of elderly primigravida**

    O09.511 **Supervision of elderly primigravida, first trimester**   M ♀

    O09.512 **Supervision of elderly primigravida, second trimester**   M ♀

    O09.513 **Supervision of elderly primigravida, third trimester**   M ♀

    O09.519 **Supervision of elderly primigravida, unspecified trimester**   M ♀ ▽

✓6ᵗʰ **O09.52** **Supervision of elderly multigravida**

    O09.521 **Supervision of elderly multigravida, first trimester**   M ♀

    O09.522 **Supervision of elderly multigravida, second trimester**   M ♀

    O09.523 **Supervision of elderly multigravida, third trimester**   M ♀

    O09.529 **Supervision of elderly multigravida, unspecified trimester**   M ♀ ▽

√5ᵗʰ **O09.6 Supervision of young primigravida and multigravida**

Supervision of pregnancy for a female less than 16 years old at expected date of delivery

√6ᵗʰ **O09.61 Supervision of young primigravida**

O09.611 Supervision of young primigravida, first trimester Ⓜ ♀

O09.612 Supervision of young primigravida, second trimester Ⓜ ♀

O09.613 Supervision of young primigravida, third trimester Ⓜ ♀

O09.619 Supervision of young primigravida, unspecified trimester Ⓜ ♀ ▽

√6ᵗʰ **O09.62 Supervision of young multigravida**

O09.621 Supervision of young multigravida, first trimester Ⓜ ♀

O09.622 Supervision of young multigravida, second trimester Ⓜ ♀

O09.623 Supervision of young multigravida, third trimester Ⓜ ♀

O09.629 Supervision of young multigravida, unspecified trimester Ⓜ ♀ ▽

√5ᵗʰ **O09.7 Supervision of high risk pregnancy due to social problems**

O09.70 Supervision of high risk pregnancy due to social problems, unspecified trimester Ⓜ ♀ ▽

O09.71 Supervision of high risk pregnancy due to social problems, first trimester Ⓜ ♀

O09.72 Supervision of high risk pregnancy due to social problems, second trimester Ⓜ ♀

O09.73 Supervision of high risk pregnancy due to social problems, third trimester Ⓜ ♀

√5ᵗʰ **O09.8 Supervision of other high risk pregnancies**

√6ᵗʰ **O09.81 Supervision of pregnancy resulting from assisted reproductive technology**

Supervision of pregnancy resulting from in-vitro fertilization

EXCLUDES 2   gestational carrier status (Z33.3)

O09.811 Supervision of pregnancy resulting from assisted reproductive technology, first trimester Ⓜ ♀

O09.812 Supervision of pregnancy resulting from assisted reproductive technology, second trimester Ⓜ ♀

O09.813 Supervision of pregnancy resulting from assisted reproductive technology, third trimester Ⓜ ♀

O09.819 Supervision of pregnancy resulting from assisted reproductive technology, unspecified trimester Ⓜ ♀ ▽

√6ᵗʰ **O09.82 Supervision of pregnancy with history of in utero procedure during previous pregnancy**

O09.821 Supervision of pregnancy with history of in utero procedure during previous pregnancy, first trimester Ⓜ ♀

O09.822 Supervision of pregnancy with history of in utero procedure during previous pregnancy, second trimester Ⓜ ♀

O09.823 Supervision of pregnancy with history of in utero procedure during previous pregnancy, third trimester Ⓜ ♀

O09.829 Supervision of pregnancy with history of in utero procedure during previous pregnancy, unspecified trimester Ⓜ ♀ ▽

EXCLUDES 1   supervision of pregnancy affected by in utero procedure during current pregnancy (O35.7)

√6ᵗʰ **O09.89 Supervision of other high risk pregnancies**

O09.891 Supervision of other high risk pregnancies, first trimester Ⓜ ♀

O09.892 Supervision of other high risk pregnancies, second trimester Ⓜ ♀

O09.893 Supervision of other high risk pregnancies, third trimester Ⓜ ♀

O09.899 Supervision of other high risk pregnancies, unspecified trimester Ⓜ ♀ ▽

√5ᵗʰ **O09.9 Supervision of high risk pregnancy, unspecified**

O09.90 Supervision of high risk pregnancy, unspecified, unspecified trimester Ⓜ ♀ ▽

O09.91 Supervision of high risk pregnancy, unspecified, first trimester Ⓜ ♀ ▽

O09.92 Supervision of high risk pregnancy, unspecified, second trimester Ⓜ ♀ ▽

O09.93 Supervision of high risk pregnancy, unspecified, third trimester Ⓜ ♀ ▽

Edema, proteinuria and hypertensive disorders in pregnancy, childbirth and the puerperium (O10-O16)

AHA: 2016,4Q,50

√4ᵗʰ **O10 Pre-existing hypertension complicating pregnancy, childbirth and the puerperium**

INCLUDES   pre-existing hypertension with pre-existing proteinuria complicating pregnancy, childbirth and the puerperium

EXCLUDES 2   *pre-existing hypertension with superimposed pre-eclampsia complicating pregnancy, childbirth and the puerperium (O11.-)*

√5ᵗʰ **O10.0 Pre-existing essential hypertension complicating pregnancy, childbirth and the puerperium**

Any condition in I10 specified as a reason for obstetric care during pregnancy, childbirth or the puerperium

√6ᵗʰ **O10.01 Pre-existing essential hypertension complicating pregnancy**

O10.011 Pre-existing essential hypertension complicating pregnancy, first trimester Ⓜ ♀

O10.012 Pre-existing essential hypertension complicating pregnancy, second trimester Ⓜ ♀

O10.013 Pre-existing essential hypertension complicating pregnancy, third trimester Ⓜ ♀

O10.019 Pre-existing essential hypertension complicating pregnancy, unspecified trimester Ⓜ ♀ ▽

O10.02 Pre-existing essential hypertension complicating childbirth Ⓜ ♀

O10.03 Pre-existing essential hypertension complicating the puerperium Ⓜ ♀

√5ᵗʰ **O10.1 Pre-existing hypertensive heart disease complicating pregnancy, childbirth and the puerperium**

Any condition in I11 specified as a reason for obstetric care during pregnancy, childbirth or the puerperium

Use additional code from I11 to identify the type of hypertensive heart disease

√6ᵗʰ **O10.11 Pre-existing hypertensive heart disease complicating pregnancy**

O10.111 Pre-existing hypertensive heart disease complicating pregnancy, first trimester Ⓜ ♀

O10.112 Pre-existing hypertensive heart disease complicating pregnancy, second trimester Ⓜ ♀

O10.113 Pre-existing hypertensive heart disease complicating pregnancy, third trimester Ⓜ ♀

O10.119 Pre-existing hypertensive heart disease complicating pregnancy, unspecified trimester Ⓜ ♀ ▽

O10.12 Pre-existing hypertensive heart disease complicating childbirth Ⓜ ♀

O10.13 Pre-existing hypertensive heart disease complicating the puerperium Ⓜ ♀

✓ Additional Character Req   ✓ˣ⁷ᵗʰ Placeholder Alert   **Manifestation**   ▽ Unspecified   ▶◀ Revised Text   ● New Code   ▲ Revised Code Title

ICD-10-CM 2019   **855**

Chapter 15. Pregnancy, Childbirth and the Puerperium

O10.2–O12.25

✓5ᵗʰ **O10.2 Pre-existing hypertensive chronic kidney disease complicating pregnancy, childbirth and the puerperium**
     Any condition in I12 specified as a reason for obstetric care during pregnancy, childbirth or the puerperium
     Use additional code from I12 to identify the type of hypertensive chronic kidney disease

     ✓6ᵗʰ **O10.21 Pre-existing hypertensive chronic kidney disease complicating pregnancy**

         O10.211 Pre-existing hypertensive chronic kidney disease complicating pregnancy, first trimester   Ⓜ ♀

         O10.212 Pre-existing hypertensive chronic kidney disease complicating pregnancy, second trimester   Ⓜ ♀

         O10.213 Pre-existing hypertensive chronic kidney disease complicating pregnancy, third trimester   Ⓜ ♀

         O10.219 Pre-existing hypertensive chronic kidney disease complicating pregnancy, unspecified trimester   Ⓜ ♀ ▽

     O10.22 Pre-existing hypertensive chronic kidney disease complicating childbirth   Ⓜ ♀

     O10.23 Pre-existing hypertensive chronic kidney disease complicating the puerperium   Ⓜ ♀

✓5ᵗʰ **O10.3 Pre-existing hypertensive heart and chronic kidney disease complicating pregnancy, childbirth and the puerperium**
     Any condition in I13 specified as a reason for obstetric care during pregnancy, childbirth or the puerperium
     Use additional code from I13 to identify the type of hypertensive heart and chronic kidney disease

     ✓6ᵗʰ **O10.31 Pre-existing hypertensive heart and chronic kidney disease complicating pregnancy**

         O10.311 Pre-existing hypertensive heart and chronic kidney disease complicating pregnancy, first trimester   Ⓜ ♀

         O10.312 Pre-existing hypertensive heart and chronic kidney disease complicating pregnancy, second trimester   Ⓜ ♀

         O10.313 Pre-existing hypertensive heart and chronic kidney disease complicating pregnancy, third trimester   Ⓜ ♀

         O10.319 Pre-existing hypertensive heart and chronic kidney disease complicating pregnancy, unspecified trimester   Ⓜ ♀ ▽

     O10.32 Pre-existing hypertensive heart and chronic kidney disease complicating childbirth   Ⓜ ♀

     O10.33 Pre-existing hypertensive heart and chronic kidney disease complicating the puerperium   Ⓜ ♀

✓5ᵗʰ **O10.4 Pre-existing secondary hypertension complicating pregnancy, childbirth and the puerperium**
     Any condition in I15 specified as a reason for obstetric care during pregnancy, childbirth or the puerperium
     Use additional code from I15 to identify the type of secondary hypertension

     ✓6ᵗʰ **O10.41 Pre-existing secondary hypertension complicating pregnancy**

         O10.411 Pre-existing secondary hypertension complicating pregnancy, first trimester   Ⓜ ♀

         O10.412 Pre-existing secondary hypertension complicating pregnancy, second trimester   Ⓜ ♀

         O10.413 Pre-existing secondary hypertension complicating pregnancy, third trimester   Ⓜ ♀

         O10.419 Pre-existing secondary hypertension complicating pregnancy, unspecified trimester   Ⓜ ♀ ▽

     O10.42 Pre-existing secondary hypertension complicating childbirth   Ⓜ ♀

     O10.43 Pre-existing secondary hypertension complicating the puerperium   Ⓜ ♀

✓5ᵗʰ **O10.9 Unspecified pre-existing hypertension complicating pregnancy, childbirth and the puerperium**

     ✓6ᵗʰ **O10.91 Unspecified pre-existing hypertension complicating pregnancy**

         O10.911 Unspecified pre-existing hypertension complicating pregnancy, first trimester   Ⓜ ♀ ▽

         O10.912 Unspecified pre-existing hypertension complicating pregnancy, second trimester   Ⓜ ♀ ▽

         O10.913 Unspecified pre-existing hypertension complicating pregnancy, third trimester   Ⓜ ♀ ▽

         O10.919 Unspecified pre-existing hypertension complicating pregnancy, unspecified trimester   Ⓜ ♀

     O10.92 Unspecified pre-existing hypertension complicating childbirth   Ⓜ ♀ ▽

     O10.93 Unspecified pre-existing hypertension complicating the puerperium   Ⓜ ♀ ▽

✓4ᵗʰ **O11 Pre-existing hypertension with pre-eclampsia**

     INCLUDES   conditions in O10 complicated by pre-eclampsia
            pre-eclampsia superimposed pre-existing in hypertension
     Use additional code from O10 to identify the type of hypertension
     DEF: Complication of pregnancy manifesting in the development of borderline hypertension, protein in the urine, and unresponsive swelling between the 20th week of pregnancy and the end of the first week following birth in mild to moderate cases. Severe preeclampsia presents with hypertension, associated with marked swelling, proteinuria, abdominal pain, and/or visual changes.

     O11.1 Pre-existing hypertension with pre-eclampsia, first trimester   Ⓜ ♀

     O11.2 Pre-existing hypertension with pre-eclampsia, second trimester   Ⓜ ♀

     O11.3 Pre-existing hypertension with pre-eclampsia, third trimester   Ⓜ ♀

     O11.4 Pre-existing hypertension with pre-eclampsia, complicating childbirth   Ⓜ ♀

     O11.5 Pre-existing hypertension with pre-eclampsia, complicating the puerperium   Ⓜ ♀

     O11.9 Pre-existing hypertension with pre-eclampsia, unspecified trimester   Ⓜ ♀ ▽

✓4ᵗʰ **O12 Gestational [pregnancy-induced] edema and proteinuria without hypertension**

     ✓5ᵗʰ **O12.0 Gestational edema**

         O12.00 Gestational edema, unspecified trimester   Ⓜ ♀ ▽

         O12.01 Gestational edema, first trimester   Ⓜ ♀

         O12.02 Gestational edema, second trimester   Ⓜ ♀

         O12.03 Gestational edema, third trimester   Ⓜ ♀

         O12.04 Gestational edema, complicating childbirth   Ⓜ ♀

         O12.05 Gestational edema, complicating the puerperium   Ⓜ ♀

     ✓5ᵗʰ **O12.1 Gestational proteinuria**

         O12.10 Gestational proteinuria, unspecified trimester   Ⓜ ♀ ▽

         O12.11 Gestational proteinuria, first trimester   Ⓜ ♀

         O12.12 Gestational proteinuria, second trimester   Ⓜ ♀

         O12.13 Gestational proteinuria, third trimester   Ⓜ ♀

         O12.14 Gestational proteinuria, complicating childbirth   Ⓜ ♀

         O12.15 Gestational proteinuria, complicating the puerperium   Ⓜ ♀

     ✓5ᵗʰ **O12.2 Gestational edema with proteinuria**

         O12.20 Gestational edema with proteinuria, unspecified trimester   Ⓜ ♀ ▽

         O12.21 Gestational edema with proteinuria, first trimester   Ⓜ ♀

         O12.22 Gestational edema with proteinuria, second trimester   Ⓜ ♀

         O12.23 Gestational edema with proteinuria, third trimester   Ⓜ ♀

         O12.24 Gestational edema with proteinuria, complicating childbirth   Ⓜ ♀

         O12.25 Gestational edema with proteinuria, complicating the puerperium   Ⓜ ♀

☑4ᵗʰ **O13 Gestational [pregnancy-induced] hypertension without significant proteinuria**

> **INCLUDES**   gestational hypertension NOS
> transient hypertension of pregnancy
> **AHA:** 2016,1Q,5

 O13.1 Gestational [pregnancy-induced] hypertension without significant proteinuria, first trimester Ⓜ ♀

 O13.2 Gestational [pregnancy-induced] hypertension without significant proteinuria, second trimester Ⓜ ♀

 O13.3 Gestational [pregnancy-induced] hypertension without significant proteinuria, third trimester Ⓜ ♀

 O13.4 Gestational [pregnancy-induced] hypertension without significant proteinuria, complicating childbirth Ⓜ ♀

 O13.5 Gestational [pregnancy-induced] hypertension without significant proteinuria, complicating the puerperium Ⓜ ♀

 O13.9 Gestational [pregnancy-induced] hypertension without significant proteinuria, unspecified trimester Ⓜ ♀ ▽

☑4ᵗʰ **O14 Pre-eclampsia**

> **EXCLUDES 1**   pre-existing hypertension with pre-eclampsia (O11)
> **DEF:** Complication of pregnancy manifesting in the development of borderline hypertension, protein in the urine, and unresponsive swelling between the 20th week of pregnancy and the end of the first week following birth in mild to moderate cases. Severe preeclampsia presents with hypertension, associated with marked swelling, proteinuria, abdominal pain, and/or visual changes.

 ☑5ᵗʰ **O14.0 Mild to moderate pre-eclampsia**

  O14.00 Mild to moderate pre-eclampsia, unspecified trimester Ⓜ ♀ ▽

  O14.02 Mild to moderate pre-eclampsia, second trimester Ⓜ ♀

  O14.03 Mild to moderate pre-eclampsia, third trimester Ⓜ ♀

  O14.04 Mild to moderate pre-eclampsia, complicating childbirth Ⓜ ♀

  O14.05 Mild to moderate pre-eclampsia, complicating the puerperium Ⓜ ♀

 ☑5ᵗʰ **O14.1 Severe pre-eclampsia**

>   **EXCLUDES 1**   HELLP syndrome (O14.2-)

  O14.10 Severe pre-eclampsia, unspecified trimester Ⓜ ♀ ▽

  O14.12 Severe pre-eclampsia, second trimester Ⓜ ♀

  O14.13 Severe pre-eclampsia, third trimester Ⓜ ♀

  O14.14 Severe pre-eclampsia complicating childbirth Ⓜ ♀

  O14.15 Severe pre-eclampsia, complicating the puerperium Ⓜ ♀

 ☑5ᵗʰ **O14.2 HELLP syndrome**

>   Severe pre-eclampsia with hemolysis, elevated liver enzymes and low platelet count (HELLP)

  O14.20 HELLP syndrome (HELLP), unspecified trimester Ⓜ ♀ ▽

  O14.22 HELLP syndrome (HELLP), second trimester Ⓜ ♀

  O14.23 HELLP syndrome (HELLP), third trimester Ⓜ ♀

  O14.24 HELLP syndrome, complicating childbirth Ⓜ ♀

  O14.25 HELLP syndrome, complicating the puerperium Ⓜ ♀

 ☑5ᵗʰ **O14.9 Unspecified pre-eclampsia**

  O14.90 Unspecified pre-eclampsia, unspecified trimester Ⓜ ♀ ▽

  O14.92 Unspecified pre-eclampsia, second trimester Ⓜ ♀ ▽

  O14.93 Unspecified pre-eclampsia, third trimester Ⓜ ♀ ▽

  O14.94 Unspecified pre-eclampsia, complicating childbirth Ⓜ ♀ ▽

  O14.95 Unspecified pre-eclampsia, complicating the puerperium Ⓜ ♀ ▽

☑4ᵗʰ **O15 Eclampsia**

> **INCLUDES**   convulsions following conditions in O10-O14 and O16
> **DEF:** Tetany and toxemia producing seizure activity or coma in a pregnant patient who most often has presented with prior preeclampsia (i.e., hypertension, albuminuria, and edema).

 ☑5ᵗʰ **O15.0 Eclampsia complicating pregnancy**

  O15.00 Eclampsia complicating pregnancy, unspecified trimester Ⓜ ♀ ▽

  O15.02 Eclampsia complicating pregnancy, second trimester Ⓜ ♀

  O15.03 Eclampsia complicating pregnancy, third trimester Ⓜ ♀

 O15.1 Eclampsia complicating labor Ⓜ ♀

 O15.2 Eclampsia complicating the puerperium Ⓜ ♀

 O15.9 Eclampsia, unspecified as to time period Ⓜ ♀ ▽
  Eclampsia NOS

☑4ᵗʰ **O16 Unspecified maternal hypertension**

 O16.1 Unspecified maternal hypertension, first trimester Ⓜ ♀ ▽

 O16.2 Unspecified maternal hypertension, second trimester Ⓜ ♀ ▽

 O16.3 Unspecified maternal hypertension, third trimester Ⓜ ♀ ▽

 O16.4 Unspecified maternal hypertension, complicating childbirth Ⓜ ♀ ▽

 O16.5 Unspecified maternal hypertension, complicating the puerperium Ⓜ ♀ ▽

 O16.9 Unspecified maternal hypertension, unspecified trimester Ⓜ ♀ ▽

Other maternal disorders predominantly related to pregnancy (O20–O29)

> **EXCLUDES 2**   maternal care related to the fetus and amniotic cavity and possible delivery problems (O30-O48)
> maternal diseases classifiable elsewhere but complicating pregnancy, labor and delivery, and the puerperium (O98-O99)

☑4ᵗʰ **O20 Hemorrhage in early pregnancy**

> **INCLUDES**   hemorrhage before completion of 20 weeks gestation
> **EXCLUDES 1**   pregnancy with abortive outcome (O00-O08)

 O20.0 Threatened abortion Ⓤ Ⓜ ♀
> Hemorrhage specified as due to threatened abortion
> **DEF:** Bloody discharge during pregnancy. The cervix may be dilated and pregnancy threatened, but the pregnancy is not terminated.

 O20.8 Other hemorrhage in early pregnancy Ⓤ Ⓜ ♀

 O20.9 Hemorrhage in early pregnancy, unspecified Ⓤ Ⓜ ♀ ▽

☑4ᵗʰ **O21 Excessive vomiting in pregnancy**

 O21.0 Mild hyperemesis gravidarum Ⓜ ♀
> Hyperemesis gravidarum, mild or unspecified, starting before the end of the 20th week of gestation

 O21.1 Hyperemesis gravidarum with metabolic disturbance Ⓜ ♀
> Hyperemesis gravidarum, starting before the end of the 20th week of gestation, with metabolic disturbance such as carbohydrate depletion
> Hyperemesis gravidarum, starting before the end of the 20th week of gestation, with metabolic disturbance such as dehydration
> Hyperemesis gravidarum, starting before the end of the 20th week of gestation, with metabolic disturbance such as electrolyte imbalance

 O21.2 Late vomiting of pregnancy Ⓜ ♀
> Excessive vomiting starting after 20 completed weeks of gestation

 O21.8 Other vomiting complicating pregnancy Ⓜ ♀
> Vomiting due to diseases classified elsewhere, complicating pregnancy
> Use additional code, to identify cause

 O21.9 Vomiting of pregnancy, unspecified Ⓜ ♀ ▽

☑4ᵗʰ **O22 Venous complications and hemorrhoids in pregnancy**

> **EXCLUDES 1**   venous complications of:
> abortion NOS (O03.9)
> ectopic or molar pregnancy (O08.7)
> failed attempted abortion (O07.35)
> induced abortion (O04.85)
> spontaneous abortion (O03.89)
> **EXCLUDES 2**   obstetric pulmonary embolism (O88.-)
> venous complications and hemorrhoids of childbirth and the puerperium (O87.-)

 ☑5ᵗʰ **O22.0 Varicose veins of lower extremity in pregnancy**

>   Varicose veins NOS in pregnancy
>   **DEF:** Distended, tortuous veins of the lower extremities associated with pregnancy.

  O22.00 Varicose veins of lower extremity in pregnancy, unspecified trimester Ⓜ ♀ ▽

☑ Additional Character Req   ☑x7ᵗʰ Placeholder Alert   **Manifestation**   ▽ Unspecified   ►◄ Revised Text   ● New Code   ▲ Revised Code Title

ICD-10-CM 2019   857

O22.01   **Varicose veins of lower extremity in pregnancy, first trimester**   M ♀

O22.02   **Varicose veins of lower extremity in pregnancy, second trimester**   M ♀

O22.03   **Varicose veins of lower extremity in pregnancy, third trimester**   M ♀

√5ᵗʰ **O22.1**   **Genital varices in pregnancy**

Perineal varices in pregnancy
Vaginal varices in pregnancy
Vulval varices in pregnancy

O22.10   **Genital varices in pregnancy, unspecified trimester**   M ♀ ▽

O22.11   **Genital varices in pregnancy, first trimester**   M ♀

O22.12   **Genital varices in pregnancy, second trimester**   M ♀

O22.13   **Genital varices in pregnancy, third trimester**   M ♀

√5ᵗʰ **O22.2**   **Superficial thrombophlebitis in pregnancy**

Phlebitis in pregnancy NOS
Thrombophlebitis of legs in pregnancy
Thrombosis in pregnancy NOS
Use additional code to identify the superficial thrombophlebitis (I80.0-)

O22.20   **Superficial thrombophlebitis in pregnancy, unspecified trimester**   M ♀ ▽

O22.21   **Superficial thrombophlebitis in pregnancy, first trimester**   M ♀

O22.22   **Superficial thrombophlebitis in pregnancy, second trimester**   M ♀

O22.23   **Superficial thrombophlebitis in pregnancy, third trimester**   M ♀

√5ᵗʰ **O22.3**   **Deep phlebothrombosis in pregnancy**

Deep vein thrombosis, antepartum
Use additional code to identify the deep vein thrombosis (I82.4-, I82.5-, I82.62-, I82.72-)
Use additional code, if applicable, for associated long-term (current) use of anticoagulants (Z79.01)

O22.30   **Deep phlebothrombosis in pregnancy, unspecified trimester**   M ♀ ▽

O22.31   **Deep phlebothrombosis in pregnancy, first trimester**   M ♀

O22.32   **Deep phlebothrombosis in pregnancy, second trimester**   M ♀

O22.33   **Deep phlebothrombosis in pregnancy, third trimester**   M ♀

√5ᵗʰ **O22.4**   **Hemorrhoids in pregnancy**

O22.40   **Hemorrhoids in pregnancy, unspecified trimester**   M ♀ ▽

O22.41   **Hemorrhoids in pregnancy, first trimester**   M ♀

O22.42   **Hemorrhoids in pregnancy, second trimester**   M ♀

O22.43   **Hemorrhoids in pregnancy, third trimester**   M ♀

√5ᵗʰ **O22.5**   **Cerebral venous thrombosis in pregnancy**

Cerebrovenous sinus thrombosis in pregnancy

O22.50   **Cerebral venous thrombosis in pregnancy, unspecified trimester**   M ♀ ▽

O22.51   **Cerebral venous thrombosis in pregnancy, first trimester**   M ♀

O22.52   **Cerebral venous thrombosis in pregnancy, second trimester**   M ♀

O22.53   **Cerebral venous thrombosis in pregnancy, third trimester**   M ♀

√5ᵗʰ **O22.8**   **Other venous complications in pregnancy**

√6ᵗʰ **O22.8X**   **Other venous complications in pregnancy**

O22.8X1   **Other venous complications in pregnancy, first trimester**   M ♀

O22.8X2   **Other venous complications in pregnancy, second trimester**   M ♀

O22.8X3   **Other venous complications in pregnancy, third trimester**   M ♀

O22.8X9   **Other venous complications in pregnancy, unspecified trimester**   M ♀ ▽

√5ᵗʰ **O22.9**   **Venous complication in pregnancy, unspecified**

Gestational phlebitis NOS
Gestational phlebopathy NOS
Gestational thrombosis NOS

O22.90   **Venous complication in pregnancy, unspecified, unspecified trimester**   M ♀ ▽

O22.91   **Venous complication in pregnancy, unspecified, first trimester**   M ♀ ▽

O22.92   **Venous complication in pregnancy, unspecified, second trimester**   M ♀ ▽

O22.93   **Venous complication in pregnancy, unspecified, third trimester**   M ♀ ▽

√4ᵗʰ **O23**   **Infections of genitourinary tract in pregnancy**

Use additional code to identify organism (B95.-, B96.-)

EXCLUDES 2   *gonococcal infections complicating pregnancy, childbirth and the puerperium (O98.2)*

infections with a predominantly sexual mode of transmission NOS complicating pregnancy, childbirth and the puerperium (O98.3)

syphilis complicating pregnancy, childbirth and the puerperium (O98.1)

tuberculosis of genitourinary system complicating pregnancy, childbirth and the puerperium (O98.0)

venereal disease NOS complicating pregnancy, childbirth and the puerperium (O98.3)

AHA: 2018,2Q,20

√5ᵗʰ **O23.0**   **Infections of kidney in pregnancy**

Pyelonephritis in pregnancy

O23.00   **Infections of kidney in pregnancy, unspecified trimester**   M ♀ ▽

O23.01   **Infections of kidney in pregnancy, first trimester**   M ♀

O23.02   **Infections of kidney in pregnancy, second trimester**   M ♀

O23.03   **Infections of kidney in pregnancy, third trimester**   M ♀

√5ᵗʰ **O23.1**   **Infections of bladder in pregnancy**

O23.10   **Infections of bladder in pregnancy, unspecified trimester**   M ♀ ▽

O23.11   **Infections of bladder in pregnancy, first trimester**   M ♀

O23.12   **Infections of bladder in pregnancy, second trimester**   M ♀

O23.13   **Infections of bladder in pregnancy, third trimester**   M ♀

√5ᵗʰ **O23.2**   **Infections of urethra in pregnancy**

O23.20   **Infections of urethra in pregnancy, unspecified trimester**   M ♀ ▽

O23.21   **Infections of urethra in pregnancy, first trimester**   M ♀

O23.22   **Infections of urethra in pregnancy, second trimester**   M ♀

O23.23   **Infections of urethra in pregnancy, third trimester**   M ♀

√5ᵗʰ **O23.3**   **Infections of other parts of urinary tract in pregnancy**

O23.30   **Infections of other parts of urinary tract in pregnancy, unspecified trimester**   M ♀ ▽

O23.31   **Infections of other parts of urinary tract in pregnancy, first trimester**   M ♀

O23.32   **Infections of other parts of urinary tract in pregnancy, second trimester**   M ♀

O23.33   **Infections of other parts of urinary tract in pregnancy, third trimester**   M ♀

√5ᵗʰ **O23.4**   **Unspecified infection of urinary tract in pregnancy**

O23.40   **Unspecified infection of urinary tract in pregnancy, unspecified trimester**   M ♀ ▽

O23.41   **Unspecified infection of urinary tract in pregnancy, first trimester**   M ♀ ▽

O23.42   **Unspecified infection of urinary tract in pregnancy, second trimester**   M ♀ ▽

O23.43   **Unspecified infection of urinary tract in pregnancy, third trimester**   M ♀ ▽

√5ᵗʰ **O23.5**   **Infections of the genital tract in pregnancy**

√6ᵗʰ **O23.51**   **Infection of cervix in pregnancy**

O23.511   **Infections of cervix in pregnancy, first trimester**   M ♀

O23.512   **Infections of cervix in pregnancy, second trimester**   M ♀

O23.513 **Infections of cervix in pregnancy, third trimester**   Ⓜ ♀

O23.519 **Infections of cervix in pregnancy, unspecified trimester**   Ⓜ ♀ ▽

√6ᵗʰ O23.52 Salpingo-oophoritis in pregnancy

     Oophoritis in pregnancy

     Salpingitis in pregnancy

O23.521 **Salpingo-oophoritis in pregnancy, first trimester**   Ⓜ ♀

O23.522 **Salpingo-oophoritis in pregnancy, second trimester**   Ⓜ ♀

O23.523 **Salpingo-oophoritis in pregnancy, third trimester**   Ⓜ ♀

O23.529 **Salpingo-oophoritis in pregnancy, unspecified trimester**   Ⓜ ♀ ▽

√6ᵗʰ O23.59 Infection of other part of genital tract in pregnancy

O23.591 **Infection of other part of genital tract in pregnancy, first trimester**   Ⓜ ♀

O23.592 **Infection of other part of genital tract in pregnancy, second trimester**   Ⓜ ♀

O23.593 **Infection of other part of genital tract in pregnancy, third trimester**   Ⓜ ♀

O23.599 **Infection of other part of genital tract in pregnancy, unspecified trimester**   Ⓜ ♀ ▽

√5ᵗʰ O23.9 **Unspecified genitourinary tract infection in pregnancy**

     Genitourinary tract infection in pregnancy NOS

O23.90 **Unspecified genitourinary tract infection in pregnancy, unspecified trimester**   Ⓜ ♀ ▽

O23.91 **Unspecified genitourinary tract infection in pregnancy, first trimester**   Ⓜ ♀ ▽

O23.92 **Unspecified genitourinary tract infection in pregnancy, second trimester**   Ⓜ ♀ ▽

O23.93 **Unspecified genitourinary tract infection in pregnancy, third trimester**   Ⓜ ♀ ▽

√4ᵗʰ O24 Diabetes mellitus in pregnancy, childbirth and the puerperium

√5ᵗʰ O24.0 Pre-existing type 1 diabetes mellitus, in pregnancy, childbirth and the puerperium

     Juvenile onset diabetes mellitus, in pregnancy, childbirth and the puerperium

     Ketosis-prone diabetes mellitus in pregnancy, childbirth and the puerperium

     Use additional code from category E10 to further identify any manifestations

√6ᵗʰ O24.01 **Pre-existing type 1 diabetes mellitus, in** pregnancy

O24.011 **Pre-existing type 1 diabetes mellitus, in pregnancy, first trimester**   🄾 Ⓜ ♀

O24.012 **Pre-existing type 1 diabetes mellitus, in pregnancy, second trimester**   🄾 Ⓜ ♀

O24.013 **Pre-existing type 1 diabetes mellitus, in pregnancy, third trimester**   🄾 Ⓜ ♀

O24.019 **Pre-existing type 1 diabetes mellitus, in pregnancy, unspecified trimester**   🄾 Ⓜ ♀ ▽

O24.02 **Pre-existing type 1 diabetes mellitus, in childbirth**   🄾 Ⓜ ♀

O24.03 **Pre-existing type 1 diabetes mellitus, in the** puerperium   🄾 Ⓜ ♀

√5ᵗʰ O24.1 Pre-existing type 2 diabetes mellitus, in pregnancy, childbirth and the puerperium

     Insulin-resistant diabetes mellitus in pregnancy, childbirth and the puerperium

     Use additional code (for):

         from category E11 to further identify any manifestations

         long-term (current) use of insulin (Z79.4)

√6ᵗʰ O24.11 **Pre-existing type 2 diabetes mellitus, in** pregnancy

O24.111 **Pre-existing type 2 diabetes mellitus, in pregnancy, first trimester**   🄾 Ⓜ ♀

O24.112 **Pre-existing type 2 diabetes mellitus, in pregnancy, second trimester**   🄾 ♀

O24.113 **Pre-existing type 2 diabetes mellitus, in pregnancy, third trimester**   🄾 Ⓜ ♀

O24.119 **Pre-existing type 2 diabetes mellitus, in pregnancy, unspecified trimester**   🄾 Ⓜ ♀ ▽

O24.12 **Pre-existing type 2 diabetes mellitus, in** childbirth   🄾 Ⓜ ♀

O24.13 **Pre-existing type 2 diabetes mellitus, in the** puerperium   🄾 Ⓜ ♀

√5ᵗʰ O24.3 Unspecified pre-existing diabetes mellitus in pregnancy, childbirth and the puerperium

     Use additional code (for):

         from category E11 to further identify any manifestation

         long-term (current) use of insulin (Z79.4)

√6ᵗʰ O24.31 **Unspecified pre-existing diabetes mellitus in** pregnancy

O24.311 **Unspecified pre-existing diabetes mellitus in pregnancy, first trimester**   🄾 Ⓜ ♀ ▽

O24.312 **Unspecified pre-existing diabetes mellitus in pregnancy, second trimester**   🄾 Ⓜ ♀ ▽

O24.313 **Unspecified pre-existing diabetes mellitus in pregnancy, third trimester**   🄾 Ⓜ ♀ ▽

O24.319 **Unspecified pre-existing diabetes mellitus in pregnancy, unspecified trimester**   🄾 Ⓜ ♀ ▽

O24.32 **Unspecified pre-existing diabetes mellitus in** childbirth   🄾 Ⓜ ♀ ▽

O24.33 **Unspecified pre-existing diabetes mellitus in the** puerperium   🄾 Ⓜ ♀ ▽

√5ᵗʰ O24.4 Gestational diabetes mellitus

     Diabetes mellitus arising in pregnancy

     Gestational diabetes mellitus NOS

     AHA: 2016,4Q,50

√6ᵗʰ O24.41 Gestational diabetes mellitus in pregnancy

O24.410 **Gestational diabetes mellitus in pregnancy, diet controlled**   Ⓜ ♀

O24.414 **Gestational diabetes mellitus in pregnancy, insulin controlled**   Ⓜ ♀

O24.415 **Gestational diabetes mellitus in pregnancy, controlled by oral hypoglycemic drugs**   Ⓜ ♀

     Gestational diabetes mellitus in pregnancy, controlled by oral antidiabetic drugs

O24.419 **Gestational diabetes mellitus in pregnancy, unspecified control**   Ⓜ ♀ ▽

     AHA: 2015,4Q,34

√6ᵗʰ O24.42 Gestational diabetes mellitus in childbirth

     AHA: 2016,1Q,5

O24.420 **Gestational diabetes mellitus in childbirth, diet controlled**   Ⓜ ♀

O24.424 **Gestational diabetes mellitus in childbirth, insulin controlled**   Ⓜ ♀

O24.425 **Gestational diabetes mellitus in childbirth, controlled by oral hypoglycemic drugs**   Ⓜ ♀

     Gestational diabetes mellitus in childbirth, controlled by oral antidiabetic drugs

O24.429 **Gestational diabetes mellitus in childbirth, unspecified control**   Ⓜ ♀ ▽

     AHA: 2015,4Q,34

√6ᵗʰ O24.43 Gestational diabetes mellitus in the puerperium

O24.430 **Gestational diabetes mellitus in the puerperium, diet controlled**   Ⓜ ♀

O24.434 **Gestational diabetes mellitus in the puerperium, insulin controlled**   Ⓜ ♀

O24.435 **Gestational diabetes mellitus in puerperium, controlled by oral hypoglycemic drugs**   Ⓜ ♀

     Gestational diabetes mellitus in puerperium, controlled by oral antidiabetic drugs

O24.439 **Gestational diabetes mellitus in the puerperium, unspecified control**   Ⓜ ♀ ▽

     AHA: 2015,4Q,34

☑ Additional Character Req   √x7ᵗʰ Placeholder Alert   Manifestation   ▽ Unspecified   ▶◀ Revised Text   ● New Code   ▲ Revised Code Title

√5ᵗʰ **O24.8 Other pre-existing diabetes mellitus in pregnancy, childbirth, and the puerperium**
Use additional code (for):
from categories E08, E09 and E13 to further identify any manifestation
long-term (current) use of insulin (Z79.4)

√6ᵗʰ **O24.81 Other pre-existing diabetes mellitus in pregnancy**
O24.811 Other pre-existing diabetes mellitus in pregnancy, **first trimester** 🄾 Ⓜ ♀
O24.812 Other pre-existing diabetes mellitus in pregnancy, **second trimester** 🄾 Ⓜ ♀
O24.813 Other pre-existing diabetes mellitus in pregnancy, **third trimester** 🄾 Ⓜ ♀
O24.819 Other pre-existing diabetes mellitus in pregnancy, **unspecified trimester** 🄾 Ⓜ ♀ ▽

O24.82 Other pre-existing diabetes mellitus in **childbirth** 🄾 Ⓜ ♀
O24.83 Other pre-existing diabetes mellitus in the **puerperium** 🄾 Ⓜ ♀

√5ᵗʰ **O24.9 Unspecified diabetes mellitus in pregnancy, childbirth and the puerperium**
Use additional code for long-term (current) use of insulin (Z79.4)

√6ᵗʰ **O24.91 Unspecified diabetes mellitus in pregnancy**
O24.911 Unspecified diabetes mellitus in pregnancy, **first trimester** Ⓜ ♀ ▽
O24.912 Unspecified diabetes mellitus in pregnancy, **second trimester** Ⓜ ♀ ▽
O24.913 Unspecified diabetes mellitus in pregnancy, **third trimester** Ⓜ ♀ ▽
O24.919 Unspecified diabetes mellitus in pregnancy, **unspecified trimester** Ⓜ ♀ ▽

O24.92 Unspecified diabetes mellitus in **childbirth** Ⓜ ♀ ▽
O24.93 Unspecified diabetes mellitus in the **puerperium** Ⓜ ♀ ▽

√4ᵗʰ **O25 Malnutrition in pregnancy, childbirth and the puerperium**

√5ᵗʰ **O25.1 Malnutrition in pregnancy**
O25.10 Malnutrition in pregnancy, **unspecified trimester** Ⓜ ♀ ▽
O25.11 Malnutrition in pregnancy, **first trimester** Ⓜ ♀
O25.12 Malnutrition in pregnancy, **second trimester** Ⓜ ♀
O25.13 Malnutrition in pregnancy, **third trimester** Ⓜ ♀

O25.2 Malnutrition in **childbirth** Ⓜ ♀
O25.3 Malnutrition in the **puerperium** Ⓜ ♀

√4ᵗʰ **O26 Maternal care for other conditions predominantly related to pregnancy**

√5ᵗʰ **O26.0 Excessive weight gain in pregnancy**
EXCLUDES 2 gestational edema (O12.0, O12.2)
O26.00 Excessive weight gain in pregnancy, **unspecified trimester** Ⓜ ♀ ▽
O26.01 Excessive weight gain in pregnancy, **first trimester** Ⓜ ♀
O26.02 Excessive weight gain in pregnancy, **second trimester** Ⓜ ♀
O26.03 Excessive weight gain in pregnancy, **third trimester** Ⓜ ♀

√5ᵗʰ **O26.1 Low weight gain in pregnancy**
O26.10 Low weight gain in pregnancy, **unspecified trimester** Ⓜ ♀ ▽
O26.11 Low weight gain in pregnancy, **first trimester** Ⓜ ♀
O26.12 Low weight gain in pregnancy, **second trimester** Ⓜ ♀
O26.13 Low weight gain in pregnancy, **third trimester** Ⓜ ♀

√5ᵗʰ **O26.2 Pregnancy care for patient with recurrent pregnancy loss**
O26.20 Pregnancy care for patient with recurrent pregnancy loss, **unspecified trimester** Ⓜ ♀ ▽
O26.21 Pregnancy care for patient with recurrent pregnancy loss, **first trimester** Ⓜ ♀
O26.22 Pregnancy care for patient with recurrent pregnancy loss, **second trimester** Ⓜ ♀
O26.23 Pregnancy care for patient with recurrent pregnancy loss, **third trimester** Ⓜ ♀

√5ᵗʰ **O26.3 Retained intrauterine contraceptive device in pregnancy**
O26.30 Retained intrauterine contraceptive device in pregnancy, **unspecified trimester** Ⓜ ♀ ▽
O26.31 Retained intrauterine contraceptive device in pregnancy, **first trimester** Ⓜ ♀
O26.32 Retained intrauterine contraceptive device in pregnancy, **second trimester** Ⓜ ♀
O26.33 Retained intrauterine contraceptive device in pregnancy, **third trimester** Ⓜ ♀

√5ᵗʰ **O26.4 Herpes gestationis**
O26.40 Herpes gestationis, **unspecified trimester** Ⓜ ♀ ▽
O26.41 Herpes gestationis, **first trimester** Ⓜ ♀
O26.42 Herpes gestationis, **second trimester** Ⓜ ♀
O26.43 Herpes gestationis, **third trimester** Ⓜ ♀

√5ᵗʰ **O26.5 Maternal hypotension syndrome**
Supine hypotensive syndrome
O26.50 Maternal hypotension syndrome, **unspecified trimester** Ⓜ ♀ ▽
O26.51 Maternal hypotension syndrome, **first trimester** Ⓜ ♀
O26.52 Maternal hypotension syndrome, **second trimester** Ⓜ ♀
O26.53 Maternal hypotension syndrome, **third trimester** Ⓜ ♀

√5ᵗʰ **O26.6 Liver and biliary tract disorders in pregnancy, childbirth and the puerperium**
Use additional code to identify the specific disorder
EXCLUDES 2 hepatorenal syndrome following labor and delivery (O90.4)

√6ᵗʰ **O26.61 Liver and biliary tract disorders in pregnancy**
O26.611 Liver and biliary tract disorders in pregnancy, **first trimester** Ⓜ ♀
O26.612 Liver and biliary tract disorders in pregnancy, **second trimester** Ⓜ ♀
O26.613 Liver and biliary tract disorders in pregnancy, **third trimester** Ⓜ ♀
O26.619 Liver and biliary tract disorders in pregnancy, **unspecified trimester** Ⓜ ♀ ▽

O26.62 Liver and biliary tract disorders in **childbirth** Ⓜ ♀
O26.63 Liver and biliary tract disorders in the **puerperium** Ⓜ ♀

√5ᵗʰ **O26.7 Subluxation of symphysis (pubis) in pregnancy, childbirth and the puerperium**
EXCLUDES 1 traumatic separation of symphysis (pubis) during childbirth (O71.6)

√6ᵗʰ **O26.71 Subluxation of symphysis (pubis) in pregnancy**
O26.711 Subluxation of symphysis (pubis) in pregnancy, **first trimester** Ⓜ ♀
O26.712 Subluxation of symphysis (pubis) in pregnancy, **second trimester** Ⓜ ♀
O26.713 Subluxation of symphysis (pubis) in pregnancy, **third trimester** Ⓜ ♀
O26.719 Subluxation of symphysis (pubis) in pregnancy, **unspecified trimester** Ⓜ ♀ ▽

O26.72 Subluxation of symphysis (pubis) in **childbirth** Ⓜ ♀
O26.73 Subluxation of symphysis (pubis) in the **puerperium** Ⓜ ♀

√5ᵗʰ **O26.8 Other specified pregnancy related conditions**

√6ᵗʰ **O26.81 Pregnancy related exhaustion and fatigue**
O26.811 Pregnancy related exhaustion and fatigue, **first trimester** Ⓜ ♀
O26.812 Pregnancy related exhaustion and fatigue, **second trimester** Ⓜ ♀
O26.813 Pregnancy related exhaustion and fatigue, **third trimester** Ⓜ ♀
O26.819 Pregnancy related exhaustion and fatigue, **unspecified trimester** Ⓜ ♀ ▽

√6ᵗʰ **O26.82 Pregnancy related peripheral neuritis**
O26.821 Pregnancy related peripheral neuritis, **first trimester** Ⓜ ♀
O26.822 Pregnancy related peripheral neuritis, **second trimester** Ⓜ ♀

O26.823   **Pregnancy related peripheral neuritis, third trimester**   Ⓜ ♀

O26.829   **Pregnancy related peripheral neuritis, unspecified trimester**   Ⓜ ♀ ▽

✓6ᵗʰ   **O26.83**   **Pregnancy related renal disease**

Use additional code to identify the specific disorder

O26.831   **Pregnancy related renal disease, first trimester**   Ⓜ ♀

O26.832   **Pregnancy related renal disease, second trimester**   Ⓜ ♀

O26.833   **Pregnancy related renal disease, third trimester**   Ⓜ ♀

O26.839   **Pregnancy related renal disease, unspecified trimester**   Ⓜ ♀ ▽

✓6ᵗʰ   **O26.84**   **Uterine size-date discrepancy complicating pregnancy**

EXCLUDES 1   encounter for suspected problem with fetal growth ruled out (Z03.74)

O26.841   **Uterine size-date discrepancy, first trimester**   Ⓜ ♀

O26.842   **Uterine size-date discrepancy, second trimester**   Ⓜ ♀

O26.843   **Uterine size-date discrepancy, third trimester**   Ⓜ ♀

O26.849   **Uterine size-date discrepancy, unspecified trimester**   Ⓜ ♀ ▽

✓6ᵗʰ   **O26.85**   **Spotting complicating pregnancy**

O26.851   **Spotting complicating pregnancy, first trimester**   Ⓜ ♀

O26.852   **Spotting complicating pregnancy, second trimester**   Ⓜ ♀

O26.853   **Spotting complicating pregnancy, third trimester**   Ⓜ ♀

O26.859   **Spotting complicating pregnancy, unspecified trimester**   Ⓜ ♀ ▽

O26.86   **Pruritic urticarial papules and plaques of pregnancy (PUPPP)**   Ⓜ ♀

Polymorphic eruption of pregnancy

✓6ᵗʰ   **O26.87**   **Cervical shortening**

EXCLUDES 1   encounter for suspected cervical shortening ruled out (Z03.75)

DEF: Cervix that has shortened to less than 25 mm before the 24th week of pregnancy. A shortened cervix is a warning sign for impending premature delivery and is treated by cervical cerclage placement or progesterone.

O26.872   **Cervical shortening, second trimester**   Ⓜ ♀

O26.873   **Cervical shortening, third trimester**   Ⓜ ♀

O26.879   **Cervical shortening, unspecified trimester**   Ⓜ ♀ ▽

✓6ᵗʰ   **O26.89**   **Other specified pregnancy related conditions**

AHA: 2015,3Q,40

O26.891   **Other specified pregnancy related conditions, first trimester**   ⓪ Ⓜ ♀

O26.892   **Other specified pregnancy related conditions, second trimester**   Ⓜ ♀

O26.893   **Other specified pregnancy related conditions, third trimester**   Ⓜ ♀

O26.899   **Other specified pregnancy related conditions, unspecified trimester**   ⓪ Ⓜ ♀ ▽

✓5ᵗʰ   **O26.9**   **Pregnancy related conditions, unspecified**

O26.90   **Pregnancy related conditions, unspecified, unspecified trimester**   ⓪ Ⓜ ♀ ▽

O26.91   **Pregnancy related conditions, unspecified, first trimester**   ⓪ Ⓜ ♀ ▽

O26.92   **Pregnancy related conditions, unspecified, second trimester**   Ⓜ ♀ ▽

O26.93   **Pregnancy related conditions, unspecified, third trimester**   Ⓜ ♀ ▽

✓4ᵗʰ   **O28**   **Abnormal findings on antenatal screening of mother**

EXCLUDES 1   diagnostic findings classified elsewhere - see Alphabetical Index

O28.0   **Abnormal hematological finding on antenatal screening of mother**   Ⓜ ♀

O28.1   **Abnormal biochemical finding on antenatal screening of mother**   Ⓜ ♀

O28.2   **Abnormal cytological finding on antenatal screening of mother**   Ⓜ ♀

O28.3   **Abnormal ultrasonic finding on antenatal screening of mother**   Ⓜ ♀

O28.4   **Abnormal radiological finding on antenatal screening of mother**   Ⓜ ♀

O28.5   **Abnormal chromosomal and genetic finding on antenatal screening of mother**   Ⓜ ♀

O28.8   **Other abnormal findings on antenatal screening of mother**   Ⓜ ♀

O28.9   **Unspecified abnormal findings on antenatal screening of mother**   Ⓜ ♀ ▽

✓4ᵗʰ   **O29**   **Complications of anesthesia during pregnancy**

INCLUDES   maternal complications arising from the administration of a general, regional or local anesthetic, analgesic or other sedation during pregnancy

Use additional code, if necessary, to identify the complication

EXCLUDES 2   complications of anesthesia during labor and delivery (O74.-)
complications of anesthesia during the puerperium (O89.-)

✓5ᵗʰ   **O29.0**   **Pulmonary complications of anesthesia during pregnancy**

✓6ᵗʰ   **O29.01**   **Aspiration pneumonitis due to anesthesia during pregnancy**

Inhalation of stomach contents or secretions NOS due to anesthesia during pregnancy
Mendelson's syndrome due to anesthesia during pregnancy

O29.011   **Aspiration pneumonitis due to anesthesia during pregnancy, first trimester**   Ⓜ ♀

O29.012   **Aspiration pneumonitis due to anesthesia during pregnancy, second trimester**   Ⓜ ♀

O29.013   **Aspiration pneumonitis due to anesthesia during pregnancy, third trimester**   Ⓜ ♀

O29.019   **Aspiration pneumonitis due to anesthesia during pregnancy, unspecified trimester**   Ⓜ ♀ ▽

✓6ᵗʰ   **O29.02**   **Pressure collapse of lung due to anesthesia during pregnancy**

O29.021   **Pressure collapse of lung due to anesthesia during pregnancy, first trimester**   Ⓜ ♀

O29.022   **Pressure collapse of lung due to anesthesia during pregnancy, second trimester**   Ⓜ ♀

O29.023   **Pressure collapse of lung due to anesthesia during pregnancy, third trimester**   Ⓜ ♀

O29.029   **Pressure collapse of lung due to anesthesia during pregnancy, unspecified trimester**   Ⓜ ♀ ▽

✓6ᵗʰ   **O29.09**   **Other pulmonary complications of anesthesia during pregnancy**

O29.091   **Other pulmonary complications of anesthesia during pregnancy, first trimester**   Ⓜ ♀

O29.092   **Other pulmonary complications of anesthesia during pregnancy, second trimester**   Ⓜ ♀

O29.093   **Other pulmonary complications of anesthesia during pregnancy, third trimester**   Ⓜ ♀

O29.099   **Other pulmonary complications of anesthesia during pregnancy, unspecified trimester**   Ⓜ ♀ ▽

✓5ᵗʰ   **O29.1**   **Cardiac complications of anesthesia during pregnancy**

✓6ᵗʰ   **O29.11**   **Cardiac arrest due to anesthesia during pregnancy**

O29.111   **Cardiac arrest due to anesthesia during pregnancy, first trimester**   Ⓜ ♀

O29.112   **Cardiac arrest due to anesthesia during pregnancy, second trimester**   Ⓜ ♀

O29.113   **Cardiac arrest due to anesthesia during pregnancy, third trimester**   Ⓜ ♀

O29.119   **Cardiac arrest due to anesthesia during pregnancy, unspecified trimester**   Ⓜ ♀ ▽

☑ Additional Character Req   ✕ˣ⁷ᵗʰ Placeholder Alert   Manifestation   ▽ Unspecified   ▶◀ Revised Text   ● New Code   ▲ Revised Code Title

√6ᵗʰ **O29.12** **Cardiac failure due to anesthesia during pregnancy**

     O29.121 Cardiac failure due to anesthesia during pregnancy, first trimester   M ♀

     O29.122 Cardiac failure due to anesthesia during pregnancy, second trimester   M ♀

     O29.123 Cardiac failure due to anesthesia during pregnancy, third trimester   M ♀

     O29.129 Cardiac failure due to anesthesia during pregnancy, unspecified trimester   M ♀ ▽

√6ᵗʰ **O29.19** **Other cardiac complications of anesthesia during pregnancy**

     O29.191 Other cardiac complications of anesthesia during pregnancy, first trimester   M ♀

     O29.192 Other cardiac complications of anesthesia during pregnancy, second trimester   M ♀

     O29.193 Other cardiac complications of anesthesia during pregnancy, third trimester   M ♀

     O29.199 Other cardiac complications of anesthesia during pregnancy, unspecified trimester   M ♀ ▽

√5ᵗʰ **O29.2** **Central nervous system complications of anesthesia during pregnancy**

√6ᵗʰ **O29.21** **Cerebral anoxia due to anesthesia during pregnancy**

     O29.211 Cerebral anoxia due to anesthesia during pregnancy, first trimester   M ♀

     O29.212 Cerebral anoxia due to anesthesia during pregnancy, second trimester   M ♀

     O29.213 Cerebral anoxia due to anesthesia during pregnancy, third trimester   M ♀

     O29.219 Cerebral anoxia due to anesthesia during pregnancy, unspecified trimester   M ♀ ▽

√6ᵗʰ **O29.29** **Other central nervous system complications of anesthesia during pregnancy**

     O29.291 Other central nervous system complications of anesthesia during pregnancy, first trimester   M ♀

     O29.292 Other central nervous system complications of anesthesia during pregnancy, second trimester   M ♀

     O29.293 Other central nervous system complications of anesthesia during pregnancy, third trimester   M ♀

     O29.299 Other central nervous system complications of anesthesia during pregnancy, unspecified trimester   M ♀ ▽

√5ᵗʰ **O29.3** **Toxic reaction to local anesthesia during pregnancy**

√6ᵗʰ **O29.3X** **Toxic reaction to local anesthesia during pregnancy**

     O29.3X1 Toxic reaction to local anesthesia during pregnancy, first trimester   M ♀

     O29.3X2 Toxic reaction to local anesthesia during pregnancy, second trimester   M ♀

     O29.3X3 Toxic reaction to local anesthesia during pregnancy, third trimester   M ♀

     O29.3X9 Toxic reaction to local anesthesia during pregnancy, unspecified trimester   M ♀ ▽

√6ᵗʰ **O29.4** **Spinal and epidural anesthesia induced headache during pregnancy**

     O29.40 Spinal and epidural anesthesia induced headache during pregnancy, unspecified trimester   M ♀ ▽

     O29.41 Spinal and epidural anesthesia induced headache during pregnancy, first trimester   M ♀

     O29.42 Spinal and epidural anesthesia induced headache during pregnancy, second trimester   M ♀

     O29.43 Spinal and epidural anesthesia induced headache during pregnancy, third trimester   M ♀

√5ᵗʰ **O29.5** **Other complications of spinal and epidural anesthesia during pregnancy**

√6ᵗʰ **O29.5X** **Other complications of spinal and epidural anesthesia during pregnancy**

     O29.5X1 Other complications of spinal and epidural anesthesia during pregnancy, first trimester   M ♀

     O29.5X2 Other complications of spinal and epidural anesthesia during pregnancy, second trimester   M ♀

     O29.5X3 Other complications of spinal and epidural anesthesia during pregnancy, third trimester   M ♀

     O29.5X9 Other complications of spinal and epidural anesthesia during pregnancy, unspecified trimester   M ♀ ▽

√5ᵗʰ **O29.6** **Failed or difficult intubation for anesthesia during pregnancy**

     O29.60 Failed or difficult intubation for anesthesia during pregnancy, unspecified trimester   M ♀ ▽

     O29.61 Failed or difficult intubation for anesthesia during pregnancy, first trimester   M ♀

     O29.62 Failed or difficult intubation for anesthesia during pregnancy, second trimester   M ♀

     O29.63 Failed or difficult intubation for anesthesia during pregnancy, third trimester   M ♀

√5ᵗʰ **O29.8** **Other complications of anesthesia during pregnancy**

√6ᵗʰ **O29.8X** **Other complications of anesthesia during pregnancy**

     O29.8X1 Other complications of anesthesia during pregnancy, first trimester   M ♀

     O29.8X2 Other complications of anesthesia during pregnancy, second trimester   M ♀

     O29.8X3 Other complications of anesthesia during pregnancy, third trimester   M ♀

     O29.8X9 Other complications of anesthesia during pregnancy, unspecified trimester   M ♀ ▽

√5ᵗʰ **O29.9** **Unspecified complication of anesthesia during pregnancy**

     O29.90 Unspecified complication of anesthesia during pregnancy, unspecified trimester   M ♀ ▽

     O29.91 Unspecified complication of anesthesia during pregnancy, first trimester   M ♀ ▽

     O29.92 Unspecified complication of anesthesia during pregnancy, second trimester   M ♀ ▽

     O29.93 Unspecified complication of anesthesia during pregnancy, third trimester   M ♀ ▽

Maternal care related to the fetus and amniotic cavity and possible delivery problems (O30-O48)

√4ᵗʰ **O30** **Multiple gestation**

     Code also any complications specific to multiple gestation

     AHA: 2016,4Q,51

√5ᵗʰ **O30.0** **Twin pregnancy**

√6ᵗʰ **O30.00** **Twin pregnancy, unspecified number of placenta and unspecified number of amniotic sacs**

     O30.001 Twin pregnancy, unspecified number of placenta and unspecified number of amniotic sacs, first trimester   M ♀ ▽

     O30.002 Twin pregnancy, unspecified number of placenta and unspecified number of amniotic sacs, second trimester   M ♀ ▽

     O30.003 Twin pregnancy, unspecified number of placenta and unspecified number of amniotic sacs, third trimester   M ♀ ▽

O30.009   **Twin pregnancy, unspecified number of placenta and unspecified number of amniotic sacs, unspecified trimester**   Ⓜ ♀ ▽

✓6ᵗʰ O30.01   **Twin pregnancy, monochorionic/monoamniotic**
Twin pregnancy, one placenta, one amniotic sac
EXCLUDES 1   conjoined twins (O30.02-)

Twin Gestation – Monochorionic/Monoamniotic

— 1 Chorionic sac
— 1 Amniotic sac
— 2 Fetuses
— 2 Umbilical cords
— 1 Placenta

O30.011   **Twin pregnancy, monochorionic/monoamniotic, first trimester**   Ⓜ ♀

O30.012   **Twin pregnancy, monochorionic/monoamniotic, second trimester**   Ⓜ ♀

O30.013   **Twin pregnancy, monochorionic/monoamniotic, third trimester**   Ⓜ ♀

O30.019   **Twin pregnancy, monochorionic/monoamniotic, unspecified trimester**   Ⓜ ♀ ▽

✓6ᵗʰ O30.02   **Conjoined twin pregnancy**

O30.021   **Conjoined twin pregnancy, first trimester**   Ⓜ ♀

O30.022   **Conjoined twin pregnancy, second trimester**   Ⓜ ♀

O30.023   **Conjoined twin pregnancy, third trimester**   Ⓜ ♀

O30.029   **Conjoined twin pregnancy, unspecified trimester**   Ⓜ ♀ ▽

✓6ᵗʰ O30.03   **Twin pregnancy, monochorionic/diamniotic**
Twin pregnancy, one placenta, two amniotic sacs

Twin Gestation – Monochorionic/Diamniotic

— 1 Chorionic sac
— 2 Amniotic sacs
— 2 Fetuses
— 2 Umbilical cords
— 1 Placenta

O30.031   **Twin pregnancy, monochorionic/diamniotic, first trimester**   Ⓜ ♀

O30.032   **Twin pregnancy, monochorionic/diamniotic, second trimester**   Ⓜ ♀

O30.033   **Twin pregnancy, monochorionic/diamniotic, third trimester**   Ⓜ ♀

O30.039   **Twin pregnancy, monochorionic/diamniotic, unspecified trimester**   Ⓜ ♀ ▽

✓6ᵗʰ O30.04   **Twin pregnancy, dichorionic/diamniotic**
Twin pregnancy, two placentae, two amniotic sacs

Twin Gestation – Dichorionic/Diamniotic

— 2 Chorionic sacs
— 2 Amniotic sacs
— 2 Fetuses
— 2 Umbilical cords
— 2 Placentas

O30.041   **Twin pregnancy, dichorionic/diamniotic, first trimester**   Ⓜ ♀

O30.042   **Twin pregnancy, dichorionic/diamniotic, second trimester**   Ⓜ ♀

O30.043   **Twin pregnancy, dichorionic/diamniotic, third trimester**   Ⓜ ♀

O30.049   **Twin pregnancy, dichorionic/diamniotic, unspecified trimester**   Ⓜ ♀ ▽

✓6ᵗʰ O30.09   **Twin pregnancy, unable to determine number of placenta and number of amniotic sacs**

O30.091   **Twin pregnancy, unable to determine number of placenta and number of amniotic sacs, first trimester**   Ⓜ ♀

O30.092   **Twin pregnancy, unable to determine number of placenta and number of amniotic sacs, second trimester**   Ⓜ ♀

O30.093   **Twin pregnancy, unable to determine number of placenta and number of amniotic sacs, third trimester**   Ⓜ ♀

O30.099   **Twin pregnancy, unable to determine number of placenta and number of amniotic sacs, unspecified trimester**   Ⓜ ♀ ▽

✓5ᵗʰ O30.1   **Triplet pregnancy**

✓6ᵗʰ O30.10   **Triplet pregnancy, unspecified number of placenta and unspecified number of amniotic sacs**
AHA: 2016,2Q,8

O30.101   **Triplet pregnancy, unspecified number of placenta and unspecified number of amniotic sacs, first trimester**   Ⓜ ♀ ▽

O30.102   **Triplet pregnancy, unspecified number of placenta and unspecified number of amniotic sacs, second trimester**   Ⓜ ♀ ▽

O30.103   **Triplet pregnancy, unspecified number of placenta and unspecified number of amniotic sacs, third trimester**   Ⓜ ♀ ▽

O30.109   **Triplet pregnancy, unspecified number of placenta and unspecified number of amniotic sacs, unspecified trimester**   Ⓜ ♀ ▽

✓6ᵗʰ O30.11   **Triplet pregnancy with two or more monochorionic fetuses**

O30.111   **Triplet pregnancy with two or more monochorionic fetuses, first trimester**   Ⓜ ♀

O30.112   **Triplet pregnancy with two or more monochorionic fetuses, second trimester**   Ⓜ ♀

✓ Additional Character Req   ✓x7ᵗʰ Placeholder Alert   Manifestation   ▽ Unspecified   ▶◀ Revised Text   ● New Code   ▲ Revised Code Title
ICD-10-CM 2019   863

O30.009–O30.112

Chapter 15. Pregnancy, Childbirth and the Puerperium

O30.113–O30.812

    O30.113 **Triplet pregnancy with two or more monochorionic fetuses, third trimester** Ⓜ ♀

    O30.119 **Triplet pregnancy with two or more monochorionic fetuses, unspecified trimester** Ⓜ ♀ ▽

✓6ᵗʰ **O30.12** **Triplet pregnancy with** two or more monoamniotic fetuses

    O30.121 **Triplet pregnancy with two or more monoamniotic fetuses, first trimester** Ⓜ ♀

    O30.122 **Triplet pregnancy with two or more monoamniotic fetuses, second trimester** Ⓜ ♀

    O30.123 **Triplet pregnancy with two or more monoamniotic fetuses, third trimester** Ⓜ ♀

    O30.129 **Triplet pregnancy with two or more monoamniotic fetuses, unspecified trimester** Ⓜ ♀ ▽

● ✓6ᵗʰ **O30.13** **Triplet pregnancy,** trichorionic/triamniotic

●   **O30.131** **Triplet pregnancy, trichorionic/triamniotic, first trimester**

●   **O30.132** **Triplet pregnancy, trichorionic/triamniotic, second trimester**

●   **O30.133** **Triplet pregnancy, trichorionic/triamniotic, third trimester**

●   **O30.139** **Triplet pregnancy, trichorionic/triamniotic, unspecified trimester** ▽

✓6ᵗʰ **O30.19** **Triplet pregnancy,** unable to determine number of placenta and number of amniotic sacs

    O30.191 **Triplet pregnancy, unable to determine number of placenta and number of amniotic sacs, first trimester** Ⓜ ♀

    O30.192 **Triplet pregnancy, unable to determine number of placenta and number of amniotic sacs, second trimester** Ⓜ ♀

    O30.193 **Triplet pregnancy, unable to determine number of placenta and number of amniotic sacs, third trimester** Ⓜ ♀

    O30.199 **Triplet pregnancy, unable to determine number of placenta and number of amniotic sacs, unspecified trimester** Ⓜ ♀ ▽

✓5ᵗʰ **O30.2** **Quadruplet** pregnancy

✓6ᵗʰ **O30.20** **Quadruplet pregnancy, unspecified number of placenta and unspecified number of amniotic sacs**

    O30.201 **Quadruplet pregnancy, unspecified number of placenta and unspecified number of amniotic sacs,** first trimester Ⓜ ♀ ▽

    O30.202 **Quadruplet pregnancy, unspecified number of placenta and unspecified number of amniotic sacs,** second trimester Ⓜ ♀ ▽

    O30.203 **Quadruplet pregnancy, unspecified number of placenta and unspecified number of amniotic sacs,** third trimester Ⓜ ♀ ▽

    O30.209 **Quadruplet pregnancy, unspecified number of placenta and unspecified number of amniotic sacs, unspecified trimester** Ⓜ ♀ ▽

✓6ᵗʰ **O30.21** **Quadruplet pregnancy with** two or more monochorionic fetuses

    O30.211 **Quadruplet pregnancy with two or more monochorionic fetuses, first trimester** Ⓜ ♀

    O30.212 **Quadruplet pregnancy with two or more monochorionic fetuses, second trimester** Ⓜ ♀

    O30.213 **Quadruplet pregnancy with two or more monochorionic fetuses, third trimester** Ⓜ ♀

    O30.219 **Quadruplet pregnancy with two or more monochorionic fetuses, unspecified trimester** Ⓜ ♀ ▽

✓6ᵗʰ **O30.22** **Quadruplet pregnancy with** two or more monoamniotic fetuses

    O30.221 **Quadruplet pregnancy with two or more monoamniotic fetuses, first trimester** Ⓜ ♀

    O30.222 **Quadruplet pregnancy with two or more monoamniotic fetuses, second trimester** Ⓜ ♀

    O30.223 **Quadruplet pregnancy with two or more monoamniotic fetuses, third trimester** Ⓜ ♀

    O30.229 **Quadruplet pregnancy with two or more monoamniotic fetuses, unspecified trimester** Ⓜ ♀ ▽

● ✓6ᵗʰ **O30.23** **Quadruplet pregnancy,** quadrachorionic/quadra-amniotic

●   **O30.231** **Quadruplet pregnancy, quadrachorionic/quadra-amniotic,** first trimester

    O30.232 **Quadruplet pregnancy, quadrachorionic/quadra-amniotic,** second trimester

●   **O30.233** **Quadruplet pregnancy, quadrachorionic/quadra-amniotic,** third trimester

●   **O30.239** **Quadruplet pregnancy, quadrachorionic/quadra-amniotic, unspecified trimester** ▽

✓6ᵗʰ **O30.29** **Quadruplet pregnancy,** unable to determine number of placenta and number of amniotic sacs

    O30.291 **Quadruplet pregnancy, unable to determine number of placenta and number of amniotic sacs,** first trimester Ⓜ ♀

    O30.292 **Quadruplet pregnancy, unable to determine number of placenta and number of amniotic sacs,** second trimester Ⓜ ♀

    O30.293 **Quadruplet pregnancy, unable to determine number of placenta and number of amniotic sacs,** third trimester Ⓜ ♀

    O30.299 **Quadruplet pregnancy, unable to determine number of placenta and number of amniotic sacs, unspecified trimester** Ⓜ ♀ ▽

✓5ᵗʰ **O30.8** **Other specified multiple gestation**

    Multiple gestation pregnancy greater then quadruplets

✓6ᵗʰ **O30.80** **Other specified multiple gestation, unspecified number of placenta and unspecified number of amniotic sacs**

    O30.801 **Other specified multiple gestation, unspecified number of placenta and unspecified number of amniotic sacs,** first trimester Ⓜ ♀ ▽

    O30.802 **Other specified multiple gestation, unspecified number of placenta and unspecified number of amniotic sacs,** second trimester Ⓜ ♀ ▽

    O30.803 **Other specified multiple gestation, unspecified number of placenta and unspecified number of amniotic sacs,** third trimester Ⓜ ♀ ▽

    O30.809 **Other specified multiple gestation, unspecified number of placenta and unspecified number of amniotic sacs, unspecified trimester** Ⓜ ♀ ▽

✓6ᵗʰ **O30.81** **Other specified multiple gestation with** two or more monochorionic fetuses

    O30.811 **Other specified multiple gestation with two or more monochorionic fetuses,** first trimester Ⓜ ♀

    O30.812 **Other specified multiple gestation with two or more monochorionic fetuses,** second trimester Ⓜ ♀

O30.813 Other specified multiple gestation with two or more monochorionic fetuses, **third trimester**   Ⓜ ♀

O30.819 Other specified multiple gestation with two or more monochorionic fetuses, **unspecified trimester**   Ⓜ ♀ ▽

✓6ᵗʰ **O30.82** Other specified multiple gestation with two or more **monoamniotic fetuses**

O30.821 Other specified multiple gestation with two or more monoamniotic fetuses, **first trimester**   Ⓜ ♀

O30.822 Other specified multiple gestation with two or more monoamniotic fetuses, **second trimester**   Ⓜ ♀

O30.823 Other specified multiple gestation with two or more monoamniotic fetuses, **third trimester**   Ⓜ ♀

O30.829 Other specified multiple gestation with two or more monoamniotic fetuses, **unspecified trimester**   Ⓜ ♀ ▽

● ✓6ᵗʰ **O30.83** Other specified multiple gestation, **number of chorions and amnions are both equal to the number of fetuses**

Pentachorionic, penta-amniotic pregnancy (quintuplets)

Hexachorionic, hexa-amniotic pregnancy (sextuplets)

Heptachorionic, hepta-amniotic pregnancy (septuplets)

● **O30.831** Other specified multiple gestation, number of chorions and amnions are both equal to the number of fetuses, **first trimester**

● **O30.832** Other specified multiple gestation, number of chorions and amnions are both equal to the number of fetuses, **second trimester**

● **O30.833** Other specified multiple gestation, number of chorions and amnions are both equal to the number of fetuses, **third trimester**

● **O30.839** Other specified multiple gestation, number of chorions and amnions are both equal to the number of fetuses, **unspecified trimester**   ▽

✓6ᵗʰ **O30.89** Other specified multiple gestation, **unable to determine** number of placenta and number of amniotic sacs

O30.891 Other specified multiple gestation, unable to determine number of placenta and number of amniotic sacs, **first trimester**   Ⓜ ♀

O30.892 Other specified multiple gestation, unable to determine number of placenta and number of amniotic sacs, **second trimester**   Ⓜ ♀

O30.893 Other specified multiple gestation, unable to determine number of placenta and number of amniotic sacs, **third trimester**   Ⓜ ♀

O30.899 Other specified multiple gestation, unable to determine number of placenta and number of amniotic sacs, **unspecified trimester**   Ⓜ ♀ ▽

✓5ᵗʰ **O30.9** Multiple gestation, unspecified

Multiple pregnancy NOS

O30.90 Multiple gestation, unspecified, **unspecified trimester**   Ⓜ ♀ ▽

O30.91 Multiple gestation, unspecified, **first trimester**   Ⓜ ♀ ▽

O30.92 Multiple gestation, unspecified, **second trimester**   Ⓜ ♀ ▽

O30.93 Multiple gestation, unspecified, **third trimester**   Ⓜ ♀ ▽

✓4ᵗʰ **O31** Complications specific to multiple gestation

EXCLUDES 2   delayed delivery of second twin, triplet, etc. (O63.2)
malpresentation of one fetus or more (O32.9)
placental transfusion syndromes (O43.0-)

AHA: 2012,4Q,107

One of the following 7th characters is to be assigned to each code under category O31. 7th character 0 is for single gestations and multiple gestations where the fetus is unspecified. 7th characters 1 through 9 are for cases of multiple gestations to identify the fetus for which the code applies. The appropriate code from category O30, Multiple gestation, must also be assigned when assigning a code from category O31 that has a 7th character of 1 through 9.

0   not applicable or unspecified
1   fetus 1
2   fetus 2
3   fetus 3
4   fetus 4
5   fetus 5
9   other fetus

✓5ᵗʰ **O31.0** Papyraceous fetus

Fetus compressus

DEF: Fetus that has died, but remains in utero for weeks before delivery, becoming compacted and mummified in appearance, with skin resembling parchment. Occurs most commonly in multigestational pregnancies. **Synonym(s):** paper doll fetus.

✓x7ᵗʰ **O31.00** Papyraceous fetus, **unspecified trimester**   Ⓜ ♀ ▽

✓x7ᵗʰ **O31.01** Papyraceous fetus, **first trimester**   Ⓜ ♀

✓x7ᵗʰ **O31.02** Papyraceous fetus, **second trimester**   Ⓜ ♀

✓x7ᵗʰ **O31.03** Papyraceous fetus, **third trimester**   Ⓜ ♀

✓5ᵗʰ **O31.1** Continuing pregnancy after spontaneous abortion of one fetus or more

✓x7ᵗʰ **O31.10** Continuing pregnancy after spontaneous abortion of one fetus or more, **unspecified trimester**   Ⓜ ♀ ▽

✓x7ᵗʰ **O31.11** Continuing pregnancy after spontaneous abortion of one fetus or more, **first trimester**   Ⓜ ♀

✓x7ᵗʰ **O31.12** Continuing pregnancy after spontaneous abortion of one fetus or more, **second trimester**   Ⓜ ♀

✓x7ᵗʰ **O31.13** Continuing pregnancy after spontaneous abortion of one fetus or more, **third trimester**   Ⓜ ♀

✓5ᵗʰ **O31.2** Continuing pregnancy after intrauterine death of one fetus or more

✓x7ᵗʰ **O31.20** Continuing pregnancy after intrauterine death of one fetus or more, **unspecified trimester**   Ⓜ ♀ ▽

✓x7ᵗʰ **O31.21** Continuing pregnancy after intrauterine death of one fetus or more, **first trimester**   Ⓜ ♀

✓x7ᵗʰ **O31.22** Continuing pregnancy after intrauterine death of one fetus or more, **second trimester**   Ⓜ ♀

✓x7ᵗʰ **O31.23** Continuing pregnancy after intrauterine death of one fetus or more, **third trimester**   Ⓜ ♀

✓5ᵗʰ **O31.3** Continuing pregnancy after elective fetal reduction of one fetus or more

Continuing pregnancy after selective termination of one fetus or more

✓x7ᵗʰ **O31.30** Continuing pregnancy after elective fetal reduction of one fetus or more, **unspecified trimester**   Ⓜ ♀ ▽

✓x7ᵗʰ **O31.31** Continuing pregnancy after elective fetal reduction of one fetus or more, **first trimester**   Ⓜ ♀

✓x7ᵗʰ **O31.32** Continuing pregnancy after elective fetal reduction of one fetus or more, **second trimester**   Ⓜ ♀

✓x7ᵗʰ **O31.33** Continuing pregnancy after elective fetal reduction of one fetus or more, **third trimester**   Ⓜ ♀

✓5ᵗʰ **O31.8** Other complications specific to multiple gestation

✓6ᵗʰ **O31.8X** Other complications specific to multiple gestation

✓7ᵗʰ **O31.8X1** Other complications specific to multiple gestation, **first trimester**   Ⓜ ♀

✓7ᵗʰ **O31.8X2** Other complications specific to multiple gestation, **second trimester**   Ⓜ ♀

✓7ᵗʰ **O31.8X3** **Other complications specific to multiple gestation, third trimester** Ⓜ ♀

✓7ᵗʰ **O31.8X9** **Other complications specific to multiple gestation, unspecified trimester** Ⓜ ♀ ▽

✓4ᵗʰ **O32** **Maternal care for malpresentation of fetus**

> **INCLUDES** the listed conditions as a reason for observation, hospitalization or other obstetric care of the mother, or for cesarean delivery before onset of labor
>
> **EXCLUDES 1** malpresentation of fetus with obstructed labor (O64.-)
>
> **AHA:** 2012,4Q,107

> One of the following 7th characters is to be assigned to each code under category O32. 7th character Ø is for single gestations and multiple gestations where the fetus is unspecified. 7th characters 1 through 9 are for cases of multiple gestations to identify the fetus for which the code applies. The appropriate code from category O3Ø, Multiple gestation, must also be assigned when assigning a code from category O32 that has a 7th character of 1 through 9.
> Ø   not applicable or unspecified
> 1   fetus 1
> 2   fetus 2
> 3   fetus 3
> 4   fetus 4
> 5   fetus 5
> 9   other fetus

Fetal Malpresentation

Breech

Shoulder
(arm prolapse)

Mother's pelvis

Compound
(extremity together with head)

Face
(mentum)

Oblique

✓x7ᵗʰ **O32.0** **Maternal care for unstable lie** Ⓜ ♀

✓x7ᵗʰ **O32.1** **Maternal care for breech presentation** Ⓜ ♀
> Maternal care for buttocks presentation
> Maternal care for complete breech
> Maternal care for frank breech
> **EXCLUDES 1** footling presentation (O32.8)
> incomplete breech (O32.8)
> **DEF:** Fetus presentation in a longitudinal lie with the buttocks or feet closest to birth canal that may require external cephalic version or cesarean delivery.

✓x7ᵗʰ **O32.2** **Maternal care for transverse and oblique lie** Ⓜ ♀
> Maternal care for oblique presentation
> Maternal care for transverse presentation

✓x7ᵗʰ **O32.3** **Maternal care for face, brow and chin presentation** Ⓜ ♀

✓x7ᵗʰ **O32.4** **Maternal care for high head at term** Ⓜ ♀
> Maternal care for failure of head to enter pelvic brim

✓x7ᵗʰ **O32.6** **Maternal care for compound presentation** Ⓜ ♀

✓x7ᵗʰ **O32.8** **Maternal care for other malpresentation of fetus** Ⓜ ♀
> Maternal care for footling presentation
> Maternal care for incomplete breech

✓x7ᵗʰ **O32.9** **Maternal care for malpresentation of fetus, unspecified** Ⓜ ♀ ▽

✓4ᵗʰ **O33** **Maternal care for disproportion**

> **INCLUDES** the listed conditions as a reason for observation, hospitalization or other obstetric care of the mother, or for cesarean delivery before onset of labor
>
> **EXCLUDES 1** disproportion with obstructed labor (O65-O66)

O33.0 **Maternal care for disproportion due to deformity of maternal pelvic bones** Ⓜ ♀
> Maternal care for disproportion due to pelvic deformity causing disproportion NOS

O33.1 **Maternal care for disproportion due to generally contracted pelvis** Ⓜ ♀
> Maternal care for disproportion due to contracted pelvis NOS causing disproportion

O33.2 **Maternal care for disproportion due to inlet contraction of pelvis** Ⓜ ♀
> Maternal care for disproportion due to inlet contraction (pelvis) causing disproportion

✓x7ᵗʰ **O33.3** **Maternal care for disproportion due to outlet contraction of pelvis** Ⓜ ♀
> Maternal care for disproportion due to mid-cavity contraction (pelvis)
> Maternal care for disproportion due to outlet contraction (pelvis)

> One of the following 7th characters is to be assigned to code O33.3. 7th character Ø is for single gestations and multiple gestations where the fetus is unspecified. 7th characters 1 through 9 are for cases of multiple gestations to identify the fetus for which the code applies. The appropriate code from category O3Ø, Multiple gestation, must also be assigned when assigning code O33.3 with a 7th character of 1 through 9.
> Ø   not applicable or unspecified
> 1   fetus 1
> 2   fetus 2
> 3   fetus 3
> 4   fetus 4
> 5   fetus 5
> 9   other fetus

✓x7ᵗʰ **O33.4** **Maternal care for disproportion of mixed maternal and fetal origin** Ⓜ ♀

> One of the following 7th characters is to be assigned to code O33.4. 7th character Ø is for single gestations and multiple gestations where the fetus is unspecified. 7th characters 1 through 9 are for cases of multiple gestations to identify the fetus for which the code applies. The appropriate code from category O3Ø, Multiple gestation, must also be assigned when assigning code O33.4 with a 7th character of 1 through 9.
> Ø   not applicable or unspecified
> 1   fetus 1
> 2   fetus 2
> 3   fetus 3
> 4   fetus 4
> 5   fetus 5
> 9   other fetus

✓x7ᵗʰ **O33.5** **Maternal care for disproportion due to unusually large fetus** Ⓜ ♀
> Maternal care for disproportion due to disproportion of fetal origin with normally formed fetus
> Maternal care for disproportion due to fetal disproportion NOS

> One of the following 7th characters is to be assigned to code O33.5. 7th character Ø is for single gestations and multiple gestations where the fetus is unspecified. 7th characters 1 through 9 are for cases of multiple gestations to identify the fetus for which the code applies. The appropriate code from category O3Ø, Multiple gestation, must also be assigned when assigning code O33.5 with a 7th character of 1 through 9.
> Ø   not applicable or unspecified
> 1   fetus 1
> 2   fetus 2
> 3   fetus 3
> 4   fetus 4
> 5   fetus 5
> 9   other fetus

√x7ᵗʰ **O33.6 Maternal care for disproportion due to hydrocephalic fetus** Ⓜ ♀

> One of the following 7th characters is to be assigned to code O33.6. 7th character Ø is for single gestations and multiple gestations where the fetus is unspecified. 7th characters 1 through 9 are for cases of multiple gestations to identify the fetus for which the code applies. The appropriate code from category O3Ø, Multiple gestation, must also be assigned when assigning code O33.6 with a 7th character of 1 through 9.
> Ø   not applicable or unspecified
> 1   fetus 1
> 2   fetus 2
> 3   fetus 3
> 4   fetus 4
> 5   fetus 5
> 9   other fetus

√x7ᵗʰ **O33.7 Maternal care for disproportion due to other fetal deformities** Ⓜ ♀

> Maternal care for disproportion due to fetal ascites
> Maternal care for disproportion due to fetal hydrops
> Maternal care for disproportion due to fetal meningomyelocele
> Maternal care for disproportion due to fetal sacral teratoma
> Maternal care for disproportion due to fetal tumor
> **EXCLUDES 1**   obstructed labor due to other fetal deformities (O66.3)
> **AHA:** 2016,4Q,51

> One of the following 7th characters is to be assigned to code O33.7. 7th character Ø is for single gestations and multiple gestations where the fetus is unspecified. 7th characters 1 through 9 are for cases of multiple gestations to identify the fetus for which the code applies. The appropriate code from category O3Ø, Multiple gestation, must also be assigned when assigning code O33.7 with a 7th character of 1 through 9.
> Ø   not applicable or unspecified
> 1   fetus 1
> 2   fetus 2
> 3   fetus 3
> 4   fetus 4
> 5   fetus 5
> 9   other fetus

O33.8 Maternal care for disproportion of other origin Ⓜ ♀

O33.9 Maternal care for disproportion, unspecified Ⓜ ♀ ▽

> Maternal care for disproportion due to cephalopelvic disproportion NOS
> Maternal care for disproportion due to fetopelvic disproportion NOS

√4ᵗʰ **O34 Maternal care for abnormality of pelvic organs**

> **INCLUDES**   the listed conditions as a reason for hospitalization or other obstetric care of the mother, or for cesarean delivery before onset of labor
> Code first any associated obstructed labor (O65.5)
> Use additional code for specific condition

√5ᵗʰ **O34.Ø Maternal care for congenital malformation of uterus**

> Maternal care for double uterus
> Maternal care for uterus bicornis

     O34.ØØ Maternal care for unspecified congenital malformation of uterus, unspecified trimester Ⓜ ♀ ▽

     O34.Ø1 Maternal care for unspecified congenital malformation of uterus, first trimester Ⓜ ♀ ▽

     O34.Ø2 Maternal care for unspecified congenital malformation of uterus, second trimester Ⓜ ♀ ▽

     O34.Ø3 Maternal care for unspecified congenital malformation of uterus, third trimester Ⓜ ♀ ▽

√5ᵗʰ **O34.1 Maternal care for benign tumor of corpus uteri**

> **EXCLUDES 2**   maternal care for benign tumor of cervix (O34.4-)
> maternal care for malignant neoplasm of uterus (O9A.1-)

     O34.1Ø Maternal care for benign tumor of corpus uteri, unspecified trimester Ⓜ ♀ ▽

     O34.11 Maternal care for benign tumor of corpus uteri, first trimester Ⓜ ♀

     O34.12 Maternal care for benign tumor of corpus uteri, second trimester Ⓜ ♀

     O34.13 Maternal care for benign tumor of corpus uteri, third trimester Ⓜ ♀

√5ᵗʰ **O34.2 Maternal care due to uterine scar from previous surgery**

> **AHA:** 2016,4Q,76

√6ᵗʰ **O34.21 Maternal care for scar from previous cesarean delivery**

> **AHA:** 2016,4Q,51-52

     O34.211 Maternal care for low transverse scar from previous cesarean delivery Ⓜ ♀

     O34.212 Maternal care for vertical scar from previous cesarean delivery Ⓜ ♀
> Maternal care for classical scar from previous cesarean delivery

     O34.219 Maternal care for unspecified type scar from previous cesarean delivery Ⓜ ♀ ▽

     O34.29 Maternal care due to uterine scar from other previous surgery Ⓜ ♀
> Maternal care due to uterine scar from other transmural uterine incision

√5ᵗʰ **O34.3 Maternal care for cervical incompetence**

> Maternal care for cerclage with or without cervical incompetence
> Maternal care for Shirodkar suture with or without cervical incompetence
> **DEF:** Inadequate functioning of the cervix marked by abnormal widening during pregnancy and causing premature birth or miscarriage.

     O34.3Ø Maternal care for cervical incompetence, unspecified trimester Ⓜ ♀ ▽

     O34.31 Maternal care for cervical incompetence, first trimester Ⓜ ♀

     O34.32 Maternal care for cervical incompetence, second trimester Ⓜ ♀

     O34.33 Maternal care for cervical incompetence, third trimester Ⓜ ♀

√5ᵗʰ **O34.4 Maternal care for other abnormalities of cervix**

     O34.4Ø Maternal care for other abnormalities of cervix, unspecified trimester Ⓜ ♀ ▽

     O34.41 Maternal care for other abnormalities of cervix, first trimester Ⓜ ♀

     O34.42 Maternal care for other abnormalities of cervix, second trimester Ⓜ ♀

     O34.43 Maternal care for other abnormalities of cervix, third trimester Ⓜ ♀

√5ᵗʰ **O34.5 Maternal care for other abnormalities of gravid uterus**

√6ᵗʰ **O34.51 Maternal care for incarceration of gravid uterus**

     O34.511 Maternal care for incarceration of gravid uterus, first trimester Ⓜ ♀

     O34.512 Maternal care for incarceration of gravid uterus, second trimester Ⓜ ♀

     O34.513 Maternal care for incarceration of gravid uterus, third trimester Ⓜ ♀

     O34.519 Maternal care for incarceration of gravid uterus, unspecified trimester Ⓜ ♀ ▽

√6ᵗʰ **O34.52 Maternal care for prolapse of gravid uterus**

     O34.521 Maternal care for prolapse of gravid uterus, first trimester Ⓜ ♀

     O34.522 Maternal care for prolapse of gravid uterus, second trimester Ⓜ ♀

     O34.523 Maternal care for prolapse of gravid uterus, third trimester Ⓜ ♀

     O34.529 Maternal care for prolapse of gravid uterus, unspecified trimester Ⓜ ♀ ▽

√6ᵗʰ **O34.53 Maternal care for retroversion of gravid uterus**

     O34.531 Maternal care for retroversion of gravid uterus, first trimester Ⓜ ♀

     O34.532 Maternal care for retroversion of gravid uterus, second trimester Ⓜ ♀

     O34.533 Maternal care for retroversion of gravid uterus, third trimester Ⓜ ♀

     O34.539 Maternal care for retroversion of gravid uterus, unspecified trimester Ⓜ ♀ ▽

✓ Additional Character Req   √x7ᵗʰ Placeholder Alert   Manifestation   ▽ Unspecified   ►◄ Revised Text   ● New Code   ▲ Revised Code Title

√6ᵗʰ O34.59 Maternal care for other abnormalities of gravid uterus

    O34.591 Maternal care for other abnormalities of gravid uterus, first trimester Ⓜ ♀

    O34.592 Maternal care for other abnormalities of gravid uterus, second trimester Ⓜ ♀

    O34.593 Maternal care for other abnormalities of gravid uterus, third trimester Ⓜ ♀

    O34.599 Maternal care for other abnormalities of gravid uterus, unspecified trimester Ⓜ ♀ ▽

√5ᵗʰ O34.6 Maternal care for abnormality of vagina

    EXCLUDES 2   *maternal care for vaginal varices in pregnancy (O22.1-)*

    O34.60 Maternal care for abnormality of vagina, unspecified trimester Ⓜ ♀ ▽

    O34.61 Maternal care for abnormality of vagina, first trimester Ⓜ ♀

    O34.62 Maternal care for abnormality of vagina, second trimester Ⓜ ♀

    O34.63 Maternal care for abnormality of vagina, third trimester Ⓜ ♀

√5ᵗʰ O34.7 Maternal care for abnormality of vulva and perineum

    EXCLUDES 2   *maternal care for perineal and vulval varices in pregnancy (O22.1-)*

    O34.70 Maternal care for abnormality of vulva and perineum, unspecified trimester Ⓜ ♀ ▽

    O34.71 Maternal care for abnormality of vulva and perineum, first trimester Ⓜ ♀

    O34.72 Maternal care for abnormality of vulva and perineum, second trimester Ⓜ ♀

    O34.73 Maternal care for abnormality of vulva and perineum, third trimester Ⓜ ♀

√5ᵗʰ O34.8 Maternal care for other abnormalities of pelvic organs

    O34.80 Maternal care for other abnormalities of pelvic organs, unspecified trimester Ⓜ ♀ ▽

    O34.81 Maternal care for other abnormalities of pelvic organs, first trimester Ⓜ ♀

    O34.82 Maternal care for other abnormalities of pelvic organs, second trimester Ⓜ ♀

    O34.83 Maternal care for other abnormalities of pelvic organs, third trimester Ⓜ ♀

√5ᵗʰ O34.9 Maternal care for abnormality of pelvic organ, unspecified

    O34.90 Maternal care for abnormality of pelvic organ, unspecified, unspecified trimester Ⓜ ♀ ▽

    O34.91 Maternal care for abnormality of pelvic organ, unspecified, first trimester Ⓜ ♀ ▽

    O34.92 Maternal care for abnormality of pelvic organ, unspecified, second trimester Ⓜ ♀ ▽

    O34.93 Maternal care for abnormality of pelvic organ, unspecified, third trimester Ⓜ ♀ ▽

√4ᵗʰ O35 Maternal care for known or suspected fetal abnormality and damage

    INCLUDES   the listed conditions in the fetus as a reason for hospitalization or other obstetric care to the mother, or for termination of pregnancy

    Code also any associated maternal condition

    EXCLUDES 1   *encounter for suspected maternal and fetal conditions ruled out (Z03.7-)*

> One of the following 7th characters is to be assigned to each code under category O35. 7th character Ø is for single gestations and multiple gestations where the fetus is unspecified. 7th characters 1 through 9 are for cases of multiple gestations to identify the fetus for which the code applies. The appropriate code from category O30, Multiple gestation, must also be assigned when assigning a code from category O35 that has a 7th character of 1 through 9.
> Ø   not applicable or unspecified
> 1   fetus 1
> 2   fetus 2
> 3   fetus 3
> 4   fetus 4
> 5   fetus 5
> 9   other fetus

√x7ᵗʰ O35.0 Maternal care for (suspected) central nervous system malformation in fetus Ⓜ ♀

    Maternal care for fetal anencephaly
    Maternal care for fetal hydrocephalus
    Maternal care for fetal spina bifida
    EXCLUDES 2   *chromosomal abnormality in fetus (O35.1)*

√x7ᵗʰ O35.1 Maternal care for (suspected) chromosomal abnormality in fetus Ⓜ ♀

√x7ᵗʰ O35.2 Maternal care for (suspected) hereditary disease in fetus Ⓜ ♀

    EXCLUDES 2   *chromosomal abnormality in fetus (O35.1)*

√x7ᵗʰ O35.3 Maternal care for (suspected) damage to fetus from viral disease in mother Ⓜ ♀

    Maternal care for damage to fetus from maternal cytomegalovirus infection
    Maternal care for damage to fetus from maternal rubella

√x7ᵗʰ O35.4 Maternal care for (suspected) damage to fetus from alcohol Ⓜ ♀

√x7ᵗʰ O35.5 Maternal care for (suspected) damage to fetus by drugs Ⓜ ♀

    Maternal care for damage to fetus from drug addiction

√x7ᵗʰ O35.6 Maternal care for (suspected) damage to fetus by radiation Ⓜ ♀

√x7ᵗʰ O35.7 Maternal care for (suspected) damage to fetus by other medical procedures Ⓜ ♀

    Maternal care for damage to fetus by amniocentesis
    Maternal care for damage to fetus by biopsy procedures
    Maternal care for damage to fetus by hematological investigation
    Maternal care for damage to fetus by intrauterine contraceptive device
    Maternal care for damage to fetus by intrauterine surgery

√x7ᵗʰ O35.8 Maternal care for other (suspected) fetal abnormality and damage Ⓜ ♀

    Maternal care for damage to fetus from maternal listeriosis
    Maternal care for damage to fetus from maternal toxoplasmosis

√x7ᵗʰ O35.9 Maternal care for (suspected) fetal abnormality and damage, unspecified Ⓜ ♀ ▽

☑4ᵗʰ **O36   Maternal care for other fetal problems**

INCLUDES   the listed conditions in the fetus as a reason for hospitalization or other obstetric care of the mother, or for termination of pregnancy

EXCLUDES 1   *encounter for suspected maternal and fetal conditions ruled out (Z03.7-)*

placental transfusion syndromes (O43.0-)

EXCLUDES 2   *labor and delivery complicated by fetal stress (O77.-)*

AHA: 2015,3Q,40

One of the following 7th characters is to be assigned to each code under category O36. 7th character 0 is for single gestations and multiple gestations where the fetus is unspecified. 7th characters 1 through 9 are for cases of multiple gestations to identify the fetus for which the code applies. The appropriate code from category O30, Multiple gestation, must also be assigned when assigning a code from category O36 that has a 7th character of 1 through 9.

0   not applicable or unspecified
1   fetus 1
2   fetus 2
3   fetus 3
4   fetus 4
5   fetus 5
9   other fetus

☑5ᵗʰ **O36.0   Maternal care for rhesus isoimmunization**

Maternal care for Rh incompatibility (with hydrops fetalis)

☑6ᵗʰ **O36.01   Maternal care for anti-D [Rh] antibodies**

AHA: 2014,4Q,17

☑7ᵗʰ **O36.011   Maternal care for anti-D [Rh] antibodies, first trimester**   0 Ⓜ ♀

☑7ᵗʰ **O36.012   Maternal care for anti-D [Rh] antibodies, second trimester**   Ⓜ ♀

☑7ᵗʰ **O36.013   Maternal care for anti-D [Rh] antibodies, third trimester**   Ⓜ ♀

☑7ᵗʰ **O36.019   Maternal care for anti-D [Rh] antibodies, unspecified trimester**   0 Ⓜ ♀ ▽

☑6ᵗʰ **O36.09   Maternal care for other rhesus isoimmunization**

☑7ᵗʰ **O36.091   Maternal care for other rhesus isoimmunization, first trimester**   0 Ⓜ ♀

☑7ᵗʰ **O36.092   Maternal care for other rhesus isoimmunization, second trimester**   Ⓜ ♀

☑7ᵗʰ **O36.093   Maternal care for other rhesus isoimmunization, third trimester**   Ⓜ ♀

☑7ᵗʰ **O36.099   Maternal care for other rhesus isoimmunization, unspecified trimester**   0 Ⓜ ♀ ▽

☑5ᵗʰ **O36.1   Maternal care for other isoimmunization**

Maternal care for ABO isoimmunization

☑6ᵗʰ **O36.11   Maternal care for Anti-A sensitization**

Maternal care for isoimmunization NOS (with hydrops fetalis)

☑7ᵗʰ **O36.111   Maternal care for Anti-A sensitization, first trimester**   Ⓜ ♀

☑7ᵗʰ **O36.112   Maternal care for Anti-A sensitization, second trimester**   Ⓜ ♀

☑7ᵗʰ **O36.113   Maternal care for Anti-A sensitization, third trimester**   Ⓜ ♀

☑7ᵗʰ **O36.119   Maternal care for Anti-A sensitization, unspecified trimester**   Ⓜ ♀ ▽

☑6ᵗʰ **O36.19   Maternal care for other isoimmunization**

Maternal care for Anti-B sensitization

☑7ᵗʰ **O36.191   Maternal care for other isoimmunization, first trimester**   Ⓜ ♀

☑7ᵗʰ **O36.192   Maternal care for other isoimmunization, second trimester**   Ⓜ ♀

☑7ᵗʰ **O36.193   Maternal care for other isoimmunization, third trimester**   Ⓜ ♀

☑7ᵗʰ **O36.199   Maternal care for other isoimmunization, unspecified trimester**   Ⓜ ♀ ▽

☑5ᵗʰ **O36.2   Maternal care for hydrops fetalis**

Maternal care for hydrops fetalis NOS

Maternal care for hydrops fetalis not associated with isoimmunization

EXCLUDES 1   *hydrops fetalis associated with ABO isoimmunization (O36.1-)*

hydrops fetalis associated with rhesus isoimmunization (O36.0-)

DEF: Hydrops fetalis: Abnormal fluid buildup in at least two of the following fetal organ spaces: the skin (edema), abdomen (ascites), around the heart (pericardia effusion), and around the lung (pleural effusion). Fluid accumulation may also occur in the mother as polyhydramnios and edema of the placenta.

☑x7ᵗʰ **O36.20   Maternal care for hydrops fetalis, unspecified trimester**   Ⓜ ♀ ▽

☑x7ᵗʰ **O36.21   Maternal care for hydrops fetalis, first trimester**   Ⓜ ♀

☑x7ᵗʰ **O36.22   Maternal care for hydrops fetalis, second trimester**   Ⓜ ♀

☑x7ᵗʰ **O36.23   Maternal care for hydrops fetalis, third trimester**   Ⓜ ♀

☑x7ᵗʰ **O36.4   Maternal care for intrauterine death**   Ⓜ ♀

Maternal care for intrauterine fetal death NOS

Maternal care for intrauterine fetal death after completion of 20 weeks of gestation

Maternal care for late fetal death

Maternal care for missed delivery

EXCLUDES 1   *missed abortion (O02.1)*

stillbirth (P95)

☑5ᵗʰ **O36.5   Maternal care for known or suspected poor fetal growth**

☑6ᵗʰ **O36.51   Maternal care for known or suspected placental insufficiency**

☑7ᵗʰ **O36.511   Maternal care for known or suspected placental insufficiency, first trimester**   Ⓜ ♀

☑7ᵗʰ **O36.512   Maternal care for known or suspected placental insufficiency, second trimester**   Ⓜ ♀

☑7ᵗʰ **O36.513   Maternal care for known or suspected placental insufficiency, third trimester**   Ⓜ ♀

☑7ᵗʰ **O36.519   Maternal care for known or suspected placental insufficiency, unspecified trimester**   Ⓜ ♀ ▽

☑6ᵗʰ **O36.59   Maternal care for other known or suspected poor fetal growth**

Maternal care for known or suspected light-for-dates NOS

Maternal care for known or suspected small-for-dates NOS

☑7ᵗʰ **O36.591   Maternal care for other known or suspected poor fetal growth, first trimester**   Ⓜ ♀

☑7ᵗʰ **O36.592   Maternal care for other known or suspected poor fetal growth, second trimester**   Ⓜ ♀

☑7ᵗʰ **O36.593   Maternal care for other known or suspected poor fetal growth, third trimester**   Ⓜ ♀

☑7ᵗʰ **O36.599   Maternal care for other known or suspected poor fetal growth, unspecified trimester**   Ⓜ ♀ ▽

☑5ᵗʰ **O36.6   Maternal care for excessive fetal growth**

Maternal care for known or suspected large-for-dates

☑x7ᵗʰ **O36.60   Maternal care for excessive fetal growth, unspecified trimester**   Ⓜ ♀ ▽

☑x7ᵗʰ **O36.61   Maternal care for excessive fetal growth, first trimester**   Ⓜ ♀

☑x7ᵗʰ **O36.62   Maternal care for excessive fetal growth, second trimester**   Ⓜ ♀

☑x7ᵗʰ **O36.63   Maternal care for excessive fetal growth, third trimester**   Ⓜ ♀

☑5ᵗʰ **O36.7   Maternal care for viable fetus in abdominal pregnancy**

☑x7ᵗʰ **O36.70   Maternal care for viable fetus in abdominal pregnancy, unspecified trimester**   Ⓜ ♀ ▽

☑x7ᵗʰ **O36.71   Maternal care for viable fetus in abdominal pregnancy, first trimester**   Ⓜ ♀

☑x7ᵗʰ **O36.72   Maternal care for viable fetus in abdominal pregnancy, second trimester**   Ⓜ ♀

☑ Additional Character Req   ☑x7ᵗʰ Placeholder Alert   Manifestation   ▽ Unspecified   ►◄ Revised Text   ● New Code   ▲ Revised Code Title

√x7ᵗʰ O36.73 Maternal care for viable fetus in abdominal pregnancy, third trimester Ⓜ ♀

√5ᵗʰ O36.8 Maternal care for other specified fetal problems

√x7ᵗʰ O36.80 Pregnancy with inconclusive fetal viability Ⓜ ♀
Encounter to determine fetal viability of pregnancy

√6ᵗʰ O36.81 Decreased fetal movements

√7ᵗʰ O36.812 Decreased fetal movements, second trimester Ⓜ ♀

√7ᵗʰ O36.813 Decreased fetal movements, third trimester Ⓜ ♀

√7ᵗʰ O36.819 Decreased fetal movements, unspecified trimester Ⓜ ♀ ▽

√6ᵗʰ O36.82 Fetal anemia and thrombocytopenia

√7ᵗʰ O36.821 Fetal anemia and thrombocytopenia, first trimester Ⓜ ♀

√7ᵗʰ O36.822 Fetal anemia and thrombocytopenia, second trimester Ⓜ ♀

√7ᵗʰ O36.823 Fetal anemia and thrombocytopenia, third trimester Ⓜ ♀

√7ᵗʰ O36.829 Fetal anemia and thrombocytopenia, unspecified trimester Ⓜ ♀ ▽

√6ᵗʰ O36.83 Maternal care for abnormalities of the fetal heart rate or rhythm
AHA: 2017,4Q,20
TIP: Assign for documented fetal tachycardia, bradycardia, decelerations, or loss of variability detected during antenatal testing.

√7ᵗʰ O36.831 Maternal care for abnormalities of the fetal heart rate or rhythm, first trimester Ⓜ ♀

√7ᵗʰ O36.832 Maternal care for abnormalities of the fetal heart rate or rhythm, second trimester Ⓜ ♀

√7ᵗʰ O36.833 Maternal care for abnormalities of the fetal heart rate or rhythm, third trimester Ⓜ ♀

√7ᵗʰ O36.839 Maternal care for abnormalities of the fetal heart rate or rhythm, unspecified trimester Ⓜ ♀ ▽

√6ᵗʰ O36.89 Maternal care for other specified fetal problems

√7ᵗʰ O36.891 Maternal care for other specified fetal problems, first trimester Ⓜ ♀

√7ᵗʰ O36.892 Maternal care for other specified fetal problems, second trimester Ⓜ ♀

√7ᵗʰ O36.893 Maternal care for other specified fetal problems, third trimester ♀

√7ᵗʰ O36.899 Maternal care for other specified fetal problems, unspecified trimester Ⓜ ♀ ▽

√5ᵗʰ O36.9 Maternal care for fetal problem, unspecified

√x7ᵗʰ O36.90 Maternal care for fetal problem, unspecified, unspecified trimester Ⓜ ♀ ▽

√x7ᵗʰ O36.91 Maternal care for fetal problem, unspecified, first trimester Ⓜ ♀ ▽

√x7ᵗʰ O36.92 Maternal care for fetal problem, unspecified, second trimester Ⓜ ♀ ▽

√x7ᵗʰ O36.93 Maternal care for fetal problem, unspecified, third trimester Ⓜ ♀ ▽

√4ᵗʰ O40 Polyhydramnios

INCLUDES   hydramnios

EXCLUDES 1   encounter for suspected maternal and fetal conditions ruled out (Z03.7-)

AHA: 2016,1Q,4
DEF: Excess amniotic fluid surrounding the fetus, typically defined as a total fluid volume of greater than 24.0 cc.

One of the following 7th characters is to be assigned to each code under category O40. 7th character 0 is for single gestations and multiple gestations where the fetus is unspecified. 7th characters 1 through 9 are for cases of multiple gestations to identify the fetus for which the code applies. The appropriate code from category O30, Multiple gestation, must also be assigned when assigning a code from category O40 that has a 7th character of 1 through 9.
0   not applicable or unspecified
1   fetus 1
2   fetus 2
3   fetus 3
4   fetus 4
5   fetus 5
9   other fetus

√x7ᵗʰ O40.1 Polyhydramnios, first trimester Ⓜ ♀

√x7ᵗʰ O40.2 Polyhydramnios, second trimester Ⓜ ♀

√x7ᵗʰ O40.3 Polyhydramnios, third trimester Ⓜ ♀

√x7ᵗʰ O40.9 Polyhydramnios, unspecified trimester Ⓜ ♀ ▽

√4ᵗʰ O41 Other disorders of amniotic fluid and membranes

EXCLUDES 1   encounter for suspected maternal and fetal conditions ruled out (Z03.7-)

One of the following 7th characters is to be assigned to each code under category O41. 7th character 0 is for single gestations and multiple gestations where the fetus is unspecified. 7th characters 1 through 9 are for cases of multiple gestations to identify the fetus for which the code applies. The appropriate code from category O30, Multiple gestation, must also be assigned when assigning a code from category O41 that has a 7th character of 1 through 9.
0   not applicable or unspecified
1   fetus 1
2   fetus 2
3   fetus 3
4   fetus 4
5   fetus 5
9   other fetus

√5ᵗʰ O41.0 Oligohydramnios
Oligohydramnios without rupture of membranes
DEF: Low amniotic fluid, occurring most frequently in the last trimester.

√x7ᵗʰ O41.00 Oligohydramnios, unspecified trimester Ⓜ ♀ ▽

√x7ᵗʰ O41.01 Oligohydramnios, first trimester Ⓜ ♀

√x7ᵗʰ O41.02 Oligohydramnios, second trimester Ⓜ ♀

√x7ᵗʰ O41.03 Oligohydramnios, third trimester Ⓜ ♀

√5ᵗʰ O41.1 Infection of amniotic sac and membranes

√6ᵗʰ O41.10 Infection of amniotic sac and membranes, unspecified

√7ᵗʰ O41.101 Infection of amniotic sac and membranes, unspecified, first trimester Ⓜ ♀ ▽

√7ᵗʰ O41.102 Infection of amniotic sac and membranes, unspecified, second trimester Ⓜ ♀ ▽

√7ᵗʰ O41.103 Infection of amniotic sac and membranes, unspecified, third trimester Ⓜ ♀ ▽

√7ᵗʰ O41.109 Infection of amniotic sac and membranes, unspecified, unspecified trimester Ⓜ ♀ ▽

√6ᵗʰ O41.12 Chorioamnionitis

√7ᵗʰ O41.121 Chorioamnionitis, first trimester Ⓜ ♀

√7ᵗʰ O41.122 Chorioamnionitis, second trimester Ⓜ ♀

√7ᵗʰ O41.123 Chorioamnionitis, third trimester Ⓜ ♀

√7ᵗʰ O41.129 Chorioamnionitis, unspecified trimester Ⓜ ♀ ▽

√6ᵗʰ O41.14 Placentitis

√7ᵗʰ O41.141 Placentitis, first trimester Ⓜ ♀

√7ᵗʰ O41.142 Placentitis, second trimester Ⓜ ♀

√7ᵗʰ **O41.143** **Placentitis,** third trimester   Ⓜ ♀

√7ᵗʰ **O41.149** **Placentitis, unspecified trimester**   Ⓜ ♀ ▽

√5ᵗʰ **O41.8** **Other specified disorders of amniotic fluid and membranes**

√6ᵗʰ **O41.8X** **Other specified disorders of amniotic fluid and membranes**

√7ᵗʰ **O41.8X1** **Other specified disorders of amniotic fluid and membranes,** first trimester   Ⓜ ♀

√7ᵗʰ **O41.8X2** **Other specified disorders of amniotic fluid and membranes,** second trimester   Ⓜ ♀

√7ᵗʰ **O41.8X3** **Other specified disorders of amniotic fluid and membranes,** third trimester   Ⓜ ♀

√7ᵗʰ **O41.8X9** **Other specified disorders of amniotic fluid and membranes, unspecified trimester**   Ⓜ ♀ ▽

√5ᵗʰ **O41.9** **Disorder of amniotic fluid and membranes, unspecified**

√x7ᵗʰ **O41.90** **Disorder of amniotic fluid and membranes, unspecified, unspecified trimester**   Ⓜ ♀ ▽

√x7ᵗʰ **O41.91** **Disorder of amniotic fluid and membranes, unspecified,** first trimester   Ⓜ ♀ ▽

√x7ᵗʰ **O41.92** **Disorder of amniotic fluid and membranes, unspecified,** second trimester   Ⓜ ♀ ▽

√x7ᵗʰ **O41.93** **Disorder of amniotic fluid and membranes, unspecified,** third trimester   Ⓜ ♀

√4ᵗʰ **O42** **Premature rupture of membranes**

AHA: 2016,1Q,3

√5ᵗʰ **O42.0** **Premature rupture of membranes,** onset of labor within 24 hours of rupture

O42.00 **Premature rupture of membranes, onset of labor within 24 hours of rupture, unspecified weeks of gestation**   Ⓜ ♀ ▽

√6ᵗʰ **O42.01** **Preterm premature rupture of membranes, onset of labor within 24 hours of rupture**

Premature rupture of membranes before 37 completed weeks of gestation

O42.011 **Preterm premature rupture of membranes, onset of labor within 24 hours of rupture,** first trimester   Ⓜ ♀

O42.012 **Preterm premature rupture of membranes, onset of labor within 24 hours of rupture,** second trimester   Ⓜ ♀

O42.013 **Preterm premature rupture of membranes, onset of labor within 24 hours of rupture,** third trimester   Ⓜ ♀

O42.019 **Preterm premature rupture of membranes, onset of labor within 24 hours of rupture, unspecified trimester**   Ⓜ ♀ ▽

O42.02 **Full-term premature rupture of membranes, onset of labor within 24 hours of rupture**   Ⓜ ♀

Premature rupture of membranes at or after 37 completed weeks of gestation, onset of labor within 24 hours of rupture

√5ᵗʰ **O42.1** **Premature rupture of membranes,** onset of labor more than 24 hours following rupture

AHA: 2016,1Q,5

O42.10 **Premature rupture of membranes, onset of labor more than 24 hours following rupture, unspecified weeks of gestation**   Ⓜ ♀ ▽

√6ᵗʰ **O42.11** **Preterm premature rupture of membranes, onset of labor more than 24 hours following rupture**

Premature rupture of membranes before 37 completed weeks of gestation

O42.111 **Preterm premature rupture of membranes, onset of labor more than 24 hours following rupture,** first trimester   Ⓜ ♀

O42.112 **Preterm premature rupture of membranes, onset of labor more than 24 hours following rupture,** second trimester   Ⓜ ♀

O42.113 **Preterm premature rupture of membranes, onset of labor more than 24 hours following rupture,** third trimester   Ⓜ ♀

O42.119 **Preterm premature rupture of membranes, onset of labor more than 24 hours following rupture, unspecified trimester**   Ⓜ ♀ ▽

O42.12 **Full-term premature rupture of membranes, onset of labor more than 24 hours following rupture**   Ⓜ ♀

Premature rupture of membranes at or after 37 completed weeks of gestation, onset of labor more than 24 hours following rupture

√5ᵗʰ **O42.9** **Premature rupture of membranes, unspecified** as to length of time between rupture and onset of labor

O42.90 **Premature rupture of membranes, unspecified as to length of time between rupture and onset of labor, unspecified weeks of gestation**   Ⓜ ♀ ▽

√6ᵗʰ **O42.91** **Preterm** premature rupture of membranes, unspecified as to length of time between rupture and onset of labor

Premature rupture of membranes before 37 completed weeks of gestation

O42.911 **Preterm premature rupture of membranes, unspecified as to length of time between rupture and onset of labor,** first trimester   Ⓜ ♀ ▽

O42.912 **Preterm premature rupture of membranes, unspecified as to length of time between rupture and onset of labor,** second trimester   Ⓜ ♀ ▽

O42.913 **Preterm premature rupture of membranes, unspecified as to length of time between rupture and onset of labor,** third trimester   Ⓜ ♀ ▽

O42.919 **Preterm premature rupture of membranes, unspecified as to length of time between rupture and onset of labor, unspecified trimester**   Ⓜ ♀ ▽

O42.92 **Full-term** premature rupture of membranes, unspecified as to length of time between rupture and onset of labor   Ⓜ ♀ ▽

Premature rupture of membranes at or after 37 completed weeks of gestation, unspecified as to length of time between rupture and onset of labor

√4ᵗʰ **O43** **Placental disorders**

EXCLUDES 2   *maternal care for poor fetal growth due to placental insufficiency (O36.5-)*

placenta previa (O44.-)

placental polyp (O90.89)

placentitis (O41.14-)

premature separation of placenta [abruptio placentae] (O45.-)

√5ᵗʰ **O43.0** **Placental transfusion syndromes**

√6ᵗʰ **O43.01** **Fetomaternal placental transfusion syndrome**

Maternofetal placental transfusion syndrome

O43.011 **Fetomaternal placental transfusion syndrome,** first trimester   🄾 Ⓜ ♀

O43.012 **Fetomaternal placental transfusion syndrome,** second trimester   Ⓜ ♀

O43.013 **Fetomaternal placental transfusion syndrome,** third trimester   Ⓜ ♀

O43.019 **Fetomaternal placental transfusion syndrome, unspecified trimester**   🄾 Ⓜ ♀ ▽

✅ Additional Character Req   √x7ᵗʰ Placeholder Alert   Manifestation   ▽ Unspecified   ►◄ Revised Text   ● New Code   ▲ Revised Code Title

ICD-10-CM 2019   **871**

√6ᵗʰ **O43.02** **Fetus-to-fetus** placental transfusion syndrome

DEF: Condition in which an imbalance in amniotic fluid occurs due to uneven blood flow between twins sharing a placenta.

Twin to Twin Transfusion Syndrome (TTTS)

Healthy twins   Twins with TTTS

O43.021 Fetus-to-fetus placental transfusion syndrome, **first trimester**   Ⓜ ♀

O43.022 Fetus-to-fetus placental transfusion syndrome, **second trimester**   Ⓜ ♀

O43.023 Fetus-to-fetus placental transfusion syndrome, **third trimester**   Ⓜ ♀

O43.029 Fetus-to-fetus placental transfusion syndrome, **unspecified trimester**   Ⓜ ♀ ▽

√5ᵗʰ **O43.1** **Malformation of placenta**

√6ᵗʰ **O43.10** **Malformation of placenta, unspecified**

Abnormal placenta NOS

O43.101 Malformation of placenta, unspecified, **first trimester**   Ⓜ ♀ ▽

O43.102 Malformation of placenta, unspecified, **second trimester**   Ⓜ ♀ ▽

O43.103 Malformation of placenta, unspecified, **third trimester**   Ⓜ ♀ ▽

O43.109 Malformation of placenta, unspecified, **unspecified trimester**   Ⓜ ♀ ▽

√6ᵗʰ **O43.11** **Circumvallate** placenta

O43.111 Circumvallate placenta, **first trimester**   Ⓜ ♀

O43.112 Circumvallate placenta, **second trimester**   Ⓜ ♀

O43.113 Circumvallate placenta, **third trimester**   Ⓜ ♀

O43.119 Circumvallate placenta, **unspecified trimester**   Ⓜ ♀ ▽

√6ᵗʰ **O43.12** **Velamentous insertion of umbilical cord**

O43.121 Velamentous insertion of umbilical cord, **first trimester**   Ⓜ ♀

O43.122 Velamentous insertion of umbilical cord, **second trimester**   Ⓜ ♀

O43.123 Velamentous insertion of umbilical cord, **third trimester**   Ⓜ ♀

O43.129 Velamentous insertion of umbilical cord, **unspecified trimester**   Ⓜ ♀ ▽

√6ᵗʰ **O43.19** **Other malformation of placenta**

O43.191 Other malformation of placenta, **first trimester**   Ⓜ ♀

O43.192 Other malformation of placenta, **second trimester**   Ⓜ ♀

O43.193 Other malformation of placenta, **third trimester**   Ⓜ ♀

O43.199 Other malformation of placenta, **unspecified trimester**   Ⓜ ♀ ▽

√5ᵗʰ **O43.2** **Morbidly adherent placenta**

Code also associated third stage postpartum hemorrhage, if applicable (O72.0)

EXCLUDES 1   retained placenta (O73.-)

√6ᵗʰ **O43.21** **Placenta accreta**

DEF: Condition where the placenta adheres too deeply to the uterine wall; often associated with placenta previa.

O43.211 Placenta accreta, **first trimester**   Ⓜ ♀

O43.212 Placenta accreta, **second trimester**   Ⓜ ♀

O43.213 Placenta accreta, **third trimester**   Ⓜ ♀

O43.219 Placenta accreta, **unspecified trimester**   Ⓜ ♀ ▽

√6ᵗʰ **O43.22** **Placenta increta**

DEF: Condition where the placenta adheres too deeply to the uterine wall and penetrates the muscle; often associated with placenta previa.

O43.221 Placenta increta, **first trimester**   Ⓜ ♀

O43.222 Placenta increta, **second trimester**   Ⓜ ♀

O43.223 Placenta increta, **third trimester**   Ⓜ ♀

O43.229 Placenta increta, **unspecified trimester**   Ⓜ ♀ ▽

√6ᵗʰ **O43.23** **Placenta percreta**

DEF: Condition where the placenta attaches through the uterine muscle and may invade other organs, resulting in antenatal complications, premature delivery, retention of all or a portion of the placenta, or postpartum bleeding.

O43.231 Placenta percreta, **first trimester**   Ⓜ ♀

O43.232 Placenta percreta, **second trimester**   Ⓜ ♀

O43.233 Placenta percreta, **third trimester**   Ⓜ ♀

O43.239 Placenta percreta, **unspecified trimester**   Ⓜ ♀ ▽

√5ᵗʰ **O43.8** **Other placental disorders**

√6ᵗʰ **O43.81** **Placental infarction**

O43.811 Placental infarction, **first trimester**   Ⓜ ♀

O43.812 Placental infarction, **second trimester**   Ⓜ ♀

O43.813 Placental infarction, **third trimester**   Ⓜ ♀

O43.819 Placental infarction, **unspecified trimester**   Ⓜ ♀ ▽

√6ᵗʰ **O43.89** **Other placental disorders**

Placental dysfunction

O43.891 Other placental disorders, **first trimester**   Ⓜ ♀

O43.892 Other placental disorders, **second trimester**   Ⓜ ♀

O43.893 Other placental disorders, **third trimester**   Ⓜ ♀

O43.899 Other placental disorders, **unspecified trimester**   Ⓜ ♀ ▽

√5ᵗʰ **O43.9** **Unspecified placental disorder**

O43.90 Unspecified placental disorder, **unspecified trimester**   Ⓜ ♀ ▽

O43.91 Unspecified placental disorder, **first trimester**   Ⓜ ♀ ▽

O43.92 Unspecified placental disorder, **second trimester**   Ⓜ ♀ ▽

O43.93 Unspecified placental disorder, **third trimester**   Ⓜ ♀ ▽

√4ᵗʰ **O44** **Placenta previa**

AHA: 2016,4Q,52-53

DEF: Placenta implanted in the lower segment of the uterus, which commonly causes hemorrhage in the last trimester of pregnancy.

√5ᵗʰ **O44.0** **Complete placenta previa NOS or without hemorrhage**

Placenta previa NOS

O44.00 Complete placenta previa NOS or without hemorrhage, **unspecified trimester**   Ⓜ ♀ ▽

O44.01 Complete placenta previa NOS or without hemorrhage, **first trimester**   Ⓜ ♀

O44.02 Complete placenta previa NOS or without hemorrhage, **second trimester**   Ⓜ ♀

O44.03   **Complete placenta previa NOS or without hemorrhage, third trimester**   M ♀

✓5ᵗʰ **O44.1**   Complete **placenta previa** with hemorrhage

> EXCLUDES 1   *labor and delivery complicated by hemorrhage from vasa previa (O69.4)*

O44.10   **Complete placenta previa with hemorrhage, unspecified trimester**   M ♀ ▽

O44.11   **Complete placenta previa with hemorrhage, first trimester**   M ♀

O44.12   **Complete placenta previa with hemorrhage, second trimester**   M ♀

O44.13   **Complete placenta previa with hemorrhage, third trimester**   M ♀

✓5ᵗʰ **O44.2**   Partial **placenta previa** without hemorrhage

> Marginal placenta previa, NOS or without hemorrhage

O44.20   **Partial placenta previa NOS or without hemorrhage, unspecified trimester**   M ♀ ▽

O44.21   **Partial placenta previa NOS or without hemorrhage, first trimester**   M ♀

O44.22   **Partial placenta previa NOS or without hemorrhage, second trimester**   M ♀

O44.23   **Partial placenta previa NOS or without hemorrhage, third trimester**   M ♀

✓5ᵗʰ **O44.3**   Partial **placenta previa** with hemorrhage

> Marginal placenta previa with hemorrhage

O44.30   **Partial placenta previa with hemorrhage, unspecified trimester**   Q M ♀ ▽

O44.31   **Partial placenta previa with hemorrhage, first trimester**   Q M ♀

O44.32   **Partial placenta previa with hemorrhage, second trimester**   M ♀

O44.33   **Partial placenta previa with hemorrhage, third trimester**   M ♀

✓5ᵗʰ **O44.4**   Low lying **placenta NOS or** without hemorrhage

> Low implantation of placenta NOS or without hemorrhage

O44.40   **Low lying placenta NOS or without hemorrhage, unspecified trimester**   M ♀ ▽

O44.41   **Low lying placenta NOS or without hemorrhage, first trimester**   M ♀

O44.42   **Low lying placenta NOS or without hemorrhage, second trimester**   M ♀

O44.43   **Low lying placenta NOS or without hemorrhage, third trimester**   M ♀

✓5ᵗʰ **O44.5**   Low lying **placenta** with hemorrhage

> Low implantation of placenta with hemorrhage

O44.50   **Low lying placenta with hemorrhage, unspecified trimester**   Q M ♀ ▽

O44.51   **Low lying placenta with hemorrhage, first trimester**   Q M ♀

O44.52   **Low lying placenta with hemorrhage, second trimester**   M ♀

O44.53   **Low lying placenta with hemorrhage, third trimester**   M ♀

✓4ᵗʰ **O45**   **Premature separation of placenta [abruptio placentae]**

✓5ᵗʰ **O45.0**   Premature separation of placenta with coagulation defect

✓6ᵗʰ **O45.00**   **Premature separation of placenta with coagulation defect, unspecified**

O45.001   **Premature separation of placenta with coagulation defect, unspecified, first trimester**   Q M ♀ ▽

O45.002   **Premature separation of placenta with coagulation defect, unspecified, second trimester**   M ♀ ▽

O45.003   **Premature separation of placenta with coagulation defect, unspecified, third trimester**   M ♀ ▽

O45.009   **Premature separation of placenta with coagulation defect, unspecified, unspecified trimester**   Q M ♀ ▽

✓6ᵗʰ **O45.01**   **Premature separation of placenta with afibrinogenemia**

> Premature separation of placenta with hypofibrinogenemia

O45.011   **Premature separation of placenta with afibrinogenemia, first trimester**   Q M ♀

O45.012   **Premature separation of placenta with afibrinogenemia, second trimester**   M ♀

O45.013   **Premature separation of placenta with afibrinogenemia, third trimester**   M ♀

O45.019   **Premature separation of placenta with afibrinogenemia, unspecified trimester**   Q M ♀ ▽

✓6ᵗʰ **O45.02**   **Premature separation of placenta with disseminated intravascular coagulation**

O45.021   **Premature separation of placenta with disseminated intravascular coagulation, first trimester**   Q M ♀

O45.022   **Premature separation of placenta with disseminated intravascular coagulation, second trimester**   M ♀

O45.023   **Premature separation of placenta with disseminated intravascular coagulation, third trimester**   M ♀

O45.029   **Premature separation of placenta with disseminated intravascular coagulation, unspecified trimester**   Q M ♀ ▽

✓6ᵗʰ **O45.09**   **Premature separation of placenta with other coagulation defect**

O45.091   **Premature separation of placenta with other coagulation defect, first trimester**   Q M ♀

O45.092   **Premature separation of placenta with other coagulation defect, second trimester**   M ♀

O45.093   **Premature separation of placenta with other coagulation defect, third trimester**   M ♀

O45.099   **Premature separation of placenta with other coagulation defect, unspecified trimester**   Q M ♀ ▽

✓5ᵗʰ **O45.8**   Other premature separation of placenta

✓6ᵗʰ **O45.8X**   **Other premature separation of placenta**

O45.8X1   **Other premature separation of placenta, first trimester**   Q M ♀

O45.8X2   **Other premature separation of placenta, second trimester**   M ♀

O45.8X3   **Other premature separation of placenta, third trimester**   M ♀

O45.8X9   **Other premature separation of placenta, unspecified trimester**   Q M ♀ ▽

✓5ᵗʰ **O45.9**   Premature separation of placenta, unspecified

> Abruptio placentae NOS

O45.90   **Premature separation of placenta, unspecified, unspecified trimester**   Q M ♀ ▽

O45.91   **Premature separation of placenta, unspecified, first trimester**   Q M ♀ ▽

O45.92   **Premature separation of placenta, unspecified, second trimester**   M ♀ ▽

O45.93   **Premature separation of placenta, unspecified, third trimester**   M ♀ ▽

✓4ᵗʰ **O46**   **Antepartum hemorrhage, not elsewhere classified**

> EXCLUDES 1   *hemorrhage in early pregnancy (O20.-)*
> *intrapartum hemorrhage NEC (O67.-)*
> *placenta previa (O44.-)*
> *premature separation of placenta [abruptio placentae] (O45.-)*

DEF: Uterine hemorrhage prior to delivery that is not related to placenta previa or abruptio placentae.

✓5ᵗʰ **O46.0**   Antepartum hemorrhage with coagulation defect

✓6ᵗʰ **O46.00**   **Antepartum hemorrhage with coagulation defect, unspecified**

O46.001   **Antepartum hemorrhage with coagulation defect, unspecified, first trimester**   Q M ♀ ▽

O46.002   **Antepartum hemorrhage with coagulation defect, unspecified, second trimester**   M ♀ ▽

O46.003   **Antepartum hemorrhage with coagulation defect, unspecified, third trimester**   M ♀ ▽

Chapter 15. Pregnancy, Childbirth and the Puerperium

O46.009 **Antepartum hemorrhage with** 🆄 Ⓜ ♀ ▽
    coagulation defect, unspecified,
    unspecified trimester

√6ᵗʰ **O46.01** **Antepartum hemorrhage** with afibrinogenemia
    Antepartum hemorrhage with hypofibrinogenemia

  O46.011 **Antepartum hemorrhage with** 🆄 Ⓜ ♀
      afibrinogenemia, first trimester

  O46.012 **Antepartum hemorrhage with** Ⓜ ♀
      afibrinogenemia, second
      trimester

  O46.013 **Antepartum hemorrhage with** Ⓜ ♀
      afibrinogenemia, third
      trimester

  O46.019 **Antepartum hemorrhage with** 🆄 Ⓜ ♀ ▽
      afibrinogenemia, unspecified
      trimester

√6ᵗʰ **O46.02** **Antepartum hemorrhage** with disseminated intravascular coagulation

  O46.021 **Antepartum hemorrhage with** 🆄 Ⓜ ♀
      disseminated intravascular
      coagulation, first trimester

  O46.022 **Antepartum hemorrhage with** Ⓜ ♀
      disseminated intravascular
      coagulation, second trimester

  O46.023 **Antepartum hemorrhage with** Ⓜ ♀
      disseminated intravascular
      coagulation, third trimester

  O46.029 **Antepartum hemorrhage with** 🆄 Ⓜ ♀ ▽
      disseminated intravascular
      coagulation, unspecified
      trimester

√6ᵗʰ **O46.09** **Antepartum hemorrhage with** other coagulation defect

  O46.091 **Antepartum hemorrhage with** 🆄 Ⓜ ♀
      other coagulation defect, first
      trimester

  O46.092 **Antepartum hemorrhage with** Ⓜ ♀
      other coagulation defect,
      second trimester

  O46.093 **Antepartum hemorrhage with** Ⓜ ♀
      other coagulation defect, third
      trimester

  O46.099 **Antepartum hemorrhage with** 🆄 Ⓜ ♀ ▽
      other coagulation defect,
      unspecified trimester

√5ᵗʰ **O46.8** **Other antepartum hemorrhage**

  √6ᵗʰ **O46.8X** **Other antepartum hemorrhage**

    O46.8X1 **Other antepartum hemorrhage,** 🆄 Ⓜ ♀
        first trimester

    O46.8X2 **Other antepartum hemorrhage,** Ⓜ ♀
        second trimester

    O46.8X3 **Other antepartum hemorrhage,** Ⓜ ♀
        third trimester

    O46.8X9 **Other antepartum hemorrhage,** 🆄 Ⓜ ♀ ▽
        unspecified trimester

√5ᵗʰ **O46.9** **Antepartum hemorrhage, unspecified**

  O46.90 **Antepartum hemorrhage, unspecified,** 🆄 Ⓜ ♀ ▽
      unspecified trimester

  O46.91 **Antepartum hemorrhage, unspecified,** 🆄 Ⓜ ♀ ▽
      first trimester

  O46.92 **Antepartum hemorrhage, unspecified,** Ⓜ ♀ ▽
      second trimester

  O46.93 **Antepartum hemorrhage, unspecified,** Ⓜ ♀ ▽
      third trimester

√4ᵗʰ **O47** **False labor**

  INCLUDES Braxton Hicks contractions
      threatened labor
  EXCLUDES 1 preterm labor (O60.-)

  √5ᵗʰ **O47.0** **False labor** before 37 completed weeks of gestation

    O47.00 **False labor before 37 completed weeks of** Ⓜ ♀ ▽
        gestation, unspecified trimester

    O47.02 **False labor before 37 completed weeks of** Ⓜ ♀
        gestation, second trimester

    O47.03 **False labor before 37 completed weeks of** Ⓜ ♀
        gestation, third trimester

  O47.1 **False labor at or after 37 completed weeks of** Ⓜ ♀
      gestation

  O47.9 **False labor, unspecified** Ⓜ ♀ ▽

√4ᵗʰ **O48** **Late pregnancy**

  O48.0 **Post-term pregnancy** Ⓜ ♀
      Pregnancy over 40 completed weeks to 42 completed weeks
      gestation

  O48.1 **Prolonged pregnancy** Ⓜ ♀
      Pregnancy which has advanced beyond 42 completed weeks
      gestation
      AHA: 2016,1Q,5

Complications of labor and delivery (O60-O77)

√4ᵗʰ **O60** **Preterm labor**

  INCLUDES onset (spontaneous) of labor before 37 completed weeks
      of gestation
  EXCLUDES 1 false labor (O47.0-)
      threatened labor NOS (O47.0-)

  √5ᵗʰ **O60.0** **Preterm labor** without delivery

    O60.00 **Preterm labor without delivery,** Ⓜ ♀ ▽
        unspecified trimester

    O60.02 **Preterm labor without delivery,** second Ⓜ ♀
        trimester

    O60.03 **Preterm labor without delivery,** third Ⓜ ♀
        trimester

  √5ᵗʰ **O60.1** **Preterm labor** with preterm delivery

    AHA: 2016,2Q,10

    One of the following 7th characters is to be assigned to each
    code under subcategory O60.1. 7th character 0 is for single
    gestations and multiple gestations where the fetus is
    unspecified. 7th characters 1 through 9 are for cases of
    multiple gestations to identify the fetus for which the code
    applies. The appropriate code from category O30, Multiple
    gestation, must also be assigned when assigning a code from
    subcategory O60.1 that has a 7th character of 1 through 9.
    0   not applicable or unspecified
    1   fetus 1
    2   fetus 2
    3   fetus 3
    4   fetus 4
    5   fetus 5
    9   other fetus

    √x7ᵗʰ **O60.10** **Preterm labor with preterm delivery,** Ⓜ ♀ ▽
        unspecified trimester
        Preterm labor with delivery NOS

    √x7ᵗʰ **O60.12** **Preterm labor** second trimester **with** Ⓜ ♀
        preterm delivery second trimester

    √x7ᵗʰ **O60.13** **Preterm labor** second trimester **with** Ⓜ ♀
        preterm delivery third trimester

    √x7ᵗʰ **O60.14** **Preterm labor** third trimester **with** Ⓜ ♀
        preterm delivery third trimester

  √5ᵗʰ **O60.2** **Term delivery with preterm labor**

    One of the following 7th characters is to be assigned to each
    code under subcategory O60.2. 7th character 0 is for single
    gestations and multiple gestations where the fetus is
    unspecified. 7th characters 1 through 9 are for cases of
    multiple gestations to identify the fetus for which the code
    applies. The appropriate code from category O30, Multiple
    gestation, must also be assigned when assigning a code from
    subcategory O60.2 that has a 7th character of 1 through 9.
    0   not applicable or unspecified
    1   fetus 1
    2   fetus 2
    3   fetus 3
    4   fetus 4
    5   fetus 5
    9   other fetus

    √x7ᵗʰ **O60.20** **Term delivery with preterm labor,** Ⓜ ♀ ▽
        unspecified trimester

    √x7ᵗʰ **O60.22** **Term delivery with preterm labor,** second Ⓜ ♀
        trimester

    √x7ᵗʰ **O60.23** **Term delivery with preterm labor,** third Ⓜ ♀
        trimester

√4ᵗʰ **O61** **Failed induction of labor**

  O61.0 **Failed** medical **induction of labor** Ⓜ ♀
      Failed induction (of labor) by oxytocin
      Failed induction (of labor) by prostaglandins

O61.1 Failed instrumental induction of labor   Ⓜ ♀
  Failed mechanical induction (of labor)
  Failed surgical induction (of labor)

O61.8 Other failed induction of labor   Ⓜ ♀

O61.9 Failed induction of labor, unspecified   Ⓜ ♀ ▽

√4ᵗʰ **O62 Abnormalities of forces of labor**
  DEF: Uterine inertia: Weak or poorly coordinated contractions of the uterus during labor.

  O62.0 Primary inadequate contractions   Ⓜ ♀
    Failure of cervical dilatation
    Primary hypotonic uterine dysfunction
    Uterine inertia during latent phase of labor

  O62.1 Secondary uterine inertia   Ⓜ ♀
    Arrested active phase of labor
    Secondary hypotonic uterine dysfunction

  O62.2 Other uterine inertia   Ⓜ ♀
    Atony of uterus without hemorrhage
    Atony of uterus NOS
    Desultory labor
    Hypotonic uterine dysfunction NOS
    Irregular labor
    Poor contractions
    Slow slope active phase of labor
    Uterine inertia NOS
    EXCLUDES 1   *atony of uterus with hemorrhage (postpartum) (O72.1)*
              postpartum atony of uterus without hemorrhage (O75.89)
    DEF: Uterine atony: Failure of the uterine muscles to contract after the fetus and placenta are delivered.

  O62.3 Precipitate labor   Ⓜ ♀
    DEF: Rapid labor with delivery occurring in three hours or less from the onset of contractions.

  O62.4 Hypertonic, incoordinate, and prolonged uterine   Ⓜ ♀
    contractions
    Cervical spasm
    Contraction ring dystocia
    Dyscoordinate labor
    Hour-glass contraction of uterus
    Hypertonic uterine dysfunction
    Incoordinate uterine action
    Tetanic contractions
    Uterine dystocia NOS
    Uterine spasm
    EXCLUDES 1   *dystocia (fetal) (maternal) NOS (O66.9)*

  O62.8 Other abnormalities of forces of labor   Ⓜ ♀
  O62.9 Abnormality of forces of labor, unspecified   Ⓜ ♀ ▽

√4ᵗʰ **O63 Long labor**

  O63.0 Prolonged first stage (of labor)   Ⓜ ♀
  O63.1 Prolonged second stage (of labor)   Ⓜ ♀
  O63.2 Delayed delivery of second twin, triplet, etc.   Ⓜ ♀
  O63.9 Long labor, unspecified   Ⓜ ♀ ▽
    Prolonged labor NOS

√4ᵗʰ **O64 Obstructed labor due to malposition and malpresentation of fetus**

One of the following 7th characters is to be assigned to each code under category O64. 7th character Ø is for single gestations and multiple gestations where the fetus is unspecified. 7th characters 1 through 9 are for cases of multiple gestations to identify the fetus for which the code applies. The appropriate code from category O30, Multiple gestation, must also be assigned when assigning a code from category O64 that has a 7th character of 1 through 9.

Ø   not applicable or unspecified
1   fetus 1
2   fetus 2
3   fetus 3
4   fetus 4
5   fetus 5
9   other fetus

Fetal Malposition

Breech

Shoulder
(arm prolapse)

Mother's pelvis

Compound
(extremity together with head)

Face
(mentum)

Oblique

√x7ᵗʰ **O64.0 Obstructed labor due to incomplete rotation of fetal**   Ⓜ ♀
    head
    Deep transverse arrest
    Obstructed labor due to persistent occipitoiliac (position)
    Obstructed labor due to persistent occipitoposterior (position)
    Obstructed labor due to persistent occipitosacral (position)
    Obstructed labor due to persistent occipitotransverse (position)

√x7ᵗʰ **O64.1 Obstructed labor due to breech presentation**   Ⓜ ♀
    Obstructed labor due to buttocks presentation
    Obstructed labor due to complete breech presentation
    Obstructed labor due to frank breech presentation

√x7ᵗʰ **O64.2 Obstructed labor due to face presentation**   Ⓜ ♀
    Obstructed labor due to chin presentation

√x7ᵗʰ **O64.3 Obstructed labor due to brow presentation**   Ⓜ ♀

√x7ᵗʰ **O64.4 Obstructed labor due to shoulder presentation**   Ⓜ ♀
    Prolapsed arm
    EXCLUDES 1   *impacted shoulders (O66.0)*
              shoulder dystocia (O66.0)

√x7ᵗʰ **O64.5 Obstructed labor due to compound presentation**   Ⓜ ♀

√x7ᵗʰ **O64.8 Obstructed labor due to other malposition and**   Ⓜ ♀
    malpresentation
    Obstructed labor due to footling presentation
    Obstructed labor due to incomplete breech presentation

√x7ᵗʰ **O64.9 Obstructed labor due to malposition and**   Ⓜ ♀ ▽
    malpresentation, unspecified

√4ᵗʰ **O65 Obstructed labor due to maternal pelvic abnormality**

  O65.0 Obstructed labor due to deformed pelvis   Ⓜ ♀
  O65.1 Obstructed labor due to generally contracted pelvis   Ⓜ ♀
  O65.2 Obstructed labor due to pelvic inlet contraction   Ⓜ ♀
  O65.3 Obstructed labor due to pelvic outlet and   Ⓜ ♀
    mid-cavity contraction
  O65.4 Obstructed labor due to fetopelvic disproportion,   Ⓜ ♀ ▽
    unspecified
    EXCLUDES 1   *dystocia due to abnormality of fetus (O66.2-O66.3)*
  O65.5 Obstructed labor due to abnormality of maternal   Ⓜ ♀
    pelvic organs
    Obstructed labor due to conditions listed in O34.-
    Use additional code to identify abnormality of pelvic organs O34.-

O65.8 **Obstructed labor due to other maternal pelvic abnormalities**   Ⓜ ♀

O65.9 **Obstructed labor due to maternal pelvic abnormality, unspecified**   Ⓜ ♀ ▽

✓4ᵗʰ O66 Other obstructed labor

O66.0 **Obstructed labor due to shoulder dystocia**   Ⓜ ♀
Impacted shoulders
DEF: Obstructed labor due to impacted fetal shoulders. It is an emergency condition that may require cesarean section, forceps delivery, vacuum extraction, or symphysiotomy.

O66.1 **Obstructed labor due to locked twins**   Ⓜ ♀

O66.2 **Obstructed labor due to unusually large fetus**   Ⓜ ♀

O66.3 **Obstructed labor due to other abnormalities of fetus**   Ⓜ ♀
Dystocia due to fetal ascites
Dystocia due to fetal hydrops
Dystocia due to fetal meningomyelocele
Dystocia due to fetal sacral teratoma
Dystocia due to fetal tumor
Dystocia due to hydrocephalic fetus
Use additional code to identify cause of obstruction

✓5ᵗʰ O66.4 Failed trial of labor

O66.40 **Failed trial of labor, unspecified**   Ⓜ ♀ ▽

O66.41 **Failed attempted vaginal birth after previous cesarean delivery**   Ⓜ ♀
Code first rupture of uterus, if applicable (O71.0-, O71.1)

O66.5 **Attempted application of vacuum extractor and forceps**   Ⓜ ♀
Attempted application of vacuum or forceps, with subsequent delivery by forceps or cesarean delivery

O66.6 **Obstructed labor due to other multiple fetuses**   Ⓜ ♀

O66.8 **Other specified obstructed labor**   Ⓜ ♀
Use additional code to identify cause of obstruction

O66.9 **Obstructed labor, unspecified**   Ⓜ ♀ ▽
Dystocia NOS
Fetal dystocia NOS
Maternal dystocia NOS

✓4ᵗʰ O67 Labor and delivery complicated by intrapartum hemorrhage, not elsewhere classified

EXCLUDES 1   antepartum hemorrhage NEC (O46.-)
    placenta previa (O44.-)
    premature separation of placenta [abruptio placentae] (O45.-)
EXCLUDES 2   postpartum hemorrhage (O72.-)

O67.0 **Intrapartum hemorrhage with coagulation defect**   Ⓜ ♀
Intrapartum hemorrhage (excessive) associated with afibrinogenemia
Intrapartum hemorrhage (excessive) associated with disseminated intravascular coagulation
Intrapartum hemorrhage (excessive) associated with hyperfibrinolysis
Intrapartum hemorrhage (excessive) associated with hypofibrinogenemia

O67.8 **Other intrapartum hemorrhage**   Ⓜ ♀
Excessive intrapartum hemorrhage

O67.9 **Intrapartum hemorrhage, unspecified**   Ⓜ ♀ ▽

O68 **Labor and delivery complicated by abnormality of fetal acid-base balance**   Ⓜ ♀
Fetal acidemia complicating labor and delivery
Fetal acidosis complicating labor and delivery
Fetal alkalosis complicating labor and delivery
Fetal metabolic acidemia complicating labor and delivery
EXCLUDES 1   fetal stress NOS (O77.9)
    labor and delivery complicated by electrocardiographic evidence of fetal stress (O77.8)
    labor and delivery complicated by ultrasonic evidence of fetal stress (O77.8)
EXCLUDES 2   abnormality in fetal heart rate or rhythm (O76)
    labor and delivery complicated by meconium in amniotic fluid (O77.0)

✓4ᵗʰ O69 Labor and delivery complicated by umbilical cord complications

AHA: 2016,1Q,5

One of the following 7th characters is to be assigned to each code under category O69. 7th character 0 is for single gestations and multiple gestations where the fetus is unspecified. 7th characters 1 through 9 are for cases of multiple gestations to identify the fetus for which the code applies. The appropriate code from category O30, Multiple gestation, must also be assigned when assigning a code from category O69 that has a 7th character of 1 through 9.
0   not applicable or unspecified
1   fetus 1
2   fetus 2
3   fetus 3
4   fetus 4
5   fetus 5
9   other fetus

✓x7ᵗʰ **O69.0** **Labor and delivery complicated by prolapse of cord**   Ⓜ ♀
DEF: Abnormal presentation of the fetus marked by a protruding umbilical cord during labor. It can cause fetal death.

✓x7ᵗʰ **O69.1** **Labor and delivery complicated by cord around neck, with compression**   Ⓜ ♀
EXCLUDES 1   labor and delivery complicated by cord around neck, without compression (O69.81)

✓x7ᵗʰ **O69.2** **Labor and delivery complicated by other cord entanglement, with compression**   Ⓜ ♀
Labor and delivery complicated by compression of cord NOS
Labor and delivery complicated by entanglement of cords of twins in monoamniotic sac
Labor and delivery complicated by knot in cord
EXCLUDES 1   labor and delivery complicated by other cord entanglement, without compression (O69.82)

✓x7ᵗʰ **O69.3** **Labor and delivery complicated by short cord**   Ⓜ ♀

✓x7ᵗʰ **O69.4** **Labor and delivery complicated by vasa previa**   Ⓜ ♀
Labor and delivery complicated by hemorrhage from vasa previa

✓x7ᵗʰ **O69.5** **Labor and delivery complicated by vascular lesion of cord**   Ⓜ ♀
Labor and delivery complicated by cord bruising
Labor and delivery complicated by cord hematoma
Labor and delivery complicated by thrombosis of umbilical vessels

✓5ᵗʰ O69.8 Labor and delivery complicated by other cord complications

✓x7ᵗʰ **O69.81** **Labor and delivery complicated by cord around neck, without compression**   Ⓜ ♀
AHA: 2016,1Q,5

✓x7ᵗʰ **O69.82** **Labor and delivery complicated by other cord entanglement, without compression**   Ⓜ ♀

✓x7ᵗʰ **O69.89** **Labor and delivery complicated by other cord complications**   Ⓜ ♀

✓x7ᵗʰ **O69.9** **Labor and delivery complicated by cord complication, unspecified**   Ⓜ ♀ ▽

✓4ᵗʰ O70 Perineal laceration during delivery

INCLUDES   episiotomy extended by laceration
EXCLUDES 1   obstetric high vaginal laceration alone (O71.4)
AHA: 2016,2Q,34; 2016,1Q,3-4,5

O70.0 **First degree perineal laceration during delivery**   Ⓜ ♀
Perineal laceration, rupture or tear involving fourchette during delivery
Perineal laceration, rupture or tear involving labia during delivery
Perineal laceration, rupture or tear involving skin during delivery
Perineal laceration, rupture or tear involving vagina during delivery
Perineal laceration, rupture or tear involving vulva during delivery
Slight perineal laceration, rupture or tear during delivery

O70.1 **Second degree perineal laceration during delivery**   Ⓜ ♀
Perineal laceration, rupture or tear during delivery as in O70.0, also involving pelvic floor
Perineal laceration, rupture or tear during delivery as in O70.0, also involving perineal muscles
Perineal laceration, rupture or tear during delivery as in O70.0, also involving vaginal muscles
EXCLUDES 1   perineal laceration involving anal sphincter (O70.2)

✓5ᵗʰ **O70.2 Third degree perineal laceration during delivery**

Perineal laceration, rupture or tear during delivery as in O70.1, also involving anal sphincter

Perineal laceration, rupture or tear during delivery as in O70.1, also involving rectovaginal septum

Perineal laceration, rupture or tear during delivery as in O70.1, also involving sphincter NOS

> EXCLUDES 1   anal sphincter tear during delivery without third degree perineal laceration (O70.4)
> perineal laceration involving anal or rectal mucosa (O70.3)

AHA: 2016,4Q,53-54

O70.20 Third degree perineal laceration during delivery, unspecified Ⓜ ♀ ▽

O70.21 Third degree perineal laceration during delivery, IIIa Ⓜ ♀

Third degree perineal laceration during delivery with less than 50% of external anal sphincter (EAS) thickness torn

O70.22 Third degree perineal laceration during delivery, IIIb Ⓜ ♀

Third degree perineal laceration during delivery with more than 50% external anal sphincter (EAS) thickness torn

O70.23 Third degree perineal laceration during delivery, IIIc Ⓜ ♀

Third degree perineal laceration during delivery with both external anal sphincter (EAS) and internal anal sphincter (IAS) torn

O70.3 Fourth degree perineal laceration during delivery Ⓜ ♀

Perineal laceration, rupture or tear during delivery as in O70.2, also involving anal mucosa

Perineal laceration, rupture or tear during delivery as in O70.2, also involving rectal mucosa

O70.4 Anal sphincter tear complicating delivery, not associated with third degree laceration Ⓜ ♀

> EXCLUDES 1   anal sphincter tear with third degree perineal laceration (O70.2)

O70.9 Perineal laceration during delivery, unspecified Ⓜ ♀ ▽

✓4ᵗʰ **O71 Other obstetric trauma**

> INCLUDES   obstetric damage from instruments

✓5ᵗʰ **O71.0 Rupture of uterus (spontaneous) before onset of labor**

> EXCLUDES 1   disruption of (current) cesarean delivery wound (O90.0)
> laceration of uterus, NEC (O71.81)

O71.00 Rupture of uterus before onset of labor, unspecified trimester Ⓜ ♀ ▽

O71.02 Rupture of uterus before onset of labor, second trimester Ⓜ ♀

O71.03 Rupture of uterus before onset of labor, third trimester Ⓜ ♀

O71.1 Rupture of uterus during labor Ⓜ ♀

Rupture of uterus not stated as occurring before onset of labor

> EXCLUDES 1   disruption of cesarean delivery wound (O90.0)
> laceration of uterus, NEC (O71.81)

O71.2 Postpartum inversion of uterus Ⓜ ♀

O71.3 Obstetric laceration of cervix Ⓜ ♀

Annular detachment of cervix

O71.4 Obstetric high vaginal laceration alone Ⓜ ♀

Laceration of vaginal wall without perineal laceration

> EXCLUDES 1   obstetric high vaginal laceration with perineal laceration (O70.-)

AHA: 2016,1Q,5

O71.5 Other obstetric injury to pelvic organs Ⓜ ♀

Obstetric injury to bladder

Obstetric injury to urethra

> EXCLUDES 2   obstetric periurethral trauma (O71.82)

AHA: 2014,4Q,18

O71.6 Obstetric damage to pelvic joints and ligaments Ⓜ ♀

Obstetric avulsion of inner symphyseal cartilage

Obstetric damage to coccyx

Obstetric traumatic separation of symphysis (pubis)

O71.7 Obstetric hematoma of pelvis Ⓜ ♀

Obstetric hematoma of perineum

Obstetric hematoma of vagina

Obstetric hematoma of vulva

✓5ᵗʰ **O71.8 Other specified obstetric trauma**

O71.81 Laceration of uterus, not elsewhere classified Ⓜ ♀

O71.82 Other specified trauma to perineum and vulva Ⓜ ♀

Obstetric periurethral trauma

AHA: 2016,1Q,4; 2014,4Q,18

O71.89 Other specified obstetric trauma Ⓜ ♀

O71.9 Obstetric trauma, unspecified Ⓜ ♀ ▽

✓4ᵗʰ **O72 Postpartum hemorrhage**

> INCLUDES   hemorrhage after delivery of fetus or infant

O72.0 Third-stage hemorrhage Ⓜ ♀

Hemorrhage associated with retained, trapped or adherent placenta

Retained placenta NOS

Code also type of adherent placenta (O43.2-)

O72.1 Other immediate postpartum hemorrhage Ⓜ ♀

Hemorrhage following delivery of placenta

Postpartum hemorrhage (atonic) NOS

Uterine atony with hemorrhage

> EXCLUDES 1   uterine atony NOS (O62.2)
> uterine atony without hemorrhage (O62.2)
> postpartum atony of uterus without hemorrhage (O75.89)

AHA: 2016,1Q,4

DEF: Uterine atony: Failure of the uterine muscles to contract after the fetus and placenta are delivered.

O72.2 Delayed and secondary postpartum hemorrhage Ⓜ ♀

Hemorrhage associated with retained portions of placenta or membranes after the first 24 hours following delivery of placenta

Retained products of conception NOS, following delivery

O72.3 Postpartum coagulation defects Ⓜ ♀

Postpartum afibrinogenemia

Postpartum fibrinolysis

✓4ᵗʰ **O73 Retained placenta and membranes, without hemorrhage**

> EXCLUDES 1   placenta accreta (O43.21-)
> placenta increta (O43.22-)
> placenta percreta (O43.23-)

DEF: Postpartum condition resulting from failure to expel placental membrane tissues due to failed contractions of the uterine wall.

O73.0 Retained placenta without hemorrhage Ⓜ ♀

Adherent placenta, without hemorrhage

Trapped placenta without hemorrhage

O73.1 Retained portions of placenta and membranes, without hemorrhage Ⓜ ♀

Retained products of conception following delivery, without hemorrhage

✓4ᵗʰ **O74 Complications of anesthesia during labor and delivery**

> INCLUDES   maternal complications arising from the administration of a general, regional or local anesthetic, analgesic or other sedation during labor and delivery

Use additional code, if applicable, to identify specific complication

O74.0 Aspiration pneumonitis due to anesthesia during labor and delivery Ⓜ ♀

Inhalation of stomach contents or secretions NOS due to anesthesia during labor and delivery

Mendelson's syndrome due to anesthesia during labor and delivery

O74.1 Other pulmonary complications of anesthesia during labor and delivery Ⓜ ♀

O74.2 Cardiac complications of anesthesia during labor and delivery Ⓜ ♀

O74.3 Central nervous system complications of anesthesia during labor and delivery Ⓜ ♀

O74.4 Toxic reaction to local anesthesia during labor and delivery Ⓜ ♀

O74.5 Spinal and epidural anesthesia-induced headache during labor and delivery Ⓜ ♀

O74.6 Other complications of spinal and epidural anesthesia during labor and delivery Ⓜ ♀

O74.7 Failed or difficult intubation for anesthesia during labor and delivery Ⓜ ♀

O74.8 Other complications of anesthesia during labor and delivery Ⓜ ♀

O74.9 Complication of anesthesia during labor and delivery, unspecified Ⓜ ♀ ▽

☑ Additional Character Req   ✓x7ᵗʰ Placeholder Alert   Manifestation   ▽ Unspecified   ▶◀ Revised Text   ● New Code   ▲ Revised Code Title

ICD-10-CM 2019   877

Chapter 15. Pregnancy, Childbirth and the Puerperium

O75–O86.03

✓4ᵗʰ **O75 Other complications of labor and delivery, not elsewhere classified**

EXCLUDES 2   *puerperal (postpartum) infection (O86.-)*
        puerperal (postpartum) sepsis (O85)

O75.0 Maternal distress during labor and delivery   Ⓜ ♀

O75.1 Shock during or following labor and delivery   Ⓜ ♀
     Obstetric shock following labor and delivery

O75.2 Pyrexia during labor, not elsewhere classified   Ⓜ ♀

O75.3 Other infection during labor   Ⓜ ♀
     Sepsis during labor
     Use additional code (B95-B97), to identify infectious agent

O75.4 Other complications of obstetric surgery and procedures   Ⓜ ♀
     Cardiac arrest following obstetric surgery or procedures
     Cardiac failure following obstetric surgery or procedures
     Cerebral anoxia following obstetric surgery or procedures
     Pulmonary edema following obstetric surgery or procedures
     Use additional code to identify specific complication

EXCLUDES 2   *complications of anesthesia during labor and delivery (O74.-)*
        disruption of obstetrical (surgical) wound (O90.0-O90.1)
        hematoma of obstetrical (surgical) wound (O90.2)
        infection of obstetrical (surgical) wound ▶(O86.0-)◀

O75.5 Delayed delivery after artificial rupture of membranes   Ⓜ ♀

✓5ᵗʰ **O75.8 Other specified complications of labor and delivery**

   O75.81 Maternal exhaustion complicating labor and delivery   Ⓜ ♀

   O75.82 Onset (spontaneous) of labor after 37 completed weeks of gestation but before 39 completed weeks gestation, with delivery by (planned) cesarean section   Ⓜ ♀
     Delivery by (planned) cesarean section occurring after 37 completed weeks of gestation but before 39 completed weeks gestation due to (spontaneous) onset of labor
     Code first to specify reason for planned cesarean section such as:
       cephalopelvic disproportion (normally formed fetus) (O33.9)
       previous cesarean delivery (O34.21)

   O75.89 Other specified complications of labor and delivery   Ⓜ ♀

O75.9 Complication of labor and delivery, unspecified   Ⓜ ♀ ▽

O76 Abnormality in fetal heart rate and rhythm complicating labor and delivery   Ⓜ ♀
     Depressed fetal heart rate tones complicating labor and delivery
     Fetal bradycardia complicating labor and delivery
     Fetal heart rate decelerations complicating labor and delivery
     Fetal heart rate irregularity complicating labor and delivery
     Fetal heart rate abnormal variability complicating labor and delivery
     Fetal tachycardia complicating labor and delivery
     Non-reassuring fetal heart rate or rhythm complicating labor and delivery

EXCLUDES 1   *fetal stress NOS (O77.9)*
        labor and delivery complicated by electrocardiographic evidence of fetal stress (O77.8)
        labor and delivery complicated by ultrasonic evidence of fetal stress (O77.8)

EXCLUDES 2   *fetal metabolic acidemia (O68)*
        other fetal stress (O77.0-O77.1)

     AHA: 2013,4Q,118

✓4ᵗʰ **O77 Other fetal stress complicating labor and delivery**

O77.0 Labor and delivery complicated by meconium in amniotic fluid   Ⓜ ♀
     AHA: 2013,4Q,117-118

O77.1 Fetal stress in labor or delivery due to drug administration   Ⓜ ♀

O77.8 Labor and delivery complicated by other evidence of fetal stress   Ⓜ ♀
     Labor and delivery complicated by electrocardiographic evidence of fetal stress
     Labor and delivery complicated by ultrasonic evidence of fetal stress

EXCLUDES 1   *abnormality of fetal acid-base balance (O68)*
        abnormality in fetal heart rate or rhythm (O76)
        fetal metabolic acidemia (O68)

O77.9 Labor and delivery complicated by fetal stress, unspecified   Ⓜ ♀ ▽

EXCLUDES 1   *abnormality of fetal acid-base balance (O68)*
        abnormality in fetal heart rate or rhythm (O76)
        fetal metabolic acidemia (O68)

Encounter for delivery (O80-O82)

O80 Encounter for full-term uncomplicated delivery   Ⓜ ♀

NOTE   Delivery requiring minimal or no assistance, with or without episiotomy, without fetal manipulation [e.g., rotation version] or instrumentation [forceps] of a spontaneous, cephalic, vaginal, full-term, single, live-born infant. This code is for use as a single diagnosis code and is not to be used with any other code from chapter 15.

     Use additional code to indicate outcome of delivery (Z37.0)
     AHA: 2016,4Q,150; 2014,2Q,9

O82 Encounter for cesarean delivery without indication   Ⓜ ♀
     Use additional code to indicate outcome of delivery (Z37.0)

Complications predominantly related to the puerperium (O85-O92)

EXCLUDES 2   *mental and behavioral disorders associated with the puerperium ▶(F53.-)◀*
        obstetrical tetanus (A34)
        puerperal osteomalacia (M83.0)

O85 Puerperal sepsis   Ⓜ ♀
     Postpartum sepsis
     Puerperal peritonitis
     Puerperal pyemia
     Use additional code (B95-B97), to identify infectious agent
     Use additional code (R65.2-) to identify severe sepsis, if applicable

EXCLUDES 1   *fever of unknown origin following delivery (O86.4)*
        genital tract infection following delivery (O86.1-)
        obstetric pyemic and septic embolism (O88.3-)
        puerperal septic thrombophlebitis (O86.81)
        urinary tract infection following delivery (O86.2-)

EXCLUDES 2   *sepsis during labor (O75.3)*

✓4ᵗʰ **O86 Other puerperal infections**
     Use additional code (B95-B97), to identify infectious agent

EXCLUDES 2   *infection during labor (O75.3)*
        obstetrical tetanus (A34)

✓5ᵗʰ **O86.0 Infection of obstetric surgical wound**
     Infected cesarean delivery wound following delivery
     Infected perineal repair following delivery

EXCLUDES 1   *▶complications of procedures, not elsewhere classified (T81.4-)◀*
        ▶postprocedural fever NOS (R50.82)◀
        ▶postprocedural retroperitoneal abscess (K68.11)◀

●   **O86.00 Infection of obstetric surgical wound, unspecified**   ▽

●   **O86.01 Infection of obstetric surgical wound, superficial incisional site**
     Subcutaneous abscess following an obstetrical procedure
     Stitch abscess following an obstetrical procedure

●   **O86.02 Infection of obstetric surgical wound, deep incisional site**
     Intramuscular abscess following an obstetrical procedure
     Sub-fascial abscess following a procedure

●   **O86.03 Infection of obstetric surgical wound, organ and space site**
     Intraabdominal abscess following an obstetrical procedure
     Subphrenic abscess following an obstetrical procedure

●   **O86.04** **Sepsis** following an obstetrical procedure
      Use additional code to identify the sepsis

●   **O86.09** **Infection** of obstetric surgical wound, other surgical site

√5ᵗʰ **O86.1** Other infection of genital tract following delivery

     O86.11 **Cervicitis** following delivery   Ⓜ ♀
     O86.12 **Endometritis** following delivery   Ⓜ ♀
     O86.13 **Vaginitis** following delivery   Ⓜ ♀
     O86.19 **Other infection** of genital tract following delivery   Ⓜ ♀

√5ᵗʰ **O86.2** Urinary tract infection following delivery

     O86.20 **Urinary tract infection** following delivery, unspecified   Ⓜ ♀ ▽
       Puerperal urinary tract infection NOS
     O86.21 **Infection of kidney** following delivery   Ⓜ ♀
     O86.22 **Infection of bladder** following delivery   Ⓜ ♀
       Infection of urethra following delivery
     O86.29 **Other** urinary tract infection following delivery   Ⓜ ♀

O86.4 **Pyrexia** of unknown origin following delivery   Ⓜ ♀
     Puerperal infection NOS following delivery
     Puerperal pyrexia NOS following delivery
     EXCLUDES 2   pyrexia during labor (O75.2)
     DEF: Fever of unknown origin experienced by the mother after childbirth.

√5ᵗʰ **O86.8** Other specified puerperal infections

     O86.81 **Puerperal** septic thrombophlebitis   Ⓜ ♀
     O86.89 **Other specified** puerperal infections   Ⓜ ♀

√4ᵗʰ **O87** Venous complications and hemorrhoids in the puerperium

     INCLUDES   venous complications in labor, delivery and the puerperium
     EXCLUDES 2   obstetric embolism (O88.-)
           puerperal septic thrombophlebitis (O86.81)
           venous complications in pregnancy (O22.-)

O87.0 **Superficial** thrombophlebitis in the puerperium   Ⓜ ♀
     Puerperal phlebitis NOS
     Puerperal thrombosis NOS

O87.1 **Deep phlebothrombosis** in the puerperium   Ⓜ ♀
     Deep vein thrombosis, postpartum
     Pelvic thrombophlebitis, postpartum
     Use additional code to identify the deep vein thrombosis (I82.4-, I82.5-, I82.62-, I82.72-)
     Use additional code, if applicable, for associated long-term (current) use of anticoagulants (Z79.01)

O87.2 **Hemorrhoids** in the puerperium   Ⓜ ♀

O87.3 **Cerebral venous thrombosis** in the puerperium   Ⓜ ♀
     Cerebrovenous sinus thrombosis in the puerperium

O87.4 **Varicose veins** of lower extremity in the puerperium   Ⓜ ♀

O87.8 **Other venous complications** in the puerperium   Ⓜ ♀
     Genital varices in the puerperium

O87.9 **Venous complication** in the puerperium, unspecified   Ⓜ ♀ ▽
     Puerperal phlebopathy NOS

√4ᵗʰ **O88** Obstetric embolism

     EXCLUDES 1   embolism complicating abortion NOS (O03.2)
           embolism complicating ectopic or molar pregnancy (O08.2)
           embolism complicating failed attempted abortion (O07.2)
           embolism complicating induced abortion (O04.7)
           embolism complicating spontaneous abortion (O03.2, O03.7)

√5ᵗʰ **O88.0** Obstetric air embolism

     DEF: Sudden blocking of the pulmonary artery or right ventricle with air or nitrogen bubbles.

   √6ᵗʰ **O88.01** Obstetric air embolism in pregnancy

       O88.011 **Air embolism** in pregnancy, first trimester   Ⓜ ♀
       O88.012 **Air embolism** in pregnancy, second trimester   Ⓜ ♀
       O88.013 **Air embolism** in pregnancy, third trimester   Ⓜ ♀
       O88.019 **Air embolism** in pregnancy, unspecified trimester   Ⓜ ♀ ▽

     O88.02 **Air embolism** in childbirth   Ⓜ ♀
     O88.03 **Air embolism** in the puerperium   Ⓜ ♀

√5ᵗʰ **O88.1** Amniotic fluid embolism
     Anaphylactoid syndrome in pregnancy

   √6ᵗʰ **O88.11** **Amniotic fluid embolism** in pregnancy

       O88.111 **Amniotic fluid embolism** in pregnancy, first trimester   Ⓜ ♀
       O88.112 **Amniotic fluid embolism** in pregnancy, second trimester   Ⓜ ♀
       O88.113 **Amniotic fluid embolism** in pregnancy, third trimester   Ⓜ ♀
       O88.119 **Amniotic fluid embolism** in pregnancy, unspecified trimester   Ⓜ ♀ ▽

     O88.12 **Amniotic fluid embolism** in childbirth   Ⓜ ♀
     O88.13 **Amniotic fluid embolism** in the puerperium   Ⓜ ♀

√5ᵗʰ **O88.2** Obstetric thromboembolism

   √6ᵗʰ **O88.21** **Thromboembolism** in pregnancy
       Obstetric (pulmonary) embolism NOS

       O88.211 **Thromboembolism** in pregnancy, first trimester   Ⓜ ♀
       O88.212 **Thromboembolism** in pregnancy, second trimester   Ⓜ ♀
       O88.213 **Thromboembolism** in pregnancy, third trimester   Ⓜ ♀
       O88.219 **Thromboembolism** in pregnancy, unspecified trimester   Ⓜ ♀ ▽

     O88.22 **Thromboembolism** in childbirth   Ⓜ ♀
     O88.23 **Thromboembolism** in the puerperium   Ⓜ ♀
       Puerperal (pulmonary) embolism NOS

√5ᵗʰ **O88.3** Obstetric pyemic and septic embolism

   √6ᵗʰ **O88.31** **Pyemic and septic embolism** in pregnancy

       O88.311 **Pyemic and septic embolism** in pregnancy, first trimester   Ⓜ ♀
       O88.312 **Pyemic and septic embolism** in pregnancy, second trimester   Ⓜ ♀
       O88.313 **Pyemic and septic embolism** in pregnancy, third trimester   Ⓜ ♀
       O88.319 **Pyemic and septic embolism** in pregnancy, unspecified trimester   Ⓜ ♀ ▽

     O88.32 **Pyemic and septic embolism** in childbirth   Ⓜ ♀
     O88.33 **Pyemic and septic embolism** in the puerperium   Ⓜ ♀

√5ᵗʰ **O88.8** Other obstetric embolism
     Obstetric fat embolism

   √6ᵗʰ **O88.81** **Other embolism** in pregnancy

       O88.811 **Other embolism** in pregnancy, first trimester   Ⓜ ♀
       O88.812 **Other embolism** in pregnancy, second trimester   Ⓜ ♀
       O88.813 **Other embolism** in pregnancy, third trimester   Ⓜ ♀
       O88.819 **Other embolism** in pregnancy, unspecified trimester   Ⓜ ♀ ▽

     O88.82 **Other embolism** in childbirth   Ⓜ ♀
     O88.83 **Other embolism** in the puerperium   Ⓜ ♀

√4ᵗʰ **O89** Complications of anesthesia during the puerperium

     INCLUDES   maternal complications arising from the administration of a general, regional or local anesthetic, analgesic or other sedation during the puerperium
     Use additional code, if applicable, to identify specific complication

√5ᵗʰ **O89.0** Pulmonary complications of anesthesia during the puerperium

     O89.01 **Aspiration pneumonitis** due to anesthesia during the puerperium   Ⓜ ♀
       Inhalation of stomach contents or secretions NOS due to anesthesia during the puerperium
       Mendelson's syndrome due to anesthesia during the puerperium

     O89.09 **Other pulmonary complications** of anesthesia during the puerperium   Ⓜ ♀

O89.1 **Cardiac complications** of anesthesia during the puerperium   Ⓜ ♀

O89.2 **Central nervous system complications** of anesthesia during the puerperium   Ⓜ ♀

O89.3 **Toxic reaction** to local anesthesia during the puerperium   Ⓜ ♀

✔ Additional Character Req   √x7ᵗʰ Placeholder Alert   **Manifestation**   ▽ Unspecified   ►◄ Revised Text   ● New Code   ▲ Revised Code Title

ICD-10-CM 2019   **879**

O86.04–O89.3

Chapter 15. Pregnancy, Childbirth and the Puerperium

O89.4 Spinal and epidural anesthesia-induced headache during the puerperium   M ♀

O89.5 Other complications of spinal and epidural anesthesia during the puerperium   M ♀

O89.6 Failed or difficult intubation for anesthesia during the puerperium   M ♀

O89.8 Other complications of anesthesia during the puerperium   M ♀

O89.9 Complication of anesthesia during the puerperium, unspecified   M ♀ ▽

✓4ᵗʰ **O90 Complications of the puerperium, not elsewhere classified**

O90.0 Disruption of cesarean delivery wound   M ♀
Dehiscence of cesarean delivery wound
    EXCLUDES 1   *rupture of uterus (spontaneous) before onset of labor (O71.0-)*
           rupture of uterus during labor (O71.1)

O90.1 Disruption of perineal obstetric wound   M ♀
Disruption of wound of episiotomy
Disruption of wound of perineal laceration
Secondary perineal tear

O90.2 Hematoma of obstetric wound   M ♀

O90.3 Peripartum cardiomyopathy   M ♀
Conditions in I42- arising during pregnancy and the puerperium
    EXCLUDES 1   *pre-existing heart disease complicating pregnancy and the puerperium (O99.4-)*
DEF: Any structural or functional abnormality of the ventricular myocardium. It is a noninflammatory disease of obscure or unknown etiology with onset during the postpartum period.

O90.4 Postpartum acute kidney failure   M ♀
Hepatorenal syndrome following labor and delivery

O90.5 Postpartum thyroiditis   M ♀

O90.6 Postpartum mood disturbance   Q M ♀
Postpartum blues
Postpartum dysphoria
Postpartum sadness
    EXCLUDES 1   *postpartum depression ▶(F53.0)◀*
           puerperal psychosis ▶(F53.1)◀

✓5ᵗʰ **O90.8** Other complications of the puerperium, not elsewhere classified

    O90.81 Anemia of the puerperium   M ♀
       Postpartum anemia NOS
         EXCLUDES 1   *pre-existing anemia complicating the puerperium (O99.03)*

    O90.89 Other complications of the puerperium, not elsewhere classified   M ♀
       Placental polyp

O90.9 Complication of the puerperium, unspecified   M ♀ ▽

✓4ᵗʰ **O91 Infections of breast associated with pregnancy, the puerperium and lactation**
Use additional code to identify infection

✓5ᵗʰ **O91.0** Infection of nipple associated with pregnancy, the puerperium and lactation

    ✓6ᵗʰ **O91.01** Infection of nipple associated with pregnancy   M ♀
       Gestational abscess of nipple
       O91.011 Infection of nipple associated with pregnancy, first trimester   M ♀
       O91.012 Infection of nipple associated with pregnancy, second trimester   M ♀
       O91.013 Infection of nipple associated with pregnancy, third trimester   M ♀
       O91.019 Infection of nipple associated with pregnancy, unspecified trimester   M ♀ ▽

    O91.02 Infection of nipple associated with the puerperium   M ♀
       Puerperal abscess of nipple

    O91.03 Infection of nipple associated with lactation   M ♀
       Abscess of nipple associated with lactation

✓5ᵗʰ **O91.1** Abscess of breast associated with pregnancy, the puerperium and lactation

    ✓6ᵗʰ **O91.11** Abscess of breast associated with pregnancy
       Gestational mammary abscess
       Gestational purulent mastitis
       Gestational subareolar abscess
       O91.111 Abscess of breast associated with pregnancy, first trimester   M ♀

       O91.112 Abscess of breast associated with pregnancy, second trimester   M ♀
       O91.113 Abscess of breast associated with pregnancy, third trimester   M ♀
       O91.119 Abscess of breast associated with pregnancy, unspecified trimester   M ♀ ▽

    O91.12 Abscess of breast associated with the puerperium   M ♀
       Puerperal mammary abscess
       Puerperal purulent mastitis
       Puerperal subareolar abscess

    O91.13 Abscess of breast associated with lactation   M ♀
       Mammary abscess associated with lactation
       Purulent mastitis associated with lactation
       Subareolar abscess associated with lactation

✓5ᵗʰ **O91.2** Nonpurulent mastitis associated with pregnancy, the puerperium and lactation

    ✓6ᵗʰ **O91.21** Nonpurulent mastitis associated with pregnancy
       Gestational interstitial mastitis
       Gestational lymphangitis of breast
       Gestational mastitis NOS
       Gestational parenchymatous mastitis
       O91.211 Nonpurulent mastitis associated with pregnancy, first trimester   M ♀
       O91.212 Nonpurulent mastitis associated with pregnancy, second trimester   M ♀
       O91.213 Nonpurulent mastitis associated with pregnancy, third trimester   M ♀
       O91.219 Nonpurulent mastitis associated with pregnancy, unspecified trimester   M ♀ ▽

    O91.22 Nonpurulent mastitis associated with the puerperium   M ♀
       Puerperal interstitial mastitis
       Puerperal lymphangitis of breast
       Puerperal mastitis NOS
       Puerperal parenchymatous mastitis

    O91.23 Nonpurulent mastitis associated with lactation   M ♀
       Interstitial mastitis associated with lactation
       Lymphangitis of breast associated with lactation
       Mastitis NOS associated with lactation
       Parenchymatous mastitis associated with lactation

✓4ᵗʰ **O92 Other disorders of breast and disorders of lactation associated with pregnancy and the puerperium**

✓5ᵗʰ **O92.0** Retracted nipple associated with pregnancy, the puerperium, and lactation

    ✓6ᵗʰ **O92.01** Retracted nipple associated with pregnancy
       O92.011 Retracted nipple associated with pregnancy, first trimester   M ♀
       O92.012 Retracted nipple associated with pregnancy, second trimester   M ♀
       O92.013 Retracted nipple associated with pregnancy, third trimester   M ♀
       O92.019 Retracted nipple associated with pregnancy, unspecified trimester   M ♀ ▽

    O92.02 Retracted nipple associated with the puerperium   M ♀

    O92.03 Retracted nipple associated with lactation   M ♀

✓5ᵗʰ **O92.1** Cracked nipple associated with pregnancy, the puerperium, and lactation
Fissure of nipple, gestational or puerperal

    ✓6ᵗʰ **O92.11** Cracked nipple associated with pregnancy
       O92.111 Cracked nipple associated with pregnancy, first trimester   M ♀
       O92.112 Cracked nipple associated with pregnancy, second trimester   M ♀
       O92.113 Cracked nipple associated with pregnancy, third trimester   M ♀
       O92.119 Cracked nipple associated with pregnancy, unspecified trimester   M ♀ ▽

    O92.12 Cracked nipple associated with the puerperium   M ♀

    O92.13 Cracked nipple associated with lactation   M ♀

√5ᵗʰ **O92.2 Other and unspecified disorders of breast associated with pregnancy and the puerperium**

     O92.20 **Unspecified disorder of breast associated with pregnancy and the puerperium** Ⓜ ♀ ▽

     O92.29 **Other disorders of breast associated with pregnancy and the puerperium** Ⓜ ♀

O92.3 Agalactia Ⓜ ♀

     Primary agalactia

     EXCLUDES 1   *elective agalactia (O92.5)*

               secondary agalactia (O92.5)

               therapeutic agalactia (O92.5)

     DEF: Absence of milk secretion in a female after delivery.

O92.4 Hypogalactia Ⓜ ♀

O92.5 Suppressed lactation Ⓜ ♀

     Elective agalactia

     Secondary agalactia

     Therapeutic agalactia

     EXCLUDES 1   *primary agalactia (O92.3)*

O92.6 Galactorrhea Ⓜ ♀

     DEF: Excessive or persistent milk secretion by the breast that may occur in the absence of nursing.

√5ᵗʰ **O92.7 Other and unspecified disorders of lactation**

     O92.70 **Unspecified disorders of lactation** Ⓜ ♀ ▽

     O92.79 **Other disorders of lactation** Ⓜ ♀

         Puerperal galactocele

Other obstetric conditions, not elsewhere classified (O94-O9A)

O94 Sequelae of complication of pregnancy, childbirth, and the puerperium Ⓜ ♀

     NOTE   This category is to be used to indicate conditions in O00-O77.-, O85-O94 and O98-O9A.- as the cause of late effects. The sequelae include conditions specified as such, or as late effects, which may occur at any time after the puerperium

     Code first condition resulting from (sequela) of complication of pregnancy, childbirth, and the puerperium

√4ᵗʰ **O98 Maternal infectious and parasitic diseases classifiable elsewhere but complicating pregnancy, childbirth and the puerperium**

     INCLUDES   the listed conditions when complicating the pregnant state, when aggravated by the pregnancy, or as a reason for obstetric care

     Use additional code (Chapter 1), to identify specific infectious or parasitic disease

     EXCLUDES 2   *herpes gestationis (O26.4-)*

               infectious carrier state (O99.82-, O99.83-)

               obstetrical tetanus (A34)

               puerperal infection (O86.-)

               puerperal sepsis (O85)

               when the reason for maternal care is that the disease is known or suspected to have affected the fetus (O35-O36)

√5ᵗʰ **O98.0 Tuberculosis complicating pregnancy, childbirth and the puerperium**

     Conditions in A15-A19

     √6ᵗʰ **O98.01** **Tuberculosis complicating pregnancy**

         O98.011 **Tuberculosis complicating pregnancy, first trimester** Ⓜ ♀

         O98.012 **Tuberculosis complicating pregnancy, second trimester** Ⓜ ♀

         O98.013 **Tuberculosis complicating pregnancy, third trimester** Ⓜ ♀

         O98.019 **Tuberculosis complicating pregnancy, unspecified trimester** Ⓜ ♀ ▽

     O98.02 **Tuberculosis complicating childbirth** Ⓜ ♀

     O98.03 **Tuberculosis complicating the puerperium** Ⓜ ♀

√5ᵗʰ **O98.1 Syphilis complicating pregnancy, childbirth and the puerperium**

     Conditions in A50-A53

     √6ᵗʰ **O98.11** **Syphilis complicating pregnancy**

         O98.111 **Syphilis complicating pregnancy, first trimester** Ⓜ ♀

         O98.112 **Syphilis complicating pregnancy, second trimester** Ⓜ ♀

         O98.113 **Syphilis complicating pregnancy, third trimester** Ⓜ ♀

         O98.119 **Syphilis complicating pregnancy, unspecified trimester** Ⓜ ♀ ▽

     O98.12 **Syphilis complicating childbirth** Ⓜ ♀

     O98.13 **Syphilis complicating the puerperium** Ⓜ ♀

√5ᵗʰ **O98.2 Gonorrhea complicating pregnancy, childbirth and the puerperium**

     Conditions in A54.-

     √6ᵗʰ **O98.21** **Gonorrhea complicating pregnancy**

         O98.211 **Gonorrhea complicating pregnancy, first trimester** Ⓜ ♀

         O98.212 **Gonorrhea complicating pregnancy, second trimester** Ⓜ ♀

         O98.213 **Gonorrhea complicating pregnancy, third trimester** Ⓜ ♀

         O98.219 **Gonorrhea complicating pregnancy, unspecified trimester** Ⓜ ♀ ▽

     O98.22 **Gonorrhea complicating childbirth** Ⓜ ♀

     O98.23 **Gonorrhea complicating the puerperium** Ⓜ ♀

√5ᵗʰ **O98.3 Other infections with a predominantly sexual mode of transmission complicating pregnancy, childbirth and the puerperium**

     Conditions in A55-A64

     √6ᵗʰ **O98.31** **Other infections with a predominantly sexual mode of transmission complicating pregnancy**

         O98.311 **Other infections with a predominantly sexual mode of transmission complicating pregnancy, first trimester** Ⓜ ♀

         O98.312 **Other infections with a predominantly sexual mode of transmission complicating pregnancy, second trimester** Ⓜ ♀

         O98.313 **Other infections with a predominantly sexual mode of transmission complicating pregnancy, third trimester** Ⓜ ♀

         O98.319 **Other infections with a predominantly sexual mode of transmission complicating pregnancy, unspecified trimester** Ⓜ ♀ ▽

     O98.32 **Other infections with a predominantly sexual mode of transmission complicating childbirth** Ⓜ ♀

     O98.33 **Other infections with a predominantly sexual mode of transmission complicating the puerperium** Ⓜ ♀

√5ᵗʰ **O98.4 Viral hepatitis complicating pregnancy, childbirth and the puerperium**

     Conditions in B15-B19

     √6ᵗʰ **O98.41** **Viral hepatitis complicating pregnancy**

         O98.411 **Viral hepatitis complicating pregnancy, first trimester** Ⓜ ♀

         O98.412 **Viral hepatitis complicating pregnancy, second trimester** Ⓜ ♀

         O98.413 **Viral hepatitis complicating pregnancy, third trimester** Ⓜ ♀

         O98.419 **Viral hepatitis complicating pregnancy, unspecified trimester** Ⓜ ♀ ▽

     O98.42 **Viral hepatitis complicating childbirth** Ⓜ ♀

     O98.43 **Viral hepatitis complicating the puerperium** Ⓜ ♀

√5ᵗʰ **O98.5 Other viral diseases complicating pregnancy, childbirth and the puerperium**

     Conditions in A80-B09, B25-B34, R87.81-, R87.82-

     EXCLUDES 1   *human immunodeficiency virus [HIV] disease complicating pregnancy, childbirth and the puerperium (O98.7-)*

     √6ᵗʰ **O98.51** **Other viral diseases complicating pregnancy**

         O98.511 **Other viral diseases complicating pregnancy, first trimester** Ⓜ ♀

         O98.512 **Other viral diseases complicating pregnancy, second trimester** Ⓜ ♀

         O98.513 **Other viral diseases complicating pregnancy, third trimester** Ⓜ ♀

         O98.519 **Other viral diseases complicating pregnancy, unspecified trimester** Ⓜ ♀ ▽

     O98.52 **Other viral diseases complicating childbirth** Ⓜ ♀

☑ Additional Character Req   √x7ᵗʰ Placeholder Alert   Manifestation   ▽ Unspecified   ►◄ Revised Text   ● New Code   ▲ Revised Code Title

ICD-10-CM 2019   **881**

O98.53   **Other viral diseases complicating the puerperium**   Ⓜ ♀

✓5ᵗʰ **O98.6**   **Protozoal diseases complicating pregnancy, childbirth and the puerperium**
     Conditions in B50-B64

   ✓6ᵗʰ **O98.61**   **Protozoal diseases complicating** pregnancy

     O98.611   **Protozoal diseases complicating pregnancy, first trimester**   Ⓜ ♀

     O98.612   **Protozoal diseases complicating pregnancy, second trimester**   Ⓜ ♀

     O98.613   **Protozoal diseases complicating pregnancy, third trimester**   Ⓜ ♀

     O98.619   **Protozoal diseases complicating pregnancy, unspecified trimester**   Ⓜ ♀ ▽

   O98.62   **Protozoal diseases complicating** childbirth   Ⓜ ♀

   O98.63   **Protozoal diseases complicating the puerperium**   Ⓜ ♀

✓5ᵗʰ **O98.7**   **Human immunodeficiency virus [HIV] disease complicating pregnancy, childbirth and the puerperium**
     Use additional code to identify the type of HIV disease:
     acquired immune deficiency syndrome (AIDS) (B20)
     asymptomatic HIV status (Z21)
     HIV positive NOS (Z21)
     symptomatic HIV disease (B20)

   ✓6ᵗʰ **O98.71**   **Human immunodeficiency virus [HIV] disease complicating** pregnancy

     O98.711   **Human immunodeficiency virus [HIV] disease complicating pregnancy, first trimester**   Ⓜ ♀

     O98.712   **Human immunodeficiency virus [HIV] disease complicating pregnancy, second trimester**   Ⓜ ♀

     O98.713   **Human immunodeficiency virus [HIV] disease complicating pregnancy, third trimester**   Ⓜ ♀

     O98.719   **Human immunodeficiency virus [HIV] disease complicating pregnancy, unspecified trimester**   Ⓜ ♀ ▽

   O98.72   **Human immunodeficiency virus [HIV] disease complicating** childbirth   Ⓜ ♀

   O98.73   **Human immunodeficiency virus [HIV] disease complicating the** puerperium   Ⓜ ♀

✓5ᵗʰ **O98.8**   **Other maternal infectious and parasitic diseases complicating pregnancy, childbirth and the puerperium**

   ✓6ᵗʰ **O98.81**   **Other maternal infectious and parasitic diseases complicating** pregnancy

     O98.811   **Other maternal infectious and parasitic diseases complicating pregnancy, first trimester**   Ⓜ ♀

     O98.812   **Other maternal infectious and parasitic diseases complicating pregnancy, second trimester**   Ⓜ ♀

     O98.813   **Other maternal infectious and parasitic diseases complicating pregnancy, third trimester**   Ⓜ ♀

     O98.819   **Other maternal infectious and parasitic diseases complicating pregnancy, unspecified trimester**   Ⓜ ♀ ▽

   O98.82   **Other maternal infectious and parasitic diseases complicating** childbirth   Ⓜ ♀

   O98.83   **Other maternal infectious and parasitic diseases complicating the** puerperium   Ⓜ ♀

✓5ᵗʰ **O98.9**   **Unspecified maternal infectious and parasitic disease complicating pregnancy, childbirth and the puerperium**

   ✓6ᵗʰ **O98.91**   **Unspecified maternal infectious and parasitic disease complicating** pregnancy

     O98.911   **Unspecified maternal infectious and parasitic disease complicating pregnancy, first trimester**   Ⓜ ♀ ▽

     O98.912   **Unspecified maternal infectious and parasitic disease complicating pregnancy, second trimester**   Ⓜ ♀ ▽

     O98.913   **Unspecified maternal infectious and parasitic disease complicating pregnancy, third trimester**   Ⓜ ♀ ▽

     O98.919   **Unspecified maternal infectious and parasitic disease complicating pregnancy, unspecified trimester**   Ⓜ ♀ ▽

   O98.92   **Unspecified maternal infectious and parasitic disease complicating** childbirth   Ⓜ ♀ ▽

   O98.93   **Unspecified maternal infectious and parasitic disease complicating the** puerperium   Ⓜ ♀ ▽

✓4ᵗʰ **O99**   **Other maternal diseases classifiable elsewhere but complicating pregnancy, childbirth and the puerperium**
     INCLUDES   conditions which complicate the pregnant state, are aggravated by the pregnancy or are a main reason for obstetric care
     Use additional code to identify specific condition
     EXCLUDES 2   when the reason for maternal care is that the condition is known or suspected to have affected the fetus (O35-O36)

✓5ᵗʰ **O99.0**   **Anemia complicating pregnancy, childbirth and the puerperium**
     Conditions in D50-D64
     EXCLUDES 1   anemia arising in the puerperium (O90.81)
             postpartum anemia NOS (O90.81)

   ✓6ᵗʰ **O99.01**   **Anemia complicating** pregnancy
     AHA: 2016,1Q,4

     O99.011   **Anemia complicating pregnancy, first trimester**   Ⓜ ♀

     O99.012   **Anemia complicating pregnancy, second trimester**   Ⓜ ♀

     O99.013   **Anemia complicating pregnancy, third trimester**   Ⓜ ♀

     O99.019   **Anemia complicating pregnancy, unspecified trimester**   Ⓜ ♀ ▽

   O99.02   **Anemia complicating** childbirth   Ⓜ ♀

   O99.03   **Anemia complicating the** puerperium   Ⓜ ♀
     EXCLUDES 1   postpartum anemia not pre-existing prior to delivery (O90.81)

✓5ᵗʰ **O99.1**   **Other diseases of the blood and blood-forming organs and certain disorders involving the immune mechanism complicating pregnancy, childbirth and the puerperium**
     Conditions in D65-D89
     EXCLUDES 1   hemorrhage with coagulation defects (O45.-, O46.0-, O67.0, O72.3)

   ✓6ᵗʰ **O99.11**   **Other diseases of the blood and blood-forming organs and certain disorders involving the immune mechanism complicating** pregnancy

     O99.111   **Other diseases of the blood and blood-forming organs and certain disorders involving the immune mechanism complicating pregnancy, first trimester**   Ⓜ ♀

     O99.112   **Other diseases of the blood and blood-forming organs and certain disorders involving the immune mechanism complicating pregnancy, second trimester**   Ⓜ ♀

     O99.113   **Other diseases of the blood and blood-forming organs and certain disorders involving the immune mechanism complicating pregnancy, third trimester**   Ⓜ ♀

     O99.119   **Other diseases of the blood and blood-forming organs and certain disorders involving the immune mechanism complicating pregnancy, unspecified trimester**   Ⓜ ♀ ▽

   O99.12   **Other diseases of the blood and blood-forming organs and certain disorders involving the immune mechanism complicating** childbirth   Ⓜ ♀

   O99.13   **Other diseases of the blood and blood-forming organs and certain disorders involving the immune mechanism complicating the** puerperium   Ⓜ ♀

✓5ᵗʰ O99.2 Endocrine, nutritional and metabolic diseases complicating pregnancy, childbirth and the puerperium
Conditions in E00-E88
> EXCLUDES 2   *diabetes mellitus (O24.-)*
> *malnutrition (O25.-)*
> *postpartum thyroiditis (O90.5)*

✓6ᵗʰ O99.21 Obesity complicating pregnancy, childbirth, and the puerperium
Use additional code to identify the type of obesity (E66.-)

O99.210 Obesity complicating pregnancy, unspecified trimester   Ⓜ ♀ ▽

O99.211 Obesity complicating pregnancy, first trimester   Ⓜ ♀

O99.212 Obesity complicating pregnancy, second trimester   Ⓜ ♀

O99.213 Obesity complicating pregnancy, third trimester   Ⓜ ♀

O99.214 Obesity complicating childbirth   Ⓜ ♀

O99.215 Obesity complicating the puerperium   Ⓜ ♀

✓6ᵗʰ O99.28 Other endocrine, nutritional and metabolic diseases complicating pregnancy, childbirth and the puerperium

O99.280 Endocrine, nutritional and metabolic diseases complicating pregnancy, unspecified trimester   Ⓜ ♀ ▽

O99.281 Endocrine, nutritional and metabolic diseases complicating pregnancy, first trimester   Ⓜ ♀

O99.282 Endocrine, nutritional and metabolic diseases complicating pregnancy, second trimester   Ⓜ ♀

O99.283 Endocrine, nutritional and metabolic diseases complicating pregnancy, third trimester   Ⓜ ♀

O99.284 Endocrine, nutritional and metabolic diseases complicating childbirth   Ⓜ ♀

O99.285 Endocrine, nutritional and metabolic diseases complicating the puerperium   Ⓜ ♀

✓5ᵗʰ O99.3 Mental disorders and diseases of the nervous system complicating pregnancy, childbirth and the puerperium

✓6ᵗʰ O99.31 Alcohol use complicating pregnancy, childbirth, and the puerperium
Use additional code(s) from F10 to identify manifestations of the alcohol use

O99.310 Alcohol use complicating pregnancy, unspecified trimester   Ⓜ ♀ ▽

O99.311 Alcohol use complicating pregnancy, first trimester   Ⓜ ♀

O99.312 Alcohol use complicating pregnancy, second trimester   Ⓜ ♀

O99.313 Alcohol use complicating pregnancy, third trimester   Ⓜ ♀

O99.314 Alcohol use complicating childbirth   Ⓜ ♀

O99.315 Alcohol use complicating the puerperium   Ⓜ ♀

✓6ᵗʰ O99.32 Drug use complicating pregnancy, childbirth, and the puerperium
Use additional code(s) from F11-F16 and F18-F19 to identify manifestations of the drug use
AHA: 2018,2Q,10

O99.320 Drug use complicating pregnancy, unspecified trimester   Ⓜ ♀ ▽

O99.321 Drug use complicating pregnancy, first trimester   Ⓜ ♀

O99.322 Drug use complicating pregnancy, second trimester   Ⓜ ♀

O99.323 Drug use complicating pregnancy, third trimester   Ⓜ ♀

O99.324 Drug use complicating childbirth   Ⓜ ♀

O99.325 Drug use complicating the puerperium   Ⓜ ♀

✓6ᵗʰ O99.33 Tobacco use disorder complicating pregnancy, childbirth, and the puerperium
Smoking complicating pregnancy, childbirth, and the puerperium
Use additional code from category F17 to identify type of tobacco nicotine dependence

O99.330 Smoking (tobacco) complicating pregnancy, unspecified trimester   Ⓜ ♀ ▽

O99.331 Smoking (tobacco) complicating pregnancy, first trimester   Ⓜ ♀

O99.332 Smoking (tobacco) complicating pregnancy, second trimester   Ⓜ ♀

O99.333 Smoking (tobacco) complicating pregnancy, third trimester   Ⓜ ♀

O99.334 Smoking (tobacco) complicating childbirth   Ⓜ ♀

O99.335 Smoking (tobacco) complicating the puerperium   Ⓜ ♀

✓6ᵗʰ O99.34 Other mental disorders complicating pregnancy, childbirth, and the puerperium
Conditions in F01-F09 and F20-F99
> EXCLUDES 2   *postpartum mood disturbance (O90.6)*
> *postnatal psychosis ►(F53.1)◄*
> *puerperal psychosis ►(F53.1)◄*

O99.340 Other mental disorders complicating pregnancy, unspecified trimester   Ⓠ Ⓜ ♀ ▽

O99.341 Other mental disorders complicating pregnancy, first trimester   Ⓠ Ⓜ ♀

O99.342 Other mental disorders complicating pregnancy, second trimester   Ⓠ Ⓜ ♀

O99.343 Other mental disorders complicating pregnancy, third trimester   Ⓠ Ⓜ ♀

O99.344 Other mental disorders complicating childbirth   Ⓜ ♀

O99.345 Other mental disorders complicating the puerperium   Ⓠ Ⓜ ♀

✓6ᵗʰ O99.35 Diseases of the nervous system complicating pregnancy, childbirth, and the puerperium
Conditions in G00-G99
> EXCLUDES 2   *pregnancy related peripheral neuritis (O26.8-)*

O99.350 Diseases of the nervous system complicating pregnancy, unspecified trimester   Ⓜ ♀ ▽

O99.351 Diseases of the nervous system complicating pregnancy, first trimester   Ⓜ ♀

O99.352 Diseases of the nervous system complicating pregnancy, second trimester   Ⓜ ♀

O99.353 Diseases of the nervous system complicating pregnancy, third trimester   Ⓜ ♀

O99.354 Diseases of the nervous system complicating childbirth   Ⓜ ♀

O99.355 Diseases of the nervous system complicating the puerperium   Ⓜ ♀

✓5ᵗʰ O99.4 Diseases of the circulatory system complicating pregnancy, childbirth and the puerperium
Conditions in I00-I99
> EXCLUDES 1   *peripartum cardiomyopathy (O90.3)*
> EXCLUDES 2   *hypertensive disorders (O10-O16)*
> *obstetric embolism (O88.-)*
> *venous complications and cerebrovenous sinus thrombosis in labor, childbirth and the puerperium (O87.-)*
> *venous complications and cerebrovenous sinus thrombosis in pregnancy (O22.-)*

AHA: 2016,2Q,8

✓6ᵗʰ O99.41 Diseases of the circulatory system complicating pregnancy

O99.411 Diseases of the circulatory system complicating pregnancy, first trimester   Ⓜ ♀

O99.412 Diseases of the circulatory system complicating pregnancy, second trimester   Ⓜ ♀

✅ Additional Character Req   ✓x7ᵗʰ Placeholder Alert   Manifestation   ▽ Unspecified   ►◄ Revised Text   ● New Code   ▲ Revised Code Title

Chapter 15. Pregnancy, Childbirth and the Puerperium

O99.413 Diseases of the circulatory system complicating pregnancy, third trimester Ⓜ ♀

O99.419 Diseases of the circulatory system complicating pregnancy, unspecified trimester Ⓜ ♀ ▽

O99.42 Diseases of the circulatory system complicating childbirth Ⓜ ♀

O99.43 Diseases of the circulatory system complicating the puerperium Ⓜ ♀

✓5ᵗʰ O99.5 Diseases of the respiratory system complicating pregnancy, childbirth and the puerperium
  Conditions in J00-J99

✓6ᵗʰ O99.51 Diseases of the respiratory system complicating pregnancy

O99.511 Diseases of the respiratory system complicating pregnancy, first trimester Ⓜ ♀

O99.512 Diseases of the respiratory system complicating pregnancy, second trimester Ⓜ ♀

O99.513 Diseases of the respiratory system complicating pregnancy, third trimester Ⓜ ♀

O99.519 Diseases of the respiratory system complicating pregnancy, unspecified trimester Ⓜ ♀ ▽

O99.52 Diseases of the respiratory system complicating childbirth Ⓜ ♀

O99.53 Diseases of the respiratory system complicating the puerperium Ⓜ ♀

✓5ᵗʰ O99.6 Diseases of the digestive system complicating pregnancy, childbirth and the puerperium
  Conditions in K00-K93
  EXCLUDES 2   hemorrhoids in pregnancy (O22.4-)
  liver and biliary tract disorders in pregnancy, childbirth and the puerperium (O26.6-)

✓6ᵗʰ O99.61 Diseases of the digestive system complicating pregnancy
  AHA: 2016,1Q,4

O99.611 Diseases of the digestive system complicating pregnancy, first trimester Ⓜ ♀

O99.612 Diseases of the digestive system complicating pregnancy, second trimester Ⓜ ♀

O99.613 Diseases of the digestive system complicating pregnancy, third trimester Ⓜ ♀

O99.619 Diseases of the digestive system complicating pregnancy, unspecified trimester Ⓜ ♀ ▽

O99.62 Diseases of the digestive system complicating childbirth Ⓜ ♀

O99.63 Diseases of the digestive system complicating the puerperium Ⓜ ♀

✓5ᵗʰ O99.7 Diseases of the skin and subcutaneous tissue complicating pregnancy, childbirth and the puerperium
  Conditions in L00-L99
  EXCLUDES 2   herpes gestationis (O26.4)
  pruritic urticarial papules and plaques of pregnancy (PUPPP) (O26.86)

✓6ᵗʰ O99.71 Diseases of the skin and subcutaneous tissue complicating pregnancy

O99.711 Diseases of the skin and subcutaneous tissue complicating pregnancy, first trimester Ⓜ ♀

O99.712 Diseases of the skin and subcutaneous tissue complicating pregnancy, second trimester Ⓜ ♀

O99.713 Diseases of the skin and subcutaneous tissue complicating pregnancy, third trimester Ⓜ ♀

O99.719 Diseases of the skin and subcutaneous tissue complicating pregnancy, unspecified trimester Ⓜ ♀ ▽

O99.72 Diseases of the skin and subcutaneous tissue complicating childbirth Ⓜ ♀

O99.73 Diseases of the skin and subcutaneous tissue complicating the puerperium Ⓜ ♀

✓5ᵗʰ O99.8 Other specified diseases and conditions complicating pregnancy, childbirth and the puerperium
  Conditions in D00-D48, H00-H95, M00-N99, and Q00-Q99
  Use additional code to identify condition
  EXCLUDES 2   genitourinary infections in pregnancy (O23.-)
  infection of genitourinary tract following delivery (O86.1-O86.3)
  malignant neoplasm complicating pregnancy, childbirth and the puerperium (O9A.1-)
  maternal care for known or suspected abnormality of maternal pelvic organs (O34.-)
  postpartum acute kidney failure (O90.4)
  traumatic injuries in pregnancy (O9A.2-)

✓6ᵗʰ O99.81 Abnormal glucose complicating pregnancy, childbirth and the puerperium
  EXCLUDES 1   gestational diabetes (O24.4-)

O99.810 Abnormal glucose complicating pregnancy Ⓜ ♀

O99.814 Abnormal glucose complicating childbirth Ⓜ ♀

O99.815 Abnormal glucose complicating the puerperium Ⓜ ♀

✓6ᵗʰ O99.82 Streptococcus B carrier state complicating pregnancy, childbirth and the puerperium
  EXCLUDES 1   carrier of streptococcus group B (GBS) in a nonpregnant woman (Z22.330)

O99.820 Streptococcus B carrier state complicating pregnancy Ⓜ ♀

O99.824 Streptococcus B carrier state complicating childbirth Ⓜ ♀

O99.825 Streptococcus B carrier state complicating the puerperium Ⓜ ♀

✓6ᵗʰ O99.83 Other infection carrier state complicating pregnancy, childbirth and the puerperium
  Use additional code to identify the carrier state (Z22.-)

O99.830 Other infection carrier state complicating pregnancy Ⓜ ♀

O99.834 Other infection carrier state complicating childbirth Ⓜ ♀

O99.835 Other infection carrier state complicating the puerperium Ⓜ ♀

✓6ᵗʰ O99.84 Bariatric surgery status complicating pregnancy, childbirth and the puerperium
  Gastric banding status complicating pregnancy, childbirth and the puerperium
  Gastric bypass status for obesity complicating pregnancy, childbirth and the puerperium
  Obesity surgery status complicating pregnancy, childbirth and the puerperium

O99.840 Bariatric surgery status complicating pregnancy, unspecified trimester Ⓜ ♀ ▽

O99.841 Bariatric surgery status complicating pregnancy, first trimester Ⓜ ♀

O99.842 Bariatric surgery status complicating pregnancy, second trimester Ⓜ ♀

O99.843 Bariatric surgery status complicating pregnancy, third trimester Ⓜ ♀

O99.844 Bariatric surgery status complicating childbirth Ⓜ ♀

O99.845 Bariatric surgery status complicating the puerperium Ⓜ ♀

O99.89 Other specified diseases and conditions complicating pregnancy, childbirth and the puerperium Ⓜ ♀

✓4ᵗʰ O9A   Maternal malignant neoplasms, traumatic injuries and abuse classifiable elsewhere but complicating pregnancy, childbirth and the puerperium

✓5ᵗʰ O9A.1   Malignant neoplasm complicating pregnancy, childbirth and the puerperium
Conditions in C00-C96
Use additional code to identify neoplasm
EXCLUDES 2   maternal care for benign tumor of corpus uteri (O34.1-)
     maternal care for benign tumor of cervix (O34.4-)
AHA: 2015,3Q,19

✓6ᵗʰ O9A.11   Malignant neoplasm complicating pregnancy

O9A.111   Malignant neoplasm complicating pregnancy, first trimester   Ⓜ ♀

O9A.112   Malignant neoplasm complicating pregnancy, second trimester   Ⓜ ♀

O9A.113   Malignant neoplasm complicating pregnancy, third trimester   Ⓜ ♀

O9A.119   Malignant neoplasm complicating pregnancy, unspecified trimester   Ⓜ ♀ ▽

O9A.12   Malignant neoplasm complicating childbirth   Ⓜ ♀

O9A.13   Malignant neoplasm complicating the puerperium   Ⓜ ♀

✓5ᵗʰ O9A.2   Injury, poisoning and certain other consequences of external causes complicating pregnancy, childbirth and the puerperium
Conditions in S00-T88, except T74 and T76
Use additional code(s) to identify the injury or poisoning
EXCLUDES 2   physical, sexual and psychological abuse complicating pregnancy, childbirth and the puerperium (O9A.3-, O9A.4-, O9A.5-)

✓6ᵗʰ O9A.21   Injury, poisoning and certain other consequences of external causes complicating pregnancy

O9A.211   Injury, poisoning and certain other consequences of external causes complicating pregnancy, first trimester   Ⓜ ♀

O9A.212   Injury, poisoning and certain other consequences of external causes complicating pregnancy, second trimester   Ⓜ ♀

O9A.213   Injury, poisoning and certain other consequences of external causes complicating pregnancy, third trimester   Ⓜ ♀

O9A.219   Injury, poisoning and certain other consequences of external causes complicating pregnancy, unspecified trimester   Ⓜ ♀ ▽

O9A.22   Injury, poisoning and certain other consequences of external causes complicating childbirth   Ⓜ ♀

O9A.23   Injury, poisoning and certain other consequences of external causes complicating the puerperium   Ⓜ ♀

✓5ᵗʰ O9A.3   Physical abuse complicating pregnancy, childbirth and the puerperium
Conditions in T74.11 or T76.11
Use additional code (if applicable):
to identify any associated current injury due to physical abuse
to identify the perpetrator of abuse (Y07.-)
EXCLUDES 2   sexual abuse complicating pregnancy, childbirth and the puerperium (O9A.4)

✓6ᵗʰ O9A.31   Physical abuse complicating pregnancy

O9A.311   Physical abuse complicating pregnancy, first trimester   Ⓜ ♀

O9A.312   Physical abuse complicating pregnancy, second trimester   Ⓜ ♀

O9A.313   Physical abuse complicating pregnancy, third trimester   Ⓜ ♀

O9A.319   Physical abuse complicating pregnancy, unspecified trimester   Ⓜ ♀ ▽

O9A.32   Physical abuse complicating childbirth   Ⓜ ♀

O9A.33   Physical abuse complicating the puerperium   Ⓜ ♀

✓5ᵗʰ O9A.4   Sexual abuse complicating pregnancy, childbirth and the puerperium
Conditions in T74.21 or T76.21
Use additional code (if applicable):
to identify any associated current injury due to sexual abuse
to identify the perpetrator of abuse (Y07.-)

✓6ᵗʰ O9A.41   Sexual abuse complicating pregnancy

O9A.411   Sexual abuse complicating pregnancy, first trimester   Ⓜ ♀

O9A.412   Sexual abuse complicating pregnancy, second trimester   Ⓜ ♀

O9A.413   Sexual abuse complicating pregnancy, third trimester   Ⓜ ♀

O9A.419   Sexual abuse complicating pregnancy, unspecified trimester   Ⓜ ♀ ▽

O9A.42   Sexual abuse complicating childbirth   Ⓜ ♀

O9A.43   Sexual abuse complicating the puerperium   Ⓜ ♀

✓5ᵗʰ O9A.5   Psychological abuse complicating pregnancy, childbirth and the puerperium
Conditions in T74.31 or T76.31
Use additional code to identify the perpetrator of abuse (Y07.-)

✓6ᵗʰ O9A.51   Psychological abuse complicating pregnancy

O9A.511   Psychological abuse complicating pregnancy, first trimester   Ⓜ ♀

O9A.512   Psychological abuse complicating pregnancy, second trimester   Ⓜ ♀

O9A.513   Psychological abuse complicating pregnancy, third trimester   Ⓜ ♀

O9A.519   Psychological abuse complicating pregnancy, unspecified trimester   Ⓜ ♀ ▽

O9A.52   Psychological abuse complicating childbirth   Ⓜ ♀

O9A.53   Psychological abuse complicating the puerperium   Ⓜ ♀

✓ Additional Character Req   ✓x7ᵗʰ Placeholder Alert   Manifestation   ▽ Unspecified   ▶◀ Revised Text   ● New Code   ▲ Revised Code Title

Chapter 16. Certain Conditions Originating in the Perinatal Period (PØØ–P96)

Chapter Specific Guidelines with Coding Examples

The chapter specific guidelines from the ICD-10-CM Official Guidelines for Coding and Reporting have been provided below. Along with these guidelines are coding examples, contained in the shaded boxes, that have been developed to help illustrate the coding and/or sequencing guidance found in these guidelines.

For coding and reporting purposes the perinatal period is defined as before birth through the 28th day following birth. The following guidelines are provided for reporting purposes

a. General perinatal rules

1) Use of Chapter 16 codes

Codes in this chapter are <u>never</u> for use on the maternal record. Codes from Chapter 15, the obstetric chapter, are never permitted on the newborn record. Chapter 16 codes may be used throughout the life of the patient if the condition is still present.

2) Principal diagnosis for birth record

When coding the birth episode in a newborn record, assign a code from category Z38, Liveborn infants according to place of birth and type of delivery, as the principal diagnosis. A code from category Z38 is assigned only once, to a newborn at the time of birth. If a newborn is transferred to another institution, a code from category Z38 should not be used at the receiving hospital.

A code from category Z38 is used only on the newborn record, not on the mother's record.

3) Use of codes from other chapters with codes from Chapter 16

Codes from other chapters may be used with codes from chapter 16 if the codes from the other chapters provide more specific detail. Codes for signs and symptoms may be assigned when a definitive diagnosis has not been established. If the reason for the encounter is a perinatal condition, the code from chapter 16 should be sequenced first.

4) Use of Chapter 16 codes after the perinatal period

Should a condition originate in the perinatal period, and continue throughout the life of the patient, the perinatal code should continue to be used regardless of the patient's age.

> A 7-year-old patient with history of birth injury that resulted in Erb's palsy is seen for subscapularis release
>
> **P14.Ø   Erb's paralysis due to birth injury**
>
> *Explanation:* Although in this instance Erb's palsy is specifically related to a birth injury, it has not resolved and continues to be a health concern. A perinatal code is appropriate even though this patient is beyond the perinatal period.

5) Birth process or community acquired conditions

If a newborn has a condition that may be either due to the birth process or community acquired and the documentation does not indicate which it is, the default is due to the birth process and the code from Chapter 16 should be used. If the condition is community-acquired, a code from Chapter 16 should not be assigned.

6) Code all clinically significant conditions

All clinically significant conditions noted on routine newborn examination should be coded. A condition is clinically significant if it requires:

clinical evaluation; or

therapeutic treatment; or

diagnostic procedures; or

extended length of hospital stay; or

increased nursing care and/or monitoring; or

has implications for future health care needs

Note: The perinatal guidelines listed above are the same as the general coding guidelines for "additional diagnoses", except for the final point regarding implications for future health care needs. Codes should be assigned for conditions that have been specified by the provider as having implications for future health care needs.

b. Observation and evaluation of newborns for suspected conditions not found

1) Use of Z05 codes

Assign a code from category Z05, Observation and evaluation of newborns and infants for suspected conditions ruled out, to identify those instances when a healthy newborn is evaluated for a suspected condition that is determined after study not to be present. Do not use a code from category Z05 when the patient has identified signs or symptoms of a suspected problem; in such cases code the sign or symptom.

2) Z05 on other than the birth record

A code from category Z05 may also be assigned as a principal or first-listed code for readmissions or encounters when the code from category Z38 code no longer applies. Codes from category Z05 are for use only for healthy newborns and infants for which no condition after study is found to be present.

3) Z05 on a birth record

A code from category Z05 is to be used as a secondary code after the code from category Z38, Liveborn infants according to place of birth and type of delivery.

> Newborn delivered via vaginal delivery; previous ultrasounds showed what appeared to be an abnormality of the right kidney. Kidney function tests were performed and ultrasounds taken and any genitourinary conditions ruled out.
>
> **Z38.ØØ   Single liveborn infant, delivered vaginally**
>
> **Z05.6   Observation and evaluation of newborn for suspected genitourinary condition ruled out**
>
> Explanation: The newborn had no signs or symptoms of kidney or other genitourinary condition but was evaluated after delivery due to the abnormal prenatal ultrasound findings. A Z code describing the type and place of birth should be coded first, followed by a Z05 category code for the work performed to rule out a suspected genitourinary condition.

c. Coding additional perinatal diagnoses

1) Assigning codes for conditions that require treatment

Assign codes for conditions that require treatment or further investigation, prolong the length of stay, or require resource utilization.

2) Codes for conditions specified as having implications for future health care needs

Assign codes for conditions that have been specified by the provider as having implications for future health care needs.

Note: This guideline should not be used for adult patients.

> An abnormal noise was heard in the left hip of a post-term newborn during a physical examination. The pediatrician would like to follow the patient after discharge as a hip click can be an early sign of hip dysplasia. The newborn was delivered via cesarean at 41 weeks.
>
> **Z38.Ø1   Single liveborn infant, delivered by cesarean**
>
> **P08.21   Post-term newborn**
>
> **R29.4   Clicking hip**
>
> *Explanation:* The abnormal hip noise or click is appended as a secondary diagnosis not only because it is an abnormal finding upon examination, but also due to its potential to be part of a bigger health issue. The hip dysplasia has not yet been diagnosed and does not warrant a code at this time.

d. Prematurity and fetal growth retardation

Providers utilize different criteria in determining prematurity. A code for prematurity should not be assigned unless it is documented. Assignment of codes in categories P05, Disorders of newborn related to slow fetal growth and fetal malnutrition, and P07, Disorders of newborn related to short gestation and low birth weight, not elsewhere classified, should be based on the recorded birth weight and estimated gestational age.

When both birth weight and gestational age are available, two codes from category P07 should be assigned, with the code for birth weight sequenced before the code for gestational age.

Chapter 16. Certain Conditions Originating in the Perinatal Period

e. Low birth weight and immaturity status

Codes from category P07, Disorders of newborn related to short gestation and low birth weight, not elsewhere classified, are for use for a child or adult who was premature or had a low birth weight as a newborn and this is affecting the patient's current health status.

See Section I.C.21. Factors influencing health status and contact with health services, Status.

A 35-year-old patient, who weighed 659 grams at birth, is seen for heart disease documented as being a consequence of the low birth weight

I51.9   **Heart disease, unspecified**

P07.02   **Extremely low birth weight newborn, 500–749 grams**

Explanation: A code from subcategories P07.0- and P07.1- is appropriate, regardless of the age of the patient, as long as the documentation provides a clear link between the patient's current illness and the low birth weight.

f. Bacterial sepsis of newborn

Category P36, Bacterial sepsis of newborn, includes congenital sepsis. If a perinate is documented as having sepsis without documentation of congenital or community acquired, the default is congenital and a code from category P36 should be assigned. If the P36 code includes the causal organism, an additional code from category B95, Streptococcus, Staphylococcus, and Enterococcus as the cause of diseases classified elsewhere, or B96, Other bacterial agents as the cause of diseases classified elsewhere, should not be assigned. If the P36 code does not include the causal organism, assign an additional code from category B96. If applicable, use additional codes to identify severe sepsis (R65.2-) and any associated acute organ dysfunction.

A full-term infant develops severe sepsis 24 hours after discharge from the hospital and is readmitted; cultures identified *E. coli* as the infective agent

P36.4   **Sepsis of newborn due to Escherichia coli**

R65.20   **Severe sepsis without septic shock**

Explanation: Even though this newborn was discharged and could have acquired *E. coli* from his/her external environment, due to the lack of documentation specifying specifically how this pathogen was acquired, the default is to code the *E. coli* sepsis as congenital. A code from chapter 1, "Certain Infectious and Parasitic Diseases," is not required because the perinatal sepsis code identifies both the sepsis and the bacteria causing the sepsis.

g. Stillbirth

Code P95, Stillbirth, is only for use in institutions that maintain separate records for stillbirths. No other code should be used with P95. Code P95 should not be used on the mother's record.

Chapter 16. Certain Conditions Originating in the Perinatal Period (P00-P96)

> **NOTE**   Codes from this chapter are for use on newborn records only, never on maternal records

> **INCLUDES**   conditions that have their origin in the fetal or perinatal period (before birth through the first 28 days after birth) even if morbidity occurs later

> **EXCLUDES 2**   congenital malformations, deformations and chromosomal abnormalities (Q00-Q99)
> endocrine, nutritional and metabolic diseases (E00-E88)
> injury, poisoning and certain other consequences of external causes (S00-T88)
> neoplasms (C00-D49)
> tetanus neonatorum (A33)

This chapter contains the following blocks:

P00-P04	Newborn affected by maternal factors and by complications of pregnancy, labor, and delivery
P05-P08	Disorders of newborn related to length of gestation and fetal growth
P09	Abnormal findings on neonatal screening
P10-P15	Birth trauma
P19-P29	Respiratory and cardiovascular disorders specific to the perinatal period
P35-P39	Infections specific to the perinatal period
P50-P61	Hemorrhagic and hematological disorders of newborn
P70-P74	Transitory endocrine and metabolic disorders specific to newborn
P76-P78	Digestive system disorders of newborn
P80-P83	Conditions involving the integument and temperature regulation of newborn
P84	Other problems with newborn
P90-P96	Other disorders originating in the perinatal period

Newborn affected by maternal factors and by complications of pregnancy, labor, and delivery (P00-P04)

> **NOTE**   These codes are for use when the listed maternal conditions are specified as the cause of confirmed morbidity or potential morbidity which have their origin in the perinatal period (before birth through the first 28 days after birth).

AHA: 2016,4Q,54-55

√4ᵗʰ **P00** **Newborn affected by maternal conditions that may be unrelated to present pregnancy**

Code first any current condition in newborn

> **EXCLUDES 2**   encounter for observation of newborn for suspected diseases and conditions ruled out (Z05.-)
> newborn affected by maternal complications of pregnancy (P01.-)
> newborn affected by maternal endocrine and metabolic disorders (P70-P74)
> newborn affected by noxious substances transmitted via placenta or breast milk (P04.-)

P00.0 **Newborn affected by maternal hypertensive disorders**
Newborn affected by maternal conditions classifiable to O10-O11, O13-O16

P00.1 **Newborn affected by maternal renal and urinary tract diseases**
Newborn affected by maternal conditions classifiable to N00-N39

P00.2 **Newborn affected by maternal infectious and parasitic diseases**
Newborn affected by maternal infectious disease classifiable to A00-B99, J09 and J10

> **EXCLUDES 1**   maternal genital tract or other localized infections (P00.8)

> **EXCLUDES 2**   infections specific to the perinatal period (P35-P39)

AHA: 2015,3Q,20

P00.3 **Newborn affected by other maternal circulatory and respiratory diseases**
Newborn affected by maternal conditions classifiable to I00-I99, J00-J99, Q20-Q34 and not included in P00.0, P00.2

P00.4 **Newborn affected by maternal nutritional disorders**
Newborn affected by maternal disorders classifiable to E40-E64
Maternal malnutrition NOS

P00.5 **Newborn affected by maternal injury**
Newborn affected by maternal conditions classifiable to O9A.2-

P00.6 **Newborn affected by surgical procedure on mother**
Newborn affected by amniocentesis

> **EXCLUDES 1**   Cesarean delivery for present delivery (P03.4)
> damage to placenta from amniocentesis, Cesarean delivery or surgical induction (P02.1)
> previous surgery to uterus or pelvic organs (P03.89)

> **EXCLUDES 2**   newborn affected by complication of (fetal) intrauterine procedure (P96.5)

P00.7 **Newborn affected by other medical procedures on mother, not elsewhere classified**
Newborn affected by radiation to mother

> **EXCLUDES 1**   damage to placenta from amniocentesis, cesarean delivery or surgical induction (P02.1)
> newborn affected by other complications of labor and delivery (P03.-)

√5ᵗʰ **P00.8** **Newborn affected by other maternal conditions**

P00.81 **Newborn affected by periodontal disease in mother**

P00.89 **Newborn affected by other maternal conditions**
Newborn affected by conditions classifiable to T80-T88
Newborn affected by maternal genital tract or other localized infections
Newborn affected by maternal systemic lupus erythematosus

P00.9 **Newborn affected by unspecified maternal condition** ▽

√4ᵗʰ **P01** **Newborn affected by maternal complications of pregnancy**

Code first any current condition in newborn

> **EXCLUDES 2**   encounter for observation of newborn for suspected diseases and conditions ruled out (Z05.-)

P01.0 **Newborn affected by incompetent cervix**

P01.1 **Newborn affected by premature rupture of membranes**

P01.2 **Newborn affected by oligohydramnios**

> **EXCLUDES 1**   oligohydramnios due to premature rupture of membranes (P01.1)

DEF: Low amniotic fluid level, resulting in underdeveloped organs in the fetus.

P01.3 **Newborn affected by polyhydramnios**
Newborn affected by hydramnios
DEF: Excess amniotic fluid surrounding the fetus, typically defined as a total fluid volume of greater than 24.0 cc.

P01.4 **Newborn affected by ectopic pregnancy**
Newborn affected by abdominal pregnancy

P01.5 **Newborn affected by multiple pregnancy**
Newborn affected by triplet (pregnancy)
Newborn affected by twin (pregnancy)

P01.6 **Newborn affected by maternal death**

P01.7 **Newborn affected by malpresentation before labor**
Newborn affected by breech presentation before labor
Newborn affected by external version before labor
Newborn affected by face presentation before labor
Newborn affected by transverse lie before labor
Newborn affected by unstable lie before labor

P01.8 **Newborn affected by other maternal complications of pregnancy**

P01.9 **Newborn affected by maternal complication of pregnancy, unspecified** ▽

√4ᵗʰ **P02** **Newborn affected by complications of placenta, cord and membranes**

Code first any current condition in newborn

> **EXCLUDES 2**   encounter for observation of newborn for suspected diseases and conditions ruled out (Z05.-)

P02.0 **Newborn affected by placenta previa**
DEF: Placenta developed in the lower segment of the uterus that can cause hemorrhaging leading to preterm delivery.

P02.1 **Newborn affected by other forms of placental separation and hemorrhage**
Newborn affected by abruptio placenta
Newborn affected by accidental hemorrhage
Newborn affected by antepartum hemorrhage
Newborn affected by damage to placenta from amniocentesis, cesarean delivery or surgical induction
Newborn affected by maternal blood loss
Newborn affected by premature separation of placenta

✔ Additional Character Req   ✔x7ᵗʰ Placeholder Alert   Manifestation   ▽ Unspecified   ▶◀ Revised Text   ● New Code   ▲ Revised Code Title

ICD-10-CM 2019   889

Chapter 16. Certain Conditions Originating in the Perinatal Period

P02.2–P04.0

✓5ᵗʰ **P02.2** **Newborn affected by other and unspecified morphological and functional abnormalities of placenta**

     P02.20 **Newborn affected by unspecified morphological and functional abnormalities of placenta** ▽

     P02.29 **Newborn affected by other morphological and functional abnormalities of placenta**
         Newborn affected by placental dysfunction
         Newborn affected by placental infarction
         Newborn affected by placental insufficiency

   P02.3 **Newborn affected by placental transfusion syndromes**
         Newborn affected by placental and cord abnormalities resulting in twin-to-twin or other transplacental transfusion

   P02.4 **Newborn affected by prolapsed cord**

   P02.5 **Newborn affected by other compression of umbilical cord**
         Newborn affected by umbilical cord (tightly) around neck
         Newborn affected by entanglement of umbilical cord
         Newborn affected by knot in umbilical cord

✓5ᵗʰ **P02.6** **Newborn affected by other and unspecified conditions of umbilical cord**

     P02.60 **Newborn affected by unspecified conditions of umbilical cord** ▽

     P02.69 **Newborn affected by other conditions of umbilical cord**
         Newborn affected by short umbilical cord
         Newborn affected by vasa previa
         EXCLUDES 1   *newborn affected by single umbilical artery (Q27.0)*

✓5ᵗʰ **P02.7** **Newborn affected by chorioamnionitis**
     ~~Newborn affected by amnionitis~~
     ~~Newborn affected by membranitis~~
     ~~Newborn affected by placentitis~~
     DEF: Inflammation of the fetal membranes due to maternal infection characterized by fetal tachycardia, respiratory distress, apnea, weak cries, and poor sucking.

●   **P02.70** **Newborn affected by fetal inflammatory response syndrome**
         Newborn affected by FIRS

●   **P02.78** **Newborn affected by other conditions from chorioamnionitis**
         Newborn affected by amnionitis
         Newborn affected by membranitis
         Newborn affected by placentitis

   P02.8 **Newborn affected by other abnormalities of membranes**

   P02.9 **Newborn affected by abnormality of membranes, unspecified** ▽

✓4ᵗʰ **P03** **Newborn affected by other complications of labor and delivery**
     Code first any current condition in newborn
     EXCLUDES 2   *encounter for observation of newborn for suspected diseases and conditions ruled out (Z05.-)*

   P03.0 **Newborn affected by breech delivery and extraction**

   P03.1 **Newborn affected by other malpresentation, malposition and disproportion during labor and delivery**
         Newborn affected by contracted pelvis
         Newborn affected by conditions classifiable to O64-O66
         Newborn affected by persistent occipitoposterior
         Newborn affected by transverse lie

   P03.2 **Newborn affected by forceps delivery**

Forceps Assisted Birth

Forceps extractor

   P03.3 **Newborn affected by delivery by vacuum extractor [ventouse]**

Vacuum Assisted Birth

Vacuum extractor

   P03.4 **Newborn affected by Cesarean delivery**

   P03.5 **Newborn affected by precipitate delivery**
     Newborn affected by rapid second stage

   P03.6 **Newborn affected by abnormal uterine contractions**
     Newborn affected by conditions classifiable to O62.-, except O62.3
     Newborn affected by hypertonic labor
     Newborn affected by uterine inertia

✓5ᵗʰ **P03.8** **Newborn affected by other specified complications of labor and delivery**

   ✓6ᵗʰ **P03.81** **Newborn affected by abnormality in fetal (intrauterine) heart rate or rhythm**
         EXCLUDES 1   *neonatal cardiac dysrhythmia (P29.1-)*

     P03.810 **Newborn affected by abnormality in fetal (intrauterine) heart rate or rhythm before the onset of labor**

     P03.811 **Newborn affected by abnormality in fetal (intrauterine) heart rate or rhythm during labor**

     P03.819 **Newborn affected by abnormality in fetal (intrauterine) heart rate or rhythm, unspecified as to time of onset** ▽

   P03.82 **Meconium passage during delivery**
         EXCLUDES 1   *meconium aspiration (P24.00, P24.01)*
                     meconium staining (P96.83)
     DEF: Fetal intestinal activity that increases in response to a fetomaternal distressed state during delivery. The anal sphincter relaxes and meconium is passed into the amniotic fluid.

   P03.89 **Newborn affected by other specified complications of labor and delivery**
     Newborn affected by abnormality of maternal soft tissues
     Newborn affected by conditions classifiable to O60-O75 and by procedures used in labor and delivery not included in P02.- and P03.0-P03.6
     Newborn affected by induction of labor

   P03.9 **Newborn affected by complication of labor and delivery, unspecified** ▽

✓4ᵗʰ **P04** **Newborn affected by noxious substances transmitted via placenta or breast milk**
     INCLUDES   nonteratogenic effects of substances transmitted via placenta
     EXCLUDES 2   *congenital malformations (Q00-Q99)*
         encounter for observation of newborn for suspected diseasesand conditions ruled out (Z05.-)
         neonatal jaundice from excessive hemolysis due to drugs or toxins transmitted from mother (P58.4)
         newborn in contact with and (suspected) exposures hazardous to health not transmitted via placenta or breast milk (Z77.-)

   P04.0 **Newborn affected by maternal anesthesia and analgesia in pregnancy, labor and delivery**
     ►Newborn affected by reactions and intoxications from maternal opiates and tranquilizers administered for procedures during pregnancy or labor and delivery◄
     EXCLUDES 2   ►*newborn affected by other maternal medication (P04.1-)*◄

√5ᵗʰ **P04.1** **Newborn affected by other maternal medication**
~~Newborn affected by cancer chemotherapy~~
~~Newborn affected by cytotoxic drugs~~
▶Code first withdrawal symptoms from maternal use of drugs of addiction, if applicable (P96.1)◀
　EXCLUDES 1　dysmorphism due to warfarin (Q86.2)
　　　fetal hydantoin syndrome (Q86.1)
　　　~~maternal use of drugs of addiction (P04.4-)~~
　EXCLUDES 2　▶maternal anesthesia and analgesia in pregnancy, labor and delivery (P04.0)◀
　　　▶maternal use of drugs of addiction (P04.4-)◀

● **P04.11** **Newborn affected by maternal antineoplastic chemotherapy**
● **P04.12** **Newborn affected by maternal cytotoxic drugs**
● **P04.13** **Newborn affected by maternal use of anticonvulsants**
● **P04.14** **Newborn affected by maternal use of opiates**
● **P04.15** **Newborn affected by maternal use of antidepressants**
● **P04.16** **Newborn affected by maternal use of amphetamines**
● **P04.17** **Newborn affected by maternal use of sedative-hypnotics**
● **P04.1A** **Newborn affected by maternal use of anxiolytics**
● **P04.18** **Newborn affected by other maternal medication**
● **P04.19** **Newborn affected by maternal use of unspecified medication** ▽

P04.2 **Newborn affected by maternal use of tobacco**
Newborn affected by exposure in utero to tobacco smoke
　EXCLUDES 2　newborn exposure to environmental tobacco smoke (P96.81)

P04.3 **Newborn affected by maternal use of alcohol**
　EXCLUDES 1　fetal alcohol syndrome (Q86.0)

√5ᵗʰ **P04.4** **Newborn affected by maternal use of drugs of addiction**
● **P04.40** **Newborn affected by maternal use of unspecified drugs of addiction** ▽
P04.41 **Newborn affected by maternal use of cocaine**
"Crack baby"
● **P04.42** **Newborn affected by maternal use of hallucinogens**
　EXCLUDES 2　newborn affected by other maternal medication (P04.1-)
P04.49 **Newborn affected by maternal use of other drugs of addiction**
　EXCLUDES 2　newborn affected by maternal anesthesia and analgesia (P04.0)
　　　withdrawal symptoms from maternal use of drugs of addiction (P96.1)

P04.5 **Newborn affected by maternal use of nutritional chemical substances**
P04.6 **Newborn affected by maternal exposure to environmental chemical substances**
√5ᵗʰ **P04.8** **Newborn affected by other maternal noxious substances**
● **P04.81** **Newborn affected by maternal use of cannabis**
● **P04.89** **Newborn affected by other maternal noxious substances**
P04.9 **Newborn affected by maternal noxious substance, unspecified** ▽

Disorders of newborn related to length of gestation and fetal growth (P05-P08)

√4ᵗʰ **P05** **Disorders of newborn related to slow fetal growth and fetal malnutrition**
AHA: 2016,4Q,55-56
√5ᵗʰ **P05.0** **Newborn light for gestational age**
Newborn light-for-dates
Weight below but length above 10th percentile for gestational age
P05.00 **Newborn light for gestational age, unspecified weight** ▽
P05.01 **Newborn light for gestational age, less than 500 grams**
P05.02 **Newborn light for gestational age, 500-749 grams**
P05.03 **Newborn light for gestational age, 750-999 grams**
P05.04 **Newborn light for gestational age, 1000-1249 grams**
P05.05 **Newborn light for gestational age, 1250-1499 grams**
P05.06 **Newborn light for gestational age, 1500-1749 grams**
P05.07 **Newborn light for gestational age, 1750-1999 grams**
P05.08 **Newborn light for gestational age, 2000-2499 grams**
P05.09 **Newborn light for gestational age, 2500 grams and over**
Newborn light for gestational age, other

√5ᵗʰ **P05.1** **Newborn small for gestational age**
Newborn small-and-light-for-dates
Newborn small-for-dates
Weight and length below 10th percentile for gestational age
P05.10 **Newborn small for gestational age, unspecified weight** ▽
P05.11 **Newborn small for gestational age, less than 500 grams**
P05.12 **Newborn small for gestational age, 500-749 grams**
P05.13 **Newborn small for gestational age, 750-999 grams**
P05.14 **Newborn small for gestational age, 1000-1249 grams**
P05.15 **Newborn small for gestational age, 1250-1499 grams**
P05.16 **Newborn small for gestational age, 1500-1749 grams**
P05.17 **Newborn small for gestational age, 1750-1999 grams**
P05.18 **Newborn small for gestational age, 2000-2499 grams**
P05.19 **Newborn small for gestational age, other**
Newborn small for gestational age, 2500 grams and over

P05.2 **Newborn affected by fetal (intrauterine) malnutrition not light or small for gestational age**
Infant, not light or small for gestational age, showing signs of fetal malnutrition, such as dry, peeling skin and loss of subcutaneous tissue
　EXCLUDES 1　newborn affected by fetal malnutrition with light for gestational age (P05.0-)
　　　newborn affected by fetal malnutrition with small for gestational age (P05.1-)

P05.9 **Newborn affected by slow intrauterine growth, unspecified** ▽
Newborn affected by fetal growth retardation NOS

√4ᵗʰ **P07** **Disorders of newborn related to short gestation and low birth weight, not elsewhere classified**
NOTE　When both birth weight and gestational age of the newborn are available, both should be coded with birth weight sequenced before gestational age
INCLUDES　the listed conditions, without further specification, as the cause of morbidity or additional care, in newborn

√5ᵗʰ **P07.0** **Extremely low birth weight newborn**
Newborn birth weight 999 g. or less
　EXCLUDES 1　low birth weight due to slow fetal growth and fetal malnutrition (P05.-)
P07.00 **Extremely low birth weight newborn, unspecified weight** ▽
P07.01 **Extremely low birth weight newborn, less than 500 grams**
P07.02 **Extremely low birth weight newborn, 500-749 grams**
P07.03 **Extremely low birth weight newborn, 750-999 grams**

√5ᵗʰ **P07.1** **Other low birth weight newborn**
Newborn birth weight 1000-2499 g.
　EXCLUDES 1　low birth weight due to slow fetal growth and fetal malnutrition (P05.-)
P07.10 **Other low birth weight newborn, unspecified weight** ▽
P07.14 **Other low birth weight newborn, 1000-1249 grams**
P07.15 **Other low birth weight newborn, 1250-1499 grams**
P07.16 **Other low birth weight newborn, 1500-1749 grams**
P07.17 **Other low birth weight newborn, 1750-1999 grams**
P07.18 **Other low birth weight newborn, 2000-2499 grams**

Chapter 16. Certain Conditions Originating in the Perinatal Period

P07.2–P11.9

✓5ᵗʰ **P07.2 Extreme immaturity of newborn**

Less than 28 completed weeks (less than 196 completed days) of gestation.

P07.20 Extreme immaturity of newborn, unspecified weeks of gestation ▽

Gestational age less than 28 completed weeks NOS

P07.21 Extreme immaturity of newborn, gestational age less than 23 completed weeks

Extreme immaturity of newborn, gestational age less than 23 weeks, 0 days

P07.22 Extreme immaturity of newborn, gestational age 23 completed weeks

Extreme immaturity of newborn, gestational age 23 weeks, 0 days through 23 weeks, 6 days

P07.23 Extreme immaturity of newborn, gestational age 24 completed weeks

Extreme immaturity of newborn, gestational age 24 weeks, 0 days through 24 weeks, 6 days

P07.24 Extreme immaturity of newborn, gestational age 25 completed weeks

Extreme immaturity of newborn, gestational age 25 weeks, 0 days through 25 weeks, 6 days

P07.25 Extreme immaturity of newborn, gestational age 26 completed weeks

Extreme immaturity of newborn, gestational age 26 weeks, 0 days through 26 weeks, 6 days

P07.26 Extreme immaturity of newborn, gestational age 27 completed weeks

Extreme immaturity of newborn, gestational age 27 weeks, 0 days through 27 weeks, 6 days

✓5ᵗʰ **P07.3 Preterm [premature] newborn [other]**

28 completed weeks or more but less than 37 completed weeks (196 completed days but less than 259 completed days) of gestation

Prematurity NOS

AHA: 2017,3Q,26

P07.30 Preterm newborn, unspecified weeks of gestation ▽

P07.31 Preterm newborn, gestational age 28 completed weeks

Preterm newborn, gestational age 28 weeks, 0 days through 28 weeks, 6 days

P07.32 Preterm newborn, gestational age 29 completed weeks

Preterm newborn, gestational age 29 weeks, 0 days through 29 weeks, 6 days

P07.33 Preterm newborn, gestational age 30 completed weeks

Preterm newborn, gestational age 30 weeks, 0 days through 30 weeks, 6 days

P07.34 Preterm newborn, gestational age 31 completed weeks

Preterm newborn, gestational age 31 weeks, 0 days through 31 weeks, 6 days

P07.35 Preterm newborn, gestational age 32 completed weeks

Preterm newborn, gestational age 32 weeks, 0 days through 32 weeks, 6 days

P07.36 Preterm newborn, gestational age 33 completed weeks

Preterm newborn, gestational age 33 weeks, 0 days through 33 weeks, 6 days

P07.37 Preterm newborn, gestational age 34 completed weeks

Preterm newborn, gestational age 34 weeks, 0 days through 34 weeks, 6 days

P07.38 Preterm newborn, gestational age 35 completed weeks

Preterm newborn, gestational age 35 weeks, 0 days through 35 weeks, 6 days

P07.39 Preterm newborn, gestational age 36 completed weeks

Preterm newborn, gestational age 36 weeks, 0 days through 36 weeks, 6 days

✓4ᵗʰ **P08 Disorders of newborn related to long gestation and high birth weight**

NOTE   When both birth weight and gestational age of the newborn are available, priority of assignment should be given to birth weight

INCLUDES   the listed conditions, without further specification, as causes of morbidity or additional care, in newborn

P08.0 Exceptionally large newborn baby

Usually implies a birth weight of 4500 g. or more

EXCLUDES 1   syndrome of infant of diabetic mother (P70.1)

syndrome of infant of mother with gestational diabetes (P70.0)

P08.1 Other heavy for gestational age newborn

Other newborn heavy- or large-for-dates regardless of period of gestation

Usually implies a birth weight of 4000 g. to 4499 g.

EXCLUDES 1   newborn with a birth weight of 4500 or more (P08.0)

syndrome of infant of diabetic mother (P70.1)

syndrome of infant of mother with gestational diabetes (P70.0).

✓5ᵗʰ **P08.2 Late newborn, not heavy for gestational age**

AHA: 2014,1Q,14

P08.21 Post-term newborn

Newborn with gestation period over 40 completed weeks to 42 completed weeks

P08.22 Prolonged gestation of newborn

Newborn with gestation period over 42 completed weeks (294 days or more), not heavy- or large-for-dates.

Postmaturity NOS

Abnormal findings on neonatal screening (P09)

P09 Abnormal findings on neonatal screening

Use additional code to identify signs, symptoms and conditions associated with the screening

EXCLUDES 2   nonspecific serologic evidence of human immunodeficiency virus [HIV] (R75)

Birth trauma (P10-P15)

✓4ᵗʰ **P10 Intracranial laceration and hemorrhage due to birth injury**

EXCLUDES 1   intracranial hemorrhage of newborn NOS (P52.9)

intracranial hemorrhage of newborn due to anoxia or hypoxia (P52.-)

nontraumatic intracranial hemorrhage of newborn (P52.-)

P10.0 Subdural hemorrhage due to birth injury

Subdural hematoma (localized) due to birth injury

EXCLUDES 1   subdural hemorrhage accompanying tentorial tear (P10.4)

P10.1 Cerebral hemorrhage due to birth injury

P10.2 Intraventricular hemorrhage due to birth injury

P10.3 Subarachnoid hemorrhage due to birth injury

P10.4 Tentorial tear due to birth injury

P10.8 Other intracranial lacerations and hemorrhages due to birth injury

P10.9 Unspecified intracranial laceration and hemorrhage due to birth injury ▽

✓4ᵗʰ **P11 Other birth injuries to central nervous system**

P11.0 Cerebral edema due to birth injury

P11.1 Other specified brain damage due to birth injury

P11.2 Unspecified brain damage due to birth injury ▽

P11.3 Birth injury to facial nerve

Facial palsy due to birth injury

P11.4 Birth injury to other cranial nerves

P11.5 Birth injury to spine and spinal cord

Fracture of spine due to birth injury

P11.9 Birth injury to central nervous system, unspecified ▽

☑4ᵗʰ **P12 Birth injury to scalp**

Birth Injuries to Scalp

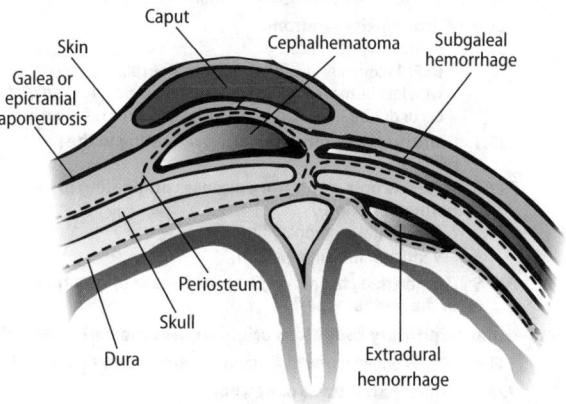

☑4ᵗʰ Caput
Cephalhematoma
Subgaleal hemorrhage
Skin
Galea or epicranial aponeurosis
Periosteum
Skull
Dura
Extradural hemorrhage

P12.0 Cephalhematoma due to birth injury
DEF: Condition that occurs in a neonate when blood vessels between the skull and periosteum rupture and blood collects in the subperiosteal space (below the periosteum). It is typically caused by prolonged labor or trauma due to instrument-assisted delivery (e.g., forceps, vacuum extraction), although in rare circumstances, it may indicate a linear skull fracture with intracranial hemorrhage.

P12.1 Chignon (from vacuum extraction) due to birth injury
DEF: Artificial swelling of the scalp that occurs when a collection of interstitial fluid and blood forms in the area of the scalp where the suction cup was applied during a vacuum-assisted delivery.

P12.2 Epicranial subaponeurotic hemorrhage due to birth injury
Subgaleal hemorrhage

P12.3 Bruising of scalp due to birth injury

P12.4 Injury of scalp of newborn due to monitoring equipment
Sampling incision of scalp of newborn
Scalp clip (electrode) injury of newborn

☑5ᵗʰ **P12.8 Other birth injuries to scalp**

P12.81 Caput succedaneum
DEF: Swelling of the scalp as a result of pressure being exerted on the head from the vaginal walls, uterus, or instrumentation used in assisting a delivery (e.g., vacuum).

P12.89 Other birth injuries to scalp

P12.9 Birth injury to scalp, unspecified   ▽

☑4ᵗʰ **P13 Birth injury to skeleton**
EXCLUDES 2 birth injury to spine (P11.5)

P13.0 Fracture of skull due to birth injury

P13.1 Other birth injuries to skull
EXCLUDES 1 cephalhematoma (P12.0)

P13.2 Birth injury to femur

P13.3 Birth injury to other long bones

P13.4 Fracture of clavicle due to birth injury

P13.8 Birth injuries to other parts of skeleton

P13.9 Birth injury to skeleton, unspecified   ▽

☑4ᵗʰ **P14 Birth injury to peripheral nervous system**

P14.0 Erb's paralysis due to birth injury
DEF: Erb's paralysis: Most common type of brachial plexus (peripheral nerve) injury in a neonate that involves nerve damage at the level of C5-C6. **Synonym(s):** Erb's palsy

P14.1 Klumpke's paralysis due to birth injury

P14.2 Phrenic nerve paralysis due to birth injury

P14.3 Other brachial plexus birth injuries

P14.8 Birth injuries to other parts of peripheral nervous system

P14.9 Birth injury to peripheral nervous system, unspecified   ▽

☑4ᵗʰ **P15 Other birth injuries**

P15.0 Birth injury to liver
Rupture of liver due to birth injury

P15.1 Birth injury to spleen
Rupture of spleen due to birth injury

P15.2 Sternomastoid injury due to birth injury

P15.3 Birth injury to eye
Subconjunctival hemorrhage due to birth injury
Traumatic glaucoma due to birth injury

P15.4 Birth injury to face
Facial congestion due to birth injury

P15.5 Birth injury to external genitalia

P15.6 Subcutaneous fat necrosis due to birth injury

P15.8 Other specified birth injuries
TIP: Use for any injury of newborn from scalpel.

P15.9 Birth injury, unspecified   ▽

Respiratory and cardiovascular disorders specific to the perinatal period (P19-P29)

☑4ᵗʰ **P19 Metabolic acidemia in newborn**
INCLUDES metabolic acidemia in newborn

P19.0 Metabolic acidemia in newborn first noted before onset of labor

P19.1 Metabolic acidemia in newborn first noted during labor

P19.2 Metabolic acidemia noted at birth

P19.9 Metabolic acidemia, unspecified   ▽

☑4ᵗʰ **P22 Respiratory distress of newborn**
EXCLUDES 1 respiratory arrest of newborn (P28.81)
respiratory failure of newborn NOS (P28.5)

P22.0 Respiratory distress syndrome of newborn
Cardiorespiratory distress syndrome of newborn
Hyaline membrane disease
Idiopathic respiratory distress syndrome [IRDS or RDS] of newborn
Pulmonary hypoperfusion syndrome
Respiratory distress syndrome, type I
DEF: Severe chest contractions upon air intake and expiratory grunting. The infant appears blue due to oxygen deficiency and has a rapid respiratory rate, formerly called hyaline membrane disease.

P22.1 Transient tachypnea of newborn
Idiopathic tachypnea of newborn
Respiratory distress syndrome, type II
Wet lung syndrome
DEF: Rapid, labored breathing of a newborn. It is a short-term problem that begins after birth and lasts about three days.

P22.8 Other respiratory distress of newborn

P22.9 Respiratory distress of newborn, unspecified   ▽

☑4ᵗʰ **P23 Congenital pneumonia**
.   INCLUDES infective pneumonia acquired in utero or during birth
EXCLUDES 1 neonatal pneumonia resulting from aspiration (P24.-)

P23.0 Congenital pneumonia due to viral agent
Use additional code (B97) to identify organism
EXCLUDES 1 congenital rubella pneumonitis (P35.0)

P23.1 Congenital pneumonia due to Chlamydia

P23.2 Congenital pneumonia due to staphylococcus

P23.3 Congenital pneumonia due to streptococcus, group B

P23.4 Congenital pneumonia due to Escherichia coli

P23.5 Congenital pneumonia due to Pseudomonas

P23.6 Congenital pneumonia due to other bacterial agents
Congenital pneumonia due to Hemophilus influenzae
Congenital pneumonia due to Klebsiella pneumoniae
Congenital pneumonia due to Mycoplasma
Congenital pneumonia due to Streptococcus, except group B
Use additional code (B95-B96) to identify organism

P23.8 Congenital pneumonia due to other organisms

P23.9 Congenital pneumonia, unspecified   ▽

☑4ᵗʰ **P24 Neonatal aspiration**
INCLUDES aspiration in utero and during delivery

☑5ᵗʰ **P24.0 Meconium aspiration**
EXCLUDES 1 meconium passage (without aspiration) during delivery (P03.82)
meconium staining (P96.83)

P24.00 Meconium aspiration without respiratory symptoms
Meconium aspiration NOS

☑ Additional Character Req   ✓x7ᵗʰ Placeholder Alert   Manifestation   ▽ Unspecified   ▶◀ Revised Text   ● New Code   ▲ Revised Code Title

P24.Ø1   **Meconium aspiration with respiratory symptoms**
Meconium aspiration pneumonia
Meconium aspiration pneumonitis
Meconium aspiration syndrome NOS
Use additional code to identify any secondary pulmonary hypertension, if applicable (I27.2-)
DEF: Aspiration of fetal intestinal material during or prior to delivery. If is usually a complication of placental insufficiency, causing pneumonitis and bronchial obstruction (inflammatory reaction of lungs).

✓5ᵗʰ **P24.1**   **Neonatal aspiration of (clear) amniotic fluid and mucus**
Neonatal aspiration of liquor (amnii)

     P24.1Ø   **Neonatal aspiration of (clear) amniotic fluid and mucus without respiratory symptoms**
Neonatal aspiration of amniotic fluid and mucus NOS

     P24.11   **Neonatal aspiration of (clear) amniotic fluid and mucus with respiratory symptoms**
Neonatal aspiration of amniotic fluid and mucus with pneumonia
Neonatal aspiration of amniotic fluid and mucus with pneumonitis
Use additional code to identify any secondary pulmonary hypertension, if applicable (I27.2-)

✓5ᵗʰ **P24.2**   **Neonatal aspiration of blood**

     P24.2Ø   **Neonatal aspiration of blood without respiratory symptoms**
Neonatal aspiration of blood NOS

     P24.21   **Neonatal aspiration of blood with respiratory symptoms**
Neonatal aspiration of blood with pneumonia
Neonatal aspiration of blood with pneumonitis
Use additional code to identify any secondary pulmonary hypertension, if applicable (I27.2-)

✓5ᵗʰ **P24.3**   **Neonatal aspiration of milk and regurgitated food**
Neonatal aspiration of stomach contents

     P24.3Ø   **Neonatal aspiration of milk and regurgitated food without respiratory symptoms**
Neonatal aspiration of milk and regurgitated food NOS

     P24.31   **Neonatal aspiration of milk and regurgitated food with respiratory symptoms**
Neonatal aspiration of milk and regurgitated food with pneumonia
Neonatal aspiration of milk and regurgitated food with pneumonitis
Use additional code to identify any secondary pulmonary hypertension, if applicable (I27.2-)

✓5ᵗʰ **P24.8**   **Other neonatal aspiration**

     P24.8Ø   **Other neonatal aspiration without respiratory symptoms**
Neonatal aspiration NEC

     P24.81   **Other neonatal aspiration with respiratory symptoms**
Neonatal aspiration pneumonia NEC
Neonatal aspiration with pneumonitis NEC
Neonatal aspiration with pneumonia NOS
Neonatal aspiration with pneumonitis NOS
Use additional code to identify any secondary pulmonary hypertension, if applicable (I27.2-)

     P24.9   **Neonatal aspiration, unspecified**   ▽

✓4ᵗʰ **P25**   **Interstitial emphysema and related conditions originating in the perinatal period**

     P25.Ø   **Interstitial emphysema originating in the perinatal period**

     P25.1   **Pneumothorax originating in the perinatal period**

     P25.2   **Pneumomediastinum originating in the perinatal period**

     P25.3   **Pneumopericardium originating in the perinatal period**

     P25.8   **Other conditions related to interstitial emphysema originating in the perinatal period**

✓4ᵗʰ **P26**   **Pulmonary hemorrhage originating in the perinatal period**
     EXCLUDES 1   *acute idiopathic hemorrhage in infants over 28 days old (RØ4.81)*

     P26.Ø   **Tracheobronchial hemorrhage originating in the perinatal period**

     P26.1   **Massive pulmonary hemorrhage originating in the perinatal period**

     P26.8   **Other pulmonary hemorrhages originating in the perinatal period**

     P26.9   **Unspecified pulmonary hemorrhage originating in the perinatal period**   ▽

✓4ᵗʰ **P27**   **Chronic respiratory disease originating in the perinatal period**
     EXCLUDES 2   *respiratory distress of newborn (P22.Ø-P22.9)*

     P27.Ø   **Wilson-Mikity syndrome**
Pulmonary dysmaturity
DEF: Pulmonary insufficiency in newborn babies, especially those with low birth weight. Rapid onset of hypercapnia and cyanosis occur during the first month of life frequently resulting in death.

     P27.1   **Bronchopulmonary dysplasia originating in the perinatal period**

     P27.8   **Other chronic respiratory diseases originating in the perinatal period**
Congenital pulmonary fibrosis
Ventilator lung in newborn

     P27.9   **Unspecified chronic respiratory disease originating in the perinatal period**   ▽

✓4ᵗʰ **P28**   **Other respiratory conditions originating in the perinatal period**
     EXCLUDES 1   *congenital malformations of the respiratory system (Q3Ø-Q34)*

     P28.Ø   **Primary atelectasis of newborn**
Primary failure to expand terminal respiratory units
Pulmonary hypoplasia associated with short gestation
Pulmonary immaturity NOS

✓5ᵗʰ **P28.1**   **Other and unspecified atelectasis of newborn**

     P28.1Ø   **Unspecified atelectasis of newborn**   ▽
Atelectasis of newborn NOS

     P28.11   **Resorption atelectasis without respiratory distress syndrome**
     EXCLUDES 1   *resorption atelectasis with respiratory distress syndrome (P22.Ø)*

     P28.19   **Other atelectasis of newborn**
Partial atelectasis of newborn
Secondary atelectasis of newborn

     P28.2   **Cyanotic attacks of newborn**
     EXCLUDES 1   *apnea of newborn (P28.3-P28.4)*

     P28.3   **Primary sleep apnea of newborn**
Central sleep apnea of newborn
Obstructive sleep apnea of newborn
Sleep apnea of newborn NOS
DEF: Unexplained cessation of breathing when a neonate makes no respiratory effort for 20 seconds or longer or when a neonate's breathing cessation is accompanied by cyanosis, bradycardia, or hypotonia.

     P28.4   **Other apnea of newborn**
Apnea of prematurity
Obstructive apnea of newborn
     EXCLUDES 1   *obstructive sleep apnea of newborn (P28.3)*

     P28.5   **Respiratory failure of newborn**
     EXCLUDES 1   *respiratory arrest of newborn (P28.81)*
                   respiratory distress of newborn (P22.Ø-)

✓5ᵗʰ **P28.8**   **Other specified respiratory conditions of newborn**

     P28.81   **Respiratory arrest of newborn**

     P28.89   **Other specified respiratory conditions of newborn**
Congenital laryngeal stridor
Sniffles in newborn
Snuffles in newborn
     EXCLUDES 1   *early congenital syphilitic rhinitis (A5Ø.Ø5)*

     P28.9   **Respiratory condition of newborn, unspecified**   ▽
Respiratory depression in newborn

✓4ᵗʰ **P29**   **Cardiovascular disorders originating in the perinatal period**
     EXCLUDES 1   *congenital malformations of the circulatory system (Q2Ø-Q28)*

     P29.Ø   **Neonatal cardiac failure**

✓5ᵗʰ **P29.1**   **Neonatal cardiac dysrhythmia**

     P29.11   **Neonatal tachycardia**

     P29.12   **Neonatal bradycardia**

     P29.2   **Neonatal hypertension**

✓5ᵗʰ **P29.3**   **Persistent fetal circulation**
AHA: 2017,4Q,20-21

     P29.3Ø   **Pulmonary hypertension of newborn**
Persistent pulmonary hypertension of newborn
DEF: Condition that occurs when pressure within the pulmonary artery is elevated and vascular resistance is observed in the lungs.

     P29.38   **Other persistent fetal circulation**
Delayed closure of ductus arteriosus

     P29.4   **Transient myocardial ischemia in newborn**

✓5ᵗʰ **P29.8** **Other cardiovascular disorders originating in the perinatal period**
    P29.81 **Cardiac arrest of newborn**
    P29.89 **Other cardiovascular disorders originating in the perinatal period**
        AHA: 2014,4Q,23
  P29.9 **Cardiovascular disorder originating in the perinatal period, unspecified** ▽

Infections specific to the perinatal period (P35-P39)

Infections acquired in utero, during birth via the umbilicus, or during the first 28 days after birth

EXCLUDES 2   *asymptomatic human immunodeficiency virus [HIV] infection status (Z21)*
    congenital gonococcal infection (A54.-)
    congenital pneumonia (P23.-)
    congenital syphilis (A50.-)
    human immunodeficiency virus [HIV] disease (B20)
    infant botulism (A48.51)
    infectious diseases not specific to the perinatal period (A00-B99, J09, J10.-)
    intestinal infectious disease (A00-A09)
    laboratory evidence of human immunodeficiency virus [HIV] (R75)
    tetanus neonatorum (A33)

✓4ᵗʰ **P35** **Congenital viral diseases**
  INCLUDES   infections acquired in utero or during birth
  P35.0 **Congenital rubella syndrome**
    Congenital rubella pneumonitis
  P35.1 **Congenital cytomegalovirus infection**
  P35.2 **Congenital herpesviral [herpes simplex] infection**
  P35.3 **Congenital viral hepatitis**
●   **P35.4** **Congenital Zika virus disease**
    Use additional code to identify manifestations of congenital Zika virus disease
  P35.8 **Other congenital viral diseases**
    Congenital varicella [chickenpox]
  P35.9 **Congenital viral disease, unspecified** ▽

✓4ᵗʰ **P36** **Bacterial sepsis of newborn**
  INCLUDES   congenital sepsis
  Use additional code(s), if applicable, to identify severe sepsis (R65.2-) and associated acute organ dysfunction(s)
  P36.0 **Sepsis of newborn due to streptococcus, group B** HCC
✓5ᵗʰ   **P36.1** **Sepsis of newborn due to other and unspecified streptococci**
    P36.10 **Sepsis of newborn due to unspecified streptococci** HCC ▽
    P36.19 **Sepsis of newborn due to other streptococci** HCC
  P36.2 **Sepsis of newborn due to Staphylococcus aureus** HCC
✓5ᵗʰ   **P36.3** **Sepsis of newborn due to other and unspecified staphylococci**
    P36.30 **Sepsis of newborn due to unspecified staphylococci** HCC ▽
    P36.39 **Sepsis of newborn due to other staphylococci** HCC
  P36.4 **Sepsis of newborn due to Escherichia coli** HCC
  P36.5 **Sepsis of newborn due to anaerobes** HCC
  P36.8 **Other bacterial sepsis of newborn** HCC
    Use additional code from category B96 to identify organism
  P36.9 **Bacterial sepsis of newborn, unspecified** HCC ▽

✓4ᵗʰ **P37** **Other congenital infectious and parasitic diseases**
  EXCLUDES 2   *congenital syphilis (A50.-)*
    infectious neonatal diarrhea (A00-A09)
    necrotizing enterocolitis in newborn (P77.-)
    noninfectious neonatal diarrhea (P78.3)
    ophthalmia neonatorum due to gonococcus (A54.31)
    tetanus neonatorum (A33)
  P37.0 **Congenital tuberculosis**
  P37.1 **Congenital toxoplasmosis**
    Hydrocephalus due to congenital toxoplasmosis
  P37.2 **Neonatal (disseminated) listeriosis**
  P37.3 **Congenital falciparum malaria**
  P37.4 **Other congenital malaria**
  P37.5 **Neonatal candidiasis**
  P37.8 **Other specified congenital infectious and parasitic diseases**
  P37.9 **Congenital infectious or parasitic disease, unspecified** ▽

✓4ᵗʰ **P38** **Omphalitis of newborn**
  EXCLUDES 1   *omphalitis not of newborn (L08.82)*
    tetanus omphalitis (A33)
    umbilical hemorrhage of newborn (P51.-)
  DEF: Omphalitis: Infection and inflammation of the umbilical stump, often due to bacteria that can spread beyond the umbilical stump to the fascia, muscle, or even the umbilical vessels.
  P38.1 **Omphalitis with mild hemorrhage**
  P38.9 **Omphalitis without hemorrhage**
    Omphalitis of newborn NOS

✓4ᵗʰ **P39** **Other infections specific to the perinatal period**
  Use additional code to identify organism or specific infection
  P39.0 **Neonatal infective mastitis**
    EXCLUDES 1   *breast engorgement of newborn (P83.4)*
        noninfective mastitis of newborn (P83.4)
  P39.1 **Neonatal conjunctivitis and dacryocystitis**
    Neonatal chlamydial conjunctivitis
    Ophthalmia neonatorum NOS
    EXCLUDES 1   *gonococcal conjunctivitis (A54.31)*
  P39.2 **Intra-amniotic infection affecting newborn, not elsewhere classified**
  P39.3 **Neonatal urinary tract infection**
  P39.4 **Neonatal skin infection**
    Neonatal pyoderma
    EXCLUDES 1   *pemphigus neonatorum (L00)*
        staphylococcal scalded skin syndrome (L00)
  P39.8 **Other specified infections specific to the perinatal period**
  P39.9 **Infection specific to the perinatal period, unspecified** ▽

Hemorrhagic and hematological disorders of newborn (P50-P61)

EXCLUDES 1   *congenital stenosis and stricture of bile ducts (Q44.3)*
    Crigler-Najjar syndrome (E80.5)
    Dubin-Johnson syndrome (E80.6)
    Gilbert syndrome (E80.4)
    hereditary hemolytic anemias (D55-D58)

✓4ᵗʰ **P50** **Newborn affected by intrauterine (fetal) blood loss**
  EXCLUDES 1   *congenital anemia from intrauterine (fetal) blood loss (P61.3)*
  P50.0 **Newborn affected by intrauterine (fetal) blood loss from vasa previa**
  P50.1 **Newborn affected by intrauterine (fetal) blood loss from ruptured cord**
  P50.2 **Newborn affected by intrauterine (fetal) blood loss from placenta**
  P50.3 **Newborn affected by hemorrhage into co-twin**
  P50.4 **Newborn affected by hemorrhage into maternal circulation**
  P50.5 **Newborn affected by intrauterine (fetal) blood loss from cut end of co-twin's cord**
  P50.8 **Newborn affected by other intrauterine (fetal) blood loss**
  P50.9 **Newborn affected by intrauterine (fetal) blood loss, unspecified** ▽
    Newborn affected by fetal hemorrhage NOS

✓4ᵗʰ **P51** **Umbilical hemorrhage of newborn**
  EXCLUDES 1   *omphalitis with mild hemorrhage (P38.1)*
    umbilical hemorrhage from cut end of co-twins cord (P50.5)
  P51.0 **Massive umbilical hemorrhage of newborn**
  P51.8 **Other umbilical hemorrhages of newborn**
    Slipped umbilical ligature NOS
  P51.9 **Umbilical hemorrhage of newborn, unspecified** ▽

✓4ᵗʰ **P52** **Intracranial nontraumatic hemorrhage of newborn**
  INCLUDES   intracranial hemorrhage due to anoxia or hypoxia
  EXCLUDES 1   *intracranial hemorrhage due to birth injury (P10.-)*
    intracranial hemorrhage due to other injury (S06.-)
  P52.0 **Intraventricular (nontraumatic) hemorrhage, grade 1, of newborn**
    Subependymal hemorrhage (without intraventricular extension)
    Bleeding into germinal matrix
  P52.1 **Intraventricular (nontraumatic) hemorrhage, grade 2, of newborn**
    Subependymal hemorrhage with intraventricular extension
    Bleeding into ventricle

✓5ᵗʰ **P52.2 Intraventricular (nontraumatic) hemorrhage, grade 3 and grade 4, of newborn**

     P52.21 Intraventricular (nontraumatic) hemorrhage, grade 3, of newborn
Subependymal hemorrhage with intraventricular extension with enlargement of ventricle

     P52.22 Intraventricular (nontraumatic) hemorrhage, grade 4, of newborn
Bleeding into cerebral cortex
Subependymal hemorrhage with intracerebral extension

P52.3 Unspecified intraventricular (nontraumatic) hemorrhage of newborn   ▽

P52.4 Intracerebral (nontraumatic) hemorrhage of newborn

P52.5 Subarachnoid (nontraumatic) hemorrhage of newborn

P52.6 Cerebellar (nontraumatic) and posterior fossa hemorrhage of newborn

P52.8 Other intracranial (nontraumatic) hemorrhages of newborn

P52.9 Intracranial (nontraumatic) hemorrhage of newborn, unspecified   ▽

P53 Hemorrhagic disease of newborn
Vitamin K deficiency of newborn

✓4ᵗʰ **P54 Other neonatal hemorrhages**

   EXCLUDES 1   *newborn affected by (intrauterine) blood loss (P50.-)*
pulmonary hemorrhage originating in the perinatal period (P26.-)

P54.0 Neonatal hematemesis
   EXCLUDES 1   *neonatal hematemesis due to swallowed maternal blood (P78.2)*

P54.1 Neonatal melena
   EXCLUDES 1   *neonatal melena due to swallowed maternal blood (P78.2)*

P54.2 Neonatal rectal hemorrhage

P54.3 Other neonatal gastrointestinal hemorrhage

P54.4 Neonatal adrenal hemorrhage

P54.5 Neonatal cutaneous hemorrhage
Neonatal bruising
Neonatal ecchymoses
Neonatal petechiae
Neonatal superficial hematomata
   EXCLUDES 2   *bruising of scalp due to birth injury (P12.3)*
cephalhematoma due to birth injury (P12.0)

P54.6 Neonatal vaginal hemorrhage   ♀
Neonatal pseudomenses

P54.8 Other specified neonatal hemorrhages

P54.9 Neonatal hemorrhage, unspecified   ▽

✓4ᵗʰ **P55 Hemolytic disease of newborn**

P55.0 Rh isoimmunization of newborn
DEF: Incompatible Rh fetal-maternal blood grouping that prematurely destroys red blood cells. Symptoms include jaundice, asphyxia, pulmonary hypertension, edema, respiratory distress, kernicterus, and coagulopathies. It is detected by a Coombs test.

P55.1 ABO isoimmunization of newborn
AHA: 2015,3Q,20

P55.8 Other hemolytic diseases of newborn

P55.9 Hemolytic disease of newborn, unspecified   ▽

✓4ᵗʰ **P56 Hydrops fetalis due to hemolytic disease**

   EXCLUDES 1   *hydrops fetalis NOS (P83.2)*

P56.0 Hydrops fetalis due to isoimmunization

✓5ᵗʰ **P56.9 Hydrops fetalis due to other and unspecified hemolytic disease**

     P56.90 Hydrops fetalis due to unspecified hemolytic disease   ▽

     P56.99 Hydrops fetalis due to other hemolytic disease

✓4ᵗʰ **P57 Kernicterus**

P57.0 Kernicterus due to isoimmunization
DEF: Complication of erythroblastosis fetalis associated with severe neural symptoms, high blood bilirubin levels, and nerve cell destruction. It results in bilirubin-pigmented gray matter of the central nervous system.

P57.8 Other specified kernicterus
   EXCLUDES 1   *Crigler-Najjar syndrome (E80.5)*

P57.9 Kernicterus, unspecified   ▽

✓4ᵗʰ **P58 Neonatal jaundice due to other excessive hemolysis**

   EXCLUDES 1   *jaundice due to isoimmunization (P55-P57)*

P58.0 Neonatal jaundice due to bruising

P58.1 Neonatal jaundice due to bleeding

P58.2 Neonatal jaundice due to infection

P58.3 Neonatal jaundice due to polycythemia

✓5ᵗʰ **P58.4 Neonatal jaundice due to drugs or toxins transmitted from mother or given to newborn**
Code first poisoning due to drug or toxin, if applicable (T36-T65 with fifth or sixth character 1-4 or 6)
Use additional code for adverse effect, if applicable, to identify drug (T36-T50 with fifth or sixth character 5)

     P58.41 Neonatal jaundice due to drugs or toxins transmitted from mother

     P58.42 Neonatal jaundice due to drugs or toxins given to newborn

P58.5 Neonatal jaundice due to swallowed maternal blood

P58.8 Neonatal jaundice due to other specified excessive hemolysis

P58.9 Neonatal jaundice due to excessive hemolysis, unspecified   ▽

✓4ᵗʰ **P59 Neonatal jaundice from other and unspecified causes**

   EXCLUDES 1   *jaundice due to inborn errors of metabolism (E70-E88)*
kernicterus (P57.-)

P59.0 Neonatal jaundice associated with preterm delivery
Hyperbilirubinemia of prematurity
Jaundice due to delayed conjugation associated with preterm delivery

P59.1 Inspissated bile syndrome
DEF: Biliary obstruction in newborn resulting from obstruction of outflow tract.

✓5ᵗʰ **P59.2 Neonatal jaundice from other and unspecified hepatocellular damage**
   EXCLUDES 1   *congenital viral hepatitis (P35.3)*

     P59.20 Neonatal jaundice from unspecified hepatocellular damage   ▽

     P59.29 Neonatal jaundice from other hepatocellular damage
Neonatal giant cell hepatitis
Neonatal (idiopathic) hepatitis

P59.3 Neonatal jaundice from breast milk inhibitor

P59.8 Neonatal jaundice from other specified causes

P59.9 Neonatal jaundice, unspecified   ▽
Neonatal physiological jaundice (intense)(prolonged) NOS
AHA: 2015,3Q,20

P60 Disseminated intravascular coagulation of newborn
Defibrination syndrome of newborn

✓4ᵗʰ **P61 Other perinatal hematological disorders**

   EXCLUDES 1   *transient hypogammaglobulinemia of infancy (D80.7)*

P61.0 Transient neonatal thrombocytopenia
Neonatal thrombocytopenia due to exchange transfusion
Neonatal thrombocytopenia due to idiopathic maternal thrombocytopenia
Neonatal thrombocytopenia due to isoimmunization
DEF: Temporary decrease in blood platelets of a newborn that is secondary to placental insufficiency.

P61.1 Polycythemia neonatorum
DEF: Abnormal increase of total red blood cells of a newborn that results in hyperviscosity, which slows the flow of blood through small blood vessels.

P61.2 Anemia of prematurity

P61.3 Congenital anemia from fetal blood loss

P61.4 Other congenital anemias, not elsewhere classified
Congenital anemia NOS

P61.5 Transient neonatal neutropenia
   EXCLUDES 1   *congenital neutropenia (nontransient) (D70.0)*
DEF: Low blood neutrophil counts of newborn that occurs due to maternal hypertension, sepsis, twin-twin transfusion, alloimmunization, and hemolytic disease.

P61.6 Other transient neonatal disorders of coagulation

P61.8 Other specified perinatal hematological disorders

P61.9 Perinatal hematological disorder, unspecified   ▽

HCC CMS-HCC   ℚ QPP   ℕ Newborn : 0   ℙ Pediatric : 0-17   𝕄 Maternity : 12-55   🄰 Adult : 15-124

Transitory endocrine and metabolic disorders specific to newborn (P70-P74)

INCLUDES transitory endocrine and metabolic disturbances caused by the infant's response to maternal endocrine and metabolic factors, or its adjustment to extrauterine environment

AHA: 2018,2Q,6

✓4ᵗʰ **P70 Transitory disorders of carbohydrate metabolism specific to newborn**

  P70.0 Syndrome of infant of mother with gestational diabetes
Newborn (with hypoglycemia) affected by maternal gestational diabetes
EXCLUDES 1 *newborn (with hypoglycemia) affected by maternal (pre-existing) diabetes mellitus (P70.1)*
syndrome of infant of a diabetic mother (P70.1)

  P70.1 Syndrome of infant of a diabetic mother
Newborn (with hypoglycemia) affected by maternal (pre-existing) diabetes mellitus
EXCLUDES 1 *newborn (with hypoglycemia) affected by maternal gestational diabetes (P70.0)*
syndrome of infant of mother with gestational diabetes (P70.0)

  P70.2 Neonatal diabetes mellitus

  P70.3 Iatrogenic neonatal hypoglycemia

  P70.4 Other neonatal hypoglycemia
Transitory neonatal hypoglycemia

  P70.8 Other transitory disorders of carbohydrate metabolism of newborn

  P70.9 Transitory disorder of carbohydrate metabolism of newborn, unspecified ▽

✓4ᵗʰ **P71 Transitory neonatal disorders of calcium and magnesium metabolism**

  P71.0 Cow's milk hypocalcemia in newborn

  P71.1 Other neonatal hypocalcemia
EXCLUDES 1 *neonatal hypoparathyroidism (P71.4)*

  P71.2 Neonatal hypomagnesemia

  P71.3 Neonatal tetany without calcium or magnesium deficiency
Neonatal tetany NOS

  P71.4 Transitory neonatal hypoparathyroidism

  P71.8 Other transitory neonatal disorders of calcium and magnesium metabolism
AHA: 2016,4Q,54

  P71.9 Transitory neonatal disorder of calcium and magnesium metabolism, unspecified ▽

✓4ᵗʰ **P72 Other transitory neonatal endocrine disorders**
EXCLUDES 1 *congenital hypothyroidism with or without goiter (E03.0-E03.1)*
dyshormogenetic goiter (E07.1)
Pendred's syndrome (E07.1)

  P72.0 Neonatal goiter, not elsewhere classified
Transitory congenital goiter with normal functioning

  P72.1 Transitory neonatal hyperthyroidism
Neonatal thyrotoxicosis

  P72.2 Other transitory neonatal disorders of thyroid function, not elsewhere classified
Transitory neonatal hypothyroidism

  P72.8 Other specified transitory neonatal endocrine disorders

  P72.9 Transitory neonatal endocrine disorder, unspecified ▽

✓4ᵗʰ **P74 Other transitory neonatal electrolyte and metabolic disturbances**

  P74.0 Late metabolic acidosis of newborn
EXCLUDES 1 *(fetal) metabolic acidosis of newborn (P19)*

  P74.1 Dehydration of newborn

  ✓5ᵗʰ **P74.2 Disturbances of sodium balance of newborn**

    P74.21 Hypernatremia of newborn

    P74.22 Hyponatremia of newborn

  ✓5ᵗʰ **P74.3 Disturbances of potassium balance of newborn**

    P74.31 Hyperkalemia of newborn

    P74.32 Hypokalemia of newborn

  ✓5ᵗʰ **P74.4 Other transitory electrolyte disturbances of newborn**

    P74.41 Alkalosis of newborn
Hyperbicarbonatemia

    ✓6ᵗʰ **P74.42 Disturbances of chlorine balance of newborn**

      P74.421 Hyperchloremia of newborn
Hyperchloremic metabolic acidosis
EXCLUDES 2 *late metabolic acidosis of the newborn (P77.0)*

      P74.422 Hypochloremia of newborn

    P74.49 Other transitory electrolyte disturbance of newborn

  P74.5 Transitory tyrosinemia of newborn

  P74.6 Transitory hyperammonemia of newborn

  P74.8 Other transitory metabolic disturbances of newborn
Amino-acid metabolic disorders described as transitory

  P74.9 Transitory metabolic disturbance of newborn, unspecified ▽

Digestive system disorders of newborn (P76-P78)

✓4ᵗʰ **P76 Other intestinal obstruction of newborn**

  P76.0 Meconium plug syndrome
Meconium ileus NOS
EXCLUDES 1 *meconium ileus in cystic fibrosis (E84.11)*
DEF: Meconium obstruction of a newborn's intestines, resulting from unusually thick or hard meconium.

  P76.1 Transitory ileus of newborn
EXCLUDES 1 *Hirschsprung's disease (Q43.1)*

  P76.2 Intestinal obstruction due to inspissated milk

  P76.8 Other specified intestinal obstruction of newborn
EXCLUDES 1 *intestinal obstruction classifiable to K56.-*

  P76.9 Intestinal obstruction of newborn, unspecified ▽

✓4ᵗʰ **P77 Necrotizing enterocolitis of newborn**
DEF: Serious intestinal infection and inflammation in preterm infants. Severity is measured by stages and may progress to life-threatening perforation or peritonitis. Resection surgical treatment may be necessary.

  P77.1 Stage 1 necrotizing enterocolitis in newborn
Necrotizing enterocolitis without pneumatosis, without perforation
DEF: Broad-spectrum symptoms with nonspecific signs, including feeding intolerance, abdominal distention, bradycardia, and metabolic abnormalities.

  P77.2 Stage 2 necrotizing enterocolitis in newborn
Necrotizing enterocolitis with pneumatosis, without perforation
DEF: Radiographic confirmation of necrotizing enterocolitis showing intestinal dilatation, fixed loops of bowels, pneumatosis intestinalis, metabolic acidosis, and thrombocytopenia.

  P77.3 Stage 3 necrotizing enterocolitis in newborn
Necrotizing enterocolitis with perforation
Necrotizing enterocolitis with pneumatosis and perforation
DEF: Advanced stage in which an infant demonstrates signs of bowel perforation, septic shock, metabolic acidosis, ascites, disseminated intravascular coagulopathy, and neutropenia.

  P77.9 Necrotizing enterocolitis in newborn, unspecified ▽
Necrotizing enterocolitis in newborn, NOS

✓4ᵗʰ **P78 Other perinatal digestive system disorders**
EXCLUDES 1 *cystic fibrosis (E84.0-E84.9)*
neonatal gastrointestinal hemorrhages (P54.0-P54.3)

  P78.0 Perinatal intestinal perforation
Meconium peritonitis

  P78.1 Other neonatal peritonitis
Neonatal peritonitis NOS

  P78.2 Neonatal hematemesis and melena due to swallowed maternal blood

  P78.3 Noninfective neonatal diarrhea
Neonatal diarrhea NOS

  ✓5ᵗʰ **P78.8 Other specified perinatal digestive system disorders**

    P78.81 Congenital cirrhosis (of liver)

    P78.82 Peptic ulcer of newborn

    P78.83 Newborn esophageal reflux
Neonatal esophageal reflux

☑ Additional Character Req   ✓x7ᵗʰ Placeholder Alert   Manifestation   ▽ Unspecified   ►◄ Revised Text   ● New Code   ▲ Revised Code Title

ICD-10-CM 2019   **897**

P78.84 **Gestational alloimmune liver disease**
GALD
Neonatal hemochromatosis
EXCLUDES 1   *hemochromatosis (E83.11-)*
AHA: 2017,4Q,21
DEF: Severe hepatic injury with onset during fetal development with manifestations beginning during fetal life. It is due to maternal antibodies to fetal hepatic cells (hepatocytes) that cross the placenta into the fetal circulation, causing hepatic cell necrosis.

P78.89 **Other specified perinatal digestive system disorders**

P78.9 **Perinatal digestive system disorder, unspecified** ▽

Conditions involving the integument and temperature regulation of newborn (P80-P83)

✓4ᵗʰ **P80 Hypothermia of newborn**
DEF: Decrease in newborn body temperature due to their larger ratio of surface area to body weight, thin skin with blood vessels close to the surface, and a limited amount of subcutaneous fat.

P80.0 **Cold injury syndrome**
Severe and usually chronic hypothermia associated with a pink flushed appearance, edema and neurological and biochemical abnormalities.
EXCLUDES 1   *mild hypothermia of newborn (P80.8)*

P80.8 **Other hypothermia of newborn**
Mild hypothermia of newborn

P80.9 **Hypothermia of newborn, unspecified** ▽

✓4ᵗʰ **P81 Other disturbances of temperature regulation of newborn**

P81.0 **Environmental hyperthermia of newborn**

P81.8 **Other specified disturbances of temperature regulation of newborn**

P81.9 **Disturbance of temperature regulation of newborn, unspecified** ▽
Fever of newborn NOS

✓4ᵗʰ **P83 Other conditions of integument specific to newborn**
EXCLUDES 1   *congenital malformations of skin and integument (Q80-Q84)*
hydrops fetalis due to hemolytic disease (P56.-)
neonatal skin infection (P39.4)
staphylococcal scalded skin syndrome (L00)
EXCLUDES 2   *cradle cap (L21.0)*
diaper [napkin] dermatitis (L22)

P83.0 **Sclerema neonatorum**
DEF: Diffuse, rapidly progressing white, waxy, nonpitting hardening of tissue, usually of legs and feet that is life-threatening. It is found in preterm or debilitated infants. Etiology is unknown.

P83.1 **Neonatal erythema toxicum**

P83.2 **Hydrops fetalis not due to hemolytic disease**
Hydrops fetalis NOS
DEF: Severe, life-threatening problem of a newborn characterized by severe edema of the entire body. It is unrelated to immune response.

✓5ᵗʰ P83.3 **Other and unspecified edema specific to newborn**
P83.30 **Unspecified edema specific to newborn** ▽
P83.39 **Other edema specific to newborn**

P83.4 **Breast engorgement of newborn**
Noninfective mastitis of newborn

P83.5 **Congenital hydrocele** ♂
DEF: Hydrocele: Serous fluid that collects in the tunica vaginalis of the scrotum along the spermatic cord in males.

P83.6 **Umbilical polyp of newborn**

✓5ᵗʰ P83.8 **Other specified conditions of integument specific to newborn**
AHA: 2017,4Q,21-22
P83.81 **Umbilical granuloma**
EXCLUDES 2   *granulomatous disorder of the skin and subcutaneous tissue, unspecified (L92.9)*
P83.88 **Other specified conditions of integument specific to newborn**
Bronze baby syndrome
Neonatal scleroderma
Urticaria neonatorum

P83.9 **Condition of the integument specific to newborn, unspecified** ▽

Other problems with newborn (P84)

P84 Other problems with newborn
Acidemia of newborn
Acidosis of newborn
Anoxia of newborn NOS
Asphyxia of newborn NOS
Hypercapnia of newborn
Hypoxemia of newborn
Hypoxia of newborn NOS
Mixed metabolic and respiratory acidosis of newborn
EXCLUDES 1   *intracranial hemorrhage due to anoxia or hypoxia (P52.-)*
hypoxic ischemic encephalopathy [HIE] (P91.6-)
late metabolic acidosis of newborn (P74.0)

Other disorders originating in the perinatal period (P90-P96)

P90 Convulsions of newborn
EXCLUDES 1   *benign myoclonic epilepsy in infancy (G40.3-)*
benign neonatal convulsions (familial) (G40.3-)

✓4ᵗʰ **P91 Other disturbances of cerebral status of newborn**
P91.0 **Neonatal cerebral ischemia**
P91.1 **Acquired periventricular cysts of newborn**
P91.2 **Neonatal cerebral leukomalacia**
Periventricular leukomalacia
P91.3 **Neonatal cerebral irritability**
P91.4 **Neonatal cerebral depression**
P91.5 **Neonatal coma**
✓5ᵗʰ P91.6 **Hypoxic ischemic encephalopathy [HIE]**
EXCLUDES 1   *neonatal cerebral depression (P91.4)*
neonatal cerebral irritability (P91.3)
neonatal coma (P91.5)
AHA: 2017,4Q,22
P91.60 **Hypoxic ischemic encephalopathy [HIE], unspecified** ▽
P91.61 **Mild hypoxic ischemic encephalopathy [HIE]**
P91.62 **Moderate hypoxic ischemic encephalopathy [HIE]**
P91.63 **Severe hypoxic ischemic encephalopathy [HIE]**
✓5ᵗʰ P91.8 **Other specified disturbances of cerebral status of newborn**
AHA: 2017,4Q,22
✓6ᵗʰ P91.81 **Neonatal encephalopathy**
P91.811 *Neonatal encephalopathy in diseases classified elsewhere*
Code first underlying condition, if known, such as:
congenital cirrhosis (of liver) ▶(P78.81)◀
intracranial nontraumatic hemorrhage of newborn (P52.-)
kernicterus (P57.-)
P91.819 **Neonatal encephalopathy, unspecified** ▽
P91.88 **Other specified disturbances of cerebral status of newborn**
P91.9 **Disturbance of cerebral status of newborn, unspecified** ▽

✓4ᵗʰ **P92 Feeding problems of newborn**
EXCLUDES 1   *eating disorders (F50.-)*
feeding problems in child over 28 days old (R63.3)
AHA: 2016,3Q,19
TIP: Continue to assign a code from this category for feeding problems in a patient greater than 28 days old when that feeding problem was initially diagnosed between day 0 and day 28. Do not assign code R63.3.
✓5ᵗʰ P92.0 **Vomiting of newborn**
EXCLUDES 1   *vomiting of child over 28 days old (R11.-)*
P92.01 **Bilious vomiting of newborn**
EXCLUDES 1   *bilious vomiting in child over 28 days old (R11.14)*
P92.09 **Other vomiting of newborn**
EXCLUDES 1   *regurgitation of food in newborn (P92.1)*
P92.1 **Regurgitation and rumination of newborn**
P92.2 **Slow feeding of newborn**
P92.3 **Underfeeding of newborn**
P92.4 **Overfeeding of newborn**

P92.5 **Neonatal difficulty in feeding at breast**
AHA: 2017,1Q,28

P92.6 **Failure to thrive in newborn**
> EXCLUDES 1   *failure to thrive in child over 28 days old (R62.51)*

P92.8 **Other feeding problems of newborn**

P92.9 **Feeding problem of newborn, unspecified**   ▽

√4ᵗʰ **P93** **Reactions and intoxications due to drugs administered to newborn**
> INCLUDES   reactions and intoxications due to drugs administered to fetus affecting newborn
> EXCLUDES 1   *jaundice due to drugs or toxins transmitted from mother or given to newborn (P58.4-)*
> *reactions and intoxications from maternal opiates, tranquilizers and other medication ▶(P04.0-P04.1, P04.4-)◀*
> *withdrawal symptoms from maternal use of drugs of addiction (P96.1)*
> *withdrawal symptoms from therapeutic use of drugs in newborn (P96.2)*

P93.0 **Grey baby syndrome**
Grey syndrome from chloramphenicol administration in newborn

P93.8 **Other reactions and intoxications due to drugs administered to newborn**
Use additional code for adverse effect, if applicable, to identify drug (T36-T50 with fifth or sixth character 5)

√4ᵗʰ **P94** **Disorders of muscle tone of newborn**

P94.0 **Transient neonatal myasthenia gravis**
> EXCLUDES 1   *myasthenia gravis (G70.0)*

P94.1 **Congenital hypertonia**

P94.2 **Congenital hypotonia**
Floppy baby syndrome, unspecified

P94.8 **Other disorders of muscle tone of newborn**

P94.9 **Disorder of muscle tone of newborn, unspecified**   ▽

P95 **Stillbirth**
Deadborn fetus NOS
Fetal death of unspecified cause
Stillbirth NOS
> EXCLUDES 1   *maternal care for intrauterine death (O36.4)*
> *missed abortion (O02.1)*
> *outcome of delivery, stillbirth (Z37.1, Z37.3, Z37.4, Z37.7)*

√4ᵗʰ **P96** **Other conditions originating in the perinatal period**

P96.0 **Congenital renal failure**
Uremia of newborn

P96.1 **Neonatal withdrawal symptoms from maternal use of drugs of addiction**
Drug withdrawal syndrome in infant of dependent mother
Neonatal abstinence syndrome
> EXCLUDES 1   *reactions and intoxications from maternal opiates and tranquilizers administered during labor and delivery (P04.0)*

P96.2 **Withdrawal symptoms from therapeutic use of drugs in newborn**

P96.3 **Wide cranial sutures of newborn**
Neonatal craniotabes

P96.5 **Complication to newborn due to (fetal) intrauterine procedure**
> EXCLUDES 2   *newborn affected by amniocentesis (P00.6)*

√5ᵗʰ **P96.8** **Other specified conditions originating in the perinatal period**

P96.81 **Exposure to (parental) (environmental) tobacco smoke in the perinatal period**
> EXCLUDES 2   *newborn affected by in utero exposure to tobacco (P04.2)*
> *exposure to environmental tobacco smoke after the perinatal period (Z77.22)*

P96.82 **Delayed separation of umbilical cord**

P96.83 **Meconium staining**
> EXCLUDES 1   *meconium aspiration (P24.00, P24.01)*
> *meconium passage during delivery (P03.82)*
> **DEF:** Meconium passed in utero causing discoloration on the fetal skin and nails or on the umbilicus. This staining may be incidental or may be an indicator of significant fetal stress that could affect outcomes.

P96.89 **Other specified conditions originating in the perinatal period**
Use additional code to specify condition

P96.9 **Condition originating in the perinatal period, unspecified**   ▽
Congenital debility NOS

☑ Additional Character Req   ✗x7ᵗʰ Placeholder Alert   Manifestation   ▽ Unspecified   ▶◀ Revised Text   ● New Code   ▲ Revised Code Title

Chapter 17. Congenital Malformations, Deformations, and Chromosomal Abnormalities (Q00–Q99)

Chapter Specific Guidelines with Coding Examples

The chapter specific guidelines from the ICD-10-CM Official Guidelines for Coding and Reporting have been provided below. Along with these guidelines are coding examples, contained in the shaded boxes, that have been developed to help illustrate the coding and/or sequencing guidance found in these guidelines.

Assign an appropriate code(s) from categories Q00–Q99, Congenital malformations, deformations, and chromosomal abnormalities when a malformation/deformation or chromosomal abnormality is documented. A malformation/deformation/or chromosomal abnormality may be the principal/first-listed diagnosis on a record or a secondary diagnosis.

When a malformation/deformation/or chromosomal abnormality does not have a unique code assignment, assign additional code(s) for any manifestations that may be present.

When the code assignment specifically identifies the malformation/deformation/or chromosomal abnormality, manifestations that are an inherent component of the anomaly should not be coded separately. Additional codes should be assigned for manifestations that are not an inherent component.

8-day-old infant with tetralogy of Fallot and pulmonary stenosis

Q21.3   Tetralogy of Fallot

Explanation: Pulmonary stenosis is inherent in the disease process of tetralogy of Fallot. When the code assignment specifically identifies the malformation/deformation/or chromosomal abnormality, manifestations that are inherent components of the anomaly should not be coded separately.

7-month-old infant with Down syndrome and common atrioventricular canal

Q90.9   Down syndrome, unspecified

Q21.2   Atrioventricular septal defect

Explanation: While a common atrioventricular canal is often associated with patients with Down syndrome, this manifestation is not an inherent component and may be reported separately. When the code assignment specifically identifies the anomaly, manifestations that are inherent components of the condition should not be coded separately. Additional codes should be assigned for manifestations that are not inherent components.

Codes from Chapter 17 may be used throughout the life of the patient. If a congenital malformation or deformity has been corrected, a personal history code should be used to identify the history of the malformation or deformity. Although present at birth, malformation/deformation/or chromosomal abnormality may not be identified until later in life. Whenever the condition is diagnosed by the physician, it is appropriate to assign a code from codes Q00-Q99. For the birth admission, the appropriate code from category Z38, Liveborn infants, according to place of birth and type of delivery, should be sequenced as the principal diagnosis, followed by any congenital anomaly codes, Q00- Q99.

Three-year-old with history of corrected ventricular septal defect

Z87.74   Personal history of (corrected) congenital malformations of heart and circulatory system

Explanation: If a congenital malformation or deformity has been corrected, a personal history code should be used to identify the history of the malformation or deformity.

Forty-year-old man with headaches diagnosed with congenital arteriovenous malformation by brain scan

Q28.2   Arteriovenous malformation of cerebral vessels

Explanation: Although present at birth, malformations may not be identified until later in life. Whenever the condition is diagnosed by the physician, it is appropriate to assign a code from the range Q00–Q99.

Newborn with anencephaly delivered vaginally in hospital

Z38.00   Single liveborn infant, delivered vaginally

Q00.0   Anencephaly

Explanation: For the birth admission, the appropriate code from category Z38 Liveborn infants, according to place of birth and type of delivery, should be sequenced as the principal diagnosis, followed by any congenital anomaly codes, Q00–Q99.

Chapter 17. Congenital Malformations, Deformations and Chromosomal Abnormalities (Q00-Q99)

NOTE ▶Codes from this chapter are not for use on maternal records◀

EXCLUDES 2   *inborn errors of metabolism (E70-E88)*

This chapter contains the following blocks:

Q00-Q07   Congenital malformations of the nervous system
Q10-Q18   Congenital malformations of eye, ear, face and neck
Q20-Q28   Congenital malformations of the circulatory system
Q30-Q34   Congenital malformations of the respiratory system
Q35-Q37   Cleft lip and cleft palate
Q38-Q45   Other congenital malformations of the digestive system
Q50-Q56   Congenital malformations of genital organs
Q60-Q64   Congenital malformations of the urinary system
Q65-Q79   Congenital malformations and deformations of the musculoskeletal system
Q80-Q89   Other congenital malformations
Q90-Q99   Chromosomal abnormalities, not elsewhere classified

Congenital malformations of the nervous system (Q00-Q07)

✓4ᵗʰ   **Q00   Anencephaly and similar malformations**

     Q00.0   Anencephaly   `HCC`
        Acephaly
        Acrania
        Amyelencephaly
        Hemianencephaly
        Hemicephaly

     Q00.1   Craniorachischisis   `HCC`
     Q00.2   Iniencephaly   `HCC`

✓4ᵗʰ   **Q01   Encephalocele**

     INCLUDES   Arnold-Chiari syndrome, type III
        encephalocystocele
        encephalomyelocele
        hydroencephalocele
        hydromeningocele, cranial
        meningocele, cerebral
        meningoencephalocele

     EXCLUDES 1   *Meckel-Gruber syndrome (Q61.9)*

     DEF: Congenital protrusion of brain tissue through a defect in the skull.

     Q01.0   Frontal encephalocele   `HCC`
     Q01.1   Nasofrontal encephalocele   `HCC`
     Q01.2   Occipital encephalocele   `HCC`
     Q01.8   Encephalocele of other sites   `HCC`
     Q01.9   Encephalocele, unspecified   `HCC` ▽

   Q02   Microcephaly   `HCC`

     INCLUDES   hydromicrocephaly
        micrencephalon

     ▶Use additional code, if applicable, to identify congenital Zika virus disease◀

     EXCLUDES 1   *Meckel-Gruber syndrome (Q61.9)*

     DEF: Congenital disorder in which the head circumference is more than two standard deviations below the mean for age, sex, race, and gestation and associated with a decreased life expectancy.

✓4ᵗʰ   **Q03   Congenital hydrocephalus**

     INCLUDES   hydrocephalus in newborn

     EXCLUDES 1   *Arnold-Chiari syndrome, type II (Q07.0-)*
        acquired hydrocephalus (G91.-)
        hydrocephalus due to congenital toxoplasmosis (P37.1)
        hydrocephalus with spina bifida (Q05.0-Q05.4)

Congenital Hydrocephalus

Pressure

Normal ventricles   Hydrocephalic ventricles

     Q03.0   Malformations of aqueduct of Sylvius   `HCC`
        Anomaly of aqueduct of Sylvius
        Obstruction of aqueduct of Sylvius, congenital
        Stenosis of aqueduct of Sylvius

     Q03.1   Atresia of foramina of Magendie and Luschka   `HCC`
        Dandy-Walker syndrome

     Q03.8   Other congenital hydrocephalus   `HCC`
     Q03.9   Congenital hydrocephalus, unspecified   `HCC` ▽

✓4ᵗʰ   **Q04   Other congenital malformations of brain**

     EXCLUDES 1   *cyclopia (Q87.0)*
        macrocephaly (Q75.3)

     Q04.0   Congenital malformations of corpus callosum   `HCC`
        Agenesis of corpus callosum

     Q04.1   Arhinencephaly   `HCC`
     Q04.2   Holoprosencephaly   `HCC`
     Q04.3   Other reduction deformities of brain   `HCC`
        Absence of part of brain
        Agenesis of part of brain
        Agyria
        Aplasia of part of brain
        Hydranencephaly
        Hypoplasia of part of brain
        Lissencephaly
        Microgyria
        Pachygyria

        EXCLUDES 1   *congenital malformations of corpus callosum (Q04.0)*

     Q04.4   Septo-optic dysplasia of brain   `HCC`
     Q04.5   Megalencephaly   `HCC`
     Q04.6   Congenital cerebral cysts   `HCC`
        Porencephaly
        Schizencephaly

        EXCLUDES 1   *acquired porencephalic cyst (G93.0)*

     Q04.8   Other specified congenital malformations of brain   `HCC`
        Arnold-Chiari syndrome, type IV
        Macrogyria

     Q04.9   Congenital malformation of brain, unspecified   `HCC` ▽
        Congenital anomaly NOS of brain
        Congenital deformity NOS of brain
        Congenital disease or lesion NOS of brain
        Multiple anomalies NOS of brain, congenital

☑4ᵗʰ **Q05 Spina bifida**

    [INCLUDES]   hydromeningocele (spinal)

                 meningocele (spinal)

                 meningomyelocele

                 myelocele

                 myelomeningocele

                 rachischisis

                 spina bifida (aperta)(cystica)

                 syringomyelocele

    Use additional code for any associated paraplegia (paraparesis) (G82.2-)

    [EXCLUDES 1]   Arnold-Chiari syndrome, type II (Q07.0-)

                 spina bifida occulta (Q76.0)

    DEF: Lack of closure in the vertebral column with protrusion of the spinal cord through the defect, often in the lumbosacral area. This condition can be recognized by the presence of alpha-fetoproteins in the amniotic fluid.

Spina Bifida

Spina bifida occulta   Meningocele   Myelomeningocele

    Q05.0 Cervical spina bifida with hydrocephalus   HCC

    Q05.1 Thoracic spina bifida with hydrocephalus   HCC

          Dorsal spina bifida with hydrocephalus

          Thoracolumbar spina bifida with hydrocephalus

    Q05.2 Lumbar spina bifida with hydrocephalus   HCC

          Lumbosacral spina bifida with hydrocephalus

    Q05.3 Sacral spina bifida with hydrocephalus   HCC

    Q05.4 Unspecified spina bifida with hydrocephalus   HCC ▽

    Q05.5 Cervical spina bifida without hydrocephalus   HCC

    Q05.6 Thoracic spina bifida without hydrocephalus   HCC

          Dorsal spina bifida NOS

          Thoracolumbar spina bifida NOS

    Q05.7 Lumbar spina bifida without hydrocephalus   HCC

          Lumbosacral spina bifida NOS

    Q05.8 Sacral spina bifida without hydrocephalus   HCC

    Q05.9 Spina bifida, unspecified   HCC ▽

☑4ᵗʰ **Q06 Other congenital malformations of spinal cord**

    Q06.0 Amyelia   HCC

    Q06.1 Hypoplasia and dysplasia of spinal cord   HCC

          Atelomyelia

          Myelatelia

          Myelodysplasia of spinal cord

    Q06.2 Diastematomyelia   HCC

          DEF: Rare congenital anomaly often associated with spina bifida. The spinal cord is separated into longitudinal halves by a bony, cartilaginous or fibrous septum, each half surrounded by a dural sac.

    Q06.3 Other congenital cauda equina malformations   HCC

    Q06.4 Hydromyelia   HCC

          Hydrorachis

    Q06.8 Other specified congenital malformations of spinal cord   HCC

    Q06.9 Congenital malformation of spinal cord, unspecified   HCC ▽

          Congenital anomaly NOS of spinal cord

          Congenital deformity NOS of spinal cord

          Congenital disease or lesion NOS of spinal cord

☑4ᵗʰ **Q07 Other congenital malformations of nervous system**

    [EXCLUDES 2]   congenital central alveolar hypoventilation syndrome (G47.35)

                 familial dysautonomia [Riley-Day] (G90.1)

                 neurofibromatosis (nonmalignant) (Q85.0-)

    ☑5ᵗʰ **Q07.0 Arnold-Chiari syndrome**

          Arnold-Chiari syndrome, type II

          [EXCLUDES 1]   Arnold-Chiari syndrome, type III (Q01.-)

                       Arnold-Chiari syndrome, type IV (Q04.8)

          DEF: Congenital malformation of the brain in which the cerebellum protrudes through the foramen magnum into the spinal canal.

          Q07.00 Arnold-Chiari syndrome without spina bifida or hydrocephalus   HCC

          Q07.01 Arnold-Chiari syndrome with spina bifida   HCC

          Q07.02 Arnold-Chiari syndrome with hydrocephalus   HCC

          Q07.03 Arnold-Chiari syndrome with spina bifida and hydrocephalus   HCC

    Q07.8 Other specified congenital malformations of nervous system   HCC

          Agenesis of nerve

          Displacement of brachial plexus

          Jaw-winking syndrome

          Marcus Gunn's syndrome

    Q07.9 Congenital malformation of nervous system, unspecified   HCC ▽

          Congenital anomaly NOS of nervous system

          Congenital deformity NOS of nervous system

          Congenital disease or lesion NOS of nervous system

Congenital malformations of eye, ear, face and neck (Q10-Q18)

    [EXCLUDES 2]   cleft lip and cleft palate (Q35-Q37)

                 congenital malformation of cervical spine (Q05.0, Q05.5, Q67.5, Q76.0-Q76.4)

                 congenital malformation of larynx (Q31.-)

                 congenital malformation of lip NEC (Q38.0)

                 congenital malformation of nose (Q30.-)

                 congenital malformation of parathyroid gland (Q89.2)

                 congenital malformation of thyroid gland (Q89.2)

☑4ᵗʰ **Q10 Congenital malformations of eyelid, lacrimal apparatus and orbit**

    [EXCLUDES 1]   cryptophthalmos NOS (Q11.2)

                 cryptophthalmos syndrome (Q87.0)

    Q10.0 Congenital ptosis

          DEF: Congenital drooping of the eyelid. Ptosis is mostly idiopathic, but may occur genetically.

    Q10.1 Congenital ectropion

    Q10.2 Congenital entropion

    Q10.3 Other congenital malformations of eyelid

          Ablepharon

          Blepharophimosis, congenital

          Coloboma of eyelid

          Congenital absence or agenesis of cilia

          Congenital absence or agenesis of eyelid

          Congenital accessory eyelid

          Congenital accessory eye muscle

          Congenital malformation of eyelid NOS

    Q10.4 Absence and agenesis of lacrimal apparatus

          Congenital absence of punctum lacrimale

    Q10.5 Congenital stenosis and stricture of lacrimal duct

    Q10.6 Other congenital malformations of lacrimal apparatus

          Congenital malformation of lacrimal apparatus NOS

    Q10.7 Congenital malformation of orbit

☑4ᵗʰ **Q11 Anophthalmos, microphthalmos and macrophthalmos**

    Q11.0 Cystic eyeball

    Q11.1 Other anophthalmos

          Anophthalmos NOS

          Agenesis of eye

          Aplasia of eye

    Q11.2 Microphthalmos

          Cryptophthalmos NOS

          Dysplasia of eye

          Hypoplasia of eye

          Rudimentary eye

          [EXCLUDES 1]   cryptophthalmos syndrome (Q87.0)

☑ Additional Character Req   ☑x7ᵗʰ Placeholder Alert   Manifestation   ▽ Unspecified   ▶◀ Revised Text   ● New Code   ▲ Revised Code Title

ICD-10-CM 2019   903

Chapter 17. Congenital Malformations, Deformations and Chromosomal Abnormalities

Q11.3–Q18.1

Q11.3 **Macrophthalmos**
     EXCLUDES 1   *macrophthalmos in congenital glaucoma (Q15.0)*

✓4ᵗʰ **Q12 Congenital lens malformations**

Q12.0 **Congenital cataract**
Q12.1 **Congenital displaced lens**
Q12.2 **Coloboma of lens**

Coloboma of Lens

Coloboma

Q12.3 **Congenital aphakia**
Q12.4 **Spherophakia**
Q12.8 **Other congenital lens malformations**
     Microphakia
Q12.9 **Congenital lens malformation, unspecified** ▽

✓4ᵗʰ **Q13 Congenital malformations of anterior segment of eye**

Q13.0 **Coloboma of iris**
     Coloboma NOS
     DEF: Defective or absent section of ocular tissue that may present as mild cupping or a small pit in the ocular disc due to extensive defects in the iris, ciliary body, choroids, and retina.
Q13.1 **Absence of iris**
     Aniridia
     Use additional code for associated glaucoma (H42)
     DEF: Incompletely formed or absent iris. It affects both eyes and is a dominant trait.
Q13.2 **Other congenital malformations of iris**
     Anisocoria, congenital
     Atresia of pupil
     Congenital malformation of iris NOS
     Corectopia
Q13.3 **Congenital corneal opacity**
Q13.4 **Other congenital corneal malformations**
     Congenital malformation of cornea NOS
     Microcornea
     Peter's anomaly
Q13.5 **Blue sclera**
✓5ᵗʰ Q13.8 **Other congenital malformations of anterior segment of eye**
     Q13.81 **Rieger's anomaly**
         Use additional code for associated glaucoma (H42)
     Q13.89 **Other congenital malformations of anterior segment of eye**
Q13.9 **Congenital malformation of anterior segment of eye, unspecified** ▽

✓4ᵗʰ **Q14 Congenital malformations of posterior segment of eye**
     EXCLUDES 2   *optic nerve hypoplasia (H47.03-)*
Q14.0 **Congenital malformation of vitreous humor**
     Congenital vitreous opacity
Q14.1 **Congenital malformation of retina**
     Congenital retinal aneurysm
Q14.2 **Congenital malformation of optic disc**
     Coloboma of optic disc
Q14.3 **Congenital malformation of choroid**
Q14.8 **Other congenital malformations of posterior segment of eye**
     Coloboma of the fundus
Q14.9 **Congenital malformation of posterior segment of eye, unspecified** ▽

✓4ᵗʰ **Q15 Other congenital malformations of eye**
     EXCLUDES 1   *congenital nystagmus (H55.01)*
         ocular albinism (E70.31-)
         optic nerve hypoplasia (H47.03-)
         retinitis pigmentosa (H35.52)
Q15.0 **Congenital glaucoma**
     Axenfeld's anomaly
     Buphthalmos
     Glaucoma of childhood
     Glaucoma of newborn
     Hydrophthalmos
     Keratoglobus, congenital, with glaucoma
     Macrocornea with glaucoma
     Macrophthalmos in congenital glaucoma
     Megalocornea with glaucoma
Q15.8 **Other specified congenital malformations of eye**
Q15.9 **Congenital malformation of eye, unspecified** ▽
     Congenital anomaly of eye
     Congenital deformity of eye

✓4ᵗʰ **Q16 Congenital malformations of ear causing impairment of hearing**
     EXCLUDES 1   *congenital deafness (H90.-)*
Q16.0 **Congenital absence of (ear) auricle**
Q16.1 **Congenital absence, atresia and stricture of auditory canal (external)**
     Congenital atresia or stricture of osseous meatus
Q16.2 **Absence of eustachian tube**
Q16.3 **Congenital malformation of ear ossicles**
     Congenital fusion of ear ossicles
Q16.4 **Other congenital malformations of middle ear**
     Congenital malformation of middle ear NOS
Q16.5 **Congenital malformation of inner ear**
     Congenital anomaly of membranous labyrinth
     Congenital anomaly of organ of Corti
Q16.9 **Congenital malformation of ear causing impairment** ▽ **of hearing, unspecified**
     Congenital absence of ear NOS

✓4ᵗʰ **Q17 Other congenital malformations of ear**
     EXCLUDES 1   *congenital malformations of ear with impairment of hearing (Q16.0-Q16.9)*
         preauricular sinus (Q18.1)
Q17.0 **Accessory auricle**
     Accessory tragus
     Polyotia
     Preauricular appendage or tag
     Supernumerary ear
     Supernumerary lobule
Q17.1 **Macrotia**
     DEF: Birth defect characterized by abnormal enlargement of the pinna of the ear.
Q17.2 **Microtia**
Q17.3 **Other misshapen ear**
     Pointed ear
Q17.4 **Misplaced ear**
     Low-set ears
     EXCLUDES 1   *cervical auricle (Q18.2)*
Q17.5 **Prominent ear**
     Bat ear
Q17.8 **Other specified congenital malformations of ear**
     Congenital absence of lobe of ear
Q17.9 **Congenital malformation of ear, unspecified** ▽
     Congenital anomaly of ear NOS

✓4ᵗʰ **Q18 Other congenital malformations of face and neck**
     EXCLUDES 1   *cleft lip and cleft palate (Q35-Q37)*
         conditions classified to Q67.0-Q67.4
         congenital malformations of skull and face bones (Q75.-)
         cyclopia (Q87.0)
         dentofacial anomalies [including malocclusion] (M26.-)
         malformation syndromes affecting facial appearance (Q87.0)
         persistent thyroglossal duct (Q89.2)
Q18.0 **Sinus, fistula and cyst of branchial cleft**
     Branchial vestige
Q18.1 **Preauricular sinus and cyst**
     Fistula of auricle, congenital
     Cervicoaural fistula

Q18.2 Other branchial cleft malformations
Branchial cleft malformation NOS
Cervical auricle
Otocephaly

Q18.3 Webbing of neck
Pterygium colli
DEF: Congenital malformation characterized by a thick, triangular skinfold that stretches from the lateral side of the neck across the shoulder. It is associated with genetic conditions such as Turner's and Noonan's syndromes.

Q18.4 Macrostomia
DEF: Rare congenital craniofacial bilateral or unilateral anomaly of the mouth due to malformed maxillary and mandibular processes. It results in an abnormally large mouth extending toward the ear.

Q18.5 Microstomia

Q18.6 Macrocheilia
Hypertrophy of lip, congenital

Q18.7 Microcheilia

Q18.8 Other specified congenital malformations of face and neck
Medial cyst of face and neck
Medial fistula of face and neck
Medial sinus of face and neck

Q18.9 Congenital malformation of face and neck, unspecified   ▽
Congenital anomaly NOS of face and neck

Congenital malformations of the circulatory system (Q20-Q28)

✓4ᵗʰ **Q20 Congenital malformations of cardiac chambers and connections**
EXCLUDES 1   *dextrocardia with situs inversus (Q89.3)*
                 mirror-image atrial arrangement with situs inversus (Q89.3)

Q20.0 Common arterial trunk
Persistent truncus arteriosus
EXCLUDES 1   *aortic septal defect (Q21.4)*

Q20.1 Double outlet right ventricle
Taussig-Bing syndrome

Q20.2 Double outlet left ventricle

Q20.3 Discordant ventriculoarterial connection
Dextrotransposition of aorta
Transposition of great vessels (complete)

Q20.4 Double inlet ventricle
Common ventricle
Cor triloculare biatriatum
Single ventricle

Q20.5 Discordant atrioventricular connection
Corrected transposition
Levotransposition
Ventricular inversion

Q20.6 Isomerism of atrial appendages
Isomerism of atrial appendages with asplenia or polysplenia

Q20.8 Other congenital malformations of cardiac chambers and connections
Cor binoculare

Q20.9 Congenital malformation of cardiac chambers and connections, unspecified   ▽

✓4ᵗʰ **Q21 Congenital malformations of cardiac septa**
EXCLUDES 1   *acquired cardiac septal defect (I51.0)*

Q21.0 Ventricular septal defect
Roger's disease

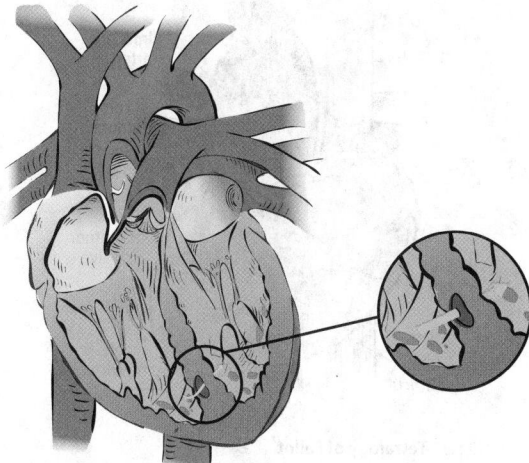

Ventricular Septal Defect

Q21.1 Atrial septal defect
Coronary sinus defect
Patent or persistent foramen ovale
Patent or persistent ostium secundum defect (type II)
Patent or persistent sinus venosus defect

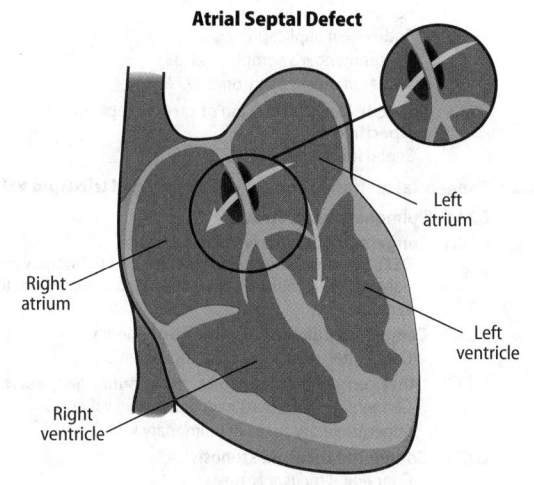

Atrial Septal Defect

Left atrium

Right atrium

Left ventricle

Right ventricle

☑ Additional Character Req   ✓x7ᵗʰ Placeholder Alert   Manifestation   ▽ Unspecified   ▶◀ Revised Text   ● New Code   ▲ Revised Code Title

Q21.2 Atrioventricular septal defect
Common atrioventricular canal
Endocardial cushion defect
Ostium primum atrial septal defect (type I)

Atrioventricular Septal Defect

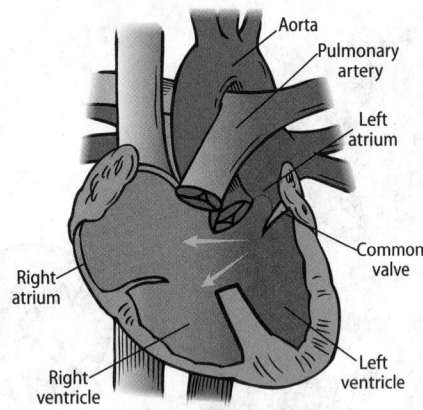

Q21.3 Tetralogy of Fallot
Ventricular septal defect with pulmonary stenosis or atresia, dextroposition of aorta and hypertrophy of right ventricle.
AHA: 2014,3Q,16

Q21.4 Aortopulmonary septal defect
Aortic septal defect
Aortopulmonary window

Q21.8 Other congenital malformations of cardiac septa
Eisenmenger's defect
Pentalogy of Fallot
Code also if applicable:
Eisenmenger's complex (I27.83)
Eisenmenger's syndrome (I27.83)

Q21.9 Congenital malformation of cardiac septum, unspecified ▽
Septal (heart) defect NOS

✓4ᵗʰ **Q22 Congenital malformations of pulmonary and tricuspid valves**

Q22.0 Pulmonary valve atresia

Q22.1 Congenital pulmonary valve stenosis
DEF: Stenosis of the opening between the pulmonary artery and right ventricle, causing obstructed blood outflow from the right ventricle.

Q22.2 Congenital pulmonary valve insufficiency
Congenital pulmonary valve regurgitation

Q22.3 Other congenital malformations of pulmonary valve
Congenital malformation of pulmonary valve NOS
Supernumerary cusps of pulmonary valve

Q22.4 Congenital tricuspid stenosis
Congenital tricuspid atresia

Q22.5 Ebstein's anomaly
DEF: Malformation of the tricuspid valve characterized by septal and posterior leaflets attaching to the wall of the right ventricle. Ebstein's anomaly causes the right ventricle to fuse with the atrium into a large right atrium and a small ventricle and leads to heart failure and abnormal cardiac rhythm.

Q22.6 Hypoplastic right heart syndrome

Q22.8 Other congenital malformations of tricuspid valve

Q22.9 Congenital malformation of tricuspid valve, unspecified ▽

✓4ᵗʰ **Q23 Congenital malformations of aortic and mitral valves**

Q23.0 Congenital stenosis of aortic valve
Congenital aortic atresia
Congenital aortic stenosis NOS
EXCLUDES 1 *congenital stenosis of aortic valve in hypoplastic left heart syndrome (Q23.4)*
congenital subaortic stenosis (Q24.4)
supravalvular aortic stenosis (congenital) (Q25.3)

Q23.1 Congenital insufficiency of aortic valve
Bicuspid aortic valve
Congenital aortic insufficiency

Q23.2 Congenital mitral stenosis
Congenital mitral atresia
DEF: Congenital stenosis of the mitral valve orifice between the left atrium and ventricle, at the supravalvular, valvular, or subvalvular levels, causing obstruction to left ventricular filling.

Q23.3 Congenital mitral insufficiency

Q23.4 Hypoplastic left heart syndrome

Q23.8 Other congenital malformations of aortic and mitral valves

Q23.9 Congenital malformation of aortic and mitral valves, unspecified ▽

✓4ᵗʰ **Q24 Other congenital malformations of heart**
EXCLUDES 1 *endocardial fibroelastosis (I42.4)*

Q24.0 Dextrocardia
EXCLUDES 1 *dextrocardia with situs inversus (Q89.3)*
isomerism of atrial appendages (with asplenia or polysplenia) (Q20.6)
mirror-image atrial arrangement with situs inversus (Q89.3)
DEF: Congenital condition in which the heart is located on the right side of the chest rather than in its normal position on the left.

Q24.1 Levocardia

Q24.2 Cor triatriatum

Q24.3 Pulmonary infundibular stenosis
Subvalvular pulmonic stenosis

Q24.4 Congenital subaortic stenosis
DEF: Congenital heart defect characterized by stenosis of the left ventricular outflow tract due to a fibrous tissue ring or septal hypertrophy below the aortic valve.

Q24.5 Malformation of coronary vessels
Congenital coronary (artery) aneurysm

Q24.6 Congenital heart block

Q24.8 Other specified congenital malformations of heart
Congenital diverticulum of left ventricle
Congenital malformation of myocardium
Congenital malformation of pericardium
Malposition of heart
Uhl's disease

Q24.9 Congenital malformation of heart, unspecified ▽
Congenital anomaly of heart
Congenital disease of heart

✓4ᵗʰ **Q25 Congenital malformations of great arteries**

Q25.0 Patent ductus arteriosus
Patent ductus Botallo
Persistent ductus arteriosus

Patent Ductus Arteriosus

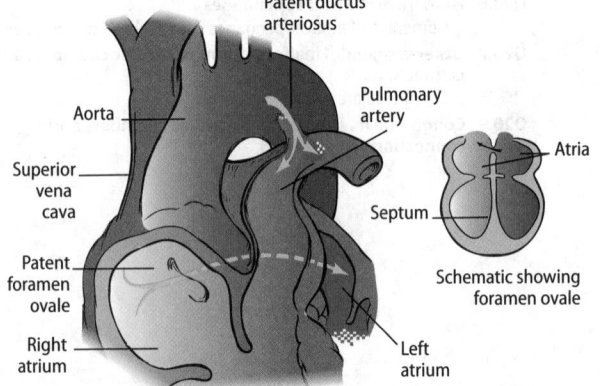

Q25.1 Coarctation of aorta
Coarctation of aorta (preductal) (postductal)
Stenosis of aorta
AHA: 2016,4Q,56-57

✓5ᵗʰ **Q25.2 Atresia of aorta**
AHA: 2016,4Q,56-57

Q25.21 Interruption of aortic arch
Atresia of aortic arch

Q25.29 Other atresia of aorta
Atresia of aorta

Chapter 17. Congenital Malformations, Deformations and Chromosomal Abnormalities

Q25.3–Q28.2

Q25.3 Supravalvular aortic stenosis
> EXCLUDES 1   *congenital aortic stenosis NOS (Q23.0)*
> *congenital stenosis of aortic valve (Q23.0)*

✓5ᵗʰ **Q25.4 Other congenital malformations of aorta**
> EXCLUDES 1   *hypoplasia of aorta in hypoplastic left heart syndrome (Q23.4)*
> **AHA:** 2016,4Q,57

Q25.40 Congenital malformation of aorta unspecified ▽

Q25.41 Absence and aplasia of aorta

Q25.42 Hypoplasia of aorta

Q25.43 Congenital aneurysm of aorta
> Congenital aneurysm of aortic root
> Congenital aneurysm of aortic sinus

Q25.44 Congenital dilation of aorta

Q25.45 Double aortic arch
> Vascular ring of aorta

Aortic Arch Anomalies

Normal aortic arch

Double aortic arch   Right aortic arch

Q25.46 Tortuous aortic arch
> Persistent convolutions of aortic arch

Q25.47 Right aortic arch
> Persistent right aortic arch

Q25.48 Anomalous origin of subclavian artery

Q25.49 Other congenital malformations of aorta
> Aortic arch
> Bovine arch

Q25.5 Atresia of pulmonary artery

Q25.6 Stenosis of pulmonary artery
> Supravalvular pulmonary stenosis

✓5ᵗʰ **Q25.7 Other congenital malformations of pulmonary artery**

Q25.71 Coarctation of pulmonary artery

Q25.72 Congenital pulmonary arteriovenous malformation
> Congenital pulmonary arteriovenous aneurysm

Q25.79 Other congenital malformations of pulmonary artery
> Aberrant pulmonary artery
> Agenesis of pulmonary artery
> Congenital aneurysm of pulmonary artery
> Congenital anomaly of pulmonary artery
> Hypoplasia of pulmonary artery

Q25.8 Other congenital malformations of other great arteries

Q25.9 Congenital malformation of great arteries, unspecified ▽

✓4ᵗʰ **Q26 Congenital malformations of great veins**

Q26.0 Congenital stenosis of vena cava
> Congenital stenosis of vena cava (inferior)(superior)

Q26.1 Persistent left superior vena cava

Q26.2 Total anomalous pulmonary venous connection
> Total anomalous pulmonary venous return [TAPVR], subdiaphragmatic
> Total anomalous pulmonary venous return [TAPVR], supradiaphragmatic

Q26.3 Partial anomalous pulmonary venous connection
> Partial anomalous pulmonary venous return

Q26.4 Anomalous pulmonary venous connection, unspecified ▽

Q26.5 Anomalous portal venous connection

Q26.6 Portal vein-hepatic artery fistula

Q26.8 Other congenital malformations of great veins
> Absence of vena cava (inferior) (superior)
> Azygos continuation of inferior vena cava
> Persistent left posterior cardinal vein
> Scimitar syndrome

Q26.9 Congenital malformation of great vein, unspecified ▽
> Congenital anomaly of vena cava (inferior) (superior) NOS

✓4ᵗʰ **Q27 Other congenital malformations of peripheral vascular system**
> EXCLUDES 2   *anomalies of cerebral and precerebral vessels (Q28.0-Q28.3)*
> *anomalies of coronary vessels (Q24.5)*
> *anomalies of pulmonary artery (Q25.5-Q25.7)*
> *congenital retinal aneurysm (Q14.1)*
> *hemangioma and lymphangioma (D18.-)*

Q27.0 Congenital absence and hypoplasia of umbilical artery
> Single umbilical artery

Q27.1 Congenital renal artery stenosis

Q27.2 Other congenital malformations of renal artery
> Congenital malformation of renal artery NOS
> Multiple renal arteries

✓5ᵗʰ **Q27.3 Arteriovenous malformation (peripheral)**
> Arteriovenous aneurysm
> EXCLUDES 1   *acquired arteriovenous aneurysm (I77.0)*
> EXCLUDES 2   *arteriovenous malformation of cerebral vessels (Q28.2)*
> *arteriovenous malformation of precerebral vessels (Q28.0)*
> **DEF:** Arteriovenous malformation: Connecting passage between an artery and a vein.

Q27.30 Arteriovenous malformation, site unspecified ▽

Q27.31 Arteriovenous malformation of vessel of upper limb

Q27.32 Arteriovenous malformation of vessel of lower limb

Q27.33 Arteriovenous malformation of digestive system vessel

Q27.34 Arteriovenous malformation of renal vessel

Q27.39 Arteriovenous malformation, other site

Q27.4 Congenital phlebectasia

Q27.8 Other specified congenital malformations of peripheral vascular system
> Absence of peripheral vascular system
> Atresia of peripheral vascular system
> Congenital aneurysm (peripheral)
> Congenital stricture, artery
> Congenital varix
> EXCLUDES 1   *arteriovenous malformation (Q27.3-)*

Q27.9 Congenital malformation of peripheral vascular system, unspecified ▽
> Anomaly of artery or vein NOS

✓4ᵗʰ **Q28 Other congenital malformations of circulatory system**
> EXCLUDES 1   *congenital aneurysm NOS (Q27.8)*
> *congenital coronary aneurysm (Q24.5)*
> *ruptured cerebral arteriovenous malformation (I60.8)*
> *ruptured malformation of precerebral vessels (I72.0)*
> EXCLUDES 2   *congenital peripheral aneurysm (Q27.8)*
> *congenital pulmonary aneurysm (Q25.79)*
> *congenital retinal aneurysm (Q14.1)*

Q28.0 Arteriovenous malformation of precerebral vessels
> Congenital arteriovenous precerebral aneurysm (nonruptured)

Q28.1 Other malformations of precerebral vessels
> Congenital malformation of precerebral vessels NOS
> Congenital precerebral aneurysm (nonruptured)

Q28.2 Arteriovenous malformation of cerebral vessels
> Arteriovenous malformation of brain NOS
> Congenital arteriovenous cerebral aneurysm (nonruptured)

Chapter 17. Congenital Malformations, Deformations and Chromosomal Abnormalities

Q25.3–Q28.2

Q28.3 Other malformations of cerebral vessels
Congenital cerebral aneurysm (nonruptured)
Congenital malformation of cerebral vessels NOS
Developmental venous anomaly

Q28.8 Other specified congenital malformations of circulatory system
Congenital aneurysm, specified site NEC
Spinal vessel anomaly

Q28.9 Congenital malformation of circulatory system, unspecified ▽

Congenital malformations of the respiratory system (Q30-Q34)

✓4ᵗʰ **Q30 Congenital malformations of nose**
EXCLUDES 1   congenital deviation of nasal septum (Q67.4)

Q30.0 Choanal atresia
Atresia of nares (anterior) (posterior)
Congenital stenosis of nares (anterior) (posterior)

Q30.1 Agenesis and underdevelopment of nose
Congenital absent of nose

Q30.2 Fissured, notched and cleft nose

Q30.3 Congenital perforated nasal septum

Q30.8 Other congenital malformations of nose
Accessory nose
Congenital anomaly of nasal sinus wall

Q30.9 Congenital malformation of nose, unspecified ▽

✓4ᵗʰ **Q31 Congenital malformations of larynx**
EXCLUDES 1   congenital laryngeal stridor NOS (P28.89)

Q31.0 Web of larynx
Glottic web of larynx
Subglottic web of larynx
Web of larynx NOS
DEF: Congenital malformation of the larynx marked by thin, translucent, or thick fibrotic membrane-like structure between the vocal folds. It is characterized by shortness of breath and stridor.

Q31.1 Congenital subglottic stenosis

Q31.2 Laryngeal hypoplasia

Q31.3 Laryngocele

Q31.5 Congenital laryngomalacia

Q31.8 Other congenital malformations of larynx
Absence of larynx
Agenesis of larynx
Atresia of larynx
Congenital cleft thyroid cartilage
Congenital fissure of epiglottis
Congenital stenosis of larynx NEC
Posterior cleft of cricoid cartilage

Q31.9 Congenital malformation of larynx, unspecified ▽

✓4ᵗʰ **Q32 Congenital malformations of trachea and bronchus**
EXCLUDES 1   congenital bronchiectasis (Q33.4)

Q32.0 Congenital tracheomalacia

Q32.1 Other congenital malformations of trachea<
Atresia of trachea
Congenital anomaly of tracheal cartilage
Congenital dilatation of trachea
Congenital malformation of trachea
Congenital stenosis of trachea
Congenital tracheocele

Q32.2 Congenital bronchomalacia

Q32.3 Congenital stenosis of bronchus

Q32.4 Other congenital malformations of bronchus
Absence of bronchus
Agenesis of bronchus
Atresia of bronchus
Congenital diverticulum of bronchus
Congenital malformation of bronchus NOS

✓4ᵗʰ **Q33 Congenital malformations of lung**

Q33.0 Congenital cystic lung
Congenital cystic lung disease
Congenital honeycomb lung
Congenital polycystic lung disease
EXCLUDES 1   cystic fibrosis (E84.0)
              cystic lung disease, acquired or unspecified (J98.4)

Q33.1 Accessory lobe of lung
Azygos lobe (fissured), lung

Q33.2 Sequestration of lung

Q33.3 Agenesis of lung
Congenital absence of lung (lobe)

Q33.4 Congenital bronchiectasis

Q33.5 Ectopic tissue in lung

Q33.6 Congenital hypoplasia and dysplasia of lung
EXCLUDES 1   pulmonary hypoplasia associated with short gestation (P28.0)

Q33.8 Other congenital malformations of lung

Q33.9 Congenital malformation of lung, unspecified ▽

✓4ᵗʰ **Q34 Other congenital malformations of respiratory system**
EXCLUDES 2   congenital central alveolar hypoventilation syndrome (G47.35)

Q34.0 Anomaly of pleura

Q34.1 Congenital cyst of mediastinum

Q34.8 Other specified congenital malformations of respiratory system
Atresia of nasopharynx

Q34.9 Congenital malformation of respiratory system, unspecified ▽
Congenital absence of respiratory system
Congenital anomaly of respiratory system NOS

Cleft lip and cleft palate (Q35-Q37)

Use additional code to identify associated malformation of the nose (Q30.2)
EXCLUDES 1   Robin syndrome (Q87.0)

✓4ᵗʰ **Q35 Cleft palate**
INCLUDES   fissure of palate
            palatoschisis
EXCLUDES 1   cleft palate with cleft lip (Q37.-)
DEF: Congenital fissure or defect of the roof of the mouth opening to the nasal cavity due to failure of embryonic cells to fuse completely.

Cleft Palate

Cleft in soft palate   Cleft in hard and soft palate

Hard palate

Soft palate

Cleft   Cleft

Q35.1 Cleft hard palate

Q35.3 Cleft soft palate

Q35.5 Cleft hard palate with cleft soft palate

Q35.7 Cleft uvula

Q35.9 Cleft palate, unspecified ▽
Cleft palate NOS

☑4ᵗʰ **Q36 Cleft lip**

   INCLUDES   cheiloschisis
                 congenital fissure of lip
                 harelip
                 labium leporinum

   EXCLUDES 1   *cleft lip with cleft palate (Q37.-)*

DEF: Congenital fissure or opening in the upper lip due to failure of embryonic cells to fuse completely.

Cleft Lip

Unilateral incomplete   Unilateral complete   Bilateral complete

Q36.0 Cleft lip, bilateral
Q36.1 Cleft lip, median
Q36.9 Cleft lip, unilateral
     Cleft lip NOS

☑4ᵗʰ **Q37 Cleft palate with cleft lip**

   INCLUDES   cheilopalatoschisis

Q37.0 Cleft hard palate with bilateral cleft lip
Q37.1 Cleft hard palate with unilateral cleft lip
     Cleft hard palate with cleft lip NOS
Q37.2 Cleft soft palate with bilateral cleft lip
Q37.3 Cleft soft palate with unilateral cleft lip
     Cleft soft palate with cleft lip NOS
Q37.4 Cleft hard and soft palate with bilateral cleft lip
Q37.5 Cleft hard and soft palate with unilateral cleft lip
     Cleft hard and soft palate with cleft lip NOS
Q37.8 Unspecified cleft palate with bilateral cleft lip ▽
Q37.9 Unspecified cleft palate with unilateral cleft lip ▽
     Cleft palate with cleft lip NOS

Other congenital malformations of the digestive system (Q38-Q45)

☑4ᵗʰ **Q38 Other congenital malformations of tongue, mouth and pharynx**

   EXCLUDES 1   *dentofacial anomalies (M26.-)*
                 macrostomia (Q18.4)
                 microstomia (Q18.5)

Q38.0 Congenital malformations of lips, not elsewhere classified
     Congenital fistula of lip
     Congenital malformation of lip NOS
     Van der Woude's syndrome
     EXCLUDES 1   *cleft lip (Q36.-)*
                   cleft lip with cleft palate (Q37.-)
                   macrocheilia (Q18.6)
                   microcheilia (Q18.7)

Q38.1 Ankyloglossia
     Tongue tie
Q38.2 Macroglossia
     Congenital hypertrophy of tongue
Q38.3 Other congenital malformations of tongue
     Aglossia
     Bifid tongue
     Congenital adhesion of tongue
     Congenital fissure of tongue
     Congenital malformation of tongue NOS
     Double tongue
     Hypoglossia
     Hypoplasia of tongue
     Microglossia
Q38.4 Congenital malformations of salivary glands and ducts
     Atresia of salivary glands and ducts
     Congenital absence of salivary glands and ducts
     Congenital accessory salivary glands and ducts
     Congenital fistula of salivary gland

Q38.5 Congenital malformations of palate, not elsewhere classified
     Congenital absence of uvula
     Congenital malformation of palate NOS
     Congenital high arched palate
     EXCLUDES 1   *cleft palate (Q35.-)*
                   cleft palate with cleft lip (Q37.-)
Q38.6 Other congenital malformations of mouth
     Congenital malformation of mouth NOS
Q38.7 Congenital pharyngeal pouch
     Congenital diverticulum of pharynx
     EXCLUDES 1   *pharyngeal pouch syndrome (D82.1)*
Q38.8 Other congenital malformations of pharynx
     Congenital malformation of pharynx NOS
     Imperforate pharynx

☑4ᵗʰ **Q39 Congenital malformations of esophagus**

Q39.0 Atresia of esophagus without fistula
     Atresia of esophagus NOS
Q39.1 Atresia of esophagus with tracheo-esophageal fistula
     Atresia of esophagus with broncho-esophageal fistula
Q39.2 Congenital tracheo-esophageal fistula without atresia
     Congenital tracheo-esophageal fistula NOS
Q39.3 Congenital stenosis and stricture of esophagus
Q39.4 Esophageal web
Q39.5 Congenital dilatation of esophagus
     Congenital cardiospasm
Q39.6 Congenital diverticulum of esophagus
     Congenital esophageal pouch
Q39.8 Other congenital malformations of esophagus
     Congenital absence of esophagus
     Congenital displacement of esophagus
     Congenital duplication of esophagus
Q39.9 Congenital malformation of esophagus, unspecified ▽

☑4ᵗʰ **Q40 Other congenital malformations of upper alimentary tract**

Q40.0 Congenital hypertrophic pyloric stenosis
     Congenital or infantile constriction
     Congenital or infantile hypertrophy
     Congenital or infantile spasm
     Congenital or infantile stenosis
     Congenital or infantile stricture
Q40.1 Congenital hiatus hernia
     Congenital displacement of cardia through esophageal hiatus
     EXCLUDES 1   *congenital diaphragmatic hernia (Q79.0)*
Q40.2 Other specified congenital malformations of stomach
     Congenital displacement of stomach
     Congenital diverticulum of stomach
     Congenital hourglass stomach
     Congenital duplication of stomach
     Megalogastria
     Microgastria
Q40.3 Congenital malformation of stomach, unspecified ▽
Q40.8 Other specified congenital malformations of upper alimentary tract
Q40.9 Congenital malformation of upper alimentary tract, unspecified ▽
     Congenital anomaly of upper alimentary tract
     Congenital deformity of upper alimentary tract

☑4ᵗʰ **Q41 Congenital absence, atresia and stenosis of small intestine**

   INCLUDES   congenital obstruction, occlusion or stricture of small intestine or intestine NOS
   EXCLUDES 1   *cystic fibrosis with intestinal manifestation (E84.11)*
                 meconium ileus NOS (without cystic fibrosis) (P76.0)

Q41.0 Congenital absence, atresia and stenosis of duodenum
Q41.1 Congenital absence, atresia and stenosis of jejunum
     Apple peel syndrome
     Imperforate jejunum
Q41.2 Congenital absence, atresia and stenosis of ileum
Q41.8 Congenital absence, atresia and stenosis of other specified parts of small intestine
Q41.9 Congenital absence, atresia and stenosis of small intestine, part unspecified ▽
     Congenital absence, atresia and stenosis of intestine NOS

☑4ᵗʰ **Q42 Congenital absence, atresia and stenosis of large intestine**

   INCLUDES   congenital obstruction, occlusion and stricture of large intestine
Q42.0 Congenital absence, atresia and stenosis of rectum with fistula

---

☑ Additional Character Req   ☑x7ᵗʰ Placeholder Alert   Manifestation   ▽ Unspecified   ►◄ Revised Text   ● New Code   ▲ Revised Code Title

Q42.1 **Congenital absence, atresia and stenosis of rectum without fistula**
　Imperforate rectum

Q42.2 **Congenital absence, atresia and stenosis of anus with fistula**

Q42.3 **Congenital absence, atresia and stenosis of anus without fistula**
　Imperforate anus

Q42.8 **Congenital absence, atresia and stenosis of other parts of large intestine**

Q42.9 **Congenital absence, atresia and stenosis of large intestine, part unspecified**　▽

√4ᵗʰ **Q43** **Other congenital malformations of intestine**

Q43.0 **Meckel's diverticulum (displaced) (hypertrophic)**
　Persistent omphalomesenteric duct
　Persistent vitelline duct
　DEF: Congenital, abnormal remnant of embryonic digestive system development that leaves a sacculation or outpouching from the wall of the small intestine near the terminal part of the ileum made of acid-secreting tissue as in the stomach.

Q43.1 **Hirschsprung's disease**
　Aganglionosis
　Congenital (aganglionic) megacolon
　DEF: Congenital enlargement or dilation of the colon, with the absence of nerve cells in a segment of colon distally that causes the inability to defecate.

Q43.2 **Other congenital functional disorders of colon**
　Congenital dilatation of colon

Q43.3 **Congenital malformations of intestinal fixation**
　Congenital omental, anomalous adhesions [bands]
　Congenital peritoneal adhesions [bands]
　Incomplete rotation of cecum and colon
　Insufficient rotation of cecum and colon
　Jackson's membrane
　Malrotation of colon
　Rotation failure of cecum and colon
　Universal mesentery

Q43.4 **Duplication of intestine**

Q43.5 **Ectopic anus**

Q43.6 **Congenital fistula of rectum and anus**
　EXCLUDES 1　congenital fistula of anus with absence, atresia and stenosis (Q42.2)
　　　congenital fistula of rectum with absence, atresia and stenosis (Q42.0)
　　　congenital rectovaginal fistula (Q52.2)
　　　congenital urethrorectal fistula (Q64.73)
　　　pilonidal fistula or sinus (L05.-)

Q43.7 **Persistent cloaca**
　Cloaca NOS

Q43.8 **Other specified congenital malformations of intestine**
　Congenital blind loop syndrome
　Congenital diverticulitis, colon
　Congenital diverticulum, intestine
　Dolichocolon
　Megaloappendix
　Megaloduodenum
　Microcolon
　Transposition of appendix
　Transposition of colon
　Transposition of intestine
　AHA: 2013,2Q,31

Q43.9 **Congenital malformation of intestine, unspecified**　▽

√4ᵗʰ **Q44** **Congenital malformations of gallbladder, bile ducts and liver**

Q44.0 **Agenesis, aplasia and hypoplasia of gallbladder**
　Congenital absence of gallbladder

Q44.1 **Other congenital malformations of gallbladder**
　Congenital malformation of gallbladder NOS
　Intrahepatic gallbladder

Q44.2 **Atresia of bile ducts**

Q44.3 **Congenital stenosis and stricture of bile ducts**

Q44.4 **Choledochal cyst**

Q44.5 **Other congenital malformations of bile ducts**
　Accessory hepatic duct
　Biliary duct duplication
　Congenital malformation of bile duct NOS
　Cystic duct duplication

Q44.6 **Cystic disease of liver**
　Fibrocystic disease of liver

Q44.7 **Other congenital malformations of liver**
　Accessory liver
　Alagille's syndrome
　Congenital absence of liver
　Congenital hepatomegaly
　Congenital malformation of liver NOS

√4ᵗʰ **Q45** **Other congenital malformations of digestive system**
　EXCLUDES 2　congenital diaphragmatic hernia (Q79.0)
　　　congenital hiatus hernia (Q40.1)

Q45.0 **Agenesis, aplasia and hypoplasia of pancreas**
　Congenital absence of pancreas

Q45.1 **Annular pancreas**

Q45.2 **Congenital pancreatic cyst**

Q45.3 **Other congenital malformations of pancreas and pancreatic duct**
　Accessory pancreas
　Congenital malformation of pancreas or pancreatic duct NOS
　EXCLUDES 1　congenital diabetes mellitus (E10.-)
　　　cystic fibrosis (E84.0-E84.9)
　　　fibrocystic disease of pancreas (E84.-)
　　　neonatal diabetes mellitus (P70.2)

Q45.8 **Other specified congenital malformations of digestive system**
　Absence (complete) (partial) of alimentary tract NOS
　Duplication of digestive system
　Malposition, congenital of digestive system

Q45.9 **Congenital malformation of digestive system, unspecified**　▽
　Congenital anomaly of digestive system
　Congenital deformity of digestive system

Congenital malformations of genital organs (Q50-Q56)

EXCLUDES 1　androgen insensitivity syndrome (E34.5-)
　　syndromes associated with anomalies in the number and form of chromosomes (Q90-Q99)

√4ᵗʰ **Q50** **Congenital malformations of ovaries, fallopian tubes and broad ligaments**

√5ᵗʰ **Q50.0** **Congenital absence of ovary**
　EXCLUDES 1　Turner's syndrome (Q96.-)

Q50.01 **Congenital absence of ovary, unilateral**　♀
Q50.02 **Congenital absence of ovary, bilateral**　♀

Q50.1 **Developmental ovarian cyst**　♀

Q50.2 **Congenital torsion of ovary**　♀

√5ᵗʰ **Q50.3** **Other congenital malformations of ovary**

Q50.31 **Accessory ovary**　♀

Q50.32 **Ovarian streak**　♀
　46, XX with streak gonads

Q50.39 **Other congenital malformation of ovary**　♀
　Congenital malformation of ovary NOS

Q50.4 **Embryonic cyst of fallopian tube**　♀
　Fimbrial cyst

Q50.5 **Embryonic cyst of broad ligament**　♀
　Epoophoron cyst
　Parovarian cyst

Q50.6 **Other congenital malformations of fallopian tube and broad ligament**
　Absence of fallopian tube and broad ligament
　Accessory fallopian tube and broad ligament
　Atresia of fallopian tube and broad ligament
　Congenital malformation of fallopian tube or broad ligament NOS

√4ᵗʰ **Q51** **Congenital malformations of uterus and cervix**

Q51.0 **Agenesis and aplasia of uterus**　♀
　Congenital absence of uterus

√5ᵗʰ **Q51.1** **Doubling of uterus with doubling of cervix and vagina**

Q51.10 **Doubling of uterus with doubling of cervix and vagina without obstruction**　♀
　Doubling of uterus with doubling of cervix and vagina NOS

Q51.11 **Doubling of uterus with doubling of cervix and vagina with obstruction**　♀

✓5ᵗʰ **Q51.2　Other doubling of uterus**
Doubling of uterus NOS
▶Septate uterus◀

● 　　　**Q51.20　Other doubling of uterus, unspecified**　　　▽
Septate uterus, unspecified

● 　　　**Q51.21　Other complete doubling of uterus**
Complete septate uterus

● 　　　**Q51.22　Other partial doubling of uterus**
Partial septate uterus

● 　　　**Q51.28　Other doubling of uterus, other specified**
Septate uterus, other specified

Q51.3　Bicornate uterus　　　♀
Bicornate uterus, complete or partial

Q51.4　Unicornate uterus　　　♀
Unicornate uterus with or without a separate uterine horn
Uterus with only one functioning horn

Q51.5　Agenesis and aplasia of cervix　　　♀
Congenital absence of cervix

Q51.6　Embryonic cyst of cervix　　　♀

Q51.7　Congenital fistulae between uterus and digestive and urinary tracts　　　♀

✓5ᵗʰ **Q51.8　Other congenital malformations of uterus and cervix**

　✓6ᵗʰ **Q51.81　Other congenital malformations of uterus**

　　　Q51.810　Arcuate uterus　　　♀
Arcuatus uterus

　　　Q51.811　Hypoplasia of uterus　　　♀

　　　Q51.818　Other congenital malformations of uterus　　　♀
Müllerian anomaly of uterus NEC

　✓6ᵗʰ **Q51.82　Other congenital malformations of cervix**

　　　Q51.820　Cervical duplication　　　♀
　　　Q51.821　Hypoplasia of cervix　　　♀
　　　Q51.828　Other congenital malformations of cervix　　　♀

Q51.9　Congenital malformation of uterus and cervix, unspecified　　　♀ ▽

✓4ᵗʰ **Q52　Other congenital malformations of female genitalia**

Q52.0　Congenital absence of vagina　　　♀
Vaginal agenesis, total or partial

✓5ᵗʰ **Q52.1　Doubling of vagina**

　　　EXCLUDES 1　　*doubling of vagina with doubling of uterus and cervix (Q51.1-)*

　　　Q52.10　Doubling of vagina, unspecified　　　♀ ▽
Septate vagina NOS

　　　Q52.11　Transverse vaginal septum　　　♀

　✓6ᵗʰ **Q52.12　Longitudinal vaginal septum**

　　　　AHA: 2016,4Q,58-59

　　　　Q52.120　Longitudinal vaginal septum, nonobstructing　　　♀

　　　　Q52.121　Longitudinal vaginal septum, obstructing, right side　　　♀

　　　　Q52.122　Longitudinal vaginal septum, obstructing, left side　　　♀

　　　　Q52.123　Longitudinal vaginal septum, microperforate, right side　　　♀

　　　　Q52.124　Longitudinal vaginal septum, microperforate, left side　　　♀

　　　　Q52.129　Other and unspecified longitudinal vaginal septum　　　♀ ▽

Q52.2　Congenital rectovaginal fistula　　　♀
　　　EXCLUDES 1　　*cloaca (Q43.7)*

Q52.3　Imperforate hymen　　　♀
DEF: Obstructive anomaly of vagina, characterized by complete closure of the membranous fold around the external opening of the vagina, obstructing the vaginal introitus.

Q52.4　Other congenital malformations of vagina　　　♀
Canal of Nuck cyst, congenital
Congenital malformation of vagina NOS
Embryonic vaginal cyst
Gartner's duct cyst

Q52.5　Fusion of labia　　　♀

Q52.6　Congenital malformation of clitoris　　　♀

✓5ᵗʰ **Q52.7　Other and unspecified congenital malformations of vulva**

　　　Q52.70　Unspecified congenital malformations of vulva　　　♀ ▽
Congenital malformation of vulva NOS

　　　Q52.71　Congenital absence of vulva　　　♀

　　　Q52.79　Other congenital malformations of vulva　　　♀
Congenital cyst of vulva

Q52.8　Other specified congenital malformations of female genitalia

Q52.9　Congenital malformation of female genitalia, unspecified　　　♀ ▽

✓4ᵗʰ **Q53　Undescended and ectopic testicle**

　✓5ᵗʰ **Q53.0　Ectopic testis**

　　　Q53.00　Ectopic testis, unspecified　　　♂ ▽
　　　Q53.01　Ectopic testis, unilateral　　　♂
　　　Q53.02　Ectopic testes, bilateral　　　♂

　✓5ᵗʰ **Q53.1　Undescended testicle, unilateral**

　　　AHA: 2017,4Q,22-23

　　　Q53.10　Unspecified undescended testicle, unilateral　　　♂ ▽

　✓6ᵗʰ **Q53.11　Abdominal testis, unilateral**

　　　　Q53.111　Unilateral intraabdominal testis　　　♂
　　　　Q53.112　Unilateral inguinal testis　　　♂

　　　Q53.12　Ectopic perineal testis, unilateral　　　♂
　　　Q53.13　Unilateral high scrotal testis　　　♂

　✓5ᵗʰ **Q53.2　Undescended testicle, bilateral**

　　　AHA: 2017,4Q,22-23

　　　Q53.20　Undescended testicle, unspecified, bilateral　　　♂ ▽

　✓6ᵗʰ **Q53.21　Abdominal testis, bilateral**

　　　　Q53.211　Bilateral intraabdominal testes　　　♂
　　　　Q53.212　Bilateral inguinal testes　　　♂

　　　Q53.22　Ectopic perineal testis, bilateral　　　♂
　　　Q53.23　Bilateral high scrotal testes　　　♂

Q53.9　Undescended testicle, unspecified　　　♂ ▽
Cryptorchism NOS

✓4ᵗʰ **Q54　Hypospadias**

　　　EXCLUDES 1　　*epispadias (Q64.0)*
DEF: Abnormal opening of the urethra on the ventral (underside) surface of the penis.

Hypospadias and Epispadias

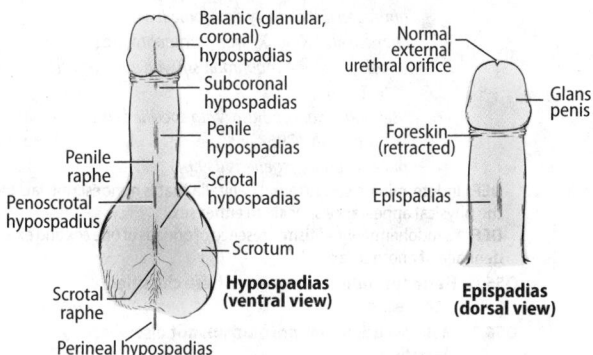

Hypospadias (ventral view)　　**Epispadias (dorsal view)**

Q54.0　Hypospadias, balanic　　　♂
Hypospadias, coronal
Hypospadias, glandular

Q54.1　Hypospadias, penile　　　♂

Q54.2　Hypospadias, penoscrotal　　　♂

Q54.3　Hypospadias, perineal　　　♂

Q54.4　Congenital chordee　　　♂
Chordee without hypospadias

Q54.8　Other hypospadias　　　♂
Hypospadias with intersex state

Q54.9　Hypospadias, unspecified　　　♂ ▽

✓4ᵗʰ **Q55　Other congenital malformations of male genital organs**

　　　EXCLUDES 1　　*congenital hydrocele (P83.5)*
　　　　　　　　　hypospadias (Q54.-)

Q55.0　Absence and aplasia of testis　　　♂
Monorchism

Chapter 17. Congenital Malformations, Deformations and Chromosomal Abnormalities

Q51.2–Q55.0

Q55.1 Hypoplasia of testis and scrotum ♂
  Fusion of testes

√5ᵗʰ **Q55.2 Other and unspecified congenital malformations of testis and scrotum**
  Q55.20 Unspecified congenital malformations of testis and scrotum ♂ ▽
    Congenital malformation of testis or scrotum NOS
  Q55.21 Polyorchism ♂
    DEF: Congenital anomaly in which there are more than two testes.
  Q55.22 Retractile testis ♂
  Q55.23 Scrotal transposition ♂
  Q55.29 Other congenital malformations of testis and scrotum ♂

Q55.3 Atresia of vas deferens ♂
  Code first any associated cystic fibrosis (E84.-)

Q55.4 Other congenital malformations of vas deferens, epididymis, seminal vesicles and prostate ♂
  Absence or aplasia of prostate
  Absence or aplasia of spermatic cord
  Congenital malformation of vas deferens, epididymis, seminal vesicles or prostate NOS

Q55.5 Congenital absence and aplasia of penis ♂
√5ᵗʰ **Q55.6 Other congenital malformations of penis**
  Q55.61 Curvature of penis (lateral) ♂
  Q55.62 Hypoplasia of penis ♂
    Micropenis
  Q55.63 Congenital torsion of penis ♂
    EXCLUDES 1 acquired torsion of penis (N48.82)
  Q55.64 Hidden penis ♂
    Buried penis
    Concealed penis
    EXCLUDES 1 acquired buried penis (N48.83)
  Q55.69 Other congenital malformation of penis ♂
    Congenital malformation of penis NOS

Q55.7 Congenital vasocutaneous fistula ♂
Q55.8 Other specified congenital malformations of male genital organs ♂
Q55.9 Congenital malformation of male genital organ, unspecified ♂ ▽
  Congenital anomaly of male genital organ
  Congenital deformity of male genital organ

√4ᵗʰ **Q56 Indeterminate sex and pseudohermaphroditism**
  EXCLUDES 1 46, XX true hermaphrodite (Q99.1)
    androgen insensitivity syndrome (E34.5-)
    chimera 46, XX/46, XY true hermaphrodite (Q99.0)
    female pseudohermaphroditism with adrenocortical disorder (E25.-)
    pseudohermaphroditism with specified chromosomal anomaly (Q96-Q99)
    pure gonadal dysgenesis (Q99.1)
  DEF: Indeterminate sex: External genitalia that is nondescript, lacking the physical appearance specific to either sex.
  DEF: Pseudohermaphroditism: Presence of gonads of one sex and external genitalia of another sex.
  Q56.0 Hermaphroditism, not elsewhere classified
    Ovotestis
  Q56.1 Male pseudohermaphroditism, not elsewhere classified ♂
    46, XY with streak gonads
    Male pseudohermaphroditism NOS
  Q56.2 Female pseudohermaphroditism, not elsewhere classified ♀
    Female pseudohermaphroditism NOS
  Q56.3 Pseudohermaphroditism, unspecified ▽
  Q56.4 Indeterminate sex, unspecified ▽
    Ambiguous genitalia

Congenital malformations of the urinary system (Q60-Q64)

√4ᵗʰ **Q60 Renal agenesis and other reduction defects of kidney**
  INCLUDES congenital absence of kidney
    congenital atrophy of kidney
    infantile atrophy of kidney
  Q60.0 Renal agenesis, unilateral
  Q60.1 Renal agenesis, bilateral
  Q60.2 Renal agenesis, unspecified ▽
  Q60.3 Renal hypoplasia, unilateral

Q60.4 Renal hypoplasia, bilateral
Q60.5 Renal hypoplasia, unspecified ▽
Q60.6 Potter's syndrome

√4ᵗʰ **Q61 Cystic kidney disease**
  EXCLUDES 1 acquired cyst of kidney (N28.1)
    Potter's syndrome (Q60.6)
  √5ᵗʰ **Q61.0 Congenital renal cyst**
    Q61.00 Congenital renal cyst, unspecified ▽
      Cyst of kidney NOS (congenital)
    Q61.01 Congenital single renal cyst
    Q61.02 Congenital multiple renal cysts
  √5ᵗʰ **Q61.1 Polycystic kidney, infantile type**
    Polycystic kidney, autosomal recessive
    Q61.11 Cystic dilatation of collecting ducts
    Q61.19 Other polycystic kidney, infantile type
  Q61.2 Polycystic kidney, adult type
    Polycystic kidney, autosomal dominant
  Q61.3 Polycystic kidney, unspecified ▽
    AHA: 2016,3Q,22
  Q61.4 Renal dysplasia
    Multicystic dysplastic kidney
    Multicystic kidney (development)
    Multicystic kidney disease
    Multicystic renal dysplasia
    EXCLUDES 1 polycystic kidney disease (Q61.11-Q61.3)
  Q61.5 Medullary cystic kidney
    Nephronopthisis
    Sponge kidney NOS
    DEF: Sponge kidney: Dilated collecting tubules that are usually asymptomatic. Calcinosis in tubules may cause renal insufficiency.
  Q61.8 Other cystic kidney diseases
    Fibrocystic kidney
    Fibrocystic renal degeneration or disease
  Q61.9 Cystic kidney disease, unspecified ▽
    Meckel-Gruber syndrome

√4ᵗʰ **Q62 Congenital obstructive defects of renal pelvis and congenital malformations of ureter**
  Q62.0 Congenital hydronephrosis
  √5ᵗʰ **Q62.1 Congenital occlusion of ureter**
    Atresia and stenosis of ureter
    Q62.10 Congenital occlusion of ureter, unspecified ▽
    Q62.11 Congenital occlusion of ureteropelvic junction
    Q62.12 Congenital occlusion of ureterovesical orifice
  Q62.2 Congenital megaureter
    Congenital dilatation of ureter
  √5ᵗʰ **Q62.3 Other obstructive defects of renal pelvis and ureter**
    Q62.31 Congenital ureterocele, orthotopic
    Q62.32 Cecoureterocele
      Ectopic ureterocele
    Q62.39 Other obstructive defects of renal pelvis and ureter
      Ureteropelvic junction obstruction NOS
  Q62.4 Agenesis of ureter
    Congenital absence ureter
  Q62.5 Duplication of ureter
    Accessory ureter
    Double ureter
  √5ᵗʰ **Q62.6 Malposition of ureter**
    Q62.60 Malposition of ureter, unspecified ▽
    Q62.61 Deviation of ureter
    Q62.62 Displacement of ureter
    Q62.63 Anomalous implantation of ureter
      Ectopia of ureter
      Ectopic ureter
    Q62.69 Other malposition of ureter
  Q62.7 Congenital vesico-uretero-renal reflux
  Q62.8 Other congenital malformations of ureter
    Anomaly of ureter NOS

√4ᵗʰ **Q63 Other congenital malformations of kidney**
  EXCLUDES 1 congenital nephrotic syndrome (N04.-)
  Q63.0 Accessory kidney
  Q63.1 Lobulated, fused and horseshoe kidney
  Q63.2 Ectopic kidney
    Congenital displaced kidney
    Malrotation of kidney

Q63.3 Hyperplastic and giant **kidney**
　Compensatory hypertrophy of kidney

Q63.8 Other specified congenital malformations of kidney
　Congenital renal calculi

Q63.9 Congenital malformation of kidney, unspecified ▽

✓4ᵗʰ **Q64** Other congenital malformations of **urinary system**

　Q64.0 **Epispadias**
　　EXCLUDES 1　hypospadias (Q54.-)

✓5ᵗʰ **Q64.1** **Exstrophy of urinary bladder**
　　Q64.10 **Exstrophy of urinary bladder, unspecified** ▽
　　　Ectopia vesicae
　　Q64.11 **Supravesical fissure of urinary bladder**
　　Q64.12 **Cloacal exstrophy of urinary bladder**
　　Q64.19 **Other exstrophy of urinary bladder**
　　　Extroversion of bladder

　Q64.2 Congenital **posterior urethral valves**

✓5ᵗʰ **Q64.3** **Other atresia and stenosis of urethra and bladder neck**
　　Q64.31 Congenital **bladder neck obstruction**
　　　Congenital obstruction of vesicourethral orifice
　　Q64.32 Congenital **stricture of urethra**
　　Q64.33 Congenital **stricture of urinary meatus**
　　Q64.39 **Other atresia and stenosis of urethra and bladder neck**
　　　Atresia and stenosis of urethra and bladder neck NOS

　Q64.4 **Malformation of urachus**
　　Cyst of urachus
　　Patent urachus
　　Prolapse of urachus

　Q64.5 Congenital **absence of bladder and urethra**

　Q64.6 Congenital **diverticulum of bladder**

✓5ᵗʰ **Q64.7** **Other and unspecified congenital malformations of bladder and urethra**
　　EXCLUDES 1　congenital prolapse of bladder (mucosa) (Q79.4)
　　Q64.70 **Unspecified congenital malformation of bladder and urethra** ▽
　　　Malformation of bladder or urethra NOS
　　Q64.71 Congenital **prolapse of urethra**
　　Q64.72 Congenital **prolapse of urinary meatus**
　　Q64.73 Congenital **urethrorectal fistula**
　　Q64.74 **Double urethra**
　　Q64.75 **Double urinary meatus**
　　Q64.79 **Other congenital malformations of bladder and urethra**

　Q64.8 Other specified congenital malformations of urinary system

　Q64.9 **Congenital malformation of urinary system, unspecified** ▽
　　Congenital anomaly NOS of urinary system
　　Congenital deformity NOS of urinary system

Congenital malformations and deformations of the musculoskeletal system (Q65-Q79)

✓4ᵗʰ **Q65** **Congenital deformities of hip**
　　EXCLUDES 1　clicking hip (R29.4)

✓5ᵗʰ **Q65.0** Congenital **dislocation of hip, unilateral**
　　Q65.00 **Congenital dislocation of unspecified hip, unilateral** ▽
　　Q65.01 Congenital dislocation of **right** hip, unilateral
　　Q65.02 Congenital dislocation of **left** hip, unilateral

　Q65.1 Congenital **dislocation of hip, bilateral**

　Q65.2 Congenital **dislocation of hip, unspecified** ▽

✓5ᵗʰ **Q65.3** Congenital **partial dislocation of hip, unilateral**
　　Q65.30 **Congenital partial dislocation of unspecified hip, unilateral** ▽
　　Q65.31 **Congenital partial dislocation of right hip, unilateral**
　　Q65.32 Congenital partial dislocation of **left** hip, unilateral

　Q65.4 Congenital **partial dislocation of hip, bilateral**

　Q65.5 Congenital **partial dislocation of hip, unspecified** ▽

　Q65.6 Congenital **unstable hip**
　　Congenital dislocatable hip

✓5ᵗʰ **Q65.8** **Other congenital deformities of hip**
　　Q65.81 Congenital **coxa valga**
　　Q65.82 Congenital **coxa vara**

　　Q65.89 **Other specified congenital deformities of hip**
　　　Anteversion of femoral neck
　　　Congenital acetabular dysplasia

　Q65.9 **Congenital deformity of hip, unspecified** ▽

✓4ᵗʰ **Q66** **Congenital deformities of feet**
　　EXCLUDES 1　reduction defects of feet (Q72.-)
　　　valgus deformities (acquired) (M21.0-)
　　　varus deformities (acquired) (M21.1-)

　Q66.0 Congenital **talipes equinovarus**

　Q66.1 Congenital **talipes calcaneovarus**

✓5ᵗʰ **Q66.2** **Congenital metatarsus (primus) varus**
　　AHA: 2016,4Q,59
　　Q66.21 **Congenital metatarsus primus varus**
　　Q66.22 **Congenital metatarsus adductus**
　　　Congenital metatarsus varus

　Q66.3 **Other congenital varus deformities of feet**
　　Hallux varus, congenital

　Q66.4 Congenital **talipes calcaneovalgus**

✓5ᵗʰ **Q66.5** Congenital **pes planus**
　　Congenital flat foot
　　Congenital rigid flat foot
　　Congenital spastic (everted) flat foot
　　EXCLUDES 1　pes planus, acquired (M21.4)
　　Q66.50 **Congenital pes planus, unspecified foot** ▽
　　Q66.51 **Congenital pes planus, right foot**
　　Q66.52 **Congenital pes planus, left foot**

　Q66.6 **Other congenital valgus deformities of feet**
　　Congenital metatarsus valgus

　Q66.7 Congenital **pes cavus**

✓5ᵗʰ **Q66.8** **Other congenital deformities of feet**
　　Q66.80 **Congenital vertical talus deformity, unspecified foot** ▽
　　Q66.81 **Congenital vertical talus deformity, right foot**
　　Q66.82 **Congenital vertical talus deformity, left foot**
　　Q66.89 **Other specified congenital deformities of feet**
　　　Congenital asymmetric talipes
　　　Congenital clubfoot NOS
　　　Congenital talipes NOS
　　　Congenital tarsal coalition
　　　Hammer toe, congenital
　　　DEF: Clubfoot: Congenital anomaly of the foot with the heel elevated and rotated outward and the toes pointing inward.

　Q66.9 Congenital **deformity of feet, unspecified** ▽

✓4ᵗʰ **Q67** **Congenital musculoskeletal deformities of head, face, spine and chest**
　　EXCLUDES 1　congenital malformation syndromes classified to Q87.-
　　　Potter's syndrome (Q60.6)

　Q67.0 Congenital **facial asymmetry**

　Q67.1 Congenital **compression facies**

　Q67.2 **Dolichocephaly**

　Q67.3 **Plagiocephaly**

　Q67.4 **Other congenital deformities of skull, face and jaw**
　　Congenital depressions in skull
　　Congenital hemifacial atrophy or hypertrophy
　　Deviation of nasal septum, congenital
　　Squashed or bent nose, congenital
　　EXCLUDES 1　dentofacial anomalies [including malocclusion] (M26.-)
　　　syphilitic saddle nose (A50.5)
　　DEF: Deviated septum: Condition in which the nasal septum, a thin wall composed of cartilage and bone that separates the two nostrils, is crooked or displaced from the midline.

　Q67.5 Congenital **deformity of spine**
　　Congenital postural scoliosis
　　Congenital scoliosis NOS
　　EXCLUDES 1　infantile idiopathic scoliosis (M41.0)
　　　scoliosis due to congenital bony malformation (Q76.3)
　　AHA: 2014,4Q,26

　Q67.6 **Pectus excavatum**
　　Congenital funnel chest

　Q67.7 **Pectus carinatum**
　　Congenital pigeon chest

☑ Additional Character Req　　✓x7ᵗʰ Placeholder Alert　　Manifestation　　▲ 　▽ Unspecified　　►◄ Revised Text　　● New Code　　▲ Revised Code Title

Chapter 17. Congenital Malformations, Deformations and Chromosomal Abnormalities

Q67.8–Q72.03

Q67.8 **Other congenital deformities of chest**
Congenital deformity of chest wall NOS

✓4ᵗʰ **Q68** **Other congenital musculoskeletal deformities**
> EXCLUDES 1   reduction defects of limb(s) (Q71-Q73)
> EXCLUDES 2   congenital myotonic chondrodystrophy (G71.13)

Q68.0 **Congenital deformity of sternocleidomastoid muscle**
Congenital contracture of sternocleidomastoid (muscle)
Congenital (sternomastoid) torticollis
Sternomastoid tumor (congenital)

Q68.1 **Congenital deformity of finger(s) and hand**
Congenital clubfinger
Spade-like hand (congenital)

Q68.2 **Congenital deformity of knee**
Congenital dislocation of knee
Congenital genu recurvatum

Q68.3 **Congenital bowing of femur**
> EXCLUDES 1   anteversion of femur (neck) (Q65.89)

Q68.4 **Congenital bowing of tibia and fibula**

Q68.5 **Congenital bowing of long bones of leg, unspecified** ▽

Q68.6 **Discoid meniscus**

Q68.8 **Other specified congenital musculoskeletal deformities**
Congenital deformity of clavicle
Congenital deformity of elbow
Congenital deformity of forearm
Congenital deformity of scapula
Congenital deformity of wrist
Congenital dislocation of elbow
Congenital dislocation of shoulder
Congenital dislocation of wrist

✓4ᵗʰ **Q69** **Polydactyly**

Q69.0 **Accessory finger(s)**

Q69.1 **Accessory thumb(s)**

Q69.2 **Accessory toe(s)**
Accessory hallux

Q69.9 **Polydactyly, unspecified** ▽
Supernumerary digit(s) NOS

✓4ᵗʰ **Q70** **Syndactyly**

✓5ᵗʰ **Q70.0** **Fused fingers**
Complex syndactyly of fingers with synostosis
Q70.00 **Fused fingers, unspecified hand** ▽
Q70.01 **Fused fingers, right hand**
Q70.02 **Fused fingers, left hand**
Q70.03 **Fused fingers, bilateral**

✓5ᵗʰ **Q70.1** **Webbed fingers**
Simple syndactyly of fingers without synostosis
Q70.10 **Webbed fingers, unspecified hand** ▽
Q70.11 **Webbed fingers, right hand**
Q70.12 **Webbed fingers, left hand**
Q70.13 **Webbed fingers, bilateral**

✓5ᵗʰ **Q70.2** **Fused toes**
Complex syndactyly of toes with synostosis
Q70.20 **Fused toes, unspecified foot** ▽
Q70.21 **Fused toes, right foot**
Q70.22 **Fused toes, left foot**
Q70.23 **Fused toes, bilateral**

✓5ᵗʰ **Q70.3** **Webbed toes**
Simple syndactyly of toes without synostosis
Q70.30 **Webbed toes, unspecified foot** ▽
Q70.31 **Webbed toes, right foot**
Q70.32 **Webbed toes, left foot**
Q70.33 **Webbed toes, bilateral**

Q70.4 **Polysyndactyly, unspecified** ▽
> EXCLUDES 1   specified syndactyly of hand and feet - code to specified conditions (Q70.0-Q70.3-)

Q70.9 **Syndactyly, unspecified** ▽
Symphalangy NOS

✓4ᵗʰ **Q71** **Reduction defects of upper limb**

✓5ᵗʰ **Q71.0** **Congenital complete absence of upper limb**
Q71.00 **Congenital complete absence of unspecified** ▽
upper limb
Q71.01 **Congenital complete absence of right upper limb**
Q71.02 **Congenital complete absence of left upper limb**
Q71.03 **Congenital complete absence of upper limb, bilateral**

✓5ᵗʰ **Q71.1** **Congenital absence of upper arm and forearm with hand present**
Q71.10 **Congenital absence of unspecified upper** ▽
arm and forearm with hand present
Q71.11 **Congenital absence of right upper arm and forearm with hand present**
Q71.12 **Congenital absence of left upper arm and forearm with hand present**
Q71.13 **Congenital absence of upper arm and forearm with hand present, bilateral**

✓5ᵗʰ **Q71.2** **Congenital absence of both forearm and hand**
Q71.20 **Congenital absence of both forearm and** ▽
hand, unspecified upper limb
Q71.21 **Congenital absence of both forearm and hand, right upper limb**
Q71.22 **Congenital absence of both forearm and hand, left upper limb**
Q71.23 **Congenital absence of both forearm and hand, bilateral**

✓5ᵗʰ **Q71.3** **Congenital absence of hand and finger**
Q71.30 **Congenital absence of unspecified hand** ▽
and finger
Q71.31 **Congenital absence of right hand and finger**
Q71.32 **Congenital absence of left hand and finger**
Q71.33 **Congenital absence of hand and finger, bilateral**

✓5ᵗʰ **Q71.4** **Longitudinal reduction defect of radius**
Clubhand (congenital)
Radial clubhand
Q71.40 **Longitudinal reduction defect of** ▽
unspecified radius
Q71.41 **Longitudinal reduction defect of right radius**
Q71.42 **Longitudinal reduction defect of left radius**
Q71.43 **Longitudinal reduction defect of radius, bilateral**

✓5ᵗʰ **Q71.5** **Longitudinal reduction defect of ulna**
Q71.50 **Longitudinal reduction defect of** ▽
unspecified ulna
Q71.51 **Longitudinal reduction defect of right ulna**
Q71.52 **Longitudinal reduction defect of left ulna**
Q71.53 **Longitudinal reduction defect of ulna, bilateral**

✓5ᵗʰ **Q71.6** **Lobster-claw hand**
Q71.60 **Lobster-claw hand, unspecified hand** ▽
Q71.61 **Lobster-claw right hand**
Q71.62 **Lobster-claw left hand**
Q71.63 **Lobster-claw hand, bilateral**

✓5ᵗʰ **Q71.8** **Other reduction defects of upper limb**
✓6ᵗʰ **Q71.81** **Congenital shortening of upper limb**
Q71.811 **Congenital shortening of right upper limb**
Q71.812 **Congenital shortening of left upper limb**
Q71.813 **Congenital shortening of upper limb, bilateral**
Q71.819 **Congenital shortening of** ▽
unspecified upper limb
✓6ᵗʰ **Q71.89** **Other reduction defects of upper limb**
Q71.891 **Other reduction defects of right upper limb**
Q71.892 **Other reduction defects of left upper limb**
Q71.893 **Other reduction defects of upper limb, bilateral**
Q71.899 **Other reduction defects of** ▽
unspecified upper limb

✓5ᵗʰ **Q71.9** **Unspecified reduction defect of upper limb**
Q71.90 **Unspecified reduction defect of unspecified** ▽
upper limb
Q71.91 **Unspecified reduction defect of right upper** ▽
limb
Q71.92 **Unspecified reduction defect of left upper** ▽
limb
Q71.93 **Unspecified reduction defect of upper limb,** ▽
bilateral

✓4ᵗʰ **Q72** **Reduction defects of lower limb**

✓5ᵗʰ **Q72.0** **Congenital complete absence of lower limb**
Q72.00 **Congenital complete absence of unspecified** ▽
lower limb
Q72.01 **Congenital complete absence of right lower limb**
Q72.02 **Congenital complete absence of left lower limb**
Q72.03 **Congenital complete absence of lower limb, bilateral**

√5ᵗʰ **Q72.1 Congenital** absence of thigh and lower leg with foot present

Q72.10 Congenital absence of unspecified thigh and lower leg with foot present ▽

Q72.11 Congenital absence of right **thigh and lower leg with foot present**

Q72.12 Congenital absence of left **thigh and lower leg with foot present**

Q72.13 Congenital absence of thigh and lower leg with foot present, bilateral

√5ᵗʰ **Q72.2 Congenital** absence of both lower leg and foot

Q72.20 Congenital absence of both lower leg and foot, unspecified lower limb ▽

Q72.21 Congenital absence of both lower leg and foot, right **lower limb**

Q72.22 Congenital absence of both lower leg and foot, left **lower limb**

Q72.23 Congenital absence of both lower leg and foot, bilateral

√5ᵗʰ **Q72.3 Congenital** absence of foot and toe(s)

Q72.30 Congenital absence of unspecified foot and toe(s) ▽

Q72.31 Congenital absence of right **foot and toe(s)**

Q72.32 Congenital absence of left **foot and toe(s)**

Q72.33 Congenital absence of foot and toe(s), bilateral

√5ᵗʰ **Q72.4 Longitudinal reduction defect of** femur

Proximal femoral focal deficiency

Q72.40 Longitudinal reduction defect of unspecified femur ▽

Q72.41 Longitudinal reduction defect of right **femur**

Q72.42 Longitudinal reduction defect of left **femur**

Q72.43 Longitudinal reduction defect of femur, bilateral

√5ᵗʰ **Q72.5 Longitudinal reduction defect of** tibia

Q72.50 Longitudinal reduction defect of unspecified tibia ▽

Q72.51 Longitudinal reduction defect of right **tibia**

Q72.52 Longitudinal reduction defect of left **tibia**

Q72.53 Longitudinal reduction defect of tibia, bilateral

√5ᵗʰ **Q72.6 Longitudinal reduction defect of** fibula

Q72.60 Longitudinal reduction defect of unspecified fibula ▽

Q72.61 Longitudinal reduction defect of right **fibula**

Q72.62 Longitudinal reduction defect of left **fibula**

Q72.63 Longitudinal reduction defect of fibula, bilateral

√5ᵗʰ **Q72.7 Split foot**

Q72.70 Split foot, unspecified lower limb ▽

Q72.71 Split foot, right **lower limb**

Q72.72 Split foot, left **lower limb**

Q72.73 Split foot, bilateral

√5ᵗʰ **Q72.8 Other reduction defects of lower limb**

√6ᵗʰ **Q72.81 Congenital** shortening **of lower limb**

Q72.811 Congenital shortening of right **lower limb**

Q72.812 Congenital shortening of left **lower limb**

Q72.813 Congenital shortening of lower limb, bilateral

Q72.819 Congenital shortening of unspecified lower limb ▽

√6ᵗʰ **Q72.89 Other reduction defects of lower limb**

Q72.891 Other reduction defects of right **lower limb**

Q72.892 Other reduction defects of left **lower limb**

Q72.893 Other reduction defects of lower limb, bilateral

Q72.899 Other reduction defects of unspecified lower limb ▽

√5ᵗʰ **Q72.9 Unspecified reduction defect of lower limb**

Q72.90 Unspecified reduction defect of unspecified lower limb ▽

Q72.91 Unspecified reduction defect of right **lower limb** ▽

Q72.92 Unspecified reduction defect of left **lower limb** ▽

Q72.93 Unspecified reduction defect of lower limb, bilateral ▽

√4ᵗʰ **Q73 Reduction defects of unspecified limb**

Q73.0 Congenital absence of unspecified limb(s) ▽

Amelia NOS

Q73.1 Phocomelia, unspecified limb(s) ▽

Phocomelia NOS

Q73.8 Other reduction defects of unspecified limb(s) ▽

Longitudinal reduction deformity of unspecified limb(s)

Ectromelia of limb NOS

Hemimelia of limb NOS

Reduction defect of limb NOS

√4ᵗʰ **Q74 Other congenital malformations of limb(s)**

EXCLUDES 1 *polydactyly (Q69.-)*

reduction defect of limb (Q71-Q73)

syndactyly (Q70.-)

Q74.0 Other congenital malformations of upper limb(s), including shoulder girdle

Accessory carpal bones

Cleidocranial dysostosis

Congenital pseudarthrosis of clavicle

Macrodactylia (fingers)

Madelung's deformity

Radioulnar synostosis

Sprengel's deformity

Triphalangeal thumb

Q74.1 Congenital malformation of knee

Congenital absence of patella

Congenital dislocation of patella

Congenital genu valgum

Congenital genu varum

Rudimentary patella

EXCLUDES 1 *congenital dislocation of knee (Q68.2)*

congenital genu recurvatum (Q68.2)

nail patella syndrome (Q87.2)

Q74.2 Other congenital malformations of lower limb(s), including pelvic girdle

Congenital fusion of sacroiliac joint

Congenital malformation of ankle joint

Congenital malformation of sacroiliac joint

EXCLUDES 1 *anteversion of femur (neck) (Q65.89)*

Q74.3 Arthrogryposis multiplex congenita

Q74.8 Other specified congenital malformations of limb(s)

Q74.9 Unspecified congenital malformation of limb(s) ▽

Congenital anomaly of limb(s) NOS

√4ᵗʰ **Q75 Other congenital malformations of** skull and face bones

EXCLUDES 1 *congenital malformation of face NOS (Q18.-)*

congenital malformation syndromes classified to Q87.-

dentofacial anomalies [including malocclusion] (M26.-)

musculoskeletal deformities of head and face (Q67.0-Q67.4)

skull defects associated with congenital anomalies of brain such as:

anencephaly (Q00.0)

encephalocele (Q01.-)

hydrocephalus (Q03.-)

microcephaly (Q02)

Q75.0 Craniosynostosis

Acrocephaly

Imperfect fusion of skull

Oxycephaly

Trigonocephaly

DEF: Congenital condition in which one or more of the cranial sutures fuse prematurely, creating a deformed or aberrant head shape.

Q75.1 Craniofacial dysostosis

Crouzon's disease

Q75.2 Hypertelorism

Q75.3 Macrocephaly

Q75.4 Mandibulofacial dysostosis

Franceschetti syndrome

Treacher Collins syndrome

Q75.5 Oculomandibular dysostosis

Q75.8 Other specified congenital malformations of skull and face bones

Absence of skull bone, congenital

Congenital deformity of forehead

Platybasia

☑ Additional Character Req   √x7ᵗʰ Placeholder Alert   Manifestation   ▽ Unspecified   ►◄ Revised Text   ● New Code   ▲ Revised Code Title

Q75.9 **Congenital malformation of skull and face bones, unspecified** ▽
　Congenital anomaly of face bones NOS
　Congenital anomaly of skull NOS

✓4ᵗʰ **Q76** **Congenital malformations of spine and bony thorax**
　EXCLUDES 1　congenital musculoskeletal deformities of spine and chest (Q67.5-Q67.8)

Q76.0 **Spina bifida occulta**
　EXCLUDES 1　meningocele (spinal) (Q05.-)
　　spina bifida (aperta) (cystica) (Q05.-)

Q76.1 **Klippel-Feil syndrome**
　Cervical fusion syndrome

Q76.2 **Congenital spondylolisthesis**
　Congenital spondylolysis
　EXCLUDES 1　spondylolisthesis (acquired) (M43.1-)
　　spondylolysis (acquired) (M43.0-)

Q76.3 **Congenital scoliosis due to congenital bony malformation**
　Hemivertebra fusion or failure of segmentation with scoliosis

✓5ᵗʰ **Q76.4** **Other congenital malformations of spine, not associated with scoliosis**

✓6ᵗʰ **Q76.41** **Congenital kyphosis**
　　Q76.411 **Congenital kyphosis, occipito-atlanto-axial region**
　　Q76.412 **Congenital kyphosis, cervical region**
　　Q76.413 **Congenital kyphosis, cervicothoracic region**
　　Q76.414 **Congenital kyphosis, thoracic region**
　　Q76.415 **Congenital kyphosis, thoracolumbar region**
　　Q76.419 **Congenital kyphosis, unspecified region** ▽

✓6ᵗʰ **Q76.42** **Congenital lordosis**
　　Q76.425 **Congenital lordosis, thoracolumbar region**
　　Q76.426 **Congenital lordosis, lumbar region**
　　Q76.427 **Congenital lordosis, lumbosacral region**
　　Q76.428 **Congenital lordosis, sacral and sacrococcygeal region**
　　Q76.429 **Congenital lordosis, unspecified region** ▽

　　Q76.49 **Other congenital malformations of spine, not associated with scoliosis**
　　　Congenital absence of vertebra NOS
　　　Congenital fusion of spine NOS
　　　Congenital malformation of lumbosacral (joint) (region) NOS
　　　Congenital malformation of spine NOS
　　　Hemivertebra NOS
　　　Malformation of spine NOS
　　　Platyspondylisis NOS
　　　Supernumerary vertebra NOS

Q76.5 **Cervical rib**
　Supernumerary rib in cervical region

Q76.6 **Other congenital malformations of ribs**
　Accessory rib
　Congenital absence of rib
　Congenital fusion of ribs
　Congenital malformation of ribs NOS
　EXCLUDES 1　short rib syndrome (Q77.2)

Q76.7 **Congenital malformation of sternum**
　Congenital absence of sternum
　Sternum bifidum

Q76.8 **Other congenital malformations of bony thorax**

Q76.9 **Congenital malformation of bony thorax, unspecified** ▽

✓4ᵗʰ **Q77** **Osteochondrodysplasia with defects of growth of tubular bones and spine**
　EXCLUDES 1　mucopolysaccharidosis (E76.0-E76.3)
　EXCLUDES 2　congenital myotonic chondrodystrophy (G71.13)

Q77.0 **Achondrogenesis**
　Hypochondrogenesis

Q77.1 **Thanatophoric short stature**

Q77.2 **Short rib syndrome**
　Asphyxiating thoracic dysplasia [Jeune]

Q77.3 **Chondrodysplasia punctata**
　EXCLUDES 1　Rhizomelic chondrodysplasia punctata (E71.43)

Q77.4 **Achondroplasia**
　Hypochondroplasia
　Osteosclerosis congenita

Q77.5 **Diastrophic dysplasia**

Q77.6 **Chondroectodermal dysplasia**
　Ellis-van Creveld syndrome

Q77.7 **Spondyloepiphyseal dysplasia**

Q77.8 **Other osteochondrodysplasia with defects of growth of tubular bones and spine**

Q77.9 **Osteochondrodysplasia with defects of growth of tubular bones and spine, unspecified** ▽

✓4ᵗʰ **Q78** **Other osteochondrodysplasias**
　EXCLUDES 2　congenital myotonic chondrodystrophy (G71.13)

Q78.0 **Osteogenesis imperfecta**
　Fragilitas ossium
　Osteopsathyrosis

Q78.1 **Polyostotic fibrous dysplasia**
　Albright(-McCune)(-Sternberg) syndrome

Q78.2 **Osteopetrosis**
　Albers-Schönberg syndrome
　Osteosclerosis NOS
　DEF: Rare congenital condition in which the bones are excessively dense, resulting from a discrepancy in the formation and breakdown of bone.

Q78.3 **Progressive diaphyseal dysplasia**
　Camurati-Engelmann syndrome

Q78.4 **Enchondromatosis**
　Maffucci's syndrome
　Ollier's disease

Q78.5 **Metaphyseal dysplasia**
　Pyle's syndrome

Q78.6 **Multiple congenital exostoses**
　Diaphyseal aclasis

Q78.8 **Other specified osteochondrodysplasias**
　Osteopoikilosis

Q78.9 **Osteochondrodysplasia, unspecified** ▽
　Chondrodystrophy NOS
　Osteodystrophy NOS

✓4ᵗʰ **Q79** **Congenital malformations of musculoskeletal system, not elsewhere classified**
　EXCLUDES 2　congenital (sternomastoid) torticollis (Q68.0)

Q79.0 **Congenital diaphragmatic hernia**
　EXCLUDES 1　congenital hiatus hernia (Q40.1)

Q79.1 **Other congenital malformations of diaphragm**
　Absence of diaphragm
　Congenital malformation of diaphragm NOS
　Eventration of diaphragm

Q79.2 **Exomphalos**
　Omphalocele
　EXCLUDES 1　umbilical hernia (K42.-)

Q79.3 **Gastroschisis**

Gastroschisis

distal

Herniated small bowel (gastroschisis)

Rectus abdominus m.

Umbilicus

skin

proximal

Defect

Q79.4 **Prune belly syndrome**
　Congenital prolapse of bladder mucosa
　Eagle-Barrett syndrome

✓5ᵗʰ **Q79.5** **Other congenital malformations of abdominal wall**
　EXCLUDES 1　umbilical hernia (K42.-)

　　Q79.51 **Congenital hernia of bladder**
　　Q79.59 **Other congenital malformations of abdominal wall**

Q79.6　Ehlers-Danlos syndrome
DEF: Connective tissue disorder that causes hyperextended skin and joints and results in fragile blood vessels with bleeding, poor wound healing, and subcutaneous pseudotumors.

Q79.8　Other congenital malformations of musculoskeletal system
Absence of muscle
Absence of tendon
Accessory muscle
Amyotrophia congenita
Congenital constricting bands
Congenital shortening of tendon
Poland syndrome

Q79.9　Congenital malformation of musculoskeletal system, unspecified ▽
Congenital anomaly of musculoskeletal system NOS
Congenital deformity of musculoskeletal system NOS

Other congenital malformations (Q80-Q89)

✓4ᵗʰ Q80　Congenital ichthyosis
　EXCLUDES 1　Refsum's disease (G60.1)
　DEF: Excessive production of skin cells resulting in red, dry, scaly skin.

Q80.0　Ichthyosis vulgaris

Q80.1　X-linked ichthyosis

Q80.2　Lamellar ichthyosis
Collodion baby

Q80.3　Congenital bullous ichthyosiform erythroderma

Q80.4　Harlequin fetus

Q80.8　Other congenital ichthyosis

Q80.9　Congenital ichthyosis, unspecified ▽

✓4ᵗʰ Q81　Epidermolysis bullosa

Q81.0　Epidermolysis bullosa simplex
　EXCLUDES 1　Cockayne's syndrome (Q87.1)

Q81.1　Epidermolysis bullosa letalis
Herlitz' syndrome

Q81.2　Epidermolysis bullosa dystrophica

Q81.8　Other epidermolysis bullosa

Q81.9　Epidermolysis bullosa, unspecified ▽

✓4ᵗʰ Q82　Other congenital malformations of skin
　EXCLUDES 1　acrodermatitis enteropathica (E83.2)
　　　congenital erythropoietic porphyria (E80.0)
　　　pilonidal cyst or sinus (L05.-)
　　　Sturge-Weber (-Dimitri) syndrome (Q85.8)

Q82.0　Hereditary lymphedema

Q82.1　Xeroderma pigmentosum

Q82.2　Congenital cutaneous mastocytosis
Congenital diffuse cutaneous mastocytosis
Congenital maculopapular cutaneous mastocytosis
Congenital urticaria pigmentosa
　EXCLUDES 1　cutaneous mastocytosis NOS (D47.01)
　　　diffuse cutaneous mastocytosis (with onset after newborn period) (D47.01)
　　　malignant mastocytosis (C96.2-)
　　　systemic mastocytosis (D47.02)
　　　urticaria pigmentosa (non-congenital) (with onset after newborn period) (D47.01)
　AHA: 2017,4Q,5

Q82.3　Incontinentia pigmenti

Q82.4　Ectodermal dysplasia (anhidrotic)
　EXCLUDES 1　Ellis-van Creveld syndrome (Q77.6)

Q82.5　Congenital non-neoplastic nevus
Birthmark NOS
Flammeus Nevus
Portwine Nevus
Sanguineous Nevus
Strawberry Nevus
Vascular Nevus NOS
Verrucous Nevus
　EXCLUDES 2　araneus nevus (I78.1)
　　　Café au lait spots (L81.3)
　　　lentigo (L81.4)
　　　melanocytic nevus (D22.-)
　　　nevus NOS (D22.-)
　　　pigmented nevus (D22.-)
　　　spider nevus (I78.1)
　　　stellar nevus (I78.1)

Q82.6　Congenital sacral dimple
Parasacral dimple
　EXCLUDES 2　pilonidal cyst with abscess (L05.01)
　　　pilonidal cyst without abscess (L05.91)
　AHA: 2016,4Q,60

Q82.8　Other specified congenital malformations of skin
Abnormal palmar creases
Accessory skin tags
Benign familial pemphigus [Hailey-Hailey]
Congenital poikiloderma
Cutis laxa (hyperelastica)
Dermatoglyphic anomalies
Inherited keratosis palmaris et plantaris
Keratosis follicularis [Darier-White]
　EXCLUDES 1　Ehlers-Danlos syndrome (Q79.6)
　AHA: 2016,1Q,17

Q82.9　Congenital malformation of skin, unspecified ▽

✓4ᵗʰ Q83　Congenital malformations of breast
　EXCLUDES 2　absence of pectoral muscle (Q79.8)
　　　hypoplasia of breast (N64.82)
　　　micromastia (N64.82)

Q83.0　Congenital absence of breast with absent nipple

Q83.1　Accessory breast
Supernumerary breast

Q83.2　Absent nipple

Q83.3　Accessory nipple
Supernumerary nipple

Q83.8　Other congenital malformations of breast

Q83.9　Congenital malformation of breast, unspecified ▽

✓4ᵗʰ Q84　Other congenital malformations of integument

Q84.0　Congenital alopecia
Congenital atrichosis

Q84.1　Congenital morphological disturbances of hair, not elsewhere classified
Beaded hair
Monilethrix
Pili annulati
　EXCLUDES 1　Menkes' kinky hair syndrome (E83.0)

Q84.2　Other congenital malformations of hair
Congenital hypertrichosis
Congenital malformation of hair NOS
Persistent lanugo

Q84.3　Anonychia
　EXCLUDES 1　nail patella syndrome (Q87.2)

Q84.4　Congenital leukonychia

Q84.5　Enlarged and hypertrophic nails
Congenital onychauxis
Pachyonychia

Q84.6　Other congenital malformations of nails
Congenital clubnail
Congenital koilonychia
Congenital malformation of nail NOS

Q84.8　Other specified congenital malformations of integument
Aplasia cutis congenita

Q84.9　Congenital malformation of integument, unspecified ▽
Congenital anomaly of integument NOS
Congenital deformity of integument NOS

√4ᵗʰ **Q85 Phakomatoses, not elsewhere classified**

EXCLUDES 1   *ataxia telangiectasia [Louis-Bar] (G11.3)*
familial dysautonomia [Riley-Day] (G90.1)

√5ᵗʰ **Q85.0 Neurofibromatosis (nonmalignant)**

Q85.00 Neurofibromatosis, unspecified HCC ▽

Q85.01 Neurofibromatosis, type 1 HCC
Von Recklinghausen disease

Q85.02 Neurofibromatosis, type 2 HCC
Acoustic neurofibromatosis
DEF: Inherited condition with cutaneous lesions, benign tumors of peripheral nerves, and bilateral 8th nerve masses.

Q85.03 Schwannomatosis HCC
DEF: Genetic mutation (SMARCB1/INI1) causing multiple benign tumors along the nerve pathways, except on the 8th cranial (vestibular) nerve.

Q85.09 Other neurofibromatosis HCC

Q85.1 Tuberous sclerosis HCC
Bourneville's disease
Epiloia

Q85.8 Other phakomatoses, not elsewhere classified HCC
Peutz-Jeghers Syndrome
Sturge-Weber(-Dimitri) syndrome
von Hippel-Lindau syndrome
EXCLUDES 1   *Meckel-Gruber syndrome (Q61.9)*

Q85.9 Phakomatosis, unspecified HCC ▽
Hamartosis NOS

√4ᵗʰ **Q86 Congenital malformation syndromes due to known exogenous causes, not elsewhere classified**

EXCLUDES 2   *iodine-deficiency-related hypothyroidism (E00-E02)*
nonteratogenic effects of substances transmitted via placenta or breast milk (P04.-)

Q86.0 Fetal alcohol syndrome (dysmorphic)

Q86.1 Fetal hydantoin syndrome
Meadow's syndrome

Q86.2 Dysmorphism due to warfarin

Q86.8 Other congenital malformation syndromes due to known exogenous causes

√4ᵗʰ **Q87 Other specified congenital malformation syndromes affecting multiple systems**
Use additional code(s) to identify all associated manifestations

Q87.0 Congenital malformation syndromes predominantly affecting facial appearance
Acrocephalopolysyndactyly
Acrocephalosyndactyly [Apert]
Cryptophthalmos syndrome
Cyclopia
Goldenhar syndrome
Moebius syndrome
Oro-facial-digital syndrome
Robin syndrome
Whistling face

Q87.1 Congenital malformation syndromes predominantly associated with short stature
Aarskog syndrome
Cockayne syndrome
De Lange syndrome
Dubowitz syndrome
Noonan syndrome
Prader-Willi syndrome
Robinow-Silverman-Smith syndrome
Russell-Silver syndrome
Seckel syndrome
EXCLUDES 1   *Ellis-van Creveld syndrome (Q77.6)*
Smith-Lemli-Opitz syndrome (E78.72)

Q87.2 Congenital malformation syndromes predominantly involving limbs
Holt-Oram syndrome
Klippel-Trenaunay-Weber syndrome
Nail patella syndrome
Rubinstein-Taybi syndrome
Sirenomelia syndrome
Thrombocytopenia with absent radius [TAR] syndrome
VATER syndrome

Q87.3 Congenital malformation syndromes involving early overgrowth
Beckwith-Wiedemann syndrome
Sotos syndrome
Weaver syndrome

√5ᵗʰ **Q87.4 Marfan's syndrome**
DEF: Disorder that affects the connective tissue of multiple systems, including disproportionally long or abnormal bone structure and eye and cardiovascular complications.

Q87.40 Marfan's syndrome, unspecified ▽

√6ᵗʰ **Q87.41 Marfan's syndrome with cardiovascular manifestations**

Q87.410 Marfan's syndrome with aortic dilation

Q87.418 Marfan's syndrome with other cardiovascular manifestations

Q87.42 Marfan's syndrome with ocular manifestations

Q87.43 Marfan's syndrome with skeletal manifestation

Q87.5 Other congenital malformation syndromes with other skeletal changes

√5ᵗʰ **Q87.8 Other specified congenital malformation syndromes, not elsewhere classified**
EXCLUDES 1   *Zellweger syndrome (E71.510)*

Q87.81 Alport syndrome
Use additional code to identify stage of chronic kidney disease (N18.1-N18.6)

Q87.82 Arterial tortuosity syndrome
AHA: 2016,4Q,60-61

Q87.89 Other specified congenital malformation syndromes, not elsewhere classified
Laurence-Moon (-Bardet)-Biedl syndrome

√4ᵗʰ **Q89 Other congenital malformations, not elsewhere classified**

√5ᵗʰ **Q89.0 Congenital absence and malformations of spleen**
EXCLUDES 1   *isomerism of atrial appendages (with asplenia or polysplenia) (Q20.6)*

Q89.01 Asplenia (congenital)

Q89.09 Congenital malformations of spleen
Congenital splenomegaly

Q89.1 Congenital malformations of adrenal gland
EXCLUDES 1   *adrenogenital disorders (E25.-)*
congenital adrenal hyperplasia (E25.0)

Q89.2 Congenital malformations of other endocrine glands
Congenital malformation of parathyroid or thyroid gland
Persistent thyroglossal duct
Thyroglossal cyst
EXCLUDES 1   *congenital goiter (E03.0)*
congenital hypothyroidism (E03.1)

Q89.3 Situs inversus
Dextrocardia with situs inversus
Mirror-image atrial arrangement with situs inversus
Situs inversus or transversus abdominalis
Situs inversus or transversus thoracis
Transposition of abdominal viscera
Transposition of thoracic viscera
EXCLUDES 1   *dextrocardia NOS (Q24.0)*
DEF: Congenital anomaly in which the internal thoracic and abdominal organs are transposed laterally and found on the opposite side from the normal position.

Q89.4 Conjoined twins
Craniopagus
Dicephaly
Pygopagus
Thoracopagus

Q89.7 Multiple congenital malformations, not elsewhere classified
Multiple congenital anomalies NOS
Multiple congenital deformities NOS
EXCLUDES 1   *congenital malformation syndromes affecting multiple systems (Q87.-)*

Q89.8 Other specified congenital malformations
Use additional code(s) to identify all associated manifestations

Q89.9 Congenital malformation, unspecified ▽
Congenital anomaly NOS
Congenital deformity NOS

Chromosomal abnormalities, not elsewhere classified (Q90–Q99)

EXCLUDES2   *mitochondrial metabolic disorders (E88.4-)*

√4ᵗʰ **Q90 Down syndrome**

Use additional code(s) to identify any associated physical conditions and degree of intellectual disabilities (F70-F79)

Q90.0 Trisomy 21, nonmosaicism (meiotic nondisjunction)
Q90.1 Trisomy 21, mosaicism (mitotic nondisjunction)
Q90.2 Trisomy 21, translocation
Q90.9 Down syndrome, unspecified   ▽
Trisomy 21 NOS

√4ᵗʰ **Q91 Trisomy 18 and Trisomy 13**

Q91.0 Trisomy 18, nonmosaicism (meiotic nondisjunction)
Q91.1 Trisomy 18, mosaicism (mitotic nondisjunction)
Q91.2 Trisomy 18, translocation
Q91.3 Trisomy 18, unspecified   ▽
Q91.4 Trisomy 13, nonmosaicism (meiotic nondisjunction)
Q91.5 Trisomy 13, mosaicism (mitotic nondisjunction)
Q91.6 Trisomy 13, translocation
Q91.7 Trisomy 13, unspecified   ▽

√4ᵗʰ **Q92 Other trisomies and partial trisomies of the autosomes, not elsewhere classified**

INCLUDES   unbalanced translocations and insertions
EXCLUDES1   *trisomies of chromosomes 13, 18, 21 (Q90-Q91)*

Q92.0 Whole chromosome trisomy, nonmosaicism (meiotic nondisjunction)
Q92.1 Whole chromosome trisomy, mosaicism (mitotic nondisjunction)
Q92.2 Partial trisomy
Less than whole arm duplicated
Whole arm or more duplicated
EXCLUDES1   *partial trisomy due to unbalanced translocation (Q92.5)*

√5ᵗʰ **Q92.6 Marker chromosomes**
Trisomies due to dicentrics
Trisomies due to extra rings
Trisomies due to isochromosomes
Individual with marker heterochromatin
Q92.61 Marker chromosomes in normal individual
Q92.62 Marker chromosomes in abnormal individual
Q92.7 Triploidy and polyploidy
Q92.8 Other specified trisomies and partial trisomies of autosomes
Duplications identified by fluorescence in situ hybridization (FISH)
Duplications identified by in situ hybridization (ISH)
Duplications seen only at prometaphase
Q92.9 Trisomy and partial trisomy of autosomes, unspecified   ▽

√4ᵗʰ **Q93 Monosomies and deletions from the autosomes, not elsewhere classified**

Q93.0 Whole chromosome monosomy, nonmosaicism (meiotic nondisjunction)
Q93.1 Whole chromosome monosomy, mosaicism (mitotic nondisjunction)
Q93.2 Chromosome replaced with ring, dicentric or isochromosome
Q93.3 Deletion of short arm of chromosome 4
Wolff-Hirschorn syndrome
Q93.4 Deletion of short arm of chromosome 5
Cri-du-chat syndrome
√5ᵗʰ **Q93.5 Other deletions of part of a chromosome**
Angelman syndrome
● **Q93.51 Angelman syndrome**
● **Q93.59 Other deletions of part of a chromosome**
Q93.7 Deletions with other complex rearrangements
Deletions due to unbalanced translocations, inversions and insertions
Code also any associated duplications due to unbalanced translocations, inversions and insertions (Q92.5)

√5ᵗʰ **Q93.8 Other deletions from the autosomes**
Q93.81 Velo-cardio-facial syndrome
Deletion 22q11.2
DEF: Microdeletion syndrome affecting multiple organs characterized by a cleft palate, heart defects, an elongated face with almond-shaped eyes, wide nose, small ears, weak immune system, weak musculature, hypothyroidism, short stature, and scoliosis. The deletion occurs at q11.2 on the long arm of the chromosome 22.
● **Q93.82 Williams syndrome**
Q93.88 Other microdeletions
Miller-Dieker syndrome
Smith-Magenis syndrome
Q93.89 Other deletions from the autosomes
Deletions identified by fluorescence in situ hybridization (FISH)
Deletions identified by in situ hybridization (ISH)
Deletions seen only at prometaphase
Q93.9 Deletion from autosomes, unspecified   ▽

√4ᵗʰ **Q95 Balanced rearrangements and structural markers, not elsewhere classified**

INCLUDES   Robertsonian and balanced reciprocal translocations and insertions

Q95.0 Balanced translocation and insertion in normal individual
Q95.1 Chromosome inversion in normal individual
Q95.2 Balanced autosomal rearrangement in abnormal individual
Q95.3 Balanced sex/autosomal rearrangement in abnormal individual
Q95.5 Individual with autosomal fragile site
Q95.8 Other balanced rearrangements and structural markers
Q95.9 Balanced rearrangement and structural marker, unspecified   ▽

√4ᵗʰ **Q96 Turner's syndrome**

EXCLUDES1   *Noonan syndrome (Q87.1)*

Q96.0 Karyotype 45, X   ♀
Q96.1 Karyotype 46, X iso (Xq)   ♀
Karyotype 46, isochromosome Xq
Q96.2 Karyotype 46, X with abnormal sex chromosome, except iso (Xq)   ♀
Karyotype 46, X with abnormal sex chromosome, except isochromosome Xq
Q96.3 Mosaicism, 45, X/46, XX or XY   ♀
Q96.4 Mosaicism, 45, X/other cell line(s) with abnormal sex chromosome   ♀
Q96.8 Other variants of Turner's syndrome   ♀
Q96.9 Turner's syndrome, unspecified   ♀ ▽

√4ᵗʰ **Q97 Other sex chromosome abnormalities, female phenotype, not elsewhere classified**

EXCLUDES1   *Turner's syndrome (Q96.-)*

Q97.0 Karyotype 47, XXX   ♀
Q97.1 Female with more than three X chromosomes   ♀
Q97.2 Mosaicism, lines with various numbers of X chromosomes   ♀
Q97.3 Female with 46, XY karyotype   ♀
Q97.8 Other specified sex chromosome abnormalities, female phenotype
Q97.9 Sex chromosome abnormality, female phenotype, unspecified   ♀ ▽

√4ᵗʰ **Q98 Other sex chromosome abnormalities, male phenotype, not elsewhere classified**

Q98.0 Klinefelter syndrome karyotype 47, XXY   ♂
Q98.1 Klinefelter syndrome, male with more than two X chromosomes   ♂
Q98.3 Other male with 46, XX karyotype   ♂
Q98.4 Klinefelter syndrome, unspecified   ♂ ▽
Q98.5 Karyotype 47, XYY
Q98.6 Male with structurally abnormal sex chromosome   ♂
Q98.7 Male with sex chromosome mosaicism   ♂
Q98.8 Other specified sex chromosome abnormalities, male phenotype   ♂
Q98.9 Sex chromosome abnormality, male phenotype, unspecified   ♂ ▽

√4ᵗʰ **Q99 Other chromosome abnormalities, not elsewhere classified**

Q99.0 Chimera 46, XX/46, XY
Chimera 46, XX/46, XY true hermaphrodite

Chapter 17. Congenital Malformations, Deformations and Chromosomal Abnormalities

Q99.1–Q99.9

Q99.1   **46, XX true hermaphrodite**
     46, XX with streak gonads
     46, XY with streak gonads
     Pure gonadal dysgenesis

Q99.2   **Fragile X chromosome**
     Fragile X syndrome

Q99.8   **Other specified chromosome abnormalities**

Q99.9   **Chromosomal abnormality, unspecified**   ▽

Chapter 18. Symptoms, Signs, and Abnormal Clinical and Laboratory Findings, Not Elsewhere Classified (R00–R99)

Chapter Specific Guidelines with Coding Examples

The chapter specific guidelines from the ICD-10-CM Official Guidelines for Coding and Reporting have been provided below. Along with these guidelines are coding examples, contained in the shaded boxes, that have been developed to help illustrate the coding and/or sequencing guidance found in these guidelines.

Chapter 18 includes symptoms, signs, abnormal results of clinical or other investigative procedures, and ill-defined conditions regarding which no diagnosis classifiable elsewhere is recorded. Signs and symptoms that point to a specific diagnosis have been assigned to a category in other chapters of the classification.

a. Use of symptom codes

Codes that describe symptoms and signs are acceptable for reporting purposes when a related definitive diagnosis has not been established (confirmed) by the provider.

Tenderness and localized pain in the right upper quadrant; based on presentation, probable gallstones

R10.11   Right upper quadrant pain

R10.811   Right upper quadrant abdominal tenderness

Explanation: Codes that describe symptoms such as abdominal pain are acceptable for reporting purposes when the provider has not established (confirmed) a definitive diagnosis.

b. Use of a symptom code with a definitive diagnosis code

Codes for signs and symptoms may be reported in addition to a related definitive diagnosis when the sign or symptom is not routinely associated with that diagnosis, such as the various signs and symptoms associated with complex syndromes. The definitive diagnosis code should be sequenced before the symptom code.

Signs or symptoms that are associated routinely with a disease process should not be assigned as additional codes, unless otherwise instructed by the classification.

Pneumonia with hemoptysis

J18.9   Pneumonia, unspecified organism

R04.2   Hemoptysis

Explanation: Codes for signs and symptoms may be reported in addition to a related definitive diagnosis when the sign or symptom is not routinely associated with that diagnosis.

Abdominal pain due to acute appendicitis

K35.80   Unspecified acute appendicitis

Explanation: Codes for signs or symptoms routinely associated with a disease process should not be assigned unless the classification instructs otherwise.

c. Combination codes that include symptoms

ICD-10-CM contains a number of combination codes that identify both the definitive diagnosis and common symptoms of that diagnosis. When using one of these combination codes, an additional code should not be assigned for the symptom.

IBS with diarrhea

K58.0   Irritable bowel syndrome, with diarrhea

Explanation: When a combination code identifies both the definitive diagnosis and the symptom, an additional code should not be assigned for the symptom.

d. Repeated falls

Code R29.6, Repeated falls, is for use for encounters when a patient has recently fallen and the reason for the fall is being investigated.

Code Z91.81, History of falling, is for use when a patient has fallen in the past and is at risk for future falls. When appropriate, both codes R29.6 and Z91.81 may be assigned together.

e. Coma scale

The coma scale codes (R40.2-) can be used in conjunction with traumatic brain injury codes, acute cerebrovascular disease or sequelae of cerebrovascular disease codes. These codes are primarily for use by trauma registries, but they may be used in any setting where this information is collected. The coma scale may also be used to assess the status of the central nervous system for other non-trauma conditions, such as monitoring patients in the intensive care unit regardless of medical condition. The coma scale codes should be sequenced after the diagnosis code(s).

These codes, one from each subcategory, are needed to complete the scale. The 7th character indicates when the scale was recorded. The 7th character should match for all three codes.

At a minimum, report the initial score documented on presentation at your facility. This may be a score from the emergency medicine technician (EMT) or in the emergency department. If desired, a facility may choose to capture multiple coma scale scores.

Assign code R40.24, Glasgow coma scale, total score, when only the total score is documented in the medical record and not the individual score(s).

Do not report codes for individual or total Glasgow coma scale scores for a patient with a medically induced coma or a sedated patient.

See Section I.B.14 for coma scale documentation by clinicians other than patient's provider

36-year-old man found down after unknown injury with skull fracture and with concussion and loss of consciousness of unknown duration. Upon hospital admission, the patient was evaluated with the following Glasgow coma scores:

Eye-opening response—3: eyes open to speech

Verbal response—3: random speech with no conversational exchange

Motor response—4: pulls limb away from painful stimulus

S02.0XXA   Fracture of vault of skull, initial encounter for closed fracture

S06.0X9A   Concussion with loss of consciousness of unspecified duration, initial encounter

R40.2133   Coma scale, eyes open, to sound, at hospital admission

R40.2233   Coma scale, best verbal response, inappropriate words, at hospital admission

R40.2343   Coma scale, best motor response, flexion withdrawal, at hospital admission

Explanation: When individual scores for the Glasgow coma scale are documented, one code from each category is needed to complete the scale. The seventh character indicates when the scale was recorded and should match for all three codes. Assign a code from subcategory R40.24- Glasgow coma scale, total score, when only the total and not the individual score(s) is documented.

f. Functional quadriplegia

GUIDELINE HAS BEEN DELETED EFFECTIVE OCTOBER 1, 2017

g. SIRS due to non-infectious process

The systemic inflammatory response syndrome (SIRS) can develop as a result of certain non-infectious disease processes, such as trauma, malignant neoplasm, or pancreatitis. When SIRS is documented with a noninfectious condition, and no subsequent infection is documented, the code for the underlying condition, such as an injury, should be assigned, followed by code R65.10, Systemic inflammatory response syndrome (SIRS) of non-infectious origin without acute organ dysfunction, or code R65.11, Systemic inflammatory response syndrome (SIRS) of non-infectious origin with acute organ dysfunction. If an associated acute organ dysfunction is documented, the appropriate code(s) for the specific type of organ dysfunction(s) should be assigned in addition to code R65.11. If acute organ dysfunction is documented, but it cannot be determined if the acute organ dysfunction is associated with SIRS or due to another condition (e.g., directly due to the trauma), the provider should be queried.

Systemic inflammatory response syndrome (SIRS) due to acute gallstone pancreatitis

K85.1Ø	**Biliary acute pancreatitis without necrosis or infection**
R65.1Ø	**Systemic inflammatory response syndrome (SIRS) of noninfectious origin without acute organ dysfunction**

Explanation: When SIRS is documented with a noninfectious condition without subsequent infection documented, the code for the underlying condition such as pancreatitis should be assigned followed by the appropriate code for SIRS of noninfectious origin, either with or without associated organ dysfunction.

h. **Death NOS**

Code R99, Ill-defined and unknown cause of mortality, is only for use in the very limited circumstance when a patient who has already died is brought into an emergency department or other healthcare facility and is pronounced dead upon arrival. It does not represent the discharge disposition of death.

i. **NIHSS stroke scale**

The NIH stroke scale (NIHSS) codes (R29.7- -) can be used in conjunction with acute stroke codes (I63) to identify the patient's neurological status and the severity of the stroke. The stroke scale codes should be sequenced after the acute stroke diagnosis code(s).

At a minimum, report the initial score documented. If desired, a facility may choose to capture multiple stroke scale scores.

See Section I.B.14 for NIHSS stroke scale documentation by clinicians other than patient's provider

Chapter 18. Symptoms, Signs and Abnormal Clinical and Laboratory Findings, Not Elsewhere Classified (R00-R99)

NOTE   This chapter includes symptoms, signs, abnormal results of clinical or other investigative procedures, and ill-defined conditions regarding which no diagnosis classifiable elsewhere is recorded.

Signs and symptoms that point rather definitely to a given diagnosis have been assigned to a category in other chapters of the classification. In general, categories in this chapter include the less well-defined conditions and symptoms that, without the necessary study of the case to establish a final diagnosis, point perhaps equally to two or more diseases or to two or more systems of the body. Practically all categories in the chapter could be designated 'not otherwise specified', 'unknown etiology' or 'transient'. The Alphabetical Index should be consulted to determine which symptoms and signs are to be allocated here and which to other chapters. The residual subcategories, numbered .8, are generally provided for other relevant symptoms that cannot be allocated elsewhere in the classification.

The conditions and signs or symptoms included in categories R00-R94 consist of:

(a) cases for which no more specific diagnosis can be made even after all the facts bearing on the case have been investigated;

(b) signs or symptoms existing at the time of initial encounter that proved to be transient and whose causes could not be determined;

(c) provisional diagnosis in a patient who failed to return for further investigation or care;

(d) cases referred elsewhere for investigation or treatment before the diagnosis was made;

(e) cases in which a more precise diagnosis was not available for any other reason;

(f) certain symptoms, for which supplementary information is provided, that represent important problems in medical care in their own right.

EXCLUDES 2   abnormal findings on antenatal screening of mother (O28.-)
certain conditions originating in the perinatal period (P04-P96)
signs and symptoms classified in the body system chapters
signs and symptoms of breast (N63, N64.5)

AHA: 2017,1Q,6,7

This chapter contains the following blocks:

R00-R09   Symptoms and signs involving the circulatory and respiratory systems
R10-R19   Symptoms and signs involving the digestive system and abdomen
R20-R23   Symptoms and signs involving the skin and subcutaneous tissue
R25-R29   Symptoms and signs involving the nervous and musculoskeletal systems
R30-R39   Symptoms and signs involving the genitourinary system
R40-R46   Symptoms and signs involving cognition, perception, emotional state and behavior
R47-R49   Symptoms and signs involving speech and voice
R50-R69   General symptoms and signs
R70-R79   Abnormal findings on examination of blood, without diagnosis
R80-R82   Abnormal findings on examination of urine, without diagnosis
R83-R89   Abnormal findings on examination of other body fluids, substances and tissues, without diagnosis
R90-R94   Abnormal findings on diagnostic imaging and in function studies, without diagnosis
R97   Abnormal tumor markers
R99   Ill-defined and unknown cause of mortality

Symptoms and signs involving the circulatory and respiratory systems (R00-R09)

✔4ᵗʰ **R00   Abnormalities of heart beat**

EXCLUDES 1   abnormalities originating in the perinatal period (P29.1-)
EXCLUDES 2   specified arrhythmias (I47-I49)

R00.0   Tachycardia, unspecified   ▽
Rapid heart beat
Sinoauricular tachycardia NOS
Sinus [sinusal] tachycardia NOS
EXCLUDES 1   neonatal tachycardia (P29.11)
paroxysmal tachycardia (I47.-)
DEF: Excessively rapid heart rate of more than 100 beats per minute.

R00.1   Bradycardia, unspecified   ▽
Sinoatrial bradycardia
Sinus bradycardia
Slow heart beat
Vagal bradycardia
Use additional code for adverse effect, if applicable, to identify drug (T36-T50 with fifth or sixth character 5)
EXCLUDES 1   neonatal bradycardia (P29.12)

R00.2   Palpitations
Awareness of heart beat

R00.8   Other abnormalities of heart beat

R00.9   Unspecified abnormalities of heart beat   ▽

✔4ᵗʰ **R01   Cardiac murmurs and other cardiac sounds**

EXCLUDES 1   cardiac murmurs and sounds originating in the perinatal period (P29.8)

R01.0   Benign and innocent cardiac murmurs
Functional cardiac murmur

R01.1   Cardiac murmur, unspecified   ▽
Cardiac bruit NOS
Heart murmur NOS
Systolic murmur NOS

R01.2   Other cardiac sounds
Cardiac dullness, increased or decreased
Precordial friction

✔4ᵗʰ **R03   Abnormal blood-pressure reading, without diagnosis**

R03.0   Elevated blood-pressure reading, without diagnosis of hypertension
NOTE   This category is to be used to record an episode of elevated blood pressure in a patient in whom no formal diagnosis of hypertension has been made, or as an isolated incidental finding.

R03.1   Nonspecific low blood-pressure reading
EXCLUDES 1   hypotension (I95.-)
maternal hypotension syndrome (O26.5-)
neurogenic orthostatic hypotension (G90.3)

✔4ᵗʰ **R04   Hemorrhage from respiratory passages**

R04.0   Epistaxis
Hemorrhage from nose
Nosebleed

R04.1   Hemorrhage from throat
EXCLUDES 2   hemoptysis (R04.2)

R04.2   Hemoptysis
Blood-stained sputum
Cough with hemorrhage
AHA: 2013,4Q,118

✔5ᵗʰ **R04.8   Hemorrhage from other sites in respiratory passages**

R04.81   Acute idiopathic pulmonary hemorrhage in infants   P
AIPHI
Acute idiopathic hemorrhage in infants over 28 days old
EXCLUDES 1   perinatal pulmonary hemorrhage (P26.-)
von Willebrand's disease (D68.0)

R04.89   Hemorrhage from other sites in respiratory passages
Pulmonary hemorrhage NOS

R04.9   Hemorrhage from respiratory passages, unspecified   ▽

R05   Cough
EXCLUDES 1   cough with hemorrhage (R04.2)
smoker's cough (J41.0)
AHA: 2016,2Q,33

✔4ᵗʰ **R06   Abnormalities of breathing**
EXCLUDES 1   acute respiratory distress syndrome (J80)
respiratory arrest (R09.2)
respiratory arrest of newborn (P28.81)
respiratory distress syndrome of newborn (P22.-)
respiratory failure (J96.-)
respiratory failure of newborn (P28.5)

✔5ᵗʰ **R06.0   Dyspnea**
EXCLUDES 1   tachypnea NOS (R06.82)
transient tachypnea of newborn (P22.1)

R06.00   Dyspnea, unspecified   ▽
AHA: 2017,1Q,26

R06.01   Orthopnea

R06.02   Shortness of breath
R06.03   Acute respiratory distress
     AHA: 2017,4Q,23
R06.09   Other forms of dyspnea

R06.1   Stridor
     EXCLUDES 1   congenital laryngeal stridor (P28.89)
              laryngismus (stridulus) (J38.5)
     DEF: Certain type of wheezing described as a loud, constant, musical sound produced when breathing with an obstructed airway, like the inspiratory sound heard when laryngeal or esophageal obstruction is present.

R06.2   Wheezing
     EXCLUDES 1   asthma (J45.-)
     AHA: 2016,2Q,33
     DEF: High-pitched whistling sound during breathing due to stenosis of the respiratory passageway. Wheezing is associated with asthma, sleep apnea, bronchiectasis, bronchiolitis, COPD, and pleural effusion.

R06.3   Periodic breathing
     Cheyne-Stokes breathing

R06.4   Hyperventilation
     EXCLUDES 1   psychogenic hyperventilation (F45.8)

R06.5   Mouth breathing
     EXCLUDES 2   dry mouth NOS (R68.2)

R06.6   Hiccough
     EXCLUDES 1   psychogenic hiccough (F45.8)

R06.7   Sneezing

√5ᵗʰ **R06.8**   Other abnormalities of breathing
     R06.81   Apnea, not elsewhere classified
         Apnea NOS
         EXCLUDES 1   apnea (of) newborn (P28.4)
                 sleep apnea (G47.3-)
                 sleep apnea of newborn (primary) (P28.3)
     R06.82   Tachypnea, not elsewhere classified
         Tachypnea NOS
         EXCLUDES 1   transitory tachypnea of newborn (P22.1)
     R06.83   Snoring
     R06.89   Other abnormalities of breathing
         Breath-holding (spells)
         Sighing

R06.9   Unspecified abnormalities of breathing   ▽

√4ᵗʰ **R07**   Pain in throat and chest
     EXCLUDES 1   epidemic myalgia (B33.0)
     EXCLUDES 2   jaw pain R68.84
              pain in breast (N64.4)

R07.0   Pain in throat
     EXCLUDES 1   chronic sore throat (J31.2)
              sore throat (acute) NOS (J02.9)
     EXCLUDES 2   dysphagia (R13.1-)
              pain in neck (M54.2)

R07.1   Chest pain on breathing
     Painful respiration

R07.2   Precordial pain
     DEF: Pain felt in the anterior (front) chest wall over the region of the heart. This type of pain is generally felt slightly to the left of the sternum, but may also extend into the surrounding chest wall region.

√5ᵗʰ **R07.8**   Other chest pain
     R07.81   Pleurodynia
         Pleurodynia NOS
         EXCLUDES 1   epidemic pleurodynia (B33.0)
     R07.82   Intercostal pain
     R07.89   Other chest pain
         Anterior chest-wall pain NOS

R07.9   Chest pain, unspecified   ▽

√4ᵗʰ **R09**   Other symptoms and signs involving the circulatory and respiratory system
     EXCLUDES 1   acute respiratory distress syndrome (J80)
              respiratory arrest of newborn (P28.81)
              respiratory distress syndrome of newborn (P22.0)
              respiratory failure (J96.-)
              respiratory failure of newborn (P28.5)

√5ᵗʰ **R09.0**   Asphyxia and hypoxemia
     EXCLUDES 1   asphyxia due to carbon monoxide (T58.-)
              asphyxia due to foreign body in respiratory tract (T17.-)
              birth (intrauterine) asphyxia (P84)
              hyperventilation (R06.4)
              traumatic asphyxia (T71.-)
     EXCLUDES 2   hypercapnia (R06.89)
     R09.01   Asphyxia
         DEF: Interference of oxygen intake due to obstruction or injury of airways resulting in a lack of oxygen perfusion to the tissues or excessive carbon dioxide in the blood. Can cause unconsciousness or death.
     R09.02   Hypoxemia
         DEF: Insufficient oxygen in the arterial blood resulting in inadequate delivery of oxygen to the body tissues.

R09.1   Pleurisy
     EXCLUDES 1   pleurisy with effusion (J90)

R09.2   Respiratory arrest   HCC
     Cardiorespiratory failure
     EXCLUDES 1   cardiac arrest (I46.-)
              respiratory arrest of newborn (P28.81)
              respiratory distress of newborn (P22.0)
              respiratory failure (J96.-)
              respiratory failure of newborn (P28.5)
              respiratory insufficiency (R06.89)
              respiratory insufficiency of newborn (P28.5)

R09.3   Abnormal sputum
     Abnormal amount of sputum
     Abnormal color of sputum
     Abnormal odor of sputum
     Excessive sputum
     EXCLUDES 1   blood-stained sputum (R04.2)

√5ᵗʰ **R09.8**   Other specified symptoms and signs involving the circulatory and respiratory systems
     R09.81   Nasal congestion
     R09.82   Postnasal drip
     R09.89   Other specified symptoms and signs involving the circulatory and respiratory systems
         Abnormal chest percussion
         Bruit (arterial)
         Chest tympany
         Choking sensation
         Feeling of foreign body in throat
         Friction sounds in chest
         Rales
         Weak pulse
         EXCLUDES 2   foreign body in throat (T17.2-)
                 wheezing (R06.2)

Symptoms and signs involving the digestive system and abdomen (R10-R19)

EXCLUDES 2   congenital or infantile pylorospasm (Q40.0)
gastrointestinal hemorrhage (K92.0-K92.2)
intestinal obstruction (K56.-)
newborn gastrointestinal hemorrhage (P54.0-P54.3)
newborn intestinal obstruction (P76.-)
pylorospasm (K31.3)
signs and symptoms involving the urinary system (R30-R39)
symptoms referable to female genital organs (N94.-)
symptoms referable to male genital organs (N48-N50)

✓4ᵗʰ **R10**   **Abdominal and pelvic pain**

    EXCLUDES 1   renal colic (N23)
    EXCLUDES 2   dorsalgia (M54.-)
               flatulence and related conditions (R14.-)

    R10.0   **Acute abdomen**   🄠
           Severe abdominal pain (generalized) (with abdominal rigidity)
           EXCLUDES 1   abdominal rigidity NOS (R19.3)
                       generalized abdominal pain NOS (R10.84)
                       localized abdominal pain (R10.1-R10.3-)

✓5ᵗʰ **R10.1**   **Pain localized to upper abdomen**

       R10.10   **Upper abdominal pain, unspecified**   🄠 ▽
       R10.11   **Right upper quadrant pain**
       R10.12   **Left upper quadrant pain**
       R10.13   **Epigastric pain**   🄠
            Dyspepsia
            EXCLUDES 1   functional dyspepsia (K30)

Abdominal Pain

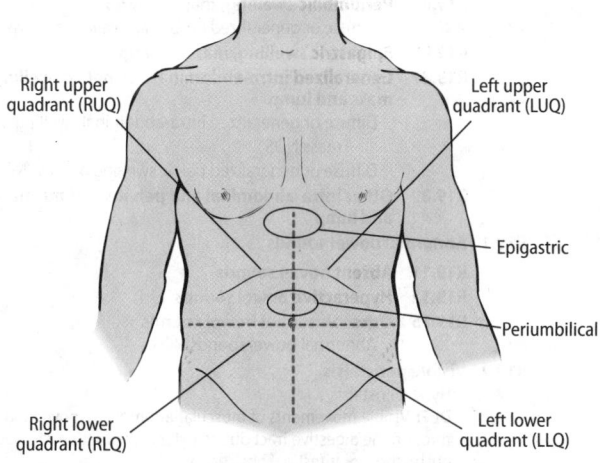

Right upper quadrant (RUQ)

Left upper quadrant (LUQ)

Epigastric

Periumbilical

Right lower quadrant (RLQ)

Left lower quadrant (LLQ)

    R10.2   **Pelvic and perineal pain**   🄠
           EXCLUDES 1   vulvodynia (N94.81)

✓5ᵗʰ **R10.3**   **Pain localized to other parts of lower abdomen**

       R10.30   **Lower abdominal pain, unspecified**   🄠 ▽
       R10.31   **Right lower quadrant pain**   🄠
       R10.32   **Left lower quadrant pain**   🄠
       R10.33   **Periumbilical pain**   🄠

✓5ᵗʰ **R10.8**   **Other abdominal pain**

       ✓6ᵗʰ **R10.81**   **Abdominal tenderness**
                Abdominal tenderness NOS
            R10.811   **Right upper quadrant abdominal tenderness**
            R10.812   **Left upper quadrant abdominal tenderness**
            R10.813   **Right lower quadrant abdominal tenderness**   🄠
            R10.814   **Left lower quadrant abdominal tenderness**   🄠
            R10.815   **Periumbilic abdominal tenderness**   🄠
            R10.816   **Epigastric abdominal tenderness**   🄠
            R10.817   **Generalized abdominal tenderness**   🄠
            R10.819   **Abdominal tenderness, unspecified site**   🄠 ▽

       ✓6ᵗʰ **R10.82**   **Rebound abdominal tenderness**
            R10.821   **Right upper quadrant rebound abdominal tenderness**
            R10.822   **Left upper quadrant rebound abdominal tenderness**
            R10.823   **Right lower quadrant rebound abdominal tenderness**   🄠
            R10.824   **Left lower quadrant rebound abdominal tenderness**   🄠
            R10.825   **Periumbilic rebound abdominal tenderness**   🄠
            R10.826   **Epigastric rebound abdominal tenderness**   🄠
            R10.827   **Generalized rebound abdominal tenderness**   🄠
            R10.829   **Rebound abdominal tenderness, unspecified site**   🄠 ▽

       R10.83   **Colic**   🄿
            Colic NOS
            Infantile colic
            EXCLUDES 1   colic in adult and child over 12 months old (R10.84)
            DEF: Inconsolable crying in an otherwise well-fed and healthy infant for more than three hours a day, three days a week, for more than three weeks.

       R10.84   **Generalized abdominal pain**   🄠
            EXCLUDES 1   generalized abdominal pain associated with acute abdomen (R10.0)

    R10.9   **Unspecified abdominal pain**   🄠 ▽

✓4ᵗʰ **R11**   **Nausea and vomiting**

    EXCLUDES 1   cyclical vomiting associated with migraine (G43.A-)
                 excessive vomiting in pregnancy (O21.-)
                 hematemesis (K92.0)
                 neonatal hematemesis (P54.0)
                 newborn vomiting (P92.0-)
                 psychogenic vomiting (F50.89)
                 vomiting associated with bulimia nervosa (F50.2)
                 vomiting following gastrointestinal surgery (K91.0)

    AHA: 2017,1Q,28
    TIP: Assign a code from this category along with K31.89 Other diseases of stomach and duodenum, to describe cyclical vomiting not due to migraine.

    R11.0   **Nausea**
           Nausea NOS
           Nausea without vomiting

✓5ᵗʰ **R11.1**   **Vomiting**

       R11.10   **Vomiting, unspecified**   ▽
            Vomiting NOS
       R11.11   **Vomiting without nausea**
       R11.12   **Projectile vomiting**
       R11.13   **Vomiting of fecal matter**
       R11.14   **Bilious vomiting**
            Bilious emesis

    R11.2   **Nausea with vomiting, unspecified**   ▽
           Persistent nausea with vomiting NOS

R12   **Heartburn**

    EXCLUDES 1   dyspepsia NOS (R10.13)
                 functional dyspepsia (K30)

✓4ᵗʰ **R13**   **Aphagia and dysphagia**

    R13.0   **Aphagia**
           Inability to swallow
           EXCLUDES 1   psychogenic aphagia (F50.9)

☑ Additional Character Req   ✓x7ᵗʰ Placeholder Alert   Manifestation   ▽ Unspecified   ▶◀ Revised Text   ● New Code   ▲ Revised Code Title

ICD-10-CM 2019   **925**

✓5ᵗʰ R13.1 Dysphagia

Code first, if applicable, dysphagia following cerebrovascular disease (I69. with final characters -91)

EXCLUDES 1   *psychogenic dysphagia (F45.8)*

Swallowing Function

Oral phase

Oropharyngeal phase

Pharyngeal phase

Pharyngoesophageal phase

R13.10 Dysphagia, unspecified ▽
Difficulty in swallowing NOS

R13.11 Dysphagia, oral phase

R13.12 Dysphagia, oropharyngeal phase

R13.13 Dysphagia, pharyngeal phase

R13.14 Dysphagia, pharyngoesophageal phase

R13.19 Other dysphagia
Cervical dysphagia
Neurogenic dysphagia

✓4ᵗʰ R14 Flatulence and related conditions

EXCLUDES 1   *psychogenic aerophagy (F45.8)*

R14.0 Abdominal distension (gaseous)
Bloating
Tympanites (abdominal) (intestinal)

R14.1 Gas pain

R14.2 Eructation

R14.3 Flatulence

✓4ᵗʰ R15 Fecal incontinence

INCLUDES   encopresis NOS

EXCLUDES 1   *fecal incontinence of nonorganic origin (F98.1)*

R15.0 Incomplete defecation

EXCLUDES 1   *constipation (K59.0-)*
fecal impaction (K56.41)

R15.1 Fecal smearing
Fecal soiling

R15.2 Fecal urgency

R15.9 Full incontinence of feces
Fecal incontinence NOS

✓4ᵗʰ R16 Hepatomegaly and splenomegaly, not elsewhere classified

R16.0 Hepatomegaly, not elsewhere classified
Hepatomegaly NOS

R16.1 Splenomegaly, not elsewhere classified
Splenomegaly NOS

R16.2 Hepatomegaly with splenomegaly, not elsewhere classified
Hepatosplenomegaly NOS

R17 Unspecified jaundice ▽

EXCLUDES 1   *neonatal jaundice (P55, P57-P59)*

✓4ᵗʰ R18 Ascites

INCLUDES   fluid in peritoneal cavity

EXCLUDES 1   *ascites in alcoholic cirrhosis (K70.31)*
ascites in alcoholic hepatitis (K70.11)
ascites in toxic liver disease with chronic active hepatitis (K71.51)

R18.0 Malignant ascites
Code first malignancy, such as:
malignant neoplasm of ovary (C56.-)
secondary malignant neoplasm of retroperitoneum and peritoneum (C78.6)

R18.8 Other ascites
Ascites NOS
Peritoneal effusion (chronic)
AHA: 2018,1Q,4

✓4ᵗʰ R19 Other symptoms and signs involving the digestive system and abdomen

EXCLUDES 1   *acute abdomen (R10.0)*

✓5ᵗʰ R19.0 Intra-abdominal and pelvic swelling, mass and lump

EXCLUDES 1   *abdominal distension (gaseous) (R14.-)*
ascites (R18.-)

R19.00 Intra-abdominal and pelvic swelling, mass and lump, unspecified site ▽

R19.01 Right upper quadrant abdominal swelling, mass and lump

R19.02 Left upper quadrant abdominal swelling, mass and lump

R19.03 Right lower quadrant abdominal swelling, mass and lump

R19.04 Left lower quadrant abdominal swelling, mass and lump

R19.05 Periumbilic swelling, mass or lump
Diffuse or generalized umbilical swelling or mass

R19.06 Epigastric swelling, mass or lump

R19.07 Generalized intra-abdominal and pelvic swelling, mass and lump
Diffuse or generalized intra-abdominal swelling or mass NOS
Diffuse or generalized pelvic swelling or mass NOS

R19.09 Other intra-abdominal and pelvic swelling, mass and lump

✓5ᵗʰ R19.1 Abnormal bowel sounds

R19.11 Absent bowel sounds

R19.12 Hyperactive bowel sounds

R19.15 Other abnormal bowel sounds
Abnormal bowel sounds NOS

R19.2 Visible peristalsis
Hyperperistalsis
DEF: Visible movements of muscular attempts to move food through the digestive tract due to pyloric obstruction, stomach obstruction, or intestinal obstruction.

✓5ᵗʰ R19.3 Abdominal rigidity

EXCLUDES 1   *abdominal rigidity with severe abdominal pain (R10.0)*

R19.30 Abdominal rigidity, unspecified site ▽

R19.31 Right upper quadrant abdominal rigidity

R19.32 Left upper quadrant abdominal rigidity

R19.33 Right lower quadrant abdominal rigidity

R19.34 Left lower quadrant abdominal rigidity

R19.35 Periumbilic abdominal rigidity

R19.36 Epigastric abdominal rigidity

R19.37 Generalized abdominal rigidity

R19.4 Change in bowel habit

EXCLUDES 1   *constipation (K59.0-)*
functional diarrhea (K59.1)

R19.5 Other fecal abnormalities
Abnormal stool color
Bulky stools
Mucus in stools
Occult blood in feces
Occult blood in stools

EXCLUDES 1   *melena (K92.1)*
neonatal melena (P54.1)

R19.6 Halitosis

R19.7   **Diarrhea, unspecified**   ▽
     Diarrhea NOS
     EXCLUDES 1   *functional diarrhea (K59.1)*
         neonatal diarrhea (P78.3)
         psychogenic diarrhea (F45.8)

R19.8   **Other specified symptoms and signs involving the digestive system and abdomen**

Symptoms and signs involving the skin and subcutaneous tissue (R20-R23)

EXCLUDES 2   *symptoms relating to breast (N64.4-N64.5)*

✓4ᵗʰ **R20**   **Disturbances of skin sensation**
     EXCLUDES 1   *dissociative anesthesia and sensory loss (F44.6)*
         psychogenic disturbances (F45.8)

R20.0   **Anesthesia of skin**
R20.1   **Hypoesthesia of skin**
R20.2   **Paresthesia of skin**
     Formication
     Pins and needles
     Tingling skin
     EXCLUDES 1   *acroparesthesia (I73.8)*

R20.3   **Hyperesthesia**
R20.8   **Other disturbances of skin sensation**
R20.9   **Unspecified disturbances of skin sensation**   ▽

R21   **Rash and other nonspecific skin eruption**
     INCLUDES   rash NOS
     EXCLUDES 1   *specified type of rash — code to condition*
         vesicular eruption (R23.8)

✓4ᵗʰ **R22**   **Localized swelling, mass and lump of skin and subcutaneous tissue**
     INCLUDES   subcutaneous nodules (localized)(superficial)
     EXCLUDES 1   *abnormal findings on diagnostic imaging (R90-R93)*
         edema (R60.-)
         enlarged lymph nodes (R59.-)
         localized adiposity (E65)
         swelling of joint (M25.4-)

R22.0   **Localized swelling, mass and lump, head**
R22.1   **Localized swelling, mass and lump, neck**
R22.2   **Localized swelling, mass and lump, trunk**
     EXCLUDES 1   *intra-abdominal or pelvic mass and lump (R19.0-)*
         intra-abdominal or pelvic swelling (R19.0-)
     EXCLUDES 2   *breast mass and lump (N63)*

✓5ᵗʰ **R22.3**   **Localized swelling, mass and lump, upper limb**
     R22.30   **Localized swelling, mass and lump, unspecified upper limb**   ▽
     R22.31   **Localized swelling, mass and lump, right upper limb**
     R22.32   **Localized swelling, mass and lump, left upper limb**
     R22.33   **Localized swelling, mass and lump, upper limb, bilateral**

✓5ᵗʰ **R22.4**   **Localized swelling, mass and lump, lower limb**
     R22.40   **Localized swelling, mass and lump, unspecified lower limb**   ▽
     R22.41   **Localized swelling, mass and lump, right lower limb**
     R22.42   **Localized swelling, mass and lump, left lower limb**
     R22.43   **Localized swelling, mass and lump, lower limb, bilateral**

R22.9   **Localized swelling, mass and lump, unspecified**   ▽

✓4ᵗʰ **R23**   **Other skin changes**
R23.0   **Cyanosis**
     EXCLUDES 1   *acrocyanosis (I73.8)*
         cyanotic attacks of newborn (P28.2)
     DEF: Bluish or purplish discoloration of the skin due to an inadequate oxygen blood level.

R23.1   **Pallor**
     Clammy skin
R23.2   **Flushing**
     Excessive blushing
     Code first, if applicable, menopausal and female climacteric states (N95.1)

R23.3   **Spontaneous ecchymoses**
     Petechiae
     EXCLUDES 1   *ecchymoses of newborn (P54.5)*
         purpura (D69.-)

R23.4   **Changes in skin texture**
     Desquamation of skin
     Induration of skin
     Scaling of skin
     EXCLUDES 1   *epidermal thickening NOS (L85.9)*

R23.8   **Other skin changes**
R23.9   **Unspecified skin changes**   ▽

Symptoms and signs involving the nervous and musculoskeletal systems (R25-R29)

✓4ᵗʰ **R25**   **Abnormal involuntary movements**
     EXCLUDES 1   *specific movement disorders (G20-G26)*
         stereotyped movement disorders (F98.4)
         tic disorders (F95.-)

R25.0   **Abnormal head movements**
R25.1   **Tremor, unspecified**   ▽
     EXCLUDES 1   *chorea NOS (G25.5)*
         essential tremor (G25.0)
         hysterical tremor (F44.4)
         intention tremor (G25.2)

R25.2   **Cramp and spasm**
     EXCLUDES 2   *carpopedal spasm (R29.0)*
         charley-horse (M62.831)
         infantile spasms (G40.4-)
         muscle spasm of back (M62.830)
         muscle spasm of calf (M62.831)

R25.3   **Fasciculation**
     Twitching NOS
R25.8   **Other abnormal involuntary movements**
R25.9   **Unspecified abnormal involuntary movements**   ▽

✓4ᵗʰ **R26**   **Abnormalities of gait and mobility**
     EXCLUDES 1   *ataxia NOS (R27.0)*
         hereditary ataxia (G11.-)
         locomotor (syphilitic) ataxia (A52.11)
         immobility syndrome (paraplegic) (M62.3)

R26.0   **Ataxic gait**
     Staggering gait
R26.1   **Paralytic gait**
     Spastic gait
R26.2   **Difficulty in walking, not elsewhere classified**
     EXCLUDES 1   *falling (R29.6)*
         unsteadiness on feet (R26.81)
     AHA: 2016,2Q,7

✓5ᵗʰ **R26.8**   **Other abnormalities of gait and mobility**
     R26.81   **Unsteadiness on feet**
     R26.89   **Other abnormalities of gait and mobility**
R26.9   **Unspecified abnormalities of gait and mobility**   ▽

✓4ᵗʰ **R27**   **Other lack of coordination**
     EXCLUDES 1   *ataxic gait (R26.0)*
         hereditary ataxia (G11.-)
         vertigo NOS (R42)

R27.0   **Ataxia, unspecified**   ▽
     EXCLUDES 1   *ataxia following cerebrovascular disease (I69. with final characters -93)*

R27.8   **Other lack of coordination**
R27.9   **Unspecified lack of coordination**   ▽

✓4ᵗʰ **R29**   **Other symptoms and signs involving the nervous and musculoskeletal systems**
R29.0   **Tetany**
     Carpopedal spasm
     EXCLUDES 1   *hysterical tetany (F44.5)*
         neonatal tetany (P71.3)
         parathyroid tetany (E20.9)
         post-thyroidectomy tetany (E89.2)
     DEF: Calcium or other mineral imbalance causing voluntary muscles such as hands, feet, or larynx to spasm rhythmically.

R29.1   **Meningismus**
R29.2   **Abnormal reflex**
     EXCLUDES 2   *abnormal pupillary reflex (H57.0)*
         hyperactive gag reflex (J39.2)
         vasovagal reaction or syncope (R55)

R29.3   **Abnormal posture**

☑ Additional Character Req   ✗7ᵗʰ Placeholder Alert   Manifestation   ▽ Unspecified   ▶◀ Revised Text   ● New Code   ▲ Revised Code Title

Chapter 18. Symptoms, Signs and Abnormal Clinical and Laboratory Findings

R29.4–R33.9

R29.4 Clicking hip
    EXCLUDES 1   congenital deformities of hip (Q65.-)

R29.5 Transient paralysis
    Code first any associated spinal cord injury (S14.0, S14.1-, S24.0, S24.1-, S34.0-, S34.1-)
    EXCLUDES 1   transient ischemic attack (G45.9)

R29.6 Repeated falls
    Falling
    Tendency to fall
    EXCLUDES 2   at risk for falling (Z91.81)
                  history of falling (Z91.81)
    AHA: 2016,2Q,6
    TIP: Code in addition to Parkinson's disease (G20), when documented.

✓5ᵗʰ **R29.7 National Institutes of Health Stroke Scale (NIHSS) score**
    Code first the type of cerebral infarction (I63.-)
    AHA: 2016,4Q,61-62

    ✓6ᵗʰ **R29.70 NIHSS score 0-9**
         R29.700 NIHSS score 0
         R29.701 NIHSS score 1
         R29.702 NIHSS score 2
         R29.703 NIHSS score 3
         R29.704 NIHSS score 4
         R29.705 NIHSS score 5
         R29.706 NIHSS score 6
         R29.707 NIHSS score 7
         R29.708 NIHSS score 8
         R29.709 NIHSS score 9

    ✓6ᵗʰ **R29.71 NIHSS score 10-19**
         R29.710 NIHSS score 10
         R29.711 NIHSS score 11
         R29.712 NIHSS score 12
         R29.713 NIHSS score 13
         R29.714 NIHSS score 14
         R29.715 NIHSS score 15
         R29.716 NIHSS score 16
         R29.717 NIHSS score 17
         R29.718 NIHSS score 18
         R29.719 NIHSS score 19

    ✓6ᵗʰ **R29.72 NIHSS score 20-29**
         R29.720 NIHSS score 20
         R29.721 NIHSS score 21
         R29.722 NIHSS score 22
         R29.723 NIHSS score 23
         R29.724 NIHSS score 24
         R29.725 NIHSS score 25
         R29.726 NIHSS score 26
         R29.727 NIHSS score 27
         R29.728 NIHSS score 28
         R29.729 NIHSS score 29

    ✓6ᵗʰ **R29.73 NIHSS score 30-39**
         R29.730 NIHSS score 30
         R29.731 NIHSS score 31
         R29.732 NIHSS score 32
         R29.733 NIHSS score 33
         R29.734 NIHSS score 34
         R29.735 NIHSS score 35
         R29.736 NIHSS score 36
         R29.737 NIHSS score 37
         R29.738 NIHSS score 38
         R29.739 NIHSS score 39

    ✓6ᵗʰ **R29.74 NIHSS score 40-42**
         R29.740 NIHSS score 40
         R29.741 NIHSS score 41
         R29.742 NIHSS score 42

✓5ᵗʰ **R29.8 Other symptoms and signs involving the nervous and musculoskeletal systems**
    ✓6ᵗʰ **R29.81 Other symptoms and signs involving the nervous system**
         R29.810 Facial weakness
             Facial droop
             EXCLUDES 1   Bell's palsy (G51.0)
                            facial weakness following cerebrovascular disease (I69. with final characters -92)

R29.818 Other symptoms and signs involving the nervous system

✓6ᵗʰ **R29.89 Other symptoms and signs involving the musculoskeletal system**
    EXCLUDES 2   pain in limb (M79.6-)

    R29.890 Loss of height
         EXCLUDES 1   osteoporosis (M80-M81)

    R29.891 Ocular torticollis
         EXCLUDES 1   congenital (sternomastoid) torticollis Q68.0
                        psychogenic torticollis (F45.8)
                        spasmodic torticollis (G24.3)
                        torticollis due to birth injury (P15.8)
                        torticollis NOS M43.6
         DEF: Abnormal head posture as a result of a contracted state of cervical muscles to correct a visual disturbance, either double vision or a visual field defect.

    R29.898 Other symptoms and signs involving the musculoskeletal system

✓5ᵗʰ **R29.9 Unspecified symptoms and signs involving the nervous and musculoskeletal systems**
    R29.90 Unspecified symptoms and signs involving the nervous system   ▽
    R29.91 Unspecified symptoms and signs involving the musculoskeletal system   ▽

Symptoms and signs involving the genitourinary system (R30-R39)

✓4ᵗʰ **R30 Pain associated with micturition**
    EXCLUDES 1   psychogenic pain associated with micturition (F45.8)

    R30.0 Dysuria
         Strangury

    R30.1 Vesical tenesmus
         DEF: Feeling of a full bladder even when there is little or no urine in the bladder.

    R30.9 Painful micturition, unspecified   ▽
         Painful urination NOS

✓4ᵗʰ **R31 Hematuria**
    EXCLUDES 1   hematuria included with underlying conditions, such as:
                 acute cystitis with hematuria (N30.01)
                 recurrent and persistent hematuria in glomerular diseases (N02.-)
    AHA: 2017,1Q,17

    R31.0 Gross hematuria

    R31.1 Benign essential microscopic hematuria

    ✓5ᵗʰ **R31.2 Other microscopic hematuria**
         AHA: 2016,4Q,62
         R31.21 Asymptomatic microscopic hematuria
             AMH
         R31.29 Other microscopic hematuria

    R31.9 Hematuria, unspecified   ▽

R32 Unspecified urinary incontinence   ◻ ▽
    Enuresis NOS
    EXCLUDES 1   functional urinary incontinence (R39.81)
                 nonorganic enuresis (F98.0)
                 stress incontinence and other specified urinary incontinence (N39.3-N39.4-)
                 urinary incontinence associated with cognitive impairment (R39.81)

✓4ᵗʰ **R33 Retention of urine**
    EXCLUDES 1   psychogenic retention of urine (F45.8)

    R33.0 Drug induced retention of urine
         Use additional code for adverse effect, if applicable, to identify drug (T36-T50 with fifth or sixth character 5)

    R33.8 Other retention of urine
         Code first, if applicable, any causal condition, such as: enlarged prostate (N40.1)

    R33.9 Retention of urine, unspecified   ▽

R34 Anuria and oliguria

> EXCLUDES 1   *anuria and oliguria complicating abortion or ectopic or molar pregnancy (O00-O07, O08.4)*
> *anuria and oliguria complicating pregnancy (O26.83-)*
> *anuria and oliguria complicating the puerperium (O90.4)*

√4ᵗʰ R35 Polyuria

> Code first, if applicable, any causal condition, such as:
> enlarged prostate (N40.1)
> EXCLUDES 1   *psychogenic polyuria (F45.8)*

R35.0 Frequency of micturition

R35.1 Nocturia

R35.8 Other polyuria
> Polyuria NOS

√4ᵗʰ R36 Urethral discharge

R36.0 Urethral discharge without blood

R36.1 Hematospermia   ♂

R36.9 Urethral discharge, unspecified   ▽
> Penile discharge NOS
> Urethrorrhea

R37 Sexual dysfunction, unspecified   ▽

√4ᵗʰ R39 Other and unspecified symptoms and signs involving the genitourinary system

R39.0 Extravasation of urine

√5ᵗʰ R39.1 Other difficulties with micturition

> Code first, if applicable, any causal condition, such as:
> enlarged prostate (N40.1)

R39.11 Hesitancy of micturition

R39.12 Poor urinary stream
> Weak urinary steam

R39.13 Splitting of urinary stream

R39.14 Feeling of incomplete bladder emptying

R39.15 Urgency of urination
> EXCLUDES 1   *urge incontinence (N39.41, N39.46)*

R39.16 Straining to void

√6ᵗʰ R39.19 Other difficulties with micturition
> AHA: 2016,4Q,63

R39.191 Need to immediately re-void

R39.192 Position dependent micturition

R39.198 Other difficulties with micturition

R39.2 Extrarenal uremia
> Prerenal uremia
> EXCLUDES 1   *uremia NOS (N19)*

√5ᵗʰ R39.8 Other symptoms and signs involving the genitourinary system
> AHA: 2017,4Q,22-23

R39.81 Functional urinary incontinence
> Urinary incontinence due to cognitive impairment, or severe physical disability or immobility
> EXCLUDES 1   *stress incontinence and other specified urinary incontinence (N39.3-N39.4-)*
> *urinary incontinence NOS (R32)*

R39.82 Chronic bladder pain
> AHA: 2016,4Q,64

R39.83 Unilateral non-palpable testicle   ♂

R39.84 Bilateral non-palpable testicles   ♂

R39.89 Other symptoms and signs involving the genitourinary system

R39.9 Unspecified symptoms and signs involving the genitourinary system   ▽

Symptoms and signs involving cognition, perception, emotional state and behavior (R40-R46)

> EXCLUDES 2   *symptoms and signs constituting part of a pattern of mental disorder (F01-F99)*

√4ᵗʰ R40 Somnolence, stupor and coma

> EXCLUDES 1   *neonatal coma (P91.5)*
> *somnolence, stupor and coma in diabetes (E08-E13)*
> *somnolence, stupor and coma in hepatic failure (K72.-)*
> *somnolence, stupor and coma in hypoglycemia (nondiabetic) (E15)*

R40.0 Somnolence
> Drowsiness
> EXCLUDES 1   *coma (R40.2-)*

R40.1 Stupor
> Catatonic stupor
> Semicoma
> EXCLUDES 1   *catatonic schizophrenia (F20.2)*
> *coma (R40.2-)*
> *depressive stupor (F31-F33)*
> *dissociative stupor (F44.2)*
> *manic stupor (F30.2)*

√5ᵗʰ R40.2 Coma

> Code first any associated:
> fracture of skull (S02.-)
> intracranial injury (S06.-)

> NOTE   One code from each subcategory, R40.21-R40.23, is required to complete the coma scale

> AHA: 2017,4Q,23-25,95; 2015,2Q,17; 2014,1Q,19

R40.20 Unspecified coma   HCC ▽
> Coma NOS
> Unconsciousness NOS

√6ᵗʰ R40.21 Coma scale, eyes open

> The following appropriate 7th character is to be added to subcategory R40.21-, R40.22-, R40.23-, and R40.24-.
> 0   unspecified time
> 1   in the field [EMT or ambulance]
> 2   at arrival to emergency department
> 3   at hospital admission
> 4   24 hours or more after hospital admission

√7ᵗʰ R40.211 Coma scale, eyes open, never   HCC
> ►Coma scale eye opening score of 1◄

√7ᵗʰ R40.212 Coma scale, eyes open, to pain   HCC
> ►Coma scale eye opening score of 2◄

√7ᵗʰ R40.213 Coma scale, eyes open, to sound
> ►Coma scale eye opening score of 3◄

√7ᵗʰ R40.214 Coma scale, eyes open, spontaneous
> ►Coma scale eye opening score of 4◄

√6ᵗʰ R40.22 Coma scale, best verbal response

√7ᵗʰ R40.221 Coma scale, best verbal response, none   HCC
> ►Coma scale verbal score of 1◄

√7ᵗʰ R40.222 Coma scale, best verbal response, incomprehensible words   HCC
> ►Coma scale verbal score of 2◄
> Incomprehensible sounds (2-5 years of age)
> Moans/grunts to pain; restless (< 2 years old)

√7ᵗʰ R40.223 Coma scale, best verbal response, inappropriate words
> ►Coma scale verbal score of 3◄
> Inappropriate crying or screaming (< 2 years of age)
> Screaming (2-5 years of age)

√7ᵗʰ R40.224 Coma scale, best verbal response, confused conversation
> ►Coma scale verbal score of 4◄
> Inappropriate words (2-5 years of age)
> Irritable cries (< 2 years of age)

√7ᵗʰ R40.225 Coma scale, best verbal response, oriented
> ►Coma scale verbal score of 5◄
> Cooing or babbling or crying appropriately (< 2 years of age)
> Uses appropriate words (2-5 years of age)

√6ᵗʰ R40.23 Coma scale, best motor response

√7ᵗʰ R40.231 Coma scale, best motor response, none   HCC
> ►Coma scale motor score of 1◄

√7ᵗʰ R40.232 Coma scale, best motor response, extension   HCC
> Abnormal extensor posturing to pain or noxious stimuli (< 2 years of age)
> ►Coma scale motor score of 2◄
> Extensor posturing to pain or noxious stimuli (2-5 years of age)

 Additional Character Req   √x 7ᵗʰ Placeholder Alert   Manifestation   ▽ Unspecified   ►◄ Revised Text   ● New Code   ▲ Revised Code Title

Chapter 18. Symptoms, Signs and Abnormal Clinical and Laboratory Findings

▲

√7ᵗʰ **R40.233 Coma scale, best motor response, abnormal flexion**
▶Abnormal flexure posturing to pain or noxious stimuli (2-5 years of age)◀
▶Coma scale motor score of 3◀
Flexion/decorticate posturing (< 2 years of age)

√7ᵗʰ **R40.234 Coma scale, best motor response, flexion withdrawal** HCC
▶Coma scale motor score of 4◀
▶Withdraws from pain or noxious stimuli (2-5 years of age)◀

√7ᵗʰ **R40.235 Coma scale, best motor response, localizes pain**
▶Coma scale motor score of 5◀
Localizes pain (2-5 years of age)
Withdraws to touch (< 2 years of age)

√7ᵗʰ **R40.236 Coma scale, best motor response, obeys commands**
▶Coma scale motor score of 6◀
Normal or spontaneous movement (< 2 years of age)
Obeys commands (2-5 years of age)

√6ᵗʰ **R40.24 Glasgow coma scale, total score**

> **NOTE** Assign a code from subcategory R40.24, when only the total coma score is documented

AHA: 2016,4Q,64-65

√7ᵗʰ **R40.241 Glasgow coma scale score 13-15**
√7ᵗʰ **R40.242 Glasgow coma scale score 9-12**
√7ᵗʰ **R40.243 Glasgow coma scale score 3-8** HCC
√7ᵗʰ **R40.244 Other coma, without documented Glasgow coma scale score, or with partial score reported** HCC

R40.3 Persistent vegetative state HCC
DEF: Persistent wakefulness without consciousness due to a nonfunctioning cerebral cortex.

R40.4 Transient alteration of awareness

√4ᵗʰ **R41 Other symptoms and signs involving cognitive functions and awareness**
EXCLUDES 1   dissociative [conversion] disorders (F44.-)
mild cognitive impairment, so stated (G31.84)

R41.0 Disorientation, unspecified ▽
Confusion NOS
Delirium NOS

R41.1 Anterograde amnesia
R41.2 Retrograde amnesia
R41.3 Other amnesia
Amnesia NOS
Memory loss NOS
EXCLUDES 1   amnestic disorder due to known physiologic condition (F04)
amnestic syndrome due to psychoactive substance use (F10-F19 with 5th character .6)
mild memory disturbance due to known physiological condition (F06.8)
transient global amnesia (G45.4)

R41.4 Neurologic neglect syndrome
Asomatognosia
Hemi-akinesia
Hemi-inattention
Hemispatial neglect
Left-sided neglect
Sensory neglect
Visuospatial neglect
EXCLUDES 1   visuospatial deficit (R41.842)

√5ᵗʰ **R41.8 Other symptoms and signs involving cognitive functions and awareness**

R41.81 Age-related cognitive decline A
Senility NOS

R41.82 Altered mental status, unspecified ▽
Change in mental status NOS
EXCLUDES 1   altered level of consciousness (R40.-)
altered mental status due to known condition - code to condition
delirium NOS (R41.0)
AHA: 2012,4Q,97

R41.83 Borderline intellectual functioning
IQ level 71 to 84
EXCLUDES 1   intellectual disabilities (F70-F79)

√6ᵗʰ **R41.84 Other specified cognitive deficit**
EXCLUDES 1   cognitive deficits as sequelae of cerebrovascular disease (I69.01-, I69.11-, I69.21-, I69.31-, I69.81-, I69.91-)

R41.840 Attention and concentration deficit
EXCLUDES 1   attention-deficit hyperactivity disorders (F90.-)
R41.841 Cognitive communication deficit
R41.842 Visuospatial deficit
R41.843 Psychomotor deficit
R41.844 Frontal lobe and executive function deficit

R41.89 Other symptoms and signs involving cognitive functions and awareness
Anosognosia

R41.9 Unspecified symptoms and signs involving cognitive functions and awareness ▽
Unspecified neurocognitive disorder

R42 Dizziness and giddiness Q
Light-headedness
Vertigo NOS
EXCLUDES 1   vertiginous syndromes (H81.-)
vertigo from infrasound (T75.23)

√4ᵗʰ **R43 Disturbances of smell and taste**

R43.0 Anosmia
DEF: Permanent or transient absence of smell that may be congenital or acquired.

R43.1 Parosmia
DEF: Abnormal perception of smell usually triggered by environmental odors.

R43.2 Parageusia
DEF: Abnormal perception of taste.

R43.8 Other disturbances of smell and taste
Mixed disturbance of smell and taste

R43.9 Unspecified disturbances of smell and taste ▽

√4ᵗʰ **R44 Other symptoms and signs involving general sensations and perceptions**
EXCLUDES 1   alcoholic hallucinations (F1.5)
hallucinations in drug psychosis (F11-F19 with .5)
hallucinations in mood disorders with psychotic symptoms (F30.2, F31.5, F32.3, F33.3)
hallucinations in schizophrenia, schizotypal and delusional disorders (F20-F29)
EXCLUDES 2   disturbances of skin sensation (R20.-)

R44.0 Auditory hallucinations
R44.1 Visual hallucinations
R44.2 Other hallucinations
R44.3 Hallucinations, unspecified ▽
R44.8 Other symptoms and signs involving general sensations and perceptions
R44.9 Unspecified symptoms and signs involving general sensations and perceptions ▽

√4ᵗʰ **R45 Symptoms and signs involving emotional state**

R45.0 Nervousness
Nervous tension
R45.1 Restlessness and agitation
R45.2 Unhappiness
R45.3 Demoralization and apathy
EXCLUDES 1   anhedonia (R45.84)
R45.4 Irritability and anger
R45.5 Hostility
R45.6 Violent behavior
R45.7 State of emotional shock and stress, unspecified ▽
√6ᵗʰ **R45.8 Other symptoms and signs involving emotional state**
R45.81 Low self-esteem

R45.82   **Worries**

R45.83   **Excessive crying of child, adolescent or adult**
EXCLUDES 1   *excessive crying of infant (baby) R68.11*

R45.84   **Anhedonia**

√6ᵗʰ **R45.85**   **Homicidal and suicidal ideations**
EXCLUDES 1   *suicide attempt (T14.91)*

     R45.850   **Homicidal ideations**

     R45.851   **Suicidal ideations**
         DEF: Thoughts of committing suicide but no actual attempt of suicide has been made.

R45.86   **Emotional lability**

R45.87   **Impulsiveness**

R45.89   **Other symptoms and signs involving emotional state**

√4ᵗʰ **R46**   **Symptoms and signs involving appearance and behavior**
EXCLUDES 1   *appearance and behavior in schizophrenia, schizotypal and delusional disorders (F20-F29)*
     mental and behavioral disorders (F01-F99)

R46.0   **Very low level of personal hygiene**

R46.1   **Bizarre personal appearance**

R46.2   **Strange and inexplicable behavior**

R46.3   **Overactivity**

R46.4   **Slowness and poor responsiveness**
EXCLUDES 1   *stupor (R40.1)*

R46.5   **Suspiciousness and marked evasiveness**

R46.6   **Undue concern and preoccupation with stressful events**

R46.7   **Verbosity and circumstantial detail obscuring reason for contact**

√5ᵗʰ **R46.8**   **Other symptoms and signs involving appearance and behavior**

     R46.81   **Obsessive-compulsive behavior**
         EXCLUDES 1   *obsessive-compulsive disorder (F42-)*

     R46.89   **Other symptoms and signs involving appearance and behavior**

Symptoms and signs involving speech and voice (R47-R49)

√4ᵗʰ **R47**   **Speech disturbances, not elsewhere classified**
EXCLUDES 1   *autism (F84.0)*
     cluttering (F80.81)
     specific developmental disorders of speech and language (F80.-)
     stuttering (F80.81)

√5ᵗʰ **R47.0**   **Dysphasia and aphasia**

     R47.01   **Aphasia**
         EXCLUDES 1   *aphasia following cerebrovascular disease (I69. with final characters -20)*
         progressive isolated aphasia (G31.01)

     R47.02   **Dysphasia**
         EXCLUDES 1   *dysphasia following cerebrovascular disease (I69. with final characters -21)*

R47.1   **Dysarthria and anarthria**
EXCLUDES 1   *dysarthria following cerebrovascular disease (I69. with final characters -22)*

√5ᵗʰ **R47.8**   **Other speech disturbances**
EXCLUDES 1   *dysarthria following cerebrovascular disease (I69. with final characters -28)*

     R47.81   **Slurred speech**

     R47.82   *Fluency disorder in conditions classified elsewhere*
         Stuttering in conditions classified elsewhere
         Code first underlying disease or condition, such as:
         Parkinson's disease (G20)
         EXCLUDES 1   *adult onset fluency disorder (F98.5)*
         childhood onset fluency disorder (F80.81)
         fluency disorder (stuttering) following cerebrovascular disease (I69. with final characters -23)

     R47.89   **Other speech disturbances**

R47.9   **Unspecified speech disturbances** ▽

√4ᵗʰ **R48**   **Dyslexia and other symbolic dysfunctions, not elsewhere classified**
EXCLUDES 1   *specific developmental disorders of scholastic skills (F81.-)*

R48.0   **Dyslexia and alexia**

R48.1   **Agnosia**
Astereognosia (astereognosis)
Autotopagnosia
EXCLUDES 1   *visual object agnosia (R48.3)*
DEF: Inability to recognize common things such as faces, objects, smells, or voices.

R48.2   **Apraxia**
EXCLUDES 1   *apraxia following cerebrovascular disease (I69. with final characters -90)*

R48.3   **Visual agnosia**
Prosopagnosia
Simultanagnosia (asimultagnosia)

R48.8   **Other symbolic dysfunctions**
Acalculia
Agraphia
AHA: 2017,1Q,27

R48.9   **Unspecified symbolic dysfunctions** ▽

√4ᵗʰ **R49**   **Voice and resonance disorders**
EXCLUDES 1   *psychogenic voice and resonance disorders (F44.4)*

R49.0   **Dysphonia**
Hoarseness

R49.1   **Aphonia**
Loss of voice

√5ᵗʰ **R49.2**   **Hypernasality and hyponasality**

     R49.21   **Hypernasality**

     R49.22   **Hyponasality**

R49.8   **Other voice and resonance disorders**

R49.9   **Unspecified voice and resonance disorder** ▽
Change in voice NOS
Resonance disorder NOS

General symptoms and signs (R50-R69)

√4ᵗʰ **R50**   **Fever of other and unknown origin**
EXCLUDES 1   *chills without fever (R68.83)*
     febrile convulsions (R56.0-)
     fever of unknown origin during labor (O75.2)
     fever of unknown origin in newborn (P81.9)
     hypothermia due to illness (R68.0)
     malignant hyperthermia due to anesthesia (T88.3)
     puerperal pyrexia NOS (O86.4)

R50.2   **Drug induced fever**
Use additional code for adverse effect, if applicable, to identify drug (T36-T50 with fifth or sixth character 5)
EXCLUDES 1   *postvaccination (postimmunization) fever (R50.83)*

√5ᵗʰ **R50.8**   **Other specified fever**

     R50.81   *Fever presenting with conditions classified elsewhere*
         Code first underlying condition when associated fever is present, such as with:
         leukemia (C91-C95)
         neutropenia (D70.-)
         sickle-cell disease (D57.-)
         AHA: 2014,4Q,22

     R50.82   **Postprocedural fever**
         EXCLUDES 1   *postprocedural infection (T81.4-)*
         posttransfusion fever (R50.84)
         postvaccination (postimmunization) fever (R50.83)

     R50.83   **Postvaccination fever**
         Postimmunization fever

     R50.84   **Febrile nonhemolytic transfusion reaction**
         FNHTR
         Posttransfusion fever

R50.9   **Fever, unspecified** ▽
Fever NOS
Fever of unknown origin [FUO]
Fever with chills
Fever with rigors
Hyperpyrexia NOS
Persistent fever
Pyrexia NOS

☑ Additional Character Req   √x7ᵗʰ Placeholder Alert   Manifestation   ▽ Unspecified   ▶◀ Revised Text   ● New Code   ▲ Revised Code Title

Chapter 18. Symptoms, Signs and Abnormal Clinical and Laboratory Findings

R51 Headache
Facial pain NOS
> EXCLUDES 1   *atypical face pain (G50.1)*
> *migraine and other headache syndromes (G43-G44)*
> *trigeminal neuralgia (G50.0)*

R52 Pain, unspecified ▽
Acute pain NOS
Generalized pain NOS
Pain NOS
> EXCLUDES 1   *acute and chronic pain, not elsewhere classified (G89.-)*
> *localized pain, unspecified type - code to pain by site, such as:*
> *abdomen pain (R10.-)*
> *back pain (M54.9)*
> *breast pain (N64.4)*
> *chest pain (R07.1-R07.9)*
> *ear pain (H92.0-)*
> *eye pain (H57.1)*
> *headache (R51)*
> *joint pain (M25.5-)*
> *limb pain (M79.6-)*
> *lumbar region pain (M54.5)*
> *pelvic and perineal pain (R10.2)*
> *renal colic (N23)*
> *shoulder pain (M25.51-)*
> *spine pain (M54.-)*
> *throat pain (R07.0)*
> *tongue pain (K14.6)*
> *tooth pain (K08.8)*
> *pain disorders exclusively related to psychological factors (F45.41)*

✓4ᵗʰ R53 Malaise and fatigue

R53.0 Neoplastic (malignant) related fatigue
Code first associated neoplasm

R53.1 Weakness
Asthenia NOS
> EXCLUDES 1   *age-related weakness (R54)*
> *muscle weakness (M62.8-)*
> *sarcopenia (M62.84)*
> *senile asthenia (R54)*

AHA: 2017,1Q,7; 2015,1Q,25

R53.2 Functional quadriplegia HCC
Complete immobility due to severe physical disability or frailty
> EXCLUDES 1   *frailty NOS (R54)*
> *hysterical paralysis (F44.4)*
> *immobility syndrome (M62.3)*
> *neurologic quadriplegia (G82.5-)*
> *quadriplegia (G82.50)*

AHA: 2016,2Q,6
DEF: Inability to move due to a nonphysiological condition, such as dementia. The patient has no mental ability to move independently.

✓5ᵗʰ R53.8 Other malaise and fatigue
> EXCLUDES 1   *combat exhaustion and fatigue (F43.0)*
> *congenital debility (P96.9)*
> *exhaustion and fatigue due to excessive exertion (T73.3)*
> *exhaustion and fatigue due to exposure (T73.2)*
> *exhaustion and fatigue due to heat (T67.-)*
> *exhaustion and fatigue due to pregnancy (O26.8-)*
> *exhaustion and fatigue due to recurrent depressive episode (F33)*
> *exhaustion and fatigue due to senile debility (R54)*

R53.81 Other malaise
Chronic debility
Debility NOS
General physical deterioration
Malaise NOS
Nervous debility
> EXCLUDES 1   *age-related physical debility (R54)*

R53.82 Chronic fatigue, unspecified ▽
Chronic fatigue syndrome NOS
> EXCLUDES 1   *postviral fatigue syndrome (G93.3)*

R53.83 Other fatigue
Fatigue NOS
Lack of energy
Lethargy
Tiredness
> EXCLUDES 2   *exhaustion and fatigue due to depressive episode (F32.-)*

R54 Age-related physical debility A
Frailty
Old age
Senescence
Senile asthenia
Senile debility
> EXCLUDES 1   *age-related cognitive decline (R41.81)*
> *sarcopenia (M62.84)*
> *senile psychosis (F03)*
> *senility NOS (R41.81)*

R55 Syncope and collapse
Blackout
Fainting
Vasovagal attack
> EXCLUDES 1   *cardiogenic shock (R57.0)*
> *carotid sinus syncope (G90.01)*
> *heat syncope (T67.1)*
> *neurocirculatory asthenia (F45.8)*
> *neurogenic orthostatic hypotension (G90.3)*
> *orthostatic hypotension (I95.1)*
> *postprocedural shock (T81.1-)*
> *psychogenic syncope (F48.8)*
> *shock NOS (R57.9)*
> *shock complicating or following abortion or ectopic or molar pregnancy (O00-O07, O08.3)*
> *shock complicating or following labor and delivery (O75.1)*
> *Stokes-Adams attack (I45.9)*
> *unconsciousness NOS (R40.2-)*

✓4ᵗʰ R56 Convulsions, not elsewhere classified
> EXCLUDES 1   *dissociative convulsions and seizures (F44.5)*
> *epileptic convulsions and seizures (G40.-)*
> *newborn convulsions and seizures (P90)*

✓5ᵗʰ R56.0 Febrile convulsions

R56.00 Simple febrile convulsions HCC
Febrile convulsion NOS
Febrile seizure NOS

R56.01 Complex febrile convulsions HCC
Atypical febrile seizure
Complex febrile seizure
Complicated febrile seizure
> EXCLUDES 1   *status epilepticus (G40.901)*

R56.1 Post traumatic seizures HCC
> EXCLUDES 1   *post traumatic epilepsy (G40.-)*

R56.9 Unspecified convulsions HCC ▽
Convulsion disorder
Fit NOS
Recurrent convulsions
Seizure(s) (convulsive) NOS

☑4ᵗʰ **R57 Shock, not elsewhere classified**

EXCLUDES 1   anaphylactic shock NOS (T78.2)

anaphylactic reaction or shock due to adverse food reaction (T78.0-)

anaphylactic shock due to adverse effect of correct drug or medicament properly administered (T88.6)

anaphylactic shock due to serum (T80.5-)

anesthetic shock (T88.3)

electric shock (T75.4)

obstetric shock (O75.1)

postprocedural shock (T81.1-)

psychic shock (F43.0)

shock complicating or following ectopic or molar pregnancy (O00–O07, O08.3)

shock due to lightning (T75.01)

traumatic shock (T79.4)

toxic shock syndrome (A48.3)

R57.0 Cardiogenic shock   HCC

EXCLUDES 2   septic shock (R65.21)

DEF: Associated with myocardial infarction, cardiac tamponade, and massive pulmonary embolism. Symptoms include mental confusion, reduced blood pressure, tachycardia, pallor, and cold, clammy skin.

R57.1 Hypovolemic shock   HCC

R57.8 Other shock   HCC

R57.9 Shock, unspecified   HCC ▽

Failure of peripheral circulation NOS ·

R58 Hemorrhage, not elsewhere classified

Hemorrhage NOS

EXCLUDES 1   hemorrhage included with underlying conditions, such as:

acute duodenal ulcer with hemorrhage (K26.0)

acute gastritis with bleeding (K29.01)

ulcerative enterocolitis with rectal bleeding (K51.01)

☑4ᵗʰ **R59 Enlarged lymph nodes**

INCLUDES   swollen glands

EXCLUDES 1   acute lymphadenitis (L04.-)

chronic lymphadenitis (I88.1)

lymphadenitis NOS (I88.9)

mesenteric (acute) (chronic) lymphadenitis (I88.0)

R59.0 Localized enlarged lymph nodes

R59.1 Generalized enlarged lymph nodes

Lymphadenopathy NOS

R59.9 Enlarged lymph nodes, unspecified   ▽

☑4ᵗʰ **R60 Edema, not elsewhere classified**

EXCLUDES 1   angioneurotic edema (T78.3)

ascites (R18.-)

cerebral edema (G93.6)

cerebral edema due to birth injury (P11.0)

edema of larynx (J38.4)

edema of nasopharynx (J39.2)

edema of pharynx (J39.2)

gestational edema (O12.0-)

hereditary edema (Q82.0)

hydrops fetalis NOS (P83.2)

hydrothorax (J94.8)

hydrops fetalis NOS (P83.2)

newborn edema (P83.3)

pulmonary edema (J81.-)

R60.0 Localized edema

R60.1 Generalized edema

EXCLUDES 2   nutritional edema (E40-E46)

R60.9 Edema, unspecified   ▽

Fluid retention NOS

R61 Generalized hyperhidrosis

Excessive sweating

Night sweats

Secondary hyperhidrosis

Code first, if applicable, menopausal and female climacteric states (N95.1)

EXCLUDES 1   focal (primary) (secondary) hyperhidrosis (L74.5-)

Frey's syndrome (L74.52)

localized (primary) (secondary) hyperhidrosis (L74.5-)

☑4ᵗʰ **R62 Lack of expected normal physiological development in childhood and adults**

EXCLUDES 1   delayed puberty (E30.0)

gonadal dysgenesis (Q99.1)

hypopituitarism (E23.0)

R62.0 Delayed milestone in childhood   ℗

Delayed attainment of expected physiological developmental stage

Late talker

Late walker

☑5ᵗʰ **R62.5 Other and unspecified lack of expected normal physiological development in childhood**

EXCLUDES 1   HIV disease resulting in failure to thrive (B20)

physical retardation due to malnutrition (E45)

R62.50 Unspecified lack of expected normal physiological development in childhood   ▽

Infantilism NOS

R62.51 Failure to thrive (child)   ℗

Failure to gain weight

EXCLUDES 1   failure to thrive in child under 28 days old (P92.6)

DEF: Organic failure to thrive (FTT): Acute or chronic illness that interferes with nutritional intake, absorption, metabolism excretion, and energy requirements.

DEF: Nonorganic failure to thrive (FTT): Symptom of neglect or abuse.

R62.52 Short stature (child)

Lack of growth

Physical retardation

Short stature NOS

EXCLUDES 1   short stature due to endocrine disorder (E34.3)

R62.59 Other lack of expected normal physiological development in childhood

R62.7 Adult failure to thrive   ▲

☑4ᵗʰ **R63 Symptoms and signs concerning food and fluid intake**

EXCLUDES 1   bulimia NOS (F50.2)

eating disorders of nonorganic origin (F50.-)

malnutrition (E40-E46)

R63.0 Anorexia

Loss of appetite

EXCLUDES 1   anorexia nervosa (F50.0-)

loss of appetite of nonorganic origin (F50.89)

R63.1 Polydipsia

Excessive thirst

R63.2 Polyphagia

Excessive eating

Hyperalimentation NOS

R63.3 Feeding difficulties

Feeding problem (elderly) (infant) NOS

Picky eater

EXCLUDES 1   eating disorders (F50.-)

feeding problems of newborn (P92.-)

infant feeding disorder of nonorganic origin (F98.2-)

AHA: 2017,1Q,28; 2016,3Q,19

TIP: Do not assign for feeding problems in a patient greater than 28 days old if the feeding problem was initially diagnosed between day 0 and day 28; use a code from category P92 instead.

R63.4 Abnormal weight loss

R63.5 Abnormal weight gain

EXCLUDES 1   excessive weight gain in pregnancy (O26.0-)

obesity (E66.-)

R63.6 Underweight

Use additional code to identify body mass index (BMI), if known (Z68.-)

EXCLUDES 1   abnormal weight loss (R63.4)

anorexia nervosa (F50.0-)

malnutrition (E40-E46)

R63.8 Other symptoms and signs concerning food and fluid intake

☑ Additional Character Req   ☑x7ᵗʰ Placeholder Alert   Manifestation   ▽ Unspecified   ►◄ Revised Text   ● New Code   ▲ Revised Code Title

ICD-10-CM 2019   **933**

R64   Cachexia   HCC
Wasting syndrome
Code first underlying condition, if known
EXCLUDES 1   *abnormal weight loss (R63.4)*
nutritional marasmus (E41)
AHA: 2017,3Q,24
TIP: Assign code E41 when emaciated or emaciation is documented in relation to malnutrition.

√4ᵗʰ **R65   Symptoms and signs specifically associated with systemic inflammation and infection**
TIP: When documentation states SIRS with an infection, assign only a code for the infection. ICD-10-CM does not offer a code for SIRS due to infectious process. If sepsis is suspected, query the provider.

√5ᵗʰ **R65.1   Systemic inflammatory response syndrome [SIRS] of non-infectious origin**
Code first underlying condition, such as:
heatstroke (T67.Ø)
injury and trauma (SØØ-T88)
EXCLUDES 1   *sepsis — code to infection*
severe sepsis (R65.2)

R65.1Ø   Systemic inflammatory response syndrome [SIRS] of non-infectious origin without acute organ dysfunction   HCC
Systemic inflammatory response syndrome (SIRS) NOS

R65.11   Systemic inflammatory response syndrome [SIRS] of non-infectious origin with acute organ dysfunction   HCC
Use additional code to identify specific acute organ dysfunction, such as:
acute kidney failure (N17.-)
acute respiratory failure (J96.Ø-)
critical illness myopathy (G72.81)
critical illness polyneuropathy (G62.81)
disseminated intravascular coagulopathy [DIC] (D65)
encephalopathy (metabolic) (septic) (G93.41)
hepatic failure (K72.Ø-)

√5ᵗʰ **R65.2   Severe sepsis**
Infection with associated acute organ dysfunction
Sepsis with acute organ dysfunction
Sepsis with multiple organ dysfunction
Systemic inflammatory response syndrome due to infectious process with acute organ dysfunction
Code first underlying infection, such as:
infection following a procedure (T81.4-)
infections following infusion, transfusion and therapeutic injection (T8Ø.2-)
puerperal sepsis (O85)
sepsis following complete or unspecified spontaneous abortion (OØ3.87)
sepsis following ectopic and molar pregnancy (OØ8.82)
sepsis following incomplete spontaneous abortion (OØ3.37)
sepsis following (induced) termination of pregnancy (OØ4.87)
sepsis NOS (A41.9)
Use additional code to identify specific acute organ dysfunction, such as:
acute kidney failure (N17.-)
acute respiratory failure (J96.Ø-)
critical illness myopathy (G72.81)
critical illness polyneuropathy (G62.81)
disseminated intravascular coagulopathy [DIC] (D65)
encephalopathy (metabolic) (septic) (G93.41)
hepatic failure (K72.Ø-)
AHA: 2017,4Q,98-99; 2016,3Q,8

R65.2Ø   Severe sepsis without septic shock   HCC
Severe sepsis NOS
AHA: 2016,3Q,14; 2013,4Q,119

R65.21   Severe sepsis with septic shock   HCC

√4ᵗʰ **R68   Other general symptoms and signs**

R68.Ø   Hypothermia, not associated with low environmental temperature
EXCLUDES 1   *hypothermia NOS (accidental) (T68)*
hypothermia due to anesthesia (T88.51)
hypothermia due to low environmental temperature (T68)
newborn hypothermia (P8Ø.-)

√5ᵗʰ **R68.1   Nonspecific symptoms peculiar to infancy**
EXCLUDES 1   *colic, infantile (R1Ø.83)*
neonatal cerebral irritability (P91.3)
teething syndrome (KØØ.7)

R68.11   Excessive crying of infant (baby)   P
EXCLUDES 1   *excessive crying of child, adolescent, or adult (R45.83)*

R68.12   Fussy infant (baby)   P
Irritable infant

R68.13   Apparent life threatening event in infant (ALTE)   P
Apparent life threatening event in newborn
Brief resolved unexplained event (BRUE)
Code first confirmed diagnosis, if known
Use additional code(s) for associated signs and symptoms if no confirmed diagnosis established, or if signs and symptoms are not associated routinely with confirmed diagnosis, or provide additional information for cause of ALTE

R68.19   Other nonspecific symptoms peculiar to infancy   P

R68.2   Dry mouth, unspecified   ▽
EXCLUDES 1   *dry mouth due to dehydration (E86.Ø)*
dry mouth due to sicca syndrome [Sjögren] (M35.Ø-)
salivary gland hyposecretion (K11.7)

R68.3   Clubbing of fingers
Clubbing of nails
EXCLUDES 1   *congenital clubfinger (Q68.1)*
DEF: Enlarged soft tissue of the distal fingers that usually occurs in heart and lung diseases.

√5ᵗʰ **R68.8   Other general symptoms and signs**

R68.81   Early satiety
DEF: Premature feeling of being full after eating only a small amount of food. The mechanism of satiety is multifactorial.

R68.82   Decreased libido   A
Decreased sexual desire

R68.83   Chills (without fever)
Chills NOS
EXCLUDES 1   *chills with fever (R5Ø.9)*

R68.84   Jaw pain
Mandibular pain
Maxilla pain
EXCLUDES 1   *temporomandibular joint arthralgia (M26.62-)*

R68.89   Other general symptoms and signs

R69   Illness, unspecified   ▽
Unknown and unspecified cases of morbidity

Abnormal findings on examination of blood, without diagnosis (R7Ø-R79)

EXCLUDES 2   *abnormal findings on antenatal screening of mother (O28.-)*
abnormalities of lipids (E78.-)
abnormalities of platelets and thrombocytes (D69.-)
abnormalities of white blood cells classified elsewhere (D7Ø-D72)
coagulation hemorrhagic disorders (D65-D68)
diagnostic abnormal findings classified elsewhere — see Alphabetical Index
hemorrhagic and hematological disorders of newborn (P5Ø-P61)

√4ᵗʰ **R7Ø   Elevated erythrocyte sedimentation rate and abnormality of plasma viscosity**
R7Ø.Ø   Elevated erythrocyte sedimentation rate
R7Ø.1   Abnormal plasma viscosity

✓4ᵗʰ **R71 Abnormality of red blood cells**

     EXCLUDES 1   anemias (D50-D64)
                            anemia of premature infant (P61.2)
                            benign (familial) polycythemia (D75.0)
                            congenital anemias (P61.2-P61.4)
                            newborn anemia due to isoimmunization (P55.-)
                            polycythemia neonatorum (P61.1)
                            polycythemia NOS (D75.1)
                            polycythemia vera (D45)
                            secondary polycythemia (D75.1)

   R71.0 Precipitous drop in hematocrit
       Drop (precipitous) in hemoglobin
       Drop in hematocrit

   R71.8 Other abnormality of red blood cells
       Abnormal red-cell morphology NOS
       Abnormal red-cell volume NOS
       Anisocytosis
       Poikilocytosis

✓4ᵗʰ **R73 Elevated blood glucose level**

     EXCLUDES 1   diabetes mellitus (E08-E13)
                            diabetes mellitus in pregnancy, childbirth and the puerperium
                              (O24.-)
                            neonatal disorders (P70.0-P70.2)
                            postsurgical hypoinsulinemia (E89.1)

   ✓5ᵗʰ **R73.0 Abnormal glucose**

       EXCLUDES 1   abnormal glucose in pregnancy (O99.81-)
                            diabetes mellitus (E08-E13)
                            dysmetabolic syndrome X (E88.81)
                            gestational diabetes (O24.4-)
                            glycosuria (R81)
                            hypoglycemia (E16.2)

     R73.01 Impaired fasting glucose
         Elevated fasting glucose

     R73.02 Impaired glucose tolerance (oral)
         Elevated glucose tolerance

     R73.03 Prediabetes
         Latent diabetes
         AHA: 2016,4Q,65

     R73.09 Other abnormal glucose
         Abnormal glucose NOS
         Abnormal non-fasting glucose tolerance

   R73.9 Hyperglycemia, unspecified ▽

✓4ᵗʰ **R74 Abnormal serum enzyme levels**

   R74.0 Nonspecific elevation of levels of transaminase and lactic acid dehydrogenase [LDH]

   R74.8 Abnormal levels of other serum enzymes
       Abnormal level of acid phosphatase
       Abnormal level of alkaline phosphatase
       Abnormal level of amylase
       Abnormal level of lipase [triacylglycerol lipase]
       TIP: Assign for documented abnormal or elevated troponin level when a definitive diagnosis has not been established.

   R74.9 Abnormal serum enzyme level, unspecified ▽

R75 Inconclusive laboratory evidence of human immunodeficiency virus [HIV]
     Nonconclusive HIV-test finding in infants
     EXCLUDES 1   asymptomatic human immunodeficiency virus [HIV] infection
                            status (Z21)
                            human immunodeficiency virus [HIV] disease (B20)
     TIP: Do not assign for patients previously diagnosed with an HIV-related illness; assign code B20 instead.

✓4ᵗʰ **R76 Other abnormal immunological findings in serum**

   R76.0 Raised antibody titer
       EXCLUDES 1   isoimmunization in pregnancy (O36.0-O36.1)
                              isoimmunization affecting newborn (P55.-)

✓5ᵗʰ **R76.1 Nonspecific reaction to test for tuberculosis**

     R76.11 Nonspecific reaction to tuberculin skin test without active tuberculosis
         Abnormal result of Mantoux test
         PPD positive
         Tuberculin (skin test) positive
         Tuberculin (skin test) reactor
         EXCLUDES 1   nonspecific reaction to cell mediated immunity measurement of gamma interferon antigen response without active tuberculosis (R76.12)

     R76.12 Nonspecific reaction to cell mediated immunity measurement of gamma interferon antigen response without active tuberculosis
         Nonspecific reaction to QuantiFERON-TB test (QFT) without active tuberculosis
         EXCLUDES 1   nonspecific reaction to tuberculin skin test without active tuberculosis (R76.11)
                            positive tuberculin skin test (R76.11)

   R76.8 Other specified abnormal immunological findings in serum
       Raised level of immunoglobulins NOS

   R76.9 Abnormal immunological finding in serum, unspecified ▽

✓4ᵗʰ **R77 Other abnormalities of plasma proteins**

     EXCLUDES 1   disorders of plasma-protein metabolism ▶(E88.0-)◀

   R77.0 Abnormality of albumin

   R77.1 Abnormality of globulin
       Hyperglobulinemia NOS

   R77.2 Abnormality of alphafetoprotein

   R77.8 Other specified abnormalities of plasma proteins

   R77.9 Abnormality of plasma protein, unspecified ▽

✓4ᵗʰ **R78 Findings of drugs and other substances, not normally found in blood**
     Use additional code to identify the any retained foreign body, if applicable (Z18.-)
     EXCLUDES 1   mental or behavioral disorders due to psychoactive substance use (F10-F19)

   R78.0 Finding of alcohol in blood
       Use additional external cause code (Y90.-), for detail regarding alcohol level

   R78.1 Finding of opiate drug in blood

   R78.2 Finding of cocaine in blood

   R78.3 Finding of hallucinogen in blood

   R78.4 Finding of other drugs of addictive potential in blood

   R78.5 Finding of other psychotropic drug in blood

   R78.6 Finding of steroid agent in blood

   ✓5ᵗʰ **R78.7 Finding of abnormal level of heavy metals in blood**

     R78.71 Abnormal lead level in blood
         EXCLUDES 1   lead poisoning (T56.0-)

     R78.79 Finding of abnormal level of heavy metals in blood

   ✓5ᵗʰ **R78.8 Finding of other specified substances, not normally found in blood**

     R78.81 Bacteremia
         EXCLUDES 1   sepsis — code to specified infection
         DEF: Laboratory finding of bacteria in the blood in the absence of two or more signs of sepsis. Transient in nature, it can progress to septicemia with a severe infectious process.

     R78.89 Finding of other specified substances, not normally found in blood
         Finding of abnormal level of lithium in blood

   R78.9 Finding of unspecified substance, not normally found in blood ▽

✓4ᵗʰ **R79　Other abnormal findings of blood chemistry**

Use additional code to identify any retained foreign body, if applicable (Z18.-)

> EXCLUDES 1　asymptomatic hyperuricemia (E79.0)
> hyperglycemia NOS (R73.9)
> hypoglycemia NOS (E16.2)
> neonatal hypoglycemia (P70.3-P70.4)
> specific findings indicating disorder of amino-acid metabolism (E70-E72)
> specific findings indicating disorder of carbohydrate metabolism (E73-E74)
> specific findings indicating disorder of lipid metabolism (E75.-)

R79.0　Abnormal level of blood mineral

Abnormal blood level of cobalt
Abnormal blood level of copper
Abnormal blood level of iron
Abnormal blood level of magnesium
Abnormal blood level of mineral NEC
Abnormal blood level of zinc

> EXCLUDES 1　abnormal level of lithium (R78.89)
> disorders of mineral metabolism (E83.-)
> neonatal hypomagnesemia (P71.2)
> nutritional mineral deficiency (E58-E61)

R79.1　Abnormal coagulation profile

Abnormal or prolonged bleeding time
Abnormal or prolonged coagulation time
Abnormal or prolonged partial thromboplastin time [PTT]
Abnormal or prolonged prothrombin time [PT]

> EXCLUDES 1　coagulation defects (D68.-)
> EXCLUDES 2　abnormality of fluid, electrolyte or acid-base balance (E86-E87)

✓5ᵗʰ **R79.8　Other specified abnormal findings of blood chemistry**

R79.81　Abnormal blood-gas level

R79.82　Elevated C-reactive protein [CRP]

R79.89　Other specified abnormal findings of blood chemistry

> TIP: Assign for positive Coombs test when not further clarified in the documentation.

R79.9　Abnormal finding of blood chemistry, unspecified　▽

Abnormal findings on examination of urine, without diagnosis (R80-R82)

> EXCLUDES 1　abnormal findings on antenatal screening of mother (O28.-)
> diagnostic abnormal findings classified elsewhere - see Alphabetical Index
> specific findings indicating disorder of amino-acid metabolism (E70-E72)
> specific findings indicating disorder of carbohydrate metabolism (E73-E74)

✓4ᵗʰ **R80　Proteinuria**

> EXCLUDES 1　gestational proteinuria (O12.1-)

R80.0　Isolated proteinuria

Idiopathic proteinuria

> EXCLUDES 1　isolated proteinuria with specific morphological lesion (N06.-)

R80.1　Persistent proteinuria, unspecified　▽

R80.2　Orthostatic proteinuria, unspecified　▽
Postural proteinuria

R80.3　Bence Jones proteinuria

R80.8　Other proteinuria

R80.9　Proteinuria, unspecified　▽
Albuminuria NOS

R81　Glycosuria

> EXCLUDES 1　renal glycosuria (E74.8)

✓4ᵗʰ **R82　Other and unspecified abnormal findings in urine**

> INCLUDES　chromoabnormalities in urine

Use additional code to identify any retained foreign body, if applicable (Z18.-)

> EXCLUDES 2　hematuria (R31.-)

R82.0　Chyluria

> EXCLUDES 1　filarial chyluria (B74.-)

R82.1　Myoglobinuria

R82.2　Biliuria

R82.3　Hemoglobinuria

> EXCLUDES 1　hemoglobinuria due to hemolysis from external causes NEC (D59.6)
> hemoglobinuria due to paroxysmal nocturnal [Marchiafava-Micheli] (D59.5)

DEF: Free hemoglobin in blood due to rapid hemolysis of red blood cells. Causes include burns, crushed injury, sickle cell anemia, thalassemia, parasitic infections, or kidney infections.

R82.4　Acetonuria

Ketonuria

DEF: Excessive excretion of acetone in urine that commonly occurs in diabetic acidosis.

R82.5　Elevated urine levels of drugs, medicaments and biological substances

Elevated urine levels of catecholamines
Elevated urine levels of indoleacetic acid
Elevated urine levels of 17-ketosteroids
Elevated urine levels of steroids

R82.6　Abnormal urine levels of substances chiefly nonmedicinal as to source

Abnormal urine level of heavy metals

✓5ᵗʰ **R82.7　Abnormal findings on microbiological examination of urine**

> EXCLUDES 1　colonization status (Z22.-)

AHA: 2016,4Q,65

R82.71　Bacteriuria

R82.79　Other abnormal findings on microbiological examination of urine
Positive culture findings of urine

R82.8　Abnormal findings on cytological and histological examination of urine

✓5ᵗʰ **R82.9　Other and unspecified abnormal findings in urine**

R82.90　Unspecified abnormal findings in urine　▽

R82.91　Other chromoabnormalities of urine
Chromoconversion (dipstick)
Idiopathic dipstick converts positive for blood with no cellular forms in sediment

> EXCLUDES 1　hemoglobinuria (R82.3)
> myoglobinuria (R82.1)

✓6ᵗʰ **R82.99　Other abnormal findings in urine**

~~Cells and casts in urine~~
~~Crystalluria~~
~~Melanuria~~

R82.991　Hypocitraturia

R82.992　Hyperoxaluria

> EXCLUDES 1　primary hyperoxaluria (E72.53)

R82.993　Hyperuricoscuria

R82.994　Hypercalciuria
Idiopathic hypercalciuria

R82.998　Other abnormal findings in urine
Cells and casts in urine
Crystalluria
Melanuria

Abnormal findings on examination of other body fluids, substances and tissues, without diagnosis (R83-R89)

EXCLUDES 1   *abnormal findings on antenatal screening of mother (O28.-)*
       diagnostic abnormal findings classified elsewhere - see Alphabetical Index

EXCLUDES 2   *abnormal findings on examination of blood, without diagnosis (R70-R79)*
       abnormal findings on examination of urine, without diagnosis (R80-R82)
       abnormal tumor markers (R97.-)

✓4ᵗʰ **R83 Abnormal findings in cerebrospinal fluid**

Cerebrospinal Fluid

Ventricles

Cerebrospinal fluid

Spinal cord

R83.0 Abnormal level of enzymes in cerebrospinal fluid
R83.1 Abnormal level of hormones in cerebrospinal fluid
R83.2 Abnormal level of other drugs, medicaments and biological substances in cerebrospinal fluid
R83.3 Abnormal level of substances chiefly nonmedicinal as to source in cerebrospinal fluid
R83.4 Abnormal immunological findings in cerebrospinal fluid
R83.5 Abnormal microbiological findings in cerebrospinal fluid
     Positive culture findings in cerebrospinal fluid
     EXCLUDES 1   *colonization status (Z22.-)*
R83.6 Abnormal cytological findings in cerebrospinal fluid
R83.8 Other abnormal findings in cerebrospinal fluid
     Abnormal chromosomal findings in cerebrospinal fluid
R83.9 Unspecified abnormal finding in cerebrospinal fluid   ▽

✓4ᵗʰ **R84 Abnormal findings in specimens from respiratory organs and thorax**
     INCLUDES   abnormal findings in bronchial washings
         abnormal findings in nasal secretions
         abnormal findings in pleural fluid
         abnormal findings in sputum
         abnormal findings in throat scrapings
     EXCLUDES 1   *blood-stained sputum (R04.2)*
R84.0 Abnormal level of enzymes in specimens from respiratory organs and thorax
R84.1 Abnormal level of hormones in specimens from respiratory organs and thorax
R84.2 Abnormal level of other drugs, medicaments and biological substances in specimens from respiratory organs and thorax
R84.3 Abnormal level of substances chiefly nonmedicinal as to source in specimens from respiratory organs and thorax
R84.4 Abnormal immunological findings in specimens from respiratory organs and thorax

R84.5 Abnormal microbiological findings in specimens from respiratory organs and thorax
     Positive culture findings in specimens from respiratory organs and thorax
     EXCLUDES 1   *colonization status (Z22.-)*
R84.6 Abnormal cytological findings in specimens from respiratory organs and thorax
R84.7 Abnormal histological findings in specimens from respiratory organs and thorax
R84.8 Other abnormal findings in specimens from respiratory organs and thorax
     Abnormal chromosomal findings in specimens from respiratory organs and thorax
R84.9 Unspecified abnormal finding in specimens from respiratory organs and thorax   ▽

✓4ᵗʰ **R85 Abnormal findings in specimens from digestive organs and abdominal cavity**
     INCLUDES   abnormal findings in peritoneal fluid
         abnormal findings in saliva
     EXCLUDES 1   *cloudy peritoneal dialysis effluent (R88.0)*
         fecal abnormalities (R19.5)
R85.0 Abnormal level of enzymes in specimens from digestive organs and abdominal cavity
R85.1 Abnormal level of hormones in specimens from digestive organs and abdominal cavity
R85.2 Abnormal level of other drugs, medicaments and biological substances in specimens from digestive organs and abdominal cavity
R85.3 Abnormal level of substances chiefly nonmedicinal as to source in specimens from digestive organs and abdominal cavity
R85.4 Abnormal immunological findings in specimens from digestive organs and abdominal cavity
R85.5 Abnormal microbiological findings in specimens from digestive organs and abdominal cavity
     Positive culture findings in specimens from digestive organs and abdominal cavity
     EXCLUDES 1   *colonization status (Z22.-)*
✓5ᵗʰ **R85.6 Abnormal cytological findings in specimens from digestive organs and abdominal cavity**
   ✓6ᵗʰ **R85.61 Abnormal cytologic smear of anus**
       EXCLUDES 1   *abnormal cytological findings in specimens from other digestive organs and abdominal cavity (R85.69)*
           anal intraepithelial neoplasia I [AIN I] (K62.82)
           anal intraepithelial neoplasia II [AIN II] (K62.82)
           anal intraepithelial neoplasia III [AIN III] (D01.3)
           carcinoma in situ of anus (histologically confirmed) (D01.3)
           dysplasia (mild) (moderate) of anus (histologically confirmed) (K62.82)
           severe dysplasia of anus (histologically confirmed) (D01.3)
       EXCLUDES 2   *anal high risk human papillomavirus (HPV) DNA test positive (R85.81)*
           anal low risk human papillomavirus (HPV) DNA test positive (R85.82)
      R85.610 Atypical squamous cells of undetermined significance on cytologic smear of anus [ASC-US]
      R85.611 Atypical squamous cells cannot exclude high grade squamous intraepithelial lesion on cytologic smear of anus [ASC-H]
      R85.612 Low grade squamous intraepithelial lesion on cytologic smear of anus [LGSIL]
      R85.613 High grade squamous intraepithelial lesion on cytologic smear of anus [HGSIL]
      R85.614 Cytologic evidence of malignancy on smear of anus
      R85.615 Unsatisfactory cytologic smear of anus
         Inadequate sample of cytologic smear of anus
      R85.616 Satisfactory anal smear but lacking transformation zone
      R85.618 Other abnormal cytological findings on specimens from anus

Chapter 18. Symptoms, Signs and Abnormal Clinical and Laboratory Findings

R85.619   **Unspecified abnormal cytological findings in specimens from anus** ▽
    Abnormal anal cytology NOS
    Atypical glandular cells of anus NOS

R85.69   **Abnormal cytological findings in specimens from other digestive organs and abdominal cavity**

R85.7   **Abnormal histological findings in specimens from digestive organs and abdominal cavity**

√5ᵗʰ   R85.8   **Other abnormal findings in specimens from digestive organs and abdominal cavity**

R85.81   **Anal high risk human papillomavirus [HPV] DNA test positive**
    EXCLUDES 1   *anogenital warts due to human papillomavirus (HPV) (A63.0)*
        condyloma acuminatum (A63.0)

R85.82   **Anal low risk human papillomavirus [HPV] DNA test positive**
    Use additional code for associated human papillomavirus (B97.7)

R85.89   **Other abnormal findings in specimens from digestive organs and abdominal cavity**
    Abnormal chromosomal findings in specimens from digestive organs and abdominal cavity

R85.9   **Unspecified abnormal finding in specimens from digestive organs and abdominal cavity** ▽

√4ᵗʰ   **R86   Abnormal findings in specimens from male genital organs**
    INCLUDES   abnormal findings in prostatic secretions
         abnormal findings in semen, seminal fluid
         abnormal spermatozoa
    EXCLUDES 1   *azoospermia (N46.0-)*
         oligospermia (N46.1-)

R86.0   **Abnormal level of enzymes in specimens from male genital organs** ♂

R86.1   **Abnormal level of hormones in specimens from male genital organs** ♂

R86.2   **Abnormal level of other drugs, medicaments and biological substances in specimens from male genital organs** ♂

R86.3   **Abnormal level of substances chiefly nonmedicinal as to source in specimens from male genital organs** ♂

R86.4   **Abnormal immunological findings in specimens from male genital organs** ♂

R86.5   **Abnormal microbiological findings in specimens from male genital organs** ♂
    Positive culture findings in specimens from male genital organs
    EXCLUDES 1   *colonization status (Z22.-)*

R86.6   **Abnormal cytological findings in specimens from male genital organs** ♂

R86.7   **Abnormal histological findings in specimens from male genital organs** ♂

R86.8   **Other abnormal findings in specimens from male genital organs** ♂
    Abnormal chromosomal findings in specimens from male genital organs

R86.9   **Unspecified abnormal finding in specimens from male genital organs** ♂ ▽

√4ᵗʰ   **R87   Abnormal findings in specimens from female genital organs**
    INCLUDES   abnormal findings in secretion and smears from cervix uteri
         abnormal findings in secretion and smears from vagina
         abnormal findings in secretion and smears from vulva

R87.0   **Abnormal level of enzymes in specimens from female genital organs** ♀

R87.1   **Abnormal level of hormones in specimens from female genital organs** ♀

R87.2   **Abnormal level of other drugs, medicaments and biological substances in specimens from female genital organs** ♀

R87.3   **Abnormal level of substances chiefly nonmedicinal as to source in specimens from female genital organs** ♀

R87.4   **Abnormal immunological findings in specimens from female genital organs** ♀

R87.5   **Abnormal microbiological findings in specimens from female genital organs** ♀
    Positive culture findings in specimens from female genital organs
    EXCLUDES 1   *colonization status (Z22.-)*

√5ᵗʰ   R87.6   **Abnormal cytological findings in specimens from female genital organs**

√6ᵗʰ   R87.61   **Abnormal cytological findings in specimens from cervix uteri**
    EXCLUDES 1   *abnormal cytological findings in specimens from other female genital organs (R87.69)*
         abnormal cytological findings in specimens from vagina (R87.62-)
         carcinoma in situ of cervix uteri (histologically confirmed) (D06.-)
         cervical intraepithelial neoplasia I [CIN I] (N87.0)
         cervical intraepithelial neoplasia II [CIN II] (N87.1)
         cervical intraepithelial neoplasia III [CIN III] (D06.-)
         dysplasia (mild) (moderate) of cervix uteri (histologically confirmed) (N87.-)
         severe dysplasia of cervix uteri (histologically confirmed) (D06.-)
    EXCLUDES 2   *cervical high risk human papillomavirus (HPV) DNA test positive (R87.810)*
         cervical low risk human papillomavirus (HPV) DNA test positive (R87.820)

R87.610   **Atypical squamous cells of undetermined significance on cytologic smear of cervix [ASC-US]** ♀

R87.611   **Atypical squamous cells cannot exclude high grade squamous intraepithelial lesion on cytologic smear of cervix [ASC-H]** ♀

R87.612   **Low grade squamous intraepithelial lesion on cytologic smear of cervix [LGSIL]** ♀

R87.613   **High grade squamous intraepithelial lesion on cytologic smear of cervix [HGSIL]** ♀

R87.614   **Cytologic evidence of malignancy on smear of cervix** ♀

R87.615   **Unsatisfactory cytologic smear of cervix** ♀
    Inadequate sample of cytologic smear of cervix

R87.616   **Satisfactory cervical smear but lacking transformation zone** ♀

R87.618   **Other abnormal cytological findings on specimens from cervix uteri** ♀

R87.619   **Unspecified abnormal cytological findings in specimens from cervix uteri** ♀ ▽
    Abnormal cervical cytology NOS
    Abnormal Papanicolaou smear of cervix NOS
    Abnormal thin preparation smear of cervix NOS
    Atypical endocervical cells of cervix NOS
    Atypical endometrial cells of cervix NOS
    Atypical glandular cells of cervix NOS

√6ᵗʰ **R87.62** **Abnormal cytological findings in specimens from vagina**
Use additional code to identify acquired absence of uterus and cervix, if applicable (Z90.71-)

EXCLUDES 1   *abnormal cytological findings in specimens from cervix uteri (R87.61-)*
abnormal cytological findings in specimens from other female genital organs (R87.69)
carcinoma in situ of vagina (histologically confirmed) (D07.2)
dysplasia (mild) (moderate) of vagina (histologically confirmed) (N89.-)
severe dysplasia of vagina (histologically confirmed) (D07.2)
vaginal intraepithelial neoplasia I [VAIN I] (N89.0)
vaginal intraepithelial neoplasia II [VAIN II] (N89.1)
vaginal intraepithelial neoplasia III [VAIN III] (D07.2)

EXCLUDES 2   *vaginal high risk human papillomavirus (HPV) DNA test positive (R87.811)*
vaginal low risk human papillomavirus (HPV) DNA test positive (R87.821)

R87.620 **Atypical squamous cells of undetermined significance on cytologic smear of vagina [ASC-US]** ♀

R87.621 **Atypical squamous cells cannot exclude high grade squamous intraepithelial lesion on cytologic smear of vagina [ASC-H]** ♀

R87.622 **Low grade squamous intraepithelial lesion on cytologic smear of vagina [LGSIL]** ♀

R87.623 **High grade squamous intraepithelial lesion on cytologic smear of vagina [HGSIL]** ♀

R87.624 **Cytologic evidence of malignancy on smear of vagina** ♀

R87.625 **Unsatisfactory cytologic smear of vagina** ♀
Inadequate sample of cytologic smear of vagina

R87.628 **Other abnormal cytological findings on specimens from vagina** ♀

R87.629 **Unspecified abnormal cytological findings in specimens from vagina** ♀ ▽
Abnormal Papanicolaou smear of vagina NOS
Abnormal thin preparation smear of vagina NOS
Abnormal vaginal cytology NOS
Atypical endocervical cells of vagina NOS
Atypical endometrial cells of vagina NOS
Atypical glandular cells of vagina NOS

R87.69 **Abnormal cytological findings in specimens from other female genital organs** ♀
Abnormal cytological findings in specimens from female genital organs NOS

EXCLUDES 1   *dysplasia of vulva (histologically confirmed) (N90.0-N90.3)*

R87.7 **Abnormal histological findings in specimens from female genital organs** ♀

EXCLUDES 1   *carcinoma in situ (histologically confirmed) of female genital organs (D06-D07.3)*
cervical intraepithelial neoplasia I [CIN I] (N87.0)
cervical intraepithelial neoplasia II [CIN II] (N87.1)
cervical intraepithelial neoplasia III [CIN III] (D06.-)
dysplasia (mild) (moderate) of cervix uteri (histologically confirmed) (N87.-)
dysplasia (mild) (moderate) of vagina (histologically confirmed) (N89.-)
severe dysplasia of cervix uteri (histologically confirmed) (D06.-)
severe dysplasia of vagina (histologically confirmed) (D07.2)
vaginal intraepithelial neoplasia I [VAIN I] (N89.0)
vaginal intraepithelial neoplasia II [VAIN II] (N89.1)
vaginal intraepithelial neoplasia III [VAIN III] (D07.2)

√5ᵗʰ **R87.8** **Other abnormal findings in specimens from female genital organs**

√6ᵗʰ **R87.81** **High risk human papillomavirus [HPV] DNA test positive from female genital organs**
EXCLUDES 1   *anogenital warts due to human papillomavirus (HPV) (A63.0)*
condyloma acuminatum (A63.0)

R87.810 **Cervical high risk human papillomavirus [HPV] DNA test positive** ♀

R87.811 **Vaginal high risk human papillomavirus [HPV] DNA test positive** ♀

√6ᵗʰ **R87.82** **Low risk human papillomavirus [HPV] DNA test positive from female genital organs**
Use additional code for associated human papillomavirus (B97.7)

R87.820 **Cervical low risk human papillomavirus [HPV] DNA test positive** ♀

R87.821 **Vaginal low risk human papillomavirus [HPV] DNA test positive** ♀

R87.89 **Other abnormal findings in specimens from female genital organs** ♀
Abnormal chromosomal findings in specimens from female genital organs

R87.9 **Unspecified abnormal finding in specimens from female genital organs** ♀ ▽

√4ᵗʰ **R88** **Abnormal findings in other body fluids and substances**

R88.0 **Cloudy (hemodialysis) (peritoneal) dialysis effluent**

R88.8 **Abnormal findings in other body fluids and substances**

√4ᵗʰ **R89** **Abnormal findings in specimens from other organs, systems and tissues**
INCLUDES   abnormal findings in nipple discharge
abnormal findings in synovial fluid
abnormal findings in wound secretions

R89.0 **Abnormal level of enzymes in specimens from other organs, systems and tissues**

R89.1 **Abnormal level of hormones in specimens from other organs, systems and tissues**

R89.2 **Abnormal level of other drugs, medicaments and biological substances in specimens from other organs, systems and tissues**

R89.3 **Abnormal level of substances chiefly nonmedicinal as to source in specimens from other organs, systems and tissues**

R89.4 **Abnormal immunological findings in specimens from other organs, systems and tissues**

R89.5 **Abnormal microbiological findings in specimens from other organs, systems and tissues**
Positive culture findings in specimens from other organs, systems and tissues
EXCLUDES 1   *colonization status (Z22.-)*

R89.6 **Abnormal cytological findings in specimens from other organs, systems and tissues**

R89.7 **Abnormal histological findings in specimens from other organs, systems and tissues**

☑ Additional Character Req   x7ᵗʰ Placeholder Alert   Manifestation   ▽ Unspecified   ►◄ Revised Text   ● New Code   ▲ Revised Code Title

Chapter 18. Symptoms, Signs and Abnormal Clinical and Laboratory Findings

R89.8   **Other abnormal findings in specimens from other organs, systems and tissues**
     Abnormal chromosomal findings in specimens from other organs, systems and tissues

R89.9   **Unspecified abnormal finding in specimens from**   ▽
     other organs, systems and tissues

Abnormal findings on diagnostic imaging and in function studies, without diagnosis (R90-R94)

INCLUDES   nonspecific abnormal findings on diagnostic imaging by computerized axial tomography [CAT scan]
     nonspecific abnormal findings on diagnostic imaging by magnetic resonance imaging [MRI][NMR]
     nonspecific abnormal findings on diagnostic imaging by positron emission tomography [PET scan]
     nonspecific abnormal findings on diagnostic imaging by thermography
     nonspecific abnormal findings on diagnostic imaging by ultrasound [echogram]
     nonspecific abnormal findings on diagnostic imaging by X-ray examination

EXCLUDES 1   abnormal findings on antenatal screening of mother (O28.-)
     diagnostic abnormal findings classified elsewhere - see Alphabetical Index

✓4ᵗʰ **R90**   **Abnormal findings on diagnostic imaging of central nervous system**

R90.0   **Intracranial space-occupying lesion found on diagnostic imaging of central nervous system**

✓5ᵗʰ **R90.8**   **Other abnormal findings on diagnostic imaging of central nervous system**

     R90.81   Abnormal echoencephalogram
     R90.82   White matter disease, unspecified   ▽
     R90.89   **Other abnormal findings on diagnostic imaging of central nervous system**
         Other cerebrovascular abnormality found on diagnostic imaging of central nervous system

✓4ᵗʰ **R91**   **Abnormal findings on diagnostic imaging of lung**

R91.1   **Solitary pulmonary nodule**
     Coin lesion lung
     Solitary pulmonary nodule, subsegmental branch of the bronchial tree

R91.8   **Other nonspecific abnormal finding of lung field**
     Lung mass NOS found on diagnostic imaging of lung
     Pulmonary infiltrate NOS
     Shadow, lung

✓4ᵗʰ **R92**   **Abnormal and inconclusive findings on diagnostic imaging of breast**

R92.0   **Mammographic microcalcification found on diagnostic imaging of breast**
     EXCLUDES 2   mammographic calcification (calculus) found on diagnostic imaging of breast (R92.1)
     DEF: Calcium and cellular debris deposits in the breast that cannot be felt but can be detected on a mammogram. The deposits can be a sign of cancer, benign conditions, or changes in the breast tissue as a result of inflammation, injury, or an obstructed duct.

R92.1   **Mammographic calcification found on diagnostic imaging of breast**
     Mammographic calculus found on diagnostic imaging of breast

R92.2   **Inconclusive mammogram**
     Dense breasts NOS
     Inconclusive mammogram NEC
     Inconclusive mammography due to dense breasts
     Inconclusive mammography NEC
     AHA: 2015,1Q,24

R92.8   **Other abnormal and inconclusive findings on diagnostic imaging of breast**

✓4ᵗʰ **R93**   **Abnormal findings on diagnostic imaging of other body structures**

R93.0   **Abnormal findings on diagnostic imaging of skull and head, not elsewhere classified**
     EXCLUDES 1   intracranial space-occupying lesion found on diagnostic imaging (R90.0)

R93.1   **Abnormal findings on diagnostic imaging of heart and coronary circulation**
     Abnormal echocardiogram NOS
     Abnormal heart shadow

R93.2   **Abnormal findings on diagnostic imaging of liver and biliary tract**
     Nonvisualization of gallbladder

R93.3   **Abnormal findings on diagnostic imaging of other parts of digestive tract**

✓5ᵗʰ **R93.4**   **Abnormal findings on diagnostic imaging of urinary organs**
     EXCLUDES 2   hypertrophy of kidney (N28.81)
     AHA: 2016,4Q,66

     R93.41   **Abnormal radiologic findings on diagnostic imaging of renal pelvis, ureter, or bladder**
         Filling defect of bladder found on diagnostic imaging
         Filling defect of renal pelvis found on diagnostic imaging
         Filling defect of ureter found on diagnostic imaging

✓6ᵗʰ   **R93.42**   **Abnormal radiologic findings on diagnostic imaging of kidney**
         R93.421   **Abnormal radiologic findings on diagnostic imaging of right kidney**
         R93.422   **Abnormal radiologic findings on diagnostic imaging of left kidney**
         R93.429   **Abnormal radiologic findings on**   ▽
            diagnostic imaging of unspecified kidney

     R93.49   **Abnormal radiologic findings on diagnostic imaging of other urinary organs**

R93.5   **Abnormal findings on diagnostic imaging of other abdominal regions, including retroperitoneum**

R93.6   **Abnormal findings on diagnostic imaging of limbs**
     EXCLUDES 2   abnormal finding in skin and subcutaneous tissue ▶(R93.8-)◀

R93.7   **Abnormal findings on diagnostic imaging of other parts of musculoskeletal system**
     EXCLUDES 2   abnormal findings on diagnostic imaging of skull (R93.0)

✓5ᵗʰ **R93.8**   **Abnormal findings on diagnostic imaging of other specified body structures**
     ~~Abnormal finding by radioisotope localization of placenta~~
     ~~Abnormal radiological finding in skin and subcutaneous tissue~~
     ~~Mediastinal shift~~

●   ✓6ᵗʰ   **R93.81**   **Abnormal radiologic findings on diagnostic imaging of testis**
●   **R93.811**   **Abnormal radiologic findings on diagnostic imaging of right testicle**
●   **R93.812**   **Abnormal radiologic findings on diagnostic imaging of left testicle**
         R93.813   **Abnormal radiologic findings on diagnostic imaging of testicles, bilateral**
●   **R93.819**   **Abnormal radiologic findings on**   ▽
            diagnostic imaging of unspecified testicle

●   **R93.89**   **Abnormal findings on diagnostic imaging of other specified body structures**
         Abnormal finding by radioisotope localization of placenta
         Abnormal radiological finding in skin and subcutaneous tissue
         Mediastinal shift

R93.9   **Diagnostic imaging inconclusive due to excess body fat of patient**

✓4ᵗʰ **R94**   **Abnormal results of function studies**
     INCLUDES   abnormal results of radionuclide [radioisotope] uptake studies
         abnormal results of scintigraphy

✓5ᵗʰ **R94.0**   **Abnormal results of function studies of central nervous system**
     R94.01   **Abnormal electroencephalogram [EEG]**
     R94.02   **Abnormal brain scan**
     R94.09   **Abnormal results of other function studies of central nervous system**

✓5ᵗʰ **R94.1**   **Abnormal results of function studies of peripheral nervous system and special senses**
     ✓6ᵗʰ   **R94.11**   **Abnormal results of function studies of eye**
         R94.110   **Abnormal electro-oculogram [EOG]**
         R94.111   **Abnormal electroretinogram [ERG]**
            Abnormal retinal function study
         R94.112   **Abnormal visually evoked potential [VEP]**
         R94.113   **Abnormal oculomotor study**
         R94.118   **Abnormal results of other function studies of eye**

√6ᵗʰ **R94.12 Abnormal results of function studies of ear and other special senses**
     AHA: 2016,3Q,17
     R94.120 Abnormal auditory function study
     R94.121 Abnormal vestibular function study
     R94.128 Abnormal results of other function studies of ear and other special senses

√6ᵗʰ **R94.13 Abnormal results of function studies of peripheral nervous system**
     R94.130 Abnormal response to nerve stimulation, unspecified ▽
     R94.131 Abnormal electromyogram [EMG]
         EXCLUDES 1   *electromyogram of eye (R94.113)*
     R94.138 Abnormal results of other function studies of peripheral nervous system

R94.2 Abnormal results of pulmonary function studies
     Reduced ventilatory capacity
     Reduced vital capacity

√5ᵗʰ **R94.3 Abnormal results of cardiovascular function studies**
     R94.30 Abnormal result of cardiovascular function study, unspecified ▽
     R94.31 Abnormal electrocardiogram [ECG] [EKG]
         EXCLUDES 1   *long QT syndrome (I45.81)*
     R94.39 Abnormal result of other cardiovascular function study
         Abnormal electrophysiological intracardiac studies
         Abnormal phonocardiogram
         Abnormal vectorcardiogram

R94.4 Abnormal results of kidney function studies
     Abnormal renal function test

R94.5 Abnormal results of liver function studies

R94.6 Abnormal results of thyroid function studies

R94.7 Abnormal results of other endocrine function studies
     EXCLUDES 2   *abnormal glucose (R73.0-)*

R94.8 Abnormal results of function studies of other organs and systems
     Abnormal basal metabolic rate [BMR]
     Abnormal bladder function test
     Abnormal splenic function test

Abnormal tumor markers (R97)

√4ᵗʰ **R97 Abnormal tumor markers**
     Elevated tumor associated antigens [TAA]
     Elevated tumor specific antigens [TSA]

R97.0 Elevated carcinoembryonic antigen [CEA]

R97.1 Elevated cancer antigen 125 [CA 125]

√5ᵗʰ **R97.2 Elevated prostate specific antigen [PSA]**
     AHA: 2016,4Q,66
     R97.20 Elevated prostate specific antigen [PSA] A ♂
     R97.21 Rising PSA following treatment for malignant neoplasm of prostate A ♂

R97.8 Other abnormal tumor markers

Ill-defined and unknown cause of mortality (R99)

R99 Ill-defined and unknown cause of mortality ▽
     Death (unexplained) NOS
     Unspecified cause of mortality

Chapter 19. Injury, Poisoning, and Certain Other Consequences of External Causes (SØØ–T88)

Chapter Specific Guidelines with Coding Examples

The chapter specific guidelines from the ICD-10-CM Official Guidelines for Coding and Reporting have been provided below. Along with these guidelines are coding examples, contained in the shaded boxes, that have been developed to help illustrate the coding and/or sequencing guidance found in these guidelines.

a. Application of 7th characters in Chapter 19

Most categories in chapter 19 have a 7th character requirement for each applicable code. Most categories in this chapter have three 7th character values (with the exception of fractures): A, initial encounter, D, subsequent encounter and S, sequela. Categories for traumatic fractures have additional 7th character values. While the patient may be seen by a new or different provider over the course of treatment for an injury, assignment of the 7th character is based on whether the patient is undergoing active treatment and not whether the provider is seeing the patient for the first time.

For complication codes, active treatment refers to treatment for the condition described by the code, even though it may be related to an earlier precipitating problem. For example, code T84.50XA, Infection and inflammatory reaction due to unspecified internal joint prosthesis, initial encounter, is used when active treatment is provided for the infection, even though the condition relates to the prosthetic device, implant or graft that was placed at a previous encounter.

7th character "A", initial encounter is used for each encounter where the patient is receiving active treatment for the condition.

> Patient evaluated after fall from a skateboard onto the sidewalk, x-rays identify a nondisplaced fracture to the distal pole of the right scaphoid bone. The patient is placed in a cast.
>
> **S62.Ø14A**   **Nondisplaced fracture of distal pole of navicular [scaphoid] bone of right wrist, initial encounter for closed fracture**
>
> **VØØ.131A**   **Fall from skateboard, initial encounter**
>
> **Y93.51**   **Activity, roller skating (inline) and skateboarding**
>
> **Y92.48Ø**   **Sidewalk as the place of occurrence of the external cause**
>
> **Y99.8**   **Other external cause status**
>
> *Explanation:* This fracture would be coded with a seventh character A for initial encounter because the patient received x-rays to identify the site of the fracture and treatment was rendered; this would be considered active treatment.

7th character "D" subsequent encounter is used for encounters after the patient has completed active treatment of the condition and is receiving routine care for the condition during the healing or recovery phase.

> Patient seen in follow-up after fall from a skateboard onto the sidewalk resulted in casting of the right arm. X-rays are taken to evaluate how well the nondisplaced fracture to the distal pole of the right scaphoid bone is healing. The physician feels the fracture is healing appropriately; no adjustments to the cast are made.
>
> **S62.Ø14D**   **Nondisplaced fracture of distal pole of navicular [scaphoid] bone of right wrist, subsequent encounter for fracture with routine healing**
>
> **VØØ.131D**   **Fall from skateboard, subsequent encounter**
>
> *Explanation:* This fracture would be coded with a seventh character D for subsequent encounter, whether the same physician who provided the initial cast application or a different physician is now seeing the patient. Although the patient received x-rays, the intent of the x-rays was to assess how the fracture was healing. There was no active treatment rendered and the visit is therefore considered a subsequent encounter.

The aftercare Z codes should not be used for aftercare for conditions such as injuries or poisonings, where 7th characters are provided to identify subsequent care. For example, for aftercare of an injury, assign the acute injury code with the 7th character "D" (subsequent encounter).

7th character "S", sequela, is for use for complications or conditions that arise as a direct result of a condition, such as scar formation after a burn.

The scars are sequelae of the burn. When using 7th character "S", it is necessary to use both the injury code that precipitated the sequela and the code for the sequela itself. The "S" is added only to the injury code, not the sequela code. The 7th character "S" identifies the injury responsible for the sequela. The specific type of sequela (e.g. scar) is sequenced first, followed by the injury code.
See Section I.B.1Ø Sequelae, (Late Effects)

> Patient with a history of a nondisplaced fracture to the distal pole of the right scaphoid bone due to a fall from a skateboard is seen for evaluation of arthritis to the right wrist that has developed as a consequence of the traumatic fracture.
>
> **M12.531**   **Traumatic arthropathy, right wrist**
>
> **S62.Ø14S**   **Nondisplaced fracture of distal pole of navicular [scaphoid] bone of right wrist, sequela**
>
> **VØØ.131S**   **Fall from skateboard, sequela**
>
> *Explanation:* The code identifying the specific sequela condition (traumatic arthritis) should be coded first followed by the injury that instigated the development of the sequela (fracture). The scaphoid fracture injury code is given a 7th character S for sequela to represent its role as the inciting injury. The fracture has healed and is not being managed or treated on this admit and therefore is not applicable as a first listed or principal diagnosis. However, it is directly related to the development of the arthritis and should be appended as a secondary code to signify this cause and effect relationship.

b. Coding of injuries

When coding injuries, assign separate codes for each injury unless a combination code is provided, in which case the combination code is assigned. **Codes from category** TØ7, Unspecified multiple injuries should not be assigned in the inpatient setting unless information for a more specific code is not available. Traumatic injury codes (SØØ-T14.9) are not to be used for normal, healing surgical wounds or to identify complications of surgical wounds.

> 11-year-old girl fell from her horse, resulting in a laceration to her right forearm with several large pieces of wooden fragments embedded in the wound as well as abrasions to her right ear; in addition, her right shoulder was dislocated
>
> **S43.ØØ4A**   **Unspecified dislocation of right shoulder joint, initial encounter**
>
> **S51.821A**   **Laceration with foreign body of right forearm, initial encounter**
>
> **SØØ.411A**   **Abrasion of right ear, initial encounter**
>
> **V8Ø.Ø1ØA**   **Animal-rider injured by fall from or being thrown from horse in noncollision accident, initial encounter**
>
> **Y93.52**   **Activity, horseback riding**
>
> *Explanation:* Each separate injury should be reported. The patient's injury to the forearm is reported with one combination code that captures both the laceration and the foreign body.

The code for the most serious injury, as determined by the provider and the focus of treatment, is sequenced first.

1) Superficial injuries

Superficial injuries such as abrasions or contusions are not coded when associated with more severe injuries of the same site.

2) Primary injury with damage to nerves/blood vessels

When a primary injury results in minor damage to peripheral nerves or blood vessels, the primary injury is sequenced first with additional code(s) for injuries to nerves and spinal cord (such as category SØ4), and/or injury to blood vessels (such as category S15). When the primary injury is to the blood vessels or nerves, that injury should be sequenced first.

c. Coding of traumatic fractures

The principles of multiple coding of injuries should be followed in coding fractures. Fractures of specified sites are coded individually by site in accordance with both the provisions within categories SØ2, S12, S22, S32, S42, S49, S52, S59, S62, S72, S79, S82, S89, S92 and the level of detail furnished by medical record content.

A fracture not indicated as open or closed should be coded to closed. A fracture not indicated whether displaced or not displaced should be coded to displaced.

More specific guidelines are as follows:

1) Initial vs. subsequent encounter for fractures

Traumatic fractures are coded using the appropriate 7th character for initial encounter (A, B, C) for each encounter where the patient is receiving active treatment for the fracture. The appropriate 7th character for initial encounter should also be assigned for a patient who delayed seeking treatment for the fracture or nonunion.

Fractures are coded using the appropriate 7th character for subsequent care for encounters after the patient has completed active treatment of the fracture and is receiving routine care for the fracture during the healing or recovery phase.

Care for complications of surgical treatment for fracture repairs during the healing or recovery phase should be coded with the appropriate complication codes.

Care of complications of fractures, such as malunion and nonunion, should be reported with the appropriate 7th character for subsequent care with nonunion (K, M, N,) or subsequent care with malunion (P, Q, R).

Malunion/nonunion: The appropriate 7th character for initial encounter should also be assigned for a patient who delayed seeking treatment for the fracture or nonunion.

Female patient fell during a forest hiking excursion almost six months ago and until recently did not feel she needed to seek medical attention for her left ankle pain; x-rays show nonunion of lateral malleolus and surgery has been scheduled

S82.62XA	Displaced fracture of lateral malleolus of left fibula, initial encounter for closed fracture
W01.0XXA	Fall on same level from slipping, tripping and stumbling without subsequent striking against object, initial encounter
Y92.821	Forest as place of occurrence of the external cause
Y93.01	Activity, walking, marching and hiking
Y99.8	Other external cause status

Explanation: A seventh character of A is used for the lateral malleolus nonunion fracture to signify that the fracture is receiving active treatment. The delayed care for the fracture has resulted in a nonunion, but capturing the nonunion in the seventh character is trumped by the provision of active care.

The open fracture designations in the assignment of the 7th character for fractures of the forearm, femur and lower leg, including ankle are based on the Gustilo open fracture classification. When the Gustilo classification type is not specified for an open fracture, the 7th character for open fracture type I or II should be assigned (B, E, H, M, Q).

A code from category M80, not a traumatic fracture code, should be used for any patient with known osteoporosis who suffers a fracture, even if the patient had a minor fall or trauma, if that fall or trauma would not usually break a normal, healthy bone.

See Section I.C.13. Osteoporosis.

The aftercare Z codes should not be used for aftercare for traumatic fractures. For aftercare of a traumatic fracture, assign the acute fracture code with the appropriate 7th character.

2) Multiple fractures sequencing

Multiple fractures are sequenced in accordance with the severity of the fracture.

d. Coding of burns and corrosions

The ICD-10-CM makes a distinction between burns and corrosions. The burn codes are for thermal burns, except sunburns, that come from a heat source, such as a fire or hot appliance. The burn codes are also for burns resulting from electricity and radiation. Corrosions are burns due to chemicals. The guidelines are the same for burns and corrosions.

Current burns (T20-T25) are classified by depth, extent and by agent (X code). Burns are classified by depth as first degree (erythema), second degree (blistering), and third degree (full-thickness involvement). Burns of the eye and internal organs (T26-T28) are classified by site, but not by degree.

1) Sequencing of burn and related condition codes

Sequence first the code that reflects the highest degree of burn when more than one burn is present.

---

a. When the reason for the admission or encounter is for treatment of external multiple burns, sequence first the code that reflects the burn of the highest degree.

b. When a patient has both internal and external burns, the circumstances of admission govern the selection of the principal diagnosis or first-listed diagnosis.

c. When a patient is admitted for burn injuries and other related conditions such as smoke inhalation and/or respiratory failure, the circumstances of admission govern the selection of the principal or first-listed diagnosis.

Patient referred for minor first-degree burns to multiple sites of her right and left hands as well as severe smoke inhalation. While she was sleeping at home, a candle on her dresser lit the bedroom curtains on fire.

T59.811A	Toxic effect of smoke, accidental (unintentional), initial encounter
J70.5	Respiratory conditions due to smoke inhalation
T23.191A	Burn of first degree of multiple sites of right wrist and hand, initial encounter
T23.192A	Burn of first degree of multiple sites of left wrist and hand, initial encounter
X08.8XXA	Exposure to other specified smoke, fire and flames, initial encounter
Y99.8	Other exteranl cause status
Y92.003	Bedroom of unspecified non-institutional (private) residence as the place of occurrence of the external cause
Y93.84	Activity, sleeping

Explanation: Based on the documentation, the inhalation injury is more severe than the first-degree burns and is sequenced first. The burns to the hands are appended as secondary diagnoses.

---

2) Burns of the same *anatomic* site

Classify burns of the same **anatomic** site **and on the same side** but of different degrees to the subcategory identifying the highest degree recorded in the diagnosis **(e.g., for second and third degree burns of right thigh, assign only code T24.311-).**

3) Non-healing burns

Non-healing burns are coded as acute burns.

Necrosis of burned skin should be coded as a non-healed burn.

4) Infected burn

For any documented infected burn site, use an additional code for the infection.

5) Assign separate codes for each burn site

When coding burns, assign separate codes for each burn site. Category T30, Burn and corrosion, body region unspecified is extremely vague and should rarely be used.

Codes for burns of "multiple sites" should only be assigned when the medical record documentation does not specify the individual sites.

Patient is treated for third-degree burns of the scalp as well as second-degree burns to the back of the right hand

| T20.35XA | Burn of third degree of scalp [any part], initial encounter |
| T23.261A | Burn of second degree of back of right hand, initial encounter |

Explanation: Two codes may be reported as the hand and face represent distinct burn sites.

---

6) Burns and corrosions classified according to extent of body surface involved

Assign codes from category T31, Burns classified according to extent of body surface involved, or T32, Corrosions classified according to extent of body surface involved, when the site of the burn is not specified or when there is a need for additional data. It is advisable to use category T31 as additional coding when needed to provide data for evaluating burn mortality, such as that needed by burn units. It is also advisable to use category T31 as an additional code for reporting purposes when there is mention of a third-degree burn involving 20 percent or more of the body surface.

Categories T31 and T32 are based on the classic "rule of nines" in estimating body surface involved: head and neck are assigned nine percent, each arm nine percent, each leg 18 percent, the anterior trunk 18 percent, posterior trunk 18 percent, and genitalia one percent. Providers may change these percentage assignments where necessary to accommodate infants and children who have proportionately larger heads than adults, and patients who have large buttocks, thighs, or abdomen that involve burns.

> Patient seen for dressing change after he accidentally spilled acetic acid on himself two days ago. The second-degree burns to his right thigh, covering about 3 percent of his body surface, are healing appropriately.
>
> | | |
> |---|---|
> | **T54.2X1D** | **Toxic effect of corrosive acids and acid-like substances, accidental (unintentional), subsequent encounter** |
> | **T24.611D** | **Corrosion of second degree of right thigh, subsequent encounter** |
> | **T32.0** | **Corrosions involving less than 10% of body surface** |
>
> *Explanation:* Code T32.0 provides additional information as to how much of the patient's body was affected by the corrosive substance.

7) Encounters for treatment of sequela of burns

Encounters for the treatment of the late effects of burns or corrosions (i.e., scars or joint contractures) should be coded with a burn or corrosion code with the 7th character "S" for sequela.

8) Sequelae with a late effect code and current burn

When appropriate, both a code for a current burn or corrosion with 7th character "A" or "D" and a burn or corrosion code with 7th character "S" may be assigned on the same record (when both a current burn and sequelae of an old burn exist). Burns and corrosions do not heal at the same rate and a current healing wound may still exist with sequela of a healed burn or corrosion.

See Section I.B.10 Sequela (Late Effects)

> Female patient seen for second-degree burn to the left ear; she also has significant scarring on her left elbow from a third-degree burn from childhood
>
> | | |
> |---|---|
> | **T20.212A** | **Burn of second degree of left ear [any part, except ear drum], initial encounter** |
> | **L90.5** | **Scar conditions and fibrosis of skin** |
> | **T22.322S** | **Burn of third degree of left elbow, sequela** |
>
> *Explanation:* The patient is being seen for management of a current second-degree burn, which is reflected in the code by appending the seventh character of A, indicating active treatment or management of this burn. The elbow scarring is a sequela of a previous third-degree burn. The sequela condition precedes the original burn injury, which is appended with a seventh character of S.

9) Use of an external cause code with burns and corrosions

An external cause code should be used with burns and corrosions to identify the source and intent of the burn, as well as the place where it occurred.

e. Adverse effects, poisoning, underdosing and toxic effects

Codes in categories T36-T65 are combination codes that include the substance that was taken as well as the intent. No additional external cause code is required for poisonings, toxic effects, adverse effects and underdosing codes.

1) Do not code directly from the Table of Drugs

Do not code directly from the Table of Drugs and Chemicals. Always refer back to the Tabular List.

2) Use as many codes as necessary to describe

Use as many codes as necessary to describe completely all drugs, medicinal or biological substances.

3) If the same code would describe the causative agent

If the same code would describe the causative agent for more than one adverse reaction, poisoning, toxic effect or underdosing, assign the code only once.

4) If two or more drugs, medicinal or biological substances

If two or more drugs, medicinal or biological substances are reported, code each individually unless a combination code is listed in the Table of Drugs and Chemicals.

5) The occurrence of drug toxicity is classified in ICD-10-CM as follows:

(a) Adverse effect

When coding an adverse effect of a drug that has been correctly prescribed and properly administered, assign the appropriate code for the nature of the adverse effect followed by the appropriate code for the adverse effect of the drug (T36-T50). The code for the drug should have a 5th or 6th character "5" (for example T36.0X5-) Examples of the nature of an adverse effect are tachycardia, delirium, gastrointestinal hemorrhaging, vomiting, hypokalemia, hepatitis, renal failure, or respiratory failure.

> Patient seen for stomach pain and jaundice, indicated by physician as possible side-effects of Inderal, recently started for hypertension. Inderal was discontinued and the patient switched to Atenolol instead.
>
> | | |
> |---|---|
> | **R10.9** | **Unspecified abdominal pain** |
> | **R17** | **Unspecified jaundice** |
> | **T44.7X5A** | **Adverse effect of beta-adrenoreceptor antagonists, initial encounter** |
> | **I10** | **Essential (primary) hypertension** |
>
> *Explanation:* The side-effects caused by the drug are listed first, followed by the code for the adverse effect of the drug to capture the specific drug that was used.

(b) Poisoning

When coding a poisoning or reaction to the improper use of a medication (e.g., overdose, wrong substance given or taken in error, wrong route of administration), first assign the appropriate code from categories T36-T50. The poisoning codes have an associated intent as their 5th or 6th character (accidental, intentional self-harm, assault and undetermined). If the intent of the poisoning is unknown or unspecified, code the intent as accidental intent. The undetermined intent is only for use if the documentation in the record specifies that the intent cannot be determined. Use additional code(s) for all manifestations of poisonings.

If there is also a diagnosis of abuse or dependence of the substance, the abuse or dependence is assigned as an additional code.

Examples of poisoning include:

   (i)   Error was made in drug prescription

        Errors made in drug prescription or in the administration of the drug by provider, nurse, patient, or other person.

   (ii   Overdose of a drug intentionally taken

        If an overdose of a drug was intentionally taken or administered and resulted in drug toxicity, it would be coded as a poisoning.

   (iii) Nonprescribed drug taken with correctly prescribed and properly administered drug

        If a nonprescribed drug or medicinal agent was taken in combination with a correctly prescribed and properly administered drug, any drug toxicity or other reaction resulting from the interaction of the two drugs would be classified as a poisoning.

   (iv) Interaction of drug(s) and alcohol

        When a reaction results from the interaction of a drug(s) and alcohol, this would be classified as poisoning.

        See Section I.C.4. if poisoning is the result of insulin pump malfunctions.

(c) Underdosing

Underdosing refers to taking less of a medication than is prescribed by a provider or a manufacturer's instruction. **Discontinuing the use of a prescribed medication on the patient's own initiative (not directed by the patient's provider) is also classified as an underdosing.** For underdosing, assign the code from categories T36-T50 (fifth or sixth character "6").

Codes for underdosing should never be assigned as principal or first-listed codes. If a patient has a relapse or exacerbation of the medical condition for which the drug is prescribed because of the reduction in dose, then the medical condition itself should be coded.

Noncompliance (Z91.12-, Z91.13- **and Z91.14-**) or complication of care (Y63.6-Y63.9) codes are to be used with an underdosing code to indicate intent, if known.

> Patient referred for atrial fibrillation with history of chronic atrial fibrillation for which she is prescribed amiodarone. Financial concerns have left the patient unable to pay for her prescriptions and she has been skipping her amiodarone dose every other day to offset the cost.
>
> **I48.2**   **Chronic atrial fibrillation**
>
> **T46.2X6A**   **Underdosing of other antidysrhythmic drugs, initial encounter**
>
> **Z91.120**   **Patient's intentional underdosing of medication regimen due to financial hardship**
>
> *Explanation:* By skipping her amiodarone pill every other day, the patient's atrial fibrillation returned. The condition for which the drug was being taken is reported first, followed by an underdosing code to show that the patient was not adhering to her prescription regiment. The Z code helps elaborate on the patient's social and/or economic circumstances that led to the patient taking less then what she was prescribed.

(d) Toxic effects

When a harmful substance is ingested or comes in contact with a person, this is classified as a toxic effect. The toxic effect codes are in categories T51-T65.

Toxic effect codes have an associated intent: accidental, intentional self-harm, assault and undetermined.

f. Adult and child abuse, neglect and other maltreatment

Sequence first the appropriate code from categories T74.- (Adult and child abuse, neglect and other maltreatment, confirmed) or T76.- (Adult and child abuse, neglect and other maltreatment, suspected) for abuse, neglect and other maltreatment, followed by any accompanying mental health or injury code(s).

If the documentation in the medical record states abuse or neglect it is coded as confirmed (T74.-). It is coded as suspected if it is documented as suspected (T76.-).

For cases of confirmed abuse or neglect an external cause code from the assault section (X92-Y09) should be added to identify the cause of any physical injuries. A perpetrator code (Y07) should be added when the perpetrator of the abuse is known. For suspected cases of abuse or neglect, do not report external cause or perpetrator code.

If a suspected case of abuse, neglect or mistreatment is ruled out during an encounter code Z04.71, Encounter for examination and observation following alleged physical adult abuse, ruled out, or code Z04.72, Encounter for examination and observation following alleged child physical abuse, ruled out, should be used, not a code from T76.

If a suspected case of alleged rape or sexual abuse is ruled out during an encounter code Z04.41, Encounter for examination and observation following alleged adult rape or code Z04.42, Encounter for examination and observation following alleged child rape, should be used, not a code from T76.

If a suspected case of forced sexual exploitation or forced labor exploitation is ruled out during an encounter, code Z04.81, Encounter for examination and observation of victim following forced sexual exploitation, or code Z04.82, Encounter for examination and observation of victim following forced labor exploitation, should be used, not a code from T76.

See Section I.C.15. Abuse in a pregnant patient.

g. Complications of care

1) General guidelines for complications of care

(a) Documentation of complications of care

See Section I.B.16. for information on documentation of complications of care.

2) Pain due to medical devices

Pain associated with devices, implants or grafts left in a surgical site (for example painful hip prosthesis) is assigned to the appropriate code(s) found in Chapter 19, Injury, poisoning, and certain other consequences of external causes. Specific codes for pain due to medical devices are found in the T code section of the ICD-10-CM. Use additional code(s) from category G89 to identify acute or chronic pain due to presence of the device, implant or graft (G89.18 or G89.28).

> Chronic left breast pain secondary to breast implant
>
> **T85.848A**   **Pain due to other internal prosthetic devices, implants and grafts, initial encounter**
>
> **N64.4**   **Mastodynia**
>
> **G89.28**   **Other chronic postprocedural pain**
>
> *Explanation:* As the pain is a complication related to the breast implant, the complication code is sequenced first. The T code does not describe the site or type of pain, so additional codes may be appended to indicate that the patient is experiencing chronic pain in the breast.

3) Transplant complications

(a) Transplant complications other than kidney

Codes under category T86, Complications of transplanted organs and tissues, are for use for both complications and rejection of transplanted organs. A transplant complication code is only assigned if the complication affects the function of the transplanted organ. Two codes are required to fully describe a transplant complication: the appropriate code from category T86 and a secondary code that identifies the complication.

Pre-existing conditions or conditions that develop after the transplant are not coded as complications unless they affect the function of the transplanted organs.

See I.C.21. for transplant organ removal status

See I.C.2. for malignant neoplasm associated with transplanted organ.

(b) Kidney transplant complications

Patients who have undergone kidney transplant may still have some form of chronic kidney disease (CKD) because the kidney transplant may not fully restore kidney function. Code T86.1- should be assigned for documented complications of a kidney transplant, such as transplant failure or rejection or other transplant complication. Code T86.1- should not be assigned for post kidney transplant patients who have chronic kidney (CKD) unless a transplant complication such as transplant failure or rejection is documented. If the documentation is unclear as to whether the patient has a complication of the transplant, query the provider.

Conditions that affect the function of the transplanted kidney, other than CKD, should be assigned a code from subcategory T86.1, Complications of transplanted organ, Kidney, and a secondary code that identifies the complication.

For patients with CKD following a kidney transplant, but who do not have a complication such as failure or rejection, *see section I.C.14. Chronic kidney disease and kidney transplant status.*

> Patient seen for chronic kidney disease stage 2; history of successful kidney transplant with no complications identified
>
> **N18.2**   **Chronic kidney disease, stage 2 (mild)**
>
> **Z94.0**   **Kidney transplant status**
>
> *Explanation:* This patient's stage 2 CKD is not indicated as being due to the transplanted kidney but instead is just the residual disease the patient had prior to the transplant.

4) Complication codes that include the external cause

As with certain other T codes, some of the complications of care codes have the external cause included in the code. The code includes the nature of the complication as well as the type of procedure that caused the complication. No external cause code indicating the type of procedure is necessary for these codes.

5) Complications of care codes within the body system chapters

Intraoperative and postprocedural complication codes are found within the body system chapters with codes specific to the organs and structures of that body system. These codes should be sequenced first, followed by a code(s) for the specific complication, if applicable.

> During a spinal fusion procedure, the surgeon inadvertently punctured the dura. The midline durotomy was repaired, and the fusion procedure was completed.
>
> **G97.41**   **Accidental puncture or laceration of dura during a procedure**
>
> *Explanation:* The accidental durotomy is not coded to an injury code in chapter 19 but instead is categorized to the nervous system chapter.

Muscle/Tendon Table

ICD-10-CM categorizes certain muscles and tendons in the upper and lower extremities by their action (e.g., extension, flexion), their anatomical location (e.g., posterior, anterior), and/or whether they are intrinsic or extrinsic to a certain anatomical area. The Muscle/Tendon Table is provided at the beginning of chapters 13 and 19 as a resource to help users when code selection depends on one or more of these characteristics. A **TIP** has been placed at those categories and/or subcategories that relate to this table. Please note that this table is not all-inclusive, and proper code assignment should be based on the provider's documentation.

Body Region	Muscle	Extensor Tendon	Flexor Tendon	Other Tendon
Shoulder				
	Deltoid	Posterior deltoid	Anterior deltoid	
	Rotator cuff			
	Infraspinatus			Infraspinatus
	Subscapularis			Subscapularis
	Supraspinatus			Supraspinatus
	Teres minor			Teres minor
	Teres major	Teres major		
Upper arm				
	Anterior muscles			
	Biceps brachii — long head		Biceps brachii — long head	
	Biceps brachii — short head		Biceps brachii — short head	
	Brachialis		Brachialis	
	Coracobrachialis		Coracobrachialis	
	Posterior muscles			
	Triceps brachii	Triceps brachii		
Forearm				
	Anterior muscles			
	Flexors			
	Deep			
	Flexor digitorum profundus		Flexor digitorum profundus	
	Flexor pollicis longus		Flexor pollicis longus	
	Intermediate			
	Flexor digitorum superficialis		Flexor digitorum superficialis	
	Superficial			
	Flexor carpi radialis		Flexor carpi radialis	
	Flexor carpi ulnaris		Flexor carpi ulnaris	
	Palmaris longus		Palmaris longus	
	Pronators			
	Pronator quadratus			Pronator quadratus
	Pronator teres			Pronator teres
	Posterior muscles			
	Extensors			
	Deep			
	Abductor pollicis longus			Abductor pollicis longus
	Extensor indicis	Extensor indicis		
	Extensor pollicis brevis	Extensor pollicis brevis		
	Extensor pollicis longus	Extensor pollicis longus		
	Superficial			
	Brachioradialis			Brachioradialis
	Extensor carpi radialis brevis	Extensor carpi radialis brevis		
	Extensor carpi radialis longus	Extensor carpi radialis longus		
	Extensor carpi ulnaris	Extensor carpi ulnaris		
	Extensor digiti minimi	Extensor digiti minimi		
	Extensor digitorum	Extensor digitorum		
	Anconeus	Anconeus		
	Supinator			Supinator

Body Region	Muscle	Extensor Tendon	Flexor Tendon	Other Tendon
Hand				
Extrinsic — attach to a site in the forearm as well as a site in the hand with action related to hand movement at the wrist				
	Extensor carpi radialis brevis	Extensor carpi radialis brevis		
	Extensor carpi radialis longus	Extensor carpie radialis longus		
	Extensor carpi ulnaris	Extensor carpi ulnaris		
	Flexor carpi radialis		Flexor carpi radialis	
	Flexor carpi ulnaris		Flexor carpi ulnaris	
	Flexor digitorum superficialis		Flexor digitorum superficialis	
	Palmaris longus		Palmaris longus	
Extrinsic — attach to a site in the forearm as well as a site in the hand with action in the hand related to finger movement				
	Adductor pollicis longus			Adductor pollicis longus
	Extensor digiti minimi	Extensor digiti minimi		
	Extensor digitorum	Extensor digitorum		
	Extensor indicis	Extensor indicis		
	Flexor digitorum profundus		Flexor digitorum profundus	
	Flexor digitorum superficialis		Flexor digitorum superficialis	
Extrinsic — attach to a site in the forearm as well as a site in the hand with action in the hand related to thumb movement				
	Extensor pollicis brevis	Extensor pollicis brevis		
	Extensor pollicis longus	Extensor pollicis longus		
	Flexor pollicis longus		Flexor pollicis longus	
Intrinsic — found within the hand only				
	Adductor pollicis			Adductor pollicis
	Dorsal interossei	Dorsal interossei	Dorsal interossei	
	Lumbricals	Lumbricals	Lumbricals	
	Palmaris brevis			Palmaris brevis
	Palmar interossei	Palmar interossei	Palmar interossei	
	Hypothenar muscles			
	Abductor digiti minimi			Abductor digiti minimi
	Flexor digiti minimi brevis		Flexor digiti minimi brevis	
	Oppenens digiti minimi		Oppenens digiti minimi	
	Thenar muscles			
	Abductor pollicis brevis			Abductor pollicis brevis
	Flexor pollicis brevis		Flexor pollicis brevis	
	Oppenens pollicis		Oppenens pollicis	
Thigh				
	Anterior muscles			
	Iliopsoas		Iliopsoas	
	Pectineus		Pectineus	
	Quadriceps	Quadriceps		
	Rectus femoris	Rectus femoris — Extends knee	Rectus femoris — Flexes hip	
	Vastus intermedius	Vastus intermedius		
	Vastus lateralis	Vastus lateralis		
	Vastus medialis	Vastus medialis		
	Sartorius		Sartorius	
	Medial muscles			
	Adductor brevis			Adductor brevis
	Adductor longus			Adductor longus
	Adductor magnus			Adductor magnus
	Gracilis			Gracilis
	Obturator externus			Obturator externus
	Posterior muscles			
	Hamstring	Hamstring — Extends hip	Hamstring — Flexes knee	
	Biceps femoris	Biceps femoris	Biceps femoris	
	Semimembranosus	Semimembranosus	Semimembranosus	
	Semitendinosus	Semitendinosus	Semitendinosus	

Body Region	Muscle	Extensor Tendon	Flexor Tendon	Other Tendon
Lower leg				
	Anterior muscles			
	Extensor digitorum longus	Extensor digitorum longus		
	Extensor hallucis longus	Extensor hallucis longus		
	Fibularis (peroneus) tertius	Fibularis (peroneus) tertius		
	Tibialis anterior	Tibialis anterior		Tibialis anterior
	Lateral muscles			
	Fibularis (peroneus) brevis		Fibularis (peroneus) brevis	
	Fibularis (peroneus) longus		Fibularis (peroneus) longus	
	Posterior muscles			
	Deep			
	Flexor digitorum longus		Flexor digitorum longus	
	Flexor hallucis longus		Flexor hallucis longus	
	Popliteus		Popliteus	
	Tibialis posterior		Tibialis posterior	
	Superficial			
	Gastrocnemius		Gastrocnemius	
	Plantaris		Plantaris	
	Soleus		Soleus	
				Calcaneal (Achilles)
Ankle/Foot				
Extrinsic — attach to a site in the lower leg as well as a site in the foot with action related to foot movement at the ankle				
	Plantaris		Plantaris	
	Soleus		Soleus	
	Tibialis anterior	Tibialis anterior		
	Tibialis posterior		Tibialis posterior	
Extrinsic — attach to a site in the lower leg as well as a site in the foot with action in the foot related to toe movement				
	Extensor digitorum longus	Extensor digitorum longus		
	Extensor hallucis longus	Extensor hallucis longus		
	Flexor digitorum longus		Flexor digitorum longus	
	Flexor hallucis longus		Flexor hallucis longus	
Intrinsic — found within the ankle/foot only				
	Dorsal muscles			
	Extensor digitorum brevis	Extensor digitorum brevis		
	Extensor hallucis brevis	Extensor hallucis brevis		
	Plantar muscles			
	Abductor digiti minimi		Abductor digiti minimi	
	Abductor hallucis		Abductor hallucis	
	Dorsal interossei	Dorsal interossei	Dorsal interossei	
	Flexor digiti minimi brevis		Flexor digiti minimi brevis	
	Flexor digitorum brevis		Flexor digitorum brevis	
	Flexor hallucis brevis		Flexor hallucis brevis	
	Lumbricals	Lumbricals	Lumbricals	
	Quadratus plantae		Quadratus plantae	
	Plantar interossei	Plantar interossei	Plantar interossei	

Chapter 19. Injury, Poisoning and Certain Other Consequences of External Causes (S00-T88)

NOTE   Use secondary code(s) from Chapter 20, External causes of morbidity, to indicate cause of injury. Codes within the T section that include the external cause do not require an additional external cause code.

Use additional code to identify any retained foreign body, if applicable (Z18.-)

EXCLUDES 1   birth trauma (P10-P15)
         obstetric trauma (O70-O71)

NOTE   The chapter uses the S-section for coding different types of injuries related to single body regions and the T-section to cover injuries to unspecified body regions as well as poisoning and certain other consequences of external causes.

AHA: 2016,2Q,3-7; 2015,4Q,35-38; 2015,3Q,37-39,40; 2015,2Q,6; 2015,1Q,3-21
TIP: The specific site of an injury can be determined from the radiology report when authenticated by a radiologist and available at the time of code assignment.

This chapter contains the following blocks:

S00-S09   Injuries to the head
S10-S19   Injuries to the neck
S20-S29   Injuries to the thorax
S30-S39   Injuries to the abdomen, lower back, lumbar spine, pelvis and external genitals
S40-S49   Injuries to the shoulder and upper arm
S50-S59   Injuries to the elbow and forearm
S60-S69   Injuries to the wrist, hand and fingers
S70-S79   Injuries to the hip and thigh
S80-S89   Injuries to the knee and lower leg
S90-S99   Injuries to the ankle and foot
T07   Injuries involving multiple body regions
T14   Injury of unspecified body region
T15-T19   Effects of foreign body entering through natural orifice
T20-T25   Burns and corrosions of external body surface, specified by site
T26-T28   Burns and corrosions confined to eye and internal organs
T30-T32   Burns and corrosions of multiple and unspecified body regions
T33-T34   Frostbite
T36-T50   Poisoning by, adverse effect of and underdosing of drugs, medicaments and biological substances
T51-T65   Toxic effects of substances chiefly nonmedicinal as to source
T66-T78   Other and unspecified effects of external causes
T79   Certain early complications of trauma
T80-T88   Complications of surgical and medical care, not elsewhere classified

Injuries to the head (S00-S09)

INCLUDES   injuries of ear
         injuries of eye
         injuries of face [any part]
         injuries of gum
         injuries of jaw
         injuries of oral cavity
         injuries of palate
         injuries of periocular area
         injuries of scalp
         injuries of temporomandibular joint area
         injuries of tongue
         injuries of tooth

Code also for any associated infection

EXCLUDES 2   burns and corrosions (T20-T32)
         effects of foreign body in ear (T16)
         effects of foreign body in larynx (T17.3)
         effects of foreign body in mouth NOS (T18.0)
         effects of foreign body in nose (T17.0-T17.1)
         effects of foreign body in pharynx (T17.2)
         effects of foreign body on external eye (T15.-)
         frostbite (T33-T34)
         insect bite or sting, venomous (T63.4)

√4ᵗʰ **S00 Superficial injury of head**

EXCLUDES 1   diffuse cerebral contusion (S06.2-)
         focal cerebral contusion (S06.3-)
         injury of eye and orbit (S05.-)
         open wound of head (S01.-)

The appropriate 7th character is to be added to each code from category S00.
A   initial encounter
D   subsequent encounter
S   sequela

√5ᵗʰ **S00.0 Superficial injury of scalp**

√x7ᵗʰ **S00.00 Unspecified superficial injury of scalp** ▽

√x7ᵗʰ **S00.01 Abrasion of scalp**

√x7ᵗʰ **S00.02 Blister (nonthermal) of scalp**

√x7ᵗʰ **S00.03 Contusion of scalp** ◖

     Bruise of scalp
     Hematoma of scalp

√x7ᵗʰ **S00.04 External constriction of part of scalp**

√x7ᵗʰ **S00.05 Superficial foreign body of scalp**
     Splinter in the scalp

√x7ᵗʰ **S00.06 Insect bite (nonvenomous) of scalp**

√x7ᵗʰ **S00.07 Other superficial bite of scalp**
     EXCLUDES 1   open bite of scalp (S01.05)

√5ᵗʰ **S00.1 Contusion of eyelid and periocular area**
     Black eye
     EXCLUDES 2   contusion of eyeball and orbital tissues (S05.1)

√x7ᵗʰ **S00.10 Contusion of unspecified eyelid and periocular area** ▽

√x7ᵗʰ **S00.11 Contusion of right eyelid and periocular area**

√x7ᵗʰ **S00.12 Contusion of left eyelid and periocular area**

√5ᵗʰ **S00.2 Other and unspecified superficial injuries of eyelid and periocular area**
     EXCLUDES 2   superficial injury of conjunctiva and cornea (S05.0-)

√6ᵗʰ **S00.20 Unspecified superficial injury of eyelid and periocular area**

√7ᵗʰ **S00.201 Unspecified superficial injury of right eyelid and periocular area** ▽

√7ᵗʰ **S00.202 Unspecified superficial injury of left eyelid and periocular area** ▽

√7ᵗʰ **S00.209 Unspecified superficial injury of unspecified eyelid and periocular area** ▽

√6ᵗʰ **S00.21 Abrasion of eyelid and periocular area**

√7ᵗʰ **S00.211 Abrasion of right eyelid and periocular area**

√7ᵗʰ **S00.212 Abrasion of left eyelid and periocular area**

√7ᵗʰ **S00.219 Abrasion of unspecified eyelid and periocular area** ▽

√6ᵗʰ **S00.22 Blister (nonthermal) of eyelid and periocular area**

√7ᵗʰ **S00.221 Blister (nonthermal) of right eyelid and periocular area**

√7ᵗʰ **S00.222 Blister (nonthermal) of left eyelid and periocular area**

√7ᵗʰ **S00.229 Blister (nonthermal) of unspecified eyelid and periocular area** ▽

√6ᵗʰ **S00.24 External constriction of eyelid and periocular area**

√7ᵗʰ **S00.241 External constriction of right eyelid and periocular area**

√7ᵗʰ **S00.242 External constriction of left eyelid and periocular area**

√7ᵗʰ **S00.249 External constriction of unspecified eyelid and periocular area** ▽

√6ᵗʰ **S00.25 Superficial foreign body of eyelid and periocular area**
     Splinter of eyelid and periocular area
     EXCLUDES 2   retained foreign body in eyelid (H02.81-)

√7ᵗʰ **S00.251 Superficial foreign body of right eyelid and periocular area**

√7ᵗʰ **S00.252 Superficial foreign body of left eyelid and periocular area**

√7ᵗʰ **S00.259 Superficial foreign body of unspecified eyelid and periocular area** ▽

√6ᵗʰ **S00.26 Insect bite (nonvenomous) of eyelid and periocular area**

√7ᵗʰ **S00.261 Insect bite (nonvenomous) of right eyelid and periocular area**

√7ᵗʰ **S00.262 Insect bite (nonvenomous) of left eyelid and periocular area**

√7ᵗʰ **S00.269 Insect bite (nonvenomous) of unspecified eyelid and periocular area** ▽

√6ᵗʰ **S00.27 Other superficial bite of eyelid and periocular area**
     EXCLUDES 1   open bite of eyelid and periocular area (S01.15)

√7ᵗʰ **S00.271 Other superficial bite of right eyelid and periocular area**

√7ᵗʰ **S00.272 Other superficial bite of left eyelid and periocular area**

√7ᵗʰ **S00.279** **Other superficial bite of unspecified eyelid and periocular area** ▽

√5ᵗʰ **S00.3** **Superficial injury of nose**

√x7ᵗʰ **S00.30** **Unspecified superficial injury of nose** ▽

√x7ᵗʰ **S00.31** **Abrasion of nose**

√x7ᵗʰ **S00.32** **Blister (nonthermal) of nose**

√x7ᵗʰ **S00.33** **Contusion of nose** 🔲
 Bruise of nose
 Hematoma of nose

√x7ᵗʰ **S00.34** **External constriction of nose**

√x7ᵗʰ **S00.35** **Superficial foreign body of nose**
 Splinter in the nose

√x7ᵗʰ **S00.36** **Insect bite (nonvenomous) of nose**

√x7ᵗʰ **S00.37** **Other superficial bite of nose**
 EXCLUDES 1 *open bite of nose (S01.25)*

√5ᵗʰ **S00.4** **Superficial injury of ear**

√6ᵗʰ **S00.40** **Unspecified superficial injury of ear**

√7ᵗʰ **S00.401** **Unspecified superficial injury of right ear** ▽

√7ᵗʰ **S00.402** **Unspecified superficial injury of left ear** ▽

√7ᵗʰ **S00.409** **Unspecified superficial injury of unspecified ear** ▽

√6ᵗʰ **S00.41** **Abrasion of ear**

√7ᵗʰ **S00.411** **Abrasion of right ear**

√7ᵗʰ **S00.412** **Abrasion of left ear**

√7ᵗʰ **S00.419** **Abrasion of unspecified ear** ▽

√6ᵗʰ **S00.42** **Blister (nonthermal) of ear**

√7ᵗʰ **S00.421** **Blister (nonthermal) of right ear**

√7ᵗʰ **S00.422** **Blister (nonthermal) of left ear**

√7ᵗʰ **S00.429** **Blister (nonthermal) of unspecified ear** ▽

√6ᵗʰ **S00.43** **Contusion of ear**
 Bruise of ear
 Hematoma of ear

√7ᵗʰ **S00.431** **Contusion of right ear** 🔲

√7ᵗʰ **S00.432** **Contusion of left ear** 🔲

√7ᵗʰ **S00.439** **Contusion of unspecified ear** 🔲 ▽

√6ᵗʰ **S00.44** **External constriction of ear**

√7ᵗʰ **S00.441** **External constriction of right ear**

√7ᵗʰ **S00.442** **External constriction of left ear**

√7ᵗʰ **S00.449** **External constriction of unspecified ear** ▽

√6ᵗʰ **S00.45** **Superficial foreign body of ear**
 Splinter in the ear

√7ᵗʰ **S00.451** **Superficial foreign body of right ear**

√7ᵗʰ **S00.452** **Superficial foreign body of left ear**

√7ᵗʰ **S00.459** **Superficial foreign body of unspecified ear** ▽

√6ᵗʰ **S00.46** **Insect bite (nonvenomous) of ear**

√7ᵗʰ **S00.461** **Insect bite (nonvenomous) of right ear**

√7ᵗʰ **S00.462** **Insect bite (nonvenomous) of left ear**

√7ᵗʰ **S00.469** **Insect bite (nonvenomous) of unspecified ear** ▽

√6ᵗʰ **S00.47** **Other superficial bite of ear**
 EXCLUDES 1 *open bite of ear (S01.35)*

√7ᵗʰ **S00.471** **Other superficial bite of right ear**

√7ᵗʰ **S00.472** **Other superficial bite of left ear**

√7ᵗʰ **S00.479** **Other superficial bite of unspecified ear** ▽

√5ᵗʰ **S00.5** **Superficial injury of lip and oral cavity**

√6ᵗʰ **S00.50** **Unspecified superficial injury of lip and oral cavity**

√7ᵗʰ **S00.501** **Unspecified superficial injury of lip** ▽

√7ᵗʰ **S00.502** **Unspecified superficial injury of oral cavity** ▽

√6ᵗʰ **S00.51** **Abrasion of lip and oral cavity**

√7ᵗʰ **S00.511** **Abrasion of lip**

√7ᵗʰ **S00.512** **Abrasion of oral cavity**

√6ᵗʰ **S00.52** **Blister (nonthermal) of lip and oral cavity**

√7ᵗʰ **S00.521** **Blister (nonthermal) of lip**

√7ᵗʰ **S00.522** **Blister (nonthermal) of oral cavity**

√6ᵗʰ **S00.53** **Contusion of lip and oral cavity**

√7ᵗʰ **S00.531** **Contusion of lip** 🔲
 Bruise of lip
 Hematoma of lip

√7ᵗʰ **S00.532** **Contusion of oral cavity** 🔲
 Bruise of oral cavity
 Hematoma of oral cavity

√6ᵗʰ **S00.54** **External constriction of lip and oral cavity**

√7ᵗʰ **S00.541** **External constriction of lip**

√7ᵗʰ **S00.542** **External constriction of oral cavity**

√6ᵗʰ **S00.55** **Superficial foreign body of lip and oral cavity**

√7ᵗʰ **S00.551** **Superficial foreign body of lip**
 Splinter of lip and oral cavity

√7ᵗʰ **S00.552** **Superficial foreign body of oral cavity**
 Splinter of lip and oral cavity

√6ᵗʰ **S00.56** **Insect bite (nonvenomous) of lip and oral cavity**

√7ᵗʰ **S00.561** **Insect bite (nonvenomous) of lip**

√7ᵗʰ **S00.562** **Insect bite (nonvenomous) of oral cavity**

√6ᵗʰ **S00.57** **Other superficial bite of lip and oral cavity**

√7ᵗʰ **S00.571** **Other superficial bite of lip**
 EXCLUDES 1 *open bite of lip (S01.551)*

√7ᵗʰ **S00.572** **Other superficial bite of oral cavity**
 EXCLUDES 1 *open bite of oral cavity (S01.552)*

√5ᵗʰ **S00.8** **Superficial injury of other parts of head**
 Superficial injuries of face [any part]

√x7ᵗʰ **S00.80** **Unspecified superficial injury of other part of head** ▽

√x7ᵗʰ **S00.81** **Abrasion of other part of head**

√x7ᵗʰ **S00.82** **Blister (nonthermal) of other part of head**

√x7ᵗʰ **S00.83** **Contusion of other part of head** 🔲
 Bruise of other part of head
 Hematoma of other part of head

√x7ᵗʰ **S00.84** **External constriction of other part of head**

√x7ᵗʰ **S00.85** **Superficial foreign body of other part of head**
 Splinter in other part of head

√x7ᵗʰ **S00.86** **Insect bite (nonvenomous) of other part of head**

√x7ᵗʰ **S00.87** **Other superficial bite of other part of head**
 EXCLUDES 1 *open bite of other part of head (S01.85)*

√5ᵗʰ **S00.9** **Superficial injury of unspecified part of head**

√x7ᵗʰ **S00.90** **Unspecified superficial injury of unspecified part of head** ▽

√x7ᵗʰ **S00.91** **Abrasion of unspecified part of head** ▽

√x7ᵗʰ **S00.92** **Blister (nonthermal) of unspecified part of head** ▽

√x7ᵗʰ **S00.93** **Contusion of unspecified part of head** 🔲 ▽
 Bruise of head
 Hematoma of head

√x7ᵗʰ **S00.94** **External constriction of unspecified part of head** ▽

√x7ᵗʰ **S00.95** **Superficial foreign body of unspecified part of head** ▽
 Splinter of head

√x7ᵗʰ **S00.96** **Insect bite (nonvenomous) of unspecified part of head** ▽

√x7ᵗʰ **S00.97** **Other superficial bite of unspecified part of head** ▽
 EXCLUDES 1 *open bite of head (S01.95)*

☑ Additional Character Req √x7ᵗʰ Placeholder Alert Manifestation ▽ Unspecified ►◄ Revised Text ● New Code ▲ Revised Code Title

Chapter 19. Injury, Poisoning and Certain Other Consequences of External Causes

S01–S01.419

√4ᵗʰ S01 Open wound of head

Code also any associated:
injury of cranial nerve (S04.-)
injury of muscle and tendon of head (S09.1-)
intracranial injury (S06.-)
wound infection

EXCLUDES 1   open skull fracture (S02.- with 7th character B)

EXCLUDES 2   injury of eye and orbit (S05.-)
traumatic amputation of part of head (S08.-)

The appropriate 7th character is to be added to each code from category S01.
A   initial encounter
D   subsequent encounter
S   sequela

√5ᵗʰ S01.0 Open wound of scalp

EXCLUDES 1   avulsion of scalp (S08.0)

√x7ᵗʰ   **S01.00 Unspecified open wound of scalp**   ▽

√x7ᵗʰ   **S01.01 Laceration without foreign body of scalp**

√x7ᵗʰ   **S01.02 Laceration with foreign body of scalp**

√x7ᵗʰ   **S01.03 Puncture wound without foreign body of scalp**

√x7ᵗʰ   **S01.04 Puncture wound with foreign body of scalp**

√x7ᵗʰ   **S01.05 Open bite of scalp**

Bite of scalp NOS

EXCLUDES 1   superficial bite of scalp (S00.06, S00.07-)

√5ᵗʰ S01.1 Open wound of eyelid and periocular area

Open wound of eyelid and periocular area with or without involvement of lacrimal passages

√6ᵗʰ   **S01.10 Unspecified open wound of eyelid and periocular area**

√7ᵗʰ   **S01.101 Unspecified open wound of right eyelid and periocular area**   ▽

√7ᵗʰ   **S01.102 Unspecified open wound of left eyelid and periocular area**   ▽

√7ᵗʰ   **S01.109 Unspecified open wound of unspecified eyelid and periocular area**   ▽

√6ᵗʰ   **S01.11 Laceration without foreign body of eyelid and periocular area**

√7ᵗʰ   **S01.111 Laceration without foreign body of right eyelid and periocular area**

√7ᵗʰ   **S01.112 Laceration without foreign body of left eyelid and periocular area**

√7ᵗʰ   **S01.119 Laceration without foreign body of unspecified eyelid and periocular area**   ▽

√6ᵗʰ   **S01.12 Laceration with foreign body of eyelid and periocular area**

√7ᵗʰ   **S01.121 Laceration with foreign body of right eyelid and periocular area**

√7ᵗʰ   **S01.122 Laceration with foreign body of left eyelid and periocular area**

√7ᵗʰ   **S01.129 Laceration with foreign body of unspecified eyelid and periocular area**   ▽

√6ᵗʰ   **S01.13 Puncture wound without foreign body of eyelid and periocular area**

√7ᵗʰ   **S01.131 Puncture wound without foreign body of right eyelid and periocular area**

√7ᵗʰ   **S01.132 Puncture wound without foreign body of left eyelid and periocular area**

√7ᵗʰ   **S01.139 Puncture wound without foreign body of unspecified eyelid and periocular area**   ▽

√6ᵗʰ   **S01.14 Puncture wound with foreign body of eyelid and periocular area**

√7ᵗʰ   **S01.141 Puncture wound with foreign body of right eyelid and periocular area**

√7ᵗʰ   **S01.142 Puncture wound with foreign body of left eyelid and periocular area**

√7ᵗʰ   **S01.149 Puncture wound with foreign body of unspecified eyelid and periocular area**   ▽

√6ᵗʰ   **S01.15 Open bite of eyelid and periocular area**

Bite of eyelid and periocular area NOS

EXCLUDES 1   superficial bite of eyelid and periocular area (S00.26, S00.27)

√7ᵗʰ   **S01.151 Open bite of right eyelid and periocular area**

√7ᵗʰ   **S01.152 Open bite of left eyelid and periocular area**

√7ᵗʰ   **S01.159 Open bite of unspecified eyelid and periocular area**   ▽

√5ᵗʰ S01.2 Open wound of nose

√x7ᵗʰ   **S01.20 Unspecified open wound of nose**   ▽

√x7ᵗʰ   **S01.21 Laceration without foreign body of nose**

√x7ᵗʰ   **S01.22 Laceration with foreign body of nose**

√x7ᵗʰ   **S01.23 Puncture wound without foreign body of nose**

√x7ᵗʰ   **S01.24 Puncture wound with foreign body of nose**

√x7ᵗʰ   **S01.25 Open bite of nose**

Bite of nose NOS

EXCLUDES 1   superficial bite of nose (S00.36, S00.37)

√5ᵗʰ S01.3 Open wound of ear

√6ᵗʰ   **S01.30 Unspecified open wound of ear**

√7ᵗʰ   **S01.301 Unspecified open wound of right ear**   ▽

√7ᵗʰ   **S01.302 Unspecified open wound of left ear**   ▽

√7ᵗʰ   **S01.309 Unspecified open wound of unspecified ear**   ▽

√6ᵗʰ   **S01.31 Laceration without foreign body of ear**

√7ᵗʰ   **S01.311 Laceration without foreign body of right ear**

√7ᵗʰ   **S01.312 Laceration without foreign body of left ear**

√7ᵗʰ   **S01.319 Laceration without foreign body of unspecified ear**   ▽

√6ᵗʰ   **S01.32 Laceration with foreign body of ear**

√7ᵗʰ   **S01.321 Laceration with foreign body of right ear**

√7ᵗʰ   **S01.322 Laceration with foreign body of left ear**

√7ᵗʰ   **S01.329 Laceration with foreign body of unspecified ear**

√6ᵗʰ   **S01.33 Puncture wound without foreign body of ear**

√7ᵗʰ   **S01.331 Puncture wound without foreign body of right ear**

√7ᵗʰ   **S01.332 Puncture wound without foreign body of left ear**

√7ᵗʰ   **S01.339 Puncture wound without foreign body of unspecified ear**   ▽

√6ᵗʰ   **S01.34 Puncture wound with foreign body of ear**

√7ᵗʰ   **S01.341 Puncture wound with foreign body of right ear**

√7ᵗʰ   **S01.342 Puncture wound with foreign body of left ear**

√7ᵗʰ   **S01.349 Puncture wound with foreign body of unspecified ear**   ▽

√6ᵗʰ   **S01.35 Open bite of ear**

Bite of ear NOS

EXCLUDES 1   superficial bite of ear (S00.46, S00.47)

√7ᵗʰ   **S01.351 Open bite of right ear**

√7ᵗʰ   **S01.352 Open bite of left ear**

√7ᵗʰ   **S01.359 Open bite of unspecified ear**   ▽

√5ᵗʰ S01.4 Open wound of cheek and temporomandibular area

√6ᵗʰ   **S01.40 Unspecified open wound of cheek and temporomandibular area**

√7ᵗʰ   **S01.401 Unspecified open wound of right cheek and temporomandibular area**   ▽

√7ᵗʰ   **S01.402 Unspecified open wound of left cheek and temporomandibular area**   ▽

√7ᵗʰ   **S01.409 Unspecified open wound of unspecified cheek and temporomandibular area**   ▽

√6ᵗʰ   **S01.41 Laceration without foreign body of cheek and temporomandibular area**

√7ᵗʰ   **S01.411 Laceration without foreign body of right cheek and temporomandibular area**

√7ᵗʰ   **S01.412 Laceration without foreign body of left cheek and temporomandibular area**

√7ᵗʰ   **S01.419 Laceration without foreign body of unspecified cheek and temporomandibular area**   ▽

√6ᵗʰ **S01.42** **Laceration with foreign body of cheek and temporomandibular area**

    √7ᵗʰ **S01.421** **Laceration with foreign body of right cheek and temporomandibular area**

    √7ᵗʰ **S01.422** **Laceration with foreign body of left cheek and temporomandibular area**

    √7ᵗʰ **S01.429** **Laceration with foreign body of unspecified cheek and temporomandibular area** ▽

√6ᵗʰ **S01.43** **Puncture wound without foreign body of cheek and temporomandibular area**

    √7ᵗʰ **S01.431** **Puncture wound without foreign body of right cheek and temporomandibular area**

    √7ᵗʰ **S01.432** **Puncture wound without foreign body of left cheek and temporomandibular area**

    √7ᵗʰ **S01.439** **Puncture wound without foreign body of unspecified cheek and temporomandibular area** ▽

√6ᵗʰ **S01.44** **Puncture wound with foreign body of cheek and temporomandibular area**

    √7ᵗʰ **S01.441** **Puncture wound with foreign body of right cheek and temporomandibular area**

    √7ᵗʰ **S01.442** **Puncture wound with foreign body of left cheek and temporomandibular area**

    √7ᵗʰ **S01.449** **Puncture wound with foreign body of unspecified cheek and temporomandibular area** ▽

√6ᵗʰ **S01.45** **Open bite of cheek and temporomandibular area**

    Bite of cheek and temporomandibular area NOS

    EXCLUDES 2   superficial bite of cheek and temporomandibular area (S00.86, S00.87)

    √7ᵗʰ **S01.451** **Open bite of right cheek and temporomandibular area**

    √7ᵗʰ **S01.452** **Open bite of left cheek and temporomandibular area**

    √7ᵗʰ **S01.459** **Open bite of unspecified cheek and temporomandibular area** ▽

√5ᵗʰ **S01.5** **Open wound of lip and oral cavity**

    EXCLUDES 2   tooth dislocation (S03.2)

         tooth fracture (S02.5)

   √6ᵗʰ **S01.50** **Unspecified open wound of lip and oral cavity**

    √7ᵗʰ **S01.501** **Unspecified open wound of lip** ▽

    √7ᵗʰ **S01.502** **Unspecified open wound of oral cavity** ▽

   √6ᵗʰ **S01.51** **Laceration of lip and oral cavity without foreign body**

    √7ᵗʰ **S01.511** **Laceration without foreign body of lip**

    √7ᵗʰ **S01.512** **Laceration without foreign body of oral cavity**

   √6ᵗʰ **S01.52** **Laceration of lip and oral cavity with foreign body**

    √7ᵗʰ **S01.521** **Laceration with foreign body of lip**

    √7ᵗʰ **S01.522** **Laceration with foreign body of oral cavity**

   √6ᵗʰ **S01.53** **Puncture wound of lip and oral cavity without foreign body**

    √7ᵗʰ **S01.531** **Puncture wound without foreign body of lip**

    √7ᵗʰ **S01.532** **Puncture wound without foreign body of oral cavity**

   √6ᵗʰ **S01.54** **Puncture wound of lip and oral cavity with foreign body**

    √7ᵗʰ **S01.541** **Puncture wound with foreign body of lip**

    √7ᵗʰ **S01.542** **Puncture wound with foreign body of oral cavity**

   √6ᵗʰ **S01.55** **Open bite of lip and oral cavity**

    √7ᵗʰ **S01.551** **Open bite of lip**

        Bite of lip NOS

        EXCLUDES 1   superficial bite of lip (S00.571)

    √7ᵗʰ **S01.552** **Open bite of oral cavity**

        Bite of oral cavity NOS

        EXCLUDES 1   superficial bite of oral cavity (S00.572)

√5ᵗʰ **S01.8** **Open wound of other parts of head**

   √x7ᵗʰ **S01.80** **Unspecified open wound of other part of head** ▽

   √x7ᵗʰ **S01.81** **Laceration without foreign body of other part of head**

   √x7ᵗʰ **S01.82** **Laceration with foreign body of other part of head**

   √x7ᵗʰ **S01.83** **Puncture wound without foreign body of other part of head**

   √x7ᵗʰ **S01.84** **Puncture wound with foreign body of other part of head**

   √x7ᵗʰ **S01.85** **Open bite of other part of head**

    Bite of other part of head NOS

    EXCLUDES 1   superficial bite of other part of head (S00.87)

√5ᵗʰ **S01.9** **Open wound of unspecified part of head**

   √x7ᵗʰ **S01.90** **Unspecified open wound of unspecified part of head** ▽

   √x7ᵗʰ **S01.91** **Laceration without foreign body of unspecified part of head** ▽

   √x7ᵗʰ **S01.92** **Laceration with foreign body of unspecified part of head** ▽

   √x7ᵗʰ **S01.93** **Puncture wound without foreign body of unspecified part of head** ▽

   √x7ᵗʰ **S01.94** **Puncture wound with foreign body of unspecified part of head** ▽

   √x7ᵗʰ **S01.95** **Open bite of unspecified part of head** ▽

    Bite of head NOS

    EXCLUDES 1   superficial bite of head NOS (S00.97)

√4ᵗʰ **S02** **Fracture of skull and facial bones**

   NOTE   A fracture not indicated as open or closed should be coded to closed.

   Code also any associated intracranial injury (S06.-)

   AHA: 2017,1Q,42; 2016,4Q,66-67

   The appropriate 7th character is to be added to each code from category S02.

   A   initial encounter for closed fracture

   B   initial encounter for open fracture

   D   subsequent encounter for fracture with routine healing

   G   subsequent encounter for fracture with delayed healing

   K   subsequent encounter for fracture with nonunion

   S   sequela

² √x7ᵗʰ **S02.0** **Fracture of vault of skull**   HCC ⓪

   Fracture of frontal bone

   Fracture of parietal bone

√5ᵗʰ **S02.1** **Fracture of base of skull**

   EXCLUDES 1   orbit NOS (S02.8)

   EXCLUDES 2   orbital floor (S02.3-)

   √6ᵗʰ **S02.10** **Unspecified fracture of base of skull**

    ² √7ᵗʰ **S02.101** **Fracture of base of skull, right side**   HCC ⓪

    ² √7ᵗʰ **S02.102** **Fracture of base of skull, left side**   HCC ⓪

    ² √7ᵗʰ **S02.109** **Fracture of base of skull, unspecified side**   HCC ⓪ ▽

   √6ᵗʰ **S02.11** **Fracture of occiput**

    ² √7ᵗʰ **S02.110** **Type I occipital condyle fracture, unspecified side**   HCC ⓪ ▽

    ² √7ᵗʰ **S02.111** **Type II occipital condyle fracture, unspecified side**   HCC ⓪ ▽

    ² √7ᵗʰ **S02.112** **Type III occipital condyle fracture, unspecified side**   HCC ⓪ ▽

    ² √7ᵗʰ **S02.113** **Unspecified occipital condyle fracture**   HCC ⓪ ▽

    ² √7ᵗʰ **S02.118** **Other fracture of occiput, unspecified side**   HCC ⓪ ▽

    ² √7ᵗʰ **S02.119** **Unspecified fracture of occiput**   HCC ⓪ ▽

    ² √7ᵗʰ **S02.11A** **Type I occipital condyle fracture, right side**   HCC ⓪

    ² √7ᵗʰ **S02.11B** **Type I occipital condyle fracture, left side**   HCC ⓪

    ² √7ᵗʰ **S02.11C** **Type II occipital condyle fracture, right side**   HCC ⓪

    ² √7ᵗʰ **S02.11D** **Type II occipital condyle fracture, left side**   HCC ⓪

    ² √7ᵗʰ **S02.11E** **Type III occipital condyle fracture, right side**   HCC ⓪

    ² √7ᵗʰ **S02.11F** **Type III occipital condyle fracture, left side**   HCC ⓪

    ² √7ᵗʰ **S02.11G** **Other fracture of occiput, right side**   HCC ⓪

    ² √7ᵗʰ **S02.11H** **Other fracture of occiput, left side**   HCC ⓪

✔ Additional Character Req   √x7ᵗʰ Placeholder Alert   Manifestation   ▽ Unspecified   ▶◀ Revised Text   ● New Code   ▲ Revised Code Title

ICD-10-CM 2019   953

² ✓7ᵗʰ **S02.19 Other fracture of base of skull**   HCC Q
- Fracture of anterior fossa of base of skull
- Fracture of ethmoid sinus
- Fracture of frontal sinus
- Fracture of middle fossa of base of skull
- Fracture of orbital roof
- Fracture of posterior fossa of base of skull
- Fracture of sphenoid
- Fracture of temporal bone

✓x7ᵗʰ **S02.2 Fracture of nasal bones**   Q

✓5ᵗʰ **S02.3 Fracture of orbital floor**
- **EXCLUDES 1**   orbit NOS (S02.8)
- **EXCLUDES 2**   orbital roof (S02.1-)

² ✓x7ᵗʰ **S02.30 Fracture of orbital floor, unspecified side**   HCC Q ▽

² ✓x7ᵗʰ **S02.31 Fracture of orbital floor, right side**   HCC Q

² ✓x7ᵗʰ **S02.32 Fracture of orbital floor, left side**   HCC Q

✓5ᵗʰ **S02.4 Fracture of malar, maxillary and zygoma bones**
- Fracture of superior maxilla
- Fracture of upper jaw (bone)
- Fracture of zygomatic process of temporal bone

✓6ᵗʰ **S02.40 Fracture of malar, maxillary and zygoma bones, unspecified**

² ✓7ᵗʰ **S02.400 Malar fracture, unspecified side**   HCC Q ▽

² ✓7ᵗʰ **S02.401 Maxillary fracture, unspecified side**   HCC Q ▽

² ✓7ᵗʰ **S02.402 Zygomatic fracture, unspecified side**   HCC Q ▽

² ✓7ᵗʰ **S02.40A Malar fracture, right side**   HCC Q

² ✓7ᵗʰ **S02.40B Malar fracture, left side**   HCC Q

² ✓7ᵗʰ **S02.40C Maxillary fracture, right side**   HCC Q

² ✓7ᵗʰ **S02.40D Maxillary fracture, left side**   HCC Q

² ✓7ᵗʰ **S02.40E Zygomatic fracture, right side**   HCC Q

² ✓7ᵗʰ **S02.40F Zygomatic fracture, left side**   HCC Q

✓6ᵗʰ **S02.41 LeFort fracture**

DEF: Named for Rene Le Fort, these fractures describe different combinations of multiple fractures that occur from significant force to the midface. A common denominator in all three types of LeFort fractures is fracture of the pterygoid processes, which are two bony plates resembling wings that extend downward from the sphenoid bone.

LeFort Fracture Types

Frontal bone   Nasal bone   Orbital floor

Type III

Type II

Type I

Maxilla

Zygomatic bone (malar) and arch

² ✓7ᵗʰ **S02.411 LeFort I fracture**   HCC Q

² ✓7ᵗʰ **S02.412 LeFort II fracture**   HCC Q

² ✓7ᵗʰ **S02.413 LeFort III fracture**   HCC Q

² ✓x7ᵗʰ **S02.42 Fracture of alveolus of maxilla**   HCC Q

✓x7ᵗʰ **S02.5 Fracture of tooth (traumatic)**
- Broken tooth
- **EXCLUDES 1**   cracked tooth (nontraumatic) (K03.81)

✓5ᵗʰ **S02.6 Fracture of mandible**
- Fracture of lower jaw (bone)

✓6ᵗʰ **S02.60 Fracture of mandible, unspecified**

² ✓7ᵗʰ **S02.600 Fracture of unspecified part of body of mandible, unspecified side**   HCC Q ▽

² ✓7ᵗʰ **S02.601 Fracture of unspecified part of body of right mandible**   HCC Q ▽

² ✓7ᵗʰ **S02.602 Fracture of unspecified part of body of left mandible**   HCC Q ▽

² ✓7ᵗʰ **S02.609 Fracture of mandible, unspecified**   HCC Q ▽

✓6ᵗʰ **S02.61 Fracture of condylar process of mandible**

² ✓7ᵗʰ **S02.610 Fracture of condylar process of mandible, unspecified side**   HCC Q ▽

² ✓7ᵗʰ **S02.611 Fracture of condylar process of right mandible**   HCC Q

² ✓7ᵗʰ **S02.612 Fracture of condylar process of left mandible**   HCC Q

✓6ᵗʰ **S02.62 Fracture of subcondylar process of mandible**

² ✓7ᵗʰ **S02.620 Fracture of subcondylar process of mandible, unspecified side**   HCC Q ▽

² ✓7ᵗʰ **S02.621 Fracture of subcondylar process of right mandible**   HCC Q

² ✓7ᵗʰ **S02.622 Fracture of subcondylar process of left mandible**   HCC Q

✓6ᵗʰ **S02.63 Fracture of coronoid process of mandible**

² ✓7ᵗʰ **S02.630 Fracture of coronoid process of mandible, unspecified side**   HCC Q ▽

² ✓7ᵗʰ **S02.631 Fracture of coronoid process of right mandible**   HCC Q

² ✓7ᵗʰ **S02.632 Fracture of coronoid process of left mandible**   HCC Q

✓6ᵗʰ **S02.64 Fracture of ramus of mandible**

² ✓7ᵗʰ **S02.640 Fracture of ramus of mandible, unspecified side**   HCC Q ▽

² ✓7ᵗʰ **S02.641 Fracture of ramus of right mandible**   HCC Q

² ✓7ᵗʰ **S02.642 Fracture of ramus of left mandible**   HCC Q

✓6ᵗʰ **S02.65 Fracture of angle of mandible**

² ✓7ᵗʰ **S02.650 Fracture of angle of mandible, unspecified side**   HCC Q ▽

² ✓7ᵗʰ **S02.651 Fracture of angle of right mandible**   HCC Q

² ✓7ᵗʰ **S02.652 Fracture of angle of left mandible**   HCC Q

² ✓x7ᵗʰ **S02.66 Fracture of symphysis of mandible**   HCC Q

✓6ᵗʰ **S02.67 Fracture of alveolus of mandible**

² ✓7ᵗʰ **S02.670 Fracture of alveolus of mandible, unspecified side**   HCC Q

² ✓7ᵗʰ **S02.671 Fracture of alveolus of right mandible**   HCC Q

² ✓7ᵗʰ **S02.672 Fracture of alveolus of left mandible**   HCC Q

² ✓x7ᵗʰ **S02.69 Fracture of mandible of other specified site**   HCC Q

✓5ᵗʰ **S02.8 Fractures of other specified skull and facial bones**
- Fracture of orbit NOS
- Fracture of palate
- **EXCLUDES 1**   fracture of orbital floor (S02.3-)
-      fracture of orbital roof (S02.1-)

² ✓x7ᵗʰ **S02.80 Fracture of other specified skull and facial bones, unspecified side**   HCC Q ▽

² ✓x7ᵗʰ **S02.81 Fracture of other specified skull and facial bones, right side**   HCC Q

² ✓x7ᵗʰ **S02.82 Fracture of other specified skull and facial bones, left side**   HCC Q

✓5ᵗʰ **S02.9 Fracture of unspecified skull and facial bones**

² ✓x7ᵗʰ **S02.91 Unspecified fracture of skull**   HCC Q ▽

² ✓x7ᵗʰ **S02.92 Unspecified fracture of facial bones**   HCC Q ▽

√4ᵗʰ **S03 Dislocation and sprain of joints and ligaments of head**

INCLUDES   avulsion of joint (capsule) or ligament of head
laceration of cartilage, joint (capsule) or ligament of head
sprain of cartilage, joint (capsule) or ligament of head
traumatic hemarthrosis of joint or ligament of head
traumatic rupture of joint or ligament of head
traumatic subluxation of joint or ligament of head
traumatic tear of joint or ligament of head

Code also any associated open wound

EXCLUDES 2   *strain of muscle or tendon of head (S09.1)*

The appropriate 7th character is to be added to each code from category S03.
A   initial encounter
D   subsequent encounter
S   sequela

√5ᵗʰ **S03.0 Dislocation of jaw**

Dislocation of jaw (cartilage) (meniscus)
Dislocation of mandible
Dislocation of temporomandibular (joint)
AHA: 2016,4Q,67

√x7ᵗʰ **S03.00 Dislocation of jaw, unspecified side** ▽

√x7ᵗʰ **S03.01 Dislocation of jaw, right side**

√x7ᵗʰ **S03.02 Dislocation of jaw, left side**

√x7ᵗʰ **S03.03 Dislocation of jaw, bilateral**

√x7ᵗʰ **S03.1 Dislocation of septal cartilage of nose**

√x7ᵗʰ **S03.2 Dislocation of tooth**

√5ᵗʰ **S03.4 Sprain of jaw**

Sprain of temporomandibular (joint) (ligament)
AHA: 2016,4Q,67

√x7ᵗʰ **S03.40 Sprain of jaw, unspecified side** ▽

√x7ᵗʰ **S03.41 Sprain of jaw, right side**

√x7ᵗʰ **S03.42 Sprain of jaw, left side**

√x7ᵗʰ **S03.43 Sprain of jaw, bilateral**

√x7ᵗʰ **S03.8 Sprain of joints and ligaments of other parts of head**

√x7ᵗʰ **S03.9 Sprain of joints and ligaments of unspecified parts of head** ▽

√4ᵗʰ **S04 Injury of cranial nerve**

The selection of side should be based on the side of the body being affected

Code first any associated intracranial injury (S06.-)
Code also any associated:
open wound of head (S01.-)
skull fracture (S02.-)

The appropriate 7th character is to be added to each code from category S04.
A   initial encounter
D   subsequent encounter
S   sequela

√5ᵗʰ **S04.0 Injury of optic nerve and pathways**

Use additional code to identify any visual field defect or blindness (H53.4-, H54.-)

√6ᵗʰ **S04.01 Injury of optic nerve**

Injury of 2nd cranial nerve

√7ᵗʰ **S04.011 Injury of optic nerve, right eye**

√7ᵗʰ **S04.012 Injury of optic nerve, left eye**

√7ᵗʰ **S04.019 Injury of optic nerve, unspecified eye** ▽

Injury of optic nerve NOS

√x7ᵗʰ **S04.02 Injury of optic chiasm**

√6ᵗʰ **S04.03 Injury of optic tract and pathways**

Injury of optic radiation

√7ᵗʰ **S04.031 Injury of optic tract and pathways, right side**

√7ᵗʰ **S04.032 Injury of optic tract and pathways, left side**

√7ᵗʰ **S04.039 Injury of optic tract and pathways, unspecified side** ▽

Injury of optic tract and pathways NOS

√6ᵗʰ **S04.04 Injury of visual cortex**

√7ᵗʰ **S04.041 Injury of visual cortex, right side**

√7ᵗʰ **S04.042 Injury of visual cortex, left side**

√7ᵗʰ **S04.049 Injury of visual cortex, unspecified side** ▽

Injury of visual cortex NOS

√5ᵗʰ **S04.1 Injury of oculomotor nerve**

Injury of 3rd cranial nerve

√x7ᵗʰ **S04.10 Injury of oculomotor nerve, unspecified side** ▽

√x7ᵗʰ **S04.11 Injury of oculomotor nerve, right side**

√x7ᵗʰ **S04.12 Injury of oculomotor nerve, left side**

√5ᵗʰ **S04.2 Injury of trochlear nerve**

Injury of 4th cranial nerve

√x7ᵗʰ **S04.20 Injury of trochlear nerve, unspecified side** ▽

√x7ᵗʰ **S04.21 Injury of trochlear nerve, right side**

√x7ᵗʰ **S04.22 Injury of trochlear nerve, left side**

√5ᵗʰ **S04.3 Injury of trigeminal nerve**

Injury of 5th cranial nerve

√x7ᵗʰ **S04.30 Injury of trigeminal nerve, unspecified side** ▽

√x7ᵗʰ **S04.31 Injury of trigeminal nerve, right side**

√x7ᵗʰ **S04.32 Injury of trigeminal nerve, left side**

√5ᵗʰ **S04.4 Injury of abducent nerve**

Injury of 6th cranial nerve

√x7ᵗʰ **S04.40 Injury of abducent nerve, unspecified side** ▽

√x7ᵗʰ **S04.41 Injury of abducent nerve, right side**

√x7ᵗʰ **S04.42 Injury of abducent nerve, left side**

√5ᵗʰ **S04.5 Injury of facial nerve**

Injury of 7th cranial nerve

√x7ᵗʰ **S04.50 Injury of facial nerve, unspecified side** ▽

√x7ᵗʰ **S04.51 Injury of facial nerve, right side**

√x7ᵗʰ **S04.52 Injury of facial nerve, left side**

√5ᵗʰ **S04.6 Injury of acoustic nerve**

Injury of auditory nerve
Injury of 8th cranial nerve

√x7ᵗʰ **S04.60 Injury of acoustic nerve, unspecified side** ▽

√x7ᵗʰ **S04.61 Injury of acoustic nerve, right side**

√x7ᵗʰ **S04.62 Injury of acoustic nerve, left side**

√5ᵗʰ **S04.7 Injury of accessory nerve**

Injury of 11th cranial nerve

√x7ᵗʰ **S04.70 Injury of accessory nerve, unspecified side** ▽

√x7ᵗʰ **S04.71 Injury of accessory nerve, right side**

√x7ᵗʰ **S04.72 Injury of accessory nerve, left side**

√5ᵗʰ **S04.8 Injury of other cranial nerves**

√6ᵗʰ **S04.81 Injury of olfactory [1st] nerve**

√7ᵗʰ **S04.811 Injury of olfactory [1st] nerve, right side**

√7ᵗʰ **S04.812 Injury of olfactory [1st] nerve, left side**

√7ᵗʰ **S04.819 Injury of olfactory [1st] nerve, unspecified side** ▽

√6ᵗʰ **S04.89 Injury of other cranial nerves**

Injury of vagus [10th] nerve

√7ᵗʰ **S04.891 Injury of other cranial nerves, right side**

√7ᵗʰ **S04.892 Injury of other cranial nerves, left side**

√7ᵗʰ **S04.899 Injury of other cranial nerves, unspecified side** ▽

√x7ᵗʰ **S04.9 Injury of unspecified cranial nerve** ▽

√4ᵗʰ **S05 Injury of eye and orbit**

INCLUDES   open wound of eye and orbit

EXCLUDES 2   *2nd cranial [optic] nerve injury (S04.0-)*
3rd cranial [oculomotor] nerve injury (S04.1-)
open wound of eyelid and periocular area (S01.1-)
orbital bone fracture (S02.1-, S02.3-, S02.8-)
superficial injury of eyelid (S00.1-S00.2)

The appropriate 7th character is to be added to each code from category S05.
A   initial encounter
D   subsequent encounter
S   sequela

√5ᵗʰ **S05.0 Injury of conjunctiva and corneal abrasion without foreign body**

EXCLUDES 1   *foreign body in conjunctival sac (T15.1)*
foreign body in cornea (T15.0)

√x7ᵗʰ **S05.00 Injury of conjunctiva and corneal abrasion without foreign body, unspecified eye** ▽

✓x7ᵗʰ **S05.01** **Injury of conjunctiva and corneal abrasion without foreign body, right eye**

✓x7ᵗʰ **S05.02** **Injury of conjunctiva and corneal abrasion without foreign body, left eye**

✓5ᵗʰ **S05.1** **Contusion of eyeball and orbital tissues**

Traumatic hyphema

EXCLUDES 2   black eye NOS (S00.1)

contusion of eyelid and periocular area (S00.1)

✓x7ᵗʰ **S05.10** **Contusion of eyeball and orbital tissues, unspecified eye** ▽

✓x7ᵗʰ **S05.11** **Contusion of eyeball and orbital tissues, right eye**

✓x7ᵗʰ **S05.12** **Contusion of eyeball and orbital tissues, left eye**

✓5ᵗʰ **S05.2** **Ocular laceration and rupture with prolapse or loss of intraocular tissue**

✓x7ᵗʰ **S05.20** **Ocular laceration and rupture with prolapse or loss of intraocular tissue, unspecified eye** ▽

✓x7ᵗʰ **S05.21** **Ocular laceration and rupture with prolapse or loss of intraocular tissue, right eye**

✓x7ᵗʰ **S05.22** **Ocular laceration and rupture with prolapse or loss of intraocular tissue, left eye**

✓5ᵗʰ **S05.3** **Ocular laceration without prolapse or loss of intraocular tissue**

Laceration of eye NOS

DEF: Tear in ocular tissue without displacing structures that is due to blunt trauma. It is characterized by pain, redness, and decreased vision.

✓x7ᵗʰ **S05.30** **Ocular laceration without prolapse or loss of intraocular tissue, unspecified eye** ▽

✓x7ᵗʰ **S05.31** **Ocular laceration without prolapse or loss of intraocular tissue, right eye**

✓x7ᵗʰ **S05.32** **Ocular laceration without prolapse or loss of intraocular tissue, left eye**

✓5ᵗʰ **S05.4** **Penetrating wound of orbit with or without foreign body**

EXCLUDES 2   retained (old) foreign body following penetrating wound in orbit (H05.5-)

✓x7ᵗʰ **S05.40** **Penetrating wound of orbit with or without foreign body, unspecified eye** ▽

✓x7ᵗʰ **S05.41** **Penetrating wound of orbit with or without foreign body, right eye**

✓x7ᵗʰ **S05.42** **Penetrating wound of orbit with or without foreign body, left eye**

✓5ᵗʰ **S05.5** **Penetrating wound with foreign body of eyeball**

EXCLUDES 2   retained (old) intraocular foreign body (H44.6-, H44.7)

✓x7ᵗʰ **S05.50** **Penetrating wound with foreign body of unspecified eyeball** ▽

✓x7ᵗʰ **S05.51** **Penetrating wound with foreign body of right eyeball**

✓x7ᵗʰ **S05.52** **Penetrating wound with foreign body of left eyeball**

✓5ᵗʰ **S05.6** **Penetrating wound without foreign body of eyeball**

Ocular penetration NOS

✓x7ᵗʰ **S05.60** **Penetrating wound without foreign body of unspecified eyeball** ▽

✓x7ᵗʰ **S05.61** **Penetrating wound without foreign body of right eyeball**

✓x7ᵗʰ **S05.62** **Penetrating wound without foreign body of left eyeball**

✓5ᵗʰ **S05.7** **Avulsion of eye**

Traumatic enucleation

✓x7ᵗʰ **S05.70** **Avulsion of unspecified eye** ▽

✓x7ᵗʰ **S05.71** **Avulsion of right eye**

✓x7ᵗʰ **S05.72** **Avulsion of left eye**

✓5ᵗʰ **S05.8** **Other injuries of eye and orbit**

Lacrimal duct injury

✓6ᵗʰ **S05.8X** **Other injuries of eye and orbit**

✓7ᵗʰ **S05.8X1** **Other injuries of right eye and orbit**

✓7ᵗʰ **S05.8X2** **Other injuries of left eye and orbit**

✓7ᵗʰ **S05.8X9** **Other injuries of unspecified eye and orbit** ▽

✓5ᵗʰ **S05.9** **Unspecified injury of eye and orbit**

Injury of eye NOS

✓x7ᵗʰ **S05.90** **Unspecified injury of unspecified eye and orbit** ▽

✓x7ᵗʰ **S05.91** **Unspecified injury of right eye and orbit** ▽

✓x7ᵗʰ **S05.92** **Unspecified injury of left eye and orbit** ▽

✓4ᵗʰ **S06** **Intracranial injury**

NOTE   7th characters D and S do not apply to codes in category S06 with 6th character 7 - death due to brain injury prior to regaining consciousness, or 8 - death due to other cause prior to regaining consciousness.

INCLUDES   traumatic brain injury

Code also any associated:

open wound of head (S01.-)

skull fracture (S02.-)

EXCLUDES 1   head injury NOS (S09.90)

AHA: 2017,4Q,25; 2017,1Q,42; 2015,3Q,37

TIP: Do not assign Z87.820 Personal history of traumatic brain injury, when residual conditions persist after an intracranial injury. The codes for the residual conditions should be first listed, followed by a code from category S06 using seventh character S to identify sequelae.

The appropriate 7th character is to be added to each code from category S06.

A   initial encounter

D   subsequent encounter

S   sequela

✓5ᵗʰ **S06.0** **Concussion**

Commotio cerebri

EXCLUDES 1   concussion with other intracranial injuries classified in subcategories S06.1- to S06.6- , S06.81- and S06.82- code to specified intracranial injury

AHA: 2016,4Q,67-68

✓6ᵗʰ **S06.0X** **Concussion**

³ ✓7ᵗʰ **S06.0X0** **Concussion without loss of consciousness** HCC Q

³ ✓7ᵗʰ **S06.0X1** **Concussion with loss of consciousness of 30 minutes or less** HCC Q

³ ✓7ᵗʰ **S06.0X9** **Concussion with loss of consciousness of unspecified duration** HCC Q ▽

Concussion NOS

✓5ᵗʰ **S06.1** **Traumatic cerebral edema**

Diffuse traumatic cerebral edema

Focal traumatic cerebral edema

✓6ᵗʰ **S06.1X** **Traumatic cerebral edema**

² ✓7ᵗʰ **S06.1X0** **Traumatic cerebral edema without loss of consciousness** HCC Q

² ✓7ᵗʰ **S06.1X1** **Traumatic cerebral edema with loss of consciousness of 30 minutes or less** HCC Q

² ✓7ᵗʰ **S06.1X2** **Traumatic cerebral edema with loss of consciousness of 31 minutes to 59 minutes** HCC Q

² ✓7ᵗʰ **S06.1X3** **Traumatic cerebral edema with loss of consciousness of 1 hour to 5 hours 59 minutes** HCC Q

² ✓7ᵗʰ **S06.1X4** **Traumatic cerebral edema with loss of consciousness of 6 hours to 24 hours** HCC Q

² ✓7ᵗʰ **S06.1X5** **Traumatic cerebral edema with loss of consciousness greater than 24 hours with return to pre-existing conscious level** HCC

² ✓7ᵗʰ **S06.1X6** **Traumatic cerebral edema with loss of consciousness greater than 24 hours without return to pre-existing conscious level with patient surviving** HCC

✓7ᵗʰ **S06.1X7** **Traumatic cerebral edema with loss of consciousness of any duration with death due to brain injury prior to regaining consciousness**

✓7ᵗʰ **S06.1X8** **Traumatic cerebral edema with loss of consciousness of any duration with death due to other cause prior to regaining consciousness**

² ✓7ᵗʰ **S06.1X9** **Traumatic cerebral edema with loss of consciousness of unspecified duration** HCC Q ▽

Traumatic cerebral edema NOS

√5ᵗʰ **S06.2** **Diffuse traumatic brain injury**

Diffuse axonal brain injury

EXCLUDES 1   traumatic diffuse cerebral edema (S06.1X-)

√6ᵗʰ **S06.2X** **Diffuse traumatic brain injury**

2 √7ᵗʰ **S06.2X0** **Diffuse traumatic brain injury** HCC Q
without loss of consciousness

2 √7ᵗʰ **S06.2X1** **Diffuse traumatic brain injury** HCC Q
**with loss of consciousness of 30
minutes or less**

2 √7ᵗʰ **S06.2X2** **Diffuse traumatic brain injury** HCC Q
**with loss of consciousness of 31
minutes to 59 minutes**

2 √7ᵗʰ **S06.2X3** **Diffuse traumatic brain injury** HCC Q
**with loss of consciousness of 1
hour to 5 hours 59 minutes**

2 √7ᵗʰ **S06.2X4** **Diffuse traumatic brain injury** HCC Q
**with loss of consciousness of 6
hours to 24 hours**

2 √7ᵗʰ **S06.2X5** **Diffuse traumatic brain injury** HCC
**with loss of consciousness greater
than 24 hours with return to
pre-existing conscious levels**

2 √7ᵗʰ **S06.2X6** **Diffuse traumatic brain injury** HCC
**with loss of consciousness greater
than 24 hours without return to
pre-existing conscious level with
patient surviving**

√7ᵗʰ **S06.2X7** **Diffuse traumatic brain injury with loss
of consciousness of any duration with
death due to brain injury prior to
regaining consciousness**

√7ᵗʰ **S06.2X8** **Diffuse traumatic brain injury with loss
of consciousness of any duration with
death due to other cause prior to
regaining consciousness**

2 √7ᵗʰ **S06.2X9** **Diffuse traumatic brain injury** HCC Q ▽
**with loss of consciousness of
unspecified duration**

Diffuse traumatic brain injury NOS

√5ᵗʰ **S06.3** **Focal traumatic brain injury**

EXCLUDES 1   any condition classifiable to S06.4-S06.6
focal cerebral edema (S06.1)

√6ᵗʰ **S06.30** **Unspecified focal traumatic brain injury**

2 √7ᵗʰ **S06.300** **Unspecified focal traumatic brain** HCC Q ▽
**injury without loss of
consciousness**

2 √7ᵗʰ **S06.301** **Unspecified focal traumatic brain** HCC Q ▽
**injury with loss of consciousness
of 30 minutes or less**

2 √7ᵗʰ **S06.302** **Unspecified focal traumatic brain** HCC Q ▽
**injury with loss of consciousness
of 31 minutes to 59 minutes**

2 √7ᵗʰ **S06.303** **Unspecified focal traumatic brain** HCC Q ▽
**injury with loss of consciousness
of 1 hour to 5 hours 59 minutes**

2 √7ᵗʰ **S06.304** **Unspecified focal traumatic brain** HCC Q ▽
**injury with loss of consciousness
of 6 hours to 24 hours**

2 √7ᵗʰ **S06.305** **Unspecified focal traumatic brain** HCC ▽
**injury with loss of consciousness
greater than 24 hours with return
to pre-existing conscious level**

2 √7ᵗʰ **S06.306** **Unspecified focal traumatic brain** HCC ▽
**injury with loss of consciousness
greater than 24 hours without
return to pre-existing conscious
level with patient surviving**

√7ᵗʰ **S06.307** **Unspecified focal traumatic brain** ▽
**injury with loss of consciousness
of any duration with death due
to brain injury prior to regaining
consciousness**

√7ᵗʰ **S06.308** **Unspecified focal traumatic brain** ▽
**injury with loss of consciousness
of any duration with death due
to other cause prior to regaining
consciousness**

2 √7ᵗʰ **S06.309** **Unspecified focal traumatic brain** HCC Q ▽
**injury with loss of consciousness
of unspecified duration**

Unspecified focal traumatic brain injury
NOS

√6ᵗʰ **S06.31** **Contusion and laceration of right cerebrum**

2 √7ᵗʰ **S06.310** **Contusion and laceration of right** HCC
**cerebrum without loss of
consciousness**

2 √7ᵗʰ **S06.311** **Contusion and laceration of right** HCC
**cerebrum with loss of
consciousness of 30 minutes or
less**

2 √7ᵗʰ **S06.312** **Contusion and laceration of right** HCC
**cerebrum with loss of
consciousness of 31 minutes to
59 minutes**

2 √7ᵗʰ **S06.313** **Contusion and laceration of right** HCC
**cerebrum with loss of
consciousness of 1 hour to 5
hours 59 minutes**

2 √7ᵗʰ **S06.314** **Contusion and laceration of right** HCC
**cerebrum with loss of
consciousness of 6 hours to 24
hours**

2 √7ᵗʰ **S06.315** **Contusion and laceration of right** HCC
**cerebrum with loss of
consciousness greater than 24
hours with return to pre-existing
conscious level**

2 √7ᵗʰ **S06.316** **Contusion and laceration of right** HCC
**cerebrum with loss of
consciousness greater than 24
hours without return to
pre-existing conscious level with
patient surviving**

√7ᵗʰ **S06.317** **Contusion and laceration of right
cerebrum with loss of consciousness of
any duration with death due to brain
injury prior to regaining consciousness**

√7ᵗʰ **S06.318** **Contusion and laceration of right
cerebrum with loss of consciousness of
any duration with death due to other
cause prior to regaining consciousness**

2 √7ᵗʰ **S06.319** **Contusion and laceration of right** HCC ▽
**cerebrum with loss of
consciousness of unspecified
duration**

Contusion and laceration of right cerebrum
NOS

√6ᵗʰ **S06.32** **Contusion and laceration of left cerebrum**

2 √7ᵗʰ **S06.320** **Contusion and laceration of left** HCC
**cerebrum without loss of
consciousness**

2 √7ᵗʰ **S06.321** **Contusion and laceration of left** HCC
**cerebrum with loss of
consciousness of 30 minutes or
less**

2 √7ᵗʰ **S06.322** **Contusion and laceration of left** HCC
**cerebrum with loss of
consciousness of 31 minutes to
59 minutes**

2 √7ᵗʰ **S06.323** **Contusion and laceration of left** HCC
**cerebrum with loss of
consciousness of 1 hour to 5
hours 59 minutes**

2 √7ᵗʰ **S06.324** **Contusion and laceration of left** HCC
**cerebrum with loss of
consciousness of 6 hours to 24
hours**

2 √7ᵗʰ **S06.325** **Contusion and laceration of left** HCC
**cerebrum with loss of
consciousness greater than 24
hours with return to pre-existing
conscious level**

2 √7ᵗʰ **S06.326** **Contusion and laceration of left** HCC
**cerebrum with loss of
consciousness greater than 24
hours without return to
pre-existing conscious level with
patient surviving**

√7ᵗʰ **S06.327** **Contusion and laceration of left cerebrum
with loss of consciousness of any duration
with death due to brain injury prior to
regaining consciousness**

√7ᵗʰ **S06.328** **Contusion and laceration of left cerebrum
with loss of consciousness of any duration
with death due to other cause prior to
regaining consciousness**

✓ Additional Character Req   ✓ₓ7ᵗʰ Placeholder Alert   Manifestation   ▽ Unspecified   ▶◀ Revised Text   ● New Code   ▲ Revised Code Title

ICD-10-CM 2019   957

2 √7ᵗʰ **S06.329** Contusion and laceration of left cerebrum with loss of consciousness of unspecified duration   HCC ▽

     Contusion and laceration of left cerebrum NOS

√6ᵗʰ **S06.33** Contusion and laceration of cerebrum, unspecified

2 √7ᵗʰ **S06.330** Contusion and laceration of cerebrum, unspecified, without loss of consciousness   HCC ▽

2 √7ᵗʰ **S06.331** Contusion and laceration of cerebrum, unspecified, with loss of consciousness of 30 minutes or less   HCC ▽

2 √7ᵗʰ **S06.332** Contusion and laceration of cerebrum, unspecified, with loss of consciousness of 31 minutes to 59 minutes   HCC ▽

2 √7ᵗʰ **S06.333** Contusion and laceration of cerebrum, unspecified, with loss of consciousness of 1 hour to 5 hours 59 minutes   HCC ▽

2 √7ᵗʰ **S06.334** Contusion and laceration of cerebrum, unspecified, with loss of consciousness of 6 hours to 24 hours   HCC ▽

2 √7ᵗʰ **S06.335** Contusion and laceration of cerebrum, unspecified, with loss of consciousness greater than 24 hours with return to pre-existing conscious level   HCC ▽

2 √7ᵗʰ **S06.336** Contusion and laceration of cerebrum, unspecified, with loss of consciousness greater than 24 hours without return to pre-existing conscious level with patient surviving   HCC ▽

√7ᵗʰ **S06.337** Contusion and laceration of cerebrum, unspecified, with loss of consciousness of any duration with death due to brain injury prior to regaining consciousness   ▽

√7ᵗʰ **S06.338** Contusion and laceration of cerebrum, unspecified, with loss of consciousness of any duration with death due to other cause prior to regaining consciousness   ▽

2 √7ᵗʰ **S06.339** Contusion and laceration of cerebrum, unspecified, with loss of consciousness of unspecified duration   HCC ▽

     Contusion and laceration of cerebrum NOS

√6ᵗʰ **S06.34** Traumatic hemorrhage of right cerebrum

     Traumatic intracerebral hemorrhage and hematoma of right cerebrum

2 √7ᵗʰ **S06.340** Traumatic hemorrhage of right cerebrum without loss of consciousness   HCC Q

2 √7ᵗʰ **S06.341** Traumatic hemorrhage of right cerebrum with loss of consciousness of 30 minutes or less   HCC Q

2 √7ᵗʰ **S06.342** Traumatic hemorrhage of right cerebrum with loss of consciousness of 31 minutes to 59 minutes   HCC Q

2 √7ᵗʰ **S06.343** Traumatic hemorrhage of right cerebrum with loss of consciousness of 1 hours to 5 hours 59 minutes   HCC Q

2 √7ᵗʰ **S06.344** Traumatic hemorrhage of right cerebrum with loss of consciousness of 6 hours to 24 hours   HCC Q

2 √7ᵗʰ **S06.345** Traumatic hemorrhage of right cerebrum with loss of consciousness greater than 24 hours with return to pre-existing conscious level   HCC

2 √7ᵗʰ **S06.346** Traumatic hemorrhage of right cerebrum with loss of consciousness greater than 24 hours without return to pre-existing conscious level with patient surviving   HCC

√7ᵗʰ **S06.347** Traumatic hemorrhage of right cerebrum with loss of consciousness of any duration with death due to brain injury prior to regaining consciousness

√7ᵗʰ **S06.348** Traumatic hemorrhage of right cerebrum with loss of consciousness of any duration with death due to other cause prior to regaining consciousness

2 √7ᵗʰ **S06.349** Traumatic hemorrhage of right cerebrum with loss of consciousness of unspecified duration   HCC Q ▽

     Traumatic hemorrhage of right cerebrum NOS

√6ᵗʰ **S06.35** Traumatic hemorrhage of left cerebrum

     Traumatic intracerebral hemorrhage and hematoma of left cerebrum

2 √7ᵗʰ **S06.350** Traumatic hemorrhage of left cerebrum without loss of consciousness   HCC Q

2 √7ᵗʰ **S06.351** Traumatic hemorrhage of left cerebrum with loss of consciousness of 30 minutes or less   HCC Q

2 √7ᵗʰ **S06.352** Traumatic hemorrhage of left cerebrum with loss of consciousness of 31 minutes to 59 minutes   HCC Q

2 √7ᵗʰ **S06.353** Traumatic hemorrhage of left cerebrum with loss of consciousness of 1 hours to 5 hours 59 minutes   HCC Q

2 √7ᵗʰ **S06.354** Traumatic hemorrhage of left cerebrum with loss of consciousness of 6 hours to 24 hours   HCC Q

2 √7ᵗʰ **S06.355** Traumatic hemorrhage of left cerebrum with loss of consciousness greater than 24 hours with return to pre-existing conscious level   HCC

2 √7ᵗʰ **S06.356** Traumatic hemorrhage of left cerebrum with loss of consciousness greater than 24 hours without return to pre-existing conscious level with patient surviving   HCC

√7ᵗʰ **S06.357** Traumatic hemorrhage of left cerebrum with loss of consciousness of any duration with death due to brain injury prior to regaining consciousness

√7ᵗʰ **S06.358** Traumatic hemorrhage of left cerebrum with loss of consciousness of any duration with death due to other cause prior to regaining consciousness

2 √7ᵗʰ **S06.359** Traumatic hemorrhage of left cerebrum with loss of consciousness of unspecified duration   HCC Q ▽

     Traumatic hemorrhage of left cerebrum NOS

√6ᵗʰ **S06.36** Traumatic hemorrhage of cerebrum, unspecified

     Traumatic intracerebral hemorrhage and hematoma, unspecified

2 √7ᵗʰ **S06.360** Traumatic hemorrhage of cerebrum, unspecified, without loss of consciousness   HCC Q ▽

2 √7ᵗʰ **S06.361** Traumatic hemorrhage of cerebrum, unspecified, with loss of consciousness of 30 minutes or less   HCC Q ▽

2 √7ᵗʰ **S06.362** Traumatic hemorrhage of cerebrum, unspecified, with loss of consciousness of 31 minutes to 59 minutes   HCC Q ▽

2 √7ᵗʰ **S06.363** Traumatic hemorrhage of cerebrum, unspecified, with loss of consciousness of 1 hours to 5 hours 59 minutes   HCC Q ▽

2 √7ᵗʰ **S06.364** Traumatic hemorrhage of cerebrum, unspecified, with loss of consciousness of 6 hours to 24 hours   HCC Q ▽

2 √7ᵗʰ **S06.365** **Traumatic hemorrhage of** HCC ▽
cerebrum, unspecified, with loss
of consciousness greater than 24
hours with return to pre-existing
conscious level

2 √7ᵗʰ **S06.366** **Traumatic hemorrhage of** HCC ▽
cerebrum, unspecified, with loss
of consciousness greater than 24
hours without return to
pre-existing conscious level with
patient surviving

√7ᵗʰ **S06.367** **Traumatic hemorrhage of** ▽
cerebrum, unspecified, with loss
of consciousness of any duration
with death due to brain injury
prior to regaining consciousness

√7ᵗʰ **S06.368** **Traumatic hemorrhage of** ▽
cerebrum, unspecified, with loss
of consciousness of any duration
with death due to other cause
prior to regaining consciousness

2 √7ᵗʰ **S06.369** **Traumatic hemorrhage of** HCC Q ▽
cerebrum, unspecified, with loss
of consciousness of unspecified
duration
> Traumatic hemorrhage of cerebrum NOS

√6ᵗʰ **S06.37** **Contusion, laceration, and hemorrhage of**
cerebellum

2 √7ᵗʰ **S06.370** **Contusion, laceration, and** HCC
hemorrhage of cerebellum
without loss of consciousness

2 √7ᵗʰ **S06.371** **Contusion, laceration, and** HCC
hemorrhage of cerebellum with
loss of consciousness of 30
minutes or less

2 √7ᵗʰ **S06.372** **Contusion, laceration, and** HCC
hemorrhage of cerebellum with
loss of consciousness of 31
minutes to 59 minutes

2 √7ᵗʰ **S06.373** **Contusion, laceration, and** HCC
hemorrhage of cerebellum with
loss of consciousness of 1 hour to
5 hours 59 minutes

2 √7ᵗʰ **S06.374** **Contusion, laceration, and** HCC
hemorrhage of cerebellum with
loss of consciousness of 6 hours
to 24 hours

2 √7ᵗʰ **S06.375** **Contusion, laceration, and** HCC
hemorrhage of cerebellum with
loss of consciousness greater than
24 hours with return to
pre-existing conscious level

2 √7ᵗʰ **S06.376** **Contusion, laceration, and** HCC
hemorrhage of cerebellum with
loss of consciousness greater than
24 hours without return to
pre-existing conscious level with
patient surviving

√7ᵗʰ **S06.377** **Contusion, laceration, and hemorrhage**
of cerebellum with loss of consciousness
of any duration with death due to brain
injury prior to regaining consciousness

√7ᵗʰ **S06.378** **Contusion, laceration, and hemorrhage**
of cerebellum with loss of consciousness
of any duration with death due to other
cause prior to regaining consciousness

2 √7ᵗʰ **S06.379** **Contusion, laceration, and** HCC ▽
hemorrhage of cerebellum with
loss of consciousness of
unspecified duration
> Contusion, laceration, and hemorrhage of
> cerebellum NOS

√6ᵗʰ **S06.38** **Contusion, laceration, and hemorrhage of**
brainstem

2 √7ᵗʰ **S06.380** **Contusion, laceration, and** HCC
hemorrhage of brainstem
without loss of consciousness

2 √7ᵗʰ **S06.381** **Contusion, laceration, and** HCC
hemorrhage of brainstem with
loss of consciousness of 30
minutes or less

2 √7ᵗʰ **S06.382** **Contusion, laceration, and** HCC
hemorrhage of brainstem with
loss of consciousness of 31
minutes to 59 minutes

2 √7ᵗʰ **S06.383** **Contusion, laceration, and** HCC
hemorrhage of brainstem with
loss of consciousness of 1 hour to
5 hours 59 minutes

2 √7ᵗʰ **S06.384** **Contusion, laceration, and** HCC
hemorrhage of brainstem with
loss of consciousness of 6 hours
to 24 hours

2 √7ᵗʰ **S06.385** **Contusion, laceration, and** HCC
hemorrhage of brainstem with
loss of consciousness greater than
24 hours with return to
pre-existing conscious level

2 √7ᵗʰ **S06.386** **Contusion, laceration, and** HCC
hemorrhage of brainstem with
loss of consciousness greater than
24 hours without return to
pre-existing conscious level with
patient surviving

√7ᵗʰ **S06.387** **Contusion, laceration, and hemorrhage**
of brainstem with loss of consciousness
of any duration with death due to brain
injury prior to regaining consciousness

√7ᵗʰ **S06.388** **Contusion, laceration, and hemorrhage**
of brainstem with loss of consciousness
of any duration with death due to other
cause prior to regaining consciousness

2 √7ᵗʰ **S06.389** **Contusion, laceration, and** HCC ▽
hemorrhage of brainstem with
loss of consciousness of
unspecified duration
> Contusion, laceration, and hemorrhage of
> brainstem NOS

√5ᵗʰ **S06.4** **Epidural hemorrhage**
Extradural hemorrhage NOS
Extradural hemorrhage (traumatic)
DEF: Epidural space: Space between the endosteum of the
cranium (skull) and the dura mater, the outermost layer of a
three-layer membrane that covers the brain.

√6ᵗʰ **S06.4X** **Epidural hemorrhage**

2 √7ᵗʰ **S06.4X0** **Epidural hemorrhage without** HCC Q
loss of consciousness

2 √7ᵗʰ **S06.4X1** **Epidural hemorrhage with loss of** HCC Q
consciousness of 30 minutes or
less

2 √7ᵗʰ **S06.4X2** **Epidural hemorrhage with loss of** HCC Q
consciousness of 31 minutes to
59 minutes

2 √7ᵗʰ **S06.4X3** **Epidural hemorrhage with loss of** HCC Q
consciousness of 1 hour to 5
hours 59 minutes

2 √7ᵗʰ **S06.4X4** **Epidural hemorrhage with loss of** HCC Q
consciousness of 6 hours to 24
hours

2 √7ᵗʰ **S06.4X5** **Epidural hemorrhage with loss of** HCC
consciousness greater than 24
hours with return to pre-existing
conscious level

2 √7ᵗʰ **S06.4X6** **Epidural hemorrhage with loss of** HCC
consciousness greater than 24
hours without return to
pre-existing conscious level with
patient surviving

√7ᵗʰ **S06.4X7** **Epidural hemorrhage with loss of**
consciousness of any duration with death
due to brain injury prior to regaining
consciousness

√7ᵗʰ **S06.4X8** **Epidural hemorrhage with loss of**
consciousness of any duration with death
due to other causes prior to regaining
consciousness

2 √7ᵗʰ **S06.4X9** **Epidural hemorrhage with loss of** HCC Q ▽
consciousness of unspecified
duration
> Epidural hemorrhage NOS

√5ᵗʰ **S06.5** **Traumatic subdural hemorrhage**
DEF: Subdural: Potential space between the dura mater and
arachnoid membrane around the brain.

√6ᵗʰ **S06.5X** **Traumatic subdural hemorrhage**

2 √7ᵗʰ **S06.5X0** **Traumatic subdural hemorrhage** HCC Q
without loss of consciousness

2 √7ᵗʰ **S06.5X1** **Traumatic subdural hemorrhage** HCC Q
with loss of consciousness of 30
minutes or less

☑ Additional Character Req   √x7ᵗʰ Placeholder Alert   **Manifestation**   ▽ Unspecified   ►◄ Revised Text   ● New Code   ▲ Revised Code Title

ICD-10-CM 2019   959

² ✓7ᵗʰ **S06.5X2 Traumatic subdural hemorrhage** HCC Q **with loss of consciousness of 31 minutes to 59 minutes**

² ✓7ᵗʰ **S06.5X3 Traumatic subdural hemorrhage** HCC Q **with loss of consciousness of 1 hour to 5 hours 59 minutes**

² ✓7ᵗʰ **S06.5X4 Traumatic subdural hemorrhage** HCC Q **with loss of consciousness of 6 hours to 24 hours**

² ✓7ᵗʰ **S06.5X5 Traumatic subdural hemorrhage** HCC **with loss of consciousness greater than 24 hours with return to pre-existing conscious level**

² ✓7ᵗʰ **S06.5X6 Traumatic subdural hemorrhage** HCC **with loss of consciousness greater than 24 hours without return to pre-existing conscious level with patient surviving**

✓7ᵗʰ **S06.5X7 Traumatic subdural hemorrhage with loss of consciousness of any duration with death due to brain injury before regaining consciousness**

✓7ᵗʰ **S06.5X8 Traumatic subdural hemorrhage with loss of consciousness of any duration with death due to other cause before regaining consciousness**

² ✓7ᵗʰ **S06.5X9 Traumatic subdural hemorrhage** HCC Q ▽ **with loss of consciousness of unspecified duration**

Traumatic subdural hemorrhage NOS

✓5ᵗʰ **S06.6 Traumatic subarachnoid hemorrhage**

DEF: Subarachnoid: Space located between the arachnoid membrane and the pia mater that contains cerebrospinal fluid.

✓6ᵗʰ **S06.6X Traumatic subarachnoid hemorrhage**

² ✓7ᵗʰ **S06.6X0 Traumatic subarachnoid hemorrhage without loss of consciousness** HCC Q

² ✓7ᵗʰ **S06.6X1 Traumatic subarachnoid hemorrhage with loss of consciousness of 30 minutes or less** HCC Q

² ✓7ᵗʰ **S06.6X2 Traumatic subarachnoid hemorrhage with loss of consciousness of 31 minutes to 59 minutes** HCC Q

² ✓7ᵗʰ **S06.6X3 Traumatic subarachnoid hemorrhage with loss of consciousness of 1 hour to 5 hours 59 minutes** HCC Q

² ✓7ᵗʰ **S06.6X4 Traumatic subarachnoid hemorrhage with loss of consciousness of 6 hours to 24 hours** HCC Q

² ✓7ᵗʰ **S06.6X5 Traumatic subarachnoid hemorrhage with loss of consciousness greater than 24 hours with return to pre-existing conscious level** HCC

² ✓7ᵗʰ **S06.6X6 Traumatic subarachnoid hemorrhage with loss of consciousness greater than 24 hours without return to pre-existing conscious level with patient surviving** HCC

✓7ᵗʰ **S06.6X7 Traumatic subarachnoid hemorrhage with loss of consciousness of any duration with death due to brain injury prior to regaining consciousness**

✓7ᵗʰ **S06.6X8 Traumatic subarachnoid hemorrhage with loss of consciousness of any duration with death due to other cause prior to regaining consciousness**

² ✓7ᵗʰ **S06.6X9 Traumatic subarachnoid hemorrhage with loss of consciousness of unspecified duration** HCC Q ▽

Traumatic subarachnoid hemorrhage NOS

✓5ᵗʰ **S06.8 Other specified intracranial injuries**

✓6ᵗʰ **S06.81 Injury of right internal carotid artery, intracranial portion, not elsewhere classified**

² ✓7ᵗʰ **S06.810 Injury of right internal carotid artery, intracranial portion, not elsewhere classified without loss of consciousness** HCC Q

² ✓7ᵗʰ **S06.811 Injury of right internal carotid artery, intracranial portion, not elsewhere classified with loss of consciousness of 30 minutes or less** HCC Q

² ✓7ᵗʰ **S06.812 Injury of right internal carotid artery, intracranial portion, not elsewhere classified with loss of consciousness of 31 minutes to 59 minutes** HCC Q

² ✓7ᵗʰ **S06.813 Injury of right internal carotid artery, intracranial portion, not elsewhere classified with loss of consciousness of 1 hour to 5 hours 59 minutes** HCC Q

² ✓7ᵗʰ **S06.814 Injury of right internal carotid artery, intracranial portion, not elsewhere classified with loss of consciousness of 6 hours to 24 hours** HCC Q

² ✓7ᵗʰ **S06.815 Injury of right internal carotid artery, intracranial portion, not elsewhere classified with loss of consciousness greater than 24 hours with return to pre-existing conscious level** HCC

² ✓7ᵗʰ **S06.816 Injury of right internal carotid artery, intracranial portion, not elsewhere classified with loss of consciousness greater than 24 hours without return to pre-existing conscious level with patient surviving** HCC

✓7ᵗʰ **S06.817 Injury of right internal carotid artery, intracranial portion, not elsewhere classified with loss of consciousness of any duration with death due to brain injury prior to regaining consciousness**

✓7ᵗʰ **S06.818 Injury of right internal carotid artery, intracranial portion, not elsewhere classified with loss of consciousness of any duration with death due to other cause prior to regaining consciousness**

² ✓7ᵗʰ **S06.819 Injury of right internal carotid artery, intracranial portion, not elsewhere classified with loss of consciousness of unspecified duration** HCC Q ▽

Injury of right internal carotid artery, intracranial portion, not elsewhere classified NOS

✓6ᵗʰ **S06.82 Injury of left internal carotid artery, intracranial portion, not elsewhere classified**

² ✓7ᵗʰ **S06.820 Injury of left internal carotid artery, intracranial portion, not elsewhere classified without loss of consciousness** HCC Q

² ✓7ᵗʰ **S06.821 Injury of left internal carotid artery, intracranial portion, not elsewhere classified with loss of consciousness of 30 minutes or less** HCC Q

² ✓7ᵗʰ **S06.822 Injury of left internal carotid artery, intracranial portion, not elsewhere classified with loss of consciousness of 31 minutes to 59 minutes** HCC Q

² ✓7ᵗʰ **S06.823 Injury of left internal carotid artery, intracranial portion, not elsewhere classified with loss of consciousness of 1 hour to 5 hours 59 minutes** HCC Q

² ✓7ᵗʰ **S06.824 Injury of left internal carotid artery, intracranial portion, not elsewhere classified with loss of consciousness of 6 hours to 24 hours** HCC Q

² ✓7ᵗʰ **S06.825 Injury of left internal carotid artery, intracranial portion, not elsewhere classified with loss of consciousness greater than 24 hours with return to pre-existing conscious level** HCC

2 √7ᵗʰ **S06.826** Injury of left internal carotid artery, intracranial portion, not elsewhere classified with loss of consciousness greater than 24 hours without return to pre-existing conscious level with patient surviving   HCC

√7ᵗʰ **S06.827** Injury of left internal carotid artery, intracranial portion, not elsewhere classified with loss of consciousness of any duration with death due to brain injury prior to regaining consciousness

√7ᵗʰ **S06.828** Injury of left internal carotid artery, intracranial portion, not elsewhere classified with loss of consciousness of any duration with death due to other cause prior to regaining consciousness

2 √7ᵗʰ **S06.829** Injury of left internal carotid artery, intracranial portion, not elsewhere classified with loss of consciousness of unspecified duration   HCC 🄾 ▽

     Injury of left internal carotid artery, intracranial portion, not elsewhere classified NOS

√6ᵗʰ **S06.89** Other specified intracranial injury

     EXCLUDES 1   concussion (S06.0X-)

2 √7ᵗʰ **S06.890** Other specified intracranial injury without loss of consciousness   HCC 🄾

2 √7ᵗʰ **S06.891** Other specified intracranial injury with loss of consciousness of 30 minutes or less   HCC 🄾

2 √7ᵗʰ **S06.892** Other specified intracranial injury with loss of consciousness of 31 minutes to 59 minutes   HCC 🄾

2 √7ᵗʰ **S06.893** Other specified intracranial injury with loss of consciousness of 1 hour to 5 hours 59 minutes   HCC 🄾

2 √7ᵗʰ **S06.894** Other specified intracranial injury with loss of consciousness of 6 hours to 24 hours   HCC 🄾

2 √7ᵗʰ **S06.895** Other specified intracranial injury with loss of consciousness greater than 24 hours with return to pre-existing conscious level   HCC

2 √7ᵗʰ **S06.896** Other specified intracranial injury with loss of consciousness greater than 24 hours without return to pre-existing conscious level with patient surviving   HCC

√7ᵗʰ **S06.897** Other specified intracranial injury with loss of consciousness of any duration with death due to brain injury prior to regaining consciousness

√7ᵗʰ **S06.898** Other specified intracranial injury with loss of consciousness of any duration with death due to other cause prior to regaining consciousness

2 √7ᵗʰ **S06.899** Other specified intracranial injury with loss of consciousness of unspecified duration   HCC 🄾 ▽

√5ᵗʰ **S06.9** Unspecified intracranial injury

     Brain injury NOS

     Head injury NOS with loss of consciousness

     Traumatic brain injury NOS

     EXCLUDES 1   conditions classifiable to S06.0- to S06.8- code to specified intracranial injury

             head injury NOS (S09.90)

√6ᵗʰ **S06.9X** Unspecified intracranial injury

2 √7ᵗʰ **S06.9X0** Unspecified intracranial injury without loss of consciousness   HCC 🄾 ▽

2 √7ᵗʰ **S06.9X1** Unspecified intracranial injury with loss of consciousness of 30 minutes or less   HCC 🄾 ▽

2 √7ᵗʰ **S06.9X2** Unspecified intracranial injury with loss of consciousness of 31 minutes to 59 minutes   HCC 🄾 ▽

2 √7ᵗʰ **S06.9X3** Unspecified intracranial injury with loss of consciousness of 1 hour to 5 hours 59 minutes   HCC 🄾 ▽

2 √7ᵗʰ **S06.9X4** Unspecified intracranial injury with loss of consciousness of 6 hours to 24 hours   HCC 🄾 ▽

2 √7ᵗʰ **S06.9X5** Unspecified intracranial injury with loss of consciousness greater than 24 hours with return to pre-existing conscious level   HCC ▽

2 √7ᵗʰ **S06.9X6** Unspecified intracranial injury with loss of consciousness greater than 24 hours without return to pre-existing conscious level with patient surviving   HCC ▽

√7ᵗʰ **S06.9X7** Unspecified intracranial injury with loss of consciousness of any duration with death due to brain injury prior to regaining consciousness ▽

√7ᵗʰ **S06.9X8** Unspecified intracranial injury with loss of consciousness of any duration with death due to other cause prior to regaining consciousness

2 √7ᵗʰ **S06.9X9** Unspecified intracranial injury with loss of consciousness of unspecified duration   HCC 🄾 ▽

√4ᵗʰ **S07** **Crushing injury of head**

     Use additional code for all associated injuries, such as:

         intracranial injuries (S06.-)

         skull fractures (S02.-)

     The appropriate 7th character is to be added to each code from category S07.

     A   initial encounter

     D   subsequent encounter

     S   sequela

√7ᵗʰ **S07.0** Crushing injury of face

√7ᵗʰ **S07.1** Crushing injury of skull

√7ᵗʰ **S07.8** Crushing injury of other parts of head

√7ᵗʰ **S07.9** Crushing injury of head, part unspecified ▽

√4ᵗʰ **S08** **Avulsion and traumatic amputation of part of head**

     An amputation not identified as partial or complete should be coded to complete

     The appropriate 7th character is to be added to each code from category S08.

     A   initial encounter

     D   subsequent encounter

     S   sequela

√7ᵗʰ **S08.0** Avulsion of scalp

√5ᵗʰ **S08.1** Traumatic amputation of ear

     √6ᵗʰ **S08.11** Complete traumatic amputation of ear

         √7ᵗʰ **S08.111** Complete traumatic amputation of right ear

         √7ᵗʰ **S08.112** Complete traumatic amputation of left ear

         √7ᵗʰ **S08.119** Complete traumatic amputation of unspecified ear ▽

     √6ᵗʰ **S08.12** Partial traumatic amputation of ear

         √7ᵗʰ **S08.121** Partial traumatic amputation of right ear

         √7ᵗʰ **S08.122** Partial traumatic amputation of left ear

         √7ᵗʰ **S08.129** Partial traumatic amputation of unspecified ear ▽

√5ᵗʰ **S08.8** Traumatic amputation of other parts of head

     √6ᵗʰ **S08.81** Traumatic amputation of nose

         √7ᵗʰ **S08.811** Complete traumatic amputation of nose

         √7ᵗʰ **S08.812** Partial traumatic amputation of nose

     √7ᵗʰ **S08.89** Traumatic amputation of other parts of head

√4ᵗʰ **S09** **Other and unspecified injuries of head**

     The appropriate 7th character is to be added to each code from category S09.

     A   initial encounter

     D   subsequent encounter

     S   sequela

√7ᵗʰ **S09.0** Injury of blood vessels of head, not elsewhere classified

     EXCLUDES 1   injury of cerebral blood vessels (S06.-)

             injury of precerebral blood vessels (S15.-)

✔ Additional Character Req   √7ᵗʰ Placeholder Alert   Manifestation   ▽ Unspecified   ▶◀ Revised Text   ● New Code   ▲ Revised Code Title

ICD-10-CM 2019   **961**

√5ᵗʰ **S09.1** **Injury of muscle and tendon of head**

Code also any associated open wound (S01.-)

EXCLUDES 2   *sprain to joints and ligament of head (S03.9)*

√x7ᵗʰ **S09.10** **Unspecified injury of muscle and tendon of head**   ◘ ▽

Injury of muscle and tendon of head NOS

√x7ᵗʰ **S09.11** **Strain of muscle and tendon of head**   ◘

√x7ᵗʰ **S09.12** **Laceration of muscle and tendon of head**

√x7ᵗʰ **S09.19** **Other specified injury of muscle and tendon of head**   ◘

√5ᵗʰ **S09.2** **Traumatic rupture of ear drum**

EXCLUDES 1   *traumatic rupture of ear drum due to blast injury (S09.31-)*

√x7ᵗʰ **S09.20** **Traumatic rupture of unspecified ear drum**   ▽

√x7ᵗʰ **S09.21** **Traumatic rupture of right ear drum**

√x7ᵗʰ **S09.22** **Traumatic rupture of left ear drum**

√5ᵗʰ **S09.3** **Other specified and unspecified injury of middle and inner ear**

EXCLUDES 1   *injury to ear NOS (S09.91-)*

EXCLUDES 2   *injury to external ear (S00.4-, S01.3-, S08.1-)*

√6ᵗʰ **S09.30** **Unspecified injury of middle and inner ear**

√7ᵗʰ **S09.301** **Unspecified injury of right middle and inner ear**   ▽

√7ᵗʰ **S09.302** **Unspecified injury of left middle and inner ear**   ▽

√7ᵗʰ **S09.309** **Unspecified injury of unspecified middle and inner ear**   ▽

√6ᵗʰ **S09.31** **Primary blast injury of ear**

Blast injury of ear NOS

√7ᵗʰ **S09.311** **Primary blast injury of right ear**

√7ᵗʰ **S09.312** **Primary blast injury of left ear**

√7ᵗʰ **S09.313** **Primary blast injury of ear, bilateral**

√7ᵗʰ **S09.319** **Primary blast injury of unspecified ear**   ▽

√6ᵗʰ **S09.39** **Other specified injury of middle and inner ear**

Secondary blast injury to ear

√7ᵗʰ **S09.391** **Other specified injury of right middle and inner ear**

√7ᵗʰ **S09.392** **Other specified injury of left middle and inner ear**

√7ᵗʰ **S09.399** **Other specified injury of unspecified middle and inner ear**   ▽

√x7ᵗʰ **S09.8** **Other specified injuries of head**   ◘

√5ᵗʰ **S09.9** **Unspecified injury of face and head**

√x7ᵗʰ **S09.90** **Unspecified injury of head**   ◘ ▽

Head injury NOS

EXCLUDES 1   *brain injury NOS (S06.9-)*

head injury NOS with loss of consciousness (S06.9-)

intracranial injury NOS (S06.9-)

√x7ᵗʰ **S09.91** **Unspecified injury of ear**   ▽

Injury of ear NOS

√x7ᵗʰ **S09.92** **Unspecified injury of nose**   ◘ ▽

Injury of nose NOS

√x7ᵗʰ **S09.93** **Unspecified injury of face**   ◘ ▽

Injury of face NOS

Injuries to the neck (S10–S19)

INCLUDES   injuries of nape

injuries of supraclavicular region

injuries of throat

EXCLUDES 2   *burns and corrosions (T20-T32)*

effects of foreign body in esophagus (T18.1)

effects of foreign body in larynx (T17.3)

effects of foreign body in pharynx (T17.2)

effects of foreign body in trachea (T17.4)

frostbite (T33-T34)

insect bite or sting, venomous (T63.4)

√4ᵗʰ **S10** **Superficial injury of neck**

The appropriate 7th character is to be added to each code from category S10.

A   initial encounter

D   subsequent encounter

S   sequela

√x7ᵗʰ **S10.0** **Contusion of throat**   ◘

Contusion of cervical esophagus

Contusion of larynx

Contusion of pharynx

Contusion of trachea

√5ᵗʰ **S10.1** **Other and unspecified superficial injuries of throat**

√x7ᵗʰ **S10.10** **Unspecified superficial injuries of throat**   ▽

√x7ᵗʰ **S10.11** **Abrasion of throat**

√x7ᵗʰ **S10.12** **Blister (nonthermal) of throat**

√x7ᵗʰ **S10.14** **External constriction of part of throat**

√x7ᵗʰ **S10.15** **Superficial foreign body of throat**

Splinter in the throat

√x7ᵗʰ **S10.16** **Insect bite (nonvenomous) of throat**

√x7ᵗʰ **S10.17** **Other superficial bite of throat**

EXCLUDES 1   *open bite of throat (S11.85)*

√5ᵗʰ **S10.8** **Superficial injury of other specified parts of neck**

√x7ᵗʰ **S10.80** **Unspecified superficial injury of other specified part of neck**   ▽

√x7ᵗʰ **S10.81** **Abrasion of other specified part of neck**

√x7ᵗʰ **S10.82** **Blister (nonthermal) of other specified part of neck**

√x7ᵗʰ **S10.83** **Contusion of other specified part of neck**   ◘

√x7ᵗʰ **S10.84** **External constriction of other specified part of neck**

√x7ᵗʰ **S10.85** **Superficial foreign body of other specified part of neck**

Splinter in other specified part of neck

√x7ᵗʰ **S10.86** **Insect bite of other specified part of neck**

√x7ᵗʰ **S10.87** **Other superficial bite of other specified part of neck**

EXCLUDES 1   *open bite of other specified parts of neck (S11.85)*

√5ᵗʰ **S10.9** **Superficial injury of unspecified part of neck**

√x7ᵗʰ **S10.90** **Unspecified superficial injury of unspecified part of neck**   ▽

√x7ᵗʰ **S10.91** **Abrasion of unspecified part of neck**   ▽

√x7ᵗʰ **S10.92** **Blister (nonthermal) of unspecified part of neck**   ▽

√x7ᵗʰ **S10.93** **Contusion of unspecified part of neck**   ◘ ▽

√x7ᵗʰ **S10.94** **External constriction of unspecified part of neck**   ▽

√x7ᵗʰ **S10.95** **Superficial foreign body of unspecified part of neck**   ▽

√x7ᵗʰ **S10.96** **Insect bite of unspecified part of neck**   ▽

√x7ᵗʰ **S10.97** **Other superficial bite of unspecified part of neck**   ▽

√4ᵗʰ **S11 Open wound of neck**

Code also any associated:
spinal cord injury (S14.0, S14.1-)
wound infection
EXCLUDES 2   open fracture of vertebra (S12.- with 7th character B)

> The appropriate 7th character is to be added to each code from category S11.
> A   initial encounter
> D   subsequent encounter
> S   sequela

√5ᵗʰ **S11.0 Open wound of larynx and trachea**

√6ᵗʰ **S11.01 Open wound of larynx**

EXCLUDES 2   open wound of vocal cord (S11.03)

√7ᵗʰ **S11.011 Laceration without foreign body of larynx**

√7ᵗʰ **S11.012 Laceration with foreign body of larynx**

√7ᵗʰ **S11.013 Puncture wound without foreign body of larynx**

√7ᵗʰ **S11.014 Puncture wound with foreign body of larynx**

√7ᵗʰ **S11.015 Open bite of larynx**

Bite of larynx NOS

√7ᵗʰ **S11.019 Unspecified open wound of larynx** ▽

√6ᵗʰ **S11.02 Open wound of trachea**

Open wound of cervical trachea
Open wound of trachea NOS
EXCLUDES 2   open wound of thoracic trachea (S27.5-)

√7ᵗʰ **S11.021 Laceration without foreign body of trachea**

√7ᵗʰ **S11.022 Laceration with foreign body of trachea**

√7ᵗʰ **S11.023 Puncture wound without foreign body of trachea**

√7ᵗʰ **S11.024 Puncture wound with foreign body of trachea**

√7ᵗʰ **S11.025 Open bite of trachea**

Bite of trachea NOS

√7ᵗʰ **S11.029 Unspecified open wound of trachea** ▽

√6ᵗʰ **S11.03 Open wound of vocal cord**

√7ᵗʰ **S11.031 Laceration without foreign body of vocal cord**

√7ᵗʰ **S11.032 Laceration with foreign body of vocal cord**

√7ᵗʰ **S11.033 Puncture wound without foreign body of vocal cord**

√7ᵗʰ **S11.034 Puncture wound with foreign body of vocal cord**

√7ᵗʰ **S11.035 Open bite of vocal cord**

Bite of vocal cord NOS

√7ᵗʰ **S11.039 Unspecified open wound of vocal cord** ▽

√5ᵗʰ **S11.1 Open wound of thyroid gland**

√x7ᵗʰ **S11.10 Unspecified open wound of thyroid gland** ▽

√x7ᵗʰ **S11.11 Laceration without foreign body of thyroid gland**

√x7ᵗʰ **S11.12 Laceration with foreign body of thyroid gland**

√x7ᵗʰ **S11.13 Puncture wound without foreign body of thyroid gland**

√x7ᵗʰ **S11.14 Puncture wound with foreign body of thyroid gland**

√x7ᵗʰ **S11.15 Open bite of thyroid gland**

Bite of thyroid gland NOS

√5ᵗʰ **S11.2 Open wound of pharynx and cervical esophagus**

EXCLUDES 1   open wound of esophagus NOS (S27.8-)

√x7ᵗʰ **S11.20 Unspecified open wound of pharynx and cervical esophagus** ▽

√x7ᵗʰ **S11.21 Laceration without foreign body of pharynx and cervical esophagus**

√x7ᵗʰ **S11.22 Laceration with foreign body of pharynx and cervical esophagus**

√x7ᵗʰ **S11.23 Puncture wound without foreign body of pharynx and cervical esophagus**

√x7ᵗʰ **S11.24 Puncture wound with foreign body of pharynx and cervical esophagus**

√x7ᵗʰ **S11.25 Open bite of pharynx and cervical esophagus**

Bite of pharynx and cervical esophagus NOS

√5ᵗʰ **S11.8 Open wound of other specified parts of neck**

√x7ᵗʰ **S11.80 Unspecified open wound of other specified part of neck** ▽

√x7ᵗʰ **S11.81 Laceration without foreign body of other specified part of neck**

√x7ᵗʰ **S11.82 Laceration with foreign body of other specified part of neck**

√x7ᵗʰ **S11.83 Puncture wound without foreign body of other specified part of neck**

√x7ᵗʰ **S11.84 Puncture wound with foreign body of other specified part of neck**

√x7ᵗʰ **S11.85 Open bite of other specified part of neck**

Bite of other specified part of neck NOS
EXCLUDES 1   superficial bite of other specified part of neck (S10.87)

√x7ᵗʰ **S11.89 Other open wound of other specified part of neck**

√5ᵗʰ **S11.9 Open wound of unspecified part of neck**

√x7ᵗʰ **S11.90 Unspecified open wound of unspecified part of neck** ▽

√x7ᵗʰ **S11.91 Laceration without foreign body of unspecified part of neck** ▽

√x7ᵗʰ **S11.92 Laceration with foreign body of unspecified part of neck** ▽

√x7ᵗʰ **S11.93 Puncture wound without foreign body of unspecified part of neck** ▽

√x7ᵗʰ **S11.94 Puncture wound with foreign body of unspecified part of neck** ▽

√x7ᵗʰ **S11.95 Open bite of unspecified part of neck** ▽

Bite of neck NOS
EXCLUDES 1   superficial bite of neck (S10.97)

√4ᵗʰ **S12 Fracture of cervical vertebra and other parts of neck**

NOTE   A fracture not indicated as displaced or nondisplaced should be coded to displaced.

A fracture not indicated as open or closed should be coded to closed.

INCLUDES   fracture of cervical neural arch
fracture of cervical spine
fracture of cervical spinous process
fracture of cervical transverse process
fracture of cervical vertebral arch
fracture of neck

Code first any associated cervical spinal cord injury (S14.0, S14.1-)
AHA: 2018,2Q,12; 2015,3Q,37-39

> The appropriate 7th character is to be added to all codes from subcategories S12.0-S12.6.
> A   initial encounter for closed fracture
> B   initial encounter for open fracture
> D   subsequent encounter for fracture with routine healing
> G   subsequent encounter for fracture with delayed healing
> K   subsequent encounter for fracture with nonunion
> S   sequela

√5ᵗʰ **S12.0 Fracture of first cervical vertebra**

Atlas

√6ᵗʰ **S12.00 Unspecified fracture of first cervical vertebra**

¹ √7ᵗʰ **S12.000 Unspecified displaced fracture of first cervical vertebra** HCC 🄾 ▽

¹ √7ᵗʰ **S12.001 Unspecified nondisplaced fracture of first cervical vertebra** HCC 🄾 ▽

¹ √x7ᵗʰ **S12.01 Stable burst fracture of first cervical vertebra** HCC 🄾

¹ √x7ᵗʰ **S12.02 Unstable burst fracture of first cervical vertebra** HCC 🄾

√6ᵗʰ **S12.03 Posterior arch fracture of first cervical vertebra**

¹ √7ᵗʰ **S12.030 Displaced posterior arch fracture of first cervical vertebra** HCC 🄾

¹ √7ᵗʰ **S12.031 Nondisplaced posterior arch fracture of first cervical vertebra** HCC 🄾

√6ᵗʰ **S12.04 Lateral mass fracture of first cervical vertebra**

¹ √7ᵗʰ **S12.040 Displaced lateral mass fracture of first cervical vertebra** HCC 🄾

¹ √7ᵗʰ **S12.041 Nondisplaced lateral mass fracture of first cervical vertebra** HCC 🄾

√6ᵗʰ **S12.09 Other fracture of first cervical vertebra**

¹ √7ᵗʰ **S12.090 Other displaced fracture of first cervical vertebra** HCC 🄾

¹ √7ᵗʰ **S12.091 Other nondisplaced fracture of first cervical vertebra** HCC 🄾

☑ Additional Character Req   √x7ᵗʰ Placeholder Alert   Manifestation   ▽ Unspecified   ►◄ Revised Text   ● New Code   ▲ Revised Code Title

ICD-10-CM 2019   963

√5ᵗʰ **S12.1** Fracture of second cervical vertebra
Axis

√6ᵗʰ **S12.10** Unspecified fracture of second cervical vertebra

[1] √7ᵗʰ **S12.100** Unspecified displaced fracture of HCC Q ▽ second cervical vertebra

[1] √7ᵗʰ **S12.101** Unspecified nondisplaced fracture of second cervical vertebra HCC Q ▽

√6ᵗʰ **S12.11** Type II dens fracture

[1] √7ᵗʰ **S12.110** Anterior displaced Type II dens fracture HCC Q

[1] √7ᵗʰ **S12.111** Posterior displaced Type II dens fracture HCC Q

[1] √7ᵗʰ **S12.112** Nondisplaced Type II dens fracture HCC Q

√6ᵗʰ **S12.12** Other dens fracture

[1] √7ᵗʰ **S12.120** Other displaced dens fracture HCC Q

[1] √7ᵗʰ **S12.121** Other nondisplaced dens fracture HCC Q

√6ᵗʰ **S12.13** Unspecified traumatic spondylolisthesis of second cervical vertebra

[1] √7ᵗʰ **S12.130** Unspecified traumatic displaced spondylolisthesis of second cervical vertebra HCC Q ▽

[1] √7ᵗʰ **S12.131** Unspecified traumatic nondisplaced spondylolisthesis of second cervical vertebra HCC Q ▽

[1] √x7ᵗʰ **S12.14** Type III traumatic spondylolisthesis of second cervical vertebra HCC Q

√6ᵗʰ **S12.15** Other traumatic spondylolisthesis of second cervical vertebra

[1] √7ᵗʰ **S12.150** Other traumatic displaced spondylolisthesis of second cervical vertebra HCC Q

[1] √7ᵗʰ **S12.151** Other traumatic nondisplaced spondylolisthesis of second cervical vertebra HCC Q

√6ᵗʰ **S12.19** Other fracture of second cervical vertebra

[1] √7ᵗʰ **S12.190** Other displaced fracture of second cervical vertebra HCC Q

[1] √7ᵗʰ **S12.191** Other nondisplaced fracture of second cervical vertebra HCC Q

√5ᵗʰ **S12.2** Fracture of third cervical vertebra

√6ᵗʰ **S12.20** Unspecified fracture of third cervical vertebra

[1] √7ᵗʰ **S12.200** Unspecified displaced fracture of third cervical vertebra HCC Q ▽

[1] √7ᵗʰ **S12.201** Unspecified nondisplaced fracture of third cervical vertebra HCC Q ▽

√6ᵗʰ **S12.23** Unspecified traumatic spondylolisthesis of third cervical vertebra

[1] √7ᵗʰ **S12.230** Unspecified traumatic displaced spondylolisthesis of third cervical vertebra HCC Q ▽

[1] √7ᵗʰ **S12.231** Unspecified traumatic nondisplaced spondylolisthesis of third cervical vertebra HCC Q ▽

[1] √x7ᵗʰ **S12.24** Type III traumatic spondylolisthesis of third cervical vertebra HCC Q

√6ᵗʰ **S12.25** Other traumatic spondylolisthesis of third cervical vertebra

[1] √7ᵗʰ **S12.250** Other traumatic displaced spondylolisthesis of third cervical vertebra HCC Q

[1] √7ᵗʰ **S12.251** Other traumatic nondisplaced spondylolisthesis of third cervical vertebra HCC Q

√6ᵗʰ **S12.29** Other fracture of third cervical vertebra

[1] √7ᵗʰ **S12.290** Other displaced fracture of third cervical vertebra HCC Q

[1] √7ᵗʰ **S12.291** Other nondisplaced fracture of third cervical vertebra HCC Q

√5ᵗʰ **S12.3** Fracture of fourth cervical vertebra

√6ᵗʰ **S12.30** Unspecified fracture of fourth cervical vertebra

[1] √7ᵗʰ **S12.300** Unspecified displaced fracture of fourth cervical vertebra HCC Q ▽

[1] √7ᵗʰ **S12.301** Unspecified nondisplaced fracture of fourth cervical vertebra HCC Q ▽

√6ᵗʰ **S12.33** Unspecified traumatic spondylolisthesis of fourth cervical vertebra

[1] √7ᵗʰ **S12.330** Unspecified traumatic displaced spondylolisthesis of fourth cervical vertebra HCC Q ▽

[1] √7ᵗʰ **S12.331** Unspecified traumatic nondisplaced spondylolisthesis of fourth cervical vertebra HCC Q ▽

[1] √x7ᵗʰ **S12.34** Type III traumatic spondylolisthesis of fourth cervical vertebra HCC Q

√6ᵗʰ **S12.35** Other traumatic spondylolisthesis of fourth cervical vertebra

[1] √7ᵗʰ **S12.350** Other traumatic displaced spondylolisthesis of fourth cervical vertebra HCC Q

[1] √7ᵗʰ **S12.351** Other traumatic nondisplaced spondylolisthesis of fourth cervical vertebra HCC Q

√6ᵗʰ **S12.39** Other fracture of fourth cervical vertebra

[1] √7ᵗʰ **S12.390** Other displaced fracture of fourth cervical vertebra HCC Q

[1] √7ᵗʰ **S12.391** Other nondisplaced fracture of fourth cervical vertebra HCC Q

√5ᵗʰ **S12.4** Fracture of fifth cervical vertebra

√6ᵗʰ **S12.40** Unspecified fracture of fifth cervical vertebra

[1] √7ᵗʰ **S12.400** Unspecified displaced fracture of fifth cervical vertebra HCC Q ▽

[1] √7ᵗʰ **S12.401** Unspecified nondisplaced fracture of fifth cervical vertebra HCC Q ▽

√6ᵗʰ **S12.43** Unspecified traumatic spondylolisthesis of fifth cervical vertebra

[1] √7ᵗʰ **S12.430** Unspecified traumatic displaced spondylolisthesis of fifth cervical vertebra HCC Q ▽

[1] √7ᵗʰ **S12.431** Unspecified traumatic nondisplaced spondylolisthesis of fifth cervical vertebra HCC Q ▽

[1] √x7ᵗʰ **S12.44** Type III traumatic spondylolisthesis of fifth cervical vertebra HCC Q

√6ᵗʰ **S12.45** Other traumatic spondylolisthesis of fifth cervical vertebra

[1] √7ᵗʰ **S12.450** Other traumatic displaced spondylolisthesis of fifth cervical vertebra HCC Q

[1] √7ᵗʰ **S12.451** Other traumatic nondisplaced spondylolisthesis of fifth cervical vertebra HCC Q

√6ᵗʰ **S12.49** Other fracture of fifth cervical vertebra

[1] √7ᵗʰ **S12.490** Other displaced fracture of fifth cervical vertebra HCC Q

[1] √7ᵗʰ **S12.491** Other nondisplaced fracture of fifth cervical vertebra HCC Q

√5ᵗʰ **S12.5** Fracture of sixth cervical vertebra

√6ᵗʰ **S12.50** Unspecified fracture of sixth cervical vertebra

[1] √7ᵗʰ **S12.500** Unspecified displaced fracture of sixth cervical vertebra HCC Q ▽

[1] √7ᵗʰ **S12.501** Unspecified nondisplaced fracture of sixth cervical vertebra HCC Q ▽

√6ᵗʰ **S12.53** Unspecified traumatic spondylolisthesis of sixth cervical vertebra

[1] √7ᵗʰ **S12.530** Unspecified traumatic displaced spondylolisthesis of sixth cervical vertebra HCC Q ▽

[1] √7ᵗʰ **S12.531** Unspecified traumatic nondisplaced spondylolisthesis of sixth cervical vertebra HCC Q ▽

[1] √x7ᵗʰ **S12.54** Type III traumatic spondylolisthesis of sixth cervical vertebra HCC Q

√6ᵗʰ **S12.55** Other traumatic spondylolisthesis of sixth cervical vertebra

[1] √7ᵗʰ **S12.550** Other traumatic displaced spondylolisthesis of sixth cervical vertebra HCC Q

[1] √7ᵗʰ **S12.551** Other traumatic nondisplaced spondylolisthesis of sixth cervical vertebra HCC Q

√6ᵗʰ **S12.59** Other fracture of sixth cervical vertebra

[1] √7ᵗʰ **S12.590** Other displaced fracture of sixth cervical vertebra HCC Q

[1] √7ᵗʰ **S12.591** Other nondisplaced fracture of sixth cervical vertebra HCC Q

√5ᵗʰ **S12.6 Fracture of seventh cervical vertebra**

√6ᵗʰ **S12.60 Unspecified fracture of seventh cervical vertebra**

¹ √7ᵗʰ **S12.600 Unspecified displaced fracture of** HCC Q ▽ **seventh cervical vertebra**

¹ √7ᵗʰ **S12.601 Unspecified nondisplaced** HCC Q ▽ **fracture of seventh cervical vertebra**

√6ᵗʰ **S12.63 Unspecified traumatic spondylolisthesis of seventh cervical vertebra**

¹ √7ᵗʰ **S12.630 Unspecified traumatic displaced** HCC Q ▽ **spondylolisthesis of seventh cervical vertebra**

¹ √7ᵗʰ **S12.631 Unspecified traumatic nondisplaced spondylolisthesis of seventh cervical vertebra** HCC Q ▽

¹ √x7ᵗʰ **S12.64 Type III traumatic spondylolisthesis of** HCC Q **seventh cervical vertebra**

√6ᵗʰ **S12.65 Other traumatic spondylolisthesis of seventh cervical vertebra**

¹ √7ᵗʰ **S12.650 Other traumatic displaced** HCC Q **spondylolisthesis of seventh cervical vertebra**

¹ √7ᵗʰ **S12.651 Other traumatic nondisplaced** HCC Q **spondylolisthesis of seventh cervical vertebra**

√6ᵗʰ **S12.69 Other fracture of seventh cervical vertebra**

¹ √7ᵗʰ **S12.690 Other displaced fracture of** HCC Q **seventh cervical vertebra**

¹ √7ᵗʰ **S12.691 Other nondisplaced fracture of** HCC Q **seventh cervical vertebra**

¹ √x7ᵗʰ **S12.8 Fracture of other parts of neck** HCC Q

Hyoid bone
Larynx
Thyroid cartilage
Trachea

The appropriate 7th character is to be added to code S12.8.
A initial encounter
D subsequent encounter
S sequela

¹ √x7ᵗʰ **S12.9 Fracture of neck, unspecified** HCC Q ▽

Fracture of neck NOS
Fracture of cervical spine NOS
Fracture of cervical vertebra NOS

The appropriate 7th character is to be added to code S12.9.
A initial encounter
D subsequent encounter
S sequela

√4ᵗʰ **S13 Dislocation and sprain of joints and ligaments at neck level**

INCLUDES avulsion of joint or ligament at neck level
laceration of cartilage, joint or ligament at neck level
sprain of cartilage, joint or ligament at neck level
traumatic hemarthrosis of joint or ligament at neck level
traumatic rupture of joint or ligament at neck level
traumatic subluxation of joint or ligament at neck level
traumatic tear of joint or ligament at neck level

Code also any associated open wound
EXCLUDES 2 strain of muscle or tendon at neck level (S16.1)

The appropriate 7th character is to be added to each code from category S13.
A initial encounter
D subsequent encounter
S sequela

√x7ᵗʰ **S13.0 Traumatic rupture of cervical intervertebral disc**

EXCLUDES 1 rupture or displacement (nontraumatic) of cervical intervertebral disc NOS (M50.-)

√5ᵗʰ **S13.1 Subluxation and dislocation of cervical vertebrae**

Code also any associated:
open wound of neck (S11.-)
spinal cord injury (S14.1-)
EXCLUDES 2 fracture of cervical vertebrae (S12.0-S12.3-)

√6ᵗʰ **S13.10 Subluxation and dislocation of unspecified cervical vertebrae**

√7ᵗʰ **S13.100 Subluxation of unspecified** ▽ **cervical vertebrae**

√7ᵗʰ **S13.101 Dislocation of unspecified cervical** ▽ **vertebrae**

√6ᵗʰ **S13.11 Subluxation and dislocation of C0/C1 cervical vertebrae**

Subluxation and dislocation of atlantooccipital joint
Subluxation and dislocation of atloidooccipital joint
Subluxation and dislocation of occipitoatloid joint

√7ᵗʰ **S13.110 Subluxation of C0/C1 cervical vertebrae**

√7ᵗʰ **S13.111 Dislocation of C0/C1 cervical vertebrae**

√6ᵗʰ **S13.12 Subluxation and dislocation of C1/C2 cervical vertebrae**

Subluxation and dislocation of atlantoaxial joint

√7ᵗʰ **S13.120 Subluxation of C1/C2 cervical vertebrae**

√7ᵗʰ **S13.121 Dislocation of C1/C2 cervical vertebrae**

√6ᵗʰ **S13.13 Subluxation and dislocation of C2/C3 cervical vertebrae**

√7ᵗʰ **S13.130 Subluxation of C2/C3 cervical vertebrae**

√7ᵗʰ **S13.131 Dislocation of C2/C3 cervical vertebrae**

√6ᵗʰ **S13.14 Subluxation and dislocation of C3/C4 cervical vertebrae**

√7ᵗʰ **S13.140 Subluxation of C3/C4 cervical vertebrae**

√7ᵗʰ **S13.141 Dislocation of C3/C4 cervical vertebrae**

√6ᵗʰ **S13.15 Subluxation and dislocation of C4/C5 cervical vertebrae**

√7ᵗʰ **S13.150 Subluxation of C4/C5 cervical vertebrae**

√7ᵗʰ **S13.151 Dislocation of C4/C5 cervical vertebrae**

√6ᵗʰ **S13.16 Subluxation and dislocation of C5/C6 cervical vertebrae**

√7ᵗʰ **S13.160 Subluxation of C5/C6 cervical vertebrae**

√7ᵗʰ **S13.161 Dislocation of C5/C6 cervical vertebrae**

√6ᵗʰ **S13.17 Subluxation and dislocation of C6/C7 cervical vertebrae**

√7ᵗʰ **S13.170 Subluxation of C6/C7 cervical vertebrae**

√7ᵗʰ **S13.171 Dislocation of C6/C7 cervical vertebrae**

√6ᵗʰ **S13.18 Subluxation and dislocation of C7/T1 cervical vertebrae**

√7ᵗʰ **S13.180 Subluxation of C7/T1 cervical vertebrae**

√7ᵗʰ **S13.181 Dislocation of C7/T1 cervical vertebrae**

√5ᵗʰ **S13.2 Dislocation of other and unspecified parts of neck**

√x7ᵗʰ **S13.20 Dislocation of unspecified parts of neck** ▽

√x7ᵗʰ **S13.29 Dislocation of other parts of neck**

√x7ᵗʰ **S13.4 Sprain of ligaments of cervical spine**

Sprain of anterior longitudinal (ligament), cervical
Sprain of atlanto-axial (joints)
Sprain of atlanto-occipital (joints)
Whiplash injury of cervical spine

√x7ᵗʰ **S13.5 Sprain of thyroid region**

Sprain of cricoarytenoid (joint) (ligament)
Sprain of cricothyroid (joint) (ligament)
Sprain of thyroid cartilage

√x7ᵗʰ **S13.8 Sprain of joints and ligaments of other parts of neck**

√x7ᵗʰ **S13.9 Sprain of joints and ligaments of unspecified parts** ▽ **of neck**

√4ᵗʰ **S14 Injury of nerves and spinal cord at neck level**

NOTE Code to highest level of cervical cord injury

Code also any associated:
fracture of cervical vertebra (S12.0- — S12.6.-)
open wound of neck (S11.-)
transient paralysis (R29.5)

The appropriate 7th character is to be added to each code from category S14.
A initial encounter
D subsequent encounter
S sequela

√x7ᵗʰ **S14.0 Concussion and edema of cervical spinal cord** HCC

√5ᵗʰ **S14.1 Other and unspecified injuries of cervical spinal cord**

√6ᵗʰ **S14.10 Unspecified injury of cervical spinal cord**

√7ᵗʰ **S14.101 Unspecified injury at C1 level of** HCC ▽ **cervical spinal cord**

√7ᵗʰ **S14.102 Unspecified injury at C2 level of** HCC ▽ **cervical spinal cord**

√7ᵗʰ **S14.103 Unspecified injury at C3 level of** HCC ▽ **cervical spinal cord**

√7ᵗʰ **S14.104 Unspecified injury at C4 level of** HCC ▽ **cervical spinal cord**

☑ Additional Character Req   √x7ᵗʰ Placeholder Alert   Manifestation   ▽ Unspecified   ▶◀ Revised Text   ● New Code   ▲ Revised Code Title

√7ᵗʰ **S14.105** **Unspecified injury at C5 level of** HCC ▽
cervical spinal cord

√7ᵗʰ **S14.106** **Unspecified injury at C6 level of** HCC ▽
cervical spinal cord

√7ᵗʰ **S14.107** **Unspecified injury at C7 level of** HCC ▽
cervical spinal cord

√7ᵗʰ **S14.108** **Unspecified injury at C8 level of** HCC ▽
cervical spinal cord

√7ᵗʰ **S14.109** **Unspecified injury at unspecified** HCC ▽
level of cervical spinal cord
Injury of cervical spinal cord NOS

√6ᵗʰ **S14.11** Complete lesion of cervical spinal cord

√7ᵗʰ **S14.111** **Complete lesion at C1 level of** HCC
cervical spinal cord

√7ᵗʰ **S14.112** **Complete lesion at C2 level of** HCC
cervical spinal cord

√7ᵗʰ **S14.113** **Complete lesion at C3 level of** HCC
cervical spinal cord

√7ᵗʰ **S14.114** **Complete lesion at C4 level of** HCC
cervical spinal cord

√7ᵗʰ **S14.115** **Complete lesion at C5 level of** HCC
cervical spinal cord

√7ᵗʰ **S14.116** **Complete lesion at C6 level of** HCC
cervical spinal cord

√7ᵗʰ **S14.117** **Complete lesion at C7 level of** HCC
cervical spinal cord

√7ᵗʰ **S14.118** **Complete lesion at C8 level of** HCC
cervical spinal cord

√7ᵗʰ **S14.119** **Complete lesion at unspecified** HCC ▽
level of cervical spinal cord

√6ᵗʰ **S14.12** Central cord syndrome of cervical spinal cord

√7ᵗʰ **S14.121** **Central cord syndrome at C1 level** HCC
of cervical spinal cord

√7ᵗʰ **S14.122** **Central cord syndrome at C2 level** HCC
of cervical spinal cord

√7ᵗʰ **S14.123** **Central cord syndrome at C3 level** HCC
of cervical spinal cord

√7ᵗʰ **S14.124** **Central cord syndrome at C4 level** HCC
of cervical spinal cord

√7ᵗʰ **S14.125** **Central cord syndrome at C5 level** HCC
of cervical spinal cord

√7ᵗʰ **S14.126** **Central cord syndrome at C6 level** HCC
of cervical spinal cord

√7ᵗʰ **S14.127** **Central cord syndrome at C7 level** HCC
of cervical spinal cord

√7ᵗʰ **S14.128** **Central cord syndrome at C8 level** HCC
of cervical spinal cord

√7ᵗʰ **S14.129** **Central cord syndrome at** HCC ▽
unspecified level of cervical
spinal cord

√6ᵗʰ **S14.13** Anterior cord syndrome of cervical spinal cord

√7ᵗʰ **S14.131** **Anterior cord syndrome at C1** HCC
level of cervical spinal cord

√7ᵗʰ **S14.132** **Anterior cord syndrome at C2** HCC
level of cervical spinal cord

√7ᵗʰ **S14.133** **Anterior cord syndrome at C3** HCC
level of cervical spinal cord

√7ᵗʰ **S14.134** **Anterior cord syndrome at C4** HCC
level of cervical spinal cord

√7ᵗʰ **S14.135** **Anterior cord syndrome at C5** HCC
level of cervical spinal cord

√7ᵗʰ **S14.136** **Anterior cord syndrome at C6** HCC
level of cervical spinal cord

√7ᵗʰ **S14.137** **Anterior cord syndrome at C7** HCC
level of cervical spinal cord

√7ᵗʰ **S14.138** **Anterior cord syndrome at C8** HCC
level of cervical spinal cord

√7ᵗʰ **S14.139** **Anterior cord syndrome at** HCC ▽
unspecified level of cervical
spinal cord

√6ᵗʰ **S14.14** Brown-Séquard syndrome of cervical spinal cord

√7ᵗʰ **S14.141** **Brown-Séquard syndrome at C1** HCC
level of cervical spinal cord

√7ᵗʰ **S14.142** **Brown-Séquard syndrome at C2** HCC
level of cervical spinal cord

√7ᵗʰ **S14.143** **Brown-Séquard syndrome at C3** HCC
level of cervical spinal cord

√7ᵗʰ **S14.144** **Brown-Séquard syndrome at C4** HCC
level of cervical spinal cord

√7ᵗʰ **S14.145** **Brown-Séquard syndrome at C5** HCC
level of cervical spinal cord

√7ᵗʰ **S14.146** **Brown-Séquard syndrome at C6** HCC
level of cervical spinal cord

√7ᵗʰ **S14.147** **Brown-Séquard syndrome at C7** HCC
level of cervical spinal cord

√7ᵗʰ **S14.148** **Brown-Séquard syndrome at C8** HCC
level of cervical spinal cord

√7ᵗʰ **S14.149** **Brown-Séquard syndrome at** HCC ▽
unspecified level of cervical
spinal cord

√6ᵗʰ **S14.15** Other incomplete lesions of cervical spinal cord
Incomplete lesion of cervical spinal cord NOS
Posterior cord syndrome of cervical spinal cord

√7ᵗʰ **S14.151** **Other incomplete lesion at C1** HCC
level of cervical spinal cord

√7ᵗʰ **S14.152** **Other incomplete lesion at C2** HCC
level of cervical spinal cord

√7ᵗʰ **S14.153** **Other incomplete lesion at C3** HCC
level of cervical spinal cord

√7ᵗʰ **S14.154** **Other incomplete lesion at C4** HCC
level of cervical spinal cord

√7ᵗʰ **S14.155** **Other incomplete lesion at C5** HCC
level of cervical spinal cord

√7ᵗʰ **S14.156** **Other incomplete lesion at C6** HCC
level of cervical spinal cord

√7ᵗʰ **S14.157** **Other incomplete lesion at C7** HCC
level of cervical spinal cord

√7ᵗʰ **S14.158** **Other incomplete lesion at C8** HCC
level of cervical spinal cord

√7ᵗʰ **S14.159** **Other incomplete lesion at** HCC ▽
unspecified level of cervical
spinal cord

√x7ᵗʰ **S14.2** **Injury of nerve root of cervical spine**

√x7ᵗʰ **S14.3** **Injury of brachial plexus**

√x7ᵗʰ **S14.4** **Injury of peripheral nerves of neck**

√x7ᵗʰ **S14.5** **Injury of cervical sympathetic nerves**

√x7ᵗʰ **S14.8** **Injury of other specified nerves of neck**

√x7ᵗʰ **S14.9** **Injury of unspecified nerves of neck** ▽

√4ᵗʰ **S15** **Injury of blood vessels at neck level**

Code also any associated open wound (S11.-)

The appropriate 7th character is to be added to each code from
category S15.
A initial encounter
D subsequent encounter
S sequela

√5ᵗʰ **S15.0** **Injury of carotid artery of neck**
Injury of carotid artery (common) (external) (internal,
extracranial portion)
Injury of carotid artery NOS
EXCLUDES 1 *injury of internal carotid artery, intracranial portion
(S06.8)*

√6ᵗʰ **S15.00** **Unspecified injury of carotid artery**

√7ᵗʰ **S15.001** **Unspecified injury of right carotid** ▽
artery

√7ᵗʰ **S15.002** **Unspecified injury of left carotid** ▽
artery

√7ᵗʰ **S15.009** **Unspecified injury of unspecified** ▽
carotid artery

√6ᵗʰ **S15.01** **Minor laceration of carotid artery**
Incomplete transection of carotid artery
Laceration of carotid artery NOS
Superficial laceration of carotid artery

√7ᵗʰ **S15.011** **Minor laceration of right carotid artery**

√7ᵗʰ **S15.012** **Minor laceration of left carotid artery**

√7ᵗʰ **S15.019** **Minor laceration of unspecified** ▽
carotid artery

√6ᵗʰ **S15.02** **Major laceration of carotid artery**
Complete transection of carotid artery
Traumatic rupture of carotid artery

√7ᵗʰ **S15.021** **Major laceration of right carotid artery**

√7ᵗʰ **S15.022** **Major laceration of left carotid artery**

√7ᵗʰ **S15.029** **Major laceration of unspecified** ▽
carotid artery

√6ᵗʰ **S15.09** **Other specified injury of carotid artery**

√7ᵗʰ **S15.091** **Other specified injury of right carotid**
artery

√7ᵗʰ **S15.092** **Other specified injury of left carotid**
artery

√7ᵗʰ **S15.099** **Other specified injury of unspecified carotid artery** ▽

√5ᵗʰ **S15.1** **Injury of vertebral artery**

  √6ᵗʰ **S15.10** **Unspecified injury of vertebral artery**

    √7ᵗʰ **S15.101** **Unspecified injury of right vertebral artery** ▽

    √7ᵗʰ **S15.102** **Unspecified injury of left vertebral artery** ▽

    √7ᵗʰ **S15.109** **Unspecified injury of unspecified vertebral artery** ▽

  √6ᵗʰ **S15.11** **Minor laceration of vertebral artery**

    Incomplete transection of vertebral artery
    Laceration of vertebral artery NOS
    Superficial laceration of vertebral artery

    √7ᵗʰ **S15.111** **Minor laceration of right vertebral artery**

    √7ᵗʰ **S15.112** **Minor laceration of left vertebral artery**

    √7ᵗʰ **S15.119** **Minor laceration of unspecified vertebral artery** ▽

  √6ᵗʰ **S15.12** **Major laceration of vertebral artery**

    Complete transection of vertebral artery
    Traumatic rupture of vertebral artery

    √7ᵗʰ **S15.121** **Major laceration of right vertebral artery**

    √7ᵗʰ **S15.122** **Major laceration of left vertebral artery**

    √7ᵗʰ **S15.129** **Major laceration of unspecified vertebral artery** ▽

  √6ᵗʰ **S15.19** **Other specified injury of vertebral artery**

    √7ᵗʰ **S15.191** **Other specified injury of right vertebral artery**

    √7ᵗʰ **S15.192** **Other specified injury of left vertebral artery**

    √7ᵗʰ **S15.199** **Other specified injury of unspecified vertebral artery** ▽

√5ᵗʰ **S15.2** **Injury of external jugular vein**

  √6ᵗʰ **S15.20** **Unspecified injury of external jugular vein**

    √7ᵗʰ **S15.201** **Unspecified injury of right external jugular vein** ▽

    √7ᵗʰ **S15.202** **Unspecified injury of left external jugular vein** ▽

    √7ᵗʰ **S15.209** **Unspecified injury of unspecified external jugular vein** ▽

  √6ᵗʰ **S15.21** **Minor laceration of external jugular vein**

    Incomplete transection of external jugular vein
    Laceration of external jugular vein NOS
    Superficial laceration of external jugular vein

    √7ᵗʰ **S15.211** **Minor laceration of right external jugular vein**

    √7ᵗʰ **S15.212** **Minor laceration of left external jugular vein**

    √7ᵗʰ **S15.219** **Minor laceration of unspecified external jugular vein** ▽

  √6ᵗʰ **S15.22** **Major laceration of external jugular vein**

    Complete transection of external jugular vein
    Traumatic rupture of external jugular vein

    √7ᵗʰ **S15.221** **Major laceration of right external jugular vein**

    √7ᵗʰ **S15.222** **Major laceration of left external jugular vein**

    √7ᵗʰ **S15.229** **Major laceration of unspecified external jugular vein** ▽

  √6ᵗʰ **S15.29** **Other specified injury of external jugular vein**

    √7ᵗʰ **S15.291** **Other specified injury of right external jugular vein**

    √7ᵗʰ **S15.292** **Other specified injury of left external jugular vein**

    √7ᵗʰ **S15.299** **Other specified injury of unspecified external jugular vein**

√5ᵗʰ **S15.3** **Injury of internal jugular vein**

  √6ᵗʰ **S15.30** **Unspecified injury of internal jugular vein**

    √7ᵗʰ **S15.301** **Unspecified injury of right internal jugular vein** ▽

    √7ᵗʰ **S15.302** **Unspecified injury of left internal jugular vein** ▽

    √7ᵗʰ **S15.309** **Unspecified injury of unspecified internal jugular vein** ▽

  √6ᵗʰ **S15.31** **Minor laceration of internal jugular vein**

    Incomplete transection of internal jugular vein
    Laceration of internal jugular vein NOS
    Superficial laceration of internal jugular vein

    √7ᵗʰ **S15.311** **Minor laceration of right internal jugular vein**

    √7ᵗʰ **S15.312** **Minor laceration of left internal jugular vein**

    √7ᵗʰ **S15.319** **Minor laceration of unspecified internal jugular vein** ▽

  √6ᵗʰ **S15.32** **Major laceration of internal jugular vein**

    Complete transection of internal jugular vein
    Traumatic rupture of internal jugular vein

    √7ᵗʰ **S15.321** **Major laceration of right internal jugular vein**

    √7ᵗʰ **S15.322** **Major laceration of left internal jugular vein**

    √7ᵗʰ **S15.329** **Major laceration of unspecified internal jugular vein** ▽

  √6ᵗʰ **S15.39** **Other specified injury of internal jugular vein**

    √7ᵗʰ **S15.391** **Other specified injury of right internal jugular vein**

    √7ᵗʰ **S15.392** **Other specified injury of left internal jugular vein**

    √7ᵗʰ **S15.399** **Other specified injury of unspecified internal jugular vein** ▽

√x7ᵗʰ **S15.8** **Injury of other specified blood vessels at neck level**

√x7ᵗʰ **S15.9** **Injury of unspecified blood vessel at neck level** ▽

√4ᵗʰ **S16** **Injury of muscle, fascia and tendon at neck level**

  Code also any associated open wound (S11.-)

  EXCLUDES 2   sprain of joint or ligament at neck level (S13.9)

  The appropriate 7th character is to be added to each code from category S16.
  A   initial encounter
  D   subsequent encounter
  S   sequela

√x7ᵗʰ **S16.1** **Strain of muscle, fascia and tendon at neck level**

√x7ᵗʰ **S16.2** **Laceration of muscle, fascia and tendon at neck level**

√x7ᵗʰ **S16.8** **Other specified injury of muscle, fascia and tendon at neck level**

√x7ᵗʰ **S16.9** **Unspecified injury of muscle, fascia and tendon at neck level** ▽

√4ᵗʰ **S17** **Crushing injury of neck**

  Use additional code for all associated injuries, such as:
  injury of blood vessels (S15.-)
  open wound of neck (S11.-)
  spinal cord injury (S14.0, S14.1-)
  vertebral fracture (S12.0- — S12.3-)

  The appropriate 7th character is to be added to each code from category S17.
  A   initial encounter
  D   subsequent encounter
  S   sequela

√x7ᵗʰ **S17.0** **Crushing injury of larynx and trachea**

√x7ᵗʰ **S17.8** **Crushing injury of other specified parts of neck**

√x7ᵗʰ **S17.9** **Crushing injury of neck, part unspecified** ▽

√4ᵗʰ **S19** **Other specified and unspecified injuries of neck**

  The appropriate 7th character is to be added to each code from category S19.
  A   initial encounter
  D   subsequent encounter
  S   sequela

√5ᵗʰ **S19.8** **Other specified injuries of neck**

  √x7ᵗʰ **S19.80** **Other specified injuries of unspecified part of neck** ▽

  √x7ᵗʰ **S19.81** **Other specified injuries of larynx**

  √x7ᵗʰ **S19.82** **Other specified injuries of cervical trachea**

    EXCLUDES 2   other specified injury of thoracic trachea (S27.5-)

  √x7ᵗʰ **S19.83** **Other specified injuries of vocal cord**

  √x7ᵗʰ **S19.84** **Other specified injuries of thyroid gland**

  √x7ᵗʰ **S19.85** **Other specified injuries of pharynx and cervical esophagus**

✓ Additional Character Req   √x7ᵗʰ Placeholder Alert   **Manifestation**   ▽ Unspecified   ►◄ Revised Text   ● New Code   ▲ Revised Code Title

ICD-10-CM 2019   **967**

√x7ᵗʰ **S19.89** **Other specified injuries of other specified part of neck**

√x7ᵗʰ **S19.9** **Unspecified injury of neck** ▽

Injuries to the thorax (S20-S29)

INCLUDES   injuries of breast
         injuries of chest (wall)
         injuries of interscapular area
EXCLUDES 2   burns and corrosions (T20-T32)
         effects of foreign body in bronchus (T17.5)
         effects of foreign body in esophagus (T18.1)
         effects of foreign body in lung (T17.8)
         effects of foreign body in trachea (T17.4)
         frostbite (T33-T34)
         injuries of axilla
         injuries of clavicle
         injuries of scapular region
         injuries of shoulder
         insect bite or sting, venomous (T63.4)

√4ᵗʰ **S20** **Superficial injury of thorax**

> The appropriate 7th character is to be added to each code from category S20.
> A   initial encounter
> D   subsequent encounter
> S   sequela

√5ᵗʰ **S20.0** **Contusion of breast**

√x7ᵗʰ **S20.00** **Contusion of breast, unspecified breast** ▽

√x7ᵗʰ **S20.01** **Contusion of right breast**

√x7ᵗʰ **S20.02** **Contusion of left breast**

√5ᵗʰ **S20.1** **Other and unspecified superficial injuries of breast**

√6ᵗʰ **S20.10** **Unspecified superficial injuries of breast**

√7ᵗʰ **S20.101** Unspecified superficial injuries of breast, right breast ▽

√7ᵗʰ **S20.102** Unspecified superficial injuries of breast, left breast ▽

√7ᵗʰ **S20.109** Unspecified superficial injuries of breast, unspecified breast ▽

√6ᵗʰ **S20.11** **Abrasion of breast**

√7ᵗʰ **S20.111** Abrasion of breast, right breast

√7ᵗʰ **S20.112** Abrasion of breast, left breast

√7ᵗʰ **S20.119** Abrasion of breast, unspecified breast ▽

√6ᵗʰ **S20.12** **Blister (nonthermal) of breast**

√7ᵗʰ **S20.121** Blister (nonthermal) of breast, right breast

√7ᵗʰ **S20.122** Blister (nonthermal) of breast, left breast

√7ᵗʰ **S20.129** Blister (nonthermal) of breast, unspecified breast ▽

√6ᵗʰ **S20.14** **External constriction of part of breast**

√7ᵗʰ **S20.141** External constriction of part of breast, right breast

√7ᵗʰ **S20.142** External constriction of part of breast, left breast

√7ᵗʰ **S20.149** External constriction of part of breast, unspecified breast ▽

√6ᵗʰ **S20.15** **Superficial foreign body of breast**
      Splinter in the breast

√7ᵗʰ **S20.151** Superficial foreign body of breast, right breast

√7ᵗʰ **S20.152** Superficial foreign body of breast, left breast

√7ᵗʰ **S20.159** Superficial foreign body of breast, unspecified breast ▽

√6ᵗʰ **S20.16** **Insect bite (nonvenomous) of breast**

√7ᵗʰ **S20.161** Insect bite (nonvenomous) of breast, right breast

√7ᵗʰ **S20.162** Insect bite (nonvenomous) of breast, left breast

√7ᵗʰ **S20.169** Insect bite (nonvenomous) of breast, unspecified breast ▽

√6ᵗʰ **S20.17** **Other superficial bite of breast**

> EXCLUDES 1   open bite of breast (S21.05-)

√7ᵗʰ **S20.171** Other superficial bite of breast, right breast

√7ᵗʰ **S20.172** Other superficial bite of breast, left breast

√7ᵗʰ **S20.179** Other superficial bite of breast, unspecified breast ▽

√5ᵗʰ **S20.2** **Contusion of thorax**

√x7ᵗʰ **S20.20** **Contusion of thorax, unspecified** ▽

√6ᵗʰ **S20.21** **Contusion of front wall of thorax**

√7ᵗʰ **S20.211** Contusion of right front wall of thorax

√7ᵗʰ **S20.212** Contusion of left front wall of thorax

√7ᵗʰ **S20.219** Contusion of unspecified front wall of thorax ▽

√6ᵗʰ **S20.22** **Contusion of back wall of thorax**

√7ᵗʰ **S20.221** Contusion of right back wall of thorax

√7ᵗʰ **S20.222** Contusion of left back wall of thorax

√7ᵗʰ **S20.229** Contusion of unspecified back wall of thorax ▽

√5ᵗʰ **S20.3** **Other and unspecified superficial injuries of front wall of thorax**

√6ᵗʰ **S20.30** **Unspecified superficial injuries of front wall of thorax**

√7ᵗʰ **S20.301** Unspecified superficial injuries of right front wall of thorax ▽

√7ᵗʰ **S20.302** Unspecified superficial injuries of left front wall of thorax ▽

√7ᵗʰ **S20.309** Unspecified superficial injuries of unspecified front wall of thorax ▽

√6ᵗʰ **S20.31** **Abrasion of front wall of thorax**

√7ᵗʰ **S20.311** Abrasion of right front wall of thorax

√7ᵗʰ **S20.312** Abrasion of left front wall of thorax

√7ᵗʰ **S20.319** Abrasion of unspecified front wall of thorax ▽

√6ᵗʰ **S20.32** **Blister (nonthermal) of front wall of thorax**

√7ᵗʰ **S20.321** Blister (nonthermal) of right front wall of thorax

√7ᵗʰ **S20.322** Blister (nonthermal) of left front wall of thorax

√7ᵗʰ **S20.329** Blister (nonthermal) of unspecified front wall of thorax ▽

√6ᵗʰ **S20.34** **External constriction of front wall of thorax**

√7ᵗʰ **S20.341** External constriction of right front wall of thorax

√7ᵗʰ **S20.342** External constriction of left front wall of thorax

√7ᵗʰ **S20.349** External constriction of unspecified front wall of thorax ▽

√6ᵗʰ **S20.35** **Superficial foreign body of front wall of thorax**
      Splinter in front wall of thorax

√7ᵗʰ **S20.351** Superficial foreign body of right front wall of thorax

√7ᵗʰ **S20.352** Superficial foreign body of left front wall of thorax

√7ᵗʰ **S20.359** Superficial foreign body of unspecified front wall of thorax ▽

√6ᵗʰ **S20.36** **Insect bite (nonvenomous) of front wall of thorax**

√7ᵗʰ **S20.361** Insect bite (nonvenomous) of right front wall of thorax

√7ᵗʰ **S20.362** Insect bite (nonvenomous) of left front wall of thorax

√7ᵗʰ **S20.369** Insect bite (nonvenomous) of unspecified front wall of thorax ▽

√6ᵗʰ **S20.37** **Other superficial bite of front wall of thorax**

> EXCLUDES 1   open bite of front wall of thorax (S21.15)

√7ᵗʰ **S20.371** Other superficial bite of right front wall of thorax

√7ᵗʰ **S20.372** Other superficial bite of left front wall of thorax

√7ᵗʰ **S20.379** Other superficial bite of unspecified front wall of thorax ▽

√5ᵗʰ **S20.4** **Other and unspecified superficial injuries of back wall of thorax**

√6ᵗʰ **S20.40** **Unspecified superficial injuries of back wall of thorax**

√7ᵗʰ **S20.401** Unspecified superficial injuries of right back wall of thorax ▽

√7ᵗʰ **S20.402** Unspecified superficial injuries of left back wall of thorax ▽

√7ᵗʰ **S20.409** Unspecified superficial injuries of unspecified back wall of thorax ▽

√6ᵗʰ **S20.41** **Abrasion of back wall of thorax**

√7ᵗʰ **S20.411** Abrasion of right back wall of thorax

√7ᵗʰ **S20.412** Abrasion of left back wall of thorax

√7ᵗʰ **S20.419** Abrasion of unspecified back wall of thorax ▽

√6ᵗʰ **S20.42** Blister (nonthermal) of back wall of thorax

    √7ᵗʰ **S20.421** Blister (nonthermal) of right back wall of thorax

    √7ᵗʰ **S20.422** Blister (nonthermal) of left back wall of thorax

    √7ᵗʰ **S20.429** Blister (nonthermal) of unspecified back wall of thorax ▽

√6ᵗʰ **S20.44** External constriction of back wall of thorax

    √7ᵗʰ **S20.441** External constriction of right back wall of thorax

    √7ᵗʰ **S20.442** External constriction of left back wall of thorax

    √7ᵗʰ **S20.449** External constriction of unspecified back wall of thorax ▽

√6ᵗʰ **S20.45** Superficial foreign body of back wall of thorax

        Splinter of back wall of thorax

    √7ᵗʰ **S20.451** Superficial foreign body of right back wall of thorax

    √7ᵗʰ **S20.452** Superficial foreign body of left back wall of thorax

    √7ᵗʰ **S20.459** Superficial foreign body of unspecified back wall of thorax ▽

√6ᵗʰ **S20.46** Insect bite (nonvenomous) of back wall of thorax

    √7ᵗʰ **S20.461** Insect bite (nonvenomous) of right back wall of thorax

    √7ᵗʰ **S20.462** Insect bite (nonvenomous) of left back wall of thorax

    √7ᵗʰ **S20.469** Insect bite (nonvenomous) of unspecified back wall of thorax ▽

√6ᵗʰ **S20.47** Other superficial bite of back wall of thorax

        EXCLUDES 1   open bite of back wall of thorax (S21.25)

    √7ᵗʰ **S20.471** Other superficial bite of right back wall of thorax

    √7ᵗʰ **S20.472** Other superficial bite of left back wall of thorax

    √7ᵗʰ **S20.479** Other superficial bite of unspecified back wall of thorax ▽

√5ᵗʰ **S20.9** Superficial injury of unspecified parts of thorax

      EXCLUDES 1   contusion of thorax NOS (S20.20)

√x7ᵗʰ **S20.90** Unspecified superficial injury of unspecified parts of thorax ▽

        Superficial injury of thoracic wall NOS

√x7ᵗʰ **S20.91** Abrasion of unspecified parts of thorax ▽

√x7ᵗʰ **S20.92** Blister (nonthermal) of unspecified parts of thorax ▽

√x7ᵗʰ **S20.94** External constriction of unspecified parts of thorax ▽

√x7ᵗʰ **S20.95** Superficial foreign body of unspecified parts of thorax ▽

        Splinter in thorax NOS

√x7ᵗʰ **S20.96** Insect bite (nonvenomous) of unspecified parts of thorax ▽

√x7ᵗʰ **S20.97** Other superficial bite of unspecified parts of thorax ▽

        EXCLUDES 1   open bite of thorax NOS (S21.95)

√4ᵗʰ **S21** Open wound of thorax

   Code also any associated injury, such as:

    injury of heart (S26.-)

    injury of intrathoracic organs (S27.-)

    rib fracture (S22.3-, S22.4-)

    spinal cord injury (S24.0-, S24.1-)

    traumatic hemopneumothorax (S27.3)

    traumatic hemothorax (S27.1)

    traumatic pneumothorax (S27.0)

    wound infection

    EXCLUDES 1   traumatic amputation (partial) of thorax (S28.1)

> The appropriate 7th character is to be added to each code from category S21.
> A   initial encounter
> D   subsequent encounter
> S   sequela

√6ᵗʰ **S21.0** Open wound of breast

   √6ᵗʰ **S21.00** Unspecified open wound of breast

      √7ᵗʰ **S21.001** Unspecified open wound of right breast ▽

√7ᵗʰ **S21.002** Unspecified open wound of left breast ▽

√7ᵗʰ **S21.009** Unspecified open wound of unspecified breast ▽

√6ᵗʰ **S21.01** Laceration without foreign body of breast

   √7ᵗʰ **S21.011** Laceration without foreign body of right breast ▽

   √7ᵗʰ **S21.012** Laceration without foreign body of left breast ▽

   √7ᵗʰ **S21.019** Laceration without foreign body of unspecified breast ▽

√6ᵗʰ **S21.02** Laceration with foreign body of breast

   √7ᵗʰ **S21.021** Laceration with foreign body of right breast ▽

   √7ᵗʰ **S21.022** Laceration with foreign body of left breast ▽

   √7ᵗʰ **S21.029** Laceration with foreign body of unspecified breast ▽

√6ᵗʰ **S21.03** Puncture wound without foreign body of breast

   √7ᵗʰ **S21.031** Puncture wound without foreign body of right breast ▽

   √7ᵗʰ **S21.032** Puncture wound without foreign body of left breast ▽

   √7ᵗʰ **S21.039** Puncture wound without foreign body of unspecified breast ▽

√6ᵗʰ **S21.04** Puncture wound with foreign body of breast

   √7ᵗʰ **S21.041** Puncture wound with foreign body of right breast ▽

   √7ᵗʰ **S21.042** Puncture wound with foreign body of left breast ▽

   √7ᵗʰ **S21.049** Puncture wound with foreign body of unspecified breast ▽

√6ᵗʰ **S21.05** Open bite of breast

      Bite of breast NOS

      EXCLUDES 1   superficial bite of breast (S20.17)

   √7ᵗʰ **S21.051** Open bite of right breast

   √7ᵗʰ **S21.052** Open bite of left breast

   √7ᵗʰ **S21.059** Open bite of unspecified breast ▽

√5ᵗʰ **S21.1** Open wound of front wall of thorax without penetration into thoracic cavity

    Open wound of chest without penetration into thoracic cavity

√6ᵗʰ **S21.10** Unspecified open wound of front wall of thorax without penetration into thoracic cavity

   √7ᵗʰ **S21.101** Unspecified open wound of right front wall of thorax without penetration into thoracic cavity ▽

   √7ᵗʰ **S21.102** Unspecified open wound of left front wall of thorax without penetration into thoracic cavity ▽

   √7ᵗʰ **S21.109** Unspecified open wound of unspecified front wall of thorax without penetration into thoracic cavity ▽

√6ᵗʰ **S21.11** Laceration without foreign body of front wall of thorax without penetration into thoracic cavity

   √7ᵗʰ **S21.111** Laceration without foreign body of right front wall of thorax without penetration into thoracic cavity

   √7ᵗʰ **S21.112** Laceration without foreign body of left front wall of thorax without penetration into thoracic cavity

   √7ᵗʰ **S21.119** Laceration without foreign body of unspecified front wall of thorax without penetration into thoracic cavity ▽

√6ᵗʰ **S21.12** Laceration with foreign body of front wall of thorax without penetration into thoracic cavity

   √7ᵗʰ **S21.121** Laceration with foreign body of right front wall of thorax without penetration into thoracic cavity

   √7ᵗʰ **S21.122** Laceration with foreign body of left front wall of thorax without penetration into thoracic cavity

   √7ᵗʰ **S21.129** Laceration with foreign body of unspecified front wall of thorax without penetration into thoracic cavity ▽

√6ᵗʰ **S21.13** Puncture wound without foreign body of front wall of thorax without penetration into thoracic cavity

   √7ᵗʰ **S21.131** Puncture wound without foreign body of right front wall of thorax without penetration into thoracic cavity

✓ Additional Character Req   √x7ᵗʰ Placeholder Alert   Manifestation   ▽ Unspecified   ▶◀ Revised Text   ● New Code   ▲ Revised Code Title

ICD-10-CM 2019   969

Chapter 19. Injury, Poisoning and Certain Other Consequences of External Causes

S21.132–S21.342

     √7ᵗʰ **S21.132** **Puncture wound without foreign body of** left **front wall of thorax without penetration into thoracic cavity**

     √7ᵗʰ **S21.139** **Puncture wound without foreign body of unspecified front wall of thorax without penetration into thoracic cavity** ▽

√6ᵗʰ **S21.14** Puncture wound with foreign body **of front wall of thorax without penetration into thoracic cavity**

     √7ᵗʰ **S21.141** **Puncture wound with foreign body of** right **front wall of thorax without penetration into thoracic cavity**

     √7ᵗʰ **S21.142** **Puncture wound with foreign body of** left **front wall of thorax without penetration into thoracic cavity**

     √7ᵗʰ **S21.149** **Puncture wound with foreign body of unspecified front wall of thorax without penetration into thoracic cavity** ▽

√6ᵗʰ **S21.15** Open bite **of front wall of thorax without penetration into thoracic cavity**

     Bite of front wall of thorax NOS

     EXCLUDES 1 *superficial bite of front wall of thorax (S20.37)*

     √7ᵗʰ **S21.151** **Open bite of** right **front wall of thorax without penetration into thoracic cavity**

     √7ᵗʰ **S21.152** **Open bite of** left **front wall of thorax without penetration into thoracic cavity**

     √7ᵗʰ **S21.159** **Open bite of unspecified front wall of thorax without penetration into thoracic cavity** ▽

√5ᵗʰ **S21.2** Open wound of back wall of thorax without penetration **into thoracic cavity**

√6ᵗʰ **S21.20** **Unspecified open wound of back wall of thorax without penetration into thoracic cavity**

     √7ᵗʰ **S21.201** **Unspecified open wound of** right **back wall of thorax without penetration into thoracic cavity** ▽

     √7ᵗʰ **S21.202** **Unspecified open wound of** left **back wall of thorax without penetration into thoracic cavity** ▽

     √7ᵗʰ **S21.209** **Unspecified open wound of unspecified back wall of thorax without penetration into thoracic cavity** ▽

√6ᵗʰ **S21.21** Laceration without foreign body **of back wall of thorax without penetration into thoracic cavity**

     √7ᵗʰ **S21.211** **Laceration without foreign body of** right **back wall of thorax without penetration into thoracic cavity**

     √7ᵗʰ **S21.212** **Laceration without foreign body of** left **back wall of thorax without penetration into thoracic cavity**

     √7ᵗʰ **S21.219** **Laceration without foreign body of unspecified back wall of thorax without penetration into thoracic cavity** ▽

√6ᵗʰ **S21.22** Laceration with foreign body **of back wall of thorax without penetration into thoracic cavity**

     √7ᵗʰ **S21.221** **Laceration with foreign body of** right **back wall of thorax without penetration into thoracic cavity**

     √7ᵗʰ **S21.222** **Laceration with foreign body of** left **back wall of thorax without penetration into thoracic cavity**

     √7ᵗʰ **S21.229** **Laceration with foreign body of unspecified back wall of thorax without penetration into thoracic cavity** ▽

√6ᵗʰ **S21.23** Puncture wound without foreign body **of back wall of thorax without penetration into thoracic cavity**

     √7ᵗʰ **S21.231** **Puncture wound without foreign body of** right **back wall of thorax without penetration into thoracic cavity**

     √7ᵗʰ **S21.232** **Puncture wound without foreign body of** left **back wall of thorax without penetration into thoracic cavity**

     √7ᵗʰ **S21.239** **Puncture wound without foreign body of unspecified back wall of thorax without penetration into thoracic cavity** ▽

√6ᵗʰ **S21.24** Puncture wound with foreign body **of back wall of thorax without penetration into thoracic cavity**

     √7ᵗʰ **S21.241** **Puncture wound with foreign body of** right **back wall of thorax without penetration into thoracic cavity**

     √7ᵗʰ **S21.242** **Puncture wound with foreign body of** left **back wall of thorax without penetration into thoracic cavity**

     √7ᵗʰ **S21.249** **Puncture wound with foreign body of unspecified back wall of thorax without penetration into thoracic cavity** ▽

√6ᵗʰ **S21.25** Open bite **of back wall of thorax without penetration into thoracic cavity**

     Bite of back wall of thorax NOS

     EXCLUDES 1 *superficial bite of back wall of thorax (S20.47)*

     √7ᵗʰ **S21.251** **Open bite of** right **back wall of thorax without penetration into thoracic cavity**

     √7ᵗʰ **S21.252** **Open bite of** left **back wall of thorax without penetration into thoracic cavity**

     √7ᵗʰ **S21.259** **Open bite of unspecified back wall of thorax without penetration into thoracic cavity** ▽

√5ᵗʰ **S21.3** Open wound of front wall of thorax with penetration **into thoracic cavity**

     Open wound of chest with penetration into thoracic cavity

√6ᵗʰ **S21.30** **Unspecified open wound of front wall of thorax with penetration into thoracic cavity**

     √7ᵗʰ **S21.301** **Unspecified open wound of** right **front wall of thorax with penetration into thoracic cavity** ▽

     √7ᵗʰ **S21.302** **Unspecified open wound of** left **front wall of thorax with penetration into thoracic cavity** ▽

     √7ᵗʰ **S21.309** **Unspecified open wound of unspecified front wall of thorax with penetration into thoracic cavity** ▽

√6ᵗʰ **S21.31** Laceration without foreign body **of front wall of thorax with penetration into thoracic cavity**

     √7ᵗʰ **S21.311** **Laceration without foreign body of** right **front wall of thorax with penetration into thoracic cavity**

     √7ᵗʰ **S21.312** **Laceration without foreign body of** left **front wall of thorax with penetration into thoracic cavity**

     √7ᵗʰ **S21.319** **Laceration without foreign body of unspecified front wall of thorax with penetration into thoracic cavity** ▽

√6ᵗʰ **S21.32** Laceration with foreign body **of front wall of thorax with penetration into thoracic cavity**

     √7ᵗʰ **S21.321** **Laceration with foreign body of** right **front wall of thorax with penetration into thoracic cavity**

     √7ᵗʰ **S21.322** **Laceration with foreign body of** left **front wall of thorax with penetration into thoracic cavity**

     √7ᵗʰ **S21.329** **Laceration with foreign body of unspecified front wall of thorax with penetration into thoracic cavity** ▽

√6ᵗʰ **S21.33** Puncture wound without foreign body **of front wall of thorax with penetration into thoracic cavity**

     √7ᵗʰ **S21.331** **Puncture wound without foreign body of** right **front wall of thorax with penetration into thoracic cavity**

     √7ᵗʰ **S21.332** **Puncture wound without foreign body of** left **front wall of thorax with penetration into thoracic cavity**

     √7ᵗʰ **S21.339** **Puncture wound without foreign body of unspecified front wall of thorax with penetration into thoracic cavity** ▽

√6ᵗʰ **S21.34** Puncture wound with foreign body **of front wall of thorax with penetration into thoracic cavity**

     √7ᵗʰ **S21.341** **Puncture wound with foreign body of** right **front wall of thorax with penetration into thoracic cavity**

     √7ᵗʰ **S21.342** **Puncture wound with foreign body of** left **front wall of thorax with penetration into thoracic cavity**

√7ᵗʰ **S21.349** Puncture wound with foreign ▽
body of unspecified front wall of
thorax with penetration into
thoracic cavity

√6ᵗʰ **S21.35** Open bite of front wall of thorax with penetration
into thoracic cavity
  EXCLUDES 1 *superficial bite of front wall of thorax*
  (S20.37)

√7ᵗʰ **S21.351** Open bite of right front wall of thorax
with penetration into thoracic cavity

√7ᵗʰ **S21.352** Open bite of left front wall of thorax with
penetration into thoracic cavity

√7ᵗʰ **S21.359** Open bite of unspecified front ▽
wall of thorax with penetration
into thoracic cavity

√5ᵗʰ **S21.4** Open wound of back wall of thorax with penetration into
thoracic cavity

√6ᵗʰ **S21.40** Unspecified open wound of back wall of thorax with
penetration into thoracic cavity

√7ᵗʰ **S21.401** Unspecified open wound of right ▽
back wall of thorax with
penetration into thoracic cavity

√7ᵗʰ **S21.402** Unspecified open wound of left ▽
back wall of thorax with
penetration into thoracic cavity

√7ᵗʰ **S21.409** Unspecified open wound of ▽
unspecified back wall of thorax
with penetration into thoracic
cavity

√6ᵗʰ **S21.41** Laceration without foreign body of back wall of
thorax with penetration into thoracic cavity

√7ᵗʰ **S21.411** Laceration without foreign body of right
back wall of thorax with penetration into
thoracic cavity

√7ᵗʰ **S21.412** Laceration without foreign body of left
back wall of thorax with penetration into
thoracic cavity

√7ᵗʰ **S21.419** Laceration without foreign body ▽
of unspecified back wall of thorax
with penetration into thoracic
cavity

√6ᵗʰ **S21.42** Laceration with foreign body of back wall of thorax
with penetration into thoracic cavity

√7ᵗʰ **S21.421** Laceration with foreign body of right
back wall of thorax with penetration into
thoracic cavity

√7ᵗʰ **S21.422** Laceration with foreign body of left back
wall of thorax with penetration into
thoracic cavity

√7ᵗʰ **S21.429** Laceration with foreign body of ▽
unspecified back wall of thorax
with penetration into thoracic
cavity

√6ᵗʰ **S21.43** Puncture wound without foreign body of back wall
of thorax with penetration into thoracic cavity

√7ᵗʰ **S21.431** Puncture wound without foreign body of
right back wall of thorax with penetration
into thoracic cavity

√7ᵗʰ **S21.432** Puncture wound without foreign body of
left back wall of thorax with penetration
into thoracic cavity

√7ᵗʰ **S21.439** Puncture wound without foreign ▽
body of unspecified back wall of
thorax with penetration into
thoracic cavity

√6ᵗʰ **S21.44** Puncture wound with foreign body of back wall of
thorax with penetration into thoracic cavity

√7ᵗʰ **S21.441** Puncture wound with foreign body of
right back wall of thorax with penetration
into thoracic cavity

√7ᵗʰ **S21.442** Puncture wound with foreign body of left
back wall of thorax with penetration into
thoracic cavity

√7ᵗʰ **S21.449** Puncture wound with foreign ▽
body of unspecified back wall of
thorax with penetration into
thoracic cavity

√6ᵗʰ **S21.45** Open bite of back wall of thorax with penetration
into thoracic cavity
  Bite of back wall of thorax NOS
  EXCLUDES 1 *superficial bite of back wall of thorax*
  (S20.47)

√7ᵗʰ **S21.451** Open bite of right back wall of thorax
with penetration into thoracic cavity

√7ᵗʰ **S21.452** Open bite of left back wall of thorax with
penetration into thoracic cavity

√7ᵗʰ **S21.459** Open bite of unspecified back ▽
wall of thorax with penetration
into thoracic cavity

√5ᵗʰ **S21.9** Open wound of unspecified part of thorax
  Open wound of thoracic wall NOS

√x7ᵗʰ **S21.90** Unspecified open wound of unspecified part ▽
of thorax

√x7ᵗʰ **S21.91** Laceration without foreign body of ▽
unspecified part of thorax

√x7ᵗʰ **S21.92** Laceration with foreign body of unspecified ▽
part of thorax

√x7ᵗʰ **S21.93** Puncture wound without foreign body of ▽
unspecified part of thorax

√x7ᵗʰ **S21.94** Puncture wound with foreign body of ▽
unspecified part of thorax

√x7ᵗʰ **S21.95** Open bite of unspecified part of thorax ▽
  EXCLUDES 1 *superficial bite of thorax (S20.97)*

√4ᵗʰ **S22** Fracture of rib(s), sternum and thoracic spine

  NOTE   A fracture not indicated as displaced or nondisplaced
  should be coded to displaced

  A fracture not indicated as open or closed should be coded
  to closed

  INCLUDES   fracture of thoracic neural arch
  fracture of thoracic spinous process
  fracture of thoracic transverse process
  fracture of thoracic vertebra
  fracture of thoracic vertebral arch

  Code first any associated:
    injury of intrathoracic organ (S27.-)
    spinal cord injury (S24.0-, S24.1-)
  EXCLUDES 1 *transection of thorax (S28.1)*
  EXCLUDES 2 *fracture of clavicle (S42.0-)*
    fracture of scapula (S42.1-)

  AHA: 2018,2Q,12; 2015,3Q,37-39

  The appropriate 7th character is to be added to each code from
  category S22.
  A   initial encounter for closed fracture
  B   initial encounter for open fracture
  D   subsequent encounter for fracture with routine healing
  G   subsequent encounter for fracture with delayed healing
  K   subsequent encounter for fracture with nonunion
  S   sequela

√5ᵗʰ **S22.0** Fracture of thoracic vertebra

√6ᵗʰ **S22.00** Fracture of unspecified thoracic vertebra

¹ √7ᵗʰ **S22.000** Wedge compression fracture of   HCC ⓪ ▽
unspecified thoracic vertebra

¹ √7ᵗʰ **S22.001** Stable burst fracture of   HCC ⓪ ▽
unspecified thoracic vertebra

¹ √7ᵗʰ **S22.002** Unstable burst fracture of   HCC ⓪ ▽
unspecified thoracic vertebra

¹ √7ᵗʰ **S22.008** Other fracture of unspecified   HCC ⓪ ▽
thoracic vertebra

¹ √7ᵗʰ **S22.009** Unspecified fracture of   HCC ⓪ ▽
unspecified thoracic vertebra

√6ᵗʰ **S22.01** Fracture of first thoracic vertebra

¹ √7ᵗʰ **S22.010** Wedge compression fracture of   HCC ⓪
first thoracic vertebra

¹ √7ᵗʰ **S22.011** Stable burst fracture of first   HCC ⓪
thoracic vertebra

¹ √7ᵗʰ **S22.012** Unstable burst fracture of first   HCC ⓪
thoracic vertebra

¹ √7ᵗʰ **S22.018** Other fracture of first thoracic   HCC ⓪
vertebra

¹ √7ᵗʰ **S22.019** Unspecified fracture of first   HCC ⓪ ▽
thoracic vertebra

√6ᵗʰ **S22.02** Fracture of second thoracic vertebra

¹ √7ᵗʰ **S22.020** Wedge compression fracture of   HCC ⓪
second thoracic vertebra

¹ √7ᵗʰ **S22.021** Stable burst fracture of second   HCC ⓪
thoracic vertebra

¹ √7ᵗʰ **S22.022** Unstable burst fracture of second   HCC ⓪
thoracic vertebra

¹ √7ᵗʰ **S22.028** Other fracture of second thoracic   HCC ⓪
vertebra

¹ √7ᵗʰ **S22.029** Unspecified fracture of second   HCC ⓪ ▽
thoracic vertebra

Chapter 19. Injury, Poisoning and Certain Other Consequences of External Causes

S22.03–S23.161

√6ᵗʰ **S22.03 Fracture of third thoracic vertebra**
- ¹ √7ᵗʰ **S22.030 Wedge compression fracture of** HCC Q
  third thoracic vertebra
- ¹ √7ᵗʰ **S22.031 Stable burst fracture of third** HCC Q
  thoracic vertebra
- ¹ √7ᵗʰ **S22.032 Unstable burst fracture of third** HCC Q
  thoracic vertebra
- ¹ √7ᵗʰ **S22.038 Other fracture of third thoracic** HCC Q
  vertebra
- ¹ √7ᵗʰ **S22.039 Unspecified fracture of third** HCC Q ▽
  thoracic vertebra

√6ᵗʰ **S22.04 Fracture of fourth thoracic vertebra**
- ¹ √7ᵗʰ **S22.040 Wedge compression fracture of** HCC Q
  fourth thoracic vertebra
- ¹ √7ᵗʰ **S22.041 Stable burst fracture of fourth** HCC Q
  thoracic vertebra
- ¹ √7ᵗʰ **S22.042 Unstable burst fracture of fourth** HCC Q
  thoracic vertebra
- ¹ √7ᵗʰ **S22.048 Other fracture of fourth thoracic** HCC Q
  vertebra
- ¹ √7ᵗʰ **S22.049 Unspecified fracture of fourth** HCC Q ▽
  thoracic vertebra

√6ᵗʰ **S22.05 Fracture of T5-T6 vertebra**
- ¹ √7ᵗʰ **S22.050 Wedge compression fracture of** HCC Q
  T5-T6 vertebra
- ¹ √7ᵗʰ **S22.051 Stable burst fracture of T5-T6** HCC Q
  vertebra
- ¹ √7ᵗʰ **S22.052 Unstable burst fracture of T5-T6** HCC Q
  vertebra
- ¹ √7ᵗʰ **S22.058 Other fracture of T5-T6 vertebra** HCC Q
- ¹ √7ᵗʰ **S22.059 Unspecified fracture of T5-T6** HCC Q ▽
  vertebra

√6ᵗʰ **S22.06 Fracture of T7-T8 vertebra**
- ¹ √7ᵗʰ **S22.060 Wedge compression fracture of** HCC Q
  T7-T8 vertebra
- ¹ √7ᵗʰ **S22.061 Stable burst fracture of T7-T8** HCC Q
  vertebra
- ¹ √7ᵗʰ **S22.062 Unstable burst fracture of T7-T8** HCC Q
  vertebra
- ¹ √7ᵗʰ **S22.068 Other fracture of T7-T8 thoracic** HCC Q
  vertebra
- ¹ √7ᵗʰ **S22.069 Unspecified fracture of T7-T8** HCC Q ▽
  vertebra

√6ᵗʰ **S22.07 Fracture of T9-T10 vertebra**
- ¹ √7ᵗʰ **S22.070 Wedge compression fracture of** HCC Q
  T9-T10 vertebra
- ¹ √7ᵗʰ **S22.071 Stable burst fracture of T9-T10** HCC Q
  vertebra
- ¹ √7ᵗʰ **S22.072 Unstable burst fracture of T9-T10** HCC Q
  vertebra
- ¹ √7ᵗʰ **S22.078 Other fracture of T9-T10 vertebra** HCC Q
- ¹ √7ᵗʰ **S22.079 Unspecified fracture of T9-T10** HCC Q ▽
  vertebra

√6ᵗʰ **S22.08 Fracture of T11-T12 vertebra**
- ¹ √7ᵗʰ **S22.080 Wedge compression fracture of** HCC Q
  T11-T12 vertebra
- ¹ √7ᵗʰ **S22.081 Stable burst fracture of T11-T12** HCC Q
  vertebra
- ¹ √7ᵗʰ **S22.082 Unstable burst fracture of** HCC Q
  T11-T12 vertebra
- ¹ √7ᵗʰ **S22.088 Other fracture of T11-T12** HCC Q
  vertebra
- ¹ √7ᵗʰ **S22.089 Unspecified fracture of T11-T12** HCC Q ▽
  vertebra

√5ᵗʰ **S22.2 Fracture of sternum**
> **DEF:** Break in flat bone (breast bone) in the anterior thorax caused by blunt trauma to the anterior chest.
- √x7ᵗʰ **S22.20 Unspecified fracture of sternum** Q ▽
- √x7ᵗʰ **S22.21 Fracture of manubrium** Q
- √x7ᵗʰ **S22.22 Fracture of body of sternum** Q
- √x7ᵗʰ **S22.23 Sternal manubrial dissociation** Q
- √x7ᵗʰ **S22.24 Fracture of xiphoid process** Q

√5ᵗʰ **S22.3 Fracture of one rib**
- √x7ᵗʰ **S22.31 Fracture of one rib, right side** Q
- √x7ᵗʰ **S22.32 Fracture of one rib, left side** Q
- √x7ᵗʰ **S22.39 Fracture of one rib, unspecified side** Q ▽

√5ᵗʰ **S22.4 Multiple fractures of ribs**
> Fractures of two or more ribs
> **EXCLUDES 1** flail chest (S22.5-)
- √x7ᵗʰ **S22.41 Multiple fractures of ribs, right side** Q
- √x7ᵗʰ **S22.42 Multiple fractures of ribs, left side** Q
- √x7ᵗʰ **S22.43 Multiple fractures of ribs, bilateral** Q
- √x7ᵗʰ **S22.49 Multiple fractures of ribs, unspecified side** Q ▽

√x7ᵗʰ **S22.5 Flail chest** Q

√x7ᵗʰ **S22.9 Fracture of bony thorax, part unspecified** Q ▽

√4ᵗʰ **S23 Dislocation and sprain of joints and ligaments of thorax**
> **INCLUDES** avulsion of joint or ligament of thorax
> laceration of cartilage, joint or ligament of thorax
> sprain of cartilage, joint or ligament of thorax
> traumatic hemarthrosis of joint or ligament of thorax
> traumatic rupture of joint or ligament of thorax
> traumatic subluxation of joint or ligament of thorax
> traumatic tear of joint or ligament of thorax
>
> Code also any associated open wound
> **EXCLUDES 2** dislocation, sprain of sternoclavicular joint (S43.2, S43.6)
> strain of muscle or tendon of thorax (S29.01-)

> The appropriate 7th character is to be added to each code from category S23.
> A initial encounter
> D subsequent encounter
> S sequela

√x7ᵗʰ **S23.0 Traumatic rupture of thoracic intervertebral disc**
> **EXCLUDES 1** rupture or displacement (nontraumatic) of thoracic intervertebral disc NOS (M51.- with fifth character 4)

√5ᵗʰ **S23.1 Subluxation and dislocation of thoracic vertebra**
> Code also any associated:
> open wound of thorax (S21.-)
> spinal cord injury (S24.0-, S24.1-)
> **EXCLUDES 2** fracture of thoracic vertebrae (S22.0-)
- √6ᵗʰ **S23.10 Subluxation and dislocation of unspecified thoracic vertebra**
  - √7ᵗʰ **S23.100 Subluxation of unspecified** ▽
    thoracic vertebra
  - √7ᵗʰ **S23.101 Dislocation of unspecified** ▽
    thoracic vertebra
- √6ᵗʰ **S23.11 Subluxation and dislocation of T1/T2 thoracic vertebra**
  - √7ᵗʰ **S23.110 Subluxation of T1/T2 thoracic vertebra**
  - √7ᵗʰ **S23.111 Dislocation of T1/T2 thoracic vertebra**
- √6ᵗʰ **S23.12 Subluxation and dislocation of T2/T3-T3/T4 thoracic vertebra**
  - √7ᵗʰ **S23.120 Subluxation of T2/T3 thoracic vertebra**
  - √7ᵗʰ **S23.121 Dislocation of T2/T3 thoracic vertebra**
  - √7ᵗʰ **S23.122 Subluxation of T3/T4 thoracic vertebra**
  - √7ᵗʰ **S23.123 Dislocation of T3/T4 thoracic vertebra**
- √6ᵗʰ **S23.13 Subluxation and dislocation of T4/T5-T5/T6 thoracic vertebra**
  - √7ᵗʰ **S23.130 Subluxation of T4/T5 thoracic vertebra**
  - √7ᵗʰ **S23.131 Dislocation of T4/T5 thoracic vertebra**
  - √7ᵗʰ **S23.132 Subluxation of T5/T6 thoracic vertebra**
  - √7ᵗʰ **S23.133 Dislocation of T5/T6 thoracic vertebra**
- √6ᵗʰ **S23.14 Subluxation and dislocation of T6/T7-T7/T8 thoracic vertebra**
  - √7ᵗʰ **S23.140 Subluxation of T6/T7 thoracic vertebra**
  - √7ᵗʰ **S23.141 Dislocation of T6/T7 thoracic vertebra**
  - √7ᵗʰ **S23.142 Subluxation of T7/T8 thoracic vertebra**
  - √7ᵗʰ **S23.143 Dislocation of T7/T8 thoracic vertebra**
- √6ᵗʰ **S23.15 Subluxation and dislocation of T8/T9-T9/T10 thoracic vertebra**
  - √7ᵗʰ **S23.150 Subluxation of T8/T9 thoracic vertebra**
  - √7ᵗʰ **S23.151 Dislocation of T8/T9 thoracic vertebra**
  - √7ᵗʰ **S23.152 Subluxation of T9/T10 thoracic vertebra**
  - √7ᵗʰ **S23.153 Dislocation of T9/T10 thoracic vertebra**
- √6ᵗʰ **S23.16 Subluxation and dislocation of T10/T11-T11/T12 thoracic vertebra**
  - √7ᵗʰ **S23.160 Subluxation of T10/T11 thoracic vertebra**
  - √7ᵗʰ **S23.161 Dislocation of T10/T11 thoracic vertebra**

√7ᵗʰ **S23.162** Subluxation of T11/T12 thoracic vertebra

√7ᵗʰ **S23.163** Dislocation of T11/T12 thoracic vertebra

√6ᵗʰ **S23.17** **Subluxation and dislocation of T12/L1 thoracic vertebra**

√7ᵗʰ **S23.170** Subluxation of T12/L1 thoracic vertebra

√7ᵗʰ **S23.171** Dislocation of T12/L1 thoracic vertebra

√5ᵗʰ **S23.2** **Dislocation of other and unspecified parts of thorax**

√x7ᵗʰ **S23.20** **Dislocation of unspecified part of thorax**   ▽

√x7ᵗʰ **S23.29** **Dislocation of other parts of thorax**

√x7ᵗʰ **S23.3** **Sprain of ligaments of thoracic spine**

√5ᵗʰ **S23.4** **Sprain of ribs and sternum**

√x7ᵗʰ **S23.41** **Sprain of ribs**

√6ᵗʰ **S23.42** **Sprain of sternum**

√7ᵗʰ **S23.420** **Sprain of sternoclavicular (joint) (ligament)**

√7ᵗʰ **S23.421** **Sprain of chondrosternal joint**

√7ᵗʰ **S23.428** **Other sprain of sternum**

√7ᵗʰ **S23.429** **Unspecified sprain of sternum**   ▽

√x7ᵗʰ **S23.8** **Sprain of other specified parts of thorax**

√x7ᵗʰ **S23.9** **Sprain of unspecified parts of thorax**   ▽

√4ᵗʰ **S24** **Injury of nerves and spinal cord at thorax level**

> **NOTE**   Code to highest level of thoracic spinal cord injury.
>
> Injuries to the spinal cord (S24.0 and S24.1) refer to the cord level and not bone level injury, and can affect nerve roots at and below the level given.

Code also any associated:
   fracture of thoracic vertebra (S22.0-)
   open wound of thorax (S21.-)
   transient paralysis (R29.5)

EXCLUDES 2   *injury of brachial plexus (S14.3)*

The appropriate 7th character is to be added to each code from category S24.
A   initial encounter
D   subsequent encounter
S   sequela

√x7ᵗʰ **S24.0** **Concussion and edema of thoracic spinal cord**   HCC

√5ᵗʰ **S24.1** **Other and unspecified injuries of thoracic spinal cord**

√6ᵗʰ **S24.10** **Unspecified injury of thoracic spinal cord**

√7ᵗʰ **S24.101** **Unspecified injury at T1 level of thoracic spinal cord**   HCC ▽

√7ᵗʰ **S24.102** **Unspecified injury at T2-T6 level of thoracic spinal cord**   HCC ▽

√7ᵗʰ **S24.103** **Unspecified injury at T7-T10 level of thoracic spinal cord**   HCC ▽

√7ᵗʰ **S24.104** **Unspecified injury at T11-T12 level of thoracic spinal cord**   HCC ▽

√7ᵗʰ **S24.109** **Unspecified injury at unspecified level of thoracic spinal cord**   HCC ▽
Injury of thoracic spinal cord NOS

√6ᵗʰ **S24.11** **Complete lesion of thoracic spinal cord**

√7ᵗʰ **S24.111** **Complete lesion at T1 level of thoracic spinal cord**   HCC

√7ᵗʰ **S24.112** **Complete lesion at T2-T6 level of thoracic spinal cord**   HCC

√7ᵗʰ **S24.113** **Complete lesion at T7-T10 level of thoracic spinal cord**   HCC

√7ᵗʰ **S24.114** **Complete lesion at T11-T12 level of thoracic spinal cord**   HCC

√7ᵗʰ **S24.119** **Complete lesion at unspecified level of thoracic spinal cord**   HCC ▽

√6ᵗʰ **S24.13** **Anterior cord syndrome of thoracic spinal cord**

√7ᵗʰ **S24.131** **Anterior cord syndrome at T1 level of thoracic spinal cord**   HCC

√7ᵗʰ **S24.132** **Anterior cord syndrome at T2-T6 level of thoracic spinal cord**   HCC

√7ᵗʰ **S24.133** **Anterior cord syndrome at T7-T10 level of thoracic spinal cord**   HCC

√7ᵗʰ **S24.134** **Anterior cord syndrome at T11-T12 level of thoracic spinal cord**   HCC

√7ᵗʰ **S24.139** **Anterior cord syndrome at unspecified level of thoracic spinal cord**   HCC ▽

√6ᵗʰ **S24.14** **Brown-Séquard syndrome of thoracic spinal cord**

√7ᵗʰ **S24.141** **Brown-Séquard syndrome at T1 level of thoracic spinal cord**   HCC

√7ᵗʰ **S24.142** **Brown-Séquard syndrome at T2-T6 level of thoracic spinal cord**   HCC

√7ᵗʰ **S24.143** **Brown-Séquard syndrome at T7-T10 level of thoracic spinal cord**   HCC

√7ᵗʰ **S24.144** **Brown-Séquard syndrome at T11-T12 level of thoracic spinal cord**   HCC

√7ᵗʰ **S24.149** **Brown-Séquard syndrome at unspecified level of thoracic spinal cord**   HCC ▽

√6ᵗʰ **S24.15** **Other incomplete lesions of thoracic spinal cord**
Incomplete lesion of thoracic spinal cord NOS
Posterior cord syndrome of thoracic spinal cord

√7ᵗʰ **S24.151** **Other incomplete lesion at T1 level of thoracic spinal cord**   HCC

√7ᵗʰ **S24.152** **Other incomplete lesion at T2-T6 level of thoracic spinal cord**   HCC

√7ᵗʰ **S24.153** **Other incomplete lesion at T7-T10 level of thoracic spinal cord**   HCC

√7ᵗʰ **S24.154** **Other incomplete lesion at T11-T12 level of thoracic spinal cord**   HCC

√7ᵗʰ **S24.159** **Other incomplete lesion at unspecified level of thoracic spinal cord**   HCC ▽

√x7ᵗʰ **S24.2** **Injury of nerve root of thoracic spine**

√x7ᵗʰ **S24.3** **Injury of peripheral nerves of thorax**

√x7ᵗʰ **S24.4** **Injury of thoracic sympathetic nervous system**
Injury of cardiac plexus
Injury of esophageal plexus
Injury of pulmonary plexus
Injury of stellate ganglion
Injury of thoracic sympathetic ganglion

√x7ᵗʰ **S24.8** **Injury of other specified nerves of thorax**

√x7ᵗʰ **S24.9** **Injury of unspecified nerve of thorax**   ▽

√4ᵗʰ **S25** **Injury of blood vessels of thorax**

Code also any associated open wound (S21.-)

The appropriate 7th character is to be added to each code from category S25.
A   initial encounter
D   subsequent encounter
S   sequela

√5ᵗʰ **S25.0** **Injury of thoracic aorta**
Injury of aorta NOS

√x7ᵗʰ **S25.00** **Unspecified injury of thoracic aorta**   ▽

√x7ᵗʰ **S25.01** **Minor laceration of thoracic aorta**
Incomplete transection of thoracic aorta
Laceration of thoracic aorta NOS
Superficial laceration of thoracic aorta

√x7ᵗʰ **S25.02** **Major laceration of thoracic aorta**
Complete transection of thoracic aorta
Traumatic rupture of thoracic aorta

√x7ᵗʰ **S25.09** **Other specified injury of thoracic aorta**

√5ᵗʰ **S25.1** **Injury of innominate or subclavian artery**

√6ᵗʰ **S25.10** **Unspecified injury of innominate or subclavian artery**

√7ᵗʰ **S25.101** **Unspecified injury of right innominate or subclavian artery**   ▽

√7ᵗʰ **S25.102** **Unspecified injury of left innominate or subclavian artery**   ▽

√7ᵗʰ **S25.109** **Unspecified injury of unspecified innominate or subclavian artery**   ▽

√6ᵗʰ **S25.11** **Minor laceration of innominate or subclavian artery**
Incomplete transection of innominate or subclavian artery
Laceration of innominate or subclavian artery NOS
Superficial laceration of innominate or subclavian artery

√7ᵗʰ **S25.111** **Minor laceration of right innominate or subclavian artery**

√7ᵗʰ **S25.112** **Minor laceration of left innominate or subclavian artery**

✓ Additional Character Req   √x7ᵗʰ Placeholder Alert   Manifestation   ▽ Unspecified   ►◄ Revised Text   ● New Code   ▲ Revised Code Title

ICD-10-CM 2019   **973**

Chapter 19. Injury, Poisoning and Certain Other Consequences of External Causes

S25.119–S25.90

√7ᵗʰ **S25.119** Minor laceration of unspecified innominate or subclavian artery ▽

√6ᵗʰ **S25.12** Major laceration of innominate or subclavian artery

    Complete transection of innominate or subclavian artery

    Traumatic rupture of innominate or subclavian artery

√7ᵗʰ **S25.121** Major laceration of right innominate or subclavian artery

√7ᵗʰ **S25.122** Major laceration of left innominate or subclavian artery

√7ᵗʰ **S25.129** Major laceration of unspecified innominate or subclavian artery ▽

√6ᵗʰ **S25.19** Other specified injury of innominate or subclavian artery

√7ᵗʰ **S25.191** Other specified injury of right innominate or subclavian artery

√7ᵗʰ **S25.192** Other specified injury of left innominate or subclavian artery

√7ᵗʰ **S25.199** Other specified injury of unspecified innominate or subclavian artery ▽

√5ᵗʰ **S25.2** Injury of superior vena cava

    Injury of vena cava NOS

√x7ᵗʰ **S25.20** Unspecified injury of superior vena cava ▽

√x7ᵗʰ **S25.21** Minor laceration of superior vena cava

    Incomplete transection of superior vena cava

    Laceration of superior vena cava NOS

    Superficial laceration of superior vena cava

√x7ᵗʰ **S25.22** Major laceration of superior vena cava

    Complete transection of superior vena cava

    Traumatic rupture of superior vena cava

√x7ᵗʰ **S25.29** Other specified injury of superior vena cava

√5ᵗʰ **S25.3** Injury of innominate or subclavian vein

√6ᵗʰ **S25.30** Unspecified injury of innominate or subclavian vein

√7ᵗʰ **S25.301** Unspecified injury of right innominate or subclavian vein ▽

√7ᵗʰ **S25.302** Unspecified injury of left innominate or subclavian vein ▽

√7ᵗʰ **S25.309** Unspecified injury of unspecified innominate or subclavian vein ▽

√6ᵗʰ **S25.31** Minor laceration of innominate or subclavian vein

    Incomplete transection of innominate or subclavian vein

    Laceration of innominate or subclavian vein NOS

    Superficial laceration of innominate or subclavian vein

√7ᵗʰ **S25.311** Minor laceration of right innominate or subclavian vein

√7ᵗʰ **S25.312** Minor laceration of left innominate or subclavian vein

√7ᵗʰ **S25.319** Minor laceration of unspecified innominate or subclavian vein ▽

√6ᵗʰ **S25.32** Major laceration of innominate or subclavian vein

    Complete transection of innominate or subclavian vein

    Traumatic rupture of innominate or subclavian vein

√7ᵗʰ **S25.321** Major laceration of right innominate or subclavian vein

√7ᵗʰ **S25.322** Major laceration of left innominate or subclavian vein

√7ᵗʰ **S25.329** Major laceration of unspecified innominate or subclavian vein ▽

√6ᵗʰ **S25.39** Other specified injury of innominate or subclavian vein

√7ᵗʰ **S25.391** Other specified injury of right innominate or subclavian vein

√7ᵗʰ **S25.392** Other specified injury of left innominate or subclavian vein

√7ᵗʰ **S25.399** Other specified injury of unspecified innominate or subclavian vein ▽

√5ᵗʰ **S25.4** Injury of pulmonary blood vessels

√6ᵗʰ **S25.40** Unspecified injury of pulmonary blood vessels

√7ᵗʰ **S25.401** Unspecified injury of right pulmonary blood vessels ▽

√7ᵗʰ **S25.402** Unspecified injury of left pulmonary blood vessels ▽

√7ᵗʰ **S25.409** Unspecified injury of unspecified pulmonary blood vessels ▽

√6ᵗʰ **S25.41** Minor laceration of pulmonary blood vessels

    Incomplete transection of pulmonary blood vessels

    Laceration of pulmonary blood vessels NOS

    Superficial laceration of pulmonary blood vessels

√7ᵗʰ **S25.411** Minor laceration of right pulmonary blood vessels

√7ᵗʰ **S25.412** Minor laceration of left pulmonary blood vessels

√7ᵗʰ **S25.419** Minor laceration of unspecified pulmonary blood vessels ▽

√6ᵗʰ **S25.42** Major laceration of pulmonary blood vessels

    Complete transection of pulmonary blood vessels

    Traumatic rupture of pulmonary blood vessels

√7ᵗʰ **S25.421** Major laceration of right pulmonary blood vessels

√7ᵗʰ **S25.422** Major laceration of left pulmonary blood vessels

√7ᵗʰ **S25.429** Major laceration of unspecified pulmonary blood vessels ▽

√6ᵗʰ **S25.49** Other specified injury of pulmonary blood vessels

√7ᵗʰ **S25.491** Other specified injury of right pulmonary blood vessels

√7ᵗʰ **S25.492** Other specified injury of left pulmonary blood vessels

√7ᵗʰ **S25.499** Other specified injury of unspecified pulmonary blood vessels ▽

√5ᵗʰ **S25.5** Injury of intercostal blood vessels

√6ᵗʰ **S25.50** Unspecified injury of intercostal blood vessels

√7ᵗʰ **S25.501** Unspecified injury of intercostal blood vessels, right side ▽

√7ᵗʰ **S25.502** Unspecified injury of intercostal blood vessels, left side ▽

√7ᵗʰ **S25.509** Unspecified injury of intercostal blood vessels, unspecified side ▽

√6ᵗʰ **S25.51** Laceration of intercostal blood vessels

√7ᵗʰ **S25.511** Laceration of intercostal blood vessels, right side

√7ᵗʰ **S25.512** Laceration of intercostal blood vessels, left side

√7ᵗʰ **S25.519** Laceration of intercostal blood vessels, unspecified side ▽

√6ᵗʰ **S25.59** Other specified injury of intercostal blood vessels

√7ᵗʰ **S25.591** Other specified injury of intercostal blood vessels, right side

√7ᵗʰ **S25.592** Other specified injury of intercostal blood vessels, left side

√7ᵗʰ **S25.599** Other specified injury of intercostal blood vessels, unspecified side ▽

√5ᵗʰ **S25.8** Injury of other blood vessels of thorax

    Injury of azygos vein

    Injury of mammary artery or vein

√6ᵗʰ **S25.80** Unspecified injury of other blood vessels of thorax

√7ᵗʰ **S25.801** Unspecified injury of other blood vessels of thorax, right side ▽

√7ᵗʰ **S25.802** Unspecified injury of other blood vessels of thorax, left side ▽

√7ᵗʰ **S25.809** Unspecified injury of other blood vessels of thorax, unspecified side ▽

√6ᵗʰ **S25.81** Laceration of other blood vessels of thorax

√7ᵗʰ **S25.811** Laceration of other blood vessels of thorax, right side

√7ᵗʰ **S25.812** Laceration of other blood vessels of thorax, left side

√7ᵗʰ **S25.819** Laceration of other blood vessels of thorax, unspecified side ▽

√6ᵗʰ **S25.89** Other specified injury of other blood vessels of thorax

√7ᵗʰ **S25.891** Other specified injury of other blood vessels of thorax, right side

√7ᵗʰ **S25.892** Other specified injury of other blood vessels of thorax, left side

√7ᵗʰ **S25.899** Other specified injury of other blood vessels of thorax, unspecified side ▽

√5ᵗʰ **S25.9** Injury of unspecified blood vessel of thorax

√x7ᵗʰ **S25.90** Unspecified injury of unspecified blood vessel of thorax ▽

√x7ᵗʰ **S25.91** Laceration of unspecified blood vessel of thorax ▽

√x7ᵗʰ **S25.99** Other specified injury of unspecified blood vessel of thorax ▽

√4ᵗʰ **S26 Injury of heart**

Code also any associated:
open wound of thorax (S21.-)
traumatic hemopneumothorax (S27.2)
traumatic hemothorax (S27.1)
traumatic pneumothorax (S27.0)

The appropriate 7th character is to be added to each code from category S26.
A   initial encounter
D   subsequent encounter
S   sequela

√5ᵗʰ **S26.0 Injury of heart** with hemopericardium

√x7ᵗʰ **S26.00** Unspecified injury of heart with hemopericardium ▽

√x7ᵗʰ **S26.01** Contusion of heart with hemopericardium

√6ᵗʰ **S26.02** Laceration of heart with hemopericardium

√7ᵗʰ **S26.020** Mild laceration of heart with hemopericardium
Laceration of heart without penetration of heart chamber

√7ᵗʰ **S26.021** Moderate laceration of heart with hemopericardium
Laceration of heart with penetration of heart chamber

√7ᵗʰ **S26.022** Major laceration of heart with hemopericardium
Laceration of heart with penetration of multiple heart chambers

√x7ᵗʰ **S26.09** Other injury of heart with hemopericardium

√5ᵗʰ **S26.1 Injury of heart** without hemopericardium

√x7ᵗʰ **S26.10** Unspecified injury of heart without hemopericardium ▽

√x7ᵗʰ **S26.11** Contusion of heart without hemopericardium

√x7ᵗʰ **S26.12** Laceration of heart without hemopericardium

√x7ᵗʰ **S26.19** Other injury of heart without hemopericardium

√5ᵗʰ **S26.9 Injury of heart, unspecified** with or without hemopericardium

√x7ᵗʰ **S26.90** Unspecified injury of heart, unspecified with or without hemopericardium ▽

√x7ᵗʰ **S26.91** Contusion of heart, unspecified with or without hemopericardium ▽
DEF: Bruising within the heart muscle, with no mention of an open wound, usually caused by blunt chest trauma in motor vehicle accidents, falling from great heights, or receiving CPR.

√x7ᵗʰ **S26.92** Laceration of heart, unspecified with or without hemopericardium ▽
Laceration of heart NOS

√x7ᵗʰ **S26.99** Other injury of heart, unspecified with or without hemopericardium ▽

√4ᵗʰ **S27 Injury of other and unspecified intrathoracic organs**

Code also any associated open wound of thorax (S21.-)

EXCLUDES 2   injury of cervical esophagus (S10-S19)
injury of trachea (cervical) (S10-S19)

The appropriate 7th character is to be added to each code from category S27.
A   initial encounter
D   subsequent encounter
S   sequela

√x7ᵗʰ **S27.0 Traumatic pneumothorax**

EXCLUDES 1   spontaneous pneumothorax (J93.-)

√x7ᵗʰ **S27.1 Traumatic hemothorax**

√x7ᵗʰ **S27.2 Traumatic hemopneumothorax**

√5ᵗʰ **S27.3 Other and unspecified injuries of lung**

√6ᵗʰ **S27.30** Unspecified injury of lung

√7ᵗʰ **S27.301** Unspecified injury of lung, unilateral ▽

√7ᵗʰ **S27.302** Unspecified injury of lung, bilateral ▽

√7ᵗʰ **S27.309** Unspecified injury of lung, unspecified ▽

√6ᵗʰ **S27.31** Primary blast injury of lung
Blast injury of lung NOS

√7ᵗʰ **S27.311** Primary blast injury of lung, unilateral

√7ᵗʰ **S27.312** Primary blast injury of lung, bilateral

√7ᵗʰ **S27.319** Primary blast injury of lung, unspecified ▽

√6ᵗʰ **S27.32** Contusion of lung
DEF: Bruising of the lung without mention of an open wound.

√7ᵗʰ **S27.321** Contusion of lung, unilateral

√7ᵗʰ **S27.322** Contusion of lung, bilateral

√7ᵗʰ **S27.329** Contusion of lung, unspecified ▽

√6ᵗʰ **S27.33** Laceration of lung

√7ᵗʰ **S27.331** Laceration of lung, unilateral

√7ᵗʰ **S27.332** Laceration of lung, bilateral

√7ᵗʰ **S27.339** Laceration of lung, unspecified ▽

√6ᵗʰ **S27.39** Other injuries of lung
Secondary blast injury of lung

√7ᵗʰ **S27.391** Other injuries of lung, unilateral

√7ᵗʰ **S27.392** Other injuries of lung, bilateral

√7ᵗʰ **S27.399** Other injuries of lung, unspecified ▽

√5ᵗʰ **S27.4 Injury of** bronchus

√6ᵗʰ **S27.40** Unspecified injury of bronchus

√7ᵗʰ **S27.401** Unspecified injury of bronchus, unilateral ▽

√7ᵗʰ **S27.402** Unspecified injury of bronchus, bilateral ▽

√7ᵗʰ **S27.409** Unspecified injury of bronchus, unspecified ▽

√6ᵗʰ **S27.41** Primary blast injury of bronchus
Blast injury of bronchus NOS

√7ᵗʰ **S27.411** Primary blast injury of bronchus, unilateral

√7ᵗʰ **S27.412** Primary blast injury of bronchus, bilateral

√7ᵗʰ **S27.419** Primary blast injury of bronchus, unspecified ▽

√6ᵗʰ **S27.42** Contusion of bronchus

√7ᵗʰ **S27.421** Contusion of bronchus, unilateral

√7ᵗʰ **S27.422** Contusion of bronchus, bilateral

√7ᵗʰ **S27.429** Contusion of bronchus, unspecified ▽

√6ᵗʰ **S27.43** Laceration of bronchus

√7ᵗʰ **S27.431** Laceration of bronchus, unilateral

√7ᵗʰ **S27.432** Laceration of bronchus, bilateral

√7ᵗʰ **S27.439** Laceration of bronchus, unspecified ▽

√6ᵗʰ **S27.49** Other injury of bronchus
Secondary blast injury of bronchus

√7ᵗʰ **S27.491** Other injury of bronchus, unilateral

√7ᵗʰ **S27.492** Other injury of bronchus, bilateral

√7ᵗʰ **S27.499** Other injury of bronchus, unspecified ▽

√5ᵗʰ **S27.5 Injury of** thoracic trachea

√x7ᵗʰ **S27.50** Unspecified injury of thoracic trachea ▽

√x7ᵗʰ **S27.51** Primary blast injury of thoracic trachea
Blast injury of thoracic trachea NOS

√x7ᵗʰ **S27.52** Contusion of thoracic trachea

√x7ᵗʰ **S27.53** Laceration of thoracic trachea

√x7ᵗʰ **S27.59** Other injury of thoracic trachea
Secondary blast injury of thoracic trachea

√5ᵗʰ **S27.6 Injury of** pleura

√x7ᵗʰ **S27.60** Unspecified injury of pleura ▽

√x7ᵗʰ **S27.63** Laceration of pleura

√x7ᵗʰ **S27.69** Other injury of pleura

√5ᵗʰ **S27.8 Injury of other specified intrathoracic organs**

√6ᵗʰ **S27.80** Injury of diaphragm

√7ᵗʰ **S27.802** Contusion of diaphragm

√7ᵗʰ **S27.803** Laceration of diaphragm

√7ᵗʰ **S27.808** Other injury of diaphragm

√7ᵗʰ **S27.809** Unspecified injury of diaphragm ▽

☑ Additional Character Req   √x7ᵗʰ Placeholder Alert   Manifestation   ▽ Unspecified   ▶◀ Revised Text   ● New Code   ▲ Revised Code Title

√6ᵗʰ **S27.81 Injury of** esophagus (thoracic part)

     √7ᵗʰ **S27.812 Contusion of** esophagus (thoracic part)

     √7ᵗʰ **S27.813 Laceration of** esophagus (thoracic part)

     √7ᵗʰ **S27.818 Other injury of** esophagus (thoracic part)

     √7ᵗʰ **S27.819 Unspecified injury of esophagus** ▽
         (thoracic part)

√6ᵗʰ **S27.89 Injury of other specified intrathoracic organs**

     Injury of lymphatic thoracic duct
     Injury of thymus gland

     √7ᵗʰ **S27.892 Contusion of other specified intrathoracic organs**

     √7ᵗʰ **S27.893 Laceration of other specified intrathoracic organs**

     √7ᵗʰ **S27.898 Other injury of other specified intrathoracic organs**

     √7ᵗʰ **S27.899 Unspecified injury of other** ▽
         specified intrathoracic organs

√x7ᵗʰ **S27.9 Injury of unspecified intrathoracic organ** ▽

√4ᵗʰ **S28 Crushing injury of thorax, and traumatic amputation of part of thorax**

     The appropriate 7th character is to be added to each code from category S28.
     A   initial encounter
     D   subsequent encounter
     S   sequela

√x7ᵗʰ **S28.0 Crushed chest**

     Use additional code for all associated injuries
     EXCLUDES 1   flail chest (S22.5)

√x7ᵗʰ **S28.1 Traumatic amputation (partial) of** part of thorax, except breast

√5ᵗʰ **S28.2 Traumatic amputation of** breast

     √6ᵗʰ **S28.21 Complete traumatic amputation of breast**

         Traumatic amputation of breast NOS

         √7ᵗʰ **S28.211 Complete traumatic amputation of** right **breast**

         √7ᵗʰ **S28.212 Complete traumatic amputation of** left **breast**

         √7ᵗʰ **S28.219 Complete traumatic amputation** ▽
            of unspecified breast

     √6ᵗʰ **S28.22 Partial traumatic amputation of breast**

         √7ᵗʰ **S28.221 Partial traumatic amputation of** right **breast**

         √7ᵗʰ **S28.222 Partial traumatic amputation of** left **breast**

         √7ᵗʰ **S28.229 Partial traumatic amputation of** ▽
            unspecified breast

√4ᵗʰ **S29 Other and unspecified injuries of thorax**

     Code also any associated open wound (S21.-)

     The appropriate 7th character is to be added to each code from category S29.
     A   initial encounter
     D   subsequent encounter
     S   sequela

√5ᵗʰ **S29.0 Injury of muscle and tendon at thorax level**

     √6ᵗʰ **S29.00 Unspecified injury of muscle and tendon of thorax**

         √7ᵗʰ **S29.001 Unspecified injury of muscle and** ▽
            tendon of front **wall of thorax**

         √7ᵗʰ **S29.002 Unspecified injury of muscle and** ▽
            tendon of back **wall of thorax**

         √7ᵗʰ **S29.009 Unspecified injury of muscle and** ▽
            tendon of unspecified wall of thorax

     √6ᵗʰ **S29.01 Strain of muscle and tendon of thorax**

         √7ᵗʰ **S29.011 Strain of muscle and tendon of** front **wall of thorax**

         √7ᵗʰ **S29.012 Strain of muscle and tendon of** back **wall of thorax**

         √7ᵗʰ **S29.019 Strain of muscle and tendon of** ▽
            unspecified wall of thorax

     √6ᵗʰ **S29.02 Laceration of muscle and tendon of thorax**

         √7ᵗʰ **S29.021 Laceration of muscle and tendon of** front **wall of thorax**

         √7ᵗʰ **S29.022 Laceration of muscle and tendon of** back **wall of thorax**

         √7ᵗʰ **S29.029 Laceration of muscle and tendon** ▽
            of unspecified wall of thorax

√6ᵗʰ **S29.09 Other injury of muscle and tendon of thorax**

     √7ᵗʰ **S29.091 Other injury of muscle and tendon of** front **wall of thorax**

     √7ᵗʰ **S29.092 Other injury of muscle and tendon of** back **wall of thorax**

     √7ᵗʰ **S29.099 Other injury of muscle and** ▽
         tendon of unspecified wall of thorax

√x7ᵗʰ **S29.8 Other specified injuries of thorax**

√x7ᵗʰ **S29.9 Unspecified injury of thorax** ▽

Injuries to the abdomen, lower back, lumbar spine, pelvis and external genitals (S30-S39)

INCLUDES   injuries to the abdominal wall
     injuries to the anus
     injuries to the buttock
     injuries to the external genitalia
     injuries to the flank
     injuries to the groin

EXCLUDES 2   burns and corrosions (T20-T32)
     effects of foreign body in anus and rectum (T18.5)
     effects of foreign body in genitourinary tract (T19.-)
     effects of foreign body in stomach, small intestine and colon (T18.2-T18.4)
     frostbite (T33-T34)
     insect bite or sting, venomous (T63.4)

√4ᵗʰ **S30 Superficial injury of abdomen, lower back, pelvis and external genitals**

     EXCLUDES 2   superficial injury of hip (S70.-)

     The appropriate 7th character is to be added to each code from category S30.
     A   initial encounter
     D   subsequent encounter
     S   sequela

√x7ᵗʰ **S30.0 Contusion of lower back and pelvis**

     Contusion of buttock

√x7ᵗʰ **S30.1 Contusion of abdominal wall**

     Contusion of flank
     Contusion of groin

√5ᵗʰ **S30.2 Contusion of external genital organs**

     √6ᵗʰ **S30.20 Contusion of unspecified external genital organ**

         √7ᵗʰ **S30.201 Contusion of unspecified external** ♂ ▽
            genital organ, male

         √7ᵗʰ **S30.202 Contusion of unspecified external** ♀ ▽
            genital organ, female

     √x7ᵗʰ **S30.21 Contusion of** penis   ♂

     √x7ᵗʰ **S30.22 Contusion of** scrotum and testes   ♂

     √x7ᵗʰ **S30.23 Contusion of** vagina and vulva   ♀

√x7ᵗʰ **S30.3 Contusion of anus**

√5ᵗʰ **S30.8 Other superficial injuries of abdomen, lower back, pelvis and external genitals**

     √6ᵗʰ **S30.81 Abrasion of abdomen, lower back, pelvis and external genitals**

         √7ᵗʰ **S30.810 Abrasion of** lower back and pelvis

         √7ᵗʰ **S30.811 Abrasion of** abdominal wall

         √7ᵗʰ **S30.812 Abrasion of** penis   ♂

         √7ᵗʰ **S30.813 Abrasion of** scrotum and testes   ♂

         √7ᵗʰ **S30.814 Abrasion of** vagina and vulva   ♀

         √7ᵗʰ **S30.815 Abrasion of unspecified** external ♂ ▽
            genital organs, male

         √7ᵗʰ **S30.816 Abrasion of unspecified** external ♀ ▽
            genital organs, female

         √7ᵗʰ **S30.817 Abrasion of** anus

     √6ᵗʰ **S30.82 Blister (nonthermal) of abdomen, lower back, pelvis and external genitals**

         √7ᵗʰ **S30.820 Blister (nonthermal) of** lower back and pelvis

         √7ᵗʰ **S30.821 Blister (nonthermal) of** abdominal wall

         √7ᵗʰ **S30.822 Blister (nonthermal) of** penis   ♂

         √7ᵗʰ **S30.823 Blister (nonthermal) of** scrotum ♂
            and testes

         √7ᵗʰ **S30.824 Blister (nonthermal) of** vagina ♀
            and vulva

         √7ᵗʰ **S30.825 Blister (nonthermal) of** ♂ ▽
            unspecified external genital organs, male

√7ᵗʰ **S30.826 Blister (nonthermal) of unspecified** external genital organs, female   ♀ ▽

√7ᵗʰ **S30.827 Blister (nonthermal) of** anus

√6ᵗʰ **S30.84 External constriction of abdomen, lower back, pelvis and external genitals**

    √7ᵗʰ **S30.840 External constriction of** lower back and pelvis

    √7ᵗʰ **S30.841 External constriction of** abdominal wall

    √7ᵗʰ **S30.842 External constriction of** penis   ♂

       Hair tourniquet syndrome of penis
       Use additional cause code to identify the constricting item (W49.0-)

    √7ᵗʰ **S30.843 External constriction of** scrotum and testes   ♂

    √7ᵗʰ **S30.844 External constriction of** vagina and vulva   ♀

    √7ᵗʰ **S30.845 External constriction of unspecified** external genital organs, male   ♂ ▽

    √7ᵗʰ **S30.846 External constriction of unspecified** external genital organs, female   ♀ ▽

√6ᵗʰ **S30.85 Superficial foreign body of abdomen, lower back, pelvis and external genitals**

       Splinter in the abdomen, lower back, pelvis and external genitals

    √7ᵗʰ **S30.850 Superficial foreign body of** lower back and pelvis

    √7ᵗʰ **S30.851 Superficial foreign body of** abdominal wall

    √7ᵗʰ **S30.852 Superficial foreign body of** penis   ♂

    √7ᵗʰ **S30.853 Superficial foreign body of** scrotum and testes   ♂

    √7ᵗʰ **S30.854 Superficial foreign body of** vagina and vulva   ♀

    √7ᵗʰ **S30.855 Superficial foreign body of unspecified** external genital organs, male   ♂ ▽

    √7ᵗʰ **S30.856 Superficial foreign body of unspecified** external genital organs, female   ♀ ▽

    √7ᵗʰ **S30.857 Superficial foreign body of** anus

√6ᵗʰ **S30.86 Insect bite (nonvenomous) of abdomen, lower back, pelvis and external genitals**

    √7ᵗʰ **S30.860 Insect bite (nonvenomous) of** lower back and pelvis

    √7ᵗʰ **S30.861 Insect bite (nonvenomous) of** abdominal wall

    √7ᵗʰ **S30.862 Insect bite (nonvenomous) of** penis   ♂

    √7ᵗʰ **S30.863 Insect bite (nonvenomous) of** scrotum and testes   ♂

    √7ᵗʰ **S30.864 Insect bite (nonvenomous) of** vagina and vulva   ♀

    √7ᵗʰ **S30.865 Insect bite (nonvenomous) of unspecified** external genital organs, male   ♂ ▽

    √7ᵗʰ **S30.866 Insect bite (nonvenomous) of unspecified** external genital organs, female   ♀ ▽

    √7ᵗʰ **S30.867 Insect bite (nonvenomous) of** anus

√6ᵗʰ **S30.87 Other superficial bite of abdomen, lower back, pelvis and external genitals**

    EXCLUDES 1   *open bite of abdomen, lower back, pelvis and external genitals (S31.05, S31.15, S31.25, S31.35, S31.45, S31.55)*

    √7ᵗʰ **S30.870 Other superficial bite of** lower back and pelvis

    √7ᵗʰ **S30.871 Other superficial bite of** abdominal wall

    √7ᵗʰ **S30.872 Other superficial bite of** penis   ♂

    √7ᵗʰ **S30.873 Other superficial bite of** scrotum and testes   ♂

    √7ᵗʰ **S30.874 Other superficial bite of** vagina and vulva   ♀

    √7ᵗʰ **S30.875 Other superficial bite of unspecified** external genital organs, male   ♂ ▽

    √7ᵗʰ **S30.876 Other superficial bite of unspecified** external genital organs, female   ♀ ▽

√7ᵗʰ **S30.877 Other superficial bite of** anus

√5ᵗʰ **S30.9 Unspecified superficial injury of abdomen, lower back, pelvis and external genitals**

    √x7ᵗʰ **S30.91 Unspecified superficial injury of** lower back and pelvis   ▽

    √x7ᵗʰ **S30.92 Unspecified superficial injury of** abdominal wall   ▽

    √x7ᵗʰ **S30.93 Unspecified superficial injury of** penis   ♂ ▽

    √x7ᵗʰ **S30.94 Unspecified superficial injury of** scrotum and testes   ♂ ▽

    √x7ᵗʰ **S30.95 Unspecified superficial injury of** vagina and vulva   ♀ ▽

    √x7ᵗʰ **S30.96 Unspecified superficial injury of unspecified** external genital organs, male   ♂ ▽

    √x7ᵗʰ **S30.97 Unspecified superficial injury of unspecified** external genital organs, female   ♀ ▽

    √x7ᵗʰ **S30.98 Unspecified superficial injury of** anus   ▽

√4ᵗʰ **S31 Open wound of abdomen, lower back, pelvis and external genitals**

    Code also any associated:
      spinal cord injury (S24.0, S24.1-, S34.0-, S34.1-)
      wound infection

    EXCLUDES 1   *traumatic amputation of part of abdomen, lower back and pelvis (S38.2-, S38.3)*

    EXCLUDES 2   *open wound of hip (S71.00–S71.02)*
              open fracture of pelvis (S32.1- — S32.9 with 7th character B)

    The appropriate 7th character is to be added to each code from category S31.
    A   initial encounter
    D   subsequent encounter
    S   sequela

√5ᵗʰ **S31.0 Open wound of lower back and pelvis**

    √6ᵗʰ **S31.00 Unspecified open wound of lower back and pelvis**

      √7ᵗʰ **S31.000 Unspecified open wound of lower back and pelvis without penetration into retroperitoneum**   ▽

         Unspecified open wound of lower back and pelvis NOS

      √7ᵗʰ **S31.001 Unspecified open wound of lower back and pelvis with penetration into retroperitoneum**   ▽

    √6ᵗʰ **S31.01 Laceration without foreign body of lower back and pelvis**

      √7ᵗʰ **S31.010 Laceration without foreign body of lower back and pelvis without penetration into retroperitoneum**

         Laceration without foreign body of lower back and pelvis NOS

      √7ᵗʰ **S31.011 Laceration without foreign body of lower back and pelvis with penetration into retroperitoneum**

    √6ᵗʰ **S31.02 Laceration with foreign body of lower back and pelvis**

      √7ᵗʰ **S31.020 Laceration with foreign body of lower back and pelvis without penetration into retroperitoneum**

         Laceration with foreign body of lower back and pelvis NOS

      √7ᵗʰ **S31.021 Laceration with foreign body of lower back and pelvis with penetration into retroperitoneum**

    √6ᵗʰ **S31.03 Puncture wound without foreign body of lower back and pelvis**

      √7ᵗʰ **S31.030 Puncture wound without foreign body of lower back and pelvis without penetration into retroperitoneum**

         Puncture wound without foreign body of lower back and pelvis NOS

      √7ᵗʰ **S31.031 Puncture wound without foreign body of lower back and pelvis with penetration into retroperitoneum**

    √6ᵗʰ **S31.04 Puncture wound with foreign body of lower back and pelvis**

      √7ᵗʰ **S31.040 Puncture wound with foreign body of lower back and pelvis without penetration into retroperitoneum**

         Puncture wound with foreign body of lower back and pelvis NOS

      √7ᵗʰ **S31.041 Puncture wound with foreign body of lower back and pelvis with penetration into retroperitoneum**

☑ Additional Character Req   √x7ᵗʰ Placeholder Alert   **Manifestation**   ▽ Unspecified   ►◄ Revised Text   ● New Code   ▲ Revised Code Title

ICD-10-CM 2019   977

Chapter 19. Injury, Poisoning and Certain Other Consequences of External Causes

S31.05–S31.151

√6ᵗʰ **S31.05** **Open bite** of lower back and pelvis

     Bite of lower back and pelvis NOS

     EXCLUDES 1   *superficial bite of lower back and pelvis (S30.860, S30.870)*

     √7ᵗʰ **S31.050** **Open bite of lower back and pelvis without penetration into retroperitoneum**

         Open bite of lower back and pelvis NOS

     √7ᵗʰ **S31.051** **Open bite of lower back and pelvis with penetration into retroperitoneum**

√5ᵗʰ **S31.1** **Open wound of** abdominal wall without penetration into peritoneal cavity

     Open wound of abdominal wall NOS

     EXCLUDES 2   *open wound of abdominal wall with penetration into peritoneal cavity (S31.6-)*

   √6ᵗʰ **S31.10** **Unspecified open wound of abdominal wall without penetration into peritoneal cavity**

     √7ᵗʰ **S31.100** **Unspecified open wound of abdominal wall, right upper quadrant without penetration into peritoneal cavity** ▽

     √7ᵗʰ **S31.101** **Unspecified open wound of abdominal wall, left upper quadrant without penetration into peritoneal cavity** ▽

     √7ᵗʰ **S31.102** **Unspecified open wound of abdominal wall, epigastric region without penetration into peritoneal cavity** ▽

     √7ᵗʰ **S31.103** **Unspecified open wound of abdominal wall, right lower quadrant without penetration into peritoneal cavity** ▽

     √7ᵗʰ **S31.104** **Unspecified open wound of abdominal wall, left lower quadrant without penetration into peritoneal cavity** ▽

     √7ᵗʰ **S31.105** **Unspecified open wound of abdominal wall, periumbilic region without penetration into peritoneal cavity** ▽

     √7ᵗʰ **S31.109** **Unspecified open wound of abdominal wall, unspecified quadrant without penetration into peritoneal cavity** ▽

         Unspecified open wound of abdominal wall NOS

   √6ᵗʰ **S31.11** **Laceration without foreign body** of abdominal wall without penetration into peritoneal cavity

     √7ᵗʰ **S31.110** **Laceration without foreign body of abdominal wall, right upper quadrant without penetration into peritoneal cavity**

     √7ᵗʰ **S31.111** **Laceration without foreign body of abdominal wall, left upper quadrant without penetration into peritoneal cavity**

     √7ᵗʰ **S31.112** **Laceration without foreign body of abdominal wall, epigastric region without penetration into peritoneal cavity**

     √7ᵗʰ **S31.113** **Laceration without foreign body of abdominal wall, right lower quadrant without penetration into peritoneal cavity**

     √7ᵗʰ **S31.114** **Laceration without foreign body of abdominal wall, left lower quadrant without penetration into peritoneal cavity**

     √7ᵗʰ **S31.115** **Laceration without foreign body of abdominal wall, periumbilic region without penetration into peritoneal cavity**

     √7ᵗʰ **S31.119** **Laceration without foreign body of abdominal wall, unspecified quadrant without penetration into peritoneal cavity** ▽

   √6ᵗʰ **S31.12** **Laceration with foreign body** of abdominal wall without penetration into peritoneal cavity

     √7ᵗʰ **S31.120** **Laceration of abdominal wall with foreign body, right upper quadrant without penetration into peritoneal cavity**

     √7ᵗʰ **S31.121** **Laceration of abdominal wall with foreign body, left upper quadrant without penetration into peritoneal cavity**

     √7ᵗʰ **S31.122** **Laceration of abdominal wall with foreign body, epigastric region without penetration into peritoneal cavity**

     √7ᵗʰ **S31.123** **Laceration of abdominal wall with foreign body, right lower quadrant without penetration into peritoneal cavity**

     √7ᵗʰ **S31.124** **Laceration of abdominal wall with foreign body, left lower quadrant without penetration into peritoneal cavity**

     √7ᵗʰ **S31.125** **Laceration of abdominal wall with foreign body, periumbilic region without penetration into peritoneal cavity**

     √7ᵗʰ **S31.129** **Laceration of abdominal wall with foreign body, unspecified quadrant without penetration into peritoneal cavity** ▽

   √6ᵗʰ **S31.13** **Puncture wound** of abdominal wall without foreign body without penetration into peritoneal cavity

     √7ᵗʰ **S31.130** **Puncture wound of abdominal wall without foreign body, right upper quadrant without penetration into peritoneal cavity**

     √7ᵗʰ **S31.131** **Puncture wound of abdominal wall without foreign body, left upper quadrant without penetration into peritoneal cavity**

     √7ᵗʰ **S31.132** **Puncture wound of abdominal wall without foreign body, epigastric region without penetration into peritoneal cavity**

     √7ᵗʰ **S31.133** **Puncture wound of abdominal wall without foreign body, right lower quadrant without penetration into peritoneal cavity**

     √7ᵗʰ **S31.134** **Puncture wound of abdominal wall without foreign body, left lower quadrant without penetration into peritoneal cavity**

     √7ᵗʰ **S31.135** **Puncture wound of abdominal wall without foreign body, periumbilic region without penetration into peritoneal cavity**

     √7ᵗʰ **S31.139** **Puncture wound of abdominal wall without foreign body, unspecified quadrant without penetration into peritoneal cavity** ▽

   √6ᵗʰ **S31.14** **Puncture wound** of abdominal wall with foreign body without penetration into peritoneal cavity

     √7ᵗʰ **S31.140** **Puncture wound of abdominal wall with foreign body, right upper quadrant without penetration into peritoneal cavity**

     √7ᵗʰ **S31.141** **Puncture wound of abdominal wall with foreign body, left upper quadrant without penetration into peritoneal cavity**

     √7ᵗʰ **S31.142** **Puncture wound of abdominal wall with foreign body, epigastric region without penetration into peritoneal cavity**

     √7ᵗʰ **S31.143** **Puncture wound of abdominal wall with foreign body, right lower quadrant without penetration into peritoneal cavity**

     √7ᵗʰ **S31.144** **Puncture wound of abdominal wall with foreign body, left lower quadrant without penetration into peritoneal cavity**

     √7ᵗʰ **S31.145** **Puncture wound of abdominal wall with foreign body, periumbilic region without penetration into peritoneal cavity**

     √7ᵗʰ **S31.149** **Puncture wound of abdominal wall with foreign body, unspecified quadrant without penetration into peritoneal cavity** ▽

   √6ᵗʰ **S31.15** **Open bite** of abdominal wall without penetration into peritoneal cavity

     Bite of abdominal wall NOS

     EXCLUDES 1   *superficial bite of abdominal wall (S30.871)*

     √7ᵗʰ **S31.150** **Open bite of abdominal wall, right upper quadrant without penetration into peritoneal cavity**

     √7ᵗʰ **S31.151** **Open bite of abdominal wall, left upper quadrant without penetration into peritoneal cavity**

√7ᵗʰ **S31.152** Open bite of abdominal wall, epigastric region without penetration into peritoneal cavity

√7ᵗʰ **S31.153** Open bite of abdominal wall, right lower quadrant without penetration into peritoneal cavity

√7ᵗʰ **S31.154** Open bite of abdominal wall, left lower quadrant without penetration into peritoneal cavity

√7ᵗʰ **S31.155** Open bite of abdominal wall, periumbilic region without penetration into peritoneal cavity

√7ᵗʰ **S31.159** Open bite of abdominal wall, unspecified quadrant without penetration into peritoneal cavity   ▽

√5ᵗʰ **S31.2 Open wound of penis**

√x7ᵗʰ **S31.20** Unspecified open wound of penis   ♂ ▽

√x7ᵗʰ **S31.21** Laceration without foreign body of penis   ♂

√x7ᵗʰ **S31.22** Laceration with foreign body of penis   ♂

√x7ᵗʰ **S31.23** Puncture wound without foreign body of penis   ♂

√x7ᵗʰ **S31.24** Puncture wound with foreign body of penis   ♂

√x7ᵗʰ **S31.25** Open bite of penis   ♂

Bite of penis NOS

EXCLUDES 1   *superficial bite of penis (S30.862, S30.872)*

√5ᵗʰ **S31.3 Open wound of scrotum and testes**

√x7ᵗʰ **S31.30** Unspecified open wound of scrotum and testes   ♂ ▽

√x7ᵗʰ **S31.31** Laceration without foreign body of scrotum and testes   ♂

√x7ᵗʰ **S31.32** Laceration with foreign body of scrotum and testes   ♂

√x7ᵗʰ **S31.33** Puncture wound without foreign body of scrotum and testes   ♂

√x7ᵗʰ **S31.34** Puncture wound with foreign body of scrotum and testes   ♂

√x7ᵗʰ **S31.35** Open bite of scrotum and testes   ♂

Bite of scrotum and testes NOS

EXCLUDES 1   *superficial bite of scrotum and testes (S30.863, S30.873)*

√5ᵗʰ **S31.4 Open wound of vagina and vulva**

EXCLUDES 1   *injury to vagina and vulva during delivery (O70.-, O71.4)*

√x7ᵗʰ **S31.40** Unspecified open wound of vagina and vulva   ♀ ▽

√x7ᵗʰ **S31.41** Laceration without foreign body of vagina and vulva   ♀

√x7ᵗʰ **S31.42** Laceration with foreign body of vagina and vulva   ♀

√x7ᵗʰ **S31.43** Puncture wound without foreign body of vagina and vulva   ♀

√x7ᵗʰ **S31.44** Puncture wound with foreign body of vagina and vulva   ♀

√x7ᵗʰ **S31.45** Open bite of vagina and vulva   ♀

Bite of vagina and vulva NOS

EXCLUDES 1   *superficial bite of vagina and vulva (S30.864, S30.874)*

√5ᵗʰ **S31.5 Open wound of unspecified external genital organs**

EXCLUDES 1   *traumatic amputation of external genital organs (S38.21, S38.22)*

√6ᵗʰ **S31.50** Unspecified open wound of unspecified external genital organs

√7ᵗʰ **S31.501** Unspecified open wound of unspecified external genital organs, male   ♂ ▽

√7ᵗʰ **S31.502** Unspecified open wound of unspecified external genital organs, female   ♀ ▽

√6ᵗʰ **S31.51** Laceration without foreign body of unspecified external genital organs

√7ᵗʰ **S31.511** Laceration without foreign body of unspecified external genital organs, male   ♂ ▽

√7ᵗʰ **S31.512** Laceration without foreign body of unspecified external genital organs, female   ♀ ▽

√6ᵗʰ **S31.52** Laceration with foreign body of unspecified external genital organs

√7ᵗʰ **S31.521** Laceration with foreign body of unspecified external genital organs, male   ♂ ▽

√7ᵗʰ **S31.522** Laceration with foreign body of unspecified external genital organs, female   ♀ ▽

√6ᵗʰ **S31.53** Puncture wound without foreign body of unspecified external genital organs

√7ᵗʰ **S31.531** Puncture wound without foreign body of unspecified external genital organs, male   ♂ ▽

√7ᵗʰ **S31.532** Puncture wound without foreign body of unspecified external genital organs, female   ♀ ▽

√6ᵗʰ **S31.54** Puncture wound with foreign body of unspecified external genital organs

√7ᵗʰ **S31.541** Puncture wound with foreign body of unspecified external genital organs, male   ♂ ▽

√7ᵗʰ **S31.542** Puncture wound with foreign body of unspecified external genital organs, female   ♀ ▽

√6ᵗʰ **S31.55** Open bite of unspecified external genital organs

Bite of unspecified external genital organs NOS

EXCLUDES 1   *superficial bite of unspecified external genital organs (S30.865, S30.866, S30.875, S30.876)*

√7ᵗʰ **S31.551** Open bite of unspecified external genital organs, male   ♂ ▽

√7ᵗʰ **S31.552** Open bite of unspecified external genital organs, female   ♀ ▽

√5ᵗʰ **S31.6 Open wound of abdominal wall with penetration into peritoneal cavity**

√6ᵗʰ **S31.60** Unspecified open wound of abdominal wall with penetration into peritoneal cavity

√7ᵗʰ **S31.600** Unspecified open wound of abdominal wall, right upper quadrant with penetration into peritoneal cavity   ▽

√7ᵗʰ **S31.601** Unspecified open wound of abdominal wall, left upper quadrant with penetration into peritoneal cavity   ▽

√7ᵗʰ **S31.602** Unspecified open wound of abdominal wall, epigastric region with penetration into peritoneal cavity   ▽

√7ᵗʰ **S31.603** Unspecified open wound of abdominal wall, right lower quadrant with penetration into peritoneal cavity   ▽

√7ᵗʰ **S31.604** Unspecified open wound of abdominal wall, left lower quadrant with penetration into peritoneal cavity   ▽

√7ᵗʰ **S31.605** Unspecified open wound of abdominal wall, periumbilic region with penetration into peritoneal cavity   ▽

√7ᵗʰ **S31.609** Unspecified open wound of abdominal wall, unspecified quadrant with penetration into peritoneal cavity   ▽

√6ᵗʰ **S31.61** Laceration without foreign body of abdominal wall with penetration into peritoneal cavity

√7ᵗʰ **S31.610** Laceration without foreign body of abdominal wall, right upper quadrant with penetration into peritoneal cavity

√7ᵗʰ **S31.611** Laceration without foreign body of abdominal wall, left upper quadrant with penetration into peritoneal cavity

√7ᵗʰ **S31.612** Laceration without foreign body of abdominal wall, epigastric region with penetration into peritoneal cavity

√7ᵗʰ **S31.613** Laceration without foreign body of abdominal wall, right lower quadrant with penetration into peritoneal cavity

√7ᵗʰ **S31.614** Laceration without foreign body of abdominal wall, left lower quadrant with penetration into peritoneal cavity

☑ Additional Character Req   √x7ᵗʰ Placeholder Alert   Manifestation   ▽ Unspecified   ▶◀ Revised Text   ● New Code   ▲ Revised Code Title

ICD-10-CM 2019   979

√7ᵗʰ **S31.615** Laceration without foreign body of abdominal wall, periumbilic region with penetration into peritoneal cavity

√7ᵗʰ **S31.619** Laceration without foreign body of abdominal wall, unspecified quadrant with penetration into peritoneal cavity ▽

√6ᵗʰ **S31.62** Laceration with foreign body of abdominal wall with penetration into peritoneal cavity

√7ᵗʰ **S31.620** Laceration with foreign body of abdominal wall, right upper quadrant with penetration into peritoneal cavity

√7ᵗʰ **S31.621** Laceration with foreign body of abdominal wall, left upper quadrant with penetration into peritoneal cavity

√7ᵗʰ **S31.622** Laceration with foreign body of abdominal wall, epigastric region with penetration into peritoneal cavity

√7ᵗʰ **S31.623** Laceration with foreign body of abdominal wall, right lower quadrant with penetration into peritoneal cavity

√7ᵗʰ **S31.624** Laceration with foreign body of abdominal wall, left lower quadrant with penetration into peritoneal cavity

√7ᵗʰ **S31.625** Laceration with foreign body of abdominal wall, periumbilic region with penetration into peritoneal cavity

√7ᵗʰ **S31.629** Laceration with foreign body of abdominal wall, unspecified quadrant with penetration into peritoneal cavity ▽

√6ᵗʰ **S31.63** Puncture wound without foreign body of abdominal wall with penetration into peritoneal cavity

√7ᵗʰ **S31.630** Puncture wound without foreign body of abdominal wall, right upper quadrant with penetration into peritoneal cavity

√7ᵗʰ **S31.631** Puncture wound without foreign body of abdominal wall, left upper quadrant with penetration into peritoneal cavity

√7ᵗʰ **S31.632** Puncture wound without foreign body of abdominal wall, epigastric region with penetration into peritoneal cavity

√7ᵗʰ **S31.633** Puncture wound without foreign body of abdominal wall, right lower quadrant with penetration into peritoneal cavity

√7ᵗʰ **S31.634** Puncture wound without foreign body of abdominal wall, left lower quadrant with penetration into peritoneal cavity

√7ᵗʰ **S31.635** Puncture wound without foreign body of abdominal wall, periumbilic region with penetration into peritoneal cavity

√7ᵗʰ **S31.639** Puncture wound without foreign body of abdominal wall, unspecified quadrant with penetration into peritoneal cavity ▽

√6ᵗʰ **S31.64** Puncture wound with foreign body of abdominal wall with penetration into peritoneal cavity

√7ᵗʰ **S31.640** Puncture wound with foreign body of abdominal wall, right upper quadrant with penetration into peritoneal cavity

√7ᵗʰ **S31.641** Puncture wound with foreign body of abdominal wall, left upper quadrant with penetration into peritoneal cavity

√7ᵗʰ **S31.642** Puncture wound with foreign body of abdominal wall, epigastric region with penetration into peritoneal cavity

√7ᵗʰ **S31.643** Puncture wound with foreign body of abdominal wall, right lower quadrant with penetration into peritoneal cavity

√7ᵗʰ **S31.644** Puncture wound with foreign body of abdominal wall, left lower quadrant with penetration into peritoneal cavity

√7ᵗʰ **S31.645** Puncture wound with foreign body of abdominal wall, periumbilic region with penetration into peritoneal cavity

√7ᵗʰ **S31.649** Puncture wound with foreign body of abdominal wall, unspecified quadrant with penetration into peritoneal cavity ▽

√6ᵗʰ **S31.65** Open bite of abdominal wall with penetration into peritoneal cavity

EXCLUDES 1 superficial bite of abdominal wall (S30.861, S30.871)

√7ᵗʰ **S31.650** Open bite of abdominal wall, right upper quadrant with penetration into peritoneal cavity

√7ᵗʰ **S31.651** Open bite of abdominal wall, left upper quadrant with penetration into peritoneal cavity

√7ᵗʰ **S31.652** Open bite of abdominal wall, epigastric region with penetration into peritoneal cavity

√7ᵗʰ **S31.653** Open bite of abdominal wall, right lower quadrant with penetration into peritoneal cavity

√7ᵗʰ **S31.654** Open bite of abdominal wall, left lower quadrant with penetration into peritoneal cavity

√7ᵗʰ **S31.655** Open bite of abdominal wall, periumbilic region with penetration into peritoneal cavity

√7ᵗʰ **S31.659** Open bite of abdominal wall, unspecified quadrant with penetration into peritoneal cavity ▽

√5ᵗʰ **S31.8** Open wound of other parts of abdomen, lower back and pelvis

√6ᵗʰ **S31.80** Open wound of unspecified buttock

√7ᵗʰ **S31.801** Laceration without foreign body of unspecified buttock ▽

√7ᵗʰ **S31.802** Laceration with foreign body of unspecified buttock ▽

√7ᵗʰ **S31.803** Puncture wound without foreign body of unspecified buttock ▽

√7ᵗʰ **S31.804** Puncture wound with foreign body of unspecified buttock ▽

√7ᵗʰ **S31.805** Open bite of unspecified buttock ▽

Bite of buttock NOS

EXCLUDES 1 superficial bite of buttock (S30.870)

√7ᵗʰ **S31.809** Unspecified open wound of unspecified buttock ▽

√6ᵗʰ **S31.81** Open wound of right buttock

√7ᵗʰ **S31.811** Laceration without foreign body of right buttock

√7ᵗʰ **S31.812** Laceration with foreign body of right buttock

√7ᵗʰ **S31.813** Puncture wound without foreign body of right buttock

√7ᵗʰ **S31.814** Puncture wound with foreign body of right buttock

√7ᵗʰ **S31.815** Open bite of right buttock

Bite of right buttock NOS

EXCLUDES 1 superficial bite of buttock (S30.870)

√7ᵗʰ **S31.819** Unspecified open wound of right buttock ▽

√6ᵗʰ **S31.82** Open wound of left buttock

√7ᵗʰ **S31.821** Laceration without foreign body of left buttock

√7ᵗʰ **S31.822** Laceration with foreign body of left buttock

√7ᵗʰ **S31.823** Puncture wound without foreign body of left buttock

√7ᵗʰ **S31.824** Puncture wound with foreign body of left buttock

√7ᵗʰ **S31.825** Open bite of left buttock

Bite of left buttock NOS

EXCLUDES 1 superficial bite of buttock (S30.870)

√7ᵗʰ **S31.829** Unspecified open wound of left buttock ▽

√6ᵗʰ **S31.83** Open wound of anus

√7ᵗʰ **S31.831** Laceration without foreign body of anus

√7ᵗʰ **S31.832** Laceration with foreign body of anus

√7ᵗʰ **S31.833** Puncture wound without foreign body of anus

√7ᵗʰ **S31.834** Puncture wound with foreign body of anus

√7ᵗʰ **S31.835** **Open bite** of anus
Bite of anus NOS
EXCLUDES 1 superficial bite of anus (S30.877)

√7ᵗʰ **S31.839** **Unspecified open wound** of anus ▽

√4ᵗʰ **S32** **Fracture of lumbar spine and pelvis**

NOTE　A fracture not indicated as displaced or nondisplaced should be coded to displaced.
A fracture not indicated as opened or closed should be coded to closed.

INCLUDES　fracture of lumbosacral neural arch
fracture of lumbosacral spinous process
fracture of lumbosacral transverse process
fracture of lumbosacral vertebra
fracture of lumbosacral vertebral arch

Code first any associated spinal cord and spinal nerve injury (S34.-)

EXCLUDES 1　transection of abdomen (S38.3)
EXCLUDES 2　fracture of hip NOS (S72.0-)

AHA: 2018,2Q,12; 2015,3Q,37-39; 2012,4Q,93

The appropriate 7th character is to be added to each code from category S32.
A　initial encounter for closed fracture
B　initial encounter for open fracture
D　subsequent encounter for fracture with routine healing
G　subsequent encounter for fracture with delayed healing
K　subsequent encounter for fracture with nonunion
S　sequela

√5ᵗʰ **S32.0** **Fracture of lumbar vertebra**
Fracture of lumbar spine NOS

√6ᵗʰ **S32.00** **Fracture of unspecified lumbar vertebra**

¹ √7ᵗʰ **S32.000** **Wedge compression fracture of** unspecified lumbar vertebra　HCC Q ▽

¹ √7ᵗʰ **S32.001** **Stable burst fracture of** unspecified lumbar vertebra　HCC Q ▽

¹ √7ᵗʰ **S32.002** **Unstable burst fracture of** unspecified lumbar vertebra　HCC Q ▽

¹ √7ᵗʰ **S32.008** **Other fracture of unspecified** lumbar vertebra　HCC Q ▽

¹ √7ᵗʰ **S32.009** **Unspecified fracture of** unspecified lumbar vertebra　HCC Q ▽

√6ᵗʰ **S32.01** **Fracture of first lumbar vertebra**

¹ √7ᵗʰ **S32.010** **Wedge compression fracture of** first lumbar vertebra　HCC Q

¹ √7ᵗʰ **S32.011** **Stable burst fracture of first** lumbar vertebra　HCC Q

¹ √7ᵗʰ **S32.012** **Unstable burst fracture of first** lumbar vertebra　HCC Q

¹ √7ᵗʰ **S32.018** **Other fracture of first lumbar** vertebra　HCC Q

¹ √7ᵗʰ **S32.019** **Unspecified fracture of first** lumbar vertebra　HCC Q ▽

√6ᵗʰ **S32.02** **Fracture of second lumbar vertebra**

¹ √7ᵗʰ **S32.020** **Wedge compression fracture of** second lumbar vertebra　HCC Q

¹ √7ᵗʰ **S32.021** **Stable burst fracture of second** lumbar vertebra　HCC Q

¹ √7ᵗʰ **S32.022** **Unstable burst fracture of second** lumbar vertebra　HCC Q

¹ √7ᵗʰ **S32.028** **Other fracture of second lumbar** vertebra　HCC Q

¹ √7ᵗʰ **S32.029** **Unspecified fracture of second** lumbar vertebra　HCC Q ▽

√6ᵗʰ **S32.03** **Fracture of third lumbar vertebra**

¹ √7ᵗʰ **S32.030** **Wedge compression fracture of** third lumbar vertebra　HCC Q

¹ √7ᵗʰ **S32.031** **Stable burst fracture of third** lumbar vertebra　HCC Q

¹ √7ᵗʰ **S32.032** **Unstable burst fracture of third** lumbar vertebra　HCC Q

¹ √7ᵗʰ **S32.038** **Other fracture of third lumbar** vertebra　HCC Q

¹ √7ᵗʰ **S32.039** **Unspecified fracture of third** lumbar vertebra　HCC Q ▽

√6ᵗʰ **S32.04** **Fracture of fourth lumbar vertebra**

¹ √7ᵗʰ **S32.040** **Wedge compression fracture of** fourth lumbar vertebra　HCC Q

¹ √7ᵗʰ **S32.041** **Stable burst fracture of fourth** lumbar vertebra　HCC Q

¹ √7ᵗʰ **S32.042** **Unstable burst fracture of fourth** lumbar vertebra　HCC Q

¹ √7ᵗʰ **S32.048** **Other fracture of fourth lumbar** vertebra　HCC Q

¹ √7ᵗʰ **S32.049** **Unspecified fracture of fourth** lumbar vertebra　HCC Q ▽

√6ᵗʰ **S32.05** **Fracture of fifth lumbar vertebra**

¹ √7ᵗʰ **S32.050** **Wedge compression fracture of** fifth lumbar vertebra　HCC Q

¹ √7ᵗʰ **S32.051** **Stable burst fracture of fifth** lumbar vertebra　HCC Q

¹ √7ᵗʰ **S32.052** **Unstable burst fracture of fifth** lumbar vertebra　HCC Q

¹ √7ᵗʰ **S32.058** **Other fracture of fifth lumbar** vertebra　HCC Q

¹ √7ᵗʰ **S32.059** **Unspecified fracture of fifth** lumbar vertebra　HCC Q ▽

√5ᵗʰ **S32.1** **Fracture of sacrum**

NOTE　For vertical fractures, code to most medial fracture extension
Use two codes if both a vertical and transverse fracture are present

Code also any associated fracture of pelvic ring (S32.8-)

¹ √x7ᵗʰ **S32.10** **Unspecified fracture of sacrum**　HCC Q ▽

√6ᵗʰ **S32.11** **Zone I fracture of sacrum**
Vertical sacral ala fracture of sacrum

Vertical Sacral Fracture Zones

Zones: ① ② ③

¹ √7ᵗʰ **S32.110** **Nondisplaced Zone I fracture of** sacrum　HCC Q

¹ √7ᵗʰ **S32.111** **Minimally displaced Zone I** fracture of sacrum　HCC Q

¹ √7ᵗʰ **S32.112** **Severely displaced Zone I fracture** of sacrum　HCC Q

¹ √7ᵗʰ **S32.119** **Unspecified Zone I fracture of** sacrum　HCC Q ▽

√6ᵗʰ **S32.12** **Zone II fracture of sacrum**
Vertical foraminal region fracture of sacrum

¹ √7ᵗʰ **S32.120** **Nondisplaced Zone II fracture of** sacrum　HCC Q

¹ √7ᵗʰ **S32.121** **Minimally displaced Zone II** fracture of sacrum　HCC Q

¹ √7ᵗʰ **S32.122** **Severely displaced Zone II** fracture of sacrum　HCC Q

¹ √7ᵗʰ **S32.129** **Unspecified Zone II fracture of** sacrum　HCC Q ▽

√6ᵗʰ **S32.13** **Zone III fracture of sacrum**
Vertical fracture into spinal canal region of sacrum

¹ √7ᵗʰ **S32.130** **Nondisplaced Zone III fracture of** sacrum　HCC Q

¹ √7ᵗʰ **S32.131** **Minimally displaced Zone III** fracture of sacrum　HCC Q

¹ √7ᵗʰ **S32.132** **Severely displaced Zone III** fracture of sacrum　HCC Q

☑ Additional Character Req　　√x7ᵗʰ Placeholder Alert　　Manifestation　　▽ Unspecified　　►◄ Revised Text　　● New Code　　▲ Revised Code Title

¹ √7ᵗʰ **S32.139** **Unspecified Zone III fracture of** HCC Q ▽
sacrum

Transverse Sacral Fracture Types

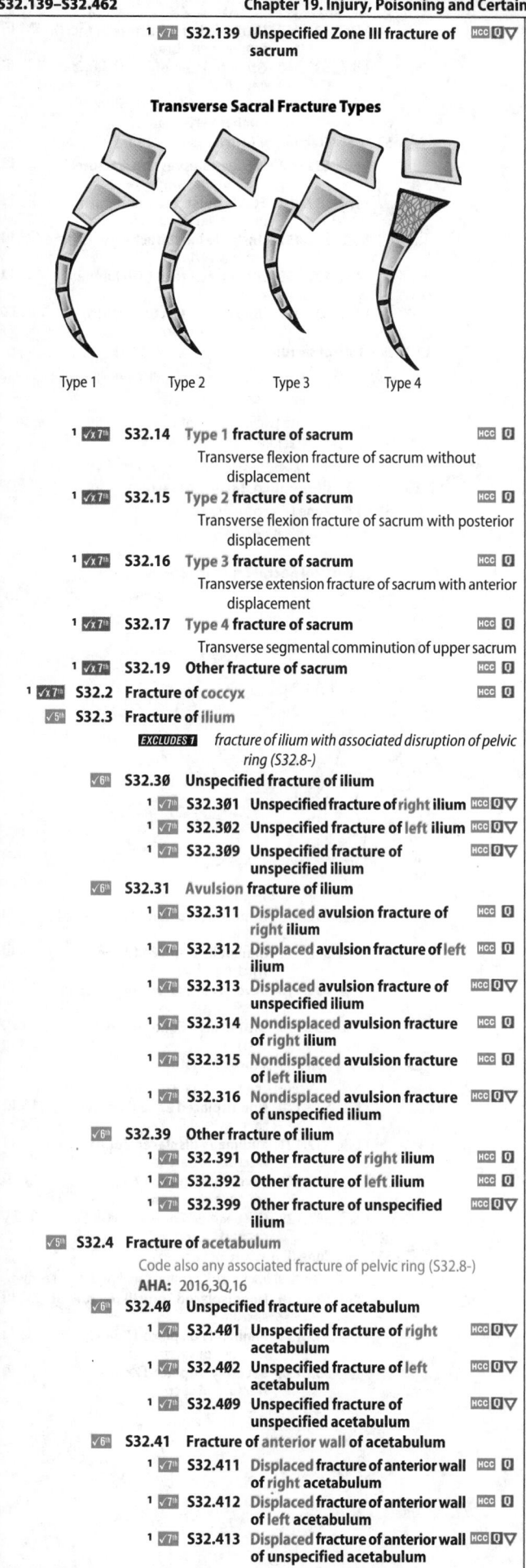

Type 1   Type 2   Type 3   Type 4

¹ √x7ᵗʰ **S32.14** **Type 1 fracture of sacrum** HCC Q
Transverse flexion fracture of sacrum without
displacement

¹ √x7ᵗʰ **S32.15** **Type 2 fracture of sacrum** HCC Q
Transverse flexion fracture of sacrum with posterior
displacement

¹ √x7ᵗʰ **S32.16** **Type 3 fracture of sacrum** HCC Q
Transverse extension fracture of sacrum with anterior
displacement

¹ √x7ᵗʰ **S32.17** **Type 4 fracture of sacrum** HCC Q
Transverse segmental comminution of upper sacrum

¹ √x7ᵗʰ **S32.19** **Other fracture of sacrum** HCC Q

¹ √x7ᵗʰ **S32.2** **Fracture of coccyx** HCC Q

√5ᵗʰ **S32.3** **Fracture of ilium**
EXCLUDES 1   *fracture of ilium with associated disruption of pelvic*
ring (S32.8-)

√6ᵗʰ **S32.30** **Unspecified fracture of ilium**
¹ √7ᵗʰ **S32.301** **Unspecified fracture of right ilium** HCC Q ▽
¹ √7ᵗʰ **S32.302** **Unspecified fracture of left ilium** HCC Q ▽
¹ √7ᵗʰ **S32.309** **Unspecified fracture of** HCC Q ▽
unspecified ilium

√6ᵗʰ **S32.31** **Avulsion fracture of ilium**
¹ √7ᵗʰ **S32.311** **Displaced avulsion fracture of** HCC Q
right ilium
¹ √7ᵗʰ **S32.312** **Displaced avulsion fracture of left** HCC Q
ilium
¹ √7ᵗʰ **S32.313** **Displaced avulsion fracture of** HCC Q ▽
unspecified ilium
¹ √7ᵗʰ **S32.314** **Nondisplaced avulsion fracture** HCC Q
of right ilium
¹ √7ᵗʰ **S32.315** **Nondisplaced avulsion fracture** HCC Q
of left ilium
¹ √7ᵗʰ **S32.316** **Nondisplaced avulsion fracture** HCC Q ▽
of unspecified ilium

√6ᵗʰ **S32.39** **Other fracture of ilium**
¹ √7ᵗʰ **S32.391** **Other fracture of right ilium** HCC Q
¹ √7ᵗʰ **S32.392** **Other fracture of left ilium** HCC Q
¹ √7ᵗʰ **S32.399** **Other fracture of unspecified** HCC Q ▽
ilium

√5ᵗʰ **S32.4** **Fracture of acetabulum**
Code also any associated fracture of pelvic ring (S32.8-)
AHA: 2016,3Q,16

√6ᵗʰ **S32.40** **Unspecified fracture of acetabulum**
¹ √7ᵗʰ **S32.401** **Unspecified fracture of right** HCC Q ▽
acetabulum
¹ √7ᵗʰ **S32.402** **Unspecified fracture of left** HCC Q ▽
acetabulum
¹ √7ᵗʰ **S32.409** **Unspecified fracture of** HCC Q ▽
unspecified acetabulum

√6ᵗʰ **S32.41** **Fracture of anterior wall of acetabulum**
¹ √7ᵗʰ **S32.411** **Displaced fracture of anterior wall** HCC Q
of right acetabulum
¹ √7ᵗʰ **S32.412** **Displaced fracture of anterior wall** HCC Q
of left acetabulum
¹ √7ᵗʰ **S32.413** **Displaced fracture of anterior wall** HCC Q ▽
of unspecified acetabulum

¹ √7ᵗʰ **S32.414** **Nondisplaced fracture of anterior** HCC Q
wall of right acetabulum
¹ √7ᵗʰ **S32.415** **Nondisplaced fracture of anterior** HCC Q
wall of left acetabulum
¹ √7ᵗʰ **S32.416** **Nondisplaced fracture of anterior** HCC Q ▽
wall of unspecified acetabulum

√6ᵗʰ **S32.42** **Fracture of posterior wall of acetabulum**
¹ √7ᵗʰ **S32.421** **Displaced fracture of posterior** HCC Q
wall of right acetabulum
¹ √7ᵗʰ **S32.422** **Displaced fracture of posterior** HCC Q
wall of left acetabulum
¹ √7ᵗʰ **S32.423** **Displaced fracture of posterior** HCC Q ▽
wall of unspecified acetabulum
¹ √7ᵗʰ **S32.424** **Nondisplaced fracture of** HCC Q
posterior wall of right
acetabulum
¹ √7ᵗʰ **S32.425** **Nondisplaced fracture of** HCC Q
posterior wall of left acetabulum
¹ √7ᵗʰ **S32.426** **Nondisplaced fracture of** HCC Q ▽
posterior wall of unspecified
acetabulum

√6ᵗʰ **S32.43** **Fracture of anterior column [iliopubic] of**
acetabulum
¹ √7ᵗʰ **S32.431** **Displaced fracture of anterior** HCC Q
column [iliopubic] of right
acetabulum
¹ √7ᵗʰ **S32.432** **Displaced fracture of anterior** HCC Q
column [iliopubic] of left
acetabulum
¹ √7ᵗʰ **S32.433** **Displaced fracture of anterior** HCC Q ▽
column [iliopubic] of unspecified
acetabulum
¹ √7ᵗʰ **S32.434** **Nondisplaced fracture of anterior** HCC Q
column [iliopubic] of right
acetabulum
¹ √7ᵗʰ **S32.435** **Nondisplaced fracture of anterior** HCC Q
column [iliopubic] of left
acetabulum
¹ √7ᵗʰ **S32.436** **Nondisplaced fracture of anterior** HCC Q ▽
column [iliopubic] of unspecified
acetabulum

√6ᵗʰ **S32.44** **Fracture of posterior column [ilioischial] of**
acetabulum
¹ √7ᵗʰ **S32.441** **Displaced fracture of posterior** HCC Q
column [ilioischial] of right
acetabulum
¹ √7ᵗʰ **S32.442** **Displaced fracture of posterior** HCC Q
column [ilioischial] of left
acetabulum
¹ √7ᵗʰ **S32.443** **Displaced fracture of posterior** HCC Q ▽
column [ilioischial] of unspecified
acetabulum
¹ √7ᵗʰ **S32.444** **Nondisplaced fracture of** HCC Q
posterior column [ilioischial] of
right acetabulum
¹ √7ᵗʰ **S32.445** **Nondisplaced fracture of** HCC Q
posterior column [ilioischial] of
left acetabulum
¹ √7ᵗʰ **S32.446** **Nondisplaced fracture of** HCC Q ▽
posterior column [ilioischial] of
unspecified acetabulum

√6ᵗʰ **S32.45** **Transverse fracture of acetabulum**
¹ √7ᵗʰ **S32.451** **Displaced transverse fracture of** HCC Q
right acetabulum
¹ √7ᵗʰ **S32.452** **Displaced transverse fracture of** HCC Q
left acetabulum
¹ √7ᵗʰ **S32.453** **Displaced transverse fracture of** HCC Q ▽
unspecified acetabulum
¹ √7ᵗʰ **S32.454** **Nondisplaced transverse fracture** HCC Q
of right acetabulum
¹ √7ᵗʰ **S32.455** **Nondisplaced transverse fracture** HCC Q
of left acetabulum
¹ √7ᵗʰ **S32.456** **Nondisplaced transverse fracture** HCC Q ▽
of unspecified acetabulum

√6ᵗʰ **S32.46** **Associated transverse-posterior fracture of**
acetabulum
¹ √7ᵗʰ **S32.461** **Displaced associated** HCC Q
transverse-posterior fracture of
right acetabulum
¹ √7ᵗʰ **S32.462** **Displaced associated** HCC Q
transverse-posterior fracture of
left acetabulum

¹ √7ᵗʰ **S32.463** Displaced associated transverse-posterior fracture of unspecified acetabulum   HCC Q ▽

¹ √7ᵗʰ **S32.464** Nondisplaced associated transverse-posterior fracture of right acetabulum   HCC Q

¹ √7ᵗʰ **S32.465** Nondisplaced associated transverse-posterior fracture of left acetabulum   HCC Q

¹ √7ᵗʰ **S32.466** Nondisplaced associated transverse-posterior fracture of unspecified acetabulum   HCC Q ▽

√6ᵗʰ **S32.47** Fracture of medial wall of acetabulum

¹ √7ᵗʰ **S32.471** Displaced fracture of medial wall of right acetabulum   HCC Q

¹ √7ᵗʰ **S32.472** Displaced fracture of medial wall of left acetabulum   HCC Q

¹ √7ᵗʰ **S32.473** Displaced fracture of medial wall of unspecified acetabulum   HCC Q ▽

¹ √7ᵗʰ **S32.474** Nondisplaced fracture of medial wall of right acetabulum   HCC Q

¹ √7ᵗʰ **S32.475** Nondisplaced fracture of medial wall of left acetabulum   HCC Q

¹ √7ᵗʰ **S32.476** Nondisplaced fracture of medial wall of unspecified acetabulum   HCC Q ▽

√6ᵗʰ **S32.48** Dome fracture of acetabulum

¹ √7ᵗʰ **S32.481** Displaced dome fracture of right acetabulum   HCC Q

¹ √7ᵗʰ **S32.482** Displaced dome fracture of left acetabulum   HCC Q

¹ √7ᵗʰ **S32.483** Displaced dome fracture of unspecified acetabulum   HCC Q ▽

¹ √7ᵗʰ **S32.484** Nondisplaced dome fracture of right acetabulum   HCC Q

¹ √7ᵗʰ **S32.485** Nondisplaced dome fracture of left acetabulum   HCC Q

¹ √7ᵗʰ **S32.486** Nondisplaced dome fracture of unspecified acetabulum   HCC Q ▽

√6ᵗʰ **S32.49** Other specified fracture of acetabulum

¹ √7ᵗʰ **S32.491** Other specified fracture of right acetabulum   HCC Q

¹ √7ᵗʰ **S32.492** Other specified fracture of left acetabulum   HCC Q

¹ √7ᵗʰ **S32.499** Other specified fracture of unspecified acetabulum   HCC Q ▽

√5ᵗʰ **S32.5** Fracture of pubis

EXCLUDES 1   fracture of pubis with associated disruption of pelvic ring (S32.8-)

√6ᵗʰ **S32.50** Unspecified fracture of pubis

¹ √7ᵗʰ **S32.501** Unspecified fracture of right pubis   HCC Q ▽

¹ √7ᵗʰ **S32.502** Unspecified fracture of left pubis   HCC Q ▽

¹ √7ᵗʰ **S32.509** Unspecified fracture of unspecified pubis   HCC Q ▽

√6ᵗʰ **S32.51** Fracture of superior rim of pubis

¹ √7ᵗʰ **S32.511** Fracture of superior rim of right pubis   HCC Q

¹ √7ᵗʰ **S32.512** Fracture of superior rim of left pubis   HCC Q

¹ √7ᵗʰ **S32.519** Fracture of superior rim of unspecified pubis   HCC Q ▽

√6ᵗʰ **S32.59** Other specified fracture of pubis

¹ √7ᵗʰ **S32.591** Other specified fracture of right pubis   HCC Q

¹ √7ᵗʰ **S32.592** Other specified fracture of left pubis   HCC Q

¹ √7ᵗʰ **S32.599** Other specified fracture of unspecified pubis   HCC Q ▽

√5ᵗʰ **S32.6** Fracture of ischium

EXCLUDES 1   fracture of ischium with associated disruption of pelvic ring (S32.8-)

√6ᵗʰ **S32.60** Unspecified fracture of ischium

¹ √7ᵗʰ **S32.601** Unspecified fracture of right ischium   HCC Q ▽

¹ √7ᵗʰ **S32.602** Unspecified fracture of left ischium   HCC Q ▽

¹ √7ᵗʰ **S32.609** Unspecified fracture of unspecified ischium   HCC Q ▽

√6ᵗʰ **S32.61** Avulsion fracture of ischium

¹ √7ᵗʰ **S32.611** Displaced avulsion fracture of right ischium   HCC Q

¹ √7ᵗʰ **S32.612** Displaced avulsion fracture of left ischium   HCC Q

¹ √7ᵗʰ **S32.613** Displaced avulsion fracture of unspecified ischium   HCC Q ▽

¹ √7ᵗʰ **S32.614** Nondisplaced avulsion fracture of right ischium   HCC Q

¹ √7ᵗʰ **S32.615** Nondisplaced avulsion fracture of left ischium   HCC Q

¹ √7ᵗʰ **S32.616** Nondisplaced avulsion fracture of unspecified ischium   HCC Q ▽

√6ᵗʰ **S32.69** Other specified fracture of ischium

¹ √7ᵗʰ **S32.691** Other specified fracture of right ischium   HCC Q

¹ √7ᵗʰ **S32.692** Other specified fracture of left ischium   HCC Q

¹ √7ᵗʰ **S32.699** Other specified fracture of unspecified ischium   HCC Q ▽

√5ᵗʰ **S32.8** Fracture of other parts of pelvis

Code also any associated:
fracture of acetabulum (S32.4-)
sacral fracture (S32.1-)

Fractures Disrupting Pelvic Circle

√6ᵗʰ **S32.81** Multiple fractures of pelvis with disruption of pelvic ring

Multiple pelvic fractures with disruption of pelvic circle

¹ √7ᵗʰ **S32.810** Multiple fractures of pelvis with stable disruption of pelvic ring   HCC Q

¹ √7ᵗʰ **S32.811** Multiple fractures of pelvis with unstable disruption of pelvic ring   HCC Q

¹ √x7ᵗʰ **S32.82** Multiple fractures of pelvis without disruption of pelvic ring   HCC Q

Multiple pelvic fractures without disruption of pelvic circle

¹ √x7ᵗʰ **S32.89** Fracture of other parts of pelvis   HCC Q

¹ √x7ᵗʰ **S32.9** Fracture of unspecified parts of lumbosacral spine and pelvis   HCC Q ▽

Fracture of lumbosacral spine NOS
Fracture of pelvis NOS
AHA: 2012,4Q,93

✓ Additional Character Req   √x7ᵗʰ Placeholder Alert   Manifestation   ▽ Unspecified   ►◄ Revised Text   ● New Code   ▲ Revised Code Title

ICD-10-CM 2019   **983**

✓4ᵗʰ **S33 Dislocation and sprain of joints and ligaments of lumbar spine and pelvis**

> **INCLUDES**   avulsion of joint or ligament of lumbar spine and pelvis
>
> laceration of cartilage, joint or ligament of lumbar spine and pelvis
>
> sprain of cartilage, joint or ligament of lumbar spine and pelvis
>
> traumatic hemarthrosis of joint or ligament of lumbar spine and pelvis
>
> traumatic rupture of joint or ligament of lumbar spine and pelvis
>
> traumatic subluxation of joint or ligament of lumbar spine and pelvis
>
> traumatic tear of joint or ligament of lumbar spine and pelvis

Code also any associated open wound

> **EXCLUDES 1**   nontraumatic rupture or displacement of lumbar intervertebral disc NOS (M51.-)
>
> obstetric damage to pelvic joints and ligaments (O71.6)
>
> **EXCLUDES 2**   dislocation and sprain of joints and ligaments of hip (S73.-)
>
> strain of muscle of lower back and pelvis (S39.Ø1-)

> The appropriate 7th character is to be added to each code from category S33.
> A   initial encounter
> D   subsequent encounter
> S   sequela

✓x 7ᵗʰ **S33.Ø Traumatic rupture of lumbar intervertebral disc**

> **EXCLUDES 1**   rupture or displacement (nontraumatic) of lumbar intervertebral disc NOS (M51.- with fifth character 6)

✓5ᵗʰ **S33.1 Subluxation and dislocation of lumbar vertebra**

> Code also any associated:
> open wound of abdomen, lower back and pelvis (S31)
> spinal cord injury (S24.Ø, S24.1-, S34.Ø-, S34.1-)
> **EXCLUDES 2**   fracture of lumbar vertebrae (S32.Ø-)

✓6ᵗʰ   **S33.1Ø Subluxation and dislocation of unspecified lumbar vertebra**

     ✓7ᵗʰ **S33.1ØØ Subluxation of unspecified lumbar vertebra** ▽

     ✓7ᵗʰ **S33.1Ø1 Dislocation of unspecified lumbar vertebra** ▽

✓6ᵗʰ   **S33.11 Subluxation and dislocation of L1/L2 lumbar vertebra**

     ✓7ᵗʰ **S33.11Ø Subluxation of L1/L2 lumbar vertebra**

     ✓7ᵗʰ **S33.111 Dislocation of L1/L2 lumbar vertebra**

✓6ᵗʰ   **S33.12 Subluxation and dislocation of L2/L3 lumbar vertebra**

     ✓7ᵗʰ **S33.12Ø Subluxation of L2/L3 lumbar vertebra**

     ✓7ᵗʰ **S33.121 Dislocation of L2/L3 lumbar vertebra**

✓6ᵗʰ   **S33.13 Subluxation and dislocation of L3/L4 lumbar vertebra**

     ✓7ᵗʰ **S33.13Ø Subluxation of L3/L4 lumbar vertebra**

     ✓7ᵗʰ **S33.131 Dislocation of L3/L4 lumbar vertebra**

✓6ᵗʰ   **S33.14 Subluxation and dislocation of L4/L5 lumbar vertebra**

     ✓7ᵗʰ **S33.14Ø Subluxation of L4/L5 lumbar vertebra**

     ✓7ᵗʰ **S33.141 Dislocation of L4/L5 lumbar vertebra**

✓x 7ᵗʰ **S33.2 Dislocation of sacroiliac and sacrococcygeal joint**

✓5ᵗʰ **S33.3 Dislocation of other and unspecified parts of lumbar spine and pelvis**

     ✓x 7ᵗʰ **S33.3Ø Dislocation of unspecified parts of lumbar spine and pelvis** ▽

     ✓x 7ᵗʰ **S33.39 Dislocation of other parts of lumbar spine and pelvis**

✓x 7ᵗʰ **S33.4 Traumatic rupture of symphysis pubis**

✓x 7ᵗʰ **S33.5 Sprain of ligaments of lumbar spine**

✓x 7ᵗʰ **S33.6 Sprain of sacroiliac joint**

✓x 7ᵗʰ **S33.8 Sprain of other parts of lumbar spine and pelvis**

✓x 7ᵗʰ **S33.9 Sprain of unspecified parts of lumbar spine and pelvis** ▽

✓4ᵗʰ **S34 Injury of lumbar and sacral spinal cord and nerves at abdomen, lower back and pelvis level**

> **NOTE**   Code to highest level of lumbar cord injury.
>
> Injuries to the spinal cord (S34.Ø and S34.1) refer to the cord level and not bone level injury, and can affect nerve roots at and below the level given.

Code also any associated:
> fracture of vertebra (S22.Ø-, S32.Ø-)
> open wound of abdomen, lower back and pelvis (S31.-)
> transient paralysis (R29.5)

> The appropriate 7th character is to be added to each code from category S34.
> A   initial encounter
> D   subsequent encounter
> S   sequela

✓5ᵗʰ **S34.Ø Concussion and edema of lumbar and sacral spinal cord**

     ✓x 7ᵗʰ **S34.Ø1 Concussion and edema of lumbar spinal cord** HCC

     ✓x 7ᵗʰ **S34.Ø2 Concussion and edema of sacral spinal cord** HCC
         Concussion and edema of conus medullaris

✓5ᵗʰ **S34.1 Other and unspecified injury of lumbar and sacral spinal cord**

     ✓6ᵗʰ **S34.1Ø Unspecified injury to lumbar spinal cord**

         ✓7ᵗʰ **S34.1Ø1 Unspecified injury to L1 level of lumbar spinal cord** HCC ▽
             Unspecified injury to lumbar spinal cord level 1

         ✓7ᵗʰ **S34.1Ø2 Unspecified injury to L2 level of lumbar spinal cord** HCC ▽
             Unspecified injury to lumbar spinal cord level 2

         ✓7ᵗʰ **S34.1Ø3 Unspecified injury to L3 level of lumbar spinal cord** HCC ▽
             Unspecified injury to lumbar spinal cord level 3

         ✓7ᵗʰ **S34.1Ø4 Unspecified injury to L4 level of lumbar spinal cord** HCC ▽
             Unspecified injury to lumbar spinal cord level 4

         ✓7ᵗʰ **S34.1Ø5 Unspecified injury to L5 level of lumbar spinal cord** HCC ▽
             Unspecified injury to lumbar spinal cord level 5

         ✓7ᵗʰ **S34.1Ø9 Unspecified injury to unspecified level of lumbar spinal cord** HCC ▽

     ✓6ᵗʰ **S34.11 Complete lesion of lumbar spinal cord**

         ✓7ᵗʰ **S34.111 Complete lesion of L1 level of lumbar spinal cord** HCC
             Complete lesion of lumbar spinal cord level 1

         ✓7ᵗʰ **S34.112 Complete lesion of L2 level of lumbar spinal cord** HCC
             Complete lesion of lumbar spinal cord level 2

         ✓7ᵗʰ **S34.113 Complete lesion of L3 level of lumbar spinal cord** HCC
             Complete lesion of lumbar spinal cord level 3

         ✓7ᵗʰ **S34.114 Complete lesion of L4 level of lumbar spinal cord** HCC
             Complete lesion of lumbar spinal cord level 4

         ✓7ᵗʰ **S34.115 Complete lesion of L5 level of lumbar spinal cord** HCC
             Complete lesion of lumbar spinal cord level 5

         ✓7ᵗʰ **S34.119 Complete lesion of unspecified level of lumbar spinal cord** HCC ▽

     ✓6ᵗʰ **S34.12 Incomplete lesion of lumbar spinal cord**

         ✓7ᵗʰ **S34.121 Incomplete lesion of L1 level of lumbar spinal cord** HCC
             Incomplete lesion of lumbar spinal cord level 1

         ✓7ᵗʰ **S34.122 Incomplete lesion of L2 level of lumbar spinal cord** HCC
             Incomplete lesion of lumbar spinal cord level 2

√7ᵗʰ **S34.123 Incomplete lesion of L3 level of lumbar spinal cord** `HCC`
Incomplete lesion of lumbar spinal cord level 3

√7ᵗʰ **S34.124 Incomplete lesion of L4 level of lumbar spinal cord** `HCC`
Incomplete lesion of lumbar spinal cord level 4

√7ᵗʰ **S34.125 Incomplete lesion of L5 level of lumbar spinal cord** `HCC`
Incomplete lesion of lumbar spinal cord level 5

√7ᵗʰ **S34.129 Incomplete lesion of unspecified level of lumbar spinal cord** `HCC` ▽

√6ᵗʰ **S34.13 Other and unspecified injury to sacral spinal cord**
Other injury to conus medullaris

√7ᵗʰ **S34.131 Complete lesion of sacral spinal cord** `HCC`
Complete lesion of conus medullaris

√7ᵗʰ **S34.132 Incomplete lesion of sacral spinal cord** `HCC`
Incomplete lesion of conus medullaris

√7ᵗʰ **S34.139 Unspecified injury to sacral spinal cord** `HCC` ▽
Unspecified injury of conus medullaris

√5ᵗʰ **S34.2 Injury of nerve root of lumbar and sacral spine**

√x7ᵗʰ **S34.21 Injury of nerve root of lumbar spine**

√x7ᵗʰ **S34.22 Injury of nerve root of sacral spine**

¹ √x7ᵗʰ **S34.3 Injury of cauda equina** `HCC`

√x7ᵗʰ **S34.4 Injury of lumbosacral plexus**

√x7ᵗʰ **S34.5 Injury of lumbar, sacral and pelvic sympathetic nerves**
Injury of celiac ganglion or plexus
Injury of hypogastric plexus
Injury of mesenteric plexus (inferior) (superior)
Injury of splanchnic nerve

√x7ᵗʰ **S34.6 Injury of peripheral nerve(s) at abdomen, lower back and pelvis level**

√x7ᵗʰ **S34.8 Injury of other nerves at abdomen, lower back and pelvis level**

√x7ᵗʰ **S34.9 Injury of unspecified nerves at abdomen, lower back and pelvis level** ▽

√4ᵗʰ **S35 Injury of blood vessels at abdomen, lower back and pelvis level**
Code also any associated open wound (S31.-)

The appropriate 7th character is to be added to each code from category S35.
A   initial encounter
D   subsequent encounter
S   sequela

√5ᵗʰ **S35.0 Injury of abdominal aorta**
EXCLUDES 1   injury of aorta NOS (S25.0)

√x7ᵗʰ **S35.00 Unspecified injury of abdominal aorta** ▽

√x7ᵗʰ **S35.01 Minor laceration of abdominal aorta**
Incomplete transection of abdominal aorta
Laceration of abdominal aorta NOS
Superficial laceration of abdominal aorta

√x7ᵗʰ **S35.02 Major laceration of abdominal aorta**
Complete transection of abdominal aorta
Traumatic rupture of abdominal aorta

√x7ᵗʰ **S35.09 Other injury of abdominal aorta**

√5ᵗʰ **S35.1 Injury of inferior vena cava**
Injury of hepatic vein
EXCLUDES 1   injury of vena cava NOS (S25.2)

√x7ᵗʰ **S35.10 Unspecified injury of inferior vena cava** ▽

√x7ᵗʰ **S35.11 Minor laceration of inferior vena cava**
Incomplete transection of inferior vena cava
Laceration of inferior vena cava NOS
Superficial laceration of inferior vena cava

√x7ᵗʰ **S35.12 Major laceration of inferior vena cava**
Complete transection of inferior vena cava
Traumatic rupture of inferior vena cava

√x7ᵗʰ **S35.19 Other injury of inferior vena cava**

√5ᵗʰ **S35.2 Injury of celiac or mesenteric artery and branches**

√6ᵗʰ **S35.21 Injury of celiac artery**

√7ᵗʰ **S35.211 Minor laceration of celiac artery**
Incomplete transection of celiac artery
Laceration of celiac artery NOS
Superficial laceration of celiac artery

√7ᵗʰ **S35.212 Major laceration of celiac artery**
Complete transection of celiac artery
Traumatic rupture of celiac artery

√7ᵗʰ **S35.218 Other injury of celiac artery**

√7ᵗʰ **S35.219 Unspecified injury of celiac artery** ▽

√6ᵗʰ **S35.22 Injury of superior mesenteric artery**

√7ᵗʰ **S35.221 Minor laceration of superior mesenteric artery**
Incomplete transection of superior mesenteric artery
Laceration of superior mesenteric artery NOS
Superficial laceration of superior mesenteric artery

√7ᵗʰ **S35.222 Major laceration of superior mesenteric artery**
Complete transection of superior mesenteric artery
Traumatic rupture of superior mesenteric artery

√7ᵗʰ **S35.228 Other injury of superior mesenteric artery**

√7ᵗʰ **S35.229 Unspecified injury of superior mesenteric artery** ▽

√6ᵗʰ **S35.23 Injury of inferior mesenteric artery**

√7ᵗʰ **S35.231 Minor laceration of inferior mesenteric artery**
Incomplete transection of inferior mesenteric artery
Laceration of inferior mesenteric artery NOS
Superficial laceration of inferior mesenteric artery

√7ᵗʰ **S35.232 Major laceration of inferior mesenteric artery**
Complete transection of inferior mesenteric artery
Traumatic rupture of inferior mesenteric artery

√7ᵗʰ **S35.238 Other injury of inferior mesenteric artery**

√7ᵗʰ **S35.239 Unspecified injury of inferior mesenteric artery** ▽

√6ᵗʰ **S35.29 Injury of branches of celiac and mesenteric artery**
Injury of gastric artery
Injury of gastroduodenal artery
Injury of hepatic artery
Injury of splenic artery

√7ᵗʰ **S35.291 Minor laceration of branches of celiac and mesenteric artery**
Incomplete transection of branches of celiac and mesenteric artery
Laceration of branches of celiac and mesenteric artery NOS
Superficial laceration of branches of celiac and mesenteric artery

√7ᵗʰ **S35.292 Major laceration of branches of celiac and mesenteric artery**
Complete transection of branches of celiac and mesenteric artery
Traumatic rupture of branches of celiac and mesenteric artery

√7ᵗʰ **S35.298 Other injury of branches of celiac and mesenteric artery**

√7ᵗʰ **S35.299 Unspecified injury of branches of celiac and mesenteric artery** ▽

√5ᵗʰ **S35.3 Injury of portal or splenic vein and branches**

√6ᵗʰ **S35.31 Injury of portal vein**

√7ᵗʰ **S35.311 Laceration of portal vein**

√7ᵗʰ **S35.318 Other specified injury of portal vein**

√7ᵗʰ **S35.319 Unspecified injury of portal vein** ▽

☑ Additional Character Req   √x7ᵗʰ Placeholder Alert   Manifestation   ▽ Unspecified   ▶◀ Revised Text   ● New Code   ▲ Revised Code Title

ICD-10-CM 2019   **985**

√6ᵗʰ **S35.32 Injury of** splenic vein
- √7ᵗʰ **S35.321 Laceration** of splenic vein
- √7ᵗʰ **S35.328 Other specified injury** of splenic vein
- √7ᵗʰ **S35.329 Unspecified injury** of splenic vein ▽

√6ᵗʰ **S35.33 Injury of** superior mesenteric vein
- √7ᵗʰ **S35.331 Laceration** of superior mesenteric vein
- √7ᵗʰ **S35.338 Other specified injury of** superior mesenteric vein
- √7ᵗʰ **S35.339 Unspecified injury of** superior mesenteric vein ▽

√6ᵗʰ **S35.34 Injury of** inferior mesenteric vein
- √7ᵗʰ **S35.341 Laceration** of inferior mesenteric vein
- √7ᵗʰ **S35.348 Other specified injury of** inferior mesenteric vein
- √7ᵗʰ **S35.349 Unspecified injury of** inferior mesenteric vein ▽

√5ᵗʰ **S35.4 Injury of** renal blood vessels
- √6ᵗʰ **S35.40 Unspecified injury of** renal blood vessel
  - √7ᵗʰ **S35.401 Unspecified injury of** right renal artery ▽
  - √7ᵗʰ **S35.402 Unspecified injury of** left renal artery ▽
  - √7ᵗʰ **S35.403 Unspecified injury of** unspecified renal artery ▽
  - √7ᵗʰ **S35.404 Unspecified injury of** right renal vein ▽
  - √7ᵗʰ **S35.405 Unspecified injury of** left renal vein ▽
  - √7ᵗʰ **S35.406 Unspecified injury of** unspecified renal vein ▽
- √6ᵗʰ **S35.41 Laceration of** renal blood vessel
  - √7ᵗʰ **S35.411 Laceration of** right renal artery
  - √7ᵗʰ **S35.412 Laceration of** left renal artery
  - √7ᵗʰ **S35.413 Laceration of** unspecified renal artery ▽
  - √7ᵗʰ **S35.414 Laceration of** right renal vein
  - √7ᵗʰ **S35.415 Laceration of** left renal vein
  - √7ᵗʰ **S35.416 Laceration of** unspecified renal vein ▽
- √6ᵗʰ **S35.49 Other specified injury of** renal blood vessel
  - √7ᵗʰ **S35.491 Other specified injury of** right renal artery
  - √7ᵗʰ **S35.492 Other specified injury of** left renal artery
  - √7ᵗʰ **S35.493 Other specified injury of** unspecified renal artery ▽
  - √7ᵗʰ **S35.494 Other specified injury of** right renal vein
  - √7ᵗʰ **S35.495 Other specified injury of** left renal vein
  - √7ᵗʰ **S35.496 Other specified injury of** unspecified renal vein ▽

√5ᵗʰ **S35.5 Injury of** iliac blood vessels
- √x7ᵗʰ **S35.50 Injury of** unspecified iliac blood vessel(s) ▽
- √6ᵗʰ **S35.51 Injury of** iliac artery or vein
  - Injury of hypogastric artery or vein
  - √7ᵗʰ **S35.511 Injury of** right iliac artery
  - √7ᵗʰ **S35.512 Injury of** left iliac artery
  - √7ᵗʰ **S35.513 Injury of** unspecified iliac artery ▽
  - √7ᵗʰ **S35.514 Injury of** right iliac vein
  - √7ᵗʰ **S35.515 Injury of** left iliac vein
  - √7ᵗʰ **S35.516 Injury of** unspecified iliac vein ▽
- √6ᵗʰ **S35.53 Injury of** uterine artery or vein
  - √7ᵗʰ **S35.531 Injury of** right uterine artery ♀
  - √7ᵗʰ **S35.532 Injury of** left uterine artery ♀
  - √7ᵗʰ **S35.533 Injury of** unspecified uterine artery ♀ ▽
  - √7ᵗʰ **S35.534 Injury of** right uterine vein ♀
  - √7ᵗʰ **S35.535 Injury of** left uterine vein ♀
  - √7ᵗʰ **S35.536 Injury of** unspecified uterine vein ♀ ▽
- √x7ᵗʰ **S35.59 Injury of** other iliac blood vessels

√5ᵗʰ **S35.8 Injury of other blood vessels at abdomen, lower back and pelvis level**
- Injury of ovarian artery or vein
- √6ᵗʰ **S35.8X Injury of other blood vessels at abdomen, lower back and pelvis level**
  - √7ᵗʰ **S35.8X1 Laceration** of other blood vessels at abdomen, lower back and pelvis level
  - √7ᵗʰ **S35.8X8 Other specified injury of** other blood vessels at abdomen, lower back and pelvis level
  - √7ᵗʰ **S35.8X9 Unspecified injury of** other blood vessels at abdomen, lower back and pelvis level ▽

√5ᵗʰ **S35.9 Injury of unspecified blood vessel at abdomen, lower back and pelvis level**
- √x7ᵗʰ **S35.90 Unspecified injury of** unspecified blood vessel at abdomen, lower back and pelvis level ▽
- √x7ᵗʰ **S35.91 Laceration** of unspecified blood vessel at abdomen, lower back and pelvis level ▽
- √x7ᵗʰ **S35.99 Other specified injury of** unspecified blood vessel at abdomen, lower back and pelvis level ▽

√4ᵗʰ **S36 Injury of intra-abdominal organs**

Code also any associated open wound (S31.-)

> The appropriate 7th character is to be added to each code from category S36.
> A initial encounter
> D subsequent encounter
> S sequela

√5ᵗʰ **S36.0 Injury of** spleen

    AHA: 2015,2Q,36; 2015,1Q,10

- √x7ᵗʰ **S36.00 Unspecified injury of** spleen ▽
- √6ᵗʰ **S36.02 Contusion of** spleen
  - √7ᵗʰ **S36.020 Minor contusion of** spleen
    - Contusion of spleen less than 2 cm
  - √7ᵗʰ **S36.021 Major contusion of** spleen
    - Contusion of spleen greater than 2 cm
  - √7ᵗʰ **S36.029 Unspecified contusion of** spleen ▽
- √6ᵗʰ **S36.03 Laceration of** spleen
  - √7ᵗʰ **S36.030 Superficial (capsular) laceration of** spleen
    - Laceration of spleen less than 1 cm
    - Minor laceration of spleen
  - √7ᵗʰ **S36.031 Moderate laceration of** spleen
    - Laceration of spleen 1 to 3 cm
  - √7ᵗʰ **S36.032 Major laceration of** spleen
    - Avulsion of spleen
    - Laceration of spleen greater than 3 cm
    - Massive laceration of spleen
    - Multiple moderate lacerations of spleen
    - Stellate laceration of spleen
  - √7ᵗʰ **S36.039 Unspecified laceration of** spleen ▽
- √x7ᵗʰ **S36.09 Other injury of** spleen

√5ᵗʰ **S36.1 Injury of** liver and gallbladder and bile duct
- √6ᵗʰ **S36.11 Injury of** liver
  - √7ᵗʰ **S36.112 Contusion of** liver
  - √7ᵗʰ **S36.113 Laceration of** liver, unspecified degree ▽
  - √7ᵗʰ **S36.114 Minor laceration of** liver
    - Laceration involving capsule only, or, without significant involvement of hepatic parenchyma [i.e., less than 1 cm deep]
  - √7ᵗʰ **S36.115 Moderate laceration of** liver
    - Laceration involving parenchyma but without major disruption of parenchyma [i.e., less than 10 cm long and less than 3 cm deep]

✓7ᵗʰ **S36.116** **Major laceration** of liver

    Laceration with significant disruption of hepatic parenchyma [i.e., greater than 10 cm long and 3 cm deep]

    Multiple moderate lacerations, with or without hematoma

    Stellate laceration of liver

✓7ᵗʰ **S36.118** **Other injury** of liver

✓7ᵗʰ **S36.119** **Unspecified injury** of liver ▽

✓6ᵗʰ **S36.12** **Injury** of **gallbladder**

    ✓7ᵗʰ **S36.122** **Contusion** of gallbladder

    ✓7ᵗʰ **S36.123** **Laceration** of gallbladder

    ✓7ᵗʰ **S36.128** **Other injury** of gallbladder

    ✓7ᵗʰ **S36.129** **Unspecified injury** of gallbladder ▽

✓x7ᵗʰ **S36.13** **Injury** of **bile duct**

✓5ᵗʰ **S36.2** **Injury** of **pancreas**

  ✓6ᵗʰ **S36.20** **Unspecified injury** of pancreas

    ✓7ᵗʰ **S36.200** **Unspecified injury** of **head** of pancreas ▽

    ✓7ᵗʰ **S36.201** **Unspecified injury** of **body** of pancreas ▽

    ✓7ᵗʰ **S36.202** **Unspecified injury** of **tail** of pancreas ▽

    ✓7ᵗʰ **S36.209** **Unspecified injury** of unspecified part of pancreas ▽

  ✓6ᵗʰ **S36.22** **Contusion** of pancreas

    ✓7ᵗʰ **S36.220** **Contusion** of **head** of pancreas

    ✓7ᵗʰ **S36.221** **Contusion** of **body** of pancreas

    ✓7ᵗʰ **S36.222** **Contusion** of **tail** of pancreas

    ✓7ᵗʰ **S36.229** **Contusion** of unspecified part of pancreas ▽

  ✓6ᵗʰ **S36.23** **Laceration** of pancreas, unspecified degree

    ✓7ᵗʰ **S36.230** **Laceration** of **head** of pancreas, unspecified degree ▽

    ✓7ᵗʰ **S36.231** **Laceration** of **body** of pancreas, unspecified degree ▽

    ✓7ᵗʰ **S36.232** **Laceration** of **tail** of pancreas, unspecified degree ▽

    ✓7ᵗʰ **S36.239** **Laceration** of unspecified part of pancreas, unspecified degree ▽

  ✓6ᵗʰ **S36.24** **Minor laceration** of pancreas

    ✓7ᵗʰ **S36.240** **Minor laceration** of **head** of pancreas

    ✓7ᵗʰ **S36.241** **Minor laceration** of **body** of pancreas

    ✓7ᵗʰ **S36.242** **Minor laceration** of **tail** of pancreas

    ✓7ᵗʰ **S36.249** **Minor laceration** of unspecified part of pancreas ▽

  ✓6ᵗʰ **S36.25** **Moderate laceration** of pancreas

    ✓7ᵗʰ **S36.250** **Moderate laceration** of **head** of pancreas

    ✓7ᵗʰ **S36.251** **Moderate laceration** of **body** of pancreas

    ✓7ᵗʰ **S36.252** **Moderate laceration** of **tail** of pancreas

    ✓7ᵗʰ **S36.259** **Moderate laceration** of unspecified part of pancreas ▽

  ✓6ᵗʰ **S36.26** **Major laceration** of pancreas

    ✓7ᵗʰ **S36.260** **Major laceration** of **head** of pancreas

    ✓7ᵗʰ **S36.261** **Major laceration** of **body** of pancreas

    ✓7ᵗʰ **S36.262** **Major laceration** of **tail** of pancreas

    ✓7ᵗʰ **S36.269** **Major laceration** of unspecified part of pancreas ▽

  ✓6ᵗʰ **S36.29** **Other injury** of pancreas

    ✓7ᵗʰ **S36.290** **Other injury** of **head** of pancreas

    ✓7ᵗʰ **S36.291** **Other injury** of **body** of pancreas

    ✓7ᵗʰ **S36.292** **Other injury** of **tail** of pancreas

    ✓7ᵗʰ **S36.299** **Other injury** of unspecified part of pancreas ▽

✓5ᵗʰ **S36.3** **Injury** of **stomach**

  ✓x7ᵗʰ **S36.30** **Unspecified injury** of stomach ▽

  ✓x7ᵗʰ **S36.32** **Contusion** of stomach

  ✓x7ᵗʰ **S36.33** **Laceration** of stomach

  ✓x7ᵗʰ **S36.39** **Other injury** of stomach

✓5ᵗʰ **S36.4** **Injury** of **small intestine**

  ✓6ᵗʰ **S36.40** **Unspecified injury** of small intestine

    ✓7ᵗʰ **S36.400** **Unspecified injury** of **duodenum** ▽

✓7ᵗʰ **S36.408** **Unspecified injury** of other part of small intestine ▽

✓7ᵗʰ **S36.409** **Unspecified injury** of unspecified part of small intestine ▽

✓6ᵗʰ **S36.41** **Primary blast** injury of small intestine

    Blast injury of small intestine NOS

    ✓7ᵗʰ **S36.410** **Primary blast injury** of **duodenum**

    ✓7ᵗʰ **S36.418** **Primary blast injury** of other part of small intestine

    ✓7ᵗʰ **S36.419** **Primary blast injury** of unspecified part of small intestine ▽

✓6ᵗʰ **S36.42** **Contusion** of small intestine

    ✓7ᵗʰ **S36.420** **Contusion** of **duodenum**

    ✓7ᵗʰ **S36.428** **Contusion** of other part of small intestine

    ✓7ᵗʰ **S36.429** **Contusion** of unspecified part of small intestine ▽

✓6ᵗʰ **S36.43** **Laceration** of small intestine

    ✓7ᵗʰ **S36.430** **Laceration** of **duodenum**

    ✓7ᵗʰ **S36.438** **Laceration** of other part of small intestine

    ✓7ᵗʰ **S36.439** **Laceration** of unspecified part of small intestine ▽

✓6ᵗʰ **S36.49** **Other injury** of small intestine

    ✓7ᵗʰ **S36.490** **Other injury** of **duodenum**

    ✓7ᵗʰ **S36.498** **Other injury** of other part of small intestine

    ✓7ᵗʰ **S36.499** **Other injury** of unspecified part of small intestine ▽

✓5ᵗʰ **S36.5** **Injury** of **colon**

    EXCLUDES 2   injury of rectum (S36.6-)

  ✓6ᵗʰ **S36.50** **Unspecified injury** of colon

    ✓7ᵗʰ **S36.500** **Unspecified injury** of **ascending [right]** colon ▽

    ✓7ᵗʰ **S36.501** **Unspecified injury** of **transverse** colon ▽

    ✓7ᵗʰ **S36.502** **Unspecified injury** of **descending [left]** colon ▽

    ✓7ᵗʰ **S36.503** **Unspecified injury** of **sigmoid** colon ▽

    ✓7ᵗʰ **S36.508** **Unspecified injury** of other part of colon ▽

    ✓7ᵗʰ **S36.509** **Unspecified injury** of unspecified part of colon ▽

  ✓6ᵗʰ **S36.51** **Primary blast** injury of colon

    Blast injury of colon NOS

    ✓7ᵗʰ **S36.510** **Primary blast injury** of **ascending [right]** colon

    ✓7ᵗʰ **S36.511** **Primary blast injury** of **transverse** colon

    ✓7ᵗʰ **S36.512** **Primary blast injury** of **descending [left]** colon

    ✓7ᵗʰ **S36.513** **Primary blast injury** of **sigmoid** colon

    ✓7ᵗʰ **S36.518** **Primary blast injury** of other part of colon

    ✓7ᵗʰ **S36.519** **Primary blast injury** of unspecified part of colon ▽

  ✓6ᵗʰ **S36.52** **Contusion** of colon

    ✓7ᵗʰ **S36.520** **Contusion** of **ascending [right]** colon

    ✓7ᵗʰ **S36.521** **Contusion** of **transverse** colon

    ✓7ᵗʰ **S36.522** **Contusion** of **descending [left]** colon

    ✓7ᵗʰ **S36.523** **Contusion** of **sigmoid** colon

    ✓7ᵗʰ **S36.528** **Contusion** of other part of colon

    ✓7ᵗʰ **S36.529** **Contusion** of unspecified part of colon ▽

  ✓6ᵗʰ **S36.53** **Laceration** of colon

    ✓7ᵗʰ **S36.530** **Laceration** of **ascending [right]** colon

    ✓7ᵗʰ **S36.531** **Laceration** of **transverse** colon

    ✓7ᵗʰ **S36.532** **Laceration** of **descending [left]** colon

    ✓7ᵗʰ **S36.533** **Laceration** of **sigmoid** colon

    ✓7ᵗʰ **S36.538** **Laceration** of other part of colon

    ✓7ᵗʰ **S36.539** **Laceration** of unspecified part of colon ▽

  ✓6ᵗʰ **S36.59** **Other injury** of colon

    Secondary blast injury of colon

    ✓7ᵗʰ **S36.590** **Other injury** of **ascending [right]** colon

    ✓7ᵗʰ **S36.591** **Other injury** of **transverse** colon

    ✓7ᵗʰ **S36.592** **Other injury** of **descending [left]** colon

---

☑ Additional Character Req   ✓x7ᵗʰ Placeholder Alert   Manifestation   ▽ Unspecified   ▶◀ Revised Text   ● New Code   ▲ Revised Code Title

Chapter 19. Injury, Poisoning and Certain Other Consequences of External Causes

S36.593–S37.511

√7ᵗʰ **S36.593** Other injury of sigmoid colon

√7ᵗʰ **S36.598** Other injury of other part of colon

√7ᵗʰ **S36.599** Other injury of unspecified part of colon ▽

√5ᵗʰ **S36.6** Injury of rectum

√x7ᵗʰ **S36.60** Unspecified injury of rectum ▽

√x7ᵗʰ **S36.61** Primary blast injury of rectum

     Blast injury of rectum NOS

√x7ᵗʰ **S36.62** Contusion of rectum

√x7ᵗʰ **S36.63** Laceration of rectum

√x7ᵗʰ **S36.69** Other injury of rectum

     Secondary blast injury of rectum

√5ᵗʰ **S36.8** Injury of other intra-abdominal organs

√x7ᵗʰ **S36.81** Injury of peritoneum

√6ᵗʰ **S36.89** Injury of other intra-abdominal organs

     Injury of retroperitoneum

√7ᵗʰ **S36.892** Contusion of other intra-abdominal organs

√7ᵗʰ **S36.893** Laceration of other intra-abdominal organs

√7ᵗʰ **S36.898** Other injury of other intra-abdominal organs

√7ᵗʰ **S36.899** Unspecified injury of other intra-abdominal organs ▽

√5ᵗʰ **S36.9** Injury of unspecified intra-abdominal organ

√x7ᵗʰ **S36.90** Unspecified injury of unspecified intra-abdominal organ ▽

√x7ᵗʰ **S36.92** Contusion of unspecified intra-abdominal organ ▽

√x7ᵗʰ **S36.93** Laceration of unspecified intra-abdominal organ ▽

√x7ᵗʰ **S36.99** Other injury of unspecified intra-abdominal organ ▽

√4ᵗʰ **S37 Injury of urinary and pelvic organs**

     Code also any associated open wound (S31.-)

     EXCLUDES 1   obstetric trauma to pelvic organs (O71.-)

     EXCLUDES 2   injury of peritoneum (S36.81)

                    injury of retroperitoneum (S36.89-)

> The appropriate 7th character is to be added to each code from category S37.
> A   initial encounter
> D   subsequent encounter
> S   sequela

√5ᵗʰ **S37.0** Injury of kidney

     EXCLUDES 2   acute kidney injury (nontraumatic) (N17.9)

√6ᵗʰ **S37.00** Unspecified injury of kidney

√7ᵗʰ **S37.001** Unspecified injury of right kidney ▽

√7ᵗʰ **S37.002** Unspecified injury of left kidney ▽

√7ᵗʰ **S37.009** Unspecified injury of unspecified kidney ▽

√6ᵗʰ **S37.01** Minor contusion of kidney

     Contusion of kidney less than 2 cm

     Contusion of kidney NOS

√7ᵗʰ **S37.011** Minor contusion of right kidney

√7ᵗʰ **S37.012** Minor contusion of left kidney

√7ᵗʰ **S37.019** Minor contusion of unspecified kidney ▽

√6ᵗʰ **S37.02** Major contusion of kidney

     Contusion of kidney greater than 2 cm

√7ᵗʰ **S37.021** Major contusion of right kidney

√7ᵗʰ **S37.022** Major contusion of left kidney

√7ᵗʰ **S37.029** Major contusion of unspecified kidney ▽

√6ᵗʰ **S37.03** Laceration of kidney, unspecified degree

√7ᵗʰ **S37.031** Laceration of right kidney, unspecified degree ▽

√7ᵗʰ **S37.032** Laceration of left kidney, unspecified degree ▽

√7ᵗʰ **S37.039** Laceration of unspecified kidney, unspecified degree ▽

√6ᵗʰ **S37.04** Minor laceration of kidney

     Laceration of kidney less than 1 cm

√7ᵗʰ **S37.041** Minor laceration of right kidney

√7ᵗʰ **S37.042** Minor laceration of left kidney

√7ᵗʰ **S37.049** Minor laceration of unspecified kidney ▽

√6ᵗʰ **S37.05** Moderate laceration of kidney

     Laceration of kidney 1 to 3 cm

√7ᵗʰ **S37.051** Moderate laceration of right kidney

√7ᵗʰ **S37.052** Moderate laceration of left kidney

√7ᵗʰ **S37.059** Moderate laceration of unspecified kidney

√6ᵗʰ **S37.06** Major laceration of kidney

     Avulsion of kidney

     Laceration of kidney greater than 3 cm

     Massive laceration of kidney

     Multiple moderate lacerations of kidney

     Stellate laceration of kidney

√7ᵗʰ **S37.061** Major laceration of right kidney

√7ᵗʰ **S37.062** Major laceration of left kidney

√7ᵗʰ **S37.069** Major laceration of unspecified kidney ▽

√6ᵗʰ **S37.09** Other injury of kidney

√7ᵗʰ **S37.091** Other injury of right kidney

√7ᵗʰ **S37.092** Other injury of left kidney

√7ᵗʰ **S37.099** Other injury of unspecified kidney ▽

√5ᵗʰ **S37.1** Injury of ureter

√x7ᵗʰ **S37.10** Unspecified injury of ureter ▽

√x7ᵗʰ **S37.12** Contusion of ureter

√x7ᵗʰ **S37.13** Laceration of ureter

√x7ᵗʰ **S37.19** Other injury of ureter

√5ᵗʰ **S37.2** Injury of bladder

√x7ᵗʰ **S37.20** Unspecified injury of bladder ▽

√x7ᵗʰ **S37.22** Contusion of bladder

√x7ᵗʰ **S37.23** Laceration of bladder

√x7ᵗʰ **S37.29** Other injury of bladder

√5ᵗʰ **S37.3** Injury of urethra

√x7ᵗʰ **S37.30** Unspecified injury of urethra ▽

√x7ᵗʰ **S37.32** Contusion of urethra

√x7ᵗʰ **S37.33** Laceration of urethra

√x7ᵗʰ **S37.39** Other injury of urethra

√5ᵗʰ **S37.4** Injury of ovary

√6ᵗʰ **S37.40** Unspecified injury of ovary

√7ᵗʰ **S37.401** Unspecified injury of ovary, unilateral ♀ ▽

√7ᵗʰ **S37.402** Unspecified injury of ovary, bilateral ♀ ▽

√7ᵗʰ **S37.409** Unspecified injury of ovary, unspecified ♀ ▽

√6ᵗʰ **S37.42** Contusion of ovary

√7ᵗʰ **S37.421** Contusion of ovary, unilateral ♀

√7ᵗʰ **S37.422** Contusion of ovary, bilateral ♀

√7ᵗʰ **S37.429** Contusion of ovary, unspecified ♀ ▽

√6ᵗʰ **S37.43** Laceration of ovary

√7ᵗʰ **S37.431** Laceration of ovary, unilateral ♀

√7ᵗʰ **S37.432** Laceration of ovary, bilateral ♀

√7ᵗʰ **S37.439** Laceration of ovary, unspecified ♀ ▽

√6ᵗʰ **S37.49** Other injury of ovary

√7ᵗʰ **S37.491** Other injury of ovary, unilateral ♀

√7ᵗʰ **S37.492** Other injury of ovary, bilateral ♀

√7ᵗʰ **S37.499** Other injury of ovary, unspecified ♀ ▽

√5ᵗʰ **S37.5** Injury of fallopian tube

√6ᵗʰ **S37.50** Unspecified injury of fallopian tube

√7ᵗʰ **S37.501** Unspecified injury of fallopian tube, unilateral ♀ ▽

√7ᵗʰ **S37.502** Unspecified injury of fallopian tube, bilateral ♀ ▽

√7ᵗʰ **S37.509** Unspecified injury of fallopian tube, unspecified ♀ ▽

√6ᵗʰ **S37.51** Primary blast injury of fallopian tube

     Blast injury of fallopian tube NOS

√7ᵗʰ **S37.511** Primary blast injury of fallopian tube, unilateral ♀

√7ᵗʰ **S37.512 Primary blast injury of fallopian tube, bilateral** ▽

√7ᵗʰ **S37.519 Primary blast injury of fallopian tube, unspecified** ♀ ▽

√6ᵗʰ **S37.52 Contusion** of fallopian tube

√7ᵗʰ **S37.521 Contusion of fallopian tube, unilateral** ♀

√7ᵗʰ **S37.522 Contusion of fallopian tube, bilateral** ♀

√7ᵗʰ **S37.529 Contusion of fallopian tube, unspecified** ♀ ▽

√6ᵗʰ **S37.53 Laceration** of fallopian tube

√7ᵗʰ **S37.531 Laceration of fallopian tube, unilateral** ♀

√7ᵗʰ **S37.532 Laceration of fallopian tube, bilateral** ♀

√7ᵗʰ **S37.539 Laceration of fallopian tube, unspecified** ♀ ▽

√6ᵗʰ **S37.59 Other injury of fallopian tube**

Secondary blast injury of fallopian tube

√7ᵗʰ **S37.591 Other injury of fallopian tube, unilateral** ♀

√7ᵗʰ **S37.592 Other injury of fallopian tube, bilateral** ♀

√7ᵗʰ **S37.599 Other injury of fallopian tube, unspecified** ♀ ▽

√5ᵗʰ **S37.6 Injury of uterus**

EXCLUDES 1   injury to gravid uterus (O9A.2-)

injury to uterus during delivery (O71.-)

√x7ᵗʰ **S37.60 Unspecified injury of uterus** ♀ ▽

√x7ᵗʰ **S37.62 Contusion of uterus** ♀

√x7ᵗʰ **S37.63 Laceration of uterus** ♀

√x7ᵗʰ **S37.69 Other injury of uterus** ♀

√5ᵗʰ **S37.8 Injury of other urinary and pelvic organs**

√6ᵗʰ **S37.81 Injury of adrenal gland**

√7ᵗʰ **S37.812 Contusion of adrenal gland**

√7ᵗʰ **S37.813 Laceration of adrenal gland**

√7ᵗʰ **S37.818 Other injury of adrenal gland**

√7ᵗʰ **S37.819 Unspecified injury of adrenal gland** ▽

√6ᵗʰ **S37.82 Injury of prostate**

√7ᵗʰ **S37.822 Contusion of prostate** ♂

√7ᵗʰ **S37.823 Laceration of prostate** ♂

√7ᵗʰ **S37.828 Other injury of prostate** ♂

√7ᵗʰ **S37.829 Unspecified injury of prostate** ♂ ▽

√6ᵗʰ **S37.89 Injury of other urinary and pelvic organ**

√7ᵗʰ **S37.892 Contusion of other urinary and pelvic organ**

√7ᵗʰ **S37.893 Laceration of other urinary and pelvic organ**

√7ᵗʰ **S37.898 Other injury of other urinary and pelvic organ**

√7ᵗʰ **S37.899 Unspecified injury of other urinary and pelvic organ** ▽

√5ᵗʰ **S37.9 Injury of unspecified urinary and pelvic organ**

√x7ᵗʰ **S37.90 Unspecified injury of unspecified urinary and pelvic organ** ▽

√x7ᵗʰ **S37.92 Contusion of unspecified urinary and pelvic organ** ▽

√x7ᵗʰ **S37.93 Laceration of unspecified urinary and pelvic organ** ▽

√x7ᵗʰ **S37.99 Other injury of unspecified urinary and pelvic organ** ▽

√4ᵗʰ **S38 Crushing injury and traumatic amputation of abdomen, lower back, pelvis and external genitals**

NOTE   An amputation not identified as partial or complete should be coded to complete

The appropriate 7th character is to be added to each code from category S38.

A   initial encounter
D   subsequent encounter
S   sequela

√5ᵗʰ **S38.0 Crushing injury of external genital organs**

Use additional code for any associated injuries

√6ᵗʰ **S38.00 Crushing injury of unspecified external genital organs**

√7ᵗʰ **S38.001 Crushing injury of unspecified external genital organs, male** ♂ ▽

√7ᵗʰ **S38.002 Crushing injury of unspecified external genital organs, female** ♀ ▽

√x7ᵗʰ **S38.01 Crushing injury of penis** ♂

√x7ᵗʰ **S38.02 Crushing injury of scrotum and testis** ♂

√x7ᵗʰ **S38.03 Crushing injury of vulva** ♀

√x7ᵗʰ **S38.1 Crushing injury of abdomen, lower back, and pelvis**

Use additional code for all associated injuries, such as:

fracture of thoracic or lumbar spine and pelvis (S22.0-, S32.-)
injury to intra-abdominal organs (S36.-)
injury to urinary and pelvic organs (S37.-)
open wound of abdominal wall (S31.-)
spinal cord injury (S34.0, S34.1-)

EXCLUDES 2   crushing injury of external genital organs (S38.0-)

√5ᵗʰ **S38.2 Traumatic amputation of external genital organs**

√6ᵗʰ **S38.21 Traumatic amputation of female external genital organs**

Traumatic amputation of clitoris
Traumatic amputation of labium (majus) (minus)
Traumatic amputation of vulva

√7ᵗʰ **S38.211 Complete traumatic amputation of female external genital organs** ♀

√7ᵗʰ **S38.212 Partial traumatic amputation of female external genital organs** ♀

√6ᵗʰ **S38.22 Traumatic amputation of penis**

√7ᵗʰ **S38.221 Complete traumatic amputation of penis** ♂

√7ᵗʰ **S38.222 Partial traumatic amputation of penis** ♂

√6ᵗʰ **S38.23 Traumatic amputation of scrotum and testis**

√7ᵗʰ **S38.231 Complete traumatic amputation of scrotum and testis** ♂

√7ᵗʰ **S38.232 Partial traumatic amputation of scrotum and testis** ♂

√x7ᵗʰ **S38.3 Transection (partial) of abdomen**

√4ᵗʰ **S39 Other and unspecified injuries of abdomen, lower back, pelvis and external genitals**

Code also any associated open wound (S31.-)

EXCLUDES 2   sprain of joints and ligaments of lumbar spine and pelvis (S33.-)

The appropriate 7th character is to be added to each code from category S39.

A   initial encounter
D   subsequent encounter
S   sequela

√5ᵗʰ **S39.0 Injury of muscle, fascia and tendon of abdomen, lower back and pelvis**

√6ᵗʰ **S39.00 Unspecified injury of muscle, fascia and tendon of abdomen, lower back and pelvis**

√7ᵗʰ **S39.001 Unspecified injury of muscle, fascia and tendon of abdomen** ▽

√7ᵗʰ **S39.002 Unspecified injury of muscle, fascia and tendon of lower back** ▽

√7ᵗʰ **S39.003 Unspecified injury of muscle, fascia and tendon of pelvis** ▽

√6ᵗʰ **S39.01 Strain of muscle, fascia and tendon of abdomen, lower back and pelvis**

√7ᵗʰ **S39.011 Strain of muscle, fascia and tendon of abdomen**

√7ᵗʰ **S39.012 Strain of muscle, fascia and tendon of lower back**

√7ᵗʰ **S39.013 Strain of muscle, fascia and tendon of pelvis**

✓ Additional Character Req   √x7ᵗʰ Placeholder Alert   Manifestation   ▽ Unspecified   ►◄ Revised Text   ● New Code   ▲ Revised Code Title

ICD-10-CM 2019   989

√6ᵗʰ **S39.02** **Laceration** of muscle, fascia and tendon of abdomen, lower back and pelvis
- √7ᵗʰ **S39.021** **Laceration of muscle, fascia and tendon of abdomen**
- √7ᵗʰ **S39.022** **Laceration of muscle, fascia and tendon of lower back**
- √7ᵗʰ **S39.023** **Laceration of muscle, fascia and tendon of pelvis**

√6ᵗʰ **S39.09** **Other injury** of muscle, fascia and tendon of abdomen, lower back and pelvis
- √7ᵗʰ **S39.091** **Other injury of muscle, fascia and tendon of abdomen**
- √7ᵗʰ **S39.092** **Other injury of muscle, fascia and tendon of lower back**
- √7ᵗʰ **S39.093** **Other injury of muscle, fascia and tendon of pelvis**

√5ᵗʰ **S39.8** **Other specified injuries** of abdomen, lower back, pelvis and external genitals
- √x7ᵗʰ **S39.81** **Other specified injuries of abdomen**
- √x7ᵗʰ **S39.82** **Other specified injuries of lower back**
- √x7ᵗʰ **S39.83** **Other specified injuries of pelvis**
- √6ᵗʰ **S39.84** **Other specified injuries of external genitals**
  - √7ᵗʰ **S39.840** **Fracture of corpus cavernosum penis**   ♂
  - √7ᵗʰ **S39.848** **Other specified injuries of external genitals**
    TIP: Assign for traumatic rupture of testis.

√5ᵗʰ **S39.9** **Unspecified injury** of abdomen, lower back, pelvis and external genitals
- √x7ᵗʰ **S39.91** **Unspecified injury of abdomen**   ▽
- √x7ᵗʰ **S39.92** **Unspecified injury of lower back**   ▽
- √x7ᵗʰ **S39.93** **Unspecified injury of pelvis**   ▽
- √x7ᵗʰ **S39.94** **Unspecified injury of external genitals**   ▽

Injuries to the shoulder and upper arm (S40-S49)

INCLUDES   injuries of axilla
injuries of scapular region
EXCLUDES 2   burns and corrosions (T20-T32)
frostbite (T33-T34)
injuries of elbow (S50-S59)
insect bite or sting, venomous (T63.4)

√4ᵗʰ **S40** **Superficial injury of shoulder and upper arm**

The appropriate 7th character is to be added to each code from category S40.
A   initial encounter
D   subsequent encounter
S   sequela

√5ᵗʰ **S40.0** **Contusion of shoulder and upper arm**
- √6ᵗʰ **S40.01** **Contusion of shoulder**
  - √7ᵗʰ **S40.011** **Contusion of right shoulder**
  - √7ᵗʰ **S40.012** **Contusion of left shoulder**
  - √7ᵗʰ **S40.019** **Contusion of unspecified shoulder**   ▽
- √6ᵗʰ **S40.02** **Contusion of upper arm**
  - √7ᵗʰ **S40.021** **Contusion of right upper arm**
  - √7ᵗʰ **S40.022** **Contusion of left upper arm**
  - √7ᵗʰ **S40.029** **Contusion of unspecified upper arm**   ▽

√5ᵗʰ **S40.2** **Other superficial injuries of shoulder**
- √6ᵗʰ **S40.21** **Abrasion of shoulder**
  - √7ᵗʰ **S40.211** **Abrasion of right shoulder**
  - √7ᵗʰ **S40.212** **Abrasion of left shoulder**
  - √7ᵗʰ **S40.219** **Abrasion of unspecified shoulder**   ▽
- √6ᵗʰ **S40.22** **Blister (nonthermal) of shoulder**
  - √7ᵗʰ **S40.221** **Blister (nonthermal) of right shoulder**
  - √7ᵗʰ **S40.222** **Blister (nonthermal) of left shoulder**
  - √7ᵗʰ **S40.229** **Blister (nonthermal) of unspecified shoulder**   ▽
- √6ᵗʰ **S40.24** **External constriction of shoulder**
  - √7ᵗʰ **S40.241** **External constriction of right shoulder**
  - √7ᵗʰ **S40.242** **External constriction of left shoulder**
  - √7ᵗʰ **S40.249** **External constriction of unspecified shoulder**   ▽

√6ᵗʰ **S40.25** **Superficial foreign body of shoulder**
Splinter in the shoulder
- √7ᵗʰ **S40.251** **Superficial foreign body of right shoulder**
- √7ᵗʰ **S40.252** **Superficial foreign body of left shoulder**
- √7ᵗʰ **S40.259** **Superficial foreign body of unspecified shoulder**   ▽

√6ᵗʰ **S40.26** **Insect bite (nonvenomous) of shoulder**
- √7ᵗʰ **S40.261** **Insect bite (nonvenomous) of right shoulder**
- √7ᵗʰ **S40.262** **Insect bite (nonvenomous) of left shoulder**
- √7ᵗʰ **S40.269** **Insect bite (nonvenomous) of unspecified shoulder**   ▽

√6ᵗʰ **S40.27** **Other superficial bite of shoulder**
EXCLUDES 1   open bite of shoulder (S41.05)
- √7ᵗʰ **S40.271** **Other superficial bite of right shoulder**
- √7ᵗʰ **S40.272** **Other superficial bite of left shoulder**
- √7ᵗʰ **S40.279** **Other superficial bite of unspecified shoulder**   ▽

√5ᵗʰ **S40.8** **Other superficial injuries of upper arm**
- √6ᵗʰ **S40.81** **Abrasion of upper arm**
  - √7ᵗʰ **S40.811** **Abrasion of right upper arm**
  - √7ᵗʰ **S40.812** **Abrasion of left upper arm**
  - √7ᵗʰ **S40.819** **Abrasion of unspecified upper arm**   ▽
- √6ᵗʰ **S40.82** **Blister (nonthermal) of upper arm**
  - √7ᵗʰ **S40.821** **Blister (nonthermal) of right upper arm**
  - √7ᵗʰ **S40.822** **Blister (nonthermal) of left upper arm**
  - √7ᵗʰ **S40.829** **Blister (nonthermal) of unspecified upper arm**   ▽
- √6ᵗʰ **S40.84** **External constriction of upper arm**
  - √7ᵗʰ **S40.841** **External constriction of right upper arm**
  - √7ᵗʰ **S40.842** **External constriction of left upper arm**
  - √7ᵗʰ **S40.849** **External constriction of unspecified upper arm**   ▽
- √6ᵗʰ **S40.85** **Superficial foreign body of upper arm**
  Splinter in the upper arm
  - √7ᵗʰ **S40.851** **Superficial foreign body of right upper arm**
  - √7ᵗʰ **S40.852** **Superficial foreign body of left upper arm**
  - √7ᵗʰ **S40.859** **Superficial foreign body of unspecified upper arm**   ▽
- √6ᵗʰ **S40.86** **Insect bite (nonvenomous) of upper arm**
  - √7ᵗʰ **S40.861** **Insect bite (nonvenomous) of right upper arm**
  - √7ᵗʰ **S40.862** **Insect bite (nonvenomous) of left upper arm**
  - √7ᵗʰ **S40.869** **Insect bite (nonvenomous) of unspecified upper arm**   ▽
- √6ᵗʰ **S40.87** **Other superficial bite of upper arm**
  EXCLUDES 1   open bite of upper arm (S41.14)
  EXCLUDES 2   other superficial bite of shoulder (S40.27-)
  - √7ᵗʰ **S40.871** **Other superficial bite of right upper arm**
  - √7ᵗʰ **S40.872** **Other superficial bite of left upper arm**
  - √7ᵗʰ **S40.879** **Other superficial bite of unspecified upper arm**   ▽

√5ᵗʰ **S40.9** **Unspecified superficial injury of shoulder and upper arm**
- √6ᵗʰ **S40.91** **Unspecified superficial injury of shoulder**
  - √7ᵗʰ **S40.911** **Unspecified superficial injury of right shoulder**   ▽
  - √7ᵗʰ **S40.912** **Unspecified superficial injury of left shoulder**   ▽
  - √7ᵗʰ **S40.919** **Unspecified superficial injury of unspecified shoulder**   ▽
- √6ᵗʰ **S40.92** **Unspecified superficial injury of upper arm**
  - √7ᵗʰ **S40.921** **Unspecified superficial injury of right upper arm**   ▽
  - √7ᵗʰ **S40.922** **Unspecified superficial injury of left upper arm**   ▽
  - √7ᵗʰ **S40.929** **Unspecified superficial injury of unspecified upper arm**   ▽

√4ᵗʰ **S41** **Open wound of shoulder and upper arm**

Code also any associated wound infection

EXCLUDES 1   *traumatic amputation of shoulder and upper arm (S48.-)*

EXCLUDES 2   *open fracture of shoulder and upper arm (S42.- with 7th character B or C)*

The appropriate 7th character is to be added to each code from category S41.
- A   initial encounter
- D   subsequent encounter
- S   sequela

√5ᵗʰ **S41.0**   **Open wound of shoulder**

√6ᵗʰ   **S41.00**   **Unspecified open wound of shoulder**

    √7ᵗʰ   **S41.001**   Unspecified open wound of right shoulder   ▽

    √7ᵗʰ   **S41.002**   Unspecified open wound of left shoulder   ▽

    √7ᵗʰ   **S41.009**   Unspecified open wound of unspecified shoulder   ▽

√6ᵗʰ   **S41.01**   **Laceration without foreign body of shoulder**

    √7ᵗʰ   **S41.011**   Laceration without foreign body of right shoulder

    √7ᵗʰ   **S41.012**   Laceration without foreign body of left shoulder

    √7ᵗʰ   **S41.019**   Laceration without foreign body of unspecified shoulder   ▽

√6ᵗʰ   **S41.02**   **Laceration with foreign body of shoulder**

    √7ᵗʰ   **S41.021**   Laceration with foreign body of right shoulder

    √7ᵗʰ   **S41.022**   Laceration with foreign body of left shoulder

    √7ᵗʰ   **S41.029**   Laceration with foreign body of unspecified shoulder   ▽

√6ᵗʰ   **S41.03**   **Puncture wound without foreign body of shoulder**

    √7ᵗʰ   **S41.031**   Puncture wound without foreign body of right shoulder

    √7ᵗʰ   **S41.032**   Puncture wound without foreign body of left shoulder

    √7ᵗʰ   **S41.039**   Puncture wound without foreign body of unspecified shoulder   ▽

√6ᵗʰ   **S41.04**   **Puncture wound with foreign body of shoulder**

    √7ᵗʰ   **S41.041**   Puncture wound with foreign body of right shoulder

    √7ᵗʰ   **S41.042**   Puncture wound with foreign body of left shoulder

    √7ᵗʰ   **S41.049**   Puncture wound with foreign body of unspecified shoulder   ▽

√6ᵗʰ   **S41.05**   **Open bite of shoulder**

    Bite of shoulder NOS

    EXCLUDES 1   *superficial bite of shoulder (S40.27)*

    √7ᵗʰ   **S41.051**   Open bite of right shoulder

    √7ᵗʰ   **S41.052**   Open bite of left shoulder

    √7ᵗʰ   **S41.059**   Open bite of unspecified shoulder   ▽

√5ᵗʰ **S41.1**   **Open wound of upper arm**

√6ᵗʰ   **S41.10**   **Unspecified open wound of upper arm**

    AHA: 2016,3Q,24

    √7ᵗʰ   **S41.101**   Unspecified open wound of right upper arm   ▽

    √7ᵗʰ   **S41.102**   Unspecified open wound of left upper arm   ▽

    √7ᵗʰ   **S41.109**   Unspecified open wound of unspecified upper arm   ▽

√6ᵗʰ   **S41.11**   **Laceration without foreign body of upper arm**

    √7ᵗʰ   **S41.111**   Laceration without foreign body of right upper arm

    √7ᵗʰ   **S41.112**   Laceration without foreign body of left upper arm

    √7ᵗʰ   **S41.119**   Laceration without foreign body of unspecified upper arm   ▽

√6ᵗʰ   **S41.12**   **Laceration with foreign body of upper arm**

    √7ᵗʰ   **S41.121**   Laceration with foreign body of right upper arm

    √7ᵗʰ   **S41.122**   Laceration with foreign body of left upper arm

    √7ᵗʰ   **S41.129**   Laceration with foreign body of unspecified upper arm   ▽

√6ᵗʰ   **S41.13**   **Puncture wound without foreign body of upper arm**

    AHA: 2016,3Q,24

    √7ᵗʰ   **S41.131**   Puncture wound without foreign body of right upper arm

    √7ᵗʰ   **S41.132**   Puncture wound without foreign body of left upper arm

    √7ᵗʰ   **S41.139**   Puncture wound without foreign body of unspecified upper arm   ▽

√6ᵗʰ   **S41.14**   **Puncture wound with foreign body of upper arm**

    AHA: 2016,3Q,24

    √7ᵗʰ   **S41.141**   Puncture wound with foreign body of right upper arm

    √7ᵗʰ   **S41.142**   Puncture wound with foreign body of left upper arm

    √7ᵗʰ   **S41.149**   Puncture wound with foreign body of unspecified upper arm   ▽

√6ᵗʰ   **S41.15**   **Open bite of upper arm**

    Bite of upper arm NOS

    EXCLUDES 1   *superficial bite of upper arm (S40.87)*

    √7ᵗʰ   **S41.151**   Open bite of right upper arm

    √7ᵗʰ   **S41.152**   Open bite of left upper arm

    √7ᵗʰ   **S41.159**   Open bite of unspecified upper arm   ▽

√4ᵗʰ **S42** **Fracture of shoulder and upper arm**

NOTE   A fracture not indicated as displaced or nondisplaced should be coded to displaced

A fracture not indicated as open or closed should be coded to closed

EXCLUDES 1   *traumatic amputation of shoulder and upper arm (S48.-)*

AHA: 2018,2Q,12; 2015,3Q,37-39

The appropriate 7th character is to be added to all codes from category S42 [unless otherwise indicated].
- A   initial encounter for closed fracture
- B   initial encounter for open fracture
- D   subsequent encounter for fracture with routine healing
- G   subsequent encounter for fracture with delayed healing
- K   subsequent encounter for fracture with nonunion
- P   subsequent encounter for fracture with malunion
- S   sequela

√5ᵗʰ **S42.0**   **Fracture of clavicle**

√6ᵗʰ   **S42.00**   **Fracture of unspecified part of clavicle**

    √7ᵗʰ   **S42.001**   Fracture of unspecified part of right clavicle   Ⓞ ▽

    √7ᵗʰ   **S42.002**   Fracture of unspecified part of left clavicle   Ⓞ ▽

    √7ᵗʰ   **S42.009**   Fracture of unspecified part of unspecified clavicle   Ⓞ ▽

     AHA: 2012,4Q,93

√6ᵗʰ   **S42.01**   **Fracture of sternal end of clavicle**

    √7ᵗʰ   **S42.011**   Anterior displaced fracture of sternal end of right clavicle   Ⓞ

    √7ᵗʰ   **S42.012**   Anterior displaced fracture of sternal end of left clavicle   Ⓞ

    √7ᵗʰ   **S42.013**   Anterior displaced fracture of sternal end of unspecified clavicle   Ⓞ ▽

     Displaced fracture of sternal end of clavicle NOS

    √7ᵗʰ   **S42.014**   Posterior displaced fracture of sternal end of right clavicle   Ⓞ

    √7ᵗʰ   **S42.015**   Posterior displaced fracture of sternal end of left clavicle   Ⓞ

    √7ᵗʰ   **S42.016**   Posterior displaced fracture of sternal end of unspecified clavicle   Ⓞ ▽

    √7ᵗʰ   **S42.017**   Nondisplaced fracture of sternal end of right clavicle   Ⓞ

    √7ᵗʰ   **S42.018**   Nondisplaced fracture of sternal end of left clavicle   Ⓞ

    √7ᵗʰ   **S42.019**   Nondisplaced fracture of sternal end of unspecified clavicle   Ⓞ ▽

√6ᵗʰ   **S42.02**   **Fracture of shaft of clavicle**

    √7ᵗʰ   **S42.021**   Displaced fracture of shaft of right clavicle   Ⓞ

    √7ᵗʰ   **S42.022**   Displaced fracture of shaft of left clavicle   Ⓞ

    √7ᵗʰ   **S42.023**   Displaced fracture of shaft of unspecified clavicle   Ⓞ ▽

☑ Additional Character Req   √x7ᵗʰ Placeholder Alert   Manifestation   ▽ Unspecified   ►◄ Revised Text   ● New Code   ▲ Revised Code Title

ICD-10-CM 2019   991

√7ᵗʰ **S42.024** Nondisplaced fracture of shaft of right clavicle ◻

√7ᵗʰ **S42.025** Nondisplaced fracture of shaft of left clavicle ◻

√7ᵗʰ **S42.026** Nondisplaced fracture of shaft of unspecified clavicle ◻ ▽

√6ᵗʰ **S42.03** Fracture of lateral end of clavicle

Fracture of acromial end of clavicle

√7ᵗʰ **S42.031** Displaced fracture of lateral end of right clavicle ◻

√7ᵗʰ **S42.032** Displaced fracture of lateral end of left clavicle ◻

√7ᵗʰ **S42.033** Displaced fracture of lateral end of unspecified clavicle ◻ ▽

√7ᵗʰ **S42.034** Nondisplaced fracture of lateral end of right clavicle ◻

√7ᵗʰ **S42.035** Nondisplaced fracture of lateral end of left clavicle ◻

√7ᵗʰ **S42.036** Nondisplaced fracture of lateral end of unspecified clavicle ◻ ▽

√5ᵗʰ **S42.1** Fracture of scapula

√6ᵗʰ **S42.10** Fracture of unspecified part of scapula

√7ᵗʰ **S42.101** Fracture of unspecified part of scapula, right shoulder ◻ ▽

√7ᵗʰ **S42.102** Fracture of unspecified part of scapula, left shoulder ◻ ▽

√7ᵗʰ **S42.109** Fracture of unspecified part of scapula, unspecified shoulder ◻ ▽

√6ᵗʰ **S42.11** Fracture of body of scapula

√7ᵗʰ **S42.111** Displaced fracture of body of scapula, right shoulder ◻

√7ᵗʰ **S42.112** Displaced fracture of body of scapula, left shoulder ◻

√7ᵗʰ **S42.113** Displaced fracture of body of scapula, unspecified shoulder ◻ ▽

√7ᵗʰ **S42.114** Nondisplaced fracture of body of scapula, right shoulder ◻

√7ᵗʰ **S42.115** Nondisplaced fracture of body of scapula, left shoulder ◻

√7ᵗʰ **S42.116** Nondisplaced fracture of body of scapula, unspecified shoulder ◻ ▽

√6ᵗʰ **S42.12** Fracture of acromial process

√7ᵗʰ **S42.121** Displaced fracture of acromial process, right shoulder ◻

√7ᵗʰ **S42.122** Displaced fracture of acromial process, left shoulder ◻

√7ᵗʰ **S42.123** Displaced fracture of acromial process, unspecified shoulder ◻ ▽

√7ᵗʰ **S42.124** Nondisplaced fracture of acromial process, right shoulder ◻

√7ᵗʰ **S42.125** Nondisplaced fracture of acromial process, left shoulder ◻

√7ᵗʰ **S42.126** Nondisplaced fracture of acromial process, unspecified shoulder ◻ ▽

√6ᵗʰ **S42.13** Fracture of coracoid process

√7ᵗʰ **S42.131** Displaced fracture of coracoid process, right shoulder ◻

√7ᵗʰ **S42.132** Displaced fracture of coracoid process, left shoulder ◻

√7ᵗʰ **S42.133** Displaced fracture of coracoid process, unspecified shoulder ◻ ▽

√7ᵗʰ **S42.134** Nondisplaced fracture of coracoid process, right shoulder ◻

√7ᵗʰ **S42.135** Nondisplaced fracture of coracoid process, left shoulder ◻

√7ᵗʰ **S42.136** Nondisplaced fracture of coracoid process, unspecified shoulder ◻ ▽

√6ᵗʰ **S42.14** Fracture of glenoid cavity of scapula

√7ᵗʰ **S42.141** Displaced fracture of glenoid cavity of scapula, right shoulder ◻

√7ᵗʰ **S42.142** Displaced fracture of glenoid cavity of scapula, left shoulder ◻

√7ᵗʰ **S42.143** Displaced fracture of glenoid cavity of scapula, unspecified shoulder ◻ ▽

√7ᵗʰ **S42.144** Nondisplaced fracture of glenoid cavity of scapula, right shoulder ◻

√7ᵗʰ **S42.145** Nondisplaced fracture of glenoid cavity of scapula, left shoulder ◻

√7ᵗʰ **S42.146** Nondisplaced fracture of glenoid cavity of scapula, unspecified shoulder ◻ ▽

√6ᵗʰ **S42.15** Fracture of neck of scapula

√7ᵗʰ **S42.151** Displaced fracture of neck of scapula, right shoulder ◻

√7ᵗʰ **S42.152** Displaced fracture of neck of scapula, left shoulder ◻

√7ᵗʰ **S42.153** Displaced fracture of neck of scapula, unspecified shoulder ◻ ▽

√7ᵗʰ **S42.154** Nondisplaced fracture of neck of scapula, right shoulder ◻

√7ᵗʰ **S42.155** Nondisplaced fracture of neck of scapula, left shoulder ◻

√7ᵗʰ **S42.156** Nondisplaced fracture of neck of scapula, unspecified shoulder ◻ ▽

√6ᵗʰ **S42.19** Fracture of other part of scapula

√7ᵗʰ **S42.191** Fracture of other part of scapula, right shoulder ◻

√7ᵗʰ **S42.192** Fracture of other part of scapula, left shoulder ◻

√7ᵗʰ **S42.199** Fracture of other part of scapula, unspecified shoulder ◻ ▽

√5ᵗʰ **S42.2** Fracture of upper end of humerus

Fracture of proximal end of humerus

EXCLUDES 2 *fracture of shaft of humerus (S42.3-)*
physeal fracture of upper end of humerus (S49.0-)

√6ᵗʰ **S42.20** Unspecified fracture of upper end of humerus

√7ᵗʰ **S42.201** Unspecified fracture of upper end of right humerus ◻ ▽

√7ᵗʰ **S42.202** Unspecified fracture of upper end of left humerus ◻ ▽

√7ᵗʰ **S42.209** Unspecified fracture of upper end of unspecified humerus ◻ ▽

√6ᵗʰ **S42.21** Unspecified fracture of surgical neck of humerus

Fracture of neck of humerus NOS

√7ᵗʰ **S42.211** Unspecified displaced fracture of surgical neck of right humerus ◻ ▽

√7ᵗʰ **S42.212** Unspecified displaced fracture of surgical neck of left humerus ◻ ▽

√7ᵗʰ **S42.213** Unspecified displaced fracture of surgical neck of unspecified humerus ◻ ▽

√7ᵗʰ **S42.214** Unspecified nondisplaced fracture of surgical neck of right humerus ◻ ▽

√7ᵗʰ **S42.215** Unspecified nondisplaced fracture of surgical neck of left humerus ◻ ▽

√7ᵗʰ **S42.216** Unspecified nondisplaced fracture of surgical neck of unspecified humerus ◻ ▽

√6ᵗʰ **S42.22** 2-part fracture of surgical neck of humerus

√7ᵗʰ **S42.221** 2-part displaced fracture of surgical neck of right humerus ◻

√7ᵗʰ **S42.222** 2-part displaced fracture of surgical neck of left humerus ◻

√7ᵗʰ **S42.223** 2-part displaced fracture of surgical neck of unspecified humerus ◻ ▽

√7ᵗʰ **S42.224** 2-part nondisplaced fracture of surgical neck of right humerus ◻

√7ᵗʰ **S42.225** 2-part nondisplaced fracture of surgical neck of left humerus ◻

√7ᵗʰ **S42.226** 2-part nondisplaced fracture of surgical neck of unspecified humerus ◻ ▽

√6ᵗʰ **S42.23** 3-part fracture of surgical neck of humerus

√7ᵗʰ **S42.231** 3-part fracture of surgical neck of right humerus ◻

√7ᵗʰ **S42.232** 3-part fracture of surgical neck of left humerus ◻

√7ᵗʰ **S42.239** 3-part fracture of surgical neck of unspecified humerus ◻ ▽

√6ᵗʰ **S42.24** 4-part fracture of surgical neck of humerus

√7ᵗʰ **S42.241** 4-part fracture of surgical neck of right humerus ◻

√7ᵗʰ **S42.242** 4-part fracture of surgical neck of left humerus ◻

√7ᵗʰ **S42.249** 4-part fracture of surgical neck of unspecified humerus ◻ ▽

√6ᵗʰ **S42.25** Fracture of greater tuberosity of humerus

√7ᵗʰ **S42.251** Displaced fracture of greater tuberosity of right humerus ◻

√7ᵗʰ **S42.252** Displaced fracture of greater tuberosity of left humerus   🔲

√7ᵗʰ **S42.253** Displaced fracture of greater tuberosity of unspecified humerus   🔲 ▽

√7ᵗʰ **S42.254** Nondisplaced fracture of greater tuberosity of right humerus   🔲

√7ᵗʰ **S42.255** Nondisplaced fracture of greater tuberosity of left humerus   🔲

√7ᵗʰ **S42.256** Nondisplaced fracture of greater tuberosity of unspecified humerus   🔲 ▽

√6ᵗʰ **S42.26** Fracture of lesser tuberosity of humerus

√7ᵗʰ **S42.261** Displaced fracture of lesser tuberosity of right humerus   🔲

√7ᵗʰ **S42.262** Displaced fracture of lesser tuberosity of left humerus   🔲

√7ᵗʰ **S42.263** Displaced fracture of lesser tuberosity of unspecified humerus   🔲 ▽

√7ᵗʰ **S42.264** Nondisplaced fracture of lesser tuberosity of right humerus   🔲

√7ᵗʰ **S42.265** Nondisplaced fracture of lesser tuberosity of left humerus   🔲

√7ᵗʰ **S42.266** Nondisplaced fracture of lesser tuberosity of unspecified humerus   🔲 ▽

√6ᵗʰ **S42.27** Torus fracture of upper end of humerus

> The appropriate 7th character is to be added to all codes in subcategory S42.27
> A initial encounter for closed fracture
> D subsequent encounter for fracture with routine healing
> G subsequent encounter for fracture with delayed healing
> K subsequent encounter for fracture with nonunion
> P subsequent encounter for fracture with malunion
> S sequela

√7ᵗʰ **S42.271** Torus fracture of upper end of right humerus   🔲

√7ᵗʰ **S42.272** Torus fracture of upper end of left humerus   🔲

√7ᵗʰ **S42.279** Torus fracture of upper end of unspecified humerus   🔲 ▽

√6ᵗʰ **S42.29** Other fracture of upper end of humerus

Fracture of anatomical neck of humerus
Fracture of articular head of humerus

√7ᵗʰ **S42.291** Other displaced fracture of upper end of right humerus   🔲

√7ᵗʰ **S42.292** Other displaced fracture of upper end of left humerus   🔲

√7ᵗʰ **S42.293** Other displaced fracture of upper end of unspecified humerus   🔲 ▽

√7ᵗʰ **S42.294** Other nondisplaced fracture of upper end of right humerus   🔲

√7ᵗʰ **S42.295** Other nondisplaced fracture of upper end of left humerus   🔲

√7ᵗʰ **S42.296** Other nondisplaced fracture of upper end of unspecified humerus   🔲 ▽

√5ᵗʰ **S42.3** Fracture of shaft of humerus

Fracture of humerus NOS
Fracture of upper arm NOS
EXCLUDES 2   physeal fractures of upper end of humerus (S49.0-)
        physeal fractures of lower end of humerus (S49.1-)

√6ᵗʰ **S42.30** Unspecified fracture of shaft of humerus

√7ᵗʰ **S42.301** Unspecified fracture of shaft of humerus, right arm   🔲 ▽

√7ᵗʰ **S42.302** Unspecified fracture of shaft of humerus, left arm   🔲 ▽

√7ᵗʰ **S42.309** Unspecified fracture of shaft of humerus, unspecified arm   🔲 ▽

√6ᵗʰ **S42.31** Greenstick fracture of shaft of humerus

> The appropriate 7th character is to be added to all codes in subcategory S42.31
> A initial encounter for closed fracture
> D subsequent encounter for fracture with routine healing
> G subsequent encounter for fracture with delayed healing
> K subsequent encounter for fracture with nonunion
> P subsequent encounter for fracture with malunion
> S sequela

√7ᵗʰ **S42.311** Greenstick fracture of shaft of humerus, right arm   🔲

√7ᵗʰ **S42.312** Greenstick fracture of shaft of humerus, left arm   🔲

√7ᵗʰ **S42.319** Greenstick fracture of shaft of humerus, unspecified arm   🔲 ▽

√6ᵗʰ **S42.32** Transverse fracture of shaft of humerus

√7ᵗʰ **S42.321** Displaced transverse fracture of shaft of humerus, right arm   🔲

√7ᵗʰ **S42.322** Displaced transverse fracture of shaft of humerus, left arm   🔲

√7ᵗʰ **S42.323** Displaced transverse fracture of shaft of humerus, unspecified arm   🔲 ▽

√7ᵗʰ **S42.324** Nondisplaced transverse fracture of shaft of humerus, right arm   🔲

√7ᵗʰ **S42.325** Nondisplaced transverse fracture of shaft of humerus, left arm   🔲

√7ᵗʰ **S42.326** Nondisplaced transverse fracture of shaft of humerus, unspecified arm   🔲 ▽

√6ᵗʰ **S42.33** Oblique fracture of shaft of humerus

√7ᵗʰ **S42.331** Displaced oblique fracture of shaft of humerus, right arm   🔲

√7ᵗʰ **S42.332** Displaced oblique fracture of shaft of humerus, left arm   🔲

√7ᵗʰ **S42.333** Displaced oblique fracture of shaft of humerus, unspecified arm   🔲 ▽

√7ᵗʰ **S42.334** Nondisplaced oblique fracture of shaft of humerus, right arm   🔲

√7ᵗʰ **S42.335** Nondisplaced oblique fracture of shaft of humerus, left arm   🔲

√7ᵗʰ **S42.336** Nondisplaced oblique fracture of shaft of humerus, unspecified arm   🔲 ▽

√6ᵗʰ **S42.34** Spiral fracture of shaft of humerus

√7ᵗʰ **S42.341** Displaced spiral fracture of shaft of humerus, right arm   🔲

√7ᵗʰ **S42.342** Displaced spiral fracture of shaft of humerus, left arm   🔲

√7ᵗʰ **S42.343** Displaced spiral fracture of shaft of humerus, unspecified arm   🔲 ▽

√7ᵗʰ **S42.344** Nondisplaced spiral fracture of shaft of humerus, right arm   🔲

√7ᵗʰ **S42.345** Nondisplaced spiral fracture of shaft of humerus, left arm   🔲

√7ᵗʰ **S42.346** Nondisplaced spiral fracture of shaft of humerus, unspecified arm   🔲 ▽

√6ᵗʰ **S42.35** Comminuted fracture of shaft of humerus

√7ᵗʰ **S42.351** Displaced comminuted fracture of shaft of humerus, right arm   🔲

√7ᵗʰ **S42.352** Displaced comminuted fracture of shaft of humerus, left arm   🔲

√7ᵗʰ **S42.353** Displaced comminuted fracture of shaft of humerus, unspecified arm   🔲 ▽

√7ᵗʰ **S42.354** Nondisplaced comminuted fracture of shaft of humerus, right arm   🔲

√7ᵗʰ **S42.355** Nondisplaced comminuted fracture of shaft of humerus, left arm   🔲

√7ᵗʰ **S42.356** Nondisplaced comminuted fracture of shaft of humerus, unspecified arm   🔲 ▽

√6ᵗʰ **S42.36 Segmental fracture of shaft of humerus**

√7ᵗʰ **S42.361 Displaced segmental fracture of shaft of humerus, right arm** ℚ

√7ᵗʰ **S42.362 Displaced segmental fracture of shaft of humerus, left arm** ℚ

√7ᵗʰ **S42.363 Displaced segmental fracture of shaft of humerus, unspecified arm** ℚ ▽

√7ᵗʰ **S42.364 Nondisplaced segmental fracture of shaft of humerus, right arm** ℚ

√7ᵗʰ **S42.365 Nondisplaced segmental fracture of shaft of humerus, left arm** ℚ

√7ᵗʰ **S42.366 Nondisplaced segmental fracture of shaft of humerus, unspecified arm** ℚ ▽

√6ᵗʰ **S42.39 Other fracture of shaft of humerus**

√7ᵗʰ **S42.391 Other fracture of shaft of right humerus** ℚ

√7ᵗʰ **S42.392 Other fracture of shaft of left humerus** ℚ

√7ᵗʰ **S42.399 Other fracture of shaft of unspecified humerus** ℚ ▽

√5ᵗʰ **S42.4 Fracture of lower end of humerus**

Fracture of distal end of humerus

EXCLUDES 2 fracture of shaft of humerus (S42.3-)

physeal fracture of lower end of humerus (S49.1-)

√6ᵗʰ **S42.40 Unspecified fracture of lower end of humerus**

Fracture of elbow NOS

√7ᵗʰ **S42.401 Unspecified fracture of lower end of right humerus** ℚ ▽

√7ᵗʰ **S42.402 Unspecified fracture of lower end of left humerus** ℚ ▽

√7ᵗʰ **S42.409 Unspecified fracture of lower end of unspecified humerus** ℚ ▽

√6ᵗʰ **S42.41 Simple supracondylar fracture without intercondylar fracture of humerus**

√7ᵗʰ **S42.411 Displaced simple supracondylar fracture without intercondylar fracture of right humerus** ℚ

√7ᵗʰ **S42.412 Displaced simple supracondylar fracture without intercondylar fracture of left humerus** ℚ

√7ᵗʰ **S42.413 Displaced simple supracondylar fracture without intercondylar fracture of unspecified humerus** ℚ ▽

√7ᵗʰ **S42.414 Nondisplaced simple supracondylar fracture without intercondylar fracture of right humerus** ℚ

√7ᵗʰ **S42.415 Nondisplaced simple supracondylar fracture without intercondylar fracture of left humerus** ℚ

√7ᵗʰ **S42.416 Nondisplaced simple supracondylar fracture without intercondylar fracture of unspecified humerus** ℚ ▽

√6ᵗʰ **S42.42 Comminuted supracondylar fracture without intercondylar fracture of humerus**

√7ᵗʰ **S42.421 Displaced comminuted supracondylar fracture without intercondylar fracture of right humerus** ℚ

√7ᵗʰ **S42.422 Displaced comminuted supracondylar fracture without intercondylar fracture of left humerus** ℚ

√7ᵗʰ **S42.423 Displaced comminuted supracondylar fracture without intercondylar fracture of unspecified humerus** ℚ ▽

√7ᵗʰ **S42.424 Nondisplaced comminuted supracondylar fracture without intercondylar fracture of right humerus** ℚ

√7ᵗʰ **S42.425 Nondisplaced comminuted supracondylar fracture without intercondylar fracture of left humerus** ℚ

√7ᵗʰ **S42.426 Nondisplaced comminuted supracondylar fracture without intercondylar fracture of unspecified humerus** ℚ ▽

√6ᵗʰ **S42.43 Fracture (avulsion) of lateral epicondyle of humerus**

√7ᵗʰ **S42.431 Displaced fracture (avulsion) of lateral epicondyle of right humerus** ℚ

√7ᵗʰ **S42.432 Displaced fracture (avulsion) of lateral epicondyle of left humerus** ℚ

√7ᵗʰ **S42.433 Displaced fracture (avulsion) of lateral epicondyle of unspecified humerus** ℚ ▽

√7ᵗʰ **S42.434 Nondisplaced fracture (avulsion) of lateral epicondyle of right humerus** ℚ

√7ᵗʰ **S42.435 Nondisplaced fracture (avulsion) of lateral epicondyle of left humerus** ℚ

√7ᵗʰ **S42.436 Nondisplaced fracture (avulsion) of lateral epicondyle of unspecified humerus** ℚ ▽

√6ᵗʰ **S42.44 Fracture (avulsion) of medial epicondyle of humerus**

√7ᵗʰ **S42.441 Displaced fracture (avulsion) of medial epicondyle of right humerus** ℚ

√7ᵗʰ **S42.442 Displaced fracture (avulsion) of medial epicondyle of left humerus** ℚ

√7ᵗʰ **S42.443 Displaced fracture (avulsion) of medial epicondyle of unspecified humerus** ℚ ▽

√7ᵗʰ **S42.444 Nondisplaced fracture (avulsion) of medial epicondyle of right humerus** ℚ

√7ᵗʰ **S42.445 Nondisplaced fracture (avulsion) of medial epicondyle of left humerus** ℚ

√7ᵗʰ **S42.446 Nondisplaced fracture (avulsion) of medial epicondyle of unspecified humerus** ℚ ▽

√7ᵗʰ **S42.447 Incarcerated fracture (avulsion) of medial epicondyle of right humerus** ℚ

√7ᵗʰ **S42.448 Incarcerated fracture (avulsion) of medial epicondyle of left humerus** ℚ

√7ᵗʰ **S42.449 Incarcerated fracture (avulsion) of medial epicondyle of unspecified humerus** ℚ ▽

√6ᵗʰ **S42.45 Fracture of lateral condyle of humerus**

Fracture of capitellum of humerus

√7ᵗʰ **S42.451 Displaced fracture of lateral condyle of right humerus** ℚ

√7ᵗʰ **S42.452 Displaced fracture of lateral condyle of left humerus** ℚ

√7ᵗʰ **S42.453 Displaced fracture of lateral condyle of unspecified humerus** ℚ ▽

√7ᵗʰ **S42.454 Nondisplaced fracture of lateral condyle of right humerus** ℚ

√7ᵗʰ **S42.455 Nondisplaced fracture of lateral condyle of left humerus** ℚ

√7ᵗʰ **S42.456 Nondisplaced fracture of lateral condyle of unspecified humerus** ℚ ▽

√6ᵗʰ **S42.46 Fracture of medial condyle of humerus**

Trochlea fracture of humerus

√7ᵗʰ **S42.461 Displaced fracture of medial condyle of right humerus** ℚ

√7ᵗʰ **S42.462 Displaced fracture of medial condyle of left humerus** ℚ

√7ᵗʰ **S42.463 Displaced fracture of medial condyle of unspecified humerus** ℚ ▽

√7ᵗʰ **S42.464 Nondisplaced fracture of medial condyle of right humerus** ℚ

√7ᵗʰ **S42.465 Nondisplaced fracture of medial condyle of left humerus** ℚ

√7ᵗʰ **S42.466 Nondisplaced fracture of medial condyle of unspecified humerus** ℚ ▽

√6ᵗʰ **S42.47 Transcondylar fracture of humerus**

√7ᵗʰ **S42.471 Displaced transcondylar fracture of right humerus** ℚ

√7ᵗʰ **S42.472 Displaced transcondylar fracture of left humerus** ℚ

√7ᵗʰ **S42.473 Displaced transcondylar fracture of unspecified humerus** ℚ ▽

√7ᵗʰ **S42.474 Nondisplaced transcondylar fracture of right humerus** ℚ

√7ᵗʰ **S42.475** **Nondisplaced** transcondylar fracture of **left** humerus   0

√7ᵗʰ **S42.476** **Nondisplaced** transcondylar fracture of unspecified humerus   0 ▽

√6ᵗʰ **S42.48** **Torus** fracture of lower end of humerus

> The appropriate 7th character is to be added to all codes in subcategory S42.48.
> A   initial encounter for closed fracture
> D   subsequent encounter for fracture with routine healing
> G   subsequent encounter for fracture with delayed healing
> K   subsequent encounter for fracture with nonunion
> P   subsequent encounter for fracture with malunion
> S   sequela

√7ᵗʰ **S42.481** **Torus** fracture of lower end of **right** humerus   0

√7ᵗʰ **S42.482** **Torus** fracture of lower end of **left** humerus   0

√7ᵗʰ **S42.489** **Torus** fracture of lower end of unspecified humerus   0 ▽

√6ᵗʰ **S42.49** **Other** fracture of lower end of humerus

√7ᵗʰ **S42.491** **Other displaced** fracture of lower end of **right** humerus   0

√7ᵗʰ **S42.492** **Other displaced** fracture of lower end of **left** humerus   0

√7ᵗʰ **S42.493** **Other displaced** fracture of lower end of unspecified humerus   0 ▽

√7ᵗʰ **S42.494** **Other nondisplaced** fracture of lower end of **right** humerus   0

√7ᵗʰ **S42.495** **Other nondisplaced** fracture of lower end of **left** humerus   0

√7ᵗʰ **S42.496** **Other nondisplaced** fracture of lower end of unspecified humerus   0 ▽

√5ᵗʰ **S42.9** **Fracture of shoulder girdle, part unspecified**

Fracture of shoulder NOS

√x7ᵗʰ **S42.90** **Fracture of unspecified shoulder girdle, part unspecified**   0 ▽

√x7ᵗʰ **S42.91** **Fracture of right shoulder girdle, part unspecified**   0 ▽

√x7ᵗʰ **S42.92** **Fracture of left shoulder girdle, part unspecified**   0 ▽

√4ᵗʰ **S43** **Dislocation and sprain of joints and ligaments of shoulder girdle**

INCLUDES   avulsion of joint or ligament of shoulder girdle
laceration of cartilage, joint or ligament of shoulder girdle
sprain of cartilage, joint or ligament of shoulder girdle
traumatic hemarthrosis of joint or ligament of shoulder girdle
traumatic rupture of joint or ligament of shoulder girdle
traumatic subluxation of joint or ligament of shoulder girdle
traumatic tear of joint or ligament of shoulder girdle

Code also any associated open wound

EXCLUDES 2   *strain of muscle, fascia and tendon of shoulder and upper arm (S46.-)*

> The appropriate 7th character is to be added to each code from category S43.
> A   initial encounter
> D   subsequent encounter
> S   sequela

√5ᵗʰ **S43.0** **Subluxation and dislocation of shoulder joint**

Dislocation of glenohumeral joint
Subluxation of glenohumeral joint

√6ᵗʰ **S43.00** **Unspecified subluxation and dislocation of shoulder joint**

Dislocation of humerus NOS
Subluxation of humerus NOS

√7ᵗʰ **S43.001** **Unspecified subluxation of right shoulder joint**   ▽

√7ᵗʰ **S43.002** **Unspecified subluxation of left shoulder joint**   ▽

√7ᵗʰ **S43.003** **Unspecified subluxation of unspecified shoulder joint**   ▽

√7ᵗʰ **S43.004** **Unspecified dislocation of right shoulder joint**   ▽

√7ᵗʰ **S43.005** **Unspecified dislocation of left shoulder joint**   ▽

√7ᵗʰ **S43.006** **Unspecified dislocation of unspecified shoulder joint**   ▽

√6ᵗʰ **S43.01** **Anterior subluxation and dislocation of humerus**

√7ᵗʰ **S43.011** **Anterior subluxation of right humerus**

√7ᵗʰ **S43.012** **Anterior subluxation of left humerus**

√7ᵗʰ **S43.013** **Anterior subluxation of unspecified humerus**   ▽

√7ᵗʰ **S43.014** **Anterior dislocation of right humerus**

√7ᵗʰ **S43.015** **Anterior dislocation of left humerus**

√7ᵗʰ **S43.016** **Anterior dislocation of unspecified humerus**   ▽

√6ᵗʰ **S43.02** **Posterior subluxation and dislocation of humerus**

√7ᵗʰ **S43.021** **Posterior subluxation of right humerus**

√7ᵗʰ **S43.022** **Posterior subluxation of left humerus**

√7ᵗʰ **S43.023** **Posterior subluxation of unspecified humerus**   ▽

√7ᵗʰ **S43.024** **Posterior dislocation of right humerus**

√7ᵗʰ **S43.025** **Posterior dislocation of left humerus**

√7ᵗʰ **S43.026** **Posterior dislocation of unspecified humerus**   ▽

√6ᵗʰ **S43.03** **Inferior subluxation and dislocation of humerus**

√7ᵗʰ **S43.031** **Inferior subluxation of right humerus**

√7ᵗʰ **S43.032** **Inferior subluxation of left humerus**

√7ᵗʰ **S43.033** **Inferior subluxation of unspecified humerus**   ▽

√7ᵗʰ **S43.034** **Inferior dislocation of right humerus**

√7ᵗʰ **S43.035** **Inferior dislocation of left humerus**

√7ᵗʰ **S43.036** **Inferior dislocation of unspecified humerus**   ▽

√6ᵗʰ **S43.08** **Other subluxation and dislocation of shoulder joint**

√7ᵗʰ **S43.081** **Other subluxation of right shoulder joint**

√7ᵗʰ **S43.082** **Other subluxation of left shoulder joint**

√7ᵗʰ **S43.083** **Other subluxation of unspecified shoulder joint**   ▽

√7ᵗʰ **S43.084** **Other dislocation of right shoulder joint**

√7ᵗʰ **S43.085** **Other dislocation of left shoulder joint**

√7ᵗʰ **S43.086** **Other dislocation of unspecified shoulder joint**   ▽

√5ᵗʰ **S43.1** **Subluxation and dislocation of acromioclavicular joint**

√6ᵗʰ **S43.10** **Unspecified dislocation of acromioclavicular joint**

√7ᵗʰ **S43.101** **Unspecified dislocation of right acromioclavicular joint**   ▽

√7ᵗʰ **S43.102** **Unspecified dislocation of left acromioclavicular joint**   ▽

√7ᵗʰ **S43.109** **Unspecified dislocation of unspecified acromioclavicular joint**   ▽

√6ᵗʰ **S43.11** **Subluxation of acromioclavicular joint**

√7ᵗʰ **S43.111** **Subluxation of right acromioclavicular joint**

√7ᵗʰ **S43.112** **Subluxation of left acromioclavicular joint**

√7ᵗʰ **S43.119** **Subluxation of unspecified acromioclavicular joint**   ▽

√6ᵗʰ **S43.12** **Dislocation of acromioclavicular joint, 100%-200% displacement**

√7ᵗʰ **S43.121** **Dislocation of right acromioclavicular joint, 100%-200% displacement**

√7ᵗʰ **S43.122** **Dislocation of left acromioclavicular joint, 100%-200% displacement**

√7ᵗʰ **S43.129** **Dislocation of unspecified acromioclavicular joint, 100%-200% displacement**   ▽

√6ᵗʰ **S43.13** **Dislocation of acromioclavicular joint, greater than 200% displacement**

√7ᵗʰ **S43.131** **Dislocation of right acromioclavicular joint, greater than 200% displacement**

√7ᵗʰ **S43.132** **Dislocation of left acromioclavicular joint, greater than 200% displacement**

√7ᵗʰ **S43.139** **Dislocation of unspecified acromioclavicular joint, greater than 200% displacement**   ▽

√6ᵗʰ **S43.14** **Inferior dislocation of acromioclavicular joint**

√7ᵗʰ **S43.141** **Inferior dislocation of right acromioclavicular joint**

√7ᵗʰ **S43.142** **Inferior dislocation of left acromioclavicular joint**

✓ Additional Character Req   √x7ᵗʰ Placeholder Alert   Manifestation   ▽ Unspecified   ▶◀ Revised Text   ● New Code   ▲ Revised Code Title

ICD-10-CM 2019   995

√7ᵗʰ **S43.149** Inferior dislocation of unspecified acromioclavicular joint ▽

√6ᵗʰ **S43.15** Posterior dislocation of acromioclavicular joint

√7ᵗʰ **S43.151** Posterior dislocation of right acromioclavicular joint

√7ᵗʰ **S43.152** Posterior dislocation of left acromioclavicular joint

√7ᵗʰ **S43.159** Posterior dislocation of unspecified acromioclavicular joint ▽

√5ᵗʰ **S43.2** Subluxation and dislocation of sternoclavicular joint

√6ᵗʰ **S43.20** Unspecified subluxation and dislocation of sternoclavicular joint

√7ᵗʰ **S43.201** Unspecified subluxation of right sternoclavicular joint ▽

√7ᵗʰ **S43.202** Unspecified subluxation of left sternoclavicular joint ▽

√7ᵗʰ **S43.203** Unspecified subluxation of unspecified sternoclavicular joint ▽

√7ᵗʰ **S43.204** Unspecified dislocation of right sternoclavicular joint ▽

√7ᵗʰ **S43.205** Unspecified dislocation of left sternoclavicular joint ▽

√7ᵗʰ **S43.206** Unspecified dislocation of unspecified sternoclavicular joint ▽

√6ᵗʰ **S43.21** Anterior subluxation and dislocation of sternoclavicular joint

√7ᵗʰ **S43.211** Anterior subluxation of right sternoclavicular joint

√7ᵗʰ **S43.212** Anterior subluxation of left sternoclavicular joint

√7ᵗʰ **S43.213** Anterior subluxation of unspecified sternoclavicular joint ▽

√7ᵗʰ **S43.214** Anterior dislocation of right sternoclavicular joint

√7ᵗʰ **S43.215** Anterior dislocation of left sternoclavicular joint

√7ᵗʰ **S43.216** Anterior dislocation of unspecified sternoclavicular joint ▽

√6ᵗʰ **S43.22** Posterior subluxation and dislocation of sternoclavicular joint

√7ᵗʰ **S43.221** Posterior subluxation of right sternoclavicular joint

√7ᵗʰ **S43.222** Posterior subluxation of left sternoclavicular joint

√7ᵗʰ **S43.223** Posterior subluxation of unspecified sternoclavicular joint ▽

√7ᵗʰ **S43.224** Posterior dislocation of right sternoclavicular joint

√7ᵗʰ **S43.225** Posterior dislocation of left sternoclavicular joint

√7ᵗʰ **S43.226** Posterior dislocation of unspecified sternoclavicular joint ▽

√5ᵗʰ **S43.3** Subluxation and dislocation of other and unspecified parts of shoulder girdle

√6ᵗʰ **S43.30** Subluxation and dislocation of unspecified parts of shoulder girdle

Dislocation of shoulder girdle NOS
Subluxation of shoulder girdle NOS

√7ᵗʰ **S43.301** Subluxation of unspecified parts of right shoulder girdle ▽

√7ᵗʰ **S43.302** Subluxation of unspecified parts of left shoulder girdle ▽

√7ᵗʰ **S43.303** Subluxation of unspecified parts of unspecified shoulder girdle ▽

√7ᵗʰ **S43.304** Dislocation of unspecified parts of right shoulder girdle ▽

√7ᵗʰ **S43.305** Dislocation of unspecified parts of left shoulder girdle ▽

√7ᵗʰ **S43.306** Dislocation of unspecified parts of unspecified shoulder girdle ▽

√6ᵗʰ **S43.31** Subluxation and dislocation of scapula

√7ᵗʰ **S43.311** Subluxation of right scapula

√7ᵗʰ **S43.312** Subluxation of left scapula

√7ᵗʰ **S43.313** Subluxation of unspecified scapula ▽

√7ᵗʰ **S43.314** Dislocation of right scapula

√7ᵗʰ **S43.315** Dislocation of left scapula

√7ᵗʰ **S43.316** Dislocation of unspecified scapula ▽

√6ᵗʰ **S43.39** Subluxation and dislocation of other parts of shoulder girdle

√7ᵗʰ **S43.391** Subluxation of other parts of right shoulder girdle

√7ᵗʰ **S43.392** Subluxation of other parts of left shoulder girdle

√7ᵗʰ **S43.393** Subluxation of other parts of unspecified shoulder girdle ▽

√7ᵗʰ **S43.394** Dislocation of other parts of right shoulder girdle

√7ᵗʰ **S43.395** Dislocation of other parts of left shoulder girdle

√7ᵗʰ **S43.396** Dislocation of other parts of unspecified shoulder girdle ▽

√5ᵗʰ **S43.4** Sprain of shoulder joint

√6ᵗʰ **S43.40** Unspecified sprain of shoulder joint

√7ᵗʰ **S43.401** Unspecified sprain of right shoulder joint ▽

√7ᵗʰ **S43.402** Unspecified sprain of left shoulder joint ▽

√7ᵗʰ **S43.409** Unspecified sprain of unspecified shoulder joint ▽

√6ᵗʰ **S43.41** Sprain of coracohumeral (ligament)

√7ᵗʰ **S43.411** Sprain of right coracohumeral (ligament)

√7ᵗʰ **S43.412** Sprain of left coracohumeral (ligament)

√7ᵗʰ **S43.419** Sprain of unspecified coracohumeral (ligament) ▽

√6ᵗʰ **S43.42** Sprain of rotator cuff capsule

EXCLUDES 1   rotator cuff syndrome (complete) (incomplete), not specified as traumatic (M75.1-)

EXCLUDES 2   injury of tendon of rotator cuff (S46.0-)

√7ᵗʰ **S43.421** Sprain of right rotator cuff capsule

√7ᵗʰ **S43.422** Sprain of left rotator cuff capsule

√7ᵗʰ **S43.429** Sprain of unspecified rotator cuff capsule ▽

√6ᵗʰ **S43.43** Superior glenoid labrum lesion

SLAP lesion
DEF: Detachment injury of the superior aspect of the glenoid labrum, which is the ring of fibrocartilage attached to the rim of the glenoid cavity of the scapula.

√7ᵗʰ **S43.431** Superior glenoid labrum lesion of right shoulder

√7ᵗʰ **S43.432** Superior glenoid labrum lesion of left shoulder

√7ᵗʰ **S43.439** Superior glenoid labrum lesion of unspecified shoulder ▽

√6ᵗʰ **S43.49** Other sprain of shoulder joint

√7ᵗʰ **S43.491** Other sprain of right shoulder joint

√7ᵗʰ **S43.492** Other sprain of left shoulder joint

√7ᵗʰ **S43.499** Other sprain of unspecified shoulder joint ▽

√5ᵗʰ **S43.5** Sprain of acromioclavicular joint

Sprain of acromioclavicular ligament

√x7ᵗʰ **S43.50** Sprain of unspecified acromioclavicular joint ▽

√x7ᵗʰ **S43.51** Sprain of right acromioclavicular joint

√x7ᵗʰ **S43.52** Sprain of left acromioclavicular joint

√5ᵗʰ **S43.6** Sprain of sternoclavicular joint

√x7ᵗʰ **S43.60** Sprain of unspecified sternoclavicular joint ▽

√x7ᵗʰ **S43.61** Sprain of right sternoclavicular joint

√x7ᵗʰ **S43.62** Sprain of left sternoclavicular joint

√5ᵗʰ **S43.8** Sprain of other specified parts of shoulder girdle

√x7ᵗʰ **S43.80** Sprain of other specified parts of unspecified shoulder girdle ▽

√x7ᵗʰ **S43.81** Sprain of other specified parts of right shoulder girdle

√x7ᵗʰ **S43.82** Sprain of other specified parts of left shoulder girdle

√5ᵗʰ **S43.9** Sprain of unspecified parts of shoulder girdle

√x7ᵗʰ **S43.90** Sprain of unspecified parts of unspecified shoulder girdle ▽

Sprain of shoulder girdle NOS

√x7ᵗʰ **S43.91** Sprain of unspecified parts of right shoulder girdle ▽

√x7ᵗʰ **S43.92** Sprain of unspecified parts of left shoulder girdle ▽

✓4th **S44 Injury of nerves at shoulder and upper arm level**

Code also any associated open wound (S41.-)

EXCLUDES 2   *injury of brachial plexus (S14.3-)*

> The appropriate 7th character is to be added to each code from category S44.
> A   initial encounter
> D   subsequent encounter
> S   sequela

✓5th **S44.0 Injury of ulnar nerve at upper arm level**

     EXCLUDES 1   *ulnar nerve NOS (S54.0)*

     ✓x7th **S44.00 Injury of ulnar nerve at upper arm level, unspecified arm** ▽

     ✓x7th **S44.01 Injury of ulnar nerve at upper arm level, right arm**

     ✓x7th **S44.02 Injury of ulnar nerve at upper arm level, left arm**

✓5th **S44.1 Injury of median nerve at upper arm level**

     EXCLUDES 1   *median nerve NOS (S54.1)*

     ✓x7th **S44.10 Injury of median nerve at upper arm level, unspecified arm** ▽

     ✓x7th **S44.11 Injury of median nerve at upper arm level, right arm**

     ✓x7th **S44.12 Injury of median nerve at upper arm level, left arm**

✓5th **S44.2 Injury of radial nerve at upper arm level**

     EXCLUDES 1   *radial nerve NOS (S54.2)*

     ✓x7th **S44.20 Injury of radial nerve at upper arm level, unspecified arm** ▽

     ✓x7th **S44.21 Injury of radial nerve at upper arm level, right arm**

     ✓x7th **S44.22 Injury of radial nerve at upper arm level, left arm**

✓5th **S44.3 Injury of axillary nerve**

     ✓x7th **S44.30 Injury of axillary nerve, unspecified arm** ▽

     ✓x7th **S44.31 Injury of axillary nerve, right arm**

     ✓x7th **S44.32 Injury of axillary nerve, left arm**

✓5th **S44.4 Injury of musculocutaneous nerve**

     ✓x7th **S44.40 Injury of musculocutaneous nerve, unspecified arm** ▽

     ✓x7th **S44.41 Injury of musculocutaneous nerve, right arm**

     ✓x7th **S44.42 Injury of musculocutaneous nerve, left arm**

✓5th **S44.5 Injury of cutaneous sensory nerve at shoulder and upper arm level**

     ✓x7th **S44.50 Injury of cutaneous sensory nerve at shoulder and upper arm level, unspecified arm** ▽

     ✓x7th **S44.51 Injury of cutaneous sensory nerve at shoulder and upper arm level, right arm**

     ✓x7th **S44.52 Injury of cutaneous sensory nerve at shoulder and upper arm level, left arm**

✓5th **S44.8 Injury of other nerves at shoulder and upper arm level**

     ✓6th **S44.8X Injury of other nerves at shoulder and upper arm level**

       ✓7th **S44.8X1 Injury of other nerves at shoulder and upper arm level, right arm**

       ✓7th **S44.8X2 Injury of other nerves at shoulder and upper arm level, left arm**

       ✓7th **S44.8X9 Injury of other nerves at shoulder and upper arm level, unspecified arm** ▽

✓5th **S44.9 Injury of unspecified nerve at shoulder and upper arm level**

     ✓x7th **S44.90 Injury of unspecified nerve at shoulder and upper arm level, unspecified arm** ▽

     ✓x7th **S44.91 Injury of unspecified nerve at shoulder and upper arm level, right arm** ▽

     ✓x7th **S44.92 Injury of unspecified nerve at shoulder and upper arm level, left arm** ▽

✓4th **S45 Injury of blood vessels at shoulder and upper arm level**

Code also any associated open wound (S41.-)

EXCLUDES 2   *injury of subclavian artery (S25.1)*
              injury of subclavian vein (S25.3)

> The appropriate 7th character is to be added to each code from category S45.
> A   initial encounter
> D   subsequent encounter
> S   sequela

✓5th **S45.0 Injury of axillary artery**

     ✓6th **S45.00 Unspecified injury of axillary artery**

       ✓7th **S45.001 Unspecified injury of axillary artery, right side** ▽

       ✓7th **S45.002 Unspecified injury of axillary artery, left side** ▽

       ✓7th **S45.009 Unspecified injury of axillary artery, unspecified side** ▽

     ✓6th **S45.01 Laceration of axillary artery**

       ✓7th **S45.011 Laceration of axillary artery, right side**

       ✓7th **S45.012 Laceration of axillary artery, left side**

       ✓7th **S45.019 Laceration of axillary artery, unspecified side** ▽

     ✓6th **S45.09 Other specified injury of axillary artery**

       ✓7th **S45.091 Other specified injury of axillary artery, right side**

       ✓7th **S45.092 Other specified injury of axillary artery, left side**

       ✓7th **S45.099 Other specified injury of axillary artery, unspecified side** ▽

✓5th **S45.1 Injury of brachial artery**

     ✓6th **S45.10 Unspecified injury of brachial artery**

       ✓7th **S45.101 Unspecified injury of brachial artery, right side** ▽

       ✓7th **S45.102 Unspecified injury of brachial artery, left side** ▽

       ✓7th **S45.109 Unspecified injury of brachial artery, unspecified side** ▽

     ✓6th **S45.11 Laceration of brachial artery**

       ✓7th **S45.111 Laceration of brachial artery, right side**

       ✓7th **S45.112 Laceration of brachial artery, left side**

       ✓7th **S45.119 Laceration of brachial artery, unspecified side** ▽

     ✓6th **S45.19 Other specified injury of brachial artery**

       ✓7th **S45.191 Other specified injury of brachial artery, right side**

       ✓7th **S45.192 Other specified injury of brachial artery, left side**

       ✓7th **S45.199 Other specified injury of brachial artery, unspecified side** ▽

✓5th **S45.2 Injury of axillary or brachial vein**

     ✓6th **S45.20 Unspecified injury of axillary or brachial vein**

       ✓7th **S45.201 Unspecified injury of axillary or brachial vein, right side** ▽

       ✓7th **S45.202 Unspecified injury of axillary or brachial vein, left side** ▽

       ✓7th **S45.209 Unspecified injury of axillary or brachial vein, unspecified side** ▽

     ✓6th **S45.21 Laceration of axillary or brachial vein**

       ✓7th **S45.211 Laceration of axillary or brachial vein, right side**

       ✓7th **S45.212 Laceration of axillary or brachial vein, left side**

       ✓7th **S45.219 Laceration of axillary or brachial vein, unspecified side** ▽

     ✓6th **S45.29 Other specified injury of axillary or brachial vein**

       ✓7th **S45.291 Other specified injury of axillary or brachial vein, right side**

       ✓7th **S45.292 Other specified injury of axillary or brachial vein, left side**

       ✓7th **S45.299 Other specified injury of axillary or brachial vein, unspecified side** ▽

✓5th **S45.3 Injury of superficial vein at shoulder and upper arm level**

     ✓6th **S45.30 Unspecified injury of superficial vein at shoulder and upper arm level**

       ✓7th **S45.301 Unspecified injury of superficial vein at shoulder and upper arm level, right arm** ▽

✓ Additional Character Req   ✓x7th Placeholder Alert   Manifestation   ▽ Unspecified   ►◄ Revised Text   ● New Code   ▲ Revised Code Title

√7ᵗʰ **S45.302** Unspecified injury of superficial vein at shoulder and upper arm level, **left** ▽

√7ᵗʰ **S45.309** Unspecified injury of superficial vein at shoulder and upper arm level, unspecified arm ▽

√6ᵗʰ **S45.31** Laceration of superficial vein at shoulder and upper arm level

√7ᵗʰ **S45.311** Laceration of superficial vein at shoulder and upper arm level, **right** arm

√7ᵗʰ **S45.312** Laceration of superficial vein at shoulder and upper arm level, **left** arm

√7ᵗʰ **S45.319** Laceration of superficial vein at shoulder and upper arm level, unspecified arm ▽

√6ᵗʰ **S45.39** Other specified injury of superficial vein at shoulder and upper arm level

√7ᵗʰ **S45.391** Other specified injury of superficial vein at shoulder and upper arm level, **right** arm

√7ᵗʰ **S45.392** Other specified injury of superficial vein at shoulder and upper arm level, **left** arm

√7ᵗʰ **S45.399** Other specified injury of superficial vein at shoulder and upper arm level, unspecified arm ▽

√5ᵗʰ **S45.8** Injury of other specified blood vessels at shoulder and upper arm level

√6ᵗʰ **S45.80** Unspecified injury of other specified blood vessels at shoulder and upper arm level

√7ᵗʰ **S45.801** Unspecified injury of other specified blood vessels at shoulder and upper arm level, **right** arm ▽

√7ᵗʰ **S45.802** Unspecified injury of other specified blood vessels at shoulder and upper arm level, **left** arm ▽

√7ᵗʰ **S45.809** Unspecified injury of other specified blood vessels at shoulder and upper arm level, unspecified arm ▽

√6ᵗʰ **S45.81** Laceration of other specified blood vessels at shoulder and upper arm level

√7ᵗʰ **S45.811** Laceration of other specified blood vessels at shoulder and upper arm level, **right** arm

√7ᵗʰ **S45.812** Laceration of other specified blood vessels at shoulder and upper arm level, **left** arm

√7ᵗʰ **S45.819** Laceration of other specified blood vessels at shoulder and upper arm level, unspecified arm ▽

√6ᵗʰ **S45.89** Other specified injury of other specified blood vessels at shoulder and upper arm level

√7ᵗʰ **S45.891** Other specified injury of other specified blood vessels at shoulder and upper arm level, **right** arm

√7ᵗʰ **S45.892** Other specified injury of other specified blood vessels at shoulder and upper arm level, **left** arm

√7ᵗʰ **S45.899** Other specified injury of other specified blood vessels at shoulder and upper arm level, unspecified arm ▽

√5ᵗʰ **S45.9** Injury of unspecified blood vessel at shoulder and upper arm level

√6ᵗʰ **S45.90** Unspecified injury of unspecified blood vessel at shoulder and upper arm level

√7ᵗʰ **S45.901** Unspecified injury of unspecified blood vessel at shoulder and upper arm level, **right** arm ▽

√7ᵗʰ **S45.902** Unspecified injury of unspecified blood vessel at shoulder and upper arm level, **left** arm ▽

√7ᵗʰ **S45.909** Unspecified injury of unspecified blood vessel at shoulder and upper arm level, unspecified arm ▽

√6ᵗʰ **S45.91** Laceration of unspecified blood vessel at shoulder and upper arm level

√7ᵗʰ **S45.911** Laceration of unspecified blood vessel at shoulder and upper arm level, **right** arm ▽

√7ᵗʰ **S45.912** Laceration of unspecified blood vessel at shoulder and upper arm level, **left** arm ▽

√7ᵗʰ **S45.919** Laceration of unspecified blood vessel at shoulder and upper arm level, unspecified arm ▽

√6ᵗʰ **S45.99** Other specified injury of unspecified blood vessel at shoulder and upper arm level

√7ᵗʰ **S45.991** Other specified injury of unspecified blood vessel at shoulder and upper arm level, **right** arm ▽

√7ᵗʰ **S45.992** Other specified injury of unspecified blood vessel at shoulder and upper arm level, **left** arm ▽

√7ᵗʰ **S45.999** Other specified injury of unspecified blood vessel at shoulder and upper arm level, unspecified arm ▽

√4ᵗʰ **S46** Injury of muscle, fascia and tendon at shoulder and upper arm level

Code also any associated open wound (S41.-)

EXCLUDES 2   injury of muscle, fascia and tendon at elbow (S56.-)
              sprain of joints and ligaments of shoulder girdle (S43.9)

TIP: Refer to the Muscle/Tendon table at the beginning of this chapter.

The appropriate 7th character is to be added to each code from category S46.
A   initial encounter
D   subsequent encounter
S   sequela

√5ᵗʰ **S46.0** Injury of muscle(s) and tendon(s) of the rotator cuff of shoulder

√6ᵗʰ **S46.00** Unspecified injury of muscle(s) and tendon(s) of the rotator cuff of shoulder

√7ᵗʰ **S46.001** Unspecified injury of muscle(s) and tendon(s) of the rotator cuff of **right** shoulder ▽

√7ᵗʰ **S46.002** Unspecified injury of muscle(s) and tendon(s) of the rotator cuff of **left** shoulder ▽

√7ᵗʰ **S46.009** Unspecified injury of muscle(s) and tendon(s) of the rotator cuff of unspecified shoulder ▽

√6ᵗʰ **S46.01** Strain of muscle(s) and tendon(s) of the rotator cuff of shoulder

√7ᵗʰ **S46.011** Strain of muscle(s) and tendon(s) of the rotator cuff of **right** shoulder

√7ᵗʰ **S46.012** Strain of muscle(s) and tendon(s) of the rotator cuff of **left** shoulder

√7ᵗʰ **S46.019** Strain of muscle(s) and tendon(s) of the rotator cuff of unspecified shoulder ▽

√6ᵗʰ **S46.02** Laceration of muscle(s) and tendon(s) of the rotator cuff of shoulder

√7ᵗʰ **S46.021** Laceration of muscle(s) and tendon(s) of the rotator cuff of **right** shoulder

√7ᵗʰ **S46.022** Laceration of muscle(s) and tendon(s) of the rotator cuff of **left** shoulder

√7ᵗʰ **S46.029** Laceration of muscle(s) and tendon(s) of the rotator cuff of unspecified shoulder ▽

√6ᵗʰ **S46.09** Other injury of muscle(s) and tendon(s) of the rotator cuff of shoulder

√7ᵗʰ **S46.091** Other injury of muscle(s) and tendon(s) of the rotator cuff of **right** shoulder

√7ᵗʰ **S46.092** Other injury of muscle(s) and tendon(s) of the rotator cuff of **left** shoulder

√7ᵗʰ **S46.099** Other injury of muscle(s) and tendon(s) of the rotator cuff of unspecified shoulder ▽

√5ᵗʰ **S46.1** Injury of muscle, fascia and tendon of long head of biceps

√6ᵗʰ **S46.10** Unspecified injury of muscle, fascia and tendon of long head of biceps

√7ᵗʰ **S46.101** Unspecified injury of muscle, fascia and tendon of long head of biceps, **right** arm ▽

√7ᵗʰ **S46.102** Unspecified injury of muscle, fascia and tendon of long head of biceps, **left** arm ▽

√7ᵗʰ **S46.109** Unspecified injury of muscle, fascia and tendon of long head of biceps, unspecified arm ▽

√6ᵗʰ **S46.11** Strain of muscle, fascia and tendon of long head of biceps

     √7ᵗʰ **S46.111** Strain of muscle, fascia and tendon of long head of biceps, right arm

     √7ᵗʰ **S46.112** Strain of muscle, fascia and tendon of long head of biceps, left arm

     √7ᵗʰ **S46.119** Strain of muscle, fascia and tendon of long head of biceps, unspecified arm ▽

√6ᵗʰ **S46.12** Laceration of muscle, fascia and tendon of long head of biceps

     √7ᵗʰ **S46.121** Laceration of muscle, fascia and tendon of long head of biceps, right arm

     √7ᵗʰ **S46.122** Laceration of muscle, fascia and tendon of long head of biceps, left arm

     √7ᵗʰ **S46.129** Laceration of muscle, fascia and tendon of long head of biceps, unspecified arm ▽

√6ᵗʰ **S46.19** Other injury of muscle, fascia and tendon of long head of biceps

     √7ᵗʰ **S46.191** Other injury of muscle, fascia and tendon of long head of biceps, right arm

     √7ᵗʰ **S46.192** Other injury of muscle, fascia and tendon of long head of biceps, left arm

     √7ᵗʰ **S46.199** Other injury of muscle, fascia and tendon of long head of biceps, unspecified arm ▽

√5ᵗʰ **S46.2** Injury of muscle, fascia and tendon of other parts of biceps

√6ᵗʰ **S46.20** Unspecified injury of muscle, fascia and tendon of other parts of biceps

     √7ᵗʰ **S46.201** Unspecified injury of muscle, fascia and tendon of other parts of biceps, right arm ▽

     √7ᵗʰ **S46.202** Unspecified injury of muscle, fascia and tendon of other parts of biceps, left arm ▽

     √7ᵗʰ **S46.209** Unspecified injury of muscle, fascia and tendon of other parts of biceps, unspecified arm ▽

√6ᵗʰ **S46.21** Strain of muscle, fascia and tendon of other parts of biceps

     √7ᵗʰ **S46.211** Strain of muscle, fascia and tendon of other parts of biceps, right arm

     √7ᵗʰ **S46.212** Strain of muscle, fascia and tendon of other parts of biceps, left arm

     √7ᵗʰ **S46.219** Strain of muscle, fascia and tendon of other parts of biceps, unspecified arm ▽

√6ᵗʰ **S46.22** Laceration of muscle, fascia and tendon of other parts of biceps

     √7ᵗʰ **S46.221** Laceration of muscle, fascia and tendon of other parts of biceps, right arm

     √7ᵗʰ **S46.222** Laceration of muscle, fascia and tendon of other parts of biceps, left arm

     √7ᵗʰ **S46.229** Laceration of muscle, fascia and tendon of other parts of biceps, unspecified arm ▽

√6ᵗʰ **S46.29** Other injury of muscle, fascia and tendon of other parts of biceps

     √7ᵗʰ **S46.291** Other injury of muscle, fascia and tendon of other parts of biceps, right arm

     √7ᵗʰ **S46.292** Other injury of muscle, fascia and tendon of other parts of biceps, left arm

     √7ᵗʰ **S46.299** Other injury of muscle, fascia and tendon of other parts of biceps, unspecified arm ▽

√5ᵗʰ **S46.3** Injury of muscle, fascia and tendon of triceps

√6ᵗʰ **S46.30** Unspecified injury of muscle, fascia and tendon of triceps

     √7ᵗʰ **S46.301** Unspecified injury of muscle, fascia and tendon of triceps, right arm ▽

     √7ᵗʰ **S46.302** Unspecified injury of muscle, fascia and tendon of triceps, left arm ▽

     √7ᵗʰ **S46.309** Unspecified injury of muscle, fascia and tendon of triceps, unspecified arm ▽

√6ᵗʰ **S46.31** Strain of muscle, fascia and tendon of triceps

     √7ᵗʰ **S46.311** Strain of muscle, fascia and tendon of triceps, right arm

     √7ᵗʰ **S46.312** Strain of muscle, fascia and tendon of triceps, left arm

     √7ᵗʰ **S46.319** Strain of muscle, fascia and tendon of triceps, unspecified arm ▽

√6ᵗʰ **S46.32** Laceration of muscle, fascia and tendon of triceps

     √7ᵗʰ **S46.321** Laceration of muscle, fascia and tendon of triceps, right arm

     √7ᵗʰ **S46.322** Laceration of muscle, fascia and tendon of triceps, left arm

     √7ᵗʰ **S46.329** Laceration of muscle, fascia and tendon of triceps, unspecified arm ▽

√6ᵗʰ **S46.39** Other injury of muscle, fascia and tendon of triceps

     √7ᵗʰ **S46.391** Other injury of muscle, fascia and tendon of triceps, right arm

     √7ᵗʰ **S46.392** Other injury of muscle, fascia and tendon of triceps, left arm

     √7ᵗʰ **S46.399** Other injury of muscle, fascia and tendon of triceps, unspecified arm ▽

√5ᵗʰ **S46.8** Injury of other muscles, fascia and tendons at shoulder and upper arm level

√6ᵗʰ **S46.80** Unspecified injury of other muscles, fascia and tendons at shoulder and upper arm level

     √7ᵗʰ **S46.801** Unspecified injury of other muscles, fascia and tendons at shoulder and upper arm level, right arm ▽

     √7ᵗʰ **S46.802** Unspecified injury of other muscles, fascia and tendons at shoulder and upper arm level, left arm ▽

     √7ᵗʰ **S46.809** Unspecified injury of other muscles, fascia and tendons at shoulder and upper arm level, unspecified arm ▽

√6ᵗʰ **S46.81** Strain of other muscles, fascia and tendons at shoulder and upper arm level

     √7ᵗʰ **S46.811** Strain of other muscles, fascia and tendons at shoulder and upper arm level, right arm

     √7ᵗʰ **S46.812** Strain of other muscles, fascia and tendons at shoulder and upper arm level, left arm

     √7ᵗʰ **S46.819** Strain of other muscles, fascia and tendons at shoulder and upper arm level, unspecified arm ▽

√6ᵗʰ **S46.82** Laceration of other muscles, fascia and tendons at shoulder and upper arm level

     √7ᵗʰ **S46.821** Laceration of other muscles, fascia and tendons at shoulder and upper arm level, right arm

     √7ᵗʰ **S46.822** Laceration of other muscles, fascia and tendons at shoulder and upper arm level, left arm

     √7ᵗʰ **S46.829** Laceration of other muscles, fascia and tendons at shoulder and upper arm level, unspecified arm ▽

√6ᵗʰ **S46.89** Other injury of other muscles, fascia and tendons at shoulder and upper arm level

     √7ᵗʰ **S46.891** Other injury of other muscles, fascia and tendons at shoulder and upper arm level, right arm

     √7ᵗʰ **S46.892** Other injury of other muscles, fascia and tendons at shoulder and upper arm level, left arm

     √7ᵗʰ **S46.899** Other injury of other muscles, fascia and tendons at shoulder and upper arm level, unspecified arm ▽

√5ᵗʰ **S46.9** Injury of unspecified muscle, fascia and tendon at shoulder and upper arm level

√6ᵗʰ **S46.90** Unspecified injury of unspecified muscle, fascia and tendon at shoulder and upper arm level

     √7ᵗʰ **S46.901** Unspecified injury of unspecified muscle, fascia and tendon at shoulder and upper arm level, right arm ▽

     √7ᵗʰ **S46.902** Unspecified injury of unspecified muscle, fascia and tendon at shoulder and upper arm level, left arm ▽

☑ Additional Character Req   √ˣ7ᵗʰ Placeholder Alert   Manifestation   ▽ Unspecified   ►◄ Revised Text   ● New Code   ▲ Revised Code Title

√7ᵗʰ **S46.909** Unspecified injury of unspecified muscle, fascia and tendon at shoulder and upper arm level, unspecified arm ▽

√6ᵗʰ **S46.91** Strain of unspecified muscle, fascia and tendon at shoulder and upper arm level

     √7ᵗʰ **S46.911** Strain of unspecified muscle, fascia and tendon at shoulder and upper arm level, right arm ▽

     √7ᵗʰ **S46.912** Strain of unspecified muscle, fascia and tendon at shoulder and upper arm level, left arm ▽

     √7ᵗʰ **S46.919** Strain of unspecified muscle, fascia and tendon at shoulder and upper arm level, unspecified arm ▽

√6ᵗʰ **S46.92** Laceration of unspecified muscle, fascia and tendon at shoulder and upper arm level

     √7ᵗʰ **S46.921** Laceration of unspecified muscle, fascia and tendon at shoulder and upper arm level, right arm ▽

     √7ᵗʰ **S46.922** Laceration of unspecified muscle, fascia and tendon at shoulder and upper arm level, left arm ▽

     √7ᵗʰ **S46.929** Laceration of unspecified muscle, fascia and tendon at shoulder and upper arm level, unspecified arm ▽

√6ᵗʰ **S46.99** Other injury of unspecified muscle, fascia and tendon at shoulder and upper arm level

     √7ᵗʰ **S46.991** Other injury of unspecified muscle, fascia and tendon at shoulder and upper arm level, right arm ▽

     √7ᵗʰ **S46.992** Other injury of unspecified muscle, fascia and tendon at shoulder and upper arm level, left arm ▽

     √7ᵗʰ **S46.999** Other injury of unspecified muscle, fascia and tendon at shoulder and upper arm level, unspecified arm ▽

√4ᵗʰ **S47** **Crushing injury of shoulder and upper arm**

Use additional code for all associated injuries

EXCLUDES 2   crushing injury of elbow (S57.0-)

The appropriate 7th character is to be added to each code from category S47.
A   initial encounter
D   subsequent encounter
S   sequela

√x7ᵗʰ **S47.1** **Crushing injury of right shoulder and upper arm**

√x7ᵗʰ **S47.2** **Crushing injury of left shoulder and upper arm**

√x7ᵗʰ **S47.9** **Crushing injury of shoulder and upper arm, unspecified arm** ▽

√4ᵗʰ **S48** **Traumatic amputation of shoulder and upper arm**

An amputation not identified as partial or complete should be coded to complete

EXCLUDES 1   traumatic amputation at elbow level (S58.0)

The appropriate 7th character is to be added to each code from category S48.
A   initial encounter
D   subsequent encounter
S   sequela

√5ᵗʰ **S48.0** **Traumatic amputation at shoulder joint**

√6ᵗʰ **S48.01** Complete traumatic amputation at shoulder joint

     2 √7ᵗʰ **S48.011** Complete traumatic amputation at right shoulder joint HCC

     2 √7ᵗʰ **S48.012** Complete traumatic amputation at left shoulder joint HCC

     2 √7ᵗʰ **S48.019** Complete traumatic amputation at unspecified shoulder joint HCC ▽

√6ᵗʰ **S48.02** Partial traumatic amputation at shoulder joint

     2 √7ᵗʰ **S48.021** Partial traumatic amputation at right shoulder joint HCC

     2 √7ᵗʰ **S48.022** Partial traumatic amputation at left shoulder joint HCC

     2 √7ᵗʰ **S48.029** Partial traumatic amputation at unspecified shoulder joint HCC ▽

√5ᵗʰ **S48.1** Traumatic amputation at level between shoulder and elbow

√6ᵗʰ **S48.11** Complete traumatic amputation at level between shoulder and elbow

     2 √7ᵗʰ **S48.111** Complete traumatic amputation at level between right shoulder and elbow HCC

     2 √7ᵗʰ **S48.112** Complete traumatic amputation at level between left shoulder and elbow HCC

     2 √7ᵗʰ **S48.119** Complete traumatic amputation at level between unspecified shoulder and elbow HCC ▽

√6ᵗʰ **S48.12** Partial traumatic amputation at level between shoulder and elbow

     2 √7ᵗʰ **S48.121** Partial traumatic amputation at level between right shoulder and elbow HCC

     2 √7ᵗʰ **S48.122** Partial traumatic amputation at level between left shoulder and elbow HCC

     2 √7ᵗʰ **S48.129** Partial traumatic amputation at level between unspecified shoulder and elbow HCC ▽

√5ᵗʰ **S48.9** Traumatic amputation of shoulder and upper arm, level unspecified

√6ᵗʰ **S48.91** Complete traumatic amputation of shoulder and upper arm, level unspecified

     2 √7ᵗʰ **S48.911** Complete traumatic amputation of right shoulder and upper arm, level unspecified HCC ▽

     2 √7ᵗʰ **S48.912** Complete traumatic amputation of left shoulder and upper arm, level unspecified HCC ▽

     2 √7ᵗʰ **S48.919** Complete traumatic amputation of unspecified shoulder and upper arm, level unspecified HCC ▽

√6ᵗʰ **S48.92** Partial traumatic amputation of shoulder and upper arm, level unspecified

     2 √7ᵗʰ **S48.921** Partial traumatic amputation of right shoulder and upper arm, level unspecified HCC ▽

     2 √7ᵗʰ **S48.922** Partial traumatic amputation of left shoulder and upper arm, level unspecified HCC ▽

     2 √7ᵗʰ **S48.929** Partial traumatic amputation of unspecified shoulder and upper arm, level unspecified HCC ▽

√4ᵗʰ **S49** **Other and unspecified injuries of shoulder and upper arm**

AHA: 2018,2Q,12; 2018,1Q,3

The appropriate 7th character is to be added to each code from subcategories S49.0 and S49.1.
A   initial encounter for closed fracture
D   subsequent encounter for fracture with routine healing
G   subsequent encounter for fracture with delayed healing
K   subsequent encounter for fracture with nonunion
P   subsequent encounter for fracture with malunion
S   sequela

√5ᵗʰ **S49.0** Physeal fracture of upper end of humerus

√6ᵗʰ **S49.00** Unspecified physeal fracture of upper end of humerus

     √7ᵗʰ **S49.001** Unspecified physeal fracture of upper end of humerus, right arm Q ▽

     √7ᵗʰ **S49.002** Unspecified physeal fracture of upper end of humerus, left arm Q ▽

     √7ᵗʰ **S49.009** Unspecified physeal fracture of upper end of humerus, unspecified arm Q ▽

√6ᵗʰ **S49.01** Salter-Harris Type I physeal fracture of upper end of humerus

     √7ᵗʰ **S49.011** Salter-Harris Type I physeal fracture of upper end of humerus, right arm Q

     √7ᵗʰ **S49.012** Salter-Harris Type I physeal fracture of upper end of humerus, left arm Q

     √7ᵗʰ **S49.019** Salter-Harris Type I physeal fracture of upper end of humerus, unspecified arm Q ▽

√6ᵗʰ **S49.02** Salter-Harris Type II physeal fracture of upper end of humerus

    √7ᵗʰ **S49.021** Salter-Harris Type II physeal fracture of upper end of humerus, **right arm**   ▢

    √7ᵗʰ **S49.022** Salter-Harris Type II physeal fracture of upper end of humerus, **left arm**   ▢

    √7ᵗʰ **S49.029** Salter-Harris Type II physeal fracture of upper end of humerus, **unspecified arm**   ▢ ▽

√6ᵗʰ **S49.03** Salter-Harris Type III physeal fracture of upper end of humerus

    √7ᵗʰ **S49.031** Salter-Harris Type III physeal fracture of upper end of humerus, **right arm**   ▢

    √7ᵗʰ **S49.032** Salter-Harris Type III physeal fracture of upper end of humerus, **left arm**   ▢

    √7ᵗʰ **S49.039** Salter-Harris Type III physeal fracture of upper end of humerus, **unspecified arm**   ▢ ▽

√6ᵗʰ **S49.04** Salter-Harris Type IV physeal fracture of upper end of humerus

    √7ᵗʰ **S49.041** Salter-Harris Type IV physeal fracture of upper end of humerus, **right arm**   ▢

    √7ᵗʰ **S49.042** Salter-Harris Type IV physeal fracture of upper end of humerus, **left arm**   ▢

    √7ᵗʰ **S49.049** Salter-Harris Type IV physeal fracture of upper end of humerus, **unspecified arm**   ▢ ▽

√6ᵗʰ **S49.09** Other physeal fracture of upper end of humerus

    √7ᵗʰ **S49.091** Other physeal fracture of upper end of humerus, **right arm**   ▢

    √7ᵗʰ **S49.092** Other physeal fracture of upper end of humerus, **left arm**   ▢

    √7ᵗʰ **S49.099** Other physeal fracture of upper end of humerus, **unspecified arm**   ▢ ▽

√5ᵗʰ **S49.1** Physeal fracture of lower end of humerus

√6ᵗʰ **S49.10** Unspecified physeal fracture of lower end of humerus

    √7ᵗʰ **S49.101** Unspecified physeal fracture of lower end of humerus, **right arm**   ▢ ▽

    √7ᵗʰ **S49.102** Unspecified physeal fracture of lower end of humerus, **left arm**   ▢ ▽

    √7ᵗʰ **S49.109** Unspecified physeal fracture of lower end of humerus, **unspecified arm**   ▢ ▽

√6ᵗʰ **S49.11** Salter-Harris Type I physeal fracture of lower end of humerus

    √7ᵗʰ **S49.111** Salter-Harris Type I physeal fracture of lower end of humerus, **right arm**   ▢

    √7ᵗʰ **S49.112** Salter-Harris Type I physeal fracture of lower end of humerus, **left arm**   ▢

    √7ᵗʰ **S49.119** Salter-Harris Type I physeal fracture of lower end of humerus, **unspecified arm**   ▢ ▽

√6ᵗʰ **S49.12** Salter-Harris Type II physeal fracture of lower end of humerus

    √7ᵗʰ **S49.121** Salter-Harris Type II physeal fracture of lower end of humerus, **right arm**   ▢

    √7ᵗʰ **S49.122** Salter-Harris Type II physeal fracture of lower end of humerus, **left arm**   ▢

    √7ᵗʰ **S49.129** Salter-Harris Type II physeal fracture of lower end of humerus, **unspecified arm**   ▢ ▽

√6ᵗʰ **S49.13** Salter-Harris Type III physeal fracture of lower end of humerus

    √7ᵗʰ **S49.131** Salter-Harris Type III physeal fracture of lower end of humerus, **right arm**   ▢

    √7ᵗʰ **S49.132** Salter-Harris Type III physeal fracture of lower end of humerus, **left arm**   ▢

    √7ᵗʰ **S49.139** Salter-Harris Type III physeal fracture of lower end of humerus, **unspecified arm**   ▢ ▽

√6ᵗʰ **S49.14** Salter-Harris Type IV physeal fracture of lower end of humerus

    √7ᵗʰ **S49.141** Salter-Harris Type IV physeal fracture of lower end of humerus, **right arm**   ▢

    √7ᵗʰ **S49.142** Salter-Harris Type IV physeal fracture of lower end of humerus, **left arm**   ▢

    √7ᵗʰ **S49.149** Salter-Harris Type IV physeal fracture of lower end of humerus, **unspecified arm**   ▢ ▽

√6ᵗʰ **S49.19** Other physeal fracture of lower end of humerus

    √7ᵗʰ **S49.191** Other physeal fracture of lower end of humerus, **right arm**   ▢

    √7ᵗʰ **S49.192** Other physeal fracture of lower end of humerus, **left arm**   ▢

    √7ᵗʰ **S49.199** Other physeal fracture of lower end of humerus, **unspecified arm**   ▢ ▽

√5ᵗʰ **S49.8** Other specified injuries of shoulder and upper arm

> The appropriate 7th character is to be added to each code in subcategory S49.8.
> A initial encounter
> D subsequent encounter
> S sequela

  √×7ᵗʰ **S49.80** Other specified injuries of shoulder and upper arm, unspecified arm   ▽

  √×7ᵗʰ **S49.81** Other specified injuries of **right** shoulder and upper arm

  √×7ᵗʰ **S49.82** Other specified injuries of **left** shoulder and upper arm

√5ᵗʰ **S49.9** Unspecified injury of shoulder and upper arm

> The appropriate 7th character is to be added to each code in subcategory S49.9.
> A initial encounter
> D subsequent encounter
> S sequela

  √×7ᵗʰ **S49.90** Unspecified injury of shoulder and upper arm, unspecified arm   ▽

  √×7ᵗʰ **S49.91** Unspecified injury of **right** shoulder and upper arm   ▽

  √×7ᵗʰ **S49.92** Unspecified injury of **left** shoulder and upper arm   ▽

Injuries to the elbow and forearm (S50-S59)

EXCLUDES 2   burns and corrosions (T20-T32)
    frostbite (T33-T34)
    injuries of wrist and hand (S60-S69)
    insect bite or sting, venomous (T63.4)

√4ᵗʰ **S50** Superficial injury of elbow and forearm

  EXCLUDES 2   superficial injury of wrist and hand (S60.-)

> The appropriate 7th character is to be added to each code from category S50.
> A initial encounter
> D subsequent encounter
> S sequela

√5ᵗʰ **S50.0** Contusion of **elbow**

  √×7ᵗʰ **S50.00** Contusion of unspecified elbow   ▽

  √×7ᵗʰ **S50.01** Contusion of **right** elbow

  √×7ᵗʰ **S50.02** Contusion of **left** elbow

√5ᵗʰ **S50.1** Contusion of **forearm**

  √×7ᵗʰ **S50.10** Contusion of unspecified forearm   ▽

  √×7ᵗʰ **S50.11** Contusion of **right** forearm

  √×7ᵗʰ **S50.12** Contusion of **left** forearm

√5ᵗʰ **S50.3** Other superficial injuries of **elbow**

  √6ᵗʰ **S50.31** Abrasion of elbow

    √7ᵗʰ **S50.311** Abrasion of **right** elbow

    √7ᵗʰ **S50.312** Abrasion of **left** elbow

    √7ᵗʰ **S50.319** Abrasion of unspecified elbow   ▽

  √6ᵗʰ **S50.32** Blister (nonthermal) of elbow

    √7ᵗʰ **S50.321** Blister (nonthermal) of **right** elbow

    √7ᵗʰ **S50.322** Blister (nonthermal) of **left** elbow

    √7ᵗʰ **S50.329** Blister (nonthermal) of unspecified elbow   ▽

√6ᵗʰ **S50.34** External constriction of elbow
- √7ᵗʰ **S50.341** External constriction of right elbow
- √7ᵗʰ **S50.342** External constriction of left elbow
- √7ᵗʰ **S50.349** External constriction of unspecified elbow ▽

√6ᵗʰ **S50.35** Superficial foreign body of elbow
Splinter in the elbow
- √7ᵗʰ **S50.351** Superficial foreign body of right elbow
- √7ᵗʰ **S50.352** Superficial foreign body of left elbow
- √7ᵗʰ **S50.359** Superficial foreign body of unspecified elbow ▽

√6ᵗʰ **S50.36** Insect bite (nonvenomous) of elbow
- √7ᵗʰ **S50.361** Insect bite (nonvenomous) of right elbow
- √7ᵗʰ **S50.362** Insect bite (nonvenomous) of left elbow
- √7ᵗʰ **S50.369** Insect bite (nonvenomous) of unspecified elbow ▽

√6ᵗʰ **S50.37** Other superficial bite of elbow
EXCLUDES 1   open bite of elbow (S51.05)
- √7ᵗʰ **S50.371** Other superficial bite of right elbow
- √7ᵗʰ **S50.372** Other superficial bite of left elbow
- √7ᵗʰ **S50.379** Other superficial bite of unspecified elbow ▽

√5ᵗʰ **S50.8** Other superficial injuries of forearm

√6ᵗʰ **S50.81** Abrasion of forearm
- √7ᵗʰ **S50.811** Abrasion of right forearm
- √7ᵗʰ **S50.812** Abrasion of left forearm
- √7ᵗʰ **S50.819** Abrasion of unspecified forearm ▽

√6ᵗʰ **S50.82** Blister (nonthermal) of forearm
- √7ᵗʰ **S50.821** Blister (nonthermal) of right forearm
- √7ᵗʰ **S50.822** Blister (nonthermal) of left forearm
- √7ᵗʰ **S50.829** Blister (nonthermal) of unspecified forearm ▽

√6ᵗʰ **S50.84** External constriction of forearm
- √7ᵗʰ **S50.841** External constriction of right forearm
- √7ᵗʰ **S50.842** External constriction of left forearm
- √7ᵗʰ **S50.849** External constriction of unspecified forearm ▽

√6ᵗʰ **S50.85** Superficial foreign body of forearm
Splinter in the forearm
- √7ᵗʰ **S50.851** Superficial foreign body of right forearm
- √7ᵗʰ **S50.852** Superficial foreign body of left forearm
- √7ᵗʰ **S50.859** Superficial foreign body of unspecified forearm ▽

√6ᵗʰ **S50.86** Insect bite (nonvenomous) of forearm
- √7ᵗʰ **S50.861** Insect bite (nonvenomous) of right forearm
- √7ᵗʰ **S50.862** Insect bite (nonvenomous) of left forearm
- √7ᵗʰ **S50.869** Insect bite (nonvenomous) of unspecified forearm ▽

√6ᵗʰ **S50.87** Other superficial bite of forearm
EXCLUDES 1   open bite of forearm (S51.85)
- √7ᵗʰ **S50.871** Other superficial bite of right forearm
- √7ᵗʰ **S50.872** Other superficial bite of left forearm
- √7ᵗʰ **S50.879** Other superficial bite of unspecified forearm ▽

√5ᵗʰ **S50.9** Unspecified superficial injury of elbow and forearm

√6ᵗʰ **S50.90** Unspecified superficial injury of elbow
- √7ᵗʰ **S50.901** Unspecified superficial injury of right elbow ▽
- √7ᵗʰ **S50.902** Unspecified superficial injury of left elbow ▽
- √7ᵗʰ **S50.909** Unspecified superficial injury of unspecified elbow ▽

√6ᵗʰ **S50.91** Unspecified superficial injury of forearm
- √7ᵗʰ **S50.911** Unspecified superficial injury of right forearm ▽
- √7ᵗʰ **S50.912** Unspecified superficial injury of left forearm ▽
- √7ᵗʰ **S50.919** Unspecified superficial injury of unspecified forearm ▽

√4ᵗʰ **S51** Open wound of elbow and forearm
Code also any associated wound infection
EXCLUDES 1   open fracture of elbow and forearm (S52.- with open fracture 7th character)
   traumatic amputation of elbow and forearm (S58.-)
EXCLUDES 2   open wound of wrist and hand (S61.-)

The appropriate 7th character is to be added to each code from category S51.
A   initial encounter
D   subsequent encounter
S   sequela

√5ᵗʰ **S51.0** Open wound of elbow

√6ᵗʰ **S51.00** Unspecified open wound of elbow
- √7ᵗʰ **S51.001** Unspecified open wound of right elbow ▽
   AHA: 2012,4Q,108
- √7ᵗʰ **S51.002** Unspecified open wound of left elbow ▽
- √7ᵗʰ **S51.009** Unspecified open wound of unspecified elbow ▽
   Open wound of elbow NOS

√6ᵗʰ **S51.01** Laceration without foreign body of elbow
- √7ᵗʰ **S51.011** Laceration without foreign body of right elbow
- √7ᵗʰ **S51.012** Laceration without foreign body of left elbow
- √7ᵗʰ **S51.019** Laceration without foreign body of unspecified elbow ▽

√6ᵗʰ **S51.02** Laceration with foreign body of elbow
- √7ᵗʰ **S51.021** Laceration with foreign body of right elbow
- √7ᵗʰ **S51.022** Laceration with foreign body of left elbow
- √7ᵗʰ **S51.029** Laceration with foreign body of unspecified elbow ▽

√6ᵗʰ **S51.03** Puncture wound without foreign body of elbow
- √7ᵗʰ **S51.031** Puncture wound without foreign body of right elbow
- √7ᵗʰ **S51.032** Puncture wound without foreign body of left elbow
- √7ᵗʰ **S51.039** Puncture wound without foreign body of unspecified elbow ▽

√6ᵗʰ **S51.04** Puncture wound with foreign body of elbow
- √7ᵗʰ **S51.041** Puncture wound with foreign body of right elbow
- √7ᵗʰ **S51.042** Puncture wound with foreign body of left elbow
- √7ᵗʰ **S51.049** Puncture wound with foreign body of unspecified elbow ▽

√6ᵗʰ **S51.05** Open bite of elbow
Bite of elbow NOS
EXCLUDES 1   superficial bite of elbow (S50.36, S50.37)
- √7ᵗʰ **S51.051** Open bite, right elbow
- √7ᵗʰ **S51.052** Open bite, left elbow
- √7ᵗʰ **S51.059** Open bite, unspecified elbow ▽

√5ᵗʰ **S51.8** Open wound of forearm
EXCLUDES 2   open wound of elbow (S51.0-)

√6ᵗʰ **S51.80** Unspecified open wound of forearm
AHA: 2016,3Q,24
- √7ᵗʰ **S51.801** Unspecified open wound of right forearm ▽
- √7ᵗʰ **S51.802** Unspecified open wound of left forearm ▽
- √7ᵗʰ **S51.809** Unspecified open wound of unspecified forearm ▽
   Open wound of forearm NOS

√6ᵗʰ **S51.81** Laceration without foreign body of forearm
- √7ᵗʰ **S51.811** Laceration without foreign body of right forearm
- √7ᵗʰ **S51.812** Laceration without foreign body of left forearm
- √7ᵗʰ **S51.819** Laceration without foreign body of unspecified forearm ▽

√6ᵗʰ **S51.82** Laceration with foreign body of forearm
- √7ᵗʰ **S51.821** Laceration with foreign body of right forearm

√7ᵗʰ **S51.822 Laceration with foreign body of** left **forearm**

√7ᵗʰ **S51.829 Laceration with foreign body of** ▽ **unspecified forearm**

√6ᵗʰ **S51.83 Puncture wound without foreign body of forearm**

AHA: 2016,3Q,24

√7ᵗʰ **S51.831 Puncture wound without foreign body of** right **forearm**

√7ᵗʰ **S51.832 Puncture wound without foreign body of** left **forearm**

√7ᵗʰ **S51.839 Puncture wound without foreign** ▽ **body of unspecified forearm**

√6ᵗʰ **S51.84 Puncture wound with foreign body of forearm**

AHA: 2016,3Q,24

√7ᵗʰ **S51.841 Puncture wound with foreign body of** right **forearm**

√7ᵗʰ **S51.842 Puncture wound with foreign body of** left **forearm**

√7ᵗʰ **S51.849 Puncture wound with foreign** ▽ **body of unspecified forearm**

√6ᵗʰ **S51.85 Open bite of forearm**

Bite of forearm NOS

EXCLUDES 1 superficial bite of forearm (S50.86, S50.87)

√7ᵗʰ **S51.851 Open bite of** right **forearm**

√7ᵗʰ **S51.852 Open bite of** left **forearm**

√7ᵗʰ **S51.859 Open bite of unspecified forearm** ▽

√4ᵗʰ **S52 Fracture of forearm**

NOTE A fracture not indicated as displaced or nondisplaced should be coded to displaced.

A fracture not indicated as open or closed should be coded to closed.

The open fracture designations are based on the Gustilo open fracture classification.

EXCLUDES 1 traumatic amputation of forearm (S58.-)
EXCLUDES 2 fracture at wrist and hand level (S62.-)

AHA: 2018,2Q,12; 2016,1Q,33; 2015,3Q,37-39

The appropriate 7th character is to be added to all codes from category S52 [unless otherwise indicated].
A initial encounter for closed fracture
B initial encounter for open fracture type I or II
   initial encounter for open fracture NOS
C initial encounter for open fracture type IIIA, IIIB, or IIIC
D subsequent encounter for closed fracture with routine healing
E subsequent encounter for open fracture type I or II with routine healing
F subsequent encounter for open fracture type IIIA, IIIB, or IIIC with routine healing
G subsequent encounter for closed fracture with delayed healing
H subsequent encounter for open fracture type I or II with delayed healing
J subsequent encounter for open fracture type IIIA, IIIB, or IIIC with delayed healing
K subsequent encounter for closed fracture with nonunion
M subsequent encounter for open fracture type I or II with nonunion
N subsequent encounter for open fracture type IIIA, IIIB, or IIIC with nonunion
P subsequent encounter for closed fracture with malunion
Q subsequent encounter for open fracture type I or II with malunion
R subsequent encounter for open fracture type IIIA, IIIB, or IIIC with malunion
S sequela

√5ᵗʰ **S52.0 Fracture of** upper end of ulna

Fracture of proximal end of ulna

EXCLUDES 2 fracture of elbow NOS (S42.40-)
            fractures of shaft of ulna (S52.2-)

√6ᵗʰ **S52.00 Unspecified fracture of upper end of ulna**

√7ᵗʰ **S52.001 Unspecified fracture of upper end** Q ▽ **of** right **ulna**

√7ᵗʰ **S52.002 Unspecified fracture of upper end** Q ▽ **of** left **ulna**

√7ᵗʰ **S52.009 Unspecified fracture of upper end** Q ▽ **of unspecified ulna**

√6ᵗʰ **S52.01 Torus fracture of upper end of ulna**

The appropriate 7th character is to be added to all codes in subcategory S52.01
A initial encounter for closed fracture
D subsequent encounter for fracture with routine healing
G subsequent encounter for fracture with delayed healing
K subsequent encounter for fracture with nonunion
P subsequent encounter for fracture with malunion
S sequela

√7ᵗʰ **S52.011 Torus fracture of upper end of** Q **right ulna**

√7ᵗʰ **S52.012 Torus fracture of upper end of** left Q **ulna**

√7ᵗʰ **S52.019 Torus fracture of upper end of** Q ▽ **unspecified ulna**

√6ᵗʰ **S52.02 Fracture of** olecranon process without intraarticular extension of ulna

√7ᵗʰ **S52.021 Displaced fracture of olecranon** Q **process without intraarticular extension of** right **ulna**

√7ᵗʰ **S52.022 Displaced fracture of olecranon** Q **process without intraarticular extension of** left **ulna**

√7ᵗʰ **S52.023 Displaced fracture of olecranon** Q ▽ **process without intraarticular extension of unspecified ulna**

√7ᵗʰ **S52.024 Nondisplaced fracture of** Q **olecranon process without intraarticular extension of** right **ulna**

√7ᵗʰ **S52.025 Nondisplaced fracture of** Q **olecranon process without intraarticular extension of** left **ulna**

√7ᵗʰ **S52.026 Nondisplaced fracture of** Q ▽ **olecranon process without intraarticular extension of unspecified ulna**

√6ᵗʰ **S52.03 Fracture of** olecranon process with intraarticular extension of ulna

√7ᵗʰ **S52.031 Displaced fracture of olecranon** Q **process with intraarticular extension of** right **ulna**

√7ᵗʰ **S52.032 Displaced fracture of olecranon** Q **process with intraarticular extension of** left **ulna**

√7ᵗʰ **S52.033 Displaced fracture of olecranon** Q ▽ **process with intraarticular extension of unspecified ulna**

√7ᵗʰ **S52.034 Nondisplaced fracture of** Q **olecranon process with intraarticular extension of** right **ulna**

√7ᵗʰ **S52.035 Nondisplaced fracture of** Q **olecranon process with intraarticular extension of** left **ulna**

√7ᵗʰ **S52.036 Nondisplaced fracture of** Q ▽ **olecranon process with intraarticular extension of unspecified ulna**

√6ᵗʰ **S52.04 Fracture of** coronoid process of ulna

√7ᵗʰ **S52.041 Displaced fracture of coronoid** Q **process of** right **ulna**

√7ᵗʰ **S52.042 Displaced fracture of coronoid** Q **process of** left **ulna**

√7ᵗʰ **S52.043 Displaced fracture of coronoid** Q ▽ **process of unspecified ulna**

√7ᵗʰ **S52.044 Nondisplaced fracture of** Q **coronoid process of** right **ulna**

√7ᵗʰ **S52.045 Nondisplaced fracture of** Q **coronoid process of** left **ulna**

√7ᵗʰ **S52.046 Nondisplaced fracture of** Q ▽ **coronoid process of unspecified ulna**

√6ᵗʰ **S52.09 Other fracture of upper end of ulna**

√7ᵗʰ **S52.091 Other fracture of upper end of** Q **right ulna**

☑ Additional Character Req   √x7ᵗʰ Placeholder Alert   **Manifestation**   ▽ Unspecified   ►◄ Revised Text   ● New Code   ▲ Revised Code Title

√7ᵗʰ **S52.092** Other fracture of upper end of left ulna   ▢

√7ᵗʰ **S52.099** Other fracture of upper end of unspecified ulna   ▢ ▽

√5ᵗʰ **S52.1** Fracture of upper end of radius

Fracture of proximal end of radius

EXCLUDES 2   physeal fractures of upper end of radius (S59.2-)

fracture of shaft of radius (S52.3-)

√6ᵗʰ **S52.10** Unspecified fracture of upper end of radius

√7ᵗʰ **S52.101** Unspecified fracture of upper end of right radius   ▢ ▽

√7ᵗʰ **S52.102** Unspecified fracture of upper end of left radius   ▢ ▽

√7ᵗʰ **S52.109** Unspecified fracture of upper end of unspecified radius   ▢ ▽

√6ᵗʰ **S52.11** Torus fracture of upper end of radius

The appropriate 7th character is to be added to all codes in subcategory S52.11
A   initial encounter for closed fracture
D   subsequent encounter for fracture with routine healing
G   subsequent encounter for fracture with delayed healing
K   subsequent encounter for fracture with nonunion
P   subsequent encounter for fracture with malunion
S   sequela

√7ᵗʰ **S52.111** Torus fracture of upper end of right radius   ▢

√7ᵗʰ **S52.112** Torus fracture of upper end of left radius   ▢

√7ᵗʰ **S52.119** Torus fracture of upper end of unspecified radius   ▢ ▽

√6ᵗʰ **S52.12** Fracture of head of radius

√7ᵗʰ **S52.121** Displaced fracture of head of right radius   ▢

√7ᵗʰ **S52.122** Displaced fracture of head of left radius   ▢

√7ᵗʰ **S52.123** Displaced fracture of head of unspecified radius   ▢ ▽

√7ᵗʰ **S52.124** Nondisplaced fracture of head of right radius   ▢

√7ᵗʰ **S52.125** Nondisplaced fracture of head of left radius   ▢

√7ᵗʰ **S52.126** Nondisplaced fracture of head of unspecified radius   ▢ ▽

√6ᵗʰ **S52.13** Fracture of neck of radius

√7ᵗʰ **S52.131** Displaced fracture of neck of right radius   ▢

√7ᵗʰ **S52.132** Displaced fracture of neck of left radius   ▢

√7ᵗʰ **S52.133** Displaced fracture of neck of unspecified radius   ▢ ▽

√7ᵗʰ **S52.134** Nondisplaced fracture of neck of right radius   ▢

√7ᵗʰ **S52.135** Nondisplaced fracture of neck of left radius   ▢

√7ᵗʰ **S52.136** Nondisplaced fracture of neck of unspecified radius   ▢ ▽

√6ᵗʰ **S52.18** Other fracture of upper end of radius

√7ᵗʰ **S52.181** Other fracture of upper end of right radius   ▢

√7ᵗʰ **S52.182** Other fracture of upper end of left radius   ▢

√7ᵗʰ **S52.189** Other fracture of upper end of unspecified radius   ▢ ▽

√5ᵗʰ **S52.2** Fracture of shaft of ulna

√6ᵗʰ **S52.20** Unspecified fracture of shaft of ulna

Fracture of ulna NOS

√7ᵗʰ **S52.201** Unspecified fracture of shaft of right ulna   ▢ ▽

√7ᵗʰ **S52.202** Unspecified fracture of shaft of left ulna   ▢ ▽

√7ᵗʰ **S52.209** Unspecified fracture of shaft of unspecified ulna   ▢ ▽

√6ᵗʰ **S52.21** Greenstick fracture of shaft of ulna

The appropriate 7th character is to be added to all codes in subcategory S52.21
A   initial encounter for closed fracture
D   subsequent encounter for fracture with routine healing
G   subsequent encounter for fracture with delayed healing
K   subsequent encounter for fracture with nonunion
P   subsequent encounter for fracture with malunion
S   sequela

√7ᵗʰ **S52.211** Greenstick fracture of shaft of right ulna   ▢

√7ᵗʰ **S52.212** Greenstick fracture of shaft of left ulna   ▢

√7ᵗʰ **S52.219** Greenstick fracture of shaft of unspecified ulna   ▢ ▽

√6ᵗʰ **S52.22** Transverse fracture of shaft of ulna

√7ᵗʰ **S52.221** Displaced transverse fracture of shaft of right ulna   ▢

√7ᵗʰ **S52.222** Displaced transverse fracture of shaft of left ulna   ▢

√7ᵗʰ **S52.223** Displaced transverse fracture of shaft of unspecified ulna   ▢ ▽

√7ᵗʰ **S52.224** Nondisplaced transverse fracture of shaft of right ulna   ▢

√7ᵗʰ **S52.225** Nondisplaced transverse fracture of shaft of left ulna   ▢

√7ᵗʰ **S52.226** Nondisplaced transverse fracture of shaft of unspecified ulna   ▢ ▽

√6ᵗʰ **S52.23** Oblique fracture of shaft of ulna

√7ᵗʰ **S52.231** Displaced oblique fracture of shaft of right ulna   ▢

√7ᵗʰ **S52.232** Displaced oblique fracture of shaft of left ulna   ▢

√7ᵗʰ **S52.233** Displaced oblique fracture of shaft of unspecified ulna   ▢ ▽

√7ᵗʰ **S52.234** Nondisplaced oblique fracture of shaft of right ulna   ▢

√7ᵗʰ **S52.235** Nondisplaced oblique fracture of shaft of left ulna   ▢

√7ᵗʰ **S52.236** Nondisplaced oblique fracture of shaft of unspecified ulna   ▢ ▽

√6ᵗʰ **S52.24** Spiral fracture of shaft of ulna

√7ᵗʰ **S52.241** Displaced spiral fracture of shaft of ulna, right arm   ▢

√7ᵗʰ **S52.242** Displaced spiral fracture of shaft of ulna, left arm   ▢

√7ᵗʰ **S52.243** Displaced spiral fracture of shaft of ulna, unspecified arm   ▢ ▽

√7ᵗʰ **S52.244** Nondisplaced spiral fracture of shaft of ulna, right arm   ▢

√7ᵗʰ **S52.245** Nondisplaced spiral fracture of shaft of ulna, left arm   ▢

√7ᵗʰ **S52.246** Nondisplaced spiral fracture of shaft of ulna, unspecified arm   ▢ ▽

√6ᵗʰ **S52.25** Comminuted fracture of shaft of ulna

√7ᵗʰ **S52.251** Displaced comminuted fracture of shaft of ulna, right arm   ▢

√7ᵗʰ **S52.252** Displaced comminuted fracture of shaft of ulna, left arm   ▢

√7ᵗʰ **S52.253** Displaced comminuted fracture of shaft of ulna, unspecified arm   ▢ ▽

√7ᵗʰ **S52.254** Nondisplaced comminuted fracture of shaft of ulna, right arm   ▢

√7ᵗʰ **S52.255** Nondisplaced comminuted fracture of shaft of ulna, left arm   ▢

√7ᵗʰ **S52.256** Nondisplaced comminuted fracture of shaft of ulna, unspecified arm   ▢ ▽

√6ᵗʰ **S52.26** Segmental fracture of shaft of ulna

√7ᵗʰ **S52.261** Displaced segmental fracture of shaft of ulna, right arm   ▢

√7ᵗʰ **S52.262** Displaced segmental fracture of shaft of ulna, left arm   ▢

√7ᵗʰ **S52.263** Displaced segmental fracture of shaft of ulna, unspecified arm   ▢ ▽

√7ᵗʰ **S52.264** Nondisplaced segmental fracture of shaft of ulna, right arm   ▢

√7ᵗʰ **S52.265** Nondisplaced segmental fracture of shaft of ulna, left arm Ⓠ

√7ᵗʰ **S52.266** Nondisplaced segmental fracture of shaft of ulna, unspecified arm Ⓠ ▽

√6ᵗʰ **S52.27** Monteggia's fracture of ulna

Fracture of upper shaft of ulna with dislocation of radial head

√7ᵗʰ **S52.271** Monteggia's fracture of right ulna Ⓠ

√7ᵗʰ **S52.272** Monteggia's fracture of left ulna Ⓠ

√7ᵗʰ **S52.279** Monteggia's fracture of unspecified ulna Ⓠ ▽

√6ᵗʰ **S52.28** Bent bone of ulna

√7ᵗʰ **S52.281** Bent bone of right ulna Ⓠ

√7ᵗʰ **S52.282** Bent bone of left ulna Ⓠ

√7ᵗʰ **S52.283** Bent bone of unspecified ulna Ⓠ ▽

√6ᵗʰ **S52.29** Other fracture of shaft of ulna

√7ᵗʰ **S52.291** Other fracture of shaft of right ulna Ⓠ

√7ᵗʰ **S52.292** Other fracture of shaft of left ulna Ⓠ

√7ᵗʰ **S52.299** Other fracture of shaft of unspecified ulna Ⓠ ▽

√5ᵗʰ **S52.3** Fracture of shaft of radius

√6ᵗʰ **S52.30** Unspecified fracture of shaft of radius

√7ᵗʰ **S52.301** Unspecified fracture of shaft of right radius Ⓠ ▽

√7ᵗʰ **S52.302** Unspecified fracture of shaft of left radius Ⓠ ▽

√7ᵗʰ **S52.309** Unspecified fracture of shaft of unspecified radius Ⓠ ▽

√6ᵗʰ **S52.31** Greenstick fracture of shaft of radius

The appropriate 7th character is to be added to all codes in subcategory S52.31.
- A initial encounter for closed fracture
- D subsequent encounter for fracture with routine healing
- G subsequent encounter for fracture with delayed healing
- K subsequent encounter for fracture with nonunion
- P subsequent encounter for fracture with malunion
- S sequela

√7ᵗʰ **S52.311** Greenstick fracture of shaft of radius, right arm Ⓠ

√7ᵗʰ **S52.312** Greenstick fracture of shaft of radius, left arm Ⓠ

√7ᵗʰ **S52.319** Greenstick fracture of shaft of radius, unspecified arm Ⓠ ▽

√6ᵗʰ **S52.32** Transverse fracture of shaft of radius

√7ᵗʰ **S52.321** Displaced transverse fracture of shaft of right radius Ⓠ

√7ᵗʰ **S52.322** Displaced transverse fracture of shaft of left radius Ⓠ

√7ᵗʰ **S52.323** Displaced transverse fracture of shaft of unspecified radius Ⓠ ▽

√7ᵗʰ **S52.324** Nondisplaced transverse fracture of shaft of right radius Ⓠ

√7ᵗʰ **S52.325** Nondisplaced transverse fracture of shaft of left radius Ⓠ

√7ᵗʰ **S52.326** Nondisplaced transverse fracture of shaft of unspecified radius Ⓠ ▽

√6ᵗʰ **S52.33** Oblique fracture of shaft of radius

√7ᵗʰ **S52.331** Displaced oblique fracture of shaft of right radius Ⓠ

√7ᵗʰ **S52.332** Displaced oblique fracture of shaft of left radius Ⓠ

√7ᵗʰ **S52.333** Displaced oblique fracture of shaft of unspecified radius Ⓠ ▽

√7ᵗʰ **S52.334** Nondisplaced oblique fracture of shaft of right radius Ⓠ

√7ᵗʰ **S52.335** Nondisplaced oblique fracture of shaft of left radius Ⓠ

√7ᵗʰ **S52.336** Nondisplaced oblique fracture of shaft of unspecified radius Ⓠ ▽

√6ᵗʰ **S52.34** Spiral fracture of shaft of radius

√7ᵗʰ **S52.341** Displaced spiral fracture of shaft of radius, right arm Ⓠ

√7ᵗʰ **S52.342** Displaced spiral fracture of shaft of radius, left arm Ⓠ

√7ᵗʰ **S52.343** Displaced spiral fracture of shaft of radius, unspecified arm Ⓠ ▽

√7ᵗʰ **S52.344** Nondisplaced spiral fracture of shaft of radius, right arm Ⓠ

√7ᵗʰ **S52.345** Nondisplaced spiral fracture of shaft of radius, left arm Ⓠ

√7ᵗʰ **S52.346** Nondisplaced spiral fracture of shaft of radius, unspecified arm Ⓠ ▽

√6ᵗʰ **S52.35** Comminuted fracture of shaft of radius

√7ᵗʰ **S52.351** Displaced comminuted fracture of shaft of radius, right arm Ⓠ

√7ᵗʰ **S52.352** Displaced comminuted fracture of shaft of radius, left arm Ⓠ

√7ᵗʰ **S52.353** Displaced comminuted fracture of shaft of radius, unspecified arm Ⓠ ▽

√7ᵗʰ **S52.354** Nondisplaced comminuted fracture of shaft of radius, right arm Ⓠ

√7ᵗʰ **S52.355** Nondisplaced comminuted fracture of shaft of radius, left arm Ⓠ

√7ᵗʰ **S52.356** Nondisplaced comminuted fracture of shaft of radius, unspecified arm Ⓠ ▽

√6ᵗʰ **S52.36** Segmental fracture of shaft of radius

√7ᵗʰ **S52.361** Displaced segmental fracture of shaft of radius, right arm Ⓠ

√7ᵗʰ **S52.362** Displaced segmental fracture of shaft of radius, left arm Ⓠ

√7ᵗʰ **S52.363** Displaced segmental fracture of shaft of radius, unspecified arm Ⓠ ▽

√7ᵗʰ **S52.364** Nondisplaced segmental fracture of shaft of radius, right arm Ⓠ

√7ᵗʰ **S52.365** Nondisplaced segmental fracture of shaft of radius, left arm Ⓠ

√7ᵗʰ **S52.366** Nondisplaced segmental fracture of shaft of radius, unspecified arm Ⓠ ▽

√6ᵗʰ **S52.37** Galeazzi's fracture

Fracture of lower shaft of radius with radioulnar joint dislocation

√7ᵗʰ **S52.371** Galeazzi's fracture of right radius Ⓠ

√7ᵗʰ **S52.372** Galeazzi's fracture of left radius Ⓠ

√7ᵗʰ **S52.379** Galeazzi's fracture of unspecified radius Ⓠ ▽

√6ᵗʰ **S52.38** Bent bone of radius

√7ᵗʰ **S52.381** Bent bone of right radius Ⓠ

√7ᵗʰ **S52.382** Bent bone of left radius Ⓠ

√7ᵗʰ **S52.389** Bent bone of unspecified radius Ⓠ ▽

√6ᵗʰ **S52.39** Other fracture of shaft of radius

√7ᵗʰ **S52.391** Other fracture of shaft of radius, right arm Ⓠ

√7ᵗʰ **S52.392** Other fracture of shaft of radius, left arm Ⓠ

√7ᵗʰ **S52.399** Other fracture of shaft of radius, unspecified arm Ⓠ ▽

√5ᵗʰ **S52.5** Fracture of lower end of radius

Fracture of distal end of radius

EXCLUDES 2   physeal fractures of lower end of radius (S59.2-)

DEF: Fracture of the distal end of the radius above the wrist, most commonly caused by a fall onto an outstretched hand.

√6ᵗʰ **S52.50** Unspecified fracture of the lower end of radius

√7ᵗʰ **S52.501** Unspecified fracture of the lower end of right radius Ⓠ ▽

√7ᵗʰ **S52.502** Unspecified fracture of the lower end of left radius Ⓠ ▽

√7ᵗʰ **S52.509** Unspecified fracture of the lower end of unspecified radius Ⓠ ▽

√6ᵗʰ **S52.51** Fracture of radial styloid process

√7ᵗʰ **S52.511** Displaced fracture of right radial styloid process Ⓠ

√7ᵗʰ **S52.512** Displaced fracture of left radial styloid process Ⓠ

√7ᵗʰ **S52.513** Displaced fracture of unspecified radial styloid process Ⓠ ▽

√7ᵗʰ **S52.514** Nondisplaced fracture of right radial styloid process Ⓠ

√7ᵗʰ **S52.515** Nondisplaced fracture of left radial styloid process Ⓠ

☑ Additional Character Req   √x7ᵗʰ Placeholder Alert   **Manifestation**   ▽ Unspecified   ►◄ Revised Text   ● New Code   ▲ Revised Code Title

ICD-10-CM 2019   **1005**

√7ᵗʰ **S52.516** Nondisplaced fracture of unspecified radial styloid process ◙ ▽

√6ᵗʰ **S52.52** Torus fracture of lower end of radius

> The appropriate 7th character is to be added to all codes in subcategory S52.52.
> A   initial encounter for closed fracture
> D   subsequent encounter for fracture with routine healing
> G   subsequent encounter for fracture with delayed healing
> K   subsequent encounter for fracture with nonunion
> P   subsequent encounter for fracture with malunion
> S   sequela

√7ᵗʰ **S52.521** Torus fracture of lower end of right radius ◙

√7ᵗʰ **S52.522** Torus fracture of lower end of left radius ◙

√7ᵗʰ **S52.529** Torus fracture of lower end of unspecified radius ◙ ▽

√6ᵗʰ **S52.53** Colles' fracture

> **AHA:** 2016,2Q,4
> **DEF:** Fracture of the radius at the wrist in which the distal fragment is pushed posteriorly. The dorsal angulation of the fragment results in the wrist cocking up.

√7ᵗʰ **S52.531** Colles' fracture of right radius ◙

√7ᵗʰ **S52.532** Colles' fracture of left radius ◙

√7ᵗʰ **S52.539** Colles' fracture of unspecified radius ◙ ▽

√6ᵗʰ **S52.54** Smith's fracture

√7ᵗʰ **S52.541** Smith's fracture of right radius ◙

√7ᵗʰ **S52.542** Smith's fracture of left radius ◙

√7ᵗʰ **S52.549** Smith's fracture of unspecified radius ◙ ▽

√6ᵗʰ **S52.55** Other extraarticular fracture of lower end of radius

√7ᵗʰ **S52.551** Other extraarticular fracture of lower end of right radius ◙

√7ᵗʰ **S52.552** Other extraarticular fracture of lower end of left radius ◙

√7ᵗʰ **S52.559** Other extraarticular fracture of lower end of unspecified radius ◙ ▽

√6ᵗʰ **S52.56** Barton's fracture

√7ᵗʰ **S52.561** Barton's fracture of right radius ◙

√7ᵗʰ **S52.562** Barton's fracture of left radius ◙

√7ᵗʰ **S52.569** Barton's fracture of unspecified radius ◙ ▽

√6ᵗʰ **S52.57** Other intraarticular fracture of lower end of radius

√7ᵗʰ **S52.571** Other intraarticular fracture of lower end of right radius ◙

√7ᵗʰ **S52.572** Other intraarticular fracture of lower end of left radius ◙

√7ᵗʰ **S52.579** Other intraarticular fracture of lower end of unspecified radius ◙ ▽

√6ᵗʰ **S52.59** Other fractures of lower end of radius

√7ᵗʰ **S52.591** Other fractures of lower end of right radius ◙

√7ᵗʰ **S52.592** Other fractures of lower end of left radius ◙

√7ᵗʰ **S52.599** Other fractures of lower end of unspecified radius ◙ ▽

√5ᵗʰ **S52.6** Fracture of lower end of ulna

√6ᵗʰ **S52.60** Unspecified fracture of lower end of ulna

√7ᵗʰ **S52.601** Unspecified fracture of lower end of right ulna ◙ ▽

√7ᵗʰ **S52.602** Unspecified fracture of lower end of left ulna ◙ ▽

√7ᵗʰ **S52.609** Unspecified fracture of lower end of unspecified ulna ◙ ▽

√6ᵗʰ **S52.61** Fracture of ulna styloid process

√7ᵗʰ **S52.611** Displaced fracture of right ulna styloid process ◙

√7ᵗʰ **S52.612** Displaced fracture of left ulna styloid process ◙

√7ᵗʰ **S52.613** Displaced fracture of unspecified ulna styloid process ◙ ▽

√7ᵗʰ **S52.614** Nondisplaced fracture of right ulna styloid process ◙

√7ᵗʰ **S52.615** Nondisplaced fracture of left ulna styloid process ◙

√7ᵗʰ **S52.616** Nondisplaced fracture of unspecified ulna styloid process ◙ ▽

√6ᵗʰ **S52.62** Torus fracture of lower end of ulna

> The appropriate 7th character is to be added to all codes in subcategory S52.62.
> A   initial encounter for closed fracture
> D   subsequent encounter for fracture with routine healing
> G   subsequent encounter for fracture with delayed healing
> K   subsequent encounter for fracture with nonunion
> P   subsequent encounter for fracture with malunion
> S   sequela

√7ᵗʰ **S52.621** Torus fracture of lower end of right ulna ◙

√7ᵗʰ **S52.622** Torus fracture of lower end of left ulna ◙

√7ᵗʰ **S52.629** Torus fracture of lower end of unspecified ulna ◙ ▽

√6ᵗʰ **S52.69** Other fracture of lower end of ulna

√7ᵗʰ **S52.691** Other fracture of lower end of right ulna ◙

√7ᵗʰ **S52.692** Other fracture of lower end of left ulna ◙

√7ᵗʰ **S52.699** Other fracture of lower end of unspecified ulna ◙ ▽

√5ᵗʰ **S52.9** Unspecified fracture of forearm

√×7ᵗʰ **S52.90** Unspecified fracture of unspecified forearm ◙ ▽

√×7ᵗʰ **S52.91** Unspecified fracture of right forearm ◙ ▽

√×7ᵗʰ **S52.92** Unspecified fracture of left forearm ◙ ▽

√4ᵗʰ **S53** Dislocation and sprain of joints and ligaments of elbow

> INCLUDES   avulsion of joint or ligament of elbow
> laceration of cartilage, joint or ligament of elbow
> sprain of cartilage, joint or ligament of elbow
> traumatic hemarthrosis of joint or ligament of elbow
> traumatic rupture of joint or ligament of elbow
> traumatic subluxation of joint or ligament of elbow
> traumatic tear of joint or ligament of elbow

Code also any associated open wound

EXCLUDES 2   strain of muscle, fascia and tendon at forearm level (S56.-)

> The appropriate 7th character is to be added to each code from category S53.
> A   initial encounter
> D   subsequent encounter
> S   sequela

√5ᵗʰ **S53.0** Subluxation and dislocation of radial head

> Dislocation of radiohumeral joint
> Subluxation of radiohumeral joint
> EXCLUDES 1   Monteggia's fracture-dislocation (S52.27-)

√6ᵗʰ **S53.00** Unspecified subluxation and dislocation of radial head

√7ᵗʰ **S53.001** Unspecified subluxation of right radial head ▽

√7ᵗʰ **S53.002** Unspecified subluxation of left radial head ▽

√7ᵗʰ **S53.003** Unspecified subluxation of unspecified radial head ▽

√7ᵗʰ **S53.004** Unspecified dislocation of right radial head ▽

√7ᵗʰ **S53.005** Unspecified dislocation of left radial head ▽

√7ᵗʰ **S53.006** Unspecified dislocation of unspecified radial head ▽

√6ᵗʰ **S53.01** Anterior subluxation and dislocation of radial head

> Anteriomedial subluxation and dislocation of radial head

√7ᵗʰ **S53.011** Anterior subluxation of right radial head

√7ᵗʰ **S53.012** Anterior subluxation of left radial head

√7ᵗʰ **S53.013** Anterior subluxation of unspecified radial head ▽

√7ᵗʰ **S53.014** Anterior dislocation of right radial head

√7ᵗʰ **S53.015** Anterior dislocation of left radial head

√7ᵗʰ **S53.016** Anterior dislocation of unspecified radial head ▽

√6ᵗʰ **S53.02** Posterior subluxation and dislocation of radial head

Posteriolateral subluxation and dislocation of radial head

√7ᵗʰ **S53.021** Posterior subluxation of right radial head

√7ᵗʰ **S53.022** Posterior subluxation of left radial head

√7ᵗʰ **S53.023** Posterior subluxation of unspecified radial head ▽

√7ᵗʰ **S53.024** Posterior dislocation of right radial head

√7ᵗʰ **S53.025** Posterior dislocation of left radial head

√7ᵗʰ **S53.026** Posterior dislocation of unspecified radial head ▽

√6ᵗʰ **S53.03** Nursemaid's elbow

√7ᵗʰ **S53.031** Nursemaid's elbow, right elbow

√7ᵗʰ **S53.032** Nursemaid's elbow, left elbow

√7ᵗʰ **S53.033** Nursemaid's elbow, unspecified elbow ▽

√6ᵗʰ **S53.09** Other subluxation and dislocation of radial head

√7ᵗʰ **S53.091** Other subluxation of right radial head

√7ᵗʰ **S53.092** Other subluxation of left radial head

√7ᵗʰ **S53.093** Other subluxation of unspecified radial head ▽

√7ᵗʰ **S53.094** Other dislocation of right radial head

√7ᵗʰ **S53.095** Other dislocation of left radial head

√7ᵗʰ **S53.096** Other dislocation of unspecified radial head ▽

√5ᵗʰ **S53.1** Subluxation and dislocation of ulnohumeral joint

Subluxation and dislocation of elbow NOS

EXCLUDES 1   dislocation of radial head alone (S53.0-)

√6ᵗʰ **S53.10** Unspecified subluxation and dislocation of ulnohumeral joint

√7ᵗʰ **S53.101** Unspecified subluxation of right ulnohumeral joint ▽

√7ᵗʰ **S53.102** Unspecified subluxation of left ulnohumeral joint ▽

√7ᵗʰ **S53.103** Unspecified subluxation of unspecified ulnohumeral joint ▽

√7ᵗʰ **S53.104** Unspecified dislocation of right ulnohumeral joint ▽

√7ᵗʰ **S53.105** Unspecified dislocation of left ulnohumeral joint ▽

√7ᵗʰ **S53.106** Unspecified dislocation of unspecified ulnohumeral joint ▽

√6ᵗʰ **S53.11** Anterior subluxation and dislocation of ulnohumeral joint

√7ᵗʰ **S53.111** Anterior subluxation of right ulnohumeral joint

√7ᵗʰ **S53.112** Anterior subluxation of left ulnohumeral joint

√7ᵗʰ **S53.113** Anterior subluxation of unspecified ulnohumeral joint ▽

√7ᵗʰ **S53.114** Anterior dislocation of right ulnohumeral joint

AHA: 2012,4Q,108

√7ᵗʰ **S53.115** Anterior dislocation of left ulnohumeral joint

√7ᵗʰ **S53.116** Anterior dislocation of unspecified ulnohumeral joint ▽

√6ᵗʰ **S53.12** Posterior subluxation and dislocation of ulnohumeral joint

√7ᵗʰ **S53.121** Posterior subluxation of right ulnohumeral joint

√7ᵗʰ **S53.122** Posterior subluxation of left ulnohumeral joint

√7ᵗʰ **S53.123** Posterior subluxation of unspecified ulnohumeral joint ▽

√7ᵗʰ **S53.124** Posterior dislocation of right ulnohumeral joint

√7ᵗʰ **S53.125** Posterior dislocation of left ulnohumeral joint

√7ᵗʰ **S53.126** Posterior dislocation of unspecified ulnohumeral joint ▽

√6ᵗʰ **S53.13** Medial subluxation and dislocation of ulnohumeral joint

√7ᵗʰ **S53.131** Medial subluxation of right ulnohumeral joint

√7ᵗʰ **S53.132** Medial subluxation of left ulnohumeral joint

√7ᵗʰ **S53.133** Medial subluxation of unspecified ulnohumeral joint ▽

√7ᵗʰ **S53.134** Medial dislocation of right ulnohumeral joint

√7ᵗʰ **S53.135** Medial dislocation of left ulnohumeral joint

√7ᵗʰ **S53.136** Medial dislocation of unspecified ulnohumeral joint ▽

√6ᵗʰ **S53.14** Lateral subluxation and dislocation of ulnohumeral joint

√7ᵗʰ **S53.141** Lateral subluxation of right ulnohumeral joint

√7ᵗʰ **S53.142** Lateral subluxation of left ulnohumeral joint

√7ᵗʰ **S53.143** Lateral subluxation of unspecified ulnohumeral joint ▽

√7ᵗʰ **S53.144** Lateral dislocation of right ulnohumeral joint

√7ᵗʰ **S53.145** Lateral dislocation of left ulnohumeral joint

√7ᵗʰ **S53.146** Lateral dislocation of unspecified ulnohumeral joint ▽

√6ᵗʰ **S53.19** Other subluxation and dislocation of ulnohumeral joint

√7ᵗʰ **S53.191** Other subluxation of right ulnohumeral joint

√7ᵗʰ **S53.192** Other subluxation of left ulnohumeral joint

√7ᵗʰ **S53.193** Other subluxation of unspecified ulnohumeral joint ▽

√7ᵗʰ **S53.194** Other dislocation of right ulnohumeral joint

√7ᵗʰ **S53.195** Other dislocation of left ulnohumeral joint

√7ᵗʰ **S53.196** Other dislocation of unspecified ulnohumeral joint ▽

√5ᵗʰ **S53.2** Traumatic rupture of radial collateral ligament

EXCLUDES 1   sprain of radial collateral ligament NOS (S53.43-)

√x7ᵗʰ **S53.20** Traumatic rupture of unspecified radial collateral ligament ▽

√x7ᵗʰ **S53.21** Traumatic rupture of right radial collateral ligament

√x7ᵗʰ **S53.22** Traumatic rupture of left radial collateral ligament

√5ᵗʰ **S53.3** Traumatic rupture of ulnar collateral ligament

EXCLUDES 1   sprain of ulnar collateral ligament (S53.44-)

√x7ᵗʰ **S53.30** Traumatic rupture of unspecified ulnar collateral ligament ▽

√x7ᵗʰ **S53.31** Traumatic rupture of right ulnar collateral ligament

√x7ᵗʰ **S53.32** Traumatic rupture of left ulnar collateral ligament

√5ᵗʰ **S53.4** Sprain of elbow

EXCLUDES 2   traumatic rupture of radial collateral ligament (S53.2-)

traumatic rupture of ulnar collateral ligament (S53.3-)

√6ᵗʰ **S53.40** Unspecified sprain of elbow

√7ᵗʰ **S53.401** Unspecified sprain of right elbow ▽

√7ᵗʰ **S53.402** Unspecified sprain of left elbow ▽

√7ᵗʰ **S53.409** Unspecified sprain of unspecified elbow ▽

Sprain of elbow NOS

√6ᵗʰ **S53.41** Radiohumeral (joint) sprain

√7ᵗʰ **S53.411** Radiohumeral (joint) sprain of right elbow

√7ᵗʰ **S53.412** Radiohumeral (joint) sprain of left elbow

√7ᵗʰ **S53.419** Radiohumeral (joint) sprain of unspecified elbow ▽

√6ᵗʰ **S53.42** Ulnohumeral (joint) sprain

√7ᵗʰ **S53.421** Ulnohumeral (joint) sprain of right elbow

√7ᵗʰ **S53.422** Ulnohumeral (joint) sprain of left elbow

√7ᵗʰ **S53.429** Ulnohumeral (joint) sprain of unspecified elbow ▽

√6ᵗʰ **S53.43** Radial collateral ligament sprain

√7ᵗʰ **S53.431** Radial collateral ligament sprain of right elbow

√7ᵗʰ **S53.432** Radial collateral ligament sprain of left elbow

---

☑ Additional Character Req   √x7ᵗʰ Placeholder Alert   Manifestation   ▽ Unspecified   ▶◀ Revised Text   ● New Code   ▲ Revised Code Title

S53.439 Radial collateral ligament sprain of unspecified elbow ▽

√6ᵗʰ **S53.44** Ulnar collateral ligament sprain

  √7ᵗʰ **S53.441** Ulnar collateral ligament sprain of right elbow

  √7ᵗʰ **S53.442** Ulnar collateral ligament sprain of left elbow

  √7ᵗʰ **S53.449** Ulnar collateral ligament sprain of unspecified elbow ▽

√6ᵗʰ **S53.49** Other sprain of elbow

  √7ᵗʰ **S53.491** Other sprain of right elbow

  √7ᵗʰ **S53.492** Other sprain of left elbow

  √7ᵗʰ **S53.499** Other sprain of unspecified elbow ▽

√4ᵗʰ **S54** Injury of nerves at forearm level

Code also any associated open wound (S51.-)

EXCLUDES 2   injury of nerves at wrist and hand level (S64.-)

The appropriate 7th character is to be added to each code from category S54.
A initial encounter
D subsequent encounter
S sequela

√5ᵗʰ **S54.0** Injury of ulnar nerve at forearm level

Injury of ulnar nerve NOS

√x7ᵗʰ **S54.00** Injury of ulnar nerve at forearm level, unspecified arm ▽

√x7ᵗʰ **S54.01** Injury of ulnar nerve at forearm level, right arm

√x7ᵗʰ **S54.02** Injury of ulnar nerve at forearm level, left arm

√5ᵗʰ **S54.1** Injury of median nerve at forearm level

Injury of median nerve NOS

√x7ᵗʰ **S54.10** Injury of median nerve at forearm level, unspecified arm ▽

√x7ᵗʰ **S54.11** Injury of median nerve at forearm level, right arm

√x7ᵗʰ **S54.12** Injury of median nerve at forearm level, left arm

√5ᵗʰ **S54.2** Injury of radial nerve at forearm level

Injury of radial nerve NOS

√x7ᵗʰ **S54.20** Injury of radial nerve at forearm level, unspecified arm ▽

√x7ᵗʰ **S54.21** Injury of radial nerve at forearm level, right arm

√x7ᵗʰ **S54.22** Injury of radial nerve at forearm level, left arm

√5ᵗʰ **S54.3** Injury of cutaneous sensory nerve at forearm level

√x7ᵗʰ **S54.30** Injury of cutaneous sensory nerve at forearm level, unspecified arm ▽

√x7ᵗʰ **S54.31** Injury of cutaneous sensory nerve at forearm level, right arm

√x7ᵗʰ **S54.32** Injury of cutaneous sensory nerve at forearm level, left arm

√5ᵗʰ **S54.8** Injury of other nerves at forearm level

√6ᵗʰ **S54.8X** Injury of other nerves at forearm level

  √7ᵗʰ **S54.8X1** Injury of other nerves at forearm level, right arm

  √7ᵗʰ **S54.8X2** Injury of other nerves at forearm level, left arm

  √7ᵗʰ **S54.8X9** Injury of other nerves at forearm level, unspecified arm ▽

√5ᵗʰ **S54.9** Injury of unspecified nerve at forearm level

√x7ᵗʰ **S54.90** Injury of unspecified nerve at forearm level, unspecified arm ▽

√x7ᵗʰ **S54.91** Injury of unspecified nerve at forearm level, right arm ▽

√x7ᵗʰ **S54.92** Injury of unspecified nerve at forearm level, left arm ▽

√4ᵗʰ **S55** Injury of blood vessels at forearm level

Code also any associated open wound (S51.-)

EXCLUDES 2   injury of blood vessels at wrist and hand level (S65.-)
         injury of brachial vessels (S45.1-S45.2)

The appropriate 7th character is to be added to each code from category S55.
A initial encounter
D subsequent encounter
S sequela

√5ᵗʰ **S55.0** Injury of ulnar artery at forearm level

√6ᵗʰ **S55.00** Unspecified injury of ulnar artery at forearm level

  √7ᵗʰ **S55.001** Unspecified injury of ulnar artery at forearm level, right arm ▽

  √7ᵗʰ **S55.002** Unspecified injury of ulnar artery at forearm level, left arm ▽

  √7ᵗʰ **S55.009** Unspecified injury of ulnar artery at forearm level, unspecified arm ▽

√6ᵗʰ **S55.01** Laceration of ulnar artery at forearm level

  √7ᵗʰ **S55.011** Laceration of ulnar artery at forearm level, right arm

  √7ᵗʰ **S55.012** Laceration of ulnar artery at forearm level, left arm

  √7ᵗʰ **S55.019** Laceration of ulnar artery at forearm level, unspecified arm ▽

√6ᵗʰ **S55.09** Other specified injury of ulnar artery at forearm level

  √7ᵗʰ **S55.091** Other specified injury of ulnar artery at forearm level, right arm

  √7ᵗʰ **S55.092** Other specified injury of ulnar artery at forearm level, left arm

  √7ᵗʰ **S55.099** Other specified injury of ulnar artery at forearm level, unspecified arm ▽

√5ᵗʰ **S55.1** Injury of radial artery at forearm level

√6ᵗʰ **S55.10** Unspecified injury of radial artery at forearm level

  √7ᵗʰ **S55.101** Unspecified injury of radial artery at forearm level, right arm

  √7ᵗʰ **S55.102** Unspecified injury of radial artery at forearm level, left arm ▽

  √7ᵗʰ **S55.109** Unspecified injury of radial artery at forearm level, unspecified arm ▽

√6ᵗʰ **S55.11** Laceration of radial artery at forearm level

  √7ᵗʰ **S55.111** Laceration of radial artery at forearm level, right arm

  √7ᵗʰ **S55.112** Laceration of radial artery at forearm level, left arm

  √7ᵗʰ **S55.119** Laceration of radial artery at forearm level, unspecified arm ▽

√6ᵗʰ **S55.19** Other specified injury of radial artery at forearm level

  √7ᵗʰ **S55.191** Other specified injury of radial artery at forearm level, right arm

  √7ᵗʰ **S55.192** Other specified injury of radial artery at forearm level, left arm

  √7ᵗʰ **S55.199** Other specified injury of radial artery at forearm level, unspecified arm ▽

√5ᵗʰ **S55.2** Injury of vein at forearm level

√6ᵗʰ **S55.20** Unspecified injury of vein at forearm level

  √7ᵗʰ **S55.201** Unspecified injury of vein at forearm level, right arm ▽

  √7ᵗʰ **S55.202** Unspecified injury of vein at forearm level, left arm ▽

  √7ᵗʰ **S55.209** Unspecified injury of vein at forearm level, unspecified arm ▽

√6ᵗʰ **S55.21** Laceration of vein at forearm level

  √7ᵗʰ **S55.211** Laceration of vein at forearm level, right arm

  √7ᵗʰ **S55.212** Laceration of vein at forearm level, left arm

  √7ᵗʰ **S55.219** Laceration of vein at forearm level, unspecified arm ▽

√6ᵗʰ **S55.29** Other specified injury of vein at forearm level

  √7ᵗʰ **S55.291** Other specified injury of vein at forearm level, right arm

  √7ᵗʰ **S55.292** Other specified injury of vein at forearm level, left arm

  √7ᵗʰ **S55.299** Other specified injury of vein at forearm level, unspecified arm ▽

√5ᵗʰ **S55.8** Injury of other blood vessels at forearm level

√6ᵗʰ **S55.80** Unspecified injury of other blood vessels at forearm level

  √7ᵗʰ **S55.801** Unspecified injury of other blood vessels at forearm level, right arm ▽

  √7ᵗʰ **S55.802** Unspecified injury of other blood vessels at forearm level, left arm ▽

  √7ᵗʰ **S55.809** Unspecified injury of other blood vessels at forearm level, unspecified arm ▽

√6ᵗʰ **S55.81** Laceration of other blood vessels at forearm level

  √7ᵗʰ **S55.811** Laceration of other blood vessels at forearm level, right arm

  √7ᵗʰ **S55.812** Laceration of other blood vessels at forearm level, left arm

√7ᵗʰ **S55.819** Laceration of other blood vessels at forearm level, unspecified arm ▽

√6ᵗʰ **S55.89** Other specified injury of other blood vessels at forearm level

　　√7ᵗʰ **S55.891** Other specified injury of other blood vessels at forearm level, right arm

　　√7ᵗʰ **S55.892** Other specified injury of other blood vessels at forearm level, left arm

　　√7ᵗʰ **S55.899** Other specified injury of other blood vessels at forearm level, unspecified arm ▽

√5ᵗʰ **S55.9** Injury of unspecified blood vessel at forearm level

　√6ᵗʰ **S55.90** Unspecified injury of unspecified blood vessel at forearm level

　　√7ᵗʰ **S55.901** Unspecified injury of unspecified blood vessel at forearm level, right arm ▽

　　√7ᵗʰ **S55.902** Unspecified injury of unspecified blood vessel at forearm level, left arm ▽

　　√7ᵗʰ **S55.909** Unspecified injury of unspecified blood vessel at forearm level, unspecified arm ▽

　√6ᵗʰ **S55.91** Laceration of unspecified blood vessel at forearm level

　　√7ᵗʰ **S55.911** Laceration of unspecified blood vessel at forearm level, right arm ▽

　　√7ᵗʰ **S55.912** Laceration of unspecified blood vessel at forearm level, left arm ▽

　　√7ᵗʰ **S55.919** Laceration of unspecified blood vessel at forearm level, unspecified arm ▽

　√6ᵗʰ **S55.99** Other specified injury of unspecified blood vessel at forearm level

　　√7ᵗʰ **S55.991** Other specified injury of unspecified blood vessel at forearm level, right arm ▽

　　√7ᵗʰ **S55.992** Other specified injury of unspecified blood vessel at forearm level, left arm ▽

　　√7ᵗʰ **S55.999** Other specified injury of unspecified blood vessel at forearm level, unspecified arm ▽

√4ᵗʰ **S56** **Injury of muscle, fascia and tendon at forearm level**

Code also any associated open wound (S51.-)

EXCLUDES 2　*injury of muscle, fascia and tendon at or below wrist (S66.-)*
sprain of joints and ligaments of elbow (S53.4-)

TIP: Refer to the Muscle/Tendon table at the beginning of this chapter

The appropriate 7th character is to be added to each code from category S56.
A　initial encounter
D　subsequent encounter
S　sequela

√5ᵗʰ **S56.0** Injury of flexor muscle, fascia and tendon of thumb at forearm level

　√6ᵗʰ **S56.00** Unspecified injury of flexor muscle, fascia and tendon of thumb at forearm level

　　√7ᵗʰ **S56.001** Unspecified injury of flexor muscle, fascia and tendon of right thumb at forearm level ▽

　　√7ᵗʰ **S56.002** Unspecified injury of flexor muscle, fascia and tendon of left thumb at forearm level ▽

　　√7ᵗʰ **S56.009** Unspecified injury of flexor muscle, fascia and tendon of unspecified thumb at forearm level ▽

　√6ᵗʰ **S56.01** Strain of flexor muscle, fascia and tendon of thumb at forearm level

　　√7ᵗʰ **S56.011** Strain of flexor muscle, fascia and tendon of right thumb at forearm level

　　√7ᵗʰ **S56.012** Strain of flexor muscle, fascia and tendon of left thumb at forearm level

　　√7ᵗʰ **S56.019** Strain of flexor muscle, fascia and tendon of unspecified thumb at forearm level ▽

　√6ᵗʰ **S56.02** Laceration of flexor muscle, fascia and tendon of thumb at forearm level

　　√7ᵗʰ **S56.021** Laceration of flexor muscle, fascia and tendon of right thumb at forearm level

　　√7ᵗʰ **S56.022** Laceration of flexor muscle, fascia and tendon of left thumb at forearm level

√7ᵗʰ **S56.029** Laceration of flexor muscle, fascia and tendon of unspecified thumb at forearm level ▽

√6ᵗʰ **S56.09** Other injury of flexor muscle, fascia and tendon of thumb at forearm level

　√7ᵗʰ **S56.091** Other injury of flexor muscle, fascia and tendon of right thumb at forearm level

　√7ᵗʰ **S56.092** Other injury of flexor muscle, fascia and tendon of left thumb at forearm level

　√7ᵗʰ **S56.099** Other injury of flexor muscle, fascia and tendon of unspecified thumb at forearm level ▽

√5ᵗʰ **S56.1** Injury of flexor muscle, fascia and tendon of other and unspecified finger at forearm level

　√6ᵗʰ **S56.10** Unspecified injury of flexor muscle, fascia and tendon of other and unspecified finger at forearm level

　　√7ᵗʰ **S56.101** Unspecified injury of flexor muscle, fascia and tendon of right index finger at forearm level ▽

　　√7ᵗʰ **S56.102** Unspecified injury of flexor muscle, fascia and tendon of left index finger at forearm level ▽

　　√7ᵗʰ **S56.103** Unspecified injury of flexor muscle, fascia and tendon of right middle finger at forearm level ▽

　　√7ᵗʰ **S56.104** Unspecified injury of flexor muscle, fascia and tendon of left middle finger at forearm level ▽

　　√7ᵗʰ **S56.105** Unspecified injury of flexor muscle, fascia and tendon of right ring finger at forearm level ▽

　　√7ᵗʰ **S56.106** Unspecified injury of flexor muscle, fascia and tendon of left ring finger at forearm level ▽

　　√7ᵗʰ **S56.107** Unspecified injury of flexor muscle, fascia and tendon of right little finger at forearm level ▽

　　√7ᵗʰ **S56.108** Unspecified injury of flexor muscle, fascia and tendon of left little finger at forearm level ▽

　　√7ᵗʰ **S56.109** Unspecified injury of flexor muscle, fascia and tendon of unspecified finger at forearm level ▽

　√6ᵗʰ **S56.11** Strain of flexor muscle, fascia and tendon of other and unspecified finger at forearm level

　　√7ᵗʰ **S56.111** Strain of flexor muscle, fascia and tendon of right index finger at forearm level

　　√7ᵗʰ **S56.112** Strain of flexor muscle, fascia and tendon of left index finger at forearm level

　　√7ᵗʰ **S56.113** Strain of flexor muscle, fascia and tendon of right middle finger at forearm level

　　√7ᵗʰ **S56.114** Strain of flexor muscle, fascia and tendon of left middle finger at forearm level

　　√7ᵗʰ **S56.115** Strain of flexor muscle, fascia and tendon of right ring finger at forearm level

　　√7ᵗʰ **S56.116** Strain of flexor muscle, fascia and tendon of left ring finger at forearm level

　　√7ᵗʰ **S56.117** Strain of flexor muscle, fascia and tendon of right little finger at forearm level

　　√7ᵗʰ **S56.118** Strain of flexor muscle, fascia and tendon of left little finger at forearm level

　　√7ᵗʰ **S56.119** Strain of flexor muscle, fascia and tendon of finger of unspecified finger at forearm level ▽

　√6ᵗʰ **S56.12** Laceration of flexor muscle, fascia and tendon of other and unspecified finger at forearm level

　　√7ᵗʰ **S56.121** Laceration of flexor muscle, fascia and tendon of right index finger at forearm level

　　√7ᵗʰ **S56.122** Laceration of flexor muscle, fascia and tendon of left index finger at forearm level

　　√7ᵗʰ **S56.123** Laceration of flexor muscle, fascia and tendon of right middle finger at forearm level

　　√7ᵗʰ **S56.124** Laceration of flexor muscle, fascia and tendon of left middle finger at forearm level

　　√7ᵗʰ **S56.125** Laceration of flexor muscle, fascia and tendon of right ring finger at forearm level

　　√7ᵗʰ **S56.126** Laceration of flexor muscle, fascia and tendon of left ring finger at forearm level

√7ᵗʰ **S56.127** Laceration of flexor muscle, fascia and tendon of **right little finger** at forearm level

√7ᵗʰ **S56.128** Laceration of flexor muscle, fascia and tendon of **left little finger** at forearm level

√7ᵗʰ **S56.129** Laceration of flexor muscle, fascia and tendon of **unspecified finger** at forearm level ▽

√6ᵗʰ **S56.19** Other injury of flexor muscle, fascia and tendon of **other and unspecified finger** at forearm level

√7ᵗʰ **S56.191** Other injury of flexor muscle, fascia and tendon of **right index finger** at forearm level

√7ᵗʰ **S56.192** Other injury of flexor muscle, fascia and tendon of **left index finger** at forearm level

√7ᵗʰ **S56.193** Other injury of flexor muscle, fascia and tendon of **right middle finger** at forearm level

√7ᵗʰ **S56.194** Other injury of flexor muscle, fascia and tendon of **left middle finger** at forearm level

√7ᵗʰ **S56.195** Other injury of flexor muscle, fascia and tendon of **right ring finger** at forearm level

√7ᵗʰ **S56.196** Other injury of flexor muscle, fascia and tendon of **left ring finger** at forearm level

√7ᵗʰ **S56.197** Other injury of flexor muscle, fascia and tendon of **right little finger** at forearm level

√7ᵗʰ **S56.198** Other injury of flexor muscle, fascia and tendon of **left little finger** at forearm level

√7ᵗʰ **S56.199** Other injury of flexor muscle, fascia and tendon of **unspecified finger** at forearm level ▽

√5ᵗʰ **S56.2** Injury of other flexor muscle, fascia and tendon at forearm level

√6ᵗʰ **S56.20** Unspecified injury of other flexor muscle, fascia and tendon at forearm level

√7ᵗʰ **S56.201** Unspecified injury of other flexor muscle, fascia and tendon at forearm level, **right arm** ▽

√7ᵗʰ **S56.202** Unspecified injury of other flexor muscle, fascia and tendon at forearm level, **left arm** ▽

√7ᵗʰ **S56.209** Unspecified injury of other flexor muscle, fascia and tendon at forearm level, **unspecified arm** ▽

√6ᵗʰ **S56.21** Strain of other flexor muscle, fascia and tendon at forearm level

√7ᵗʰ **S56.211** Strain of other flexor muscle, fascia and tendon at forearm level, **right arm**

√7ᵗʰ **S56.212** Strain of other flexor muscle, fascia and tendon at forearm level, **left arm**

√7ᵗʰ **S56.219** Strain of other flexor muscle, fascia and tendon at forearm level, **unspecified arm** ▽

√6ᵗʰ **S56.22** Laceration of other flexor muscle, fascia and tendon at forearm level

√7ᵗʰ **S56.221** Laceration of other flexor muscle, fascia and tendon at forearm level, **right arm**

√7ᵗʰ **S56.222** Laceration of other flexor muscle, fascia and tendon at forearm level, **left arm**

√7ᵗʰ **S56.229** Laceration of other flexor muscle, fascia and tendon at forearm level, **unspecified arm** ▽

√6ᵗʰ **S56.29** Other injury of other flexor muscle, fascia and tendon at forearm level

√7ᵗʰ **S56.291** Other injury of other flexor muscle, fascia and tendon at forearm level, **right arm**

√7ᵗʰ **S56.292** Other injury of other flexor muscle, fascia and tendon at forearm level, **left arm**

√7ᵗʰ **S56.299** Other injury of other flexor muscle, fascia and tendon at forearm level, **unspecified arm** ▽

√5ᵗʰ **S56.3** Injury of **extensor or abductor** muscles, fascia and tendons of **thumb** at forearm level

√6ᵗʰ **S56.30** Unspecified injury of extensor or abductor muscles, fascia and tendons of thumb at forearm level

√7ᵗʰ **S56.301** Unspecified injury of extensor or abductor muscles, fascia and tendons of **right thumb** at forearm level ▽

√7ᵗʰ **S56.302** Unspecified injury of extensor or abductor muscles, fascia and tendons of **left thumb** at forearm level ▽

√7ᵗʰ **S56.309** Unspecified injury of extensor or abductor muscles, fascia and tendons of **unspecified thumb** at forearm level ▽

√6ᵗʰ **S56.31** Strain of extensor or abductor muscles, fascia and tendons of thumb at forearm level

√7ᵗʰ **S56.311** Strain of extensor or abductor muscles, fascia and tendons of **right thumb** at forearm level

√7ᵗʰ **S56.312** Strain of extensor or abductor muscles, fascia and tendons of **left thumb** at forearm level

√7ᵗʰ **S56.319** Strain of extensor or abductor muscles, fascia and tendons of **unspecified thumb** at forearm level ▽

√6ᵗʰ **S56.32** Laceration of extensor or abductor muscles, fascia and tendons of thumb at forearm level

√7ᵗʰ **S56.321** Laceration of extensor or abductor muscles, fascia and tendons of **right thumb** at forearm level

√7ᵗʰ **S56.322** Laceration of extensor or abductor muscles, fascia and tendons of **left thumb** at forearm level

√7ᵗʰ **S56.329** Laceration of extensor or abductor muscles, fascia and tendons of **unspecified thumb** at forearm level ▽

√6ᵗʰ **S56.39** Other injury of extensor or abductor muscles, fascia and tendons of thumb at forearm level

√7ᵗʰ **S56.391** Other injury of extensor or abductor muscles, fascia and tendons of **right thumb** at forearm level

√7ᵗʰ **S56.392** Other injury of extensor or abductor muscles, fascia and tendons of **left thumb** at forearm level

√7ᵗʰ **S56.399** Other injury of extensor or abductor muscles, fascia and tendons of **unspecified thumb** at forearm level ▽

√5ᵗʰ **S56.4** Injury of **extensor** muscle, fascia and tendon of other and unspecified **finger** at forearm level

√6ᵗʰ **S56.40** Unspecified injury of extensor muscle, fascia and tendon of other and unspecified finger at forearm level

√7ᵗʰ **S56.401** Unspecified injury of extensor muscle, fascia and tendon of **right index finger** at forearm level ▽

√7ᵗʰ **S56.402** Unspecified injury of extensor muscle, fascia and tendon of **left index finger** at forearm level ▽

√7ᵗʰ **S56.403** Unspecified injury of extensor muscle, fascia and tendon of **right middle finger** at forearm level ▽

√7ᵗʰ **S56.404** Unspecified injury of extensor muscle, fascia and tendon of **left middle finger** at forearm level ▽

√7ᵗʰ **S56.405** Unspecified injury of extensor muscle, fascia and tendon of **right ring finger** at forearm level ▽

√7ᵗʰ **S56.406** Unspecified injury of extensor muscle, fascia and tendon of **left ring finger** at forearm level ▽

√7ᵗʰ **S56.407** Unspecified injury of extensor muscle, fascia and tendon of **right little finger** at forearm level ▽

√7ᵗʰ **S56.408** Unspecified injury of extensor muscle, fascia and tendon of **left little finger** at forearm level ▽

√7ᵗʰ **S56.409** Unspecified injury of extensor muscle, fascia and tendon of **unspecified finger** at forearm level ▽

√6ᵗʰ **S56.41** Strain of extensor muscle, fascia and tendon of other and unspecified finger at forearm level

√7ᵗʰ **S56.411** Strain of extensor muscle, fascia and tendon of **right index finger** at forearm level

√7ᵗʰ **S56.412** Strain of extensor muscle, fascia and tendon of **left index finger** at forearm level

√7ᵗʰ **S56.413** Strain of extensor muscle, fascia and tendon of right middle finger at forearm level

√7ᵗʰ **S56.414** Strain of extensor muscle, fascia and tendon of left middle finger at forearm level

√7ᵗʰ **S56.415** Strain of extensor muscle, fascia and tendon of right ring finger at forearm level

√7ᵗʰ **S56.416** Strain of extensor muscle, fascia and tendon of left ring finger at forearm level

√7ᵗʰ **S56.417** Strain of extensor muscle, fascia and tendon of right little finger at forearm level

√7ᵗʰ **S56.418** Strain of extensor muscle, fascia and tendon of left little finger at forearm level

√7ᵗʰ **S56.419** Strain of extensor muscle, fascia and tendon of finger, unspecified finger at forearm level ▽

√6ᵗʰ **S56.42** Laceration of extensor muscle, fascia and tendon of other and unspecified finger at forearm level

√7ᵗʰ **S56.421** Laceration of extensor muscle, fascia and tendon of right index finger at forearm level

√7ᵗʰ **S56.422** Laceration of extensor muscle, fascia and tendon of left index finger at forearm level

√7ᵗʰ **S56.423** Laceration of extensor muscle, fascia and tendon of right middle finger at forearm level

√7ᵗʰ **S56.424** Laceration of extensor muscle, fascia and tendon of left middle finger at forearm level

√7ᵗʰ **S56.425** Laceration of extensor muscle, fascia and tendon of right ring finger at forearm level

√7ᵗʰ **S56.426** Laceration of extensor muscle, fascia and tendon of left ring finger at forearm level

√7ᵗʰ **S56.427** Laceration of extensor muscle, fascia and tendon of right little finger at forearm level

√7ᵗʰ **S56.428** Laceration of extensor muscle, fascia and tendon of left little finger at forearm level

√7ᵗʰ **S56.429** Laceration of extensor muscle, fascia and tendon of unspecified finger at forearm level ▽

√6ᵗʰ **S56.49** Other injury of extensor muscle, fascia and tendon of other and unspecified finger at forearm level

√7ᵗʰ **S56.491** Other injury of extensor muscle, fascia and tendon of right index finger at forearm level

√7ᵗʰ **S56.492** Other injury of extensor muscle, fascia and tendon of left index finger at forearm level

√7ᵗʰ **S56.493** Other injury of extensor muscle, fascia and tendon of right middle finger at forearm level

√7ᵗʰ **S56.494** Other injury of extensor muscle, fascia and tendon of left middle finger at forearm level

√7ᵗʰ **S56.495** Other injury of extensor muscle, fascia and tendon of right ring finger at forearm level

√7ᵗʰ **S56.496** Other injury of extensor muscle, fascia and tendon of left ring finger at forearm level

√7ᵗʰ **S56.497** Other injury of extensor muscle, fascia and tendon of right little finger at forearm level

√7ᵗʰ **S56.498** Other injury of extensor muscle, fascia and tendon of left little finger at forearm level

√7ᵗʰ **S56.499** Other injury of extensor muscle, fascia and tendon of unspecified finger at forearm level ▽

√5ᵗʰ **S56.5** Injury of other extensor muscle, fascia and tendon at forearm level

√6ᵗʰ **S56.50** Unspecified injury of other extensor muscle, fascia and tendon at forearm level

√7ᵗʰ **S56.501** Unspecified injury of other extensor muscle, fascia and tendon at forearm level, right arm ▽

√7ᵗʰ **S56.502** Unspecified injury of other extensor muscle, fascia and tendon at forearm level, left arm ▽

√7ᵗʰ **S56.509** Unspecified injury of other extensor muscle, fascia and tendon at forearm level, unspecified arm ▽

√6ᵗʰ **S56.51** Strain of other extensor muscle, fascia and tendon at forearm level

√7ᵗʰ **S56.511** Strain of other extensor muscle, fascia and tendon at forearm level, right arm

√7ᵗʰ **S56.512** Strain of other extensor muscle, fascia and tendon at forearm level, left arm

√7ᵗʰ **S56.519** Strain of other extensor muscle, fascia and tendon at forearm level, unspecified arm ▽

√6ᵗʰ **S56.52** Laceration of other extensor muscle, fascia and tendon at forearm level

√7ᵗʰ **S56.521** Laceration of other extensor muscle, fascia and tendon at forearm level, right arm

√7ᵗʰ **S56.522** Laceration of other extensor muscle, fascia and tendon at forearm level, left arm

√7ᵗʰ **S56.529** Laceration of other extensor muscle, fascia and tendon at forearm level, unspecified arm ▽

√6ᵗʰ **S56.59** Other injury of other extensor muscle, fascia and tendon at forearm level

√7ᵗʰ **S56.591** Other injury of other extensor muscle, fascia and tendon at forearm level, right arm

√7ᵗʰ **S56.592** Other injury of other extensor muscle, fascia and tendon at forearm level, left arm

√7ᵗʰ **S56.599** Other injury of other extensor muscle, fascia and tendon at forearm level, unspecified arm ▽

√5ᵗʰ **S56.8** Injury of other muscles, fascia and tendons at forearm level

√6ᵗʰ **S56.80** Unspecified injury of other muscles, fascia and tendons at forearm level

√7ᵗʰ **S56.801** Unspecified injury of other muscles, fascia and tendons at forearm level, right arm ▽

√7ᵗʰ **S56.802** Unspecified injury of other muscles, fascia and tendons at forearm level, left arm ▽

√7ᵗʰ **S56.809** Unspecified injury of other muscles, fascia and tendons at forearm level, unspecified arm ▽

√6ᵗʰ **S56.81** Strain of other muscles, fascia and tendons at forearm level

√7ᵗʰ **S56.811** Strain of other muscles, fascia and tendons at forearm level, right arm

√7ᵗʰ **S56.812** Strain of other muscles, fascia and tendons at forearm level, left arm

√7ᵗʰ **S56.819** Strain of other muscles, fascia and tendons at forearm level, unspecified arm

√6ᵗʰ **S56.82** Laceration of other muscles, fascia and tendons at forearm level

√7ᵗʰ **S56.821** Laceration of other muscles, fascia and tendons at forearm level, right arm

√7ᵗʰ **S56.822** Laceration of other muscles, fascia and tendons at forearm level, left arm

√7ᵗʰ **S56.829** Laceration of other muscles, fascia and tendons at forearm level, unspecified arm ▽

√6ᵗʰ **S56.89** Other injury of other muscles, fascia and tendons at forearm level

√7ᵗʰ **S56.891** Other injury of other muscles, fascia and tendons at forearm level, right arm

√7ᵗʰ **S56.892** Other injury of other muscles, fascia and tendons at forearm level, left arm

√7ᵗʰ **S56.899** Other injury of other muscles, fascia and tendons at forearm level, unspecified arm ▽

√5ᵗʰ **S56.9** Injury of unspecified muscles, fascia and tendons at forearm level

√6ᵗʰ **S56.90** Unspecified injury of unspecified muscles, fascia and tendons at forearm level

√7ᵗʰ **S56.901** Unspecified injury of unspecified muscles, fascia and tendons at forearm level, right arm ▽

☑ Additional Character Req   √✗7ᵗʰ Placeholder Alert   Manifestation   ▽ Unspecified   ▶◀ Revised Text   ● New Code   ▲ Revised Code Title

ICD-10-CM 2019   1011

√7ᵗʰ **S56.902** Unspecified injury of unspecified muscles, fascia and tendons at forearm level, left arm ▽

√7ᵗʰ **S56.909** Unspecified injury of unspecified muscles, fascia and tendons at forearm level, unspecified arm ▽

√6ᵗʰ **S56.91** Strain of unspecified muscles, fascia and tendons at forearm level

√7ᵗʰ **S56.911** Strain of unspecified muscles, fascia and tendons at forearm level, right arm ▽

√7ᵗʰ **S56.912** Strain of unspecified muscles, fascia and tendons at forearm level, left arm ▽

√7ᵗʰ **S56.919** Strain of unspecified muscles, fascia and tendons at forearm level, unspecified arm ▽

√6ᵗʰ **S56.92** Laceration of unspecified muscles, fascia and tendons at forearm level

√7ᵗʰ **S56.921** Laceration of unspecified muscles, fascia and tendons at forearm level, right arm ▽

√7ᵗʰ **S56.922** Laceration of unspecified muscles, fascia and tendons at forearm level, left arm ▽

√7ᵗʰ **S56.929** Laceration of unspecified muscles, fascia and tendons at forearm level, unspecified arm ▽

√6ᵗʰ **S56.99** Other injury of unspecified muscles, fascia and tendons at forearm level

√7ᵗʰ **S56.991** Other injury of unspecified muscles, fascia and tendons at forearm level, right arm ▽

√7ᵗʰ **S56.992** Other injury of unspecified muscles, fascia and tendons at forearm level, left arm ▽

√7ᵗʰ **S56.999** Other injury of unspecified muscles, fascia and tendons at forearm level, unspecified arm ▽

√4ᵗʰ **S57 Crushing injury of elbow and forearm**

Use additional code(s) for all associated injuries

EXCLUDES 2 *crushing injury of wrist and hand (S67.-)*

The appropriate 7th character is to be added to each code from category S57.
A   initial encounter
D   subsequent encounter
S   sequela

√5ᵗʰ **S57.0** Crushing injury of elbow

√x7ᵗʰ **S57.00** Crushing injury of unspecified elbow ▽

√x7ᵗʰ **S57.01** Crushing injury of right elbow

√x7ᵗʰ **S57.02** Crushing injury of left elbow

√5ᵗʰ **S57.8** Crushing injury of forearm

√x7ᵗʰ **S57.80** Crushing injury of unspecified forearm ▽

√x7ᵗʰ **S57.81** Crushing injury of right forearm

√x7ᵗʰ **S57.82** Crushing injury of left forearm

√4ᵗʰ **S58 Traumatic amputation of elbow and forearm**

An amputation not identified as partial or complete should be coded to complete

EXCLUDES 1 *traumatic amputation of wrist and hand (S68.-)*

The appropriate 7th character is to be added to each code from category S58.
A   initial encounter
D   subsequent encounter
S   sequela

√5ᵗʰ **S58.0** Traumatic amputation at elbow level

√6ᵗʰ **S58.01** Complete traumatic amputation at elbow level

² √7ᵗʰ **S58.011** Complete traumatic amputation at elbow level, right arm HCC

² √7ᵗʰ **S58.012** Complete traumatic amputation at elbow level, left arm HCC

² √7ᵗʰ **S58.019** Complete traumatic amputation at elbow level, unspecified arm HCC ▽

√6ᵗʰ **S58.02** Partial traumatic amputation at elbow level

² √7ᵗʰ **S58.021** Partial traumatic amputation at elbow level, right arm HCC

² √7ᵗʰ **S58.022** Partial traumatic amputation at elbow level, left arm HCC

² √7ᵗʰ **S58.029** Partial traumatic amputation at elbow level, unspecified arm HCC ▽

√5ᵗʰ **S58.1** Traumatic amputation at level between elbow and wrist

√6ᵗʰ **S58.11** Complete traumatic amputation at level between elbow and wrist

² √7ᵗʰ **S58.111** Complete traumatic amputation at level between elbow and wrist, right arm HCC

² √7ᵗʰ **S58.112** Complete traumatic amputation at level between elbow and wrist, left arm HCC

² √7ᵗʰ **S58.119** Complete traumatic amputation at level between elbow and wrist, unspecified arm HCC ▽

√6ᵗʰ **S58.12** Partial traumatic amputation at level between elbow and wrist

² √7ᵗʰ **S58.121** Partial traumatic amputation at level between elbow and wrist, right arm HCC

² √7ᵗʰ **S58.122** Partial traumatic amputation at level between elbow and wrist, left arm HCC

² √7ᵗʰ **S58.129** Partial traumatic amputation at level between elbow and wrist, unspecified arm HCC ▽

√5ᵗʰ **S58.9** Traumatic amputation of forearm, level unspecified

EXCLUDES 1 *traumatic amputation of wrist (S68.-)*

√6ᵗʰ **S58.91** Complete traumatic amputation of forearm, level unspecified

² √7ᵗʰ **S58.911** Complete traumatic amputation of right forearm, level unspecified HCC ▽

² √7ᵗʰ **S58.912** Complete traumatic amputation of left forearm, level unspecified HCC ▽

² √7ᵗʰ **S58.919** Complete traumatic amputation of unspecified forearm, level unspecified HCC ▽

√6ᵗʰ **S58.92** Partial traumatic amputation of forearm, level unspecified

² √7ᵗʰ **S58.921** Partial traumatic amputation of right forearm, level unspecified HCC ▽

² √7ᵗʰ **S58.922** Partial traumatic amputation of left forearm, level unspecified HCC ▽

² √7ᵗʰ **S58.929** Partial traumatic amputation of unspecified forearm, level unspecified HCC ▽

√4ᵗʰ **S59 Other and unspecified injuries of elbow and forearm**

EXCLUDES 2 *other and unspecified injuries of wrist and hand (S69.-)*

AHA: 2018,2Q,12; 2018,1Q,3; 2015,3Q,37-39

The appropriate 7th character is to be added to each code from subcategories S59.0, S59.1, and S59.2.
A   initial encounter for closed fracture
D   subsequent encounter for fracture with routine healing
G   subsequent encounter for fracture with delayed healing
K   subsequent encounter for fracture with nonunion
P   subsequent encounter for fracture with malunion
S   sequela

√5ᵗʰ **S59.0** Physeal fracture of lower end of ulna

√6ᵗʰ **S59.00** Unspecified physeal fracture of lower end of ulna

√7ᵗʰ **S59.001** Unspecified physeal fracture of lower end of ulna, right arm Q ▽

√7ᵗʰ **S59.002** Unspecified physeal fracture of lower end of ulna, left arm Q ▽

√7ᵗʰ **S59.009** Unspecified physeal fracture of lower end of ulna, unspecified arm Q ▽

√6ᵗʰ **S59.01** Salter-Harris Type I physeal fracture of lower end of ulna

√7ᵗʰ **S59.011** Salter-Harris Type I physeal fracture of lower end of ulna, right arm Q

√7ᵗʰ **S59.012** Salter-Harris Type I physeal fracture of lower end of ulna, left arm Q

√7ᵗʰ **S59.019** Salter-Harris Type I physeal fracture of lower end of ulna, unspecified arm Q ▽

√6ᵗʰ **S59.02** Salter-Harris Type II physeal fracture of lower end of ulna

√7ᵗʰ **S59.021** Salter-Harris Type II physeal fracture of lower end of ulna, right arm Q

√7ᵗʰ **S59.022** Salter-Harris Type II physeal fracture of lower end of ulna, left arm

√7ᵗʰ **S59.029** Salter-Harris Type II physeal fracture of lower end of ulna, unspecified arm

√6ᵗʰ **S59.03** Salter-Harris Type III physeal fracture of lower end of ulna

√7ᵗʰ **S59.031** Salter-Harris Type III physeal fracture of lower end of ulna, right arm

√7ᵗʰ **S59.032** Salter-Harris Type III physeal fracture of lower end of ulna, left arm

√7ᵗʰ **S59.039** Salter-Harris Type III physeal fracture of lower end of ulna, unspecified arm

√6ᵗʰ **S59.04** Salter-Harris Type IV physeal fracture of lower end of ulna

√7ᵗʰ **S59.041** Salter-Harris Type IV physeal fracture of lower end of ulna, right arm

√7ᵗʰ **S59.042** Salter-Harris Type IV physeal fracture of lower end of ulna, left arm

√7ᵗʰ **S59.049** Salter-Harris Type IV physeal fracture of lower end of ulna, unspecified arm

√6ᵗʰ **S59.09** Other physeal fracture of lower end of ulna

√7ᵗʰ **S59.091** Other physeal fracture of lower end of ulna, right arm

√7ᵗʰ **S59.092** Other physeal fracture of lower end of ulna, left arm

√7ᵗʰ **S59.099** Other physeal fracture of lower end of ulna, unspecified arm

√5ᵗʰ **S59.1** Physeal fracture of upper end of radius

√6ᵗʰ **S59.10** Unspecified physeal fracture of upper end of radius

√7ᵗʰ **S59.101** Unspecified physeal fracture of upper end of radius, right arm

√7ᵗʰ **S59.102** Unspecified physeal fracture of upper end of radius, left arm

√7ᵗʰ **S59.109** Unspecified physeal fracture of upper end of radius, unspecified arm

√6ᵗʰ **S59.11** Salter-Harris Type I physeal fracture of upper end of radius

√7ᵗʰ **S59.111** Salter-Harris Type I physeal fracture of upper end of radius, right arm

√7ᵗʰ **S59.112** Salter-Harris Type I physeal fracture of upper end of radius, left arm

√7ᵗʰ **S59.119** Salter-Harris Type I physeal fracture of upper end of radius, unspecified arm

√6ᵗʰ **S59.12** Salter-Harris Type II physeal fracture of upper end of radius

√7ᵗʰ **S59.121** Salter-Harris Type II physeal fracture of upper end of radius, right arm

√7ᵗʰ **S59.122** Salter-Harris Type II physeal fracture of upper end of radius, left arm

√7ᵗʰ **S59.129** Salter-Harris Type II physeal fracture of upper end of radius, unspecified arm

√6ᵗʰ **S59.13** Salter-Harris Type III physeal fracture of upper end of radius

√7ᵗʰ **S59.131** Salter-Harris Type III physeal fracture of upper end of radius, right arm

√7ᵗʰ **S59.132** Salter-Harris Type III physeal fracture of upper end of radius, left arm

√7ᵗʰ **S59.139** Salter-Harris Type III physeal fracture of upper end of radius, unspecified arm

√6ᵗʰ **S59.14** Salter-Harris Type IV physeal fracture of upper end of radius

√7ᵗʰ **S59.141** Salter-Harris Type IV physeal fracture of upper end of radius, right arm

√7ᵗʰ **S59.142** Salter-Harris Type IV physeal fracture of upper end of radius, left arm

√7ᵗʰ **S59.149** Salter-Harris Type IV physeal fracture of upper end of radius, unspecified arm

√6ᵗʰ **S59.19** Other physeal fracture of upper end of radius

√7ᵗʰ **S59.191** Other physeal fracture of upper end of radius, right arm

√7ᵗʰ **S59.192** Other physeal fracture of upper end of radius, left arm

√7ᵗʰ **S59.199** Other physeal fracture of upper end of radius, unspecified arm

√5ᵗʰ **S59.2** Physeal fracture of lower end of radius

√6ᵗʰ **S59.20** Unspecified physeal fracture of lower end of radius

√7ᵗʰ **S59.201** Unspecified physeal fracture of lower end of radius, right arm

√7ᵗʰ **S59.202** Unspecified physeal fracture of lower end of radius, left arm

√7ᵗʰ **S59.209** Unspecified physeal fracture of lower end of radius, unspecified arm

√6ᵗʰ **S59.21** Salter-Harris Type I physeal fracture of lower end of radius

√7ᵗʰ **S59.211** Salter-Harris Type I physeal fracture of lower end of radius, right arm

√7ᵗʰ **S59.212** Salter-Harris Type I physeal fracture of lower end of radius, left arm

√7ᵗʰ **S59.219** Salter-Harris Type I physeal fracture of lower end of radius, unspecified arm

√6ᵗʰ **S59.22** Salter-Harris Type II physeal fracture of lower end of radius

√7ᵗʰ **S59.221** Salter-Harris Type II physeal fracture of lower end of radius, right arm

√7ᵗʰ **S59.222** Salter-Harris Type II physeal fracture of lower end of radius, left arm

√7ᵗʰ **S59.229** Salter-Harris Type II physeal fracture of lower end of radius, unspecified arm

√6ᵗʰ **S59.23** Salter-Harris Type III physeal fracture of lower end of radius

√7ᵗʰ **S59.231** Salter-Harris Type III physeal fracture of lower end of radius, right arm

√7ᵗʰ **S59.232** Salter-Harris Type III physeal fracture of lower end of radius, left arm

√7ᵗʰ **S59.239** Salter-Harris Type III physeal fracture of lower end of radius, unspecified arm

√6ᵗʰ **S59.24** Salter-Harris Type IV physeal fracture of lower end of radius

√7ᵗʰ **S59.241** Salter-Harris Type IV physeal fracture of lower end of radius, right arm

√7ᵗʰ **S59.242** Salter-Harris Type IV physeal fracture of lower end of radius, left arm

√7ᵗʰ **S59.249** Salter-Harris Type IV physeal fracture of lower end of radius, unspecified arm

√6ᵗʰ **S59.29** Other physeal fracture of lower end of radius

√7ᵗʰ **S59.291** Other physeal fracture of lower end of radius, right arm

√7ᵗʰ **S59.292** Other physeal fracture of lower end of radius, left arm

√7ᵗʰ **S59.299** Other physeal fracture of lower end of radius, unspecified arm

√5ᵗʰ **S59.8** Other specified injuries of elbow and forearm

The appropriate 7th character is to be added to each code in subcategory S59.8.
A   initial encounter
D   subsequent encounter
S   sequela

√6ᵗʰ **S59.80** Other specified injuries of elbow

√7ᵗʰ **S59.801** Other specified injuries of right elbow

√7ᵗʰ **S59.802** **Other specified injuries of left elbow**

√7ᵗʰ **S59.809** **Other specified injuries of unspecified elbow** ▽

√6ᵗʰ **S59.81** **Other specified injuries of forearm**

√7ᵗʰ **S59.811** **Other specified injuries right forearm**

√7ᵗʰ **S59.812** **Other specified injuries left forearm**

√7ᵗʰ **S59.819** **Other specified injuries unspecified forearm** ▽

√5ᵗʰ **S59.9** **Unspecified injury of elbow and forearm**

> The appropriate 7th character is to be added to each code in subcategory S59.9.
> A   initial encounter
> D   subsequent encounter
> S   sequela

√6ᵗʰ **S59.90** **Unspecified injury of elbow**

√7ᵗʰ **S59.901** **Unspecified injury of right elbow** ▽

√7ᵗʰ **S59.902** **Unspecified injury of left elbow** ▽

√7ᵗʰ **S59.909** **Unspecified injury of unspecified elbow** ▽

√6ᵗʰ **S59.91** **Unspecified injury of forearm**

√7ᵗʰ **S59.911** **Unspecified injury of right forearm** ▽

√7ᵗʰ **S59.912** **Unspecified injury of left forearm** ▽

√7ᵗʰ **S59.919** **Unspecified injury of unspecified forearm** ▽

Injuries to the wrist, hand and fingers (S60-S69)

EXCLUDES 2   *burns and corrosions (T20-T32)*
frostbite (T33-T34)
insect bite or sting, venomous (T63.4)

√4ᵗʰ **S60** **Superficial injury of wrist, hand and fingers**

> The appropriate 7th character is to be added to each code from category S60.
> A   initial encounter
> D   subsequent encounter
> S   sequela

√5ᵗʰ **S60.0** **Contusion of finger without damage to nail**

EXCLUDES 1   *contusion involving nail (matrix) (S60.1)*

√x7ᵗʰ **S60.00** **Contusion of unspecified finger without damage to nail** ▽
Contusion of finger(s) NOS

√6ᵗʰ **S60.01** **Contusion of thumb without damage to nail**

√7ᵗʰ **S60.011** **Contusion of right thumb without damage to nail**

√7ᵗʰ **S60.012** **Contusion of left thumb without damage to nail**

√7ᵗʰ **S60.019** **Contusion of unspecified thumb without damage to nail** ▽

√6ᵗʰ **S60.02** **Contusion of index finger without damage to nail**

√7ᵗʰ **S60.021** **Contusion of right index finger without damage to nail**

√7ᵗʰ **S60.022** **Contusion of left index finger without damage to nail**

√7ᵗʰ **S60.029** **Contusion of unspecified index finger without damage to nail** ▽

√6ᵗʰ **S60.03** **Contusion of middle finger without damage to nail**

√7ᵗʰ **S60.031** **Contusion of right middle finger without damage to nail**

√7ᵗʰ **S60.032** **Contusion of left middle finger without damage to nail**

√7ᵗʰ **S60.039** **Contusion of unspecified middle finger without damage to nail** ▽

√6ᵗʰ **S60.04** **Contusion of ring finger without damage to nail**

√7ᵗʰ **S60.041** **Contusion of right ring finger without damage to nail**

√7ᵗʰ **S60.042** **Contusion of left ring finger without damage to nail**

√7ᵗʰ **S60.049** **Contusion of unspecified ring finger without damage to nail** ▽

√6ᵗʰ **S60.05** **Contusion of little finger without damage to nail**

√7ᵗʰ **S60.051** **Contusion of right little finger without damage to nail**

√7ᵗʰ **S60.052** **Contusion of left little finger without damage to nail**

√7ᵗʰ **S60.059** **Contusion of unspecified little finger without damage to nail** ▽

√5ᵗʰ **S60.1** **Contusion of finger with damage to nail**

√x7ᵗʰ **S60.10** **Contusion of unspecified finger with damage to nail** ▽

√6ᵗʰ **S60.11** **Contusion of thumb with damage to nail**

√7ᵗʰ **S60.111** **Contusion of right thumb with damage to nail**

√7ᵗʰ **S60.112** **Contusion of left thumb with damage to nail**

√7ᵗʰ **S60.119** **Contusion of unspecified thumb with damage to nail** ▽

√6ᵗʰ **S60.12** **Contusion of index finger with damage to nail**

√7ᵗʰ **S60.121** **Contusion of right index finger with damage to nail**

√7ᵗʰ **S60.122** **Contusion of left index finger with damage to nail**

√7ᵗʰ **S60.129** **Contusion of unspecified index finger with damage to nail** ▽

√6ᵗʰ **S60.13** **Contusion of middle finger with damage to nail**

√7ᵗʰ **S60.131** **Contusion of right middle finger with damage to nail**

√7ᵗʰ **S60.132** **Contusion of left middle finger with damage to nail**

√7ᵗʰ **S60.139** **Contusion of unspecified middle finger with damage to nail** ▽

√6ᵗʰ **S60.14** **Contusion of ring finger with damage to nail**

√7ᵗʰ **S60.141** **Contusion of right ring finger with damage to nail**

√7ᵗʰ **S60.142** **Contusion of left ring finger with damage to nail**

√7ᵗʰ **S60.149** **Contusion of unspecified ring finger with damage to nail** ▽

√6ᵗʰ **S60.15** **Contusion of little finger with damage to nail**

√7ᵗʰ **S60.151** **Contusion of right little finger with damage to nail**

√7ᵗʰ **S60.152** **Contusion of left little finger with damage to nail**

√7ᵗʰ **S60.159** **Contusion of unspecified little finger with damage to nail** ▽

√5ᵗʰ **S60.2** **Contusion of wrist and hand**

EXCLUDES 2   *contusion of fingers (S60.0-, S60.1-)*

√6ᵗʰ **S60.21** **Contusion of wrist**

√7ᵗʰ **S60.211** **Contusion of right wrist**

√7ᵗʰ **S60.212** **Contusion of left wrist**

√7ᵗʰ **S60.219** **Contusion of unspecified wrist** ▽

√6ᵗʰ **S60.22** **Contusion of hand**

√7ᵗʰ **S60.221** **Contusion of right hand**

√7ᵗʰ **S60.222** **Contusion of left hand**

√7ᵗʰ **S60.229** **Contusion of unspecified hand** ▽

√5ᵗʰ **S60.3** **Other superficial injuries of thumb**

√6ᵗʰ **S60.31** **Abrasion of thumb**

√7ᵗʰ **S60.311** **Abrasion of right thumb**

√7ᵗʰ **S60.312** **Abrasion of left thumb**

√7ᵗʰ **S60.319** **Abrasion of unspecified thumb** ▽

√6ᵗʰ **S60.32** **Blister (nonthermal) of thumb**

√7ᵗʰ **S60.321** **Blister (nonthermal) of right thumb**

√7ᵗʰ **S60.322** **Blister (nonthermal) of left thumb**

√7ᵗʰ **S60.329** **Blister (nonthermal) of unspecified thumb** ▽

√6ᵗʰ **S60.34** **External constriction of thumb**

> Hair tourniquet syndrome of thumb
> Use additional cause code to identify the constricting item (W49.0-)

√7ᵗʰ **S60.341** **External constriction of right thumb**

√7ᵗʰ **S60.342** **External constriction of left thumb**

√7ᵗʰ **S60.349** **External constriction of unspecified thumb** ▽

√6ᵗʰ **S60.35** **Superficial foreign body of thumb**

> Splinter in the thumb

√7ᵗʰ **S60.351** **Superficial foreign body of right thumb**

√7ᵗʰ **S60.352** **Superficial foreign body of left thumb**

√7ᵗʰ **S60.359** **Superficial foreign body of unspecified thumb** ▽

√6ᵗʰ **S60.36** **Insect bite (nonvenomous) of thumb**

√7ᵗʰ **S60.361** **Insect bite (nonvenomous) of right thumb**

√7ᵗʰ **S60.362** Insect bite (nonvenomous) of left thumb

√7ᵗʰ **S60.369** Insect bite (nonvenomous) of unspecified thumb ▽

√6ᵗʰ **S60.37** Other superficial bite of thumb

EXCLUDES 1   open bite of thumb (S61.05-, S61.15-)

√7ᵗʰ **S60.371** Other superficial bite of right thumb

√7ᵗʰ **S60.372** Other superficial bite of left thumb

√7ᵗʰ **S60.379** Other superficial bite of unspecified thumb ▽

√6ᵗʰ **S60.39** Other superficial injuries of thumb

√7ᵗʰ **S60.391** Other superficial injuries of right thumb

√7ᵗʰ **S60.392** Other superficial injuries of left thumb

√7ᵗʰ **S60.399** Other superficial injuries of unspecified thumb ▽

√5ᵗʰ **S60.4** Other superficial injuries of other fingers

√6ᵗʰ **S60.41** Abrasion of fingers

√7ᵗʰ **S60.410** Abrasion of right index finger

√7ᵗʰ **S60.411** Abrasion of left index finger

√7ᵗʰ **S60.412** Abrasion of right middle finger

√7ᵗʰ **S60.413** Abrasion of left middle finger

√7ᵗʰ **S60.414** Abrasion of right ring finger

√7ᵗʰ **S60.415** Abrasion of left ring finger

√7ᵗʰ **S60.416** Abrasion of right little finger

√7ᵗʰ **S60.417** Abrasion of left little finger

√7ᵗʰ **S60.418** Abrasion of other finger

Abrasion of specified finger with unspecified laterality

√7ᵗʰ **S60.419** Abrasion of unspecified finger ▽

√6ᵗʰ **S60.42** Blister (nonthermal) of fingers

√7ᵗʰ **S60.420** Blister (nonthermal) of right index finger

√7ᵗʰ **S60.421** Blister (nonthermal) of left index finger

√7ᵗʰ **S60.422** Blister (nonthermal) of right middle finger

√7ᵗʰ **S60.423** Blister (nonthermal) of left middle finger

√7ᵗʰ **S60.424** Blister (nonthermal) of right ring finger

√7ᵗʰ **S60.425** Blister (nonthermal) of left ring finger

√7ᵗʰ **S60.426** Blister (nonthermal) of right little finger

√7ᵗʰ **S60.427** Blister (nonthermal) of left little finger

√7ᵗʰ **S60.428** Blister (nonthermal) of other finger

Blister (nonthermal) of specified finger with unspecified laterality

√7ᵗʰ **S60.429** Blister (nonthermal) of unspecified finger ▽

√6ᵗʰ **S60.44** External constriction of fingers

Hair tourniquet syndrome of finger

Use additional cause code to identify the constricting item (W49.0-)

√7ᵗʰ **S60.440** External constriction of right index finger

√7ᵗʰ **S60.441** External constriction of left index finger

√7ᵗʰ **S60.442** External constriction of right middle finger

√7ᵗʰ **S60.443** External constriction of left middle finger

√7ᵗʰ **S60.444** External constriction of right ring finger

√7ᵗʰ **S60.445** External constriction of left ring finger

√7ᵗʰ **S60.446** External constriction of right little finger

√7ᵗʰ **S60.447** External constriction of left little finger

√7ᵗʰ **S60.448** External constriction of other finger

External constriction of specified finger with unspecified laterality

√7ᵗʰ **S60.449** External constriction of unspecified finger ▽

√6ᵗʰ **S60.45** Superficial foreign body of fingers

Splinter in the finger(s)

√7ᵗʰ **S60.450** Superficial foreign body of right index finger

√7ᵗʰ **S60.451** Superficial foreign body of left index finger

√7ᵗʰ **S60.452** Superficial foreign body of right middle finger

√7ᵗʰ **S60.453** Superficial foreign body of left middle finger

√7ᵗʰ **S60.454** Superficial foreign body of right ring finger

√7ᵗʰ **S60.455** Superficial foreign body of left ring finger

√7ᵗʰ **S60.456** Superficial foreign body of right little finger

√7ᵗʰ **S60.457** Superficial foreign body of left little finger

√7ᵗʰ **S60.458** Superficial foreign body of other finger

Superficial foreign body of specified finger with unspecified laterality

√7ᵗʰ **S60.459** Superficial foreign body of unspecified finger ▽

√6ᵗʰ **S60.46** Insect bite (nonvenomous) of fingers

√7ᵗʰ **S60.460** Insect bite (nonvenomous) of right index finger

√7ᵗʰ **S60.461** Insect bite (nonvenomous) of left index finger

√7ᵗʰ **S60.462** Insect bite (nonvenomous) of right middle finger

√7ᵗʰ **S60.463** Insect bite (nonvenomous) of left middle finger

√7ᵗʰ **S60.464** Insect bite (nonvenomous) of right ring finger

√7ᵗʰ **S60.465** Insect bite (nonvenomous) of left ring finger

√7ᵗʰ **S60.466** Insect bite (nonvenomous) of right little finger

√7ᵗʰ **S60.467** Insect bite (nonvenomous) of left little finger

√7ᵗʰ **S60.468** Insect bite (nonvenomous) of other finger

Insect bite (nonvenomous) of specified finger with unspecified laterality

√7ᵗʰ **S60.469** Insect bite (nonvenomous) of unspecified finger ▽

√6ᵗʰ **S60.47** Other superficial bite of fingers

EXCLUDES 1   open bite of fingers (S61.25-, S61.35-)

√7ᵗʰ **S60.470** Other superficial bite of right index finger

√7ᵗʰ **S60.471** Other superficial bite of left index finger

√7ᵗʰ **S60.472** Other superficial bite of right middle finger

√7ᵗʰ **S60.473** Other superficial bite of left middle finger

√7ᵗʰ **S60.474** Other superficial bite of right ring finger

√7ᵗʰ **S60.475** Other superficial bite of left ring finger

√7ᵗʰ **S60.476** Other superficial bite of right little finger

√7ᵗʰ **S60.477** Other superficial bite of left little finger

√7ᵗʰ **S60.478** Other superficial bite of other finger

Other superficial bite of specified finger with unspecified laterality

√7ᵗʰ **S60.479** Other superficial bite of unspecified finger ▽

√5ᵗʰ **S60.5** Other superficial injuries of hand

EXCLUDES 2   superficial injuries of fingers (S60.3-, S60.4-)

√6ᵗʰ **S60.51** Abrasion of hand

√7ᵗʰ **S60.511** Abrasion of right hand

√7ᵗʰ **S60.512** Abrasion of left hand

√7ᵗʰ **S60.519** Abrasion of unspecified hand ▽

√6ᵗʰ **S60.52** Blister (nonthermal) of hand

√7ᵗʰ **S60.521** Blister (nonthermal) of right hand

√7ᵗʰ **S60.522** Blister (nonthermal) of left hand

√7ᵗʰ **S60.529** Blister (nonthermal) of unspecified hand ▽

√6ᵗʰ **S60.54** External constriction of hand

√7ᵗʰ **S60.541** External constriction of right hand

√7ᵗʰ **S60.542** External constriction of left hand

√7ᵗʰ **S60.549** External constriction of unspecified hand ▽

√6ᵗʰ **S60.55** Superficial foreign body of hand

Splinter in the hand

√7ᵗʰ **S60.551** Superficial foreign body of right hand

√7ᵗʰ **S60.552** Superficial foreign body of left hand

√7ᵗʰ **S60.559** Superficial foreign body of unspecified hand ▽

√6ᵗʰ **S60.56** Insect bite (nonvenomous) of hand

√7ᵗʰ **S60.561** Insect bite (nonvenomous) of right hand

☑ Additional Character Req   √x7ᵗʰ Placeholder Alert   Manifestation   ▽ Unspecified   ►◄ Revised Text   ● New Code   ▲ Revised Code Title

√7ᵗʰ **S60.562** Insect bite (nonvenomous) of left hand
√7ᵗʰ **S60.569** Insect bite (nonvenomous) of unspecified hand ▽
√6ᵗʰ **S60.57** Other superficial bite of hand
    EXCLUDES 1   open bite of hand (S61.45-)
√7ᵗʰ **S60.571** Other superficial bite of hand of right hand
√7ᵗʰ **S60.572** Other superficial bite of hand of left hand
√7ᵗʰ **S60.579** Other superficial bite of hand of unspecified hand ▽

√5ᵗʰ **S60.8** Other superficial injuries of wrist
√6ᵗʰ **S60.81** Abrasion of wrist
√7ᵗʰ **S60.811** Abrasion of right wrist
√7ᵗʰ **S60.812** Abrasion of left wrist
√7ᵗʰ **S60.819** Abrasion of unspecified wrist ▽
√6ᵗʰ **S60.82** Blister (nonthermal) of wrist
√7ᵗʰ **S60.821** Blister (nonthermal) of right wrist
√7ᵗʰ **S60.822** Blister (nonthermal) of left wrist
√7ᵗʰ **S60.829** Blister (nonthermal) of unspecified wrist ▽
√6ᵗʰ **S60.84** External constriction of wrist
√7ᵗʰ **S60.841** External constriction of right wrist
√7ᵗʰ **S60.842** External constriction of left wrist
√7ᵗʰ **S60.849** External constriction of unspecified wrist ▽
√6ᵗʰ **S60.85** Superficial foreign body of wrist
    Splinter in the wrist
√7ᵗʰ **S60.851** Superficial foreign body of right wrist
√7ᵗʰ **S60.852** Superficial foreign body of left wrist
√7ᵗʰ **S60.859** Superficial foreign body of unspecified wrist ▽
√6ᵗʰ **S60.86** Insect bite (nonvenomous) of wrist
√7ᵗʰ **S60.861** Insect bite (nonvenomous) of right wrist
√7ᵗʰ **S60.862** Insect bite (nonvenomous) of left wrist
√7ᵗʰ **S60.869** Insect bite (nonvenomous) of unspecified wrist ▽
√6ᵗʰ **S60.87** Other superficial bite of wrist
    EXCLUDES 1   open bite of wrist (S61.55)
√7ᵗʰ **S60.871** Other superficial bite of right wrist
√7ᵗʰ **S60.872** Other superficial bite of left wrist
√7ᵗʰ **S60.879** Other superficial bite of unspecified wrist ▽

√5ᵗʰ **S60.9** Unspecified superficial injury of wrist, hand and fingers
√6ᵗʰ **S60.91** Unspecified superficial injury of wrist
√7ᵗʰ **S60.911** Unspecified superficial injury of right wrist ▽
√7ᵗʰ **S60.912** Unspecified superficial injury of left wrist ▽
√7ᵗʰ **S60.919** Unspecified superficial injury of unspecified wrist ▽
√6ᵗʰ **S60.92** Unspecified superficial injury of hand
√7ᵗʰ **S60.921** Unspecified superficial injury of right hand ▽
√7ᵗʰ **S60.922** Unspecified superficial injury of left hand ▽
√7ᵗʰ **S60.929** Unspecified superficial injury of unspecified hand ▽
√6ᵗʰ **S60.93** Unspecified superficial injury of thumb
√7ᵗʰ **S60.931** Unspecified superficial injury of right thumb ▽
√7ᵗʰ **S60.932** Unspecified superficial injury of left thumb ▽
√7ᵗʰ **S60.939** Unspecified superficial injury of unspecified thumb ▽
√6ᵗʰ **S60.94** Unspecified superficial injury of other fingers
√7ᵗʰ **S60.940** Unspecified superficial injury of right index finger ▽
√7ᵗʰ **S60.941** Unspecified superficial injury of left index finger ▽
√7ᵗʰ **S60.942** Unspecified superficial injury of right middle finger ▽
√7ᵗʰ **S60.943** Unspecified superficial injury of left middle finger ▽
√7ᵗʰ **S60.944** Unspecified superficial injury of right ring finger ▽

√7ᵗʰ **S60.945** Unspecified superficial injury of left ring finger ▽
√7ᵗʰ **S60.946** Unspecified superficial injury of right little finger ▽
√7ᵗʰ **S60.947** Unspecified superficial injury of left little finger ▽
√7ᵗʰ **S60.948** Unspecified superficial injury of other finger
    Unspecified superficial injury of specified finger with unspecified laterality
√7ᵗʰ **S60.949** Unspecified superficial injury of unspecified finger ▽

√4ᵗʰ **S61** Open wound of wrist, hand and fingers
    Code also any associated wound infection
    EXCLUDES 1   open fracture of wrist, hand and finger (S62.- with 7th character B)
          traumatic amputation of wrist and hand (S68.-)

The appropriate 7th character is to be added to each code from category S61.
A   initial encounter
D   subsequent encounter
S   sequela

√5ᵗʰ **S61.0** Open wound of thumb without damage to nail
    EXCLUDES 1   open wound of thumb with damage to nail (S61.1-)
√6ᵗʰ **S61.00** Unspecified open wound of thumb without damage to nail
√7ᵗʰ **S61.001** Unspecified open wound of right thumb without damage to nail ▽
√7ᵗʰ **S61.002** Unspecified open wound of left thumb without damage to nail ▽
√7ᵗʰ **S61.009** Unspecified open wound of unspecified thumb without damage to nail ▽
√6ᵗʰ **S61.01** Laceration without foreign body of thumb without damage to nail
√7ᵗʰ **S61.011** Laceration without foreign body of right thumb without damage to nail
√7ᵗʰ **S61.012** Laceration without foreign body of left thumb without damage to nail
√7ᵗʰ **S61.019** Laceration without foreign body of unspecified thumb without damage to nail ▽
√6ᵗʰ **S61.02** Laceration with foreign body of thumb without damage to nail
√7ᵗʰ **S61.021** Laceration with foreign body of right thumb without damage to nail
√7ᵗʰ **S61.022** Laceration with foreign body of left thumb without damage to nail
√7ᵗʰ **S61.029** Laceration with foreign body of unspecified thumb without damage to nail ▽
√6ᵗʰ **S61.03** Puncture wound without foreign body of thumb without damage to nail
√7ᵗʰ **S61.031** Puncture wound without foreign body of right thumb without damage to nail
√7ᵗʰ **S61.032** Puncture wound without foreign body of left thumb without damage to nail
√7ᵗʰ **S61.039** Puncture wound without foreign body of unspecified thumb without damage to nail ▽
√6ᵗʰ **S61.04** Puncture wound with foreign body of thumb without damage to nail
√7ᵗʰ **S61.041** Puncture wound with foreign body of right thumb without damage to nail
√7ᵗʰ **S61.042** Puncture wound with foreign body of left thumb without damage to nail
√7ᵗʰ **S61.049** Puncture wound with foreign body of unspecified thumb without damage to nail ▽
√6ᵗʰ **S61.05** Open bite of thumb without damage to nail
    Bite of thumb NOS
    EXCLUDES 1   superficial bite of thumb (S60.36-, S60.37-)
√7ᵗʰ **S61.051** Open bite of right thumb without damage to nail
√7ᵗʰ **S61.052** Open bite of left thumb without damage to nail
√7ᵗʰ **S61.059** Open bite of unspecified thumb without damage to nail ▽

✓5ᵗʰ **S61.1** Open wound of thumb with damage to nail

    ✓6ᵗʰ **S61.10** Unspecified open wound of thumb with damage to nail

       ✓7ᵗʰ **S61.101** Unspecified open wound of right thumb with damage to nail ▽

       ✓7ᵗʰ **S61.102** Unspecified open wound of left thumb with damage to nail ▽

       ✓7ᵗʰ **S61.109** Unspecified open wound of unspecified thumb with damage to nail ▽

    ✓6ᵗʰ **S61.11** Laceration without foreign body of thumb with damage to nail

       ✓7ᵗʰ **S61.111** Laceration without foreign body of right thumb with damage to nail

       ✓7ᵗʰ **S61.112** Laceration without foreign body of left thumb with damage to nail

       ✓7ᵗʰ **S61.119** Laceration without foreign body of unspecified thumb with damage to nail ▽

    ✓6ᵗʰ **S61.12** Laceration with foreign body of thumb with damage to nail

       ✓7ᵗʰ **S61.121** Laceration with foreign body of right thumb with damage to nail

       ✓7ᵗʰ **S61.122** Laceration with foreign body of left thumb with damage to nail

       ✓7ᵗʰ **S61.129** Laceration with foreign body of unspecified thumb with damage to nail ▽

    ✓6ᵗʰ **S61.13** Puncture wound without foreign body of thumb with damage to nail

       ✓7ᵗʰ **S61.131** Puncture wound without foreign body of right thumb with damage to nail

       ✓7ᵗʰ **S61.132** Puncture wound without foreign body of left thumb with damage to nail

       ✓7ᵗʰ **S61.139** Puncture wound without foreign body of unspecified thumb with damage to nail ▽

    ✓6ᵗʰ **S61.14** Puncture wound with foreign body of thumb with damage to nail

       ✓7ᵗʰ **S61.141** Puncture wound with foreign body of right thumb with damage to nail

       ✓7ᵗʰ **S61.142** Puncture wound with foreign body of left thumb with damage to nail

       ✓7ᵗʰ **S61.149** Puncture wound with foreign body of unspecified thumb with damage to nail ▽

    ✓6ᵗʰ **S61.15** Open bite of thumb with damage to nail

       Bite of thumb with damage to nail NOS

       EXCLUDES 1   superficial bite of thumb (S60.36-, S60.37-)

       ✓7ᵗʰ **S61.151** Open bite of right thumb with damage to nail

       ✓7ᵗʰ **S61.152** Open bite of left thumb with damage to nail

       ✓7ᵗʰ **S61.159** Open bite of unspecified thumb with damage to nail ▽

✓5ᵗʰ **S61.2** Open wound of other finger without damage to nail

    EXCLUDES 1   open wound of finger involving nail (matrix) (S61.3-)

    EXCLUDES 2   open wound of thumb without damage to nail (S61.0-)

    ✓6ᵗʰ **S61.20** Unspecified open wound of other finger without damage to nail

       ✓7ᵗʰ **S61.200** Unspecified open wound of right index finger without damage to nail ▽

       ✓7ᵗʰ **S61.201** Unspecified open wound of left index finger without damage to nail ▽

       ✓7ᵗʰ **S61.202** Unspecified open wound of right middle finger without damage to nail ▽

       ✓7ᵗʰ **S61.203** Unspecified open wound of left middle finger without damage to nail ▽

       ✓7ᵗʰ **S61.204** Unspecified open wound of right ring finger without damage to nail ▽

       ✓7ᵗʰ **S61.205** Unspecified open wound of left ring finger without damage to nail ▽

       ✓7ᵗʰ **S61.206** Unspecified open wound of right little finger without damage to nail ▽

       ✓7ᵗʰ **S61.207** Unspecified open wound of left little finger without damage to nail ▽

       ✓7ᵗʰ **S61.208** Unspecified open wound of other finger without damage to nail ▽

       Unspecified open wound of specified finger with unspecified laterality without damage to nail

       ✓7ᵗʰ **S61.209** Unspecified open wound of unspecified finger without damage to nail ▽

    ✓6ᵗʰ **S61.21** Laceration without foreign body of finger without damage to nail

       ✓7ᵗʰ **S61.210** Laceration without foreign body of right index finger without damage to nail

       ✓7ᵗʰ **S61.211** Laceration without foreign body of left index finger without damage to nail

       ✓7ᵗʰ **S61.212** Laceration without foreign body of right middle finger without damage to nail

       ✓7ᵗʰ **S61.213** Laceration without foreign body of left middle finger without damage to nail

       ✓7ᵗʰ **S61.214** Laceration without foreign body of right ring finger without damage to nail

       ✓7ᵗʰ **S61.215** Laceration without foreign body of left ring finger without damage to nail

       ✓7ᵗʰ **S61.216** Laceration without foreign body of right little finger without damage to nail

       ✓7ᵗʰ **S61.217** Laceration without foreign body of left little finger without damage to nail

       ✓7ᵗʰ **S61.218** Laceration without foreign body of other finger without damage to nail

       Laceration without foreign body of specified finger with unspecified laterality without damage to nail

       ✓7ᵗʰ **S61.219** Laceration without foreign body of unspecified finger without damage to nail ▽

    ✓6ᵗʰ **S61.22** Laceration with foreign body of finger without damage to nail

       ✓7ᵗʰ **S61.220** Laceration with foreign body of right index finger without damage to nail

       ✓7ᵗʰ **S61.221** Laceration with foreign body of left index finger without damage to nail

       ✓7ᵗʰ **S61.222** Laceration with foreign body of right middle finger without damage to nail

       ✓7ᵗʰ **S61.223** Laceration with foreign body of left middle finger without damage to nail

       ✓7ᵗʰ **S61.224** Laceration with foreign body of right ring finger without damage to nail

       ✓7ᵗʰ **S61.225** Laceration with foreign body of left ring finger without damage to nail

       ✓7ᵗʰ **S61.226** Laceration with foreign body of right little finger without damage to nail

       ✓7ᵗʰ **S61.227** Laceration with foreign body of left little finger without damage to nail

       ✓7ᵗʰ **S61.228** Laceration with foreign body of other finger without damage to nail

       Laceration with foreign body of specified finger with unspecified laterality without damage to nail

       ✓7ᵗʰ **S61.229** Laceration with foreign body of unspecified finger without damage to nail ▽

    ✓6ᵗʰ **S61.23** Puncture wound without foreign body of finger without damage to nail

       ✓7ᵗʰ **S61.230** Puncture wound without foreign body of right index finger without damage to nail

       ✓7ᵗʰ **S61.231** Puncture wound without foreign body of left index finger without damage to nail

       ✓7ᵗʰ **S61.232** Puncture wound without foreign body of right middle finger without damage to nail

       ✓7ᵗʰ **S61.233** Puncture wound without foreign body of left middle finger without damage to nail

       ✓7ᵗʰ **S61.234** Puncture wound without foreign body of right ring finger without damage to nail

       ✓7ᵗʰ **S61.235** Puncture wound without foreign body of left ring finger without damage to nail

       ✓7ᵗʰ **S61.236** Puncture wound without foreign body of right little finger without damage to nail

       ✓7ᵗʰ **S61.237** Puncture wound without foreign body of left little finger without damage to nail

---

☑ Additional Character Req   ✓ᴀ7ᵗʰ Placeholder Alert   Manifestation   ▽ Unspecified   ►◄ Revised Text   ● New Code   ▲ Revised Code Title

Chapter 19. Injury, Poisoning and Certain Other Consequences of External Causes

√7ᵗʰ **S61.238 Puncture wound without foreign body of other finger without damage to nail**
Puncture wound without foreign body of specified finger with unspecified laterality without damage to nail

√7ᵗʰ **S61.239 Puncture wound without foreign body of unspecified finger without damage to nail** ▽

√6ᵗʰ **S61.24 Puncture wound with foreign body of finger without damage to nail**

√7ᵗʰ **S61.240 Puncture wound with foreign body of right index finger without damage to nail**

√7ᵗʰ **S61.241 Puncture wound with foreign body of left index finger without damage to nail**

√7ᵗʰ **S61.242 Puncture wound with foreign body of right middle finger without damage to nail**

√7ᵗʰ **S61.243 Puncture wound with foreign body of left middle finger without damage to nail**

√7ᵗʰ **S61.244 Puncture wound with foreign body of right ring finger without damage to nail**

√7ᵗʰ **S61.245 Puncture wound with foreign body of left ring finger without damage to nail**

√7ᵗʰ **S61.246 Puncture wound with foreign body of right little finger without damage to nail**

√7ᵗʰ **S61.247 Puncture wound with foreign body of left little finger without damage to nail**

√7ᵗʰ **S61.248 Puncture wound with foreign body of other finger without damage to nail**
Puncture wound with foreign body of specified finger with unspecified laterality without damage to nail

√7ᵗʰ **S61.249 Puncture wound with foreign body of unspecified finger without damage to nail** ▽

√6ᵗʰ **S61.25 Open bite of finger without damage to nail**
Bite of finger without damage to nail NOS
EXCLUDES 1   superficial bite of finger (S60.46-, S60.47-)

√7ᵗʰ **S61.250 Open bite of right index finger without damage to nail**

√7ᵗʰ **S61.251 Open bite of left index finger without damage to nail**

√7ᵗʰ **S61.252 Open bite of right middle finger without damage to nail**

√7ᵗʰ **S61.253 Open bite of left middle finger without damage to nail**

√7ᵗʰ **S61.254 Open bite of right ring finger without damage to nail**

√7ᵗʰ **S61.255 Open bite of left ring finger without damage to nail**

√7ᵗʰ **S61.256 Open bite of right little finger without damage to nail**

√7ᵗʰ **S61.257 Open bite of left little finger without damage to nail**

√7ᵗʰ **S61.258 Open bite of other finger without damage to nail**
Open bite of specified finger with unspecified laterality without damage to nail

√7ᵗʰ **S61.259 Open bite of unspecified finger without damage to nail** ▽

√5ᵗʰ **S61.3 Open wound of other finger with damage to nail**

√6ᵗʰ **S61.30 Unspecified open wound of finger with damage to nail**

√7ᵗʰ **S61.300 Unspecified open wound of right index finger with damage to nail** ▽

√7ᵗʰ **S61.301 Unspecified open wound of left index finger with damage to nail** ▽

√7ᵗʰ **S61.302 Unspecified open wound of right middle finger with damage to nail** ▽

√7ᵗʰ **S61.303 Unspecified open wound of left middle finger with damage to nail** ▽

√7ᵗʰ **S61.304 Unspecified open wound of right ring finger with damage to nail** ▽

√7ᵗʰ **S61.305 Unspecified open wound of left ring finger with damage to nail** ▽

√7ᵗʰ **S61.306 Unspecified open wound of right little finger with damage to nail** ▽

√7ᵗʰ **S61.307 Unspecified open wound of left little finger with damage to nail** ▽

√7ᵗʰ **S61.308 Unspecified open wound of other finger with damage to nail** ▽
Unspecified open wound of specified finger with unspecified laterality with damage to nail

√7ᵗʰ **S61.309 Unspecified open wound of unspecified finger with damage to nail** ▽

√6ᵗʰ **S61.31 Laceration without foreign body of finger with damage to nail**

√7ᵗʰ **S61.310 Laceration without foreign body of right index finger with damage to nail**

√7ᵗʰ **S61.311 Laceration without foreign body of left index finger with damage to nail**

√7ᵗʰ **S61.312 Laceration without foreign body of right middle finger with damage to nail**

√7ᵗʰ **S61.313 Laceration without foreign body of left middle finger with damage to nail**

√7ᵗʰ **S61.314 Laceration without foreign body of right ring finger with damage to nail**

√7ᵗʰ **S61.315 Laceration without foreign body of left ring finger with damage to nail**

√7ᵗʰ **S61.316 Laceration without foreign body of right little finger with damage to nail**

√7ᵗʰ **S61.317 Laceration without foreign body of left little finger with damage to nail**

√7ᵗʰ **S61.318 Laceration without foreign body of other finger with damage to nail**
Laceration without foreign body of specified finger with unspecified laterality with damage to nail

√7ᵗʰ **S61.319 Laceration without foreign body of unspecified finger with damage to nail** ▽

√6ᵗʰ **S61.32 Laceration with foreign body of finger with damage to nail**

√7ᵗʰ **S61.320 Laceration with foreign body of right index finger with damage to nail**

√7ᵗʰ **S61.321 Laceration with foreign body of left index finger with damage to nail**

√7ᵗʰ **S61.322 Laceration with foreign body of right middle finger with damage to nail**

√7ᵗʰ **S61.323 Laceration with foreign body of left middle finger with damage to nail**

√7ᵗʰ **S61.324 Laceration with foreign body of right ring finger with damage to nail**

√7ᵗʰ **S61.325 Laceration with foreign body of left ring finger with damage to nail**

√7ᵗʰ **S61.326 Laceration with foreign body of right little finger with damage to nail**

√7ᵗʰ **S61.327 Laceration with foreign body of left little finger with damage to nail**

√7ᵗʰ **S61.328 Laceration with foreign body of other finger with damage to nail**
Laceration with foreign body of specified finger with unspecified laterality with damage to nail

√7ᵗʰ **S61.329 Laceration with foreign body of unspecified finger with damage to nail** ▽

√6ᵗʰ **S61.33 Puncture wound without foreign body of finger with damage to nail**

√7ᵗʰ **S61.330 Puncture wound without foreign body of right index finger with damage to nail**

√7ᵗʰ **S61.331 Puncture wound without foreign body of left index finger with damage to nail**

√7ᵗʰ **S61.332 Puncture wound without foreign body of right middle finger with damage to nail**

√7ᵗʰ **S61.333 Puncture wound without foreign body of left middle finger with damage to nail**

√7ᵗʰ **S61.334 Puncture wound without foreign body of right ring finger with damage to nail**

√7ᵗʰ **S61.335 Puncture wound without foreign body of left ring finger with damage to nail**

√7ᵗʰ **S61.336 Puncture wound without foreign body of right little finger with damage to nail**

√7ᵗʰ **S61.337 Puncture wound without foreign body of left little finger with damage to nail**

√7ᵗʰ **S61.338** **Puncture wound without foreign body of other finger with damage to nail**
Puncture wound without foreign body of specified finger with unspecified laterality with damage to nail

√7ᵗʰ **S61.339** **Puncture wound without foreign body of unspecified finger with damage to nail** ▽

√6ᵗʰ **S61.34** **Puncture wound with foreign body of finger with damage to nail**

√7ᵗʰ **S61.340** **Puncture wound with foreign body of right index finger with damage to nail**

√7ᵗʰ **S61.341** **Puncture wound with foreign body of left index finger with damage to nail**

√7ᵗʰ **S61.342** **Puncture wound with foreign body of right middle finger with damage to nail**

√7ᵗʰ **S61.343** **Puncture wound with foreign body of left middle finger with damage to nail**

√7ᵗʰ **S61.344** **Puncture wound with foreign body of right ring finger with damage to nail**

√7ᵗʰ **S61.345** **Puncture wound with foreign body of left ring finger with damage to nail**

√7ᵗʰ **S61.346** **Puncture wound with foreign body of right little finger with damage to nail**

√7ᵗʰ **S61.347** **Puncture wound with foreign body of left little finger with damage to nail**

√7ᵗʰ **S61.348** **Puncture wound with foreign body of other finger with damage to nail**
Puncture wound with foreign body of specified finger with unspecified laterality with damage to nail

√7ᵗʰ **S61.349** **Puncture wound with foreign body of unspecified finger with damage to nail** ▽

√6ᵗʰ **S61.35** **Open bite of finger with damage to nail**
Bite of finger with damage to nail NOS
EXCLUDES 1 *superficial bite of finger (S60.46-, S60.47-)*

√7ᵗʰ **S61.350** **Open bite of right index finger with damage to nail**

√7ᵗʰ **S61.351** **Open bite of left index finger with damage to nail**

√7ᵗʰ **S61.352** **Open bite of right middle finger with damage to nail**

√7ᵗʰ **S61.353** **Open bite of left middle finger with damage to nail**

√7ᵗʰ **S61.354** **Open bite of right ring finger with damage to nail**

√7ᵗʰ **S61.355** **Open bite of left ring finger with damage to nail**

√7ᵗʰ **S61.356** **Open bite of right little finger with damage to nail**

√7ᵗʰ **S61.357** **Open bite of left little finger with damage to nail**

√7ᵗʰ **S61.358** **Open bite of other finger with damage to nail**
Open bite of specified finger with unspecified laterality with damage to nail

√7ᵗʰ **S61.359** **Open bite of unspecified finger with damage to nail** ▽

√5ᵗʰ **S61.4** **Open wound of hand**

√6ᵗʰ **S61.40** **Unspecified open wound of hand**

√7ᵗʰ **S61.401** **Unspecified open wound of right hand** ▽

√7ᵗʰ **S61.402** **Unspecified open wound of left hand** ▽

√7ᵗʰ **S61.409** **Unspecified open wound of unspecified hand** ▽

√6ᵗʰ **S61.41** **Laceration without foreign body of hand**

√7ᵗʰ **S61.411** **Laceration without foreign body of right hand**

√7ᵗʰ **S61.412** **Laceration without foreign body of left hand**

√7ᵗʰ **S61.419** **Laceration without foreign body of unspecified hand** ▽

√6ᵗʰ **S61.42** **Laceration with foreign body of hand**

√7ᵗʰ **S61.421** **Laceration with foreign body of right hand**

√7ᵗʰ **S61.422** **Laceration with foreign body of left hand**

√7ᵗʰ **S61.429** **Laceration with foreign body of unspecified hand** ▽

√6ᵗʰ **S61.43** **Puncture wound without foreign body of hand**

√7ᵗʰ **S61.431** **Puncture wound without foreign body of right hand**

√7ᵗʰ **S61.432** **Puncture wound without foreign body of left hand**

√7ᵗʰ **S61.439** **Puncture wound without foreign body of unspecified hand** ▽

√6ᵗʰ **S61.44** **Puncture wound with foreign body of hand**

√7ᵗʰ **S61.441** **Puncture wound with foreign body of right hand**

√7ᵗʰ **S61.442** **Puncture wound with foreign body of left hand**

√7ᵗʰ **S61.449** **Puncture wound with foreign body of unspecified hand** ▽

√6ᵗʰ **S61.45** **Open bite of hand**
Bite of hand NOS
EXCLUDES 1 *superficial bite of hand (S60.56-, S60.57-)*

√7ᵗʰ **S61.451** **Open bite of right hand**

√7ᵗʰ **S61.452** **Open bite of left hand**

√7ᵗʰ **S61.459** **Open bite of unspecified hand** ▽

√5ᵗʰ **S61.5** **Open wound of wrist**

√6ᵗʰ **S61.50** **Unspecified open wound of wrist**

√7ᵗʰ **S61.501** **Unspecified open wound of right wrist** ▽

√7ᵗʰ **S61.502** **Unspecified open wound of left wrist** ▽

√7ᵗʰ **S61.509** **Unspecified open wound of unspecified wrist** ▽

√6ᵗʰ **S61.51** **Laceration without foreign body of wrist**

√7ᵗʰ **S61.511** **Laceration without foreign body of right wrist**

√7ᵗʰ **S61.512** **Laceration without foreign body of left wrist**

√7ᵗʰ **S61.519** **Laceration without foreign body of unspecified wrist** ▽

√6ᵗʰ **S61.52** **Laceration with foreign body of wrist**

√7ᵗʰ **S61.521** **Laceration with foreign body of right wrist**

√7ᵗʰ **S61.522** **Laceration with foreign body of left wrist**

√7ᵗʰ **S61.529** **Laceration with foreign body of unspecified wrist** ▽

√6ᵗʰ **S61.53** **Puncture wound without foreign body of wrist**

√7ᵗʰ **S61.531** **Puncture wound without foreign body of right wrist**

√7ᵗʰ **S61.532** **Puncture wound without foreign body of left wrist**

√7ᵗʰ **S61.539** **Puncture wound without foreign body of unspecified wrist** ▽

√6ᵗʰ **S61.54** **Puncture wound with foreign body of wrist**

√7ᵗʰ **S61.541** **Puncture wound with foreign body of right wrist**

√7ᵗʰ **S61.542** **Puncture wound with foreign body of left wrist**

√7ᵗʰ **S61.549** **Puncture wound with foreign body of unspecified wrist** ▽

√6ᵗʰ **S61.55** **Open bite of wrist**
Bite of wrist NOS
EXCLUDES 1 *superficial bite of wrist (S60.86-, S60.87-)*

√7ᵗʰ **S61.551** **Open bite of right wrist**

√7ᵗʰ **S61.552** **Open bite of left wrist**

√7ᵗʰ **S61.559** **Open bite of unspecified wrist** ▽

☑ Additional Character Req	√x7ᵗʰ Placeholder Alert	Manifestation	▽ Unspecified	▶◀ Revised Text	● New Code	▲ Revised Code Title

Chapter 19. Injury, Poisoning and Certain Other Consequences of External Causes

S62–S62.145

√4ᵗʰ **S62 Fracture at wrist and hand level**

> **NOTE**   A fracture not indicated as displaced or nondisplaced should be coded to displaced
>
> A fracture not indicated as open or closed should be coded to closed

> **EXCLUDES 1**   *traumatic amputation of wrist and hand (S68.-)*
> **EXCLUDES 2**   *fracture of distal parts of ulna and radius (S52.-)*

> **AHA:** 2018,2Q,12; 2015,3Q,37-39

> The appropriate 7th character is to be added to each code from category S62.
> A   initial encounter for closed fracture
> B   initial encounter for open fracture
> D   subsequent encounter for fracture with routine healing
> G   subsequent encounter for fracture with delayed healing
> K   subsequent encounter for fracture with nonunion
> P   subsequent encounter for fracture with malunion
> S   sequela

√5ᵗʰ **S62.0 Fracture of navicular [scaphoid] bone of wrist**

    √6ᵗʰ **S62.00 Unspecified fracture of navicular [scaphoid] bone of wrist**

       √7ᵗʰ **S62.001 Unspecified fracture of navicular [scaphoid] bone of right wrist** ◨ ▽

       √7ᵗʰ **S62.002 Unspecified fracture of navicular [scaphoid] bone of left wrist** ◨ ▽
           AHA: 2012,4Q,106

       √7ᵗʰ **S62.009 Unspecified fracture of navicular [scaphoid] bone of unspecified wrist** ◨ ▽

    √6ᵗʰ **S62.01 Fracture of distal pole of navicular [scaphoid] bone of wrist**

       Fracture of volar tuberosity of navicular [scaphoid] bone of wrist

       √7ᵗʰ **S62.011 Displaced fracture of distal pole of navicular [scaphoid] bone of right wrist** ◨

       √7ᵗʰ **S62.012 Displaced fracture of distal pole of navicular [scaphoid] bone of left wrist** ◨

       √7ᵗʰ **S62.013 Displaced fracture of distal pole of navicular [scaphoid] bone of unspecified wrist** ◨ ▽

       √7ᵗʰ **S62.014 Nondisplaced fracture of distal pole of navicular [scaphoid] bone of right wrist** ◨

       √7ᵗʰ **S62.015 Nondisplaced fracture of distal pole of navicular [scaphoid] bone of left wrist** ◨

       √7ᵗʰ **S62.016 Nondisplaced fracture of distal pole of navicular [scaphoid] bone of unspecified wrist** ◨ ▽

    √6ᵗʰ **S62.02 Fracture of middle third of navicular [scaphoid] bone of wrist**

       √7ᵗʰ **S62.021 Displaced fracture of middle third of navicular [scaphoid] bone of right wrist** ◨

       √7ᵗʰ **S62.022 Displaced fracture of middle third of navicular [scaphoid] bone of left wrist** ◨

       √7ᵗʰ **S62.023 Displaced fracture of middle third of navicular [scaphoid] bone of unspecified wrist** ◨ ▽

       √7ᵗʰ **S62.024 Nondisplaced fracture of middle third of navicular [scaphoid] bone of right wrist** ◨

       √7ᵗʰ **S62.025 Nondisplaced fracture of middle third of navicular [scaphoid] bone of left wrist** ◨

       √7ᵗʰ **S62.026 Nondisplaced fracture of middle third of navicular [scaphoid] bone of unspecified wrist** ◨ ▽

    √6ᵗʰ **S62.03 Fracture of proximal third of navicular [scaphoid] bone of wrist**

       √7ᵗʰ **S62.031 Displaced fracture of proximal third of navicular [scaphoid] bone of right wrist** ◨

       √7ᵗʰ **S62.032 Displaced fracture of proximal third of navicular [scaphoid] bone of left wrist** ◨

       √7ᵗʰ **S62.033 Displaced fracture of proximal third of navicular [scaphoid] bone of unspecified wrist** ◨ ▽

       √7ᵗʰ **S62.034 Nondisplaced fracture of proximal third of navicular [scaphoid] bone of right wrist** ◨

       √7ᵗʰ **S62.035 Nondisplaced fracture of proximal third of navicular [scaphoid] bone of left wrist** ◨

       √7ᵗʰ **S62.036 Nondisplaced fracture of proximal third of navicular [scaphoid] bone of unspecified wrist** ◨ ▽

√5ᵗʰ **S62.1 Fracture of other and unspecified carpal bone(s)**

> **EXCLUDES 2**   *fracture of scaphoid of wrist (S62.0-)*

    √6ᵗʰ **S62.10 Fracture of unspecified carpal bone**

       Fracture of wrist NOS

       √7ᵗʰ **S62.101 Fracture of unspecified carpal bone, right wrist** ◨ ▽

       √7ᵗʰ **S62.102 Fracture of unspecified carpal bone, left wrist** ◨ ▽
           AHA: 2012,4Q,95

       √7ᵗʰ **S62.109 Fracture of unspecified carpal bone, unspecified wrist** ◨ ▽

    √6ᵗʰ **S62.11 Fracture of triquetrum [cuneiform] bone of wrist**

       √7ᵗʰ **S62.111 Displaced fracture of triquetrum [cuneiform] bone, right wrist** ◨

       √7ᵗʰ **S62.112 Displaced fracture of triquetrum [cuneiform] bone, left wrist** ◨

       √7ᵗʰ **S62.113 Displaced fracture of triquetrum [cuneiform] bone, unspecified wrist** ◨ ▽

       √7ᵗʰ **S62.114 Nondisplaced fracture of triquetrum [cuneiform] bone, right wrist** ◨

       √7ᵗʰ **S62.115 Nondisplaced fracture of triquetrum [cuneiform] bone, left wrist** ◨

       √7ᵗʰ **S62.116 Nondisplaced fracture of triquetrum [cuneiform] bone, unspecified wrist** ◨ ▽

    √6ᵗʰ **S62.12 Fracture of lunate [semilunar]**

       √7ᵗʰ **S62.121 Displaced fracture of lunate [semilunar], right wrist** ◨

       √7ᵗʰ **S62.122 Displaced fracture of lunate [semilunar], left wrist** ◨

       √7ᵗʰ **S62.123 Displaced fracture of lunate [semilunar], unspecified wrist** ◨ ▽

       √7ᵗʰ **S62.124 Nondisplaced fracture of lunate [semilunar], right wrist** ◨

       √7ᵗʰ **S62.125 Nondisplaced fracture of lunate [semilunar], left wrist** ◨

       √7ᵗʰ **S62.126 Nondisplaced fracture of lunate [semilunar], unspecified wrist** ◨ ▽

    √6ᵗʰ **S62.13 Fracture of capitate [os magnum] bone**

       √7ᵗʰ **S62.131 Displaced fracture of capitate [os magnum] bone, right wrist** ◨

       √7ᵗʰ **S62.132 Displaced fracture of capitate [os magnum] bone, left wrist** ◨

       √7ᵗʰ **S62.133 Displaced fracture of capitate [os magnum] bone, unspecified wrist** ◨ ▽

       √7ᵗʰ **S62.134 Nondisplaced fracture of capitate [os magnum] bone, right wrist** ◨

       √7ᵗʰ **S62.135 Nondisplaced fracture of capitate [os magnum] bone, left wrist** ◨

       √7ᵗʰ **S62.136 Nondisplaced fracture of capitate [os magnum] bone, unspecified wrist** ◨ ▽

    √6ᵗʰ **S62.14 Fracture of body of hamate [unciform] bone**

       Fracture of hamate [unciform] bone NOS

       √7ᵗʰ **S62.141 Displaced fracture of body of hamate [unciform] bone, right wrist** ◨

       √7ᵗʰ **S62.142 Displaced fracture of body of hamate [unciform] bone, left wrist** ◨

       √7ᵗʰ **S62.143 Displaced fracture of body of hamate [unciform] bone, unspecified wrist** ◨ ▽

       √7ᵗʰ **S62.144 Nondisplaced fracture of body of hamate [unciform] bone, right wrist** ◨

       √7ᵗʰ **S62.145 Nondisplaced fracture of body of hamate [unciform] bone, left wrist** ◨

S62.146 Nondisplaced fracture of body of hamate [unciform] bone, unspecified wrist

S62.15 Fracture of hook process of hamate [unciform] bone
    Fracture of unciform process of hamate [unciform] bone

S62.151 Displaced fracture of hook process of hamate [unciform] bone, right wrist

S62.152 Displaced fracture of hook process of hamate [unciform] bone, left wrist

S62.153 Displaced fracture of hook process of hamate [unciform] bone, unspecified wrist

S62.154 Nondisplaced fracture of hook process of hamate [unciform] bone, right wrist

S62.155 Nondisplaced fracture of hook process of hamate [unciform] bone, left wrist

S62.156 Nondisplaced fracture of hook process of hamate [unciform] bone, unspecified wrist

S62.16 Fracture of pisiform

S62.161 Displaced fracture of pisiform, right wrist

S62.162 Displaced fracture of pisiform, left wrist

S62.163 Displaced fracture of pisiform, unspecified wrist

S62.164 Nondisplaced fracture of pisiform, right wrist

S62.165 Nondisplaced fracture of pisiform, left wrist

S62.166 Nondisplaced fracture of pisiform, unspecified wrist

S62.17 Fracture of trapezium [larger multangular]

S62.171 Displaced fracture of trapezium [larger multangular], right wrist

S62.172 Displaced fracture of trapezium [larger multangular], left wrist

S62.173 Displaced fracture of trapezium [larger multangular], unspecified wrist

S62.174 Nondisplaced fracture of trapezium [larger multangular], right wrist

S62.175 Nondisplaced fracture of trapezium [larger multangular], left wrist

S62.176 Nondisplaced fracture of trapezium [larger multangular], unspecified wrist

S62.18 Fracture of trapezoid [smaller multangular]

S62.181 Displaced fracture of trapezoid [smaller multangular], right wrist

S62.182 Displaced fracture of trapezoid [smaller multangular], left wrist

S62.183 Displaced fracture of trapezoid [smaller multangular], unspecified wrist

S62.184 Nondisplaced fracture of trapezoid [smaller multangular], right wrist

S62.185 Nondisplaced fracture of trapezoid [smaller multangular], left wrist

S62.186 Nondisplaced fracture of trapezoid [smaller multangular], unspecified wrist

S62.2 Fracture of first metacarpal bone

S62.20 Unspecified fracture of first metacarpal bone

S62.201 Unspecified fracture of first metacarpal bone, right hand

S62.202 Unspecified fracture of first metacarpal bone, left hand

S62.209 Unspecified fracture of first metacarpal bone, unspecified hand

S62.21 Bennett's fracture
    DEF: Intra-articular, two-part fracture at the base of the first metacarpal bone (thumb) on the ulnar side at the carpometacarpal (CMC) joint.

S62.211 Bennett's fracture, right hand

S62.212 Bennett's fracture, left hand

S62.213 Bennett's fracture, unspecified hand

S62.22 Rolando's fracture
    DEF: Comminuted, three part intra-articular fracture at the base of the thumb metacarpal.

S62.221 Displaced Rolando's fracture, right hand

S62.222 Displaced Rolando's fracture, left hand

S62.223 Displaced Rolando's fracture, unspecified hand

S62.224 Nondisplaced Rolando's fracture, right hand

S62.225 Nondisplaced Rolando's fracture, left hand

S62.226 Nondisplaced Rolando's fracture, unspecified hand

S62.23 Other fracture of base of first metacarpal bone

S62.231 Other displaced fracture of base of first metacarpal bone, right hand

S62.232 Other displaced fracture of base of first metacarpal bone, left hand

S62.233 Other displaced fracture of base of first metacarpal bone, unspecified hand

S62.234 Other nondisplaced fracture of base of first metacarpal bone, right hand

S62.235 Other nondisplaced fracture of base of first metacarpal bone, left hand

S62.236 Other nondisplaced fracture of base of first metacarpal bone, unspecified hand

S62.24 Fracture of shaft of first metacarpal bone

S62.241 Displaced fracture of shaft of first metacarpal bone, right hand

S62.242 Displaced fracture of shaft of first metacarpal bone, left hand

S62.243 Displaced fracture of shaft of first metacarpal bone, unspecified hand

S62.244 Nondisplaced fracture of shaft of first metacarpal bone, right hand

S62.245 Nondisplaced fracture of shaft of first metacarpal bone, left hand

S62.246 Nondisplaced fracture of shaft of first metacarpal bone, unspecified hand

S62.25 Fracture of neck of first metacarpal bone

S62.251 Displaced fracture of neck of first metacarpal bone, right hand

S62.252 Displaced fracture of neck of first metacarpal bone, left hand

S62.253 Displaced fracture of neck of first metacarpal bone, unspecified hand

S62.254 Nondisplaced fracture of neck of first metacarpal bone, right hand

S62.255 Nondisplaced fracture of neck of first metacarpal bone, left hand

S62.256 Nondisplaced fracture of neck of first metacarpal bone, unspecified hand

S62.29 Other fracture of first metacarpal bone

S62.291 Other fracture of first metacarpal bone, right hand

S62.292 Other fracture of first metacarpal bone, left hand

S62.299 Other fracture of first metacarpal bone, unspecified hand

✓ Additional Character Req   ✓x7ᵗʰ Placeholder Alert   Manifestation   ▽ Unspecified   ▶◀ Revised Text   ● New Code   ▲ Revised Code Title

ICD-10-CM 2019   **1021**

√5ᵗʰ **S62.3** **Fracture of other and unspecified metacarpal bone**

       EXCLUDES 2   *fracture of first metacarpal bone (S62.2-)*

   √6ᵗʰ **S62.30** **Unspecified fracture of other metacarpal bone**

     √7ᵗʰ **S62.300** **Unspecified fracture of second metacarpal bone, right hand** Q ▽

     √7ᵗʰ **S62.301** **Unspecified fracture of second metacarpal bone, left hand** Q ▽

     √7ᵗʰ **S62.302** **Unspecified fracture of third metacarpal bone, right hand** Q ▽

     √7ᵗʰ **S62.303** **Unspecified fracture of third metacarpal bone, left hand** Q ▽

     √7ᵗʰ **S62.304** **Unspecified fracture of fourth metacarpal bone, right hand** Q ▽

     √7ᵗʰ **S62.305** **Unspecified fracture of fourth metacarpal bone, left hand** Q ▽

     √7ᵗʰ **S62.306** **Unspecified fracture of fifth metacarpal bone, right hand** Q ▽

     √7ᵗʰ **S62.307** **Unspecified fracture of fifth metacarpal bone, left hand** Q ▽

     √7ᵗʰ **S62.308** **Unspecified fracture of other metacarpal bone** Q ▽

       Unspecified fracture of specified metacarpal bone with unspecified laterality

     √7ᵗʰ **S62.309** **Unspecified fracture of unspecified metacarpal bone** Q ▽

   √6ᵗʰ **S62.31** **Displaced fracture of base of other metacarpal bone**

     √7ᵗʰ **S62.310** **Displaced fracture of base of second metacarpal bone, right hand** Q

     √7ᵗʰ **S62.311** **Displaced fracture of base of second metacarpal bone, left hand** Q

     √7ᵗʰ **S62.312** **Displaced fracture of base of third metacarpal bone, right hand** Q

     √7ᵗʰ **S62.313** **Displaced fracture of base of third metacarpal bone, left hand** Q

     √7ᵗʰ **S62.314** **Displaced fracture of base of fourth metacarpal bone, right hand** Q

     √7ᵗʰ **S62.315** **Displaced fracture of base of fourth metacarpal bone, left hand** Q

     √7ᵗʰ **S62.316** **Displaced fracture of base of fifth metacarpal bone, right hand** Q

     √7ᵗʰ **S62.317** **Displaced fracture of base of fifth metacarpal bone, left hand** Q

     √7ᵗʰ **S62.318** **Displaced fracture of base of other metacarpal bone** Q

       Displaced fracture of base of specified metacarpal bone with unspecified laterality

     √7ᵗʰ **S62.319** **Displaced fracture of base of unspecified metacarpal bone** Q ▽

   √6ᵗʰ **S62.32** **Displaced fracture of shaft of other metacarpal bone**

     √7ᵗʰ **S62.320** **Displaced fracture of shaft of second metacarpal bone, right hand** Q

     √7ᵗʰ **S62.321** **Displaced fracture of shaft of second metacarpal bone, left hand** Q

     √7ᵗʰ **S62.322** **Displaced fracture of shaft of third metacarpal bone, right hand** Q

     √7ᵗʰ **S62.323** **Displaced fracture of shaft of third metacarpal bone, left hand** Q

     √7ᵗʰ **S62.324** **Displaced fracture of shaft of fourth metacarpal bone, right hand** Q

     √7ᵗʰ **S62.325** **Displaced fracture of shaft of fourth metacarpal bone, left hand** Q

     √7ᵗʰ **S62.326** **Displaced fracture of shaft of fifth metacarpal bone, right hand** Q

     √7ᵗʰ **S62.327** **Displaced fracture of shaft of fifth metacarpal bone, left hand** Q

     √7ᵗʰ **S62.328** **Displaced fracture of shaft of other metacarpal bone** Q

       Displaced fracture of shaft of specified metacarpal bone with unspecified laterality

     √7ᵗʰ **S62.329** **Displaced fracture of shaft of unspecified metacarpal bone** Q ▽

   √6ᵗʰ **S62.33** **Displaced fracture of neck of other metacarpal bone**

     √7ᵗʰ **S62.330** **Displaced fracture of neck of second metacarpal bone, right hand** Q

     √7ᵗʰ **S62.331** **Displaced fracture of neck of second metacarpal bone, left hand** Q

     √7ᵗʰ **S62.332** **Displaced fracture of neck of third metacarpal bone, right hand** Q

     √7ᵗʰ **S62.333** **Displaced fracture of neck of third metacarpal bone, left hand** Q

     √7ᵗʰ **S62.334** **Displaced fracture of neck of fourth metacarpal bone, right hand** Q

     √7ᵗʰ **S62.335** **Displaced fracture of neck of fourth metacarpal bone, left hand** Q

     √7ᵗʰ **S62.336** **Displaced fracture of neck of fifth metacarpal bone, right hand** Q

     √7ᵗʰ **S62.337** **Displaced fracture of neck of fifth metacarpal bone, left hand** Q

     √7ᵗʰ **S62.338** **Displaced fracture of neck of other metacarpal bone** Q

       Displaced fracture of neck of specified metacarpal bone with unspecified laterality

     √7ᵗʰ **S62.339** **Displaced fracture of neck of unspecified metacarpal bone** Q ▽

   √6ᵗʰ **S62.34** **Nondisplaced fracture of base of other metacarpal bone**

     √7ᵗʰ **S62.340** **Nondisplaced fracture of base of second metacarpal bone, right hand** Q

     √7ᵗʰ **S62.341** **Nondisplaced fracture of base of second metacarpal bone, left hand** Q

     √7ᵗʰ **S62.342** **Nondisplaced fracture of base of third metacarpal bone, right hand** Q

     √7ᵗʰ **S62.343** **Nondisplaced fracture of base of third metacarpal bone, left hand** Q

     √7ᵗʰ **S62.344** **Nondisplaced fracture of base of fourth metacarpal bone, right hand** Q

     √7ᵗʰ **S62.345** **Nondisplaced fracture of base of fourth metacarpal bone, left hand** Q

     √7ᵗʰ **S62.346** **Nondisplaced fracture of base of fifth metacarpal bone, right hand** Q

     √7ᵗʰ **S62.347** **Nondisplaced fracture of base of fifth metacarpal bone, left hand** Q

     √7ᵗʰ **S62.348** **Nondisplaced fracture of base of other metacarpal bone** Q

       Nondisplaced fracture of base of specified metacarpal bone with unspecified laterality

     √7ᵗʰ **S62.349** **Nondisplaced fracture of base of unspecified metacarpal bone** Q ▽

   √6ᵗʰ **S62.35** **Nondisplaced fracture of shaft of other metacarpal bone**

     √7ᵗʰ **S62.350** **Nondisplaced fracture of shaft of second metacarpal bone, right hand** Q

     √7ᵗʰ **S62.351** **Nondisplaced fracture of shaft of second metacarpal bone, left hand** Q

     √7ᵗʰ **S62.352** **Nondisplaced fracture of shaft of third metacarpal bone, right hand** Q

     √7ᵗʰ **S62.353** **Nondisplaced fracture of shaft of third metacarpal bone, left hand** Q

     √7ᵗʰ **S62.354** **Nondisplaced fracture of shaft of fourth metacarpal bone, right hand** Q

     √7ᵗʰ **S62.355** **Nondisplaced fracture of shaft of fourth metacarpal bone, left hand** Q

     √7ᵗʰ **S62.356** **Nondisplaced fracture of shaft of fifth metacarpal bone, right hand** Q

     √7ᵗʰ **S62.357** **Nondisplaced fracture of shaft of fifth metacarpal bone, left hand** Q

     √7ᵗʰ **S62.358** **Nondisplaced fracture of shaft of other metacarpal bone** Q

       Nondisplaced fracture of shaft of specified metacarpal bone with unspecified laterality

     √7ᵗʰ **S62.359** **Nondisplaced fracture of shaft of unspecified metacarpal bone** Q ▽

√6ᵗʰ **S62.36** **Nondisplaced fracture of neck of other metacarpal bone**

    √7ᵗʰ **S62.360** **Nondisplaced fracture of neck of second metacarpal bone, right hand** ⓪

    √7ᵗʰ **S62.361** **Nondisplaced fracture of neck of second metacarpal bone, left hand** ⓪

    √7ᵗʰ **S62.362** **Nondisplaced fracture of neck of third metacarpal bone, right hand** ⓪

    √7ᵗʰ **S62.363** **Nondisplaced fracture of neck of third metacarpal bone, left hand** ⓪

    √7ᵗʰ **S62.364** **Nondisplaced fracture of neck of fourth metacarpal bone, right hand** ⓪

    √7ᵗʰ **S62.365** **Nondisplaced fracture of neck of fourth metacarpal bone, left hand** ⓪

    √7ᵗʰ **S62.366** **Nondisplaced fracture of neck of fifth metacarpal bone, right hand** ⓪

    √7ᵗʰ **S62.367** **Nondisplaced fracture of neck of fifth metacarpal bone, left hand** ⓪

    √7ᵗʰ **S62.368** **Nondisplaced fracture of neck of other metacarpal bone** ⓪
       Nondisplaced fracture of neck of specified metacarpal bone with unspecified laterality

    √7ᵗʰ **S62.369** **Nondisplaced fracture of neck of unspecified metacarpal bone** ⓪ ▽

√6ᵗʰ **S62.39** **Other fracture of other metacarpal bone**

    √7ᵗʰ **S62.390** **Other fracture of second metacarpal bone, right hand** ⓪

    √7ᵗʰ **S62.391** **Other fracture of second metacarpal bone, left hand** ⓪

    √7ᵗʰ **S62.392** **Other fracture of third metacarpal bone, right hand** ⓪

    √7ᵗʰ **S62.393** **Other fracture of third metacarpal bone, left hand** ⓪

    √7ᵗʰ **S62.394** **Other fracture of fourth metacarpal bone, right hand** ⓪

    √7ᵗʰ **S62.395** **Other fracture of fourth metacarpal bone, left hand** ⓪

    √7ᵗʰ **S62.396** **Other fracture of fifth metacarpal bone, right hand** ⓪

    √7ᵗʰ **S62.397** **Other fracture of fifth metacarpal bone, left hand** ⓪

    √7ᵗʰ **S62.398** **Other fracture of other metacarpal bone** ⓪
       Other fracture of specified metacarpal bone with unspecified laterality

    √7ᵗʰ **S62.399** **Other fracture of unspecified metacarpal bone** ⓪ ▽

√5ᵗʰ **S62.5** **Fracture of thumb**

    √6ᵗʰ **S62.50** **Fracture of unspecified phalanx of thumb**

       √7ᵗʰ **S62.501** **Fracture of unspecified phalanx of right thumb** ▽

       √7ᵗʰ **S62.502** **Fracture of unspecified phalanx of left thumb** ▽

       √7ᵗʰ **S62.509** **Fracture of unspecified phalanx of unspecified thumb** ▽

    √6ᵗʰ **S62.51** **Fracture of proximal phalanx of thumb**

       √7ᵗʰ **S62.511** **Displaced fracture of proximal phalanx of right thumb**

       √7ᵗʰ **S62.512** **Displaced fracture of proximal phalanx of left thumb**

       √7ᵗʰ **S62.513** **Displaced fracture of proximal phalanx of unspecified thumb** ▽

       √7ᵗʰ **S62.514** **Nondisplaced fracture of proximal phalanx of right thumb**

       √7ᵗʰ **S62.515** **Nondisplaced fracture of proximal phalanx of left thumb**

       √7ᵗʰ **S62.516** **Nondisplaced fracture of proximal phalanx of unspecified thumb** ▽

    √6ᵗʰ **S62.52** **Fracture of distal phalanx of thumb**

       √7ᵗʰ **S62.521** **Displaced fracture of distal phalanx of right thumb**

       √7ᵗʰ **S62.522** **Displaced fracture of distal phalanx of left thumb**

       √7ᵗʰ **S62.523** **Displaced fracture of distal phalanx of unspecified thumb** ▽

       √7ᵗʰ **S62.524** **Nondisplaced fracture of distal phalanx of right thumb**

       √7ᵗʰ **S62.525** **Nondisplaced fracture of distal phalanx of left thumb**

       √7ᵗʰ **S62.526** **Nondisplaced fracture of distal phalanx of unspecified thumb** ▽

√5ᵗʰ **S62.6** **Fracture of other and unspecified finger(s)**

    EXCLUDES 2   *fracture of thumb (S62.5-)*

    √6ᵗʰ **S62.60** **Fracture of unspecified phalanx of finger**

       √7ᵗʰ **S62.600** **Fracture of unspecified phalanx of right index finger** ▽

       √7ᵗʰ **S62.601** **Fracture of unspecified phalanx of left index finger** ▽

       √7ᵗʰ **S62.602** **Fracture of unspecified phalanx of right middle finger** ▽

       √7ᵗʰ **S62.603** **Fracture of unspecified phalanx of left middle finger** ▽

       √7ᵗʰ **S62.604** **Fracture of unspecified phalanx of right ring finger** ▽

       √7ᵗʰ **S62.605** **Fracture of unspecified phalanx of left ring finger** ▽

       √7ᵗʰ **S62.606** **Fracture of unspecified phalanx of right little finger** ▽

       √7ᵗʰ **S62.607** **Fracture of unspecified phalanx of left little finger** ▽

       √7ᵗʰ **S62.608** **Fracture of unspecified phalanx of other finger** ▽
          Fracture of unspecified phalanx of specified finger with unspecified laterality

       √7ᵗʰ **S62.609** **Fracture of unspecified phalanx of unspecified finger** ▽

    √6ᵗʰ **S62.61** **Displaced fracture of proximal phalanx of finger**

       √7ᵗʰ **S62.610** **Displaced fracture of proximal phalanx of right index finger**

       √7ᵗʰ **S62.611** **Displaced fracture of proximal phalanx of left index finger**

       √7ᵗʰ **S62.612** **Displaced fracture of proximal phalanx of right middle finger**

       √7ᵗʰ **S62.613** **Displaced fracture of proximal phalanx of left middle finger**

       √7ᵗʰ **S62.614** **Displaced fracture of proximal phalanx of right ring finger**

       √7ᵗʰ **S62.615** **Displaced fracture of proximal phalanx of left ring finger**

       √7ᵗʰ **S62.616** **Displaced fracture of proximal phalanx of right little finger**

       √7ᵗʰ **S62.617** **Displaced fracture of proximal phalanx of left little finger**

       √7ᵗʰ **S62.618** **Displaced fracture of proximal phalanx of other finger**
          Displaced fracture of proximal phalanx of specified finger with unspecified laterality

       √7ᵗʰ **S62.619** **Displaced fracture of proximal phalanx of unspecified finger** ▽

    √6ᵗʰ **S62.62** **Displaced fracture of middle phalanx of finger**

       √7ᵗʰ **S62.620** **Displaced fracture of middle phalanx of right index finger**

       √7ᵗʰ **S62.621** **Displaced fracture of middle phalanx of left index finger**

       √7ᵗʰ **S62.622** **Displaced fracture of middle phalanx of right middle finger**

       √7ᵗʰ **S62.623** **Displaced fracture of middle phalanx of left middle finger**

       √7ᵗʰ **S62.624** **Displaced fracture of middle phalanx of right ring finger**

       √7ᵗʰ **S62.625** **Displaced fracture of middle phalanx of left ring finger**

▲   √7ᵗʰ **S62.626** **Displaced fracture of middle phalanx of right little finger**

▲   √7ᵗʰ **S62.627** **Displaced fracture of middle phalanx of left little finger**

▲   √7ᵗʰ **S62.628** **Displaced fracture of middle phalanx of other finger**
          ▶Displaced fracture of middle phalanx of specified finger with unspecified laterality◀

▲   √7ᵗʰ **S62.629** **Displaced fracture of middle phalanx of unspecified finger** ▽

    √6ᵗʰ **S62.63** **Displaced fracture of distal phalanx of finger**

       √7ᵗʰ **S62.630** **Displaced fracture of distal phalanx of right index finger**

☑ Additional Character Req   √x7ᵗʰ Placeholder Alert   Manifestation   ▽ Unspecified   ▶◀ Revised Text   ● New Code   ▲ Revised Code Title

ICD-10-CM 2019   **1023**

(left margin, vertical) Chapter 19. Injury, Poisoning and Certain Other Consequences of External Causes

(left margin, vertical, bottom) S62.631–S63.024

√7ᵗʰ **S62.631 Displaced fracture of distal phalanx of left index finger**

√7ᵗʰ **S62.632 Displaced fracture of distal phalanx of right middle finger**

√7ᵗʰ **S62.633 Displaced fracture of distal phalanx of left middle finger**

√7ᵗʰ **S62.634 Displaced fracture of distal phalanx of right ring finger**

√7ᵗʰ **S62.635 Displaced fracture of distal phalanx of left ring finger**

√7ᵗʰ **S62.636 Displaced fracture of distal phalanx of right little finger**

√7ᵗʰ **S62.637 Displaced fracture of distal phalanx of left little finger**

√7ᵗʰ **S62.638 Displaced fracture of distal phalanx of other finger**
Displaced fracture of distal phalanx of specified finger with unspecified laterality

√7ᵗʰ **S62.639 Displaced fracture of distal phalanx of unspecified finger** ▽

√6ᵗʰ **S62.64 Nondisplaced fracture of proximal phalanx of finger**

√7ᵗʰ **S62.640 Nondisplaced fracture of proximal phalanx of right index finger**

√7ᵗʰ **S62.641 Nondisplaced fracture of proximal phalanx of left index finger**

√7ᵗʰ **S62.642 Nondisplaced fracture of proximal phalanx of right middle finger**

√7ᵗʰ **S62.643 Nondisplaced fracture of proximal phalanx of left middle finger**

√7ᵗʰ **S62.644 Nondisplaced fracture of proximal phalanx of right ring finger**

√7ᵗʰ **S62.645 Nondisplaced fracture of proximal phalanx of left ring finger**

√7ᵗʰ **S62.646 Nondisplaced fracture of proximal phalanx of right little finger**

√7ᵗʰ **S62.647 Nondisplaced fracture of proximal phalanx of left little finger**

√7ᵗʰ **S62.648 Nondisplaced fracture of proximal phalanx of other finger**
Nondisplaced fracture of proximal phalanx of specified finger with unspecified laterality

√7ᵗʰ **S62.649 Nondisplaced fracture of proximal phalanx of unspecified finger** ▽

√6ᵗʰ **S62.65 Nondisplaced fracture of middle phalanx of finger**

√7ᵗʰ **S62.650 Nondisplaced fracture of middle phalanx of right index finger**

√7ᵗʰ **S62.651 Nondisplaced fracture of middle phalanx of left index finger**

√7ᵗʰ **S62.652 Nondisplaced fracture of middle phalanx of right middle finger**

√7ᵗʰ **S62.653 Nondisplaced fracture of middle phalanx of left middle finger**

▲ √7ᵗʰ **S62.654 Nondisplaced fracture of middle phalanx of right ring finger**

▲ √7ᵗʰ **S62.655 Nondisplaced fracture of middle phalanx of left ring finger**

▲ √7ᵗʰ **S62.656 Nondisplaced fracture of middle phalanx of right little finger**

▲ √7ᵗʰ **S62.657 Nondisplaced fracture of middle phalanx of left little finger**

▲ √7ᵗʰ **S62.658 Nondisplaced fracture of middle phalanx of other finger**
►Nondisplaced fracture of middle phalanx of specified finger with unspecified laterality◄

▲ √7ᵗʰ **S62.659 Nondisplaced fracture of middle phalanx of unspecified finger** ▽

√6ᵗʰ **S62.66 Nondisplaced fracture of distal phalanx of finger**

√7ᵗʰ **S62.660 Nondisplaced fracture of distal phalanx of right index finger**

√7ᵗʰ **S62.661 Nondisplaced fracture of distal phalanx of left index finger**

√7ᵗʰ **S62.662 Nondisplaced fracture of distal phalanx of right middle finger**

√7ᵗʰ **S62.663 Nondisplaced fracture of distal phalanx of left middle finger**

√7ᵗʰ **S62.664 Nondisplaced fracture of distal phalanx of right ring finger**

√7ᵗʰ **S62.665 Nondisplaced fracture of distal phalanx of left ring finger**

√7ᵗʰ **S62.666 Nondisplaced fracture of distal phalanx of right little finger**

√7ᵗʰ **S62.667 Nondisplaced fracture of distal phalanx of left little finger**

√7ᵗʰ **S62.668 Nondisplaced fracture of distal phalanx of other finger**
Nondisplaced fracture of distal phalanx of specified finger with unspecified laterality

√7ᵗʰ **S62.669 Nondisplaced fracture of distal phalanx of unspecified finger** ▽

√5ᵗʰ **S62.9 Unspecified fracture of wrist and hand**

√x7ᵗʰ **S62.90 Unspecified fracture of unspecified wrist and hand** ◨ ▽

√x7ᵗʰ **S62.91 Unspecified fracture of right wrist and hand** ◨ ▽

√x7ᵗʰ **S62.92 Unspecified fracture of left wrist and hand** ◨ ▽

√4ᵗʰ **S63 Dislocation and sprain of joints and ligaments at wrist and hand level**

INCLUDES avulsion of joint or ligament at wrist and hand level
laceration of cartilage, joint or ligament at wrist and hand level
sprain of cartilage, joint or ligament at wrist and hand level
traumatic hemarthrosis of joint or ligament at wrist and hand level
traumatic rupture of joint or ligament at wrist and hand level
traumatic subluxation of joint or ligament at wrist and hand level
traumatic tear of joint or ligament at wrist and hand level

Code also any associated open wound

EXCLUDES 2 *strain of muscle, fascia and tendon of wrist and hand (S66.-)*

The appropriate 7th character is to be added to each code from category S63.
A   initial encounter
D   subsequent encounter
S   sequela

√5ᵗʰ **S63.0 Subluxation and dislocation of wrist and hand joints**

√6ᵗʰ **S63.00 Unspecified subluxation and dislocation of wrist and hand**
Dislocation of carpal bone NOS
Dislocation of distal end of radius NOS
Subluxation of carpal bone NOS
Subluxation of distal end of radius NOS

√7ᵗʰ **S63.001 Unspecified subluxation of right wrist and hand** ▽

√7ᵗʰ **S63.002 Unspecified subluxation of left wrist and hand** ▽

√7ᵗʰ **S63.003 Unspecified subluxation of unspecified wrist and hand** ▽

√7ᵗʰ **S63.004 Unspecified dislocation of right wrist and hand** ▽

√7ᵗʰ **S63.005 Unspecified dislocation of left wrist and hand** ▽

√7ᵗʰ **S63.006 Unspecified dislocation of unspecified wrist and hand** ▽

√6ᵗʰ **S63.01 Subluxation and dislocation of distal radioulnar joint**

√7ᵗʰ **S63.011 Subluxation of distal radioulnar joint of right wrist**

√7ᵗʰ **S63.012 Subluxation of distal radioulnar joint of left wrist**

√7ᵗʰ **S63.013 Subluxation of distal radioulnar joint of unspecified wrist** ▽

√7ᵗʰ **S63.014 Dislocation of distal radioulnar joint of right wrist**

√7ᵗʰ **S63.015 Dislocation of distal radioulnar joint of left wrist**

√7ᵗʰ **S63.016 Dislocation of distal radioulnar joint of unspecified wrist** ▽

√6ᵗʰ **S63.02 Subluxation and dislocation of radiocarpal joint**

√7ᵗʰ **S63.021 Subluxation of radiocarpal joint of right wrist**

√7ᵗʰ **S63.022 Subluxation of radiocarpal joint of left wrist**

√7ᵗʰ **S63.023 Subluxation of radiocarpal joint of unspecified wrist** ▽

√7ᵗʰ **S63.024 Dislocation of radiocarpal joint of right wrist**

√7ᵗʰ **S63.025** Dislocation of radiocarpal joint of left wrist

√7ᵗʰ **S63.026** Dislocation of radiocarpal joint of unspecified wrist ▽

√6ᵗʰ **S63.03** Subluxation and dislocation of midcarpal joint

√7ᵗʰ **S63.031** Subluxation of midcarpal joint of right wrist

√7ᵗʰ **S63.032** Subluxation of midcarpal joint of left wrist

√7ᵗʰ **S63.033** Subluxation of midcarpal joint of unspecified wrist ▽

√7ᵗʰ **S63.034** Dislocation of midcarpal joint of right wrist

√7ᵗʰ **S63.035** Dislocation of midcarpal joint of left wrist

√7ᵗʰ **S63.036** Dislocation of midcarpal joint of unspecified wrist ▽

√6ᵗʰ **S63.04** Subluxation and dislocation of carpometacarpal joint of thumb

> EXCLUDES 2   interphalangeal subluxation and dislocation of thumb (S63.1-)

√7ᵗʰ **S63.041** Subluxation of carpometacarpal joint of right thumb

√7ᵗʰ **S63.042** Subluxation of carpometacarpal joint of left thumb

√7ᵗʰ **S63.043** Subluxation of carpometacarpal joint of unspecified thumb ▽

√7ᵗʰ **S63.044** Dislocation of carpometacarpal joint of right thumb

√7ᵗʰ **S63.045** Dislocation of carpometacarpal joint of left thumb

√7ᵗʰ **S63.046** Dislocation of carpometacarpal joint of unspecified thumb ▽

√6ᵗʰ **S63.05** Subluxation and dislocation of other carpometacarpal joint

> EXCLUDES 2   subluxation and dislocation of carpometacarpal joint of thumb (S63.04-)

√7ᵗʰ **S63.051** Subluxation of other carpometacarpal joint of right hand

√7ᵗʰ **S63.052** Subluxation of other carpometacarpal joint of left hand

√7ᵗʰ **S63.053** Subluxation of other carpometacarpal joint of unspecified hand ▽

√7ᵗʰ **S63.054** Dislocation of other carpometacarpal joint of right hand

√7ᵗʰ **S63.055** Dislocation of other carpometacarpal joint of left hand

√7ᵗʰ **S63.056** Dislocation of other carpometacarpal joint of unspecified hand ▽

√6ᵗʰ **S63.06** Subluxation and dislocation of metacarpal (bone), proximal end

√7ᵗʰ **S63.061** Subluxation of metacarpal (bone), proximal end of right hand

√7ᵗʰ **S63.062** Subluxation of metacarpal (bone), proximal end of left hand

√7ᵗʰ **S63.063** Subluxation of metacarpal (bone), proximal end of unspecified hand ▽

√7ᵗʰ **S63.064** Dislocation of metacarpal (bone), proximal end of right hand

√7ᵗʰ **S63.065** Dislocation of metacarpal (bone), proximal end of left hand

√7ᵗʰ **S63.066** Dislocation of metacarpal (bone), proximal end of unspecified hand ▽

√6ᵗʰ **S63.07** Subluxation and dislocation of distal end of ulna

√7ᵗʰ **S63.071** Subluxation of distal end of right ulna

√7ᵗʰ **S63.072** Subluxation of distal end of left ulna

√7ᵗʰ **S63.073** Subluxation of distal end of unspecified ulna ▽

√7ᵗʰ **S63.074** Dislocation of distal end of right ulna

√7ᵗʰ **S63.075** Dislocation of distal end of left ulna

√7ᵗʰ **S63.076** Dislocation of distal end of unspecified ulna ▽

√6ᵗʰ **S63.09** Other subluxation and dislocation of wrist and hand

√7ᵗʰ **S63.091** Other subluxation of right wrist and hand

√7ᵗʰ **S63.092** Other subluxation of left wrist and hand

√7ᵗʰ **S63.093** Other subluxation of unspecified wrist and hand ▽

√7ᵗʰ **S63.094** Other dislocation of right wrist and hand

√7ᵗʰ **S63.095** Other dislocation of left wrist and hand

√7ᵗʰ **S63.096** Other dislocation of unspecified wrist and hand ▽

√5ᵗʰ **S63.1** Subluxation and dislocation of thumb

√6ᵗʰ **S63.10** Unspecified subluxation and dislocation of thumb

√7ᵗʰ **S63.101** Unspecified subluxation of right thumb ▽

√7ᵗʰ **S63.102** Unspecified subluxation of left thumb ▽

√7ᵗʰ **S63.103** Unspecified subluxation of unspecified thumb ▽

√7ᵗʰ **S63.104** Unspecified dislocation of right thumb ▽

√7ᵗʰ **S63.105** Unspecified dislocation of left thumb ▽

√7ᵗʰ **S63.106** Unspecified dislocation of unspecified thumb ▽

√6ᵗʰ **S63.11** Subluxation and dislocation of metacarpophalangeal joint of thumb

√7ᵗʰ **S63.111** Subluxation of metacarpophalangeal joint of right thumb

√7ᵗʰ **S63.112** Subluxation of metacarpophalangeal joint of left thumb

√7ᵗʰ **S63.113** Subluxation of metacarpophalangeal joint of unspecified thumb

√7ᵗʰ **S63.114** Dislocation of metacarpophalangeal joint of right thumb

√7ᵗʰ **S63.115** Dislocation of metacarpophalangeal joint of left thumb

√7ᵗʰ **S63.116** Dislocation of metacarpophalangeal joint of unspecified thumb ▽

√6ᵗʰ **S63.12** Subluxation and dislocation of interphalangeal joint of thumb

√7ᵗʰ **S63.121** Subluxation of interphalangeal joint of right thumb

√7ᵗʰ **S63.122** Subluxation of interphalangeal joint of left thumb

√7ᵗʰ **S63.123** Subluxation of interphalangeal joint of unspecified thumb

√7ᵗʰ **S63.124** Dislocation of interphalangeal joint of right thumb

√7ᵗʰ **S63.125** Dislocation of interphalangeal joint of left thumb

√7ᵗʰ **S63.126** Dislocation of interphalangeal joint of unspecified thumb ▽

√5ᵗʰ **S63.2** Subluxation and dislocation of other finger(s)

> EXCLUDES 2   subluxation and dislocation of thumb (S63.1-)

√6ᵗʰ **S63.20** Unspecified subluxation of other finger

√7ᵗʰ **S63.200** Unspecified subluxation of right index finger ▽

√7ᵗʰ **S63.201** Unspecified subluxation of left index finger ▽

√7ᵗʰ **S63.202** Unspecified subluxation of right middle finger ▽

√7ᵗʰ **S63.203** Unspecified subluxation of left middle finger ▽

√7ᵗʰ **S63.204** Unspecified subluxation of right ring finger ▽

√7ᵗʰ **S63.205** Unspecified subluxation of left ring finger ▽

√7ᵗʰ **S63.206** Unspecified subluxation of right little finger ▽

√7ᵗʰ **S63.207** Unspecified subluxation of left little finger ▽

√7ᵗʰ **S63.208** Unspecified subluxation of other finger ▽

> Unspecified subluxation of specified finger with unspecified laterality

√7ᵗʰ **S63.209** Unspecified subluxation of unspecified finger ▽

√6ᵗʰ **S63.21** Subluxation of metacarpophalangeal joint of finger

√7ᵗʰ **S63.210** Subluxation of metacarpophalangeal joint of right index finger

√7ᵗʰ **S63.211** Subluxation of metacarpophalangeal joint of left index finger

√7ᵗʰ **S63.212** Subluxation of metacarpophalangeal joint of right middle finger

☑ Additional Character Req   √x7ᵗʰ Placeholder Alert   Manifestation   ▽ Unspecified   ►◄ Revised Text   ● New Code   ▲ Revised Code Title

ICD-10-CM 2019   1025

√7ᵗʰ **S63.213 Subluxation of metacarpophalangeal joint of left middle finger**

√7ᵗʰ **S63.214 Subluxation of metacarpophalangeal joint of right ring finger**

√7ᵗʰ **S63.215 Subluxation of metacarpophalangeal joint of left ring finger**

√7ᵗʰ **S63.216 Subluxation of metacarpophalangeal joint of right little finger**

√7ᵗʰ **S63.217 Subluxation of metacarpophalangeal joint of left little finger**

√7ᵗʰ **S63.218 Subluxation of metacarpophalangeal joint of other finger**
Subluxation of metacarpophalangeal joint of specified finger with unspecified laterality

√7ᵗʰ **S63.219 Subluxation of metacarpophalangeal joint of unspecified finger** ▽

√6ᵗʰ **S63.22 Subluxation of unspecified interphalangeal joint of finger**

√7ᵗʰ **S63.220 Subluxation of unspecified interphalangeal joint of right index finger** ▽

√7ᵗʰ **S63.221 Subluxation of unspecified interphalangeal joint of left index finger** ▽

√7ᵗʰ **S63.222 Subluxation of unspecified interphalangeal joint of right middle finger** ▽

√7ᵗʰ **S63.223 Subluxation of unspecified interphalangeal joint of left middle finger** ▽

√7ᵗʰ **S63.224 Subluxation of unspecified interphalangeal joint of right ring finger** ▽

√7ᵗʰ **S63.225 Subluxation of unspecified interphalangeal joint of left ring finger** ▽

√7ᵗʰ **S63.226 Subluxation of unspecified interphalangeal joint of right little finger** ▽

√7ᵗʰ **S63.227 Subluxation of unspecified interphalangeal joint of left little finger** ▽

√7ᵗʰ **S63.228 Subluxation of unspecified interphalangeal joint of other finger** ▽
Subluxation of unspecified interphalangeal joint of specified finger with unspecified laterality

√7ᵗʰ **S63.229 Subluxation of unspecified interphalangeal joint of unspecified finger** ▽

√6ᵗʰ **S63.23 Subluxation of proximal interphalangeal joint of finger**

√7ᵗʰ **S63.230 Subluxation of proximal interphalangeal joint of right index finger**

√7ᵗʰ **S63.231 Subluxation of proximal interphalangeal joint of left index finger**

√7ᵗʰ **S63.232 Subluxation of proximal interphalangeal joint of right middle finger**

√7ᵗʰ **S63.233 Subluxation of proximal interphalangeal joint of left middle finger**

√7ᵗʰ **S63.234 Subluxation of proximal interphalangeal joint of right ring finger**

√7ᵗʰ **S63.235 Subluxation of proximal interphalangeal joint of left ring finger**

√7ᵗʰ **S63.236 Subluxation of proximal interphalangeal joint of right little finger**

√7ᵗʰ **S63.237 Subluxation of proximal interphalangeal joint of left little finger**

√7ᵗʰ **S63.238 Subluxation of proximal interphalangeal joint of other finger**
Subluxation of proximal interphalangeal joint of specified finger with unspecified laterality

√7ᵗʰ **S63.239 Subluxation of proximal interphalangeal joint of unspecified finger** ▽

√6ᵗʰ **S63.24 Subluxation of distal interphalangeal joint of finger**

√7ᵗʰ **S63.240 Subluxation of distal interphalangeal joint of right index finger**

√7ᵗʰ **S63.241 Subluxation of distal interphalangeal joint of left index finger**

√7ᵗʰ **S63.242 Subluxation of distal interphalangeal joint of right middle finger**

√7ᵗʰ **S63.243 Subluxation of distal interphalangeal joint of left middle finger**

√7ᵗʰ **S63.244 Subluxation of distal interphalangeal joint of right ring finger**

√7ᵗʰ **S63.245 Subluxation of distal interphalangeal joint of left ring finger**

√7ᵗʰ **S63.246 Subluxation of distal interphalangeal joint of right little finger**

√7ᵗʰ **S63.247 Subluxation of distal interphalangeal joint of left little finger**

√7ᵗʰ **S63.248 Subluxation of distal interphalangeal joint of other finger**
Subluxation of distal interphalangeal joint of specified finger with unspecified laterality

√7ᵗʰ **S63.249 Subluxation of distal interphalangeal joint of unspecified finger** ▽

√6ᵗʰ **S63.25 Unspecified dislocation of other finger**

√7ᵗʰ **S63.250 Unspecified dislocation of right index finger** ▽

√7ᵗʰ **S63.251 Unspecified dislocation of left index finger** ▽

√7ᵗʰ **S63.252 Unspecified dislocation of right middle finger** ▽

√7ᵗʰ **S63.253 Unspecified dislocation of left middle finger** ▽

√7ᵗʰ **S63.254 Unspecified dislocation of right ring finger** ▽

√7ᵗʰ **S63.255 Unspecified dislocation of left ring finger** ▽

√7ᵗʰ **S63.256 Unspecified dislocation of right little finger** ▽

√7ᵗʰ **S63.257 Unspecified dislocation of left little finger** ▽

√7ᵗʰ **S63.258 Unspecified dislocation of other finger** ▽
Unspecified dislocation of specified finger with unspecified laterality

√7ᵗʰ **S63.259 Unspecified dislocation of unspecified finger** ▽
Unspecified dislocation of unspecified finger with unspecified laterality

√6ᵗʰ **S63.26 Dislocation of metacarpophalangeal joint of finger**

√7ᵗʰ **S63.260 Dislocation of metacarpophalangeal joint of right index finger**

√7ᵗʰ **S63.261 Dislocation of metacarpophalangeal joint of left index finger**

√7ᵗʰ **S63.262 Dislocation of metacarpophalangeal joint of right middle finger**

√7ᵗʰ **S63.263 Dislocation of metacarpophalangeal joint of left middle finger**

√7ᵗʰ **S63.264 Dislocation of metacarpophalangeal joint of right ring finger**

√7ᵗʰ **S63.265 Dislocation of metacarpophalangeal joint of left ring finger**

√7ᵗʰ **S63.266 Dislocation of metacarpophalangeal joint of right little finger**

√7ᵗʰ **S63.267 Dislocation of metacarpophalangeal joint of left little finger**

√7ᵗʰ **S63.268 Dislocation of metacarpophalangeal joint of other finger**
Dislocation of metacarpophalangeal joint of specified finger with unspecified laterality

√7ᵗʰ **S63.269 Dislocation of metacarpophalangeal joint of unspecified finger** ▽

√6ᵗʰ **S63.27 Dislocation of unspecified interphalangeal joint of finger**

√7ᵗʰ **S63.270 Dislocation of unspecified interphalangeal joint of right index finger** ▽

√7ᵗʰ **S63.271 Dislocation of unspecified interphalangeal joint of left index finger** ▽

√7ᵗʰ **S63.272 Dislocation of unspecified interphalangeal joint of right middle finger** ▽

√7ᵗʰ **S63.273** **Dislocation of unspecified interphalangeal joint of left middle finger** ▽

√7ᵗʰ **S63.274** **Dislocation of unspecified interphalangeal joint of right ring finger** ▽

√7ᵗʰ **S63.275** **Dislocation of unspecified interphalangeal joint of left ring finger** ▽

√7ᵗʰ **S63.276** **Dislocation of unspecified interphalangeal joint of right little finger** ▽

√7ᵗʰ **S63.277** **Dislocation of unspecified interphalangeal joint of left little finger** ▽

√7ᵗʰ **S63.278** **Dislocation of unspecified interphalangeal joint of other finger** ▽
     Dislocation of unspecified interphalangeal joint of specified finger with unspecified laterality

√7ᵗʰ **S63.279** **Dislocation of unspecified interphalangeal joint of unspecified finger** ▽
     Dislocation of unspecified interphalangeal joint of unspecified finger without specified laterality

√6ᵗʰ **S63.28** **Dislocation of proximal interphalangeal joint of finger**

√7ᵗʰ **S63.280** **Dislocation of proximal interphalangeal joint of right index finger**

√7ᵗʰ **S63.281** **Dislocation of proximal interphalangeal joint of left index finger**

√7ᵗʰ **S63.282** **Dislocation of proximal interphalangeal joint of right middle finger**

√7ᵗʰ **S63.283** **Dislocation of proximal interphalangeal joint of left middle finger**

√7ᵗʰ **S63.284** **Dislocation of proximal interphalangeal joint of right ring finger**

√7ᵗʰ **S63.285** **Dislocation of proximal interphalangeal joint of left ring finger**

√7ᵗʰ **S63.286** **Dislocation of proximal interphalangeal joint of right little finger**

√7ᵗʰ **S63.287** **Dislocation of proximal interphalangeal joint of left little finger**

√7ᵗʰ **S63.288** **Dislocation of proximal interphalangeal joint of other finger**
     Dislocation of proximal interphalangeal joint of specified finger with unspecified laterality

√7ᵗʰ **S63.289** **Dislocation of proximal interphalangeal joint of unspecified finger** ▽

√6ᵗʰ **S63.29** **Dislocation of distal interphalangeal joint of finger**

√7ᵗʰ **S63.290** **Dislocation of distal interphalangeal joint of right index finger**

√7ᵗʰ **S63.291** **Dislocation of distal interphalangeal joint of left index finger**

√7ᵗʰ **S63.292** **Dislocation of distal interphalangeal joint of right middle finger**

√7ᵗʰ **S63.293** **Dislocation of distal interphalangeal joint of left middle finger**

√7ᵗʰ **S63.294** **Dislocation of distal interphalangeal joint of right ring finger**

√7ᵗʰ **S63.295** **Dislocation of distal interphalangeal joint of left ring finger**

√7ᵗʰ **S63.296** **Dislocation of distal interphalangeal joint of right little finger**

√7ᵗʰ **S63.297** **Dislocation of distal interphalangeal joint of left little finger**

√7ᵗʰ **S63.298** **Dislocation of distal interphalangeal joint of other finger**
     Dislocation of distal interphalangeal joint of specified finger with unspecified laterality

√7ᵗʰ **S63.299** **Dislocation of distal interphalangeal joint of unspecified finger** ▽

√5ᵗʰ **S63.3** **Traumatic rupture of ligament of wrist**

√6ᵗʰ **S63.30** **Traumatic rupture of unspecified ligament of wrist**

√7ᵗʰ **S63.301** **Traumatic rupture of unspecified ligament of right wrist** ▽

√7ᵗʰ **S63.302** **Traumatic rupture of unspecified ligament of left wrist** ▽

√7ᵗʰ **S63.309** **Traumatic rupture of unspecified ligament of unspecified wrist** ▽

√6ᵗʰ **S63.31** **Traumatic rupture of collateral ligament of wrist**

√7ᵗʰ **S63.311** **Traumatic rupture of collateral ligament of right wrist**

√7ᵗʰ **S63.312** **Traumatic rupture of collateral ligament of left wrist**

√7ᵗʰ **S63.319** **Traumatic rupture of collateral ligament of unspecified wrist** ▽

√6ᵗʰ **S63.32** **Traumatic rupture of radiocarpal ligament**

√7ᵗʰ **S63.321** **Traumatic rupture of right radiocarpal ligament**

√7ᵗʰ **S63.322** **Traumatic rupture of left radiocarpal ligament**

√7ᵗʰ **S63.329** **Traumatic rupture of unspecified radiocarpal ligament** ▽

√6ᵗʰ **S63.33** **Traumatic rupture of ulnocarpal (palmar) ligament**

√7ᵗʰ **S63.331** **Traumatic rupture of right ulnocarpal (palmar) ligament**

√7ᵗʰ **S63.332** **Traumatic rupture of left ulnocarpal (palmar) ligament**

√7ᵗʰ **S63.339** **Traumatic rupture of unspecified ulnocarpal (palmar) ligament** ▽

√6ᵗʰ **S63.39** **Traumatic rupture of other ligament of wrist**

√7ᵗʰ **S63.391** **Traumatic rupture of other ligament of right wrist**

√7ᵗʰ **S63.392** **Traumatic rupture of other ligament of left wrist**

√7ᵗʰ **S63.399** **Traumatic rupture of other ligament of unspecified wrist** ▽

√5ᵗʰ **S63.4** **Traumatic rupture of ligament of finger at metacarpophalangeal and interphalangeal joint(s)**

√6ᵗʰ **S63.40** **Traumatic rupture of unspecified ligament of finger at metacarpophalangeal and interphalangeal joint**

√7ᵗʰ **S63.400** **Traumatic rupture of unspecified ligament of right index finger at metacarpophalangeal and interphalangeal joint** ▽

√7ᵗʰ **S63.401** **Traumatic rupture of unspecified ligament of left index finger at metacarpophalangeal and interphalangeal joint** ▽

√7ᵗʰ **S63.402** **Traumatic rupture of unspecified ligament of right middle finger at metacarpophalangeal and interphalangeal joint** ▽

√7ᵗʰ **S63.403** **Traumatic rupture of unspecified ligament of left middle finger at metacarpophalangeal and interphalangeal joint** ▽

√7ᵗʰ **S63.404** **Traumatic rupture of unspecified ligament of right ring finger at metacarpophalangeal and interphalangeal joint** ▽

√7ᵗʰ **S63.405** **Traumatic rupture of unspecified ligament of left ring finger at metacarpophalangeal and interphalangeal joint** ▽

√7ᵗʰ **S63.406** **Traumatic rupture of unspecified ligament of right little finger at metacarpophalangeal and interphalangeal joint** ▽

√7ᵗʰ **S63.407** **Traumatic rupture of unspecified ligament of left little finger at metacarpophalangeal and interphalangeal joint** ▽

√7ᵗʰ **S63.408** **Traumatic rupture of unspecified ligament of other finger at metacarpophalangeal and interphalangeal joint** ▽
     Traumatic rupture of unspecified ligament of specified finger with unspecified laterality at metacarpophalangeal and interphalangeal joint

√7ᵗʰ **S63.409** **Traumatic rupture of unspecified ligament of unspecified finger at metacarpophalangeal and interphalangeal joint** ▽

✓6ᵗʰ **S63.41   Traumatic rupture of collateral ligament of finger at metacarpophalangeal and interphalangeal joint**

✓7ᵗʰ **S63.410   Traumatic rupture of collateral ligament of right index finger at metacarpophalangeal and interphalangeal joint**

✓7ᵗʰ **S63.411   Traumatic rupture of collateral ligament of left index finger at metacarpophalangeal and interphalangeal joint**

✓7ᵗʰ **S63.412   Traumatic rupture of collateral ligament of right middle finger at metacarpophalangeal and interphalangeal joint**

✓7ᵗʰ **S63.413   Traumatic rupture of collateral ligament of left middle finger at metacarpophalangeal and interphalangeal joint**

✓7ᵗʰ **S63.414   Traumatic rupture of collateral ligament of right ring finger at metacarpophalangeal and interphalangeal joint**

✓7ᵗʰ **S63.415   Traumatic rupture of collateral ligament of left ring finger at metacarpophalangeal and interphalangeal joint**

✓7ᵗʰ **S63.416   Traumatic rupture of collateral ligament of right little finger at metacarpophalangeal and interphalangeal joint**

✓7ᵗʰ **S63.417   Traumatic rupture of collateral ligament of left little finger at metacarpophalangeal and interphalangeal joint**

✓7ᵗʰ **S63.418   Traumatic rupture of collateral ligament of other finger at metacarpophalangeal and interphalangeal joint**

Traumatic rupture of collateral ligament of specified finger with unspecified laterality at metacarpophalangeal and interphalangeal joint

✓7ᵗʰ **S63.419   Traumatic rupture of collateral ligament of unspecified finger at metacarpophalangeal and interphalangeal joint**   ▽

✓6ᵗʰ **S63.42   Traumatic rupture of palmar ligament of finger at metacarpophalangeal and interphalangeal joint**

✓7ᵗʰ **S63.420   Traumatic rupture of palmar ligament of right index finger at metacarpophalangeal and interphalangeal joint**

✓7ᵗʰ **S63.421   Traumatic rupture of palmar ligament of left index finger at metacarpophalangeal and interphalangeal joint**

✓7ᵗʰ **S63.422   Traumatic rupture of palmar ligament of right middle finger at metacarpophalangeal and interphalangeal joint**

✓7ᵗʰ **S63.423   Traumatic rupture of palmar ligament of left middle finger at metacarpophalangeal and interphalangeal joint**

✓7ᵗʰ **S63.424   Traumatic rupture of palmar ligament of right ring finger at metacarpophalangeal and interphalangeal joint**

✓7ᵗʰ **S63.425   Traumatic rupture of palmar ligament of left ring finger at metacarpophalangeal and interphalangeal joint**

✓7ᵗʰ **S63.426   Traumatic rupture of palmar ligament of right little finger at metacarpophalangeal and interphalangeal joint**

✓7ᵗʰ **S63.427   Traumatic rupture of palmar ligament of left little finger at metacarpophalangeal and interphalangeal joint**

✓7ᵗʰ **S63.428   Traumatic rupture of palmar ligament of other finger at metacarpophalangeal and interphalangeal joint**

Traumatic rupture of palmar ligament of specified finger with unspecified laterality at metacarpophalangeal and interphalangeal joint

✓7ᵗʰ **S63.429   Traumatic rupture of palmar ligament of unspecified finger at metacarpophalangeal and interphalangeal joint**   ▽

✓6ᵗʰ **S63.43   Traumatic rupture of volar plate of finger at metacarpophalangeal and interphalangeal joint**

✓7ᵗʰ **S63.430   Traumatic rupture of volar plate of right index finger at metacarpophalangeal and interphalangeal joint**

✓7ᵗʰ **S63.431   Traumatic rupture of volar plate of left index finger at metacarpophalangeal and interphalangeal joint**

✓7ᵗʰ **S63.432   Traumatic rupture of volar plate of right middle finger at metacarpophalangeal and interphalangeal joint**

✓7ᵗʰ **S63.433   Traumatic rupture of volar plate of left middle finger at metacarpophalangeal and interphalangeal joint**

✓7ᵗʰ **S63.434   Traumatic rupture of volar plate of right ring finger at metacarpophalangeal and interphalangeal joint**

✓7ᵗʰ **S63.435   Traumatic rupture of volar plate of left ring finger at metacarpophalangeal and interphalangeal joint**

✓7ᵗʰ **S63.436   Traumatic rupture of volar plate of right little finger at metacarpophalangeal and interphalangeal joint**

✓7ᵗʰ **S63.437   Traumatic rupture of volar plate of left little finger at metacarpophalangeal and interphalangeal joint**

✓7ᵗʰ **S63.438   Traumatic rupture of volar plate of other finger at metacarpophalangeal and interphalangeal joint**

Traumatic rupture of volar plate of specified finger with unspecified laterality at metacarpophalangeal and interphalangeal joint

✓7ᵗʰ **S63.439   Traumatic rupture of volar plate of unspecified finger at metacarpophalangeal and interphalangeal joint**   ▽

✓6ᵗʰ **S63.49   Traumatic rupture of other ligament of finger at metacarpophalangeal and interphalangeal joint**

✓7ᵗʰ **S63.490   Traumatic rupture of other ligament of right index finger at metacarpophalangeal and interphalangeal joint**

✓7ᵗʰ **S63.491   Traumatic rupture of other ligament of left index finger at metacarpophalangeal and interphalangeal joint**

✓7ᵗʰ **S63.492   Traumatic rupture of other ligament of right middle finger at metacarpophalangeal and interphalangeal joint**

✓7ᵗʰ **S63.493   Traumatic rupture of other ligament of left middle finger at metacarpophalangeal and interphalangeal joint**

✓7ᵗʰ **S63.494   Traumatic rupture of other ligament of right ring finger at metacarpophalangeal and interphalangeal joint**

✓7ᵗʰ **S63.495   Traumatic rupture of other ligament of left ring finger at metacarpophalangeal and interphalangeal joint**

✓7ᵗʰ **S63.496   Traumatic rupture of other ligament of right little finger at metacarpophalangeal and interphalangeal joint**

✓7ᵗʰ **S63.497   Traumatic rupture of other ligament of left little finger at metacarpophalangeal and interphalangeal joint**

✓7ᵗʰ **S63.498   Traumatic rupture of other ligament of other finger at metacarpophalangeal and interphalangeal joint**

Traumatic rupture of ligament of specified finger with unspecified laterality at metacarpophalangeal and interphalangeal joint

✓7ᵗʰ **S63.499   Traumatic rupture of other ligament of unspecified finger at metacarpophalangeal and interphalangeal joint**   ▽

✓5ᵗʰ **S63.5   Other and unspecified sprain of wrist**

✓6ᵗʰ **S63.50   Unspecified sprain of wrist**

✓7ᵗʰ **S63.501   Unspecified sprain of right wrist**   ▽

✓7ᵗʰ **S63.502   Unspecified sprain of left wrist**   ▽

✓7ᵗʰ **S63.509   Unspecified sprain of unspecified wrist**   ▽

√6ᵗʰ **S63.51** Sprain of carpal (joint)
- √7ᵗʰ **S63.511** Sprain of carpal joint of right wrist
- √7ᵗʰ **S63.512** Sprain of carpal joint of left wrist
- √7ᵗʰ **S63.519** Sprain of carpal joint of unspecified wrist ▽

√6ᵗʰ **S63.52** Sprain of radiocarpal joint
> *EXCLUDES 1*   *traumatic rupture of radiocarpal ligament (S63.32-)*
- √7ᵗʰ **S63.521** Sprain of radiocarpal joint of right wrist
- √7ᵗʰ **S63.522** Sprain of radiocarpal joint of left wrist
- √7ᵗʰ **S63.529** Sprain of radiocarpal joint of unspecified wrist ▽

√6ᵗʰ **S63.59** Other specified sprain of wrist
- √7ᵗʰ **S63.591** Other specified sprain of right wrist
- √7ᵗʰ **S63.592** Other specified sprain of left wrist
- √7ᵗʰ **S63.599** Other specified sprain of unspecified wrist ▽

√5ᵗʰ **S63.6** Other and unspecified sprain of finger(s)
> *EXCLUDES 1*   *traumatic rupture of ligament of finger at metacarpophalangeal and interphalangeal joint(s) (S63.4-)*

√6ᵗʰ **S63.60** Unspecified sprain of thumb
- √7ᵗʰ **S63.601** Unspecified sprain of right thumb ▽
- √7ᵗʰ **S63.602** Unspecified sprain of left thumb ▽
- √7ᵗʰ **S63.609** Unspecified sprain of unspecified thumb ▽

√6ᵗʰ **S63.61** Unspecified sprain of other and unspecified finger(s)
- √7ᵗʰ **S63.610** Unspecified sprain of right index finger ▽
- √7ᵗʰ **S63.611** Unspecified sprain of left index finger ▽
- √7ᵗʰ **S63.612** Unspecified sprain of right middle finger ▽
- √7ᵗʰ **S63.613** Unspecified sprain of left middle finger ▽
- √7ᵗʰ **S63.614** Unspecified sprain of right ring finger ▽
- √7ᵗʰ **S63.615** Unspecified sprain of left ring finger ▽
- √7ᵗʰ **S63.616** Unspecified sprain of right little finger ▽
- √7ᵗʰ **S63.617** Unspecified sprain of left little finger ▽
- √7ᵗʰ **S63.618** Unspecified sprain of other finger ▽
  > Unspecified sprain of specified finger with unspecified laterality
- √7ᵗʰ **S63.619** Unspecified sprain of unspecified finger ▽

√6ᵗʰ **S63.62** Sprain of interphalangeal joint of thumb
- √7ᵗʰ **S63.621** Sprain of interphalangeal joint of right thumb
- √7ᵗʰ **S63.622** Sprain of interphalangeal joint of left thumb
- √7ᵗʰ **S63.629** Sprain of interphalangeal joint of unspecified thumb ▽

√6ᵗʰ **S63.63** Sprain of interphalangeal joint of other and unspecified finger(s)
- √7ᵗʰ **S63.630** Sprain of interphalangeal joint of right index finger
- √7ᵗʰ **S63.631** Sprain of interphalangeal joint of left index finger
- √7ᵗʰ **S63.632** Sprain of interphalangeal joint of right middle finger
- √7ᵗʰ **S63.633** Sprain of interphalangeal joint of left middle finger
- √7ᵗʰ **S63.634** Sprain of interphalangeal joint of right ring finger
- √7ᵗʰ **S63.635** Sprain of interphalangeal joint of left ring finger
- √7ᵗʰ **S63.636** Sprain of interphalangeal joint of right little finger
- √7ᵗʰ **S63.637** Sprain of interphalangeal joint of left little finger
- √7ᵗʰ **S63.638** Sprain of interphalangeal joint of other finger
- √7ᵗʰ **S63.639** Sprain of interphalangeal joint of unspecified finger ▽

√6ᵗʰ **S63.64** Sprain of metacarpophalangeal joint of thumb
- √7ᵗʰ **S63.641** Sprain of metacarpophalangeal joint of right thumb
- √7ᵗʰ **S63.642** Sprain of metacarpophalangeal joint of left thumb
- √7ᵗʰ **S63.649** Sprain of metacarpophalangeal joint of unspecified thumb ▽

√6ᵗʰ **S63.65** Sprain of metacarpophalangeal joint of other and unspecified finger(s)
- √7ᵗʰ **S63.650** Sprain of metacarpophalangeal joint of right index finger
- √7ᵗʰ **S63.651** Sprain of metacarpophalangeal joint of left index finger
- √7ᵗʰ **S63.652** Sprain of metacarpophalangeal joint of right middle finger
- √7ᵗʰ **S63.653** Sprain of metacarpophalangeal joint of left middle finger
- √7ᵗʰ **S63.654** Sprain of metacarpophalangeal joint of right ring finger
- √7ᵗʰ **S63.655** Sprain of metacarpophalangeal joint of left ring finger
- √7ᵗʰ **S63.656** Sprain of metacarpophalangeal joint of right little finger
- √7ᵗʰ **S63.657** Sprain of metacarpophalangeal joint of left little finger
- √7ᵗʰ **S63.658** Sprain of metacarpophalangeal joint of other finger
  > Sprain of metacarpophalangeal joint of specified finger with unspecified laterality
- √7ᵗʰ **S63.659** Sprain of metacarpophalangeal joint of unspecified finger ▽

√6ᵗʰ **S63.68** Other sprain of thumb
- √7ᵗʰ **S63.681** Other sprain of right thumb
- √7ᵗʰ **S63.682** Other sprain of left thumb
- √7ᵗʰ **S63.689** Other sprain of unspecified thumb ▽

√6ᵗʰ **S63.69** Other sprain of other and unspecified finger(s)
- √7ᵗʰ **S63.690** Other sprain of right index finger
- √7ᵗʰ **S63.691** Other sprain of left index finger
- √7ᵗʰ **S63.692** Other sprain of right middle finger
- √7ᵗʰ **S63.693** Other sprain of left middle finger
- √7ᵗʰ **S63.694** Other sprain of right ring finger
- √7ᵗʰ **S63.695** Other sprain of left ring finger
- √7ᵗʰ **S63.696** Other sprain of right little finger
- √7ᵗʰ **S63.697** Other sprain of left little finger
- √7ᵗʰ **S63.698** Other sprain of other finger
  > Other sprain of specified finger with unspecified laterality
- √7ᵗʰ **S63.699** Other sprain of unspecified finger ▽

√5ᵗʰ **S63.8** Sprain of other part of wrist and hand
√6ᵗʰ **S63.8X** Sprain of other part of wrist and hand
- √7ᵗʰ **S63.8X1** Sprain of other part of right wrist and hand
- √7ᵗʰ **S63.8X2** Sprain of other part of left wrist and hand
- √7ᵗʰ **S63.8X9** Sprain of other part of unspecified wrist and hand ▽

√5ᵗʰ **S63.9** Sprain of unspecified part of wrist and hand
- √x7ᵗʰ **S63.90** Sprain of unspecified part of unspecified wrist and hand ▽
- √x7ᵗʰ **S63.91** Sprain of unspecified part of right wrist and hand ▽
- √x7ᵗʰ **S63.92** Sprain of unspecified part of left wrist and hand ▽

√4ᵗʰ **S64 Injury of nerves at wrist and hand level**
> Code also any associated open wound (S61.-)

> The appropriate 7th character is to be added to each code from category S64.
> A   initial encounter
> D   subsequent encounter
> S   sequela

√5ᵗʰ **S64.0** Injury of ulnar nerve at wrist and hand level
- √x7ᵗʰ **S64.00** Injury of ulnar nerve at wrist and hand level of unspecified arm ▽
- √x7ᵗʰ **S64.01** Injury of ulnar nerve at wrist and hand level of right arm

✓x7ᵗʰ **S64.02** **Injury of ulnar nerve at wrist and hand level of** left **arm**

✓5ᵗʰ **S64.1** **Injury of** median **nerve at wrist and hand level**

     ✓x7ᵗʰ **S64.10** **Injury of median nerve at wrist and hand level of unspecified arm** ▽

     ✓x7ᵗʰ **S64.11** **Injury of median nerve at wrist and hand level of** right **arm**

     ✓x7ᵗʰ **S64.12** **Injury of median nerve at wrist and hand level of** left **arm**

✓5ᵗʰ **S64.2** **Injury of** radial **nerve at wrist and hand level**

     ✓x7ᵗʰ **S64.20** **Injury of radial nerve at wrist and hand level of unspecified arm** ▽

     ✓x7ᵗʰ **S64.21** **Injury of radial nerve at wrist and hand level of** right **arm**

     ✓x7ᵗʰ **S64.22** **Injury of radial nerve at wrist and hand level of** left **arm**

✓5ᵗʰ **S64.3** **Injury of** digital **nerve of** thumb

     ✓x7ᵗʰ **S64.30** **Injury of digital nerve of unspecified thumb** ▽

     ✓x7ᵗʰ **S64.31** **Injury of digital nerve of** right **thumb**

     ✓x7ᵗʰ **S64.32** **Injury of digital nerve of** left **thumb**

✓5ᵗʰ **S64.4** **Injury of** digital **nerve of other and unspecified** finger

     ✓x7ᵗʰ **S64.40** **Injury of digital nerve of unspecified finger** ▽

     ✓6ᵗʰ **S64.49** **Injury of digital nerve of other finger**

         ✓7ᵗʰ **S64.490** **Injury of digital nerve of** right index **finger**

         ✓7ᵗʰ **S64.491** **Injury of digital nerve of** left index **finger**

         ✓7ᵗʰ **S64.492** **Injury of digital nerve of** right middle **finger**

         ✓7ᵗʰ **S64.493** **Injury of digital nerve of** left middle **finger**

         ✓7ᵗʰ **S64.494** **Injury of digital nerve of** right ring **finger**

         ✓7ᵗʰ **S64.495** **Injury of digital nerve of** left ring **finger**

         ✓7ᵗʰ **S64.496** **Injury of digital nerve of** right little **finger**

         ✓7ᵗʰ **S64.497** **Injury of digital nerve of** left little **finger**

         ✓7ᵗʰ **S64.498** **Injury of digital nerve of other finger**

             Injury of digital nerve of specified finger with unspecified laterality

✓5ᵗʰ **S64.8** **Injury of other nerves at wrist and hand level**

     ✓6ᵗʰ **S64.8X** **Injury of other nerves at wrist and hand level**

         ✓7ᵗʰ **S64.8X1** **Injury of other nerves at wrist and hand level of** right **arm**

         ✓7ᵗʰ **S64.8X2** **Injury of other nerves at wrist and hand level of** left **arm**

         ✓7ᵗʰ **S64.8X9** **Injury of other nerves at wrist and hand level of unspecified arm** ▽

✓5ᵗʰ **S64.9** **Injury of unspecified nerve at wrist and hand level**

     ✓x7ᵗʰ **S64.90** **Injury of unspecified nerve at wrist and hand level of unspecified arm** ▽

     ✓x7ᵗʰ **S64.91** **Injury of unspecified nerve at wrist and hand level of** right **arm** ▽

     ✓x7ᵗʰ **S64.92** **Injury of unspecified nerve at wrist and hand level of** left **arm** ▽

✓4ᵗʰ **S65** **Injury of blood vessels at wrist and hand level**

     Code also any associated open wound (S61.-)

     The appropriate 7th character is to be added to each code from category S65.
     A   initial encounter
     D   subsequent encounter
     S   sequela

✓5ᵗʰ **S65.0** **Injury of** ulnar artery **at wrist and hand level**

     ✓6ᵗʰ **S65.00** **Unspecified injury of ulnar artery at wrist and hand level**

         ✓7ᵗʰ **S65.001** **Unspecified injury of ulnar artery at wrist and hand level of** right **arm** ▽

         ✓7ᵗʰ **S65.002** **Unspecified injury of ulnar artery at wrist and hand level of** left **arm** ▽

         ✓7ᵗʰ **S65.009** **Unspecified injury of ulnar artery at wrist and hand level of unspecified arm** ▽

     ✓6ᵗʰ **S65.01** Laceration **of ulnar artery at wrist and hand level**

         ✓7ᵗʰ **S65.011** **Laceration of ulnar artery at wrist and hand level of** right **arm**

         ✓7ᵗʰ **S65.012** **Laceration of ulnar artery at wrist and hand level of** left **arm**

         ✓7ᵗʰ **S65.019** **Laceration of ulnar artery at wrist and hand level of unspecified arm** ▽

     ✓6ᵗʰ **S65.09** **Other specified injury of ulnar artery at wrist and hand level**

         ✓7ᵗʰ **S65.091** **Other specified injury of ulnar artery at wrist and hand level of** right **arm**

         ✓7ᵗʰ **S65.092** **Other specified injury of ulnar artery at wrist and hand level of** left **arm**

         ✓7ᵗʰ **S65.099** **Other specified injury of ulnar artery at wrist and hand level of unspecified arm** ▽

✓5ᵗʰ **S65.1** **Injury of** radial artery **at wrist and hand level**

     ✓6ᵗʰ **S65.10** **Unspecified injury of radial artery at wrist and hand level**

         ✓7ᵗʰ **S65.101** **Unspecified injury of radial artery at wrist and hand level of** right **arm** ▽

         ✓7ᵗʰ **S65.102** **Unspecified injury of radial artery at wrist and hand level of** left **arm** ▽

         ✓7ᵗʰ **S65.109** **Unspecified injury of radial artery at wrist and hand level of unspecified arm** ▽

     ✓6ᵗʰ **S65.11** **Laceration of radial artery at wrist and hand level**

         ✓7ᵗʰ **S65.111** **Laceration of radial artery at wrist and hand level of** right **arm**

         ✓7ᵗʰ **S65.112** **Laceration of radial artery at wrist and hand level of** left **arm**

         ✓7ᵗʰ **S65.119** **Laceration of radial artery at wrist and hand level of unspecified arm** ▽

     ✓6ᵗʰ **S65.19** **Other specified injury of radial artery at wrist and hand level**

         ✓7ᵗʰ **S65.191** **Other specified injury of radial artery at wrist and hand level of** right **arm**

         ✓7ᵗʰ **S65.192** **Other specified injury of radial artery at wrist and hand level of** left **arm**

         ✓7ᵗʰ **S65.199** **Other specified injury of radial artery at wrist and hand level of unspecified arm** ▽

✓5ᵗʰ **S65.2** **Injury of** superficial palmar arch

     ✓6ᵗʰ **S65.20** **Unspecified injury of superficial palmar arch**

         ✓7ᵗʰ **S65.201** **Unspecified injury of superficial palmar arch of** right **hand** ▽

         ✓7ᵗʰ **S65.202** **Unspecified injury of superficial palmar arch of** left **hand** ▽

         ✓7ᵗʰ **S65.209** **Unspecified injury of superficial palmar arch of unspecified hand** ▽

     ✓6ᵗʰ **S65.21** **Laceration of superficial palmar arch**

         ✓7ᵗʰ **S65.211** **Laceration of superficial palmar arch of** right **hand**

         ✓7ᵗʰ **S65.212** **Laceration of superficial palmar arch of** left **hand**

         ✓7ᵗʰ **S65.219** **Laceration of superficial palmar arch of unspecified hand** ▽

     ✓6ᵗʰ **S65.29** **Other specified injury of superficial palmar arch**

         ✓7ᵗʰ **S65.291** **Other specified injury of superficial palmar arch of** right **hand**

         ✓7ᵗʰ **S65.292** **Other specified injury of superficial palmar arch of** left **hand**

         ✓7ᵗʰ **S65.299** **Other specified injury of superficial palmar arch of unspecified hand** ▽

✓5ᵗʰ **S65.3** **Injury of** deep palmar arch

     ✓6ᵗʰ **S65.30** **Unspecified injury of deep palmar arch**

         ✓7ᵗʰ **S65.301** **Unspecified injury of deep palmar arch of** right **hand** ▽

         ✓7ᵗʰ **S65.302** **Unspecified injury of deep palmar arch of** left **hand** ▽

         ✓7ᵗʰ **S65.309** **Unspecified injury of deep palmar arch of unspecified hand** ▽

     ✓6ᵗʰ **S65.31** **Laceration of deep palmar arch**

         ✓7ᵗʰ **S65.311** **Laceration of deep palmar arch of** right **hand**

         ✓7ᵗʰ **S65.312** **Laceration of deep palmar arch of** left **hand**

         ✓7ᵗʰ **S65.319** **Laceration of deep palmar arch of unspecified hand** ▽

     ✓6ᵗʰ **S65.39** **Other specified injury of deep palmar arch**

         ✓7ᵗʰ **S65.391** **Other specified injury of deep palmar arch of** right **hand**

         ✓7ᵗʰ **S65.392** **Other specified injury of deep palmar arch of** left **hand**

√7ᵗʰ **S65.399** Other specified injury of deep palmar arch of unspecified hand ▽

√5ᵗʰ **S65.4** **Injury of blood vessel of thumb**

  √6ᵗʰ **S65.40** Unspecified injury of blood vessel of thumb

    √7ᵗʰ **S65.401** Unspecified injury of blood vessel of right thumb ▽

    √7ᵗʰ **S65.402** Unspecified injury of blood vessel of left thumb ▽

    √7ᵗʰ **S65.409** Unspecified injury of blood vessel of unspecified thumb ▽

  √6ᵗʰ **S65.41** Laceration of blood vessel of thumb

    √7ᵗʰ **S65.411** Laceration of blood vessel of right thumb

    √7ᵗʰ **S65.412** Laceration of blood vessel of left thumb

    √7ᵗʰ **S65.419** Laceration of blood vessel of unspecified thumb ▽

  √6ᵗʰ **S65.49** Other specified injury of blood vessel of thumb

    √7ᵗʰ **S65.491** Other specified injury of blood vessel of right thumb

    √7ᵗʰ **S65.492** Other specified injury of blood vessel of left thumb

    √7ᵗʰ **S65.499** Other specified injury of blood vessel of unspecified thumb ▽

√5ᵗʰ **S65.5** **Injury of blood vessel of other and unspecified finger**

  √6ᵗʰ **S65.50** Unspecified injury of blood vessel of other and unspecified finger

    √7ᵗʰ **S65.500** Unspecified injury of blood vessel of right index finger ▽

    √7ᵗʰ **S65.501** Unspecified injury of blood vessel of left index finger ▽

    √7ᵗʰ **S65.502** Unspecified injury of blood vessel of right middle finger ▽

    √7ᵗʰ **S65.503** Unspecified injury of blood vessel of left middle finger ▽

    √7ᵗʰ **S65.504** Unspecified injury of blood vessel of right ring finger ▽

    √7ᵗʰ **S65.505** Unspecified injury of blood vessel of left ring finger ▽

    √7ᵗʰ **S65.506** Unspecified injury of blood vessel of right little finger ▽

    √7ᵗʰ **S65.507** Unspecified injury of blood vessel of left little finger ▽

    √7ᵗʰ **S65.508** Unspecified injury of blood vessel of other finger ▽

        Unspecified injury of blood vessel of specified finger with unspecified laterality

    √7ᵗʰ **S65.509** Unspecified injury of blood vessel of unspecified finger ▽

  √6ᵗʰ **S65.51** Laceration of blood vessel of other and unspecified finger

    √7ᵗʰ **S65.510** Laceration of blood vessel of right index finger

    √7ᵗʰ **S65.511** Laceration of blood vessel of left index finger

    √7ᵗʰ **S65.512** Laceration of blood vessel of right middle finger

    √7ᵗʰ **S65.513** Laceration of blood vessel of left middle finger

    √7ᵗʰ **S65.514** Laceration of blood vessel of right ring finger

    √7ᵗʰ **S65.515** Laceration of blood vessel of left ring finger

    √7ᵗʰ **S65.516** Laceration of blood vessel of right little finger

    √7ᵗʰ **S65.517** Laceration of blood vessel of left little finger

    √7ᵗʰ **S65.518** Laceration of blood vessel of other finger

        Laceration of blood vessel of specified finger with unspecified laterality

    √7ᵗʰ **S65.519** Laceration of blood vessel of unspecified finger ▽

  √6ᵗʰ **S65.59** Other specified injury of blood vessel of other and unspecified finger

    √7ᵗʰ **S65.590** Other specified injury of blood vessel of right index finger

    √7ᵗʰ **S65.591** Other specified injury of blood vessel of left index finger

    √7ᵗʰ **S65.592** Other specified injury of blood vessel of right middle finger

    √7ᵗʰ **S65.593** Other specified injury of blood vessel of left middle finger

    √7ᵗʰ **S65.594** Other specified injury of blood vessel of right ring finger

    √7ᵗʰ **S65.595** Other specified injury of blood vessel of left ring finger

    √7ᵗʰ **S65.596** Other specified injury of blood vessel of right little finger

    √7ᵗʰ **S65.597** Other specified injury of blood vessel of left little finger

    √7ᵗʰ **S65.598** Other specified injury of blood vessel of other finger

        Other specified injury of blood vessel of specified finger with unspecified laterality

    √7ᵗʰ **S65.599** Other specified injury of blood vessel of unspecified finger ▽

√5ᵗʰ **S65.8** **Injury of other blood vessels at wrist and hand level**

  √6ᵗʰ **S65.80** Unspecified injury of other blood vessels at wrist and hand level

    √7ᵗʰ **S65.801** Unspecified injury of other blood vessels at wrist and hand level of right arm ▽

    √7ᵗʰ **S65.802** Unspecified injury of other blood vessels at wrist and hand level of left arm ▽

    √7ᵗʰ **S65.809** Unspecified injury of other blood vessels at wrist and hand level of unspecified arm ▽

  √6ᵗʰ **S65.81** Laceration of other blood vessels at wrist and hand level

    √7ᵗʰ **S65.811** Laceration of other blood vessels at wrist and hand level of right arm

    √7ᵗʰ **S65.812** Laceration of other blood vessels at wrist and hand level of left arm

    √7ᵗʰ **S65.819** Laceration of other blood vessels at wrist and hand level of unspecified arm ▽

  √6ᵗʰ **S65.89** Other specified injury of other blood vessels at wrist and hand level

    √7ᵗʰ **S65.891** Other specified injury of other blood vessels at wrist and hand level of right arm

    √7ᵗʰ **S65.892** Other specified injury of other blood vessels at wrist and hand level of left arm

    √7ᵗʰ **S65.899** Other specified injury of other blood vessels at wrist and hand level of unspecified arm ▽

√5ᵗʰ **S65.9** **Injury of unspecified blood vessel at wrist and hand level**

  √6ᵗʰ **S65.90** Unspecified injury of unspecified blood vessel at wrist and hand level

    √7ᵗʰ **S65.901** Unspecified injury of unspecified blood vessel at wrist and hand level of right arm ▽

    √7ᵗʰ **S65.902** Unspecified injury of unspecified blood vessel at wrist and hand level of left arm ▽

    √7ᵗʰ **S65.909** Unspecified injury of unspecified blood vessel at wrist and hand level of unspecified arm ▽

  √6ᵗʰ **S65.91** Laceration of unspecified blood vessel at wrist and hand level

    √7ᵗʰ **S65.911** Laceration of unspecified blood vessel at wrist and hand level of right arm ▽

    √7ᵗʰ **S65.912** Laceration of unspecified blood vessel at wrist and hand level of left arm ▽

    √7ᵗʰ **S65.919** Laceration of unspecified blood vessel at wrist and hand level of unspecified arm ▽

  √6ᵗʰ **S65.99** Other specified injury of unspecified blood vessel at wrist and hand level

    √7ᵗʰ **S65.991** Other specified injury of unspecified blood vessel at wrist and hand of right arm ▽

    √7ᵗʰ **S65.992** Other specified injury of unspecified blood vessel at wrist and hand of left arm ▽

    √7ᵗʰ **S65.999** Other specified injury of unspecified blood vessel at wrist and hand of unspecified arm ▽

☑ Additional Character Req   √x7ᵗʰ Placeholder Alert   Manifestation   ▽ Unspecified   ►◄ Revised Text   ● New Code   ▲ Revised Code Title

Chapter 19. Injury, Poisoning and Certain Other Consequences of External Causes

S66–S66.127

√4ᵗʰ **S66 Injury of muscle, fascia and tendon at wrist and hand level**

Code also any associated open wound (S61.-)

EXCLUDES 2   *sprain of joints and ligaments of wrist and hand (S63.-)*

TIP: Refer to the Muscle/Tendon table at the beginning of this chapter.

The appropriate 7th character is to be added to each code from category S66.

A   initial encounter
D   subsequent encounter
S   sequela

√5ᵗʰ **S66.0 Injury of long flexor muscle, fascia and tendon of thumb at wrist and hand level**

√6ᵗʰ **S66.00 Unspecified injury of long flexor muscle, fascia and tendon of thumb at wrist and hand level**

√7ᵗʰ **S66.001 Unspecified injury of long flexor muscle, fascia and tendon of right thumb at wrist and hand level** ▽

√7ᵗʰ **S66.002 Unspecified injury of long flexor muscle, fascia and tendon of left thumb at wrist and hand level** ▽

√7ᵗʰ **S66.009 Unspecified injury of long flexor muscle, fascia and tendon of unspecified thumb at wrist and hand level** ▽

√6ᵗʰ **S66.01 Strain of long flexor muscle, fascia and tendon of thumb at wrist and hand level**

√7ᵗʰ **S66.011 Strain of long flexor muscle, fascia and tendon of right thumb at wrist and hand level**

√7ᵗʰ **S66.012 Strain of long flexor muscle, fascia and tendon of left thumb at wrist and hand level**

√7ᵗʰ **S66.019 Strain of long flexor muscle, fascia and tendon of unspecified thumb at wrist and hand level** ▽

√6ᵗʰ **S66.02 Laceration of long flexor muscle, fascia and tendon of thumb at wrist and hand level**

√7ᵗʰ **S66.021 Laceration of long flexor muscle, fascia and tendon of right thumb at wrist and hand level**

√7ᵗʰ **S66.022 Laceration of long flexor muscle, fascia and tendon of left thumb at wrist and hand level**

√7ᵗʰ **S66.029 Laceration of long flexor muscle, fascia and tendon of unspecified thumb at wrist and hand level** ▽

√6ᵗʰ **S66.09 Other specified injury of long flexor muscle, fascia and tendon of thumb at wrist and hand level**

√7ᵗʰ **S66.091 Other specified injury of long flexor muscle, fascia and tendon of right thumb at wrist and hand level**

√7ᵗʰ **S66.092 Other specified injury of long flexor muscle, fascia and tendon of left thumb at wrist and hand level**

√7ᵗʰ **S66.099 Other specified injury of long flexor muscle, fascia and tendon of unspecified thumb at wrist and hand level** ▽

√5ᵗʰ **S66.1 Injury of flexor muscle, fascia and tendon of other and unspecified finger at wrist and hand level**

EXCLUDES 2   *Injury of long flexor muscle, fascia and tendon of thumb at wrist and hand level (S66.0-)*

√6ᵗʰ **S66.10 Unspecified injury of flexor muscle, fascia and tendon of other and unspecified finger at wrist and hand level**

√7ᵗʰ **S66.100 Unspecified injury of flexor muscle, fascia and tendon of right index finger at wrist and hand level** ▽

√7ᵗʰ **S66.101 Unspecified injury of flexor muscle, fascia and tendon of left index finger at wrist and hand level** ▽

√7ᵗʰ **S66.102 Unspecified injury of flexor muscle, fascia and tendon of right middle finger at wrist and hand level** ▽

√7ᵗʰ **S66.103 Unspecified injury of flexor muscle, fascia and tendon of left middle finger at wrist and hand level** ▽

√7ᵗʰ **S66.104 Unspecified injury of flexor muscle, fascia and tendon of right ring finger at wrist and hand level** ▽

√7ᵗʰ **S66.105 Unspecified injury of flexor muscle, fascia and tendon of left ring finger at wrist and hand level** ▽

√7ᵗʰ **S66.106 Unspecified injury of flexor muscle, fascia and tendon of right little finger at wrist and hand level** ▽

√7ᵗʰ **S66.107 Unspecified injury of flexor muscle, fascia and tendon of left little finger at wrist and hand level** ▽

√7ᵗʰ **S66.108 Unspecified injury of flexor muscle, fascia and tendon of other finger at wrist and hand level**

Unspecified injury of flexor muscle, fascia and tendon of specified finger with unspecified laterality at wrist and hand level

√7ᵗʰ **S66.109 Unspecified injury of flexor muscle, fascia and tendon of unspecified finger at wrist and hand level** ▽

√6ᵗʰ **S66.11 Strain of flexor muscle, fascia and tendon of other and unspecified finger at wrist and hand level**

√7ᵗʰ **S66.110 Strain of flexor muscle, fascia and tendon of right index finger at wrist and hand level**

√7ᵗʰ **S66.111 Strain of flexor muscle, fascia and tendon of left index finger at wrist and hand level**

√7ᵗʰ **S66.112 Strain of flexor muscle, fascia and tendon of right middle finger at wrist and hand level**

√7ᵗʰ **S66.113 Strain of flexor muscle, fascia and tendon of left middle finger at wrist and hand level**

√7ᵗʰ **S66.114 Strain of flexor muscle, fascia and tendon of right ring finger at wrist and hand level**

√7ᵗʰ **S66.115 Strain of flexor muscle, fascia and tendon of left ring finger at wrist and hand level**

√7ᵗʰ **S66.116 Strain of flexor muscle, fascia and tendon of right little finger at wrist and hand level**

√7ᵗʰ **S66.117 Strain of flexor muscle, fascia and tendon of left little finger at wrist and hand level**

√7ᵗʰ **S66.118 Strain of flexor muscle, fascia and tendon of other finger at wrist and hand level**

Strain of flexor muscle, fascia and tendon of specified finger with unspecified laterality at wrist and hand level

√7ᵗʰ **S66.119 Strain of flexor muscle, fascia and tendon of unspecified finger at wrist and hand level** ▽

√6ᵗʰ **S66.12 Laceration of flexor muscle, fascia and tendon of other and unspecified finger at wrist and hand level**

√7ᵗʰ **S66.120 Laceration of flexor muscle, fascia and tendon of right index finger at wrist and hand level**

√7ᵗʰ **S66.121 Laceration of flexor muscle, fascia and tendon of left index finger at wrist and hand level**

√7ᵗʰ **S66.122 Laceration of flexor muscle, fascia and tendon of right middle finger at wrist and hand level**

√7ᵗʰ **S66.123 Laceration of flexor muscle, fascia and tendon of left middle finger at wrist and hand level**

√7ᵗʰ **S66.124 Laceration of flexor muscle, fascia and tendon of right ring finger at wrist and hand level**

√7ᵗʰ **S66.125 Laceration of flexor muscle, fascia and tendon of left ring finger at wrist and hand level**

√7ᵗʰ **S66.126 Laceration of flexor muscle, fascia and tendon of right little finger at wrist and hand level**

√7ᵗʰ **S66.127 Laceration of flexor muscle, fascia and tendon of left little finger at wrist and hand level**

    ✓7ᵗʰ **S66.128** **Laceration of flexor muscle, fascia and tendon of other finger at wrist and hand level**
       Laceration of flexor muscle, fascia and tendon of specified finger with unspecified laterality at wrist and hand level

    ✓7ᵗʰ **S66.129** **Laceration of flexor muscle, fascia and tendon of unspecified finger at wrist and hand level** ▽

✓6ᵗʰ **S66.19** **Other injury of flexor muscle, fascia and tendon of other and unspecified finger at wrist and hand level**

    ✓7ᵗʰ **S66.190** **Other injury of flexor muscle, fascia and tendon of right index finger at wrist and hand level**

    ✓7ᵗʰ **S66.191** **Other injury of flexor muscle, fascia and tendon of left index finger at wrist and hand level**

    ✓7ᵗʰ **S66.192** **Other injury of flexor muscle, fascia and tendon of right middle finger at wrist and hand level**

    ✓7ᵗʰ **S66.193** **Other injury of flexor muscle, fascia and tendon of left middle finger at wrist and hand level**

    ✓7ᵗʰ **S66.194** **Other injury of flexor muscle, fascia and tendon of right ring finger at wrist and hand level**

    ✓7ᵗʰ **S66.195** **Other injury of flexor muscle, fascia and tendon of left ring finger at wrist and hand level**

    ✓7ᵗʰ **S66.196** **Other injury of flexor muscle, fascia and tendon of right little finger at wrist and hand level**

    ✓7ᵗʰ **S66.197** **Other injury of flexor muscle, fascia and tendon of left little finger at wrist and hand level**

    ✓7ᵗʰ **S66.198** **Other injury of flexor muscle, fascia and tendon of other finger at wrist and hand level**
       Other injury of flexor muscle, fascia and tendon of specified finger with unspecified laterality at wrist and hand level

    ✓7ᵗʰ **S66.199** **Other injury of flexor muscle, fascia and tendon of unspecified finger at wrist and hand level** ▽

✓5ᵗʰ **S66.2** **Injury of extensor muscle, fascia and tendon of thumb at wrist and hand level**

✓6ᵗʰ **S66.20** **Unspecified injury of extensor muscle, fascia and tendon of thumb at wrist and hand level**

    ✓7ᵗʰ **S66.201** **Unspecified injury of extensor muscle, fascia and tendon of right thumb at wrist and hand level** ▽

    ✓7ᵗʰ **S66.202** **Unspecified injury of extensor muscle, fascia and tendon of left thumb at wrist and hand level** ▽

    ✓7ᵗʰ **S66.209** **Unspecified injury of extensor muscle, fascia and tendon of unspecified thumb at wrist and hand level** ▽

✓6ᵗʰ **S66.21** **Strain of extensor muscle, fascia and tendon of thumb at wrist and hand level**

    ✓7ᵗʰ **S66.211** **Strain of extensor muscle, fascia and tendon of right thumb at wrist and hand level**

    ✓7ᵗʰ **S66.212** **Strain of extensor muscle, fascia and tendon of left thumb at wrist and hand level**

    ✓7ᵗʰ **S66.219** **Strain of extensor muscle, fascia and tendon of unspecified thumb at wrist and hand level** ▽

✓6ᵗʰ **S66.22** **Laceration of extensor muscle, fascia and tendon of thumb at wrist and hand level**

    ✓7ᵗʰ **S66.221** **Laceration of extensor muscle, fascia and tendon of right thumb at wrist and hand level**

    ✓7ᵗʰ **S66.222** **Laceration of extensor muscle, fascia and tendon of left thumb at wrist and hand level**

    ✓7ᵗʰ **S66.229** **Laceration of extensor muscle, fascia and tendon of unspecified thumb at wrist and hand level** ▽

✓6ᵗʰ **S66.29** **Other specified injury of extensor muscle, fascia and tendon of thumb at wrist and hand level**

    ✓7ᵗʰ **S66.291** **Other specified injury of extensor muscle, fascia and tendon of right thumb at wrist and hand level**

    ✓7ᵗʰ **S66.292** **Other specified injury of extensor muscle, fascia and tendon of left thumb at wrist and hand level**

    ✓7ᵗʰ **S66.299** **Other specified injury of extensor muscle, fascia and tendon of unspecified thumb at wrist and hand level** ▽

✓5ᵗʰ **S66.3** **Injury of extensor muscle, fascia and tendon of other and unspecified finger at wrist and hand level**
    EXCLUDES 2   *injury of extensor muscle, fascia and tendon of thumb at wrist and hand level (S66.2-)*

✓6ᵗʰ **S66.30** **Unspecified injury of extensor muscle, fascia and tendon of other and unspecified finger at wrist and hand level**

    ✓7ᵗʰ **S66.300** **Unspecified injury of extensor muscle, fascia and tendon of right index finger at wrist and hand level** ▽

    ✓7ᵗʰ **S66.301** **Unspecified injury of extensor muscle, fascia and tendon of left index finger at wrist and hand level** ▽

    ✓7ᵗʰ **S66.302** **Unspecified injury of extensor muscle, fascia and tendon of right middle finger at wrist and hand level** ▽

    ✓7ᵗʰ **S66.303** **Unspecified injury of extensor muscle, fascia and tendon of left middle finger at wrist and hand level** ▽

    ✓7ᵗʰ **S66.304** **Unspecified injury of extensor muscle, fascia and tendon of right ring finger at wrist and hand level** ▽

    ✓7ᵗʰ **S66.305** **Unspecified injury of extensor muscle, fascia and tendon of left ring finger at wrist and hand level** ▽

    ✓7ᵗʰ **S66.306** **Unspecified injury of extensor muscle, fascia and tendon of right little finger at wrist and hand level** ▽

    ✓7ᵗʰ **S66.307** **Unspecified injury of extensor muscle, fascia and tendon of left little finger at wrist and hand level** ▽

    ✓7ᵗʰ **S66.308** **Unspecified injury of extensor muscle, fascia and tendon of other finger at wrist and hand level** ▽
       Unspecified injury of extensor muscle, fascia and tendon of specified finger with unspecified laterality at wrist and hand level

    ✓7ᵗʰ **S66.309** **Unspecified injury of extensor muscle, fascia and tendon of unspecified finger at wrist and hand level** ▽

✓6ᵗʰ **S66.31** **Strain of extensor muscle, fascia and tendon of other and unspecified finger at wrist and hand level**

    ✓7ᵗʰ **S66.310** **Strain of extensor muscle, fascia and tendon of right index finger at wrist and hand level**

    ✓7ᵗʰ **S66.311** **Strain of extensor muscle, fascia and tendon of left index finger at wrist and hand level**

    ✓7ᵗʰ **S66.312** **Strain of extensor muscle, fascia and tendon of right middle finger at wrist and hand level**

    ✓7ᵗʰ **S66.313** **Strain of extensor muscle, fascia and tendon of left middle finger at wrist and hand level**

    ✓7ᵗʰ **S66.314** **Strain of extensor muscle, fascia and tendon of right ring finger at wrist and hand level**

    ✓7ᵗʰ **S66.315** **Strain of extensor muscle, fascia and tendon of left ring finger at wrist and hand level**

    ✓7ᵗʰ **S66.316** **Strain of extensor muscle, fascia and tendon of right little finger at wrist and hand level**

✓7ᵗʰ **S66.317** Strain of extensor muscle, fascia and tendon of left little finger at wrist and hand level

✓7ᵗʰ **S66.318** Strain of extensor muscle, fascia and tendon of other finger at wrist and hand level

Strain of extensor muscle, fascia and tendon of specified finger with unspecified laterality at wrist and hand level

✓7ᵗʰ **S66.319** Strain of extensor muscle, fascia and tendon of unspecified finger at wrist and hand level ▽

✓6ᵗʰ **S66.32** Laceration of extensor muscle, fascia and tendon of other and unspecified finger at wrist and hand level

✓7ᵗʰ **S66.320** Laceration of extensor muscle, fascia and tendon of right index finger at wrist and hand level

✓7ᵗʰ **S66.321** Laceration of extensor muscle, fascia and tendon of left index finger at wrist and hand level

✓7ᵗʰ **S66.322** Laceration of extensor muscle, fascia and tendon of right middle finger at wrist and hand level

✓7ᵗʰ **S66.323** Laceration of extensor muscle, fascia and tendon of left middle finger at wrist and hand level

✓7ᵗʰ **S66.324** Laceration of extensor muscle, fascia and tendon of right ring finger at wrist and hand level

✓7ᵗʰ **S66.325** Laceration of extensor muscle, fascia and tendon of left ring finger at wrist and hand level

✓7ᵗʰ **S66.326** Laceration of extensor muscle, fascia and tendon of right little finger at wrist and hand level

✓7ᵗʰ **S66.327** Laceration of extensor muscle, fascia and tendon of left little finger at wrist and hand level

✓7ᵗʰ **S66.328** Laceration of extensor muscle, fascia and tendon of other finger at wrist and hand level

Laceration of extensor muscle, fascia and tendon of specified finger with unspecified laterality at wrist and hand level

✓7ᵗʰ **S66.329** Laceration of extensor muscle, fascia and tendon of unspecified finger at wrist and hand level ▽

✓6ᵗʰ **S66.39** Other injury of extensor muscle, fascia and tendon of other and unspecified finger at wrist and hand level

✓7ᵗʰ **S66.390** Other injury of extensor muscle, fascia and tendon of right index finger at wrist and hand level

✓7ᵗʰ **S66.391** Other injury of extensor muscle, fascia and tendon of left index finger at wrist and hand level

✓7ᵗʰ **S66.392** Other injury of extensor muscle, fascia and tendon of right middle finger at wrist and hand level

✓7ᵗʰ **S66.393** Other injury of extensor muscle, fascia and tendon of left middle finger at wrist and hand level

✓7ᵗʰ **S66.394** Other injury of extensor muscle, fascia and tendon of right ring finger at wrist and hand level

✓7ᵗʰ **S66.395** Other injury of extensor muscle, fascia and tendon of left ring finger at wrist and hand level

✓7ᵗʰ **S66.396** Other injury of extensor muscle, fascia and tendon of right little finger at wrist and hand level

✓7ᵗʰ **S66.397** Other injury of extensor muscle, fascia and tendon of left little finger at wrist and hand level

✓7ᵗʰ **S66.398** Other injury of extensor muscle, fascia and tendon of other finger at wrist and hand level

Other injury of extensor muscle, fascia and tendon of specified finger with unspecified laterality at wrist and hand level

✓7ᵗʰ **S66.399** Other injury of extensor muscle, fascia and tendon of unspecified finger at wrist and hand level ▽

✓5ᵗʰ **S66.4** Injury of intrinsic muscle, fascia and tendon of thumb at wrist and hand level

✓6ᵗʰ **S66.40** Unspecified injury of intrinsic muscle, fascia and tendon of thumb at wrist and hand level

✓7ᵗʰ **S66.401** Unspecified injury of intrinsic muscle, fascia and tendon of right thumb at wrist and hand level ▽

✓7ᵗʰ **S66.402** Unspecified injury of intrinsic muscle, fascia and tendon of left thumb at wrist and hand level ▽

✓7ᵗʰ **S66.409** Unspecified injury of intrinsic muscle, fascia and tendon of unspecified thumb at wrist and hand level ▽

✓6ᵗʰ **S66.41** Strain of intrinsic muscle, fascia and tendon of thumb at wrist and hand level

✓7ᵗʰ **S66.411** Strain of intrinsic muscle, fascia and tendon of right thumb at wrist and hand level

✓7ᵗʰ **S66.412** Strain of intrinsic muscle, fascia and tendon of left thumb at wrist and hand level

✓7ᵗʰ **S66.419** Strain of intrinsic muscle, fascia and tendon of unspecified thumb at wrist and hand level ▽

✓6ᵗʰ **S66.42** Laceration of intrinsic muscle, fascia and tendon of thumb at wrist and hand level

✓7ᵗʰ **S66.421** Laceration of intrinsic muscle, fascia and tendon of right thumb at wrist and hand level

✓7ᵗʰ **S66.422** Laceration of intrinsic muscle, fascia and tendon of left thumb at wrist and hand level

✓7ᵗʰ **S66.429** Laceration of intrinsic muscle, fascia and tendon of unspecified thumb at wrist and hand level ▽

✓6ᵗʰ **S66.49** Other specified injury of intrinsic muscle, fascia and tendon of thumb at wrist and hand level

✓7ᵗʰ **S66.491** Other specified injury of intrinsic muscle, fascia and tendon of right thumb at wrist and hand level

✓7ᵗʰ **S66.492** Other specified injury of intrinsic muscle, fascia and tendon of left thumb at wrist and hand level

✓7ᵗʰ **S66.499** Other specified injury of intrinsic muscle, fascia and tendon of unspecified thumb at wrist and hand level ▽

✓5ᵗʰ **S66.5** Injury of intrinsic muscle, fascia and tendon of other and unspecified finger at wrist and hand level

EXCLUDES 2 *injury of intrinsic muscle, fascia and tendon of thumb at wrist and hand level (S66.4-)*

✓6ᵗʰ **S66.50** Unspecified injury of intrinsic muscle, fascia and tendon of other and unspecified finger at wrist and hand level

✓7ᵗʰ **S66.500** Unspecified injury of intrinsic muscle, fascia and tendon of right index finger at wrist and hand level ▽

✓7ᵗʰ **S66.501** Unspecified injury of intrinsic muscle, fascia and tendon of left index finger at wrist and hand level ▽

✓7ᵗʰ **S66.502** Unspecified injury of intrinsic muscle, fascia and tendon of right middle finger at wrist and hand level ▽

✓7ᵗʰ **S66.503** Unspecified injury of intrinsic muscle, fascia and tendon of left middle finger at wrist and hand level ▽

✓7ᵗʰ **S66.504** Unspecified injury of intrinsic muscle, fascia and tendon of right ring finger at wrist and hand level ▽

√7ᵗʰ **S66.505** Unspecified injury of intrinsic muscle, fascia and tendon of left ring finger at wrist and hand level ▽

√7ᵗʰ **S66.506** Unspecified injury of intrinsic muscle, fascia and tendon of right little finger at wrist and hand level ▽

√7ᵗʰ **S66.507** Unspecified injury of intrinsic muscle, fascia and tendon of left little finger at wrist and hand level ▽

√7ᵗʰ **S66.508** Unspecified injury of intrinsic muscle, fascia and tendon of other finger at wrist and hand level ▽

Unspecified injury of intrinsic muscle, fascia and tendon of specified finger with unspecified laterality at wrist and hand level

√7ᵗʰ **S66.509** Unspecified injury of intrinsic muscle, fascia and tendon of unspecified finger at wrist and hand level ▽

√6ᵗʰ **S66.51** Strain of intrinsic muscle, fascia and tendon of other and unspecified finger at wrist and hand level

√7ᵗʰ **S66.510** Strain of intrinsic muscle, fascia and tendon of right index finger at wrist and hand level

√7ᵗʰ **S66.511** Strain of intrinsic muscle, fascia and tendon of left index finger at wrist and hand level

√7ᵗʰ **S66.512** Strain of intrinsic muscle, fascia and tendon of right middle finger at wrist and hand level

√7ᵗʰ **S66.513** Strain of intrinsic muscle, fascia and tendon of left middle finger at wrist and hand level

√7ᵗʰ **S66.514** Strain of intrinsic muscle, fascia and tendon of right ring finger at wrist and hand level

√7ᵗʰ **S66.515** Strain of intrinsic muscle, fascia and tendon of left ring finger at wrist and hand level

√7ᵗʰ **S66.516** Strain of intrinsic muscle, fascia and tendon of right little finger at wrist and hand level

√7ᵗʰ **S66.517** Strain of intrinsic muscle, fascia and tendon of left little finger at wrist and hand level

√7ᵗʰ **S66.518** Strain of intrinsic muscle, fascia and tendon of other finger at wrist and hand level

Strain of intrinsic muscle, fascia and tendon of specified finger with unspecified laterality at wrist and hand level

√7ᵗʰ **S66.519** Strain of intrinsic muscle, fascia and tendon of unspecified finger at wrist and hand level ▽

√6ᵗʰ **S66.52** Laceration of intrinsic muscle, fascia and tendon of other and unspecified finger at wrist and hand level

√7ᵗʰ **S66.520** Laceration of intrinsic muscle, fascia and tendon of right index finger at wrist and hand level

√7ᵗʰ **S66.521** Laceration of intrinsic muscle, fascia and tendon of left index finger at wrist and hand level

√7ᵗʰ **S66.522** Laceration of intrinsic muscle, fascia and tendon of right middle finger at wrist and hand level

√7ᵗʰ **S66.523** Laceration of intrinsic muscle, fascia and tendon of left middle finger at wrist and hand level

√7ᵗʰ **S66.524** Laceration of intrinsic muscle, fascia and tendon of right ring finger at wrist and hand level

√7ᵗʰ **S66.525** Laceration of intrinsic muscle, fascia and tendon of left ring finger at wrist and hand level

√7ᵗʰ **S66.526** Laceration of intrinsic muscle, fascia and tendon of right little finger at wrist and hand level

√7ᵗʰ **S66.527** Laceration of intrinsic muscle, fascia and tendon of left little finger at wrist and hand level

√7ᵗʰ **S66.528** Laceration of intrinsic muscle, fascia and tendon of other finger at wrist and hand level

Laceration of intrinsic muscle, fascia and tendon of specified finger with unspecified laterality at wrist and hand level

√7ᵗʰ **S66.529** Laceration of intrinsic muscle, fascia and tendon of unspecified finger at wrist and hand level ▽

√6ᵗʰ **S66.59** Other injury of intrinsic muscle, fascia and tendon of other and unspecified finger at wrist and hand level

√7ᵗʰ **S66.590** Other injury of intrinsic muscle, fascia and tendon of right index finger at wrist and hand level

√7ᵗʰ **S66.591** Other injury of intrinsic muscle, fascia and tendon of left index finger at wrist and hand level

√7ᵗʰ **S66.592** Other injury of intrinsic muscle, fascia and tendon of right middle finger at wrist and hand level

√7ᵗʰ **S66.593** Other injury of intrinsic muscle, fascia and tendon of left middle finger at wrist and hand level

√7ᵗʰ **S66.594** Other injury of intrinsic muscle, fascia and tendon of right ring finger at wrist and hand level

√7ᵗʰ **S66.595** Other injury of intrinsic muscle, fascia and tendon of left ring finger at wrist and hand level

√7ᵗʰ **S66.596** Other injury of intrinsic muscle, fascia and tendon of right little finger at wrist and hand level

√7ᵗʰ **S66.597** Other injury of intrinsic muscle, fascia and tendon of left little finger at wrist and hand level

√7ᵗʰ **S66.598** Other injury of intrinsic muscle, fascia and tendon of other finger at wrist and hand level

Other injury of intrinsic muscle, fascia and tendon of specified finger with unspecified laterality at wrist and hand level

√7ᵗʰ **S66.599** Other injury of intrinsic muscle, fascia and tendon of unspecified finger at wrist and hand level ▽

√5ᵗʰ **S66.8** Injury of other specified muscles, fascia and tendons at wrist and hand level

√6ᵗʰ **S66.80** Unspecified injury of other specified muscles, fascia and tendons at wrist and hand level

√7ᵗʰ **S66.801** Unspecified injury of other specified muscles, fascia and tendons at wrist and hand level, right hand ▽

√7ᵗʰ **S66.802** Unspecified injury of other specified muscles, fascia and tendons at wrist and hand level, left hand ▽

√7ᵗʰ **S66.809** Unspecified injury of other specified muscles, fascia and tendons at wrist and hand level, unspecified hand ▽

√6ᵗʰ **S66.81** Strain of other specified muscles, fascia and tendons at wrist and hand level

√7ᵗʰ **S66.811** Strain of other specified muscles, fascia and tendons at wrist and hand level, right hand

√7ᵗʰ **S66.812** Strain of other specified muscles, fascia and tendons at wrist and hand level, left hand

√7ᵗʰ **S66.819** Strain of other specified muscles, fascia and tendons at wrist and hand level, unspecified hand ▽

√6ᵗʰ **S66.82** Laceration of other specified muscles, fascia and tendons at wrist and hand level

√7ᵗʰ **S66.821** Laceration of other specified muscles, fascia and tendons at wrist and hand level, right hand

√7ᵗʰ **S66.822** Laceration of other specified muscles, fascia and tendons at wrist and hand level, left hand

✅ Additional Character Req   √x7ᵗʰ Placeholder Alert   Manifestation   ▽ Unspecified   ▶◀ Revised Text   ● New Code   ▲ Revised Code Title

ICD-10-CM 2019   1035

Chapter 19. Injury, Poisoning and Certain Other Consequences of External Causes

√7ᵗʰ **S66.829** Laceration of other specified muscles, fascia and tendons at wrist and hand level, unspecified hand ▽

√6ᵗʰ **S66.89** Other injury of other specified muscles, fascia and tendons at wrist and hand level

√7ᵗʰ **S66.891** Other injury of other specified muscles, fascia and tendons at wrist and hand level, right hand

√7ᵗʰ **S66.892** Other injury of other specified muscles, fascia and tendons at wrist and hand level, left hand

√7ᵗʰ **S66.899** Other injury of other specified muscles, fascia and tendons at wrist and hand level, unspecified hand ▽

√5ᵗʰ **S66.9** Injury of unspecified muscle, fascia and tendon at wrist and hand level

√6ᵗʰ **S66.90** Unspecified injury of unspecified muscle, fascia and tendon at wrist and hand level

√7ᵗʰ **S66.901** Unspecified injury of unspecified muscle, fascia and tendon at wrist and hand level, right hand ▽

√7ᵗʰ **S66.902** Unspecified injury of unspecified muscle, fascia and tendon at wrist and hand level, left hand ▽

√7ᵗʰ **S66.909** Unspecified injury of unspecified muscle, fascia and tendon at wrist and hand level, unspecified hand ▽

√6ᵗʰ **S66.91** Strain of unspecified muscle, fascia and tendon at wrist and hand level

√7ᵗʰ **S66.911** Strain of unspecified muscle, fascia and tendon at wrist and hand level, right hand ▽

√7ᵗʰ **S66.912** Strain of unspecified muscle, fascia and tendon at wrist and hand level, left hand ▽

√7ᵗʰ **S66.919** Strain of unspecified muscle, fascia and tendon at wrist and hand level, unspecified hand ▽

√6ᵗʰ **S66.92** Laceration of unspecified muscle, fascia and tendon at wrist and hand level

√7ᵗʰ **S66.921** Laceration of unspecified muscle, fascia and tendon at wrist and hand level, right hand ▽

√7ᵗʰ **S66.922** Laceration of unspecified muscle, fascia and tendon at wrist and hand level, left hand ▽

√7ᵗʰ **S66.929** Laceration of unspecified muscle, fascia and tendon at wrist and hand level, unspecified hand ▽

√6ᵗʰ **S66.99** Other injury of unspecified muscle, fascia and tendon at wrist and hand level

√7ᵗʰ **S66.991** Other injury of unspecified muscle, fascia and tendon at wrist and hand level, right hand ▽

√7ᵗʰ **S66.992** Other injury of unspecified muscle, fascia and tendon at wrist and hand level, left hand ▽

√7ᵗʰ **S66.999** Other injury of unspecified muscle, fascia and tendon at wrist and hand level, unspecified hand ▽

√4ᵗʰ **S67** Crushing injury of wrist, hand and fingers

Use additional code for all associated injuries, such as:
   fracture of wrist and hand (S62.-)
   open wound of wrist and hand (S61.-)

The appropriate 7th character is to be added to each code from category S67.
A   initial encounter
D   subsequent encounter
S   sequela

√5ᵗʰ **S67.0** Crushing injury of thumb

√x7ᵗʰ **S67.00** Crushing injury of unspecified thumb ▽

√x7ᵗʰ **S67.01** Crushing injury of right thumb

√x7ᵗʰ **S67.02** Crushing injury of left thumb

√5ᵗʰ **S67.1** Crushing injury of other and unspecified finger(s)

EXCLUDES 2   *crushing injury of thumb (S67.0-)*

√x7ᵗʰ **S67.10** Crushing injury of unspecified finger(s) ▽

√6ᵗʰ **S67.19** Crushing injury of other finger(s)

√7ᵗʰ **S67.190** Crushing injury of right index finger

√7ᵗʰ **S67.191** Crushing injury of left index finger

√7ᵗʰ **S67.192** Crushing injury of right middle finger

√7ᵗʰ **S67.193** Crushing injury of left middle finger

√7ᵗʰ **S67.194** Crushing injury of right ring finger

√7ᵗʰ **S67.195** Crushing injury of left ring finger

√7ᵗʰ **S67.196** Crushing injury of right little finger

√7ᵗʰ **S67.197** Crushing injury of left little finger

√7ᵗʰ **S67.198** Crushing injury of other finger
Crushing injury of specified finger with unspecified laterality

√5ᵗʰ **S67.2** Crushing injury of hand

EXCLUDES 2   *crushing injury of fingers (S67.1-)*
           crushing injury of thumb (S67.0-)

√x7ᵗʰ **S67.20** Crushing injury of unspecified hand ▽

√x7ᵗʰ **S67.21** Crushing injury of right hand

√x7ᵗʰ **S67.22** Crushing injury of left hand

√5ᵗʰ **S67.3** Crushing injury of wrist

√x7ᵗʰ **S67.30** Crushing injury of unspecified wrist ▽

√x7ᵗʰ **S67.31** Crushing injury of right wrist

√x7ᵗʰ **S67.32** Crushing injury of left wrist

√5ᵗʰ **S67.4** Crushing injury of wrist and hand

EXCLUDES 1   *crushing injury of hand alone (S67.2-)*
           crushing injury of wrist alone (S67.3-)
EXCLUDES 2   *crushing injury of fingers (S67.1-)*
           crushing injury of thumb (S67.0-)

√x7ᵗʰ **S67.40** Crushing injury of unspecified wrist and hand ▽

√x7ᵗʰ **S67.41** Crushing injury of right wrist and hand

√x7ᵗʰ **S67.42** Crushing injury of left wrist and hand

√5ᵗʰ **S67.9** Crushing injury of unspecified part(s) of wrist, hand and fingers

√x7ᵗʰ **S67.90** Crushing injury of unspecified part(s) of unspecified wrist, hand and fingers ▽

√x7ᵗʰ **S67.91** Crushing injury of unspecified part(s) of right wrist, hand and fingers ▽

√x7ᵗʰ **S67.92** Crushing injury of unspecified part(s) of left wrist, hand and fingers ▽

√4ᵗʰ **S68** Traumatic amputation of wrist, hand and fingers

An amputation not identified as partial or complete should be coded to complete.

The appropriate 7th character is to be added to each code from category S68.
A   initial encounter
D   subsequent encounter
S   sequela

√5ᵗʰ **S68.0** Traumatic metacarpophalangeal amputation of thumb
Traumatic amputation of thumb NOS

√6ᵗʰ **S68.01** Complete traumatic metacarpophalangeal amputation of thumb

³ √7ᵗʰ **S68.011** Complete traumatic metacarpophalangeal amputation of right thumb   HCC

³ √7ᵗʰ **S68.012** Complete traumatic metacarpophalangeal amputation of left thumb   HCC

³ √7ᵗʰ **S68.019** Complete traumatic metacarpophalangeal amputation of unspecified thumb   HCC ▽

√6ᵗʰ **S68.02** Partial traumatic metacarpophalangeal amputation of thumb

³ √7ᵗʰ **S68.021** Partial traumatic metacarpophalangeal amputation of right thumb   HCC

³ √7ᵗʰ **S68.022** Partial traumatic metacarpophalangeal amputation of left thumb   HCC

³ √7ᵗʰ **S68.029** Partial traumatic metacarpophalangeal amputation of unspecified thumb   HCC ▽

√5ᵗʰ **S68.1** **Traumatic metacarpophalangeal amputation of other and unspecified finger**

Traumatic amputation of finger NOS

EXCLUDES 2   traumatic metacarpophalangeal amputation of thumb (S68.0-)

√6ᵗʰ **S68.11** **Complete traumatic metacarpophalangeal amputation of other and unspecified finger**

³ √7ᵗʰ **S68.110** Complete traumatic metacarpophalangeal amputation of right index finger   HCC

³ √7ᵗʰ **S68.111** Complete traumatic metacarpophalangeal amputation of left index finger   HCC

³ √7ᵗʰ **S68.112** Complete traumatic metacarpophalangeal amputation of right middle finger   HCC

³ √7ᵗʰ **S68.113** Complete traumatic metacarpophalangeal amputation of left middle finger   HCC

³ √7ᵗʰ **S68.114** Complete traumatic metacarpophalangeal amputation of right ring finger   HCC

³ √7ᵗʰ **S68.115** Complete traumatic metacarpophalangeal amputation of left ring finger   HCC

³ √7ᵗʰ **S68.116** Complete traumatic metacarpophalangeal amputation of right little finger   HCC

³ √7ᵗʰ **S68.117** Complete traumatic metacarpophalangeal amputation of left little finger   HCC

³ √7ᵗʰ **S68.118** Complete traumatic metacarpophalangeal amputation of other finger   HCC

Complete traumatic metacarpophalangeal amputation of specified finger with unspecified laterality

³ √7ᵗʰ **S68.119** Complete traumatic metacarpophalangeal amputation of unspecified finger   HCC ▽

√6ᵗʰ **S68.12** **Partial traumatic metacarpophalangeal amputation of other and unspecified finger**

³ √7ᵗʰ **S68.120** Partial traumatic metacarpophalangeal amputation of right index finger   HCC

³ √7ᵗʰ **S68.121** Partial traumatic metacarpophalangeal amputation of left index finger   HCC

³ √7ᵗʰ **S68.122** Partial traumatic metacarpophalangeal amputation of right middle finger   HCC

³ √7ᵗʰ **S68.123** Partial traumatic metacarpophalangeal amputation of left middle finger   HCC

³ √7ᵗʰ **S68.124** Partial traumatic metacarpophalangeal amputation of right ring finger   HCC

³ √7ᵗʰ **S68.125** Partial traumatic metacarpophalangeal amputation of left ring finger   HCC

³ √7ᵗʰ **S68.126** Partial traumatic metacarpophalangeal amputation of right little finger   HCC

³ √7ᵗʰ **S68.127** Partial traumatic metacarpophalangeal amputation of left little finger   HCC

³ √7ᵗʰ **S68.128** Partial traumatic metacarpophalangeal amputation of other finger   HCC

Partial traumatic metacarpophalangeal amputation of specified finger with unspecified laterality

³ √7ᵗʰ **S68.129** Partial traumatic metacarpophalangeal amputation of unspecified finger   HCC ▽

√5ᵗʰ **S68.4** **Traumatic amputation of hand at wrist level**

Traumatic amputation of hand NOS

Traumatic amputation of wrist

√6ᵗʰ **S68.41** **Complete traumatic amputation of hand at wrist level**

² √7ᵗʰ **S68.411** Complete traumatic amputation of right hand at wrist level   HCC

² √7ᵗʰ **S68.412** Complete traumatic amputation of left hand at wrist level   HCC

² √7ᵗʰ **S68.419** Complete traumatic amputation of unspecified hand at wrist level   HCC ▽

√6ᵗʰ **S68.42** **Partial traumatic amputation of hand at wrist level**

² √7ᵗʰ **S68.421** Partial traumatic amputation of right hand at wrist level   HCC

² √7ᵗʰ **S68.422** Partial traumatic amputation of left hand at wrist level   HCC

² √7ᵗʰ **S68.429** Partial traumatic amputation of unspecified hand at wrist level   HCC ▽

√5ᵗʰ **S68.5** **Traumatic transphalangeal amputation of thumb**

Traumatic interphalangeal joint amputation of thumb

√6ᵗʰ **S68.51** **Complete traumatic transphalangeal amputation of thumb**

³ √7ᵗʰ **S68.511** Complete traumatic transphalangeal amputation of right thumb   HCC

³ √7ᵗʰ **S68.512** Complete traumatic transphalangeal amputation of left thumb   HCC

³ √7ᵗʰ **S68.519** Complete traumatic transphalangeal amputation of unspecified thumb   HCC ▽

√6ᵗʰ **S68.52** **Partial traumatic transphalangeal amputation of thumb**

³ √7ᵗʰ **S68.521** Partial traumatic transphalangeal amputation of right thumb   HCC

³ √7ᵗʰ **S68.522** Partial traumatic transphalangeal amputation of left thumb   HCC

³ √7ᵗʰ **S68.529** Partial traumatic transphalangeal amputation of unspecified thumb   HCC ▽

√5ᵗʰ **S68.6** **Traumatic transphalangeal amputation of other and unspecified finger**

√6ᵗʰ **S68.61** **Complete traumatic transphalangeal amputation of other and unspecified finger(s)**

³ √7ᵗʰ **S68.610** Complete traumatic transphalangeal amputation of right index finger   HCC

³ √7ᵗʰ **S68.611** Complete traumatic transphalangeal amputation of left index finger   HCC

³ √7ᵗʰ **S68.612** Complete traumatic transphalangeal amputation of right middle finger   HCC

³ √7ᵗʰ **S68.613** Complete traumatic transphalangeal amputation of left middle finger   HCC

³ √7ᵗʰ **S68.614** Complete traumatic transphalangeal amputation of right ring finger   HCC

³ √7ᵗʰ **S68.615** Complete traumatic transphalangeal amputation of left ring finger   HCC

³ √7ᵗʰ **S68.616** Complete traumatic transphalangeal amputation of right little finger   HCC

³ √7ᵗʰ **S68.617** Complete traumatic transphalangeal amputation of left little finger   HCC

³ √7ᵗʰ **S68.618** Complete traumatic transphalangeal amputation of other finger   HCC

Complete traumatic transphalangeal amputation of specified finger with unspecified laterality

³ √7ᵗʰ **S68.619** Complete traumatic transphalangeal amputation of unspecified finger   HCC ▽

√6ᵗʰ **S68.62** **Partial traumatic transphalangeal amputation of other and unspecified finger**

³ √7ᵗʰ **S68.620** Partial traumatic transphalangeal amputation of right index finger   HCC

³ √7ᵗʰ **S68.621** Partial traumatic transphalangeal amputation of left index finger   HCC

³ √7ᵗʰ **S68.622** Partial traumatic transphalangeal amputation of right middle finger   HCC

³ √7ᵗʰ **S68.623** Partial traumatic transphalangeal amputation of left middle finger   HCC

³ √7ᵗʰ **S68.624** Partial traumatic transphalangeal amputation of right ring finger   HCC

³ √7ᵗʰ **S68.625** Partial traumatic transphalangeal amputation of left ring finger   HCC

³ √7ᵗʰ **S68.626** Partial traumatic transphalangeal amputation of right little finger   HCC

☑ Additional Character Req   √x7ᵗʰ Placeholder Alert   Manifestation   ▽ Unspecified   ▶◀ Revised Text   ● New Code   ▲ Revised Code Title

³ ✓7ᵗʰ **S68.627 Partial traumatic transphalangeal** ᴴᶜᶜ
  amputation of left little finger

³ ✓7ᵗʰ **S68.628 Partial traumatic transphalangeal** ᴴᶜᶜ
  amputation of other finger
    Partial traumatic transphalangeal
    amputation of specified finger with
    unspecified laterality

³ ✓7ᵗʰ **S68.629 Partial traumatic transphalangeal** ᴴᶜᶜ ▽
  amputation of unspecified finger

✓5ᵗʰ **S68.7 Traumatic transmetacarpal amputation of hand**

✓6ᵗʰ **S68.71 Complete traumatic transmetacarpal amputation**
  of hand

² ✓7ᵗʰ **S68.711 Complete traumatic** ᴴᶜᶜ
  transmetacarpal amputation of
  right hand

² ✓7ᵗʰ **S68.712 Complete traumatic** ᴴᶜᶜ
  transmetacarpal amputation of
  left hand

² ✓7ᵗʰ **S68.719 Complete traumatic** ᴴᶜᶜ ▽
  transmetacarpal amputation of
  unspecified hand

✓6ᵗʰ **S68.72 Partial traumatic transmetacarpal amputation of**
  hand

² ✓7ᵗʰ **S68.721 Partial traumatic transmetacarpal** ᴴᶜᶜ
  amputation of right hand

² ✓7ᵗʰ **S68.722 Partial traumatic transmetacarpal** ᴴᶜᶜ
  amputation of left hand

² ✓7ᵗʰ **S68.729 Partial traumatic transmetacarpal** ᴴᶜᶜ ▽
  amputation of unspecified hand

✓4ᵗʰ **S69 Other and unspecified injuries of wrist, hand and finger(s)**

The appropriate 7th character is to be added to each code from
category S69.
  A   initial encounter
  D   subsequent encounter
  S   sequela

✓5ᵗʰ **S69.8 Other specified injuries of wrist, hand and finger(s)**

✓x7ᵗʰ **S69.80 Other specified injuries of unspecified wrist,** ▽
  hand and finger(s)

✓x7ᵗʰ **S69.81 Other specified injuries of right wrist, hand and**
  finger(s)

✓x7ᵗʰ **S69.82 Other specified injuries of left wrist, hand and**
  finger(s)

✓5ᵗʰ **S69.9 Unspecified injury of wrist, hand and finger(s)**

✓x7ᵗʰ **S69.90 Unspecified injury of unspecified wrist,** ▽
  hand and finger(s)

✓x7ᵗʰ **S69.91 Unspecified injury of right wrist, hand and** ▽
  finger(s)

✓x7ᵗʰ **S69.92 Unspecified injury of left wrist, hand and** ▽
  finger(s)

Injuries to the hip and thigh (S70-S79)

EXCLUDES 2 *burns and corrosions (T20-T32)*
          frostbite (T33-T34)
          snake bite (T63.0-)
          venomous insect bite or sting (T63.4-)

✓4ᵗʰ **S70 Superficial injury of hip and thigh**

The appropriate 7th character is to be added to each code from
category S70.
  A   initial encounter
  D   subsequent encounter
  S   sequela

✓5ᵗʰ **S70.0 Contusion of hip**

✓x7ᵗʰ **S70.00 Contusion of unspecified hip** ▽

✓x7ᵗʰ **S70.01 Contusion of right hip**

✓x7ᵗʰ **S70.02 Contusion of left hip**

✓5ᵗʰ **S70.1 Contusion of thigh**

✓x7ᵗʰ **S70.10 Contusion of unspecified thigh** ▽

✓x7ᵗʰ **S70.11 Contusion of right thigh**

✓x7ᵗʰ **S70.12 Contusion of left thigh**

✓5ᵗʰ **S70.2 Other superficial injuries of hip**

✓6ᵗʰ **S70.21 Abrasion of hip**

✓7ᵗʰ **S70.211 Abrasion, right hip**

✓7ᵗʰ **S70.212 Abrasion, left hip**

✓7ᵗʰ **S70.219 Abrasion, unspecified hip** ▽

✓6ᵗʰ **S70.22 Blister (nonthermal) of hip**

✓7ᵗʰ **S70.221 Blister (nonthermal), right hip**

✓7ᵗʰ **S70.222 Blister (nonthermal), left hip**

✓7ᵗʰ **S70.229 Blister (nonthermal), unspecified** ▽
  hip

✓6ᵗʰ **S70.24 External constriction of hip**

✓7ᵗʰ **S70.241 External constriction, right hip**

✓7ᵗʰ **S70.242 External constriction, left hip**

✓7ᵗʰ **S70.249 External constriction, unspecified** ▽
  hip

✓6ᵗʰ **S70.25 Superficial foreign body of hip**
    Splinter in the hip

✓7ᵗʰ **S70.251 Superficial foreign body, right hip**

✓7ᵗʰ **S70.252 Superficial foreign body, left hip**

✓7ᵗʰ **S70.259 Superficial foreign body,** ▽
  unspecified hip

✓6ᵗʰ **S70.26 Insect bite (nonvenomous) of hip**

✓7ᵗʰ **S70.261 Insect bite (nonvenomous), right hip**

✓7ᵗʰ **S70.262 Insect bite (nonvenomous), left hip**

✓7ᵗʰ **S70.269 Insect bite (nonvenomous),** ▽
  unspecified hip

✓6ᵗʰ **S70.27 Other superficial bite of hip**
    EXCLUDES 1 *open bite of hip (S71.05-)*

✓7ᵗʰ **S70.271 Other superficial bite of hip, right hip**

✓7ᵗʰ **S70.272 Other superficial bite of hip, left hip**

✓7ᵗʰ **S70.279 Other superficial bite of hip,** ▽
  unspecified hip

✓5ᵗʰ **S70.3 Other superficial injuries of thigh**

✓6ᵗʰ **S70.31 Abrasion of thigh**

✓7ᵗʰ **S70.311 Abrasion, right thigh**

✓7ᵗʰ **S70.312 Abrasion, left thigh**

✓7ᵗʰ **S70.319 Abrasion, unspecified thigh** ▽

✓6ᵗʰ **S70.32 Blister (nonthermal) of thigh**

✓7ᵗʰ **S70.321 Blister (nonthermal), right thigh**

✓7ᵗʰ **S70.322 Blister (nonthermal), left thigh**

✓7ᵗʰ **S70.329 Blister (nonthermal), unspecified** ▽
  thigh

✓6ᵗʰ **S70.34 External constriction of thigh**

✓7ᵗʰ **S70.341 External constriction, right thigh**

✓7ᵗʰ **S70.342 External constriction, left thigh**

✓7ᵗʰ **S70.349 External constriction, unspecified** ▽
  thigh

✓6ᵗʰ **S70.35 Superficial foreign body of thigh**
    Splinter in the thigh

✓7ᵗʰ **S70.351 Superficial foreign body, right thigh**

✓7ᵗʰ **S70.352 Superficial foreign body, left thigh**

✓7ᵗʰ **S70.359 Superficial foreign body,** ▽
  unspecified thigh

✓6ᵗʰ **S70.36 Insect bite (nonvenomous) of thigh**

✓7ᵗʰ **S70.361 Insect bite (nonvenomous), right thigh**

✓7ᵗʰ **S70.362 Insect bite (nonvenomous), left thigh**

✓7ᵗʰ **S70.369 Insect bite (nonvenomous),** ▽
  unspecified thigh

✓6ᵗʰ **S70.37 Other superficial bite of thigh**
    EXCLUDES 1 *open bite of thigh (S71.15)*

✓7ᵗʰ **S70.371 Other superficial bite of right thigh**

✓7ᵗʰ **S70.372 Other superficial bite of left thigh**

✓7ᵗʰ **S70.379 Other superficial bite of** ▽
  unspecified thigh

✓5ᵗʰ **S70.9 Unspecified superficial injury of hip and thigh**

✓6ᵗʰ **S70.91 Unspecified superficial injury of hip**

✓7ᵗʰ **S70.911 Unspecified superficial injury of** ▽
  right hip

✓7ᵗʰ **S70.912 Unspecified superficial injury of** ▽
  left hip

✓7ᵗʰ **S70.919 Unspecified superficial injury of** ▽
  unspecified hip

✓6ᵗʰ **S70.92 Unspecified superficial injury of thigh**

✓7ᵗʰ **S70.921 Unspecified superficial injury of** ▽
  right thigh

✓7ᵗʰ **S70.922 Unspecified superficial injury of** ▽
  left thigh

    √7ᵗʰ **S70.929** **Unspecified superficial injury of** unspecified thigh ▽

√4ᵗʰ **S71** **Open wound of hip and thigh**

    Code also any associated wound infection

    EXCLUDES 1   open fracture of hip and thigh (S72.-)

                   traumatic amputation of hip and thigh (S78.-)

    EXCLUDES 2   bite of venomous animal (T63.-)

                   open wound of ankle, foot and toes (S91.-)

                   open wound of knee and lower leg (S81.-)

> The appropriate 7th character is to be added to each code from category S71.
> A   initial encounter
> D   subsequent encounter
> S   sequela

√5ᵗʰ **S71.0** **Open wound of hip**

   √6ᵗʰ **S71.00** **Unspecified open wound of hip**

      √7ᵗʰ **S71.001** **Unspecified open wound, right** hip ▽

      √7ᵗʰ **S71.002** **Unspecified open wound, left** hip ▽

      √7ᵗʰ **S71.009** **Unspecified open wound, unspecified hip** ▽

   √6ᵗʰ **S71.01** Laceration without foreign body of hip

      √7ᵗʰ **S71.011** **Laceration without foreign body, right** hip

      √7ᵗʰ **S71.012** **Laceration without foreign body, left** hip

      √7ᵗʰ **S71.019** **Laceration without foreign body, unspecified hip** ▽

   √6ᵗʰ **S71.02** Laceration with foreign body of hip

      √7ᵗʰ **S71.021** **Laceration with foreign body, right** hip

      √7ᵗʰ **S71.022** **Laceration with foreign body, left** hip

      √7ᵗʰ **S71.029** **Laceration with foreign body, unspecified hip** ▽

   √6ᵗʰ **S71.03** Puncture wound without foreign body of hip

      √7ᵗʰ **S71.031** **Puncture wound without foreign body, right** hip

      √7ᵗʰ **S71.032** **Puncture wound without foreign body, left** hip

      √7ᵗʰ **S71.039** **Puncture wound without foreign body, unspecified hip** ▽

   √6ᵗʰ **S71.04** Puncture wound with foreign body of hip

      √7ᵗʰ **S71.041** **Puncture wound with foreign body, right** hip

      √7ᵗʰ **S71.042** **Puncture wound with foreign body, left** hip

      √7ᵗʰ **S71.049** **Puncture wound with foreign body, unspecified hip** ▽

   √6ᵗʰ **S71.05** **Open bite of hip**

       Bite of hip NOS

       EXCLUDES 1   superficial bite of hip (S70.26, S70.27)

      √7ᵗʰ **S71.051** **Open bite, right** hip

      √7ᵗʰ **S71.052** **Open bite, left** hip

      √7ᵗʰ **S71.059** **Open bite, unspecified hip** ▽

√5ᵗʰ **S71.1** **Open wound of thigh**

   √6ᵗʰ **S71.10** **Unspecified open wound of thigh**

      AHA: 2016,3Q,24

      √7ᵗʰ **S71.101** **Unspecified open wound, right** thigh ▽

      √7ᵗʰ **S71.102** **Unspecified open wound, left** thigh ▽

      √7ᵗʰ **S71.109** **Unspecified open wound, unspecified thigh** ▽

   √6ᵗʰ **S71.11** Laceration without foreign body of thigh

      √7ᵗʰ **S71.111** **Laceration without foreign body, right** thigh

      √7ᵗʰ **S71.112** **Laceration without foreign body, left** thigh

      √7ᵗʰ **S71.119** **Laceration without foreign body, unspecified thigh** ▽

   √6ᵗʰ **S71.12** Laceration with foreign body of thigh

      √7ᵗʰ **S71.121** **Laceration with foreign body, right thigh**

      √7ᵗʰ **S71.122** **Laceration with foreign body, left thigh**

      √7ᵗʰ **S71.129** **Laceration with foreign body, unspecified thigh** ▽

   √6ᵗʰ **S71.13** **Puncture wound without foreign body** of thigh

      AHA: 2016,3Q,24

      √7ᵗʰ **S71.131** **Puncture wound without foreign body, right thigh**

      √7ᵗʰ **S71.132** **Puncture wound without foreign body, left thigh**

      √7ᵗʰ **S71.139** **Puncture wound without foreign body, unspecified thigh** ▽

   √6ᵗʰ **S71.14** **Puncture wound with foreign body** of thigh

      AHA: 2016,3Q,24

      √7ᵗʰ **S71.141** **Puncture wound with foreign body, right thigh**

      √7ᵗʰ **S71.142** **Puncture wound with foreign body, left thigh**

      √7ᵗʰ **S71.149** **Puncture wound with foreign body, unspecified thigh** ▽

   √6ᵗʰ **S71.15** **Open bite of thigh**

       Bite of thigh NOS

       EXCLUDES 1   superficial bite of thigh (S70.37-)

      √7ᵗʰ **S71.151** **Open bite, right thigh**

      √7ᵗʰ **S71.152** **Open bite, left thigh**

      √7ᵗʰ **S71.159** **Open bite, unspecified thigh** ▽

√4ᵗʰ **S72** **Fracture of femur**

   NOTE   A fracture not indicated as displaced or nondisplaced should be coded to displaced.

         A fracture not indicated as open or closed should be coded to closed.

         The open fracture designations are based on the Gustilo open fracture classification.

   EXCLUDES 1   traumatic amputation of hip and thigh (S78.-)

   EXCLUDES 2   fracture of lower leg and ankle (S82.-)

              fracture of foot (S92.-)

              periprosthetic fracture of prosthetic implant of hip (M97.0-)

AHA: 2018,2Q,12; 2016,1Q,33; 2015,3Q,37-39; 2015,1Q,17; 2013,4Q,128

> The appropriate 7th character is to be added to all codes from category S72 [unless otherwise indicated].
> A   initial encounter for closed fracture
> B   initial encounter for open fracture type I or II
>   initial encounter for open fracture NOS
> C   initial encounter for open fracture type IIIA, IIIB, or IIIC
> D   subsequent encounter for closed fracture with routine healing
> E   subsequent encounter for open fracture type I or II with routine healing
> F   subsequent encounter for open fracture type IIIA, IIIB, or IIIC with routine healing
> G   subsequent encounter for closed fracture with delayed healing
> H   subsequent encounter for open fracture type I or II with delayed healing
> J   subsequent encounter for open fracture type IIIA, IIIB, or IIIC with delayed healing
> K   subsequent encounter for closed fracture with nonunion
> M   subsequent encounter for open fracture type I or II with nonunion
> N   subsequent encounter for open fracture type IIIA, IIIB, or IIIC with nonunion
> P   subsequent encounter for closed fracture with malunion
> Q   subsequent encounter for open fracture type I or II with malunion
> R   subsequent encounter for open fracture type IIIA, IIIB, or IIIC with malunion
> S   sequela

√5ᵗʰ **S72.0** **Fracture of head and neck of femur**

      EXCLUDES 2   physeal fracture of upper end of femur (S79.0-)

      AHA: 2016,3Q,16

   √6ᵗʰ **S72.00** **Fracture of unspecified part of neck of femur**

       Fracture of hip NOS

       Fracture of neck of femur NOS

      ¹ √7ᵗʰ **S72.001** **Fracture of unspecified part of neck of right femur** HCC 0 ▽

      ¹ √7ᵗʰ **S72.002** **Fracture of unspecified part of neck of left femur** HCC 0 ▽

      ¹ √7ᵗʰ **S72.009** **Fracture of unspecified part of neck of unspecified femur** HCC 0 ▽

   √6ᵗʰ **S72.01** **Unspecified intracapsular fracture of femur**

       Subcapital fracture of femur

      ¹ √7ᵗʰ **S72.011** **Unspecified intracapsular fracture of right femur** HCC 0 ▽

☑ Additional Character Req   √x7ᵗʰ Placeholder Alert   Manifestation   ▽ Unspecified   ▶◀ Revised Text   ● New Code   ▲ Revised Code Title

ICD-10-CM 2019   **1039**

¹ √7ᵗʰ **S72.012** **Unspecified intracapsular fracture of left femur** HCC Q ▽

¹ √7ᵗʰ **S72.019** **Unspecified intracapsular fracture of unspecified femur** HCC Q ▽

√6ᵗʰ **S72.02** **Fracture of epiphysis (separation) (upper) of femur**

Transepiphyseal fracture of femur

EXCLUDES 1   *capital femoral epiphyseal fracture (pediatric) of femur (S79.01-)*
Salter-Harris Type I physeal fracture of upper end of femur (S79.01-)

¹ √7ᵗʰ **S72.021** **Displaced fracture of epiphysis (separation) (upper) of right femur** HCC Q

¹ √7ᵗʰ **S72.022** **Displaced fracture of epiphysis (separation) (upper) of left femur** HCC Q

¹ √7ᵗʰ **S72.023** **Displaced fracture of epiphysis (separation) (upper) of unspecified femur** HCC Q ▽

¹ √7ᵗʰ **S72.024** **Nondisplaced fracture of epiphysis (separation) (upper) of right femur** HCC Q

¹ √7ᵗʰ **S72.025** **Nondisplaced fracture of epiphysis (separation) (upper) of left femur** HCC Q

¹ √7ᵗʰ **S72.026** **Nondisplaced fracture of epiphysis (separation) (upper) of unspecified femur** HCC Q ▽

√6ᵗʰ **S72.03** **Midcervical fracture of femur**

Transcervical fracture of femur NOS

¹ √7ᵗʰ **S72.031** **Displaced midcervical fracture of right femur** HCC Q

¹ √7ᵗʰ **S72.032** **Displaced midcervical fracture of left femur** HCC Q

¹ √7ᵗʰ **S72.033** **Displaced midcervical fracture of unspecified femur** HCC Q ▽

¹ √7ᵗʰ **S72.034** **Nondisplaced midcervical fracture of right femur** HCC Q

¹ √7ᵗʰ **S72.035** **Nondisplaced midcervical fracture of left femur** HCC Q

¹ √7ᵗʰ **S72.036** **Nondisplaced midcervical fracture of unspecified femur** HCC Q ▽

√6ᵗʰ **S72.04** **Fracture of base of neck of femur**

Cervicotrochanteric fracture of femur

¹ √7ᵗʰ **S72.041** **Displaced fracture of base of neck of right femur** HCC Q

¹ √7ᵗʰ **S72.042** **Displaced fracture of base of neck of left femur** HCC Q

¹ √7ᵗʰ **S72.043** **Displaced fracture of base of neck of unspecified femur** HCC Q ▽

¹ √7ᵗʰ **S72.044** **Nondisplaced fracture of base of neck of right femur** HCC Q

¹ √7ᵗʰ **S72.045** **Nondisplaced fracture of base of neck of left femur** HCC Q

¹ √7ᵗʰ **S72.046** **Nondisplaced fracture of base of neck of unspecified femur** HCC Q ▽

√6ᵗʰ **S72.05** **Unspecified fracture of head of femur**

Fracture of head of femur NOS

¹ √7ᵗʰ **S72.051** **Unspecified fracture of head of right femur** HCC Q ▽

¹ √7ᵗʰ **S72.052** **Unspecified fracture of head of left femur** HCC Q ▽

¹ √7ᵗʰ **S72.059** **Unspecified fracture of head of unspecified femur** HCC Q ▽

√6ᵗʰ **S72.06** **Articular fracture of head of femur**

¹ √7ᵗʰ **S72.061** **Displaced articular fracture of head of right femur** HCC Q

¹ √7ᵗʰ **S72.062** **Displaced articular fracture of head of left femur** HCC Q

¹ √7ᵗʰ **S72.063** **Displaced articular fracture of head of unspecified femur** HCC Q ▽

¹ √7ᵗʰ **S72.064** **Nondisplaced articular fracture of head of right femur** HCC Q

¹ √7ᵗʰ **S72.065** **Nondisplaced articular fracture of head of left femur** HCC Q

¹ √7ᵗʰ **S72.066** **Nondisplaced articular fracture of head of unspecified femur** HCC Q ▽

√6ᵗʰ **S72.09** **Other fracture of head and neck of femur**

¹ √7ᵗʰ **S72.091** **Other fracture of head and neck of right femur** HCC Q

¹ √7ᵗʰ **S72.092** **Other fracture of head and neck of left femur** HCC Q

¹ √7ᵗʰ **S72.099** **Other fracture of head and neck of unspecified femur** HCC Q ▽

√5ᵗʰ **S72.1** **Pertrochanteric fracture**

AHA: 2016,3Q,16

√6ᵗʰ **S72.10** **Unspecified trochanteric fracture of femur**

Fracture of trochanter NOS

¹ √7ᵗʰ **S72.101** **Unspecified trochanteric fracture of right femur** HCC Q ▽

¹ √7ᵗʰ **S72.102** **Unspecified trochanteric fracture of left femur** HCC Q ▽

¹ √7ᵗʰ **S72.109** **Unspecified trochanteric fracture of unspecified femur** HCC Q ▽

√6ᵗʰ **S72.11** **Fracture of greater trochanter of femur**

¹ √7ᵗʰ **S72.111** **Displaced fracture of greater trochanter of right femur** HCC Q

¹ √7ᵗʰ **S72.112** **Displaced fracture of greater trochanter of left femur** HCC Q

¹ √7ᵗʰ **S72.113** **Displaced fracture of greater trochanter of unspecified femur** HCC Q ▽

¹ √7ᵗʰ **S72.114** **Nondisplaced fracture of greater trochanter of right femur** HCC Q

¹ √7ᵗʰ **S72.115** **Nondisplaced fracture of greater trochanter of left femur** HCC Q

¹ √7ᵗʰ **S72.116** **Nondisplaced fracture of greater trochanter of unspecified femur** HCC Q ▽

√6ᵗʰ **S72.12** **Fracture of lesser trochanter of femur**

¹ √7ᵗʰ **S72.121** **Displaced fracture of lesser trochanter of right femur** HCC Q

¹ √7ᵗʰ **S72.122** **Displaced fracture of lesser trochanter of left femur** HCC Q

¹ √7ᵗʰ **S72.123** **Displaced fracture of lesser trochanter of unspecified femur** HCC Q ▽

¹ √7ᵗʰ **S72.124** **Nondisplaced fracture of lesser trochanter of right femur** HCC Q

¹ √7ᵗʰ **S72.125** **Nondisplaced fracture of lesser trochanter of left femur** HCC Q

¹ √7ᵗʰ **S72.126** **Nondisplaced fracture of lesser trochanter of unspecified femur** HCC Q ▽

√6ᵗʰ **S72.13** **Apophyseal fracture of femur**

EXCLUDES 1   *chronic (nontraumatic) slipped upper femoral epiphysis (M93.0-)*

¹ √7ᵗʰ **S72.131** **Displaced apophyseal fracture of right femur** HCC Q

¹ √7ᵗʰ **S72.132** **Displaced apophyseal fracture of left femur** HCC Q

¹ √7ᵗʰ **S72.133** **Displaced apophyseal fracture of unspecified femur** HCC Q ▽

¹ √7ᵗʰ **S72.134** **Nondisplaced apophyseal fracture of right femur** HCC Q

¹ √7ᵗʰ **S72.135** **Nondisplaced apophyseal fracture of left femur** HCC Q

¹ √7ᵗʰ **S72.136** **Nondisplaced apophyseal fracture of unspecified femur** HCC Q ▽

√6ᵗʰ **S72.14** **Intertrochanteric fracture of femur**

¹ √7ᵗʰ **S72.141** **Displaced intertrochanteric fracture of right femur** HCC Q

¹ √7ᵗʰ **S72.142** **Displaced intertrochanteric fracture of left femur** HCC Q

¹ √7ᵗʰ **S72.143** **Displaced intertrochanteric fracture of unspecified femur** HCC Q ▽

¹ √7ᵗʰ **S72.144** **Nondisplaced intertrochanteric fracture of right femur** HCC Q

¹ √7ᵗʰ **S72.145** **Nondisplaced intertrochanteric fracture of left femur** HCC Q

¹ √7ᵗʰ **S72.146** **Nondisplaced intertrochanteric fracture of unspecified femur** HCC Q ▽

√5ᵗʰ **S72.2** **Subtrochanteric fracture of femur**

¹ √x7ᵗʰ **S72.21** **Displaced subtrochanteric fracture of right femur** HCC Q

¹ √x7ᵗʰ **S72.22** **Displaced subtrochanteric fracture of left femur** HCC Q

¹ √x7ᵗʰ **S72.23** **Displaced subtrochanteric fracture of unspecified femur** HCC Q ▽

¹ √x7ᵗʰ **S72.24** **Nondisplaced subtrochanteric fracture of right femur** HCC Q

¹ √x7ᵗʰ **S72.25** **Nondisplaced subtrochanteric fracture of left femur** HCC Q

¹ √x7ᵗʰ **S72.26** **Nondisplaced subtrochanteric fracture of unspecified femur** HCC Q ▽

✓5ᵗʰ **S72.3 Fracture of shaft of femur**

  ✓6ᵗʰ **S72.30 Unspecified fracture of shaft of femur**

    ¹ ✓7ᵗʰ **S72.301 Unspecified fracture of shaft of right femur** HCC Q ▽

    ¹ ✓7ᵗʰ **S72.302 Unspecified fracture of shaft of left femur** HCC Q ▽

    ¹ ✓7ᵗʰ **S72.309 Unspecified fracture of shaft of unspecified femur** HCC Q ▽

  ✓6ᵗʰ **S72.32 Transverse fracture of shaft of femur**

    ¹ ✓7ᵗʰ **S72.321 Displaced transverse fracture of shaft of right femur** HCC Q

    ¹ ✓7ᵗʰ **S72.322 Displaced transverse fracture of shaft of left femur** HCC Q

    ¹ ✓7ᵗʰ **S72.323 Displaced transverse fracture of shaft of unspecified femur** HCC Q ▽

    ¹ ✓7ᵗʰ **S72.324 Nondisplaced transverse fracture of shaft of right femur** HCC Q

    ¹ ✓7ᵗʰ **S72.325 Nondisplaced transverse fracture of shaft of left femur** HCC Q

    ¹ ✓7ᵗʰ **S72.326 Nondisplaced transverse fracture of shaft of unspecified femur** HCC Q ▽

  ✓6ᵗʰ **S72.33 Oblique fracture of shaft of femur**

    ¹ ✓7ᵗʰ **S72.331 Displaced oblique fracture of shaft of right femur** HCC Q

    ¹ ✓7ᵗʰ **S72.332 Displaced oblique fracture of shaft of left femur** HCC Q

    ¹ ✓7ᵗʰ **S72.333 Displaced oblique fracture of shaft of unspecified femur** HCC Q ▽

    ¹ ✓7ᵗʰ **S72.334 Nondisplaced oblique fracture of shaft of right femur** HCC Q

    ¹ ✓7ᵗʰ **S72.335 Nondisplaced oblique fracture of shaft of left femur** HCC Q

    ¹ ✓7ᵗʰ **S72.336 Nondisplaced oblique fracture of shaft of unspecified femur** HCC Q ▽

  ✓6ᵗʰ **S72.34 Spiral fracture of shaft of femur**

    ¹ ✓7ᵗʰ **S72.341 Displaced spiral fracture of shaft of right femur** HCC Q

    ¹ ✓7ᵗʰ **S72.342 Displaced spiral fracture of shaft of left femur** HCC Q

    ¹ ✓7ᵗʰ **S72.343 Displaced spiral fracture of shaft of unspecified femur** HCC Q ▽

    ¹ ✓7ᵗʰ **S72.344 Nondisplaced spiral fracture of shaft of right femur** HCC Q

    ¹ ✓7ᵗʰ **S72.345 Nondisplaced spiral fracture of shaft of left femur** HCC Q

    ¹ ✓7ᵗʰ **S72.346 Nondisplaced spiral fracture of shaft of unspecified femur** HCC Q ▽

  ✓6ᵗʰ **S72.35 Comminuted fracture of shaft of femur**

    ¹ ✓7ᵗʰ **S72.351 Displaced comminuted fracture of shaft of right femur** HCC Q

    ¹ ✓7ᵗʰ **S72.352 Displaced comminuted fracture of shaft of left femur** HCC Q

    ¹ ✓7ᵗʰ **S72.353 Displaced comminuted fracture of shaft of unspecified femur** HCC Q ▽

    ¹ ✓7ᵗʰ **S72.354 Nondisplaced comminuted fracture of shaft of right femur** HCC Q

    ¹ ✓7ᵗʰ **S72.355 Nondisplaced comminuted fracture of shaft of left femur** HCC Q

    ¹ ✓7ᵗʰ **S72.356 Nondisplaced comminuted fracture of shaft of unspecified femur** HCC Q ▽

  ✓6ᵗʰ **S72.36 Segmental fracture of shaft of femur**

    ¹ ✓7ᵗʰ **S72.361 Displaced segmental fracture of shaft of right femur** HCC Q

    ¹ ✓7ᵗʰ **S72.362 Displaced segmental fracture of shaft of left femur** HCC Q

    ¹ ✓7ᵗʰ **S72.363 Displaced segmental fracture of shaft of unspecified femur** HCC Q ▽

    ¹ ✓7ᵗʰ **S72.364 Nondisplaced segmental fracture of shaft of right femur** HCC Q

    ¹ ✓7ᵗʰ **S72.365 Nondisplaced segmental fracture of shaft of left femur** HCC Q

    ¹ ✓7ᵗʰ **S72.366 Nondisplaced segmental fracture of shaft of unspecified femur** HCC Q ▽

  ✓6ᵗʰ **S72.39 Other fracture of shaft of femur**

    ¹ ✓7ᵗʰ **S72.391 Other fracture of shaft of right femur** HCC Q

    ¹ ✓7ᵗʰ **S72.392 Other fracture of shaft of left femur** HCC Q

    ¹ ✓7ᵗʰ **S72.399 Other fracture of shaft of unspecified femur** HCC Q ▽

✓5ᵗʰ **S72.4 Fracture of lower end of femur**

  Fracture of distal end of femur

  EXCLUDES 2   fracture of shaft of femur (S72.3-)

                physeal fracture of lower end of femur (S79.1-)

  AHA: 2016,4Q,42

  ✓6ᵗʰ **S72.40 Unspecified fracture of lower end of femur**

    AHA: 2018,1Q,21; 2016,4Q,42

    ¹ ✓7ᵗʰ **S72.401 Unspecified fracture of lower end of right femur** HCC Q ▽

    ¹ ✓7ᵗʰ **S72.402 Unspecified fracture of lower end of left femur** HCC Q ▽

    ¹ ✓7ᵗʰ **S72.409 Unspecified fracture of lower end of unspecified femur** HCC Q ▽

  ✓6ᵗʰ **S72.41 Unspecified condyle fracture of lower end of femur**

    Condyle fracture of femur NOS

    ¹ ✓7ᵗʰ **S72.411 Displaced unspecified condyle fracture of lower end of right femur** HCC Q ▽

    ¹ ✓7ᵗʰ **S72.412 Displaced unspecified condyle fracture of lower end of left femur** HCC Q ▽

    ¹ ✓7ᵗʰ **S72.413 Displaced unspecified condyle fracture of lower end of unspecified femur** HCC Q ▽

    ¹ ✓7ᵗʰ **S72.414 Nondisplaced unspecified condyle fracture of lower end of right femur** HCC Q ▽

    ¹ ✓7ᵗʰ **S72.415 Nondisplaced unspecified condyle fracture of lower end of left femur** HCC Q ▽

    ¹ ✓7ᵗʰ **S72.416 Nondisplaced unspecified condyle fracture of lower end of unspecified femur** HCC Q ▽

  ✓6ᵗʰ **S72.42 Fracture of lateral condyle of femur**

    ¹ ✓7ᵗʰ **S72.421 Displaced fracture of lateral condyle of right femur** HCC Q

    ¹ ✓7ᵗʰ **S72.422 Displaced fracture of lateral condyle of left femur** HCC Q

    ¹ ✓7ᵗʰ **S72.423 Displaced fracture of lateral condyle of unspecified femur** HCC Q ▽

    ¹ ✓7ᵗʰ **S72.424 Nondisplaced fracture of lateral condyle of right femur** HCC Q

    ¹ ✓7ᵗʰ **S72.425 Nondisplaced fracture of lateral condyle of left femur** HCC Q

    ¹ ✓7ᵗʰ **S72.426 Nondisplaced fracture of lateral condyle of unspecified femur** HCC Q ▽

  ✓6ᵗʰ **S72.43 Fracture of medial condyle of femur**

    ¹ ✓7ᵗʰ **S72.431 Displaced fracture of medial condyle of right femur** HCC Q

    ¹ ✓7ᵗʰ **S72.432 Displaced fracture of medial condyle of left femur** HCC Q

    ¹ ✓7ᵗʰ **S72.433 Displaced fracture of medial condyle of unspecified femur** HCC Q ▽

    ¹ ✓7ᵗʰ **S72.434 Nondisplaced fracture of medial condyle of right femur** HCC Q

    ¹ ✓7ᵗʰ **S72.435 Nondisplaced fracture of medial condyle of left femur** HCC Q

    ¹ ✓7ᵗʰ **S72.436 Nondisplaced fracture of medial condyle of unspecified femur** HCC Q ▽

  ✓6ᵗʰ **S72.44 Fracture of lower epiphysis (separation) of femur**

    EXCLUDES 1   Salter-Harris Type I physeal fracture of lower end of femur (S79.11-)

    ¹ ✓7ᵗʰ **S72.441 Displaced fracture of lower epiphysis (separation) of right femur** HCC Q

    ¹ ✓7ᵗʰ **S72.442 Displaced fracture of lower epiphysis (separation) of left femur** HCC Q

    ¹ ✓7ᵗʰ **S72.443 Displaced fracture of lower epiphysis (separation) of unspecified femur** HCC Q ▽

    ¹ ✓7ᵗʰ **S72.444 Nondisplaced fracture of lower epiphysis (separation) of right femur** HCC Q

    ¹ ✓7ᵗʰ **S72.445 Nondisplaced fracture of lower epiphysis (separation) of left femur** HCC Q

    ¹ ✓7ᵗʰ **S72.446 Nondisplaced fracture of lower epiphysis (separation) of unspecified femur** HCC Q ▽

☑ Additional Character Req   ✓x7ᵗʰ Placeholder Alert   Manifestation   ▽ Unspecified   ►◄ Revised Text   ● New Code   ▲ Revised Code Title

√6th **S72.45** **Supracondylar fracture without intracondylar extension of lower end of femur**
Supracondylar fracture of lower end of femur NOS
> EXCLUDES 1   supracondylar fracture with intracondylar extension of lower end of femur (S72.46-)

1 √7th **S72.451** **Displaced supracondylar fracture without intracondylar extension of lower end of right femur** HCC Q

1 √7th **S72.452** **Displaced supracondylar fracture without intracondylar extension of lower end of left femur** HCC Q

1 √7th **S72.453** **Displaced supracondylar fracture without intracondylar extension of lower end of unspecified femur** HCC Q ▽

1 √7th **S72.454** **Nondisplaced supracondylar fracture without intracondylar extension of lower end of right femur** HCC Q

1 √7th **S72.455** **Nondisplaced supracondylar fracture without intracondylar extension of lower end of left femur** HCC Q

1 √7th **S72.456** **Nondisplaced supracondylar fracture without intracondylar extension of lower end of unspecified femur** HCC Q ▽

√6th **S72.46** **Supracondylar fracture with intracondylar extension of lower end of femur**
> EXCLUDES 1   supracondylar fracture without intracondylar extension of lower end of femur (S72.45-)

1 √7th **S72.461** **Displaced supracondylar fracture with intracondylar extension of lower end of right femur** HCC Q

1 √7th **S72.462** **Displaced supracondylar fracture with intracondylar extension of lower end of left femur** HCC Q

1 √7th **S72.463** **Displaced supracondylar fracture with intracondylar extension of lower end of unspecified femur** HCC Q ▽

1 √7th **S72.464** **Nondisplaced supracondylar fracture with intracondylar extension of lower end of right femur** HCC Q

1 √7th **S72.465** **Nondisplaced supracondylar fracture with intracondylar extension of lower end of left femur** HCC Q

1 √7th **S72.466** **Nondisplaced supracondylar fracture with intracondylar extension of lower end of unspecified femur** HCC Q ▽

√6th **S72.47** **Torus fracture of lower end of femur**

> The appropriate 7th character is to be added to all codes in subcategory S72.47.
> A   initial encounter for closed fracture
> D   subsequent encounter for fracture with routine healing
> G   subsequent encounter for fracture with delayed healing
> K   subsequent encounter for fracture with nonunion
> P   subsequent encounter for fracture with malunion
> S   sequela

1 √7th **S72.471** **Torus fracture of lower end of right femur** HCC Q

1 √7th **S72.472** **Torus fracture of lower end of left femur** HCC Q

1 √7th **S72.479** **Torus fracture of lower end of unspecified femur** HCC Q ▽

√6th **S72.49** **Other fracture of lower end of femur**

1 √7th **S72.491** **Other fracture of lower end of right femur** HCC Q

1 √7th **S72.492** **Other fracture of lower end of left femur** HCC Q

1 √7th **S72.499** **Other fracture of lower end of unspecified femur** HCC Q ▽

√5th **S72.8** **Other fracture of femur**

√6th **S72.8X** **Other fracture of femur**

1 √7th **S72.8X1** **Other fracture of right femur** HCC Q

1 √7th **S72.8X2** **Other fracture of left femur** HCC Q

1 √7th **S72.8X9** **Other fracture of unspecified femur** HCC Q ▽

√5th **S72.9** **Unspecified fracture of femur**
Fracture of thigh NOS
Fracture of upper leg NOS
> EXCLUDES 1   fracture of hip NOS (S72.00-, S72.01-)

1 √x7th **S72.90** **Unspecified fracture of unspecified femur** HCC Q ▽
AHA: 2012,4Q,93

1 √x7th **S72.91** **Unspecified fracture of right femur** HCC Q ▽

1 √x7th **S72.92** **Unspecified fracture of left femur** HCC Q ▽

√4th **S73** **Dislocation and sprain of joint and ligaments of hip**
> INCLUDES   avulsion of joint or ligament of hip
> laceration of cartilage, joint or ligament of hip
> sprain of cartilage, joint or ligament of hip
> traumatic hemarthrosis of joint or ligament of hip
> traumatic rupture of joint or ligament of hip
> traumatic subluxation of joint or ligament of hip
> traumatic tear of joint or ligament of hip

Code also any associated open wound
> EXCLUDES 2   strain of muscle, fascia and tendon of hip and thigh (S76.-)

> The appropriate 7th character is to be added to each code from category S73.
> A   initial encounter
> D   subsequent encounter
> S   sequela

√5th **S73.0** **Subluxation and dislocation of hip**
> EXCLUDES 2   dislocation and subluxation of hip prosthesis (T84.020, T84.021)

√6th **S73.00** **Unspecified subluxation and dislocation of hip**
Dislocation of hip NOS
Subluxation of hip NOS

1 √7th **S73.001** **Unspecified subluxation of right hip** HCC ▽

1 √7th **S73.002** **Unspecified subluxation of left hip** HCC ▽

1 √7th **S73.003** **Unspecified subluxation of unspecified hip** HCC ▽

1 √7th **S73.004** **Unspecified dislocation of right hip** HCC ▽

1 √7th **S73.005** **Unspecified dislocation of left hip** HCC ▽

1 √7th **S73.006** **Unspecified dislocation of unspecified hip** HCC ▽

√6th **S73.01** **Posterior subluxation and dislocation of hip**

1 √7th **S73.011** **Posterior subluxation of right hip** HCC

1 √7th **S73.012** **Posterior subluxation of left hip** HCC

1 √7th **S73.013** **Posterior subluxation of unspecified hip** HCC ▽

1 √7th **S73.014** **Posterior dislocation of right hip** HCC

1 √7th **S73.015** **Posterior dislocation of left hip** HCC

1 √7th **S73.016** **Posterior dislocation of unspecified hip** HCC ▽

√6th **S73.02** **Obturator subluxation and dislocation of hip**

1 √7th **S73.021** **Obturator subluxation of right hip** HCC

1 √7th **S73.022** **Obturator subluxation of left hip** HCC

1 √7th **S73.023** **Obturator subluxation of unspecified hip** HCC ▽

1 √7th **S73.024** **Obturator dislocation of right hip** HCC

1 √7th **S73.025** **Obturator dislocation of left hip** HCC

1 √7th **S73.026** **Obturator dislocation of unspecified hip** HCC ▽

√6th **S73.03** **Other anterior subluxation and dislocation of hip**

1 √7th **S73.031** **Other anterior subluxation of right hip** HCC

1 √7th **S73.032** **Other anterior subluxation of left hip** HCC

1 √7th **S73.033** **Other anterior subluxation of unspecified hip** HCC ▽

1 √7th **S73.034** **Other anterior dislocation of right hip** HCC

1 √7th **S73.035** **Other anterior dislocation of left hip** HCC

1 √7th **S73.036** **Other anterior dislocation of unspecified hip** HCC ▽

√6ᵗʰ **S73.04** **Central** subluxation and dislocation of hip

¹ √7ᵗʰ **S73.041** **Central subluxation** of **right** hip `HCC`

¹ √7ᵗʰ **S73.042** **Central subluxation** of **left** hip `HCC`

¹ √7ᵗʰ **S73.043** **Central subluxation** of **unspecified** hip `HCC` ▽

¹ √7ᵗʰ **S73.044** **Central dislocation** of **right** hip `HCC`

¹ √7ᵗʰ **S73.045** **Central dislocation** of **left** hip `HCC`

¹ √7ᵗʰ **S73.046** **Central dislocation** of **unspecified** hip `HCC` ▽

√5ᵗʰ **S73.1** **Sprain** of hip

AHA: 2014,4Q,25

√6ᵗʰ **S73.10** **Unspecified sprain** of hip

√7ᵗʰ **S73.101** **Unspecified sprain** of **right** hip ▽

√7ᵗʰ **S73.102** **Unspecified sprain** of **left** hip ▽

√7ᵗʰ **S73.109** **Unspecified sprain** of **unspecified** hip ▽

√6ᵗʰ **S73.11** **Iliofemoral ligament** sprain of hip

√7ᵗʰ **S73.111** **Iliofemoral ligament sprain** of **right** hip

√7ᵗʰ **S73.112** **Iliofemoral ligament sprain** of **left** hip

√7ᵗʰ **S73.119** **Iliofemoral ligament sprain** of **unspecified** hip ▽

√6ᵗʰ **S73.12** **Ischiocapsular (ligament)** sprain of hip

√7ᵗʰ **S73.121** **Ischiocapsular ligament sprain** of **right** hip

√7ᵗʰ **S73.122** **Ischiocapsular ligament sprain** of **left** hip

√7ᵗʰ **S73.129** **Ischiocapsular ligament sprain** of **unspecified** hip ▽

√6ᵗʰ **S73.19** **Other sprain** of hip

√7ᵗʰ **S73.191** **Other sprain** of **right** hip

√7ᵗʰ **S73.192** **Other sprain** of **left** hip

√7ᵗʰ **S73.199** **Other sprain** of **unspecified** hip ▽

√4ᵗʰ **S74** **Injury of nerves at hip and thigh level**

Code also any associated open wound (S71.-)

EXCLUDES 2   *injury of nerves at ankle and foot level (S94.-)*

injury of nerves at lower leg level (S84.-)

The appropriate 7th character is to be added to each code from category S74.

A   initial encounter

D   subsequent encounter

S   sequela

√5ᵗʰ **S74.0** **Injury of sciatic nerve** at hip and thigh level

√x7ᵗʰ **S74.00** **Injury of sciatic nerve** at hip and thigh level, **unspecified leg** ▽

√x7ᵗʰ **S74.01** **Injury of sciatic nerve** at hip and thigh level, **right leg**

√x7ᵗʰ **S74.02** **Injury of sciatic nerve** at hip and thigh level, **left leg**

√5ᵗʰ **S74.1** **Injury of femoral nerve** at hip and thigh level

√x7ᵗʰ **S74.10** **Injury of femoral nerve** at hip and thigh level, **unspecified leg** ▽

√x7ᵗʰ **S74.11** **Injury of femoral nerve** at hip and thigh level, **right leg**

√x7ᵗʰ **S74.12** **Injury of femoral nerve** at hip and thigh level, **left leg**

√5ᵗʰ **S74.2** **Injury of cutaneous sensory nerve** at hip and thigh level

√x7ᵗʰ **S74.20** **Injury of cutaneous sensory nerve** at hip and thigh level, **unspecified leg** ▽

√x7ᵗʰ **S74.21** **Injury of cutaneous sensory nerve** at hip and high level, **right leg**

√x7ᵗʰ **S74.22** **Injury of cutaneous sensory nerve** at hip and thigh level, **left leg**

√5ᵗʰ **S74.8** **Injury of other nerves** at hip and thigh level

√6ᵗʰ **S74.8X** **Injury of other nerves** at hip and thigh level

√7ᵗʰ **S74.8X1** **Injury of other nerves** at hip and thigh level, **right leg**

√7ᵗʰ **S74.8X2** **Injury of other nerves** at hip and thigh level, **left leg**

√7ᵗʰ **S74.8X9** **Injury of other nerves** at hip and thigh level, **unspecified leg** ▽

√5ᵗʰ **S74.9** **Injury of unspecified nerve** at hip and thigh level

√x7ᵗʰ **S74.90** **Injury of unspecified nerve** at hip and thigh level, **unspecified leg** ▽

√x7ᵗʰ **S74.91** **Injury of unspecified nerve** at hip and thigh level, **right leg** ▽

√x7ᵗʰ **S74.92** **Injury of unspecified nerve** at hip and thigh level, **left leg** ▽

√4ᵗʰ **S75** **Injury of blood vessels at hip and thigh level**

Code also any associated open wound (S71.-)

EXCLUDES 2   *injury of blood vessels at lower leg level (S85.-)*

injury of popliteal artery (S85.0)

The appropriate 7th character is to be added to each code from category S75.

A   initial encounter

D   subsequent encounter

S   sequela

√5ᵗʰ **S75.0** **Injury of femoral artery**

√6ᵗʰ **S75.00** **Unspecified injury of femoral artery**

√7ᵗʰ **S75.001** **Unspecified injury of femoral artery, right leg** ▽

√7ᵗʰ **S75.002** **Unspecified injury of femoral artery, left leg** ▽

√7ᵗʰ **S75.009** **Unspecified injury of femoral artery, unspecified leg** ▽

√6ᵗʰ **S75.01** **Minor laceration** of femoral artery

Incomplete transection of femoral artery

Laceration of femoral artery NOS

Superficial laceration of femoral artery

√7ᵗʰ **S75.011** **Minor laceration of femoral artery, right leg**

√7ᵗʰ **S75.012** **Minor laceration of femoral artery, left leg**

√7ᵗʰ **S75.019** **Minor laceration of femoral artery, unspecified leg** ▽

√6ᵗʰ **S75.02** **Major laceration** of femoral artery

Complete transection of femoral artery

Traumatic rupture of femoral artery

√7ᵗʰ **S75.021** **Major laceration of femoral artery, right leg**

√7ᵗʰ **S75.022** **Major laceration of femoral artery, left leg**

√7ᵗʰ **S75.029** **Major laceration of femoral artery, unspecified leg** ▽

√6ᵗʰ **S75.09** **Other specified injury** of femoral artery

√7ᵗʰ **S75.091** **Other specified injury of femoral artery, right leg**

√7ᵗʰ **S75.092** **Other specified injury of femoral artery, left leg**

√7ᵗʰ **S75.099** **Other specified injury of femoral artery, unspecified leg** ▽

√5ᵗʰ **S75.1** **Injury of femoral vein** at hip and thigh level

√6ᵗʰ **S75.10** **Unspecified injury of femoral vein** at hip and thigh level

√7ᵗʰ **S75.101** **Unspecified injury of femoral vein at hip and thigh level, right leg** ▽

√7ᵗʰ **S75.102** **Unspecified injury of femoral vein at hip and thigh level, left leg** ▽

√7ᵗʰ **S75.109** **Unspecified injury of femoral vein at hip and thigh level, unspecified leg** ▽

√6ᵗʰ **S75.11** **Minor laceration** of femoral vein at hip and thigh level

Incomplete transection of femoral vein at hip and thigh level

Laceration of femoral vein at hip and thigh level NOS

Superficial laceration of femoral vein at hip and thigh level

√7ᵗʰ **S75.111** **Minor laceration of femoral vein at hip and thigh level, right leg**

√7ᵗʰ **S75.112** **Minor laceration of femoral vein at hip and thigh level, left leg**

√7ᵗʰ **S75.119** **Minor laceration of femoral vein at hip and thigh level, unspecified leg** ▽

√6ᵗʰ **S75.12** **Major laceration** of femoral vein at hip and thigh level

Complete transection of femoral vein at hip and thigh level

Traumatic rupture of femoral vein at hip and thigh level

√7ᵗʰ **S75.121** **Major laceration of femoral vein at hip and thigh level, right leg**

√7ᵗʰ **S75.122** **Major laceration of femoral vein at hip and thigh level, left leg**

☑ Additional Character Req   √x7ᵗʰ Placeholder Alert   Manifestation   ▽ Unspecified   ▶◀ Revised Text   ● New Code   ▲ Revised Code Title

ICD-10-CM 2019   1043

Chapter 19. Injury, Poisoning and Certain Other Consequences of External Causes

S75.129–S76.029

✓7ᵗʰ **S75.129** Major laceration of femoral vein at hip and thigh level, unspecified leg ▽

✓6ᵗʰ **S75.19** Other specified injury of femoral vein at hip and thigh level

     ✓7ᵗʰ **S75.191** Other specified injury of femoral vein at hip and thigh level, right leg

     ✓7ᵗʰ **S75.192** Other specified injury of femoral vein at hip and thigh level, left leg

     ✓7ᵗʰ **S75.199** Other specified injury of femoral vein at hip and thigh level, unspecified leg ▽

✓5ᵗʰ **S75.2** Injury of greater saphenous vein at hip and thigh level

     EXCLUDES 1   greater saphenous vein NOS (S85.3)

✓6ᵗʰ **S75.20** Unspecified injury of greater saphenous vein at hip and thigh level

     ✓7ᵗʰ **S75.201** Unspecified injury of greater saphenous vein at hip and thigh level, right leg ▽

     ✓7ᵗʰ **S75.202** Unspecified injury of greater saphenous vein at hip and thigh level, left leg ▽

     ✓7ᵗʰ **S75.209** Unspecified injury of greater saphenous vein at hip and thigh level, unspecified leg ▽

✓6ᵗʰ **S75.21** Minor laceration of greater saphenous vein at hip and thigh level

     Incomplete transection of greater saphenous vein at hip and thigh level

     Laceration of greater saphenous vein at hip and thigh level NOS

     Superficial laceration of greater saphenous vein at hip and thigh level

     ✓7ᵗʰ **S75.211** Minor laceration of greater saphenous vein at hip and thigh level, right leg

     ✓7ᵗʰ **S75.212** Minor laceration of greater saphenous vein at hip and thigh level, left leg

     ✓7ᵗʰ **S75.219** Minor laceration of greater saphenous vein at hip and thigh level, unspecified leg ▽

✓6ᵗʰ **S75.22** Major laceration of greater saphenous vein at hip and thigh level

     Complete transection of greater saphenous vein at hip and thigh level

     Traumatic rupture of greater saphenous vein at hip and thigh level

     ✓7ᵗʰ **S75.221** Major laceration of greater saphenous vein at hip and thigh level, right leg

     ✓7ᵗʰ **S75.222** Major laceration of greater saphenous vein at hip and thigh level, left leg

     ✓7ᵗʰ **S75.229** Major laceration of greater saphenous vein at hip and thigh level, unspecified leg ▽

✓6ᵗʰ **S75.29** Other specified injury of greater saphenous vein at hip and thigh level

     ✓7ᵗʰ **S75.291** Other specified injury of greater saphenous vein at hip and thigh level, right leg

     ✓7ᵗʰ **S75.292** Other specified injury of greater saphenous vein at hip and thigh level, left leg

     ✓7ᵗʰ **S75.299** Other specified injury of greater saphenous vein at hip and thigh level, unspecified leg ▽

✓5ᵗʰ **S75.8** Injury of other blood vessels at hip and thigh level

✓6ᵗʰ **S75.80** Unspecified injury of other blood vessels at hip and thigh level

     ✓7ᵗʰ **S75.801** Unspecified injury of other blood vessels at hip and thigh level, right leg ▽

     ✓7ᵗʰ **S75.802** Unspecified injury of other blood vessels at hip and thigh level, left leg ▽

     ✓7ᵗʰ **S75.809** Unspecified injury of other blood vessels at hip and thigh level, unspecified leg ▽

✓6ᵗʰ **S75.81** Laceration of other blood vessels at hip and thigh level

     ✓7ᵗʰ **S75.811** Laceration of other blood vessels at hip and thigh level, right leg

     ✓7ᵗʰ **S75.812** Laceration of other blood vessels at hip and thigh level, left leg

✓7ᵗʰ **S75.819** Laceration of other blood vessels at hip and thigh level, unspecified leg ▽

✓6ᵗʰ **S75.89** Other specified injury of other blood vessels at hip and thigh level

     ✓7ᵗʰ **S75.891** Other specified injury of other blood vessels at hip and thigh level, right leg

     ✓7ᵗʰ **S75.892** Other specified injury of other blood vessels at hip and thigh level, left leg

     ✓7ᵗʰ **S75.899** Other specified injury of other blood vessels at hip and thigh level, unspecified leg ▽

✓5ᵗʰ **S75.9** Injury of unspecified blood vessel at hip and thigh level

✓6ᵗʰ **S75.90** Unspecified injury of unspecified blood vessel at hip and thigh level

     ✓7ᵗʰ **S75.901** Unspecified injury of unspecified blood vessel at hip and thigh level, right leg ▽

     ✓7ᵗʰ **S75.902** Unspecified injury of unspecified blood vessel at hip and thigh level, left leg ▽

     ✓7ᵗʰ **S75.909** Unspecified injury of unspecified blood vessel at hip and thigh level, unspecified leg ▽

✓6ᵗʰ **S75.91** Laceration of unspecified blood vessel at hip and thigh level

     ✓7ᵗʰ **S75.911** Laceration of unspecified blood vessel at hip and thigh level, right leg ▽

     ✓7ᵗʰ **S75.912** Laceration of unspecified blood vessel at hip and thigh level, left leg ▽

     ✓7ᵗʰ **S75.919** Laceration of unspecified blood vessel at hip and thigh level, unspecified leg ▽

✓6ᵗʰ **S75.99** Other specified injury of unspecified blood vessel at hip and thigh level

     ✓7ᵗʰ **S75.991** Other specified injury of unspecified blood vessel at hip and thigh level, right leg ▽

     ✓7ᵗʰ **S75.992** Other specified injury of unspecified blood vessel at hip and thigh level, left leg ▽

     ✓7ᵗʰ **S75.999** Other specified injury of unspecified blood vessel at hip and thigh level, unspecified leg ▽

✓4ᵗʰ **S76** Injury of muscle, fascia and tendon at hip and thigh level

     Code also any associated open wound (S71.-)

     EXCLUDES 2   injury of muscle, fascia and tendon at lower leg level (S86) sprain of joint and ligament of hip (S73.1)

     TIP: Refer to the Muscle/Tendon table at the beginning of this chapter.

     The appropriate 7th character is to be added to each code from category S76.
     A   initial encounter
     D   subsequent encounter
     S   sequela

✓5ᵗʰ **S76.0** Injury of muscle, fascia and tendon of hip

✓6ᵗʰ **S76.00** Unspecified injury of muscle, fascia and tendon of hip

     ✓7ᵗʰ **S76.001** Unspecified injury of muscle, fascia and tendon of right hip ▽

     ✓7ᵗʰ **S76.002** Unspecified injury of muscle, fascia and tendon of left hip ▽

     ✓7ᵗʰ **S76.009** Unspecified injury of muscle, fascia and tendon of unspecified hip ▽

✓6ᵗʰ **S76.01** Strain of muscle, fascia and tendon of hip

     ✓7ᵗʰ **S76.011** Strain of muscle, fascia and tendon of right hip

     ✓7ᵗʰ **S76.012** Strain of muscle, fascia and tendon of left hip

     ✓7ᵗʰ **S76.019** Strain of muscle, fascia and tendon of unspecified hip ▽

✓6ᵗʰ **S76.02** Laceration of muscle, fascia and tendon of hip

     ✓7ᵗʰ **S76.021** Laceration of muscle, fascia and tendon of right hip

     ✓7ᵗʰ **S76.022** Laceration of muscle, fascia and tendon of left hip

     ✓7ᵗʰ **S76.029** Laceration of muscle, fascia and tendon of unspecified hip ▽

√6ᵗʰ **S76.09** Other specified injury of muscle, fascia and tendon of hip

    √7ᵗʰ **S76.091** Other specified injury of muscle, fascia and tendon of right hip

    √7ᵗʰ **S76.092** Other specified injury of muscle, fascia and tendon of left hip

    √7ᵗʰ **S76.099** Other specified injury of muscle, fascia and tendon of unspecified hip ▽

√5ᵗʰ **S76.1** Injury of quadriceps muscle, fascia and tendon

    Injury of patellar ligament (tendon)

  √6ᵗʰ **S76.10** Unspecified injury of quadriceps muscle, fascia and tendon

    √7ᵗʰ **S76.101** Unspecified injury of right quadriceps muscle, fascia and tendon ▽

    √7ᵗʰ **S76.102** Unspecified injury of left quadriceps muscle, fascia and tendon ▽

    √7ᵗʰ **S76.109** Unspecified injury of unspecified quadriceps muscle, fascia and tendon ▽

  √6ᵗʰ **S76.11** Strain of quadriceps muscle, fascia and tendon

    √7ᵗʰ **S76.111** Strain of right quadriceps muscle, fascia and tendon

    √7ᵗʰ **S76.112** Strain of left quadriceps muscle, fascia and tendon

    √7ᵗʰ **S76.119** Strain of unspecified quadriceps muscle, fascia and tendon ▽

  √6ᵗʰ **S76.12** Laceration of quadriceps muscle, fascia and tendon

    √7ᵗʰ **S76.121** Laceration of right quadriceps muscle, fascia and tendon

    √7ᵗʰ **S76.122** Laceration of left quadriceps muscle, fascia and tendon

    √7ᵗʰ **S76.129** Laceration of unspecified quadriceps muscle, fascia and tendon ▽

  √6ᵗʰ **S76.19** Other specified injury of quadriceps muscle, fascia and tendon

    √7ᵗʰ **S76.191** Other specified injury of right quadriceps muscle, fascia and tendon

    √7ᵗʰ **S76.192** Other specified injury of left quadriceps muscle, fascia and tendon

    √7ᵗʰ **S76.199** Other specified injury of unspecified quadriceps muscle, fascia and tendon ▽

√5ᵗʰ **S76.2** Injury of adductor muscle, fascia and tendon of thigh

  √6ᵗʰ **S76.20** Unspecified injury of adductor muscle, fascia and tendon of thigh

    √7ᵗʰ **S76.201** Unspecified injury of adductor muscle, fascia and tendon of right thigh ▽

    √7ᵗʰ **S76.202** Unspecified injury of adductor muscle, fascia and tendon of left thigh ▽

    √7ᵗʰ **S76.209** Unspecified injury of adductor muscle, fascia and tendon of unspecified thigh ▽

  √6ᵗʰ **S76.21** Strain of adductor muscle, fascia and tendon of thigh

    √7ᵗʰ **S76.211** Strain of adductor muscle, fascia and tendon of right thigh

    √7ᵗʰ **S76.212** Strain of adductor muscle, fascia and tendon of left thigh

    √7ᵗʰ **S76.219** Strain of adductor muscle, fascia and tendon of unspecified thigh ▽

  √6ᵗʰ **S76.22** Laceration of adductor muscle, fascia and tendon of thigh

    √7ᵗʰ **S76.221** Laceration of adductor muscle, fascia and tendon of right thigh

    √7ᵗʰ **S76.222** Laceration of adductor muscle, fascia and tendon of left thigh

    √7ᵗʰ **S76.229** Laceration of adductor muscle, fascia and tendon of unspecified thigh ▽

  √6ᵗʰ **S76.29** Other injury of adductor muscle, fascia and tendon of thigh

    √7ᵗʰ **S76.291** Other injury of adductor muscle, fascia and tendon of right thigh

    √7ᵗʰ **S76.292** Other injury of adductor muscle, fascia and tendon of left thigh

    √7ᵗʰ **S76.299** Other injury of adductor muscle, fascia and tendon of unspecified thigh ▽

√5ᵗʰ **S76.3** Injury of muscle, fascia and tendon of the posterior muscle group at thigh level

  √6ᵗʰ **S76.30** Unspecified injury of muscle, fascia and tendon of the posterior muscle group at thigh level

    √7ᵗʰ **S76.301** Unspecified injury of muscle, fascia and tendon of the posterior muscle group at thigh level, right thigh ▽

    √7ᵗʰ **S76.302** Unspecified injury of muscle, fascia and tendon of the posterior muscle group at thigh level, left thigh ▽

    √7ᵗʰ **S76.309** Unspecified injury of muscle, fascia and tendon of the posterior muscle group at thigh level, unspecified thigh ▽

  √6ᵗʰ **S76.31** Strain of muscle, fascia and tendon of the posterior muscle group at thigh level

    √7ᵗʰ **S76.311** Strain of muscle, fascia and tendon of the posterior muscle group at thigh level, right thigh

    √7ᵗʰ **S76.312** Strain of muscle, fascia and tendon of the posterior muscle group at thigh level, left thigh

    √7ᵗʰ **S76.319** Strain of muscle, fascia and tendon of the posterior muscle group at thigh level, unspecified thigh ▽

  √6ᵗʰ **S76.32** Laceration of muscle, fascia and tendon of the posterior muscle group at thigh level

    √7ᵗʰ **S76.321** Laceration of muscle, fascia and tendon of the posterior muscle group at thigh level, right thigh

    √7ᵗʰ **S76.322** Laceration of muscle, fascia and tendon of the posterior muscle group at thigh level, left thigh

    √7ᵗʰ **S76.329** Laceration of muscle, fascia and tendon of the posterior muscle group at thigh level, unspecified thigh ▽

  √6ᵗʰ **S76.39** Other specified injury of muscle, fascia and tendon of the posterior muscle group at thigh level

    √7ᵗʰ **S76.391** Other specified injury of muscle, fascia and tendon of the posterior muscle group at thigh level, right thigh

    √7ᵗʰ **S76.392** Other specified injury of muscle, fascia and tendon of the posterior muscle group at thigh level, left thigh

    √7ᵗʰ **S76.399** Other specified injury of muscle, fascia and tendon of the posterior muscle group at thigh level, unspecified thigh ▽

√5ᵗʰ **S76.8** Injury of other specified muscles, fascia and tendons at thigh level

  √6ᵗʰ **S76.80** Unspecified injury of other specified muscles, fascia and tendons at thigh level

    √7ᵗʰ **S76.801** Unspecified injury of other specified muscles, fascia and tendons at thigh level, right thigh ▽

    √7ᵗʰ **S76.802** Unspecified injury of other specified muscles, fascia and tendons at thigh level, left thigh ▽

    √7ᵗʰ **S76.809** Unspecified injury of other specified muscles, fascia and tendons at thigh level, unspecified thigh ▽

  √6ᵗʰ **S76.81** Strain of other specified muscles, fascia and tendons at thigh level

    √7ᵗʰ **S76.811** Strain of other specified muscles, fascia and tendons at thigh level, right thigh

    √7ᵗʰ **S76.812** Strain of other specified muscles, fascia and tendons at thigh level, left thigh

    √7ᵗʰ **S76.819** Strain of other specified muscles, fascia and tendons at thigh level, unspecified thigh ▽

  √6ᵗʰ **S76.82** Laceration of other specified muscles, fascia and tendons at thigh level

    √7ᵗʰ **S76.821** Laceration of other specified muscles, fascia and tendons at thigh level, right thigh

---

☑ Additional Character Req   √x7ᵗʰ Placeholder Alert   Manifestation   ▽ Unspecified   ►◄ Revised Text   ● New Code   ▲ Revised Code Title

☑7ᵗʰ **S76.822 Laceration of other specified muscles, fascia and tendons at thigh level, left thigh**

☑7ᵗʰ **S76.829 Laceration of other specified muscles, fascia and tendons at thigh level, unspecified thigh** ▽

☑6ᵗʰ **S76.89 Other injury of other specified muscles, fascia and tendons at thigh level**

☑7ᵗʰ **S76.891 Other injury of other specified muscles, fascia and tendons at thigh level, right thigh**

☑7ᵗʰ **S76.892 Other injury of other specified muscles, fascia and tendons at thigh level, left thigh**

☑7ᵗʰ **S76.899 Other injury of other specified muscles, fascia and tendons at thigh level, unspecified thigh** ▽

☑5ᵗʰ **S76.9 Injury of unspecified muscles, fascia and tendons at thigh level**

☑6ᵗʰ **S76.90 Unspecified injury of unspecified muscles, fascia and tendons at thigh level**

☑7ᵗʰ **S76.901 Unspecified injury of unspecified muscles, fascia and tendons at thigh level, right thigh** ▽

☑7ᵗʰ **S76.902 Unspecified injury of unspecified muscles, fascia and tendons at thigh level, left thigh** ▽

☑7ᵗʰ **S76.909 Unspecified injury of unspecified muscles, fascia and tendons at thigh level, unspecified thigh** ▽

☑6ᵗʰ **S76.91 Strain of unspecified muscles, fascia and tendons at thigh level**

☑7ᵗʰ **S76.911 Strain of unspecified muscles, fascia and tendons at thigh level, right thigh** ▽

☑7ᵗʰ **S76.912 Strain of unspecified muscles, fascia and tendons at thigh level, left thigh** ▽

☑7ᵗʰ **S76.919 Strain of unspecified muscles, fascia and tendons at thigh level, unspecified thigh** ▽

☑6ᵗʰ **S76.92 Laceration of unspecified muscles, fascia and tendons at thigh level**

☑7ᵗʰ **S76.921 Laceration of unspecified muscles, fascia and tendons at thigh level, right thigh** ▽

☑7ᵗʰ **S76.922 Laceration of unspecified muscles, fascia and tendons at thigh level, left thigh** ▽

☑7ᵗʰ **S76.929 Laceration of unspecified muscles, fascia and tendons at thigh level, unspecified thigh** ▽

☑6ᵗʰ **S76.99 Other specified injury of unspecified muscles, fascia and tendons at thigh level**

☑7ᵗʰ **S76.991 Other specified injury of unspecified muscles, fascia and tendons at thigh level, right thigh** ▽

☑7ᵗʰ **S76.992 Other specified injury of unspecified muscles, fascia and tendons at thigh level, left thigh** ▽

☑7ᵗʰ **S76.999 Other specified injury of unspecified muscles, fascia and tendons at thigh level, unspecified thigh** ▽

☑4ᵗʰ **S77 Crushing injury of hip and thigh**

Use additional code(s) for all associated injuries

EXCLUDES 2   crushing injury of ankle and foot (S97.-)
crushing injury of lower leg (S87.-)

The appropriate 7th character is to be added to each code from category S77.
A   initial encounter
D   subsequent encounter
S   sequela

☑5ᵗʰ **S77.0 Crushing injury of hip**

☑x7ᵗʰ **S77.00 Crushing injury of unspecified hip** ▽

☑x7ᵗʰ **S77.01 Crushing injury of right hip**

☑x7ᵗʰ **S77.02 Crushing injury of left hip**

☑5ᵗʰ **S77.1 Crushing injury of thigh**

☑x7ᵗʰ **S77.10 Crushing injury of unspecified thigh** ▽

☑x7ᵗʰ **S77.11 Crushing injury of right thigh**

☑x7ᵗʰ **S77.12 Crushing injury of left thigh**

☑5ᵗʰ **S77.2 Crushing injury of hip with thigh**

☑x7ᵗʰ **S77.20 Crushing injury of unspecified hip with thigh** ▽

☑x7ᵗʰ **S77.21 Crushing injury of right hip with thigh**

☑x7ᵗʰ **S77.22 Crushing injury of left hip with thigh**

☑4ᵗʰ **S78 Traumatic amputation of hip and thigh**

An amputation not identified as partial or complete should be coded to complete

EXCLUDES 1   traumatic amputation of knee (S88.0-)

The appropriate 7th character is to be added to each code from category S78.
A   initial encounter
D   subsequent encounter
S   sequela

☑5ᵗʰ **S78.0 Traumatic amputation at hip joint**

☑6ᵗʰ **S78.01 Complete traumatic amputation at hip joint**

☑7ᵗʰ **S78.011 Complete traumatic amputation at right hip joint** HCC

☑7ᵗʰ **S78.012 Complete traumatic amputation at left hip joint** HCC

☑7ᵗʰ **S78.019 Complete traumatic amputation at unspecified hip joint** HCC ▽

☑6ᵗʰ **S78.02 Partial traumatic amputation at hip joint**

☑7ᵗʰ **S78.021 Partial traumatic amputation at right hip joint** HCC

☑7ᵗʰ **S78.022 Partial traumatic amputation at left hip joint** HCC

☑7ᵗʰ **S78.029 Partial traumatic amputation at unspecified hip joint** HCC ▽

☑5ᵗʰ **S78.1 Traumatic amputation at level between hip and knee**

EXCLUDES 1   traumatic amputation of knee (S88.0-)

☑6ᵗʰ **S78.11 Complete traumatic amputation at level between hip and knee**

☑7ᵗʰ **S78.111 Complete traumatic amputation at level between right hip and knee** HCC

☑7ᵗʰ **S78.112 Complete traumatic amputation at level between left hip and knee** HCC

☑7ᵗʰ **S78.119 Complete traumatic amputation at level between unspecified hip and knee** HCC ▽

☑6ᵗʰ **S78.12 Partial traumatic amputation at level between hip and knee**

☑7ᵗʰ **S78.121 Partial traumatic amputation at level between right hip and knee** HCC

☑7ᵗʰ **S78.122 Partial traumatic amputation at level between left hip and knee** HCC

☑7ᵗʰ **S78.129 Partial traumatic amputation at level between unspecified hip and knee** HCC ▽

☑5ᵗʰ **S78.9 Traumatic amputation of hip and thigh, level unspecified**

☑6ᵗʰ **S78.91 Complete traumatic amputation of hip and thigh, level unspecified**

☑7ᵗʰ **S78.911 Complete traumatic amputation of right hip and thigh, level unspecified** HCC ▽

☑7ᵗʰ **S78.912 Complete traumatic amputation of left hip and thigh, level unspecified** HCC ▽

☑7ᵗʰ **S78.919 Complete traumatic amputation of unspecified hip and thigh, level unspecified** HCC ▽

☑6ᵗʰ **S78.92 Partial traumatic amputation of hip and thigh, level unspecified**

☑7ᵗʰ **S78.921 Partial traumatic amputation of right hip and thigh, level unspecified** HCC ▽

☑7ᵗʰ **S78.922 Partial traumatic amputation of left hip and thigh, level unspecified** HCC ▽

☑7ᵗʰ **S78.929 Partial traumatic amputation of unspecified hip and thigh, level unspecified** HCC ▽

✓4ᵗʰ **S79 Other and unspecified injuries of hip and thigh**

> **NOTE**   A fracture not indicated as open or closed should be coded to closed

AHA: 2018,2Q,12; 2018,1Q,3; 2015,3Q,37-39

The appropriate 7th character is to be added to each code from subcategories S79.0 and S79.1.
A   initial encounter for closed fracture
D   subsequent encounter for fracture with routine healing
G   subsequent encounter for fracture with delayed healing
K   subsequent encounter for fracture with nonunion
P   subsequent encounter for fracture with malunion
S   sequela

✓5ᵗʰ **S79.0 Physeal fracture of upper end of femur**

> *EXCLUDES 1*   apophyseal fracture of upper end of femur (S72.13-)
> nontraumatic slipped upper femoral epiphysis (M93.0-)

   ✓6ᵗʰ **S79.00 Unspecified physeal fracture of upper end of femur**

     1 ✓7ᵗʰ **S79.001 Unspecified physeal fracture of upper end of right femur** HCC Q ▽

     1 ✓7ᵗʰ **S79.002 Unspecified physeal fracture of upper end of left femur** HCC Q ▽

     1 ✓7ᵗʰ **S79.009 Unspecified physeal fracture of upper end of unspecified femur** HCC Q ▽

   ✓6ᵗʰ **S79.01 Salter-Harris Type I physeal fracture of upper end of femur**

     Acute on chronic slipped capital femoral epiphysis (traumatic)
     Acute slipped capital femoral epiphysis (traumatic)
     Capital femoral epiphyseal fracture

> *EXCLUDES 1*   chronic slipped upper femoral epiphysis (nontraumatic) (M93.02-)

     1 ✓7ᵗʰ **S79.011 Salter-Harris Type I physeal fracture of upper end of right femur** HCC Q

     1 ✓7ᵗʰ **S79.012 Salter-Harris Type I physeal fracture of upper end of left femur** HCC Q

     1 ✓7ᵗʰ **S79.019 Salter-Harris Type I physeal fracture of upper end of unspecified femur** HCC Q ▽

   ✓6ᵗʰ **S79.09 Other physeal fracture of upper end of femur**

     1 ✓7ᵗʰ **S79.091 Other physeal fracture of upper end of right femur** HCC Q

     1 ✓7ᵗʰ **S79.092 Other physeal fracture of upper end of left femur** HCC Q

     1 ✓7ᵗʰ **S79.099 Other physeal fracture of upper end of unspecified femur** HCC Q ▽

✓5ᵗʰ **S79.1 Physeal fracture of lower end of femur**

   ✓6ᵗʰ **S79.10 Unspecified physeal fracture of lower end of femur**

     1 ✓7ᵗʰ **S79.101 Unspecified physeal fracture of lower end of right femur** HCC Q ▽

     1 ✓7ᵗʰ **S79.102 Unspecified physeal fracture of lower end of left femur** HCC Q ▽

     1 ✓7ᵗʰ **S79.109 Unspecified physeal fracture of lower end of unspecified femur** HCC Q ▽

   ✓6ᵗʰ **S79.11 Salter-Harris Type I physeal fracture of lower end of femur**

     1 ✓7ᵗʰ **S79.111 Salter-Harris Type I physeal fracture of lower end of right femur** HCC Q

     1 ✓7ᵗʰ **S79.112 Salter-Harris Type I physeal fracture of lower end of left femur** HCC Q

     1 ✓7ᵗʰ **S79.119 Salter-Harris Type I physeal fracture of lower end of unspecified femur** HCC Q ▽

   ✓6ᵗʰ **S79.12 Salter-Harris Type II physeal fracture of lower end of femur**

     1 ✓7ᵗʰ **S79.121 Salter-Harris Type II physeal fracture of lower end of right femur** HCC Q

     1 ✓7ᵗʰ **S79.122 Salter-Harris Type II physeal fracture of lower end of left femur** HCC Q

     1 ✓7ᵗʰ **S79.129 Salter-Harris Type II physeal fracture of lower end of unspecified femur** HCC Q ▽

   ✓6ᵗʰ **S79.13 Salter-Harris Type III physeal fracture of lower end of femur**

     1 ✓7ᵗʰ **S79.131 Salter-Harris Type III physeal fracture of lower end of right femur** HCC Q

     1 ✓7ᵗʰ **S79.132 Salter-Harris Type III physeal fracture of lower end of left femur** HCC Q

     1 ✓7ᵗʰ **S79.139 Salter-Harris Type III physeal fracture of lower end of unspecified femur** HCC Q ▽

   ✓6ᵗʰ **S79.14 Salter-Harris Type IV physeal fracture of lower end of femur**

     1 ✓7ᵗʰ **S79.141 Salter-Harris Type IV physeal fracture of lower end of right femur** HCC Q

     1 ✓7ᵗʰ **S79.142 Salter-Harris Type IV physeal fracture of lower end of left femur** HCC Q

     1 ✓7ᵗʰ **S79.149 Salter-Harris Type IV physeal fracture of lower end of unspecified femur** HCC Q ▽

   ✓6ᵗʰ **S79.19 Other physeal fracture of lower end of femur**

     1 ✓7ᵗʰ **S79.191 Other physeal fracture of lower end of right femur** HCC Q

     1 ✓7ᵗʰ **S79.192 Other physeal fracture of lower end of left femur** HCC Q

     1 ✓7ᵗʰ **S79.199 Other physeal fracture of lower end of unspecified femur** HCC Q ▽

✓5ᵗʰ **S79.8 Other specified injuries of hip and thigh**

The appropriate 7th character is to be added to each code in subcategory S79.8.
A   initial encounter
D   subsequent encounter
S   sequela

   ✓6ᵗʰ **S79.81 Other specified injuries of hip**

     ✓7ᵗʰ **S79.811 Other specified injuries of right hip**

     ✓7ᵗʰ **S79.812 Other specified injuries of left hip**

     ✓7ᵗʰ **S79.819 Other specified injuries of unspecified hip** ▽

   ✓6ᵗʰ **S79.82 Other specified injuries of thigh**

     ✓7ᵗʰ **S79.821 Other specified injuries of right thigh**

     ✓7ᵗʰ **S79.822 Other specified injuries of left thigh**

     ✓7ᵗʰ **S79.829 Other specified injuries of unspecified thigh** ▽

✓5ᵗʰ **S79.9 Unspecified injury of hip and thigh**

The appropriate 7th character is to be added to each code in subcategory S79.9.
A   initial encounter
D   subsequent encounter
S   sequela

   ✓6ᵗʰ **S79.91 Unspecified injury of hip**

     ✓7ᵗʰ **S79.911 Unspecified injury of right hip** ▽

     ✓7ᵗʰ **S79.912 Unspecified injury of left hip** ▽

     ✓7ᵗʰ **S79.919 Unspecified injury of unspecified hip** ▽

   ✓6ᵗʰ **S79.92 Unspecified injury of thigh**

     ✓7ᵗʰ **S79.921 Unspecified injury of right thigh** ▽

     ✓7ᵗʰ **S79.922 Unspecified injury of left thigh** ▽

     ✓7ᵗʰ **S79.929 Unspecified injury of unspecified thigh** ▽

Injuries to the knee and lower leg (S80-S89)

> *EXCLUDES 2*   burns and corrosions (T20-T32)
> frostbite (T33-T34)
> injuries of ankle and foot, except fracture of ankle and malleolus (S90-S99)
> insect bite or sting, venomous (T63.4)

✓4ᵗʰ **S80 Superficial injury of knee and lower leg**

> *EXCLUDES 2*   superficial injury of ankle and foot (S90.-)

The appropriate 7th character is to be added to each code from category S80.
A   initial encounter
D   subsequent encounter
S   sequela

✓5ᵗʰ **S80.0 Contusion of knee**

   ✓x7ᵗʰ **S80.00 Contusion of unspecified knee** ▽

   ✓x7ᵗʰ **S80.01 Contusion of right knee**

   ✓x7ᵗʰ **S80.02 Contusion of left knee**

✓5ᵗʰ **S80.1 Contusion of lower leg**

   ✓x7ᵗʰ **S80.10 Contusion of unspecified lower leg** ▽

√x7ᵗʰ **S80.11** Contusion of right lower leg

√x7ᵗʰ **S80.12** Contusion of left lower leg

√5ᵗʰ **S80.2** Other superficial injuries of knee

√6ᵗʰ **S80.21** Abrasion of knee

√7ᵗʰ **S80.211** Abrasion, right knee

√7ᵗʰ **S80.212** Abrasion, left knee

√7ᵗʰ **S80.219** Abrasion, unspecified knee ▽

√6ᵗʰ **S80.22** Blister (nonthermal) of knee

√7ᵗʰ **S80.221** Blister (nonthermal), right knee

√7ᵗʰ **S80.222** Blister (nonthermal), left knee

√7ᵗʰ **S80.229** Blister (nonthermal), unspecified knee ▽

√6ᵗʰ **S80.24** External constriction of knee

√7ᵗʰ **S80.241** External constriction, right knee

√7ᵗʰ **S80.242** External constriction, left knee

√7ᵗʰ **S80.249** External constriction, unspecified knee ▽

√6ᵗʰ **S80.25** Superficial foreign body of knee

Splinter in the knee

√7ᵗʰ **S80.251** Superficial foreign body, right knee

√7ᵗʰ **S80.252** Superficial foreign body, left knee

√7ᵗʰ **S80.259** Superficial foreign body, unspecified knee ▽

√6ᵗʰ **S80.26** Insect bite (nonvenomous) of knee

√7ᵗʰ **S80.261** Insect bite (nonvenomous), right knee

√7ᵗʰ **S80.262** Insect bite (nonvenomous), left knee

√7ᵗʰ **S80.269** Insect bite (nonvenomous), unspecified knee ▽

√6ᵗʰ **S80.27** Other superficial bite of knee

EXCLUDES 1   open bite of knee (S81.05-)

√7ᵗʰ **S80.271** Other superficial bite of right knee

√7ᵗʰ **S80.272** Other superficial bite of left knee

√7ᵗʰ **S80.279** Other superficial bite of unspecified knee ▽

√5ᵗʰ **S80.8** Other superficial injuries of lower leg

√6ᵗʰ **S80.81** Abrasion of lower leg

√7ᵗʰ **S80.811** Abrasion, right lower leg

√7ᵗʰ **S80.812** Abrasion, left lower leg

√7ᵗʰ **S80.819** Abrasion, unspecified lower leg ▽

√6ᵗʰ **S80.82** Blister (nonthermal) of lower leg

√7ᵗʰ **S80.821** Blister (nonthermal), right lower leg

√7ᵗʰ **S80.822** Blister (nonthermal), left lower leg

√7ᵗʰ **S80.829** Blister (nonthermal), unspecified lower leg ▽

√6ᵗʰ **S80.84** External constriction of lower leg

√7ᵗʰ **S80.841** External constriction, right lower leg

√7ᵗʰ **S80.842** External constriction, left lower leg

√7ᵗʰ **S80.849** External constriction, unspecified lower leg ▽

√6ᵗʰ **S80.85** Superficial foreign body of lower leg

Splinter in the lower leg

√7ᵗʰ **S80.851** Superficial foreign body, right lower leg

√7ᵗʰ **S80.852** Superficial foreign body, left lower leg

√7ᵗʰ **S80.859** Superficial foreign body, unspecified lower leg ▽

√6ᵗʰ **S80.86** Insect bite (nonvenomous) of lower leg

√7ᵗʰ **S80.861** Insect bite (nonvenomous), right lower leg

√7ᵗʰ **S80.862** Insect bite (nonvenomous), left lower leg

√7ᵗʰ **S80.869** Insect bite (nonvenomous), unspecified lower leg ▽

√6ᵗʰ **S80.87** Other superficial bite of lower leg

EXCLUDES 1   open bite of lower leg (S81.85-)

√7ᵗʰ **S80.871** Other superficial bite, right lower leg

√7ᵗʰ **S80.872** Other superficial bite, left lower leg

√7ᵗʰ **S80.879** Other superficial bite, unspecified lower leg ▽

√5ᵗʰ **S80.9** Unspecified superficial injury of knee and lower leg

√6ᵗʰ **S80.91** Unspecified superficial injury of knee

√7ᵗʰ **S80.911** Unspecified superficial injury of right knee ▽

√7ᵗʰ **S80.912** Unspecified superficial injury of left knee ▽

√7ᵗʰ **S80.919** Unspecified superficial injury of unspecified knee ▽

√6ᵗʰ **S80.92** Unspecified superficial injury of lower leg

√7ᵗʰ **S80.921** Unspecified superficial injury of right lower leg ▽

√7ᵗʰ **S80.922** Unspecified superficial injury of left lower leg ▽

√7ᵗʰ **S80.929** Unspecified superficial injury of unspecified lower leg ▽

√4ᵗʰ **S81** Open wound of knee and lower leg

Code also any associated wound infection

EXCLUDES 1   open fracture of knee and lower leg (S82.-)

        traumatic amputation of lower leg (S88.-)

EXCLUDES 2   open wound of ankle and foot (S91.-)

The appropriate 7th character is to be added to each code from category S81.

A   initial encounter

D   subsequent encounter

S   sequela

√5ᵗʰ **S81.0** Open wound of knee

√6ᵗʰ **S81.00** Unspecified open wound of knee

√7ᵗʰ **S81.001** Unspecified open wound, right knee ▽

√7ᵗʰ **S81.002** Unspecified open wound, left knee ▽

√7ᵗʰ **S81.009** Unspecified open wound, unspecified knee ▽

√6ᵗʰ **S81.01** Laceration without foreign body of knee

√7ᵗʰ **S81.011** Laceration without foreign body, right knee

√7ᵗʰ **S81.012** Laceration without foreign body, left knee

√7ᵗʰ **S81.019** Laceration without foreign body, unspecified knee ▽

√6ᵗʰ **S81.02** Laceration with foreign body of knee

√7ᵗʰ **S81.021** Laceration with foreign body, right knee

√7ᵗʰ **S81.022** Laceration with foreign body, left knee

√7ᵗʰ **S81.029** Laceration with foreign body, unspecified knee ▽

√6ᵗʰ **S81.03** Puncture wound without foreign body of knee

√7ᵗʰ **S81.031** Puncture wound without foreign body, right knee

√7ᵗʰ **S81.032** Puncture wound without foreign body, left knee

√7ᵗʰ **S81.039** Puncture wound without foreign body, unspecified knee ▽

√6ᵗʰ **S81.04** Puncture wound with foreign body of knee

√7ᵗʰ **S81.041** Puncture wound with foreign body, right knee

√7ᵗʰ **S81.042** Puncture wound with foreign body, left knee

√7ᵗʰ **S81.049** Puncture wound with foreign body, unspecified knee ▽

√6ᵗʰ **S81.05** Open bite of knee

Bite of knee NOS

EXCLUDES 1   superficial bite of knee (S80.27-)

√7ᵗʰ **S81.051** Open bite, right knee

√7ᵗʰ **S81.052** Open bite, left knee

√7ᵗʰ **S81.059** Open bite, unspecified knee ▽

√5ᵗʰ **S81.8** Open wound of lower leg

√6ᵗʰ **S81.80** Unspecified open wound of lower leg

AHA: 2016,3Q,24

√7ᵗʰ **S81.801** Unspecified open wound, right lower leg ▽

√7ᵗʰ **S81.802** Unspecified open wound, left lower leg ▽

√7ᵗʰ **S81.809** Unspecified open wound, unspecified lower leg ▽

√6ᵗʰ **S81.81** Laceration without foreign body of lower leg

√7ᵗʰ **S81.811** Laceration without foreign body, right lower leg

√7ᵗʰ **S81.812** Laceration without foreign body, left lower leg

√7ᵗʰ **S81.819** Laceration without foreign body, unspecified lower leg ▽

√6ᵗʰ **S81.82** **Laceration with foreign body of lower leg**

    √7ᵗʰ **S81.821** **Laceration with foreign body, right lower leg**

    √7ᵗʰ **S81.822** **Laceration with foreign body, left lower leg**

    √7ᵗʰ **S81.829** **Laceration with foreign body, unspecified lower leg** ▽

√6ᵗʰ **S81.83** **Puncture wound without foreign body of lower leg**

    AHA: 2016,3Q,24

    √7ᵗʰ **S81.831** **Puncture wound without foreign body, right lower leg**

    √7ᵗʰ **S81.832** **Puncture wound without foreign body, left lower leg**

    √7ᵗʰ **S81.839** **Puncture wound without foreign body, unspecified lower leg** ▽

√6ᵗʰ **S81.84** **Puncture wound with foreign body of lower leg**

    AHA: 2016,3Q,24

    √7ᵗʰ **S81.841** **Puncture wound with foreign body, right lower leg**

    √7ᵗʰ **S81.842** **Puncture wound with foreign body, left lower leg**

    √7ᵗʰ **S81.849** **Puncture wound with foreign body, unspecified lower leg** ▽

√6ᵗʰ **S81.85** **Open bite of lower leg**

    Bite of lower leg NOS

      EXCLUDES 1   *superficial bite of lower leg (S80.86-, S80.87-)*

    √7ᵗʰ **S81.851** **Open bite, right lower leg**

    √7ᵗʰ **S81.852** **Open bite, left lower leg**

    √7ᵗʰ **S81.859** **Open bite, unspecified lower leg** ▽

√4ᵗʰ **S82** **Fracture of lower leg, including ankle**

    NOTE   A fracture not indicated as displaced or nondisplaced should be coded to displaced

        A fracture not indicated as open or closed should be coded to closed

        The open fracture designations are based on the Gustilo open fracture classification.

    INCLUDES   fracture of malleolus

    EXCLUDES 1   *traumatic amputation of lower leg (S88.-)*

    EXCLUDES 2   *fracture of foot, except ankle (S92.-)*

        periprosthetic fracture of prosthetic implant of knee (M97.0-)

    AHA: 2018,2Q,12; 2016,1Q,33; 2015,3Q,37-39

The appropriate 7th character is to be added to all codes from category S82 [unless otherwise indicated].

A   initial encounter for closed fracture

B   initial encounter for open fracture type I or II

    initial encounter for open fracture NOS

C   initial encounter for open fracture type IIIA, IIIB, or IIIC

D   subsequent encounter for closed fracture with routine healing

E   subsequent encounter for open fracture type I or II with routine healing

F   subsequent encounter for open fracture type IIIA, IIIB, or IIIC with routine healing

G   subsequent encounter for closed fracture with delayed healing

H   subsequent encounter for open fracture type I or II with delayed healing

J   subsequent encounter for open fracture type IIIA, IIIB, or IIIC with delayed healing

K   subsequent encounter for closed fracture with nonunion

M   subsequent encounter for open fracture type I or II with nonunion

N   subsequent encounter for open fracture type IIIA, IIIB, or IIIC with nonunion

P   subsequent encounter for closed fracture with malunion

Q   subsequent encounter for open fracture type I or II with malunion

R   subsequent encounter for open fracture type IIIA, IIIB, or IIIC with malunion

S   sequela

√5ᵗʰ **S82.0** **Fracture of patella**

    Knee cap

√6ᵗʰ **S82.00** **Unspecified fracture of patella**

    √7ᵗʰ **S82.001** **Unspecified fracture of right patella** 🅠 ▽

    √7ᵗʰ **S82.002** **Unspecified fracture of left patella** 🅠 ▽

    √7ᵗʰ **S82.009** **Unspecified fracture of unspecified patella** 🅠 ▽

√6ᵗʰ **S82.01** **Osteochondral fracture of patella**

    √7ᵗʰ **S82.011** **Displaced osteochondral fracture of right patella** 🅠

    √7ᵗʰ **S82.012** **Displaced osteochondral fracture of left patella** 🅠

    √7ᵗʰ **S82.013** **Displaced osteochondral fracture of unspecified patella** 🅠 ▽

    √7ᵗʰ **S82.014** **Nondisplaced osteochondral fracture of right patella** 🅠

    √7ᵗʰ **S82.015** **Nondisplaced osteochondral fracture of left patella** 🅠

    √7ᵗʰ **S82.016** **Nondisplaced osteochondral fracture of unspecified patella** 🅠 ▽

√6ᵗʰ **S82.02** **Longitudinal fracture of patella**

    √7ᵗʰ **S82.021** **Displaced longitudinal fracture of right patella** 🅠

    √7ᵗʰ **S82.022** **Displaced longitudinal fracture of left patella** 🅠

    √7ᵗʰ **S82.023** **Displaced longitudinal fracture of unspecified patella** 🅠 ▽

    √7ᵗʰ **S82.024** **Nondisplaced longitudinal fracture of right patella** 🅠

    √7ᵗʰ **S82.025** **Nondisplaced longitudinal fracture of left patella** 🅠

    √7ᵗʰ **S82.026** **Nondisplaced longitudinal fracture of unspecified patella** 🅠 ▽

√6ᵗʰ **S82.03** **Transverse fracture of patella**

    √7ᵗʰ **S82.031** **Displaced transverse fracture of right patella** 🅠

    √7ᵗʰ **S82.032** **Displaced transverse fracture of left patella** 🅠

    √7ᵗʰ **S82.033** **Displaced transverse fracture of unspecified patella** 🅠 ▽

    √7ᵗʰ **S82.034** **Nondisplaced transverse fracture of right patella** 🅠

    √7ᵗʰ **S82.035** **Nondisplaced transverse fracture of left patella** 🅠

    √7ᵗʰ **S82.036** **Nondisplaced transverse fracture of unspecified patella** 🅠 ▽

√6ᵗʰ **S82.04** **Comminuted fracture of patella**

    √7ᵗʰ **S82.041** **Displaced comminuted fracture of right patella** 🅠

    √7ᵗʰ **S82.042** **Displaced comminuted fracture of left patella** 🅠

    √7ᵗʰ **S82.043** **Displaced comminuted fracture of unspecified patella** 🅠 ▽

    √7ᵗʰ **S82.044** **Nondisplaced comminuted fracture of right patella** 🅠

    √7ᵗʰ **S82.045** **Nondisplaced comminuted fracture of left patella** 🅠

    √7ᵗʰ **S82.046** **Nondisplaced comminuted fracture of unspecified patella** 🅠 ▽

√6ᵗʰ **S82.09** **Other fracture of patella**

    √7ᵗʰ **S82.091** **Other fracture of right patella** 🅠

    √7ᵗʰ **S82.092** **Other fracture of left patella** 🅠

    √7ᵗʰ **S82.099** **Other fracture of unspecified patella** 🅠 ▽

√5ᵗʰ **S82.1** **Fracture of upper end of tibia**

    Fracture of proximal end of tibia

    EXCLUDES 2   *fracture of shaft of tibia (S82.2-)*

        physeal fracture of upper end of tibia (S89.0-)

√6ᵗʰ **S82.10** **Unspecified fracture of upper end of tibia**

    √7ᵗʰ **S82.101** **Unspecified fracture of upper end of right tibia** 🅠 ▽

    √7ᵗʰ **S82.102** **Unspecified fracture of upper end of left tibia** 🅠 ▽

    √7ᵗʰ **S82.109** **Unspecified fracture of upper end of unspecified tibia** 🅠 ▽

√6ᵗʰ **S82.11** **Fracture of tibial spine**

    √7ᵗʰ **S82.111** **Displaced fracture of right tibial spine** 🅠

    √7ᵗʰ **S82.112** **Displaced fracture of left tibial spine** 🅠

    √7ᵗʰ **S82.113** **Displaced fracture of unspecified tibial spine** 🅠 ▽

    √7ᵗʰ **S82.114** **Nondisplaced fracture of right tibial spine** 🅠

    √7ᵗʰ **S82.115** **Nondisplaced fracture of left tibial spine** 🅠

✔ Additional Character Req   √x7ᵗʰ Placeholder Alert   Manifestation   ▽ Unspecified   ▶◀ Revised Text   ● New Code   ▲ Revised Code Title

ICD-10-CM 2019   1049

Chapter 19. Injury, Poisoning and Certain Other Consequences of External Causes

S82.116–S82.292

√7th **S82.116** Nondisplaced fracture of unspecified tibial spine ⓠ ▽

√6th **S82.12** Fracture of lateral condyle of tibia

√7th **S82.121** Displaced fracture of lateral condyle of right tibia ⓠ

√7th **S82.122** Displaced fracture of lateral condyle of left tibia ⓠ

√7th **S82.123** Displaced fracture of lateral condyle of unspecified tibia ⓠ ▽

√7th **S82.124** Nondisplaced fracture of lateral condyle of right tibia ⓠ

√7th **S82.125** Nondisplaced fracture of lateral condyle of left tibia ⓠ

√7th **S82.126** Nondisplaced fracture of lateral condyle of unspecified tibia ⓠ ▽

√6th **S82.13** Fracture of medial condyle of tibia

√7th **S82.131** Displaced fracture of medial condyle of right tibia ⓠ

√7th **S82.132** Displaced fracture of medial condyle of left tibia ⓠ

√7th **S82.133** Displaced fracture of medial condyle of unspecified tibia ⓠ ▽

√7th **S82.134** Nondisplaced fracture of medial condyle of right tibia ⓠ

√7th **S82.135** Nondisplaced fracture of medial condyle of left tibia ⓠ

√7th **S82.136** Nondisplaced fracture of medial condyle of unspecified tibia ⓠ ▽

√6th **S82.14** Bicondylar fracture of tibia

Fracture of tibial plateau NOS

√7th **S82.141** Displaced bicondylar fracture of right tibia ⓠ

√7th **S82.142** Displaced bicondylar fracture of left tibia ⓠ

√7th **S82.143** Displaced bicondylar fracture of unspecified tibia ⓠ ▽

√7th **S82.144** Nondisplaced bicondylar fracture of right tibia ⓠ

√7th **S82.145** Nondisplaced bicondylar fracture of left tibia ⓠ

√7th **S82.146** Nondisplaced bicondylar fracture of unspecified tibia ⓠ ▽

√6th **S82.15** Fracture of tibial tuberosity

√7th **S82.151** Displaced fracture of right tibial tuberosity ⓠ

√7th **S82.152** Displaced fracture of left tibial tuberosity ⓠ

√7th **S82.153** Displaced fracture of unspecified tibial tuberosity ⓠ ▽

√7th **S82.154** Nondisplaced fracture of right tibial tuberosity ⓠ

√7th **S82.155** Nondisplaced fracture of left tibial tuberosity ⓠ

√7th **S82.156** Nondisplaced fracture of unspecified tibial tuberosity ⓠ ▽

√6th **S82.16** Torus fracture of upper end of tibia

> The appropriate 7th character is to be added to all codes in subcategory S82.16.
> A   initial encounter for closed fracture
> D   subsequent encounter for fracture with routine healing
> G   subsequent encounter for fracture with delayed healing
> K   subsequent encounter for fracture with nonunion
> P   subsequent encounter for fracture with malunion
> S   sequela

√7th **S82.161** Torus fracture of upper end of right tibia ⓠ

√7th **S82.162** Torus fracture of upper end of left tibia ⓠ

√7th **S82.169** Torus fracture of upper end of unspecified tibia ⓠ ▽

√6th **S82.19** Other fracture of upper end of tibia

√7th **S82.191** Other fracture of upper end of right tibia ⓠ

√7th **S82.192** Other fracture of upper end of left tibia ⓠ

√7th **S82.199** Other fracture of upper end of unspecified tibia ⓠ ▽

√5th **S82.2** Fracture of shaft of tibia

√6th **S82.20** Unspecified fracture of shaft of tibia

Fracture of tibia NOS

√7th **S82.201** Unspecified fracture of shaft of right tibia ⓠ ▽

√7th **S82.202** Unspecified fracture of shaft of left tibia ⓠ ▽

√7th **S82.209** Unspecified fracture of shaft of unspecified tibia ⓠ ▽

√6th **S82.22** Transverse fracture of shaft of tibia

√7th **S82.221** Displaced transverse fracture of shaft of right tibia ⓠ

√7th **S82.222** Displaced transverse fracture of shaft of left tibia ⓠ

√7th **S82.223** Displaced transverse fracture of shaft of unspecified tibia ⓠ ▽

√7th **S82.224** Nondisplaced transverse fracture of shaft of right tibia ⓠ

√7th **S82.225** Nondisplaced transverse fracture of shaft of left tibia ⓠ

√7th **S82.226** Nondisplaced transverse fracture of shaft of unspecified tibia ⓠ ▽

√6th **S82.23** Oblique fracture of shaft of tibia

√7th **S82.231** Displaced oblique fracture of shaft of right tibia ⓠ

√7th **S82.232** Displaced oblique fracture of shaft of left tibia ⓠ

√7th **S82.233** Displaced oblique fracture of shaft of unspecified tibia ⓠ ▽

√7th **S82.234** Nondisplaced oblique fracture of shaft of right tibia ⓠ

√7th **S82.235** Nondisplaced oblique fracture of shaft of left tibia ⓠ

√7th **S82.236** Nondisplaced oblique fracture of shaft of unspecified tibia ⓠ ▽

√6th **S82.24** Spiral fracture of shaft of tibia

Toddler fracture

√7th **S82.241** Displaced spiral fracture of shaft of right tibia ⓠ

√7th **S82.242** Displaced spiral fracture of shaft of left tibia ⓠ

√7th **S82.243** Displaced spiral fracture of shaft of unspecified tibia ⓠ ▽

√7th **S82.244** Nondisplaced spiral fracture of shaft of right tibia ⓠ

√7th **S82.245** Nondisplaced spiral fracture of shaft of left tibia ⓠ

√7th **S82.246** Nondisplaced spiral fracture of shaft of unspecified tibia ⓠ ▽

√6th **S82.25** Comminuted fracture of shaft of tibia

√7th **S82.251** Displaced comminuted fracture of shaft of right tibia ⓠ

√7th **S82.252** Displaced comminuted fracture of shaft of left tibia ⓠ

√7th **S82.253** Displaced comminuted fracture of shaft of unspecified tibia ⓠ ▽

√7th **S82.254** Nondisplaced comminuted fracture of shaft of right tibia ⓠ

√7th **S82.255** Nondisplaced comminuted fracture of shaft of left tibia ⓠ

√7th **S82.256** Nondisplaced comminuted fracture of shaft of unspecified tibia ⓠ ▽

√6th **S82.26** Segmental fracture of shaft of tibia

√7th **S82.261** Displaced segmental fracture of shaft of right tibia ⓠ

√7th **S82.262** Displaced segmental fracture of shaft of left tibia ⓠ

√7th **S82.263** Displaced segmental fracture of shaft of unspecified tibia ⓠ ▽

√7th **S82.264** Nondisplaced segmental fracture of shaft of right tibia ⓠ

√7th **S82.265** Nondisplaced segmental fracture of shaft of left tibia ⓠ

√7th **S82.266** Nondisplaced segmental fracture of shaft of unspecified tibia ⓠ ▽

√6th **S82.29** Other fracture of shaft of tibia

√7th **S82.291** Other fracture of shaft of right tibia ⓠ

√7th **S82.292** Other fracture of shaft of left tibia ⓠ

√7ʰ **S82.299** **Other fracture of shaft of unspecified tibia** ▯ ▽

√5ʰ **S82.3** **Fracture of lower end of tibia**

EXCLUDES 1   bimalleolar fracture of lower leg (S82.84-)
fracture of medial malleolus alone (S82.5-)
Maisonneuve's fracture (S82.86-)
pilon fracture of distal tibia (S82.87-)
trimalleolar fractures of lower leg (S82.85-)

√6ʰ **S82.30** **Unspecified fracture of lower end of tibia**

√7ʰ **S82.301** **Unspecified fracture of lower end of right tibia** ▯ ▽

√7ʰ **S82.302** **Unspecified fracture of lower end of left tibia** ▯ ▽

√7ʰ **S82.309** **Unspecified fracture of lower end of unspecified tibia** ▯ ▽

√6ʰ **S82.31** **Torus fracture of lower end of tibia**

The appropriate 7th character is to be added to all codes in subcategory S82.31.
A   initial encounter for closed fracture
D   subsequent encounter for fracture with routine healing
G   subsequent encounter for fracture with delayed healing
K   subsequent encounter for fracture with nonunion
P   subsequent encounter for fracture with malunion
S   sequela

√7ʰ **S82.311** **Torus fracture of lower end of right tibia** ▯

√7ʰ **S82.312** **Torus fracture of lower end of left tibia** ▯

√7ʰ **S82.319** **Torus fracture of lower end of unspecified tibia** ▯ ▽

√6ʰ **S82.39** **Other fracture of lower end of tibia**

AHA: 2015,1Q,25

√7ʰ **S82.391** **Other fracture of lower end of right tibia** ▯

√7ʰ **S82.392** **Other fracture of lower end of left tibia** ▯

√7ʰ **S82.399** **Other fracture of lower end of unspecified tibia** ▯ ▽

√5ʰ **S82.4** **Fracture of shaft of fibula**

EXCLUDES 2   fracture of lateral malleolus alone (S82.6-)

√6ʰ **S82.40** **Unspecified fracture of shaft of fibula**

√7ʰ **S82.401** **Unspecified fracture of shaft of right fibula** ▯ ▽

√7ʰ **S82.402** **Unspecified fracture of shaft of left fibula** ▯ ▽

√7ʰ **S82.409** **Unspecified fracture of shaft of unspecified fibula** ▯ ▽

√6ʰ **S82.42** **Transverse fracture of shaft of fibula**

√7ʰ **S82.421** **Displaced transverse fracture of shaft of right fibula** ▯

√7ʰ **S82.422** **Displaced transverse fracture of shaft of left fibula** ▯

√7ʰ **S82.423** **Displaced transverse fracture of shaft of unspecified fibula** ▯ ▽

√7ʰ **S82.424** **Nondisplaced transverse fracture of shaft of right fibula** ▯

√7ʰ **S82.425** **Nondisplaced transverse fracture of shaft of left fibula** ▯

√7ʰ **S82.426** **Nondisplaced transverse fracture of shaft of unspecified fibula** ▯ ▽

√6ʰ **S82.43** **Oblique fracture of shaft of fibula**

√7ʰ **S82.431** **Displaced oblique fracture of shaft of right fibula** ▯

√7ʰ **S82.432** **Displaced oblique fracture of shaft of left fibula** ▯

√7ʰ **S82.433** **Displaced oblique fracture of shaft of unspecified fibula** ▯ ▽

√7ʰ **S82.434** **Nondisplaced oblique fracture of shaft of right fibula** ▯

√7ʰ **S82.435** **Nondisplaced oblique fracture of shaft of left fibula** ▯

√7ʰ **S82.436** **Nondisplaced oblique fracture of shaft of unspecified fibula** ▯ ▽

√6ʰ **S82.44** **Spiral fracture of shaft of fibula**

√7ʰ **S82.441** **Displaced spiral fracture of shaft of right fibula** ▯

√7ʰ **S82.442** **Displaced spiral fracture of shaft of left fibula** ▯

√7ʰ **S82.443** **Displaced spiral fracture of shaft of unspecified fibula** ▯ ▽

√7ʰ **S82.444** **Nondisplaced spiral fracture of shaft of right fibula** ▯

√7ʰ **S82.445** **Nondisplaced spiral fracture of shaft of left fibula** ▯

√7ʰ **S82.446** **Nondisplaced spiral fracture of shaft of unspecified fibula** ▯ ▽

√6ʰ **S82.45** **Comminuted fracture of shaft of fibula**

√7ʰ **S82.451** **Displaced comminuted fracture of shaft of right fibula** ▯

√7ʰ **S82.452** **Displaced comminuted fracture of shaft of left fibula** ▯

√7ʰ **S82.453** **Displaced comminuted fracture of shaft of unspecified fibula** ▯ ▽

√7ʰ **S82.454** **Nondisplaced comminuted fracture of shaft of right fibula** ▯

√7ʰ **S82.455** **Nondisplaced comminuted fracture of shaft of left fibula** ▯

√7ʰ **S82.456** **Nondisplaced comminuted fracture of shaft of unspecified fibula** ▯ ▽

√6ʰ **S82.46** **Segmental fracture of shaft of fibula**

√7ʰ **S82.461** **Displaced segmental fracture of shaft of right fibula** ▯

√7ʰ **S82.462** **Displaced segmental fracture of shaft of left fibula** ▯

√7ʰ **S82.463** **Displaced segmental fracture of shaft of unspecified fibula** ▯ ▽

√7ʰ **S82.464** **Nondisplaced segmental fracture of shaft of right fibula** ▯

√7ʰ **S82.465** **Nondisplaced segmental fracture of shaft of left fibula** ▯

√7ʰ **S82.466** **Nondisplaced segmental fracture of shaft of unspecified fibula** ▯ ▽

√6ʰ **S82.49** **Other fracture of shaft of fibula**

√7ʰ **S82.491** **Other fracture of shaft of right fibula** ▯

√7ʰ **S82.492** **Other fracture of shaft of left fibula** ▯

√7ʰ **S82.499** **Other fracture of shaft of unspecified fibula** ▯ ▽

√5ʰ **S82.5** **Fracture of medial malleolus**

EXCLUDES 1   pilon fracture of distal tibia (S82.87-)
Salter-Harris type III of lower end of tibia (S89.13-)
Salter-Harris type IV of lower end of tibia (S89.14-)

√x 7ʰ **S82.51** **Displaced fracture of medial malleolus of right tibia** ▯

√x 7ʰ **S82.52** **Displaced fracture of medial malleolus of left tibia** ▯

√x 7ʰ **S82.53** **Displaced fracture of medial malleolus of unspecified tibia** ▯ ▽

√x 7ʰ **S82.54** **Nondisplaced fracture of medial malleolus of right tibia** ▯

√x 7ʰ **S82.55** **Nondisplaced fracture of medial malleolus of left tibia** ▯

√x 7ʰ **S82.56** **Nondisplaced fracture of medial malleolus of unspecified tibia** ▯ ▽

√5ʰ **S82.6** **Fracture of lateral malleolus**

EXCLUDES 1   pilon fracture of distal tibia (S82.87-)

√x 7ʰ **S82.61** **Displaced fracture of lateral malleolus of right fibula** ▯

√x 7ʰ **S82.62** **Displaced fracture of lateral malleolus of left fibula** ▯

√x 7ʰ **S82.63** **Displaced fracture of lateral malleolus of unspecified fibula** ▯ ▽

√x 7ʰ **S82.64** **Nondisplaced fracture of lateral malleolus of right fibula** ▯

√x 7ʰ **S82.65** **Nondisplaced fracture of lateral malleolus of left fibula** ▯

√x 7ʰ **S82.66** **Nondisplaced fracture of lateral malleolus of unspecified fibula** ▯ ▽

☑ Additional Character Req   √x 7ʰ Placeholder Alert   Manifestation   ▽ Unspecified   ►◄ Revised Text   ● New Code   ▲ Revised Code Title

Chapter 19. Injury, Poisoning and Certain Other Consequences of External Causes

S82.8–S82.876

✓5ᵗʰ **S82.8** **Other fractures of lower leg**

✓6ᵗʰ   **S82.81** **Torus fracture of upper end of fibula**

The appropriate 7th character is to be added to all codes in subcategory S82.81

A   initial encounter for closed fracture
D   subsequent encounter for fracture with routine healing
G   subsequent encounter for fracture with delayed healing
K   subsequent encounter for fracture with nonunion
P   subsequent encounter for fracture with malunion
S   sequela

✓7ᵗʰ **S82.811** Torus fracture of upper end of right fibula   ◘

✓7ᵗʰ **S82.812** Torus fracture of upper end of left fibula   ◘

✓7ᵗʰ **S82.819** Torus fracture of upper end of unspecified fibula   ◘ ▽

✓6ᵗʰ   **S82.82** **Torus fracture of lower end of fibula**

The appropriate 7th character is to be added to all codes in subcategory S82.82.

A   initial encounter for closed fracture
D   subsequent encounter for fracture with routine healing
G   subsequent encounter for fracture with delayed healing
K   subsequent encounter for fracture with nonunion
P   subsequent encounter for fracture with malunion
S   sequela

✓7ᵗʰ **S82.821** Torus fracture of lower end of right fibula   ◘

✓7ᵗʰ **S82.822** Torus fracture of lower end of left fibula   ◘

✓7ᵗʰ **S82.829** Torus fracture of lower end of unspecified fibula   ◘ ▽

✓6ᵗʰ   **S82.83** **Other fracture of upper and lower end of fibula**

AHA: 2015,1Q,25

✓7ᵗʰ **S82.831** Other fracture of upper and lower end of right fibula   ◘

✓7ᵗʰ **S82.832** Other fracture of upper and lower end of left fibula   ◘

✓7ᵗʰ **S82.839** Other fracture of upper and lower end of unspecified fibula   ◘ ▽

✓6ᵗʰ **S82.84** **Bimalleolar fracture of lower leg**

Right Bimalleolar Fracture

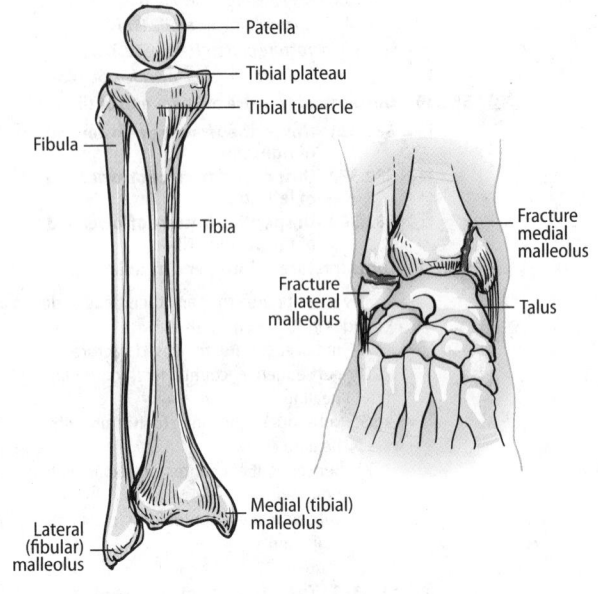

Patella
Tibial plateau
Tibial tubercle
Fibula
Tibia
Lateral (fibular) malleolus
Medial (tibial) malleolus
Fracture medial malleolus
Fracture lateral malleolus
Talus

✓7ᵗʰ **S82.841** Displaced bimalleolar fracture of right lower leg   ◘

✓7ᵗʰ **S82.842** Displaced bimalleolar fracture of left lower leg   ◘

✓7ᵗʰ **S82.843** Displaced bimalleolar fracture of unspecified lower leg   ◘ ▽

✓7ᵗʰ **S82.844** Nondisplaced bimalleolar fracture of right lower leg   ◘

✓7ᵗʰ **S82.845** Nondisplaced bimalleolar fracture of left lower leg   ◘

✓7ᵗʰ **S82.846** Nondisplaced bimalleolar fracture of unspecified lower leg   ◘ ▽

✓6ᵗʰ **S82.85** **Trimalleolar fracture of lower leg**

✓7ᵗʰ **S82.851** Displaced trimalleolar fracture of right lower leg   ◘

✓7ᵗʰ **S82.852** Displaced trimalleolar fracture of left lower leg   ◘

✓7ᵗʰ **S82.853** Displaced trimalleolar fracture of unspecified lower leg   ◘ ▽

✓7ᵗʰ **S82.854** Nondisplaced trimalleolar fracture of right lower leg   ◘

✓7ᵗʰ **S82.855** Nondisplaced trimalleolar fracture of left lower leg   ◘

✓7ᵗʰ **S82.856** Nondisplaced trimalleolar fracture of unspecified lower leg   ◘ ▽

✓6ᵗʰ **S82.86** **Maisonneuve's fracture**

✓7ᵗʰ **S82.861** Displaced Maisonneuve's fracture of right leg   ◘

✓7ᵗʰ **S82.862** Displaced Maisonneuve's fracture of left leg   ◘

✓7ᵗʰ **S82.863** Displaced Maisonneuve's fracture of unspecified leg   ◘ ▽

✓7ᵗʰ **S82.864** Nondisplaced Maisonneuve's fracture of right leg   ◘

✓7ᵗʰ **S82.865** Nondisplaced Maisonneuve's fracture of left leg   ◘

✓7ᵗʰ **S82.866** Nondisplaced Maisonneuve's fracture of unspecified leg   ◘ ▽

✓6ᵗʰ **S82.87** **Pilon fracture of tibia**

✓7ᵗʰ **S82.871** Displaced pilon fracture of right tibia   ◘

✓7ᵗʰ **S82.872** Displaced pilon fracture of left tibia   ◘

✓7ᵗʰ **S82.873** Displaced pilon fracture of unspecified tibia   ◘ ▽

✓7ᵗʰ **S82.874** Nondisplaced pilon fracture of right tibia   ◘

✓7ᵗʰ **S82.875** Nondisplaced pilon fracture of left tibia   ◘

✓7ᵗʰ **S82.876** Nondisplaced pilon fracture of unspecified tibia   ◘ ▽

√6th **S82.89   Other fractures of lower leg**
         Fracture of ankle NOS
         √7th **S82.891   Other fracture of right lower leg**   🔲
         √7th **S82.892   Other fracture of left lower leg**   🔲
         √7th **S82.899   Other fracture of unspecified**   🔲 ▽
                      lower leg

√5th **S82.9   Unspecified fracture of lower leg**
      √x7th **S82.90   Unspecified fracture of unspecified lower**   🔲 ▽
                  leg
      √x7th **S82.91   Unspecified fracture of right lower leg**   🔲 ▽
      √x7th **S82.92   Unspecified fracture of left lower leg**   🔲 ▽

√4th **S83   Dislocation and sprain of joints and ligaments of knee**
      INCLUDES   avulsion of joint or ligament of knee
                 laceration of cartilage, joint or ligament of knee
                 sprain of cartilage, joint or ligament of knee
                 traumatic hemarthrosis of joint or ligament of knee
                 traumatic rupture of joint or ligament of knee
                 traumatic subluxation of joint or ligament of knee
                 traumatic tear of joint or ligament of knee
      Code also any associated open wound
      EXCLUDES 1   derangement of patella (M22.0-M22.3)
                   injury of patellar ligament (tendon) (S76.1-)
                   internal derangement of knee (M23.-)
                   old dislocation of knee (M23.8X)
                   pathological dislocation of knee (M24.36)
                   recurrent dislocation of knee (M22.0)
      EXCLUDES 2   strain of muscle, fascia and tendon of lower leg (S86.-)

      The appropriate 7th character is to be added to each code from
      category S83.
      A   initial encounter
      D   subsequent encounter
      S   sequela

√5th **S83.0   Subluxation and dislocation of patella**
      √6th **S83.00   Unspecified subluxation and dislocation of patella**
            √7th **S83.001   Unspecified subluxation of right**   ▽
                        patella
            √7th **S83.002   Unspecified subluxation of left**   ▽
                        patella
            √7th **S83.003   Unspecified subluxation of**   ▽
                        unspecified patella
            √7th **S83.004   Unspecified dislocation of right**   ▽
                        patella
            √7th **S83.005   Unspecified dislocation of left**   ▽
                        patella
            √7th **S83.006   Unspecified dislocation of**   ▽
                        unspecified patella
      √6th **S83.01   Lateral subluxation and dislocation of patella**
            √7th **S83.011   Lateral subluxation of right patella**
            √7th **S83.012   Lateral subluxation of left patella**
            √7th **S83.013   Lateral subluxation of**   ▽
                        unspecified patella
            √7th **S83.014   Lateral dislocation of right patella**
            √7th **S83.015   Lateral dislocation of left patella**
            √7th **S83.016   Lateral dislocation of unspecified**   ▽
                        patella
      √6th **S83.09   Other subluxation and dislocation of patella**
            √7th **S83.091   Other subluxation of right patella**
            √7th **S83.092   Other subluxation of left patella**
            √7th **S83.093   Other subluxation of unspecified**   ▽
                        patella
            √7th **S83.094   Other dislocation of right patella**
            √7th **S83.095   Other dislocation of left patella**
            √7th **S83.096   Other dislocation of unspecified**   ▽
                        patella

√5th **S83.1   Subluxation and dislocation of knee**
      EXCLUDES 2   instability of knee prosthesis (T84.022, T84.023)
      √6th **S83.10   Unspecified subluxation and dislocation of knee**
            √7th **S83.101   Unspecified subluxation of right**   ▽
                        knee
            √7th **S83.102   Unspecified subluxation of left**   ▽
                        knee
            √7th **S83.103   Unspecified subluxation of**   ▽
                        unspecified knee
            √7th **S83.104   Unspecified dislocation of right**   ▽
                        knee

            √7th **S83.105   Unspecified dislocation of left**   ▽
                        knee
            √7th **S83.106   Unspecified dislocation of**   ▽
                        unspecified knee
      √6th **S83.11   Anterior subluxation and dislocation of proximal**
                  end of tibia
                  Posterior subluxation and dislocation of distal end of
                      femur
            √7th **S83.111   Anterior subluxation of proximal end of**
                        tibia, right knee
            √7th **S83.112   Anterior subluxation of proximal end of**
                        tibia, left knee
            √7th **S83.113   Anterior subluxation of proximal**   ▽
                        end of tibia, unspecified knee
            √7th **S83.114   Anterior dislocation of proximal end of**
                        tibia, right knee
            √7th **S83.115   Anterior dislocation of proximal end of**
                        tibia, left knee
            √7th **S83.116   Anterior dislocation of proximal**   ▽
                        end of tibia, unspecified knee
      √6th **S83.12   Posterior subluxation and dislocation of proximal**
                  end of tibia
                  Anterior dislocation of distal end of femur
            √7th **S83.121   Posterior subluxation of proximal end of**
                        tibia, right knee
            √7th **S83.122   Posterior subluxation of proximal end of**
                        tibia, left knee
            √7th **S83.123   Posterior subluxation of proximal**   ▽
                        end of tibia, unspecified knee
            √7th **S83.124   Posterior dislocation of proximal end of**
                        tibia, right knee
            √7th **S83.125   Posterior dislocation of proximal end of**
                        tibia, left knee
            √7th **S83.126   Posterior dislocation of proximal**   ▽
                        end of tibia, unspecified knee
      √6th **S83.13   Medial subluxation and dislocation of proximal end**
                  of tibia
            √7th **S83.131   Medial subluxation of proximal end of**
                        tibia, right knee
            √7th **S83.132   Medial subluxation of proximal end of**
                        tibia, left knee
            √7th **S83.133   Medial subluxation of proximal**   ▽
                        end of tibia, unspecified knee
            √7th **S83.134   Medial dislocation of proximal end of**
                        tibia, right knee
            √7th **S83.135   Medial dislocation of proximal end of**
                        tibia, left knee
            √7th **S83.136   Medial dislocation of proximal**   ▽
                        end of tibia, unspecified knee
      √6th **S83.14   Lateral subluxation and dislocation of proximal end**
                  of tibia
            √7th **S83.141   Lateral subluxation of proximal end of**
                        tibia, right knee
            √7th **S83.142   Lateral subluxation of proximal end of**
                        tibia, left knee
            √7th **S83.143   Lateral subluxation of proximal**   ▽
                        end of tibia, unspecified knee
            √7th **S83.144   Lateral dislocation of proximal end of**
                        tibia, right knee
            √7th **S83.145   Lateral dislocation of proximal end of**
                        tibia, left knee
            √7th **S83.146   Lateral dislocation of proximal**   ▽
                        end of tibia, unspecified knee
      √6th **S83.19   Other subluxation and dislocation of knee**
            √7th **S83.191   Other subluxation of right knee**
            √7th **S83.192   Other subluxation of left knee**
            √7th **S83.193   Other subluxation of unspecified**   ▽
                        knee
            √7th **S83.194   Other dislocation of right knee**
            √7th **S83.195   Other dislocation of left knee**
            √7th **S83.196   Other dislocation of unspecified**   ▽
                        knee

√5th **S83.2   Tear of meniscus, current injury**
      EXCLUDES 1   old bucket-handle tear (M23.2)
      √6th **S83.20   Tear of unspecified meniscus, current injury**
                  Tear of meniscus of knee NOS
            √7th **S83.200   Bucket-handle tear of unspecified**   ▽
                        meniscus, current injury, right
                        knee
            √7th **S83.201   Bucket-handle tear of unspecified**   ▽
                        meniscus, current injury, left knee

☑ Additional Character Req   √x7th Placeholder Alert   Manifestation   ▽ Unspecified   ►◄ Revised Text   ● New Code   ▲ Revised Code Title

Chapter 19. Injury, Poisoning and Certain Other Consequences of External Causes

S83.202–S83.92

- √7ᵗʰ **S83.202** Bucket-handle tear of unspecified meniscus, current injury, unspecified knee ▽
- √7ᵗʰ **S83.203** Other tear of unspecified meniscus, current injury, right knee ▽
- √7ᵗʰ **S83.204** Other tear of unspecified meniscus, current injury, left knee ▽
- √7ᵗʰ **S83.205** Other tear of unspecified meniscus, current injury, unspecified knee ▽
- √7ᵗʰ **S83.206** Unspecified tear of unspecified meniscus, current injury, right knee ▽
- √7ᵗʰ **S83.207** Unspecified tear of unspecified meniscus, current injury, left knee ▽
- √7ᵗʰ **S83.209** Unspecified tear of unspecified meniscus, current injury, unspecified knee ▽

√6ᵗʰ **S83.21** Bucket-handle tear of medial meniscus, current injury
- √7ᵗʰ **S83.211** Bucket-handle tear of medial meniscus, current injury, right knee
- √7ᵗʰ **S83.212** Bucket-handle tear of medial meniscus, current injury, left knee
- √7ᵗʰ **S83.219** Bucket-handle tear of medial meniscus, current injury, unspecified knee ▽

√6ᵗʰ **S83.22** Peripheral tear of medial meniscus, current injury
- √7ᵗʰ **S83.221** Peripheral tear of medial meniscus, current injury, right knee
- √7ᵗʰ **S83.222** Peripheral tear of medial meniscus, current injury, left knee
- √7ᵗʰ **S83.229** Peripheral tear of medial meniscus, current injury, unspecified knee ▽

√6ᵗʰ **S83.23** Complex tear of medial meniscus, current injury
- √7ᵗʰ **S83.231** Complex tear of medial meniscus, current injury, right knee
- √7ᵗʰ **S83.232** Complex tear of medial meniscus, current injury, left knee
- √7ᵗʰ **S83.239** Complex tear of medial meniscus, current injury, unspecified knee ▽

√6ᵗʰ **S83.24** Other tear of medial meniscus, current injury
- √7ᵗʰ **S83.241** Other tear of medial meniscus, current injury, right knee
- √7ᵗʰ **S83.242** Other tear of medial meniscus, current injury, left knee
- √7ᵗʰ **S83.249** Other tear of medial meniscus, current injury, unspecified knee ▽

√6ᵗʰ **S83.25** Bucket-handle tear of lateral meniscus, current injury
- √7ᵗʰ **S83.251** Bucket-handle tear of lateral meniscus, current injury, right knee
- √7ᵗʰ **S83.252** Bucket-handle tear of lateral meniscus, current injury, left knee
- √7ᵗʰ **S83.259** Bucket-handle tear of lateral meniscus, current injury, unspecified knee ▽

√6ᵗʰ **S83.26** Peripheral tear of lateral meniscus, current injury
- √7ᵗʰ **S83.261** Peripheral tear of lateral meniscus, current injury, right knee
- √7ᵗʰ **S83.262** Peripheral tear of lateral meniscus, current injury, left knee
- √7ᵗʰ **S83.269** Peripheral tear of lateral meniscus, current injury, unspecified knee ▽

√6ᵗʰ **S83.27** Complex tear of lateral meniscus, current injury
- √7ᵗʰ **S83.271** Complex tear of lateral meniscus, current injury, right knee
- √7ᵗʰ **S83.272** Complex tear of lateral meniscus, current injury, left knee
- √7ᵗʰ **S83.279** Complex tear of lateral meniscus, current injury, unspecified knee ▽

√6ᵗʰ **S83.28** Other tear of lateral meniscus, current injury
- √7ᵗʰ **S83.281** Other tear of lateral meniscus, current injury, right knee
- √7ᵗʰ **S83.282** Other tear of lateral meniscus, current injury, left knee
- √7ᵗʰ **S83.289** Other tear of lateral meniscus, current injury, unspecified knee ▽

√5ᵗʰ **S83.3** Tear of articular cartilage of knee, current
- √x7ᵗʰ **S83.30** Tear of articular cartilage of unspecified knee, current ▽
- √x7ᵗʰ **S83.31** Tear of articular cartilage of right knee, current
- √x7ᵗʰ **S83.32** Tear of articular cartilage of left knee, current

√5ᵗʰ **S83.4** Sprain of collateral ligament of knee
- √6ᵗʰ **S83.40** Sprain of unspecified collateral ligament of knee
  - √7ᵗʰ **S83.401** Sprain of unspecified collateral ligament of right knee ▽
  - √7ᵗʰ **S83.402** Sprain of unspecified collateral ligament of left knee ▽
  - √7ᵗʰ **S83.409** Sprain of unspecified collateral ligament of unspecified knee ▽
- √6ᵗʰ **S83.41** Sprain of medial collateral ligament of knee
  - Sprain of tibial collateral ligament
  - √7ᵗʰ **S83.411** Sprain of medial collateral ligament of right knee
  - √7ᵗʰ **S83.412** Sprain of medial collateral ligament of left knee
  - √7ᵗʰ **S83.419** Sprain of medial collateral ligament of unspecified knee ▽
- √6ᵗʰ **S83.42** Sprain of lateral collateral ligament of knee
  - Sprain of fibular collateral ligament
  - √7ᵗʰ **S83.421** Sprain of lateral collateral ligament of right knee
  - √7ᵗʰ **S83.422** Sprain of lateral collateral ligament of left knee
  - √7ᵗʰ **S83.429** Sprain of lateral collateral ligament of unspecified knee ▽

√5ᵗʰ **S83.5** Sprain of cruciate ligament of knee
- **AHA:** 2016,2Q,3
- √6ᵗʰ **S83.50** Sprain of unspecified cruciate ligament of knee
  - √7ᵗʰ **S83.501** Sprain of unspecified cruciate ligament of right knee ▽
  - √7ᵗʰ **S83.502** Sprain of unspecified cruciate ligament of left knee ▽
  - √7ᵗʰ **S83.509** Sprain of unspecified cruciate ligament of unspecified knee ▽
- √6ᵗʰ **S83.51** Sprain of anterior cruciate ligament of knee
  - √7ᵗʰ **S83.511** Sprain of anterior cruciate ligament of right knee
  - √7ᵗʰ **S83.512** Sprain of anterior cruciate ligament of left knee
  - √7ᵗʰ **S83.519** Sprain of anterior cruciate ligament of unspecified knee ▽
- √6ᵗʰ **S83.52** Sprain of posterior cruciate ligament of knee
  - √7ᵗʰ **S83.521** Sprain of posterior cruciate ligament of right knee
  - √7ᵗʰ **S83.522** Sprain of posterior cruciate ligament of left knee
  - √7ᵗʰ **S83.529** Sprain of posterior cruciate ligament of unspecified knee ▽

√5ᵗʰ **S83.6** Sprain of the superior tibiofibular joint and ligament
- √x7ᵗʰ **S83.60** Sprain of the superior tibiofibular joint and ligament, unspecified knee ▽
- √x7ᵗʰ **S83.61** Sprain of the superior tibiofibular joint and ligament, right knee
- √x7ᵗʰ **S83.62** Sprain of the superior tibiofibular joint and ligament, left knee

√5ᵗʰ **S83.8** Sprain of other specified parts of knee
- √6ᵗʰ **S83.8X** Sprain of other specified parts of knee
  - √7ᵗʰ **S83.8X1** Sprain of other specified parts of right knee
  - √7ᵗʰ **S83.8X2** Sprain of other specified parts of left knee
  - √7ᵗʰ **S83.8X9** Sprain of other specified parts of unspecified knee ▽

√5ᵗʰ **S83.9** Sprain of unspecified site of knee
- √x7ᵗʰ **S83.90** Sprain of unspecified site of unspecified knee ▽
- √x7ᵗʰ **S83.91** Sprain of unspecified site of right knee ▽
- √x7ᵗʰ **S83.92** Sprain of unspecified site of left knee ▽

√4ᵗʰ **S84 Injury of nerves at lower leg level**

Code also any associated open wound (S81.-)

EXCLUDES 2   injury of nerves at ankle and foot level (S94.-)

The appropriate 7th character is to be added to each code from category S84.
A   initial encounter
D   subsequent encounter
S   sequela

√5ᵗʰ   **S84.0 Injury of tibial nerve at lower leg level**

√x7ᵗʰ   **S84.00 Injury of tibial nerve at lower leg level, unspecified leg** ▽

√x7ᵗʰ   **S84.01 Injury of tibial nerve at lower leg level, right leg**

√x7ᵗʰ   **S84.02 Injury of tibial nerve at lower leg level, left leg**

√5ᵗʰ   **S84.1 Injury of peroneal nerve at lower leg level**

√x7ᵗʰ   **S84.10 Injury of peroneal nerve at lower leg level, unspecified leg** ▽

√x7ᵗʰ   **S84.11 Injury of peroneal nerve at lower leg level, right leg**

√x7ᵗʰ   **S84.12 Injury of peroneal nerve at lower leg level, left leg**

√5ᵗʰ   **S84.2 Injury of cutaneous sensory nerve at lower leg level**

√x7ᵗʰ   **S84.20 Injury of cutaneous sensory nerve at lower leg level, unspecified leg** ▽

√x7ᵗʰ   **S84.21 Injury of cutaneous sensory nerve at lower leg level, right leg**

√x7ᵗʰ   **S84.22 Injury of cutaneous sensory nerve at lower leg level, left leg**

√5ᵗʰ   **S84.8 Injury of other nerves at lower leg level**

√6ᵗʰ   **S84.80 Injury of other nerves at lower leg level**

√7ᵗʰ   **S84.801 Injury of other nerves at lower leg level, right leg**

√7ᵗʰ   **S84.802 Injury of other nerves at lower leg level, left leg**

√7ᵗʰ   **S84.809 Injury of other nerves at lower leg level, unspecified leg** ▽

√5ᵗʰ   **S84.9 Injury of unspecified nerve at lower leg level**

√x7ᵗʰ   **S84.90 Injury of unspecified nerve at lower leg level, unspecified leg** ▽

√x7ᵗʰ   **S84.91 Injury of unspecified nerve at lower leg level, right leg** ▽

√x7ᵗʰ   **S84.92 Injury of unspecified nerve at lower leg level, left leg** ▽

√4ᵗʰ **S85 Injury of blood vessels at lower leg level**

Code also any associated open wound (S81.-)

EXCLUDES 2   injury of blood vessels at ankle and foot level (S95.-)

The appropriate 7th character is to be added to each code from category S85.
A   initial encounter
D   subsequent encounter
S   sequela

√5ᵗʰ   **S85.0 Injury of popliteal artery**

√6ᵗʰ   **S85.00 Unspecified injury of popliteal artery**

√7ᵗʰ   **S85.001 Unspecified injury of popliteal artery, right leg** ▽

√7ᵗʰ   **S85.002 Unspecified injury of popliteal artery, left leg** ▽

√7ᵗʰ   **S85.009 Unspecified injury of popliteal artery, unspecified leg** ▽

√6ᵗʰ   **S85.01 Laceration of popliteal artery**

√7ᵗʰ   **S85.011 Laceration of popliteal artery, right leg**

√7ᵗʰ   **S85.012 Laceration of popliteal artery, left leg**

√7ᵗʰ   **S85.019 Laceration of popliteal artery, unspecified leg** ▽

√6ᵗʰ   **S85.09 Other specified injury of popliteal artery**

√7ᵗʰ   **S85.091 Other specified injury of popliteal artery, right leg**

√7ᵗʰ   **S85.092 Other specified injury of popliteal artery, left leg**

√7ᵗʰ   **S85.099 Other specified injury of popliteal artery, unspecified leg** ▽

√5ᵗʰ   **S85.1 Injury of tibial artery**

√6ᵗʰ   **S85.10 Unspecified injury of unspecified tibial artery**

Injury of tibial artery NOS

√7ᵗʰ   **S85.101 Unspecified injury of unspecified tibial artery, right leg** ▽

√7ᵗʰ   **S85.102 Unspecified injury of unspecified tibial artery, left leg** ▽

√7ᵗʰ   **S85.109 Unspecified injury of unspecified tibial artery, unspecified leg** ▽

√6ᵗʰ   **S85.11 Laceration of unspecified tibial artery**

√7ᵗʰ   **S85.111 Laceration of unspecified tibial artery, right leg** ▽

√7ᵗʰ   **S85.112 Laceration of unspecified tibial artery, left leg** ▽

√7ᵗʰ   **S85.119 Laceration of unspecified tibial artery, unspecified leg** ▽

√6ᵗʰ   **S85.12 Other specified injury of unspecified tibial artery**

√7ᵗʰ   **S85.121 Other specified injury of unspecified tibial artery, right leg** ▽

√7ᵗʰ   **S85.122 Other specified injury of unspecified tibial artery, left leg** ▽

√7ᵗʰ   **S85.129 Other specified injury of unspecified tibial artery, unspecified leg** ▽

√6ᵗʰ   **S85.13 Unspecified injury of anterior tibial artery**

√7ᵗʰ   **S85.131 Unspecified injury of anterior tibial artery, right leg** ▽

√7ᵗʰ   **S85.132 Unspecified injury of anterior tibial artery, left leg** ▽

√7ᵗʰ   **S85.139 Unspecified injury of anterior tibial artery, unspecified leg** ▽

√6ᵗʰ   **S85.14 Laceration of anterior tibial artery**

√7ᵗʰ   **S85.141 Laceration of anterior tibial artery, right leg**

√7ᵗʰ   **S85.142 Laceration of anterior tibial artery, left leg**

√7ᵗʰ   **S85.149 Laceration of anterior tibial artery, unspecified leg** ▽

√6ᵗʰ   **S85.15 Other specified injury of anterior tibial artery**

√7ᵗʰ   **S85.151 Other specified injury of anterior tibial artery, right leg**

√7ᵗʰ   **S85.152 Other specified injury of anterior tibial artery, left leg**

√7ᵗʰ   **S85.159 Other specified injury of anterior tibial artery, unspecified leg** ▽

√6ᵗʰ   **S85.16 Unspecified injury of posterior tibial artery**

√7ᵗʰ   **S85.161 Unspecified injury of posterior tibial artery, right leg** ▽

√7ᵗʰ   **S85.162 Unspecified injury of posterior tibial artery, left leg** ▽

√7ᵗʰ   **S85.169 Unspecified injury of posterior tibial artery, unspecified leg** ▽

√6ᵗʰ   **S85.17 Laceration of posterior tibial artery**

√7ᵗʰ   **S85.171 Laceration of posterior tibial artery, right leg**

√7ᵗʰ   **S85.172 Laceration of posterior tibial artery, left leg**

√7ᵗʰ   **S85.179 Laceration of posterior tibial artery, unspecified leg** ▽

√6ᵗʰ   **S85.18 Other specified injury of posterior tibial artery**

√7ᵗʰ   **S85.181 Other specified injury of posterior tibial artery, right leg**

√7ᵗʰ   **S85.182 Other specified injury of posterior tibial artery, left leg**

√7ᵗʰ   **S85.189 Other specified injury of posterior tibial artery, unspecified leg** ▽

√5ᵗʰ   **S85.2 Injury of peroneal artery**

√6ᵗʰ   **S85.20 Unspecified injury of peroneal artery**

√7ᵗʰ   **S85.201 Unspecified injury of peroneal artery, right leg** ▽

√7ᵗʰ   **S85.202 Unspecified injury of peroneal artery, left leg** ▽

√7ᵗʰ   **S85.209 Unspecified injury of peroneal artery, unspecified leg** ▽

√6ᵗʰ   **S85.21 Laceration of peroneal artery**

√7ᵗʰ   **S85.211 Laceration of peroneal artery, right leg**

√7ᵗʰ   **S85.212 Laceration of peroneal artery, left leg**

√7ᵗʰ   **S85.219 Laceration of peroneal artery, unspecified leg** ▽

√6ᵗʰ   **S85.29 Other specified injury of peroneal artery**

√7ᵗʰ   **S85.291 Other specified injury of peroneal artery, right leg**

√7ᵗʰ   **S85.292 Other specified injury of peroneal artery, left leg**

√7ᵗʰ   **S85.299 Other specified injury of peroneal artery, unspecified leg** ▽

✔ Additional Character Req   √x7ᵗʰ Placeholder Alert   Manifestation   ▽ Unspecified   ►◄ Revised Text   ● New Code   ▲ Revised Code Title

ICD-10-CM 2019   1055

Chapter 19. Injury, Poisoning and Certain Other Consequences of External Causes

S84–S85.299

√5ᵗʰ **S85.3** **Injury of greater saphenous vein at lower leg level**

Injury of greater saphenous vein NOS
Injury of saphenous vein NOS

√6ᵗʰ **S85.30** **Unspecified injury of greater saphenous vein at lower leg level**

√7ᵗʰ **S85.301** Unspecified injury of greater saphenous vein at lower leg level, right leg ▽

√7ᵗʰ **S85.302** Unspecified injury of greater saphenous vein at lower leg level, left leg ▽

√7ᵗʰ **S85.309** Unspecified injury of greater saphenous vein at lower leg level, unspecified leg ▽

√6ᵗʰ **S85.31** **Laceration of greater saphenous vein at lower leg level**

√7ᵗʰ **S85.311** Laceration of greater saphenous vein at lower leg level, right leg

√7ᵗʰ **S85.312** Laceration of greater saphenous vein at lower leg level, left leg

√7ᵗʰ **S85.319** Laceration of greater saphenous vein at lower leg level, unspecified leg ▽

√6ᵗʰ **S85.39** **Other specified injury of greater saphenous vein at lower leg level**

√7ᵗʰ **S85.391** Other specified injury of greater saphenous vein at lower leg level, right leg

√7ᵗʰ **S85.392** Other specified injury of greater saphenous vein at lower leg level, left leg

√7ᵗʰ **S85.399** Other specified injury of greater saphenous vein at lower leg level, unspecified leg ▽

√5ᵗʰ **S85.4** **Injury of lesser saphenous vein at lower leg level**

√6ᵗʰ **S85.40** **Unspecified injury of lesser saphenous vein at lower leg level**

√7ᵗʰ **S85.401** Unspecified injury of lesser saphenous vein at lower leg level, right leg ▽

√7ᵗʰ **S85.402** Unspecified injury of lesser saphenous vein at lower leg level, left leg ▽

√7ᵗʰ **S85.409** Unspecified injury of lesser saphenous vein at lower leg level, unspecified leg ▽

√6ᵗʰ **S85.41** **Laceration of lesser saphenous vein at lower leg level**

√7ᵗʰ **S85.411** Laceration of lesser saphenous vein at lower leg level, right leg

√7ᵗʰ **S85.412** Laceration of lesser saphenous vein at lower leg level, left leg

√7ᵗʰ **S85.419** Laceration of lesser saphenous vein at lower leg level, unspecified leg ▽

√6ᵗʰ **S85.49** **Other specified injury of lesser saphenous vein at lower leg level**

√7ᵗʰ **S85.491** Other specified injury of lesser saphenous vein at lower leg level, right leg

√7ᵗʰ **S85.492** Other specified injury of lesser saphenous vein at lower leg level, left leg

√7ᵗʰ **S85.499** Other specified injury of lesser saphenous vein at lower leg level, unspecified leg ▽

√5ᵗʰ **S85.5** **Injury of popliteal vein**

√6ᵗʰ **S85.50** **Unspecified injury of popliteal vein**

√7ᵗʰ **S85.501** Unspecified injury of popliteal vein, right leg ▽

√7ᵗʰ **S85.502** Unspecified injury of popliteal vein, left leg ▽

√7ᵗʰ **S85.509** Unspecified injury of popliteal vein, unspecified leg ▽

√6ᵗʰ **S85.51** **Laceration of popliteal vein**

√7ᵗʰ **S85.511** Laceration of popliteal vein, right leg

√7ᵗʰ **S85.512** Laceration of popliteal vein, left leg

√7ᵗʰ **S85.519** Laceration of popliteal vein, unspecified leg ▽

√6ᵗʰ **S85.59** **Other specified injury of popliteal vein**

√7ᵗʰ **S85.591** Other specified injury of popliteal vein, right leg

√7ᵗʰ **S85.592** Other specified injury of popliteal vein, left leg

√7ᵗʰ **S85.599** Other specified injury of popliteal vein, unspecified leg ▽

√5ᵗʰ **S85.8** **Injury of other blood vessels at lower leg level**

√6ᵗʰ **S85.80** **Unspecified injury of other blood vessels at lower leg level**

√7ᵗʰ **S85.801** Unspecified injury of other blood vessels at lower leg level, right leg ▽

√7ᵗʰ **S85.802** Unspecified injury of other blood vessels at lower leg level, left leg ▽

√7ᵗʰ **S85.809** Unspecified injury of other blood vessels at lower leg level, unspecified leg ▽

√6ᵗʰ **S85.81** **Laceration of other blood vessels at lower leg level**

√7ᵗʰ **S85.811** Laceration of other blood vessels at lower leg level, right leg

√7ᵗʰ **S85.812** Laceration of other blood vessels at lower leg level, left leg

√7ᵗʰ **S85.819** Laceration of other blood vessels at lower leg level, unspecified leg ▽

√6ᵗʰ **S85.89** **Other specified injury of other blood vessels at lower leg level**

√7ᵗʰ **S85.891** Other specified injury of other blood vessels at lower leg level, right leg

√7ᵗʰ **S85.892** Other specified injury of other blood vessels at lower leg level, left leg

√7ᵗʰ **S85.899** Other specified injury of other blood vessels at lower leg level, unspecified leg ▽

√5ᵗʰ **S85.9** **Injury of unspecified blood vessel at lower leg level**

√6ᵗʰ **S85.90** **Unspecified injury of unspecified blood vessel at lower leg level**

√7ᵗʰ **S85.901** Unspecified injury of unspecified blood vessel at lower leg level, right leg ▽

√7ᵗʰ **S85.902** Unspecified injury of unspecified blood vessel at lower leg level, left leg ▽

√7ᵗʰ **S85.909** Unspecified injury of unspecified blood vessel at lower leg level, unspecified leg ▽

√6ᵗʰ **S85.91** **Laceration of unspecified blood vessel at lower leg level**

√7ᵗʰ **S85.911** Laceration of unspecified blood vessel at lower leg level, right leg ▽

√7ᵗʰ **S85.912** Laceration of unspecified blood vessel at lower leg level, left leg ▽

√7ᵗʰ **S85.919** Laceration of unspecified blood vessel at lower leg level, unspecified leg ▽

√6ᵗʰ **S85.99** **Other specified injury of unspecified blood vessel at lower leg level**

√7ᵗʰ **S85.991** Other specified injury of unspecified blood vessel at lower leg level, right leg ▽

√7ᵗʰ **S85.992** Other specified injury of unspecified blood vessel at lower leg level, left leg ▽

√7ᵗʰ **S85.999** Other specified injury of unspecified blood vessel at lower leg level, unspecified leg ▽

√4ᵗʰ **S86** **Injury of muscle, fascia and tendon at lower leg level**

Code also any associated open wound (S81.-)

EXCLUDES 2 injury of muscle, fascia and tendon at ankle (S96.-)
injury of patellar ligament (tendon) (S76.1-)
sprain of joints and ligaments of knee (S83.-)

TIP: Refer to the Muscle/Tendon table at the beginning of this chapter.

The appropriate 7th character is to be added to each code from category S86.
A   initial encounter
D   subsequent encounter
S   sequela

√5ᵗʰ **S86.0** **Injury of Achilles tendon**

√6ᵗʰ **S86.00** **Unspecified injury of Achilles tendon**

√7ᵗʰ **S86.001** Unspecified injury of right Achilles tendon ▽

√7ᵗʰ **S86.002** Unspecified injury of left Achilles tendon ▽

√7ᵗʰ **S86.009** Unspecified injury of unspecified Achilles tendon ▽

√6ᵗʰ **S86.01** Strain of Achilles tendon
   √7ᵗʰ **S86.011** Strain of right Achilles tendon
   √7ᵗʰ **S86.012** Strain of left Achilles tendon
   √7ᵗʰ **S86.019** Strain of unspecified Achilles tendon ▽

√6ᵗʰ **S86.02** Laceration of Achilles tendon
   √7ᵗʰ **S86.021** Laceration of right Achilles tendon
   √7ᵗʰ **S86.022** Laceration of left Achilles tendon
   √7ᵗʰ **S86.029** Laceration of unspecified Achilles tendon ▽

√6ᵗʰ **S86.09** Other specified injury of Achilles tendon
   √7ᵗʰ **S86.091** Other specified injury of right Achilles tendon
   √7ᵗʰ **S86.092** Other specified injury of left Achilles tendon
   √7ᵗʰ **S86.099** Other specified injury of unspecified Achilles tendon ▽

√5ᵗʰ **S86.1** Injury of other muscle(s) and tendon(s) of posterior muscle group at lower leg level
√6ᵗʰ **S86.10** Unspecified injury of other muscle(s) and tendon(s) of posterior muscle group at lower leg level
   √7ᵗʰ **S86.101** Unspecified injury of other muscle(s) and tendon(s) of posterior muscle group at lower leg level, right leg ▽
   √7ᵗʰ **S86.102** Unspecified injury of other muscle(s) and tendon(s) of posterior muscle group at lower leg level, left leg ▽
   √7ᵗʰ **S86.109** Unspecified injury of other muscle(s) and tendon(s) of posterior muscle group at lower leg level, unspecified leg ▽

√6ᵗʰ **S86.11** Strain of other muscle(s) and tendon(s) of posterior muscle group at lower leg level
   √7ᵗʰ **S86.111** Strain of other muscle(s) and tendon(s) of posterior muscle group at lower leg level, right leg
   √7ᵗʰ **S86.112** Strain of other muscle(s) and tendon(s) of posterior muscle group at lower leg level, left leg
   √7ᵗʰ **S86.119** Strain of other muscle(s) and tendon(s) of posterior muscle group at lower leg level, unspecified leg ▽

√6ᵗʰ **S86.12** Laceration of other muscle(s) and tendon(s) of posterior muscle group at lower leg level
   √7ᵗʰ **S86.121** Laceration of other muscle(s) and tendon(s) of posterior muscle group at lower leg level, right leg
   √7ᵗʰ **S86.122** Laceration of other muscle(s) and tendon(s) of posterior muscle group at lower leg level, left leg
   √7ᵗʰ **S86.129** Laceration of other muscle(s) and tendon(s) of posterior muscle group at lower leg level, unspecified leg ▽

√6ᵗʰ **S86.19** Other injury of other muscle(s) and tendon(s) of posterior muscle group at lower leg level
   √7ᵗʰ **S86.191** Other injury of other muscle(s) and tendon(s) of posterior muscle group at lower leg level, right leg
   √7ᵗʰ **S86.192** Other injury of other muscle(s) and tendon(s) of posterior muscle group at lower leg level, left leg
   √7ᵗʰ **S86.199** Other injury of other muscle(s) and tendon(s) of posterior muscle group at lower leg level, unspecified leg ▽

√5ᵗʰ **S86.2** Injury of muscle(s) and tendon(s) of anterior muscle group at lower leg level
√6ᵗʰ **S86.20** Unspecified injury of muscle(s) and tendon(s) of anterior muscle group at lower leg level
   √7ᵗʰ **S86.201** Unspecified injury of muscle(s) and tendon(s) of anterior muscle group at lower leg level, right leg ▽
   √7ᵗʰ **S86.202** Unspecified injury of muscle(s) and tendon(s) of anterior muscle group at lower leg level, left leg ▽
   √7ᵗʰ **S86.209** Unspecified injury of muscle(s) and tendon(s) of anterior muscle group at lower leg level, unspecified leg ▽

√6ᵗʰ **S86.21** Strain of muscle(s) and tendon(s) of anterior muscle group at lower leg level
   √7ᵗʰ **S86.211** Strain of muscle(s) and tendon(s) of anterior muscle group at lower leg level, right leg
   √7ᵗʰ **S86.212** Strain of muscle(s) and tendon(s) of anterior muscle group at lower leg level, left leg
   √7ᵗʰ **S86.219** Strain of muscle(s) and tendon(s) of anterior muscle group at lower leg level, unspecified leg ▽

√6ᵗʰ **S86.22** Laceration of muscle(s) and tendon(s) of anterior muscle group at lower leg level
   √7ᵗʰ **S86.221** Laceration of muscle(s) and tendon(s) of anterior muscle group at lower leg level, right leg
   √7ᵗʰ **S86.222** Laceration of muscle(s) and tendon(s) of anterior muscle group at lower leg level, left leg
   √7ᵗʰ **S86.229** Laceration of muscle(s) and tendon(s) of anterior muscle group at lower leg level, unspecified leg ▽

√6ᵗʰ **S86.29** Other injury of muscle(s) and tendon(s) of anterior muscle group at lower leg level
   √7ᵗʰ **S86.291** Other injury of muscle(s) and tendon(s) of anterior muscle group at lower leg level, right leg
   √7ᵗʰ **S86.292** Other injury of muscle(s) and tendon(s) of anterior muscle group at lower leg level, left leg
   √7ᵗʰ **S86.299** Other injury of muscle(s) and tendon(s) of anterior muscle group at lower leg level, unspecified leg ▽

√5ᵗʰ **S86.3** Injury of muscle(s) and tendon(s) of peroneal muscle group at lower leg level
√6ᵗʰ **S86.30** Unspecified injury of muscle(s) and tendon(s) of peroneal muscle group at lower leg level
   √7ᵗʰ **S86.301** Unspecified injury of muscle(s) and tendon(s) of peroneal muscle group at lower leg level, right leg ▽
   √7ᵗʰ **S86.302** Unspecified injury of muscle(s) and tendon(s) of peroneal muscle group at lower leg level, left leg ▽
   √7ᵗʰ **S86.309** Unspecified injury of muscle(s) and tendon(s) of peroneal muscle group at lower leg level, unspecified leg ▽

√6ᵗʰ **S86.31** Strain of muscle(s) and tendon(s) of peroneal muscle group at lower leg level
   √7ᵗʰ **S86.311** Strain of muscle(s) and tendon(s) of peroneal muscle group at lower leg level, right leg
   √7ᵗʰ **S86.312** Strain of muscle(s) and tendon(s) of peroneal muscle group at lower leg level, left leg
   √7ᵗʰ **S86.319** Strain of muscle(s) and tendon(s) of peroneal muscle group at lower leg level, unspecified leg ▽

√6ᵗʰ **S86.32** Laceration of muscle(s) and tendon(s) of peroneal muscle group at lower leg level
   √7ᵗʰ **S86.321** Laceration of muscle(s) and tendon(s) of peroneal muscle group at lower leg level, right leg
   √7ᵗʰ **S86.322** Laceration of muscle(s) and tendon(s) of peroneal muscle group at lower leg level, left leg
   √7ᵗʰ **S86.329** Laceration of muscle(s) and tendon(s) of peroneal muscle group at lower leg level, unspecified leg ▽

√6ᵗʰ **S86.39** Other injury of muscle(s) and tendon(s) of peroneal muscle group at lower leg level
   √7ᵗʰ **S86.391** Other injury of muscle(s) and tendon(s) of peroneal muscle group at lower leg level, right leg
   √7ᵗʰ **S86.392** Other injury of muscle(s) and tendon(s) of peroneal muscle group at lower leg level, left leg
   √7ᵗʰ **S86.399** Other injury of muscle(s) and tendon(s) of peroneal muscle group at lower leg level, unspecified leg ▽

| ☑ Additional Character Req | ☑x7ᵗʰ Placeholder Alert | Manifestation | ▽ Unspecified | ►◄ Revised Text | ● New Code | ▲ Revised Code Title |

√5ᵗʰ **S86.8** **Injury of other muscles and tendons at lower leg level**

√6ᵗʰ **S86.80** **Unspecified injury of other muscles and tendons at lower leg level**

√7ᵗʰ **S86.801** **Unspecified injury of other muscle(s) and tendon(s) at lower leg level, right leg** ▽

√7ᵗʰ **S86.802** **Unspecified injury of other muscle(s) and tendon(s) at lower leg level, left leg** ▽

√7ᵗʰ **S86.809** **Unspecified injury of other muscle(s) and tendon(s) at lower leg level, unspecified leg** ▽

√6ᵗʰ **S86.81** **Strain of other muscles and tendons at lower leg level**

√7ᵗʰ **S86.811** **Strain of other muscle(s) and tendon(s) at lower leg level, right leg**

√7ᵗʰ **S86.812** **Strain of other muscle(s) and tendon(s) at lower leg level, left leg**

√7ᵗʰ **S86.819** **Strain of other muscle(s) and tendon(s) at lower leg level, unspecified leg** ▽

√6ᵗʰ **S86.82** **Laceration of other muscles and tendons at lower leg level**

√7ᵗʰ **S86.821** **Laceration of other muscle(s) and tendon(s) at lower leg level, right leg**

√7ᵗʰ **S86.822** **Laceration of other muscle(s) and tendon(s) at lower leg level, left leg**

√7ᵗʰ **S86.829** **Laceration of other muscle(s) and tendon(s) at lower leg level, unspecified leg** ▽

√6ᵗʰ **S86.89** **Other injury of other muscles and tendons at lower leg level**

√7ᵗʰ **S86.891** **Other injury of other muscle(s) and tendon(s) at lower leg level, right leg**

√7ᵗʰ **S86.892** **Other injury of other muscle(s) and tendon(s) at lower leg level, left leg**

√7ᵗʰ **S86.899** **Other injury of other muscle(s) and tendon(s) at lower leg level, unspecified leg** ▽

√5ᵗʰ **S86.9** **Injury of unspecified muscle and tendon at lower leg level**

√6ᵗʰ **S86.90** **Unspecified injury of unspecified muscle and tendon at lower leg level**

√7ᵗʰ **S86.901** **Unspecified injury of unspecified muscle(s) and tendon(s) at lower leg level, right leg** ▽

√7ᵗʰ **S86.902** **Unspecified injury of unspecified muscle(s) and tendon(s) at lower leg level, left leg** ▽

√7ᵗʰ **S86.909** **Unspecified injury of unspecified muscle(s) and tendon(s) at lower leg level, unspecified leg** ▽

√6ᵗʰ **S86.91** **Strain of unspecified muscle and tendon at lower leg level**

√7ᵗʰ **S86.911** **Strain of unspecified muscle(s) and tendon(s) at lower leg level, right leg** ▽

√7ᵗʰ **S86.912** **Strain of unspecified muscle(s) and tendon(s) at lower leg level, left leg** ▽

√7ᵗʰ **S86.919** **Strain of unspecified muscle(s) and tendon(s) at lower leg level, unspecified leg** ▽

√6ᵗʰ **S86.92** **Laceration of unspecified muscle and tendon at lower leg level**

√7ᵗʰ **S86.921** **Laceration of unspecified muscle(s) and tendon(s) at lower leg level, right leg** ▽

√7ᵗʰ **S86.922** **Laceration of unspecified muscle(s) and tendon(s) at lower leg level, left leg** ▽

√7ᵗʰ **S86.929** **Laceration of unspecified muscle(s) and tendon(s) at lower leg level, unspecified leg** ▽

√6ᵗʰ **S86.99** **Other injury of unspecified muscle and tendon at lower leg level**

√7ᵗʰ **S86.991** **Other injury of unspecified muscle(s) and tendon(s) at lower leg level, right leg** ▽

√7ᵗʰ **S86.992** **Other injury of unspecified muscle(s) and tendon(s) at lower leg level, left leg** ▽

√7ᵗʰ **S86.999** **Other injury of unspecified muscle(s) and tendon(s) at lower leg level, unspecified leg** ▽

√4ᵗʰ **S87** **Crushing injury of lower leg**

Use additional code(s) for all associated injuries

EXCLUDES 2   *crushing injury of ankle and foot (S97.-)*

The appropriate 7th character is to be added to each code from category S87.
A   initial encounter
D   subsequent encounter
S   sequela

√5ᵗʰ **S87.0** **Crushing injury of knee**

√×7ᵗʰ **S87.00** **Crushing injury of unspecified knee** ▽

√×7ᵗʰ **S87.01** **Crushing injury of right knee**

√×7ᵗʰ **S87.02** **Crushing injury of left knee**

√5ᵗʰ **S87.8** **Crushing injury of lower leg**

√×7ᵗʰ **S87.80** **Crushing injury of unspecified lower leg** ▽

√×7ᵗʰ **S87.81** **Crushing injury of right lower leg**

√×7ᵗʰ **S87.82** **Crushing injury of left lower leg**

√4ᵗʰ **S88** **Traumatic amputation of lower leg**

An amputation not identified as partial or complete should be coded to complete

EXCLUDES 1   *traumatic amputation of ankle and foot (S98.-)*

The appropriate 7th character is to be added to each code from category S88.
A   initial encounter
D   subsequent encounter
S   sequela

√5ᵗʰ **S88.0** **Traumatic amputation at knee level**

√6ᵗʰ **S88.01** **Complete traumatic amputation at knee level**

√7ᵗʰ **S88.011** **Complete traumatic amputation at knee level, right lower leg** HCC

√7ᵗʰ **S88.012** **Complete traumatic amputation at knee level, left lower leg** HCC

√7ᵗʰ **S88.019** **Complete traumatic amputation at knee level, unspecified lower leg** HCC ▽

√6ᵗʰ **S88.02** **Partial traumatic amputation at knee level**

√7ᵗʰ **S88.021** **Partial traumatic amputation at knee level, right lower leg** HCC

√7ᵗʰ **S88.022** **Partial traumatic amputation at knee level, left lower leg** HCC

√7ᵗʰ **S88.029** **Partial traumatic amputation at knee level, unspecified lower leg** HCC ▽

√5ᵗʰ **S88.1** **Traumatic amputation at level between knee and ankle**

√6ᵗʰ **S88.11** **Complete traumatic amputation at level between knee and ankle**

√7ᵗʰ **S88.111** **Complete traumatic amputation at level between knee and ankle, right lower leg** HCC

√7ᵗʰ **S88.112** **Complete traumatic amputation at level between knee and ankle, left lower leg** HCC

√7ᵗʰ **S88.119** **Complete traumatic amputation at level between knee and ankle, unspecified lower leg** HCC ▽

√6ᵗʰ **S88.12** **Partial traumatic amputation at level between knee and ankle**

√7ᵗʰ **S88.121** **Partial traumatic amputation at level between knee and ankle, right lower leg** HCC

√7ᵗʰ **S88.122** **Partial traumatic amputation at level between knee and ankle, left lower leg** HCC

√7ᵗʰ **S88.129** **Partial traumatic amputation at level between knee and ankle, unspecified lower leg** HCC ▽

√5ᵗʰ **S88.9** **Traumatic amputation of lower leg, level unspecified**

√6ᵗʰ **S88.91** **Complete traumatic amputation of lower leg, level unspecified**

√7ᵗʰ **S88.911** **Complete traumatic amputation of right lower leg, level unspecified** HCC ▽

√7ᵗʰ **S88.912** **Complete traumatic amputation of left lower leg, level unspecified** HCC ▽

√7ᵗʰ **S88.919** **Complete traumatic amputation of unspecified lower leg, level unspecified** HCC ▽

HCC CMS-HCC	Q QPP	N Newborn : 0	P Pediatric : 0-17	M Maternity : 12-55	A Adult : 15-124

√6ᵗʰ **S88.92** Partial traumatic amputation of lower leg, level unspecified

     √7ᵗʰ **S88.921** Partial traumatic amputation of HCC ▽ right lower leg, level unspecified

     √7ᵗʰ **S88.922** Partial traumatic amputation of HCC ▽ left lower leg, level unspecified

     √7ᵗʰ **S88.929** Partial traumatic amputation of HCC ▽ unspecified lower leg, level unspecified

√4ᵗʰ **S89** Other and unspecified injuries of lower leg

   NOTE   A fracture not indicated as open or closed should be coded to closed.

   EXCLUDES 2   *other and unspecified injuries of ankle and foot (S99.-)*

   AHA: 2018,2Q,12; 2018,1Q,3; 2015,3Q,37-39

The appropriate 7th character is to be added to each code from subcategories S89.0, S89.1, S89.2, and S89.3.
A   initial encounter for closed fracture
D   subsequent encounter for fracture with routine healing
G   subsequent encounter for fracture with delayed healing
K   subsequent encounter for fracture with nonunion
P   subsequent encounter for fracture with malunion
S   sequela

√5ᵗʰ **S89.0** Physeal fracture of upper end of tibia

   √6ᵗʰ **S89.00** Unspecified physeal fracture of upper end of tibia

     √7ᵗʰ **S89.001** Unspecified physeal fracture of [Q] ▽ upper end of right tibia

     √7ᵗʰ **S89.002** Unspecified physeal fracture of [Q] ▽ upper end of left tibia

     √7ᵗʰ **S89.009** Unspecified physeal fracture of [Q] ▽ upper end of unspecified tibia

   √6ᵗʰ **S89.01** Salter-Harris Type I physeal fracture of upper end of tibia

     √7ᵗʰ **S89.011** Salter-Harris Type I physeal [Q] fracture of upper end of right tibia

     √7ᵗʰ **S89.012** Salter-Harris Type I physeal [Q] fracture of upper end of left tibia

     √7ᵗʰ **S89.019** Salter-Harris Type I physeal [Q] ▽ fracture of upper end of unspecified tibia

   √6ᵗʰ **S89.02** Salter-Harris Type II physeal fracture of upper end of tibia

     √7ᵗʰ **S89.021** Salter-Harris Type II physeal [Q] fracture of upper end of right tibia

     √7ᵗʰ **S89.022** Salter-Harris Type II physeal [Q] fracture of upper end of left tibia

     √7ᵗʰ **S89.029** Salter-Harris Type II physeal [Q] ▽ fracture of upper end of unspecified tibia

   √6ᵗʰ **S89.03** Salter-Harris Type III physeal fracture of upper end of tibia

     √7ᵗʰ **S89.031** Salter-Harris Type III physeal [Q] fracture of upper end of right tibia

     √7ᵗʰ **S89.032** Salter-Harris Type III physeal [Q] fracture of upper end of left tibia

     √7ᵗʰ **S89.039** Salter-Harris Type III physeal [Q] ▽ fracture of upper end of unspecified tibia

   √6ᵗʰ **S89.04** Salter-Harris Type IV physeal fracture of upper end of tibia

     √7ᵗʰ **S89.041** Salter-Harris Type IV physeal [Q] fracture of upper end of right tibia

     √7ᵗʰ **S89.042** Salter-Harris Type IV physeal [Q] fracture of upper end of left tibia

     √7ᵗʰ **S89.049** Salter-Harris Type IV physeal [Q] ▽ fracture of upper end of unspecified tibia

   √6ᵗʰ **S89.09** Other physeal fracture of upper end of tibia

     √7ᵗʰ **S89.091** Other physeal fracture of upper [Q] end of right tibia

     √7ᵗʰ **S89.092** Other physeal fracture of upper [Q] end of left tibia

     √7ᵗʰ **S89.099** Other physeal fracture of upper [Q] ▽ end of unspecified tibia

√5ᵗʰ **S89.1** Physeal fracture of lower end of tibia

   √6ᵗʰ **S89.10** Unspecified physeal fracture of lower end of tibia

     √7ᵗʰ **S89.101** Unspecified physeal fracture of [Q] ▽ lower end of right tibia

     √7ᵗʰ **S89.102** Unspecified physeal fracture of [Q] ▽ lower end of left tibia

     √7ᵗʰ **S89.109** Unspecified physeal fracture of [Q] ▽ lower end of unspecified tibia

   √6ᵗʰ **S89.11** Salter-Harris Type I physeal fracture of lower end of tibia

     √7ᵗʰ **S89.111** Salter-Harris Type I physeal [Q] fracture of lower end of right tibia

     √7ᵗʰ **S89.112** Salter-Harris Type I physeal [Q] fracture of lower end of left tibia

     √7ᵗʰ **S89.119** Salter-Harris Type I physeal [Q] ▽ fracture of lower end of unspecified tibia

   √6ᵗʰ **S89.12** Salter-Harris Type II physeal fracture of lower end of tibia

     √7ᵗʰ **S89.121** Salter-Harris Type II physeal [Q] fracture of lower end of right tibia

     √7ᵗʰ **S89.122** Salter-Harris Type II physeal [Q] fracture of lower end of left tibia

     √7ᵗʰ **S89.129** Salter-Harris Type II physeal [Q] ▽ fracture of lower end of unspecified tibia

   √6ᵗʰ **S89.13** Salter-Harris Type III physeal fracture of lower end of tibia

     EXCLUDES 1 *fracture of medial malleolus (adult) (S82.5-)*

     √7ᵗʰ **S89.131** Salter-Harris Type III physeal [Q] fracture of lower end of right tibia

     √7ᵗʰ **S89.132** Salter-Harris Type III physeal [Q] fracture of lower end of left tibia

     √7ᵗʰ **S89.139** Salter-Harris Type III physeal [Q] ▽ fracture of lower end of unspecified tibia

   √6ᵗʰ **S89.14** Salter-Harris Type IV physeal fracture of lower end of tibia

     EXCLUDES 1 *fracture of medial malleolus (adult) (S82.5-)*

     √7ᵗʰ **S89.141** Salter-Harris Type IV physeal [Q] fracture of lower end of right tibia

     √7ᵗʰ **S89.142** Salter-Harris Type IV physeal [Q] fracture of lower end of left tibia

     √7ᵗʰ **S89.149** Salter-Harris Type IV physeal [Q] ▽ fracture of lower end of unspecified tibia

   √6ᵗʰ **S89.19** Other physeal fracture of lower end of tibia

     √7ᵗʰ **S89.191** Other physeal fracture of lower [Q] end of right tibia

     √7ᵗʰ **S89.192** Other physeal fracture of lower [Q] end of left tibia

     √7ᵗʰ **S89.199** Other physeal fracture of lower [Q] ▽ end of unspecified tibia

√5ᵗʰ **S89.2** Physeal fracture of upper end of fibula

   √6ᵗʰ **S89.20** Unspecified physeal fracture of upper end of fibula

     √7ᵗʰ **S89.201** Unspecified physeal fracture of [Q] ▽ upper end of right fibula

     √7ᵗʰ **S89.202** Unspecified physeal fracture of [Q] ▽ upper end of left fibula

     √7ᵗʰ **S89.209** Unspecified physeal fracture of [Q] ▽ upper end of unspecified fibula

   √6ᵗʰ **S89.21** Salter-Harris Type I physeal fracture of upper end of fibula

     √7ᵗʰ **S89.211** Salter-Harris Type I physeal [Q] fracture of upper end of right fibula

     √7ᵗʰ **S89.212** Salter-Harris Type I physeal [Q] fracture of upper end of left fibula

     √7ᵗʰ **S89.219** Salter-Harris Type I physeal [Q] ▽ fracture of upper end of unspecified fibula

   √6ᵗʰ **S89.22** Salter-Harris Type II physeal fracture of upper end of fibula

     √7ᵗʰ **S89.221** Salter-Harris Type II physeal [Q] fracture of upper end of right fibula

     √7ᵗʰ **S89.222** Salter-Harris Type II physeal [Q] fracture of upper end of left fibula

---

☑ Additional Character Req   √ₓ7ᵗʰ Placeholder Alert   Manifestation   ▽ Unspecified   ►◄ Revised Text   ● New Code   ▲ Revised Code Title

Chapter 19. Injury, Poisoning and Certain Other Consequences of External Causes

S89.229–S90.426

   ✓7ᵗʰ **S89.229** **Salter-Harris Type II physeal fracture of upper end of unspecified fibula** ◨ ▽

  ✓6ᵗʰ **S89.29** **Other physeal fracture of upper end of fibula**

   ✓7ᵗʰ **S89.291** **Other physeal fracture of upper end of right fibula** ◨

   ✓7ᵗʰ **S89.292** **Other physeal fracture of upper end of left fibula** ◨

   ✓7ᵗʰ **S89.299** **Other physeal fracture of upper end of unspecified fibula** ◨ ▽

✓5ᵗʰ **S89.3** **Physeal fracture of lower end of fibula**

  ✓6ᵗʰ **S89.30** **Unspecified physeal fracture of lower end of fibula**

   ✓7ᵗʰ **S89.301** **Unspecified physeal fracture of lower end of right fibula** ◨ ▽

   ✓7ᵗʰ **S89.302** **Unspecified physeal fracture of lower end of left fibula** ◨ ▽

   ✓7ᵗʰ **S89.309** **Unspecified physeal fracture of lower end of unspecified fibula** ◨ ▽

  ✓6ᵗʰ **S89.31** **Salter-Harris Type I physeal fracture of lower end of fibula**

   ✓7ᵗʰ **S89.311** **Salter-Harris Type I physeal fracture of lower end of right fibula** ◨

   ✓7ᵗʰ **S89.312** **Salter-Harris Type I physeal fracture of lower end of left fibula** ◨

   ✓7ᵗʰ **S89.319** **Salter-Harris Type I physeal fracture of lower end of unspecified fibula** ◨ ▽

  ✓6ᵗʰ **S89.32** **Salter-Harris Type II physeal fracture of lower end of fibula**

   ✓7ᵗʰ **S89.321** **Salter-Harris Type II physeal fracture of lower end of right fibula** ◨

   ✓7ᵗʰ **S89.322** **Salter-Harris Type II physeal fracture of lower end of left fibula** ◨

   ✓7ᵗʰ **S89.329** **Salter-Harris Type II physeal fracture of lower end of unspecified fibula** ◨ ▽

  ✓6ᵗʰ **S89.39** **Other physeal fracture of lower end of fibula**

   ✓7ᵗʰ **S89.391** **Other physeal fracture of lower end of right fibula** ◨

   ✓7ᵗʰ **S89.392** **Other physeal fracture of lower end of left fibula** ◨

   ✓7ᵗʰ **S89.399** **Other physeal fracture of lower end of unspecified fibula** ◨ ▽

✓5ᵗʰ **S89.8** **Other specified injuries of lower leg**

The appropriate 7th character is to be added to each code in subcategory S89.8.
A initial encounter
D subsequent encounter
S sequela

  ✓x7ᵗʰ **S89.80** **Other specified injuries of unspecified lower leg** ▽

  ✓x7ᵗʰ **S89.81** **Other specified injuries of right lower leg**

  ✓x7ᵗʰ **S89.82** **Other specified injuries of left lower leg**

✓5ᵗʰ **S89.9** **Unspecified injury of lower leg**

The appropriate 7th character is to be added to each code in subcategory S89.9.
A initial encounter
D subsequent encounter
S sequela

  ✓x7ᵗʰ **S89.90** **Unspecified injury of unspecified lower leg** ▽

  ✓x7ᵗʰ **S89.91** **Unspecified injury of right lower leg** ▽

  ✓x7ᵗʰ **S89.92** **Unspecified injury of left lower leg** ▽

Injuries to the ankle and foot (S90-S99)

EXCLUDES 2   *burns and corrosions (T20-T32)*
fracture of ankle and malleolus (S82.-)
frostbite (T33-T34)
insect bite or sting, venomous (T63.4)

✓4ᵗʰ **S90** **Superficial injury of ankle, foot and toes**

The appropriate 7th character is to be added to each code from category S90.
A initial encounter
D subsequent encounter
S sequela

✓5ᵗʰ **S90.0** **Contusion of ankle**

  ✓x7ᵗʰ **S90.00** **Contusion of unspecified ankle** ▽

  ✓x7ᵗʰ **S90.01** **Contusion of right ankle**

  ✓x7ᵗʰ **S90.02** **Contusion of left ankle**

✓5ᵗʰ **S90.1** **Contusion of toe without damage to nail**

  ✓6ᵗʰ **S90.11** **Contusion of great toe without damage to nail**

   ✓7ᵗʰ **S90.111** **Contusion of right great toe without damage to nail**

   ✓7ᵗʰ **S90.112** **Contusion of left great toe without damage to nail**

   ✓7ᵗʰ **S90.119** **Contusion of unspecified great toe without damage to nail** ▽

  ✓6ᵗʰ **S90.12** **Contusion of lesser toe without damage to nail**

   ✓7ᵗʰ **S90.121** **Contusion of right lesser toe(s) without damage to nail**

   ✓7ᵗʰ **S90.122** **Contusion of left lesser toe(s) without damage to nail**

   ✓7ᵗʰ **S90.129** **Contusion of unspecified lesser toe(s) without damage to nail** ▽
Contusion of toe NOS

✓5ᵗʰ **S90.2** **Contusion of toe with damage to nail**

  ✓6ᵗʰ **S90.21** **Contusion of great toe with damage to nail**

   ✓7ᵗʰ **S90.211** **Contusion of right great toe with damage to nail**

   ✓7ᵗʰ **S90.212** **Contusion of left great toe with damage to nail**

   ✓7ᵗʰ **S90.219** **Contusion of unspecified great toe with damage to nail** ▽

  ✓6ᵗʰ **S90.22** **Contusion of lesser toe with damage to nail**

   ✓7ᵗʰ **S90.221** **Contusion of right lesser toe(s) with damage to nail**

   ✓7ᵗʰ **S90.222** **Contusion of left lesser toe(s) with damage to nail**

   ✓7ᵗʰ **S90.229** **Contusion of unspecified lesser toe(s) with damage to nail** ▽

✓5ᵗʰ **S90.3** **Contusion of foot**

EXCLUDES 2   *contusion of toes (S90.1-, S90.2-)*

  ✓x7ᵗʰ **S90.30** **Contusion of unspecified foot** ▽
Contusion of foot NOS

  ✓x7ᵗʰ **S90.31** **Contusion of right foot**

  ✓x7ᵗʰ **S90.32** **Contusion of left foot**

✓5ᵗʰ **S90.4** **Other superficial injuries of toe**

  ✓6ᵗʰ **S90.41** **Abrasion of toe**

   ✓7ᵗʰ **S90.411** **Abrasion, right great toe**

   ✓7ᵗʰ **S90.412** **Abrasion, left great toe**

   ✓7ᵗʰ **S90.413** **Abrasion, unspecified great toe** ▽

   ✓7ᵗʰ **S90.414** **Abrasion, right lesser toe(s)**

   ✓7ᵗʰ **S90.415** **Abrasion, left lesser toe(s)**

   ✓7ᵗʰ **S90.416** **Abrasion, unspecified lesser toe(s)** ▽

  ✓6ᵗʰ **S90.42** **Blister (nonthermal) of toe**

   ✓7ᵗʰ **S90.421** **Blister (nonthermal), right great toe**

   ✓7ᵗʰ **S90.422** **Blister (nonthermal), left great toe**

   ✓7ᵗʰ **S90.423** **Blister (nonthermal), unspecified great toe** ▽

   ✓7ᵗʰ **S90.424** **Blister (nonthermal), right lesser toe(s)**

   ✓7ᵗʰ **S90.425** **Blister (nonthermal), left lesser toe(s)**

   ✓7ᵗʰ **S90.426** **Blister (nonthermal), unspecified lesser toe(s)** ▽

√6ᵗʰ **S90.44** **External constriction** of toe
    Hair tourniquet syndrome of toe
    √7ᵗʰ **S90.441** **External constriction, right great toe**
    √7ᵗʰ **S90.442** **External constriction, left great toe**
    √7ᵗʰ **S90.443** **External constriction, unspecified great toe** ▽
    √7ᵗʰ **S90.444** **External constriction, right lesser toe(s)**
    √7ᵗʰ **S90.445** **External constriction, left lesser toe(s)**
    √7ᵗʰ **S90.446** **External constriction, unspecified lesser toe(s)** ▽

√6ᵗʰ **S90.45** **Superficial foreign body** of toe
    Splinter in the toe
    √7ᵗʰ **S90.451** **Superficial foreign body, right great toe**
    √7ᵗʰ **S90.452** **Superficial foreign body, left great toe**
    √7ᵗʰ **S90.453** **Superficial foreign body, unspecified great toe** ▽
    √7ᵗʰ **S90.454** **Superficial foreign body, right lesser toe(s)**
    √7ᵗʰ **S90.455** **Superficial foreign body, left lesser toe(s)**
    √7ᵗʰ **S90.456** **Superficial foreign body, unspecified lesser toe(s)** ▽

√6ᵗʰ **S90.46** **Insect bite (nonvenomous)** of toe
    √7ᵗʰ **S90.461** **Insect bite (nonvenomous), right great toe**
    √7ᵗʰ **S90.462** **Insect bite (nonvenomous), left great toe**
    √7ᵗʰ **S90.463** **Insect bite (nonvenomous), unspecified great toe** ▽
    √7ᵗʰ **S90.464** **Insect bite (nonvenomous), right lesser toe(s)**
    √7ᵗʰ **S90.465** **Insect bite (nonvenomous), left lesser toe(s)**
    √7ᵗʰ **S90.466** **Insect bite (nonvenomous), unspecified lesser toe(s)** ▽

√6ᵗʰ **S90.47** **Other superficial bite** of toe
    EXCLUDES 1   open bite of toe (S91.15-, S91.25-)
    √7ᵗʰ **S90.471** **Other superficial bite of right great toe**
    √7ᵗʰ **S90.472** **Other superficial bite of left great toe**
    √7ᵗʰ **S90.473** **Other superficial bite of unspecified great toe** ▽
    √7ᵗʰ **S90.474** **Other superficial bite of right lesser toe(s)**
    √7ᵗʰ **S90.475** **Other superficial bite of left lesser toe(s)**
    √7ᵗʰ **S90.476** **Other superficial bite of unspecified lesser toe(s)** ▽

√5ᵗʰ **S90.5** **Other superficial injuries** of ankle
√6ᵗʰ **S90.51** **Abrasion** of ankle
    √7ᵗʰ **S90.511** **Abrasion, right ankle**
    √7ᵗʰ **S90.512** **Abrasion, left ankle**
    √7ᵗʰ **S90.519** **Abrasion, unspecified ankle** ▽

√6ᵗʰ **S90.52** **Blister (nonthermal)** of ankle
    √7ᵗʰ **S90.521** **Blister (nonthermal), right ankle**
    √7ᵗʰ **S90.522** **Blister (nonthermal), left ankle**
    √7ᵗʰ **S90.529** **Blister (nonthermal), unspecified ankle** ▽

√6ᵗʰ **S90.54** **External constriction** of ankle
    √7ᵗʰ **S90.541** **External constriction, right ankle**
    √7ᵗʰ **S90.542** **External constriction, left ankle**
    √7ᵗʰ **S90.549** **External constriction, unspecified ankle** ▽

√6ᵗʰ **S90.55** **Superficial foreign body** of ankle
    Splinter in the ankle
    √7ᵗʰ **S90.551** **Superficial foreign body, right ankle**
    √7ᵗʰ **S90.552** **Superficial foreign body, left ankle**
    √7ᵗʰ **S90.559** **Superficial foreign body, unspecified ankle** ▽

√6ᵗʰ **S90.56** **Insect bite (nonvenomous)** of ankle
    √7ᵗʰ **S90.561** **Insect bite (nonvenomous), right ankle**
    √7ᵗʰ **S90.562** **Insect bite (nonvenomous), left ankle**
    √7ᵗʰ **S90.569** **Insect bite (nonvenomous), unspecified ankle** ▽

√6ᵗʰ **S90.57** **Other superficial bite** of ankle
    EXCLUDES 1   open bite of ankle (S91.05-)
    √7ᵗʰ **S90.571** **Other superficial bite of ankle, right ankle**
    √7ᵗʰ **S90.572** **Other superficial bite of ankle, left ankle**

    √7ᵗʰ **S90.579** **Other superficial bite of ankle, unspecified ankle** ▽

√5ᵗʰ **S90.8** **Other superficial injuries** of foot
√6ᵗʰ **S90.81** **Abrasion** of foot
    √7ᵗʰ **S90.811** **Abrasion, right foot**
    √7ᵗʰ **S90.812** **Abrasion, left foot**
    √7ᵗʰ **S90.819** **Abrasion, unspecified foot** ▽

√6ᵗʰ **S90.82** **Blister (nonthermal)** of foot
    √7ᵗʰ **S90.821** **Blister (nonthermal), right foot**
    √7ᵗʰ **S90.822** **Blister (nonthermal), left foot**
    √7ᵗʰ **S90.829** **Blister (nonthermal), unspecified foot** ▽

√6ᵗʰ **S90.84** **External constriction** of foot
    √7ᵗʰ **S90.841** **External constriction, right foot**
    √7ᵗʰ **S90.842** **External constriction, left foot**
    √7ᵗʰ **S90.849** **External constriction, unspecified foot** ▽

√6ᵗʰ **S90.85** **Superficial foreign body** of foot
    Splinter in the foot
    √7ᵗʰ **S90.851** **Superficial foreign body, right foot**
    √7ᵗʰ **S90.852** **Superficial foreign body, left foot**
    √7ᵗʰ **S90.859** **Superficial foreign body, unspecified foot** ▽

√6ᵗʰ **S90.86** **Insect bite (nonvenomous)** of foot
    √7ᵗʰ **S90.861** **Insect bite (nonvenomous), right foot**
    √7ᵗʰ **S90.862** **Insect bite (nonvenomous), left foot**
    √7ᵗʰ **S90.869** **Insect bite (nonvenomous), unspecified foot** ▽

√6ᵗʰ **S90.87** **Other superficial bite** of foot
    EXCLUDES 1   open bite of foot (S91.35-)
    √7ᵗʰ **S90.871** **Other superficial bite of right foot**
    √7ᵗʰ **S90.872** **Other superficial bite of left foot**
    √7ᵗʰ **S90.879** **Other superficial bite of unspecified foot** ▽

√5ᵗʰ **S90.9** **Unspecified superficial injury** of ankle, foot and toe
√6ᵗʰ **S90.91** **Unspecified superficial injury** of ankle
    √7ᵗʰ **S90.911** **Unspecified superficial injury of right ankle** ▽
    √7ᵗʰ **S90.912** **Unspecified superficial injury of left ankle** ▽
    √7ᵗʰ **S90.919** **Unspecified superficial injury of unspecified ankle** ▽

√6ᵗʰ **S90.92** **Unspecified superficial injury** of foot
    √7ᵗʰ **S90.921** **Unspecified superficial injury of right foot** ▽
    √7ᵗʰ **S90.922** **Unspecified superficial injury of left foot** ▽
    √7ᵗʰ **S90.929** **Unspecified superficial injury of unspecified foot** ▽

√6ᵗʰ **S90.93** **Unspecified superficial injury** of toes
    √7ᵗʰ **S90.931** **Unspecified superficial injury of right great toe** ▽
    √7ᵗʰ **S90.932** **Unspecified superficial injury of left great toe** ▽
    √7ᵗʰ **S90.933** **Unspecified superficial injury of unspecified great toe** ▽
    √7ᵗʰ **S90.934** **Unspecified superficial injury of right lesser toe(s)** ▽
    √7ᵗʰ **S90.935** **Unspecified superficial injury of left lesser toe(s)** ▽
    √7ᵗʰ **S90.936** **Unspecified superficial injury of unspecified lesser toe(s)** ▽

☑ Additional Character Req   √x7ᵗʰ Placeholder Alert   Manifestation   ▽ Unspecified   ▶◀ Revised Text   ● New Code   ▲ Revised Code Title

√4ᵗʰ S91   Open wound of ankle, foot and toes

Code also any associated wound infection

EXCLUDES 1   open fracture of ankle, foot and toes (S92.- with 7th character B)

traumatic amputation of ankle and foot (S98.-)

The appropriate 7th character is to be added to each code from category S91.
A   initial encounter
D   subsequent encounter
S   sequela

√5ᵗʰ S91.0   Open wound of ankle

   √6ᵗʰ S91.00   Unspecified open wound of ankle

     √7ᵗʰ S91.001   Unspecified open wound, right ankle ▽

     √7ᵗʰ S91.002   Unspecified open wound, left ankle ▽

     √7ᵗʰ S91.009   Unspecified open wound, unspecified ankle ▽

   √6ᵗʰ S91.01   Laceration without foreign body of ankle

     √7ᵗʰ S91.011   Laceration without foreign body, right ankle

     √7ᵗʰ S91.012   Laceration without foreign body, left ankle

     √7ᵗʰ S91.019   Laceration without foreign body, unspecified ankle ▽

   √6ᵗʰ S91.02   Laceration with foreign body of ankle

     √7ᵗʰ S91.021   Laceration with foreign body, right ankle

     √7ᵗʰ S91.022   Laceration with foreign body, left ankle

     √7ᵗʰ S91.029   Laceration with foreign body, unspecified ankle ▽

   √6ᵗʰ S91.03   Puncture wound without foreign body of ankle

     √7ᵗʰ S91.031   Puncture wound without foreign body, right ankle

     √7ᵗʰ S91.032   Puncture wound without foreign body, left ankle

     √7ᵗʰ S91.039   Puncture wound without foreign body, unspecified ankle ▽

   √6ᵗʰ S91.04   Puncture wound with foreign body of ankle

     √7ᵗʰ S91.041   Puncture wound with foreign body, right ankle

     √7ᵗʰ S91.042   Puncture wound with foreign body, left ankle

     √7ᵗʰ S91.049   Puncture wound with foreign body, unspecified ankle ▽

   √6ᵗʰ S91.05   Open bite of ankle

     EXCLUDES 1   superficial bite of ankle (S90.56-, S90.57-)

     √7ᵗʰ S91.051   Open bite, right ankle

     √7ᵗʰ S91.052   Open bite, left ankle

     √7ᵗʰ S91.059   Open bite, unspecified ankle ▽

√5ᵗʰ S91.1   Open wound of toe without damage to nail

   √6ᵗʰ S91.10   Unspecified open wound of toe without damage to nail

     √7ᵗʰ S91.101   Unspecified open wound of right great toe without damage to nail ▽

     √7ᵗʰ S91.102   Unspecified open wound of left great toe without damage to nail ▽

     √7ᵗʰ S91.103   Unspecified open wound of unspecified great toe without damage to nail ▽

     √7ᵗʰ S91.104   Unspecified open wound of right lesser toe(s) without damage to nail ▽

     √7ᵗʰ S91.105   Unspecified open wound of left lesser toe(s) without damage to nail ▽

     √7ᵗʰ S91.106   Unspecified open wound of unspecified lesser toe(s) without damage to nail ▽

     √7ᵗʰ S91.109   Unspecified open wound of unspecified toe(s) without damage to nail ▽

   √6ᵗʰ S91.11   Laceration without foreign body of toe without damage to nail

     √7ᵗʰ S91.111   Laceration without foreign body of right great toe without damage to nail

     √7ᵗʰ S91.112   Laceration without foreign body of left great toe without damage to nail

     √7ᵗʰ S91.113   Laceration without foreign body of unspecified great toe without damage to nail ▽

     √7ᵗʰ S91.114   Laceration without foreign body of right lesser toe(s) without damage to nail

     √7ᵗʰ S91.115   Laceration without foreign body of left lesser toe(s) without damage to nail

     √7ᵗʰ S91.116   Laceration without foreign body of unspecified lesser toe(s) without damage to nail ▽

     √7ᵗʰ S91.119   Laceration without foreign body of unspecified toe without damage to nail ▽

   √6ᵗʰ S91.12   Laceration with foreign body of toe without damage to nail

     √7ᵗʰ S91.121   Laceration with foreign body of right great toe without damage to nail

     √7ᵗʰ S91.122   Laceration with foreign body of left great toe without damage to nail

     √7ᵗʰ S91.123   Laceration with foreign body of unspecified great toe without damage to nail ▽

     √7ᵗʰ S91.124   Laceration with foreign body of right lesser toe(s) without damage to nail

     √7ᵗʰ S91.125   Laceration with foreign body of left lesser toe(s) without damage to nail

     √7ᵗʰ S91.126   Laceration with foreign body of unspecified lesser toe(s) without damage to nail ▽

     √7ᵗʰ S91.129   Laceration with foreign body of unspecified toe(s) without damage to nail ▽

   √6ᵗʰ S91.13   Puncture wound without foreign body of toe without damage to nail

     √7ᵗʰ S91.131   Puncture wound without foreign body of right great toe without damage to nail

     √7ᵗʰ S91.132   Puncture wound without foreign body of left great toe without damage to nail

     √7ᵗʰ S91.133   Puncture wound without foreign body of unspecified great toe without damage to nail ▽

     √7ᵗʰ S91.134   Puncture wound without foreign body of right lesser toe(s) without damage to nail

     √7ᵗʰ S91.135   Puncture wound without foreign body of left lesser toe(s) without damage to nail

     √7ᵗʰ S91.136   Puncture wound without foreign body of unspecified lesser toe(s) without damage to nail ▽

     √7ᵗʰ S91.139   Puncture wound without foreign body of unspecified toe(s) without damage to nail ▽

   √6ᵗʰ S91.14   Puncture wound with foreign body of toe without damage to nail

     √7ᵗʰ S91.141   Puncture wound with foreign body of right great toe without damage to nail

     √7ᵗʰ S91.142   Puncture wound with foreign body of left great toe without damage to nail

     √7ᵗʰ S91.143   Puncture wound with foreign body of unspecified great toe without damage to nail ▽

     √7ᵗʰ S91.144   Puncture wound with foreign body of right lesser toe(s) without damage to nail

     √7ᵗʰ S91.145   Puncture wound with foreign body of left lesser toe(s) without damage to nail

     √7ᵗʰ S91.146   Puncture wound with foreign body of unspecified lesser toe(s) without damage to nail

     √7ᵗʰ S91.149   Puncture wound with foreign body of unspecified toe(s) without damage to nail ▽

   √6ᵗʰ S91.15   Open bite of toe without damage to nail

     Bite of toe NOS

     EXCLUDES 1   superficial bite of toe (S90.46-, S90.47-)

     √7ᵗʰ S91.151   Open bite of right great toe without damage to nail

     √7ᵗʰ S91.152   Open bite of left great toe without damage to nail

     √7ᵗʰ S91.153   Open bite of unspecified great toe without damage to nail ▽

     √7ᵗʰ S91.154   Open bite of right lesser toe(s) without damage to nail

     √7ᵗʰ S91.155   Open bite of left lesser toe(s) without damage to nail

√7ᵗʰ **S91.156** Open bite of unspecified lesser toe(s) without damage to nail ▽

√7ᵗʰ **S91.159** Open bite of unspecified toe(s) without damage to nail ▽

√5ᵗʰ **S91.2** Open wound of toe with damage to nail

  √6ᵗʰ **S91.20** Unspecified open wound of toe with damage to nail

    √7ᵗʰ **S91.201** Unspecified open wound of right great toe with damage to nail ▽

    √7ᵗʰ **S91.202** Unspecified open wound of left great toe with damage to nail ▽

    √7ᵗʰ **S91.203** Unspecified open wound of unspecified great toe with damage to nail ▽

    √7ᵗʰ **S91.204** Unspecified open wound of right lesser toe(s) with damage to nail ▽

    √7ᵗʰ **S91.205** Unspecified open wound of left lesser toe(s) with damage to nail ▽

    √7ᵗʰ **S91.206** Unspecified open wound of unspecified lesser toe(s) with damage to nail ▽

    √7ᵗʰ **S91.209** Unspecified open wound of unspecified toe(s) with damage to nail ▽

  √6ᵗʰ **S91.21** Laceration without foreign body of toe with damage to nail

    √7ᵗʰ **S91.211** Laceration without foreign body of right great toe with damage to nail

    √7ᵗʰ **S91.212** Laceration without foreign body of left great toe with damage to nail

    √7ᵗʰ **S91.213** Laceration without foreign body of unspecified great toe with damage to nail ▽

    √7ᵗʰ **S91.214** Laceration without foreign body of right lesser toe(s) with damage to nail ▽

    √7ᵗʰ **S91.215** Laceration without foreign body of left lesser toe(s) with damage to nail ▽

    √7ᵗʰ **S91.216** Laceration without foreign body of unspecified lesser toe(s) with damage to nail ▽

    √7ᵗʰ **S91.219** Laceration without foreign body of unspecified toe(s) with damage to nail ▽

  √6ᵗʰ **S91.22** Laceration with foreign body of toe with damage to nail

    √7ᵗʰ **S91.221** Laceration with foreign body of right great toe with damage to nail

    √7ᵗʰ **S91.222** Laceration with foreign body of left great toe with damage to nail

    √7ᵗʰ **S91.223** Laceration with foreign body of unspecified great toe with damage to nail ▽

    √7ᵗʰ **S91.224** Laceration with foreign body of right lesser toe(s) with damage to nail

    √7ᵗʰ **S91.225** Laceration with foreign body of left lesser toe(s) with damage to nail

    √7ᵗʰ **S91.226** Laceration with foreign body of unspecified lesser toe(s) with damage to nail ▽

    √7ᵗʰ **S91.229** Laceration with foreign body of unspecified toe(s) with damage to nail ▽

  √6ᵗʰ **S91.23** Puncture wound without foreign body of toe with damage to nail

    √7ᵗʰ **S91.231** Puncture wound without foreign body of right great toe with damage to nail

    √7ᵗʰ **S91.232** Puncture wound without foreign body of left great toe with damage to nail

    √7ᵗʰ **S91.233** Puncture wound without foreign body of unspecified great toe with damage to nail ▽

    √7ᵗʰ **S91.234** Puncture wound without foreign body of right lesser toe(s) with damage to nail

    √7ᵗʰ **S91.235** Puncture wound without foreign body of left lesser toe(s) with damage to nail

    √7ᵗʰ **S91.236** Puncture wound without foreign body of unspecified lesser toe(s) with damage to nail ▽

    √7ᵗʰ **S91.239** Puncture wound without foreign body of unspecified toe(s) with damage to nail ▽

  √6ᵗʰ **S91.24** Puncture wound with foreign body of toe with damage to nail

    √7ᵗʰ **S91.241** Puncture wound with foreign body of right great toe with damage to nail

    √7ᵗʰ **S91.242** Puncture wound with foreign body of left great toe with damage to nail

    √7ᵗʰ **S91.243** Puncture wound with foreign body of unspecified great toe with damage to nail ▽

    √7ᵗʰ **S91.244** Puncture wound with foreign body of right lesser toe(s) with damage to nail

    √7ᵗʰ **S91.245** Puncture wound with foreign body of left lesser toe(s) with damage to nail

    √7ᵗʰ **S91.246** Puncture wound with foreign body of unspecified lesser toe(s) with damage to nail ▽

    √7ᵗʰ **S91.249** Puncture wound with foreign body of unspecified toe(s) with damage to nail ▽

  √6ᵗʰ **S91.25** Open bite of toe with damage to nail

Bite of toe with damage to nail NOS

EXCLUDES 1   *superficial bite of toe (S90.46-, S90.47-)*

    √7ᵗʰ **S91.251** Open bite of right great toe with damage to nail

    √7ᵗʰ **S91.252** Open bite of left great toe with damage to nail

    √7ᵗʰ **S91.253** Open bite of unspecified great toe with damage to nail ▽

    √7ᵗʰ **S91.254** Open bite of right lesser toe(s) with damage to nail

    √7ᵗʰ **S91.255** Open bite of left lesser toe(s) with damage to nail

    √7ᵗʰ **S91.256** Open bite of unspecified lesser toe(s) with damage to nail ▽

    √7ᵗʰ **S91.259** Open bite of unspecified toe(s) with damage to nail ▽

√5ᵗʰ **S91.3** Open wound of foot

  √6ᵗʰ **S91.30** Unspecified open wound of foot

    √7ᵗʰ **S91.301** Unspecified open wound, right foot ▽

    √7ᵗʰ **S91.302** Unspecified open wound, left foot ▽

    √7ᵗʰ **S91.309** Unspecified open wound, unspecified foot ▽

  √6ᵗʰ **S91.31** Laceration without foreign body of foot

    √7ᵗʰ **S91.311** Laceration without foreign body, right foot

    √7ᵗʰ **S91.312** Laceration without foreign body, left foot

    √7ᵗʰ **S91.319** Laceration without foreign body, unspecified foot ▽

  √6ᵗʰ **S91.32** Laceration with foreign body of foot

    √7ᵗʰ **S91.321** Laceration with foreign body, right foot

    √7ᵗʰ **S91.322** Laceration with foreign body, left foot

    √7ᵗʰ **S91.329** Laceration with foreign body, unspecified foot ▽

  √6ᵗʰ **S91.33** Puncture wound without foreign body of foot

    √7ᵗʰ **S91.331** Puncture wound without foreign body, right foot

    √7ᵗʰ **S91.332** Puncture wound without foreign body, left foot

    √7ᵗʰ **S91.339** Puncture wound without foreign body, unspecified foot ▽

  √6ᵗʰ **S91.34** Puncture wound with foreign body of foot

    √7ᵗʰ **S91.341** Puncture wound with foreign body, right foot

    √7ᵗʰ **S91.342** Puncture wound with foreign body, left foot

    √7ᵗʰ **S91.349** Puncture wound with foreign body, unspecified foot ▽

  √6ᵗʰ **S91.35** Open bite of foot

EXCLUDES 1   *superficial bite of foot (S90.86-, S90.87-)*

    √7ᵗʰ **S91.351** Open bite, right foot

    √7ᵗʰ **S91.352** Open bite, left foot

    √7ᵗʰ **S91.359** Open bite, unspecified foot ▽

✔ Additional Character Req	√x7ᵗʰ Placeholder Alert	**Manifestation**	▽ Unspecified	▶◀ Revised Text	● New Code	▲ Revised Code Title

ICD-10-CM 2019   **1063**

✓4ᵗʰ S92 Fracture of foot and toe, except ankle

> **NOTE** A fracture not indicated as displaced or nondisplaced should be coded to displaced
>
> A fracture not indicated as open or closed should be coded to closed.

EXCLUDES 1   *traumatic amputation of ankle and foot (S98.-)*

EXCLUDES 2   *fracture of ankle (S82.-)*

           fracture of malleolus (S82.-)

AHA: 2018,2Q,12; 2015,3Q,37-39

The appropriate 7th character is to be added to each code from category S92.

A   initial encounter for closed fracture
B   initial encounter for open fracture
D   subsequent encounter for fracture with routine healing
G   subsequent encounter for fracture with delayed healing
K   subsequent encounter for fracture with nonunion
P   subsequent encounter for fracture with malunion
S   sequela

✓5ᵗʰ S92.0 Fracture of calcaneus

Heel bone
Os calcis

EXCLUDES 2   *physeal fracture of calcaneus (S99.0-)*

✓6ᵗʰ S92.00 Unspecified fracture of calcaneus

- ✓7ᵗʰ S92.001 Unspecified fracture of right calcaneus ▫ ▽
- ✓7ᵗʰ S92.002 Unspecified fracture of left calcaneus ▫ ▽
- ✓7ᵗʰ S92.009 Unspecified fracture of unspecified calcaneus ▫ ▽

✓6ᵗʰ S92.01 Fracture of body of calcaneus

- ✓7ᵗʰ S92.011 Displaced fracture of body of right calcaneus ▫
- ✓7ᵗʰ S92.012 Displaced fracture of body of left calcaneus ▫
- ✓7ᵗʰ S92.013 Displaced fracture of body of unspecified calcaneus ▫ ▽
- ✓7ᵗʰ S92.014 Nondisplaced fracture of body of right calcaneus ▫
- ✓7ᵗʰ S92.015 Nondisplaced fracture of body of left calcaneus ▫
- ✓7ᵗʰ S92.016 Nondisplaced fracture of body of unspecified calcaneus ▫ ▽

✓6ᵗʰ S92.02 Fracture of anterior process of calcaneus

- ✓7ᵗʰ S92.021 Displaced fracture of anterior process of right calcaneus ▫
- ✓7ᵗʰ S92.022 Displaced fracture of anterior process of left calcaneus ▫
- ✓7ᵗʰ S92.023 Displaced fracture of anterior process of unspecified calcaneus ▫ ▽
- ✓7ᵗʰ S92.024 Nondisplaced fracture of anterior process of right calcaneus ▫
- ✓7ᵗʰ S92.025 Nondisplaced fracture of anterior process of left calcaneus ▫
- ✓7ᵗʰ S92.026 Nondisplaced fracture of anterior process of unspecified calcaneus ▫ ▽

✓6ᵗʰ S92.03 Avulsion fracture of tuberosity of calcaneus

- ✓7ᵗʰ S92.031 Displaced avulsion fracture of tuberosity of right calcaneus ▫
- ✓7ᵗʰ S92.032 Displaced avulsion fracture of tuberosity of left calcaneus ▫
- ✓7ᵗʰ S92.033 Displaced avulsion fracture of tuberosity of unspecified calcaneus ▫ ▽
- ✓7ᵗʰ S92.034 Nondisplaced avulsion fracture of tuberosity of right calcaneus ▫
- ✓7ᵗʰ S92.035 Nondisplaced avulsion fracture of tuberosity of left calcaneus ▫
- ✓7ᵗʰ S92.036 Nondisplaced avulsion fracture of tuberosity of unspecified calcaneus ▫ ▽

✓6ᵗʰ S92.04 Other fracture of tuberosity of calcaneus

- ✓7ᵗʰ S92.041 Displaced other fracture of tuberosity of right calcaneus ▫
- ✓7ᵗʰ S92.042 Displaced other fracture of tuberosity of left calcaneus ▫
- ✓7ᵗʰ S92.043 Displaced other fracture of tuberosity of unspecified calcaneus ▫ ▽
- ✓7ᵗʰ S92.044 Nondisplaced other fracture of tuberosity of right calcaneus ▫
- ✓7ᵗʰ S92.045 Nondisplaced other fracture of tuberosity of left calcaneus ▫
- ✓7ᵗʰ S92.046 Nondisplaced other fracture of tuberosity of unspecified calcaneus ▫ ▽

✓6ᵗʰ S92.05 Other extraarticular fracture of calcaneus

- ✓7ᵗʰ S92.051 Displaced other extraarticular fracture of right calcaneus ▫
- ✓7ᵗʰ S92.052 Displaced other extraarticular fracture of left calcaneus ▫
- ✓7ᵗʰ S92.053 Displaced other extraarticular fracture of unspecified calcaneus ▫ ▽
- ✓7ᵗʰ S92.054 Nondisplaced other extraarticular fracture of right calcaneus ▫
- ✓7ᵗʰ S92.055 Nondisplaced other extraarticular fracture of left calcaneus ▫
- ✓7ᵗʰ S92.056 Nondisplaced other extraarticular fracture of unspecified calcaneus ▫ ▽

✓6ᵗʰ S92.06 Intraarticular fracture of calcaneus

- ✓7ᵗʰ S92.061 Displaced intraarticular fracture of right calcaneus ▫
- ✓7ᵗʰ S92.062 Displaced intraarticular fracture of left calcaneus ▫
- ✓7ᵗʰ S92.063 Displaced intraarticular fracture of unspecified calcaneus ▫ ▽
- ✓7ᵗʰ S92.064 Nondisplaced intraarticular fracture of right calcaneus ▫
- ✓7ᵗʰ S92.065 Nondisplaced intraarticular fracture of left calcaneus ▫
- ✓7ᵗʰ S92.066 Nondisplaced intraarticular fracture of unspecified calcaneus ▫ ▽

✓5ᵗʰ S92.1 Fracture of talus

Astragalus

✓6ᵗʰ S92.10 Unspecified fracture of talus

- ✓7ᵗʰ S92.101 Unspecified fracture of right talus ▫ ▽
- ✓7ᵗʰ S92.102 Unspecified fracture of left talus ▫ ▽
- ✓7ᵗʰ S92.109 Unspecified fracture of unspecified talus ▫ ▽

✓6ᵗʰ S92.11 Fracture of neck of talus

- ✓7ᵗʰ S92.111 Displaced fracture of neck of right talus ▫
- ✓7ᵗʰ S92.112 Displaced fracture of neck of left talus ▫
- ✓7ᵗʰ S92.113 Displaced fracture of neck of unspecified talus ▫ ▽
- ✓7ᵗʰ S92.114 Nondisplaced fracture of neck of right talus ▫
- ✓7ᵗʰ S92.115 Nondisplaced fracture of neck of left talus ▫
- ✓7ᵗʰ S92.116 Nondisplaced fracture of neck of unspecified talus ▫ ▽

✓6ᵗʰ S92.12 Fracture of body of talus

- ✓7ᵗʰ S92.121 Displaced fracture of body of right talus ▫
- ✓7ᵗʰ S92.122 Displaced fracture of body of left talus ▫
- ✓7ᵗʰ S92.123 Displaced fracture of body of unspecified talus ▫ ▽
- ✓7ᵗʰ S92.124 Nondisplaced fracture of body of right talus ▫
- ✓7ᵗʰ S92.125 Nondisplaced fracture of body of left talus ▫
- ✓7ᵗʰ S92.126 Nondisplaced fracture of body of unspecified talus ▫ ▽

✓6ᵗʰ S92.13 Fracture of posterior process of talus

- ✓7ᵗʰ S92.131 Displaced fracture of posterior process of right talus ▫
- ✓7ᵗʰ S92.132 Displaced fracture of posterior process of left talus ▫
- ✓7ᵗʰ S92.133 Displaced fracture of posterior process of unspecified talus ▫ ▽
- ✓7ᵗʰ S92.134 Nondisplaced fracture of posterior process of right talus ▫
- ✓7ᵗʰ S92.135 Nondisplaced fracture of posterior process of left talus ▫
- ✓7ᵗʰ S92.136 Nondisplaced fracture of posterior process of unspecified talus ▫ ▽

√6ᵗʰ **S92.14** **Dome** fracture of talus

     EXCLUDES 1   osteochondritis dissecans (M93.2)

   √7ᵗʰ **S92.141** **Displaced dome fracture of right** talus   Q

   √7ᵗʰ **S92.142** **Displaced dome fracture of left** talus   Q

   √7ᵗʰ **S92.143** **Displaced dome fracture of unspecified talus**   Q ▽

   √7ᵗʰ **S92.144** **Nondisplaced dome fracture of right talus**   Q

   √7ᵗʰ **S92.145** **Nondisplaced dome fracture of left talus**   Q

   √7ᵗʰ **S92.146** **Nondisplaced dome fracture of unspecified talus**   Q ▽

√6ᵗʰ **S92.15** **Avulsion** fracture (chip fracture) of talus

   √7ᵗʰ **S92.151** **Displaced avulsion fracture (chip fracture) of right talus**   Q

   √7ᵗʰ **S92.152** **Displaced avulsion fracture (chip fracture) of left talus**   Q

   √7ᵗʰ **S92.153** **Displaced avulsion fracture (chip fracture) of unspecified talus**   Q ▽

   √7ᵗʰ **S92.154** **Nondisplaced avulsion fracture (chip fracture) of right talus**   Q

   √7ᵗʰ **S92.155** **Nondisplaced avulsion fracture (chip fracture) of left talus**   Q

   √7ᵗʰ **S92.156** **Nondisplaced avulsion fracture (chip fracture) of unspecified talus**   Q ▽

√6ᵗʰ **S92.19** **Other** fracture of talus

   √7ᵗʰ **S92.191** **Other fracture of right talus**   Q

   √7ᵗʰ **S92.192** **Other fracture of left talus**   Q

   √7ᵗʰ **S92.199** **Other fracture of unspecified talus**   Q ▽

√5ᵗʰ **S92.2** **Fracture of other and unspecified tarsal bone(s)**

√6ᵗʰ **S92.20** **Fracture of unspecified tarsal bone(s)**

   √7ᵗʰ **S92.201** **Fracture of unspecified tarsal bone(s) of right foot**   Q ▽

   √7ᵗʰ **S92.202** **Fracture of unspecified tarsal bone(s) of left foot**   Q ▽

   √7ᵗʰ **S92.209** **Fracture of unspecified tarsal bone(s) of unspecified foot**   Q ▽

√6ᵗʰ **S92.21** **Fracture of cuboid bone**

   √7ᵗʰ **S92.211** **Displaced fracture of cuboid bone of right foot**   Q

   √7ᵗʰ **S92.212** **Displaced fracture of cuboid bone of left foot**   Q

   √7ᵗʰ **S92.213** **Displaced fracture of cuboid bone of unspecified foot**   Q ▽

   √7ᵗʰ **S92.214** **Nondisplaced fracture of cuboid bone of right foot**   Q

   √7ᵗʰ **S92.215** **Nondisplaced fracture of cuboid bone of left foot**   Q

   √7ᵗʰ **S92.216** **Nondisplaced fracture of cuboid bone of unspecified foot**   Q ▽

√6ᵗʰ **S92.22** **Fracture of lateral cuneiform**

   √7ᵗʰ **S92.221** **Displaced fracture of lateral cuneiform of right foot**   Q

   √7ᵗʰ **S92.222** **Displaced fracture of lateral cuneiform of left foot**   Q

   √7ᵗʰ **S92.223** **Displaced fracture of lateral cuneiform of unspecified foot**   Q ▽

   √7ᵗʰ **S92.224** **Nondisplaced fracture of lateral cuneiform of right foot**   Q

   √7ᵗʰ **S92.225** **Nondisplaced fracture of lateral cuneiform of left foot**   Q

   √7ᵗʰ **S92.226** **Nondisplaced fracture of lateral cuneiform of unspecified foot**   Q ▽

√6ᵗʰ **S92.23** **Fracture of intermediate cuneiform**

   √7ᵗʰ **S92.231** **Displaced fracture of intermediate cuneiform of right foot**   Q

   √7ᵗʰ **S92.232** **Displaced fracture of intermediate cuneiform of left foot**   Q

   √7ᵗʰ **S92.233** **Displaced fracture of intermediate cuneiform of unspecified foot**   Q ▽

   √7ᵗʰ **S92.234** **Nondisplaced fracture of intermediate cuneiform of right foot**   Q

   √7ᵗʰ **S92.235** **Nondisplaced fracture of intermediate cuneiform of left foot**   Q

   √7ᵗʰ **S92.236** **Nondisplaced fracture of intermediate cuneiform of unspecified foot**   Q ▽

√6ᵗʰ **S92.24** **Fracture of medial cuneiform**

   √7ᵗʰ **S92.241** **Displaced fracture of medial cuneiform of right foot**   Q

   √7ᵗʰ **S92.242** **Displaced fracture of medial cuneiform of left foot**   Q

   √7ᵗʰ **S92.243** **Displaced fracture of medial cuneiform of unspecified foot**   Q ▽

   √7ᵗʰ **S92.244** **Nondisplaced fracture of medial cuneiform of right foot**   Q

   √7ᵗʰ **S92.245** **Nondisplaced fracture of medial cuneiform of left foot**   Q

   √7ᵗʰ **S92.246** **Nondisplaced fracture of medial cuneiform of unspecified foot**   Q ▽

√6ᵗʰ **S92.25** **Fracture of navicular [scaphoid] of foot**

   √7ᵗʰ **S92.251** **Displaced fracture of navicular [scaphoid] of right foot**   Q

   √7ᵗʰ **S92.252** **Displaced fracture of navicular [scaphoid] of left foot**   Q

   √7ᵗʰ **S92.253** **Displaced fracture of navicular [scaphoid] of unspecified foot**   Q ▽

   √7ᵗʰ **S92.254** **Nondisplaced fracture of navicular [scaphoid] of right foot**   Q

   √7ᵗʰ **S92.255** **Nondisplaced fracture of navicular [scaphoid] of left foot**   Q

   √7ᵗʰ **S92.256** **Nondisplaced fracture of navicular [scaphoid] of unspecified foot**   Q ▽

√5ᵗʰ **S92.3** **Fracture of metatarsal bone(s)**

     EXCLUDES 2   physeal fracture of metatarsal (S99.1-)

     AHA: 2018,1Q,3

√6ᵗʰ **S92.30** **Fracture of unspecified metatarsal bone(s)**

   √7ᵗʰ **S92.301** **Fracture of unspecified metatarsal bone(s), right foot**   Q ▽

   √7ᵗʰ **S92.302** **Fracture of unspecified metatarsal bone(s), left foot**   Q ▽

   √7ᵗʰ **S92.309** **Fracture of unspecified metatarsal bone(s), unspecified foot**   Q ▽

√6ᵗʰ **S92.31** **Fracture of first metatarsal bone**

   √7ᵗʰ **S92.311** **Displaced fracture of first metatarsal bone, right foot**   Q

   √7ᵗʰ **S92.312** **Displaced fracture of first metatarsal bone, left foot**   Q

   √7ᵗʰ **S92.313** **Displaced fracture of first metatarsal bone, unspecified foot**   Q ▽

   √7ᵗʰ **S92.314** **Nondisplaced fracture of first metatarsal bone, right foot**   Q

   √7ᵗʰ **S92.315** **Nondisplaced fracture of first metatarsal bone, left foot**   Q

   √7ᵗʰ **S92.316** **Nondisplaced fracture of first metatarsal bone, unspecified foot**   Q ▽

√6ᵗʰ **S92.32** **Fracture of second metatarsal bone**

   √7ᵗʰ **S92.321** **Displaced fracture of second metatarsal bone, right foot**   Q

   √7ᵗʰ **S92.322** **Displaced fracture of second metatarsal bone, left foot**   Q

   √7ᵗʰ **S92.323** **Displaced fracture of second metatarsal bone, unspecified foot**   Q ▽

   √7ᵗʰ **S92.324** **Nondisplaced fracture of second metatarsal bone, right foot**   Q

   √7ᵗʰ **S92.325** **Nondisplaced fracture of second metatarsal bone, left foot**   Q

   √7ᵗʰ **S92.326** **Nondisplaced fracture of second metatarsal bone, unspecified foot**   Q ▽

√6ᵗʰ **S92.33** **Fracture of third metatarsal bone**

   √7ᵗʰ **S92.331** **Displaced fracture of third metatarsal bone, right foot**   Q

   √7ᵗʰ **S92.332** **Displaced fracture of third metatarsal bone, left foot**   Q

   √7ᵗʰ **S92.333** **Displaced fracture of third metatarsal bone, unspecified foot**   Q ▽

   √7ᵗʰ **S92.334** **Nondisplaced fracture of third metatarsal bone, right foot**   Q

   √7ᵗʰ **S92.335** **Nondisplaced fracture of third metatarsal bone, left foot**   Q

☑ Additional Character Req   ☑7ᵗʰ Placeholder Alert   Manifestation   ▽ Unspecified   ►◄ Revised Text   ● New Code   ▲ Revised Code Title

ICD-10-CM 2019   **1065**

✓7ᵗʰ **S92.336** Nondisplaced fracture of third metatarsal bone, unspecified foot ▢ ▽

✓6ᵗʰ **S92.34** Fracture of fourth metatarsal bone

   ✓7ᵗʰ **S92.341** Displaced fracture of fourth metatarsal bone, right foot ▢

   ✓7ᵗʰ **S92.342** Displaced fracture of fourth metatarsal bone, left foot ▢

   ✓7ᵗʰ **S92.343** Displaced fracture of fourth metatarsal bone, unspecified foot ▢ ▽

   ✓7ᵗʰ **S92.344** Nondisplaced fracture of fourth metatarsal bone, right foot ▢

   ✓7ᵗʰ **S92.345** Nondisplaced fracture of fourth metatarsal bone, left foot ▢

   ✓7ᵗʰ **S92.346** Nondisplaced fracture of fourth metatarsal bone, unspecified foot ▢ ▽

✓6ᵗʰ **S92.35** Fracture of fifth metatarsal bone

   ✓7ᵗʰ **S92.351** Displaced fracture of fifth metatarsal bone, right foot ▢

   ✓7ᵗʰ **S92.352** Displaced fracture of fifth metatarsal bone, left foot ▢

   ✓7ᵗʰ **S92.353** Displaced fracture of fifth metatarsal bone, unspecified foot ▢ ▽

   ✓7ᵗʰ **S92.354** Nondisplaced fracture of fifth metatarsal bone, right foot ▢

   ✓7ᵗʰ **S92.355** Nondisplaced fracture of fifth metatarsal bone, left foot ▢

   ✓7ᵗʰ **S92.356** Nondisplaced fracture of fifth metatarsal bone, unspecified foot ▢ ▽

✓5ᵗʰ **S92.4** Fracture of great toe

   EXCLUDES 2   *physeal fracture of phalanx of toe (S99.2-)*

✓6ᵗʰ **S92.40** Unspecified fracture of great toe

   ✓7ᵗʰ **S92.401** Displaced unspecified fracture of right great toe ▽

   ✓7ᵗʰ **S92.402** Displaced unspecified fracture of left great toe ▽

   ✓7ᵗʰ **S92.403** Displaced unspecified fracture of unspecified great toe ▽

   ✓7ᵗʰ **S92.404** Nondisplaced unspecified fracture of right great toe ▽

   ✓7ᵗʰ **S92.405** Nondisplaced unspecified fracture of left great toe ▽

   ✓7ᵗʰ **S92.406** Nondisplaced unspecified fracture of unspecified great toe ▽

✓6ᵗʰ **S92.41** Fracture of proximal phalanx of great toe

   ✓7ᵗʰ **S92.411** Displaced fracture of proximal phalanx of right great toe

   ✓7ᵗʰ **S92.412** Displaced fracture of proximal phalanx of left great toe

   ✓7ᵗʰ **S92.413** Displaced fracture of proximal phalanx of unspecified great toe ▽

   ✓7ᵗʰ **S92.414** Nondisplaced fracture of proximal phalanx of right great toe

   ✓7ᵗʰ **S92.415** Nondisplaced fracture of proximal phalanx of left great toe

   ✓7ᵗʰ **S92.416** Nondisplaced fracture of proximal phalanx of unspecified great toe ▽

✓6ᵗʰ **S92.42** Fracture of distal phalanx of great toe

   ✓7ᵗʰ **S92.421** Displaced fracture of distal phalanx of right great toe

   ✓7ᵗʰ **S92.422** Displaced fracture of distal phalanx of left great toe

   ✓7ᵗʰ **S92.423** Displaced fracture of distal phalanx of unspecified great toe ▽

   ✓7ᵗʰ **S92.424** Nondisplaced fracture of distal phalanx of right great toe

   ✓7ᵗʰ **S92.425** Nondisplaced fracture of distal phalanx of left great toe

   ✓7ᵗʰ **S92.426** Nondisplaced fracture of distal phalanx of unspecified great toe ▽

✓6ᵗʰ **S92.49** Other fracture of great toe

   ✓7ᵗʰ **S92.491** Other fracture of right great toe

   ✓7ᵗʰ **S92.492** Other fracture of left great toe

   ✓7ᵗʰ **S92.499** Other fracture of unspecified great toe ▽

✓5ᵗʰ **S92.5** Fracture of lesser toe(s)

   EXCLUDES 2   *physeal fracture of phalanx of toe (S99.2-)*

✓6ᵗʰ **S92.50** Unspecified fracture of lesser toe(s)

   ✓7ᵗʰ **S92.501** Displaced unspecified fracture of right lesser toe(s) ▽

✓7ᵗʰ **S92.502** Displaced unspecified fracture of left lesser toe(s) ▽

✓7ᵗʰ **S92.503** Displaced unspecified fracture of unspecified lesser toe(s) ▽

✓7ᵗʰ **S92.504** Nondisplaced unspecified fracture of right lesser toe(s) ▽

✓7ᵗʰ **S92.505** Nondisplaced unspecified fracture of left lesser toe(s) ▽

✓7ᵗʰ **S92.506** Nondisplaced unspecified fracture of unspecified lesser toe(s) ▽

✓6ᵗʰ **S92.51** Fracture of proximal phalanx of lesser toe(s)

   ✓7ᵗʰ **S92.511** Displaced fracture of proximal phalanx of right lesser toe(s)

   ✓7ᵗʰ **S92.512** Displaced fracture of proximal phalanx of left lesser toe(s)

   ✓7ᵗʰ **S92.513** Displaced fracture of proximal phalanx of unspecified lesser toe(s) ▽

   ✓7ᵗʰ **S92.514** Nondisplaced fracture of proximal phalanx of right lesser toe(s)

   ✓7ᵗʰ **S92.515** Nondisplaced fracture of proximal phalanx of left lesser toe(s))

   ✓7ᵗʰ **S92.516** Nondisplaced fracture of proximal phalanx of unspecified lesser toe(s) ▽

✓6ᵗʰ **S92.52** Fracture of middle phalanx of lesser toe(s)

   ✓7ᵗʰ **S92.521** Displaced fracture of middle phalanx of right lesser toe(s)

   ✓7ᵗʰ **S92.522** Displaced fracture of middle phalanx of left lesser toe(s)

   ✓7ᵗʰ **S92.523** Displaced fracture of middle phalanx of unspecified lesser toe(s) ▽

   ✓7ᵗʰ **S92.524** Nondisplaced fracture of middle phalanx of right lesser toe(s)

   ✓7ᵗʰ **S92.525** Nondisplaced fracture of middle phalanx of left lesser toe(s)

   ✓7ᵗʰ **S92.526** Nondisplaced fracture of middle phalanx of unspecified lesser toe(s) ▽

✓6ᵗʰ **S92.53** Fracture of distal phalanx of lesser toe(s)

   ✓7ᵗʰ **S92.531** Displaced fracture of distal phalanx of right lesser toe(s)

   ✓7ᵗʰ **S92.532** Displaced fracture of distal phalanx of left lesser toe(s)

   ✓7ᵗʰ **S92.533** Displaced fracture of distal phalanx of unspecified lesser toe(s) ▽

   ✓7ᵗʰ **S92.534** Nondisplaced fracture of distal phalanx of right lesser toe(s)

   ✓7ᵗʰ **S92.535** Nondisplaced fracture of distal phalanx of left lesser toe(s)

   ✓7ᵗʰ **S92.536** Nondisplaced fracture of distal phalanx of unspecified lesser toe(s) ▽

✓6ᵗʰ **S92.59** Other fracture of lesser toe(s)

   ✓7ᵗʰ **S92.591** Other fracture of right lesser toe(s)

   ✓7ᵗʰ **S92.592** Other fracture of left lesser toe(s)

   ✓7ᵗʰ **S92.599** Other fracture of unspecified lesser toe(s) ▽

✓5ᵗʰ **S92.8** Other fracture of foot, except ankle

✓6ᵗʰ **S92.81** Other fracture of foot

   Sesamoid fracture of foot

   AHA: 2016,4Q,68

   ✓7ᵗʰ **S92.811** Other fracture of right foot ▢

   ✓7ᵗʰ **S92.812** Other fracture of left foot ▢

   ✓7ᵗʰ **S92.819** Other fracture of unspecified foot ▢ ▽

✓5ᵗʰ **S92.9** Unspecified fracture of foot and toe

✓6ᵗʰ **S92.90** Unspecified fracture of foot

   ✓7ᵗʰ **S92.901** Unspecified fracture of right foot ▢ ▽

   ✓7ᵗʰ **S92.902** Unspecified fracture of left foot ▢ ▽

   ✓7ᵗʰ **S92.909** Unspecified fracture of unspecified foot ▢ ▽

✓6ᵗʰ **S92.91** Unspecified fracture of toe

   ✓7ᵗʰ **S92.911** Unspecified fracture of right toe(s) ▽

   ✓7ᵗʰ **S92.912** Unspecified fracture of left toe(s) ▽

√7ᵗʰ **S92.919** **Unspecified fracture of unspecified toe(s)** ▽

√4ᵗʰ **S93** **Dislocation and sprain of joints and ligaments at ankle, foot and toe level**

> INCLUDES   avulsion of joint or ligament of ankle, foot and toe
> laceration of cartilage, joint or ligament of ankle, foot and toe
> sprain of cartilage, joint or ligament of ankle, foot and toe
> traumatic hemarthrosis of joint or ligament of ankle, foot and toe
> traumatic rupture of joint or ligament of ankle, foot and toe
> traumatic subluxation of joint or ligament of ankle, foot and toe
> traumatic tear of joint or ligament of ankle, foot and toe

Code also any associated open wound

> EXCLUDES 2   strain of muscle and tendon of ankle and foot (S96.-)

> The appropriate 7th character is to be added to each code from category S93.
> A   initial encounter
> D   subsequent encounter
> S   sequela

√5ᵗʰ **S93.0** **Subluxation and dislocation of ankle joint**

Subluxation and dislocation of astragalus
Subluxation and dislocation of fibula, lower end
Subluxation and dislocation of talus
Subluxation and dislocation of tibia, lower end

√x7ᵗʰ **S93.01** **Subluxation** of **right** ankle joint

√x7ᵗʰ **S93.02** **Subluxation** of **left** ankle joint

√x7ᵗʰ **S93.03** **Subluxation** of **unspecified** ankle joint ▽

√x7ᵗʰ **S93.04** **Dislocation** of **right** ankle joint

√x7ᵗʰ **S93.05** **Dislocation** of **left** ankle joint

√x7ᵗʰ **S93.06** **Dislocation** of **unspecified** ankle joint ▽

√5ᵗʰ **S93.1** **Subluxation and dislocation of** toe

√6ᵗʰ **S93.10** **Unspecified subluxation and dislocation of toe**

Dislocation of toe NOS
Subluxation of toe NOS

√7ᵗʰ **S93.101** **Unspecified** subluxation of **right** toe(s) ▽

√7ᵗʰ **S93.102** **Unspecified** subluxation of **left** toe(s) ▽

√7ᵗʰ **S93.103** **Unspecified** subluxation of **unspecified** toe(s) ▽

√7ᵗʰ **S93.104** **Unspecified** dislocation of **right** toe(s) ▽

√7ᵗʰ **S93.105** **Unspecified** dislocation of **left** toe(s) ▽

√7ᵗʰ **S93.106** **Unspecified** dislocation of **unspecified** toe(s) ▽

√6ᵗʰ **S93.11** **Dislocation of** interphalangeal joint

√7ᵗʰ **S93.111** **Dislocation of interphalangeal joint of right great** toe

√7ᵗʰ **S93.112** **Dislocation of interphalangeal joint of left great** toe

√7ᵗʰ **S93.113** **Dislocation of interphalangeal joint of unspecified great toe** ▽

√7ᵗʰ **S93.114** **Dislocation of interphalangeal joint of right lesser** toe(s)

√7ᵗʰ **S93.115** **Dislocation of interphalangeal joint of left lesser** toe(s)

√7ᵗʰ **S93.116** **Dislocation of interphalangeal joint of unspecified lesser toe(s)** ▽

√7ᵗʰ **S93.119** **Dislocation of interphalangeal joint of unspecified toe(s)** ▽

√6ᵗʰ **S93.12** **Dislocation of** metatarsophalangeal joint

√7ᵗʰ **S93.121** **Dislocation of metatarsophalangeal joint of right great toe**

√7ᵗʰ **S93.122** **Dislocation of metatarsophalangeal joint of left great toe**

√7ᵗʰ **S93.123** **Dislocation of metatarsophalangeal joint of unspecified great toe** ▽

√7ᵗʰ **S93.124** **Dislocation of metatarsophalangeal joint of right lesser** toe(s)

√7ᵗʰ **S93.125** **Dislocation of metatarsophalangeal joint of left lesser** toe(s)

√7ᵗʰ **S93.126** **Dislocation of metatarsophalangeal joint of unspecified lesser toe(s)** ▽

√7ᵗʰ **S93.129** **Dislocation of metatarsophalangeal joint of unspecified toe(s)** ▽

√6ᵗʰ **S93.13** **Subluxation of** interphalangeal joint

√7ᵗʰ **S93.131** **Subluxation of interphalangeal joint of right great** toe

√7ᵗʰ **S93.132** **Subluxation of interphalangeal joint of left great** toe

√7ᵗʰ **S93.133** **Subluxation of interphalangeal joint of unspecified great toe**

√7ᵗʰ **S93.134** **Subluxation of interphalangeal joint of right lesser** toe(s)

√7ᵗʰ **S93.135** **Subluxation of interphalangeal joint of left lesser** toe(s)

√7ᵗʰ **S93.136** **Subluxation of interphalangeal joint of unspecified lesser toe(s)** ▽

√7ᵗʰ **S93.139** **Subluxation of interphalangeal joint of unspecified toe(s)** ▽

√6ᵗʰ **S93.14** **Subluxation of** metatarsophalangeal joint

√7ᵗʰ **S93.141** **Subluxation of metatarsophalangeal joint of right great** toe

√7ᵗʰ **S93.142** **Subluxation of metatarsophalangeal joint of left great** toe

√7ᵗʰ **S93.143** **Subluxation of metatarsophalangeal joint of unspecified great toe** ▽

√7ᵗʰ **S93.144** **Subluxation of metatarsophalangeal joint of right lesser** toe(s)

√7ᵗʰ **S93.145** **Subluxation of metatarsophalangeal joint of left lesser** toe(s)

√7ᵗʰ **S93.146** **Subluxation of metatarsophalangeal joint of unspecified lesser toe(s)** ▽

√7ᵗʰ **S93.149** **Subluxation of metatarsophalangeal joint of unspecified toe(s)** ▽

√5ᵗʰ **S93.3** **Subluxation and dislocation of** foot

> EXCLUDES 2   dislocation of toe (S93.1-)

√6ᵗʰ **S93.30** **Unspecified subluxation and dislocation of foot**

Dislocation of foot NOS
Subluxation of foot NOS

√7ᵗʰ **S93.301** **Unspecified** subluxation of **right** foot ▽

√7ᵗʰ **S93.302** **Unspecified** subluxation of **left** foot ▽

√7ᵗʰ **S93.303** **Unspecified** subluxation of **unspecified** foot ▽

√7ᵗʰ **S93.304** **Unspecified** dislocation of **right** foot ▽

√7ᵗʰ **S93.305** **Unspecified** dislocation of **left** foot ▽

√7ᵗʰ **S93.306** **Unspecified** dislocation of **unspecified** foot ▽

√6ᵗʰ **S93.31** **Subluxation and dislocation of** tarsal joint

√7ᵗʰ **S93.311** **Subluxation** of tarsal joint of **right** foot

√7ᵗʰ **S93.312** **Subluxation** of tarsal joint of **left** foot

√7ᵗʰ **S93.313** **Subluxation** of tarsal joint of **unspecified** foot ▽

√7ᵗʰ **S93.314** **Dislocation** of tarsal joint of **right** foot

√7ᵗʰ **S93.315** **Dislocation** of tarsal joint of **left** foot

√7ᵗʰ **S93.316** **Dislocation** of tarsal joint of **unspecified** foot ▽

√6ᵗʰ **S93.32** **Subluxation and dislocation of** tarsometatarsal joint

√7ᵗʰ **S93.321** **Subluxation** of tarsometatarsal joint of **right** foot

√7ᵗʰ **S93.322** **Subluxation** of tarsometatarsal joint of **left** foot

√7ᵗʰ **S93.323** **Subluxation** of tarsometatarsal joint of **unspecified** foot ▽

√7ᵗʰ **S93.324** **Dislocation** of tarsometatarsal joint of **right** foot

√7ᵗʰ **S93.325** **Dislocation** of tarsometatarsal joint of **left** foot

√7ᵗʰ **S93.326** **Dislocation** of tarsometatarsal joint of **unspecified** foot ▽

☑ Additional Character Req   √x7ᵗʰ Placeholder Alert   Manifestation   ▽ Unspecified   ►◄ Revised Text   ● New Code   ▲ Revised Code Title

√6ᵗʰ **S93.33** Other subluxation and dislocation of foot

  √7ᵗʰ **S93.331** Other subluxation of right foot

  √7ᵗʰ **S93.332** Other subluxation of left foot

  √7ᵗʰ **S93.333** Other subluxation of unspecified foot ▽

  √7ᵗʰ **S93.334** Other dislocation of right foot

  √7ᵗʰ **S93.335** Other dislocation of left foot

  √7ᵗʰ **S93.336** Other dislocation of unspecified foot ▽

√5ᵗʰ **S93.4** Sprain of ankle

  EXCLUDES 2   injury of Achilles tendon (S86.0-)

  √6ᵗʰ **S93.40** Sprain of unspecified ligament of ankle

    Sprain of ankle NOS

    Sprained ankle NOS

    √7ᵗʰ **S93.401** Sprain of unspecified ligament of right ankle ▽

    √7ᵗʰ **S93.402** Sprain of unspecified ligament of left ankle ▽

    √7ᵗʰ **S93.409** Sprain of unspecified ligament of unspecified ankle ▽

  √6ᵗʰ **S93.41** Sprain of calcaneofibular ligament

    √7ᵗʰ **S93.411** Sprain of calcaneofibular ligament of right ankle

    √7ᵗʰ **S93.412** Sprain of calcaneofibular ligament of left ankle

    √7ᵗʰ **S93.419** Sprain of calcaneofibular ligament of unspecified ankle ▽

  √6ᵗʰ **S93.42** Sprain of deltoid ligament

    √7ᵗʰ **S93.421** Sprain of deltoid ligament of right ankle

    √7ᵗʰ **S93.422** Sprain of deltoid ligament of left ankle

    √7ᵗʰ **S93.429** Sprain of deltoid ligament of unspecified ankle ▽

  √6ᵗʰ **S93.43** Sprain of tibiofibular ligament

    √7ᵗʰ **S93.431** Sprain of tibiofibular ligament of right ankle

    √7ᵗʰ **S93.432** Sprain of tibiofibular ligament of left ankle

    √7ᵗʰ **S93.439** Sprain of tibiofibular ligament of unspecified ankle ▽

  √6ᵗʰ **S93.49** Sprain of other ligament of ankle

    Sprain of internal collateral ligament

    Sprain of talofibular ligament

    √7ᵗʰ **S93.491** Sprain of other ligament of right ankle

    √7ᵗʰ **S93.492** Sprain of other ligament of left ankle

    √7ᵗʰ **S93.499** Sprain of other ligament of unspecified ankle ▽

√5ᵗʰ **S93.5** Sprain of toe

  √6ᵗʰ **S93.50** Unspecified sprain of toe

    √7ᵗʰ **S93.501** Unspecified sprain of right great toe ▽

    √7ᵗʰ **S93.502** Unspecified sprain of left great toe ▽

    √7ᵗʰ **S93.503** Unspecified sprain of unspecified great toe ▽

    √7ᵗʰ **S93.504** Unspecified sprain of right lesser toe(s) ▽

    √7ᵗʰ **S93.505** Unspecified sprain of left lesser toe(s) ▽

    √7ᵗʰ **S93.506** Unspecified sprain of unspecified lesser toe(s) ▽

    √7ᵗʰ **S93.509** Unspecified sprain of unspecified toe(s) ▽

  √6ᵗʰ **S93.51** Sprain of interphalangeal joint of toe

    √7ᵗʰ **S93.511** Sprain of interphalangeal joint of right great toe

    √7ᵗʰ **S93.512** Sprain of interphalangeal joint of left great toe

    √7ᵗʰ **S93.513** Sprain of interphalangeal joint of unspecified great toe ▽

    √7ᵗʰ **S93.514** Sprain of interphalangeal joint of right lesser toe(s)

    √7ᵗʰ **S93.515** Sprain of interphalangeal joint of left lesser toe(s)

    √7ᵗʰ **S93.516** Sprain of interphalangeal joint of unspecified lesser toe(s) ▽

    √7ᵗʰ **S93.519** Sprain of interphalangeal joint of unspecified toe(s) ▽

√6ᵗʰ **S93.52** Sprain of metatarsophalangeal joint of toe

  √7ᵗʰ **S93.521** Sprain of metatarsophalangeal joint of right great toe

  √7ᵗʰ **S93.522** Sprain of metatarsophalangeal joint of left great toe

  √7ᵗʰ **S93.523** Sprain of metatarsophalangeal joint of unspecified great toe ▽

  √7ᵗʰ **S93.524** Sprain of metatarsophalangeal joint of right lesser toe(s)

  √7ᵗʰ **S93.525** Sprain of metatarsophalangeal joint of left lesser toe(s)

  √7ᵗʰ **S93.526** Sprain of metatarsophalangeal joint of unspecified lesser toe(s) ▽

  √7ᵗʰ **S93.529** Sprain of metatarsophalangeal joint of unspecified toe(s) ▽

√5ᵗʰ **S93.6** Sprain of foot

  EXCLUDES 2   sprain of metatarsophalangeal joint of toe (S93.52-)

    sprain of toe (S93.5-)

  √6ᵗʰ **S93.60** Unspecified sprain of foot

    √7ᵗʰ **S93.601** Unspecified sprain of right foot ▽

    √7ᵗʰ **S93.602** Unspecified sprain of left foot ▽

    √7ᵗʰ **S93.609** Unspecified sprain of unspecified foot ▽

  √6ᵗʰ **S93.61** Sprain of tarsal ligament of foot

    √7ᵗʰ **S93.611** Sprain of tarsal ligament of right foot

    √7ᵗʰ **S93.612** Sprain of tarsal ligament of left foot

    √7ᵗʰ **S93.619** Sprain of tarsal ligament of unspecified foot ▽

  √6ᵗʰ **S93.62** Sprain of tarsometatarsal ligament of foot

    √7ᵗʰ **S93.621** Sprain of tarsometatarsal ligament of right foot

    √7ᵗʰ **S93.622** Sprain of tarsometatarsal ligament of left foot

    √7ᵗʰ **S93.629** Sprain of tarsometatarsal ligament of unspecified foot ▽

  √6ᵗʰ **S93.69** Other sprain of foot

    √7ᵗʰ **S93.691** Other sprain of right foot

    √7ᵗʰ **S93.692** Other sprain of left foot

    √7ᵗʰ **S93.699** Other sprain of unspecified foot ▽

√4ᵗʰ **S94** Injury of nerves at ankle and foot level

Code also any associated open wound (S91.-)

> The appropriate 7th character is to be added to each code from category S94.
> A   initial encounter
> D   subsequent encounter
> S   sequela

√5ᵗʰ **S94.0** Injury of lateral plantar nerve

  √×7ᵗʰ **S94.00** Injury of lateral plantar nerve, unspecified leg ▽

  √×7ᵗʰ **S94.01** Injury of lateral plantar nerve, right leg

  √×7ᵗʰ **S94.02** Injury of lateral plantar nerve, left leg

√5ᵗʰ **S94.1** Injury of medial plantar nerve

  √×7ᵗʰ **S94.10** Injury of medial plantar nerve, unspecified leg ▽

  √×7ᵗʰ **S94.11** Injury of medial plantar nerve, right leg

  √×7ᵗʰ **S94.12** Injury of medial plantar nerve, left leg

√5ᵗʰ **S94.2** Injury of deep peroneal nerve at ankle and foot level

  Injury of terminal, lateral branch of deep peroneal nerve

  √×7ᵗʰ **S94.20** Injury of deep peroneal nerve at ankle and foot level, unspecified leg ▽

  √×7ᵗʰ **S94.21** Injury of deep peroneal nerve at ankle and foot level, right leg

  √×7ᵗʰ **S94.22** Injury of deep peroneal nerve at ankle and foot level, left leg

√5ᵗʰ **S94.3** Injury of cutaneous sensory nerve at ankle and foot level

  √×7ᵗʰ **S94.30** Injury of cutaneous sensory nerve at ankle and foot level, unspecified leg ▽

  √×7ᵗʰ **S94.31** Injury of cutaneous sensory nerve at ankle and foot level, right leg

  √×7ᵗʰ **S94.32** Injury of cutaneous sensory nerve at ankle and foot level, left leg

√5ᵗʰ **S94.8** Injury of other nerves at ankle and foot level

  √6ᵗʰ **S94.8X** Injury of other nerves at ankle and foot level

    √7ᵗʰ **S94.8X1** Injury of other nerves at ankle and foot level, right leg

✓x7ᵗʰ **S94.8X2** Injury of other nerves at ankle and foot level, **left** leg

✓x7ᵗʰ **S94.8X9** Injury of other nerves at ankle and foot level, unspecified leg ▽

✓5ᵗʰ **S94.9** Injury of unspecified nerve at ankle and foot level

   ✓x7ᵗʰ **S94.90** Injury of unspecified nerve at ankle and foot level, unspecified leg ▽

   ✓x7ᵗʰ **S94.91** Injury of unspecified nerve at ankle and foot level, **right** leg ▽

   ✓x7ᵗʰ **S94.92** Injury of unspecified nerve at ankle and foot level, **left** leg ▽

✓4ᵗʰ **S95** **Injury of blood vessels at ankle and foot level**

   Code also any associated open wound (S91.-)

   EXCLUDES 2   *injury of posterior tibial artery and vein (S85.1-, S85.8-)*

   The appropriate 7th character is to be added to each code from category S95.
   A   initial encounter
   D   subsequent encounter
   S   sequela

   ✓5ᵗʰ **S95.0** Injury of **dorsal artery** of foot

     ✓6ᵗʰ **S95.00** Unspecified injury of dorsal artery of foot

       ✓7ᵗʰ **S95.001** Unspecified injury of dorsal artery of **right** foot ▽

       ✓7ᵗʰ **S95.002** Unspecified injury of dorsal artery of **left** foot ▽

       ✓7ᵗʰ **S95.009** Unspecified injury of dorsal artery of unspecified foot ▽

     ✓6ᵗʰ **S95.01** Laceration of dorsal artery of foot

       ✓7ᵗʰ **S95.011** Laceration of dorsal artery of **right** foot

       ✓7ᵗʰ **S95.012** Laceration of dorsal artery of **left** foot

       ✓7ᵗʰ **S95.019** Laceration of dorsal artery of unspecified foot ▽

     ✓6ᵗʰ **S95.09** Other specified injury of dorsal artery of foot

       ✓7ᵗʰ **S95.091** Other specified injury of dorsal artery of **right** foot

       ✓7ᵗʰ **S95.092** Other specified injury of dorsal artery of **left** foot

       ✓7ᵗʰ **S95.099** Other specified injury of dorsal artery of unspecified foot ▽

   ✓5ᵗʰ **S95.1** Injury of **plantar artery** of foot

     ✓6ᵗʰ **S95.10** Unspecified injury of plantar artery of foot

       ✓7ᵗʰ **S95.101** Unspecified injury of plantar artery of **right** foot ▽

       ✓7ᵗʰ **S95.102** Unspecified injury of plantar artery of **left** foot ▽

       ✓7ᵗʰ **S95.109** Unspecified injury of plantar artery of unspecified foot ▽

     ✓6ᵗʰ **S95.11** Laceration of plantar artery of foot

       ✓7ᵗʰ **S95.111** Laceration of plantar artery of **right** foot

       ✓7ᵗʰ **S95.112** Laceration of plantar artery of **left** foot

       ✓7ᵗʰ **S95.119** Laceration of plantar artery of unspecified foot ▽

     ✓6ᵗʰ **S95.19** Other specified injury of plantar artery of foot

       ✓7ᵗʰ **S95.191** Other specified injury of plantar artery of **right** foot

       ✓7ᵗʰ **S95.192** Other specified injury of plantar artery of **left** foot

       ✓7ᵗʰ **S95.199** Other specified injury of plantar artery of unspecified foot ▽

   ✓5ᵗʰ **S95.2** Injury of **dorsal vein** of foot

     ✓6ᵗʰ **S95.20** Unspecified injury of dorsal vein of foot

       ✓7ᵗʰ **S95.201** Unspecified injury of dorsal vein of **right** foot ▽

       ✓7ᵗʰ **S95.202** Unspecified injury of dorsal vein of **left** foot ▽

       ✓7ᵗʰ **S95.209** Unspecified injury of dorsal vein of unspecified foot ▽

     ✓6ᵗʰ **S95.21** Laceration of dorsal vein of foot

       ✓7ᵗʰ **S95.211** Laceration of dorsal vein of **right** foot

       ✓7ᵗʰ **S95.212** Laceration of dorsal vein of **left** foot

       ✓7ᵗʰ **S95.219** Laceration of dorsal vein of unspecified foot ▽

     ✓6ᵗʰ **S95.29** Other specified injury of dorsal vein of foot

       ✓7ᵗʰ **S95.291** Other specified injury of dorsal vein of **right** foot

       ✓7ᵗʰ **S95.292** Other specified injury of dorsal vein of **left** foot

       ✓7ᵗʰ **S95.299** Other specified injury of dorsal vein of unspecified foot ▽

✓5ᵗʰ **S95.8** Injury of other blood vessels at ankle and foot level

   ✓6ᵗʰ **S95.80** Unspecified injury of other blood vessels at ankle and foot level

     ✓7ᵗʰ **S95.801** Unspecified injury of other blood vessels at ankle and foot level, **right** leg ▽

     ✓7ᵗʰ **S95.802** Unspecified injury of other blood vessels at ankle and foot level, **left** leg ▽

     ✓7ᵗʰ **S95.809** Unspecified injury of other blood vessels at ankle and foot level, unspecified leg ▽

   ✓6ᵗʰ **S95.81** Laceration of other blood vessels at ankle and foot level

     ✓7ᵗʰ **S95.811** Laceration of other blood vessels at ankle and foot level, **right** leg

     ✓7ᵗʰ **S95.812** Laceration of other blood vessels at ankle and foot level, **left** leg

     ✓7ᵗʰ **S95.819** Laceration of other blood vessels at ankle and foot level, unspecified leg ▽

   ✓6ᵗʰ **S95.89** Other specified injury of other blood vessels at ankle and foot level

     ✓7ᵗʰ **S95.891** Other specified injury of other blood vessels at ankle and foot level, **right** leg

     ✓7ᵗʰ **S95.892** Other specified injury of other blood vessels at ankle and foot level, **left** leg

     ✓7ᵗʰ **S95.899** Other specified injury of other blood vessels at ankle and foot level, unspecified leg ▽

✓5ᵗʰ **S95.9** Injury of unspecified blood vessel at ankle and foot level

   ✓6ᵗʰ **S95.90** Unspecified injury of unspecified blood vessel at ankle and foot level

     ✓7ᵗʰ **S95.901** Unspecified injury of unspecified blood vessel at ankle and foot level, **right** leg ▽

     ✓7ᵗʰ **S95.902** Unspecified injury of unspecified blood vessel at ankle and foot level, **left** leg ▽

     ✓7ᵗʰ **S95.909** Unspecified injury of unspecified blood vessel at ankle and foot level, unspecified leg ▽

   ✓6ᵗʰ **S95.91** Laceration of unspecified blood vessel at ankle and foot level

     ✓7ᵗʰ **S95.911** Laceration of unspecified blood vessel at ankle and foot level, **right** leg ▽

     ✓7ᵗʰ **S95.912** Laceration of unspecified blood vessel at ankle and foot level, **left** leg ▽

     ✓7ᵗʰ **S95.919** Laceration of unspecified blood vessel at ankle and foot level, unspecified leg ▽

   ✓6ᵗʰ **S95.99** Other specified injury of unspecified blood vessel at ankle and foot level

     ✓7ᵗʰ **S95.991** Other specified injury of unspecified blood vessel at ankle and foot level, **right** leg ▽

     ✓7ᵗʰ **S95.992** Other specified injury of unspecified blood vessel at ankle and foot level, **left** leg ▽

     ✓7ᵗʰ **S95.999** Other specified injury of unspecified blood vessel at ankle and foot level, unspecified leg ▽

✓ Additional Character Req   ✓x7ᵗʰ Placeholder Alert   Manifestation   ▽ Unspecified   ►◄ Revised Text   ● New Code   ▲ Revised Code Title

ICD-10-CM 2019   **1069**

Chapter 19. Injury, Poisoning and Certain Other Consequences of External Causes

S96–S96.802

√4ᵗʰ **S96 Injury of muscle and tendon at ankle and foot level**

Code also any associated open wound (S91.-)

EXCLUDES 2   injury of Achilles tendon (S86.0-)

sprain of joints and ligaments of ankle and foot (S93.-)

TIP: Refer to the Muscle/Tendon table at the beginning of this chapter,

The appropriate 7th character is to be added to each code from category S96.

A   initial encounter

D   subsequent encounter

S   sequela

√5ᵗʰ **S96.0 Injury of muscle and tendon of long flexor muscle of toe at ankle and foot level**

√6ᵗʰ   **S96.00 Unspecified injury of muscle and tendon of long flexor muscle of toe at ankle and foot level**

√7ᵗʰ   **S96.001 Unspecified injury of muscle and tendon of long flexor muscle of toe at ankle and foot level, right foot** ▽

√7ᵗʰ   **S96.002 Unspecified injury of muscle and tendon of long flexor muscle of toe at ankle and foot level, left foot** ▽

√7ᵗʰ   **S96.009 Unspecified injury of muscle and tendon of long flexor muscle of toe at ankle and foot level, unspecified foot** ▽

√6ᵗʰ   **S96.01 Strain of muscle and tendon of long flexor muscle of toe at ankle and foot level**

√7ᵗʰ   **S96.011 Strain of muscle and tendon of long flexor muscle of toe at ankle and foot level, right foot**

√7ᵗʰ   **S96.012 Strain of muscle and tendon of long flexor muscle of toe at ankle and foot level, left foot**

√7ᵗʰ   **S96.019 Strain of muscle and tendon of long flexor muscle of toe at ankle and foot level, unspecified foot** ▽

√6ᵗʰ   **S96.02 Laceration of muscle and tendon of long flexor muscle of toe at ankle and foot level**

√7ᵗʰ   **S96.021 Laceration of muscle and tendon of long flexor muscle of toe at ankle and foot level, right foot**

√7ᵗʰ   **S96.022 Laceration of muscle and tendon of long flexor muscle of toe at ankle and foot level, left foot**

√7ᵗʰ   **S96.029 Laceration of muscle and tendon of long flexor muscle of toe at ankle and foot level, unspecified foot** ▽

√6ᵗʰ   **S96.09 Other injury of muscle and tendon of long flexor muscle of toe at ankle and foot level**

√7ᵗʰ   **S96.091 Other injury of muscle and tendon of long flexor muscle of toe at ankle and foot level, right foot**

√7ᵗʰ   **S96.092 Other injury of muscle and tendon of long flexor muscle of toe at ankle and foot level, left foot**

√7ᵗʰ   **S96.099 Other injury of muscle and tendon of long flexor muscle of toe at ankle and foot level, unspecified foot** ▽

√5ᵗʰ **S96.1 Injury of muscle and tendon of long extensor muscle of toe at ankle and foot level**

√6ᵗʰ   **S96.10 Unspecified injury of muscle and tendon of long extensor muscle of toe at ankle and foot level**

√7ᵗʰ   **S96.101 Unspecified injury of muscle and tendon of long extensor muscle of toe at ankle and foot level, right foot** ▽

√7ᵗʰ   **S96.102 Unspecified injury of muscle and tendon of long extensor muscle of toe at ankle and foot level, left foot** ▽

√7ᵗʰ   **S96.109 Unspecified injury of muscle and tendon of long extensor muscle of toe at ankle and foot level, unspecified foot** ▽

√6ᵗʰ   **S96.11 Strain of muscle and tendon of long extensor muscle of toe at ankle and foot level**

√7ᵗʰ   **S96.111 Strain of muscle and tendon of long extensor muscle of toe at ankle and foot level, right foot**

√7ᵗʰ   **S96.112 Strain of muscle and tendon of long extensor muscle of toe at ankle and foot level, left foot**

√7ᵗʰ   **S96.119 Strain of muscle and tendon of long extensor muscle of toe at ankle and foot level, unspecified foot** ▽

√6ᵗʰ   **S96.12 Laceration of muscle and tendon of long extensor muscle of toe at ankle and foot level**

√7ᵗʰ   **S96.121 Laceration of muscle and tendon of long extensor muscle of toe at ankle and foot level, right foot**

√7ᵗʰ   **S96.122 Laceration of muscle and tendon of long extensor muscle of toe at ankle and foot level, left foot**

√7ᵗʰ   **S96.129 Laceration of muscle and tendon of long extensor muscle of toe at ankle and foot level, unspecified foot** ▽

√6ᵗʰ   **S96.19 Other specified injury of muscle and tendon of long extensor muscle of toe at ankle and foot level**

√7ᵗʰ   **S96.191 Other specified injury of muscle and tendon of long extensor muscle of toe at ankle and foot level, right foot**

√7ᵗʰ   **S96.192 Other specified injury of muscle and tendon of long extensor muscle of toe at ankle and foot level, left foot**

√7ᵗʰ   **S96.199 Other specified injury of muscle and tendon of long extensor muscle of toe at ankle and foot level, unspecified foot** ▽

√5ᵗʰ **S96.2 Injury of intrinsic muscle and tendon at ankle and foot level**

√6ᵗʰ   **S96.20 Unspecified injury of intrinsic muscle and tendon at ankle and foot level**

√7ᵗʰ   **S96.201 Unspecified injury of intrinsic muscle and tendon at ankle and foot level, right foot** ▽

√7ᵗʰ   **S96.202 Unspecified injury of intrinsic muscle and tendon at ankle and foot level, left foot** ▽

√7ᵗʰ   **S96.209 Unspecified injury of intrinsic muscle and tendon at ankle and foot level, unspecified foot** ▽

√6ᵗʰ   **S96.21 Strain of intrinsic muscle and tendon at ankle and foot level**

√7ᵗʰ   **S96.211 Strain of intrinsic muscle and tendon at ankle and foot level, right foot**

√7ᵗʰ   **S96.212 Strain of intrinsic muscle and tendon at ankle and foot level, left foot**

√7ᵗʰ   **S96.219 Strain of intrinsic muscle and tendon at ankle and foot level, unspecified foot** ▽

√6ᵗʰ   **S96.22 Laceration of intrinsic muscle and tendon at ankle and foot level**

√7ᵗʰ   **S96.221 Laceration of intrinsic muscle and tendon at ankle and foot level, right foot**

√7ᵗʰ   **S96.222 Laceration of intrinsic muscle and tendon at ankle and foot level, left foot**

√7ᵗʰ   **S96.229 Laceration of intrinsic muscle and tendon at ankle and foot level, unspecified foot** ▽

√6ᵗʰ   **S96.29 Other specified injury of intrinsic muscle and tendon at ankle and foot level**

√7ᵗʰ   **S96.291 Other specified injury of intrinsic muscle and tendon at ankle and foot level, right foot**

√7ᵗʰ   **S96.292 Other specified injury of intrinsic muscle and tendon at ankle and foot level, left foot**

√7ᵗʰ   **S96.299 Other specified injury of intrinsic muscle and tendon at ankle and foot level, unspecified foot** ▽

√5ᵗʰ **S96.8 Injury of other specified muscles and tendons at ankle and foot level**

√6ᵗʰ   **S96.80 Unspecified injury of other specified muscles and tendons at ankle and foot level**

√7ᵗʰ   **S96.801 Unspecified injury of other specified muscles and tendons at ankle and foot level, right foot** ▽

√7ᵗʰ   **S96.802 Unspecified injury of other specified muscles and tendons at ankle and foot level, left foot** ▽

√7ᵗʰ S96.809 Unspecified injury of other ▽
specified muscles and tendons at
ankle and foot level, unspecified
foot

√6ᵗʰ S96.81 Strain of other specified muscles and tendons at
ankle and foot level

√7ᵗʰ S96.811 Strain of other specified muscles and
tendons at ankle and foot level, right foot

√7ᵗʰ S96.812 Strain of other specified muscles and
tendons at ankle and foot level, left foot

√7ᵗʰ S96.819 Strain of other specified muscles ▽
and tendons at ankle and foot
level, unspecified foot

√6ᵗʰ S96.82 Laceration of other specified muscles and tendons
at ankle and foot level

√7ᵗʰ S96.821 Laceration of other specified muscles and
tendons at ankle and foot level, right foot

√7ᵗʰ S96.822 Laceration of other specified muscles and
tendons at ankle and foot level, left foot

√7ᵗʰ S96.829 Laceration of other specified ▽
muscles and tendons at ankle and
foot level, unspecified foot

√6ᵗʰ S96.89 Other specified injury of other specified muscles
and tendons at ankle and foot level

√7ᵗʰ S96.891 Other specified injury of other specified
muscles and tendons at ankle and foot
level, right foot

√7ᵗʰ S96.892 Other specified injury of other specified
muscles and tendons at ankle and foot
level, left foot

√7ᵗʰ S96.899 Other specified injury of other ▽
specified muscles and tendons at
ankle and foot level, unspecified
foot

√5ᵗʰ S96.9 Injury of unspecified muscle and tendon at ankle and foot
level

√6ᵗʰ S96.90 Unspecified injury of unspecified muscle and
tendon at ankle and foot level

√7ᵗʰ S96.901 Unspecified injury of unspecified ▽
muscle and tendon at ankle and
foot level, right foot

√7ᵗʰ S96.902 Unspecified injury of unspecified ▽
muscle and tendon at ankle and
foot level, left foot

√7ᵗʰ S96.909 Unspecified injury of unspecified ▽
muscle and tendon at ankle and
foot level, unspecified foot

√6ᵗʰ S96.91 Strain of unspecified muscle and tendon at ankle
and foot level

√7ᵗʰ S96.911 Strain of unspecified muscle and ▽
tendon at ankle and foot level,
right foot

√7ᵗʰ S96.912 Strain of unspecified muscle and ▽
tendon at ankle and foot level,
left foot

√7ᵗʰ S96.919 Strain of unspecified muscle and ▽
tendon at ankle and foot level,
unspecified foot

√6ᵗʰ S96.92 Laceration of unspecified muscle and tendon at
ankle and foot level

√7ᵗʰ S96.921 Laceration of unspecified muscle ▽
and tendon at ankle and foot
level, right foot

√7ᵗʰ S96.922 Laceration of unspecified muscle ▽
and tendon at ankle and foot
level, left foot

√7ᵗʰ S96.929 Laceration of unspecified muscle ▽
and tendon at ankle and foot
level, unspecified foot

√6ᵗʰ S96.99 Other specified injury of unspecified muscle and
tendon at ankle and foot level

√7ᵗʰ S96.991 Other specified injury of ▽
unspecified muscle and tendon
at ankle and foot level, right foot

√7ᵗʰ S96.992 Other specified injury of ▽
unspecified muscle and tendon
at ankle and foot level, left foot

√7ᵗʰ S96.999 Other specified injury of ▽
unspecified muscle and tendon
at ankle and foot level,
unspecified foot

√4ᵗʰ **S97 Crushing injury of ankle and foot**

Use additional code(s) for all associated injuries

The appropriate 7th character is to be added to each code from
category S97.
A initial encounter
D subsequent encounter
S sequela

√5ᵗʰ S97.0 Crushing injury of ankle

√x7ᵗʰ S97.00 Crushing injury of unspecified ankle ▽

√x7ᵗʰ S97.01 Crushing injury of right ankle

√x7ᵗʰ S97.02 Crushing injury of left ankle

√5ᵗʰ S97.1 Crushing injury of toe

√6ᵗʰ S97.10 Crushing injury of unspecified toe(s)

√7ᵗʰ S97.101 Crushing injury of unspecified ▽
right toe(s)

√7ᵗʰ S97.102 Crushing injury of unspecified left ▽
toe(s)

√7ᵗʰ S97.109 Crushing injury of unspecified ▽
toe(s)
Crushing injury of toe NOS

√6ᵗʰ S97.11 Crushing injury of great toe

√7ᵗʰ S97.111 Crushing injury of right great toe

√7ᵗʰ S97.112 Crushing injury of left great toe

√7ᵗʰ S97.119 Crushing injury of unspecified ▽
great toe

√6ᵗʰ S97.12 Crushing injury of lesser toe(s)

√7ᵗʰ S97.121 Crushing injury of right lesser toe(s)

√7ᵗʰ S97.122 Crushing injury of left lesser toe(s)

√7ᵗʰ S97.129 Crushing injury of unspecified ▽
lesser toe(s)

√5ᵗʰ S97.8 Crushing injury of foot

√x7ᵗʰ S97.80 Crushing injury of unspecified foot ▽
Crushing injury of foot NOS

√x7ᵗʰ S97.81 Crushing injury of right foot

√x7ᵗʰ S97.82 Crushing injury of left foot

√4ᵗʰ **S98 Traumatic amputation of ankle and foot**

An amputation not identified as partial or complete should be coded
to complete

The appropriate 7th character is to be added to each code from
category S98.
A initial encounter
D subsequent encounter
S sequela

√5ᵗʰ S98.0 Traumatic amputation of foot at ankle level

√6ᵗʰ S98.01 Complete traumatic amputation of foot at ankle
level

√7ᵗʰ S98.011 Complete traumatic amputation HCC
of right foot at ankle level

√7ᵗʰ S98.012 Complete traumatic amputation HCC
of left foot at ankle level

√7ᵗʰ S98.019 Complete traumatic amputation HCC ▽
of unspecified foot at ankle level

√6ᵗʰ S98.02 Partial traumatic amputation of foot at ankle level

√7ᵗʰ S98.021 Partial traumatic amputation of HCC
right foot at ankle level

√7ᵗʰ S98.022 Partial traumatic amputation of HCC
left foot at ankle level

√7ᵗʰ S98.029 Partial traumatic amputation of HCC ▽
unspecified foot at ankle level

√5ᵗʰ S98.1 Traumatic amputation of one toe

√6ᵗʰ S98.11 Complete traumatic amputation of great toe

√7ᵗʰ S98.111 Complete traumatic amputation HCC
of right great toe

√7ᵗʰ S98.112 Complete traumatic amputation HCC
of left great toe

√7ᵗʰ S98.119 Complete traumatic amputation HCC ▽
of unspecified great toe

√6ᵗʰ S98.12 Partial traumatic amputation of great toe

√7ᵗʰ S98.121 Partial traumatic amputation of HCC
right great toe

√7ᵗʰ S98.122 Partial traumatic amputation of HCC
left great toe

√7ᵗʰ S98.129 Partial traumatic amputation of HCC ▽
unspecified great toe

☑ Additional Character Req   √x7ᵗʰ Placeholder Alert   Manifestation   ▽ Unspecified   ▶◀ Revised Text   ● New Code   ▲ Revised Code Title

Chapter 19. Injury, Poisoning and Certain Other Consequences of External Causes

S98.13–S99.119

√6ᵗʰ **S98.13** Complete **traumatic amputation of** one lesser toe
Traumatic amputation of toe NOS

     √7ᵗʰ **S98.131** **Complete traumatic amputation** HCC
of one right **lesser toe**

     √7ᵗʰ **S98.132** **Complete traumatic amputation** HCC
of one left **lesser toe**

     √7ᵗʰ **S98.139** **Complete traumatic amputation** HCC ▽
of one unspecified **lesser toe**

√6ᵗʰ **S98.14** Partial **traumatic amputation of** one lesser toe

     √7ᵗʰ **S98.141** **Partial traumatic amputation of** HCC
one right **lesser toe**

     √7ᵗʰ **S98.142** **Partial traumatic amputation of** HCC
one left **lesser toe**

     √7ᵗʰ **S98.149** **Partial traumatic amputation of** HCC ▽
one unspecified **lesser toe**

√5ᵗʰ **S98.2** **Traumatic amputation of** two or more lesser toes

     √6ᵗʰ **S98.21** Complete **traumatic amputation of two or more lesser toes**

         √7ᵗʰ **S98.211** **Complete traumatic amputation** HCC
of two or more right **lesser toes**

         √7ᵗʰ **S98.212** **Complete traumatic amputation** HCC
of two or more left **lesser toes**

         √7ᵗʰ **S98.219** **Complete traumatic amputation** HCC ▽
of two or more unspecified lesser
toes

     √6ᵗʰ **S98.22** Partial **traumatic amputation of two or more lesser toes**

         √7ᵗʰ **S98.221** **Partial traumatic amputation of** HCC
two or more right **lesser toes**

         √7ᵗʰ **S98.222** **Partial traumatic amputation of** HCC
two or more left **lesser toes**

         √7ᵗʰ **S98.229** **Partial traumatic amputation of** HCC ▽
two or more unspecified lesser
toes

√5ᵗʰ **S98.3** **Traumatic amputation of** midfoot

     √6ᵗʰ **S98.31** Complete **traumatic amputation of midfoot**

         √7ᵗʰ **S98.311** **Complete traumatic amputation** HCC
of right **midfoot**

         √7ᵗʰ **S98.312** **Complete traumatic amputation** HCC
of left **midfoot**

         √7ᵗʰ **S98.319** **Complete traumatic amputation** HCC ▽
of unspecified **midfoot**

     √6ᵗʰ **S98.32** Partial **traumatic amputation of midfoot**

         √7ᵗʰ **S98.321** **Partial traumatic amputation of** HCC
right **midfoot**

         √7ᵗʰ **S98.322** **Partial traumatic amputation of** HCC
left **midfoot**

         √7ᵗʰ **S98.329** **Partial traumatic amputation of** HCC ▽
unspecified **midfoot**

√5ᵗʰ **S98.9** **Traumatic amputation of** foot, level unspecified

     √6ᵗʰ **S98.91** Complete **traumatic amputation of foot, level unspecified**

         √7ᵗʰ **S98.911** **Complete traumatic amputation** HCC ▽
of right **foot, level unspecified**

         √7ᵗʰ **S98.912** **Complete traumatic amputation** HCC ▽
of left **foot, level unspecified**

         √7ᵗʰ **S98.919** **Complete traumatic amputation** HCC ▽
of unspecified **foot, level
unspecified**

     √6ᵗʰ **S98.92** Partial **traumatic amputation of foot, level unspecified**

         √7ᵗʰ **S98.921** **Partial traumatic amputation of** HCC ▽
right **foot, level unspecified**

         √7ᵗʰ **S98.922** **Partial traumatic amputation of** HCC ▽
left **foot, level unspecified**

         √7ᵗʰ **S98.929** **Partial traumatic amputation of** HCC ▽
unspecified **foot, level
unspecified**

√4ᵗʰ **S99** **Other and unspecified injuries of ankle and foot**

     AHA: 2018,2Q,12; 2018,1Q,3; 2016,4Q,68-69

√5ᵗʰ **S99.0** **Physeal fracture of** calcaneus

> The appropriate 7th character is to be added to each code
> from subcategory S99.0.
> A   initial encounter for closed fracture
> B   initial encounter for open fracture
> D   subsequent encounter for fracture with routine healing
> G   subsequent encounter for fracture with delayed healing
> K   subsequent encounter for fracture with nonunion
> P   subsequent encounter for fracture with malunion
> S   sequela

     √6ᵗʰ **S99.00** **Unspecified physeal fracture of** calcaneus

         √7ᵗʰ **S99.001** **Unspecified physeal fracture of** Q ▽
right **calcaneus**

         √7ᵗʰ **S99.002** **Unspecified physeal fracture of** Q ▽
left **calcaneus**

         √7ᵗʰ **S99.009** **Unspecified physeal fracture of** Q
unspecified **calcaneus**

     √6ᵗʰ **S99.01** Salter-Harris Type I **physeal fracture of calcaneus**

         √7ᵗʰ **S99.011** **Salter-Harris Type I physeal** Q
fracture of right **calcaneus**

         √7ᵗʰ **S99.012** **Salter-Harris Type I physeal** Q
fracture of left **calcaneus**

         √7ᵗʰ **S99.019** **Salter-Harris Type I physeal** Q ▽
fracture of unspecified **calcaneus**

     √6ᵗʰ **S99.02** Salter-Harris Type II **physeal fracture of calcaneus**

         √7ᵗʰ **S99.021** **Salter-Harris Type II physeal** Q
fracture of right **calcaneus**

         √7ᵗʰ **S99.022** **Salter-Harris Type II physeal** Q
fracture of left **calcaneus**

         √7ᵗʰ **S99.029** **Salter-Harris Type II physeal** Q ▽
fracture of unspecified **calcaneus**

     √6ᵗʰ **S99.03** Salter-Harris Type III **physeal fracture of calcaneus**

         √7ᵗʰ **S99.031** **Salter-Harris Type III physeal** Q
fracture of right **calcaneus**

         √7ᵗʰ **S99.032** **Salter-Harris Type III physeal** Q
fracture of left **calcaneus**

         √7ᵗʰ **S99.039** **Salter-Harris Type III physeal** Q ▽
fracture of unspecified **calcaneus**

     √6ᵗʰ **S99.04** Salter-Harris Type IV **physeal fracture of calcaneus**

         √7ᵗʰ **S99.041** **Salter-Harris Type IV physeal** Q
fracture of right **calcaneus**

         √7ᵗʰ **S99.042** **Salter-Harris Type IV physeal** Q
fracture of left **calcaneus**

         √7ᵗʰ **S99.049** **Salter-Harris Type IV physeal** Q ▽
fracture of unspecified **calcaneus**

     √6ᵗʰ **S99.09** Other **physeal fracture of calcaneus**

         √7ᵗʰ **S99.091** **Other physeal fracture of** right Q
calcaneus

         √7ᵗʰ **S99.092** **Other physeal fracture of** left Q
calcaneus

         √7ᵗʰ **S99.099** **Other physeal fracture of** Q ▽
unspecified **calcaneus**

√5ᵗʰ **S99.1** **Physeal fracture of** metatarsal

> The appropriate 7th character is to be added to each code
> from subcategory S99.1
> A   initial encounter for closed fracture
> B   initial encounter for open fracture
> D   subsequent encounter for fracture with routine healing
> G   subsequent encounter for fracture with delayed healing
> K   subsequent encounter for fracture with nonunion
> P   subsequent encounter for fracture with malunion
> S   sequela

     √6ᵗʰ **S99.10** **Unspecified physeal fracture of metatarsal**

▲

         √7ᵗʰ **S99.101** **Unspecified physeal fracture of** Q ▽
right **metatarsal**

         √7ᵗʰ **S99.102** **Unspecified physeal fracture of** Q ▽
left **metatarsal**

         √7ᵗʰ **S99.109** **Unspecified physeal fracture of** Q ▽
unspecified **metatarsal**

     √6ᵗʰ **S99.11** Salter-Harris Type I **physeal fracture of metatarsal**

         √7ᵗʰ **S99.111** **Salter-Harris Type I physeal** Q
fracture of right **metatarsal**

         √7ᵗʰ **S99.112** **Salter-Harris Type I physeal** Q
fracture of left **metatarsal**

         √7ᵗʰ **S99.119** **Salter-Harris Type I physeal** Q ▽
fracture of unspecified **metatarsal**

√6ᵗʰ **S99.12** Salter-Harris Type II physeal fracture of metatarsal

     √7ᵗʰ **S99.121** Salter-Harris Type II physeal fracture of **right** metatarsal   Q

     √7ᵗʰ **S99.122** Salter-Harris Type II physeal fracture of **left** metatarsal   Q

     √7ᵗʰ **S99.129** Salter-Harris Type II physeal fracture of unspecified metatarsal   Q ▽

√6ᵗʰ **S99.13** Salter-Harris Type III physeal fracture of metatarsal

     √7ᵗʰ **S99.131** Salter-Harris Type III physeal fracture of **right** metatarsal   Q

     √7ᵗʰ **S99.132** Salter-Harris Type III physeal fracture of **left** metatarsal   Q

     √7ᵗʰ **S99.139** Salter-Harris Type III physeal fracture of unspecified metatarsal   Q ▽

√6ᵗʰ **S99.14** Salter-Harris Type IV physeal fracture of metatarsal

     √7ᵗʰ **S99.141** Salter-Harris Type IV physeal fracture of **right** metatarsal   Q

     √7ᵗʰ **S99.142** Salter-Harris Type IV physeal fracture of **left** metatarsal   Q

     √7ᵗʰ **S99.149** Salter-Harris Type IV physeal fracture of unspecified metatarsal   Q ▽

√6ᵗʰ **S99.19** Other physeal fracture of metatarsal

     √7ᵗʰ **S99.191** Other physeal fracture of **right** metatarsal   Q

     √7ᵗʰ **S99.192** Other physeal fracture of **left** metatarsal   Q

     √7ᵗʰ **S99.199** Other physeal fracture of unspecified metatarsal   Q ▽

√5ᵗʰ **S99.2** Physeal fracture of **phalanx of toe**

> The appropriate 7th character is to be added to each code from subcategories S99.2.
> A   initial encounter for closed fracture
> B   initial encounter for open fracture
> D   subsequent encounter for fracture with routine healing
> G   subsequent encounter for fracture with delayed healing
> K   subsequent encounter for fracture with nonunion
> P   subsequent encounter for fracture with malunion
> S   sequela

√6ᵗʰ **S99.20** Unspecified physeal fracture of phalanx of toe

     √7ᵗʰ **S99.201** Unspecified physeal fracture of phalanx of **right** toe   ▽

     √7ᵗʰ **S99.202** Unspecified physeal fracture of phalanx of **left** toe   ▽

     √7ᵗʰ **S99.209** Unspecified physeal fracture of phalanx of unspecified toe   ▽

√6ᵗʰ **S99.21** Salter-Harris Type I physeal fracture of phalanx of toe

     √7ᵗʰ **S99.211** Salter-Harris Type I physeal fracture of phalanx of **right** toe

     √7ᵗʰ **S99.212** Salter-Harris Type I physeal fracture of phalanx of **left** toe

     √7ᵗʰ **S99.219** Salter-Harris Type I physeal fracture of phalanx of unspecified toe   ▽

√6ᵗʰ **S99.22** Salter-Harris Type II physeal fracture of phalanx of toe

     √7ᵗʰ **S99.221** Salter-Harris Type II physeal fracture of phalanx of **right** toe

     √7ᵗʰ **S99.222** Salter-Harris Type II physeal fracture of phalanx of **left** toe

     √7ᵗʰ **S99.229** Salter-Harris Type II physeal fracture of phalanx of unspecified toe   ▽

√6ᵗʰ **S99.23** Salter-Harris Type III physeal fracture of phalanx of toe

     √7ᵗʰ **S99.231** Salter-Harris Type III physeal fracture of phalanx of **right** toe

     √7ᵗʰ **S99.232** Salter-Harris Type III physeal fracture of phalanx of **left** toe

     √7ᵗʰ **S99.239** Salter-Harris Type III physeal fracture of phalanx of unspecified toe   ▽

√6ᵗʰ **S99.24** Salter-Harris Type IV physeal fracture of phalanx of toe

     √7ᵗʰ **S99.241** Salter-Harris Type IV physeal fracture of phalanx of **right** toe

     √7ᵗʰ **S99.242** Salter-Harris Type IV physeal fracture of phalanx of **left** toe

     √7ᵗʰ **S99.249** Salter-Harris Type IV physeal fracture of phalanx of unspecified toe   ▽

√6ᵗʰ **S99.29** Other physeal fracture of phalanx of toe

     √7ᵗʰ **S99.291** Other physeal fracture of phalanx of **right** toe

     √7ᵗʰ **S99.292** Other physeal fracture of phalanx of **left** toe

     √7ᵗʰ **S99.299** Other physeal fracture of phalanx of unspecified toe   ▽

√5ᵗʰ **S99.8** Other specified injuries of ankle and foot

> The appropriate 7th character is to be added to each code from subcategory S99.8.
> A   initial encounter
> D   subsequent encounter
> S   sequela

√6ᵗʰ **S99.81** Other specified injuries of ankle

     √7ᵗʰ **S99.811** Other specified injuries of **right** ankle

     √7ᵗʰ **S99.812** Other specified injuries of **left** ankle

     √7ᵗʰ **S99.819** Other specified injuries of unspecified ankle   ▽

√6ᵗʰ **S99.82** Other specified injuries of foot

     √7ᵗʰ **S99.821** Other specified injuries of **right** foot

     √7ᵗʰ **S99.822** Other specified injuries of **left** foot

     √7ᵗʰ **S99.829** Other specified injuries of unspecified foot   ▽

√5ᵗʰ **S99.9** Unspecified injury of ankle and foot

> The appropriate 7th character is to be added to each code from subcategory S99.9.
> A   initial encounter
> D   subsequent encounter
> S   sequela

√6ᵗʰ **S99.91** Unspecified injury of ankle

     √7ᵗʰ **S99.911** Unspecified injury of **right** ankle   ▽

     √7ᵗʰ **S99.912** Unspecified injury of **left** ankle   ▽

     √7ᵗʰ **S99.919** Unspecified injury of unspecified ankle   ▽

√6ᵗʰ **S99.92** Unspecified injury of foot

     √7ᵗʰ **S99.921** Unspecified injury of **right** foot   ▽

     √7ᵗʰ **S99.922** Unspecified injury of **left** foot   ▽

     √7ᵗʰ **S99.929** Unspecified injury of unspecified foot   ▽

Injury, Poisoning And Certain Other Consequences of External Causes (T07-T88)

Injuries involving multiple body regions (T07)

> **EXCLUDES 1**   burns and corrosions (T20-T32)
>   frostbite (T33-T34)
>   insect bite or sting, venomous (T63.4)
>   sunburn (L55.-)

√x7ᵗʰ **T07** Unspecified multiple injuries   ▽

     EXCLUDES 1   injury NOS (T14.90)

     AHA: 2017,4Q,26

> The appropriate 7th character is to be added to code T07.
> A   initial encounter
> D   subsequent encounter
> S   sequela

☑ Additional Character Req   ✓x7ᵗʰ Placeholder Alert   Manifestation   ▽ Unspecified   ►◄ Revised Text   ● New Code   ▲ Revised Code Title

ICD-10-CM 2019   **1073**

Injury of unspecified body region (T14)

✓4ᵗʰ T14 Injury of unspecified body region
  EXCLUDES 1 *multiple unspecified injuries (T07)*
  AHA: 2017,4Q,26

  The appropriate 7th character is to be added to each code from category T14.
  A   initial encounter
  D   subsequent encounter
  S   sequela

✓x7ᵗʰ T14.8 Other injury of unspecified body region
  Abrasion NOS
  Contusion NOS
  Crush injury NOS
  Fracture NOS
  Skin injury NOS
  Vascular injury NOS
  Wound NOS

✓5ᵗʰ T14.9 Unspecified injury
  ✓x7ᵗʰ T14.90 Injury, unspecified ▽
    Injury NOS
  ✓x7ᵗʰ T14.91 Suicide attempt HCC
    Attempted suicide NOS

Effects of foreign body entering through natural orifice (T15-T19)

EXCLUDES 2 *foreign body accidentally left in operation wound (T81.5-)*
  foreign body in penetrating wound - See open wound by body region
  residual foreign body in soft tissue (M79.5)
  splinter, without open wound - See superficial injury by body region

✓4ᵗʰ T15 Foreign body on external eye
  EXCLUDES 2 *foreign body in penetrating wound of orbit and eye ball (S05.4-, S05.5-)*
    open wound of eyelid and periocular area (S01.1-)
    retained foreign body in eyelid (H02.8-)
    retained (old) foreign body in penetrating wound of orbit and eye ball (H05.5-, H44.6-, H44.7-)
    superficial foreign body of eyelid and periocular area (S00.25-)

  The appropriate 7th character is to be added to each code from category T15.
  A   initial encounter
  D   subsequent encounter
  S   sequela

✓5ᵗʰ T15.0 Foreign body in cornea
  ✓x7ᵗʰ T15.00 Foreign body in cornea, unspecified eye ▽
  ✓x7ᵗʰ T15.01 Foreign body in cornea, right eye
  ✓x7ᵗʰ T15.02 Foreign body in cornea, left eye

✓5ᵗʰ T15.1 Foreign body in conjunctival sac
  ✓x7ᵗʰ T15.10 Foreign body in conjunctival sac, unspecified eye ▽
  ✓x7ᵗʰ T15.11 Foreign body in conjunctival sac, right eye
  ✓x7ᵗʰ T15.12 Foreign body in conjunctival sac, left eye

✓5ᵗʰ T15.8 Foreign body in other and multiple parts of external eye
  Foreign body in lacrimal punctum
  ✓x7ᵗʰ T15.80 Foreign body in other and multiple parts of external eye, unspecified eye ▽
  ✓x7ᵗʰ T15.81 Foreign body in other and multiple parts of external eye, right eye
  ✓x7ᵗʰ T15.82 Foreign body in other and multiple parts of external eye, left eye

✓5ᵗʰ T15.9 Foreign body on external eye, part unspecified
  ✓x7ᵗʰ T15.90 Foreign body on external eye, part unspecified, unspecified eye ▽
  ✓x7ᵗʰ T15.91 Foreign body on external eye, part unspecified, right eye ▽
  ✓x7ᵗʰ T15.92 Foreign body on external eye, part unspecified, left eye ▽

✓4ᵗʰ T16 Foreign body in ear
  INCLUDES foreign body in auditory canal

  The appropriate 7th character is to be added to each code from category T16.
  A   initial encounter
  D   subsequent encounter
  S   sequela

✓x7ᵗʰ T16.1 Foreign body in right ear
✓x7ᵗʰ T16.2 Foreign body in left ear
✓x7ᵗʰ T16.9 Foreign body in ear, unspecified ear ▽

✓4ᵗʰ T17 Foreign body in respiratory tract
  The appropriate 7th character is to be added to each code from category T17.
  A   initial encounter
  D   subsequent encounter
  S   sequela

✓x7ᵗʰ T17.0 Foreign body in nasal sinus
✓x7ᵗʰ T17.1 Foreign body in nostril
  Foreign body in nose NOS
✓5ᵗʰ T17.2 Foreign body in pharynx
  Foreign body in nasopharynx
  Foreign body in throat NOS
  ✓6ᵗʰ T17.20 Unspecified foreign body in pharynx
    ✓7ᵗʰ T17.200 Unspecified foreign body in pharynx causing asphyxiation ▽
    ✓7ᵗʰ T17.208 Unspecified foreign body in pharynx causing other injury ▽
  ✓6ᵗʰ T17.21 Gastric contents in pharynx
    Aspiration of gastric contents into pharynx
    Vomitus in pharynx
    ✓7ᵗʰ T17.210 Gastric contents in pharynx causing asphyxiation
    ✓7ᵗʰ T17.218 Gastric contents in pharynx causing other injury
  ✓6ᵗʰ T17.22 Food in pharynx
    Bones in pharynx
    Seeds in pharynx
    ✓7ᵗʰ T17.220 Food in pharynx causing asphyxiation
    ✓7ᵗʰ T17.228 Food in pharynx causing other injury
  ✓6ᵗʰ T17.29 Other foreign object in pharynx
    ✓7ᵗʰ T17.290 Other foreign object in pharynx causing asphyxiation
    ✓7ᵗʰ T17.298 Other foreign object in pharynx causing other injury
✓5ᵗʰ T17.3 Foreign body in larynx
  ✓6ᵗʰ T17.30 Unspecified foreign body in larynx
    ✓7ᵗʰ T17.300 Unspecified foreign body in larynx causing asphyxiation ▽
    ✓7ᵗʰ T17.308 Unspecified foreign body in larynx causing other injury ▽
  ✓6ᵗʰ T17.31 Gastric contents in larynx
    Aspiration of gastric contents into larynx
    Vomitus in larynx
    ✓7ᵗʰ T17.310 Gastric contents in larynx causing asphyxiation
    ✓7ᵗʰ T17.318 Gastric contents in larynx causing other injury
  ✓6ᵗʰ T17.32 Food in larynx
    Bones in larynx
    Seeds in larynx
    ✓7ᵗʰ T17.320 Food in larynx causing asphyxiation
    ✓7ᵗʰ T17.328 Food in larynx causing other injury
  ✓6ᵗʰ T17.39 Other foreign object in larynx
    ✓7ᵗʰ T17.390 Other foreign object in larynx causing asphyxiation
    ✓7ᵗʰ T17.398 Other foreign object in larynx causing other injury
✓5ᵗʰ T17.4 Foreign body in trachea
  ✓6ᵗʰ T17.40 Unspecified foreign body in trachea
    ✓7ᵗʰ T17.400 Unspecified foreign body in trachea causing asphyxiation ▽
    ✓7ᵗʰ T17.408 Unspecified foreign body in trachea causing other injury ▽

√6ᵗʰ **T17.41** Gastric contents in trachea
    Aspiration of gastric contents into trachea
    Vomitus in trachea
      √7ᵗʰ **T17.410** Gastric contents in trachea causing asphyxiation
      √7ᵗʰ **T17.418** Gastric contents in trachea causing other injury

√6ᵗʰ **T17.42** Food in trachea
    Bones in trachea
    Seeds in trachea
      √7ᵗʰ **T17.420** Food in trachea causing asphyxiation
      √7ᵗʰ **T17.428** Food in trachea causing other injury

√6ᵗʰ **T17.49** Other foreign object in trachea
      √7ᵗʰ **T17.490** Other foreign object in trachea causing asphyxiation
      √7ᵗʰ **T17.498** Other foreign object in trachea causing other injury

√5ᵗʰ **T17.5** Foreign body in bronchus

√6ᵗʰ **T17.50** Unspecified foreign body in bronchus
      √7ᵗʰ **T17.500** Unspecified foreign body in bronchus causing asphyxiation   ▽
      √7ᵗʰ **T17.508** Unspecified foreign body in bronchus causing other injury   ▽

√6ᵗʰ **T17.51** Gastric contents in bronchus
    Aspiration of gastric contents into bronchus
    Vomitus in bronchus
      √7ᵗʰ **T17.510** Gastric contents in bronchus causing asphyxiation
      √7ᵗʰ **T17.518** Gastric contents in bronchus causing other injury

√6ᵗʰ **T17.52** Food in bronchus
    Bones in bronchus
    Seeds in bronchus
      √7ᵗʰ **T17.520** Food in bronchus causing asphyxiation
      √7ᵗʰ **T17.528** Food in bronchus causing other injury

√6ᵗʰ **T17.59** Other foreign object in bronchus
      √7ᵗʰ **T17.590** Other foreign object in bronchus causing asphyxiation
      √7ᵗʰ **T17.598** Other foreign object in bronchus causing other injury

√5ᵗʰ **T17.8** Foreign body in other parts of respiratory tract
    Foreign body in bronchioles
    Foreign body in lung

√6ᵗʰ **T17.80** Unspecified foreign body in other parts of respiratory tract
      √7ᵗʰ **T17.800** Unspecified foreign body in other parts of respiratory tract causing asphyxiation   ▽
      √7ᵗʰ **T17.808** Unspecified foreign body in other parts of respiratory tract causing other injury   ▽

√6ᵗʰ **T17.81** Gastric contents in other parts of respiratory tract
    Aspiration of gastric contents into other parts of respiratory tract
    Vomitus in other parts of respiratory tract
      √7ᵗʰ **T17.810** Gastric contents in other parts of respiratory tract causing asphyxiation
      √7ᵗʰ **T17.818** Gastric contents in other parts of respiratory tract causing other injury

√6ᵗʰ **T17.82** Food in other parts of respiratory tract
    Bones in other parts of respiratory tract
    Seeds in other parts of respiratory tract
      √7ᵗʰ **T17.820** Food in other parts of respiratory tract causing asphyxiation
      √7ᵗʰ **T17.828** Food in other parts of respiratory tract causing other injury

√6ᵗʰ **T17.89** Other foreign object in other parts of respiratory tract
      √7ᵗʰ **T17.890** Other foreign object in other parts of respiratory tract causing asphyxiation
      √7ᵗʰ **T17.898** Other foreign object in other parts of respiratory tract causing other injury

√5ᵗʰ **T17.9** Foreign body in respiratory tract, part unspecified

√6ᵗʰ **T17.90** Unspecified foreign body in respiratory tract, part unspecified
      √7ᵗʰ **T17.900** Unspecified foreign body in respiratory tract, part unspecified causing asphyxiation   ▽

      √7ᵗʰ **T17.908** Unspecified foreign body in respiratory tract, part unspecified causing other injury   ▽

√6ᵗʰ **T17.91** Gastric contents in respiratory tract, part unspecified
    Aspiration of gastric contents into respiratory tract, part unspecified
    Vomitus in trachea respiratory tract, part unspecified
      √7ᵗʰ **T17.910** Gastric contents in respiratory tract, part unspecified causing asphyxiation   ▽
      √7ᵗʰ **T17.918** Gastric contents in respiratory tract, part unspecified causing other injury   ▽

√6ᵗʰ **T17.92** Food in respiratory tract, part unspecified
    Bones in respiratory tract, part unspecified
    Seeds in respiratory tract, part unspecified
      √7ᵗʰ **T17.920** Food in respiratory tract, part unspecified causing asphyxiation   ▽
      √7ᵗʰ **T17.928** Food in respiratory tract, part unspecified causing other injury   ▽

√6ᵗʰ **T17.99** Other foreign object in respiratory tract, part unspecified
      √7ᵗʰ **T17.990** Other foreign object in respiratory tract, part unspecified in causing asphyxiation   ▽
      √7ᵗʰ **T17.998** Other foreign object in respiratory tract, part unspecified causing other injury   ▽

√4ᵗʰ **T18** Foreign body in alimentary tract
    EXCLUDES 2   *foreign body in pharynx (T17.2-)*

> The appropriate 7th character is to be added to each code from category T18.
> A   initial encounter
> D   subsequent encounter
> S   sequela

√x7ᵗʰ **T18.0** Foreign body in mouth

√5ᵗʰ **T18.1** Foreign body in esophagus
    EXCLUDES 2   *foreign body in respiratory tract (T17.-)*

√6ᵗʰ **T18.10** Unspecified foreign body in esophagus
      √7ᵗʰ **T18.100** Unspecified foreign body in esophagus causing compression of trachea   ▽
        Unspecified foreign body in esophagus causing obstruction of respiration
      √7ᵗʰ **T18.108** Unspecified foreign body in esophagus causing other injury   ▽

√6ᵗʰ **T18.11** Gastric contents in esophagus
    Vomitus in esophagus
      √7ᵗʰ **T18.110** Gastric contents in esophagus causing compression of trachea
        Gastric contents in esophagus causing obstruction of respiration
      √7ᵗʰ **T18.118** Gastric contents in esophagus causing other injury

√6ᵗʰ **T18.12** Food in esophagus
    Bones in esophagus
    Seeds in esophagus
      √7ᵗʰ **T18.120** Food in esophagus causing compression of trachea
        Food in esophagus causing obstruction of respiration
      √7ᵗʰ **T18.128** Food in esophagus causing other injury

√6ᵗʰ **T18.19** Other foreign object in esophagus
    AHA: 2015,1Q,23
      √7ᵗʰ **T18.190** Other foreign object in esophagus causing compression of trachea
        Other foreign body in esophagus causing obstruction of respiration
      √7ᵗʰ **T18.198** Other foreign object in esophagus causing other injury

√x7ᵗʰ **T18.2** Foreign body in stomach

√x7ᵗʰ **T18.3** Foreign body in small intestine

√x7ᵗʰ **T18.4** Foreign body in colon

√x7ᵗʰ **T18.5** Foreign body in anus and rectum
    Foreign body in rectosigmoid (junction)

√x7ᵗʰ **T18.8** Foreign body in other parts of alimentary tract

---

√x7ᵗʰ **T18.9** **Foreign body of alimentary tract, part unspecified** ▽
     Foreign body in digestive system NOS
     Swallowed foreign body NOS

√4ᵗʰ **T19** **Foreign body in genitourinary tract**
     EXCLUDES 2   complications due to implanted mesh (T83.7-)
        mechanical complications of contraceptive device
          (intrauterine) (vaginal) (T83.3-)
        presence of contraceptive device (intrauterine) (vaginal)
          (Z97.5)

     The appropriate 7th character is to be added to each code from category T19.
     A   initial encounter
     D   subsequent encounter
     S   sequela

√x7ᵗʰ **T19.0** **Foreign body in urethra**

√x7ᵗʰ **T19.1** **Foreign body in bladder**

√x7ᵗʰ **T19.2** **Foreign body in vulva and vagina** ♀

√x7ᵗʰ **T19.3** **Foreign body in uterus** ♀

√x7ᵗʰ **T19.4** **Foreign body in penis** ♂

√x7ᵗʰ **T19.8** **Foreign body in other parts of genitourinary tract**

√x7ᵗʰ **T19.9** **Foreign body in genitourinary tract, part unspecified** ▽

Burns and corrosions (T20-T32)

INCLUDES   burns (thermal) from electrical heating appliances
        burns (thermal) from electricity
        burns (thermal) from flame
        burns (thermal) from friction
        burns (thermal) from hot air and hot gases
        burns (thermal) from hot objects
        burns (thermal) from lightning
        burns (thermal) from radiation
        chemical burn [corrosion] (external) (internal)
        scalds
EXCLUDES 2   erythema [dermatitis] ab igne (L59.0)
        radiation-related disorders of the skin and subcutaneous tissue
          (L55-L59)
        sunburn (L55.-)
AHA: 2016,2Q,4

Burns and corrosions of external body surface, specified by site (T20-T25)

INCLUDES   burns and corrosions of first degree [erythema]
        burns and corrosions of second degree [blisters] [epidermal loss]
        burns and corrosions of third degree [deep necrosis of underlying
          tissue] [full-thickness skin loss]
Use additional code from category T31 or T32 to identify extent of body surface involved

√4ᵗʰ **T20** **Burn and corrosion of head, face, and neck**
     EXCLUDES 2   burn and corrosion of ear drum (T28.41, T28.91)
        burn and corrosion of eye and adnexa (T26.-)
        burn and corrosion of mouth and pharynx (T28.0)
     AHA: 2015,1Q,18-19

     The appropriate 7th character is to be added to each code from category T20.
     A   initial encounter
     D   subsequent encounter
     S   sequela

√5ᵗʰ **T20.0** **Burn of unspecified degree of head, face, and neck**
     Use additional external cause code to identify the source, place and intent of the burn (X00-X19, X75-X77, X96-X98, Y92)

√x7ᵗʰ **T20.00** **Burn of unspecified degree of head, face, and neck, unspecified site** ▽

√6ᵗʰ **T20.01** **Burn of unspecified degree of ear [any part, except ear drum]**
     EXCLUDES 2   burn of ear drum (T28.41-)

√7ᵗʰ **T20.011** **Burn of unspecified degree of right ear [any part, except ear drum]** ▽

√7ᵗʰ **T20.012** **Burn of unspecified degree of left ear [any part, except ear drum]** ▽

√7ᵗʰ **T20.019** **Burn of unspecified degree of unspecified ear [any part, except ear drum]** ▽

√x7ᵗʰ **T20.02** **Burn of unspecified degree of lip(s)** ▽

√x7ᵗʰ **T20.03** **Burn of unspecified degree of chin** ▽

√x7ᵗʰ **T20.04** **Burn of unspecified degree of nose (septum)** ▽

√x7ᵗʰ **T20.05** **Burn of unspecified degree of scalp [any part]** ▽

√x7ᵗʰ **T20.06** **Burn of unspecified degree of forehead and cheek** ▽

√x7ᵗʰ **T20.07** **Burn of unspecified degree of neck** ▽

√x7ᵗʰ **T20.09** **Burn of unspecified degree of multiple sites of head, face, and neck** ▽

√5ᵗʰ **T20.1** **Burn of first degree of head, face, and neck**
     Use additional external cause code to identify the source, place and intent of the burn (X00-X19, X75-X77, X96-X98, Y92)

√x7ᵗʰ **T20.10** **Burn of first degree of head, face, and neck, unspecified site** ▽

√6ᵗʰ **T20.11** **Burn of first degree of ear [any part, except ear drum]**
     EXCLUDES 2   burn of ear drum (T28.41-)

√7ᵗʰ **T20.111** **Burn of first degree of right ear [any part, except ear drum]**

√7ᵗʰ **T20.112** **Burn of first degree of left ear [any part, except ear drum]**

√7ᵗʰ **T20.119** **Burn of first degree of unspecified ear [any part, except ear drum]** ▽

√x7ᵗʰ **T20.12** **Burn of first degree of lip(s)**

√x7ᵗʰ **T20.13** **Burn of first degree of chin**

√x7ᵗʰ **T20.14** **Burn of first degree of nose (septum)**

√x7ᵗʰ **T20.15** **Burn of first degree of scalp [any part]**

√x7ᵗʰ **T20.16** **Burn of first degree of forehead and cheek**

√x7ᵗʰ **T20.17** **Burn of first degree of neck**

√x7ᵗʰ **T20.19** **Burn of first degree of multiple sites of head, face, and neck**

Degree of Burns

Normal   First Degree Burn
Second Degree Burn   Third Degree Burn

(Epidermis, Dermis, Subcutaneous)

√5ᵗʰ **T20.2** **Burn of second degree of head, face, and neck**
     Use additional external cause code to identify the source, place and intent of the burn (X00-X19, X75-X77, X96-X98, Y92)

√x7ᵗʰ **T20.20** **Burn of second degree of head, face, and neck, unspecified site** ▽

√6ᵗʰ **T20.21** **Burn of second degree of ear [any part, except ear drum]**
     EXCLUDES 2   burn of ear drum (T28.41-)

√7ᵗʰ **T20.211** **Burn of second degree of right ear [any part, except ear drum]**

√7ᵗʰ **T20.212** **Burn of second degree of left ear [any part, except ear drum]**

√7ᵗʰ **T20.219** **Burn of second degree of unspecified ear [any part, except ear drum]** ▽

√x7ᵗʰ **T20.22** **Burn of second degree of lip(s)**

√x7ᵗʰ **T20.23** **Burn of second degree of chin**

√x7ᵗʰ **T20.24** **Burn of second degree of nose (septum)**

√x7ᵗʰ **T20.25** **Burn of second degree of scalp [any part]**

√x7ᵗʰ **T20.26** **Burn of second degree of forehead and cheek**

√x7ᵗʰ **T20.27** **Burn of second degree of neck**

√x7ᵗʰ **T20.29** Burn of second degree of multiple sites of head, face, and neck

√5ᵗʰ **T20.3** Burn of third degree of head, face, and neck

Use additional external cause code to identify the source, place and intent of the burn (X00-X19, X75-X77, X96-X98, Y92)

√x7ᵗʰ **T20.30** Burn of third degree of head, face, and neck, unspecified site

√6ᵗʰ **T20.31** Burn of third degree of ear [any part, except ear drum]

EXCLUDES 2 burn of ear drum (T28.41-)

AHA: 2015,1Q,18

√7ᵗʰ **T20.311** Burn of third degree of right ear [any part, except ear drum]

√7ᵗʰ **T20.312** Burn of third degree of left ear [any part, except ear drum]

√7ᵗʰ **T20.319** Burn of third degree of unspecified ear [any part, except ear drum] ▽

√x7ᵗʰ **T20.32** Burn of third degree of lip(s)

√x7ᵗʰ **T20.33** Burn of third degree of chin

√x7ᵗʰ **T20.34** Burn of third degree of nose (septum)

√x7ᵗʰ **T20.35** Burn of third degree of scalp [any part]

√x7ᵗʰ **T20.36** Burn of third degree of forehead and cheek

√x7ᵗʰ **T20.37** Burn of third degree of neck

√x7ᵗʰ **T20.39** Burn of third degree of multiple sites of head, face, and neck

√5ᵗʰ **T20.4** Corrosion of unspecified degree of head, face, and neck

Code first (T51-T65) to identify chemical and intent
Use additional external cause code to identify place (Y92)

√x7ᵗʰ **T20.40** Corrosion of unspecified degree of head, face, and neck, unspecified site ▽

√6ᵗʰ **T20.41** Corrosion of unspecified degree of ear [any part, except ear drum]

EXCLUDES 2 corrosion of ear drum (T28.91-)

√7ᵗʰ **T20.411** Corrosion of unspecified degree of right ear [any part, except ear drum] ▽

√7ᵗʰ **T20.412** Corrosion of unspecified degree of left ear [any part, except ear drum] ▽

√7ᵗʰ **T20.419** Corrosion of unspecified degree of unspecified ear [any part, except ear drum] ▽

√x7ᵗʰ **T20.42** Corrosion of unspecified degree of lip(s) ▽

√x7ᵗʰ **T20.43** Corrosion of unspecified degree of chin ▽

√x7ᵗʰ **T20.44** Corrosion of unspecified degree of nose (septum) ▽

√x7ᵗʰ **T20.45** Corrosion of unspecified degree of scalp [any part] ▽

√x7ᵗʰ **T20.46** Corrosion of unspecified degree of forehead and cheek ▽

√x7ᵗʰ **T20.47** Corrosion of unspecified degree of neck ▽

√x7ᵗʰ **T20.49** Corrosion of unspecified degree of multiple sites of head, face, and neck ▽

√5ᵗʰ **T20.5** Corrosion of first degree of head, face, and neck

Code first (T51-T65) to identify chemical and intent
Use additional external cause code to identify place (Y92)

√x7ᵗʰ **T20.50** Corrosion of first degree of head, face, and neck, unspecified site ▽

√6ᵗʰ **T20.51** Corrosion of first degree of ear [any part, except ear drum]

EXCLUDES 2 corrosion of ear drum (T28.91-)

√7ᵗʰ **T20.511** Corrosion of first degree of right ear [any part, except ear drum]

√7ᵗʰ **T20.512** Corrosion of first degree of left ear [any part, except ear drum]

√7ᵗʰ **T20.519** Corrosion of first degree of unspecified ear [any part, except ear drum] ▽

√x7ᵗʰ **T20.52** Corrosion of first degree of lip(s)

√x7ᵗʰ **T20.53** Corrosion of first degree of chin

√x7ᵗʰ **T20.54** Corrosion of first degree of nose (septum)

√x7ᵗʰ **T20.55** Corrosion of first degree of scalp [any part]

√x7ᵗʰ **T20.56** Corrosion of first degree of forehead and cheek

√x7ᵗʰ **T20.57** Corrosion of first degree of neck

√x7ᵗʰ **T20.59** Corrosion of first degree of multiple sites of head, face, and neck

√5ᵗʰ **T20.6** Corrosion of second degree of head, face, and neck

Code first (T51-T65) to identify chemical and intent
Use additional external cause code to identify place (Y92)

√x7ᵗʰ **T20.60** Corrosion of second degree of head, face, and neck, unspecified site ▽

√6ᵗʰ **T20.61** Corrosion of second degree of ear [any part, except ear drum]

EXCLUDES 2 corrosion of ear drum (T28.91-)

√7ᵗʰ **T20.611** Corrosion of second degree of right ear [any part, except ear drum]

√7ᵗʰ **T20.612** Corrosion of second degree of left ear [any part, except ear drum]

√7ᵗʰ **T20.619** Corrosion of second degree of unspecified ear [any part, except ear drum] ▽

√x7ᵗʰ **T20.62** Corrosion of second degree of lip(s)

√x7ᵗʰ **T20.63** Corrosion of second degree of chin

√x7ᵗʰ **T20.64** Corrosion of second degree of nose (septum)

√x7ᵗʰ **T20.65** Corrosion of second degree of scalp [any part]

√x7ᵗʰ **T20.66** Corrosion of second degree of forehead and cheek

√x7ᵗʰ **T20.67** Corrosion of second degree of neck

√x7ᵗʰ **T20.69** Corrosion of second degree of multiple sites of head, face, and neck

√5ᵗʰ **T20.7** Corrosion of third degree of head, face, and neck

Code first (T51-T65) to identify chemical and intent
Use additional external cause code to identify place (Y92)

√x7ᵗʰ **T20.70** Corrosion of third degree of head, face, and neck, unspecified site ▽

√6ᵗʰ **T20.71** Corrosion of third degree of ear [any part, except ear drum]

EXCLUDES 2 corrosion of ear drum (T28.91-)

√7ᵗʰ **T20.711** Corrosion of third degree of right ear [any part, except ear drum]

√7ᵗʰ **T20.712** Corrosion of third degree of left ear [any part, except ear drum]

√7ᵗʰ **T20.719** Corrosion of third degree of unspecified ear [any part, except ear drum] ▽

√x7ᵗʰ **T20.72** Corrosion of third degree of lip(s)

√x7ᵗʰ **T20.73** Corrosion of third degree of chin

√x7ᵗʰ **T20.74** Corrosion of third degree of nose (septum)

√x7ᵗʰ **T20.75** Corrosion of third degree of scalp [any part]

√x7ᵗʰ **T20.76** Corrosion of third degree of forehead and cheek

√x7ᵗʰ **T20.77** Corrosion of third degree of neck

√x7ᵗʰ **T20.79** Corrosion of third degree of multiple sites of head, face, and neck

√4ᵗʰ **T21** Burn and corrosion of trunk

INCLUDES burns and corrosion of hip region

EXCLUDES 2 burns and corrosion of axilla (T22.- with fifth character 4)

burns and corrosion of scapular region (T22.- with fifth character 6)

burns and corrosion of shoulder (T22.- with fifth character 5)

The appropriate 7th character is to be added to each code from category T21.
A initial encounter
D subsequent encounter
S sequela

√5ᵗʰ **T21.0** Burn of unspecified degree of trunk

Use additional external cause code to identify the source, place and intent of the burn (X00-X19, X75-X77, X96-X98, Y92)

√x7ᵗʰ **T21.00** Burn of unspecified degree of trunk, unspecified site ▽

√x7ᵗʰ **T21.01** Burn of unspecified degree of chest wall ▽

Burn of unspecified degree of breast

√x7ᵗʰ **T21.02** Burn of unspecified degree of abdominal wall ▽

Burn of unspecified degree of flank
Burn of unspecified degree of groin

√x7ᵗʰ **T21.03** Burn of unspecified degree of upper back ▽

Burn of unspecified degree of interscapular region

√x7ᵗʰ **T21.04** Burn of unspecified degree of lower back ▽

√x7ᵗʰ **T21.05** Burn of unspecified degree of buttock ▽

Burn of unspecified degree of anus

☑ Additional Character Req √x7ᵗʰ Placeholder Alert Manifestation ▽ Unspecified ►◄ Revised Text ● New Code ▲ Revised Code Title

√x7ᵗʰ **T21.06** **Burn of unspecified degree of** male genital region ♂ ▽
  Burn of unspecified degree of penis
  Burn of unspecified degree of scrotum
  Burn of unspecified degree of testis

√x7ᵗʰ **T21.07** **Burn of unspecified degree of** female genital region ♀ ▽
  Burn of unspecified degree of labium (majus) (minus)
  Burn of unspecified degree of perineum
  Burn of unspecified degree of vulva
  EXCLUDES 2   burn of vagina (T28.3)

√x7ᵗʰ **T21.09** **Burn of unspecified degree of other site of trunk** ▽

√5ᵗʰ **T21.1** **Burn of** first degree **of trunk**
  Use additional external cause code to identify the source, place and intent of the burn (X00-X19, X75-X77, X96-X98, Y92)

√x7ᵗʰ **T21.10** **Burn of first degree of trunk, unspecified site** ▽

√x7ᵗʰ **T21.11** **Burn of first degree of** chest wall
  Burn of first degree of breast

√x7ᵗʰ **T21.12** **Burn of first degree of** abdominal wall
  Burn of first degree of flank
  Burn of first degree of groin

√x7ᵗʰ **T21.13** **Burn of first degree of** upper back
  Burn of first degree of interscapular region

√x7ᵗʰ **T21.14** **Burn of first degree of** lower back

√x7ᵗʰ **T21.15** **Burn of first degree of** buttock
  Burn of first degree of anus

√x7ᵗʰ **T21.16** **Burn of first degree of** male genital region ♂
  Burn of first degree of penis
  Burn of first degree of scrotum
  Burn of first degree of testis

√x7ᵗʰ **T21.17** **Burn of first degree of** female genital region ♀
  Burn of first degree of labium (majus) (minus)
  Burn of first degree of perineum
  Burn of first degree of vulva
  EXCLUDES 2   burn of vagina (T28.3)

√x7ᵗʰ **T21.19** **Burn of first degree of other site of trunk**

√5ᵗʰ **T21.2** **Burn of** second degree **of trunk**
  Use additional external cause code to identify the source, place and intent of the burn (X00-X19, X75-X77, X96-X98, Y92)

√x7ᵗʰ **T21.20** **Burn of second degree of trunk, unspecified site** ▽

√x7ᵗʰ **T21.21** **Burn of second degree of** chest wall
  Burn of second degree of breast

√x7ᵗʰ **T21.22** **Burn of second degree of** abdominal wall
  Burn of second degree of flank
  Burn of second degree of groin

√x7ᵗʰ **T21.23** **Burn of second degree of** upper back
  Burn of second degree of interscapular region

√x7ᵗʰ **T21.24** **Burn of second degree of** lower back

√x7ᵗʰ **T21.25** **Burn of second degree of** buttock
  Burn of second degree of anus

√x7ᵗʰ **T21.26** **Burn of second degree of** male genital region ♂
  Burn of second degree of penis
  Burn of second degree of scrotum
  Burn of second degree of testis

√x7ᵗʰ **T21.27** **Burn of second degree of** female genital region ♀
  Burn of second degree of labium (majus) (minus)
  Burn of second degree of perineum
  Burn of second degree of vulva
  EXCLUDES 2   burn of vagina (T28.3)

√x7ᵗʰ **T21.29** **Burn of second degree of other site of trunk**

√5ᵗʰ **T21.3** **Burn of** third degree **of trunk**
  Use additional external cause code to identify the source, place and intent of the burn (X00-X19, X75-X77, X96-X98, Y92)

√x7ᵗʰ **T21.30** **Burn of third degree of trunk, unspecified site** ▽

√x7ᵗʰ **T21.31** **Burn of third degree of** chest wall
  Burn of third degree of breast
  AHA: 2016,2Q,5

√x7ᵗʰ **T21.32** **Burn of third degree of** abdominal wall
  Burn of third degree of flank
  Burn of third degree of groin

√x7ᵗʰ **T21.33** **Burn of third degree of** upper back
  Burn of third degree of interscapular region

√x7ᵗʰ **T21.34** **Burn of third degree of** lower back

√x7ᵗʰ **T21.35** **Burn of third degree of** buttock
  Burn of third degree of anus

√x7ᵗʰ **T21.36** **Burn of third degree of** male genital region ♂
  Burn of third degree of penis
  Burn of third degree of scrotum
  Burn of third degree of testis

√x7ᵗʰ **T21.37** **Burn of third degree of** female genital region ♀
  Burn of third degree of labium (majus) (minus)
  Burn of third degree of perineum
  Burn of third degree of vulva
  EXCLUDES 2   burn of vagina (T28.3)

√x7ᵗʰ **T21.39** **Burn of third degree of other site of trunk**

√5ᵗʰ **T21.4** **Corrosion of unspecified degree of trunk**
  Code first (T51-T65) to identify chemical and intent
  Use additional external cause code to identify place (Y92)

√x7ᵗʰ **T21.40** **Corrosion of unspecified degree of trunk, unspecified site** ▽

√x7ᵗʰ **T21.41** **Corrosion of unspecified degree of** chest wall ▽
  Corrosion of unspecified degree of breast

√x7ᵗʰ **T21.42** **Corrosion of unspecified degree of** abdominal wall ▽
  Corrosion of unspecified degree of flank
  Corrosion of unspecified degree of groin

√x7ᵗʰ **T21.43** **Corrosion of unspecified degree of** upper back ▽
  Corrosion of unspecified degree of interscapular region

√x7ᵗʰ **T21.44** **Corrosion of unspecified degree of** lower back ▽

√x7ᵗʰ **T21.45** **Corrosion of unspecified degree of** buttock ▽
  Corrosion of unspecified degree of anus

√x7ᵗʰ **T21.46** **Corrosion of unspecified degree of** male genital region ♂ ▽
  Corrosion of unspecified degree of penis
  Corrosion of unspecified degree of scrotum
  Corrosion of unspecified degree of testis

√x7ᵗʰ **T21.47** **Corrosion of unspecified degree of** female genital region ♀ ▽
  Corrosion of unspecified degree of labium (majus) (minus)
  Corrosion of unspecified degree of perineum
  Corrosion of unspecified degree of vulva
  EXCLUDES 2   corrosion of vagina (T28.8)

√x7ᵗʰ **T21.49** **Corrosion of unspecified degree of other site of trunk** ▽

√5ᵗʰ **T21.5** **Corrosion of** first degree **of trunk**
  Code first (T51-T65) to identify chemical and intent
  Use additional external cause code to identify place (Y92)

√x7ᵗʰ **T21.50** **Corrosion of first degree of trunk, unspecified site** ▽

√x7ᵗʰ **T21.51** **Corrosion of first degree of** chest wall
  Corrosion of first degree of breast

√x7ᵗʰ **T21.52** **Corrosion of first degree of** abdominal wall
  Corrosion of first degree of flank
  Corrosion of first degree of groin

√x7ᵗʰ **T21.53** **Corrosion of first degree of** upper back
  Corrosion of first degree of interscapular region

√x7ᵗʰ **T21.54** **Corrosion of first degree of** lower back

√x7ᵗʰ **T21.55** **Corrosion of first degree of** buttock
  Corrosion of first degree of anus

√x7ᵗʰ **T21.56** **Corrosion of first degree of** male genital region ♂
  Corrosion of first degree of penis
  Corrosion of first degree of scrotum
  Corrosion of first degree of testis

√x7ᵗʰ **T21.57** **Corrosion of first degree of female genital region** ♀
Corrosion of first degree of labium (majus) (minus)
Corrosion of first degree of perineum
Corrosion of first degree of vulva
EXCLUDES 2 corrosion of vagina (T28.8)

√x7ᵗʰ **T21.59** **Corrosion of first degree of other site of trunk**

√5ᵗʰ **T21.6** **Corrosion of second degree of trunk**
Code first (T51-T65) to identify chemical and intent
Use additional external cause code to identify place (Y92)

√x7ᵗʰ **T21.60** **Corrosion of second degree of trunk, unspecified site** ▽

√x7ᵗʰ **T21.61** **Corrosion of second degree of chest wall**
Corrosion of second degree of breast

√x7ᵗʰ **T21.62** **Corrosion of second degree of abdominal wall**
Corrosion of second degree of flank
Corrosion of second degree of groin

√x7ᵗʰ **T21.63** **Corrosion of second degree of upper back**
Corrosion of second degree of interscapular region

√x7ᵗʰ **T21.64** **Corrosion of second degree of lower back**

√x7ᵗʰ **T21.65** **Corrosion of second degree of buttock**
Corrosion of second degree of anus

√x7ᵗʰ **T21.66** **Corrosion of second degree of male genital region** ♂
Corrosion of second degree of penis
Corrosion of second degree of scrotum
Corrosion of second degree of testis

√x7ᵗʰ **T21.67** **Corrosion of second degree of female genital region** ♀
Corrosion of second degree of labium (majus) (minus)
Corrosion of second degree of perineum
Corrosion of second degree of vulva
EXCLUDES 2 corrosion of vagina (T28.8)

√x7ᵗʰ **T21.69** **Corrosion of second degree of other site of trunk**

√5ᵗʰ **T21.7** **Corrosion of third degree of trunk**
Code first (T51-T65) to identify chemical and intent
Use additional external cause code to identify place (Y92)

√x7ᵗʰ **T21.70** **Corrosion of third degree of trunk, unspecified site** ▽

√x7ᵗʰ **T21.71** **Corrosion of third degree of chest wall**
Corrosion of third degree of breast

√x7ᵗʰ **T21.72** **Corrosion of third degree of abdominal wall**
Corrosion of third degree of flank
Corrosion of third degree of groin

√x7ᵗʰ **T21.73** **Corrosion of third degree of upper back**
Corrosion of third degree of interscapular region

√x7ᵗʰ **T21.74** **Corrosion of third degree of lower back**

√x7ᵗʰ **T21.75** **Corrosion of third degree of buttock**
Corrosion of third degree of anus

√x7ᵗʰ **T21.76** **Corrosion of third degree of male genital region** ♂
Corrosion of third degree of penis
Corrosion of third degree of scrotum
Corrosion of third degree of testis

√x7ᵗʰ **T21.77** **Corrosion of third degree of female genital region** ♀
Corrosion of third degree of labium (majus) (minus)
Corrosion of third degree of perineum
Corrosion of third degree of vulva
EXCLUDES 2 corrosion of vagina (T28.8)

√x7ᵗʰ **T21.79** **Corrosion of third degree of other site of trunk**

√4ᵗʰ **T22** **Burn and corrosion of shoulder and upper limb, except wrist and hand**
EXCLUDES 2 burn and corrosion of interscapular region (T21.-)
burn and corrosion of wrist and hand (T23.-)

The appropriate 7th character is to be added to each code from category T22.
A initial encounter
D subsequent encounter
S sequela

√5ᵗʰ **T22.0** **Burn of unspecified degree of shoulder and upper limb, except wrist and hand**
Use additional external cause code to identify the source, place and intent of the burn (X00-X19, X75-X77, X96-X98, Y92)

√6ᵗʰ **T22.00** **Burn of unspecified degree of shoulder and upper limb, except wrist and hand, unspecified site** ▽

√6ᵗʰ **T22.01** **Burn of unspecified degree of forearm**
√7ᵗʰ **T22.011** **Burn of unspecified degree of right forearm** ▽
√7ᵗʰ **T22.012** **Burn of unspecified degree of left forearm** ▽
√7ᵗʰ **T22.019** **Burn of unspecified degree of unspecified forearm** ▽

√6ᵗʰ **T22.02** **Burn of unspecified degree of elbow**
√7ᵗʰ **T22.021** **Burn of unspecified degree of right elbow** ▽
√7ᵗʰ **T22.022** **Burn of unspecified degree of left elbow** ▽
√7ᵗʰ **T22.029** **Burn of unspecified degree of unspecified elbow** ▽

√6ᵗʰ **T22.03** **Burn of unspecified degree of upper arm**
√7ᵗʰ **T22.031** **Burn of unspecified degree of right upper arm** ▽
√7ᵗʰ **T22.032** **Burn of unspecified degree of left upper arm** ▽
√7ᵗʰ **T22.039** **Burn of unspecified degree of unspecified upper arm** ▽

√6ᵗʰ **T22.04** **Burn of unspecified degree of axilla**
√7ᵗʰ **T22.041** **Burn of unspecified degree of right axilla** ▽
√7ᵗʰ **T22.042** **Burn of unspecified degree of left axilla** ▽
√7ᵗʰ **T22.049** **Burn of unspecified degree of unspecified axilla** ▽

√6ᵗʰ **T22.05** **Burn of unspecified degree of shoulder**
√7ᵗʰ **T22.051** **Burn of unspecified degree of right shoulder** ▽
√7ᵗʰ **T22.052** **Burn of unspecified degree of left shoulder** ▽
√7ᵗʰ **T22.059** **Burn of unspecified degree of unspecified shoulder** ▽

√6ᵗʰ **T22.06** **Burn of unspecified degree of scapular region**
√7ᵗʰ **T22.061** **Burn of unspecified degree of right scapular region** ▽
√7ᵗʰ **T22.062** **Burn of unspecified degree of left scapular region** ▽
√7ᵗʰ **T22.069** **Burn of unspecified degree of unspecified scapular region** ▽

√6ᵗʰ **T22.09** **Burn of unspecified degree of multiple sites of shoulder and upper limb, except wrist and hand**
√7ᵗʰ **T22.091** **Burn of unspecified degree of multiple sites of right shoulder and upper limb, except wrist and hand** ▽
√7ᵗʰ **T22.092** **Burn of unspecified degree of multiple sites of left shoulder and upper limb, except wrist and hand** ▽
√7ᵗʰ **T22.099** **Burn of unspecified degree of multiple sites of unspecified shoulder and upper limb, except wrist and hand** ▽

√5ᵗʰ **T22.1** **Burn of first degree of shoulder and upper limb, except wrist and hand**
Use additional external cause code to identify the source, place and intent of the burn (X00-X19, X75-X77, X96-X98, Y92)

√x7ᵗʰ **T22.10** **Burn of first degree of shoulder and upper limb, except wrist and hand, unspecified site** ▽

√✔ Additional Character Req   √x7ᵗʰ Placeholder Alert   Manifestation   ▽ Unspecified   ►◄ Revised Text   ● New Code   ▲ Revised Code Title

Chapter 19. Injury, Poisoning and Certain Other Consequences of External Causes

T22.11–T22.40

√6ᵗʰ **T22.11 Burn of first degree of forearm**
- √7ᵗʰ **T22.111** Burn of first degree of **right** forearm
- √7ᵗʰ **T22.112** Burn of first degree of **left** forearm
- √7ᵗʰ **T22.119** Burn of first degree of unspecified forearm ▽

√6ᵗʰ **T22.12 Burn of first degree of elbow**
- √7ᵗʰ **T22.121** Burn of first degree of **right** elbow
- √7ᵗʰ **T22.122** Burn of first degree of **left** elbow
- √7ᵗʰ **T22.129** Burn of first degree of unspecified elbow ▽

√6ᵗʰ **T22.13 Burn of first degree of upper arm**
- √7ᵗʰ **T22.131** Burn of first degree of **right** upper arm
- √7ᵗʰ **T22.132** Burn of first degree of **left** upper arm
- √7ᵗʰ **T22.139** Burn of first degree of unspecified upper arm ▽

√6ᵗʰ **T22.14 Burn of first degree of axilla**
- √7ᵗʰ **T22.141** Burn of first degree of **right** axilla
- √7ᵗʰ **T22.142** Burn of first degree of **left** axilla
- √7ᵗʰ **T22.149** Burn of first degree of unspecified axilla ▽

√6ᵗʰ **T22.15 Burn of first degree of shoulder**
- √7ᵗʰ **T22.151** Burn of first degree of **right** shoulder
- √7ᵗʰ **T22.152** Burn of first degree of **left** shoulder
- √7ᵗʰ **T22.159** Burn of first degree of unspecified shoulder ▽

√6ᵗʰ **T22.16 Burn of first degree of scapular region**
- √7ᵗʰ **T22.161** Burn of first degree of **right** scapular region
- √7ᵗʰ **T22.162** Burn of first degree of **left** scapular region
- √7ᵗʰ **T22.169** Burn of first degree of unspecified scapular region ▽

√6ᵗʰ **T22.19 Burn of first degree of multiple sites of shoulder and upper limb, except wrist and hand**
- √7ᵗʰ **T22.191** Burn of first degree of multiple sites of **right** shoulder and upper limb, except wrist and hand
- √7ᵗʰ **T22.192** Burn of first degree of multiple sites of **left** shoulder and upper limb, except wrist and hand
- √7ᵗʰ **T22.199** Burn of first degree of multiple sites of unspecified shoulder and upper limb, except wrist and hand ▽

√5ᵗʰ **T22.2 Burn of second degree of shoulder and upper limb, except wrist and hand**
> Use additional external cause code to identify the source, place and intent of the burn (X00-X19, X75-X77, X96-X98, Y92)

√x7ᵗʰ **T22.20** Burn of second degree of shoulder and upper limb, except wrist and hand, unspecified site ▽

√6ᵗʰ **T22.21 Burn of second degree of forearm**
- √7ᵗʰ **T22.211** Burn of second degree of **right** forearm
- √7ᵗʰ **T22.212** Burn of second degree of **left** forearm
- √7ᵗʰ **T22.219** Burn of second degree of unspecified forearm ▽

√6ᵗʰ **T22.22 Burn of second degree of elbow**
- √7ᵗʰ **T22.221** Burn of second degree of **right** elbow
- √7ᵗʰ **T22.222** Burn of second degree of **left** elbow
- √7ᵗʰ **T22.229** Burn of second degree of unspecified elbow ▽

√6ᵗʰ **T22.23 Burn of second degree of upper arm**
- √7ᵗʰ **T22.231** Burn of second degree of **right** upper arm
- √7ᵗʰ **T22.232** Burn of second degree of **left** upper arm
- √7ᵗʰ **T22.239** Burn of second degree of unspecified upper arm ▽

√6ᵗʰ **T22.24 Burn of second degree of axilla**
- √7ᵗʰ **T22.241** Burn of second degree of **right** axilla
- √7ᵗʰ **T22.242** Burn of second degree of **left** axilla
- √7ᵗʰ **T22.249** Burn of second degree of unspecified axilla ▽

√6ᵗʰ **T22.25 Burn of second degree of shoulder**
- √7ᵗʰ **T22.251** Burn of second degree of **right** shoulder
- √7ᵗʰ **T22.252** Burn of second degree of **left** shoulder
- √7ᵗʰ **T22.259** Burn of second degree of unspecified shoulder ▽

√6ᵗʰ **T22.26 Burn of second degree of scapular region**
- √7ᵗʰ **T22.261** Burn of second degree of **right** scapular region
- √7ᵗʰ **T22.262** Burn of second degree of **left** scapular region
- √7ᵗʰ **T22.269** Burn of second degree of unspecified scapular region ▽

√6ᵗʰ **T22.29 Burn of second degree of multiple sites of shoulder and upper limb, except wrist and hand**
- √7ᵗʰ **T22.291** Burn of second degree of multiple sites of **right** shoulder and upper limb, except wrist and hand
- √7ᵗʰ **T22.292** Burn of second degree of multiple sites of **left** shoulder and upper limb, except wrist and hand
- √7ᵗʰ **T22.299** Burn of second degree of multiple sites of unspecified shoulder and upper limb, except wrist and hand ▽

√5ᵗʰ **T22.3 Burn of third degree of shoulder and upper limb, except wrist and hand**
> Use additional external cause code to identify the source, place and intent of the burn (X00-X19, X75-X77, X96-X98, Y92)

√x7ᵗʰ **T22.30** Burn of third degree of shoulder and upper limb, except wrist and hand, unspecified site ▽

√6ᵗʰ **T22.31 Burn of third degree of forearm**
- √7ᵗʰ **T22.311** Burn of third degree of **right** forearm
- √7ᵗʰ **T22.312** Burn of third degree of **left** forearm
- √7ᵗʰ **T22.319** Burn of third degree of unspecified forearm ▽

√6ᵗʰ **T22.32 Burn of third degree of elbow**
- √7ᵗʰ **T22.321** Burn of third degree of **right** elbow
- √7ᵗʰ **T22.322** Burn of third degree of **left** elbow
- √7ᵗʰ **T22.329** Burn of third degree of unspecified elbow ▽

√6ᵗʰ **T22.33 Burn of third degree of upper arm**
- √7ᵗʰ **T22.331** Burn of third degree of **right** upper arm
- √7ᵗʰ **T22.332** Burn of third degree of **left** upper arm
- √7ᵗʰ **T22.339** Burn of third degree of unspecified upper arm ▽

√6ᵗʰ **T22.34 Burn of third degree of axilla**
- √7ᵗʰ **T22.341** Burn of third degree of **right** axilla
- √7ᵗʰ **T22.342** Burn of third degree of **left** axilla
- √7ᵗʰ **T22.349** Burn of third degree of unspecified axilla ▽

√6ᵗʰ **T22.35 Burn of third degree of shoulder**
- √7ᵗʰ **T22.351** Burn of third degree of **right** shoulder
- √7ᵗʰ **T22.352** Burn of third degree of **left** shoulder
- √7ᵗʰ **T22.359** Burn of third degree of unspecified shoulder ▽

√6ᵗʰ **T22.36 Burn of third degree of scapular region**
- √7ᵗʰ **T22.361** Burn of third degree of **right** scapular region
- √7ᵗʰ **T22.362** Burn of third degree of **left** scapular region
- √7ᵗʰ **T22.369** Burn of third degree of unspecified scapular region ▽

√6ᵗʰ **T22.39 Burn of third degree of multiple sites of shoulder and upper limb, except wrist and hand**
- √7ᵗʰ **T22.391** Burn of third degree of multiple sites of **right** shoulder and upper limb, except wrist and hand
- √7ᵗʰ **T22.392** Burn of third degree of multiple sites of **left** shoulder and upper limb, except wrist and hand
- √7ᵗʰ **T22.399** Burn of third degree of multiple sites of unspecified shoulder and upper limb, except wrist and hand ▽

√5ᵗʰ **T22.4 Corrosion of unspecified degree of shoulder and upper limb, except wrist and hand**
> Code first (T51-T65) to identify chemical and intent
> Use additional external cause code to identify place (Y92)

√x7ᵗʰ **T22.40** Corrosion of unspecified degree of shoulder and upper limb, except wrist and hand, unspecified site ▽

√6ᵗʰ **T22.41** Corrosion of unspecified degree of forearm

  √7ᵗʰ **T22.411** Corrosion of unspecified degree of right forearm ▽

  √7ᵗʰ **T22.412** Corrosion of unspecified degree of left forearm ▽

  √7ᵗʰ **T22.419** Corrosion of unspecified degree of unspecified forearm ▽

√6ᵗʰ **T22.42** Corrosion of unspecified degree of elbow

  √7ᵗʰ **T22.421** Corrosion of unspecified degree of right elbow ▽

  √7ᵗʰ **T22.422** Corrosion of unspecified degree of left elbow ▽

  √7ᵗʰ **T22.429** Corrosion of unspecified degree of unspecified elbow ▽

√6ᵗʰ **T22.43** Corrosion of unspecified degree of upper arm

  √7ᵗʰ **T22.431** Corrosion of unspecified degree of right upper arm ▽

  √7ᵗʰ **T22.432** Corrosion of unspecified degree of left upper arm ▽

  √7ᵗʰ **T22.439** Corrosion of unspecified degree of unspecified upper arm ▽

√6ᵗʰ **T22.44** Corrosion of unspecified degree of axilla

  √7ᵗʰ **T22.441** Corrosion of unspecified degree of right axilla ▽

  √7ᵗʰ **T22.442** Corrosion of unspecified degree of left axilla ▽

  √7ᵗʰ **T22.449** Corrosion of unspecified degree of unspecified axilla ▽

√6ᵗʰ **T22.45** Corrosion of unspecified degree of shoulder

  √7ᵗʰ **T22.451** Corrosion of unspecified degree of right shoulder ▽

  √7ᵗʰ **T22.452** Corrosion of unspecified degree of left shoulder ▽

  √7ᵗʰ **T22.459** Corrosion of unspecified degree of unspecified shoulder ▽

√6ᵗʰ **T22.46** Corrosion of unspecified degree of scapular region

  √7ᵗʰ **T22.461** Corrosion of unspecified degree of right scapular region ▽

  √7ᵗʰ **T22.462** Corrosion of unspecified degree of left scapular region ▽

  √7ᵗʰ **T22.469** Corrosion of unspecified degree of unspecified scapular region ▽

√6ᵗʰ **T22.49** Corrosion of unspecified degree of multiple sites of shoulder and upper limb, except wrist and hand

  √7ᵗʰ **T22.491** Corrosion of unspecified degree of multiple sites of right shoulder and upper limb, except wrist and hand ▽

  √7ᵗʰ **T22.492** Corrosion of unspecified degree of multiple sites of left shoulder and upper limb, except wrist and hand ▽

  √7ᵗʰ **T22.499** Corrosion of unspecified degree of multiple sites of unspecified shoulder and upper limb, except wrist and hand ▽

√5ᵗʰ **T22.5** Corrosion of first degree of shoulder and upper limb, except wrist and hand

  Code first (T51-T65) to identify chemical and intent

  Use additional external cause code to identify place (Y92)

√x7ᵗʰ **T22.50** Corrosion of first degree of shoulder and upper limb, except wrist and hand unspecified site ▽

√6ᵗʰ **T22.51** Corrosion of first degree of forearm

  √7ᵗʰ **T22.511** Corrosion of first degree of right forearm

  √7ᵗʰ **T22.512** Corrosion of first degree of left forearm

  √7ᵗʰ **T22.519** Corrosion of first degree of unspecified forearm ▽

√6ᵗʰ **T22.52** Corrosion of first degree of elbow

  √7ᵗʰ **T22.521** Corrosion of first degree of right elbow

  √7ᵗʰ **T22.522** Corrosion of first degree of left elbow

  √7ᵗʰ **T22.529** Corrosion of first degree of unspecified elbow ▽

√6ᵗʰ **T22.53** Corrosion of first degree of upper arm

  √7ᵗʰ **T22.531** Corrosion of first degree of right upper arm

  √7ᵗʰ **T22.532** Corrosion of first degree of left upper arm

  √7ᵗʰ **T22.539** Corrosion of first degree of unspecified upper arm ▽

√6ᵗʰ **T22.54** Corrosion of first degree of axilla

  √7ᵗʰ **T22.541** Corrosion of first degree of right axilla

  √7ᵗʰ **T22.542** Corrosion of first degree of left axilla

  √7ᵗʰ **T22.549** Corrosion of first degree of unspecified axilla ▽

√6ᵗʰ **T22.55** Corrosion of first degree of shoulder

  √7ᵗʰ **T22.551** Corrosion of first degree of right shoulder

  √7ᵗʰ **T22.552** Corrosion of first degree of left shoulder

  √7ᵗʰ **T22.559** Corrosion of first degree of unspecified shoulder ▽

√6ᵗʰ **T22.56** Corrosion of first degree of scapular region

  √7ᵗʰ **T22.561** Corrosion of first degree of right scapular region

  √7ᵗʰ **T22.562** Corrosion of first degree of left scapular region

  √7ᵗʰ **T22.569** Corrosion of first degree of unspecified scapular region ▽

√6ᵗʰ **T22.59** Corrosion of first degree of multiple sites of shoulder and upper limb, except wrist and hand

  √7ᵗʰ **T22.591** Corrosion of first degree of multiple sites of right shoulder and upper limb, except wrist and hand

  √7ᵗʰ **T22.592** Corrosion of first degree of multiple sites of left shoulder and upper limb, except wrist and hand

  √7ᵗʰ **T22.599** Corrosion of first degree of multiple sites of unspecified shoulder and upper limb, except wrist and hand ▽

√5ᵗʰ **T22.6** Corrosion of second degree of shoulder and upper limb, except wrist and hand

  Code first (T51-T65) to identify chemical and intent

  Use additional external cause code to identify place (Y92)

√x7ᵗʰ **T22.60** Corrosion of second degree of shoulder and upper limb, except wrist and hand, unspecified site ▽

√6ᵗʰ **T22.61** Corrosion of second degree of forearm

  √7ᵗʰ **T22.611** Corrosion of second degree of right forearm

  √7ᵗʰ **T22.612** Corrosion of second degree of left forearm

  √7ᵗʰ **T22.619** Corrosion of second degree of unspecified forearm ▽

√6ᵗʰ **T22.62** Corrosion of second degree of elbow

  √7ᵗʰ **T22.621** Corrosion of second degree of right elbow

  √7ᵗʰ **T22.622** Corrosion of second degree of left elbow

  √7ᵗʰ **T22.629** Corrosion of second degree of unspecified elbow ▽

√6ᵗʰ **T22.63** Corrosion of second degree of upper arm

  √7ᵗʰ **T22.631** Corrosion of second degree of right upper arm

  √7ᵗʰ **T22.632** Corrosion of second degree of left upper arm

  √7ᵗʰ **T22.639** Corrosion of second degree of unspecified upper arm ▽

√6ᵗʰ **T22.64** Corrosion of second degree of axilla

  √7ᵗʰ **T22.641** Corrosion of second degree of right axilla

  √7ᵗʰ **T22.642** Corrosion of second degree of left axilla

  √7ᵗʰ **T22.649** Corrosion of second degree of unspecified axilla ▽

√6ᵗʰ **T22.65** Corrosion of second degree of shoulder

  √7ᵗʰ **T22.651** Corrosion of second degree of right shoulder

  √7ᵗʰ **T22.652** Corrosion of second degree of left shoulder

  √7ᵗʰ **T22.659** Corrosion of second degree of unspecified shoulder ▽

√6ᵗʰ **T22.66** Corrosion of second degree of scapular region

  √7ᵗʰ **T22.661** Corrosion of second degree of right scapular region

  √7ᵗʰ **T22.662** Corrosion of second degree of left scapular region

  √7ᵗʰ **T22.669** Corrosion of second degree of unspecified scapular region ▽

√6ᵗʰ **T22.69** Corrosion of second degree of multiple sites of shoulder and upper limb, except wrist and hand

  √7ᵗʰ **T22.691** Corrosion of second degree of multiple sites of right shoulder and upper limb, except wrist and hand

☑ Additional Character Req   √x7ᵗʰ Placeholder Alert   Manifestation   ▽ Unspecified   ▶◀ Revised Text   ● New Code   ▲ Revised Code Title

ICD-10-CM 2019   1081

☑7ᵗʰ **T22.692** Corrosion of second degree of multiple sites of left shoulder and upper limb, except wrist and hand

☑7ᵗʰ **T22.699** Corrosion of second degree of multiple sites of unspecified shoulder and upper limb, except wrist and hand ▽

☑5ᵗʰ **T22.7** Corrosion of third degree of shoulder and upper limb, except wrist and hand

    Code first (T51-T65) to identify chemical and intent

    Use additional external cause code to identify place (Y92)

☑x7ᵗʰ **T22.70** Corrosion of third degree of shoulder and upper limb, except wrist and hand, unspecified site ▽

☑6ᵗʰ **T22.71** Corrosion of third degree of forearm

   ☑7ᵗʰ **T22.711** Corrosion of third degree of right forearm

   ☑7ᵗʰ **T22.712** Corrosion of third degree of left forearm

   ☑7ᵗʰ **T22.719** Corrosion of third degree of unspecified forearm ▽

☑6ᵗʰ **T22.72** Corrosion of third degree of elbow

   ☑7ᵗʰ **T22.721** Corrosion of third degree of right elbow

   ☑7ᵗʰ **T22.722** Corrosion of third degree of left elbow

   ☑7ᵗʰ **T22.729** Corrosion of third degree of unspecified elbow ▽

☑6ᵗʰ **T22.73** Corrosion of third degree of upper arm

   ☑7ᵗʰ **T22.731** Corrosion of third degree of right upper arm

   ☑7ᵗʰ **T22.732** Corrosion of third degree of left upper arm

   ☑7ᵗʰ **T22.739** Corrosion of third degree of unspecified upper arm ▽

☑6ᵗʰ **T22.74** Corrosion of third degree of axilla

   ☑7ᵗʰ **T22.741** Corrosion of third degree of right axilla

   ☑7ᵗʰ **T22.742** Corrosion of third degree of left axilla

   ☑7ᵗʰ **T22.749** Corrosion of third degree of unspecified axilla ▽

☑6ᵗʰ **T22.75** Corrosion of third degree of shoulder

   ☑7ᵗʰ **T22.751** Corrosion of third degree of right shoulder

   ☑7ᵗʰ **T22.752** Corrosion of third degree of left shoulder

   ☑7ᵗʰ **T22.759** Corrosion of third degree of unspecified shoulder ▽

☑6ᵗʰ **T22.76** Corrosion of third degree of scapular region

   ☑7ᵗʰ **T22.761** Corrosion of third degree of right scapular region

   ☑7ᵗʰ **T22.762** Corrosion of third degree of left scapular region

   ☑7ᵗʰ **T22.769** Corrosion of third degree of unspecified scapular region ▽

☑6ᵗʰ **T22.79** Corrosion of third degree of multiple sites of shoulder and upper limb, except wrist and hand

   ☑7ᵗʰ **T22.791** Corrosion of third degree of multiple sites of right shoulder and upper limb, except wrist and hand

   ☑7ᵗʰ **T22.792** Corrosion of third degree of multiple sites of left shoulder and upper limb, except wrist and hand

   ☑7ᵗʰ **T22.799** Corrosion of third degree of multiple sites of unspecified shoulder and upper limb, except wrist and hand ▽

☑4ᵗʰ **T23** **Burn and corrosion of wrist and hand**

AHA: 2015,1Q,19

The appropriate 7th character is to be added to each code from category T23.

A   initial encounter

D   subsequent encounter

S   sequela

☑5ᵗʰ **T23.0** Burn of unspecified degree of wrist and hand

    Use additional external cause code to identify the source, place and intent of the burn (X00-X19, X75-X77, X96-X98, Y92)

☑6ᵗʰ **T23.00** Burn of unspecified degree of hand, unspecified site

   ☑7ᵗʰ **T23.001** Burn of unspecified degree of right hand, unspecified site ▽

   ☑7ᵗʰ **T23.002** Burn of unspecified degree of left hand, unspecified site ▽

   ☑7ᵗʰ **T23.009** Burn of unspecified degree of unspecified hand, unspecified site ▽

☑6ᵗʰ **T23.01** Burn of unspecified degree of thumb (nail)

   ☑7ᵗʰ **T23.011** Burn of unspecified degree of right thumb (nail) ▽

   ☑7ᵗʰ **T23.012** Burn of unspecified degree of left thumb (nail) ▽

   ☑7ᵗʰ **T23.019** Burn of unspecified degree of unspecified thumb (nail) ▽

☑6ᵗʰ **T23.02** Burn of unspecified degree of single finger (nail) except thumb

   ☑7ᵗʰ **T23.021** Burn of unspecified degree of single right finger (nail) except thumb ▽

   ☑7ᵗʰ **T23.022** Burn of unspecified degree of single left finger (nail) except thumb ▽

   ☑7ᵗʰ **T23.029** Burn of unspecified degree of unspecified single finger (nail) except thumb ▽

☑6ᵗʰ **T23.03** Burn of unspecified degree of multiple fingers (nail), not including thumb

   ☑7ᵗʰ **T23.031** Burn of unspecified degree of multiple right fingers (nail), not including thumb ▽

   ☑7ᵗʰ **T23.032** Burn of unspecified degree of multiple left fingers (nail), not including thumb ▽

   ☑7ᵗʰ **T23.039** Burn of unspecified degree of unspecified multiple fingers (nail), not including thumb ▽

☑6ᵗʰ **T23.04** Burn of unspecified degree of multiple fingers (nail), including thumb

   ☑7ᵗʰ **T23.041** Burn of unspecified degree of multiple right fingers (nail), including thumb ▽

   ☑7ᵗʰ **T23.042** Burn of unspecified degree of multiple left fingers (nail), including thumb ▽

   ☑7ᵗʰ **T23.049** Burn of unspecified degree of unspecified multiple fingers (nail), including thumb ▽

☑6ᵗʰ **T23.05** Burn of unspecified degree of palm

   ☑7ᵗʰ **T23.051** Burn of unspecified degree of right palm ▽

   ☑7ᵗʰ **T23.052** Burn of unspecified degree of left palm ▽

   ☑7ᵗʰ **T23.059** Burn of unspecified degree of unspecified palm ▽

☑6ᵗʰ **T23.06** Burn of unspecified degree of back of hand

   ☑7ᵗʰ **T23.061** Burn of unspecified degree of back of right hand ▽

   ☑7ᵗʰ **T23.062** Burn of unspecified degree of back of left hand ▽

   ☑7ᵗʰ **T23.069** Burn of unspecified degree of back of unspecified hand ▽

☑6ᵗʰ **T23.07** Burn of unspecified degree of wrist

   ☑7ᵗʰ **T23.071** Burn of unspecified degree of right wrist ▽

   ☑7ᵗʰ **T23.072** Burn of unspecified degree of left wrist ▽

   ☑7ᵗʰ **T23.079** Burn of unspecified degree of unspecified wrist ▽

☑6ᵗʰ **T23.09** Burn of unspecified degree of multiple sites of wrist and hand

   ☑7ᵗʰ **T23.091** Burn of unspecified degree of multiple sites of right wrist and hand ▽

   ☑7ᵗʰ **T23.092** Burn of unspecified degree of multiple sites of left wrist and hand ▽

   ☑7ᵗʰ **T23.099** Burn of unspecified degree of multiple sites of unspecified wrist and hand ▽

☑5ᵗʰ **T23.1** Burn of first degree of wrist and hand

    Use additional external cause code to identify the source, place and intent of the burn (X00-X19, X75-X77, X96-X98, Y92)

☑6ᵗʰ **T23.10** Burn of first degree of hand, unspecified site

   ☑7ᵗʰ **T23.101** Burn of first degree of right hand, unspecified site ▽

    √7ᵗʰ **T23.102** Burn of first degree of left hand, unspecified site ▽

    √7ᵗʰ **T23.109** Burn of first degree of unspecified hand, unspecified site ▽

√6ᵗʰ **T23.11** Burn of first degree of thumb (nail)

    √7ᵗʰ **T23.111** Burn of first degree of right thumb (nail)

    √7ᵗʰ **T23.112** Burn of first degree of left thumb (nail)

    √7ᵗʰ **T23.119** Burn of first degree of unspecified thumb (nail) ▽

√6ᵗʰ **T23.12** Burn of first degree of single finger (nail) except thumb

    √7ᵗʰ **T23.121** Burn of first degree of single right finger (nail) except thumb

    √7ᵗʰ **T23.122** Burn of first degree of single left finger (nail) except thumb

    √7ᵗʰ **T23.129** Burn of first degree of unspecified single finger (nail) except thumb ▽

√6ᵗʰ **T23.13** Burn of first degree of multiple fingers (nail), not including thumb

    √7ᵗʰ **T23.131** Burn of first degree of multiple right fingers (nail), not including thumb

    √7ᵗʰ **T23.132** Burn of first degree of multiple left fingers (nail), not including thumb

    √7ᵗʰ **T23.139** Burn of first degree of unspecified multiple fingers (nail), not including thumb ▽

√6ᵗʰ **T23.14** Burn of first degree of multiple fingers (nail), including thumb

    √7ᵗʰ **T23.141** Burn of first degree of multiple right fingers (nail), including thumb

    √7ᵗʰ **T23.142** Burn of first degree of multiple left fingers (nail), including thumb

    √7ᵗʰ **T23.149** Burn of first degree of unspecified multiple fingers (nail), including thumb ▽

√6ᵗʰ **T23.15** Burn of first degree of palm

    √7ᵗʰ **T23.151** Burn of first degree of right palm

    √7ᵗʰ **T23.152** Burn of first degree of left palm

    √7ᵗʰ **T23.159** Burn of first degree of unspecified palm ▽

√6ᵗʰ **T23.16** Burn of first degree of back of hand

    √7ᵗʰ **T23.161** Burn of first degree of back of right hand

    √7ᵗʰ **T23.162** Burn of first degree of back of left hand

    √7ᵗʰ **T23.169** Burn of first degree of back of unspecified hand ▽

√6ᵗʰ **T23.17** Burn of first degree of wrist

    √7ᵗʰ **T23.171** Burn of first degree of right wrist

    √7ᵗʰ **T23.172** Burn of first degree of left wrist

    √7ᵗʰ **T23.179** Burn of first degree of unspecified wrist ▽

√6ᵗʰ **T23.19** Burn of first degree of multiple sites of wrist and hand

    √7ᵗʰ **T23.191** Burn of first degree of multiple sites of right wrist and hand

    √7ᵗʰ **T23.192** Burn of first degree of multiple sites of left wrist and hand

    √7ᵗʰ **T23.199** Burn of first degree of multiple sites of unspecified wrist and hand ▽

√5ᵗʰ **T23.2** Burn of second degree of wrist and hand

Use additional external cause code to identify the source, place and intent of the burn (X00-X19, X75-X77, X96-X98, Y92)

√6ᵗʰ **T23.20** Burn of second degree of hand, unspecified site

    √7ᵗʰ **T23.201** Burn of second degree of right hand, unspecified site ▽

    √7ᵗʰ **T23.202** Burn of second degree of left hand, unspecified site ▽

    √7ᵗʰ **T23.209** Burn of second degree of unspecified hand, unspecified site ▽

√6ᵗʰ **T23.21** Burn of second degree of thumb (nail)

    √7ᵗʰ **T23.211** Burn of second degree of right thumb (nail)

    √7ᵗʰ **T23.212** Burn of second degree of left thumb (nail)

    √7ᵗʰ **T23.219** Burn of second degree of unspecified thumb (nail) ▽

√6ᵗʰ **T23.22** Burn of second degree of single finger (nail) except thumb

    √7ᵗʰ **T23.221** Burn of second degree of single right finger (nail) except thumb

    √7ᵗʰ **T23.222** Burn of second degree of single left finger (nail) except thumb

    √7ᵗʰ **T23.229** Burn of second degree of unspecified single finger (nail) except thumb ▽

√6ᵗʰ **T23.23** Burn of second degree of multiple fingers (nail), not including thumb

    √7ᵗʰ **T23.231** Burn of second degree of multiple right fingers (nail), not including thumb

    √7ᵗʰ **T23.232** Burn of second degree of multiple left fingers (nail), not including thumb

    √7ᵗʰ **T23.239** Burn of second degree of unspecified multiple fingers (nail), not including thumb ▽

√6ᵗʰ **T23.24** Burn of second degree of multiple fingers (nail), including thumb

    √7ᵗʰ **T23.241** Burn of second degree of multiple right fingers (nail), including thumb

    √7ᵗʰ **T23.242** Burn of second degree of multiple left fingers (nail), including thumb

    √7ᵗʰ **T23.249** Burn of second degree of unspecified multiple fingers (nail), including thumb ▽

√6ᵗʰ **T23.25** Burn of second degree of palm

    √7ᵗʰ **T23.251** Burn of second degree of right palm

    √7ᵗʰ **T23.252** Burn of second degree of left palm

    √7ᵗʰ **T23.259** Burn of second degree of unspecified palm ▽

√6ᵗʰ **T23.26** Burn of second degree of back of hand

    √7ᵗʰ **T23.261** Burn of second degree of back of right hand

    √7ᵗʰ **T23.262** Burn of second degree of back of left hand

    √7ᵗʰ **T23.269** Burn of second degree of back of unspecified hand ▽

√6ᵗʰ **T23.27** Burn of second degree of wrist

    √7ᵗʰ **T23.271** Burn of second degree of right wrist

    √7ᵗʰ **T23.272** Burn of second degree of left wrist

    √7ᵗʰ **T23.279** Burn of second degree of unspecified wrist ▽

√6ᵗʰ **T23.29** Burn of second degree of multiple sites of wrist and hand

    √7ᵗʰ **T23.291** Burn of second degree of multiple sites of right wrist and hand

    √7ᵗʰ **T23.292** Burn of second degree of multiple sites of left wrist and hand

    √7ᵗʰ **T23.299** Burn of second degree of multiple sites of unspecified wrist and hand ▽

√5ᵗʰ **T23.3** Burn of third degree of wrist and hand

Use additional external cause code to identify the source, place and intent of the burn (X00-X19, X75-X77, X96-X98, Y92)

√6ᵗʰ **T23.30** Burn of third degree of hand, unspecified site

AHA: 2016,2Q,5

    √7ᵗʰ **T23.301** Burn of third degree of right hand, unspecified site ▽

    √7ᵗʰ **T23.302** Burn of third degree of left hand, unspecified site ▽

    √7ᵗʰ **T23.309** Burn of third degree of unspecified hand, unspecified site ▽

√6ᵗʰ **T23.31** Burn of third degree of thumb (nail)

    √7ᵗʰ **T23.311** Burn of third degree of right thumb (nail)

    √7ᵗʰ **T23.312** Burn of third degree of left thumb (nail)

    √7ᵗʰ **T23.319** Burn of third degree of unspecified thumb (nail) ▽

√6ᵗʰ **T23.32** Burn of third degree of single finger (nail) except thumb

    √7ᵗʰ **T23.321** Burn of third degree of single right finger (nail) except thumb

    √7ᵗʰ **T23.322** Burn of third degree of single left finger (nail) except thumb

    √7ᵗʰ **T23.329** Burn of third degree of unspecified single finger (nail) except thumb ▽

☑ Additional Character Req   ⱽˣ⁷ᵗʰ Placeholder Alert   Manifestation   ▽ Unspecified   ►◄ Revised Text   ● New Code   ▲ Revised Code Title

ICD-10-CM 2019

1083

Chapter 19. Injury, Poisoning and Certain Other Consequences of External Causes

T23.33–T23.539

√6ᵗʰ **T23.33** Burn of third degree of multiple fingers (nail), not including thumb
- √7ᵗʰ **T23.331** Burn of third degree of multiple right fingers (nail), not including thumb
- √7ᵗʰ **T23.332** Burn of third degree of multiple left fingers (nail), not including thumb
- √7ᵗʰ **T23.339** Burn of third degree of unspecified multiple fingers (nail), not including thumb ▽

√6ᵗʰ **T23.34** Burn of third degree of multiple fingers (nail), including thumb
- √7ᵗʰ **T23.341** Burn of third degree of multiple right fingers (nail), including thumb
- √7ᵗʰ **T23.342** Burn of third degree of multiple left fingers (nail), including thumb
- √7ᵗʰ **T23.349** Burn of third degree of unspecified multiple fingers (nail), including thumb ▽

√6ᵗʰ **T23.35** Burn of third degree of palm
- √7ᵗʰ **T23.351** Burn of third degree of right palm
- √7ᵗʰ **T23.352** Burn of third degree of left palm
- √7ᵗʰ **T23.359** Burn of third degree of unspecified palm ▽

√6ᵗʰ **T23.36** Burn of third degree of back of hand
- √7ᵗʰ **T23.361** Burn of third degree of back of right hand
- √7ᵗʰ **T23.362** Burn of third degree of back of left hand
- √7ᵗʰ **T23.369** Burn of third degree of back of unspecified hand ▽

√6ᵗʰ **T23.37** Burn of third degree of wrist
- √7ᵗʰ **T23.371** Burn of third degree of right wrist
- √7ᵗʰ **T23.372** Burn of third degree of left wrist
- √7ᵗʰ **T23.379** Burn of third degree of unspecified wrist ▽

√6ᵗʰ **T23.39** Burn of third degree of multiple sites of wrist and hand
- √7ᵗʰ **T23.391** Burn of third degree of multiple sites of right wrist and hand
- √7ᵗʰ **T23.392** Burn of third degree of multiple sites of left wrist and hand
- √7ᵗʰ **T23.399** Burn of third degree of multiple sites of unspecified wrist and hand ▽

√5ᵗʰ **T23.4** Corrosion of unspecified degree of wrist and hand

    Code first (T51-T65) to identify chemical and intent
    Use additional external cause code to identify place (Y92)

√6ᵗʰ **T23.40** Corrosion of unspecified degree of hand, unspecified site
- √7ᵗʰ **T23.401** Corrosion of unspecified degree of right hand, unspecified site ▽
- √7ᵗʰ **T23.402** Corrosion of unspecified degree of left hand, unspecified site ▽
- √7ᵗʰ **T23.409** Corrosion of unspecified degree of unspecified hand, unspecified site ▽

√6ᵗʰ **T23.41** Corrosion of unspecified degree of thumb (nail)
- √7ᵗʰ **T23.411** Corrosion of unspecified degree of right thumb (nail) ▽
- √7ᵗʰ **T23.412** Corrosion of unspecified degree of left thumb (nail) ▽
- √7ᵗʰ **T23.419** Corrosion of unspecified degree of unspecified thumb (nail) ▽

√6ᵗʰ **T23.42** Corrosion of unspecified degree of single finger (nail) except thumb
- √7ᵗʰ **T23.421** Corrosion of unspecified degree of single right finger (nail) except thumb ▽
- √7ᵗʰ **T23.422** Corrosion of unspecified degree of single left finger (nail) except thumb ▽
- √7ᵗʰ **T23.429** Corrosion of unspecified degree of unspecified single finger (nail) except thumb ▽

√6ᵗʰ **T23.43** Corrosion of unspecified degree of multiple fingers (nail), not including thumb
- √7ᵗʰ **T23.431** Corrosion of unspecified degree of multiple right fingers (nail), not including thumb ▽
- √7ᵗʰ **T23.432** Corrosion of unspecified degree of multiple left fingers (nail), not including thumb ▽

√7ᵗʰ **T23.439** Corrosion of unspecified degree of unspecified multiple fingers (nail), not including thumb ▽

√6ᵗʰ **T23.44** Corrosion of unspecified degree of multiple fingers (nail), including thumb
- √7ᵗʰ **T23.441** Corrosion of unspecified degree of multiple right fingers (nail), including thumb ▽
- √7ᵗʰ **T23.442** Corrosion of unspecified degree of multiple left fingers (nail), including thumb ▽
- √7ᵗʰ **T23.449** Corrosion of unspecified degree of unspecified multiple fingers (nail), including thumb ▽

√6ᵗʰ **T23.45** Corrosion of unspecified degree of palm
- √7ᵗʰ **T23.451** Corrosion of unspecified degree of right palm ▽
- √7ᵗʰ **T23.452** Corrosion of unspecified degree of left palm ▽
- √7ᵗʰ **T23.459** Corrosion of unspecified degree of unspecified palm ▽

√6ᵗʰ **T23.46** Corrosion of unspecified degree of back of hand
- √7ᵗʰ **T23.461** Corrosion of unspecified degree of back of right hand ▽
- √7ᵗʰ **T23.462** Corrosion of unspecified degree of back of left hand ▽
- √7ᵗʰ **T23.469** Corrosion of unspecified degree of back of unspecified hand ▽

√6ᵗʰ **T23.47** Corrosion of unspecified degree of wrist
- √7ᵗʰ **T23.471** Corrosion of unspecified degree of right wrist ▽
- √7ᵗʰ **T23.472** Corrosion of unspecified degree of left wrist ▽
- √7ᵗʰ **T23.479** Corrosion of unspecified degree of unspecified wrist ▽

√6ᵗʰ **T23.49** Corrosion of unspecified degree of multiple sites of wrist and hand
- √7ᵗʰ **T23.491** Corrosion of unspecified degree of multiple sites of right wrist and hand ▽
- √7ᵗʰ **T23.492** Corrosion of unspecified degree of multiple sites of left wrist and hand ▽
- √7ᵗʰ **T23.499** Corrosion of unspecified degree of multiple sites of unspecified wrist and hand ▽

√5ᵗʰ **T23.5** Corrosion of first degree of wrist and hand

    Code first (T51-T65) to identify chemical and intent
    Use additional external cause code to identify place (Y92)

√6ᵗʰ **T23.50** Corrosion of first degree of hand, unspecified site
- √7ᵗʰ **T23.501** Corrosion of first degree of right hand, unspecified site ▽
- √7ᵗʰ **T23.502** Corrosion of first degree of left hand, unspecified site ▽
- √7ᵗʰ **T23.509** Corrosion of first degree of unspecified hand, unspecified site ▽

√6ᵗʰ **T23.51** Corrosion of first degree of thumb (nail)
- √7ᵗʰ **T23.511** Corrosion of first degree of right thumb (nail)
- √7ᵗʰ **T23.512** Corrosion of first degree of left thumb (nail)
- √7ᵗʰ **T23.519** Corrosion of first degree of unspecified thumb (nail) ▽

√6ᵗʰ **T23.52** Corrosion of first degree of single finger (nail) except thumb
- √7ᵗʰ **T23.521** Corrosion of first degree of single right finger (nail) except thumb
- √7ᵗʰ **T23.522** Corrosion of first degree of single left finger (nail) except thumb
- √7ᵗʰ **T23.529** Corrosion of first degree of unspecified single finger (nail) except thumb ▽

√6ᵗʰ **T23.53** Corrosion of first degree of multiple fingers (nail), not including thumb
- √7ᵗʰ **T23.531** Corrosion of first degree of multiple right fingers (nail), not including thumb
- √7ᵗʰ **T23.532** Corrosion of first degree of multiple left fingers (nail), not including thumb
- √7ᵗʰ **T23.539** Corrosion of first degree of unspecified multiple fingers (nail), not including thumb ▽

√6ᵗʰ **T23.54** **Corrosion of first degree of** multiple fingers (nail), including thumb

　√7ᵗʰ **T23.541** Corrosion of first degree of multiple right fingers (nail), including thumb

　√7ᵗʰ **T23.542** Corrosion of first degree of multiple left fingers (nail), including thumb

　√7ᵗʰ **T23.549** Corrosion of first degree of unspecified multiple fingers (nail), including thumb　▽

√6ᵗʰ **T23.55** **Corrosion of first degree of** palm

　√7ᵗʰ **T23.551** Corrosion of first degree of right palm

　√7ᵗʰ **T23.552** Corrosion of first degree of left palm

　√7ᵗʰ **T23.559** Corrosion of first degree of unspecified palm　▽

√6ᵗʰ **T23.56** **Corrosion of first degree of** back of hand

　√7ᵗʰ **T23.561** Corrosion of first degree of back of right hand

　√7ᵗʰ **T23.562** Corrosion of first degree of back of left hand

　√7ᵗʰ **T23.569** Corrosion of first degree of back of unspecified hand　▽

√6ᵗʰ **T23.57** **Corrosion of first degree of** wrist

　√7ᵗʰ **T23.571** Corrosion of first degree of right wrist

　√7ᵗʰ **T23.572** Corrosion of first degree of left wrist

　√7ᵗʰ **T23.579** Corrosion of first degree of unspecified wrist　▽

√6ᵗʰ **T23.59** **Corrosion of first degree of** multiple sites of wrist and hand

　√7ᵗʰ **T23.591** Corrosion of first degree of multiple sites of right wrist and hand

　√7ᵗʰ **T23.592** Corrosion of first degree of multiple sites of left wrist and hand

　√7ᵗʰ **T23.599** Corrosion of first degree of multiple sites of unspecified wrist and hand　▽

√5ᵗʰ **T23.6** **Corrosion of** second degree **of wrist and hand**

Code first (T51-T65) to identify chemical and intent

Use additional external cause code to identify place (Y92)

√6ᵗʰ **T23.60** **Corrosion of second degree of hand, unspecified site**

　√7ᵗʰ **T23.601** Corrosion of second degree of right hand, unspecified site　▽

　√7ᵗʰ **T23.602** Corrosion of second degree of left hand, unspecified site　▽

　√7ᵗʰ **T23.609** Corrosion of second degree of unspecified hand, unspecified site　▽

√6ᵗʰ **T23.61** **Corrosion of second degree of** thumb (nail)

　√7ᵗʰ **T23.611** Corrosion of second degree of right thumb (nail)

　√7ᵗʰ **T23.612** Corrosion of second degree of left thumb (nail)

　√7ᵗʰ **T23.619** Corrosion of second degree of unspecified thumb (nail)　▽

√6ᵗʰ **T23.62** **Corrosion of second degree of** single finger (nail) except thumb

　√7ᵗʰ **T23.621** Corrosion of second degree of single right finger (nail) except thumb

　√7ᵗʰ **T23.622** Corrosion of second degree of single left finger (nail) except thumb

　√7ᵗʰ **T23.629** Corrosion of second degree of unspecified single finger (nail) except thumb　▽

√6ᵗʰ **T23.63** **Corrosion of second degree of** multiple fingers (nail), not including thumb

　√7ᵗʰ **T23.631** Corrosion of second degree of multiple right fingers (nail), not including thumb

　√7ᵗʰ **T23.632** Corrosion of second degree of multiple left fingers (nail), not including thumb

　√7ᵗʰ **T23.639** Corrosion of second degree of unspecified multiple fingers (nail), not including thumb　▽

√6ᵗʰ **T23.64** **Corrosion of second degree of** multiple fingers (nail), including thumb

　√7ᵗʰ **T23.641** Corrosion of second degree of multiple right fingers (nail), including thumb

　√7ᵗʰ **T23.642** Corrosion of second degree of multiple left fingers (nail), including thumb

　√7ᵗʰ **T23.649** Corrosion of second degree of unspecified multiple fingers (nail), including thumb　▽

√6ᵗʰ **T23.65** **Corrosion of second degree of** palm

　√7ᵗʰ **T23.651** Corrosion of second degree of right palm

　√7ᵗʰ **T23.652** Corrosion of second degree of left palm

　√7ᵗʰ **T23.659** Corrosion of second degree of unspecified palm　▽

√6ᵗʰ **T23.66** **Corrosion of second degree of** back of hand

　√7ᵗʰ **T23.661** Corrosion of second degree back of right hand

　√7ᵗʰ **T23.662** Corrosion of second degree back of left hand

　√7ᵗʰ **T23.669** Corrosion of second degree back of unspecified hand　▽

√6ᵗʰ **T23.67** **Corrosion of second degree of** wrist

　√7ᵗʰ **T23.671** Corrosion of second degree of right wrist

　√7ᵗʰ **T23.672** Corrosion of second degree of left wrist

　√7ᵗʰ **T23.679** Corrosion of second degree of unspecified wrist　▽

√6ᵗʰ **T23.69** **Corrosion of second degree of** multiple sites of wrist and hand

　√7ᵗʰ **T23.691** Corrosion of second degree of multiple sites of right wrist and hand

　√7ᵗʰ **T23.692** Corrosion of second degree of multiple sites of left wrist and hand

　√7ᵗʰ **T23.699** Corrosion of second degree of multiple sites of unspecified wrist and hand　▽

√5ᵗʰ **T23.7** **Corrosion of** third degree **of wrist and hand**

Code first (T51-T65) to identify chemical and intent

Use additional external cause code to identify place (Y92)

√6ᵗʰ **T23.70** **Corrosion of third degree of hand, unspecified site**

　√7ᵗʰ **T23.701** Corrosion of third degree of right hand, unspecified site　▽

　√7ᵗʰ **T23.702** Corrosion of third degree of left hand, unspecified site　▽

　√7ᵗʰ **T23.709** Corrosion of third degree of unspecified hand, unspecified site　▽

√6ᵗʰ **T23.71** **Corrosion of third degree of** thumb (nail)

　√7ᵗʰ **T23.711** Corrosion of third degree of right thumb (nail)

　√7ᵗʰ **T23.712** Corrosion of third degree of left thumb (nail)

　√7ᵗʰ **T23.719** Corrosion of third degree of unspecified thumb (nail)　▽

√6ᵗʰ **T23.72** **Corrosion of third degree of** single finger (nail) except thumb

　√7ᵗʰ **T23.721** Corrosion of third degree of single right finger (nail) except thumb

　√7ᵗʰ **T23.722** Corrosion of third degree of single left finger (nail) except thumb

　√7ᵗʰ **T23.729** Corrosion of third degree of unspecified single finger (nail) except thumb　▽

√6ᵗʰ **T23.73** **Corrosion of third degree of** multiple fingers (nail), not including thumb

　√7ᵗʰ **T23.731** Corrosion of third degree of multiple right fingers (nail), not including thumb

　√7ᵗʰ **T23.732** Corrosion of third degree of multiple left fingers (nail), not including thumb

　√7ᵗʰ **T23.739** Corrosion of third degree of unspecified multiple fingers (nail), not including thumb　▽

√6ᵗʰ **T23.74** **Corrosion of third degree of** multiple fingers (nail), including thumb

　√7ᵗʰ **T23.741** Corrosion of third degree of multiple right fingers (nail), including thumb

　√7ᵗʰ **T23.742** Corrosion of third degree of multiple left fingers (nail), including thumb

　√7ᵗʰ **T23.749** Corrosion of third degree of unspecified multiple fingers (nail), including thumb　▽

√6ᵗʰ **T23.75** **Corrosion of third degree of** palm

　√7ᵗʰ **T23.751** Corrosion of third degree of right palm

　√7ᵗʰ **T23.752** Corrosion of third degree of left palm

　√7ᵗʰ **T23.759** Corrosion of third degree of unspecified palm　▽

√6ᵗʰ **T23.76** **Corrosion of third degree of** back of hand

　√7ᵗʰ **T23.761** Corrosion of third degree of back of right hand

☑ Additional Character Req　　√x7ᵗʰ Placeholder Alert　　Manifestation　　▽ Unspecified　　►◄ Revised Text　　● New Code　　▲ Revised Code Title

ICD-10-CM 2019　　**1085**

√7ᵗʰ **T23.762** Corrosion of third degree of back of left hand

√7ᵗʰ **T23.769** Corrosion of third degree back of unspecified hand ▽

√6ᵗʰ **T23.77** Corrosion of third degree of wrist

√7ᵗʰ **T23.771** Corrosion of third degree of right wrist

√7ᵗʰ **T23.772** Corrosion of third degree of left wrist

√7ᵗʰ **T23.779** Corrosion of third degree of unspecified wrist ▽

√6ᵗʰ **T23.79** Corrosion of third degree of multiple sites of wrist and hand

√7ᵗʰ **T23.791** Corrosion of third degree of multiple sites of right wrist and hand

√7ᵗʰ **T23.792** Corrosion of third degree of multiple sites of left wrist and hand

√7ᵗʰ **T23.799** Corrosion of third degree of multiple sites of unspecified wrist and hand ▽

√4ᵗʰ **T24** **Burn and corrosion of lower limb, except ankle and foot**

EXCLUDES 2   burn and corrosion of ankle and foot (T25.-)

burn and corrosion of hip region (T21.-)

The appropriate 7th character is to be added to each code from category T24.
A   initial encounter
D   subsequent encounter
S   sequela

√5ᵗʰ **T24.0** **Burn of unspecified degree of lower limb, except ankle and foot**

Use additional external cause code to identify the source, place and intent of the burn (X00-X19, X75-X77, X96-X98, Y92)

√6ᵗʰ **T24.00** Burn of unspecified degree of unspecified site of lower limb, except ankle and foot

√7ᵗʰ **T24.001** Burn of unspecified degree of unspecified site of right lower limb, except ankle and foot ▽

√7ᵗʰ **T24.002** Burn of unspecified degree of unspecified site of left lower limb, except ankle and foot ▽

√7ᵗʰ **T24.009** Burn of unspecified degree of unspecified site of unspecified lower limb, except ankle and foot ▽

√6ᵗʰ **T24.01** Burn of unspecified degree of thigh

√7ᵗʰ **T24.011** Burn of unspecified degree of right thigh ▽

√7ᵗʰ **T24.012** Burn of unspecified degree of left thigh ▽

√7ᵗʰ **T24.019** Burn of unspecified degree of unspecified thigh ▽

√6ᵗʰ **T24.02** Burn of unspecified degree of knee

√7ᵗʰ **T24.021** Burn of unspecified degree of right knee ▽

√7ᵗʰ **T24.022** Burn of unspecified degree of left knee ▽

√7ᵗʰ **T24.029** Burn of unspecified degree of unspecified knee ▽

√6ᵗʰ **T24.03** Burn of unspecified degree of lower leg

√7ᵗʰ **T24.031** Burn of unspecified degree of right lower leg ▽

√7ᵗʰ **T24.032** Burn of unspecified degree of left lower leg ▽

√7ᵗʰ **T24.039** Burn of unspecified degree of unspecified lower leg ▽

√6ᵗʰ **T24.09** Burn of unspecified degree of multiple sites of lower limb, except ankle and foot

√7ᵗʰ **T24.091** Burn of unspecified degree of multiple sites of right lower limb, except ankle and foot ▽

√7ᵗʰ **T24.092** Burn of unspecified degree of multiple sites of left lower limb, except ankle and foot ▽

√7ᵗʰ **T24.099** Burn of unspecified degree of multiple sites of unspecified lower limb, except ankle and foot ▽

√5ᵗʰ **T24.1** **Burn of first degree of lower limb, except ankle and foot**

Use additional external cause code to identify the source, place and intent of the burn (X00-X19, X75-X77, X96-X98, Y92)

√6ᵗʰ **T24.10** Burn of first degree of unspecified site of lower limb, except ankle and foot

√7ᵗʰ **T24.101** Burn of first degree of unspecified site of right lower limb, except ankle and foot ▽

√7ᵗʰ **T24.102** Burn of first degree of unspecified site of left lower limb, except ankle and foot ▽

√7ᵗʰ **T24.109** Burn of first degree of unspecified site of unspecified lower limb, except ankle and foot ▽

√6ᵗʰ **T24.11** Burn of first degree of thigh

√7ᵗʰ **T24.111** Burn of first degree of right thigh

√7ᵗʰ **T24.112** Burn of first degree of left thigh

√7ᵗʰ **T24.119** Burn of first degree of unspecified thigh ▽

√6ᵗʰ **T24.12** Burn of first degree of knee

√7ᵗʰ **T24.121** Burn of first degree of right knee

√7ᵗʰ **T24.122** Burn of first degree of left knee

√7ᵗʰ **T24.129** Burn of first degree of unspecified knee ▽

√6ᵗʰ **T24.13** Burn of first degree of lower leg

√7ᵗʰ **T24.131** Burn of first degree of right lower leg

√7ᵗʰ **T24.132** Burn of first degree of left lower leg

√7ᵗʰ **T24.139** Burn of first degree of unspecified lower leg ▽

√6ᵗʰ **T24.19** Burn of first degree of multiple sites of lower limb, except ankle and foot

√7ᵗʰ **T24.191** Burn of first degree of multiple sites of right lower limb, except ankle and foot

√7ᵗʰ **T24.192** Burn of first degree of multiple sites of left lower limb, except ankle and foot

√7ᵗʰ **T24.199** Burn of first degree of multiple sites of unspecified lower limb, except ankle and foot ▽

√5ᵗʰ **T24.2** **Burn of second degree of lower limb, except ankle and foot**

Use additional external cause code to identify the source, place and intent of the burn (X00-X19, X75-X77, X96-X98, Y92)

√6ᵗʰ **T24.20** Burn of second degree of unspecified site of lower limb, except ankle and foot

√7ᵗʰ **T24.201** Burn of second degree of unspecified site of right lower limb, except ankle and foot ▽

√7ᵗʰ **T24.202** Burn of second degree of unspecified site of left lower limb, except ankle and foot ▽

√7ᵗʰ **T24.209** Burn of second degree of unspecified site of unspecified lower limb, except ankle and foot ▽

√6ᵗʰ **T24.21** Burn of second degree of thigh

√7ᵗʰ **T24.211** Burn of second degree of right thigh

√7ᵗʰ **T24.212** Burn of second degree of left thigh

√7ᵗʰ **T24.219** Burn of second degree of unspecified thigh ▽

√6ᵗʰ **T24.22** Burn of second degree of knee

√7ᵗʰ **T24.221** Burn of second degree of right knee

√7ᵗʰ **T24.222** Burn of second degree of left knee

√7ᵗʰ **T24.229** Burn of second degree of unspecified knee ▽

√6ᵗʰ **T24.23** Burn of second degree of lower leg

√7ᵗʰ **T24.231** Burn of second degree of right lower leg

√7ᵗʰ **T24.232** Burn of second degree of left lower leg

√7ᵗʰ **T24.239** Burn of second degree of unspecified lower leg ▽

√6ᵗʰ **T24.29** Burn of second degree of multiple sites of lower limb, except ankle and foot

√7ᵗʰ **T24.291** Burn of second degree of multiple sites of right lower limb, except ankle and foot

√7ᵗʰ **T24.292** Burn of second degree of multiple sites of left lower limb, except ankle and foot

√7ᵗʰ **T24.299** Burn of second degree of multiple sites of unspecified lower limb, except ankle and foot ▽

✓5ᵗʰ **T24.3** **Burn of** third degree **of lower limb, except ankle and foot**

Use additional external cause code to identify the source, place and intent of the burn (X00-X19, X75-X77, X96-X98, Y92)

  ✓6ᵗʰ **T24.30** **Burn of third degree of unspecified site of lower limb, except ankle and foot**

    ✓7ᵗʰ **T24.301** Burn of third degree of unspecified site of right lower limb, except ankle and foot ▽

    ✓7ᵗʰ **T24.302** Burn of third degree of unspecified site of left lower limb, except ankle and foot ▽

    ✓7ᵗʰ **T24.309** Burn of third degree of unspecified site of unspecified lower limb, except ankle and foot ▽

  ✓6ᵗʰ **T24.31** **Burn of third degree of** thigh

    ✓7ᵗʰ **T24.311** Burn of third degree of right thigh

    ✓7ᵗʰ **T24.312** Burn of third degree of left thigh

    ✓7ᵗʰ **T24.319** Burn of third degree of unspecified thigh ▽

  ✓6ᵗʰ **T24.32** **Burn of third degree of** knee

    ✓7ᵗʰ **T24.321** Burn of third degree of right knee

    ✓7ᵗʰ **T24.322** Burn of third degree of left knee

    ✓7ᵗʰ **T24.329** Burn of third degree of unspecified knee ▽

  ✓6ᵗʰ **T24.33** **Burn of third degree of** lower leg

    ✓7ᵗʰ **T24.331** Burn of third degree of right lower leg

    ✓7ᵗʰ **T24.332** Burn of third degree of left lower leg

    ✓7ᵗʰ **T24.339** Burn of third degree of unspecified lower leg ▽

  ✓6ᵗʰ **T24.39** **Burn of third degree** multiple sites **of lower limb, except ankle and foot**

AHA: 2016,2Q,4

    ✓7ᵗʰ **T24.391** Burn of third degree of multiple sites of right lower limb, except ankle and foot

    ✓7ᵗʰ **T24.392** Burn of third degree of multiple sites of left lower limb, except ankle and foot

    ✓7ᵗʰ **T24.399** Burn of third degree of multiple sites of unspecified lower limb, except ankle and foot ▽

✓5ᵗʰ **T24.4** **Corrosion of unspecified degree of lower limb, except ankle and foot**

Code first (T51-T65) to identify chemical and intent

Use additional external cause code to identify place (Y92)

  ✓6ᵗʰ **T24.40** **Corrosion of unspecified degree of unspecified site of lower limb, except ankle and foot**

    ✓7ᵗʰ **T24.401** Corrosion of unspecified degree of unspecified site of right lower limb, except ankle and foot ▽

    ✓7ᵗʰ **T24.402** Corrosion of unspecified degree of unspecified site of left lower limb, except ankle and foot ▽

    ✓7ᵗʰ **T24.409** Corrosion of unspecified degree of unspecified site of unspecified lower limb, except ankle and foot ▽

  ✓6ᵗʰ **T24.41** **Corrosion of unspecified degree of** thigh

    ✓7ᵗʰ **T24.411** Corrosion of unspecified degree of right thigh ▽

    ✓7ᵗʰ **T24.412** Corrosion of unspecified degree of left thigh ▽

    ✓7ᵗʰ **T24.419** Corrosion of unspecified degree of unspecified thigh ▽

  ✓6ᵗʰ **T24.42** **Corrosion of unspecified degree of** knee

    ✓7ᵗʰ **T24.421** Corrosion of unspecified degree of right knee ▽

    ✓7ᵗʰ **T24.422** Corrosion of unspecified degree of left knee ▽

    ✓7ᵗʰ **T24.429** Corrosion of unspecified degree of unspecified knee ▽

  ✓6ᵗʰ **T24.43** **Corrosion of unspecified degree of** lower leg

    ✓7ᵗʰ **T24.431** Corrosion of unspecified degree of right lower leg ▽

    ✓7ᵗʰ **T24.432** Corrosion of unspecified degree of left lower leg ▽

    ✓7ᵗʰ **T24.439** Corrosion of unspecified degree of unspecified lower leg ▽

  ✓6ᵗʰ **T24.49** **Corrosion of unspecified degree of** multiple sites **of lower limb, except ankle and foot**

    ✓7ᵗʰ **T24.491** Corrosion of unspecified degree of multiple sites of right lower limb, except ankle and foot ▽

    ✓7ᵗʰ **T24.492** Corrosion of unspecified degree of multiple sites of left lower limb, except ankle and foot ▽

    ✓7ᵗʰ **T24.499** Corrosion of unspecified degree of multiple sites of unspecified lower limb, except ankle and foot ▽

✓5ᵗʰ **T24.5** **Corrosion of** first degree **of lower limb, except ankle and foot**

Code first (T51-T65) to identify chemical and intent

Use additional external cause code to identify place (Y92)

  ✓6ᵗʰ **T24.50** **Corrosion of first degree of unspecified site of lower limb, except ankle and foot**

    ✓7ᵗʰ **T24.501** Corrosion of first degree of unspecified site of right lower limb, except ankle and foot ▽

    ✓7ᵗʰ **T24.502** Corrosion of first degree of unspecified site of left lower limb, except ankle and foot ▽

    ✓7ᵗʰ **T24.509** Corrosion of first degree of unspecified site of unspecified lower limb, except ankle and foot ▽

  ✓6ᵗʰ **T24.51** **Corrosion of first degree of** thigh

    ✓7ᵗʰ **T24.511** Corrosion of first degree of right thigh

    ✓7ᵗʰ **T24.512** Corrosion of first degree of left thigh

    ✓7ᵗʰ **T24.519** Corrosion of first degree of unspecified thigh ▽

  ✓6ᵗʰ **T24.52** **Corrosion of first degree of** knee

    ✓7ᵗʰ **T24.521** Corrosion of first degree of right knee

    ✓7ᵗʰ **T24.522** Corrosion of first degree of left knee

    ✓7ᵗʰ **T24.529** Corrosion of first degree of unspecified knee ▽

  ✓6ᵗʰ **T24.53** **Corrosion of first degree of** lower leg

    ✓7ᵗʰ **T24.531** Corrosion of first degree of right lower leg

    ✓7ᵗʰ **T24.532** Corrosion of first degree of left lower leg

    ✓7ᵗʰ **T24.539** Corrosion of first degree of unspecified lower leg ▽

  ✓6ᵗʰ **T24.59** **Corrosion of first degree of** multiple sites **of lower limb, except ankle and foot**

    ✓7ᵗʰ **T24.591** Corrosion of first degree of multiple sites of right lower limb, except ankle and foot

    ✓7ᵗʰ **T24.592** Corrosion of first degree of multiple sites of left lower limb, except ankle and foot

    ✓7ᵗʰ **T24.599** Corrosion of first degree of multiple sites of unspecified lower limb, except ankle and foot ▽

✓5ᵗʰ **T24.6** **Corrosion of** second degree **of lower limb, except ankle and foot**

Code first (T51-T65) to identify chemical and intent

Use additional external cause code to identify place (Y92)

  ✓6ᵗʰ **T24.60** **Corrosion of second degree of unspecified site of lower limb, except ankle and foot**

    ✓7ᵗʰ **T24.601** Corrosion of second degree of unspecified site of right lower limb, except ankle and foot ▽

    ✓7ᵗʰ **T24.602** Corrosion of second degree of unspecified site of left lower limb, except ankle and foot ▽

    ✓7ᵗʰ **T24.609** Corrosion of second degree of unspecified site of unspecified lower limb, except ankle and foot ▽

  ✓6ᵗʰ **T24.61** **Corrosion of second degree of** thigh

    ✓7ᵗʰ **T24.611** Corrosion of second degree of right thigh

    ✓7ᵗʰ **T24.612** Corrosion of second degree of left thigh

    ✓7ᵗʰ **T24.619** Corrosion of second degree of unspecified thigh ▽

  ✓6ᵗʰ **T24.62** **Corrosion of second degree of** knee

    ✓7ᵗʰ **T24.621** Corrosion of second degree of right knee

    ✓7ᵗʰ **T24.622** Corrosion of second degree of left knee

    ✓7ᵗʰ **T24.629** Corrosion of second degree of unspecified knee ▽

  ✓6ᵗʰ **T24.63** **Corrosion of second degree of** lower leg

    ✓7ᵗʰ **T24.631** Corrosion of second degree of right lower leg

    ✓7ᵗʰ **T24.632** Corrosion of second degree of left lower leg

    ✓7ᵗʰ **T24.639** Corrosion of second degree of unspecified lower leg ▽

☑ Additional Character Req   ✓x7ᵗʰ Placeholder Alert   Manifestation   ▽ Unspecified   ▶◀ Revised Text   ● New Code   ▲ Revised Code Title

√6ᵗʰ T24.69 Corrosion of second degree of multiple sites of lower limb, except ankle and foot

√7ᵗʰ **T24.691** Corrosion of second degree of multiple sites of right lower limb, except ankle and foot

√7ᵗʰ **T24.692** Corrosion of second degree of multiple sites of left lower limb, except ankle and foot

√7ᵗʰ **T24.699** Corrosion of second degree of multiple sites of unspecified lower limb, except ankle and foot ▽

√5ᵗʰ T24.7 Corrosion of third degree of lower limb, except ankle and foot

Code first (T51-T65) to identify chemical and intent
Use additional external cause code to identify place (Y92)

√6ᵗʰ T24.70 Corrosion of third degree of unspecified site of lower limb, except ankle and foot

√7ᵗʰ **T24.701** Corrosion of third degree of unspecified site of right lower limb, except ankle and foot ▽

√7ᵗʰ **T24.702** Corrosion of third degree of unspecified site of left lower limb, except ankle and foot ▽

√7ᵗʰ **T24.709** Corrosion of third degree of unspecified site of unspecified lower limb, except ankle and foot ▽

√6ᵗʰ T24.71 Corrosion of third degree of thigh

√7ᵗʰ **T24.711** Corrosion of third degree of right thigh

√7ᵗʰ **T24.712** Corrosion of third degree of left thigh

√7ᵗʰ **T24.719** Corrosion of third degree of unspecified thigh ▽

√6ᵗʰ T24.72 Corrosion of third degree of knee

√7ᵗʰ **T24.721** Corrosion of third degree of right knee

√7ᵗʰ **T24.722** Corrosion of third degree of left knee

√7ᵗʰ **T24.729** Corrosion of third degree of unspecified knee ▽

√6ᵗʰ T24.73 Corrosion of third degree of lower leg

√7ᵗʰ **T24.731** Corrosion of third degree of right lower leg

√7ᵗʰ **T24.732** Corrosion of third degree of left lower leg

√7ᵗʰ **T24.739** Corrosion of third degree of unspecified lower leg ▽

√6ᵗʰ T24.79 Corrosion of third degree of multiple sites of lower limb, except ankle and foot

√7ᵗʰ **T24.791** Corrosion of third degree of multiple sites of right lower limb, except ankle and foot

√7ᵗʰ **T24.792** Corrosion of third degree of multiple sites of left lower limb, except ankle and foot

√7ᵗʰ **T24.799** Corrosion of third degree of multiple sites of unspecified lower limb, except ankle and foot ▽

√4ᵗʰ T25 Burn and corrosion of ankle and foot

The appropriate 7th character is to be added to each code from category T25.
A   initial encounter
D   subsequent encounter
S   sequela

√5ᵗʰ T25.0 Burn of unspecified degree of ankle and foot

Use additional external cause code to identify the source, place and intent of the burn (X00-X19, X75-X77, X96-X98, Y92)

√6ᵗʰ T25.01 Burn of unspecified degree of ankle

√7ᵗʰ **T25.011** Burn of unspecified degree of right ankle ▽

√7ᵗʰ **T25.012** Burn of unspecified degree of left ankle ▽

√7ᵗʰ **T25.019** Burn of unspecified degree of unspecified ankle ▽

√6ᵗʰ T25.02 Burn of unspecified degree of foot

EXCLUDES 2   burn of unspecified degree of toe(s) (nail) (T25.03-)

√7ᵗʰ **T25.021** Burn of unspecified degree of right foot ▽

√7ᵗʰ **T25.022** Burn of unspecified degree of left foot ▽

√7ᵗʰ **T25.029** Burn of unspecified degree of unspecified foot ▽

√6ᵗʰ T25.03 Burn of unspecified degree of toe(s) (nail)

√7ᵗʰ **T25.031** Burn of unspecified degree of right toe(s) (nail) ▽

√7ᵗʰ **T25.032** Burn of unspecified degree of left toe(s) (nail) ▽

√7ᵗʰ **T25.039** Burn of unspecified degree of unspecified toe(s) (nail) ▽

√6ᵗʰ T25.09 Burn of unspecified degree of multiple sites of ankle and foot

√7ᵗʰ **T25.091** Burn of unspecified degree of multiple sites of right ankle and foot ▽

√7ᵗʰ **T25.092** Burn of unspecified degree of multiple sites of left ankle and foot ▽

√7ᵗʰ **T25.099** Burn of unspecified degree of multiple sites of unspecified ankle and foot ▽

√5ᵗʰ T25.1 Burn of first degree of ankle and foot

Use additional external cause code to identify the source, place and intent of the burn (X00-X19, X75-X77, X96-X98, Y92)

√6ᵗʰ T25.11 Burn of first degree of ankle

√7ᵗʰ **T25.111** Burn of first degree of right ankle

√7ᵗʰ **T25.112** Burn of first degree of left ankle

√7ᵗʰ **T25.119** Burn of first degree of unspecified ankle ▽

√6ᵗʰ T25.12 Burn of first degree of foot

EXCLUDES 2   burn of first degree of toe(s) (nail) (T25.13-)

√7ᵗʰ **T25.121** Burn of first degree of right foot

√7ᵗʰ **T25.122** Burn of first degree of left foot

√7ᵗʰ **T25.129** Burn of first degree of unspecified foot ▽

√6ᵗʰ T25.13 Burn of first degree of toe(s) (nail)

√7ᵗʰ **T25.131** Burn of first degree of right toe(s) (nail)

√7ᵗʰ **T25.132** Burn of first degree of left toe(s) (nail)

√7ᵗʰ **T25.139** Burn of first degree of unspecified toe(s) (nail) ▽

√6ᵗʰ T25.19 Burn of first degree of multiple sites of ankle and foot

√7ᵗʰ **T25.191** Burn of first degree of multiple sites of right ankle and foot

√7ᵗʰ **T25.192** Burn of first degree of multiple sites of left ankle and foot

√7ᵗʰ **T25.199** Burn of first degree of multiple sites of unspecified ankle and foot ▽

√5ᵗʰ T25.2 Burn of second degree of ankle and foot

Use additional external cause code to identify the source, place and intent of the burn (X00-X19, X75-X77, X96-X98, Y92)

√6ᵗʰ T25.21 Burn of second degree of ankle

√7ᵗʰ **T25.211** Burn of second degree of right ankle

√7ᵗʰ **T25.212** Burn of second degree of left ankle

√7ᵗʰ **T25.219** Burn of second degree of unspecified ankle ▽

√6ᵗʰ T25.22 Burn of second degree of foot

EXCLUDES 2   burn of second degree of toe(s) (nail) (T25.23-)

√7ᵗʰ **T25.221** Burn of second degree of right foot

√7ᵗʰ **T25.222** Burn of second degree of left foot

√7ᵗʰ **T25.229** Burn of second degree of unspecified foot ▽

√6ᵗʰ T25.23 Burn of second degree of toe(s) (nail)

√7ᵗʰ **T25.231** Burn of second degree of right toe(s) (nail)

√7ᵗʰ **T25.232** Burn of second degree of left toe(s) (nail)

√7ᵗʰ **T25.239** Burn of second degree of unspecified toe(s) (nail) ▽

√6ᵗʰ T25.29 Burn of second degree of multiple sites of ankle and foot

√7ᵗʰ **T25.291** Burn of second degree of multiple sites of right ankle and foot

√7ᵗʰ **T25.292** Burn of second degree of multiple sites of left ankle and foot

√7ᵗʰ **T25.299** Burn of second degree of multiple sites of unspecified ankle and foot ▽

√5ᵗʰ **T25.3** **Burn of third degree of ankle and foot**

Use additional external cause code to identify the source, place and intent of the burn (X00-X19, X75-X77, X96-X98, Y92)

√6ᵗʰ **T25.31** **Burn of third degree of ankle**

√7ᵗʰ **T25.311** **Burn of third degree of right ankle**

√7ᵗʰ **T25.312** **Burn of third degree of left ankle**

√7ᵗʰ **T25.319** **Burn of third degree of unspecified ankle** ▽

√6ᵗʰ **T25.32** **Burn of third degree of foot**

EXCLUDES 2   *burn of third degree of toe(s) (nail) (T25.33-)*

√7ᵗʰ **T25.321** **Burn of third degree of right foot**

√7ᵗʰ **T25.322** **Burn of third degree of left foot**

√7ᵗʰ **T25.329** **Burn of third degree of unspecified foot** ▽

√6ᵗʰ **T25.33** **Burn of third degree of toe(s) (nail)**

√7ᵗʰ **T25.331** **Burn of third degree of right toe(s) (nail)**

√7ᵗʰ **T25.332** **Burn of third degree of left toe(s) (nail)**

√7ᵗʰ **T25.339** **Burn of third degree of unspecified toe(s) (nail)** ▽

√6ᵗʰ **T25.39** **Burn of third degree of multiple sites of ankle and foot**

√7ᵗʰ **T25.391** **Burn of third degree of multiple sites of right ankle and foot**

√7ᵗʰ **T25.392** **Burn of third degree of multiple sites of left ankle and foot**

√7ᵗʰ **T25.399** **Burn of third degree of multiple sites of unspecified ankle and foot** ▽

√5ᵗʰ **T25.4** **Corrosion of unspecified degree of ankle and foot**

Code first (T51-T65) to identify chemical and intent
Use additional external cause code to identify place (Y92)

√6ᵗʰ **T25.41** **Corrosion of unspecified degree of ankle**

√7ᵗʰ **T25.411** **Corrosion of unspecified degree of right ankle** ▽

√7ᵗʰ **T25.412** **Corrosion of unspecified degree of left ankle** ▽

√7ᵗʰ **T25.419** **Corrosion of unspecified degree of unspecified ankle** ▽

√6ᵗʰ **T25.42** **Corrosion of unspecified degree of foot**

EXCLUDES 2   *corrosion of unspecified degree of toe(s) (nail) (T25.43-)*

√7ᵗʰ **T25.421** **Corrosion of unspecified degree of right foot** ▽

√7ᵗʰ **T25.422** **Corrosion of unspecified degree of left foot** ▽

√7ᵗʰ **T25.429** **Corrosion of unspecified degree of unspecified foot** ▽

√6ᵗʰ **T25.43** **Corrosion of unspecified degree of toe(s) (nail)**

√7ᵗʰ **T25.431** **Corrosion of unspecified degree of right toe(s) (nail)** ▽

√7ᵗʰ **T25.432** **Corrosion of unspecified degree of left toe(s) (nail)** ▽

√7ᵗʰ **T25.439** **Corrosion of unspecified degree of unspecified toe(s) (nail)** ▽

√6ᵗʰ **T25.49** **Corrosion of unspecified degree of multiple sites of ankle and foot**

√7ᵗʰ **T25.491** **Corrosion of unspecified degree of multiple sites of right ankle and foot** ▽

√7ᵗʰ **T25.492** **Corrosion of unspecified degree of multiple sites of left ankle and foot** ▽

√7ᵗʰ **T25.499** **Corrosion of unspecified degree of multiple sites of unspecified ankle and foot** ▽

√5ᵗʰ **T25.5** **Corrosion of first degree of ankle and foot**

Code first (T51-T65) to identify chemical and intent
Use additional external cause code to identify place (Y92)

√6ᵗʰ **T25.51** **Corrosion of first degree of ankle**

√7ᵗʰ **T25.511** **Corrosion of first degree of right ankle**

√7ᵗʰ **T25.512** **Corrosion of first degree of left ankle**

√7ᵗʰ **T25.519** **Corrosion of first degree of unspecified ankle** ▽

√6ᵗʰ **T25.52** **Corrosion of first degree of foot**

EXCLUDES 2   *corrosion of first degree of toe(s) (nail) (T25.53-)*

√7ᵗʰ **T25.521** **Corrosion of first degree of right foot**

√7ᵗʰ **T25.522** **Corrosion of first degree of left foot**

√7ᵗʰ **T25.529** **Corrosion of first degree of unspecified foot** ▽

√6ᵗʰ **T25.53** **Corrosion of first degree of toe(s) (nail)**

√7ᵗʰ **T25.531** **Corrosion of first degree of right toe(s) (nail)**

√7ᵗʰ **T25.532** **Corrosion of first degree of left toe(s) (nail)**

√7ᵗʰ **T25.539** **Corrosion of first degree of unspecified toe(s) (nail)** ▽

√6ᵗʰ **T25.59** **Corrosion of first degree of multiple sites of ankle and foot**

√7ᵗʰ **T25.591** **Corrosion of first degree of multiple sites of right ankle and foot**

√7ᵗʰ **T25.592** **Corrosion of first degree of multiple sites of left ankle and foot**

√7ᵗʰ **T25.599** **Corrosion of first degree of multiple sites of unspecified ankle and foot** ▽

√5ᵗʰ **T25.6** **Corrosion of second degree of ankle and foot**

Code first (T51-T65) to identify chemical and intent
Use additional external cause code to identify place (Y92)

√6ᵗʰ **T25.61** **Corrosion of second degree of ankle**

√7ᵗʰ **T25.611** **Corrosion of second degree of right ankle**

√7ᵗʰ **T25.612** **Corrosion of second degree of left ankle**

√7ᵗʰ **T25.619** **Corrosion of second degree of unspecified ankle** ▽

√6ᵗʰ **T25.62** **Corrosion of second degree of foot**

EXCLUDES 2   *corrosion of second degree of toe(s) (nail) (T25.63-)*

√7ᵗʰ **T25.621** **Corrosion of second degree of right foot**

√7ᵗʰ **T25.622** **Corrosion of second degree of left foot**

√7ᵗʰ **T25.629** **Corrosion of second degree of unspecified foot** ▽

√6ᵗʰ **T25.63** **Corrosion of second degree of toe(s) (nail)**

√7ᵗʰ **T25.631** **Corrosion of second degree of right toe(s) (nail)**

√7ᵗʰ **T25.632** **Corrosion of second degree of left toe(s) (nail)**

√7ᵗʰ **T25.639** **Corrosion of second degree of unspecified toe(s) (nail)** ▽

√6ᵗʰ **T25.69** **Corrosion of second degree of multiple sites of ankle and foot**

√7ᵗʰ **T25.691** **Corrosion of second degree of right ankle and foot**

√7ᵗʰ **T25.692** **Corrosion of second degree of left ankle and foot**

√7ᵗʰ **T25.699** **Corrosion of second degree of unspecified ankle and foot** ▽

√5ᵗʰ **T25.7** **Corrosion of third degree of ankle and foot**

Code first (T51-T65) to identify chemical and intent
Use additional external cause code to identify place (Y92)

√6ᵗʰ **T25.71** **Corrosion of third degree of ankle**

√7ᵗʰ **T25.711** **Corrosion of third degree of right ankle**

√7ᵗʰ **T25.712** **Corrosion of third degree of left ankle**

√7ᵗʰ **T25.719** **Corrosion of third degree of unspecified ankle** ▽

√6ᵗʰ **T25.72** **Corrosion of third degree of foot**

EXCLUDES 2   *corrosion of third degree of toe(s) (nail) (T25.73-)*

√7ᵗʰ **T25.721** **Corrosion of third degree of right foot**

√7ᵗʰ **T25.722** **Corrosion of third degree of left foot**

√7ᵗʰ **T25.729** **Corrosion of third degree of unspecified foot** ▽

√6ᵗʰ **T25.73** **Corrosion of third degree of toe(s) (nail)**

√7ᵗʰ **T25.731** **Corrosion of third degree of right toe(s) (nail)**

√7ᵗʰ **T25.732** **Corrosion of third degree of left toe(s) (nail)**

√7ᵗʰ **T25.739** **Corrosion of third degree of unspecified toe(s) (nail)** ▽

☑ Additional Character Req   √x7ᵗʰ Placeholder Alert   Manifestation   ▽ Unspecified   ▶◀ Revised Text   ● New Code   ▲ Revised Code Title

ICD-10-CM 2019

1089

Chapter 19. Injury, Poisoning and Certain Other Consequences of External Causes

√6ᵗʰ **T25.79** Corrosion of third degree of multiple sites of ankle and foot
- √7ᵗʰ **T25.791** Corrosion of third degree of multiple sites of right ankle and foot
- √7ᵗʰ **T25.792** Corrosion of third degree of multiple sites of left ankle and foot
- √7ᵗʰ **T25.799** Corrosion of third degree of multiple sites of unspecified ankle and foot ▽

Burns and corrosions confined to eye and internal organs (T26-T28)

√4ᵗʰ **T26 Burn and corrosion confined to eye and adnexa**

The appropriate 7th character is to be added to each code from category T26.
A   initial encounter
D   subsequent encounter
S   sequela

√5ᵗʰ **T26.0 Burn of** eyelid and periocular area
Use additional external cause code to identify the source, place and intent of the burn (X00-X19, X75-X77, X96-X98, Y92)
- √7ᵗʰ **T26.00** Burn of unspecified eyelid and periocular area ▽
- √7ᵗʰ **T26.01** Burn of right eyelid and periocular area
- √7ᵗʰ **T26.02** Burn of left eyelid and periocular area

√5ᵗʰ **T26.1 Burn of** cornea and conjunctival sac
Use additional external cause code to identify the source, place and intent of the burn (X00-X19, X75-X77, X96-X98, Y92)
- √7ᵗʰ **T26.10** Burn of cornea and conjunctival sac, unspecified eye ▽
- √7ᵗʰ **T26.11** Burn of cornea and conjunctival sac, right eye
- √7ᵗʰ **T26.12** Burn of cornea and conjunctival sac, left eye

√5ᵗʰ **T26.2 Burn with resulting** rupture and destruction of eyeball
Use additional external cause code to identify the source, place and intent of the burn (X00-X19, X75-X77, X96-X98, Y92)
- √7ᵗʰ **T26.20** Burn with resulting rupture and destruction of unspecified eyeball ▽
- √7ᵗʰ **T26.21** Burn with resulting rupture and destruction of right eyeball
- √7ᵗʰ **T26.22** Burn with resulting rupture and destruction of left eyeball

√5ᵗʰ **T26.3 Burns of other specified parts of eye and adnexa**
Use additional external cause code to identify the source, place and intent of the burn (X00-X19, X75-X77, X96-X98, Y92)
- √7ᵗʰ **T26.30** Burns of other specified parts of unspecified eye and adnexa ▽
- √7ᵗʰ **T26.31** Burns of other specified parts of right eye and adnexa
- √7ᵗʰ **T26.32** Burns of other specified parts of left eye and adnexa

√5ᵗʰ **T26.4 Burn of eye and adnexa, part unspecified**
Use additional external cause code to identify the source, place and intent of the burn (X00-X19, X75-X77, X96-X98, Y92)
- √7ᵗʰ **T26.40** Burn of unspecified eye and adnexa, part unspecified ▽
- √7ᵗʰ **T26.41** Burn of right eye and adnexa, part unspecified ▽
- √7ᵗʰ **T26.42** Burn of left eye and adnexa, part unspecified ▽

√5ᵗʰ **T26.5 Corrosion of** eyelid and periocular area
Code first (T51-T65) to identify chemical and intent
Use additional external cause code to identify place (Y92)
- √7ᵗʰ **T26.50** Corrosion of unspecified eyelid and periocular area ▽
- √7ᵗʰ **T26.51** Corrosion of right eyelid and periocular area
- √7ᵗʰ **T26.52** Corrosion of left eyelid and periocular area

√5ᵗʰ **T26.6 Corrosion of** cornea and conjunctival sac
Code first (T51-T65) to identify chemical and intent
Use additional external cause code to identify place (Y92)
- √7ᵗʰ **T26.60** Corrosion of cornea and conjunctival sac, unspecified eye ▽
- √7ᵗʰ **T26.61** Corrosion of cornea and conjunctival sac, right eye
- √7ᵗʰ **T26.62** Corrosion of cornea and conjunctival sac, left eye

√5ᵗʰ **T26.7 Corrosion with resulting** rupture and destruction of eyeball
Code first (T51-T65) to identify chemical and intent
Use additional external cause code to identify place (Y92)
- √7ᵗʰ **T26.70** Corrosion with resulting rupture and destruction of unspecified eyeball ▽
- √7ᵗʰ **T26.71** Corrosion with resulting rupture and destruction of right eyeball
- √7ᵗʰ **T26.72** Corrosion with resulting rupture and destruction of left eyeball

√5ᵗʰ **T26.8 Corrosions of other specified parts of eye and adnexa**
Code first (T51-T65) to identify chemical and intent
Use additional external cause code to identify place (Y92)
- √7ᵗʰ **T26.80** Corrosions of other specified parts of unspecified eye and adnexa ▽
- √7ᵗʰ **T26.81** Corrosions of other specified parts of right eye and adnexa
- √7ᵗʰ **T26.82** Corrosions of other specified parts of left eye and adnexa

√5ᵗʰ **T26.9 Corrosion of eye and adnexa, part unspecified**
Code first (T51-T65) to identify chemical and intent
Use additional external cause code to identify place (Y92)
- √7ᵗʰ **T26.90** Corrosion of unspecified eye and adnexa, part unspecified ▽
- √7ᵗʰ **T26.91** Corrosion of right eye and adnexa, part unspecified ▽
- √7ᵗʰ **T26.92** Corrosion of left eye and adnexa, part unspecified ▽

√4ᵗʰ **T27 Burn and corrosion of respiratory tract**
Use additional external cause code to identify the source and intent of the burn (X00-X19, X75-X77, X96-X98)
Use additional external cause code to identify place (Y92)

The appropriate 7th character is to be added to each code from category T27.
A   initial encounter
D   subsequent encounter
S   sequela

- √7ᵗʰ **T27.0 Burn of** larynx and trachea
- √7ᵗʰ **T27.1 Burn involving** larynx and trachea with lung
- √7ᵗʰ **T27.2 Burn of other parts of respiratory tract**
  Burn of thoracic cavity
- √7ᵗʰ **T27.3 Burn of respiratory tract, part unspecified** ▽
- √7ᵗʰ **T27.4 Corrosion of larynx and trachea**
  Code first (T51-T65) to identify chemical and intent
- √7ᵗʰ **T27.5 Corrosion involving** larynx and trachea with lung
- √7ᵗʰ **T27.6 Corrosion of other parts of respiratory tract**
  Code first (T51-T65) to identify chemical and intent
- √7ᵗʰ **T27.7 Corrosion of respiratory tract, part unspecified** ▽
  Code first (T51-T65) to identify chemical and intent

√4ᵗʰ **T28 Burn and corrosion of other internal organs**
Use additional external cause code to identify the source and intent of the burn (X00-X19, X75-X77, X96-X98)
Use additional external cause code to identify place (Y92)

The appropriate 7th character is to be added to each code from category T28.
A   initial encounter
D   subsequent encounter
S   sequela

- √7ᵗʰ **T28.0 Burn of** mouth and pharynx
- √7ᵗʰ **T28.1 Burn of** esophagus
- √7ᵗʰ **T28.2 Burn of other parts of alimentary tract**
- √7ᵗʰ **T28.3 Burn of internal genitourinary organs**
- √5ᵗʰ **T28.4 Burns of other and unspecified internal organs**
  Code first (T51-T65) to identify chemical and intent
  - √7ᵗʰ **T28.40** Burn of unspecified internal organ ▽
  - √6ᵗʰ **T28.41 Burn of** ear drum
    - √7ᵗʰ **T28.411** Burn of right ear drum
    - √7ᵗʰ **T28.412** Burn of left ear drum
    - √7ᵗʰ **T28.419** Burn of unspecified ear drum ▽
  - √7ᵗʰ **T28.49** Burn of other internal organ
- √7ᵗʰ **T28.5 Corrosion of mouth and pharynx**
  Code first (T51-T65) to identify chemical and intent

√x7ᵗʰ **T28.6** **Corrosion of esophagus**
     Code first (T51-T65) to identify chemical and intent

√x7ᵗʰ **T28.7** **Corrosion of other parts of alimentary tract**
     Code first (T51-T65) to identify chemical and intent

√x7ᵗʰ **T28.8** **Corrosion of internal genitourinary organs**
     Code first (T51-T65) to identify chemical and intent

√5ᵗʰ **T28.9** **Corrosions of other and unspecified internal organs**
     Code first (T51-T65) to identify chemical and intent

    √x7ᵗʰ **T28.90** **Corrosions of unspecified internal organs** ▽

    √6ᵗʰ **T28.91** **Corrosions of ear drum**

       √7ᵗʰ **T28.911** **Corrosions of right ear drum**

       √7ᵗʰ **T28.912** **Corrosions of left ear drum**

       √7ᵗʰ **T28.919** **Corrosions of unspecified ear drum** ▽

    √x7ᵗʰ **T28.99** **Corrosions of other internal organs**

Burns and corrosions of multiple and unspecified body regions (T30-T32)

√4ᵗʰ **T30** **Burn and corrosion, body region unspecified**

    T30.0 **Burn of unspecified body region, unspecified degree** ▽
     This code is not for inpatient use. Code to specified site and degree of burns
     Burn NOS
     Multiple burns NOS

    T30.4 **Corrosion of unspecified body region, unspecified degree** ▽
     This code is not for inpatient use. Code to specified site and degree of corrosion
     Corrosion NOS
     Multiple corrosion NOS

√4ᵗʰ **T31** **Burns classified according to extent of body surface involved**

    NOTE   This category is to be used as the primary code only when the site of the burn is unspecified. It should be used as a supplementary code with categories T20-T25 when the site is specified.

    T31.0 **Burns involving less than 10% of body surface**

√5ᵗʰ **T31.1** **Burns involving 10-19% of body surface**

    T31.10 **Burns involving 10-19% of body surface with 0% to 9% third degree burns**
     Burns involving 10-19% of body surface NOS

    T31.11 **Burns involving 10-19% of body surface with 10-19% third degree burns** HCC

√5ᵗʰ **T31.2** **Burns involving 20-29% of body surface**

    T31.20 **Burns involving 20-29% of body surface with 0% to 9% third degree burns**
     Burns involving 20-29% of body surface NOS

    T31.21 **Burns involving 20-29% of body surface with 10-19% third degree burns** HCC

    T31.22 **Burns involving 20-29% of body surface with 20-29% third degree burns** HCC

√5ᵗʰ **T31.3** **Burns involving 30-39% of body surface**

    T31.30 **Burns involving 30-39% of body surface with 0% to 9% third degree burns**
     Burns involving 30-39% of body surface NOS

    T31.31 **Burns involving 30-39% of body surface with 10-19% third degree burns** HCC

    T31.32 **Burns involving 30-39% of body surface with 20-29% third degree burns** HCC

    T31.33 **Burns involving 30-39% of body surface with 30-39% third degree burns** HCC

√5ᵗʰ **T31.4** **Burns involving 40-49% of body surface**

    T31.40 **Burns involving 40-49% of body surface with 0% to 9% third degree burns**
     Burns involving 40-49% of body surface NOS

    T31.41 **Burns involving 40-49% of body surface with 10-19% third degree burns** HCC

    T31.42 **Burns involving 40-49% of body surface with 20-29% third degree burns** HCC

    T31.43 **Burns involving 40-49% of body surface with 30-39% third degree burns** HCC

    T31.44 **Burns involving 40-49% of body surface with 40-49% third degree burns** HCC

√5ᵗʰ **T31.5** **Burns involving 50-59% of body surface**

    T31.50 **Burns involving 50-59% of body surface with 0% to 9% third degree burns**
     Burns involving 50-59% of body surface NOS

    T31.51 **Burns involving 50-59% of body surface with 10-19% third degree burns** HCC

    T31.52 **Burns involving 50-59% of body surface with 20-29% third degree burns** HCC

    T31.53 **Burns involving 50-59% of body surface with 30-39% third degree burns** HCC

    T31.54 **Burns involving 50-59% of body surface with 40-49% third degree burns** HCC

    T31.55 **Burns involving 50-59% of body surface with 50-59% third degree burns** HCC

√5ᵗʰ **T31.6** **Burns involving 60-69% of body surface**

    T31.60 **Burns involving 60-69% of body surface with 0% to 9% third degree burns**
     Burns involving 60-69% of body surface NOS

    T31.61 **Burns involving 60-69% of body surface with 10-19% third degree burns** HCC

    T31.62 **Burns involving 60-69% of body surface with 20-29% third degree burns** HCC

    T31.63 **Burns involving 60-69% of body surface with 30-39% third degree burns** HCC

    T31.64 **Burns involving 60-69% of body surface with 40-49% third degree burns** HCC

    T31.65 **Burns involving 60-69% of body surface with 50-59% third degree burns** HCC

    T31.66 **Burns involving 60-69% of body surface with 60-69% third degree burns** HCC

√5ᵗʰ **T31.7** **Burns involving 70-79% of body surface**

    T31.70 **Burns involving 70-79% of body surface with 0% to 9% third degree burns**
     Burns involving 70-79% of body surface NOS

    T31.71 **Burns involving 70-79% of body surface with 10-19% third degree burns** HCC

    T31.72 **Burns involving 70-79% of body surface with 20-29% third degree burns** HCC

    T31.73 **Burns involving 70-79% of body surface with 30-39% third degree burns** HCC

    T31.74 **Burns involving 70-79% of body surface with 40-49% third degree burns** HCC

    T31.75 **Burns involving 70-79% of body surface with 50-59% third degree burns** HCC

    T31.76 **Burns involving 70-79% of body surface with 60-69% third degree burns** HCC

    T31.77 **Burns involving 70-79% of body surface with 70-79% third degree burns** HCC

√5ᵗʰ **T31.8** **Burns involving 80-89% of body surface**

    T31.80 **Burns involving 80-89% of body surface with 0% to 9% third degree burns**
     Burns involving 80-89% of body surface NOS

    T31.81 **Burns involving 80-89% of body surface with 10-19% third degree burns** HCC

    T31.82 **Burns involving 80-89% of body surface with 20-29% third degree burns** HCC

    T31.83 **Burns involving 80-89% of body surface with 30-39% third degree burns** HCC

    T31.84 **Burns involving 80-89% of body surface with 40-49% third degree burns** HCC

    T31.85 **Burns involving 80-89% of body surface with 50-59% third degree burns** HCC

    T31.86 **Burns involving 80-89% of body surface with 60-69% third degree burns** HCC

    T31.87 **Burns involving 80-89% of body surface with 70-79% third degree burns** HCC

    T31.88 **Burns involving 80-89% of body surface with 80-89% third degree burns** HCC

√5ᵗʰ **T31.9** **Burns involving 90% or more of body surface**

    T31.90 **Burns involving 90% or more of body surface with 0% to 9% third degree burns**
     Burns involving 90% or more of body surface NOS

    T31.91 **Burns involving 90% or more of body surface with 10-19% third degree burns** HCC

    T31.92 **Burns involving 90% or more of body surface with 20-29% third degree burns** HCC

    T31.93 **Burns involving 90% or more of body surface with 30-39% third degree burns** HCC

    T31.94 **Burns involving 90% or more of body surface with 40-49% third degree burns** HCC

Chapter 19. Injury, Poisoning and Certain Other Consequences of External Causes

T28.6–T31.94

T31.95 Burns involving 90% or more of body surface with 50-59% third degree burns   HCC

T31.96 Burns involving 90% or more of body surface with 60-69% third degree burns   HCC

T31.97 Burns involving 90% or more of body surface with 70-79% third degree burns   HCC

T31.98 Burns involving 90% or more of body surface with 80-89% third degree burns   HCC

T31.99 Burns involving 90% or more of body surface with 90% or more third degree burns   HCC

Rule of Nines Estimation of Total Body Surface Burned

Head and neck 9%

Each arm 9%

Anterior trunk 18%

Posterior trunk 18%

Genitalia 1%

Anterior leg 9%

Posterior leg 9%

√4th T32 Corrosions classified according to extent of body surface involved

NOTE   This category is to be used as the primary code only when the site of the corrosion is unspecified. It may be used as a supplementary code with categories T20-T25 when the site is specified.

T32.0 Corrosions involving less than 10% of body surface

√5th T32.1 Corrosions involving 10-19% of body surface

    T32.10 Corrosions involving 10-19% of body surface with 0% to 9% third degree corrosion
       Corrosions involving 10-19% of body surface NOS

    T32.11 Corrosions involving 10-19% of body surface with 10-19% third degree corrosion   HCC

√5th T32.2 Corrosions involving 20-29% of body surface

    T32.20 Corrosions involving 20-29% of body surface with 0% to 9% third degree corrosion

    T32.21 Corrosions involving 20-29% of body surface with 10-19% third degree corrosion   HCC

    T32.22 Corrosions involving 20-29% of body surface with 20-29% third degree corrosion   HCC

√5th T32.3 Corrosions involving 30-39% of body surface

    T32.30 Corrosions involving 30-39% of body surface with 0% to 9% third degree corrosion

    T32.31 Corrosions involving 30-39% of body surface with 10-19% third degree corrosion   HCC

    T32.32 Corrosions involving 30-39% of body surface with 20-29% third degree corrosion   HCC

    T32.33 Corrosions involving 30-39% of body surface with 30-39% third degree corrosion   HCC

√5th T32.4 Corrosions involving 40-49% of body surface

    T32.40 Corrosions involving 40-49% of body surface with 0% to 9% third degree corrosion

    T32.41 Corrosions involving 40-49% of body surface with 10-19% third degree corrosion   HCC

    T32.42 Corrosions involving 40-49% of body surface with 20-29% third degree corrosion   HCC

    T32.43 Corrosions involving 40-49% of body surface with 30-39% third degree corrosion   HCC

    T32.44 Corrosions involving 40-49% of body surface with 40-49% third degree corrosion   HCC

√5th T32.5 Corrosions involving 50-59% of body surface

    T32.50 Corrosions involving 50-59% of body surface with 0% to 9% third degree corrosion

    T32.51 Corrosions involving 50-59% of body surface with 10-19% third degree corrosion   HCC

    T32.52 Corrosions involving 50-59% of body surface with 20-29% third degree corrosion   HCC

T32.53 Corrosions involving 50-59% of body surface with 30-39% third degree corrosion   HCC

T32.54 Corrosions involving 50-59% of body surface with 40-49% third degree corrosion   HCC

T32.55 Corrosions involving 50-59% of body surface with 50-59% third degree corrosion   HCC

√5th T32.6 Corrosions involving 60-69% of body surface

    T32.60 Corrosions involving 60-69% of body surface with 0% to 9% third degree corrosion

    T32.61 Corrosions involving 60-69% of body surface with 10-19% third degree corrosion   HCC

    T32.62 Corrosions involving 60-69% of body surface with 20-29% third degree corrosion   HCC

    T32.63 Corrosions involving 60-69% of body surface with 30-39% third degree corrosion   HCC

    T32.64 Corrosions involving 60-69% of body surface with 40-49% third degree corrosion   HCC

    T32.65 Corrosions involving 60-69% of body surface with 50-59% third degree corrosion   HCC

    T32.66 Corrosions involving 60-69% of body surface with 60-69% third degree corrosion   HCC

√5th T32.7 Corrosions involving 70-79% of body surface

    T32.70 Corrosions involving 70-79% of body surface with 0% to 9% third degree corrosion

    T32.71 Corrosions involving 70-79% of body surface with 10-19% third degree corrosion   HCC

    T32.72 Corrosions involving 70-79% of body surface with 20-29% third degree corrosion   HCC

    T32.73 Corrosions involving 70-79% of body surface with 30-39% third degree corrosion   HCC

    T32.74 Corrosions involving 70-79% of body surface with 40-49% third degree corrosion   HCC

    T32.75 Corrosions involving 70-79% of body surface with 50-59% third degree corrosion   HCC

    T32.76 Corrosions involving 70-79% of body surface with 60-69% third degree corrosion   HCC

    T32.77 Corrosions involving 70-79% of body surface with 70-79% third degree corrosion   HCC

√5th T32.8 Corrosions involving 80-89% of body surface

    T32.80 Corrosions involving 80-89% of body surface with 0% to 9% third degree corrosion

    T32.81 Corrosions involving 80-89% of body surface with 10-19% third degree corrosion   HCC

    T32.82 Corrosions involving 80-89% of body surface with 20-29% third degree corrosion   HCC

    T32.83 Corrosions involving 80-89% of body surface with 30-39% third degree corrosion   HCC

    T32.84 Corrosions involving 80-89% of body surface with 40-49% third degree corrosion   HCC

    T32.85 Corrosions involving 80-89% of body surface with 50-59% third degree corrosion   HCC

    T32.86 Corrosions involving 80-89% of body surface with 60-69% third degree corrosion   HCC

    T32.87 Corrosions involving 80-89% of body surface with 70-79% third degree corrosion   HCC

    T32.88 Corrosions involving 80-89% of body surface with 80-89% third degree corrosion   HCC

√5th T32.9 Corrosions involving 90% or more of body surface

    T32.90 Corrosions involving 90% or more of body surface with 0% to 9% third degree corrosion

    T32.91 Corrosions involving 90% or more of body surface with 10-19% third degree corrosion   HCC

    T32.92 Corrosions involving 90% or more of body surface with 20-29% third degree corrosion   HCC

    T32.93 Corrosions involving 90% or more of body surface with 30-39% third degree corrosion   HCC

    T32.94 Corrosions involving 90% or more of body surface with 40-49% third degree corrosion   HCC

    T32.95 Corrosions involving 90% or more of body surface with 50-59% third degree corrosion   HCC

    T32.96 Corrosions involving 90% or more of body surface with 60-69% third degree corrosion   HCC

    T32.97 Corrosions involving 90% or more of body surface with 70-79% third degree corrosion   HCC

    T32.98 Corrosions involving 90% or more of body surface with 80-89% third degree corrosion   HCC

    T32.99 Corrosions involving 90% or more of body surface with 90% or more third degree corrosion   HCC

Frostbite (T33-T34)

EXCLUDES 2   *hypothermia and other effects of reduced temperature (T68, T69.-)*

√4ᵗʰ **T33 Superficial frostbite**

> INCLUDES   frostbite with partial thickness skin loss
>
> The appropriate 7th character is to be added to each code from category T33.
> A   initial encounter
> D   subsequent encounter
> S   sequela

√5ᵗʰ **T33.0 Superficial frostbite of head**
- √6ᵗʰ **T33.01 Superficial frostbite of ear**
  - √7ᵗʰ **T33.011 Superficial frostbite of right ear**
  - √7ᵗʰ **T33.012 Superficial frostbite of left ear**
  - √7ᵗʰ **T33.019 Superficial frostbite of unspecified ear** ▽
- √x7ᵗʰ **T33.02 Superficial frostbite of nose**
- √x7ᵗʰ **T33.09 Superficial frostbite of other part of head**

√x7ᵗʰ **T33.1 Superficial frostbite of neck**

√x7ᵗʰ **T33.2 Superficial frostbite of thorax**

√x7ᵗʰ **T33.3 Superficial frostbite of abdominal wall, lower back and pelvis**

√5ᵗʰ **T33.4 Superficial frostbite of arm**
> EXCLUDES 2   *superficial frostbite of wrist and hand (T33.5-)*
- √x7ᵗʰ **T33.40 Superficial frostbite of unspecified arm** ▽
- √x7ᵗʰ **T33.41 Superficial frostbite of right arm**
- √x7ᵗʰ **T33.42 Superficial frostbite of left arm**

√5ᵗʰ **T33.5 Superficial frostbite of wrist, hand, and fingers**
- √6ᵗʰ **T33.51 Superficial frostbite of wrist**
  - √7ᵗʰ **T33.511 Superficial frostbite of right wrist**
  - √7ᵗʰ **T33.512 Superficial frostbite of left wrist**
  - √7ᵗʰ **T33.519 Superficial frostbite of unspecified wrist** ▽
- √6ᵗʰ **T33.52 Superficial frostbite of hand**
  > EXCLUDES 2   *superficial frostbite of fingers (T33.53-)*
  - √7ᵗʰ **T33.521 Superficial frostbite of right hand**
  - √7ᵗʰ **T33.522 Superficial frostbite of left hand**
  - √7ᵗʰ **T33.529 Superficial frostbite of unspecified hand** ▽
- √6ᵗʰ **T33.53 Superficial frostbite of finger(s)**
  - √7ᵗʰ **T33.531 Superficial frostbite of right finger(s)**
  - √7ᵗʰ **T33.532 Superficial frostbite of left finger(s)**
  - √7ᵗʰ **T33.539 Superficial frostbite of unspecified finger(s)** ▽

√5ᵗʰ **T33.6 Superficial frostbite of hip and thigh**
- √x7ᵗʰ **T33.60 Superficial frostbite of unspecified hip and thigh** ▽
- √x7ᵗʰ **T33.61 Superficial frostbite of right hip and thigh**
- √x7ᵗʰ **T33.62 Superficial frostbite of left hip and thigh**

√5ᵗʰ **T33.7 Superficial frostbite of knee and lower leg**
> EXCLUDES 2   *superficial frostbite of ankle and foot (T33.8-)*
- √x7ᵗʰ **T33.70 Superficial frostbite of unspecified knee and lower leg** ▽
- √x7ᵗʰ **T33.71 Superficial frostbite of right knee and lower leg**
- √x7ᵗʰ **T33.72 Superficial frostbite of left knee and lower leg**

√5ᵗʰ **T33.8 Superficial frostbite of ankle, foot, and toe(s)**
- √6ᵗʰ **T33.81 Superficial frostbite of ankle**
  - √7ᵗʰ **T33.811 Superficial frostbite of right ankle**
  - √7ᵗʰ **T33.812 Superficial frostbite of left ankle**
  - √7ᵗʰ **T33.819 Superficial frostbite of unspecified ankle** ▽
- √6ᵗʰ **T33.82 Superficial frostbite of foot**
  - √7ᵗʰ **T33.821 Superficial frostbite of right foot**
  - √7ᵗʰ **T33.822 Superficial frostbite of left foot**
  - √7ᵗʰ **T33.829 Superficial frostbite of unspecified foot** ▽
- √6ᵗʰ **T33.83 Superficial frostbite of toe(s)**
  - √7ᵗʰ **T33.831 Superficial frostbite of right toe(s)**
  - √7ᵗʰ **T33.832 Superficial frostbite of left toe(s)**
  - √7ᵗʰ **T33.839 Superficial frostbite of unspecified toe(s)** ▽

√5ᵗʰ **T33.9 Superficial frostbite of other and unspecified sites**
- √x7ᵗʰ **T33.90 Superficial frostbite of unspecified sites** ▽
  Superficial frostbite NOS
- √x7ᵗʰ **T33.99 Superficial frostbite of other sites**
  Superficial frostbite of leg NOS
  Superficial frostbite of trunk NOS

√4ᵗʰ **T34 Frostbite with tissue necrosis**

> The appropriate 7th character is to be added to each code from category T34.
> A   initial encounter
> D   subsequent encounter
> S   sequela

√5ᵗʰ **T34.0 Frostbite with tissue necrosis of head**
- √6ᵗʰ **T34.01 Frostbite with tissue necrosis of ear**
  - √7ᵗʰ **T34.011 Frostbite with tissue necrosis of right ear**
  - √7ᵗʰ **T34.012 Frostbite with tissue necrosis of left ear**
  - √7ᵗʰ **T34.019 Frostbite with tissue necrosis of unspecified ear** ▽
- √x7ᵗʰ **T34.02 Frostbite with tissue necrosis of nose**
- √x7ᵗʰ **T34.09 Frostbite with tissue necrosis of other part of head**

√x7ᵗʰ **T34.1 Frostbite with tissue necrosis of neck**

√x7ᵗʰ **T34.2 Frostbite with tissue necrosis of thorax**

√x7ᵗʰ **T34.3 Frostbite with tissue necrosis of abdominal wall, lower back and pelvis**

√5ᵗʰ **T34.4 Frostbite with tissue necrosis of arm**
> EXCLUDES 2   *frostbite with tissue necrosis of wrist and hand (T34.5-)*
- √x7ᵗʰ **T34.40 Frostbite with tissue necrosis of unspecified arm** ▽
- √x7ᵗʰ **T34.41 Frostbite with tissue necrosis of right arm**
- √x7ᵗʰ **T34.42 Frostbite with tissue necrosis of left arm**

√5ᵗʰ **T34.5 Frostbite with tissue necrosis of wrist, hand, and finger(s)**
- √6ᵗʰ **T34.51 Frostbite with tissue necrosis of wrist**
  - √7ᵗʰ **T34.511 Frostbite with tissue necrosis of right wrist**
  - √7ᵗʰ **T34.512 Frostbite with tissue necrosis of left wrist**
  - √7ᵗʰ **T34.519 Frostbite with tissue necrosis of unspecified wrist** ▽
- √6ᵗʰ **T34.52 Frostbite with tissue necrosis of hand**
  > EXCLUDES 2   *frostbite with tissue necrosis of finger(s) (T34.53-)*
  - √7ᵗʰ **T34.521 Frostbite with tissue necrosis of right hand**
  - √7ᵗʰ **T34.522 Frostbite with tissue necrosis of left hand**
  - √7ᵗʰ **T34.529 Frostbite with tissue necrosis of unspecified hand** ▽
- √6ᵗʰ **T34.53 Frostbite with tissue necrosis of finger(s)**
  - √7ᵗʰ **T34.531 Frostbite with tissue necrosis of right finger(s)**
  - √7ᵗʰ **T34.532 Frostbite with tissue necrosis of left finger(s)**
  - √7ᵗʰ **T34.539 Frostbite with tissue necrosis of unspecified finger(s)** ▽

√5ᵗʰ **T34.6 Frostbite with tissue necrosis of hip and thigh**
- √x7ᵗʰ **T34.60 Frostbite with tissue necrosis of unspecified hip and thigh** ▽
- √x7ᵗʰ **T34.61 Frostbite with tissue necrosis of right hip and thigh**
- √x7ᵗʰ **T34.62 Frostbite with tissue necrosis of left hip and thigh**

√5ᵗʰ **T34.7 Frostbite with tissue necrosis of knee and lower leg**
> EXCLUDES 2   *frostbite with tissue necrosis of ankle and foot (T34.8-)*
- √x7ᵗʰ **T34.70 Frostbite with tissue necrosis of unspecified knee and lower leg** ▽
- √x7ᵗʰ **T34.71 Frostbite with tissue necrosis of right knee and lower leg**
- √x7ᵗʰ **T34.72 Frostbite with tissue necrosis of left knee and lower leg**

√5ᵗʰ **T34.8 Frostbite with tissue necrosis of ankle, foot, and toe(s)**
- √6ᵗʰ **T34.81 Frostbite with tissue necrosis of ankle**
  - √7ᵗʰ **T34.811 Frostbite with tissue necrosis of right ankle**
  - √7ᵗʰ **T34.812 Frostbite with tissue necrosis of left ankle**
  - √7ᵗʰ **T34.819 Frostbite with tissue necrosis of unspecified ankle** ▽

☑ Additional Character Req   √x7ᵗʰ Placeholder Alert   Manifestation   ▽ Unspecified   ▶◀ Revised Text   ● New Code   ▲ Revised Code Title

ICD-10-CM 2019   **1093**

√6ᵗʰ **T34.82** Frostbite with tissue necrosis of foot
- √7ᵗʰ **T34.821** Frostbite with tissue necrosis of right foot
- √7ᵗʰ **T34.822** Frostbite with tissue necrosis of left foot
- √7ᵗʰ **T34.829** Frostbite with tissue necrosis of unspecified foot ▽

√6ᵗʰ **T34.83** Frostbite with tissue necrosis of toe(s)
- √7ᵗʰ **T34.831** Frostbite with tissue necrosis of right toe(s)
- √7ᵗʰ **T34.832** Frostbite with tissue necrosis of left toe(s)
- √7ᵗʰ **T34.839** Frostbite with tissue necrosis of unspecified toe(s) ▽

√5ᵗʰ **T34.9** Frostbite with tissue necrosis of other and unspecified sites
- √×7ᵗʰ **T34.90** Frostbite with tissue necrosis of unspecified sites ▽
  Frostbite with tissue necrosis NOS
- √×7ᵗʰ **T34.99** Frostbite with tissue necrosis of other sites
  Frostbite with tissue necrosis of leg NOS
  Frostbite with tissue necrosis of trunk NOS

Poisoning by, adverse effects of and underdosing of drugs, medicaments and biological substances (T36-T50)

INCLUDES adverse effect of correct substance properly administered
poisoning by overdose of substance
poisoning by wrong substance given or taken in error
underdosing by (inadvertently) (deliberately) taking less substance than prescribed or instructed

Code first, for adverse effects, the nature of the adverse effect, such as:
adverse effect NOS (T88.7)
aspirin gastritis (K29.-)
blood disorders (D56-D76)
contact dermatitis (L23-L25)
dermatitis due to substances taken internally (L27.-)
nephropathy (N14.0-N14.2)

NOTE The drug giving rise to the adverse effect should be identified by use of codes from categories T36-T50 with fifth or sixth character 5.

Use additional code(s) to specify:
manifestations of poisoning
underdosing or failure in dosage during medical and surgical care (Y63.6, Y63.8-Y63.9)
underdosing of medication regimen (Z91.12-, Z91.13-)

EXCLUDES 1 toxic reaction to local anesthesia in pregnancy (O29.3-)
EXCLUDES 2 abuse and dependence of psychoactive substances (F10-F19)
abuse of non-dependence-producing substances (F55.-)
drug reaction and poisoning affecting newborn (P00-P96)
pathological drug intoxication (inebriation) (F10-F19)

AHA: 2016,2Q,8; 2015,3Q,22

√4ᵗʰ **T36 Poisoning by, adverse effect of and underdosing of systemic antibiotics**

EXCLUDES 1 antineoplastic antibiotics (T45.1-)
locally applied antibiotic NEC (T49.0)
topically used antibiotic for ear, nose and throat (T49.6)
topically used antibiotic for eye (T49.5)

The appropriate 7th character is to be added to each code from category T36.
A initial encounter
D subsequent encounter
S sequela

√5ᵗʰ **T36.0** Poisoning by, adverse effect of and underdosing of penicillins
- √6ᵗʰ **T36.0X** Poisoning by, adverse effect of and underdosing of penicillins
  - √7ᵗʰ **T36.0X1** Poisoning by penicillins, accidental (unintentional)
    Poisoning by penicillins NOS
  - 2 √7ᵗʰ **T36.0X2** Poisoning by penicillins, intentional self-harm HCC
  - √7ᵗʰ **T36.0X3** Poisoning by penicillins, assault
  - √7ᵗʰ **T36.0X4** Poisoning by penicillins, undetermined
  - √7ᵗʰ **T36.0X5** Adverse effect of penicillins
  - √7ᵗʰ **T36.0X6** Underdosing of penicillins

√5ᵗʰ **T36.1** Poisoning by, adverse effect of and underdosing of cephalosporins and other beta-lactam antibiotics
- √6ᵗʰ **T36.1X** Poisoning by, adverse effect of and underdosing of cephalosporins and other beta-lactam antibiotics
  - √7ᵗʰ **T36.1X1** Poisoning by cephalosporins and other beta-lactam antibiotics, accidental (unintentional)
    Poisoning by cephalosporins and other beta-lactam antibiotics NOS
  - 2 √7ᵗʰ **T36.1X2** Poisoning by cephalosporins and other beta-lactam antibiotics, intentional self-harm HCC
  - √7ᵗʰ **T36.1X3** Poisoning by cephalosporins and other beta-lactam antibiotics, assault
  - √7ᵗʰ **T36.1X4** Poisoning by cephalosporins and other beta-lactam antibiotics, undetermined
  - √7ᵗʰ **T36.1X5** Adverse effect of cephalosporins and other beta-lactam antibiotics
  - √7ᵗʰ **T36.1X6** Underdosing of cephalosporins and other beta-lactam antibiotics

√5ᵗʰ **T36.2** Poisoning by, adverse effect of and underdosing of chloramphenicol group
- √6ᵗʰ **T36.2X** Poisoning by, adverse effect of and underdosing of chloramphenicol group
  - √7ᵗʰ **T36.2X1** Poisoning by chloramphenicol group, accidental (unintentional)
    Poisoning by chloramphenicol group NOS
  - 2 **T36.2X2** Poisoning by chloramphenicol group, intentional self-harm HCC
  - √7ᵗʰ **T36.2X3** Poisoning by chloramphenicol group, assault
  - √7ᵗʰ **T36.2X4** Poisoning by chloramphenicol group, undetermined
  - √7ᵗʰ **T36.2X5** Adverse effect of chloramphenicol group
  - √7ᵗʰ **T36.2X6** Underdosing of chloramphenicol group

√5ᵗʰ **T36.3** Poisoning by, adverse effect of and underdosing of macrolides
- √6ᵗʰ **T36.3X** Poisoning by, adverse effect of and underdosing of macrolides
  - √7ᵗʰ **T36.3X1** Poisoning by macrolides, accidental (unintentional)
    Poisoning by macrolides NOS
  - 2 √7ᵗʰ **T36.3X2** Poisoning by macrolides, intentional self-harm HCC
  - √7ᵗʰ **T36.3X3** Poisoning by macrolides, assault
  - √7ᵗʰ **T36.3X4** Poisoning by macrolides, undetermined
  - √7ᵗʰ **T36.3X5** Adverse effect of macrolides
  - √7ᵗʰ **T36.3X6** Underdosing of macrolides

√5ᵗʰ **T36.4** Poisoning by, adverse effect of and underdosing of tetracyclines
- √6ᵗʰ **T36.4X** Poisoning by, adverse effect of and underdosing of tetracyclines
  - √7ᵗʰ **T36.4X1** Poisoning by tetracyclines, accidental (unintentional)
    Poisoning by tetracyclines NOS
  - 2 √7ᵗʰ **T36.4X2** Poisoning by tetracyclines, intentional self-harm HCC
  - √7ᵗʰ **T36.4X3** Poisoning by tetracyclines, assault
  - √7ᵗʰ **T36.4X4** Poisoning by tetracyclines, undetermined
  - √7ᵗʰ **T36.4X5** Adverse effect of tetracyclines
  - √7ᵗʰ **T36.4X6** Underdosing of tetracyclines

√5ᵗʰ **T36.5** Poisoning by, adverse effect of and underdosing of aminoglycosides
  Poisoning by, adverse effect of and underdosing of streptomycin
- √6ᵗʰ **T36.5X** Poisoning by, adverse effect of and underdosing of aminoglycosides
  - √7ᵗʰ **T36.5X1** Poisoning by aminoglycosides, accidental (unintentional)
    Poisoning by aminoglycosides NOS
  - 2 √7ᵗʰ **T36.5X2** Poisoning by aminoglycosides, intentional self-harm HCC
  - √7ᵗʰ **T36.5X3** Poisoning by aminoglycosides, assault
  - √7ᵗʰ **T36.5X4** Poisoning by aminoglycosides, undetermined
  - √7ᵗʰ **T36.5X5** Adverse effect of aminoglycosides
  - √7ᵗʰ **T36.5X6** Underdosing of aminoglycosides

√5ᵗʰ **T36.6** Poisoning by, adverse effect of and underdosing of rifampicins

　√6ᵗʰ **T36.6X** Poisoning by, adverse effect of and underdosing of rifampicins

　　√7ᵗʰ **T36.6X1** Poisoning by rifampicins, accidental (unintentional)
　　　　Poisoning by rifampicins NOS

　　² √7ᵗʰ **T36.6X2** Poisoning by rifampicins, intentional self-harm　HCC

　　√7ᵗʰ **T36.6X3** Poisoning by rifampicins, assault

　　√7ᵗʰ **T36.6X4** Poisoning by rifampicins, undetermined

　　√7ᵗʰ **T36.6X5** Adverse effect of rifampicins

　　√7ᵗʰ **T36.6X6** Underdosing of rifampicins

√5ᵗʰ **T36.7** Poisoning by, adverse effect of and underdosing of antifungal antibiotics, systemically used

　√6ᵗʰ **T36.7X** Poisoning by, adverse effect of and underdosing of antifungal antibiotics, systemically used

　　√7ᵗʰ **T36.7X1** Poisoning by antifungal antibiotics, systemically used, accidental (unintentional)
　　　　Poisoning by antifungal antibiotics, systemically used NOS

　　² √7ᵗʰ **T36.7X2** Poisoning by antifungal antibiotics, systemically used, intentional self-harm　HCC

　　√7ᵗʰ **T36.7X3** Poisoning by antifungal antibiotics, systemically used, assault

　　√7ᵗʰ **T36.7X4** Poisoning by antifungal antibiotics, systemically used, undetermined

　　√7ᵗʰ **T36.7X5** Adverse effect of antifungal antibiotics, systemically used

　　√7ᵗʰ **T36.7X6** Underdosing of antifungal antibiotics, systemically used

√5ᵗʰ **T36.8** Poisoning by, adverse effect of and underdosing of other systemic antibiotics

　√6ᵗʰ **T36.8X** Poisoning by, adverse effect of and underdosing of other systemic antibiotics
　　　AHA: 2017,1Q,39

　　√7ᵗʰ **T36.8X1** Poisoning by other systemic antibiotics, accidental (unintentional)
　　　　Poisoning by other systemic antibiotics NOS

　　² √7ᵗʰ **T36.8X2** Poisoning by other systemic antibiotics, intentional self-harm　HCC

　　√7ᵗʰ **T36.8X3** Poisoning by other systemic antibiotics, assault

　　√7ᵗʰ **T36.8X4** Poisoning by other systemic antibiotics, undetermined

　　√7ᵗʰ **T36.8X5** Adverse effect of other systemic antibiotics

　　√7ᵗʰ **T36.8X6** Underdosing of other systemic antibiotics

√5ᵗʰ **T36.9** Poisoning by, adverse effect of and underdosing of unspecified systemic antibiotic

　√x7ᵗʰ **T36.91** Poisoning by unspecified systemic antibiotic, accidental (unintentional)　▽
　　　Poisoning by systemic antibiotic NOS

　² √x7ᵗʰ **T36.92** Poisoning by unspecified systemic antibiotic, intentional self-harm　HCC ▽

　√x7ᵗʰ **T36.93** Poisoning by unspecified systemic antibiotic, assault　▽

　√x7ᵗʰ **T36.94** Poisoning by unspecified systemic antibiotic, undetermined　▽

　√x7ᵗʰ **T36.95** Adverse effect of unspecified systemic antibiotic　▽

　√x7ᵗʰ **T36.96** Underdosing of unspecified systemic antibiotic　▽

▲√4ᵗʰ **T37** Poisoning by, adverse effect of and underdosing of other systemic anti-infectives and antiparasitics

　　EXCLUDES 1　anti-infectives topically used for ear, nose and throat (T49.6-)
　　　　anti-infectives topically used for eye (T49.5-)
　　　　locally applied anti-infectives NEC (T49.0-)

　The appropriate 7th character is to be added to each code from category T37.
　A　initial encounter
　D　subsequent encounter
　S　sequela

√5ᵗʰ **T37.0** Poisoning by, adverse effect of and underdosing of sulfonamides

　√6ᵗʰ **T37.0X** Poisoning by, adverse effect of and underdosing of sulfonamides

　　√7ᵗʰ **T37.0X1** Poisoning by sulfonamides, accidental (unintentional)
　　　　Poisoning by sulfonamides NOS

　　² √7ᵗʰ **T37.0X2** Poisoning by sulfonamides, intentional self-harm　HCC

　　√7ᵗʰ **T37.0X3** Poisoning by sulfonamides, assault

　　√7ᵗʰ **T37.0X4** Poisoning by sulfonamides, undetermined

　　√7ᵗʰ **T37.0X5** Adverse effect of sulfonamides

　　√7ᵗʰ **T37.0X6** Underdosing of sulfonamides

√5ᵗʰ **T37.1** Poisoning by, adverse effect of and underdosing of antimycobacterial drugs

　　EXCLUDES 1　rifampicins (T36.6-)
　　　　streptomycin (T36.5-)

　√6ᵗʰ **T37.1X** Poisoning by, adverse effect of and underdosing of antimycobacterial drugs

　　√7ᵗʰ **T37.1X1** Poisoning by antimycobacterial drugs, accidental (unintentional)
　　　　Poisoning by antimycobacterial drugs NOS

　　² √7ᵗʰ **T37.1X2** Poisoning by antimycobacterial drugs, intentional self-harm　HCC

　　√7ᵗʰ **T37.1X3** Poisoning by antimycobacterial drugs, assault

　　√7ᵗʰ **T37.1X4** Poisoning by antimycobacterial drugs, undetermined

　　√7ᵗʰ **T37.1X5** Adverse effect of antimycobacterial drugs

　　√7ᵗʰ **T37.1X6** Underdosing of antimycobacterial drugs

√5ᵗʰ **T37.2** Poisoning by, adverse effect of and underdosing of antimalarials and drugs acting on other blood protozoa

　　EXCLUDES 1　hydroxyquinoline derivatives (T37.8-)

　√6ᵗʰ **T37.2X** Poisoning by, adverse effect of and underdosing of antimalarials and drugs acting on other blood protozoa

　　√7ᵗʰ **T37.2X1** Poisoning by antimalarials and drugs acting on other blood protozoa, accidental (unintentional)
　　　　Poisoning by antimalarials and drugs acting on other blood protozoa NOS

　　² √7ᵗʰ **T37.2X2** Poisoning by antimalarials and drugs acting on other blood protozoa, intentional self-harm　HCC

　　√7ᵗʰ **T37.2X3** Poisoning by antimalarials and drugs acting on other blood protozoa, assault

　　√7ᵗʰ **T37.2X4** Poisoning by antimalarials and drugs acting on other blood protozoa, undetermined

　　√7ᵗʰ **T37.2X5** Adverse effect of antimalarials and drugs acting on other blood protozoa

　　√7ᵗʰ **T37.2X6** Underdosing of antimalarials and drugs acting on other blood protozoa

√5ᵗʰ **T37.3** Poisoning by, adverse effect of and underdosing of other antiprotozoal drugs

　√6ᵗʰ **T37.3X** Poisoning by, adverse effect of and underdosing of other antiprotozoal drugs

　　√7ᵗʰ **T37.3X1** Poisoning by other antiprotozoal drugs, accidental (unintentional)
　　　　Poisoning by other antiprotozoal drugs NOS

　　² √7ᵗʰ **T37.3X2** Poisoning by other antiprotozoal drugs, intentional self-harm　HCC

　　√7ᵗʰ **T37.3X3** Poisoning by other antiprotozoal drugs, assault

　　√7ᵗʰ **T37.3X4** Poisoning by other antiprotozoal drugs, undetermined

　　√7ᵗʰ **T37.3X5** Adverse effect of other antiprotozoal drugs

☑ Additional Character Req　　√x7ᵗʰ Placeholder Alert　　Manifestation　　▽ Unspecified　　▶◀ Revised Text　　● New Code　　▲ Revised Code Title

ICD-10-CM 2019

1095

Chapter 19. Injury, Poisoning and Certain Other Consequences of External Causes

T36.6–T37.3X5

     √7ᵗʰ **T37.3X6** Underdosing of other antiprotozoal drugs

√5ᵗʰ **T37.4** Poisoning by, adverse effect of and underdosing of anthelmintics

   √6ᵗʰ **T37.4X** Poisoning by, adverse effect of and underdosing of anthelmintics

     √7ᵗʰ **T37.4X1** Poisoning by anthelmintics, accidental (unintentional)

       Poisoning by anthelmintics NOS

     2 √7ᵗʰ **T37.4X2** Poisoning by anthelmintics, intentional self-harm   HCC

     √7ᵗʰ **T37.4X3** Poisoning by anthelmintics, assault

     √7ᵗʰ **T37.4X4** Poisoning by anthelmintics, undetermined

     √7ᵗʰ **T37.4X5** Adverse effect of anthelmintics

     √7ᵗʰ **T37.4X6** Underdosing of anthelmintics

√5ᵗʰ **T37.5** Poisoning by, adverse effect of and underdosing of antiviral drugs

    EXCLUDES 1   amantadine (T42.8-)

           cytarabine (T45.1-)

   √6ᵗʰ **T37.5X** Poisoning by, adverse effect of and underdosing of antiviral drugs

     √7ᵗʰ **T37.5X1** Poisoning by antiviral drugs, accidental (unintentional)

       Poisoning by antiviral drugs NOS

     2 √7ᵗʰ **T37.5X2** Poisoning by antiviral drugs, intentional self-harm   HCC

     √7ᵗʰ **T37.5X3** Poisoning by antiviral drugs, assault

     √7ᵗʰ **T37.5X4** Poisoning by antiviral drugs, undetermined

     √7ᵗʰ **T37.5X5** Adverse effect of antiviral drugs

     √7ᵗʰ **T37.5X6** Underdosing of antiviral drugs

√5ᵗʰ **T37.8** Poisoning by, adverse effect of and underdosing of other specified systemic anti-infectives and antiparasitics

    Poisoning by, adverse effect of and underdosing of hydroxyquinoline derivatives

    EXCLUDES 1   antimalarial drugs (T37.2-)

   √6ᵗʰ **T37.8X** Poisoning by, adverse effect of and underdosing of other specified systemic anti-infectives and antiparasitics

     √7ᵗʰ **T37.8X1** Poisoning by other specified systemic anti-infectives and antiparasitics, accidental (unintentional)

       Poisoning by other specified systemic anti-infectives and antiparasitics NOS

     2 √7ᵗʰ **T37.8X2** Poisoning by other specified systemic anti-infectives and antiparasitics, intentional self-harm   HCC

     √7ᵗʰ **T37.8X3** Poisoning by other specified systemic anti-infectives and antiparasitics, assault

     √7ᵗʰ **T37.8X4** Poisoning by other specified systemic anti-infectives and antiparasitics, undetermined

     √7ᵗʰ **T37.8X5** Adverse effect of other specified systemic anti-infectives and antiparasitics

     √7ᵗʰ **T37.8X6** Underdosing of other specified systemic anti-infectives and antiparasitics

√5ᵗʰ **T37.9** Poisoning by, adverse effect of and underdosing of unspecified systemic anti-infective and antiparasitics

   √x7ᵗʰ **T37.91** Poisoning by unspecified systemic anti-infective and antiparasitics, accidental (unintentional)   ▽

     Poisoning by, adverse effect of and underdosing of systemic anti-infective and antiparasitics NOS

   2 √x7ᵗʰ **T37.92** Poisoning by unspecified systemic anti-infective and antiparasitics, intentional self-harm   HCC ▽

   √x7ᵗʰ **T37.93** Poisoning by unspecified systemic anti-infective and antiparasitics, assault   ▽

   √x7ᵗʰ **T37.94** Poisoning by unspecified systemic anti-infective and antiparasitics, undetermined   ▽

   √x7ᵗʰ **T37.95** Adverse effect of unspecified systemic anti-infective and antiparasitic   ▽

   √x7ᵗʰ **T37.96** Underdosing of unspecified systemic anti-infectives and antiparasitics   ▽

√4ᵗʰ **T38** Poisoning by, adverse effect of and underdosing of hormones and their synthetic substitutes and antagonists, not elsewhere classified

    EXCLUDES 1   mineralocorticoids and their antagonists (T50.0-)

           oxytocic hormones (T48.0-)

           parathyroid hormones and derivatives (T50.9-)

> The appropriate 7th character is to be added to each code from category T38.
> A   initial encounter
> D   subsequent encounter
> S   sequela

√5ᵗʰ **T38.0** Poisoning by, adverse effect of and underdosing of glucocorticoids and synthetic analogues

    EXCLUDES 1   glucocorticoids, topically used (T49.-)

   √6ᵗʰ **T38.0X** Poisoning by, adverse effect of and underdosing of glucocorticoids and synthetic analogues

     √7ᵗʰ **T38.0X1** Poisoning by glucocorticoids and synthetic analogues, accidental (unintentional)

       Poisoning by glucocorticoids and synthetic analogues NOS

     2 √7ᵗʰ **T38.0X2** Poisoning by glucocorticoids and synthetic analogues, intentional self-harm   HCC

     √7ᵗʰ **T38.0X3** Poisoning by glucocorticoids and synthetic analogues, assault

     √7ᵗʰ **T38.0X4** Poisoning by glucocorticoids and synthetic analogues, undetermined

     √7ᵗʰ **T38.0X5** Adverse effect of glucocorticoids and synthetic analogues

     √7ᵗʰ **T38.0X6** Underdosing of glucocorticoids and synthetic analogues

√5ᵗʰ **T38.1** Poisoning by, adverse effect of and underdosing of thyroid hormones and substitutes

   √6ᵗʰ **T38.1X** Poisoning by, adverse effect of and underdosing of thyroid hormones and substitutes

     √7ᵗʰ **T38.1X1** Poisoning by thyroid hormones and substitutes, accidental (unintentional)

       Poisoning by thyroid hormones and substitutes NOS

     2 √7ᵗʰ **T38.1X2** Poisoning by thyroid hormones and substitutes, intentional self-harm   HCC

     √7ᵗʰ **T38.1X3** Poisoning by thyroid hormones and substitutes, assault

     √7ᵗʰ **T38.1X4** Poisoning by thyroid hormones and substitutes, undetermined

     √7ᵗʰ **T38.1X5** Adverse effect of thyroid hormones and substitutes

     √7ᵗʰ **T38.1X6** Underdosing of thyroid hormones and substitutes

√5ᵗʰ **T38.2** Poisoning by, adverse effect of and underdosing of antithyroid drugs

   √6ᵗʰ **T38.2X** Poisoning by, adverse effect of and underdosing of antithyroid drugs

     √7ᵗʰ **T38.2X1** Poisoning by antithyroid drugs, accidental (unintentional)

       Poisoning by antithyroid drugs NOS

     2 √7ᵗʰ **T38.2X2** Poisoning by antithyroid drugs, intentional self-harm   HCC

     √7ᵗʰ **T38.2X3** Poisoning by antithyroid drugs, assault

     √7ᵗʰ **T38.2X4** Poisoning by antithyroid drugs, undetermined

     √7ᵗʰ **T38.2X5** Adverse effect of antithyroid drugs

     √7ᵗʰ **T38.2X6** Underdosing of antithyroid drugs

√5ᵗʰ **T38.3** Poisoning by, adverse effect of and underdosing of insulin and oral hypoglycemic [antidiabetic] drugs

   √6ᵗʰ **T38.3X** Poisoning by, adverse effect of and underdosing of insulin and oral hypoglycemic [antidiabetic] drugs

     √7ᵗʰ **T38.3X1** Poisoning by insulin and oral hypoglycemic [antidiabetic] drugs, accidental (unintentional)

       Poisoning by insulin and oral hypoglycemic [antidiabetic] drugs NOS

     2 √7ᵗʰ **T38.3X2** Poisoning by insulin and oral hypoglycemic [antidiabetic] drugs, intentional self-harm   HCC

√7ᵗʰ **T38.3X3** **Poisoning by insulin and oral hypoglycemic [antidiabetic] drugs,** assault

√7ᵗʰ **T38.3X4** **Poisoning by insulin and oral hypoglycemic [antidiabetic] drugs,** undetermined

√7ᵗʰ **T38.3X5** Adverse effect **of insulin and oral hypoglycemic [antidiabetic] drugs**

√7ᵗʰ **T38.3X6** Underdosing **of insulin and oral hypoglycemic [antidiabetic] drugs**

√5ᵗʰ **T38.4** **Poisoning by, adverse effect of and underdosing of oral contraceptives**

Poisoning by, adverse effect of and underdosing of multiple- and single-ingredient oral contraceptive preparations

√6ᵗʰ **T38.4X** **Poisoning by, adverse effect of and underdosing of oral contraceptives**

√7ᵗʰ **T38.4X1** **Poisoning by oral contraceptives,** accidental **(unintentional)**

Poisoning by oral contraceptives NOS

² √7ᵗʰ **T38.4X2** **Poisoning by oral contraceptives,** intentional self-harm   HCC

√7ᵗʰ **T38.4X3** **Poisoning by oral contraceptives,** assault

√7ᵗʰ **T38.4X4** **Poisoning by oral contraceptives,** undetermined

√7ᵗʰ **T38.4X5** Adverse effect **of oral contraceptives**

√7ᵗʰ **T38.4X6** Underdosing **of oral contraceptives**

√5ᵗʰ **T38.5** **Poisoning by, adverse effect of and underdosing of other estrogens and progestogens**

Poisoning by, adverse effect of and underdosing of estrogens and progestogens mixtures and substitutes

√6ᵗʰ **T38.5X** **Poisoning by, adverse effect of and underdosing of other estrogens and progestogens**

√7ᵗʰ **T38.5X1** **Poisoning by other estrogens and progestogens,** accidental **(unintentional)**

Poisoning by other estrogens and progestogens NOS

² √7ᵗʰ **T38.5X2** **Poisoning by other estrogens and progestogens,** intentional self-harm   HCC

√7ᵗʰ **T38.5X3** **Poisoning by other estrogens and progestogens,** assault

√7ᵗʰ **T38.5X4** **Poisoning by other estrogens and progestogens,** undetermined

√7ᵗʰ **T38.5X5** Adverse effect **of other estrogens and progestogens**

√7ᵗʰ **T38.5X6** Underdosing **of other estrogens and progestogens**

√5ᵗʰ **T38.6** **Poisoning by, adverse effect of and underdosing of antigonadotrophins, antiestrogens, antiandrogens, not elsewhere classified**

Poisoning by, adverse effect of and underdosing of tamoxifen

√6ᵗʰ **T38.6X** **Poisoning by, adverse effect of and underdosing of antigonadotrophins, antiestrogens, antiandrogens, not elsewhere classified**

√7ᵗʰ **T38.6X1** **Poisoning by antigonadotrophins, antiestrogens, antiandrogens, not elsewhere classified,** accidental **(unintentional)**

Poisoning by antigonadotrophins, antiestrogens, antiandrogens, not elsewhere classified NOS

² √7ᵗʰ **T38.6X2** **Poisoning by antigonadotrophins, antiestrogens, antiandrogens, not elsewhere classified,** intentional self-harm   HCC

√7ᵗʰ **T38.6X3** **Poisoning by antigonadotrophins, antiestrogens, antiandrogens, not elsewhere classified,** assault

√7ᵗʰ **T38.6X4** **Poisoning by antigonadotrophins, antiestrogens, antiandrogens, not elsewhere classified,** undetermined

√7ᵗʰ **T38.6X5** Adverse effect **of antigonadotrophins, antiestrogens, antiandrogens, not elsewhere classified**

√7ᵗʰ **T38.6X6** Underdosing **of antigonadotrophins, antiestrogens, antiandrogens, not elsewhere classified**

√5ᵗʰ **T38.7** **Poisoning by, adverse effect of and underdosing of androgens and anabolic congeners**

√6ᵗʰ **T38.7X** **Poisoning by, adverse effect of and underdosing of androgens and anabolic congeners**

√7ᵗʰ **T38.7X1** **Poisoning by androgens and anabolic congeners,** accidental **(unintentional)**

Poisoning by androgens and anabolic congeners NOS

² √7ᵗʰ **T38.7X2** **Poisoning by androgens and anabolic congeners,** intentional self-harm   HCC

√7ᵗʰ **T38.7X3** **Poisoning by androgens and anabolic congeners,** assault

√7ᵗʰ **T38.7X4** **Poisoning by androgens and anabolic congeners,** undetermined

√7ᵗʰ **T38.7X5** Adverse effect **of androgens and anabolic congeners**

√7ᵗʰ **T38.7X6** Underdosing **of androgens and anabolic congeners**

√5ᵗʰ **T38.8** **Poisoning by, adverse effect of and underdosing of other and unspecified hormones and synthetic substitutes**

√6ᵗʰ **T38.80** **Poisoning by, adverse effect of and underdosing of unspecified hormones and synthetic substitutes**

√7ᵗʰ **T38.801** **Poisoning by unspecified hormones and synthetic substitutes,** accidental **(unintentional)** ▽

Poisoning by unspecified hormones and synthetic substitutes NOS

² √7ᵗʰ **T38.802** **Poisoning by unspecified hormones and synthetic substitutes,** intentional self-harm   HCC ▽

√7ᵗʰ **T38.803** **Poisoning by unspecified hormones and synthetic substitutes,** assault ▽

√7ᵗʰ **T38.804** **Poisoning by unspecified hormones and synthetic substitutes,** undetermined ▽

√7ᵗʰ **T38.805** Adverse effect **of unspecified hormones and synthetic substitutes** ▽

√7ᵗʰ **T38.806** Underdosing **of unspecified hormones and synthetic substitutes** ▽

√6ᵗʰ **T38.81** **Poisoning by, adverse effect of and underdosing of anterior pituitary [adenohypophyseal] hormones**

√7ᵗʰ **T38.811** **Poisoning by anterior pituitary [adenohypophyseal] hormones,** accidental **(unintentional)**

Poisoning by anterior pituitary [adenohypophyseal] hormones NOS

² √7ᵗʰ **T38.812** **Poisoning by anterior pituitary [adenohypophyseal] hormones,** intentional self-harm   HCC

√7ᵗʰ **T38.813** **Poisoning by anterior pituitary [adenohypophyseal] hormones,** assault

√7ᵗʰ **T38.814** **Poisoning by anterior pituitary [adenohypophyseal] hormones,** undetermined

√7ᵗʰ **T38.815** Adverse effect **of anterior pituitary [adenohypophyseal] hormones**

√7ᵗʰ **T38.816** Underdosing **of anterior pituitary [adenohypophyseal] hormones**

√6ᵗʰ **T38.89** **Poisoning by, adverse effect of and underdosing of other hormones and synthetic substitutes**

√7ᵗʰ **T38.891** **Poisoning by other hormones and synthetic substitutes,** accidental **(unintentional)**

Poisoning by other hormones and synthetic substitutes NOS

² √7ᵗʰ **T38.892** **Poisoning by other hormones and synthetic substitutes,** intentional self-harm   HCC

√7ᵗʰ **T38.893** **Poisoning by other hormones and synthetic substitutes,** assault

√7ᵗʰ **T38.894** **Poisoning by other hormones and synthetic substitutes,** undetermined

√7ᵗʰ **T38.895** Adverse effect **of other hormones and synthetic substitutes**

√7ᵗʰ **T38.896** Underdosing **of other hormones and synthetic substitutes**

☑ Additional Character Req   √ₓ7ᵗʰ Placeholder Alert   Manifestation   ▽ Unspecified   ►◄ Revised Text   ● New Code   ▲ Revised Code Title

ICD-10-CM 2019

1097

T38.9 Poisoning by, adverse effect of and underdosing of other and unspecified hormone antagonists

  T38.90 Poisoning by, adverse effect of and underdosing of unspecified hormone antagonists

    T38.901 Poisoning by unspecified hormone antagonists, accidental (unintentional)
      Poisoning by unspecified hormone antagonists NOS ▽

    T38.902 Poisoning by unspecified hormone antagonists, intentional self-harm ▽ HCC

    T38.903 Poisoning by unspecified hormone antagonists, assault ▽

    T38.904 Poisoning by unspecified hormone antagonists, undetermined ▽

    T38.905 Adverse effect of unspecified hormone antagonists ▽

    T38.906 Underdosing of unspecified hormone antagonists ▽

  T38.99 Poisoning by, adverse effect of and underdosing of other hormone antagonists

    T38.991 Poisoning by other hormone antagonists, accidental (unintentional)
      Poisoning by other hormone antagonists NOS

    T38.992 Poisoning by other hormone antagonists, intentional self-harm HCC

    T38.993 Poisoning by other hormone antagonists, assault

    T38.994 Poisoning by other hormone antagonists, undetermined

    T38.995 Adverse effect of other hormone antagonists

    T38.996 Underdosing of other hormone antagonists

T39 Poisoning by, adverse effect of and underdosing of nonopioid analgesics, antipyretics and antirheumatics

> The appropriate 7th character is to be added to each code from category T39.
> A   initial encounter
> D   subsequent encounter
> S   sequela

  T39.0 Poisoning by, adverse effect of and underdosing of salicylates

    T39.01 Poisoning by, adverse effect of and underdosing of aspirin
      Poisoning by, adverse effect of and underdosing of acetylsalicylic acid

      T39.011 Poisoning by aspirin, accidental (unintentional)

      T39.012 Poisoning by aspirin, intentional self-harm HCC

      T39.013 Poisoning by aspirin, assault

      T39.014 Poisoning by aspirin, undetermined

      T39.015 Adverse effect of aspirin
        AHA: 2016,1Q,15

      T39.016 Underdosing of aspirin

    T39.09 Poisoning by, adverse effect of and underdosing of other salicylates

      T39.091 Poisoning by salicylates, accidental (unintentional)
        Poisoning by salicylates NOS

      T39.092 Poisoning by salicylates, intentional self-harm HCC

      T39.093 Poisoning by salicylates, assault

      T39.094 Poisoning by salicylates, undetermined

      T39.095 Adverse effect of salicylates

      T39.096 Underdosing of salicylates

  T39.1 Poisoning by, adverse effect of and underdosing of 4-Aminophenol derivatives

    T39.1X Poisoning by, adverse effect of and underdosing of 4-Aminophenol derivatives

      T39.1X1 Poisoning by 4-Aminophenol derivatives, accidental (unintentional)
        Poisoning by 4-Aminophenol derivatives NOS

      T39.1X2 Poisoning by 4-Aminophenol derivatives, intentional self-harm HCC

      T39.1X3 Poisoning by 4-Aminophenol derivatives, assault

      T39.1X4 Poisoning by 4-Aminophenol derivatives, undetermined

      T39.1X5 Adverse effect of 4-Aminophenol derivatives

      T39.1X6 Underdosing of 4-Aminophenol derivatives

  T39.2 Poisoning by, adverse effect of and underdosing of pyrazolone derivatives

    T39.2X Poisoning by, adverse effect of and underdosing of pyrazolone derivatives

      T39.2X1 Poisoning by pyrazolone derivatives, accidental (unintentional)
        Poisoning by pyrazolone derivatives NOS

      T39.2X2 Poisoning by pyrazolone derivatives, intentional self-harm HCC

      T39.2X3 Poisoning by pyrazolone derivatives, assault

      T39.2X4 Poisoning by pyrazolone derivatives, undetermined

      T39.2X5 Adverse effect of pyrazolone derivatives

      T39.2X6 Underdosing of pyrazolone derivatives

  T39.3 Poisoning by, adverse effect of and underdosing of other nonsteroidal anti-inflammatory drugs [NSAID]

    T39.31 Poisoning by, adverse effect of and underdosing of propionic acid derivatives
      Poisoning by, adverse effect of and underdosing of fenoprofen
      Poisoning by, adverse effect of and underdosing of flurbiprofen
      Poisoning by, adverse effect of and underdosing of ibuprofen
      Poisoning by, adverse effect of and underdosing of ketoprofen
      Poisoning by, adverse effect of and underdosing of naproxen
      Poisoning by, adverse effect of and underdosing of oxaprozin

      T39.311 Poisoning by propionic acid derivatives, accidental (unintentional)

      T39.312 Poisoning by propionic acid derivatives, intentional self-harm HCC

      T39.313 Poisoning by propionic acid derivatives, assault

      T39.314 Poisoning by propionic acid derivatives, undetermined

      T39.315 Adverse effect of propionic acid derivatives

      T39.316 Underdosing of propionic acid derivatives

    T39.39 Poisoning by, adverse effect of and underdosing of other nonsteroidal anti-inflammatory drugs [NSAID]

      T39.391 Poisoning by other nonsteroidal anti-inflammatory drugs [NSAID], accidental (unintentional)
        Poisoning by other nonsteroidal anti-inflammatory drugs NOS

      T39.392 Poisoning by other nonsteroidal anti-inflammatory drugs [NSAID], intentional self-harm HCC

      T39.393 Poisoning by other nonsteroidal anti-inflammatory drugs [NSAID], assault

      T39.394 Poisoning by other nonsteroidal anti-inflammatory drugs [NSAID], undetermined

      T39.395 Adverse effect of other nonsteroidal anti-inflammatory drugs [NSAID]

      T39.396 Underdosing of other nonsteroidal anti-inflammatory drugs [NSAID]

√5ᵗʰ **T39.4** **Poisoning by, adverse effect of and underdosing of antirheumatics, not elsewhere classified**

> EXCLUDES 1   poisoning by, adverse effect of and underdosing of glucocorticoids (T38.0-)
>
> poisoning by, adverse effect of and underdosing of salicylates (T39.0-)

√6ᵗʰ **T39.4X** **Poisoning by, adverse effect of and underdosing of antirheumatics, not elsewhere classified**

√7ᵗʰ **T39.4X1** **Poisoning by antirheumatics, not elsewhere classified, accidental (unintentional)**

> Poisoning by antirheumatics, not elsewhere classified NOS

² √7ᵗʰ **T39.4X2** **Poisoning by antirheumatics, not elsewhere classified, intentional self-harm**   HCC

√7ᵗʰ **T39.4X3** **Poisoning by antirheumatics, not elsewhere classified, assault**

√7ᵗʰ **T39.4X4** **Poisoning by antirheumatics, not elsewhere classified, undetermined**

√7ᵗʰ **T39.4X5** **Adverse effect of antirheumatics, not elsewhere classified**

√7ᵗʰ **T39.4X6** **Underdosing of antirheumatics, not elsewhere classified**

√5ᵗʰ **T39.8** **Poisoning by, adverse effect of and underdosing of other nonopioid analgesics and antipyretics, not elsewhere classified**

√6ᵗʰ **T39.8X** **Poisoning by, adverse effect of and underdosing of other nonopioid analgesics and antipyretics, not elsewhere classified**

√7ᵗʰ **T39.8X1** **Poisoning by other nonopioid analgesics and antipyretics, not elsewhere classified, accidental (unintentional)**

> Poisoning by other nonopioid analgesics and antipyretics, not elsewhere classified NOS

² √7ᵗʰ **T39.8X2** **Poisoning by other nonopioid analgesics and antipyretics, not elsewhere classified, intentional self-harm**   HCC

√7ᵗʰ **T39.8X3** **Poisoning by other nonopioid analgesics and antipyretics, not elsewhere classified, assault**

√7ᵗʰ **T39.8X4** **Poisoning by other nonopioid analgesics and antipyretics, not elsewhere classified, undetermined**

√7ᵗʰ **T39.8X5** **Adverse effect of other nonopioid analgesics and antipyretics, not elsewhere classified**

√7ᵗʰ **T39.8X6** **Underdosing of other nonopioid analgesics and antipyretics, not elsewhere classified**

√5ᵗʰ **T39.9** **Poisoning by, adverse effect of and underdosing of unspecified nonopioid analgesic, antipyretic and antirheumatic**

√x7ᵗʰ **T39.91** **Poisoning by unspecified nonopioid analgesic, antipyretic and antirheumatic, accidental (unintentional)**   ▽

> Poisoning by nonopioid analgesic, antipyretic and antirheumatic NOS

² √x7ᵗʰ **T39.92** **Poisoning by unspecified nonopioid analgesic, antipyretic and antirheumatic, intentional self-harm**   HCC ▽

√x7ᵗʰ **T39.93** **Poisoning by unspecified nonopioid analgesic, antipyretic and antirheumatic, assault**   ▽

√x7ᵗʰ **T39.94** **Poisoning by unspecified nonopioid analgesic, antipyretic and antirheumatic, undetermined**   ▽

√x7ᵗʰ **T39.95** **Adverse effect of unspecified nonopioid analgesic, antipyretic and antirheumatic**   ▽

√x7ᵗʰ **T39.96** **Underdosing of unspecified nonopioid analgesic, antipyretic and antirheumatic**   ▽

√4ᵗʰ **T40** **Poisoning by, adverse effect of and underdosing of narcotics and psychodysleptics [hallucinogens]**

> EXCLUDES 2   drug dependence and related mental and behavioral disorders due to psychoactive substance use (F10.-F19.-)

> The appropriate 7th character is to be added to each code from category T40.
> A   initial encounter
> D   subsequent encounter
> S   sequela

√5ᵗʰ **T40.0** **Poisoning by, adverse effect of and underdosing of opium**

√6ᵗʰ **T40.0X** **Poisoning by, adverse effect of and underdosing of opium**

√7ᵗʰ **T40.0X1** **Poisoning by opium, accidental (unintentional)**

> Poisoning by opium NOS

² √7ᵗʰ **T40.0X2** **Poisoning by opium, intentional self-harm**   HCC

√7ᵗʰ **T40.0X3** **Poisoning by opium, assault**

√7ᵗʰ **T40.0X4** **Poisoning by opium, undetermined**

√7ᵗʰ **T40.0X5** **Adverse effect of opium**

√7ᵗʰ **T40.0X6** **Underdosing of opium**

√5ᵗʰ **T40.1** **Poisoning by and adverse effect of heroin**

√6ᵗʰ **T40.1X** **Poisoning by and adverse effect of heroin**

√7ᵗʰ **T40.1X1** **Poisoning by heroin, accidental (unintentional)**

> Poisoning by heroin NOS

² √7ᵗʰ **T40.1X2** **Poisoning by heroin, intentional self-harm**   HCC

√7ᵗʰ **T40.1X3** **Poisoning by heroin, assault**

√7ᵗʰ **T40.1X4** **Poisoning by heroin, undetermined**

√5ᵗʰ **T40.2** **Poisoning by, adverse effect of and underdosing of other opioids**

√6ᵗʰ **T40.2X** **Poisoning by, adverse effect of and underdosing of other opioids**

√7ᵗʰ **T40.2X1** **Poisoning by other opioids, accidental (unintentional)**

> Poisoning by other opioids NOS

² √7ᵗʰ **T40.2X2** **Poisoning by other opioids, intentional self-harm**   HCC

√7ᵗʰ **T40.2X3** **Poisoning by other opioids, assault**

√7ᵗʰ **T40.2X4** **Poisoning by other opioids, undetermined**

√7ᵗʰ **T40.2X5** **Adverse effect of other opioids**

√7ᵗʰ **T40.2X6** **Underdosing of other opioids**

√5ᵗʰ **T40.3** **Poisoning by, adverse effect of and underdosing of methadone**

√6ᵗʰ **T40.3X** **Poisoning by, adverse effect of and underdosing of methadone**

√7ᵗʰ **T40.3X1** **Poisoning by methadone, accidental (unintentional)**

> Poisoning by methadone NOS

² √7ᵗʰ **T40.3X2** **Poisoning by methadone, intentional self-harm**   HCC

√7ᵗʰ **T40.3X3** **Poisoning by methadone, assault**

√7ᵗʰ **T40.3X4** **Poisoning by methadone, undetermined**

√7ᵗʰ **T40.3X5** **Adverse effect of methadone**

√7ᵗʰ **T40.3X6** **Underdosing of methadone**

√5ᵗʰ **T40.4** **Poisoning by, adverse effect of and underdosing of other synthetic narcotics**

√6ᵗʰ **T40.4X** **Poisoning by, adverse effect of and underdosing of other synthetic narcotics**

√7ᵗʰ **T40.4X1** **Poisoning by other synthetic narcotics, accidental (unintentional)**

> Poisoning by other synthetic narcotics NOS

² √7ᵗʰ **T40.4X2** **Poisoning by other synthetic narcotics, intentional self-harm**   HCC

√7ᵗʰ **T40.4X3** **Poisoning by other synthetic narcotics, assault**

√7ᵗʰ **T40.4X4** **Poisoning by other synthetic narcotics, undetermined**

√7ᵗʰ **T40.4X5** **Adverse effect of other synthetic narcotics**

√7ᵗʰ **T40.4X6** **Underdosing of other synthetic narcotics**

☑ Additional Character Req   √x7ᵗʰ Placeholder Alert   Manifestation   ▽ Unspecified   ►◄ Revised Text   ● New Code   ▲ Revised Code Title

√5ᵗʰ **T40.5** Poisoning by, adverse effect of and underdosing of cocaine

    √6ᵗʰ **T40.5X** Poisoning by, adverse effect of and underdosing of cocaine

       √7ᵗʰ **T40.5X1** Poisoning by cocaine, accidental (unintentional)
          Poisoning by cocaine NOS
          AHA: 2016,2Q,8

       ² √7ᵗʰ **T40.5X2** Poisoning by cocaine, intentional self-harm   HCC

       √7ᵗʰ **T40.5X3** Poisoning by cocaine, assault

       √7ᵗʰ **T40.5X4** Poisoning by cocaine, undetermined

       √7ᵗʰ **T40.5X5** Adverse effect of cocaine

       √7ᵗʰ **T40.5X6** Underdosing of cocaine

√5ᵗʰ **T40.6** Poisoning by, adverse effect of and underdosing of other and unspecified narcotics

    √6ᵗʰ **T40.60** Poisoning by, adverse effect of and underdosing of unspecified narcotics

       √7ᵗʰ **T40.601** Poisoning by unspecified narcotics, accidental (unintentional) ▽
          Poisoning by narcotics NOS

       ² √7ᵗʰ **T40.602** Poisoning by unspecified narcotics, intentional self-harm   HCC ▽

       √7ᵗʰ **T40.603** Poisoning by unspecified narcotics, assault ▽

       √7ᵗʰ **T40.604** Poisoning by unspecified narcotics, undetermined ▽

       √7ᵗʰ **T40.605** Adverse effect of unspecified narcotics ▽

       √7ᵗʰ **T40.606** Underdosing of unspecified narcotics ▽

    √6ᵗʰ **T40.69** Poisoning by, adverse effect of and underdosing of other narcotics

       √7ᵗʰ **T40.691** Poisoning by other narcotics, accidental (unintentional)
          Poisoning by other narcotics NOS

       ² √7ᵗʰ **T40.692** Poisoning by other narcotics, intentional self-harm   HCC

       √7ᵗʰ **T40.693** Poisoning by other narcotics, assault

       √7ᵗʰ **T40.694** Poisoning by other narcotics, undetermined

       √7ᵗʰ **T40.695** Adverse effect of other narcotics

       √7ᵗʰ **T40.696** Underdosing of other narcotics

√5ᵗʰ **T40.7** Poisoning by, adverse effect of and underdosing of cannabis (derivatives)

    √6ᵗʰ **T40.7X** Poisoning by, adverse effect of and underdosing of cannabis (derivatives)

       √7ᵗʰ **T40.7X1** Poisoning by cannabis (derivatives), accidental (unintentional)
          Poisoning by cannabis NOS

       ² √7ᵗʰ **T40.7X2** Poisoning by cannabis (derivatives), intentional self-harm   HCC

       √7ᵗʰ **T40.7X3** Poisoning by cannabis (derivatives), assault

       √7ᵗʰ **T40.7X4** Poisoning by cannabis (derivatives), undetermined

       √7ᵗʰ **T40.7X5** Adverse effect of cannabis (derivatives)

       √7ᵗʰ **T40.7X6** Underdosing of cannabis (derivatives)

√5ᵗʰ **T40.8** Poisoning by and adverse effect of lysergide [LSD]

    √6ᵗʰ **T40.8X** Poisoning by and adverse effect of lysergide [LSD]

       √7ᵗʰ **T40.8X1** Poisoning by lysergide [LSD], accidental (unintentional)
          Poisoning by lysergide [LSD] NOS

       ² √7ᵗʰ **T40.8X2** Poisoning by lysergide [LSD], intentional self-harm   HCC

       √7ᵗʰ **T40.8X3** Poisoning by lysergide [LSD], assault

       √7ᵗʰ **T40.8X4** Poisoning by lysergide [LSD], undetermined

√5ᵗʰ **T40.9** Poisoning by, adverse effect of and underdosing of other and unspecified psychodysleptics [hallucinogens]

    √6ᵗʰ **T40.90** Poisoning by, adverse effect of and underdosing of unspecified psychodysleptics [hallucinogens]

       √7ᵗʰ **T40.901** Poisoning by unspecified psychodysleptics [hallucinogens], accidental (unintentional) ▽

       ² √7ᵗʰ **T40.902** Poisoning by unspecified psychodysleptics [hallucinogens], intentional self-harm   HCC ▽

       √7ᵗʰ **T40.903** Poisoning by unspecified psychodysleptics [hallucinogens], assault ▽

       √7ᵗʰ **T40.904** Poisoning by unspecified psychodysleptics [hallucinogens], undetermined ▽

       √7ᵗʰ **T40.905** Adverse effect of unspecified psychodysleptics [hallucinogens] ▽

       √7ᵗʰ **T40.906** Underdosing of unspecified psychodysleptics ▽

    √6ᵗʰ **T40.99** Poisoning by, adverse effect of and underdosing of other psychodysleptics [hallucinogens]

       √7ᵗʰ **T40.991** Poisoning by other psychodysleptics [hallucinogens], accidental (unintentional)
          Poisoning by other psychodysleptics [hallucinogens] NOS

       ² √7ᵗʰ **T40.992** Poisoning by other psychodysleptics [hallucinogens], intentional self-harm   HCC

       √7ᵗʰ **T40.993** Poisoning by other psychodysleptics [hallucinogens], assault

       √7ᵗʰ **T40.994** Poisoning by other psychodysleptics [hallucinogens], undetermined

       √7ᵗʰ **T40.995** Adverse effect of other psychodysleptics [hallucinogens]

       √7ᵗʰ **T40.996** Underdosing of other psychodysleptics

√4ᵗʰ **T41** Poisoning by, adverse effect of and underdosing of anesthetics and therapeutic gases

    EXCLUDES 1   benzodiazepines (T42.4-)
          cocaine (T40.5-)
          complications of anesthesia during labor and delivery (O74.-)
          complications of anesthesia during pregnancy (O29.-)
          complications of anesthesia during the puerperium (O89.-)
          opioids (T40.0-T40.2-)

> The appropriate 7th character is to be added to each code from category T41.
> A   initial encounter
> D   subsequent encounter
> S   sequela

√5ᵗʰ **T41.0** Poisoning by, adverse effect of and underdosing of inhaled anesthetics

    EXCLUDES 1   oxygen (T41.5-)

    √6ᵗʰ **T41.0X** Poisoning by, adverse effect of and underdosing of inhaled anesthetics

       √7ᵗʰ **T41.0X1** Poisoning by inhaled anesthetics, accidental (unintentional)
          Poisoning by inhaled anesthetics NOS

       ² √7ᵗʰ **T41.0X2** Poisoning by inhaled anesthetics, intentional self-harm   HCC

       √7ᵗʰ **T41.0X3** Poisoning by inhaled anesthetics, assault

       √7ᵗʰ **T41.0X4** Poisoning by inhaled anesthetics, undetermined

       √7ᵗʰ **T41.0X5** Adverse effect of inhaled anesthetics

       √7ᵗʰ **T41.0X6** Underdosing of inhaled anesthetics

√5ᵗʰ **T41.1** Poisoning by, adverse effect of and underdosing of intravenous anesthetics
    Poisoning by, adverse effect of and underdosing of thiobarbiturates

    √6ᵗʰ **T41.1X** Poisoning by, adverse effect of and underdosing of intravenous anesthetics

       √7ᵗʰ **T41.1X1** Poisoning by intravenous anesthetics, accidental (unintentional)
          Poisoning by intravenous anesthetics NOS

       ² √7ᵗʰ **T41.1X2** Poisoning by intravenous anesthetics, intentional self-harm   HCC

       √7ᵗʰ **T41.1X3** Poisoning by intravenous anesthetics, assault

       √7ᵗʰ **T41.1X4** Poisoning by intravenous anesthetics, undetermined

       √7ᵗʰ **T41.1X5** Adverse effect of intravenous anesthetics

       √7ᵗʰ **T41.1X6** Underdosing of intravenous anesthetics

√5ᵗʰ **T41.2** **Poisoning by, adverse effect of and underdosing of other and unspecified general anesthetics**

    √6ᵗʰ **T41.20** **Poisoning by, adverse effect of and underdosing of unspecified general anesthetics**

       √7ᵗʰ **T41.201** **Poisoning by unspecified general anesthetics, accidental (unintentional)** ▽

          Poisoning by general anesthetics NOS

       ² √7ᵗʰ **T41.202** **Poisoning by unspecified general anesthetics, intentional self-harm** HCC ▽

       √7ᵗʰ **T41.203** **Poisoning by unspecified general anesthetics, assault** ▽

       √7ᵗʰ **T41.204** **Poisoning by unspecified general anesthetics, undetermined** ▽

       √7ᵗʰ **T41.205** **Adverse effect of unspecified general anesthetics** ▽

          AHA: 2016,4Q,73

       √7ᵗʰ **T41.206** **Underdosing of unspecified general anesthetics** ▽

    √6ᵗʰ **T41.29** **Poisoning by, adverse effect of and underdosing of other general anesthetics**

       √7ᵗʰ **T41.291** **Poisoning by other general anesthetics, accidental (unintentional)**

          Poisoning by other general anesthetics NOS

       ² √7ᵗʰ **T41.292** **Poisoning by other general anesthetics, intentional self-harm** HCC

       √7ᵗʰ **T41.293** **Poisoning by other general anesthetics, assault**

       √7ᵗʰ **T41.294** **Poisoning by other general anesthetics, undetermined**

       √7ᵗʰ **T41.295** **Adverse effect of other general anesthetics**

       √7ᵗʰ **T41.296** **Underdosing of other general anesthetics**

√5ᵗʰ **T41.3** **Poisoning by, adverse effect of and underdosing of local anesthetics**

    Cocaine (topical)

    EXCLUDES 2   poisoning by cocaine used as a central nervous system stimulant (T40.5X1-T40.5X4)

    √6ᵗʰ **T41.3X** **Poisoning by, adverse effect of and underdosing of local anesthetics**

       √7ᵗʰ **T41.3X1** **Poisoning by local anesthetics, accidental (unintentional)**

          Poisoning by local anesthetics NOS

       ² √7ᵗʰ **T41.3X2** **Poisoning by local anesthetics, intentional self-harm** HCC

       √7ᵗʰ **T41.3X3** **Poisoning by local anesthetics, assault**

       √7ᵗʰ **T41.3X4** **Poisoning by local anesthetics, undetermined**

       √7ᵗʰ **T41.3X5** **Adverse effect of local anesthetics**

       √7ᵗʰ **T41.3X6** **Underdosing of local anesthetics**

√5ᵗʰ **T41.4** **Poisoning by, adverse effect of and underdosing of unspecified anesthetic**

    √x7ᵗʰ **T41.41** **Poisoning by unspecified anesthetic, accidental (unintentional)** ▽

       Poisoning by anesthetic NOS

    ² √x7ᵗʰ **T41.42** **Poisoning by unspecified anesthetic, intentional self-harm** HCC ▽

    √x7ᵗʰ **T41.43** **Poisoning by unspecified anesthetic, assault** ▽

    √x7ᵗʰ **T41.44** **Poisoning by unspecified anesthetic, undetermined** ▽

    √x7ᵗʰ **T41.45** **Adverse effect of unspecified anesthetic** ▽

    √x7ᵗʰ **T41.46** **Underdosing of unspecified anesthetics** ▽

√5ᵗʰ **T41.5** **Poisoning by, adverse effect of and underdosing of therapeutic gases**

    √6ᵗʰ **T41.5X** **Poisoning by, adverse effect of and underdosing of therapeutic gases**

       √7ᵗʰ **T41.5X1** **Poisoning by therapeutic gases, accidental (unintentional)**

          Poisoning by therapeutic gases NOS

       ² √7ᵗʰ **T41.5X2** **Poisoning by therapeutic gases, intentional self-harm** HCC

       √7ᵗʰ **T41.5X3** **Poisoning by therapeutic gases, assault**

       √7ᵗʰ **T41.5X4** **Poisoning by therapeutic gases, undetermined**

       √7ᵗʰ **T41.5X5** **Adverse effect of therapeutic gases**

       √7ᵗʰ **T41.5X6** **Underdosing of therapeutic gases**

√4ᵗʰ **T42** **Poisoning by, adverse effect of and underdosing of antiepileptic, sedative- hypnotic and antiparkinsonism drugs**

    EXCLUDES 2   drug dependence and related mental and behavioral disorders due to psychoactive substance use (F10.- — F19.-)

    The appropriate 7th character is to be added to each code from category T42.
    A   initial encounter
    D   subsequent encounter
    S   sequela

√5ᵗʰ **T42.0** **Poisoning by, adverse effect of and underdosing of hydantoin derivatives**

    √6ᵗʰ **T42.0X** **Poisoning by, adverse effect of and underdosing of hydantoin derivatives**

       √7ᵗʰ **T42.0X1** **Poisoning by hydantoin derivatives, accidental (unintentional)**

          Poisoning by hydantoin derivatives NOS

       ² √7ᵗʰ **T42.0X2** **Poisoning by hydantoin derivatives, intentional self-harm** HCC

       √7ᵗʰ **T42.0X3** **Poisoning by hydantoin derivatives, assault**

       √7ᵗʰ **T42.0X4** **Poisoning by hydantoin derivatives, undetermined**

       √7ᵗʰ **T42.0X5** **Adverse effect of hydantoin derivatives**

       √7ᵗʰ **T42.0X6** **Underdosing of hydantoin derivatives**

√5ᵗʰ **T42.1** **Poisoning by, adverse effect of and underdosing of iminostilbenes**

    Poisoning by, adverse effect of and underdosing of carbamazepine

    √6ᵗʰ **T42.1X** **Poisoning by, adverse effect of and underdosing of iminostilbenes**

       √7ᵗʰ **T42.1X1** **Poisoning by iminostilbenes, accidental (unintentional)**

          Poisoning by iminostilbenes NOS

       ² √7ᵗʰ **T42.1X2** **Poisoning by iminostilbenes, intentional self-harm** HCC

       √7ᵗʰ **T42.1X3** **Poisoning by iminostilbenes, assault**

       √7ᵗʰ **T42.1X4** **Poisoning by iminostilbenes, undetermined**

       √7ᵗʰ **T42.1X5** **Adverse effect of iminostilbenes**

       √7ᵗʰ **T42.1X6** **Underdosing of iminostilbenes**

√5ᵗʰ **T42.2** **Poisoning by, adverse effect of and underdosing of succinimides and oxazolidinediones**

    √6ᵗʰ **T42.2X** **Poisoning by, adverse effect of and underdosing of succinimides and oxazolidinediones**

       √7ᵗʰ **T42.2X1** **Poisoning by succinimides and oxazolidinediones, accidental (unintentional)**

          Poisoning by succinimides and oxazolidinediones NOS

       ² √7ᵗʰ **T42.2X2** **Poisoning by succinimides and oxazolidinediones, intentional self-harm** HCC

       √7ᵗʰ **T42.2X3** **Poisoning by succinimides and oxazolidinediones, assault**

       √7ᵗʰ **T42.2X4** **Poisoning by succinimides and oxazolidinediones, undetermined**

       √7ᵗʰ **T42.2X5** **Adverse effect of succinimides and oxazolidinediones**

       √7ᵗʰ **T42.2X6** **Underdosing of succinimides and oxazolidinediones**

√5ᵗʰ **T42.3** **Poisoning by, adverse effect of and underdosing of barbiturates**

    EXCLUDES 1   poisoning by, adverse effect of and underdosing of thiobarbiturates (T41.1-)

    √6ᵗʰ **T42.3X** **Poisoning by, adverse effect of and underdosing of barbiturates**

       √7ᵗʰ **T42.3X1** **Poisoning by barbiturates, accidental (unintentional)**

          Poisoning by barbiturates NOS

       ² √7ᵗʰ **T42.3X2** **Poisoning by barbiturates, intentional self-harm** HCC

       √7ᵗʰ **T42.3X3** **Poisoning by barbiturates, assault**

       √7ᵗʰ **T42.3X4** **Poisoning by barbiturates, undetermined**

       √7ᵗʰ **T42.3X5** **Adverse effect of barbiturates**

       √7ᵗʰ **T42.3X6** **Underdosing of barbiturates**

☑ Additional Character Req   √x7ᵗʰ Placeholder Alert   Manifestation   ▽ Unspecified   ►◄ Revised Text   ● New Code   ▲ Revised Code Title

Chapter 19. Injury, Poisoning and Certain Other Consequences of External Causes

T42.4–T43.026

√5ᵗʰ **T42.4 Poisoning by, adverse effect of and underdosing of benzodiazepines**

  √6ᵗʰ **T42.4X Poisoning by, adverse effect of and underdosing of benzodiazepines**

    √7ᵗʰ **T42.4X1 Poisoning by benzodiazepines, accidental (unintentional)**
       Poisoning by benzodiazepines NOS

    2 √7ᵗʰ **T42.4X2 Poisoning by benzodiazepines, intentional self-harm**   HCC

    √7ᵗʰ **T42.4X3 Poisoning by benzodiazepines, assault**

    √7ᵗʰ **T42.4X4 Poisoning by benzodiazepines, undetermined**

    √7ᵗʰ **T42.4X5 Adverse effect of benzodiazepines**

    √7ᵗʰ **T42.4X6 Underdosing of benzodiazepines**

√5ᵗʰ **T42.5 Poisoning by, adverse effect of and underdosing of mixed antiepileptics**

  √6ᵗʰ **T42.5X Poisoning by, adverse effect of and underdosing of antiepileptics**

    √7ᵗʰ **T42.5X1 Poisoning by mixed antiepileptics, accidental (unintentional)**
       Poisoning by mixed antiepileptics NOS

    2 √7ᵗʰ **T42.5X2 Poisoning by mixed antiepileptics, intentional self-harm**   HCC

    √7ᵗʰ **T42.5X3 Poisoning by mixed antiepileptics, assault**

    √7ᵗʰ **T42.5X4 Poisoning by mixed antiepileptics, undetermined**

    √7ᵗʰ **T42.5X5 Adverse effect of mixed antiepileptics**

    √7ᵗʰ **T42.5X6 Underdosing of mixed antiepileptics**

√5ᵗʰ **T42.6 Poisoning by, adverse effect of and underdosing of other antiepileptic and sedative-hypnotic drugs**

   Poisoning by, adverse effect of and underdosing of methaqualone

   Poisoning by, adverse effect of and underdosing of valproic acid

    EXCLUDES 1   poisoning by, adverse effect of and underdosing of carbamazepine (T42.1-)

  √6ᵗʰ **T42.6X Poisoning by, adverse effect of and underdosing of other antiepileptic and sedative-hypnotic drugs**

    √7ᵗʰ **T42.6X1 Poisoning by other antiepileptic and sedative-hypnotic drugs, accidental (unintentional)**
       Poisoning by other antiepileptic and sedative-hypnotic drugs NOS

    2 √7ᵗʰ **T42.6X2 Poisoning by other antiepileptic and sedative-hypnotic drugs, intentional self-harm**   HCC

    √7ᵗʰ **T42.6X3 Poisoning by other antiepileptic and sedative-hypnotic drugs, assault**

    √7ᵗʰ **T42.6X4 Poisoning by other antiepileptic and sedative-hypnotic drugs, undetermined**

    √7ᵗʰ **T42.6X5 Adverse effect of other antiepileptic and sedative-hypnotic drugs**

    √7ᵗʰ **T42.6X6 Underdosing of other antiepileptic and sedative-hypnotic drugs**

√5ᵗʰ **T42.7 Poisoning by, adverse effect of and underdosing of unspecified antiepileptic and sedative-hypnotic drugs**

  √x7ᵗʰ **T42.71 Poisoning by unspecified antiepileptic and sedative-hypnotic drugs, accidental (unintentional)** ▽
     Poisoning by antiepileptic and sedative-hypnotic drugs NOS

  2 √x7ᵗʰ **T42.72 Poisoning by unspecified antiepileptic and sedative-hypnotic drugs, intentional self-harm**   HCC ▽

  √x7ᵗʰ **T42.73 Poisoning by unspecified antiepileptic and sedative-hypnotic drugs, assault** ▽

  √x7ᵗʰ **T42.74 Poisoning by unspecified antiepileptic and sedative-hypnotic drugs, undetermined** ▽

  √x7ᵗʰ **T42.75 Adverse effect of unspecified antiepileptic and sedative-hypnotic drugs** ▽

  √x7ᵗʰ **T42.76 Underdosing of unspecified antiepileptic and sedative-hypnotic drugs** ▽

√5ᵗʰ **T42.8 Poisoning by, adverse effect of and underdosing of antiparkinsonism drugs and other central muscle-tone depressants**

   Poisoning by, adverse effect of and underdosing of amantadine

  √6ᵗʰ **T42.8X Poisoning by, adverse effect of and underdosing of antiparkinsonism drugs and other central muscle-tone depressants**

    √7ᵗʰ **T42.8X1 Poisoning by antiparkinsonism drugs and other central muscle-tone depressants, accidental (unintentional)**
       Poisoning by antiparkinsonism drugs and other central muscle-tone depressants NOS

    2 √7ᵗʰ **T42.8X2 Poisoning by antiparkinsonism drugs and other central muscle-tone depressants, intentional self-harm**   HCC

    √7ᵗʰ **T42.8X3 Poisoning by antiparkinsonism drugs and other central muscle-tone depressants, assault**

    √7ᵗʰ **T42.8X4 Poisoning by antiparkinsonism drugs and other central muscle-tone depressants, undetermined**

    √7ᵗʰ **T42.8X5 Adverse effect of antiparkinsonism drugs and other central muscle-tone depressants**

    √7ᵗʰ **T42.8X6 Underdosing of antiparkinsonism drugs and other central muscle-tone depressants**

√4ᵗʰ **T43 Poisoning by, adverse effect of and underdosing of psychotropic drugs, not elsewhere classified**

  EXCLUDES 1   appetite depressants (T50.5-)
     barbiturates (T42.3-)
     benzodiazepines (T42.4-)
     methaqualone (T42.6-)
     psychodysleptics [hallucinogens] (T40.7-T40.9-)

  EXCLUDES 2   drug dependence and related mental and behavioral disorders due to psychoactive substance use (F10.- – F19.-)

> The appropriate 7th character is to be added to each code from category T43.
> A   initial encounter
> D   subsequent encounter
> S   sequela

√5ᵗʰ **T43.0 Poisoning by, adverse effect of and underdosing of tricyclic and tetracyclic antidepressants**

  √6ᵗʰ **T43.01 Poisoning by, adverse effect of and underdosing of tricyclic antidepressants**

    √7ᵗʰ **T43.011 Poisoning by tricyclic antidepressants, accidental (unintentional)**
       Poisoning by tricyclic antidepressants NOS

    2 √7ᵗʰ **T43.012 Poisoning by tricyclic antidepressants, intentional self-harm**   HCC

    √7ᵗʰ **T43.013 Poisoning by tricyclic antidepressants, assault**

    √7ᵗʰ **T43.014 Poisoning by tricyclic antidepressants, undetermined**

    √7ᵗʰ **T43.015 Adverse effect of tricyclic antidepressants**

    √7ᵗʰ **T43.016 Underdosing of tricyclic antidepressants**

  √6ᵗʰ **T43.02 Poisoning by, adverse effect of and underdosing of tetracyclic antidepressants**

    √7ᵗʰ **T43.021 Poisoning by tetracyclic antidepressants, accidental (unintentional)**
       Poisoning by tetracyclic antidepressants NOS

    2 √7ᵗʰ **T43.022 Poisoning by tetracyclic antidepressants, intentional self-harm**   HCC

    √7ᵗʰ **T43.023 Poisoning by tetracyclic antidepressants, assault**

    √7ᵗʰ **T43.024 Poisoning by tetracyclic antidepressants, undetermined**

    √7ᵗʰ **T43.025 Adverse effect of tetracyclic antidepressants**

    √7ᵗʰ **T43.026 Underdosing of tetracyclic antidepressants**

√5ᵗʰ **T43.1** **Poisoning by, adverse effect of and underdosing of monoamine-oxidase-inhibitor antidepressants**

√6ᵗʰ **T43.1X** **Poisoning by, adverse effect of and underdosing of** monoamine-oxidase-inhibitor antidepressants

√7ᵗʰ **T43.1X1** **Poisoning by monoamine-oxidase-inhibitor antidepressants, accidental (unintentional)**
Poisoning by monoamine-oxidase-inhibitor antidepressants NOS

2 √7ᵗʰ **T43.1X2** **Poisoning by monoamine-oxidase-inhibitor antidepressants, intentional self-harm**   HCC

√7ᵗʰ **T43.1X3** **Poisoning by monoamine-oxidase-inhibitor antidepressants, assault**

√7ᵗʰ **T43.1X4** **Poisoning by monoamine-oxidase-inhibitor antidepressants, undetermined**

√7ᵗʰ **T43.1X5** **Adverse effect of monoamine-oxidase-inhibitor antidepressants**

√7ᵗʰ **T43.1X6** Underdosing of monoamine-oxidase-inhibitor antidepressants

√5ᵗʰ **T43.2** **Poisoning by, adverse effect of and underdosing of other and unspecified antidepressants**

√6ᵗʰ **T43.20** **Poisoning by, adverse effect of and underdosing of unspecified antidepressants**

√7ᵗʰ **T43.201** **Poisoning by unspecified antidepressants, accidental (unintentional)** ▽
Poisoning by antidepressants NOS

2 √7ᵗʰ **T43.202** **Poisoning by unspecified antidepressants, intentional self-harm**   HCC ▽

√7ᵗʰ **T43.203** **Poisoning by unspecified antidepressants, assault** ▽

√7ᵗʰ **T43.204** **Poisoning by unspecified antidepressants, undetermined** ▽

√7ᵗʰ **T43.205** **Adverse effect of unspecified antidepressants** ▽
Antidepressant discontinuation syndrome

√7ᵗʰ **T43.206** Underdosing of unspecified antidepressants ▽

√6ᵗʰ **T43.21** **Poisoning by, adverse effect of and underdosing of selective serotonin and norepinephrine reuptake inhibitors**
Poisoning by, adverse effect of and underdosing of SSNRI antidepressants

√7ᵗʰ **T43.211** **Poisoning by selective serotonin and norepinephrine reuptake inhibitors, accidental (unintentional)**

2 √7ᵗʰ **T43.212** **Poisoning by selective serotonin and norepinephrine reuptake inhibitors, intentional self-harm**   HCC

√7ᵗʰ **T43.213** **Poisoning by selective serotonin and norepinephrine reuptake inhibitors, assault**

√7ᵗʰ **T43.214** **Poisoning by selective serotonin and norepinephrine reuptake inhibitors, undetermined**

√7ᵗʰ **T43.215** **Adverse effect of selective serotonin and norepinephrine reuptake inhibitors**

√7ᵗʰ **T43.216** Underdosing of selective serotonin and norepinephrine reuptake inhibitors

√6ᵗʰ **T43.22** **Poisoning by, adverse effect of and underdosing of selective serotonin reuptake inhibitors**
Poisoning by, adverse effect of and underdosing of SSRI antidepressants

√7ᵗʰ **T43.221** **Poisoning by selective serotonin reuptake inhibitors, accidental (unintentional)**

2 √7ᵗʰ **T43.222** **Poisoning by selective serotonin reuptake inhibitors, intentional self-harm**   HCC

√7ᵗʰ **T43.223** **Poisoning by selective serotonin reuptake inhibitors, assault**

√7ᵗʰ **T43.224** **Poisoning by selective serotonin reuptake inhibitors, undetermined**

√7ᵗʰ **T43.225** **Adverse effect of selective serotonin reuptake inhibitors**

√7ᵗʰ **T43.226** Underdosing of selective serotonin reuptake inhibitors

√6ᵗʰ **T43.29** **Poisoning by, adverse effect of and underdosing of other antidepressants**

√7ᵗʰ **T43.291** **Poisoning by other antidepressants, accidental (unintentional)**
Poisoning by other antidepressants NOS

2 √7ᵗʰ **T43.292** **Poisoning by other antidepressants, intentional self-harm**   HCC

√7ᵗʰ **T43.293** **Poisoning by other antidepressants, assault**

√7ᵗʰ **T43.294** **Poisoning by other antidepressants, undetermined**

√7ᵗʰ **T43.295** **Adverse effect of other antidepressants**

√7ᵗʰ **T43.296** Underdosing of other antidepressants

√5ᵗʰ **T43.3** **Poisoning by, adverse effect of and underdosing of phenothiazine antipsychotics and neuroleptics**

√6ᵗʰ **T43.3X** **Poisoning by, adverse effect of and underdosing of** phenothiazine antipsychotics and neuroleptics

√7ᵗʰ **T43.3X1** **Poisoning by phenothiazine antipsychotics and neuroleptics, accidental (unintentional)**
Poisoning by phenothiazine antipsychotics and neuroleptics NOS

2 √7ᵗʰ **T43.3X2** **Poisoning by phenothiazine antipsychotics and neuroleptics, intentional self-harm**   HCC

√7ᵗʰ **T43.3X3** **Poisoning by phenothiazine antipsychotics and neuroleptics, assault**

√7ᵗʰ **T43.3X4** **Poisoning by phenothiazine antipsychotics and neuroleptics, undetermined**

√7ᵗʰ **T43.3X5** **Adverse effect of phenothiazine antipsychotics and neuroleptics**

√7ᵗʰ **T43.3X6** Underdosing of phenothiazine antipsychotics and neuroleptics

√5ᵗʰ **T43.4** **Poisoning by, adverse effect of and underdosing of butyrophenone and thiothixene neuroleptics**

√6ᵗʰ **T43.4X** **Poisoning by, adverse effect of and underdosing of** butyrophenone and thiothixene neuroleptics

√7ᵗʰ **T43.4X1** **Poisoning by butyrophenone and thiothixene neuroleptics, accidental (unintentional)**
Poisoning by butyrophenone and thiothixene neuroleptics NOS

2 √7ᵗʰ **T43.4X2** **Poisoning by butyrophenone and thiothixene neuroleptics, intentional self-harm**   HCC

√7ᵗʰ **T43.4X3** **Poisoning by butyrophenone and thiothixene neuroleptics, assault**

√7ᵗʰ **T43.4X4** **Poisoning by butyrophenone and thiothixene neuroleptics, undetermined**

√7ᵗʰ **T43.4X5** **Adverse effect of butyrophenone and thiothixene neuroleptics**

√7ᵗʰ **T43.4X6** Underdosing of butyrophenone and thiothixene neuroleptics

√5ᵗʰ **T43.5** **Poisoning by, adverse effect of and underdosing of other and unspecified antipsychotics and neuroleptics**

EXCLUDES 1   poisoning by, adverse effect of and underdosing of rauwolfia (T46.5-)

√6ᵗʰ **T43.50** **Poisoning by, adverse effect of and underdosing of unspecified antipsychotics and neuroleptics**

√7ᵗʰ **T43.501** **Poisoning by unspecified antipsychotics and neuroleptics, accidental (unintentional)** ▽
Poisoning by antipsychotics and neuroleptics NOS

2 √7ᵗʰ **T43.502** **Poisoning by unspecified antipsychotics and neuroleptics, intentional self-harm**   HCC ▽

√7ᵗʰ **T43.503** **Poisoning by unspecified antipsychotics and neuroleptics, assault** ▽

√7ᵗʰ **T43.504** **Poisoning by unspecified antipsychotics and neuroleptics, undetermined** ▽

√7ᵗʰ **T43.505** **Adverse effect of unspecified antipsychotics and neuroleptics** ▽

√7ᵗʰ **T43.506** Underdosing of unspecified antipsychotics and neuroleptics ▽

√6ᵗʰ **T43.59** **Poisoning by, adverse effect of and underdosing of other antipsychotics and neuroleptics**

AHA: 2017,1Q,40

√7ᵗʰ **T43.591** **Poisoning by other antipsychotics and neuroleptics, accidental (unintentional)**

Poisoning by other antipsychotics and neuroleptics NOS

2 √7ᵗʰ **T43.592** **Poisoning by other antipsychotics and neuroleptics, intentional self-harm** HCC

√7ᵗʰ **T43.593** **Poisoning by other antipsychotics and neuroleptics, assault**

√7ᵗʰ **T43.594** **Poisoning by other antipsychotics and neuroleptics, undetermined**

√7ᵗʰ **T43.595** **Adverse effect of other antipsychotics and neuroleptics**

√7ᵗʰ **T43.596** **Underdosing of other antipsychotics and neuroleptics**

√5ᵗʰ **T43.6** **Poisoning by, adverse effect of and underdosing of psychostimulants**

EXCLUDES 1 *poisoning by, adverse effect of and underdosing of cocaine (T40.5-)*

√6ᵗʰ **T43.60** **Poisoning by, adverse effect of and underdosing of unspecified psychostimulant**

√7ᵗʰ **T43.601** **Poisoning by unspecified psychostimulants, accidental (unintentional)** ▽

Poisoning by psychostimulants NOS

2 √7ᵗʰ **T43.602** **Poisoning by unspecified psychostimulants, intentional self-harm** HCC ▽

√7ᵗʰ **T43.603** **Poisoning by unspecified psychostimulants, assault** ▽

√7ᵗʰ **T43.604** **Poisoning by unspecified psychostimulants, undetermined** ▽

√7ᵗʰ **T43.605** **Adverse effect of unspecified psychostimulants** ▽

√7ᵗʰ **T43.606** **Underdosing of unspecified psychostimulants** ▽

√6ᵗʰ **T43.61** **Poisoning by, adverse effect of and underdosing of caffeine**

√7ᵗʰ **T43.611** **Poisoning by caffeine, accidental (unintentional)**

Poisoning by caffeine NOS

2 √7ᵗʰ **T43.612** **Poisoning by caffeine, intentional self-harm** HCC

√7ᵗʰ **T43.613** **Poisoning by caffeine, assault**

√7ᵗʰ **T43.614** **Poisoning by caffeine, undetermined**

√7ᵗʰ **T43.615** **Adverse effect of caffeine**

√7ᵗʰ **T43.616** **Underdosing of caffeine**

√6ᵗʰ **T43.62** **Poisoning by, adverse effect of and underdosing of amphetamines**

Poisoning by, adverse effect of and underdosing of methamphetamines

√7ᵗʰ **T43.621** **Poisoning by amphetamines, accidental (unintentional)**

Poisoning by amphetamines NOS

2 √7ᵗʰ **T43.622** **Poisoning by amphetamines, intentional self-harm** HCC

√7ᵗʰ **T43.623** **Poisoning by amphetamines, assault**

√7ᵗʰ **T43.624** **Poisoning by amphetamines, undetermined**

√7ᵗʰ **T43.625** **Adverse effect of amphetamines**

√7ᵗʰ **T43.626** **Underdosing of amphetamines**

√6ᵗʰ **T43.63** **Poisoning by, adverse effect of and underdosing of methylphenidate**

√7ᵗʰ **T43.631** **Poisoning by methylphenidate, accidental (unintentional)**

Poisoning by methylphenidate NOS

2 √7ᵗʰ **T43.632** **Poisoning by methylphenidate, intentional self-harm** HCC

√7ᵗʰ **T43.633** **Poisoning by methylphenidate, assault**

√7ᵗʰ **T43.634** **Poisoning by methylphenidate, undetermined**

√7ᵗʰ **T43.635** **Adverse effect of methylphenidate**

√7ᵗʰ **T43.636** **Underdosing of methylphenidate**

√6ᵗʰ **T43.64** **Poisoning by ecstasy**

Poisoning by MDMA

Poisoning by 3,4-methylenedioxymethamphetamine

√7ᵗʰ **T43.641** **Poisoning by ecstasy, accidental (unintentional)**

Poisoning by ecstasy NOS

√7ᵗʰ **T43.642** **Poisoning by ecstasy, intentional self-harm**

√7ᵗʰ **T43.643** **Poisoning by ecstasy, assault**

√7ᵗʰ **T43.644** **Poisoning by ecstasy, undetermined**

√6ᵗʰ **T43.69** **Poisoning by, adverse effect of and underdosing of other psychostimulants**

√7ᵗʰ **T43.691** **Poisoning by other psychostimulants, accidental (unintentional)**

Poisoning by other psychostimulants NOS

2 √7ᵗʰ **T43.692** **Poisoning by other psychostimulants, intentional self-harm** HCC

√7ᵗʰ **T43.693** **Poisoning by other psychostimulants, assault**

√7ᵗʰ **T43.694** **Poisoning by other psychostimulants, undetermined**

√7ᵗʰ **T43.695** **Adverse effect of other psychostimulants**

√7ᵗʰ **T43.696** **Underdosing of other psychostimulants**

√5ᵗʰ **T43.8** **Poisoning by, adverse effect of and underdosing of other psychotropic drugs**

√6ᵗʰ **T43.8X** **Poisoning by, adverse effect of and underdosing of other psychotropic drugs**

√7ᵗʰ **T43.8X1** **Poisoning by other psychotropic drugs, accidental (unintentional)**

Poisoning by other psychotropic drugs NOS

2 √7ᵗʰ **T43.8X2** **Poisoning by other psychotropic drugs, intentional self-harm** HCC

√7ᵗʰ **T43.8X3** **Poisoning by other psychotropic drugs, assault**

√7ᵗʰ **T43.8X4** **Poisoning by other psychotropic drugs, undetermined**

√7ᵗʰ **T43.8X5** **Adverse effect of other psychotropic drugs**

√7ᵗʰ **T43.8X6** **Underdosing of other psychotropic drugs**

√5ᵗʰ **T43.9** **Poisoning by, adverse effect of and underdosing of unspecified psychotropic drug**

√x7ᵗʰ **T43.91** **Poisoning by unspecified psychotropic drug, accidental (unintentional)** ▽

Poisoning by psychotropic drug NOS

2 √x7ᵗʰ **T43.92** **Poisoning by unspecified psychotropic drug, intentional self-harm** HCC ▽

√x7ᵗʰ **T43.93** **Poisoning by unspecified psychotropic drug, assault** ▽

√x7ᵗʰ **T43.94** **Poisoning by unspecified psychotropic drug, undetermined** ▽

√x7ᵗʰ **T43.95** **Adverse effect of unspecified psychotropic drug** ▽

√x7ᵗʰ **T43.96** **Underdosing of unspecified psychotropic drug** ▽

√4ᵗʰ **T44** **Poisoning by, adverse effect of and underdosing of drugs primarily affecting the autonomic nervous system**

The appropriate 7th character is to be added to each code from category T44.

A   initial encounter
D   subsequent encounter
S   sequela

√5ᵗʰ **T44.0** **Poisoning by, adverse effect of and underdosing of anticholinesterase agents**

√6ᵗʰ **T44.0X** **Poisoning by, adverse effect of and underdosing of anticholinesterase agents**

√7ᵗʰ **T44.0X1** **Poisoning by anticholinesterase agents, accidental (unintentional)**

Poisoning by anticholinesterase agents NOS

2 √7ᵗʰ **T44.0X2** **Poisoning by anticholinesterase agents, intentional self-harm** HCC

√7ᵗʰ **T44.0X3** **Poisoning by anticholinesterase agents, assault**

√7ᵗʰ **T44.0X4** **Poisoning by anticholinesterase agents, undetermined**

√7ᵗʰ **T44.0X5** **Adverse effect of anticholinesterase agents**

√7ᵗʰ **T44.0X6** **Underdosing of anticholinesterase agents**

√5ᵗʰ **T44.1** **Poisoning by, adverse effect of and underdosing of other parasympathomimetics [cholinergics]**

  √6ᵗʰ **T44.1X** **Poisoning by, adverse effect of and underdosing of other parasympathomimetics [cholinergics]**

    √7ᵗʰ **T44.1X1** **Poisoning by other parasympathomimetics [cholinergics], accidental (unintentional)**
Poisoning by other parasympathomimetics [cholinergics] NOS

    ² √7ᵗʰ **T44.1X2** **Poisoning by other parasympathomimetics [cholinergics], intentional self-harm**   HCC

    √7ᵗʰ **T44.1X3** **Poisoning by other parasympathomimetics [cholinergics], assault**

    √7ᵗʰ **T44.1X4** **Poisoning by other parasympathomimetics [cholinergics], undetermined**

    √7ᵗʰ **T44.1X5** **Adverse effect of other parasympathomimetics [cholinergics]**

    √7ᵗʰ **T44.1X6** **Underdosing of other parasympathomimetics**

√5ᵗʰ **T44.2** **Poisoning by, adverse effect of and underdosing of ganglionic blocking drugs**

  √6ᵗʰ **T44.2X** **Poisoning by, adverse effect of and underdosing of ganglionic blocking drugs**

    √7ᵗʰ **T44.2X1** **Poisoning by ganglionic blocking drugs, accidental (unintentional)**
Poisoning by ganglionic blocking drugs NOS

    ² √7ᵗʰ **T44.2X2** **Poisoning by ganglionic blocking drugs, intentional self-harm**   HCC

    √7ᵗʰ **T44.2X3** **Poisoning by ganglionic blocking drugs, assault**

    √7ᵗʰ **T44.2X4** **Poisoning by ganglionic blocking drugs, undetermined**

    √7ᵗʰ **T44.2X5** **Adverse effect of ganglionic blocking drugs**

    √7ᵗʰ **T44.2X6** **Underdosing of ganglionic blocking drugs**

√5ᵗʰ **T44.3** **Poisoning by, adverse effect of and underdosing of other parasympatholytics [anticholinergics and antimuscarinics] and spasmolytics**
Poisoning by, adverse effect of and underdosing of papaverine

  √6ᵗʰ **T44.3X** **Poisoning by, adverse effect of and underdosing of other parasympatholytics [anticholinergics and antimuscarinics] and spasmolytics**

    √7ᵗʰ **T44.3X1** **Poisoning by other parasympatholytics [anticholinergics and antimuscarinics] and spasmolytics, accidental (unintentional)**
Poisoning by other parasympatholytics [anticholinergics and antimuscarinics] and spasmolytics NOS

    ² √7ᵗʰ **T44.3X2** **Poisoning by other parasympatholytics [anticholinergics and antimuscarinics] and spasmolytics, intentional self-harm**   HCC

    √7ᵗʰ **T44.3X3** **Poisoning by other parasympatholytics [anticholinergics and antimuscarinics] and spasmolytics, assault**

    √7ᵗʰ **T44.3X4** **Poisoning by other parasympatholytics [anticholinergics and antimuscarinics] and spasmolytics, undetermined**

    √7ᵗʰ **T44.3X5** **Adverse effect of other parasympatholytics [anticholinergics and antimuscarinics] and spasmolytics**

    √7ᵗʰ **T44.3X6** **Underdosing of other parasympatholytics [anticholinergics and antimuscarinics] and spasmolytics**

√5ᵗʰ **T44.4** **Poisoning by, adverse effect of and underdosing of predominantly alpha-adrenoreceptor agonists**
Poisoning by, adverse effect of and underdosing of metaraminol

  √6ᵗʰ **T44.4X** **Poisoning by, adverse effect of and underdosing of predominantly alpha-adrenoreceptor agonists**

    √7ᵗʰ **T44.4X1** **Poisoning by predominantly alpha-adrenoreceptor agonists, accidental (unintentional)**
Poisoning by predominantly alpha-adrenoreceptor agonists NOS

    ² √7ᵗʰ **T44.4X2** **Poisoning by predominantly alpha-adrenoreceptor agonists, intentional self-harm**   HCC

    √7ᵗʰ **T44.4X3** **Poisoning by predominantly alpha-adrenoreceptor agonists, assault**

    √7ᵗʰ **T44.4X4** **Poisoning by predominantly alpha-adrenoreceptor agonists, undetermined**

    √7ᵗʰ **T44.4X5** **Adverse effect of predominantly alpha-adrenoreceptor agonists**

    √7ᵗʰ **T44.4X6** **Underdosing of predominantly alpha-adrenoreceptor agonists**

√5ᵗʰ **T44.5** **Poisoning by, adverse effect of and underdosing of predominantly beta-adrenoreceptor agonists**

   EXCLUDES 1   *poisoning by, adverse effect of and underdosing of beta-adrenoreceptor agonists used in asthma therapy (T48.6-)*

  √6ᵗʰ **T44.5X** **Poisoning by, adverse effect of and underdosing of predominantly beta-adrenoreceptor agonists**

    √7ᵗʰ **T44.5X1** **Poisoning by predominantly beta-adrenoreceptor agonists, accidental (unintentional)**
Poisoning by predominantly beta-adrenoreceptor agonists NOS

    ² √7ᵗʰ **T44.5X2** **Poisoning by predominantly beta-adrenoreceptor agonists, intentional self-harm**   HCC

    √7ᵗʰ **T44.5X3** **Poisoning by predominantly beta-adrenoreceptor agonists, assault**

    √7ᵗʰ **T44.5X4** **Poisoning by predominantly beta-adrenoreceptor agonists, undetermined**

    √7ᵗʰ **T44.5X5** **Adverse effect of predominantly beta-adrenoreceptor agonists**

    √7ᵗʰ **T44.5X6** **Underdosing of predominantly beta-adrenoreceptor agonists**

√5ᵗʰ **T44.6** **Poisoning by, adverse effect of and underdosing of alpha-adrenoreceptor antagonists**

   EXCLUDES 1   *poisoning by, adverse effect of and underdosing of ergot alkaloids (T48.0)*

  √6ᵗʰ **T44.6X** **Poisoning by, adverse effect of and underdosing of alpha-adrenoreceptor antagonists**

    √7ᵗʰ **T44.6X1** **Poisoning by alpha-adrenoreceptor antagonists, accidental (unintentional)**
Poisoning by alpha-adrenoreceptor antagonists NOS

    ² √7ᵗʰ **T44.6X2** **Poisoning by alpha-adrenoreceptor antagonists, intentional self-harm**   HCC

    √7ᵗʰ **T44.6X3** **Poisoning by alpha-adrenoreceptor antagonists, assault**

    √7ᵗʰ **T44.6X4** **Poisoning by alpha-adrenoreceptor antagonists, undetermined**

    √7ᵗʰ **T44.6X5** **Adverse effect of alpha-adrenoreceptor antagonists**

    √7ᵗʰ **T44.6X6** **Underdosing of alpha-adrenoreceptor antagonists**

√5ᵗʰ **T44.7** **Poisoning by, adverse effect of and underdosing of beta-adrenoreceptor antagonists**

  √6ᵗʰ **T44.7X** **Poisoning by, adverse effect of and underdosing of beta-adrenoreceptor antagonists**

    √7ᵗʰ **T44.7X1** **Poisoning by beta-adrenoreceptor antagonists, accidental (unintentional)**
Poisoning by beta-adrenoreceptor antagonists NOS

    ² √7ᵗʰ **T44.7X2** **Poisoning by beta-adrenoreceptor antagonists, intentional self-harm**   HCC

    √7ᵗʰ **T44.7X3** **Poisoning by beta-adrenoreceptor antagonists, assault**

    √7ᵗʰ **T44.7X4** **Poisoning by beta-adrenoreceptor antagonists, undetermined**

    √7ᵗʰ **T44.7X5** **Adverse effect of beta-adrenoreceptor antagonists**

    √7ᵗʰ **T44.7X6** **Underdosing of beta-adrenoreceptor antagonists**

√ Additional Character Req   √x7ᵗʰ Placeholder Alert   Manifestation   ▽ Unspecified   ►◄ Revised Text   ● New Code   ▲ Revised Code Title

Chapter 19. Injury, Poisoning and Certain Other Consequences of External Causes

√5ᵗʰ **T44.8 Poisoning by, adverse effect of and underdosing of centrally-acting and adrenergic-neuron- blocking agents**

> EXCLUDES 1   poisoning by, adverse effect of and underdosing of clonidine (T46.5)
>
> poisoning by, adverse effect of and underdosing of guanethidine (T46.5)

√6ᵗʰ **T44.8X Poisoning by, adverse effect of and underdosing of centrally-acting and adrenergic- neuron-blocking agents**

√7ᵗʰ **T44.8X1 Poisoning by centrally-acting and adrenergic-neuron-blocking agents, accidental (unintentional)**

> Poisoning by centrally-acting and adrenergic-neuron-blocking agents NOS

² √7ᵗʰ **T44.8X2 Poisoning by centrally-acting and adrenergic-neuron-blocking agents, intentional self-harm**   HCC

√7ᵗʰ **T44.8X3 Poisoning by centrally-acting and adrenergic-neuron-blocking agents, assault**

√7ᵗʰ **T44.8X4 Poisoning by centrally-acting and adrenergic-neuron-blocking agents, undetermined**

√7ᵗʰ **T44.8X5 Adverse effect of centrally-acting and adrenergic-neuron-blocking agents**

√7ᵗʰ **T44.8X6 Underdosing of centrally-acting and adrenergic-neuron-blocking agents**

√5ᵗʰ **T44.9 Poisoning by, adverse effect of and underdosing of other and unspecified drugs primarily affecting the autonomic nervous system**

> Poisoning by, adverse effect of and underdosing of drug stimulating both alpha and beta-adrenoreceptors

√6ᵗʰ **T44.90 Poisoning by, adverse effect of and underdosing of unspecified drugs primarily affecting the autonomic nervous system**

√7ᵗʰ **T44.901 Poisoning by unspecified drugs primarily affecting the autonomic nervous system, accidental (unintentional)**   ▽

> Poisoning by unspecified drugs primarily affecting the autonomic nervous system NOS

² √7ᵗʰ **T44.902 Poisoning by unspecified drugs primarily affecting the autonomic nervous system, intentional self-harm**   HCC ▽

√7ᵗʰ **T44.903 Poisoning by unspecified drugs primarily affecting the autonomic nervous system, assault**   ▽

√7ᵗʰ **T44.904 Poisoning by unspecified drugs primarily affecting the autonomic nervous system, undetermined**   ▽

√7ᵗʰ **T44.905 Adverse effect of unspecified drugs primarily affecting the autonomic nervous system**   ▽

√7ᵗʰ **T44.906 Underdosing of unspecified drugs primarily affecting the autonomic nervous system**   ▽

√6ᵗʰ **T44.99 Poisoning by, adverse effect of and underdosing of other drugs primarily affecting the autonomic nervous system**

√7ᵗʰ **T44.991 Poisoning by other drug primarily affecting the autonomic nervous system, accidental (unintentional)**

> Poisoning by other drugs primarily affecting the autonomic nervous system NOS

² √7ᵗʰ **T44.992 Poisoning by other drug primarily affecting the autonomic nervous system, intentional self-harm**   HCC

√7ᵗʰ **T44.993 Poisoning by other drug primarily affecting the autonomic nervous system, assault**

√7ᵗʰ **T44.994 Poisoning by other drug primarily affecting the autonomic nervous system, undetermined**

√7ᵗʰ **T44.995 Adverse effect of other drug primarily affecting the autonomic nervous system**

√7ᵗʰ **T44.996 Underdosing of other drug primarily affecting the autonomic nervous system**

√4ᵗʰ **T45 Poisoning by, adverse effect of and underdosing of primarily systemic and hematological agents, not elsewhere classified**

> The appropriate 7th character is to be added to each code from category T45.
> A   initial encounter
> D   subsequent encounter
> S   sequela

√5ᵗʰ **T45.0 Poisoning by, adverse effect of and underdosing of antiallergic and antiemetic drugs**

> EXCLUDES 1   poisoning by, adverse effect of and underdosing of phenothiazine-based neuroleptics (T43.3)

√6ᵗʰ **T45.0X Poisoning by, adverse effect of and underdosing of antiallergic and antiemetic drugs**

√7ᵗʰ **T45.0X1 Poisoning by antiallergic and antiemetic drugs, accidental (unintentional)**

> Poisoning by antiallergic and antiemetic drugs NOS

² √7ᵗʰ **T45.0X2 Poisoning by antiallergic and antiemetic drugs, intentional self-harm**   HCC

√7ᵗʰ **T45.0X3 Poisoning by antiallergic and antiemetic drugs, assault**

√7ᵗʰ **T45.0X4 Poisoning by antiallergic and antiemetic drugs, undetermined**

√7ᵗʰ **T45.0X5 Adverse effect of antiallergic and antiemetic drugs**

√7ᵗʰ **T45.0X6 Underdosing of antiallergic and antiemetic drugs**

√5ᵗʰ **T45.1 Poisoning by, adverse effect of and underdosing of antineoplastic and immunosuppressive drugs**

> EXCLUDES 1   poisoning by, adverse effect of and underdosing of tamoxifen (T38.6)

> AHA: 2014,4Q,22

√6ᵗʰ **T45.1X Poisoning by, adverse effect of and underdosing of antineoplastic and immunosuppressive drugs**

√7ᵗʰ **T45.1X1 Poisoning by antineoplastic and immunosuppressive drugs, accidental (unintentional)**

> Poisoning by antineoplastic and immunosuppressive drugs NOS

² √7ᵗʰ **T45.1X2 Poisoning by antineoplastic and immunosuppressive drugs, intentional self-harm**   HCC

√7ᵗʰ **T45.1X3 Poisoning by antineoplastic and immunosuppressive drugs, assault**

√7ᵗʰ **T45.1X4 Poisoning by antineoplastic and immunosuppressive drugs, undetermined**

√7ᵗʰ **T45.1X5 Adverse effect of antineoplastic and immunosuppressive drugs**

√7ᵗʰ **T45.1X6 Underdosing of antineoplastic and immunosuppressive drugs**

√5ᵗʰ **T45.2 Poisoning by, adverse effect of and underdosing of vitamins**

> EXCLUDES 2   poisoning by, adverse effect of and underdosing of iron (T45.4)
>
> poisoning by, adverse effect of and underdosing of nicotinic acid (derivatives) (T46.7)
>
> poisoning by, adverse effect of and underdosing of vitamin K (T45.7)

√6ᵗʰ **T45.2X Poisoning by, adverse effect of and underdosing of vitamins**

√7ᵗʰ **T45.2X1 Poisoning by vitamins, accidental (unintentional)**

> Poisoning by vitamins NOS

² √7ᵗʰ **T45.2X2 Poisoning by vitamins, intentional self-harm**   HCC

√7ᵗʰ **T45.2X3 Poisoning by vitamins, assault**

√7ᵗʰ **T45.2X4 Poisoning by vitamins, undetermined**

√7ᵗʰ **T45.2X5 Adverse effect of vitamins**

√7ᵗʰ **T45.2X6 Underdosing of vitamins**

> EXCLUDES 1   vitamin deficiencies (E50-E56)

√5ᵗʰ **T45.3 Poisoning by, adverse effect of and underdosing of enzymes**

√6ᵗʰ **T45.3X Poisoning by, adverse effect of and underdosing of enzymes**

√7ᵗʰ **T45.3X1 Poisoning by enzymes, accidental (unintentional)**

> Poisoning by enzymes NOS

² √7ᵗʰ **T45.3X2 Poisoning by enzymes, intentional self-harm**   HCC

√7ᵗʰ **T45.3X3 Poisoning by enzymes, assault**

☑7ᵗʰ **T45.3X4** **Poisoning by enzymes,** undetermined

☑7ᵗʰ **T45.3X5** **Adverse effect** of enzymes

☑7ᵗʰ **T45.3X6** **Underdosing** of enzymes

☑5ᵗʰ **T45.4** **Poisoning by, adverse effect of and underdosing of iron and its compounds**

  ☑6ᵗʰ **T45.4X** **Poisoning by, adverse effect of and underdosing of iron and its compounds**

    ☑7ᵗʰ **T45.4X1** **Poisoning by iron and its compounds,** accidental **(unintentional)**

        Poisoning by iron and its compounds NOS

    ² ☑7ᵗʰ **T45.4X2** **Poisoning by iron and its compounds, intentional self-harm** ᴴᶜᶜ

    ☑7ᵗʰ **T45.4X3** **Poisoning by iron and its compounds, assault**

    ☑7ᵗʰ **T45.4X4** **Poisoning by iron and its compounds, undetermined**

    ☑7ᵗʰ **T45.4X5** **Adverse effect** of iron and its compounds

    ☑7ᵗʰ **T45.4X6** **Underdosing** of iron and its compounds

        EXCLUDES 1   iron deficiency (E61.1)

☑5ᵗʰ **T45.5** **Poisoning by, adverse effect of and underdosing of anticoagulants and antithrombotic drugs**

  ☑6ᵗʰ **T45.51** **Poisoning by, adverse effect of and underdosing of anticoagulants**

    ☑7ᵗʰ **T45.511** **Poisoning by anticoagulants,** accidental **(unintentional)**

        Poisoning by anticoagulants NOS

    ² ☑7ᵗʰ **T45.512** **Poisoning by anticoagulants, intentional self-harm** ᴴᶜᶜ

    ☑7ᵗʰ **T45.513** **Poisoning by anticoagulants, assault**

    ☑7ᵗʰ **T45.514** **Poisoning by anticoagulants, undetermined**

    ☑7ᵗʰ **T45.515** **Adverse effect** of anticoagulants

        AHA: 2016,1Q,14; 2013,2Q,34

    ☑7ᵗʰ **T45.516** **Underdosing** of anticoagulants

  ☑6ᵗʰ **T45.52** **Poisoning by, adverse effect of and underdosing of antithrombotic drugs**

    Poisoning by, adverse effect of and underdosing of antiplatelet drugs

    EXCLUDES 2   poisoning by, adverse effect of and underdosing of aspirin (T39.Ø1-)

               poisoning by, adverse effect of and underdosing of acetylsalicylic acid (T39.Ø1-)

    ☑7ᵗʰ **T45.521** **Poisoning by antithrombotic drugs,** accidental **(unintentional)**

        Poisoning by antithrombotic drug NOS

    ² ☑7ᵗʰ **T45.522** **Poisoning by antithrombotic drugs, intentional self-harm** ᴴᶜᶜ

    ☑7ᵗʰ **T45.523** **Poisoning by antithrombotic drugs, assault**

    ☑7ᵗʰ **T45.524** **Poisoning by antithrombotic drugs, undetermined**

    ☑7ᵗʰ **T45.525** **Adverse effect** of antithrombotic drugs

        AHA: 2016,1Q,15

    ☑7ᵗʰ **T45.526** **Underdosing** of antithrombotic drugs

☑5ᵗʰ **T45.6** **Poisoning by, adverse effect of and underdosing of fibrinolysis-affecting drugs**

  ☑6ᵗʰ **T45.6Ø** **Poisoning by, adverse effect of and underdosing of unspecified fibrinolysis-affecting drugs**

    ☑7ᵗʰ **T45.6Ø1** **Poisoning by unspecified fibrinolysis-affecting drugs, accidental (unintentional)** ▽

        Poisoning by fibrinolysis-affecting drug NOS

    ² ☑7ᵗʰ **T45.6Ø2** **Poisoning by unspecified fibrinolysis-affecting drugs, intentional self-harm** ᴴᶜᶜ ▽

    ☑7ᵗʰ **T45.6Ø3** **Poisoning by unspecified fibrinolysis-affecting drugs, assault** ▽

    ☑7ᵗʰ **T45.6Ø4** **Poisoning by unspecified fibrinolysis-affecting drugs, undetermined** ▽

    ☑7ᵗʰ **T45.6Ø5** **Adverse effect** of unspecified fibrinolysis-affecting drugs ▽

    ☑7ᵗʰ **T45.6Ø6** **Underdosing** of unspecified fibrinolysis-affecting drugs ▽

  ☑6ᵗʰ **T45.61** **Poisoning by, adverse effect of and underdosing of thrombolytic drugs**

    ☑7ᵗʰ **T45.611** **Poisoning by thrombolytic drug, accidental (unintentional)**

        Poisoning by thrombolytic drug NOS

    ² ☑7ᵗʰ **T45.612** **Poisoning by thrombolytic drug, intentional self-harm** ᴴᶜᶜ

    ☑7ᵗʰ **T45.613** **Poisoning by thrombolytic drug,** assault

    ☑7ᵗʰ **T45.614** **Poisoning by thrombolytic drug, undetermined**

    ☑7ᵗʰ **T45.615** **Adverse effect** of thrombolytic drugs

        AHA: 2017,2Q,9

    ☑7ᵗʰ **T45.616** **Underdosing** of thrombolytic drugs

  ☑6ᵗʰ **T45.62** **Poisoning by, adverse effect of and underdosing of hemostatic drugs**

    ☑7ᵗʰ **T45.621** **Poisoning by hemostatic drug, accidental (unintentional)**

        Poisoning by hemostatic drug NOS

    ² ☑7ᵗʰ **T45.622** **Poisoning by hemostatic drug, intentional self-harm** ᴴᶜᶜ

    ☑7ᵗʰ **T45.623** **Poisoning by hemostatic drug,** assault

    ☑7ᵗʰ **T45.624** **Poisoning by hemostatic drug, undetermined**

    ☑7ᵗʰ **T45.625** **Adverse effect** of hemostatic drug

    ☑7ᵗʰ **T45.626** **Underdosing** of hemostatic drugs

  ☑6ᵗʰ **T45.69** **Poisoning by, adverse effect of and underdosing of other fibrinolysis-affecting drugs**

    ☑7ᵗʰ **T45.691** **Poisoning by other fibrinolysis-affecting drugs,** accidental **(unintentional)**

        Poisoning by other fibrinolysis-affecting drug NOS

    ² ☑7ᵗʰ **T45.692** **Poisoning by other fibrinolysis-affecting drugs, intentional self-harm** ᴴᶜᶜ

    ☑7ᵗʰ **T45.693** **Poisoning by other fibrinolysis-affecting drugs, assault**

    ☑7ᵗʰ **T45.694** **Poisoning by other fibrinolysis-affecting drugs, undetermined**

    ☑7ᵗʰ **T45.695** **Adverse effect** of other fibrinolysis-affecting drugs

    ☑7ᵗʰ **T45.696** **Underdosing** of other fibrinolysis-affecting drugs

☑5ᵗʰ **T45.7** **Poisoning by, adverse effect of and underdosing of anticoagulant antagonists, vitamin K and other coagulants**

  ☑6ᵗʰ **T45.7X** **Poisoning by, adverse effect of and underdosing of anticoagulant antagonists, vitamin K and other coagulants**

    ☑7ᵗʰ **T45.7X1** **Poisoning by anticoagulant antagonists, vitamin K and other coagulants, accidental (unintentional)**

        Poisoning by anticoagulant antagonists, vitamin K and other coagulants NOS

    ² ☑7ᵗʰ **T45.7X2** **Poisoning by anticoagulant antagonists, vitamin K and other coagulants,** intentional self-harm ᴴᶜᶜ

    ☑7ᵗʰ **T45.7X3** **Poisoning by anticoagulant antagonists, vitamin K and other coagulants,** assault

    ☑7ᵗʰ **T45.7X4** **Poisoning by anticoagulant antagonists, vitamin K and other coagulants, undetermined**

    ☑7ᵗʰ **T45.7X5** **Adverse effect** of anticoagulant antagonists, vitamin K and other coagulants

    ☑7ᵗʰ **T45.7X6** **Underdosing** of anticoagulant antagonist, vitamin K and other coagulants

        EXCLUDES 1   vitamin K deficiency (E56.1)

☑ Additional Character Req   ☑✗7ᵗʰ Placeholder Alert   Manifestation   ▽ Unspecified   ►◄ Revised Text   ● New Code   ▲ Revised Code Title

ICD-10-CM 2019   **1107**

√5ᵗʰ **T45.8** **Poisoning by, adverse effect of and underdosing of other primarily systemic and hematological agents**

Poisoning by, adverse effect of and underdosing of liver preparations and other antianemic agents

Poisoning by, adverse effect of and underdosing of natural blood and blood products

Poisoning by, adverse effect of and underdosing of plasma substitute

EXCLUDES 2   *poisoning by, adverse effect of and underdosing of immunoglobulin (T50.Z1)*

poisoning by, adverse effect of and underdosing of iron (T45.4)

transfusion reactions (T80.-)

√6ᵗʰ **T45.8X** **Poisoning by, adverse effect of and underdosing of other primarily systemic and hematological agents**

√7ᵗʰ **T45.8X1** **Poisoning by other primarily systemic and hematological agents, accidental (unintentional)**

Poisoning by other primarily systemic and hematological agents NOS

2 √7ᵗʰ **T45.8X2** **Poisoning by other primarily systemic and hematological agents, intentional self-harm** HCC

√7ᵗʰ **T45.8X3** **Poisoning by other primarily systemic and hematological agents, assault**

√7ᵗʰ **T45.8X4** **Poisoning by other primarily systemic and hematological agents, undetermined**

√7ᵗʰ **T45.8X5** **Adverse effect of other primarily systemic and hematological agents**

AHA: 2016,4Q,42

√7ᵗʰ **T45.8X6** **Underdosing of other primarily systemic and hematological agents**

√5ᵗʰ **T45.9** **Poisoning by, adverse effect of and underdosing of unspecified primarily systemic and hematological agent**

√x7ᵗʰ **T45.91** **Poisoning by unspecified primarily systemic and hematological agent, accidental (unintentional)** ▽

Poisoning by primarily systemic and hematological agent NOS

2 √x7ᵗʰ **T45.92** **Poisoning by unspecified primarily systemic and hematological agent, intentional self-harm** HCC ▽

√x7ᵗʰ **T45.93** **Poisoning by unspecified primarily systemic and hematological agent, assault** ▽

√x7ᵗʰ **T45.94** **Poisoning by unspecified primarily systemic and hematological agent, undetermined** ▽

√x7ᵗʰ **T45.95** **Adverse effect of unspecified primarily systemic and hematological agent** ▽

√x7ᵗʰ **T45.96** **Underdosing of unspecified primarily systemic and hematological agent** ▽

√4ᵗʰ **T46** **Poisoning by, adverse effect of and underdosing of agents primarily affecting the cardiovascular system**

EXCLUDES 1   *poisoning by, adverse effect of and underdosing of metaraminol (T44.4)*

The appropriate 7th character is to be added to each code from category T46.

A   initial encounter
D   subsequent encounter
S   sequela

√5ᵗʰ **T46.0** **Poisoning by, adverse effect of and underdosing of cardiac-stimulant glycosides and drugs of similar action**

√6ᵗʰ **T46.0X** **Poisoning by, adverse effect of and underdosing of cardiac-stimulant glycosides and drugs of similar action**

√7ᵗʰ **T46.0X1** **Poisoning by cardiac-stimulant glycosides and drugs of similar action, accidental (unintentional)**

Poisoning by cardiac-stimulant glycosides and drugs of similar action NOS

2 √7ᵗʰ **T46.0X2** **Poisoning by cardiac-stimulant glycosides and drugs of similar action, intentional self-harm** HCC

√7ᵗʰ **T46.0X3** **Poisoning by cardiac-stimulant glycosides and drugs of similar action, assault**

√7ᵗʰ **T46.0X4** **Poisoning by cardiac-stimulant glycosides and drugs of similar action, undetermined**

√7ᵗʰ **T46.0X5** **Adverse effect of cardiac-stimulant glycosides and drugs of similar action**

√7ᵗʰ **T46.0X6** **Underdosing of cardiac-stimulant glycosides and drugs of similar action**

√5ᵗʰ **T46.1** **Poisoning by, adverse effect of and underdosing of calcium-channel blockers**

√6ᵗʰ **T46.1X** **Poisoning by, adverse effect of and underdosing of calcium-channel blockers**

√7ᵗʰ **T46.1X1** **Poisoning by calcium-channel blockers, accidental (unintentional)**

Poisoning by calcium-channel blockers NOS

2 √7ᵗʰ **T46.1X2** **Poisoning by calcium-channel blockers, intentional self-harm** HCC

√7ᵗʰ **T46.1X3** **Poisoning by calcium-channel blockers, assault**

√7ᵗʰ **T46.1X4** **Poisoning by calcium-channel blockers, undetermined**

√7ᵗʰ **T46.1X5** **Adverse effect of calcium-channel blockers**

√7ᵗʰ **T46.1X6** **Underdosing of calcium-channel blockers**

√5ᵗʰ **T46.2** **Poisoning by, adverse effect of and underdosing of other antidysrhythmic drugs, not elsewhere classified**

EXCLUDES 1   *poisoning by, adverse effect of and underdosing of beta-adrenoreceptor antagonists (T44.7-)*

√6ᵗʰ **T46.2X** **Poisoning by, adverse effect of and underdosing of other antidysrhythmic drugs**

√7ᵗʰ **T46.2X1** **Poisoning by other antidysrhythmic drugs, accidental (unintentional)**

Poisoning by other antidysrhythmic drugs NOS

2 √7ᵗʰ **T46.2X2** **Poisoning by other antidysrhythmic drugs, intentional self-harm** HCC

√7ᵗʰ **T46.2X3** **Poisoning by other antidysrhythmic drugs, assault**

√7ᵗʰ **T46.2X4** **Poisoning by other antidysrhythmic drugs, undetermined**

√7ᵗʰ **T46.2X5** **Adverse effect of other antidysrhythmic drugs**

√7ᵗʰ **T46.2X6** **Underdosing of other antidysrhythmic drugs**

√5ᵗʰ **T46.3** **Poisoning by, adverse effect of and underdosing of coronary vasodilators**

Poisoning by, adverse effect of and underdosing of dipyridamole

EXCLUDES 1   *poisoning by, adverse effect of and underdosing of calcium-channel blockers (T46.1)*

√6ᵗʰ **T46.3X** **Poisoning by, adverse effect of and underdosing of coronary vasodilators**

√7ᵗʰ **T46.3X1** **Poisoning by coronary vasodilators, accidental (unintentional)**

Poisoning by coronary vasodilators NOS

2 √7ᵗʰ **T46.3X2** **Poisoning by coronary vasodilators, intentional self-harm** HCC

√7ᵗʰ **T46.3X3** **Poisoning by coronary vasodilators, assault**

√7ᵗʰ **T46.3X4** **Poisoning by coronary vasodilators, undetermined**

√7ᵗʰ **T46.3X5** **Adverse effect of coronary vasodilators**

√7ᵗʰ **T46.3X6** **Underdosing of coronary vasodilators**

√5ᵗʰ **T46.4** **Poisoning by, adverse effect of and underdosing of angiotensin-converting-enzyme inhibitors**

√6ᵗʰ **T46.4X** **Poisoning by, adverse effect of and underdosing of angiotensin-converting-enzyme inhibitors**

√7ᵗʰ **T46.4X1** **Poisoning by angiotensin-converting-enzyme inhibitors, accidental (unintentional)**

Poisoning by angiotensin-converting-enzyme inhibitors NOS

2 √7ᵗʰ **T46.4X2** **Poisoning by angiotensin-converting-enzyme inhibitors, intentional self-harm** HCC

√7ᵗʰ **T46.4X3** **Poisoning by angiotensin-converting-enzyme inhibitors, assault**

√7ᵗʰ **T46.4X4** **Poisoning by angiotensin-converting-enzyme inhibitors, undetermined**

√7ᵗʰ **T46.4X5** **Adverse effect of angiotensin-converting-enzyme inhibitors**

√7ᵗʰ **T46.4X6** Underdosing of angiotensin-converting-enzyme inhibitors

√5ᵗʰ **T46.5** Poisoning by, adverse effect of and underdosing of other antihypertensive drugs

EXCLUDES 2 *poisoning by, adverse effect of and underdosing of beta-adrenoreceptor antagonists (T44.7)*
poisoning by, adverse effect of and underdosing of calcium-channel blockers (T46.1)
poisoning by, adverse effect of and underdosing of diuretics (T50.0-T50.2)

√6ᵗʰ **T46.5X** Poisoning by, adverse effect of and underdosing of other antihypertensive drugs

√7ᵗʰ **T46.5X1** Poisoning by other antihypertensive drugs, accidental (unintentional)
Poisoning by other antihypertensive drugs NOS

2 √7ᵗʰ **T46.5X2** Poisoning by other antihypertensive drugs, intentional self-harm HCC

√7ᵗʰ **T46.5X3** Poisoning by other antihypertensive drugs, assault

√7ᵗʰ **T46.5X4** Poisoning by other antihypertensive drugs, undetermined

√7ᵗʰ **T46.5X5** Adverse effect of other antihypertensive drugs

√7ᵗʰ **T46.5X6** Underdosing of other antihypertensive drugs

√5ᵗʰ **T46.6** Poisoning by, adverse effect of and underdosing of antihyperlipidemic and antiarteriosclerotic drugs

√6ᵗʰ **T46.6X** Poisoning by, adverse effect of and underdosing of antihyperlipidemic and antiarteriosclerotic drugs

√7ᵗʰ **T46.6X1** Poisoning by antihyperlipidemic and antiarteriosclerotic drugs, accidental (unintentional)
Poisoning by antihyperlipidemic and antiarteriosclerotic drugs NOS

2 √7ᵗʰ **T46.6X2** Poisoning by antihyperlipidemic and antiarteriosclerotic drugs, intentional self-harm HCC

√7ᵗʰ **T46.6X3** Poisoning by antihyperlipidemic and antiarteriosclerotic drugs, assault

√7ᵗʰ **T46.6X4** Poisoning by antihyperlipidemic and antiarteriosclerotic drugs, undetermined

√7ᵗʰ **T46.6X5** Adverse effect of antihyperlipidemic and antiarteriosclerotic drugs

√7ᵗʰ **T46.6X6** Underdosing of antihyperlipidemic and antiarteriosclerotic drugs

√5ᵗʰ **T46.7** Poisoning by, adverse effect of and underdosing of peripheral vasodilators

Poisoning by, adverse effect of and underdosing of nicotinic acid (derivatives)

EXCLUDES 1 *poisoning by, adverse effect of and underdosing of papaverine (T44.3)*

√6ᵗʰ **T46.7X** Poisoning by, adverse effect of and underdosing of peripheral vasodilators

√7ᵗʰ **T46.7X1** Poisoning by peripheral vasodilators, accidental (unintentional)
Poisoning by peripheral vasodilators NOS

2 √7ᵗʰ **T46.7X2** Poisoning by peripheral vasodilators, intentional self-harm HCC

√7ᵗʰ **T46.7X3** Poisoning by peripheral vasodilators, assault

√7ᵗʰ **T46.7X4** Poisoning by peripheral vasodilators, undetermined

√7ᵗʰ **T46.7X5** Adverse effect of peripheral vasodilators

√7ᵗʰ **T46.7X6** Underdosing of peripheral vasodilators

√5ᵗʰ **T46.8** Poisoning by, adverse effect of and underdosing of antivaricose drugs, including sclerosing agents

√6ᵗʰ **T46.8X** Poisoning by, adverse effect of and underdosing of antivaricose drugs, including sclerosing agents

√7ᵗʰ **T46.8X1** Poisoning by antivaricose drugs, including sclerosing agents, accidental (unintentional)
Poisoning by antivaricose drugs, including sclerosing agents NOS

2 √7ᵗʰ **T46.8X2** Poisoning by antivaricose drugs, including sclerosing agents, intentional self-harm HCC

√7ᵗʰ **T46.8X3** Poisoning by antivaricose drugs, including sclerosing agents, assault

√7ᵗʰ **T46.8X4** Poisoning by antivaricose drugs, including sclerosing agents, undetermined

√7ᵗʰ **T46.8X5** Adverse effect of antivaricose drugs, including sclerosing agents

√7ᵗʰ **T46.8X6** Underdosing of antivaricose drugs, including sclerosing agents

√5ᵗʰ **T46.9** Poisoning by, adverse effect of and underdosing of other and unspecified agents primarily affecting the cardiovascular system

√6ᵗʰ **T46.90** Poisoning by, adverse effect of and underdosing of unspecified agents primarily affecting the cardiovascular system

√7ᵗʰ **T46.901** Poisoning by unspecified agents primarily affecting the cardiovascular system, accidental (unintentional) ▽

2 √7ᵗʰ **T46.902** Poisoning by unspecified agents primarily affecting the cardiovascular system, intentional self-harm HCC ▽

√7ᵗʰ **T46.903** Poisoning by unspecified agents primarily affecting the cardiovascular system, assault ▽

√7ᵗʰ **T46.904** Poisoning by unspecified agents primarily affecting the cardiovascular system, undetermined ▽

√7ᵗʰ **T46.905** Adverse effect of unspecified agents primarily affecting the cardiovascular system ▽

√7ᵗʰ **T46.906** Underdosing of unspecified agents primarily affecting the cardiovascular system ▽

√6ᵗʰ **T46.99** Poisoning by, adverse effect of and underdosing of other agents primarily affecting the cardiovascular system

√7ᵗʰ **T46.991** Poisoning by other agents primarily affecting the cardiovascular system, accidental (unintentional)

2 √7ᵗʰ **T46.992** Poisoning by other agents primarily affecting the cardiovascular system, intentional self-harm HCC

√7ᵗʰ **T46.993** Poisoning by other agents primarily affecting the cardiovascular system, assault

√7ᵗʰ **T46.994** Poisoning by other agents primarily affecting the cardiovascular system, undetermined

√7ᵗʰ **T46.995** Adverse effect of other agents primarily affecting the cardiovascular system

√7ᵗʰ **T46.996** Underdosing of other agents primarily affecting the cardiovascular system

√4ᵗʰ **T47** Poisoning by, adverse effect of and underdosing of agents primarily affecting the gastrointestinal system

The appropriate 7th character is to be added to each code from category T47.
A initial encounter
D subsequent encounter
S sequela

√5ᵗʰ **T47.0** Poisoning by, adverse effect of and underdosing of histamine H2-receptor blockers

√6ᵗʰ **T47.0X** Poisoning by, adverse effect of and underdosing of histamine H2-receptor blockers

√7ᵗʰ **T47.0X1** Poisoning by histamine H2-receptor blockers, accidental (unintentional)
Poisoning by histamine H2-receptor blockers NOS

2 √7ᵗʰ **T47.0X2** Poisoning by histamine H2-receptor blockers, intentional self-harm HCC

√7ᵗʰ **T47.0X3** Poisoning by histamine H2-receptor blockers, assault

√7ᵗʰ **T47.0X4** Poisoning by histamine H2-receptor blockers, undetermined

√7ᵗʰ **T47.0X5** Adverse effect of histamine H2-receptor blockers

√7ᵗʰ **T47.0X6** Underdosing of histamine H2-receptor blockers

Chapter 19. Injury, Poisoning and Certain Other Consequences of External Causes

T47.1–T47.96

√5ᵗʰ **T47.1** **Poisoning by, adverse effect of and underdosing of other antacids and anti-gastric-secretion drugs**

√6ᵗʰ **T47.1X** **Poisoning by, adverse effect of and underdosing of other antacids and anti-gastric-secretion drugs**

√7ᵗʰ **T47.1X1** **Poisoning by other antacids and anti-gastric-secretion drugs, accidental (unintentional)**
Poisoning by other antacids and anti-gastric-secretion drugs NOS

2 √7ᵗʰ **T47.1X2** **Poisoning by other antacids and anti-gastric-secretion drugs, intentional self-harm** HCC

√7ᵗʰ **T47.1X3** **Poisoning by other antacids and anti-gastric-secretion drugs, assault**

√7ᵗʰ **T47.1X4** **Poisoning by other antacids and anti-gastric-secretion drugs, undetermined**

√7ᵗʰ **T47.1X5** **Adverse effect of other antacids and anti-gastric-secretion drugs**

√7ᵗʰ **T47.1X6** **Underdosing of other antacids and anti-gastric-secretion drugs**

√5ᵗʰ **T47.2** **Poisoning by, adverse effect of and underdosing of stimulant laxatives**

√6ᵗʰ **T47.2X** **Poisoning by, adverse effect of and underdosing of stimulant laxatives**

√7ᵗʰ **T47.2X1** **Poisoning by stimulant laxatives, accidental (unintentional)**
Poisoning by stimulant laxatives NOS

2 √7ᵗʰ **T47.2X2** **Poisoning by stimulant laxatives, intentional self-harm** HCC

√7ᵗʰ **T47.2X3** **Poisoning by stimulant laxatives, assault**

√7ᵗʰ **T47.2X4** **Poisoning by stimulant laxatives, undetermined**

√7ᵗʰ **T47.2X5** **Adverse effect of stimulant laxatives**

√7ᵗʰ **T47.2X6** **Underdosing of stimulant laxatives**

√5ᵗʰ **T47.3** **Poisoning by, adverse effect of and underdosing of saline and osmotic laxatives**

√6ᵗʰ **T47.3X** **Poisoning by and adverse effect of saline and osmotic laxatives**

√7ᵗʰ **T47.3X1** **Poisoning by saline and osmotic laxatives, accidental (unintentional)**
Poisoning by saline and osmotic laxatives NOS

2 √7ᵗʰ **T47.3X2** **Poisoning by saline and osmotic laxatives, intentional self-harm** HCC

√7ᵗʰ **T47.3X3** **Poisoning by saline and osmotic laxatives, assault**

√7ᵗʰ **T47.3X4** **Poisoning by saline and osmotic laxatives, undetermined**

√7ᵗʰ **T47.3X5** **Adverse effect of saline and osmotic laxatives**

√7ᵗʰ **T47.3X6** **Underdosing of saline and osmotic laxatives**

√5ᵗʰ **T47.4** **Poisoning by, adverse effect of and underdosing of other laxatives**

√6ᵗʰ **T47.4X** **Poisoning by, adverse effect of and underdosing of other laxatives**

√7ᵗʰ **T47.4X1** **Poisoning by other laxatives, accidental (unintentional)**
Poisoning by other laxatives NOS

2 √7ᵗʰ **T47.4X2** **Poisoning by other laxatives, intentional self-harm** HCC

√7ᵗʰ **T47.4X3** **Poisoning by other laxatives, assault**

√7ᵗʰ **T47.4X4** **Poisoning by other laxatives, undetermined**

√7ᵗʰ **T47.4X5** **Adverse effect of other laxatives**

√7ᵗʰ **T47.4X6** **Underdosing of other laxatives**

√5ᵗʰ **T47.5** **Poisoning by, adverse effect of and underdosing of digestants**

√6ᵗʰ **T47.5X** **Poisoning by, adverse effect of and underdosing of digestants**

√7ᵗʰ **T47.5X1** **Poisoning by digestants, accidental (unintentional)**
Poisoning by digestants NOS

2 √7ᵗʰ **T47.5X2** **Poisoning by digestants, intentional self-harm** HCC

√7ᵗʰ **T47.5X3** **Poisoning by digestants, assault**

√7ᵗʰ **T47.5X4** **Poisoning by digestants, undetermined**

√7ᵗʰ **T47.5X5** **Adverse effect of digestants**

√7ᵗʰ **T47.5X6** **Underdosing of digestants**

√5ᵗʰ **T47.6** **Poisoning by, adverse effect of and underdosing of antidiarrheal drugs**

EXCLUDES 2   *poisoning by, adverse effect of and underdosing of systemic antibiotics and other anti-infectives (T36-T37)*

√6ᵗʰ **T47.6X** **Poisoning by, adverse effect of and underdosing of antidiarrheal drugs**

√7ᵗʰ **T47.6X1** **Poisoning by antidiarrheal drugs, accidental (unintentional)**
Poisoning by antidiarrheal drugs NOS

2 √7ᵗʰ **T47.6X2** **Poisoning by antidiarrheal drugs, intentional self-harm** HCC

√7ᵗʰ **T47.6X3** **Poisoning by antidiarrheal drugs, assault**

√7ᵗʰ **T47.6X4** **Poisoning by antidiarrheal drugs, undetermined**

√7ᵗʰ **T47.6X5** **Adverse effect of antidiarrheal drugs**

√7ᵗʰ **T47.6X6** **Underdosing of antidiarrheal drugs**

√5ᵗʰ **T47.7** **Poisoning by, adverse effect of and underdosing of emetics**

√6ᵗʰ **T47.7X** **Poisoning by, adverse effect of and underdosing of emetics**

√7ᵗʰ **T47.7X1** **Poisoning by emetics, accidental (unintentional)**
Poisoning by emetics NOS

2 √7ᵗʰ **T47.7X2** **Poisoning by emetics, intentional self-harm** HCC

√7ᵗʰ **T47.7X3** **Poisoning by emetics, assault**

√7ᵗʰ **T47.7X4** **Poisoning by emetics, undetermined**

√7ᵗʰ **T47.7X5** **Adverse effect of emetics**

√7ᵗʰ **T47.7X6** **Underdosing of emetics**

√5ᵗʰ **T47.8** **Poisoning by, adverse effect of and underdosing of other agents primarily affecting gastrointestinal system**

√6ᵗʰ **T47.8X** **Poisoning by, adverse effect of and underdosing of other agents primarily affecting gastrointestinal system**

√7ᵗʰ **T47.8X1** **Poisoning by other agents primarily affecting gastrointestinal system, accidental (unintentional)**
Poisoning by other agents primarily affecting gastrointestinal system NOS

2 √7ᵗʰ **T47.8X2** **Poisoning by other agents primarily affecting gastrointestinal system, intentional self-harm** HCC

√7ᵗʰ **T47.8X3** **Poisoning by other agents primarily affecting gastrointestinal system, assault**

√7ᵗʰ **T47.8X4** **Poisoning by other agents primarily affecting gastrointestinal system, undetermined**

√7ᵗʰ **T47.8X5** **Adverse effect of other agents primarily affecting gastrointestinal system**

√7ᵗʰ **T47.8X6** **Underdosing of other agents primarily affecting gastrointestinal system**

√5ᵗʰ **T47.9** **Poisoning by, adverse effect of and underdosing of unspecified agents primarily affecting the gastrointestinal system**

√7ᵗʰ **T47.91** **Poisoning by unspecified agents primarily affecting the gastrointestinal system, accidental (unintentional)** ▽
Poisoning by agents primarily affecting the gastrointestinal system NOS

2 √x7ᵗʰ **T47.92** **Poisoning by unspecified agents primarily affecting the gastrointestinal system, intentional self-harm** HCC ▽

√x7ᵗʰ **T47.93** **Poisoning by unspecified agents primarily affecting the gastrointestinal system, assault** ▽

√x7ᵗʰ **T47.94** **Poisoning by unspecified agents primarily affecting the gastrointestinal system, undetermined** ▽

√x7ᵗʰ **T47.95** **Adverse effect of unspecified agents primarily affecting the gastrointestinal system** ▽

√x7ᵗʰ **T47.96** **Underdosing of unspecified agents primarily affecting the gastrointestinal system** ▽

✓4ᵗʰ **T48** **Poisoning by, adverse effect of and underdosing of agents primarily acting on smooth and skeletal muscles and the respiratory system**

> The appropriate 7th character is to be added to each code from category T48.
> A initial encounter
> D subsequent encounter
> S sequela

✓5ᵗʰ **T48.0** **Poisoning by, adverse effect of and underdosing of oxytocic drugs**

> *EXCLUDES 1* poisoning by, adverse effect of and underdosing of estrogens, progestogens and antagonists (T38.4-T38.6)

 ✓6ᵗʰ **T48.0X** **Poisoning by, adverse effect of and underdosing of oxytocic drugs**

  ✓7ᵗʰ **T48.0X1** **Poisoning by oxytocic drugs, accidental (unintentional)**
   Poisoning by oxytocic drugs NOS

  ² ✓7ᵗʰ **T48.0X2** **Poisoning by oxytocic drugs, intentional self-harm** ᴴᶜᶜ

  ✓7ᵗʰ **T48.0X3** **Poisoning by oxytocic drugs, assault**

  ✓7ᵗʰ **T48.0X4** **Poisoning by oxytocic drugs, undetermined**

  ✓7ᵗʰ **T48.0X5** **Adverse effect of oxytocic drugs**

  ✓7ᵗʰ **T48.0X6** **Underdosing of oxytocic drugs**

✓5ᵗʰ **T48.1** **Poisoning by, adverse effect of and underdosing of skeletal muscle relaxants [neuromuscular blocking agents]**

 ✓6ᵗʰ **T48.1X** **Poisoning by, adverse effect of and underdosing of skeletal muscle relaxants [neuromuscular blocking agents]**

  ✓7ᵗʰ **T48.1X1** **Poisoning by skeletal muscle relaxants [neuromuscular blocking agents], accidental (unintentional)**
   Poisoning by skeletal muscle relaxants [neuromuscular blocking agents] NOS

  ² ✓7ᵗʰ **T48.1X2** **Poisoning by skeletal muscle relaxants [neuromuscular blocking agents], intentional self-harm** ᴴᶜᶜ

  ✓7ᵗʰ **T48.1X3** **Poisoning by skeletal muscle relaxants [neuromuscular blocking agents], assault**

  ✓7ᵗʰ **T48.1X4** **Poisoning by skeletal muscle relaxants [neuromuscular blocking agents], undetermined**

  ✓7ᵗʰ **T48.1X5** **Adverse effect of skeletal muscle relaxants [neuromuscular blocking agents]**

  ✓7ᵗʰ **T48.1X6** **Underdosing of skeletal muscle relaxants [neuromuscular blocking agents]**

✓5ᵗʰ **T48.2** **Poisoning by, adverse effect of and underdosing of other and unspecified drugs acting on muscles**

 ✓6ᵗʰ **T48.20** **Poisoning by, adverse effect of and underdosing of unspecified drugs acting on muscles**

  ✓7ᵗʰ **T48.201** **Poisoning by unspecified drugs acting on muscles, accidental (unintentional)** ▽
   Poisoning by unspecified drugs acting on muscles NOS

  ² ✓7ᵗʰ **T48.202** **Poisoning by unspecified drugs acting on muscles, intentional self-harm** ᴴᶜᶜ ▽

  ✓7ᵗʰ **T48.203** **Poisoning by unspecified drugs acting on muscles, assault** ▽

  ✓7ᵗʰ **T48.204** **Poisoning by unspecified drugs acting on muscles, undetermined** ▽

  ✓7ᵗʰ **T48.205** **Adverse effect of unspecified drugs acting on muscles** ▽

  ✓7ᵗʰ **T48.206** **Underdosing of unspecified drugs acting on muscles** ▽

 ✓6ᵗʰ **T48.29** **Poisoning by, adverse effect of and underdosing of other drugs acting on muscles**

  ✓7ᵗʰ **T48.291** **Poisoning by other drugs acting on muscles, accidental (unintentional)**
   Poisoning by other drugs acting on muscles NOS

  ² ✓7ᵗʰ **T48.292** **Poisoning by other drugs acting on muscles, intentional self-harm** ᴴᶜᶜ

  ✓7ᵗʰ **T48.293** **Poisoning by other drugs acting on muscles, assault**

  ✓7ᵗʰ **T48.294** **Poisoning by other drugs acting on muscles, undetermined**

  ✓7ᵗʰ **T48.295** **Adverse effect of other drugs acting on muscles**

  ✓7ᵗʰ **T48.296** **Underdosing of other drugs acting on muscles**

✓5ᵗʰ **T48.3** **Poisoning by, adverse effect of and underdosing of antitussives**

 ✓6ᵗʰ **T48.3X** **Poisoning by, adverse effect of and underdosing of antitussives**

  ✓7ᵗʰ **T48.3X1** **Poisoning by antitussives, accidental (unintentional)**
   Poisoning by antitussives NOS

  ² ✓7ᵗʰ **T48.3X2** **Poisoning by antitussives, intentional self-harm** ᴴᶜᶜ

  ✓7ᵗʰ **T48.3X3** **Poisoning by antitussives, assault**

  ✓7ᵗʰ **T48.3X4** **Poisoning by antitussives, undetermined**

  ✓7ᵗʰ **T48.3X5** **Adverse effect of antitussives**

  ✓7ᵗʰ **T48.3X6** **Underdosing of antitussives**

✓5ᵗʰ **T48.4** **Poisoning by, adverse effect of and underdosing of expectorants**

 ✓6ᵗʰ **T48.4X** **Poisoning by, adverse effect of and underdosing of expectorants**

  ✓7ᵗʰ **T48.4X1** **Poisoning by expectorants, accidental (unintentional)**
   Poisoning by expectorants NOS

  ² ✓7ᵗʰ **T48.4X2** **Poisoning by expectorants, intentional self-harm** ᴴᶜᶜ

  ✓7ᵗʰ **T48.4X3** **Poisoning by expectorants, assault**

  ✓7ᵗʰ **T48.4X4** **Poisoning by expectorants, undetermined**

  ✓7ᵗʰ **T48.4X5** **Adverse effect of expectorants**

  ✓7ᵗʰ **T48.4X6** **Underdosing of expectorants**

✓5ᵗʰ **T48.5** **Poisoning by, adverse effect of and underdosing of other anti-common-cold drugs**

> Poisoning by, adverse effect of and underdosing of decongestants
> *EXCLUDES 2* poisoning by, adverse effect of and underdosing of antipyretics, NEC (T39.9-)
> poisoning by, adverse effect of and underdosing of non-steroidal antiinflammatory drugs (T39.3-)
> poisoning by, adverse effect of and underdosing of salicylates (T39.0-)

 ✓6ᵗʰ **T48.5X** **Poisoning by, adverse effect of and underdosing of other anti-common-cold drugs**

  ✓7ᵗʰ **T48.5X1** **Poisoning by other anti-common-cold drugs, accidental (unintentional)**
   Poisoning by other anti-common-cold drugs NOS

  ² ✓7ᵗʰ **T48.5X2** **Poisoning by other anti-common-cold drugs, intentional self-harm** ᴴᶜᶜ

  ✓7ᵗʰ **T48.5X3** **Poisoning by other anti-common-cold drugs, assault**

  ✓7ᵗʰ **T48.5X4** **Poisoning by other anti-common-cold drugs, undetermined**

  ✓7ᵗʰ **T48.5X5** **Adverse effect of other anti-common-cold drugs**

  ✓7ᵗʰ **T48.5X6** **Underdosing of other anti-common-cold drugs**

✓5ᵗʰ **T48.6** **Poisoning by, adverse effect of and underdosing of antiasthmatics, not elsewhere classified**

> Poisoning by, adverse effect of and underdosing of beta-adrenoreceptor agonists used in asthma therapy
> *EXCLUDES 1* poisoning by, adverse effect of and underdosing of anterior pituitary [adenohypophyseal] hormones (T38.8)
> poisoning by, adverse effect of and underdosing of beta-adrenoreceptor agonists not used in asthma therapy (T44.5)

 ✓6ᵗʰ **T48.6X** **Poisoning by, adverse effect of and underdosing of antiasthmatics**

  ✓7ᵗʰ **T48.6X1** **Poisoning by antiasthmatics, accidental (unintentional)**
   Poisoning by antiasthmatics NOS

  ² ✓7ᵗʰ **T48.6X2** **Poisoning by antiasthmatics, intentional self-harm** ᴴᶜᶜ

  ✓7ᵗʰ **T48.6X3** **Poisoning by antiasthmatics, assault**

  ✓7ᵗʰ **T48.6X4** **Poisoning by antiasthmatics, undetermined**

  ✓7ᵗʰ **T48.6X5** **Adverse effect of antiasthmatics**

✓ Additional Character Req ✓x7ᵗʰ Placeholder Alert Manifestation ▽ Unspecified ►◄ Revised Text ● New Code ▲ Revised Code Title

✓7ᵗʰ **T48.6X6** Underdosing of antiasthmatics

✓5ᵗʰ **T48.9** Poisoning by, adverse effect of and underdosing of other and unspecified agents primarily acting on the respiratory system

     ✓6ᵗʰ **T48.90** Poisoning by, adverse effect of and underdosing of unspecified agents primarily acting on the respiratory system

         ✓7ᵗʰ **T48.901** Poisoning by unspecified agents primarily acting on the respiratory system, accidental (unintentional) ▽

         2 ✓7ᵗʰ **T48.902** Poisoning by unspecified agents primarily acting on the respiratory system, intentional self-harm   HCC ▽

         ✓7ᵗʰ **T48.903** Poisoning by unspecified agents primarily acting on the respiratory system, assault ▽

         ✓7ᵗʰ **T48.904** Poisoning by unspecified agents primarily acting on the respiratory system, undetermined ▽

         ✓7ᵗʰ **T48.905** Adverse effect of unspecified agents primarily acting on the respiratory system ▽

         ✓7ᵗʰ **T48.906** Underdosing of unspecified agents primarily acting on the respiratory system ▽

     ✓6ᵗʰ **T48.99** Poisoning by, adverse effect of and underdosing of other agents primarily acting on the respiratory system

         ✓7ᵗʰ **T48.991** Poisoning by other agents primarily acting on the respiratory system, accidental (unintentional)

         2 ✓7ᵗʰ **T48.992** Poisoning by other agents primarily acting on the respiratory system, intentional self-harm   HCC

         ✓7ᵗʰ **T48.993** Poisoning by other agents primarily acting on the respiratory system, assault

         ✓7ᵗʰ **T48.994** Poisoning by other agents primarily acting on the respiratory system, undetermined

         ✓7ᵗʰ **T48.995** Adverse effect of other agents primarily acting on the respiratory system

         ✓7ᵗʰ **T48.996** Underdosing of other agents primarily acting on the respiratory system

✓4ᵗʰ **T49** Poisoning by, adverse effect of and underdosing of topical agents primarily affecting skin and mucous membrane and by ophthalmological, otorhinolaryngological and dental drugs

     INCLUDES   poisoning by, adverse effect of and underdosing of glucocorticoids, topically used

> The appropriate 7th character is to be added to each code from category T49.
> A   initial encounter
> D   subsequent encounter
> S   sequela

✓5ᵗʰ **T49.0** Poisoning by, adverse effect of and underdosing of local antifungal, anti-infective and anti-inflammatory drugs

     ✓6ᵗʰ **T49.0X** Poisoning by, adverse effect of and underdosing of local antifungal, anti-infective and anti-inflammatory drugs

         ✓7ᵗʰ **T49.0X1** Poisoning by local antifungal, anti-infective and anti-inflammatory drugs, accidental (unintentional)
             Poisoning by local antifungal, anti-infective and anti-inflammatory drugs NOS

         2 ✓7ᵗʰ **T49.0X2** Poisoning by local antifungal, anti-infective and anti-inflammatory drugs, intentional self-harm   HCC

         ✓7ᵗʰ **T49.0X3** Poisoning by local antifungal, anti-infective and anti-inflammatory drugs, assault

         ✓7ᵗʰ **T49.0X4** Poisoning by local antifungal, anti-infective and anti-inflammatory drugs, undetermined

         ✓7ᵗʰ **T49.0X5** Adverse effect of local antifungal, anti-infective and anti-inflammatory drugs

         ✓7ᵗʰ **T49.0X6** Underdosing of local antifungal, anti-infective and anti-inflammatory drugs

✓5ᵗʰ **T49.1** Poisoning by, adverse effect of and underdosing of antipruritics

     ✓6ᵗʰ **T49.1X** Poisoning by, adverse effect of and underdosing of antipruritics

         ✓7ᵗʰ **T49.1X1** Poisoning by antipruritics, accidental (unintentional)
             Poisoning by antipruritics NOS

         2 ✓7ᵗʰ **T49.1X2** Poisoning by antipruritics, intentional self-harm   HCC

         ✓7ᵗʰ **T49.1X3** Poisoning by antipruritics, assault

         ✓7ᵗʰ **T49.1X4** Poisoning by antipruritics, undetermined

         ✓7ᵗʰ **T49.1X5** Adverse effect of antipruritics

         ✓7ᵗʰ **T49.1X6** Underdosing of antipruritics

✓5ᵗʰ **T49.2** Poisoning by, adverse effect of and underdosing of local astringents and local detergents

     ✓6ᵗʰ **T49.2X** Poisoning by, adverse effect of and underdosing of local astringents and local detergents

         ✓7ᵗʰ **T49.2X1** Poisoning by local astringents and local detergents, accidental (unintentional)
             Poisoning by local astringents and local detergents NOS

         2 ✓7ᵗʰ **T49.2X2** Poisoning by local astringents and local detergents, intentional self-harm   HCC

         ✓7ᵗʰ **T49.2X3** Poisoning by local astringents and local detergents, assault

         ✓7ᵗʰ **T49.2X4** Poisoning by local astringents and local detergents, undetermined

         ✓7ᵗʰ **T49.2X5** Adverse effect of local astringents and local detergents

         ✓7ᵗʰ **T49.2X6** Underdosing of local astringents and local detergents

✓5ᵗʰ **T49.3** Poisoning by, adverse effect of and underdosing of emollients, demulcents and protectants

     ✓6ᵗʰ **T49.3X** Poisoning by, adverse effect of and underdosing of emollients, demulcents and protectants

         ✓7ᵗʰ **T49.3X1** Poisoning by emollients, demulcents and protectants, accidental (unintentional)
             Poisoning by emollients, demulcents and protectants NOS

         2 ✓7ᵗʰ **T49.3X2** Poisoning by emollients, demulcents and protectants, intentional self-harm   HCC

         ✓7ᵗʰ **T49.3X3** Poisoning by emollients, demulcents and protectants, assault

         ✓7ᵗʰ **T49.3X4** Poisoning by emollients, demulcents and protectants, undetermined

         ✓7ᵗʰ **T49.3X5** Adverse effect of emollients, demulcents and protectants

         ✓7ᵗʰ **T49.3X6** Underdosing of emollients, demulcents and protectants

✓5ᵗʰ **T49.4** Poisoning by, adverse effect of and underdosing of keratolytics, keratoplastics, and other hair treatment drugs and preparations

     ✓6ᵗʰ **T49.4X** Poisoning by, adverse effect of and underdosing of keratolytics, keratoplastics, and other hair treatment drugs and preparations

         ✓7ᵗʰ **T49.4X1** Poisoning by keratolytics, keratoplastics, and other hair treatment drugs and preparations, accidental (unintentional)
             Poisoning by keratolytics, keratoplastics, and other hair treatment drugs and preparations NOS

         2 ✓7ᵗʰ **T49.4X2** Poisoning by keratolytics, keratoplastics, and other hair treatment drugs and preparations, intentional self-harm   HCC

         ✓7ᵗʰ **T49.4X3** Poisoning by keratolytics, keratoplastics, and other hair treatment drugs and preparations, assault

         ✓7ᵗʰ **T49.4X4** Poisoning by keratolytics, keratoplastics, and other hair treatment drugs and preparations, undetermined

         ✓7ᵗʰ **T49.4X5** Adverse effect of keratolytics, keratoplastics, and other hair treatment drugs and preparations

         ✓7ᵗʰ **T49.4X6** Underdosing of keratolytics, keratoplastics, and other hair treatment drugs and preparations

☑5ᵗʰ T49.5 Poisoning by, adverse effect of and underdosing of ophthalmological drugs and preparations

     ☑6ᵗʰ T49.5X Poisoning by, adverse effect of and underdosing of ophthalmological drugs and preparations

         ☑7ᵗʰ T49.5X1 Poisoning by ophthalmological drugs and preparations, accidental (unintentional)

             Poisoning by ophthalmological drugs and preparations NOS

         ² **☑7ᵗʰ T49.5X2** Poisoning by ophthalmological drugs and preparations, intentional self-harm   HCC

         ☑7ᵗʰ T49.5X3 Poisoning by ophthalmological drugs and preparations, assault

         ☑7ᵗʰ T49.5X4 Poisoning by ophthalmological drugs and preparations, undetermined

         ☑7ᵗʰ T49.5X5 Adverse effect of ophthalmological drugs and preparations

         ☑7ᵗʰ T49.5X6 Underdosing of ophthalmological drugs and preparations

☑5ᵗʰ T49.6 Poisoning by, adverse effect of and underdosing of otorhinolaryngological drugs and preparations

     ☑6ᵗʰ T49.6X Poisoning by, adverse effect of and underdosing of otorhinolaryngological drugs and preparations

         ☑7ᵗʰ T49.6X1 Poisoning by otorhinolaryngological drugs and preparations, accidental (unintentional)

             Poisoning by otorhinolaryngological drugs and preparations NOS

         ² **☑7ᵗʰ T49.6X2** Poisoning by otorhinolaryngological drugs and preparations, intentional self-harm   HCC

         ☑7ᵗʰ T49.6X3 Poisoning by otorhinolaryngological drugs and preparations, assault

         ☑7ᵗʰ T49.6X4 Poisoning by otorhinolaryngological drugs and preparations, undetermined

         ☑7ᵗʰ T49.6X5 Adverse effect of otorhinolaryngological drugs and preparations

         ☑7ᵗʰ T49.6X6 Underdosing of otorhinolaryngological drugs and preparations

☑5ᵗʰ T49.7 Poisoning by, adverse effect of and underdosing of dental drugs, topically applied

     ☑6ᵗʰ T49.7X Poisoning by, adverse effect of and underdosing of dental drugs, topically applied

         ☑7ᵗʰ T49.7X1 Poisoning by dental drugs, topically applied, accidental (unintentional)

             Poisoning by dental drugs, topically applied NOS

         ² **☑7ᵗʰ T49.7X2** Poisoning by dental drugs, topically applied, intentional self-harm   HCC

         ☑7ᵗʰ T49.7X3 Poisoning by dental drugs, topically applied, assault

         ☑7ᵗʰ T49.7X4 Poisoning by dental drugs, topically applied, undetermined

         ☑7ᵗʰ T49.7X5 Adverse effect of dental drugs, topically applied

         ☑7ᵗʰ T49.7X6 Underdosing of dental drugs, topically applied

☑5ᵗʰ T49.8 Poisoning by, adverse effect of and underdosing of other topical agents

     Poisoning by, adverse effect of and underdosing of spermicides

     ☑6ᵗʰ T49.8X Poisoning by, adverse effect of and underdosing of other topical agents

         ☑7ᵗʰ T49.8X1 Poisoning by other topical agents, accidental (unintentional)

             Poisoning by other topical agents NOS

         ² **☑7ᵗʰ T49.8X2** Poisoning by other topical agents, intentional self-harm   HCC

         ☑7ᵗʰ T49.8X3 Poisoning by other topical agents, assault

         ☑7ᵗʰ T49.8X4 Poisoning by other topical agents, undetermined

         ☑7ᵗʰ T49.8X5 Adverse effect of other topical agents

         ☑7ᵗʰ T49.8X6 Underdosing of other topical agents

☑5ᵗʰ T49.9 Poisoning by, adverse effect of and underdosing of unspecified topical agent

     ☑x7ᵗʰ T49.91 Poisoning by unspecified topical agent, accidental (unintentional)   ▽

     ² **☑x7ᵗʰ T49.92** Poisoning by unspecified topical agent, intentional self-harm   HCC ▽

     ☑x7ᵗʰ T49.93 Poisoning by unspecified topical agent, assault   ▽

     ☑x7ᵗʰ T49.94 Poisoning by unspecified topical agent, undetermined   ▽

     ☑x7ᵗʰ T49.95 Adverse effect of unspecified topical agent   ▽

     ☑x7ᵗʰ T49.96 Underdosing of unspecified topical agent   ▽

☑4ᵗʰ T50 Poisoning by, adverse effect of and underdosing of diuretics and other and unspecified drugs, medicaments and biological substances

> The appropriate 7th character is to be added to each code from category T50.
> A initial encounter
> D subsequent encounter
> S sequela

☑5ᵗʰ T50.0 Poisoning by, adverse effect of and underdosing of mineralocorticoids and their antagonists

     ☑6ᵗʰ T50.0X Poisoning by, adverse effect of and underdosing of mineralocorticoids and their antagonists

         ☑7ᵗʰ T50.0X1 Poisoning by mineralocorticoids and their antagonists, accidental (unintentional)

             Poisoning by mineralocorticoids and their antagonists NOS

         ² **☑7ᵗʰ T50.0X2** Poisoning by mineralocorticoids and their antagonists, intentional self-harm   HCC

         ☑7ᵗʰ T50.0X3 Poisoning by mineralocorticoids and their antagonists, assault

         ☑7ᵗʰ T50.0X4 Poisoning by mineralocorticoids and their antagonists, undetermined

         ☑7ᵗʰ T50.0X5 Adverse effect of mineralocorticoids and their antagonists

         ☑7ᵗʰ T50.0X6 Underdosing of mineralocorticoids and their antagonists

☑5ᵗʰ T50.1 Poisoning by, adverse effect of and underdosing of loop [high-ceiling] diuretics

     ☑6ᵗʰ T50.1X Poisoning by, adverse effect of and underdosing of loop [high-ceiling] diuretics

         ☑7ᵗʰ T50.1X1 Poisoning by loop [high-ceiling] diuretics, accidental (unintentional)

             Poisoning by loop [high-ceiling] diuretics NOS

         ² **☑7ᵗʰ T50.1X2** Poisoning by loop [high-ceiling] diuretics, intentional self-harm   HCC

         ☑7ᵗʰ T50.1X3 Poisoning by loop [high-ceiling] diuretics, assault

         ☑7ᵗʰ T50.1X4 Poisoning by loop [high-ceiling] diuretics, undetermined

         ☑7ᵗʰ T50.1X5 Adverse effect of loop [high-ceiling] diuretics

         ☑7ᵗʰ T50.1X6 Underdosing of loop [high-ceiling] diuretics

☑5ᵗʰ T50.2 Poisoning by, adverse effect of and underdosing of carbonic-anhydrase inhibitors, benzothiadiazides and other diuretics

     Poisoning by, adverse effect of and underdosing of acetazolamide

     ☑6ᵗʰ T50.2X Poisoning by, adverse effect of and underdosing of carbonic-anhydrase inhibitors, benzothiadiazides and other diuretics

         ☑7ᵗʰ T50.2X1 Poisoning by carbonic-anhydrase inhibitors, benzothiadiazides and other diuretics, accidental (unintentional)

             Poisoning by carbonic-anhydrase inhibitors, benzothiadiazides and other diuretics NOS

         ² **☑7ᵗʰ T50.2X2** Poisoning by carbonic-anhydrase inhibitors, benzothiadiazides and other diuretics, intentional self-harm   HCC

         ☑7ᵗʰ T50.2X3 Poisoning by carbonic-anhydrase inhibitors, benzothiadiazides and other diuretics, assault

         ☑7ᵗʰ T50.2X4 Poisoning by carbonic-anhydrase inhibitors, benzothiadiazides and other diuretics, undetermined

         ☑7ᵗʰ T50.2X5 Adverse effect of carbonic-anhydrase inhibitors, benzothiadiazides and other diuretics

         ☑7ᵗʰ T50.2X6 Underdosing of carbonic-anhydrase inhibitors, benzothiadiazides and other diuretics

---

☑ Additional Character Req   ☑x7ᵗʰ Placeholder Alert   Manifestation   ▽ Unspecified   ▶◀ Revised Text   ● New Code   ▲ Revised Code Title

√5ᵗʰ **T50.3 Poisoning by, adverse effect of and underdosing of electrolytic, caloric and water-balance agents**

Poisoning by, adverse effect of and underdosing of oral rehydration salts

√6ᵗʰ **T50.3X Poisoning by, adverse effect of and underdosing of electrolytic, caloric and water-balance agents**

√7ᵗʰ **T50.3X1 Poisoning by electrolytic, caloric and water-balance agents, accidental (unintentional)**

Poisoning by electrolytic, caloric and water-balance agents NOS

2 √7ᵗʰ **T50.3X2 Poisoning by electrolytic, caloric and water-balance agents, intentional self-harm** HCC

√7ᵗʰ **T50.3X3 Poisoning by electrolytic, caloric and water-balance agents, assault**

√7ᵗʰ **T50.3X4 Poisoning by electrolytic, caloric and water-balance agents, undetermined**

√7ᵗʰ **T50.3X5 Adverse effect of electrolytic, caloric and water-balance agents**

√7ᵗʰ **T50.3X6 Underdosing of electrolytic, caloric and water-balance agents**

√5ᵗʰ **T50.4 Poisoning by, adverse effect of and underdosing of drugs affecting uric acid metabolism**

√6ᵗʰ **T50.4X Poisoning by, adverse effect of and underdosing of drugs affecting uric acid metabolism**

√7ᵗʰ **T50.4X1 Poisoning by drugs affecting uric acid metabolism, accidental (unintentional)**

Poisoning by drugs affecting uric acid metabolism NOS

2 √7ᵗʰ **T50.4X2 Poisoning by drugs affecting uric acid metabolism, intentional self-harm** HCC

√7ᵗʰ **T50.4X3 Poisoning by drugs affecting uric acid metabolism, assault**

√7ᵗʰ **T50.4X4 Poisoning by drugs affecting uric acid metabolism, undetermined**

√7ᵗʰ **T50.4X5 Adverse effect of drugs affecting uric acid metabolism**

√7ᵗʰ **T50.4X6 Underdosing of drugs affecting uric acid metabolism**

√5ᵗʰ **T50.5 Poisoning by, adverse effect of and underdosing of appetite depressants**

√6ᵗʰ **T50.5X Poisoning by, adverse effect of and underdosing of appetite depressants**

√7ᵗʰ **T50.5X1 Poisoning by appetite depressants, accidental (unintentional)**

Poisoning by appetite depressants NOS

2 √7ᵗʰ **T50.5X2 Poisoning by appetite depressants, intentional self-harm** HCC

√7ᵗʰ **T50.5X3 Poisoning by appetite depressants, assault**

√7ᵗʰ **T50.5X4 Poisoning by appetite depressants, undetermined**

√7ᵗʰ **T50.5X5 Adverse effect of appetite depressants**

√7ᵗʰ **T50.5X6 Underdosing of appetite depressants**

√5ᵗʰ **T50.6 Poisoning by, adverse effect of and underdosing of antidotes and chelating agents**

Poisoning by, adverse effect of and underdosing of alcohol deterrents

√6ᵗʰ **T50.6X Poisoning by, adverse effect of and underdosing of antidotes and chelating agents**

√7ᵗʰ **T50.6X1 Poisoning by antidotes and chelating agents, accidental (unintentional)**

Poisoning by antidotes and chelating agents NOS

2 √7ᵗʰ **T50.6X2 Poisoning by antidotes and chelating agents, intentional self-harm** HCC

√7ᵗʰ **T50.6X3 Poisoning by antidotes and chelating agents, assault**

√7ᵗʰ **T50.6X4 Poisoning by antidotes and chelating agents, undetermined**

√7ᵗʰ **T50.6X5 Adverse effect of antidotes and chelating agents**

√7ᵗʰ **T50.6X6 Underdosing of antidotes and chelating agents**

√5ᵗʰ **T50.7 Poisoning by, adverse effect of and underdosing of analeptics and opioid receptor antagonists**

√6ᵗʰ **T50.7X Poisoning by, adverse effect of and underdosing of analeptics and opioid receptor antagonists**

√7ᵗʰ **T50.7X1 Poisoning by analeptics and opioid receptor antagonists, accidental (unintentional)**

Poisoning by analeptics and opioid receptor antagonists NOS

2 √7ᵗʰ **T50.7X2 Poisoning by analeptics and opioid receptor antagonists, intentional self-harm** HCC

√7ᵗʰ **T50.7X3 Poisoning by analeptics and opioid receptor antagonists, assault**

√7ᵗʰ **T50.7X4 Poisoning by analeptics and opioid receptor antagonists, undetermined**

√7ᵗʰ **T50.7X5 Adverse effect of analeptics and opioid receptor antagonists**

√7ᵗʰ **T50.7X6 Underdosing of analeptics and opioid receptor antagonists**

√5ᵗʰ **T50.8 Poisoning by, adverse effect of and underdosing of diagnostic agents**

√6ᵗʰ **T50.8X Poisoning by, adverse effect of and underdosing of diagnostic agents**

√7ᵗʰ **T50.8X1 Poisoning by diagnostic agents, accidental (unintentional)**

Poisoning by diagnostic agents NOS

2 √7ᵗʰ **T50.8X2 Poisoning by diagnostic agents, intentional self-harm** HCC

√7ᵗʰ **T50.8X3 Poisoning by diagnostic agents, assault**

√7ᵗʰ **T50.8X4 Poisoning by diagnostic agents, undetermined**

√7ᵗʰ **T50.8X5 Adverse effect of diagnostic agents**

√7ᵗʰ **T50.8X6 Underdosing of diagnostic agents**

√5ᵗʰ **T50.A Poisoning by, adverse effect of and underdosing of bacterial vaccines**

√6ᵗʰ **T50.A1 Poisoning by, adverse effect of and underdosing of pertussis vaccine, including combinations with a pertussis component**

√7ᵗʰ **T50.A11 Poisoning by pertussis vaccine, including combinations with a pertussis component, accidental (unintentional)**

2 √7ᵗʰ **T50.A12 Poisoning by pertussis vaccine, including combinations with a pertussis component, intentional self-harm** HCC

√7ᵗʰ **T50.A13 Poisoning by pertussis vaccine, including combinations with a pertussis component, assault**

√7ᵗʰ **T50.A14 Poisoning by pertussis vaccine, including combinations with a pertussis component, undetermined**

√7ᵗʰ **T50.A15 Adverse effect of pertussis vaccine, including combinations with a pertussis component**

√7ᵗʰ **T50.A16 Underdosing of pertussis vaccine, including combinations with a pertussis component**

√6ᵗʰ **T50.A2 Poisoning by, adverse effect of and underdosing of mixed bacterial vaccines without a pertussis component**

√7ᵗʰ **T50.A21 Poisoning by mixed bacterial vaccines without a pertussis component, accidental (unintentional)**

2 √7ᵗʰ **T50.A22 Poisoning by mixed bacterial vaccines without a pertussis component, intentional self-harm** HCC

√7ᵗʰ **T50.A23 Poisoning by mixed bacterial vaccines without a pertussis component, assault**

√7ᵗʰ **T50.A24 Poisoning by mixed bacterial vaccines without a pertussis component, undetermined**

√7ᵗʰ **T50.A25 Adverse effect of mixed bacterial vaccines without a pertussis component**

√7ᵗʰ **T50.A26 Underdosing of mixed bacterial vaccines without a pertussis component**

√6ᵗʰ **T50.A9 Poisoning by, adverse effect of and underdosing of other bacterial vaccines**

√7ᵗʰ **T50.A91 Poisoning by other bacterial vaccines, accidental (unintentional)**

2 √7ᵗʰ **T50.A92 Poisoning by other bacterial vaccines, intentional self-harm** HCC

√7ᵗʰ **T50.A93** Poisoning by other bacterial vaccines, assault

√7ᵗʰ **T50.A94** Poisoning by other bacterial vaccines, undetermined

√7ᵗʰ **T50.A95** Adverse effect of other bacterial vaccines

√7ᵗʰ **T50.A96** Underdosing of other bacterial vaccines

√5ᵗʰ **T50.B** Poisoning by, adverse effect of and underdosing of viral vaccines

√6ᵗʰ **T50.B1** Poisoning by, adverse effect of and underdosing of smallpox vaccines

√7ᵗʰ **T50.B11** Poisoning by smallpox vaccines, accidental (unintentional)

² √7ᵗʰ **T50.B12** Poisoning by smallpox vaccines, intentional self-harm   HCC

√7ᵗʰ **T50.B13** Poisoning by smallpox vaccines, assault

√7ᵗʰ **T50.B14** Poisoning by smallpox vaccines, undetermined

√7ᵗʰ **T50.B15** Adverse effect of smallpox vaccines

√7ᵗʰ **T50.B16** Underdosing of smallpox vaccines

√6ᵗʰ **T50.B9** Poisoning by, adverse effect of and underdosing of other viral vaccines

√7ᵗʰ **T50.B91** Poisoning by other viral vaccines, accidental (unintentional)

² √7ᵗʰ **T50.B92** Poisoning by other viral vaccines, intentional self-harm   HCC

√7ᵗʰ **T50.B93** Poisoning by other viral vaccines, assault

√7ᵗʰ **T50.B94** Poisoning by other viral vaccines, undetermined

√7ᵗʰ **T50.B95** Adverse effect of other viral vaccines

√7ᵗʰ **T50.B96** Underdosing of other viral vaccines

√5ᵗʰ **T50.Z** Poisoning by, adverse effect of and underdosing of other vaccines and biological substances

√6ᵗʰ **T50.Z1** Poisoning by, adverse effect of and underdosing of immunoglobulin

√7ᵗʰ **T50.Z11** Poisoning by immunoglobulin, accidental (unintentional)

² √7ᵗʰ **T50.Z12** Poisoning by immunoglobulin, intentional self-harm   HCC

√7ᵗʰ **T50.Z13** Poisoning by immunoglobulin, assault

√7ᵗʰ **T50.Z14** Poisoning by immunoglobulin, undetermined

√7ᵗʰ **T50.Z15** Adverse effect of immunoglobulin

√7ᵗʰ **T50.Z16** Underdosing of immunoglobulin

√6ᵗʰ **T50.Z9** Poisoning by, adverse effect of and underdosing of other vaccines and biological substances

√7ᵗʰ **T50.Z91** Poisoning by other vaccines and biological substances, accidental (unintentional)

² √7ᵗʰ **T50.Z92** Poisoning by other vaccines and biological substances, intentional self-harm   HCC

√7ᵗʰ **T50.Z93** Poisoning by other vaccines and biological substances, assault

√7ᵗʰ **T50.Z94** Poisoning by other vaccines and biological substances, undetermined

√7ᵗʰ **T50.Z95** Adverse effect of other vaccines and biological substances

√7ᵗʰ **T50.Z96** Underdosing of other vaccines and biological substances

√5ᵗʰ **T50.9** Poisoning by, adverse effect of and underdosing of other and unspecified drugs, medicaments and biological substances

AHA: 2016,1Q,38; 2015,1Q,21

√6ᵗʰ **T50.90** Poisoning by, adverse effect of and underdosing of unspecified drugs, medicaments and biological substances

√7ᵗʰ **T50.901** Poisoning by unspecified drugs, medicaments and biological substances, accidental (unintentional)   ▽

² √7ᵗʰ **T50.902** Poisoning by unspecified drugs, medicaments and biological substances, intentional self-harm   HCC ▽

√7ᵗʰ **T50.903** Poisoning by unspecified drugs, medicaments and biological substances, assault   ▽

√7ᵗʰ **T50.904** Poisoning by unspecified drugs, medicaments and biological substances, undetermined   ▽

√7ᵗʰ **T50.905** Adverse effect of unspecified drugs, medicaments and biological substances   ▽

√7ᵗʰ **T50.906** Underdosing of unspecified drugs, medicaments and biological substances   ▽

√6ᵗʰ **T50.99** Poisoning by, adverse effect of and underdosing of other drugs, medicaments and biological substances

√7ᵗʰ **T50.991** Poisoning by other drugs, medicaments and biological substances, accidental (unintentional)

² √7ᵗʰ **T50.992** Poisoning by other drugs, medicaments and biological substances, intentional self-harm   HCC

√7ᵗʰ **T50.993** Poisoning by other drugs, medicaments and biological substances, assault

√7ᵗʰ **T50.994** Poisoning by other drugs, medicaments and biological substances, undetermined

√7ᵗʰ **T50.995** Adverse effect of other drugs, medicaments and biological substances

√7ᵗʰ **T50.996** Underdosing of other drugs, medicaments and biological substances

Toxic effects of substances chiefly nonmedicinal as to source (T51-T65)

NOTE   When no intent is indicated code to accidental. Undetermined intent is only for use when there is specific documentation in the record that the intent of the toxic effect cannot be determined.

Use additional code(s) for all associated manifestations of toxic effect, such as:
personal history of foreign body fully removed (Z87.821)
respiratory conditions due to external agents (J60-J70)
to identify any retained foreign body, if applicable (Z18.-)

EXCLUDES 1   contact with and (suspected) exposure to toxic substances (Z77.-)

AHA: 2017,1Q,39-40

√4ᵗʰ **T51** Toxic effect of alcohol

> The appropriate 7th character is to be added to each code from category T51.
> A   initial encounter
> D   subsequent encounter
> S   sequela

√5ᵗʰ **T51.0** Toxic effect of ethanol

Toxic effect of ethyl alcohol

EXCLUDES 2   acute alcohol intoxication or "hangover" effects (F10.129, F10.229, F10.929)
drunkenness (F10.129, F10.229, F10.929)
pathological alcohol intoxication (F10.129, F10.229, F10.929)

√6ᵗʰ **T51.0X** Toxic effect of ethanol

√7ᵗʰ **T51.0X1** Toxic effect of ethanol, accidental (unintentional)

Toxic effect of ethanol NOS

² √7ᵗʰ **T51.0X2** Toxic effect of ethanol, intentional self-harm   HCC

√7ᵗʰ **T51.0X3** Toxic effect of ethanol, assault

√7ᵗʰ **T51.0X4** Toxic effect of ethanol, undetermined

√5ᵗʰ **T51.1** Toxic effect of methanol

Toxic effect of methyl alcohol

√6ᵗʰ **T51.1X** Toxic effect of methanol

√7ᵗʰ **T51.1X1** Toxic effect of methanol, accidental (unintentional)

Toxic effect of methanol NOS

² √7ᵗʰ **T51.1X2** Toxic effect of methanol, intentional self-harm   HCC

√7ᵗʰ **T51.1X3** Toxic effect of methanol, assault

√7ᵗʰ **T51.1X4** Toxic effect of methanol, undetermined

√5ᵗʰ **T51.2** Toxic effect of 2-Propanol

Toxic effect of isopropyl alcohol

√6ᵗʰ **T51.2X** Toxic effect of 2-Propanol

√7ᵗʰ **T51.2X1** Toxic effect of 2-Propanol, accidental (unintentional)

Toxic effect of 2-Propanol NOS

² √7ᵗʰ **T51.2X2** Toxic effect of 2-Propanol, intentional self-harm   HCC

√7ᵗʰ **T51.2X3** Toxic effect of 2-Propanol, assault

√7ᵗʰ **T51.2X4** Toxic effect of 2-Propanol, undetermined

✔ Additional Character Req   √x7ᵗʰ Placeholder Alert   Manifestation   ▽ Unspecified   ►◄ Revised Text   ● New Code   ▲ Revised Code Title

ICD-10-CM 2019   1115

Chapter 19. Injury, Poisoning and Certain Other Consequences of External Causes

T51.3–T53.1X4

√5th **T51.3** **Toxic effect of fusel oil**
     Toxic effect of amyl alcohol
     Toxic effect of butyl [1-butanol] alcohol
     Toxic effect of propyl [1-propanol] alcohol

     √6th **T51.3X** **Toxic effect of fusel oil**
         √7th **T51.3X1** **Toxic effect of fusel oil, accidental (unintentional)**
             Toxic effect of fusel oil NOS
         2 √7th **T51.3X2** **Toxic effect of fusel oil, intentional self-harm** HCC
         √7th **T51.3X3** **Toxic effect of fusel oil, assault**
         √7th **T51.3X4** **Toxic effect of fusel oil, undetermined**

√5th **T51.8** **Toxic effect of other alcohols**
     √6th **T51.8X** **Toxic effect of other alcohols**
         √7th **T51.8X1** **Toxic effect of other alcohols, accidental (unintentional)**
             Toxic effect of other alcohols NOS
         2 √7th **T51.8X2** **Toxic effect of other alcohols, intentional self-harm** HCC
         √7th **T51.8X3** **Toxic effect of other alcohols, assault**
         √7th **T51.8X4** **Toxic effect of other alcohols, undetermined**

√5th **T51.9** **Toxic effect of unspecified alcohol**
     √x7th **T51.91** **Toxic effect of unspecified alcohol, accidental (unintentional)** ▽
     2 √x7th **T51.92** **Toxic effect of unspecified alcohol, intentional self-harm** HCC ▽
     √x7th **T51.93** **Toxic effect of unspecified alcohol, assault** ▽
     √x7th **T51.94** **Toxic effect of unspecified alcohol, undetermined** ▽

√4th **T52** **Toxic effect of organic solvents**
     EXCLUDES 1   halogen derivatives of aliphatic and aromatic hydrocarbons (T53.-)

     The appropriate 7th character is to be added to each code from category T52.
     A   initial encounter
     D   subsequent encounter
     S   sequela

     √5th **T52.0** **Toxic effects of petroleum products**
         Toxic effects of ether petroleum
         Toxic effects of gasoline [petrol]
         Toxic effects of kerosene [paraffin oil]
         Toxic effects of naphtha petroleum
         Toxic effects of paraffin wax
         Toxic effects of spirit petroleum

         √6th **T52.0X** **Toxic effects of petroleum products**
             √7th **T52.0X1** **Toxic effect of petroleum products, accidental (unintentional)**
                 Toxic effects of petroleum products NOS
             2 √7th **T52.0X2** **Toxic effect of petroleum products, intentional self-harm** HCC
             √7th **T52.0X3** **Toxic effect of petroleum products, assault**
             √7th **T52.0X4** **Toxic effect of petroleum products, undetermined**

     √5th **T52.1** **Toxic effects of benzene**
         EXCLUDES 1   homologues of benzene (T52.2)
                      nitroderivatives and aminoderivatives of benzene and its homologues (T65.3)

         √6th **T52.1X** **Toxic effects of benzene**
             √7th **T52.1X1** **Toxic effect of benzene, accidental (unintentional)**
                 Toxic effects of benzene NOS
             2 √7th **T52.1X2** **Toxic effect of benzene, intentional self-harm** HCC
             √7th **T52.1X3** **Toxic effect of benzene, assault**
             √7th **T52.1X4** **Toxic effect of benzene, undetermined**

     √5th **T52.2** **Toxic effects of homologues of benzene**
         Toxic effects of toluene [methylbenzene]
         Toxic effects of xylene [dimethylbenzene]

         √6th **T52.2X** **Toxic effects of homologues of benzene**
             √7th **T52.2X1** **Toxic effect of homologues of benzene, accidental (unintentional)**
                 Toxic effects of homologues of benzene NOS

         2 √7th **T52.2X2** **Toxic effect of homologues of benzene, intentional self-harm** HCC
         √7th **T52.2X3** **Toxic effect of homologues of benzene, assault**
         √7th **T52.2X4** **Toxic effect of homologues of benzene, undetermined**

     √5th **T52.3** **Toxic effects of glycols**
         √6th **T52.3X** **Toxic effects of glycols**
             √7th **T52.3X1** **Toxic effect of glycols, accidental (unintentional)**
                 Toxic effects of glycols NOS
             2 √7th **T52.3X2** **Toxic effect of glycols, intentional self-harm** HCC
             √7th **T52.3X3** **Toxic effect of glycols, assault**
             √7th **T52.3X4** **Toxic effect of glycols, undetermined**

     √5th **T52.4** **Toxic effects of ketones**
         √6th **T52.4X** **Toxic effects of ketones**
             √7th **T52.4X1** **Toxic effect of ketones, accidental (unintentional)**
                 Toxic effects of ketones NOS
             2 √7th **T52.4X2** **Toxic effect of ketones, intentional self-harm** HCC
             √7th **T52.4X3** **Toxic effect of ketones, assault**
             √7th **T52.4X4** **Toxic effect of ketones, undetermined**

     √5th **T52.8** **Toxic effects of other organic solvents**
         √6th **T52.8X** **Toxic effect of other organic solvents**
             √7th **T52.8X1** **Toxic effect of other organic solvents, accidental (unintentional)**
                 Toxic effects of other organic solvents NOS
             2 √7th **T52.8X2** **Toxic effect of other organic solvents, intentional self-harm** HCC
             √7th **T52.8X3** **Toxic effect of other organic solvents, assault**
             √7th **T52.8X4** **Toxic effect of other organic solvents, undetermined**

     √5th **T52.9** **Toxic effects of unspecified organic solvent**
         √x7th **T52.91** **Toxic effect of unspecified organic solvent, accidental (unintentional)** ▽
         2 √x7th **T52.92** **Toxic effect of unspecified organic solvent, intentional self-harm** HCC ▽
         √x7th **T52.93** **Toxic effect of unspecified organic solvent, assault** ▽
         √x7th **T52.94** **Toxic effect of unspecified organic solvent, undetermined** ▽

√4th **T53** **Toxic effect of halogen derivatives of aliphatic and aromatic hydrocarbons**
     The appropriate 7th character is to be added to each code from category T53.
     A   initial encounter
     D   subsequent encounter
     S   sequela

     √5th **T53.0** **Toxic effects of carbon tetrachloride**
         Toxic effects of tetrachloromethane
         √6th **T53.0X** **Toxic effects of carbon tetrachloride**
             √7th **T53.0X1** **Toxic effect of carbon tetrachloride, accidental (unintentional)**
                 Toxic effects of carbon tetrachloride NOS
             2 √7th **T53.0X2** **Toxic effect of carbon tetrachloride, intentional self-harm** HCC
             √7th **T53.0X3** **Toxic effect of carbon tetrachloride, assault**
             √7th **T53.0X4** **Toxic effect of carbon tetrachloride, undetermined**

     √5th **T53.1** **Toxic effects of chloroform**
         Toxic effects of trichloromethane
         √6th **T53.1X** **Toxic effects of chloroform**
             √7th **T53.1X1** **Toxic effect of chloroform, accidental (unintentional)**
                 Toxic effects of chloroform NOS
             2 √7th **T53.1X2** **Toxic effect of chloroform, intentional self-harm** HCC
             √7th **T53.1X3** **Toxic effect of chloroform, assault**
             √7th **T53.1X4** **Toxic effect of chloroform, undetermined**

√5ᵗʰ **T53.2 Toxic effects of trichloroethylene**
Toxic effects of trichloroethene

√6ᵗʰ **T53.2X Toxic effects of** trichloroethylene

√7ᵗʰ **T53.2X1 Toxic effect of trichloroethylene, accidental (unintentional)**
Toxic effects of trichloroethylene NOS

² √7ᵗʰ **T53.2X2 Toxic effect of trichloroethylene, intentional self-harm** HCC

√7ᵗʰ **T53.2X3 Toxic effect of trichloroethylene,** assault

√7ᵗʰ **T53.2X4 Toxic effect of trichloroethylene, undetermined**

√5ᵗʰ **T53.3 Toxic effects of tetrachloroethylene**
Toxic effects of perchloroethylene
Toxic effect of tetrachloroethene

√6ᵗʰ **T53.3X Toxic effects of** tetrachloroethylene

√7ᵗʰ **T53.3X1 Toxic effect of tetrachloroethylene, accidental (unintentional)**
Toxic effects of tetrachloroethylene NOS

² √7ᵗʰ **T53.3X2 Toxic effect of tetrachloroethylene, intentional self-harm** HCC

√7ᵗʰ **T53.3X3 Toxic effect of tetrachloroethylene, assault**

√7ᵗʰ **T53.3X4 Toxic effect of tetrachloroethylene, undetermined**

√5ᵗʰ **T53.4 Toxic effects of dichloromethane**
Toxic effects of methylene chloride

√6ᵗʰ **T53.4X Toxic effects of** dichloromethane

√7ᵗʰ **T53.4X1 Toxic effect of dichloromethane, accidental (unintentional)**
Toxic effects of dichloromethane NOS

² √7ᵗʰ **T53.4X2 Toxic effect of dichloromethane, intentional self-harm** HCC

√7ᵗʰ **T53.4X3 Toxic effect of dichloromethane,** assault

√7ᵗʰ **T53.4X4 Toxic effect of dichloromethane, undetermined**

√5ᵗʰ **T53.5 Toxic effects of chlorofluorocarbons**

√6ᵗʰ **T53.5X Toxic effects of** chlorofluorocarbons

√7ᵗʰ **T53.5X1 Toxic effect of chlorofluorocarbons, accidental (unintentional)**
Toxic effects of chlorofluorocarbons NOS

² √7ᵗʰ **T53.5X2 Toxic effect of chlorofluorocarbons, intentional self-harm** HCC

√7ᵗʰ **T53.5X3 Toxic effect of chlorofluorocarbons, assault**

√7ᵗʰ **T53.5X4 Toxic effect of chlorofluorocarbons, undetermined**

√5ᵗʰ **T53.6 Toxic effects of other halogen derivatives of aliphatic hydrocarbons**

√6ᵗʰ **T53.6X Toxic effects of** other halogen derivatives of aliphatic hydrocarbons

√7ᵗʰ **T53.6X1 Toxic effect of other halogen derivatives of aliphatic hydrocarbons, accidental (unintentional)**
Toxic effects of other halogen derivatives of aliphatic hydrocarbons NOS

² √7ᵗʰ **T53.6X2 Toxic effect of other halogen derivatives of aliphatic hydrocarbons, intentional self-harm** HCC

√7ᵗʰ **T53.6X3 Toxic effect of other halogen derivatives of aliphatic hydrocarbons, assault**

√7ᵗʰ **T53.6X4 Toxic effect of other halogen derivatives of aliphatic hydrocarbons, undetermined**

√5ᵗʰ **T53.7 Toxic effects of other halogen derivatives of aromatic hydrocarbons**

√6ᵗʰ **T53.7X Toxic effects of** other halogen derivatives of aromatic hydrocarbons

√7ᵗʰ **T53.7X1 Toxic effect of other halogen derivatives of aromatic hydrocarbons, accidental (unintentional)**
Toxic effects of other halogen derivatives of aromatic hydrocarbons NOS

² √7ᵗʰ **T53.7X2 Toxic effect of other halogen derivatives of aromatic hydrocarbons, intentional self-harm** HCC

√7ᵗʰ **T53.7X3 Toxic effect of other halogen derivatives of aromatic hydrocarbons, assault**

√7ᵗʰ **T53.7X4 Toxic effect of other halogen derivatives of aromatic hydrocarbons, undetermined**

√5ᵗʰ **T53.9 Toxic effects of unspecified halogen derivatives of aliphatic and aromatic hydrocarbons**

√x7ᵗʰ **T53.91 Toxic effect of unspecified halogen derivatives of aliphatic and aromatic hydrocarbons, accidental (unintentional)** ▽

² √x7ᵗʰ **T53.92 Toxic effect of unspecified halogen derivatives of aliphatic and aromatic hydrocarbons, intentional self-harm** HCC ▽

√x7ᵗʰ **T53.93 Toxic effect of unspecified halogen derivatives of aliphatic and aromatic hydrocarbons, assault** ▽

√x7ᵗʰ **T53.94 Toxic effect of unspecified halogen derivatives of aliphatic and aromatic hydrocarbons, undetermined** ▽

√4ᵗʰ **T54 Toxic effect of corrosive substances**

The appropriate 7th character is to be added to each code from category T54.
A   initial encounter
D   subsequent encounter
S   sequela

√5ᵗʰ **T54.0 Toxic effects of phenol and phenol homologues**

√6ᵗʰ **T54.0X Toxic effects of** phenol and phenol homologues

√7ᵗʰ **T54.0X1 Toxic effect of phenol and phenol homologues, accidental (unintentional)**
Toxic effects of phenol and phenol homologues NOS

² √7ᵗʰ **T54.0X2 Toxic effect of phenol and phenol homologues, intentional self-harm** HCC

√7ᵗʰ **T54.0X3 Toxic effect of phenol and phenol homologues, assault**

√7ᵗʰ **T54.0X4 Toxic effect of phenol and phenol homologues, undetermined**

√5ᵗʰ **T54.1 Toxic effects of other corrosive organic compounds**

√6ᵗʰ **T54.1X Toxic effects of other corrosive organic compounds**

√7ᵗʰ **T54.1X1 Toxic effect of other corrosive organic compounds, accidental (unintentional)**
Toxic effects of other corrosive organic compounds NOS

² √7ᵗʰ **T54.1X2 Toxic effect of other corrosive organic compounds, intentional self-harm** HCC

√7ᵗʰ **T54.1X3 Toxic effect of other corrosive organic compounds, assault**

√7ᵗʰ **T54.1X4 Toxic effect of other corrosive organic compounds, undetermined**

√5ᵗʰ **T54.2 Toxic effects of corrosive acids and acid-like substances**
Toxic effects of hydrochloric acid
Toxic effects of sulfuric acid

√6ᵗʰ **T54.2X Toxic effects of** corrosive acids and acid-like substances

√7ᵗʰ **T54.2X1 Toxic effect of corrosive acids and acid-like substances, accidental (unintentional)**
Toxic effects of corrosive acids and acid-like substances NOS

² √7ᵗʰ **T54.2X2 Toxic effect of corrosive acids and acid-like substances, intentional self-harm** HCC

√7ᵗʰ **T54.2X3 Toxic effect of corrosive acids and acid-like substances, assault**

√7ᵗʰ **T54.2X4 Toxic effect of corrosive acids and acid-like substances, undetermined**

√5ᵗʰ **T54.3 Toxic effects of corrosive alkalis and alkali-like substances**
Toxic effects of potassium hydroxide
Toxic effects of sodium hydroxide

√6ᵗʰ **T54.3X Toxic effects of** corrosive alkalis and alkali-like substances

√7ᵗʰ **T54.3X1 Toxic effect of corrosive alkalis and alkali-like substances, accidental (unintentional)**
Toxic effects of corrosive alkalis and alkali-like substances NOS

² √7ᵗʰ **T54.3X2 Toxic effect of corrosive alkalis and alkali-like substances, intentional self-harm** HCC

√7ᵗʰ **T54.3X3 Toxic effect of corrosive alkalis and alkali-like substances, assault**

√7th **T54.3X4** Toxic effect of corrosive alkalis and alkali-like substances, **undetermined**

√5th **T54.9** **Toxic effects of unspecified corrosive substance**

   √x7th **T54.91** **Toxic effect of unspecified corrosive substance, accidental (unintentional)** ▽

   2 √x7th **T54.92** **Toxic effect of unspecified corrosive substance, intentional self-harm** HCC ▽

   √x7th **T54.93** **Toxic effect of unspecified corrosive substance, assault** ▽

   √x7th **T54.94** **Toxic effect of unspecified corrosive substance, undetermined** ▽

√4th **T55** **Toxic effect of soaps and detergents**

> The appropriate 7th character is to be added to each code from category T55.
> A   initial encounter
> D   subsequent encounter
> S   sequela

√5th **T55.0** **Toxic effect of soaps**

   √6th **T55.0X** **Toxic effect of soaps**

     √7th **T55.0X1** **Toxic effect of soaps, accidental (unintentional)**
       Toxic effect of soaps NOS

     2 √7th **T55.0X2** **Toxic effect of soaps, intentional self-harm** HCC

     √7th **T55.0X3** **Toxic effect of soaps, assault**

     √7th **T55.0X4** **Toxic effect of soaps, undetermined**

√5th **T55.1** **Toxic effect of detergents**

   √6th **T55.1X** **Toxic effect of detergents**

     √7th **T55.1X1** **Toxic effect of detergents, accidental (unintentional)**
       Toxic effect of detergents NOS

     2 √7th **T55.1X2** **Toxic effect of detergents, intentional self-harm** HCC

     √7th **T55.1X3** **Toxic effect of detergents, assault**

     √7th **T55.1X4** **Toxic effect of detergents, undetermined**

√4th **T56** **Toxic effect of metals**

> INCLUDES   toxic effects of fumes and vapors of metals
>   toxic effects of metals from all sources, except medicinal substances
>
> Use additional code to identify any retained metal foreign body, if applicable (Z18.0-, T18.1-)
>
> EXCLUDES 1   *arsenic and its compounds (T57.0)*
>   *manganese and its compounds (T57.2)*

> The appropriate 7th character is to be added to each code from category T56.
> A   initial encounter
> D   subsequent encounter
> S   sequela

√5th **T56.0** **Toxic effects of lead and its compounds**

   √6th **T56.0X** **Toxic effects of lead and its compounds**

     √7th **T56.0X1** **Toxic effect of lead and its compounds, accidental (unintentional)**
       Toxic effects of lead and its compounds NOS

     2 √7th **T56.0X2** **Toxic effect of lead and its compounds, intentional self-harm** HCC

     √7th **T56.0X3** **Toxic effect of lead and its compounds, assault**

     √7th **T56.0X4** **Toxic effect of lead and its compounds, undetermined**

√5th **T56.1** **Toxic effects of mercury and its compounds**

   √6th **T56.1X** **Toxic effects of mercury and its compounds**

     √7th **T56.1X1** **Toxic effect of mercury and its compounds, accidental (unintentional)**
       Toxic effects of mercury and its compounds NOS

     2 √7th **T56.1X2** **Toxic effect of mercury and its compounds, intentional self-harm** HCC

     √7th **T56.1X3** **Toxic effect of mercury and its compounds, assault**

     √7th **T56.1X4** **Toxic effect of mercury and its compounds, undetermined**

√5th **T56.2** **Toxic effects of chromium and its compounds**

   √6th **T56.2X** **Toxic effects of chromium and its compounds**

     √7th **T56.2X1** **Toxic effect of chromium and its compounds, accidental (unintentional)**
       Toxic effects of chromium and its compounds NOS

     2 √7th **T56.2X2** **Toxic effect of chromium and its compounds, intentional self-harm** HCC

     √7th **T56.2X3** **Toxic effect of chromium and its compounds, assault**

     √7th **T56.2X4** **Toxic effect of chromium and its compounds, undetermined**

√5th **T56.3** **Toxic effects of cadmium and its compounds**

   √6th **T56.3X** **Toxic effects of cadmium and its compounds**

     √7th **T56.3X1** **Toxic effect of cadmium and its compounds, accidental (unintentional)**
       Toxic effects of cadmium and its compounds NOS

     2 √7th **T56.3X2** **Toxic effect of cadmium and its compounds, intentional self-harm** HCC

     √7th **T56.3X3** **Toxic effect of cadmium and its compounds, assault**

     √7th **T56.3X4** **Toxic effect of cadmium and its compounds, undetermined**

√5th **T56.4** **Toxic effects of copper and its compounds**

   √6th **T56.4X** **Toxic effects of copper and its compounds**

     √7th **T56.4X1** **Toxic effect of copper and its compounds, accidental (unintentional)**
       Toxic effect of copper and its compounds NOS

     2 √7th **T56.4X2** **Toxic effect of copper and its compounds, intentional self-harm** HCC

     √7th **T56.4X3** **Toxic effect of copper and its compounds, assault**

     √7th **T56.4X4** **Toxic effect of copper and its compounds, undetermined**

√5th **T56.5** **Toxic effects of zinc and its compounds**

   √6th **T56.5X** **Toxic effects of zinc and its compounds**

     √7th **T56.5X1** **Toxic effect of zinc and its compounds, accidental (unintentional)**
       Toxic effects of zinc and its compounds NOS

     2 √7th **T56.5X2** **Toxic effect of zinc and its compounds, intentional self-harm** HCC

     √7th **T56.5X3** **Toxic effect of zinc and its compounds, assault**

     √7th **T56.5X4** **Toxic effect of zinc and its compounds, undetermined**

√5th **T56.6** **Toxic effects of tin and its compounds**

   √6th **T56.6X** **Toxic effects of tin and its compounds**

     √7th **T56.6X1** **Toxic effect of tin and its compounds, accidental (unintentional)**
       Toxic effects of tin and its compounds NOS

     2 √7th **T56.6X2** **Toxic effect of tin and its compounds, intentional self-harm** HCC

     √7th **T56.6X3** **Toxic effect of tin and its compounds, assault**

     √7th **T56.6X4** **Toxic effect of tin and its compounds, undetermined**

√5th **T56.7** **Toxic effects of beryllium and its compounds**

   √6th **T56.7X** **Toxic effects of beryllium and its compounds**

     √7th **T56.7X1** **Toxic effect of beryllium and its compounds, accidental (unintentional)**
       Toxic effects of beryllium and its compounds NOS

     2 √7th **T56.7X2** **Toxic effect of beryllium and its compounds, intentional self-harm** HCC

     √7th **T56.7X3** **Toxic effect of beryllium and its compounds, assault**

     √7th **T56.7X4** **Toxic effect of beryllium and its compounds, undetermined**

√5ᵗʰ **T56.8**   **Toxic effects of other metals**

     √6ᵗʰ **T56.81**   **Toxic effect of thallium**

         √7ᵗʰ **T56.811**   **Toxic effect of thallium, accidental (unintentional)**
                  Toxic effect of thallium NOS

         ² √7ᵗʰ **T56.812**   **Toxic effect of thallium, intentional self-harm**   HCC

         √7ᵗʰ **T56.813**   **Toxic effect of thallium, assault**

         √7ᵗʰ **T56.814**   **Toxic effect of thallium, undetermined**

     √6ᵗʰ **T56.89**   **Toxic effects of other metals**

         √7ᵗʰ **T56.891**   **Toxic effect of other metals, accidental (unintentional)**
                  Toxic effects of other metals NOS

         ² √7ᵗʰ **T56.892**   **Toxic effect of other metals, intentional self-harm**   HCC

         √7ᵗʰ **T56.893**   **Toxic effect of other metals, assault**

         √7ᵗʰ **T56.894**   **Toxic effect of other metals, undetermined**

√5ᵗʰ **T56.9**   **Toxic effects of unspecified metal**

     √x7ᵗʰ **T56.91**   **Toxic effect of unspecified metal, accidental (unintentional)**   ▽

     ² √x7ᵗʰ **T56.92**   **Toxic effect of unspecified metal, intentional self-harm**   HCC ▽

     √x7ᵗʰ **T56.93**   **Toxic effect of unspecified metal, assault**   ▽

     √x7ᵗʰ **T56.94**   **Toxic effect of unspecified metal, undetermined**   ▽

√4ᵗʰ **T57**   **Toxic effect of other inorganic substances**

> The appropriate 7th character is to be added to each code from category T57.
> A   initial encounter
> D   subsequent encounter
> S   sequela

√5ᵗʰ **T57.0**   **Toxic effect of arsenic and its compounds**

     √6ᵗʰ **T57.0X**   **Toxic effect of arsenic and its compounds**

         √7ᵗʰ **T57.0X1**   **Toxic effect of arsenic and its compounds, accidental (unintentional)**
                  Toxic effect of arsenic and its compounds NOS

         ² √7ᵗʰ **T57.0X2**   **Toxic effect of arsenic and its compounds, intentional self-harm**   HCC

         √7ᵗʰ **T57.0X3**   **Toxic effect of arsenic and its compounds, assault**

         √7ᵗʰ **T57.0X4**   **Toxic effect of arsenic and its compounds, undetermined**

√5ᵗʰ **T57.1**   **Toxic effect of phosphorus and its compounds**

     EXCLUDES 1   organophosphate insecticides (T60.0)

     √6ᵗʰ **T57.1X**   **Toxic effect of phosphorus and its compounds**

         √7ᵗʰ **T57.1X1**   **Toxic effect of phosphorus and its compounds, accidental (unintentional)**
                  Toxic effect of phosphorus and its compounds NOS

         ² √7ᵗʰ **T57.1X2**   **Toxic effect of phosphorus and its compounds, intentional self-harm**   HCC

         √7ᵗʰ **T57.1X3**   **Toxic effect of phosphorus and its compounds, assault**

         √7ᵗʰ **T57.1X4**   **Toxic effect of phosphorus and its compounds, undetermined**

√5ᵗʰ **T57.2**   **Toxic effect of manganese and its compounds**

     √6ᵗʰ **T57.2X**   **Toxic effect of manganese and its compounds**

         √7ᵗʰ **T57.2X1**   **Toxic effect of manganese and its compounds, accidental (unintentional)**
                  Toxic effect of manganese and its compounds NOS

         ² √7ᵗʰ **T57.2X2**   **Toxic effect of manganese and its compounds, intentional self-harm**   HCC

         √7ᵗʰ **T57.2X3**   **Toxic effect of manganese and its compounds, assault**

         √7ᵗʰ **T57.2X4**   **Toxic effect of manganese and its compounds, undetermined**

√5ᵗʰ **T57.3**   **Toxic effect of hydrogen cyanide**

     √6ᵗʰ **T57.3X**   **Toxic effect of hydrogen cyanide**

         √7ᵗʰ **T57.3X1**   **Toxic effect of hydrogen cyanide, accidental (unintentional)**
                  Toxic effect of hydrogen cyanide NOS

         ² √7ᵗʰ **T57.3X2**   **Toxic effect of hydrogen cyanide, intentional self-harm**   HCC

         √7ᵗʰ **T57.3X3**   **Toxic effect of hydrogen cyanide, assault**

         √7ᵗʰ **T57.3X4**   **Toxic effect of hydrogen cyanide, undetermined**

√5ᵗʰ **T57.8**   **Toxic effect of other specified inorganic substances**

     √6ᵗʰ **T57.8X**   **Toxic effect of other specified inorganic substances**

         √7ᵗʰ **T57.8X1**   **Toxic effect of other specified inorganic substances, accidental (unintentional)**
                  Toxic effect of other specified inorganic substances NOS

         ² √7ᵗʰ **T57.8X2**   **Toxic effect of other specified inorganic substances, intentional self-harm**   HCC

         √7ᵗʰ **T57.8X3**   **Toxic effect of other specified inorganic substances, assault**

         √7ᵗʰ **T57.8X4**   **Toxic effect of other specified inorganic substances, undetermined**

√5ᵗʰ **T57.9**   **Toxic effect of unspecified inorganic substance**

     √x7ᵗʰ **T57.91**   **Toxic effect of unspecified inorganic substance, accidental (unintentional)**   ▽

     ² √x7ᵗʰ **T57.92**   **Toxic effect of unspecified inorganic substance, intentional self-harm**   HCC ▽

     √x7ᵗʰ **T57.93**   **Toxic effect of unspecified inorganic substance, assault**   ▽

     √x7ᵗʰ **T57.94**   **Toxic effect of unspecified inorganic substance, undetermined**   ▽

√4ᵗʰ **T58**   **Toxic effect of carbon monoxide**

> INCLUDES   asphyxiation from carbon monoxide
>   toxic effect of carbon monoxide from all sources

> The appropriate 7th character is to be added to each code from category T58.
> A   initial encounter
> D   subsequent encounter
> S   sequela

√5ᵗʰ **T58.0**   **Toxic effect of carbon monoxide from motor vehicle exhaust**
         Toxic effect of exhaust gas from gas engine
         Toxic effect of exhaust gas from motor pump

     √x7ᵗʰ **T58.01**   **Toxic effect of carbon monoxide from motor vehicle exhaust, accidental (unintentional)**

     ² √x7ᵗʰ **T58.02**   **Toxic effect of carbon monoxide from motor vehicle exhaust, intentional self-harm**   HCC

     √x7ᵗʰ **T58.03**   **Toxic effect of carbon monoxide from motor vehicle exhaust, assault**

     √x7ᵗʰ **T58.04**   **Toxic effect of carbon monoxide from motor vehicle exhaust, undetermined**

√5ᵗʰ **T58.1**   **Toxic effect of carbon monoxide from utility gas**
         Toxic effect of acetylene
         Toxic effect of gas NOS used for lighting, heating, cooking
         Toxic effect of water gas

     √x7ᵗʰ **T58.11**   **Toxic effect of carbon monoxide from utility gas, accidental (unintentional)**

     ² √x7ᵗʰ **T58.12**   **Toxic effect of carbon monoxide from utility gas, intentional self-harm**   HCC

     √x7ᵗʰ **T58.13**   **Toxic effect of carbon monoxide from utility gas, assault**

     √x7ᵗʰ **T58.14**   **Toxic effect of carbon monoxide from utility gas, undetermined**

√5ᵗʰ **T58.2**   **Toxic effect of carbon monoxide from incomplete combustion of other domestic fuels**
         Toxic effect of carbon monoxide from incomplete combustion of coal, coke, kerosene, wood

     √6ᵗʰ **T58.2X**   **Toxic effect of carbon monoxide from incomplete combustion of other domestic fuels**

         √7ᵗʰ **T58.2X1**   **Toxic effect of carbon monoxide from incomplete combustion of other domestic fuels, accidental (unintentional)**

         ² √7ᵗʰ **T58.2X2**   **Toxic effect of carbon monoxide from incomplete combustion of other domestic fuels, intentional self-harm**   HCC

         √7ᵗʰ **T58.2X3**   **Toxic effect of carbon monoxide from incomplete combustion of other domestic fuels, assault**

☑ Additional Character Req   √x7ᵗʰ Placeholder Alert   **Manifestation**   ▽ Unspecified   ▶◀ Revised Text   ● New Code   ▲ Revised Code Title

ICD-10-CM 2019   **1119**

✓7ᵗʰ **T58.2X4** **Toxic effect of carbon monoxide from incomplete combustion of other domestic fuels,** undetermined

✓5ᵗʰ **T58.8** **Toxic effect of carbon monoxide from other source**

Toxic effect of carbon monoxide from blast furnace gas

Toxic effect of carbon monoxide from fuels in industrial use

Toxic effect of carbon monoxide from kiln vapor

✓6ᵗʰ **T58.8X** **Toxic effect of carbon monoxide from other source**

✓7ᵗʰ **T58.8X1** **Toxic effect of carbon monoxide from other source,** accidental (unintentional)

² ✓7ᵗʰ **T58.8X2** **Toxic effect of carbon monoxide from other source,** intentional self-harm   HCC

✓7ᵗʰ **T58.8X3** **Toxic effect of carbon monoxide from other source,** assault

✓7ᵗʰ **T58.8X4** **Toxic effect of carbon monoxide from other source,** undetermined

✓5ᵗʰ **T58.9** **Toxic effect of carbon monoxide from unspecified source**

✓x7ᵗʰ **T58.91** **Toxic effect of carbon monoxide from unspecified source,** accidental (unintentional) ▽

² ✓x7ᵗʰ **T58.92** **Toxic effect of carbon monoxide from unspecified source,** intentional self-harm   HCC ▽

✓x7ᵗʰ **T58.93** **Toxic effect of carbon monoxide from unspecified source,** assault ▽

✓x7ᵗʰ **T58.94** **Toxic effect of carbon monoxide from unspecified source,** undetermined ▽

✓4ᵗʰ **T59** **Toxic effect of other gases, fumes and vapors**

INCLUDES   aerosol propellants

EXCLUDES 1   *chlorofluorocarbons (T53.5)*

The appropriate 7th character is to be added to each code from category T59.

A   initial encounter

D   subsequent encounter

S   sequela

✓5ᵗʰ **T59.Ø** **Toxic effect of nitrogen oxides**

✓6ᵗʰ **T59.ØX** **Toxic effect of nitrogen oxides**

✓7ᵗʰ **T59.ØX1** **Toxic effect of nitrogen oxides,** accidental (unintentional)

Toxic effect of nitrogen oxides NOS

² ✓7ᵗʰ **T59.ØX2** **Toxic effect of nitrogen oxides,** intentional self-harm   HCC

✓7ᵗʰ **T59.ØX3** **Toxic effect of nitrogen oxides,** assault

✓7ᵗʰ **T59.ØX4** **Toxic effect of nitrogen oxides,** undetermined

✓5ᵗʰ **T59.1** **Toxic effect of sulfur dioxide**

✓6ᵗʰ **T59.1X** **Toxic effect of sulfur dioxide**

✓7ᵗʰ **T59.1X1** **Toxic effect of sulfur dioxide,** accidental (unintentional)

Toxic effect of sulfur dioxide NOS

² ✓7ᵗʰ **T59.1X2** **Toxic effect of sulfur dioxide,** intentional self-harm   HCC

✓7ᵗʰ **T59.1X3** **Toxic effect of sulfur dioxide,** assault

✓7ᵗʰ **T59.1X4** **Toxic effect of sulfur dioxide,** undetermined

✓5ᵗʰ **T59.2** **Toxic effect of formaldehyde**

✓6ᵗʰ **T59.2X** **Toxic effect of formaldehyde**

✓7ᵗʰ **T59.2X1** **Toxic effect of formaldehyde,** accidental (unintentional)

Toxic effect of formaldehyde NOS

² ✓7ᵗʰ **T59.2X2** **Toxic effect of formaldehyde,** intentional self-harm   HCC

✓7ᵗʰ **T59.2X3** **Toxic effect of formaldehyde,** assault

✓7ᵗʰ **T59.2X4** **Toxic effect of formaldehyde,** undetermined

✓5ᵗʰ **T59.3** **Toxic effect of lacrimogenic gas**

Toxic effect of tear gas

✓6ᵗʰ **T59.3X** **Toxic effect of lacrimogenic gas**

✓7ᵗʰ **T59.3X1** **Toxic effect of lacrimogenic gas,** accidental (unintentional)

Toxic effect of lacrimogenic gas NOS

² ✓7ᵗʰ **T59.3X2** **Toxic effect of lacrimogenic gas,** intentional self-harm   HCC

✓7ᵗʰ **T59.3X3** **Toxic effect of lacrimogenic gas,** assault

✓7ᵗʰ **T59.3X4** **Toxic effect of lacrimogenic gas,** undetermined

✓5ᵗʰ **T59.4** **Toxic effect of chlorine gas**

✓6ᵗʰ **T59.4X** **Toxic effect of chlorine gas**

✓7ᵗʰ **T59.4X1** **Toxic effect of chlorine gas,** accidental (unintentional)

Toxic effect of chlorine gas NOS

² ✓7ᵗʰ **T59.4X2** **Toxic effect of chlorine gas,** intentional self-harm   HCC

✓7ᵗʰ **T59.4X3** **Toxic effect of chlorine gas,** assault

✓7ᵗʰ **T59.4X4** **Toxic effect of chlorine gas,** undetermined

✓5ᵗʰ **T59.5** **Toxic effect of fluorine gas and hydrogen fluoride**

✓6ᵗʰ **T59.5X** **Toxic effect of fluorine gas and hydrogen fluoride**

✓7ᵗʰ **T59.5X1** **Toxic effect of fluorine gas and hydrogen fluoride,** accidental (unintentional)

Toxic effect of fluorine gas and hydrogen fluoride NOS

² ✓7ᵗʰ **T59.5X2** **Toxic effect of fluorine gas and hydrogen fluoride,** intentional self-harm   HCC

✓7ᵗʰ **T59.5X3** **Toxic effect of fluorine gas and hydrogen fluoride,** assault

✓7ᵗʰ **T59.5X4** **Toxic effect of fluorine gas and hydrogen fluoride,** undetermined

✓5ᵗʰ **T59.6** **Toxic effect of hydrogen sulfide**

✓6ᵗʰ **T59.6X** **Toxic effect of hydrogen sulfide**

✓7ᵗʰ **T59.6X1** **Toxic effect of hydrogen sulfide,** accidental (unintentional)

Toxic effect of hydrogen sulfide NOS

² ✓7ᵗʰ **T59.6X2** **Toxic effect of hydrogen sulfide,** intentional self-harm   HCC

✓7ᵗʰ **T59.6X3** **Toxic effect of hydrogen sulfide,** assault

✓7ᵗʰ **T59.6X4** **Toxic effect of hydrogen sulfide,** undetermined

✓5ᵗʰ **T59.7** **Toxic effect of carbon dioxide**

✓6ᵗʰ **T59.7X** **Toxic effect of carbon dioxide**

✓7ᵗʰ **T59.7X1** **Toxic effect of carbon dioxide,** accidental (unintentional)

Toxic effect of carbon dioxide NOS

² ✓7ᵗʰ **T59.7X2** **Toxic effect of carbon dioxide,** intentional self-harm   HCC

✓7ᵗʰ **T59.7X3** **Toxic effect of carbon dioxide,** assault

✓7ᵗʰ **T59.7X4** **Toxic effect of carbon dioxide,** undetermined

✓5ᵗʰ **T59.8** **Toxic effect of other specified gases, fumes and vapors**

✓6ᵗʰ **T59.81** **Toxic effect of smoke**

Smoke inhalation

EXCLUDES 2   *toxic effect of cigarette (tobacco) smoke (T65.22-)*

✓7ᵗʰ **T59.811** **Toxic effect of smoke,** accidental (unintentional)

Toxic effect of smoke NOS

AHA: 2013,4Q,121

² ✓7ᵗʰ **T59.812** **Toxic effect of smoke,** intentional self-harm   HCC

✓7ᵗʰ **T59.813** **Toxic effect of smoke,** assault

✓7ᵗʰ **T59.814** **Toxic effect of smoke,** undetermined

✓6ᵗʰ **T59.89** **Toxic effect of other specified gases, fumes and vapors**

✓7ᵗʰ **T59.891** **Toxic effect of other specified gases, fumes and vapors,** accidental (unintentional)

² ✓7ᵗʰ **T59.892** **Toxic effect of other specified gases, fumes and vapors,** intentional self-harm   HCC

✓7ᵗʰ **T59.893** **Toxic effect of other specified gases, fumes and vapors,** assault

✓7ᵗʰ **T59.894** **Toxic effect of other specified gases, fumes and vapors,** undetermined

✓5ᵗʰ **T59.9** **Toxic effect of unspecified gases, fumes and vapors**

✓x7ᵗʰ **T59.91** **Toxic effect of unspecified gases, fumes and vapors,** accidental (unintentional) ▽

² ✓x7ᵗʰ **T59.92** **Toxic effect of unspecified gases, fumes and vapors,** intentional self-harm   HCC ▽

✓x7ᵗʰ **T59.93** **Toxic effect of unspecified gases, fumes and vapors,** assault ▽

✓x7ᵗʰ **T59.94** **Toxic effect of unspecified gases, fumes and vapors,** undetermined ▽

√4ᵗʰ **T60 Toxic effect of pesticides**

INCLUDES   toxic effect of wood preservatives

The appropriate 7th character is to be added to each code from category T60.
A   initial encounter
D   subsequent encounter
S   sequela

√5ᵗʰ **T60.0 Toxic effect of organophosphate and carbamate insecticides**

√6ᵗʰ **T60.0X Toxic effect of organophosphate and carbamate insecticides**

√7ᵗʰ **T60.0X1 Toxic effect of organophosphate and carbamate insecticides, accidental (unintentional)**
Toxic effect of organophosphate and carbamate insecticides NOS

2 √7ᵗʰ **T60.0X2 Toxic effect of organophosphate and carbamate insecticides, intentional self-harm**   HCC

√7ᵗʰ **T60.0X3 Toxic effect of organophosphate and carbamate insecticides, assault**

√7ᵗʰ **T60.0X4 Toxic effect of organophosphate and carbamate insecticides, undetermined**

√5ᵗʰ **T60.1 Toxic effect of halogenated insecticides**

EXCLUDES 1   chlorinated hydrocarbon (T53.-)

√6ᵗʰ **T60.1X Toxic effect of halogenated insecticides**

√7ᵗʰ **T60.1X1 Toxic effect of halogenated insecticides, accidental (unintentional)**
Toxic effect of halogenated insecticides NOS

2 √7ᵗʰ **T60.1X2 Toxic effect of halogenated insecticides, intentional self-harm**   HCC

√7ᵗʰ **T60.1X3 Toxic effect of halogenated insecticides, assault**

√7ᵗʰ **T60.1X4 Toxic effect of halogenated insecticides, undetermined**

√5ᵗʰ **T60.2 Toxic effect of other insecticides**

√6ᵗʰ **T60.2X Toxic effect of other insecticides**

√7ᵗʰ **T60.2X1 Toxic effect of other insecticides, accidental (unintentional)**
Toxic effect of other insecticides NOS

2 √7ᵗʰ **T60.2X2 Toxic effect of other insecticides, intentional self-harm**   HCC

√7ᵗʰ **T60.2X3 Toxic effect of other insecticides, assault**

√7ᵗʰ **T60.2X4 Toxic effect of other insecticides, undetermined**

√5ᵗʰ **T60.3 Toxic effect of herbicides and fungicides**

√6ᵗʰ **T60.3X Toxic effect of herbicides and fungicides**

√7ᵗʰ **T60.3X1 Toxic effect of herbicides and fungicides, accidental (unintentional)**
Toxic effect of herbicides and fungicides NOS

2 √7ᵗʰ **T60.3X2 Toxic effect of herbicides and fungicides, intentional self-harm**   HCC

√7ᵗʰ **T60.3X3 Toxic effect of herbicides and fungicides, assault**

√7ᵗʰ **T60.3X4 Toxic effect of herbicides and fungicides, undetermined**

√5ᵗʰ **T60.4 Toxic effect of rodenticides**

EXCLUDES 1   strychnine and its salts (T65.1)
thallium (T56.81-)

√6ᵗʰ **T60.4X Toxic effect of rodenticides**

√7ᵗʰ **T60.4X1 Toxic effect of rodenticides, accidental (unintentional)**
Toxic effect of rodenticides NOS

2 √7ᵗʰ **T60.4X2 Toxic effect of rodenticides, intentional self-harm**   HCC

√7ᵗʰ **T60.4X3 Toxic effect of rodenticides, assault**

√7ᵗʰ **T60.4X4 Toxic effect of rodenticides, undetermined**

√5ᵗʰ **T60.8 Toxic effect of other pesticides**

√6ᵗʰ **T60.8X Toxic effect of other pesticides**

√7ᵗʰ **T60.8X1 Toxic effect of other pesticides, accidental (unintentional)**
Toxic effect of other pesticides NOS

2 √7ᵗʰ **T60.8X2 Toxic effect of other pesticides, intentional self-harm**   HCC

√7ᵗʰ **T60.8X3 Toxic effect of other pesticides, assault**

√7ᵗʰ **T60.8X4 Toxic effect of other pesticides, undetermined**

√5ᵗʰ **T60.9 Toxic effect of unspecified pesticide**

√x7ᵗʰ **T60.91 Toxic effect of unspecified pesticide, accidental (unintentional)**   ▽

2 √x7ᵗʰ **T60.92 Toxic effect of unspecified pesticide, intentional self-harm**   HCC ▽

√x7ᵗʰ **T60.93 Toxic effect of unspecified pesticide, assault**   ▽

√x7ᵗʰ **T60.94 Toxic effect of unspecified pesticide, undetermined**   ▽

√4ᵗʰ **T61 Toxic effect of noxious substances eaten as seafood**

EXCLUDES 1   allergic reaction to food, such as:
anaphylactic reaction or shock due to adverse food reaction (T78.0-)
bacterial foodborne intoxications (A05.-)
dermatitis (L23.6, L25.4, L27.2)
food protein-induced enterocolitis syndrome (K52.21)
food protein-induced enteropathy (K52.22)
gastroenteritis (noninfective) (K52.29)
toxic effect of aflatoxin and other mycotoxins (T64)
toxic effect of cyanides (T65.0-)
toxic effect of harmful algae bloom (T65.82-)
toxic effect of hydrogen cyanide (T57.3-)
toxic effect of mercury (T56.1-)
toxic effect of red tide (T65.82-)

The appropriate 7th character is to be added to each code from category T61.
A   initial encounter
D   subsequent encounter
S   sequela

√5ᵗʰ **T61.0 Ciguatera fish poisoning**

√x7ᵗʰ **T61.01 Ciguatera fish poisoning, accidental (unintentional)**

2 √x7ᵗʰ **T61.02 Ciguatera fish poisoning, intentional self-harm**   HCC

√x7ᵗʰ **T61.03 Ciguatera fish poisoning, assault**

√x7ᵗʰ **T61.04 Ciguatera fish poisoning, undetermined**

√5ᵗʰ **T61.1 Scombroid fish poisoning**
Histamine-like syndrome

√x7ᵗʰ **T61.11 Scombroid fish poisoning, accidental (unintentional)**

2 √x7ᵗʰ **T61.12 Scombroid fish poisoning, intentional self-harm**   HCC

√x7ᵗʰ **T61.13 Scombroid fish poisoning, assault**

√x7ᵗʰ **T61.14 Scombroid fish poisoning, undetermined**

√5ᵗʰ **T61.7 Other fish and shellfish poisoning**

√6ᵗʰ **T61.77 Other fish poisoning**

√7ᵗʰ **T61.771 Other fish poisoning, accidental (unintentional)**

2 √7ᵗʰ **T61.772 Other fish poisoning, intentional self-harm**   HCC

√7ᵗʰ **T61.773 Other fish poisoning, assault**

√7ᵗʰ **T61.774 Other fish poisoning, undetermined**

√6ᵗʰ **T61.78 Other shellfish poisoning**

√7ᵗʰ **T61.781 Other shellfish poisoning, accidental (unintentional)**

2 √7ᵗʰ **T61.782 Other shellfish poisoning, intentional self-harm**   HCC

√7ᵗʰ **T61.783 Other shellfish poisoning, assault**

√7ᵗʰ **T61.784 Other shellfish poisoning, undetermined**

√5ᵗʰ **T61.8 Toxic effect of other seafood**

√6ᵗʰ **T61.8X Toxic effect of other seafood**

√7ᵗʰ **T61.8X1 Toxic effect of other seafood, accidental (unintentional)**

2 √7ᵗʰ **T61.8X2 Toxic effect of other seafood, intentional self-harm**   HCC

√7ᵗʰ **T61.8X3 Toxic effect of other seafood, assault**

√7ᵗʰ **T61.8X4 Toxic effect of other seafood, undetermined**

√5ᵗʰ **T61.9 Toxic effect of unspecified seafood**

√x7ᵗʰ **T61.91 Toxic effect of unspecified seafood, accidental (unintentional)**   ▽

2 √x7ᵗʰ **T61.92 Toxic effect of unspecified seafood, intentional self-harm**   HCC ▽

√x7ᵗʰ **T61.93 Toxic effect of unspecified seafood, assault**   ▽

Chapter 19. Injury, Poisoning and Certain Other Consequences of External Causes

T60–T61.93

√x7ᵗʰ **T61.94 Toxic effect of unspecified seafood,** ▽
     undetermined

√4ᵗʰ **T62 Toxic effect of other noxious substances eaten as food**

> **EXCLUDES 1**   allergic reaction to food, such as:
> anaphylactic shock (reaction) due to adverse food reaction (T78.0-)
> bacterial food borne intoxications (A05.-)
> dermatitis (L23.6, L25.4, L27.2)
> food protein-induced enterocolitis syndrome (K52.21)
> food protein-induced enteropathy (K52.22)
> gastroenteritis (noninfective) (K52.29)
> toxic effect of aflatoxin and other mycotoxins (T64)
> toxic effect of cyanides (T65.0-)
> toxic effect of hydrogen cyanide (T57.3-)
> toxic effect of mercury (T56.1-)

> The appropriate 7th character is to be added to each code from category T62.
> A   initial encounter
> D   subsequent encounter
> S   sequela

√5ᵗʰ **T62.0 Toxic effect of ingested mushrooms**

   √6ᵗʰ **T62.0X Toxic effect of ingested mushrooms**

     √7ᵗʰ **T62.0X1 Toxic effect of ingested mushrooms, accidental (unintentional)**
       Toxic effect of ingested mushrooms NOS

     2 √7ᵗʰ **T62.0X2 Toxic effect of ingested mushrooms, intentional self-harm** HCC

     √7ᵗʰ **T62.0X3 Toxic effect of ingested mushrooms, assault**

     √7ᵗʰ **T62.0X4 Toxic effect of ingested mushrooms, undetermined**

√5ᵗʰ **T62.1 Toxic effect of ingested berries**

   √6ᵗʰ **T62.1X Toxic effect of ingested berries**

     √7ᵗʰ **T62.1X1 Toxic effect of ingested berries, accidental (unintentional)**
       Toxic effect of ingested berries NOS

     2 √7ᵗʰ **T62.1X2 Toxic effect of ingested berries, intentional self-harm** HCC

     √7ᵗʰ **T62.1X3 Toxic effect of ingested berries, assault**

     √7ᵗʰ **T62.1X4 Toxic effect of ingested berries, undetermined**

√5ᵗʰ **T62.2 Toxic effect of other ingested (parts of) plant(s)**

   √6ᵗʰ **T62.2X Toxic effect of other ingested (parts of) plant(s)**

     √7ᵗʰ **T62.2X1 Toxic effect of other ingested (parts of) plant(s), accidental (unintentional)**
       Toxic effect of other ingested (parts of) plant(s) NOS

     2 √7ᵗʰ **T62.2X2 Toxic effect of other ingested (parts of) plant(s), intentional self-harm** HCC

     √7ᵗʰ **T62.2X3 Toxic effect of other ingested (parts of) plant(s), assault**

     √7ᵗʰ **T62.2X4 Toxic effect of other ingested (parts of) plant(s), undetermined**

√5ᵗʰ **T62.8 Toxic effect of other specified noxious substances eaten as food**

   √6ᵗʰ **T62.8X Toxic effect of other specified noxious substances eaten as food**

     √7ᵗʰ **T62.8X1 Toxic effect of other specified noxious substances eaten as food, accidental (unintentional)**
       Toxic effect of other specified noxious substances eaten as food NOS

     2 √7ᵗʰ **T62.8X2 Toxic effect of other specified noxious substances eaten as food, intentional self-harm** HCC

     √7ᵗʰ **T62.8X3 Toxic effect of other specified noxious substances eaten as food, assault**

     √7ᵗʰ **T62.8X4 Toxic effect of other specified noxious substances eaten as food, undetermined**

√5ᵗʰ **T62.9 Toxic effect of unspecified noxious substance eaten as food**

   √x7ᵗʰ **T62.91 Toxic effect of unspecified noxious** ▽
     substance eaten as food, accidental (unintentional)
       Toxic effect of unspecified noxious substance eaten as food NOS

2 √x7ᵗʰ **T62.92 Toxic effect of unspecified noxious** HCC ▽
     substance eaten as food, intentional self-harm

√x7ᵗʰ **T62.93 Toxic effect of unspecified noxious** ▽
     substance eaten as food, assault

√x7ᵗʰ **T62.94 Toxic effect of unspecified noxious** ▽
     substance eaten as food, undetermined

√4ᵗʰ **T63 Toxic effect of contact with venomous animals and plants**

> **INCLUDES**   bite or touch of venomous animal
> pricked or stuck by thorn or leaf
> **EXCLUDES 2**   ingestion of toxic animal or plant (T61.-, T62.-)

> The appropriate 7th character is to be added to each code from category T63.
> A   initial encounter
> D   subsequent encounter
> S   sequela

√5ᵗʰ **T63.0 Toxic effect of snake venom**

   √6ᵗʰ **T63.00 Toxic effect of unspecified snake venom**

     √7ᵗʰ **T63.001 Toxic effect of unspecified snake** ▽
     venom, accidental (unintentional)
       Toxic effect of unspecified snake venom NOS

     2 √7ᵗʰ **T63.002 Toxic effect of unspecified snake** HCC ▽
     venom, intentional self-harm

     √7ᵗʰ **T63.003 Toxic effect of unspecified snake** ▽
     venom, assault

     √7ᵗʰ **T63.004 Toxic effect of unspecified snake** ▽
     venom, undetermined

   √6ᵗʰ **T63.01 Toxic effect of rattlesnake venom**

     √7ᵗʰ **T63.011 Toxic effect of rattlesnake venom, accidental (unintentional)**
       Toxic effect of rattlesnake venom NOS

     2 √7ᵗʰ **T63.012 Toxic effect of rattlesnake venom,** HCC
     intentional self-harm

     √7ᵗʰ **T63.013 Toxic effect of rattlesnake venom, assault**

     √7ᵗʰ **T63.014 Toxic effect of rattlesnake venom, undetermined**

   √6ᵗʰ **T63.02 Toxic effect of coral snake venom**

     √7ᵗʰ **T63.021 Toxic effect of coral snake venom, accidental (unintentional)**
       Toxic effect of coral snake venom NOS

     2 √7ᵗʰ **T63.022 Toxic effect of coral snake venom,** HCC
     intentional self-harm

     √7ᵗʰ **T63.023 Toxic effect of coral snake venom, assault**

     √7ᵗʰ **T63.024 Toxic effect of coral snake venom, undetermined**

   √6ᵗʰ **T63.03 Toxic effect of taipan venom**

     √7ᵗʰ **T63.031 Toxic effect of taipan venom, accidental (unintentional)**
       Toxic effect of taipan venom NOS

     2 √7ᵗʰ **T63.032 Toxic effect of taipan venom,** HCC
     intentional self-harm

     √7ᵗʰ **T63.033 Toxic effect of taipan venom, assault**

     √7ᵗʰ **T63.034 Toxic effect of taipan venom, undetermined**

   √6ᵗʰ **T63.04 Toxic effect of cobra venom**

     √7ᵗʰ **T63.041 Toxic effect of cobra venom, accidental (unintentional)**
       Toxic effect of cobra venom NOS

     2 √7ᵗʰ **T63.042 Toxic effect of cobra venom,** HCC
     intentional self-harm

     √7ᵗʰ **T63.043 Toxic effect of cobra venom, assault**

     √7ᵗʰ **T63.044 Toxic effect of cobra venom, undetermined**

   √6ᵗʰ **T63.06 Toxic effect of venom of other North and South American snake**

     √7ᵗʰ **T63.061 Toxic effect of venom of other North and South American snake, accidental (unintentional)**
       Toxic effect of venom of other North and South American snake NOS

     2 √7ᵗʰ **T63.062 Toxic effect of venom of other** HCC
     North and South American snake, intentional self-harm

     √7ᵗʰ **T63.063 Toxic effect of venom of other North and South American snake, assault**

     √7ᵗʰ **T63.064 Toxic effect of venom of other North and South American snake, undetermined**

✓6ᵗʰ **T63.07 Toxic effect of venom of** other Australian snake

  ✓7ᵗʰ **T63.071 Toxic effect of venom of other Australian snake,** accidental (unintentional)
    Toxic effect of venom of other Australian snake NOS

  ² ✓7ᵗʰ **T63.072 Toxic effect of venom of other Australian snake,** intentional self-harm   HCC

  ✓7ᵗʰ **T63.073 Toxic effect of venom of other Australian snake,** assault

  ✓7ᵗʰ **T63.074 Toxic effect of venom of other Australian snake,** undetermined

✓6ᵗʰ **T63.08 Toxic effect of venom of** other African and Asian snake

  ✓7ᵗʰ **T63.081 Toxic effect of venom of other African and Asian snake,** accidental (unintentional)
    Toxic effect of venom of other African and Asian snake NOS

  ² ✓7ᵗʰ **T63.082 Toxic effect of venom of other African and Asian snake,** intentional self-harm   HCC

  ✓7ᵗʰ **T63.083 Toxic effect of venom of other African and Asian snake,** assault

  ✓7ᵗʰ **T63.084 Toxic effect of venom of other African and Asian snake,** undetermined

✓6ᵗʰ **T63.09 Toxic effect of venom of** other snake

  ✓7ᵗʰ **T63.091 Toxic effect of venom of other snake,** accidental (unintentional)
    Toxic effect of venom of other snake NOS

  ² ✓7ᵗʰ **T63.092 Toxic effect of venom of other snake,** intentional self-harm   HCC

  ✓7ᵗʰ **T63.093 Toxic effect of venom of other snake,** assault

  ✓7ᵗʰ **T63.094 Toxic effect of venom of other snake,** undetermined

✓5ᵗʰ **T63.1 Toxic effect of venom of other reptiles**

  ✓6ᵗʰ **T63.11 Toxic effect of venom of** gila monster

    ✓7ᵗʰ **T63.111 Toxic effect of venom of gila monster,** accidental (unintentional)
      Toxic effect of venom of gila monster NOS

    ² ✓7ᵗʰ **T63.112 Toxic effect of venom of gila monster,** intentional self-harm   HCC

    ✓7ᵗʰ **T63.113 Toxic effect of venom of gila monster,** assault

    ✓7ᵗʰ **T63.114 Toxic effect of venom of gila monster,** undetermined

  ✓6ᵗʰ **T63.12 Toxic effect of venom of** other venomous lizard

    ✓7ᵗʰ **T63.121 Toxic effect of venom of other venomous lizard,** accidental (unintentional)
      Toxic effect of venom of other venomous lizard NOS

    ² ✓7ᵗʰ **T63.122 Toxic effect of venom of other venomous lizard,** intentional self-harm   HCC

    ✓7ᵗʰ **T63.123 Toxic effect of venom of other venomous lizard,** assault

    ✓7ᵗʰ **T63.124 Toxic effect of venom of other venomous lizard,** undetermined

  ✓6ᵗʰ **T63.19 Toxic effect of venom of** other reptiles

    ✓7ᵗʰ **T63.191 Toxic effect of venom of other reptiles,** accidental (unintentional)
      Toxic effect of venom of other reptiles NOS

    ² ✓7ᵗʰ **T63.192 Toxic effect of venom of other reptiles,** intentional self-harm   HCC

    ✓7ᵗʰ **T63.193 Toxic effect of venom of other reptiles,** assault

    ✓7ᵗʰ **T63.194 Toxic effect of venom of other reptiles,** undetermined

✓5ᵗʰ **T63.2 Toxic effect of venom of scorpion**

  ✓6ᵗʰ **T63.2X Toxic effect of** venom of scorpion

    ✓7ᵗʰ **T63.2X1 Toxic effect of venom of scorpion,** accidental (unintentional)
      Toxic effect of venom of scorpion NOS

    ² ✓7ᵗʰ **T63.2X2 Toxic effect of venom of scorpion,** intentional self-harm   HCC

    ✓7ᵗʰ **T63.2X3 Toxic effect of venom of scorpion,** assault

    ✓7ᵗʰ **T63.2X4 Toxic effect of venom of scorpion,** undetermined

✓5ᵗʰ **T63.3 Toxic effect of** venom of spider

  ✓6ᵗʰ **T63.30 Toxic effect of unspecified spider venom**

    ✓7ᵗʰ **T63.301 Toxic effect of unspecified spider venom,** accidental (unintentional) ▽

    ² ✓7ᵗʰ **T63.302 Toxic effect of unspecified spider venom,** intentional self-harm   HCC ▽

    ✓7ᵗʰ **T63.303 Toxic effect of unspecified spider venom,** assault ▽

    ✓7ᵗʰ **T63.304 Toxic effect of unspecified spider venom,** undetermined ▽

  ✓6ᵗʰ **T63.31 Toxic effect of venom of** black widow spider

    ✓7ᵗʰ **T63.311 Toxic effect of venom of black widow spider,** accidental (unintentional)

    ² ✓7ᵗʰ **T63.312 Toxic effect of venom of black widow spider,** intentional self-harm   HCC

    ✓7ᵗʰ **T63.313 Toxic effect of venom of black widow spider,** assault

    ✓7ᵗʰ **T63.314 Toxic effect of venom of black widow spider,** undetermined

  ✓6ᵗʰ **T63.32 Toxic effect of venom of** tarantula

    ✓7ᵗʰ **T63.321 Toxic effect of venom of tarantula,** accidental (unintentional)

    ² ✓7ᵗʰ **T63.322 Toxic effect of venom of tarantula,** intentional self-harm   HCC

    ✓7ᵗʰ **T63.323 Toxic effect of venom of tarantula,** assault

    ✓7ᵗʰ **T63.324 Toxic effect of venom of tarantula,** undetermined

  ✓6ᵗʰ **T63.33 Toxic effect of venom of** brown recluse spider

    ✓7ᵗʰ **T63.331 Toxic effect of venom of brown recluse spider,** accidental (unintentional)

    ² ✓7ᵗʰ **T63.332 Toxic effect of venom of brown recluse spider,** intentional self-harm   HCC

    ✓7ᵗʰ **T63.333 Toxic effect of venom of brown recluse spider,** assault

    ✓7ᵗʰ **T63.334 Toxic effect of venom of brown recluse spider,** undetermined

  ✓6ᵗʰ **T63.39 Toxic effect of venom of** other spider

    ✓7ᵗʰ **T63.391 Toxic effect of venom of other spider,** accidental (unintentional)

    ² ✓7ᵗʰ **T63.392 Toxic effect of venom of other spider,** intentional self-harm   HCC

    ✓7ᵗʰ **T63.393 Toxic effect of venom of other spider,** assault

    ✓7ᵗʰ **T63.394 Toxic effect of venom of other spider,** undetermined

✓5ᵗʰ **T63.4 Toxic effect of venom of other arthropods**

  ✓6ᵗʰ **T63.41 Toxic effect of venom of** centipedes and venomous millipedes

    ✓7ᵗʰ **T63.411 Toxic effect of venom of centipedes and venomous millipedes,** accidental (unintentional)

    ² ✓7ᵗʰ **T63.412 Toxic effect of venom of centipedes and venomous millipedes,** intentional self-harm   HCC

    ✓7ᵗʰ **T63.413 Toxic effect of venom of centipedes and venomous millipedes,** assault

    ✓7ᵗʰ **T63.414 Toxic effect of venom of centipedes and venomous millipedes,** undetermined

  ✓6ᵗʰ **T63.42 Toxic effect of venom of** ants

    ✓7ᵗʰ **T63.421 Toxic effect of venom of ants,** accidental (unintentional)

    ² ✓7ᵗʰ **T63.422 Toxic effect of venom of ants,** intentional self-harm   HCC

    ✓7ᵗʰ **T63.423 Toxic effect of venom of ants,** assault

    ✓7ᵗʰ **T63.424 Toxic effect of venom of ants,** undetermined

  ✓6ᵗʰ **T63.43 Toxic effect of venom of** caterpillars

    ✓7ᵗʰ **T63.431 Toxic effect of venom of caterpillars,** accidental (unintentional)

    ² ✓7ᵗʰ **T63.432 Toxic effect of venom of caterpillars,** intentional self-harm   HCC

    ✓7ᵗʰ **T63.433 Toxic effect of venom of caterpillars,** assault

    ✓7ᵗʰ **T63.434 Toxic effect of venom of caterpillars,** undetermined

  ✓6ᵗʰ **T63.44 Toxic effect of venom of** bees

    ✓7ᵗʰ **T63.441 Toxic effect of venom of bees,** accidental (unintentional)

✓ Additional Character Req   ✓x7ᵗʰ Placeholder Alert   Manifestation   ▽ Unspecified   ▶◀ Revised Text   ● New Code   ▲ Revised Code Title

² ✓7ᵗʰ **T63.442 Toxic effect of venom of bees,** HCC
    intentional self-harm

✓7ᵗʰ **T63.443 Toxic effect of venom of bees, assault**

✓7ᵗʰ **T63.444 Toxic effect of venom of bees,**
    undetermined

✓6ᵗʰ **T63.45 Toxic effect of venom of hornets**

✓7ᵗʰ **T63.451 Toxic effect of venom of hornets,**
    accidental (unintentional)

² ✓7ᵗʰ **T63.452 Toxic effect of venom of hornets,** HCC
    intentional self-harm

✓7ᵗʰ **T63.453 Toxic effect of venom of hornets, assault**

✓7ᵗʰ **T63.454 Toxic effect of venom of hornets,**
    undetermined

✓6ᵗʰ **T63.46 Toxic effect of venom of wasps**

    Toxic effect of yellow jacket

✓7ᵗʰ **T63.461 Toxic effect of venom of wasps, accidental**
    (unintentional)

² ✓7ᵗʰ **T63.462 Toxic effect of venom of wasps,** HCC
    intentional self-harm

✓7ᵗʰ **T63.463 Toxic effect of venom of wasps, assault**

✓7ᵗʰ **T63.464 Toxic effect of venom of wasps,**
    undetermined

✓6ᵗʰ **T63.48 Toxic effect of venom of other arthropod**

✓7ᵗʰ **T63.481 Toxic effect of venom of other arthropod,**
    accidental (unintentional)

² ✓7ᵗʰ **T63.482 Toxic effect of venom of other** HCC
    arthropod, intentional self-harm

✓7ᵗʰ **T63.483 Toxic effect of venom of other arthropod,**
    assault

✓7ᵗʰ **T63.484 Toxic effect of venom of other arthropod,**
    undetermined

✓5ᵗʰ **T63.5 Toxic effect of contact with venomous fish**

    EXCLUDES 2   *poisoning by ingestion of fish (T61.-)*

✓6ᵗʰ **T63.51 Toxic effect of contact with stingray**

✓7ᵗʰ **T63.511 Toxic effect of contact with stingray,**
    accidental (unintentional)

² ✓7ᵗʰ **T63.512 Toxic effect of contact with** HCC
    stingray, intentional self-harm

✓7ᵗʰ **T63.513 Toxic effect of contact with stingray,**
    assault

✓7ᵗʰ **T63.514 Toxic effect of contact with stingray,**
    undetermined

✓6ᵗʰ **T63.59 Toxic effect of contact with other venomous fish**

✓7ᵗʰ **T63.591 Toxic effect of contact with other**
    venomous fish, accidental (unintentional)

² ✓7ᵗʰ **T63.592 Toxic effect of contact with other** HCC
    venomous fish, intentional
    self-harm

✓7ᵗʰ **T63.593 Toxic effect of contact with other**
    venomous fish, assault

✓7ᵗʰ **T63.594 Toxic effect of contact with other**
    venomous fish, undetermined

✓5ᵗʰ **T63.6 Toxic effect of contact with other venomous marine animals**

    EXCLUDES 1   *sea-snake venom (T63.09)*

    EXCLUDES 2   *poisoning by ingestion of shellfish (T61.78-)*

✓6ᵗʰ **T63.61 Toxic effect of contact with Portugese Man-o-war**

    Toxic effect of contact with bluebottle

✓7ᵗʰ **T63.611 Toxic effect of contact with Portugese**
    Man-o-war, accidental (unintentional)

² ✓7ᵗʰ **T63.612 Toxic effect of contact with** HCC
    Portugese Man-o-war, intentional
    self-harm

✓7ᵗʰ **T63.613 Toxic effect of contact with Portugese**
    Man-o-war, assault

✓7ᵗʰ **T63.614 Toxic effect of contact with Portugese**
    Man-o-war, undetermined

✓6ᵗʰ **T63.62 Toxic effect of contact with other jellyfish**

✓7ᵗʰ **T63.621 Toxic effect of contact with other jellyfish,**
    accidental (unintentional)

² ✓7ᵗʰ **T63.622 Toxic effect of contact with other** HCC
    jellyfish, intentional self-harm

✓7ᵗʰ **T63.623 Toxic effect of contact with other jellyfish,**
    assault

✓7ᵗʰ **T63.624 Toxic effect of contact with other jellyfish,**
    undetermined

✓6ᵗʰ **T63.63 Toxic effect of contact with sea anemone**

✓7ᵗʰ **T63.631 Toxic effect of contact with sea anemone,**
    accidental (unintentional)

² ✓7ᵗʰ **T63.632 Toxic effect of contact with sea** HCC
    anemone, intentional self-harm

✓7ᵗʰ **T63.633 Toxic effect of contact with sea anemone,**
    assault

✓7ᵗʰ **T63.634 Toxic effect of contact with sea anemone,**
    undetermined

✓6ᵗʰ **T63.69 Toxic effect of contact with other venomous marine animals**

✓7ᵗʰ **T63.691 Toxic effect of contact with other**
    venomous marine animals, accidental
    (unintentional)

² ✓7ᵗʰ **T63.692 Toxic effect of contact with other** HCC
    venomous marine animals,
    intentional self-harm

✓7ᵗʰ **T63.693 Toxic effect of contact with other**
    venomous marine animals, assault

✓7ᵗʰ **T63.694 Toxic effect of contact with other**
    venomous marine animals, undetermined

✓5ᵗʰ **T63.7 Toxic effect of contact with venomous plant**

✓6ᵗʰ **T63.71 Toxic effect of contact with venomous marine plant**

✓7ᵗʰ **T63.711 Toxic effect of contact with venomous**
    marine plant, accidental (unintentional)

² ✓7ᵗʰ **T63.712 Toxic effect of contact with** HCC
    venomous marine plant,
    intentional self-harm

✓7ᵗʰ **T63.713 Toxic effect of contact with venomous**
    marine plant, assault

✓7ᵗʰ **T63.714 Toxic effect of contact with venomous**
    marine plant, undetermined

✓6ᵗʰ **T63.79 Toxic effect of contact with other venomous plant**

✓7ᵗʰ **T63.791 Toxic effect of contact with other**
    venomous plant, accidental
    (unintentional)

² ✓7ᵗʰ **T63.792 Toxic effect of contact with other** HCC
    venomous plant, intentional
    self-harm

✓7ᵗʰ **T63.793 Toxic effect of contact with other**
    venomous plant, assault

✓7ᵗʰ **T63.794 Toxic effect of contact with other**
    venomous plant, undetermined

✓5ᵗʰ **T63.8 Toxic effect of contact with other venomous animals**

✓6ᵗʰ **T63.81 Toxic effect of contact with venomous frog**

    EXCLUDES 1   *contact with nonvenomous frog (W62.0)*

✓7ᵗʰ **T63.811 Toxic effect of contact with venomous**
    frog, accidental (unintentional)

² ✓7ᵗʰ **T63.812 Toxic effect of contact with** HCC
    venomous frog, intentional
    self-harm

✓7ᵗʰ **T63.813 Toxic effect of contact with venomous**
    frog, assault

✓7ᵗʰ **T63.814 Toxic effect of contact with venomous**
    frog, undetermined

✓6ᵗʰ **T63.82 Toxic effect of contact with venomous toad**

    EXCLUDES 1   *contact with nonvenomous toad (W62.1)*

✓7ᵗʰ **T63.821 Toxic effect of contact with venomous**
    toad, accidental (unintentional)

² ✓7ᵗʰ **T63.822 Toxic effect of contact with** HCC
    venomous toad, intentional
    self-harm

✓7ᵗʰ **T63.823 Toxic effect of contact with venomous**
    toad, assault

✓7ᵗʰ **T63.824 Toxic effect of contact with venomous**
    toad, undetermined

✓6ᵗʰ **T63.83 Toxic effect of contact with other venomous amphibian**

    EXCLUDES 1   *contact with nonvenomous amphibian*
    (W62.9)

✓7ᵗʰ **T63.831 Toxic effect of contact with other**
    venomous amphibian, accidental
    (unintentional)

² ✓7ᵗʰ **T63.832 Toxic effect of contact with other** HCC
    venomous amphibian, intentional
    self-harm

✓7ᵗʰ **T63.833 Toxic effect of contact with other**
    venomous amphibian, assault

✓7ᵗʰ **T63.834 Toxic effect of contact with other**
    venomous amphibian, undetermined

✓6ᵗʰ **T63.89 Toxic effect of contact with other venomous animals**

✓7ᵗʰ **T63.891 Toxic effect of contact with other**
    venomous animals, accidental
    (unintentional)

² √7ᵗʰ **T63.892** Toxic effect of contact with other venomous animals, **intentional self-harm** `HCC`

√7ᵗʰ **T63.893** Toxic effect of contact with other venomous animals, **assault**

√7ᵗʰ **T63.894** Toxic effect of contact with other venomous animals, **undetermined**

√5ᵗʰ **T63.9** **Toxic effect of contact with unspecified venomous animal**

√x7ᵗʰ **T63.91** Toxic effect of contact with unspecified venomous animal, **accidental (unintentional)** ▽

² √x7ᵗʰ **T63.92** Toxic effect of contact with unspecified venomous animal, **intentional self-harm** `HCC` ▽

√x7ᵗʰ **T63.93** Toxic effect of contact with unspecified venomous animal, **assault** ▽

√x7ᵗʰ **T63.94** Toxic effect of contact with unspecified venomous animal, **undetermined** ▽

√4ᵗʰ **T64** **Toxic effect of aflatoxin and other mycotoxin food contaminants**

> The appropriate 7th character is to be added to each code from category T64.
> A   initial encounter
> D   subsequent encounter
> S   sequela

√5ᵗʰ **T64.0** **Toxic effect of aflatoxin**

√x7ᵗʰ **T64.01** Toxic effect of aflatoxin, **accidental (unintentional)**

² √x7ᵗʰ **T64.02** Toxic effect of aflatoxin, **intentional self-harm** `HCC`

√x7ᵗʰ **T64.03** Toxic effect of aflatoxin, **assault**

√x7ᵗʰ **T64.04** Toxic effect of aflatoxin, **undetermined**

√5ᵗʰ **T64.8** **Toxic effect of other mycotoxin food contaminants**

√x7ᵗʰ **T64.81** Toxic effect of other mycotoxin food contaminants, **accidental (unintentional)**

² √x7ᵗʰ **T64.82** Toxic effect of other mycotoxin food contaminants, **intentional self-harm** `HCC`

√x7ᵗʰ **T64.83** Toxic effect of other mycotoxin food contaminants, **assault**

√x7ᵗʰ **T64.84** Toxic effect of other mycotoxin food contaminants, **undetermined**

√4ᵗʰ **T65** **Toxic effect of other and unspecified substances**

> The appropriate 7th character is to be added to each code from category T65.
> A   initial encounter
> D   subsequent encounter
> S   sequela

√5ᵗʰ **T65.0** **Toxic effect of cyanides**

> **EXCLUDES 1**   hydrogen cyanide (T57.3-)

√6ᵗʰ **T65.0X** **Toxic effect of cyanides**

√7ᵗʰ **T65.0X1** Toxic effect of cyanides, **accidental (unintentional)**
Toxic effect of cyanides NOS

² √7ᵗʰ **T65.0X2** Toxic effect of cyanides, **intentional self-harm** `HCC`

√7ᵗʰ **T65.0X3** Toxic effect of cyanides, **assault**

√7ᵗʰ **T65.0X4** Toxic effect of cyanides, **undetermined**

√5ᵗʰ **T65.1** **Toxic effect of strychnine and its salts**

√6ᵗʰ **T65.1X** **Toxic effect of strychnine and its salts**

√7ᵗʰ **T65.1X1** Toxic effect of strychnine and its salts, **accidental (unintentional)**
Toxic effect of strychnine and its salts NOS

² √7ᵗʰ **T65.1X2** Toxic effect of strychnine and its salts, **intentional self-harm** `HCC`

√7ᵗʰ **T65.1X3** Toxic effect of strychnine and its salts, **assault**

√7ᵗʰ **T65.1X4** Toxic effect of strychnine and its salts, **undetermined**

√5ᵗʰ **T65.2** **Toxic effect of tobacco and nicotine**

> **EXCLUDES 2**   nicotine dependence (F17.-)

√6ᵗʰ **T65.21** **Toxic effect of chewing tobacco**

√7ᵗʰ **T65.211** Toxic effect of chewing tobacco, **accidental (unintentional)**
Toxic effect of chewing tobacco NOS

² √7ᵗʰ **T65.212** Toxic effect of chewing tobacco, **intentional self-harm** `HCC`

√7ᵗʰ **T65.213** Toxic effect of chewing tobacco, **assault**

√7ᵗʰ **T65.214** Toxic effect of chewing tobacco, **undetermined**

√6ᵗʰ **T65.22** **Toxic effect of tobacco cigarettes**
Toxic effect of tobacco smoke
Use additional code for exposure to second hand tobacco smoke (Z57.31, Z77.22)

√7ᵗʰ **T65.221** Toxic effect of tobacco cigarettes, **accidental (unintentional)**
Toxic effect of tobacco cigarettes NOS

² √7ᵗʰ **T65.222** Toxic effect of tobacco cigarettes, **intentional self-harm** `HCC`

√7ᵗʰ **T65.223** Toxic effect of tobacco cigarettes, **assault**

√7ᵗʰ **T65.224** Toxic effect of tobacco cigarettes, **undetermined**

√6ᵗʰ **T65.29** **Toxic effect of other tobacco and nicotine**

√7ᵗʰ **T65.291** Toxic effect of other tobacco and nicotine, **accidental (unintentional)**
Toxic effect of other tobacco and nicotine NOS

² √7ᵗʰ **T65.292** Toxic effect of other tobacco and nicotine, **intentional self-harm** `HCC`

√7ᵗʰ **T65.293** Toxic effect of other tobacco and nicotine, **assault**

√7ᵗʰ **T65.294** Toxic effect of other tobacco and nicotine, **undetermined**

√5ᵗʰ **T65.3** **Toxic effect of nitroderivatives and aminoderivatives of benzene and its homologues**
Toxic effect of anilin [benzenamine]
Toxic effect of nitrobenzene
Toxic effect of trinitrotoluene

√6ᵗʰ **T65.3X** **Toxic effect of nitroderivatives and aminoderivatives of benzene and its homologues**

√7ᵗʰ **T65.3X1** Toxic effect of nitroderivatives and aminoderivatives of benzene and its homologues, **accidental (unintentional)**
Toxic effect of nitroderivatives and aminoderivatives of benzene and its homologues NOS

² √7ᵗʰ **T65.3X2** Toxic effect of nitroderivatives and aminoderivatives of benzene and its homologues, **intentional self-harm** `HCC`

√7ᵗʰ **T65.3X3** Toxic effect of nitroderivatives and aminoderivatives of benzene and its homologues, **assault**

√7ᵗʰ **T65.3X4** Toxic effect of nitroderivatives and aminoderivatives of benzene and its homologues, **undetermined**

√5ᵗʰ **T65.4** **Toxic effect of carbon disulfide**

√6ᵗʰ **T65.4X** **Toxic effect of carbon disulfide**

√7ᵗʰ **T65.4X1** Toxic effect of carbon disulfide, **accidental (unintentional)**
Toxic effect of carbon disulfide NOS

² √7ᵗʰ **T65.4X2** Toxic effect of carbon disulfide, **intentional self-harm** `HCC`

√7ᵗʰ **T65.4X3** Toxic effect of carbon disulfide, **assault**

√7ᵗʰ **T65.4X4** Toxic effect of carbon disulfide, **undetermined**

√5ᵗʰ **T65.5** **Toxic effect of nitroglycerin and other nitric acids and esters**
Toxic effect of 1,2,3-Propanetriol trinitrate

√6ᵗʰ **T65.5X** **Toxic effect of nitroglycerin and other nitric acids and esters**

√7ᵗʰ **T65.5X1** Toxic effect of nitroglycerin and other nitric acids and esters, **accidental (unintentional)**
Toxic effect of nitroglycerin and other nitric acids and esters NOS

² √7ᵗʰ **T65.5X2** Toxic effect of nitroglycerin and other nitric acids and esters, **intentional self-harm** `HCC`

√7ᵗʰ **T65.5X3** Toxic effect of nitroglycerin and other nitric acids and esters, **assault**

√7ᵗʰ **T65.5X4** Toxic effect of nitroglycerin and other nitric acids and esters, **undetermined**

√5ᵗʰ **T65.6** **Toxic effect of paints and dyes, not elsewhere classified**

√6ᵗʰ **T65.6X** **Toxic effect of paints and dyes, not elsewhere classified**

√7ᵗʰ **T65.6X1** Toxic effect of paints and dyes, not elsewhere classified, **accidental (unintentional)**
Toxic effect of paints and dyes NOS

✓ Additional Character Req   √x7ᵗʰ Placeholder Alert   Manifestation   ▽ Unspecified   ▶◀ Revised Text   ● New Code   ▲ Revised Code Title

²　√7ᵗʰ　**T65.6X2** **Toxic effect of paints and dyes, not elsewhere classified, intentional self-harm** ᴴᶜᶜ

√7ᵗʰ　**T65.6X3** **Toxic effect of paints and dyes, not elsewhere classified, assault**

√7ᵗʰ　**T65.6X4** **Toxic effect of paints and dyes, not elsewhere classified, undetermined**

√5ᵗʰ　**T65.8** **Toxic effect of other specified substances**

√6ᵗʰ　**T65.81** **Toxic effect of latex**

√7ᵗʰ　**T65.811** **Toxic effect of latex, accidental (unintentional)**
Toxic effect of latex NOS

²　√7ᵗʰ　**T65.812** **Toxic effect of latex, intentional self-harm** ᴴᶜᶜ

√7ᵗʰ　**T65.813** **Toxic effect of latex, assault**

√7ᵗʰ　**T65.814** **Toxic effect of latex, undetermined**

√6ᵗʰ　**T65.82** **Toxic effect of harmful algae and algae toxins**
Toxic effect of (harmful) algae bloom NOS
Toxic effect of blue-green algae bloom
Toxic effect of brown tide
Toxic effect of cyanobacteria bloom
Toxic effect of Florida red tide
Toxic effect of pfiesteria piscicida
Toxic effect of red tide

√7ᵗʰ　**T65.821** **Toxic effect of harmful algae and algae toxins, accidental (unintentional)**
Toxic effect of harmful algae and algae toxins NOS

²　√7ᵗʰ　**T65.822** **Toxic effect of harmful algae and algae toxins, intentional self-harm** ᴴᶜᶜ

√7ᵗʰ　**T65.823** **Toxic effect of harmful algae and algae toxins, assault**

√7ᵗʰ　**T65.824** **Toxic effect of harmful algae and algae toxins, undetermined**

√6ᵗʰ　**T65.83** **Toxic effect of fiberglass**

√7ᵗʰ　**T65.831** **Toxic effect of fiberglass, accidental (unintentional)**
Toxic effect of fiberglass NOS

²　√7ᵗʰ　**T65.832** **Toxic effect of fiberglass, intentional self-harm** ᴴᶜᶜ

√7ᵗʰ　**T65.833** **Toxic effect of fiberglass, assault**

√7ᵗʰ　**T65.834** **Toxic effect of fiberglass, undetermined**

√6ᵗʰ　**T65.89** **Toxic effect of other specified substances**

√7ᵗʰ　**T65.891** **Toxic effect of other specified substances, accidental (unintentional)**
Toxic effect of other specified substances NOS

AHA: 2018,1Q,5

²　√7ᵗʰ　**T65.892** **Toxic effect of other specified substances, intentional self-harm** ᴴᶜᶜ

√7ᵗʰ　**T65.893** **Toxic effect of other specified substances, assault**

√7ᵗʰ　**T65.894** **Toxic effect of other specified substances, undetermined**

√5ᵗʰ　**T65.9** **Toxic effect of unspecified substance**

√x7ᵗʰ　**T65.91** **Toxic effect of unspecified substance, accidental (unintentional)** ▽
Poisoning NOS

²　√x7ᵗʰ　**T65.92** **Toxic effect of unspecified substance, intentional self-harm** ᴴᶜᶜ ▽

√x7ᵗʰ　**T65.93** **Toxic effect of unspecified substance, assault** ▽

√x7ᵗʰ　**T65.94** **Toxic effect of unspecified substance, undetermined** ▽

Other and unspecified effects of external causes (T66-T78)

√x7ᵗʰ **T66** **Radiation sickness, unspecified** ▽

EXCLUDES 1　specified adverse effects of radiation, such as:
burns (T20-T31)
leukemia (C91-C95)
radiation gastroenteritis and colitis (K52.0)
radiation pneumonitis (J70.0)
radiation related disorders of the skin and subcutaneous tissue (L55-L59)
radiation sunburn (L55.-)

The appropriate 7th character is to be added to code T66.
A initial encounter
D subsequent encounter
S sequela

√4ᵗʰ **T67** **Effects of heat and light**

EXCLUDES 1　erythema [dermatitis] ab igne (L59.0)
malignant hyperpyrexia due to anesthesia (T88.3)
radiation-related disorders of the skin and subcutaneous tissue (L55-L59)

EXCLUDES 2　burns (T20-T31)
sunburn (L55.-)
sweat disorder due to heat (L74-L75)

The appropriate 7th character is to be added to each code from category T67.
A initial encounter
D subsequent encounter
S sequela

√x7ᵗʰ **T67.0** **Heatstroke and sunstroke**
Heat apoplexy
Heat pyrexia
Siriasis
Thermoplegia
Use additional code(s) to identify any associated complications of heatstroke, such as:
coma and stupor (R40.-)
systemic inflammatory response syndrome (R65.1-)
DEF: Headache, vertigo, cramps, and elevated body temperature due to prolonged exposure to high environmental temperatures that requires emergency intervention.

√x7ᵗʰ **T67.1** **Heat syncope**
Heat collapse

√x7ᵗʰ **T67.2** **Heat cramp**

√x7ᵗʰ **T67.3** **Heat exhaustion, anhydrotic**
Heat prostration due to water depletion
EXCLUDES 1　heat exhaustion due to salt depletion (T67.4)

√x7ᵗʰ **T67.4** **Heat exhaustion due to salt depletion**
Heat prostration due to salt (and water) depletion

√x7ᵗʰ **T67.5** **Heat exhaustion, unspecified** ▽
Heat prostration NOS

√x7ᵗʰ **T67.6** **Heat fatigue, transient**

√x7ᵗʰ **T67.7** **Heat edema**

√x7ᵗʰ **T67.8** **Other effects of heat and light**

√x7ᵗʰ **T67.9** **Effect of heat and light, unspecified** ▽

√x7ᵗʰ **T68** **Hypothermia**
Accidental hypothermia
Hypothermia NOS
Use additional code to identify source of exposure:
exposure to excessive cold of man-made origin (W93)
exposure to excessive cold of natural origin (X31)
EXCLUDES 1　hypothermia following anesthesia (T88.51)
hypothermia not associated with low environmental temperature (R68.0)
hypothermia of newborn (P80.-)
EXCLUDES 2　frostbite (T33-T34)

The appropriate 7th character is to be added to code T68.
A initial encounter
D subsequent encounter
S sequela

✓4ᵗʰ **T69 Other effects of reduced temperature**

Use additional code to identify source of exposure:
exposure to excessive cold of man-made origin (W93)
exposure to excessive cold of natural origin (X31)

EXCLUDES 2   frostbite (T33-T34)

The appropriate 7th character is to be added to each code from category T69.
A   initial encounter
D   subsequent encounter
S   sequela

✓5ᵗʰ **T69.0 Immersion hand and foot**

    ✓6ᵗʰ **T69.01 Immersion hand**

       ✓7ᵗʰ **T69.011 Immersion hand, right hand**

       ✓7ᵗʰ **T69.012 Immersion hand, left hand**

       ✓7ᵗʰ **T69.019 Immersion hand, unspecified hand** ▽

    ✓6ᵗʰ **T69.02 Immersion foot**

       Trench foot

       ✓7ᵗʰ **T69.021 Immersion foot, right foot**

       ✓7ᵗʰ **T69.022 Immersion foot, left foot**

       ✓7ᵗʰ **T69.029 Immersion foot, unspecified foot** ▽

✓x7ᵗʰ **T69.1 Chilblains**

DEF: Red, swollen, itchy skin primarily affecting the fingers and toes, nose and ears, and legs. Chilblains follows damp-cold exposure, and can also be associated with pruritus and a burning feeling.

✓x7ᵗʰ **T69.8 Other specified effects of reduced temperature**

✓x7ᵗʰ **T69.9 Effect of reduced temperature, unspecified** ▽

✓4ᵗʰ **T70 Effects of air pressure and water pressure**

The appropriate 7th character is to be added to each code from category T70.
A   initial encounter
D   subsequent encounter
S   sequela

✓x7ᵗʰ **T70.0 Otitic barotrauma**

Aero-otitis media
Effects of change in ambient atmospheric pressure or water pressure on ears

✓x7ᵗʰ **T70.1 Sinus barotrauma**

Aerosinusitis
Effects of change in ambient atmospheric pressure on sinuses

✓5ᵗʰ **T70.2 Other and unspecified effects of high altitude**

    EXCLUDES 2   polycythemia due to high altitude (D75.1)

    ✓x7ᵗʰ **T70.20 Unspecified effects of high altitude** ▽

    ✓x7ᵗʰ **T70.29 Other effects of high altitude**

       Alpine sickness
       Anoxia due to high altitude
       Barotrauma NOS
       Hypobaropathy
       Mountain sickness

✓x7ᵗʰ **T70.3 Caisson disease [decompression sickness]**

Compressed-air disease
Diver's palsy or paralysis
DEF: Rapid reduction in air pressure while breathing compressed air. Symptoms include skin lesions, joint pains, and respiratory and neurological problems.

✓x7ᵗʰ **T70.4 Effects of high-pressure fluids**

Hydraulic jet injection (industrial)
Pneumatic jet injection (industrial)
Traumatic jet injection (industrial)

✓x7ᵗʰ **T70.8 Other effects of air pressure and water pressure**

✓x7ᵗʰ **T70.9 Effect of air pressure and water pressure, unspecified** ▽

✓4ᵗʰ **T71 Asphyxiation**

Mechanical suffocation
Traumatic suffocation

EXCLUDES 1   acute respiratory distress (syndrome) (J80)
       anoxia due to high altitude (T70.2)
       asphyxia NOS (R09.01)
       asphyxia from carbon monoxide (T58.-)
       asphyxia from inhalation of food or foreign body (T17.-)
       asphyxia from other gases, fumes and vapors (T59.-)
       respiratory distress (syndrome) in newborn (P22.-)

The appropriate 7th character is to be added to each code from category T71.
A   initial encounter
D   subsequent encounter
S   sequela

✓5ᵗʰ **T71.1 Asphyxiation due to mechanical threat to breathing**

Suffocation due to mechanical threat to breathing

    ✓6ᵗʰ **T71.11 Asphyxiation due to smothering under pillow**

       ✓7ᵗʰ **T71.111 Asphyxiation due to smothering under pillow, accidental**

          Asphyxiation due to smothering under pillow NOS

       ² ✓7ᵗʰ **T71.112 Asphyxiation due to smothering** HCC **under pillow, intentional self-harm**

       ✓7ᵗʰ **T71.113 Asphyxiation due to smothering under pillow, assault**

       ✓7ᵗʰ **T71.114 Asphyxiation due to smothering under pillow, undetermined**

    ✓6ᵗʰ **T71.12 Asphyxiation due to plastic bag**

       ✓7ᵗʰ **T71.121 Asphyxiation due to plastic bag, accidental**

          Asphyxiation due to plastic bag NOS

       ² ✓7ᵗʰ **T71.122 Asphyxiation due to plastic bag,** HCC **intentional self-harm**

       ✓7ᵗʰ **T71.123 Asphyxiation due to plastic bag, assault**

       ✓7ᵗʰ **T71.124 Asphyxiation due to plastic bag, undetermined**

    ✓6ᵗʰ **T71.13 Asphyxiation due to being trapped in bed linens**

       ✓7ᵗʰ **T71.131 Asphyxiation due to being trapped in bed linens, accidental**

          Asphyxiation due to being trapped in bed linens NOS

       ² ✓7ᵗʰ **T71.132 Asphyxiation due to being** HCC **trapped in bed linens, intentional self-harm**

       ✓7ᵗʰ **T71.133 Asphyxiation due to being trapped in bed linens, assault**

       ✓7ᵗʰ **T71.134 Asphyxiation due to being trapped in bed linens, undetermined**

    ✓6ᵗʰ **T71.14 Asphyxiation due to smothering under another person's body (in bed)**

       ✓7ᵗʰ **T71.141 Asphyxiation due to smothering under another person's body (in bed), accidental**

          Asphyxiation due to smothering under another person's body (in bed) NOS

       ✓7ᵗʰ **T71.143 Asphyxiation due to smothering under another person's body (in bed), assault**

       ✓7ᵗʰ **T71.144 Asphyxiation due to smothering under another person's body (in bed), undetermined**

    ✓6ᵗʰ **T71.15 Asphyxiation due to smothering in furniture**

       ✓7ᵗʰ **T71.151 Asphyxiation due to smothering in furniture, accidental**

          Asphyxiation due to smothering in furniture NOS

       ² ✓7ᵗʰ **T71.152 Asphyxiation due to smothering** HCC **in furniture, intentional self-harm**

       ✓7ᵗʰ **T71.153 Asphyxiation due to smothering in furniture, assault**

       ✓7ᵗʰ **T71.154 Asphyxiation due to smothering in furniture, undetermined**

☑ Additional Character Req   ✓x7ᵗʰ Placeholder Alert   Manifestation   ▽ Unspecified   ▶◀ Revised Text   ● New Code   ▲ Revised Code Title

Chapter 19. Injury, Poisoning and Certain Other Consequences of External Causes

✓6ᵗʰ T71.16 Asphyxiation due to hanging

Hanging by window shade cord
Use additional code for any associated injuries, such as:
  crushing injury of neck (S17.-)
  fracture of cervical vertebrae (S12.0-S12.2-)
  open wound of neck (S11.-)

     ✓7ᵗʰ **T71.161 Asphyxiation due to hanging,** accidental
         Asphyxiation due to hanging NOS
         Hanging NOS

     ² ✓7ᵗʰ **T71.162 Asphyxiation due to hanging,**   HCC
         intentional self-harm

     ✓7ᵗʰ **T71.163 Asphyxiation due to hanging,** assault

     ✓7ᵗʰ **T71.164 Asphyxiation due to hanging,**
         undetermined

✓6ᵗʰ T71.19 Asphyxiation due to mechanical threat to breathing due to other causes

     ✓7ᵗʰ **T71.191 Asphyxiation due to mechanical threat to breathing due to other causes,** accidental
         Asphyxiation due to other causes NOS

     ² ✓7ᵗʰ **T71.192 Asphyxiation due to mechanical threat to breathing due to other causes, intentional self-harm**   HCC

     ✓7ᵗʰ **T71.193 Asphyxiation due to mechanical threat to breathing due to other causes,** assault

     ✓7ᵗʰ **T71.194 Asphyxiation due to mechanical threat to breathing due to other causes, undetermined**

✓5ᵗʰ T71.2 Asphyxiation due to systemic oxygen deficiency due to low oxygen content in ambient air

Suffocation due to systemic oxygen deficiency due to low oxygen content in ambient air

     ✓x7ᵗʰ **T71.20 Asphyxiation due to systemic oxygen deficiency due to low oxygen content in ambient air due to unspecified cause**   ▽

     ✓x7ᵗʰ **T71.21 Asphyxiation due to cave-in or falling earth**
         Use additional code for any associated cataclysm (X34-X38)

     ✓6ᵗʰ **T71.22 Asphyxiation due to** being trapped in a car trunk

       ✓7ᵗʰ **T71.221 Asphyxiation due to being trapped in a car trunk,** accidental

       ² ✓7ᵗʰ **T71.222 Asphyxiation due to being trapped in a car trunk, intentional self-harm**   HCC

       ✓7ᵗʰ **T71.223 Asphyxiation due to being trapped in a car trunk,** assault

       ✓7ᵗʰ **T71.224 Asphyxiation due to being trapped in a car trunk,** undetermined

     ✓6ᵗʰ **T71.23 Asphyxiation due to being** trapped in a (discarded) refrigerator

       ✓7ᵗʰ **T71.231 Asphyxiation due to being trapped in a (discarded) refrigerator,** accidental

       ² ✓7ᵗʰ **T71.232 Asphyxiation due to being trapped in a (discarded) refrigerator, intentional self-harm**   HCC

       ✓7ᵗʰ **T71.233 Asphyxiation due to being trapped in a (discarded) refrigerator,** assault

       ✓7ᵗʰ **T71.234 Asphyxiation due to being trapped in a (discarded) refrigerator,** undetermined

     ✓x7ᵗʰ **T71.29 Asphyxiation due to being trapped in other low oxygen environment**

✓x7ᵗʰ T71.9 Asphyxiation due to unspecified cause   ▽

Suffocation (by strangulation) due to unspecified cause
Suffocation NOS
Systemic oxygen deficiency due to low oxygen content in ambient air due to unspecified cause
Systemic oxygen deficiency due to mechanical threat to breathing due to unspecified cause
Traumatic asphyxia NOS

✓4ᵗʰ T73 Effects of other deprivation

The appropriate 7th character is to be added to each code from category T73.
A   initial encounter
D   subsequent encounter
S   sequela

     ✓x7ᵗʰ **T73.0 Starvation**
         Deprivation of food

     ✓x7ᵗʰ **T73.1 Deprivation of water**

     ✓x7ᵗʰ **T73.2 Exhaustion due to exposure**

     ✓x7ᵗʰ **T73.3 Exhaustion due to excessive exertion**
         Exhaustion due to overexertion

     ✓x7ᵗʰ **T73.8 Other effects of deprivation**

     ✓x7ᵗʰ **T73.9 Effect of deprivation, unspecified**   ▽

✓4ᵗʰ T74 Adult and child abuse, neglect and other maltreatment, confirmed

Use additional code, if applicable, to identify any associated current injury
Use additional external cause code to identify perpetrator, if known (Y07.-)
EXCLUDES 1   abuse and maltreatment in pregnancy (O9A.3-, O9A.4-, O9A.5-)
          adult and child maltreatment, suspected (T76.-)

The appropriate 7th character is to be added to each code from category T74.
A   initial encounter
D   subsequent encounter
S   sequela

     ✓5ᵗʰ **T74.0 Neglect or abandonment, confirmed**

       ✓x7ᵗʰ **T74.01 Adult neglect or abandonment, confirmed**   Ⓐ

       ✓x7ᵗʰ **T74.02 Child neglect or abandonment, confirmed**   Ⓟ

     ✓5ᵗʰ **T74.1 Physical abuse, confirmed**
         EXCLUDES 2   sexual abuse (T74.2-)

       ✓x7ᵗʰ **T74.11 Adult physical abuse, confirmed**   Ⓐ

       ✓x7ᵗʰ **T74.12 Child physical abuse, confirmed**   Ⓟ
         EXCLUDES 2   shaken infant syndrome (T74.4)

     ✓5ᵗʰ **T74.2 Sexual abuse, confirmed**
         Rape, confirmed
         Sexual assault, confirmed

       ✓x7ᵗʰ **T74.21 Adult sexual abuse, confirmed**   Ⓐ

       ✓x7ᵗʰ **T74.22 Child sexual abuse, confirmed**   Ⓟ

     ✓5ᵗʰ **T74.3 Psychological abuse, confirmed**
         ►Bullying and intimidation, confirmed◄
         ►Intimidation through social media, confirmed◄

       ✓x7ᵗʰ **T74.31 Adult psychological abuse, confirmed**   Ⓐ

       ✓x7ᵗʰ **T74.32 Child psychological abuse, confirmed**   Ⓟ

     ✓x7ᵗʰ **T74.4 Shaken infant syndrome**   Ⓟ

     ✓5ᵗʰ **T74.5 Forced sexual exploitation, confirmed**

       ✓x7ᵗʰ **T74.51 Adult forced sexual exploitation, confirmed**

       ✓x7ᵗʰ **T74.52 Child sexual exploitation, confirmed**

     ✓5ᵗʰ **T74.6 Forced labor exploitation, confirmed**

       ✓x7ᵗʰ **T74.61 Adult forced labor exploitation, confirmed**

       ✓x7ᵗʰ **T74.62 Child forced labor exploitation, confirmed**

     ✓5ᵗʰ **T74.9 Unspecified maltreatment, confirmed**

       ✓x7ᵗʰ **T74.91 Unspecified adult maltreatment, confirmed**   Ⓐ ▽

       ✓x7ᵗʰ **T74.92 Unspecified child maltreatment, confirmed**   Ⓟ ▽

✓4ᵗʰ T75 Other and unspecified effects of other external causes

EXCLUDES 1   adverse effects NEC (T78.-)
EXCLUDES 2   burns (electric) (T20-T31)

The appropriate 7th character is to be added to each code from category T75.
A   initial encounter
D   subsequent encounter
S   sequela

     ✓5ᵗʰ **T75.0 Effects of lightning**
         Struck by lightning

       ✓x7ᵗʰ **T75.00 Unspecified effects of lightning**   ▽
         Struck by lightning NOS

       ✓x7ᵗʰ **T75.01 Shock due to being struck by lightning**

√x7ᵗʰ **T75.09　Other effects of lightning**
Use additional code for other effects of lightning

√x7ᵗʰ **T75.1　Unspecified effects of drowning and nonfatal submersion**　▽
Immersion
EXCLUDES 1　specified effects of drowning - code to effects

√5ᵗʰ **T75.2　Effects of vibration**

√x7ᵗʰ **T75.20　Unspecified effects of vibration**　▽

√x7ᵗʰ **T75.21　Pneumatic hammer syndrome**

√x7ᵗʰ **T75.22　Traumatic vasospastic syndrome**

√x7ᵗʰ **T75.23　Vertigo from infrasound**
EXCLUDES 1　vertigo NOS (R42)

√x7ᵗʰ **T75.29　Other effects of vibration**

√x7ᵗʰ **T75.3　Motion sickness**
Airsickness
Seasickness
Travel sickness
Use additional external cause code to identify vehicle or type of motion (Y92.81-, Y93.5-)

√x7ᵗʰ **T75.4　Electrocution**
Shock from electric current
Shock from electroshock gun (taser)

√5ᵗʰ **T75.8　Other specified effects of external causes**

√x7ᵗʰ **T75.81　Effects of abnormal gravitation [G] forces**

√x7ᵗʰ **T75.82　Effects of weightlessness**

√x7ᵗʰ **T75.89　Other specified effects of external causes**

√4ᵗʰ **T76　Adult and child abuse, neglect and other maltreatment, suspected**
Use additional code, if applicable, to identify any associated current injury
EXCLUDES 1　adult and child maltreatment, confirmed (T74.-)
suspected abuse and maltreatment in pregnancy (O9A.3-, O9A.4-, O9A.5-)
suspected adult physical abuse, ruled out (Z04.71)
suspected adult sexual abuse, ruled out (Z04.41)
suspected child physical abuse, ruled out (Z04.72)
suspected child sexual abuse, ruled out (Z04.42)

The appropriate 7th character is to be added to each code from category T76.
A　initial encounter
D　subsequent encounter
S　sequela

√5ᵗʰ **T76.0　Neglect or abandonment, suspected**

√x7ᵗʰ **T76.01　Adult neglect or abandonment, suspected**　Ⓐ

√x7ᵗʰ **T76.02　Child neglect or abandonment, suspected**　Ⓟ

√5ᵗʰ **T76.1　Physical abuse, suspected**

√x7ᵗʰ **T76.11　Adult physical abuse, suspected**　Ⓐ

√x7ᵗʰ **T76.12　Child physical abuse, suspected**　Ⓟ

√5ᵗʰ **T76.2　Sexual abuse, suspected**
Rape, suspected
EXCLUDES 1　alleged abuse, ruled out (Z04.7)

√x7ᵗʰ **T76.21　Adult sexual abuse, suspected**　Ⓐ

√x7ᵗʰ **T76.22　Child sexual abuse, suspected**　Ⓟ

√5ᵗʰ **T76.3　Psychological abuse, suspected**
▶Bullying and intimidation, suspected◀
▶Intimidation through social media, suspected◀

√x7ᵗʰ **T76.31　Adult psychological abuse, suspected**　Ⓐ

√x7ᵗʰ **T76.32　Child psychological abuse, suspected**　Ⓟ

● √5ᵗʰ **T76.5　Forced sexual exploitation, suspected**

● √x7ᵗʰ **T76.51　Adult forced sexual exploitation, suspected**

● √x7ᵗʰ **T76.52　Child sexual exploitation, suspected**

● √5ᵗʰ **T76.6　Forced labor exploitation, suspected**

● √x7ᵗʰ **T76.61　Adult forced labor exploitation, suspected**

● √x7ᵗʰ **T76.62　Child forced labor exploitation, suspected**

√5ᵗʰ **T76.9　Unspecified maltreatment, suspected**

√x7ᵗʰ **T76.91　Unspecified adult maltreatment, suspected**　Ⓐ ▽

√x7ᵗʰ **T76.92　Unspecified child maltreatment, suspected**　Ⓟ ▽

√4ᵗʰ **T78　Adverse effects, not elsewhere classified**
EXCLUDES 2　complications of surgical and medical care NEC (T80-T88)

The appropriate 7th character is to be added to each code from category T78.
A　initial encounter
D　subsequent encounter
S　sequela

√5ᵗʰ **T78.0　Anaphylactic reaction due to food**
Anaphylactic reaction due to adverse food reaction
Anaphylactic shock or reaction due to nonpoisonous foods
Anaphylactoid reaction due to food

√x7ᵗʰ **T78.00　Anaphylactic reaction due to unspecified food**　▽

√x7ᵗʰ **T78.01　Anaphylactic reaction due to peanuts**

√x7ᵗʰ **T78.02　Anaphylactic reaction due to shellfish (crustaceans)**

√x7ᵗʰ **T78.03　Anaphylactic reaction due to other fish**

√x7ᵗʰ **T78.04　Anaphylactic reaction due to fruits and vegetables**

√x7ᵗʰ **T78.05　Anaphylactic reaction due to tree nuts and seeds**
EXCLUDES 2　anaphylactic reaction due to peanuts (T78.01)

√x7ᵗʰ **T78.06　Anaphylactic reaction due to food additives**

√x7ᵗʰ **T78.07　Anaphylactic reaction due to milk and dairy products**

√x7ᵗʰ **T78.08　Anaphylactic reaction due to eggs**

√x7ᵗʰ **T78.09　Anaphylactic reaction due to other food products**

√x7ᵗʰ **T78.1　Other adverse food reactions, not elsewhere classified**
Use additional code to identify the type of reaction, if applicable
EXCLUDES 1　anaphylactic reaction or shock due to adverse food reaction (T78.0-)
anaphylactic reaction due to food (T78.0-)
bacterial food borne intoxications (A05.-)
EXCLUDES 2　allergic and dietetic gastroenteritis and colitis (K52.29)
allergic rhinitis due to food (J30.5)
dermatitis due to food in contact with skin (L23.6, L24.6, L25.4)
dermatitis due to ingested food (L27.2)
food protein-induced enterocolitis syndrome (K52.21)
food protein-induced enteropathy (K52.22)

√x7ᵗʰ **T78.2　Anaphylactic shock, unspecified**　▽
Allergic shock
Anaphylactic reaction
Anaphylaxis
EXCLUDES 1　anaphylactic reaction or shock due to adverse effect of correct medicinal substance properly administered (T88.6)
anaphylactic reaction or shock due to adverse food reaction (T78.0-)
anaphylactic reaction or shock due to serum (T80.5-)

√x7ᵗʰ **T78.3　Angioneurotic edema**
Allergic angioedema
Giant urticaria
Quincke's edema
EXCLUDES 1　serum urticaria (T80.6-)
urticaria (L50.-)

√5ᵗʰ **T78.4　Other and unspecified allergy**
EXCLUDES 1　specified types of allergic reaction such as:
allergic diarrhea (K52.29)
allergic gastroenteritis and colitis (K52.29)
dermatitis (L23-L25, L27.-)
food protein-induced enterocolitis syndrome (K52.21)
food protein-induced enteropathy (K52.22)
hay fever (J30.1)

√x7ᵗʰ **T78.40　Allergy, unspecified**　▽
Allergic reaction NOS
Hypersensitivity NOS

√x7ᵗʰ **T78.41　Arthus phenomenon**
Arthus reaction

√x7ᵗʰ **T78.49　Other allergy**

√x7ᵗʰ **T78.8　Other adverse effects, not elsewhere classified**

Chapter 19. Injury, Poisoning and Certain Other Consequences of External Causes

T79–T79.9

Certain early complications of trauma (T79)

✓4ᵗʰ **T79 Certain early complications of trauma, not elsewhere classified**

> **EXCLUDES 2**   acute respiratory distress syndrome (J80)
>
> complications occurring during or following medical procedures (T80-T88)
>
> complications of surgical and medical care NEC (T80-T88)
>
> newborn respiratory distress syndrome (P22.0)

> The appropriate 7th character is to be added to each code from category T79.
> A   initial encounter
> D   subsequent encounter
> S   sequela

¹ ✓x7ᵗʰ **T79.0 Air embolism (traumatic)**   HCC

> **EXCLUDES 1**   air embolism complicating abortion or ectopic or molar pregnancy (O00-O07, O08.2)
>
> air embolism complicating pregnancy, childbirth and the puerperium (O88.0)
>
> air embolism following infusion, transfusion, and therapeutic injection (T80.0)
>
> air embolism following procedure NEC (T81.7-)

> **DEF:** Arterial or venous obstruction due to the introduction of air bubbles into the blood vessels following surgery or trauma.

¹ ✓x7ᵗʰ **T79.1 Fat embolism (traumatic)**   HCC

> **EXCLUDES 1**   fat embolism complicating:
>
> abortion or ectopic or molar pregnancy (O00-O07, O08.2)
>
> pregnancy, childbirth and the puerperium (O88.8)

> **DEF:** Arterial blockage due to the entrance of fat into the circulatory system after a fracture of the large bones or administration of corticosteroids.

¹ ✓x7ᵗʰ **T79.2 Traumatic secondary and recurrent hemorrhage and seroma**   HCC

¹ ✓x7ᵗʰ **T79.4 Traumatic shock**   HCC

> Shock (immediate) (delayed) following injury

> **EXCLUDES 1**   anaphylactic shock due to adverse food reaction (T78.0-)
>
> anaphylactic shock due to correct medicinal substance properly administered (T88.6)
>
> anaphylactic shock due to serum (T80.5-)
>
> anaphylactic shock NOS (T78.2)
>
> anesthetic shock (T88.2)
>
> electric shock (T75.4)
>
> nontraumatic shock NEC (R57.-)
>
> obstetric shock (O75.1)
>
> postprocedural shock (T81.1-)
>
> septic shock (R65.21)
>
> shock complicating abortion or ectopic or molar pregnancy (O00-O07, O08.3)
>
> shock due to lightning (T75.01)
>
> shock NOS (R57.9)

¹ ✓x7ᵗʰ **T79.5 Traumatic anuria**   HCC

> Crush syndrome
> Renal failure following crushing

¹ ✓x7ᵗʰ **T79.6 Traumatic ischemia of muscle**   HCC

> Traumatic rhabdomyolysis
> Volkmann's ischemic contracture

> **EXCLUDES 2**   anterior tibial syndrome (M76.8)
>
> compartment syndrome (traumatic) (T79.A-)
>
> nontraumatic ischemia of muscle (M62.2-)

¹ ✓x7ᵗʰ **T79.7 Traumatic subcutaneous emphysema**   HCC

> **EXCLUDES 1**   emphysema NOS (J43)
>
> emphysema (subcutaneous) resulting from a procedure (T81.82)

✓5ᵗʰ **T79.A Traumatic compartment syndrome**

> **EXCLUDES 1**   fibromyalgia (M79.7)
>
> nontraumatic compartment syndrome (M79.A-)
>
> traumatic ischemic infarction of muscle (T79.6)

> **DEF:** Compression of nerves and blood vessels within an enclosed muscle space due to previous trauma, which leads to impaired blood flow and muscle and nerve damage.

¹ ✓x7ᵗʰ **T79.A0 Compartment syndrome, unspecified**   HCC ▽

> Compartment syndrome NOS

✓6ᵗʰ **T79.A1 Traumatic compartment syndrome of upper extremity**

> Traumatic compartment syndrome of shoulder, arm, forearm, wrist, hand, and fingers

¹ ✓7ᵗʰ **T79.A11 Traumatic compartment syndrome of right upper extremity**   HCC

¹ ✓7ᵗʰ **T79.A12 Traumatic compartment syndrome of left upper extremity**   HCC

¹ ✓7ᵗʰ **T79.A19 Traumatic compartment syndrome of unspecified upper extremity**   HCC ▽

✓6ᵗʰ **T79.A2 Traumatic compartment syndrome of lower extremity**

> Traumatic compartment syndrome of hip, buttock, thigh, leg, foot, and toes

¹ ✓7ᵗʰ **T79.A21 Traumatic compartment syndrome of right lower extremity**   HCC

¹ ✓7ᵗʰ **T79.A22 Traumatic compartment syndrome of left lower extremity**   HCC

¹ ✓7ᵗʰ **T79.A29 Traumatic compartment syndrome of unspecified lower extremity**   HCC ▽

¹ ✓x7ᵗʰ **T79.A3 Traumatic compartment syndrome of abdomen**   HCC

¹ ✓x7ᵗʰ **T79.A9 Traumatic compartment syndrome of other sites**   HCC

¹ ✓x7ᵗʰ **T79.8 Other early complications of trauma**   HCC

¹ ✓x7ᵗʰ **T79.9 Unspecified early complication of trauma**   HCC ▽

Complications of surgical and medical care, not elsewhere classified (T80-T88)

Use additional code for adverse effect, if applicable, to identify drug (T36-T50 with fifth or sixth character 5)

Use additional code(s) to identify the specified condition resulting from the complication

Use additional code to identify devices involved and details of circumstances (Y62-Y82)

EXCLUDES 2　*any encounters with medical care for postprocedural conditions in which no complications are present, such as:*
　artificial opening status (Z93.-)
　closure of external stoma (Z43.-)
　fitting and adjustment of external prosthetic device (Z44.-)
burns and corrosions from local applications and irradiation (T20-T32)
complications of surgical procedures during pregnancy, childbirth and the puerperium (O00-O9A)
mechanical complication of respirator [ventilator] (J95.850)
poisoning and toxic effects of drugs and chemicals (T36-T65 with fifth or sixth character 1-4 or 6)
postprocedural fever (R50.82)
specified complications classified elsewhere, such as:
　cerebrospinal fluid leak from spinal puncture (G97.0)
　colostomy malfunction (K94.0-)
　disorders of fluid and electrolyte imbalance (E86-E87)
　functional disturbances following cardiac surgery (I97.0-I97.1)
　intraoperative and postprocedural complications of specified body systems (D78.-, E36.-, E89.-, G97.3-, G97.4, H59.3-, H59.-, H95.2-, H95.3, I97.4-, I97.5, J95.6-, J95.7, K91.6-, L76.-, M96.-, N99.-)
　ostomy complications (J95.0-, K94.-, N99.5-)
　postgastric surgery syndromes (K91.1)
　postlaminectomy syndrome NEC (M96.1)
　postmastectomy lymphedema syndrome (I97.2)
　postsurgical blind-loop syndrome (K91.2)
　ventilator associated pneumonia (J95.851)

AHA:　2015,1Q,15

✓4ᵗʰ **T80　Complications following infusion, transfusion and therapeutic injection**

INCLUDES　complications following perfusion

EXCLUDES 2　*bone marrow transplant rejection (T86.01)*
febrile nonhemolytic transfusion reaction (R50.84)
fluid overload due to transfusion (E87.71)
posttransfusion purpura (D69.51)
transfusion associated circulatory overload (TACO) (E87.71)
transfusion (red blood cell) associated hemochromatosis (E83.111)
transfusion related acute lung injury (TRALI) (J95.84)

The appropriate 7th character is to be added to each code from category T80.
　A　initial encounter
　D　subsequent encounter
　S　sequela

✓x7ᵗʰ **T80.0　Air embolism following infusion, transfusion and therapeutic injection**

✓x7ᵗʰ **T80.1　Vascular complications following infusion, transfusion and therapeutic injection**

Use additional code to identify the vascular complication

EXCLUDES 2　*extravasation of vesicant agent (T80.81-)*
infiltration of vesicant agent (T80.81-)
postprocedural vascular complications (T81.7-)
vascular complications specified as due to prosthetic devices, implants and grafts (T82.8-, T83.8-, T84.8-, T85.8-)

✓5ᵗʰ **T80.2　Infections following infusion, transfusion and therapeutic injection**

Use additional code to identify the specific infection, such as: sepsis (A41.9)

Use additional code (R65.2-) to identify severe sepsis, if applicable

EXCLUDES 2　*infections specified as due to prosthetic devices, implants and grafts (T82.6-T82.7, T83.5-T83.6, T84.5-T84.7, T85.7)*
postprocedural infections (T81.4-)

✓6ᵗʰ **T80.21　Infection due to central venous catheter**

Infection due to pulmonary artery catheter (Swan-Ganz catheter)

✓7ᵗʰ **T80.211　Bloodstream infection due to central venous catheter**

Catheter-related bloodstream infection (CRBSI) NOS

Central line-associated bloodstream infection (CLABSI)

Bloodstream infection due to Hickman catheter

Bloodstream infection due to peripherally inserted central catheter (PICC)

Bloodstream infection due to portacath (port-a-cath)

Bloodstream infection due to pulmonary artery catheter

Bloodstream infection due to triple lumen catheter

Bloodstream infection due to umbilical venous catheter

✓7ᵗʰ **T80.212　Local infection due to central venous catheter**

Exit or insertion site infection

Local infection due to Hickman catheter

Local infection due to peripherally inserted central catheter (PICC)

Local infection due to portacath (port-a-cath)

Local infection due to pulmonary artery catheter

Local infection due to triple lumen catheter

Local infection due to umbilical venous catheter

Port or reservoir infection

Tunnel infection

✓7ᵗʰ **T80.218　Other infection due to central venous catheter**

Other central line-associated infection

Other infection due to Hickman catheter

Other infection due to peripherally inserted central catheter (PICC)

Other infection due to portacath (port-a-cath)

Other infection due to pulmonary artery catheter

Other infection due to triple lumen catheter

Other infection due to umbilical venous catheter

✓7ᵗʰ **T80.219　Unspecified infection due to central venous catheter**　▽

Central line-associated infection NOS

Unspecified infection due to Hickman catheter

Unspecified infection due to peripherally inserted central catheter (PICC)

Unspecified infection due to portacath (port-a-cath)

Unspecified infection due to pulmonary artery catheter

Unspecified infection due to triple lumen catheter

Unspecified infection due to umbilical venous catheter

✓x7ᵗʰ **T80.22　Acute infection following transfusion, infusion, or injection of blood and blood products**

✓x7ᵗʰ **T80.29　Infection following other infusion, transfusion and therapeutic injection**

Chapter 19. Injury, Poisoning and Certain Other Consequences of External Causes

T80.3–T80.69

✓5ᵗʰ **T80.3** **ABO incompatibility** reaction due to transfusion of blood or blood products

     EXCLUDES 1 ▶*minor blood group antigens reactions (Duffy) (E) (K) (Kell) (Kidd) (Lewis) (M) (N) (P) (S) (T80.A-)*◀

   ✓x7ᵗʰ **T80.30** **ABO incompatibility reaction due to** ▽
       transfusion of blood or blood products, unspecified
       ABO incompatibility blood transfusion NOS
       Reaction to ABO incompatibility from transfusion NOS

   ✓6ᵗʰ **T80.31** **ABO incompatibility** with hemolytic transfusion reaction

     ✓7ᵗʰ **T80.310** **ABO incompatibility with** acute **hemolytic transfusion reaction**
         ABO incompatibility with hemolytic transfusion reaction less than 24 hours after transfusion
         Acute hemolytic transfusion reaction (AHTR) due to ABO incompatibility

     ✓7ᵗʰ **T80.311** **ABO incompatibility with** delayed **hemolytic transfusion reaction**
         ABO incompatibility with hemolytic transfusion reaction 24 hours or more after transfusion
         Delayed hemolytic transfusion reaction (DHTR) due to ABO incompatibility

     ✓7ᵗʰ **T80.319** **ABO incompatibility with** ▽ **hemolytic transfusion reaction, unspecified**
         ABO incompatibility with hemolytic transfusion reaction at unspecified time after transfusion
         Hemolytic transfusion reaction (HTR) due to ABO incompatibility NOS

   ✓x7ᵗʰ **T80.39** **Other ABO incompatibility reaction due to transfusion of blood or blood products**
       Delayed serologic transfusion reaction (DSTR) from ABO incompatibility
       Other ABO incompatible blood transfusion
       Other reaction to ABO incompatible blood transfusion

✓5ᵗʰ **T80.4** **Rh incompatibility** reaction due to transfusion of blood or blood products
     Reaction due to incompatibility of Rh antigens (C) (c) (D) (E) (e)

   ✓x7ᵗʰ **T80.40** **Rh incompatibility reaction due to** ▽ **transfusion of blood or blood products, unspecified**
       Reaction due to Rh factor in transfusion NOS
       Rh incompatible blood transfusion NOS

   ✓6ᵗʰ **T80.41** **Rh incompatibility** with hemolytic transfusion reaction

     ✓7ᵗʰ **T80.410** **Rh incompatibility with** acute **hemolytic transfusion reaction**
         Acute hemolytic transfusion reaction (AHTR) due to Rh incompatibility
         Rh incompatibility with hemolytic transfusion reaction less than 24 hours after transfusion

     ✓7ᵗʰ **T80.411** **Rh incompatibility with** delayed **hemolytic transfusion reaction**
         Delayed hemolytic transfusion reaction (DHTR) due to Rh incompatibility
         Rh incompatibility with hemolytic transfusion reaction 24 hours or more after transfusion

     ✓7ᵗʰ **T80.419** **Rh incompatibility with hemolytic** ▽ **transfusion reaction, unspecified**
         Rh incompatibility with hemolytic transfusion reaction at unspecified time after transfusion
         Hemolytic transfusion reaction (HTR) due to Rh incompatibility NOS

   ✓x7ᵗʰ **T80.49** **Other Rh incompatibility reaction due to transfusion of blood or blood products**
       Delayed serologic transfusion reaction (DSTR) from Rh incompatibility
       Other reaction to Rh incompatible blood transfusion

✓5ᵗʰ **T80.A** **Non-ABO incompatibility** reaction due to transfusion of blood or blood products
     Reaction due to incompatibility of minor antigens (Duffy) (Kell) (Kidd) (Lewis) (M) (N) (P) (S)

   ✓x7ᵗʰ **T80.A0** **Non-ABO incompatibility reaction due to** ▽ **transfusion of blood or blood products, unspecified**
       Non-ABO antigen incompatibility reaction from transfusion NOS

   ✓6ᵗʰ **T80.A1** **Non-ABO incompatibility** with hemolytic transfusion reaction

     ✓7ᵗʰ **T80.A10** **Non-ABO incompatibility with** acute **hemolytic transfusion reaction**
         Acute hemolytic transfusion reaction (AHTR) due to non-ABO incompatibility
         Non-ABO incompatibility with hemolytic transfusion reaction less than 24 hours after transfusion

     ✓7ᵗʰ **T80.A11** **Non-ABO incompatibility with** delayed **hemolytic transfusion reaction**
         Delayed hemolytic transfusion reaction (DHTR) due to non-ABO incompatibility
         Non-ABO incompatibility with hemolytic transfusion reaction 24 or more hours after transfusion

     ✓7ᵗʰ **T80.A19** **Non-ABO incompatibility with** ▽ **hemolytic transfusion reaction, unspecified**
         Hemolytic transfusion reaction (HTR) due to non-ABO incompatibility NOS
         Non-ABO incompatibility with hemolytic transfusion reaction at unspecified time after transfusion

   ✓x7ᵗʰ **T80.A9** **Other non-ABO incompatibility reaction due to transfusion of blood or blood products**
       Delayed serologic transfusion reaction (DSTR) from non-ABO incompatibility
       Other reaction to non-ABO incompatible blood transfusion

✓5ᵗʰ **T80.5** **Anaphylactic reaction due to serum**
     Allergic shock due to serum
     Anaphylactic shock due to serum
     Anaphylactoid reaction due to serum
     Anaphylaxis due to serum
     EXCLUDES 1 *ABO incompatibility reaction due to transfusion of blood or blood products (T80.3-)*
         allergic reaction or shock NOS (T78.2)
         anaphylactic reaction or shock NOS (T78.2)
         anaphylactic reaction or shock due to adverse effect of correct medicinal substance properly administered (T88.6)
         other serum reaction (T80.6-)
     DEF: Life-threatening hypersensitivity to a foreign serum causing respiratory distress, vascular collapse, and shock.

   ✓x7ᵗʰ **T80.51** **Anaphylactic reaction** due to administration of blood and blood products

   ✓x7ᵗʰ **T80.52** **Anaphylactic reaction** due to vaccination

   ✓x7ᵗʰ **T80.59** **Anaphylactic reaction** due to other serum

✓5ᵗʰ **T80.6** **Other serum reactions**
     Intoxication by serum
     Protein sickness
     Serum rash
     Serum sickness
     Serum urticaria
     EXCLUDES 2 *serum hepatitis (B16-B19)*
     DEF: Serum sickness: Hypersensitivity to a foreign serum that causes fever, hives, swelling, and lymphadenopathy.

   ✓x7ᵗʰ **T80.61** **Other serum reaction** due to administration of blood and blood products

   ✓x7ᵗʰ **T80.62** **Other serum reaction** due to vaccination

   ✓x7ᵗʰ **T80.69** **Other serum reaction due to other serum**
       Code also, if applicable, arthropathy in hypersensitivity reactions classified elsewhere (M36.4)

√5ᵗʰ **T80.8 Other complications following infusion, transfusion and therapeutic injection**

√6ᵗʰ **T80.81 Extravasation of vesicant agent**

Infiltration of vesicant agent

√7ᵗʰ **T80.810 Extravasation of vesicant antineoplastic chemotherapy**

Infiltration of vesicant antineoplastic chemotherapy

√7ᵗʰ **T80.818 Extravasation of other vesicant agent**

Infiltration of other vesicant agent

√x7ᵗʰ **T80.89 Other complications following infusion, transfusion and therapeutic injection**

Delayed serologic transfusion reaction (DSTR), unspecified incompatibility

Use additional code to identify graft-versus-host reaction, if applicable, (D89.81-)

√5ᵗʰ **T80.9 Unspecified complication following infusion, transfusion and therapeutic injection**

√x7ᵗʰ **T80.90 Unspecified complication** following infusion and therapeutic injection ▽

√6ᵗʰ **T80.91 Hemolytic transfusion reaction, unspecified incompatibility**

EXCLUDES 1   ABO incompatibility with hemolytic transfusion reaction (T80.31-)
non-ABO incompatibility with hemolytic transfusion reaction (T80.A1-)
Rh incompatibility with hemolytic transfusion reaction (T80.41-)

√7ᵗʰ **T80.910 Acute hemolytic transfusion reaction, unspecified incompatibility** ▽

√7ᵗʰ **T80.911 Delayed hemolytic transfusion reaction, unspecified incompatibility** ▽

√7ᵗʰ **T80.919 Hemolytic transfusion reaction, unspecified incompatibility, unspecified as acute or delayed** ▽

Hemolytic transfusion reaction NOS

√x7ᵗʰ **T80.92 Unspecified transfusion reaction** ▽

Transfusion reaction NOS

√4ᵗʰ **T81 Complications of procedures, not elsewhere classified**

Use additional code for adverse effect, if applicable, to identify drug (T36-T50 with fifth or sixth character 5)

EXCLUDES 2   complications following immunization (T88.0-T88.1)
complications following infusion, transfusion and therapeutic injection (T80.-)
complications of transplanted organs and tissue (T86.-)
specified complications classified elsewhere, such as:
complication of prosthetic devices, implants and grafts (T82-T85)
dermatitis due to drugs and medicaments (L23.3, L24.4, L25.1, L27.0-L27.1)
endosseous dental implant failure (M27.6-)
floppy iris syndrome (IFIS) (intraoperative) (H21.81)
intraoperative and postprocedural complications of specific body system (D78.-, E36.-, E89.-, G97.3-, G97.4, H59.3-, H59.-, H95.2-, H95.3, I97.4-, I97.5, J95, K91.-, L76.-, M96.-, N99.-)
ostomy complications (J95.0-, K94.-, N99.5-)
plateau iris syndrome (post-iridectomy) (postprocedural) H21.82
poisoning and toxic effects of drugs and chemicals (T36-T65 with fifth or sixth character 1-4 or 6)

The appropriate 7th character is to be added to each code from category T81.
A   initial encounter
D   subsequent encounter
S   sequela

√5ᵗʰ **T81.1 Postprocedural shock**

Shock during or resulting from a procedure, not elsewhere classified

EXCLUDES 1   anaphylactic shock due to correct substance properly administered (T88.6)
anaphylactic shock due to serum (T80.5-)
anaphylactic shock NOS (T78.2)
anesthetic shock (T88.2)
electric shock (T75.4)
obstetric shock (O75.1)
septic shock (R65.21)
shock following abortion or ectopic or molar pregnancy (O00-O07, O08.3)
traumatic shock (T79.4)

√x7ᵗʰ **T81.10 Postprocedural shock unspecified** ▽

Collapse NOS during or resulting from a procedure, not elsewhere classified
Postprocedural failure of peripheral circulation
Postprocedural shock NOS

▲   ¹ √x7ᵗʰ **T81.11 Postprocedural cardiogenic shock** HCC

¹ √x7ᵗʰ **T81.12 Postprocedural septic shock** HCC

Postprocedural endotoxic shock resulting from a procedure, not elsewhere classified
Postprocedural gram-negative shock resulting from a procedure, not elsewhere classified
Code first underlying infection
Use additional code, to identify any associated acute organ dysfunction, if applicable

√x7ᵗʰ **T81.19 Other postprocedural shock**

Postprocedural hypovolemic shock

√5ᵗʰ **T81.3 Disruption of wound, not elsewhere classified**

Disruption of any suture materials or other closure methods

EXCLUDES 1   breakdown (mechanical) of permanent sutures (T85.612)
displacement of permanent sutures (T85.622)
disruption of cesarean delivery wound (O90.0)
disruption of perineal obstetric wound (O90.1)
mechanical complication of permanent sutures NEC (T85.692)

AHA: 2014,1Q,23

√x7ᵗʰ **T81.30 Disruption of wound, unspecified** ▽

Disruption of wound NOS

☑ Additional Character Req   √x7ᵗʰ Placeholder Alert   Manifestation   ▽ Unspecified   ▶◀ Revised Text   ● New Code   ▲ Revised Code Title

ICD-10-CM 2019   1133

√x7ᵗʰ **T81.31 Disruption of external operation (surgical) wound, not elsewhere classified**
Dehiscence of operation wound NOS
Disruption of operation wound NOS
Disruption or dehiscence of closure of cornea
Disruption or dehiscence of closure of mucosa
Disruption or dehiscence of closure of skin and subcutaneous tissue
Full-thickness skin disruption or dehiscence
Superficial disruption or dehiscence of operation wound
EXCLUDES 1   dehiscence of amputation stump (T87.81)

√x7ᵗʰ **T81.32 Disruption of internal operation (surgical) wound, not elsewhere classified**
Deep disruption or dehiscence of operation wound NOS
Disruption or dehiscence of closure of internal organ or other internal tissue
Disruption or dehiscence of closure of muscle or muscle flap
Disruption or dehiscence of closure of ribs or rib cage
Disruption or dehiscence of closure of skull or craniotomy
Disruption or dehiscence of closure of sternum or sternotomy
Disruption or dehiscence of closure of tendon or ligament
Disruption or dehiscence of closure of superficial or muscular fascia
AHA: 2017,3Q,4

√x7ᵗʰ **T81.33 Disruption of traumatic injury wound repair**
Disruption or dehiscence of closure of traumatic laceration (external) (internal)

√5ᵗʰ **T81.4 Infection following a procedure**
~~Intra-abdominal abscess following a procedure~~
~~Postprocedural infection, not elsewhere classified~~
~~Sepsis following a procedure~~
~~Stitch abscess following a procedure~~
~~Subphrenic abscess following a procedure~~
Wound abscess following a procedure
Use additional code to identify infection
Use additional code (R65.2-) to identify severe sepsis, if applicable
EXCLUDES 1   ~~obstetric surgical wound infection (O86.0)~~
~~postprocedural fever NOS (R50.82)~~
~~postprocedural retroperitoneal abscess (K68.11)~~
EXCLUDES 2   bleb associated endophthalmitis (H59.4-)
infection due to infusion, transfusion and therapeutic injection (T80.2-)
infection due to prosthetic devices, implants and grafts (T82.6-T82.7, T83.5-T83.6, T84.5-T84.7, T85.7)
▶obstetric surgical wound infection (O86.0-)◀
▶postprocedural fever NOS (R50.82)◀
▶postprocedural retroperitoneal abscess (K68.11)◀
AHA: 2014,1Q,23

● √x7ᵗʰ **T81.40 Infection following a procedure, unspecified** ▽
● √x7ᵗʰ **T81.41 Infection following a procedure, superficial incisional surgical site**
Subcutaneous abscess following a procedure
Stitch abscess following a procedure
● √x7ᵗʰ **T81.42 Infection following a procedure, deep incisional surgical site**
Intra-muscular abscess following a procedure
● √x7ᵗʰ **T81.43 Infection following a procedure, organ and space surgical site**
Intra-abdominal abscess following a procedure
Subphrenic abscess following a procedure
● √x7ᵗʰ **T81.44 Sepsis following a procedure**
Use additional code to identify the sepsis
● √x7ᵗʰ **T81.49 Infection following a procedure, other surgical site**

√5ᵗʰ **T81.5 Complications of foreign body accidentally left in body following procedure**
AHA: 2014,4Q,24

√6ᵗʰ **T81.50 Unspecified complication of foreign body accidentally left in body following procedure**
√7ᵗʰ **T81.500 Unspecified complication of foreign body accidentally left in body following surgical operation** ▽
√7ᵗʰ **T81.501 Unspecified complication of foreign body accidentally left in body following infusion or transfusion** ▽
√7ᵗʰ **T81.502 Unspecified complication of foreign body accidentally left in body following kidney dialysis** HCC ▽
√7ᵗʰ **T81.503 Unspecified complication of foreign body accidentally left in body following injection or immunization** ▽
√7ᵗʰ **T81.504 Unspecified complication of foreign body accidentally left in body following endoscopic examination** ▽
√7ᵗʰ **T81.505 Unspecified complication of foreign body accidentally left in body following heart catheterization** ▽
√7ᵗʰ **T81.506 Unspecified complication of foreign body accidentally left in body following aspiration, puncture or other catheterization** ▽
√7ᵗʰ **T81.507 Unspecified complication of foreign body accidentally left in body following removal of catheter or packing** ▽
√7ᵗʰ **T81.508 Unspecified complication of foreign body accidentally left in body following other procedure** ▽
√7ᵗʰ **T81.509 Unspecified complication of foreign body accidentally left in body following unspecified procedure** ▽

√6ᵗʰ **T81.51 Adhesions due to foreign body accidentally left in body following procedure**
√7ᵗʰ **T81.510 Adhesions due to foreign body accidentally left in body following surgical operation**
√7ᵗʰ **T81.511 Adhesions due to foreign body accidentally left in body following infusion or transfusion**
√7ᵗʰ **T81.512 Adhesions due to foreign body accidentally left in body following kidney dialysis** HCC
√7ᵗʰ **T81.513 Adhesions due to foreign body accidentally left in body following injection or immunization**
√7ᵗʰ **T81.514 Adhesions due to foreign body accidentally left in body following endoscopic examination**
√7ᵗʰ **T81.515 Adhesions due to foreign body accidentally left in body following heart catheterization**
√7ᵗʰ **T81.516 Adhesions due to foreign body accidentally left in body following aspiration, puncture or other catheterization**
√7ᵗʰ **T81.517 Adhesions due to foreign body accidentally left in body following removal of catheter or packing**
√7ᵗʰ **T81.518 Adhesions due to foreign body accidentally left in body following other procedure**
√7ᵗʰ **T81.519 Adhesions due to foreign body accidentally left in body following unspecified procedure** ▽

√6ᵗʰ **T81.52 Obstruction due to foreign body accidentally left in body following procedure**
√7ᵗʰ **T81.520 Obstruction due to foreign body accidentally left in body following surgical operation**
√7ᵗʰ **T81.521 Obstruction due to foreign body accidentally left in body following infusion or transfusion**

Chapter 19. Injury, Poisoning and Certain Other Consequences of External Causes

√7ᵗʰ **T81.522** Obstruction due to foreign body accidentally left in body following kidney dialysis `HCC`

√7ᵗʰ **T81.523** Obstruction due to foreign body accidentally left in body following injection or immunization

√7ᵗʰ **T81.524** Obstruction due to foreign body accidentally left in body following endoscopic examination

√7ᵗʰ **T81.525** Obstruction due to foreign body accidentally left in body following heart catheterization

√7ᵗʰ **T81.526** Obstruction due to foreign body accidentally left in body following aspiration, puncture or other catheterization

√7ᵗʰ **T81.527** Obstruction due to foreign body accidentally left in body following removal of catheter or packing

√7ᵗʰ **T81.528** Obstruction due to foreign body accidentally left in body following other procedure

√7ᵗʰ **T81.529** Obstruction due to foreign body accidentally left in body following unspecified procedure ▽

√6ᵗʰ **T81.53** Perforation due to foreign body accidentally left in body following procedure

√7ᵗʰ **T81.530** Perforation due to foreign body accidentally left in body following surgical operation

√7ᵗʰ **T81.531** Perforation due to foreign body accidentally left in body following infusion or transfusion

√7ᵗʰ **T81.532** Perforation due to foreign body accidentally left in body following kidney dialysis `HCC`

√7ᵗʰ **T81.533** Perforation due to foreign body accidentally left in body following injection or immunization

√7ᵗʰ **T81.534** Perforation due to foreign body accidentally left in body following endoscopic examination

√7ᵗʰ **T81.535** Perforation due to foreign body accidentally left in body following heart catheterization

√7ᵗʰ **T81.536** Perforation due to foreign body accidentally left in body following aspiration, puncture or other catheterization

√7ᵗʰ **T81.537** Perforation due to foreign body accidentally left in body following removal of catheter or packing

√7ᵗʰ **T81.538** Perforation due to foreign body accidentally left in body following other procedure

√7ᵗʰ **T81.539** Perforation due to foreign body accidentally left in body following unspecified procedure ▽

√6ᵗʰ **T81.59** Other complications of foreign body accidentally left in body following procedure

    EXCLUDES 2   obstruction or perforation due to prosthetic devices and implants intentionally left in body (T82.0-T82.5, T83.0-T83.4, T83.7, T84.0-T84.4, T85.0-T85.6)

√7ᵗʰ **T81.590** Other complications of foreign body accidentally left in body following surgical operation

√7ᵗʰ **T81.591** Other complications of foreign body accidentally left in body following infusion or transfusion

√7ᵗʰ **T81.592** Other complications of foreign body accidentally left in body following kidney dialysis `HCC`

√7ᵗʰ **T81.593** Other complications of foreign body accidentally left in body following injection or immunization

√7ᵗʰ **T81.594** Other complications of foreign body accidentally left in body following endoscopic examination

√7ᵗʰ **T81.595** Other complications of foreign body accidentally left in body following heart catheterization

√7ᵗʰ **T81.596** Other complications of foreign body accidentally left in body following aspiration, puncture or other catheterization

√7ᵗʰ **T81.597** Other complications of foreign body accidentally left in body following removal of catheter or packing

√7ᵗʰ **T81.598** Other complications of foreign body accidentally left in body following other procedure

√7ᵗʰ **T81.599** Other complications of foreign body accidentally left in body following unspecified procedure ▽

√5ᵗʰ **T81.6** Acute reaction to foreign substance accidentally left during a procedure

    EXCLUDES 2   complications of foreign body accidentally left in body cavity or operation wound following procedure (T81.5-)

√x7ᵗʰ **T81.60** Unspecified acute reaction to foreign substance accidentally left during a procedure ▽

√x7ᵗʰ **T81.61** Aseptic peritonitis due to foreign substance accidentally left during a procedure
    Chemical peritonitis

√x7ᵗʰ **T81.69** Other acute reaction to foreign substance accidentally left during a procedure

√5ᵗʰ **T81.7** Vascular complications following a procedure, not elsewhere classified
    Air embolism following procedure NEC
    Phlebitis or thrombophlebitis resulting from a procedure
    EXCLUDES 1   embolism complicating abortion or ectopic or molar pregnancy (O00-O07, O08.2)
     embolism complicating pregnancy, childbirth and the puerperium (O88.-)
     traumatic embolism (T79.0)
    EXCLUDES 2   embolism due to prosthetic devices, implants and grafts (T82.8-, T83.81, T84.8-, T85.81-)
     embolism following infusion, transfusion and therapeutic injection (T80.0)

√6ᵗʰ **T81.71** Complication of artery following a procedure, not elsewhere classified

√7ᵗʰ **T81.710** Complication of mesenteric artery following a procedure, not elsewhere classified

√7ᵗʰ **T81.711** Complication of renal artery following a procedure, not elsewhere classified

√7ᵗʰ **T81.718** Complication of other artery following a procedure, not elsewhere classified

√7ᵗʰ **T81.719** Complication of unspecified artery following a procedure, not elsewhere classified ▽

√x7ᵗʰ **T81.72** Complication of vein following a procedure, not elsewhere classified

√5ᵗʰ **T81.8** Other complications of procedures, not elsewhere classified
    EXCLUDES 2   hypothermia following anesthesia (T88.51)
     malignant hyperpyrexia due to anesthesia (T88.3)

√x7ᵗʰ **T81.81** Complication of inhalation therapy

√x7ᵗʰ **T81.82** Emphysema (subcutaneous) resulting from a procedure

√x7ᵗʰ **T81.83** Persistent postprocedural fistula
    AHA: 2017,3Q,3-4

√x7ᵗʰ **T81.89** Other complications of procedures, not elsewhere classified
    Use additional code to specify complication, such as:
    postprocedural delirium (F05)
    AHA: 2014,1Q,23

√x7ᵗʰ **T81.9** Unspecified complication of procedure ▽

√4ᵗʰ T82 Complications of cardiac and vascular prosthetic devices, implants and grafts

> EXCLUDES 2   *failure and rejection of transplanted organs and tissue (T86.-)*

> The appropriate 7th character is to be added to each code from category T82.
> A   initial encounter
> D   subsequent encounter
> S   sequela

√5ᵗʰ T82.0 Mechanical complication of heart valve prosthesis

Mechanical complication of artificial heart valve

> EXCLUDES 1   *mechanical complication of biological heart valve graft (T82.22-)*

√x7ᵗʰ T82.01 Breakdown (mechanical) of heart valve prosthesis

√x7ᵗʰ T82.02 Displacement of heart valve prosthesis

Malposition of heart valve prosthesis

√x7ᵗʰ T82.03 Leakage of heart valve prosthesis

√x7ᵗʰ T82.09 Other mechanical complication of heart valve prosthesis

Obstruction (mechanical) of heart valve prosthesis
Perforation of heart valve prosthesis
Protrusion of heart valve prosthesis

√5ᵗʰ T82.1 Mechanical complication of cardiac electronic device

√6ᵗʰ T82.11 Breakdown (mechanical) of cardiac electronic device

√7ᵗʰ T82.110 Breakdown (mechanical) of cardiac electrode

√7ᵗʰ T82.111 Breakdown (mechanical) of cardiac pulse generator (battery)

√7ᵗʰ T82.118 Breakdown (mechanical) of other cardiac electronic device

√7ᵗʰ T82.119 Breakdown (mechanical) of unspecified cardiac electronic device ▽

√6ᵗʰ T82.12 Displacement of cardiac electronic device

Malposition of cardiac electronic device

√7ᵗʰ T82.120 Displacement of cardiac electrode

√7ᵗʰ T82.121 Displacement of cardiac pulse generator (battery)

√7ᵗʰ T82.128 Displacement of other cardiac electronic device

√7ᵗʰ T82.129 Displacement of unspecified cardiac electronic device ▽

√6ᵗʰ T82.19 Other mechanical complication of cardiac electronic device

Leakage of cardiac electronic device
Obstruction of cardiac electronic device
Perforation of cardiac electronic device
Protrusion of cardiac electronic device

√7ᵗʰ T82.190 Other mechanical complication of cardiac electrode

√7ᵗʰ T82.191 Other mechanical complication of cardiac pulse generator (battery)

√7ᵗʰ T82.198 Other mechanical complication of other cardiac electronic device

√7ᵗʰ T82.199 Other mechanical complication of unspecified cardiac device ▽

√5ᵗʰ T82.2 Mechanical complication of coronary artery bypass graft and biological heart valve graft

> EXCLUDES 1   *mechanical complication of artificial heart valve prosthesis (T82.0-)*

√6ᵗʰ T82.21 Mechanical complication of coronary artery bypass graft

√7ᵗʰ T82.211 Breakdown (mechanical) of coronary artery bypass graft

√7ᵗʰ T82.212 Displacement of coronary artery bypass graft

Malposition of coronary artery bypass graft

√7ᵗʰ T82.213 Leakage of coronary artery bypass graft

√7ᵗʰ T82.218 Other mechanical complication of coronary artery bypass graft

Obstruction, mechanical of coronary artery bypass graft
Perforation of coronary artery bypass graft
Protrusion of coronary artery bypass graft

√6ᵗʰ T82.22 Mechanical complication of biological heart valve graft

√7ᵗʰ T82.221 Breakdown (mechanical) of biological heart valve graft

√7ᵗʰ T82.222 Displacement of biological heart valve graft

Malposition of biological heart valve graft

√7ᵗʰ T82.223 Leakage of biological heart valve graft

√7ᵗʰ T82.228 Other mechanical complication of biological heart valve graft

Obstruction of biological heart valve graft
Perforation of biological heart valve graft
Protrusion of biological heart valve graft

√5ᵗʰ T82.3 Mechanical complication of other vascular grafts

√6ᵗʰ T82.31 Breakdown (mechanical) of other vascular grafts

¹ √7ᵗʰ T82.310 Breakdown (mechanical) of aortic (bifurcation) graft (replacement) HCC

¹ √7ᵗʰ T82.311 Breakdown (mechanical) of carotid arterial graft (bypass) HCC

¹ √7ᵗʰ T82.312 Breakdown (mechanical) of femoral arterial graft (bypass) HCC

¹ √7ᵗʰ T82.318 Breakdown (mechanical) of other vascular grafts HCC

¹ √7ᵗʰ T82.319 Breakdown (mechanical) of unspecified vascular grafts HCC ▽

√6ᵗʰ T82.32 Displacement of other vascular grafts

Malposition of other vascular grafts

¹ √7ᵗʰ T82.320 Displacement of aortic (bifurcation) graft (replacement) HCC

¹ √7ᵗʰ T82.321 Displacement of carotid arterial graft (bypass) HCC

¹ √7ᵗʰ T82.322 Displacement of femoral arterial graft (bypass) HCC

¹ √7ᵗʰ T82.328 Displacement of other vascular grafts HCC

¹ √7ᵗʰ T82.329 Displacement of unspecified vascular grafts HCC ▽

√6ᵗʰ T82.33 Leakage of other vascular grafts

¹ √7ᵗʰ T82.330 Leakage of aortic (bifurcation) graft (replacement) HCC

¹ √7ᵗʰ T82.331 Leakage of carotid arterial graft (bypass) HCC

¹ √7ᵗʰ T82.332 Leakage of femoral arterial graft (bypass) HCC

¹ √7ᵗʰ T82.338 Leakage of other vascular grafts HCC

¹ √7ᵗʰ T82.339 Leakage of unspecified vascular graft HCC ▽

√6ᵗʰ T82.39 Other mechanical complication of other vascular grafts

Obstruction (mechanical) of other vascular grafts
Perforation of other vascular grafts
Protrusion of other vascular grafts

¹ √7ᵗʰ T82.390 Other mechanical complication of aortic (bifurcation) graft (replacement) HCC

¹ √7ᵗʰ T82.391 Other mechanical complication of carotid arterial graft (bypass) HCC

¹ √7ᵗʰ T82.392 Other mechanical complication of femoral arterial graft (bypass) HCC

¹ √7ᵗʰ T82.398 Other mechanical complication of other vascular grafts HCC

¹ √7ᵗʰ T82.399 Other mechanical complication of unspecified vascular grafts HCC ▽

√5ᵗʰ T82.4 Mechanical complication of vascular dialysis catheter

Mechanical complication of hemodialysis catheter

> EXCLUDES 1   *mechanical complication of intraperitoneal dialysis catheter (T85.62)*

√x7ᵗʰ T82.41 Breakdown (mechanical) of vascular dialysis catheter HCC

√x7ᵗʰ T82.42 Displacement of vascular dialysis catheter HCC

Malposition of vascular dialysis catheter

√x7ᵗʰ T82.43 Leakage of vascular dialysis catheter HCC

√x7ᵗʰ T82.49 Other complication of vascular dialysis catheter HCC

Obstruction (mechanical) of vascular dialysis catheter
Perforation of vascular dialysis catheter
Protrusion of vascular dialysis catheter

√5ᵗʰ **T82.5 Mechanical complication of other cardiac and vascular devices and implants**

> **EXCLUDES 2**   mechanical complication of epidural and subdural infusion catheter (T85.61)

  √6ᵗʰ **T82.51 Breakdown (mechanical) of other cardiac and vascular devices and implants**

    ¹ √7ᵗʰ **T82.510 Breakdown (mechanical) of surgically created arteriovenous fistula**   HCC

    ¹ √7ᵗʰ **T82.511 Breakdown (mechanical) of surgically created arteriovenous shunt**

    √7ᵗʰ **T82.512 Breakdown (mechanical) of artificial heart**

    ¹ √7ᵗʰ **T82.513 Breakdown (mechanical) of balloon (counterpulsation) device**   HCC

    ¹ √7ᵗʰ **T82.514 Breakdown (mechanical) of infusion catheter**

    ¹ √7ᵗʰ **T82.515 Breakdown (mechanical) of umbrella device**   HCC

    ¹ √7ᵗʰ **T82.518 Breakdown (mechanical) of other cardiac and vascular devices and implants**   HCC

    √7ᵗʰ **T82.519 Breakdown (mechanical) of unspecified cardiac and vascular devices and implants**   ▽

  √6ᵗʰ **T82.52 Displacement of other cardiac and vascular devices and implants**

> Malposition of other cardiac and vascular devices and implants

    ¹ √7ᵗʰ **T82.520 Displacement of surgically created arteriovenous fistula**   HCC

    ¹ √7ᵗʰ **T82.521 Displacement of surgically created arteriovenous shunt**   HCC

    √7ᵗʰ **T82.522 Displacement of artificial heart**

    ¹ √7ᵗʰ **T82.523 Displacement of balloon (counterpulsation) device**   HCC

    ¹ √7ᵗʰ **T82.524 Displacement of infusion catheter**   HCC

    ¹ √7ᵗʰ **T82.525 Displacement of umbrella device**   HCC

    ¹ √7ᵗʰ **T82.528 Displacement of other cardiac and vascular devices and implants**   HCC

    √7ᵗʰ **T82.529 Displacement of unspecified cardiac and vascular devices and implants**   ▽

  √6ᵗʰ **T82.53 Leakage of other cardiac and vascular devices and implants**

    ¹ √7ᵗʰ **T82.530 Leakage of surgically created arteriovenous fistula**   HCC

    ¹ √7ᵗʰ **T82.531 Leakage of surgically created arteriovenous shunt**   HCC

    √7ᵗʰ **T82.532 Leakage of artificial heart**

    ¹ √7ᵗʰ **T82.533 Leakage of balloon (counterpulsation) device**   HCC

    ¹ √7ᵗʰ **T82.534 Leakage of infusion catheter**   HCC

    ¹ √7ᵗʰ **T82.535 Leakage of umbrella device**   HCC

    ¹ √7ᵗʰ **T82.538 Leakage of other cardiac and vascular devices and implants**   HCC

    √7ᵗʰ **T82.539 Leakage of unspecified cardiac and vascular devices and implants**   ▽

  √6ᵗʰ **T82.59 Other mechanical complication of other cardiac and vascular devices and implants**

> Obstruction (mechanical) of other cardiac and vascular devices and implants
>
> Perforation of other cardiac and vascular devices and implants
>
> Protrusion of other cardiac and vascular devices and implants

    ¹ √7ᵗʰ **T82.590 Other mechanical complication of surgically created arteriovenous fistula**   HCC

    ¹ √7ᵗʰ **T82.591 Other mechanical complication of surgically created arteriovenous shunt**   HCC

    √7ᵗʰ **T82.592 Other mechanical complication of artificial heart**

    ¹ √7ᵗʰ **T82.593 Other mechanical complication of balloon (counterpulsation) device**   HCC

    ¹ √7ᵗʰ **T82.594 Other mechanical complication of infusion catheter**   HCC

    ¹ √7ᵗʰ **T82.595 Other mechanical complication of umbrella device**   HCC

    ¹ √7ᵗʰ **T82.598 Other mechanical complication of other cardiac and vascular devices and implants**   HCC

    √7ᵗʰ **T82.599 Other mechanical complication of unspecified cardiac and vascular devices and implants**   ▽

¹ √x7ᵗʰ **T82.6 Infection and inflammatory reaction due to cardiac valve prosthesis**   HCC

> Use additional code to identify infection

¹ √x7ᵗʰ **T82.7 Infection and inflammatory reaction due to other cardiac and vascular devices, implants and grafts**   HCC

> Use additional code to identify infection

√5ᵗʰ **T82.8 Other specified complications of cardiac and vascular prosthetic devices, implants and grafts**

> **AHA:** 2016,4Q,70

  √6ᵗʰ **T82.81 Embolism due to cardiac and vascular prosthetic devices, implants and grafts**

    √7ᵗʰ **T82.817 Embolism due to cardiac prosthetic devices, implants and grafts**

    ¹ √7ᵗʰ **T82.818 Embolism due to vascular prosthetic devices, implants and grafts**   HCC

  √6ᵗʰ **T82.82 Fibrosis due to cardiac and vascular prosthetic devices, implants and grafts**

    √7ᵗʰ **T82.827 Fibrosis due to cardiac prosthetic devices, implants and grafts**

    ¹ √7ᵗʰ **T82.828 Fibrosis due vascular prosthetic devices, implants and grafts**   HCC

  √6ᵗʰ **T82.83 Hemorrhage due to cardiac and vascular prosthetic devices, implants and grafts**

    √7ᵗʰ **T82.837 Hemorrhage due to cardiac prosthetic devices, implants and grafts**

    ¹ √7ᵗʰ **T82.838 Hemorrhage due to vascular prosthetic devices, implants and grafts**   HCC

  √6ᵗʰ **T82.84 Pain due to cardiac and vascular prosthetic devices, implants and grafts**

    √7ᵗʰ **T82.847 Pain due to cardiac prosthetic devices, implants and grafts**

    ¹ √7ᵗʰ **T82.848 Pain due to vascular prosthetic devices, implants and grafts**   HCC

  √6ᵗʰ **T82.85 Stenosis due to cardiac and vascular prosthetic devices, implants and grafts**

    √7ᵗʰ **T82.855 Stenosis of coronary artery stent**

> In-stent stenosis (restenosis) of coronary artery stent
>
> Restenosis of coronary artery stent

    ¹ √7ᵗʰ **T82.856 Stenosis of peripheral vascular stent**   HCC

> In-stent stenosis (restenosis) of peripheral vascular stent
>
> Restenosis of peripheral vascular stent

    √7ᵗʰ **T82.857 Stenosis of other cardiac prosthetic devices, implants and grafts**

    ¹ √7ᵗʰ **T82.858 Stenosis of other vascular prosthetic devices, implants and grafts**   HCC

  √6ᵗʰ **T82.86 Thrombosis of cardiac and vascular prosthetic devices, implants and grafts**

    √7ᵗʰ **T82.867 Thrombosis due to cardiac prosthetic devices, implants and grafts**

    ¹ √7ᵗʰ **T82.868 Thrombosis due to vascular prosthetic devices, implants and grafts**   HCC

  √6ᵗʰ **T82.89 Other specified complication of cardiac and vascular prosthetic devices, implants and grafts**

    √7ᵗʰ **T82.897 Other specified complication of cardiac prosthetic devices, implants and grafts**

    ¹ √7ᵗʰ **T82.898 Other specified complication of vascular prosthetic devices, implants and grafts**   HCC

√x7ᵗʰ **T82.9 Unspecified complication of cardiac and vascular prosthetic device, implant and graft**   ▽

☑ Additional Character Req   √x7ᵗʰ Placeholder Alert   Manifestation   ▽ Unspecified   ▶◀ Revised Text   ● New Code   ▲ Revised Code Title

✓4ᵗʰ **T83 Complications of genitourinary prosthetic devices, implants and grafts**

> EXCLUDES 2 *failure and rejection of transplanted organs and tissue (T86.-)*

> **AHA:** 2016,4Q,70-71

> The appropriate 7th character is to be added to each code from category T83.
> A initial encounter
> D subsequent encounter
> S sequela

✓5ᵗʰ **T83.0 Mechanical complication of** urinary catheter

> EXCLUDES 2 *complications of stoma of urinary tract (N99.5-)*

✓6ᵗʰ **T83.01 Breakdown (mechanical) of urinary catheter**

1 ✓7ᵗʰ **T83.010 Breakdown (mechanical) of** cystostomy **catheter** HCC

1 ✓7ᵗʰ **T83.011 Breakdown (mechanical) of** indwelling urethral **catheter** HCC

1 ✓7ᵗʰ **T83.012 Breakdown (mechanical) of** nephrostomy **catheter** HCC

1 ✓7ᵗʰ **T83.018 Breakdown (mechanical) of other urinary catheter** HCC
> Breakdown (mechanical) of Hopkins catheter
> Breakdown (mechanical) of ileostomy catheter
> Breakdown (mechanical) urostomy catheter

✓6ᵗʰ **T83.02 Displacement of urinary catheter**
> Malposition of urinary catheter

1 ✓7ᵗʰ **T83.020 Displacement of** cystostomy **catheter** HCC

1 ✓7ᵗʰ **T83.021 Displacement of** indwelling urethral **catheter** HCC

1 ✓7ᵗʰ **T83.022 Displacement of** nephrostomy **catheter** HCC

1 ✓7ᵗʰ **T83.028 Displacement of other urinary catheter** HCC
> Displacement of Hopkins catheter
> Displacement of ileostomy catheter
> Displacement of urostomy catheter

✓6ᵗʰ **T83.03 Leakage of urinary catheter**

1 ✓7ᵗʰ **T83.030 Leakage of** cystostomy **catheter** HCC

1 ✓7ᵗʰ **T83.031 Leakage of** indwelling urethral **catheter** HCC

1 ✓7ᵗʰ **T83.032 Leakage of** nephrostomy **catheter** HCC

1 ✓7ᵗʰ **T83.038 Leakage of other urinary catheter** HCC
> Leakage of Hopkins catheter
> Leakage of ileostomy catheter
> Leakage of urostomy catheter

✓6ᵗʰ **T83.09 Other mechanical complication of urinary catheter**
> Obstruction (mechanical) of urinary catheter
> Perforation of urinary catheter
> Protrusion of urinary catheter

1 ✓7ᵗʰ **T83.090 Other mechanical complication of** cystostomy **catheter** HCC

1 ✓7ᵗʰ **T83.091 Other mechanical complication of** indwelling urethral **catheter** HCC

1 ✓7ᵗʰ **T83.092 Other mechanical complication of** nephrostomy **catheter** HCC

1 ✓7ᵗʰ **T83.098 Other mechanical complication of other urinary catheter** HCC
> Other mechanical complication of Hopkins catheter
> Other mechanical complication of ileostomy catheter
> Other mechanical complication of urostomy catheter

✓5ᵗʰ **T83.1 Mechanical complication of other urinary devices and implants**

✓6ᵗʰ **T83.11 Breakdown (mechanical) of other urinary devices and implants**

1 ✓7ᵗʰ **T83.110 Breakdown (mechanical) of urinary** electronic stimulator device HCC
> EXCLUDES 2 *breakdown (mechanical) of electrode (lead) for sacral nerve neurostimulator (T85.111)*
> *breakdown (mechanical) of implanted electronic sacral neurostimulator, pulse generator or receiver (T85.113)*

1 ✓7ᵗʰ **T83.111 Breakdown (mechanical) of** implanted urinary sphincter HCC

1 ✓7ᵗʰ **T83.112 Breakdown (mechanical) of** indwelling ureteral stent HCC

1 ✓7ᵗʰ **T83.113 Breakdown (mechanical) of other urinary stents** HCC
> Breakdown (mechanical) of ileal conduit stent
> Breakdown (mechanical) of nephroureteral stent

1 ✓7ᵗʰ **T83.118 Breakdown (mechanical) of other urinary devices and implants** HCC

✓6ᵗʰ **T83.12 Displacement of other urinary devices and implants**
> Malposition of other urinary devices and implants

1 ✓7ᵗʰ **T83.120 Displacement of urinary** electronic stimulator device HCC
> EXCLUDES 2 *displacement of electrode (lead) for sacral nerve neurostimulator (T85.121)*
> *displacement of implanted electronic sacral neurostimulator, pulse generator or receiver (T85.123)*

1 ✓7ᵗʰ **T83.121 Displacement of** implanted urinary sphincter HCC

1 ✓7ᵗʰ **T83.122 Displacement of** indwelling ureteral stent HCC

1 ✓7ᵗʰ **T83.123 Displacement of other urinary stents** HCC
> Displacement of ileal conduit stent
> Displacement of nephroureteral stent

1 ✓7ᵗʰ **T83.128 Displacement of other urinary devices and implants** HCC

✓6ᵗʰ **T83.19 Other mechanical complication of other urinary devices and implants**
> Leakage of other urinary devices and implants
> Obstruction (mechanical) of other urinary devices and implants
> Perforation of other urinary devices and implants
> Protrusion of other urinary devices and implants

1 ✓7ᵗʰ **T83.190 Other mechanical complication of urinary** electronic stimulator device HCC
> EXCLUDES 2 *other mechanical complication of electrode (lead) for sacral nerve neurostimulator (T85.191)*
> *other mechanical complication of implanted electronic sacral neurostimulator, pulse generator or receiver (T85.193)*

1 ✓7ᵗʰ **T83.191 Other mechanical complication of** implanted urinary sphincter HCC

1 ✓7ᵗʰ **T83.192 Other mechanical complication of** indwelling ureteral stent HCC

1 ✓7ᵗʰ **T83.193 Other mechanical complication of other urinary stent** HCC
> Other mechanical complication of ileal conduit stent
> Other mechanical complication of nephroureteral stent

¹ √7ᵗʰ **T83.198 Other mechanical complication of other urinary devices and implants** `HCC`

√5ᵗʰ **T83.2 Mechanical complication of graft of urinary organ**

¹ √x7ᵗʰ **T83.21 Breakdown (mechanical) of graft of urinary organ** `HCC`

¹ √x7ᵗʰ **T83.22 Displacement of graft of urinary organ** `HCC`
     Malposition of graft of urinary organ

¹ √x7ᵗʰ **T83.23 Leakage of graft of urinary organ** `HCC`

¹ √x7ᵗʰ **T83.24 Erosion of graft of urinary organ** `HCC`

¹ √x7ᵗʰ **T83.25 Exposure of graft of urinary organ** `HCC`

¹ √x7ᵗʰ **T83.29 Other mechanical complication of graft of urinary organ** `HCC`
     Obstruction (mechanical) of graft of urinary organ
     Perforation of graft of urinary organ
     Protrusion of graft of urinary organ

√5ᵗʰ **T83.3 Mechanical complication of intrauterine contraceptive device**

√7ᵗʰ **T83.31 Breakdown (mechanical) of intrauterine contraceptive device** ♀

√x7ᵗʰ **T83.32 Displacement of intrauterine contraceptive device** ♀
     Malposition of intrauterine contraceptive device
     Missing string of intrauterine contraceptive device
     AHA: 2018,1Q,5

√x7ᵗʰ **T83.39 Other mechanical complication of intrauterine contraceptive device** ♀
     Leakage of intrauterine contraceptive device
     Obstruction (mechanical) of intrauterine contraceptive device
     Perforation of intrauterine contraceptive device
     Protrusion of intrauterine contraceptive device

√5ᵗʰ **T83.4 Mechanical complication of other prosthetic devices, implants and grafts of genital tract**

√6ᵗʰ **T83.41 Breakdown (mechanical) of other prosthetic devices, implants and grafts of genital tract**

¹ √7ᵗʰ **T83.410 Breakdown (mechanical) of implanted penile prosthesis** `HCC` ♂
     Breakdown (mechanical) of penile prosthesis cylinder
     Breakdown (mechanical) of penile prosthesis pump
     Breakdown (mechanical) of penile prosthesis reservoir

¹ √7ᵗʰ **T83.411 Breakdown (mechanical) of implanted testicular prosthesis** `HCC`

¹ √7ᵗʰ **T83.418 Breakdown (mechanical) of other prosthetic devices, implants and grafts of genital tract** `HCC`

√6ᵗʰ **T83.42 Displacement of other prosthetic devices, implants and grafts of genital tract**
     Malposition of other prosthetic devices, implants and grafts of genital tract

¹ √7ᵗʰ **T83.420 Displacement of implanted penile prosthesis** `HCC` ♂
     Displacement of penile prosthesis cylinder
     Displacement of penile prosthesis pump
     Displacement of penile prosthesis reservoir

¹ √7ᵗʰ **T83.421 Displacement of implanted testicular prosthesis** `HCC`

¹ √7ᵗʰ **T83.428 Displacement of other prosthetic devices, implants and grafts of genital tract** `HCC`
     AHA: 2018,1Q,5

√6ᵗʰ **T83.49 Other mechanical complication of other prosthetic devices, implants and grafts of genital tract**
     Leakage of other prosthetic devices, implants and grafts of genital tract
     Obstruction, mechanical of other prosthetic devices, implants and grafts of genital tract
     Perforation of other prosthetic devices, implants and grafts of genital tract
     Protrusion of other prosthetic devices, implants and grafts of genital tract

¹ √7ᵗʰ **T83.490 Other mechanical complication of implanted penile prosthesis** `HCC` ♂
     Other mechanical complication of penile prosthesis cylinder
     Other mechanical complication of penile prosthesis pump
     Other mechanical complication of penile prosthesis reservoir

¹ √7ᵗʰ **T83.491 Other mechanical complication of implanted testicular prosthesis** `HCC`

¹ √7ᵗʰ **T83.498 Other mechanical complication of other prosthetic devices, implants and grafts of genital tract** `HCC`

√5ᵗʰ **T83.5 Infection and inflammatory reaction due to prosthetic device, implant and graft in urinary system**
     Use additional code to identify infection

√6ᵗʰ **T83.51 Infection and inflammatory reaction due to urinary catheter**
     `EXCLUDES 2` complications of stoma of urinary tract (N99.5-)

¹ √7ᵗʰ **T83.510 Infection and inflammatory reaction due to cystostomy catheter** `HCC`

¹ √7ᵗʰ **T83.511 Infection and inflammatory reaction due to indwelling urethral catheter** `HCC`

¹ √7ᵗʰ **T83.512 Infection and inflammatory reaction due to nephrostomy catheter** `HCC`

¹ √7ᵗʰ **T83.518 Infection and inflammatory reaction due to other urinary catheter** `HCC`
     Infection and inflammatory reaction due to Hopkins catheter
     Infection and inflammatory reaction due to ileostomy catheter
     Infection and inflammatory reaction due to urostomy catheter

√6ᵗʰ **T83.59 Infection and inflammatory reaction due to prosthetic device, implant and graft in urinary system**

¹ √7ᵗʰ **T83.590 Infection and inflammatory reaction due to implanted urinary neurostimulation device** `HCC`
     `EXCLUDES 2` infection and inflammatory reaction due to electrode lead of sacral nerve neurostimulator (T85.732)
     infection and inflammatory reaction due to pulse generator or receiver of sacral nerve neurostimulator (T85.734)

¹ √7ᵗʰ **T83.591 Infection and inflammatory reaction due to implanted urinary sphincter** `HCC`

¹ √7ᵗʰ **T83.592 Infection and inflammatory reaction due to indwelling ureteral stent** `HCC`

¹ √7ᵗʰ **T83.593 Infection and inflammatory reaction due to other urinary stents** `HCC`
     Infection and inflammatory reaction due to ileal conduit stents
     Infection and inflammatory reaction due to nephroureteral stent

¹ √7ᵗʰ **T83.598 Infection and inflammatory reaction due to other prosthetic device, implant and graft in urinary system** `HCC`

Chapter 19. Injury, Poisoning and Certain Other Consequences of External Causes

T83.6–T84.052

√5ᵗʰ **T83.6** **Infection and inflammatory reaction due to prosthetic device, implant and graft in genital tract**
Use additional code to identify infection

     1 √x7ᵗʰ **T83.61** **Infection and inflammatory reaction due to implanted penile prosthesis** HCC
Infection and inflammatory reaction due to penile prosthesis cylinder
Infection and inflammatory reaction due to penile prosthesis pump
Infection and inflammatory reaction due to penile prosthesis reservoir

     1 √x7ᵗʰ **T83.62** **Infection and inflammatory reaction due to implanted testicular prosthesis** HCC

     1 √x7ᵗʰ **T83.69** **Infection and inflammatory reaction due to other prosthetic device, implant and graft in genital tract** HCC

√5ᵗʰ **T83.7** **Complications due to implanted mesh and other prosthetic materials**

     √6ᵗʰ **T83.71** **Erosion of implanted mesh and other prosthetic materials**

       1 √7ᵗʰ **T83.711** **Erosion of implanted vaginal mesh to surrounding organ or tissue** HCC ♀
Erosion of implanted vaginal mesh into pelvic floor muscles

       1 √7ᵗʰ **T83.712** **Erosion of implanted urethral mesh to surrounding organ or tissue** HCC
Erosion of implanted female urethral sling
Erosion of implanted male urethral sling
Erosion of implanted urethral mesh into pelvic floor muscles

       1 √7ᵗʰ **T83.713** **Erosion of implanted urethral bulking agent to surrounding organ or tissue** HCC

       1 √7ᵗʰ **T83.714** **Erosion of implanted ureteral bulking agent to surrounding organ or tissue** HCC

       1 √7ᵗʰ **T83.718** **Erosion of other implanted mesh to organ or tissue** HCC

       1 √7ᵗʰ **T83.719** **Erosion of other prosthetic materials to surrounding organ or tissue** HCC

     √6ᵗʰ **T83.72** **Exposure of implanted mesh and other prosthetic materials into surrounding organ or tissue**
Extrusion of implanted mesh

       1 √7ᵗʰ **T83.721** **Exposure of implanted vaginal mesh into vagina** HCC ♀
Exposure of implanted vaginal mesh through vaginal wall

       1 √7ᵗʰ **T83.722** **Exposure of implanted urethral mesh into urethra** HCC
Exposure of implanted female urethral sling
Exposure of implanted male urethral sling
Exposure of implanted urethral mesh through urethral wall

       1 √7ᵗʰ **T83.723** **Exposure of implanted urethral bulking agent into urethra** HCC

       1 √7ᵗʰ **T83.724** **Exposure of implanted ureteral bulking agent into ureter** HCC

       1 √7ᵗʰ **T83.728** **Exposure of other implanted mesh into organ or tissue** HCC

       1 √7ᵗʰ **T83.729** **Exposure of other prosthetic materials into organ or tissue** HCC

     1 √x7ᵗʰ **T83.79** **Other specified complications due to other genitourinary prosthetic materials** HCC

√5ᵗʰ **T83.8** **Other specified complications of genitourinary prosthetic devices, implants and grafts**

     1 √x7ᵗʰ **T83.81** **Embolism due to genitourinary prosthetic devices, implants and grafts** HCC

     1 √x7ᵗʰ **T83.82** **Fibrosis due to genitourinary prosthetic devices, implants and grafts** HCC

     1 √x7ᵗʰ **T83.83** **Hemorrhage due to genitourinary prosthetic devices, implants and grafts** HCC

     1 √x7ᵗʰ **T83.84** **Pain due to genitourinary prosthetic devices, implants and grafts** HCC

     1 √x7ᵗʰ **T83.85** **Stenosis due to genitourinary prosthetic devices, implants and grafts** HCC

     1 √x7ᵗʰ **T83.86** **Thrombosis due to genitourinary prosthetic devices, implants and grafts** HCC

     1 √x7ᵗʰ **T83.89** **Other specified complication of genitourinary prosthetic devices, implants and grafts** HCC

     1 √x7ᵗʰ **T83.9** **Unspecified complication of genitourinary prosthetic device, implant and graft** HCC ▽

√4ᵗʰ **T84** **Complications of internal orthopedic prosthetic devices, implants and grafts**
EXCLUDES 2   failure and rejection of transplanted organs and tissues (T86.-)
fracture of bone following insertion of orthopedic implant, joint prosthesis or bone plate (M96.6)

The appropriate 7th character is to be added to each code from category T84.
A   initial encounter
D   subsequent encounter
S   sequela

√5ᵗʰ **T84.0** **Mechanical complication of internal joint prosthesis**

     √6ᵗʰ **T84.01** **Broken internal joint prosthesis**
Breakage (fracture) of prosthetic joint
Broken prosthetic joint implant
EXCLUDES 1   periprosthetic joint implant fracture (M97-)
AHA: 2016,4Q,42

       1 √7ᵗʰ **T84.010** **Broken internal right hip prosthesis** HCC

       1 √7ᵗʰ **T84.011** **Broken internal left hip prosthesis** HCC

       1 √7ᵗʰ **T84.012** **Broken internal right knee prosthesis** HCC

       1 √7ᵗʰ **T84.013** **Broken internal left knee prosthesis** HCC

       1 √7ᵗʰ **T84.018** **Broken internal joint prosthesis, other site** HCC
Use additional code to identify the joint (Z96.6-)

       1 √7ᵗʰ **T84.019** **Broken internal joint prosthesis, unspecified site** HCC ▽

     √6ᵗʰ **T84.02** **Dislocation of internal joint prosthesis**
Instability of internal joint prosthesis
Subluxation of internal joint prosthesis

       1 √7ᵗʰ **T84.020** **Dislocation of internal right hip prosthesis** HCC

       1 √7ᵗʰ **T84.021** **Dislocation of internal left hip prosthesis** HCC

       1 √7ᵗʰ **T84.022** **Instability of internal right knee prosthesis** HCC

       1 √7ᵗʰ **T84.023** **Instability of internal left knee prosthesis** HCC

       1 √7ᵗʰ **T84.028** **Dislocation of other internal joint prosthesis** HCC
Use additional code to identify the joint (Z96.6-)

       1 √7ᵗʰ **T84.029** **Dislocation of unspecified internal joint prosthesis** HCC ▽

     √6ᵗʰ **T84.03** **Mechanical loosening of internal prosthetic joint**
Aseptic loosening of prosthetic joint

       1 √7ᵗʰ **T84.030** **Mechanical loosening of internal right hip prosthetic joint** HCC

       1 √7ᵗʰ **T84.031** **Mechanical loosening of internal left hip prosthetic joint** HCC

       1 √7ᵗʰ **T84.032** **Mechanical loosening of internal right knee prosthetic joint** HCC

       1 √7ᵗʰ **T84.033** **Mechanical loosening of internal left knee prosthetic joint** HCC

       1 √7ᵗʰ **T84.038** **Mechanical loosening of other internal prosthetic joint** HCC
Use additional code to identify the joint (Z96.6-)

       1 √7ᵗʰ **T84.039** **Mechanical loosening of unspecified internal prosthetic joint** HCC ▽

     √6ᵗʰ **T84.05** **Periprosthetic osteolysis of internal prosthetic joint**
Use additional code to identify major osseous defect, if applicable (M89.7-)

       1 √7ᵗʰ **T84.050** **Periprosthetic osteolysis of internal prosthetic right hip joint** HCC

       1 √7ᵗʰ **T84.051** **Periprosthetic osteolysis of internal prosthetic left hip joint** HCC

       1 √7ᵗʰ **T84.052** **Periprosthetic osteolysis of internal prosthetic right knee joint** HCC

¹ √7ᵗʰ **T84.053** Periprosthetic osteolysis of internal prosthetic left knee joint   HCC

¹ √7ᵗʰ **T84.058** Periprosthetic osteolysis of other internal prosthetic joint   HCC

    Use additional code to identify the joint (Z96.6-)

¹ √7ᵗʰ **T84.059** Periprosthetic osteolysis of unspecified internal prosthetic joint   HCC ▽

√6ᵗʰ **T84.06** Wear of articular bearing surface of internal prosthetic joint

¹ √7ᵗʰ **T84.060** Wear of articular bearing surface of internal prosthetic right hip joint   HCC

¹ √7ᵗʰ **T84.061** Wear of articular bearing surface of internal prosthetic left hip joint   HCC

¹ √7ᵗʰ **T84.062** Wear of articular bearing surface of internal prosthetic right knee joint   HCC

¹ √7ᵗʰ **T84.063** Wear of articular bearing surface of internal prosthetic left knee joint   HCC

¹ √7ᵗʰ **T84.068** Wear of articular bearing surface of other internal prosthetic joint   HCC

    Use additional code to identify the joint (Z96.6-)

¹ √7ᵗʰ **T84.069** Wear of articular bearing surface of unspecified internal prosthetic joint   HCC ▽

√6ᵗʰ **T84.09** Other mechanical complication of internal joint prosthesis

    Prosthetic joint implant failure NOS

¹ √7ᵗʰ **T84.090** Other mechanical complication of internal right hip prosthesis   HCC

¹ √7ᵗʰ **T84.091** Other mechanical complication of internal left hip prosthesis   HCC

¹ √7ᵗʰ **T84.092** Other mechanical complication of internal right knee prosthesis   HCC

¹ √7ᵗʰ **T84.093** Other mechanical complication of internal left knee prosthesis   HCC

¹ √7ᵗʰ **T84.098** Other mechanical complication of other internal joint prosthesis   HCC

    Use additional code to identify the joint (Z96.6-)

¹ √7ᵗʰ **T84.099** Other mechanical complication of unspecified internal joint prosthesis   HCC ▽

√5ᵗʰ **T84.1** Mechanical complication of internal fixation device of bones of limb

    EXCLUDES 2   mechanical complication of internal fixation device of bones of feet (T84.2-)

          mechanical complication of internal fixation device of bones of fingers (T84.2-)

          mechanical complication of internal fixation device of bones of hands (T84.2-)

          mechanical complication of internal fixation device of bones of toes (T84.2-)

√6ᵗʰ **T84.11** Breakdown (mechanical) of internal fixation device of bones of limb

¹ √7ᵗʰ **T84.110** Breakdown (mechanical) of internal fixation device of right humerus   HCC

¹ √7ᵗʰ **T84.111** Breakdown (mechanical) of internal fixation device of left humerus   HCC

¹ √7ᵗʰ **T84.112** Breakdown (mechanical) of internal fixation device of bone of right forearm   HCC

¹ √7ᵗʰ **T84.113** Breakdown (mechanical) of internal fixation device of bone of left forearm   HCC

¹ √7ᵗʰ **T84.114** Breakdown (mechanical) of internal fixation device of right femur   HCC

¹ √7ᵗʰ **T84.115** Breakdown (mechanical) of internal fixation device of left femur   HCC

¹ √7ᵗʰ **T84.116** Breakdown (mechanical) of internal fixation device of bone of right lower leg   HCC

¹ √7ᵗʰ **T84.117** Breakdown (mechanical) of internal fixation device of bone of left lower leg   HCC

¹ √7ᵗʰ **T84.119** Breakdown (mechanical) of internal fixation device of unspecified bone of limb   HCC ▽

√6ᵗʰ **T84.12** Displacement of internal fixation device of bones of limb

    Malposition of internal fixation device of bones of limb

¹ √7ᵗʰ **T84.120** Displacement of internal fixation device of right humerus   HCC

¹ √7ᵗʰ **T84.121** Displacement of internal fixation device of left humerus   HCC

¹ √7ᵗʰ **T84.122** Displacement of internal fixation device of bone of right forearm   HCC

¹ √7ᵗʰ **T84.123** Displacement of internal fixation device of bone of left forearm   HCC

¹ √7ᵗʰ **T84.124** Displacement of internal fixation device of right femur   HCC

¹ √7ᵗʰ **T84.125** Displacement of internal fixation device of left femur   HCC

¹ √7ᵗʰ **T84.126** Displacement of internal fixation device of bone of right lower leg   HCC

¹ √7ᵗʰ **T84.127** Displacement of internal fixation device of bone of left lower leg   HCC

¹ √7ᵗʰ **T84.129** Displacement of internal fixation device of unspecified bone of limb   HCC ▽

√6ᵗʰ **T84.19** Other mechanical complication of internal fixation device of bones of limb

    Obstruction (mechanical) of internal fixation device of bones of limb

    Perforation of internal fixation device of bones of limb

    Protrusion of internal fixation device of bones of limb

¹ √7ᵗʰ **T84.190** Other mechanical complication of internal fixation device of right humerus   HCC

¹ √7ᵗʰ **T84.191** Other mechanical complication of internal fixation device of left humerus   HCC

¹ √7ᵗʰ **T84.192** Other mechanical complication of internal fixation device of bone of right forearm   HCC

¹ √7ᵗʰ **T84.193** Other mechanical complication of internal fixation device of bone of left forearm   HCC

¹ √7ᵗʰ **T84.194** Other mechanical complication of internal fixation device of right femur   HCC

¹ √7ᵗʰ **T84.195** Other mechanical complication of internal fixation device of left femur   HCC

¹ √7ᵗʰ **T84.196** Other mechanical complication of internal fixation device of bone of right lower leg   HCC

¹ √7ᵗʰ **T84.197** Other mechanical complication of internal fixation device of bone of left lower leg   HCC

¹ √7ᵗʰ **T84.199** Other mechanical complication of internal fixation device of unspecified bone of limb   HCC ▽

√5ᵗʰ **T84.2** Mechanical complication of internal fixation device of other bones

√6ᵗʰ **T84.21** Breakdown (mechanical) of internal fixation device of other bones

¹ √7ᵗʰ **T84.210** Breakdown (mechanical) of internal fixation device of bones of hand and fingers   HCC

¹ √7ᵗʰ **T84.213** Breakdown (mechanical) of internal fixation device of bones of foot and toes   HCC

¹ √7ᵗʰ **T84.216** Breakdown (mechanical) of internal fixation device of vertebrae   HCC

¹ √7ᵗʰ **T84.218** Breakdown (mechanical) of internal fixation device of other bones   HCC

√6ᵗʰ **T84.22** Displacement of internal fixation device of other bones

    Malposition of internal fixation device of other bones

¹ √7ᵗʰ **T84.220** Displacement of internal fixation device of bones of hand and fingers   HCC

¹ √7ᵗʰ **T84.223** Displacement of internal fixation device of bones of foot and toes   HCC

☑ Additional Character Req   √x7ᵗʰ Placeholder Alert   Manifestation   ▽ Unspecified   ▶◀ Revised Text   ● New Code   ▲ Revised Code Title

¹ √7ᵗʰ **T84.226** **Displacement of internal fixation device of** vertebrae   HCC

¹ √7ᵗʰ **T84.228** **Displacement of internal fixation device of other bones**   HCC

√6ᵗʰ **T84.29** **Other mechanical complication of internal fixation device of other bones**

Obstruction (mechanical) of internal fixation device of other bones

Perforation of internal fixation device of other bones

Protrusion of internal fixation device of other bones

¹ √7ᵗʰ **T84.290** **Other mechanical complication of internal fixation device of bones of** hand and fingers   HCC

¹ √7ᵗʰ **T84.293** **Other mechanical complication of internal fixation device of bones of** foot and toes   HCC

¹ √7ᵗʰ **T84.296** **Other mechanical complication of internal fixation device of** vertebrae   HCC

¹ √7ᵗʰ **T84.298** **Other mechanical complication of internal fixation device of other bones**   HCC

√5ᵗʰ **T84.3** **Mechanical complication of other bone devices, implants and grafts**

EXCLUDES 2   *other complications of bone graft (T86.83-)*

√6ᵗʰ **T84.31** **Breakdown (mechanical) of other bone devices, implants and grafts**

¹ √7ᵗʰ **T84.310** **Breakdown (mechanical) of electronic bone stimulator**   HCC

¹ √7ᵗʰ **T84.318** **Breakdown (mechanical) of other bone devices, implants and grafts**   HCC

√6ᵗʰ **T84.32** **Displacement of other bone devices, implants and grafts**

Malposition of other bone devices, implants and grafts

¹ √7ᵗʰ **T84.320** **Displacement of** electronic bone stimulator   HCC

¹ √7ᵗʰ **T84.328** **Displacement of other bone devices, implants and grafts**   HCC

AHA: 2014,4Q,28

√6ᵗʰ **T84.39** **Other mechanical complication of other bone devices, implants and grafts**

Obstruction (mechanical) of other bone devices, implants and grafts

Perforation of other bone devices, implants and grafts

Protrusion of other bone devices, implants and grafts

¹ √7ᵗʰ **T84.390** **Other mechanical complication of** electronic bone stimulator   HCC

¹ √7ᵗʰ **T84.398** **Other mechanical complication of other bone devices, implants and grafts**   HCC

√5ᵗʰ **T84.4** **Mechanical complication of other internal orthopedic devices, implants and grafts**

√6ᵗʰ **T84.41** **Breakdown (mechanical) of other internal orthopedic devices, implants and grafts**

¹ √7ᵗʰ **T84.410** **Breakdown (mechanical) of** muscle and tendon graft   HCC

¹ √7ᵗʰ **T84.418** **Breakdown (mechanical) of other internal orthopedic devices, implants and grafts**   HCC

√6ᵗʰ **T84.42** **Displacement of other internal orthopedic devices, implants and grafts**

Malposition of other internal orthopedic devices, implants and grafts

¹ √7ᵗʰ **T84.420** **Displacement of** muscle and tendon graft   HCC

¹ √7ᵗʰ **T84.428** **Displacement of other internal orthopedic devices, implants and grafts**   HCC

√6ᵗʰ **T84.49** **Other mechanical complication of other internal orthopedic devices, implants and grafts**

Mechanical complication of other internal orthopedic devices, implants and grafts NOS

Obstruction (mechanical) of other internal orthopedic devices, implants and grafts

Perforation of other internal orthopedic devices, implants and grafts

Protrusion of other internal orthopedic devices, implants and grafts

¹ √7ᵗʰ **T84.490** **Other mechanical complication of** muscle and tendon graft   HCC

¹ √7ᵗʰ **T84.498** **Other mechanical complication of other internal orthopedic devices, implants and grafts**   HCC

√5ᵗʰ **T84.5** **Infection and inflammatory reaction due to** internal joint prosthesis

Use additional code to identify infection

AHA: 2015,1Q,16

¹ √x7ᵗʰ **T84.50** **Infection and inflammatory reaction due to unspecified internal joint prosthesis**   HCC ▽

¹ √x7ᵗʰ **T84.51** **Infection and inflammatory reaction due to internal** right hip **prosthesis**   HCC

¹ √x7ᵗʰ **T84.52** **Infection and inflammatory reaction due to internal** left hip **prosthesis**   HCC

¹ √x7ᵗʰ **T84.53** **Infection and inflammatory reaction due to internal** right knee **prosthesis**   HCC

¹ √x7ᵗʰ **T84.54** **Infection and inflammatory reaction due to internal** left knee **prosthesis**   HCC

¹ √x7ᵗʰ **T84.59** **Infection and inflammatory reaction due to other internal joint prosthesis**   HCC

√5ᵗʰ **T84.6** **Infection and inflammatory reaction due to** internal fixation device

Use additional code to identify infection

¹ √x7ᵗʰ **T84.60** **Infection and inflammatory reaction due to internal fixation device of unspecified site**   HCC ▽

√6ᵗʰ **T84.61** **Infection and inflammatory reaction due to internal fixation device of** arm

¹ √7ᵗʰ **T84.610** **Infection and inflammatory reaction due to internal fixation device of** right humerus   HCC

¹ √7ᵗʰ **T84.611** **Infection and inflammatory reaction due to internal fixation device of** left humerus   HCC

¹ √7ᵗʰ **T84.612** **Infection and inflammatory reaction due to internal fixation device of** right radius   HCC

¹ √7ᵗʰ **T84.613** **Infection and inflammatory reaction due to internal fixation device of** left radius   HCC

¹ √7ᵗʰ **T84.614** **Infection and inflammatory reaction due to internal fixation device of** right ulna   HCC

¹ √7ᵗʰ **T84.615** **Infection and inflammatory reaction due to internal fixation device of** left ulna   HCC

¹ √7ᵗʰ **T84.619** **Infection and inflammatory reaction due to internal fixation device of unspecified bone of arm**   HCC ▽

√6ᵗʰ **T84.62** **Infection and inflammatory reaction due to internal fixation device of** leg

¹ √7ᵗʰ **T84.620** **Infection and inflammatory reaction due to internal fixation device of** right femur   HCC

¹ √7ᵗʰ **T84.621** **Infection and inflammatory reaction due to internal fixation device of** left femur   HCC

¹ √7ᵗʰ **T84.622** **Infection and inflammatory reaction due to internal fixation device of** right tibia   HCC

¹ √7ᵗʰ **T84.623** **Infection and inflammatory reaction due to internal fixation device of** left tibia   HCC

¹ √7ᵗʰ **T84.624** **Infection and inflammatory reaction due to internal fixation device of** right fibula   HCC

¹ √7ᵗʰ **T84.625** **Infection and inflammatory reaction due to internal fixation device of** left fibula   HCC

¹ √7ᵗʰ **T84.629** **Infection and inflammatory reaction due to internal fixation device of unspecified bone of leg**   HCC ▽

¹ √x7ᵗʰ **T84.63** **Infection and inflammatory reaction due to internal fixation device of** spine   HCC

¹ √x7ᵗʰ **T84.69** **Infection and inflammatory reaction due to internal fixation device of other site**   HCC

¹ √x7ᵗʰ **T84.7** **Infection and inflammatory reaction due to other internal orthopedic prosthetic devices, implants and grafts**   HCC

Use additional code to identify infection

√5ᵗʰ **T84.8** **Other specified complications of internal orthopedic prosthetic devices, implants and grafts**

¹ √x7ᵗʰ **T84.81** **Embolism due to internal orthopedic prosthetic devices, implants and grafts**   HCC

¹ √x7ᵗʰ **T84.82** **Fibrosis due to internal orthopedic prosthetic devices, implants and grafts**   HCC

---

¹ √x7ᵗʰ **T84.83** **Hemorrhage** due to internal orthopedic prosthetic devices, implants and grafts   HCC

¹ √x7ᵗʰ **T84.84** **Pain** due to internal orthopedic prosthetic devices, implants and grafts   HCC

¹ √x7ᵗʰ **T84.85** **Stenosis** due to internal orthopedic prosthetic devices, implants and grafts   HCC

¹ √x7ᵗʰ **T84.86** **Thrombosis** due to internal orthopedic prosthetic devices, implants and grafts   HCC

¹ √x7ᵗʰ **T84.89** **Other specified complication** of internal orthopedic prosthetic devices, implants and grafts   HCC

¹ √x7ᵗʰ **T84.9** **Unspecified complication** of internal orthopedic prosthetic device, implant and graft   HCC ▽

√4ᵗʰ **T85 Complications of other internal prosthetic devices, implants and grafts**

> EXCLUDES 2   *failure and rejection of transplanted organs and tissue (T86.-)*
>
> **AHA:** 2016,4Q,71-72

> The appropriate 7th character is to be added to each code from category T85.
> A   initial encounter
> D   subsequent encounter
> S   sequela

√5ᵗʰ **T85.0** **Mechanical complication of** ventricular intracranial (communicating) shunt

¹ √x7ᵗʰ **T85.01** **Breakdown (mechanical) of** ventricular intracranial (communicating) shunt   HCC

¹ √x7ᵗʰ **T85.02** **Displacement of** ventricular intracranial (communicating) shunt   HCC

> Malposition of ventricular intracranial (communicating) shunt

¹ √x7ᵗʰ **T85.03** **Leakage of** ventricular intracranial (communicating) shunt   HCC

¹ √x7ᵗʰ **T85.09** **Other mechanical complication of** ventricular intracranial (communicating) shunt   HCC

> Obstruction (mechanical) of ventricular intracranial (communicating) shunt
>
> Perforation of ventricular intracranial (communicating) shunt
>
> Protrusion of ventricular intracranial (communicating) shunt

√5ᵗʰ **T85.1** **Mechanical complication of** implanted electronic stimulator of nervous system

√6ᵗʰ **T85.11** **Breakdown (mechanical) of implanted electronic stimulator of nervous system**

¹ √7ᵗʰ **T85.110** **Breakdown (mechanical) of implanted electronic neurostimulator of brain electrode (lead)**   HCC

¹ √7ᵗʰ **T85.111** **Breakdown (mechanical) of implanted electronic neurostimulator of peripheral nerve electrode (lead)**   HCC

> Breakdown of electrode (lead) for cranial nerve neurostimulators
>
> Breakdown of electrode (lead) for gastric neurostimulator
>
> Breakdown of electrode (lead) for sacral nerve neurostimulator
>
> Breakdown of electrode (lead) for vagal nerve neurostimulators

¹ √7ᵗʰ **T85.112** **Breakdown (mechanical) of implanted electronic neurostimulator of spinal cord electrode (lead)**   HCC

¹ √7ᵗʰ **T85.113** **Breakdown (mechanical) of implanted electronic neurostimulator, generator**   HCC

> ▶Breakdown (mechanical) of implanted electronic neurostimulator generator, brain, peripheral, gastric, spinal◀
>
> Breakdown (mechanical) of implanted electronic sacral neurostimulator, pulse generator or receiver

¹ √7ᵗʰ **T85.118** **Breakdown (mechanical) of other implanted electronic stimulator of nervous system**   HCC

√6ᵗʰ **T85.12** **Displacement of implanted electronic stimulator of nervous system**

> Malposition of implanted electronic stimulator of nervous system

¹ √7ᵗʰ **T85.120** **Displacement of implanted electronic neurostimulator of brain electrode (lead)**   HCC

¹ √7ᵗʰ **T85.121** **Displacement of implanted electronic neurostimulator of peripheral nerve electrode (lead)**   HCC

> Displacement of electrode (lead) for cranial nerve neurostimulators
>
> Displacement of electrode (lead) for gastric neurostimulator
>
> Displacement of electrode (lead) for sacral nerve neurostimulator
>
> Displacement of electrode (lead) for vagal nerve neurostimulators

¹ √7ᵗʰ **T85.122** **Displacement of implanted electronic neurostimulator of spinal cord electrode (lead)**   HCC

¹ √7ᵗʰ **T85.123** **Displacement of implanted electronic neurostimulator, generator**   HCC

> Displacement of implanted electronic neurostimulator generator, brain, peripheral, gastric, spinal
>
> Displacement of implanted electronic sacral neurostimulator, pulse generator or receiver

¹ √7ᵗʰ **T85.128** **Displacement of other implanted electronic stimulator of nervous system**   HCC

√6ᵗʰ **T85.19** **Other mechanical complication of implanted electronic stimulator of nervous system**

> Leakage of implanted electronic stimulator of nervous system
>
> Obstruction (mechanical) of implanted electronic stimulator of nervous system
>
> Perforation of implanted electronic stimulator of nervous system
>
> Protrusion of implanted electronic stimulator of nervous system

¹ √7ᵗʰ **T85.190** **Other mechanical complication of implanted electronic neurostimulator of brain electrode (lead)**   HCC

¹ √7ᵗʰ **T85.191** **Other mechanical complication of implanted electronic neurostimulator of peripheral nerve electrode (lead)**   HCC

> Other mechanical complication of electrode (lead) for cranial nerve neurostimulators
>
> Other mechanical complication of electrode (lead) for gastric neurostimulator
>
> Other mechanical complication of electrode (lead) for sacral nerve neurostimulator
>
> Other mechanical complication of electrode (lead) for vagal nerve neurostimulators

¹ √7ᵗʰ **T85.192** **Other mechanical complication of implanted electronic neurostimulator of spinal cord electrode (lead)**   HCC

¹ √7ᵗʰ **T85.193** **Other mechanical complication of implanted electronic neurostimulator, generator**   HCC

> Other mechanical complication of implanted electronic neurostimulator generator, brain, peripheral, gastric, spinal
>
> Other mechanical complication of implanted electronic sacral neurostimulator, pulse generator or receiver

¹ √7ᵗʰ **T85.199** **Other mechanical complication of other implanted electronic stimulator of nervous system**   HCC

☑ Additional Character Req   √x7ᵗʰ Placeholder Alert   Manifestation   ▽ Unspecified   ▶◀ Revised Text   ● New Code   ▲ Revised Code Title

ICD-10-CM 2019

1143

Chapter 19. Injury, Poisoning and Certain Other Consequences of External Causes

T85.2–T85.621

√5th **T85.2** Mechanical complication of intraocular lens
- √x7th **T85.21** Breakdown (mechanical) of intraocular lens
- √x7th **T85.22** Displacement of intraocular lens
  - Malposition of intraocular lens
- √x7th **T85.29** Other mechanical complication of intraocular lens
  - Obstruction (mechanical) of intraocular lens
  - Perforation of intraocular lens
  - Protrusion of intraocular lens

√5th **T85.3** Mechanical complication of other ocular prosthetic devices, implants and grafts
- EXCLUDES 2 *other complications of corneal graft (T86.84-)*
- √6th **T85.31** Breakdown (mechanical) of other ocular prosthetic devices, implants and grafts
  - √7th **T85.310** Breakdown (mechanical) of prosthetic orbit of right eye
  - √7th **T85.311** Breakdown (mechanical) of prosthetic orbit of left eye
  - √7th **T85.318** Breakdown (mechanical) of other ocular prosthetic devices, implants and grafts
- √6th **T85.32** Displacement of other ocular prosthetic devices, implants and grafts
  - Malposition of other ocular prosthetic devices, implants and grafts
  - √7th **T85.320** Displacement of prosthetic orbit of right eye
  - √7th **T85.321** Displacement of prosthetic orbit of left eye
  - √7th **T85.328** Displacement of other ocular prosthetic devices, implants and grafts
- √6th **T85.39** Other mechanical complication of other ocular prosthetic devices, implants and grafts
  - Obstruction (mechanical) of other ocular prosthetic devices, implants and grafts
  - Perforation of other ocular prosthetic devices, implants and grafts
  - Protrusion of other ocular prosthetic devices, implants and grafts
  - √7th **T85.390** Other mechanical complication of prosthetic orbit of right eye
  - √7th **T85.391** Other mechanical complication of prosthetic orbit of left eye
  - √7th **T85.398** Other mechanical complication of other ocular prosthetic devices, implants and grafts

√5th **T85.4** Mechanical complication of breast prosthesis and implant
- √x7th **T85.41** Breakdown (mechanical) of breast prosthesis and implant
- √x7th **T85.42** Displacement of breast prosthesis and implant
  - Malposition of breast prosthesis and implant
- √x7th **T85.43** Leakage of breast prosthesis and implant
- √x7th **T85.44** Capsular contracture of breast implant
- √x7th **T85.49** Other mechanical complication of breast prosthesis and implant
  - Obstruction (mechanical) of breast prosthesis and implant
  - Perforation of breast prosthesis and implant
  - Protrusion of breast prosthesis and implant

√5th **T85.5** Mechanical complication of gastrointestinal prosthetic devices, implants and grafts
- √6th **T85.51** Breakdown (mechanical) of gastrointestinal prosthetic devices, implants and grafts
  - √7th **T85.510** Breakdown (mechanical) of bile duct prosthesis
  - √7th **T85.511** Breakdown (mechanical) of esophageal anti-reflux device
  - √7th **T85.518** Breakdown (mechanical) of other gastrointestinal prosthetic devices, implants and grafts
- √6th **T85.52** Displacement of gastrointestinal prosthetic devices, implants and grafts
  - Malposition of gastrointestinal prosthetic devices, implants and grafts
  - √7th **T85.520** Displacement of bile duct prosthesis
  - √7th **T85.521** Displacement of esophageal anti-reflux device
  - √7th **T85.528** Displacement of other gastrointestinal prosthetic devices, implants and grafts

√6th **T85.59** Other mechanical complication of gastrointestinal prosthetic devices, implants and
- Obstruction, mechanical of gastrointestinal prosthetic devices, implants and grafts
- Perforation of gastrointestinal prosthetic devices, implants and grafts
- Protrusion of gastrointestinal prosthetic devices, implants and grafts
  - √7th **T85.590** Other mechanical complication of bile duct prosthesis
  - √7th **T85.591** Other mechanical complication of esophageal anti-reflux device
  - √7th **T85.598** Other mechanical complication of other gastrointestinal prosthetic devices, implants and grafts

√5th **T85.6** Mechanical complication of other specified internal and external prosthetic devices, implants and grafts
- √6th **T85.61** Breakdown (mechanical) of other specified internal prosthetic devices, implants and grafts
  - √7th **T85.610** Breakdown (mechanical) of cranial or spinal infusion catheter
    - Breakdown (mechanical) of epidural infusion catheter
    - Breakdown (mechanical) of intrathecal infusion catheter
    - Breakdown (mechanical) of subarachnoid infusion catheter
    - Breakdown (mechanical) of subdural infusion catheter
  - √7th **T85.611** Breakdown (mechanical) of intraperitoneal dialysis catheter [HCC]
    - EXCLUDES 1 *mechanical complication of vascular dialysis catheter (T82.4-)*
  - √7th **T85.612** Breakdown (mechanical) of permanent sutures
    - EXCLUDES 1 *mechanical complication of permanent (wire) suture used in bone repair (T84.1-T84.2)*
  - √7th **T85.613** Breakdown (mechanical) of artificial skin graft and decellularized allodermis
    - Failure of artificial skin graft and decellularized allodermis
    - Non-adherence of artificial skin graft and decellularized allodermis
    - Poor incorporation of artificial skin graft and decellularized allodermis
    - Shearing of artificial skin graft and decellularized allodermis
  - √7th **T85.614** Breakdown (mechanical) of insulin pump
  - 1 √7th **T85.615** Breakdown (mechanical) of other nervous system device, implant or graft [HCC]
    - Breakdown (mechanical) of intrathecal infusion pump
  - √7th **T85.618** Breakdown (mechanical) of other specified internal prosthetic devices, implants and grafts
- √6th **T85.62** Displacement of other specified internal prosthetic devices, implants and grafts
  - Malposition of other specified internal prosthetic devices, implants and grafts
  - √7th **T85.620** Displacement of cranial or spinal infusion catheter
    - Displacement of epidural infusion catheter
    - Displacement of intrathecal infusion catheter
    - Displacement of subarachnoid infusion catheter
    - Displacement of subdural infusion catheter
  - √7th **T85.621** Displacement of intraperitoneal dialysis catheter [HCC]
    - EXCLUDES 1 *mechanical complication of vascular dialysis catheter (T82.4-)*

√7ᵗʰ **T85.622 Displacement of permanent sutures**
     EXCLUDES 1   *mechanical complication of permanent (wire) suture used in bone repair (T84.1-T84.2)*

√7ᵗʰ **T85.623 Displacement of artificial skin graft and decellularized allodermis**
     Dislodgement of artificial skin graft and decellularized allodermis

√7ᵗʰ **T85.624 Displacement of insulin pump**

1 √7ᵗʰ **T85.625 Displacement of other nervous system device, implant or graft** HCC
     Displacement of intrathecal infusion pump

√7ᵗʰ **T85.628 Displacement of other specified internal prosthetic devices, implants and grafts**

√6ᵗʰ **T85.63 Leakage of other specified internal prosthetic devices, implants and grafts**

√7ᵗʰ **T85.630 Leakage of cranial or spinal infusion catheter**
     Leakage of epidural infusion catheter
     Leakage of intrathecal infusion catheter infusion catheter
     Leakage of subdural infusion catheter
     Leakage of subarachnoid infusion catheter

√7ᵗʰ **T85.631 Leakage of intraperitoneal dialysis catheter** HCC
     EXCLUDES 1   *mechanical complication of vascular dialysis catheter (T82.4)*

√7ᵗʰ **T85.633 Leakage of insulin pump**

1 √7ᵗʰ **T85.635 Leakage of other nervous system device, implant or graft** HCC
     Leakage of intrathecal infusion pump

√7ᵗʰ **T85.638 Leakage of other specified internal prosthetic devices, implants and grafts**

√6ᵗʰ **T85.69 Other mechanical complication of other specified internal prosthetic devices, implants and grafts**
     Obstruction, mechanical of other specified internal prosthetic devices, implants and grafts
     Perforation of other specified internal prosthetic devices, implants and grafts
     Protrusion of other specified internal prosthetic devices, implants and grafts

√7ᵗʰ **T85.690 Other mechanical complication of cranial or spinal infusion catheter**
     Other mechanical complication of epidural infusion catheter
     Other mechanical complication of intrathecal infusion catheter
     Other mechanical complication of subarachnoid infusion catheter
     Other mechanical complication of subdural infusion catheter

√7ᵗʰ **T85.691 Other mechanical complication of intraperitoneal dialysis catheter** HCC
     EXCLUDES 1   *mechanical complication of vascular dialysis catheter (T82.4)*

√7ᵗʰ **T85.692 Other mechanical complication of permanent sutures**
     EXCLUDES 1   *mechanical complication of permanent (wire) suture used in bone repair (T84.1-T84.2)*

√7ᵗʰ **T85.693 Other mechanical complication of artificial skin graft and decellularized allodermis**

√7ᵗʰ **T85.694 Other mechanical complication of insulin pump**

1 √7ᵗʰ **T85.695 Other mechanical complication of other nervous system device, implant or graft** HCC
     Other mechanical complication of intrathecal infusion pump

√7ᵗʰ **T85.698 Other mechanical complication of other specified internal prosthetic devices, implants and grafts**
     Mechanical complication of nonabsorbable surgical material NOS

√5ᵗʰ **T85.7 Infection and inflammatory reaction due to other internal prosthetic devices, implants and grafts**
     Use additional code to identify infection

√x7ᵗʰ **T85.71 Infection and inflammatory reaction due to peritoneal dialysis catheter** HCC

1 √x7ᵗʰ **T85.72 Infection and inflammatory reaction due to insulin pump** HCC

√6ᵗʰ **T85.73 Infection and inflammatory reaction due to nervous system devices, implants and graft**

1 √7ᵗʰ **T85.730 Infection and inflammatory reaction due to ventricular intracranial (communicating) shunt** HCC

1 √7ᵗʰ **T85.731 Infection and inflammatory reaction due to implanted electronic neurostimulator of brain, electrode (lead)** HCC

1 √7ᵗʰ **T85.732 Infection and inflammatory reaction due to implanted electronic neurostimulator of peripheral nerve, electrode (lead)** HCC
     Infection and inflammatory reaction due to electrode (lead) for cranial nerve neurostimulators
     Infection and inflammatory reaction due to electrode (lead) for gastric neurostimulator
     Infection and inflammatory reaction due to electrode (lead) for sacral nerve neurostimulator
     Infection and inflammatory reaction due to electrode (lead) for vagal nerve neurostimulators

1 √7ᵗʰ **T85.733 Infection and inflammatory reaction due to implanted electronic neurostimulator of spinal cord, electrode (lead)** HCC

1 √7ᵗʰ **T85.734 Infection and inflammatory reaction due to implanted electronic neurostimulator, generator** HCC
     Generator pocket infection

1 √7ᵗʰ **T85.735 Infection and inflammatory reaction due to cranial or spinal infusion catheter** HCC
     Infection and inflammatory reaction due to epidural catheter
     Infection and inflammatory reaction due to intrathecal infusion catheter
     Infection and inflammatory reaction due to subarachnoid catheter
     Infection and inflammatory reaction due to subdural catheter

1 √7ᵗʰ **T85.738 Infection and inflammatory reaction due to other nervous system device, implant or graft** HCC
     Infection and inflammatory reaction due to intrathecal infusion pump

1 √x7ᵗʰ **T85.79 Infection and inflammatory reaction due to other internal prosthetic devices, implants and grafts** HCC

√5ᵗʰ **T85.8 Other specified complications of internal prosthetic devices, implants and grafts, not elsewhere classified**

√6ᵗʰ **T85.81 Embolism due to internal prosthetic devices, implants and grafts, not elsewhere classified**

1 √7ᵗʰ **T85.810 Embolism due to nervous system prosthetic devices, implants and grafts** HCC

√7ᵗʰ **T85.818 Embolism due to other internal prosthetic devices, implants and grafts**

√6ᵗʰ **T85.82 Fibrosis due to internal prosthetic devices, implants and grafts, not elsewhere classified**

1 √7ᵗʰ **T85.820 Fibrosis due to nervous system prosthetic devices, implants and grafts** HCC

√7ᵗʰ **T85.828 Fibrosis due to other internal prosthetic devices, implants and grafts**

✓6th T85.83 **Hemorrhage due to internal prosthetic devices, implants and grafts, not elsewhere classified**

   1 ✓7th T85.830 **Hemorrhage due to nervous system prosthetic devices, implants and grafts** HCC

   ✓7th T85.838 **Hemorrhage due to other internal prosthetic devices, implants and grafts**

✓6th T85.84 **Pain due to internal prosthetic devices, implants and grafts, not elsewhere classified**

   1 ✓7th T85.840 **Pain due to nervous system prosthetic devices, implants and grafts** HCC

   ✓7th T85.848 **Pain due to other internal prosthetic devices, implants and grafts**

✓6th T85.85 **Stenosis due to internal prosthetic devices, implants and grafts, not elsewhere classified**

   1 ✓7th T85.850 **Stenosis due to nervous system prosthetic devices, implants and grafts** HCC

   ✓7th T85.858 **Stenosis due to other internal prosthetic devices, implants and grafts**

✓6th T85.86 **Thrombosis due to internal prosthetic devices, implants and grafts, not elsewhere classified**

   1 ✓7th T85.860 **Thrombosis due to nervous system prosthetic devices, implants and grafts** HCC

   ✓7th T85.868 **Thrombosis due to other internal prosthetic devices, implants and grafts**

✓6th T85.89 **Other specified complication of internal prosthetic devices, implants and grafts, not elsewhere classified**

   Erosion or breakdown of subcutaneous device pocket

   1 ✓7th T85.890 **Other specified complication of nervous system prosthetic devices, implants and grafts** HCC

   ✓7th T85.898 **Other specified complication of other internal prosthetic devices, implants and grafts**

✓x7th T85.9 **Unspecified complication of internal prosthetic device, implant and graft** ▽

   Complication of internal prosthetic device, implant and graft NOS

✓4th T86 **Complications of transplanted organs and tissue**

   Use additional code to identify other transplant complications, such as:
   graft-versus-host disease (D89.81-)
   malignancy associated with organ transplant (C80.2)
   post-transplant lymphoproliferative disorders (PTLD) (D47.Z1)

✓5th T86.0 **Complications of bone marrow transplant**

   T86.00 **Unspecified complication of bone marrow transplant** HCC ▽

   T86.01 **Bone marrow transplant rejection** HCC

   T86.02 **Bone marrow transplant failure** HCC

   T86.03 **Bone marrow transplant infection** HCC

   T86.09 **Other complications of bone marrow transplant** HCC

✓5th T86.1 **Complications of kidney transplant**

   T86.10 **Unspecified complication of kidney transplant** ▽

   T86.11 **Kidney transplant rejection**

   T86.12 **Kidney transplant failure**
     AHA: 2013,1Q,24

   T86.13 **Kidney transplant infection**
     Use additional code to specify infection

   T86.19 **Other complication of kidney transplant**

✓5th T86.2 **Complications of heart transplant**

   EXCLUDES 1   complication of:
     artificial heart device (T82.5)
     heart-lung transplant (T86.3)

   T86.20 **Unspecified complication of heart transplant** HCC ▽

   T86.21 **Heart transplant rejection** HCC

   T86.22 **Heart transplant failure** HCC

   T86.23 **Heart transplant infection** HCC
     Use additional code to specify infection

   ✓6th T86.29 **Other complications of heart transplant**

     T86.290 **Cardiac allograft vasculopathy** HCC
      EXCLUDES 1   atherosclerosis of coronary arteries (I25.75-, I25.76-, I25.81-)

     T86.298 **Other complications of heart transplant** HCC

✓5th T86.3 **Complications of heart-lung transplant**

   T86.30 **Unspecified complication of heart-lung transplant** HCC ▽

   T86.31 **Heart-lung transplant rejection** HCC

   T86.32 **Heart-lung transplant failure** HCC

   T86.33 **Heart-lung transplant infection** HCC
     Use additional code to specify infection

   T86.39 **Other complications of heart-lung transplant**

✓5th T86.4 **Complications of liver transplant**

   T86.40 **Unspecified complication of liver transplant** HCC ▽

   T86.41 **Liver transplant rejection** HCC

   T86.42 **Liver transplant failure** HCC

   T86.43 **Liver transplant infection** HCC
     Use additional code to identify infection, such as:
     cytomegalovirus (CMV) infection (B25.-)

   T86.49 **Other complications of liver transplant** HCC

T86.5 **Complications of stem cell transplant**

   Complications from stem cells from peripheral blood
   Complications from stem cells from umbilical cord

✓5th T86.8 **Complications of other transplanted organs and tissues**

   ✓6th T86.81 **Complications of lung transplant**

     EXCLUDES 1   complication of heart-lung transplant (T86.3-)

     T86.810 **Lung transplant rejection** HCC

     T86.811 **Lung transplant failure** HCC

     T86.812 **Lung transplant infection** HCC
      Use additional code to specify infection

     T86.818 **Other complications of lung transplant** HCC

     T86.819 **Unspecified complication of lung transplant** HCC ▽

   ✓6th T86.82 **Complications of skin graft (allograft) (autograft)**

     EXCLUDES 2   complication of artificial skin graft (T85.693)

     T86.820 **Skin graft (allograft) rejection**

     T86.821 **Skin graft (allograft) (autograft) failure**

     T86.822 **Skin graft (allograft) (autograft) infection**
      Use additional code to specify infection

     T86.828 **Other complications of skin graft (allograft) (autograft)**

     T86.829 **Unspecified complication of skin graft (allograft) (autograft)** ▽

   ✓6th T86.83 **Complications of bone graft**

     EXCLUDES 2   mechanical complications of bone graft (T84.3-)

     T86.830 **Bone graft rejection**

     T86.831 **Bone graft failure**

     T86.832 **Bone graft infection**
      Use additional code to specify infection

     T86.838 **Other complications of bone graft**

     T86.839 **Unspecified complication of bone graft** ▽

   ✓6th T86.84 **Complications of corneal transplant**

     EXCLUDES 2   mechanical complications of corneal graft (T85.3-)

     T86.840 **Corneal transplant rejection**

     T86.841 **Corneal transplant failure**

     T86.842 **Corneal transplant infection** HCC
      Use additional code to specify infection

     T86.848 **Other complications of corneal transplant**

     T86.849 **Unspecified complication of corneal transplant** ▽

   ✓6th T86.85 **Complication of intestine transplant**

     T86.850 **Intestine transplant rejection** HCC

     T86.851 **Intestine transplant failure** HCC

     T86.852 **Intestine transplant infection** HCC
      Use additional code to specify infection

     T86.858 **Other complications of intestine transplant** HCC

     T86.859 **Unspecified complication of intestine transplant** HCC ▽

   ✓6th T86.89 **Complications of other transplanted tissue**

     Transplant failure or rejection of pancreas

     T86.890 **Other transplanted tissue rejection**

     T86.891 **Other transplanted tissue failure**

      T86.892   **Other transplanted tissue** infection
          Use additional code to specify infection

      T86.898   **Other complications of other transplanted tissue**

      T86.899   **Unspecified complication of other transplanted tissue** ▽

✓5ᵗʰ **T86.9**   **Complication of unspecified transplanted organ and tissue**

      T86.90   **Unspecified complication of unspecified transplanted organ and tissue** ▽

      T86.91   **Unspecified transplanted organ and tissue rejection** ▽

      T86.92   **Unspecified transplanted organ and tissue failure** ▽

      T86.93   **Unspecified transplanted organ and tissue infection** ▽
          Use additional code to specify infection

      T86.99   **Other complications of unspecified transplanted organ and tissue** ▽

✓4ᵗʰ **T87**   **Complications peculiar to reattachment and amputation**

  ✓5ᵗʰ **T87.0**   **Complications of reattached (part of)** upper extremity

    ✓6ᵗʰ **T87.0X**   **Complications of reattached (part of) upper extremity**

      T87.0X1   **Complications of reattached (part of)** right **upper extremity** HCC

      T87.0X2   **Complications of reattached (part of)** left **upper extremity** HCC

      T87.0X9   **Complications of reattached (part of) unspecified upper extremity** HCC ▽

  ✓5ᵗʰ **T87.1**   **Complications of reattached (part of)** lower extremity

    ✓6ᵗʰ **T87.1X**   **Complications of reattached (part of) lower extremity**

      T87.1X1   **Complications of reattached (part of)** right **lower extremity** HCC

      T87.1X2   **Complications of reattached (part of)** left **lower extremity** HCC

      T87.1X9   **Complications of reattached (part of) unspecified lower extremity** HCC ▽

  T87.2   **Complications of other reattached body part** HCC

  ✓5ᵗʰ **T87.3**   **Neuroma of amputation stump**
      DEF: Non-neoplastic tumor generated at the proximal end of severed, partially transected, or injured nerve following amputation.

    T87.30   **Neuroma of amputation stump, unspecified extremity** HCC ▽

    T87.31   **Neuroma of amputation stump,** right upper **extremity** HCC

    T87.32   **Neuroma of amputation stump,** left upper **extremity** HCC

    T87.33   **Neuroma of amputation stump,** right lower **extremity** HCC

    T87.34   **Neuroma of amputation stump,** left lower **extremity** HCC

  ✓5ᵗʰ **T87.4**   **Infection of amputation stump**

    T87.40   **Infection of amputation stump, unspecified extremity** HCC ▽

    T87.41   **Infection of amputation stump,** right upper **extremity** HCC

    T87.42   **Infection of amputation stump,** left upper **extremity** HCC

    T87.43   **Infection of amputation stump,** right lower **extremity** HCC

    T87.44   **Infection of amputation stump,** left lower **extremity** HCC

  ✓5ᵗʰ **T87.5**   **Necrosis of amputation stump**

    T87.50   **Necrosis of amputation stump, unspecified extremity** HCC ▽

    T87.51   **Necrosis of amputation stump,** right upper **extremity** HCC

    T87.52   **Necrosis of amputation stump,** left upper **extremity** HCC

    T87.53   **Necrosis of amputation stump,** right lower **extremity** HCC

    T87.54   **Necrosis of amputation stump,** left lower **extremity** HCC

  ✓5ᵗʰ **T87.8**   **Other complications of amputation stump**

    T87.81   **Dehiscence of amputation stump** HCC

    T87.89   **Other complications of amputation stump** HCC
       Amputation stump contracture
       Amputation stump contracture of next proximal joint
       Amputation stump flexion
       Amputation stump edema
       Amputation stump hematoma
       EXCLUDES 2   *phantom limb syndrome (G54.6-G54.7)*

  T87.9   **Unspecified complications of amputation stump** HCC ▽

✓4ᵗʰ **T88**   **Other complications of surgical and medical care, not elsewhere classified**

    EXCLUDES 2   *complication following infusion, transfusion and therapeutic injection (T80.-)*
         complication following procedure NEC (T81.-)
         complications of anesthesia in labor and delivery (O74.-)
         complications of anesthesia in pregnancy (O29.-)
         complications of anesthesia in puerperium (O89.-)
         complications of devices, implants and grafts (T82-T85)
         complications of obstetric surgery and procedure (O75.4)
         dermatitis due to drugs and medicaments (L23.3, L24.4, L25.1, L27.0-L27.1)
         poisoning and toxic effects of drugs and chemicals (T36-T65 with fifth or sixth character 1-4 or 6)
         specified complications classified elsewhere

> The appropriate 7th character is to be added to each code from category T88.
> A   initial encounter
> D   subsequent encounter
> S   sequela

  ✓x7ᵗʰ **T88.0**   **Infection following immunization**
       Sepsis following immunization

  ✓x7ᵗʰ **T88.1**   **Other complications following immunization, not elsewhere classified**
       Generalized vaccinia
       Rash following immunization
       EXCLUDES 1   *vaccinia not from vaccine (B08.011)*
       EXCLUDES 2   *anaphylactic shock due to serum (T80.5-)*
          other serum reactions (T80.6-)
          postimmunization arthropathy (M02.2)
          postimmunization encephalitis (G04.02)
          postimmunization fever (R50.83)

  ✓x7ᵗʰ **T88.2**   **Shock due to anesthesia**
       Use additional code for adverse effect, if applicable, to identify drug (T41.- with fifth or sixth character 5)
       EXCLUDES 1   *complications of anesthesia (in):*
          labor and delivery (O74.-)
          postprocedural shock NOS (T81.1-)
          pregnancy (O29.-)
          puerperium (O89.-)

  ✓x7ᵗʰ **T88.3**   **Malignant hyperthermia due to anesthesia**
       Use additional code for adverse effect, if applicable, to identify drug (T41.- with fifth or sixth character 5)

  ✓x7ᵗʰ **T88.4**   **Failed or difficult intubation**

  ✓5ᵗʰ **T88.5**   **Other complications of anesthesia**
       Use additional code for adverse effect, if applicable, to identify drug (T41.- with fifth or sixth character 5)

    ✓x7ᵗʰ **T88.51**   **Hypothermia following anesthesia**

    ✓x7ᵗʰ **T88.52**   **Failed moderate sedation during procedure**
       Failed conscious sedation during procedure
       EXCLUDES 2   *personal history of failed moderate sedation (Z92.83)*

    ✓x7ᵗʰ **T88.53**   **Unintended awareness under general anesthesia during procedure**
       EXCLUDES 2   *personal history of unintended awareness under general anesthesia (Z92.84)*
       AHA: 2016,4Q,72-73

    ✓x7ᵗʰ **T88.59**   **Other complications of anesthesia**

☑ Additional Character Req   ✓x7ᵗʰ Placeholder Alert   Manifestation   ▽ Unspecified   ▶◀ Revised Text   ● New Code   ▲ Revised Code Title

ICD-10-CM 2019   1147

√x7ᵗʰ **T88.6 Anaphylactic reaction due to adverse effect of correct drug or medicament properly administered**

Anaphylactic shock due to adverse effect of correct drug or medicament properly administered

Anaphylactoid reaction NOS

Use additional code for adverse effect, if applicable, to identify drug (T36-T50 with fifth or sixth character 5)

> **EXCLUDES 1**   *anaphylactic reaction due to serum (T80.5-)*
> *anaphylactic shock or reaction due to adverse food reaction (T78.0-)*

√x7ᵗʰ **T88.7 Unspecified adverse effect of drug or medicament**   ▽

Drug hypersensitivity NOS

Drug reaction NOS

Use additional code for adverse effect, if applicable, to identify drug (T36-T50 with fifth or sixth character 5)

> **EXCLUDES 1**   *specified adverse effects of drugs and medicaments (A00-R94 and T80-T88.6, T88.8)*

√x7ᵗʰ **T88.8 Other specified complications of surgical and medical care, not elsewhere classified**

Use additional code to identify the complication

√x7ᵗʰ **T88.9 Complication of surgical and medical care, unspecified**   ▽

Chapter 20. External Causes of Morbidity (V00–Y99)

Chapter Specific Guidelines with Coding Examples

The chapter specific guidelines from the ICD-10-CM Official Guidelines for Coding and Reporting have been provided below. Along with these guidelines are coding examples, contained in the shaded boxes, that have been developed to help illustrate the coding and/or sequencing guidance found in these guidelines.

The external causes of morbidity codes should never be sequenced as the first-listed or principal diagnosis.

External cause codes are intended to provide data for injury research and evaluation of injury prevention strategies. These codes capture how the injury or health condition happened (cause), the intent (unintentional or accidental; or intentional, such as suicide or assault), the place where the event occurred the activity of the patient at the time of the event, and the person's status (e.g., civilian, military).

There is no national requirement for mandatory ICD-10-CM external cause code reporting. Unless a provider is subject to a state-based external cause code reporting mandate or these codes are required by a particular payer, reporting of ICD-10-CM codes in Chapter 20, External Causes of Morbidity, is not required. In the absence of a mandatory reporting requirement, providers are encouraged to voluntarily report external cause codes, as they provide valuable data for injury research and evaluation of injury prevention strategies.

a. General external cause coding guidelines

1) Used with any code in the range of A00.0–T88.9, Z00–Z99

An external cause code may be used with any code in the range of A00.0-T88.9, Z00-Z99, classification that represents a health condition due to an external cause. Though they are most applicable to injuries, they are also valid for use with such things as infections or diseases due to an external source, and other health conditions, such as a heart attack that occurs during strenuous physical activity.

Actinic reticuloid due to tanning bed use	
L57.1	**Actinic reticuloid**
W89.1XXA	**Exposure to tanning bed, initial encounter**

Explanation: An external cause code may be used with any code in the range of A00.0–T88.9, Z00–Z99, classifications that describe health conditions due to an external cause. Code W89.1 Exposure to tanning bed requires a seventh character of A to report this initial encounter, with a placeholder X for the fifth and sixth characters.

2) External cause code used for length of treatment

Assign the external cause code, with the appropriate 7th character (initial encounter, subsequent encounter or sequela) for each encounter for which the injury or condition is being treated.

Most categories in chapter 20 have a 7th character requirement for each applicable code. Most categories in this chapter have three 7th character values: A, initial encounter, D, subsequent encounter and S, sequela. While the patient may be seen by a new or different provider over the course of treatment for an injury or condition, assignment of the 7th character for external cause should match the 7th character of the code assigned for the associated injury or condition for the encounter.

3) Use the full range of external cause codes

Use the full range of external cause codes to completely describe the cause, the intent, the place of occurrence, and if applicable, the activity of the patient at the time of the event, and the patient's status, for all injuries, and other health conditions due to an external cause.

4) Assign as many external cause codes as necessary

Assign as many external cause codes as necessary to fully explain each cause. If only one external code can be recorded, assign the code most related to the principal diagnosis.

5) The selection of the appropriate external cause code

The selection of the appropriate external cause code is guided by the Alphabetic Index of External Causes and by Inclusion and Exclusion notes in the Tabular List.

6) External cause code can never be a principal diagnosis

An external cause code can never be a principal (first-listed) diagnosis.

7) Combination external cause codes

Certain of the external cause codes are combination codes that identify sequential events that result in an injury, such as a fall which results in striking against an object. The injury may be due to either event or both.

The combination external cause code used should correspond to the sequence of events regardless of which caused the most serious injury.

Toddler tripped and fell while walking and struck his head on an end table, sustaining a scalp contusion	
S00.03XA	**Contusion of scalp, initial encounter**
W01.190A	**Fall on same level from slipping, tripping and stumbling with subsequent striking against furniture, initial encounter**

Explanation: Combination external cause codes identify sequential events that result in an injury, such as a fall resulting in striking against an object. The injury may be due to either or both events.

8) No external cause code needed in certain circumstances

No external cause code from Chapter 20 is needed if the external cause and intent are included in a code from another chapter (e.g. T36.0X1- Poisoning by penicillins, accidental (unintentional)).

b. Place of occurrence guideline

Codes from category Y92, Place of occurrence of the external cause, are secondary codes for use after other external cause codes to identify the location of the patient at the time of injury or other condition.

Generally, a place of occurrence code is assigned only once, at the initial encounter for treatment. However, in the rare instance that a new injury occurs during hospitalization, an additional place of occurrence code may be assigned. No 7th characters are used for Y92.

Do not use place of occurrence code Y92.9 if the place is not stated or is not applicable.

A farmer was working in his barn and sustained a foot contusion when the horse stepped on his left foot	
S90.32XA	**Contusion of left foot, initial encounter**
W55.19XA	**Other contact with horse, initial encounter**
Y92.71	**Barn as the place of occurrence of the external cause**

Explanation: A place-of-occurrence code from category Y92 is assigned at the initial encounter to identify the location of the patient at the time the injury occurred.

c. Activity code

Assign a code from category Y93, Activity code, to describe the activity of the patient at the time the injury or other health condition occurred.

An activity code is used only once, at the initial encounter for treatment. Only one code from Y93 should be recorded on a medical record.

The activity codes are not applicable to poisonings, adverse effects, misadventures or sequela.

Do not assign Y93.9, Unspecified activity, if the activity is not stated.

A code from category Y93 is appropriate for use with external cause and intent codes if identifying the activity provides additional information about the event.

Ranch hand who was grooming a horse sustained a foot contusion when the horse stepped on his left foot	
S90.32XA	**Contusion of left foot, initial encounter**
W55.19XA	**Other contact with horse, initial encounter**
Y93.K3	**Activity, grooming and shearing an animal**

Explanation: One activity code from category Y93 is assigned at the initial encounter only to describe the activity of the patient at the time the injury occurred.

d. Place of occurrence, activity, and status codes used with other external cause code

When applicable, place of occurrence, activity, and external cause status codes are sequenced after the main external cause code(s). Regardless of the number of external cause codes assigned, generally there should be only one place of occurrence code, one activity code, and one external cause status code assigned to an encounter. However, in the rare instance that a new injury occurs during hospitalization, an additional place of occurrence code may be assigned.

e. If the reporting format limits the number of external cause codes

If the reporting format limits the number of external cause codes that can be used in reporting clinical data, report the code for the cause/intent most related to the principal diagnosis. If the format permits capture of additional external cause codes, the cause/intent, including medical misadventures, of the additional events should be reported rather than the codes for place, activity, or external status.

f. Multiple external cause coding guidelines

More than one external cause code is required to fully describe the external cause of an illness or injury. The assignment of external cause codes should be sequenced in the following priority:

If two or more events cause separate injuries, an external cause code should be assigned for each cause. The first-listed external cause code will be selected in the following order:

External codes for child and adult abuse take priority over all other external cause codes.

See Section I.C.19., Child and Adult abuse guidelines.

External cause codes for terrorism events take priority over all other external cause codes except child and adult abuse.

External cause codes for cataclysmic events take priority over all other external cause codes except child and adult abuse and terrorism.

External cause codes for transport accidents take priority over all other external cause codes except cataclysmic events, child and adult abuse and terrorism.

Activity and external cause status codes are assigned following all causal (intent) external cause codes.

The first-listed external cause code should correspond to the cause of the most serious diagnosis due to an assault, accident, or self-harm, following the order of hierarchy listed above..

> 30-year-old man accidentally discharged his hunting rifle, sustaining an open gunshot wound, with no retained bullet fragments, to the right thigh, which caused him to fall down the stairs, resulting in closed displaced comminuted fracture of his left radial shaft
>
> | S71.131A | Puncture wound without foreign body, right thigh, initial encounter |
> |---|---|
> | S52.352A | Displaced comminuted fracture of shaft of radius, left arm, initial encounter for closed fracture |
> | W33.02XA | Accidental discharge of hunting rifle, initial encounter |
> | W10.9XXA | Fall (on) (from) unspecified stairs and steps, initial encounter |
>
> *Explanation:* If two or more events cause separate injuries, an external cause code should be assigned for each cause.

g. Child and adult abuse guideline

Adult and child abuse, neglect and maltreatment are classified as assault. Any of the assault codes may be used to indicate the external cause of any injury resulting from the confirmed abuse.

For confirmed cases of abuse, neglect and maltreatment, when the perpetrator is known, a code from Y07, Perpetrator of maltreatment and neglect, should accompany any other assault codes.

See Section I.C.19. Adult and child abuse, neglect and other maltreatment

h. Unknown or undetermined intent guideline

If the intent (accident, self-harm, assault) of the cause of an injury or other condition is unknown or unspecified, code the intent as accidental intent. All transport accident categories assume accidental intent.

1) Use of undetermined intent

External cause codes for events of undetermined intent are only for use if the documentation in the record specifies that the intent cannot be determined.

i. Sequelae (late effects) of external cause guidelines

1) Sequelae external cause codes

Sequela are reported using the external cause code with the 7th character "S" for sequela. These codes should be used with any report of a late effect or sequela resulting from a previous injury.

See Section I.B.10 Sequela (Late Effects)

2) Sequela external cause code with a related current injury

A sequela external cause code should never be used with a related current nature of injury code.

3) Use of sequela external cause codes for subsequent visits

Use a late effect external cause code for subsequent visits when a late effect of the initial injury is being treated. Do not use a late effect external cause code for subsequent visits for follow-up care (e.g., to assess healing, to receive rehabilitative therapy) of the injury when no late effect of the injury has been documented.

j. Terrorism guidelines

1) Cause of injury identified by the Federal Government (FBI) as terrorism

When the cause of an injury is identified by the Federal Government (FBI) as terrorism, the first-listed external cause code should be a code from category Y38, Terrorism. The definition of terrorism employed by the FBI is found at the inclusion note at the beginning of category Y38. Use additional code for place of occurrence (Y92.-). More than one Y38 code may be assigned if the injury is the result of more than one mechanism of terrorism.

2) Cause of an injury is suspected to be the result of terrorism

When the cause of an injury is suspected to be the result of terrorism a code from category Y38 should not be assigned. Suspected cases should be classified as assault.

3) Code Y38.9, Terrorism, secondary effects

Assign code Y38.9, Terrorism, secondary effects, for conditions occurring subsequent to the terrorist event. This code should not be assigned for conditions that are due to the initial terrorist act.

It is acceptable to assign code Y38.9 with another code from Y38 if there is an injury due to the initial terrorist event and an injury that is a subsequent result of the terrorist event.

k. External cause status

A code from category Y99, External cause status, should be assigned whenever any other external cause code is assigned for an encounter, including an Activity code, except for the events noted below. Assign a code from category Y99, External cause status, to indicate the work status of the person at the time the event occurred. The status code indicates whether the event occurred during military activity, whether a non-military person was at work, whether an individual including a student or volunteer was involved in a non-work activity at the time of the causal event.

A code from Y99, External cause status, should be assigned, when applicable, with other external cause codes, such as transport accidents and falls. The external cause status codes are not applicable to poisonings, adverse effects, misadventures or late effects.

Do not assign a code from category Y99 if no other external cause codes (cause, activity) are applicable for the encounter.

An external cause status code is used only once, at the initial encounter for treatment. Only one code from Y99 should be recorded on a medical record.

Do not assign code Y99.9, Unspecified external cause status, if the status is not stated.

Chapter 20. External Causes of Morbidity (V00-Y99)

NOTE This chapter permits the classification of environmental events and circumstances as the cause of injury, and other adverse effects. Where a code from this section is applicable, it is intended that it shall be used secondary to a code from another chapter of the Classification indicating the nature of the condition. Most often, the condition will be classifiable to Chapter 19, Injury, poisoning and certain other consequences of external causes (S00-T88). Other conditions that may be stated to be due to external causes are classified in Chapters I to XVIII. For these conditions, codes from Chapter 20 should be used to provide additional information as to the cause of the condition.

This chapter contains the following blocks:

V00-X58	Accidents
V00-V99	Transport accidents
V00-V09	Pedestrian injured in transport accident
V10-V19	Pedal cycle rider injured in transport accident
V20-V29	Motorcycle rider injured in transport accident
V30-V39	Occupant of three-wheeled motor vehicle injured in transport accident
V40-V49	Car occupant injured in transport accident
V50-V59	Occupant of pick-up truck or van injured in transport accident
V60-V69	Occupant of heavy transport vehicle injured in transport accident
V70-V79	Bus occupant injured in transport accident
V80-V89	Other land transport accidents
V90-V94	Water transport accidents
V95-V97	Air and space transport accidents
V98-V99	Other and unspecified transport accidents
W00-X58	Other external causes of accidental injury
W00-W19	Slipping, tripping, stumbling and falls
W20-W49	Exposure to inanimate mechanical forces
W50-W64	Exposure to animate mechanical forces
W65-W74	Accidental non-transport drowning and submersion
W85-W99	Exposure to electric current, radiation and extreme ambient air temperature and pressure
X00-X08	Exposure to smoke, fire and flames
X10-X19	Contact with heat and hot substances
X30-X39	Exposure to forces of nature
▶X50◀	▶Overexertion and strenuous or repetitive movements◀
X52-X58	Accidental exposure to other specified factors
X71-X83	Intentional self-harm
X92-Y09	Assault
Y21-Y33	Event of undetermined intent
Y35-Y38	Legal intervention, operations of war, military operations, and terrorism
Y62-Y84	Complications of medical and surgical care
Y62-Y69	Misadventures to patients during surgical and medical care
Y70-Y82	Medical devices associated with adverse incidents in diagnostic and therapeutic use
Y83-Y84	Surgical and other medical procedures as the cause of abnormal reaction of the patient, or of later complication, without mention of misadventure at the time of the procedure
Y90-Y99	Supplementary factors related to causes of morbidity classified elsewhere

Accidents (V00-X58)

AHA: 2018,2Q,7-8

Transport accidents (V00-V99)

NOTE This section is structured in 12 groups. Those relating to land transport accidents (V00-V89) reflect the victim's mode of transport and are subdivided to identify the victim's 'counterpart' or the type of event. The vehicle of which the injured person is an occupant is identified in the first two characters since it is seen as the most important factor to identify for prevention purposes. A transport accident is one in which the vehicle involved must be moving or running or in use for transport purposes at the time of the accident.

Use additional code to identify:
airbag injury (W22.1)
type of street or road (Y92.4-)
use of cellular telephone and other electronic equipment at the time of the transport accident (Y93.C-)

EXCLUDES 1 agricultural vehicles in stationary use or maintenance (W31.-)
assault by crashing of motor vehicle (Y03.-)
automobile or motor cycle in stationary use or maintenance - code to type of accident
crashing of motor vehicle, undetermined intent (Y32)
intentional self-harm by crashing of motor vehicle (X82)

EXCLUDES 2 transport accidents due to cataclysm (X34-X38)

NOTE Definitions related to transport accidents:

(a) A transport accident (V00-V99) is any accident involving a device designed primarily for, or used at the time primarily for, conveying persons or good from one place to another.

(b) A public highway [trafficway] or street is the entire width between property lines (or other boundary lines) of land open to the public as a matter of right or custom for purposes of moving persons or property from one place to another. A roadway is that part of the public highway designed, improved and customarily used for vehicular traffic.

(c) A traffic accident is any vehicle accident occurring on the public highway [i.e. originating on, terminating on, or involving a vehicle partially on the highway]. A vehicle accident is assumed to have occurred on the public highway unless another place is specified, except in the case of accidents involving only off-road motor vehicles, which are classified as nontraffic accidents unless the contrary is stated.

(d) A nontraffic accident is any vehicle accident that occurs entirely in any place other than a public highway.

(e) ▶A pedestrian is any person involved in an accident who was not at the time of the accident riding in or on a motor vehicle, railway train, streetcar or animal-drawn or other vehicle, or on a pedal cycle or animal. This includes, a person changing a tire, working on a parked car, or a person on foot. It also includes the user of a pedestrian conveyance such as a baby stroller, ice-skates, skis, sled, roller skates, a skateboard, nonmotorized or motorized wheelchair, motorized mobility scooter, or nonmotorized scooter.◀

(f) A driver is an occupant of a transport vehicle who is operating or intending to operate it.

(g) A passenger is any occupant of a transport vehicle other than the driver, except a person traveling on the outside of the vehicle.

(h) A person on the outside of a vehicle is any person being transported by a vehicle but not occupying the space normally reserved for the driver or passengers, or the space intended for the transport of property. This includes a person travelling on the bodywork, bumper, fender, roof, running board or step of a vehicle, as well as, hanging on the outside of the vehicle.

(i) A pedal cycle is any land transport vehicle operated solely by nonmotorized pedals including a bicycle or tricycle.

(j) A pedal cyclist is any person riding a pedal cycle or in a sidecar or trailer attached to a pedal cycle.

(k) A motorcycle is a two-wheeled motor vehicle with one or two riding saddles and sometimes with a third wheel for the support of a sidecar. The sidecar is considered part of the motorcycle. This includes a moped, motor scooter, or motorized bicycle.

(l) A motorcycle rider is any person riding a motorcycle or in a sidecar or trailer attached to the motorcycle.

(m) A three-wheeled motor vehicle is a motorized tricycle designed primarily for on-road use. This includes a motor-driven tricycle, a motorized rickshaw, or a three-wheeled motor car.

(n) A car [automobile] is a four-wheeled motor vehicle designed primarily for carrying up to 7 persons. A trailer being towed by the car is considered part of the car. It does not include a van or minivan - see definition (o).

(o) A pick-up truck or van is a four or six-wheeled motor vehicle designed for carrying passengers as well as property or cargo weighing less than the local limit for classification as a heavy goods vehicle, and not requiring a special driver's license. This includes a minivan and a sport-utility vehicle (SUV).

(p) A heavy transport vehicle is a motor vehicle designed primarily for carrying property, meeting local criteria for classification as a heavy goods vehicle in terms of weight and requiring a special driver's license.

(q) A bus (coach) is a motor vehicle designed or adapted primarily for carrying more than 10 passengers, and requiring a special driver's license.

(r) A railway train or railway vehicle is any device, with or without freight or passenger cars couple to it, designed for traffic on a railway track. This includes subterranean (subways) or elevated trains.

(s) A streetcar, is a device designed and used primarily for transporting passengers within a municipality, running on rails, usually subject to normal traffic control signals, and operated principally on a right-of-way that forms part of the roadway. This includes a tram or trolley that runs on rails. A trailer being towed by a streetcar is considered part of the streetcar.

(t) A special vehicle mainly used on industrial premises is a motor vehicle designed primarily for use within the buildings and premises of industrial or commercial establishments. This includes battery-powered airport passenger vehicles or baggage/mail trucks, forklifts, coal-cars in a coal mine, logging cars and trucks used in mines or quarries.

(u) A special vehicle mainly used in agriculture is a motor vehicle designed specifically for use in farming and agriculture

✓ Additional Character Req   ✓x7ᵗʰ Placeholder Alert   ~~Manifestation~~   ▽ Unspecified   ▶◀ Revised Text   ● New Code   ▲ Revised Code Title

ICD-10-CM 2019

1151

(horticulture), to work the land, tend and harvest crops and transport materials on the farm. This includes harvesters, farm machinery and tractor and trailers.

(v) A special construction vehicle is a motor vehicle designed specifically for use on construction and demolition sites. This includes bulldozers, diggers, earth levellers, dump trucks, backhoes, front-end loaders, pavers, and mechanical shovels.

(w) A special all-terrain vehicle is a motor vehicle of special design to enable it to negotiate over rough or soft terrain, snow or sand. Examples of special design are high construction, special wheels and tires, tracks, and support on a cushion of air. This includes snow mobiles, All-terrain vehicles (ATV), and dune buggies. It does not include passenger vehicle designated as Sport Utility Vehicles. (SUV)

(x) A watercraft is any device designed for transporting passengers or goods on water. This includes motor or sailboats, ships, and hovercraft.

(y) An aircraft is any device for transporting passengers or goods in the air. This includes hot-air balloons, gliders, helicopters and airplanes.

(z) A military vehicle is any motorized vehicle operating on a public roadway owned by the military and being operated by a member of the military.

AHA: 2018,2Q,7-8

Pedestrian injured in transport accident (V00-V09)

INCLUDES   person changing tire on transport vehicle
person examining engine of vehicle broken down in (on side of) road

EXCLUDES 1   fall due to non-transport collision with other person (W03)
pedestrian on foot falling (slipping) on ice and snow (W00.-)
struck or bumped by another person (W51)

The appropriate 7th character is to be added to each code from categories V00-V09.
A   initial encounter
D   subsequent encounter
S   sequela

✓4ᵗʰ **V00   Pedestrian conveyance accident**

Use additional place of occurrence and activity external cause codes, if known (Y92.-, Y93.-)

EXCLUDES 1   collision with another person without fall (W51)
fall due to person on foot colliding with another person on foot (W03)
fall from non-moving wheelchair, nonmotorized scooter and motorized mobility scooter without collision (W05.-)
pedestrian (conveyance) collision with other land transport vehicle (V01-V09)
pedestrian on foot falling (slipping) on ice and snow (W00.-)

✓5ᵗʰ **V00.0   Pedestrian on foot injured in collision with pedestrian conveyance**

✓x7ᵗʰ   **V00.01   Pedestrian on foot injured in collision with roller-skater**

✓x7ᵗʰ   **V00.02   Pedestrian on foot injured in collision with skateboarder**

✓x7ᵗʰ   **V00.09   Pedestrian on foot injured in collision with other pedestrian conveyance**

✓5ᵗʰ **V00.1   Rolling-type pedestrian conveyance accident**

EXCLUDES 1   ▶accident with baby stroller◀ (V00.82-)
accident with motorized mobility scooter (V00.83-)
accident with wheelchair (powered) (V00.81-)

✓6ᵗʰ   **V00.11   In-line roller-skate accident**

✓7ᵗʰ   **V00.111   Fall from in-line roller-skates**

✓7ᵗʰ   **V00.112   In-line roller-skater colliding with stationary object**

✓7ᵗʰ   **V00.118   Other in-line roller-skate accident**

EXCLUDES 1   roller-skater collision with other land transport vehicle (V01-V09 with 5th character 1)

✓6ᵗʰ   **V00.12   Non-in-line roller-skate accident**

✓7ᵗʰ   **V00.121   Fall from non-in-line roller-skates**

✓7ᵗʰ   **V00.122   Non-in-line roller-skater colliding with stationary object**

✓7ᵗʰ   **V00.128   Other non-in-line roller-skating accident**

EXCLUDES 1   roller-skater collision with other land transport vehicle (V01-V09 with 5th character 1)

✓6ᵗʰ **V00.13   Skateboard accident**

✓7ᵗʰ   **V00.131   Fall from skateboard**

✓7ᵗʰ   **V00.132   Skateboarder colliding with stationary object**

✓7ᵗʰ   **V00.138   Other skateboard accident**

EXCLUDES 1   skateboarder collision with other land transport vehicle (V01-V09 with 5th character 2)

✓6ᵗʰ **V00.14   Scooter (nonmotorized) accident**

EXCLUDES 1   ▶motor scooter accident◀ (V20-V29)

✓7ᵗʰ   **V00.141   Fall from scooter (nonmotorized)**

✓7ᵗʰ   **V00.142   Scooter (nonmotorized) colliding with stationary object**

✓7ᵗʰ   **V00.148   Other scooter (nonmotorized) accident**

EXCLUDES 1   scooter (nonmotorized) collision with other land transport vehicle (V01-V09 with fifth character 9)

✓6ᵗʰ **V00.15   Heelies accident**

Rolling shoe
Wheeled shoe
Wheelies accident

✓7ᵗʰ   **V00.151   Fall from heelies**

✓7ᵗʰ   **V00.152   Heelies colliding with stationary object**

✓7ᵗʰ   **V00.158   Other heelies accident**

✓6ᵗʰ **V00.18   Accident on other rolling-type pedestrian conveyance**

✓7ᵗʰ   **V00.181   Fall from other rolling-type pedestrian conveyance**

✓7ᵗʰ   **V00.182   Pedestrian on other rolling-type pedestrian conveyance colliding with stationary object**

✓7ᵗʰ   **V00.188   Other accident on other rolling-type pedestrian conveyance**

✓5ᵗʰ **V00.2   Gliding-type pedestrian conveyance accident**

✓6ᵗʰ   **V00.21   Ice-skates accident**

✓7ᵗʰ   **V00.211   Fall from ice-skates**

✓7ᵗʰ   **V00.212   Ice-skater colliding with stationary object**

✓7ᵗʰ   **V00.218   Other ice-skates accident**

EXCLUDES 1   ice-skater collision with other land transport vehicle ▶(V01-V09 with 5th character 9)◀

✓6ᵗʰ   **V00.22   Sled accident**

✓7ᵗʰ   **V00.221   Fall from sled**

✓7ᵗʰ   **V00.222   Sledder colliding with stationary object**

✓7ᵗʰ   **V00.228   Other sled accident**

EXCLUDES 1   sled collision with other land transport vehicle ▶(V01-V09 with 5th character 9)◀

✓6ᵗʰ   **V00.28   Other gliding-type pedestrian conveyance accident**

✓7ᵗʰ   **V00.281   Fall from other gliding-type pedestrian conveyance**

✓7ᵗʰ   **V00.282   Pedestrian on other gliding-type pedestrian conveyance colliding with stationary object**

✓7ᵗʰ   **V00.288   Other accident on other gliding-type pedestrian conveyance**

EXCLUDES 1   gliding-type pedestrian conveyance collision with other land transport vehicle ▶(V01-V09 with 5th character 9)◀

✓5ᵗʰ **V00.3   Flat-bottomed pedestrian conveyance accident**

✓6ᵗʰ   **V00.31   Snowboard accident**

✓7ᵗʰ   **V00.311   Fall from snowboard**

✓7ᵗʰ   **V00.312   Snowboarder colliding with stationary object**

√7ᵗʰ **V00.318 Other snowboard accident**

> *EXCLUDES 1*   *snowboarder collision with other land transport vehicle ▶(V01-V09 with 5th character 9)◄*

√6ᵗʰ **V00.32 Snow-ski accident**

√7ᵗʰ **V00.321 Fall from snow-skis**

√7ᵗʰ **V00.322 Snow-skier colliding with stationary object**

√7ᵗʰ **V00.328 Other snow-ski accident**

> *EXCLUDES 1*   *snow-skier collision with other land transport vehicle ▶(V01-V09 with 5th character 9)◄*

√6ᵗʰ **V00.38 Other flat-bottomed pedestrian conveyance accident**

√7ᵗʰ **V00.381 Fall from other flat-bottomed pedestrian conveyance**

√7ᵗʰ **V00.382 Pedestrian on other flat-bottomed pedestrian conveyance colliding with stationary object**

√7ᵗʰ **V00.388 Other accident on other flat-bottomed pedestrian conveyance**

√5ᵗʰ **V00.8 Accident on other pedestrian conveyance**

√6ᵗʰ **V00.81 Accident with wheelchair (powered)**

√7ᵗʰ **V00.811 Fall from moving wheelchair (powered)**

> *EXCLUDES 1*   *fall from non-moving wheelchair (W05.0)*

√7ᵗʰ **V00.812 Wheelchair (powered) colliding with stationary object**

√7ᵗʰ **V00.818 Other accident with wheelchair (powered)**

▲ √6ᵗʰ **V00.82 Accident with baby stroller**

▲ √7ᵗʰ **V00.821 Fall from baby stroller**

▲ √7ᵗʰ **V00.822 Baby stroller colliding with stationary object**

▲ √7ᵗʰ **V00.828 Other accident with baby stroller**

√6ᵗʰ **V00.83 Accident with motorized mobility scooter**

√7ᵗʰ **V00.831 Fall from motorized mobility scooter**

> *EXCLUDES 1*   *fall from non-moving motorized mobility scooter (W05.2)*

√7ᵗʰ **V00.832 Motorized mobility scooter colliding with stationary object**

√7ᵗʰ **V00.838 Other accident with motorized mobility scooter**

√6ᵗʰ **V00.89 Accident on other pedestrian conveyance**

√7ᵗʰ **V00.891 Fall from other pedestrian conveyance**

√7ᵗʰ **V00.892 Pedestrian on other pedestrian conveyance colliding with stationary object**

√7ᵗʰ **V00.898 Other accident on other pedestrian conveyance**

> *EXCLUDES 1*   *other pedestrian (conveyance) collision with other land transport vehicle ▶(V01-V09 with 5th character 9)◄*

√4ᵗʰ **V01 Pedestrian injured in collision with pedal cycle**

√5ᵗʰ **V01.0 Pedestrian injured in collision with pedal cycle in nontraffic accident**

√x7ᵗʰ **V01.00 Pedestrian on foot injured in collision with pedal cycle in nontraffic accident**

> Pedestrian NOS injured in collision with pedal cycle in nontraffic accident

√x7ᵗʰ **V01.01 Pedestrian on roller-skates injured in collision with pedal cycle in nontraffic accident**

√x7ᵗʰ **V01.02 Pedestrian on skateboard injured in collision with pedal cycle in nontraffic accident**

√x7ᵗʰ **V01.09 Pedestrian with other conveyance injured in collision with pedal cycle in nontraffic accident**

> ▶Pedestrian with baby stroller injured in collision with pedal cycle in nontraffic accident◄
>
> Pedestrian on ice-skates injured in collision with pedal cycle in nontraffic accident
>
> Pedestrian on nonmotorized scooter injured in collision with pedal cycle in nontraffic accident
>
> Pedestrian on sled injured in collision with pedal cycle in nontraffic accident
>
> Pedestrian on snowboard injured in collision with pedal cycle in nontraffic accident
>
> Pedestrian on snow-skis injured in collision with pedal cycle in nontraffic accident
>
> Pedestrian in wheelchair (powered) injured in collision with pedal cycle in nontraffic accident
>
> Pedestrian in motorized mobility scooter injured in collision with pedal cycle in nontraffic accident

√5ᵗʰ **V01.1 Pedestrian injured in collision with pedal cycle in traffic accident**

√x7ᵗʰ **V01.10 Pedestrian on foot injured in collision with pedal cycle in traffic accident**

> Pedestrian NOS injured in collision with pedal cycle in traffic accident

√x7ᵗʰ **V01.11 Pedestrian on roller-skates injured in collision with pedal cycle in traffic accident**

√x7ᵗʰ **V01.12 Pedestrian on skateboard injured in collision with pedal cycle in traffic accident**

√x7ᵗʰ **V01.19 Pedestrian with other conveyance injured in collision with pedal cycle in traffic accident**

> ▶Pedestrian with baby stroller injured in collision with pedal cycle in traffic accident◄
>
> Pedestrian on ice-skates injured in collision with pedal cycle in traffic accident
>
> Pedestrian on nonmotorized scooter injured in collision with pedal cycle in traffic accident
>
> Pedestrian on sled injured in collision with pedal cycle in traffic accident
>
> Pedestrian on snowboard injured in collision with pedal cycle in traffic accident
>
> Pedestrian on snow-skis injured in collision with pedal cycle in traffic accident
>
> Pedestrian in wheelchair (powered) injured in collision with pedal cycle in traffic accident
>
> Pedestrian in motorized mobility scooter injured in collision with pedal cycle in traffic accident

√5ᵗʰ **V01.9 Pedestrian injured in collision with pedal cycle, unspecified whether traffic or nontraffic accident**

√x7ᵗʰ **V01.90 Pedestrian on foot injured in collision with pedal cycle, unspecified whether traffic or nontraffic accident**   ▽

> Pedestrian NOS injured in collision with pedal cycle, unspecified whether traffic or nontraffic accident

√x7ᵗʰ **V01.91 Pedestrian on roller-skates injured in collision with pedal cycle, unspecified whether traffic or nontraffic accident**   ▽

√x7ᵗʰ **V01.92 Pedestrian on skateboard injured in collision with pedal cycle, unspecified whether traffic or nontraffic accident**   ▽

√x7ᵗʰ **V01.99 Pedestrian with other conveyance injured in collision with pedal cycle, unspecified whether traffic or nontraffic accident** ▽
► Pedestrian with baby stroller injured in collision with pedal cycle, unspecified whether traffic or nontraffic accident ◄
Pedestrian on ice-skates injured in collision with pedal cycle unspecified, whether traffic or nontraffic accident
Pedestrian on nonmotorized scooter injured in collision with pedal cycle, unspecified whether traffic or nontraffic accident
Pedestrian on sled injured in collision with pedal cycle unspecified, whether traffic or nontraffic accident
Pedestrian on snowboard injured in collision with pedal cycle, unspecified whether traffic or nontraffic accident
Pedestrian on snow-skis injured in collision with pedal cycle, unspecified whether traffic or nontraffic accident
Pedestrian in wheelchair (powered) injured in collision with pedal cycle, unspecified whether traffic or nontraffic accident
Pedestrian in motorized mobility scooter injured in collision with pedal cycle, unspecified whether traffic or nontraffic accident

√4ᵗʰ **V02 Pedestrian injured in collision with two- or three-wheeled motor vehicle**

√5ᵗʰ **V02.0 Pedestrian injured in collision with two- or three-wheeled motor vehicle in nontraffic accident**

√x7ᵗʰ **V02.00 Pedestrian on foot injured in collision with two- or three-wheeled motor vehicle in nontraffic accident**
Pedestrian NOS injured in collision with two- or three-wheeled motor vehicle in nontraffic accident

√x7ᵗʰ **V02.01 Pedestrian on roller-skates injured in collision with two- or three-wheeled motor vehicle in nontraffic accident**

√x7ᵗʰ **V02.02 Pedestrian on skateboard injured in collision with two- or three-wheeled motor vehicle in nontraffic accident**

√x7ᵗʰ **V02.09 Pedestrian with other conveyance injured in collision with two- or three-wheeled motor vehicle in nontraffic accident**
► Pedestrian with baby stroller injured in collision with two- or three-wheeled motor vehicle in nontraffic accident ◄
Pedestrian on ice-skates injured in collision with two- or three-wheeled motor vehicle in nontraffic accident
Pedestrian on nonmotorized scooter injured in collision with two- or three-wheeled motor vehicle in nontraffic accident
Pedestrian on sled injured in collision with two- or three-wheeled motor vehicle in nontraffic accident
Pedestrian on snowboard injured in collision with two- or three-wheeled motor vehicle in nontraffic accident
Pedestrian on snow-skis injured in collision with two- or three-wheeled motor vehicle in nontraffic accident
Pedestrian in wheelchair (powered) injured in collision with two- or three-wheeled motor vehicle in nontraffic accident
Pedestrian in motorized mobility scooter injured in collision with two- or three-wheeled motor vehicle in nontraffic accident

√5ᵗʰ **V02.1 Pedestrian injured in collision with two- or three-wheeled motor vehicle in traffic accident**

√x7ᵗʰ **V02.10 Pedestrian on foot injured in collision with two- or three-wheeled motor vehicle in traffic accident**
Pedestrian NOS injured in collision with two- or three-wheeled motor vehicle in traffic accident

√x7ᵗʰ **V02.11 Pedestrian on roller-skates injured in collision with two- or three-wheeled motor vehicle in traffic accident**

√x7ᵗʰ **V02.12 Pedestrian on skateboard injured in collision with two- or three-wheeled motor vehicle in traffic accident**

√x7ᵗʰ **V02.19 Pedestrian with other conveyance injured in collision with two- or three-wheeled motor vehicle in traffic accident**
► Pedestrian with baby stroller injured in collision with two- or three-wheeled motor vehicle in traffic accident ◄
Pedestrian on ice-skates injured in collision with two- or three-wheeled motor vehicle in traffic accident
Pedestrian on nonmotorized scooter injured in collision with two- or three-wheeled motor vehicle in traffic accident
Pedestrian on sled injured in collision with two- or three-wheeled motor vehicle in traffic accident
Pedestrian on snowboard injured in collision with two- or three-wheeled motor vehicle in traffic accident
Pedestrian on snow-skis injured in collision with two- or three-wheeled motor vehicle in traffic accident
Pedestrian in wheelchair (powered) injured in collision with two- or three-wheeled motor vehicle in traffic accident
Pedestrian in motorized mobility scooter injued in collision with two- or three-wheeled motor vehicle in traffic accident

√5ᵗʰ **V02.9 Pedestrian injured in collision with two- or three-wheeled motor vehicle, unspecified whether traffic or nontraffic accident**

√x7ᵗʰ **V02.90 Pedestrian on foot injured in collision with two- or three-wheeled motor vehicle, unspecified whether traffic or nontraffic accident** ▽
Pedestrian NOS injured in collision with two- or three-wheeled motor vehicle, unspecified whether traffic or nontraffic accident

√x7ᵗʰ **V02.91 Pedestrian on roller-skates injured in collision with two- or three-wheeled motor vehicle, unspecified whether traffic or nontraffic accident** ▽

√x7ᵗʰ **V02.92 Pedestrian on skateboard injured in collision with two- or three-wheeled motor vehicle, unspecified whether traffic or nontraffic accident** ▽

√x7ᵗʰ **V02.99 Pedestrian with other conveyance injured in collision with two- or three-wheeled motor vehicle, unspecified whether traffic or nontraffic accident** ▽
► Pedestrian with baby stroller injured in collision with two- or three-wheeled motor vehicle, unspecified whether traffic or nontraffic accident ◄
Pedestrian on ice-skates injured in collision with two- or three-wheeled motor vehicle, unspecified whether traffic or nontraffic accident
Pedestrian on nonmotorized scooter injured in collision with two- or three-wheeled motor vehicle, unspecified whether traffic or nontraffic accident
Pedestrian on sled injured in collision with two- or three-wheeled motor vehicle, unspecified whether traffic or nontraffic accident
Pedestrian on snowboard injured in collision with two- or three-wheeled motor vehicle, unspecified whether traffic or nontraffic accident
Pedestrian on snow-skis injured in collision with two- or three-wheeled motor vehicle, unspecified whether traffic or nontraffic accident
Pedestrian in wheelchair (powered) injured in collision with two- or three-wheeled motor vehicle, unspecified whether traffic or nontraffic accident
Pedestrian in motorized mobility scooter injured in collision with two- or three wheeled motor vehicle, unspecified whether traffic or nontraffic accident

✓4ᵗʰ **V03 Pedestrian injured in collision with car, pick-up truck or van**

  ✓5ᵗʰ **V03.0 Pedestrian injured in collision with car, pick-up truck or van in nontraffic accident**

    ✓x7ᵗʰ **V03.00 Pedestrian on foot injured in collision with car, pick-up truck or van in nontraffic accident**
      Pedestrian NOS injured in collision with car, pick-up truck or van in nontraffic accident

    ✓x7ᵗʰ **V03.01 Pedestrian on roller-skates injured in collision with car, pick-up truck or van in nontraffic accident**

    ✓x7ᵗʰ **V03.02 Pedestrian on skateboard injured in collision with car, pick-up truck or van in nontraffic accident**

    ✓x7ᵗʰ **V03.09 Pedestrian with other conveyance injured in collision with car, pick-up truck or van in nontraffic accident**
      ►Pedestrian with baby stroller injured in collision with car, pick-up truck or van in nontraffic accident◄
      Pedestrian on ice-skates injured in collision with car, pick-up truck or van in nontraffic accident
      Pedestrian on nonmotorized scooter injured in collision with car, pick-up truck or van in nontraffic accident
      Pedestrian on sled injured in collision with car, pick-up truck or van in nontraffic accident
      Pedestrian on snowboard injured in collision with car, pick-up truck or van in nontraffic accident
      Pedestrian on snow-skis injured in collision with car, pick-up truck or van in nontraffic accident
      Pedestrian in wheelchair (powered) injured in collision with car, pick-up truck or van in nontraffic accident
      Pedestrian on motorized mobility scooter injured in collision with car, pick-up truck or van in nontraffic accident

  ✓5ᵗʰ **V03.1 Pedestrian injured in collision with car, pick-up truck or van in traffic accident**

    ✓x7ᵗʰ **V03.10 Pedestrian on foot injured in collision with car, pick-up truck or van in traffic accident**
      Pedestrian NOS injured in collision with car, pick-up truck or van in traffic accident

    ✓x7ᵗʰ **V03.11 Pedestrian on roller-skates injured in collision with car, pick-up truck or van in traffic accident**

    ✓x7ᵗʰ **V03.12 Pedestrian on skateboard injured in collision with car, pick-up truck or van in traffic accident**

    ✓x7ᵗʰ **V03.19 Pedestrian with other conveyance injured in collision with car, pick-up truck or van in traffic accident**
      ►Pedestrian with baby stroller injured in collision with car, pick-up truck or van in traffic accident◄
      Pedestrian on ice-skates injured in collision with car, pick-up truck or van in traffic accident
      Pedestrian on nonmotorized scooter injured in collision with car, pick-up truck or van in traffic accident
      Pedestrian on sled injured in collision with car, pick-up truck or van in traffic accident
      Pedestrian on snowboard injured in collision with car, pick-up truck or van in traffic accident
      Pedestrian on snow-skis injured in collision with car, pick-up truck or van in traffic accident
      Pedestrian in wheelchair (powered) injured in collision with car, pick-up truck or van in traffic accident
      Pedestrian in motorized mobility scooter injured in collision with car, pick-up truck or van in traffic accident

  ✓5ᵗʰ **V03.9 Pedestrian injured in collision with car, pick-up truck or van, unspecified whether traffic or nontraffic accident**

    ✓x7ᵗʰ **V03.90 Pedestrian on foot injured in collision with car, pick-up truck or van, unspecified whether traffic or nontraffic accident** ▽
      Pedestrian NOS injured in collision with car, pick-up truck or van, unspecified whether traffic or nontraffic accident

    ✓x7ᵗʰ **V03.91 Pedestrian on roller-skates injured in collision with car, pick-up truck or van, unspecified whether traffic or nontraffic accident** ▽

    ✓x7ᵗʰ **V03.92 Pedestrian on skateboard injured in collision with car, pick-up truck or van, unspecified whether traffic or nontraffic accident** ▽

    ✓x7ᵗʰ **V03.99 Pedestrian with other conveyance injured in collision with car, pick-up truck or van, unspecified whether traffic or nontraffic accident** ▽
      ►Pedestrian with baby stroller injured in collision with car, pick-up truck or van, unspecified whether traffic or nontraffic accident◄
      Pedestrian on ice-skates injured in collision with car, pick-up truck or van, unspecified whether traffic or nontraffic accident
      Pedestrian on nonmotorized scooter injured in collision with car, pick-up truck or van, unspecified whether traffic or nontraffic accident
      Pedestrian on sled injured in collision with car, pick-up truck or van in nontraffic accident
      Pedestrian on snowboard injured in collision with car, pick-up truck or van, unspecified whether traffic or nontraffic accident
      Pedestrian on snow-skis injured in collision with car, pick-up truck or van, unspecified whether traffic or nontraffic accident
      Pedestrian in wheelchair (powered) injured in collision with car, pick-up truck or van, unspecified whether traffic or nontraffic accident
      Pedestrian in motorized mobility scooter injured in collision with car, pick-up truck or van, unspecified whether traffic or nontraffic accident

✓4ᵗʰ **V04 Pedestrian injured in collision with heavy transport vehicle or bus**

  EXCLUDES 1   *pedestrian injured in collision with military vehicle (V09.01, V09.21)*

  ✓5ᵗʰ **V04.0 Pedestrian injured in collision with heavy transport vehicle or bus in nontraffic accident**

    ✓x7ᵗʰ **V04.00 Pedestrian on foot injured in collision with heavy transport vehicle or bus in nontraffic accident**
      Pedestrian NOS injured in collision with heavy transport vehicle or bus in nontraffic accident

    ✓x7ᵗʰ **V04.01 Pedestrian on roller-skates injured in collision with heavy transport vehicle or bus in nontraffic accident**

    ✓x7ᵗʰ **V04.02 Pedestrian on skateboard injured in collision with heavy transport vehicle or bus in nontraffic accident**

    ✓x7ᵗʰ **V04.09 Pedestrian with other conveyance injured in collision with heavy transport vehicle or bus in nontraffic accident**
      ►Pedestrian with baby stroller injured in collision with heavy transport vehicle or bus in nontraffic accident◄
      Pedestrian on ice-skates injured in collision with heavy transport vehicle or bus in nontraffic accident
      Pedestrian on nonmotorized scooter injured in collision with heavy transport vehicle or bus in nontraffic accident
      Pedestrian on sled injured in collision with heavy transport vehicle or bus in nontraffic accident
      Pedestrian on snowboard injured in collision with heavy transport vehicle or bus in nontraffic accident
      Pedestrian on snow-skis injured in collision with heavy transport vehicle or bus in nontraffic accident
      Pedestrian in wheelchair (powered) injured in collision with heavy transport vehicle or bus in nontraffic accident
      Pedestrian in motorized mobility scooter injured in collision with heavy transport vehicle or bus in nontraffic accident

  ✓5ᵗʰ **V04.1 Pedestrian injured in collision with heavy transport vehicle or bus in traffic accident**

    ✓x7ᵗʰ **V04.10 Pedestrian on foot injured in collision with heavy transport vehicle or bus in traffic accident**
      Pedestrian NOS injured in collision with heavy transport vehicle or bus in traffic accident

    ✓x7ᵗʰ **V04.11 Pedestrian on roller-skates injured in collision with heavy transport vehicle or bus in traffic accident**

    ✓x7ᵗʰ **V04.12 Pedestrian on skateboard injured in collision with heavy transport vehicle or bus in traffic accident**

✅ Additional Character Req   ✓x7ᵗʰ Placeholder Alert   Manifestation   ▽ Unspecified   ►◄ Revised Text   ● New Code   ▲ Revised Code Title

√x7ᵗʰ **V04.19** **Pedestrian with other conveyance injured in collision with heavy transport vehicle or bus in traffic accident**
▶Pedestrian with baby stroller injured in collision with heavy transport vehicle or bus in traffic accident◄
Pedestrian on ice-skates injured in collision with heavy transport vehicle or bus in traffic accident
Pedestrian on nonmotorized scooter injured in collision with heavy transport vehicle or bus in traffic accident
Pedestrian on sled injured in collision with heavy transport vehicle or bus in traffic accident
Pedestrian on snowboard injured in collision with heavy transport vehicle or bus in traffic accident
Pedestrian on snow-skis injured in collision with heavy transport vehicle or bus in traffic accident
Pedestrian in wheelchair (powered) injured in collision with heavy transport vehicle or bus in traffic accident
Pedestrian in motorized mobility scooter injured in collision with heavy transport vehicle or bus in traffic accident

√5ᵗʰ **V04.9** **Pedestrian injured in collision with heavy transport vehicle or bus, unspecified whether traffic or nontraffic accident**

√x7ᵗʰ **V04.90** **Pedestrian on foot injured in collision with heavy transport vehicle or bus, unspecified whether traffic or nontraffic accident** ▽
Pedestrian NOS injured in collision with heavy transport vehicle or bus, unspecified whether traffic or nontraffic accident

√x7ᵗʰ **V04.91** **Pedestrian on roller-skates injured in collision with heavy transport vehicle or bus, unspecified whether traffic or nontraffic accident** ▽

√x7ᵗʰ **V04.92** **Pedestrian on skateboard injured in collision with heavy transport vehicle or bus, unspecified whether traffic or nontraffic accident** ▽

√x7ᵗʰ **V04.99** **Pedestrian with other conveyance injured in collision with heavy transport vehicle or bus, unspecified whether traffic or nontraffic accident** ▽
▶Pedestrian with baby stroller injured in collision with heavy transport vehicle or bus, unspecified whether traffic or nontraffic accident◄
Pedestrian on ice-skates injured in collision with heavy transport vehicle or bus, unspecified whether traffic or nontraffic accident
Pedestrian on nonmotorized scooter injured in collision with heavy transport vehicle or bus, unspecified whether traffic or nontraffic accident
Pedestrian on sled injured in collision with heavy transport vehicle or bus, unspecified whether traffic or nontraffic accident
Pedestrian on snowboard injured in collision with heavy transport vehicle or bus, unspecified whether traffic or nontraffic accident
Pedestrian on snow-skis injured in collision with heavy transport vehicle or bus, unspecified whether traffic or nontraffic accident
Pedestrian in wheelchair (powered) injured in collision with heavy transport vehicle or bus, unspecified whether traffic or nontraffic accident
Pedestrian in motorized mobility scooter injured in collision with heavy transport vehicle or bus, unspecified whether traffic or nontraffic accident

√4ᵗʰ **V05** **Pedestrian injured in collision with railway train or railway vehicle**

√5ᵗʰ **V05.0** **Pedestrian injured in collision with railway train or railway vehicle in nontraffic accident**

√x7ᵗʰ **V05.00** **Pedestrian on foot injured in collision with railway train or railway vehicle in nontraffic accident**
Pedestrian NOS injured in collision with railway train or railway vehicle in nontraffic accident

√x7ᵗʰ **V05.01** **Pedestrian on roller-skates injured in collision with railway train or railway vehicle in nontraffic accident**

√x7ᵗʰ **V05.02** **Pedestrian on skateboard injured in collision with railway train or railway vehicle in nontraffic accident**

√x7ᵗʰ **V05.09** **Pedestrian with other conveyance injured in collision with railway train or railway vehicle in nontraffic accident**
▶Pedestrian with baby stroller injured in collision with railway train or railway vehicle in nontraffic accident◄
Pedestrian on ice-skates injured in collision with railway train or railway vehicle in nontraffic accident
Pedestrian on nonmotorized scooter injured in collision with railway train or railway vehicle in nontraffic accident
Pedestrian on sled injured in collision with railway train or railway vehicle in nontraffic accident
Pedestrian on snowboard injured in collision with railway train or railway vehicle in nontraffic accident
Pedestrian on snow-skis injured in collision with railway train or railway vehicle in nontraffic accident
Pedestrian in wheelchair (powered) injured in collision with railway train or railway vehicle in nontraffic accident
Pedestrian in motorized mobility scooter injured in collision with railway train or railway vehicle in nontraffic accident

√5ᵗʰ **V05.1** **Pedestrian injured in collision with railway train or railway vehicle in traffic accident**

√x7ᵗʰ **V05.10** **Pedestrian on foot injured in collision with railway train or railway vehicle in traffic accident**
Pedestrian NOS injured in collision with railway train or railway vehicle in traffic accident

√x7ᵗʰ **V05.11** **Pedestrian on roller-skates injured in collision with railway train or railway vehicle in traffic accident**

√x7ᵗʰ **V05.12** **Pedestrian on skateboard injured in collision with railway train or railway vehicle in traffic accident**

√x7ᵗʰ **V05.19** **Pedestrian with other conveyance injured in collision with railway train or railway vehicle in traffic accident**
▶Pedestrian with baby stroller injured in collision with railway train or railway vehicle in traffic accident◄
Pedestrian on ice-skates injured in collision with railway train or railway vehicle in traffic accident
Pedestrian on nonmotorized scooter injured in collision with railway train or railway vehicle in traffic accident
Pedestrian on sled injured in collision with railway train or railway vehicle in traffic accident
Pedestrian on snowboard injured in collision with railway train or railway vehicle in traffic accident
Pedestrian on snow-skis injured in collision with railway train or railway vehicle in traffic accident
Pedestrian in wheelchair (powered) injured in collision with railway train or railway vehicle in traffic accident
Pedestrian in motorized mobility scooter injured in collision with railway train or railway vehicle in traffic accident

√5ᵗʰ **V05.9** **Pedestrian injured in collision with railway train or railway vehicle, unspecified whether traffic or nontraffic accident**

√x7ᵗʰ **V05.90** **Pedestrian on foot injured in collision with railway train or railway vehicle, unspecified whether traffic or nontraffic accident** ▽
Pedestrian NOS injured in collision with railway train or railway vehicle, unspecified whether traffic or nontraffic accident

√x7ᵗʰ **V05.91** **Pedestrian on roller-skates injured in collision with railway train or railway vehicle, unspecified whether traffic or nontraffic accident** ▽

√x7ᵗʰ **V05.92** **Pedestrian on skateboard injured in collision with railway train or railway vehicle, unspecified whether traffic or nontraffic accident** ▽

√x7ᵗʰ **V05.99** **Pedestrian with other conveyance injured in collision with railway train or railway vehicle, unspecified whether traffic or nontraffic accident** ▽

▶Pedestrian with baby stroller injured in collision with railway train or railway vehicle, unspecified whether traffic or nontraffic◀

Pedestrian on ice-skates injured in collision with railway train or railway vehicle, unspecified whether traffic or nontraffic

Pedestrian on nonmotorized scooter injured in collision with railway train or railway vehicle, unspecified whether traffic or nontraffic

Pedestrian on sled injured in collision with railway train or railway vehicle, unspecified whether traffic or nontraffic

Pedestrian on snowboard injured in collision with railway train or railway vehicle, unspecified whether traffic or nontraffic

Pedestrian on snow-skis injured in collision with railway train or railway vehicle, unspecified whether traffic or nontraffic

Pedestrian in wheelchair (powered) injured in collision with railway train or railway vehicle, unspecified whether traffic or nontraffic

Pedestrian in motorized mobility scooter injured in collision with railway train or railway vehicle, unspecified whether traffic or nontraffic

√4ᵗʰ **V06** **Pedestrian injured in collision with other nonmotor vehicle**

INCLUDES   collision with animal-drawn vehicle, animal being ridden, nonpowered streetcar

EXCLUDES 1   *pedestrian injured in collision with pedestrian conveyance (V00.0-)*

√5ᵗʰ **V06.0** **Pedestrian injured in collision with other nonmotor vehicle in nontraffic accident**

√x7ᵗʰ **V06.00** **Pedestrian on foot injured in collision with other nonmotor vehicle in nontraffic accident**

Pedestrian NOS injured in collision with other nonmotor vehicle in nontraffic accident

√x7ᵗʰ **V06.01** **Pedestrian on roller-skates injured in collision with other nonmotor vehicle in nontraffic accident**

√x7ᵗʰ **V06.02** **Pedestrian on skateboard injured in collision with other nonmotor vehicle in nontraffic accident**

√x7ᵗʰ **V06.09** **Pedestrian with other conveyance injured in collision with other nonmotor vehicle in nontraffic accident**

▶Pedestrian with baby stroller injured in collision with other nonmotor vehicle in nontraffic accident◀

Pedestrian on ice-skates injured in collision with other nonmotor vehicle in nontraffic accident

Pedestrian on nonmotorized scooter injured in collision with other nonmotor vehicle in nontraffic accident

Pedestrian on sled injured in collision with other nonmotor vehicle in nontraffic accident

Pedestrian on snowboard injured in collision with other nonmotor vehicle in nontraffic accident

Pedestrian on snow-skis injured in collision with other nonmotor vehicle in nontraffic accident

Pedestrian in wheelchair (powered) injured in collision with other nonmotor vehicle in nontraffic accident

Pedestrian in motorized mobility scooter injured in collision with other nonmotor vehicle in nontraffic accident

√5ᵗʰ **V06.1** **Pedestrian injured in collision with other nonmotor vehicle in traffic accident**

√x7ᵗʰ **V06.10** **Pedestrian on foot injured in collision with other nonmotor vehicle in traffic accident**

Pedestrian NOS injured in collision with other nonmotor vehicle in traffic accident

√x7ᵗʰ **V06.11** **Pedestrian on roller-skates injured in collision with other nonmotor vehicle in traffic accident**

√x7ᵗʰ **V06.12** **Pedestrian on skateboard injured in collision with other nonmotor vehicle in traffic accident**

√x7ᵗʰ **V06.19** **Pedestrian with other conveyance injured in collision with other nonmotor vehicle in traffic accident**

▶Pedestrian with baby stroller injured in collision with other nonmotor vehicle in nontraffic accident◀

Pedestrian on ice-skates injured in collision with other nonmotor vehicle in traffic accident

Pedestrian on nonmotorized scooter injured in collision with other nonmotor vehicle in traffic accident

Pedestrian on sled injured in collision with other nonmotor vehicle in traffic accident

Pedestrian on snowboard injured in collision with other nonmotor vehicle in traffic accident

Pedestrian on snow-skis injured in collision with other nonmotor vehicle in traffic accident

Pedestrian in wheelchair (powered) injured in collision with other nonmotor vehicle in traffic accident

Pedestrian in motorized mobility scooter injured in collision with other nonmotor vehicle in traffic accident

√5ᵗʰ **V06.9** **Pedestrian injured in collision with other nonmotor vehicle, unspecified whether traffic or nontraffic accident**

√x7ᵗʰ **V06.90** **Pedestrian on foot injured in collision with other nonmotor vehicle, unspecified whether traffic or nontraffic accident** ▽

Pedestrian NOS injured in collision with other nonmotor vehicle, unspecified whether traffic or nontraffic accident

√x7ᵗʰ **V06.91** **Pedestrian on roller-skates injured in collision with other nonmotor vehicle, unspecified whether traffic or nontraffic accident** ▽

√x7ᵗʰ **V06.92** **Pedestrian on skateboard injured in collision with other nonmotor vehicle, unspecified whether traffic or nontraffic accident** ▽

√x7ᵗʰ **V06.99** **Pedestrian with other conveyance injured in collision with other nonmotor vehicle, unspecified whether traffic or nontraffic accident** ▽

▶Pedestrian with baby stroller injured in collision with other nonmotor vehicle, unspecified whether traffic or nontraffic accident◀

Pedestrian on ice-skates injured in collision with other nonmotor vehicle, unspecified whether traffic or nontraffic accident

Pedestrian on nonmotorized scooter injured in collision with other nonmotor vehicle, unspecified whether traffic or nontraffic accident

Pedestrian on sled injured in collision with other nonmotor vehicle, unspecified whether traffic or nontraffic accident

Pedestrian on snowboard injured in collision with other nonmotor vehicle, unspecified whether traffic or nontraffic accident

Pedestrian on snow-skis injured in collision with other nonmotor vehicle, unspecified whether traffic or nontraffic accident

Pedestrian in wheelchair (powered) injured in collision with other nonmotor vehicle, unspecified whether traffic or nontraffic accident

Pedestrian in motorized mobility scooter injured in collision with other nonmotorized vehicle, unspecified whether traffic or nontraffic accident

√4ᵗʰ **V09** **Pedestrian injured in other and unspecified transport accidents**

√5ᵗʰ **V09.0** **Pedestrian injured in nontraffic accident involving other and unspecified motor vehicles**

√x7ᵗʰ **V09.00** **Pedestrian injured in nontraffic accident involving unspecified motor vehicles** ▽

√x7ᵗʰ **V09.01** **Pedestrian injured in nontraffic accident involving military vehicle**

√x7ᵗʰ **V09.09** **Pedestrian injured in nontraffic accident involving other motor vehicles**

Pedestrian injured in nontraffic accident by special vehicle

√x7ᵗʰ **V09.1** **Pedestrian injured in unspecified nontraffic accident** ▽

☑ Additional Character Req   √x7ᵗʰ Placeholder Alert   Manifestation   ▽ Unspecified   ▶◀ Revised Text   ● New Code   ▲ Revised Code Title

ICD-10-CM 2019   1157

✓5ᵗʰ **V09.2** **Pedestrian injured in traffic accident involving other and unspecified motor vehicles**

✓x7ᵗʰ **V09.20** Pedestrian injured in traffic accident involving unspecified motor vehicles ▽

✓x7ᵗʰ **V09.21** Pedestrian injured in traffic accident involving military vehicle

✓x7ᵗʰ **V09.29** Pedestrian injured in traffic accident involving other motor vehicles

✓x7ᵗʰ **V09.3** Pedestrian injured in unspecified traffic accident ▽

✓x7ᵗʰ **V09.9** Pedestrian injured in unspecified transport accident ▽

Pedal cycle rider injured in transport accident (V10-V19)

INCLUDES   any non-motorized vehicle, excluding an animal-drawn vehicle, or a sidecar or trailer attached to the pedal cycle

EXCLUDES 2   rupture of pedal cycle tire (W37.0)

The appropriate 7th character is to be added to each code from categories V10-V19.
A   initial encounter
D   subsequent encounter
S   sequela

✓4ᵗʰ **V10** **Pedal cycle rider injured in collision with pedestrian or animal**

EXCLUDES 1   pedal cycle rider collision with animal-drawn vehicle or animal being ridden (V16.-)

✓x7ᵗʰ **V10.0** Pedal cycle driver injured in collision with pedestrian or animal in nontraffic accident

✓x7ᵗʰ **V10.1** Pedal cycle passenger injured in collision with pedestrian or animal in nontraffic accident

✓x7ᵗʰ **V10.2** Unspecified pedal cyclist injured in collision with pedestrian or animal in nontraffic accident ▽

✓x7ᵗʰ **V10.3** Person boarding or alighting a pedal cycle injured in collision with pedestrian or animal

✓x7ᵗʰ **V10.4** Pedal cycle driver injured in collision with pedestrian or animal in traffic accident

✓x7ᵗʰ **V10.5** Pedal cycle passenger injured in collision with pedestrian or animal in traffic accident

✓x7ᵗʰ **V10.9** Unspecified pedal cyclist injured in collision with pedestrian or animal in traffic accident ▽

✓4ᵗʰ **V11** **Pedal cycle rider injured in collision with other pedal cycle**

✓x7ᵗʰ **V11.0** Pedal cycle driver injured in collision with other pedal cycle in nontraffic accident

✓x7ᵗʰ **V11.1** Pedal cycle passenger injured in collision with other pedal cycle in nontraffic accident

✓x7ᵗʰ **V11.2** Unspecified pedal cyclist injured in collision with other pedal cycle in nontraffic accident ▽

✓x7ᵗʰ **V11.3** Person boarding or alighting a pedal cycle injured in collision with other pedal cycle

✓x7ᵗʰ **V11.4** Pedal cycle driver injured in collision with other pedal cycle in traffic accident

✓x7ᵗʰ **V11.5** Pedal cycle passenger injured in collision with other pedal cycle in traffic accident

✓x7ᵗʰ **V11.9** Unspecified pedal cyclist injured in collision with other pedal cycle in traffic accident ▽

✓4ᵗʰ **V12** **Pedal cycle rider injured in collision with two- or three-wheeled motor vehicle**

✓x7ᵗʰ **V12.0** Pedal cycle driver injured in collision with two- or three-wheeled motor vehicle in nontraffic accident

✓x7ᵗʰ **V12.1** Pedal cycle passenger injured in collision with two- or three-wheeled motor vehicle in nontraffic accident

✓x7ᵗʰ **V12.2** Unspecified pedal cyclist injured in collision with two- or three-wheeled motor vehicle in nontraffic accident ▽

✓x7ᵗʰ **V12.3** Person boarding or alighting a pedal cycle injured in collision with two- or three-wheeled motor vehicle

✓x7ᵗʰ **V12.4** Pedal cycle driver injured in collision with two- or three-wheeled motor vehicle in traffic accident

✓x7ᵗʰ **V12.5** Pedal cycle passenger injured in collision with two- or three-wheeled motor vehicle in traffic accident

✓x7ᵗʰ **V12.9** Unspecified pedal cyclist injured in collision with two- or three-wheeled motor vehicle in traffic accident ▽

✓4ᵗʰ **V13** **Pedal cycle rider injured in collision with car, pick-up truck or van**

✓x7ᵗʰ **V13.0** Pedal cycle driver injured in collision with car, pick-up truck or van in nontraffic accident

✓x7ᵗʰ **V13.1** Pedal cycle passenger injured in collision with car, pick-up truck or van in nontraffic accident

✓x7ᵗʰ **V13.2** Unspecified pedal cyclist injured in collision with car, pick-up truck or van in nontraffic accident ▽

✓x7ᵗʰ **V13.3** Person boarding or alighting a pedal cycle injured in collision with car, pick-up truck or van

✓x7ᵗʰ **V13.4** Pedal cycle driver injured in collision with car, pick-up truck or van in traffic accident

✓x7ᵗʰ **V13.5** Pedal cycle passenger injured in collision with car, pick-up truck or van in traffic accident

✓x7ᵗʰ **V13.9** Unspecified pedal cyclist injured in collision with car, pick-up truck or van in traffic accident ▽

✓4ᵗʰ **V14** **Pedal cycle rider injured in collision with heavy transport vehicle or bus**

EXCLUDES 1   pedal cycle rider injured in collision with military vehicle (V19.81)

✓x7ᵗʰ **V14.0** Pedal cycle driver injured in collision with heavy transport vehicle or bus in nontraffic accident

✓x7ᵗʰ **V14.1** Pedal cycle passenger injured in collision with heavy transport vehicle or bus in nontraffic accident

✓x7ᵗʰ **V14.2** Unspecified pedal cyclist injured in collision with heavy transport vehicle or bus in nontraffic accident ▽

✓x7ᵗʰ **V14.3** Person boarding or alighting a pedal cycle injured in collision with heavy transport vehicle or bus

✓x7ᵗʰ **V14.4** Pedal cycle driver injured in collision with heavy transport vehicle or bus in traffic accident

✓x7ᵗʰ **V14.5** Pedal cycle passenger injured in collision with heavy transport vehicle or bus in traffic accident

✓x7ᵗʰ **V14.9** Unspecified pedal cyclist injured in collision with heavy transport vehicle or bus in traffic accident ▽

✓4ᵗʰ **V15** **Pedal cycle rider injured in collision with railway train or railway vehicle**

✓x7ᵗʰ **V15.0** Pedal cycle driver injured in collision with railway train or railway vehicle in nontraffic accident

✓x7ᵗʰ **V15.1** Pedal cycle passenger injured in collision with railway train or railway vehicle in nontraffic accident

✓x7ᵗʰ **V15.2** Unspecified pedal cyclist injured in collision with railway train or railway vehicle in nontraffic accident ▽

✓x7ᵗʰ **V15.3** Person boarding or alighting a pedal cycle injured in collision with railway train or railway vehicle

✓x7ᵗʰ **V15.4** Pedal cycle driver injured in collision with railway train or railway vehicle in traffic accident

✓x7ᵗʰ **V15.5** Pedal cycle passenger injured in collision with railway train or railway vehicle in traffic accident

✓x7ᵗʰ **V15.9** Unspecified pedal cyclist injured in collision with railway train or railway vehicle in traffic accident ▽

✓4ᵗʰ **V16** **Pedal cycle rider injured in collision with other nonmotor vehicle**

INCLUDES   collision with animal-drawn vehicle, animal being ridden, streetcar

✓x7ᵗʰ **V16.0** Pedal cycle driver injured in collision with other nonmotor vehicle in nontraffic accident

✓x7ᵗʰ **V16.1** Pedal cycle passenger injured in collision with other nonmotor vehicle in nontraffic accident

✓x7ᵗʰ **V16.2** Unspecified pedal cyclist injured in collision with other nonmotor vehicle in nontraffic accident ▽

✓x7ᵗʰ **V16.3** Person boarding or alighting a pedal cycle injured in collision with other nonmotor vehicle in nontraffic accident

✓x7ᵗʰ **V16.4** Pedal cycle driver injured in collision with other nonmotor vehicle in traffic accident

✓x7ᵗʰ **V16.5** Pedal cycle passenger injured in collision with other nonmotor vehicle in traffic accident

✓x7ᵗʰ **V16.9** Unspecified pedal cyclist injured in collision with other nonmotor vehicle in traffic accident ▽

✓4ᵗʰ **V17** **Pedal cycle rider injured in collision with fixed or stationary object**

✓x7ᵗʰ **V17.0** Pedal cycle driver injured in collision with fixed or stationary object in nontraffic accident

✓x7ᵗʰ **V17.1** Pedal cycle passenger injured in collision with fixed or stationary object in nontraffic accident

✓x7ᵗʰ **V17.2** Unspecified pedal cyclist injured in collision with fixed or stationary object in nontraffic accident ▽

✓x7ᵗʰ **V17.3** Person boarding or alighting a pedal cycle injured in collision with fixed or stationary object

✓x7ᵗʰ **V17.4** Pedal cycle driver injured in collision with fixed or stationary object in traffic accident

✓x7ᵗʰ **V17.5** Pedal cycle passenger injured in collision with fixed or stationary object in traffic accident

✓x7ᵗʰ **V17.9** Unspecified pedal cyclist injured in collision with fixed or stationary object in traffic accident ▽

✓4ᵗʰ **V18** **Pedal cycle rider injured in noncollision transport accident**

INCLUDES   fall or thrown from pedal cycle (without antecedent collision)
         overturning pedal cycle NOS
         overturning pedal cycle without collision

✓x7ᵗʰ **V18.0** Pedal cycle driver injured in noncollision transport accident in nontraffic accident

√x7ᵗʰ **V18.1** Pedal cycle passenger injured in noncollision transport accident in nontraffic accident

√x7ᵗʰ **V18.2** Unspecified pedal cyclist injured in noncollision transport accident in nontraffic accident ▽

√x7ᵗʰ **V18.3** Person boarding or alighting a pedal cycle injured in noncollision transport accident

√x7ᵗʰ **V18.4** Pedal cycle driver injured in noncollision transport accident in traffic accident

√x7ᵗʰ **V18.5** Pedal cycle passenger injured in noncollision transport accident in traffic accident

√x7ᵗʰ **V18.9** Unspecified pedal cyclist injured in noncollision transport accident in traffic accident ▽

√4ᵗʰ **V19 Pedal cycle rider injured in other and unspecified transport accidents**

√5ᵗʰ **V19.0** Pedal cycle driver injured in collision with other and unspecified motor vehicles in nontraffic accident

√x7ᵗʰ **V19.00** Pedal cycle driver injured in collision with unspecified motor vehicles in nontraffic accident ▽

√x7ᵗʰ **V19.09** Pedal cycle driver injured in collision with other motor vehicles in nontraffic accident

√5ᵗʰ **V19.1** Pedal cycle passenger injured in collision with other and unspecified motor vehicles in nontraffic accident

√x7ᵗʰ **V19.10** Pedal cycle passenger injured in collision with unspecified motor vehicles in nontraffic accident ▽

√x7ᵗʰ **V19.19** Pedal cycle passenger injured in collision with other motor vehicles in nontraffic accident

√5ᵗʰ **V19.2** Unspecified pedal cyclist injured in collision with other and unspecified motor vehicles in nontraffic accident

√x7ᵗʰ **V19.20** Unspecified pedal cyclist injured in collision with unspecified motor vehicles in nontraffic accident ▽
Pedal cycle collision NOS, nontraffic

√x7ᵗʰ **V19.29** Unspecified pedal cyclist injured in collision with other motor vehicles in nontraffic accident ▽

√x7ᵗʰ **V19.3** Pedal cyclist (driver) (passenger) injured in unspecified nontraffic accident ▽
Pedal cycle accident NOS, nontraffic
Pedal cyclist injured in nontraffic accident NOS

√5ᵗʰ **V19.4** Pedal cycle driver injured in collision with other and unspecified motor vehicles in traffic accident

√x7ᵗʰ **V19.40** Pedal cycle driver injured in collision with unspecified motor vehicles in traffic accident ▽

√x7ᵗʰ **V19.49** Pedal cycle driver injured in collision with other motor vehicles in traffic accident

√5ᵗʰ **V19.5** Pedal cycle passenger injured in collision with other and unspecified motor vehicles in traffic accident

√x7ᵗʰ **V19.50** Pedal cycle passenger injured in collision with unspecified motor vehicles in traffic accident ▽

√x7ᵗʰ **V19.59** Pedal cycle passenger injured in collision with other motor vehicles in traffic accident

√5ᵗʰ **V19.6** Unspecified pedal cyclist injured in collision with other and unspecified motor vehicles in traffic accident

√x7ᵗʰ **V19.60** Unspecified pedal cyclist injured in collision with unspecified motor vehicles in traffic accident ▽
Pedal cycle collision NOS (traffic)

√x7ᵗʰ **V19.69** Unspecified pedal cyclist injured in collision with other motor vehicles in traffic accident ▽

√5ᵗʰ **V19.8** Pedal cyclist (driver) (passenger) injured in other specified transport accidents

√x7ᵗʰ **V19.81** Pedal cyclist (driver) (passenger) injured in transport accident with military vehicle

√x7ᵗʰ **V19.88** Pedal cyclist (driver) (passenger) injured in other specified transport accidents

√x7ᵗʰ **V19.9** Pedal cyclist (driver) (passenger) injured in unspecified traffic accident ▽
Pedal cycle accident NOS

Motorcycle rider injured in transport accident (V20-V29)

INCLUDES   moped
                motorcycle with sidecar
                motorized bicycle
                motor scooter

EXCLUDES 1   *three-wheeled motor vehicle (V30-V39)*

The appropriate 7th character is to be added to each code from categories V20-V29.
A   initial encounter
D   subsequent encounter
S   sequela

√4ᵗʰ **V20 Motorcycle rider injured in collision with pedestrian or animal**

EXCLUDES 1   *motorcycle rider collision with animal-drawn vehicle or animal being ridden (V26.-)*

√x7ᵗʰ **V20.0** Motorcycle driver injured in collision with pedestrian or animal in nontraffic accident

√x7ᵗʰ **V20.1** Motorcycle passenger injured in collision with pedestrian or animal in nontraffic accident

√x7ᵗʰ **V20.2** Unspecified motorcycle rider injured in collision with pedestrian or animal in nontraffic accident ▽

√x7ᵗʰ **V20.3** Person boarding or alighting a motorcycle injured in collision with pedestrian or animal

√x7ᵗʰ **V20.4** Motorcycle driver injured in collision with pedestrian or animal in traffic accident

√x7ᵗʰ **V20.5** Motorcycle passenger injured in collision with pedestrian or animal in traffic accident

√x7ᵗʰ **V20.9** Unspecified motorcycle rider injured in collision with pedestrian or animal in traffic accident ▽

√4ᵗʰ **V21 Motorcycle rider injured in collision with pedal cycle**

√x7ᵗʰ **V21.0** Motorcycle driver injured in collision with pedal cycle in nontraffic accident

√x7ᵗʰ **V21.1** Motorcycle passenger injured in collision with pedal cycle in nontraffic accident

√x7ᵗʰ **V21.2** Unspecified motorcycle rider injured in collision with pedal cycle in nontraffic accident ▽

√x7ᵗʰ **V21.3** Person boarding or alighting a motorcycle injured in collision with pedal cycle

√x7ᵗʰ **V21.4** Motorcycle driver injured in collision with pedal cycle in traffic accident

√x7ᵗʰ **V21.5** Motorcycle passenger injured in collision with pedal cycle in traffic accident

√x7ᵗʰ **V21.9** Unspecified motorcycle rider injured in collision with pedal cycle in traffic accident ▽

√4ᵗʰ **V22 Motorcycle rider injured in collision with two- or three-wheeled motor vehicle**

√x7ᵗʰ **V22.0** Motorcycle driver injured in collision with two- or three-wheeled motor vehicle in nontraffic accident

√x7ᵗʰ **V22.1** Motorcycle passenger injured in collision with two- or three-wheeled motor vehicle in nontraffic accident

√x7ᵗʰ **V22.2** Unspecified motorcycle rider injured in collision with two- or three-wheeled motor vehicle in nontraffic accident ▽

√x7ᵗʰ **V22.3** Person boarding or alighting a motorcycle injured in collision with two- or three-wheeled motor vehicle

√x7ᵗʰ **V22.4** Motorcycle driver injured in collision with two- or three-wheeled motor vehicle in traffic accident

√x7ᵗʰ **V22.5** Motorcycle passenger injured in collision with two- or three-wheeled motor vehicle in traffic accident

√x7ᵗʰ **V22.9** Unspecified motorcycle rider injured in collision with two- or three-wheeled motor vehicle in traffic accident ▽

√4ᵗʰ **V23 Motorcycle rider injured in collision with car, pick-up truck or van**

√x7ᵗʰ **V23.0** Motorcycle driver injured in collision with car, pick-up truck or van in nontraffic accident

√x7ᵗʰ **V23.1** Motorcycle passenger injured in collision with car, pick-up truck or van in nontraffic accident

√x7ᵗʰ **V23.2** Unspecified motorcycle rider injured in collision with car, pick-up truck or van in nontraffic accident ▽

√x7ᵗʰ **V23.3** Person boarding or alighting a motorcycle injured in collision with car, pick-up truck or van

√x7ᵗʰ **V23.4** Motorcycle driver injured in collision with car, pick-up truck or van in traffic accident

√x7ᵗʰ **V23.5** Motorcycle passenger injured in collision with car, pick-up truck or van in traffic accident

√x7ᵗʰ **V23.9** Unspecified motorcycle rider injured in collision with car, pick-up truck or van in traffic accident ▽

Chapter 20. External Causes of Morbidity

V24–V29.9

✓4ᵗʰ **V24** Motorcycle rider injured in collision with heavy transport vehicle or bus

    EXCLUDES 1   motorcycle rider injured in collision with military vehicle (V29.81)

✓x7ᵗʰ **V24.0** Motorcycle driver injured in collision with heavy transport vehicle or bus in nontraffic accident

✓x7ᵗʰ **V24.1** Motorcycle passenger injured in collision with heavy transport vehicle or bus in nontraffic accident

✓x7ᵗʰ **V24.2** Unspecified motorcycle rider injured in collision with heavy transport vehicle or bus in nontraffic accident ▽

✓x7ᵗʰ **V24.3** Person boarding or alighting a motorcycle injured in collision with heavy transport vehicle or bus

✓x7ᵗʰ **V24.4** Motorcycle driver injured in collision with heavy transport vehicle or bus in traffic accident

✓x7ᵗʰ **V24.5** Motorcycle passenger injured in collision with heavy transport vehicle or bus in traffic accident

✓x7ᵗʰ **V24.9** Unspecified motorcycle rider injured in collision with heavy transport vehicle or bus in traffic accident ▽

✓4ᵗʰ **V25** Motorcycle rider injured in collision with railway train or railway vehicle

✓x7ᵗʰ **V25.0** Motorcycle driver injured in collision with railway train or railway vehicle in nontraffic accident

✓x7ᵗʰ **V25.1** Motorcycle passenger injured in collision with railway train or railway vehicle in nontraffic accident

✓x7ᵗʰ **V25.2** Unspecified motorcycle rider injured in collision with railway train or railway vehicle in nontraffic accident ▽

✓x7ᵗʰ **V25.3** Person boarding or alighting a motorcycle injured in collision with railway train or railway vehicle

✓x7ᵗʰ **V25.4** Motorcycle driver injured in collision with railway train or railway vehicle in traffic accident

✓x7ᵗʰ **V25.5** Motorcycle passenger injured in collision with railway train or railway vehicle in traffic accident

✓x7ᵗʰ **V25.9** Unspecified motorcycle rider injured in collision with railway train or railway vehicle in traffic accident ▽

✓4ᵗʰ **V26** Motorcycle rider injured in collision with other nonmotor vehicle

    INCLUDES   collision with animal-drawn vehicle, animal being ridden, streetcar

✓x7ᵗʰ **V26.0** Motorcycle driver injured in collision with other nonmotor vehicle in nontraffic accident

✓x7ᵗʰ **V26.1** Motorcycle passenger injured in collision with other nonmotor vehicle in nontraffic accident

✓x7ᵗʰ **V26.2** Unspecified motorcycle rider injured in collision with other nonmotor vehicle in nontraffic accident ▽

✓x7ᵗʰ **V26.3** Person boarding or alighting a motorcycle injured in collision with other nonmotor vehicle

✓x7ᵗʰ **V26.4** Motorcycle driver injured in collision with other nonmotor vehicle in traffic accident

✓x7ᵗʰ **V26.5** Motorcycle passenger injured in collision with other nonmotor vehicle in traffic accident

✓x7ᵗʰ **V26.9** Unspecified motorcycle rider injured in collision with other nonmotor vehicle in traffic accident ▽

✓4ᵗʰ **V27** Motorcycle rider injured in collision with fixed or stationary object

✓x7ᵗʰ **V27.0** Motorcycle driver injured in collision with fixed or stationary object in nontraffic accident

✓x7ᵗʰ **V27.1** Motorcycle passenger injured in collision with fixed or stationary object in nontraffic accident

✓x7ᵗʰ **V27.2** Unspecified motorcycle rider injured in collision with fixed or stationary object in nontraffic accident ▽

✓x7ᵗʰ **V27.3** Person boarding or alighting a motorcycle injured in collision with fixed or stationary object

✓x7ᵗʰ **V27.4** Motorcycle driver injured in collision with fixed or stationary object in traffic accident

✓x7ᵗʰ **V27.5** Motorcycle passenger injured in collision with fixed or stationary object in traffic accident

✓x7ᵗʰ **V27.9** Unspecified motorcycle rider injured in collision with fixed or stationary object in traffic accident ▽

✓4ᵗʰ **V28** Motorcycle rider injured in noncollision transport accident

    INCLUDES   fall or thrown from motorcycle (without antecedent collision)
                 overturning motorcycle NOS
                 overturning motorcycle without collision

✓x7ᵗʰ **V28.0** Motorcycle driver injured in noncollision transport accident in nontraffic accident

✓x7ᵗʰ **V28.1** Motorcycle passenger injured in noncollision transport accident in nontraffic accident

✓x7ᵗʰ **V28.2** Unspecified motorcycle rider injured in noncollision transport accident in nontraffic accident ▽

✓x7ᵗʰ **V28.3** Person boarding or alighting a motorcycle injured in noncollision transport accident

✓x7ᵗʰ **V28.4** Motorcycle driver injured in noncollision transport accident in traffic accident

✓x7ᵗʰ **V28.5** Motorcycle passenger injured in noncollision transport accident in traffic accident

✓x7ᵗʰ **V28.9** Unspecified motorcycle rider injured in noncollision transport accident in traffic accident ▽

✓4ᵗʰ **V29** Motorcycle rider injured in other and unspecified transport accidents

✓5ᵗʰ **V29.0** Motorcycle driver injured in collision with other and unspecified motor vehicles in nontraffic accident

✓x7ᵗʰ **V29.00** Motorcycle driver injured in collision with unspecified motor vehicles in nontraffic accident ▽

✓x7ᵗʰ **V29.09** Motorcycle driver injured in collision with other motor vehicles in nontraffic accident

✓5ᵗʰ **V29.1** Motorcycle passenger injured in collision with other and unspecified motor vehicles in nontraffic accident

✓x7ᵗʰ **V29.10** Motorcycle passenger injured in collision with unspecified motor vehicles in nontraffic accident ▽

✓x7ᵗʰ **V29.19** Motorcycle passenger injured in collision with other motor vehicles in nontraffic accident

✓5ᵗʰ **V29.2** Unspecified motorcycle rider injured in collision with other and unspecified motor vehicles in nontraffic accident

✓x7ᵗʰ **V29.20** Unspecified motorcycle rider injured in collision with unspecified motor vehicles in nontraffic accident ▽

Motorcycle collision NOS, nontraffic

✓x7ᵗʰ **V29.29** Unspecified motorcycle rider injured in collision with other motor vehicles in nontraffic accident ▽

✓x7ᵗʰ **V29.3** Motorcycle rider (driver) (passenger) injured in unspecified nontraffic accident ▽

Motorcycle accident NOS, nontraffic
Motorcycle rider injured in nontraffic accident NOS

✓5ᵗʰ **V29.4** Motorcycle driver injured in collision with other and unspecified motor vehicles in traffic accident

✓x7ᵗʰ **V29.40** Motorcycle driver injured in collision with unspecified motor vehicles in traffic accident ▽

✓x7ᵗʰ **V29.49** Motorcycle driver injured in collision with other motor vehicles in traffic accident

✓5ᵗʰ **V29.5** Motorcycle passenger injured in collision with other and unspecified motor vehicles in traffic accident

✓x7ᵗʰ **V29.50** Motorcycle passenger injured in collision with unspecified motor vehicles in traffic accident ▽

✓x7ᵗʰ **V29.59** Motorcycle passenger injured in collision with other motor vehicles in traffic accident

✓5ᵗʰ **V29.6** Unspecified motorcycle rider injured in collision with other and unspecified motor vehicles in traffic accident

✓x7ᵗʰ **V29.60** Unspecified motorcycle rider injured in collision with unspecified motor vehicles in traffic accident ▽

Motorcycle collision NOS (traffic)

✓x7ᵗʰ **V29.69** Unspecified motorcycle rider injured in collision with other motor vehicles in traffic accident ▽

✓5ᵗʰ **V29.8** Motorcycle rider (driver) (passenger) injured in other specified transport accidents

✓x7ᵗʰ **V29.81** Motorcycle rider (driver) (passenger) injured in transport accident with military vehicle

✓x7ᵗʰ **V29.88** Motorcycle rider (driver) (passenger) injured in other specified transport accidents

✓x7ᵗʰ **V29.9** Motorcycle rider (driver) (passenger) injured in unspecified traffic accident ▽

Motorcycle accident NOS

Occupant of three-wheeled motor vehicle injured in transport accident (V30-V39)

INCLUDES	motorized tricycle
	motorized rickshaw
	three-wheeled motor car
EXCLUDES 1	all-terrain vehicles (V86.-)
	motorcycle with sidecar (V20-V29)
	vehicle designed primarily for off-road use (V86.-)

The appropriate 7th character is to be added to each code from categories V30-V39.
A   initial encounter
D   subsequent encounter
S   sequela

√4ᵗʰ **V30 Occupant of three-wheeled motor vehicle injured in collision with pedestrian or animal**

     EXCLUDES 1   *three-wheeled motor vehicle collision with animal-drawn vehicle or animal being ridden (V36.-)*

√x7ᵗʰ **V30.0** Driver of three-wheeled motor vehicle injured in collision with pedestrian or animal in nontraffic accident

√x7ᵗʰ **V30.1** Passenger in three-wheeled motor vehicle injured in collision with pedestrian or animal in nontraffic accident

√x7ᵗʰ **V30.2** Person on outside of three-wheeled motor vehicle injured in collision with pedestrian or animal in nontraffic accident

√x7ᵗʰ **V30.3** Unspecified occupant of three-wheeled motor vehicle injured in collision with pedestrian or animal in nontraffic accident ▽

√x7ᵗʰ **V30.4** Person boarding or alighting a three-wheeled motor vehicle injured in collision with pedestrian or animal

√x7ᵗʰ **V30.5** Driver of three-wheeled motor vehicle injured in collision with pedestrian or animal in traffic accident

√x7ᵗʰ **V30.6** Passenger in three-wheeled motor vehicle injured in collision with pedestrian or animal in traffic accident

√x7ᵗʰ **V30.7** Person on outside of three-wheeled motor vehicle injured in collision with pedestrian or animal in traffic accident

√x7ᵗʰ **V30.9** Unspecified occupant of three-wheeled motor vehicle injured in collision with pedestrian or animal in traffic accident ▽

√4ᵗʰ **V31 Occupant of three-wheeled motor vehicle injured in collision with pedal cycle**

√x7ᵗʰ **V31.0** Driver of three-wheeled motor vehicle injured in collision with pedal cycle in nontraffic accident

√x7ᵗʰ **V31.1** Passenger in three-wheeled motor vehicle injured in collision with pedal cycle in nontraffic accident

√x7ᵗʰ **V31.2** Person on outside of three-wheeled motor vehicle injured in collision with pedal cycle in nontraffic accident

√x7ᵗʰ **V31.3** Unspecified occupant of three-wheeled motor vehicle injured in collision with pedal cycle in nontraffic accident ▽

√x7ᵗʰ **V31.4** Person boarding or alighting a three-wheeled motor vehicle injured in collision with pedal cycle

√x7ᵗʰ **V31.5** Driver of three-wheeled motor vehicle injured in collision with pedal cycle in traffic accident

√x7ᵗʰ **V31.6** Passenger in three-wheeled motor vehicle injured in collision with pedal cycle in traffic accident

√x7ᵗʰ **V31.7** Person on outside of three-wheeled motor vehicle injured in collision with pedal cycle in traffic accident

√x7ᵗʰ **V31.9** Unspecified occupant of three-wheeled motor vehicle injured in collision with pedal cycle in traffic accident ▽

√4ᵗʰ **V32 Occupant of three-wheeled motor vehicle injured in collision with two- or three-wheeled motor vehicle**

√x7ᵗʰ **V32.0** Driver of three-wheeled motor vehicle injured in collision with two- or three-wheeled motor vehicle in nontraffic accident

√x7ᵗʰ **V32.1** Passenger in three-wheeled motor vehicle injured in collision with two- or three-wheeled motor vehicle in nontraffic accident

√x7ᵗʰ **V32.2** Person on outside of three-wheeled motor vehicle injured in collision with two- or three-wheeled motor vehicle in nontraffic accident

√x7ᵗʰ **V32.3** Unspecified occupant of three-wheeled motor vehicle injured in collision with two- or three-wheeled motor vehicle in nontraffic accident ▽

√x7ᵗʰ **V32.4** Person boarding or alighting a three-wheeled motor vehicle injured in collision with two- or three-wheeled motor vehicle

√x7ᵗʰ **V32.5** Driver of three-wheeled motor vehicle injured in collision with two- or three-wheeled motor vehicle in traffic accident

√x7ᵗʰ **V32.6** Passenger in three-wheeled motor vehicle injured in collision with two- or three-wheeled motor vehicle in traffic accident

√x7ᵗʰ **V32.7** Person on outside of three-wheeled motor vehicle injured in collision with two- or three-wheeled motor vehicle in traffic accident

√x7ᵗʰ **V32.9** Unspecified occupant of three-wheeled motor vehicle injured in collision with two- or three-wheeled motor vehicle in traffic accident ▽

√4ᵗʰ **V33 Occupant of three-wheeled motor vehicle injured in collision with car, pick-up truck or van**

√x7ᵗʰ **V33.0** Driver of three-wheeled motor vehicle injured in collision with car, pick-up truck or van in nontraffic accident

√x7ᵗʰ **V33.1** Passenger in three-wheeled motor vehicle injured in collision with car, pick-up truck or van in nontraffic accident

√x7ᵗʰ **V33.2** Person on outside of three-wheeled motor vehicle injured in collision with car, pick-up truck or van in nontraffic accident

√x7ᵗʰ **V33.3** Unspecified occupant of three-wheeled motor vehicle injured in collision with car, pick-up truck or van in nontraffic accident ▽

√x7ᵗʰ **V33.4** Person boarding or alighting a three-wheeled motor vehicle injured in collision with car, pick-up truck or van

√x7ᵗʰ **V33.5** Driver of three-wheeled motor vehicle injured in collision with car, pick-up truck or van in traffic accident

√x7ᵗʰ **V33.6** Passenger in three-wheeled motor vehicle injured in collision with car, pick-up truck or van in traffic accident

√x7ᵗʰ **V33.7** Person on outside of three-wheeled motor vehicle injured in collision with car, pick-up truck or van in traffic accident

√x7ᵗʰ **V33.9** Unspecified occupant of three-wheeled motor vehicle injured in collision with car, pick-up truck or van in traffic accident ▽

√4ᵗʰ **V34 Occupant of three-wheeled motor vehicle injured in collision with heavy transport vehicle or bus**

     EXCLUDES 1   *occupant of three-wheeled motor vehicle injured in collision with military vehicle (V39.81)*

√x7ᵗʰ **V34.0** Driver of three-wheeled motor vehicle injured in collision with heavy transport vehicle or bus in nontraffic accident

√x7ᵗʰ **V34.1** Passenger in three-wheeled motor vehicle injured in collision with heavy transport vehicle or bus in nontraffic accident

√x7ᵗʰ **V34.2** Person on outside of three-wheeled motor vehicle injured in collision with heavy transport vehicle or bus in nontraffic accident

√x7ᵗʰ **V34.3** Unspecified occupant of three-wheeled motor vehicle injured in collision with heavy transport vehicle or bus in nontraffic accident ▽

√x7ᵗʰ **V34.4** Person boarding or alighting a three-wheeled motor vehicle injured in collision with heavy transport vehicle or bus

√x7ᵗʰ **V34.5** Driver of three-wheeled motor vehicle injured in collision with heavy transport vehicle or bus in traffic accident

√x7ᵗʰ **V34.6** Passenger in three-wheeled motor vehicle injured in collision with heavy transport vehicle or bus in traffic accident

√x7ᵗʰ **V34.7** Person on outside of three-wheeled motor vehicle injured in collision with heavy transport vehicle or bus in traffic accident

√x7ᵗʰ **V34.9** Unspecified occupant of three-wheeled motor vehicle injured in collision with heavy transport vehicle or bus in traffic accident ▽

√4ᵗʰ **V35 Occupant of three-wheeled motor vehicle injured in collision with railway train or railway vehicle**

√x7ᵗʰ **V35.0** Driver of three-wheeled motor vehicle injured in collision with railway train or railway vehicle in nontraffic accident

√x7ᵗʰ **V35.1** Passenger in three-wheeled motor vehicle injured in collision with railway train or railway vehicle in nontraffic accident

√x7ᵗʰ **V35.2** Person on outside of three-wheeled motor vehicle injured in collision with railway train or railway vehicle in nontraffic accident

√x7ᵗʰ **V35.3** Unspecified occupant of three-wheeled motor vehicle injured in collision with railway train or railway vehicle in nontraffic accident ▽

√x7ᵗʰ **V35.4** Person boarding or alighting a three-wheeled motor vehicle injured in collision with railway train or railway vehicle

√x7ᵗʰ **V35.5** Driver of three-wheeled motor vehicle injured in collision with railway train or railway vehicle in traffic accident

√x7ᵗʰ **V35.6** Passenger in three-wheeled motor vehicle injured in collision with railway train or railway vehicle in traffic accident

√x7ᵗʰ **V35.7** Person on outside of three-wheeled motor vehicle injured in collision with railway train or railway vehicle in traffic accident

√x7ᵗʰ **V35.9** Unspecified occupant of three-wheeled motor vehicle injured in collision with railway train or railway vehicle in traffic accident ▽

☑ Additional Character Req   √x7ᵗʰ Placeholder Alert   Manifestation   ▽ Unspecified   ►◄ Revised Text   ● New Code   ▲ Revised Code Title

Chapter 20. External Causes of Morbidity

V36–V39.9

V36   **Occupant of three-wheeled motor vehicle injured in collision with other nonmotor vehicle**
> INCLUDES   collision with animal-drawn vehicle, animal being ridden, streetcar

   √x7ᵗʰ   **V36.Ø**   Driver of three-wheeled motor vehicle injured in collision with other nonmotor vehicle in nontraffic accident

   √x7ᵗʰ   **V36.1**   Passenger in three-wheeled motor vehicle injured in collision with other nonmotor vehicle in nontraffic accident

   √x7ᵗʰ   **V36.2**   Person on outside of three-wheeled motor vehicle injured in collision with other nonmotor vehicle in nontraffic accident

   √x7ᵗʰ   **V36.3**   Unspecified occupant of three-wheeled motor vehicle injured in collision with other nonmotor vehicle in nontraffic accident   ▽

   √x7ᵗʰ   **V36.4**   Person boarding or alighting a three-wheeled motor vehicle injured in collision with other nonmotor vehicle

   √x7ᵗʰ   **V36.5**   Driver of three-wheeled motor vehicle injured in collision with other nonmotor vehicle in traffic accident

   √x7ᵗʰ   **V36.6**   Passenger in three-wheeled motor vehicle injured in collision with other nonmotor vehicle in traffic accident

   √x7ᵗʰ   **V36.7**   Person on outside of three-wheeled motor vehicle injured in collision with other nonmotor vehicle in traffic accident

   √x7ᵗʰ   **V36.9**   Unspecified occupant of three-wheeled motor vehicle injured in collision with other nonmotor vehicle in traffic accident   ▽

√4ᵗʰ V37   **Occupant of three-wheeled motor vehicle injured in collision with fixed or stationary object**

   √x7ᵗʰ   **V37.Ø**   Driver of three-wheeled motor vehicle injured in collision with fixed or stationary object in nontraffic accident

   √x7ᵗʰ   **V37.1**   Passenger in three-wheeled motor vehicle injured in collision with fixed or stationary object in nontraffic accident

   √x7ᵗʰ   **V37.2**   Person on outside of three-wheeled motor vehicle injured in collision with fixed or stationary object in nontraffic accident

   √x7ᵗʰ   **V37.3**   Unspecified occupant of three-wheeled motor vehicle injured in collision with fixed or stationary object in nontraffic accident   ▽

   √x7ᵗʰ   **V37.4**   Person boarding or alighting a three-wheeled motor vehicle injured in collision with fixed or stationary object

   √x7ᵗʰ   **V37.5**   Driver of three-wheeled motor vehicle injured in collision with fixed or stationary object in traffic accident

   √x7ᵗʰ   **V37.6**   Passenger in three-wheeled motor vehicle injured in collision with fixed or stationary object in traffic accident

   √x7ᵗʰ   **V37.7**   Person on outside of three-wheeled motor vehicle injured in collision with fixed or stationary object in traffic accident

   √x7ᵗʰ   **V37.9**   Unspecified occupant of three-wheeled motor vehicle injured in collision with fixed or stationary object in traffic accident   ▽

√4ᵗʰ V38   **Occupant of three-wheeled motor vehicle injured in noncollision transport accident**
> INCLUDES   fall or thrown from three-wheeled motor vehicle
> overturning of three-wheeled motor vehicle NOS
> overturning of three-wheeled motor vehicle without collision

   √x7ᵗʰ   **V38.Ø**   Driver of three-wheeled motor vehicle injured in noncollision transport accident in nontraffic accident

   √x7ᵗʰ   **V38.1**   Passenger in three-wheeled motor vehicle injured in noncollision transport accident in nontraffic accident

   √x7ᵗʰ   **V38.2**   Person on outside of three-wheeled motor vehicle injured in noncollision transport accident in nontraffic accident

   √x7ᵗʰ   **V38.3**   Unspecified occupant of three-wheeled motor vehicle injured in noncollision transport accident in nontraffic accident   ▽

   √x7ᵗʰ   **V38.4**   Person boarding or alighting a three-wheeled motor vehicle injured in noncollision transport accident

   √x7ᵗʰ   **V38.5**   Driver of three-wheeled motor vehicle injured in noncollision transport accident in traffic accident

   √x7ᵗʰ   **V38.6**   Passenger in three-wheeled motor vehicle injured in noncollision transport accident in traffic accident

   √x7ᵗʰ   **V38.7**   Person on outside of three-wheeled motor vehicle injured in noncollision transport accident in traffic accident

   √x7ᵗʰ   **V38.9**   Unspecified occupant of three-wheeled motor vehicle injured in noncollision transport accident in traffic accident   ▽

√4ᵗʰ V39   **Occupant of three-wheeled motor vehicle injured in other and unspecified transport accidents**

   √5ᵗʰ   **V39.Ø**   Driver of three-wheeled motor vehicle injured in collision with other and unspecified motor vehicles in nontraffic accident

     √x7ᵗʰ   **V39.ØØ**   Driver of three-wheeled motor vehicle injured in collision with unspecified motor vehicles in nontraffic accident   ▽

     √x7ᵗʰ   **V39.Ø9**   Driver of three-wheeled motor vehicle injured in collision with other motor vehicles in nontraffic accident

   √5ᵗʰ   **V39.1**   Passenger in three-wheeled motor vehicle injured in collision with other and unspecified motor vehicles in nontraffic accident

     √x7ᵗʰ   **V39.1Ø**   Passenger in three-wheeled motor vehicle injured in collision with unspecified motor vehicles in nontraffic accident   ▽

     √x7ᵗʰ   **V39.19**   Passenger in three-wheeled motor vehicle injured in collision with other motor vehicles in nontraffic accident

   √5ᵗʰ   **V39.2**   Unspecified occupant of three-wheeled motor vehicle injured in collision with other and unspecified motor vehicles in nontraffic accident

     √x7ᵗʰ   **V39.2Ø**   Unspecified occupant of three-wheeled motor vehicle injured in collision with unspecified motor vehicles in nontraffic accident   ▽
> Collision NOS involving three-wheeled motor vehicle, nontraffic

     √x7ᵗʰ   **V39.29**   Unspecified occupant of three-wheeled motor vehicle injured in collision with other motor vehicles in nontraffic accident   ▽

   √x7ᵗʰ   **V39.3**   Occupant (driver) (passenger) of three-wheeled motor vehicle injured in unspecified nontraffic accident   ▽
> Accident NOS involving three-wheeled motor vehicle, nontraffic
> Occupant of three-wheeled motor vehicle injured in nontraffic accident NOS

   √5ᵗʰ   **V39.4**   Driver of three-wheeled motor vehicle injured in collision with other and unspecified motor vehicles in traffic accident

     √x7ᵗʰ   **V39.4Ø**   Driver of three-wheeled motor vehicle injured in collision with unspecified motor vehicles in traffic accident   ▽

     √x7ᵗʰ   **V39.49**   Driver of three-wheeled motor vehicle injured in collision with other motor vehicles in traffic accident

   √5ᵗʰ   **V39.5**   Passenger in three-wheeled motor vehicle injured in collision with other and unspecified motor vehicles in traffic accident

     √x7ᵗʰ   **V39.5Ø**   Passenger in three-wheeled motor vehicle injured in collision with unspecified motor vehicles in traffic accident   ▽

     √x7ᵗʰ   **V39.59**   Passenger in three-wheeled motor vehicle injured in collision with other motor vehicles in traffic accident

   √5ᵗʰ   **V39.6**   Unspecified occupant of three-wheeled motor vehicle injured in collision with other and unspecified motor vehicles in traffic accident

     √x7ᵗʰ   **V39.6Ø**   Unspecified occupant of three-wheeled motor vehicle injured in collision with unspecified motor vehicles in traffic accident   ▽
> Collision NOS involving three-wheeled motor vehicle (traffic)

     √x7ᵗʰ   **V39.69**   Unspecified occupant of three-wheeled motor vehicle injured in collision with other motor vehicles in traffic accident   ▽

   √5ᵗʰ   **V39.8**   Occupant (driver) (passenger) of three-wheeled motor vehicle injured in other specified transport accidents

     √x7ᵗʰ   **V39.81**   Occupant (driver) (passenger) of three-wheeled motor vehicle injured in transport accident with military vehicle

     √x7ᵗʰ   **V39.89**   Occupant (driver) (passenger) of three-wheeled motor vehicle injured in other specified transport accidents

   √x7ᵗʰ   **V39.9**   Occupant (driver) (passenger) of three-wheeled motor vehicle injured in unspecified traffic accident   ▽
> Accident NOS involving three-wheeled motor vehicle

Car occupant injured in transport accident (V40-V49)

INCLUDES   a four-wheeled motor vehicle designed primarily for carrying passengers
automobile (pulling a trailer or camper)

EXCLUDES 1   bus (V50-V59)
minibus (V50-V59)
minivan (V50-V59)
motorcoach (V70-V79)
pick-up truck (V50-V59)
sport utility vehicle (SUV) (V50-V59)

The appropriate 7th character is to be added to each code from categories V40-V49.
A   initial encounter
D   subsequent encounter
S   sequela

✓4th **V40   Car occupant injured in collision with pedestrian or animal**

EXCLUDES 1   car collision with animal-drawn vehicle or animal being ridden (V46.-)

✓x7th   **V40.0   Car driver injured in collision with pedestrian or animal in nontraffic accident**

✓x7th   **V40.1   Car passenger injured in collision with pedestrian or animal in nontraffic accident**

✓x7th   **V40.2   Person on outside of car injured in collision with pedestrian or animal in nontraffic accident**

✓x7th   **V40.3   Unspecified car occupant injured in collision with   ▽ pedestrian or animal in nontraffic accident**

✓x7th   **V40.4   Person boarding or alighting a car injured in collision with pedestrian or animal**

✓x7th   **V40.5   Car driver injured in collision with pedestrian or animal in traffic accident**

✓x7th   **V40.6   Car passenger injured in collision with pedestrian or animal in traffic accident**

✓x7th   **V40.7   Person on outside of car injured in collision with pedestrian or animal in traffic accident**

✓x7th   **V40.9   Unspecified car occupant injured in collision with   ▽ pedestrian or animal in traffic accident**

✓4th **V41   Car occupant injured in collision with pedal cycle**

✓x7th   **V41.0   Car driver injured in collision with pedal cycle in nontraffic accident**

✓x7th   **V41.1   Car passenger injured in collision with pedal cycle in nontraffic accident**

✓x7th   **V41.2   Person on outside of car injured in collision with pedal cycle in nontraffic accident**

✓x7th   **V41.3   Unspecified car occupant injured in collision with   ▽ pedal cycle in nontraffic accident**

✓x7th   **V41.4   Person boarding or alighting a car injured in collision with pedal cycle**

✓x7th   **V41.5   Car driver injured in collision with pedal cycle in traffic accident**

✓x7th   **V41.6   Car passenger injured in collision with pedal cycle in traffic accident**

✓x7th   **V41.7   Person on outside of car injured in collision with pedal cycle in traffic accident**

✓x7th   **V41.9   Unspecified car occupant injured in collision with   ▽ pedal cycle in traffic accident**

✓4th **V42   Car occupant injured in collision with two- or three-wheeled motor vehicle**

✓x7th   **V42.0   Car driver injured in collision with two- or three-wheeled motor vehicle in nontraffic accident**

✓x7th   **V42.1   Car passenger injured in collision with two- or three-wheeled motor vehicle in nontraffic accident**

✓x7th   **V42.2   Person on outside of car injured in collision with two- or three-wheeled motor vehicle in nontraffic accident**

✓x7th   **V42.3   Unspecified car occupant injured in collision with   ▽ two- or three-wheeled motor vehicle in nontraffic accident**

✓x7th   **V42.4   Person boarding or alighting a car injured in collision with two- or three-wheeled motor vehicle**

✓x7th   **V42.5   Car driver injured in collision with two- or three-wheeled motor vehicle in traffic accident**

✓x7th   **V42.6   Car passenger injured in collision with two- or three-wheeled motor vehicle in traffic accident**

✓x7th   **V42.7   Person on outside of car injured in collision with two- or three-wheeled motor vehicle in traffic accident**

✓x7th   **V42.9   Unspecified car occupant injured in collision with   ▽ two- or three-wheeled motor vehicle in traffic accident**

✓4th **V43   Car occupant injured in collision with car, pick-up truck or van**

✓5th   **V43.0   Car driver injured in collision with car, pick-up truck or van in nontraffic accident**

✓x7th   **V43.01   Car driver injured in collision with sport utility vehicle in nontraffic accident**

✓x7th   **V43.02   Car driver injured in collision with other type car in nontraffic accident**

✓x7th   **V43.03   Car driver injured in collision with pick-up truck in nontraffic accident**

✓x7th   **V43.04   Car driver injured in collision with van in nontraffic accident**

✓5th   **V43.1   Car passenger injured in collision with car, pick-up truck or van in nontraffic accident**

✓x7th   **V43.11   Car passenger injured in collision with sport utility vehicle in nontraffic accident**

✓x7th   **V43.12   Car passenger injured in collision with other type car in nontraffic accident**

✓x7th   **V43.13   Car passenger injured in collision with pick-up in nontraffic accident**

✓x7th   **V43.14   Car passenger injured in collision with van in nontraffic accident**

✓5th   **V43.2   Person on outside of car injured in collision with car, pick-up truck or van in nontraffic accident**

✓x7th   **V43.21   Person on outside of car injured in collision with sport utility vehicle in nontraffic accident**

✓x7th   **V43.22   Person on outside of car injured in collision with other type car in nontraffic accident**

✓x7th   **V43.23   Person on outside of car injured in collision with pick-up truck in nontraffic accident**

✓x7th   **V43.24   Person on outside of car injured in collision with van in nontraffic accident**

✓5th   **V43.3   Unspecified car occupant injured in collision with car, pick-up truck or van in nontraffic accident**

✓x7th   **V43.31   Unspecified car occupant injured in collision   ▽ with sport utility vehicle in nontraffic accident**

✓x7th   **V43.32   Unspecified car occupant injured in collision   ▽ with other type car in nontraffic accident**

✓x7th   **V43.33   Unspecified car occupant injured in collision   ▽ with pick-up truck in nontraffic accident**

✓x7th   **V43.34   Unspecified car occupant injured in collision   ▽ with van in nontraffic accident**

✓5th   **V43.4   Person boarding or alighting a car injured in collision with car, pick-up truck or van**

✓x7th   **V43.41   Person boarding or alighting a car injured in collision with sport utility vehicle**

✓x7th   **V43.42   Person boarding or alighting a car injured in collision with other type car**

✓x7th   **V43.43   Person boarding or alighting a car injured in collision with pick-up truck**

✓x7th   **V43.44   Person boarding or alighting a car injured in collision with van**

✓5th   **V43.5   Car driver injured in collision with car, pick-up truck or van in traffic accident**

✓x7th   **V43.51   Car driver injured in collision with sport utility vehicle in traffic accident**

✓x7th   **V43.52   Car driver injured in collision with other type car in traffic accident**

✓x7th   **V43.53   Car driver injured in collision with pick-up truck in traffic accident**

✓x7th   **V43.54   Car driver injured in collision with van in traffic accident**

✓5th   **V43.6   Car passenger injured in collision with car, pick-up truck or van in traffic accident**

✓x7th   **V43.61   Car passenger injured in collision with sport utility vehicle in traffic accident**

✓x7th   **V43.62   Car passenger injured in collision with other type car in traffic accident**

✓x7th   **V43.63   Car passenger injured in collision with pick-up truck in traffic accident**

✓x7th   **V43.64   Car passenger injured in collision with van in traffic accident**

✓5th   **V43.7   Person on outside of car injured in collision with car, pick-up truck or van in traffic accident**

✓x7th   **V43.71   Person on outside of car injured in collision with sport utility vehicle in traffic accident**

✓x7th   **V43.72   Person on outside of car injured in collision with other type car in traffic accident**

✓x7th   **V43.73   Person on outside of car injured in collision with pick-up truck in traffic accident**

✓x7th   **V43.74   Person on outside of car injured in collision with van in traffic accident**

| ✓ Additional Character Req | ✓x7th Placeholder Alert | Manifestation | ▽ Unspecified | ►◄ Revised Text | ● New Code | ▲ Revised Code Title |

ICD-10-CM 2019   1163

√5ᵗʰ **V43.9** Unspecified car occupant injured in collision with car, pick-up truck or van **in traffic accident**

    √x7ᵗʰ **V43.91** Unspecified car occupant injured in collision with sport utility vehicle **in traffic accident** ▽

    √x7ᵗʰ **V43.92** Unspecified car occupant injured in collision with other type car **in traffic accident** ▽

    √x7ᵗʰ **V43.93** Unspecified car occupant injured in collision with pick-up truck **in traffic accident** ▽

    √x7ᵗʰ **V43.94** Unspecified car occupant injured in collision with van **in traffic accident** ▽

√4ᵗʰ **V44** Car occupant injured in collision with heavy transport vehicle or bus

    EXCLUDES 1   car occupant injured in collision with military vehicle (V49.81)

    √x7ᵗʰ **V44.0** Car driver injured in collision with heavy transport vehicle or bus **in nontraffic accident**

    √x7ᵗʰ **V44.1** Car passenger injured in collision with heavy transport vehicle or bus **in nontraffic accident**

    √x7ᵗʰ **V44.2** Person on outside of car injured in collision with heavy transport vehicle or bus **in nontraffic accident**

    √x7ᵗʰ **V44.3** Unspecified car occupant injured in collision with heavy transport vehicle or bus **in nontraffic accident** ▽

    √x7ᵗʰ **V44.4** Person boarding or alighting a car injured in collision with heavy transport vehicle or bus

    √x7ᵗʰ **V44.5** Car driver injured in collision with heavy transport vehicle or bus **in traffic accident**

    √x7ᵗʰ **V44.6** Car passenger injured in collision with heavy transport vehicle or bus **in traffic accident**

    √x7ᵗʰ **V44.7** Person on outside of car injured in collision with heavy transport vehicle or bus **in traffic accident**

    √x7ᵗʰ **V44.9** Unspecified car occupant injured in collision with heavy transport vehicle or bus **in traffic accident** ▽

√4ᵗʰ **V45** Car occupant injured in collision with railway train or railway vehicle

    √x7ᵗʰ **V45.0** Car driver injured in collision with railway train or railway vehicle **in nontraffic accident**

    √x7ᵗʰ **V45.1** Car passenger injured in collision with railway train or railway vehicle **in nontraffic accident**

    √x7ᵗʰ **V45.2** Person on outside of car injured in collision with railway train or railway vehicle **in nontraffic accident**

    √x7ᵗʰ **V45.3** Unspecified car occupant injured in collision with railway train or railway vehicle **in nontraffic accident** ▽

    √x7ᵗʰ **V45.4** Person boarding or alighting a car injured in collision with railway train or railway vehicle

    √x7ᵗʰ **V45.5** Car driver injured in collision with railway train or railway vehicle **in traffic accident**

    √x7ᵗʰ **V45.6** Car passenger injured in collision with railway train or railway vehicle **in traffic accident**

    √x7ᵗʰ **V45.7** Person on outside of car injured in collision with railway train or railway vehicle **in traffic accident**

    √x7ᵗʰ **V45.9** Unspecified car occupant injured in collision with railway train or railway vehicle **in traffic accident** ▽

√4ᵗʰ **V46** Car occupant injured in collision with other nonmotor vehicle

    INCLUDES   collision with animal-drawn vehicle, animal being ridden, streetcar

    √x7ᵗʰ **V46.0** Car driver injured in collision with other nonmotor vehicle **in nontraffic accident**

    √x7ᵗʰ **V46.1** Car passenger injured in collision with other nonmotor vehicle **in nontraffic accident**

    √x7ᵗʰ **V46.2** Person on outside of car injured in collision with other nonmotor vehicle **in nontraffic accident**

    √x7ᵗʰ **V46.3** Unspecified car occupant injured in collision with other nonmotor vehicle **in nontraffic accident** ▽

    √x7ᵗʰ **V46.4** Person boarding or alighting a car injured in collision with other nonmotor vehicle

    √x7ᵗʰ **V46.5** Car driver injured in collision with other nonmotor vehicle **in traffic accident**

    √x7ᵗʰ **V46.6** Car passenger injured in collision with other nonmotor vehicle **in traffic accident**

    √x7ᵗʰ **V46.7** Person on outside of car injured in collision with other nonmotor vehicle **in traffic accident**

    √x7ᵗʰ **V46.9** Unspecified car occupant injured in collision with other nonmotor vehicle **in traffic accident** ▽

√4ᵗʰ **V47** Car occupant injured in collision with fixed or stationary object

    AHA: 2016,4Q,73

    √x7ᵗʰ **V47.0** Car driver injured in collision with fixed or stationary object **in nontraffic accident**

    √x7ᵗʰ **V47.1** Car passenger injured in collision with fixed or stationary object **in nontraffic accident**

    √x7ᵗʰ **V47.2** Person on outside of car injured in collision with fixed or stationary object **in nontraffic accident**

    √x7ᵗʰ **V47.3** Unspecified car occupant injured in collision with fixed or stationary object **in nontraffic accident** ▽

    √x7ᵗʰ **V47.4** Person boarding or alighting a car injured in collision with fixed or stationary object

    √x7ᵗʰ **V47.5** Car driver injured in collision with fixed or stationary object **in traffic accident**

    √x7ᵗʰ **V47.6** Car passenger injured in collision with fixed or stationary object **in traffic accident**

    √x7ᵗʰ **V47.7** Person on outside of car injured in collision with fixed or stationary object **in traffic accident**

    √x7ᵗʰ **V47.9** Unspecified car occupant injured in collision with fixed or stationary object **in traffic accident** ▽

√4ᵗʰ **V48** Car occupant injured in noncollision transport accident

    INCLUDES   overturning car NOS

                 overturning car without collision

    √x7ᵗʰ **V48.0** Car driver injured in noncollision transport accident **in nontraffic accident**

    √x7ᵗʰ **V48.1** Car passenger injured in noncollision transport accident **in nontraffic accident**

    √x7ᵗʰ **V48.2** Person on outside of car injured in noncollision transport accident **in nontraffic accident**

    √x7ᵗʰ **V48.3** Unspecified car occupant injured in noncollision transport accident **in nontraffic accident** ▽

    √x7ᵗʰ **V48.4** Person boarding or alighting a car injured in noncollision transport accident

    √x7ᵗʰ **V48.5** Car driver injured in noncollision transport accident **in traffic accident**

    √x7ᵗʰ **V48.6** Car passenger injured in noncollision transport accident **in traffic accident**

    √x7ᵗʰ **V48.7** Person on outside of car injured in noncollision transport accident **in traffic accident**

    √x7ᵗʰ **V48.9** Unspecified car occupant injured in noncollision transport accident **in traffic accident** ▽

√4ᵗʰ **V49** Car occupant injured in other and unspecified transport accidents

    √5ᵗʰ **V49.0** Driver injured in collision with other and unspecified motor vehicles **in nontraffic accident**

       √x7ᵗʰ **V49.00** Driver injured in collision with unspecified motor vehicles in nontraffic accident ▽

       √x7ᵗʰ **V49.09** Driver injured in collision with other motor vehicles in nontraffic accident

    √5ᵗʰ **V49.1** Passenger injured in collision with other and unspecified motor vehicles **in nontraffic accident**

       √x7ᵗʰ **V49.10** Passenger injured in collision with unspecified motor vehicles in nontraffic accident ▽

       √x7ᵗʰ **V49.19** Passenger injured in collision with other motor vehicles in nontraffic accident

    √5ᵗʰ **V49.2** Unspecified car occupant injured in collision with other and unspecified motor vehicles **in nontraffic accident**

       √x7ᵗʰ **V49.20** Unspecified car occupant injured in collision with unspecified motor vehicles in nontraffic accident ▽

          Car collision NOS, nontraffic

       √x7ᵗʰ **V49.29** Unspecified car occupant injured in collision with other motor vehicles in nontraffic accident ▽

    √x7ᵗʰ **V49.3** Car occupant (driver) (passenger) injured in unspecified nontraffic accident ▽

       Car accident NOS, nontraffic

       Car occupant injured in nontraffic accident NOS

    √5ᵗʰ **V49.4** Driver injured in collision with other and unspecified motor vehicles **in traffic accident**

       √x7ᵗʰ **V49.40** Driver injured in collision with unspecified motor vehicles in traffic accident ▽

       √x7ᵗʰ **V49.49** Driver injured in collision with other motor vehicles in traffic accident

    √5ᵗʰ **V49.5** Passenger injured in collision with other and unspecified motor vehicles **in traffic accident**

       √x7ᵗʰ **V49.50** Passenger injured in collision with unspecified motor vehicles in traffic accident ▽

       √x7ᵗʰ **V49.59** Passenger injured in collision with other motor vehicles in traffic accident

    √5ᵗʰ **V49.6** Unspecified car occupant injured in collision with other and unspecified motor vehicles **in traffic accident**

       √x7ᵗʰ **V49.60** Unspecified car occupant injured in collision with unspecified motor vehicles in traffic accident ▽

          Car collision NOS (traffic)

       √x7ᵗʰ **V49.69** Unspecified car occupant injured in collision with other motor vehicles in traffic accident ▽

√5ᵗʰ **V49.8** Car occupant (driver) (passenger) injured in other specified transport accidents

  √x7ᵗʰ **V49.81** Car occupant (driver) (passenger) injured in transport accident with military vehicle

  √x7ᵗʰ **V49.88** Car occupant (driver) (passenger) injured in other specified transport accidents

√x7ᵗʰ **V49.9** Car occupant (driver) (passenger) injured in unspecified traffic accident ▽

  Car accident NOS

Occupant of pick-up truck or van injured in transport accident (V50-V59)

INCLUDES   a four or six wheel motor vehicle designed primarily for carrying passengers and property but weighing less than the local limit for classification as a heavy goods vehicle

  minibus
  minivan
  sport utility vehicle (SUV)
  truck
  van

EXCLUDES 1   *heavy transport vehicle (V60-V69)*

The appropriate 7th character is to be added to each code from categories V50-V59.
A   initial encounter
D   subsequent encounter
S   sequela

√4ᵗʰ **V50** Occupant of pick-up truck or van injured in collision with pedestrian or animal

  EXCLUDES 1   *pick-up truck or van collision with animal-drawn vehicle or animal being ridden (V56.-)*

√x7ᵗʰ **V50.0** Driver of pick-up truck or van injured in collision with pedestrian or animal in nontraffic accident

√x7ᵗʰ **V50.1** Passenger in pick-up truck or van injured in collision with pedestrian or animal in nontraffic accident

√x7ᵗʰ **V50.2** Person on outside of pick-up truck or van injured in collision with pedestrian or animal in nontraffic accident

√x7ᵗʰ **V50.3** Unspecified occupant of pick-up truck or van injured in collision with pedestrian or animal in nontraffic accident ▽

√x7ᵗʰ **V50.4** Person boarding or alighting a pick-up truck or van injured in collision with pedestrian or animal

√x7ᵗʰ **V50.5** Driver of pick-up truck or van injured in collision with pedestrian or animal in traffic accident

√x7ᵗʰ **V50.6** Passenger in pick-up truck or van injured in collision with pedestrian or animal in traffic accident

√x7ᵗʰ **V50.7** Person on outside of pick-up truck or van injured in collision with pedestrian or animal in traffic accident

√x7ᵗʰ **V50.9** Unspecified occupant of pick-up truck or van injured in collision with pedestrian or animal in traffic accident ▽

√4ᵗʰ **V51** Occupant of pick-up truck or van injured in collision with pedal cycle

√x7ᵗʰ **V51.0** Driver of pick-up truck or van injured in collision with pedal cycle in nontraffic accident

√x7ᵗʰ **V51.1** Passenger in pick-up truck or van injured in collision with pedal cycle in nontraffic accident

√x7ᵗʰ **V51.2** Person on outside of pick-up truck or van injured in collision with pedal cycle in nontraffic accident

√x7ᵗʰ **V51.3** Unspecified occupant of pick-up truck or van injured in collision with pedal cycle in nontraffic accident ▽

√x7ᵗʰ **V51.4** Person boarding or alighting a pick-up truck or van injured in collision with pedal cycle

√x7ᵗʰ **V51.5** Driver of pick-up truck or van injured in collision with pedal cycle in traffic accident

√x7ᵗʰ **V51.6** Passenger in pick-up truck or van injured in collision with pedal cycle in traffic accident

√x7ᵗʰ **V51.7** Person on outside of pick-up truck or van injured in collision with pedal cycle in traffic accident

√x7ᵗʰ **V51.9** Unspecified occupant of pick-up truck or van injured in collision with pedal cycle in traffic accident ▽

√4ᵗʰ **V52** Occupant of pick-up truck or van injured in collision with two- or three-wheeled motor vehicle

√x7ᵗʰ **V52.0** Driver of pick-up truck or van injured in collision with two- or three-wheeled motor vehicle in nontraffic accident

√x7ᵗʰ **V52.1** Passenger in pick-up truck or van injured in collision with two- or three-wheeled motor vehicle in nontraffic accident

√x7ᵗʰ **V52.2** Person on outside of pick-up truck or van injured in collision with two- or three-wheeled motor vehicle in nontraffic accident

√x7ᵗʰ **V52.3** Unspecified occupant of pick-up truck or van injured in collision with two- or three-wheeled motor vehicle in nontraffic accident ▽

√x7ᵗʰ **V52.4** Person boarding or alighting a pick-up truck or van injured in collision with two- or three-wheeled motor vehicle

√x7ᵗʰ **V52.5** Driver of pick-up truck or van injured in collision with two- or three-wheeled motor vehicle in traffic accident

√x7ᵗʰ **V52.6** Passenger in pick-up truck or van injured in collision with two- or three-wheeled motor vehicle in traffic accident

√x7ᵗʰ **V52.7** Person on outside of pick-up truck or van injured in collision with two- or three-wheeled motor vehicle in traffic accident

√x7ᵗʰ **V52.9** Unspecified occupant of pick-up truck or van injured in collision with two- or three-wheeled motor vehicle in traffic accident ▽

√4ᵗʰ **V53** Occupant of pick-up truck or van injured in collision with car, pick-up truck or van

√x7ᵗʰ **V53.0** Driver of pick-up truck or van injured in collision with car, pick-up truck or van in nontraffic accident

√x7ᵗʰ **V53.1** Passenger in pick-up truck or van injured in collision with car, pick-up truck or van in nontraffic accident

√x7ᵗʰ **V53.2** Person on outside of pick-up truck or van injured in collision with car, pick-up truck or van in nontraffic accident

√x7ᵗʰ **V53.3** Unspecified occupant of pick-up truck or van injured in collision with car, pick-up truck or van in nontraffic accident ▽

√x7ᵗʰ **V53.4** Person boarding or alighting a pick-up truck or van injured in collision with car, pick-up truck or van

√x7ᵗʰ **V53.5** Driver of pick-up truck or van injured in collision with car, pick-up truck or van in traffic accident

√x7ᵗʰ **V53.6** Passenger in pick-up truck or van injured in collision with car, pick-up truck or van in traffic accident

√x7ᵗʰ **V53.7** Person on outside of pick-up truck or van injured in collision with car, pick-up truck or van in traffic accident

√x7ᵗʰ **V53.9** Unspecified occupant of pick-up truck or van injured in collision with car, pick-up truck or van in traffic accident ▽

√4ᵗʰ **V54** Occupant of pick-up truck or van injured in collision with heavy transport vehicle or bus

  EXCLUDES 1   *occupant of pick-up truck or van injured in collision with military vehicle (V59.81)*

√x7ᵗʰ **V54.0** Driver of pick-up truck or van injured in collision with heavy transport vehicle or bus in nontraffic accident

√x7ᵗʰ **V54.1** Passenger in pick-up truck or van injured in collision with heavy transport vehicle or bus in nontraffic accident

√x7ᵗʰ **V54.2** Person on outside of pick-up truck or van injured in collision with heavy transport vehicle or bus in nontraffic accident

√x7ᵗʰ **V54.3** Unspecified occupant of pick-up truck or van injured in collision with heavy transport vehicle or bus in nontraffic accident ▽

√x7ᵗʰ **V54.4** Person boarding or alighting a pick-up truck or van injured in collision with heavy transport vehicle or bus

√x7ᵗʰ **V54.5** Driver of pick-up truck or van injured in collision with heavy transport vehicle or bus in traffic accident

√x7ᵗʰ **V54.6** Passenger in pick-up truck or van injured in collision with heavy transport vehicle or bus in traffic accident

√x7ᵗʰ **V54.7** Person on outside of pick-up truck or van injured in collision with heavy transport vehicle or bus in traffic accident

√x7ᵗʰ **V54.9** Unspecified occupant of pick-up truck or van injured in collision with heavy transport vehicle or bus in traffic accident ▽

√4ᵗʰ **V55** Occupant of pick-up truck or van injured in collision with railway train or railway vehicle

√x7ᵗʰ **V55.0** Driver of pick-up truck or van injured in collision with railway train or railway vehicle in nontraffic accident

√x7ᵗʰ **V55.1** Passenger in pick-up truck or van injured in collision with railway train or railway vehicle in nontraffic accident

√x7ᵗʰ **V55.2** Person on outside of pick-up truck or van injured in collision with railway train or railway vehicle in nontraffic accident

√x7ᵗʰ **V55.3** Unspecified occupant of pick-up truck or van injured in collision with railway train or railway vehicle in nontraffic accident ▽

√x7ᵗʰ **V55.4** Person boarding or alighting a pick-up truck or van injured in collision with railway train or railway vehicle

√x7ᵗʰ **V55.5** Driver of pick-up truck or van injured in collision with railway train or railway vehicle in traffic accident

√x7ᵗʰ **V55.6** Passenger in pick-up truck or van injured in collision with railway train or railway vehicle in traffic accident

√x7ᵗʰ **V55.7** Person on outside of pick-up truck or van injured in collision with railway train or railway vehicle in traffic accident

---

✓ Additional Character Req   √x7ᵗʰ Placeholder Alert   Manifestation   ▽ Unspecified   ►◄ Revised Text   ● New Code   ▲ Revised Code Title

√x7th **V55.9** **Unspecified occupant** of pick-up truck or van injured in collision with railway train or railway vehicle in traffic accident ▽

√4th **V56** **Occupant of pick-up truck or van injured in collision with other nonmotor vehicle**
> INCLUDES   collision with animal-drawn vehicle, animal being ridden, streetcar

√x7th **V56.0** **Driver** of pick-up truck or van injured in collision with other nonmotor vehicle in nontraffic accident

√x7th **V56.1** **Passenger** in pick-up truck or van injured in collision with other nonmotor vehicle in nontraffic accident

√x7th **V56.2** **Person on outside** of pick-up truck or van injured in collision with other nonmotor vehicle in nontraffic accident

√x7th **V56.3** **Unspecified occupant** of pick-up truck or van injured in collision with other nonmotor vehicle in nontraffic accident ▽

√x7th **V56.4** **Person boarding or alighting** a pick-up truck or van injured in collision with other nonmotor vehicle

√x7th **V56.5** **Driver** of pick-up truck or van injured in collision with other nonmotor vehicle in traffic accident

√x7th **V56.6** **Passenger** in pick-up truck or van injured in collision with other nonmotor vehicle in traffic accident

√x7th **V56.7** **Person on outside** of pick-up truck or van injured in collision with other nonmotor vehicle in traffic accident

√x7th **V56.9** **Unspecified occupant** of pick-up truck or van injured in collision with other nonmotor vehicle in traffic accident ▽

√4th **V57** **Occupant of pick-up truck or van injured in collision with fixed or stationary object**

√x7th **V57.0** **Driver** of pick-up truck or van injured in collision with fixed or stationary object in nontraffic accident

√x7th **V57.1** **Passenger** in pick-up truck or van injured in collision with fixed or stationary object in nontraffic accident

√x7th **V57.2** **Person on outside** of pick-up truck or van injured in collision with fixed or stationary object in nontraffic accident

√x7th **V57.3** **Unspecified occupant** of pick-up truck or van injured in collision with fixed or stationary object in nontraffic accident ▽

√x7th **V57.4** **Person boarding or alighting** a pick-up truck or van injured in collision with fixed or stationary object

√x7th **V57.5** **Driver** of pick-up truck or van injured in collision with fixed or stationary object in traffic accident

√x7th **V57.6** **Passenger** in pick-up truck or van injured in collision with fixed or stationary object in traffic accident

√x7th **V57.7** **Person on outside** of pick-up truck or van injured in collision with fixed or stationary object in traffic accident

√x7th **V57.9** **Unspecified occupant** of pick-up truck or van injured in collision with fixed or stationary object in traffic accident ▽

√4th **V58** **Occupant of pick-up truck or van injured in noncollision transport accident**
> INCLUDES   overturning pick-up truck or van NOS
> overturning pick-up truck or van without collision

√x7th **V58.0** **Driver** of pick-up truck or van injured in noncollision transport accident in nontraffic accident

√x7th **V58.1** **Passenger** in pick-up truck or van injured in noncollision transport accident in nontraffic accident

√x7th **V58.2** **Person on outside** of pick-up truck or van injured in noncollision transport accident in nontraffic accident

√x7th **V58.3** **Unspecified occupant** of pick-up truck or van injured in noncollision transport accident in nontraffic accident ▽

√x7th **V58.4** **Person boarding or alighting** a pick-up truck or van injured in noncollision transport accident

√x7th **V58.5** **Driver** of pick-up truck or van injured in noncollision transport accident in traffic accident

√x7th **V58.6** **Passenger** in pick-up truck or van injured in noncollision transport accident in traffic accident

√x7th **V58.7** **Person on outside** of pick-up truck or van injured in noncollision transport accident in traffic accident

√x7th **V58.9** **Unspecified occupant** of pick-up truck or van injured in noncollision transport accident in traffic accident ▽

√4th **V59** **Occupant of pick-up truck or van injured in other and unspecified transport accidents**

√5th **V59.0** **Driver** of pick-up truck or van injured in collision with other and unspecified motor vehicles in nontraffic accident

√x7th   **V59.00** **Driver** of pick-up truck or van injured in collision with unspecified motor vehicles in nontraffic accident ▽

√x7th   **V59.09** **Driver** of pick-up truck or van injured in collision with other motor vehicles in nontraffic accident

√5th **V59.1** **Passenger** in pick-up truck or van injured in collision with other and unspecified motor vehicles in nontraffic accident

√x7th   **V59.10** **Passenger** in pick-up truck or van injured in collision with unspecified motor vehicles in nontraffic accident ▽

√x7th   **V59.19** **Passenger** in pick-up truck or van injured in collision with other motor vehicles in nontraffic accident

√5th **V59.2** **Unspecified occupant** of pick-up truck or van injured in collision with other and unspecified motor vehicles in nontraffic accident

√x7th   **V59.20** **Unspecified occupant** of pick-up truck or van injured in collision with unspecified motor vehicles in nontraffic accident ▽
> Collision NOS involving pick-up truck or van, nontraffic

√x7th   **V59.29** **Unspecified occupant** of pick-up truck or van injured in collision with other motor vehicles in nontraffic accident ▽

√x7th **V59.3** **Occupant (driver) (passenger)** of pick-up truck or van injured in unspecified nontraffic accident ▽
> Accident NOS involving pick-up truck or van, nontraffic
> Occupant of pick-up truck or van injured in nontraffic accident NOS

√5th **V59.4** **Driver** of pick-up truck or van injured in collision with other and unspecified motor vehicles in traffic accident

√x7th   **V59.40** **Driver** of pick-up truck or van injured in collision with unspecified motor vehicles in traffic accident ▽

√x7th   **V59.49** **Driver** of pick-up truck or van injured in collision with other motor vehicles in traffic accident

√5th **V59.5** **Passenger** in pick-up truck or van injured in collision with other and unspecified motor vehicles in traffic accident

√x7th   **V59.50** **Passenger** in pick-up truck or van injured in collision with unspecified motor vehicles in traffic accident ▽

√x7th   **V59.59** **Passenger** in pick-up truck or van injured in collision with other motor vehicles in traffic accident

√5th **V59.6** **Unspecified occupant** of pick-up truck or van injured in collision with other and unspecified motor vehicles in traffic accident

√x7th   **V59.60** **Unspecified occupant** of pick-up truck or van injured in collision with unspecified motor vehicles in traffic accident ▽
> Collision NOS involving pick-up truck or van (traffic)

√x7th   **V59.69** **Unspecified occupant** of pick-up truck or van injured in collision with other motor vehicles in traffic accident ▽

√5th **V59.8** **Occupant (driver) (passenger)** of pick-up truck or van injured in other specified transport accidents

√x7th   **V59.81** **Occupant (driver) (passenger)** of pick-up truck or van injured in transport accident with military vehicle

√x7th   **V59.88** **Occupant (driver) (passenger)** of pick-up truck or van injured in other specified transport accidents

√x7th **V59.9** **Occupant (driver) (passenger)** of pick-up truck or van injured in unspecified traffic accident ▽
> Accident NOS involving pick-up truck or van

Occupant of heavy transport vehicle injured in transport accident (V60-V69)

> INCLUDES   18 wheeler
> armored car
> panel truck
> EXCLUDES 1   *bus*
> *motorcoach*

The appropriate 7th character is to be added to each code from categories V60-V69.
A   initial encounter
D   subsequent encounter
S   sequela

√4th **V60** **Occupant of heavy transport vehicle injured in collision with pedestrian or animal**
> EXCLUDES 1   *heavy transport vehicle collision with animal-drawn vehicle or animal being ridden (V66.-)*

√x7th **V60.0** **Driver** of heavy transport vehicle injured in collision with pedestrian or animal in nontraffic accident

√x7th **V60.1** **Passenger** in heavy transport vehicle injured in collision with pedestrian or animal in nontraffic accident

√x7th **V60.2** **Person on outside** of heavy transport vehicle injured in collision with pedestrian or animal in nontraffic accident

√x7ᵗʰ **V60.3** Unspecified occupant of heavy transport vehicle injured in collision with pedestrian or animal in nontraffic accident ▽

√x7ᵗʰ **V60.4** Person boarding or alighting a heavy transport vehicle injured in collision with pedestrian or animal

√x7ᵗʰ **V60.5** Driver of heavy transport vehicle injured in collision with pedestrian or animal in traffic accident

√x7ᵗʰ **V60.6** Passenger in heavy transport vehicle injured in collision with pedestrian or animal in traffic accident

√x7ᵗʰ **V60.7** Person on outside of heavy transport vehicle injured in collision with pedestrian or animal in traffic accident

√x7ᵗʰ **V60.9** Unspecified occupant of heavy transport vehicle injured in collision with pedestrian or animal in traffic accident ▽

√4ᵗʰ **V61** Occupant of heavy transport vehicle injured in collision with pedal cycle

√x7ᵗʰ **V61.0** Driver of heavy transport vehicle injured in collision with pedal cycle in nontraffic accident

√x7ᵗʰ **V61.1** Passenger in heavy transport vehicle injured in collision with pedal cycle in nontraffic accident

√x7ᵗʰ **V61.2** Person on outside of heavy transport vehicle injured in collision with pedal cycle in nontraffic accident

√x7ᵗʰ **V61.3** Unspecified occupant of heavy transport vehicle injured in collision with pedal cycle in nontraffic accident ▽

√x7ᵗʰ **V61.4** Person boarding or alighting a heavy transport vehicle injured in collision with pedal cycle while boarding or alighting

√x7ᵗʰ **V61.5** Driver of heavy transport vehicle injured in collision with pedal cycle in traffic accident

√x7ᵗʰ **V61.6** Passenger in heavy transport vehicle injured in collision with pedal cycle in traffic accident

√x7ᵗʰ **V61.7** Person on outside of heavy transport vehicle injured in collision with pedal cycle in traffic accident

√x7ᵗʰ **V61.9** Unspecified occupant of heavy transport vehicle injured in collision with pedal cycle in traffic accident ▽

√4ᵗʰ **V62** Occupant of heavy transport vehicle injured in collision with two- or three-wheeled motor vehicle

√x7ᵗʰ **V62.0** Driver of heavy transport vehicle injured in collision with two- or three-wheeled motor vehicle in nontraffic accident

√x7ᵗʰ **V62.1** Passenger in heavy transport vehicle injured in collision with two- or three-wheeled motor vehicle in nontraffic accident

√x7ᵗʰ **V62.2** Person on outside of heavy transport vehicle injured in collision with two- or three-wheeled motor vehicle in nontraffic accident

√x7ᵗʰ **V62.3** Unspecified occupant of heavy transport vehicle injured in collision with two- or three-wheeled motor vehicle in nontraffic accident ▽

√x7ᵗʰ **V62.4** Person boarding or alighting a heavy transport vehicle injured in collision with two- or three-wheeled motor vehicle

√x7ᵗʰ **V62.5** Driver of heavy transport vehicle injured in collision with two- or three-wheeled motor vehicle in traffic accident

√x7ᵗʰ **V62.6** Passenger in heavy transport vehicle injured in collision with two- or three-wheeled motor vehicle in traffic accident

√x7ᵗʰ **V62.7** Person on outside of heavy transport vehicle injured in collision with two- or three-wheeled motor vehicle in traffic accident

√x7ᵗʰ **V62.9** Unspecified occupant of heavy transport vehicle injured in collision with two- or three-wheeled motor vehicle in traffic accident ▽

√4ᵗʰ **V63** Occupant of heavy transport vehicle injured in collision with car, pick-up truck or van

√x7ᵗʰ **V63.0** Driver of heavy transport vehicle injured in collision with car, pick-up truck or van in nontraffic accident

√x7ᵗʰ **V63.1** Passenger in heavy transport vehicle injured in collision with car, pick-up truck or van in nontraffic accident

√x7ᵗʰ **V63.2** Person on outside of heavy transport vehicle injured in collision with car, pick-up truck or van in nontraffic accident

√x7ᵗʰ **V63.3** Unspecified occupant of heavy transport vehicle injured in collision with car, pick-up truck or van in nontraffic accident ▽

√x7ᵗʰ **V63.4** Person boarding or alighting a heavy transport vehicle injured in collision with car, pick-up truck or van

√x7ᵗʰ **V63.5** Driver of heavy transport vehicle injured in collision with car, pick-up truck or van in traffic accident

√x7ᵗʰ **V63.6** Passenger in heavy transport vehicle injured in collision with car, pick-up truck or van in traffic accident

√x7ᵗʰ **V63.7** Person on outside of heavy transport vehicle injured in collision with car, pick-up truck or van in traffic accident

√x7ᵗʰ **V63.9** Unspecified occupant of heavy transport vehicle injured in collision with car, pick-up truck or van in traffic accident ▽

√4ᵗʰ **V64** Occupant of heavy transport vehicle injured in collision with heavy transport vehicle or bus
> EXCLUDES 1 occupant of heavy transport vehicle injured in collision with military vehicle (V69.81)

√x7ᵗʰ **V64.0** Driver of heavy transport vehicle injured in collision with heavy transport vehicle or bus in nontraffic accident

√x7ᵗʰ **V64.1** Passenger in heavy transport vehicle injured in collision with heavy transport vehicle or bus in nontraffic accident

√x7ᵗʰ **V64.2** Person on outside of heavy transport vehicle injured in collision with heavy transport vehicle or bus in nontraffic accident

√x7ᵗʰ **V64.3** Unspecified occupant of heavy transport vehicle injured in collision with heavy transport vehicle or bus in nontraffic accident ▽

√x7ᵗʰ **V64.4** Person boarding or alighting a heavy transport vehicle injured in collision with heavy transport vehicle or bus while boarding or alighting

√x7ᵗʰ **V64.5** Driver of heavy transport vehicle injured in collision with heavy transport vehicle or bus in traffic accident

√x7ᵗʰ **V64.6** Passenger in heavy transport vehicle injured in collision with heavy transport vehicle or bus in traffic accident

√x7ᵗʰ **V64.7** Person on outside of heavy transport vehicle injured in collision with heavy transport vehicle or bus in traffic accident

√x7ᵗʰ **V64.9** Unspecified occupant of heavy transport vehicle injured in collision with heavy transport vehicle or bus in traffic accident ▽

√4ᵗʰ **V65** Occupant of heavy transport vehicle injured in collision with railway train or railway vehicle

√x7ᵗʰ **V65.0** Driver of heavy transport vehicle injured in collision with railway train or railway vehicle in nontraffic accident

√x7ᵗʰ **V65.1** Passenger in heavy transport vehicle injured in collision with railway train or railway vehicle in nontraffic accident

√x7ᵗʰ **V65.2** Person on outside of heavy transport vehicle injured in collision with railway train or railway vehicle in nontraffic accident

√x7ᵗʰ **V65.3** Unspecified occupant of heavy transport vehicle injured in collision with railway train or railway vehicle in nontraffic accident ▽

√x7ᵗʰ **V65.4** Person boarding or alighting a heavy transport vehicle injured in collision with railway train or railway vehicle

√x7ᵗʰ **V65.5** Driver of heavy transport vehicle injured in collision with railway train or railway vehicle in traffic accident

√x7ᵗʰ **V65.6** Passenger in heavy transport vehicle injured in collision with railway train or railway vehicle in traffic accident

√x7ᵗʰ **V65.7** Person on outside of heavy transport vehicle injured in collision with railway train or railway vehicle in traffic accident

√x7ᵗʰ **V65.9** Unspecified occupant of heavy transport vehicle injured in collision with railway train or railway vehicle in traffic accident ▽

√4ᵗʰ **V66** Occupant of heavy transport vehicle injured in collision with other nonmotor vehicle
> INCLUDES collision with animal-drawn vehicle, animal being ridden, streetcar

√x7ᵗʰ **V66.0** Driver of heavy transport vehicle injured in collision with other nonmotor vehicle in nontraffic accident

√x7ᵗʰ **V66.1** Passenger in heavy transport vehicle injured in collision with other nonmotor vehicle in nontraffic accident

√x7ᵗʰ **V66.2** Person on outside of heavy transport vehicle injured in collision with other nonmotor vehicle in nontraffic accident

√x7ᵗʰ **V66.3** Unspecified occupant of heavy transport vehicle injured in collision with other nonmotor vehicle in nontraffic accident ▽

√x7ᵗʰ **V66.4** Person boarding or alighting a heavy transport vehicle injured in collision with other nonmotor vehicle

√x7ᵗʰ **V66.5** Driver of heavy transport vehicle injured in collision with other nonmotor vehicle in traffic accident

√x7ᵗʰ **V66.6** Passenger in heavy transport vehicle injured in collision with other nonmotor vehicle in traffic accident

√x7ᵗʰ **V66.7** Person on outside of heavy transport vehicle injured in collision with other nonmotor vehicle in traffic accident

√x7ᵗʰ **V66.9** Unspecified occupant of heavy transport vehicle injured in collision with other nonmotor vehicle in traffic accident ▽

Chapter 20. External Causes of Morbidity (side tab)

V67–V71.5 (side tab)

✓4ᵗʰ **V67** **Occupant of heavy transport vehicle injured in collision with fixed or stationary object**

✓x7ᵗʰ **V67.Ø** Driver of heavy transport vehicle injured in collision with fixed or stationary object in nontraffic accident

✓x7ᵗʰ **V67.1** Passenger in heavy transport vehicle injured in collision with fixed or stationary object in nontraffic accident

✓x7ᵗʰ **V67.2** Person on outside of heavy transport vehicle injured in collision with fixed or stationary object in nontraffic accident

✓x7ᵗʰ **V67.3** Unspecified occupant of heavy transport vehicle injured in collision with fixed or stationary object in nontraffic accident ▽

✓x7ᵗʰ **V67.4** Person boarding or alighting a heavy transport vehicle injured in collision with fixed or stationary object

✓x7ᵗʰ **V67.5** Driver of heavy transport vehicle injured in collision with fixed or stationary object in traffic accident

✓x7ᵗʰ **V67.6** Passenger in heavy transport vehicle injured in collision with fixed or stationary object in traffic accident

✓x7ᵗʰ **V67.7** Person on outside of heavy transport vehicle injured in collision with fixed or stationary object in traffic accident

✓x7ᵗʰ **V67.9** Unspecified occupant of heavy transport vehicle injured in collision with fixed or stationary object in traffic accident ▽

✓4ᵗʰ **V68** **Occupant of heavy transport vehicle injured in noncollision transport accident**

   INCLUDES   overturning heavy transport vehicle NOS
          overturning heavy transport vehicle without collision

✓x7ᵗʰ **V68.Ø** Driver of heavy transport vehicle injured in noncollision transport accident in nontraffic accident

✓x7ᵗʰ **V68.1** Passenger in heavy transport vehicle injured in noncollision transport accident in nontraffic accident

✓x7ᵗʰ **V68.2** Person on outside of heavy transport vehicle injured in noncollision transport accident in nontraffic accident

✓x7ᵗʰ **V68.3** Unspecified occupant of heavy transport vehicle injured in noncollision transport accident in nontraffic accident ▽

✓x7ᵗʰ **V68.4** Person boarding or alighting a heavy transport vehicle injured in noncollision transport accident

✓x7ᵗʰ **V68.5** Driver of heavy transport vehicle injured in noncollision transport accident in traffic accident

✓x7ᵗʰ **V68.6** Passenger in heavy transport vehicle injured in noncollision transport accident in traffic accident

✓x7ᵗʰ **V68.7** Person on outside of heavy transport vehicle injured in noncollision transport accident in traffic accident

✓x7ᵗʰ **V68.9** Unspecified occupant of heavy transport vehicle injured in noncollision transport accident in traffic accident ▽

✓4ᵗʰ **V69** **Occupant of heavy transport vehicle injured in other and unspecified transport accidents**

✓5ᵗʰ **V69.Ø** Driver of heavy transport vehicle injured in collision with other and unspecified motor vehicles in nontraffic accident

✓x7ᵗʰ **V69.ØØ** Driver of heavy transport vehicle injured in collision with unspecified motor vehicles in nontraffic accident ▽

✓x7ᵗʰ **V69.Ø9** Driver of heavy transport vehicle injured in collision with other motor vehicles in nontraffic accident

✓5ᵗʰ **V69.1** Passenger in heavy transport vehicle injured in collision with other and unspecified motor vehicles in nontraffic accident

✓x7ᵗʰ **V69.1Ø** Passenger in heavy transport vehicle injured in collision with unspecified motor vehicles in nontraffic accident ▽

✓x7ᵗʰ **V69.19** Passenger in heavy transport vehicle injured in collision with other motor vehicles in nontraffic accident

✓5ᵗʰ **V69.2** Unspecified occupant of heavy transport vehicle injured in collision with other and unspecified motor vehicles in nontraffic accident

✓x7ᵗʰ **V69.2Ø** Unspecified occupant of heavy transport vehicle injured in collision with unspecified motor vehicles in nontraffic accident ▽
        Collision NOS involving heavy transport vehicle, nontraffic

✓x7ᵗʰ **V69.29** Unspecified occupant of heavy transport vehicle injured in collision with other motor vehicles in nontraffic accident ▽

✓x7ᵗʰ **V69.3** Occupant (driver) (passenger) of heavy transport vehicle injured in unspecified nontraffic accident ▽
        Accident NOS involving heavy transport vehicle, nontraffic
        Occupant of heavy transport vehicle injured in nontraffic accident NOS

✓5ᵗʰ **V69.4** Driver of heavy transport vehicle injured in collision with other and unspecified motor vehicles in traffic accident

✓x7ᵗʰ **V69.4Ø** Driver of heavy transport vehicle injured in collision with unspecified motor vehicles in traffic accident ▽

✓x7ᵗʰ **V69.49** Driver of heavy transport vehicle injured in collision with other motor vehicles in traffic accident

✓5ᵗʰ **V69.5** Passenger in heavy transport vehicle injured in collision with other and unspecified motor vehicles in traffic accident

✓x7ᵗʰ **V69.5Ø** Passenger in heavy transport vehicle injured in collision with unspecified motor vehicles in traffic accident ▽

✓x7ᵗʰ **V69.59** Passenger in heavy transport vehicle injured in collision with other motor vehicles in traffic accident

✓5ᵗʰ **V69.6** Unspecified occupant of heavy transport vehicle injured in collision with other and unspecified motor vehicles in traffic accident

✓x7ᵗʰ **V69.6Ø** Unspecified occupant of heavy transport vehicle injured in collision with unspecified motor vehicles in traffic accident ▽
        Collision NOS involving heavy transport vehicle (traffic)

✓x7ᵗʰ **V69.69** Unspecified occupant of heavy transport vehicle injured in collision with other motor vehicles in traffic accident ▽

✓5ᵗʰ **V69.8** Occupant (driver) (passenger) of heavy transport vehicle injured in other specified transport accidents

✓x7ᵗʰ **V69.81** Occupant (driver) (passenger) of heavy transport vehicle injured in transport accidents with military vehicle

✓x7ᵗʰ **V69.88** Occupant (driver) (passenger) of heavy transport vehicle injured in other specified transport accidents

✓x7ᵗʰ **V69.9** Occupant (driver) (passenger) of heavy transport vehicle injured in unspecified traffic accident ▽
        Accident NOS involving heavy transport vehicle

Bus occupant injured in transport accident (V7Ø-V79)

INCLUDES   motorcoach
EXCLUDES 1   minibus (V5Ø-V59)

The appropriate 7th character is to be added to each code from categories V7Ø-V79.
A   initial encounter
D   subsequent encounter
S   sequela

✓4ᵗʰ **V7Ø** **Bus occupant injured in collision with pedestrian or animal**

   EXCLUDES 1   bus collision with animal-drawn vehicle or animal being ridden (V76.-)

✓x7ᵗʰ **V7Ø.Ø** Driver of bus injured in collision with pedestrian or animal in nontraffic accident

✓x7ᵗʰ **V7Ø.1** Passenger on bus injured in collision with pedestrian or animal in nontraffic accident

✓x7ᵗʰ **V7Ø.2** Person on outside of bus injured in collision with pedestrian or animal in nontraffic accident

✓x7ᵗʰ **V7Ø.3** Unspecified occupant of bus injured in collision with pedestrian or animal in nontraffic accident ▽

✓x7ᵗʰ **V7Ø.4** Person boarding or alighting from bus injured in collision with pedestrian or animal

✓x7ᵗʰ **V7Ø.5** Driver of bus injured in collision with pedestrian or animal in traffic accident

✓x7ᵗʰ **V7Ø.6** Passenger on bus injured in collision with pedestrian or animal in traffic accident

✓x7ᵗʰ **V7Ø.7** Person on outside of bus injured in collision with pedestrian or animal in traffic accident

✓x7ᵗʰ **V7Ø.9** Unspecified occupant of bus injured in collision with pedestrian or animal in traffic accident ▽

✓4ᵗʰ **V71** **Bus occupant injured in collision with pedal cycle**

✓x7ᵗʰ **V71.Ø** Driver of bus injured in collision with pedal cycle in nontraffic accident

✓x7ᵗʰ **V71.1** Passenger on bus injured in collision with pedal cycle in nontraffic accident

✓x7ᵗʰ **V71.2** Person on outside of bus injured in collision with pedal cycle in nontraffic accident

✓x7ᵗʰ **V71.3** Unspecified occupant of bus injured in collision with pedal cycle in nontraffic accident ▽

✓x7ᵗʰ **V71.4** Person boarding or alighting from bus injured in collision with pedal cycle

✓x7ᵗʰ **V71.5** Driver of bus injured in collision with pedal cycle in traffic accident

✓x7ᵗʰ **V71.6** Passenger on bus injured in collision with pedal cycle in traffic accident

✓x7ᵗʰ **V71.7** Person on outside of bus injured in collision with pedal cycle in traffic accident

✓x7ᵗʰ **V71.9** Unspecified occupant of bus injured in collision with pedal cycle in traffic accident   ▽

✓4ᵗʰ **V72** Bus occupant injured in collision with two- or three-wheeled motor vehicle

✓x7ᵗʰ **V72.0** Driver of bus injured in collision with two- or three-wheeled motor vehicle in nontraffic accident

✓x7ᵗʰ **V72.1** Passenger on bus injured in collision with two- or three-wheeled motor vehicle in nontraffic accident

✓x7ᵗʰ **V72.2** Person on outside of bus injured in collision with two- or three-wheeled motor vehicle in nontraffic accident

✓x7ᵗʰ **V72.3** Unspecified occupant of bus injured in collision with two- or three-wheeled motor vehicle in nontraffic accident   ▽

✓x7ᵗʰ **V72.4** Person boarding or alighting from bus injured in collision with two- or three-wheeled motor vehicle

✓x7ᵗʰ **V72.5** Driver of bus injured in collision with two- or three-wheeled motor vehicle in traffic accident

✓x7ᵗʰ **V72.6** Passenger on bus injured in collision with two- or three-wheeled motor vehicle in traffic accident

✓x7ᵗʰ **V72.7** Person on outside of bus injured in collision with two- or three-wheeled motor vehicle in traffic accident

✓x7ᵗʰ **V72.9** Unspecified occupant of bus injured in collision with two- or three-wheeled motor vehicle in traffic accident   ▽

✓4ᵗʰ **V73** Bus occupant injured in collision with car, pick-up truck or van

✓x7ᵗʰ **V73.0** Driver of bus injured in collision with car, pick-up truck or van in nontraffic accident

✓x7ᵗʰ **V73.1** Passenger on bus injured in collision with car, pick-up truck or van in nontraffic accident

✓x7ᵗʰ **V73.2** Person on outside of bus injured in collision with car, pick-up truck or van in nontraffic accident

✓x7ᵗʰ **V73.3** Unspecified occupant of bus injured in collision with car, pick-up truck or van in nontraffic accident   ▽

✓x7ᵗʰ **V73.4** Person boarding or alighting from bus injured in collision with car, pick-up truck or van

✓x7ᵗʰ **V73.5** Driver of bus injured in collision with car, pick-up truck or van in traffic accident

✓x7ᵗʰ **V73.6** Passenger on bus injured in collision with car, pick-up truck or van in traffic accident

✓x7ᵗʰ **V73.7** Person on outside of bus injured in collision with car, pick-up truck or van in traffic accident

✓x7ᵗʰ **V73.9** Unspecified occupant of bus injured in collision with car, pick-up truck or van in traffic accident   ▽

✓4ᵗʰ **V74** Bus occupant injured in collision with heavy transport vehicle or bus

EXCLUDES 1   *bus occupant injured in collision with military vehicle (V79.81)*

✓x7ᵗʰ **V74.0** Driver of bus injured in collision with heavy transport vehicle or bus in nontraffic accident

✓x7ᵗʰ **V74.1** Passenger on bus injured in collision with heavy transport vehicle or bus in nontraffic accident

✓x7ᵗʰ **V74.2** Person on outside of bus injured in collision with heavy transport vehicle or bus in nontraffic accident

✓x7ᵗʰ **V74.3** Unspecified occupant of bus injured in collision with heavy transport vehicle or bus in nontraffic accident   ▽

✓x7ᵗʰ **V74.4** Person boarding or alighting from bus injured in collision with heavy transport vehicle or bus

✓x7ᵗʰ **V74.5** Driver of bus injured in collision with heavy transport vehicle or bus in traffic accident

✓x7ᵗʰ **V74.6** Passenger on bus injured in collision with heavy transport vehicle or bus in traffic accident

✓x7ᵗʰ **V74.7** Person on outside of bus injured in collision with heavy transport vehicle or bus in traffic accident

✓x7ᵗʰ **V74.9** Unspecified occupant of bus injured in collision with heavy transport vehicle or bus in traffic accident   ▽

✓4ᵗʰ **V75** Bus occupant injured in collision with railway train or railway vehicle

✓x7ᵗʰ **V75.0** Driver of bus injured in collision with railway train or railway vehicle in nontraffic accident

✓x7ᵗʰ **V75.1** Passenger on bus injured in collision with railway train or railway vehicle in nontraffic accident

✓x7ᵗʰ **V75.2** Person on outside of bus injured in collision with railway train or railway vehicle in nontraffic accident

✓x7ᵗʰ **V75.3** Unspecified occupant of bus injured in collision with railway train or railway vehicle in nontraffic accident   ▽

✓x7ᵗʰ **V75.4** Person boarding or alighting from bus injured in collision with railway train or railway vehicle

✓x7ᵗʰ **V75.5** Driver of bus injured in collision with railway train or railway vehicle in traffic accident

✓x7ᵗʰ **V75.6** Passenger on bus injured in collision with railway train or railway vehicle in traffic accident

✓x7ᵗʰ **V75.7** Person on outside of bus injured in collision with railway train or railway vehicle in traffic accident

✓x7ᵗʰ **V75.9** Unspecified occupant of bus injured in collision with railway train or railway vehicle in traffic accident   ▽

✓4ᵗʰ **V76** Bus occupant injured in collision with other nonmotor vehicle

INCLUDES   collision with animal-drawn vehicle, animal being ridden, streetcar

✓x7ᵗʰ **V76.0** Driver of bus injured in collision with other nonmotor vehicle in nontraffic accident

✓x7ᵗʰ **V76.1** Passenger on bus injured in collision with other nonmotor vehicle in nontraffic accident

✓x7ᵗʰ **V76.2** Person on outside of bus injured in collision with other nonmotor vehicle in nontraffic accident

✓x7ᵗʰ **V76.3** Unspecified occupant of bus injured in collision with other nonmotor vehicle in nontraffic accident   ▽

✓x7ᵗʰ **V76.4** Person boarding or alighting from bus injured in collision with other nonmotor vehicle

✓x7ᵗʰ **V76.5** Driver of bus injured in collision with other nonmotor vehicle in traffic accident

✓x7ᵗʰ **V76.6** Passenger on bus injured in collision with other nonmotor vehicle in traffic accident

✓x7ᵗʰ **V76.7** Person on outside of bus injured in collision with other nonmotor vehicle in traffic accident

✓x7ᵗʰ **V76.9** Unspecified occupant of bus injured in collision with other nonmotor vehicle in traffic accident   ▽

✓4ᵗʰ **V77** Bus occupant injured in collision with fixed or stationary object

✓x7ᵗʰ **V77.0** Driver of bus injured in collision with fixed or stationary object in nontraffic accident

✓x7ᵗʰ **V77.1** Passenger on bus injured in collision with fixed or stationary object in nontraffic accident

✓x7ᵗʰ **V77.2** Person on outside of bus injured in collision with fixed or stationary object in nontraffic accident

✓x7ᵗʰ **V77.3** Unspecified occupant of bus injured in collision with fixed or stationary object in nontraffic accident   ▽

✓x7ᵗʰ **V77.4** Person boarding or alighting from bus injured in collision with fixed or stationary object

✓x7ᵗʰ **V77.5** Driver of bus injured in collision with fixed or stationary object in traffic accident

✓x7ᵗʰ **V77.6** Passenger on bus injured in collision with fixed or stationary object in traffic accident

✓x7ᵗʰ **V77.7** Person on outside of bus injured in collision with fixed or stationary object in traffic accident

✓x7ᵗʰ **V77.9** Unspecified occupant of bus injured in collision with fixed or stationary object in traffic accident   ▽

✓4ᵗʰ **V78** Bus occupant injured in noncollision transport accident

INCLUDES   overturning bus NOS

overturning bus without collision

✓x7ᵗʰ **V78.0** Driver of bus injured in noncollision transport accident in nontraffic accident

✓x7ᵗʰ **V78.1** Passenger on bus injured in noncollision transport accident in nontraffic accident

✓x7ᵗʰ **V78.2** Person on outside of bus injured in noncollision transport accident in nontraffic accident

✓x7ᵗʰ **V78.3** Unspecified occupant of bus injured in noncollision transport accident in nontraffic accident   ▽

✓x7ᵗʰ **V78.4** Person boarding or alighting from bus injured in noncollision transport accident

✓x7ᵗʰ **V78.5** Driver of bus injured in noncollision transport accident in traffic accident

✓x7ᵗʰ **V78.6** Passenger on bus injured in noncollision transport accident in traffic accident

✓x7ᵗʰ **V78.7** Person on outside of bus injured in noncollision transport accident in traffic accident

✓x7ᵗʰ **V78.9** Unspecified occupant of bus injured in noncollision transport accident in traffic accident   ▽

✓4ᵗʰ **V79** Bus occupant injured in other and unspecified transport accidents

✓5ᵗʰ **V79.0** Driver of bus injured in collision with other and unspecified motor vehicles in nontraffic accident

✓x7ᵗʰ **V79.00** Driver of bus injured in collision with unspecified motor vehicles in nontraffic accident   ▽

✓x7ᵗʰ **V79.09** Driver of bus injured in collision with other motor vehicles in nontraffic accident

---

✅ Additional Character Req   ✓x7ᵗʰ Placeholder Alert   Manifestation   ▽ Unspecified   ▶◀ Revised Text   ● New Code   ▲ Revised Code Title

Chapter 20. External Causes of Morbidity

V79.1–V80.82

√5ᵗʰ **V79.1** Passenger on bus injured in collision with other and unspecified motor vehicles in nontraffic accident

    √x7ᵗʰ **V79.10** Passenger on bus injured in collision with unspecified motor vehicles in nontraffic accident ▽

    √x7ᵗʰ **V79.19** Passenger on bus injured in collision with other motor vehicles in nontraffic accident

√5ᵗʰ **V79.2** Unspecified bus occupant injured in collision with other and unspecified motor vehicles in nontraffic accident

    √x7ᵗʰ **V79.20** Unspecified bus occupant injured in collision with unspecified motor vehicles in nontraffic accident ▽

        Bus collision NOS, nontraffic

    √x7ᵗʰ **V79.29** Unspecified bus occupant injured in collision with other motor vehicles in nontraffic accident ▽

√5ᵗʰ **V79.3** Bus occupant (driver) (passenger) injured in unspecified nontraffic accident ▽

    Bus accident NOS, nontraffic

    Bus occupant injured in nontraffic accident NOS

√5ᵗʰ **V79.4** Driver of bus injured in collision with other and unspecified motor vehicles in traffic accident

    √x7ᵗʰ **V79.40** Driver of bus injured in collision with unspecified motor vehicles in traffic accident ▽

    √x7ᵗʰ **V79.49** Driver of bus injured in collision with other motor vehicles in traffic accident

√5ᵗʰ **V79.5** Passenger on bus injured in collision with other and unspecified motor vehicles in traffic accident

    √x7ᵗʰ **V79.50** Passenger on bus injured in collision with unspecified motor vehicles in traffic accident ▽

    √x7ᵗʰ **V79.59** Passenger on bus injured in collision with other motor vehicles in traffic accident

√5ᵗʰ **V79.6** Unspecified bus occupant injured in collision with other and unspecified motor vehicles in traffic accident

    √x7ᵗʰ **V79.60** Unspecified bus occupant injured in collision with unspecified motor vehicles in traffic accident ▽

        Bus collision NOS (traffic)

    √x7ᵗʰ **V79.69** Unspecified bus occupant injured in collision with other motor vehicles in traffic accident ▽

√5ᵗʰ **V79.8** Bus occupant (driver) (passenger) injured in other specified transport accidents

    √x7ᵗʰ **V79.81** Bus occupant (driver) (passenger) injured in transport accidents with military vehicle

    √x7ᵗʰ **V79.88** Bus occupant (driver) (passenger) injured in other specified transport accidents

√x7ᵗʰ **V79.9** Bus occupant (driver) (passenger) injured in unspecified traffic accident ▽

    Bus accident NOS

Other land transport accidents (V80-V89)

The appropriate 7th character is to be added to each code from categories V80-V89.
A   initial encounter
D subsequent encounter
S sequela

√4ᵗʰ **V80** Animal-rider or occupant of animal-drawn vehicle injured in transport accident

  √5ᵗʰ **V80.0** Animal-rider or occupant of animal drawn vehicle injured by fall from or being thrown from animal or animal-drawn vehicle in noncollision accident

    √6ᵗʰ **V80.01** Animal-rider injured by fall from or being thrown from animal in noncollision accident

       √7ᵗʰ **V80.010** Animal-rider injured by fall from or being thrown from horse in noncollision accident

       √7ᵗʰ **V80.018** Animal-rider injured by fall from or being thrown from other animal in noncollision accident

    √x7ᵗʰ **V80.02** Occupant of animal-drawn vehicle injured by fall from or being thrown from animal-drawn vehicle in noncollision accident

        Overturning animal-drawn vehicle NOS

        Overturning animal-drawn vehicle without collision

√5ᵗʰ **V80.1** Animal-rider or occupant of animal-drawn vehicle injured in collision with pedestrian or animal

    EXCLUDES 1 animal-rider or animal-drawn vehicle collision with animal-drawn vehicle or animal being ridden (V80.7)

  √x7ᵗʰ **V80.11** Animal-rider injured in collision with pedestrian or animal

  √x7ᵗʰ **V80.12** Occupant of animal-drawn vehicle injured in collision with pedestrian or animal

√5ᵗʰ **V80.2** Animal-rider or occupant of animal-drawn vehicle injured in collision with pedal cycle

  √x7ᵗʰ **V80.21** Animal-rider injured in collision with pedal cycle

  √x7ᵗʰ **V80.22** Occupant of animal-drawn vehicle injured in collision with pedal cycle

√5ᵗʰ **V80.3** Animal-rider or occupant of animal-drawn vehicle injured in collision with two- or three-wheeled motor vehicle

  √x7ᵗʰ **V80.31** Animal-rider injured in collision with two- or three-wheeled motor vehicle

  √x7ᵗʰ **V80.32** Occupant of animal-drawn vehicle injured in collision with two- or three-wheeled motor vehicle

√5ᵗʰ **V80.4** Animal-rider or occupant of animal-drawn vehicle injured in collision with car, pick-up truck, van, heavy transport vehicle or bus

    EXCLUDES 1 animal-rider injured in collision with military vehicle (V80.910)

        occupant of animal-drawn vehicle injured in collision with military vehicle (V80.920)

  √x7ᵗʰ **V80.41** Animal-rider injured in collision with car, pick-up truck, van, heavy transport vehicle or bus

  √x7ᵗʰ **V80.42** Occupant of animal-drawn vehicle injured in collision with car, pick-up truck, van, heavy transport vehicle or bus

√5ᵗʰ **V80.5** Animal-rider or occupant of animal-drawn vehicle injured in collision with other specified motor vehicle

  √x7ᵗʰ **V80.51** Animal-rider injured in collision with other specified motor vehicle

  √x7ᵗʰ **V80.52** Occupant of animal-drawn vehicle injured in collision with other specified motor vehicle

√5ᵗʰ **V80.6** Animal-rider or occupant of animal-drawn vehicle injured in collision with railway train or railway vehicle

  √x7ᵗʰ **V80.61** Animal-rider injured in collision with railway train or railway vehicle

  √x7ᵗʰ **V80.62** Occupant of animal-drawn vehicle injured in collision with railway train or railway vehicle

√5ᵗʰ **V80.7** Animal-rider or occupant of animal-drawn vehicle injured in collision with other nonmotor vehicles

  √6ᵗʰ **V80.71** Animal-rider or occupant of animal-drawn vehicle injured in collision with animal being ridden

    √7ᵗʰ **V80.710** Animal-rider injured in collision with other animal being ridden

    √7ᵗʰ **V80.711** Occupant of animal-drawn vehicle injured in collision with animal being ridden

  √6ᵗʰ **V80.72** Animal-rider or occupant of animal-drawn vehicle injured in collision with other animal-drawn vehicle

    √7ᵗʰ **V80.720** Animal-rider injured in collision with animal-drawn vehicle

    √7ᵗʰ **V80.721** Occupant of animal-drawn vehicle injured in collision with other animal-drawn vehicle

  √6ᵗʰ **V80.73** Animal-rider or occupant of animal-drawn vehicle injured in collision with streetcar

    √7ᵗʰ **V80.730** Animal-rider injured in collision with streetcar

    √7ᵗʰ **V80.731** Occupant of animal-drawn vehicle injured in collision with streetcar

  √6ᵗʰ **V80.79** Animal-rider or occupant of animal-drawn vehicle injured in collision with other nonmotor vehicles

    √7ᵗʰ **V80.790** Animal-rider injured in collision with other nonmotor vehicles

    √7ᵗʰ **V80.791** Occupant of animal-drawn vehicle injured in collision with other nonmotor vehicles

√5ᵗʰ **V80.8** Animal-rider or occupant of animal-drawn vehicle injured in collision with fixed or stationary object

  √x7ᵗʰ **V80.81** Animal-rider injured in collision with fixed or stationary object

  √x7ᵗʰ **V80.82** Occupant of animal-drawn vehicle injured in collision with fixed or stationary object

√5ᵗʰ **V80.9** **Animal-rider or occupant of animal-drawn vehicle injured in other and unspecified transport accidents**

    √6ᵗʰ **V80.91** Animal-rider injured in other and unspecified transport accidents

        √7ᵗʰ **V80.910** Animal-rider injured in transport accident with military vehicle

        √7ᵗʰ **V80.918** Animal-rider injured in other transport accident

        √7ᵗʰ **V80.919** Animal-rider injured in unspecified transport accident   ▽
             Animal rider accident NOS

    √6ᵗʰ **V80.92** Occupant of animal-drawn vehicle injured in other and unspecified transport accidents

        √7ᵗʰ **V80.920** Occupant of animal-drawn vehicle injured in transport accident with military vehicle

        √7ᵗʰ **V80.928** Occupant of animal-drawn vehicle injured in other transport accident

        √7ᵗʰ **V80.929** Occupant of animal-drawn vehicle injured in unspecified transport accident   ▽
             Animal-drawn vehicle accident NOS

√4ᵗʰ **V81** **Occupant of railway train or railway vehicle injured in transport accident**

    INCLUDES   derailment of railway train or railway vehicle
             person on outside of train

    EXCLUDES 1   streetcar (V82.-)

  √x7ᵗʰ **V81.0** **Occupant of railway train or railway vehicle injured in collision with motor vehicle in nontraffic accident**

    EXCLUDES 1   occupant of railway train or railway vehicle injured due to collision with military vehicle (V81.83)

  √x7ᵗʰ **V81.1** **Occupant of railway train or railway vehicle injured in collision with motor vehicle in traffic accident**

    EXCLUDES 1   occupant of railway train or railway vehicle injured due to collision with military vehicle (V81.83)

  √x7ᵗʰ **V81.2** **Occupant of railway train or railway vehicle injured in collision with or hit by rolling stock**

  √x7ᵗʰ **V81.3** **Occupant of railway train or railway vehicle injured in collision with other object**
             Railway collision NOS

  √x7ᵗʰ **V81.4** **Person injured while boarding or alighting from railway train or railway vehicle**

  √x7ᵗʰ **V81.5** **Occupant of railway train or railway vehicle injured by fall in railway train or railway vehicle**

  √x7ᵗʰ **V81.6** **Occupant of railway train or railway vehicle injured by fall from railway train or railway vehicle**

  √x7ᵗʰ **V81.7** **Occupant of railway train or railway vehicle injured in derailment without antecedent collision**

  √5ᵗʰ **V81.8** **Occupant of railway train or railway vehicle injured in other specified railway accidents**

    √x7ᵗʰ **V81.81** Occupant of railway train or railway vehicle injured due to explosion or fire on train

    √x7ᵗʰ **V81.82** Occupant of railway train or railway vehicle injured due to object falling onto train
             Occupant of railway train or railway vehicle injured due to falling earth onto train
             Occupant of railway train or railway vehicle injured due to falling rocks onto train
             Occupant of railway train or railway vehicle injured due to falling snow onto train
             Occupant of railway train or railway vehicle injured due to falling trees onto train

    √x7ᵗʰ **V81.83** Occupant of railway train or railway vehicle injured due to collision with military vehicle

    √x7ᵗʰ **V81.89** Occupant of railway train or railway vehicle injured due to other specified railway accident

  √x7ᵗʰ **V81.9** **Occupant of railway train or railway vehicle injured in unspecified railway accident**   ▽
             Railway accident NOS

√4ᵗʰ **V82** **Occupant of powered streetcar injured in transport accident**

    INCLUDES   interurban electric car
             person on outside of streetcar
             tram (car)
             trolley (car)

    EXCLUDES 1   bus (V70-V79)
             motorcoach (V70-V79)
             nonpowered streetcar (V76.-)
             train (V81.-)

  √x7ᵗʰ **V82.0** **Occupant of streetcar injured in collision with motor vehicle in nontraffic accident**

  √x7ᵗʰ **V82.1** **Occupant of streetcar injured in collision with motor vehicle in traffic accident**

  √x7ᵗʰ **V82.2** **Occupant of streetcar injured in collision with or hit by rolling stock**

  √x7ᵗʰ **V82.3** **Occupant of streetcar injured in collision with other object**
    EXCLUDES 1   collision with animal-drawn vehicle or animal being ridden (V82.8)

  √x7ᵗʰ **V82.4** **Person injured while boarding or alighting from streetcar**

  √x7ᵗʰ **V82.5** **Occupant of streetcar injured by fall in streetcar**
    EXCLUDES 1   fall in streetcar:
                 while boarding or alighting (V82.4)
                 with antecedent collision (V82.0-V82.3)

  √x7ᵗʰ **V82.6** **Occupant of streetcar injured by fall from streetcar**
    EXCLUDES 1   fall from streetcar:
                 while boarding or alighting (V82.4)
                 with antecedent collision (V82.0-V82.3)

  √x7ᵗʰ **V82.7** **Occupant of streetcar injured in derailment without antecedent collision**
    EXCLUDES 1   occupant of streetcar injured in derailment with antecedent collision (V82.0-V82.3)

  √x7ᵗʰ **V82.8** **Occupant of streetcar injured in other specified transport accidents**
             Streetcar collision with military vehicle
             Streetcar collision with train or nonmotor vehicles

  √x7ᵗʰ **V82.9** **Occupant of streetcar injured in unspecified traffic accident**   ▽
             Streetcar accident NOS

√4ᵗʰ **V83** **Occupant of special vehicle mainly used on industrial premises injured in transport accident**

    INCLUDES   battery-powered airport passenger vehicle
             battery-powered truck (baggage) (mail)
             coal-car in mine
             forklift (truck)
             logging car
             self-propelled industrial truck
             station baggage truck (powered)
             tram, truck, or tub (powered) in mine or quarry

    EXCLUDES 1   special construction vehicles (V85.-)
             special industrial vehicle in stationary use or maintenance (W31.-)

  √x7ᵗʰ **V83.0** **Driver of special industrial vehicle injured in traffic accident**

  √x7ᵗʰ **V83.1** **Passenger of special industrial vehicle injured in traffic accident**

  √x7ᵗʰ **V83.2** **Person on outside of special industrial vehicle injured in traffic accident**

  √x7ᵗʰ **V83.3** **Unspecified occupant of special industrial vehicle injured in traffic accident**   ▽

  √x7ᵗʰ **V83.4** **Person injured while boarding or alighting from special industrial vehicle**

  √x7ᵗʰ **V83.5** **Driver of special industrial vehicle injured in nontraffic accident**

  √x7ᵗʰ **V83.6** **Passenger of special industrial vehicle injured in nontraffic accident**

  √x7ᵗʰ **V83.7** **Person on outside of special industrial vehicle injured in nontraffic accident**

  √x7ᵗʰ **V83.9** **Unspecified occupant of special industrial vehicle injured in nontraffic accident**   ▽
             Special-industrial-vehicle accident NOS

√4ᵗʰ **V84** **Occupant of special vehicle mainly used in agriculture injured in transport accident**

    INCLUDES   self-propelled farm machinery
             tractor (and trailer)

    EXCLUDES 1   animal-powered farm machinery accident (W30.8-)
             contact with combine harvester (W30.0)
             special agricultural vehicle in stationary use or maintenance (W30.-)

  √x7ᵗʰ **V84.0** **Driver of special agricultural vehicle injured in traffic accident**

  √x7ᵗʰ **V84.1** **Passenger of special agricultural vehicle injured in traffic accident**

  √x7ᵗʰ **V84.2** **Person on outside of special agricultural vehicle injured in traffic accident**

  √x7ᵗʰ **V84.3** **Unspecified occupant of special agricultural vehicle injured in traffic accident**   ▽

  √x7ᵗʰ **V84.4** **Person injured while boarding or alighting from special agricultural vehicle**

  √x7ᵗʰ **V84.5** **Driver of special agricultural vehicle injured in nontraffic accident**

√ Additional Character Req   √x7ᵗʰ Placeholder Alert   Manifestation   ▽ Unspecified   ►◄ Revised Text   ● New Code   ▲ Revised Code Title

√x7ᵗʰ **V84.6** Passenger of special agricultural vehicle injured in nontraffic accident

√x7ᵗʰ **V84.7** Person on outside of special agricultural vehicle injured in nontraffic accident

√x7ᵗʰ **V84.9** Unspecified occupant of special agricultural vehicle injured in nontraffic accident ▽
Special-agricultural vehicle accident NOS

√4ᵗʰ **V85** Occupant of special construction vehicle injured in transport accident

INCLUDES   bulldozer
digger
dump truck
earth-leveller
mechanical shovel
road-roller

EXCLUDES 1   special industrial vehicle (V83.-)
special construction vehicle in stationary use or maintenance (W31.-)

√x7ᵗʰ **V85.0** Driver of special construction vehicle injured in traffic accident

√x7ᵗʰ **V85.1** Passenger of special construction vehicle injured in traffic accident

√x7ᵗʰ **V85.2** Person on outside of special construction vehicle injured in traffic accident

√x7ᵗʰ **V85.3** Unspecified occupant of special construction vehicle injured in traffic accident ▽

√x7ᵗʰ **V85.4** Person injured while boarding or alighting from special construction vehicle

√x7ᵗʰ **V85.5** Driver of special construction vehicle injured in nontraffic accident

√x7ᵗʰ **V85.6** Passenger of special construction vehicle injured in nontraffic accident

√x7ᵗʰ **V85.7** Person on outside of special construction vehicle injured in nontraffic accident

√x7ᵗʰ **V85.9** Unspecified occupant of special construction vehicle injured in nontraffic accident ▽
Special-construction-vehicle accident NOS

√4ᵗʰ **V86** Occupant of special all-terrain or other off-road motor vehicle, injured in transport accident

EXCLUDES 1   special all-terrain vehicle in stationary use or maintenance (W31.-)
sport-utility vehicle (V50-V59)
three-wheeled motor vehicle designed for on-road use (V30-V39)

AHA: 2017,4Q,26

√5ᵗʰ **V86.0** Driver of special all-terrain or other off-road motor vehicle injured in traffic accident

√x7ᵗʰ **V86.01** Driver of ambulance or fire engine injured in traffic accident

√x7ᵗʰ **V86.02** Driver of snowmobile injured in traffic accident

√x7ᵗʰ **V86.03** Driver of dune buggy injured in traffic accident

√x7ᵗʰ **V86.04** Driver of military vehicle injured in traffic accident

√x7ᵗʰ **V86.05** Driver of 3- or 4- wheeled all-terrain vehicle (ATV) injured in traffic accident

√x7ᵗʰ **V86.06** Driver of dirt bike or motor/cross bike injured in traffic accident

√x7ᵗʰ **V86.09** Driver of other special all-terrain or other off-road motor vehicle injured in traffic accident
Driver of dirt bike injured in traffic accident
Driver of go cart injured in traffic accident
Driver of golf cart injured in traffic accident

√5ᵗʰ **V86.1** Passenger of special all-terrain or other off-road motor vehicle injured in traffic accident

√x7ᵗʰ **V86.11** Passenger of ambulance or fire engine injured in traffic accident

√x7ᵗʰ **V86.12** Passenger of snowmobile injured in traffic accident

√x7ᵗʰ **V86.13** Passenger of dune buggy injured in traffic accident

√x7ᵗʰ **V86.14** Passenger of military vehicle injured in traffic accident

√x7ᵗʰ **V86.15** Passenger of 3- or 4- wheeled all-terrain vehicle (ATV) injured in traffic accident

√x7ᵗʰ **V86.16** Passenger of dirt bike or motor/cross bike injured in traffic accident

√x7ᵗʰ **V86.19** Passenger of other special all-terrain or other off-road motor vehicle injured in traffic accident
Passenger of dirt bike injured in traffic accident
Passenger of go cart injured in traffic accident
Passenger of golf cart injured in traffic accident

√5ᵗʰ **V86.2** Person on outside of special all-terrain or other off-road motor vehicle injured in traffic accident

√x7ᵗʰ **V86.21** Person on outside of ambulance or fire engine injured in traffic accident

√x7ᵗʰ **V86.22** Person on outside of snowmobile injured in traffic accident

√x7ᵗʰ **V86.23** Person on outside of dune buggy injured in traffic accident

√x7ᵗʰ **V86.24** Person on outside of military vehicle injured in traffic accident

√x7ᵗʰ **V86.25** Person on outside of 3- or 4- wheeled all-terrain vehicle (ATV) injured in traffic accident

√x7ᵗʰ **V86.26** Person on outside of dirt bike or motor/cross bike injured in traffic accident

√x7ᵗʰ **V86.29** Person on outside of other special all-terrain or other off-road motor vehicle injured in traffic accident
Person on outside of dirt bike injured in traffic accident
Person on outside of go cart in traffic accident
Person on outside of golf cart in traffic accident

√5ᵗʰ **V86.3** Unspecified occupant of special all-terrain or other off-road motor vehicle injured in traffic accident

√x7ᵗʰ **V86.31** Unspecified occupant of ambulance or fire engine injured in traffic accident ▽

√x7ᵗʰ **V86.32** Unspecified occupant of snowmobile injured in traffic accident ▽

√x7ᵗʰ **V86.33** Unspecified occupant of dune buggy injured in traffic accident ▽

√x7ᵗʰ **V86.34** Unspecified occupant of military vehicle injured in traffic accident ▽

√x7ᵗʰ **V86.35** Unspecified occupant of 3- or 4- wheeled all-terrain vehicle (ATV) injured in traffic accident ▽

√x7ᵗʰ **V86.36** Unspecified occupant of dirt bike or motor/cross bike injured in traffic accident ▽

√x7ᵗʰ **V86.39** Unspecified occupant of other special all-terrain or other off-road motor vehicle injured in traffic accident ▽
Unspecified occupant of dirt bike injured in traffic accident
Unspecified occupant of go cart injured in traffic accident
Unspecified occupant of golf cart injured in traffic accident

√5ᵗʰ **V86.4** Person injured while boarding or alighting from special all-terrain or other off-road motor vehicle

√x7ᵗʰ **V86.41** Person injured while boarding or alighting from ambulance or fire engine

√x7ᵗʰ **V86.42** Person injured while boarding or alighting from snowmobile

√x7ᵗʰ **V86.43** Person injured while boarding or alighting from dune buggy

√x7ᵗʰ **V86.44** Person injured while boarding or alighting from military vehicle

√x7ᵗʰ **V86.45** Person injured while boarding or alighting from a 3- or 4- wheeled all-terrain vehicle (ATV)

√x7ᵗʰ **V86.46** Person injured while boarding or alighting from a dirt bike or motor/cross bike

√x7ᵗʰ **V86.49** Person injured while boarding or alighting from other special all-terrain or other off-road motor vehicle
Person injured while boarding or alighting from dirt bike
Person injured while boarding or alighting from go cart
Person injured while boarding or alighting from golf cart

√5ᵗʰ **V86.5** Driver of special all-terrain or other off-road motor vehicle injured in nontraffic accident

√x7ᵗʰ **V86.51** Driver of ambulance or fire engine injured in nontraffic accident

√x7ᵗʰ **V86.52** Driver of snowmobile injured in nontraffic accident

√x7ᵗʰ **V86.53** Driver of dune buggy injured in nontraffic accident

✓x7th **V86.54** Driver of military vehicle injured in nontraffic accident

✓x7th **V86.55** Driver of 3- or 4- wheeled all-terrain vehicle (ATV) injured in nontraffic accident

✓x7th **V86.56** Driver of dirt bike or motor/cross bike injured in nontraffic accident

✓x7th **V86.59** Driver of other special all-terrain or other off-road motor vehicle injured in nontraffic accident
Driver of dirt bike injured in nontraffic accident
Driver of go cart injured in nontraffic accident
Driver of golf cart injured in nontraffic accident

✓5th **V86.6** Passenger of special all-terrain or other off-road motor vehicle injured in nontraffic accident

✓x7th **V86.61** Passenger of ambulance or fire engine injured in nontraffic accident

✓x7th **V86.62** Passenger of snowmobile injured in nontraffic accident

✓x7th **V86.63** Passenger of dune buggy injured in nontraffic accident

✓x7th **V86.64** Passenger of military vehicle injured in nontraffic accident

✓x7th **V86.65** Passenger of 3- or 4- wheeled all-terrain vehicle (ATV) injured in nontraffic accident

✓x7th **V86.66** Passenger of dirt bike or motor/cross bike injured in nontraffic accident

✓x7th **V86.69** Passenger of other special all-terrain or other off-road motor vehicle injured in nontraffic accident
Passenger of dirt bike injured in nontraffic accident
Passenger of go cart injured in nontraffic accident
Passenger of golf cart injured in nontraffic accident

✓5th **V86.7** Person on outside of special all-terrain or other off-road motor vehicle injured in nontraffic accident

✓x7th **V86.71** Person on outside of ambulance or fire engine injured in nontraffic accident

✓x7th **V86.72** Person on outside of snowmobile injured in nontraffic accident

✓x7th **V86.73** Person on outside of dune buggy injured in nontraffic accident

✓x7th **V86.74** Person on outside of military vehicle injured in nontraffic accident

✓x7th **V86.75** Person on outside of 3- or 4- wheeled all-terrain vehicle (ATV) injured in nontraffic accident

✓x7th **V86.76** Person on outside of dirt bike or motor/cross bike injured in nontraffic accident

✓x7th **V86.79** Person on outside of other special all-terrain or other off-road motor vehicles injured in nontraffic accident
Person on outside of dirt bike injured in nontraffic accident
Person on outside of go cart injured in nontraffic accident
Person on outside of golf cart injured in nontraffic accident

✓5th **V86.9** Unspecified occupant of special all-terrain or other off-road motor vehicle injured in nontraffic accident

✓x7th **V86.91** Unspecified occupant of ambulance or fire engine injured in nontraffic accident ▽

✓x7th **V86.92** Unspecified occupant of snowmobile injured in nontraffic accident ▽

✓x7th **V86.93** Unspecified occupant of dune buggy injured in nontraffic accident ▽

✓x7th **V86.94** Unspecified occupant of military vehicle injured in nontraffic accident ▽

✓x7th **V86.95** Unspecified occupant of 3- or 4- wheeled all-terrain vehicle (ATV) injured in nontraffic accident ▽

✓x7th **V86.96** Unspecified occupant of dirt bike or motor/cross bike injured in nontraffic accident ▽

✓x7th **V86.99** Unspecified occupant of other special all-terrain or other off-road motor vehicle injured in nontraffic accident ▽
Off-road motor-vehicle accident NOS
Other motor-vehicle accident NOS
Unspecified occupant of go cart injured in nontraffic accident
Unspecified occupant of golf cart injured in nontraffic accident

✓4th **V87** Traffic accident of specified type but victim's mode of transport unknown
EXCLUDES 1   collision involving:
pedal cycle (V10-V19)
pedestrian (V01-V09)

✓x7th **V87.0** Person injured in collision between car and two- or three-wheeled powered vehicle (traffic)

✓x7th **V87.1** Person injured in collision between other motor vehicle and two- or three-wheeled motor vehicle (traffic)

✓x7th **V87.2** Person injured in collision between car and pick-up truck or van (traffic)

✓x7th **V87.3** Person injured in collision between car and bus (traffic)

✓x7th **V87.4** Person injured in collision between car and heavy transport vehicle (traffic)

✓x7th **V87.5** Person injured in collision between heavy transport vehicle and bus (traffic)

✓x7th **V87.6** Person injured in collision between railway train or railway vehicle and car (traffic)

✓x7th **V87.7** Person injured in collision between other specified motor vehicles (traffic)

✓x7th **V87.8** Person injured in other specified noncollision transport accidents involving motor vehicle (traffic)

✓x7th **V87.9** Person injured in other specified (collision)(noncollision) transport accidents involving nonmotor vehicle (traffic)

✓4th **V88** Nontraffic accident of specified type but victim's mode of transport unknown
EXCLUDES 1   collision involving:
pedal cycle (V10-V19)
pedestrian (V01-V09)

✓x7th **V88.0** Person injured in collision between car and two- or three-wheeled motor vehicle, nontraffic

✓x7th **V88.1** Person injured in collision between other motor vehicle and two- or three-wheeled motor vehicle, nontraffic

✓x7th **V88.2** Person injured in collision between car and pick-up truck or van, nontraffic

✓x7th **V88.3** Person injured in collision between car and bus, nontraffic

✓x7th **V88.4** Person injured in collision between car and heavy transport vehicle, nontraffic

✓x7th **V88.5** Person injured in collision between heavy transport vehicle and bus, nontraffic

✓x7th **V88.6** Person injured in collision between railway train or railway vehicle and car, nontraffic

✓x7th **V88.7** Person injured in collision between other specified motor vehicle, nontraffic

✓x7th **V88.8** Person injured in other specified noncollision transport accidents involving motor vehicle, nontraffic

✓x7th **V88.9** Person injured in other specified (collision)(noncollision) transport accidents involving nonmotor vehicle, nontraffic

✓4th **V89** Motor- or nonmotor-vehicle accident, type of vehicle unspecified

✓x7th **V89.0** Person injured in unspecified motor-vehicle accident, nontraffic ▽
Motor-vehicle accident NOS, nontraffic

✓x7th **V89.1** Person injured in unspecified nonmotor-vehicle accident, nontraffic ▽
Nonmotor-vehicle accident NOS (nontraffic)

✓x7th **V89.2** Person injured in unspecified motor-vehicle accident, traffic ▽
Motor-vehicle accident [MVA] NOS
Road (traffic) accident [RTA] NOS

✓x7th **V89.3** Person injured in unspecified nonmotor-vehicle accident, traffic ▽
Nonmotor-vehicle traffic accident NOS

✓x7th **V89.9** Person injured in unspecified vehicle accident ▽
Collision NOS

Chapter 20. External Causes of Morbidity

V90–V90.39

Water transport accidents (V90-V94)

The appropriate 7th character is to be added to each code from categories V90-V94.
A   initial encounter
D   subsequent encounter
S   sequela

√4ᵗʰ **V90**   **Drowning and submersion due to accident to watercraft**

> EXCLUDES 1   civilian water transport accident involving military watercraft (V94.81-)
> fall into water not from watercraft (W16.-)
> military watercraft accident in military or war operations (Y36.0-, Y37.0-)
> water-transport-related drowning or submersion without accident to watercraft (V92.-)

√5ᵗʰ **V90.0**   **Drowning and submersion due to watercraft overturning**

√x7ᵗʰ **V90.00**   **Drowning and submersion due to merchant ship overturning**

√x7ᵗʰ **V90.01**   **Drowning and submersion due to passenger ship overturning**
> Drowning and submersion due to Ferry-boat overturning
> Drowning and submersion due to Liner overturning

√x7ᵗʰ **V90.02**   **Drowning and submersion due to fishing boat overturning**

√x7ᵗʰ **V90.03**   **Drowning and submersion due to other powered watercraft overturning**
> Drowning and submersion due to Hovercraft (on open water) overturning
> Drowning and submersion due to Jet ski overturning

√x7ᵗʰ **V90.04**   **Drowning and submersion due to sailboat overturning**

√x7ᵗʰ **V90.05**   **Drowning and submersion due to canoe or kayak overturning**

√x7ᵗʰ **V90.06**   **Drowning and submersion due to (nonpowered) inflatable craft overturning**

√x7ᵗʰ **V90.08**   **Drowning and submersion due to other unpowered watercraft overturning**
> Drowning and submersion due to windsurfer overturning

√x7ᵗʰ **V90.09**   **Drowning and submersion due to unspecified watercraft overturning** ▽
> Drowning and submersion due to boat NOS overturning
> Drowning and submersion due to ship NOS overturning
> Drowning and submersion due to watercraft NOS overturning

√5ᵗʰ **V90.1**   **Drowning and submersion due to watercraft sinking**

√x7ᵗʰ **V90.10**   **Drowning and submersion due to merchant ship sinking**

√x7ᵗʰ **V90.11**   **Drowning and submersion due to passenger ship sinking**
> Drowning and submersion due to Ferry-boat sinking
> Drowning and submersion due to Liner sinking

√x7ᵗʰ **V90.12**   **Drowning and submersion due to fishing boat sinking**

√x7ᵗʰ **V90.13**   **Drowning and submersion due to other powered watercraft sinking**
> Drowning and submersion due to Hovercraft (on open water) sinking
> Drowning and submersion due to Jet ski sinking

√x7ᵗʰ **V90.14**   **Drowning and submersion due to sailboat sinking**

√x7ᵗʰ **V90.15**   **Drowning and submersion due to canoe or kayak sinking**

√x7ᵗʰ **V90.16**   **Drowning and submersion due to (nonpowered) inflatable craft sinking**

√x7ᵗʰ **V90.18**   **Drowning and submersion due to other unpowered watercraft sinking**

√x7ᵗʰ **V90.19**   **Drowning and submersion due to unspecified watercraft sinking** ▽
> Drowning and submersion due to boat NOS sinking
> Drowning and submersion due to ship NOS sinking
> Drowning and submersion due to watercraft NOS sinking

√5ᵗʰ **V90.2**   **Drowning and submersion due to falling or jumping from burning watercraft**

√x7ᵗʰ **V90.20**   **Drowning and submersion due to falling or jumping from burning merchant ship**

√x7ᵗʰ **V90.21**   **Drowning and submersion due to falling or jumping from burning passenger ship**
> Drowning and submersion due to falling or jumping from burning Ferry-boat
> Drowning and submersion due to falling or jumping from burning Liner

√x7ᵗʰ **V90.22**   **Drowning and submersion due to falling or jumping from burning fishing boat**

√x7ᵗʰ **V90.23**   **Drowning and submersion due to other burning powered watercraft**
> Drowning and submersion due to falling and jumping from burning Hovercraft (on open water)
> Drowning and submersion due to falling and jumping from burning Jet ski

√x7ᵗʰ **V90.24**   **Drowning and submersion due to falling or jumping from burning sailboat**

√x7ᵗʰ **V90.25**   **Drowning and submersion due to falling or jumping from burning canoe or kayak**

√x7ᵗʰ **V90.26**   **Drowning and submersion due to falling or jumping from burning (nonpowered) inflatable craft**

√x7ᵗʰ **V90.27**   **Drowning and submersion due to falling or jumping from burning water-skis**

√x7ᵗʰ **V90.28**   **Drowning and submersion due to other burning unpowered watercraft**
> Drowning and submersion due to falling and jumping from burning surf-board
> Drowning and submersion due to falling and jumping from burning windsurfer

√x7ᵗʰ **V90.29**   **Drowning and submersion due to falling or jumping from unspecified burning watercraft** ▽
> Drowning and submersion due to falling or jumping from burning boat NOS
> Drowning and submersion due to falling or jumping from burning ship NOS
> Drowning and submersion due to falling or jumping from burning watercraft NOS

√5ᵗʰ **V90.3**   **Drowning and submersion due to falling or jumping from crushed watercraft**

√x7ᵗʰ **V90.30**   **Drowning and submersion due to falling or jumping from crushed merchant ship**

√x7ᵗʰ **V90.31**   **Drowning and submersion due to falling or jumping from crushed passenger ship**
> Drowning and submersion due to falling and jumping from crushed Ferry boat
> Drowning and submersion due to falling and jumping from crushed Liner

√x7ᵗʰ **V90.32**   **Drowning and submersion due to falling or jumping from crushed fishing boat**

√x7ᵗʰ **V90.33**   **Drowning and submersion due to falling or jumping from other crushed powered watercraft**
> Drowning and submersion due to falling and jumping from crushed Hovercraft
> Drowning and submersion due to falling and jumping from crushed Jet ski

√x7ᵗʰ **V90.34**   **Drowning and submersion due to falling or jumping from crushed sailboat**

√x7ᵗʰ **V90.35**   **Drowning and submersion due to falling or jumping from crushed canoe or kayak**

√x7ᵗʰ **V90.36**   **Drowning and submersion due to falling or jumping from crushed (nonpowered) inflatable craft**

√x7ᵗʰ **V90.37**   **Drowning and submersion due to falling or jumping from crushed water-skis**

√x7ᵗʰ **V90.38**   **Drowning and submersion due to falling or jumping from other crushed unpowered watercraft**
> Drowning and submersion due to falling and jumping from crushed surf-board
> Drowning and submersion due to falling and jumping from crushed windsurfer

√x7ᵗʰ **V90.39**   **Drowning and submersion due to falling or jumping from crushed unspecified watercraft** ▽
> Drowning and submersion due to falling and jumping from crushed boat NOS
> Drowning and submersion due to falling and jumping from crushed ship NOS
> Drowning and submersion due to falling and jumping from crushed watercraft NOS

✓5ᵗʰ V90.8 Drowning and submersion due to other accident to watercraft

  ✓7ᵗʰ **V90.80 Drowning and submersion due to other accident to merchant ship**

  ✓7ᵗʰ **V90.81 Drowning and submersion due to other accident to passenger ship**
    Drowning and submersion due to other accident to Ferry-boat
    Drowning and submersion due to other accident to Liner

  ✓7ᵗʰ **V90.82 Drowning and submersion due to other accident to fishing boat**

  ✓7ᵗʰ **V90.83 Drowning and submersion due to other accident to other powered watercraft**
    Drowning and submersion due to other accident to Hovercraft (on open water)
    Drowning and submersion due to other accident to Jet ski

  ✓7ᵗʰ **V90.84 Drowning and submersion due to other accident to sailboat**

  ✓7ᵗʰ **V90.85 Drowning and submersion due to other accident to canoe or kayak**

  ✓7ᵗʰ **V90.86 Drowning and submersion due to other accident to (nonpowered) inflatable craft**

  ✓7ᵗʰ **V90.87 Drowning and submersion due to other accident to water-skis**

  ✓7ᵗʰ **V90.88 Drowning and submersion due to other accident to other unpowered watercraft**
    Drowning and submersion due to other accident to surf-board
    Drowning and submersion due to other accident to windsurfer

  ✓7ᵗʰ **V90.89 Drowning and submersion due to other accident to unspecified watercraft** ▽
    Drowning and submersion due to other accident to boat NOS
    Drowning and submersion due to other accident to ship NOS
    Drowning and submersion due to other accident to watercraft NOS

✓4ᵗʰ V91 Other injury due to accident to watercraft
  INCLUDES any injury except drowning and submersion as a result of an accident to watercraft
  EXCLUDES 1 civilian water transport accident involving military watercraft (V94.81-)
    military watercraft accident in military or war operations (Y36, Y37.-)
  EXCLUDES 2 drowning and submersion due to accident to watercraft (V90.-)

✓5ᵗʰ V91.0 Burn due to watercraft on fire
  EXCLUDES 1 burn from localized fire or explosion on board ship without accident to watercraft (V93.-)

  ✓7ᵗʰ **V91.00 Burn due to merchant ship on fire**

  ✓7ᵗʰ **V91.01 Burn due to passenger ship on fire**
    Burn due to Ferry-boat on fire
    Burn due to Liner on fire

  ✓7ᵗʰ **V91.02 Burn due to fishing boat on fire**

  ✓7ᵗʰ **V91.03 Burn due to other powered watercraft on fire**
    Burn due to Hovercraft (on open water) on fire
    Burn due to Jet ski on fire

  ✓7ᵗʰ **V91.04 Burn due to sailboat on fire**

  ✓7ᵗʰ **V91.05 Burn due to canoe or kayak on fire**

  ✓7ᵗʰ **V91.06 Burn due to (nonpowered) inflatable craft on fire**

  ✓7ᵗʰ **V91.07 Burn due to water-skis on fire**

  ✓7ᵗʰ **V91.08 Burn due to other unpowered watercraft on fire**

  ✓7ᵗʰ **V91.09 Burn due to unspecified watercraft on fire** ▽
    Burn due to boat NOS on fire
    Burn due to ship NOS on fire
    Burn due to watercraft NOS on fire

✓5ᵗʰ V91.1 Crushed between watercraft and other watercraft or other object due to collision
  Crushed by lifeboat after abandoning ship in a collision
  NOTE Select the specified type of watercraft that the victim was on at the time of the collision

  ✓7ᵗʰ **V91.10 Crushed between merchant ship and other watercraft or other object due to collision**

  ✓7ᵗʰ **V91.11 Crushed between passenger ship and other watercraft or other object due to collision**
    Crushed between Ferry-boat and other watercraft or other object due to collision
    Crushed between Liner and other watercraft or other object due to collision

  ✓7ᵗʰ **V91.12 Crushed between fishing boat and other watercraft or other object due to collision**

  ✓7ᵗʰ **V91.13 Crushed between other powered watercraft and other watercraft or other object due to collision**
    Crushed between Hovercraft (on open water) and other watercraft or other object due to collision
    Crushed between Jet ski and other watercraft or other object due to collision

  ✓7ᵗʰ **V91.14 Crushed between sailboat and other watercraft or other object due to collision**

  ✓7ᵗʰ **V91.15 Crushed between canoe or kayak and other watercraft or other object due to collision**

  ✓7ᵗʰ **V91.16 Crushed between (nonpowered) inflatable craft and other watercraft or other object due to collision**

  ✓7ᵗʰ **V91.18 Crushed between other unpowered watercraft and other watercraft or other object due to collision**
    Crushed between surfboard and other watercraft or other object due to collision
    Crushed between windsurfer and other watercraft or other object due to collision

  ✓7ᵗʰ **V91.19 Crushed between unspecified watercraft and other watercraft or other object due to collision** ▽
    Crushed between boat NOS and other watercraft or other object due to collision
    Crushed between ship NOS and other watercraft or other object due to collision
    Crushed between watercraft NOS and other watercraft or other object due to collision

✓5ᵗʰ V91.2 Fall due to collision between watercraft and other watercraft or other object
  Fall while remaining on watercraft after collision
  NOTE Select the specified type of watercraft that the victim was on at the time of the collision
  EXCLUDES 1 crushed between watercraft and other watercraft and other object due to collision (V91.1-)
    drowning and submersion due to falling from crushed watercraft (V90.3-)

  ✓7ᵗʰ **V91.20 Fall due to collision between merchant ship and other watercraft or other object**

  ✓7ᵗʰ **V91.21 Fall due to collision between passenger ship and other watercraft or other object**
    Fall due to collision between Ferry-boat and other watercraft or other object
    Fall due to collision between Liner and other watercraft or other object

  ✓7ᵗʰ **V91.22 Fall due to collision between fishing boat and other watercraft or other object**

  ✓7ᵗʰ **V91.23 Fall due to collision between other powered watercraft and other watercraft or other object**
    Fall due to collision between Hovercraft (on open water) and other watercraft or other object
    Fall due to collision between Jet ski and other watercraft or other object

  ✓7ᵗʰ **V91.24 Fall due to collision between sailboat and other watercraft or other object**

  ✓7ᵗʰ **V91.25 Fall due to collision between canoe or kayak and other watercraft or other object**

  ✓7ᵗʰ **V91.26 Fall due to collision between (nonpowered) inflatable craft and other watercraft or other object**

  ✓7ᵗʰ **V91.29 Fall due to collision between unspecified watercraft and other watercraft or other object** ▽
    Fall due to collision between boat NOS and other watercraft or other object
    Fall due to collision between ship NOS and other watercraft or other object
    Fall due to collision between watercraft NOS and other watercraft or other object

☑5ᵗʰ **V91.3** **Hit or struck by falling object due to accident to watercraft**

Hit or struck by falling object (part of damaged watercraft or other object) after falling or jumping from damaged watercraft

EXCLUDES 2   *drowning or submersion due to fall or jumping from damaged watercraft (V90.2-, V90.3-)*

√x7ᵗʰ **V91.3Ø** **Hit or struck by falling object due to accident to merchant ship**

√x7ᵗʰ **V91.31** **Hit or struck by falling object due to accident to passenger ship**

Hit or struck by falling object due to accident to Ferry-boat

Hit or struck by falling object due to accident to Liner

√x7ᵗʰ **V91.32** **Hit or struck by falling object due to accident to fishing boat**

√x7ᵗʰ **V91.33** **Hit or struck by falling object due to accident to other powered watercraft**

Hit or struck by falling object due to accident to Hovercraft (on open water)

Hit or struck by falling object due to accident to Jet ski

√x7ᵗʰ **V91.34** **Hit or struck by falling object due to accident to sailboat**

√x7ᵗʰ **V91.35** **Hit or struck by falling object due to accident to canoe or kayak**

√x7ᵗʰ **V91.36** **Hit or struck by falling object due to accident to (nonpowered) inflatable craft**

√x7ᵗʰ **V91.37** **Hit or struck by falling object due to accident to water-skis**

Hit by water-skis after jumping off of waterskis

√x7ᵗʰ **V91.38** **Hit or struck by falling object due to accident to other unpowered watercraft**

Hit or struck by surf-board after falling off damaged surf-board

Hit or struck by object after falling off damaged windsurfer

√x7ᵗʰ **V91.39** **Hit or struck by falling object due to accident to unspecified watercraft**   ▽

Hit or struck by falling object due to accident to boat NOS

Hit or struck by falling object due to accident to ship NOS

Hit or struck by falling object due to accident to watercraft NOS

☑5ᵗʰ **V91.8** **Other injury due to other accident to watercraft**

√x7ᵗʰ **V91.8Ø** **Other injury due to other accident to merchant ship**

√x7ᵗʰ **V91.81** **Other injury due to other accident to passenger ship**

Other injury due to other accident to Ferry-boat

Other injury due to other accident to Liner

√x7ᵗʰ **V91.82** **Other injury due to other accident to fishing boat**

√x7ᵗʰ **V91.83** **Other injury due to other accident to other powered watercraft**

Other injury due to other accident to Hovercraft (on open water)

Other injury due to other accident to Jet ski

√x7ᵗʰ **V91.84** **Other injury due to other accident to sailboat**

√x7ᵗʰ **V91.85** **Other injury due to other accident to canoe or kayak**

√x7ᵗʰ **V91.86** **Other injury due to other accident to (nonpowered) inflatable craft**

√x7ᵗʰ **V91.87** **Other injury due to other accident to water-skis**

√x7ᵗʰ **V91.88** **Other injury due to other accident to other unpowered watercraft**

Other injury due to other accident to surf-board

Other injury due to other accident to windsurfer

√x7ᵗʰ **V91.89** **Other injury due to other accident to unspecified watercraft**   ▽

Other injury due to other accident to boat NOS

Other injury due to other accident to ship NOS

Other injury due to other accident to watercraft NOS

☑4ᵗʰ **V92** **Drowning and submersion due to accident on board watercraft, without accident to watercraft**

EXCLUDES 1   *civilian water transport accident involving military watercraft (V94.81-)*

drowning or submersion due to accident to watercraft (V90-V91)

drowning or submersion of diver who voluntarily jumps from boat not involved in an accident (W16.711, W16.721)

fall into water without watercraft (W16.-)

military watercraft accident in military or war operations (Y36, Y37)

☑5ᵗʰ **V92.Ø** **Drowning and submersion due to fall off watercraft**

Drowning and submersion due to fall from gangplank of watercraft

Drowning and submersion due to fall overboard watercraft

EXCLUDES 2   *hitting head on object or bottom of body of water due to fall from watercraft (V94.Ø-)*

√x7ᵗʰ **V92.ØØ** **Drowning and submersion due to fall off merchant ship**

√x7ᵗʰ **V92.Ø1** **Drowning and submersion due to fall off passenger ship**

Drowning and submersion due to fall off Ferry-boat

Drowning and submersion due to fall off Liner

√x7ᵗʰ **V92.Ø2** **Drowning and submersion due to fall off fishing boat**

√x7ᵗʰ **V92.Ø3** **Drowning and submersion due to fall off other powered watercraft**

Drowning and submersion due to fall off Hovercraft (on open water)

Drowning and submersion due to fall off Jet ski

√x7ᵗʰ **V92.Ø4** **Drowning and submersion due to fall off sailboat**

√x7ᵗʰ **V92.Ø5** **Drowning and submersion due to fall off canoe or kayak**

√x7ᵗʰ **V92.Ø6** **Drowning and submersion due to fall off (nonpowered) inflatable craft**

√x7ᵗʰ **V92.Ø7** **Drowning and submersion due to fall off water-skis**

EXCLUDES 1   *drowning and submersion due to falling off burning water-skis (V90.27)*

drowning and submersion due to falling off crushed water-skis (V90.37)

hit by boat while water-skiing NOS (V94.X)

√x7ᵗʰ **V92.Ø8** **Drowning and submersion due to fall off other unpowered watercraft**

Drowning and submersion due to fall off surf-board

Drowning and submersion due to fall off windsurfer

EXCLUDES 1   *drowning and submersion due to fall off burning unpowered watercraft (V90.28)*

drowning and submersion due to fall off crushed unpowered watercraft (V90.38)

drowning and submersion due to fall off damaged unpowered watercraft (V90.88)

drowning and submersion due to rider of nonpowered watercraft being hit by other watercraft (V94.-)

other injury due to rider of nonpowered watercraft being hit by other watercraft (V94.-)

√x7ᵗʰ **V92.Ø9** **Drowning and submersion due to fall off unspecified watercraft**   ▽

Drowning and submersion due to fall off boat NOS

Drowning and submersion due to fall off ship

Drowning and submersion due to fall off watercraft NOS

☑5ᵗʰ **V92.1** **Drowning and submersion due to being thrown overboard by motion of watercraft**

EXCLUDES 1   *drowning and submersion due to fall off surf-board (V92.08)*

drowning and submersion due to fall off water-skis (V92.07)

drowning and submersion due to fall off windsurfer (V92.08)

√x7ᵗʰ **V92.1Ø** **Drowning and submersion due to being thrown overboard by motion of merchant ship**

√x7ᵗʰ **V92.11** **Drowning and submersion due to being thrown overboard by motion of** passenger ship

Drowning and submersion due to being thrown overboard by motion of Ferry-boat

Drowning and submersion due to being thrown overboard by motion of Liner

√x7ᵗʰ **V92.12** **Drowning and submersion due to being thrown overboard by motion of** fishing boat

√x7ᵗʰ **V92.13** **Drowning and submersion due to being thrown overboard by motion of other** powered **watercraft**

Drowning and submersion due to being thrown overboard by motion of Hovercraft

√x7ᵗʰ **V92.14** **Drowning and submersion due to being thrown overboard by motion of** sailboat

√x7ᵗʰ **V92.15** **Drowning and submersion due to being thrown overboard by motion of** canoe or kayak

√x7ᵗʰ **V92.16** **Drowning and submersion due to being thrown overboard by motion of (nonpowered)** inflatable craft

√x7ᵗʰ **V92.19** **Drowning and submersion due to being thrown overboard by motion of unspecified watercraft** ▽

Drowning and submersion due to being thrown overboard by motion of boat NOS

Drowning and submersion due to being thrown overboard by motion of ship NOS

Drowning and submersion due to being thrown overboard by motion of watercraft NOS

√5ᵗʰ **V92.2** **Drowning and submersion due to being** washed overboard **from watercraft**

Code first any associated cataclysm (X37.0-)

√x7ᵗʰ **V92.20** **Drowning and submersion due to being washed overboard from** merchant ship

√x7ᵗʰ **V92.21** **Drowning and submersion due to being washed overboard from** passenger ship

Drowning and submersion due to being washed overboard from Ferry-boat

Drowning and submersion due to being washed overboard from Liner

√x7ᵗʰ **V92.22** **Drowning and submersion due to being washed overboard from** fishing boat

√x7ᵗʰ **V92.23** **Drowning and submersion due to being washed overboard from other** powered **watercraft**

Drowning and submersion due to being washed overboard from Hovercraft (on open water)

Drowning and submersion due to being washed overboard from Jet ski

√x7ᵗʰ **V92.24** **Drowning and submersion due to being washed overboard from** sailboat

√x7ᵗʰ **V92.25** **Drowning and submersion due to being washed overboard from** canoe or kayak

√x7ᵗʰ **V92.26** **Drowning and submersion due to being washed overboard from (nonpowered)** inflatable craft

√x7ᵗʰ **V92.27** **Drowning and submersion due to being washed overboard from** water-skis

EXCLUDES 1   *drowning and submersion due to fall off water-skis (V92.07)*

√x7ᵗʰ **V92.28** **Drowning and submersion due to being washed overboard from other** unpowered **watercraft**

Drowning and submersion due to being washed overboard from surf-board

Drowning and submersion due to being washed overboard from windsurfer

√x7ᵗʰ **V92.29** **Drowning and submersion due to being washed overboard from unspecified watercraft** ▽

Drowning and submersion due to being washed overboard from boat NOS

Drowning and submersion due to being washed overboard from ship NOS

Drowning and submersion due to being washed overboard from watercraft NOS

√4ᵗʰ **V93** **Other injury due to accident on board watercraft, without accident to watercraft**

EXCLUDES 1   *civilian water transport accident involving military watercraft (V94.81-)*

other injury due to accident to watercraft (V91.-)

military watercraft accident in military or war operations (Y36, Y37.-)

EXCLUDES 2   *drowning and submersion due to accident on board watercraft, without accident to watercraft (V92.-)*

√5ᵗʰ **V93.0** **Burn due to localized fire on board watercraft**

EXCLUDES 1   *burn due to watercraft on fire (V91.0-)*

√x7ᵗʰ **V93.00** **Burn due to localized fire on board** merchant vessel

√x7ᵗʰ **V93.01** **Burn due to localized fire on board** passenger vessel

Burn due to localized fire on board Ferry-boat

Burn due to localized fire on board Liner

√x7ᵗʰ **V93.02** **Burn due to localized fire on board** fishing boat

√x7ᵗʰ **V93.03** **Burn due to localized fire on board other** powered **watercraft**

Burn due to localized fire on board Hovercraft

Burn due to localized fire on board Jet ski

√x7ᵗʰ **V93.04** **Burn due to localized fire on board** sailboat

√x7ᵗʰ **V93.09** **Burn due to localized fire on board unspecified watercraft** ▽

Burn due to localized fire on board boat NOS

Burn due to localized fire on board ship NOS

Burn due to localized fire on board watercraft NOS

√5ᵗʰ **V93.1** **Other burn on board watercraft**

Burn due to source other than fire on board watercraft

EXCLUDES 1   *burn due to watercraft on fire (V91.0-)*

√x7ᵗʰ **V93.10** **Other burn on board** merchant vessel

√x7ᵗʰ **V93.11** **Other burn on board** passenger vessel

Other burn on board Ferry-boat

Other burn on board Liner

√x7ᵗʰ **V93.12** **Other burn on board** fishing boat

√x7ᵗʰ **V93.13** **Other burn on board other** powered **watercraft**

Other burn on board Hovercraft

Other burn on board Jet ski

√x7ᵗʰ **V93.14** **Other burn on board** sailboat

√x7ᵗʰ **V93.19** **Other burn on board unspecified watercraft** ▽

Other burn on board boat NOS

Other burn on board ship NOS

Other burn on board watercraft NOS

√5ᵗʰ **V93.2** **Heat exposure on board watercraft**

EXCLUDES 1   *exposure to man-made heat not aboard watercraft (W92)*

exposure to natural heat while on board watercraft (X30)

exposure to sunlight while on board watercraft (X32)

EXCLUDES 2   *burn due to fire on board watercraft (V93.0-)*

√x7ᵗʰ **V93.20** **Heat exposure on board** merchant ship

√x7ᵗʰ **V93.21** **Heat exposure on board** passenger ship

Heat exposure on board Ferry-boat

Heat exposure on board Liner

√x7ᵗʰ **V93.22** **Heat exposure on board** fishing boat

√x7ᵗʰ **V93.23** **Heat exposure on board other** powered **watercraft**

Heat exposure on board hovercraft

√x7ᵗʰ **V93.24** **Heat exposure on board** sailboat

√x7ᵗʰ **V93.29** **Heat exposure on board unspecified watercraft** ▽

Heat exposure on board boat NOS

Heat exposure on board ship NOS

Heat exposure on board watercraft NOS

√5ᵗʰ **V93.3** **Fall on board watercraft**

EXCLUDES 1   *fall due to collision of watercraft (V91.2-)*

√x7ᵗʰ **V93.30** **Fall on board** merchant ship

√x7ᵗʰ **V93.31** **Fall on board** passenger ship

Fall on board Ferry-boat

Fall on board Liner

√x7ᵗʰ **V93.32** **Fall on board** fishing boat

√x7ᵗʰ **V93.33** **Fall on board other** powered **watercraft**

Fall on board Hovercraft (on open water)

Fall on board Jet ski

√x7ᵗʰ **V93.34** **Fall on board** sailboat

☑ Additional Character Req   √x7ᵗʰ Placeholder Alert   Manifestation   ▽ Unspecified   ►◄ Revised Text   ● New Code   ▲ Revised Code Title

ICD-10-CM 2019   1177

V92.11–V93.34

Chapter 20. External Causes of Morbidity *(left margin)*

V93.35–V94.9 *(left margin)*

√x7ᵗʰ **V93.35 Fall on board** canoe or kayak

√x7ᵗʰ **V93.36 Fall on board (nonpowered)** inflatable craft

√x7ᵗʰ **V93.38 Fall on board other** unpowered **watercraft**

√x7ᵗʰ **V93.39 Fall on board unspecified watercraft** ▽

     Fall on board boat NOS

     Fall on board ship NOS

     Fall on board watercraft NOS

√5ᵗʰ **V93.4 Struck by falling object on board watercraft**

     Hit by falling object on board watercraft

     EXCLUDES 1 *struck by falling object due to accident to watercraft (V91.3)*

√x7ᵗʰ **V93.40 Struck by falling object on** merchant ship

√x7ᵗʰ **V93.41 Struck by falling object on** passenger ship

     Struck by falling object on Ferry-boat

     Struck by falling object on Liner

√x7ᵗʰ **V93.42 Struck by falling object on** fishing boat

√x7ᵗʰ **V93.43 Struck by falling object on other** powered **watercraft**

     Struck by falling object on Hovercraft

√x7ᵗʰ **V93.44 Struck by falling object on** sailboat

√x7ᵗʰ **V93.48 Struck by falling object on other** unpowered **watercraft**

√x7ᵗʰ **V93.49 Struck by falling object on unspecified watercraft** ▽

√5ᵗʰ **V93.5 Explosion on board watercraft**

     Boiler explosion on steamship

     EXCLUDES 2 *fire on board watercraft (V93.0-)*

√x7ᵗʰ **V93.50 Explosion on board** merchant ship

√x7ᵗʰ **V93.51 Explosion on board** passenger ship

     Explosion on board Ferry-boat

     Explosion on board Liner

√x7ᵗʰ **V93.52 Explosion on board** fishing boat

√x7ᵗʰ **V93.53 Explosion on board other** powered **watercraft**

     Explosion on board Hovercraft

     Explosion on board Jet ski

√x7ᵗʰ **V93.54 Explosion on board** sailboat

√x7ᵗʰ **V93.59 Explosion on board unspecified watercraft** ▽

     Explosion on board boat NOS

     Explosion on board ship NOS

     Explosion on board watercraft NOS

√5ᵗʰ **V93.6 Machinery accident on board watercraft**

     EXCLUDES 1 *machinery explosion on board watercraft (V93.4-)*

                    machinery fire on board watercraft (V93.0-)

√x7ᵗʰ **V93.60 Machinery accident on board** merchant ship

√x7ᵗʰ **V93.61 Machinery accident on board** passenger ship

     Machinery accident on board Ferry-boat

     Machinery accident on board Liner

√x7ᵗʰ **V93.62 Machinery accident on board** fishing boat

√x7ᵗʰ **V93.63 Machinery accident on board other** powered **watercraft**

     Machinery accident on board Hovercraft

√x7ᵗʰ **V93.64 Machinery accident on board** sailboat

√x7ᵗʰ **V93.69 Machinery accident on board unspecified watercraft** ▽

     Machinery accident on board boat NOS

     Machinery accident on board ship NOS

     Machinery accident on board watercraft NOS

√5ᵗʰ **V93.8 Other injury due to other accident on board watercraft**

     Accidental poisoning by gases or fumes on watercraft

√x7ᵗʰ **V93.80 Other injury due to other accident on board** merchant ship

√x7ᵗʰ **V93.81 Other injury due to other accident on board** passenger ship

     Other injury due to other accident on board Ferry-boat

     Other injury due to other accident on board Liner

√x7ᵗʰ **V93.82 Other injury due to other accident on board** fishing boat

√x7ᵗʰ **V93.83 Other injury due to other accident on board other** powered **watercraft**

     Other injury due to other accident on board Hovercraft

     Other injury due to other accident on board Jet ski

√x7ᵗʰ **V93.84 Other injury due to other accident on board** sailboat

√x7ᵗʰ **V93.85 Other injury due to other accident on board** canoe or kayak

√x7ᵗʰ **V93.86 Other injury due to other accident on board (nonpowered)** inflatable craft

√x7ᵗʰ **V93.87 Other injury due to other accident on board** water-skis

     Hit or struck by object while waterskiing

√x7ᵗʰ **V93.88 Other injury due to other accident on board other** unpowered **watercraft**

     Hit or struck by object while surfing

     Hit or struck by object while on board windsurfer

√x7ᵗʰ **V93.89 Other injury due to other accident on board unspecified watercraft** ▽

     Other injury due to other accident on board boat NOS

     Other injury due to other accident on board ship NOS

     Other injury due to other accident on board watercraft NOS

√4ᵗʰ **V94 Other and unspecified water transport accidents**

     EXCLUDES 1 *military watercraft accidents in military or war operations (Y36, Y37)*

√x7ᵗʰ **V94.0 Hitting object or bottom of body of water due to fall from watercraft**

     EXCLUDES 2 *drowning and submersion due to fall from watercraft (V92.0-)*

√5ᵗʰ **V94.1 Bather struck by watercraft**

     Swimmer hit by watercraft

√x7ᵗʰ **V94.11 Bather struck by** powered **watercraft**

√x7ᵗʰ **V94.12 Bather struck by** nonpowered **watercraft**

√5ᵗʰ **V94.2 Rider of nonpowered watercraft struck by other watercraft**

√x7ᵗʰ **V94.21 Rider of nonpowered watercraft struck by other** nonpowered **watercraft**

     Canoer hit by other nonpowered watercraft

     Surfer hit by other nonpowered watercraft

     Windsurfer hit by other nonpowered watercraft

√x7ᵗʰ **V94.22 Rider of nonpowered watercraft struck by** powered **watercraft**

     Canoer hit by motorboat

     Surfer hit by motorboat

     Windsurfer hit by motorboat

√5ᵗʰ **V94.3 Injury to rider of (inflatable) watercraft being pulled behind other watercraft**

√x7ᵗʰ **V94.31 Injury to rider of (inflatable)** recreational **watercraft being pulled behind other watercraft**

     Injury to rider of inner-tube pulled behind motor boat

√x7ᵗʰ **V94.32 Injury to rider of** non-recreational **watercraft being pulled behind other watercraft**

     Injury to occupant of dingy being pulled behind boat or ship

     Injury to occupant of life-raft being pulled behind boat or ship

√x7ᵗʰ **V94.4 Injury to barefoot water-skier**

     Injury to person being pulled behind boat or ship

√5ᵗʰ **V94.8 Other water transport accident**

√6ᵗʰ **V94.81 Water transport accident involving military watercraft**

√7ᵗʰ **V94.810 Civilian watercraft involved in water transport accident with military watercraft**

     Passenger on civilian watercraft injured due to accident with military watercraft

√7ᵗʰ **V94.811 Civilian in water injured by military watercraft**

√7ᵗʰ **V94.818 Other water transport accident involving military watercraft**

√x7ᵗʰ **V94.89 Other water transport accident**

√x7ᵗʰ **V94.9 Unspecified water transport accident** ▽

     Water transport accident NOS

Air and space transport accidents (V95-V97)

EXCLUDES 1   *military aircraft accidents in military or war operations (Y36, Y37)*

The appropriate 7th character is to be added to each code from categories V95-V97.
A   initial encounter
D   subsequent encounter
S   sequela

√4ᵗʰ **V95   Accident to powered aircraft causing injury to occupant**

  √5ᵗʰ **V95.0   Helicopter accident injuring occupant**

    √x7ᵗʰ **V95.00   Unspecified helicopter accident injuring occupant** ▽

    √x7ᵗʰ **V95.01   Helicopter crash injuring occupant**

    √x7ᵗʰ **V95.02   Forced landing of helicopter injuring occupant**

    √x7ᵗʰ **V95.03   Helicopter collision injuring occupant**
      Helicopter collision with any object, fixed, movable or moving

    √x7ᵗʰ **V95.04   Helicopter fire injuring occupant**

    √x7ᵗʰ **V95.05   Helicopter explosion injuring occupant**

    √x7ᵗʰ **V95.09   Other helicopter accident injuring occupant**

  √5ᵗʰ **V95.1   Ultralight, microlight or powered-glider accident injuring occupant**

    √x7ᵗʰ **V95.10   Unspecified ultralight, microlight or powered-glider accident injuring occupant** ▽

    √x7ᵗʰ **V95.11   Ultralight, microlight or powered-glider crash injuring occupant**

    √x7ᵗʰ **V95.12   Forced landing of ultralight, microlight or powered-glider injuring occupant**

    √x7ᵗʰ **V95.13   Ultralight, microlight or powered-glider collision injuring occupant**
      Ultralight, microlight or powered-glider collision with any object, fixed, movable or moving .

    √x7ᵗʰ **V95.14   Ultralight, microlight or powered-glider fire injuring occupant**

    √x7ᵗʰ **V95.15   Ultralight, microlight or powered-glider explosion injuring occupant**

    √x7ᵗʰ **V95.19   Other ultralight, microlight or powered-glider accident injuring occupant**

  √5ᵗʰ **V95.2   Other private fixed-wing aircraft accident injuring occupant**

    √x7ᵗʰ **V95.20   Unspecified accident to other private fixed-wing aircraft, injuring occupant** ▽

    √x7ᵗʰ **V95.21   Other private fixed-wing aircraft crash injuring occupant**

    √x7ᵗʰ **V95.22   Forced landing of other private fixed-wing aircraft injuring occupant**

    √x7ᵗʰ **V95.23   Other private fixed-wing aircraft collision injuring occupant**
      Other private fixed-wing aircraft collision with any object, fixed, movable or moving

    √x7ᵗʰ **V95.24   Other private fixed-wing aircraft fire injuring occupant**

    √x7ᵗʰ **V95.25   Other private fixed-wing aircraft explosion injuring occupant**

    √x7ᵗʰ **V95.29   Other accident to other private fixed-wing aircraft injuring occupant**

  √5ᵗʰ **V95.3   Commercial fixed-wing aircraft accident injuring occupant**

    √x7ᵗʰ **V95.30   Unspecified accident to commercial fixed-wing aircraft injuring occupant** ▽

    √x7ᵗʰ **V95.31   Commercial fixed-wing aircraft crash injuring occupant**

    √x7ᵗʰ **V95.32   Forced landing of commercial fixed-wing aircraft injuring occupant**

    √x7ᵗʰ **V95.33   Commercial fixed-wing aircraft collision injuring occupant**
      Commercial fixed-wing aircraft collision with any object, fixed, movable or moving

    √x7ᵗʰ **V95.34   Commercial fixed-wing aircraft fire injuring occupant**

    √x7ᵗʰ **V95.35   Commercial fixed-wing aircraft explosion injuring occupant**

    √x7ᵗʰ **V95.39   Other accident to commercial fixed-wing aircraft injuring occupant**

  √5ᵗʰ **V95.4   Spacecraft accident injuring occupant**

    √x7ᵗʰ **V95.40   Unspecified spacecraft accident injuring occupant** ▽

    √x7ᵗʰ **V95.41   Spacecraft crash injuring occupant**

    √x7ᵗʰ **V95.42   Forced landing of spacecraft injuring occupant**

    √x7ᵗʰ **V95.43   Spacecraft collision injuring occupant**
      Spacecraft collision with any object, fixed, moveable or moving

    √x7ᵗʰ **V95.44   Spacecraft fire injuring occupant**

    √x7ᵗʰ **V95.45   Spacecraft explosion injuring occupant**

    √x7ᵗʰ **V95.49   Other spacecraft accident injuring occupant**

  √x7ᵗʰ **V95.8   Other powered aircraft accidents injuring occupant**

  √x7ᵗʰ **V95.9   Unspecified aircraft accident injuring occupant** ▽
    Aircraft accident NOS
    Air transport accident NOS

√4ᵗʰ **V96   Accident to nonpowered aircraft causing injury to occupant**

  √5ᵗʰ **V96.0   Balloon accident injuring occupant**

    √x7ᵗʰ **V96.00   Unspecified balloon accident injuring occupant** ▽

    √x7ᵗʰ **V96.01   Balloon crash injuring occupant**

    √x7ᵗʰ **V96.02   Forced landing of balloon injuring occupant**

    √x7ᵗʰ **V96.03   Balloon collision injuring occupant**
      Balloon collision with any object, fixed, moveable or moving

    √x7ᵗʰ **V96.04   Balloon fire injuring occupant**

    √x7ᵗʰ **V96.05   Balloon explosion injuring occupant**

    √x7ᵗʰ **V96.09   Other balloon accident injuring occupant**

  √5ᵗʰ **V96.1   Hang-glider accident injuring occupant**

    √x7ᵗʰ **V96.10   Unspecified hang-glider accident injuring occupant** ▽

    √x7ᵗʰ **V96.11   Hang-glider crash injuring occupant**

    √x7ᵗʰ **V96.12   Forced landing of hang-glider injuring occupant**

    √x7ᵗʰ **V96.13   Hang-glider collision injuring occupant**
      Hang-glider collision with any object, fixed, moveable or moving

    √x7ᵗʰ **V96.14   Hang-glider fire injuring occupant**

    √x7ᵗʰ **V96.15   Hang-glider explosion injuring occupant**

    √x7ᵗʰ **V96.19   Other hang-glider accident injuring occupant**

  √5ᵗʰ **V96.2   Glider (nonpowered) accident injuring occupant**

    √x7ᵗʰ **V96.20   Unspecified glider (nonpowered) accident injuring occupant** ▽

    √x7ᵗʰ **V96.21   Glider (nonpowered) crash injuring occupant**

    √x7ᵗʰ **V96.22   Forced landing of glider (nonpowered) injuring occupant**

    √x7ᵗʰ **V96.23   Glider (nonpowered) collision injuring occupant**
      Glider (nonpowered) collision with any object, fixed, moveable or moving

    √x7ᵗʰ **V96.24   Glider (nonpowered) fire injuring occupant**

    √x7ᵗʰ **V96.25   Glider (nonpowered) explosion injuring occupant**

    √x7ᵗʰ **V96.29   Other glider (nonpowered) accident injuring occupant**

  √x7ᵗʰ **V96.8   Other nonpowered-aircraft accidents injuring occupant**
    Kite carrying a person accident injuring occupant

  √x7ᵗʰ **V96.9   Unspecified nonpowered-aircraft accident injuring occupant** ▽
    Nonpowered-aircraft accident NOS

√4ᵗʰ **V97   Other specified air transport accidents**

  √x7ᵗʰ **V97.0   Occupant of aircraft injured in other specified air transport accidents**
    Fall in, on or from aircraft in air transport accident
    EXCLUDES 1   *accident while boarding or alighting aircraft (V97.1)*

  √x7ᵗʰ **V97.1   Person injured while boarding or alighting from aircraft**

  √5ᵗʰ **V97.2   Parachutist accident**

    √x7ᵗʰ **V97.21   Parachutist entangled in object**
      Parachutist landing in tree

    √x7ᵗʰ **V97.22   Parachutist injured on landing**

    √x7ᵗʰ **V97.29   Other parachutist accident**

  √5ᵗʰ **V97.3   Person on ground injured in air transport accident**

    √x7ᵗʰ **V97.31   Hit by object falling from aircraft**
      Hit by crashing aircraft
      Injured by aircraft hitting house
      Injured by aircraft hitting car

    √x7ᵗʰ **V97.32   Injured by rotating propeller**

    √x7ᵗʰ **V97.33   Sucked into jet engine**

✔ Additional Character Req   √x7ᵗʰ Placeholder Alert   Manifestation   ▽ Unspecified   ►◄ Revised Text   ● New Code   ▲ Revised Code Title

ICD-10-CM 2019   1179

√x7ᵗʰ **V97.39** **Other injury to person on ground due to air transport accident**

√5ᵗʰ **V97.8** **Other air transport accidents, not elsewhere classified**

     EXCLUDES 1   *aircraft accident NOS (V95.9)*

         exposure to changes in air pressure during ascent or descent (W94.-)

√6ᵗʰ **V97.81** **Air transport accident involving military aircraft**

     √7ᵗʰ **V97.810** **Civilian aircraft involved in air transport accident with military aircraft**

         Passenger in civilian aircraft injured due to accident with military aircraft

     √7ᵗʰ **V97.811** **Civilian injured by military aircraft**

     √7ᵗʰ **V97.818** **Other air transport accident involving military aircraft**

√x7ᵗʰ **V97.89** **Other air transport accidents, not elsewhere classified**

         Injury from machinery on aircraft

Other and unspecified transport accidents (V98-V99)

     EXCLUDES 1   *vehicle accident, type of vehicle unspecified (V89.-)*

The appropriate 7th character is to be added to each code from categories V98-V99.
A   initial encounter
D   subsequent encounter
S   sequela

√4ᵗʰ **V98** **Other specified transport accidents**

√x7ᵗʰ **V98.0** **Accident to, on or involving cable-car, not on rails**

         Caught or dragged by cable-car, not on rails
         Fall or jump from cable-car, not on rails
         Object thrown from or in cable-car, not on rails

√x7ᵗʰ **V98.1** **Accident to, on or involving land-yacht**

√x7ᵗʰ **V98.2** **Accident to, on or involving ice yacht**

√x7ᵗʰ **V98.3** **Accident to, on or involving ski lift**

         Accident to, on or involving ski chair-lift
         Accident to, on or involving ski-lift with gondola

√x7ᵗʰ **V98.8** **Other specified transport accidents**

√x7ᵗʰ **V99** **Unspecified transport accident** ▽

Other External Causes of Accidental Injury (W00-X58)

Slipping, tripping, stumbling and falls (W00-W19)

     EXCLUDES 1   *assault involving a fall (Y01-Y02)*
         fall from animal (V80.-)
         fall (in) (from) machinery (in operation) (W28-W31)
         fall (in) (from) transport vehicle (V01-V99)
         intentional self-harm involving a fall (X80-X81)

     EXCLUDES 2   *at risk for fall (history of fall) Z91.81*
         fall (in) (from) burning building (X00.-)
         fall into fire (X00-X04, X08)

The appropriate 7th character is to be added to each code from categories W00-W19.
A   initial encounter
D   subsequent encounter
S   sequela

√4ᵗʰ **W00** **Fall due to ice and snow**

     INCLUDES   pedestrian on foot falling (slipping) on ice and snow

     EXCLUDES 1   *fall on (from) ice and snow involving pedestrian conveyance (V00.-)*

         fall from stairs and steps not due to ice and snow (W10.-)

     AHA: 2016,2Q,4

√x7ᵗʰ **W00.0** **Fall on same level due to ice and snow**

√x7ᵗʰ **W00.1** **Fall from stairs and steps due to ice and snow**

√x7ᵗʰ **W00.2** **Other fall from one level to another due to ice and snow**

√x7ᵗʰ **W00.9** **Unspecified fall due to ice and snow** ▽

√4ᵗʰ **W01** **Fall on same level from slipping, tripping and stumbling**

     INCLUDES   fall on moving sidewalk

     EXCLUDES 1   *fall due to bumping (striking) against object (W18.0-)*
         fall in shower or bathtub (W18.2-)
         fall on same level NOS (W18.30)
         fall on same level from slipping, tripping and stumbling due to ice or snow (W00.0)
         fall off or from toilet (W18.1-)
         slipping, tripping and stumbling NOS (W18.40)
         slipping, tripping and stumbling without falling (W18.4-)

√x7ᵗʰ **W01.0** **Fall on same level from slipping, tripping and stumbling without subsequent striking against object**

         Falling over animal

√5ᵗʰ **W01.1** **Fall on same level from slipping, tripping and stumbling with subsequent striking against object**

√x7ᵗʰ **W01.10** **Fall on same level from slipping, tripping and stumbling with subsequent striking against unspecified object** ▽

√6ᵗʰ **W01.11** **Fall on same level from slipping, tripping and stumbling with subsequent striking against sharp object**

     √7ᵗʰ **W01.110** **Fall on same level from slipping, tripping and stumbling with subsequent striking against sharp glass**

     √7ᵗʰ **W01.111** **Fall on same level from slipping, tripping and stumbling with subsequent striking against power tool or machine**

     √7ᵗʰ **W01.118** **Fall on same level from slipping, tripping and stumbling with subsequent striking against other sharp object**

     √7ᵗʰ **W01.119** **Fall on same level from slipping, tripping and stumbling with subsequent striking against unspecified sharp object** ▽

√6ᵗʰ **W01.19** **Fall on same level from slipping, tripping and stumbling with subsequent striking against other object**

     √7ᵗʰ **W01.190** **Fall on same level from slipping, tripping and stumbling with subsequent striking against furniture**

     √7ᵗʰ **W01.198** **Fall on same level from slipping, tripping and stumbling with subsequent striking against other object**

√x7ᵗʰ **W03** **Other fall on same level due to collision with another person**

     Fall due to non-transport collision with other person

     EXCLUDES 1   *collision with another person without fall (W51)*
         crushed or pushed by a crowd or human stampede (W52)
         fall involving pedestrian conveyance (V00-V09)
         fall due to ice or snow (W00)
         fall on same level NOS (W18.30)

     AHA: 2012,4Q,108

√x7ᵗʰ **W04** **Fall while being carried or supported by other persons**

     Accidentally dropped while being carried

√4ᵗʰ **W05** **Fall from non-moving wheelchair, nonmotorized scooter and motorized mobility scooter**

     EXCLUDES 1   *fall from moving wheelchair (powered) (V00.811)*
         fall from moving motorized mobility scooter (V00.831)
         fall from nonmotorized scooter (V00.141)

√x7ᵗʰ **W05.0** **Fall from non-moving wheelchair**

√x7ᵗʰ **W05.1** **Fall from non-moving nonmotorized scooter**

√x7ᵗʰ **W05.2** **Fall from non-moving motorized mobility scooter**

√x7ᵗʰ **W06** **Fall from bed**

√x7ᵗʰ **W07** **Fall from chair**

√x7ᵗʰ **W08** **Fall from other furniture**

√4ᵗʰ **W09** **Fall on and from playground equipment**

     EXCLUDES 1   *fall involving recreational machinery (W31)*

√x7ᵗʰ **W09.0** **Fall on or from playground slide**

√x7ᵗʰ **W09.1** **Fall from playground swing**

√x7ᵗʰ **W09.2** **Fall on or from jungle gym**

√x7ᵗʰ **W09.8** **Fall on or from other playground equipment**

√4ᵗʰ **W10** **Fall on and from stairs and steps**

     EXCLUDES 1   *Fall from stairs and steps due to ice and snow (W00.1)*

√x7ᵗʰ **W10.0** **Fall (on)(from) escalator**

√x7ᵗʰ **W10.1** **Fall (on)(from) sidewalk curb**

√x7ᵗʰ **W10.2** **Fall (on)(from) incline**
Fall (on) (from) ramp

√x7ᵗʰ **W10.8** **Fall (on) (from) other stairs and steps**

√x7ᵗʰ **W10.9** **Fall (on) (from) unspecified stairs and steps** ▽

√x7ᵗʰ **W11** **Fall on and from ladder**

√x7ᵗʰ **W12** **Fall on and from scaffolding**

√4ᵗʰ **W13** **Fall from, out of or through building or structure**

√x7ᵗʰ **W13.0** **Fall from, out of or through balcony**
Fall from, out of or through railing

√x7ᵗʰ **W13.1** **Fall from, out of or through bridge**

√x7ᵗʰ **W13.2** **Fall from, out of or through roof**

√x7ᵗʰ **W13.3** **Fall through floor**

√x7ᵗʰ **W13.4** **Fall from, out of or through window**
EXCLUDES 2   *fall with subsequent striking against sharp glass (W01.110)*

√x7ᵗʰ **W13.8** **Fall from, out of or through other building or structure**
Fall from, out of or through viaduct
Fall from, out of or through wall
Fall from, out of or through flag-pole

√x7ᵗʰ **W13.9** **Fall from, out of or through building, not otherwise specified** ▽
EXCLUDES 1   *collapse of a building or structure (W20.-)*
fall or jump from burning building or structure (X00.-)

√x7ᵗʰ **W14** **Fall from tree**

√x7ᵗʰ **W15** **Fall from cliff**

√4ᵗʰ **W16** **Fall, jump or diving into water**
EXCLUDES 1   *accidental non-watercraft drowning and submersion not involving fall (W65-W74)*
effects of air pressure from diving (W94.-)
fall into water from watercraft (V90-V94)
hitting an object or against bottom when falling from watercraft (V94.0)
EXCLUDES 2   *striking or hitting diving board (W21.4)*

√5ᵗʰ **W16.0** **Fall into swimming pool**
Fall into swimming pool NOS
EXCLUDES 1   *fall into empty swimming pool (W17.3)*

√6ᵗʰ **W16.01** **Fall into swimming pool striking water surface**

√7ᵗʰ **W16.011** **Fall into swimming pool striking water surface causing drowning and submersion**
EXCLUDES 1   *drowning and submersion while in swimming pool without fall (W67)*

√7ᵗʰ **W16.012** **Fall into swimming pool striking water surface causing other injury**

√6ᵗʰ **W16.02** **Fall into swimming pool striking bottom**

√7ᵗʰ **W16.021** **Fall into swimming pool striking bottom causing drowning and submersion**
EXCLUDES 1   *drowning and submersion while in swimming pool without fall (W67)*

√7ᵗʰ **W16.022** **Fall into swimming pool striking bottom causing other injury**

√6ᵗʰ **W16.03** **Fall into swimming pool striking wall**

√7ᵗʰ **W16.031** **Fall into swimming pool striking wall causing drowning and submersion**
EXCLUDES 1   *drowning and submersion while in swimming pool without fall (W67)*

√7ᵗʰ **W16.032** **Fall into swimming pool striking wall causing other injury**

√5ᵗʰ **W16.1** **Fall into natural body of water**
Fall into lake
Fall into open sea
Fall into river
Fall into stream

√6ᵗʰ **W16.11** **Fall into natural body of water striking water surface**

√7ᵗʰ **W16.111** **Fall into natural body of water striking water surface causing drowning and submersion**
EXCLUDES 1   *drowning and submersion while in natural body of water without fall (W69)*

√7ᵗʰ **W16.112** **Fall into natural body of water striking water surface causing other injury**

√6ᵗʰ **W16.12** **Fall into natural body of water striking bottom**

√7ᵗʰ **W16.121** **Fall into natural body of water striking bottom causing drowning and submersion**
EXCLUDES 1   *drowning and submersion while in natural body of water without fall (W69)*

√7ᵗʰ **W16.122** **Fall into natural body of water striking bottom causing other injury**

√6ᵗʰ **W16.13** **Fall into natural body of water striking side**

√7ᵗʰ **W16.131** **Fall into natural body of water striking side causing drowning and submersion**
EXCLUDES 1   *drowning and submersion while in natural body of water without fall (W69)*

√7ᵗʰ **W16.132** **Fall into natural body of water striking side causing other injury**

√5ᵗʰ **W16.2** **Fall in (into) filled bathtub or bucket of water**

√6ᵗʰ **W16.21** **Fall in (into) filled bathtub**
EXCLUDES 1   *fall into empty bathtub (W18.2)*

√7ᵗʰ **W16.211** **Fall in (into) filled bathtub causing drowning and submersion**
EXCLUDES 1   *drowning and submersion while in filled bathtub without fall (W65)*

√7ᵗʰ **W16.212** **Fall in (into) filled bathtub causing other injury**

√6ᵗʰ **W16.22** **Fall in (into) bucket of water**

√7ᵗʰ **W16.221** **Fall in (into) bucket of water causing drowning and submersion**

√7ᵗʰ **W16.222** **Fall in (into) bucket of water causing other injury**

√5ᵗʰ **W16.3** **Fall into other water**
Fall into fountain
Fall into reservoir

√6ᵗʰ **W16.31** **Fall into other water striking water surface**

√7ᵗʰ **W16.311** **Fall into other water striking water surface causing drowning and submersion**
EXCLUDES 1   *drowning and submersion while in other water without fall (W73)*

√7ᵗʰ **W16.312** **Fall into other water striking water surface causing other injury**

√6ᵗʰ **W16.32** **Fall into other water striking bottom**

√7ᵗʰ **W16.321** **Fall into other water striking bottom causing drowning and submersion**
EXCLUDES 1   *drowning and submersion while in other water without fall (W73)*

√7ᵗʰ **W16.322** **Fall into other water striking bottom causing other injury**

√6ᵗʰ **W16.33** **Fall into other water striking wall**

√7ᵗʰ **W16.331** **Fall into other water striking wall causing drowning and submersion**
EXCLUDES 1   *drowning and submersion while in other water without fall (W73)*

√7ᵗʰ **W16.332** **Fall into other water striking wall causing other injury**

√5ᵗʰ **W16.4** **Fall into unspecified water**

√x7ᵗʰ **W16.41** **Fall into unspecified water causing drowning and submersion** ▽

☑ Additional Character Req   √x7ᵗʰ Placeholder Alert   Manifestation   ▽ Unspecified   ▶◀ Revised Text   ● New Code   ▲ Revised Code Title

Chapter 20. External Causes of Morbidity

W16.42–W18.11

√x7ᵗʰ **W16.42 Fall into unspecified water causing other injury** ▽

√5ᵗʰ **W16.5 Jumping or diving into** swimming pool

    √6ᵗʰ **W16.51 Jumping or diving into swimming pool striking water surface**

        √7ᵗʰ **W16.511 Jumping or diving into swimming pool striking water surface causing drowning and submersion**

             EXCLUDES 1   *drowning and submersion while in swimming pool without jumping or diving (W67)*

        √7ᵗʰ **W16.512 Jumping or diving into swimming pool striking water surface causing other injury**

    √6ᵗʰ **W16.52 Jumping or diving into swimming pool striking bottom**

        √7ᵗʰ **W16.521 Jumping or diving into swimming pool striking bottom causing drowning and submersion**

             EXCLUDES 1   *drowning and submersion while in swimming pool without jumping or diving (W67)*

        √7ᵗʰ **W16.522 Jumping or diving into swimming pool striking bottom causing other injury**

    √6ᵗʰ **W16.53 Jumping or diving into swimming pool striking wall**

        √7ᵗʰ **W16.531 Jumping or diving into swimming pool striking wall causing drowning and submersion**

             EXCLUDES 1   *drowning and submersion while in swimming pool without jumping or diving (W67)*

        √7ᵗʰ **W16.532 Jumping or diving into swimming pool striking wall causing other injury**

√5ᵗʰ **W16.6 Jumping or diving into** natural body of water

     Jumping or diving into lake

     Jumping or diving into open sea

     Jumping or diving into river

     Jumping or diving into stream

    √6ᵗʰ **W16.61 Jumping or diving into natural body of water striking water surface**

        √7ᵗʰ **W16.611 Jumping or diving into natural body of water striking water surface causing drowning and submersion**

             EXCLUDES 1   *drowning and submersion while in natural body of water without jumping or diving (W69)*

        √7ᵗʰ **W16.612 Jumping or diving into natural body of water striking water surface causing other injury**

    √6ᵗʰ **W16.62 Jumping or diving into natural body of water striking bottom**

        √7ᵗʰ **W16.621 Jumping or diving into natural body of water striking bottom causing drowning and submersion**

             EXCLUDES 1   *drowning and submersion while in natural body of water without jumping or diving (W69)*

        √7ᵗʰ **W16.622 Jumping or diving into natural body of water striking bottom causing other injury**

√5ᵗʰ **W16.7 Jumping or diving** from boat

     EXCLUDES 1   *fall from boat into water - see watercraft accident (V90-V94)*

    √6ᵗʰ **W16.71 Jumping or diving from boat striking water surface**

        √7ᵗʰ **W16.711 Jumping or diving from boat striking water surface causing drowning and submersion**

        √7ᵗʰ **W16.712 Jumping or diving from boat striking water surface causing other injury**

    √6ᵗʰ **W16.72 Jumping or diving from boat striking bottom**

        √7ᵗʰ **W16.721 Jumping or diving from boat striking bottom causing drowning and submersion**

        √7ᵗʰ **W16.722 Jumping or diving from boat striking bottom causing other injury**

√5ᵗʰ **W16.8 Jumping or diving into other water**

     Jumping or diving into fountain

     Jumping or diving into reservoir

    √6ᵗʰ **W16.81 Jumping or diving into other water striking water surface**

        √7ᵗʰ **W16.811 Jumping or diving into other water striking water surface causing drowning and submersion**

             EXCLUDES 1   *drowning and submersion while in other water without jumping or diving (W73)*

        √7ᵗʰ **W16.812 Jumping or diving into other water striking water surface causing other injury**

    √6ᵗʰ **W16.82 Jumping or diving into other water striking bottom**

        √7ᵗʰ **W16.821 Jumping or diving into other water striking bottom causing drowning and submersion**

             EXCLUDES 1   *drowning and submersion while in other water without jumping or diving (W73)*

        √7ᵗʰ **W16.822 Jumping or diving into other water striking bottom causing other injury**

    √6ᵗʰ **W16.83 Jumping or diving into other water striking wall**

        √7ᵗʰ **W16.831 Jumping or diving into other water striking wall causing drowning and submersion**

             EXCLUDES 1   *drowning and submersion while in other water without jumping or diving (W73)*

        √7ᵗʰ **W16.832 Jumping or diving into other water striking wall causing other injury**

√5ᵗʰ **W16.9 Jumping or diving into unspecified water**

    √x7ᵗʰ **W16.91 Jumping or diving into unspecified water causing drowning and submersion** ▽

    √x7ᵗʰ **W16.92 Jumping or diving into unspecified water causing other injury** ▽

√4ᵗʰ **W17 Other fall from one level to another**

    √x7ᵗʰ **W17.0 Fall into well**

    √x7ᵗʰ **W17.1 Fall into storm drain or manhole**

    √x7ᵗʰ **W17.2 Fall into hole**

         Fall into pit

    √x7ᵗʰ **W17.3 Fall into empty swimming pool**

         EXCLUDES 1   *fall into filled swimming pool (W16.0-)*

    √x7ᵗʰ **W17.4 Fall from dock**

    √5ᵗʰ **W17.8 Other fall from one level to another**

        √x7ᵗʰ **W17.81 Fall down embankment (hill)**

        √x7ᵗʰ **W17.82 Fall from (out of) grocery cart**

             Fall due to grocery cart tipping over

        √x7ᵗʰ **W17.89 Other fall from one level to another**

             Fall from cherry picker

             Fall from lifting device

             Fall from mobile elevated work platform [MEWP]

             Fall from sky lift

             AHA: 2015,2Q,6

√4ᵗʰ **W18 Other slipping, tripping and stumbling and falls**

    √5ᵗʰ **W18.0 Fall due to bumping against object**

         Striking against object with subsequent fall

         EXCLUDES 1   *fall on same level due to slipping, tripping, or stumbling with subsequent striking against object (W01.1-)*

        √x7ᵗʰ **W18.00 Striking against unspecified object with subsequent fall** ▽

        √x7ᵗʰ **W18.01 Striking against sports equipment with subsequent fall**

        √x7ᵗʰ **W18.02 Striking against glass with subsequent fall**

        √x7ᵗʰ **W18.09 Striking against other object with subsequent fall**

    √5ᵗʰ **W18.1 Fall from or off toilet**

        √x7ᵗʰ **W18.11 Fall from or off toilet without subsequent striking against object**

             Fall from (off) toilet NOS

√x7th **W18.12 Fall from or off toilet** with subsequent striking against object

√x7th **W18.2 Fall in (into) shower or empty bathtub**

     EXCLUDES 1   *fall in full bathtub causing drowning or submersion (W16.21-)*

√5th **W18.3 Other and unspecified fall on same level**

√x7th **W18.30 Fall on same level, unspecified** ▽

√x7th **W18.31 Fall on same level due to stepping on an object**

       Fall on same level due to stepping on an animal

       EXCLUDES 1   *slipping, tripping and stumbling without fall due to stepping on animal (W18.41)*

√x7th **W18.39 Other fall on same level**

√5th **W18.4 Slipping, tripping and stumbling without falling**

     EXCLUDES 1   *collision with another person without fall (W51)*

√x7th **W18.40 Slipping, tripping and stumbling without falling, unspecified** ▽

√x7th **W18.41 Slipping, tripping and stumbling without falling due to** stepping on object

       Slipping, tripping and stumbling without falling due to stepping on animal

       EXCLUDES 1   *slipping, tripping and stumbling with fall due to stepping on animal (W18.31)*

√x7th **W18.42 Slipping, tripping and stumbling without falling due to** stepping into hole or opening

√x7th **W18.43 Slipping, tripping and stumbling without falling due to** stepping from one level to another

√x7th **W18.49 Other slipping, tripping and stumbling without falling**

√x7th **W19 Unspecified fall** ▽

     Accidental fall NOS

     AHA: 2012,4Q,95

Exposure to inanimate mechanical forces (W20-W49)

     EXCLUDES 1   *assault (X92-Y09)*

       contact or collision with animals or persons (W50-W64)

       exposure to inanimate mechanical forces involving military or war operations (Y36.-, Y37.-)

       intentional self-harm (X71-X83)

The appropriate 7th character is to be added to each code from categories W20-W49.
A   initial encounter
D   subsequent encounter
S   sequela

√4th **W20 Struck by thrown, projected or falling object**

     Code first any associated:
     cataclysm (X34-X39)
     lightning strike (T75.00)

     EXCLUDES 1   *falling object in machinery accident (W24, W28-W31)*

       falling object in transport accident (V01-V99)

       object set in motion by explosion (W35-W40)

       object set in motion by firearm (W32-W34)

       struck by thrown sports equipment (W21.-)

√x7th **W20.0 Struck by falling object in cave-in**

     EXCLUDES 2   *asphyxiation due to cave-in (T71.21)*

√x7th **W20.1 Struck by object due to collapse of building**

     EXCLUDES 1   *struck by object due to collapse of burning building (X00.2, X02.2)*

√x7th **W20.8 Other cause of strike by thrown, projected or falling object**

     EXCLUDES 1   *struck by thrown sports equipment (W21.-)*

√4th **W21 Striking against or struck by sports equipment**

     EXCLUDES 1   *assault with sports equipment (Y08.0-)*

       striking against or struck by sports equipment with subsequent fall (W18.01)

√5th **W21.0 Struck by** hit or thrown ball

√x7th **W21.00 Struck by hit or thrown ball, unspecified type** ▽

√x7th **W21.01 Struck by** football

√x7th **W21.02 Struck by** soccer ball

√x7th **W21.03 Struck by** baseball

√x7th **W21.04 Struck by** golf ball

√x7th **W21.05 Struck by** basketball

√x7th **W21.06 Struck by** volleyball

√x7th **W21.07 Struck by** softball

√x7th **W21.09 Struck by other hit or thrown ball**

√5th **W21.1 Struck by** bat, racquet or club

√x7th **W21.11 Struck by** baseball bat

√x7th **W21.12 Struck by** tennis racquet

√x7th **W21.13 Struck by** golf club

√x7th **W21.19 Struck by other bat, racquet or club**

√5th **W21.2 Struck by** hockey stick or puck

√6th **W21.21 Struck by** hockey stick

√7th **W21.210 Struck by** ice hockey stick

√7th **W21.211 Struck by** field hockey stick

√6th **W21.22 Struck by** hockey puck

√7th **W21.220 Struck by** ice hockey puck

√7th **W21.221 Struck by** field hockey puck

√5th **W21.3 Struck by sports** foot wear

√x7th **W21.31 Struck by shoe** cleats

       Stepped on by shoe cleats

√x7th **W21.32 Struck by skate** blades

       Skated over by skate blades

√x7th **W21.39 Struck by other sports foot wear**

√x7th **W21.4 Striking against** diving board

     Use additional code for subsequent falling into water, if applicable (W16.-)

√5th **W21.8 Striking against or struck by other sports equipment**

√x7th **W21.81 Striking against or struck by** football helmet

√x7th **W21.89 Striking against or struck by other sports equipment**

√x7th **W21.9 Striking against or struck by unspecified sports equipment** ▽

√4th **W22 Striking against or struck by other objects**

     EXCLUDES 1   *striking against or struck by object with subsequent fall (W18.09)*

√5th **W22.0 Striking against** stationary object

     EXCLUDES 1   *striking against stationary sports equipment (W21.8)*

√x7th **W22.01 Walked into** wall

√x7th **W22.02 Walked into** lamppost

√x7th **W22.03 Walked into** furniture

√6th **W22.04 Striking against wall of** swimming pool

√7th **W22.041 Striking against wall of swimming pool causing** drowning and submersion

       EXCLUDES 1   *drowning and submersion while swimming without striking against wall (W67)*

√7th **W22.042 Striking against wall of swimming pool causing other injury**

√x7th **W22.09 Striking against other stationary object**

√5th **W22.1 Striking against or struck by** automobile airbag

√x7th **W22.10 Striking against or struck by unspecified automobile airbag** ▽

√x7th **W22.11 Striking against or struck by** driver side automobile airbag

√x7th **W22.12 Striking against or struck by** front passenger side automobile airbag

√x7th **W22.19 Striking against or struck by other automobile airbag**

√x7th **W22.8 Striking against or struck by other objects**

     Striking against or struck by object NOS

     EXCLUDES 1   *struck by thrown, projected or falling object (W20.-)*

√4th **W23 Caught, crushed, jammed or pinched in or between objects**

     EXCLUDES 1   *injury caused by cutting or piercing instruments (W25-W27)*

       injury caused by firearms malfunction (W32.1, W33.1-, W34.1-)

       injury caused by lifting and transmission devices (W24.-)

       injury caused by machinery (W28-W31)

       injury caused by nonpowered hand tools (W27.-)

       injury caused by transport vehicle being used as a means of transportation (V01-V99)

       injury caused by struck by thrown, projected or falling object (W20.-)

√x7th **W23.0 Caught, crushed, jammed, or pinched between** moving objects

---

☑ Additional Character Req   √x7th Placeholder Alert   Manifestation   ▽ Unspecified   ►◄ Revised Text   ● New Code   ▲ Revised Code Title

Chapter 20. External Causes of Morbidity

√x7ᵗʰ **W23.1** **Caught, crushed, jammed, or pinched between stationary objects**

√4ᵗʰ **W24** **Contact with lifting and transmission devices, not elsewhere classified**
> *EXCLUDES 1*   *transport accidents (V01-V99)*

√x7ᵗʰ **W24.0** **Contact with lifting devices, not elsewhere classified**
> Contact with chain hoist
> Contact with drive belt
> Contact with pulley (block)

√x7ᵗʰ **W24.1** **Contact with transmission devices, not elsewhere classified**
> Contact with transmission belt or cable

√x7ᵗʰ **W25** **Contact with sharp glass**
> Code first any associated:
> injury due to flying glass from explosion or firearm discharge (W32-W40)
> transport accident (V00-V99)
> *EXCLUDES 1*   *fall on same level due to slipping, tripping and stumbling with subsequent striking against sharp glass (W01.10)*
> *striking against sharp glass with subsequent fall (W18.02)*
> *EXCLUDES 2*   *glass embedded in skin (W45)*

√4ᵗʰ **W26** **Contact with other sharp objects**
> *EXCLUDES 2*   *sharp object(s) embedded in skin (W45)*
> **AHA:** 2016,4Q,73

√x7ᵗʰ **W26.0** **Contact with knife**
> *EXCLUDES 1*   *contact with electric knife (W29.1)*

√x7ᵗʰ **W26.1** **Contact with sword or dagger**

√x7ᵗʰ **W26.2** **Contact with edge of stiff paper**
> Paper cut

√x7ᵗʰ **W26.8** **Contact with other sharp object(s), not elsewhere classified**
> Contact with tin can lid

√x7ᵗʰ **W26.9** **Contact with unspecified sharp object(s)** ▽

√4ᵗʰ **W27** **Contact with nonpowered hand tool**

√x7ᵗʰ **W27.0** **Contact with workbench tool**
> Contact with auger
> Contact with axe
> Contact with chisel
> Contact with handsaw
> Contact with screwdriver

√x7ᵗʰ **W27.1** **Contact with garden tool**
> Contact with hoe
> Contact with nonpowered lawn mower
> Contact with pitchfork
> Contact with rake

√x7ᵗʰ **W27.2** **Contact with scissors**

√x7ᵗʰ **W27.3** **Contact with needle (sewing)**
> *EXCLUDES 1*   *contact with hypodermic needle (W46.-)*

√x7ᵗʰ **W27.4** **Contact with kitchen utensil**
> Contact with fork
> Contact with ice-pick
> Contact with can-opener NOS

√x7ᵗʰ **W27.5** **Contact with paper-cutter**

√x7ᵗʰ **W27.8** **Contact with other nonpowered hand tool**
> Contact with nonpowered sewing machine
> Contact with shovel

√x7ᵗʰ **W28** **Contact with powered lawn mower**
> Powered lawn mower (commercial) (residential)
> *EXCLUDES 1*   *contact with nonpowered lawn mower (W27.1)*
> *EXCLUDES 2*   *exposure to electric current (W86.-)*

√4ᵗʰ **W29** **Contact with other powered hand tools and household machinery**
> *EXCLUDES 1*   *contact with commercial machinery (W31.82)*
> *contact with hot household appliance (X15)*
> *contact with nonpowered hand tool (W27.-)*
> *exposure to electric current (W86)*

√x7ᵗʰ **W29.0** **Contact with powered kitchen appliance**
> Contact with blender
> Contact with can-opener
> Contact with garbage disposal
> Contact with mixer

√x7ᵗʰ **W29.1** **Contact with electric knife**

√x7ᵗʰ **W29.2** **Contact with other powered household machinery**
> Contact with electric fan
> Contact with powered dryer (clothes) (powered) (spin)
> Contact with washing-machine
> Contact with sewing machine

√x7ᵗʰ **W29.3** **Contact with powered garden and outdoor hand tools and machinery**
> Contact with chainsaw
> Contact with edger
> Contact with garden cultivator (tiller)
> Contact with hedge trimmer
> Contact with other powered garden tool
> *EXCLUDES 1*   *contact with powered lawn mower (W28)*

√x7ᵗʰ **W29.4** **Contact with nail gun**

√x7ᵗʰ **W29.8** **Contact with other powered hand tools and household machinery**
> Contact with do-it-yourself tool NOS

√4ᵗʰ **W30** **Contact with agricultural machinery**
> *INCLUDES*   animal-powered farm machine
> *EXCLUDES 1*   *agricultural transport vehicle accident (V01-V99)*
> *explosion of grain store (W40.8)*
> *exposure to electric current (W86.-)*

√x7ᵗʰ **W30.0** **Contact with combine harvester**
> Contact with reaper
> Contact with thresher

√x7ᵗʰ **W30.1** **Contact with power take-off devices (PTO)**

√x7ᵗʰ **W30.2** **Contact with hay derrick**

√x7ᵗʰ **W30.3** **Contact with grain storage elevator**
> *EXCLUDES 1*   *explosion of grain store (W40.8)*

√5ᵗʰ **W30.8** **Contact with other specified agricultural machinery**

√x7ᵗʰ **W30.81** **Contact with agricultural transport vehicle in stationary use**
> Contact with agricultural transport vehicle under repair, not on public roadway
> *EXCLUDES 1*   *agricultural transport vehicle accident (V01-V99)*

√x7ᵗʰ **W30.89** **Contact with other specified agricultural machinery**

√x7ᵗʰ **W30.9** **Contact with unspecified agricultural machinery** ▽
> Contact with farm machinery NOS

√4ᵗʰ **W31** **Contact with other and unspecified machinery**
> *EXCLUDES 1*   *contact with agricultural machinery (W30.-)*
> *contact with machinery in transport under own power or being towed by a vehicle (V01-V99)*
> *exposure to electric current (W86)*

√x7ᵗʰ **W31.0** **Contact with mining and earth-drilling machinery**
> Contact with bore or drill (land) (seabed)
> Contact with shaft hoist
> Contact with shaft lift
> Contact with undercutter

√x7ᵗʰ **W31.1** **Contact with metalworking machines**
> Contact with abrasive wheel
> Contact with forging machine
> Contact with lathe
> Contact with mechanical shears
> Contact with metal drilling machine
> Contact with milling machine
> Contact with power press
> Contact with rolling-mill
> Contact with metal sawing machine

√x7ᵗʰ **W31.2** **Contact with powered woodworking and forming machines**
> Contact with band saw
> Contact with bench saw
> Contact with circular saw
> Contact with molding machine
> Contact with overhead plane
> Contact with powered saw
> Contact with radial saw
> Contact with sander
> *EXCLUDES 1*   *nonpowered woodworking tools (W27.0)*

√x7ᵗʰ **W31.3** **Contact with prime movers**
    Contact with gas turbine
    Contact with internal combustion engine
    Contact with steam engine
    Contact with water driven turbine

√5ᵗʰ **W31.8** **Contact with other specified machinery**

  √x7ᵗʰ **W31.81** **Contact with recreational machinery**
      Contact with roller coaster

  √x7ᵗʰ **W31.82** **Contact with other commercial machinery**
      Contact with commercial electric fan
      Contact with commercial kitchen appliances
      Contact with commercial powered dryer (clothes)
        (powered) (spin)
      Contact with commercial washing-machine
      Contact with commercial sewing machine
      EXCLUDES 1   *contact with household machinery (W29.-)*
                contact with powered lawn mower (W28)

  √x7ᵗʰ **W31.83** **Contact with special construction vehicle in stationary use**
      Contact with special construction vehicle under repair,
        not on public roadway
      EXCLUDES 1   *special construction vehicle accident (V01-V99)*

  √x7ᵗʰ **W31.89** **Contact with other specified machinery**

√x7ᵗʰ **W31.9** **Contact with unspecified machinery**   ▽
    Contact with machinery NOS

√4ᵗʰ **W32** **Accidental handgun discharge and malfunction**

  INCLUDES   accidental discharge and malfunction of gun for single
       hand use
      accidental discharge and malfunction of pistol
      accidental discharge and malfunction of revolver
      handgun discharge and malfunction NOS

  EXCLUDES 1   *accidental airgun discharge and malfunction (W34.010, W34.110)*
      accidental BB gun discharge and malfunction (W34.010, W34.110)
      accidental pellet gun discharge and malfunction (W34.010, W34.110)
      accidental shotgun discharge and malfunction (W33.01, W33.11)
      assault by handgun discharge (X93)
      handgun discharge involving legal intervention (Y35.0-)
      handgun discharge involving military or war operations (Y36.4-)
      intentional self-harm by handgun discharge (X72)
      Very pistol discharge and malfunction (W34.09, W34.19)

√x7ᵗʰ **W32.0** **Accidental handgun discharge**

√x7ᵗʰ **W32.1** **Accidental handgun malfunction**
    Injury due to explosion of handgun (parts)
    Injury due to malfunction of mechanism or component of
      handgun
    Injury due to recoil of handgun
    Powder burn from handgun

√4ᵗʰ **W33** **Accidental rifle, shotgun and larger firearm discharge and malfunction**

  INCLUDES   rifle, shotgun and larger firearm discharge and malfunction
      NOS

  EXCLUDES 1   *accidental airgun discharge and malfunction (W34.010, W34.110)*
      accidental BB gun discharge and malfunction (W34.010, W34.110)
      accidental handgun discharge and malfunction (W32.-)
      accidental pellet gun discharge and malfunction (W34.010, W34.110)
      assault by rifle, shotgun and larger firearm discharge (X94)
      firearm discharge involving legal intervention (Y35.0-)
      firearm discharge involving military or war operations (Y36.4-)
      intentional self-harm by rifle, shotgun and larger firearm discharge (X73)

√5ᵗʰ **W33.0** **Accidental rifle, shotgun and larger firearm discharge**

  √x7ᵗʰ **W33.00** **Accidental discharge of unspecified larger firearm**   ▽
      Discharge of unspecified larger firearm NOS

  √x7ᵗʰ **W33.01** **Accidental discharge of shotgun**
      Discharge of shotgun NOS

  √x7ᵗʰ **W33.02** **Accidental discharge of hunting rifle**
      Discharge of hunting rifle NOS

  √x7ᵗʰ **W33.03** **Accidental discharge of machine gun**
      Discharge of machine gun NOS

  √x7ᵗʰ **W33.09** **Accidental discharge of other larger firearm**
      Discharge of other larger firearm NOS

√5ᵗʰ **W33.1** **Accidental rifle, shotgun and larger firearm malfunction**
    Injury due to explosion of rifle, shotgun and larger firearm
      (parts)
    Injury due to malfunction of mechanism or component of rifle,
      shotgun and larger firearm
    Injury due to piercing, cutting, crushing or pinching due to (by)
      slide trigger mechanism, scope or other gun part
    Injury due to recoil of rifle, shotgun and larger firearm
    Powder burn from rifle, shotgun and larger firearm

  √x7ᵗʰ **W33.10** **Accidental malfunction of unspecified larger firearm**   ▽
      Malfunction of unspecified larger firearm NOS

  √x7ᵗʰ **W33.11** **Accidental malfunction of shotgun**
      Malfunction of shotgun NOS

  √x7ᵗʰ **W33.12** **Accidental malfunction of hunting rifle**
      Malfunction of hunting rifle NOS

  √x7ᵗʰ **W33.13** **Accidental malfunction of machine gun**
      Malfunction of machine gun NOS

  √x7ᵗʰ **W33.19** **Accidental malfunction of other larger firearm**
      Malfunction of other larger firearm NOS

√4ᵗʰ **W34** **Accidental discharge and malfunction from other and unspecified firearms and guns**

  √5ᵗʰ **W34.0** **Accidental discharge from other and unspecified firearms and guns**

    √x7ᵗʰ **W34.00** **Accidental discharge from unspecified firearms or gun**   ▽
        Discharge from firearm NOS
        Gunshot wound NOS
        Shot NOS

    √6ᵗʰ **W34.01** **Accidental discharge of gas, air or spring-operated guns**

      √7ᵗʰ **W34.010** **Accidental discharge of airgun**
          Accidental discharge of BB gun
          Accidental discharge of pellet gun

      √7ᵗʰ **W34.011** **Accidental discharge of paintball gun**
          Accidental injury due to paintball discharge

      √7ᵗʰ **W34.018** **Accidental discharge of other gas, air or spring-operated gun**

    √x7ᵗʰ **W34.09** **Accidental discharge from other specified firearms**
      Accidental discharge from Very pistol [flare]

  √5ᵗʰ **W34.1** **Accidental malfunction from other and unspecified firearms and guns**

    √x7ᵗʰ **W34.10** **Accidental malfunction from unspecified firearms or gun**   ▽
        Firearm malfunction NOS

    √6ᵗʰ **W34.11** **Accidental malfunction of gas, air or spring-operated guns**

      √7ᵗʰ **W34.110** **Accidental malfunction of airgun**
          Accidental malfunction of BB gun
          Accidental malfunction of pellet gun

      √7ᵗʰ **W34.111** **Accidental malfunction of paintball gun**
          Accidental injury due to paintball gun malfunction

      √7ᵗʰ **W34.118** **Accidental malfunction of other gas, air or spring-operated gun**

    √x7ᵗʰ **W34.19** **Accidental malfunction from other specified firearms**
      Accidental malfunction from Very pistol [flare]

√x7ᵗʰ **W35** **Explosion and rupture of boiler**
  EXCLUDES 1   *explosion and rupture of boiler on watercraft (V93.4)*

√4ᵗʰ **W36** **Explosion and rupture of gas cylinder**

  √x7ᵗʰ **W36.1** **Explosion and rupture of aerosol can**

  √x7ᵗʰ **W36.2** **Explosion and rupture of air tank**

  √x7ᵗʰ **W36.3** **Explosion and rupture of pressurized-gas tank**

  √x7ᵗʰ **W36.8** **Explosion and rupture of other gas cylinder**

✓ Additional Character Req   √x7ᵗʰ Placeholder Alert   Manifestation   ▽ Unspecified   ▶◀ Revised Text   ● New Code   ▲ Revised Code Title

Chapter 20. External Causes of Morbidity

W36.9–W55.21

√x7ᵗʰ **W36.9** **Explosion and rupture of** unspecified gas cylinder ▽

√4ᵗʰ **W37** **Explosion and rupture of** pressurized tire, pipe or hose

√x7ᵗʰ **W37.0** **Explosion of** bicycle tire

√x7ᵗʰ **W37.8** **Explosion and rupture of other pressurized tire, pipe or hose**

√x7ᵗʰ **W38** **Explosion and rupture of other specified** pressurized devices

√x7ᵗʰ **W39** **Discharge of** firework

√4ᵗʰ **W40** **Explosion of other materials**

> **EXCLUDES 1**   assault by explosive material (X96)
> explosion involving legal intervention (Y35.1-)
> explosion involving military or war operations (Y36.0-, Y36.2-)
> intentional self-harm by explosive material (X75)

√x7ᵗʰ **W40.0** **Explosion of** blasting material

Explosion of blasting cap
Explosion of detonator
Explosion of dynamite
Explosion of explosive (any) used in blasting operations

√x7ᵗʰ **W40.1** **Explosion of** explosive gases

Explosion of acetylene
Explosion of butane
Explosion of coal gas
Explosion in mine NOS
Explosion of explosive gas
Explosion of fire damp
Explosion of gasoline fumes
Explosion of methane
Explosion of propane

√x7ᵗʰ **W40.8** **Explosion of other specified explosive materials**

Explosion in dump NOS
Explosion in factory NOS
Explosion in grain store
Explosion in munitions

> **EXCLUDES 1**   explosion involving legal intervention (Y35.1-)
> explosion involving military or war operations (Y36.0-, Y36.2-)

√x7ᵗʰ **W40.9** **Explosion of unspecified explosive materials** ▽

Explosion NOS

√4ᵗʰ **W42** **Exposure to noise**

√x7ᵗʰ **W42.0** **Exposure to supersonic waves**

√x7ᵗʰ **W42.9** **Exposure to other noise**

Exposure to sound waves NOS

√4ᵗʰ **W45** **Foreign body or object entering through skin**

> **INCLUDES**   foreign body or object embedded in skin
> nail embedded in skin
> **EXCLUDES 2**   contact with hand tools (nonpowered) (powered) (W27-W29)
> contact with other sharp objects (W26.-)
> contact with sharp glass (W25.-)
> struck by objects (W20-W22)

√x7ᵗʰ **W45.0** **Nail entering through skin**

√x7ᵗʰ **W45.8** **Other foreign body or object entering through skin**

Splinter in skin NOS

√4ᵗʰ **W46** **Contact with hypodermic needle**

√x7ᵗʰ **W46.0** **Contact with hypodermic needle**

Hypodermic needle stick NOS

√x7ᵗʰ **W46.1** **Contact with** contaminated **hypodermic needle**

√4ᵗʰ **W49** **Exposure to other inanimate mechanical forces**

> **INCLUDES**   exposure to abnormal gravitational [G] forces
> exposure to inanimate mechanical forces NEC
> **EXCLUDES 1**   exposure to inanimate mechanical forces involving military or war operations (Y36.-, Y37.-)

√5ᵗʰ **W49.0** **Item causing** external constriction

√x7ᵗʰ **W49.01** **Hair causing external constriction**

√x7ᵗʰ **W49.02** **String or thread causing external constriction**

√x7ᵗʰ **W49.03** **Rubber band causing external constriction**

√x7ᵗʰ **W49.04** **Ring or other jewelry causing external constriction**

√x7ᵗʰ **W49.09** **Other specified item causing external constriction**

√x7ᵗʰ **W49.9** **Exposure to other inanimate mechanical forces**

Exposure to animate mechanical forces (W50-W64)

> **EXCLUDES 1**   toxic effect of contact with venomous animals and plants (T63.-)

The appropriate 7th character is to be added to each code from categories W50-W64.
A   initial encounter
D   subsequent encounter
S   sequela

√4ᵗʰ **W50** **Accidental hit, strike, kick, twist, bite or scratch by another person**

> **INCLUDES**   hit, strike, kick, twist, bite, or scratch by another person NOS
> **EXCLUDES 1**   assault by bodily force (Y04)
> struck by objects (W20-W22)

√x7ᵗʰ **W50.0** **Accidental hit or strike by another person**

Hit or strike by another person NOS

√x7ᵗʰ **W50.1** **Accidental kick by another person**

Kick by another person NOS

√x7ᵗʰ **W50.2** **Accidental twist by another person**

Twist by another person NOS

√x7ᵗʰ **W50.3** **Accidental bite by another person**

Human bite
Bite by another person NOS

√x7ᵗʰ **W50.4** **Accidental scratch by another person**

Scratch by another person NOS

√x7ᵗʰ **W51** **Accidental striking against or bumped into by another person**

> **EXCLUDES 1**   assault by striking against or bumping into by another person (Y04.2)
> fall due to collision with another person (W03)

√x7ᵗʰ **W52** **Crushed, pushed or stepped on by crowd or human stampede**

Crushed, pushed or stepped on by crowd or human stampede with or without fall

√4ᵗʰ **W53** **Contact with rodent**

> **INCLUDES**   contact with saliva, feces or urine of rodent

√5ᵗʰ **W53.0** **Contact with** mouse

√x7ᵗʰ **W53.01** **Bitten by mouse**

√x7ᵗʰ **W53.09** **Other contact with mouse**

√5ᵗʰ **W53.1** **Contact with** rat

√x7ᵗʰ **W53.11** **Bitten by rat**

√x7ᵗʰ **W53.19** **Other contact with rat**

√5ᵗʰ **W53.2** **Contact with** squirrel

√x7ᵗʰ **W53.21** **Bitten by squirrel**

√x7ᵗʰ **W53.29** **Other contact with squirrel**

√5ᵗʰ **W53.8** **Contact with other rodent**

√x7ᵗʰ **W53.81** **Bitten by other rodent**

√x7ᵗʰ **W53.89** **Other contact with other rodent**

√4ᵗʰ **W54** **Contact with dog**

> **INCLUDES**   contact with saliva, feces or urine of dog

√x7ᵗʰ **W54.0** **Bitten by dog**

√x7ᵗʰ **W54.1** **Struck by dog**

Knocked over by dog

√x7ᵗʰ **W54.8** **Other contact with dog**

√4ᵗʰ **W55** **Contact with other mammals**

> **INCLUDES**   contact with saliva, feces or urine of mammal
> **EXCLUDES 1**   animal being ridden - see transport accidents
> bitten or struck by dog (W54)
> bitten or struck by rodent (W53.-)
> contact with marine mammals (W56.-)

√5ᵗʰ **W55.0** **Contact with** cat

√x7ᵗʰ **W55.01** **Bitten by cat**

√x7ᵗʰ **W55.03** **Scratched by cat**

√x7ᵗʰ **W55.09** **Other contact with cat**

√5ᵗʰ **W55.1** **Contact with** horse

√x7ᵗʰ **W55.11** **Bitten by horse**

√x7ᵗʰ **W55.12** **Struck by horse**

√x7ᵗʰ **W55.19** **Other contact with horse**

√5ᵗʰ **W55.2** **Contact with** cow

Contact with bull

√x7ᵗʰ **W55.21** **Bitten by cow**

W55.22 Struck by cow
   Gored by bull
W55.29 Other contact with cow
W55.3 Contact with other hoof stock
   Contact with goats
   Contact with sheep
   W55.31 Bitten by other hoof stock
   W55.32 Struck by other hoof stock
      Gored by goat
      Gored by ram
   W55.39 Other contact with other hoof stock
W55.4 Contact with pig
   W55.41 Bitten by pig
   W55.42 Struck by pig
   W55.49 Other contact with pig
W55.5 Contact with raccoon
   W55.51 Bitten by raccoon
   W55.52 Struck by raccoon
   W55.59 Other contact with raccoon
W55.8 Contact with other mammals
   W55.81 Bitten by other mammals
   W55.82 Struck by other mammals
   W55.89 Other contact with other mammals

W56 Contact with nonvenomous marine animal
   EXCLUDES 1 contact with venomous marine animal (T63.-)
   W56.0 Contact with dolphin
      W56.01 Bitten by dolphin
      W56.02 Struck by dolphin
      W56.09 Other contact with dolphin
   W56.1 Contact with sea lion
      W56.11 Bitten by sea lion
      W56.12 Struck by sea lion
      W56.19 Other contact with sea lion
   W56.2 Contact with orca
      Contact with killer whale
      W56.21 Bitten by orca
      W56.22 Struck by orca
      W56.29 Other contact with orca
   W56.3 Contact with other marine mammals
      W56.31 Bitten by other marine mammals
      W56.32 Struck by other marine mammals
      W56.39 Other contact with other marine mammals
   W56.4 Contact with shark
      W56.41 Bitten by shark
      W56.42 Struck by shark
      W56.49 Other contact with shark
   W56.5 Contact with other fish
      W56.51 Bitten by other fish
      W56.52 Struck by other fish
      W56.59 Other contact with other fish
   W56.8 Contact with other nonvenomous marine animals
      W56.81 Bitten by other nonvenomous marine animals
      W56.82 Struck by other nonvenomous marine animals
      W56.89 Other contact with other nonvenomous marine animals

W57 Bitten or stung by nonvenomous insect and other nonvenomous arthropods
   EXCLUDES 1 contact with venomous insects and arthropods (T63.2-, T63.3-, T63.4-)

W58 Contact with crocodile or alligator
   W58.0 Contact with alligator
      W58.01 Bitten by alligator
      W58.02 Struck by alligator
      W58.03 Crushed by alligator
      W58.09 Other contact with alligator

W58.1 Contact with crocodile
   W58.11 Bitten by crocodile
   W58.12 Struck by crocodile
   W58.13 Crushed by crocodile
   W58.19 Other contact with crocodile

W59 Contact with other nonvenomous reptiles
   EXCLUDES 1 contact with venomous reptile (T63.0-, T63.1-)
   W59.0 Contact with nonvenomous lizards
      W59.01 Bitten by nonvenomous lizards
      W59.02 Struck by nonvenomous lizards
      W59.09 Other contact with nonvenomous lizards
         Exposure to nonvenomous lizards
   W59.1 Contact with nonvenomous snakes
      W59.11 Bitten by nonvenomous snake
      W59.12 Struck by nonvenomous snake
      W59.13 Crushed by nonvenomous snake
      W59.19 Other contact with nonvenomous snake
   W59.2 Contact with turtles
      EXCLUDES 1 contact with tortoises (W59.8-)
      W59.21 Bitten by turtle
      W59.22 Struck by turtle
      W59.29 Other contact with turtle
         Exposure to turtles
   W59.8 Contact with other nonvenomous reptiles
      W59.81 Bitten by other nonvenomous reptiles
      W59.82 Struck by other nonvenomous reptiles
      W59.83 Crushed by other nonvenomous reptiles
      W59.89 Other contact with other nonvenomous reptiles

W60 Contact with nonvenomous plant thorns and spines and sharp leaves
   EXCLUDES 1 contact with venomous plants (T63.7-)

W61 Contact with birds (domestic) (wild)
   INCLUDES contact with excreta of birds
   W61.0 Contact with parrot
      W61.01 Bitten by parrot
      W61.02 Struck by parrot
      W61.09 Other contact with parrot
         Exposure to parrots
   W61.1 Contact with macaw
      W61.11 Bitten by macaw
      W61.12 Struck by macaw
      W61.19 Other contact with macaw
         Exposure to macaws
   W61.2 Contact with other psittacines
      W61.21 Bitten by other psittacines
      W61.22 Struck by other psittacines
      W61.29 Other contact with other psittacines
         Exposure to other psittacines
   W61.3 Contact with chicken
      W61.32 Struck by chicken
      W61.33 Pecked by chicken
      W61.39 Other contact with chicken
         Exposure to chickens
   W61.4 Contact with turkey
      W61.42 Struck by turkey
      W61.43 Pecked by turkey
      W61.49 Other contact with turkey
   W61.5 Contact with goose
      W61.51 Bitten by goose
      W61.52 Struck by goose
      W61.59 Other contact with goose
   W61.6 Contact with duck
      W61.61 Bitten by duck
      W61.62 Struck by duck
      W61.69 Other contact with duck

☑ Additional Character Req   ✓x7th Placeholder Alert   Manifestation   ▽ Unspecified   ►◄ Revised Text   ● New Code   ▲ Revised Code Title

√5ᵗʰ **W61.9** **Contact with other birds**

    √x7ᵗʰ **W61.91** **Bitten by other birds**

    √x7ᵗʰ **W61.92** **Struck by other birds**

    √x7ᵗʰ **W61.99** **Other contact with other birds**
              Contact with bird NOS

√4ᵗʰ **W62** **Contact with nonvenomous amphibians**

     EXCLUDES 1   *contact with venomous amphibians (T63.81-R63.83)*

√x7ᵗʰ **W62.0** **Contact with nonvenomous frogs**

√x7ᵗʰ **W62.1** **Contact with nonvenomous toads**

√x7ᵗʰ **W62.9** **Contact with other nonvenomous amphibians**

√x7ᵗʰ **W64** **Exposure to other animate mechanical forces**

     INCLUDES   exposure to nonvenomous animal NOS

     EXCLUDES 1   *contact with venomous animal (T63.-)*

Accidental non-transport drowning and submersion (W65-W74)

     EXCLUDES 1   *accidental drowning and submersion due to fall into water (W16.-)*
                  accidental drowning and submersion due to water transport accident (V90.-, V92.-)

     EXCLUDES 2   *accidental drowning and submersion due to cataclysm (X34-X39)*

The appropriate 7th character is to be added to each code from categories W65-W74.
A   initial encounter
D   subsequent encounter
S   sequela

√x7ᵗʰ **W65** **Accidental drowning and submersion while in bath-tub**

     EXCLUDES 1   *accidental drowning and submersion due to fall in (into) bathtub (W16.211)*

√x7ᵗʰ **W67** **Accidental drowning and submersion while in swimming-pool**

     EXCLUDES 1   *accidental drowning and submersion due to fall into swimming pool (W16.011, W16.021, W16.031)*
                  accidental drowning and submersion due to striking into wall of swimming pool (W22.041)

√x7ᵗʰ **W69** **Accidental drowning and submersion while in natural water**
     Accidental drowning and submersion while in lake
     Accidental drowning and submersion while in open sea
     Accidental drowning and submersion while in river
     Accidental drowning and submersion while in stream

     EXCLUDES 1   *accidental drowning and submersion due to fall into natural body of water (W16.111, W16.121, W16.131)*

√x7ᵗʰ **W73** **Other specified cause of accidental non-transport drowning and submersion**
     Accidental drowning and submersion while in quenching tank
     Accidental drowning and submersion while in reservoir

     EXCLUDES 1   *accidental drowning and submersion due to fall into other water (W16.311, W16.321, W16.331)*

√x7ᵗʰ **W74** **Unspecified cause of accidental drowning and submersion**   ▽
     Drowning NOS

Exposure to electric current, radiation and extreme ambient air temperature and pressure (W85-W99)

     EXCLUDES 1   exposure to:
              failure in dosage of radiation or temperature during surgical and medical care (Y63.2-Y63.5)
              lightning (T75.0-)
              natural cold (X31)
              natural heat (X30)
              natural radiation NOS (X39)
              radiological procedure and radiotherapy (Y84.2)
              sunlight (X32)

AHA: 2018,2Q,7-8

The appropriate 7th character is to be added to each code from categories W85-W99.
A   initial encounter
D   subsequent encounter
S   sequela

√x7ᵗʰ **W85** **Exposure to electric transmission lines**
     Broken power line

√4ᵗʰ **W86** **Exposure to other specified electric current**

    √x7ᵗʰ **W86.0** **Exposure to domestic wiring and appliances**

    √x7ᵗʰ **W86.1** **Exposure to industrial wiring, appliances and electrical machinery**
            Exposure to conductors
            Exposure to control apparatus
            Exposure to electrical equipment and machinery
            Exposure to transformers

    √x7ᵗʰ **W86.8** **Exposure to other electric current**
            Exposure to wiring and appliances in or on farm (not farmhouse)
            Exposure to wiring and appliances outdoors
            Exposure to wiring and appliances in or on public building
            Exposure to wiring and appliances in or on residential institutions
            Exposure to wiring and appliances in or on schools

√4ᵗʰ **W88** **Exposure to ionizing radiation**

     EXCLUDES 1   *exposure to sunlight (X32)*

√x7ᵗʰ **W88.0** **Exposure to X-rays**

√x7ᵗʰ **W88.1** **Exposure to radioactive isotopes**

√x7ᵗʰ **W88.8** **Exposure to other ionizing radiation**

√4ᵗʰ **W89** **Exposure to man-made visible and ultraviolet light**

     INCLUDES   exposure to welding light (arc)

     EXCLUDES 1   *exposure to sunlight (X32)*

√x7ᵗʰ **W89.0** **Exposure to welding light (arc)**

√x7ᵗʰ **W89.1** **Exposure to tanning bed**

√x7ᵗʰ **W89.8** **Exposure to other man-made visible and ultraviolet light**

√x7ᵗʰ **W89.9** **Exposure to unspecified man-made visible and**   ▽
            ultraviolet light

√4ᵗʰ **W90** **Exposure to other nonionizing radiation**

     EXCLUDES 1   *exposure to sunlight (X32)*

√x7ᵗʰ **W90.0** **Exposure to radiofrequency**

√x7ᵗʰ **W90.1** **Exposure to infrared radiation**

√x7ᵗʰ **W90.2** **Exposure to laser radiation**

√x7ᵗʰ **W90.8** **Exposure to other nonionizing radiation**

√x7ᵗʰ **W92** **Exposure to excessive heat of man-made origin**

√4ᵗʰ **W93** **Exposure to excessive cold of man-made origin**

    √5ᵗʰ **W93.0** **Contact with or inhalation of dry ice**

        √x7ᵗʰ **W93.01** **Contact with dry ice**

        √x7ᵗʰ **W93.02** **Inhalation of dry ice**

    √5ᵗʰ **W93.1** **Contact with or inhalation of liquid air**

        √x7ᵗʰ **W93.11** **Contact with liquid air**
                 Contact with liquid hydrogen
                 Contact with liquid nitrogen

        √x7ᵗʰ **W93.12** **Inhalation of liquid air**
                 Inhalation of liquid hydrogen
                 Inhalation of liquid nitrogen

    √x7ᵗʰ **W93.2** **Prolonged exposure in deep freeze unit or refrigerator**

    √x7ᵗʰ **W93.8** **Exposure to other excessive cold of man-made origin**

√4ᵗʰ **W94** **Exposure to high and low air pressure and changes in air pressure**

    √x7ᵗʰ **W94.0** **Exposure to prolonged high air pressure**

    √5ᵗʰ **W94.1** **Exposure to prolonged low air pressure**

        √x7ᵗʰ **W94.11** **Exposure to residence or prolonged visit at high altitude**

        √x7ᵗʰ **W94.12** **Exposure to other prolonged low air pressure**

    √5ᵗʰ **W94.2** **Exposure to rapid changes in air pressure during ascent**

        √x7ᵗʰ **W94.21** **Exposure to reduction in atmospheric pressure while surfacing from deep-water diving**

        √x7ᵗʰ **W94.22** **Exposure to reduction in atmospheric pressure while surfacing from underground**

        √x7ᵗʰ **W94.23** **Exposure to sudden change in air pressure in aircraft during ascent**

        √x7ᵗʰ **W94.29** **Exposure to other rapid changes in air pressure during ascent**

    √5ᵗʰ **W94.3** **Exposure to rapid changes in air pressure during descent**

        √x7ᵗʰ **W94.31** **Exposure to sudden change in air pressure in aircraft during descent**

        √x7ᵗʰ **W94.32** **Exposure to high air pressure from rapid descent in water**

        √x7ᵗʰ **W94.39** **Exposure to other rapid changes in air pressure during descent**

√x7ᵗʰ **W99** **Exposure to other man-made environmental factors**

Exposure to smoke, fire and flames (X00-X08)

EXCLUDES 1   arson (X97)

EXCLUDES 2   explosions (W35-W40)
           lightning (T75.0-)
           transport accident (V01-V99)

AHA: 2018,2Q,7-8

The appropriate 7th character is to be added to each code from categories X00-X08.
A   initial encounter
D   subsequent encounter
S   sequela

✓4th **X00** **Exposure to uncontrolled fire in building or structure**

     INCLUDES   conflagration in building or structure

     Code first any associated cataclysm

     EXCLUDES 2   exposure to ignition or melting of nightwear (X05)
               exposure to ignition or melting of other clothing and apparel (X06.-)
               exposure to other specified smoke, fire and flames (X08.-)

     AHA: 2016,2Q,5

   ✓x7th **X00.0** **Exposure to flames in uncontrolled fire in building or structure**

   ✓x7th **X00.1** **Exposure to smoke in uncontrolled fire in building or structure**

   ✓x7th **X00.2** **Injury due to collapse of burning building or structure in uncontrolled fire**

         EXCLUDES 1   injury due to collapse of building not on fire (W20.1)

   ✓x7th **X00.3** **Fall from burning building or structure in uncontrolled fire**

   ✓x7th **X00.4** **Hit by object from burning building or structure in uncontrolled fire**

   ✓x7th **X00.5** **Jump from burning building or structure in uncontrolled fire**

   ✓x7th **X00.8** **Other exposure to uncontrolled fire in building or structure**

✓4th **X01** **Exposure to uncontrolled fire, not in building or structure**

     INCLUDES   exposure to forest fire

   ✓x7th **X01.0** **Exposure to flames in uncontrolled fire, not in building or structure**

   ✓x7th **X01.1** **Exposure to smoke in uncontrolled fire, not in building or structure**

   ✓x7th **X01.3** **Fall due to uncontrolled fire, not in building or structure**

   ✓x7th **X01.4** **Hit by object due to uncontrolled fire, not in building or structure**

   ✓x7th **X01.8** **Other exposure to uncontrolled fire, not in building or structure**

✓4th **X02** **Exposure to controlled fire in building or structure**

     INCLUDES   exposure to fire in fireplace
               exposure to fire in stove

   ✓x7th **X02.0** **Exposure to flames in controlled fire in building or structure**

   ✓x7th **X02.1** **Exposure to smoke in controlled fire in building or structure**

   ✓x7th **X02.2** **Injury due to collapse of burning building or structure in controlled fire**

         EXCLUDES 1   injury due to collapse of building not on fire (W20.1)

   ✓x7th **X02.3** **Fall from burning building or structure in controlled fire**

   ✓x7th **X02.4** **Hit by object from burning building or structure in controlled fire**

   ✓x7th **X02.5** **Jump from burning building or structure in controlled fire**

   ✓x7th **X02.8** **Other exposure to controlled fire in building or structure**

✓4th **X03** **Exposure to controlled fire, not in building or structure**

     INCLUDES   exposure to bon fire
               exposure to camp-fire
               exposure to trash fire

   ✓x7th **X03.0** **Exposure to flames in controlled fire, not in building or structure**

   ✓x7th **X03.1** **Exposure to smoke in controlled fire, not in building or structure**

   ✓x7th **X03.3** **Fall due to controlled fire, not in building or structure**

   ✓x7th **X03.4** **Hit by object due to controlled fire, not in building or structure**

   ✓x7th **X03.8** **Other exposure to controlled fire, not in building or structure**

✓x7th **X04** **Exposure to ignition of highly flammable material**

     Exposure to ignition of gasoline
     Exposure to ignition of kerosene
     Exposure to ignition of petrol

     EXCLUDES 2   exposure to ignition or melting of nightwear (X05)
               exposure to ignition or melting of other clothing and apparel (X06)

     AHA: 2016,2Q,4

✓x7th **X05** **Exposure to ignition or melting of nightwear**

     EXCLUDES 2   exposure to uncontrolled fire in building or structure (X00.-)
               exposure to uncontrolled fire, not in building or structure (X01.-)
               exposure to controlled fire in building or structure (X02.-)
               exposure to controlled fire, not in building or structure (X03.-)
               exposure to ignition of highly flammable materials (X04.-)

✓4th **X06** **Exposure to ignition or melting of other clothing and apparel**

     EXCLUDES 2   exposure to uncontrolled fire in building or structure (X00.-)
               exposure to uncontrolled fire, not in building or structure (X01.-)
               exposure to controlled fire in building or structure (X02.-)
               exposure to controlled fire, not in building or structure (X03.-)
               exposure to ignition of highly flammable materials (X04.-)

   ✓x7th **X06.0** **Exposure to ignition of plastic jewelry**

   ✓x7th **X06.1** **Exposure to melting of plastic jewelry**

   ✓x7th **X06.2** **Exposure to ignition of other clothing and apparel**

   ✓x7th **X06.3** **Exposure to melting of other clothing and apparel**

✓4th **X08** **Exposure to other specified smoke, fire and flames**

   ✓5th **X08.0** **Exposure to bed fire**

         Exposure to mattress fire

     ✓x7th **X08.00** **Exposure to bed fire due to unspecified burning material**   ▽

     ✓x7th **X08.01** **Exposure to bed fire due to burning cigarette**

     ✓x7th **X08.09** **Exposure to bed fire due to other burning material**

   ✓5th **X08.1** **Exposure to sofa fire**

     ✓x7th **X08.10** **Exposure to sofa fire due to unspecified burning material**   ▽

     ✓x7th **X08.11** **Exposure to sofa fire due to burning cigarette**

     ✓x7th **X08.19** **Exposure to sofa fire due to other burning material**

   ✓5th **X08.2** **Exposure to other furniture fire**

     ✓x7th **X08.20** **Exposure to other furniture fire due to unspecified burning material**   ▽

     ✓x7th **X08.21** **Exposure to other furniture fire due to burning cigarette**

     ✓x7th **X08.29** **Exposure to other furniture fire due to other burning material**

   ✓x7th **X08.8** **Exposure to other specified smoke, fire and flames**

Contact with heat and hot substances (X10-X19)

EXCLUDES 1   exposure to excessive natural heat (X30)
               exposure to fire and flames (X00-X08)

AHA: 2018,2Q,7-8

The appropriate 7th character is to be added to each code from categories X10-X19.
A   initial encounter
D   subsequent encounter
S   sequela

✓4th **X10** **Contact with hot drinks, food, fats and cooking oils**

   ✓x7th **X10.0** **Contact with hot drinks**

   ✓x7th **X10.1** **Contact with hot food**

   ✓x7th **X10.2** **Contact with fats and cooking oils**

✓4th **X11** **Contact with hot tap-water**

     INCLUDES   contact with boiling tap-water
               contact with boiling water NOS

     EXCLUDES 1   contact with water heated on stove (X12)

   ✓x7th **X11.0** **Contact with hot water in bath or tub**

         EXCLUDES 1   contact with running hot water in bath or tub (X11.1)

   ✓x7th **X11.1** **Contact with running hot water**

         Contact with hot water running out of hose
         Contact with hot water running out of tap

✓ Additional Character Req   ✓x7th Placeholder Alert   Manifestation   ▽ Unspecified   ►◄ Revised Text   ● New Code   ▲ Revised Code Title

ICD-10-CM 2019   **1189**

√x7ᵗʰ **X11.8 Contact with other hot tap-water**
     Contact with hot water in bucket
     Contact with hot tap-water NOS

√x7ᵗʰ **X12 Contact with other hot fluids**
     Contact with water heated on stove
     EXCLUDES 1   *hot (liquid) metals (X18)*

√4ᵗʰ **X13 Contact with steam and other hot vapors**
     √x7ᵗʰ **X13.0 Inhalation of steam and other hot vapors**
     √x7ᵗʰ **X13.1 Other contact with steam and other hot vapors**

√4ᵗʰ **X14 Contact with hot air and other hot gases**
     √x7ᵗʰ **X14.0 Inhalation of hot air and gases**
     √x7ᵗʰ **X14.1 Other contact with hot air and other hot gases**

√4ᵗʰ **X15 Contact with hot household appliances**
     EXCLUDES 1   *contact with heating appliances (X16)*
                    contact with powered household appliances (W29.-)
                    exposure to controlled fire in building or structure due to household appliance (X02.8)
                    exposure to household appliances electrical current (W86.0)
     √x7ᵗʰ **X15.0 Contact with hot stove (kitchen)**
     √x7ᵗʰ **X15.1 Contact with hot toaster**
     √x7ᵗʰ **X15.2 Contact with hotplate**
     √x7ᵗʰ **X15.3 Contact with hot saucepan or skillet**
     √x7ᵗʰ **X15.8 Contact with other hot household appliances**
          Contact with cooker
          Contact with kettle
          Contact with light bulbs

√x7ᵗʰ **X16 Contact with hot heating appliances, radiators and pipes**
     EXCLUDES 1   *contact with powered appliances (W29.-)*
                    exposure to controlled fire in building or structure due to appliance (X02.8)
                    exposure to industrial appliances electrical current (W86.1)

√x7ᵗʰ **X17 Contact with hot engines, machinery and tools**
     EXCLUDES 1   *contact with hot heating appliances, radiators and pipes (X16)*
                    contact with hot household appliances (X15)

√x7ᵗʰ **X18 Contact with other hot metals**
     Contact with liquid metal

√x7ᵗʰ **X19 Contact with other heat and hot substances**
     EXCLUDES 1   *objects that are not normally hot, e.g., an object made hot by a house fire (X00-X08)*

Exposure to forces of nature (X30-X39)

AHA: 2018,2Q,7-8

The appropriate 7th character is to be added to each code from categories X30-X39.
A   initial encounter
D   subsequent encounter
S   sequela

√x7ᵗʰ **X30 Exposure to excessive natural heat**
     Exposure to excessive heat as the cause of sunstroke
     Exposure to heat NOS
     EXCLUDES 1   *excessive heat of man-made origin (W92)*
                    exposure to man-made radiation (W89)
                    exposure to sunlight (X32)
                    exposure to tanning bed (W89)

√x7ᵗʰ **X31 Exposure to excessive natural cold**
     Excessive cold as the cause of chilblains NOS
     Excessive cold as the cause of immersion foot or hand
     Exposure to cold NOS
     Exposure to weather conditions
     EXCLUDES 1   *cold of man-made origin (W93.-)*
                    contact with or inhalation of dry ice (W93.-)
                    contact with or inhalation of liquefied gas (W93.-)

√x7ᵗʰ **X32 Exposure to sunlight**
     EXCLUDES 1   *man-made radiation (tanning bed) (W89)*
     EXCLUDES 2   *radiation-related disorders of the skin and subcutaneous tissue (L55-L59)*

√x7ᵗʰ **X34 Earthquake**
     EXCLUDES 2   *tidal wave (tsunami) due to earthquake (X37.41)*

√x7ᵗʰ **X35 Volcanic eruption**
     EXCLUDES 2   *tidal wave (tsunami) due to volcanic eruption (X37.41)*

√4ᵗʰ **X36 Avalanche, landslide and other earth movements**
     INCLUDES   victim of mudslide of cataclysmic nature
     EXCLUDES 1   *earthquake (X34)*
     EXCLUDES 2   *transport accident involving collision with avalanche or landslide not in motion (V01-V99)*
     √x7ᵗʰ **X36.0 Collapse of dam or man-made structure causing earth movement**
     √x7ᵗʰ **X36.1 Avalanche, landslide, or mudslide**

√4ᵗʰ **X37 Cataclysmic storm**
     √x7ᵗʰ **X37.0 Hurricane**
          Storm surge
          Typhoon
     √x7ᵗʰ **X37.1 Tornado**
          Cyclone
          Twister
     √x7ᵗʰ **X37.2 Blizzard (snow)(ice)**
     √x7ᵗʰ **X37.3 Dust storm**
     √5ᵗʰ **X37.4 Tidalwave**
         √x7ᵗʰ **X37.41 Tidal wave due to earthquake or volcanic eruption**
              Tidal wave NOS
              Tsunami
         √x7ᵗʰ **X37.42 Tidal wave due to storm**
         √x7ᵗʰ **X37.43 Tidal wave due to landslide**
     √x7ᵗʰ **X37.8 Other cataclysmic storms**
          Cloudburst
          Torrential rain
         EXCLUDES 2   *flood (X38)*
     √x7ᵗʰ **X37.9 Unspecified cataclysmic storm**   ▽
          Storm NOS
         EXCLUDES 2   *collapse of dam or man-made structure causing earth movement ▶(X36.0)◀*

√x7ᵗʰ **X38 Flood**
     Flood arising from remote storm
     Flood of cataclysmic nature arising from melting snow
     Flood resulting directly from storm
     EXCLUDES 1   *collapse of dam or man-made structure causing earth movement ▶(X36.0)◀*
                    tidal wave NOS (X37.41)
                    tidal wave caused by storm ▶(X37.42)◀

√4ᵗʰ **X39 Exposure to other forces of nature**
     √5ᵗʰ **X39.0 Exposure to natural radiation**
         EXCLUDES 1   *▶contact with and (suspected) exposure to radon and other naturally occurring radiation◀ (Z77.123)*
                    exposure to man-made radiation (W88-W90)
                    exposure to sunlight (X32)
         √x7ᵗʰ **X39.01 Exposure to radon**
         √x7ᵗʰ **X39.08 Exposure to other natural radiation**
     √x7ᵗʰ **X39.8 Other exposure to forces of nature**

Overexertion and strenuous or repetitive movements (X50)

√4ᵗʰ **X50 Overexertion and strenuous or repetitive movements**
     AHA: 2018,2Q,7-8; 2016,4Q,73-74

The appropriate 7th character is to be added to each code from category X50.
A   initial encounter
D   subsequent encounter
S   sequela

     √x7ᵗʰ **X50.0 Overexertion from strenuous movement or load**
          Lifting heavy objects
          Lifting weights

√x7ᵗʰ **X50.1 Overexertion from prolonged static or awkward postures**
Prolonged bending
Prolonged kneeling
Prolonged reaching
Prolonged sitting
Prolonged standing
Prolonged twisting
Static bending
Static kneeling
Static reaching
Static sitting
Static standing
Static twisting

√x7ᵗʰ **X50.3 Overexertion from repetitive movements**
Use of hand as hammer
EXCLUDES 2   overuse from prolonged static or awkward postures (X50.1)

√x7ᵗʰ **X50.9 Other and unspecified overexertion or strenuous movements or postures**   ▽
Contact pressure
Contact stress

Accidental exposure to other specified factors (X52-X58)

AHA: 2018,2Q,7-8

The appropriate 7th character is to be added to each code from categories X52-X58.
A   initial encounter
D   subsequent encounter
S   sequela

√x7ᵗʰ **X52 Prolonged stay in weightless environment**
Weightlessness in spacecraft (simulator)

√x7ᵗʰ **X58 Exposure to other specified factors**
Accident NOS
Exposure NOS

Intentional self-harm (X71-X83)

Purposely self-inflicted injury
Suicide (attempted)

The appropriate 7th character is to be added to each code from categories X71-X83.
A   initial encounter
D   subsequent encounter
S   sequela

√4ᵗʰ **X71 Intentional self-harm by drowning and submersion**

√x7ᵗʰ **X71.0 Intentional self-harm by drowning and submersion while in bathtub**   HCC

√x7ᵗʰ **X71.1 Intentional self-harm by drowning and submersion while in swimming pool**   HCC

√x7ᵗʰ **X71.2 Intentional self-harm by drowning and submersion after jump into swimming pool**   HCC

√x7ᵗʰ **X71.3 Intentional self-harm by drowning and submersion in natural water**   HCC

√x7ᵗʰ **X71.8 Other intentional self-harm by drowning and submersion**   HCC

√x7ᵗʰ **X71.9 Intentional self-harm by drowning and submersion, unspecified**   HCC ▽

√x7ᵗʰ **X72 Intentional self-harm by handgun discharge**   HCC
Intentional self-harm by gun for single hand use
Intentional self-harm by pistol
Intentional self-harm by revolver
EXCLUDES 1   Very pistol (X74.8)

√4ᵗʰ **X73 Intentional self-harm by rifle, shotgun and larger firearm discharge**
EXCLUDES 1   airgun (X74.01)

√x7ᵗʰ **X73.0 Intentional self-harm by shotgun discharge**   HCC

√x7ᵗʰ **X73.1 Intentional self-harm by hunting rifle discharge**   HCC

√x7ᵗʰ **X73.2 Intentional self-harm by machine gun discharge**   HCC

√x7ᵗʰ **X73.8 Intentional self-harm by other larger firearm discharge**   HCC

√x7ᵗʰ **X73.9 Intentional self-harm by unspecified larger firearm discharge**   HCC ▽

√4ᵗʰ **X74 Intentional self-harm by other and unspecified firearm and gun discharge**

√5ᵗʰ **X74.0 Intentional self-harm by gas, air or spring-operated guns**

√x7ᵗʰ **X74.01 Intentional self-harm by airgun**   HCC
Intentional self-harm by BB gun discharge
Intentional self-harm by pellet gun discharge

√x7ᵗʰ **X74.02 Intentional self-harm by paintball gun**   HCC

√x7ᵗʰ **X74.09 Intentional self-harm by other gas, air or spring-operated gun**   HCC

√x7ᵗʰ **X74.8 Intentional self-harm by other firearm discharge**   HCC
Intentional self-harm by Very pistol [flare] discharge

√x7ᵗʰ **X74.9 Intentional self-harm by unspecified firearm discharge**   HCC ▽

√x7ᵗʰ **X75 Intentional self-harm by explosive material**   HCC

√x7ᵗʰ **X76 Intentional self-harm by smoke, fire and flames**   HCC

√4ᵗʰ **X77 Intentional self-harm by steam, hot vapors and hot objects**

√x7ᵗʰ **X77.0 Intentional self-harm by steam or hot vapors**   HCC

√x7ᵗʰ **X77.1 Intentional self-harm by hot tap water**   HCC

√x7ᵗʰ **X77.2 Intentional self-harm by other hot fluids**   HCC

√x7ᵗʰ **X77.3 Intentional self-harm by hot household appliances**   HCC

√x7ᵗʰ **X77.8 Intentional self-harm by other hot objects**   HCC

√x7ᵗʰ **X77.9 Intentional self-harm by unspecified hot objects**   HCC ▽

√4ᵗʰ **X78 Intentional self-harm by sharp object**

√x7ᵗʰ **X78.0 Intentional self-harm by sharp glass**   HCC

√x7ᵗʰ **X78.1 Intentional self-harm by knife**   HCC

√x7ᵗʰ **X78.2 Intentional self-harm by sword or dagger**   HCC

√x7ᵗʰ **X78.8 Intentional self-harm by other sharp object**   HCC

√x7ᵗʰ **X78.9 Intentional self-harm by unspecified sharp object**   HCC ▽

√x7ᵗʰ **X79 Intentional self-harm by blunt object**   HCC

√x7ᵗʰ **X80 Intentional self-harm by jumping from a high place**   HCC
Intentional fall from one level to another

√4ᵗʰ **X81 Intentional self-harm by jumping or lying in front of moving object**

√x7ᵗʰ **X81.0 Intentional self-harm by jumping or lying in front of motor vehicle**   HCC

√x7ᵗʰ **X81.1 Intentional self-harm by jumping or lying in front of (subway) train**   HCC

√x7ᵗʰ **X81.8 Intentional self-harm by jumping or lying in front of other moving object**   HCC

√4ᵗʰ **X82 Intentional self-harm by crashing of motor vehicle**

√x7ᵗʰ **X82.0 Intentional collision of motor vehicle with other motor vehicle**   HCC

√x7ᵗʰ **X82.1 Intentional collision of motor vehicle with train**   HCC

√x7ᵗʰ **X82.2 Intentional collision of motor vehicle with tree**   HCC

√x7ᵗʰ **X82.8 Other intentional self-harm by crashing of motor vehicle**   HCC

√4ᵗʰ **X83 Intentional self-harm by other specified means**
EXCLUDES 1   intentional self-harm by poisoning or contact with toxic substance - see Table of Drugs and Chemicals

√x7ᵗʰ **X83.0 Intentional self-harm by crashing of aircraft**   HCC

√x7ᵗʰ **X83.1 Intentional self-harm by electrocution**   HCC

√x7ᵗʰ **X83.2 Intentional self-harm by exposure to extremes of cold**   HCC

√x7ᵗʰ **X83.8 Intentional self-harm by other specified means**   HCC

Assault (X92-Y09)

INCLUDES   homicide
injuries inflicted by another person with intent to injure or kill, by any means
EXCLUDES 1   injuries due to legal intervention (Y35.-)
injuries due to operations of war (Y36.-)
injuries due to terrorism (Y38.-)

The appropriate 7th character is to be added to each code from categories X92-Y04 and Y08.
A   initial encounter
D   subsequent encounter
S   sequela

√4ᵗʰ **X92 Assault by drowning and submersion**

√x7ᵗʰ **X92.0 Assault by drowning and submersion while in bathtub**

√x7ᵗʰ **X92.1 Assault by drowning and submersion while in swimming pool**

Chapter 20. External Causes of Morbidity

X92.2–Y07.436

- ✓x7ᵗʰ **X92.2** **Assault by drowning and submersion** after push into swimming pool
- ✓x7ᵗʰ **X92.3** **Assault by drowning and submersion** in natural water
- ✓x7ᵗʰ **X92.8** **Other assault by drowning and submersion**
- ✓x7ᵗʰ **X92.9** **Assault by drowning and submersion, unspecified** ▽

✓x7ᵗʰ **X93 Assault by handgun discharge**
    Assault by discharge of gun for single hand use
    Assault by discharge of pistol
    Assault by discharge of revolver
    EXCLUDES 1   Very pistol (X95.8)

✓4ᵗʰ **X94 Assault by rifle, shotgun and larger firearm discharge**
    EXCLUDES 1   airgun (X95.01)
- ✓x7ᵗʰ **X94.0** **Assault by shotgun**
- ✓x7ᵗʰ **X94.1** **Assault by hunting rifle**
- ✓x7ᵗʰ **X94.2** **Assault by machine gun**
- ✓x7ᵗʰ **X94.8** **Assault by other larger firearm discharge**
- ✓x7ᵗʰ **X94.9** **Assault by unspecified larger firearm discharge** ▽

✓4ᵗʰ **X95 Assault by other and unspecified firearm and gun discharge**
- ✓5ᵗʰ **X95.0** **Assault by gas, air or spring-operated guns**
  - ✓x7ᵗʰ **X95.01** **Assault by airgun discharge**
        Assault by BB gun discharge
        Assault by pellet gun discharge
  - ✓x7ᵗʰ **X95.02** **Assault by paintball gun discharge**
  - ✓x7ᵗʰ **X95.09** **Assault by other gas, air or spring-operated gun**
- ✓x7ᵗʰ **X95.8** **Assault by other firearm discharge**
      Assault by Very pistol [flare] discharge
- ✓x7ᵗʰ **X95.9** **Assault by unspecified firearm discharge** ▽

✓4ᵗʰ **X96 Assault by explosive material**
    EXCLUDES 1   incendiary device (X97)
               terrorism involving explosive material (Y38.2-)
- ✓x7ᵗʰ **X96.0** **Assault by antipersonnel bomb**
      EXCLUDES 1   antipersonnel bomb use in military or war (Y36.2-)
- ✓x7ᵗʰ **X96.1** **Assault by gasoline bomb**
- ✓x7ᵗʰ **X96.2** **Assault by letter bomb**
- ✓x7ᵗʰ **X96.3** **Assault by fertilizer bomb**
- ✓x7ᵗʰ **X96.4** **Assault by pipe bomb**
- ✓x7ᵗʰ **X96.8** **Assault by other specified explosive**
- ✓x7ᵗʰ **X96.9** **Assault by unspecified explosive** ▽

✓x7ᵗʰ **X97 Assault by smoke, fire and flames**
    Assault by arson
    Assault by cigarettes
    Assault by incendiary device

✓4ᵗʰ **X98 Assault by steam, hot vapors and hot objects**
- ✓x7ᵗʰ **X98.0** **Assault by steam or hot vapors**
- ✓x7ᵗʰ **X98.1** **Assault by hot tap water**
- ✓x7ᵗʰ **X98.2** **Assault by hot fluids**
- ✓x7ᵗʰ **X98.3** **Assault by hot household appliances**
- ✓x7ᵗʰ **X98.8** **Assault by other hot objects**
- ✓x7ᵗʰ **X98.9** **Assault by unspecified hot objects** ▽

✓4ᵗʰ **X99 Assault by sharp object**
    EXCLUDES 1   assault by strike by sports equipment (Y08.0-)
- ✓x7ᵗʰ **X99.0** **Assault by sharp glass**
- ✓x7ᵗʰ **X99.1** **Assault by knife**
- ✓x7ᵗʰ **X99.2** **Assault by sword or dagger**
- ✓x7ᵗʰ **X99.8** **Assault by other sharp object**
- ✓x7ᵗʰ **X99.9** **Assault by unspecified sharp object** ▽
      Assault by stabbing NOS

✓x7ᵗʰ **Y00 Assault by blunt object**
    EXCLUDES 1   assault by strike by sports equipment (Y08.0-)

✓x7ᵗʰ **Y01 Assault by pushing from high place**

✓4ᵗʰ **Y02 Assault by pushing or placing victim in front of moving object**
- ✓x7ᵗʰ **Y02.0** **Assault by pushing or placing victim in front of motor vehicle**
- ✓x7ᵗʰ **Y02.1** **Assault by pushing or placing victim in front of (subway) train**

- ✓x7ᵗʰ **Y02.8** **Assault by pushing or placing victim in front of other moving object**

✓4ᵗʰ **Y03 Assault by crashing of motor vehicle**
- ✓x7ᵗʰ **Y03.0** **Assault by being hit or run over by motor vehicle**
- ✓x7ᵗʰ **Y03.8** **Other assault by crashing of motor vehicle**

✓4ᵗʰ **Y04 Assault by bodily force**
    EXCLUDES 1   assault by:
               submersion (X92.-)
               use of weapon (X93-X95, X99, Y00)
- ✓x7ᵗʰ **Y04.0** **Assault by unarmed brawl or fight**
- ✓x7ᵗʰ **Y04.1** **Assault by human bite**
- ✓x7ᵗʰ **Y04.2** **Assault by strike against or bumped into by another person**
- ✓x7ᵗʰ **Y04.8** **Assault by other bodily force**
      Assault by bodily force NOS

✓4ᵗʰ **Y07 Perpetrator of assault, maltreatment and neglect**
    NOTE   Codes from this category are for use only in cases of confirmed abuse (T74.-)
           Selection of the correct perpetrator code is based on the relationship between the perpetrator and the victim
    INCLUDES   perpetrator of abandonment
               perpetrator of emotional neglect
               perpetrator of mental cruelty
               perpetrator of physical abuse
               perpetrator of physical neglect
               perpetrator of sexual abuse
               perpetrator of torture

- ✓5ᵗʰ **Y07.0** **Spouse or partner, perpetrator of maltreatment and neglect**
      Spouse or partner, perpetrator of maltreatment and neglect against spouse or partner
  - **Y07.01** **Husband, perpetrator of maltreatment and neglect**
  - **Y07.02** **Wife, perpetrator of maltreatment and neglect**
  - **Y07.03** **Male partner, perpetrator of maltreatment and neglect**
  - **Y07.04** **Female partner, perpetrator of maltreatment and neglect**
- ✓5ᵗʰ **Y07.1** **Parent (adoptive) (biological), perpetrator of maltreatment and neglect**
  - **Y07.11** **Biological father, perpetrator of maltreatment and neglect**
  - **Y07.12** **Biological mother, perpetrator of maltreatment and neglect**
  - **Y07.13** **Adoptive father, perpetrator of maltreatment and neglect**
  - **Y07.14** **Adoptive mother, perpetrator of maltreatment and neglect**
- ✓5ᵗʰ **Y07.4** **Other family member, perpetrator of maltreatment and neglect**
  - ✓6ᵗʰ **Y07.41** **Sibling, perpetrator of maltreatment and neglect**
        EXCLUDES 1   stepsibling, perpetrator of maltreatment and neglect (Y07.435, Y07.436)
    - **Y07.410** **Brother, perpetrator of maltreatment and neglect**
    - **Y07.411** **Sister, perpetrator of maltreatment and neglect**
  - ✓6ᵗʰ **Y07.42** **Foster parent, perpetrator of maltreatment and neglect**
    - **Y07.420** **Foster father, perpetrator of maltreatment and neglect**
    - **Y07.421** **Foster mother, perpetrator of maltreatment and neglect**
  - ✓6ᵗʰ **Y07.43** **Stepparent or stepsibling, perpetrator of maltreatment and neglect**
    - **Y07.430** **Stepfather, perpetrator of maltreatment and neglect**
    - **Y07.432** **Male friend of parent (co-residing in household), perpetrator of maltreatment and neglect**
    - **Y07.433** **Stepmother, perpetrator of maltreatment and neglect**
    - **Y07.434** **Female friend of parent (co-residing in household), perpetrator of maltreatment and neglect**
    - **Y07.435** **Stepbrother, perpetrator or maltreatment and neglect**
    - **Y07.436** **Stepsister, perpetrator of maltreatment and neglect**

☑6ᵗʰ **Y07.49** **Other family member, perpetrator of maltreatment and neglect**

Y07.490 Male cousin, perpetrator of maltreatment and neglect

Y07.491 Female cousin, perpetrator of maltreatment and neglect

Y07.499 Other family member, perpetrator of maltreatment and neglect

☑5ᵗʰ **Y07.5** Non-family member, perpetrator of maltreatment and neglect

Y07.50 **Unspecified non-family member, perpetrator of maltreatment and neglect** ▽

☑6ᵗʰ **Y07.51** Daycare provider, perpetrator of maltreatment and neglect

Y07.510 At-home childcare provider, perpetrator of maltreatment and neglect

Y07.511 Daycare center childcare provider, perpetrator of maltreatment and neglect

Y07.512 At-home adultcare provider, perpetrator of maltreatment and neglect

Y07.513 Adultcare center provider, perpetrator of maltreatment and neglect

Y07.519 **Unspecified daycare provider, perpetrator of maltreatment and neglect** ▽

☑6ᵗʰ **Y07.52** Healthcare provider, perpetrator of maltreatment and neglect

Y07.521 Mental health provider, perpetrator of maltreatment and neglect

Y07.528 **Other therapist or healthcare provider, perpetrator of maltreatment and neglect**
Nurse perpetrator of maltreatment and neglect
Occupational therapist perpetrator of maltreatment and neglect
Physical therapist perpetrator of maltreatment and neglect
Speech therapist perpetrator of maltreatment and neglect

Y07.529 **Unspecified healthcare provider, perpetrator of maltreatment and neglect** ▽

Y07.53 Teacher or instructor, perpetrator of maltreatment and neglect
Coach, perpetrator of maltreatment and neglect

Y07.59 Other non-family member, perpetrator of maltreatment and neglect

● **Y07.6** Multiple perpetrators of maltreatment and neglect

Y07.9 Unspecified perpetrator of maltreatment and neglect ▽

☑4ᵗʰ **Y08** **Assault by other specified means**

☑5ᵗʰ **Y08.0** **Assault by strike by sport equipment**

☑x7ᵗʰ **Y08.01** **Assault by strike by hockey stick**

☑x7ᵗʰ **Y08.02** **Assault by strike by baseball bat**

☑x7ᵗʰ **Y08.09** **Assault by strike by other specified type of sport equipment**

☑5ᵗʰ **Y08.8** **Assault by other specified means**

☑x7ᵗʰ **Y08.81** **Assault by crashing of aircraft**

☑x7ᵗʰ **Y08.89** **Assault by other specified means**

Y09 **Assault by unspecified means** ▽
Assassination (attempted) NOS
Homicide (attempted) NOS
Manslaughter (attempted) NOS
Murder (attempted) NOS

Event of undetermined intent (Y21-Y33)

Undetermined intent is only for use when there is specific documentation in the record that the intent of the injury cannot be determined. If no such documentation is present, code to accidental (unintentional).

The appropriate 7th character is to be added to each code from categories Y21-Y33.
A   initial encounter
D   subsequent encounter
S   sequela

☑4ᵗʰ **Y21** **Drowning and submersion, undetermined intent**

☑x7ᵗʰ **Y21.0** **Drowning and submersion while in bathtub, undetermined intent**

☑x7ᵗʰ **Y21.1** **Drowning and submersion after fall into bathtub, undetermined intent**

☑x7ᵗʰ **Y21.2** **Drowning and submersion** while in swimming pool, **undetermined intent**

☑x7ᵗʰ **Y21.3** **Drowning and submersion** after fall into swimming pool, **undetermined intent**

☑x7ᵗʰ **Y21.4** **Drowning and submersion** in natural water, **undetermined intent**

☑x7ᵗʰ **Y21.8** **Other drowning and submersion, undetermined intent**

☑x7ᵗʰ **Y21.9** **Unspecified drowning and submersion, undetermined intent** ▽

☑x7ᵗʰ **Y22** **Handgun discharge, undetermined intent**
Discharge of gun for single hand use, undetermined intent
Discharge of pistol, undetermined intent
Discharge of revolver, undetermined intent
EXCLUDES 2 Very pistol (Y24.8)

☑4ᵗʰ **Y23** **Rifle, shotgun and larger firearm discharge, undetermined intent**
EXCLUDES 2 airgun (Y24.0)

☑x7ᵗʰ **Y23.0** Shotgun **discharge, undetermined intent**

☑x7ᵗʰ **Y23.1** Hunting rifle **discharge, undetermined intent**

☑x7ᵗʰ **Y23.2** Military firearm **discharge, undetermined intent**

☑x7ᵗʰ **Y23.3** Machine gun **discharge, undetermined intent**

☑x7ᵗʰ **Y23.8** **Other larger firearm discharge, undetermined intent**

☑x7ᵗʰ **Y23.9** **Unspecified larger firearm discharge, undetermined intent** ▽

☑4ᵗʰ **Y24** **Other and unspecified firearm discharge, undetermined intent**

☑x7ᵗʰ **Y24.0** Airgun **discharge, undetermined intent**
BB gun discharge, undetermined intent
Pellet gun discharge, undetermined intent

☑x7ᵗʰ **Y24.8** **Other firearm discharge, undetermined intent**
Paintball gun discharge, undetermined intent
Very pistol [flare] discharge, undetermined intent

☑x7ᵗʰ **Y24.9** **Unspecified firearm discharge, undetermined intent** ▽

☑x7ᵗʰ **Y25** **Contact with explosive material, undetermined intent**

☑x7ᵗʰ **Y26** **Exposure to smoke, fire and flames, undetermined intent**

☑4ᵗʰ **Y27** **Contact with steam, hot vapors and hot objects, undetermined intent**

☑x7ᵗʰ **Y27.0** **Contact with** steam and hot vapors, **undetermined intent**

☑x7ᵗʰ **Y27.1** **Contact with hot** tap water, **undetermined intent**

☑x7ᵗʰ **Y27.2** **Contact with hot** fluids, **undetermined intent**

☑x7ᵗʰ **Y27.3** **Contact with hot** household appliance, **undetermined intent**

☑x7ᵗʰ **Y27.8** **Contact with other hot** objects, **undetermined intent**

☑x7ᵗʰ **Y27.9** **Contact with unspecified hot objects, undetermined intent** ▽

☑4ᵗʰ **Y28** **Contact with sharp object, undetermined intent**

☑x7ᵗʰ **Y28.0** **Contact with sharp** glass, **undetermined intent**

☑x7ᵗʰ **Y28.1** **Contact with** knife, **undetermined intent**

☑x7ᵗʰ **Y28.2** **Contact with** sword or dagger, **undetermined intent**

☑x7ᵗʰ **Y28.8** **Contact with other sharp object, undetermined intent**

☑x7ᵗʰ **Y28.9** **Contact with unspecified sharp object, undetermined intent** ▽

☑x7ᵗʰ **Y29** **Contact with blunt object, undetermined intent**

☑x7ᵗʰ **Y30** **Falling, jumping or pushed from a high place, undetermined intent**
Victim falling from one level to another, undetermined intent

☑x7ᵗʰ **Y31** **Falling, lying or running before or into moving object, undetermined intent**

☑x7ᵗʰ **Y32** **Crashing of motor vehicle, undetermined intent**

☑x7ᵗʰ **Y33** **Other specified events, undetermined intent**

Legal intervention, operations of war, military operations, and terrorism (Y35-Y38)

The appropriate 7th character is to be added to each code from categories Y35-Y38.
A   initial encounter
D   subsequent encounter
S   sequela

√4ᵗʰ **Y35   Legal intervention**

INCLUDES   any injury sustained as a result of an encounter with any law enforcement official, serving in any capacity at the time of the encounter, whether on-duty or off-duty. Includes injury to law enforcement official, suspect and bystander

√5ᵗʰ **Y35.0   Legal intervention involving firearm discharge**

√6ᵗʰ **Y35.00   Legal intervention involving unspecified firearm discharge**
Legal intervention involving gunshot wound
Legal intervention involving shot NOS

√7ᵗʰ **Y35.001   Legal intervention involving unspecified firearm discharge, law enforcement official injured** ▽

√7ᵗʰ **Y35.002   Legal intervention involving unspecified firearm discharge, bystander injured** ▽

√7ᵗʰ **Y35.003   Legal intervention involving unspecified firearm discharge, suspect injured** ▽

√6ᵗʰ **Y35.01   Legal intervention involving injury by machine gun**

√7ᵗʰ **Y35.011   Legal intervention involving injury by machine gun, law enforcement official injured**

√7ᵗʰ **Y35.012   Legal intervention involving injury by machine gun, bystander injured**

√7ᵗʰ **Y35.013   Legal intervention involving injury by machine gun, suspect injured**

√6ᵗʰ **Y35.02   Legal intervention involving injury by handgun**

√7ᵗʰ **Y35.021   Legal intervention involving injury by handgun, law enforcement official injured**

√7ᵗʰ **Y35.022   Legal intervention involving injury by handgun, bystander injured**

√7ᵗʰ **Y35.023   Legal intervention involving injury by handgun, suspect injured**

√6ᵗʰ **Y35.03   Legal intervention involving injury by rifle pellet**

√7ᵗʰ **Y35.031   Legal intervention involving injury by rifle pellet, law enforcement official injured**

√7ᵗʰ **Y35.032   Legal intervention involving injury by rifle pellet, bystander injured**

√7ᵗʰ **Y35.033   Legal intervention involving injury by rifle pellet, suspect injured**

√6ᵗʰ **Y35.04   Legal intervention involving injury by rubber bullet**

√7ᵗʰ **Y35.041   Legal intervention involving injury by rubber bullet, law enforcement official injured**

√7ᵗʰ **Y35.042   Legal intervention involving injury by rubber bullet, bystander injured**

√7ᵗʰ **Y35.043   Legal intervention involving injury by rubber bullet, suspect injured**

√6ᵗʰ **Y35.09   Legal intervention involving other firearm discharge**

√7ᵗʰ **Y35.091   Legal intervention involving other firearm discharge, law enforcement official injured**

√7ᵗʰ **Y35.092   Legal intervention involving other firearm discharge, bystander injured**

√7ᵗʰ **Y35.093   Legal intervention involving other firearm discharge, suspect injured**

√5ᵗʰ **Y35.1   Legal intervention involving explosives**

√6ᵗʰ **Y35.10   Legal intervention involving unspecified explosives**

√7ᵗʰ **Y35.101   Legal intervention involving unspecified explosives, law enforcement official injured** ▽

√7ᵗʰ **Y35.102   Legal intervention involving unspecified explosives, bystander injured** ▽

√7ᵗʰ **Y35.103   Legal intervention involving unspecified explosives, suspect injured** ▽

√6ᵗʰ **Y35.11   Legal intervention involving injury by dynamite**

√7ᵗʰ **Y35.111   Legal intervention involving injury by dynamite, law enforcement official injured**

√7ᵗʰ **Y35.112   Legal intervention involving injury by dynamite, bystander injured**

√7ᵗʰ **Y35.113   Legal intervention involving injury by dynamite, suspect injured**

√6ᵗʰ **Y35.12   Legal intervention involving injury by explosive shell**

√7ᵗʰ **Y35.121   Legal intervention involving injury by explosive shell, law enforcement official injured**

√7ᵗʰ **Y35.122   Legal intervention involving injury by explosive shell, bystander injured**

√7ᵗʰ **Y35.123   Legal intervention involving injury by explosive shell, suspect injured**

√6ᵗʰ **Y35.19   Legal intervention involving other explosives**
Legal intervention involving injury by grenade
Legal intervention involving injury by mortar bomb

√7ᵗʰ **Y35.191   Legal intervention involving other explosives, law enforcement official injured**

√7ᵗʰ **Y35.192   Legal intervention involving other explosives, bystander injured**

√7ᵗʰ **Y35.193   Legal intervention involving other explosives, suspect injured**

√5ᵗʰ **Y35.2   Legal intervention involving gas**
Legal intervention involving asphyxiation by gas
Legal intervention involving poisoning by gas

√6ᵗʰ **Y35.20   Legal intervention involving unspecified gas**

√7ᵗʰ **Y35.201   Legal intervention involving unspecified gas, law enforcement official injured** ▽

√7ᵗʰ **Y35.202   Legal intervention involving unspecified gas, bystander injured** ▽

√7ᵗʰ **Y35.203   Legal intervention involving unspecified gas, suspect injured** ▽

√6ᵗʰ **Y35.21   Legal intervention involving injury by tear gas**

√7ᵗʰ **Y35.211   Legal intervention involving injury by tear gas, law enforcement official injured**

√7ᵗʰ **Y35.212   Legal intervention involving injury by tear gas, bystander injured**

√7ᵗʰ **Y35.213   Legal intervention involving injury by tear gas, suspect injured**

√6ᵗʰ **Y35.29   Legal intervention involving other gas**

√7ᵗʰ **Y35.291   Legal intervention involving other gas, law enforcement official injured**

√7ᵗʰ **Y35.292   Legal intervention involving other gas, bystander injured**

√7ᵗʰ **Y35.293   Legal intervention involving other gas, suspect injured**

√5ᵗʰ **Y35.3   Legal intervention involving blunt objects**
Legal intervention involving being hit or struck by blunt object

√6ᵗʰ **Y35.30   Legal intervention involving unspecified blunt objects**

√7ᵗʰ **Y35.301   Legal intervention involving unspecified blunt objects, law enforcement official injured** ▽

√7ᵗʰ **Y35.302   Legal intervention involving unspecified blunt objects, bystander injured** ▽

√7ᵗʰ **Y35.303   Legal intervention involving unspecified blunt objects, suspect injured** ▽

√6ᵗʰ **Y35.31   Legal intervention involving baton**

√7ᵗʰ **Y35.311   Legal intervention involving baton, law enforcement official injured**

√7ᵗʰ **Y35.312   Legal intervention involving baton, bystander injured**

√7ᵗʰ **Y35.313   Legal intervention involving baton, suspect injured**

√6ᵗʰ **Y35.39   Legal intervention involving other blunt objects**

√7ᵗʰ **Y35.391   Legal intervention involving other blunt objects, law enforcement official injured**

√7ᵗʰ **Y35.392   Legal intervention involving other blunt objects, bystander injured**

√7ᵗʰ **Y35.393   Legal intervention involving other blunt objects, suspect injured**

√5ᵗʰ **Y35.4 Legal intervention involving** sharp objects

Legal intervention involving being cut by sharp objects

Legal intervention involving being stabbed by sharp objects

√6ᵗʰ **Y35.40 Legal intervention involving unspecified sharp objects**

√7ᵗʰ **Y35.401 Legal intervention involving unspecified sharp objects,** law enforcement official **injured** ▽

√7ᵗʰ **Y35.402 Legal intervention involving unspecified sharp objects,** bystander **injured** ▽

√7ᵗʰ **Y35.403 Legal intervention involving unspecified sharp objects,** suspect **injured** ▽

√6ᵗʰ **Y35.41 Legal intervention involving** bayonet

√7ᵗʰ **Y35.411 Legal intervention involving bayonet,** law enforcement official **injured**

√7ᵗʰ **Y35.412 Legal intervention involving bayonet,** bystander **injured**

√7ᵗʰ **Y35.413 Legal intervention involving bayonet,** suspect **injured**

√6ᵗʰ **Y35.49 Legal intervention involving other sharp objects**

√7ᵗʰ **Y35.491 Legal intervention involving other sharp objects,** law enforcement official **injured**

√7ᵗʰ **Y35.492 Legal intervention involving other sharp objects,** bystander **injured**

√7ᵗʰ **Y35.493 Legal intervention involving other sharp objects,** suspect **injured**

√5ᵗʰ **Y35.8 Legal intervention involving other specified means**

√6ᵗʰ **Y35.81 Legal intervention involving** manhandling

√7ᵗʰ **Y35.811 Legal intervention involving manhandling,** law enforcement official **injured**

√7ᵗʰ **Y35.812 Legal intervention involving manhandling,** bystander **injured**

√7ᵗʰ **Y35.813 Legal intervention involving manhandling,** suspect **injured**

√6ᵗʰ **Y35.89 Legal intervention involving other specified means**

√7ᵗʰ **Y35.891 Legal intervention involving other specified means,** law enforcement official **injured**

√7ᵗʰ **Y35.892 Legal intervention involving other specified means,** bystander **injured**

√7ᵗʰ **Y35.893 Legal intervention involving other specified means,** suspect **injured**

AHA: 2018,1Q,5

√5ᵗʰ **Y35.9 Legal intervention, means unspecified**

√x7ᵗʰ **Y35.91 Legal intervention, means unspecified,** law enforcement official **injured** ▽

√x7ᵗʰ **Y35.92 Legal intervention, means unspecified,** bystander **injured** ▽

√x7ᵗʰ **Y35.93 Legal intervention, means unspecified,** suspect **injured** ▽

√4ᵗʰ **Y36 Operations of war**

INCLUDES injuries to military personnel and civilians caused by war, civil insurrection, and peacekeeping missions

EXCLUDES 1 injury to military personnel occurring during peacetime military operations (Y37.-)

military vehicles involved in transport accidents with non-military vehicle during peacetime (V09.01, V09.21, V19.81, V29.81, V39.81, V49.81, V59.81, V69.81, V79.81)

AHA: 2014,3Q,4

√5ᵗʰ **Y36.0 War operations involving** explosion of marine weapons

√6ᵗʰ **Y36.00 War operations involving explosion of unspecified marine weapon**

War operations involving underwater blast NOS

√7ᵗʰ **Y36.000 War operations involving explosion of unspecified marine weapon,** military personnel ▽

√7ᵗʰ **Y36.001 War operations involving explosion of unspecified marine weapon,** civilian ▽

√6ᵗʰ **Y36.01 War operations involving explosion of** depth-charge

√7ᵗʰ **Y36.010 War operations involving explosion of depth-charge,** military personnel

√7ᵗʰ **Y36.011 War operations involving explosion of depth-charge,** civilian

√6ᵗʰ **Y36.02 War operations involving explosion of** marine mine

War operations involving explosion of marine mine, at sea or in harbor

√7ᵗʰ **Y36.020 War operations involving explosion of marine mine,** military personnel

√7ᵗʰ **Y36.021 War operations involving explosion of marine mine,** civilian

√6ᵗʰ **Y36.03 War operations involving explosion of** sea-based artillery shell

√7ᵗʰ **Y36.030 War operations involving explosion of sea-based artillery shell,** military personnel

√7ᵗʰ **Y36.031 War operations involving explosion of sea-based artillery shell,** civilian

√6ᵗʰ **Y36.04 War operations involving explosion of** torpedo

√7ᵗʰ **Y36.040 War operations involving explosion of torpedo,** military personnel

√7ᵗʰ **Y36.041 War operations involving explosion of torpedo,** civilian

√6ᵗʰ **Y36.05 War operations involving** accidental detonation of onboard marine weapons

√7ᵗʰ **Y36.050 War operations involving accidental detonation of onboard marine weapons,** military personnel

√7ᵗʰ **Y36.051 War operations involving accidental detonation of onboard marine weapons,** civilian

√6ᵗʰ **Y36.09 War operations involving explosion of other marine weapons**

√7ᵗʰ **Y36.090 War operations involving explosion of other marine weapons,** military personnel

√7ᵗʰ **Y36.091 War operations involving explosion of other marine weapons,** civilian

√5ᵗʰ **Y36.1 War operations involving** destruction of aircraft

√6ᵗʰ **Y36.10 War operations involving unspecified destruction of aircraft**

√7ᵗʰ **Y36.100 War operations involving unspecified destruction of aircraft,** military personnel ▽

√7ᵗʰ **Y36.101 War operations involving unspecified destruction of aircraft,** civilian ▽

√6ᵗʰ **Y36.11 War operations involving destruction of aircraft due to** enemy fire or explosives

War operations involving destruction of aircraft due to air to air missile

War operations involving destruction of aircraft due to explosive placed on aircraft

War operations involving destruction of aircraft due to rocket propelled grenade [RPG]

War operations involving destruction of aircraft due to small arms fire

War operations involving destruction of aircraft due to surface to air missile

√7ᵗʰ **Y36.110 War operations involving destruction of aircraft due to enemy fire or explosives,** military personnel

√7ᵗʰ **Y36.111 War operations involving destruction of aircraft due to enemy fire or explosives,** civilian

√6ᵗʰ **Y36.12 War operations involving destruction of aircraft due to** collision with other aircraft

√7ᵗʰ **Y36.120 War operations involving destruction of aircraft due to collision with other aircraft,** military personnel

√7ᵗʰ **Y36.121 War operations involving destruction of aircraft due to collision with other aircraft,** civilian

√6ᵗʰ **Y36.13 War operations involving destruction of aircraft due to** onboard fire

√7ᵗʰ **Y36.130 War operations involving destruction of aircraft due to onboard fire,** military personnel

√7ᵗʰ **Y36.131 War operations involving destruction of aircraft due to onboard fire,** civilian

√6ᵗʰ **Y36.14 War operations involving destruction of aircraft due to** accidental detonation of onboard munitions and explosives

√7ᵗʰ **Y36.140 War operations involving destruction of aircraft due to accidental detonation of onboard munitions and explosives,** military personnel

✔ Additional Character Req   √x7ᵗʰ Placeholder Alert   Manifestation   ▽ Unspecified   ►◄ Revised Text   ● New Code   ▲ Revised Code Title

✓7ᵗʰ **Y36.141 War operations involving destruction of aircraft due to accidental detonation of onboard munitions and explosives, civilian**

✓6ᵗʰ **Y36.19 War operations involving other destruction of aircraft**

✓7ᵗʰ **Y36.190 War operations involving other destruction of aircraft, military personnel**

✓7ᵗʰ **Y36.191 War operations involving other destruction of aircraft, civilian**

✓5ᵗʰ **Y36.2 War operations involving other explosions and fragments**

EXCLUDES 1   *war operations involving explosion of aircraft (Y36.1-)*
war operations involving explosion of marine weapons (Y36.0-)
war operations involving explosion of nuclear weapons (Y36.5-)
war operations involving explosion occurring after cessation of hostilities (Y36.8-)

✓6ᵗʰ **Y36.20 War operations involving unspecified explosion and fragments**

War operations involving air blast NOS
War operations involving blast NOS
War operations involving blast fragments NOS
War operations involving blast wave NOS
War operations involving blast wind NOS
War operations involving explosion NOS
War operations involving explosion of bomb NOS

✓7ᵗʰ **Y36.200 War operations involving unspecified explosion and fragments, military personnel** ▽

✓7ᵗʰ **Y36.201 War operations involving unspecified explosion and fragments, civilian** ▽

✓6ᵗʰ **Y36.21 War operations involving explosion of aerial bomb**

✓7ᵗʰ **Y36.210 War operations involving explosion of aerial bomb, military personnel**

✓7ᵗʰ **Y36.211 War operations involving explosion of aerial bomb, civilian**

✓6ᵗʰ **Y36.22 War operations involving explosion of guided missile**

✓7ᵗʰ **Y36.220 War operations involving explosion of guided missile, military personnel**

✓7ᵗʰ **Y36.221 War operations involving explosion of guided missile, civilian**

✓6ᵗʰ **Y36.23 War operations involving explosion of improvised explosive device [IED]**

War operations involving explosion of person-borne improvised explosive device [IED]
War operations involving explosion of vehicle-borne improvised explosive device [IED]
War operations involving explosion of roadside improvised explosive device [IED]

✓7ᵗʰ **Y36.230 War operations involving explosion of improvised explosive device [IED], military personnel**

✓7ᵗʰ **Y36.231 War operations involving explosion of improvised explosive device [IED], civilian**

✓6ᵗʰ **Y36.24 War operations involving explosion due to accidental detonation and discharge of own munitions or munitions launch device**

✓7ᵗʰ **Y36.240 War operations involving explosion due to accidental detonation and discharge of own munitions or munitions launch device, military personnel**

✓7ᵗʰ **Y36.241 War operations involving explosion due to accidental detonation and discharge of own munitions or munitions launch device, civilian**

✓6ᵗʰ **Y36.25 War operations involving fragments from munitions**

✓7ᵗʰ **Y36.250 War operations involving fragments from munitions, military personnel**

✓7ᵗʰ **Y36.251 War operations involving fragments from munitions, civilian**

✓6ᵗʰ **Y36.26 War operations involving fragments of improvised explosive device [IED]**

War operations involving fragments of person-borne improvised explosive device [IED]
War operations involving fragments of vehicle-borne improvised explosive device [IED]
War operations involving fragments of roadside improvised explosive device [IED]

✓7ᵗʰ **Y36.260 War operations involving fragments of improvised explosive device [IED], military personnel**

✓7ᵗʰ **Y36.261 War operations involving fragments of improvised explosive device [IED], civilian**

✓6ᵗʰ **Y36.27 War operations involving fragments from weapons**

✓7ᵗʰ **Y36.270 War operations involving fragments from weapons, military personnel**

✓7ᵗʰ **Y36.271 War operations involving fragments from weapons, civilian**

✓6ᵗʰ **Y36.29 War operations involving other explosions and fragments**

War operations involving explosion of grenade
War operations involving explosions of land mine
War operations involving shrapnel NOS

✓7ᵗʰ **Y36.290 War operations involving other explosions and fragments, military personnel**

✓7ᵗʰ **Y36.291 War operations involving other explosions and fragments, civilian**

✓5ᵗʰ **Y36.3 War operations involving fires, conflagrations and hot substances**

War operations involving smoke, fumes, and heat from fires, conflagrations and hot substances

EXCLUDES 1   *war operations involving fires and conflagrations aboard military aircraft (Y36.1-)*
war operations involving fires and conflagrations aboard military watercraft (Y36.0-)
war operations involving fires and conflagrations caused indirectly by conventional weapons (Y36.2-)
war operations involving fires and thermal effects of nuclear weapons (Y36.53-)

✓6ᵗʰ **Y36.30 War operations involving unspecified fire, conflagration and hot substance**

✓7ᵗʰ **Y36.300 War operations involving unspecified fire, conflagration and hot substance, military personnel** ▽

✓7ᵗʰ **Y36.301 War operations involving unspecified fire, conflagration and hot substance, civilian** ▽

✓6ᵗʰ **Y36.31 War operations involving gasoline bomb**

War operations involving incendiary bomb
War operations involving petrol bomb

✓7ᵗʰ **Y36.310 War operations involving gasoline bomb, military personnel**

✓7ᵗʰ **Y36.311 War operations involving gasoline bomb, civilian**

✓6ᵗʰ **Y36.32 War operations involving incendiary bullet**

✓7ᵗʰ **Y36.320 War operations involving incendiary bullet, military personnel**

✓7ᵗʰ **Y36.321 War operations involving incendiary bullet, civilian**

✓6ᵗʰ **Y36.33 War operations involving flamethrower**

✓7ᵗʰ **Y36.330 War operations involving flamethrower, military personnel**

✓7ᵗʰ **Y36.331 War operations involving flamethrower, civilian**

✓6ᵗʰ **Y36.39 War operations involving other fires, conflagrations and hot substances**

✓7ᵗʰ **Y36.390 War operations involving other fires, conflagrations and hot substances, military personnel**

✓7ᵗʰ **Y36.391 War operations involving other fires, conflagrations and hot substances, civilian**

✓5ᵗʰ **Y36.4 War operations involving firearm discharge and other forms of conventional warfare**

✓6ᵗʰ **Y36.41 War operations involving rubber bullets**

✓7ᵗʰ **Y36.410 War operations involving rubber bullets, military personnel**

✓7ᵗʰ **Y36.411** War operations involving rubber bullets, civilian

✓6ᵗʰ **Y36.42** War operations involving firearms pellets

  ✓7ᵗʰ **Y36.420** War operations involving firearms pellets, military personnel

  ✓7ᵗʰ **Y36.421** War operations involving firearms pellets, civilian

✓6ᵗʰ **Y36.43** War operations involving other firearms discharge

War operations involving bullets NOS

> **EXCLUDES 1**   war operations involving munitions fragments (Y36.25-)
> war operations involving incendiary bullets (Y36.32-)

  ✓7ᵗʰ **Y36.430** War operations involving other firearms discharge, military personnel

  ✓7ᵗʰ **Y36.431** War operations involving other firearms discharge, civilian

✓6ᵗʰ **Y36.44** War operations involving unarmed hand to hand combat

> **EXCLUDES 1**   war operations involving combat using blunt or piercing object (Y36.45-)
> war operations involving intentional restriction of air and airway (Y36.46-)
> war operations involving unintentional restriction of air and airway (Y36.47-)

  ✓7ᵗʰ **Y36.440** War operations involving unarmed hand to hand combat, military personnel

  ✓7ᵗʰ **Y36.441** War operations involving unarmed hand to hand combat, civilian

✓6ᵗʰ **Y36.45** War operations involving combat using blunt or piercing object

  ✓7ᵗʰ **Y36.450** War operations involving combat using blunt or piercing object, military personnel

  ✓7ᵗʰ **Y36.451** War operations involving combat using blunt or piercing object, civilian

✓6ᵗʰ **Y36.46** War operations involving intentional restriction of air and airway

  ✓7ᵗʰ **Y36.460** War operations involving intentional restriction of air and airway, military personnel

  ✓7ᵗʰ **Y36.461** War operations involving intentional restriction of air and airway, civilian

✓6ᵗʰ **Y36.47** War operations involving unintentional restriction of air and airway

  ✓7ᵗʰ **Y36.470** War operations involving unintentional restriction of air and airway, military personnel

  ✓7ᵗʰ **Y36.471** War operations involving unintentional restriction of air and airway, civilian

✓6ᵗʰ **Y36.49** War operations involving other forms of conventional warfare

  ✓7ᵗʰ **Y36.490** War operations involving other forms of conventional warfare, military personnel

  ✓7ᵗʰ **Y36.491** War operations involving other forms of conventional warfare, civilian

✓5ᵗʰ **Y36.5** War operations involving nuclear weapons

War operations involving dirty bomb NOS

✓6ᵗʰ **Y36.50** War operations involving unspecified effect of nuclear weapon

  ✓7ᵗʰ **Y36.500** War operations involving unspecified effect of nuclear weapon, military personnel ▽

  ✓7ᵗʰ **Y36.501** War operations involving unspecified effect of nuclear weapon, civilian ▽

✓6ᵗʰ **Y36.51** War operations involving direct blast effect of nuclear weapon

War operations involving blast pressure of nuclear weapon

  ✓7ᵗʰ **Y36.510** War operations involving direct blast effect of nuclear weapon, military personnel

  ✓7ᵗʰ **Y36.511** War operations involving direct blast effect of nuclear weapon, civilian

✓6ᵗʰ **Y36.52** War operations involving indirect blast effect of nuclear weapon

War operations involving being thrown by blast of nuclear weapon

War operations involving being struck or crushed by blast debris of nuclear weapon

  ✓7ᵗʰ **Y36.520** War operations involving indirect blast effect of nuclear weapon, military personnel

  ✓7ᵗʰ **Y36.521** War operations involving indirect blast effect of nuclear weapon, civilian

✓6ᵗʰ **Y36.53** War operations involving thermal radiation effect of nuclear weapon

War operations involving direct heat from nuclear weapon

War operation involving fireball effects from nuclear weapon

  ✓7ᵗʰ **Y36.530** War operations involving thermal radiation effect of nuclear weapon, military personnel

  ✓7ᵗʰ **Y36.531** War operations involving thermal radiation effect of nuclear weapon, civilian

✓6ᵗʰ **Y36.54** War operation involving nuclear radiation effects of nuclear weapon

War operation involving acute radiation exposure from nuclear weapon

War operation involving exposure to immediate ionizing radiation from nuclear weapon

War operation involving fallout exposure from nuclear weapon

War operation involving secondary effects of nuclear weapons

  ✓7ᵗʰ **Y36.540** War operation involving nuclear radiation effects of nuclear weapon, military personnel

  ✓7ᵗʰ **Y36.541** War operation involving nuclear radiation effects of nuclear weapon, civilian

✓6ᵗʰ **Y36.59** War operation involving other effects of nuclear weapons

  ✓7ᵗʰ **Y36.590** War operation involving other effects of nuclear weapons, military personnel

  ✓7ᵗʰ **Y36.591** War operation involving other effects of nuclear weapons, civilian

✓5ᵗʰ **Y36.6** War operations involving biological weapons

✓6ᵗʰ **Y36.6X** War operations involving biological weapons

  ✓7ᵗʰ **Y36.6X0** War operations involving biological weapons, military personnel

  ✓7ᵗʰ **Y36.6X1** War operations involving biological weapons, civilian

✓5ᵗʰ **Y36.7** War operations involving chemical weapons and other forms of unconventional warfare

> **EXCLUDES 1**   war operations involving incendiary devices (Y36.3-, Y36.5-)

✓6ᵗʰ **Y36.7X** War operations involving chemical weapons and other forms of unconventional warfare

  ✓7ᵗʰ **Y36.7X0** War operations involving chemical weapons and other forms of unconventional warfare, military personnel

  ✓7ᵗʰ **Y36.7X1** War operations involving chemical weapons and other forms of unconventional warfare, civilian

✓5ᵗʰ **Y36.8** War operations occurring after cessation of hostilities

War operations classifiable to categories Y36.0-Y36.8 but occurring after cessation of hostilities

✓6ᵗʰ **Y36.81** Explosion of mine placed during war operations but exploding after cessation of hostilities

  ✓7ᵗʰ **Y36.810** Explosion of mine placed during war operations but exploding after cessation of hostilities, military personnel

  ✓7ᵗʰ **Y36.811** Explosion of mine placed during war operations but exploding after cessation of hostilities, civilian

✓6ᵗʰ **Y36.82** Explosion of bomb placed during war operations but exploding after cessation of hostilities

  ✓7ᵗʰ **Y36.820** Explosion of bomb placed during war operations but exploding after cessation of hostilities, military personnel

✓ Additional Character Req   ✓x7ᵗʰ Placeholder Alert   Manifestation   ▽ Unspecified   ▶◀ Revised Text   ● New Code   ▲ Revised Code Title

ICD-10-CM 2019   1197

√7ᵗʰ **Y36.821** **Explosion of bomb placed during war operations but exploding after cessation of hostilities,** civilian

√6ᵗʰ **Y36.88** **Other war operations occurring after cessation of hostilities**

√7ᵗʰ **Y36.880** **Other war operations occurring after cessation of hostilities,** military personnel

√7ᵗʰ **Y36.881** **Other war operations occurring after cessation of hostilities,** civilian

√6ᵗʰ **Y36.89** **Unspecified war operations occurring after cessation of hostilities**

√7ᵗʰ **Y36.890** **Unspecified war operations occurring after cessation of hostilities,** military personnel ▽

√7ᵗʰ **Y36.891** **Unspecified war operations occurring after cessation of hostilities,** civilian ▽

√5ᵗʰ **Y36.9** **Other and unspecified war operations**

√x7ᵗʰ **Y36.90** **War operations, unspecified** ▽

√x7ᵗʰ **Y36.91** **War operations involving unspecified weapon of mass destruction [WMD]** ▽

√x7ᵗʰ **Y36.92** **War operations involving** friendly fire

√4ᵗʰ **Y37** **Military operations**

INCLUDES   injuries to military personnel and civilians occurring during peacetime on military property and during routine military exercises and operations

EXCLUDES 1   *military aircraft involved in aircraft accident with civilian aircraft (V97.81-)*

military vehicles involved in transport accident with civilian vehicle (V09.01, V09.21, V19.81, V29.81, V39.81, V49.81, V59.81, V69.81, V79.81)

military watercraft involved in water transport accident with civilian watercraft (V94.81-)

war operations (Y36.-)

√5ᵗʰ **Y37.0** **Military operations involving** explosion of marine weapons

√6ᵗʰ **Y37.00** **Military operations involving explosion of unspecified marine weapon**

Military operations involving underwater blast NOS

√7ᵗʰ **Y37.000** **Military operations involving explosion of unspecified marine weapon,** military personnel ▽

√7ᵗʰ **Y37.001** **Military operations involving explosion of unspecified marine weapon,** civilian ▽

√6ᵗʰ **Y37.01** **Military operations involving explosion of depth-charge**

√7ᵗʰ **Y37.010** **Military operations involving explosion of depth-charge,** military personnel

√7ᵗʰ **Y37.011** **Military operations involving explosion of depth-charge,** civilian

√6ᵗʰ **Y37.02** **Military operations involving explosion of** marine mine

Military operations involving explosion of marine mine, at sea or in harbor

√7ᵗʰ **Y37.020** **Military operations involving explosion of marine mine,** military personnel

√7ᵗʰ **Y37.021** **Military operations involving explosion of marine mine,** civilian

√6ᵗʰ **Y37.03** **Military operations involving explosion of** sea-based artillery shell

√7ᵗʰ **Y37.030** **Military operations involving explosion of sea-based artillery shell,** military personnel

√7ᵗʰ **Y37.031** **Military operations involving explosion of sea-based artillery shell,** civilian

√6ᵗʰ **Y37.04** **Military operations involving explosion of** torpedo

√7ᵗʰ **Y37.040** **Military operations involving explosion of torpedo,** military personnel

√7ᵗʰ **Y37.041** **Military operations involving explosion of torpedo,** civilian

√6ᵗʰ **Y37.05** **Military operations involving accidental detonation of** onboard marine weapons

√7ᵗʰ **Y37.050** **Military operations involving accidental detonation of onboard marine weapons,** military personnel

√7ᵗʰ **Y37.051** **Military operations involving accidental detonation of onboard marine weapons,** civilian

√6ᵗʰ **Y37.09** **Military operations involving explosion of other marine weapons**

√7ᵗʰ **Y37.090** **Military operations involving explosion of other marine weapons,** military personnel

√7ᵗʰ **Y37.091** **Military operations involving explosion of other marine weapons,** civilian

√5ᵗʰ **Y37.1** **Military operations involving** destruction of aircraft

√6ᵗʰ **Y37.10** **Military operations involving unspecified destruction of aircraft**

√7ᵗʰ **Y37.100** **Military operations involving unspecified destruction of aircraft,** military personnel ▽

√7ᵗʰ **Y37.101** **Military operations involving unspecified destruction of aircraft,** civilian ▽

√6ᵗʰ **Y37.11** **Military operations involving destruction of aircraft due to enemy fire or explosives**

Military operations involving destruction of aircraft due to air to air missile

Military operations involving destruction of aircraft due to explosive placed on aircraft

Military operations involving destruction of aircraft due to rocket propelled grenade [RPG]

Military operations involving destruction of aircraft due to small arms fire

Military operations involving destruction of aircraft due to surface to air missile

√7ᵗʰ **Y37.110** **Military operations involving destruction of aircraft due to enemy fire or explosives,** military personnel

√7ᵗʰ **Y37.111** **Military operations involving destruction of aircraft due to enemy fire or explosives,** civilian

√6ᵗʰ **Y37.12** **Military operations involving destruction of aircraft due to collision with other aircraft**

√7ᵗʰ **Y37.120** **Military operations involving destruction of aircraft due to collision with other aircraft,** military personnel

√7ᵗʰ **Y37.121** **Military operations involving destruction of aircraft due to collision with other aircraft,** civilian

√6ᵗʰ **Y37.13** **Military operations involving destruction of aircraft due to onboard fire**

√7ᵗʰ **Y37.130** **Military operations involving destruction of aircraft due to onboard fire,** military personnel

√7ᵗʰ **Y37.131** **Military operations involving destruction of aircraft due to onboard fire,** civilian

√6ᵗʰ **Y37.14** **Military operations involving destruction of aircraft due to** accidental detonation of onboard munitions and explosives

√7ᵗʰ **Y37.140** **Military operations involving destruction of aircraft due to accidental detonation of onboard munitions and explosives, military personnel**

√7ᵗʰ **Y37.141** **Military operations involving destruction of aircraft due to accidental detonation of onboard munitions and explosives, civilian**

√6ᵗʰ **Y37.19** **Military operations involving other destruction of aircraft**

√7ᵗʰ **Y37.190** **Military operations involving other destruction of aircraft,** military personnel

√7ᵗʰ **Y37.191** **Military operations involving other destruction of aircraft,** civilian

√5ᵗʰ **Y37.2** **Military operations involving** other explosions and fragments

     EXCLUDES 1   *military operations involving explosion of aircraft (Y37.1-)*

           military operations involving explosion of marine weapons (Y37.0-)

           military operations involving explosion of nuclear weapons (Y37.5-)

   √6ᵗʰ **Y37.20** **Military operations involving unspecified explosion and fragments**

       Military operations involving air blast NOS

       Military operations involving blast NOS

       Military operations involving blast fragments NOS

       Military operations involving blast wave NOS

       Military operations involving blast wind NOS

       Military operations involving explosion NOS

       Military operations involving explosion of bomb NOS

     √7ᵗʰ **Y37.200** **Military operations involving unspecified explosion and fragments, military personnel** ▽

     √7ᵗʰ **Y37.201** **Military operations involving unspecified explosion and fragments, civilian** ▽

   √6ᵗʰ **Y37.21** **Military operations involving explosion of** aerial bomb

     √7ᵗʰ **Y37.210** **Military operations involving explosion of aerial bomb, military personnel**

     √7ᵗʰ **Y37.211** **Military operations involving explosion of aerial bomb, civilian**

   √6ᵗʰ **Y37.22** **Military operations involving explosion of** guided missile

     √7ᵗʰ **Y37.220** **Military operations involving explosion of guided missile, military personnel**

     √7ᵗʰ **Y37.221** **Military operations involving explosion of guided missile, civilian**

   √6ᵗʰ **Y37.23** **Military operations involving explosion of** improvised explosive device [IED]

       Military operations involving explosion of person-borne improvised explosive device [IED]

       Military operations involving explosion of vehicle-borne improvised explosive device [IED]

       Military operations involving explosion of roadside improvised explosive device [IED]

     √7ᵗʰ **Y37.230** **Military operations involving explosion of improvised explosive device [IED], military personnel**

     √7ᵗʰ **Y37.231** **Military operations involving explosion of improvised explosive device [IED], civilian**

   √6ᵗʰ **Y37.24** **Military operations involving explosion** due to accidental detonation and discharge of own munitions or munitions launch device

     √7ᵗʰ **Y37.240** **Military operations involving explosion due to accidental detonation and discharge of own munitions or munitions launch device, military personnel**

     √7ᵗʰ **Y37.241** **Military operations involving explosion due to accidental detonation and discharge of own munitions or munitions launch device, civilian**

   √6ᵗʰ **Y37.25** **Military operations involving** fragments from munitions

     √7ᵗʰ **Y37.250** **Military operations involving fragments from munitions, military personnel**

     √7ᵗʰ **Y37.251** **Military operations involving fragments from munitions, civilian**

   √6ᵗʰ **Y37.26** **Military operations involving** fragments of improvised explosive device [IED]

       Military operations involving fragments of person-borne improvised explosive device [IED]

       Military operations involving fragments of vehicle-borne improvised explosive device [IED]

       Military operations involving fragments of roadside improvised explosive device [IED]

     √7ᵗʰ **Y37.260** **Military operations involving fragments of improvised explosive device [IED], military personnel**

     √7ᵗʰ **Y37.261** **Military operations involving fragments of improvised explosive device [IED], civilian**

   √6ᵗʰ **Y37.27** **Military operations involving** fragments from weapons

     √7ᵗʰ **Y37.270** **Military operations involving fragments from weapons, military personnel**

     √7ᵗʰ **Y37.271** **Military operations involving fragments from weapons, civilian**

   √6ᵗʰ **Y37.29** **Military operations involving other explosions and fragments**

       Military operations involving explosion of grenade

       Military operations involving explosions of land mine

       Military operations involving shrapnel NOS

     √7ᵗʰ **Y37.290** **Military operations involving other explosions and fragments, military personnel**

     √7ᵗʰ **Y37.291** **Military operations involving other explosions and fragments, civilian**

√5ᵗʰ **Y37.3** **Military operations involving** fires, conflagrations and hot substances

     Military operations involving smoke, fumes, and heat from fires, conflagrations and hot substances

     EXCLUDES 1   *military operations involving fires and conflagrations aboard military aircraft (Y37.1-)*

           military operations involving fires and conflagrations aboard military watercraft (Y37.0-)

           military operations involving fires and conflagrations caused indirectly by conventional weapons (Y37.2-)

           military operations involving fires and thermal effects of nuclear weapons (Y36.53-)

   √6ᵗʰ **Y37.30** **Military operations involving unspecified fire, conflagration and hot substance**

     √7ᵗʰ **Y37.300** **Military operations involving unspecified fire, conflagration and hot substance, military personnel** ▽

     √7ᵗʰ **Y37.301** **Military operations involving unspecified fire, conflagration and hot substance, civilian** ▽

   √6ᵗʰ **Y37.31** **Military operations involving** gasoline bomb

       Military operations involving incendiary bomb

       Military operations involving petrol bomb

     √7ᵗʰ **Y37.310** **Military operations involving gasoline bomb, military personnel**

     √7ᵗʰ **Y37.311** **Military operations involving gasoline bomb, civilian**

   √6ᵗʰ **Y37.32** **Military operations involving** incendiary bullet

     √7ᵗʰ **Y37.320** **Military operations involving incendiary bullet, military personnel**

     √7ᵗʰ **Y37.321** **Military operations involving incendiary bullet, civilian**

   √6ᵗʰ **Y37.33** **Military operations involving** flamethrower

     √7ᵗʰ **Y37.330** **Military operations involving flamethrower, military personnel**

     √7ᵗʰ **Y37.331** **Military operations involving flamethrower, civilian**

   √6ᵗʰ **Y37.39** **Military operations involving other fires, conflagrations and hot substances**

     √7ᵗʰ **Y37.390** **Military operations involving other fires, conflagrations and hot substances, military personnel**

     √7ᵗʰ **Y37.391** **Military operations involving other fires, conflagrations and hot substances, civilian**

√5ᵗʰ **Y37.4** **Military operations involving firearm discharge and other forms of conventional warfare**

   √6ᵗʰ **Y37.41** **Military operations involving** rubber bullets

     √7ᵗʰ **Y37.410** **Military operations involving rubber bullets, military personnel**

     √7ᵗʰ **Y37.411** **Military operations involving rubber bullets, civilian**

   √6ᵗʰ **Y37.42** **Military operations involving** firearms pellets

     √7ᵗʰ **Y37.420** **Military operations involving firearms pellets, military personnel**

     √7ᵗʰ **Y37.421** **Military operations involving firearms pellets, civilian**

☑ Additional Character Req   √x7ᵗʰ Placeholder Alert   Manifestation   ▽ Unspecified   ►◄ Revised Text   ● New Code   ▲ Revised Code Title

ICD-10-CM 2019

1199

Y37.2–Y37.421

√6ᵗʰ **Y37.43** **Military operations involving other firearms discharge**
Military operations involving bullets NOS
EXCLUDES 1 *military operations involving munitions fragments (Y37.25-)*
military operations involving incendiary bullets (Y37.32-)

√7ᵗʰ **Y37.430** **Military operations involving other firearms discharge, military personnel**
√7ᵗʰ **Y37.431** **Military operations involving other firearms discharge, civilian**

√6ᵗʰ **Y37.44** **Military operations involving unarmed hand to hand combat**
EXCLUDES 1 *military operations involving combat using blunt or piercing object (Y37.45-)*
military operations involving intentional restriction of air and airway (Y37.46-)
military operations involving unintentional restriction of air and airway (Y37.47-)

√7ᵗʰ **Y37.440** **Military operations involving unarmed hand to hand combat, military personnel**
√7ᵗʰ **Y37.441** **Military operations involving unarmed hand to hand combat, civilian**

√6ᵗʰ **Y37.45** **Military operations involving combat using blunt or piercing object**
√7ᵗʰ **Y37.450** **Military operations involving combat using blunt or piercing object, military personnel**
√7ᵗʰ **Y37.451** **Military operations involving combat using blunt or piercing object, civilian**

√6ᵗʰ **Y37.46** **Military operations involving intentional restriction of air and airway**
√7ᵗʰ **Y37.460** **Military operations involving intentional restriction of air and airway, military personnel**
√7ᵗʰ **Y37.461** **Military operations involving intentional restriction of air and airway, civilian**

√6ᵗʰ **Y37.47** **Military operations involving unintentional restriction of air and airway**
√7ᵗʰ **Y37.470** **Military operations involving unintentional restriction of air and airway, military personnel**
√7ᵗʰ **Y37.471** **Military operations involving unintentional restriction of air and airway, civilian**

√6ᵗʰ **Y37.49** **Military operations involving other forms of conventional warfare**
√7ᵗʰ **Y37.490** **Military operations involving other forms of conventional warfare, military personnel**
√7ᵗʰ **Y37.491** **Military operations involving other forms of conventional warfare, civilian**

√5ᵗʰ **Y37.5** **Military operations involving nuclear weapons**
Military operation involving dirty bomb NOS

√6ᵗʰ **Y37.50** **Military operations involving unspecified effect of nuclear weapon**
√7ᵗʰ **Y37.500** **Military operations involving unspecified effect of nuclear weapon, military personnel** ▽
√7ᵗʰ **Y37.501** **Military operations involving unspecified effect of nuclear weapon, civilian** ▽

√6ᵗʰ **Y37.51** **Military operations involving direct blast effect of nuclear weapon**
Military operations involving blast pressure of nuclear weapon
√7ᵗʰ **Y37.510** **Military operations involving direct blast effect of nuclear weapon, military personnel**
√7ᵗʰ **Y37.511** **Military operations involving direct blast effect of nuclear weapon, civilian**

√6ᵗʰ **Y37.52** **Military operations involving indirect blast effect of nuclear weapon**
Military operations involving being thrown by blast of nuclear weapon
Military operations involving being struck or crushed by blast debris of nuclear weapon
√7ᵗʰ **Y37.520** **Military operations involving indirect blast effect of nuclear weapon, military personnel**
√7ᵗʰ **Y37.521** **Military operations involving indirect blast effect of nuclear weapon, civilian**

√6ᵗʰ **Y37.53** **Military operations involving thermal radiation effect of nuclear weapon**
Military operations involving direct heat from nuclear weapon
Military operation involving fireball effects from nuclear weapon
√7ᵗʰ **Y37.530** **Military operations involving thermal radiation effect of nuclear weapon, military personnel**
√7ᵗʰ **Y37.531** **Military operations involving thermal radiation effect of nuclear weapon, civilian**

√6ᵗʰ **Y37.54** **Military operation involving nuclear radiation effects of nuclear weapon**
Military operation involving acute radiation exposure from nuclear weapon
Military operation involving exposure to immediate ionizing radiation from nuclear weapon
Military operation involving fallout exposure from nuclear weapon
Military operation involving secondary effects of nuclear weapons
√7ᵗʰ **Y37.540** **Military operation involving nuclear radiation effects of nuclear weapon, military personnel**
√7ᵗʰ **Y37.541** **Military operation involving nuclear radiation effects of nuclear weapon, civilian**

√6ᵗʰ **Y37.59** **Military operation involving other effects of nuclear weapons**
√7ᵗʰ **Y37.590** **Military operation involving other effects of nuclear weapons, military personnel**
√7ᵗʰ **Y37.591** **Military operation involving other effects of nuclear weapons, civilian**

√5ᵗʰ **Y37.6** **Military operations involving biological weapons**
√6ᵗʰ **Y37.6X** **Military operations involving biological weapons**
√7ᵗʰ **Y37.6X0** **Military operations involving biological weapons, military personnel**
√7ᵗʰ **Y37.6X1** **Military operations involving biological weapons, civilian**

√5ᵗʰ **Y37.7** **Military operations involving chemical weapons and other forms of unconventional warfare**
EXCLUDES 1 *military operations involving incendiary devices (Y36.3-, Y36.5-)*
√6ᵗʰ **Y37.7X** **Military operations involving chemical weapons and other forms of unconventional warfare**
√7ᵗʰ **Y37.7X0** **Military operations involving chemical weapons and other forms of unconventional warfare, military personnel**
√7ᵗʰ **Y37.7X1** **Military operations involving chemical weapons and other forms of unconventional warfare, civilian**

√5ᵗʰ **Y37.9** **Other and unspecified military operations**
√x7ᵗʰ **Y37.90** **Military operations, unspecified** ▽
√x7ᵗʰ **Y37.91** **Military operations involving unspecified weapon of mass destruction [WMD]** ▽
√x7ᵗʰ **Y37.92** **Military operations involving friendly fire**

√4ᵗʰ **Y38 Terrorism**
NOTE These codes are for use to identify injuries resulting from the unlawful use of force or violence against persons or property to intimidate or coerce a Government, the civilian population, or any segment thereof, in furtherance of political or social objective
Use additional code for place of occurrence (Y92.-)

√5ᵗʰ **Y38.0** **Terrorism involving explosion of marine weapons**
Terrorism involving depth-charge
Terrorism involving marine mine
Terrorism involving mine NOS, at sea or in harbor
Terrorism involving sea-based artillery shell
Terrorism involving torpedo
Terrorism involving underwater blast
√6ᵗʰ **Y38.0X** **Terrorism involving explosion of marine weapons**
√7ᵗʰ **Y38.0X1** **Terrorism involving explosion of marine weapons, public safety official injured**
√7ᵗʰ **Y38.0X2** **Terrorism involving explosion of marine weapons, civilian injured**

√7ᵗʰ **Y38.ØX3** **Terrorism involving explosion of marine weapons,** terrorist **injured**

√5ᵗʰ **Y38.1** **Terrorism involving destruction of aircraft**

Terrorism involving aircraft burned
Terrorism involving aircraft exploded
Terrorism involving aircraft being shot down
Terrorism involving aircraft used as a weapon

√6ᵗʰ **Y38.1X** **Terrorism involving** destruction of aircraft

√7ᵗʰ **Y38.1X1** **Terrorism involving destruction of aircraft,** public safety official **injured**

√7ᵗʰ **Y38.1X2** **Terrorism involving destruction of aircraft,** civilian **injured**

√7ᵗʰ **Y38.1X3** **Terrorism involving destruction of aircraft,** terrorist **injured**

√5ᵗʰ **Y38.2** **Terrorism involving other explosions and fragments**

Terrorism involving antipersonnel (fragments) bomb
Terrorism involving blast NOS
Terrorism involving explosion NOS
Terrorism involving explosion of breech block
Terrorism involving explosion of cannon block
Terrorism involving explosion (fragments) of artillery shell
Terrorism involving explosion (fragments) of bomb
Terrorism involving explosion (fragments) of grenade
Terrorism involving explosion (fragments) of guided missile
Terrorism involving explosion (fragments) of land mine
Terrorism involving explosion of mortar bomb
Terrorism involving explosion of munitions
Terrorism involving explosion (fragments) of rocket
Terrorism involving explosion (fragments) of shell
Terrorism involving shrapnel
Terrorism involving mine NOS, on land

EXCLUDES 1   *terrorism involving explosion of nuclear weapon (Y38.5)*

terrorism involving suicide bomber (Y38.81)

√6ᵗʰ **Y38.2X** **Terrorism involving other explosions and fragments**

√7ᵗʰ **Y38.2X1** **Terrorism involving other explosions and fragments,** public safety official **injured**

√7ᵗʰ **Y38.2X2** **Terrorism involving other explosions and fragments,** civilian **injured**

√7ᵗʰ **Y38.2X3** **Terrorism involving other explosions and fragments,** terrorist **injured**

√5ᵗʰ **Y38.3** **Terrorism involving fires, conflagration and hot substances**

Terrorism involving conflagration NOS
Terrorism involving fire NOS
Terrorism involving petrol bomb

EXCLUDES 1   *terrorism involving fire or heat of nuclear weapon (Y38.5)*

√6ᵗʰ **Y38.3X** **Terrorism involving** fires, conflagration and hot substances

√7ᵗʰ **Y38.3X1** **Terrorism involving fires, conflagration and hot substances,** public safety official **injured**

√7ᵗʰ **Y38.3X2** **Terrorism involving fires, conflagration and hot substances,** civilian **injured**

√7ᵗʰ **Y38.3X3** **Terrorism involving fires, conflagration and hot substances,** terrorist **injured**

√5ᵗʰ **Y38.4** **Terrorism involving firearms**

Terrorism involving carbine bullet
Terrorism involving machine gun bullet
Terrorism involving pellets (shotgun)
Terrorism involving pistol bullet
Terrorism involving rifle bullet
Terrorism involving rubber (rifle) bullet

√6ᵗʰ **Y38.4X** **Terrorism involving** firearms

√7ᵗʰ **Y38.4X1** **Terrorism involving firearms,** public safety official **injured**

√7ᵗʰ **Y38.4X2** **Terrorism involving firearms,** civilian **injured**

√7ᵗʰ **Y38.4X3** **Terrorism involving firearms,** terrorist **injured**

√5ᵗʰ **Y38.5** **Terrorism involving nuclear weapons**

Terrorism involving blast effects of nuclear weapon
Terrorism involving exposure to ionizing radiation from nuclear weapon
Terrorism involving fireball effect of nuclear weapon
Terrorism involving heat from nuclear weapon

√6ᵗʰ **Y38.5X** **Terrorism involving** nuclear weapons

√7ᵗʰ **Y38.5X1** **Terrorism involving nuclear weapons,** public safety official **injured**

√7ᵗʰ **Y38.5X2** **Terrorism involving nuclear weapons,** civilian **injured**

√7ᵗʰ **Y38.5X3** **Terrorism involving nuclear weapons,** terrorist **injured**

√5ᵗʰ **Y38.6** **Terrorism involving biological weapons**

Terrorism involving anthrax
Terrorism involving cholera
Terrorism involving smallpox

√6ᵗʰ **Y38.6X** **Terrorism involving** biological weapons

√7ᵗʰ **Y38.6X1** **Terrorism involving biological weapons,** public safety official **injured**

√7ᵗʰ **Y38.6X2** **Terrorism involving biological weapons,** civilian **injured**

√7ᵗʰ **Y38.6X3** **Terrorism involving biological weapons,** terrorist **injured**

√5ᵗʰ **Y38.7** **Terrorism involving chemical weapons**

Terrorism involving gases, fumes, chemicals
Terrorism involving hydrogen cyanide
Terrorism involving phosgene
Terrorism involving sarin

√6ᵗʰ **Y38.7X** **Terrorism involving** chemical weapons

√7ᵗʰ **Y38.7X1** **Terrorism involving chemical weapons,** public safety official **injured**

√7ᵗʰ **Y38.7X2** **Terrorism involving chemical weapons,** civilian **injured**

√7ᵗʰ **Y38.7X3** **Terrorism involving chemical weapons,** terrorist **injured**

√5ᵗʰ **Y38.8** **Terrorism involving other and unspecified means**

√x7ᵗʰ **Y38.8Ø** **Terrorism involving unspecified means** ▽

Terrorism NOS

√6ᵗʰ **Y38.81** **Terrorism involving** suicide bomber

√7ᵗʰ **Y38.811** **Terrorism involving suicide bomber,** public safety official **injured**

√7ᵗʰ **Y38.812** **Terrorism involving suicide bomber,** civilian **injured**

√6ᵗʰ **Y38.89** **Terrorism involving other means**

Terrorism involving drowning and submersion
Terrorism involving lasers
Terrorism involving piercing or stabbing instruments

√7ᵗʰ **Y38.891** **Terrorism involving other means,** public safety official **injured**

√7ᵗʰ **Y38.892** **Terrorism involving other means,** civilian **injured**

√7ᵗʰ **Y38.893** **Terrorism involving other means,** terrorist **injured**

√5ᵗʰ **Y38.9** **Terrorism, secondary effects**

NOTE   This code is for use to identify conditions occurring subsequent to a terrorist attack not those that are due to the initial terrorist attack

√6ᵗʰ **Y38.9X** **Terrorism,** secondary effects

√7ᵗʰ **Y38.9X1** **Terrorism, secondary effects,** public safety official **injured**

√7ᵗʰ **Y38.9X2** **Terrorism, secondary effects,** civilian **injured**

✓ Additional Character Req   √x7ᵗʰ Placeholder Alert   Manifestation   ▽ Unspecified   ▶◀ Revised Text   ● New Code   ▲ Revised Code Title

ICD-10-CM 2019   1201

Y38.ØX3-Y38.9X2

Complications of Medical and Surgical Care (Y62-Y84)

> **INCLUDES**   complications of medical devices
> surgical and medical procedures as the cause of abnormal reaction of the patient, or of later complication, without mention of misadventure at the time of the procedure

Misadventures to patients during surgical and medical care (Y62-Y69)

> **EXCLUDES 1**   *surgical and medical procedures as the cause of abnormal reaction of the patient, without mention of misadventure at the time of the procedure (Y83-Y84)*
> **EXCLUDES 2**   *breakdown or malfunctioning of medical device (during procedure) (after implantation) (ongoing use) (Y70-Y82)*

✓4ᵗʰ Y62 Failure of sterile precautions during surgical and medical care

Y62.0 Failure of sterile precautions during surgical operation

Y62.1 Failure of sterile precautions during infusion or transfusion

Y62.2 Failure of sterile precautions during kidney dialysis and other perfusion   HCC

Y62.3 Failure of sterile precautions during injection or immunization

Y62.4 Failure of sterile precautions during endoscopic examination

Y62.5 Failure of sterile precautions during heart catheterization

Y62.6 Failure of sterile precautions during aspiration, puncture and other catheterization

Y62.8 Failure of sterile precautions during other surgical and medical care

Y62.9 Failure of sterile precautions during unspecified surgical and medical care   ▽

✓4ᵗʰ Y63 Failure in dosage during surgical and medical care

> **EXCLUDES 2**   *accidental overdose of drug or wrong drug given in error (T36-T50)*

Y63.0 Excessive amount of blood or other fluid given during transfusion or infusion

Y63.1 Incorrect dilution of fluid used during infusion

Y63.2 Overdose of radiation given during therapy

Y63.3 Inadvertent exposure of patient to radiation during medical care

Y63.4 Failure in dosage in electroshock or insulin-shock therapy

Y63.5 Inappropriate temperature in local application and packing

Y63.6 Underdosing and nonadministration of necessary drug, medicament or biological substance

Y63.8 Failure in dosage during other surgical and medical care

Y63.9 Failure in dosage during unspecified surgical and medical care   ▽

✓4ᵗʰ Y64 Contaminated medical or biological substances

Y64.0 Contaminated medical or biological substance, transfused or infused

Y64.1 Contaminated medical or biological substance, injected or used for immunization

Y64.8 Contaminated medical or biological substance administered by other means

Y64.9 Contaminated medical or biological substance administered by unspecified means   ▽
Administered contaminated medical or biological substance NOS

✓4ᵗʰ Y65 Other misadventures during surgical and medical care

Y65.0 Mismatched blood in transfusion

Y65.1 Wrong fluid used in infusion

Y65.2 Failure in suture or ligature during surgical operation

Y65.3 Endotracheal tube wrongly placed during anesthetic procedure

Y65.4 Failure to introduce or to remove other tube or instrument

✓5ᵗʰ Y65.5 Performance of wrong procedure (operation)

     Y65.51 Performance of wrong procedure (operation) on correct patient
         Wrong device implanted into correct surgical site
         EXCLUDES 1   *performance of correct procedure (operation) on wrong side or body part (Y65.53)*

     Y65.52 Performance of procedure (operation) on patient not scheduled for surgery
         Performance of procedure (operation) intended for another patient
         Performance of procedure (operation) on wrong patient

     Y65.53 Performance of correct procedure (operation) on wrong side or body part
         Performance of correct procedure (operation) on wrong side
         Performance of correct procedure (operation) on wrong site

Y65.8 Other specified misadventures during surgical and medical care

Y66 Nonadministration of surgical and medical care
Premature cessation of surgical and medical care

> **EXCLUDES 1**   *DNR status (Z66)*
> *palliative care (Z51.5)*

Y69 Unspecified misadventure during surgical and medical care   ▽

Medical devices associated with adverse incidents in diagnostic and therapeutic use (Y70-Y82)

> **INCLUDES**   breakdown or malfunction of medical devices (during use) (after implantation) (ongoing use)
> **EXCLUDES 2**   ~~breakdown or malfunctioning of medical device (after implantation) (during procedure) (ongoing use) (Y70-Y82)~~
> *later complications following use of medical devices without breakdown or malfunctioning of device (Y83-Y84)*
> *misadventure to patients during surgical and medical care, classifiable to (Y62-Y69)*
> *surgical and other medical procedures as the cause of abnormal reaction of the patient, or of later complication, without mention of misadventure at the time of the procedure (Y83-Y84)*

✓4ᵗʰ Y70 Anesthesiology devices associated with adverse incidents

Y70.0 Diagnostic and monitoring anesthesiology devices associated with adverse incidents

Y70.1 Therapeutic (nonsurgical) and rehabilitative anesthesiology devices associated with adverse incidents

Y70.2 Prosthetic and other implants, materials and accessory anesthesiology devices associated with adverse incidents

Y70.3 Surgical instruments, materials and anesthesiology devices (including sutures) associated with adverse incidents

Y70.8 Miscellaneous anesthesiology devices associated with adverse incidents, not elsewhere classified

✓4ᵗʰ Y71 Cardiovascular devices associated with adverse incidents

Y71.0 Diagnostic and monitoring cardiovascular devices associated with adverse incidents

Y71.1 Therapeutic (nonsurgical) and rehabilitative cardiovascular devices associated with adverse incidents

Y71.2 Prosthetic and other implants, materials and accessory cardiovascular devices associated with adverse incidents

Y71.3 Surgical instruments, materials and cardiovascular devices (including sutures) associated with adverse incidents

Y71.8 Miscellaneous cardiovascular devices associated with adverse incidents, not elsewhere classified

✓4ᵗʰ Y72 Otorhinolaryngological devices associated with adverse incidents

Y72.0 Diagnostic and monitoring otorhinolaryngological devices associated with adverse incidents

Y72.1 Therapeutic (nonsurgical) and rehabilitative otorhinolaryngological devices associated with adverse incidents

Y72.2 Prosthetic and other implants, materials and accessory otorhinolaryngological devices associated with adverse incidents

Y72.3 Surgical instruments, materials and otorhinolaryngological devices (including sutures) associated with adverse incidents

Y72.8 Miscellaneous otorhinolaryngological devices associated with adverse incidents, not elsewhere classified

✓4ᵗʰ Y73 Gastroenterology and urology devices associated with adverse incidents

Y73.0 Diagnostic and monitoring gastroenterology and urology devices associated with adverse incidents

Y73.1 Therapeutic (nonsurgical) and rehabilitative gastroenterology and urology devices associated with adverse incidents

Y73.2 Prosthetic and other implants, materials and accessory gastroenterology and urology devices associated with adverse incidents

Y73.3 Surgical instruments, materials and gastroenterology and urology devices (including sutures) associated with adverse incidents

Y73.8 Miscellaneous gastroenterology and urology devices associated with adverse incidents, not elsewhere classified

☑4ᵗʰ **Y74** **General hospital** and personal-use devices associated with adverse incidents

    Y74.0 Diagnostic and monitoring general hospital and personal-use devices associated with adverse incidents

    Y74.1 Therapeutic (nonsurgical) and rehabilitative general hospital and personal-use devices associated with adverse incidents

    Y74.2 Prosthetic and other implants, materials and accessory general hospital and personal-use devices associated with adverse incidents

    Y74.3 Surgical instruments, materials and general hospital and personal-use devices (including sutures) associated with adverse incidents

    Y74.8 Miscellaneous general hospital and personal-use devices associated with adverse incidents, not elsewhere classified

☑4ᵗʰ **Y75** **Neurological** devices associated with adverse incidents

    Y75.0 Diagnostic and monitoring neurological devices associated with adverse incidents

    Y75.1 Therapeutic (nonsurgical) and rehabilitative neurological devices associated with adverse incidents

    Y75.2 Prosthetic and other implants, materials and neurological devices associated with adverse incidents

    Y75.3 Surgical instruments, materials and neurological devices (including sutures) associated with adverse incidents

    Y75.8 Miscellaneous neurological devices associated with adverse incidents, not elsewhere classified

☑4ᵗʰ **Y76** **Obstetric and gynecological** devices associated with adverse incidents

    Y76.0 Diagnostic and monitoring obstetric and gynecological devices associated with adverse incidents ♀

    Y76.1 Therapeutic (nonsurgical) and rehabilitative obstetric and gynecological devices associated with adverse incidents ♀

    Y76.2 Prosthetic and other implants, materials and accessory obstetric and gynecological devices associated with adverse incidents ♀

    Y76.3 Surgical instruments, materials and obstetric and gynecological devices (including sutures) associated with adverse incidents ♀

    Y76.8 Miscellaneous obstetric and gynecological devices associated with adverse incidents, not elsewhere classified ♀

☑4ᵗʰ **Y77** **Ophthalmic** devices associated with adverse incidents

    Y77.0 Diagnostic and monitoring ophthalmic devices associated with adverse incidents

    Y77.1 Therapeutic (nonsurgical) and rehabilitative ophthalmic devices associated with adverse incidents

    Y77.2 Prosthetic and other implants, materials and accessory ophthalmic devices associated with adverse incidents

    Y77.3 Surgical instruments, materials and ophthalmic devices (including sutures) associated with adverse incidents

    Y77.8 Miscellaneous ophthalmic devices associated with adverse incidents, not elsewhere classified

☑4ᵗʰ **Y78** **Radiological** devices associated with adverse incidents

    Y78.0 Diagnostic and monitoring radiological devices associated with adverse incidents

    Y78.1 Therapeutic (nonsurgical) and rehabilitative radiological devices associated with adverse incidents

    Y78.2 Prosthetic and other implants, materials and accessory radiological devices associated with adverse incidents

    Y78.3 Surgical instruments, materials and radiological devices (including sutures) associated with adverse incidents

    Y78.8 Miscellaneous radiological devices associated with adverse incidents, not elsewhere classified

☑4ᵗʰ **Y79** **Orthopedic** devices associated with adverse incidents

    Y79.0 Diagnostic and monitoring orthopedic devices associated with adverse incidents

    Y79.1 Therapeutic (nonsurgical) and rehabilitative orthopedic devices associated with adverse incidents

    Y79.2 Prosthetic and other implants, materials and accessory orthopedic devices associated with adverse incidents

    Y79.3 Surgical instruments, materials and orthopedic devices (including sutures) associated with adverse incidents

    Y79.8 Miscellaneous orthopedic devices associated with adverse incidents, not elsewhere classified

☑4ᵗʰ **Y80** **Physical medicine** devices associated with adverse incidents

    Y80.0 Diagnostic and monitoring physical medicine devices associated with adverse incidents

    Y80.1 Therapeutic (nonsurgical) and rehabilitative physical medicine devices associated with adverse incidents

    Y80.2 Prosthetic and other implants, materials and accessory physical medicine devices associated with adverse incidents

    Y80.3 Surgical instruments, materials and physical medicine devices (including sutures) associated with adverse incidents

    Y80.8 Miscellaneous physical medicine devices associated with adverse incidents, not elsewhere classified

☑4ᵗʰ **Y81** **General- and plastic-surgery** devices associated with adverse incidents

    Y81.0 Diagnostic and monitoring general- and plastic-surgery devices associated with adverse incidents

    Y81.1 Therapeutic (nonsurgical) and rehabilitative general- and plastic-surgery devices associated with adverse incidents

    Y81.2 Prosthetic and other implants, materials and accessory general- and plastic-surgery devices associated with adverse incidents

    Y81.3 Surgical instruments, materials and general- and plastic-surgery devices (including sutures) associated with adverse incidents

    Y81.8 Miscellaneous general- and plastic-surgery devices associated with adverse incidents, not elsewhere classified

☑4ᵗʰ **Y82** **Other and unspecified** medical devices associated with adverse incidents

    Y82.8 Other medical devices associated with adverse incidents

    Y82.9 Unspecified medical devices associated with adverse incidents ▽

Surgical and other medical procedures as the cause of abnormal reaction of the patient, or of later complication, without mention of misadventure at the time of the procedure (Y83-Y84)

EXCLUDES 1   misadventures to patients during surgical and medical care, classifiable to (Y62-Y69)

EXCLUDES 2   breakdown or malfunctioning of medical device (during procedure) (after implantation) (ongoing use) (Y70-Y82)

☑4ᵗʰ **Y83** **Surgical operation** and other **surgical procedures** as the cause of abnormal reaction of the patient, or of later complication, without mention of misadventure at the time of the procedure

    Y83.0 Surgical operation with transplant of whole organ as the cause of abnormal reaction of the patient, or of later complication, without mention of misadventure at the time of the procedure

    Y83.1 Surgical operation with implant of artificial internal device as the cause of abnormal reaction of the patient, or of later complication, without mention of misadventure at the time of the procedure

    Y83.2 Surgical operation with anastomosis, bypass or graft as the cause of abnormal reaction of the patient, or of later complication, without mention of misadventure at the time of the procedure

    Y83.3 Surgical operation with formation of external stoma as the cause of abnormal reaction of the patient, or of later complication, without mention of misadventure at the time of the procedure

    Y83.4 Other reconstructive surgery as the cause of abnormal reaction of the patient, or of later complication, without mention of misadventure at the time of the procedure

    Y83.5 Amputation of limb(s) as the cause of abnormal reaction of the patient, or of later complication, without mention of misadventure at the time of the procedure

    Y83.6 Removal of other organ (partial) (total) as the cause of abnormal reaction of the patient, or of later complication, without mention of misadventure at the time of the procedure

    Y83.8 Other surgical procedures as the cause of abnormal reaction of the patient, or of later complication, without mention of misadventure at the time of the procedure

    Y83.9 Surgical procedure, unspecified as the cause of abnormal reaction of the patient, or of later complication, without mention of misadventure at the time of the procedure ▽

☑4ᵗʰ **Y84** **Other medical procedures** as the cause of abnormal reaction of the patient, or of later complication, without mention of misadventure at the time of the procedure

    Y84.0 Cardiac catheterization as the cause of abnormal reaction of the patient, or of later complication, without mention of misadventure at the time of the procedure

    Y84.1 Kidney dialysis as the cause of abnormal reaction of the patient, or of later complication, without mention of misadventure at the time of the procedure

☑ Additional Character Req   ✓x7ᵗʰ Placeholder Alert   Manifestation   ▽ Unspecified   ▶◀ Revised Text   ● New Code   ▲ Revised Code Title

ICD-10-CM 2019   1203

Chapter 20. External Causes of Morbidity

Y84.2 Radiological procedure and radiotherapy as the cause of abnormal reaction of the patient, or of later complication, without mention of misadventure at the time of the procedure
     AHA: 2017,1Q,33

Y84.3 Shock therapy as the cause of abnormal reaction of the patient, or of later complication, without mention of misadventure at the time of the procedure

Y84.4 Aspiration of fluid as the cause of abnormal reaction of the patient, or of later complication, without mention of misadventure at the time of the procedure

Y84.5 Insertion of gastric or duodenal sound as the cause of abnormal reaction of the patient, or of later complication, without mention of misadventure at the time of the procedure

Y84.6 Urinary catheterization as the cause of abnormal reaction of the patient, or of later complication, without mention of misadventure at the time of the procedure

Y84.7 Blood-sampling as the cause of abnormal reaction of the patient, or of later complication, without mention of misadventure at the time of the procedure

Y84.8 Other medical procedures as the cause of abnormal reaction of the patient, or of later complication, without mention of misadventure at the time of the procedure
     AHA: 2014,4Q,24

Y84.9 Medical procedure, unspecified as the cause of abnormal reaction of the patient, or of later complication, without mention of misadventure at the time of the procedure ▽

Supplementary factors related to causes of morbidity classified elsewhere (Y90-Y99)

NOTE These categories may be used to provide supplementary information concerning causes of morbidity. They are not to be used for single-condition coding.

√4ᵗʰ Y90 Evidence of alcohol involvement determined by blood alcohol level
Code first any associated alcohol related disorders (F10)

Y90.0 Blood alcohol level of less than 20 mg/100 ml

Y90.1 Blood alcohol level of 20-39 mg/100 ml

Y90.2 Blood alcohol level of 40-59 mg/100 ml

Y90.3 Blood alcohol level of 60-79 mg/100 ml

Y90.4 Blood alcohol level of 80-99 mg/100 ml

Y90.5 Blood alcohol level of 100-119 mg/100 ml

Y90.6 Blood alcohol level of 120-199 mg/100 ml

Y90.7 Blood alcohol level of 200-239 mg/100 ml

Y90.8 Blood alcohol level of 240 mg/100 ml or more

Y90.9 Presence of alcohol in blood, level not specified ▽

√4ᵗʰ Y92 Place of occurrence of the external cause
The following category is for use, when relevant, to identify the place of occurrence of the external cause. Use in conjunction with an activity code.
Place of occurrence should be recorded only at the initial encounter for treatment

√5ᵗʰ Y92.0 Non-institutional (private) residence as the place of occurrence of the external cause
     EXCLUDES 1 abandoned or derelict house (Y92.89)
          home under construction but not yet occupied (Y92.6-)
          institutional place of residence (Y92.1-)

     √6ᵗʰ Y92.00 Unspecified non-institutional (private) residence as the place of occurrence of the external cause

▲   **Y92.000** Kitchen of unspecified non-institutional (private) residence as the place of occurrence of the external cause ▽

         Y92.001 Dining room of unspecified non-institutional (private) residence as the place of occurrence of the external cause ▽

         Y92.002 Bathroom of unspecified non-institutional (private) residence single-family (private) house as the place of occurrence of the external cause ▽

         Y92.003 Bedroom of unspecified non-institutional (private) residence as the place of occurrence of the external cause ▽

Y92.007 Garden or yard of unspecified non-institutional (private) residence as the place of occurrence of the external cause ▽

Y92.008 Other place in unspecified non-institutional (private) residence as the place of occurrence of the external cause ▽

Y92.009 Unspecified place in unspecified non-institutional (private) residence as the place of occurrence of the external cause ▽
     Home (NOS) as the place of occurrence of the external cause

√6ᵗʰ Y92.01 Single-family non-institutional (private) house as the place of occurrence of the external cause
     Farmhouse as the place of occurrence of the external cause
     EXCLUDES 1 barn (Y92.71)
          chicken coop or hen house (Y92.72)
          farm field (Y92.73)
          orchard (Y92.74)
          single family mobile home or trailer (Y92.02-)
          slaughter house (Y92.86)

     Y92.010 Kitchen of single-family (private) house as the place of occurrence of the external cause

     Y92.011 Dining room of single-family (private) house as the place of occurrence of the external cause

     Y92.012 Bathroom of single-family (private) house as the place of occurrence of the external cause

     Y92.013 Bedroom of single-family (private) house as the place of occurrence of the external cause

     Y92.014 Private driveway to single-family (private) house as the place of occurrence of the external cause

     Y92.015 Private garage of single-family (private) house as the place of occurrence of the external cause

     Y92.016 Swimming-pool in single-family (private) house or garden as the place of occurrence of the external cause

     Y92.017 Garden or yard in single-family (private) house as the place of occurrence of the external cause

     Y92.018 Other place in single-family (private) house as the place of occurrence of the external cause

     Y92.019 Unspecified place in single-family (private) house as the place of occurrence of the external cause ▽

√6ᵗʰ Y92.02 Mobile home as the place of occurrence of the external cause

     Y92.020 Kitchen in mobile home as the place of occurrence of the external cause

     Y92.021 Dining room in mobile home as the place of occurrence of the external cause

     Y92.022 Bathroom in mobile home as the place of occurrence of the external cause

     Y92.023 Bedroom in mobile home as the place of occurrence of the external cause

     Y92.024 Driveway of mobile home as the place of occurrence of the external cause

     Y92.025 Garage of mobile home as the place of occurrence of the external cause

     Y92.026 Swimming-pool of mobile home as the place of occurrence of the external cause

     Y92.027 Garden or yard of mobile home as the place of occurrence of the external cause

     Y92.028 Other place in mobile home as the place of occurrence of the external cause

     Y92.029 Unspecified place in mobile home as the place of occurrence of the external cause ▽

✓6ᵗʰ **Y92.03** Apartment as the place of occurrence of the external cause
> Condominium as the place of occurrence of the external cause
> Co-op apartment as the place of occurrence of the external cause

     Y92.030 Kitchen in apartment as the place of occurrence of the external cause

     Y92.031 Bathroom in apartment as the place of occurrence of the external cause

     Y92.032 Bedroom in apartment as the place of occurrence of the external cause

     Y92.038 Other place in apartment as the place of occurrence of the external cause

     Y92.039 Unspecified place in apartment ▽ as the place of occurrence of the external cause

✓6ᵗʰ **Y92.04** Boarding-house as the place of occurrence of the external cause

     Y92.040 Kitchen in boarding-house as the place of occurrence of the external cause

     Y92.041 Bathroom in boarding-house as the place of occurrence of the external cause

     Y92.042 Bedroom in boarding-house as the place of occurrence of the external cause

     Y92.043 Driveway of boarding-house as the place of occurrence of the external cause

     Y92.044 Garage of boarding-house as the place of occurrence of the external cause

     Y92.045 Swimming-pool of boarding-house as the place of occurrence of the external cause

     Y92.046 Garden or yard of boarding-house as the place of occurrence of the external cause

     Y92.048 Other place in boarding-house as the place of occurrence of the external cause

     Y92.049 Unspecified place in ▽ boarding-house as the place of occurrence of the external cause

✓6ᵗʰ **Y92.09** Other non-institutional residence as the place of occurrence of the external cause
> **AHA:** 2017,2Q,10

     Y92.090 Kitchen in other non-institutional residence as the place of occurrence of the external cause

     Y92.091 Bathroom in other non-institutional residence as the place of occurrence of the external cause

     Y92.092 Bedroom in other non-institutional residence as the place of occurrence of the external cause

     Y92.093 Driveway of other non-institutional residence as the place of occurrence of the external cause

     Y92.094 Garage of other non-institutional residence as the place of occurrence of the external cause

     Y92.095 Swimming-pool of other non-institutional residence as the place of occurrence of the external cause

     Y92.096 Garden or yard of other non-institutional residence as the place of occurrence of the external cause

     Y92.098 Other place in other non-institutional residence as the place of occurrence of the external cause

     Y92.099 Unspecified place in other ▽ non-institutional residence as the place of occurrence of the external cause

✓5ᵗʰ **Y92.1** Institutional (nonprivate) residence as the place of occurrence of the external cause

     Y92.10 Unspecified residential institution as the ▽ place of occurrence of the external cause

✓6ᵗʰ **Y92.11** Children's home and orphanage as the place of occurrence of the external cause

     Y92.110 Kitchen in children's home and orphanage as the place of occurrence of the external cause

     Y92.111 Bathroom in children's home and orphanage as the place of occurrence of the external cause

     Y92.112 Bedroom in children's home and orphanage as the place of occurrence of the external cause

     Y92.113 Driveway of children's home and orphanage as the place of occurrence of the external cause

     Y92.114 Garage of children's home and orphanage as the place of occurrence of the external cause

     Y92.115 Swimming-pool of children's home and orphanage as the place of occurrence of the external cause

     Y92.116 Garden or yard of children's home and orphanage as the place of occurrence of the external cause

     Y92.118 Other place in children's home and orphanage as the place of occurrence of the external cause

     Y92.119 Unspecified place in children's ▽ home and orphanage as the place of occurrence of the external cause

✓6ᵗʰ **Y92.12** Nursing home as the place of occurrence of the external cause
> Home for the sick as the place of occurrence of the external cause
> Hospice as the place of occurrence of the external cause
> **AHA:** 2017,2Q,10

     Y92.120 Kitchen in nursing home as the place of occurrence of the external cause

     Y92.121 Bathroom in nursing home as the place of occurrence of the external cause

     Y92.122 Bedroom in nursing home as the place of occurrence of the external cause

     Y92.123 Driveway of nursing home as the place of occurrence of the external cause

     Y92.124 Garage of nursing home as the place of occurrence of the external cause

     Y92.125 Swimming-pool of nursing home as the place of occurrence of the external cause

     Y92.126 Garden or yard of nursing home as the place of occurrence of the external cause

     Y92.128 Other place in nursing home as the place of occurrence of the external cause

     Y92.129 Unspecified place in nursing ▽ home as the place of occurrence of the external cause

✓6ᵗʰ **Y92.13** Military base as the place of occurrence of the external cause
> EXCLUDES 1   military training grounds (Y92.84)

     Y92.130 Kitchen on military base as the place of occurrence of the external cause

     Y92.131 Mess hall on military base as the place of occurrence of the external cause

     Y92.133 Barracks on military base as the place of occurrence of the external cause

     Y92.135 Garage on military base as the place of occurrence of the external cause

     Y92.136 Swimming-pool on military base as the place of occurrence of the external cause

     Y92.137 Garden or yard on military base as the place of occurrence of the external cause

     Y92.138 Other place on military base as the place of occurrence of the external cause

     Y92.139 Unspecified place military base ▽ as the place of occurrence of the external cause

✓6ᵗʰ **Y92.14** Prison as the place of occurrence of the external cause

     Y92.140 Kitchen in prison as the place of occurrence of the external cause

     Y92.141 Dining room in prison as the place of occurrence of the external cause

     Y92.142 Bathroom in prison as the place of occurrence of the external cause

     Y92.143 Cell of prison as the place of occurrence of the external cause

     Y92.146 Swimming-pool of prison as the place of occurrence of the external cause

     Y92.147 Courtyard of prison as the place of occurrence of the external cause

     Y92.148 Other place in prison as the place of occurrence of the external cause

     Y92.149 Unspecified place in prison as the ▽ place of occurrence of the external cause

✔ Additional Character Req   ✓x7ᵗʰ Placeholder Alert   Manifestation   ▽ Unspecified   ▶◀ Revised Text   ● New Code   ▲ Revised Code Title

ICD-10-CM 2019   1205

Chapter 20. External Causes of Morbidity

Y92.15–Y92.243

√6ᵗʰ **Y92.15** **Reform school** as the place of occurrence of the external cause
     Y92.150 **Kitchen** in reform school as the place of occurrence of the external cause
     Y92.151 **Dining room** in reform school as the place of occurrence of the external cause
     Y92.152 **Bathroom** in reform school as the place of occurrence of the external cause
     Y92.153 **Bedroom** in reform school as the place of occurrence of the external cause
     Y92.154 **Driveway** of reform school as the place of occurrence of the external cause
     Y92.155 **Garage** of reform school as the place of occurrence of the external cause
     Y92.156 **Swimming-pool** of reform school as the place of occurrence of the external cause
     Y92.157 **Garden or yard** of reform school as the place of occurrence of the external cause
     Y92.158 **Other place** in reform school as the place of occurrence of the external cause
     Y92.159 **Unspecified place** in reform school as the place of occurrence of the external cause ▽

√6ᵗʰ **Y92.16** **School dormitory** as the place of occurrence of the external cause
     EXCLUDES 1 *reform school as the place of occurrence of the external cause (Y92.15-)*
         school buildings and grounds as the place of occurrence of the external cause (Y92.2-)
         school sports and athletic areas as the place of occurrence of the external cause (Y92.3-)
     Y92.160 **Kitchen** in school dormitory as the place of occurrence of the external cause
     Y92.161 **Dining room** in school dormitory as the place of occurrence of the external cause
     Y92.162 **Bathroom** in school dormitory as the place of occurrence of the external cause
     Y92.163 **Bedroom** in school dormitory as the place of occurrence of the external cause
     Y92.168 **Other place** in school dormitory as the place of occurrence of the external cause
     Y92.169 **Unspecified place** in school dormitory as the place of occurrence of the external cause ▽

√6ᵗʰ **Y92.19** **Other specified residential institution** as the place of occurrence of the external cause
     AHA: 2017,2Q,10
     Y92.190 **Kitchen** in other specified residential institution as the place of occurrence of the external cause
     Y92.191 **Dining room** in other specified residential institution as the place of occurrence of the external cause
     Y92.192 **Bathroom** in other specified residential institution as the place of occurrence of the external cause
     Y92.193 **Bedroom** in other specified residential institution as the place of occurrence of the external cause
     Y92.194 **Driveway** of other specified residential institution as the place of occurrence of the external cause
     Y92.195 **Garage** of other specified residential institution as the place of occurrence of the external cause
     Y92.196 **Pool** of other specified residential institution as the place of occurrence of the external cause
     Y92.197 **Garden or yard** of other specified residential institution as the place of occurrence of the external cause
     Y92.198 **Other place** in other specified residential institution as the place of occurrence of the external cause
     Y92.199 **Unspecified place** in other specified residential institution as the place of occurrence of the external cause ▽

√5ᵗʰ **Y92.2** **School, other institution and public administrative area** as the place of occurrence of the external cause
     Building and adjacent grounds used by the general public or by a particular group of the public
     EXCLUDES 1 *building under construction as the place of occurrence of the external cause (Y92.6)*
         residential institution as the place of occurrence of the external cause (Y92.1)
         school dormitory as the place of occurrence of the external cause (Y92.16-)
         sports and athletics area of schools as the place of occurrence of the external cause (Y92.3-)

√6ᵗʰ **Y92.21** **School (private) (public) (state)** as the place of occurrence of the external cause
     Y92.210 **Daycare center** as the place of occurrence of the external cause
     Y92.211 **Elementary school** as the place of occurrence of the external cause
         Kindergarten as the place of occurrence of the external cause
     Y92.212 **Middle school** as the place of occurrence of the external cause
     Y92.213 **High school** as the place of occurrence of the external cause
         AHA: 2012,4Q,108
     Y92.214 **College** as the place of occurrence of the external cause
         University as the place of occurrence of the external cause
     Y92.215 **Trade school** as the place of occurrence of the external cause
     Y92.218 **Other school** as the place of occurrence of the external cause
     Y92.219 **Unspecified school** as the place of occurrence of the external cause ▽

Y92.22 **Religious institution** as the place of occurrence of the external cause
     Church as the place of occurrence of the external cause
     Mosque as the place of occurrence of the external cause
     Synagogue as the place of occurrence of the external cause

√6ᵗʰ **Y92.23** **Hospital** as the place of occurrence of the external cause
     EXCLUDES 1 *ambulatory (outpatient) health services establishments (Y92.53-)*
         home for the sick as the place of occurrence of the external cause (Y92.12-)
         hospice as the place of occurrence of the external cause (Y92.12-)
         nursing home as the place of occurrence of the external cause (Y92.12-)
     Y92.230 **Patient room** in hospital as the place of occurrence of the external cause
     Y92.231 **Patient bathroom** in hospital as the place of occurrence of the external cause
     Y92.232 **Corridor** of hospital as the place of occurrence of the external cause
     Y92.233 **Cafeteria** of hospital as the place of occurrence of the external cause
     Y92.234 **Operating room** of hospital as the place of occurrence of the external cause
     Y92.238 **Other place** in hospital as the place of occurrence of the external cause
     Y92.239 **Unspecified place** in hospital as the place of occurrence of the external cause ▽

√6ᵗʰ **Y92.24** **Public administrative building** as the place of occurrence of the external cause
     Y92.240 **Courthouse** as the place of occurrence of the external cause
     Y92.241 **Library** as the place of occurrence of the external cause
     Y92.242 **Post office** as the place of occurrence of the external cause
     Y92.243 **City hall** as the place of occurrence of the external cause

Y92.248 **Other public administrative building** as the place of occurrence of the external cause

✓6ᵗʰ **Y92.25** **Cultural building** as the place of occurrence of the external cause

   Y92.250 **Art Gallery** as the place of occurrence of the external cause

   Y92.251 **Museum** as the place of occurrence of the external cause

   Y92.252 **Music hall** as the place of occurrence of the external cause

   Y92.253 **Opera house** as the place of occurrence of the external cause

   Y92.254 **Theater (live)** as the place of occurrence of the external cause

   Y92.258 **Other cultural public building** as the place of occurrence of the external cause

Y92.26 **Movie house or cinema** as the place of occurrence of the external cause

Y92.29 **Other specified public building** as the place of occurrence of the external cause

   Assembly hall as the place of occurrence of the external cause

   Clubhouse as the place of occurrence of the external cause

✓5ᵗʰ **Y92.3** **Sports and athletics area** as the place of occurrence of the external cause

✓6ᵗʰ **Y92.31** **Athletic court** as the place of occurrence of the external cause

   EXCLUDES 1   *tennis court in private home or garden (Y92.09)*

   Y92.310 **Basketball court** as the place of occurrence of the external cause

   Y92.311 **Squash court** as the place of occurrence of the external cause

   Y92.312 **Tennis court** as the place of occurrence of the external cause

   Y92.318 **Other athletic court** as the place of occurrence of the external cause

✓6ᵗʰ **Y92.32** **Athletic field** as the place of occurrence of the external cause

   Y92.320 **Baseball field** as the place of occurrence of the external cause

   Y92.321 **Football field** as the place of occurrence of the external cause

   Y92.322 **Soccer field** as the place of occurrence of the external cause

   Y92.328 **Other athletic field** as the place of occurrence of the external cause

      Cricket field as the place of occurrence of the external cause

      Hockey field as the place of occurrence of the external cause

✓6ᵗʰ **Y92.33** **Skating rink** as the place of occurrence of the external cause

   Y92.330 **Ice skating rink (indoor) (outdoor)** as the place of occurrence of the external cause

   Y92.331 **Roller skating rink** as the place of occurrence of the external cause

Y92.34 **Swimming pool (public)** as the place of occurrence of the external cause

   EXCLUDES 1   *swimming pool in private home or garden (Y92.016)*

Y92.39 **Other specified sports and athletic area** as the place of occurrence of the external cause

   Golf-course as the place of occurrence of the external cause

   Gymnasium as the place of occurrence of the external cause

   Riding-school as the place of occurrence of the external cause

   Stadium as the place of occurrence of the external cause

✓5ᵗʰ **Y92.4** **Street, highway and other paved roadways** as the place of occurrence of the external cause

   EXCLUDES 1   *private driveway of residence (Y92.014, Y92.024, Y92.043, Y92.093, Y92.113, Y92.123, Y92.154, Y92.194)*

✓6ᵗʰ **Y92.41** **Street and highway** as the place of occurrence of the external cause

   Y92.410 **Unspecified street and highway** as the place of occurrence of the external cause ▽

      Road NOS as the place of occurrence of the external cause

   Y92.411 **Interstate** highway as the place of occurrence of the external cause

      Freeway as the place of occurrence of the external cause

      Motorway as the place of occurrence of the external cause

   Y92.412 **Parkway** as the place of occurrence of the external cause

   Y92.413 **State road** as the place of occurrence of the external cause

   Y92.414 **Local residential or business street** as the place of occurrence of the external cause

   Y92.415 **Exit ramp or entrance ramp** of street or highway as the place of occurrence of the external cause

✓6ᵗʰ **Y92.48** **Other paved roadways** as the place of occurrence of the external cause

   Y92.480 **Sidewalk** as the place of occurrence of the external cause

   Y92.481 **Parking lot** as the place of occurrence of the external cause

   Y92.482 **Bike path** as the place of occurrence of the external cause

   Y92.488 **Other paved roadways** as the place of occurrence of the external cause

✓5ᵗʰ **Y92.5** **Trade and service area** as the place of occurrence of the external cause

   EXCLUDES 1   *garage in private home (Y92.015)*

      schools and other public administration buildings (Y92.2-)

✓6ᵗʰ **Y92.51** **Private commercial establishments** as the place of occurrence of the external cause

   Y92.510 **Bank** as the place of occurrence of the external cause

   Y92.511 **Restaurant or café** as the place of occurrence of the external cause

   Y92.512 **Supermarket, store or market** as the place of occurrence of the external cause

   Y92.513 **Shop (commercial)** as the place of occurrence of the external cause

✓6ᵗʰ **Y92.52** **Service areas** as the place of occurrence of the external cause

   Y92.520 **Airport** as the place of occurrence of the external cause

   Y92.521 **Bus station** as the place of occurrence of the external cause

   Y92.522 **Railway station** as the place of occurrence of the external cause

   Y92.523 **Highway rest stop** as the place of occurrence of the external cause

   Y92.524 **Gas station** as the place of occurrence of the external cause

      Petroleum station as the place of occurrence of the external cause

      Service station as the place of occurrence of the external cause

✓6ᵗʰ **Y92.53** **Ambulatory health services establishments** as the place of occurrence of the external cause

   Y92.530 **Ambulatory surgery center** as the place of occurrence of the external cause

      Outpatient surgery center, including that connected with a hospital as the place of occurrence of the external cause

      Same day surgery center, including that connected with a hospital as the place of occurrence of the external cause

☑ Additional Character Req   ✓x7ᵗʰ Placeholder Alert   Manifestation   ▽ Unspecified   ▶◀ Revised Text   ● New Code   ▲ Revised Code Title

ICD-10-CM 2019   1207

Y92.531   **Health care provider office as the place of occurrence of the external cause**
     Physician office as the place of occurrence of the external cause

Y92.532   **Urgent care center as the place of occurrence of the external cause**

Y92.538   **Other ambulatory health services establishments as the place of occurrence of the external cause**

Y92.59   **Other trade areas as the place of occurrence of the external cause**
     Office building as the place of occurrence of the external cause
     Casino as the place of occurrence of the external cause
     Garage (commercial) as the place of occurrence of the external cause
     Hotel as the place of occurrence of the external cause
     Radio or television station as the place of occurrence of the external cause
     Shopping mall as the place of occurrence of the external cause
     Warehouse as the place of occurrence of the external cause

✓5ᵗʰ **Y92.6**   **Industrial and construction area as the place of occurrence of the external cause**

Y92.61   **Building [any] under construction as the place of occurrence of the external cause**

Y92.62   **Dock or shipyard as the place of occurrence of the external cause**
     Dockyard as the place of occurrence of the external cause
     Dry dock as the place of occurrence of the external cause
     Shipyard as the place of occurrence of the external cause

Y92.63   **Factory as the place of occurrence of the external cause**
     Factory building as the place of occurrence of the external cause
     Factory premises as the place of occurrence of the external cause
     Industrial yard as the place of occurrence of the external cause

Y92.64   **Mine or pit as the place of occurrence of the external cause**
     Mine as the place of occurrence of the external cause

Y92.65   **Oil rig as the place of occurrence of the external cause**
     Pit (coal) (gravel) (sand) as the place of occurrence of the external cause

Y92.69   **Other specified industrial and construction area as the place of occurrence of the external cause**
     Gasworks as the place of occurrence of the external cause
     Power-station (coal) (nuclear) (oil) as the place of occurrence of the external cause
     Tunnel under construction as the place of occurrence of the external cause
     Workshop as the place of occurrence of the external cause

✓5ᵗʰ **Y92.7**   **Farm as the place of occurrence of the external cause**
     Ranch as the place of occurrence of the external cause
     EXCLUDES 1   *farmhouse and home premises of farm (Y92.0̸1-)*

Y92.71   **Barn as the place of occurrence of the external cause**

Y92.72   **Chicken coop as the place of occurrence of the external cause**
     Hen house as the place of occurrence of the external cause

Y92.73   **Farm field as the place of occurrence of the external cause**

Y92.74   **Orchard as the place of occurrence of the external cause**

Y92.79   **Other farm location as the place of occurrence of the external cause**

✓5ᵗʰ **Y92.8**   **Other places as the place of occurrence of the external cause**

✓6ᵗʰ **Y92.81**   **Transport vehicle as the place of occurrence of the external cause**
     EXCLUDES 1   *transport accidents (V0̸0̸-V99)*

Y92.810   **Car as the place of occurrence of the external cause**

Y92.811   **Bus as the place of occurrence of the external cause**

Y92.812   **Truck as the place of occurrence of the external cause**

Y92.813   **Airplane as the place of occurrence of the external cause**

Y92.814   **Boat as the place of occurrence of the external cause**

Y92.815   **Train as the place of occurrence of the external cause**

Y92.816   **Subway car as the place of occurrence of the external cause**

Y92.818   **Other transport vehicle as the place of occurrence of the external cause**

✓6ᵗʰ **Y92.82**   **Wilderness area**

Y92.820   **Desert as the place of occurrence of the external cause**

Y92.821   **Forest as the place of occurrence of the external cause**

Y92.828   **Other wilderness area as the place of occurrence of the external cause**
     Swamp as the place of occurrence of the external cause
     Mountain as the place of occurrence of the external cause
     Marsh as the place of occurrence of the external cause
     Prairie as the place of occurrence of the external cause

✓6ᵗʰ **Y92.83**   **Recreation area as the place of occurrence of the external cause**

Y92.830   **Public park as the place of occurrence of the external cause**

Y92.831   **Amusement park as the place of occurrence of the external cause**

Y92.832   **Beach as the place of occurrence of the external cause**
     Seashore as the place of occurrence of the external cause

Y92.833   **Campsite as the place of occurrence of the external cause**

Y92.834   **Zoological garden (Zoo) as the place of occurrence of the external cause**

Y92.838   **Other recreation area as the place of occurrence of the external cause**

Y92.84   **Military training ground as the place of occurrence of the external cause**

Y92.85   **Railroad track as the place of occurrence of the external cause**

Y92.86   **Slaughter house as the place of occurrence of the external cause**

Y92.89   **Other specified places as the place of occurrence of the external cause**
     Derelict house as the place of occurrence of the external cause

Y92.9   **Unspecified place or not applicable**   ▽

✓4ᵗʰ Y93   Activity codes

NOTE   Category Y93 is provided for use to indicate the activity of the person seeking healthcare for an injury or health condition, such as a heart attack while shoveling snow, which resulted from, or was contributed to, by the activity. These codes are appropriate for use for both acute injuries, such as those from chapter 19, and conditions that are due to the long-term, cumulative effects of an activity, such as those from chapter 13. They are also appropriate for use with external cause codes for cause and intent if identifying the activity provides additional information on the event. These codes should be used in conjunction with codes for external cause status (Y99) and place of occurrence (Y92).

This section contains the following broad activity categories:

Y93.0	Activities involving walking and running
Y93.1	Activities involving water and water craft
Y93.2	Activities involving ice and snow
Y93.3	Activities involving climbing, rappelling, and jumping off
Y93.4	Activities involving dancing and other rhythmic movement
Y93.5	Activities involving other sports and athletics played individually
Y93.6	Activities involving other sports and athletics played as a team or group
Y93.7	Activities involving other specified sports and athletics
Y93.A	Activities involving other cardiorespiratory exercise
Y93.B	Activities involving other muscle strengthening exercises
Y93.C	Activities involving computer technology and electronic devices
Y93.D	Activities involving arts and handcrafts
Y93.E	Activities involving personal hygiene and interior property and clothing maintenance
Y93.F	Activities involving caregiving
Y93.G	Activities involving food preparation, cooking and grilling
Y93.H	Activities involving exterior property and land maintenance, building and construction
Y93.I	Activities involving roller coasters and other types of external motion
Y93.J	Activities involving playing musical instrument
Y93.K	Activities involving animal care
Y93.8	Activities, other specified
Y93.9	Activity, unspecified

✓5ᵗʰ Y93.0   Activities involving walking and running

> **EXCLUDES 1**   activity, walking an animal (Y93.K1)
> activity, walking or running on a treadmill (Y93.A1)

Y93.01   **Activity, walking, marching and hiking**
Activity, walking, marching and hiking on level or elevated terrain
> **EXCLUDES 1**   activity, mountain climbing (Y93.31)

Y93.02   **Activity, running**

✓5ᵗʰ Y93.1   Activities involving water and water craft

> **EXCLUDES 1**   activities involving ice (Y93.2-)

Y93.11   **Activity, swimming**

Y93.12   **Activity, springboard and platform diving**

Y93.13   **Activity, water polo**

Y93.14   **Activity, water aerobics and water exercise**

Y93.15   **Activity, underwater diving and snorkeling**
Activity, SCUBA diving

Y93.16   **Activity, rowing, canoeing, kayaking, rafting and tubing**
Activity, canoeing, kayaking, rafting and tubing in calm and turbulent water

Y93.17   **Activity, water skiing and wake boarding**

Y93.18   **Activity, surfing, windsurfing and boogie boarding**
Activity, water sliding

Y93.19   **Activity, other involving water and watercraft**
Activity involving water NOS
Activity, parasailing
Activity, water survival training and testing

✓5ᵗʰ Y93.2   Activities involving ice and snow

> **EXCLUDES 1**   activity, shoveling ice and snow (Y93.H1)

Y93.21   **Activity, ice skating**
Activity, figure skating (singles) (pairs)
Activity, ice dancing
> **EXCLUDES 1**   activity, ice hockey (Y93.22)

Y93.22   **Activity, ice hockey**

▲ **Y93.23**   **Activity, snow (alpine) (downhill) skiing, snowboarding, sledding, toboganing and snow tubing**
> **EXCLUDES 1**   activity, cross country skiing (Y93.24)

Y93.24   **Activity, cross country skiing**
Activity, nordic skiing

Y93.29   **Activity, other involving ice and snow**
Activity involving ice and snow NOS

✓5ᵗʰ Y93.3   Activities involving climbing, rappelling and jumping off

> **EXCLUDES 1**   activity, hiking on level or elevated terrain (Y93.01)
> activity, jumping rope (Y93.56)
> activity, trampoline jumping (Y93.44)

Y93.31   **Activity, mountain climbing, rock climbing and wall climbing** .

Y93.32   **Activity, rappelling**

Y93.33   **Activity, BASE jumping**
Activity, Building, Antenna, Span, Earth jumping

Y93.34   **Activity, bungee jumping**

Y93.35   **Activity, hang gliding**

Y93.39   **Activity, other involving climbing, rappelling and jumping off**

✓5ᵗʰ Y93.4   Activities involving dancing and other rhythmic movement

> **EXCLUDES 1**   activity, martial arts (Y93.75)

Y93.41   **Activity, dancing**
AHA: 2012,4Q,108

Y93.42   **Activity, yoga**

Y93.43   **Activity, gymnastics**
Activity, rhythmic gymnastics
> **EXCLUDES 1**   activity, trampolining (Y93.44)

Y93.44   **Activity, trampolining**

Y93.45   **Activity, cheerleading**

Y93.49   **Activity, other involving dancing and other rhythmic movements**

✓5ᵗʰ Y93.5   Activities involving other sports and athletics played individually

> **EXCLUDES 1**   activity, dancing (Y93.41)
> activity, gymnastic (Y93.43)
> activity, trampoline (Y93.44)
> activity, yoga (Y93.42)

Y93.51   **Activity, roller skating (inline) and skateboarding**

Y93.52   **Activity, horseback riding**

Y93.53   **Activity, golf**

Y93.54   **Activity, bowling**

Y93.55   **Activity, bike riding**

Y93.56   **Activity, jumping rope**

Y93.57   **Activity, non-running track and field events**
> **EXCLUDES 1**   activity, running (any form) (Y93.02)

Y93.59   **Activity, other involving other sports and athletics played individually**
> **EXCLUDES 1**   activities involving climbing, rappelling, and jumping (Y93.3-)
> activities involving ice and snow (Y93.2-)
> activities involving walking and running (Y93.0-)
> activities involving water and watercraft (Y93.1-)

✓5ᵗʰ Y93.6   Activities involving other sports and athletics played as a team or group

> **EXCLUDES 1**   activity, ice hockey (Y93.22)
> activity, water polo (Y93.13)

Y93.61   **Activity, American tackle football**
Activity, football NOS

Y93.62   **Activity, American flag or touch football**

Y93.63   **Activity, rugby**

Y93.64   **Activity, baseball**
Activity, softball

Y93.65   **Activity, lacrosse and field hockey**

Y93.66   **Activity, soccer**

Y93.67   **Activity, basketball**

Y93.68   **Activity, volleyball (beach) (court)**

☑ Additional Character Req   ✓x7ᵗʰ Placeholder Alert   Manifestation   ▽ Unspecified   ►◄ Revised Text   ● New Code   ▲ Revised Code Title

Chapter 20. External Causes of Morbidity

Y93.6A–Y93.84

Y93.6A   **Activity, physical games generally associated with school recess, summer camp and children**
Activity, capture the flag
Activity, dodge ball
Activity, four square
Activity, kickball

Y93.69   **Activity, other involving other sports and athletics played as a team or group**
Activity, cricket

✓5ᵗʰ **Y93.7**   **Activities involving other specified sports and athletics**

Y93.71   **Activity, boxing**

Y93.72   **Activity, wrestling**

Y93.73   **Activity, racquet and hand sports**
Activity, handball
Activity, racquetball
Activity, squash
Activity, tennis

Y93.74   **Activity, frisbee**
Activity, ultimate frisbee

Y93.75   **Activity, martial arts**
Activity, combatives

Y93.79   **Activity, other specified sports and athletics**
EXCLUDES 1   *sports and athletics activities specified in categories Y93.0-Y93.6*

✓5ᵗʰ **Y93.A**   **Activities involving other cardiorespiratory exercise**
Activities involving physical training

Y93.A1   **Activity, exercise machines primarily for cardiorespiratory conditioning**
Activity, elliptical and stepper machines
Activity, stationary bike
Activity, treadmill

Y93.A2   **Activity, calisthenics**
Activity, jumping jacks
Activity, warm up and cool down

Y93.A3   **Activity, aerobic and step exercise**

Y93.A4   **Activity, circuit training**

Y93.A5   **Activity, obstacle course**
Activity, challenge course
Activity, confidence course

Y93.A6   **Activity, grass drills**
Activity, guerilla drills

Y93.A9   **Activity, other involving cardiorespiratory exercise**
EXCLUDES 1   *activities involving cardiorespiratory exercise specified in categories Y93.0-Y93.7*

✓5ᵗʰ **Y93.B**   **Activities involving other muscle strengthening exercises**

Y93.B1   **Activity, exercise machines primarily for muscle strengthening**

Y93.B2   **Activity, push-ups, pull-ups, sit-ups**

Y93.B3   **Activity, free weights**
Activity, barbells
Activity, dumbbells

Y93.B4   **Activity, pilates**

Y93.B9   **Activity, other involving muscle strengthening exercises**
EXCLUDES 1   *activities involving muscle strengthening specified in categories Y93.0-Y93.A*

✓5ᵗʰ **Y93.C**   **Activities involving computer technology and electronic devices**
EXCLUDES 1   *activity, electronic musical keyboard or instruments (Y93.J-)*

Y93.C1   **Activity, computer keyboarding**
Activity, electronic game playing using keyboard or other stationary device

Y93.C2   **Activity, hand held interactive electronic device**
Activity, cellular telephone and communication device
Activity, electronic game playing using interactive device
EXCLUDES 1   *activity, electronic game playing using keyboard or other stationary device (Y93.C1)*

Y93.C9   **Activity, other involving computer technology and electronic devices**

✓5ᵗʰ **Y93.D**   **Activities involving arts and handcrafts**
EXCLUDES 1   *activities involving playing musical instrument (Y93.J-)*

Y93.D1   **Activity, knitting and crocheting**

Y93.D2   **Activity, sewing**

Y93.D3   **Activity, furniture building and finishing**
Activity, furniture repair

Y93.D9   **Activity, other involving arts and handcrafts**

✓5ᵗʰ **Y93.E**   **Activities involving personal hygiene and interior property and clothing maintenance**
EXCLUDES 1   *activities involving cooking and grilling (Y93.G-)*
activities involving exterior property and land maintenance, building and construction (Y93.H-)
activities involving caregiving (Y93.F-)
activity, dishwashing (Y93.G1)
activity, food preparation (Y93.G1)
activity, gardening (Y93.H2)

Y93.E1   **Activity, personal bathing and showering**

Y93.E2   **Activity, laundry**

Y93.E3   **Activity, vacuuming**

Y93.E4   **Activity, ironing**

Y93.E5   **Activity, floor mopping and cleaning**

Y93.E6   **Activity, residential relocation**
Activity, packing up and unpacking involved in moving to a new residence

Y93.E8   **Activity, other personal hygiene**

Y93.E9   **Activity, other interior property and clothing maintenance**

✓5ᵗʰ **Y93.F**   **Activities involving caregiving**
Activity involving the provider of caregiving

Y93.F1   **Activity, caregiving, bathing**

Y93.F2   **Activity, caregiving, lifting**

Y93.F9   **Activity, other caregiving**

✓5ᵗʰ **Y93.G**   **Activities involving food preparation, cooking and grilling**

Y93.G1   **Activity, food preparation and clean up**
Activity, dishwashing

Y93.G2   **Activity, grilling and smoking food**

Y93.G3   **Activity, cooking and baking**
Activity, use of stove, oven and microwave oven

Y93.G9   **Activity, other involving cooking and grilling**

✓5ᵗʰ **Y93.H**   **Activities involving exterior property and land maintenance, building and construction**

Y93.H1   **Activity, digging, shoveling and raking**
Activity, dirt digging
Activity, raking leaves
Activity, snow shoveling

Y93.H2   **Activity, gardening and landscaping**
Activity, pruning, trimming shrubs, weeding

Y93.H3   **Activity, building and construction**

Y93.H9   **Activity, other involving exterior property and land maintenance, building and construction**

✓5ᵗʰ **Y93.I**   **Activities involving roller coasters and other types of external motion**

Y93.I1   **Activity, rollercoaster riding**

Y93.I9   **Activity, other involving external motion**

✓5ᵗʰ **Y93.J**   **Activities involving playing musical instrument**
Activity involving playing electric musical instrument

Y93.J1   **Activity, piano playing**
Activity, musical keyboard (electronic) playing

Y93.J2   **Activity, drum and other percussion instrument playing**

Y93.J3   **Activity, string instrument playing**

Y93.J4   **Activity, winds and brass instrument playing**

✓5ᵗʰ **Y93.K**   **Activities involving animal care**
EXCLUDES 1   *activity, horseback riding (Y93.52)*

Y93.K1   **Activity, walking an animal**

Y93.K2   **Activity, milking an animal**

Y93.K3   **Activity, grooming and shearing an animal**

Y93.K9   **Activity, other involving animal care**

✓5ᵗʰ **Y93.8**   **Activities, other specified**

Y93.81   **Activity, refereeing a sports activity**

Y93.82   **Activity, spectator at an event**

Y93.83   **Activity, rough housing and horseplay**

Y93.84   **Activity, sleeping**

Chapter 20. External Causes of Morbidity

      Y93.85 **Activity, choking game**
           Activity, blackout game
           Activity, fainting game
           Activity, pass out game
           AHA: 2016,4Q,74-76
      Y93.89 **Activity, other specified**
    Y93.9 **Activity, unspecified** ▽

  Y95 **Nosocomial condition**
      AHA: 2013,4Q,119

✓4ᵗʰ **Y99** **External cause status**

        NOTE   A single code from category Y99 should be used in
               conjunction with the external cause code(s) assigned to a
               record to indicate the status of the person at the time the
               event occurred.

    Y99.0 **Civilian activity done for income or pay**
        Civilian activity done for financial or other compensation
        EXCLUDES 1   *military activity (Y99.1)*
                     volunteer activity (Y99.2)

    Y99.1 **Military activity**
        EXCLUDES 1   *activity of off duty military personnel (Y99.8)*

    Y99.2 **Volunteer activity**
        EXCLUDES 1   *activity of child or other family member assisting in*
                     compensated work of other family member
                     (Y99.8)

    Y99.8 **Other external cause status**
        Activity NEC
        Activity of child or other family member assisting in
            compensated work of other family member
        Hobby not done for income
        Leisure activity
        Off-duty activity of military personnel
        Recreation or sport not for income or while a student
        Student activity
        EXCLUDES 1   *civilian activity done for income or compensation*
                     (Y99.0)
                     military activity (Y99.1)
        AHA: 2012,4Q,108

    Y99.9 **Unspecified external cause status** ▽

Chapter 21. Factors Influencing Health Status and Contact with Health Services (Z00–Z99)

Chapter Specific Guidelines with Coding Examples

The chapter specific guidelines from the ICD-10-CM Official Guidelines for Coding and Reporting have been provided below. Along with these guidelines are coding examples, contained in the shaded boxes, that have been developed to help illustrate the coding and/or sequencing guidance found in these guidelines.

Note: The chapter specific guidelines provide additional information about the use of Z codes for specified encounters.

a. Use of Z codes in any healthcare setting

Z codes are for use in any healthcare setting. Z codes may be used as either a first-listed (principal diagnosis code in the inpatient setting) or secondary code, depending on the circumstances of the encounter. Certain Z codes may only be used as first-listed or principal diagnosis.

> Patient with middle lobe lung cancer presents for initiation of chemotherapy
>
> **Z51.11**   **Encounter for antineoplastic chemotherapy**
>
> **C34.2**   **Malignant neoplasm of middle lobe, bronchus or lung**
>
> *Explanation:* A Z code can be used as first-listed in this situation based on guidelines in this chapter as well as chapter 2, "Neoplasms."

> Patient has chronic lymphocytic leukemia for which the patient had previous chemotherapy and is now in remission
>
> **C91.11**   **Chronic lymphocytic leukemia of B-cell type in remission**
>
> **Z92.21**   **Personal history of antineoplastic chemotherapy**
>
> *Explanation:*The personal history Z code is used to describe a secondary (supplementary) diagnosis to identify that this patient has had chemotherapy in the past.

b. Z codes indicate a reason for an encounter

Z codes are not procedure codes. A corresponding procedure code must accompany a Z code to describe any procedure performed.

c. Categories of Z codes

1) Contact/exposure

Category Z20 indicates contact with, and suspected exposure to, communicable diseases. These codes are for patients who do not show any sign or symptom of a disease but are suspected to have been exposed to it by close personal contact with an infected individual or are in an area where a disease is epidemic.

Category Z77, Other contact with and (suspected) exposures hazardous to health, indicates contact with and suspected exposures hazardous to health.

Contact/exposure codes may be used as a first-listed code to explain an encounter for testing, or, more commonly, as a secondary code to identify a potential risk.

2) Inoculations and vaccinations

Code Z23 is for encounters for inoculations and vaccinations. It indicates that a patient is being seen to receive a prophylactic inoculation against a disease. Procedure codes are required to identify the actual administration of the injection and the type(s) of immunizations given. Code Z23 may be used as a secondary code if the inoculation is given as a routine part of preventive health care, such as a well-baby visit.

3) Status

Status codes indicate that a patient is either a carrier of a disease or has the sequelae or residual of a past disease or condition. This includes such things as the presence of prosthetic or mechanical devices resulting from past treatment. A status code is informative, because the status may affect the course of treatment and its outcome. A status code is distinct from a history code. The history code indicates that the patient no longer has the condition.

A status code should not be used with a diagnosis code from one of the body system chapters, if the diagnosis code includes the information provided by the status code. For example, code Z94.1, Heart transplant status, should not be used with a code from subcategory T86.2, Complications of heart transplant. The status code does not provide additional information. The complication code indicates that the patient is a heart transplant patient.

For encounters for weaning from a mechanical ventilator, assign a code from subcategory J96.1, Chronic respiratory failure, followed by code Z99.11, Dependence on respirator [ventilator] status.

The status Z codes/categories are:

Z14	Genetic carrier

Genetic carrier status indicates that a person carries a gene, associated with a particular disease, which may be passed to offspring who may develop that disease. The person does not have the disease and is not at risk of developing the disease.

Z15	Genetic susceptibility to disease

Genetic susceptibility indicates that a person has a gene that increases the risk of that person developing the disease.

Codes from category Z15 should not be used as principal or first-listed codes. If the patient has the condition to which he/she is susceptible, and that condition is the reason for the encounter, the code for the current condition should be sequenced first. If the patient is being seen for follow-up after completed treatment for this condition, and the condition no longer exists, a follow-up code should be sequenced first, followed by the appropriate personal history and genetic susceptibility codes. If the purpose of the encounter is genetic counseling associated with procreative management, code Z31.5, Encounter for genetic counseling, should be assigned as the first-listed code, followed by a code from category Z15. Additional codes should be assigned for any applicable family or personal history.

Z16	Resistance to antimicrobial drugs

This code indicates that a patient has a condition that is resistant to antimicrobial drug treatment. Sequence the infection code first.

Z17	Estrogen receptor status
Z18	Retained foreign body fragments
Z19	Hormone sensitivity malignancy status
Z21	Asymptomatic HIV infection status

This code indicates that a patient has tested positive for HIV but has manifested no signs or symptoms of the disease.

Z22	Carrier of infectious disease

Carrier status indicates that a person harbors the specific organisms of a disease without manifest symptoms and is capable of transmitting the infection.

Z28.3	Underimmunization status
Z33.1	Pregnant state, incidental

This code is a secondary code only for use when the pregnancy is in no way complicating the reason for visit. Otherwise, a code from the obstetric chapter is required.

Z66	Do not resuscitate

This code may be used when it is documented by the provider that a patient is on do not resuscitate status at any time during the stay.

Z67	Blood type
Z68	Body mass index (BMI)

BMI codes should only be assigned when the associated diagnosis (such as overweight or obesity) meets the definition of a reportable diagnosis (see Section III, Reporting Additional Diagnoses). **Do not assign BMI codes during pregnancy.** *See Section I.B.14 for BMI documentation by clinicians other than the patient's provider.*

Z74.01	Bed confinement status
Z76.82	Awaiting organ transplant status
Z78	Other specified health status

Code Z78.1, Physical restraint status, may be used when it is documented by the provider that a patient has been put in restraints during the current encounter. Please note that this code should not be reported when it is documented by the provider that a patient is temporarily restrained during a procedure.

Z79	Long-term (current) drug therapy

Codes from this category indicate a patient's continuous use of a prescribed drug (including such things as aspirin therapy) for the long-term treatment of a condition or for prophylactic use. It is not for use for patients who have addictions to drugs. This subcategory is not for use of medications for detoxification or maintenance programs to prevent withdrawal symptoms in patients with drug dependence (e.g., methadone maintenance for opiate dependence). Assign the appropriate code for the drug dependence instead.

Assign a code from Z79 if the patient is receiving a medication for an extended period as a prophylactic measure (such as for the prevention of deep vein thrombosis) or as treatment of a chronic condition (such as arthritis) or a disease requiring a lengthy course of treatment (such as cancer). Do not assign a code from category Z79 for medication being administered for a brief period of time to treat an acute illness or injury (such as a course of antibiotics to treat acute bronchitis).

Z88   Allergy status to drugs, medicaments and biological substances

Except: Z88.9, Allergy status to unspecified drugs, medicaments and biological substances status

Z89   Acquired absence of limb

Z90   Acquired absence of organs, not elsewhere classified

Z91.0-   Allergy status, other than to drugs and biological substances

Z92.82   Status post administration of tPA (rtPA) in a different facility within the last 24 hours prior to admission to a current facility

Assign code Z92.82, Status post administration of tPA (rtPA) in a different facility within the last 24 hours prior to admission to current facility, as a secondary diagnosis when a patient is received by transfer into a facility and documentation indicates they were administered tissue plasminogen activator (tPA) within the last 24 hours prior to admission to the current facility.

This guideline applies even if the patient is still receiving the tPA at the time they are received into the current facility.

The appropriate code for the condition for which the tPA was administered (such as cerebrovascular disease or myocardial infarction) should be assigned first.

Code Z92.82 is only applicable to the receiving facility record and not to the transferring facility record.

Z93   Artificial opening status

Z94   Transplanted organ and tissue status

Z95   Presence of cardiac and vascular implants and grafts

Z96   Presence of other functional implants

Z97   Presence of other devices

Z98   Other postprocedural states

Assign code Z98.85, Transplanted organ removal status, to indicate that a transplanted organ has been previously removed. This code should not be assigned for the encounter in which the transplanted organ is removed. The complication necessitating removal of the transplant organ should be assigned for that encounter.

See section I.C19. for information on the coding of organ transplant complications.

Z99   Dependence on enabling machines and devices, not elsewhere classified

Note: Categories Z89-Z90 and Z93-Z99 are for use only if there are no complications or malfunctions of the organ or tissue replaced, the amputation site or the equipment on which the patient is dependent.

4) History (of)

There are two types of history Z codes, personal and family. Personal history codes explain a patient's past medical condition that no longer exists and is not receiving any treatment, but that has the potential for recurrence, and therefore may require continued monitoring.

Family history codes are for use when a patient has a family member(s) who has had a particular disease that causes the patient to be at higher risk of also contracting the disease.

Personal history codes may be used in conjunction with follow-up codes and family history codes may be used in conjunction with screening codes to explain the need for a test or procedure. History codes are also acceptable on any medical record regardless of the reason for visit. A history of an illness, even if no longer present, is important information that may alter the type of treatment ordered.

The history Z code categories are:

Z80   Family history of primary malignant neoplasm

Z81   Family history of mental and behavioral disorders

Z82   Family history of certain disabilities and chronic diseases (leading to disablement)

Z83   Family history of other specific disorders

Z84   Family history of other conditions

Z85   Personal history of malignant neoplasm

Z86   Personal history of certain other diseases

Z87   Personal history of other diseases and conditions

Z91.4-   Personal history of psychological trauma, not elsewhere classified

Z91.5   Personal history of self-harm

Z91.81   History of falling

Z91.82   Personal history of military deployment

Z92   Personal history of medical treatment

Except: Z92.0, Personal history of contraception

Except: Z92.82, Status post administration of tPA (rtPA) in a different facility within the last 24 hours prior to admission to a current facility

5) Screening

Screening is the testing for disease or disease precursors in seemingly well individuals so that early detection and treatment can be provided for those who test positive for the disease (e.g., screening mammogram).

The testing of a person to rule out or confirm a suspected diagnosis because the patient has some sign or symptom is a diagnostic examination, not a screening. In these cases, the sign or symptom is used to explain the reason for the test.

A screening code may be a first-listed code if the reason for the visit is specifically the screening exam. It may also be used as an additional code if the screening is done during an office visit for other health problems. A screening code is not necessary if the screening is inherent to a routine examination, such as a pap smear done during a routine pelvic examination.

Should a condition be discovered during the screening then the code for the condition may be assigned as an additional diagnosis.

> Prostate screening of healthy 50-year-old male patient; PSA noted to be elevated but normal digital rectal exam
>
> **Z12.5**   **Encounter for screening for malignant neoplasm of prostate**
>
> **R97.20**   **Elevated prostate specific antigen [PSA]**
>
> *Explanation:* The patient had no signs or symptoms of any prostate-related illness prior to coming in for the screening. The screening code is appropriately used as the first-listed code to signify that this was for routine screening. The elevated PSA is reported as a secondary diagnosis to reflect that an abnormal lab value was found as a result of the screening procedure(s).

The Z code indicates that a screening exam is planned. A procedure code is required to confirm that the screening was performed.

The screening Z codes/categories:

Z11   Encounter for screening for infectious and parasitic diseases

Z12   Encounter for screening for malignant neoplasms

Z13   Encounter for screening for other diseases and disorders

Except: Z13.9, Encounter for screening, unspecified

Z36   Encounter for antenatal screening for mother

6) Observation

There are three observation Z code categories. They are for use in very limited circumstances when a person is being observed for a suspected condition that is ruled out. The observation codes are not for use if an injury or illness or any signs or symptoms related to the suspected condition are present. In such cases the diagnosis/symptom code is used with the corresponding external cause code.

The observation codes are to be used as principal diagnosis only. The only exception to this is when the principal diagnosis is required to be a code from category Z38, Liveborn infants according to place of birth and type of delivery. Then a code from category Z05, Encounter for observation and evaluation of newborn for suspected diseases and conditions ruled out, is sequenced after the Z38 code. Additional codes may be used in addition to the observation code but only if they are unrelated to the suspected condition being observed.

Codes from subcategory Z03.7, Encounter for suspected maternal and fetal conditions ruled out, may either be used as a first-listed or as an additional code assignment depending on the case. They are for use in very limited circumstances on a maternal record when an encounter is for a suspected maternal or fetal condition that is ruled out during that encounter (for example, a maternal or fetal condition may be suspected due to an abnormal test result). These codes should not be used when the condition is confirmed. In those cases, the confirmed condition should be coded. In addition, these codes are not for use if an illness or any signs or symptoms related to the suspected condition or problem are present. In such cases the diagnosis/symptom code is used.

Additional codes may be used in addition to the code from subcategory Z03.7, but only if they are unrelated to the suspected condition being evaluated.

Codes from subcategory Z03.7 may not be used for encounters for antenatal screening of mother. *See Section I.C.21. Screening.*

For encounters for suspected fetal condition that are inconclusive following testing and evaluation, assign the appropriate code from category O35, O36, O40 or O41.

The observation Z code categories:

Z03	Encounter for medical observation for suspected diseases and conditions ruled out
Z04	Encounter for examination and observation for other reasons
	Except: Z04.9, Encounter for examination and observation for unspecified reason
Z05	Encounter for observation and evaluation of newborn for suspected diseases and conditions ruled out

7) Aftercare

Aftercare visit codes cover situations when the initial treatment of a disease has been performed and the patient requires continued care during the healing or recovery phase, or for the long-term consequences of the disease. The aftercare Z code should not be used if treatment is directed at a current, acute disease. The diagnosis code is to be used in these cases. Exceptions to this rule are codes Z51.0, Encounter for antineoplastic radiation therapy, and codes from subcategory Z51.1, Encounter for antineoplastic chemotherapy and immunotherapy. These codes are to be first-listed, followed by the diagnosis code when a patient's encounter is solely to receive radiation therapy, chemotherapy, or immunotherapy for the treatment of a neoplasm. If the reason for the encounter is more than one type of antineoplastic therapy, code Z51.0 and a code from subcategory Z51.1 may be assigned together, in which case one of these codes would be reported as a secondary diagnosis.

The aftercare Z codes should also not be used for aftercare for injuries. For aftercare of an injury, assign the acute injury code with the appropriate 7th character (for subsequent encounter).

The aftercare codes are generally first-listed to explain the specific reason for the encounter. An aftercare code may be used as an additional code when some type of aftercare is provided in addition to the reason for admission and no diagnosis code is applicable. An example of this would be the closure of a colostomy during an encounter for treatment of another condition.

Aftercare codes should be used in conjunction with other aftercare codes or diagnosis codes to provide better detail on the specifics of an aftercare encounter visit, unless otherwise directed by the classification. Should a patient receive multiple types of antineoplastic therapy during the same encounter, code Z51.0, Encounter for antineoplastic radiation therapy, and codes from subcategory Z51.1, Encounter for antineoplastic chemotherapy and immunotherapy, may be used together on a record. The sequencing of multiple aftercare codes depends on the circumstances of the encounter.

> Patient presents for third round of gemcitabine and first dose of antineoplastic radiation therapy for advanced pancreatic carcinoma
>
> **Z51.11**   **Encounter for antineoplastic chemotherapy**
>
> **Z51.0**   **Encounter for antineoplastic radiation therapy**
>
> **C25.9**   **Malignant neoplasm of pancreas, unspecified**
>
> *Explanation:* Gemcitabine is an antineoplastic chemotherapy. Since the encounter was solely to administer antineoplastic treatment, both forms of treatment are reported and either code can be the first-listed diagnosis, followed by the neoplastic condition code. Aftercare codes are typically not assigned for current treatment of disease; however, Z51.0 and subcategory Z51.1 are an exception to this standard.

Certain aftercare Z code categories need a secondary diagnosis code to describe the resolving condition or sequelae. For others, the condition is included in the code title.

Additional Z code aftercare category terms include fitting and adjustment, and attention to artificial openings.

Status Z codes may be used with aftercare Z codes to indicate the nature of the aftercare. For example code Z95.1, Presence of aortocoronary bypass graft, may be used with code Z48.812, Encounter for surgical

aftercare following surgery on the circulatory system, to indicate the surgery for which the aftercare is being performed. A status code should not be used when the aftercare code indicates the type of status, such as using Z43.0, Encounter for attention to tracheostomy, with Z93.0, Tracheostomy status.

The aftercare Z category/codes:

Z42	Encounter for plastic and reconstructive surgery following medical procedure or healed injury
Z43	Encounter for attention to artificial openings
Z44	Encounter for fitting and adjustment of external prosthetic device
Z45	Encounter for adjustment and management of implanted device
Z46	Encounter for fitting and adjustment of other devices
Z47	Orthopedic aftercare
Z48	Encounter for other postprocedural aftercare
Z49	Encounter for care involving renal dialysis
Z51	Encounter for other aftercare and medical care

8) Follow-up

The follow-up codes are used to explain continuing surveillance following completed treatment of a disease, condition, or injury. They imply that the condition has been fully treated and no longer exists. They should not be confused with aftercare codes, or injury codes with a 7th character for subsequent encounter, that explain ongoing care of a healing condition or its sequelae. Follow-up codes may be used in conjunction with history codes to provide the full picture of the healed condition and its treatment. The follow-up code is sequenced first, followed by the history code.

A follow-up code may be used to explain multiple visits. Should a condition be found to have recurred on the follow-up visit, then the diagnosis code for the condition should be assigned in place of the follow-up code.

The follow-up Z code categories:

Z08	Encounter for follow-up examination after completed treatment for malignant neoplasm
Z09	Encounter for follow-up examination after completed treatment for conditions other than malignant neoplasm
Z39	Encounter for maternal postpartum care and examination

> Follow-up for patient several months after completing a regime of IV antibiotics for recurrent pneumonia; lungs are clear and pneumonia is resolved
>
> **Z09**   **Encounter for follow-up examination after completed treatment for conditions other than malignant neoplasm**
>
> **Z87.01**   **Personal history of pneumonia (recurrent)**
>
> *Explanation:* Code Z09 identifies the follow-up visit as being unrelated to a malignant neoplasm, and code Z87 describes the condition that has now resolved.

> Follow-up for patient several months after completing a regime of IV antibiotics for recurrent pneumonia; pneumonia has recurred, and a new antibiotic regimen has been prescribed
>
> **J18.9**   **Pneumonia, unspecified organism**
>
> *Explanation:* Since the follow-up exam for pneumonia determined that the pneumonia was not resolved or recurred, code Z09 Encounter for follow-up examination after completed treatment for conditions other than malignant neoplasm, no longer applies. Instead the first-listed code describes the pneumonia.

9) Donor

Codes in category Z52, Donors of organs and tissues, are used for living individuals who are donating blood or other body tissue. These codes are only for individuals donating for others, not for self-donations. They are not used to identify cadaveric donations.

10) Counseling

Counseling Z codes are used when a patient or family member receives assistance in the aftermath of an illness or injury, or when support is required in coping with family or social problems.

The counseling Z codes/categories:

Z30.0-	Encounter for general counseling and advice on contraception
Z31.5	Encounter for procreative genetic counseling
Z31.6-	Encounter for general counseling and advice on procreation

Z32.2   Encounter for childbirth instruction

Z32.3   Encounter for childcare instruction

Z69   Encounter for mental health services for victim and perpetrator of abuse

Z70   Counseling related to sexual attitude, behavior and orientation

Z71   Persons encountering health services for other counseling and medical advice, not elsewhere classified

Z76.81   Expectant mother prebirth pediatrician visit

11) Encounters for obstetrical and reproductive services

See Section I.C.15. Pregnancy, Childbirth, and the Puerperium, for further instruction on the use of these codes.

Z codes for pregnancy are for use in those circumstances when none of the problems or complications included in the codes from the Obstetrics chapter exist (a routine prenatal visit or postpartum care). Codes in category Z34, Encounter for supervision of normal pregnancy, are always first-listed and are not to be used with any other code from the OB chapter.

Codes in category Z3A, Weeks of gestation, may be assigned to provide additional information about the pregnancy. Category Z3A codes should not be assigned for pregnancies with abortive outcomes (categories O00-O08), elective termination of pregnancy (code Z33.2), nor for postpartum conditions, as category Z3A is not applicable to these conditions. The date of the admission should be used to determine weeks of gestation for inpatient admissions that encompass more than one gestational week.

The outcome of delivery, category Z37, should be included on all maternal delivery records. It is always a secondary code. Codes in category Z37 should not be used on the newborn record.

Z codes for family planning (contraceptive) or procreative management and counseling should be included on an obstetric record either during the pregnancy or the postpartum stage, if applicable.

Z codes/categories for obstetrical and reproductive services:

Z30   Encounter for contraceptive management

Z31   Encounter for procreative management

Z32.2   Encounter for childbirth instruction

Z32.3   Encounter for childcare instruction

Z33   Pregnant state

Z34   Encounter for supervision of normal pregnancy

Z36   Encounter for antenatal screening of mother

Z3A   Weeks of gestation

Z37   Outcome of delivery

Z39   Encounter for maternal postpartum care and examination

Z76.81   Expectant mother prebirth pediatrician visit

12) Newborns and infants

See Section I.C.16. Newborn (Perinatal) Guidelines, for further instruction on the use of these codes.

Newborn Z codes/categories:

Z76.1   Encounter for health supervision and care of foundling

Z00.1-   Encounter for routine child health examination

Z38   Liveborn infants according to place of birth and type of delivery

13) Routine and administrative examinations

The Z codes allow for the description of encounters for routine examinations, such as, a general check-up, or, examinations for administrative purposes, such as, a pre-employment physical. The codes are not to be used if the examination is for diagnosis of a suspected condition or for treatment purposes. In such cases the diagnosis code is used. During a routine exam, should a diagnosis or condition be discovered, it should be coded as an additional code. Pre-existing and chronic conditions and history codes may also be included as additional codes as long as the examination is for administrative purposes and not focused on any particular condition.

Some of the codes for routine health examinations distinguish between "with" and "without" abnormal findings. Code assignment depends on the information that is known at the time the encounter is being coded. For example, if no abnormal findings were found during the examination, but the encounter is being coded before test results are back, it is acceptable to assign the code for "without abnormal findings." When assigning a code for "with abnormal findings," additional code(s) should be assigned to identify the specific abnormal finding(s).

12-month-old boy presented for well-child visit; pediatrician notices some eczema on the child's scalp and back of the knees

Z00.121   Encounter for routine child health examination with abnormal findings

L30.9   Dermatitis, unspecified

Explanation: The Z code identifying that this is a routine well-child visit is reported first. Because an abnormal finding (eczema) was documented, a code for this condition may also be appended.

Pre-operative examination and pre-procedural laboratory examination Z codes are for use only in those situations when a patient is being cleared for a procedure or surgery and no treatment is given.

The Z codes/categories for routine and administrative examinations:

Z00   Encounter for general examination without complaint, suspected or reported diagnosis

Z01   Encounter for other special examination without complaint, suspected or reported diagnosis

Z02   Encounter for administrative examination

         Except: Z02.9, Encounter for administrative examinations, unspecified

Z32.0-   Encounter for pregnancy test

14) Miscellaneous Z codes

The miscellaneous Z codes capture a number of other health care encounters that do not fall into one of the other categories. Certain of these codes identify the reason for the encounter; others are for use as additional codes that provide useful information on circumstances that may affect a patient's care and treatment.

Prophylactic organ removal

For encounters specifically for prophylactic removal of an organ (such as prophylactic removal of breasts due to a genetic susceptibility to cancer or a family history of cancer), the principal or first-listed code should be a code from category Z40, Encounter for prophylactic surgery, followed by the appropriate codes to identify the associated risk factor (such as genetic susceptibility or family history).

If the patient has a malignancy of one site and is having prophylactic removal at another site to prevent either a new primary malignancy or metastatic disease, a code for the malignancy should also be assigned in addition to a code from subcategory Z40.0, Encounter for prophylactic surgery for risk factors related to malignant neoplasms. A Z40.0 code should not be assigned if the patient is having organ removal for treatment of a malignancy, such as the removal of the testes for the treatment of prostate cancer.

Miscellaneous Z codes/categories:

Z28   Immunization not carried out

         Except: Z28.3, Underimmunization status

Z29   Encounter for other prophylactic measures

Z40   Encounter for prophylactic surgery

Z41   Encounter for procedures for purposes other than remedying health state

         Except: Z41.9, Encounter for procedure for purposes other than remedying health state, unspecified

Z53   Persons encountering health services for specific procedures and treatment, not carried out

Z55   Problems related to education and literacy

Z56   Problems related to employment and unemployment

Z57   Occupational exposure to risk factors

Z58   Problems related to physical environment

Z59   Problems related to housing and economic circumstances

Z60   Problems related to social environment

Z62   Problems related to upbringing

Z63   Other problems related to primary support group, including family circumstances

Z64   Problems related to certain psychosocial circumstances

Z65   Problems related to other psychosocial circumstances

Z72	Problems related to lifestyle
	Note: These codes should be assigned only when the documentation specifies that the patient has an associated problem
Z73	Problems related to life management difficulty
Z74	Problems related to care provider dependency
	Except: Z74.Ø1, Bed confinement status
Z75	Problems related to medical facilities and other health care
Z76.Ø	Encounter for issue of repeat prescription
Z76.3	Healthy person accompanying sick person
Z76.4	Other boarder to healthcare facility
Z76.5	Malingerer [conscious simulation]
Z91.1-	Patient's noncompliance with medical treatment and regimen
Z91.83	Wandering in diseases classified elsewhere
Z91.84-	Oral health risk factors
Z91.89	Other specified personal risk factors, not elsewhere classified

See Section I.B.14 for Z55-Z65 Persons with potential health hazards related to socioeconomic and psychosocial circumstances, documentation by clinicians other than the patient's provider

15) Nonspecific Z codes

Certain Z codes are so non-specific, or potentially redundant with other codes in the classification, that there can be little justification for their use in the inpatient setting. Their use in the outpatient setting should be limited to those instances when there is no further documentation to permit more precise coding. Otherwise, any sign or symptom or any other reason for visit that is captured in another code should be used.

Nonspecific Z codes/categories:

ZØ2.9	Encounter for administrative examinations, unspecified
ZØ4.9	Encounter for examination and observation for unspecified reason
Z13.9	Encounter for screening, unspecified
Z41.9	Encounter for procedure for purposes other than remedying health state, unspecified
Z52.9	Donor of unspecified organ or tissue
Z86.59	Personal history of other mental and behavioral disorders
Z88.9	Allergy status to unspecified drugs, medicaments and biological substances status
Z92.Ø	Personal history of contraception

16) Z codes that may only be principal/first-listed diagnosis

The following Z codes/categories may only be reported as the principal/first-listed diagnosis, except when there are multiple encounters on the same day and the medical records for the encounters are combined:

ZØØ	Encounter for general examination without complaint, suspected or reported diagnosis
	Except: ZØØ.6
ZØ1	Encounter for other special examination without complaint, suspected or reported diagnosis
ZØ2	Encounter for administrative examination
ZØ3	Encounter for medical observation for suspected diseases and conditions ruled out
ZØ4	Encounter for examination and observation for other reasons

Z33.2	Encounter for elective termination of pregnancy
Z31.81	Encounter for male factor infertility in female patient
Z31.83	Encounter for assisted reproductive fertility procedure cycle
Z31.84	Encounter for fertility preservation procedure
Z34	Encounter for supervision of normal pregnancy
Z39	Encounter for maternal postpartum care and examination
Z38	Liveborn infants according to place of birth and type of delivery
Z4Ø	Encounter for prophylactic surgery
Z42	Encounter for plastic and reconstructive surgery following medical procedure or healed injury
Z51.Ø	Encounter for antineoplastic radiation therapy
Z51.1-	Encounter for antineoplastic chemotherapy and immunotherapy
Z52	Donors of organs and tissues
	Except: Z52.9, Donor of unspecified organ or tissue
Z76.1	Encounter for health supervision and care of foundling
Z76.2	Encounter for health supervision and care of other healthy infant and child
Z99.12	Encounter for respirator [ventilator] dependence during power failure

---

Female patient seen at 32 weeks' gestation to check the progress of her first pregnancy

Z34.Ø3   **Encounter for supervision of normal first pregnancy, third trimester**

Z3A.32   **32 weeks gestation of pregnancy**

Explanation: Category Z34 is appropriate as a first-listed diagnosis. Category Z3A helps to clarify at which point in the pregnancy the patient was provided supervision.

Chapter 21. Factors Influencing Health Status and Contact With Health Services (Z00-Z99)

NOTE Z codes represent reasons for encounters. A corresponding procedure code must accompany a Z code if a procedure is performed. Categories Z00-Z99 are provided for occasions when circumstances other than a disease, injury or external cause classifiable to categories A00-Y89 are recorded as "diagnoses" or "problems." This can arise in two main ways:

(a) When a person who may or may not be sick encounters the health services for some specific purpose, such as to receive limited care or service for a current condition, to donate an organ or tissue, to receive prophylactic vaccination (immunization), or to discuss a problem which is in itself not a disease or injury.

(b) When some circumstance or problem is present which influences the person's health status but is not in itself a current illness or injury.

This chapter contains the following blocks:

Z00-Z13　Persons encountering health services for examinations
Z14-Z15　Genetic carrier and genetic susceptibility to disease
Z16　Resistance to antimicrobial drugs
Z17　Estrogen receptor status
Z18　Retained foreign body fragments
▶Z19◀　▶Hormone sensitivity malignancy status◀
Z20-Z29　Persons with potential health hazards related to communicable diseases
Z30-Z39　Persons encountering health services in circumstances related to reproduction
Z40-Z53　Encounters for other specific health care
Z55-Z65　Persons with potential health hazards related to socioeconomic and psychosocial circumstances
Z66　Do not resuscitate status
Z67　Blood type
Z68　Body mass index (BMI)
Z69-Z76　Persons encountering health services in other circumstances
Z77-Z99　Persons with potential health hazards related to family and personal history and certain conditions influencing health status

Persons encountering health services for examinations (Z00-Z13)

NOTE Nonspecific abnormal findings disclosed at the time of these examinations are classified to categories R70-R94.

EXCLUDES 1 examinations related to pregnancy and reproduction (Z30-Z36, Z39.-)

Z00 Encounter for general examination without complaint, suspected or reported diagnosis
　EXCLUDES 1 encounter for examination for administrative purposes (Z02.-)
　EXCLUDES 2 encounter for pre-procedural examinations (Z01.81-)
　　special screening examinations (Z11-Z13)
　AHA: 2017,4Q,95

Z00.0 Encounter for general adult medical examination
Encounter for adult periodic examination (annual) (physical) and any associated laboratory and radiologic examinations
　EXCLUDES 1 encounter for examination of sign or symptom - code to sign or symptom
　　general health check-up of infant or child (Z00.12-)

Z00.00 Encounter for general adult medical examination without abnormal findings
Encounter for adult health check-up NOS
AHA: 2016,1Q,36

Z00.01 Encounter for general adult medical examination with abnormal findings
Use additional code to identify abnormal findings
AHA: 2016,1Q,35-36

Z00.1 Encounter for newborn, infant and child health examinations

Z00.11 Newborn health examination
Health check for child under 29 days old
Use additional code to identify any abnormal findings
　EXCLUDES 1 health check for child over 28 days old (Z00.12-)

Z00.110 Health examination for newborn under 8 days old
Health check for newborn under 8 days old

Z00.111 Health examination for newborn 8 to 28 days old
Health check for newborn 8 to 28 days old
Newborn weight check

Z00.12 Encounter for routine child health examination
~~Encounter for development testing of infant or child~~
Health check (routine) for child over 28 days old
▶Immunizations appropriate for age◀
▶Routine developmental screening of infant or child◀
▶Routine vison and hearing testing◀
　EXCLUDES 1 health check for child under 29 days old (Z00.11-)
　　health supervision of foundling or other healthy infant or child (Z76.1-Z76.2)
　　newborn health examination (Z00.11-)

Z00.121 Encounter for routine child health examination with abnormal findings
Use additional code to identify abnormal findings
AHA: 2016,1Q,34-35

Z00.129 Encounter for routine child health examination without abnormal findings
Encounter for routine child health examination NOS
AHA: 2016,1Q,34

Z00.2 Encounter for examination for period of rapid growth in childhood

Z00.3 Encounter for examination for adolescent development state
Encounter for puberty development state

Z00.5 Encounter for examination of potential donor of organ and tissue

Z00.6 Encounter for examination for normal comparison and control in clinical research program
Examination of participant or control in clinical research program

Z00.7 Encounter for examination for period of delayed growth in childhood

Z00.70 Encounter for examination for period of delayed growth in childhood without abnormal findings

Z00.71 Encounter for examination for period of delayed growth in childhood with abnormal findings
Use additional code to identify abnormal findings

Z00.8 Encounter for other general examination
Encounter for health examination in population surveys

Z01 Encounter for other special examination without complaint, suspected or reported diagnosis
　INCLUDES routine examination of specific system
　NOTE Codes from category Z01 represent the reason for the encounter. A separate procedure code is required to identify any examinations or procedures performed
　EXCLUDES 1 encounter for examination for administrative purposes (Z02.-)
　　encounter for examination for suspected conditions, proven not to exist (Z03.-)
　　encounter for laboratory and radiologic examinations as a component of general medical examinations (Z00.0-)
　　encounter for laboratory, radiologic and imaging examinations for sign(s) and symptom(s) - code to the sign(s) or symptom(s)
　EXCLUDES 2 screening examinations (Z11-Z13)

Z01.0 Encounter for examination of eyes and vision
　EXCLUDES 1 examination for driving license (Z02.4)

Z01.00 Encounter for examination of eyes and vision without abnormal findings
Encounter for examination of eyes and vision NOS

Z01.01 Encounter for examination of eyes and vision with abnormal findings
Use additional code to identify abnormal findings
AHA: 2016,4Q,21

Z01.1 Encounter for examination of ears and hearing

Z01.10 Encounter for examination of ears and hearing without abnormal findings
Encounter for examination of ears and hearing NOS
AHA: 2016,4Q,24

✓6ᵗʰ **Z01.11** **Encounter for examination of ears and hearing** with **abnormal findings**
AHA: 2016,3Q,17-18

Z01.110 **Encounter for hearing examination following** failed **hearing screening** `PDx`

Z01.118 **Encounter for examination of ears and hearing with other abnormal findings** `PDx`
Use additional code to identify abnormal findings

Z01.12 **Encounter for hearing conservation and treatment** `PDx`

✓5ᵗʰ **Z01.2** **Encounter for dental examination and cleaning**

Z01.20 **Encounter for dental examination and cleaning** without **abnormal findings** `PDx`
Encounter for dental examination and cleaning NOS

Z01.21 **Encounter for dental examination and cleaning with abnormal findings** `PDx`
Use additional code to identify abnormal findings

✓5ᵗʰ **Z01.3** **Encounter for examination of** blood pressure

Z01.30 **Encounter for examination of blood pressure** without **abnormal findings** `PDx`
Encounter for examination of blood pressure NOS

Z01.31 **Encounter for examination of blood pressure with abnormal findings** `PDx`
Use additional code to identify abnormal findings

✓5ᵗʰ **Z01.4** **Encounter for** gynecological **examination**

EXCLUDES 2   *pregnancy examination or test (Z32.0-)*
routine examination for contraceptive maintenance (Z30.4-)

✓6ᵗʰ **Z01.41** **Encounter for** routine **gynecological examination**
Encounter for general gynecological examination with or without cervical smear
Encounter for gynecological examination (general) (routine) NOS
Encounter for pelvic examination (annual) (periodic)
Use additional code:
for screening for human papillomavirus, if applicable, (Z11.51)
for screening vaginal pap smear, if applicable (Z12.72)
to identify acquired absence of uterus, if applicable (Z90.71-)

EXCLUDES 1   *gynecologic examination status-post hysterectomy for malignant condition (Z08)*
screening cervical pap smear not a part of a routine gynecological examination (Z12.4)

Z01.411 **Encounter for gynecological examination (general) (routine) with abnormal findings** `PDx` ♀
Use additional code to identify abnormal findings

Z01.419 **Encounter for gynecological examination (general) (routine) without abnormal findings** `PDx` ♀

Z01.42 **Encounter for** cervical smear to confirm findings **of recent normal smear following initial abnormal smear** `PDx` ♀

✓5ᵗʰ **Z01.8** **Encounter for other specified special examinations**

✓6ᵗʰ **Z01.81** **Encounter for** preprocedural **examinations**
Encounter for preoperative examinations
Encounter for radiological and imaging examinations as part of preprocedural examination
TIP: Assign a code for the condition necessitating surgery and any findings as additional diagnoses.

Z01.810 **Encounter for preprocedural cardiovascular examination** `PDx`

Z01.811 **Encounter for preprocedural respiratory examination** `PDx`

Z01.812 **Encounter for preprocedural laboratory examination** `PDx`
Blood and urine tests prior to treatment or procedure

Z01.818 **Encounter for other preprocedural examination** `PDx`
Encounter for preprocedural examination NOS
Encounter for examinations prior to antineoplastic chemotherapy

Z01.82 **Encounter for** allergy testing `PDx`
EXCLUDES 1   *encounter for antibody response examination (Z01.84)*

Z01.83 **Encounter for** blood typing `PDx`
Encounter for Rh typing

Z01.84 **Encounter for** antibody response **examination** `PDx`
Encounter for immunity status testing
EXCLUDES 1   *encounter for allergy testing (Z01.82)*

Z01.89 **Encounter for other specified special examinations** `PDx`

✓4ᵗʰ **Z02** **Encounter for** administrative **examination**

Z02.0 **Encounter for examination for** admission to educational institution `PDx`
Encounter for examination for admission to preschool (education)
Encounter for examination for re-admission to school following illness or medical treatment

Z02.1 **Encounter for** pre-employment **examination** `PDx`

Z02.2 **Encounter for examination for** admission to residential institution `PDx`
EXCLUDES 1   *examination for admission to prison (Z02.89)*

Z02.3 **Encounter for examination for** recruitment to armed forces `PDx`

Z02.4 **Encounter for examination for** driving license `PDx`

Z02.5 **Encounter for examination for** participation in sport `PDx`
EXCLUDES 1   *blood-alcohol and blood-drug test (Z02.83)*

Z02.6 **Encounter for examination for** insurance purposes `PDx`

✓5ᵗʰ **Z02.7** **Encounter for** issue of medical certificate
EXCLUDES 1   *encounter for general medical examination (Z00-Z01, Z02.0-Z02.6, Z02.8-Z02.9)*

Z02.71 **Encounter for** disability determination `PDx`
Encounter for issue of medical certificate of incapacity
Encounter for issue of medical certificate of invalidity

Z02.79 **Encounter for issue of other medical certificate** `PDx`

✓5ᵗʰ **Z02.8** **Encounter for other administrative examinations**

Z02.81 **Encounter for** paternity testing `PDx`

Z02.82 **Encounter for** adoption services `PDx`

Z02.83 **Encounter for** blood-alcohol and blood-drug test `PDx`
Use additional code for findings of alcohol or drugs in blood (R78.-)

Z02.89 **Encounter for other administrative examinations** `PDx`
Encounter for examination for admission to prison
Encounter for examination for admission to summer camp
Encounter for immigration examination
Encounter for naturalization examination
Encounter for premarital examination
EXCLUDES 1   *health supervision of foundling or other healthy infant or child (Z76.1-Z76.2)*

Z02.9 **Encounter for administrative examinations, unspecified** `PDx` ▽

✓ Additional Character Req	✓x7ᵗʰ Placeholder Alert	Manifestation	▽ Unspecified	►◄ Revised Text	● New Code ▲ Revised Code Title

✓4ᵗʰ **Z03 Encounter for** medical observation **for suspected diseases and conditions ruled out**

> **NOTE**   This category is to be used when a person without a diagnosis is suspected of having an abnormal condition, without signs or symptoms, which requires study, but after examination and observation, is ruled out. This category is also for use for administrative and legal observation status.
>
> **EXCLUDES 1**   *contact with and (suspected) exposures hazardous to health (Z77.-)*
> *encounter for observation and evaluation of newborn for suspected diseases and conditions ruled out ▶(Z05.-)◀*
> *person with feared complaint in whom no diagnosis is made (Z71.1)*
> *signs or symptoms under study - code to signs or symptoms*

AHA: 2018,2Q,7-8; 2017,4Q,27

Z03.6 Encounter for observation for suspected toxic effect **from ingested substance ruled out** `PDx`
> Encounter for observation for suspected adverse effect from drug
> Encounter for observation for suspected poisoning

✓5ᵗʰ **Z03.7 Encounter for suspected** maternal and fetal conditions **ruled out**
> Encounter for suspected maternal and fetal conditions not found
>
> **EXCLUDES 1**   *known or suspected fetal anomalies affecting management of mother, not ruled out (O26.-, O35.-, O36.-, O40.-, O41.-)*

     Z03.71 Encounter for suspected problem with amniotic cavity and membrane ruled out `PDx` `M` ♀
> Encounter for suspected oligohydramnios ruled out
> Encounter for suspected polyhydramnios ruled out

     Z03.72 Encounter for suspected placental **problem ruled out** `PDx` `M` ♀

     Z03.73 Encounter for suspected fetal anomaly **ruled out** `PDx` `M` ♀

     Z03.74 Encounter for suspected problem with fetal growth ruled out `PDx` `M` ♀

     Z03.75 Encounter for suspected cervical shortening **ruled out** `PDx` `M` ♀

     Z03.79 Encounter for other suspected maternal and fetal conditions ruled out `PDx` ♀

✓5ᵗʰ **Z03.8 Encounter for** observation **for other suspected diseases and conditions ruled out**

     ✓6ᵗʰ **Z03.81 Encounter for observation for suspected** exposure **to biological agents ruled out**

         Z03.810 Encounter for observation for suspected exposure to anthrax **ruled out** `PDx`

         Z03.818 Encounter for observation for suspected exposure to other biological agents ruled out `PDx`

     Z03.89 Encounter for observation for other suspected diseases and conditions ruled out `PDx`

✓4ᵗʰ **Z04 Encounter for examination and observation for other reasons**

> **INCLUDES**   encounter for examination for medicolegal reasons
>
> This category is to be used when a person without a diagnosis is suspected of having an abnormal condition, without signs or symptoms, which requires study, but after examination and observation, is ruled-out. This category is also for use for administrative and legal observation status.

AHA: 2018,2Q,7-8

Z04.1 Encounter for examination and observation following transport accident `PDx`
> **EXCLUDES 1**   *encounter for examination and observation following work accident (Z04.2)*
>
> **AHA:** 2018,2Q,8

Z04.2 Encounter for examination and observation following work accident `PDx`

Z04.3 Encounter for examination and observation following other accident `PDx`

✓5ᵗʰ **Z04.4 Encounter for examination and observation following** alleged **rape**
> Encounter for examination and observation of victim following alleged rape
> Encounter for examination and observation of victim following alleged sexual abuse

     Z04.41 Encounter for examination and observation following alleged adult **rape** `PDx` `A`
> Suspected adult rape, ruled out
> Suspected adult sexual abuse, ruled out

     Z04.42 Encounter for examination and observation following alleged child **rape** `PDx` `P`
> Suspected child rape, ruled out
> Suspected child sexual abuse, ruled out

Z04.6 Encounter for general psychiatric examination, **requested by authority** `PDx`

✓5ᵗʰ **Z04.7 Encounter for examination and observation following** alleged **physical abuse**

     Z04.71 Encounter for examination and observation following alleged adult **physical abuse** `PDx` `A`
> Suspected adult physical abuse, ruled out
>
> **EXCLUDES 1**   *confirmed case of adult physical abuse (T74.-)*
> *encounter for examination and observation following alleged adult sexual abuse (Z04.41)*
> *suspected case of adult physical abuse, not ruled out (T76.-)*

     Z04.72 Encounter for examination and observation following alleged child **physical abuse** `PDx` `P`
> Suspected child physical abuse, ruled out
>
> **EXCLUDES 1**   *confirmed case of child physical abuse (T74.-)*
> *encounter for examination and observation following alleged child sexual abuse (Z04.42)*
> *suspected case of child physical abuse, not ruled out (T76.-)*

✓5ᵗʰ **Z04.8 Encounter for examination and observation for** other **specified reasons**
> Encounter for examination and observation for request for expert evidence

     ● **Z04.81 Encounter for examination and observation of victim following forced sexual exploitation**

     ● **Z04.82 Encounter for examination and observation of victim following forced labor exploitation**

     ● **Z04.89 Encounter for examination and observation for other specified reasons**

Z04.9 Encounter for examination and observation for unspecified reason `PDx` ▽
> Encounter for observation NOS

✓4ᵗʰ **Z05 Encounter for observation and evaluation of newborn for suspected diseases and conditions ruled out**
> This category is to be used for newborns, within the neonatal period (the first 28 days of life), who are suspected of having an abnormal condition, but without signs or symptoms, and which, after examination and observation, is ruled out.
>
> **AHA:** 2017,4Q,27; 2016,4Q,77

Z05.0 Observation and evaluation of newborn for suspected cardiac **condition ruled out**

Z05.1 Observation and evaluation of newborn for suspected infectious **condition ruled out**

Z05.2 Observation and evaluation of newborn for suspected neurological **condition ruled out**

Z05.3 Observation and evaluation of newborn for suspected respiratory **condition ruled out**

✓5ᵗʰ **Z05.4 Observation and evaluation of newborn for suspected** genetic, metabolic or immunologic **condition ruled out**

     Z05.41 Observation and evaluation of newborn for suspected genetic **condition ruled out**
> **AHA:** 2016,4Q,55

     Z05.42 Observation and evaluation of newborn for suspected metabolic **condition ruled out**

     Z05.43 Observation and evaluation of newborn for suspected immunologic **condition ruled out**

Z05.5 Observation and evaluation of newborn for suspected gastrointestinal **condition ruled out**

`HCC` CMS-HCC   `PDx` Primary Dx Only   `Q` QPP   `N` Newborn : 0   `P` Pediatric : 0-17   `M` Maternity : 12-55   `A` Adult : 15-124

1220   **ICD-10-CM 2019**

Z05.6 Observation and evaluation of newborn for suspected genitourinary condition ruled out

√5ᵗʰ **Z05.7** Observation and evaluation of newborn for suspected skin, subcutaneous, musculoskeletal and connective tissue condition ruled out

Z05.71 Observation and evaluation of newborn for suspected skin and subcutaneous tissue condition ruled out

Z05.72 Observation and evaluation of newborn for suspected musculoskeletal condition ruled out

Z05.73 Observation and evaluation of newborn for suspected connective tissue condition ruled out

Z05.8 Observation and evaluation of newborn for other specified suspected condition ruled out

Z05.9 Observation and evaluation of newborn for unspecified suspected condition ruled out ▽

Z08 Encounter for follow-up examination after completed treatment for malignant neoplasm
  Medical surveillance following completed treatment
  Use additional code to identify any acquired absence of organs (Z90.-)
  Use additional code to identify the personal history of malignant neoplasm (Z85.-)
  EXCLUDES 1 aftercare following medical care (Z43-Z49, Z51)

Z09 Encounter for follow-up examination after completed treatment for conditions other than malignant neoplasm
  Medical surveillance following completed treatment
  Use additional code to identify any applicable history of disease code (Z86.-. Z87.-)
  EXCLUDES 1 aftercare following medical care (Z43-Z49, Z51)
            surveillance of contraception (Z30.4-)
            surveillance of prosthetic and other medical devices (Z44-Z46)
  AHA: 2017,1Q,9; 2015,1Q,8

√4ᵗʰ **Z11** Encounter for screening for infectious and parasitic diseases
  Screening is the testing for disease or disease precursors in asymptomatic individuals so that early detection and treatment can be provided for those who test positive for the disease.
  EXCLUDES 1 encounter for diagnostic examination - code to sign or symptom

Z11.0 Encounter for screening for intestinal infectious diseases

Z11.1 Encounter for screening for respiratory tuberculosis

Z11.2 Encounter for screening for other bacterial diseases

Z11.3 Encounter for screening for infections with a predominantly sexual mode of transmission
  EXCLUDES 2 encounter for screening for human immunodeficiency virus [HIV] (Z11.4)
            encounter for screening for human papillomavirus (Z11.51)

Z11.4 Encounter for screening for human immunodeficiency virus [HIV]

√5ᵗʰ **Z11.5** Encounter for screening for other viral diseases
  EXCLUDES 2 encounter for screening for viral intestinal disease (Z11.0)

Z11.51 Encounter for screening for human papillomavirus (HPV)

Z11.59 Encounter for screening for other viral diseases

Z11.6 Encounter for screening for other protozoal diseases and helminthiases
  EXCLUDES 2 encounter for screening for protozoal intestinal disease (Z11.0)

Z11.8 Encounter for screening for other infectious and parasitic diseases
  Encounter for screening for chlamydia
  Encounter for screening for rickettsial
  Encounter for screening for spirochetal
  Encounter for screening for mycoses

Z11.9 Encounter for screening for infectious and parasitic diseases, unspecified ▽

√4ᵗʰ **Z12** Encounter for screening for malignant neoplasms
  Screening is the testing for disease or disease precursors in asymptomatic individuals so that early detection and treatment can be provided for those who test positive for the disease.
  Use additional code to identify any family history of malignant neoplasm (Z80.-)
  EXCLUDES 1 encounter for diagnostic examination - code to sign or symptom

Z12.0 Encounter for screening for malignant neoplasm of stomach

Z12.1 Encounter for screening for malignant neoplasm of intestinal tract
  AHA: 2017,1Q,8,9

Z12.10 Encounter for screening for malignant neoplasm of intestinal tract, unspecified ▽

Z12.11 Encounter for screening for malignant neoplasm of colon 0
  Encounter for screening colonoscopy NOS
  AHA: 2018,1Q,6
  TIP: Surveillance colonoscopies are a type of screening exam used to screen for malignancies in those patients with history of polyps and/or cancer (previously removed).

Z12.12 Encounter for screening for malignant neoplasm of rectum
  AHA: 2018,1Q,6

Z12.13 Encounter for screening for malignant neoplasm of small intestine

Z12.2 Encounter for screening for malignant neoplasm of respiratory organs

√5ᵗʰ **Z12.3** Encounter for screening for malignant neoplasm of breast

Z12.31 Encounter for screening mammogram for malignant neoplasm of breast 0
  EXCLUDES 1 inconclusive mammogram (R92.2)
  AHA: 2015,1Q,24

Z12.39 Encounter for other screening for malignant neoplasm of breast

Z12.4 Encounter for screening for malignant neoplasm of cervix ♀
  Encounter for screening pap smear for malignant neoplasm of cervix
  EXCLUDES 1 when screening is part of general gynecological examination (Z01.4-)
  EXCLUDES 2 encounter for screening for human papillomavirus (Z11.51)

Z12.5 Encounter for screening for malignant neoplasm of prostate ♂

Z12.6 Encounter for screening for malignant neoplasm of bladder

√5ᵗʰ **Z12.7** Encounter for screening for malignant neoplasm of other genitourinary organs

Z12.71 Encounter for screening for malignant neoplasm of testis ♂

Z12.72 Encounter for screening for malignant neoplasm of vagina ♀
  Vaginal pap smear status-post hysterectomy for non-malignant condition
  Use additional code to identify acquired absence of uterus (Z90.71-)
  EXCLUDES 1 vaginal pap smear status-post hysterectomy for malignant conditions (Z08)

Z12.73 Encounter for screening for malignant neoplasm of ovary ♀

Z12.79 Encounter for screening for malignant neoplasm of other genitourinary organs

√5ᵗʰ **Z12.8** Encounter for screening for malignant neoplasm of other sites

Z12.81 Encounter for screening for malignant neoplasm of oral cavity

Z12.82 Encounter for screening for malignant neoplasm of nervous system

Z12.83 Encounter for screening for malignant neoplasm of skin

Z12.89 Encounter for screening for malignant neoplasm of other sites

Z12.9 Encounter for screening for malignant neoplasm, site unspecified ▽

√4ᵗʰ **Z13** Encounter for screening for other diseases and disorders
  Screening is the testing for disease or disease precursors in asymptomatic individuals so that early detection and treatment can be provided for those who test positive for the disease.
  EXCLUDES 1 encounter for diagnostic examination - code to sign or symptom

Z13.0 Encounter for screening for diseases of the blood and blood-forming organs and certain disorders involving the immune mechanism

Z13.1 Encounter for screening for diabetes mellitus

√5ᵗʰ **Z13.2** Encounter for screening for nutritional, metabolic and other endocrine disorders

Z13.21 Encounter for screening for nutritional disorder

Chapter 21. Factors Influencing Health Status and Contact With Health Services

√6ᵗʰ **Z13.22 Encounter for screening for** metabolic **disorder**

Z13.220 Encounter for screening for lipoid **disorders**
Encounter for screening for cholesterol level
Encounter for screening for hypercholesterolemia
Encounter for screening for hyperlipidemia

Z13.228 Encounter for screening for other metabolic disorders

Z13.29 Encounter for screening for other suspected endocrine disorder
EXCLUDES 1   encounter for screening for diabetes mellitus (Z13.1)

● √5ᵗʰ **Z13.3 Encounter for screening examination for** mental health and behavioral **disorders**

● **Z13.30 Encounter for screening examination for** mental health and behavioral disorders, unspecified   ▽

● **Z13.31 Encounter for screening for** depression
Encounter for screening for depression, adult
Encounter for screening for depression for child or adolescent

● **Z13.32 Encounter for screening for** maternal depression
Encounter for screening for perinatal depression

● **Z13.39 Encounter for screening examination for other** mental health and behavioral disorders
Encounter for screening for alcoholism
Encounter for screening for intellectual disabilities

√5ᵗʰ **Z13.4 Encounter for screening for certain** developmental **disorders in** childhood
▶Encounter for development testing of infant or child◀
Encounter for screening for developmental handicaps in early childhood
EXCLUDES 1   routine development testing of infant or child (Z00.1-)
EXCLUDES 2   ▶encounter for routine child health examination (Z00.12-)◀

● **Z13.40 Encounter for screening for unspecified** developmental delays   ▽

● **Z13.41 Encounter for** autism **screening**

● **Z13.42 Encounter for screening for** global developmental delays **(milestones)**
Encounter for screening for developmental handicaps in early childhood

● **Z13.49 Encounter for screening for other developmental** delays

Z13.5 Encounter for screening for eye and ear **disorders**
EXCLUDES 2   encounter for general hearing examination (Z01.1-)
encounter for general vision examination (Z01.0-)
AHA: 2016,3Q,17

Z13.6 Encounter for screening for cardiovascular **disorders**

√5ᵗʰ **Z13.7 Encounter for screening for** genetic and chromosomal **anomalies**
EXCLUDES 1   genetic testing for procreative management (Z31.4-)

Z13.71 Encounter for nonprocreative screening for genetic disease carrier status

Z13.79 Encounter for other screening for genetic and chromosomal anomalies

√5ᵗʰ **Z13.8 Encounter for screening for other specified diseases and** disorders
EXCLUDES 2   screening for malignant neoplasms (Z12.-)

√6ᵗʰ **Z13.81 Encounter for screening for** digestive system disorders

Z13.810 Encounter for screening for upper gastrointestinal disorder

Z13.811 Encounter for screening for lower gastrointestinal disorder
EXCLUDES 1   encounter for screening for intestinal infectious disease (Z11.0)

Z13.818 Encounter for screening for other digestive system disorders

√6ᵗʰ **Z13.82 Encounter for screening for** musculoskeletal disorder

Z13.820 Encounter for screening for osteoporosis

Z13.828 Encounter for screening for other musculoskeletal disorder

Z13.83 Encounter for screening for respiratory disorder NEC
EXCLUDES 1   encounter for screening for respiratory tuberculosis (Z11.1)

Z13.84 Encounter for screening for dental **disorders**

√6ᵗʰ **Z13.85 Encounter for screening for** nervous system **disorders**

Z13.850 Encounter for screening for traumatic brain injury

Z13.858 Encounter for screening for other nervous system disorders

Z13.88 Encounter for screening for disorder due to exposure to contaminants
EXCLUDES 1   those exposed to contaminants without suspected disorders (Z57.-, Z77.-)

Z13.89 Encounter for screening for other disorder
Encounter for screening for genitourinary disorders

Z13.9 Encounter for screening, unspecified   ▽

Genetic carrier and genetic susceptibility to disease (Z14-Z15)

√4ᵗʰ **Z14 Genetic carrier**
DEF: Individuals carrying a gene mutation associated with a certain disease that typically do not develop the disease but are able to pass the mutated genes to offspring.

√5ᵗʰ **Z14.0 Hemophilia A carrier**

Z14.01 Asymptomatic hemophilia A carrier

Z14.02 Symptomatic hemophilia A carrier

Z14.1 Cystic fibrosis carrier

Z14.8 Genetic carrier of other disease

√4ᵗʰ **Z15 Genetic susceptibility to disease**
INCLUDES   confirmed abnormal gene
Use additional code, if applicable, for any associated family history of the disease (Z80-Z84)
EXCLUDES 1   chromosomal anomalies (Q90-Q99)

√5ᵗʰ **Z15.0 Genetic susceptibility to** malignant neoplasm
Code first, if applicable, any current malignant neoplasm (C00-C75, C81-C96)
Use additional code, if applicable, for any personal history of malignant neoplasm (Z85.-)

Z15.01 Genetic susceptibility to malignant neoplasm of breast

Z15.02 Genetic susceptibility to malignant neoplasm of ovary   ♀

Z15.03 Genetic susceptibility to malignant neoplasm of prostate   ♂

Z15.04 Genetic susceptibility to malignant neoplasm of endometrium   ♀

Z15.09 Genetic susceptibility to other malignant neoplasm

√5ᵗʰ **Z15.8 Genetic susceptibility to other disease**

Z15.81 Genetic susceptibility to multiple endocrine neoplasia [MEN]
EXCLUDES 1   multiple endocrine neoplasia [MEN] syndromes (E31.2-)

Z15.89 Genetic susceptibility to other disease

Resistance to antimicrobial drugs (Z16)

√4ᵗʰ **Z16 Resistance to antimicrobial drugs**
NOTE   The codes in this category are provided for use as additional codes to identify the resistance and non-responsiveness of a condition to antimicrobial drugs.
Code first the infection
EXCLUDES 1   Methicillin resistant Staphylococcus aureus infection (A49.02)
Methicillin resistant Staphylococcus aureus pneumonia (J15.212)
sepsis due to Methicillin resistant Staphylococcus aureus (A41.02)

√5ᵗʰ **Z16.1 Resistance to** beta lactam **antibiotics**

Z16.10 Resistance to unspecified beta lactam antibiotics   ▽

Z16.11 Resistance to penicillins
Resistance to amoxicillin
Resistance to ampicillin

Z16.12 **Extended spectrum beta lactamase (ESBL) resistance**
> EXCLUDES 2 *Methicillin resistant Staphylococcus aureus infection in diseases classified elsewhere (B95.62)*

Z16.19 **Resistance to other specified beta lactam antibiotics**
Resistance to cephalosporins

√5ᵗʰ **Z16.2** **Resistance to other antibiotics**

Z16.20 **Resistance to unspecified antibiotic** ▽
Resistance to antibiotics NOS

Z16.21 **Resistance to vancomycin**

Z16.22 **Resistance to vancomycin related antibiotics**

Z16.23 **Resistance to quinolones and fluoroquinolones**

Z16.24 **Resistance to multiple antibiotics**

Z16.29 **Resistance to other single specified antibiotic**
Resistance to aminoglycosides
Resistance to macrolides
Resistance to sulfonamides
Resistance to tetracyclines

√5ᵗʰ **Z16.3** **Resistance to other antimicrobial drugs**
> EXCLUDES 1 *resistance to antibiotics (Z16.1-, Z16.2-)*

Z16.30 **Resistance to unspecified antimicrobial drugs** ▽
Drug resistance NOS

Z16.31 **Resistance to antiparasitic drug(s)**
Resistance to quinine and related compounds

Z16.32 **Resistance to antifungal drug(s)**

Z16.33 **Resistance to antiviral drug(s)**

√6ᵗʰ **Z16.34** **Resistance to antimycobacterial drug(s)**
Resistance to tuberculostatics

Z16.341 **Resistance to single antimycobacterial drug**
Resistance to antimycobacterial drug NOS

Z16.342 **Resistance to multiple antimycobacterial drugs**

Z16.35 **Resistance to multiple antimicrobial drugs**
> EXCLUDES 1 *resistance to multiple antibiotics only (Z16.24)*

Z16.39 **Resistance to other specified antimicrobial drug**

Estrogen receptor status (Z17)

√4ᵗʰ **Z17** **Estrogen receptor status**
Code first malignant neoplasm of breast (C50.-)
DEF: Receptor status of breast cancer cells for the hormone estrogen that is used to help determine treatment and evaluate prognosis. ER+ breast cancer responds to hormone therapies while ER- breast cancer does not.

Z17.0 **Estrogen receptor positive status [ER+]**

Z17.1 **Estrogen receptor negative status [ER-]**

Retained foreign body fragments (Z18)

√4ᵗʰ **Z18** **Retained foreign body fragments**
> INCLUDES embedded fragment (status)
> embedded splinter (status)
> retained foreign body status
> EXCLUDES 1 *artificial joint prosthesis status (Z96.6-)*
> *foreign body accidentally left during a procedure (T81.5-)*
> *foreign body entering through orifice (T15-T19)*
> *in situ cardiac device (Z95.-)*
> *organ or tissue replaced by means other than transplant (Z96.-, Z97.-)*
> *organ or tissue replaced by transplant (Z94.-)*
> *personal history of retained foreign body fully removed Z87.821*
> *superficial foreign body (non-embedded splinter) - code to superficial foreign body, by site*

DEF: Embedded or retained fragment, splinter, or foreign body, natural or synthetic that can cause infection.

√5ᵗʰ **Z18.0** **Retained radioactive fragments**

Z18.01 **Retained depleted uranium fragments**

Z18.09 **Other retained radioactive fragments**
Other retained depleted isotope fragments
Retained nontherapeutic radioactive fragments

√5ᵗʰ **Z18.1** **Retained metal fragments**
> EXCLUDES 1 *retained radioactive metal fragments (Z18.01-Z18.09)*

Z18.10 **Retained metal fragments, unspecified** ▽
Retained metal fragment NOS

Z18.11 **Retained magnetic metal fragments**

Z18.12 **Retained nonmagnetic metal fragments**

Z18.2 **Retained plastic fragments**
Acrylics fragments
▶Diethylhexyl phthalates fragments◀
Isocyanate fragments

√5ᵗʰ **Z18.3** **Retained organic fragments**

Z18.31 **Retained animal quills or spines**

Z18.32 **Retained tooth**

Z18.33 **Retained wood fragments**

Z18.39 **Other retained organic fragments**

√5ᵗʰ **Z18.8** **Other specified retained foreign body**

Z18.81 **Retained glass fragments**

Z18.83 **Retained stone or crystalline fragments**
Retained concrete or cement fragments

Z18.89 **Other specified retained foreign body fragments**

Z18.9 **Retained foreign body fragments, unspecified material** ▽

Hormone sensitivity malignancy status (Z19)

√4ᵗʰ **Z19** **Hormone sensitivity malignancy status**
Code first malignant neoplasm - see Table of Neoplasms, by site, malignant
AHA: 2016,4Q,76

Z19.1 **Hormone sensitive malignancy status**

Z19.2 **Hormone resistant malignancy status**
Castrate resistant prostate malignancy status

Persons with potential health hazards related to communicable diseases (Z20-Z29)

√4ᵗʰ **Z20** **Contact with and (suspected) exposure to communicable diseases**
> EXCLUDES 1 *carrier of infectious disease (Z22.-)*
> *diagnosed current infectious or parasitic disease - see Alphabetic Index*
> EXCLUDES 2 *personal history of infectious and parasitic diseases (Z86.1-)*

√5ᵗʰ **Z20.0** **Contact with and (suspected) exposure to intestinal infectious diseases**

Z20.01 **Contact with and (suspected) exposure to intestinal infectious diseases due to Escherichia coli (E. coli)**

Z20.09 **Contact with and (suspected) exposure to other intestinal infectious diseases**

Z20.1 **Contact with and (suspected) exposure to tuberculosis**

Z20.2 **Contact with and (suspected) exposure to infections with a predominantly sexual mode of transmission**

Z20.3 **Contact with and (suspected) exposure to rabies**

Z20.4 **Contact with and (suspected) exposure to rubella**

Z20.5 **Contact with and (suspected) exposure to viral hepatitis**

Z20.6 **Contact with and (suspected) exposure to human immunodeficiency virus [HIV]**
> EXCLUDES 1 *asymptomatic human immunodeficiency virus [HIV] HIV infection status (Z21)*

Z20.7 **Contact with and (suspected) exposure to pediculosis, acariasis and other infestations**

√5ᵗʰ **Z20.8** **Contact with and (suspected) exposure to other communicable diseases**

√6ᵗʰ **Z20.81** **Contact with and (suspected) exposure to other bacterial communicable diseases**

Z20.810 **Contact with and (suspected) exposure to anthrax**

Z20.811 **Contact with and (suspected) exposure to meningococcus**

Z20.818 **Contact with and (suspected) exposure to other bacterial communicable diseases**

√6ᵗʰ **Z20.82** **Contact with and (suspected) exposure to other viral communicable diseases**

Z20.820 **Contact with and (suspected) exposure to varicella**

Z20.821 **Contact with and (suspected) exposure to Zika virus**

Z20.828 **Contact with and (suspected) exposure to other viral communicable diseases**

Z20.89   **Contact with and (suspected) exposure to other communicable diseases**

Z20.9   **Contact with and (suspected) exposure to unspecified communicable disease** ▽

Z21   **Asymptomatic human immunodeficiency virus [HIV] infection status**   HCC

HIV positive NOS

Code first human immunodeficiency virus [HIV] disease complicating pregnancy, childbirth and the puerperium, if applicable (O98.7-)

EXCLUDES 1   *acquired immunodeficiency syndrome (B20)*

contact with human immunodeficiency virus [HIV] (Z20.6)

exposure to human immunodeficiency virus [HIV] (Z20.6)

human immunodeficiency virus [HIV] disease (B20)

inconclusive laboratory evidence of human immunodeficiency virus [HIV] (R75)

DEF: Phase of human immunodeficiency virus (HIV) infection with no clinical symptoms. This phase may last for 10 years or more.

✓4ᵗʰ **Z22**   **Carrier of infectious disease**

INCLUDES   colonization status

suspected carrier

EXCLUDES 2   *carrier of viral hepatitis (B18.-)*

Z22.0   **Carrier of typhoid**

Z22.1   **Carrier of other intestinal infectious diseases**

Z22.2   **Carrier of diphtheria**

✓5ᵗʰ **Z22.3**   **Carrier of other specified bacterial diseases**

Z22.31   **Carrier of bacterial disease due to meningococci**

✓6ᵗʰ **Z22.32**   **Carrier of bacterial disease due to staphylococci**

Z22.321   **Carrier or suspected carrier of Methicillin susceptible Staphylococcus aureus**

MSSA colonization

Z22.322   **Carrier or suspected carrier of Methicillin resistant Staphylococcus aureus**

MRSA colonization

DEF: Carriers (colonization) of methicillin resistant *Staphylococcus aureus* (MRSA) have MRSA on their skin or in their body but do not exhibit signs of infection. These individuals are able to pass MRSA on to others who may develop an infection.

✓6ᵗʰ **Z22.33**   **Carrier of bacterial disease due to streptococci**

Z22.330   **Carrier of Group B streptococcus**

EXCLUDES 1   *carrier of streptococcus group B (GBS) complicating pregnancy, childbirth and the puerperium (O99.82-)*

Z22.338   **Carrier of other streptococcus**

Z22.39   **Carrier of other specified bacterial diseases**

Z22.4   **Carrier of infections with a predominantly sexual mode of transmission**

Z22.6   **Carrier of human T-lymphotropic virus type-1 [HTLV-1] infection**

Z22.8   **Carrier of other infectious diseases**

Z22.9   **Carrier of infectious disease, unspecified** ▽

Z23   **Encounter for immunization**

Code first any routine childhood examination

NOTE   Procedure codes are required to identify the types of immunizations given

✓4ᵗʰ **Z28**   **Immunization not carried out and underimmunization status**

INCLUDES   vaccination not carried out

✓5ᵗʰ **Z28.0**   **Immunization not carried out because of contraindication**

DEF: Contraindication: Situation where a drug, surgery, or other procedure may negatively affect or cause harm to a patient.

Z28.01   **Immunization not carried out because of acute illness of patient**

Z28.02   **Immunization not carried out because of chronic illness or condition of patient**

Z28.03   **Immunization not carried out because of immune compromised state of patient**

Z28.04   **Immunization not carried out because of patient allergy to vaccine or component**

Z28.09   **Immunization not carried out because of other contraindication**

Z28.1   **Immunization not carried out because of patient decision for reasons of belief or group pressure**

Immunization not carried out because of religious belief

✓5ᵗʰ **Z28.2**   **Immunization not carried out because of patient decision for other and unspecified reason**

Z28.20   **Immunization not carried out because of patient decision for unspecified reason** ▽

Z28.21   **Immunization not carried out because of patient refusal**

Z28.29   **Immunization not carried out because of patient decision for other reason**

Z28.3   **Underimmunization status**

Delinquent immunization status

Lapsed immunization schedule status

✓5ᵗʰ **Z28.8**   **Immunization not carried out for other reason**

Z28.81   **Immunization not carried out due to patient having had the disease**

Z28.82   **Immunization not carried out because of caregiver refusal**

Immunization not carried out because of guardian refusal

Immunization not carried out because of parent refusal

EXCLUDES 1   *immunization not carried out because of caregiver refusal because of religious belief (Z28.1)*

Z28.83   **Immunization not carried out due to unavailability of vaccine**

Delay in delivery of vaccine

Lack of availability of vaccine

Manufacturer delay of vaccine

Z28.89   **Immunization not carried out for other reason**

Z28.9   **Immunization not carried out for unspecified reason** ▽

✓4ᵗʰ **Z29**   **Encounter for other prophylactic measures**

EXCLUDES 1   *desensitization to allergens (Z51.6)*

prophylactic surgery (Z40.-)

AHA: 2016,4Q,78-79

✓5ᵗʰ **Z29.1**   **Encounter for prophylactic immunotherapy**

Encounter for administration of immunoglobulin

Z29.11   **Encounter for prophylactic immunotherapy for respiratory syncytial virus (RSV)**

Z29.12   **Encounter for prophylactic antivenin**

Z29.13   **Encounter for prophylactic Rho(D) immune globulin**

Z29.14   **Encounter for prophylactic rabies immune globin**

Z29.3   **Encounter for prophylactic fluoride administration**

Z29.8   **Encounter for other specified prophylactic measures**

Z29.9   **Encounter for prophylactic measures, unspecified** ▽

Persons encountering health services in circumstances related to reproduction (Z30-Z39)

✓4ᵗʰ **Z30**   **Encounter for contraceptive management**

AHA: 2016,4Q,78

DEF: Contraceptive management to prevent pregnancy. Methods include oral medications, intrauterine devices, and surgical procedures for males and females (sterilization).

✓5ᵗʰ **Z30.0**   **Encounter for general counseling and advice on contraception**

✓6ᵗʰ **Z30.01**   **Encounter for initial prescription of contraceptives**

EXCLUDES 1   *encounter for surveillance of contraceptives (Z30.4-)*

Z30.011   **Encounter for initial prescription of contraceptive pills**   ♀

Z30.012   **Encounter for prescription of emergency contraception**   ♀

Encounter for postcoital contraception

Z30.013   **Encounter for initial prescription of injectable contraceptive**   ♀

Z30.014   **Encounter for initial prescription of intrauterine contraceptive device**   ♀

EXCLUDES 1   *encounter for insertion of intrauterine contraceptive device (Z30.430, Z30.432)*

Z30.015   **Encounter for initial prescription of vaginal ring hormonal contraceptive**

Z30.016   **Encounter for initial prescription of transdermal patch hormonal contraceptive device**

Z30.017 Encounter for initial prescription of implantable subdermal contraceptive

Z30.018 Encounter for initial prescription of other contraceptives ♀

Encounter for initial prescription of barrier contraception

Encounter for initial prescription of diaphragm

Z30.019 Encounter for initial prescription of contraceptives, unspecified ♀ ▽

Z30.02 Counseling and instruction in natural family planning to avoid pregnancy

Z30.09 Encounter for other general counseling and advice on contraception

Encounter for family planning advice NOS

Z30.2 Encounter for sterilization

√5ᵗʰ **Z30.4** Encounter for surveillance of contraceptives

Z30.40 Encounter for surveillance of contraceptives, unspecified ▽

Z30.41 Encounter for surveillance of contraceptive pills ♀

Encounter for repeat prescription for contraceptive pill

Z30.42 Encounter for surveillance of injectable contraceptive ♀

√6ᵗʰ **Z30.43** Encounter for surveillance of intrauterine contraceptive device

Z30.430 Encounter for insertion of intrauterine contraceptive device ♀

Z30.431 Encounter for routine checking of intrauterine contraceptive device ♀

Z30.432 Encounter for removal of intrauterine contraceptive device ♀

Z30.433 Encounter for removal and reinsertion of intrauterine contraceptive device ♀

Encounter for replacement of intrauterine contraceptive device

Z30.44 Encounter for surveillance of vaginal ring hormonal contraceptive device ♀

Z30.45 Encounter for surveillance of transdermal patch hormonal contraceptive device ♀

Z30.46 Encounter for surveillance of implantable subdermal contraceptive ♀

Encounter for checking, reinsertion or removal of implantable subdermal contraceptive

Z30.49 Encounter for surveillance of other contraceptives ♀

Encounter for surveillance of barrier contraception

Encounter for surveillance of diaphragm

Z30.8 Encounter for other contraceptive management

Encounter for postvasectomy sperm count

Encounter for routine examination for contraceptive maintenance

EXCLUDES 1   sperm count following sterilization reversal (Z31.42)

sperm count for fertility testing (Z31.41)

Z30.9 Encounter for contraceptive management, unspecified ▽

√4ᵗʰ **Z31** Encounter for procreative management

EXCLUDES 1   complications associated with artificial fertilization (N98.-)

female infertility (N97.-)

male infertility (N46.-)

Z31.0 Encounter for reversal of previous sterilization

√5ᵗʰ **Z31.4** Encounter for procreative investigation and testing

EXCLUDES 1   postvasectomy sperm count (Z30.8)

Z31.41 Encounter for fertility testing

Encounter for fallopian tube patency testing

Encounter for sperm count for fertility testing

Z31.42 Aftercare following sterilization reversal

Sperm count following sterilization reversal

√6ᵗʰ **Z31.43** Encounter for genetic testing of female for procreative management ♀

Use additional code for recurrent pregnancy loss, if applicable (N96, O26.2-)

EXCLUDES 1   nonprocreative genetic testing (Z13.7-)

Z31.430 Encounter of female for testing for genetic disease carrier status for procreative management ♀

Z31.438 Encounter for other genetic testing of female for procreative management ♀

√6ᵗʰ **Z31.44** Encounter for genetic testing of male for procreative management

EXCLUDES 1   nonprocreative genetic testing (Z13.7-)

Z31.440 Encounter of male for testing for genetic disease carrier status for procreative management ♂

Z31.441 Encounter for testing of male partner of patient with recurrent pregnancy loss A ♂

Z31.448 Encounter for other genetic testing of male for procreative management A ♂

Z31.49 Encounter for other procreative investigation and testing

Z31.5 Encounter for procreative genetic counseling

AHA: 2017,4Q,27

√5ᵗʰ **Z31.6** Encounter for general counseling and advice on procreation

Z31.61 Procreative counseling and advice using natural family planning

Z31.62 Encounter for fertility preservation counseling

Encounter for fertility preservation counseling prior to cancer therapy

Encounter for fertility preservation counseling prior to surgical removal of gonads

Z31.69 Encounter for other general counseling and advice on procreation

Z31.7 Encounter for procreative management and counseling for gestational carrier

EXCLUDES 1   pregnant state, gestational carrier (Z33.3)

AHA: 2016,4Q,78

√5ᵗʰ **Z31.8** Encounter for other procreative management

Z31.81 Encounter for male factor infertility in female patient PDx ♀

Z31.82 Encounter for Rh incompatibility status ♀

AHA: 2015,3Q,40; 2014,4Q,17

Z31.83 Encounter for assisted reproductive fertility procedure cycle PDx ♀

Patient undergoing in vitro fertilization cycle

Use additional code to identify the type of infertility

EXCLUDES 1   pre-cycle diagnosis and testing - code to reason for encounter

Z31.84 Encounter for fertility preservation procedure PDx

Encounter for fertility preservation procedure prior to cancer therapy

Encounter for fertility preservation procedure prior to surgical removal of gonads

Z31.89 Encounter for other procreative management

Z31.9 Encounter for procreative management, unspecified ▽

√4ᵗʰ **Z32** Encounter for pregnancy test and childbirth and childcare instruction

√5ᵗʰ **Z32.0** Encounter for pregnancy test

Z32.00 Encounter for pregnancy test, result unknown ♀

Encounter for pregnancy test NOS

Z32.01 Encounter for pregnancy test, result positive M ♀

Z32.02 Encounter for pregnancy test, result negative ♀

Z32.2 Encounter for childbirth instruction

Z32.3 Encounter for childcare instruction

Encounter for prenatal or postpartum childcare instruction

✔ Additional Character Req   √x7ᵗʰ Placeholder Alert   Manifestation   ▽ Unspecified   ►◄ Revised Text   ● New Code   ▲ Revised Code Title

ICD-10-CM 2019   1225

Z33 Pregnant state

Z33.1 Pregnant state, incidental Ⓜ ♀
Pregnant state NOS
EXCLUDES 1 complications of pregnancy (O00-O9A)
pregnant state, gestational carrier (Z33.3)

Z33.2 Encounter for elective termination of pregnancy PDx Ⓜ ♀
EXCLUDES 1 early fetal death with retention of dead fetus (O02.1)
late fetal death (O36.4)
spontaneous abortion (O03)
TIP: Do not assign a code from category Z3A with this code.

Z33.3 Pregnant state, gestational carrier Ⓜ ♀
EXCLUDES 1 encounter for procreative management and
counseling for gestational carrier (Z31.7)
AHA: 2016,4Q,78

Z34 Encounter for supervision of normal pregnancy
EXCLUDES 1 any complication of pregnancy (O00-O9A)
encounter for pregnancy test (Z32.0-)
encounter for supervision of high risk pregnancy (O09.-)
AHA: 2014,4Q,17

Z34.0 Encounter for supervision of normal first pregnancy
Z34.00 Encounter for supervision of normal first PDx Ⓜ ♀ ▽ pregnancy, unspecified trimester
Z34.01 Encounter for supervision of normal first PDx Ⓜ ♀ pregnancy, first trimester
Z34.02 Encounter for supervision of normal first PDx Ⓜ ♀ pregnancy, second trimester
Z34.03 Encounter for supervision of normal first PDx Ⓜ ♀ pregnancy, third trimester

Z34.8 Encounter for supervision of other normal pregnancy
Z34.80 Encounter for supervision of other normal PDx Ⓜ ♀ ▽ pregnancy, unspecified trimester
Z34.81 Encounter for supervision of other normal PDx Ⓜ ♀ pregnancy, first trimester
Z34.82 Encounter for supervision of other normal PDx Ⓜ ♀ pregnancy, second trimester
Z34.83 Encounter for supervision of other normal PDx Ⓜ ♀ pregnancy, third trimester

Z34.9 Encounter for supervision of normal pregnancy, unspecified
Z34.90 Encounter for supervision of normal PDx Ⓜ ♀ ▽ pregnancy, unspecified, unspecified trimester
Z34.91 Encounter for supervision of normal PDx Ⓜ ♀ ▽ pregnancy, unspecified, first trimester
Z34.92 Encounter for supervision of normal PDx Ⓜ ♀ ▽ pregnancy, unspecified, second trimester
Z34.93 Encounter for supervision of normal PDx Ⓜ ♀ ▽ pregnancy, unspecified, third trimester

Z36 Encounter for antenatal screening of mother
INCLUDES encounter for placental sample (taken vaginally)
screening is the testing for disease or disease precursors
in asymptomatic individuals so that early detection
and treatment can be provided for those who test
positive for the disease.
EXCLUDES 1 diagnostic examination - code to sign or symptom
encounter for suspected maternal and fetal conditions ruled
out (Z03.7-)
suspected fetal condition affecting management of pregnancy
- code to condition in Chapter 15
EXCLUDES 2 abnormal findings on antenatal screening of mother (O28.-)
genetic counseling and testing (Z31.43-, Z31.5)
routine prenatal care (Z34)
AHA: 2017,4Q,28

Z36.0 Encounter for antenatal screening for chromosomal anomalies Ⓜ ♀

Z36.1 Encounter for antenatal screening for raised alphafetoprotein level Ⓜ ♀
Encounter for antenatal screening for elevated maternal serum alphafetoprotein level
DEF: High levels of alpha-fetoprotein (AFP) that may indicate a possibility of spina bifida and other neural tube defects, anencephaly, or omphalocele in the fetus.

Z36.2 Encounter for other antenatal screening follow-up Ⓜ ♀
Non-visualized anatomy on a previous scan

Z36.3 Encounter for antenatal screening for malformations Ⓜ ♀
Screening for a suspected anomaly

Z36.4 Encounter for antenatal screening for fetal growth retardation Ⓜ ♀
Intrauterine growth restriction (IUGR)/small-for-dates

Z36.5 Encounter for antenatal screening for isoimmunization Ⓜ ♀

Z36.8 Encounter for other antenatal screening
Z36.81 Encounter for antenatal screening for hydrops fetalis Ⓜ ♀
DEF: Hydrops fetalis: Abnormal accumulation of fluid in two or more parts of the fetus, such as ascites, effusion of the pleural or pericardial tissues, or edema.
Z36.82 Encounter for antenatal screening for nuchal translucency Ⓜ ♀
Z36.83 Encounter for fetal screening for congenital cardiac abnormalities Ⓜ ♀
Z36.84 Encounter for antenatal screening for fetal lung maturity Ⓜ ♀
Z36.85 Encounter for antenatal screening for Streptococcus B Ⓜ ♀
Z36.86 Encounter for antenatal screening for cervical length Ⓜ ♀
Screening for risk of pre-term labor
Z36.87 Encounter for antenatal screening for uncertain dates Ⓜ ♀
Z36.88 Encounter for antenatal screening for fetal macrosomia Ⓜ ♀
Screening for large-for-dates
Z36.89 Encounter for other specified antenatal screening Ⓜ ♀
Z36.8A Encounter for antenatal screening for other genetic defects Ⓜ ♀

Z36.9 Encounter for antenatal screening, unspecified Ⓜ ♀ ▽

Z3A Weeks of gestation
NOTE Codes from category Z3A are for use, only on the maternal record, to indicate the weeks of gestation of the pregnancy, if known.
Code first complications of pregnancy, childbirth and the puerperium (O09-O9A)
AHA: 2016,2Q,34; 2014,3Q,17; 2014,2Q,9; 2013,2Q,33
TIP: Do not assign a code from this category with codes from categories O00-O08 or code Z33.2.

Z3A.0 Weeks of gestation of pregnancy, unspecified or less than 10 weeks
Z3A.00 Weeks of gestation of pregnancy not specified Ⓜ ♀ ▽
Z3A.01 Less than 8 weeks gestation of pregnancy Ⓜ ♀
Z3A.08 8 weeks gestation of pregnancy Ⓜ ♀
Z3A.09 9 weeks gestation of pregnancy Ⓜ ♀

Z3A.1 Weeks of gestation of pregnancy, weeks 10-19
Z3A.10 10 weeks gestation of pregnancy Ⓜ ♀
Z3A.11 11 weeks gestation of pregnancy Ⓜ ♀
Z3A.12 12 weeks gestation of pregnancy Ⓜ ♀
Z3A.13 13 weeks gestation of pregnancy Ⓜ ♀
Z3A.14 14 weeks gestation of pregnancy Ⓜ ♀
Z3A.15 15 weeks gestation of pregnancy Ⓜ ♀
Z3A.16 16 weeks gestation of pregnancy Ⓜ ♀
Z3A.17 17 weeks gestation of pregnancy Ⓜ ♀
Z3A.18 18 weeks gestation of pregnancy Ⓜ ♀
Z3A.19 19 weeks gestation of pregnancy Ⓜ ♀

Z3A.2 Weeks of gestation of pregnancy, weeks 20-29
Z3A.20 20 weeks gestation of pregnancy Ⓜ ♀
Z3A.21 21 weeks gestation of pregnancy Ⓜ ♀
Z3A.22 22 weeks gestation of pregnancy Ⓜ ♀
Z3A.23 23 weeks gestation of pregnancy Ⓜ ♀
Z3A.24 24 weeks gestation of pregnancy Ⓜ ♀
Z3A.25 25 weeks gestation of pregnancy Ⓜ ♀
Z3A.26 26 weeks gestation of pregnancy Ⓜ ♀
Z3A.27 27 weeks gestation of pregnancy Ⓜ ♀
Z3A.28 28 weeks gestation of pregnancy Ⓜ ♀
Z3A.29 29 weeks gestation of pregnancy Ⓜ ♀

Z3A.3 Weeks of gestation of pregnancy, weeks 30-39
Z3A.30 30 weeks gestation of pregnancy Ⓜ ♀
Z3A.31 31 weeks gestation of pregnancy Ⓜ ♀
Z3A.32 32 weeks gestation of pregnancy Ⓜ ♀
Z3A.33 33 weeks gestation of pregnancy Ⓜ ♀
Z3A.34 34 weeks gestation of pregnancy Ⓜ ♀
Z3A.35 35 weeks gestation of pregnancy Ⓜ ♀
Z3A.36 36 weeks gestation of pregnancy Ⓜ ♀

Z3A.37 37 weeks gestation of pregnancy M ♀
Z3A.38 38 weeks gestation of pregnancy M ♀
Z3A.39 39 weeks gestation of pregnancy M ♀

✓5ᵗʰ **Z3A.4 Weeks of gestation of pregnancy, weeks 40 or greater**
   AHA: 2014,4Q,23
   Z3A.40 40 weeks gestation of pregnancy M ♀
   Z3A.41 41 weeks gestation of pregnancy M ♀
   Z3A.42 42 weeks gestation of pregnancy M ♀
   Z3A.49 Greater than 42 weeks gestation of pregnancy M ♀

✓4ᵗʰ **Z37 Outcome of delivery**
   This category is intended for use as an additional code to identify the outcome of delivery on the mother's record. It is not for use on the newborn record.
   EXCLUDES 1 stillbirth (P95)

   Z37.0 Single live birth M ♀
      AHA: 2016,2Q,34; 2014,2Q,9
   Z37.1 Single stillbirth M ♀
   Z37.2 Twins, both liveborn M ♀
   Z37.3 Twins, one liveborn and one stillborn M ♀
   Z37.4 Twins, both stillborn M ♀
✓5ᵗʰ **Z37.5 Other multiple births, all liveborn**
      Z37.50 Multiple births, unspecified, all liveborn M ♀ ▽
      Z37.51 Triplets, all liveborn M ♀
      Z37.52 Quadruplets, all liveborn M ♀
      Z37.53 Quintuplets, all liveborn M ♀
      Z37.54 Sextuplets, all liveborn M ♀
      Z37.59 Other multiple births, all liveborn M ♀
✓5ᵗʰ **Z37.6 Other multiple births, some liveborn**
      Z37.60 Multiple births, unspecified, some liveborn M ♀ ▽
      Z37.61 Triplets, some liveborn M ♀
      Z37.62 Quadruplets, some liveborn M ♀
      Z37.63 Quintuplets, some liveborn M ♀
      Z37.64 Sextuplets, some liveborn M ♀
      Z37.69 Other multiple births, some liveborn M ♀
   Z37.7 Other multiple births, all stillborn M ♀
   Z37.9 Outcome of delivery, unspecified M ♀ ▽
      Multiple birth NOS
      Single birth NOS

✓4ᵗʰ **Z38 Liveborn infants according to place of birth and type of delivery**
   This category is for use as the principal code on the initial record of a newborn baby. It is to be used for the initial birth record only. It is not to be used on the mother's record.
   AHA: 2017,2Q,5-7; 2016,3Q,18; 2015,2Q,15
   TIP: For attending physician services, a code from this category can be reported as first listed every time the physician visits the newborn during the birth admission.

✓5ᵗʰ **Z38.0 Single liveborn infant, born in hospital**
      Single liveborn infant, born in birthing center or other health care facility
      Z38.00 Single liveborn infant, delivered vaginally PDx N
      Z38.01 Single liveborn infant, delivered by cesarean PDx N
   Z38.1 Single liveborn infant, born outside hospital PDx N
   Z38.2 Single liveborn infant, unspecified as to place of birth PDx N ▽
      Single liveborn infant NOS
✓5ᵗʰ **Z38.3 Twin liveborn infant, born in hospital**
      Z38.30 Twin liveborn infant, delivered vaginally PDx N
      Z38.31 Twin liveborn infant, delivered by cesarean PDx N
   Z38.4 Twin liveborn infant, born outside hospital PDx N
   Z38.5 Twin liveborn infant, unspecified as to place of birth PDx N ▽
✓5ᵗʰ **Z38.6 Other multiple liveborn infant, born in hospital**
      Z38.61 Triplet liveborn infant, delivered vaginally PDx N
      Z38.62 Triplet liveborn infant, delivered by cesarean PDx N
      Z38.63 Quadruplet liveborn infant, delivered vaginally PDx N
      Z38.64 Quadruplet liveborn infant, delivered by cesarean PDx N
      Z38.65 Quintuplet liveborn infant, delivered vaginally PDx N
      Z38.66 Quintuplet liveborn infant, delivered by cesarean PDx N

      Z38.68 Other multiple liveborn infant, delivered vaginally PDx N
      Z38.69 Other multiple liveborn infant, delivered by cesarean PDx N
   Z38.7 Other multiple liveborn infant, born outside hospital PDx N
   Z38.8 Other multiple liveborn infant, unspecified as to place of birth PDx N ▽

✓4ᵗʰ **Z39 Encounter for maternal postpartum care and examination**
   Z39.0 Encounter for care and examination of mother immediately after delivery PDx M ♀
      Care and observation in uncomplicated cases when the delivery occurs outside a healthcare facility
      EXCLUDES 1 care for postpartum complication - see Alphabetic index
   Z39.1 Encounter for care and examination of lactating mother PDx M ♀
      Encounter for supervision of lactation
      EXCLUDES 1 disorders of lactation (O92.-)
   Z39.2 Encounter for routine postpartum follow-up PDx M

Encounters for other specific health care (Z40–Z53)

   Categories Z40-Z53 are intended for use to indicate a reason for care. They may be used for patients who have already been treated for a disease or injury, but who are receiving aftercare or prophylactic care, or care to consolidate the treatment, or to deal with a residual state
   EXCLUDES 2 follow-up examination for medical surveillance after treatment (Z08-Z09)

✓4ᵗʰ **Z40 Encounter for prophylactic surgery**
   EXCLUDES 1 organ donations (Z52.-)
            therapeutic organ removal - code to condition
✓5ᵗʰ **Z40.0 Encounter for prophylactic surgery for risk factors related to malignant neoplasms**
      Admission for prophylactic organ removal
      Use additional code to identify risk factor
      AHA: 2017,4Q,28-29
      Z40.00 Encounter for prophylactic removal of unspecified organ PDx ▽
      Z40.01 Encounter for prophylactic removal of breast PDx
      Z40.02 Encounter for prophylactic removal of ovary(s) PDx ♀
              Encounter for prophylactic removal of ovary(s) and fallopian tube(s)
      Z40.03 Encounter for prophylactic removal of fallopian tube(s) PDx ♀
      Z40.09 Encounter for prophylactic removal of other organ PDx
   Z40.8 Encounter for other prophylactic surgery PDx
   Z40.9 Encounter for prophylactic surgery, unspecified PDx ▽

✓4ᵗʰ **Z41 Encounter for procedures for purposes other than remedying health state**
   Z41.1 Encounter for cosmetic surgery
      Encounter for cosmetic breast implant
      Encounter for cosmetic procedure
      EXCLUDES 1 encounter for plastic and reconstructive surgery following medical procedure or healed injury (Z42.-)
               encounter for post-mastectomy breast implantation (Z42.1)
   Z41.2 Encounter for routine and ritual male circumcision ♂
   Z41.3 Encounter for ear piercing
   Z41.8 Encounter for other procedures for purposes other than remedying health state
   Z41.9 Encounter for procedure for purposes other than remedying health state, unspecified ▽

✓4ᵗʰ **Z42 Encounter for plastic and reconstructive surgery following medical procedure or healed injury**
   EXCLUDES 1 encounter for cosmetic plastic surgery (Z41.1)
            encounter for plastic surgery for treatment of current injury - code to relevent injury
   Z42.1 Encounter for breast reconstruction following mastectomy PDx ▲
      EXCLUDES 1 deformity and disproportion of reconstructed breast (N65.1-)

✓ Additional Character Req   ✓x7ᵗʰ Placeholder Alert   **Manifestation**   ▽ Unspecified   ▶◀ Revised Text   ● New Code   ▲ Revised Code Title

Z42.8 Encounter for other plastic and reconstructive surgery following medical procedure or healed injury [PDx]
> **AHA:** 2017,1Q,42

√4ᵗʰ **Z43** Encounter for attention to artificial openings
> [INCLUDES] closure of artificial openings
> passage of sounds or bougies through artificial openings
> reforming artificial openings
> removal of catheter from artificial openings
> toilet or cleansing of artificial openings
>
> [EXCLUDES 1] complications of external stoma (J95.0-, K94.-, N99.5-)
> [EXCLUDES 2] fitting and adjustment of prosthetic and other devices (Z44-Z46)

Z43.0 Encounter for attention to tracheostomy [HCC]
Z43.1 Encounter for attention to gastrostomy [HCC]
> [EXCLUDES 2] artificial opening status only, without need for care (Z93.-)

Z43.2 Encounter for attention to ileostomy [HCC]
Z43.3 Encounter for attention to colostomy [HCC]
Z43.4 Encounter for attention to other artificial openings of digestive tract [HCC]
Z43.5 Encounter for attention to cystostomy [HCC]
Z43.6 Encounter for attention to other artificial openings of urinary tract [HCC]
> Encounter for attention to nephrostomy
> Encounter for attention to ureterostomy
> Encounter for attention to urethrostomy

Z43.7 Encounter for attention to artificial vagina
Z43.8 Encounter for attention to other artificial openings [HCC]
Z43.9 Encounter for attention to unspecified artificial opening [HCC] ▽

√4ᵗʰ **Z44** Encounter for fitting and adjustment of external prosthetic device
> [INCLUDES] removal or replacement of external prosthetic device
> [EXCLUDES 1] malfunction or other complications of device - see Alphabetical Index
> presence of prosthetic device (Z97.-)

√5ᵗʰ **Z44.0** Encounter for fitting and adjustment of artificial arm
> √6ᵗʰ **Z44.00** Encounter for fitting and adjustment of unspecified artificial arm
> > **Z44.001** Encounter for fitting and adjustment of unspecified right artificial arm ▽
> > **Z44.002** Encounter for fitting and adjustment of unspecified left artificial arm ▽
> > **Z44.009** Encounter for fitting and adjustment of unspecified artificial arm, unspecified arm ▽
>
> √6ᵗʰ **Z44.01** Encounter for fitting and adjustment of complete artificial arm
> > **Z44.011** Encounter for fitting and adjustment of complete right artificial arm
> > **Z44.012** Encounter for fitting and adjustment of complete left artificial arm
> > **Z44.019** Encounter for fitting and adjustment of complete artificial arm, unspecified arm ▽
>
> √6ᵗʰ **Z44.02** Encounter for fitting and adjustment of partial artificial arm
> > **Z44.021** Encounter for fitting and adjustment of partial artificial right arm
> > **Z44.022** Encounter for fitting and adjustment of partial artificial left arm
> > **Z44.029** Encounter for fitting and adjustment of partial artificial arm, unspecified arm ▽

√5ᵗʰ **Z44.1** Encounter for fitting and adjustment of artificial leg
> √6ᵗʰ **Z44.10** Encounter for fitting and adjustment of unspecified artificial leg
> > **Z44.101** Encounter for fitting and adjustment of unspecified right artificial leg [HCC] ▽
> > **Z44.102** Encounter for fitting and adjustment of unspecified left artificial leg [HCC] ▽
> > **Z44.109** Encounter for fitting and adjustment of unspecified artificial leg, unspecified leg [HCC] ▽

√6ᵗʰ **Z44.11** Encounter for fitting and adjustment of complete artificial leg
> > **Z44.111** Encounter for fitting and adjustment of complete right artificial leg [HCC]
> > **Z44.112** Encounter for fitting and adjustment of complete left artificial leg [HCC]
> > **Z44.119** Encounter for fitting and adjustment of complete artificial leg, unspecified leg [HCC] ▽

√6ᵗʰ **Z44.12** Encounter for fitting and adjustment of partial artificial leg
> > **Z44.121** Encounter for fitting and adjustment of partial artificial right leg [HCC]
> > **Z44.122** Encounter for fitting and adjustment of partial artificial left leg [HCC]
> > **Z44.129** Encounter for fitting and adjustment of partial artificial leg, unspecified leg [HCC] ▽

√5ᵗʰ **Z44.2** Encounter for fitting and adjustment of artificial eye
> [EXCLUDES 1] mechanical complication of ocular prosthesis (T85.3)
> **Z44.20** Encounter for fitting and adjustment of artificial eye, unspecified ▽
> **Z44.21** Encounter for fitting and adjustment of artificial right eye
> **Z44.22** Encounter for fitting and adjustment of artificial left eye

√5ᵗʰ **Z44.3** Encounter for fitting and adjustment of external breast prosthesis
> [EXCLUDES 1] complications of breast implant (T85.4-)
> encounter for adjustment or removal of breast implant (Z45.81-)
> encounter for initial breast implant insertion for cosmetic breast augmentation (Z41.1)
> encounter for breast reconstruction following mastectomy (Z42.1)
>
> **Z44.30** Encounter for fitting and adjustment of external breast prosthesis, unspecified breast ▽
> **Z44.31** Encounter for fitting and adjustment of external right breast prosthesis
> **Z44.32** Encounter for fitting and adjustment of external left breast prosthesis

Z44.8 Encounter for fitting and adjustment of other external prosthetic devices
Z44.9 Encounter for fitting and adjustment of unspecified external prosthetic device ▽

√4ᵗʰ **Z45** Encounter for adjustment and management of implanted device
> [INCLUDES] removal or replacement of implanted device
> [EXCLUDES 1] malfunction or other complications of device - see Alphabetical Index
> [EXCLUDES 2] encounter for fitting and adjustment of non-implanted device (Z46.-)

√5ᵗʰ **Z45.0** Encounter for adjustment and management of cardiac device
> √6ᵗʰ **Z45.01** Encounter for adjustment and management of cardiac pacemaker
> > Encounter for adjustment and management of cardiac resynchronization therapy pacemaker (CRT-P)
> > [EXCLUDES 1] encounter for adjustment and management of automatic implantable cardiac defibrillator with synchronous cardiac pacemaker (Z45.02)
> >
> > **TIP:** Assign an additional code for the condition the pacemaker is controlling (e.g., sick sinus syndrome) only when the interrogation of the pacemaker identifies a problem with this condition.
> >
> > **Z45.010** Encounter for checking and testing of cardiac pacemaker pulse generator [battery]
> > > Encounter for replacing cardiac pacemaker pulse generator [battery]

[HCC] CMS-HCC   [PDx] Primary Dx Only   [Q] QPP   [N] Newborn : 0   [P] Pediatric : 0-17   [M] Maternity : 12-55   [A] Adult : 15-124

1228   ICD-10-CM 2019

Z45.018 Encounter for adjustment and management of other part of cardiac pacemaker
EXCLUDES 2 presence of prosthetic and other devices (Z95-Z97)

Z45.02 Encounter for adjustment and management of automatic implantable cardiac defibrillator
Encounter for adjustment and management of automatic implantable cardiac defibrillator with synchronous cardiac pacemaker
Encounter for adjustment and management of cardiac resynchronization therapy defibrillator (CRT-D)

Z45.09 Encounter for adjustment and management of other cardiac device

Z45.1 Encounter for adjustment and management of infusion pump

Z45.2 Encounter for adjustment and management of vascular access device
Encounter for adjustment and management of vascular catheters
EXCLUDES 1 encounter for adjustment and management of renal dialysis catheter (Z49.01)

✓5ᵗʰ **Z45.3 Encounter for adjustment and management of implanted devices of the special senses**

Z45.31 Encounter for adjustment and management of implanted visual substitution device

✓6ᵗʰ **Z45.32 Encounter for adjustment and management of implanted hearing device**
EXCLUDES 1 encounter for fitting and adjustment of hearing aide (Z46.1)

Z45.320 Encounter for adjustment and management of bone conduction device

Z45.321 Encounter for adjustment and management of cochlear device

Z45.328 Encounter for adjustment and management of other implanted hearing device

✓5ᵗʰ **Z45.4 Encounter for adjustment and management of implanted nervous system device**

Z45.41 Encounter for adjustment and management of cerebrospinal fluid drainage device
Encounter for adjustment and management of cerebral ventricular (communicating) shunt

Z45.42 Encounter for adjustment and management of neuropacemaker (brain) (peripheral nerve) (spinal cord)

Z45.49 Encounter for adjustment and management of other implanted nervous system device
AHA: 2014,3Q,19

✓5ᵗʰ **Z45.8 Encounter for adjustment and management of other implanted devices**

✓6ᵗʰ **Z45.81 Encounter for adjustment or removal of breast implant**
Encounter for elective implant exchange (different material) (different size)
Encounter removal of tissue expander without synchronous insertion of permanent implant
EXCLUDES 1 complications of breast implant (T85.4-)
encounter for initial breast implant insertion for cosmetic breast augmentation (Z41.1)
encounter for breast reconstruction following mastectomy (Z42.1)

Z45.811 Encounter for adjustment or removal of right breast implant

Z45.812 Encounter for adjustment or removal of left breast implant

Z45.819 Encounter for adjustment or removal of unspecified breast implant ▽

Z45.82 Encounter for adjustment or removal of myringotomy device (stent) (tube)

Z45.89 Encounter for adjustment and management of other implanted devices
AHA: 2014,4Q,26-28

Z45.9 Encounter for adjustment and management of unspecified implanted device ▽

✓4ᵗʰ **Z46 Encounter for fitting and adjustment of other devices**
INCLUDES removal or replacement of other device
EXCLUDES 1 malfunction or other complications of device - see Alphabetical Index
EXCLUDES 2 encounter for fitting and management of implanted devices (Z45.-)
issue of repeat prescription only (Z76.0)
presence of prosthetic and other devices (Z95-Z97)

Z46.0 Encounter for fitting and adjustment of spectacles and contact lenses

Z46.1 Encounter for fitting and adjustment of hearing aid
EXCLUDES 1 encounter for adjustment and management of implanted hearing device (Z45.32-)

Z46.2 Encounter for fitting and adjustment of other devices related to nervous system and special senses
EXCLUDES 2 encounter for adjustment and management of implanted nervous system device (Z45.4-)
encounter for adjustment and management of implanted visual substitution device (Z45.31)

Z46.3 Encounter for fitting and adjustment of dental prosthetic device
Encounter for fitting and adjustment of dentures

Z46.4 Encounter for fitting and adjustment of orthodontic device

✓5ᵗʰ **Z46.5 Encounter for fitting and adjustment of other gastrointestinal appliance and device**
EXCLUDES 1 encounter for attention to artificial openings of digestive tract (Z43.1-Z43.4)

Z46.51 Encounter for fitting and adjustment of gastric lap band

Z46.59 Encounter for fitting and adjustment of other gastrointestinal appliance and device

Z46.6 Encounter for fitting and adjustment of urinary device
EXCLUDES 2 attention to artificial openings of urinary tract (Z43.5, Z43.6)

✓5ᵗʰ **Z46.8 Encounter for fitting and adjustment of other specified devices**

Z46.81 Encounter for fitting and adjustment of insulin pump
Encounter for insulin pump instruction and training
Encounter for insulin pump titration

Z46.82 Encounter for fitting and adjustment of non-vascular catheter

Z46.89 Encounter for fitting and adjustment of other specified devices
Encounter for fitting and adjustment of wheelchair

Z46.9 Encounter for fitting and adjustment of unspecified device ▽

✓4ᵗʰ **Z47 Orthopedic aftercare**
EXCLUDES 1 aftercare for healing fracture - code to fracture with 7th character D

Z47.1 Aftercare following joint replacement surgery
Use additional code to identify the joint (Z96.6-)

Z47.2 Encounter for removal of internal fixation device
EXCLUDES 1 encounter for adjustment of internal fixation device for fracture treatment - code to fracture with appropriate 7th character
encounter for removal of external fixation device - code to fracture with 7th character D
infection or inflammatory reaction to internal fixation device (T84.6-)
mechanical complication of internal fixation device (T84.1-)

✓5ᵗʰ **Z47.3 Aftercare following explantation of joint prosthesis**
Aftercare following explantation of joint prosthesis, staged procedure
Encounter for joint prosthesis insertion following prior explantation of joint prosthesis
AHA: 2015,1Q,16

Z47.31 Aftercare following explantation of shoulder joint prosthesis
EXCLUDES 1 acquired absence of shoulder joint following prior explantation of shoulder joint prosthesis (Z89.23-)
shoulder joint prosthesis explantation status (Z89.23-)

Z47.32 Aftercare following explantation of hip joint prosthesis

> EXCLUDES 1   *acquired absence of hip joint following prior explantation of hip joint prosthesis (Z89.62-)*
> *hip joint prosthesis explantation status (Z89.62-)*

Z47.33 Aftercare following explantation of knee joint prosthesis

> EXCLUDES 1   *acquired absence of knee joint following prior explantation of knee prosthesis (Z89.52-)*
> *knee joint prosthesis explantation status (Z89.52-)*

√5ᵗʰ **Z47.8 Encounter for other orthopedic aftercare**

Z47.81 Encounter for orthopedic aftercare following surgical amputation
> Use additional code to identify the limb amputated (Z89.-)

Z47.82 Encounter for orthopedic aftercare following scoliosis surgery

Z47.89 Encounter for other orthopedic aftercare
> AHA: 2015,1Q,8

√4ᵗʰ **Z48 Encounter for other postprocedural aftercare**

> EXCLUDES 1   *encounter for aftercare following injury - code to Injury, by site, with appropriate 7th character for subsequent encounter*
> *encounter for follow-up examination after completed treatment (Z08-Z09)*
> EXCLUDES 2   *encounter for attention to artificial openings (Z43.-)*
> *encounter for fitting and adjustment of prosthetic and other devices (Z44-Z46)*

> AHA: 2015,4Q,38; 2015,1Q,6-7

√5ᵗʰ **Z48.0 Encounter for attention to dressings, sutures and drains**

> EXCLUDES 1   *encounter for planned postprocedural wound closure (Z48.1)*

Z48.00 Encounter for change or removal of nonsurgical wound dressing
> Encounter for change or removal of wound dressing NOS

Z48.01 Encounter for change or removal of surgical wound dressing

Z48.02 Encounter for removal of sutures
> Encounter for removal of staples

Z48.03 Encounter for change or removal of drains

Z48.1 Encounter for planned postprocedural wound closure

> EXCLUDES 1   *encounter for attention to dressings and sutures (Z48.0-)*

√5ᵗʰ **Z48.2 Encounter for aftercare following organ transplant**

Z48.21 Encounter for aftercare following heart transplant HCC

Z48.22 Encounter for aftercare following kidney transplant

Z48.23 Encounter for aftercare following liver transplant HCC

Z48.24 Encounter for aftercare following lung transplant HCC

√6ᵗʰ **Z48.28 Encounter for aftercare following multiple organ transplant**

Z48.280 Encounter for aftercare following heart-lung transplant HCC

Z48.288 Encounter for aftercare following multiple organ transplant

√6ᵗʰ **Z48.29 Encounter for aftercare following other organ transplant**

Z48.290 Encounter for aftercare following bone marrow transplant HCC

Z48.298 Encounter for aftercare following other organ transplant

Z48.3 Aftercare following surgery for neoplasm
> Use additional code to identify the neoplasm

√5ᵗʰ **Z48.8 Encounter for other specified postprocedural aftercare**

√6ᵗʰ **Z48.81 Encounter for surgical aftercare following surgery on specified body systems**

> NOTE   These codes identify the body system requiring aftercare. They are for use in conjunction with other aftercare codes to fully explain the aftercare encounter. The condition treated should also be coded if still present.

> EXCLUDES 1   *aftercare for injury- code the injury with 7th character D*
> *aftercare following surgery for neoplasm (Z48.3)*
> EXCLUDES 2   *aftercare following organ transplant (Z48.2-)*
> *orthopedic aftercare (Z47.-)*

> AHA: 2015,4Q,38

Z48.810 Encounter for surgical aftercare following surgery on the sense organs

Z48.811 Encounter for surgical aftercare following surgery on the nervous system
> EXCLUDES 2   *encounter for surgical aftercare following surgery on the sense organs (Z48.810)*

Z48.812 Encounter for surgical aftercare following surgery on the circulatory system
> AHA: 2012,4Q,96

Z48.813 Encounter for surgical aftercare following surgery on the respiratory system

Z48.814 Encounter for surgical aftercare following surgery on the teeth or oral cavity

Z48.815 Encounter for surgical aftercare following surgery on the digestive system

Z48.816 Encounter for surgical aftercare following surgery on the genitourinary system
> EXCLUDES 1   *encounter for aftercare following sterilization reversal (Z31.42)*

Z48.817 Encounter for surgical aftercare following surgery on the skin and subcutaneous tissue

Z48.89 Encounter for other specified surgical aftercare

√4ᵗʰ **Z49 Encounter for care involving renal dialysis**

> Code also associated end stage renal disease (N18.6)

√5ᵗʰ **Z49.0 Preparatory care for renal dialysis**

> Encounter for dialysis instruction and training

Z49.01 Encounter for fitting and adjustment of extracorporeal dialysis catheter HCC
> Removal or replacement of renal dialysis catheter
> Toilet or cleansing of renal dialysis catheter

Z49.02 Encounter for fitting and adjustment of peritoneal dialysis catheter HCC

√5ᵗʰ **Z49.3 Encounter for adequacy testing for dialysis**

Z49.31 Encounter for adequacy testing for hemodialysis HCC

Z49.32 Encounter for adequacy testing for peritoneal dialysis HCC
> Encounter for peritoneal equilibration test

√4ᵗʰ **Z51 Encounter for other aftercare and medical care**

> Code also condition requiring care
> EXCLUDES 1   *follow-up examination after treatment (Z08-Z09)*

Z51.0 Encounter for antineoplastic radiation therapy PDx
> AHA: 2017,4Q,103
> TIP: Do not assign when admission is for insertion/implantation of radioactive elements. Assign a code for the malignancy instead. Any complications related to the radioactive elements should be assigned as secondary diagnoses.

√5ᵗʰ **Z51.1 Encounter for antineoplastic chemotherapy and immunotherapy**
> EXCLUDES 2   *encounter for chemotherapy and immunotherapy for nonneoplastic condition - code to condition*

Z51.11 Encounter for antineoplastic chemotherapy PDx
> AHA: 2015,3Q,19

Z51.12 Encounter for antineoplastic immunotherapy PDx

Z51.5 Encounter for palliative care
   AHA: 2017,1Q,48
Z51.6 Encounter for desensitization to allergens
   AHA: 2016,4Q,77
√5ᵗʰ **Z51.8 Encounter for other specified aftercare**
   EXCLUDES 1 holiday relief care (Z75.5)
   Z51.81 Encounter for therapeutic drug level monitoring
      Code also any long-term (current) drug therapy (Z79.-)
      EXCLUDES 1 encounter for blood-drug test for administrative or medicolegal reasons (Z02.83)
      DEF: Drug monitoring: Measurement of the level of a specific drug in the body or measurement of a specific function to assess effectiveness of a drug.
   Z51.89 Encounter for other specified aftercare
      AHA: 2012,4Q,95-97

√4ᵗʰ **Z52 Donors of organs and tissues**
   INCLUDES autologous and other living donors
   EXCLUDES 1 cadaveric donor - omit code
              examination of potential donor (Z00.5)
   AHA: 2012,4Q,99
√5ᵗʰ **Z52.0 Blood donor**
   √6ᵗʰ **Z52.00 Unspecified blood donor**
      Z52.000 Unspecified donor, whole blood PDx ▽
      Z52.001 Unspecified donor, stem cells PDx ▽
      Z52.008 Unspecified donor, other blood PDx ▽
   √6ᵗʰ **Z52.01 Autologous blood donor**
      Z52.010 Autologous donor, whole blood PDx
      Z52.011 Autologous donor, stem cells PDx
      Z52.018 Autologous donor, other blood PDx
   √6ᵗʰ **Z52.09 Other blood donor**
      Volunteer donor
      Z52.090 Other blood donor, whole blood PDx
      Z52.091 Other blood donor, stem cells PDx
      Z52.098 Other blood donor, other blood PDx
√5ᵗʰ **Z52.1 Skin donor**
   Z52.10 Skin donor, unspecified PDx ▽
   Z52.11 Skin donor, autologous PDx
   Z52.19 Skin donor, other PDx
√5ᵗʰ **Z52.2 Bone donor**
   Z52.20 Bone donor, unspecified PDx ▽
   Z52.21 Bone donor, autologous PDx
   Z52.29 Bone donor, other PDx
   Z52.3 Bone marrow donor PDx
   Z52.4 Kidney donor PDx
   Z52.5 Cornea donor PDx
   Z52.6 Liver donor PDx
√5ᵗʰ **Z52.8 Donor of other specified organs or tissues**
   √6ᵗʰ **Z52.81 Egg (Oocyte) donor**
      Z52.810 Egg (Oocyte) donor under age 35, anonymous recipient PDx ♀
         Egg donor under age 35 NOS
      Z52.811 Egg (Oocyte) donor under age 35, designated recipient PDx ♀
      Z52.812 Egg (Oocyte) donor age 35 and over, anonymous recipient PDx ♀
         Egg donor age 35 and over NOS
      Z52.813 Egg (Oocyte) donor age 35 and over, designated recipient PDx ♀
      Z52.819 Egg (Oocyte) donor, unspecified PDx ♀ ▽
   Z52.89 Donor of other specified organs or tissues PDx
   Z52.9 Donor of unspecified organ or tissue ▽
      Donor NOS

√4ᵗʰ **Z53 Persons encountering health services for specific procedures and treatment, not carried out**
√5ᵗʰ **Z53.0 Procedure and treatment not carried out because of contraindication**
   Z53.01 Procedure and treatment not carried out due to patient smoking
   Z53.09 Procedure and treatment not carried out because of other contraindication
Z53.1 Procedure and treatment not carried out because of patient's decision for reasons of belief and group pressure

√5ᵗʰ **Z53.2 Procedure and treatment not carried out because of patient's decision for other and unspecified reasons**
   Z53.20 Procedure and treatment not carried out because of patient's decision for unspecified reasons ▽
   Z53.21 Procedure and treatment not carried out due to patient leaving prior to being seen by health care provider
   Z53.29 Procedure and treatment not carried out because of patient's decision for other reasons
√5ᵗʰ **Z53.3 Procedure converted to open procedure**
   AHA: 2016,4Q,79
   Z53.31 Laparoscopic surgical procedure converted to open procedure
   Z53.32 Thoracoscopic surgical procedure converted to open procedure
   Z53.33 Arthroscopic surgical procedure converted to open procedure
   Z53.39 Other specified procedure converted to open procedure
Z53.8 Procedure and treatment not carried out for other reasons
Z53.9 Procedure and treatment not carried out, unspecified reason ▽

Persons with potential health hazards related to socioeconomic and psychosocial circumstances (Z55-Z65)

AHA: 2018,1Q,18
TIP: Codes from this code block can be assigned based on documentation from clinicians other than the diagnosing provider.

√4ᵗʰ **Z55 Problems related to education and literacy**
   EXCLUDES 1 disorders of psychological development (F80-F89)
   Z55.0 Illiteracy and low-level literacy
   Z55.1 Schooling unavailable and unattainable
   Z55.2 Failed school examinations
   Z55.3 Underachievement in school
   Z55.4 Educational maladjustment and discord with teachers and classmates
   Z55.8 Other problems related to education and literacy
      Problems related to inadequate teaching
   Z55.9 Problems related to education and literacy, unspecified ▽
      Academic problems NOS

√4ᵗʰ **Z56 Problems related to employment and unemployment**
   EXCLUDES 2 occupational exposure to risk factors (Z57.-)
              problems related to housing and economic circumstances (Z59.-)
   Z56.0 Unemployment, unspecified ▽
   Z56.1 Change of job ▲
   Z56.2 Threat of job loss
   Z56.3 Stressful work schedule
   Z56.4 Discord with boss and workmates
   Z56.5 Uncongenial work environment
      Difficult conditions at work
   Z56.6 Other physical and mental strain related to work
   √5ᵗʰ **Z56.8 Other problems related to employment**
      Z56.81 Sexual harassment on the job
      Z56.82 Military deployment status
         Individual (civilian or military) currently deployed in theater or in support of military war, peacekeeping and humanitarian operations
      Z56.89 Other problems related to employment
   Z56.9 Unspecified problems related to employment ▽
      Occupational problems NOS

√4ᵗʰ **Z57 Occupational exposure to risk factors**
   Z57.0 Occupational exposure to noise
   Z57.1 Occupational exposure to radiation
   Z57.2 Occupational exposure to dust
   √5ᵗʰ **Z57.3 Occupational exposure to other air contaminants**
      Z57.31 Occupational exposure to environmental tobacco smoke
         EXCLUDES 2 exposure to environmental tobacco smoke (Z77.22)
      Z57.39 Occupational exposure to other air contaminants

Z57.4   **Occupational exposure to toxic agents in agriculture**
Occupational exposure to solids, liquids, gases or vapors in agriculture

Z57.5   **Occupational exposure to toxic agents in other industries**
Occupational exposure to solids, liquids, gases or vapors in other industries

Z57.6   **Occupational exposure to extreme temperature**

Z57.7   **Occupational exposure to vibration**

Z57.8   **Occupational exposure to other risk factors**

Z57.9   **Occupational exposure to unspecified risk factor** ▽

✓4ᵗʰ **Z59**   **Problems related to housing and economic circumstances**
EXCLUDES 2   problems related to upbringing (Z62.-)

Z59.0   **Homelessness**

Z59.1   **Inadequate housing**
Lack of heating
Restriction of space
Technical defects in home preventing adequate care
Unsatisfactory surroundings
EXCLUDES 1   problems related to the natural and physical environment (Z77.1-)

Z59.2   **Discord with neighbors, lodgers and landlord**

Z59.3   **Problems related to living in residential institution**
Boarding-school resident
EXCLUDES 1   institutional upbringing (Z62.2)

Z59.4   **Lack of adequate food and safe drinking water**
Inadequate drinking water supply
EXCLUDES 1   effects of hunger (T73.0)
inappropriate diet or eating habits (Z72.4)
malnutrition (E40-E46)

Z59.5   **Extreme poverty**

Z59.6   **Low income**

Z59.7   **Insufficient social insurance and welfare support**

Z59.8   **Other problems related to housing and economic circumstances**
Foreclosure on loan
Isolated dwelling
Problems with creditors

Z59.9   **Problem related to housing and economic circumstances, unspecified** ▽

✓4ᵗʰ **Z60**   **Problems related to social environment**

Z60.0   **Problems of adjustment to life-cycle transitions**
Empty nest syndrome
Phase of life problem
Problem with adjustment to retirement [pension]

Z60.2   **Problems related to living alone**

Z60.3   **Acculturation difficulty**
Problem with migration
Problem with social transplantation
DEF: Problem adapting to a different culture or environment not based on any coexisting mental disorder.

Z60.4   **Social exclusion and rejection**
Exclusion and rejection on the basis of personal characteristics, such as unusual physical appearance, illness or behavior.
EXCLUDES 1   target of adverse discrimination such as for racial or religious reasons (Z60.5)

Z60.5   **Target of (perceived) adverse discrimination and persecution**
EXCLUDES 1   social exclusion and rejection (Z60.4)

Z60.8   **Other problems related to social environment**

Z60.9   **Problem related to social environment, unspecified** ▽

✓4ᵗʰ **Z62**   **Problems related to upbringing**
INCLUDES   current and past negative life events in childhood
current and past problems of a child related to upbringing
EXCLUDES 2   maltreatment syndrome (T74.-)
problems related to housing and economic circumstances (Z59.-)

Z62.0   **Inadequate parental supervision and control**

Z62.1   **Parental overprotection**

✓5ᵗʰ **Z62.2**   **Upbringing away from parents**
EXCLUDES 1   problems with boarding school (Z59.3)

Z62.21   **Child in welfare custody** ℗
Child in care of non-parental family member
Child in foster care
EXCLUDES 2   problem for parent due to child in welfare custody (Z63.5)

Z62.22   **Institutional upbringing**
Child living in orphanage or group home

Z62.29   **Other upbringing away from parents**

Z62.3   **Hostility towards and scapegoating of child** ℗

Z62.6   **Inappropriate (excessive) parental pressure**

✓5ᵗʰ **Z62.8**   **Other specified problems related to upbringing**

✓6ᵗʰ **Z62.81**   **Personal history of abuse in childhood**

Z62.810   **Personal history of physical and sexual abuse in childhood**
EXCLUDES 1   current child physical abuse (T74.12, T76.12)
current child sexual abuse (T74.22, T76.22)

Z62.811   **Personal history of psychological abuse in childhood**
EXCLUDES 1   current child psychological abuse (T74.32, T76.32)

Z62.812   **Personal history of neglect in childhood**
EXCLUDES 1   current child neglect (T74.02, T76.02)

Z62.813   **Personal history of forced labor or sexual exploitation in childhood**

Z62.819   **Personal history of unspecified abuse in childhood** ▽
EXCLUDES 1   current child abuse NOS (T74.92, T76.92)

✓6ᵗʰ **Z62.82**   **Parent-child conflict**

Z62.820   **Parent-biological child conflict**
Parent-child problem NOS

Z62.821   **Parent-adopted child conflict**

Z62.822   **Parent-foster child conflict**

✓6ᵗʰ **Z62.89**   **Other specified problems related to upbringing**

Z62.890   **Parent-child estrangement NEC**

Z62.891   **Sibling rivalry**

Z62.898   **Other specified problems related to upbringing**

Z62.9   **Problem related to upbringing, unspecified** ▽

✓4ᵗʰ **Z63**   **Other problems related to primary support group, including family circumstances**
EXCLUDES 2   maltreatment syndrome (T74.-, T76)
parent-child problems (Z62.-)
problems related to negative life events in childhood (Z62.-)
problems related to upbringing (Z62.-)

Z63.0   **Problems in relationship with spouse or partner**
Relationship distress with spouse or intimate partner
EXCLUDES 1   counseling for spousal or partner abuse problems (Z69.1)
counseling related to sexual attitude, behavior, and orientation (Z70.-)

Z63.1   **Problems in relationship with in-laws**

✓5ᵗʰ **Z63.3**   **Absence of family member**
EXCLUDES 1   absence of family member due to disappearance and death (Z63.4)
absence of family member due to separation and divorce (Z63.5)

Z63.31   **Absence of family member due to military deployment**
Individual or family affected by other family member being on military deployment
EXCLUDES 1   family disruption due to return of family member from military deployment (Z63.71)

Z63.32   **Other absence of family member**

Z63.4   **Disappearance and death of family member**
Assumed death of family member
Bereavement
AHA: 2014,1Q,25

Z63.5   **Disruption of family by separation and divorce**
Marital estrangement

Z63.6   **Dependent relative needing care at home**

✓5ᵗʰ **Z63.7**   **Other stressful life events affecting family and household**

Z63.71   **Stress on family due to return of family member from military deployment**
Individual or family affected by family member having returned from military deployment (current or past conflict)

Z63.72   **Alcoholism and drug addiction in family**

Z63.79 Other stressful life events affecting family and household
Anxiety (normal) about sick person in family
Health problems within family
Ill or disturbed family member
Isolated family

Z63.8 Other specified problems related to primary support group
Family discord NOS
Family estrangement NOS
High expressed emotional level within family
Inadequate family support NOS
Inadequate or distorted communication within family

Z63.9 Problem related to primary support group, unspecified   ▽
Relationship disorder NOS

✓4th **Z64 Problems related to certain psychosocial circumstances**

Z64.0 Problems related to unwanted pregnancy ♀
Z64.1 Problems related to multiparity ♀
Z64.4 Discord with counselors
Discord with probation officer
Discord with social worker

✓4th **Z65 Problems related to other psychosocial circumstances**

Z65.0 Conviction in civil and criminal proceedings without imprisonment
Z65.1 Imprisonment and other incarceration
Z65.2 Problems related to release from prison
Z65.3 Problems related to other legal circumstances
Arrest
Child custody or support proceedings
Litigation
Prosecution
Z65.4 Victim of crime and terrorism
Victim of torture
Z65.5 Exposure to disaster, war and other hostilities
> EXCLUDES 1   target of perceived discrimination or persecution (Z60.5)
Z65.8 Other specified problems related to psychosocial circumstances
Religious or spiritual problem
Z65.9 Problem related to unspecified psychosocial circumstances   ▽

Do not resuscitate status (Z66)

Z66 Do not resuscitate
DNR status
DEF: Medical order written by a physician that instructs others not to perform cardiopulmonary resuscitation (CPR), intubation, or advanced life support (ACLS). It prevents unnecessary invasive treatment to prolong life should breathing stop or cardiac arrest occur.

Blood type (Z67)

✓4th **Z67 Blood type**
AHA: 2015,3Q,40

Blood Types

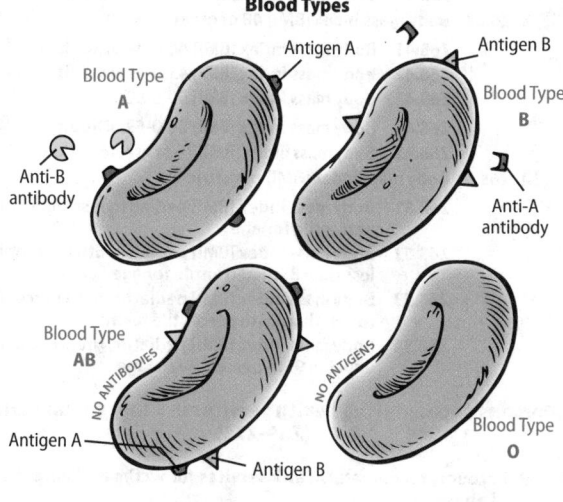
Antigen A
Antigen B
Blood Type A
Blood Type B
Anti-B antibody
Anti-A antibody
Blood Type AB
NO ANTIBODIES
NO ANTIGENS
Blood Type O
Antigen A
Antigen B

✓5th **Z67.1 Type A blood**
    Z67.10 Type A blood, Rh positive
    Z67.11 Type A blood, Rh negative
✓5th **Z67.2 Type B blood**
    Z67.20 Type B blood, Rh positive
    Z67.21 Type B blood, Rh negative
✓5th **Z67.3 Type AB blood**
    Z67.30 Type AB blood, Rh positive
    Z67.31 Type AB blood, Rh negative
✓5th **Z67.4 Type O blood**
    Z67.40 Type O blood, Rh positive
    Z67.41 Type O blood, Rh negative
✓5th **Z67.9 Unspecified blood type**
    Z67.90 Unspecified blood type, Rh positive   ▽
    Z67.91 Unspecified blood type, Rh negative   ▽

Body mass index [BMI] (Z68)

✓4th **Z68 Body mass index [BMI]**
Kilograms per meters squared
> NOTE   BMI adult codes are for use for persons 21 years of age or older
> BMI pediatric codes are for use for persons 2-20 years of age. These percentiles are based on the growth charts published by the Centers for Disease Control and Prevention (CDC)

AHA: 2017,1Q,39
DEF: Index used to help determine whether an individual is underweight, a healthy weight, overweight, or obese.
TIP: A BMI code may be assigned to support an associated condition based on medical record documentation from clinicians who are not the patient's provider.

Z68.1 Body mass index [BMI] 19.9 or less, adult   A
✓5th **Z68.2 Body mass index [BMI] 20-29, adult**
    Z68.20 Body mass index [BMI] 20.0-20.9, adult   A
    Z68.21 Body mass index [BMI] 21.0-21.9, adult   A
    Z68.22 Body mass index [BMI] 22.0-22.9, adult   A
    Z68.23 Body mass index [BMI] 23.0-23.9, adult   A
    Z68.24 Body mass index [BMI] 24.0-24.9, adult   A
    Z68.25 Body mass index [BMI] 25.0-25.9, adult   A
    Z68.26 Body mass index [BMI] 26.0-26.9, adult   A
    Z68.27 Body mass index [BMI] 27.0-27.9, adult   A
    Z68.28 Body mass index [BMI] 28.0-28.9, adult   A
    Z68.29 Body mass index [BMI] 29.0-29.9, adult   A
✓5th **Z68.3 Body mass index [BMI] 30-39, adult**
    Z68.30 Body mass index [BMI] 30.0-30.9, adult   A
    Z68.31 Body mass index [BMI] 31.0-31.9, adult   A
    Z68.32 Body mass index [BMI] 32.0-32.9, adult   A

Z68.33 Body mass index [BMI] 33.0-33.9, **adult** Ⓐ
Z68.34 Body mass index [BMI] 34.0-34.9, **adult** Ⓐ
Z68.35 Body mass index [BMI] 35.0-35.9, **adult** Ⓐ
Z68.36 Body mass index [BMI] 36.0-36.9, **adult** Ⓐ
Z68.37 Body mass index [BMI] 37.0-37.9, **adult** Ⓐ
Z68.38 Body mass index [BMI] 38.0-38.9, **adult** Ⓐ
Z68.39 Body mass index [BMI] 39.0-39.9, **adult** Ⓐ

√5ᵗʰ **Z68.4** Body mass index [BMI] 40 or greater, **adult**

Z68.41 Body mass index [BMI] 40.0-44.9, **adult** ᴴᶜᶜ Ⓐ
Z68.42 Body mass index [BMI] 45.0-49.9, **adult** ᴴᶜᶜ Ⓐ
Z68.43 Body mass index [BMI] 50-59.9, **adult** ᴴᶜᶜ Ⓐ
Z68.44 Body mass index [BMI] 60.0-69.9, **adult** ᴴᶜᶜ Ⓐ
Z68.45 Body mass index [BMI] 70 or greater, **adult** ᴴᶜᶜ Ⓐ

√5ᵗʰ **Z68.5** Body mass index [BMI] pediatric

Z68.51 Body mass index [BMI] pediatric, less than 5th percentile for age
Z68.52 Body mass index [BMI] pediatric, 5th percentile to less than 85th percentile for age
Z68.53 Body mass index [BMI] pediatric, 85th percentile to less than 95th percentile for age
Z68.54 Body mass index [BMI] pediatric, greater than or equal to 95th percentile for age

Persons encountering health services in other circumstances (Z69-Z76)

√4ᵗʰ **Z69** Encounter for mental health services for victim and perpetrator of abuse

INCLUDES　counseling for victims and perpetrators of abuse

√5ᵗʰ **Z69.0** Encounter for mental health services for child abuse problems

√6ᵗʰ **Z69.01** Encounter for mental health services for parental child abuse

Z69.010 Encounter for mental health services for victim of parental child abuse Ⓟ
Encounter for mental health services for victim of child abuse by parent
Encounter for mental health services for victim of child neglect by parent
Encounter for mental health services for victim of child psychological abuse by parent
Encounter for mental health services for victim of child sexual abuse by parent

Z69.011 Encounter for mental health services for perpetrator of parental child abuse
Encounter for mental health services for perpetrator of parental child neglect
Encounter for mental health services for perpetrator of parental child psychological abuse
Encounter for mental health services for perpetrator of parental child sexual abuse

EXCLUDES 1　encounter for mental health services for non-parental child abuse (Z69.02-)

√6ᵗʰ **Z69.02** Encounter for mental health services for non-parental child abuse

Z69.020 Encounter for mental health services for victim of non-parental child abuse Ⓟ
Encounter for mental health services for victim of non-parental child neglect
Encounter for mental health services for victim of non-parental child psychological abuse
Encounter for mental health services for victim of non-parental child sexual abuse

Z69.021 Encounter for mental health services for perpetrator of non-parental child abuse
Encounter for mental health services for perpetrator of non-parental child neglect
Encounter for mental health services for perpetrator of non-parental child psychological abuse
Encounter for mental health services for perpetrator of non-parental child sexual abuse

√5ᵗʰ **Z69.1** Encounter for mental health services for spousal or partner abuse problems

Z69.11 Encounter for mental health services for victim of spousal or partner abuse
Encounter for mental health services for victim of spouse or partner neglect
Encounter for mental health services for victim of spouse or partner psychological abuse
Encounter for mental health services for victim of spouse or partner violence, physical

Z69.12 Encounter for mental health services for perpetrator of spousal or partner abuse
Encounter for mental health services for perpetrator of spouse or partner neglect
Encounter for mental health services for perpetrator of spouse or partner psychological abuse
Encounter for mental health services for perpetrator of spouse or partner violence, physical
Encounter for mental health services for perpetrator of spouse or partner violence, sexual

√5ᵗʰ **Z69.8** Encounter for mental health services for victim or perpetrator of other abuse

Z69.81 Encounter for mental health services for victim of other abuse
Encounter for mental health services for perpetrator of non-spousal adult abuse
Encounter for mental health services for victim of non-spousal adult abuse
Encounter for mental health services for victim of spouse or partner violence, sexual
Encounter for rape victim counseling

Z69.82 Encounter for mental health services for perpetrator of other abuse

√4ᵗʰ **Z70** Counseling related to sexual attitude, behavior and orientation

INCLUDES　encounter for mental health services for sexual attitude, behavior and orientation

EXCLUDES 2　contraceptive or procreative counseling (Z30-Z31)

Z70.0 Counseling related to sexual attitude

Z70.1 Counseling related to patient's sexual behavior and orientation
Patient concerned regarding impotence
Patient concerned regarding non-responsiveness
Patient concerned regarding promiscuity
Patient concerned regarding sexual orientation

Z70.2 Counseling related to sexual behavior and orientation of third party
Advice sought regarding sexual behavior and orientation of child
Advice sought regarding sexual behavior and orientation of partner
Advice sought regarding sexual behavior and orientation of spouse

Z70.3 Counseling related to combined concerns regarding sexual attitude, behavior and orientation

Z70.8 Other sex counseling
Encounter for sex education

Z70.9 Sex counseling, unspecified　　▽

☑4th **Z71 Persons encountering health services for other counseling and medical advice, not elsewhere classified**

     EXCLUDES 2   *contraceptive or procreation counseling (Z30-Z31)*

           sex counseling (Z70.-)

   Z71.0 Person encountering health services to consult on behalf of another person

     Person encountering health services to seek advice or treatment for non-attending third party

     EXCLUDES 2   *anxiety (normal) about sick person in family (Z63.7)*

           expectant (adoptive) parent(s) pre-birth pediatrician visit (Z76.81)

   Z71.1 Person with feared health complaint in whom no diagnosis is made

     Person encountering health services with feared condition which was not demonstrated

     Person encountering health services in which problem was normal state

     "Worried well"

     EXCLUDES 1   *medical observation for suspected diseases and conditions proven not to exist (Z03.-)*

   Z71.2 Person consulting for explanation of examination or test findings

   Z71.3 Dietary counseling and surveillance

     Use additional code for any associated underlying medical condition

     Use additional code to identify body mass index (BMI), if known (Z68.-)

☑5th   **Z71.4 Alcohol abuse counseling and surveillance**

     Use additional code for alcohol abuse or dependence (F10.-)

     Z71.41 Alcohol abuse counseling and surveillance of alcoholic

     Z71.42 Counseling for family member of alcoholic

         Counseling for significant other, partner, or friend of alcoholic

☑5th   **Z71.5 Drug abuse counseling and surveillance**

     Use additional code for drug abuse or dependence (F11-F16, F18-F19)

     Z71.51 Drug abuse counseling and surveillance of drug abuser

     Z71.52 Counseling for family member of drug abuser

         Counseling for significant other, partner, or friend of drug abuser

   Z71.6 Tobacco abuse counseling

     Use additional code for nicotine dependence (F17.-)

   Z71.7 Human immunodeficiency virus [HIV] counseling

☑5th   **Z71.8 Other specified counseling**

     EXCLUDES 2   *counseling for contraception (Z30.0-)*

     AHA: 2017,4Q,27

     Z71.81 Spiritual or religious counseling

     Z71.82 Exercise counseling

     Z71.83 Encounter for nonprocreative genetic counseling

         EXCLUDES 1   *counseling for procreative genetics (Z31.5)*

             counseling for procreative management (Z31.6)

     Z71.89 Other specified counseling

   Z71.9 Counseling, unspecified   ▽

     Encounter for medical advice NOS

☑4th **Z72 Problems related to lifestyle**

     EXCLUDES 2   *problems related to life-management difficulty (Z73.-)*

           problems related to socioeconomic and psychosocial circumstances (Z55-Z65)

   Z72.0 Tobacco use

     Tobacco use NOS

     EXCLUDES 1   *history of tobacco dependence (Z87.891)*

           nicotine dependence (F17.2-)

           tobacco dependence (F17.2-)

           tobacco use during pregnancy (O99.33-)

   Z72.3 Lack of physical exercise

   Z72.4 Inappropriate diet and eating habits

     EXCLUDES 1   *behavioral eating disorders of infancy or childhood (F98.2-F98.3)*

           eating disorders (F50.-)

           lack of adequate food (Z59.4)

           malnutrition and other nutritional deficiencies (E40-E64)

☑5th   **Z72.5 High risk sexual behavior**

     Promiscuity

     EXCLUDES 1   *paraphilias (F65)*

     Z72.51 High risk heterosexual behavior

     Z72.52 High risk homosexual behavior

     Z72.53 High risk bisexual behavior

   Z72.6 Gambling and betting

     EXCLUDES 1   *compulsive or pathological gambling (F63.0)*

☑5th   **Z72.8 Other problems related to lifestyle**

☑6th   **Z72.81 Antisocial behavior**

         EXCLUDES 1   *conduct disorders (F91.-)*

         Z72.810 Child and adolescent antisocial behavior   P

           Antisocial behavior (child) (adolescent) without manifest psychiatric disorder

           Delinquency NOS

           Group delinquency

           Offenses in the context of gang membership

           Stealing in company with others

           Truancy from school

         Z72.811 Adult antisocial behavior   A

           Adult antisocial behavior without manifest psychiatric disorder

☑6th   **Z72.82 Problems related to sleep**

         Z72.820 Sleep deprivation

           Lack of adequate sleep

           EXCLUDES 1   *insomnia (G47.0-)*

         Z72.821 Inadequate sleep hygiene

           Bad sleep habits

           Irregular sleep habits

           Unhealthy sleep wake schedule

           EXCLUDES 1   *insomnia (F51.0-, G47.0-)*

     Z72.89 Other problems related to lifestyle

         Self-damaging behavior

   Z72.9 Problem related to lifestyle, unspecified   ▽

☑4th **Z73 Problems related to life management difficulty**

     EXCLUDES 2   *problems related to socioeconomic and psychosocial circumstances (Z55-Z65)*

     DEF: State of emotional, mental, and physical exhaustion causing difficulties in managing personal, school, or work circumstances. It is usually due to prolonged stress or poor interpersonal relationship skills or parenting skills.

   Z73.0 Burn-out

   Z73.1 Type A behavior pattern

   Z73.2 Lack of relaxation and leisure

   Z73.3 Stress, not elsewhere classified

     Physical and mental strain NOS

     EXCLUDES 1   *stress related to employment or unemployment (Z56.-)*

   Z73.4 Inadequate social skills, not elsewhere classified

   Z73.5 Social role conflict, not elsewhere classified

   Z73.6 Limitation of activities due to disability

     EXCLUDES 1   *care-provider dependency (Z74.-)*

☑5th   **Z73.8 Other problems related to life management difficulty**

☑6th   **Z73.81 Behavioral insomnia of childhood**

         DEF: Behaviors on the part of the child or caregivers that cause negative compliance with a child's sleep schedule resulting in lack of adequate sleep.

         Z73.810 Behavioral insomnia of childhood, sleep-onset association type   P

         Z73.811 Behavioral insomnia of childhood, limit setting type   P

         Z73.812 Behavioral insomnia of childhood, combined type   P

         Z73.819 Behavioral insomnia of childhood, unspecified type   P ▽

     Z73.82 Dual sensory impairment

     Z73.89 Other problems related to life management difficulty

   Z73.9 Problem related to life management difficulty, unspecified   ▽

☑ Additional Character Req   ✓x7th Placeholder Alert   Manifestation   ▽ Unspecified   ▶◀ Revised Text   ● New Code   ▲ Revised Code Title

ICD-10-CM 2019   1235

Chapter 21. Factors Influencing Health Status and Contact With Health Services

✓4ᵗʰ **Z74 Problems related to care provider dependency**

EXCLUDES 2   *dependence on enabling machines or devices NEC (Z99.-)*

✓5ᵗʰ **Z74.0 Reduced mobility**

Z74.01   Bed confinement status
Bedridden

Z74.09   Other reduced mobility
Chair ridden
Reduced mobility NOS
EXCLUDES 2   *wheelchair dependence (Z99.3)*

Z74.1   Need for assistance with personal care

Z74.2   Need for assistance at home and no other household member able to render care

Z74.3   Need for continuous supervision

Z74.8   Other problems related to care provider dependency

Z74.9   Problem related to care provider dependency, ▽
unspecified

✓4ᵗʰ **Z75 Problems related to medical facilities and other health care**

Z75.0   Medical services not available in home
EXCLUDES 1   *no other household member able to render care (Z74.2)*

Z75.1   Person awaiting admission **to adequate facility elsewhere**

Z75.2   Other waiting period for investigation and treatment

Z75.3   Unavailability and inaccessibility of health-care facilities
EXCLUDES 1   *bed unavailable (Z75.1)*

Z75.4   Unavailability and inaccessibility of other helping agencies

Z75.5   Holiday relief care

Z75.8   Other problems related to medical facilities and other health care

Z75.9   Unspecified problem related to medical facilities ▽
and other health care

✓4ᵗʰ **Z76 Persons encountering health services in other circumstances**

Z76.0   Encounter for issue of repeat prescription
Encounter for issue of repeat prescription for appliance
Encounter for issue of repeat prescription for medicaments
Encounter for issue of repeat prescription for spectacles
EXCLUDES 2   *issue of medical certificate (Z02.7)*
   repeat prescription for contraceptive (Z30.4-)

Z76.1   Encounter for health supervision and care of PDx
foundling

Z76.2   Encounter for health supervision and care of other PDx P
healthy infant and child
Encounter for medical or nursing care or supervision of healthy infant under circumstances such as adverse socioeconomic conditions at home
Encounter for medical or nursing care or supervision of healthy infant under circumstances such as awaiting foster or adoptive placement
Encounter for medical or nursing care or supervision of healthy infant under circumstances such as maternal illness
Encounter for medical or nursing care or supervision of healthy infant under circumstances such as number of children at home preventing or interfering with normal care

Z76.3   Healthy person accompanying sick person

Z76.4   Other boarder to healthcare facility
EXCLUDES 1   *homelessness (Z59.0)*

Z76.5   Malingerer [conscious simulation]
Person feigning illness (with obvious motivation)
EXCLUDES 1   *factitious disorder ▶(F68.1-, F68.A)◀*
   peregrinating patient (F68.1-)
DEF: Act of intentionally exaggerating an illness or disability in order to receive personal gain or to avoid punishment or responsibility.

✓6ᵗʰ **Z76.8   Persons encountering health services in other specified circumstances**

Z76.81   Expectant parent(s) prebirth pediatrician visit
Pre-adoption pediatrician visit for adoptive parent(s)

Z76.82   Awaiting organ transplant status
Patient waiting for organ availability

Z76.89   Persons encountering health services in other specified circumstances
Persons encountering health services NOS
AHA: 2014,2Q,10

Persons with potential health hazards related to family and personal history and certain conditions influencing health status (Z77-Z99)

Code also any follow-up examination (Z08-Z09)

✓4ᵗʰ **Z77 Other contact with and (suspected) exposures hazardous to health**

INCLUDES   contact with and (suspected) exposures to potential hazards to health

EXCLUDES 2   *contact with and (suspected) exposure to communicable diseases (Z20.-)*
   exposure to (parental) (environmental) tobacco smoke in the perinatal period (P96.81)
   newborn affected by noxious substances transmitted via placenta or breast milk (P04.-)
   occupational exposure to risk factors (Z57.-)
   retained foreign body (Z18.-)
   retained foreign body fully removed (Z87.821)
   toxic effects of substances chiefly nonmedicinal as to source (T51-T65)

✓5ᵗʰ **Z77.0   Contact with and (suspected) exposure to** hazardous, chiefly nonmedicinal, chemicals

✓6ᵗʰ **Z77.01   Contact with and (suspected) exposure to hazardous** metals

Z77.010   Contact with and (suspected) exposure to arsenic

Z77.011   Contact with and (suspected) exposure to lead

Z77.012   Contact with and (suspected) exposure to uranium
EXCLUDES 1   *retained depleted uranium fragments (Z18.01)*

Z77.018   Contact with and (suspected) exposure to other hazardous metals
Contact with and (suspected) exposure to chromium compounds
Contact with and (suspected) exposure to nickel dust

✓6ᵗʰ **Z77.02   Contact with and (suspected) exposure to hazardous** aromatic compounds

Z77.020   Contact with and (suspected) exposure to aromatic amines

Z77.021   Contact with and (suspected) exposure to benzene

Z77.028   Contact with and (suspected) exposure to other hazardous aromatic compounds
Aromatic dyes NOS
Polycyclic aromatic hydrocarbons

✓6ᵗʰ **Z77.09   Contact with and (suspected) exposure to other hazardous, chiefly** nonmedicinal, chemicals

Z77.090   Contact with and (suspected) exposure to asbestos

Z77.098   Contact with and (suspected) exposure to other hazardous, chiefly nonmedicinal, chemicals
Dyes NOS

✓5ᵗʰ **Z77.1   Contact with and (suspected) exposure to** environmental pollution and hazards in the physical environment

✓6ᵗʰ **Z77.11   Contact with and (suspected) exposure to** environmental pollution

Z77.110   Contact with and (suspected) exposure to air pollution

Z77.111   Contact with and (suspected) exposure to water pollution

Z77.112   Contact with and (suspected) exposure to soil pollution

Z77.118   Contact with and (suspected) exposure to other environmental pollution

✓6ᵗʰ **Z77.12   Contact with and (suspected) exposure to** hazards in the physical environment

Z77.120   Contact with and (suspected) exposure to mold (toxic)

Z74–Z77.120

Z77.121 Contact with and (suspected) exposure to harmful algae and algae toxins
Contact with and (suspected) exposure to (harmful) algae bloom NOS
Contact with and (suspected) exposure to blue-green algae bloom
Contact with and (suspected) exposure to brown tide
Contact with and (suspected) exposure to cyanobacteria bloom
Contact with and (suspected) exposure to Florida red tide
Contact with and (suspected) exposure to pfiesteria piscicida
Contact with and (suspected) exposure to red tide

Z77.122 Contact with and (suspected) exposure to noise

Z77.123 Contact with and (suspected) exposure to radon and other naturally occurring radiation
EXCLUDES 2   radiation exposure as the cause of a confirmed condition (W88-W90, X39.0-)
radiation sickness NOS (T66)

Z77.128 Contact with and (suspected) exposure to other hazards in the physical environment

▲ √5ᵗʰ **Z77.2 Contact with and (suspected) exposure to other hazardous substances**

Z77.21 Contact with and (suspected) exposure to potentially hazardous body fluids

Z77.22 Contact with and (suspected) exposure to environmental tobacco smoke (acute) (chronic)
Exposure to second hand tobacco smoke (acute) (chronic)
Passive smoking (acute) (chronic)
EXCLUDES 1   nicotine dependence (F17.-)
tobacco use (Z72.0)
EXCLUDES 2   occupational exposure to environmental tobacco smoke (Z57.31)

▲ **Z77.29 Contact with and (suspected) exposure to other hazardous substances**
AHA: 2016,2Q,33

Z77.9 Other contact with and (suspected) exposures hazardous to health

√4ᵗʰ **Z78 Other specified health status**
EXCLUDES 2   asymptomatic human immunodeficiency virus [HIV] infection status (Z21)
postprocedural status (Z93-Z99)
sex reassignment status (Z87.890)

Z78.0 Asymptomatic menopausal state   Ⓐ ♀
Menopausal state NOS
Postmenopausal status NOS
EXCLUDES 2   symptomatic menopausal state (N95.1)

Z78.1 Physical restraint status
EXCLUDES 1   physical restraint due to a procedure - omit code
DEF: Application of mechanical restraining devices or manual restraints to limit physical mobility of a patient.

Z78.9 Other specified health status

√4ᵗʰ **Z79 Long term (current) drug therapy**
INCLUDES   long term (current) drug use for prophylactic purposes
Code also any therapeutic drug level monitoring (Z51.81)
EXCLUDES 2   drug abuse and dependence (F11-F19)
drug use complicating pregnancy, childbirth, and the puerperium (O99.32-)
long term (current) use of oral antidiabetic drugs (Z79.84)
long term (current) use of oral hypoglycemic drugs (Z79.84)

√5ᵗʰ **Z79.0 Long term (current) use of anticoagulants and antithrombotics/antiplatelets**
EXCLUDES 2   long term (current) use of aspirin (Z79.82)

Z79.01 Long term (current) use of anticoagulants

Z79.02 Long term (current) use of antithrombotics/antiplatelets

Z79.1 Long term (current) use of non-steroidal anti-inflammatories (NSAID)
EXCLUDES 2   long term (current) use of aspirin (Z79.82)

Z79.2 Long term (current) use of antibiotics

Z79.3 Long term (current) use of hormonal contraceptives
Long term (current) use of birth control pill or patch

Z79.4 Long term (current) use of insulin   HCC
TIP: When both long-term (current) insulin and long-term (current) oral hypoglycemic use is documented, assign only a code for the long-term insulin use.

√5ᵗʰ **Z79.5 Long term (current) use of steroids**

Z79.51 Long term (current) use of inhaled steroids

Z79.52 Long term (current) use of systemic steroids

√5ᵗʰ **Z79.8 Other long term (current) drug therapy**

√6ᵗʰ **Z79.81 Long term (current) use of agents affecting estrogen receptors and estrogen levels**
Code first, if applicable:
malignant neoplasm of breast (C50.-)
malignant neoplasm of prostate (C61)
Use additional code, if applicable, to identify:
estrogen receptor positive status (Z17.0)
family history of breast cancer (Z80.3)
genetic susceptibility to malignant neoplasm (cancer) (Z15.0-)
personal history of breast cancer (Z85.3)
personal history of prostate cancer (Z85.46)
postmenopausal status (Z78.0)
EXCLUDES 1   hormone replacement therapy (Z79.890)

Z79.810 Long term (current) use of selective estrogen receptor modulators (SERMs)
Long term (current) use of raloxifene (Evista)
Long term (current) use of tamoxifen (Nolvadex)
Long term (current) use of toremifene (Fareston)

Z79.811 Long term (current) use of aromatase inhibitors
Long term (current) use of anastrozole (Arimidex)
Long term (current) use of exemestane (Aromasin)
Long term (current) use of letrozole (Femara)

Z79.818 Long term (current) use of other agents affecting estrogen receptors and estrogen levels
Long term (current) use of estrogen receptor downregulators
Long term (current) use of fulvestrant (Faslodex)
Long term (current) use of gonadotropin-releasing hormone (GnRH) agonist
Long term (current) use of goserelin acetate (Zoladex)
Long term (current) use of leuprolide acetate (leuprorelin) (Lupron)
Long term (current) use of megestrol acetate (Megace)

Z79.82 Long term (current) use of aspirin

Z79.83 Long term (current) use of bisphosphonates
AHA: 2016,4Q,42

Z79.84 Long term (current) use of oral hypoglycemic drugs
Long term (current) use of oral antidiabetic drugs
EXCLUDES 2   long term (current) use of insulin (Z79.4)
AHA: 2016,4Q,76
TIP: When both long-term (current) insulin and long-term (current) oral hypoglycemic use is documented, assign only code Z79.4 for the long-term insulin use.

√6ᵗʰ **Z79.89 Other long term (current) drug therapy**

Z79.890 Hormone replacement therapy

Z79.891 Long term (current) use of opiate analgesic
Long term (current) use of methadone for pain management
EXCLUDES 1   methadone use NOS (F11.9-)
use of methodone for treatment of heroin addiction (F11.2-)

Z79.899   **Other long term (current) drug therapy**
AHA: 2015,4Q,34; 2015,3Q,21

✓4ᵗʰ **Z80**   **Family history of primary malignant neoplasm**

Z80.0   **Family history of malignant neoplasm of digestive organs**
Conditions classifiable to C15-C26
AHA: 2018,1Q,6

Z80.1   **Family history of malignant neoplasm of trachea, bronchus and lung**
Conditions classifiable to C33-C34

Z80.2   **Family history of malignant neoplasm of other respiratory and intrathoracic organs**
Conditions classifiable to C30-C32, C37-C39

Z80.3   **Family history of malignant neoplasm of breast**
Conditions classifiable to C50.-

✓5ᵗʰ **Z80.4**   **Family history of malignant neoplasm of genital organs**
Conditions classifiable to C51-C63

     Z80.41   **Family history of malignant neoplasm of ovary**
     Z80.42   **Family history of malignant neoplasm of prostate**
     Z80.43   **Family history of malignant neoplasm of testis**
     Z80.49   **Family history of malignant neoplasm of other genital organs**

✓5ᵗʰ **Z80.5**   **Family history of malignant neoplasm of urinary tract**
Conditions classifiable to C64-C68

     Z80.51   **Family history of malignant neoplasm of kidney**
     Z80.52   **Family history of malignant neoplasm of bladder**
     Z80.59   **Family history of malignant neoplasm of other urinary tract organ**

Z80.6   **Family history of leukemia**
Conditions classifiable to C91-C95

Z80.7   **Family history of other malignant neoplasms of lymphoid, hematopoietic and related tissues**
Conditions classifiable to C81-C90, C96.-

Z80.8   **Family history of malignant neoplasm of other organs or systems**
Conditions classifiable to C00-C14, C40-C49, C69-C79

Z80.9   **Family history of malignant neoplasm, unspecified**   ▽
Conditions classifiable to C80.1

✓4ᵗʰ **Z81**   **Family history of mental and behavioral disorders**

Z81.0   **Family history of intellectual disabilities**
Conditions classifiable to F70-F79

Z81.1   **Family history of alcohol abuse and dependence**
Conditions classifiable to F10.-

Z81.2   **Family history of tobacco abuse and dependence**
Conditions classifiable to F17.-

Z81.3   **Family history of other psychoactive substance abuse and dependence**
Conditions classifiable to F11-F16, F18-F19

Z81.4   **Family history of other substance abuse and dependence**
Conditions classifiable to F55

Z81.8   **Family history of other mental and behavioral disorders**
Conditions classifiable elsewhere in F01-F99

✓4ᵗʰ **Z82**   **Family history of certain disabilities and chronic diseases (leading to disablement)**

Z82.0   **Family history of epilepsy and other diseases of the nervous system**
Conditions classifiable to G00-G99

Z82.1   **Family history of blindness and visual loss**
Conditions classifiable to H54.-

Z82.2   **Family history of deafness and hearing loss**
Conditions classifiable to H90-H91

Z82.3   **Family history of stroke**
Conditions classifiable to I60-I64

✓5ᵗʰ **Z82.4**   **Family history of ischemic heart disease and other diseases of the circulatory system**
Conditions classifiable to I00-I52, I65-I99

     Z82.41   **Family history of sudden cardiac death**
     Z82.49   **Family history of ischemic heart disease and other diseases of the circulatory system**

Z82.5   **Family history of asthma and other chronic lower respiratory diseases**
Conditions classifiable to J40-J47
EXCLUDES 2   family history of other diseases of the respiratory system (Z83.6)

✓5ᵗʰ **Z82.6**   **Family history of arthritis and other diseases of the musculoskeletal system and connective tissue**
Conditions classifiable to M00-M99

     Z82.61   **Family history of arthritis**

     Z82.62   **Family history of osteoporosis**
     Z82.69   **Family history of other diseases of the musculoskeletal system and connective tissue**

✓5ᵗʰ **Z82.7**   **Family history of congenital malformations, deformations and chromosomal abnormalities**
Conditions classifiable to Q00-Q99

     Z82.71   **Family history of polycystic kidney**
     Z82.79   **Family history of other congenital malformations, deformations and chromosomal abnormalities**

Z82.8   **Family history of other disabilities and chronic diseases leading to disablement, not elsewhere classified**

✓4ᵗʰ **Z83**   **Family history of other specific disorders**
EXCLUDES 2   contact with and (suspected) exposure to communicable disease in the family (Z20.-)

Z83.0   **Family history of human immunodeficiency virus [HIV] disease**
Conditions classifiable to B20

Z83.1   **Family history of other infectious and parasitic diseases**
Conditions classifiable to A00-B19, B25-B94, B99

Z83.2   **Family history of diseases of the blood and blood-forming organs and certain disorders involving the immune mechanism**
Conditions classifiable to D50-D89

Z83.3   **Family history of diabetes mellitus**
Conditions classifiable to E08-E13

✓5ᵗʰ **Z83.4**   **Family history of other endocrine, nutritional and metabolic diseases**
Conditions classifiable to E00-E07, E15-E88

     Z83.41   **Family history of multiple endocrine neoplasia [MEN] syndrome**
     Z83.42   **Family history of familial hypercholesterolemia**
         AHA: 2016,4Q,77

• ✓6ᵗʰ   **Z83.43**   **Family history of other disorder of lipoprotein metabolism and other lipidemias**
•   **Z83.430**   **Family history of elevated lipoprotein(a)**
               Family history of elevated Lp(a)
•   **Z83.438**   **Family history of other disorder of lipoprotein metabolism and other lipidemia**
               Family history of familial combined hyperlipidemia

     Z83.49   **Family history of other endocrine, nutritional and metabolic diseases**

✓5ᵗʰ **Z83.5**   **Family history of eye and ear disorders**

   ✓6ᵗʰ   **Z83.51**   **Family history of eye disorders**
         Conditions classifiable to H00-H53, H55-H59
         EXCLUDES 2   family history of blindness and visual loss (Z82.1)

         Z83.511   **Family history of glaucoma**
         Z83.518   **Family history of other specified eye disorder**

     Z83.52   **Family history of ear disorders**
         Conditions classifiable to H60-H83, H92-H95
         EXCLUDES 2   family history of deafness and hearing loss (Z82.2)

Z83.6   **Family history of other diseases of the respiratory system**
Conditions classifiable to J00-J39, J60-J99
EXCLUDES 2   family history of asthma and other chronic lower respiratory diseases (Z82.5)

✓5ᵗʰ **Z83.7**   **Family history of diseases of the digestive system**
Conditions classifiable to K00-K93

     Z83.71   **Family history of colonic polyps**
         EXCLUDES 2   family history of malignant neoplasm of digestive organs (Z80.0)

     Z83.79   **Family history of other diseases of the digestive system**

✓4ᵗʰ **Z84**   **Family history of other conditions**

Z84.0   **Family history of diseases of the skin and subcutaneous tissue**
Conditions classifiable to L00-L99

Z84.1   **Family history of disorders of kidney and ureter**
Conditions classifiable to N00-N29

Z84.2   **Family history of other diseases of the genitourinary system**
Conditions classifiable to N30-N99

Z84.3   **Family history of consanguinity**

✓5ᵗʰ **Z84.8**   **Family history of other specified conditions**

     Z84.81   **Family history of carrier of genetic disease**

Z84.82 Family history of sudden infant death syndrome
Family history of SIDS
AHA: 2016,4Q,77

Z84.89 Family history of other specified conditions

☑4ᵗʰ **Z85 Personal history of malignant neoplasm**

Code first any follow-up examination after treatment of malignant neoplasm (Z08)
Use additional code to identify:
alcohol use and dependence (F10.-)
exposure to environmental tobacco smoke (Z77.22)
history of tobacco dependence (Z87.891)
occupational exposure to environmental tobacco smoke (Z57.31)
tobacco dependence (F17.-)
tobacco use (Z72.0)

EXCLUDES 2   *personal history of benign neoplasm (Z86.01-)*
personal history of carcinoma-in-situ (Z86.00-)

☑5ᵗʰ **Z85.0 Personal history of malignant neoplasm of** digestive organs
AHA: 2017,1Q,9

Z85.00 Personal history of malignant neoplasm ▽
of unspecified digestive organ

Z85.01 Personal history of malignant neoplasm of
esophagus
Conditions classifiable to C15

☑6ᵗʰ **Z85.02 Personal history of malignant neoplasm of** stomach

Z85.020 Personal history of malignant carcinoid
tumor of stomach
Conditions classifiable to C7A.092

Z85.028 Personal history of other malignant
neoplasm of stomach
Conditions classifiable to C16

☑6ᵗʰ **Z85.03 Personal history of malignant neoplasm of** large
intestine

Z85.030 Personal history of malignant carcinoid
tumor of large intestine
Conditions classifiable to C7A.022-C7A.025,
C7A.029

Z85.038 Personal history of other malignant
neoplasm of large intestine
Conditions classifiable to C18

☑6ᵗʰ **Z85.04 Personal history of malignant neoplasm of** rectum,
rectosigmoid junction, and anus

Z85.040 Personal history of malignant carcinoid
tumor of rectum
Conditions classifiable to C7A.026

Z85.048 Personal history of other malignant
neoplasm of rectum, rectosigmoid
junction, and anus
Conditions classifiable to C19-C21

Z85.05 Personal history of malignant neoplasm of liver
Conditions classifiable to C22

☑6ᵗʰ **Z85.06 Personal history of malignant neoplasm of** small
intestine

Z85.060 Personal history of malignant carcinoid
tumor of small intestine
Conditions classifiable to C7A.01-

Z85.068 Personal history of other malignant
neoplasm of small intestine
Conditions classifiable to C17

Z85.07 Personal history of malignant neoplasm of pancreas
Conditions classifiable to C25

Z85.09 Personal history of malignant neoplasm of other
digestive organs

☑5ᵗʰ **Z85.1 Personal history of malignant neoplasm of** trachea, bronchus
and lung

☑6ᵗʰ **Z85.11 Personal history of malignant neoplasm of**
bronchus and lung

Z85.110 Personal history of malignant carcinoid
tumor of bronchus and lung
Conditions classifiable to C7A.090

Z85.118 Personal history of other malignant
neoplasm of bronchus and lung
Conditions classifiable to C34

Z85.12 Personal history of malignant neoplasm of trachea
Conditions classifiable to C33

☑5ᵗʰ **Z85.2 Personal history of malignant neoplasm of other** respiratory
and intrathoracic organs

Z85.20 Personal history of malignant neoplasm ▽
of unspecified respiratory organ

Z85.21 Personal history of malignant neoplasm of larynx
Conditions classifiable to C32

Z85.22 Personal history of malignant neoplasm of nasal
cavities, middle ear, and accessory sinuses
Conditions classifiable to C30-C31

☑6ᵗʰ **Z85.23 Personal history of malignant neoplasm of** thymus

Z85.230 Personal history of malignant carcinoid
tumor of thymus
Conditions classifiable to C7A.091

Z85.238 Personal history of other malignant
neoplasm of thymus
Conditions classifiable to C37

Z85.29 Personal history of malignant neoplasm of other
respiratory and intrathoracic organs

Z85.3 Personal history of malignant neoplasm of breast
Conditions classifiable to C50.-

☑5ᵗʰ **Z85.4 Personal history of malignant neoplasm of** genital organs
Conditions classifiable to C51-C63

Z85.40 Personal history of malignant neoplasm ♀ ▽
of unspecified female genital organ

Z85.41 Personal history of malignant neoplasm ♀
of cervix uteri

Z85.42 Personal history of malignant neoplasm ♀
of other parts of uterus

Z85.43 Personal history of malignant neoplasm ♀
of ovary

Z85.44 Personal history of malignant neoplasm ♀
of other female genital organs

Z85.45 Personal history of malignant neoplasm ♂ ▽
of unspecified male genital organ

Z85.46 Personal history of malignant neoplasm ♂
of prostate

Z85.47 Personal history of malignant neoplasm ♂
of testis

Z85.48 Personal history of malignant neoplasm ♂
of epididymis

Z85.49 Personal history of malignant neoplasm ♂
of other male genital organs

☑5ᵗʰ **Z85.5 Personal history of malignant neoplasm of** urinary tract
Conditions classifiable to C64-C68

Z85.50 Personal history of malignant neoplasm ▽
of unspecified urinary tract organ

Z85.51 Personal history of malignant neoplasm of bladder

☑6ᵗʰ **Z85.52 Personal history of malignant neoplasm of** kidney

EXCLUDES 1   *personal history of malignant neoplasm*
of renal pelvis (Z85.53)

Z85.520 Personal history of malignant carcinoid
tumor of kidney
Conditions classifiable to C7A.093

Z85.528 Personal history of other malignant
neoplasm of kidney
Conditions classifiable to C64

Z85.53 Personal history of malignant neoplasm of renal
pelvis

Z85.54 Personal history of malignant neoplasm of ureter

Z85.59 Personal history of malignant neoplasm of other
urinary tract organ

Z85.6 Personal history of leukemia
Conditions classifiable to C91-C95

EXCLUDES 1   *leukemia in remission C91.0-C95.9 with 5th*
character 1

☑5ᵗʰ **Z85.7 Personal history of other malignant neoplasms of** lymphoid,
hematopoietic and related tissues

Z85.71 Personal history of Hodgkin lymphoma
Conditions classifiable to C81

Z85.72 Personal history of non-Hodgkin lymphomas
Conditions classifiable to C82-C85

Z85.79 Personal history of other malignant neoplasms of
lymphoid, hematopoietic and related tissues
Conditions classifiable to C88-C90, C96

EXCLUDES 1   *multiple myeloma in remission (C90.01)*
plasma cell leukemia in remission (C90.11)
plasmacytoma in remission (C90.21)

Chapter 21. Factors Influencing Health Status and Contact With Health Services

Z84.82–Z85.79

✓5ᵗʰ **Z85.8 Personal history of malignant neoplasms of other organs and systems**
  Conditions classifiable to C00-C14, C40-C49, C69-C75, C7A.098, C76-C79

  ✓6ᵗʰ **Z85.81 Personal history of malignant neoplasm of lip, oral cavity, and pharynx**
    Z85.810 Personal history of malignant neoplasm of tongue
    Z85.818 Personal history of malignant neoplasm of other sites of lip, oral cavity, and pharynx
    Z85.819 Personal history of malignant neoplasm of unspecified site of lip, oral cavity, and pharynx

  ✓6ᵗʰ **Z85.82 Personal history of malignant neoplasm of skin**
    Z85.820 Personal history of malignant melanoma of skin
      Conditions classifiable to C43
    Z85.821 Personal history of Merkel cell carcinoma
      Conditions classifiable to C4A
    Z85.828 Personal history of other malignant neoplasm of skin
      Conditions classifiable to C44

  ✓6ᵗʰ **Z85.83 Personal history of malignant neoplasm of bone and soft tissue**
    Z85.830 Personal history of malignant neoplasm of bone
    Z85.831 Personal history of malignant neoplasm of soft tissue
      EXCLUDES 2 personal history of malignant neoplasm of skin (Z85.82-)

  ✓6ᵗʰ **Z85.84 Personal history of malignant neoplasm of eye and nervous tissue**
    Z85.840 Personal history of malignant neoplasm of eye
    Z85.841 Personal history of malignant neoplasm of brain
    Z85.848 Personal history of malignant neoplasm of other parts of nervous tissue

  ✓6ᵗʰ **Z85.85 Personal history of malignant neoplasm of endocrine glands**
    Z85.850 Personal history of malignant neoplasm of thyroid
    Z85.858 Personal history of malignant neoplasm of other endocrine glands

  Z85.89 Personal history of malignant neoplasm of other organs and systems

Z85.9 Personal history of malignant neoplasm, unspecified
  Conditions classifiable to C7A.00, C80.1

✓4ᵗʰ **Z86 Personal history of certain other diseases**
  Code first any follow-up examination after treatment (Z09)

  ✓5ᵗʰ **Z86.0 Personal history of in-situ and benign neoplasms and neoplasms of uncertain behavior**
    EXCLUDES 2 personal history of malignant neoplasms (Z85.-)
    AHA: 2017,1Q,9

    ✓6ᵗʰ **Z86.00 Personal history of in-situ neoplasm**
      Conditions classifiable to D00-D09
      Z86.000 Personal history of in-situ neoplasm of breast
      Z86.001 Personal history of in-situ neoplasm of cervix uteri
        Personal history of cervical intraepithelial neoplasia III [CIN III]
      Z86.008 Personal history of in-situ neoplasm of other site
        Personal history of vaginal intraepithelial neoplasia III [VAIN III]
        Personal history of vulvar intraepithelial neoplasia III [VIN III]

    ✓6ᵗʰ **Z86.01 Personal history of benign neoplasm**
      Z86.010 Personal history of colonic polyps
        AHA: 2017,1Q,14
      Z86.011 Personal history of benign neoplasm of the brain
      Z86.012 Personal history of benign carcinoid tumor

    Z86.018 Personal history of other benign neoplasm
      AHA: 2017,1Q,14
    Z86.03 Personal history of neoplasm of uncertain behavior

  ✓5ᵗʰ **Z86.1 Personal history of infectious and parasitic diseases**
    Conditions classifiable to A00-B89, B99
    EXCLUDES 1 personal history of infectious diseases specific to a body system
      sequelae of infectious and parasitic diseases (B90-B94)
    Z86.11 Personal history of tuberculosis
    Z86.12 Personal history of poliomyelitis
    Z86.13 Personal history of malaria
    Z86.14 Personal history of Methicillin resistant Staphylococcus aureus infection
      Personal history of MRSA infection
    Z86.19 Personal history of other infectious and parasitic diseases

  Z86.2 Personal history of diseases of the blood and blood-forming organs and certain disorders involving the immune mechanism
    Conditions classifiable to D50-D89

  ✓5ᵗʰ **Z86.3 Personal history of endocrine, nutritional and metabolic diseases**
    Conditions classifiable to E00-E88
    Z86.31 Personal history of diabetic foot ulcer
      EXCLUDES 2 current diabetic foot ulcer (E08.621, E09.621, E10.621, E11.621, E13.621)
    Z86.32 Personal history of gestational diabetes ♀
      Personal history of conditions classifiable to O24.4-
      EXCLUDES 1 gestational diabetes mellitus in current pregnancy (O24.4-)
    Z86.39 Personal history of other endocrine, nutritional and metabolic disease

  ✓5ᵗʰ **Z86.5 Personal history of mental and behavioral disorders**
    Conditions classifiable to F40-F59
    Z86.51 Personal history of combat and operational stress reaction
    Z86.59 Personal history of other mental and behavioral disorders

  ✓5ᵗʰ **Z86.6 Personal history of diseases of the nervous system and sense organs**
    Conditions classifiable to G00-G99, H00-H95
    Z86.61 Personal history of infections of the central nervous system
      Personal history of encephalitis
      Personal history of meningitis
    Z86.69 Personal history of other diseases of the nervous system and sense organs
      AHA: 2016,4Q,24

  ✓5ᵗʰ **Z86.7 Personal history of diseases of the circulatory system**
    Conditions classifiable to I00-I99
    EXCLUDES 2 old myocardial infarction (I25.2)
      personal history of anaphylactic shock (Z87.892)
      postmyocardial infarction syndrome (I24.1)
    ✓6ᵗʰ **Z86.71 Personal history of venous thrombosis and embolism**
      Z86.711 Personal history of pulmonary embolism
      Z86.718 Personal history of other venous thrombosis and embolism
    Z86.72 Personal history of thrombophlebitis
    Z86.73 Personal history of transient ischemic attack (TIA), and cerebral infarction without residual deficits
      Personal history of prolonged reversible ischemic neurological deficit (PRIND)
      Personal history of stroke NOS without residual deficits
      EXCLUDES 1 personal history of traumatic brain injury (Z87.820)
        sequelae of cerebrovascular disease (I69.-)
      AHA: 2012,4Q,92
    Z86.74 Personal history of sudden cardiac arrest
      Personal history of sudden cardiac death successfully resuscitated
    Z86.79 Personal history of other diseases of the circulatory system

HCC CMS-HCC   PDx Primary Dx Only   Q QPP   N Newborn : 0   P Pediatric : 0-17   M Maternity : 12-55   A Adult : 15-124

✓4ᵗʰ **Z87** **Personal history of other diseases and conditions**

    Code first any follow-up examination after treatment (Z09)

✓5ᵗʰ **Z87.0** **Personal history of diseases of the respiratory system**

    Conditions classifiable to J00–J99

    Z87.01 **Personal history of pneumonia (recurrent)**

    Z87.09 **Personal history of other diseases of the respiratory system**

✓5ᵗʰ **Z87.1** **Personal history of diseases of the digestive system**

    Conditions classifiable to K00–K93

    Z87.11 **Personal history of peptic ulcer disease**

    Z87.19 **Personal history of other diseases of the digestive system**

        AHA: 2017,1Q,14

Z87.2 **Personal history of diseases of the skin and subcutaneous tissue**

    Conditions classifiable to L00–L99

        EXCLUDES 2   *personal history of diabetic foot ulcer (Z86.31)*

✓5ᵗʰ **Z87.3** **Personal history of diseases of the musculoskeletal system and connective tissue**

    Conditions classifiable to M00–M99

        EXCLUDES 2   *personal history of (healed) traumatic fracture (Z87.81)*

✓6ᵗʰ **Z87.31** **Personal history of (healed) nontraumatic fracture**

    Z87.310 **Personal history of (healed) osteoporosis fracture**

        Personal history of (healed) fragility fracture

        Personal history of (healed) collapsed vertebra due to osteoporosis

        TIP: Assign for history of osteoporosis fractures that have resolved, even when a code from category M80 indicating current osteoporosis fracture is also reported.

    Z87.311 **Personal history of (healed) other pathological fracture**

        Personal history of (healed) collapsed vertebra NOS

        EXCLUDES 2   *personal history of osteoporosis fracture (Z87.310)*

    Z87.312 **Personal history of (healed) stress fracture**

        Personal history of (healed) fatigue fracture

    Z87.39 **Personal history of other diseases of the musculoskeletal system and connective tissue**

✓5ᵗʰ **Z87.4** **Personal history of diseases of the genitourinary system**

    Conditions classifiable to N00–N99

✓6ᵗʰ **Z87.41** **Personal history of dysplasia of the female genital tract**

        EXCLUDES 1   *personal history of intraepithelial neoplasia III of female genital tract (Z86.001, Z86.008)*

           personal history of malignant neoplasm of female genital tract (Z85.40-Z85.44)

    Z87.410 **Personal history of cervical dysplasia** ♀

    Z87.411 **Personal history of vaginal dysplasia** ♀

    Z87.412 **Personal history of vulvar dysplasia** ♀

    Z87.42 **Personal history of other diseases of the female genital tract** ♀

✓6ᵗʰ **Z87.43** **Personal history of diseases of the male genital organs**

    Z87.430 **Personal history of prostatic dysplasia** ♂

        EXCLUDES 1   *personal history of malignant neoplasm of prostate (Z85.46)*

    Z87.438 **Personal history of other diseases of male genital organs** ♂

✓6ᵗʰ **Z87.44** **Personal history of diseases of the urinary system**

        EXCLUDES 1   *personal history of malignant neoplasm of cervix uteri (Z85.41)*

    Z87.440 **Personal history of urinary (tract) infections**

    Z87.441 **Personal history of nephrotic syndrome**

    Z87.442 **Personal history of urinary calculi**

        Personal history of kidney stones

    Z87.448 **Personal history of other diseases of urinary system**

✓5ᵗʰ **Z87.5** **Personal history of complications of pregnancy, childbirth and the puerperium**

    Conditions classifiable to O00–O9A

        EXCLUDES 2   *recurrent pregnancy loss (N96)*

    Z87.51 **Personal history of pre-term labor** ♀

        EXCLUDES 1   *current pregnancy with history of pre-term labor (O09.21-)*

    Z87.59 **Personal history of other complications of pregnancy, childbirth and the puerperium** ♀

        Personal history of trophoblastic disease

✓5ᵗʰ **Z87.7** **Personal history of (corrected) congenital malformations**

    Conditions classifiable to Q00–Q89 that have been repaired or corrected

        EXCLUDES 1   *congenital malformations that have been partially corrected or repair but which still require medical treatment - code to condition*

        EXCLUDES 2   *other postprocedural states (Z98.-)*

           personal history of medical treatment (Z92.-)

           presence of cardiac and vascular implants and grafts (Z95.-)

           presence of other devices (Z97.-)

           presence of other functional implants (Z96.-)

           transplanted organ and tissue status (Z94.-)

✓6ᵗʰ **Z87.71** **Personal history of (corrected) congenital malformations of genitourinary system**

    Z87.710 **Personal history of (corrected) hypospadias** ♂

    Z87.718 **Personal history of other specified (corrected) congenital malformations of genitourinary system**

✓6ᵗʰ **Z87.72** **Personal history of (corrected) congenital malformations of nervous system and sense organs**

    Z87.720 **Personal history of (corrected) congenital malformations of eye**

    Z87.721 **Personal history of (corrected) congenital malformations of ear**

    Z87.728 **Personal history of other specified (corrected) congenital malformations of nervous system and sense organs**

✓6ᵗʰ **Z87.73** **Personal history of (corrected) congenital malformations of digestive system**

    Z87.730 **Personal history of (corrected) cleft lip and palate**

    Z87.738 **Personal history of other specified (corrected) congenital malformations of digestive system**

    Z87.74 **Personal history of (corrected) congenital malformations of heart and circulatory system**

    Z87.75 **Personal history of (corrected) congenital malformations of respiratory system**

    Z87.76 **Personal history of (corrected) congenital malformations of integument, limbs and musculoskeletal system**

✓6ᵗʰ **Z87.79** **Personal history of other (corrected) congenital malformations**

    Z87.790 **Personal history of (corrected) congenital malformations of face and neck**

    Z87.798 **Personal history of other (corrected) congenital malformations**

✓5ᵗʰ **Z87.8** **Personal history of other specified conditions**

        EXCLUDES 2   *personal history of self harm (Z91.5)*

    Z87.81 **Personal history of (healed) traumatic fracture**

        EXCLUDES 2   *personal history of (healed) nontraumatic fracture (Z87.31-)*

✓6ᵗʰ **Z87.82** **Personal history of other (healed) physical injury and trauma**

    Conditions classifiable to S00–T88, except traumatic fractures

    Z87.820 **Personal history of traumatic brain injury**

        EXCLUDES 1   *personal history of transient ischemic attack (TIA), and cerebral infarction without residual deficits (Z86.73)*

☑ Additional Character Req   ✓x7ᵗʰ Placeholder Alert   Manifestation   ▽ Unspecified   ▶◀ Revised Text   ● New Code   ▲ Revised Code Title

ICD-10-CM 2019   **1241**

Z87.821 **Personal history of** retained foreign body fully removed

Z87.828 **Personal history of other (healed) physical injury and trauma**

√6ᵗʰ   **Z87.89 Personal history of other specified conditions**

Z87.890 **Personal history of** sex reassignment

Z87.891 **Personal history of** nicotine dependence

    EXCLUDES 1   current nicotine dependence (F17.2-)

    AHA: 2017,2Q,27

Z87.892 **Personal history of** anaphylaxis

    Code also allergy status such as:

      allergy status to drugs, medicaments and biological substances (Z88.-)

      allergy status, other than to drugs and biological substances (Z91.0-)

Z87.898 **Personal history of other specified conditions**

    AHA: 2013,1Q,21

√4ᵗʰ   **Z88 Allergy status to drugs, medicaments and biological substances**

    EXCLUDES 2   allergy status, other than to drugs and biological substances (Z91.0-)

    AHA: 2015,3Q,23

Z88.0 Allergy status to penicillin

Z88.1 Allergy status to other antibiotic agents status

Z88.2 Allergy status to sulfonamides **status**

Z88.3 Allergy status to other anti-infective agents status

Z88.4 Allergy status to anesthetic **agent status**

Z88.5 Allergy status to narcotic **agent status**

Z88.6 Allergy status to analgesic **agent status**

Z88.7 Allergy status to serum and vaccine **status**

Z88.8 Allergy status to other drugs, medicaments and biological substances status

Z88.9 Allergy status to unspecified drugs, medicaments and biological substances status ▽

√4ᵗʰ   **Z89 Acquired absence of limb**

    INCLUDES   amputation status

      postprocedural loss of limb

      post-traumatic loss of limb

    EXCLUDES 1   acquired deformities of limbs (M20-M21)

      congenital absence of limbs (Q71-Q73)

√5ᵗʰ   **Z89.0 Acquired absence of** thumb and other finger(s)

√6ᵗʰ   **Z89.01 Acquired absence of** thumb

Z89.011 **Acquired absence of** right thumb

Z89.012 **Acquired absence of** left thumb

Z89.019 **Acquired absence of unspecified thumb** ▽

√6ᵗʰ   **Z89.02 Acquired absence of other** finger(s)

    EXCLUDES 2   acquired absence of thumb (Z89.01-)

Z89.021 **Acquired absence of** right finger(s)

Z89.022 **Acquired absence of** left finger(s)

Z89.029 **Acquired absence of unspecified finger(s)** ▽

√5ᵗʰ   **Z89.1 Acquired absence of** hand and wrist

√6ᵗʰ   **Z89.11 Acquired absence of** hand

Z89.111 **Acquired absence of** right hand

Z89.112 **Acquired absence of** left hand

Z89.119 **Acquired absence of unspecified hand** ▽

√6ᵗʰ   **Z89.12 Acquired absence of** wrist

    Disarticulation at wrist

Z89.121 **Acquired absence of** right wrist

Z89.122 **Acquired absence of** left wrist

Z89.129 **Acquired absence of unspecified wrist** ▽

√5ᵗʰ   **Z89.2 Acquired absence of** upper limb above wrist

√6ᵗʰ   **Z89.20 Acquired absence of upper limb, unspecified level**

Z89.201 **Acquired absence of** right upper limb, unspecified level ▽

Z89.202 **Acquired absence of** left upper limb, unspecified level ▽

Z89.209 **Acquired absence of unspecified upper limb, unspecified level** ▽

    Acquired absence of arm NOS

√6ᵗʰ   **Z89.21 Acquired absence of** upper limb below elbow

Z89.211 **Acquired absence of** right upper limb below elbow

Z89.212 **Acquired absence of** left upper limb below elbow

Z89.219 **Acquired absence of unspecified upper limb below elbow** ▽

√6ᵗʰ   **Z89.22 Acquired absence of** upper limb above elbow

    Disarticulation at elbow

Z89.221 **Acquired absence of** right upper limb above elbow

Z89.222 **Acquired absence of** left upper limb above elbow

Z89.229 **Acquired absence of unspecified upper limb above elbow** ▽

√6ᵗʰ   **Z89.23 Acquired absence of** shoulder

    Acquired absence of shoulder joint following explantation of shoulder joint prosthesis, with or without presence of antibiotic-impregnated cement spacer

Z89.231 **Acquired absence of** right shoulder

Z89.232 **Acquired absence of** left shoulder

Z89.239 **Acquired absence of unspecified shoulder** ▽

√5ᵗʰ   **Z89.4 Acquired absence of** toe(s), foot, and ankle

√6ᵗʰ   **Z89.41 Acquired absence of** great toe

Z89.411 **Acquired absence of** right great toe   HCC

Z89.412 **Acquired absence of** left great toe   HCC

Z89.419 **Acquired absence of unspecified great toe**   HCC ▽

√6ᵗʰ   **Z89.42 Acquired absence of other** toe(s)

    EXCLUDES 2   acquired absence of great toe (Z89.41-)

Z89.421 **Acquired absence of other** right toe(s)   HCC

Z89.422 **Acquired absence of other** left toe(s)   HCC

Z89.429 **Acquired absence of other toe(s), unspecified side**   HCC ▽

√6ᵗʰ   **Z89.43 Acquired absence of** foot

Z89.431 **Acquired absence of** right foot   HCC

Z89.432 **Acquired absence of** left foot   HCC

Z89.439 **Acquired absence of unspecified foot**   HCC ▽

√6ᵗʰ   **Z89.44 Acquired absence of** ankle

    Disarticulation of ankle

Z89.441 **Acquired absence of** right ankle   HCC

Z89.442 **Acquired absence of** left ankle   HCC

Z89.449 **Acquired absence of unspecified ankle**   HCC ▽

√5ᵗʰ   **Z89.5 Acquired absence of leg below knee**

√6ᵗʰ   **Z89.51 Acquired absence of** leg below knee

Z89.511 **Acquired absence of** right leg below knee   HCC

Z89.512 **Acquired absence of** left leg below knee   HCC

Z89.519 **Acquired absence of unspecified leg below knee**   HCC ▽

√6ᵗʰ   **Z89.52 Acquired absence of** knee

    Acquired absence of knee joint following explantation of knee joint prosthesis, with or without presence of antibiotic-impregnated cement spacer

Z89.521 **Acquired absence of** right knee

Z89.522 **Acquired absence of** left knee

Z89.529 **Acquired absence of unspecified knee** ▽

√5ᵗʰ   **Z89.6 Acquired absence of leg above knee**

√6ᵗʰ   **Z89.61 Acquired absence of** leg above knee

    Acquired absence of leg NOS

    Disarticulation at knee

Z89.611 **Acquired absence of** right leg above knee   HCC

Z89.612 **Acquired absence of** left leg above knee   HCC

Z89.619 **Acquired absence of unspecified leg above knee**   HCC ▽

√6ᵗʰ **Z89.62** **Acquired absence of hip**
Acquired absence of hip joint following explantation of hip joint prosthesis, with or without presence of antibiotic-impregnated cement spacer
Disarticulation at hip

     Z89.621 Acquired absence of right hip joint
     Z89.622 Acquired absence of left hip joint
     Z89.629 Acquired absence of unspecified hip joint   ▽

Z89.9 **Acquired absence of limb, unspecified**   ▽

√4ᵗʰ **Z90** **Acquired absence of organs, not elsewhere classified**
     INCLUDES   postprocedural or post-traumatic loss of body part NEC
     EXCLUDES 1   congenital absence - see Alphabetical Index
     EXCLUDES 2   postprocedural absence of endocrine glands (E89.-)

√5ᵗʰ **Z90.0** **Acquired absence of part of head and neck**
     Z90.01 **Acquired absence of eye**
     Z90.02 **Acquired absence of larynx**
     Z90.09 **Acquired absence of other part of head and neck**
         Acquired absence of nose
         EXCLUDES 2   teeth (K08.1)

√5ᵗʰ **Z90.1** **Acquired absence of breast and nipple**
     Z90.10 **Acquired absence of unspecified breast and nipple**   ▽
     Z90.11 **Acquired absence of right breast and nipple**
     Z90.12 **Acquired absence of left breast and nipple**
     Z90.13 **Acquired absence of bilateral breasts and nipples**

Z90.2 **Acquired absence of lung [part of]**
Z90.3 **Acquired absence of stomach [part of]**

√5ᵗʰ **Z90.4** **Acquired absence of other specified parts of digestive tract**
√6ᵗʰ   **Z90.41** **Acquired absence of pancreas**
     Code also exocrine pancreatic insufficiency (K86.81)
     Use additional code to identify any associated:
     insulin use (Z79.4)
     diabetes mellitus, postpancreatectomy (E13.-)
     Z90.410 **Acquired total absence of pancreas**
         Acquired absence of pancreas NOS
     Z90.411 **Acquired partial absence of pancreas**
     Z90.49 **Acquired absence of other specified parts of digestive tract**

Z90.5 **Acquired absence of kidney**
Z90.6 **Acquired absence of other parts of urinary tract**
     Acquired absence of bladder

√5ᵗʰ **Z90.7** **Acquired absence of genital organ(s)**
     EXCLUDES 1   personal history of sex reassignment (Z87.890)
     EXCLUDES 2   female genital mutilation status (N90.81-)

√6ᵗʰ   **Z90.71** **Acquired absence of cervix and uterus**
     Z90.710 **Acquired absence of both cervix and uterus**   ♀
         Acquired absence of uterus NOS
         Status post total hysterectomy
     Z90.711 **Acquired absence of uterus with remaining cervical stump**   ♀
         Status post partial hysterectomy with remaining cervical stump
     Z90.712 **Acquired absence of cervix with remaining uterus**   ♀

√6ᵗʰ   **Z90.72** **Acquired absence of ovaries**
     Z90.721 **Acquired absence of ovaries, unilateral**   ♀
     Z90.722 **Acquired absence of ovaries, bilateral**   ♀

Z90.79 **Acquired absence of other genital organ(s)**

√5ᵗʰ **Z90.8** **Acquired absence of other organs**
     Z90.81 **Acquired absence of spleen**
     Z90.89 **Acquired absence of other organs**

√4ᵗʰ **Z91** **Personal risk factors, not elsewhere classified**
     EXCLUDES 2   contact with and (suspected) exposures hazardous to health (Z77.-)
         exposure to pollution and other problems related to physical environment (Z77.1-)
         female genital mutilation status (N90.81-)
         personal history of physical injury and trauma (Z87.81, Z87.82-)
         occupational exposure to risk factors (Z57.-)

√5ᵗʰ **Z91.0** **Allergy status, other than to drugs and biological substances**
     EXCLUDES 2   allergy status to drugs, medicaments, and biological substances (Z88.-)

√6ᵗʰ   **Z91.01** **Food allergy status**
     EXCLUDES 2   food additives allergy status (Z91.02)
     Z91.010 **Allergy to peanuts**
     Z91.011 **Allergy to milk products**
         EXCLUDES 1   lactose intolerance (E73.-)
     Z91.012 **Allergy to eggs**
     Z91.013 **Allergy to seafood**
         Allergy to shellfish
         Allergy to octopus or squid ink
     Z91.018 **Allergy to other foods**
         Allergy to nuts other than peanuts

Z91.02 **Food additives allergy status**

√6ᵗʰ   **Z91.03** **Insect allergy status**
     Z91.030 **Bee allergy status**
     Z91.038 **Other insect allergy status**

√6ᵗʰ   **Z91.04** **Nonmedicinal substance allergy status**
     Z91.040 **Latex allergy status**
         Latex sensitivity status
     Z91.041 **Radiographic dye allergy status**
         Allergy status to contrast media used for diagnostic X-ray procedure
     Z91.048 **Other nonmedicinal substance allergy status**

Z91.09 **Other allergy status, other than to drugs and biological substances**

√5ᵗʰ **Z91.1** **Patient's noncompliance with medical treatment and regimen**
     Z91.11 **Patient's noncompliance with dietary regimen**

√6ᵗʰ   **Z91.12** **Patient's intentional underdosing of medication regimen**
     Code first underdosing of medication (T36-T50) with fifth or sixth character 6
     EXCLUDES 1   adverse effect of prescribed drug taken as directed - code to adverse effect
         poisoning (overdose) - code to poisoning
     Z91.120 **Patient's intentional underdosing of medication regimen due to financial hardship**
     Z91.128 **Patient's intentional underdosing of medication regimen for other reason**

√6ᵗʰ   **Z91.13** **Patient's unintentional underdosing of medication regimen**
     Code first underdosing of medication (T36-T50) with fifth or sixth character 6
     EXCLUDES 1   adverse effect of prescribed drug taken as directed - code to adverse effect
         poisoning (overdose) - code to poisoning
     Z91.130 **Patient's unintentional underdosing of medication regimen due to age-related debility**
     Z91.138 **Patient's unintentional underdosing of medication regimen for other reason**

Z91.14 **Patient's other noncompliance with medication regimen**
     Patient's underdosing of medication NOS

Z91.15 **Patient's noncompliance with renal dialysis**   HCC

Z91.19 **Patient's noncompliance with other medical treatment and regimen**
     Nonadherence to medical treatment

Chapter 21. Factors Influencing Health Status and Contact With Health Services

Z91.4–Z94.9

✓5ᵗʰ **Z91.4 Personal history of psychological trauma, not elsewhere classified**

   ✓6ᵗʰ **Z91.41 Personal history of adult abuse** A

      EXCLUDES 2   *personal history of abuse in childhood (Z62.81-)*

     Z91.410 Personal history of adult physical and sexual abuse A

       EXCLUDES 1   *current adult physical abuse (T74.11, T76.11)*

        current adult sexual abuse (T74.21, T76.11)

     Z91.411 Personal history of adult psychological abuse A

     Z91.412 Personal history of adult neglect A

       EXCLUDES 1   *current adult neglect (T74.01, T76.01)*

     Z91.419 Personal history of unspecified adult abuse A ▽

   Z91.42 Personal history of forced labor or sexual exploitation

   Z91.49 Other personal history of psychological trauma, not elsewhere classified

  Z91.5 Personal history of self-harm

   Personal history of parasuicide

   Personal history of self-poisoning

   Personal history of suicide attempt

✓5ᵗʰ **Z91.8 Other specified personal risk factors, not elsewhere classified**

  Z91.81 History of falling

   At risk for falling

  Z91.82 Personal history of military deployment A

   Individual (civilian or military) with past history of military war, peacekeeping and humanitarian deployment (current or past conflict)

   Returned from military deployment

  Z91.83 *Wandering in diseases classified elsewhere*

   Code first underlying disorder such as:

   Alzheimer's disease (G30.-)

   autism or pervasive developmental disorder (F84.-)

   intellectual disabilities (F70-F79)

   unspecified dementia with behavioral disturbance (F03.9-)

  ✓6ᵗʰ **Z91.84 Oral health risk factors**

   AHA: 2017,4Q,29

   Z91.841 Risk for dental caries, low

   Z91.842 Risk for dental caries, moderate

   Z91.843 Risk for dental caries, high

   Z91.849 Unspecified risk for dental caries ▽

  Z91.89 Other specified personal risk factors, not elsewhere classified

   AHA: 2017,1Q,45

✓4ᵗʰ **Z92 Personal history of medical treatment**

  EXCLUDES 2   *postprocedural states (Z98.-)*

  Z92.0 Personal history of contraception

   EXCLUDES 1   *counseling or management of current contraceptive practices (Z30.-)*

   long term (current) use of contraception (Z79.3)

   presence of (intrauterine) contraceptive device (Z97.5)

✓5ᵗʰ **Z92.2 Personal history of drug therapy**

  EXCLUDES 2   *long term (current) drug therapy (Z79.-)*

  Z92.21 Personal history of antineoplastic chemotherapy

  Z92.22 Personal history of monoclonal drug therapy

  Z92.23 Personal history of estrogen therapy

  ✓6ᵗʰ **Z92.24 Personal history of steroid therapy**

   Z92.240 Personal history of inhaled steroid therapy

   Z92.241 Personal history of systemic steroid therapy

    Personal history of steroid therapy NOS

  Z92.25 Personal history of immunosupression therapy

   EXCLUDES 2   *personal history of steroid therapy (Z92.24)*

  Z92.29 Personal history of other drug therapy

Z92.3 Personal history of irradiation

  Personal history of exposure to therapeutic radiation

  EXCLUDES 1   *exposure to radiation in the physical environment (Z77.12)*

   occupational exposure to radiation (Z57.1)

✓5ᵗʰ **Z92.8 Personal history of other medical treatment**

  Z92.81 Personal history of extracorporeal membrane oxygenation (ECMO)

  Z92.82 Status post administration of tPA (rtPA) in a different facility within the last 24 hours prior to admission to current facility

   Code first condition requiring tPA administration, such as:

   acute cerebral infarction (I63.-)

   acute myocardial infarction (I21.-, I22.-)

   AHA: 2013,4Q,124

  Z92.83 Personal history of failed moderate sedation

   Personal history of failed conscious sedation

   EXCLUDES 2   *failed moderate sedation during procedure (T88.52)*

  Z92.84 Personal history of unintended awareness under general anesthesia

   EXCLUDES 2   *unintended awareness under general anesthesia during procedure (T88.53)*

   AHA: 2016,4Q,72-73,77

  Z92.89 Personal history of other medical treatment

✓4ᵗʰ **Z93 Artificial opening status**

  EXCLUDES 1   *artificial openings requiring attention or management (Z43.-)*

   complications of external stoma (J95.0-, K94.-, N99.5-)

  Z93.0 Tracheostomy status HCC

   AHA: 2013,4Q,129

  Z93.1 Gastrostomy status HCC

  Z93.2 Ileostomy status HCC

  Z93.3 Colostomy status HCC

  Z93.4 Other artificial openings of gastrointestinal tract status HCC

  ✓5ᵗʰ **Z93.5 Cystostomy status** HCC ▽

   Z93.50 Unspecified cystostomy status HCC

   Z93.51 Cutaneous-vesicostomy status HCC

   Z93.52 Appendico-vesicostomy status HCC

   Z93.59 Other cystostomy status HCC

  Z93.6 Other artificial openings of urinary tract status HCC

   Nephrostomy status

   Ureterostomy status

   Urethrostomy status

  Z93.8 Other artificial opening status HCC

  Z93.9 Artificial opening status, unspecified HCC ▽

✓4ᵗʰ **Z94 Transplanted organ and tissue status**

  INCLUDES   organ or tissue replaced by heterogenous or homogenous transplant

  EXCLUDES 1   *complications of transplanted organ or tissue - see Alphabetical Index*

  EXCLUDES 2   *presence of vascular grafts (Z95.-)*

  Z94.0 Kidney transplant status

  Z94.1 Heart transplant status HCC

   EXCLUDES 1   *artificial heart status (Z95.812)*

   heart-valve replacement status (Z95.2-Z95.4)

  Z94.2 Lung transplant status HCC

  Z94.3 Heart and lungs transplant status HCC

  Z94.4 Liver transplant status HCC

  Z94.5 Skin transplant status

   Autogenous skin transplant status

  Z94.6 Bone transplant status

  Z94.7 Corneal transplant status

  ✓5ᵗʰ **Z94.8 Other transplanted organ and tissue status**

   Z94.81 Bone marrow transplant status HCC

   Z94.82 Intestine transplant status HCC

   Z94.83 Pancreas transplant status HCC

   Z94.84 Stem cells transplant status HCC

   Z94.89 Other transplanted organ and tissue status

  Z94.9 Transplanted organ and tissue status, unspecified ▽

√4ᵗʰ **Z95 Presence of cardiac and vascular implants and grafts**

    EXCLUDES 2   *complications of cardiac and vascular devices, implants and grafts (T82.-)*

    Z95.0 Presence of cardiac pacemaker
      Presence of cardiac resynchronization therapy (CRT-P) pacemaker
      EXCLUDES 1   *adjustment or management of cardiac device (Z45.0-)*
           adjustment or management of cardiac pacemaker (Z45.0)
           presence of automatic (implantable) cardiac defibrillator with synchronous cardiac pacemaker (Z95.810)

    Z95.1 Presence of aortocoronary bypass graft
      Presence of coronary artery bypass graft

    Z95.2 Presence of prosthetic heart valve
      Presence of heart valve NOS

    Z95.3 Presence of xenogenic heart valve

    Z95.4 Presence of other heart-valve replacement

    Z95.5 Presence of coronary angioplasty implant and graft
      EXCLUDES 1   *coronary angioplasty status without implant and graft (Z98.61)*

√5ᵗʰ **Z95.8 Presence of other cardiac and vascular implants and grafts**

    √6ᵗʰ **Z95.81 Presence of other cardiac implants and grafts**

       Z95.810 Presence of automatic (implantable) cardiac defibrillator
          Presence of automatic (implantable) cardiac defibrillator with synchronous cardiac pacemaker
          Presence of cardiac resynchronization therapy defibrillator (CRT-D)
          ►Presence of cardioverter-defibrillator (ICD)◄

       Z95.811 Presence of heart assist device   HCC
       Z95.812 Presence of fully implantable artificial heart   HCC
       Z95.818 Presence of other cardiac implants and grafts

    √6ᵗʰ **Z95.82 Presence of other vascular implants and grafts**

       Z95.820 Peripheral vascular angioplasty status with implants and grafts
          EXCLUDES 1   *peripheral vascular angioplasty without implant and graft (Z98.62)*

       Z95.828 Presence of other vascular implants and grafts
          Presence of intravascular prosthesis NEC

    Z95.9 Presence of cardiac and vascular implant and graft, unspecified   ▽

√4ᵗʰ **Z96 Presence of other functional implants**

    EXCLUDES 2   *complications of internal prosthetic devices, implants and grafts (T82-T85)*
          fitting and adjustment of prosthetic and other devices (Z44-Z46)

    Z96.0 Presence of urogenital implants

    Z96.1 Presence of intraocular lens
      Presence of pseudophakia

√5ᵗʰ **Z96.2 Presence of otological and audiological implants**

    Z96.20 Presence of otological and audiological implant, unspecified   ▽

    Z96.21 Cochlear implant status

    Z96.22 Myringotomy tube(s) status

    Z96.29 Presence of other otological and audiological implants
      Presence of bone-conduction hearing device
      Presence of eustachian tube stent
      Stapes replacement

    Z96.3 Presence of artificial larynx

√5ᵗʰ **Z96.4 Presence of endocrine implants**

    Z96.41 Presence of insulin pump (external) (internal)

    Z96.49 Presence of other endocrine implants

    Z96.5 Presence of tooth-root and mandibular implants

√5ᵗʰ **Z96.6 Presence of orthopedic joint implants**

    Z96.60 Presence of unspecified orthopedic joint implant   ▽

    √6ᵗʰ **Z96.61 Presence of artificial shoulder joint**

       Z96.611 Presence of right artificial shoulder joint
       Z96.612 Presence of left artificial shoulder joint
       Z96.619 Presence of unspecified artificial shoulder joint   ▽

    √6ᵗʰ **Z96.62 Presence of artificial elbow joint**

       Z96.621 Presence of right artificial elbow joint
       Z96.622 Presence of left artificial elbow joint
       Z96.629 Presence of unspecified artificial elbow joint   ▽

    √6ᵗʰ **Z96.63 Presence of artificial wrist joint**

       Z96.631 Presence of right artificial wrist joint
       Z96.632 Presence of left artificial wrist joint
       Z96.639 Presence of unspecified artificial wrist joint   ▽

    √6ᵗʰ **Z96.64 Presence of artificial hip joint**

      Hip-joint replacement (partial) (total)

       Z96.641 Presence of right artificial hip joint
       Z96.642 Presence of left artificial hip joint
       Z96.643 Presence of artificial hip joint, bilateral
       Z96.649 Presence of unspecified artificial hip joint   ▽

    √6ᵗʰ **Z96.65 Presence of artificial knee joint**

       Z96.651 Presence of right artificial knee joint
       Z96.652 Presence of left artificial knee joint
       Z96.653 Presence of artificial knee joint, bilateral
       Z96.659 Presence of unspecified artificial knee joint   ▽

    √6ᵗʰ **Z96.66 Presence of artificial ankle joint**

       Z96.661 Presence of right artificial ankle joint
       Z96.662 Presence of left artificial ankle joint
       Z96.669 Presence of unspecified artificial ankle joint   ▽

    √6ᵗʰ **Z96.69 Presence of other orthopedic joint implants**

       Z96.691 Finger-joint replacement of right hand
       Z96.692 Finger-joint replacement of left hand
       Z96.693 Finger-joint replacement, bilateral
       Z96.698 Presence of other orthopedic joint implants

    Z96.7 Presence of other bone and tendon implants
      Presence of skull plate

√5ᵗʰ **Z96.8 Presence of other specified functional implants**

    Z96.81 Presence of artificial skin

    Z96.89 Presence of other specified functional implants

    Z96.9 Presence of functional implant, unspecified   ▽

√4ᵗʰ **Z97 Presence of other devices**

    EXCLUDES 1   *complications of internal prosthetic devices, implants and grafts (T82-T85)*
          fitting and adjustment of prosthetic and other devices (Z44-Z46)
    EXCLUDES 2   *presence of cerebrospinal fluid drainage device (Z98.2)*

    Z97.0 Presence of artificial eye

√5ᵗʰ **Z97.1 Presence of artificial limb (complete) (partial)**

    Z97.10 Presence of artificial limb (complete) (partial), unspecified   ▽

    Z97.11 Presence of artificial right arm (complete) (partial)

    Z97.12 Presence of artificial left arm (complete) (partial)

    Z97.13 Presence of artificial right leg (complete) (partial)

    Z97.14 Presence of artificial left leg (complete) (partial)

    Z97.15 Presence of artificial arms, bilateral (complete) (partial)

    Z97.16 Presence of artificial legs, bilateral (complete) (partial)

    Z97.2 Presence of dental prosthetic device (complete) (partial)
      Presence of dentures (complete) (partial)

    Z97.3 Presence of spectacles and contact lenses

    Z97.4 Presence of external hearing-aid

    Z97.5 Presence of (intrauterine) contraceptive device   ♀
      EXCLUDES 1   *checking, reinsertion or removal of implantable subdermal contraceptive (Z30.46)*
          checking, reinsertion or removal of intrauterine contraceptive device (Z30.43-)

    Z97.8 Presence of other specified devices

☑ Additional Character Req   √x7ᵗʰ Placeholder Alert   Manifestation   ▽ Unspecified   ►◄ Revised Text   ● New Code   ▲ Revised Code Title

ICD-10-CM 2019   1245

Chapter 21. Factors Influencing Health Status and Contact With Health Services

Z98–Z99.89

√4th **Z98 Other postprocedural states**

EXCLUDES 2   *aftercare (Z43-Z49, Z51)*
follow-up medical care (Z08-Z09)
postprocedural complication - see Alphabetical Index

Z98.0 Intestinal bypass and anastomosis status

EXCLUDES 2   *bariatric surgery status (Z98.84)*
gastric bypass status (Z98.84)
obesity surgery status (Z98.84)

Z98.1 Arthrodesis status

Z98.2 Presence of cerebrospinal fluid drainage device
Presence of CSF shunt

Z98.3 Post therapeutic collapse of lung status
Code first underlying disease

√5th **Z98.4 Cataract extraction status**

Use additional code to identify intraocular lens implant status (Z96.1)

EXCLUDES 1   *aphakia (H27.0)*

Z98.41 Cataract extraction status, right eye

Z98.42 Cataract extraction status, left eye

Z98.49 Cataract extraction status, unspecified eye ▽

√5th **Z98.5 Sterilization status**

EXCLUDES 1   *female infertility (N97.-)*
male infertility (N46.-)

Z98.51 Tubal ligation status ♀

Z98.52 Vasectomy status A ♂

√5th **Z98.6 Angioplasty status**

Z98.61 Coronary angioplasty status

EXCLUDES 1   *coronary angioplasty status with implant and graft (Z95.5)*

Z98.62 Peripheral vascular angioplasty status

EXCLUDES 1   *peripheral vascular angioplasty status with implant and graft (Z95.820)*

√5th **Z98.8 Other specified postprocedural states**

√6th **Z98.81 Dental procedure status**

Z98.810 Dental sealant status

Z98.811 Dental restoration status
Dental crown status
Dental fillings status

Z98.818 Other dental procedure status

Z98.82 Breast implant status

EXCLUDES 1   *breast implant removal status (Z98.86)*

Z98.83 Filtering (vitreous) bleb after glaucoma surgery status

EXCLUDES 1   *inflammation (infection) of postprocedural bleb (H59.4-)*

Z98.84 Bariatric surgery status
Gastric banding status
Gastric bypass status for obesity
Obesity surgery status

EXCLUDES 1   *bariatric surgery status complicating pregnancy, childbirth, or the puerperium (O99.84)*

EXCLUDES 2   *intestinal bypass and anastomosis status (Z98.0)*

Z98.85 Transplanted organ removal status
Transplanted organ previously removed due to complication, failure, rejection or infection

EXCLUDES 1   *encounter for removal of transplanted organ - code to complication of transplanted organ (T86.-)*

Z98.86 Personal history of breast implant removal

√6th **Z98.87 Personal history of in utero procedure** ♀

Z98.870 Personal history of in utero procedure during pregnancy ♀

EXCLUDES 2   *complications from in utero procedure for current pregnancy (O35.7)*
supervision of current pregnancy with history of in utero procedure during previous pregnancy (O09.82-)

Z98.871 Personal history of in utero procedure while a fetus

√6th **Z98.89 Other specified postprocedural states**

Z98.890 Other specified postprocedural states
Personal history of surgery, not elsewhere classified

Z98.891 History of uterine scar from previous surgery

EXCLUDES 1   *maternal care due to uterine scar from previous surgery (O34.2-)*

AHA: 2016,4Q,51-52,76

√4th **Z99 Dependence on enabling machines and devices, not elsewhere classified**

EXCLUDES 1   *cardiac pacemaker status (Z95.0)*

Z99.0 Dependence on aspirator

√5th **Z99.1 Dependence on respirator**
Dependence on ventilator

Z99.11 Dependence on respirator [ventilator] status HCC

AHA: 2015,1Q,21

Z99.12 Encounter for respirator [ventilator] dependence during power failure HCC PDx

EXCLUDES 1   *mechanical complication of respirator [ventilator] (J95.850)*

Z99.2 Dependence on renal dialysis HCC
Hemodialysis status
Peritoneal dialysis status
Presence of arteriovenous shunt for dialysis
Renal dialysis status NOS

EXCLUDES 1   *encounter for fitting and adjustment of dialysis catheter (Z49.0-)*

EXCLUDES 2   *noncompliance with renal dialysis (Z91.15)*

AHA: 2016,1Q,12; 2013,4Q,125

Z99.3 Dependence on wheelchair
Wheelchair confinement status
Code first cause of dependence, such as:
muscular dystrophy ▶(G71.0-)◀
obesity (E66.-)

√5th **Z99.8 Dependence on other enabling machines and devices**

Z99.81 Dependence on supplemental oxygen
Dependence on long-term oxygen

AHA: 2013,4Q,129

Z99.89 Dependence on other enabling machines and devices
Dependence on machine or device NOS

Notes

Notes

Appendixes

Appendix A: 10 Steps to Correct Coding

Follow the 10 steps below to correctly code encounters for health care services.

Step 1: Identify the reason for the visit or encounter (i.e., a sign, symptom, diagnosis and/or condition).

The medical record documentation should accurately reflect the patient's condition, using terminology that includes specific diagnoses and symptoms or clearly states the reasons for the encounter.

Choosing the main term that best describes the reason chiefly responsible for the service provided is the most important step in coding. If symptoms are present and documented but a definitive diagnosis has not yet been determined, code the symptoms. **For outpatient cases, do not code conditions that are referred to as "rule out," "suspected," "probable," or "questionable."** Diagnoses often are not established at the time of the initial encounter/visit and may require two or more visits to be established. Code only what is documented in the available records and only to the highest degree of certainty known at the time of the patient's visit, unless it is an inpatient medical record, in which case uncertain diagnoses may be reported if documented at the time of discharge.

Step 2: After selecting the reason for the encounter, always consult the alphabetic index before verifying code selection in the tabular section.

The most critical rule is to begin code selection in the *alphabetic index*. Never turn first to the tabular list. The index provides cross-references, essential and nonessential modifiers, and inclusion terms not found in the tabular list. To prevent coding errors, always use both the alphabetic index (to identify a code) and the tabular list (to verify a code), as the index does not include the important instructional notes found in the tabular list. An added benefit of using the tabular list, which groups like things together, is that while looking at one code in the list, a coder might see a more specific one that would have been missed had the coder relied solely on the alphabetic index. Additionally, many of the codes require a fourth, fifth, sixth, or seventh, character to be valid, and many of these characters can be found only in the tabular list.

Step 3: Locate the main term entry.

The alphabetic index is a listing of conditions, which may be expressed as nouns or eponyms, with critical use of adjectives. Some conditions known by several names have multiple main entries. Reasons for encounters may be located under general terms such as admission, encounter, and examination. Other general terms such as history of, status post, or presence (of) are used to locate factors influencing health.

Step 4: Read cross-references listed with the main term or the subterm.

Cross-references such as *"see"* and *"see also"* are identified by italicized type and should always be checked to ensure that all alternative terms are researched.

Step 5: Review entries for modifiers.

Nonessential modifiers are the terms in parentheses following the main term entry. These parenthetical terms are supplementary words or explanatory information that may or may not appear in the diagnostic statement and do not affect code selection. The subterms listed under the main term are essential modifiers that do affect coding assignment. Each line of indent represents a more specific code entry. The nonessential modifiers apply to the subterms following a main term except when they are mutually exclusive, in which case the subterm takes precedence. For example, if "acute" is listed as a nonessential modifier but there is a subentry for "chronic," then the nonessential modifier of "acute" does not apply.

Step 6: Interpret abbreviations, cross-references, default codes, additional characters, and brackets.

The abbreviation NEC (not elsewhere classified) that follows some main terms or subterms indicates that there is no specific code for the condition even though the medical documentation may be very specific. The code next to the main term is called the default code. It represents the condition most commonly associated with the main term or the unspecified code for the main term. Additional characters may be required to construct the code; the tabular list must be referenced to determine what those specific characters should be. The alphabetic index uses brackets [ ] to enclose manifestation codes that can be used only as secondary codes to the underlying condition code immediately preceding it. Both codes must be reported in this multiple-coding situation.

Step 7: Choose a potential code and locate it in the tabular list.

The coder must follow any Includes, Excludes 1 and Excludes 2 notes, and other instructional notes, such as "Code first" and "Use additional code," listed in the tabular list for the chapter, category, subcategory, and subclassification level of code selection that direct the coder to use a different or additional code. Any codes in the tabular range, A00.- through T88.9-, may be used to identify the diagnostic reason for the encounter. The tabular list encompasses many codes describing disease and injury classifications (e.g., infectious and parasitic diseases, neoplasms, symptoms, nervous and circulatory system etc.).

Codes that describe symptoms and signs, as opposed to definitive diagnoses, should be used for reporting purposes when an established diagnosis has not been made (confirmed) by the physician. Chapter 18 of the ICD-10-CM code book, "Symptoms, Signs, and Abnormal Clinical and Laboratory Findings, Not Elsewhere Classified" (codes R00.-–R99), contains many, but not all, codes for symptoms.

ICD-10-CM classifies encounters with health care providers for circumstances other than a disease or injury using codes in chapter 21, "Factors Influencing Health Status and Contact with Health Services" (codes Z00–Z99). Circumstances other than a disease or injury often are recorded as chiefly responsible for the encounter.

Step 8: Determine whether the code is at the highest level of specificity.

A code is invalid if it has not been coded to the full number of characters (greatest level of specificity) required. Codes in ICD-10-CM can contain from three up to seven alphanumeric characters. A three-character code is to be used only if the category is not further subdivided into four-, five-, six-, or seven-character codes. Placeholder character X is used both to allow for future expansion and as a placeholder for empty characters in a code that requires a seventh character but has no fourth, fifth, or sixth character. Certain categories require seventh characters that apply to all codes in that category. Always check the category level for applicable seventh characters for that category.

Step 9: Assign the code.

Having reviewed all relevant information concerning the possible code choices, assign the code that most completely describes the condition.

Repeat steps one through nine for all additional documented conditions that meet the following criteria:

- Conditions that currently exist at the time of the visit
- Conditions that require or affect patient care, treatment, or management

Step 10: Sequence codes correctly.

Sequencing is the order in which the codes are listed on the claim. List first the ICD-10-CM code for the diagnosis, condition, problem, or other reason for the encounter/visit, which is shown in the medical record to be chiefly responsible for the services provided. List additional codes that describe any coexisting conditions. Follow the official coding guidelines (see section II, "Selection of Principal Diagnosis"; section III, "Reporting Additional Diagnoses"; and section IV, "Diagnostic Coding and Reporting Guidelines for Outpatient Services") on proper sequencing of codes.

Coding Examples

Diagnosis: Anorexia

Step 1: The reason for the encounter was the condition, anorexia.

Step 2: Consult the alphabetic index.

Step 3: Locate the main term "Anorexia."

Step 4: There are no cross-references to check.

Step 5: Note that there are two possible subterms (essential modifiers), "hysterical" and "nervosa," neither of which is documented in this instance and therefore cannot be used in code selection. The code listed next to the main term is called the default code selection.

Step 6: There are no abbreviations, cross-references, additional character icons, or brackets.

Step 7: Turn to code R63.Ø in the tabular list and read the instructional notes. In this case the Excludes 1 note indicates that anorexia nervosa and loss of appetite determined to be of nonorganic origin should be coded to a code from chapter 5. The diagnostic statement does not indicate nonorganic origin.

Step 8: There is no further division of the category past the fourth character subcategory. Therefore, the subcategory code level is the highest level of specificity.

Step 9: The default code, R63.Ø Anorexia, is the correct code selection

Step 10: Since anorexia is listed as the chief reason for the health care encounter, the first-listed, or principal, diagnosis is R63.Ø. Note that this is a chapter 18 symptom code but can be assigned since the provider did not establish a more definitive diagnosis.

Diagnosis: Acute bronchitis

Step 1: The reason for the encounter was the condition, acute bronchitis.

Step 2: Consult the alphabetic index.

Step 3: Locate the main term "Bronchitis."

Step 4: There are cross-references to interpret.

Step 5: Review entries for modifiers. Since "acute" is not listed as a nonessential modifier, read past the "with" modifier until you find the subterm "acute or subacute" with a nonessential modifier of "with bronchospasm or obstruction," code J2Ø.9.

Step 6: There are no abbreviations, cross-references, additional character icons, or brackets.

Step 7: Since there are no more appropriate subterms, turn to code J2Ø.9 in the tabular list. The Includes note under category J2Ø does refer to other alternative terms for acute bronchitis. Note that the inclusion term list is not exhaustive but is only a representative selection of diagnoses that are included in the subcategory. The Excludes 1 note refers bronchitis and tracheobronchitis NOS to category J4Ø. There are several Excludes 2 notes that, if applicable, can be coded in addition to this code.

Step 8: Note that the subcategories included in J2Ø represent acute bronchitis due to various infectious organisms that would be selected if identified in the documentation. In this case, the organism was not identified and there is no further division of the category past the fourth character subcategory. Therefore, the subcategory code level is the highest level of specificity.

Step 9: Assign code J2Ø.9 Acute bronchitis, unspecified.

Step 10: Repeat steps 1-9 for any additional code assignments.

Diagnosis: Infectious diarrhea

Step 1: The reason for the encounter was the condition, infectious diarrhea.

Step 2: Consult the alphabetic index.

Step 3: Locate the main term "Diarrhea" in the alphabetic index.

Step 4: There are no cross-references to check.

Step 5: Review entries for modifiers. Note that the nonessential modifiers (in parentheses) after the main term do not include the term "infectious," which means that the coder should search the subterms for the term "infectious." The subterm "infectious" refers to code AØ9.

Step 6: There are no abbreviations, cross-references, additional character icons, or brackets.

Step 7: Locate code AØ9 in the tabular list, and read all instructional notes under the main category and subcategories. The Includes notes does not list the term "infectious diarrhea" under code AØ9; however, as instructed by the alphabetic index, you should code the condition to AØ9. The ICD-10-CM code book implies that infectious diarrhea is the same as infectious gastroenteritis, enteritis, and colitis.

Step 8: There is no further division of the category past the third-character category level. Therefore, the category code level is the highest level of specificity. The final code assignment would be AØ9.

Step 9: Assign code AØ9 Infectious gastroenteritis and colitis, unspecified.

Step 10: Since infectious diarrhea is listed as the chief reason for the health care encounter, the first-listed, or principal, diagnosis is AØ9.

Diagnosis: Decubitus ulcer of right elbow with skin loss and necrosis of subcutaneous tissue

Step 1: The reason for the encounter was the condition, decubitus ulcer.

Step 2: Consult the alphabetic index.

Step 3: Locate the main term "Ulcer" in the alphabetic index.

Step 4: There are no cross-references to check.

Step 5: This entry does not have any important nonessential modifiers; however, there are other terms such as ulcerated, ulcerating, etc., that are included as main terms. Locate the subterm "decubitus" and note that there is an italicized cross-reference to "see Ulcer, pressure, by site." Go to the subterm "pressure" and locate "elbow," which refers to code L89.Ø-.

Step 6: Note that the code L89.Ø is followed by a dash and an additional character icon, which indicate that more characters are required. From here, the tabular list can be consulted at code L89.Ø-.

Step 7: Locate code L89.Ø in the tabular list, and check the category level L89 for any instructional, Includes, and Excludes 1 and 2 notes. Note that "decubitus" is an Includes note under L89 Pressure ulcer. Excludes 2 notes indicate that if this were documented as a diabetic pressure ulcer, it would be necessary to use a code from chapter 4.

Step 8: Read through the subcategory codes under L89.Ø and note that the fifth character describes laterality. Locate the right elbow at subcategory L89.Ø1. See that an additional sixth character is now needed to complete the code. The sixth character specifies the stage of the ulcer, which can be determined either by the specific documentation of the stage (e.g., stage 1, stage 2) or in this case, a description that matches one of the Includes notes that follow each stage code. For example, the description in this case of "skin loss and necrosis of the subcutaneous tissue" matches the Includes notes under L89.Ø13 Pressure ulcer of right elbow, stage 3.

Step 9: Assign code L89.Ø13 Pressure ulcer of right elbow, stage 3

Step 10: Since the decubitus ulcer is listed as the chief reason for the health care encounter, the first-listed, or principal, diagnosis is L89.Ø13. However, according to the Code first instructional note at the L89 category level, gangrene would be sequenced before the pressure ulcer if it were documented.

Diagnosis: First visit for bimalleolar fracture of the right ankle due to trauma

Step 1: The reason for the encounter was the condition, bimalleolar fracture of the right ankle.

Step 2: Consult the alphabetic index.

Step 3: Locate the main term "Fracture" in the alphabetic index.

Step 4: Note that the first main term for Fracture is pathological with cross-reference to "see also Fracture, traumatic." Locate the main term "Fracture, traumatic."

Step 5: Review entries for nonessential modifiers. Locate the subterms "ankle," "bimalleolar." Note that "displaced" is a nonessential modifier following "bimalleolar," indicating that S82.84- is the default code unless the fracture is specified as nondisplaced.

Step 6: Note that code S82.84- is followed by a dash and an additional character icon, both of which indicate that more characters are required. From here, the tabular list can be consulted at code S82.84.

Step 7: Locate code S82.84 Bimalleolar fracture of lower leg, in the tabular list and check the category level S82 for any instructional, Includes, and Excludes 1 and 2 notes. See the instructional notes indicating that fractures not specified as displaced or nondisplaced default to displaced, and fractures not designated as open or closed default to closed. See also the list of appropriate seventh characters to be added to all codes from category S82.

Step 8: Read through the subcategory codes under S82.84, and note that the sixth character specifies displaced or nondisplaced and laterality. Locate the displaced bimalleolar fracture of the right lower leg at code S82.841. See that an additional seventh character is still needed to complete the code. The seventh character specifies the type of encounter and whether the fracture is open or closed. Use character A listed in the box at the category level to describe initial encounter, closed fracture.

Step 9: Assign code S82.841A Displaced bimalleolar fracture of right lower leg, initial encounter for closed fracture.

Step 10: Since this is an injury code, code additionally any external cause, place of occurrence, and activity codes, with the injury (fracture) sequenced first.

A09	Infectious gastroenteritis and colitis, unspecified
A33	Tetanus neonatorum
A34	Obstetrical tetanus
A35	Other tetanus
A46	Erysipelas
A55	Chlamydial lymphogranuloma (venereum)
A57	Chancroid
A58	Granuloma inguinale
A64	Unspecified sexually transmitted disease
A65	Nonvenereal syphilis
A70	Chlamydia psittaci infections
A78	Q fever
A86	Unspecified viral encephalitis
A89	Unspecified viral infection of central nervous system
A90	Dengue fever [classical dengue]
A91	Dengue hemorrhagic fever
A94	Unspecified arthropod-borne viral fever
A99	Unspecified viral hemorrhagic fever
B03	Smallpox
B04	Monkeypox
B09	Unspecified viral infection characterized by skin and mucous membrane lesions
B20	Human immunodeficiency virus [HIV] disease
B49	Unspecified mycosis
B54	Unspecified malaria
B59	Pneumocystosis
B64	Unspecified protozoal disease
B72	Dracunculiasis
B75	Trichinellosis
B79	Trichuriasis
B80	Enterobiasis
B86	Scabies
B89	Unspecified parasitic disease
B91	Sequelae of poliomyelitis
B92	Sequelae of leprosy
C01	Malignant neoplasm of base of tongue
C07	Malignant neoplasm of parotid gland
C12	Malignant neoplasm of pyriform sinus
C19	Malignant neoplasm of rectosigmoid junction
C20	Malignant neoplasm of rectum
C23	Malignant neoplasm of gallbladder
C33	Malignant neoplasm of trachea
C37	Malignant neoplasm of thymus
C52	Malignant neoplasm of vagina
C55	Malignant neoplasm of uterus, part unspecified
C58	Malignant neoplasm of placenta
C61	Malignant neoplasm of prostate
C73	Malignant neoplasm of thyroid gland
D34	Benign neoplasm of thyroid gland
D45	Polycythemia vera
D62	Acute posthemorrhagic anemia
D65	Disseminated intravascular coagulation [defibrination syndrome]
D66	Hereditary factor VIII deficiency
D67	Hereditary factor IX deficiency
D71	Functional disorders of polymorphonuclear neutrophils
D77	Other disorders of blood and blood-forming organs in diseases classified elsewhere
E02	Subclinical iodine-deficiency hypothyroidism
E15	Nondiabetic hypoglycemic coma
E35	Disorders of endocrine glands in diseases classified elsewhere
E40	Kwashiorkor
E41	Nutritional marasmus
E42	Marasmic kwashiorkor
E43	Unspecified severe protein-calorie malnutrition
E45	Retarded development following protein-calorie malnutrition
E46	Unspecified protein-calorie malnutrition
E52	Niacin deficiency [pellagra]
E54	Ascorbic acid deficiency
E58	Dietary calcium deficiency
E59	Dietary selenium deficiency
E60	Dietary zinc deficiency
E65	Localized adiposity
E68	Sequelae of hyperalimentation
F04	Amnestic disorder due to known physiological condition
F05	Delirium due to known physiological condition
F09	Unspecified mental disorder due to known physiological condition
F21	Schizotypal disorder
F22	Delusional disorders
F23	Brief psychotic disorder
F24	Shared psychotic disorder
F28	Other psychotic disorder not due to a substance or known physiological condition
F29	Unspecified psychosis not due to a substance or known physiological condition
F39	Unspecified mood [affective] disorder
F54	Psychological and behavioral factors associated with disorders or diseases classified elsewhere
F59	Unspecified behavioral syndromes associated with physiological disturbances and physical factors
F66	Other sexual disorders
F69	Unspecified disorder of adult personality and behavior
F70	Mild intellectual disabilities
F71	Moderate intellectual disabilities
F72	Severe intellectual disabilities
F73	Profound intellectual disabilities
F78	Other intellectual disabilities
F79	Unspecified intellectual disabilities
F82	Specific developmental disorder of motor function
F88	Other disorders of psychological development
F89	Unspecified disorder of psychological development
F99	Mental disorder, not otherwise specified
G01	Meningitis in bacterial diseases classified elsewhere
G02	Meningitis in other infectious and parasitic diseases classified elsewhere
G07	Intracranial and intraspinal abscess and granuloma in diseases classified elsewhere
G08	Intracranial and intraspinal phlebitis and thrombophlebitis
G09	Sequelae of inflammatory diseases of central nervous system
G10	Huntington's disease
G14	Postpolio syndrome
G20	Parkinson's disease
G26	Extrapyramidal and movement disorders in diseases classified elsewhere
G35	Multiple sclerosis
G53	Cranial nerve disorders in diseases classified elsewhere
G55	Nerve root and plexus compressions in diseases classified elsewhere
G59	Mononeuropathy in diseases classified elsewhere
G63	Polyneuropathy in diseases classified elsewhere
G64	Other disorders of peripheral nervous system
G92	Toxic encephalopathy
G94	Other disorders of brain in diseases classified elsewhere
H22	Disorders of iris and ciliary body in diseases classified elsewhere
H28	Cataract in diseases classified elsewhere
H32	Chorioretinal disorders in diseases classified elsewhere
H36	Retinal disorders in diseases classified elsewhere
H42	Glaucoma in diseases classified elsewhere
I00	Rheumatic fever without heart involvement
I10	Essential (primary) hypertension
I32	Pericarditis in diseases classified elsewhere
I38	Endocarditis, valve unspecified

I39	Endocarditis and heart valve disorders in diseases classified elsewhere
I41	Myocarditis in diseases classified elsewhere
I43	Cardiomyopathy in diseases classified elsewhere
I52	Other heart disorders in diseases classified elsewhere
I76	Septic arterial embolism
I81	Portal vein thrombosis
I96	Gangrene, not elsewhere classified
J00	Acute nasopharyngitis (common cold)
J13	Pneumonia due to Streptococcus pneumoniae
J14	Pneumonia due to Hemophilus influenzae
J17	Pneumonia in diseases classified elsewhere
J22	Unspecified acute lower respiratory infection
J36	Peritonsillar abscess
J40	Bronchitis, not specified as acute or chronic
J42	Unspecified chronic bronchitis
J60	Coalworker's pneumoconiosis
J61	Pneumoconiosis due to asbestos and other mineral fibers
J64	Unspecified pneumoconiosis
J65	Pneumoconiosis associated with tuberculosis
J80	Acute respiratory distress syndrome
J82	Pulmonary eosinophilia, not elsewhere classified
J90	Pleural effusion, not elsewhere classified
J99	Respiratory disorders in diseases classified elsewhere
K23	Disorders of esophagus in diseases classified elsewhere
K30	Functional dyspepsia
K36	Other appendicitis
K37	Unspecified appendicitis
K67	Disorders of peritoneum in infectious diseases classified elsewhere
K77	Liver disorders in diseases classified elsewhere
K87	Disorders of gallbladder, biliary tract and pancreas in diseases classified elsewhere
L00	Staphylococcal scalded skin syndrome
L14	Bullous disorders in diseases classified elsewhere
L22	Diaper dermatitis
L26	Exfoliative dermatitis
L42	Pityriasis rosea
L45	Papulosquamous disorders in diseases classified elsewhere
L52	Erythema nodosum
L54	Erythema in diseases classified elsewhere
L62	Nail disorders in diseases classified elsewhere
L80	Vitiligo
L83	Acanthosis nigricans
L84	Corns and callosities
L86	Keratoderma in diseases classified elsewhere
L88	Pyoderma gangrenosum
L99	Other disorders of skin and subcutaneous tissue in diseases classified elsewhere
N08	Glomerular disorders in diseases classified elsewhere
N10	Acute tubulo-interstitial nephritis
N12	Tubulo-interstitial nephritis, not specified as acute or chronic
N16	Renal tubulo-interstitial disorders in diseases classified elsewhere
N19	Unspecified kidney failure
N22	Calculus of urinary tract in diseases classified elsewhere
N23	Unspecified renal colic
N29	Other disorders of kidney and ureter in diseases classified elsewhere
N33	Bladder disorders in diseases classified elsewhere
N37	Urethral disorders in diseases classified elsewhere
N51	Disorders of male genital organs in diseases classified elsewhere
N62	Hypertrophy of breast
N72	Inflammatory disease of cervix uteri
N74	Female pelvic inflammatory disorders in diseases classified elsewhere
N86	Erosion and ectropion of cervix uteri
N96	Recurrent pregnancy loss
O68	Labor and delivery complicated by abnormality of fetal acid-base balance
O76	Abnormality in fetal heart rate and rhythm complicating labor and delivery
O80	Encounter for full-term uncomplicated delivery
O82	Encounter for cesarean delivery without indication
O85	Puerperal sepsis
O94	Sequelae of complication of pregnancy, childbirth, and the puerperium
P09	Abnormal findings on neonatal screening
P53	Hemorrhagic disease of newborn
P60	Disseminated intravascular coagulation of newborn
P84	Other problems with newborn
P90	Convulsions of newborn
P95	Stillbirth
Q02	Microcephaly
R05	Cough
R12	Heartburn
R17	Unspecified jaundice
R21	Rash and other nonspecific skin eruption
R32	Unspecified urinary incontinence
R34	Anuria and oliguria
R37	Sexual dysfunction, unspecified
R42	Dizziness and giddiness
R51	Headache
R52	Pain, unspecified
R54	Age-related physical debility
R55	Syncope and collapse
R58	Hemorrhage, not elsewhere classified
R61	Generalized hyperhidrosis
R64	Cachexia
R69	Illness, unspecified
R75	Inconclusive laboratory evidence of human immunodeficiency virus [HIV]
R81	Glycosuria
R99	Ill-defined and unknown cause of mortality
Y09	Assault by unspecified means
Y66	Nonadministration of surgical and medical care
Y69	Unspecified misadventure during surgical and medical care
Y95	Nosocomial condition
Z08	Encounter for follow-up examination after completed treatment for malignant neoplasm
Z09	Encounter for follow-up examination after completed treatment for conditions other than malignant neoplasm
Z21	Asymptomatic human immunodeficiency virus [HIV] infection status
Z23	Encounter for immunization
Z66	Do not resuscitate

Appendix C: Pharmacology List 2019

This section enables the coder to quickly review drugs, drug actions, and indications that are often associated with overlooked or undocumented diagnoses. The coder should review the patient's medication record and know what condition the physician is treating with the prescribed medication based on documentation in the medical record. When documentation is lacking, the coder can reference this section to locate the drug, determine the drug action, confirm drug indications, and when necessary query the physician.

Drug	Z Code	Drug Action/Classification	Indications
Abilify [aripiprazole]		Antipsychotic	Depression, bipolar disorder, schizophrenia, autism symptoms
Abstral [fentanyl citrate]	Z79.891	Analgesic, narcotic	Breakthrough cancer pain
Acarbose [acarbose]	Z79.84	Oral hypoglycemic	Diabetes mellitus
Accupril [quinapril hydrochloride]		ACE inhibitor	Congestive heart failure; hypertension
Acetaminophen with codeine [acetominophen/codeine phosphate]	Z79.891	Analgesic, narcotic	Pain, moderate to severe
Actemra [tocilizumab]		Antirheumatic	Rheumatoid arthritis
Actimmune [interferon gamma-1b]	Z79.899	Antineoplastic interferons; antiviral interferons	Chronic granulomatous disease; malignant osteopetrosis
Activella [estradiol/norethindrone acetate]	Z79.890	Estrogen therapy	Menopause symptoms; vaginal and vulvar atrophy; osteoporosis prevention
Actonel [risedronate sodium]	Z79.83	Biophosphonate	Decrease in bone loss in multiple myeloma patients; Paget's disease; hyperparathyroidism; osteoporosis
Actoplus Met [metformin hydrochloride/pioglitazone hydrochloride]	Z79.84	Oral hypoglycemic	Diabetes mellitus
Actos [pioglitazone hydrochloride]	Z79.84	Oral hypoglycemic	Diabetes mellitus
Aczone [dapsone]		Acne agent, topical	Acne vulgaris
Adalat CC [nifedipine]		Calcium channel blocker	Vasospastic angina; chronic stable angina; hypertension
Advair [fluticasone propionate/salmeterol xinafoate]	Z79.51	Corticosteroid -inhaled; antiasthmatic	Prophylaxis and treatment of asthma and COPD
Advil [ibuprofen]	Z79.1	Nonsteroidal anti-inflammatory drug (NSAID)	Pain or fever relief
Aerospan [flunisolide]	Z79.51	Corticosteroid -inhaled; antiasthmatic	Prophylaxis and treatment of asthma
Afrezza [human insulin recombinant]	Z79.4	Insulin -inhaled	Diabetes mellitus
Aggrastat [tirofiban hydrochloride]	Z79.02	Antiplatelet	Unstable angina; heart attacks
Aggrenox [aspirin/dipyridamole]	Z79.02	Antiplatelet	Lessening of the chance of heart attack or stroke
Aldactone [spironolactone]		Cardiovascular agent; antihypertensive agent; diuretic; electrolytic and renal agent	Severe heart failure; ascites associated with cirrhosis; hypokalemia
Aleve [naproxen sodium]	Z79.1	Nonsteroidal anti-inflammatory drug (NSAID)	Reduction of temporary aches and pains
Allegra [fexofenadine hydrochloride]		Antihistamine	Seasonal allergic rhinitis
Allopurinol [allopurinol]		Antigout	Gouty arthritis, renal calculus, hyperuricemia, hyperuricemia secondary to leukemia, hyperuricemia secondary to lymphoma
Alora [estradiol]	Z79.890	Estrogen therapy	Menopause symptoms
Alphagan P [brimonidine tartrate]		Antiglaucoma agent (ophthalmic); antihypertensive, ocular	Open angle glaucoma or another condition in which pressure in the eye is too high (ocular hypertension)
Alprazolam [alprazolam]		Antianxiety; sedative/hypnotic	
Altabax [retapamulin]	Z79.2	Antibiotic, topical	Skin infections
Altace [ramipril]		ACE inhibitor	Congestive heart failure; hypertension
Altavera [ethinyl estradiol/levonorgestrel]	Z79.3	Contraceptive	Prevention of pregnancy
Alvesco [ciclesonide]	Z79.51	Corticosteroid -inhaled; antiasthmatic	Prophylaxis and treatment of asthma
Alyacen [ethinyl estradiol/norethindrone]	Z79.3	Contraceptive	Prevention of pregnancy
Amaryl [glimepiride]	Z79.84	Oral hypoglycemic	Diabetes mellitus
Ambien [zolpidem tartrate]		CNS depressant; anoxiolytic/sedative/hypnotic	Insomnia
A-Methapred [methylprednisolone sodium succinate]	Z79.52	Corticosteroid	Severe inflammation
Amikacin [amikacin sulfate]	Z79.2	Antibiotic	Gram-negative bacterial infections such as *Pseudomonas, Escherichia coli (E. coli), Proteus, Klebsiella-Enterobacter-Serratia*

Drug	Z Code	Drug Action/Classification	Indications
Aminophylline [aminophylline]		Bronchodilator, pulmonary vasodilator, smooth muscle relaxant	Relief and/or prevention of symptoms from asthma and reversible bronchospasms in bronchitis and emphysema
Amitriptyline hydrochloride [amitriptyline hydrochloride]		Antidepressant	Depression
Amoxicillin [amoxicillin]	Z79.2	Antibiotic	Treatment of infections with a broad spectrum of bactericidal activity against many gram-positive and gram-negative micro-organisms; otitis media, gonorrhea, skin, respiratory, gastrointestinal, and genitourinary infections
Ampicillin [ampicillin sodium]	Z79.2	Antibiotic	Bacterial infections
Ampyra [dalfampridine]		Potassium channel blocker	Improvement in walking in patients with multiple sclerosis
Amrix [cyclobenzaprine hydrochloride]		Muscle relaxant	Adjunct to rest and physical therapy for muscle spasms
Anaprox [naproxen sodium]	Z79.1	Nonsteroidal anti-inflammatory drug (NSAID)	Pain, inflammation or fever relief
Anastrozole [anastrozole]	Z79.811	Aromatase inhibitor	Postmenopausal breast cancer
Ancef [cefazolin sodium]	Z79.2	Antibiotic	Respiratory tract infections due to *Streptococcus pneumoniae*, *Klebsiella* species, *Haemophilus influenzae (H. influenzae)*, *Staphylococcus aureus*, and group A betahemolytic streptococci; urinary tract infections due to *E. coli, Proteus mirabilis, Klebsiella* species and some strains of Enterobacter and enterococci; skin and skin structure infections, biliary tract infections, bone and joint infections, genital infections, septicemia, and endocarditis
Androderm [testosterone]	Z79.890	Testosterone therapy -topical	Primary hypogonadism, hypogonadotropic hypogonadism
AndroGel [testosterone]	Z79.890	Testosterone therapy -topical	Primary hypogonadism, hypogonadotropic hypogonadism
Angeliq [drospirenone/estradiol]	Z79.890	Estrogen therapy	Menopause symptoms
Angiomax [bivalirudin]	Z79.02	Antithrombotic	Prevention of blood clots
Antabuse [disulfiram]		Alcohol treatment	Alcoholism
Antineoplastic/chemotherapy	Z79.899	Antineoplastic	Cancer
Anzemet [dolasetron mesylate]		Antiemetic/ antinauseant	Nausea/vomiting following surgery or from effects of chemotherapy or cancer
Apidra [insulin glulisine recombinant]	Z79.4	Insulin	Diabetes mellitus
Aranelle [ethinyl estradiol/norethindrone]	Z79.3	Contraceptive	Prevention of pregnancy; acne
Aranesp [darbepoetin alfa]		Erythropoiesis-stimulating agent (ESA)	Treatment of lower than normal blood cells (anemia) from disorders such as CKD and neoplasms
Argatroban [argatroban]	Z79.02	Antithrombotic	Prophylaxis and treatment of venous thrombosis in thrombocytopenia patients
Aricept [donepezil hydrochloride]		Acetylcholinesterase/cholinesterase inhibitors	Symptoms of mild to moderate Alzheimer's disease; can improve thinking ability in some patients
Arimidex [anastrozole]	Z79.811	Aromatase inhibitor	Postmenopausal breast cancer
Aristospan [triamcinolone hexacetonide]	Z79.52	Corticosteroid	Severe inflammation
Arixtra [fondaparinux sodium]	Z79.01	Anticoagulant	Venous thrombosis and pulmonary embolism
Arnuity Ellipta [fluticasone furoate]	Z79.51	Corticosteroid -inhaled; antiasthmatic	Prophylaxis and treatment of asthma
Aromasin [exemestane]	Z79.811	Aromatase inhibitor	Postmenopausal breast cancer
Arthrotec [diclofenac sodium/misoprostol]	Z79.1	Non-steroidal anti-inflammatory drug (NSAID)-prostaglandin combo	Treatment of patients with arthritis who may develop stomach ulcers from taking nonsteroidal anti-inflammatory drugs (NSAIDs) alone; used to help relieve some symptoms of arthritis, such as inflammation, swelling, stiffness, and joint pain
Asacol HD [mesalamine]		Antiinflammatory	Ulcerative colitis
Ashlyna [ethinyl estradiol/levonorgestrel]	Z79.3	Contraceptive	Prevention of pregnancy
Asmanex [mometasone furoate]	Z79.51	Corticosteroid -inhaled; antiasthmatic	Prophylaxis and treatment of asthma
Astagraf XL [tacrolimus]	Z79.899	Immunosuppressant	Prophylaxis of organ transplant rejection
Astramorph [morphine sulfate]	Z79.891	Analgesic, narcotic	Pain
Atelvia [risedronate sodium]	Z79.83	Bisphosphonate	Prevention of thinning of the bones (osteoporosis)
Atenolol [atenolol]		Beta blocker	Angina pectoris; hypertension; acute myocardial infarction
Ativan [lorazepam]		Antianxiety; sedative/hypnotic	Anxiety disorder associated with depressive symptoms; controls tension, agitation, irritability, and insomnia
Atrovent [ipratropium bromide]		Antiasthmatic/bronchodilator	Chronic bronchitis, emphysema; bronchial asthma

Drug	Z Code	Drug Action/Classification	Indications
Augmentin [amoxicillin/clavulanate potassium]	Z79.2	Antibiotic	Middle ear, lower respiratory, sinus, skin and skin structures, and urinary tract infections
Avandamet [rosiglitazone maleate/metformin hydrochloride]	Z79.84	Oral hypoglycemic	Diabetes mellitus
Avandia [rosiglitazone maleate]	Z79.84	Oral hypoglycemic	Diabetes mellitus
Avapro [irbesartan]		Antihypertensive	Hypertension
Avelox [moxifloxacin hydrochloride]	Z79.2	Antibiotic	Bacterial infections, specifically pneumonia; skin; intra-abdominal; plague; acute sinusitis; acute chronic bronchitis
Aviane [ethinyl estradiol/levonorgestrel]	Z79.3	Contraceptive	Prevention of pregnancy
Avonex [interferon beta-1a]	Z79.899	Antiviral	Treatment of relapsing multiple sclerosis
Axid AR [nizatidine]		Histamine H2-receptor antagonist	Acid/peptic disorder; gastroesophageal reflux; duodenal, gastric, and peptic ulcers
Aygestin [norethindrone acetate]	Z79.3	Contraceptive	Prevention of pregnancy; menstrual disorders
Azactam [aztreonam]	Z79.2	Antibiotic	Severe bacterial infections
Azithromycin [azithromycin]	Z79.2	Antibiotic	Bacterial infections
Bactrim [sulfamethoxazole/trimethoprim]	Z79.2	Antibiotic	Treatment of urinary tract infections, acute otitis media, acute exacerbation of chronic bronchitis, shigellosis, and *pneumocystis carinii*
Bactroban [mupirocin]	Z79.2	Antibiotic, topical	Impetigo; *Staphylococcus* infection of skin
Balziva [ethinyl estradiol/norethindrone]	Z79.3	Contraceptive	Prevention of pregnancy
Basaglar [insulin glargine]	Z79.4	Insulin	Diabetes mellitus
Bayer [acetylsalicylic acid]	Z79.82	Aspirin	Prophylaxis and treatment of heart attacks, angina or strokes; reduction of fever, pain and inflammation
Beconase AQ [beclomethasone dipropionate monohydrate]		Corticosteroid -inhaled/nasal	Perennial and seasonal allergies; vasomotor rhinitis
Bekyree [desogestrel/ethinyl estradiol]	Z79.3	Contraceptive	Prevention of pregnancy
Betoptic [betaxolol hydrochloride]		Beta blocker; ophthalmic glaucoma agent	Lowering of intraocular pressure; also used for treatment of ocular hypertension and chronic open-angle glaucoma
Beyaz [drospirenone/ethinyl estradiol/levomefolate calcium]	Z79.3	Contraceptive	Prevention of pregnancy; acne
Biaxin [clarithromycin]	Z79.2	Antibiotic	Acid/peptic disorder or ulcer, acute exacerbation chronic bronchitis, human immunodeficiency virus, lower and upper respiratory tract infection, sinus infection, prophylaxis mycobacterium avium complex, pharyngitis, pneumonia, tonsillitis
Biltricide [praziquantel]		Antiparasitic	Infections from Schistosoma species and liver flukes
Binosto [alendronate sodium]	Z79.83	Bisphosphonate	Prevention of thinning of the bones (osteoporosis)
Boniva [ibandronate sodium]	Z79.83	Bisphosphonate	Prevention of thinning of the bones (osteoporosis)
Brevicon [ethinyl estradiol/norethindrone]	Z79.3	Contraceptive	Prevention of pregnancy; acne
Briellyn [ethinyl estradiol/norethindrone]	Z79.3	Contraceptive	Prevention of pregnancy
Brilinta [ticagrelor]	Z79.02	Antiplatelet	Unstable angina; heart attacks; prevention of blood clots
Brisdelle [paroxetine]		Selective serotonin reuptake inhibitor (SSRI)	Vasomotor symptoms related to menopause
Buprenex [buprenorphine hydrochloride]	Z79.891	Analgesic, narcotic	Moderate to severe pain
Buprenorphine HCl [buprenorphine hydrochloride]	Z79.891	Analgesic, narcotic	Moderate to severe pain
Buspirone [buspirone hydrochloride]		Antianxiety	Generalized anxiety disorder
Butorphanol tartrate [butorphanol tartrate]	Z79.891	Analgesic, narcotic	Moderate to severe postsurgical pain
Butrans [buprenorphine]	Z79.891	Analgesic, narcotic	Chronic pain
Calan [verapamil hydrochloride]		Calcium channel blocker	Angina pectoris at rest and chronic stable, arrhythmia, atrial fibrillation, atrial flutter, paroxysmal supraventricular tachycardia, ventricular arrhythmia, Hypertension
Caldolor [ibuprofen]	Z79.1	Nonsteroidal anti-inflammatory drug (NSAID)	Pain or fever relief
Cambia [diclofenac potassium]	Z79.1	Nonsteroidal anti-inflammatory drug (NSAID)	Migraine headaches
Camila [norethindrone]	Z79.3	Contraceptive	Prevention of pregnancy; menstrual disorders

Drug	Z Code	Drug Action/Classification	Indications
Cardizem CD [diltiazem hydrochloride]		Calcium channel blocker	Chronic stable angina, atrial fibrillation, atrial flutter, hypertension, paroxysmal supraventricular tachycardia
Cardura [doxazosin mesylate]		Antihypertensive	Benign prostatic hyperplasia; hypertension
Catapres [clonidine hydrochloride]		Antihypertensive	Hypertension
Cefprozil [cefprozil]	Z79.2	Antibiotic	Acute exacerbation and chronic bronchitis, lower respiratory tract infection, upper respiratory tract infection, pharyngitis, tonsillitis
Ceftin [cefuroxime axetil]	Z79.2	Antibiotic	Acute exacerbation and chronic bronchitis, middle ear infection, sexually transmitted gonorrhea infection, upper respiratory tract infection, urinary tract infection, pharyngitis, tonsillitis
Ceftriaxone [ceftriaxone sodium]	Z79.2	Antibiotic	Bacterial infections
Celebrex [celecoxib]	Z79.1	Nonsteroidal anti-inflammatory drug (NSAID)	Relief of some symptoms caused by arthritis, such as inflammation, swelling, stiffness, and joint pain
Celestone Soluspan [betamethasone acetate/betamethasone sodium phosphate]	Z79.52	Corticosteroid; antiasthmatic	Asthma; severe inflammation
Celexa [citalopram hydrobromide]		Antidepressant	Depression
Cellcept [mycophenolate mofetil]	Z79.899	Immunosuppressant	Prophylaxis of organ transplant rejection
Centany [mupirocin]	Z79.2	Antibiotic	Skin infections
Cephalexin [cephalexin]	Z79.2	Antibiotic	Bacterial infections
Chantix [varenicline tartrate]		Smoking cessation aid	Nicotine addiction, smoking
Cipro [ciprofloxacin hydrochloride]	Z79.2	Antibiotic	Cystitis, infectious diarrhea, gonorrhea, bone and joint infection, gastrointestinal tract infection, lower and upper respiratory tract infection, sinus infection, urinary tract infection, nosocomial pneumonia, chronic prostatitis
Ciprofloxacin [ciprofloxacin]	Z79.2	Antibiotic	Bacterial infections
Clarithromycin [clarithromycin]	Z79.2	Antibiotic	Skin and respiratory bacterial infections
Claritin [loratadine]		Antihistamine	Seasonal allergic rhinitis; chronic idiopathic urticaria
Cleocin [clindamycin phosphate]	Z79.2	Antibiotic	Bacterial infections
Climara [estradiol]	Z79.890	Estrogen therapy	Osteoporosis prevention and to treat menopausal symptoms; vaginal and vulvar atrophy; hypoestrogenism; ovarian failure
Clindamycin [clindamycin phosphate]	Z79.2	Antibiotic	Bacterial infections
Clonazepam [clonazepam]		Anticonvulsant	Absence, akinetic and myoclonic epilepsy, Lennox-Gastaut syndrome
Clonidine [clonidine hydrochloride]		Antihypertensive	Hypertension
Clopidogrel bisulfate [clopidogrel bisulfate]	Z79.02	Antiplatelet	Unstable angina; heart attacks; prevention of blood clots
Codeine [codeine sulfate]	Z79.891	Analgesic, narcotic	Mild to moderate pain
Cogentin [benztropine mesylate]		Antiparkinsonism	Parkinson's disease
Colace [docusate sodium]		Gastrointestinal agent; laxative, stool softener	Constipation
Colocort [hydrocortisone]	Z79.52	Corticosteroid	Inflammation of the colon
CombiPatch [ethinyl estradiol/norethindrone acetate]	Z79.890	Estrogen therapy	Menopause symptoms; vaginal and vulvar atrophy; osteoporosis prevention
Combivent [ipratropium bromide/albuterol sulfate]		Antiasthmatic/bronchodilator	Chronic bronchitis, emphysema; bronchial asthma
Compro [prochlorperazine]		Antiemetic; antipsychotic	Nausea, vomiting, and manic phase of bipolar syndrome or schizophrenia
Copaxone [glatiramer acetate]		Immunostimulant	Multiple sclerosis
Coreg [carvedilol]		Beta blocker	Hypertension; chronic heart failure; left ventricular dysfunction following myocardial infarction
Coreg CR [carvedilol phosphate]		Beta blocker	Hypertension; chronic heart failure; left ventricular dysfunction following myocardial infarction
Cortef [hydrocortisone]	Z79.52	Corticosteroid	Severe inflammation
Cortenema [hydrocortisone]	Z79.52	Corticosteroid	Inflammation of the colon
Cortifoam [hydrocortisone acetate]	Z79.52	Corticosteroid	Colon and rectum inflammation
Cortisone acetate [cortisone acetate]	Z79.52	Corticosteroid	Inflammation
Cortisporin [hydrocortisone acetate/neomycin sulfate/polymyxin B sulfate]		Topical anti-infective, topical steroid	Dermatosis

Drug	Z Code	Drug Action/Classification	Indications
Coumadin [warfarin sodium]	Z79.Ø1	Anticoagulant	Prophylaxis and treatment of venous thrombosis, treatment of atrial fibrillation with embolization (pulmonary embolism), arrhythmias, myocardial infarction, and stroke prevention
Cozaar [losartan potassium]		Antihypertensive	Hypertension
Crestor [rosuvastatin calcium]		HMG-CoA reductase inhibitor (statin)	Hypercholesterolemia; hyperlipidemia; hyperproteinemia
Crixivan [indinavir sulfate]		HIV inhibitor	HIV, asymptomatic HIV
Cryselle [ethinyl estradiol/norgestrel]	Z79.3	Contraceptive	Prevention of pregnancy
Cyclafem [ethinyl estradiol/norethindrone]	Z79.3	Contraceptive	Prevention of pregnancy
Cyclessa [desogestrel/ethinyl estradiol]	Z79.3	Contraceptive	Prevention of pregnancy
Cyclosporine [cyclosporine]	Z79.899	Immunosuppressant	Prophylaxis of organ transplant rejection
Cymbalta [duloxetine]		Antidepressant, serotonin and norepinephrine reuptake inhibitor (SNRI)	Major depressive disorder; general anxiety disorder; fibromyalgia; diabetic peripheral neuropathy; chronic musculoskeletal pain
Cytomel [liothyronine sodium]		Thyroid hormone	Hypothyroidism or prevention of euthyroid goiters
Daptomycin [daptomycin]	Z79.2	Antibiotic	Skin and underlying tissue bacterial infections
Dasetta [ethinyl estradiol/norethindrone]	Z79.3	Contraceptive	Prevention of pregnancy
Daypro [oxaprozin]	Z79.1	Nonsteroidal anti-inflammatory drug (NSAID)	Osteoarthritis and rheumatoid arthritis
Daysee [ethinyl estradiol/levonorgestrel]	Z79.3	Contraceptive	Prevention of pregnancy
Delestrogen [estradiol valerate]	Z79.89Ø	Estrogen therapy	Menopause symptoms
Demerol [meperidine hydrochloride]	Z79.891	Analgesic, narcotic	Moderate to severe pain
Depakote [divalproex sodium]		Anticonvulsant	Bipolar affective disorder; complex absence, complex partial and mixed pattern epilepsy; migraine headache
Depo-Medrol [methylprednisolone acetate]	Z79.52	Corticosteroid	Arthritis; joint disorders
Depo-Provera [medroxyprogesterone acetate]	Z79.3, Z79.89Ø	Antineoplastic; contraceptive; progestin	Amenorrhea; carcinoma, endometrium, adjunct; carcinoma, renal; Prevention of pregnancy; hemorrhage
Depo-SubQ Provera [medroxyprogesterone acetate]	Z79.3	Contraceptive	Prevention of pregnancy; menstrual disorder pain
Desogen [desogestrel/ethinyl estradiol]	Z79.3	Contraceptive	Prevention of pregnancy
Detrol [tolterodine tartrate]		Muscarinic receptor antagonist	Overactive bladders in patients with urinary frequency, urgency, or urge incontinence
Dexamethasone Intensol [dexamethasone]	Z79.52	Corticosteroid	Arthritis; allergic disorders; breathing disorders; lupus
Dexilant [dexlansoprazole]		Proton pump inhibitor	Healing of erosive esophagitis; relieve of heartburn; treatment of non-erosive gastroesophageal reflux disease
Diabinese [chlorpropamide]	Z79.84	Oral hypoglycemic	Diabetes mellitus
Diaβeta [glyburide]	Z79.84	Oral hypoglycemic	Diabetes mellitus
Diclegis [doxylamine succinate/pyridoxine hydrochloride]		Antiemetic	Nausea/vomiting in pregnancy
Didronel [etidronate disodium]	Z79.83	Bisphosphonate	Paget's disease and irregular bone growth
Dificid [fidaxomicin]	Z79.2	Antibiotic	*Clostridium difficile*
Diflucan [fluconazole]		Antifungal	Oropharyngeal and esophageal candidiasis and cryptococcal meningitis in AIDS patients
Digoxin [digoxin]		Cardiotonic glycoside	Heart failure, atrial flutter, atrial fibrillation, and supraventricular tachycardia
Dilantin [phenytoin sodium]		Anticonvulsant	Grand mal and psychomotor seizures
Dilaudid [hydromorphone hydrochloride]	Z79.891	Analgesic, narcotic	Moderate to severe pain
Diovan [valsartan]		ACE inhibitor	Hypertension
Divigel [estradiol]	Z79.89Ø	Estrogen therapy -topical	Menopause symptoms
Dolophine HCl [methadone hydrochloride]	Z79.891	Analgesic, narcotic	Pain; treatment of opioid addiction
Doxycycline [doxycycline]	Z79.2	Antibiotic	Bacterial infections; acne
Duavee [bazedoxifene acetate/conjugated estrogens]	Z79.89Ø	Estrogen therapy	Menopause symptoms; osteoporosis prevention

Appendix C: Pharmacology List 2019

Drug	Z Code	Drug Action/Classification	Indications
Duetact [glimepiride/pioglitazone hydrochloride]	Z79.84	Oral hypoglycemic	Diabetes mellitus
Duexis [famotidine/ibuprofen]	Z79.1	Nonsteroidal anti-inflammatory drug (NSAID)	Symptomatic treatment of osteoarthritis and rheumatoid arthritis; reduce risk of ulcers
Dulera [formoterol fumarate/mometasone furoate]	Z79.51	Corticosteroid -inhaled; antiasthmatic	Prophylaxis and treatment of asthma
Duragesic [fentanyl]	Z79.891	Analgesic, narcotic	Chronic pain
Duramorph [morphine sulfate]	Z79.891	Analgesic, narcotic	Moderate to severe pain
Durlaza [aspirin]	Z79.82	Aspirin	Prevention of heart attack, stroke, angina
Dyloject [diclofenac sodium]	Z79.1	Nonsteroidal anti-inflammatory drug (NSAID)	Pain relief
Dynacin [minocycline hydrochloride]	Z79.2	Antibiotic	Severe acne treatment
E.E.S. [erythromycin ethylsuccinate]	Z79.2	Antibiotic	Bacterial infections
Effexor XR [venlafaxine hydrochloride]		Antidepressant, serotonin and norepinephrine reuptake inhibitors (SNRIs)	Major depressive disorder; social anxiety disorder; panic disorder
Effient [prasugrel hydrochloride]	Z79.02	Antiplatelet	Lessening of the chance of heart attack or stroke
Elestrin [estradiol]	Z79.890	Estrogen therapy	Menopause symptoms
Eligard [leuprolide acetate]	Z79.818	Agents affecting estrogen receptors and estrogen levels	Palliative treatment of prostate cancer symptoms
Elinest [norgestrel/ethinyl estradiol]	Z79.3	Contraceptive	Prevention of pregnancy
Eliquis [apixaban]	Z79.01	Anticoagulant	Venous thrombosis
Embeda [morphine sulfate/naltrexone hydrochloride]	Z79.891	Analgesic, narcotic	Moderate to severe pain
Emoquette [ethinyl estradiol/desogestrel]	Z79.3	Contraceptive	Prevention of pregnancy
Enbrel [etanercept]	Z79.899	Antirheumatic	Rheumatoid arthritis; polyarticular juvenile idiopathic arthritis; psoriatic arthritis; ankylosing spondylitis, plaque psoriasis
Enpresse [ethinyl estradiol/levonorgestrel]	Z79.3	Contraceptive	Prevention of pregnancy
Enskyce [desogestrel/ethinyl estradiol]	Z79.3	Contraceptive	Prevention of pregnancy
Entocort EC [budesonide]	Z79.52	Corticosteroid	Crohn's disease; ulcerative colitis
Entyvio [vedolizumab]	Z79.899	Immunosuppressant	Ulcerative colitis; Crohn's disease
Envarsus XR [tacrolimus]	Z79.899	Immunosuppressant	Prophylaxis of organ transplant rejection
Epinephrine [epinephrine]		Bronchodilator, cardiotonic	Most commonly, relief of distress due to bronchospasm and restoration of cardiac rhythm in cardiac arrest
Epivir, Epivir-HBV [lamivudine]		HIV and HBV inhibitor	HIV, hepatitis B (HBV), asymptomatic HIV
Errin [norethindrone]	Z79.3	Contraceptive	Prevention of pregnancy
Ertapenem [ertapenem sodium]	Z79.2	Antibiotic	Stomach, urinary tract, pelvis, skin and lung infections
ERYC [erythromycin]	Z79.2	Antibiotic	Respiratory tract infections
Erygel [erythromycin]	Z79.2	Antibiotic, topical	Bacterial skin infections
EryPed [erythromycin ethylsuccinate]	Z79.2	Antibiotic	Bacterial infections; rheumatic fever attacks
Ery-Tab [erythromycin]	Z79.2	Antibiotic	Bacterial infections
Erythrocin [erythromycin lactobionate]	Z79.2	Antibiotic	Bacterial infections
Erythromycin [erythromycin]	Z79.2	Antibiotic	Respiratory tract infections
Estarylla [ethinyl estradiol/norgestimate]	Z79.3	Contraceptive	Prevention of pregnancy
Estrace [estradiol]	Z79.890	Estrogen therapy	Vaginal cream for treatment of vaginal and vulvar atrophy
Estraderm [estradiol]	Z79.890	Estrogen therapy	Osteoporosis prevention and to treat menopausal symptoms, vaginal and vulvar atrophy, hypoestrogenism, ovarian failure
Estrasorb [estradiol hemihydrate]	Z79.890	Estrogen therapy -topical	Menopause symptoms
EstroGel [estradiol]	Z79.890	Estrogen therapy -topical	Menopause symptoms
Estrostep Fe [ethinyl estradiol/norethindrone acetate]	Z79.3	Contraceptive	Prevention of pregnancy
Evista [raloxifene hydrochloride]	Z79.810	Selective estrogen receptor modulator (SERM)	Prevention of thinning of the bones (osteoporosis) only in postmenopausal women
Exalgo [hydromorphone hydrochloride]	Z79.891	Analgesic, narcotic	Moderate to severe pain
Exemestane [exemestane]	Z79.811	Aromatase inhibitor	Postmenopausal breast cancer
Factive [gemifloxacin mesylate]	Z79.2	Antibiotic	Bacterial lung infections

Drug	Z Code	Drug Action/Classification	Indications
Falmina [ethinyl estradiol/levonorgestrel]	Z79.3	Contraceptive	Prevention of pregnancy
Fareston [toremifene citrate]	Z79.810	Selective estrogen receptor modulator (SERM)	Treatment of metastatic breast cancer in postmenopausal women
Farxiga [dapagliflozin propanediol]	Z79.84	Oral hypoglycemic	Diabetes mellitus
Faslodex [fulvestrant]	Z79.818	Agents affecting estrogen receptors and estrogen levels	Hormone-related breast cancer; metastatic breast cancer
Feldene [piroxicam]	Z79.1	Nonsteroidal anti-inflammatory drug (NSAID)	Treatment of pain and inflammation due to arthritis
Femara [letrozole]	Z79.811	Aromatase inhibitor	Postmenopausal breast cancer
Femcon Fe [ethinyl estradiol/norethindrone]	Z79.3	Contraceptive	Prevention of pregnancy; acne
Femhrt [ethinyl estradiol/norethindrone acetate]	Z79.3, Z79.890	Contraceptive; estrogen therapy	Prevention of pregnancy; menopause symptoms; osteoporosis prevention
Femring [estradiol acetate]	Z79.890	Estrogen therapy	Osteoporosis prevention and to treat menopausal symptoms; hypoestrogenism; ovarian failure
Femtrace [estradiol acetate]	Z79.890	Estrogen therapy	Menopause symptoms
Fentanyl [fentanyl]	Z79.891	Analgesic, narcotic	Postprocedural or chronic pain
Fentora [fentanyl citrate]	Z79.891	Analgesic, narcotic	Breakthrough cancer pain
Fioricet with codeine [acetaminophen/butalbital/caffeine/codeine phosphate]	Z79.891	Analgesic, narcotic	Tension headaches
Flagyl [metronidazole]	Z79.2	Antibiotic	Bacterial infections
Flavoxate hydrochloride [flavoxate hydrochloride]		Urinary tract spasmolytic	Relief of dysuria, urgency, nocturia, suprapubic pain, frequency, and incontinence associated with cystitis, prostatitis, urethritis, and urethrocystitis/urethrotrigonitis
Flomax [tamsulosin hydrochloride]		Antiadrenergic	Benign prostatic hyperplasia
Flonase allergy relief [fluticasone propionate]		Corticosteroid -inhaled/nasal	Perennial and seasonal allergic rhinitis
Flovent HFA [fluticasone propionate]	Z79.51	Corticosteroid -inhaled; antiasthmatic	Asthma
Fortamet [metformin hydrochloride]	Z79.84	Oral hypoglycemic	Diabetes mellitus
Fortaz [ceftazidime]	Z79.2	Antibiotic	Pneumonia and lower respiratory infections
Fosamax [alendronate sodium]	Z79.83	Biophosphonate	Osteoporosis; Paget's disease
Fosinopril sodium [fosinopril sodium]		ACE inhibitor	Hypertension
Fosrenol [lanthanum carbonate]		Phosphate binder	End-stage renal disease (ESRD)
Fragmin [dalteparin sodium]	Z79.01	Anticoagulant	Prophylaxis and treatment of blood clots
Fulyzaq [crofelemer]		Antidiarrheal	Diarrhea occurring in HIV/AIDs patient's on anti-retroviral therapy
Gengraf [cyclosporine]	Z79.899	Immunosuppressant	Prophylaxis of organ transplant rejection
Gentamicin sulfate [gentamicin sulfate]	Z79.2	Antibiotic	Severe bacterial infections
Gildagia [ethinyl estradiol/norethindrone]	Z79.3	Contraceptive	Prevention of pregnancy
Gildess [ethinyl estradiol/norethindrone acetate]	Z79.3	Contraceptive	Prevention of pregnancy
Glimepiride [glimepiride]	Z79.84	Oral hypoglycemic	Diabetes mellitus
Glucophage [metformin hydrochloride]	Z79.84	Oral hypoglycemic	Diabetes mellitus
Glucotrol [glipizide]	Z79.84	Oral hypoglycemic	Diabetes mellitus
Glucovance [glyburide/metformin hydrochloride]	Z79.84	Oral hypoglycemic	Diabetes mellitus
Glumetza [metformin hydrochloride]	Z79.84	Oral hypoglycemic	Diabetes mellitus
Glyburide (micronized) [glyburide]	Z79.84	Oral hypoglycemic	Diabetes mellitus
Glynase [glyburide]	Z79.84	Oral hypoglycemic	Diabetes mellitus
Glyset [miglitol]	Z79.84	Oral hypoglycemic	Diabetes mellitus
Harvoni [ledipasvir/sofosbuvir]	Z79.899	Antiviral	Chronic hepatitis C
Heparin sodium [heparin sodium]	Z79.01	Anticoagulant	Prophylaxis and treatment of venous thrombosis, pulmonary embolism; prevention of cerebral thrombosis, and treatment of consumptive coagulopathies
Humalog [insulin lispro recombinant]	Z79.4	Insulin	Diabetes mellitus

Drug	Z Code	Drug Action/Classification	Indications
Humira [adalimumab]	Z79.899	Antirheumatic	Rheumatoid arthritis; juvenile idiopathic arthritis; psoriatic arthritis; Crohn's disease; ulcerative colitis; plaque psoriasis; hidradenitis suppurativa; uveitis
Humulin [insulin recombinant]	Z79.4	Insulin	Diabetes mellitus
Hydrochlorothiazide [hydrochlorothiazide]		Diuretic; antihypertensive	Management of hypertension and in adjunctive therapy for edema associated with congestive heart failure; hepatic cirrhosis; corticosteroid, and estrogen therapy
Hydrocodone [acetaminophen/hydrocodone bitartrate]	Z79.891	Analgesic, narcotic	Moderate to severe pain
Hydrocodone bitartrate and acetaminophen [acetaminophen/ hydrocodone bitartrate]	Z79.891	Analgesic, narcotic	Pain, moderate to severe
Hydrocortisone [hydrocortisone]	Z79.52	Corticosteroid	Addison's disease; arthritis; immune disorders; allergies; breathing problems
Hydromorphone HCl [hydromorphone hydrochloride]	Z79.891	Analgesic, narcotic	Moderate to severe pain
Hyzaar [hydrochlorothiazide/ losartan potassium]		Antihypertensive	Hypertension
Ibuprofen [ibuprofen]	Z79.1	Nonsteroidal anti-inflammatory drug (NSAID)	Pain or fever relief
Imitrex [sumatriptan succinate]		Antimigraine	Migraine headache
Imuran [azathioprine]	Z79.899	Immunosuppressant	Rheumatoid arthritis
Inderal [propranolol hydrochloride]		Beta blocker	Angina pectoris; hypertension; cardiac arrhythmias
Indocin [indomethacin]	Z79.1	Nonsteroidal anti-inflammatory drug (NSAID)	Treatment of pain and inflammation
Integrilin [eptifibatide]	Z79.02	Antiplatelet	Unstable angina; heart attacks; prevention of blood clots
Intron [interferon alfa 2-b]	Z79.899	Antineoplastic interferons; antiviral interferons	Cancer; hepatitis
Introvale [levonorgestrel/ethinyl estradiol]	Z79.3	Contraceptive	Prevention of pregnancy
Invanz [ertapeneum sodium]	Z79.2	Antibiotic	Stomach, urinary tract, pelvis, skin and lung infections
Invokamet [canagliflozin/metformin hydrochloride]	Z79.84	Oral hypoglycemic	Diabetes mellitus
Invokana [canagliflozin]	Z79.84	Oral hypoglycemic	Diabetes mellitus
Iprivask [desirudin recombinant]	Z79.02	Antithrombotic	Prophylaxis and treatment of venous thrombosis and pulmonary embolism
Isoniazid [isoniazid]	Z79.2	Antibiotic	Tuberculosis
Isopto carpine [pilocarpine hydrochloride]		Cholinergic parasympathomimetic agent	Reduction of intraocular pressure in open-angle glaucoma or ocular hypertension; management of acute angle-closure glaucoma
Isordil [isosorbide dinitrate]		Smooth muscle relaxant	Acute anginal attacks
Isuprel [isoproterenol hydrochloride]		Adrenergic agent	Bronchodilator for asthma, chronic pulmonary emphysema, bronchitis, and other conditions accompanied by bronchospasm; can be used in cardiogenic shock cases
Jantoven [warfarin sodium]	Z79.01	Anticoagulant	Prophylaxis and treatment of venous thrombosis, pulmonary embolism; prevention of cerebral thrombosis, and treatment of consumptive coagulopathies
Janumet [metformin hydrochloride/sitagliptin phosphate]	Z79.84	Oral hypoglycemic	Diabetes mellitus
Januvia [sitagliptin phosphate]	Z79.84	Oral hypoglycemic	Diabetes mellitus
Jencycla [norethindrone]	Z79.3	Contraceptive	Prevention of pregnancy
Jentadueto [linagliptin/metformin hydrochloride]]	Z79.84	Oral hypoglycemic	Diabetes mellitus
Junel [ethinyl estradiol/norethindrone acetate]	Z79.3	Contraceptive	Prevention of pregnancy
Kadian [morphine sulfate]	Z79.891	Analgesic, narcotic	Moderate to severe pain
Kariva [desogestrel/ethinyl estradiol]	Z79.3	Contraceptive	Prevention of pregnancy
Kazano [alogliptin benzoate/metformin hydrochloride]	Z79.84	Oral hypoglycemic	Diabetes mellitus
Keflex [cephalexin]	Z79.2	Antibiotic	Bone, middle ear, skin and skin structures, upper respiratory tract and urinary tract infections; acute prostatitis

Drug	Z Code	Drug Action/Classification	Indications
Kefzol [cefazolin sodium]	Z79.2	Antibiotic	Skin, ear, urinary tract and upper respiratory bacterial infections
Kelnor [ethynodiol diacetate/ethinyl estradiol]	Z79.3	Contraceptive	Prevention of pregnancy
Kenalog-10; Kenalog-40 [triamcinolone acetonide]	Z79.52	Corticosteroid	Gouty arthritis; bursitis; tenosynovitis; epicondylitis; rheumatoid arthritis; synovitis; osteoarthritis
Kimidess [ethinyl estradiol/desogestrel]	Z79.3	Contraceptive	Prevention of pregnancy
Klaron [sulfacetamide sodium]	Z79.2	Antibiotic, topical	Acne vulgaris
Klonopin [clonazepam]		Anticonvulsant; CNS depressant	Epilepsy; seizures; panic disorder
Klor-Con [potassium chloride]		Replaces potassium and maintains potassium level	Hypokalemia
Kombiglyze [metformin hydrochloride/saxagliptin hydrochloride]	Z79.84	Oral hypoglycemic	Diabetes mellitus
K-Tab [potassium chloride]		Replaces potassium and maintains potassium level	Hypokalemia
Kurvelo [ethinyl estradiol/levonorgestrel]	Z79.3	Contraceptive	Prevention of pregnancy; menstrual disorders
Kyleena [levonorgestrel]	Z79.3	Contraceptive	Prevention of pregnancy
Lamisil [terbinafine hydrochloride]		Antifungal	*Tinea cruris* (jock itch), *T. pedis* (athlete's foot), *T. corporis* (ringworm)
Lanoxin [digoxin]		Cardiotonic glycoside	Congestive heart failure
Lantus [insulin glargine recombinant]	Z79.4	Insulin	Diabetes mellitus
Larin [ethinyl estradiol/norethindrone acetate]	Z79.3	Contraceptive	Prevention of pregnancy
Lasix [furosemide]		Antihypertensive; diuretic	Management of edema associated with congestive heart failure, renal disease, including nephrotic syndrome and hypertension
Lescol [fluvastatin sodium]		HMG-CoA reductase inhibitor (statin)	Hypercholesterolemia; hyperlipidemia; hyperlipoproteinemia
Lessina [ethinyl estradiol/levonorgestrel]	Z79.3	Contraceptive	Prevention of pregnancy
Letrozole [letrozole]	Z79.811	Aromatase inhibitor	Postmenopausal breast cancer
Levaquin [levofloxacin]	Z79.2	Antibiotic	Acute exacerbation chronic bronchitis; cellulitis; furuncle; impetigo; infections of the lower and upper respiratory tract, sinus, skin and skin structures, and urinary tract; pneumonia, community-acquired; pyoderma
Levemir [insulin detemir recombinant]	Z79.4	Insulin	Diabetes mellitus
Levonest [levonorgestrel/ethinyl estradiol]	Z79.3	Contraceptive	Prevention of pregnancy; menstrual disorders; acne
Levora [levonorgestrel/ethinyl estradiol]	Z79.3	Contraceptive	Prevention of pregnancy
Levothroid [levothyroxine sodium]		Thyroid hormone	Hypothyroidism
Levoxyl [levothyroxine sodium]		Thyroid hormone	Euthyroid goiter; hypothyroidism
Lexapro [escitalopram oxalate]		Antidepressant, selective serotonin reuptake inhibitor (SSRI)	Depression; anxiety
Lialda [mesalamine]		Antiinflammatory	Ulcerative colitis
Librium [chlordiazepoxide hydrochloride]		Antianxiety	Acute withdrawal symptoms, especially from alcohol, or for other anxiety-producing conditions
Lidocaine hydrochloride [lidocaine hydrochloride]		Antiarrhythmic	Management of ventricular arrhythmias or during cardiac manipulation, such as cardiac surgery
Liletta [levonorgestrel]	Z79.3	Contraceptive	Intrauterine device to Prevention of pregnancy
Lincocin [lincocin hydrochloride]	Z79.2	Antibiotic	Severe bacterial infections
Lipitor [atorvastatin calcium]		HMG-CoA reductase inhibitor (statin)	Hypercholesterolemia; hyperlipidemia; hyperproteinemia
Lithium [lithium carbonate]		Antimanic	Control of manic episodes in bipolar disorders
Lo Loestrin Fe [ethinyl estradiol/norethindrone acetate]	Z79.3	Contraceptive	Prevention of pregnancy
Lo Minastrin Fe [ethinyl estradiol/norethindrone acetate]	Z79.3	Contraceptive	Prevention of pregnancy
Locoid [hydrocotisone butyrate]	Z79.52	Corticosteroid -topical	Atopic dermatitis; other dermatoses
Loestrin [ethinyl estradiol/norethindrone acetate]	Z79.3	Contraceptive	Prevention of pregnancy
Lomotil [diphenoxylate hydrochloride/atropine sulfate]		Antidiarrheal	Symptoms of chronic and functional diarrhea

Drug	Z Code	Drug Action/Classification	Indications
Lopid [gemfibrozil]		Lipid regulating agent	Hypercholesterolemia, hyperlipidemia, hyperlipoproteinemia, hypertriglyceridemia
Lopressor [metoprolol tartrate]		Beta blocker	Angina pectoris; hypertension; acute myocardial infarction
Lorazepam [lorazepam]		Antianxiety; sedative/hypnotic	Anxiety disorder associated with depressive symptoms; controls tension, agitation, irritability, and insomnia
Loryna [drospirenone/ethinyl estradiol]	Z79.3	Contraceptive	Prevention of pregnancy
LoSeasonique [ethinyl estradiol/levonorgestrel]	Z79.3	Contraceptive	Prevention of pregnancy
Lotensin [benazepril hydrochloride]		ACE inhibitor	Hypertension
Lotrel [amlodipine besylate/benazepril hydrochloride]		Antihypertensive	Hypertension
Lotrisone [clotrimazole/ betamethasone dipropionate]		Antifungal-corticosteroid	Relief of redness, swelling, itching, and other discomfort of fungus infections
Lovastatin [lovastatin]		HMG-CoA reductase inhibitor (statin)	Hypercholesterolemia; hyperlipidemia; hyperlipoproteinemia
Lovenox [enoxaparin sodium]	Z79.01	Anticoagulant	Prophylaxis and treatment of venous thrombosis and pulmonary embolism
Low-Ogestrel [norgestrel/ethinyl estradiol]	Z79.3	Contraceptive	Prevention of pregnancy
Lupron [leuprolide acetate]	Z79.818	Agents affecting estrogen receptors and estrogen levels	Endometriosis symptoms; uterine fibroids
Macrobid [nitrofuantoin]	Z79.2	Antibiotic	Urinary tract infections
Macrodantin [nitrofurantoin]	Z79.2	Antibiotic	Urinary tract infections
Marlissa [ethinyl estradiol/levonorgestrel]	Z79.3	Contraceptive	Prevention of pregnancy
Maxipime [cefepime hydrochloride]	Z79.2	Antibiotic	Bacterial infections
Meclizine hydrochloride [meclizine hydrochloride]		Antihistamine	Nausea and vomiting, and dizziness associated with motion sickness
Medrol [methylprednisolone]	Z79.52	Corticosteroid	Endocrine, rheumatic, hematologic disorders; collagen, dermatological, ophthalmic, respiratory, neoplastic, gastrointestinal, nervous system disorders; allergic and edematous states
Mefoxin [cefoxitin sodium]	Z79.2	Antibiotic	Bacterial infections
Megace ES [megestrol acetate]	Z79.818	Agents affecting estrogen receptors and estrogen levels	Endometrial or advanced breast cancers; weight loss due to AIDS
Menest [esteriefied estrogens]	Z79.890	Estrogen therapy	Menopause symptoms; ovarian failure
Menostar [estradiol]	Z79.890	Estrogen therapy	Menopause symptoms; osteoporosis prevention
Mepron [atovaquone]	Z79.2	Antibiotic	Pneumonia due to *penumocystis jiroveci*
Merrem [meropenem]	Z79.2	Antibiotic	Bacterial infections of skin or stomach; bacterial meningitis
Metformin [metformin hydrochloride]	Z79.84	Oral hypoglycemic	Diabetes mellitus
Methadone HCl [methadone hydrochloride]	Z79.891	Analgesic, narcotic	Pain; treatment of opioid addiction
Methadose [methadone hydrochloride]	Z79.891	Analgesic, narcotic	Acute and chronic pain
Methergine [methylergonovine maleate]		Oxytocic agent	Routine management of postpartum hemorrhage after delivery of placenta
Methylprednisolone [methylprednisolone]	Z79.52	Corticosteroid	Inflammatory disorders
Metro [metronidazole]	Z79.2	Antibiotic	Bacterial infections
Metronidazole [metronidazole]	Z79.2	Antibiotic	Bacterial infections
Miacalcin [calcitonin salmon]		Calcitonin; a peptide hormone	Hypercalcemia, osteoporosis, postmenopausal symptoms, Paget's disease
Microgestin [ethinyl estradiol/norethindrone acetate]	Z79.3	Contraceptive	Prevention of pregnancy
Micronor [norethindrone]	Z79.3	Contraceptive	Prevention of pregnancy
Minastrin [ethinyl estradiol/norethindrone acetate]	Z79.3	Contraceptive	Prevention of pregnancy
Minivelle [estradiol]	Z79.890	Estrogen therapy	Menopause symptoms; osteoporosis prevention
Minocin [minocycline hydrochloride]	Z79.2	Antibiotic	Bacterial infections; acne
Mirena [levonorgestrel]	Z79.3	Contraceptive	Intrauterine device for prevention of pregnancy; menstrual disorders

Drug	Z Code	Drug Action/Classification	Indications
Mobic [meloxicam]	Z79.1	Nonsteroidal anti-inflammatory drug (NSAID)	Treatment of pain and inflammation due to osteoarthritis and rheumatoid arthritis
Modicon [ethinyl estradiol/norethindrone]	Z79.3	Contraceptive	Prevention of pregnancy
Monoclonal antibodies	Z79.899	Monoclonal antibodies	Cancer; prophylaxis of organ transplant rejection
Monodox [doxycycline]	Z79.2	Antibiotic	Bacterial infections; acne
Monoket [isosorbide mononitrate]		Antianginal; coronary vasodilator, nitrate	Angina pectoris
Mono-Linyah [norgestimate/ethinyl estradiol]	Z79.3	Contraceptive	Prevention of pregnancy; menstrual disorders; acne
Monurol [fosfomycin tromethamine]	Z79.2	Antibiotic	Bacterial bladder infections
Morphine [morphine sulfate]	Z79.891	Analgesic, narcotic	Moderate to severe pain
Motrin IB [ibuprofen]	Z79.1	Nonsteroidal anti-inflammatory drug (NSAID)	Pain or fever relief
Moxatag [amoxicillin]	Z79.2	Antibiotic	Bacterial tonsillitis and pharyngitis
MS Contin [morphine sulfate]	Z79.891	Analgesic, narcotic	Moderate to severe pain
Multaq [dronedarone hydrochloride]		Cardiac rhythm regulator	Treatment of patients with recent episodes of atrial fibrillation or atrial flutter
Mycobutin [rifabutin]	Z79.2	Antibiotic	Mycobacterium avium complex (MAC) prophylactic in HIV patients
Myzilra [ethinyl estradiol/levonorgestrel]	Z79.3	Contraceptive	Prevention of pregnancy
Nabumetone [nabumetone]	Z79.1	Non-steroidal anti-inflammatory drug (NSAID)	Osteoarthritis and rheumatoid arthritis
Nalfon [fenoprofen calcium]	Z79.1	Nonsteroidal anti-inflammatory drug (NSAID)	Pain or inflammation relief
Namzaric [memantine/donepezil hydrochlroides]		Acetylcholinesterase/cholinesterase inhibitors	Dementia due to Alzheimer's
Naprelan [naproxen sodium]	Z79.1	Nonsteroidal anti-inflammatory drug (NSAID)	Pain or inflammation relief
Naprosyn [naproxen]	Z79.1	Nonsteroidal anti-inflammatory drug (NSAID)	Rheumatoid, gouty arthritis and osteoarthritis; ankylosing spondylitis; bursitis; dysmenorrhea; pain, mild to moderate; tendonitis
Natazia [estradiol valerate/dienogest]	Z79.3	Contraceptive	Prevention of pregnancy; menstrual disorders
Nebupent [pentamidine isethionate]	Z79.2	Antibiotic	Severe bacterial lung infection in high risk patients with HIV
Nefazodone hydrochloride [nefazodone hydrochloride]		Antidepressant	Depression
Nembutal sodium [pentobarbital sodium]		Sedative/hypnotic	Adjunct medication in diagnostic procedures or for emergency use with convulsive disorders
NeoProfen [ibuprofen lysine]	Z79.1	Nonsteroidal anti-inflammatory drug (NSAID)	Pain or fever relief
Neoral [cyclosporine]	Z79.899	Immunosuppressant	Prophylaxis of organ transplant rejection
Neurontin [gabapentin]		Anticonvulsant	Epilepsy, partial
Nexium [esomeprazole magnesium]		Proton pump inhibitor	Gastroesophageal reflux disease (GERD), erosive esophagitis
Nexplanon [etonogestrel]	Z79.3	Contraceptive	Implantable device used for prevention of pregnancy
Nitrofurantoin [nitrofurantoin]	Z79.2	Antibiotic	Bacterial urinary tract infections
Nitropress [sodium nitroprusside]		Vasodilator	Potent, rapid action in reducing blood pressure in hypertensive crisis or for controlling bleeding during anesthesia by producing controlled hypotension
Nitrostat [nitroglycerin]		Muscle relaxant; antianginal; antihypertensive; coronary vasodilator	Prophylaxis and treatment of angina pectoris; heart failure associated with myocardial infarction; hypertension, perioperative; surgery, adjunct
Norco [acetaminophen/hydrocodone bitartrate]	Z79.891	Analgesic, narcotic	Moderate to severe pain
Norinyl [mestranol/norethisterone]	Z79.3	Contraceptive	Prevention of pregnancy
Norpace [disopyramide phosphate]		Antiarrhythmic	Coronary artery disease, for prevention, recurrence and control of unifocal, multifocal, and paired PVCs
Nor-QD [norethindrone]	Z79.3	Contraceptive	Prevention of pregnancy
Nortrel [ethinyl estradiol/norethindrone]	Z79.3	Contraceptive	Prevention of pregnancy
Norvasc [amlodipine besylate]		Calcium channel blocker	Hypertension, chronic stable angina, and vasospastic angina
Novolin [insulin recombinant]	Z79.4	Insulin	Diabetes mellitus

Drug	Z Code	Drug Action/Classification	Indications
NovoLog [insulin recombinant]	Z79.4	Insulin	Diabetes mellitus
Nucynta [tapentadol hydrochloride]	Z79.891	Analgesic, narcotic	Moderate to severe pain
NuvaRing [etonogestrel/ethinyl estradiol]	Z79.3	Contraceptive	Vaginal ring to Prevention of pregnancy
Ogestrel [norgestrel/ethinyl estradiol]	Z79.3	Contraceptive	Prevention of pregnancy
Onglyza [saxagliptin hydrochloride]	Z79.84	Oral hypoglycemic	Diabetes mellitus
Opana [oxymorphone hydrochloride]	Z79.891	Analgesic, narcotic	Moderate to severe pain
Oracea [doxycycline]	Z79.2	Antibiotic	Rosacea
Orapred ODT [prednisolone sodium phosphate]	Z79.52	Corticosteroid	Inflammatory disorders
Orbactiv [oritavancin diphosphate]	Z79.2	Antibiotic	Bacterial skin infections
Orencia [abatacept]	Z79.899	Antirheumatic	Rheumatoid arthritis; polyarticular juvenile idiopathic arthritis; psoriatic arthritis
Orphenadrine citrate [orphenadrine citrate]		Muscle relaxant	Acute spasms, tension, and post-trauma cases
Orsythia [ethinyl estradiol/levonorgestrel]	Z79.3	Contraceptive	Prevention of pregnancy
Ortho Cyclen [ethinyl estradiol/norgestimate]	Z79.3	Contraceptive	Prevention of pregnancy
Ortho-Novum [norethindrone/ethinyl estradiol]	Z79.3	Contraceptive	Prevention of pregnancy
Ortho-Tri-Cyclen [ethinyl estradiol/norgestimate]	Z79.3	Contraceptive	Prevention of pregnancy
Oseni [alogliptin benzoate/pioglitazone hydrochloride]	Z79.84	Oral hypoglycemic	Diabetes mellitus
Osphena [ospemifene]	Z79.810, Z79.890	Selective estrogen receptor modulator (SERM)	Postmenopausal dyspareunia due to vaginal atrophy; osteoporosis prevention and treatment of menopausal symptoms
Otezla [apremilast]	Z79.899	Antirheumatic	Psoriatic arthritis; plaque psoriasis
Oxandrin [oxandrolone]	Z79.890	Testosterone therapy	Promotes weight gain; bone pain due to osteoporosis
Oxazepam [oxazepam]		Antianxiety	Anxiety, tension, and alcohol withdrawal
Oxycodone HCl [oxycodone hydrochloride]	Z79.891	Analgesic, narcotic	Moderate to severe pain
OxyContin [oxycodone hydrochloride]	Z79.891	Analgesic, narcotic	Moderate to severe pain
Pavabid [papaverine hydrochloride]		Vasodilator	Relief of cerebral and peripheral ischemia
Paxil [paroxetine hydrochloride]		Antidepressant	Anxiety with panic disorder and depression; obsessive-compulsive disorder
PCE [erythromycin]	Z79.2	Antibiotic	Bacterial infections
PediaPred [prednisolone sodium phosphate]	Z79.52	Corticosteroid	Inflammatory disorders
Pegintron [peginterferon alfa-2b]	Z79.899	Antiviral	Hepatitis C
Penicillin-VK [penicillin V potassium]	Z79.2	Antibiotic	Chorea, prevention; endocarditis, prevention, secondary to tooth extraction; erysipelas; infections of the skin and skin structures, upper respiratory tract; rheumatic fever, prophylaxis; scarlet fever; Vincent's gingivitis; Vincent's pharyngitis
Pentam [pentamidine isethionate]	Z79.2	Antibiotic	Severe bacterial lung infections
Pepcid [famotidine]		Histamine H2-receptor inhibitor	Acid/peptic disorder; adenoma, secretory; gastroesophageal reflux; duodenal and gastric ulcer; Zollinger-Ellison syndrome
Percocet [oxycodone hydrochloride/acetaminophen]	Z79.891	Analgesic, narcotic	Pain, moderate to severe
Persantine [dipyridamole]	Z79.02	Antiplatelet	Therapy for chronic angina pectoris, preventing clots post heart valve surgery
Pfizerpen [penicillin g potassium]	Z79.2	Antibiotic	Severe bacterial infections
Phenobarbital [phenobarbital sodium]		Anticonvulsant	Grand mal epilepsy
Philith [ethinyl estradiol/norethindrone]	Z79.3	Contraceptive	Prevention of pregnancy
Pimtrea [desogestrel/ethinyl estradiol]	Z79.3	Contraceptive	Prevention of pregnancy
Pirmella [ethinyl estradiol/norethindrone]	Z79.3	Contraceptive	Prevention of pregnancy
Pitocin [oxytocin]		Uterotonic	Induction or stimulation of labor at term

Drug	Z Code	Drug Action/Classification	Indications
Plan B One-Step [levonorgestrel]	Z79.3	Contraceptive	Prevention of pregnancy
Plasmanate [plasma, plasma protein fraction]		Blood volume expander	Hypovolemic shock, burn patients, and hemorrhages when whole blood is unavailable
Plavix [clopidogrel bisulfate]	Z79.02	Antiplatelet	Lessening of the chance of heart attack or stroke
Ponstel [mefenamic acid]	Z79.1	Nonsteroidal anti-inflammatory drug (NSAID)	Treatment of pain
Portia [ethinyl estradiol/levonorgestrel]	Z79.3	Contraceptive	Prevention of pregnancy
Pradaxa [dabigatran etexilate mesylate]	Z79.02	Antithrombotic	Prophylaxis and treatment of blood clots in patients with atrial fibrillation
Prandimet [metformin hydrochloride/repaglinide]	Z79.84	Oral hypoglycemic	Diabetes mellitus
Prandin [repaglinide]	Z79.84	Oral hypoglycemic	Diabetes mellitus
Pravachol [pravastatin sodium]		HMG-CoA reductase inhibitor (statin)	Hypercholesterolemia; hyperlipidemia; hyperlipoproteinemia
Precose [acarbose]	Z79.84	Oral hypoglycemic	Diabetes mellitus
Prednisolone [prednisolone]	Z79.52	Corticosteroid	Inflammatory disorders
Prednisone [prednisone]	Z79.52	Corticosteroid	Used for its immunosuppressant effects and for relief of inflammation; used in arthritis, polymyositis and other systemic diseases
Pregnyl [chorionic gonadotropin]		Gonadotropic hormone	Prepubertal cryptorchidism; hypogonadism; corpus luteum insufficiency and infertility
Prelone [prednisolone]	Z79.52	Corticosteroid	Inflammatory disorders
Premarin [conjugated estrogens]	Z79.890	Estorgen therapy	Vasomotor symptoms associated with menopause; atrophic vaginitis; kraurosis vulvae, female hypogonadism; primary ovarian failure
Prempro [conjugated estrogens/medroxyprogesterone acetate]	Z79.890	Estrogen/progesterone therapy	Menopause; osteoporosis; atrophic vaginitis
Prevacid [lansoprazole]		Proton pump inhibitor	Acid/peptic disorder, erosive esophagitis, duodenal ulcer, Zollinger-Ellison syndrome
Previfem [ethinyl estradiol/norgestimate]	Z79.3	Contraceptive	Prevention of pregnancy
Prezista [darunavir ethanolate]	Z79.899	Antiviral	HIV
Priftin [rifapentine]	Z79.2	Antibiotic	Tuberculosis
Prilosec [omeprazole magnesium]		Proton pump inhibitor	Acid/peptic disorder; endocrine adenoma; erosive esophagitis; systemic mastocytosis; gastroesophageal reflux; duodenal, peptic and gastric ulcer; Zollinger-Ellison syndrome
Primaxin [cilastatin sodium/imipenem]	Z79.2	Antibiotic	Skin, stomach, female reproductive organs or lower respiratory tract infections
Prinivil [lisinopril]		ACE inhibitor	Congestive heart failure; hypertension
Procardia [nifedipine]		Calcium channel blocker	Management of vasospastic angina and chronic stable angina, hypertension
Prograf [tacrolimus]	Z79.899	Immunosuppressant	Prophylaxis of organ transplant rejection
Promethazine hydrochloride [promethazine hydrochloride]		Anesthesia, adjunct to; antiemetic; antihistamine; antitussive/expectorant; sedative/hypnotic; vertigo/motion sickness/vomiting	Anesthesia; adjunct; angioedema; conjunctivitis; dermographism; hypersensitivity, motion sickness; pain; perennial, seasonal, and allergic rhinitis; sedation, obstetrical; urticaria
Protonix [pantoprazole]		Proton pump inhibitor	Short-term treatment and maintenance therapy of erosive esophagitis associated with gastroesophageal reflux disease (GERD)
Protopic [tacrolimus]	Z79.899	Immunosuppressant	Atomic dermatitis (eczema)
Proventil-HFA [albuterol sulfate]		Antiasthmatic/bronchodilator	Asthma
Provera [medroxyprogesterone acetate]	Z79.3, Z79.890	Antineoplastic; contraceptive; progestin	Amenorrhea; carcinoma, endometrium, adjunct; carcinoma, renal; Prevention of pregnancy; hemorrhage
Prozac [fluoxetine hydrochloride]		Selective serotonin reuptake inhibitor (SSRI)	Bulimia nervosa; depression; obsessive-compulsive disorder
Pulmicort [budesonide]	Z79.51	Corticosteroid -inhaled; antiasthmatic	Prophylaxis and treatment of asthma
Qnasl [beclomethasone dipropionate]		Corticosteroid -inhaled/nasal	Perennial and seasonal allergies; vasomotor rhinitis
Qtern [dapagliflozin propanediol/saxagliptin hydrochloride]	Z79.84	Oral hypoglycemic	Diabetes mellitus
Quartette [levonorgestrel/ethinyl estradiol]	Z79.3	Contraceptive	Prevention of pregnancy

Drug	Z Code	Drug Action/Classification	Indications
Quasense [ethinyl estradiol/levonorgestrel]	Z79.3	Contraceptive	Prevention of pregnancy
Quinidine gluconate [quinidine gluconate]		Antiarrhythmic	Management of cardiac arrhythmias
Qvar [beclomethasone dipropionate]	Z79.51	Corticosteroid -inhaled; antiasthmatic	Prophylaxis and treatment of asthma
Raloxifene [raloxifene hydrochloride]	Z79.810	Selective estrogen receptor modulator (SERM)	Prevention of thinning of the bones (osteoporosis) only in postmenopausal women
Rapaflo [silodosin]		Antiadrenergic	Benign prostatic hyperplasia
Rapamune [sirolimus]	Z79.899	Immunosuppressant	Prophylaxis of organ transplant rejection
Rayos [prednisone]	Z79.52	Corticosteroid; antiasthmatic	Arthritis; blood disorders; allergies; asthma
Rebetol [ribavirin]	Z79.899	Antiviral	Chronic hepatitis C
Rebif [interferon beta-1a]	Z79.899	Antiviral	Treatment of relapsing multiple sclerosis
Reclast [zoledronic acid]	Z79.83	Bisphosphonate	Prevention of thinning of the bones (osteoporosis); Paget's disease; bone cancer
Relenza [zanamivir]		Antiviral	Treat and prevent influenza A and B
Renvela [sevelamer carbonate]		Phosphate binder	Chronic kidney disease (CKD) on dialysis
Repaglinide [repaglinide]	Z79.84	Oral hypoglycemic	Diabetes mellitus
Reprexain [hydrocodone bitartrate/ibuprofen]	Z79.891	Analgesic, narcotic; nonsteroidal anti-inflammatory drug (NSAID)	Pain, inflammation or fever relief
Restasis [cyclosporine ophthalmic emulsion]		Antiinflammatory, ophthalmic	Ocular inflammation due to keratoconjunctivitis sicca
Restoril [temazepam]		Sedative/hypnotic	Insomnia
Retrovir [zidovudine]		Antiretroviral	Indicated in symptomatic HIV infection
Rifadin [rifampin]	Z79.2	Antibiotic	Tuberculosis
Rimactane [rifampin]	Z79.2	Antibiotic	Tuberculosis
Riomet [metformin hydrochloride]	Z79.84	Oral hypoglycemic	Diabetes mellitus
Risperdal [risperidone]		Antipsychotic/antimanic	Schizophrenia; bipolar I disorder
Ritalin [methylphenidate hydrochloride]		CNS stimulant	Depression; hyperkinetic activity in children
Roxicet [oxycodone hydrochloride/acetaminophen]	Z79.891	Analgesic, narcotic	Pain, moderate to severe
Roxicodone [oxycodone hydrochloride]	Z79.891	Analgesic, narcotic	Pain relief
Ryzodeg [insulin aspart/insulin degludec]	Z79.4	Insulin	Diabetes mellitus
Sabril [vigabatrin]		Anticonvulsant	Refractory complex partial seizures
Safyral [drospirenone/ethinyl estradiol/levomefolate calcium]	Z79.3	Contraceptive	Prevention of pregnancy
Sandimmune [cyclosporine]	Z79.899	Immunosuppressant	Prophylaxis of organ transplant rejection
Sarafem [fluoxetine hydrochloride]		Selective serotonin reuptake inhibitor (SSRI)	Premenstrual dysphoric disorder (PMDD)
Savaysa [edoxaban tosylate]	Z79.01	Anticoagulant	Prophylaxis and treatment of venous thrombosis, pulmonary embolism; prevention of blood clots due to atrial fibrillation
Seasonale [levonorgestrel/ethinyl estradiol]	Z79.3	Contraceptive	Prevention of pregnancy
Seasonique [ethinyl estradiol/levonorgestrel]	Z79.3	Contraceptive	Prevention of pregnancy
Selfemra [fluoxetine hydrochloride]		Selective serotonin reuptake inhibitor (SSRI)	Premenstrual dysphoric disorder (PMDD)
Septra [sulfamethoxazole trimethoprim]	Z79.2	Antibiotic	Urinary tract infections, acute otitis media, acute exacerbations of chronic bronchitis, and shigellosis
Serevent [salmeterol xinafoate]		Bronchodilator	Asthma
Seromycin [cycloserine]	Z79.2	Antibiotic	Tuberculosis; urinary tract infections
Seroquel XR [quetiapine fumarate]		Antipsychotic	Schizophrenia; bipolar disorder; major depressive disorder
Setlakin [ethinyl estradiol/levonorgestrel]	Z79.3	Contraceptive	Prevention of pregnancy
Silvadene [silver sulfadiazine]	Z79.2	Antibiotic, topical	Wound sepsis due to second/third degree burns
Simulect [basiliximab]	Z79.899	Immunosuppressant	Prophylaxis of organ transplant rejection
Sinemet [carbidopa/levodopa]		Antiparkinsonian	Parkinson's disease
Singulair [montelukast sodium]		Antiasthmatic	Asthma; exercise-induced bronchoconstriction; perennial and seasonal allergic rhinitis

Drug	Z Code	Drug Action/Classification	Indications
Sirolimus [sirolimus]	Z79.899	Immunosuppressant	Prophylaxis of organ transplant rejection
Sitagliptin [sitagliptin/metformin hydrochloride]	Z79.84	Oral hypoglycemic	Diabetes mellitus
Sivextro [tedizolid phosphate]	Z79.2	Antibiotic	Skin infections including MRSA
Skyla [levonorgestrel]	Z79.3	Contraceptive	Intrauterine device to Prevention of pregnancy
Solodyn [minocycline hydrochloride]	Z79.2	Antibiotic	Bacterial infections
Soltamox [tamoxifen citrate]	Z79.810	Selective estrogen receptor modulator (SERM)	Breast cancer
Solu-Cortef [hydrocortisone sodium succinate]	Z79.52	Corticosteroid; antiasthmatic	Asthma; severe inflammation; allergic reactions
Solu-Medrol [methylprednisolone sodium succinate]	Z79.52	Corticosteroid	Anti-inflammatory and antiallergenic for shock and ulcerative colitis
Spiriva [tiotropium bromide]		Antiasthmatic/bronchodilator	Chronic obstructive pulmonary disease (COPD); asthma
Sprintec [norgestimate/ethinyl estradiol]	Z79.3	Contraceptive	Prevention of pregnancy
Starlix [nateglinide]	Z79.84	Oral hypoglycemic	Diabetes mellitus
Strattera [atomexetine hydrochloride]		CNS stimulant	Attention deficit hyperactivity disorder (ADHD)
Streptomycin sulfate [streptomycin sulfate]	Z79.2	Antibiotic	Severe bacterial infections
Sublimaze [fentanyl citrate]	Z79.891	Analgesic, narcotic	Pain relief
Supprelin LA [histrelin acetate]	Z79.818	Agents affecting estrogen receptors and estrogen levels	Precocious puberty
Suprax [cefixime]	Z79.2	Antibiotic	Bacterial infections
Sustiva [efavirenz]	Z79.899	Antiviral	HIV/AIDs
Syeda [drospirenone/ethinyl estradiol]	Z79.3	Contraceptive	Prevention of pregnancy
Sylatron [peginterferon alfa-2b]	Z79.899	Antineoplastic interferons; antiviral interferons	Prevention of recurrent malignant melanoma
Symbicort [budesonide/formoterol fumarate dihydrate]	Z79.51	Corticosteroid -inhaled; antiasthmatic	Prophylaxis and treatment of asthma and COPD
Symbyax [olanzapine/fluoxetine]		Antidepressant	Acute depressive episodes associated with bipolar I disorder; treatment resistant depression
Synarel [nafarelin acetate]	Z79.818	Agents affecting estrogen receptors and estrogen levels	Endometriosis symptoms; precocious puberty
Synercid [dalfopristin/quinupristin]	Z79.2	Antibiotic	Severe blood infections
Synjardy [empagliflozin/metformin hydrochloride]	Z79.84	Oral hypoglycemic	Diabetes mellitus
Synthroid [levothyroxine sodium]		Thyroid hormone	Hypothyroidism
Tacrolimus [tacrolimus]	Z79.899	Immunosuppressant	Prophylaxis of organ transplant rejection
Tamiflu [oseltamivir phosphate]		Antiviral	Treatment and prevention of influenza A and B
Tamoxifen [tamoxifen citrate]	Z79.810	Selective estrogen receptor modulator (SERM)	Metastatic breast cancer in postmenopausal women
Tazicef [ceftazidime]	Z79.2	Antibiotic	Confirmed or suspected bacterial infections
Teflaro [ceftaroline fosamil]	Z79.2	Antibiotic	Bacterial skin infections; pneumonia
Tegretol [carbamazepine]		Anticonvulsant; analgesic	Epilepsy, especially with complex symptomatology; specific analgesic for trigeminal neuralgia
Tenormin [atenolol]		Beta blocker	Angina pectoris; hypertension; acute myocardial infarction
Terazosin hydrochloride [terazosin hydrochloride]		Antiadrenergic	Benign prostatic hypertrophy; hypertension
Testim [testosterone]	Z79.890	Testosterone therapy -topical	Primary hypogonadism; hypogonadotropic hypogonadism
Tetracycline HCl [tetracycline hydrochloride]	Z79.2	Antibiotic	Bacterial infections
Tiazac [diltiazem hydrochloride]		Calcium channel blocker	Chronic stable angina, atrial fibrillation, atrial flutter, hypertension, paroxysmal supraventricular tachycardia
Tivorbex [indomethacin]	Z79.1	Nonsteroidal anti-inflammatory drug (NSAID)	Treatment of pain, inflammation and joint stiffness
Tobradex [tobramycin/dexamethasone]		Aminoglycoside ocular anti-infective; anti-inflammatory	Infectious conjunctivitis; dermatosis, corticosteroid-responsive with secondary infection; foreign body in eye; corneal inflammation; uveitis

Drug	Z Code	Drug Action/Classification	Indications
Tobramycin [dexamethasone/tobramycin]	Z79.2	Antibiotic	Bacterial eye infections
Topamax [topiramate]		Anticonvulsant	Epilepsy; primary generalized tonic-clonic seizures; seizures associated with Lennox-Gastaut syndrome; migraine headache
Toprol-XL [metoprolol succinate]		Beta blocker	Angina pectoris; hypertension
Toremifene [toremifene citrate]	Z79.810	Selective estrogen receptor modulator (SERM)	Metastatic breast cancer in postmenopausal women
Torisel [temsirolimus]	Z79.899	Antineoplastic	Renal cell carcinoma
Toujeo Solostar [insulin glargine recombinant]	Z79.4	Insulin	Diabetes mellitus
Trazodone hydrochloride [trazodone hydrochloride]		Antidepressant	Depression
Trelstar [triptorelin pamoate]	Z79.818	Agents affecting estrogen receptors and estrogen levels	Palliative treatment of prostate cancer symptoms
Tresiba [insulin degludec]	Z79.4	Insulin	Diabetes mellitus
Triamterene and hydrochlorothiazide [triamterene/ hydrochlorothiazide]		Antihypertensive; diuretic	Edema; hypertension
Tri-Estarylla [ethinyl estradiol/norgestimate]	Z79.3	Contraceptive	Prevention of pregnancy; acne
Tri-Legest [ethinyl estradiol/norethindrone acetate]	Z79.3	Contraceptive	Prevention of pregnancy
Tri-Linyah [ethinyl estradiol/norgestimate]	Z79.3	Contraceptive	Prevention of pregnancy
Tri-Lo-Estarylla [ethinyl estradiol/norgestimate]	Z79.3	Contraceptive	Prevention of pregnancy
Tri-Lo-Sprintec [ethinyl estradiol/norgestimate]	Z79.3	Contraceptive	Prevention of pregnancy
Trimethoprim [trimethoprim]	Z79.2	Antibiotic	Acute exacerbation chronic bronchitis; travelers' diarrhea; infections of the middle, lower respiratory tract, and urinary tract; pneumonia, pneumocystis; shigellosis
Tri-Norinyl [ethinyl estradiol/norethindrone]	Z79.3	Contraceptive	Prevention of pregnancy
Tri-Previfem [ethinyl estradiol/norgestimate]	Z79.3	Contraceptive	Prevention of pregnancy
Triptodur [triptorelin]	Z79.818	Agents affecting estrogen receptors and estrogen levels	Precocious puberty
Tri-Sprintec [ethinyl estradiol/norgestimate]	Z79.3	Contraceptive	Prevention of pregnancy; acne
Trivora [ethinyl estradiol/ levonorgestrel]	Z79.3	Contraceptive	Prevention of pregnancy
Trokendi XR [topiramate]		Anticonvulsant	Epilepsy; primary generalized tonic-clonic seizures; seizures associated with Lennox-Gastaut syndrome; migraine headache
Trulicity [dulaglutide]		Antidiabetic -injectable	Diabetes mellitus
Truvada [emtricitabine/ tenofovir disoproxil fumarate]	Z79.899	Antiviral	Treatment and prevention of HIV
Tygacil [tigecycline]	Z79.2	Antibiotic	Bacterial skin or digestive system infections; pneumonia
Tylenol with codeine [acetaminophen/codeine phosphate]	Z79.891	Analgesic, narcotic	Pain and cough
Ultram [tramadol hydrochloride]	Z79.891	Analgesic, non-narcotic (opiate, narcotic-like)	Moderate to severe pain
Unasyn [ampicillin sodium/sulbactam sodium]	Z79.2	Antibiotic	Bacterial infections
Vagifem [estradiol]	Z79.890	Estrogen therapy	Menopause symptoms
Valium [diazepam]		Antianxiety; muscle relaxant; anticonvulsant	Anxiety, tension, withdrawal from alcohol, muscle spasms and anticonvulsant therapy; epilepsy, generalized tonic-clonic; status epilepticus; stiff-man syndrome; tetanus
Vancocin HCl [vancomycin hydrochloride]	Z79.2	Antibiotic	Severe bacterial infections
Vancomycin HCl [vancomycin hydrochloride]	Z79.2	Antibiotic	Severe bacterial infections
Vantas [histrelin acetate]	Z79.818	Agents affecting estrogen receptors and estrogen levels	Palliative treatment of prostate cancer symptoms
Vasotec [enalaprilat maleate]		ACE inhibitor	Congestive heart failure; hypertension

Drug	Z Code	Drug Action/Classification	Indications
Velivet [desogestrel/ethinyl estradiol]	Z79.3	Contraceptive	Prevention of pregnancy
Venlafaxine hydrochloride [venlafaxine hydrochloride]		Antidepressant, serotonin and norepinephrine reuptake inhibitor (SNRI)	Major depressive disorder; social anxiety disorder; panic disorder
Ventolin HFA [albuterol sulfate]		Antiasthmatic/bronchodilator	Asthma
Verapamil HCL [verapamil hydrochloride]		Calcium channel blocker	Angina pectoris, chronic stable angina, atrial fibrillation, atrial flutter, paroxysmal supraventricular tachycardia, ventricular arrhythmia, hypertension
Viagra [sildenafil citrate]		Phosphodiesterase-5 (PDE5) inhibitor	Erectile dysfunction
Vibativ [telavancin hydrochloride]	Z79.2	Antibiotic	Pneumonia; severe bacterial skin infections
Vibramycin [doxycycline calcium]	Z79.2	Antibiotic	Bacterial infections
Vicoprofen [hydrocodone bitartrate/ibuprofen]	Z79.891	Analgesic, narcotic; nonsteroidal anti-inflammatory drug (NSAID)	Pain, inflammation or fever relief
Victoza [liraglutide recombinant]		Antidiabetic -injectable	Diabetes mellitus
Vienva [ethinyl estradiol/levonorgestrel]	Z79.3	Contraceptive	Prevention of pregnancy
Viorele [desogestrel/ethinyl estradiol]	Z79.3	Contraceptive	Prevention of pregnancy
Virazole [ribavirin]	Z79.899	Antiviral	Respiratory syncytial virus (RSV)
Viread [tenofovir disoproxil fumarate]	Z79.899	Antiviral	HIV; chronic hepatitis B
Vistaril [hydroxyzine pamoate]		Antianxiety; antiemetic	Treatment of nausea and vomiting, for reducing narcotic requirement in surgery and as tranquilizer for tension, anxiety, or agitation states
Vivelle [estradiol]	Z79.890	Estrogen therapy	Menopause symptoms; osteoporosis prevention
Voltaren [diclofenac sodium]	Z79.1	Nonsteroidal anti-inflammatory drug (NSAID)	Treatment of pain, inflammation and joint stiffness due to arthritis
Vytorin [ezetimibe/simvastatin]		Antihyperlipidemic	Primary or mixed hyperlipidemia; homozygous familial hypercholesterolemia
Warfarin [warfarin sodium]	Z79.01	Anticoagulant	Prophylaxis and treatment of venous thrombosis, treatment of atrial fibrillation with embolization (pulmonary embolism), arrhythmias, myocardial infarction, and stroke prevention
Wellbutrin SR, Wellbutrin XL [bupropion hydrochloride]		Antidepressant	Depression
Wera [ethinyl estradiol/norethindrone]	Z79.3	Contraceptive	Prevention of pregnancy
Xalatan [latanoprost]		Prostaglandin F2α analogue	Glaucoma, open-angle; ocular hypertension
Xanax, Xanax XR [alprazolam]		Antianxiety; sedative/hypnotic	Anxiety disorders with panic disorder and depression
Xarelto [rivaraxaban]	Z79.01	Anticoagulant	Prophylaxis and treatment of venous thrombosis, pulmonary embolism; prevention of blood clots due to atrial fibrillation
Xeljanz [tofacitinib]	Z79.899	Antirheumatic	Rheumatoid arthritis; psoriatic arthritis
Xifaxan [rifaximin]	Z79.2	Antibiotic	*E. coli* diarrhea
Xigduo [dapagliflozin propanediol/metformin hydrochloride]	Z79.84	Oral hypoglycemic	Diabetes mellitus
Xigris [drotrecogin alfa]		Biologic response modifier	Severe sepsis
Xyrem [sodium oxybate]		CNS depressant; anxiolytic/sedative/hypnotic	Cataplexy and/or excessive daytime sleepiness in narcolepsy
Xyzal [levocetirizine dihydrochloride]		Antihistamine	Perennial allergic rhinitis; chronic idiopathic urticaria
Yasmin [drospirenone/ethinyl estradiol]	Z79.3	Contraceptive	Prevention of pregnancy
Yaz [drospirenone/ethinyl estradiol]	Z79.3	Contraceptive	Prevention of pregnancy; menstrual disorders
Zantac [ranitidine hydrochloride]		Histamine H2-receptors inhibitor	Acid/peptic disorder, erosive esophagitis, gastrointestinal hypersecretion, mastocytosis, gastroesophageal reflux, peptic ulcer, Zollinger-Ellison syndrome
Zerbaxa [ceftolozane sulfate/tazobactam sodium]	Z79.2	Antibiotic	Complicated urinary tract and intra-abdominal infections
Zestoretic [lisinopril/hydrochlorothiazide]		ACE inhibitor	Congestive heart failure; hypertension
Zestril [lisinopril]		ACE inhibitor	Congestive heart failure; hypertension
Ziac [bisoprolol fumarate/hydrochlorothiazide]		Antihypertensive	Hypertension
Zinacef [cefuroxime sodium]	Z79.2	Antibiotic	Bacterial infections
Zipsor [diclofenac potassium]	Z79.1	Nonsteroidal anti-inflammatory drug (NSAID)	Pain and inflammation relief

Drug	Z Code	Drug Action/Classification	Indications
Zithromax [azithromycin]	Z79.2	Antibiotic	Infections of the cervix, lower respiratory tract, skin and skin structures, urethra, nongonococcal; mycobacterium avium complex; pharyngitis, streptococcal pneumonia; tonsillitis
Zmax [azithromycin]	Z79.2	Antibiotic	Pneumonia; sinusitis
Zocor [simvastatin]		HMG-CoA reductase inhibitor (statin)	Hypercholesterolemia; hyperlipidemia; hyperlipoproteinemia; hypertriglyceridemia
Zoladex [goserelin acetate]	Z79.818	Agents affecting estrogen receptors and estrogen levels	Palliative treatment of prostate cancer and breast cancer symptoms; endometriosis
Zoloft [sertraline hydrochloride]		Antidepressant	Anxiety with panic disorder and depression; obsessive-compulsive disorder
Zometa [zoledronic acid]	Z79.83	Bisphosphonate	Multiple myeloma; Paget's disease
Zorvolex [diclofenac]	Z79.1	Nonsteroidal anti-inflammatory drug (NSAID)	Pain, inflammation or fever relief
Zosyn [piperacillin sodium/tazobactam sodium]	Z79.2	Antibiotic	Bacterial infections
Zovia [ethynodiol diacetate/ethinyl estradiol]	Z79.3	Contraceptive	Prevention of pregnancy
Zovirax [acyclovir]		Antiviral	Genital herpes and herpes zoster infections
Zyban [bupropion hydrochloride]		Smoking cessation aid	Nicotine addiction, smoking
Zyflo [zileuton]		Antiasthmatic	Asthma
Zyloprim [allopurinol]		Antigout	Gouty arthritis, renal calculus, hyperuricemia, hyperuricemia secondary to leukemia, hyperuricemia secondary to lymphoma
Zyprexa [olanzapine]		Antipsychotic/antimanic	Psychotic disorders; schizophrenia
Zyrtec [cetirizine hydrochloride]		Antihistamine	Perennial and seasonal allergic rhinitis; chronic urticaria
Zyvox [linezolid]	Z79.2	Antibiotic	Severe bacterial infections

Appendix D: Z Codes for Long-Term Drug Use with Associated Drugs

Z79.Ø1 Long term (current) use of anticoagulants
- Arixtra
- Coumadin
- Eliquis
- Fragmin
- Heparin
- Jantoven
- Lovenox
- Savaysa
- Warfarin
- Xarelto

Z79.Ø2 Long term (current) use of antithrombotics/antiplatelets
- Aggrastat
- Aggrenox
- Angiomax
- Argatroban
- Brilinta
- Clopidogrel bisulfate
- Effient
- Integrilin
- Iprivask
- Persantine
- Plavix
- Pradaxa

Z79.1 Long term (current) use of non-steroidal anti-inflammatories (NSAID)
- Advil
- Aleve
- Anaprox
- Arthrotec
- Caldolor
- Cambia
- Celebrex
- Daypro
- Duexis
- Dyloject
- Feldene
- Ibuprofen
- Indocin
- Mobic
- Motrin IB
- Nabumetone
- Nalfon
- Naprelan
- Naprosyn
- NeoProfen
- Ponstel
- Tivorbex
- Voltaren
- Zipsor
- Zorvolex

Z79.2 Long term (current) use of antibiotics
- Altabax
- Amikacin
- Amoxicillin
- Ampicillin
- Ancef
- Augmentin
- Avelox
- Azactam
- Azithromycin
- Bactrim
- Bactroban
- Biaxin
- Cefprozil
- Ceftin
- Ceftriaxone
- Centany
- Cephalexin
- Cipro
- Ciprofloxacin
- Clarithromycin
- Cleocin
- Clindamycin
- Daptomycin
- Dificid
- Doxycycline
- Dynacin
- E.E.S.
- Ertapenem
- ERYC
- Erygel
- EryPed
- Ery-Tab
- Erythrocin
- Erythromycin
- Factive
- Flagyl
- Fortaz
- Gentamicin sulfate
- Invanz
- Isoniazid
- Keflex
- Kefzol
- Klaron
- Levaquin
- Lincocin
- Macrobid
- Macrodantin
- Maxipime
- Mefoxin
- Mepron
- Merrem
- Metro
- Metronidazole
- Minocin
- Monodox
- Monurol
- Moxatag
- Mycobutin
- Nebupent
- Nitrofurantoin
- Oracea
- Orbactiv
- PCE
- Penicillin-VK
- Pentam
- Pfizerpen
- Priftin
- Primaxin
- Rifadin
- Rimactane
- Septra
- Seromycin
- Silvadene
- Sivextro
- Solodyn
- Streptomycin sulfate
- Suprax
- Synercid
- Tazicef
- Teflaro
- Tetracycline HCl
- Tobramycin
- Trimethoprim
- Tygacil
- Unasyn
- Vancocin HCl
- Vancomycin HCl
- Vibativ
- Vibramycin
- Xifaxan
- Zerbaxa
- Zinacef
- Zithromax
- Zmax
- Zosyn
- Zyvox

Z79.3 Long term (current) use of hormonal contraceptives
- Altavera
- Alyacen
- Aranelle
- Ashlyna
- Aviane
- Aygestin
- Balziva
- Bekyree

Beyaz
Brevicon
Briellyn
Camila
Cryselle
Cyclafem
Cyclessa
Dasetta
Daysee
Depo-Provera
Depo-SubQ Provera
Desogen
Elinest
Emoquette
Enpresse
Enskyce
Errin
Estarylla
Estrostep Fe
Falmina
Femcon Fe
Femhrt
Gildagia
Gildess
Introvale
Jencycla
Junel
Kariva
Kelnor
Kimidess
Kurvelo
Kyleena
Larin
Lessina
Levonest
Levora
Liletta
Lo Loestrin Fe
Lo Minastrin Fe
Loestrin
Loryna
LoSeasonique
Low-Ogestrel
Marlissa
Microgestin
Micronor
Minastrin
Mirena
Modicon
Mono-Linyah
Myzilra
Natazia
Nexplanon
Norinyl
Nor-QD
Nortrel

NuvaRing
Ogestrel
Orsythia
Ortho Cyclen
Ortho-Novum
Ortho-Tri-Cyclen
Philith
Pimtrea
Pirmella
Plan B One-Step
Portia
Previfem
Provera
Quartette
Quasense
Safyral
Seasonale
Seasonique
Setlakin
Skyla
Sprintec
Syeda
Tri-Estarylla
Tri-Legest
Tri-Linyah
Tri-Lo-Estarylla
Tri-Lo-Sprintec
Tri-Norinyl
Tri-Previfem
Tri-Sprintec
Trivora
Velivet
Vienva
Viorele
Wera
Yasmin
Yaz
Zovia

Z79.4   Long term (current) use of insulin
Afrezza
Apidra
Basaglar
Humalog
Humulin
Lantus
Levemir
Novolin
NovoLog
Ryzodeg
Toujeo Solostar
Tresiba

Z79.51   Long term (current) use of inhaled steroids
Advair
Aerospan

Alvesco
Arnuity Ellipta
Asmanex
Dulera
Flovent
Pulmicort
Qvar
Symbicort

Z79.52   Long term (current) use of systemic steroids
A-Methapred
Aristospan
Celestone Soluspan
Colocort
Cortef
Cortenema
Cortifoam
Cortisone acetate
Depo-Medrol
Dexamethasone Intensol
Entocort EC
Hydrocortisone
Kenalog-10
Kenalog-40
Locoid
Medrol
Methylprednisolone
Orapred ODT
PediaPred
Prednisolone
Prednisone
Prelone
Rayos
Solu-Cortef
Solu-Medrol

Z79.810 Long term (current) use of selective estrogen receptor modulators (SERMs)
Evista
Fareston
Osphena
Raloxifene
Soltamox
Tamoxifen
Toremifene

Z79.811 Long term (current) use of aromatase inhibitors
Anastrozole
Arimidex
Aromasin
Exemestane
Femara
Letrozole

Z79.818 Long term (current) use of other agents affecting estrogen receptors and estrogen levels
Eligard
Faslodex
Lupron
Megace ES
Supprelin LA
Synarel
Trelstar
Triptodur
Vantas
Zoladex

Z79.82 Long term (current) use of aspirin
Bayer
Durlaza

Z79.83 Long term (current) use of bisphosphonates
Actonel
Atelvia
Binosto
Boniva
Didronel
Fosamax
Reclast
Zometa

Z79.84 Long term (current) use of oral hypoglycemic drugs
Acarbose
Actoplus Met
Actos
Amaryl
Avandamet
Avandia
Diabinese
DiaBeta
Duetact
Farxiga
Fortamet
Glimepiride
Glucophage
Glucotrol
Glucovance
Glumetza
Glyburide
Glynase
Glyset
Invokamet
Invokana
Janumet
Januvia
Jentadueto
Kazano
Kombiglyze
Metformin

Onglyza
Oseni
PrandiMet
Prandin
Precose
Qtern
Repaglinide
Riomet
Sitagliptin
Starlix
Synjardy
Xigduo

Z79.890 Hormone replacement therapy
Activella
Alora
Androderm
AndroGel
Angeliq
Climara
CombiPatch
Delestrogen
Divigel
Duavee
Elestrin
Estrace
Estraderm
Estrasorb
EstroGel
Femhrt
Femring
Femtrace
Menest
Menostar
Minivelle
Osphena
Oxandrin
Premarin
Prempro
Provera
Testim
Vagifem
Vivelle

Z79.891 Long term (current) use of opiate analgesic
Abstral
Acetaminophen with codeine
Astramorph
Buprenex
Buprenorphine HCl
Butorphanol tartrate
Butrans
Codeine
Demerol
Dilaudid
Dolophine HCl

Duragesic
Duramorph
Embeda
Exalgo
Fentanyl
Fentora
Fioricet with codeine
Hydrocodone
Hydrocodone bitartrate and acetaminophen
Hydromorphone HCl
Kadian
Methadone HCl
Methadose
Morphine
MS Contin
Norco
Nucynta
Opana
Oxycodone HCl
OxyContin
Percocet
Reprexain
Roxicet
Roxicodone
Sublimaze
Tylenol with codeine
Ultram
Vicoprofen

Z79.899 Other long term (current) drug therapy
Actimmune
Antineoplastic/chemotherapy
Astagraf XL
Avonex
Cellcept
Cyclosporine
Enbrel
Entyvio
Envarsus XR
Gengraf
Harvoni
Humira
Imuran
Intron
Monoclonal antibodies
Neoral
Orencia
Otezla
Pegintron
Prezista
Prograf
Protopic
Rapamune
Rebetol

Appendix D: Z Codes for Long-Term Drug Use with Associated Drugs

Rebif
Sandimmune
Simulect
Sirolimus
Sustiva
Sylatron
Tacrolimus
Torisel
Truvada
Virazole
Viread
Xeljanz

Z00.00	Z01.21	Z02.5	Z04.1	Z34.81	Z38.65	Z51.11	Z52.5
Z00.01	Z01.30	Z02.6	Z04.2	Z34.82	Z38.66	Z51.12	Z52.6
Z00.110	Z01.31	Z02.71	Z04.3	Z34.83	Z38.68	Z52.000	Z52.810
Z00.111	Z01.411	Z02.79	Z04.41	Z34.90	Z38.69	Z52.001	Z52.811
Z00.121	Z01.419	Z02.81	Z04.42	Z34.91	Z38.7	Z52.008	Z52.812
Z00.129	Z01.42	Z02.82	Z04.6	Z34.92	Z38.8	Z52.010	Z52.813
Z00.2	Z01.810	Z02.83	Z04.71	Z34.93	Z39.0	Z52.011	Z52.819
Z00.3	Z01.811	Z02.89	Z04.72	Z38.00	Z39.1	Z52.018	Z52.89
Z00.5	Z01.812	Z02.9	Z04.8	Z38.01	Z39.2	Z52.090	Z76.1
Z00.70	Z01.818	Z03.6	Z04.9	Z38.1	Z40.00	Z52.091	Z76.2
Z00.71	Z01.82	Z03.71	Z31.81	Z38.2	Z40.01	Z52.098	Z99.12
Z00.8	Z01.83	Z03.72	Z31.83	Z38.30	Z40.02	Z52.10	
Z01.00	Z01.84	Z03.73	Z31.84	Z38.31	Z40.03	Z52.11	
Z01.01	Z01.89	Z03.74	Z33.2	Z38.4	Z40.09	Z52.19	
Z01.10	Z02.0	Z03.75	Z34.00	Z38.5	Z40.8	Z52.20	
Z01.110	Z02.1	Z03.79	Z34.01	Z38.61	Z40.9	Z52.21	
Z01.118	Z02.2	Z03.810	Z34.02	Z38.62	Z42.1	Z52.29	
Z01.12	Z02.3	Z03.818	Z34.03	Z38.63	Z42.8	Z52.3	
Z01.20	Z02.4	Z03.89	Z34.80	Z38.64	Z51.0	Z52.4	

Appendix F: Centers for Medicare & Medicaid Services Hierarchical Condition Categories (CMS-HCC)

In the 1970s, Medicare began demonstration projects that contracted with health maintenance organizations (HMOs) to provide care for Medicare beneficiaries in exchange for prospective payments. In 1985, this project changed from demonstration status to a regular part of the Medicare program, Medicare Part C. The Balanced Budget Act (BBA) of 1997 named Medicare's Part C managed care program Medicare+Choice, and the Medicare Modernization Act (MMA) of 2003 again renamed it to Medicare Advantage (MA).

Medicare is one of the world's largest health insurance programs, and about one-third of the beneficiaries on Medicare are enrolled in a MA private health care plan. Due to the great variance in the health status of Medicare beneficiaries, risk adjustment provides a means of adequately compensating those plans with large numbers of seriously ill patients while not overburdening other plans that have healthier individuals. Medicare Advantage (MA) plans have been using the Hierarchical Condition Category (HCC) risk adjustment model since 2004.

The Risk Adjustment Model

The primary purpose of a risk adjustment model is to predict (on average) the future health care costs for specific consortiums enrolled in Medicare Advantage (MA) health plans. CMS is then able to provide capitation payments to these private health plans. Capitation payments are an incentive for health plans to enroll not only healthier individuals but those with chronic conditions or who are more seriously ill by removing some of the financial burden.

The MA risk adjustment model uses HCCs to assess the disease burden of its enrollees. HCC diagnostic groupings were created after examining claims data so that enrollees with similar disease processes, and consequently similar health care expenditures, could be pooled into a larger data set in which an average expenditure rate could be determined. The medical conditions included in HCC categories are those that were determined to most predictably affect the health status and health care costs of any individual. Several important principles to the risk adjustment model and the development of the HCC categories include but are not limited to:

1. The HCC diagnostic categories should be clinically meaningful.
   - Diagnostic categories are well-defined.
   - Clinically specific diseases or medical conditions are grouped to each category.
2. The HCC diagnostic categories should predict medical expenditures.
   - The diagnoses grouped to a specific category should have as close to the same cost burden not only in the current year but also in the future.
3. The HCC diagnostic categories should have adequate sample sizes and discretionary categories excluded to be as accurate and stable in their estimate of costs as possible.
   - A diagnostic category that groups extremely rare diseases or conditions would not be reliably effective in determining current or future costs.
   - Codes that are not credible as cost predictors or may be subject to coding variation should be excluded, when possible.
4. The HCC diagnostic categories should be both hierarchical and additive.
   - Hierarchical measurement is used within a specific disease process.
   - Disease processes that are unrelated to each other are measured additively.
5. The diagnostic classification should encourage specificity and should not reward coding proliferation.
   - More diagnosis codes and vague diagnosis codes do not equal greater disease burden.

More than 9,000 ICD-10-CM diagnosis codes map to 79 HCCs in the current risk adjustment model. Diagnoses are excluded from mapping when they do not predict future cost or are vague or variable in diagnosis, coding, or treatment, such as symptoms or osteoarthritis. Also excluded are diagnosis codes from laboratories, radiology, and home health claims.

Risk Adjustment Factors

The CMS-HCC risk adjustment model uses "risk adjustment factors" to calculate a risk score for each member. This score summarizes that particular patient's expected cost of care relative to other members'. Each member's risk score is based on demographic and health status information and is calculated as the sum of these demographic and health factors weighted by their estimated marginal contributions to total risk. The model also takes into account where the patient resides (community or institutional), Medicaid eligibility (full or partial benefits), the patient's Medicare enrollment status (new or established), age, disability status, whether the patient is frail or has end-stage renal disease (ESRD), and even prescription drug use.

No procedure codes, ICD-10-PCS or CPT, are included in the MA risk adjustment model. The model relies solely on diagnostic and demographic data. Not all ICD-10-CM diagnoses map to an HCC, and there is no specific code sequencing involved. The CMS-HCC model is additive as well as hierarchical. The additive functionality allows a patient to have more than one HCC category assigned, providing a more complete clinical picture and prediction of resource consumption. The hierarchical aspect of the model provides a means of ranking diagnoses that are similar in disease process, by severity. The hierarchy of the condition categories ensures the patient's conditions are classified to the most severe condition within the related group. Less severe conditions within a particular hierarchy are superseded by more severe diagnoses within the same group. The hierarchy and additive relationship permits this model to characterize the person's illness level within each disease process, while still allowing the effects of unrelated disease processes to be counted in the patient's overall score.

Certain combinations of coexisting diagnoses for an individual can increase medical costs. The CMS-HCC model adjusts for these higher costs by the addition of "disease interaction" factors. For each patient, multiple HCCs assigned, along with demographic and disease interaction factors, are used to calculate a single, combined risk adjustment factor (RAF). The RAF score for an individual member represents all of the HCCs that have been submitted from all sources for that member to CMS during the course of an entire calendar year.

There are separate CMS-HCC models for new enrollees and continuing enrollees. The new enrollee model uses demographic factors only, such as age, sex, and disability status, and is used when the enrollee has less than 12 months of medical history. The community model accounts for age, sex, original reason for Medicare entitlement (age or disability), Medicaid eligibility, and clinical conditions as measured by HCCs. In the second step, expected costs are adjusted for outliers based on the member's risk score and whether the patient has ESRD.

Demographic data (age, sex, eligibility) as well as health status (diagnoses codes submitted on claims to CMS) of an MA population are used to determine the reimbursement to the health plan to care for their members.

RAF scores, which range from 0.118 to 2.4888, indicate patient health status. A RAF score of 1.0 or below is the benchmark CMS uses to indicate the average healthy patient with the same demographic and diagnostic factors. These patients are expected to use average or lower-than-average resources. When the RAF score is higher than 1.0, CMS considers the patient to be sicker than the average patient with the same criteria and expects greater-than-average resource utilization.

A low RAF score may accurately indicate a healthier patient, but it may also falsely indicate a healthier patient due to incomplete or inaccurate coding, incomplete or insufficient record documentation, or patients who fail to complete an annual assessment.

A high RAF score may accurately indicate a sicker patient, or it may be falsely inflated from overcoding due to diagnoses that are reported but not documented, or from copying and pasting from previous encounters or problem lists of resolved conditions.

Documentation Requirements

Payment is made per HCC category (not per diagnosis code). No matter how many times in the year the diagnosis codes are reported, a single payment is made to the MA plan each year. Each year the list of HCCs and the RAF for each patient is "reset." This means the annual health assessment is extremely important, and adequate documentation is critical. Accurate risk adjustment payment relies on complete medical record documentation and diagnosis coding. CMS requires that all applicable diagnosis codes be reported and that all diagnoses be reported to the highest level of specificity and that these be substantiated by the medical record.

CMS's Guiding Principle:

The risk adjustment diagnosis must be based on clinical medical record documentation from a face-to-face encounter, coded according to the *ICD-10-CM Guidelines for Coding and Reporting*; assigned based on dates of service within the data collection period, submitted to the MA organization from an appropriate risk adjustment provider type and an appropriate risk adjustment physician data source.

Appendix F: Centers for Medicare & Medicaid Services Hierarchical Condition Categories (CMS-HCC)

A "face-to-face" health service encounter between a patient and healthcare provider describes an encounter between the patient and the provider (MD, DO), including qualified nonphysician practitioners (NPP) (e.g. nurse practitioner or physician's assistant), which is face-to-face with the patient. CMS provides a current listing of acceptable physician specialty types for risk adjustment data submission within the 2012 Regional Technical Assistance Participant Guide. The only exception to the face-to-face encounter requirement is pathology services (professional component only). Currently, CMS does not provide a listing of all services that are considered face-to-face visits for risk adjustment data, but does provide guidance on what types of services are not acceptable for risk adjustment in the Participant Guide. For example, diagnostic radiology does not qualify because diagnostic radiologists typically do not document confirmed diagnoses. Other examples of services that are not acceptable include diagnostic reports that have not been interpreted, such as laboratory reports.

It is essential that the medical record documentation show evidence by provider authentication that the direct face-to-face service was personally furnished by the physician or qualified NPP. Examples of these services include office visits, hospital visits, preoperative anesthesia assessment, and surgical and invasive procedures.

Risk adjustment relies on annual health information. Each enrollee is assigned an individual risk score based on the health status information obtained from the diagnosis codes on the claims. The CMS-HCC model relies on ICD-10-CM coding specificity for accurate risk adjustment by using the most specific code available that is substantiated by the documentation in the medical record. Providers should fully document and accurately code the evaluation and management of all severe and chronic conditions to ensure a full, complete, and accurate clinical record of the patient's condition and reflect the work involved in caring for the patient, particularly those with complex and challenging health issues. All conditions affecting the treatment or management of the patient's health should be documented at least once a year, as applicable to care provided, to accurately describe the true complexity and severity of the patient's health. If the diagnosis coding on the claim is not accurate or complete, the claim may indicate that the provider did much less medical decision-making, evaluation, and management than was actually performed.

Documentation for a valid reportable diagnosis must clearly indicate evidence of M.E.A.T., for each diagnosis:

M   monitored
E   evaluated
A   assessed
T   treated

Documentation to support or validate risk adjustment conditions may be found anywhere in the note for the face-to-face encounter. It is important to ensure that the note accurately reflects all chronic conditions that affect the health and care of the patient. Each encounter must be unique and reflect only that visit as it occurred. Chronic conditions require long-term attention and management, and should be reported when treated but are often inadequately documented due to familiarity with the patient. Insufficient documentation influences the assignment of diagnosis codes and directly affects the patient's risk score.

Documentation should be concise, include the reason for the face-to-face visit, and support the need for the patient to be monitored, evaluated, assessed, and/or treated for the conditions listed through clinical rationale and/or plan of care described in clear (legible) notes. Each page of progress notes should be properly authenticated and include the patient's name and the date.

Providers should document each clinical diagnosis to the highest degree of specificity per encounter, including all complications and/or manifestations, including clear links to causal conditions. Only confirmed conditions should be documented—no rule-out conditions or abnormal findings without clinical significance. All known conditions, including chronic conditions, that affect the care and treatment of the patient at least once per year should be noted.

Providers should specifically document the condition and test or report results, and document the status of any changes to the condition, using terminology such as decreased, increased, worsening, improving, or unchanged. Documentation should include supporting evidence of the results or plan of care.

Documentation Tips
- Document all cause-and-effect relationships.
- Report the most specific diagnosis code available that is supported by the documentation.
- Include all current diagnoses as part of the current medical decision-making, and document for every visit.
- Identify diagnoses that are current or chronic problems rather than a past medical history or previous resolved condition.

- Document history of heart attack, status codes, etc., that affect the patient's care as "history of" or "PMH" when they no longer exist or are not current conditions.
- Ensure each progress note has the date, signature, and credentials/specialty.
- Document the thought processes used to assess each condition.
- Know high revenue HCCs that are often undiagnosed or undercoded.
- Avoid "unspecified" codes.
- Ensure the codes reported are accurate.
- Ensure each encounter is billed.
- Review rejection reports, and audit reports to assess risks.

Audits
Because reimbursement is by patient, rather than based on an average of the entire population, and is based upon documentation, there is the potential for upcoding. Audits are conducted by the MA plan and CMS recovery auditors.

Initial Validation Audit (IVA)
CMS requires that the MA plan validate HCCs. This is usually performed by an independent auditor working with the plan or a contracted vendor to validate the MA plan's data submitted to CMS.

The MA plan submits the one best medical record that supports each HCC identified for the beneficiary.

Risk Adjustment Data Validation Audit
Risk adjustment data validation (RADV) audits were introduced in 2011 and updated for 2015. They are performed by CMS to validate the integrity and accuracy of risk-adjusted payments by verifying that the diagnosis codes the MA plans submit are supported by the medical record documentation for a member.

MA plans can be selected by CMS for RADV audits annually and if chosen are required to submit their members' medical records to CMS. Providers are required to assist the MA plan by providing the medical record documentation included in the audit. Even though each diagnosis needs to be reported only once in a calendar year, during a RADV audit up to five dates of service may be submitted to support any one HCC.

To be validated, medical record documentation must meet certain criteria and standards. Even if the diagnosis is documented and coded correctly, any deficiency in the documentation can make the encounter and the HCC invalid. Diagnoses that cannot be validated are considered payment errors. The results of the audit are communicated to the MA plan, which then communicates these results to the provider. Under- and overpayments are subject to payment adjustment. The results of RADV audits can be extrapolated over the MA plan population to calculate potential payment errors and overpayments/recoupments. Regulations include a RADV appeal process, a document dispute process, and a procedure for obtaining physician-signature attestations.

The following items are reviewed during the validation process:
- The record is for the correct enrollee.
- The record is from the correct calendar year for the payment year being audited.
- The record is legible.
- The date of service is present on the records and is for a face-to-face visit.
- The record is from a valid provider type.
- Valid credentials and/or a valid physician specialty are documented on the record.
- The record contains a signature from an acceptable type of physician.
- There is a diagnosis on the record.
- The diagnosis supports an HCC.
- The diagnosis supports the submitted HCC.

Mitigate audit risk by coding each reportable diagnosis each time it meets reporting guidelines. Audit regularly to assess areas of risk and in need of improvement and to capture conditions documented but not coded. Check for additional qualifying HCCs. Ensure claims are submitted and that corrected claims are submitted when indicated. There are three claims submission deadlines: January, March, and September. CMS adjusts each member's risk score twice a year, with the final reconciliation in August of the year after the plan year.

If providers emphasize correct coding and documentation and perform internal audits to determine where the risks are and prepare for audits, incorrect payment is less likely.

Appendix G: Centers for Medicare & Medicaid Services Quality Payment Program

In 2015, in an effort to repeal the faulty Medicare sustainable growth rate (SGR), focus on quality of patient outcomes, and control Medicare spending, Congress passed the Medicare Access and CHIP Reauthorization Act (MACRA), which included sweeping changes for practitioners who provide services reimbursed under the Medicare physician fee schedule (MPFS). MACRA repealed the Medicare SGR methodology used for updating the MPFS and replaced it with the Quality Payment Program (QPP).

Under the QPP, providers who demonstrate success at controlling costs while providing high-quality care to their patients are eligible to earn increased payments. Clinicians who successfully report on determined criteria receive a larger payment. Those who do not participate at all or do not fulfill the defined requirements receive a negative payment adjustment of 5 percent of Medicare Part B reimbursements based on 2018 performance to be applied in 2020; future payment adjustments will rise to as high as +/– 9 percent through the 2020 performance year and will be applied in 2022.

[H2]Passage of the Medicare Access and CHIP Reauthorization Act of 2015

The final rule for implementing MACRA was published November 4, 2016. The final rule primarily provides details on how the QPP was to be implemented, including requiring the secretary of Health and Human Services (HHS) to sunset the value-based (VM) modifier incentive program, the Medicare electronic health record (EHR) incentive program, and the Physician Quality Reporting System (PQRS), and incorporates these incentive programs into the QPP.

[H2]Replacement of the Sustainable Growth Rate

Under the SGR, if overall physician costs were higher than a targeted Medicare expenditure, payments were reduced across the board. With the SGR method, payments to clinicians would have resulted in substantial cuts.

Because the QPP replaces the SGR methodology, the following revisions are detailed in MACRA:

- Establishes conversion factor updates:
  - a Medicare physician fee schedule conversion factor adjustment of 0.5 percent for 2016–2019 and a conversion factor adjustment of 0.00 percent for 2020–2025
  - the qualifying participant (QP) alternative payment models (APM) conversion factor of 0.75 percent and a nonqualifying provider APM conversion factor of 0.25 percent for 2026 and each subsequent year

Under the QPP, the Centers for Medicare and Medicaid Services (CMS) aims to:

- Support quality of patient care improvement by focusing on better outcomes for patients, decreasing provider burden, and preserving the independent clinical practice
- Promote the adoption of APMs, which align incentives across healthcare stakeholders
- Advance existing efforts of delivery system reform, including ensuring a smooth transition to a new system that promotes high-quality, efficient care through unification of CMS legacy programs such as the EHR incentive program

Quality Payment Program Established

The MACRA final rule established the Quality Payment Program (QPP) effective January 1, 2017. Within the QPP there are two interrelated pathways: advanced alternative payment models (APM) and the Merit-based Incentive Payment System (MIPS).

MACRA promotes provider participation in many APMs, including the Shared Saving Program and medical home models. CMS indicates that the QPP provides clinicians with new opportunities to improve care delivery with the agency supporting and rewarding providers who find new ways to engage patients, families, and caregivers and to improve care coordination and population health management. In addition, CMS stresses that the QPP is a flexible program and allows providers to "choose their pace."

Eligible clinicians (EC) must select which track/pathway—MIPS or advanced APMs—they will participate in based on the practice size, specialty, location, and patient population. Unlike previous quality initiatives, a provider does not have to enroll in the QPP. However, groups wishing to participate in the MIPS program via the Consumer Assessment of Healthcare Providers and Systems (CAHPS) for MIPS survey measures or CMS Web Interface (WI) do have a June 30 deadline each year. The CAHPS for MIPS survey is an optional quality measure that groups participating in MIPS can elect to administer. In the quality performance category, it counts as a patient experience measure. In addition, MIPS-eligible

clinicians may also be awarded points under the improvement activities performance category for administering the survey.

Merit-based Incentive Payment System

MIPS is the track for clinicians who opt to participate in traditional Medicare as opposed to participating through an advanced APM. In doing so, clinicians may earn a payment adjustment related to evidence-based and practice-specific quality data. As a result, depending on the degree and success of performance in all four categories for CY 2018, clinicians receive one of the following:

- Positive payment adjustment in which additional compensation is received
- Neutral payment adjustment that neither increases nor reduces Medicare payments
- Negative payment adjustment of up to 5 percent of Medicare payment furnished in calendar year (CY) 2020

Participation in the MIPS track is determined based on the amount billed to Medicare and the number of beneficiaries seen per year. The following provider types are eligible for participation IF:

- Medicare billings are equal to or greater than $90,000

  AND
- Care is provided to 200 or more Medicare patients each year

For the first and second years, the following provider types are considered ECs:

- Physicians (MD, DO, DDS, DMD, DPM, OD, DC)
- Physician assistants (PA)
- Nurse practitioners (NP)
- Clinical nurse specialists (CNS)
- Certified registered nurse anesthetists (CRNA)
- Any clinician group that includes one of the professionals listed above

Anatomy of MIPS

MIPS incorporates pieces of three former Medicare reporting programs:

- Physician Quality Reporting System (PQRS)
- Medicare EHR Incentive Program/meaningful use
- Value-based payment modifier

Under these programs, clinicians would have likely faced a negative payment adjustment as high as 9 percent starting in 2022; with the MACRA legislation, these programs have ended, the payment adjustments in the early years of the QPP have been reduced, and reporting requirements have been streamlined. Clinicians who have previously participated in any of the three programs will certainly see similarities as a number of requirements should be familiar.

A measurement-based regime creates a single reporting framework for physicians that comprise four performance categories:

- Quality—replaces the PQRS
- Improvement Activities (IA)—implemented in 2017
- Advancing Care Information (ACI)—replaces the Medicare EHR Incentive Program, aka "meaningful use"
- Cost—replaces the value-based modifier

Each of the four performance categories has been weighted, with greatest emphasis placed on the Quality category at 50 percent, ACI is second at 25 percent, IA at 15 percent, and cost at 10 percent.

The 2018 MIPS performance threshold equates to 15 points out of a possible 100 points. Simply put, eligible clinicians are required to score 15 points to avoid the negative 5 percent payment adjustment.

Quality Performance

Under the MIPS Quality performance category, ECs and groups must select six measures from a listing of more than 270 measures, with at least one of the six measures being an outcome measure. Patient outcomes such as mortality, whether a patient is readmitted to the hospital, and the patient's experience are areas that CMS and the healthcare industry seek to improve. An outcome measure is the way CMS can quantify changes in the health of an individual, groups of individuals, and even certain populations that they can attribute back to a specific intervention or series of interventions.

Quality measures are tools for quantifying, or measuring, healthcare processes and patient outcomes and perceptions, as well as organizational structure and/or systems linked to the ability to provide high-quality healthcare. These measures play an important role under the MIPS. Reporting should be done on a minimum of half of the EC's or group practice's Medicare Part B patients. Each measure is worth up to 10 points and is compared to a national benchmark.

Improvement Activities

The IA category assesses to what degree a clinician participates in activities designed to improve clinical practices. ECs are required to attest that they have participated in a minimum of four improvement activities from an expanded inventory of more than 100 activities across nine subcategories for 90 consecutive days. These nine subcategories include:

- Expanded practice access
- Population management
- Care coordination
- Beneficiary engagement
- Patient safety and practice assessment
- Participation in an APM
- Achieving health equity
- Integrating behavioral and mental health
- Emergency preparedness and response

This category was created with some inherent flexibility; for example, for groups with 15 or fewer participants, nonpatient-facing clinicians (e.g., pathologists), or those ECs in a rural or health professional shortage area (HPSA) are required to declare participation in only up to two activities for at least 90 consecutive days.

Advancing Care Information

This performance category replaces the Medicare EHR Incentive Program, commonly known as "meaningful use." CMS wants to encourage and promote the use of certified EHR technology (CEHRT) among providers and, in particular, the use of interoperability and sharing of information among clinicians and between providers and patients.

All MIPS ECs are required to use CEHRT to report the ACI performance category. For those ECs who do not have a certified EHR system, specific criteria must be met to qualify to have the ACI performance category reweighted to 0 percent and not be included in the EC's total score.

Cost

In this performance category, CMS determines an EC or group practice's cost score by calculating data from two measures previously included in the value-based payment modifier that involves the total cost of care for attributed beneficiaries and what Medicare spends per beneficiary. This amount is the total of both Medicare Part A and B payments from three days before through 30 days after a beneficiary has had an inpatient hospitalization episode. CMS then determines which ECs and practices have an adequate number of beneficiaries and hospitalizations associated with them. This number is compared with national benchmarks with one point being given for year-over-year improvement.

Quality and resource use reports (QRUR) are confidential feedback reports that provide information about the resources used (cost) and the quality of care provided by physicians and group practices to Medicare fee-for-service (FFS) patients. The reports are shared with clinicians under CMS's Physician Feedback Program and provide comparative performance data that clinicians can use to help improve care provided to Medicare Part B beneficiaries.

MIPS Scoring

CMS uses scoring to determine an EC's successful participation in the QPP and thereby determine if the clinician's reimbursement will be negative, neutral, or positive.

The scoring methodology is a unified approach across all performance categories, allowing eligible clinicians to understand what is expected so they can perform successfully in the MIPS.

For more information and details on QPP go to: https://qpp.cms.gov.

Illustrations

Chapter 3. Diseases of the Blood and Blood-forming Organs and Certain Disorders Involving the Immune Mechanism (D50–D89)

Red Blood Cells

White Blood Cell

Platelet

Coagulation

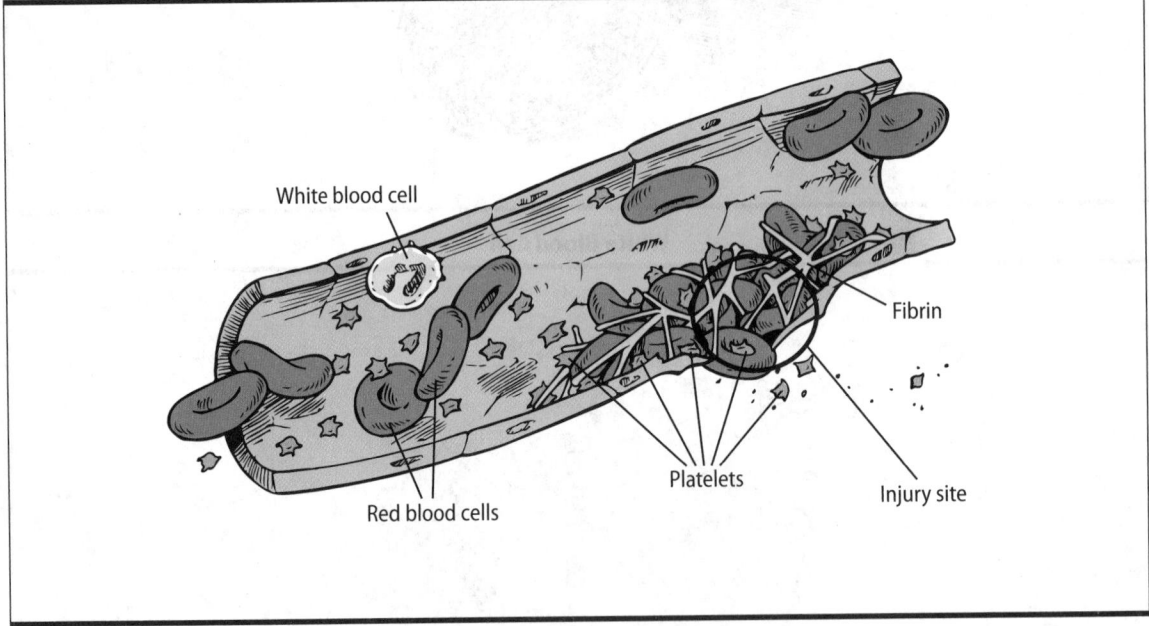

White blood cell

Fibrin

Platelets

Injury site

Red blood cells

Spleen Anatomical Location and External Structures

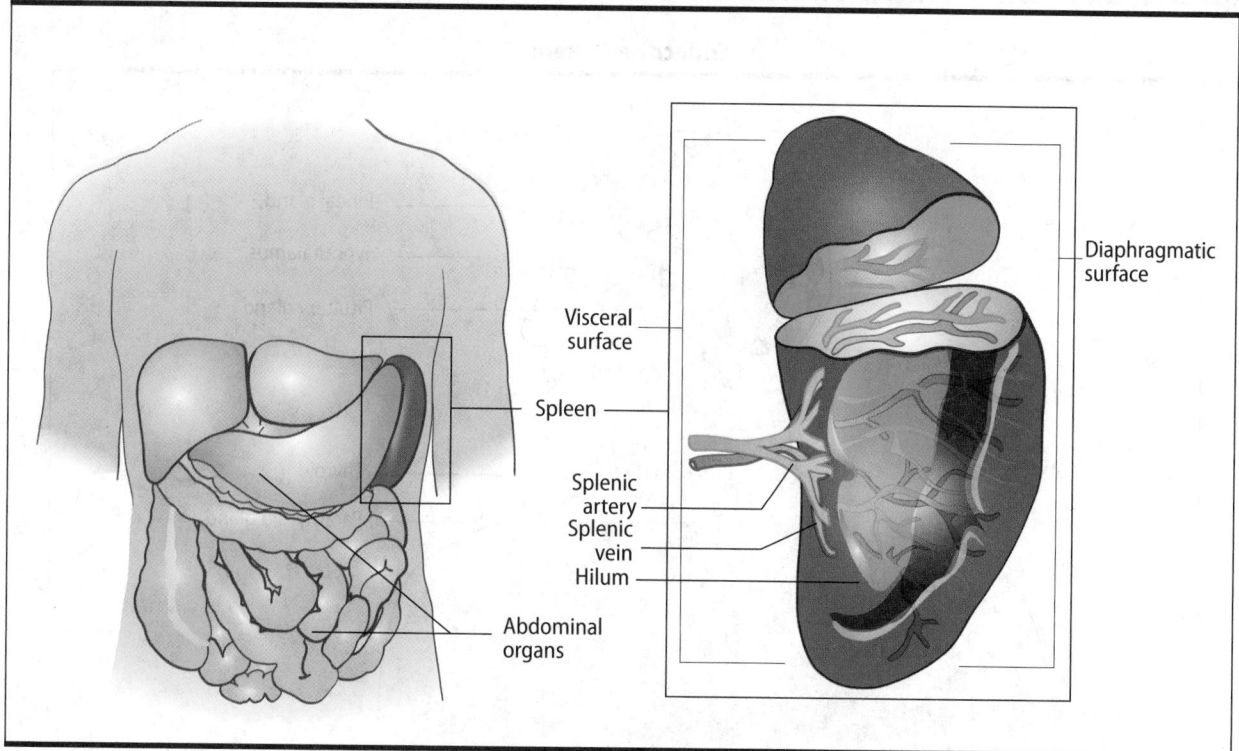

Spleen Interior Structures

Chapter 4. Endocrine, Nutritional and Metabolic Diseases (E00–E89)

Endocrine System

Thyroid

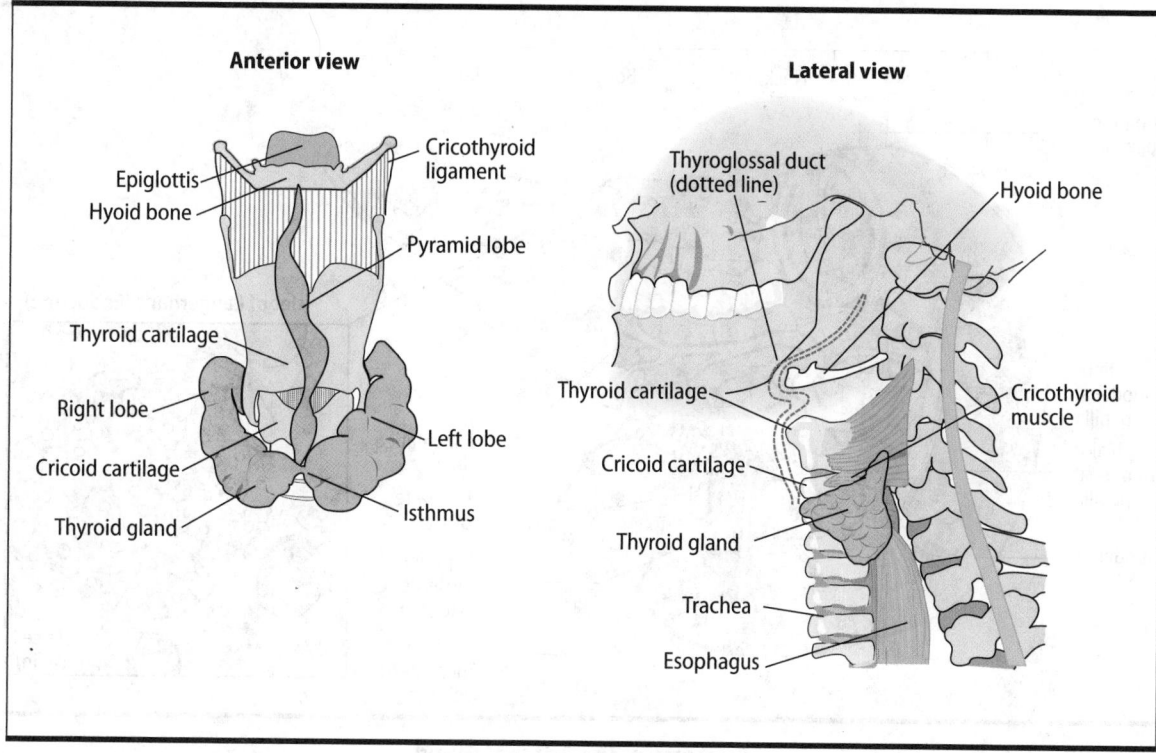

Thyroid and Parathyroid Glands

Posterior view

- Epiglottis
- Pharynx
- Thyroid gland
- Parathyroid gland

Pancreas

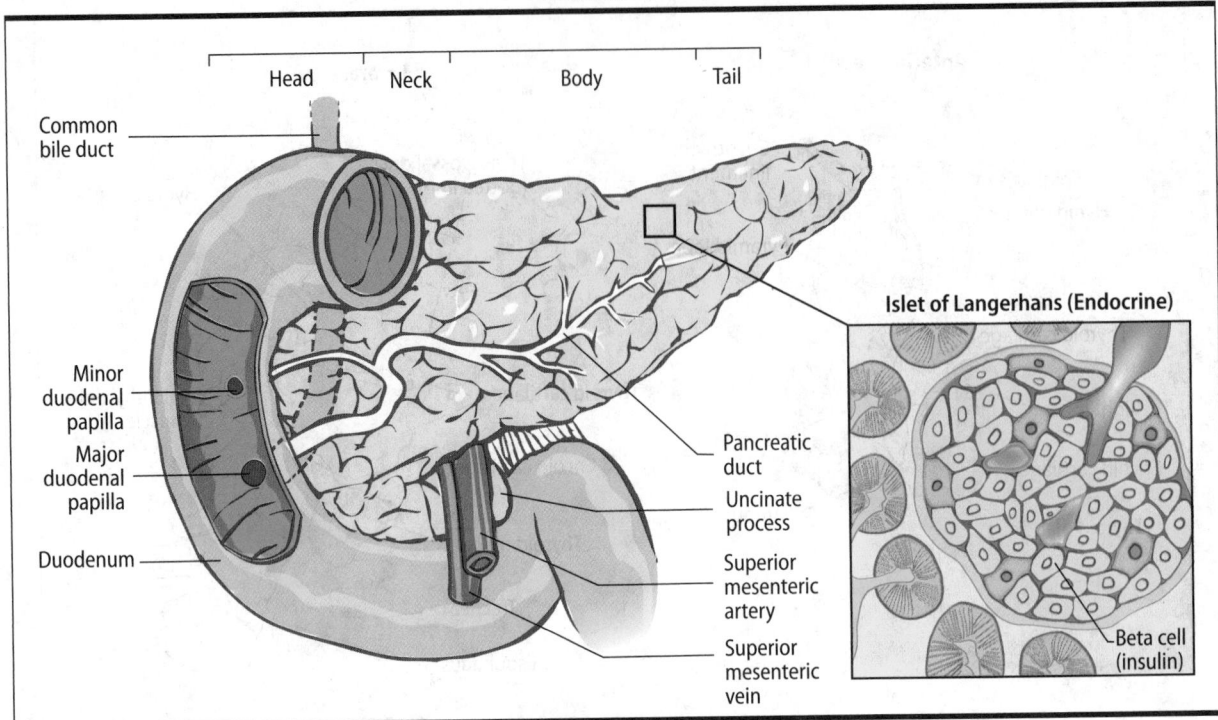

Anatomy of the Adrenal Gland

Structure of an Ovary

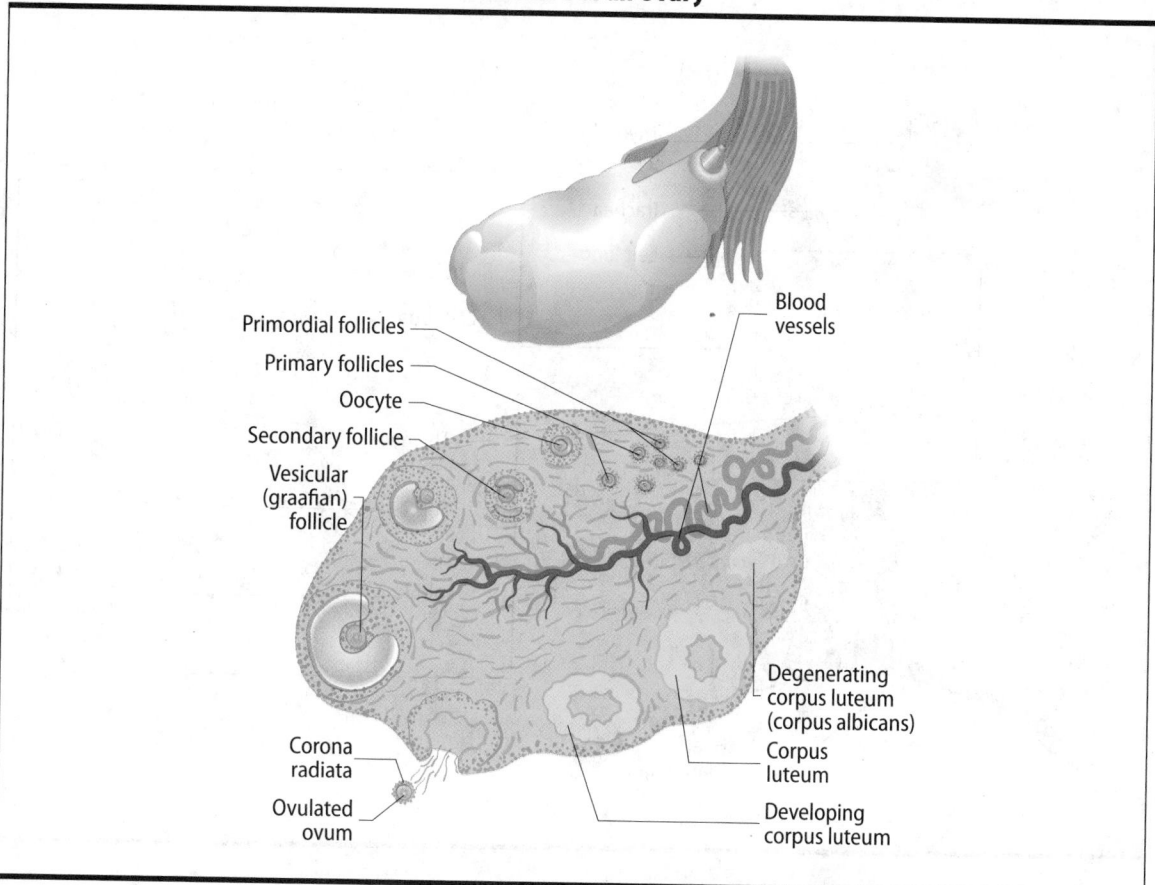

Testis and Associated Structures

Thymus

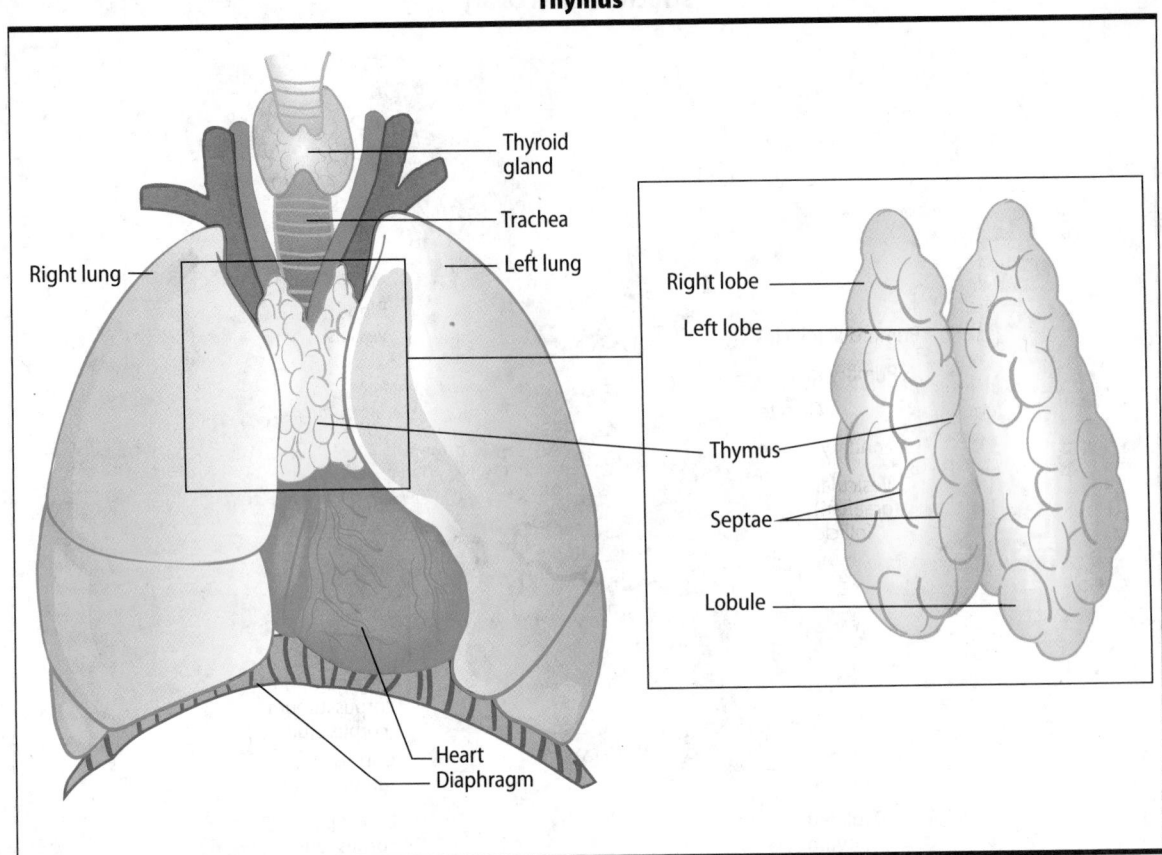

Chapter 6. Diseases of the Nervous System (GØØ–G99)

Brain

Cranial Nerves

Peripheral Nervous System

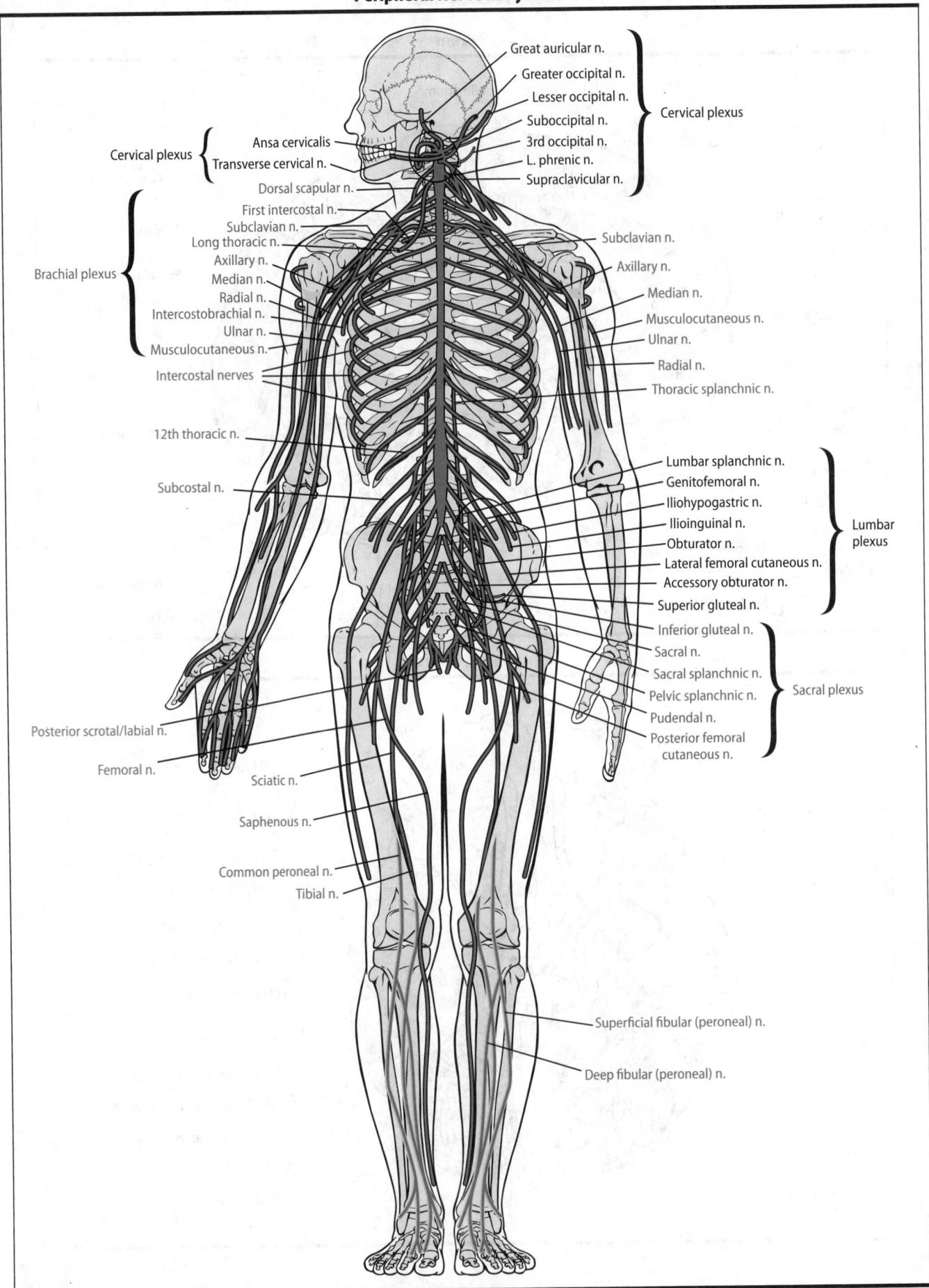

Spinal Cord and Spinal Nerves

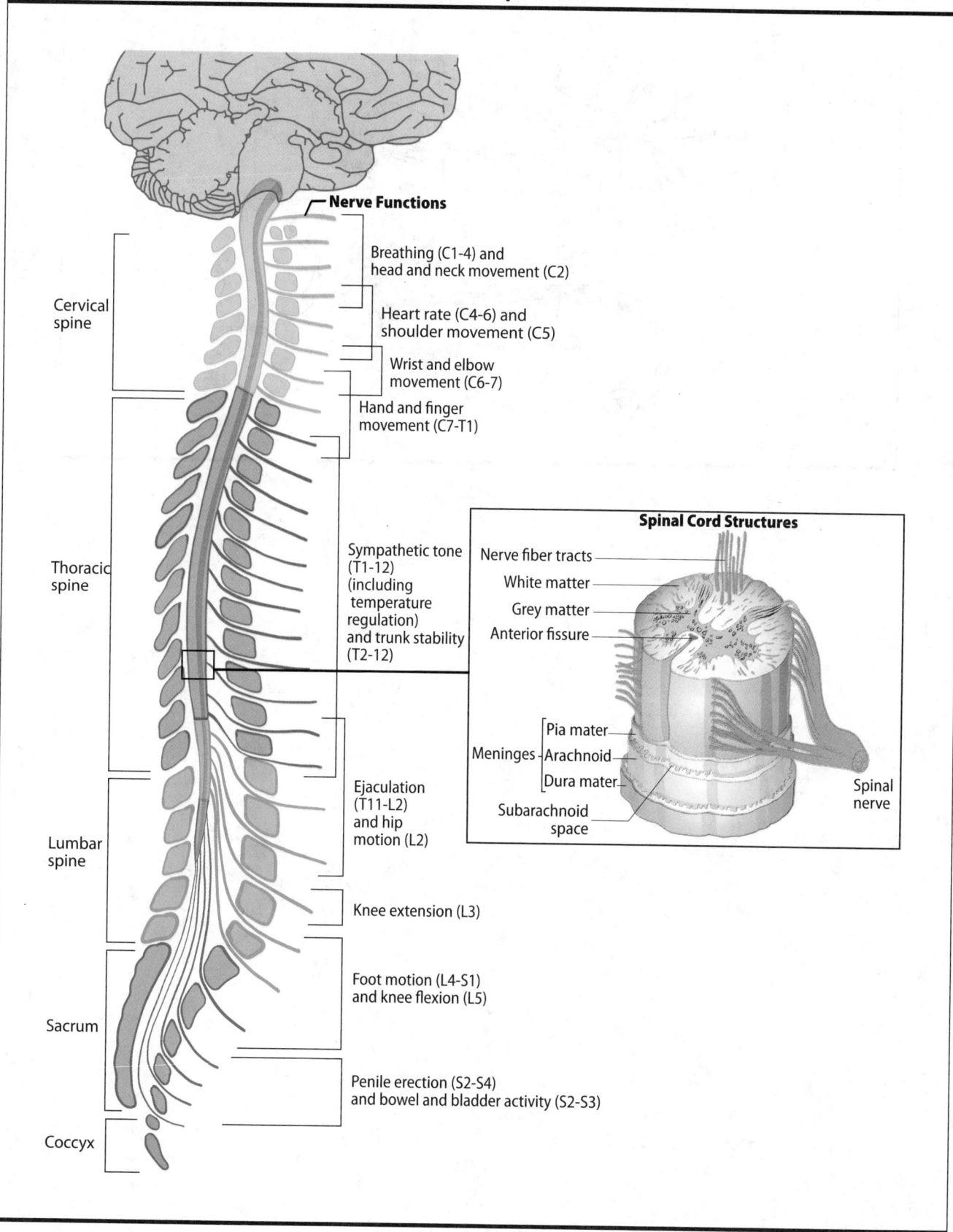

Nerve Functions

Breathing (C1-4) and head and neck movement (C2)

Heart rate (C4-6) and shoulder movement (C5)

Wrist and elbow movement (C6-7)

Hand and finger movement (C7-T1)

Cervical spine

Thoracic spine

Sympathetic tone (T1-12) (including temperature regulation) and trunk stability (T2-12)

Ejaculation (T11-L2) and hip motion (L2)

Lumbar spine

Knee extension (L3)

Foot motion (L4-S1) and knee flexion (L5)

Sacrum

Penile erection (S2-S4) and bowel and bladder activity (S2-S3)

Coccyx

Spinal Cord Structures

Nerve fiber tracts
White matter
Grey matter
Anterior fissure

Meninges — Pia mater
Arachnoid
Dura mater

Subarachnoid space

Spinal nerve

Nerve Cell

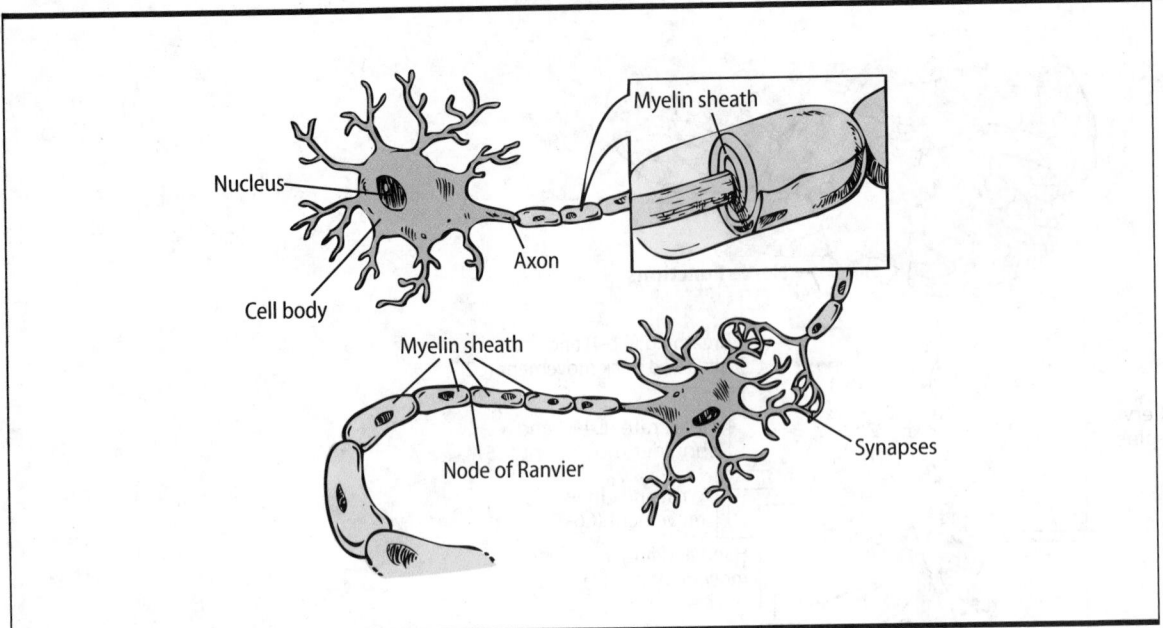

Chapter 7. Diseases of the Eye and Adnexa (HØØ–H59)

Eye

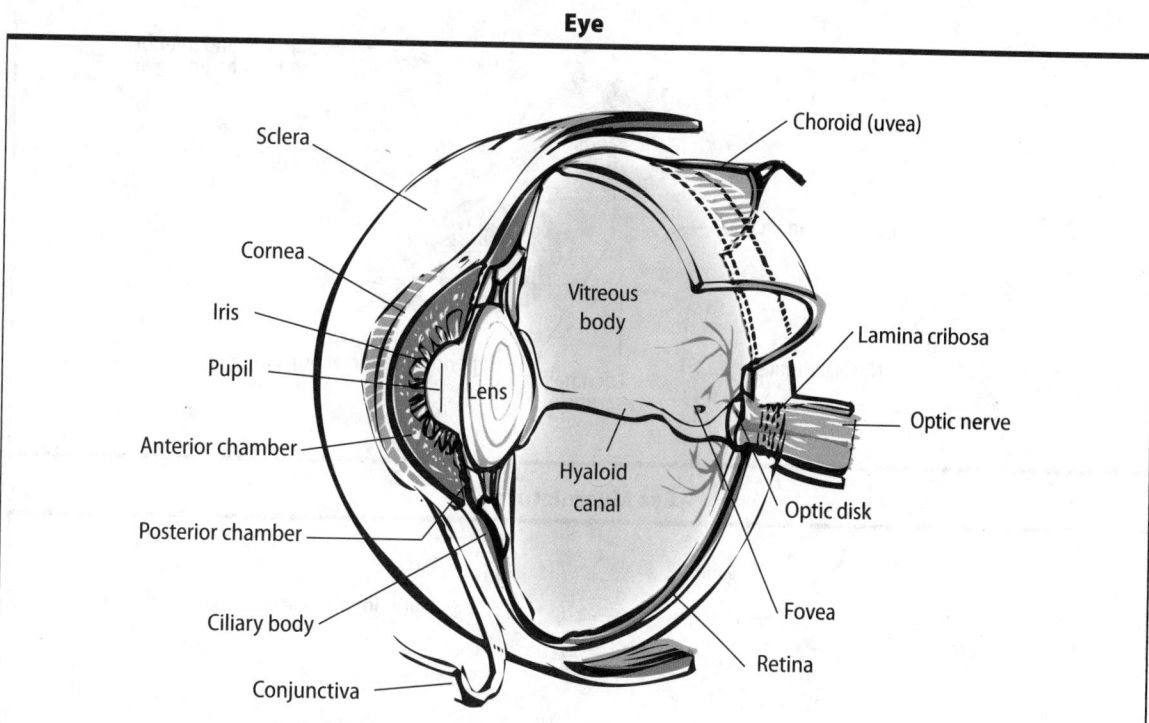

Posterior Pole of Globe/Flow of Aqueous Humor

Lacrimal System

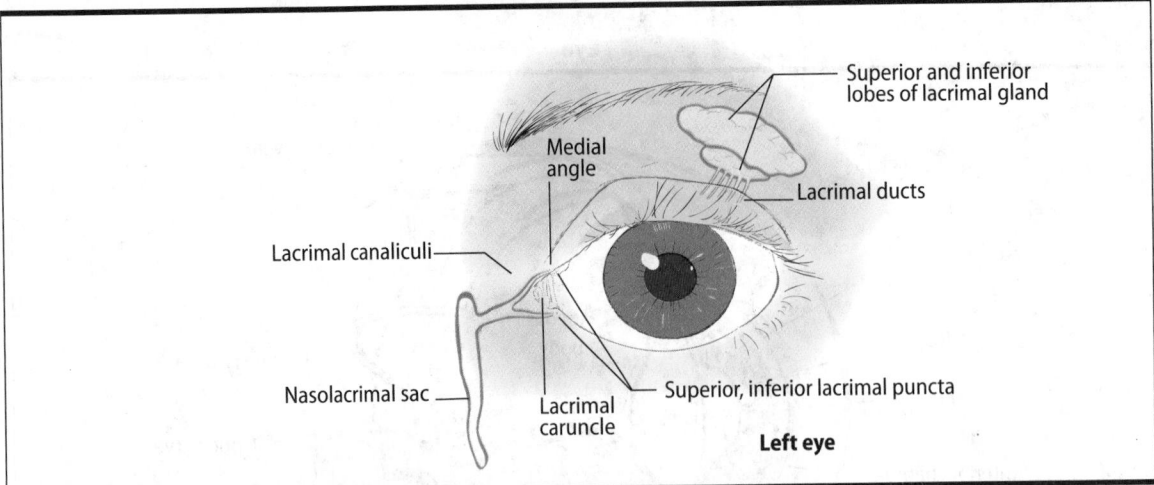

Superior and inferior lobes of lacrimal gland

Medial angle

Lacrimal ducts

Lacrimal canaliculi

Lacrimal caruncle

Superior, inferior lacrimal puncta

Nasolacrimal sac

Left eye

Eye Musculature

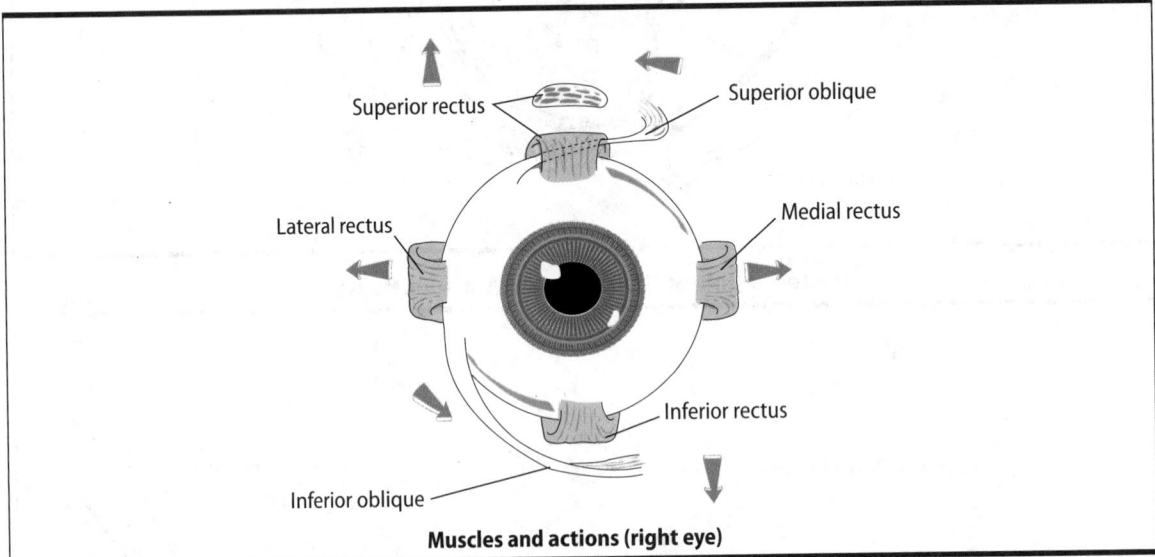

Superior rectus

Superior oblique

Lateral rectus

Medial rectus

Inferior rectus

Inferior oblique

Muscles and actions (right eye)

Eyelid Structures

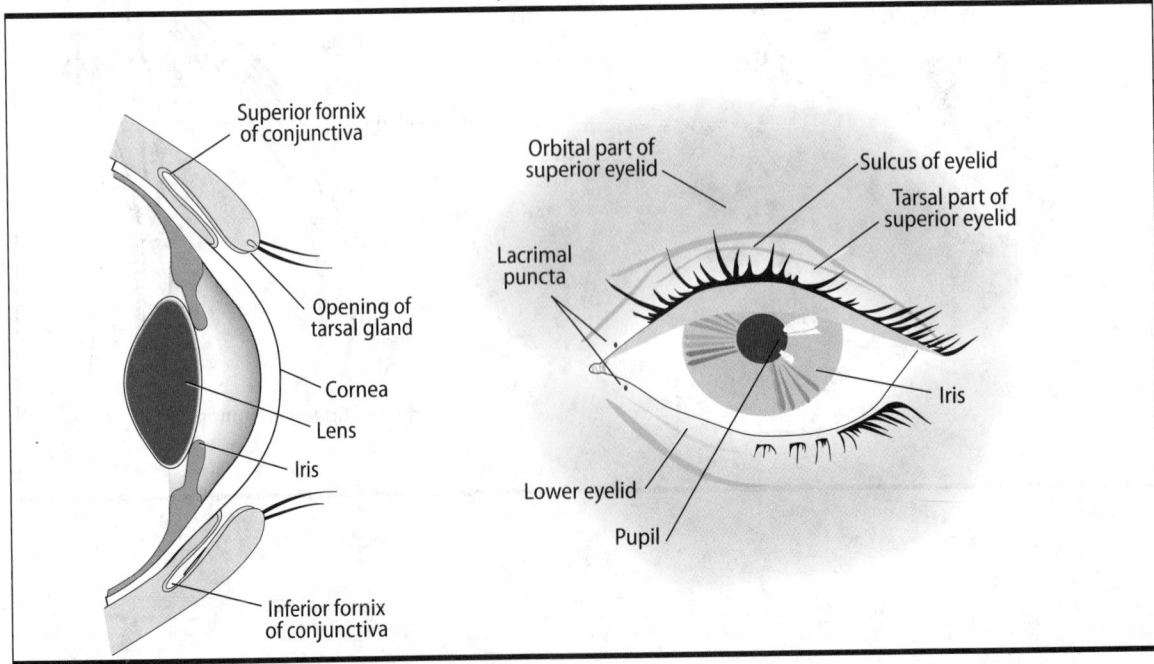

Superior fornix of conjunctiva

Orbital part of superior eyelid

Sulcus of eyelid

Tarsal part of superior eyelid

Lacrimal puncta

Opening of tarsal gland

Cornea

Lens

Iris

Iris

Lower eyelid

Pupil

Inferior fornix of conjunctiva

Chapter 8. Diseases of the Ear and Mastoid Process (H60–H95)

Ear Anatomy

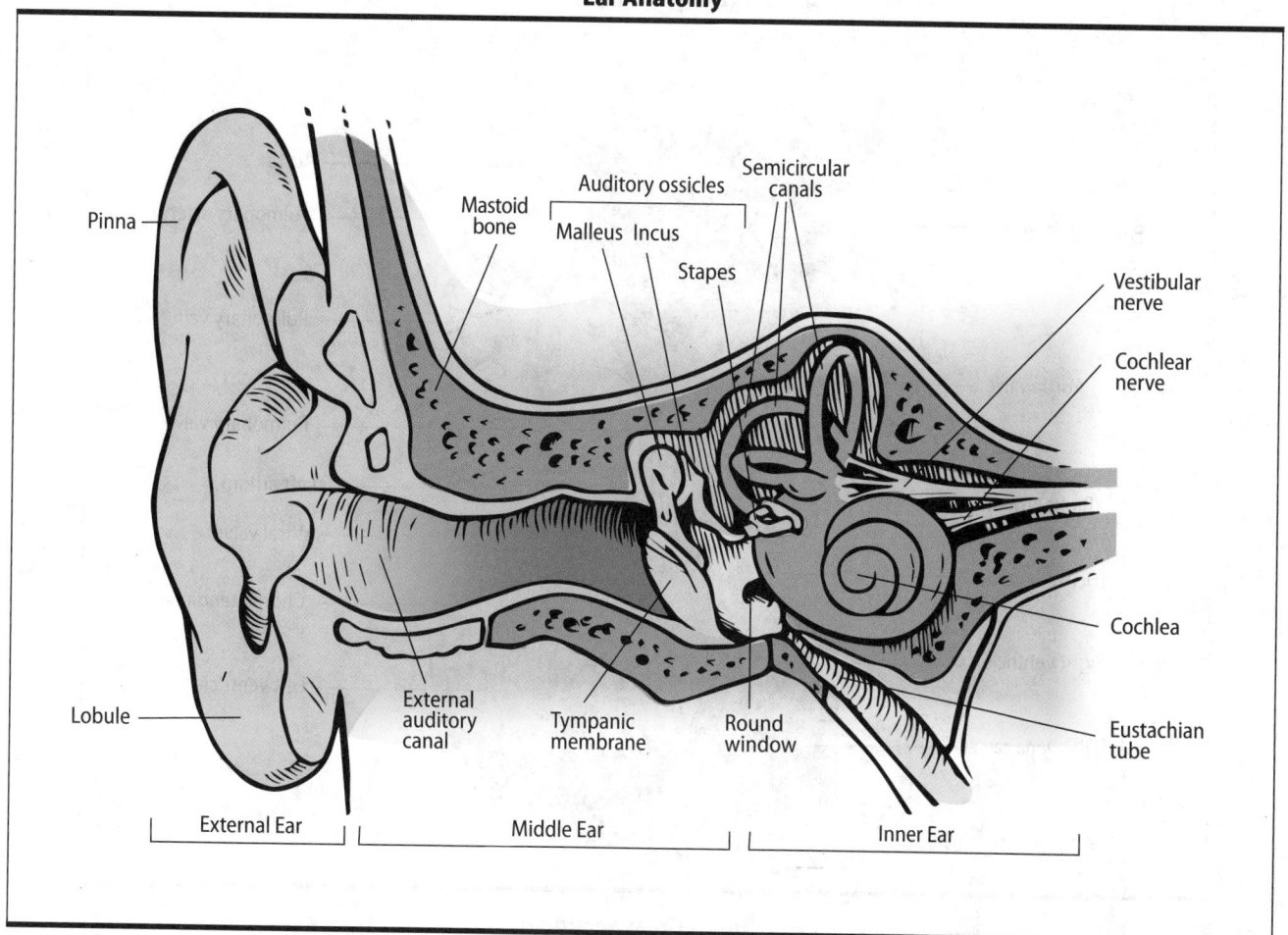

Chapter 9. Diseases of the Circulatory System (IØØ–I99)

Anatomy of the Heart

- Superior vena cava
- Aortic valve
- Right atrium
- Tricuspid valve
- Right ventricle
- Inferior vena cava
- Aorta
- Pulmonary artery
- Pulmonary vein
- Pulmonary valve
- Left atrium
- Mitral valve
- Chorda tendinae
- Left ventricle

Heart Cross Section

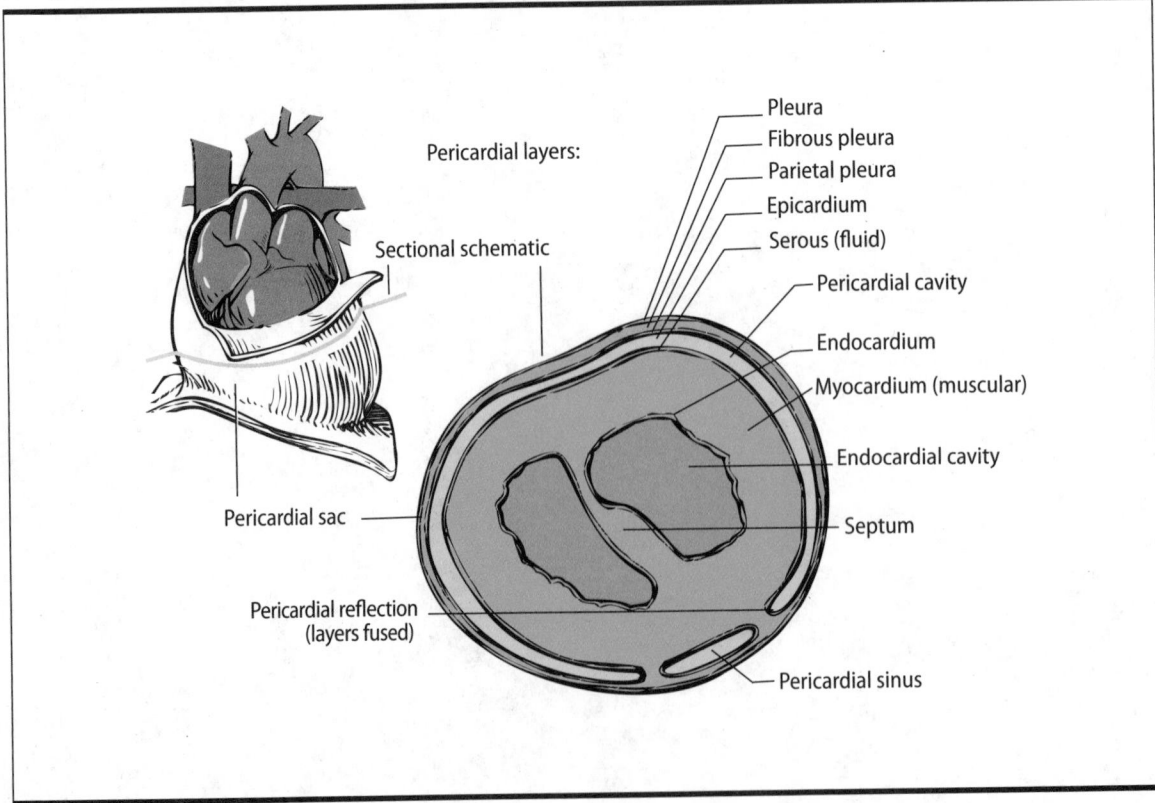

Pericardial layers:

Sectional schematic

- Pleura
- Fibrous pleura
- Parietal pleura
- Epicardium
- Serous (fluid)
- Pericardial cavity
- Endocardium
- Myocardium (muscular)
- Endocardial cavity
- Septum
- Pericardial sac
- Pericardial reflection (layers fused)
- Pericardial sinus

Heart Valves

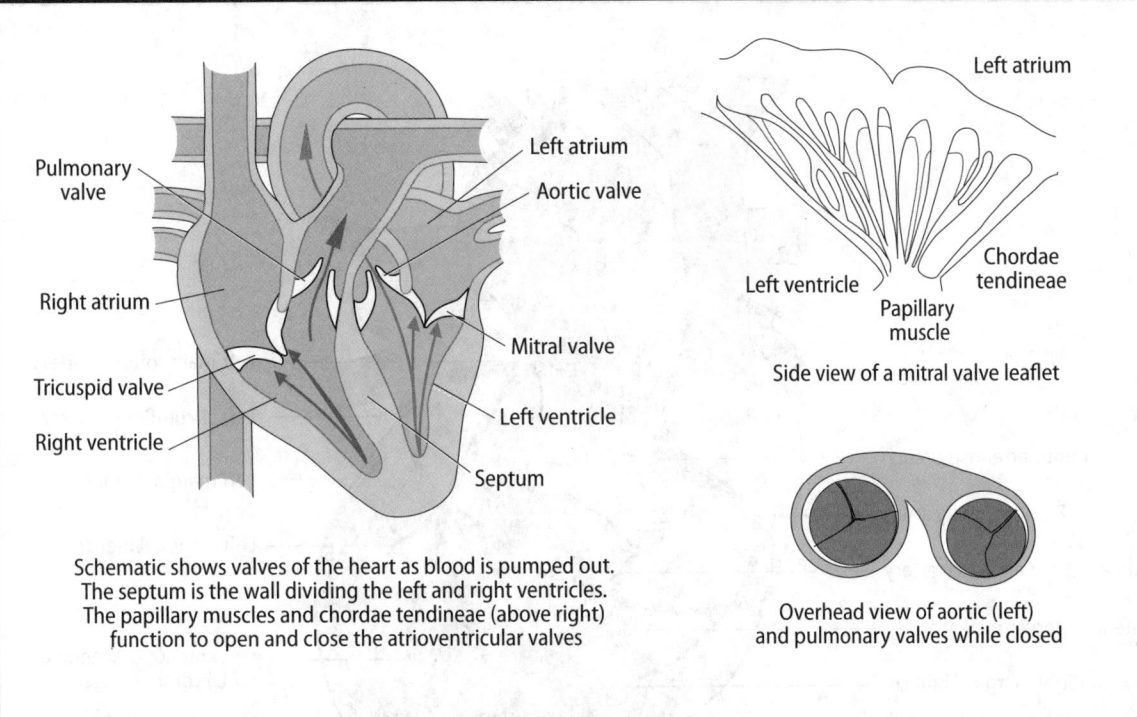

Pulmonary valve

Left atrium

Aortic valve

Right atrium

Mitral valve

Tricuspid valve

Left ventricle

Right ventricle

Septum

Left atrium

Left ventricle

Chordae tendineae

Papillary muscle

Side view of a mitral valve leaflet

Schematic shows valves of the heart as blood is pumped out.
The septum is the wall dividing the left and right ventricles.
The papillary muscles and chordae tendineae (above right)
function to open and close the atrioventricular valves

Overhead view of aortic (left)
and pulmonary valves while closed

Heart Conduction System

Sinoatrial node (pacemaker)

Atrioventricular node

Atrioventricular bundle (of His)

Left bundle branch

Right bundle branch

Purkinje fibers

Coronary Arteries

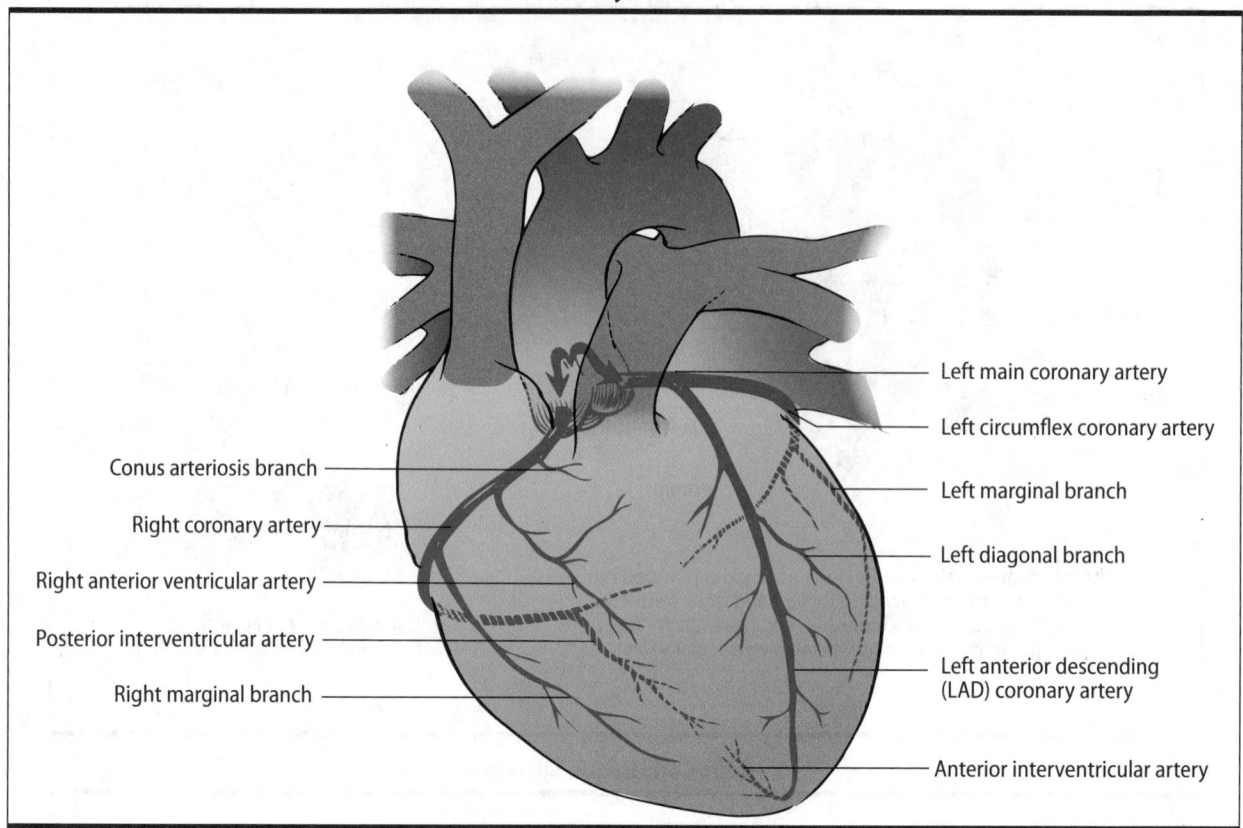

- Left main coronary artery
- Left circumflex coronary artery
- Left marginal branch
- Left diagonal branch
- Left anterior descending (LAD) coronary artery
- Anterior interventricular artery

- Conus arteriosis branch
- Right coronary artery
- Right anterior ventricular artery
- Posterior interventricular artery
- Right marginal branch

Arteries

Veins

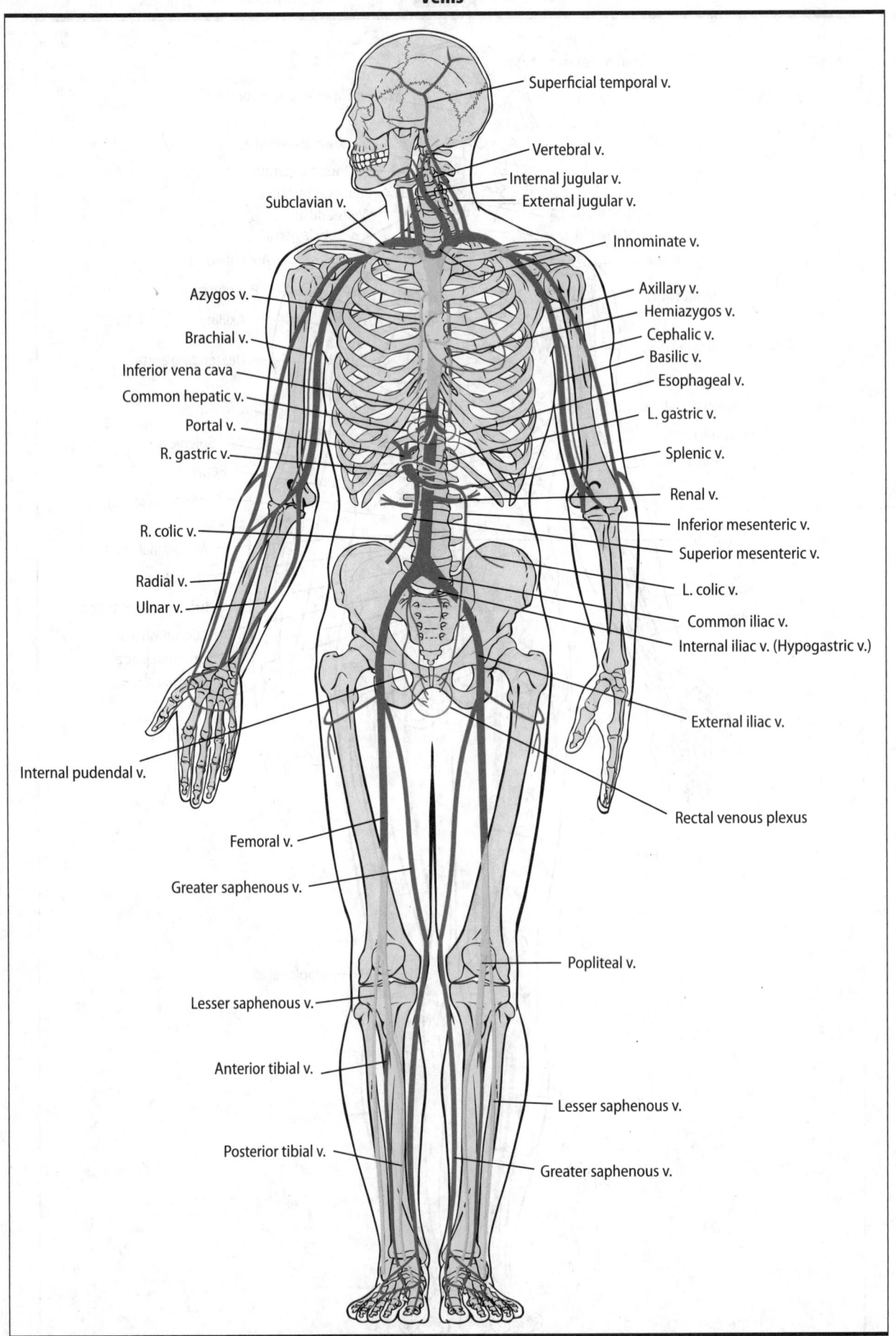

Superficial temporal v.

Vertebral v.

Internal jugular v.

External jugular v.

Subclavian v.

Innominate v.

Axillary v.

Azygos v.

Hemiazygos v.

Brachial v.

Cephalic v.

Basilic v.

Inferior vena cava

Esophageal v.

Common hepatic v.

L. gastric v.

Portal v.

R. gastric v.

Splenic v.

Renal v.

R. colic v.

Inferior mesenteric v.

Superior mesenteric v.

Radial v.

L. colic v.

Ulnar v.

Common iliac v.

Internal iliac v. (Hypogastric v.)

External iliac v.

Internal pudendal v.

Rectal venous plexus

Femoral v.

Greater saphenous v.

Popliteal v.

Lesser saphenous v.

Anterior tibial v.

Lesser saphenous v.

Posterior tibial v.

Greater saphenous v.

Internal Carotid and Vertebral Arteries and Branches

Side View

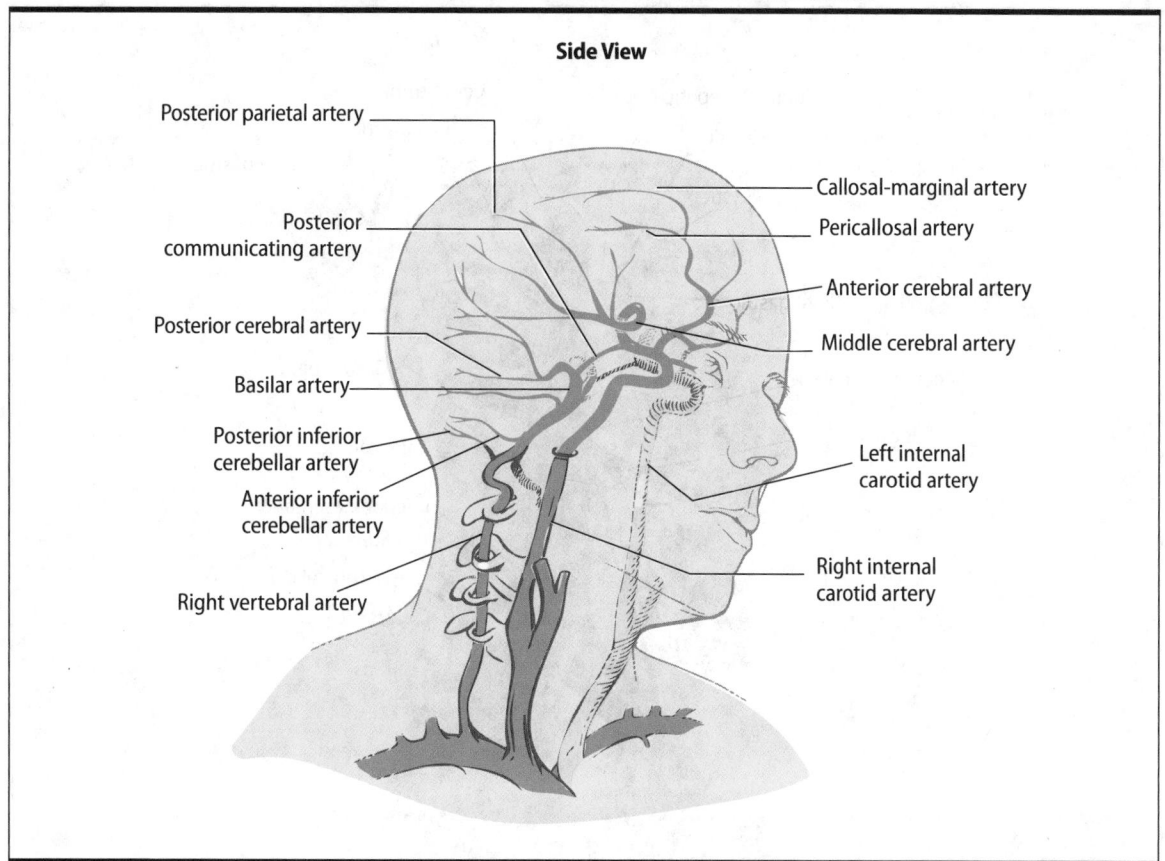

External Carotid Artery and Branches

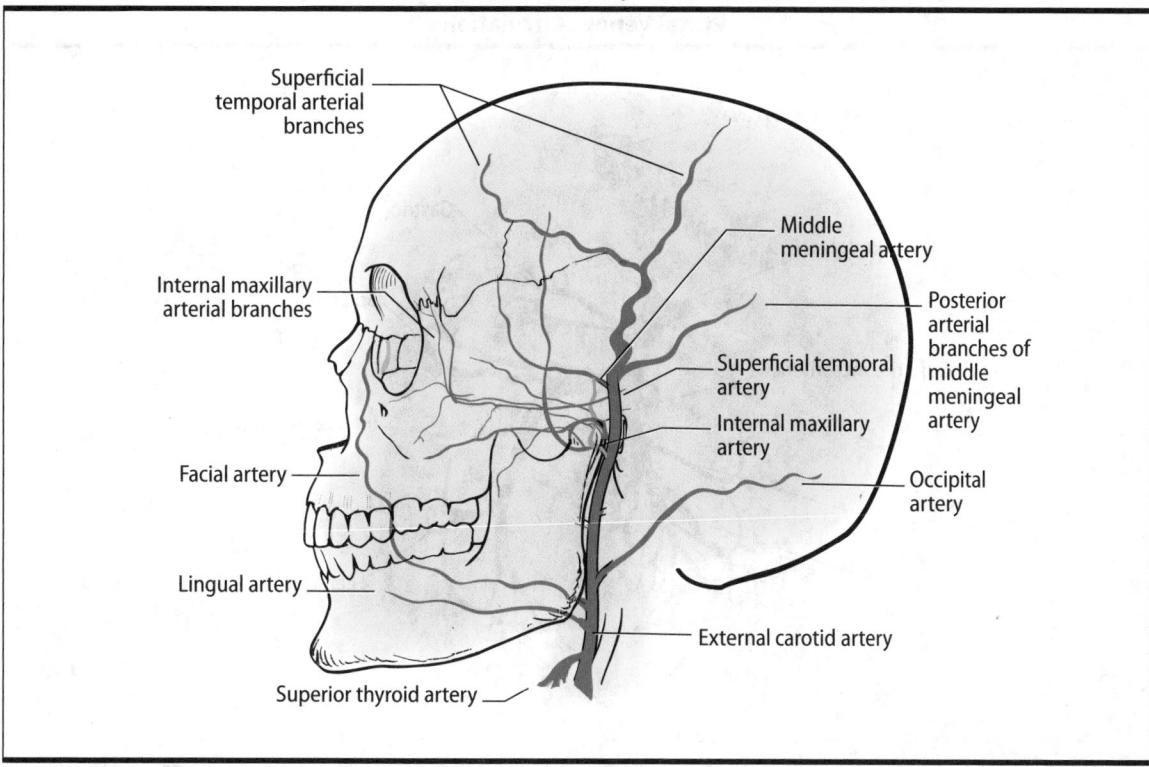

Branches of Abdominal Aorta

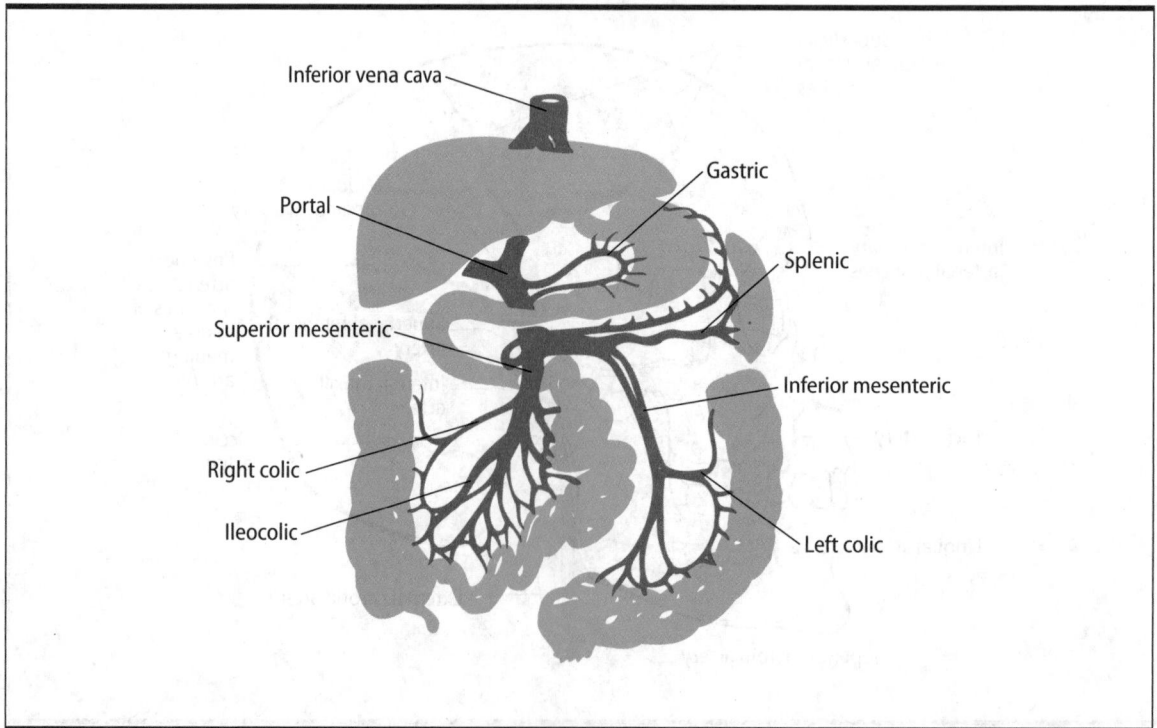

Portal Venous Circulation

Lymphatic System

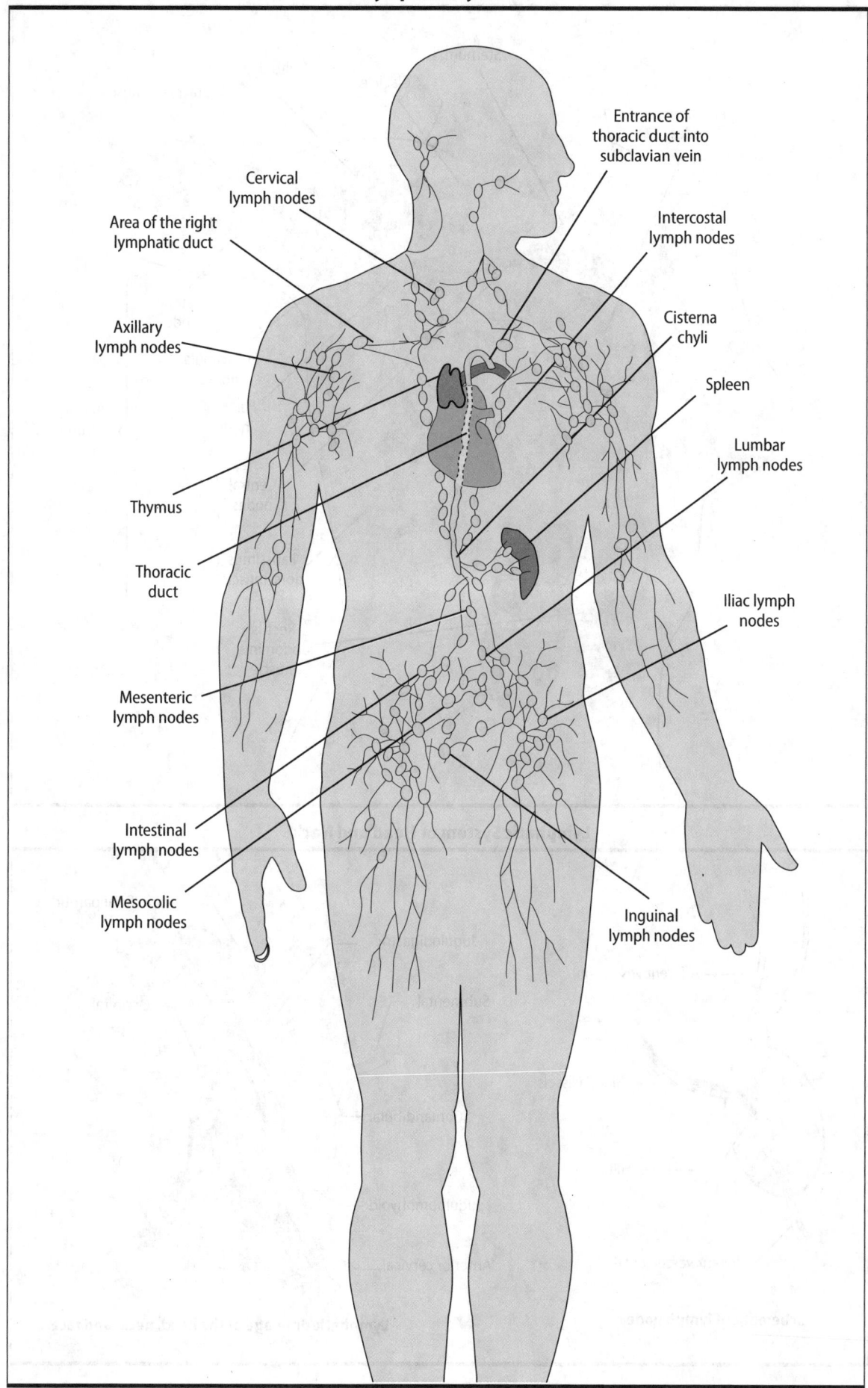

Axillary Lymph Nodes

Sternum

Parasternal nodes

Clavicle

Deltoid muscle

Brachialis muscle

Lateral nodes

Subscapular nodes

Pectoral nodes

Axillary lymph nodes

Central nodes

Latissimus dorsi muscle

Rectus abdominis muscle

Lymphatic System of Head and Neck

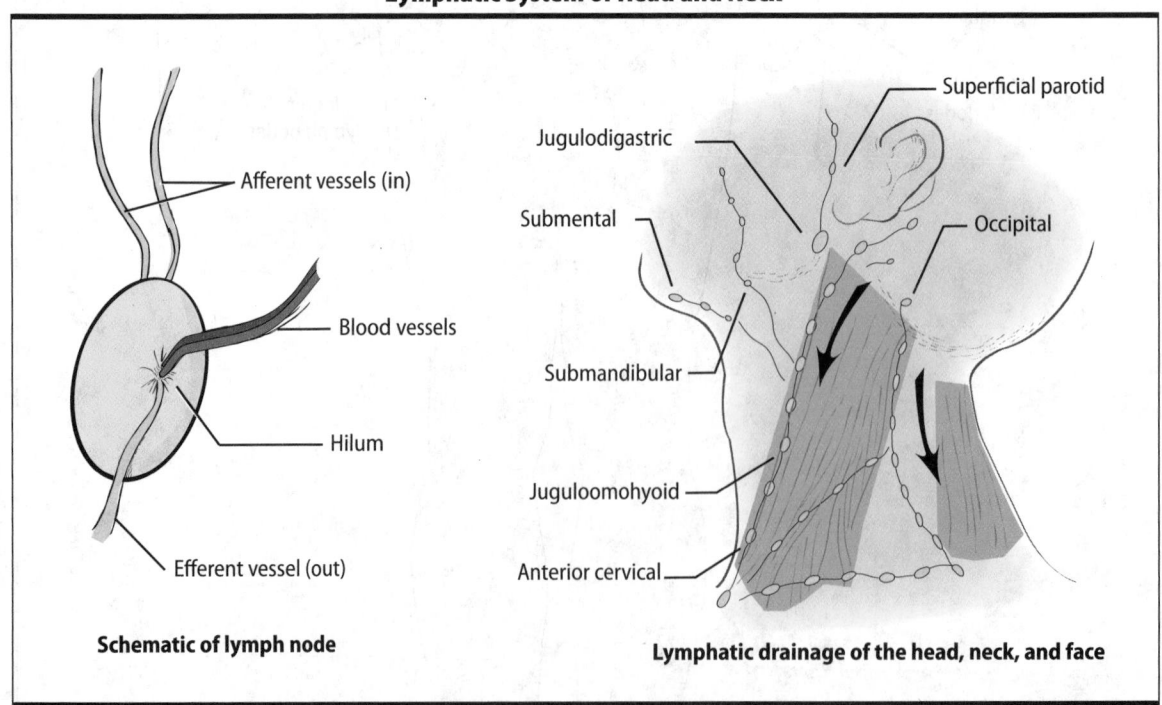

Afferent vessels (in)

Blood vessels

Hilum

Efferent vessel (out)

Schematic of lymph node

Jugulodigastric

Superficial parotid

Submental

Occipital

Submandibular

Juguloomohyoid

Anterior cervical

Lymphatic drainage of the head, neck, and face

Lymphatic Capillaries

Schematic of lymphatic capillaries

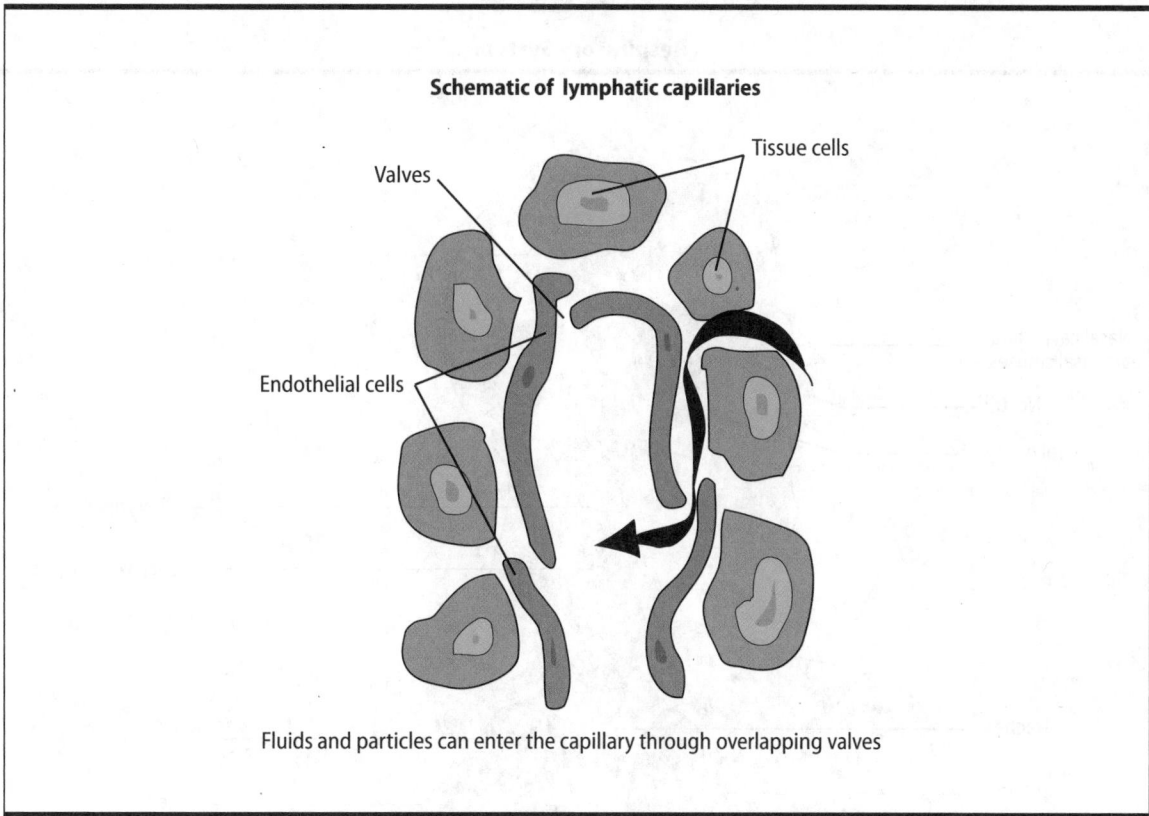

Fluids and particles can enter the capillary through overlapping valves

Lymphatic Drainage

Lymphatic drainage of the colon follows blood supply

Chapter 10. Diseases of the Respiratory System (J00–J99)

Respiratory System

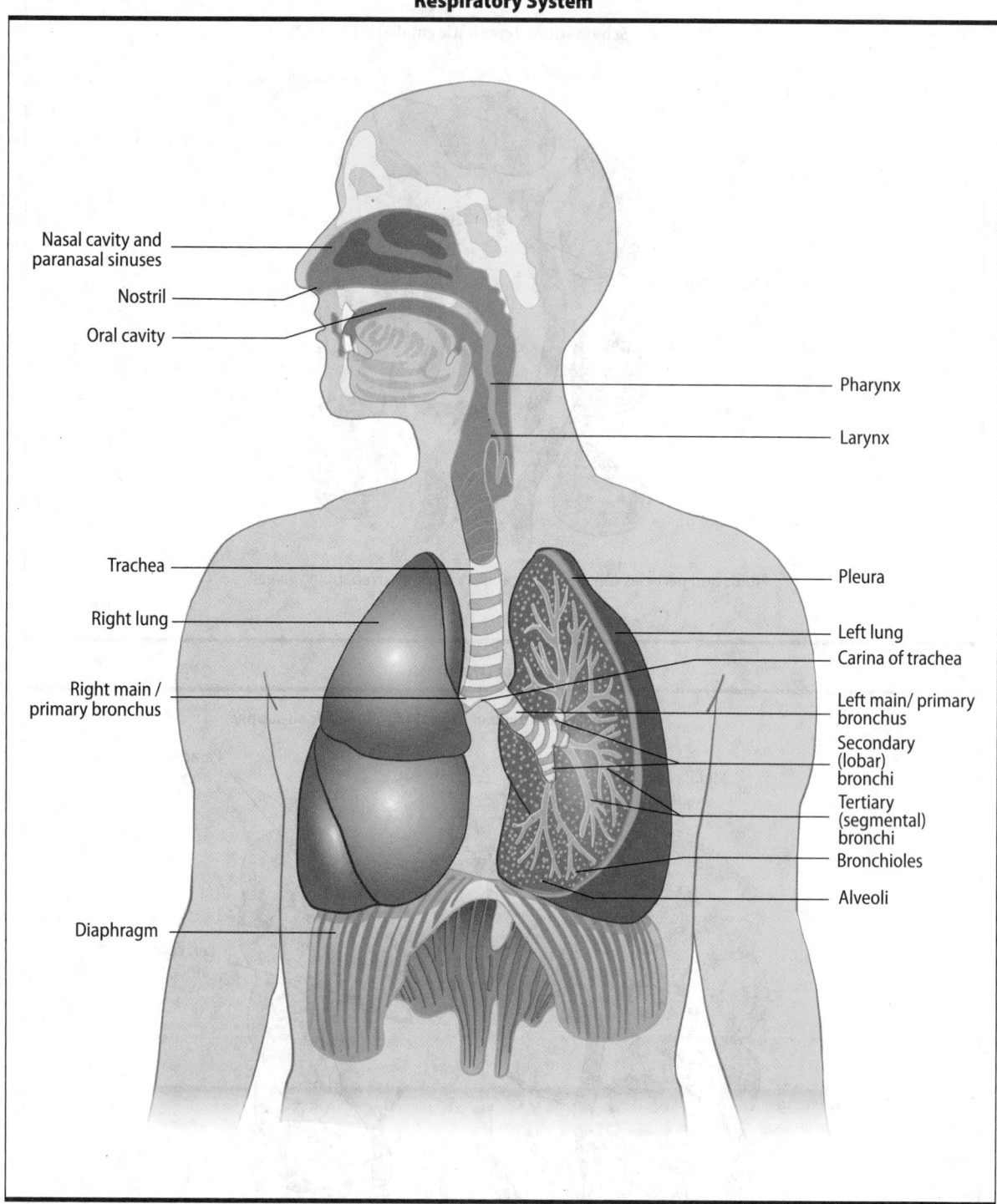

- Nasal cavity and paranasal sinuses
- Nostril
- Oral cavity
- Pharynx
- Larynx
- Trachea
- Right lung
- Pleura
- Left lung
- Carina of trachea
- Right main / primary bronchus
- Left main/ primary bronchus
- Secondary (lobar) bronchi
- Tertiary (segmental) bronchi
- Bronchioles
- Alveoli
- Diaphragm

Upper Respiratory System

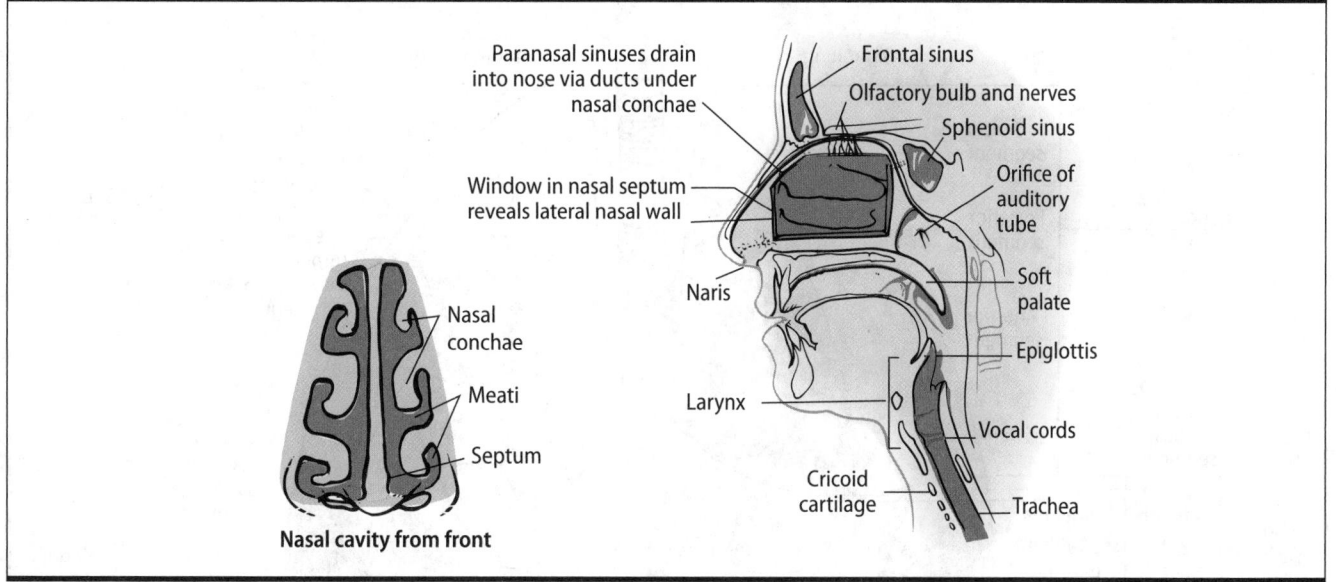

Paranasal sinuses drain into nose via ducts under nasal conchae

Frontal sinus

Olfactory bulb and nerves

Sphenoid sinus

Window in nasal septum reveals lateral nasal wall

Orifice of auditory tube

Naris

Soft palate

Nasal conchae

Epiglottis

Meati

Larynx

Vocal cords

Septum

Cricoid cartilage

Trachea

Nasal cavity from front

Lower Respiratory System

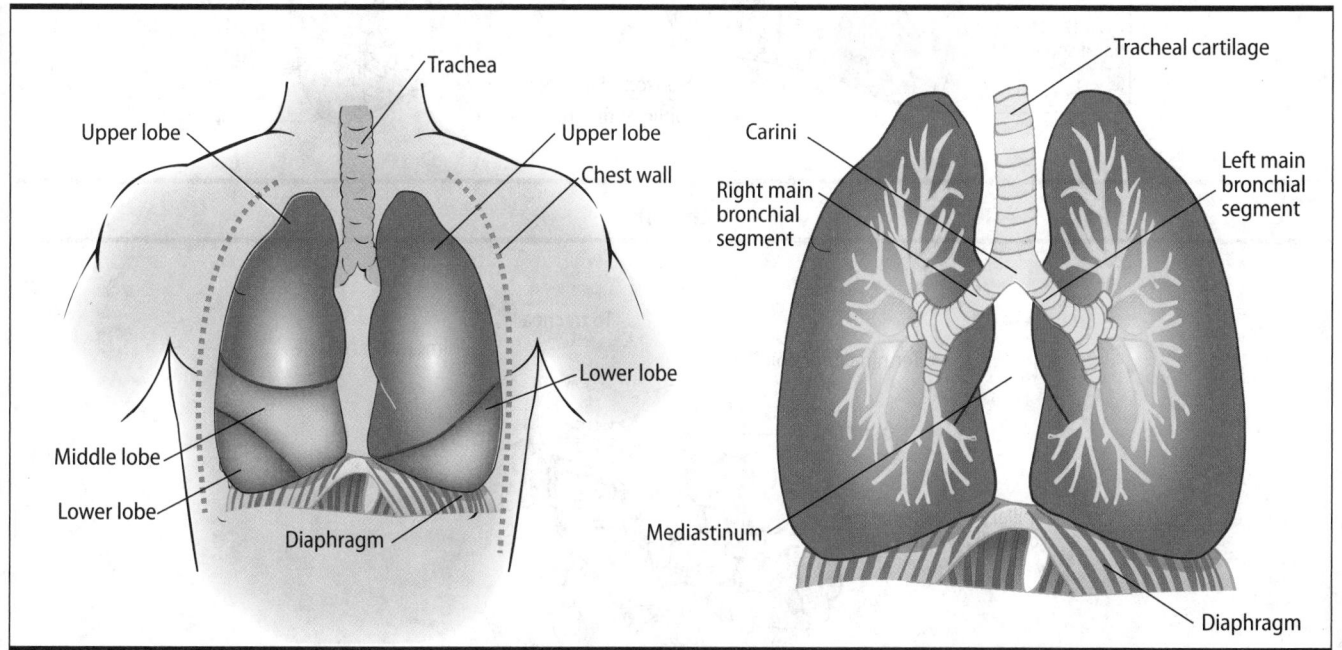

Trachea

Tracheal cartilage

Upper lobe

Upper lobe

Carini

Chest wall

Left main bronchial segment

Right main bronchial segment

Lower lobe

Middle lobe

Lower lobe

Diaphragm

Mediastinum

Diaphragm

Paranasal Sinuses

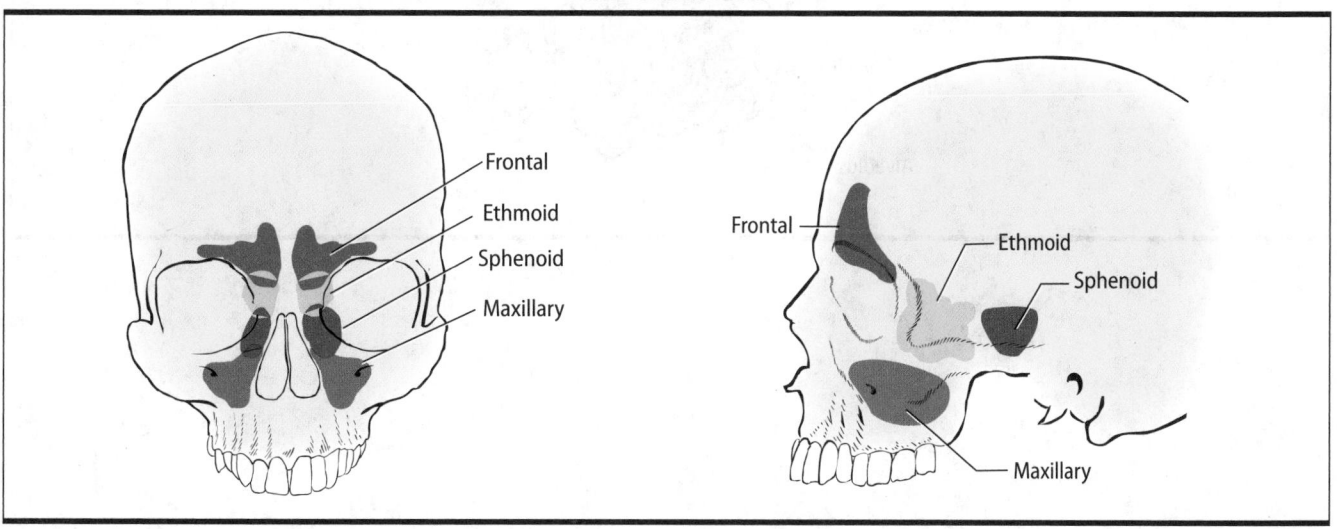

Frontal

Ethmoid

Sphenoid

Maxillary

Frontal

Ethmoid

Sphenoid

Maxillary

Lung Segments

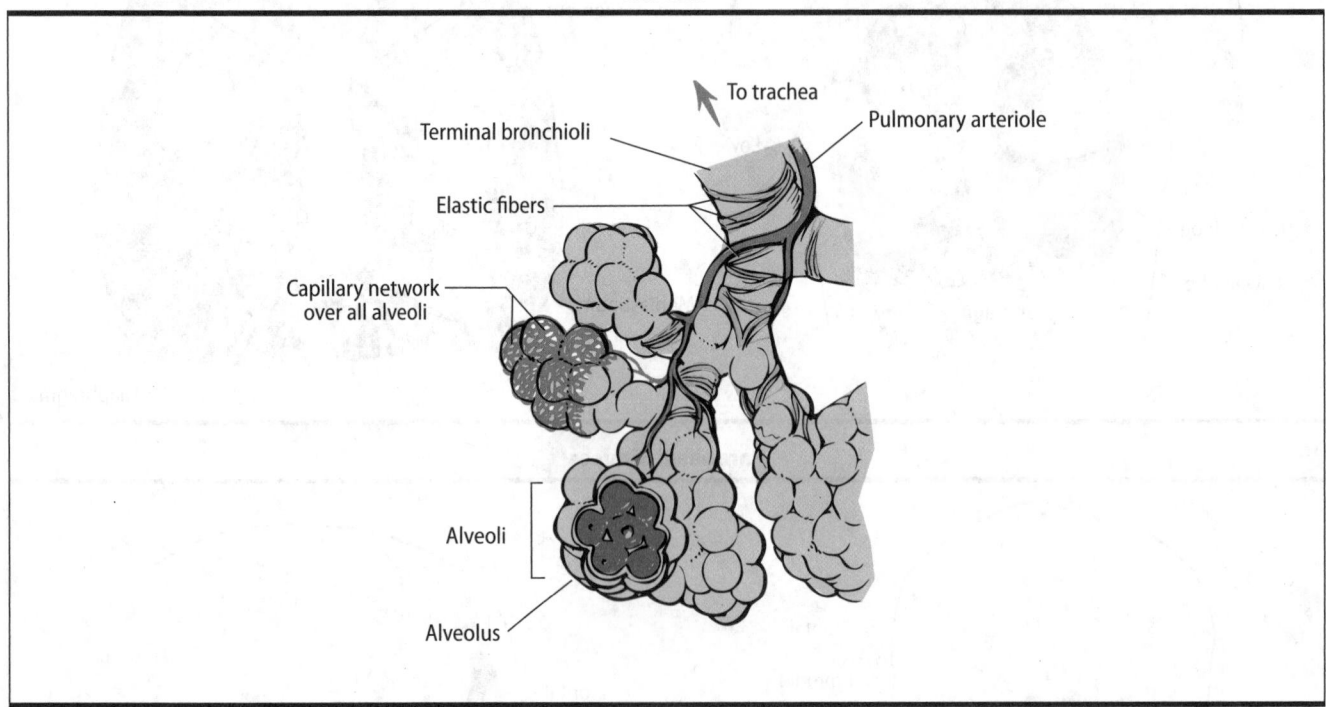

Right lung

Left lung

Apical segment

Apical-posterior segment

Anterior segment

Superior lobe

Posterior segment

Superior lobe

Superior lingular segment

Inferior lingular segment

Anterior segment

Medial basal segment

Lateral segment

Superior basal segment

Middle lobe

Superior segment

Posterior basal segment

Lateral basal segment

Inferior lobe

Inferior lobe

Anterior medial segment

Anterior basal segment

Horizontal fissure

Oblique fissures

Alveoli

To trachea

Terminal bronchioli

Pulmonary arteriole

Elastic fibers

Capillary network over all alveoli

Alveoli

Alveolus

Chapter 11. Diseases of the Digestive System (K00–K95)

Digestive System

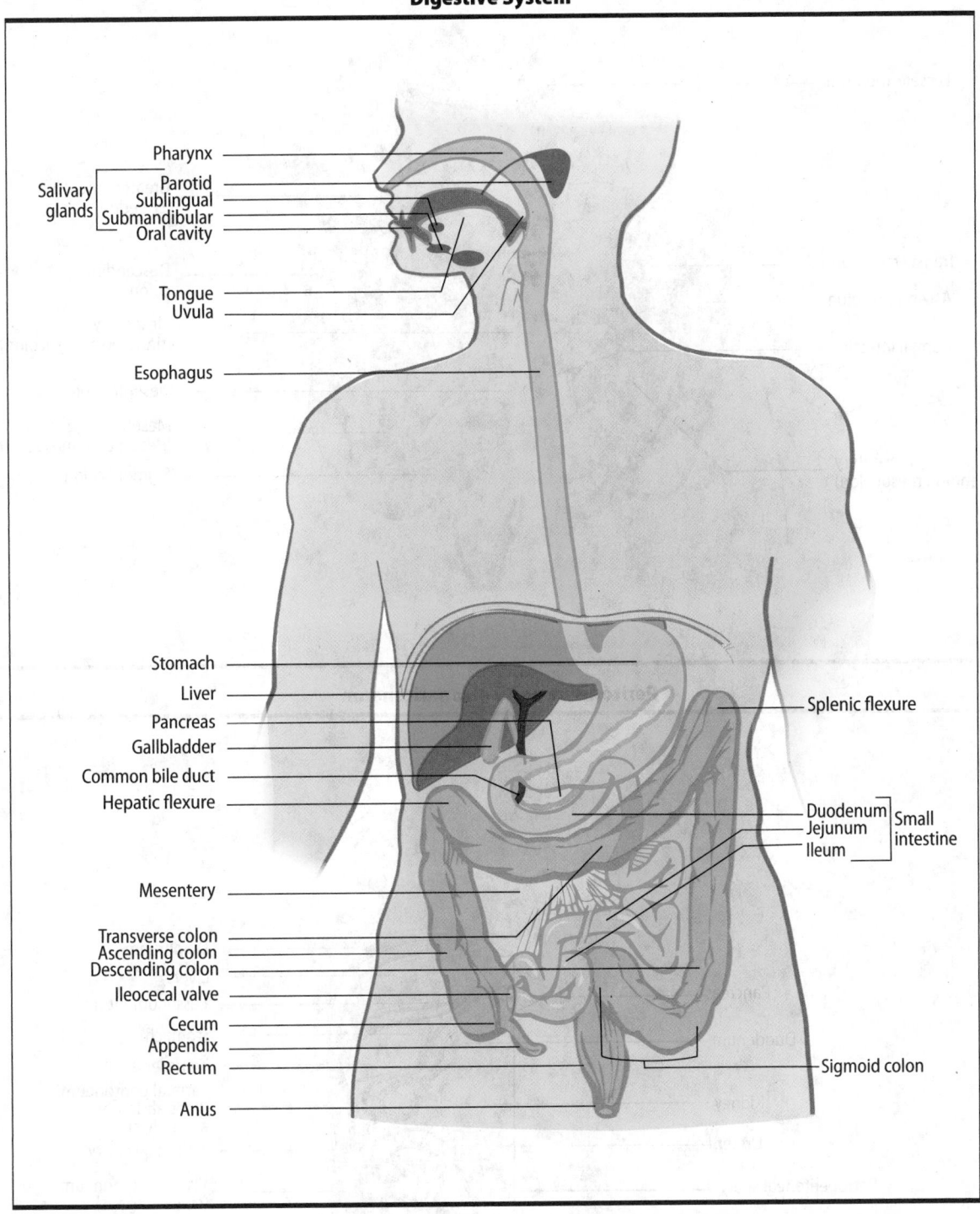

Omentum and Mesentery

Lesser omentum

Greater omentum (cut edge)

Transverse colon

Descending colon

Ascending colon

Mesentery (transverse mesocolon)

Small intestine

Mesentery proper

Mesentery (descending mesocolon)

Mesentery (ascending mesocolon)

Sigmoid colon

Peritoneum and Retroperitoneum

Pancreas

Diaphragm

Liver

Duodenum

Lesser omentum

Stomach

Kidney

Transverse colon

Parietal peritoneum (lines abdomen and pelvis)

Ureter

Peritoneal cavity

Retroperitoneal space

Visceral peritoneum (covers organs)

Mesentery

Greater omentum

Small intestine

Sigmoid colon

Bladder

Rectum

Chapter 12. Diseases of the Skin and Subcutaneous Tissue (L00–L99)

Nail Anatomy

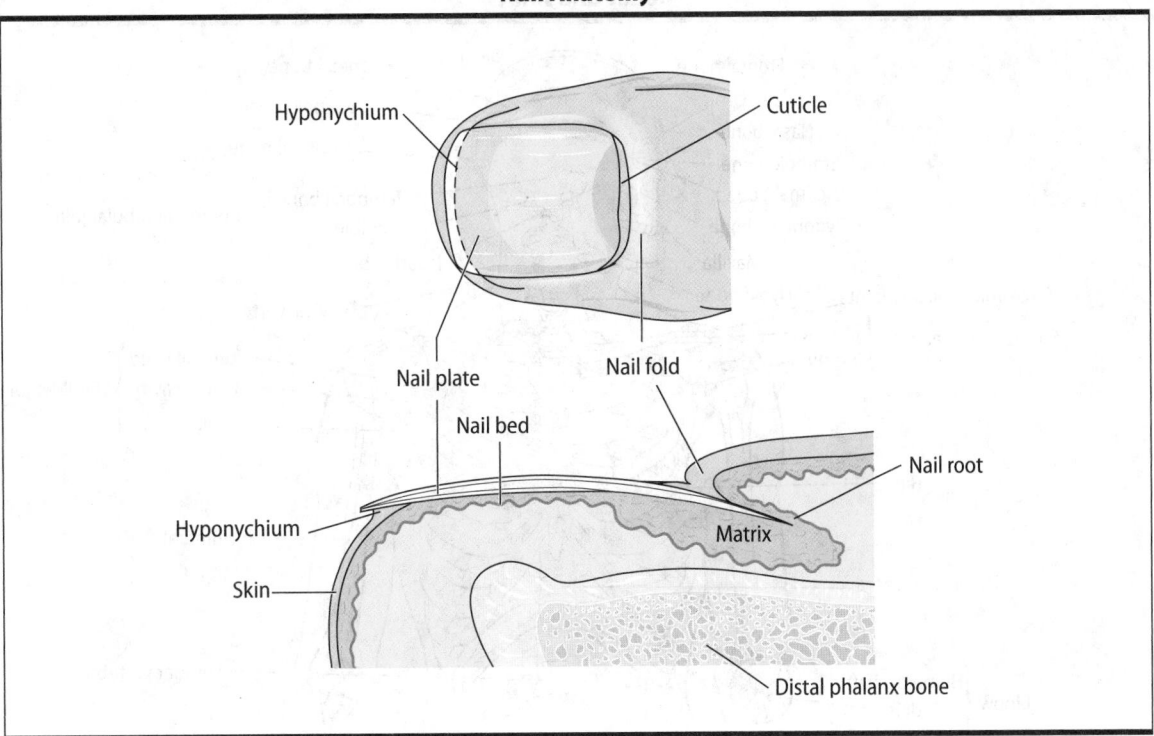

Hyponychium

Cuticle

Nail plate

Nail fold

Nail bed

Nail root

Hyponychium

Matrix

Skin

Distal phalanx bone

Skin and Subcutaneous Tissue

Hair

Basal layer

Layer corneal

Epidermis

Hair shaft

Dermis

Sebaceous gland

Bulb

Hypodermis
(subcutaneous layer)

Hair follicles

Sweat (eccrine gland)

Sensory nerve

Adipose tissue

Blood vessels

Chapter 13. Diseases of the Musculoskeletal System and Connective Tissue (MØØ–M99)

Bones and Joints

Shoulder Anterior View

Shoulder Posterior View

Elbow Anterior View

Shoulder Posterior View

Hand

Hip Anterior View

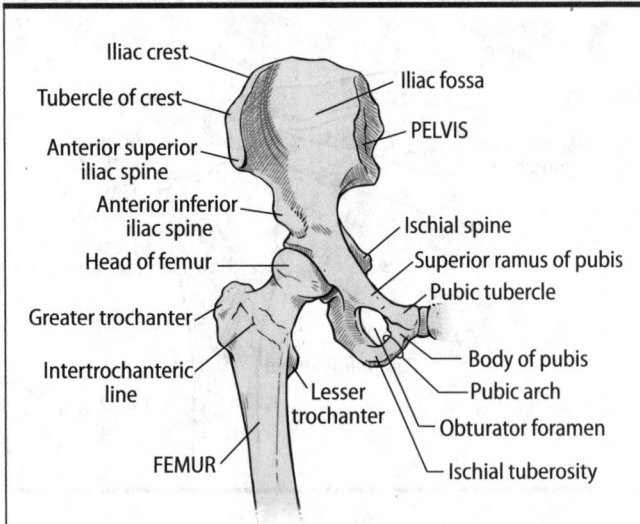

Iliac crest
Tubercle of crest
Anterior superior iliac spine
Anterior inferior iliac spine
Head of femur
Greater trochanter
Intertrochanteric line
Lesser trochanter
FEMUR

Iliac fossa
PELVIS
Ischial spine
Superior ramus of pubis
Pubic tubercle
Body of pubis
Pubic arch
Obturator foramen
Ischial tuberosity

Hip Posterior View

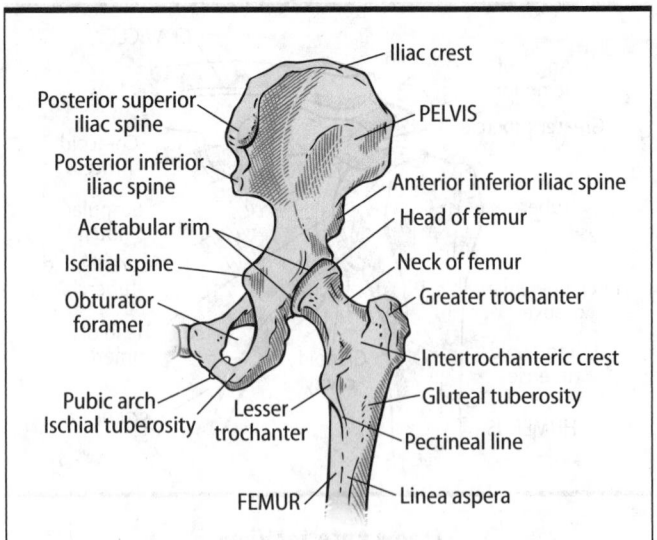

Posterior superior iliac spine
Posterior inferior iliac spine
Acetabular rim
Ischial spine
Obturator foramen
Pubic arch
Ischial tuberosity
Lesser trochanter
FEMUR

Iliac crest
PELVIS
Anterior inferior iliac spine
Head of femur
Neck of femur
Greater trochanter
Intertrochanteric crest
Gluteal tuberosity
Pectineal line
Linea aspera

Knee Anterior View

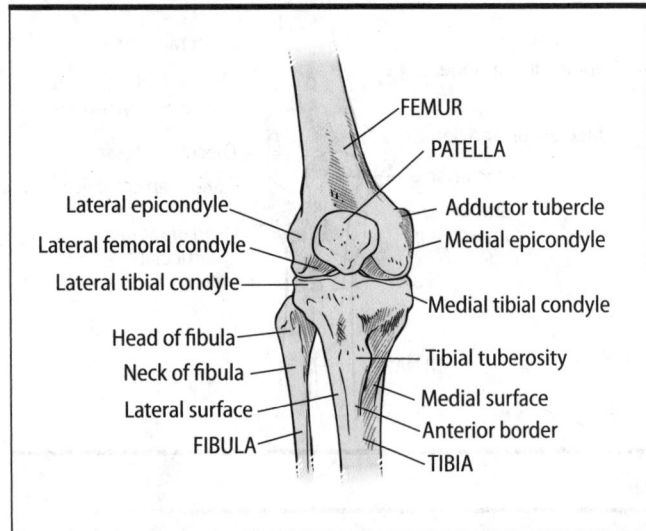

Lateral epicondyle
Lateral femoral condyle
Lateral tibial condyle
Head of fibula
Neck of fibula
Lateral surface
FIBULA

FEMUR
PATELLA
Adductor tubercle
Medial epicondyle
Medial tibial condyle
Tibial tuberosity
Medial surface
Anterior border
TIBIA

Knee Posterior View

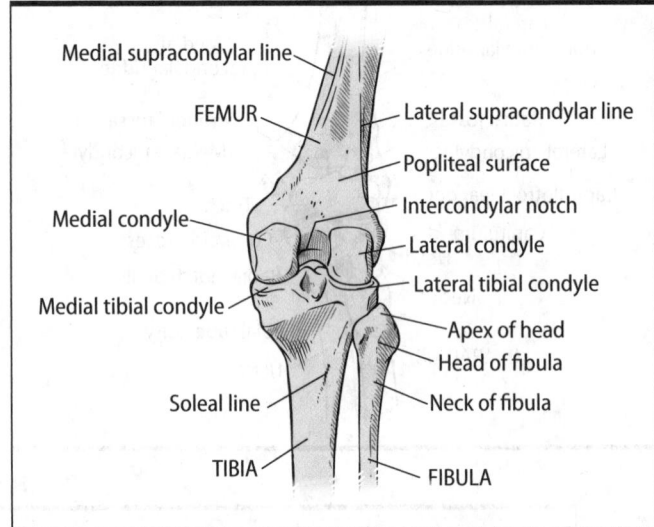

Medial supracondylar line
FEMUR
Medial condyle
Medial tibial condyle
Soleal line
TIBIA

Lateral supracondylar line
Popliteal surface
Intercondylar notch
Lateral condyle
Lateral tibial condyle
Apex of head
Head of fibula
Neck of fibula
FIBULA

Foot

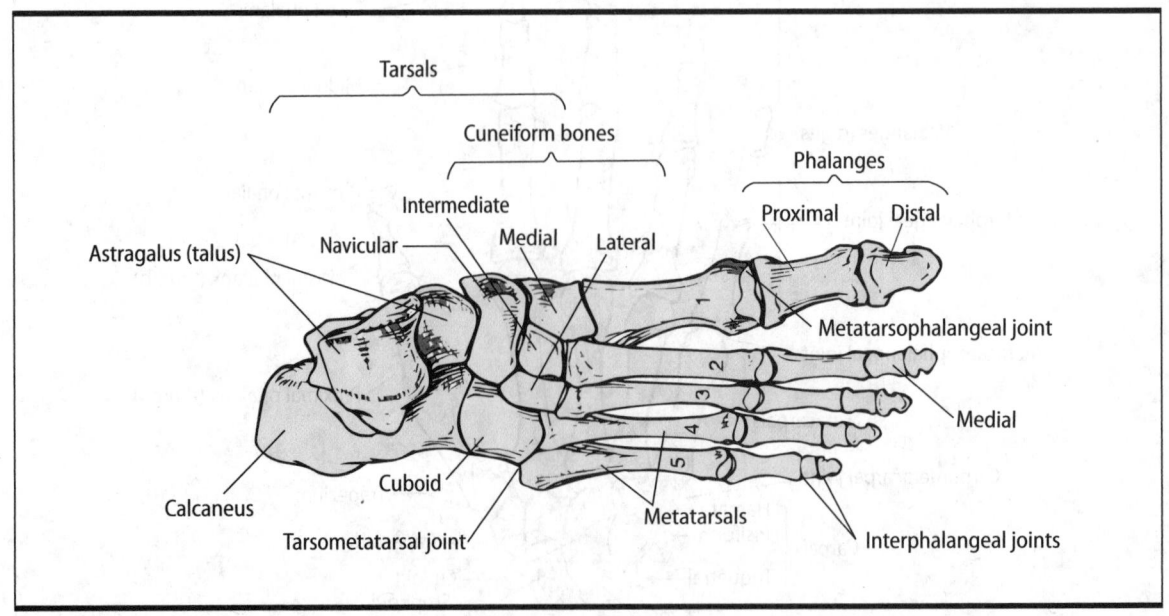

Tarsals
Cuneiform bones
Phalanges
Intermediate
Medial
Lateral
Proximal
Distal
Astragalus (talus)
Navicular
Metatarsophalangeal joint
Medial
Calcaneus
Cuboid
Metatarsals
Tarsometatarsal joint
Interphalangeal joints

Muscles

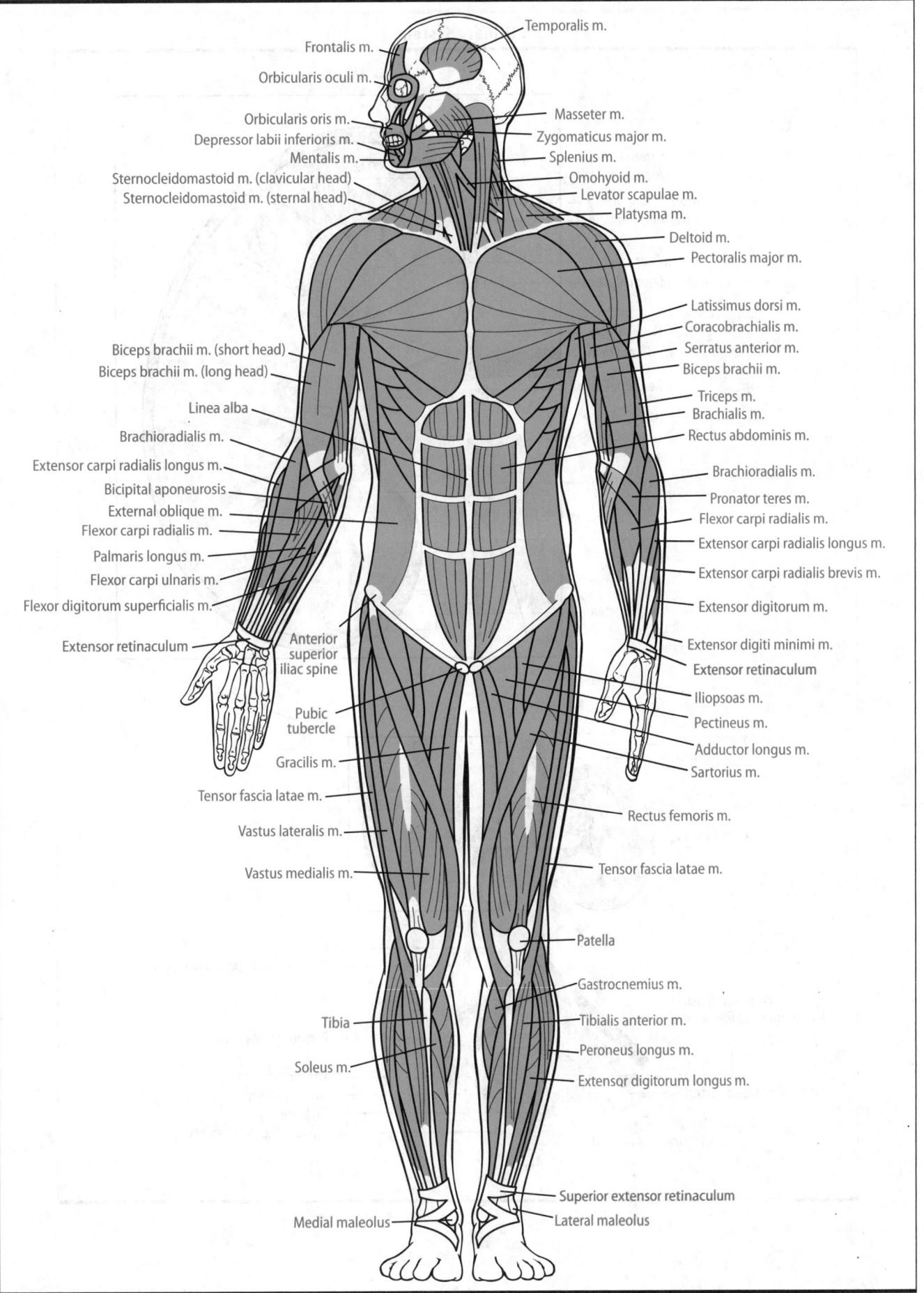

Chapter 14. Diseases of the Genitourinary System (NØØ–N99)

Urinary System

Male Genitourinary System

Female Internal Genitalia

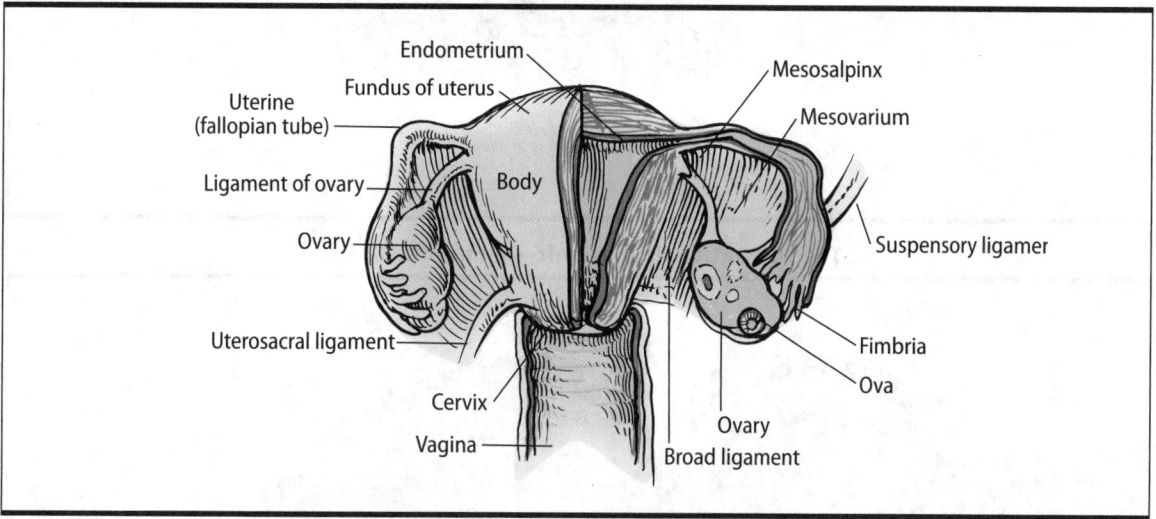

Female Genitourinary Tract Lateral View

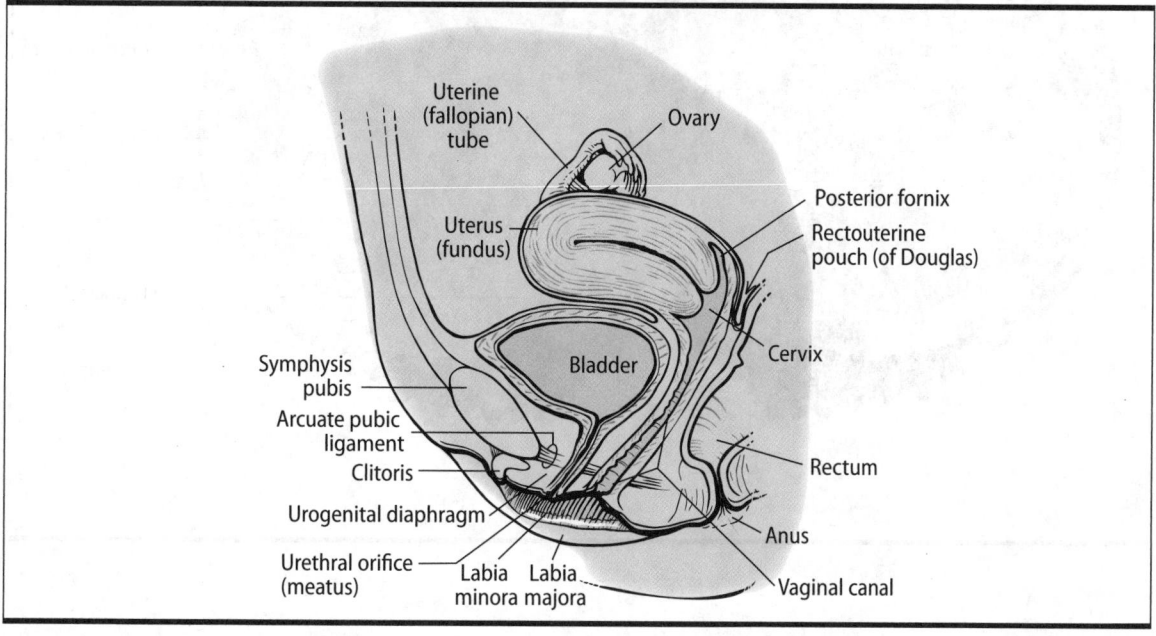

Chapter 15. Pregnancy, Childbirth and the Puerperium (O00–O9A)

Term Pregnancy – Single Gestation

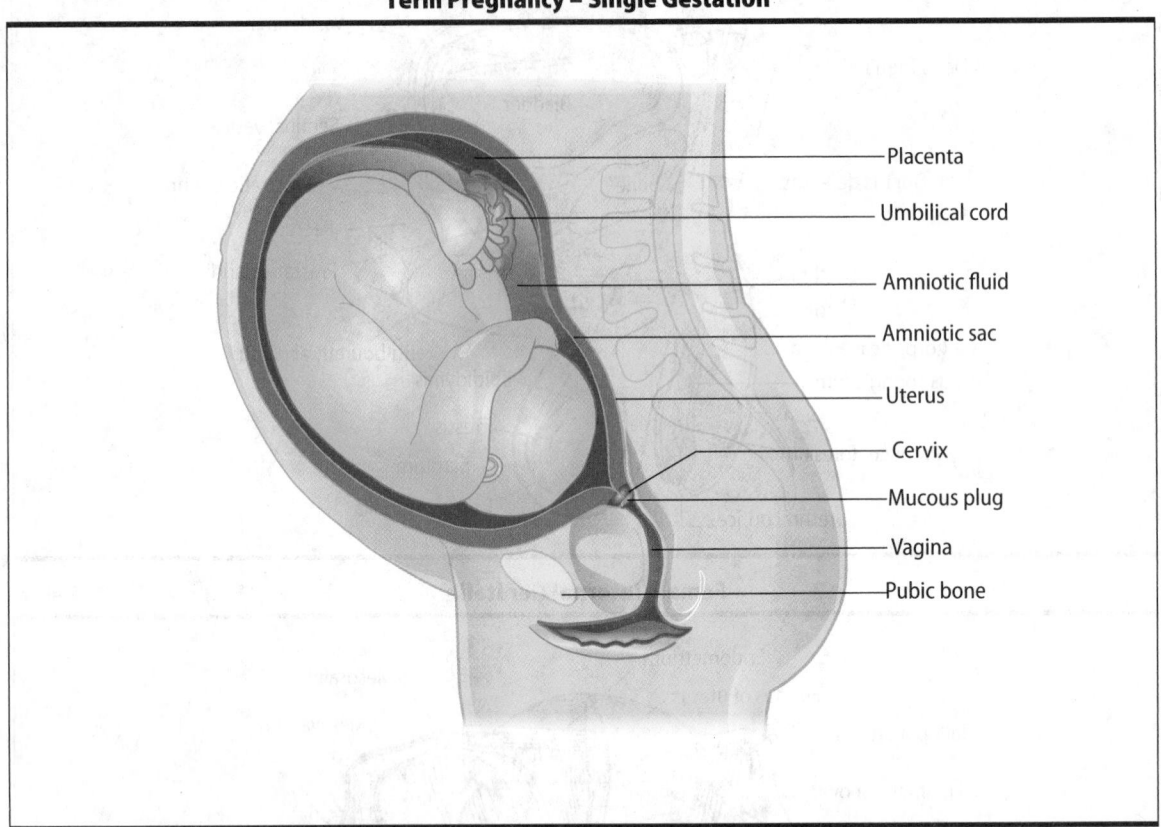

Placenta

Umbilical cord

Amniotic fluid

Amniotic sac

Uterus

Cervix

Mucous plug

Vagina

Pubic bone

Twin Gestation–Dichorionic–Diamniotic (DI-DI)

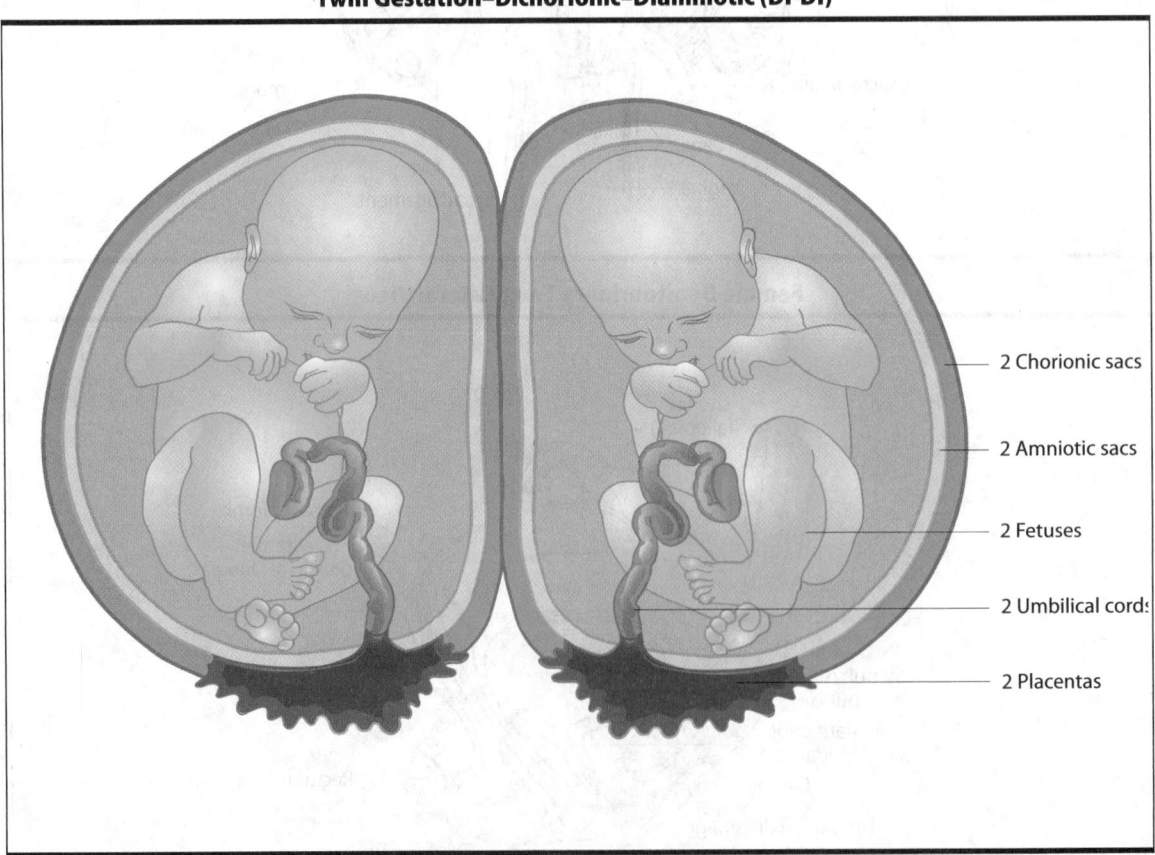

2 Chorionic sacs

2 Amniotic sacs

2 Fetuses

2 Umbilical cords

2 Placentas

Twin Gestation–Monochorionic–Diamniotic (MO-DI)

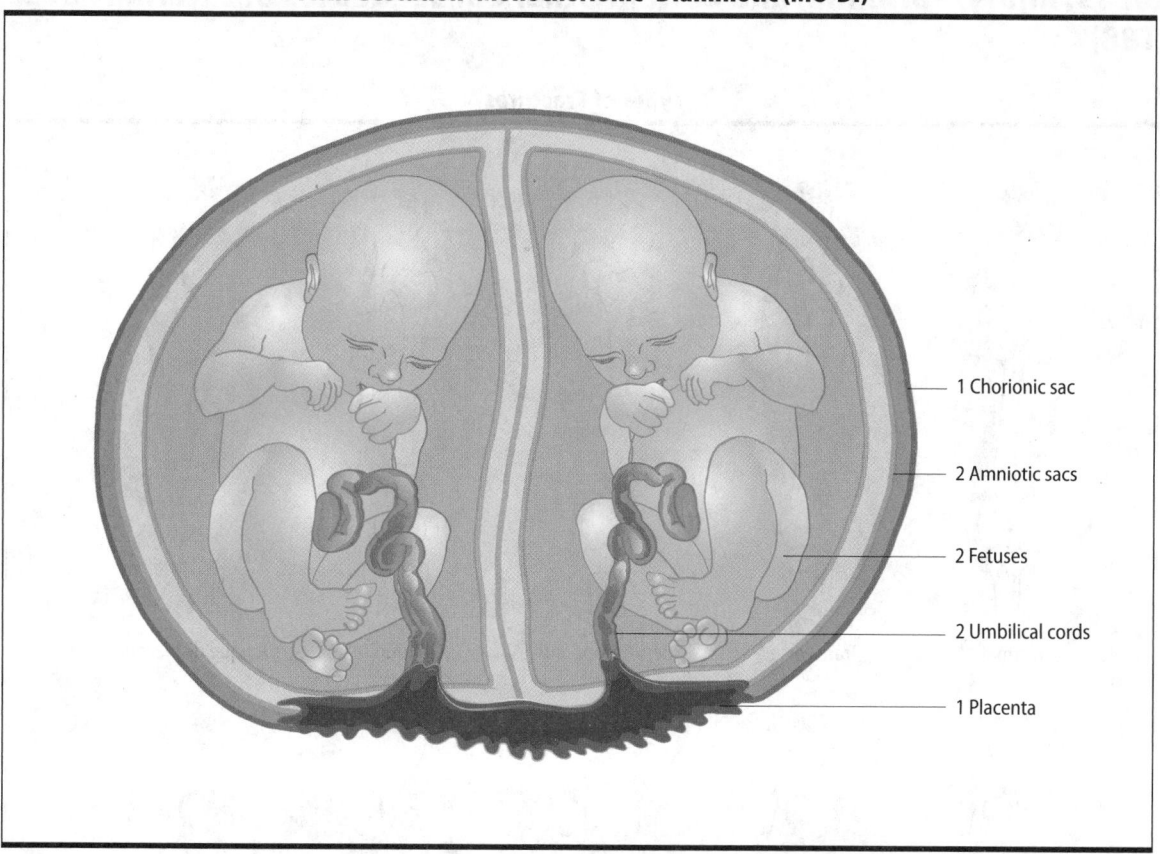

1 Chorionic sac

2 Amniotic sacs

2 Fetuses

2 Umbilical cords

1 Placenta

Twin Gestation–Monochorionic–Monoamniotic (MO-MO)

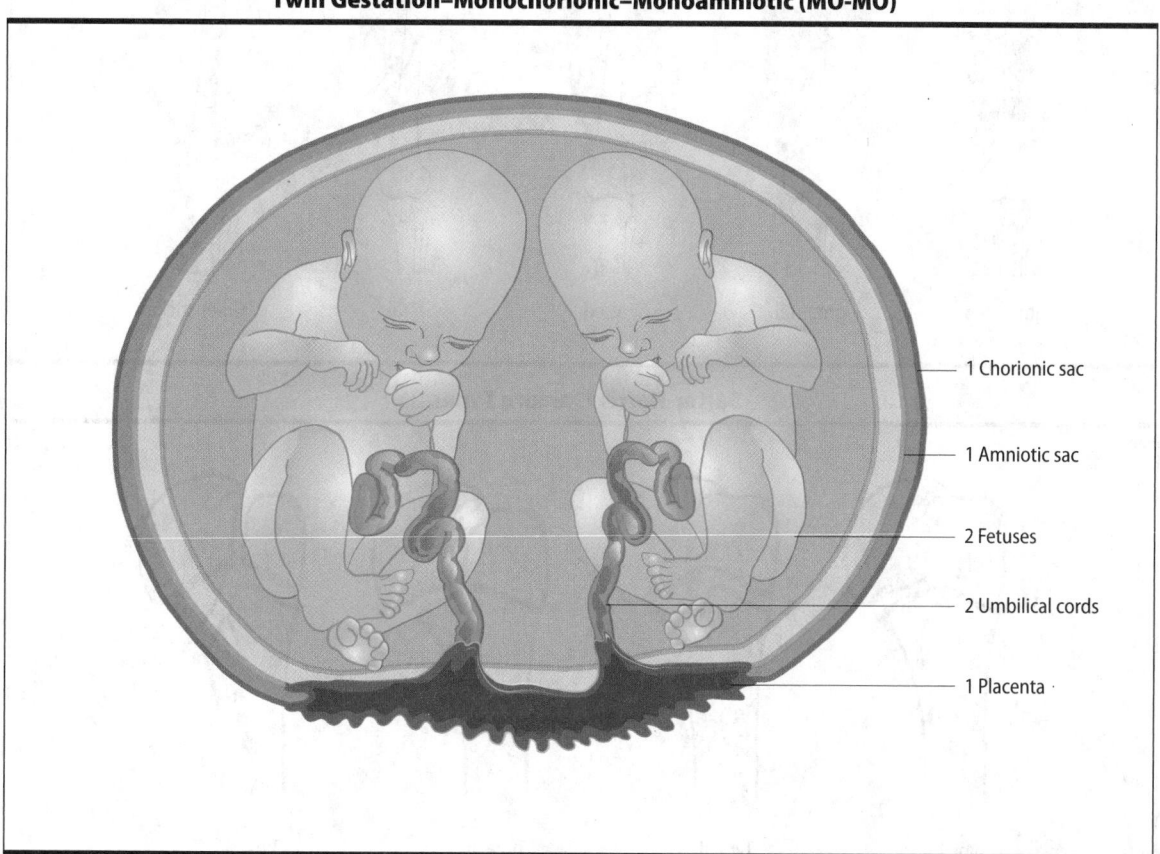

1 Chorionic sac

1 Amniotic sac

2 Fetuses

2 Umbilical cords

1 Placenta

Chapter 19. Injury, Poisoning and Certain Other Consequences of External Causes (S00–T88)

Types of Fractures

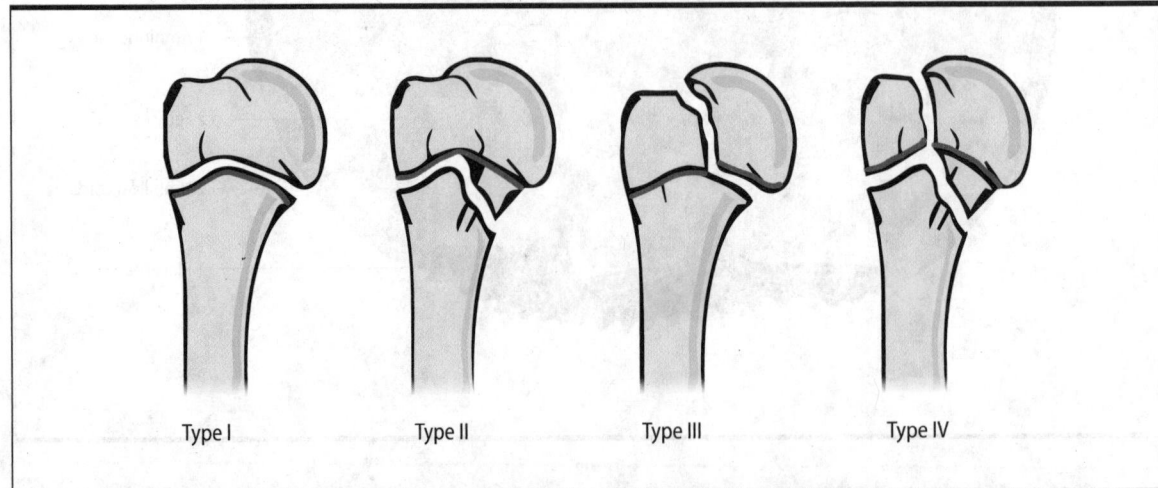

Salter-Harris Fracture Types